THIRD EDITION

TEXTBOOK OF CARDIOVASCULAR MEDICINE

THIRD EDITION

TEXTBOOK OF CARDIOVASCULAR MEDICINE

Editor

Eric J. Topol, MD
Professor, Department of Genetics
Case Western Reserve University
Cleveland, Ohio

Associate Editors

Robert M. Califf, MD
Vice Chancellor for Clinical Research
Duke University
Durham, North Carolina

Eric N. Prystowsky, MD
Consulting Professor of Medicine
Duke University Medical Center
Durham, North Carolina
Director, Clinical Electrophysiology Laboratory
St. Vincent
Indianapolis, Indiana

James D. Thomas, MD
Professor, Department of Biomedical Engineering
Case Western Reserve University
Cleveland, Ohio
Charles and Lorraine Chair of Cardiovascular Imaging
Department of Cardiovascular Medicine
Cleveland Clinic
Cleveland, Ohio

Paul D. Thompson, MD
Professor of Medicine
University of Connecticut School of Medicine
Director of Cardiology
Cardiology Division
Hartford Hospital
Hartford, Connecticut

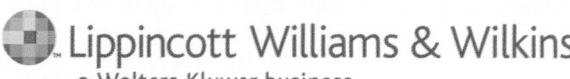

Lippincott Williams & Wilkins
a Wolters Kluwer business
Philadelphia • Baltimore • New York • London
Buenos Aires • Hong Kong • Sydney • Tokyo

Acquisitions Editor: Fran Destefano
Managing Editor: Joanne Bersin
Marketing Manager: Angela Panetta
Production Editor: Dave Murphy
Designer: Risa Clow
Compositor: TechBooks
Printer: R. R. Donnelley—Willard

530 Walnut St.
Philadelphia, PA 19106

Printed in the United States of America

Library of Congress Cataloging-in-Publication Data

Textbook of cardiovascular medicine / editor, Eric J. Topol; associate editors, Robert M. Califf... [et al.]. — 3rd ed.
p. ; cm.
Includes bibliographical references and index.
ISBN-13: 978-0-7817-7012-5
ISBN-10: 0-7817-7012-2
1. Cardiology. 2. Cardiovascular system—Diseases. I. Topol, Eric J., 1954–. II. Califf, Robert M.
[DNLM: 1. Cardiovascular Diseases. 2. Cardiology. WG 100 T3545 2007]
RC667.T44 2007
616.1′2—dc22

2006024342

To purchase additional copies of this book, call our customer service department at (800) 638-3030 or fax orders to (301) 824-7390. International customers should call (301) 714-2324.

Visit Lippincott Williams & Wilkins on the Internet: http://www.LWW.com. Lippincott Williams & Wilkins customer service representatives are available from 8:30 am to 6:00 pm, EST.

01 02 03 04 05
1 2 3 4 5 6 7 8 9 10

This book is dedicated to my family (Susan, Sarah and Evan) who have provided immense support and encouragement throughout my career

CONTRIBUTING AUTHORS

Philip A. Ades, MD
Professor of Medicine
Division of Cardiology
University of Vermont College of Medicine
Director, Cardiac Rehabilitation and Prevention
Department of Medicine
Fletcher-Allen HealthCare
Burlington, VT

Karen P. Alexander, MD
Assistant Professor
Department of Cardiology/Medicine
Duke University
Department of Cardiology/Medicine
Duke University Medical Center
Durham, NC

Amjad Al Mahameed, MD
Associate Staff
Department of Cardiovascular Medicine
Cleveland Clinic
Director, Vascular Medicine Research
Department of Cardiovascular Medicine
Cleveland Clinic
Cleveland, OH

Mark E. Anderson, MD, PhD
Potter-Lambert Chair in Cardiology
Director of Cardiology
Associate Director, Cardiovascular Center
Department of Medicine
The Carver College of Medicine
The University of Iowa
Iowa City, IA

Brian H. Annex, MD
Professor of Medicine
Department of Medicine
Duke University and Durham VA Medical Center
Director, Vascular Medicine
Department of Medicine
Duke University Medical Center
Durham NC

Rene A. Arcilla, MD
Emeritus Professor
Department of Pediatrics
University of Chicago
Emeritus Director
Heart Institute for Children
Advocate Hope Children's Hospital
Oak Lawn, IL

Doron Aronson, MD
Senior Lecturer
Rappaport Faculty of Medicine
Technion Medical School
Director, Cardiac Intermediate Unit
Department of Cardiology
Rambam Medical Center
Haifa, Israel

Craig R. Asher, MD
Staff Cardiologist
Department of Cardiology
Cleveland Clinic Florida
Weston, FL

Eric H. Awtry, MD
Assistant Professor
Department of Medicine
Boston University School of Medicine
Director of Education
Division of Cardiology
Boston Medical Center
Boston, MA

Johannes Backs, MD
Postdoctoral Research Fellow
Department of Molecular Biology
University of Texas Southwestern
Medical Center at Dallas
Resident
Department of Cardiology
University of Heidelberg
Heidelberg, Germany

Gary J. Balady, MD
Professor of Medicine
Department of Medicine
Boston University School of Medicine
Director, Preventive Cardiology
Department of Medicine, Section of Cardiology
Boston Medical Center
Boston, MA

Joaquin Barnoya, MD, MPH
Assistant Adjunct Professor
Department of Epidemiology
University of California, San Francisco
Director of Research and Education
Department of Pediatrics
Unidad de Cirugis Cardiovascular
Guatemala City, Gautemala

John R. Bartholomew, MD
Assistant Clinical Professor
Department of Medicine
Penn State College of Medicine
Section Head—Vascular Medicine
Department of Cardiovascular Medicine
Cleveland Clinic
Cleveland, OH

Rhonda Bassel-Duby, PhD
Associate Professor
Department of Molecular Biology
University of Texas Southwestern Medical Center
Dallas, TX

Craig T. Basson, MD, PhD
Professor; Director, Cardiovascular Research
Division of Cardiology, Department of Medicine
Weill Medical College of Cornell University
Attending Physician
Department of Cardiology, Medicine
New York Presbyterian Hospital
Cornell Medical Center
New York, NY

Kenneth L. Baughman, MD
Professor
Department of Medicine
Harvard Medical School
Director, Advanced Heart Disease Section
Department of Medicine/Cardiovascular Disease
Brigham and Women's Hospital
Boston, MA

Christophe Bauters, MD
Professor, Department of Cardiology
Lille University
Chief, Department of Heart Failure
Hôpital Cardiologique
Lille, France

Richard C. Becker, MD
Professor of Medicine
Department of Medicine
Duke University College of Medicine
Director, Cardiovascular Thrombosis Center
Duke University Medical Center
Durham, NC

Robert H. Beekman III, MD
Professor of Pediatrics
Department of Pediatric Cardiology
University of Cincinnati School of Medicine
Director of Cardiology
Department of Pediatric Cardiology
Cincinnati Children's Hospital Medical Center
Cincinnati, OH

Susan M. Begelman, MD, RVT
Medical Director, Noninvasive Vascular Laboratory
Department of Cardiovascular Medicine
Cleveland Clinic
Cleveland, OH

David G. Benditt, MD
Professor
Department of Medicine
University of Minnesota
Director, Cardiac Arrhythmia Service
University of Minnesota Hospital—Fairview
Minneapolis, MN

Ronald Berger, MD, PhD
Professor
Department of Medicine, Biomedical Engineering
Johns Hopkins University
Director of Electrophysiology Training Program
Department of Medicine
Johns Hopkins Hospital
Baltimore, MD

Michael E. Bertrand, MD
Professor of Cardiology
University of Lille 2
Lille Heart Institute
Lille, France

Mandeep Bhargava, MD
Department of Cardiovascular Medicine
Cleveland Clinic
Cleveland, OH

Deepak L. Bhatt, MD
Associate Professor of Medicine
Department of Cardiovascular Medicine
Cleveland Clinic
Staff Physician
Department of Cardiovascular Medicine
Cleveland Clinic
Cleveland, OH

Eugene H. Blackstone, MD
Director, Clinical Research
Department of Thoracic and Cardiovascular Surgery
Cleveland Clinic
Cleveland, OH

Burns C. Blaxall, PhD
Assistant Professor
Cardiovascular Research Institute
University of Rochester Medical Center
Rochester, NY

Robert C. Block, MD
Preventive Cardiology Post-doctoral Fellow
Department of Community and Preventive Medicine
University of Rochester School of Medicine and Dentistry
Clinical Instructor
General Medicine Unit
Strong Memorial Hospital
Rochester, NY

David A. Bluemke, MD, PhD, MsB
Associate Professor
Department of Radiology and Medicine
Johns Hopkins University School of Medicine
Clinical Director, MRI
Russell R. Morgan Department of Radiology and Radiological Science
Johns Hopkins Hospital
Baltimore, MD

Meredith Bond, PhD
Professor and Chair
Department of Physiology
University of Maryland School of Medicine
Baltimore, MD

Lawrence M. Boxt, MD
Professor of Clinical Radiology
Department of Radiology
Albert Einstein College of Medicine
Chief of Cardiac MRI and CT
Department of Cardiology
Northshore University Hospital
Manhasset, NY

Andrew Boyle, MD
Assistant Professor
Department of Medicine
University of Minnesota
Medical Director
Department of Inpatient Cardiology
University of Minnesota Medical Center at Fairview
Minneapolis, MN

M. Elizabeth Brickner, MD
Associate Professor
Department of Internal Medicine
University of Texas, Southwestern Medical Center
Dallas, TX

Matthew M. Burg, PhD
Associate Clinical Professor of Medicine
Department of Medicine, Section of Cardiovascular Medicine
Yale University School of Medicine
Associate Clinical Professor of Medicine
Department of Medicine, Division of General Medicine
Columbia University School of Medicine
New York, NY

Allen Burke, MD
Associate Professor
Department of Pathology
University of Maryland
Deputy Director, CVPath
International Registry of Pathology
Gaithersburg, MD

Robert M. Califf, MD
Vice Chancellor for Clinical Research
Duke University
Durham, NC

Hugh Calkins, MD
Professor of Medicine
Johns Hopkins University
Director of the Arrhythmia Services and Clinical Electrophysiology Laboratory
Johns Hopkins Hospital
Baltimore, MD

Blase A. Carabello, MD
Professor of Medicine
Department of Medicine
Baylor College of Medicine
Medical Care Line Executive
Department of Medicine
Michael E. DeBakey Veterans Affairs Medical Center
Houston, TX

Fabio Cattaneo, MD
Consultant
Clinica Luganese Moncucco
Lugano, Switzerland

Manuel D. Cerquiera, MD
Chairman, Department of Molecular and Functional Imaging
Cleveland Clinic
Professor of Radiology
Cleveland Clinic Lerner College of Medicine of Case Western Reserve University
Cleveland, OH

Kanu Chatterjee, MD
Ernest Gallo Distinguished Professor of Medicine
Department of Medicine
University of California, San Francisco
Professor of Medicine
Department of Medicine
Moffitt-Long Hospital, UCSF
San Francisco, CA

Melvin D. Cheitlin, MACC
Emeritus Professor of Medicine
Department of Medicine
University of California, San Francisco
Former Chief of Cardiology
Department of Medicine
San Francisco General Hospital
San Francisco, CA

Derek P. Chew, MBBS, MPH
Associate Professor
Department of Medicine
Flinders University
Director, Cardiac Intensive Care
Department of Cardiovascular Medicine
Flinders Medical Centre
South Australia, Australia

G. Ralph Corey, MD
Professor of Medicine and Infectious Disease
Department of Medicine
Duke University Medical Center
Durham, NC

Mark A. Creager, MD
Professor of Medicine
Department of Medicine
Harvard Medical School
Director, Advanced Heart Disease
Department of Medicine
Brigham and Women's Hospital
Boston, MA

Michael H. Criqui, MD, MPH
Professor
Department of Family and Preventive Medicine
Department of Medicine
University of California San Diego
School of Medicine
La Jolla, CA

Lori B. Daniels, MD
Department of Medicine, Division of Cardiology
University of California, San Diego
Department of Medicine, Division of Cardiology
University of California, San Diego Medical Center
San Diego, CA

Dawood Darbar, MD
Assistant Professor
Department of Medicine
Vanderbilt University School of Medicine
Director, Vanderbilt Arrhythmia Service
Vanderbilt University Medical Center
Vanderbilt Heart Institute
Nashville, TN

John R. Davies, MD
Division of Cardiovascular Medicine
Addenbrooke's Hospital
Cambridge University
Cambridge, UK

Steven B. Deitelzweig, MD
Member, Section of Vascular Medicine
Section Head, Hospital-Based Internal Medicine
Ochsner Clinic Foundation
New Orleans, LA

Milind Y. Desai, MD
Departments of Cardiovascular Medicine and Radiology
Cleveland Clinic
Cleveland, OH

Angela Dispenzieri, MD
Associate Professor
Department of Medicine, Division of Hematology
Mayo Clinic
Department of Medicine, Division of Hematology
Rochester Methodist Hospital
Rochester, MN

Ellen A. Dornelas, PhD
Assistant Professor
Department of Medicine
University of Connecticut School of Medicine
Director of Behavioral Health Programs
Department of Preventive Cardiology
Hartford Hospital
Hartford, CT

John S. Douglas, Jr., MD
Professor of Medicine
Department of Medicine
Emory University School of Medicine
Director of Interventional Cardiology
Division of Cardiology
Emory University Hospital
Atlanta, GA

Sarfraz Durrani, MD
Fellow, Electrophysiology
Department of Cardiology
Duke University Medical Center
Durham, NC

Perry M. Elliott, MD
Senior Lecturer
Department of Medicine
University College London
Consultant Cardiologist
The Heart Hospital
London, UK

John Ellis, MD
Professor, Department of Anesthesia & Critical Care
The University of Chicago
Chicago, IL

Robert C. Elston, MD
Department of Epidemiology and Biostatistics
Case Western Reserve University
Cleveland, OH

N. A. Mark Estes, MD
Professor of Medicine
Tufts University
Director of the Electrophysiology
Division of Cardiology
Tufts New England Medical Center
Boston, MA

John D. Fisher, MD
Professor of Medicine
Albert Einstein College of Medicine
Director, Arrhythmia Services
Department of Medicine, Cardiology
Montefiore Medical Center
Bronx, NY

Frank A. Flachskampf, MD
Professor of Internal Medicine
University of Erlangen
Chief, Department of Internal Medicine/Cardiology
Asklepios Klinik Hamburg
Hamburg, Germany

Joe Foss, MD
Director of Clinical Research
The Department of General Anesthesiology
Cleveland Clinic
Cleveland, Ohio

Vance G. Fowler, Jr., MD, MHS
Associate Professor
Department of Medicine
Division of Infectious Diseases
Duke University Medical Center
Durham, NC

Keith A. A. Fox, MB, ChB
Professor of Cardiology
Department of Cardiovascular Research
University of Edinburgh
Consultant Cardiologist
Department of Cardiology
Royal Infirmary of Edinburgh
Edinburgh, UK

Gary S. Francis, MD
Professor of Medicine
Department of Cardiology
Cleveland Clinic, Lerner College of Medicine of Case Western University
Head, Clinical Cardiology Section
Department of Cardiology
Cleveland Clinic
Cleveland, OH

Anthony J. Furlan, MD
Head, Section of Stroke and Neurocritical Care
Department of Neurology
Cleveland Clinic
Cleveland, OH

Mario J. Garcia, MD
Professor of Medicine
Cleveland Clinic Lerner College of Medicine of Case Western Reserve University
Director, Cardiac Imaging
Department of Cardiovascular Medicine
Cleveland Clinic
Cleveland, OH

A. Marc Gillinov, MD
Staff Surgeon and Surgical Director
Center for Atrial Fibrillation
Department of Thoracic and Cardiovascular Surgery
Cleveland Clinic
Cleveland, OH

Stanton A. Glantz, PhD
Professor
Department of Medicine, Cardiology
University of California, San Francisco
San Francisco, CA

Nicola J. Goodson, MRCP, PhD
Senior Lecturer in Rheumatology
Academic Rheumatology Unit, Division of Infection and Immunity
University Hospital Aintree, Liverpool University
Honorary Consultant Rheumatologist
Rheumatology Department
University Hospital Aintree
Liverpool, UK

Heather L. Gornik, MD
Associate Staff Physician
Sections of Clinical Cardiology and Vascular Medicine
Department of Cardiovascular Medicine
Cleveland Clinic
Cleveland, OH

Augustus O. Grant, MB, ChB, PhD
Professor of Medicine
Department of Medicine
Duke University
Professor
Department of Medicine
Duke University Medical Center
Durham, NC

Philip Greenland, MD
Harry W. Dingman Professor
Department of Preventive Medicine and Medicine
Northwestern University Feinberg School of Medicine
Cardiology Consultant
Department of Medicine
Northwestern Memorial Hospital
Chicago, IL

Brian P. Griffin, MD
Department of Cardiovascular Medicine
Cleveland Clinic
Cleveland, OH

Richard A. Grimm, DO
Director, Echocardiography Laboratory
Department of Cardiovascular Medicine
Cleveland Clinic
Cleveland, OH

Christian Gring, MD
Imaging Section, Cardiology Division,
Cleveland Clinic
Cleveland, OH

Madhu Gupta, MSc, PhD
Director, Molecular Cardiology
The Heart Institute for Children
Hope Children's Hospital
Palos Heights, IL

Mahesh P. Gupta, PhD
Associate Professor
Department of Surgery
The University of Chicago
Chicago, IL

Garrie J. Haas, MD
Associate Professor of Clinical Medicine
Department of Medicine/Division of Cardiovascular Medicine
The Ohio State University Medical Center
Columbus, OH

David E. Haines, MD
Director
Heart Rhythm Center
William Beaumont Hospital
Royal Oak, MI

Rainer Hambrecht, MD
Associate Professor
Department of Cardiology
University of Leipzig
Vice-Director
Heart Center
Leipzig, Germany

Stephen C. Hammill, MD
Professor
Department of Medicine
Mayo Clinic College of Medicine
Director, Heart Rhythm Services
Division of Cardiovascular Diseases
Mayo Clinic
Rochester, MN

Heather Cohen Henri, MD
Clinical Instructor of Medicine
Department of Medicine
Stanford University Medical Center
Clinical Instructor of Medicine
Department of Medicine
Stanford Hospital and Clinics
Palo Alto, CA

Frederick A. Heupler, Jr., MD
Quality Assurance Officer
Department of Cardiovascular Medicine
Cleveland Clinic
Cleveland, OH

L. David Hillis, MD
Daniel W. Foster Distinguished Chair in Internal Medicine
Vice-Chair, Department of Medicine
University of Texas Southwestern Medical Center
Dallas, TX

Judith S. Hochman, MD
Harold Snyder Family Professor of Cardiology
Clinical Chief, The Leon H. Charney Department of Cardiology
Director, Cardiovascular Clinical Research
Department of Cardiology/Medicine
New York University School of Medicine
New York, NY

Katherine J. Hoercher, RN
Director of Research
Kaufman Center for Heart Failure
Cleveland Clinic
Cleveland, OH

Judith Hsia, MD
Professor
Department of Medicine
George Washington University
Washington, DC

G. Chad Hughes, MD
Assistant Professor
Department of Surgery
Duke University
Durham, NC

Srinivas Iyengar, MD
Clinical Instructor
Department of Cardiology
The Ohio State University
Heart Failure Fellow
Department of Cardiology
The Ohio State University Medical Center
Columbus, OH

Michael R. Jaff, DO
Assistant Professor
Department of Medicine
Harvard Medical School
Director, Vascular Medicine
Department of Cardiovascular Medicine
Massachusetts General Hospital
Boston, MA

Jean Jeudy, Jr., MD
Department of Diagnostic Radiology
Division of Cardiothoracic Imaging
University of Maryland Medical System
Assistant Professor
University of Maryland School of Medicine
Baltimore, MD

Prince Kannankeril, MD, MSCI
Assistant Professor
Department of Pediatrics
Vanderbilt University
Assistant Professor
Department of Pediatrics
Vanderbilt Children's Hospital
Nashville, TN

Samir R. Kapadia, MD
Associate Professor
Department of Medicine
Cleveland Clinic Lerner College of Medicine of Case Western Reserve University
Director, Interventional Cardiology Fellowship
Department of Cardiovascular Medicine
Cleveland Clinic
Cleveland, OH

David Kass, MD
Abraham and Virginia Weiss Professor of Cardiology
Professor of Medicine
Professor of Biomedical Engineering
Department of Medicine
Johns Hopkins University Medical Institutions
Baltimore, MD

Amos Katz, MD
Associate Professor
Cardiology Department
Faculty of Health Sciences
Ben-Gurion University of the Negev
Chief, Department of Cardiology
Barilai Medical Center
Ashkelon, Israel

Arnold M. Katz, MD
Professor Emeritus
Department of Medicine
University of Connecticut
Visiting Professor
Department of Medicine and Physiology
Department Medical School
Lebanon, NH

David E. Kelley, MD
Professor of Medicine
Department of Medicine, Division of Endocrinology and Metabolism
University of Pittsburgh
Pittsburgh, PA

Allan L. Klein, MD
Professor of Medicine
Department of Cardiovascular Medicine
Cleveland Clinic Lerner College of Medicine of Case Western Reserve University
Director, Cardiovascular Imaging Research
Department of Cardiovascular Medicine
Cleveland Clinic
Cleveland, OH

Liviu Klein, MD, MS
Fellow in Cardiovascular Disease
Division of Cardiology
Northwestern University Feinberg School of Medicine
Bluhm Cardiovascular Institute
Northwestern Memorial Hospital
Chicago, IL

Robert A. Kloner, MD, PhD
Professor of Medicine
Division of Cardiovascular Medicine
Keck School of Medicine at the University of Southern California
Director of Research
Heart Institute
Good Samaritan Hospital
Los Angeles, CA

Robert H. Knopp, MD
Professor of Medicine
Department of Medicine
University of Washington
Chief
Division of Metabolism, Endocrinology and Nutrition
Harborview Medical Center
Seattle, WA

Andrew Krumerman, MD
Assistant Professor of Medicine
Department of Medicine
Albert Einstein College of Medicine
Attending Electrophysiologist
Division of Cardiology
Montefiore Medical Center
Bronx, NY

Richard A. Lange, MD
Professor
Department of Internal Medicine
Johns Hopkins Medical Institution
Chief of Clinical Cardiology
Department of Internal Medicine
The Johns Hopkins Hospital
Baltimore, MD

Daniel Laskowitz, MD, MHS
Associate Professor of Medicine (Neurology)
Department of Medicine
Duke University School of Medicine
Durham, NC

Michael S. Lauer, MD
Professor of Medicine, Epidemiology and Biostatistics
Cleveland Clinic Lerner College of Medicine of Case Western Reserve University
Clinical Cardiologist
Department of Cardiovascular Medicine
Cleveland Clinic
Cleveland, OH

Julie Laveglia, RN, BSN
Staff Nurse
Coronary Intensive Care Unit
Cleveland Clinic
Cleveland OH

Jennifer S. Li, MD, MHS
Associate Professor
Department of Pediatrics
Duke University Medical Center
Durham, NC

Joao A. C. Lima, MD, MBA
Associate Professor of Medicine and Radiology
Department of Medicine
Johns Hopkins University
Director of Cardiovascular Imaging
Department of Medicine
Johns Hopkins Hospital
Baltimore, MD

Aldons J. Lusis, PhD
Professor
Department of Medicine/Division of Cardiology, Department of Human Genetics; Department of Microbiology, Immunology and Molecular Genetics
UCLA
Los Angeles, CA

John S. MacGregor, MD, PhD
Professor of Medicine
Department of Medicine
University of California San Francisco
Director, Cardiac Catheterization Laboratory and Interventional Cardiology
San Francisco General Hospital
San Francisco, CA

Kenneth W. Mahaffey, MD
Associate Professor of Medicine
Department of Cardiology
Duke Clinical Research Institute
Associate Professor of Medicine
Department of Cardiology
Duke University Medical Center
Durham, NC

JoAnn E. Manson, MD, DrPH
Elizabeth F. Brigham Professor of Women's Health and Professor of Medicine
Harvard Medical School
Chief, Division of Preventive Medicine and Co-Director of the Connors Center for Women's Health and Gender Biology
Brigham and Women's Hospital
Harvard Medical School
Boston, MA

Srinivas Mantha, MD
Professor
Department of Anesthesiology and Intensive Care
Nizam's Institute of Medical Science
Hyderabad, India

Daniel B. Mark, MD, MPH
Director, Outcomes Research
Duke Clinical Research Institute
Professor of Medicine
Duke University Medical Center
Durham, NC

Anjli Maroo, MD, RVT
Fellow, Section of Interventional Cardiology
Department of Cardiovascular Medicine
Cleveland Clinic
Cleveland, OH

Oscar C. Marroquin, MD
Assistant Professor
Department of Medicine
University of Pittsburgh
Attending Cardiologist
Cardiovascular Institute
University of Pittsburgh Medical Center
Pittsburgh, PA

Thomas H. Marwick, MB, BS, PhD
Professor of Medicine
School of Medicine (Southern Division)
University of Queensland
Princess Alexandra Hospital
Director of Echocardiology
Department of Cardiology
Princess Alexandra Hospital
Brisbane, Australia

William J. McKenna, BA, MD, DSc
Professor of Cardiology
Department of Medicine
University College London
Clinical Director
The Heart Hospital
University College London Hospitals NHS Trust
London, UK

Dennis M. McNamara, MD
Associate Professor
Cardiovascular Institute
University of Pittsburgh
Director, Heart Failure and Transplantation Program
University of Pittsburgh Medical Center
Pittsburgh, PA

Bernhard Meier, MD
Professor and Head of Cardiology
Department of Cardiology
University Hospital Bern
Chairman
Department of Cardiology
University Hospital Bern
Bern, Switzerland

Fred Morady, MD
Professor
Department of Medicine
University of Michigan Hospital
Director
Clinical Electrophysiology Service
University of Michigan Hospital
Ann Arbor, MI

Srinivas Murali, MD
Professor of Medicine
Drexel University College of Medicine
Director, Division of Cardiovascular Medicine
Director, Gerald McGinness Cardiovascular Institute
Allegheny General Hospital
Pittsburgh, PA

Ross T. Murphy, MD, MRCPI
Consultant Cardiologist
St. James' Hospital
Dublin, Ireland

Elizabeth G. Nabel, MD
Director
National Heart, Lung, and Blood Institute, NIH
Bethesda, MD

Gerald V. Naccarelli, MD
Bernard Trabin Chair in Cardiology
Professor of Medicine
Chief, Division of Cardiology
Department of Medicine
Penn State University College of Medicine
Chief
Division of Cardiology
The Milton S. Hershey Medical Center
Hershey, PA

L. Kristin Newby, MD, MHS
Associate Professor of Medicine
Department of Medicine/Division of Cardiology
Duke University Medical Center
Durham, NC

Christopher M. O'Connor, MD
Professor of Medicine
Division of Cardiovascular Medicine
Duke University Health System
Chief, Division of Clinical Pharmacology
Duke University Health System
Durham, NC

Peter M. Okin, MD
Professor of Medicine
Division of Cardiology, Department of Medicine
Weill Medical College of Cornell University
Attending Physician
Division of Cardiology, Department of Medicine
New York Presbyterian Hospital
New York, NY

Jeffrey W. Olin, DO
Professor of Medicine (Cardiology)
Zena and Michael A. Wiener Cardiovascular Institute and Marie-Josée and Henry R. Kravis Center for Cardiovascular Health
Mount Sinai School of Medicine
Director, Vascular Medicine
Zena and Michael A. Wiener Cardiovascular Institute and Marie-Josée and Henry R. Kravis Center for Cardiovascular Health
Mount Sinai School of Medicine
New York, NY

Eric N. Olson, PhD
Professor and Chair
Department of Molecular Biology
University of Texas Southwestern Medical Center
Dallas, TX

Joseph P. Ornato, MD
Professor and Chairman
Department of Emergency Medicine
Virginia Commonwealth University Medical Center
Richmond, VA

Douglas L. Packer, MD
Professor of Medicine
Consultant, Department of Internal Medicine
Division of Cardiovascular Diseases
Co-Director Applied Basic Electrophysiology Laboratory
Department of Internal Medicine, Division of Cardiovascular Diseases, Heart Rhythm Services
Mayo Clinic College of Medicine
Professor of Medicine
Consultant, Department of Internal Medicine
Division of Cardiovascular Diseases
Director, Heart Rhythm Services
Department of Internal Medicine, Division of Cardiovascular Diseases, Heart Rhythm Services
St. Mary's Hospital
Rochester, MN

Pathmaja Paramsothy, MD
Acting Assistant Professor of Medicine
Department of Internal Medicine/Division of Cardiology
University of Washington/Harborview Medical Center
Seattle, WA

Thomas A. Pearson, MD, MPH, PhD
Senior Associate Dean for Clinical Research
Albert D. Kaiser Professor and Chair
Department of Community and Preventive Medicine
University of Rochester
Director, Strong Preventive Cardiology Clinic
University of Rochester Medical Center
Rochester, NY

Mary Ann Peberty, MD
Associate Professor of Medicine and Emergency Medicine
Department of Emergency Medicine and
The Department of Internal Medicine (Cardiology)
Virginia Commonwealth University Health System—
Medical College of Virginia
Richmond, VA

Frank Pelosi, Jr., MD
Assistant Professor of Medicine
Department of Internal Medicine
University of Michigan Health System
Ann Arbor, MI

Marc S. Penn, MD, PhD
Director, Experimental Animal Lab
Associate Director, Cardiovascular Medicine Fellowship
Department of Cardiovascular Medicine
Cleveland Clinic
Cleveland, OH

Eric D. Peterson, MD, MPH
Associate Professor
Department of Medicine/Division of Cardiology
Duke University Medical Center
Associate Vice Chair for Quality
Department of Medicine/Division of Cardiology
Duke University Medical Center
Durham, NC

Eric N. Prystowsky, MD
Consulting Professor of Medicine
Duke University Medical Center
Director, Clinical Electrophysiology Laboratory
St. Vincent
Indianapolis, IN

Reed E. Pyeritz, MD, PhD
Professor of Medicine and Genetics
University of Pennsylvania School of Medicine
Chief, Medical Genetics
Hospital of the University of Pennsylvania
Philadelphia, PA

Marlene Rabinovitch, MD
Dwight and Vera Dunlevie Professor of Pediatric Cardiology
Research Director of Wall Center for Pulmonary Vascular Diseases
Department of Pediatrics
Stanford University School of Medicine
Staff Cardiologist
Department of Pediatrics
Lucile Packard Children's Hospital
Stanford, CA

Daniel J. Rader, MD
Professor
Department of Medicine
University of Pennsylvania School of Medicine
Director, Preventive Cardiovascular Medicine
Department of Medicine
University of Pennsylvania Health System
Philadelphia, PA

Satish R. Raj, MD, MSCI
Assistant Professor
Department of Medicine and Pharmacology
Vanderbilt University School of Medicine
Attending Physician
Department of Medicine
Vanderbilt University Hospital
Nashville, TN

Norman B. Ratliff, MD
Section Head, Autopsy Service
Professor of Pathology
Cleveland Clinic
Cleveland, OH

Elliot J. Rayfield, MD
Clinical Professor
Department of Medicine
Mount Sinai School of Medicine
Attending Physician
Department of Medicine
Mount Sinai Hospital
New York, NY

Dale G. Renlund, MD
Professor
Department of Internal Medicine
University of Utah School of Medicine
Director
Heart Failure Prevention and Treatment Program
Department of Cardiology
LDS Hospital
Salt Lake City, UT

Shereif H. Rezkalla, MD
Clinical Professor of Medicine
University of Wisconsin Medical School
Director of Cardiovascular Research
Department of Cardiology
Mansfield Clinic
Marshfield, WI

David Robertson, MD
Elton Yates Professor of Medicine, Pharmacology and Neurology
General Clinical Research Center
Vanderbilt University
Nashville, TN

Dan M. Roden, MD
Director, Oates Institute for Experimental Therapeutics
Vanderbilt University School of Medicine
Nashville, TN

E. Rene Rodriguez, MD
Adjunct Associate Professor of Pathology
Department of Pathology
Johns Hopkins University School of Medicine
Staff
Department of Anatomic Pathology
Cleveland Clinic
Cleveland, OH

Leonardo Rodriguez, MD
Program Director Advanced Imaging Fellowship
Cardiovascular Imaging Section
Cleveland Clinic
Staff
Department of Cardiovascular Medicine
Cleveland Clinic
Cleveland, OH

Marco Roffi, MD
Staff Cardiologist
Department of Cardiology
University Hospital
Zurich, Switzerland

Michael F. Roizen, MD
Chairman, Division of Anesthesiology
Critical Care Medicine and Comprehensive Pain Management
Cleveland Clinic
Cleveland, OH

James H. F. Rudd, MD, PhD
British Heart Foundation International Research Fellow
Imaging Science Laboratory
Mount Sinai School of Medicine
Specialist Registrar
Department of Cardiovascular Medicine
Addenbrooke's and Papworth Hospitals
New York, NY

Peter Rudd, MD
Professor and Chief, General Internal Medicine
Department of Medicine
Stanford University School of Medicine
Department of Medicine
Stanford Hospital and Clinics
Stanford, CA

Joseph F. Sabik III, MD
Program Director, Thoracic Surgery Residency
Department of Thoracic and Cardiovascular Surgery
Cleveland Clinic
Cleveland, OH

Markus Schwaiger, MD
Professor, Department of Medicine
Technische Universitaet Muenchen
Chairman, Department of Nuclear Medicine
Klinikum R.D. Isar D. Tu Muenchen
Muenchen, Germany

Robert A. Schweikert, MD
Staff
Department of Cardiovascular Medicine
Cleveland Clinic
Cleveland, OH

Christine E. Seidman, MD
Department of Genetics
Harvard Medical School
Boston, MA

Srijita Sen-Chowdhry, MA
Fellow in Cardiology
Centre for Cardiology in The Young
University College, London

Elena B. Sgarbossa, MD
Weston, FL

Cathy A. Sila, MD
Cleveland Clinic
Cleveland, OH

Nicholas G. Smedira, MD
Surgical Director, Kaufman Center for Heart Failure
Department of Cardiovascular and Thoracic Surgery
Cleveland Clinic
Cleveland, OH

Daniel H. Solomon, MD, MPH
Assistant Professor
Department of Medicine
Harvard Medical School
Assistant Professor
Division of Rheumatology
Brigham and Women's Hospital
Boston, MA

David Spragg, MD
Department of Medicine, Cardiology
The Johns Hopkins Medical Institutions
Johns Hopkins University
Baltimore, MD

Randall C. Starling, MD, MPH
Head, Section of Heart Failure and Cardiac Transplant Medicine
Medical Director, Kaufman Center for Heart Failure
Department of Cardiovascular Medicine
Cleveland Clinic
Cleveland, OH

William J. Stewart, MD
Associate Professor of Medicine
Department of Cardiovascular Medicine
Cleveland Clinic Lerner College of Medicine
Staff Physician
Department of Cardiovascular Medicine
Cleveland Clinic
Cleveland, OH

Neil J. Stone, MD
Professor of Clinical Medicine (Cardiology)
Feinberg School of Medicine
Northwestern University
Medical Director, Vascular Center of the Bluhm
Cardiovascular Institute and Attending Physician
Northwestern Memorial Hospital
Chicago, IL

Lynda A. Szczech, MD, MSCE
Associate Professor of Medicine
Department of Medicine/Nephrology
Duke University Medical Center/DCRI
Durham, NC

Carmela D. Tan, MD
Associate Staff
Department of Anatomic Pathology
Cleveland Clinic
Cleveland, OH

W. H. Wilson Tang, MD
Assistant Professor
Department of Medicine
Cleveland Clinic Lerner College of Medicine of Case
Western Reserve University
Staff Physician
Department of Cardiovascular Medicine
Cleveland Clinic
Cleveland, OH

Victor F. Tapson, MD
Professor of Medicine
Director, Center for Pulmonary Vascular Disease
Division of Pulmonary and Critical Care Medicine
Duke University Medical Center
Durham, NC

Mark B. Taubman, MD
Director, Cardiovascular Research Institute
University of Rochester Medical Center
Paul N. Yu Professor and Chief of Cardiology
Department of Medicine/Cardiology
Strong Memorial Hospital
Rochester, NY

David O. Taylor, MD
Professor of Medicine
Department of Cardiovascular Medicine
Cleveland Clinic
Cleveland, OH

Patrick Tchou, MD
Co-Section Head, Section of Cardiac
Electrophysiology and Pacing
Department of Cardiovascular Medicine
Cleveland Clinic
Cleveland, OH

Ayalew Tefferi, MD
Professor
Department of Hematology
Mayo Clinic
Consultant
Department of Hematology
Mayo Clinic
Rochester, MN

James D. Thomas, MD
Professor, Department of Biomedical Engineering
Case Western Reserve University
Charles and Lorraine Chair of Cardiovascular
Imaging
Department of Cardiovascular Medicine
Cleveland Clinic
Cleveland, OH

Paul D. Thompson, MD
Professor of Medicine
University of Connecticut School of Medicine
Director of Cardiology
Cardiology Division
Hartford Hospital
Hartford, CT

Xian-Li Tian, MD
Department of Molecular Cardiology
Lerner Research Institute
Cleveland Clinic
Cleveland, OH

E. Murat Tuzcu, MD
Professor of Medicine
Department of Cardiovascular Medicine
Cleveland Clinic Lerner College of Medicine of
Case Western Reserve University
Interventional Cardiologist
Department of Cardiovascular Medicine
Cleveland Clinic
Cleveland, OH

Alec S. Vahanian, MD
Professor
Department of Cardiology
Paris Université VII
Chief
Department of Cardiology
Hôpital Bichat
Paris, France

Eric Van Belle, MD, PhD
Professor of Medicine
Cardiology Department
University of Lille II Medical School
Associate Director of the Cardiac Catheterization and
Interventional Cardiology Unit
Cardiology Department
Centre Hospitalier Regional de Lille
Lille, France

Frans J. Van de Werf, MD, PhD
Professor of Cardiology
Department of Cardiology
University of Leuven
Chief, Department of Cardiology
Gasthuisberg University Hospital
Leuven, Belgium

George F. Van Hare, MD
Professor of Pediatrics
Department of Pediatric Cardiology
Stanford University
Director, Pediatric Arrhythmia Center at UCSF
Stanford
Lucille Packard Children's Hospital
Palo Alto, CA

Renu Virmani, MD
Medical Director, CVPath Institute, Inc.
Clinical Research Professor, Department of Pathology
Vanderbilt University School of Medicine
Clinical Professor, Department of Pathology
Georgetown University School of Medicine
Clinical Professor, Department of Pathology
University of Maryland School of Medicine
Clinical Professor, Department of Pathology
Uniformed University of Health Sciences
Clinical Professor, Department of Pathology
George Washington School of Medicine

Galen Wagner, MD
Associate Professor
Department of Medicine
Duke University Medical Center
Director, ECG Core Lab
Duke University Medical Center
Durham, NC

Qing Wang, MD
Associate Professor
Department of Molecular Medicine
Cleveland Clinic Lerner College of Medicine of Case Western Reserve University
Full Staff
Department of Molecular Cardiology
Lerner Research Institute
Cleveland Clinic
Cleveland, OH

Peter L. Weissberg, MD
Medical Director
British Heart Foundation
Professor of Cardiology
Centre for Clinical Investigation
Addenbrooke's Hospital
London, United Kingdom

Harvey D. White, MB, ChB, DSc
Honorary Clinical Professor
Department of Medicine
University of Auckland
Director of Coronary Care and Cardiovascular Research
Green Lane Cardiovascular Service
Auckland City Hospital
Auckland, New Zealand

Richard D. White, MD
Professor and Chairman, Department of Radiology
University of Florida-Shands Jacksonville
Jacksonville, FL

David Wilber, MD
Professor
Department of Medicine
Loyola University Chicago
Director
Division of Cardiology
Loyola University Medical Center
Maywood, IL

Bruce L. Wilkoff, MD
Professor of Medicine
Department of Cardiovascular Medicine
Cleveland Clinic Lerner College of Medicine of Case Western Reserve University
Director, Cardiac Pacing and Tachyarrhythmia Devices
Department of Cardiovascular Medicine
Cleveland Clinic
Cleveland, OH

Deborah L. Wolbrette, MD
Associate Professor
Department of Medicine, Division of Cardiology
Penn State's Milton S. Hershey College of Medicine
Director of Pacing and Electrocardiography
Heart and Vascular Institute
The Milton S. Hershey Medical Center
Hershey, PA

Jay S. Yadav, MD
Director, Vascular Intervention
Department of Cardiovascular Medicine
Cleveland Clinic
Cleveland, OH

James B. Young, MD
Professor
Division of Medicine
Cleveland Clinic Lerner College of Medicine of Case Western Reserve University
Chairman
Division of Medicine
Cleveland Clinic
Cleveland, OH

Sibylle Zeigler, MD
Klinikum rechts der Isar
der Technischen Universität München
Nuklearmedizinische Klinik und Poliklinik

PREFACE

The success of the first edition of this Textbook was largely predicated on fulfilling its mission: "building a new, authoritative reference textbook in the field of cardiovascular medicine . . . based on the radical changes that have taken place in the past decade." These changes not only included coverage of the largest specialty within medicine, but also the fully transformed electronic capabilities that have become both pervasive and prosaic. The CD-ROM version of the earlier editions of the Textbook received significant recognition and acclaim. This has now evolved, in this 3rd edition, into a DVD with over 1000 digital images and multimedia video clips to bring the text alive.

The field of cardiovascular medicine has gone through some radical changes since the last edition. These include the use of multidetector CT angiography to eventually replace diagnostic cardiac catheterization, the routine use of drug-eluting stents for percutaneous coronary intervention, the use of pulmonary vein isolation procedures to ablate atrial fibrillation, the more wide scale acceptance of statins, ACE inhibitors and defibrillators, and resynchronization therapy for the treatment of heart failure. We are right at the cusp of breakthroughs in the genomics of complex cardiovascular traits, such as myocardial infarction and valvular heart disease, and for this reason the molecular cardiovascular content has been emphasized. All of these marked changes in the field have been highlighted in this edition. There are new chapters covering women and heart disease, prevention of heart failure, stem cells and myocardial regeneration, cardiac resynchronization, peri-operative management, percutaneous valve repair and intracardiac procedures as well as several others that capture the advances in molecular cardiology.

The book and DVD are fully hybridized. As in the past, we have more chapters than are presented in the hard copy, and have 20 chapters on the DVD to reduce the bulk of the text, to provide a comprehensive resource and preserve the valuable information on such topics as congenital heart disease, sudden death, mechanisms and genetics of arrhythmias, pan-coverage of molecular cardiology, databases in cardiology, pharmacology, the importance of chest X-rays for clinical assessment, electrophysiologic testing, both invasively and non-invasively.

In order to execute this prodigious effort, we relied on more than 200 expert contributing authors from all over the world. On behalf of all the Section Editors and authors, we hope that this initiative will prove useful in day-to-day care of patients with cardiovascular disease, serve as a stimulus for future research in basic and clinical science, and provide a utilitarian reference source for all health care professionals, trainees, scientists and biomedical researchers active in the field of cardiovascular medicine in the 21st century. Hopefully, in some way, all of the effort and expertise brought together here will help advance our field.

Eric J. Topol, MD

ACKNOWLEDGMENTS

As in the first and second editions, this project was overwhelming and consumptive and, without question, one of the most challenging and enormous undertakings that I have ever encountered. In order for it to be accomplished, a huge number of dedicated individuals came together in a highly synergistic fashion. The people behind the project include the superb Section Editors, Robert Califf, Paul Thompson, Eric Prystowsky, and Jim Thomas, over 200 contributing authors from all over the world, and two project teams. One, based at Cleveland Clinic, included Donna Wasiewicz-Bressan, Managing Editor; Milind Desai, DVD Director; Suzanne Turner, Charlene Surace, Mary Ann Citraro, and Marion Tomasko, graphic artists; with extensive DVD contributions from Timothy Crowe in production, Manuel Cerqueira for nuclear scintigraphy, Mina Chung for electrophysiologic tracings, Heather Gornik for peripheral vascular disease graphics, Wael Jaber for cardiovascular imaging, Samir Kapadia for interventional cardiology procedures, Richard Krasuski for congenital heart disease, Rene Rodriguez and Carmella Tan for cardiovascular pathology, Tom Mihaljevic, Nicholas Smedira, Marc Gillinov and Lars Svensson for their contributions from cardiac surgical operations. Heart sounds were collected by Deb Mukherjee, Steve Lin, Khaldoun Tarakji, and Raymond Migrino. The hyperlinks from book to DVD were provided by a superb team of fellows including Mark Iler, Daniel Sauri, John Zakaib, Bret Rogers, Ronan Curtin, Anthony Bavry, Boris Lowe, Chris Gring, Thomas Callahan, and Ross Murphy. The other group, based at Lippincott Williams & Wilkins Publishers and its production subsidiary Techbooks, included Fran DeStefano, and the editorial and production teams of Joanne Bersin, Dave Murphy, and Max Leckrone. Only with the tight collaboration and dedication of all the editors, authors, and the project teams could such a vast endeavor come together so successfully. My personal appreciation to all of these people runs very deep, and cannot be adequately expressed in words.

CONTENTS

SECTION ONE ■ PREVENTIVE CARDIOLOGY
PAUL D. THOMPSON

SECTION TWO ■ CLINICAL CARDIOLOGY
ROBERT M. CALIFF

SECTION THREE ■ CARDIOVASCULAR IMAGING
JAMES THOMAS

SECTION SIX ■ HEART FAILURE AND TRANSPLANTATION
ERIC J. TOPOL

SECTION SEVEN ■ MOLECULAR CARDIOLOGY
ERIC J. TOPOL

SECTION EIGHT ■ VASCULAR BIOLOGY AND MEDICINE

ERIC J. TOPOL

THIRD
EDITION

TEXTBOOK OF CARDIOVASCULAR MEDICINE

SECTION ONE
PREVENTIVE CARDIOLOGY

PAUL D. THOMPSON, M.D.

CHAPTER 1 ■ ATHEROSCLEROTIC BIOLOGY AND EPIDEMIOLOGY OF DISEASE

JAMES H.F. RUDD, JOHN R. DAVIES, AND PETER L. WEISSBERG

EPIDEMIOLOGY OF CARDIOVASCULAR DISEASE

Atherosclerosis, with its complications, is the leading cause of mortality and morbidity in the developed world. In the United States, a snapshot of the population reveals that 60 million adults currently suffer from atherosclerotic cardiovascular disease, which accounts for 42% of all deaths annually, at a cost to the nation of $128 billion. Fortunately, despite this catastrophic burden of disease, much evidence has emerged over the last decade suggesting that the progression of atherosclerosis can be slowed or even reversed in many people with appropriate lifestyle and drug interventions.

The origin of the current epidemic of cardiovascular disease can be traced back to the time of industrialization in the 1700s. The three factors largely responsible for this were an increase in the use of tobacco products, reduced physical activity, and the adoption of a diet high in fat, calories, and cholesterol. This rising tide of cardiovascular disease continued into the twentieth century, but began to recede when data from the Framingham study identified a number of modifiable risk factors for cardiovascular disease, including cigarette smoking, hypertension, and hypercholesterolemia (1).

The number of deaths per 100,000 attributable to cardiovascular disease peaked in the Western world in 1964 to 1965, since which time there has been a gradual decline in death rates (Fig. 1.1) (2). The age-adjusted coronary heart disease (CHD) mortality in the United States dropped by more than 40% and cerebrovascular disease mortality by more than 50%, with the greatest reductions being seen among whites and men. This reduction has occurred despite a quadrupling of the proportion of the population older than 65 years of age and has been due to a number of factors, particularly major health promotion campaigns aimed at reducing the prevalence of Framingham risk factors. Indeed, there has been a substantial change in the prevalence of population cardiovascular risk factors over the last 30 years (Table 1.1). The war is not won, however, and the decline in the death rate from cardiovascular disease slowed in the 1990s (Fig. 1.2). This is likely owing to a large increase in the prevalence of both obesity and type 2 diabetes mellitus, as well as a resurgence of cigarette smoking in some sectors of society (3). Female death rates from cardiovascular disease overtook male death rates in 1984 and have shown a smaller decline over the last 30 years (4). The consequences of atherosclerosis are also beginning to be felt in less well-developed regions of the globe (5), with death from atherosclerotic cardiovascular disease set to replace infection as the leading cause of death in the Third World in the near future. This phenomenon is further illustrated by the increase in CHD mortality in countries of Eastern and Central Europe (most notably countries of the former Soviet Union). For example, in the Ukraine the age standardized death rate in the year 2000 was just over 800 per 100,000 people representing an increase of over 60% when compared to 1990 (6).

A further note of caution should also be struck. Western countries are experiencing a dramatic increase in the prevalence of heart failure. In the United States, almost 5 million people carry a diagnosis of heart failure (7), thus singling it out as an emerging epidemic (8). However, the determinants of this epidemic have yet to be fully elucidated, with some epidemiologic studies pointing toward hypertension as the driving factor (9) and others suggesting CHD as the predominant cause (10).

BIOLOGY OF ATHEROSCLEROSIS

Traditionally, atherosclerosis has been viewed as a degenerative disease, affecting predominantly older people, slowly progressing over many years, and eventually leading to symptoms through mechanical effects of blood flow. The perceived insidious and relentless nature of its development has meant that

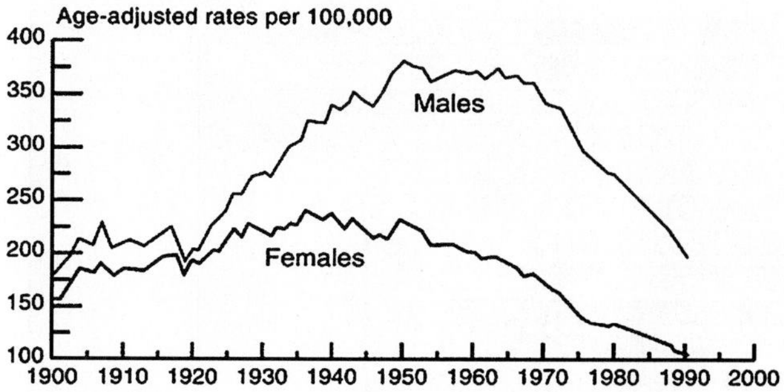

FIGURE 1.1. Trends in death rates for heart diseases: United States, 1900–1991. (*Source:* Feinleib M. Trends in heart disease in the United States [review]. *Am J Med Sci* 1995;310[Suppl 1]:S8–S14, with permission.)

a somewhat pessimistic view of the potential to modify its progression by medical therapy has held sway. There has been little emphasis on the diagnosis and treatment of high-risk asymptomatic patients. Disease management has instead been dominated by interventional revascularization approaches, targeting the largest and most visible or symptomatic lesions with coronary angioplasty or bypass surgery.

Recently, for several reasons, this defeatist view of the pathogenesis and progression of atherosclerosis has begun to change. First, careful descriptive studies of the underlying pathology of atherosclerosis have revealed that atherosclerotic plaques differ in their cellular composition and that the cell types predominating in the plaque can determine the risk of fatal clinical events. A high degree of plaque inflammation is particularly dangerous. Second, recent epidemiologic work has identified many new potentially modifiable risk factors for atherosclerosis, above and beyond those highlighted as a result of the Framingham study (11). The third and most important reason is because several large-scale clinical trials have reported that drugs—in particular, the HMG-CoA reductase inhibitors (statins)—are able to reduce the number of clinical events in patients with established atherosclerosis and do so without necessarily affecting the size of atherosclerotic plaques. These three strands of evidence have shown that, rather than being an irreversibly progressive disease, atherosclerosis is a dynamic, inflammatory process that may be amenable to medical therapy. Understanding the cellular and molecular interactions that determine the development and progression of atherosclerosis brings with it opportunities to develop novel therapeutic agents targeting key molecular and cellular interactions in its etiology. In addition, the recognition that the clinical consequences of atherosclerosis depend almost entirely on plaque composition argues for a new approach to diagnosis, with less emphasis placed on the degree of lumen narrowing and more interest in the cellular composition of the plaque.

TABLE 1.1

TEMPORAL CHANGES IN CORONARY RISK FACTORS

Cigarette smoking	1960	Men, 55%; women, 33%
	1990	Men, 30%; women, 27%
Undiagnosed hypertension	1960	52%
	1980	29%
Mean serum cholesterol	1960	225 mg/dL
	1990	208 mg/dL
Diabetes mellitus	1970	2.6%
	1990	9.1%
Sedentary lifestyle	1970	41%
	1985	27%
Obesity	1960	25%
	1990	38%

From Miller M, Vogel RA. *The practice of coronary disease prevention.* Baltimore: Williams & Wilkins, 1996.

NORMAL ARTERY

The healthy artery consists of three histologically distinct layers. Innermost and surrounding the lumen is the tunica intima, which comprises a single layer of endothelial cells in close proximity to the internal elastic lamina. The tunica media surrounds the internal elastic lamina, and its composition varies depending on the type of artery. The tunica media of the smallest arterial vessels, arterioles, comprises a single layer of vascular smooth muscle cells (VSMCs). Small arteries have a similar structure but with a thicker layer of medial VSMCs. Arterioles and small arteries are termed *resistance vessels* because they contribute vascular resistance and, hence, directly affect blood pressure. At the opposite end of the spectrum are large elastic or conduit arteries, named for the high proportion of elastin in the tunica media. The tunica media of all arteries is contained within a connective tissue layer that contains blood vessels and nerves and that is known as the *tunica adventitia.* In normal arteries, the vessel lumen diameter can be altered by contraction and relaxation of the medial VSMCs in response to a variety of systemic and locally released signals.

ATHEROSCLEROTIC VESSEL

Atherosclerosis is primarily a disease affecting the intimal layer of elastic arteries. For reasons that remain largely unknown, some arterial beds appear more prone than others. Coronary, carotid, cerebral, and renal arteries and the aorta are most often involved. The arteries supplying the lower limbs are also vulnerable to disease. Interestingly, the internal mammary artery is almost always spared, making it an invaluable vessel for coronary bypass surgery.

Atherosclerotic lesions develop over many years and pass through several overlapping stages. Histologically, the earliest lesion is a subendothelial accumulation of lipid-laden macrophage foam cells and associated T lymphocytes known as a *fatty streak.* Fatty streaks are asymptomatic and nonstenotic. Postmortem examinations have shown that they are present in the aorta at the end of the first decade of life, are present in the coronary arteries by the second, and begin to appear in the cerebral circulation by the third decade. With time, the lesion progresses and the core of the early plaque becomes necrotic, containing cellular debris, crystalline cholesterol, and inflammatory cells, particularly macrophage foam cells. This necrotic core becomes bounded on its luminal aspect by an endothelialized fibrous cap, consisting of VSMCs embedded in an extensive collagenous extracellular matrix. Inflammatory cells are also present in the fibrous cap, concentrated particularly in the "shoulder" regions, where T cells, mast cells, and especially macrophages have a tendency to accumulate. Advanced lesions may become increasingly complex, showing evidence of calcification, ulceration, new microvessel formation, and rupture or erosion (12). Microvessels within the plaque may play important roles in the formation of macrophage-rich vulnerable atheroma by providing an extended surface area of activated endothelial cells to hasten recruitment of further inflammatory cells as well as by promotion of intraplaque hemorrhage (13).

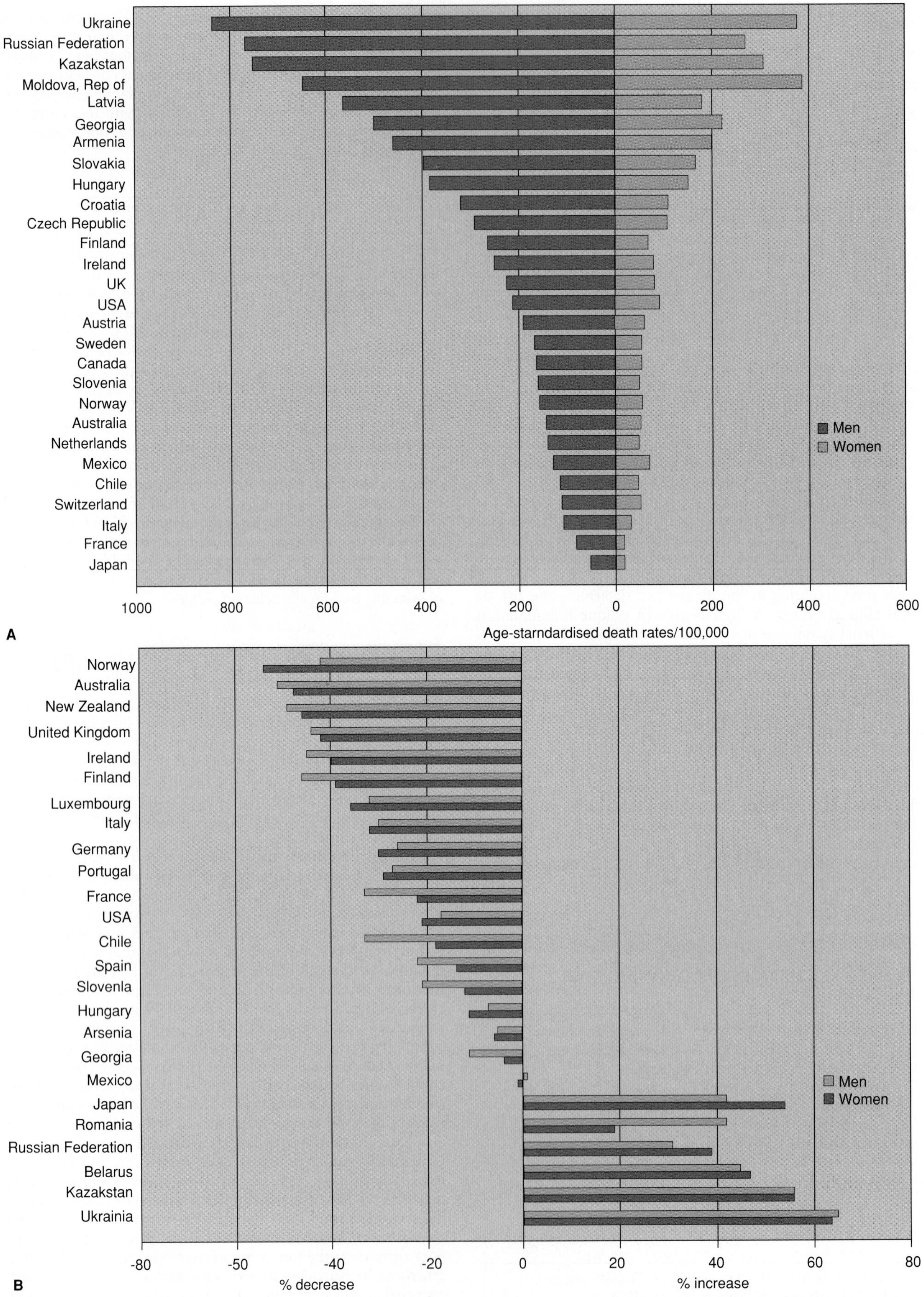

FIGURE 1.2. A. Death rates from CHD, men and women aged 35–74, 2000, selected countries. B. Changes in death rates from CHD, men and women aged 35–74, between 1990 and 2000, selected countries.

Thus, the composition of atherosclerotic plaques is variable, dynamic and complex, and it is the interaction between the various cell types within a plaque that determines the progression, complications, and outcome of the disease.

CELLULAR ROLES IN ATHEROGENESIS

Endothelial Cells

The endothelium plays a central role in maintaining vascular health by virtue of its vital anti-inflammatory and anticoagulant properties. Many of these characteristics are mediated by the nitric oxide (NO) molecule. This molecule was discovered in the 1980s, having been isolated from lipopolysaccharide-primed macrophages (14). NO is synthesized by endothelial cells under the control of the enzyme endothelial NO synthase (NOS) and has a number of anti-atherogenic properties. First, it acts as a powerful inhibitor of platelet aggregation on endothelial cells. Second, it can reduce inflammatory cell recruitment into the intima by abrogating the expression of genes involved in this process, such as those encoding intercellular adhesion molecule-1 (ICAM-1), vascular cell adhesion molecule-1 (VCAM-1), P-selectin, and monocyte chemoattractant protein-1 (MCP-1) (15–17). There is some evidence that NO may also reduce lipid entry into the arterial intima (18). NO is also a potent anti-inflammatory molecule and, depending on concentration, may be a scavenger or a producer of potentially destructive oxygen free radicals, such as peroxynitrite (19–21). The earliest detectable manifestation of atherosclerosis is a decrease in the bioavailability of NO in response to pharmacologic or hemodynamic stimuli (22). This may occur for two reasons. Either there may be decreased manufacture of NO because of endothelial cell dysfunction, or increased NO breakdown may take place. There is evidence that both mechanisms may be important in different situations (23). Many atherosclerosis risk factors can lead to impaired endothelial function and reduced NO bioavailability. For example, hyperlipidemic patients have reduced NO-dependent vasodilatation, which is reversed when patients are treated with lipid-lowering medication (24). Diabetics also have impaired endothelial function, occurring primarily as a result of impaired NO production. There is, however, some evidence to suggest that increased oxidative stress leading to enhanced NO breakdown may also be a factor in early endothelial dysfunction (25). Similarly, other risk factors for atherosclerosis, such as hypertension and cigarette smoking, are associated with reduced NO bioavailability (26,27). In cigarette smokers, endothelial impairment is thought to be caused by enhanced NO degradation by oxygen-derived free-radical agents such as the superoxide ion. There are also other consequences of an increased reactivity between NO and superoxide species. The product of their interaction, ONOO– (peroxynitrite), is a powerful oxidizing agent and can reach high concentrations in atherosclerotic lesions. This may result in cellular oxidative injury.

Another consequence of endothelial cell dysfunction that occurs in early atherosclerosis is the expression of surface-bound selectins and adhesion molecules, including P-selectin, ICAM-1, and VCAM-1. These molecules attract and capture circulating inflammatory cells and facilitate their migration into the subendothelial space (22). Normal endothelial cells do not express these molecules, but their appearance may be induced by abnormal arterial shear stress, subendothelial oxidized lipid, and, in diabetic patients, the presence of advanced glycosylation products in the arterial wall. The importance of selectins and adhesion molecules in the development of atherosclerosis is demonstrated in experiments using mice, which lack their expression. These animals develop smaller lesions with a lower lipid content and fewer inflammatory cells than control mice when fed a lipid-rich diet (28). Animal models have reinforced the importance of inflammatory cell recruitment to the pathogenesis of atherosclerosis, but because inflammatory cells are never seen in the intima in the absence of lipid, the results suggest that subendothelial lipid accumulation is also necessary for the development of atherosclerosis.

The tendency for atherosclerosis to occur preferentially in particular sites may be explained by subtle variations in endothelial function. This is probably caused by variations in local blood flow patterns, especially conditions of low flow, which can influence expression of a number of endothelial cell genes, including those encoding ICAM-1 and endothelial NOS (29,30). In addition to flow speed, flow type can have a direct effect on cell morphology. In areas of laminar flow (atheroprotective flow), endothelial cells tend to have an ellipsoid shape, contrasting with the situation found at vessel branch points and curves, where turbulent flow (atherogenic flow) induces a conformational change toward polygonal-shaped cells (31). Such cells have an increased permeability to low-density lipoprotein (LDL) cholesterol and may promote lesion formation (32).

These data are consistent with the idea that the primary event in atherogenesis is endothelial dysfunction. The endothelium can be damaged by a variety of means, leading to dysfunction and, by unknown mechanisms, subsequent subendothelial lipid accumulation. In this situation, the normal homeostatic features of the endothelium break down; it becomes more adhesive to inflammatory cells and platelets, it loses its anticoagulant properties, and there is reduced bioavailability of NO. Importantly, endothelial function is improved by drugs that have been shown to substantially reduce death from vascular disease, including statins and angiotensin-converting enzyme inhibitors (33,34).

Inflammatory Cells

LDL from the circulation is able to diffuse passively through the tight junctions that bind neighboring endothelial cells. The rate of passive diffusion is increased when circulating levels of LDL are elevated. In addition, other lipid fractions may be important in atherosclerosis. Lipoprotein(a) has the same basic molecular structure as LDL, with an additional apolipoprotein(a) element attached by a disulfide bridge. It has been shown to be highly atherogenic (35), accumulate in the arterial wall in a manner similar to LDL (36), impair vessel fibrinolysis (37), and stimulate smooth muscle cell proliferation (38). The accumulation of subendothelial lipids, particularly when at least partly oxidized, is thought to stimulate the local inflammatory reaction that initiates and maintains activation of overlying endothelial cells. The activated cells express a variety of selectins and adhesion molecules and also produce a number of chemokines—in particular, MCP-1, whose expression is upregulated by the presence of oxidized LDL in the subendothelial space (39). Interestingly, the protective effect of high-density lipoprotein (HDL) against atherosclerotic vascular disease may be partly explained by its ability to block endothelial cell expression of adhesion molecules (40,41). Chemokines are proinflammatory cytokines responsible for chemoattraction, migration, and subsequent activation of leukocytes. Mice lacking the MCP-1 gene develop smaller atherosclerotic lesions than normal animals (42). The first stage of inflammatory cell recruitment to the intima is the initiation of "rolling" of monocytes and T cells along the endothelial cell layer. This phenomenon is mediated by the selectin molecules, which selectively bind ligands found on these inflammatory cells. The subsequent firm adhesion to and migration of leukocytes through the endothelial cell layer depends on the endothelial expression of adhesion molecules such as ICAM-1 and VCAM-1 and their binding to appropriate receptors on inflammatory cells. Once present in the intima, monocytes differentiate into macrophages under the influence of chemokines such as macrophage colony-stimulating factor. Such molecules also stimulate the expression of the scavenger receptors that allow macrophages to ingest oxidized lipids and to develop into macrophage foam cells, the predominant cell in an early atherosclerotic lesion. The formation of scavenger receptors is also regulated by peroxisome proliferator-activated receptor-γ (PPAR-γ a nuclear transcription factor expressed at high levels in foam cells) (43). PPAR-γ agonists (glitazones), which are used to treat patients with type 2 diabetes, have been shown to have many anti-atherogenic effects, including increasing production of NO (44), decreased endothelial inflammatory cell recruitment and reduced vascular endothelial growth factor (VEGF) expression (45). Also, PPAR-γ agonists can reduce the lipid content of plaques by enhancing reverse cholesterol transport from plaque to liver. Positive results with these drugs in patients with type 2 diabetes are emerging. As well as reducing matrix metalloproteinase (MMP) 9 levels, glitazones also significantly ameliorated C-reactive protein (CRP) and CD40 ligand levels, as well as causing direct plaque regression in a rabbit atheroma model (46). Clearly their use in large clinical trials in patients without diabetes as anti-atheroma drugs is awaited with interest.

In early atherosclerosis at least, the macrophage can be thought of as performing a predominantly beneficial role as a "neutralizer" of potentially harmful oxidized lipid components in the vessel wall. However, macrophage foam cells also synthesize a variety of proinflammatory cytokines and growth factors that contribute both beneficially and detrimentally to the evolution of the plaque. Some of these factors are chemoattractant (osteopontin) and growth-enhancing (platelet-derived growth factor) for VSMCs (12,47). Under the influence of these cytokines, VSMCs migrate from the media to the intima, where they adopt a synthetic phenotype, well-suited to matrix production and protective fibrous cap formation.

However, activated macrophages have a high rate of apoptosis. Once dead, they release their lipid content, which becomes part of the core of the plaque, thereby contributing to its enlargement. The apoptotic cells also contain high concentrations of tissue factor, which may invoke thrombosis if exposed to circulating platelets (48). Interestingly, the selective glycoprotein 2b3a receptor antagonist abciximab has been shown to have an effect on the levels of tissue factor found in monocytes. In an in vitro study by Steiner (49), the drug attenuated both the amount of tissue factor and its RNA levels. As tissue factor is a potent instigator of the clotting cascade, this role may explain part of the protective effect of abciximab on the microcirculation of patients with acute coronary syndromes (50).

It is now generally recognized that the pathologic progression and consequences of atherosclerotic lesions are determined by dynamic interactions between inflammatory cells recruited in response to subendothelial lipid accumulation, and the local reparative "wound healing" response of surrounding VSMCs.

Vascular Smooth Muscle Cells

VSMCs reside mostly in the media of healthy adult arteries, where their role is to regulate vascular tone. Thus, medial VSMCs contain large amounts of contractile proteins, including myosin, α-actin, and tropomyosin. Continued expression of this "contractile" phenotype is maintained by the influence of extracellular proteins in the media, which act via integrins in the VSMC membrane. In atherosclerosis, however, the cells become influenced by cytokines produced by activated macrophages and endothelial cells. Under these influences, VSMCs migrate to the intima and undergo a phenotypic change characterized by a reduction in content of contractile proteins and a large increase in the number of synthetic organelles. This migration of VSMCs from the media to the intima, and the consequent change from a contractile to a "synthetic" phenotype, was previously thought to be a crucial step in the development of atherosclerosis in the modified response to injury hypothesis discussed previously. More recently, it has been recognized that intimal VSMCs in atherosclerotic plaques bear a remarkable similarity to VSMCs found in the early developing blood vessels (51), suggesting that intimal VSMCs may be performing a beneficial, reparative role rather than a destructive one in atherosclerosis. VSMCs are well-equipped for this action. First, they can express the proteinases that they require to break free from the medial basement membrane and allow them to migrate to the site of inflammation or injury in response to chemokines. Second, they can produce various growth factors, including VEGF and platelet-derived growth factor, that act in an autocrine loop to facilitate their proliferation at the site of injury. Finally, and most important, they produce large quantities of matrix proteins, in particular glycosaminoglycans, elastin, and collagen isoforms 1 and 3, necessary to repair the vessel and form a fibrous cap over the lipid-rich core of the lesion. This fibrous cap separates the highly thrombogenic lipid-rich plaque core from circulating platelets and the proteins of the coagulation cascade and also confers structural stability to the atherosclerotic lesion. And because the VSMC is the only cell capable of synthesizing this cap, it follows that VSMCs play a pivotal role in maintaining plaque stability and protecting against the potentially fatal thrombotic consequences of atherosclerosis (52).

CELLULAR INTERACTIONS AND LESION STABILITY

Generally, early atherosclerosis progresses without symptoms until a lesion declares itself in one of two ways. As discussed, macrophage foam cells may undergo apoptosis, especially in the presence of high concentrations of oxidized LDL. Their cellular remnants then become part of an enlarging lipid-rich core. Plaque size thus increases, and there may be a consequent reduction in vessel lumen area. At times of increased demand, such as exercise, this may be sufficient to cause ischemic symptoms such as angina. More hazardous is if the plaque presents with disruption of the fibrous cap, leading to exposure of the thrombogenic lipid core. This is likely to result in subsequent platelet accumulation and activation, fibrin deposition, and intravascular thrombosis. Depending on factors such as collateral blood supply, extent of arterial thrombus, and local fibrinolytic activity, the end result may be arterial occlusion and downstream necrosis.

By studying the pathology of ruptured plaques, several characteristics have been identified that seem to be predictive of the risk of rupture in individual lesions (53). Plaques that are vulnerable to rupture tend to have thin fibrous caps (<65 μm) with a high ratio of inflammatory cells to VSMCs and contain a lipid core that occupies more than 50% of the volume of the plaque. Of these, the most important is the cellular composition of the fibrous cap. Plaques containing a heavy inflammatory cell infiltrate and relatively few VSMCs have the highest risk of rupture (54). Interestingly, in the coronary tree, such high-risk plaques are usually located in the proximal portions of the main arteries (55). Recently, evidence of the importance of intraplaque hemorrhage from microvessels in plaque destabilization has emerged. It is thought that the leaking vessels initiate platelet and red cell phagocytosis by plaque macrophages, causing them to become activated and tipping the balance toward plaque rupture (56).

Inflammatory cells in plaques act to promote plaque rupture by a number of synergistic mechanisms. First, activated T cells produce proinflammatory cytokines, typified by IFN-γ, that directly inhibit VSMC proliferation (57) and almost completely shut down collagen synthesis (58,59). Thus, VSMCs in the vicinity of activated T cells in plaques are poorly able to lay down or repair extracellular matrix. Second, macrophage-derived inflammatory cytokines, in particular interleukin-1β and tumor necrosis factor-α along with IFN-γ from T cells, are synergistically cytotoxic for VSMCs, causing depletion in cell number by apoptosis (60). These cytokines are found at high levels in vulnerable plaques (61). Third, activated macrophages can induce VSMC apoptosis by direct cell–cell contact (62). Finally, and probably most important, macrophages secrete a variety of matrix metalloproteinases that degrade the matrix components of the fibrous cap by proteolytic cleavage of its protein components (52). The production of matrix metalloproteinases is upregulated by inflammatory mediators such as tumor necrosis factor-α. As well as being under threat from such an array of insults, VSMCs themselves within the fibrous cap of a mature plaque have a reduced ability to proliferate (63,64) and an enhanced susceptibility to apoptosis (65). Thus, inflammatory cells can destroy the fabric of the fibrous cap, and resident VSMCs are poorly equipped to compensate, particularly in the presence of inhibitory inflammatory cytokines. It is important to note that all of these features can be present in small, hemodynamically insignificant plaques that are clinically silent and angiographically invisible. Thus, plaque composition is far more important than plaque size in determining outcome.

INFLAMMATORY MARKERS IN ATHEROSCLEROSIS

The cell biology of plaque development and subsequent rupture illustrates that atherosclerosis is fundamentally an inflammatory condition. Confirmation of this inflammatory basis has come from several studies of different patient populations that have all demonstrated a correlation between levels of markers of systemic inflammation, principally CRP, and risk of a clinical event owing to plaque rupture (66–70). However, unlike in other systemic inflammatory conditions, such as rheumatoid arthritis, levels of CRP in atherosclerosis are characteristically not elevated above the conventional normal range, and a correlation between CRP level and coronary events was demonstrated only after development of a highly sensitive assay for CRP that was capable of measuring levels below the lower limit of detection of conventional assays. The risk of clinical events associated with an elevated CRP seems to be independent of the presence of other Framingham risk factors for atherosclerosis. Elevated CRP also predicts near-term plaque rupture events as well those up to 20 years in the future, suggesting that inflammation is important in both early and late atherosclerosis (71). Additionally, CRP level accurately indicates the likelihood of sudden cardiac death, a condition usually associated with multiple atherosclerotic plaque ruptures (72). However, despite initial enthusiasm, large meta-analyses have suggested that the relative risk of a cardiovascular event is increased by only approximately 1.5 times in those people with a baseline elevated CRP (above 3 mg/dL) (73,74). With such a modest predictive value, it may be that the routine measurement of CRP alone in asymptomatic patients is not yet justified for accurate disease prediction.

Similar, although less compelling, correlations with clinical events have also been published for other markers of inflammation, including soluble ICAM-1, VCAM-1, P-selectin, and interleukin-6 (the primary driver of CRP production) (75–78). Results of these studies have been interpreted by some as indicating that atherosclerosis arises as a consequence of a systemic inflammatory process (e.g., chronic infection) and by others that it reflects the inflammatory processes of atherosclerosis itself. However, there is accumulating evidence in favor of the latter interpretation.

TWO FORMS OF PLAQUE DISRUPTION: FIBROUS CAP RUPTURE AND ENDOTHELIAL EROSION

Atherosclerotic plaques become life threatening when they initiate clot formation in the vessel lumen and disturb blood flow. This can occur in two different ways. Either there can be fibrous cap rupture, with consequent exposure of the thrombogenic extracellular matrix of the cap and the tissue factor–rich lipid core to circulating blood, or less commonly, there is erosion of the endothelial cells covering the fibrous cap, also potentially leading to the formation of a platelet-rich thrombus. Endothelial erosion probably accounts for approximately 30% of acute coronary syndromes overall and seems particularly common in women (79). Both forms of plaque disruption invariably lead to local platelet accumulation and activation. This may result in triggering of the clotting cascade, thrombus formation, and, if extensive, complete vessel occlusion. Platelet-rich thrombus contains chemokines and mitogens, in particular platelet-derived growth factor and thrombin that induce migration and proliferation of VSMCs from the arterial media to the plaque and transforming growth factor-β that contributes to healing of the disrupted lesion (80). Platelets also express CD40 on their cell membrane, which causes local endothelial cell activation, resulting in the recruitment of more inflammatory cells to the lesion and perpetuating the cycle of inflammation, rupture, and thrombosis. However, fibrous cap rupture or erosion does not invariably lead to vessel occlusion. Up to 70% of plaques causing high-grade stenosis contain histologic evidence of previous subclinical plaque rupture with subsequent repair (81). This is particularly likely to occur if high blood flow through the vessel prevents the accumulation of a large occlusive thrombus. Thus, nonocclusive plaque rupture induces formation of a new fibrous cap over the organizing thrombus, which restabilizes the lesion but at the expense of increasing its size. Because this occurs suddenly, there is little opportunity for adaptive remodeling of the artery, and the healed lesion may now impede flow sufficiently to produce ischemic symptoms. This explains why patients who have previously had normal exercise tolerance may suddenly develop symptoms of stable angina pectoris. It also follows that if lesions can grow as a consequence of repeated episodes of silent rupture and repair, an inhibition of plaque rupture rate will reduce progression of atherosclerosis. Therefore, atheromatous plaques may become larger by two methods. The first is a gradual increase in size as a consequence of macrophage foam cell accumulation and incorporation of apoptotic cells into an enlarging necrotic lipid-laden plaque core. The second is a stepwise increase in size because of repeated, often silent episodes of plaque rupture or erosion with subsequent VSMC-driven repair.

BALANCE OF ATHEROSCLEROSIS: THERAPEUTIC IMPLICATIONS

Atherosclerosis is a dynamic process in which the balance between the destructive influence of inflammatory cells and the reactive, stabilizing effects of VSMCs determines outcome (Fig. 1.3). This balance can be tipped toward plaque rupture by factors such as an atherogenic lipoprotein profile, high levels of lipid oxidation, local free radical generation, and genetic variability in expression and activity of certain central inflammatory molecules. For example, an association between plaque progression and a polymorphism in the stromelysin-1 gene promoter has been described (82). Until recently, it was also thought that infectious organisms might be involved in atherosclerosis, either as plaque initiators or as having some role in initiating plaque rupture. *Chlamydia pneumoniae* is found in plaques, localizing at high concentrations within macrophages, but is rarely found in normal arteries (83). Although these data imply a pathologic association between the

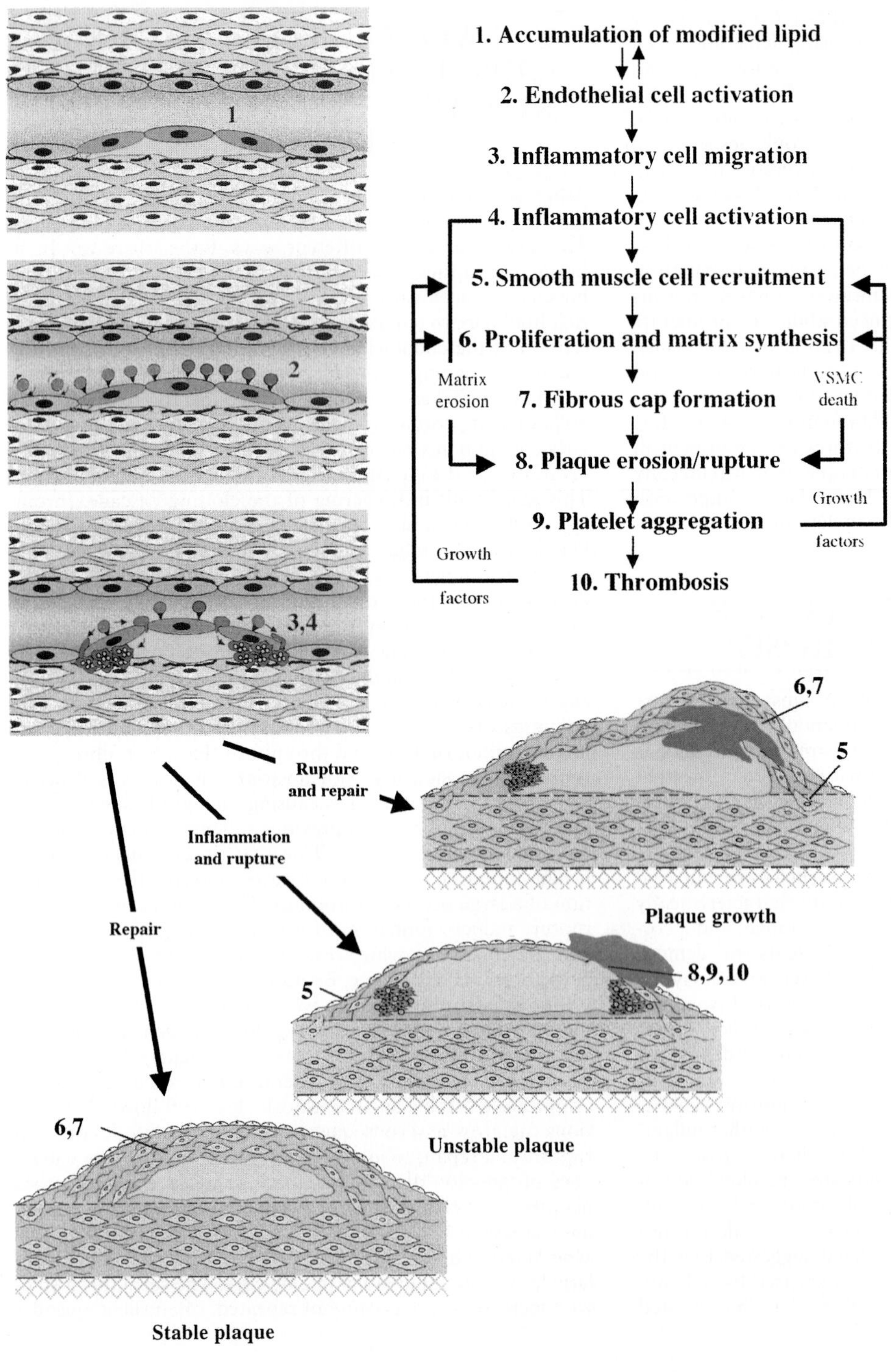

FIGURE 1.3. Cellular interactions in the development and progression of atherosclerosis. (*Source:* Weissberg PL. Atherogenesis: current understanding of the causes of atheroma. *Heart* 2000;83:247–252, with permission.)

presence of chlamydia infection and atherosclerosis, neither a causative role nor an association between serum markers of infection and ischemic heart disease has been established. Although animal work has shown that healthy rabbits nasally inoculated with chlamydia develop extensive atherosclerosis (84), the situation appears to be somewhat different in humans. Two large prospective studies and an extensive meta-analysis of previous data failed to show any association between serum markers of infection with chlamydia and incidence of or mortality from ischemic heart disease (85,86). These results effectively excluded a strong association but allowed the possibility of a weaker link. This hypothesis has now been effectively rejected after several negative trials of antibiotics in coronary artery disease (87–89).

The balance can be tipped toward plaque stability by a reduction in plaque inflammation or an increase in VSMC-driven repair. Lipid reduction, by whatever means, reduces clinical events. Evidence that this may be due to a plaque-stabilizing effect comes from animal studies that showed that statins reduced inflammatory cell and increased VSMC content of plaques (90,91), changes that would be expected to enhance stability. Dietary lipid lowering in rabbits also reduced the number of microvessels in the aortic intima, suggesting another mechanism of favorably altering the biology of plaques (92).

More important, however, evidence from human clinical studies also points to a plaque-stabilizing effect of statins. Despite angiographic studies showing that statins produce only a small, hemodynamically insignificant reduction in lumen stenosis (93,94), more sensitive intravascular ultrasound studies have shown beyond doubt that statins can halt lesion enlargement in the coronary arteries, with the most benefit being seen with higher doses of the most potent drugs (95). Statins can also reduce new lesion formation, and, importantly, the number of new vessel occlusions. These arise after a plaque ruptures, leading to an occlusive thrombus in the context of a well-collateralized myocardial circulation. This seems to imply that statins stabilize plaques by reducing rupture rate. This conclusion is supported by the results of all the large primary and secondary prevention studies, which have demonstrated that statins (pravastatin, simvastatin, and lovastatin) produce major reductions in events owing to plaque rupture, such as myocardial infarction and stroke (34,96–99). Because statins have only a modest effect on plaque size but cause profound reductions in the number of clinical events, these studies highlight the inadequacy of angiography for the prediction of clinical events and suggest that statins have beneficial effects on plaque inflammation in addition to, or as a result of, their lipid-lowering effects. Importantly, this notion is supported by the observation that the reduction in clinical events due to statin therapy is accompanied by a parallel reduction in CRP levels that is unlikely to be caused by effects of statins on nonatherosclerotic inflammation (100,101). Also, in the first study of its kind, it has been shown that statins reduce inflammation and increase plaque collagen content in human carotid artery atherosclerosis (102). However, the various statins do differ in their anti-inflammatory effect; in the REVERSAL study, atorvastatin achieved a far greater reduction in CRP than pravastatin (95); whether this has important clinical relevance is not yet known.

Statin drugs may help to stabilize plaques in a number of different ways. It is known that they can exert direct effects on endothelial cell function, inflammatory cell number and activity, VSMC proliferation, platelet aggregation, and thrombus formation (103–107). Evidence that non–lipid-lowering effects may be important in vivo comes from animal studies in which pravastatin caused beneficial changes in plaque composition (but not size), even when lipid levels were maintained at pretreatment levels (91). Additionally, in mice, simvastatin has direct anti-inflammatory effects comparable to those of indomethacin (108). Recently, a newly recognized effect of statins as immune modulators has been described, whereby major histocompatibility complex class II–mediated T-cell activation is reduced by a variety of statins (109). However, the matter of non–lipid-lowering effects of statins is not yet proven beyond doubt: several of the pleiotropic anti-inflammatory effects of statins (decreased expression of MMPs, and tissue factor) occur in animals on a lipid-lowering diet alone, without exposure to drugs of any kind (110). In addition, the administration of other forms of anti-inflammatory drugs to patients with atherosclerosis does not seem to confer any clinical benefit and may do harm; the cyclooxygenase-2 (COX-2) class of drugs are a case in point, causing a doubling of the rate of myocardial infarction in one study (111).

RESTENOSIS

Restenosis describes the late loss of gain in lumen diameter achieved immediately after balloon dilatation of an atherosclerotic plaque. For many years, it has been thought of as an undesirable response to vascular injury. However, in effect, it represents an extreme form of plaque stabilization. Whether performed on a stable or unstable plaque, balloon angioplasty causes endothelial disruption and often substantial damage to the full thickness of the vessel wall. The initial thrombotic response that would otherwise lead to early vessel occlusion is prevented by antiplatelet and antithrombotic therapy. There then follows a reparative response driven by medial VSMCs and adventitial myofibroblasts. The former form a matrix-rich neointima over the exposed plaque, whereas the latter produce a collagenous matrix in the adventitia. The net result is that the adventitial reaction "splints" the vessel and prevents the positive remodeling that would normally allow expansion of the vessel to accommodate the neointima. However, although this phenomenon may lead to angiographic or clinical restenosis, much more important, it renders the lesion stable, making the likelihood of a further plaque rupture at that site extremely remote. In effect, by stimulating a vigorous VSMC repair response, balloon angioplasty tips "the balance of atherosclerosis" in favor of plaque stability. This phenomenon undoubtedly underlies the success of angioplasty in the treatment of acute myocardial infarction. Most of the adverse effects of the response to balloon angioplasty on remodeling can be countered by deployment of a stent, particularly the drug-eluting variety, where significant restenosis is rarely encountered. The drugs used to coat the stents are antiproliferative agents, and are highly effective at eliminating restenosis (112). However, by impairing the synthetic ability of the VSMCs of the cap, there have been reports of early thrombotic occlusions of treated arteries, although longer term analysis of the data suggest that this is not frequent (113). Nevertheless, drug-eluting stents are likely to become universally used in the catheter laboratory in the near future.

CONTROVERSIES AND PERSONAL PERSPECTIVES

Many issues concerning the initiation and progression of atherosclerosis remain to be resolved. In particular, controversy persists over the extent to which endothelial dysfunction precedes or is the consequence of intimal lipid accumulation; the relative contributions of endothelial erosion and plaque rupture to clinical events; and the extent to which statins achieve their plaque-stabilizing effects directly via lipid lowering or by their so-called pleiotropic effects on the intercellular interactions that lead to plaque rupture. Integral to this last issue is the outstanding question of what is the optimal level of lipid reduction. In other words, is lower LDL always better?

Despite these controversies, it is certain that drug treatment will become increasingly prominent in the management of patients with, and at high risk of developing, atherosclerosis. Improvements in drug design will come from a number of complementary approaches. First, improvement will come by modifications of existing molecules, based on understanding how currently available drugs such as statins and angiotensin-converting enzyme inhibitors influence plaque progression. This will include evaluation of how other lipid-modifying strategies, such as inhibiting cholesterol absorption in the gut and modifying the balance between pro- and anti-atherogenic lipoproteins and triglycerides, might influence the atherosclerotic process. Second, improvements will come by targeting molecular interactions known to be involved in atherogenesis. Likely candidates include endothelial adhesion molecules, MMPs, inflammatory cytokines and their signaling molecules, in particular, nuclear factor-κ B and its downstream transcriptional activators. Here the challenge lies in identifying pathways or molecular species that are specific for atherosclerosis whose modification will not compromise the normal inflammatory response to pathogens. This approach will include developing regulators of VSMC behavior, such as modulators of transforming growth factor-β–driven matrix production, that may lead to enhanced maintenance of the fibrous cap. Another important example includes establishing the role of drugs targeting peroxisome proliferator–activated receptors in modifying inflammation and the vascular consequences of the metabolic syndrome that links insulin resistance, diabetes, hypertension, and dyslipidemia with premature atherosclerosis. The third approach is to use new technologies such as proteomics to design new therapeutic molecules and gene array technologies to identify new molecular targets in vascular disease. In addition, as a consequence of sequencing the human genome, a number of "orphan" receptors have already been identified that might provide vascular-specific targets for novel therapies. Finally, local drug delivery to high-risk plaques with drug-eluting stents has been proposed as a means of reducing risk of rupture (plaque passivation) (115,116). This approach will need better methods of identifying high-risk plaques, which will probably include invasive imaging data derived from IVUS and thermography coupled with noninvasive methods such as high-resolution molecular magnetic resonance imaging and possibly Fluorodeoxyglucose positron emission tomography (FDG-PET) (117,118).

THE FUTURE

It is almost inconceivable that advances in our understanding of the atherosclerotic disease process will not lead to the development of new anti-atheroma drugs that will act synergistically with statins and angiotensin-converting enzyme inhibitors. For example, a novel HDL-like molecule has recently been shown to reduce atheroma burden when given by intravenous infusion over 5 weeks to a high-risk group of patients (114). Furthermore, we predict that advances in genetics and diagnostics will combine with therapeutic advances to produce substantial reductions in premature cardiovascular deaths. Thus, new gene polymorphisms and mutations will be identified that confer increased likelihood either of developing atheroma or of experiencing its consequences. This will lead, in turn, to better prescription of lifestyle modifications and better targeting of current and new therapies for primary prevention of cardiovascular events. This approach will be led by new diagnostic tests—based on specific circulating markers of vascular inflammation and imaging of the inflammatory process underlying plaque rupture—that will allow better preclinical diagnosis of patients at greatest risk of cardiovascular events and subsequent monitoring of plaque-modifying therapies.

References

1. Wong ND, Wilson PW, Kannel WB. Serum cholesterol as a prognostic factor after myocardial infarction: the Framingham Study. *Ann Intern Med* 1991;115:687–693.
2. National Heart, Lung, and Blood Institute (NHLBI). *NHLBI fact book fiscal year 1997*. Bethesda, MD: NHBLI, 1998.
3. Cooper R, Cutler J, Desvigne-Nickens P, et al. Trends and disparities in coronary heart disease, stroke, and other cardiovascular diseases in the United States: findings of the national conference on cardiovascular disease prevention. *Circulation* 2000;102:3137–3147.
4. McGovern PG, Pankow JS, Shahar E, et al. Recent trends in acute coronary heart disease—mortality, morbidity, medical care, and risk factors. The Minnesota Heart Survey Investigators. *N Engl J Med* 1996;334:884–890.
5. Reddy KS, Yusuf S. Emerging epidemic of cardiovascular disease in developing countries. *Circulation* 1998;97:596–601.
6. British Heart Foundation Health Promotion Research Group. *Coronary heart disease statistics*. London: British Heart Foundation, 2005:1–200.
7. Hunt SA, Baker DW, Chin MH, et al. ACC/AHA guidelines for the evaluation and management of chronic heart failure in the adult: executive summary. A report of the American College of Cardiology/American Heart Association Task Force on Practice Guidelines (Committee to revise the 1995 Guidelines for the Evaluation and Management of Heart Failure). *J Am Coll Cardiol* 2001;38:2101–2113.
8. Braunwald E. Shattuck lecture—cardiovascular medicine at the turn of the millennium: triumphs, concerns, and opportunities. *N Engl J Med* 1997; 337:1360–1369.
9. Ho KK, Pinsky JL, Kannel WB, et al. The epidemiology of heart failure: the Framingham Study. *J Am Coll Cardiol* 1993;22:6A–13A.
10. Gheorghiade M, Bonow RO. Chronic heart failure in the United States: a manifestation of coronary artery disease. *Circulation* 1998;97:282–289.
11. Fruchart JC, Nierman MC, Stroes ES, et al. New risk factors for atherosclerosis and patient risk assessment. *Circulation* 2004;109:III15-III19.
12. Shanahan CM, Cary NR, Metcalfe JC, et al. High expression of genes for calcification-regulating proteins in human atherosclerotic plaques. *J Clin Invest* 1994;93:2393–2402.
13. Aikawa M, Sugiyama S, Hill CC, et al. Lipid lowering reduces oxidative stress and endothelial cell activation in rabbit atheroma. *Circulation* 2002;106:1390–1396.
14. Palmer RM, Ferrige AG, Moncada S. Nitric oxide release accounts for the biological activity of endothelium-derived relaxing factor. *Nature* 1987; 327:524–526.
15. Gauthier TW, Scalia R, Murohara T, et al. Nitric oxide protects against leukocyte-endothelium interactions in the early stages of hypercholesterolemia. *Arterioscler Thromb Vasc Biol* 1995;15:1652–1659.
16. Tsao PS, Buitrago R, Chan JR, et al. Fluid flow inhibits endothelial adhesiveness. Nitric oxide and transcriptional regulation of VCAM-1. *Circulation* 1996;94:1682–1689.
17. Tsao PS, Wang B, Buitrago R, et al. Nitric oxide regulates monocyte chemotactic protein-1. *Circulation* 1997;96:934–940.
18. Cardona-Sanclemente LE, Born GV. Effect of inhibition of nitric oxide synthesis on the uptake of LDL and fibrinogen by arterial walls and other organs of the rat. *Br J Pharmacol* 1995;114:1490–1494.
19. Anggard E. Nitric oxide: mediator, murderer, and medicine [see comments]. *Lancet* 1994;343:1199–1206.
20. Bhagat K, Vallance P. Nitric oxide 9 years on. *J R Soc Med* 1996;89:667–673.
21. Hobbs AJ, Higgs A, Moncada S. Inhibition of nitric oxide synthase as a potential therapeutic target. *Annu Rev Pharmacol Toxicol* 1999;39:191–220.
22. Ross R. Atherosclerosis-an inflammatory disease. *N Engl J Med* 1999;340: 115–126.
23. Li H, Forstermann U. Nitric oxide in the pathogenesis of vascular disease. *J Pathol* 2000;190:244–254.
24. Stroes ES, Koomans HA, de Bruin TW, et al. Vascular function in the forearm of hypercholesterolaemic patients off and on lipid-lowering medication. *Lancet* 1995;346:467–471.
25. Williams SB, Cusco JA, Roddy MA, et al. Impaired nitric oxide-mediated vasodilation in patients with non-insulin-dependent diabetes mellitus. *J Am Coll Cardiol* 1996;27:567–574.
26. Heitzer T, Just H, Munzel T. Antioxidant vitamin C improves endothelial dysfunction in chronic smokers [see comments]. *Circulation* 1996;94: 6–9.

27. Panza JA, Garcia CE, Kilcoyne CM, et al. Impaired endothelium-dependent vasodilation in patients with essential hypertension. Evidence that nitric oxide abnormality is not localized to a single signal transduction pathway. *Circulation* 1995;91:1732–1738.
28. Nakashima Y, Plump AS, Raines EW, et al. ApoE-deficient mice develop lesions of all phases of atherosclerosis throughout the arterial tree. *Arterioscler Thromb* 1994;14:133–140.
29. Resnick N, Yahav H, Khachigian LM, et al. Endothelial gene regulation by laminar shear stress. *Adv Exp Med Biol* 1997;430:155–164.
30. Topper JN, Cai J, Falb D, et al. Identification of vascular endothelial genes differentially responsive to fluid mechanical stimuli: cyclooxygenase-2, manganese superoxide dismutase, and endothelial cell nitric oxide synthase are selectively up-regulated by steady laminar shear stress. *Proc Natl Acad Sci U S A* 1996;93:10417–10422.
31. Cunningham KS, Gotlieb AI. The role of shear stress in the pathogenesis of atherosclerosis. *Lab Invest* 2005;85:9–23.
32. Gimbrone MA, Jr. Vascular endothelium, hemodynamic forces, and atherogenesis. *Am J Pathol* 1999;155:1–5.
33. Yusuf S, Sleight P, Pogue J, et al. Effects of an angiotensin-converting-enzyme inhibitor, ramipril, on cardiovascular events in high-risk patients. The Heart Outcomes Prevention Evaluation Study Investigators. *N Engl J Med* 2000;342:145–153.
34. LIPID Study Group. Prevention of cardiovascular events and death with pravastatin in patients with coronary heart disease and a broad range of initial cholesterol levels. The Long-Term Intervention with Pravastatin in Ischaemic Disease (LIPID) Study Group. *N Engl J Med* 1998;339:1349–1357.
35. Poon M, Zhang X, Dunsky KG, et al. Apolipoprotein(a) induces monocyte chemotactic activity in human vascular endothelial cells. *Circulation* 1997;96:2514–2519.
36. Rath M, Niendorf A, Reblin T, et al. Detection and quantification of lipoprotein(a) in the arterial wall of 107 coronary bypass patients. *Arteriosclerosis* 1989;9:579–592.
37. Loscalzo J, Weinfeld M, Fless GM, et al. Lipoprotein(a), fibrin binding, and plasminogen activation. *Arteriosclerosis* 1990;10:240–245.
38. Grainger DJ, Kirschenlohr HL, Metcalfe JC, et al. Proliferation of human smooth muscle cells promoted by lipoprotein(a). *Science* 1993;260:1655–1658.
39. Boring L, Gosling J, Cleary M, et al. Decreased lesion formation in CCR2-/- mice reveals a role for chemokines in the initiation of atherosclerosis. *Nature* 1998;394:894–897.
40. Xia P, Vadas MA, Rye KA, et al. High density lipoproteins (HDL) interrupt the sphingosine kinase signaling pathway. A possible mechanism for protection against atherosclerosis by HDL. *J Biol Chem* 1999;274:33143–33147.
41. Calabresi L, Franceschini G, Sirtori CR, et al. Inhibition of VCAM-1 expression in endothelial cells by reconstituted high density lipoproteins. *Biochem Biophys Res Commun* 1997;238:61–65.
42. Gosling J, Slaymaker S, Gu L, et al. MCP-1 deficiency reduces susceptibility to atherosclerosis in mice that overexpress human apolipoprotein B. *J Clin Invest* 1999;103:773–778.
43. Tontonoz P, Nagy L, Alvarez JG, et al. PPARgamma promotes monocyte/macrophage differentiation and uptake of oxidized LDL. *Cell* 1998;93:241–252.
44. Calnek DS, Mazzella L, Roser S, et al. Peroxisome proliferator-activated receptor gamma ligands increase release of nitric oxide from endothelial cells. *Arterioscler Thromb Vasc Biol* 2003;23:52–57.
45. Panigrahy D, Singer S, Shen LQ, et al. PPARgamma ligands inhibit primary tumor growth and metastasis by inhibiting angiogenesis. *J Clin Invest* 2002;110:923–932.
46. Corti R, Osende JI, Fallon JT, et al. The selective peroxisomal proliferator-activated receptor-gamma agonist has an additive effect on plaque regression in combination with simvastatin in experimental atherosclerosis: in vivo study by high-resolution magnetic resonance imaging. *J Am Coll Cardiol* 2004;43:464–473.
47. Liaw L, Almeida M, Hart CE, et al. Osteopontin promotes vascular cell adhesion and spreading and is chemotactic for smooth muscle cells in vitro. *Circ Res* 1994;74:214–224.
48. Zaman AG, Helft G, Worthley SG, et al. The role of plaque rupture and thrombosis in coronary artery disease. *Atherosclerosis* 2000;149:251–266.
49. Steiner S, Seidinger D, Huber K, et al. Effect of glycoprotein IIb/IIIa antagonist abciximab on monocyte-platelet aggregates and tissue factor expression. *Arterioscler Thromb Vasc Biol* 2003;23:1697–1702.
50. CAPTURE investigators. Randomised placebo-controlled trial of abciximab before and during coronary intervention in refractory unstable angina: the CAPTURE Study. *Lancet* 1997;349:1429–1435.
51. Shanahan CM, Weissberg PL. Smooth muscle cell heterogeneity: patterns of gene expression in vascular smooth muscle cells in vitro and in vivo. *Arterioscler Thromb Vasc Biol* 1998;18:333–338.
52. Libby P. Molecular bases of the acute coronary syndromes. *Circulation* 1995;91:2844–2850.
53. Galis ZS, Sukhova GK, Lark MW, et al. Increased expression of matrix metalloproteinases and matrix degrading activity in vulnerable regions of human atherosclerotic plaques. *J Clin Invest* 1994;94:2493–2503.
54. Davies MJ. Stability and instability: two faces of coronary atherosclerosis. The Paul Dudley White Lecture 1995. *Circulation* 1996;94:2013–2020.
55. Kolodgie FD, Virmani R, Burke AP, et al. Pathologic assessment of the vulnerable human coronary plaque. *Heart* 2004;90:1385–1391.
56. Kockx MM, Cromheeke KM, Knaapen MW, et al. Phagocytosis and macrophage activation associated with hemorrhagic microvessels in human atherosclerosis. *Arterioscler Thromb Vasc Biol* 2003;23:440–446.
57. Warner SJ, Friedman GB, Libby P. Immune interferon inhibits proliferation and induces 2′-5′-oligoadenylate synthetase gene expression in human vascular smooth muscle cells. *J Clin Invest* 1989;83:1174–1182.
58. Amento EP, Ehsani N, Palmer H, et al. Cytokines and growth factors positively and negatively regulate interstitial collagen gene expression in human vascular smooth muscle cells. *Arterioscler Thromb* 1991;11:1223–1230.
59. Libby P, Sukhova G, Lee RT, et al. Cytokines regulate vascular functions related to stability of the atherosclerotic plaque. *J Cardiovasc Pharmacol* 1995;25[Suppl 2]:S9–S12.
60. Geng YJ, Wu Q, Muszynski M, et al. Apoptosis of vascular smooth muscle cells induced by in vitro stimulation with interferon-gamma, tumor necrosis factor-alpha, and interleukin-1 beta. *Arterioscler Thromb Vasc Biol* 1996;16:19–27.
61. Sukhova GK, Schonbeck U, Rabkin E, et al. Evidence for increased collagenolysis by interstitial collagenases-1 and -3 in vulnerable human atheromatous plaques. *Circulation* 1999;99:2503–2509.
62. Boyle JJ, Bowyer DE, Weissberg PL, et al. Human blood-derived macrophages induce apoptosis in human plaque-derived vascular smooth muscle cells by Fas-ligand/Fas interactions. *Arterioscler Thromb Vasc Biol* 2001;21:1402–1407.
63. Bennett MR, Macdonald K, Chan SW, et al. Cooperative interactions between RB and p53 regulate cell proliferation, cell senescence, and apoptosis in human vascular smooth muscle cells from atherosclerotic plaques. *Circ Res* 1998;82:704–712.
64. Ross R, Wight TN, Strandness E, et al. Human atherosclerosis. I. Cell constitution and characteristics of advanced lesions of the superficial femoral artery. *Am J Pathol* 1984;114:79–93.
65. Bennett MR, Littlewood TD, Schwartz SM, et al. Increased sensitivity of human vascular smooth muscle cells from atherosclerotic plaques to p53-mediated apoptosis. *Circ Res* 1997;81:591–599.
66. Ridker PM, Cushman M, Stampfer MJ, et al. Inflammation, aspirin, and the risk of cardiovascular disease in apparently healthy men. *N Engl J Med* 1997;336:973–979.
67. Ridker PM, Hennekens CH, Buring JE, et al. C-reactive protein and other markers of inflammation in the prediction of cardiovascular disease in women. *N Engl J Med* 2000;342:836–843.
68. Ridker PM. High-sensitivity C-reactive protein: potential adjunct for global risk assessment in the primary prevention of cardiovascular disease. *Circulation* 2001;103:1813–1818.
69. Sacks FM, Ridker PM. Lipid lowering and beyond: results from the CARE study on lipoproteins and inflammation. Cholesterol and Recurrent Events. *Herz* 1999;24:51–56.
70. Ridker PM, Cook N. Clinical usefulness of very high and very low levels of C-reactive protein across the full range of Framingham Risk Scores. *Circulation* 2004;109:1955–1959.
71. Sakkinen P, Abbott RD, Curb JD, et al. C-reactive protein and myocardial infarction. *J Clin Epidemiol* 2002;55:445–451.
72. Albert CM, Ma J, Rifai N, et al. Prospective study of C-reactive protein, homocysteine, and plasma lipid levels as predictors of sudden cardiac death. *Circulation* 2002;105:2595–2599.
73. Pepys MB. CRP or not CRP? That is the question. *Arterioscler Thromb Vasc Biol* 2005;25:1091–1094.
74. Danesh J, Wheeler JG, Hirschfield GM, et al. C-reactive protein and other circulating markers of inflammation in the prediction of coronary heart disease. *N Engl J Med* 2004;350:1387–1397.
75. Ridker PM, Hennekens CH, Roitman-Johnson B, et al. Plasma concentration of soluble intercellular adhesion molecule 1 and risks of future myocardial infarction in apparently healthy men [see comments]. *Lancet* 1998;351:88–92.
76. Ridker PM, Buring JE, Rifai N. Soluble P-selectin and the risk of future cardiovascular events. *Circulation* 2001;103:491–495.
77. Peter K, Weirich U, Nordt TK, et al. Soluble vascular cell adhesion molecule-1 (VCAM-1) as potential marker of atherosclerosis. *Thromb Haemost* 1999;82[Suppl 1]:38–43.
78. Ridker PM, Rifai N, Stampfer MJ, et al. Plasma concentration of interleukin-6 and the risk of future myocardial infarction among apparently healthy men. *Circulation* 2000;101:1767–1772.
79. Farb A, Burke AP, Tang AL, et al. Coronary plaque erosion without rupture into a lipid core. A frequent cause of coronary thrombosis in sudden coronary death. *Circulation* 1996;93:1354–1363.
80. McNamara CA, Sarembock IJ, Bachhuber BG, et al. Thrombin and vascular smooth muscle cell proliferation: implications for atherosclerosis and restenosis. *Semin Thromb Hemost* 1996;22:139–144.
81. Davies MJ. Acute coronary thrombosis—the role of plaque disruption and its initiation and prevention. *Eur Heart J* 1995;16[Suppl L]:3–7.
82. Ye S, Eriksson P, Hamsten A, et al. Progression of coronary atherosclerosis is associated with a common genetic variant of the human stromelysin-1 promoter which results in reduced gene expression. *J Biol Chem* 1996;271:13055–13060.
83. Kol A, Sukhova GK, Lichtman AH, et al. Chlamydial heat shock protein 60 localizes in human atheroma and regulates macrophage tumor

necrosis factor-alpha and matrix metalloproteinase expression. *Circulation* 1998;98:300–307.
84. Muhlestein JB, Anderson JL, Hammond EH, et al. Infection with *Chlamydia pneumoniae* accelerates the development of atherosclerosis and treatment with azithromycin prevents it in a rabbit model. *Circulation* 1998; 97:633–636.
85. Danesh J, Whincup P, Walker M, et al. *Chlamydia pneumoniae* IgG titres and coronary heart disease: prospective study and meta-analysis [see comments]. *BMJ* 2000;321:208–213.
86. Wald NJ, Law MR, Morris JK, et al. *Chlamydia pneumoniae* infection and mortality from ischaemic heart disease: large prospective study [see comments]. *BMJ* 2000;321:204–207.
87. O'Connor CM, Dunne MW, Pfeffer MA, et al. Azithromycin for the secondary prevention of coronary heart disease events: the WIZARD study: a randomized controlled trial. *JAMA* 2003;290:1459–1466.
88. Cannon CP, Braunwald E, McCabe CH, et al. Intensive versus moderate lipid lowering with statins after acute coronary syndromes. *N Engl J Med* 2004;350:1495–1504.
89. Zahn R, Schneider S, Frilling B, et al. Antibiotic therapy after acute myocardial infarction: a prospective randomized study. *Circulation* 2003;107: 1253–1259.
90. Shiomi M, Ito T, Tsukada T, et al. Reduction of serum cholesterol levels alters lesional composition of atherosclerotic plaques. Effect of pravastatin sodium on atherosclerosis in mature WHHL rabbits. *Arterioscler Thromb Vasc Biol* 1995;15:1938–1944.
91. Williams JK, Sukhova GK, Herrington DM, et al. Pravastatin has cholesterol-lowering independent effects on the artery wall of atherosclerotic monkeys. *J Am Coll Cardiol* 1998;31:684–691.
92. Aikawa M, Rabkin E, Okada Y, et al. Lipid lowering by diet reduces matrix metalloproteinase activity and increases collagen content of rabbit atheroma: a potential mechanism of lesion stabilization [see comments]. *Circulation* 1998;97:2433–2444.
93. Pitt B, Mancini GB, Ellis SG, et al. Pravastatin Limitation of Atherosclerosis in the Coronary arteries (PLAC I): reduction in atherosclerosis progression and clinical events. PLAC I investigation. *J Am Coll Cardiol* 1995;26:1133–1139.
94. MAAS Investigators. Effect of simvastatin on coronary atheroma: the Multicentre Anti- Atheroma Study (MAAS). *Lancet* 1994;344:633–638.
95. Nissen SE, Tuzcu EM, Schoenhagen P, et al. Statin therapy, LDL cholesterol, C-reactive protein, and coronary artery disease. *N Engl J Med* 2005;352: 29–38.
96. Sacks FM, Pfeffer MA, Moye LA, et al. The effect of pravastatin on coronary events after myocardial infarction in patients with average cholesterol levels. Cholesterol and Recurrent Events trial investigators. *N Engl J Med* 1996;335:1001–1009.
97. Shepherd J, Cobbe SM, Ford I, et al. Prevention of coronary heart disease with pravastatin in men with hypercholesterolemia. West of Scotland Coronary Prevention Study Group. *N Engl J Med* 1995;333:1301–1307.
98. Downs JR, Clearfield M, Weis S, et al. Primary prevention of acute coronary events with lovastatin in men and women with average cholesterol levels: results of AFCAPS/TexCAPS. Air Force/Texas Coronary Atherosclerosis Prevention Study. *JAMA* 1998;279:1615–1622.
99. 4S Study. Randomised trial of cholesterol lowering in 4444 patients with coronary heart disease: the Scandinavian Simvastatin Survival Study (4S). *Lancet* 1994;344:1383–1389.
100. Jialal I, Stein D, Balis D, et al. Effect of hydroxymethyl glutaryl coenzyme a reductase inhibitor therapy on high sensitive C-reactive protein levels. *Circulation* 2001;103:1933–1935.
101. Ridker PM, Rifai N, Pfeffer MA, et al. Inflammation, pravastatin, and the risk of coronary events after myocardial infarction in patients with average cholesterol levels. Cholesterol and Recurrent Events (CARE) investigators. *Circulation* 1998;98:839–844.
102. Crisby M, Nordin-Fredriksson G, Shah PK, et al. Pravastatin treatment increases collagen content and decreases lipid content, inflammation, metalloproteinases, and cell death in human carotid plaques: implications for plaque stabilization. *Circulation* 2001;103:926–933.
103. Katznelson S, Wang XM, Chia D, et al. The inhibitory effects of pravastatin on natural killer cell activity in vivo and on cytotoxic T lymphocyte activity in vitro. *J Heart Lung Transplant* 1998;17:335–340.
104. Lacoste L, Lam JY, Hung J, et al. Hyperlipidemia and coronary disease. Correction of the increased thrombogenic potential with cholesterol reduction [see comments]. *Circulation* 1995;92:3172–3177.
105. Negre-Aminou P, van Vliet AK, van Erck M, et al. Inhibition of proliferation of human smooth muscle cells by various HMG-CoA reductase inhibitors; comparison with other human cell types. *Biochim Biophys Acta* 1997;1345:259–268.
106. Rosenson RS, Tangney CC. Antiatherothrombotic properties of statins: implications for cardiovascular event reduction [see comments]. *JAMA* 1998;279:1643–1650.
107. Treasure CB, Klein JL, Weintraub WS, et al. Beneficial effects of cholesterol-lowering therapy on the coronary endothelium in patients with coronary artery disease. *N Engl J Med* 1995;332:481–487.
108. Sparrow CP, Burton CA, Hernandez M, et al. Simvastatin has anti-inflammatory and antiatherosclerotic activities independent of plasma cholesterol lowering. *Arterioscler Thromb Vasc Biol* 2001;21:115–121.
109. Kwak B, Mulhaupt F, Myit S, et al. Statins as a newly recognized type of immunomodulator. *Nat Med* 2000;6:1399–1402.
110. Schonbeck U, Libby P. Inflammation, immunity, and HMG-CoA reductase inhibitors: statins as antiinflammatory agents? *Circulation* 2004;109:II18-II26.
111. Mukherjee D, Nissen SE, Topol EJ. Risk of cardiovascular events associated with selective COX-2 inhibitors. *JAMA* 2001;286:954–959.
112. Sousa JE, Costa MA, Abizaid A, et al. Four-year angiographic and intravascular ultrasound follow-up of patients treated with sirolimus-eluting stents. *Circulation* 2005;111:2326–2329.
113. Babapulle MN, Joseph L, Belisle P, et al. A hierarchical Bayesian meta-analysis of randomised clinical trials of drug-eluting stents. *Lancet* 2004; 364:583–591.
114. Assmann G, Gotto AM, Jr. HDL cholesterol and protective factors in atherosclerosis. *Circulation* 2004;109:III8–III14.
115. Meier B. Plaque sealing by coronary angioplasty. *Heart* 2004;90:1395–1398.
116. Spratt JC, Camenzind E. Plaque stabilisation by systemic and local drug administration. *Heart* 2004;90:1392–1394.
117. Davies JR, Rudd JH, Weissberg PL. Molecular and metabolic imaging of atherosclerosis. *J Nucl Med* 2004;45:1898–1907.
118. Rudd JHF, Warburton EA, Fryer TD, et al. Imaging atherosclerotic plaque inflammation with [18F]-fluorodeoxyglucose positron emission tomography. *Circulation* 2002;105:2708–2711.

CHAPTER 2 ■ DIET AND NUTRITIONAL ISSUES

NEIL J. STONE

OVERVIEW

Diet and nutritional issues play an important role in the primary and secondary prevention of coronary heart disease (CHD). Atherogenic diet, sedentary lifestyle, and weight gain can lead to both abnormal lipid and metabolic profiles as well as increased CHD risk. Adoption of a healthy lifestyle has beneficial effects on the lipid profile and is a crucial part of the treatment of individuals who have multiple metabolic risk factors ("the metabolic syndrome"). Moreover, data on the value of diet and lifestyle in reducing oxidant stress, thrombotic tendencies, chronic inflammation, and ischemic sudden death continue to emerge.

The American Heart Association's (AHA) recommended population or "healthy" diet focuses on healthy eating patterns and foods. It recommends an overall healthy eating pattern with general advice that should help physicians to counsel on obesity, hypertension, and hypercholesterolemia. For individuals who have medical problems that necessitate consumption of a therapeutic cardiovascular diet, consultation with a dietitian for medical nutrition therapy is recommended for guidance in making the necessary lifestyle changes. To reduce levels of low-density lipoprotein cholesterol (LDL-C), the earlier AHA Step II diet restricted saturated fatty acids to less than 7% of energy and dietary cholesterol to less than 200 mg/d. The current AHA dietary module to reduce LDL-C preserves this recommendation and also recommends a reduction in trans fatty acids (TFAs). For individuals with multiple metabolic risk factors and obesity, treatment begins with caloric restriction and increased energy expenditure. For those with elevated blood pressure, a low-sodium regimen with increased emphasis on fruits and vegetables, nonfat dairy products, and weight reduction, if needed, is recommended.

The response to diet is variable and increasingly is shown to be genetically based. Therapeutic diets that reduce risk factors must be targeted to the specific characteristics of the individual (e.g., high LDL-C level, metabolic syndrome, hypertension). These individual characteristics may also underlie individual responsiveness to diet.

Understanding the response of the individual to various dietary components is useful, because some people may use the therapeutic diet to reach their LDL-C goal or reduce their need for medication to reach LDL-C goals. The response of LDL-C to dietary cholesterol is highly variable. People with combined forms of hyperlipidemia may be the most sensitive to diet. Dietary options such as plant sterol and stanol esters taken as margarines reduce cholesterol absorption significantly and can reduce LDL-C by 10% or more. Most saturated fats raise blood cholesterol, although stearic acid is an important exception. It is converted to oleic acid and is essentially neutral in lowering blood cholesterol. Because saturated fats play a major role in raising LDL-C, restriction of saturated fats along with weight control are the hallmarks of effective cholesterol-lowering diets. Other factors are important. TFAs, when consumed in high amounts, can raise LDL-C, lower high-density lipoprotein cholesterol (HDL-C) and lipoprotein (a) [Lp(a)]. Sources high in TFAs, such as hydrogenated vegetable oils in stick margarine, cookies, biscuits, and cakes, should be avoided. Butter contains cholesterol and saturated fat and is cholesterol raising compared with soft margarine. Therapeutic diets should be low in both saturated fatty acids and TFAs.

Mediterranean-style diets have proven to be both attainable and effective in reducing health risks over the long term. The use of monounsaturated fats such as canola and olive oil in place of saturated fats in this kind of diet is especially beneficial in those with metabolic syndrome or diabetes. A diet with unsaturated fats does not lower HDL-C as much as when additional carbohydrate is used to lower saturated fat intake. Regardless of the fats used, calories must be counted as excess calories—unsaturated or not—can lead to weight gain, higher triglycerides (TG) and lower HDL-C. Reducing excess body weight can be a crucial factor in improving lipid profile. The addition of regular exercise to changes in diet can be particularly beneficial in helping a patient maintain weight loss. Recent data suggest that omega-3 fatty acids play a cardioprotective role. Marine sources of omega-3 fatty acids appear to reduce cardiovascular events by a nonlipid mechanism, most likely anti-arrhythmic in nature. Plant sources of omega 3-fatty acids rich in linolenic acid as seen in canola and safflower oils, English walnuts, and flaxseed may also contribute increased omega-3 fatty acid blood levels and reduced cardiac events.

Alone or in combination, vitamins cannot be recommended for reduction of cardiovascular risk. Indeed, mega-vitamin combinations may interfere with the beneficial action of niacin on HDL-C and angiographic progression. Diets that emphasize sources of antioxidants in fruits, vegetables, nuts, and whole-grain products are recommended.

GLOSSARY

α-Linolenic acid: Plant-based omega-3 polyunsaturated fatty acid (PUFA).

BMI (body mass index): Calculated as weight/height^2. This index minimizes the effect of height on body weight and has become the preferred index for categorizing levels of obesity.

Cis: Naturally occurring double bonds that produce a bend in the molecule that impairs crystallization.

DASH diet: Dietary Alternative to Stop Hypertension diet focuses on including more fruit, vegetables, grains; low-fat and fat-free dairy products; and fish, poultry, legumes, and lean meats. It also advocates sodium restriction, which has been shown to be especially effective in those with hypertension, African Americans, and women.

Dietary cholesterol: A crucial waxy substance found in animal cells. Response to its ingestion is highly variable.

Docosahexanoic acid (DHA): Marine omega-3 fatty acid.

Eicosapentanoic acid (EPA): Marine omega-3 fatty acid.

Glycemic index/load: A measure of the carbohydrate and insulin response to intake of particular carbohydrate. Foods with the highest glycemic index promote the highest postprandial glucose rises. Glycemic load is the product of the glycemic index and the total carbohydrate consumed. Carrots have a high glycemic index, but a small amount on your salad would not constitute a high glycemic load.

Insulin resistance: Increased insulin levels relative to glucose levels. In some studies, this is an independent predictor of CAD risk. It is associated with atherogenic dyslipidemia, hypertension, and visceral obesity.

Linoleic acid: Major human PUFA; an essential fatty acid.

Mediterranean diet pyramid: Graphic summary of eating style that excludes all fats but olive and canola oils; recommends fish, poultry, with red meat sparingly, and includes physical activity and consumption of wine in moderation.

Metabolic syndrome: Describes easily measured metabolic risk factors that are related to both insulin resistance and/or obesity, these include abdominal obesity, high TG levels, low HDL-c levels, hypertension, glucose intolerance of diabetes, hypercoagulability and increased inflammation. An important clinical construct because all of the variables in metabolic syndrome improve with weight loss obtained with diet and exercise.

Monounsaturated fatty acids (MUFA): Fatty acids, such as oleic acid, whose carbon chains have one double bond. Foods high in monounsaturated fats include canola and olive oil.

Oleic acid: A monounsaturated fatty acid.

Omega-3 or *n*-3 polyunsaturated fatty acid (PUFA): Fatty acids whose first double bond is three carbon atoms from the methyl end of the fatty-acid chain. Marine (fish) sources rich in EPA and DHA and plant sources rich in α-linolenic acid such as flaxseed, canola, and soybean oil, and walnuts represent *n*-3 fatty acids.

Omega-6 or *n*-6 polyunsaturated fatty acid (PUFA): PUFAs whose first double bond is six carbon atoms from the methyl end of the fatty-acid chain. Linoleic acid is an *n*-6 PUFA.

Partial hydrogenation: A process whereby hydrogen atoms are added to fatty acids. Produces TFAs.

Plant sterol/stanol esters: Sitosterol, campesterol, and stigmasterol are the most abundant plant sterols with cellular functions in plants analogous to cholesterol's cellular role in animals. Stanols are saturated sterols with no double bonds in their multiring nuclear structure. Foods enriched with plant stanol or sterol esters lower serum cholesterol levels by reducing intestinal absorption of cholesterol.

Polyunsaturated fatty acids (PUFAs): Fatty acids whose carbon chains have one or more double bonds.

Saturated fatty acids: Fatty acids whose carbon chains have no double bonds.

Soluble or viscous fiber: Form of fiber that binds bile acids in the intestine and lowers cholesterol.

***Trans* fatty acids:** Fatty acid configuration in which the molecule is straightened out, leading to a more densely packed form. Solid at room temperatures.

USDA: United States Department of Agriculture.

DIETARY PRESCRIPTION AND LIFESTYLE CHANGES TO REDUCE CORONARY HEART DISEASE

The contemporary practice of preventive cardiology requires an understanding of diet and lifestyle prescriptions both in the prevention and treatment of CHD. An essential component is restriction of fatty acids that raise LDL-C. Epidemiologic, clinical trial, and nonhuman primate evidence demonstrate a consistent relationship between increased intakes of saturated dietary fat, elevated blood cholesterol, and CHD (1). Therapeutic diets that require additional LDL-C lowering can emphasize not only restriction of dietary saturated fat, but also sources of TFA and dietary cholesterol. The use of plant sterol/stanols and soluble fiber can result in even more LDL-C lowering. These strategies may permit LDL-C goals to be realized without starting or adding LDL-C–lowering medication.

In addition, the development of atherogenic dyslipidemia characterized by high TG, low HDL-C and small, dense LDL-C (2) requires a specific focus on improving the atherogenic

TABLE 2.1

NUTRITIONAL FACTORS TO LOWER LDL-C

1. Reduce Saturated fats
2. Reduce TFAs
3. Reduce dietary cholesterol
4. Utilize plant-based interventions
   - -Increased dietary fiber, especially viscous sources
   - -Plant sterols/stanols
   - -Nuts (avoiding caloric excess with these)
   - -Soy protein with isoflavones (to substitute for saturated fats)

Abbreviation: TFA, trans fatty acid.

diet, sedentary behaviors, and weight gain associated with this pattern. For individuals with impaired glucose tolerance, an important component of the metabolic syndrome, the prescription of lifestyle change that embraces a healthy diet, regular exercise, and weight loss may be particularly effective in preventing the progression to diabetes and the increased CHD risk that this entails (3,4). A recent evidence-based review of popular diets for cardiovascular disease (CVD) felt that there was a consistent basic science and clinical trial base to support the benefit of the Mediterranean-style diet for cardioprotection (5). Therapeutic diets and associated preventive measures such as weight reduction and/or smoking cessation have resulted in significant reductions in total mortality (6), CHD death (7,8), angiographic progression (9,10), and angina (11). Careful reviews of clinical trials and diets (5,12) emphasize the key role of omega 3 fatty acids in improving CHD survival in high-risk populations. Thus, a dietary prescription can be thought of as having these components:

- Dietary alterations to achieve optimal LDL-C lowering (Table 2.1)
- Emphasis on weight control, regular physical activity, and if needed, use of unsaturated fats rather than carbohydrates to improve glycemia
- Inclusion of healthy foods such as fruits and vegetables, marine and plant sources of omega 3 fatty acids, and dietary fiber
- Restriction of sodium if hypertension is a consideration

Therapeutic Diets Recommended by AHA, NCEP, DASH, Dietary Guidelines 2005

The AHA Dietary Guidelines known as "Revision 2000" (13) stress three underlying principles. First, there are dietary patterns that all individuals can follow throughout their life span that promote and encourage cardiovascular health. This includes particular emphasis on patterns that help individuals avoid obesity. Second, the focus should shift to healthy dietary practices over an extended period of time, rather than insisting on "perfection" with each meal. This allows for the inclusion of a wide variety of healthy foods and avoids restricting the diet to repetitious and unsatisfying dietary experiences. Finally, the guidelines form a framework on which specific recommendations can be made to individuals, based on their health and risk factor status, and appropriately modified by their dietary preferences and cultural background.

The NCEP Adult Treatment Panel III guidelines (1) advocate saturated fat and dietary cholesterol restrictions similar to prior dietary recommendations. Their dietary recommendations extend beyond these, however, with specific nutritional and lifestyle options for those who need more intensive nutritional efforts to more optimally lower LDL-C or who require an approach that more specifically targets the metabolic syndrome (Table 2.2). The program called Dietary Approaches to Stop Hypertension (DASH) provided dietary recommendations for individuals with high blood pressure (14) that emphasized more fruit, vegetables, and grains with low-fat and fat-free dairy products along with fish, poultry, legumes, and lean meats. The first DASH trial's results (at a sodium level of 3 g/d) were extended by the DASH-sodium trial (15) that looked at the DASH diet over a range of sodium intakes (3.5, 2.3, and 1.2 g/d). At each of these three levels of sodium intake, systolic and diastolic pressure was lower among patients following the DASH diet than among those assigned to the control diet. Moreover, the trial showed that in certain groups (African Americans, women, those with hypertension versus high-normal pressure), blood pressure reductions achieved with DASH-sodium were of a magnitude heretofore seen only with blood pressure–lowering drugs.

Essential Resources for Nutritional and Lifestyle Measures in Practice

Cardiologists interested in preventive nutritional and lifestyle measures for their patients should read and obtain copies of three invaluable sources of reference. The first is the published guidelines for obesity (16) that provide practical information on how to deal with obesity in clinical practice. The second is the Dietary Guidelines 2005 for Americans. It can be accessed on line at http://www.healthierus.gov/dietaryguidelines and is worth reviewing (17). The third is an article entitled "The escalating pandemics of obesity and sedentary lifestyle. A call to action for clinicians" (18). It provides a useful blueprint for not only identifying those at risk, but employing behavioral strategies to help improve your effectiveness with such patients.

EFFICACY OF DIETS IN AFFECTING LIPID LEVELS

Clinical and Biologic Factors

Any critical analysis of diet must consider the various factors that influence the results of dietary change. Outpatient studies of restriction of saturated fat and dietary cholesterol have shown that individual responsiveness can be highly variable (19,20). Not surprising to most clinicians is that compliance to diet and changes in body weight explain much of the variance. The importance of critical analysis of diet studies was shown in the Minnesota Coronary Survey Dietary Trial. Here the regression toward the mean phenomenon helps to explain why subjects with high initial serum cholesterol levels had an 18% reduction in serum cholesterol levels, whereas those with lower levels had an 11% reduction (21).

Genetic factors must always be considered. In familial hypercholesterolemia (FH), affected heterozygous children are unlikely to normalize their cholesterol values by diet alone (22). In striking contrast, children with skin and tendon xanthomas and elevated cholesterols who resemble those with FH may have a remarkable response to diet if instead they are homozygous for sitosterolemia, where increased plant sterol absorption is present (23). Polymorphisms within genes that affect apoproteins (especially apolipoprotein E), LDL subclasses, and enzymes such as hepatic lipase also contribute to heterogeneity in the dietary response (24–26).

TABLE 2.2

CLINICAL APPROACHES TO DIET, ACTIVITY, AND WEIGHT LOSS

Population approach		Clinical approach
Diet	■ Briefly assess dietary intake of saturated fat and cholesterol. ■ Promote U.S. Dietary Guidelines (population diet) using pamphlets/handouts and food guide pyramid—emphasize food portions. ■ Provide shopping and food preparation pamphlets/handouts highlighting low saturated fat foods including reduced fat dairy products, leaner meats, lower fat ground meat, and reduced fat baked goods. Make full use of office personnel to promote public health message	Promote ATP III TLC diet by ■ Individualized diet counseling that provides acceptable substitutions for favorite foods contributing to a patient's elevated LDL level—counseling often best performed by a registered dietitian ■ Reinforcement of dietary principles during follow-up visits at which LDL response to diet is assessed ■ Consideration of readiness to change and level of motivation
Physical activity	■ Promote regular physical activity by taking a physical activity history ■ Provide pamphlets/advice regarding general principles of physical activity ■ Recommend 30 min/d of regular, moderate-intensity activity	Follow Surgeon General recommendations for physical activity (U.S. Department of Health and Human Services. Physical activity and health. . . 1996b). Promote regular physical activity for individuals using: ■ Specific recommendations to increase physical activity based on a patient's cardiac status, age, and other factors ■ Specific advice regarding how physical activity could be integrated into the patient 's lifestyle ■ Follow-up visits to monitor physical activity level, and follow-up counseling regarding barriers to daily physical activity
Body weight	■ Ensure that weight, height, and waist circumference are measured at every visit Promote prevention of weight gain: ■ Provide access to tables identifying height/weight categories for BMI in waiting room or exam room ■ Provide literature relating BMI to health outcomes ■ Provide literature explaining use of nutrition fact labeling to identify calorie content and recommended portion sizes of foods	■ Follow OEI guidelines for weight management (NIH [16,17]) Promote prevention of weight gain: ■ Calculate BMI for every patient at every visit ■ Anticipate high-risk times for weight gain (perimenopausal years, times of significant life stress) and counsel patient on ways to prevent weight gain ■ Follow-up visits to discuss success of weight gain prevention strategies Discuss 10% weight loss goals for persons who are overweight: ■ Discuss lifestyle patterns that promote weight loss Portion control Daily physical activity Follow-up visits to examine weight/BMI and discuss barriers to adherence

Adapted from reference 1 (ATP III).
Abbreviations: ATP, Adult Treatment panel; BMI, body mass index; LDL, low-density lipoprotein; OEI, Obesity Education Initiative; TLC, therapeutic lifestyle changes.

USING DIET TO ALTER RISK FOR CORONARY HEART DISEASE

Effect of Dietary Factors on Lipids and Coronary Heart Disease

In published landmark studies, Keys et al. (27) and Hegsted et al. (28) quantified the response of serum cholesterol levels in humans to consumption of varying proportions of dietary fat and cholesterol. They demonstrated that saturated fatty acids (C12:0 to C16:0) are approximately twice as potent in raising cholesterol as polyunsaturated fats are in lowering them. Both investigators showed an independent effect of dietary cholesterol on serum cholesterol, although monounsaturated fats (*cis* C18:1) were believed to have no specific independent effect. These equations do not take into account the effects of behenic acid (22:0), caprylic acid (8:0), and capric acid (10:0), which are cholesterol raising, or the effects of TFAs in industrialized societies (29).

CHOLESTEROL-RAISING FACTORS: DIETARY CHOLESTEROL

Since pioneering experiments in rabbits almost a century ago, we have known that dietary cholesterol causes marked elevations of blood cholesterol in laboratory animals. In contrast, dietary cholesterol causes a variable response in blood cholesterol when tested in humans (30). If one looks only at tightly controlled studies, on average, the response of blood cholesterol to dietary cholesterol is approximately 10 mg/dL per 100 mg dietary cholesterol per 1,000 Kcal (31).

Mechanism

The most significant quantitative response to dietary cholesterol is the suppression of hepatic cholesterol synthesis (32). Also, the effect of dietary cholesterol on receptor-mediated LDL clearance is strikingly affected by the proportion of saturated fat fed.

Feeding Studies

Age, gender, and race can determine response to dietary cholesterol. Dietary studies performed in healthy young men and women showed that consumption of one or two eggs daily when added to a low saturated fat diet may have only a small effect on blood cholesterol values (33,34). Young men respond to egg ingestion by a rise in LDL-C; in young women, although there is a significant increase in LDL-C, there is an increase in HDL-C as well. Caucasians respond with higher blood cholesterol responses than non-Caucasians (35).

Dietary Cholesterol and Coronary Heart Disease

Men traditionally have higher dietary cholesterol intakes than women. Although there has been a steady decline in dietary cholesterol intakes over the past several decades, the recent focus on low-carbohydrate diets has shifted dieters to diets that remain high in sources of dietary cholesterol and saturated fats. Although studies of low-carbohydrate diets do not show worsening of LDL-C even at 1 year (36), the concern is that higher cholesterol intakes still place patients at long-term CHD risk. Four cohort studies reported on by Stamler and Shekelle (37) noted an association between dietary cholesterol and risk for CHD independent of the serum cholesterol level. Although food frequency records in men and women followed prospectively indicated that one egg per day did not increase CHD risk, this was not true for diabetic men and women in these cohorts (38). For those with hypercholesterolemia, ATP III recommends that less than 200 mg/d of dietary cholesterol should be consumed to maximize the amount of LDL-C lowering that can be achieved through reduction in dietary cholesterol (1).

Plant Stanol and Sterol Esters

Cholesterol is the sterol component of mammalian cell membranes. Plant sterols such as sitosterol, campesterol, and stigmasterol are structurally similar and their ingestion by humans can inhibit cholesterol absorption (39,40), Stanols are saturated sterols without double bonds in the sterol ring structure.

Mechanism of Action. Plant sterol and stanol esters compete with dietary cholesterol for absorption via mixed micelles. Usually, only a small amount of plant sterols and even less of plant stanols are absorbed. Ingestion of products enriched with plant sterol/stanol esters does not cause fat malabsorption.

Feeding Studies. The efficacy of the plant sterol and stanol esters in lowering cholesterol appears to be similar. Meta-analysis shows that the dose–response relation is continuous up to a dose of about 2 g of plant sterol or stanol per day, although there is considerable variability of response (39,40). The reduction in the concentration of LDL-C at each dose is significantly greater in older people than in younger people. Levels of TG and HDL-C are not affected. A randomized clinical trial in the United States suggested a dose-dependent response with 3 g/d lowered LDL-C 10.1% with no significant reduction in serum vitamin A or 25 hydroxyvitamin D levels (41). Consumption of plant sterol or stanol ester enriched products appears to be generally safe, but there is a reduction in β-carotene absorption. The AHA has expressed concern with the use of these products in children and pregnant women (42). A workshop of experts convened in 2001 noted that "safety testing of sterols and stanols has exceeded that of ordinary food-stuffs that are eaten widely and generally recognized as safe. Adverse effects of the absorption of plant sterols into the circulation appear largely hypothetical in adults" (40).

Plant Sterols/Stanols and Coronary Heart Disease

Based on their proven ability to lower LDL-C, Law (39) suggested that a reduction of CHD of about 25% could be expected with regular dietary supplementation with plant stanol esters. A subgroup analysis of the Scandinavian Simvastatin Survival Study indicated that CHD subjects with evidence for low cholesterol absorption, but not high absorption, experienced reduced CHD events during simvastatin treatment. This suggested a combined role for plant sterols and statins in those with high cholesterol absorption and low synthesis (43).

There has been concern that elevated plant sterol concentrations could increase risk of CHD. Wilund and associates (44) found no association between plant sterol levels and subclinical atherosclerosis in humans. This was supported by studies in wild-type and hypercholesterolemic mice with greater than 20-fold normal levels of plant sterols. On the other hand, a recent study of surgically obtained carotid specimens showed that the higher the ratio of absorbed sterols to absorbed cholesterol, the higher the ratio of both in the arterial specimens obtained (45). It is not known if this is clinically a significant problem.

Cholesterol-Raising Fatty Acids

Saturated Fatty Acids

The major saturated fats in the diet are lauric (C12:0), myristic (C14:0), palmitic (C16:0), and stearic (C18:0) (Fig. 2.1). They have no double bonds and are solid at room temperature. The major foods that are rich in saturated fats primarily include those of animal origin, such as meat fats and dairy fats, and selected vegetable fats, such as coconut, palm kernel, palm oils, and vegetable shortening. Palmitic acid is the predominant saturated fat in animal and dairy fats, whereas lauric acid is the predominant fat in coconut oil and palm kernel oil. Stearic acid is found in cocoa butter, which is most often consumed as chocolate.

Mechanism. Detailed studies looking at mechanism have determined that saturated fats suppress LDL-receptor activity thereby raising LDL-C (46).

Feeding Studies. A multicenter, randomized, crossover-design trial in 103 healthy adults 22 to 67 years old showed that

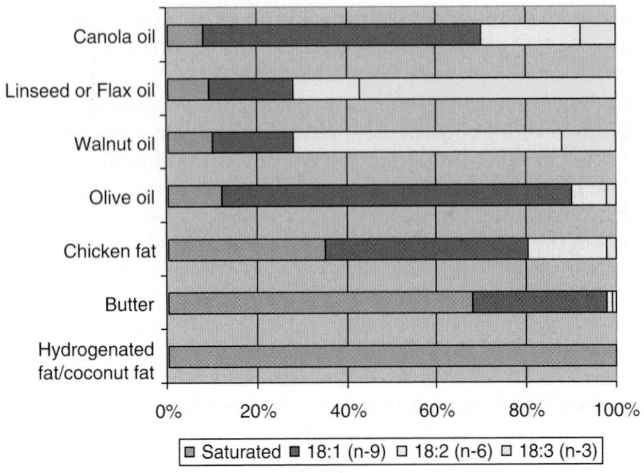

FIGURE 2.1. Fatty acid composition of commonly used oils. (*Source:* From deLorgeril M, Salen P, Laporte F, de Leiris J. Alpha-linolenic acid in the prevention and treatment of coronary heart disease. *Eur Heart J Suppl* 2001;3[Suppl D]:D26–D32.)

compared to an average American diet with 15% of energy as saturated fatty acids, lowering saturated fatty acids to 6.1% reduced LDL-C by 11% (47). In a single-center study from Seattle in men and women with both hypercholesterolemia alone and combined hyperlipidemia, reduction in saturated fat resulted in LDL-C declines of approximately 8% (48).

Although most studies examined saturated fat in total, there are important differences among saturated fatty acids. Stearic acid (18:0), the second most abundant saturated fatty acid in animal fats, is not a cholesterol-raising fatty acid and does not raise LDL-C relative to oleic acid (49). This may explain why substitution of a milk chocolate bar for a high-carbohydrate snack did not affect the LDL-lowering response to a standard diet (50).

Saturated Fats and Coronary Heart Disease

Epidemiologic Data

The Seven Countries Study showed a direct relationship between saturated fat intake and rates of CHD (51). In that trial, Finland had the highest rate of CAD mortality, Mediterranean groups far lower, and the Japanese with low intakes of total and saturated fat, had the lowest rates of CHD. Twenty-five–year follow-up of these 12,763 middle-aged men belonging to 16 cohorts in seven countries confirmed a positive association of animal fat (butter, lard, margarine, and meat) and a negative association of vegetable foods groups (except potatoes) with CHD rates (52). Yet saturated fat intake does not explain the lower rate of CHD in France. The inverse association between wine ethanol and CHD has been one possible explanation for what has become known as the "French paradox" (52). Law and Wald (53) noted that serum HDL-C levels explained little of the difference and offered a time-lag observation, suggesting that consumption of animal fat increased more recently in France than in Britain and that this accounted for the difference.

Clinical Trial Data

The evidence that lowering serum cholesterol levels by decreasing intakes of saturated fatty acids reduces CHD events was demonstrated in a meta-analysis by Gordon (54) that reviewed six robust dietary trials with 6,356 subjects. It showed that lowering serum cholesterol levels by reducing the intake of saturated fatty acids significantly lowered the incidence of CHD by 24%. Two informative diet trials with angiographic endpoints were the St. Thomas Atherosclerosis Trial (STARS) and Heidelberg trials (9,10). In STARS, CHD subjects were randomly assigned to received treatment with usual care, diet, or diet and cholestyramine resin (10). The diet restricted total fat intake to 27% of total energy and saturated fat intake to 8% to 10% of energy and was high in fiber, chiefly pectin. The primary end point of this angiographic trial was the per-patient change in the mean absolute width of coronary segments. Progression of angiographic CAD correlated significantly with in-trial plasma total cholesterol, LDL-C, apolipoprotein B, and Lp(a) levels. By multiple regression analysis, LDL-C level was the best predictor of change in the diameter of the coronary vessel.

The Heidelberg trial (10) showed the benefit of combining diet and exercise. Subjects underwent total fat restriction to less than 20% of calories resulted in initial LDL-C level decrease of 25% in subjects after 3 weeks on a metabolic ward. Although adherence to the diet fell markedly after the metabolic ward phase, the intervention group participated in intensive physical exercise. When follow-up angiograms were reviewed, a significant decrease in progression and an increase in regression were seen in the intervention group.

Trans Fatty Acids. Saturated fatty acids are not the only cholesterol-raising fatty acids. TFAs are found in meat and dairy products as a byproduct of fermentation in ruminant animals and also in products with partially hydrogenated oils. The most common TFA in the American diet is elaidic acid, the *trans* isomer of oleic acid, which is found in stick margarines and shortenings, milk, butter, cheese, commercially processed baked goods such as donuts and cookies, and vegetable oils used (and often reused) for frying.

Feeding Studies. When TFAs are ingested as 7.7% or more of energy, they raise total cholesterol, LDL-C and Lp(a), and lower HDL-C, but do not lower necessarily lower HDL-C or raise Lp(a) at lower levels of intake (55,56).

Mechanisms. The food industry uses partial hydrogenation to improve the texture of foods as well as to increase the oxidative and thermal stability of vegetable oils. It accomplishes this by converting the naturally occurring *cis* double bonds, which produce a bend in the molecule, impairing crystallization and keeping the oil liquid, to their straighter *trans* isomers, which can be more tightly packed and hence solid at room temperature.

Trans Fatty Acids and Coronary Heart Disease

Willet and colleagues (57) determined from dietary questionnaires given to participants in the Nurses Health Study that intake of *trans* isomers, after adjustment for age and total energy intake, was directly related to risk of CAD. They noted that consumption of foods that are major sources of TFA, such as margarine, cookies (biscuits), cake, and white bread, were each significantly associated with higher risks of CAD. Margarines are now available without TFA.

Cholesterol-Lowering Fatty Acids

Unsaturated Fatty Acids

Unsaturated fatty acids lower LDL-C levels when they are exchanged for saturated fatty acids in the diet. The more unsaturated a fatty acid, the more liquid it tends to be at room temperature. The two major groups are the PUFAs and the monounsaturated fatty acids (MUFAs). A recent meta-analysis found no significant differences in total cholesterol, LDL-C, and HDL-C levels when MUFAs and PUFAs are directly compared (58). There may be, however, significant differences with respect to oxidation and coagulation parameters.

Polyunsaturated Fatty Acids

PUFAs are not a homogenous class, but are divided into two groups by the position of the first double bond from the terminal end of the carbon chain. Examples of *n*-6 fatty PUFAs include corn, sunflower, safflower, sesame, and cottonseed oils. The major *n*-6 PUFA, linoleic acid (18:2) is an 18-carbon "essential" fatty acid that cannot be synthesized by the body. Linoleic acid is needed for normal immune response, and essential fatty acid deficiency impairs B- and T-cell–mediated responses (59). Although an essential fatty acid, there are cautions to the use of high amounts of *n*-6 PUFA. In one clinical study, excess PUFA intake was shown to have unwelcome side effects such as weight gain and cholelithiasis (60). It is reassuring, nonetheless, that the 10.5-year follow-up of the large Multiple Risk Factor Intervention Trial (MRFIT) showed no adverse effects of a high PUFA intake in men (61).

n-3 Polyunsaturated Fatty Acids or Omega-3 Fatty Acids. The *n*-3 PUFAs are often referred to as *marine lipids or omega-3 fatty acids.* Fatty fish are rich sources of marine *n*-3 PUFAs. When taken as fish oil capsules, marine *n*-3 PUFAS lower TG in dose-related fashion (62). In clinical trials of MI survivors, LDL-C actually rises slightly (10). The effect on TG is substantial at doses of 2 to 3 g/d of *n*-3 PUFAs and they are recommended as part of the treatment strategy for those with severe hypertriglyceridemia. Although HDL-C levels rise slightly, it is not a major effect. α-Linolenic acid is a plant-based *n*-3 PUFA. Common sources of α-linolenic acid are tofu, soybean and canola oil, nuts, and flax seed. These are healthy additions to the diets of vegetarians and those who do not eat seafood; however, α-linolenic acid does not lower TG levels significantly.

Polyunsaturated Fatty Acids and Coronary Heart Disease. The *n*-6 PUFA appear to reduce risk of CHD more than MUFA in older epidemiologic trials (13). This was also seen in human primate studies. Omega-3 fatty acids may reduce risk of CHD by lowering serum TG levels, decreasing thrombotic tendency, improving endothelial dysfunction, and preventing fatal cardiac arrhythmias. The latter quality appears independent of its effects on lipids (62).

n-3 Polyunsaturated Fatty Acids, Coronary Heart Disease, and Sudden Death. Observational studies comparing Greenland Inuit with their Danish counterparts suggested that a fish-based diet was cardioprotective (63). The Inuit diet, rich in seal and whale, provided a strikingly higher intake of *n*-3 PUFA. This was associated with lower values for total cholesterol, TG, LDL-C, and VLDL-C, increased values for HDL-C and bleeding times, and lower rates of CHD. Although studies of fish intake and CHD events have not been entirely consistent (62), emerging prospective and clinical trial data suggests clinical benefit when sources of omega-3 fatty acids are consumed. For example, blood levels of *n*-3 fatty acids were strongly associated with a decreased risk of sudden cardiac death in men (64). In addition, two or more servings of fish per week was associated with 30% lower risk of CHD (and especially CHD death) in female nurses (65).

The Diet and Reinfarction Trial (DART) noted that men who were instructed to eat fish after they had experienced MI showed a 29% decline in all-cause mortality compared with those in the placebo group (7). The mechanism for this beneficial effect was independent of lipid levels. In this trial, a group of the men (25%) who could not tolerate fish were given 875 mg of fish oil in capsule form. The Gruppo Italiano per lo Studio della Sopravvivenza nell'Infarto Miocardio (GISSI)–Prevenzione Trial, a large-scale open-label, randomized, controlled trial involving 11,324 MI survivors, demonstrated that 875-mg fish oil capsules, but not vitamin E, reduced the primary cumulative end point of all-cause mortality, nonfatal MI, and nonfatal stroke (8). Neither intervention significantly reduced the other primary end point, the cumulative rate of cardiovascular death, nonfatal MI, and nonfatal stroke. Analysis of secondary end points suggested that the benefit of *n*-3 supplementation was due to reduction of mortality and not in reduction of nonfatal MI.

These studies were complemented by a carefully done population-based case-control study from Seattle and King County, Washington (66). Among 334 patients who had experienced primary cardiac arrest, the monthly intake of *n*-3 PUFAs was significantly less than that seen in age- and gender-matched community controls. The equivalent of one fatty-fish meal per week was associated with a 50% reduction in the risk for primary cardiac arrest after adjustment for potential confounding factors. These findings were consistent with experimental evidence suggesting that the *n*-3 PUFAs have an important effect on the vulnerability to ventricular fibrillation in the setting of myocardial ischemia (67). Nonetheless, enough questions remain in terms of patient selection in post-MI survivors that a call for additional clinical trials of *n*-3 fatty acids has been made (68).

The evidence for plant sources of *n*-3 fatty acids is not as robust as that for marine sources. In the prospective Nurses Health Study, investigators found that a higher intake of oil and vinegar salad dressing, an important source of α-linolenic acid, was associated with reduced risk of fatal ischemic heart disease (IHD) when women who were almost frequent users were compared to those who were not (69). Also in Costa Rica, where fish intake is low, adipose tissue α-linolenic acid was inversely related to nonfatal acute MI, especially after correcting for TFA (70). In contrast, α-linolenic acid intake was not associated with a reduction in 10-year risk of CHD incidence in the Zutphen Elderly Study where fish intake is high, even though investigators corrected for TFA (7). The AHA guidelines for omega 3 intake are given in Table 2.3.

TABLE 2.3

OMEGA 3 FATTY ACID RECOMMENDATIONS FROM AHA

Population	Recommendations for omega-3 fatty acids
Patient without documented CHD	Eat a variety of (preferably oil) fish at least twice a week; include oils and foods high in α-linolenic acid
Patient with documented CHD	Consume ~1 g EPA plus DHA/d, preferably, from oil fish. EPA + DHA supplements could be considered in consultation with the physician
Patients needing TG lowering	2–4 g/d of EPA + DHA provided as capsules under a physician's care

Abbreviations: CHD, coronary heart disease; DHA, docosahexanoic acid; EPA, eicosapentanoic acid; TG, triglycerides.
Source: Kris-Etherton PM, Harris WS, Appel LJ; American Heart Association. Nutrition Committee. Fish consumption, fish oil, omega-3 fatty acids, and cardiovascular disease. Circulation. 2002 Nov 19;106(21):2747–2757.

Monounsaturated Fatty Acids

MUFAs can be considered to replace saturated fat in the diet (71). This class of fatty acids has only one double bond. Oleic acid is representative of the *cis* (hydrogen atoms are on the same side) forms of MUFA. Common sources include canola (rapeseed) oil, olive oil, peanut oil, almonds, and avocados.

Mechanism. In contrast to PUFAs, MUFAs do not appear to lower HDL-C when added to the diet (71). Most important, LDL isolated from subjects on diets rich in MUFA is less susceptible to oxidation than LDL from subjects on diets rich in PUFAs (72).

Feeding Studies. Grundy (73) noted that a high-carbohydrate diet raises TG and lowers HDL-C, whereas a MUFA diet did not. Mensink and Katan (74) used olive-oil–enriched foods in studying 57 outpatient volunteers to show that an olive-oil–rich diet caused a specific fall in non-HDL cholesterol and did not significantly change TG.

Gardner and Kraemer (75) used a meta-analysis of 14 studies to demonstrate that there were no significant differences in lipids when a high MUFA diet was compared with a high PUFA diet. Nonetheless, a double-blind, five-period cross-over design study of subjects with normal cholesterol and HDL-C demonstrated that high MUFA diets lowered LDL-C by 14%, similar to that seen with the low saturated fat diet (76). TG, however, were higher with the low saturated fat diets than with the high MUFA diets. HDL-C was maintained by the high MUFA diets, whereas it was lowered by 4% by the AAD. Thus, with respect to HDL-C and TG, the high MUFA diets had a more favorable response on these important cardiac risk factors.

MUFA and CHD

Five prospective cohort studies demonstrated a consistent inverse association between nut consumption and risk of CHD. The fats in nuts are either MUFA or PUFA fats that lower LDL-C. Hu and Stampfer (77) estimated from their data in the Nurses Health Study that substitution of the fat from 1 ounce of nuts for equivalent energy from carbohydrate in an average diet was associated with a 30% reduction in CHD risk and the substitution of nut fat for saturated fat was associated with 45% reduction in risk. The challenge, of course, is to substitute nuts for saturated fats, not add them so that the diet is increased in caloric density.

Mediterranean Diet and CHD

There is controversy as to whether the Mediterranean diet's healthful effects are due to increased MUFA from olive oil, *n*-3 fatty acids from fish intake, antioxidants from fruits and vegetables, low saturated fat intake, or modest alcohol ingestion. Indeed, the answer may be that the dietary pattern rather than an individual food source may be the answer. An informative observational study of the Mediterranean diet was undertaken by Greek investigators in 1,302 Greek men and women with CHD who completed a validated food frequency questionnaire on usual dietary intakes during the year preceding enrollment and had a Mediterranean diet score calculated that ranged from 0 (minimal adherence to the traditional Mediterranean diet) to 9 (maximal adherence to the traditional Mediterranean diet) (78). After a mean follow-up of 45.4 months, each two-point increment on the adherence scale was associated with a 27% lower mortality rate among persons with prevalent CHD at enrollment. Associations between individual food groups contributing to the Mediterranean diet score and mortality were generally not significant. A prior study in 22,043 Greek subjects who completed a similar Mediterranean Diet score showed that greater compliance with the Mediterranean Diet score was associated with reductions in CHD and cancer mortality (79).

The Lyon Trial compared a "Mediterranean-type" diet rich in linolenic acid with the AHA Step 1 diet in 605 subjects with previous MI (80). It supplied a canola oil-based margarine to the intervention group that was not only high in oleic acid, but more so in α-linolenic acid. The intervention group diet also differed from the control group by being lower in saturated fat and cholesterol and higher in fiber. There was no significant difference in alcohol ingestion between the groups. The control group had a total and saturated fat intake higher than that recommended baseline AHA Step I diet. Despite a lack of improvement in body mass index (BMI) and lipid profiles, there was a striking difference in mortality with eight sudden deaths in the control group and none in the treatment group. A follow-up of the original results showed that the significant difference in CHD end points was maintained at 47 months (81). This trial emphasizes that dietary patterns rather than single nutrient substitution may be more relevant to understanding a healthy diet. In this study there were several interventions employed including more *n*-3 fatty acids as α-linolenic acid, more fiber, more MUFAs, and less saturated fatty acids and dietary cholesterol.

The Indo-Mediterranean trial was a randomized single-blind trial in 1,000 South Asian subjects with or at high risk for CHD (82). The intervention group ate a diet rich in whole grains, fruits, vegetables, walnuts, and almonds. The controls consumed a diet that was called "prudent" but actually had was much higher in saturated fats (12.5% on average) than allowed by any AHA diet (AHA diets have been <10% or <7% of total calories). The Mediterranean-style diet group had an on-trial saturated fat consumption of 8.2% and had a twofold increase in α-linolenic acid in contrast to the control group. The treatment regimen was associated with significant reductions in sudden death nonfatal MI at 2 years follow-up.

Low-Fat, High-Carbohydrate Diets

A diet low in fat and high in complex carbohydrates is typical of an "Asian-style" diet. Often the percentage of energy that comes from carbohydrates is 60% to 65%, allowing total fat calories to be as low as 15% to 20% of total energy. Thus, intakes of saturated fat and dietary cholesterol are very low.

Low-Fat Diets and CHD

The value of a low-fat vegetarian-style diet as part of a comprehensive lifestyle intervention that includes exercise was examined in the Lifestyle Heart Trial (11). In this small, but provocative study, a highly motivated group of patients with symptomatic coronary disease consumed a diet in which fewer than 10% of calories came from fat and no cholesterol was allowed. The treatment group lost 22 lb, whereas the control group, who were on what was essentially a Step II diet, did not lose any weight. The intervention subjects showed a decline in LDL-C levels of 37.8%, to 100 mg per dL.

At the end of 1 year, the intensively treated group had decreased progression and/or regression of angiographic CAD compared with the control group. At the end of 5 years, improvement was documented by both angiography and decreased size and severity of perfusion abnormalities on rest-dipyridamole positron emission tomography (83). The small sample size, the difficulties caused when 49% of the subjects refused to participate after randomization, and the multiple interventions preclude any generalizations about the value of the very-low-fat diet to the average coronary patient that might be based on the results of this study.

The Stanford Coronary Risk Intervention Project was a 4-year multifactor intervention trial. The study used serial, quantitative coronary angiography in 300 men and women to show a significant reduction in new lesion formation in the coronary arteries of those randomly assigned to the risk-reduction group, compared with that in the usual-care group (84). All risk-reduction group subjects were instructed to consume a low-fat, low-cholesterol, and high-carbohydrate diet, with a goal of intake of less than 20% of energy from fat, less than 6% of energy from saturated fat, and less than 75 mg of cholesterol per day. Increased physical activity and a specific endurance exercise training program were recommended. Multiple regression analysis identified in-study dietary fat intake as the best correlate with new lesion formation. Participants randomly assigned to the risk-reduction group preferentially increased complex carbohydrate intake to offset reduction in dietary fat restriction. The authors suggested that the reduction in dietary fat accomplished by subjects in their study decreased the rate of new lesion formation by mechanisms not limited to LDL-C reduction.

Dietary Fiber

Fiber, or nondigestible plant-based carbohydrate, is an important part of a balanced diet (85). In terms of optimal cholesterol lowering, it is useful to think of fiber in terms of its viscous (formerly *soluble*) and nonviscous (*insoluble*) forms. Nonviscous fiber aids in the treatment of constipation but is not lipid lowering. The ATP III panel suggested increased amounts of dietary viscous fiber as a way to achieve optimal lowering of LDL-C (1). Jenkins et al. (86) showed the value of a dietary portfolio of LDL-C–lowering foods in a study of 46 hyperlipidemic adults fed either a diet very low in saturated fat, the diet plus a lovastatin 20 mg/d or a diet high in plant sterols, soy protein, viscous fibers, and almonds. The dietary portfolio lowered LDL-C, TC/HDL, and high-sensitivity C reactive protein (CRP) similar to the diet and lovastatin group. Both were significantly treatment regimens improved significantly from the control diet.

Gardner et al. (87) utilized a plant-based strategy in hypercholesterolemic adults to obtain significantly greater reduction in LDL-C levels than with a usual low-fat diet. Their plant-based modifications to the low-fat diet included a higher content of soy, fiber, garlic, and plant sterols as compared with those who consumed the more convenience food–based low (30% of calories) total fat diet (87). An accompanying editorial pointed noted that because the plant-based intervention achieved an additional reduction in LDL-C of 4.7% over the 4.6% reduction obtained with diet by the control group, that this 9.3% total reduction in LDL-C from baseline was large enough to reduce all-cause mortality if sustained over time (88). Dietary fiber supplementation may improve blood pressure as well, a meta-analysis of placebo controlled studies suggested that the effect is small, but larger in those over 40 and in hypertensives versus normotensives (89).

Fiber and Coronary Heart Disease

The relationship between total and soluble dietary fiber intake and the risk of CHD and CVD was examined in the 9,776 healthy adults who participated in the National Health and Nutrition Examination Survey (NHANES) I Epidemiologic Follow-up Study (89). Based on 24-hour dietary recall, subjects consuming more than 4.0 g of soluble fiber per 1,735 kcal (upper quartile) had a 15% lower risk of CHD, a 24% lower CHD mortality, a 10% lower risk of CVD, a 12% lower CVD mortality, and an 11% lower total mortality compared with those consuming fewer than 1.3 g of soluble fiber per 1,735 kcal (lower quartile). Data from 10 prospective cohort studies from the United States and Europe representing a 6- to 10-year follow-up of 91,058 men and 245,186 women were analyzed to determine the relation to CHD of dietary fiber and its subtypes (90). After adjustment for demographics, BMI, and lifestyle factors, each 10-g/d increment of energy-adjusted and measurement error–corrected total dietary fiber was associated with a 14% decrease in risk of all CHD events and a 27% reduction in CHD death. Using uncorrected data, cereal and fruit, but not vegetable, intake was correlated with risk of CHD.

Other Dietary Factors and Lipids

Vegetable Protein

Soy protein has been consumed worldwide for centuries, and some Asian populations are known to consume 20 g/d of soy protein in products such as soy milk, tempeh, and tofu (91). The mechanism by which soy lowers LDL-C are still unclear, but it appears that the isoflavone fraction is important in this regard. Soy products may be useful in replacing products high in saturated fat. Nonetheless, LDL-C–lowering obtained with soy is likely to be only modest (92).

Coffee

There has been considerable interest in whether coffee has deleterious effects on the coronary risk profile. This may depend on whether the coffee is filtered coffee or boiled (93). Boiled coffee is consumed in Scandinavia, France, and Turkey and contains the diterpene lipids cafestol and kahweol. Diterpenes are extracted by hot water but are retained by a paper filter. When present, the diterpenes raise cholesterol by 6% to 10%, with lower values seen with longer duration of observation.

Coffee and CHD. Prospective cohort data with 2- to 10-year follow-ups support the contention that two to five cups of filtered coffee daily is not likely to increase CHD events significantly (94–96). In the absence of a placebo-controlled, clinical trial to eliminate unknown confounding variables, it appears that individuals who drink, on average, one to two cups of filtered coffee per day probably incur little change in lipid levels or CHD rates, as long as the coffee consumption is neither associated with the use of dairy creamers nor accompanied by cigarette smoking.

Garlic

The use of garlic to reduce LDL-C has produced inconsistent results. Allicin, the sulfur-rich component of garlic that provides its characteristic odor, is believed to be the active lipid-lowering compound in garlic (97). However, the lack of significant reductions of LDL-C in at least six well-designed trials indicates that it cannot be considered an effective LDL-C–lowering substance (98).

Dietary Factors That Affect HDL-C and Triglyceride Levels

The dietary factors that alter HDL-C and TG levels are not the same as those that alter LDL-C levels. Major factors are excess dietary energy, high carbohydrate intake, alcohol, and fish oil.

Knuiman and colleagues (99) reviewed epidemiologic data on the relationship between diet and HDL-C levels and concluded that three partly opposing dietary factors determine the ratio of total cholesterol to HDL-C in an adult population.

They convincingly argued that the proportion of energy from saturated fat raised total cholesterol and LDL-C levels, the proportion of energy from total fat raised HDL-C levels, and an excess in dietary energy, which produces obesity, lowered HDL-C levels. In addition, weight loss markedly affects TG levels and can improve HDL-C levels. A meta-analysis of studies on the effects of weight loss on lipid and lipoprotein levels showed a significant negative correlation between weight loss and total cholesterol, LDL-C, and TG levels (100). HDL-C levels decreased during the active weight loss phase but increased by 0.009 mmol/L with every kilogram of weight loss when weight was maintained.

High-carbohydrate, low-fat diets reduce HDL-C by decreasing HDL apolipoprotein transport rates (101). Foods with high glycemic index/load (see glossary) can increase postprandial glucose as well as increase TG, lower HDL-C, or raise apo B (102). Ludwig and Jenkins (102) emphasized that we need to look beyond macronutrient amounts and focus on nutrient quality. They noted that just as high-fat diets do not necessarily increase LDL-C, so, too high-carbohydrate diets do not necessarily increase TG. Although alcohol raises TG concentrations, it also raises HDL-C. The Framingham Offspring Study's analysis of 1,584 middle-aged men and 1,639 middle-aged women showed that TG levels, BMI, and alcohol intake all contributed significantly to fasting HDL-C and apoprotein A-I variability. Finally, as noted, marine sources of omega 3 fatty acids lower TG in dose-dependent fashion with mild increases in HDL-C (62).

ANTIOXIDANTS, VITAMINS, AND CORONARY HEART DISEASE

Ever since oxidation of LDL by cells in the arterial wall was proposed as a pivotal step in the initiation of the early lesions seen in coronary atherosclerosis (103), there has been great interest in antioxidant vitamins such as vitamins E, C, and β-carotene. Vitamin E (α-tocopherol), is carried on LDL and is a potent lipid-soluble antioxidant. Food sources of vitamin E include seed oils, nuts, avocados, whole-grain and fortified cereals, eggs, and green vegetables. β-Carotene is lipid soluble. Food sources included carrots and boiled broccoli. Vitamin C is water soluble and widely available in fruits and vegetables, but losses of vitamin C can occur with cooking.

Antioxidant Vitamins and Coronary Artery Disease

Vitamin E use is common. A cross-sectional analysis from the 1999–2000 National Health and Nutrition Examination Survey estimated that 11% of adults take Vitamin E supplements (104). Yet use of antioxidant vitamins have not proven effective in reducing risk of CVD (105). Indeed, a recent meta-analysis of the dose–response relationship between vitamin E supplementation and total mortality by using data from randomized, controlled trials not only showed no benefit, but suggested that vitamin E levels of 400 IU or greater may be associated with increased mortality (106). An important caveat is that trials that used high doses tested adults with chronic diseases and thus, this meta-analysis finding may not be easily generalized to the population as a whole.

β-Carotene and Coronary Artery Disease

A large clinical trial using β-carotene supplementation showed no beneficial effects on cancer or CVD and did not confirm the suggestions of an increased risk of lung cancer in former smokers in two smaller trials (107–109).

Vitamin C and Vitamin Cocktails

Nine prospective cohort studies with information on intakes of vitamin E, carotenoids, and vitamin C were pooled to examine relationships with CHD events occurring over a 10-year period. Among the 293,172 subjects free of CHD at baseline, only high-dose vitamin C appeared to reduce CHD events in significant fashion when contrasted with those who didn't take vitamin C (110). A caution regarding the pooled use of antioxidants was seen in the HATS trial that randomized subjects with a 2 × 2 factorial design to a combination that included either a cocktail of 800 IU of vitamin E (as D-α-tocopherol), 1,000 mg of vitamin C, 25 mg of natural β-carotene, and 100 μg of selenium, simvastatin–niacin, cocktail, or drug placebos. Those subjects who received the vitamin cocktail as well as the niacin–simvastatin therapy had the protective increase in HDL_2 seen with simvastatin plus niacin attenuated (along with angiographic benefits) as contrasted to those given the placebo cocktail (111).

At this time the scientific data do not justify the use of vitamin supplements in the prevention or treatment of CHD (112).

CONCLUSIONS

How can cardiologists best advise their patients on the use of diet and lifestyle to reduce risks of CHD? Put simply, the major nutritional factors that make the most difference in improving CHD risk are caloric intake/energy balance to avoid overweight/obesity, LDL-raising fatty acids (especially saturated fats and TFAs), and beneficial fatty acids (unsaturated fatty acids, especially omega 3 fatty acids). At every visit, I suggest the cardiologist advise his or her patients to "Eat less and move more!" Advice to realign caloric intake to one's physical activity and shift to higher fiber and omega 3 fatty acid dietary sources and away from high animal and dairy fat is supported by a growing amount of evidence. Point out that avoiding all carbohydrates reduces the intake of vitamins, minerals, and fiber that are provided by healthful carbohydrates such as whole grains, fruits, and vegetables. One way to accomplish much of this is for physicians to counsel patients on lifestyle patterns such as a Mediterranean-style diet and regular exercise (Fig. 2.2). This advice is affordable, feasible,

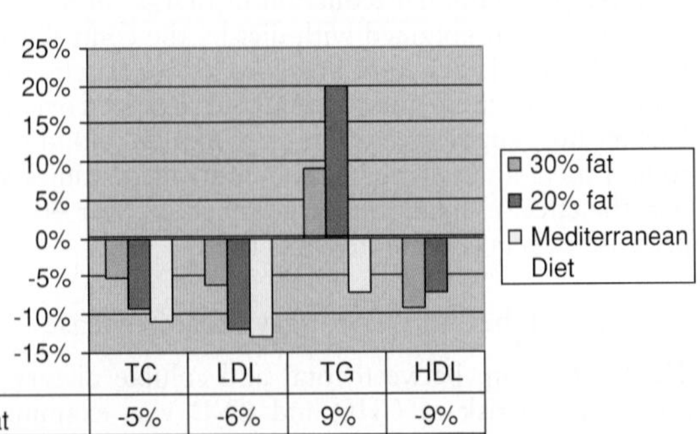

	TC	LDL	TG	HDL
30% fat	-5%	-6%	9%	-9%
20% fat	-9%	-12%	20%	-7%
Mediterranean Diet	-11%	-13%	-7%	0

FIGURE 2.2. Effect of dietary changes versus the standard Western diet. Sacks FM, Katan M. Randomized clinical trials on the effects of dietary fat and carbohydrate on plasma lipoprotein and cardiovascular disease. (*Source: Am J Med* 2002;113[Suppl 9B]:13S–24S.)

and associated with beneficial health outcomes over the long term. Indeed, a focus on a healthy lifestyle should become an integral part of every patient–physician interaction. Weight loss plans that provide benefit only over the short term should take a back seat to more healthful, long-term options. Referral to dietitians for medical nutritional consultation cannot be emphasized strongly enough. Reducing out-of-pocket payment for unproven vitamin supplements may help to provide funds for needed professional nutritional assistance.

CONTROVERSIES AND PERSONAL PERSPECTIVES

A number of pyramids are now offered to Americans to consider. The USDA, DASH, Mediterranean diet, and Mayo Clinic pyramids are examples of what is available (5,14,18). These can be very helpful in education efforts to the general public (Fig. 2.3). Most important, the physician should take advantage of the patient's readiness to change. For example, a patient with elevated LDL-C and metabolic syndrome who is recovered from recent bypass surgery needs to understand why he or she required such a technically complex and expensive intervention. This may be especially effective in the hospital setting.

Many physicians are under the false impression that nutritional advice just does not work in clinical practice. I am concerned that many find it easier to advocate fad diets rather than stress the evidence-based nutritional principles mentioned in this chapter. My experience in preventive cardiology for the past three decades has found these principles invaluable. Find out if the patient is ready to change and realize that failure is much less likely when individualized counseling and follow-up are provided and the focus is on lifestyle (diet and exercise) instead of on single dietary components. A useful approach to nutritional counseling for physicians is given in Table 2.4.

THE FUTURE

As we approach the year 2010, the United States is well on its way to attaining an even lower overall serum cholesterol level through improved diet. The ongoing challenge in health care will be to develop innovative programs to help patients improve nutritional quality while at the same time controlling nutritional quantity! Healthcare organizations need to consider innovative way to provide lifestyle counseling. Instead of a doctor–patient visit, it may be more productive to have a doctor, nurse, and dietitian meet with 10 to 14 patients in a 1-hour group session that encourages participation and problem solving. Finally, exciting advances in medical genetics hold the promise of more targeted nutritional advice, not only for the general population, but particularly for those at high risk for heart disease and stroke.

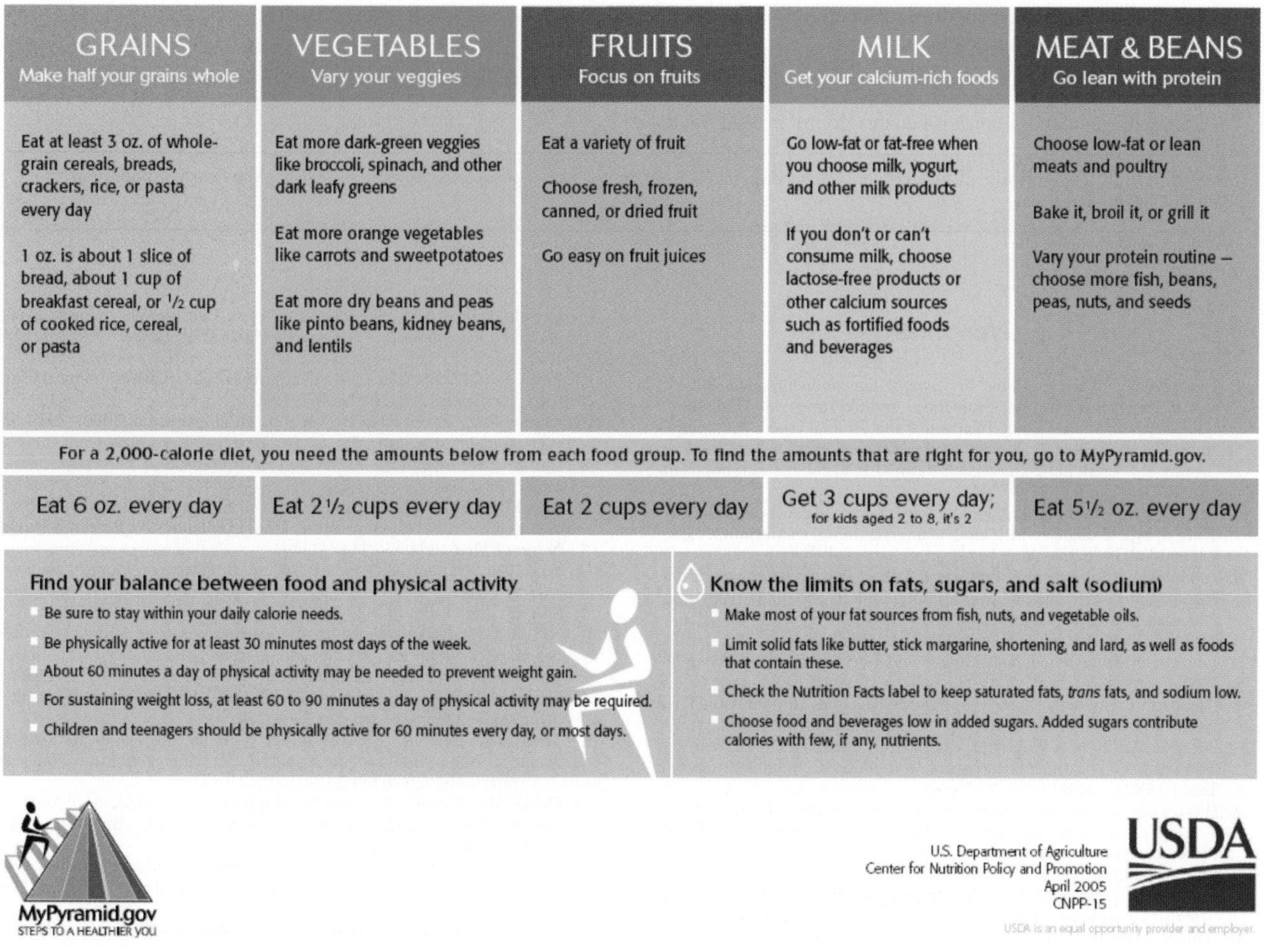
GRAINS
Make half your grains whole
Eat at least 3 oz. of whole-grain cereals, breads, crackers, rice, or pasta every day
1 oz. is about 1 slice of bread, about 1 cup of breakfast cereal, or 1/2 cup of cooked rice, cereal, or pasta
VEGETABLES
Vary your veggies
Eat more dark-green veggies like broccoli, spinach, and other dark leafy greens
Eat more orange vegetables like carrots and sweetpotatoes
Eat more dry beans and peas like pinto beans, kidney beans, and lentils
FRUITS
Focus on fruits
Eat a variety of fruit
Choose fresh, frozen, canned, or dried fruit
Go easy on fruit juices
MILK
Get your calcium-rich foods
Go low-fat or fat-free when you choose milk, yogurt, and other milk products
If you don't or can't consume milk, choose lactose-free products or other calcium sources such as fortified foods and beverages
MEAT & BEANS
Go lean with protein
Choose low-fat or lean meats and poultry
Bake it, broil it, or grill it
Vary your protein routine – choose more fish, beans, peas, nuts, and seeds
For a 2,000-calorie diet, you need the amounts below from each food group. To find the amounts that are right for you, go to MyPyramid.gov.
Eat 6 oz. every day
Eat 2 1/2 cups every day
Eat 2 cups every day
Get 3 cups every day; for kids aged 2 to 8, it's 2
Eat 5 1/2 oz. every day
Find your balance between food and physical activity
Be sure to stay within your daily calorie needs.
Be physically active for at least 30 minutes most days of the week.
About 60 minutes a day of physical activity may be needed to prevent weight gain.
For sustaining weight loss, at least 60 to 90 minutes a day of physical activity may be required.
Children and teenagers should be physically active for 60 minutes every day, or most days.
Know the limits on fats, sugars, and salt (sodium)
Make most of your fat sources from fish, nuts, and vegetable oils.
Limit solid fats like butter, stick margarine, shortening, and lard, as well as foods that contain these.
Check the Nutrition Facts label to keep saturated fats, trans fats, and sodium low.
Choose food and beverages low in added sugars. Added sugars contribute calories with few, if any, nutrients.
MyPyramid.gov
STEPS TO A HEALTHIER YOU
U.S. Department of Agriculture
Center for Nutrition Policy and Promotion
April 2005
CNPP-15
USDA
USDA is an equal opportunity provider and employer.

FIGURE 2.3. 2005 Recommendations for health eating. (*Source:* USDA Center for Nutrition Policy and Promotion.)

TABLE 2.4

NUTRITIONAL DECISIONS IN HYPERCHOLESTEROLEMIA

1. Assess lipid/metabolic status
   Elevated LDL-C — Metabolic Syndrome (3/5 for diagnosis)
   –Increased waist circumference
   –Elevated TG
   –Reduced HDL-C
   –Elevated BP
   –Impaired fasting glucose
2. Assess CHD risk factors and CHD risk status (clinical data; use Framingham score)
3. Set goals for therapy
   a. LDL-C to goal
   b. Reduce metabolic syndrome risk factors with lifestyle change, including DASH diet if hypertensive (and if needed, medications)
4. Discuss whether patient is ready to change atherogenic lifestyle
   a. If not ready for lifestyle change, let patient know help is available when he or she is ready
   b. Consider focusing on eating healthier at just one meal (e.g., breakfast)
5. Emphasize therapeutic lifestyle change ("Move more, eat less"); focus on
   –Atherogenic diet
   More fiber sources, fruits, vegetables, fish, legumes, nuts, whole grains
   Decrease or substitute for large portions, fatty cuts of meat, fried foods, commercial baked goods, and high-fat dairy products
   –Sedentary behavior
   Encourage adding exercise into the daily routine; do more each day
   –Weight gain
   Start with avoiding further weight gain/reduced calories if overweight/obese
6. Get help
   Registered dietitians to provide medical nutrition consultation
7. Use monitors
   –Keep a diet diary
   –Use pedometer to increase steps per day
8. Give feedback
   –Check waist circumference, risk factors after appropriate interval
9. Discuss unproven measures to avoid
   –Megavitamins
   –Fad diets
   –Aspirin for men and women if benefits do not exceed the risks

Abbreviations: BP, blood pressure; CHD, coronary heart disease; HDL-C, high-density lipoprotein cholesterol; LDL-C, low-density lipoprotein cholesterol; TG, triglycerides.

References

1. Third Report of the National Cholesterol Education Program (NCEP) Expert Panel on Detection, Evaluation, and Treatment of High Blood Cholesterol in Adults. Adult Treatment Panel III final report. *Circulation* 2002;106:3143–3421.
2. Grundy SM. Small LDL, atherogenic dyslipidemia, and the metabolic syndrome. *Circulation* 1997;95:1–4.
3. The Diabetes Prevention Program Research Group. Reduction in the incidence of type 2 diabetes with lifestyle intervention or metformin. *N Engl J Med* 2002;346:393–403.
4. Tuomilehto J, Lindstrom J, Eriksson JG, et al. Prevention of type 2 diabetes mellitus by changes in lifestyle among subjects with impaired glucose tolerance. *N Engl J Med* 2001;344:1343–1350.
5. Parikh P, McDaniel MC, Ashen MD, et al. Diets and cardiovascular disease. An evidence-based assessment. *J Am Coll Cardiol* 2005;45:1379–1387.
6. Hjermann I, Holme I, Leren P. Oslo Study Diet and Anti-Smoking Trial: results after 102 months. *Am J Med* 1986;80[Suppl 2A]:7–12.
7. Burr ML, Fehily AM, Gilbert JF, et al. Effects of changes in fat, fish, and fibre intakes on death and myocardial reinfarction: Diet and Reinfarction Trial (DART). *Lancet* 1989;2:757–761.
8. Dietary supplementation with *n*-3 polyunsaturated fatty acids and vitamin E after myocardial infarction: results of the GISSI-Prevenzione trial. GISSI-Prevenzione Investigators. *Lancet* 1999;354:447–455.
9. Watts GF, Lewis B, Brunt JNH, et al. Effects of coronary artery disease of lipid lowering diet, or diet plus cholestyramine in the St. Thomas Atherosclerosis Regression Study (STARS). *Lancet* 1992;339:563–569.
10. Schuler G, Hambrecht R, Schlierf G, et al. Regular physical exercise and low-fat diet: effects of progression on coronary artery disease. *Circulation* 1992;86:1–11.
11. Ornish D, Brown SE, Scherwitz LW, et al. Can lifestyle changes reverse coronary heart disease? The Lifestyle Heart Trial. *Lancet* 1990;335:129–133.
12. Brousseau ME, Schaefer EJ. Diet and coronary heart disease: clinical trials. *Curr Atheroscler Rep* 2000;2:487–493.
13. Krause RM, Eckel RH, Howard B, et al. Revision 2000: AHA dietary guidelines; a statement for healthcare professionals from the Nutrition Committee of the American Heart Association. *Circulation* 2000; 102:2296–2311.
14. Appel LJ, Moore TJ, Obarzanek E, et al. A clinical trial of the effects of dietary patterns on blood pressure. DASH Collaborative Research Group. *N Engl J Med* 1997;336:1117–1124.
15. Sacks FM, Svetkey LP, Vollmer WM, et al. Effects on blood pressure of reduced dietary sodium and the Dietary Approaches to Stop Hypertension (DASH) diet. *N Engl J Med* 2001;344:3–10.
16. NHLBI Obesity Education Initiative. *Summary report: Strategy development workshop for public education on weight and obesity.* NIH publication 94-3314. Bethesda, MD: National Institutes of Health, 1994: 139.
17. Dietary Guidelines for America 2005. Available: www.healthierus.gov/dietaryguidelines. Accessed August 1, 2005.
18. Manson JE, Skerrett PJ, Greenland P, VanItallie TB. The escalating pandemics of obesity and sedentary lifestyle. A call to action for clinicians. *Arch Intern Med* 2004;164:249–258.
19. Denke MA, Grundy SM. Individual responses to a cholesterol-lowering diet in 50 men with moderate hypercholesterolemia. *Arch Intern Med* 1994;154:317–325.
20. Denke MA. Review of human studies evaluating individual dietary responsiveness in patients with hypercholesterolemia. *Am J Clin Nutr* 1995;62:471S–477S.
21. Denke MA, Frantz ID Jr. Response to a cholesterol-lowering diet efficacy is greater in hypercholesterolemic subjects even after adjustment for regression to the mean. *Am J Med* 1993;94:626–631.

22. Goldstein JL, Hobbs HH, Brown MS. Familial hypercholesterolemia. In: Scriver CR, Beaudet AL, Valle D, Sly WS, eds. *The metabolic basis of inherited disease,* 8th ed. New York: McGraw-Hill.
23. Kwiterovich PO, Virgil DG, Schweitzer A, et al. Response of obligate heterozygotes for phytosterolemia to a low-fat diet and to a plant sterol ester dietary challenge. *J Lipid Res* 2003;44:1143–1155.
24. Lopez-Miranda J, Ordovas JM, Mata P, et al. Effect of apolipoprotein E phenotype on diet-induced lowering of plasma low density lipoprotein cholesterol. *J Lipid Res* 1994;35:1965–1975.
25. Krauss RM, Dreon DM. Low-density-lipoprotein subclasses and response to a low-fat diet in healthy men. *Am J Clin Nutr* 1995;62:478S–487S.
26. Fisler JS, Warden CH. Dietary fat and genotype: toward individualized prescriptions for lifestyle changes. *Am J Clin Nutr* 2005;81:1255–1256.
27. Keys A, Anderson JT, Grande F. Prediction of serum-cholesterol responses of man to changes in fats in the diet. *Lancet* 1957;2:959–966.
28. Hegsted DM, McGandy RB, Myers ML, et al. Quantitative effects of dietary fat on serum cholesterol levels in man. *Am J Clin Nutr* 1995;17:281–295.
29. Cater NB, Denke MA. Behenic acid is a cholesterol-raising saturated fatty acid. *Am J Clin Nutr* 2001;73:41–44.
30. McNamara DJ, Kolb R, Parker TS, et al. Heterogeneity of cholesterol homeostasis in man: Response to changes in dietary fat quality and cholesterol quantity. *J Clin Invest* 1987;79:1729–1739.
31. Grundy SM, Barrett-Connor E, Rudel LL, et al. Workshop on the impact of dietary cholesterol on plasma lipoproteins and atherogenesis. *Arteriosclerosis* 1988;8:95–101.
32. Woolett LA, Spady DK, Dietschy JM. Mechanisms by which saturated triacylglycerols elevate the plasma low density lipoprotein-cholesterol concentration in hamsters: Differential effects of fatty acid chain length. *J Clin Invest* 1989;84:119–128.
33. Ginsberg HN, Karmally W, Siddiqui M, et al. A dose-response study of the effects of dietary cholesterol on fasting and postprandial lipid and lipoprotein metabolism in healthy young men. *Arterioscler Thromb* 1994;14:576–586.
34. Ginsberg HN, Karmally W, Siddiqui M, et al. Increases in dietary cholesterol are associated with modest increases in both LDL and HDL cholesterol in healthy women. *Arterioscler Thromb Vasc Biol* 1995;15:169–178.
35. Fielding CJ, Havel RJ, Todd KM, et al. Effects of dietary cholesterol and fat saturation on plasma lipoproteins in an ethnically diverse population of healthy young men. *J Clin Invest* 1995;95:611–618.
36. Stern L, Iqbal N, Seshadri P, et al. The effects of low-carbohydrate versus conventional weight loss diets in severely obese adults: one-year follow-up of a randomized trial. *Ann Intern Med* 2004;140:778–785.
37. Stamler J, Shekelle R. Dietary cholesterol and human coronary heart disease. *Arch Pathol Lab Med* 1988;112:1032–1040.
38. Hu F, Stampfer MJ, Rimm EB, et al. A prospective study of egg consumption and risk of cardiovascular disease in men and women. *JAMA* 1999;281:1387–1394.
39. Law M. Plant sterol and stanol margarines in health. *BMJ* 2000;320:861–864.
40. Katan MB, Grundy SM, Jones P, et al. Stresa workshop participants. Efficacy and safety of plant stanols and sterols in the management of blood cholesterol levels. *Mayo Clin Proc* 2003;78:965–978.
41. Nguyen TT, Dale LC, von Bergmann K, et al. Cholesterol-lowering effect of stanol ester in a US population of mildly hypercholesterolemic men and women: a randomized controlled trial. *Mayo Clin Proc* 1999;74:1198–1206.
42. Lichtenstein AH, Deckelbaum RJ, for the American Heart Association Nutrition Committee. Stanol/sterol ester-containing foods and blood cholesterol levels. A statement for healthcare professionals from the Nutrition Committee of the Council on Nutrition, Physical Activity and Metabolism of the American Heart Association. *Circulation* 2001;103:1177–1179.
43. Miettinen TA, Strandberg TE, Gylling H. Noncholesterol sterols and cholesterol lowering by long-term simvastatin treatment in coronary patients: relation to basal serum cholestanol. *Arterioscler Thromb Vasc Biol* 2000;20:1340–1346.
44. Wilund KR, Yu L, Xu F, Vega GL, et al. No association between plasma levels of plant sterols and atherosclerosis in mice and men. *Arterioscler Thromb Vasc Biol* 2004;24:2326–2332.
45. Miettinen TA, Railo M, Lepantalo M, Gylling H. Plant sterols in serum and in atherosclerotic plaques of patients undergoing carotid endarterectomy. *J Am Coll Cardiol* 2005;45:1794–1801.
46. Woolett LA, Spady DK, Dietschy JM. Mechanisms by which saturated triacylglycerols elevate the plasma low density lipoprotein–cholesterol concentration in hamsters: differential effects of fatty acid chain length. *J Clin Invest* 1989;84:119–128.
47. Ginsberg HN, Kris-Etherton P, Dennis B. Effects of reducing dietary saturated fatty acids on plasma lipids and lipoproteins in healthy subjects: the Delta Study, Protocol 1. DELTA Research Group. *Arterioscler Thromb Vasc Biol* 1998;18:441–449.
48. Walden CE, Retzlaff BM, Buck BL, et al. Lipoprotein lipid response to the National Cholesterol Education Program Step II diet by hypercholesterolemic and combined hyperlipidemic women and men. *Arterioscler Thromb Vasc Biol* 1997;17:375–382.
49. Grundy SM. Influence of stearic acid on cholesterol metabolism relative to other long-chain fatty acids. *Am J Clin Nutr* 1994;60[Suppl 6]:986S–990S.
50. Kris-Etherton PM, Derr JA, Mustad VA, et al. Effects of a milk chocolate bar per day substituted for a high-carbohydrate snack in young men on an NCEP/AHA Step 1 Diet. *Am J Clin Nutr* 1994;60[6 Suppl]:1037S–1042S.
51. Keys A. *Seven countries: a multivariate analysis of death and coronary heart disease.* Cambridge, MA: Harvard University Press, 1980.
52. Criqui MH, Ringel BL. Does diet or alcohol explain the French paradox? *Lancet* 1994;344:1719–1723.
53. Law M, Wald N. Why heart disease mortality is low in France: the time lag explanation. *BMJ* 1999;318:1471–1480.
54. Gordon DJ. Cholesterol lowering and total mortality. In: Rifkind BM, ed. *Lowering cholesterol in high-risk individuals and populations.* New York: Marcel Dekker, 1995: 33.
55. Judd JT, Clevidence BA, Muesing RA, et al. Dietary *trans* fatty acids: effects on plasma lipids and lipoproteins of healthy men and women. *Am J Clin Nutr* 1994;59:861–886.
56. Mensink RP, Katan MB. Effect of dietary trans fatty acids on high-density and low-density lipoprotein cholesterol levels in healthy subjects. *N Engl J Med* 1990;323:439–445.
57. Willett WC, Stampfer MJ, Manson JE, et al. Intake of *trans* fatty acids and risk of coronary heart disease among women. *Lancet* 1993;341:581–585.
58. Gardner CD, Kraemer HC. Monounsaturated versus polyunsaturated dietary fat and serum lipids: a meta-analysis. *Arterioscler Thromb Vasc Biol* 1995;15:1917–1927.
59. Meydani SN, Lichtenstein AH, White PJ, et al. Food use and health effects of soybean and sunflower oils. *J Am Coll Nutr* 1991;10:406–428.
60. Sturdevant RAL, Pearce ML, Dayton S. Increased prevalence of cholelithiasis in men ingesting a serum cholesterol lowering diet. *N Engl J Med* 1973;288:24–27.
61. Dolecek TA. Epidemiological evidence of relationships between dietary polyunsaturated fatty acids and mortality in the multiple risk factor intervention trial. *Proc Soc Exp Biol Med* 1992;200:177–182.
62. Kris-Etherton PM, Harris WS, Appel LJ. American Heart Association. Nutrition Committee. Fish consumption, fish oil, omega-3 fatty acids, and cardiovascular disease. *Circulation* 2002;106:2747–2757.
63. Dyerberg J, Bang HO. Haemostatic function and platelet polyunsaturated fatty acids in Eskimos. *Lancet* 1979;2:433–435.
64. Albert CM, Campos H, Stampfer MJ, et al. Blood levels of long-chain n-3 fatty acids and the risk of sudden death. *N Engl J Med* 2002;346:1113–1118.
65. Hu FB, Bronner L, Willett WC, et al. Fish and omega-3 fatty acid and risk of coronary heart disease in women. *JAMA* 2002;287:1815–1821.
66. Siscovick DS, Raghunathan TE, King I, et al. Dietary intake and cell membrane levels of long-chain n-3 polyunsaturated fatty acids and the risk of primary cardiac arrest. *JAMA* 1995;274:1363–1367.
67. Billman GE, Hallaq H, Leaf A. Prevention of ischemia-induced ventricular fibrillation by n-3 fatty acids. *Proc Natl Acad Sci U S A* 1994;91:4427–4430.
68. Grundy SM: N-3 fatty acids: priority for myocardial infarction clinical trials. *Circulation* 2003;107:1834–1836.
69. Hu FB, Stampfer MJ, Manson JE, et al. Dietary intake of alpha-linolenic acid and risk of fatal ischemic heart disease among women. *Am J Clin Nutr* 1999;69:890–897.
70. Baylin A, Kabagambe EK, Ascherio A, et al. Adipose tissue alpha-linolenic acid and nonfatal acute myocardial infarction in Costa Rica. *Circulation* 2003;107:1586–1591.
71. Kris-Etherton P. Monounsaturated fats and the risk of cardiovascular disease. *Circulation* 1999;100:1253–1258.
72. Reaven P, Parthasarathy S, Grasse BJ, et al. Effects of oleate-rich and linoleate-rich diets on the susceptibility of low density lipoprotein to oxidative modification in mildly hypercholesterolemic subjects. *J Clin Invest* 1993;91:668–676.
73. Grundy SM. Comparison of monounsaturated fatty acids and carbohydrates for lowering plasma cholesterol. *N Engl J Med* 1986;3143:745–748.
74. Mensink RP, Katan MB. Effect of monounsaturated fatty acids versus complex carbohydrates on high density lipoproteins in healthy men and women. *Lancet* 1987;1:125–129.
75. Gardner CD, Kraemer HC. Monounsaturated versus polyunsaturated dietary fat and serum lipids: a meta-analysis. *Arterioscler Thromb Vasc Biol* 1995;15:1917–1927.
76. Kris-Etherton P, Pearson TA, Wan Y, et al. High-monounsaturated fatty acid diets lower both cholesterol and triacylglycerol concentrations. *Am J Clin Nutr* 1999;70:1009–1015.
77. Hu FB, Stampfer MJ. Nut consumption and risk of coronary heart disease: a review of epidemiologic evidence. *Curr Atheroscler Rep* 1999;1:204–209.
78. Trichopoulou A, Bamia C, Trichopoulos D. Mediterranean diet and survival among patients with coronary heart disease in Greece. *Arch Intern Med* 2005;165:929–935.
79. Trichopoulou A, Costacou T, Bamia C, Trichopoulos D. Adherence to a Mediterranean diet and survival in a Greek population. *N Engl J Med* 2003;348:2599–2608.
80. de Lorgeril M, Renaud S, Marnelle N, et al. Mediterranean alpha-linolenic acid rich diet in secondary prevention of coronary heart disease. *Lancet* 1994;343:1454–1459.

81. de Lorgeril M. Mediterranean diet, traditional risk factors, and the rate of cardiovascular complications after myocardial infarction: final report of the Lyon Diet Heart Study. *Circulation* 1999;99:779–785.
82. Singh RB, Dubnov G, Niaz MA, et al. Effect of an Indo-Mediterranean diet on progression of coronary artery disease in high risk patients (Indo-Mediterranean Diet Heart Study): a randomised single-blind trial. *Lancet* 2002;360:1455–1461.
83. Gould KL, Ornish D, Scherwitz L, et al. Changes in myocardial perfusion abnormalities by positron emission tomography after long-term, intense risk factor modification. *JAMA* 1995;274:894–901.
84. Quinn TG, Alderman EL, McMillan A, et al. Development of new coronary atherosclerotic lesions during a 4-year multifactor risk reduction program: the Stanford Risk Intervention Project (SCRIP). SCRIP Investigators. *J Am Coll Cardiol* 1994;24:900–908.
85. Van Horn L. Fiber, lipids, and coronary heart disease. Nutrition Committee. *Circulation* 1997;95:2701–2704.
86. Jenkins DJ, Kendall CW, Marchie A, et al. Effects of a dietary portfolio of cholesterol-lowering foods vs lovastatin on serum lipids and C-reactive protein. *JAMA* 2003;290:502–510.
87. Gardner CD, Coulston A, Chatterjee L, et al. The effect of a plant-based diet on plasma lipids in hypercholesterolemic adults: a randomized trial. *Ann Intern Med* 2005;142:725–733.
88. Jenkins DJA, Kendall CWC, Marchie A. Diet and cholesterol reduction. *Ann Intern Med* 2005;142:793–795.
89. Streppel MT, Arends LR, van't Veer P, et al. Dietary fiber and blood pressure: a meta-analysis of randomized placebo-controlled trials. *Arch Intern Med* 2005;165:150–156.
90. Pereira MA, O'Reilly E, Augustsson K, et al. Dietary fiber and risk of coronary heart disease: a pooled analysis of cohort studies. *Arch Intern Med* 2004;164:370–376.
91. Erdman JW. Control of serum lipids with soy protein. *N Engl J Med* 1995;333:313–315.
92. Lichtenstein AH. Got soy? *Am J Clin Nutr* 2001;73:667–668.
93. Urgert R, Katan MB. The cholesterol-raising factor from coffee beans. *Annu Rev Nutr* 1997;17:305–324.
94. Grobbee DE, Rimm EB, Giovannucci E, et al. Coffee, caffeine, and cardiovascular disease in men. *N Engl J Med* 1990;323:1026–1032.
95. Willett W, Stampfer MJ, Manson JE, et al. Coffee consumption and coronary heart disease in women: a ten-year followup. *JAMA* 1996;275:458–462.
96. LaCroix AZ, Mead LA, Liang KY, et al. Coffee consumption and the incidence of coronary heart disease. *N Engl J Med* 1986;315:377–382.
97. Kerckhoffs DA, Brouns F, Hornstra G, Mensink RP. Effects on the human serum lipoprotein profile of β-glucan, soy protein and isoflavones, plant sterols and stanols, garlic and tocotrienols. *J Nutr* 2002;132:2494–2505.
98. Isaacsohn JL, Moser M, Stein EA, et al. Garlic powder and plasma lipids and lipoproteins: a multicenter, randomized, placebo-controlled trial. *Arch Intern Med* 1998;158:1189–1194.
99. Knuiman JT, West CE, Katan MB, et al. Total cholesterol and high density lipoprotein cholesterol levels in populations differing in fat and carbohydrate intake. *Arteriosclerosis* 1987;7:612–619.
100. Dattilo AM, Kris-Etherton PM. Effects of weight reduction on blood lipids and lipoproteins: a meta-analysis. *Am J Clin Nutr* 1992;56:320–328.
101. Brinton EA, Eisenberg S, Breslow JL. A low-fat diet decreases high density lipoprotein (HDL) cholesterol levels by decreasing HDL apolipoprotein transport rates. *J Clin Invest* 1990;85:1.
102. Ludwig DS, Jenkins DJ. Carbohydrates and the postprandial state: have our cake and eat it too? *Am J Clin Nutr* 2004;80:797–798.
103. Steinberg D, Parthasarathy S, Carew TE, et al. Beyond cholesterol: modifications of low-density lipoprotein that increase its atherogenicity. *N Engl J Med* 1989;320:915–924.
104. Ford ES, Ajani UA, Mokdad AH. Brief communication: the prevalence of high intake of vitamin e from the use of supplements among U.S. adults. *Ann Intern Med* 2005;143:116–120.
105. Vivekananthan DP, Penn MS, Sapp SK, et al. Use of antioxidant vitamins for the prevention of cardiovascular disease: meta-analysis of randomised trials. *Lancet* 2003;361:2017–2023.
106. Miller ER, Pastor-Barriuso R, Dalal, D, et al. Meta-Analysis: High-dosage vitamin E supplementation may increase all-cause mortality. *Ann Intern Med* 2005;142:37–46.
107. Hennekens CH, Buring JE, Manson JE, et al. Lack of effect of long-term supplementation with beta carotene on the incidence of malignant neoplasms and cardiovascular disease. *N Engl J Med* 1996;334:1145–1149.
108. Omenn GS, Goodman GE, Thornquist MD, et al. Effects of a combination of beta carotene vitamin A on lung cancer and cardiovascular disease. *N Engl J Med* 1996;334:1150–1155.
109. The effect of vitamin E and beta carotene on the incidence of lung cancer and other cancers in male smokers. Alpha Tocopherol, Beta Carotene Prevention Study Group. *N Engl J Med* 1994;330:1029–1035.
110. Knekt P, Ritz J, Pereira MA, et al. Antioxidant vitamins and coronary heart disease risk: a pooled analysis of 9 cohorts. *Am J Clin Nutr* 2004;80:1508–1520.
111. Brown BG, Zhao XQ, Chait A, et al. Simvastatin and niacin, antioxidant vitamins, or the combination for the prevention of coronary disease. *N Engl J Med* 2001;345:1583–1592.
112. Kris-Etherton PM, Lichtenstein AH, Howard BV, et al. Nutrition Committee of the American Heart Association Council on Nutrition, Physical Activity, and Metabolism. Antioxidant vitamin supplements and cardiovascular disease. *Circulation* 2004;110:637–641.

CHAPTER 3 ■ OBESITY AND METABOLIC SYNDROME

OSCAR C. MARROQUIN AND DAVID E. KELLEY

INTRODUCTION

Obesity now looms as a major public health challenge for developed societies. Cardiovascular disease (CVD) is one of the major comorbidities of obesity. The relationship between obesity and CVD is the focus of this chapter. Physicians need to integrate an assessment of obesity into patient evaluation and also promote its treatment. These principles pertain to the management of many cardiovascular illnesses and emphatically to the promotion of cardiovascular health. One of the goals of this chapter is to outline current practices for the assessment of obesity. These are simple and straightforward. The pathophysiology that links obesity with the metabolic syndrome will also be addressed, stressing the importance of regional distribution of adiposity as well as the roles of adipose tissue as an endocrine organ and a source of low-grade inflammation. Central adiposity and the closely associated phenomena of increased fat content within liver and skeletal muscle are at the core of the metabolic syndrome and insulin resistance. Delineation of the metabolic syndrome was a major step forward in the conceptualization of how insulin resistance and obesity contribute to risk for CVD. Recently, controversy has arisen as to whether the metabolic syndrome actually constitutes a treatable disease entity.

The second main aim of this chapter is to examine the mechanisms and manifestations of CVD in obesity. There are multiple pathways through which increased risk occurs. Risks for CVD associated with obesity and insulin resistance coalesce into propensity for the formation, progression, and, likely, the fragility of atherosclerotic plaques, and thus into an increased risk for coronary thrombosis and myocardial infarction. However, this is not the singular manifestation of obesity-related risk for CVD. Obesity-related risk for cardiovascular disease is also manifest as congestive heart failure, endothelial dysfunction, arterial stiffness, hypertension, and perturbations of substrate metabolism within cardiac myocytes, and these aspects will also be addressed in this chapter.

EPIDEMIOLOGY

During the last several decades, the prevalence of obesity has increased to epidemic proportions. The prevalence of obesity among U.S. adults increased from 12% in 1991 to 21.3% in 2002 (Fig. 3.1) (1). In 2002, 58% of adult Americans (66% of men and 50% of women) were overweight (2). Overweight is defined as a body mass index (BMI) above 25 kg/m^2 but less than 30 kg/m^2, and obesity is defined as a BMI of 30 kg/m^2 or greater. The prevalence of class III obesity, a BMI greater than 40 kg/m^2, increased from 0.9% in 1991 to 2.4% in 2002 (3). There are ethnic differences in obesity. African Americans and Hispanics have higher rates of obesity than do non-Hispanic whites, whereas the prevalence of obesity is lower among Asian Americans (4), although the BMI at which obesity-related comorbidities may develop appears to be lower in Asian Americans, so cut-points for "at-risk" BMI are lower. Of particular concern is the widespread increase in the prevalence of overweight and obesity among school-age children as well as adolescents and young adults (5,6). These trends have been observed in the United States (2,5,6), Great Britain (7), and Asia (8), where similar behavioral factors affecting diet and physical activity are presumably at work.

CLINICAL ASSESSMENT OF OBESITY

In the United States, the National Institutes of Health bases its classification of body weight on the concept of body mass index (9). The BMI is calculated by dividing the body weight in kilograms by the square of the height in meters (Table 3.1).

A lean BMI is 25 kg/m^2 or less. Although a lean body weight is regarded as "normal," as pointed out earlier, this is maintained in only a minority of adults in the United States. In children and adolescents, no specific BMI values have been set

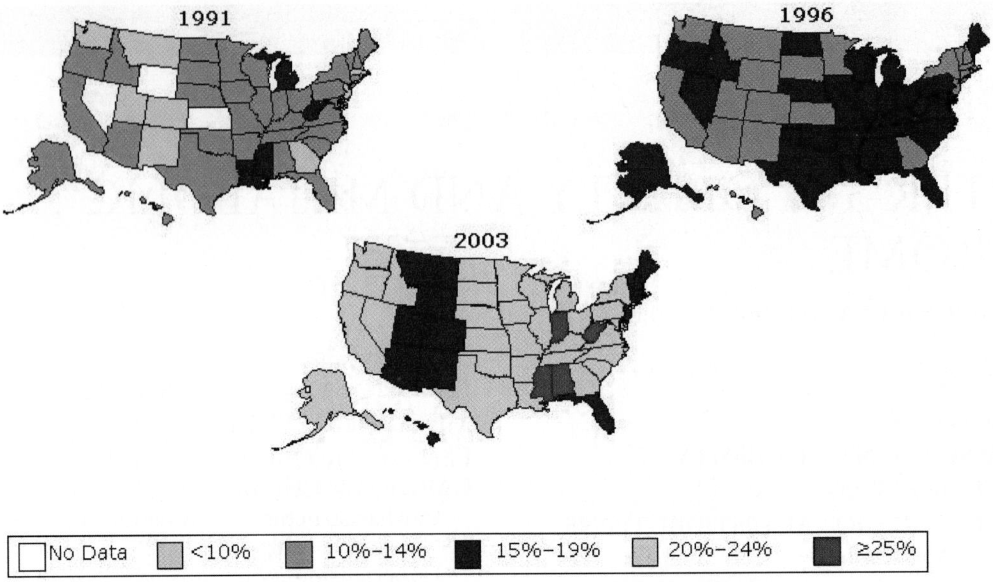

FIGURE 3.1. Obesity trends among U.S. adults for the years 1991, 1996, and 2003. Obesity is defined as a body mass index of ≥30, or about 30 pounds overweight for a person of height 5 feet 4 inches. (From *Behavioral risk factor surveillance system*, Centers for Disease Control, Atlanta, GA.)

to identify obesity and overweight; however, BMI at or greater than the 95th percentile for sex- and age-specific distribution has been used to identify overweight (2).

In addition to measuring height and weight (and thereby determining BMI), measuring waist circumference is also recommended. At any BMI, a higher waist circumference identifies increased metabolic risk. Although the relationship is a continuum, a cut-point for waist circumference is greater than 102 cm (>40 inches) for men and greater than 88 cm (>35 inches) for women. Measuring waist circumference takes into account the distribution of adipose tissue. For example, for the same level of BMI, the cardiovascular risk may be significantly lower in a person in whom excess body fat is predominantly in a gluteal-femoral distribution rather than upper body, abdominal adiposity (10–12).

ASSESSMENT OF FAT MASS

More-precise measurements of the amount of body fat and more exact ascertainment of its distribution generally exceed cost constraints as well as practical needs for clinical care. In a research setting, there are several methods that can be used to accurately assess fat mass and ascertain the distribution of adipose tissue, including assessments of the lipid content of liver and skeletal muscle. Estimation of fat mass (and of fat-free mass) is usually obtained using dual-energy x-ray absorptiometry (DXA). A limitation is that DXA is not adequate for severe obesity due to the size constraint of the scanning table. The use of underwater weighing to estimate fat mass has waned with the widespread availability of DXA. Air-displacement systems that permit determination of body density have become available. Thus, calculation of fat mass is beginning to be more common (e.g., the BOD POD technology; Life Measurement Inc., Concord, CA). Bioimpedance can be used to estimate total body water based on resistance to a very small amount of transmitted electrical current. Using assumptions about tissue hydration, one can estimate fat-free mass and fat mass. This last point is crucial for understanding the limitations of bioimpedance because rapid shifts in fluid balance, as might occur with treatment of congestive heart failure, can render these estimations inaccurate.

TABLE 3.1

CLINICAL CLASSIFICATION OF OBESITY

Category	Range of body mass index (kg/m^2)
Normal weight	≤25.0
Overweight	25.1–29.9
Class I obesity	30.0–34.9
Class II obesity	35.0–39.9
Class III obesity	≥40.0

ASSESSMENT OF REGIONAL DISTRIBUTIONS OF ADIPOSE TISSUE

The importance of adipose tissue distribution in relation to metabolic risk was recognized by Vague et al. (13) more than a half century ago. This perspective has been substantiated by the findings obtained using modern bioimaging technologies for body composition, such as computed tomography (CT), magnetic resonance imaging (MRI), and magnetic resonance spectroscopy (MRS). Abdominal CT or MRI, most commonly performed using a cross-sectional image centered at the L4–5 disc space, is generally used to measure visceral abdominal adiposity (visceral adipose tissue, VAT) and subcutaneous abdominal adiposity (SAT) (Fig. 3.2) (14–16). Visceral adiposity generally is greater in men than in women and increases with aging and after menopause in women. As a percentage of total abdominal adiposity and in relation to BMI, VAT varies across races, being higher in Asians, lower in Africans, and intermediate in those of European ancestry. Visceral adiposity is the sum of omental, mesenteric, and perinephric adipose tissue, essentially all adipose tissue beneath the abdominal wall musculature.

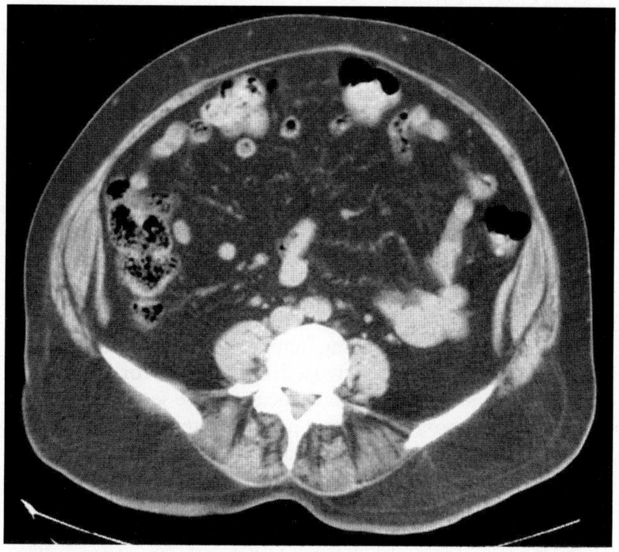

FIGURE 3.2. Cross-sectional image abdominal CT at the L4–5 disk space to measure visceral adiposity.

In general, the amount of VAT correlates well with severity of insulin resistance and with dyslipidemia (14–16). That visceral adiposity correlates with metabolic syndrome more strongly than does an overall index of obesity such as BMI or systemic fat mass is an intriguing because the volume of VAT generally represents only about 10% of systemic adipose tissue. It remains incompletely understood why this relatively small mass of VAT correlates so well with systemic manifestations of insulin resistance, including various risk factors for CVD. VAT, or at least a portion of VAT, releases free fatty acids (FFAs) into the portal circulation (17). The strong association between VAT and severity of dyslipidemia may relate in part to this portal delivery of fatty acids, although this is a difficult concept to test in humans due to inaccessibility of portal sampling. Adipocytes within VAT do have a higher rate of lipolysis and are less responsive to suppression of lipolysis by insulin (18,19). Nonetheless, this explanation is at best only partial satisfactory because a majority of systemic FFA flux derives from subcutaneous adipose tissue and in particular abdominal subcutaneous adipose tissue (20).

The strong correlation between VAT and insulin resistance has been an impetus to regard regional depots of adipose tissue as distinct or individual "miniorgans," each with important individual contributions. This discussion needs to take into account not only "metabolically adverse" depots such as VAT, but also "metabolically protective" depots. Gluteal-femoral adiposity poses little risk for insulin resistance; in fact, this depot appears to mitigate risk (21–23). A metabolic basis appears to be that adipocytes within the subcutaneous adipose tissue of the gluteal-femoral region has a lower rate of lipolysis than adipocytes of omental and mesenteric adipose tissue and of adipocytes within subcutaneous adipose tissue of the abdomen. Indeed, metabolic risk associated with gluteal-femoral adiposity appears to be associated with paucity rather than an excess (21–23). A decrease in gluteal-femoral adiposity is a risk factor for hyperglycemia and type 2 diabetes (24–26). Recent studies from the author's laboratory indicates that matched for BMI and fat mass, men and women with type 2 diabetes have less gluteal-femoral adiposity. Also of interest is that in response to the peroxisome proliferator activated receptor (PPAR)-γ glitazones, insulin sensitivity of gluteal-femoral adipose tissue is increased in patients with type 2 diabetes, and this increase correlates strongly with improved systemic insulin sensitivity (27).

A few clinical investigations reported that abdominal subcutaneous adiposity is more strongly related to insulin resistance than visceral adiposity (28–30), although most studies found a stronger association for visceral adiposity (31–33). There may be several reasons for this ambiguity. First, there are two layers that comprise abdominal subcutaneous adipose tissue, and these differ in metabolism and association with insulin resistance (34). The outer layer, termed superficial abdominal subcutaneous adipose tissue, is larger in women than in men and seems similar to gluteal-femoral adiposity; it seems to be benign or even protective against insulin resistance. The inner layer, termed deep abdominal subcutaneous adipose tissue, is larger in men than in women, and correlates much more strongly with insulin resistance, and in a manner quite similar to that of VAT (34). Thus, part of the reason for differing patterns of association between abdominal subcutaneous adipose tissue and insulin resistance may relate to differing proportions of the superficial and deep layers. A second reason for potential ambiguity concerning the relationship between abdominal subcutaneous adiposity and insulin resistance concerns the effects of adipocyte size. Preceding the contemporary emphasis on characterizing obesity by assessing patterns of adipose tissue distribution, obesity research centered on assessments of adipocyte size and number (35). Obesity is associated with larger adipocytes (36,37). Adipocyte size in abdominal subcutaneous adipose tissue is a risk factor for type 2 diabetes even after adjustment for effects of overall obesity and central adiposity (38,39). Large adipocytes have higher rates of lipolysis and may have altered patterns of adipokine secretion that contribute to insulin resistance.

In certain respects, the differing relationships between superficial and deep abdominal subcutaneous adipose tissue with insulin resistance are analogous to the differing relationships of VAT and subcutaneous adipose tissue with insulin resistance. This comparison can be further developed by considering the role of intermuscular adipose tissue in the leg. Most of the adipose tissue in the leg is contained in subcutaneous adipose tissue, and as discussed earlier, this is gluteal-femoral adipose tissue, which is actually protective against insulin resistance. A smaller proportion, approximately 5% to 15%, concerns adipose tissue located immediately adjacent to muscle and beneath the fascia. The amount of subfascial adipose tissue correlates with insulin resistance (40). At the whole-body level, the amount of subfascial adipose tissue surrounding skeletal muscle may approximate the amount of VAT. It is not clear how subfascial adipose tissue surrounding skeletal muscle contributes to insulin resistance. Insulin regulation of lipolysis may be different in this depot than in subcutaneous adipose tissue, potentially exposing muscle to high concentrations of fatty acids and interfering with glucose uptake. Another possibility is endocrine activity of subfascial adipose tissue, although there are little direct data testing this hypothesis.

METABOLIC BASIS OF OBESITY-RELATED INSULIN RESISTANCE

Studies of the relationship between insulin resistance and the topography of adipose tissue distribution are quite interesting for probing the relationship between body composition and metabolic complications of obesity. However, these investigations do not of themselves delineate the mechanisms by which adiposity triggers insulin resistance. There are several mechanisms that can be considered: the effects of fatty acids, adipokines, and inflammation. These are not mutually exclusive. It is likely that all are operative and interactive. Another important consideration concerns the accumulation of fat within liver and skeletal muscle.

Glucose and Fatty Acid Competition

Most tissues, and perhaps especially skeletal muscle and cardiac muscle, can oxidize and store both fatty acids and glucose. Indeed, these two substrates compete for utilization, and this competition, or at least uncontrolled competition, is central to the pathogenesis of insulin resistance. More than 40 years ago, Randle and colleagues established in a series of biochemical studies that fatty acids compete with glucose for utilization by skeletal muscle and that increased availability of fatty acids induces resistance to the effect of insulin in stimulating glucose metabolism by skeletal muscle (41). One of the key functions of insulin is to control this competition and keep this within healthy boundaries. Increases of insulin, as are triggered in response to increases in plasma glucose from food ingestion, suppresses lipolysis in adipocytes, dramatically lowers plasma FFA, and lessens competition to the utilization of glucose. Normally, in the transition from the fasted to the fed state, adipose tissue shifts from FFA efflux to FFA uptake. and systemically the marker of this transition from catabolism to anabolism is a pronounced suppression of plasma fatty acid levels (42). In metabolic studies, elevation of plasma FFA above fasting levels, as can be achieved by lipid infusions, induces fairly severe insulin resistance (43–45). The metabolic profile of impaired glucose metabolism that is induced is characterized by decreased glucose transport, reduction of glucose oxidation, and impaired stimulation of glycogen formation. This metabolic profile matches precisely the abnormalities that characterize those found in type 2 diabetes and in obesity (46). Moreover, the induction of insulin resistance does not even require "elevation" of fatty acids. A decade ago, in the author's laboratory, a metabolic investigation in healthy, lean volunteers revealed that simply preventing the normal suppression of plasma FFA that occurs in response to insulin is sufficient to induce skeletal muscle insulin resistance (45). Thus, a key aspect of the normal response of muscle to increased glucose uptake in response to insulin is contingent on the effectiveness with which insulin suppresses plasma fatty acids. In obesity and in type 2 diabetes, this ability of insulin to suppress fatty acids is blunted. Plasma fatty acid levels during insulin infusion have repeatedly been shown to correlate in a robust manner with the severity of resistance to the ability of insulin to stimulate glucose uptake (47,48). After weight loss there is improved insulin suppression of lipolysis and plasma FFA, and this is a key response that contributes to the improvement of glucose metabolism after weight loss (47). Pharmacologic suppression of lipolysis in patients with type 2 diabetes has been shown to acutely improve insulin resistance (49).

There are regional differences across depots of adipose tissue in responsiveness to insulin in suppressing lipolysis. Adipocytes from omentum and mesenteric adipose tissue have higher basal rates of lipolysis and suppress less in response to insulin than adipocytes from gluteal femoral adipose tissue (18,50). Thus, regional differences in adipocyte metabolism with regard to insulin sensitivity of lipolysis may be an important mechanism accounting for differing relationships of these depots to systemic insulin sensitivity. The majority of systemic fatty acid flux derives from abdominal subcutaneous adipose tissue (20,51). This reflects both the greater absolute amount of adiposity in this depot than in VAT and the regional differences in adipocyte metabolism mentioned earlier. Treatment of patients with type 2 diabetes with glitazones, such as pioglitazone or rosiglitazone, typically induces modest weight gain, some of which is increased adiposity. There is also some repartitioning of the distribution of adipose tissue that occurs. Despite weight gain, there is a modest decrease in VAT, of approximately 10%, and a relative increase in subcutaneous adipose tissue. Along with this shift in the distribution of adipose tissue, there is a decrease in hepatic steatosis.

Endocrine Activity of Adipose Tissue

Adipose tissue is an incredibly active endocrine tissue. Identification of leptin and the finding that its tissue of origin is adipose tissue have profoundly increased our respect for this tissue. Suddenly, it was perceived that this otherwise seemingly lifeless and inert depository was in fact actively attempting to manage its resources by influencing neural pathways of appetite regulation and by cellular signaling modifying energy expenditure and fat oxidation in liver and skeletal muscle. The potent effects of leptin deficiency and equally potent effects of its replacement in conditions of leptin deficiency indicate the potency and primacy of this signaling pathway. Leptin resistance is a major barrier to obesity management (52). Leptin increases in direct proportion to fat mass, most particularly in direct proportion to subcutaneous adiposity, but another important adipokine, adiponectin, follows an opposite pattern. Adiponectin, which improves insulin sensitivity and may protect against CVD by salutary effects on vascular endothelium, decreases as individuals become more obese. It is thought, although not firmly established, that VAT is the main source of adiponectin, and thus an expanded VAT mass is associated with lower production of adiponectin. The manner in which this is regulated is unclear, but it may relate to fat cell size and interaction with secretion of other adipokines. It is interesting that a transgenic mouse overexpressing adiponectin is massively obese due to greatly expanded subcutaneous adiposity, yet it does not manifest insulin resistance. There is a growing list of adipokines that influence insulin sensitivity. These include resistin, visastin, acylation-stimulating protein (ASP), and others (53). One that has received recent attention is retinol-binding protein. In a transgenic animal model in which insulin resistance of adipose tissue was induced by knocking out GLUT 4, the glucose transporter that is predominant in adipose tissue, the animals developed insulin resistance of muscle and liver and manifested higher circulating levels of retinol-binding protein (54). This is of interest because of role of the retinoic acid X receptor as a transcription factor for pathways influencing insulin sensitivity. Another emerging area concerns the role of endocannabinoids, a pathway that also influences appetite and energy expenditure (55). This has emerged as a therapeutic target for the treatment of obesity. Rimonabant, an antagonist to endocannabinoid signaling, ameliorates the metabolic syndrome and induces weight loss (56).

Inflammation and Adipose Tissue

Inflammation plays an important role in the development of atherosclerosis. C-reactive protein (CRP), which is the best studied of the inflammatory markers related to risk for CVD, is produced in the liver, and its expression is under the transcriptional control of interleukin-6 and tumor necrosis factor-α. One of the main mechanisms by which obesity may influence levels of CRP is through production of cytokines by adipose tissue that regulate hepatic production of CRP (57). Visceral adiposity is strongly associated with plasma levels of CRP, as is BMI. Adipocytes are not the only cells within adipose tissue that secrete products influencing inflammation and insulin resistance. Macrophages can be found in adipose tissue, and are present in greater amounts in obesity (58). It seems likely that chemokines generated by adipocytes attract monocytes and macrophages, which in turn augment production of inflammatory cytokines. Thus, there appears to be at least a rough parallel with the attraction of these cell types into the atherosclerotic plaque within the vessel wall on formation of fat-laden foam cells. In adipose tissue, production of cytokines such as interleukin-6 and tumor necrosis factor-α likely derive substantially, perhaps predominately, from the macrophages within adipose tissue rather than directly from adipocytes (58). Cytokines can induce insulin resistance. For example, tumor necrosis factor-α induces phosphorylation of serine residues on the insulin receptor, impairing tyrosine phosphorylation triggered by insulin binding and thereby interfering with insulin signal transduction.

The emerging recognition of the connections between inflammation and obesity is providing important new insight into the pathogenesis of the metabolic syndrome. Survival of organisms relies both on capacity to fight infection and capacity to store nutrients, so the two pathways are both integral to survival. These metabolic and inflammation pathways may have evolved with close interdependence, sharing signaling proteins and transcription factors. It has been postulated that one of the cellular targets of PPAR-γ agonists are macrophages and that an effect of this treatment is to suppress macrophage activity within adipose tissue. The concept that adipose tissue in obesity is a source of low-grade inflammation provides another strong link between adiposity and the metabolic syndrome. Markers of inflammation, notably CRP, help to identify individuals at risk for CVD. Whether targeting inflammatory adipose tissue even without inducing weight loss will modulate risk for CVD is an important research question.

ECTOPIC FAT IN LIVER AND MUSCLE

Skeletal muscle and liver normally contain small amounts of triglyceride, far less than is contained in adipose tissue. In obesity, these repositories can be greatly increased. Hepatic steatosis occurs commonly in obesity, especially in visceral obesity and especially in type 2 diabetes (59), and it is strongly correlated with insulin resistance. In patients with type 2 diabetes, the amount of insulin required to achieve glycemic control is correlated with the amount of hepatic steatosis (60), indicating the importance of this depot to the pathogenesis of hepatic insulin resistance. Hepatic steatosis is correlated with the severity of dyslipidemia. In obesity, the intracellular content of lipid in skeletal muscle is increased and correlates with severity of insulin resistance. Muscle lipid content is increased in type 2 diabetes and in first-degree relatives of these patients. Elevated fatty acid delivery is a key factor leading to hepatic steatosis and increased muscle lipid content. With regard to muscle, there is increasing evidence of mitochondrial dysfunction in obesity and type 2 diabetes, which contributes to inefficient fat oxidation and partitioning of fatty acids into triglyceride (61). However, it is not clear that it is the accumulation of triglyceride that mediates insulin resistance. There is a conundrum in that triglyceride content in skeletal muscle is elevated in lean, endurance-trained athletes, who maintain very high levels of insulin sensitivity. Instead of triglyceride, other lipid moieties may actually mediate insulin resistance. One candidate for this may be diacylglycerol. It has been postulated that diacylglycerol activates certain isoforms of protein kinase C and that this in turn inhibits insulin signaling (62). Intracellular lipid may also induce a low-grade inflammatory condition within hepatocytes and myocytes.

METABOLIC SYNDROME

Many ascribe the formulation of the concept of the metabolic syndrome to Reaven's seminal Banting lecture in 1988 (63). In a recent review article, Reaven outlined the roots of the concept of the metabolic syndrome beginning with clinical observations and studies concerning "insulin insensitivity" by Himsworth and Kerr (64) in the 1930s, a decade after the clinical introduction of insulin. Recognition of an insulin-resistant and as well an insulin-deficient form of diabetes mellitus emerged in the 1960s, and it is now widely accepted that insulin resistance is a major risk factor for type 2 diabetes. Nearly 30 years ago, clinical investigations supported a strong link between insulin resistance and hypertriglyceridemia (and low high-density-lipoprotein [HDL] cholesterol). The connection to CVD was also perceived at this time by Albrink and Mann (65) and others. Later, it was recognized that many individuals with essential hypertension manifested insulin resistance (66). Thus, by 1988 there was already a strong body of evidence that insulin resistance was related to type 2 diabetes mellitus and impaired glucose tolerance, hyperlipidemia, small, dense low-density-lipoprotein (LDL) cholesterol, and hypertension. This concept is well established. Although it is not used diagnostically, the metabolic syndrome has also been linked with prothrombotic and proinflammatory states (67). What has proven more challenging has been to arrive at accepted cut-points that clinically identify the presence of the insulin resistance or metabolic syndrome.

The metabolic syndrome represents a constellation of several established and emerging risk factors predisposing to CVD and its complications. A universally accepted definition of the metabolic syndrome does not exist. It is well established that its key components are abdominal obesity, atherogenic dyslipidemia, hypertension, glucose intolerance, and proinflammatory and prothrombotic states (67,68). The two most commonly used definitions of the metabolic syndrome are those proposed by the World Health Organization (WHO) (69,70) and the Third Report of the National Cholesterol Education Program Expert Panel on Detection, Evaluation, and Treatment of High Blood Cholesterol in Adults (Adult Treatment Panel III [ATP III]) (Table 3.2) (71). The defining criteria are based on levels of waist circumference, serum triglycerides, blood HDL-cholesterol level, blood pressure, serum glucose. Although the use of the two criteria (WHO and ATP III) correctly classified 86% of subjects as having or not having the syndrome, the estimates differed substantially for some populations, such as African Americans and Indian Asians (72).

Data suggest that the metabolic syndrome is highly prevalent in the adult population. Using data from the third National Health and Nutrition Examination Survey (NHANES III), Ford et al. showed that approximately 47 million U.S. residents have the metabolic syndrome, that the age-adjusted prevalence of the syndrome is 23.7%, and that it increases substantially with age (73).

The increased risk of incident diabetes and CVD in persons who have the metabolic syndrome is well established (74–77). In patients with established coronary artery disease (CAD) the metabolic syndrome appears to be highly prevalent (>50%), and compared to patients who do not have the syndrome, these patients usually have worse coronary artery disease, more atherogenic dyslipidemia and a higher incidence of prior myocardial infarction (77). In addition, patients with the metabolic syndrome have a proinflammatory state manifested by elevated levels of proinflammatory cytokines such as interleukin-6 and nonspecific markers of inflammation such as C-reactive protein (76,78) as well as low levels of protective and antiinflammatory substances such as adiponectin (79). It is well accepted that all these factors, which are discussed in more

TABLE 3.2

METABOLIC SYNDROME: DIAGNOSTIC CRITERIA

ATP III criteria for diagnosing the metabolic syndrome: The presence of three or more of the following makes the diagnosis.	WHO criteria for the diagnosis of the metabolic syndrome: The presence of two or more of the following in a patient with diabetes, glucose intolerance, impaired fasting glucose, or insulin resistance makes the diagnosis.
Abdominal obesity: waist circumference of ≥88 cm in women and ≥102 cm in men Hypertriglyceridemia: ≥150 mg/dL Low HDL cholesterol: ≥40 mg/dL in men and ≥50 mg/dL in women Hypertension: ≥130/85 mm Hg High fasting glucose: ≥110 mg/dL	Hypertension: ≥160/90 mm Hg Hyperlipidemia: triglycerides of ≥150 mg/dL or HDL cholesterol ≥35 mg/dL in men or ≥39 in women Central obesity: waist-to-hip ratio of ≥0.90 in men or ≥0.85 in women or a BMI ≥30 kg/m^2 Microalbuminuria: urinary albumin excretion rate at ≥20 mg/min or an albumin-to-creatinine ratio of ≥20 mg/g

ATP III, Third Report of the National Cholesterol Education Program Expert Panel on Detection, Evaluation, and Treatment of High Blood Cholesterol in Adults (Adult Treatment Panel III; HDL, high-density lipoprotein; WHO, World Heath Organization.

detail in other chapters of this book, are markers associated with adverse cardiovascular risk. Their role in the development of the CVD associated with obesity and the metabolic syndrome remains controversial.

In general, obesity and the metabolic syndrome predict a poor cardiovascular outcome. Two large longitudinal studies in men without CVD at baseline showed that the metabolic syndrome is associated with an adverse cardiovascular outcome. In the first, using WHO criteria for the syndrome, Isomaa et al. showed that there was a threefold increase in the risk for coronary heart disease and stroke and a higher cardiovascular mortality associated with the metabolic syndrome compared to metabolic-normal controls (75). In the other study, Lakka et al., followed 1,209 Finnish men for 11 years and found that the metabolic syndrome was associated with a significantly increased cardiovascular mortality (80). Furthermore, using both WHO and ATP III definitions, and after adjusting for conventional cardiovascular risk factors, the authors found that the metabolic syndrome was also associated with a greater-than-threefold increase in mortality when compared to patients without the syndrome.

The adverse cardiovascular risk associated with the metabolic syndrome has also been confirmed in women. Using data from the Women's Ischemia Syndrome Evaluation (WISE) study, Marroquin et al. showed that women with the metabolic syndrome had a lower 4-year survival than women with normal metabolic status (94.3% vs. 97.8%, respectively) (76). Interestingly, in women who had significant angiographic CAD at study entry, the presence of the metabolic syndrome was associated with a greater-than-fourfold increase in mortality at 4 years, which was similar in magnitude to the risk conferred by diagnosed and treated diabetes mellitus in that population.

EFFECTS OF OBESITY ON THE CARDIOVASCULAR SYSTEM

Cardiac Structure and Function

Obesity is characterized by expansion of fat mass as well as of skeletal muscle, viscera, and skin, all of which increase oxygen consumption (81). Although it is metabolically active, adipose tissue oxygen consumption is lower than for lean tissue, and hence total-body oxygen consumption expressed per kilogram of body weight in the obese is lower than in leaner persons (82). Obesity is also accompanied by expansion of extracellular volume, which comprises the intravascular and interstitial fluid spaces. Total blood volume and plasma volume generally increase in proportion to the degree of overweight (83,84). This leads to increased left ventricular (LV) filling, resulting increased stroke volume. The increase in cardiac output is generally in proportion to excess weight, reflecting the interrelationships among weight, blood volume, stroke volume, and cardiac output (83,84).

The initial response to increased metabolic demand and total blood volume is increased LV filling, leading to chamber dilation, which, over time, increases myocardial wall stress, which in turn leads to LV mass growth. In turn, the process of hypertrophy and dilation occurring together results in preserved cavity radius and wall thickness, yielding normal wall stress (85). When obesity and arterial hypertension coexist, however, there is a relative increase in LV mass in relation to the degree of dilation, resulting in increased wall stress.

Congestive Heart Failure

When the hypertrophic response is commensurate to left ventricular dilation, filling pressures and wall stress are normalized by increased ventricular mass, and systolic function is maintained (86). Under these circumstances, however, left ventricular diastolic dysfunction is likely to occur. Diminished ventricular compliance results in impaired accommodation of volume during diastole, resulting in diastolic dysfunction (87). Factors associated with the latter include the degree and duration of being overweight, the degree of volume expansion, and the adverse loading conditions imposed by hypertension (87).

When left ventricular filling exceeds favorable loading conditions and hypertrophy does not keep pace to normalize resultant wall stress, ventricular contractility is impaired and systolic dysfunction ensues. Studies have demonstrated that there is an inverse relationship between LV ejection fraction and BMI as well as duration of obesity (86).

Hypertension

Studies have suggested that important differences exist in the characteristics of hypertension between obese and lean individuals. In obese hypertensive patients, the hypertension is characterized principally by an increase in stroke volume (cardiac output) but normal peripheral resistance. In lean hypertensive patients, cardiac output is normal, but peripheral resistance is increased (88,89). Perhaps the most striking difference between obese and lean hypertensive patients is that obese hypertensive patients actually have a better long-term prognosis in terms of cardiovascular mortality and morbidity (90). It should be emphasized, however, that even though obese patients appear to have better outcomes than lean patients, they still have a poorer prognosis than normotensive controls (90).

Endothelial Dysfunction

It is well known that most patients with the metabolic syndrome have a cluster of established coronary risk factors, such as hyperglycemia, atherogenic dyslipidemia, and hypertension. These abnormalities together have a greater impact on endothelial function than any one alone (91). Although the precise mechanisms by which the metabolic syndrome produce endothelial dysfunction are not well understood, it is well accepted that hyperglycemia, hyperinsulinemia, oxidative stress, and a prothrombotic and proinflammatory state probably contribute to the vascular damage associated with the metabolic syndrome. The insulin-resistant state activates the sympathoadrenal system as well as the renin–angiotensin system, which in turn can lead to a variety of vascular abnormalities, including endothelial dysfunction (91).

Several studies have shown that obesity and the metabolic syndrome are associated with endothelial dysfunction as measured by impaired endothelial-dependent vasodilation (92,93). The individual contributions of each of the components of the metabolic syndrome to endothelial function are difficult to ascertain; however, when endothelial dysfunction is present in patients with diabetes mellitus (DM), the degree of dysfunction is greater in patients with type 2 DM than in patients with type 1 DM, suggesting that factors other than hyperglycemia alone, such as the insulin resistance that is the primary abnormality in the metabolic syndrome and the associated dyslipidemia, might play a role (94,95). This is further supported by studies using euglycemic hyperinsulinemic clamps, in which insulin resistance is closely related to endothelial dysfunction (96,97).

Although in the normal physiologic state, insulin stimulates nitric oxide (NO) synthesis and enhances NO-mediated vasodilation, this action is reversed or blunted in insulin-resistant states (93,98). Besides decreased synthesis and responsiveness to NO, insulin-resistant states have been associated with increased levels of endothelin-1 (ET-1), a potent vasoconstrictor and proatherosclerotic vascular hormone associated with endothelial dysfunction and hypertension (99).

Insulin resistance–induced hyperglycemia can also play a role in the development of endothelial dysfunction through a variety of molecular changes. One of them, the production of advanced glycation end products (AGEs), which increase the ability of LDL cholesterol to become oxidated, result in release of interleukin-1 (IL-1) and tumor necrosis factor-α (TNF-α) and growth factors that can stimulate the migration and proliferation of smooth muscle cells, resulting in endothelial dysfunction and early atherosclerosis (100). Other pathways by which insulin resistance–induced hyperglycemia can induce endothelial dysfunction include the polyol pathway, which leads to depletion of the reduced form of nicotinamide adenine dinucleotide phosphate (NADPH), which in turn is essential for the regeneration of antioxidant molecules and a cofactor of the endothelial nitric oxide synthase (eNOS), and the activation of the protein kinase C (PKC) pathway through increases in the synthesis of diacylglycerol. The activation of the PKC pathway can lead to decreases in eNOS and increases in the production of ET-1 (101). In addition, this pathway can lead to production of vascular endothelial growth factor (VGEF) and the production of prothrombotic factors such as von Willebrand (vWB) factor, plasminogen activator inhibitor-1 (PAI-1), and fibrinogen (102).

Finally, the oxidative stress commonly seen in states of insulin resistance such as the metabolic syndrome are known to activate many of the cellular pathways that lead to endothelial dysfunction and remodeling. Increases in reactive oxygen species (ROS) such as superoxide and hydrogen peroxide inactivate NO and generate peroxynitrite, which causes lipid peroxidation with enhanced formation of AGE, resulting in endothelial dysfunction (103).

CONTROVERSIES AND PERSONAL PERSPECTIVES

An issue of contention is whether the clinical definitions of the metabolic syndrome (as shown in Table 3.2) add to risk identification more than consideration of the various risk factors considered separately. Two frameworks are commonly employed to assess cardiovascular-related risk among the obese. The first is the Framingham Risk Score, which estimates the 10-year risk of incident CHD. This score is based on age, gender, blood pressure, LDL and HDL cholesterol, and smoking history, and was derived from a primarily white population (104). Obesity-related risk is represented by the weight-related factors of diabetes, hypertension, and hyperlipidemia. The second model is that of the metabolic syndrome, a clustering of cardiovascular risk factors with underlying pathophysiology thought to be linked with insulin resistance.

Both models have limitations. For example, the ability of the Framingham score to predict an individual's risk is often relatively low, and it tends to underestimate risk among people with diabetes (105), a major weight-related health complication. However, the addition of metabolic syndrome to these calculations has not been shown to increase predictive ability for CVD risk (e.g., sensitivity for the metabolic syndrome was 67.3%, for the Framingham risk score it was 81.4%, and for the two combined it was 81.4%) (106). In addition, a recent statement from the American Diabetes Association and the European Association for the Study of Diabetes suggests that the metabolic syndrome is imprecisely defined, lacks evidence regarding pathogenesis, and may not be a valuable marker of CVD risk (107). However, others argue that obesity is a major driving force behind cardiovascular risk factor clustering and that the accumulation of risk among obese patients should not be overlooked (108).

THE FUTURE

Insulin resistance has been recognized for nearly eight decades, and the concept of a metabolic syndrome, or more appropriately dysmetabolic syndrome, has been articulated for two decades. What is needed is an efficient and accurate of incorporating these concepts into clinical practice, especially from a diagnostic perspective and with regard to monitoring response to treatment. Conformity in the assay of insulin would be a big step forward, but the logistic challenges of achieving a standardized assay as well as defining the appropriate testing conditions (e.g., after an overnight fast) have yet to be resolved.

Another major goal is to develop clinical evidence regarding the impact of intentional weight loss on cardiovascular morbidity and mortality. We have learned a great deal about the effect of intentional weight loss on CVD risk factors and are increasing our understanding of its effects on subclinical CVD. However, outcome data are not readily available regarding intentional weight loss. The National Institutes of Health is conducting a multicenter clinical investigation addressing this issue in type 2 diabetes mellitus, the Action for Health in Diabetes (Look AHEAD) study. It should be completed in 2010 and will provide the first set of outcome data regarding long-term effects of interventions to achieve moderate weight loss along with increased physical activity and CVD outcomes in overweight and obese men and women with type 2 diabetes mellitus. It is hoped that we will begin to develop effective interventions for obesity and insulin resistance and learn to integrate these into a comprehensive program for preventing and treating CVD.

References

1. Mokdad AH, Serdula MK, Dietz WH, et al. The continuing epidemic of obesity in the United States. *JAMA* 2000;284:1650–1651.
2. National Center for Health Statistics. Centers for disease control and prevention. Overweight and Obesity: US Obesity trends 1985–2003. Available at http://www.cdc.gov/nccdphp/dnpa/obesity/trend/maps/index.htm. Accessed August 1, 2005.
3. Freedman DS, Khan LK, Serdula MK, et al. Trends and correlates of class 3 obesity in the United States from 1990 through 2000. *JAMA* 2002;288: 1758–1761.
4. Hedley AA, Ogden CL, Johnson CL, et al. Prevalence of overweight and obesity among US children, adolescents, and adults, 1999–2002. *JAMA* 2004;291:2847–2850.
5. Melnik TA, Rhoades SJ, Wales KR, et al. Overweight school children in New York City: prevalence estimates and characteristics. *Int J Obes Relat Metab Disord* 1998;22:7–13.
6. Ogden CL, Troiano RP, Briefel RR, et al. Prevalence of overweight among preschool children in the United States, 1971 through 1994. *Pediatrics* 1997;99:E1.
7. Ehtisham S, Barrett TG, Shaw NJ. Type 2 diabetes mellitus in UK children—an emerging problem. *Diabet Med* 2000;17:867–871.
8. Kitagawa T, Owada M, Urakami T, Yamauchi K. Increased incidence of non–insulin dependent diabetes mellitus among Japanese schoolchildren correlates with an increased intake of animal protein and fat. *Clin Pediatr (Phila)* 1998;37:111–115.
9. National Institutes of Health, National Heart, Lung and Blood Institute. *Clinical guidelines on the identification, evaluation, and treatment of overweight and obesity in adults.* Bethesda, MD: U.S. Department of Health and Human Services, 1998.
10. Bjorntorp P. Abdominal obesity and the metabolic syndrome. *Ann Med* 1992;24:465–468.
11. Despres JP. Abdominal obesity as important component of insulin-resistance syndrome. *Nutrition* 1993;9:452–459.
12. Eckel RH, Krauss RM. American Heart Association call to action: obesity as a major risk factor for coronary heart disease. AHA Nutrition Committee. *Circulation* 1998;97:2099–2100.
13. Vague J. Sexual differentiation, a factor affecting the forms of obesity. *Presse Med* 1947;30:339–340.
14. Despres JP, Lemieux S, Lamarche B, et al. The insulin resistance-dyslipidemic syndrome: contribution of visceral obesity and therapeutic implications. *Int J Obes Relat Metab Disord* 1995;19(Suppl 1):S76–S86.
15. Goodpaster BH. Measuring body fat distribution and content in humans. *Curr Opin Clin Nutr Metab Care* 2002;5:481–487.
16. Seidell JC, Bjorntorp P, Sjostrom L, et al. Visceral fat accumulation in men is positively associated with insulin, glucose, and C-peptide levels, but negatively with testosterone levels. *Metabolism* 1990;39:897–901.
17. Bjorntorp P. "Portal" adipose tissue as a generator of risk factors for cardiovascular disease and diabetes. *Arteriosclerosis* 1990;10:493–496.
18. Lofgren P, Hoffstedt J, Ryden M, et al. Major gender differences in the lipolytic capacity of abdominal subcutaneous fat cells in obesity observed before and after long-term weight reduction. *J Clin Endocrinol Metab* 2002;87:764–771.
19. Elbers JM, de Jong S, Teerlink T, et al. Changes in fat cell size and in vitro lipolytic activity of abdominal and gluteal adipocytes after a one-year cross-sex hormone administration in transsexuals. *Metabolism* 1999;48: 1371–1377.
20. Basu A, Basu R, Shah P, et al. Systemic and regional free fatty acid metabolism in type 2 diabetes. *Am J Physiol Endocrinol Metab* 2001;280: E1000–E1006.
21. Goodpaster BH, Krishnaswami S, Harris TB, et al. Obesity, regional body fat distribution, and the metabolic syndrome in older men and women. *Arch Intern Med* 2005;165:777–783.
22. Seidell JC, Han TS, Feskens EJ, Lean ME. Narrow hips and broad waist circumferences independently contribute to increased risk of non–insulin-dependent diabetes mellitus. *J Intern Med* 1997;242:401–406.
23. Seidell JC, Perusse L, Despres JP, Bouchard C. Waist and hip circumferences have independent and opposite effects on cardiovascular disease risk factors: the Quebec Family Study. *Am J Clin Nutr* 2001;74:315–321.
24. Snijder MB, Dekker JM, Visser M, et al. Associations of hip and thigh circumferences independent of waist circumference with the incidence of type 2 diabetes: the Hoorn Study. *Am J Clin Nutr* 2003;77:1192–1197.
25. Snijder MB, Dekker JM, Visser M, et al. Larger thigh and hip circumferences are associated with better glucose tolerance: the Hoorn study. *Obes Res* 2003;11:104–111.
26. Snijder MB, Visser M, Dekker JM, et al. Low subcutaneous thigh fat is a risk factor for unfavourable glucose and lipid levels, independently of high abdominal fat. The Health ABC Study. *Diabetologia* 2005;48:301–308.
27. Virtanen KA, Hallsten K, Parkkola R, et al. Differential effects of rosiglitazone and metformin on adipose tissue distribution and glucose uptake in type 2 diabetic subjects. *Diabetes* 2003;52:283–290.
28. Abate N, Garg A, Peshock RM, et al. Relationship of generalized and regional adiposity to insulin sensitivity in men with NIDDM. *Diabetes* 1996;45:1684–1693.
29. Abate N, Garg A, Peshock RM, et al. Relationships of generalized and regional adiposity to insulin sensitivity in men. *J Clin Invest* 1995;96:88–98.
30. Garg A. Regional adiposity and insulin resistance. *J Clin Endocrinol Metab* 2004;89:4206–4210.
31. Cnop M, Landchild MJ, Vidal J, et al. The concurrent accumulation of intra-abdominal and subcutaneous fat explains the association between insulin resistance and plasma leptin concentrations: distinct metabolic effects of two fat compartments. *Diabetes* 200251:1005–1015.
32. Kelley DE, Williams KV, Price JC, et al. Plasma fatty acids, adiposity, and variance of skeletal muscle insulin resistance in type 2 diabetes mellitus. *J Clin Endocrinol Metab* 2001;86:5412–5419.
33. Ross R, Aru J, Freeman J, et al. Abdominal adiposity and insulin resistance in obese men. *Am J Physiol Endocrinol Metab* 2002;282:E657–E663.
34. Kelley DE, Thaete FL, Troost F, et al. Subdivisions of subcutaneous abdominal adipose tissue and insulin resistance. *Am J Physiol Endocrinol Metab* 2000;278:E941–E948.
35. Salans LB, Cushman SW, Weismann RE. Studies of human adipose tissue. Adipose cell size and number in nonobese and obese patients. *J Clin Invest* 1973;52:929–941.
36. Kirtland J, Gurr MI. Adipose tissue cellularity: a review. 2. The relationship between cellularity and obesity. *Int J Obes* 1979;3:15–55.
37. Sjostrom L, Bjorntorp P. Body composition and adipose cellularity in human obesity. *Acta Med Scand* 1974;195:201–211.
38. Weyer C, Foley JE, Bogardus C, et al. Enlarged subcutaneous abdominal adipocyte size, but not obesity itself, predicts type II diabetes independent of insulin resistance. *Diabetologia* 2000;43:1498–1506.
39. Weyer C, Wolford JK, Hanson RL, et al. Subcutaneous abdominal adipocyte size, a predictor of type 2 diabetes, is linked to chromosome 1q21–q23 and is associated with a common polymorphism in LMNA in Pima Indians. *Mol Genet Metab* 2001;72:231–238.
40. Goodpaster BH, Thaete FL, Kelley DE. Thigh adipose tissue distribution is associated with insulin resistance in obesity and in type 2 diabetes mellitus. *Am J Clin Nutr* 2000;71:885–892.
41. Randle P, Garland P, Hales C, Newsholme E. The glucose fatty acid cycle. Its role in insulin sensitivity and the metabolic disturbances of diabetes mellitus. *Lancet* 1963: 785–789.
42. Frayn K. Adipose tissue as a buffer for daily lipid flux. *Diabetologia* 2002;45:1201–1210.
43. Boden G. Role of fatty acids in the pathogenesis of insulin resistance in NIDDM. *Diabetes* 1997;46:3–10.
44. Boden G, Chen X. Effects of fat on glucose uptake and utilization in patients with non–insulin-dependent diabetes mellitus. *J Clin Invest* 1995;96:1261–1268.
45. Kelley D, Mokan M, Simoneau JA, Mandarino L. Interaction between glucose and free fatty acid metabolism in human skeletal muscle. *J Clin Invest* 1993;92:93–98.
46. Kelley D, Mokan M, Mandarino L. Intracellular defects in glucose metabolism in obese patients with noninsulin-dependent diabetes mellitus. *Diabetes* 1992;41:698–706.
47. Kelley DE, Goodpaster B, Wing RR, Simoneau JA. Skeletal muscle fatty acid metabolism in association with insulin resistance, obesity, and weight loss. *Am J Physiol* 1999;277:E1130–E1141.
48. Kelley DE, Williams KV, Price JC, et al. Plasma fatty acids, adiposity, and variance of skeletal muscle insulin resistance in type 2 diabetes mellitus. *J Clin Endocrinol Metab* 2001;86:5412–5419.
49. Santomauro A, Boden G, Silva M, et al. Overnight lowering of free fatty acids with Acipimox improves insulin resistance and glucose tolerance in obese diabetic and nondiabetic subjects. *Diabetes* 1999;48:1836–1841.
50. Montague C, O'Rahilly S. The perils of portliness: causes and consequences of visceral adiposity. *Diabetes* 2000;49:883–888.
51. Jensen M, Haymond M, Rizza R, et al. Influence of body fat distribution of free fatty acid metabolism in obesity. *J Clin Invest* 1989;83:1168–1173.
52. Munzberg H, Myers M. Molecular and anatomical determinants of central leptin resistance. *Nat Neurosci* 2005;8:566–570.
53. Havel P. Update on adipocyte hormones: regulation of energy balance and carbohydrate/lipid metabolism. *Diabetes* 2004;53:S143–S151.
54. Tamori Y, Sakaue H, Kasuga M. RBP4, an unexpected adipokine. *Nat Med* 2006;12:30–31.
55. Bensaid M, Gary-Bobo M, Esclangon A, et al. The cannabinoid CB1 receptor antagonist SR14176 increases Acrp30 mRNA expression in adipose

tissue of obese fa/fa rats and in cultured adipocyte cells. *Mol Pharmacol* 2003;63:908–914.
56. Jbilo O, Ravinet-Trillou C, Arnone M, Buisson I, et al. The CB1 receptor antagonist rimonabant reverses the diet-induced obesity phenotype through the regulation of lipolysis and energy balance. *FASEB J* 2005;19: 1567–1569.
57. Yudkin JS, Stehouwer CD, Emeis JJ, Coppack SW. C-reactive protein in healthy subjects: associations with obesity, insulin resistance, and endothelial dysfunction: a potential role for cytokines originating from adipose tissue? *Arterioscler Thromb Vasc Biol* 1999;19:972–978.
58. Weisberg SP, McCann D, Desai M, et al. Obesity is associated with macrophage accumulation in adipose tissue. *J Clin Invest* 2003;112: 1796–1808.
59. Kelley D, McKolanis T, Hegazi R, et al. Fatty liver in type 2 diabetes mellitus: relation to regional adiposity, fatty acids, and insulin resistance. *Am J Physiol (Endocrinol Metab)* 2003;285:E906–E916.
60. Seppala-Lindroos A, Vehkavaara S, Hakkinen AM, et al. Fat accumulation in the liver is associated with defects in insulin suppression of glucose production and serum free fatty acids independent of obesity in normal men. *J Clin Endocrinol Metab* 2002;87:3023–3028.
61. Kelley D, He J, Menshikova E, Ritov V. Dysfunction of mitochondria in human skeletal muscle in type 2 diabetes mellitus. *Diabetes* 2002;51: 2944–2950.
62. Shulman G. Cellular mechanisms of insulin resistance. *J Clin Invest* 2000; 106:171–176.
63. Reaven G. Role of insulin resistance in human disease. *Diabetes* 1988; 37:1595–1607.
64. Himsworth H, Kerr R. Insulin-sensitive and insulin-insensitive types of diabetes mellitus. *Clin Sci* 1939;4:119–152.
65. Albrink MJ, Mann EB. Serum triglycerides in coronary artery disease. *Trans Assoc Am Physicians* 1958;71:162–173.
66. Ferrannini E, Buzzigoli G, Bonadonna R, et al. Insulin resistance in essential hypertension. *N Engl J Med* 1987;317:350–357.
67. Eckel RH, Grundy SM, Zimmet PZ. The metabolic syndrome. *Lancet* 2005;365:1415–1428.
68. Grundy SM, Brewer Jr HB, Cleeman JI, et al. Definition of metabolic syndrome: report of the National Heart, Lung, and Blood Institute/American Heart Association conference on scientific issues related to definition. *Circulation* 2004;109:433–438.
69. Alberti KG, Zimmet PZ. Definition, diagnosis and classification of diabetes mellitus and its complications. Part 1: diagnosis and classification of diabetes mellitus provisional report of a WHO consultation. *Diabet Med* 1998;15:539–553.
70. Einhorn D, Reaven GM, Cobin RH, et al. American College of Endocrinology position statement on the insulin resistance syndrome. *Endocr Pract* 2003;9:237–252.
71. Third Report of the National Cholesterol Education Program (NCEP) Expert Panel on Detection, Evaluation and Treatment of High Blood Cholesterol in Adults (Adult Treatment Panel III) final report. *Circulation* 2002;106:3143–3421.
72. Ford ES, Giles WH. A comparison of the prevalence of the metabolic syndrome using two proposed definitions. *Diabetes Care* 2003;26:575–581.
73. Ford ES, Giles WH, Dietz WH. Prevalence of the metabolic syndrome among US adults: findings from the third National Health and Nutrition Examination Survey. *JAMA* 2002;287:356–359.
74. Hanson RL, Imperatore G, Bennett PH, Knowler WC. Components of the "metabolic syndrome" and incidence of type 2 diabetes. *Diabetes* 2002;51:3120–3127.
75. Isomaa B, Almgren P, Tuomi T, et al. Cardiovascular morbidity and mortality associated with the metabolic syndrome. *Diabetes Care* 2001;24: 683–689.
76. Marroquin OC, Kip KE, Kelley DE, et al. Metabolic syndrome modifies the cardiovascular risk associated with angiographic coronary artery disease in women: a report from the Women's Ischemia Syndrome Evaluation. *Circulation* 2004;109:714–721.
77. Solymoss BC, Bourassa MG, Lesperance J, et al. Incidence and clinical characteristics of the metabolic syndrome in patients with coronary artery disease. *Coron Artery Dis* 2003;14:207–212.
78. Ridker PM, Buring JE, Cook NR, Rifai N. C-reactive protein, the metabolic syndrome, and risk of incident cardiovascular events: an 8-year follow-up of 14,719 initially healthy American women. *Circulation* 2003;107:391–397.
79. Pischon T, Girman CJ, Hotamisligil GS, et al. Plasma adiponectin levels and risk of myocardial infarction in men. *JAMA* 2004;291:1730–1737.
80. Lakka HM, Laaksonen DE, Lakka TA, et al. The metabolic syndrome and total and cardiovascular disease mortality in middle-aged men. *JAMA* 2002;288:2709–2716.
81. Ravussin E. Energy expenditure and body weight. In: Brownell K, Fairburn CG, eds. *Eating disorders and obesity.* New York: Guilford Press, 1995: 32–37.
82. Frayn K. Studies of human adipose tissue in vivo. In: Kinney JM, Tucker HN, eds. *Energy metabolism: tissue determinants and cellular corollaries.* New York: Raven Press, 1992: 267–291.
83. de Divitiis O, Fazio S, Petitto M, et al. Obesity and cardiac function. *Circulation* 1981;64:477–482.
84. Messerli FH, Ventura HO, Reisin E, et al. Borderline hypertension and obesity: two prehypertensive states with elevated cardiac output. *Circulation* 1982;66:55–60.
85. Wikstrand J, Pettersson P, Bjorntorp P. Body fat distribution and left ventricular morphology and function in obese females. *J Hypertens* 1993;11:1259–1266.
86. Alpert MA. Obesity cardiomyopathy: pathophysiology and evolution of the clinical syndrome. *Am J Med Sci* 2001;321:225–236.
87. Alpert MA, Lambert CR, Terry BE, et al. Interrelationship of left ventricular mass, systolic function and diastolic filling in normotensive morbidly obese patients. *Int J Obes Relat Metab Disord* 1995;19:550–557.
88. Licata G, Scaglione R, Capuana G, et al. Hypertension in obese subjects: distinct hypertensive subgroup. *J Hum Hypertens* 1990;4:37–41.
89. Schemeided R, Messerli F. Does obesity influence early target organ damage in hypertensive patients? *Circulation* 1993;87:1482–1488.
90. Barrett-Connor E, Khaw KT. Is hypertension more benign when associated with obesity? *Circulation* 1985;72:53–60.
91. Deedwania PC. The deadly quartet revisited. *Am J Med* 1998;105:1S–3S.
92. Lavrenic A, Salobir B, Keber I. Physical training improves flow-mediated dilation in patients with the polymetabolic syndrome. *Arterioscler Thromb Vasc Biol* 2000;20:551–555.
93. Steinberg HO, Chaker H, Leaming R, et al. Obesity/insulin resistance is associated with endothelial dysfunction. Implications for the syndrome of insulin resistance. *J Clin Invest* 1996;97:2601–2610.
94. Avogaro A, Piarulli F, Valerio A, et al. Forearm nitric oxide balance, vascular relaxation, and glucose metabolism in NIDDM patients. *Diabetes* 1997;46:1040–1046.
95. Vehkavaara S, Seppala-Lindroos A, Westervacka J, et al. In vivo endothelial function characterizes patients with impaired fasting glucose. *Diabetes Care* 1999;22:2055–2060.
96. Lteif AA, Han K, Mather KJ. Obesity, insulin resistance, and the metabolic syndrome: determinants of endothelial dysfunction in whites and blacks. *Circulation* 2005;112:32–38.
97. Petrie JR, Ueda S, Webb DJ, et al. Endothelial nitric oxide production and insulin sensitivity. A physiological link with implications for pathogenesis of cardiovascular disease. *Circulation* 1996;93:1331–1333.
98. Steinberg HO, Brechtel G, Johnson A, et al. Insulin-mediated skeletal muscle vasodilation is nitric oxide dependent. A novel action of insulin to increase nitric oxide release. *J Clin Invest* 1994;94:1172–1179.
99. Ferri C, Bellini C, Desideri G, et al. Plasma endothelin-1 levels in obese hypertensive and normotensive men. *Diabetes* 1995;44:431–436.
100. Bucala R, Tracey KJ, Cerami A. Advanced glycosylation products quench nitric oxide and mediate defective endothelium-dependent vasodilatation in experimental diabetes. *J Clin Invest* 1991;87:432–438.
101. Park JY, Takahara N, Gabriele A, et al. Induction of endothelin-1 expression by glucose: an effect of protein kinase C activation. *Diabetes* 2000; 49:1239–1248.
102. Williams B. Factors regulating the expression of vascular permeability/ vascular endothelial growth factor by human vascular tissues. *Diabetologia* 1997;40(Suppl 2):S118–S120.
103. Tesfamariam B. Free radicals in diabetic endothelial cell dysfunction. *Free Radic Biol Med* 1994;16:383–391.
104. Wilson PWF, D'Agostino RB, Levy D, et al. Prediction of coronary heart disease using risk factor categories. *Circulation* 1998;97:1837–1847.
105. McEwan P, Williams JE, Griffiths JD, et al. Evaluating the performance of the Framingham risk equations in a population with diabetes. *Diabet Med* 2004;21:318–323.
106. Stern MP, Williams K, Gonzalez-Villalpando C, et al. Does the metabolic syndrome improve identification of individuals at risk of type 2 diabetes and/or cardiovascular disease? *Diabetes Care* 2004;27:2676–2681.
107. Kahn R, Buse J, Ferrannini E, Stern M. The metabolic syndrome: time for a critical appraisal: joint statement from the American Diabetes Association and the European Association for the Study of Diabetes. *Diabetes Care* 2005;28:2289–2304.
108. Frantz S. Groups question existence of metabolic syndrome. *Nat Rev Drug Discov* 2005;4:796–797.

CHAPTER 4 ■ DIABETES

DORON ARONSON AND ELLIOT J. RAYFIELD

EPIDEMIOLOGY

In the past two decades, there has been an explosive increase in the number of people diagnosed with diabetes worldwide. The diabetes epidemic relates particularly to type 2 diabetes, and is taking place both in developed and developing countries. The World Health Organization estimates that the global number of people with diabetes will rise from the current estimate of 150 to 220 million in 2010, and 300 million in 2025 (1,2).

In the United States, almost 8% of the adult population and 19% of the population older than the age of 65 years have diabetes (3), and 800,000 new cases of diabetes are diagnosed per year. Approximately 90% of patients with diabetes have type 2 diabetes, which is now being diagnosed in young people, including adolescents (4). On the basis of fasting plasma glucose levels, one third to one half of cases of type 2 diabetes are undiagnosed and untreated (5).

Impaired glucose tolerance (IGT) is defined as hyperglycemia with glucose values intermediate between normal and diabetes, and affects at least 200 million people worldwide. Approximately 40% of subjects with IGT progress to diabetes over 5 to 10 years (1).

The decline in heart disease mortality in the general American population has been attributed to the reduction in cardiovascular risk factors and improvement in treatment of heart disease. Recent data from the Framingham Heart Study indicate that patients with diabetes have benefited in a similar manner to those without diabetes during the decline in cardiovascular event rates in the US population over the last several decades. Adults with diabetes have experienced a 50% reduction in the rate of incident cardiovascular disease (CVD), although patients with diabetes remained at a consistent, approximately twofold excess of cardiovascular events compared with those without (6).

Both type 1 and type 2 diabetes are powerful and independent risk factors for coronary artery disease (CAD), stroke, and peripheral arterial disease (7). Atherosclerosis accounts for 65% to 80% of all deaths among North American diabetic patients, compared with one third of all deaths in the general North American population (8). More then 75% of all hospitalizations for diabetic complications are attributable to CVD (8). A history of diabetes is equivalent in risk for death to a history of myocardial infarction, and the combination compounds the risk (9).

Coronary Artery Disease in Type I Diabetes

In type I diabetes, atherosclerosis occurs earlier in life, is more diffuse, and leads to higher case fatality and shorter survival (10). The earliest manifestations of CAD occur late in the third decade or in the fourth decade of life regardless of whether diabetes developed early in childhood or in late adolescence (11). The risk increases rapidly after the age of 40, and by the age of 55 years, 35% of patients with type 1 diabetes die of CAD. The protection from CAD observed in nondiabetic women is lost in women with type 1 diabetes (11,12).

The degree of chronic hyperglycemia is related to the progression of CAD in type 1 diabetes (10). Uncontrolled diabetes is associated with greater progression of surrogate markers of atherosclerosis such as carotid IMT (13) and of coronary artery calcifications (14).

The risk of CAD increases dramatically in the subset of type 1 diabetic patients which develop diabetic nephropathy (11,15). Data from the Steno Memorial Hospital showed that in patients with persistent proteinuria the relative mortality from CVD was 37 times that in the general population while in patients without proteinuria cardiovascular mortality was only 4.2 times higher (15). When nephropathy is superimposed on diabetes, some of the atherogenic mechanisms present in diabetes (hypertension, lipid abnormalities, and a hypercoagulable state) are accentuated (16). Nephropathy also results in accelerated accumulation of advanced glycosylation end products (AGEs) in the circulation and tissue that parallels the severity of renal functional impairment (17).

Coronary Artery Disease in Type 2 Diabetes

The relative risk of CVD in type 2 diabetes compared to the general population is increased two- to fourfold (18). The increased cardiovascular risk is particularly striking in women. A number of studies reported a disproportionate impact of CAD in diabetic women compared with diabetic men (19). Indeed, the usual protection that premenopausal women have against atherosclerosis is almost completely lost when diabetes is present.

LIPOPROTEIN DISORDERS

The metabolic abnormalities associated with type 1 and type 2 diabetes results in changes in the transport, composition, and metabolism of lipoproteins. Lipoprotein metabolism is influenced by several factors including type of diabetes, glycemic control, obesity, insulin resistance, the presence of diabetic nephropathy, and genetic background (20). Abnormalities in plasma lipoprotein concentrations are commonly observed in diabetic individuals, and have a profound impact on the on the atherosclerotic process.

Lipoprotein Profile in Type 1 Diabetes

Glycemic control is the chief determinant of lipoproteins profile in patients with type 1 diabetes. In well to moderately controlled diabetes, lipoprotein levels are usually within the normal range. In patients with poor control, triglycerides are markedly elevated, low-density lipoprotein (LDL) is modesty increased (usually when HbA1c >11%), and high-density lipoprotein (HDL) levels are decreased (Table 4.1). Hypertriglyceridemia and hypercholesterolemia are readily reversible with intensive insulin therapy, and HDL levels may be higher than in normal controls (21).

Lipoprotein Profile in Type 2 Diabetes

The dyslipidemia in type 2 diabetes results from a complex interaction between an insulin-resistant state, obesity, and hyperglycemia (20), and is often present for years before the development of fasting hyperglycemia and the diagnosis of type 2 diabetes. The typical lipoprotein profile associated with type 2 diabetes includes high triglycerides, low HDL, and normal LDL levels (see Table 4.1). However, the composition of LDL particles is altered, resulting in a preponderance of small, triglyceride-enriched and cholesterol-depleted particles (small, dense LDL). This lipoprotein profile has been termed *atherogenic lipoprotein phenotype*, and is also characteristic of the metabolic syndrome and obesity (22,23).

The most consistent change is an increase in very low-density lipoprotein (VLDL) triglyceride levels (24,25). HDL levels are typically 25% to 30% lower than in nondiabetics and are commonly associated with other lipid and lipoprotein abnormalities, particularly high triglyceride levels.

Very Low-Density Lipoprotein Metabolism in Diabetes

Hypertriglyceridemia in type 2 diabetes results from high fasting and postprandial triglyceride-rich lipoproteins, especially VLDL (24), which is the consequence of both overproduction and impaired catabolism of VLDL (25). Increased VLDL production is almost uniformly present in patients with type 2

TABLE 4.1

LIPOPROTEIN ABNORMALITIES IN DIABETES

	Type 1 diabetes		Type 2 diabetes		
Lipoprotein	Conventional therapy	Intensive therapy	Poor control	Good control	Atherogenic modifications
VLDL-TG	Normal or increased	Decreased	Increased	Normal or increased	Cholesteryl ester rich VLDL
LDL	Normal or increased	Normal or decreased	Normal	Normal	Glycosylation of LDL Apo B increases uptake through the scavenger receptor LDL susceptible to oxidative modification High proportion of small dense LDL
HDL	Normal	Increased	Decreased	Normal or decreased	Decreased HDL Increased CETP activity

Abbreviations: CETP, cholesteryl ester transfer protein; HDL, high-density lipoprotein; LDL, low-density lipoprotein; VLDL-TG, very low-density lipoprotein.

Diabetes

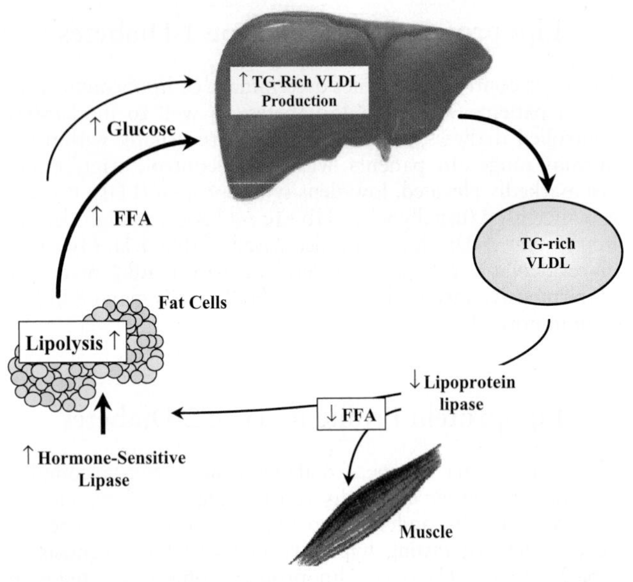

FIGURE 4.1. Mechanism of increased VLDL triglyceride in diabetes: in the setting of insulin deficiency or insulin resistance higher rates of glucose and FFAs flux to the liver lead to enhanced VLDL production and secretion. Decreased LPL activity contributes to the accumulation of these particles in the plasma.

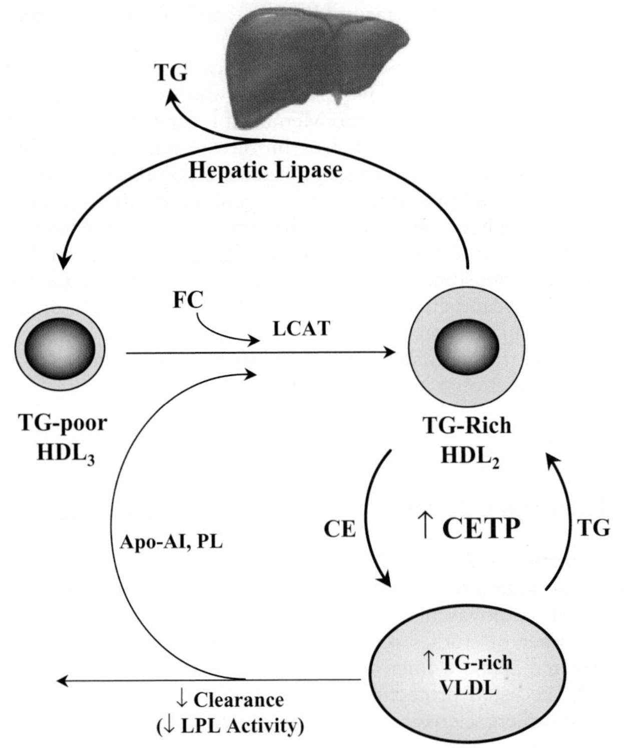

FIGURE 4.2. Mechanism of decreased HDL in diabetes: the rate of HDL_2 formation is dependent on the rate of flux of surface components from lipolysis of triglyceride-rich lipoproteins. Inefficient LPL-mediated triglyceride-rich lipoprotein catabolism reduces the rate of HDL_2 formation. Excess of triglyceride-rich lipoproteins enhances CETP, resulting in the formation of HDL_2, which is a triglyceride-rich particle that efficiently interacts with hepatic lipase. The result is the predominance of the small and dense HDL_3 in diabetic patients. A similar mechanism governs the predominance of small, dense species of LDL.

diabetes and hypertriglyceridemia, owing to an increase in free fatty acids (FFA) flux to the liver (25). Because maintenance of stored fat in adipose tissue depends on the suppression of hormone-sensitive lipase by insulin, insulin deficiency, or resistance results in increased hormone-sensitive lipase activity and excessive release of FFA from adipocytes. Because FFA availability is a major determinant of VLDL production by the liver, VLDL overproduction and hypertriglyceridemia ensues (25,26) (Fig. 4.1).

In type 2 patients with more severe hypertriglyceridemia, VLDL clearance by lipoprotein lipase (LPL), the rate-limiting enzyme responsible for the removal of plasma triglyceride-rich lipoproteins, is also impaired (24). LPL requires insulin for maintenance of normal tissue levels, and its activity is low in patients with poorly controlled type 2 diabetes (24). The result is enzymatic activity insufficient to match the overproduction rate, with further accumulation of VLDL triglyceride.

Increased fatty acid flux to the liver also results in the production of large triglyceride-rich VLDL particles because the size of VLDL is also mainly determined by the amount of triglyceride available. VLDL size is an important determinant of its metabolic fate (see below).

High-Density Lipoprotein Metabolism

Decreased HDL levels in diabetes are closely related to the abnormal metabolism of triglyceride-rich lipoproteins (24–26) (Fig. 4.2). During lipolysis of chylomicrons and VLDL, surface components (free cholesterol, redundant phospholipids, and apolipoproteins) are transferred into the HDL fraction. These components may enter nascent discoid HDL particles secreted by the liver. The free cholesterol is esterified by lecithin cholesterol acyl transferase to generate mature spherical HDL. Alternatively, these surface components may be incorporated into preexisting HDL particles. The latter process results in an increase in size and decrease in density of HDL particles, leading to the conversion of preexisting HDL_3 (triglyceride depleted) to HDL_2.

In diabetes, decreased HDL synthesis is related to the decreased LPL activity because the rate of HDL_2 formation depends on the rate of flux of surface components from lipolysis of triglyceride-rich lipoprotein (see Figure 4.2). When LPL-mediated VLDL catabolism is inefficient, less surface material is transferred to HDL, impairing HDL formation.

Increased catabolism of HDL in diabetes also occurs because increased secretion of VLDL into plasma promotes the transfer of triglycerides from these lipoproteins to HDL in exchange for cholesteryl ester. This exchange occurs in plasma, and is facilitated by cholesteryl ester transfer protein (CETP), generating a triglyceride-enriched (and cholesteryl ester–depleted) HDL_2. This particle is highly susceptible to catabolism by hepatic triglyceride lipase (HTGL), an enzyme found primarily on endothelial cells of hepatic sinusoids (25). HTGL has both triglyceride hydrolase and phospholipase activity, and generates smaller HDL_3 particle, which are depleted in triglycerides and phospholipids (see Fig. 4.2).

Low-Density Lipoprotein Metabolism

In diabetes, although the absolute number of LDL particles is normal, alterations in LDL clearance and susceptibility to oxidative modification result in an increase in LDL atherogenic potential. The composition of LDL particles is altered, resulting in a preponderance of small, triglyceride-enriched and cholesterol depleted particles (22,23). These particles are more susceptible to oxidative modification, are particularly prone to induce endothelial dysfunction, and easily penetrate the arterial wall.

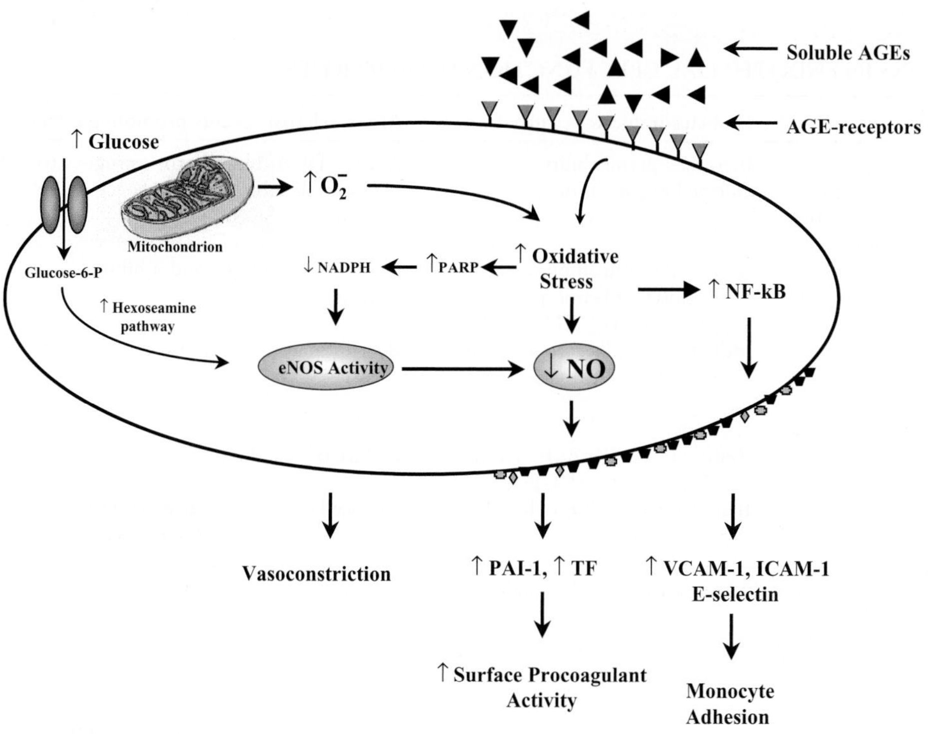

FIGURE 4.3. Potential mechanisms of endothelial dysfunction in diabetes. Diabetes leads to reduced NO bioavailability and NF-κB activation, resulting in perturbations in vascular tone, increased procoagulant activity and increased expression of adhesion molecules on endothelial cells. *Abbreviations:* TF, tissue factor; ICAM, intracellular adhesion molecule; NF-κB, nuclear factor-κB; PAI-1, plasminogen activator inhibitor-1; PARP, poly(ADP-ribose) polymerase; VCAM, vascular cell adhesion molecule.

The formation of small, dense LDL in diabetes occurs in a similar fashion to the increased formation of small and dense HDL_3, as described. CETP mediates the exchange of triglyceride from VLDL for cholesteryl ester in LDL. If sufficient LDL cholesteryl ester is replaced by triglyceride from VLDL then when the particle comes into contact with hepatic lipase, hydrolysis of newly acquired triglyceride in LDL and HDL by HTGL in turn decreases the size of LDL particles (27). The symmetry of the mechanisms for the formation of small, dense species of LDL and HDL (see Figure 4.2) helps to explain why low HDL levels and a preponderance of small, dense LDL are associated with diabetes and the metabolic syndrome and why HDL cholesterol level is strongly correlated with LDL size (27).

The glycosylation process (see Advanced Glycosylation End Products) occurs both on the apoprotein B (Apo B) (28) and phospholipid (29) components of LDL. Glycosylation of LDL Apo B occurs within the putative LDL receptor–binding domain, and impairs LDL-receptor–mediated LDL clearance.

Advanced glycosylation of an amine-containing phospholipids component of LDL is accompanied by progressive oxidative modification of unsaturated fatty acid residues and confers increased susceptibility of LDL to oxidative modification (29).

ENDOTHELIAL CELL DYSFUNCTION

Endothelial dysfunction can promote both the formation of atherosclerotic plaques, and the occurrence of acute events. One of the hallmarks of vascular disease in diabetes is endothelial dysfunction, which contributes to the initiation, progression, and clinical presentation of the atherosclerotic process in these patients.

Impaired Endothelium-Dependent Vasodilation

Impaired endothelium-dependent relaxation is a consistent finding in animal models and in human diabetes (30–32). The alterations in nitric oxide (NO) regulation in diabetes are complex and involve increased reactive oxygen species (ROS) (33,34), quenching of bioactive NO by glucose (35), changes in endothelial NO synthase (eNOS) levels or its cofactors (36,37), and perturbations in eNOS activation (38,39) (Fig. 4.3). Consequently, multiple abnormalities in endothelial cell function have been described in association with diabetes (Table 4.2).

Hyperglycemia Impairs Endothelium-Dependent Vasodilation

Hyperglycemia appears to be a primary mediator of endothelial dysfunction in diabetes. A short exposure (several hours) to high glucose concentrations is sufficient to induce impaired endothelium-dependent relaxation (30).

There is abundant evidence supporting the importance of ROS in inducing and maintaining endothelial dysfunction in diabetes (34,39,40). The excess of superoxide in endothelial cells (33,38,39) can directly inhibit two critical endothelial enzymes, eNOS and prostacyclin synthase (34,41). In addition to can reduce eNOS activity through activation of the hexosamine pathway (38,39).

Diabetes-related oxidative stress also induces DNA single-strand breakage leading to the activation of the nuclear enzyme poly(ADP-ribose) polymerase (PARP). The result of this process is rapid depletion of endothelial energy sources, including NADPH. Because eNOS is an NADPH-dependent enzyme, it activity is suppressed (36,37). A PARP inhibitor can maintain normal vascular responsiveness, despite the persistence of severe hyperglycemia (37).

TABLE 4.2

DIABETES-RELATED ALTERATIONS IN ENDOTHELIAL CELL FUNCTIONAL PROPERTIES

Endothelial function	Effectors	Diabetes-induced perturbations	Atherosclerosis/events promoting effects
Selective permeability barrier	Continuous endothelium with tight junctions in the lateral borders	Increased permeability Delayed regeneration	Allow LDL or bloodborne mitogens to reach the subendothelial space
Provides a nonthrombogenic surface	NO, PGI_2 t-PA, HS, thrombomodulin TF	Reduced antithrombotic and fibrinolytic phenotype ($\downarrow$NO, $\downarrow PGI_2$, $\uparrow$PAI-1, $\uparrow$TF)	Promote thrombosis and inhibit fibrinolysis
Provides a nonadherent surface for circulating leukocytes	NO	Induction of adhesion molecules (e.g., VCAM-1, E-selectin)	Recruit macrophages into the vascular wall
Regulation of vascular tone	NO, PGI_2, ET-1	Reduced vasodilator function ($\downarrow$NO, $\downarrow PGI_2$, $\uparrow$ET-1)	Failure of vasodilation
Secrete growth inhibitors	NO, HS	Inactivation of NO; reduced NO production	Reduced antiproliferative activity of NO on vascular smooth muscle cells

Abbreviations: AGEs, advanced glycosylation end products; NO, nitric oxide; ET-1, endothelin-1; HS, heparan sulfate; PGI_2, prostacyclin; TF, tissue factor; VCAM-1, vascular cell adhesion molecule-1.

DIABETES AS A PROTHROMBOTIC STATE

Local and systemic thrombogenic risk factors at the time of plaque disruption may determine the degree of thrombus formation, and hence, the clinical outcome. Diabetes is characterized by a variety of alterations in platelet function as well as in the coagulation and fibrinolytic systems that combine to produce a prothrombotic state (Table 4.3).

Platelet Aggregation

Platelets from diabetic subjects exhibit enhanced adhesiveness and hyperaggregability in response to both strong (e.g.,

TABLE 4.3

COAGULATION AND FIBRINOLYTIC ABNORMALITIES OF PROGNOSTIC SIGNIFICANCE IN DIABETES

Factor	Prognostic significance	Diabetes effect
Platelet hyperactivity	Spontaneous platelet aggregation in vitro predicts coronary events and mortality in patients surviving myocardial infarction	Platelet hyperaggregability in response to agonists and increase fractions of circulating activated platelets
vWF	Increased concentrations of endothelium-derived vWF derived reflect endothelial perturbation, and is associated with subsequent myocardial infarction	Elevated vWF levels, especially in the presence of vascular complications and endothelial dysfunction or insulin resistance. Confers a high risk for cardiovascular events
Fibrinogen	High fibrinogen levels associated with increased risk for reinfarction and death	Increased in diabetic patients
Factor VII	High levels of factor VII coagulant activity is associated with increased risk for coronary events	Elevated and correlates with glycemic control and microalbuminuria
PAI-1	Reduced fibrinolytic capacity owing to increased plasma PAI-1 levels is predisposed to myocardial infarction in postinfarction patients or patients with angina	Elevated PAI-1 levels occur as a result of obesity or hyperglycemia
CD 40 ligand	Involved in the induction of adhesion molecules and the release of cytokines and tissue factor	Increased
TF	Expressed in coronary atherosclerotic plaques and may account for the magnitude of the thrombotic responses to rupture of coronary atherosclerotic plaques	AGE-RAGE interaction induces cell surface expression of TF

Abbreviations: AGE, advanced glycosylation end products; RAGE, receptor for advanced glycosylation end products; TF, tissue factor; vWF, von Willebrand factor; PAI-1, plasminogen activator inhibitor 1.

thrombin, TxA_2) and weak (e.g., ADP, epinephrine, collagen) agonists (42). Shear-induced platelet adhesion and aggregation is increased in diabetic patients (43). Platelet hypersensitivity is more evident in diabetic patients with vascular complications. However, it is also observed in newly diagnosed diabetic patients, suggesting that altered platelet function may be a consequence of metabolic changes secondary to the diabetic state (44).

The CD40 ligand is rapidly presented to platelet surface after platelet activation and is involved in the induction of adhesion molecules and the release of cytokines and tissue factor. CD40 ligand is elevated in patients with diabetes and can be reduced by thiazolidinediones (45).

Increased numbers of GPIb (the von Willebrand receptor, to which platelets are exposed at injury sites) and GPIIb–IIIa (the fibrinogen receptor) have been found in patients with diabetes (46). Elevated fractions of $CD62^+/CD63^+$ (activated) platelets circulate in diabetic patients in the absence of clinically detectable vascular lesions (47,48).

The mechanism for these abnormalities is not well understood. There is a significant correlation between glucose levels and platelet-dependent thrombosis (49). Increased oxidant stress might lead to enhanced generation of certain isoprostanes, which induce platelet activation (50). In addition, hyperglycemia increases mitochondrial ROS generation in human platelets, leading to increased platelet aggregation through the activation of intracellular signaling systems (51).

Platelets from patients with diabetes may be less sensitive to aspirin (52,53). A high proportion of nonresponders to the standard clopidogrel loading dose among patients with diabetes has also been described (54).

Alterations in Coagulation Factors

In diabetic patients plasma concentrations of vWF are elevated, and are closely associated with the presence of vascular complications and endothelial dysfunction (55). Fibrinogen levels are often increased in diabetes, and this elevation is associated with poor glycemic control (56). However, the association between diabetes and elevated fibrinogen may be partly related to the presence of vascular disease at the clinical or preclinical stage (57). Fibrinogen levels may fall with intensive insulin therapy (58), although this finding is not consistent, and transient elevation of fibrinogen with intensive insulin therapy has been reported (59).

Plasma factor VII levels have been shown to increase in normal subjects following a meal (60). Plasma levels of factor VII increase in normal subjects in response to moderate hyperglycemia, but not during hyperinsulinemia with euglycemia (61). Plasma factor VII levels decrease with improved with glycemic control (58).

HYPERGLYCEMIA AS AN ATHEROGENIC FACTOR

Prolonged exposure to hyperglycemia is a primary casual factor in the pathogenesis of diabetic microvascular complications and contributes to macrovascular complications (62). Under hyperglycemic conditions, most cells are able to reduce glucose transport across the cell membrane, thereby maintaining constant intracellular glucose concentrations. Diabetes selectively damages cells such as endothelial cell and mesangial cells, whose glucose transport rate does not decline rapidly in response to hyperglycemia, leading to high intracellular glucose (34). Hyperglycemia induces a large number of alterations in vascular tissue that potentially promote accelerated atherosclerosis. Several major mechanisms have emerged that encompass most of the pathologic alterations observed in the vasculature of diabetic animals and humans: (1) nonenzymatic glycosylation of proteins and lipids, (2) protein kinase C (PKC) activation, (3) Increased flux through the hexosamine pathway, and (4) increased oxidative stress.

Advanced Glycosylation End Products

One of the important mechanisms responsible for the accelerated atherosclerosis in diabetes is the nonenzymatic reaction between glucose and proteins or lipoproteins in arterial walls, collectively known as Maillard, or browning reaction (63) (Fig. 4.4). Glucose forms chemically reversible early glycosylation products with reactive amino groups of proteins (Schiff bases). Over a period of days, the unstable Schiff base subsequently rearranges to form the more stable Amadori-type early glycosylation products. Formation of Amadori product from the Schiff base is slower but much faster than the reverse reaction, and therefore tend to accumulate on proteins. Equilibrium levels of Amadori products are reached in weeks (see Figure 4.4).

Some of the early glycosylation products on long-lived proteins (e.g., vessel wall collagen) continue to undergo complex series of chemical rearrangements in vivo to form complex compounds and crosslinks known as advanced AGEs (63,64) (see Figure 4.4). An important distinction of AGEs compared with

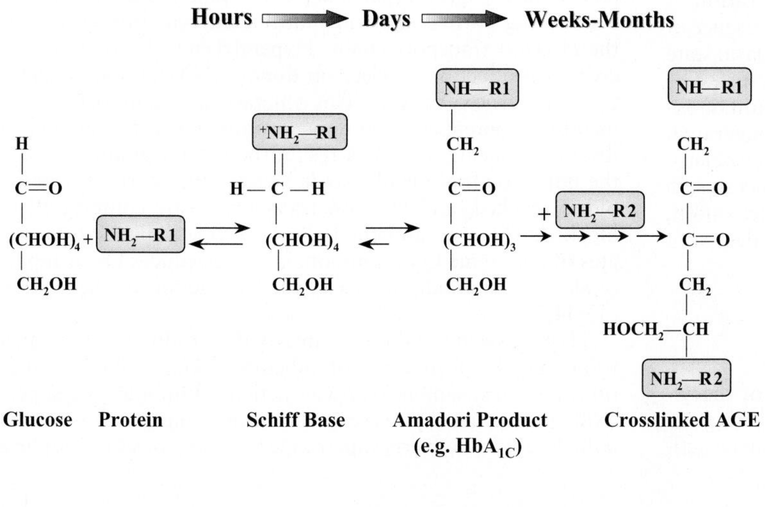

FIGURE 4.4. Formation of advanced AGEs. The process can be inhibited by aminoguanidine, which reacts with Amadori products and prevents the development of more advanced products. AGE crosslink breakers bind to a fully formed AGE and create a ring prone to a sequence of spontaneous break. The result is a severing of AGE cross bridges between collagen and other macromolecules (see text for details).

the Amadori products is that once formed, advanced AGE–protein adducts are stable and virtually irreversible. The degree of nonenzymatic glycation is determined mainly by the glucose concentration and time of exposure. Therefore, AGEs accumulate continuously on long-lived vessel wall proteins with aging and at an accelerated rate in diabetes (64). However, another critical factor to the formation of AGEs is the tissue microenvironment redox potential. Thus, situations in which the local redox potential has been shifted to favor oxidant stress, AGEs formation increases substantially (33,65).

AGEs can accelerate the atherosclerotic process by diverse mechanisms. Glycosylation of proteins and lipoproteins can interfere with their normal function by disrupting molecular conformation, alter proteins involved in gene transcription, reduce degradative capacity, and interfere with receptor recognition.

The Advanced Glycosylation End Products Receptor Mediates Inflammation

The pathophysiologic significance of AGEs stems not only from their ability to modify the functional properties of proteins, but also to their ability to interact with AGE-binding proteins or AGE receptors. The presence of a specific AGE receptor (RAGE) has been demonstrated in all cells relevant to the atherosclerotic process including monocyte-derived macrophages, endothelial cells, and smooth muscle cells (65,66). In diabetic vasculature, cells expressing high levels of RAGE are often proximal to areas in which AGEs are abundant (65).

AGE interaction with RAGE on endothelial cells results in the induction of oxidative stress and consequently of the transcription factor NF-κB (67,68) and increases the expression of adhesion molecules (69) (see Figure 4.3). In addition, RAGE-mediated monocyte–macrophage interaction with AGEs results also in the production of proinflammatory cytokines such as tumor necrosis factor-α and platelet-derived growth factor (70).

Engagement of AGEs with their specific receptors results in reduced endothelial barrier function, with increased permeability of endothelial cell monolayers (71). Thus, the interaction of AGEs with RAGE-bearing endothelial cells can promote initiating events in atherogenesis such as increased lipid entry into the subendothelium and adhesive interactions of monocytes with the endothelial surface with subsequent transendothelial migration. In animal models, blockade of AGE–RAGE interaction using a truncated soluble extracellular domain of RAGE resulted in a striking suppression of atherosclerotic lesion formation, with lesions largely arrested at the fatty streak stage with a large reduction in complex lesions (72).

Schmidt et al. proposed the following *two-hit model* for RAGE-mediated perturbations in diabetic vasculature (65,66). In the setting of hyperglycemia, formation and deposition of AGEs in tissues and vasculature is accelerated. The presence of AGEs (RAGE ligands) in the vasculature results in a basal state of increased RAGE expression and activation (first hit). The superimposition of another stimulus, such as deposition of oxidized lipoproteins or inflammation, results in an exaggerated, chronic inflammation and promotes accelerated atherosclerosis (second hit). In contrast to other inflammatory processes, in which a negative feedback loop terminates cellular activation, RAGE activation appears to result in a smoldering degree of cellular stimulation (65,66,69).

Protein Kinase C

Intracellular hyperglycemia increases the synthesis of diacylglycerol (DAG), the major endogenous cellular activating cofactor for PKC. The elevation of DAG and subsequent activation of PKC in the vasculature can be maintained chronically (73). The PKC system is ubiquitously distributed in cells and is involved in the transcription of several growth factors, and in signal transduction in response to growth factors (74). In endothelial cells, PKC activation decreases NO bioavailability and decreases eNOS (7,75). Furthermore, PKC activation in endothelial cells results in upregulation of adhesion molecules and activation of proinflammatory genes (76). In vascular smooth muscle cells, PKC activation has been shown to modulate growth rate, DNA synthesis, and growth factor receptor turnover (73).

The Hexosamine Pathway

Shunting of excess intracellular glucose into the hexosamine pathway may contribute to diabetic macrovascular disease. In this pathway, fructose-6-phosphate derived from glycolysis provides substrate to reactions that require UDP-*N*-acetylglucosamine, such as proteoglycan synthesis and the formation of *O*-linked glycoproteins (34,75).

O-glycosylation typically involves the addition of a single sugar, usually *N*-acetylglucosamine (abbreviated GlcNAc) to the protein's serine and threonine residues. Serine/threonine phosphorylation is a critical step in the regulation of various enzymes.

Many transcription factors and other nuclear and cytoplasmic proteins are dynamically modified by *O*-linked GlcNAc, and show reciprocal modification by phosphorylation (75). For example, hyperglycemia increases eNOS-associated *O*-GlcANc, resulting in a parallel decrease in eNOS serine phosphorylation (which results in enzyme activation) and therefore a decrease in eNOS activity (39). This pathway is also involved in hyperglycemia-induced increase in the transcription of transforming growth factor-β and PAI-1 (34,77).

Oxidative Stress

Oxidative damage to arterial wall proteins occurs even with short-term exposure to hyperglycemia in the diabetic range (78). Importantly, there appears to be a tight pathogenic link between hyperglycemia-induced oxidant stress and other hyperglycemia-dependent mechanisms of vascular damage described above, namely AGEs formation, PKC activation, and increased flux through the hexosamine pathway (33,34) (Fig. 4.5).

Hyperglycemia can increase oxidative stress through several pathways (Figure 4.5). A major mechanism appears to be the overproduction of the superoxide anion (O_2^-) by the mitochondrial electron transport chain (33,34). Physiologic generation of O_2 species (particularly the superoxide radical) occurs during normal electron shuttling by cytochromes within the electron transport chain. Hyperglycemia leads to an increased production of electron donors (NADH and $FADH_2$) by the tricarboxylic cycle. This generates a high mitochondrial membrane potential by pumping protons across the mitochondrial inner membrane. As a result, the voltage gradient across the mitochondrial membrane increases until a critical threshold is reached, and electron transport inside complex III is blocked. This increases the half-life of free radical intermediates of coenzyme Q (ubiquinone), which reduces O_2 to superoxide, and markedly increases the production of superoxide (33,34,75,77).

Hyperglycemia-induced superoxide production activates promotes the formation of advanced AGEs, PKC activation, and hexosamine pathway activity. Inhibition of superoxide production by overexpression of manganese dismutase (which rapidly converts superoxide to H_2O_2) or of uncoupling

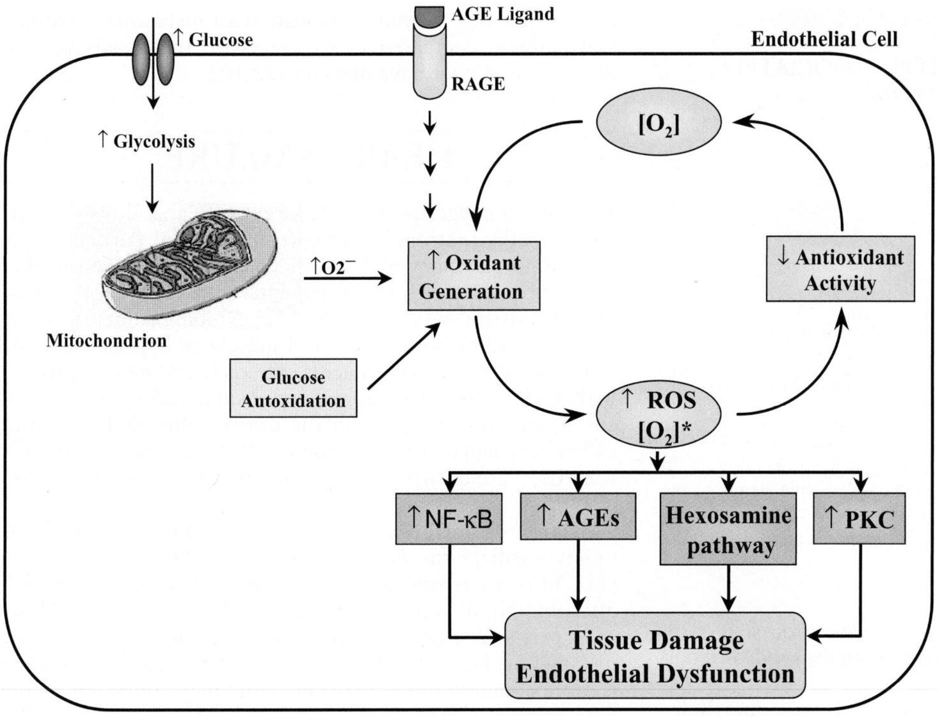

FIGURE 4.5. Relationship between rates of oxidant generation, antioxidant activity, oxidative stress, and oxidative damage in diabetes. $[O_2]^*$ represents various forms of reactive oxygen species [ROS]. The overall rate of formation of oxidative products leading to oxidative tissue damage is dependent on ambient levels of both $[O_2]^*$ and substrate. Increased generation of $[O_2]^*$ depends on several sources including glucose autoxidation, increased mitochondrial superoxide production, and as a result of the receptor for advanced AGEs activation. $[O_2]^*$ deactivation is reduced because antioxidant defenses are compromised in diabetes. Note that oxidative stress also promotes other hyperglycemia-induced mechanisms of tissue damage. Oxidative stress activates PKC and accelerates the formation of advanced glycosylation end products (AGEs).

protein-1 (which collapses the proton electromechanical gradients) prevents hyperglycemia-induced superoxide overproduction. Concomitantly, increased intracellular AGE formation, PKC activation, and increased hexosamine formation are prevented (33,34,75).

Diabetes and Inflammation

Inflammatory markers are increased in patients with diabetes (79,80), and their level generally correlate with the degree of glycemic control (81). The metabolic syndrome is associated with a proinflammatory state (see The Metabolic Syndrome). Another important modulator of inflammation in patients with diabetes is hyperglycemia, which promotes inflammation via AGEs formation (see Advanced Glycosylation End Products), but can also induce cytokine secretion by several cell types is hyperglycemia (82). In monocytes, chronic hyperglycemia causes a dramatic increase in the release of cytokines (83). Furthermore, recent studies have shown that hyperglycemia, but not hyperinsulinemia, leads to the induction and secretion of acute phase reactants by adipocytes by promoting intracellular oxidative stress (84,85). Thus, hyperglycemia might amplify inflammation (marked by a high concentration of C-reactive protein [CRP]) and promote atherosclerosis and plaque vulnerability.

Insulin-sensitizing interventions such as thiazolidinediones reduced CRP in patients with diabetes (86,87). However, the effect of antihyperglycemic therapy on the level of inflammatory markers is more complex. In the Diabetes Control and Complications Trial of patients with type 1 diabetes, there was a significant reduction of sICAM-1 but no overall treatment effect of intensive insulin regimen on CRP level. Furthermore, there was a significant rise in CRP levels among intensively treated patients who gained the most weight (88). Thus, given the robust proinflammatory effect of obesity, weight gain may mitigate the beneficial effect of intensive insulin therapy on inflammation.

THE METABOLIC SYNDROME

The metabolic syndrome is a cluster of cardiovascular risk factors that frequently coincides with insulin resistance and hyperglycemia. The metabolic syndrome is a common condition, associated with genetic predisposition, sedentary lifestyle, obesity, and aging. Using the NCEP/ATP-III criteria (Table 4.4), it is estimated that one out of four adults living in the United States merits the diagnosis (89).

The primary importance of the metabolic syndrome lays in the fact that each of its components is an established risk factor for CAD. The metabolic syndrome is associated with a two to threefold increase in cardiovascular mortality and 1.5- to 2.0-fold increase in all-cause mortality (90,91). Alone, each component of the cluster conveys increased CAD risk. However, the notion that it is a useful marker of cardiovascular risk beyond the risk associated with each of its individual components is uncertain (92). Furthermore, because the treatment of

TABLE 4.4

ATP III CRITERIA FOR IDENTIFICATION OF THE METABOLIC SYNDROME (209)

Abdominal obesity (waist circumference)	
Men	>102 cm (40 in)
Women	>88 cm (35 in)
Triglycerides	≥150 mg/dL
HDL cholesterol	
Men	<40 mg/dL
Women	<50 mg/dL
Blood pressure	≥130/≥85 mm Hg
Fasting glucose	≥110 mg/dL

Abbreviation: HDL, high-density lipoprotein.

TABLE 4.5

CARDIOVASCULAR RISK FACTORS ASSOCIATED WITH THE METABOLIC SYNDROME

Hypertension
Abdominal obesity
Dyslipidemia
Increased VLDL triglycerides
Decreased HDL
Small, dense atherogenic LDL particles
Postprandial lipemia
Prothrombotic state—elevated PAI-1 and fibrinogen
Endothelial dysfunction
Chronic subclinical inflammation—elevated cytokines and CRP

Abbreviations: CRP, C-reactive protein; HDL, high-density lipoprotein; LDL, low-density lipoprotein; PAI-1, plasminogen activator inhibitor 1; VLDL, very low-density lipoprotein.

the syndrome is no different than the treatment for each of its components, the medical value of diagnosing the syndrome has been questioned (92–94).

The pathophysiologic processes that lead to the metabolic syndrome are primarily related to obesity and insulin resistance. Both genetic and acquired causes contribute to the syndrome, and much of the heterogeneity in the manifestations of the syndrome is related to fact that its components (e.g., lipoprotein abnormalities) are regulated by factors other than insulin resistance.

Beyond the association with classical CAD risk factors, it is now recognized that the metabolic syndrome is associated with nontransitional risk factors for CAD including inflammation, prothrombotic state, and endothelial dysfunction (Table 4.5). An important mechanism for the chronic inflammation associated with the metabolic syndrome appears to be inflammatory cell infiltration with increased production of inflammatory cytokines in adipose tissue (95,96). Both tumor necrosis factor-α and interleukin-6 are expressed in and released by adipose tissue (97,98). There is a close relationship between circulating CRP and cytokine concentrations (97) and between CRP concentrations and anthropometric measures of obesity (97,99,100). Because the synthesis of CRP by the liver is predominantly regulated by interleukin-6, it is believed that interleukin-6 originating from adipose tissue contributes to the raised CRP concentrations in obese insulin-resistant subjects. Fatty infiltration to the liver, a common complication of obesity, may stimulates hepatic cytokine production, which could further contribute to low-grade inflammation (101).

Although insulin resistance is strongly associated with atherogenic dyslipidemia and a proinflammatory state (102), it is less tightly associated with hypertension and a prothrombotic state (103). Furthermore, insulin resistance or hyperinsulinemia may not be present in subjects with the syndrome (92). Whereas the mechanistic link between insulin resistance and dyslipidemia is sufficiently clear (see Lipoprotein Disorders in Diabetes), the mechanism underlying the proinflammatory state is largely unknown. It has been suggested that insulin suppresses several proinflammatory transcription factors, such as the nuclear factor (NF)-κB. Thus, impaired insulin action owing to insulin resistance would result in activation of proinflammatory transcription factors and an increase in the expression of inflammatory gene products (104).

Insulin resistant individuals who go on to develop type 2 diabetes become exposed to the atherogenic effects of hyperglycemia. Therefore, the risk for cardiovascular and all-cause mortality is higher among patients with metabolic syndrome and diabetes compared to patients with the metabolic syndrome who do not have diabetes (92,105).

HEART FAILURE

The risk for congestive heart failure (CHF) and idiopathic cardiomyopathy is strongly increased in diabetes, particularly in women. In patients with CHF, diabetes is an independent predictor of poor prognosis in patients with CHF (106). Additionally, patients with advanced CHF exhibit insulin resistance, characterized by both fasting and stimulated hyperinsulinemia (107), and glucose intolerance is extremely common in patients with CHF (108). The severity of insulin resistance in CHF correlates with the symptomatic status rather than measures of left ventricular (LV) function (108). Consequently, patients with CHF are at increased risk of developing type 2 diabetes (109).

Diabetes is a strong predictor of the development of CHF after myocardial infarction, even after controlling for infarct size (110,111). LV remodeling, an important determinant of CHF after infarction, is not increased in diabetes (112,113). However, persistence of echocardiographic evidence for diastolic dysfunction beyond the acute phase of myocardial ischemia is more common in diabetes (113) and may contribute to the development of late CHF.

Pathogenesis of Diabetic Cardiomyopathy

The cardiomyopathic process associated with diabetes mellitus manifests initially as diminished LV compliance in the presence of normal LV systolic function. Diastolic abnormalities occur in 27% to 69% of asymptomatic diabetic patients (114,115).

The pathogenesis of diabetic cardiomyopathy is multifactorial and results from both metabolic and structural alterations. Metabolic abnormalities such as hyperglycemia (116) and insulin resistance (117) have been associated with LV mass and risk of symptomatic CHF. Recent studies indicate that the oxidative stress in diabetes promotes myocyte apoptosis and contribute to the development of diabetic cardiomyopathy (118).

Role of Advanced Glycosylation End Products

Part of the normal aging process of humans is the gradual decrease in the elasticity of the cardiovascular system, which leads to increased arterial as well as to LV stiffness. Diabetic patients have increased arterial stiffness compared to nondiabetic individuals and manifest diminished LV compliance at a young age (114,119).

Several investigators have demonstrated that diabetes has several features of accelerated aging both at the tissue level and at the level of collagen itself (120). Among the structural alterations associated with AGEs formation are collagen-to-collagen cross-linking (64,121) (Fig. 4.6), which alters the structure and function of this protein leading to tissue rigidity (121).

Recent studies have used the newly developed an AGE "breaker" compound (122). Treatment of rats with streptozotocin-induced diabetes with the AGE breaker ALT-711 (alagebrium) for 1 to 3 weeks reversed the diabetes-induced increase of large artery stiffness (123). Similarly, ALT-711 therapy resulted in a significant reduction in age-related LV stiffness in dogs (124). Preliminary studies have shown the efficacy of ALT-711 in humans (125). Alagebrium is currently being

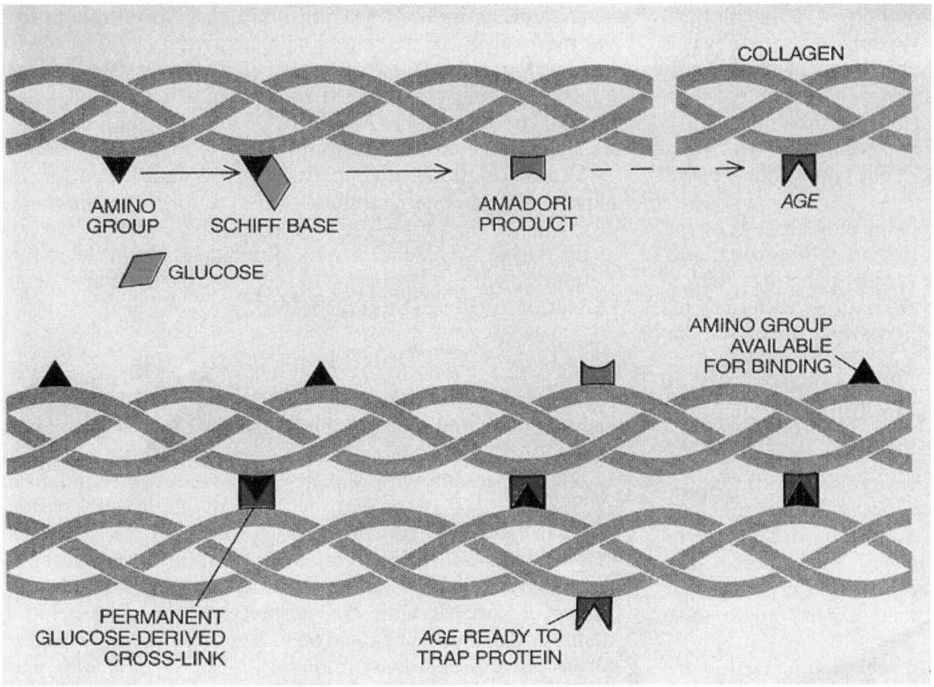

FIGURE 4.6. Schematic description of the formation of collagen cross links. Glucose attaches to an amino group (NH_2) of a protein (*top*), such as collagen to form a Schiff base, which is subsequently transforms itself into an Amadori product (see Figure 4.4 for chemical structure). The latter can pass through several incompletely understood steps (*broken arrows*) to become an AGE. AGEs can react with free amino groups on an adjacent protein to form cross-links (*bottom*). Cross-linking can lead to decreased compliance of large vessels and of the myocardium (see text for details). Reproduced from Cerami et al. (210) with permission.

evaluated in patients with heart failure and evidence of diastolic dysfunction.

ACUTE CORONARY SYNDROMES IN PATIENTS WITH DIABETES

Acute coronary syndromes (ACS) represent a major cause of death in patients with diabetes. Whether presenting with unstable angina (126,127), acute myocardial infarction (110), or cardiogenic shock (128), patients with diabetes have a higher mortality in the acute phase, and worse long-term outcome.

Diabetes is associated with multiple alterations that promote vascular inflammation, potentially leading to plaque instability and disruption. Higher proportion of ulcerated plaque (94% versus 60%) and intracoronary thrombi (94% versus 55%) are observed by angioscopy in patients with diabetes presenting with unstable angina (129). Coronary tissue obtained from culprit lesions of patients with diabetes and unstable angina or myocardial infarction exhibit a larger content of lipid-rich atheroma, macrophage infiltration, and a higher incidence of coronary thrombus that occupies a larger area (130).

Unstable Angina

Of all patients presenting with non–ST-segment elevation ACS, 20% to 25% have diabetes (126). Diabetes is an important risk factor for an adverse outcome in this setting, with higher 30-day and 1-year mortality (126,127). In a meta-analysis of six large-scale ACS trials, patients with diabetes had a twofold higher mortality (127).

Retrospective analyses suggest that therapy with platelet glycoprotein IIb/IIIa inhibitors may improve the outcome of patients with diabetes and ACS (127). However, a randomized trial found a neutral effect of abciximab in patients with diabetes undergoing elective percutaneous coronary intervention (PCI) who received a 600-mg bolus dose of clopidogrel before PCI (131).

ST-Elevation Infarction

The in-hospital mortality from myocardial infarction in patients with diabetes is 1.5- to 2-fold higher than in nondiabetic patients (110,132). In the GUSTO-I trial, 30-day mortality was highest among diabetic patients treated with insulin (12.5%) compared with non–insulin-treated diabetic (9.7%) and nondiabetic (6.2%) patients (132). Diabetic women have a particularly poor prognosis, with an almost twofold increase in mortality compared with diabetic men (110).

The excess in-hospital mortality associated with diabetes correlates primarily with an increased incidence of CHF (110). However, there is no evidence that diabetes is associated with larger infarctions, and systolic function is similar in patients with and without diabetes (110,112). These observations led to the suggestion that preexisting diastolic dysfunction (see Arterial Stiffness and Diastolic Dysfunction in Diabetes) is a major culprit of the congestive symptoms (112).

Other contributing mechanisms to the worse clinical outcome of patients with diabetes in the acute phase of infarction include (a) the diffuse nature of coronary atherosclerosis in diabetes, (b) reduced ability to develop collateral blood vessels in the presence of CAD (133), and (c) an abnormal pattern of exogenous substrate use in the setting of ischemia and postreperfusion period leading to increased oxygen consumption by the myocardium.

Diabetic patients surviving the acute phase of myocardial infarction suffer from high late mortality rates, which are mainly related to recurrent myocardial infarction and the development of new CHF (110,134,135).

Fibrinolytic Therapy and Primary Angioplasty

Patients with diabetes treated with fibrinolytic agents benefit by the same mortality reduction as nondiabetic patients (110,136). Importantly, no increase in serious bleeding complications or stroke has been observed in diabetics (136,137), and retinal bleeding is extremely uncommon (138).

Primary PCI has emerged as the preferred reperfusion strategy in patients with acute ST-elevation infarction, and appears to be an effective alternative to thrombolysis in diabetic patients (128,139,140). In the CAPTIM trial (141), there was a trend toward improved outcome among patients with diabetes who were randomized to primary angioplasty compared with those randomized to prehospital fibrinolytic therapy (relative risk for the primary endpoint of death, recurrent myocardial infarction and stroke at 30 days 2.47; 95% confidence interval 0.91–6.74).

However, patients with diabetes remain at increased risk for adverse outcomes after primary PCI compared with patients without diabetes (142,143). Despite excellent angiographic results and restoration of epicardial flow, patients with diabetes are more likely to have abnormal myocardial microvascular perfusion (144).

Glucose–Insulin–Potassium Infusions and Glycemic Control

A large randomized controlled trial including over 20,000 patients with acute ST-elevation infarction found a neutral effect of glucose–insulin–potassium (GIK) infusion with regard to mortality, cardiac arrest and cardiogenic shock (145). The Dutch Glucose–Insulin–Potassium Study found no significant benefit of GIK in patients undergoing primary angioplasty (146).

Metabolic derangements during myocardial infarction are particularly evident in patients with diabetes, who already have diminished capability to secrete insulin, diminished utilization of glucose for production of energy-rich phosphates, and excessive oxidation of FFA. However, in the DIGAMI-2 study GIK infusion did not affect the outcome of patients with diabetes and acute myocardial infarction, although the study was terminated prematurely owing to slow patient recruitment rate, and failed to achieve satisfactory glycemic control (147).

CORONARY REVASCULARIZATION

Angioplasty in patients with diabetes is associated with unique problems including higher periprocedural complication rates, a greater incidence of restenosis, and adverse long-term outcome after PCI. Therefore, the decision regarding optimal revascularization method requires special attention in these patients.

Coronary Angioplasty

As many as 25% of PCIs involve patients with diabetes. Procedural success rates and completeness of revascularization are similar in patients with and without diabetes (148–150). In-hospital complications (death, infarction, and need for emergency surgery) rates have been reported to be higher in patients with diabetes PCI (148,150). Although these differences are small, periprocedural complications are poorly tolerated by patients with diabetes, leading to a higher rate of periprocedural death (151).

Greater restenosis rates and adverse long-term outcome, especially in the presence of multivessel disease, have been consistently reported in patients with diabetes. Angiographic restenosis rates of 37% to 50% have been reported following successful stenting among patients with diabetes (152,153), frequently leading to bypass grafting for symptomatic relief (150,153,154). The high incidence of restenosis in diabetic patients is associated with a greater need for repeat revascularization, high cardiac event rate, and lower overall survival rates, especially in the presence of multivessel disease (153,155,156).

Increased restenosis rates in patients with diabetes appear to be related to exaggerated intimal proliferation at the site of angioplasty-induced arterial injury (157). Multiple potential mechanisms related either to hyperglycemia (158,159) or insulin resistance (160,161) contribute to exaggerated intimal hyperplasia following arterial injury in patients with diabetes. Recent data suggest that AGEs–RAGE interaction following arterial injury may contribute to restenosis in diabetes (162,163).

Vessel occlusion at angioplasty sites was observed in 15% of patients with diabetes, ranging from 11% for a one-site procedure to 37% for a three-site procedure. This complication was associated with a reduction in LV ejection fraction at follow-up. Restenosis with vessel occlusion appears to be a major determinant of long-term mortality (164).

Drug-Eluting Stents

Analysis of the diabetic subgroup in the SIRIUS trial (165) demonstrated that sirolimus-eluting stents reduced the relative incidence of in-lesion angiographic restenosis from 59.5% to 17.6% in patients with diabetes (65% reduction) and from 30.7% to 6.1% in patients without diabetes (80% reduction). In both patients with and without diabetes, sirolimus-eluting stents transformed restenosis from diffuse to focal pattern. However, the absolute late loss and restenosis remain higher in patients with diabetes receiving sirolimus-eluting stents, and diabetes remained an independent predictor of Target lesion revascularization (TLR) (OR 1.65, $P = .03$). Furthermore, in insulin-requiring patients, the angiographic in-segment restenosis rate was 35% in the sirolimus-eluting stents arm and 50% in the bare metal stent (BMS) arm (165). Analysis of the diabetic subgroup in the RAVEL trial also supports the superiority of the sirolimus-eluting stents for the treatment of noncomplex lesions in patients with diabetes (166).

In the TAXUS-IV randomized trial, the relative and absolute magnitude of the paclitaxel-eluting stent in patients with diabetes was comparable to that of nondiabetics. Moreover, diffuse in-stent restenosis was reduced by more than 90% in patients with diabetes receiving the paclitaxel-eluting stent, such that when angiographic restenosis did occur, it was predominantly focal in nature (167). In a randomized trial comparing the efficacy of the sirolimus-eluting stent and the paclitaxel-eluting stent in patients with diabetes, the paclitaxel stent was associated with a higher rate of in-segment late luminal loss as well as an increased risk of angiographic restenosis (168). However, these studies were not powered to show significant reductions in clinical endpoints.

Drug-eluting stents are considered by many to be the standard of care for patients with diabetes undergoing PCI. However, patients with the most complex diabetes (e.g., those with multivessel and diffuse disease) were excluded from enrollment in the drug-eluting stent trials, and angiographic follow-up was incomplete.

Coronary Artery Bypass Grafting Operation

Patients with diabetes undergoing coronary artery bypass grafting (CABG) surgery have higher rates of wound infection involving both sternotomy and graft harvest sites, increased incidence of acute renal failure, and prolonged postoperative stay (169,170). Higher rates of postoperative death and stroke have also been reported (171). Aggressive, perioperative glucose control through the use of continuous, IV insulin infusion reduces the incidence of deep wound infection (170,172,173) and perioperative morbidity (173).

Despite smaller distal vessels and vessels judged to be of poorer quality in the diabetic population, diabetes does not appear to adversely affect patency of internal mammary or vein grafts (174,175). The large long-term survival benefit conveyed by internal mammary grafting in patients with diabetes (149) also suggests high patency rates, similar to the nondiabetic population.

The relative survival benefit of CABG surgery versus medical therapy is comparable in diabetic and nondiabetic patients (170). However, long-term survival rate after bypass surgery remains lower in diabetic then in nondiabetic patients (169–171,176).

Multivessel Angioplasty Versus Coronary Artery Bypass Grafting

The Bypass Angioplasty Revascularization Investigation (BARI) study enrolled 1,829 patients with angiographically documented multivessel CAD and either clinically severe angina or objective evidence of marked myocardial ischemia requiring revascularization. At 5 years, there was a near doubling of mortality among diabetics on insulin or oral therapy assigned to multivessel angioplasty compared with those assigned to surgery (35% versus 19%, $P = .003$). In contrast, the 5-year mortality in nondiabetics and diabetics not on drug treatment was 9% with both revascularization strategies (177). The 5.4-year cardiac mortality rates was 3.5-fold higher in the percutaneous transluminal coronary angioplasty (PTCA) group (20.6 % versus 5.8%) (149). The survival benefit of CABG was limited to the 81% diabetic patients receiving an internal mammary graft. Cardiac mortality after was 2.9% when internal mammary graft was used and 18.2% when only vein grafts were used. The latter rate was similar to patients receiving PTCA (20.6%) (149).

The results of other randomized trials comparing multivessel angioplasty to CABG are consistent with the BARI findings. Long-term follow-up of patients participating in the Emory Angioplasty versus Surgery Trial (EAST) demonstrated an improved outcome in diabetic patients randomized to CABG (75.5% versus 60.1% with PTCA at 8 years) (178).

The Arterial Revascularization Therapy Study compared stenting and CABG for the treatment of patients with multivessel coronary disease. The incidence of 5-year mortality in patients with diabetes assigned to multivessel stenting was 5.1% higher (179). Based on the available evidence, surgery should continue to be viewed as the preferred therapy for diabetic patients with multivessel disease when using bare metal stents. However, the difference in outcomes seen between bare metal stents versus CABG for the treatment of multivessel disease is likely to narrow substantially with the advent of drug-eluting stents.

Mechanism of Coronary Artery Bypass Grafting Protection

The BARI investigators have identified two mechanisms for the protective effect of CABG in diabetes. First, a strong protective effect with respect to survival in a small group of patients who sustained a Q-wave myocardial infarction, accounting for about 50% of the overall reduction in mortality attributable to the procedure. Second, a moderate constant reduction in mortality throughout follow-up that occurred in the majority of diabetic patients who remained free of myocardial infarction during follow-up. A steadily increasing advantage of CABG compared with PTCA was also apparent at 7-year follow-up (180).

The protective effects of CABG may be related to the increased restenosis rates following angioplasty in diabetes and incomplete revascularization associated with multivessel angioplasty (155,181). In the BARI study population, 3.1 grafts were placed per patient undergoing CABG, whereas the mean number of successfully treated lesions in the PTCA group was 2.0 (149). Together with the high restenosis rate, it is likely that a higher proportion of the myocardium remains unrevascularized in patients with diabetes. The impact of incomplete revascularization may be even more severe in view of the more diffuse and distal CAD, poor collateral development (133), and microcirculatory dysfunction in diabetes.

DIABETIC AUTONOMIC NEUROPATHY AND THE HEART

Although clinically apparent autonomic neuropathy (e.g., orthostatic hypotension, gastroparesis) generally occur only in patients with diabetes of long duration, subclinical diabetic autonomic neuropathy, mainly in the form of cardiac autonomic neuropathy (CAN), evolves early in the course of diabetes (182). CAN is extremely common in both type 1 and type 2 diabetes, affecting up to 60% of unselected populations (182,183). Cardiovascular risk factors may accelerate the adverse effectsof hyperglycemia on the peripheral nerves in patients with diabetes (184).

CAN involves parasympathetic dysfunction as well as derangements of adrenergic cardiac innervation (182,185). Reduced heart rate variability is a hallmark and earliest indicator of CAN in diabetic patients and may confer a higher risk for arrhythmic events (182,183). Patients with autonomic neuropathy have a decreased myocardial perfusion reserve capacity when challenged with a vasodilatator, possibly because of defective myocardial sympathetic vasodilatation (186).

Autonomic neuropathy with involvement of the sensory supply to the heart may lead to painless infarction and ischemic episodes in diabetics (187). Several studies have correlated abnormalities in autonomic function in patients with silent ischemia (182).

THERAPY

Prevention of CVD in patients with diabetes requires intensified multifactorial intervention comprising behavioral modification and pharmacologic therapies aimed at several modifiable risk factors, including control of glycemia, blood pressure, and blood lipid levels, as well as smoking cessation (188). Long-term, intensified intervention involving multiple risk factors has been shown to reduce the risk of cardiovascular events in patients with type 2 diabetes (189). However, despite these evidence-based guidelines, only a small fraction (3% to 12%) of adults diagnosed with diabetes in the United States are achieving the currently recommended level of control (190).

Dyslipidemia

Nonpharmacologic strategies to treat dyslipidemia in diabetes include dietary modification, weight loss, physical exercise, and improved glycemic control (21). In patients with type 1 diabetes, optimal glycemic control should result in normal or below-normal lipoprotein levels, and prevent the atherogenic state associated with lipoprotein glycosylation. Improved diabetic control in type 2 diabetes is beneficial but not always associated with reversal of lipoprotein abnormalities (21).

Pharmacologic Therapy

Recent publications have argued against the relevance the traditional classification to primary and secondary CVD prevention in diabetes (21). The rationale for this approach is that patients with diabetes have a relatively high 10-year risk of developing CVD. In addition, the onset of CVD in patients with diabetes carries a poor prognosis, both at the time of an acute event and in the post-event period (21,110,191). These considerations led to the recommendation that LDL cholesterol should

TABLE 4.6

STANDARDS OF MEDICAL CARE IN PATIENTS WITH DIABETES (188,191,198)

Indications for initial treatment and goals for adult hypertensive diabetic patient			
	Systolic	**Diastolic**	
Goal (mm Hg)	130<	<80	
Behavioral therapy alone (maximum 3 months) then add pharmacologic treatment	130–139	80–89	
Behavioral therapy and pharmacologic treatment	≥140	≥90	
Target lipid levels and treatment priorities for adult patients with diabetes[b]			
ORDER OF PRIORITIES			
I. LDL cholesterol lowering			
II. HDL cholesterol raising			
III. Triglyceride lowering			
	Target lipid levels		
LDL cholesterol			
Known CVD[a]	<70 mg/dL (1.8 mmol/L)		
Without overt CAD[b]	<100 mg/dL (2.6 mmol/L)		
HDL cholesterol	Men: >40 mg/dL (1.15 mmol/L) Women: >50 mg/dL (1.40 mmol/L)		
Triglycerides	<150 mg/dL (1.7 mmol/L)		
Glycemic control for nonpregnant individuals with diabetes[c]			
	Normal	**Goal**	**Additional action suggested[d]**
Average preprandial glucose (mg/dL)	<110	90–130	<90/>150
Average bedtime glucose (mg/dL)	<120	10–150	<110/>180
HbA1c (%)	<6	<7	8>

[a]Initiation of statin therapy regardless of baseline LDL-C levels.
[b]At age ≥40, statin therapy is recommended regardless baseline LDL levels.
[c]Values calibrated to plasma glucose. Whole blood values are 10 mg/dL lower.
[d]Values above/below these levels are not "goals" nor are they "acceptable" in most patients. They are an indication for a significant change in the treatment plan. A1c is referenced to a nondiabetic range of 4.0% to 6.0% (mean 5.0%, SD 0.5%).

be lowered to below 100 mg/dL in diabetic subjects without prior CAD (21,188,191).

The first priority of pharmacologic therapy is to lower LDL cholesterol followed by an emphasis on HDL cholesterol and lastly on triglyceride levels (188) (Table 4.6). The Heart Protection Study (HPS) demonstrated that in people with diabetes over the age of 40 years with a total cholesterol above 135 mg/dL, LDL reduction of approximately 30% from baseline with simvastatin was associated with about a 25% reduction in the first event rate for major CVD events independent of baseline LDL, preexisting vascular disease, type or duration of diabetes, or adequacy of glycemic control (192). In HPS, patients with both diabetes and CVD obtained the greatest benefit from statin therapy. Therefore, the presence of this combination supports initiation of statin therapy regardless of baseline LDL-C levels, with a goal of achieving LDL-C to below 70 mg/dL (191).

It remains unclear whether LDL-lowering drugs are indicated when the baseline LDL-C is less than 100 mg/dL in this group and whether the less than 70 mg/dL should be used. However, recent data from the Collaborative Atorvastatin Diabetes Study (CARDS) challenges the use of a particular threshold level of LDL-C as a sole arbiter of which patient with type 2 diabetes should receive statin treatment (193). In this study, a 26% reduction in major cardiovascular events occurred in patients with baseline LDL-C concentrations below 100 mg/dL. Based on HPS and CARDS, the American Diabetes Association recommends statin therapy to achieve an LDL reduction of about 30% to 40% regardless of baseline LDL in patients over the age of 40 years without overt CVD (188) (Table 4.6).

The fibric acid derivatives are effective in the treatment of hypertriglyceridemia in diabetic patients and do not adversely affect glucose metabolism. Fenofibrate has been shown to reduce the angiographic progression of CAD in type 2 diabetes (194).

The use of nicotinic acid has been discouraged in patients with diabetes owing to possible deterioration in glycemic control (21). However, at modest doses (750 to 2000 mg/d), significant benefit with regard to LDL, HDL, and triglyceride levels are accompanied by only modest changes in glucose that are generally amenable to adjustments of diabetes therapy (188,195).

Hypertension

The combined presence of hypertension and diabetes considerably accelerates the development of both macrovascular and microvascular diabetic complications. Controlling blood pressure levels has been shown to reduce the incidence of CVD by 33% to 50% in patients with diabetes and hypertension (196). For people with diabetes, the blood pressure goal to reduce cardiovascular risk was defined as below 130/85 mm Hg by the Joint National Committee on Prevention, Detection, Evaluation, and Treatment of High Blood Pressure (JNC 7) (197). In addition, because of the high cardiovascular risk associated with blood pressure of 130/80 mm Hg or higher in patients with diabetes, this value is considered to be the cut point for defining hypertension, rather than 140/90 mm Hg, as in the general population.

The American Diabetes Association recommends a more aggressive program of blood pressure reduction, aiming for a target of less than 130/80 mm Hg in patients with diabetes (188,198) (Table 4.6). This goal requires multiple drug antihypertensive therapy with two or three antihypertensive agents in patients with diabetes (199,200).

Pharmacologic Therapy

Current evidence suggests that, for the prevention of cardiovascular events, angiotensin-converting enzyme (ACE) inhibitors diuretics, β-adrenergic blockers and calcium antagonists effectively reduce mortality and morbidity in patients with diabetes and hypertension. However, there is no clear proof that one class of drugs is better than another (198). However, because of the large number of studies in patients with diabetes demonstrating improvement in both microvascular and macrovascular outcomes, it is now an established practice to begin antihypertensive drug therapy in patients with diabetes with an ACE inhibitor even in the absence of microalbuminuria (198). Angiotensin II receptor blockers can be considered equal to ACE inhibitors in patients with type 2 diabetes (201).

Thiazides are often effective antihypertensive agents in diabetes, and are considered an appropriate choice for a second or third drug (198). Because in the United Kingdom Prospective Diabetes Study (UKPDS) no difference was found between atenolol and captopril in improving multiple diabetes-related endpoints (199), β-blockers are also appropriate choice for a second drug. Calcium channel blockers contribute to improvements in outcomes when combined with ACE inhibitors to achieve low-targeted blood pressure (202). It is important to emphasize that aggressive blood pressure reduction may be more important than the specific drug regimen being used (198).

Glycemic Control

Prospective randomized controlled studies have shown that achieving glycemic control is associated with decreased rate of retinopathy, nephropathy and neuropathy (203). The effects of improved glycemic control on cardiovascular outcomes are less impressive. However, tight control retards the development of atherosclerosis in type 1 patients as measured by the development of carotid intimal media thickening (13).

In the UKPDS, the intensive-treatment group demonstrated a 16% risk reduction ($P = .052$) for fatal and nonfatal myocardial infarction (203). However, epidemiologic analysis of the UKPDS cohort showed a statistically significant effect of HbA1c lowering with an approximate 14% reduction in all-cause mortality and myocardial infarction for every 1% reduction in HbA1c (204). The current recommendations of the American Diabetes Association for glycemic control are summarized in Table 4.6.

However, the insulin-sensitizing thiazolidinediones are agonists of the nuclear receptor peroxisomal proliferation activating receptor-γ that in vitro can decrease proinflammatory functions of macrophages and smooth muscle cells. Thus, these agents may have direct effects on key processes in atherosclerosis (205).

Prevention of Type 2 Diabetes

Randomized controlled trials have shown that the onset of type 2 diabetes can be prevented or delayed with lifestyle modifications or pharmacologic interventions (206,207). In the Diabetes Prevention Program, metformin was about half as effective as diet and exercise in delaying the onset of diabetes. This effect was obtained with modest weight loss (5%–10% of body weight) and modest physical activity (30 minutes daily). The greater benefit of weight loss and physical inactivity strongly suggests that lifestyle modification should be the first choice to prevent or delay diabetes (208).

CONTROVERSIES AND PERSONAL PERSPECTIVES

In recent years, diabetes has become a major research focus in the field of preventive and clinical cardiology. The recognition that CVD in patients with diabetes is associated with unique problems led to the design of clinical trails addressing specific therapeutic questions in patients with diabetes. These research efforts, together with the advent of effective therapies, resulted in a substantial reduction in rate of incident CVD among patients with diabetes. However, despite substantial progress, patients with diabetes remain at a consistent, approximately twofold excess of cardiovascular events, and the onset of CVD in patients with diabetes carries a poor prognosis, both at the time of an acute event and in the post-event period. The predicted increase in the number of patients with diabetes indicates that diabetes and atherosclerosis will continue to be of major concern to physicians and the health care system.

Randomized primary prevention trials have clearly shown that glycemic control reduces the incidence of microvascular complications in both type 1 and type 2 diabetes. However, the effect on macrovascular complications was modest. It is possible that a long time is necessary for the reversal of established hyperglycemia-induced vascular pathology. Furthermore, in diabetic patients with functioning pancreatic transplants renal pathology continues to progress for at least 5 years after diabetes has been cured. The mechanism for these observations is unclear, but may be related to a slow replacement of glycosylated molecules or because phenotypic alterations in vascular cells may persist despite the return of normoglycemia (the so-called memory effect).

Lipid lowering and aggressive blood pressure reduction appear to be more efficacious than glycemic control as primary prevention in patients with diabetes. Additionally, improvement in insulin resistance appears to inhibit the atherogenic processes in the vascular wall independent of metabolic control. Given the complexity and multiple mechanisms that contribute to the pathogenesis of atherosclerosis in diabetes, a multifactorial intervention approach is logical, and provides the best evidence-based treatment plan for preventing cardiac events.

The diffuse nature of the atherosclerotic process in diabetic patients is often emphasized. However, the striking excess of coronary events in diabetic patients with or without established CAD appears to be out of proportion to the severity of atherosclerosis. These observations raise the possibility that unique pathogenic mechanisms in diabetes operate to weaken plaque stability.

THE FUTURE

Current lines of investigation focus of several interactions between diabetes and mechanisms of atherosclerosis. There is growing evidence regarding the critical role of oxidative stress and particularly hyperglycemia-induced reactive oxygen production in the pathogenesis of diabetic complications. Importantly, oxidant stress augments other hyperglycemia-dependent mechanisms of vascular damage, including AGEs formation, PKC activation, increased flux through the hexosamine pathway, and endothelial dysfunction. Conventional antioxidants appear to be ineffective in reducing the amount of superoxide that is continuously produced under hyperglycemic conditions. New types of antioxidants, catalytic antioxidants such as a superoxide dismutase/catalase mimetic are currently being studied.

Markers of inflammation are associated with insulin resistance and the development of type 2 diabetes and are raised in patients with type 2 diabetes. Understanding the complex relationship between inflammation and diabetes may improve our understanding of diabetic vascular disease. There is little understanding of the factors that abnormal hemostatic and fibrinolytic function observed in patients with diabetes. Finally, the pathogenesis, natural history, and clinical significance of diabetic cardiomyopathy remain to be determined.

Although there is growing evidence for the use of drug-eluting stents in patients with diabetes undergoing PCI, it is less clear whether these improvements reached the stage where PCI can challenge surgery as the optimal revascularization strategy in patients with diabetes and multivessel disease. Prospective studies designed specifically to address this question are under way.

Prevention of both type 1 and type 2 diabetes is a major focus of basic and clinical investigations. Screening of the human genome for susceptibility genes for diabetes can identify regions of genetic susceptibility, after which the final localization of disease genes can be carried out, followed by sequencing of candidate genes to identify the specific mutations. Multiple molecular defects can lead to type 2 diabetes and the molecular details of several rare forms of type 2 diabetes have already been identified.

References

1. Zimmet P, Alberti KG, Shaw J. Global and societal implications of the diabetes epidemic. *Nature* 2001;414:782–787.
2. King H, Aubert RE, Herman WH. Global burden of diabetes, 1995–2025: prevalence, numerical estimates, and projections [see comments]. *Diabetes Care* 1998;21:1414–1431.
3. Harris MI. Diabetes in America: epidemiology and scope of the problem. *Diabetes Care* 1998;21[Suppl 3]:C11–14.
4. Sinha R, Fisch G, Teague B, et al. Prevalence of impaired glucose tolerance among children and adolescents with marked obesity. *N Engl J Med* 2002;346:802–810.
5. Howard BV, Rodriguez BL, Bennett PH, et al. Prevention Conference VI: Diabetes and Cardiovascular Disease: Writing Group I: epidemiology. *Circulation* 2002;105:e132–137.
6. Fox CS, Coady S, Sorlie PD, et al. Trends in cardiovascular complications of diabetes. *JAMA* 2004;292:2495–2499.
7. Beckman JA, Creager MA, Libby P. Diabetes and atherosclerosis: epidemiology, pathophysiology, and management. *JAMA* 2002;287:2570–2581.
8. American Diabetes Association. Consensus Statement: role of cardiovascular risk factors in prevention and treatment of macrovascular disease in diabetes. *Diabetes Care* 1993;16:72–78.
9. Haffner SM, Lehto S, Ronnemaa T, et al. Mortality from coronary heart disease in subjects with type 2 diabetes and in nondiabetic subjects with and without prior myocardial infarction. *N Engl J Med* 1998;339:229–234.
10. Libby P, Nathan DM, Abraham K, et al. Report of the National Heart, Lung, and Blood Institute-National Institute of Diabetes and Digestive and Kidney Diseases Working Group on Cardiovascular Complications of Type 1 Diabetes Mellitus. *Circulation* 2005;111:3489–3493.
11. Krolewski AS, Kosinski EJ, Warram JH, et al. Magnitude and determinants of coronary artery disease in juvenile- onset, insulin-dependent diabetes mellitus. *Am J Cardiol* 1987;59:750–755.
12. Laing SP, Swerdlow AJ, Slater SD, et al. Mortality from heart disease in a cohort of 23,000 patients with insulin-treated diabetes. *Diabetologia* 2003;46:760–765.
13. Nathan DM, Lachin J, Cleary P, et al. Intensive diabetes therapy and carotid intima-media thickness in type 1 diabetes mellitus. *N Engl J Med* 2003;348:2294–2303.
14. Snell-Bergeon JK, Hokanson JE, Jensen L, et al. Progression of coronary artery calcification in type 1 diabetes: the importance of glycemic control. *Diabetes Care* 2003;26:2923–2928.
15. Borch-Johnsen K, Kreiner S. Proteinuria: value as predictor of cardiovascular mortality in insulin dependent diabetes mellitus. *Br Med J (Clin Res Ed)* 1987;294:1651–1654.
16. Deckert T, Kofoed-Enevoldsen A, Norgaard K, et al. Microalbuminuria. Implications for micro- and macrovascular disease. *Diabetes Care* 1992;15:1181–1191.
17. Makita Z, Radoff S, Rayfield EJ, et al. Advanced glycosylation end products in patients with diabetic nephropathy [see comments]. *N Engl J Med* 1991;325:836–842.
18. Stamler J, Vaccaro O, Neaton JD, et al. Diabetes, other risk factors, and 12-yr cardiovascular mortality for men screened in the Multiple Risk Factor Intervention Trial. *Diabetes Care* 1993;16:434–444.
19. Barrett-Connor EL, Cohn BA, Wingard DL, et al. Why is diabetes mellitus a stronger risk factor for fatal ischemic heart disease in women than in men? The Rancho Bernardo Study [published erratum appears in *JAMA* 1991;265:3249]. *JAMA* 1991;265:627–631.
20. Ginsberg HN. Lipoprotein physiology in nondiabetic and diabetic states. Relationship to atherogenesis. *Diabetes Care* 1991;14:839–855.
21. Haffner SM. Management of dyslipidemia in adults with diabetes. *Diabetes Care* 1998;21:160–178.
22. Selby JV, Austin MA, Newman B, et al. LDL subclass phenotypes and the insulin resistance syndrome in women. *Circulation* 1993;88:381–387.
23. Haffner SM, D'Agostino R Jr, Goff D, et al. LDL size in African Americans, Hispanics, and non-Hispanic whites: the insulin resistance atherosclerosis study. *Arterioscler Thromb Vasc Biol* 1999;19:2234–2240.
24. Syvanne M, Taskinen MR. Lipids and lipoproteins as coronary risk factors in non-insulin-dependent diabetes mellitus. *Lancet* 1997;350:SI20–SI23.
25. Ginsberg HN. Diabetic dyslipidemia: basic mechanisms underlying the common hypertriglyceridemia and low HDL cholesterol levels. *Diabetes* 1996;45[Suppl 3]:S27–30.
26. Ginsberg HN. Insulin resistance and cardiovascular disease. *J Clin Invest* 2000;106:453–458.
27. Packard CJ, Shepherd J. Lipoprotein heterogeneity and apolipoprotein B metabolism. *Arterioscler Thromb Vasc Biol* 1997;17:3542–3556.
28. Bucala R, Mitchell R, Arnold K, et al. Identification of the major site of apolipoprotein B modification by advanced glycosylation end products blocking uptake by the low density lipoprotein receptor. *J Biol Chem* 1995;270:10828–10832.
29. Bucala R, Makita Z, Koschinsky T, et al. Lipid advanced glycosylation: pathway for lipid oxidation in vivo. *Proc Natl Acad Sci USA* 1993;90: 6434–6438.
30. Williams SB, Goldfine AB, Timimi FK, et al. Acute hyperglycemia attenuates endothelium-dependent vasodilation in humans in vivo. *Circulation* 1998;97:1695–1701.
31. De Vriese AS, Verbeuren TJ, Van de Voorde J, et al. Endothelial dysfunction in diabetes. *Br J Pharmacol* 2000;130:963–974.
32. Calles-Escandon J, Cipolla M. Diabetes and endothelial dysfunction: a clinical perspective. *Endocr Rev* 2001;22:36–52.
33. Nishikawa T, Edelstein D, Du XL, et al. Normalizing mitochondrial superoxide production blocks three pathways of hyperglycaemic damage. *Nature* 2000;404:787–790.
34. Brownlee M. The pathobiology of diabetic complications: a unifying mechanism. *Diabetes* 2005;54:1615–1625.
35. Brodsky SV, Morrishow AM, Dharia N, et al. Glucose scavenging of nitric oxide. *Am J Physiol Renal Physiol* 2001;280:F480–F486.
36. Garcia Soriano F, Virag L, Jagtap P, et al. Diabetic endothelial dysfunction: the role of poly(ADP-ribose) polymerase activation. *Nat Med* 2001;7:108–113.
37. Soriano FG, Pacher P, Mabley J, et al. Rapid reversal of the diabetic endothelial dysfunction by pharmacological inhibition of poly(ADP-ribose) polymerase. *Circ Res* 2001;89:684–691.
38. Guzik TJ, Mussa S, Gastaldi D, et al. Mechanisms of increased vascular superoxide production in human diabetes mellitus: role of NAD(P)H oxidase and endothelial nitric oxide synthase. *Circulation* 2002;105:1656–1662.
39. Du XL, Edelstein D, Dimmeler S, et al. Hyperglycemia inhibits endothelial nitric oxide synthase activity by posttranslational modification at the Akt site. *J Clin Invest* 2001;108:1341–1348.
40. Rosen P, Nawroth PP, King G, et al. The role of oxidative stress in the onset and progression of diabetes and its complications: a summary of a Congress Series sponsored by UNESCO-MCBN, the American Diabetes Association and the German Diabetes Society. *Diabetes Metab Res Rev* 2001;17:189–212.
41. Kobayashi T, Tahara Y, Matsumoto M, et al. Roles of thromboxane A(2) and prostacyclin in the development of atherosclerosis in apoE-deficient mice. *J Clin Invest* 2004;114:784–794.
42. Vinik AI, Erbas T, Park TS, et al. Platelet dysfunction in type 2 diabetes. *Diabetes Care* 2001;24:1476–1485.
43. Knobler H, Savion N, Shenkman B, et al. Shear-induced platelet adhesion and aggregation on subendothelium are increased in diabetic patients. *Thromb Res* 1998;90:181–190.
44. Davi G, Gresele P, Violi F, et al. Diabetes mellitus, hypercholesterolemia, and hypertension but not vascular disease per se are associated with persistent platelet activation in vivo. Evidence derived from the study of peripheral arterial disease. *Circulation* 1997;96:69–75.
45. Marx N, Imhof A, Froehlich J, et al. Effect of rosiglitazone treatment on soluble CD40L in patients with type 2 diabetes and coronary artery disease. *Circulation* 2003;107:1954–1957.
46. Tschoepe D, Roesen P, Kaufmann L, et al. Evidence for abnormal platelet glycoprotein expression in diabetes mellitus. *Eur J Clin Invest* 1990;20: 166–170.

47. Tschoepe D, Driesch E, Schwippert B, et al. Exposure of adhesion molecules on activated platelets in patients with newly diagnosed IDDM is not normalized by near-normoglycemia. *Diabetes* 1995;44:890–894.
48. Tschoepe D, Roesen P, Schwippert B, et al. Platelets in diabetes: the role in the hemostatic regulation in atherosclerosis. *Semin Thromb Hemost* 1993;19:122–128.
49. Shechter M, Merz CN, Paul-Labrador MJ, et al. Blood glucose and platelet-dependent thrombosis in patients with coronary artery disease. *J Am Coll Cardiol* 2000;35:300–307.
50. Davi G, Ciabattoni G, Consoli A, et al. In vivo formation of 8-iso-prostaglandin f2alpha and platelet activation in diabetes mellitus: effects of improved metabolic control and vitamin E supplementation [see comments]. *Circulation* 1999;99:224–229.
51. Yamagishi SI, Edelstein D, Du XL, et al. Hyperglycemia potentiates collagen-induced platelet activation through mitochondrial superoxide overproduction. *Diabetes* 2001;50:1491–1494.
52. Watala C, Golanski J, Pluta J, et al. Reduced sensitivity of platelets from type 2 diabetic patients to acetylsalicylic acid (aspirin)-its relation to metabolic control. *Thromb Res* 2004;113:101–113.
53. Watala C, Pluta J, Golanski J, et al. Increased protein glycation in diabetes mellitus is associated with decreased aspirin-mediated protein acetylation and reduced sensitivity of blood platelets to aspirin. *J Mol Med* 2005; 83:148–158.
54. Angiolillo DJ, Fernandez-Ortiz A, Bernardo E, et al. Platelet function profiles in patients with type 2 diabetes and coronary artery disease on combined aspirin and clopidogrel treatment. *Diabetes* 2005;54:2430–2435.
55. Stehouwer CD, Nauta JJ, Zeldenrust GC, et al. Urinary albumin excretion, cardiovascular disease, and endothelial dysfunction in non-insulin-dependent diabetes mellitus. *Lancet* 1992;340:319–323.
56. Kannel WB, D'Agostino RB, Wilson PW, et al. Diabetes, fibrinogen, and risk of cardiovascular disease: the Framingham experience. *Am Heart J* 1990;120:672–676.
57. Vague P, Juhan-Vague I. Fibrinogen, fibrinolysis and diabetes mellitus: a comment. *Diabetologia* 1997;40:738–740.
58. D'Elia JA, Weinrauch LA, Gleason RE, et al. Fibrinogen and factor VII levels improve with glycemic control in patients with type 1 diabetes mellitus who have microvascular complications. *Arch Intern Med* 2001;161: 98–101.
59. Emanuele N, Azad N, Abraira C, et al. Effect of intensive glycemic control on fibrinogen, lipids, and lipoproteins: Veterans Affairs Cooperative Study in Type II Diabetes Mellitus. *Arch Intern Med* 1998;158:2485–2490.
60. Kapur R, Hoffman CJ, Bhushan V, et al. Postprandial elevation of activated factor VII in young adults. *Arterioscler Thromb Vasc Biol* 1996;16:1327–1332.
61. Rao AK, Chouhan V, Chen X, et al. Activation of the tissue factor pathway of blood coagulation during prolonged hyperglycemia in young healthy men. *Diabetes* 1999;48:1156–1161.
62. The Diabetes Control and Complications Trial Research Group. The effect of intensive treatment of diabetes on the development and progression of long-term complications in insulin-dependent diabetes mellitus. *N Engl J Med* 1993;329:977–986.
63. Ulrich P, Cerami A. Protein glycation, diabetes, and aging. *Recent Prog Horm Res* 2001;56:1–21.
64. Brownlee M, Cerami A, Vlassara H. Advanced glycosylation end products in tissue and the biochemical basis of diabetic complications. *N Engl J Med* 1988;318:1315–1321.
65. Schmidt AM, Yan SD, Wautier JL, et al. Activation of receptor for advanced glycation end products: a mechanism for chronic vascular dysfunction in diabetic vasculopathy and atherosclerosis. *Circ Res* 1999;84:489–497.
66. Schmidt AM, Yan SD, Yan SF, et al. The multiligand receptor RAGE as a progression factor amplifying immune and inflammatory responses. *J Clin Invest* 2001;108:949–955.
67. Yan SD, Schmidt AM, Anderson GM, et al. Enhanced cellular oxidant stress by the interaction of advanced glycation end products with their receptors/binding proteins. *J Biol Chem* 1994;269:9889–9897.
68. Wautier JL, Wautier MP, Schmidt AM, et al. Advanced glycation end products (AGEs) on the surface of diabetic erythrocytes bind to the vessel wall via a specific receptor inducing oxidant stress in the vasculature: a link between surface-associated AGEs and diabetic complications. *Proc Natl Acad Sci U S A* 1994;91:7742–7746.
69. Basta G, Lazzerini G, Massaro M, et al. Advanced glycation end products activate endothelium through signal-transduction receptor RAGE: a mechanism for amplification of inflammatory responses. *Circulation* 2002; 105:816–822.
70. Vlassara H, Brownlee M, Manogue KR, et al. Cachectin/TNF and IL-1 induced by glucose-modified proteins: role in normal tissue remodeling. *Science* 1988;240:1546–1548.
71. Wautier JL, Zoukourian C, Chappey O, et al. Receptor-mediated endothelial cell dysfunction in diabetic vasculopathy. Soluble receptor for advanced glycation end products blocks hyperpermeability in diabetic rats. *J Clin Invest* 1996;97:238–243.
72. Park L, Raman KG, Lee KJ, et al. Suppression of accelerated diabetic atherosclerosis by the soluble receptor for advanced glycation endproducts. *Nat Med* 1998;4:1025–1031.
73. Koya D, King GL. Protein kinase C activation and the development of diabetic complications. *Diabetes* 1998;47:859–866.
74. Koya D, Haneda M, Nakagawa H, et al. Amelioration of accelerated diabetic mesangial expansion by treatment with a PKC beta inhibitor in diabetic db/db mice, a rodent model for type 2 diabetes. *FASEB J* 2000;14:439–447.
75. Brownlee M. Biochemistry and molecular cell biology of diabetic complications. *Nature* 2001;414:813–820.
76. Kouroedov A, Eto M, Joch H, et al. Selective inhibition of protein kinase Cbeta2 prevents acute effects of high glucose on vascular cell adhesion molecule-1 expression in human endothelial cells. *Circulation* 2004;110:91–96.
77. Du XL, Edelstein D, Rossetti L, et al. Hyperglycemia-induced mitochondrial superoxide overproduction activates the hexosamine pathway and induces plasminogen activator inhibitor-1 expression by increasing Sp1 glycosylation. *Proc Natl Acad Sci U S A* 2000;97:12222–12226.
78. Pennathur S, Wagner JD, Leeuwenburgh C, et al. A hydroxyl radical-like species oxidizes cynomolgus monkey artery wall proteins in early diabetic vascular disease. *J Clin Invest* 2001;107:853–860.
79. Aronson D, Bartha P, Zinder O, et al. Association between fasting glucose and C-reactive protein in middle-aged subjects. *Diabet Med* 2004;21: 39–44.
80. Meigs JB, Hu FB, Rifai N, et al. Biomarkers of endothelial dysfunction and risk of type 2 diabetes mellitus. *JAMA* 2004;291:1978–1986.
81. King DE, Mainous AG 3rd, Buchanan TA, et al. C-reactive protein and glycemic control in adults with diabetes. *Diabetes Care* 2003;26: 1535–1539.
82. Esposito K, Nappo F, Marfella R, et al. Inflammatory cytokine concentrations are acutely increased by hyperglycemia in humans: role of oxidative stress. *Circulation* 2002;106:2067–2072.
83. Guha M, Bai W, Nadler JL, et al. Molecular mechanisms of tumor necrosis factor alpha gene expression in monocytic cells via hyperglycemia-induced oxidant stress-dependent and—independent pathways. *J Biol Chem* 2000;275:17728–17739.
84. Lin Y, Berg AH, Iyengar P, et al. The hyperglycemia-induced inflammatory response in adipocytes: the role of reactive oxygen species. *J Biol Chem* 2005;280:4617–4626.
85. Lin Y, Rajala MW, Berger JP, et al. Hyperglycemia-induced production of acute phase reactants in adipose tissue. *J Biol Chem* 2001;276:42077–42083.
86. Haffner SM, Greenberg AS, Weston WM, et al. Effect of rosiglitazone treatment on nontraditional markers of cardiovascular disease in patients with type 2 diabetes mellitus. *Circulation* 2002;106:679–684.
87. Pfutzner A, Marx N, Lubben G, et al. Improvement of cardiovascular risk markers by pioglitazone is independent from glycemic control: results from the pioneer study. *J Am Coll Cardiol* 2005;45:1925–1931.
88. Schaumberg DA, Glynn RJ, Jenkins AJ, et al. Effect of intensive glycemic control on levels of markers of inflammation in type 1 diabetes mellitus in the diabetes control and complications trial. *Circulation* 2005;111:2446–2453.
89. Ford ES, Giles WH, Dietz WH. Prevalence of the metabolic syndrome among US adults: findings from the third National Health and Nutrition Examination Survey. *JAMA* 2002;287:356–359.
90. Hunt KJ, Resendez RG, Williams K, et al. National Cholesterol Education Program versus World Health Organization metabolic syndrome in relation to all-cause and cardiovascular mortality in the San Antonio Heart Study. *Circulation* 2004;110:1251–1257.
91. Isomaa B, Almgren P, Tuomi T, et al. Cardiovascular morbidity and mortality associated with the metabolic syndrome. *Diabetes Care* 2001;24: 683–689.
92. Kahn R, Buse J, Ferrannini E, et al. The metabolic syndrome: time for a critical appraisal Joint statement from the American Diabetes Association and the European Association for the Study of Diabetes. *Diabetologia* 2005;48:1684–1699.
93. Gale EA. The myth of the metabolic syndrome. *Diabetologia* 2005;48:1679–1683.
94. Reaven GM. The metabolic syndrome: requiescat in pace. *Clin Chem* 2005;51:931–938.
95. Wellen KE, Hotamisligil GS. Obesity-induced inflammatory changes in adipose tissue. *J Clin Invest* 2003;112:1785–1788.
96. Weisberg SP, McCann D, Desai M, et al. Obesity is associated with macrophage accumulation in adipose tissue. *J Clin Invest* 2003;112: 1796–1808.
97. Yudkin JS, Stehouwer CD, Emeis JJ, et al. C-reactive protein in healthy subjects: associations with obesity, insulin resistance, and endothelial dysfunction: a potential role for cytokines originating from adipose tissue? *Arterioscler Thromb Vasc Biol* 1999;19:972–978.
98. Hotamisligil GS, Arner P, Caro JF, et al. Increased adipose tissue expression of tumor necrosis factor-alpha in human obesity and insulin resistance. *J Clin Invest* 1995;95:2409–2415.
99. Greenfield JR, Samaras K, Jenkins AB, et al. Obesity is an important determinant of baseline serum C-reactive protein concentration in monozygotic twins, independent of genetic influences. *Circulation* 2004;109: 3022–3028.
100. Aronson D, Bartha P, Zinder O, et al. Obesity is the major determinant of elevated C-reactive protein in subjects with the metabolic syndrome. *Int J Obes Relat Metab Disord* 2004;28:674–679.

101. Kerner A, Avizohar O, Sella R, et al. Association between elevated liver enzymes and C-reactive protein: possible hepatic contribution to systemic inflammation in the metabolic syndrome. *Arterioscler Thromb Vasc Biol* 2005;25:193–197.
102. Festa A, D'Agostino R Jr, Howard G, et al. Chronic subclinical inflammation as part of the insulin resistance syndrome: the Insulin Resistance Atherosclerosis Study (IRAS). *Circulation* 2000;102:42–47.
103. Grundy SM, Hansen B, Smith SC Jr, et al. Clinical management of metabolic syndrome: report of the American Heart Association/National Heart, Lung, and Blood Institute/American Diabetes Association conference on scientific issues related to management. *Circulation* 2004;109: 551–556.
104. Dandona P, Aljada A, Chaudhuri A, et al. Metabolic syndrome: a comprehensive perspective based on interactions between obesity, diabetes, and inflammation. *Circulation* 2005;111:1448–1454.
105. Malik S, Wong ND, Franklin SS, et al. Impact of the metabolic syndrome on mortality from coronary heart disease, cardiovascular disease, and all causes in United States adults. *Circulation* 2004;110:1245–1250.
106. Ho KK, Anderson KM, Kannel WB, et al. Survival after the onset of congestive heart failure in Framingham Heart Study subjects [see comments]. *Circulation* 1993;88:107–115.
107. Witteles RM, Tang WH, Jamali AH, et al. Insulin resistance in idiopathic dilated cardiomyopathy: a possible etiologic link. *J Am Coll Cardiol* 2004;44:78–81.
108. Suskin N, McKelvie RS, Burns RJ, et al. Glucose and insulin abnormalities relate to functional capacity in patients with congestive heart failure. *Eur Heart J* 2000;21:1368–1375.
109. Tenenbaum A, Motro M, Fisman EZ, et al. Functional class in patients with heart failure is associated with the development of diabetes. *Am J Med* 2003;114:271–275.
110. Aronson D, Rayfield EJ, Chesebro JH. Mechanisms determining course and outcome of diabetic patients who have had acute myocardial infarction. *Ann Intern Med* 1997;126:296–306.
111. Lewis EF, Moye LA, Rouleau JL, et al. Predictors of late development of heart failure in stable survivors of myocardial infarction: the CARE study. *J Am Coll Cardiol* 2003;42:1446–1453.
112. Solomon SD, St John Sutton M, Lamas GA, et al. Ventricular remodeling does not accompany the development of heart failure in diabetic patients after myocardial infarction. *Circulation* 2002;106:1251–1255.
113. Carrabba N, Valenti R, Parodi G, et al. Left ventricular remodeling and heart failure in diabetic patients treated with primary angioplasty for acute myocardial infarction. *Circulation* 2004;110:1974–1979.
114. Zarich SW, Arbuckle BE, Cohen LR, et al. Diastolic abnormalities in young asymptomatic diabetic patients assessed by pulsed Doppler echocardiography. *J Am Coll Cardiol* 1988;12:114–120.
115. Paillole C, Dahan M, Paycha F, et al. Prevalence and significance of left ventricular filling abnormalities determined by Doppler echocardiography in young type I (insulin- dependent) diabetic patients. *Am J Cardiol* 1989;64:1010–1016.
116. Rutter MK, Parise H, Benjamin EJ, et al. Impact of glucose intolerance and insulin resistance on cardiac structure and function: sex-related differences in the Framingham Heart Study. *Circulation* 2003;107:448–454.
117. Verdecchia P, Reboldi G, Schillaci G, et al. Circulating insulin and insulin growth factor-1 are independent determinants of left ventricular mass and geometry in essential hypertension. *Circulation* 1999;100:1802–1807.
118. Frustaci A, Kajstura J, Chimenti C, et al. Myocardial cell death in human diabetes. *Circ Res* 2000;87:1123–1132.
119. Aronson D. Cross-linking of glycated collagen in the pathogenesis of arterial and myocardial stiffening of aging and diabetes. *J Hypertens* 2003;21:3–12.
120. Monnier VM, Kohn RR, Cerami A. Accelerated age-related browning of human collagen in diabetes mellitus. *Proc Natl Acad Sci U S A* 1984; 81:583–587.
121. Brownlee M, Vlassara H, Kooney A, et al. Aminoguanidine prevents diabetes-induced arterial wall protein cross-linking. *Science* 1986; 232:1629–1632.
122. Vasan S, Zhang X, Zhang X, et al. An agent cleaving glucose-derived protein crosslinks in vitro and in vivo [see comments]. *Nature* 1996;382: 275–278.
123. Wolffenbuttel BH, Boulanger CM, Crijns FR, et al. Breakers of advanced glycation end products restore large artery properties in experimental diabetes. *Proc Natl Acad Sci U S A* 1998;95:4630–4634.
124. Asif M, Egan J, Vasan S, et al. An advanced glycation endproduct cross-link breaker can reverse age-related increases in myocardial stiffness [published erratum appears in *Proc Natl Acad Sci U S A* 2000;97:5679]. *Proc Natl Acad Sci U S A* 2000;97:2809–2813.
125. Kass DA, Shapiro EP, Kawaguchi M, et al. Improved arterial compliance by a novel advanced glycation end-product crosslink breaker. *Circulation* 2001;104:1464–1470.
126. Malmberg K, Yusuf S, Gerstein HC, et al. Impact of diabetes on long-term prognosis in patients with unstable angina and non-Q-wave myocardial infarction: results of the OASIS (Organization to Assess Strategies for Ischemic Syndromes) Registry. *Circulation* 2000;102:1014–1019.
127. Roffi M, Chew DP, Mukherjee D, et al. Platelet glycoprotein IIb/IIIa inhibitors reduce mortality in diabetic patients with non-ST-segment-elevation acute coronary syndromes. *Circulation* 2001;104:2767–2771.
128. Shindler DM, Palmeri ST, Antonelli TA, et al. Diabetes mellitus in cardiogenic shock complicating acute myocardial infarction: a report from the SHOCK Trial Registry. SHould we emergently revascularize Occluded Coronaries for cardiogenic shocK? *J Am Coll Cardiol* 2000;36:1097–1103.
129. Silva JA, Escobar A, Collins TJ, et al. Unstable angina. A comparison of angioscopic findings between diabetic and nondiabetic patients. *Circulation* 1995;92:1731–1736.
130. Moreno PR, Murcia AM, Palacios IF, et al. Coronary composition and macrophage infiltration in atherectomy specimens from patients with diabetes mellitus. *Circulation* 2000;102:2180–2184.
131. Mehilli J, Kastrati A, Schuhlen H, et al. Randomized clinical trial of abciximab in diabetic patients undergoing elective percutaneous coronary interventions after treatment with a high loading dose of clopidogrel. *Circulation* 2004;110:3627–3635.
132. Mak KH, Moliterno DJ, Granger CB, et al. Influence of diabetes mellitus on clinical outcome in the thrombolytic era of acute myocardial infarction. GUSTO-I Investigators. Global Utilization of Streptokinase and Tissue Plasminogen Activator for Occluded Coronary Arteries. *J Am Coll Cardiol.* 1997;30:171–179.
133. Abaci A, Oguzhan A, Kahraman S, et al. Effect of diabetes mellitus on formation of coronary collateral vessels. *Circulation* 1999;99:2239–2242.
134. Zuanetti G, Latini R, Maggioni AP, et al. Influence of diabetes on mortality in acute myocardial infarction: data from the GISSI-2 study. *J Am Coll Cardiol* 1993;22:1788–1794.
135. Goldberg RB, Mellies MJ, Sacks FM, et al. Cardiovascular events and their reduction with pravastatin in diabetic and glucose-intolerant myocardial infarction survivors with average cholesterol levels: subgroup analyses in the cholesterol and recurrent events (CARE) trial. The Care Investigators. *Circulation* 1998;98:2513–2519.
136. Fibrinolytic Therapy Trialists' (FTT) Collaborative Group. Indications for fibrinolytic therapy in suspected acute myocardial infarction: collaborative overview of early mortality and major morbidity results from all randomized trials of more then 1000 patients. *Lancet* 1994;343:311–322.
137. Granger CB, Califf RM, Young S, et al. Outcome of patients with diabetes mellitus and acute myocardial infarction treated with thrombolytic agents. The Thrombolysis and Angioplasty in Myocardial Infarction (TAMI) Study Group. *J Am Coll Cardiol* 1993;21:920–925.
138. Mahaffey KW, Granger CB, Toth CA, et al. Diabetic retinopathy should not be a contraindication to thrombolytic. *J Am Coll Cardiol* 1997;30:1606–1610.
139. Hasdai D, Granger CB, Srivatsa SS, et al. Diabetes mellitus and outcome after primary coronary angioplasty for acute myocardial infarction: lessons from the GUSTO-IIb Angioplasty Substudy. Global Use of Strategies to Open Occluded Arteries in Acute Coronary Syndromes [see comments]. *J Am Coll Cardiol* 2000;35:1502–1512.
140. Hsu LF, Mak KH, Lau KW, et al. Clinical outcomes of patients with diabetes mellitus and acute myocardial infarction treated with primary angioplasty or fibrinolysis. *Heart* 2002;88:260–265.
141. Bonnefoy E, Steg PG, Chabaud S, et al. Is primary angioplasty more effective than prehospital fibrinolysis in diabetics with acute myocardial infarction? Data from the CAPTIM randomized clinical trial. *Eur Heart J* 2005;26:1712–1718.
142. Stuckey TD, Stone GW, Cox DA, et al. Impact of stenting and abciximab in patients with diabetes mellitus undergoing primary angioplasty in acute myocardial infarction (the CADILLAC trial). *Am J Cardiol* 2005;95: 1–7.
143. Harjai KJ, Stone GW, Boura J, et al. Comparison of outcomes of diabetic and nondiabetic patients undergoing primary angioplasty for acute myocardial infarction. *Am J Cardiol* 2003;91:1041–1045.
144. Prasad A, Stone GW, Stuckey TD, et al. Impact of diabetes mellitus on myocardial perfusion after primary angioplasty in patients with acute myocardial infarction. *J Am Coll Cardiol* 2005;45:508–514.
145. Mehta SR, Yusuf S, Diaz R, et al. Effect of glucose-insulin-potassium infusion on mortality in patients with acute ST-segment elevation myocardial infarction: the CREATE-ECLA randomized controlled trial. *JAMA* 2005;293:437–446.
146. van der Horst IC, Zijlstra F, van't Hof AW, et al. Glucose-insulin-potassium infusion inpatients treated with primary angioplasty for acute myocardial infarction: the glucose-insulin-potassium study: a randomized trial. *J Am Coll Cardiol* 2003;42:784–791.
147. Malmberg K, Ryden L, Wedel H, et al. Intense metabolic control by means of insulin in patients with diabetes mellitus and acute myocardial infarction (DIGAMI 2): effects on mortality and morbidity. *Eur Heart J* 2005;26:650–661.
148. Kip KE, Faxon DP, Detre KM, et al. Coronary angioplasty in diabetic patients. The National Heart, Lung, and Blood Institute Percutaneous Transluminal Coronary Angioplasty Registry [see comments]. *Circulation* 1996;94:1818–1825.
149. The Bypass Angioplasty Revascularization Investigation (BARI). Influence of diabetes on 5-year mortality and morbidity in a randomized trial comparing CABG and PTCA in patients with multivessel disease [see comments]. *Circulation* 1997;96:1761–1769.
150. Abizaid A, Mintz GS, Pichard AD, et al. Clinical, intravascular ultrasound, and quantitative angiographic determinants of the coronary flow reserve

before and after percutaneous transluminal coronary angioplasty. *Am J Cardiol* 1998;82:423–428.
151. Goldberg S, Savage MP, Fischman DL. The interventional cardiologist and the diabetic patient. Have we pushed the envelope too far or not far enough? [editorial; comment]. *Circulation* 1996;94:1804–1806.
152. Kastrati A, Schomig A, Elezi S, et al. Predictive factors of restenosis after coronary stent placement. *J Am Coll Cardiol* 1997;30:1428–1436.
153. Elezi S, Kastrati A, Pache J, et al. Diabetes mellitus and the clinical and angiographic outcome after coronary stent placement. *J Am Coll Cardiol* 1998;32:1866–1873.
154. Schofer J, Schluter M, Rau T, et al. Influence of treatment modality on angiographic outcome after coronary stenting in diabetic patients: a controlled study. *J Am Coll Cardiol* 2000;35:1554–1559.
155. Gum P, O'Keefe JJ, Borkon A, et al. Bypass surgery versus coronary angioplasty for revascularization of treated diabetic patients. *Circulation* 1997;96:II7–II10.
156. Abizaid A, Kornowski R, Mintz GS, et al. The influence of diabetes mellitus on acute and late clinical outcomes following coronary stent implantation. *J Am Coll Cardiol* 1998;32:584–589.
157. Kornowski R, Mintz GS, Kent KM, et al. Increased restenosis in diabetes mellitus after coronary interventions is due to exaggerated intimal hyperplasia. A serial intravascular ultrasound study. *Circulation* 1997;95:1366–1369.
158. Aronson D, Bloomgarden Z, Rayfield EJ. Potential mechanisms promoting restenosis in diabetic patients. *J Am Coll Cardiol* 1996;27:528–535.
159. Aronson D. Potential role of advanced glycosylation end products in promoting restenosis in diabetes and renal failure. *Med Hypotheses* 2002;59: 297–301.
160. Park SH, Marso SP, Zhou Z, et al. Neointimal hyperplasia after arterial injury is increased in a rat model of non-insulin-dependent diabetes mellitus. *Circulation* 2001;104:815–819.
161. Indolfi C, Torella D, Cavuto L, et al. Effects of balloon injury on neointimal hyperplasia in streptozotocin-induced diabetes and in hyperinsulinemic nondiabetic pancreatic islet-transplanted rats. *Circulation* 2001;103:2980–2986.
162. Sakaguchi T, Yan SF, Yan SD, et al. Central role of RAGE-dependent neointimal expansion in arterial restenosis. *J Clin Invest* 2003;111: 959–972.
163. Zhou Z, Wang K, Penn MS, et al. Receptor for AGE (RAGE) mediates neointimal formation in response to arterial injury. *Circulation* 2003;107:2238–2343.
164. Van Belle E, Ketelers R, Bauters C, et al. Patency of percutaneous transluminal coronary angioplasty sites at 6-month angiographic follow-up: a key determinant of survival in diabetics after coronary balloon angioplasty. *Circulation* 2001;103:1218–1224.
165. Moussa I, Leon MB, Baim DS, et al. Impact of sirolimus-eluting stents on outcome in diabetic patients: a SIRIUS (SIRolImUS-coated Bx Velocity balloon-expandable stent in the treatment of patients with de novo coronary artery lesions) substudy. *Circulation* 2004;109:2273–2278.
166. Abizaid A, Costa MA, Blanchard D, et al. Sirolimus-eluting stents inhibit neointimal hyperplasia in diabetic patients. Insights from the RAVEL Trial. *Eur Heart J* 2004;25:107–112.
167. Hermiller JB, Raizner A, Cannon L, et al. Outcomes with the polymer-based paclitaxel-eluting TAXUS stent in patients with diabetes mellitus: the TAXUS-IV trial. *J Am Coll Cardiol* 2005;45:1172–1179.
168. Dibra A, Kastrati A, Mehilli J, et al. Paclitaxel-eluting or sirolimus-eluting stents to prevent restenosis in diabetic patients. *N Engl J Med* 2005;353: 663–670.
169. Kubal C, Srinivasan AK, Grayson AD, et al. Effect of risk-adjusted diabetes on mortality and morbidity after coronary artery bypass surgery. *Ann Thorac Surg* 2005;79:1570–1576.
170. Eagle KA, Guyton RA, Davidoff R, et al. ACC/AHA 2004 guideline update for coronary artery bypass graft surgery: summary article. A report of the American College of Cardiology/American Heart Association Task Force on Practice Guidelines (Committee to Update the 1999 Guidelines for Coronary Artery Bypass Graft Surgery). *J Am Coll Cardiol* 2004;44:1146–1154, e213–e310.
171. Thourani VH, Weintraub WS, Stein B, et al. Influence of diabetes mellitus on early and late outcome after coronary artery bypass grafting. *Ann Thorac Surg* 1999;67:1045–1052.
172. Zerr KJ, Furnary AP, Grunkemeier GL, et al. Glucose control lowers the risk of wound infection in diabetics after open heart operations. *Ann Thorac Surg* 1997;63:356–361.
173. Lazar HL, Chipkin SR, Fitzgerald CA, et al. Tight glycemic control in diabetic coronary artery bypass graft patients improves perioperative outcomes and decreases recurrent ischemic events. *Circulation* 2004;109:1497–1502.
174. Hoogwerf BJ, Waness A, Cressman M, et al. Effects of aggressive cholesterol lowering and low-dose anticoagulation on clinical and angiographic outcomes in patients with diabetes: the Post Coronary Artery Bypass Graft Trial. *Diabetes* 1999;48:1289–1294.
175. Schwartz L, Kip KE, Frye RL, et al. Coronary bypass graft patency in patients with diabetes in the Bypass Angioplasty Revascularization Investigation (BARI). *Circulation* 2002;106:2652–2658.
176. Barsness GW, Peterson ED, Ohman EM, et al. Relationship between diabetes mellitus and long-term survival after coronary bypass and angioplasty. *Circulation* 1997;96:2551–2556.
177. The Bypass Angioplasty Revascularization Investigation (BARI) Investigators. Comparison of coronary bypass surgery with angioplasty in patients with multivessel disease. *N Engl J Med* 1996;335:217–225.
178. King SB 3rd, Kosinski AS, Guyton RA, et al. Eight-year mortality in the Emory Angioplasty versus Surgery Trial (EAST) [see comments]. *J Am Coll Cardiol* 2000;35:1116–1121.
179. Serruys PW, Ong AT, van Herwerden LA, et al. Five-year outcomes after coronary stenting versus bypass surgery for the treatment of multivessel disease: the final analysis of the Arterial Revascularization Therapies Study (ARTS) randomized trial. *J Am Coll Cardiol* 2005;46:575–581.
180. The BARI Investigators. Seven-year outcome in the Bypass Angioplasty Revascularization Investigation (BARI) by treatment and diabetic status [see comments]. *J Am Coll Cardiol* 2000;35:1122–1129.
181. Detre KM, Lombardero MS, Brooks MM, et al. The effect of previous coronary-artery bypass surgery on the prognosis of patients with diabetes who have acute myocardial infarction. Bypass Angioplasty Revascularization Investigation Investigators [see comments]. *N Engl J Med* 2000; 342:989–997.
182. Aronson D. Pharmacologic modulation of autonomic tone: implications for the diabetic patient. *Diabetologia* 1997;40:476–481.
183. Toyry JP, Niskanen LK, Mantysaari MJ, et al. Occurrence, predictors, and clinical significance of autonomic neuropathy in NIDDM. Ten-year follow-up from the diagnosis. *Diabetes* 1996;45:308–315.
184. Tesfaye S, Chaturvedi N, Eaton SE, et al. Vascular risk factors and diabetic neuropathy. *N Engl J Med* 2005;352:341–350.
185. Kreiner G, Wolzt M, Fasching P, et al. Myocardial m-[123I]iodobenzylguanidine scintigraphy for the assessment of adrenergic cardiac innervation in patients with IDDM. Comparison with cardiovascular reflex tests and relationship to left ventricular function. *Diabetes* 1995;44:543–549.
186. Taskiran M, Fritz-Hansen T, Rasmussen V, et al. Decreased myocardial perfusion reserve in diabetic autonomic neuropathy. *Diabetes* 2002; 51: 3306–310.
187. Milan Study on Atherosclerosis and Diabetes (MiSAD) Group. Prevalence of unrecognized silent myocardial ischemia and its association with atherosclerotic risk factors in noninsulin-dependent diabetes mellitus. *Am J Cardiol* 1997;79:134–139.
188. American Diabetes Association. Standards of medical care in diabetes. *Diabetes Care* 2005;28[Suppl 1]:S4–S36.
189. Gaede P, Vedel P, Larsen N, et al. Multifactorial intervention and cardiovascular disease in patients with type 2 diabetes. *N Engl J Med* 2003;348:383–393.
190. Saydah SH, Fradkin J, Cowie CC. Poor control of risk factors for vascular disease among adults with previously diagnosed diabetes. *JAMA* 2004;291:335–342.
191. Grundy SM, Cleeman JI, Merz CN, et al. Implications of recent clinical trials for the National Cholesterol Education Program Adult Treatment Panel III guidelines. *Circulation* 2004;110:227–239.
192. Collins R, Armitage J, Parish S, et al. MRC/BHF Heart Protection Study of cholesterol-lowering with simvastatin in 5963 people with diabetes: a randomised placebo-controlled trial. *Lancet* 2003;361:2005–2016.
193. Colhoun HM, Betteridge DJ, Durrington PN, et al. Primary prevention of cardiovascular disease with atorvastatin in type 2 diabetes in the Collaborative Atorvastatin Diabetes Study (CARDS): multicentre randomised placebo-controlled trial. *Lancet* 2004;364:685–696.
194. Effect of fenofibrate on progression of coronary-artery disease in type 2 diabetes: the Diabetes Atherosclerosis Intervention Study, a randomised study. *Lancet* 2001;357:905–910.
195. Elam MB, Hunninghake DB, Davis KB, et al. Effect of niacin on lipid and lipoprotein levels and glycemic control in patients with diabetes and peripheral arterial disease: the ADMIT study: a randomized trial. Arterial Disease Multiple Intervention Trial. *JAMA* 2000;284:1263–1270.
196. National Diabetes Information Clearinghouse. *Diabetes statistics* [NIH Publication 02-3892]. Bethesda, MD: National Institutes of Health, 2000.
197. Chobanian AV, Bakris GL, Black HR, et al. The Seventh Report of the Joint National Committee on Prevention, Detection, Evaluation, and Treatment of High Blood Pressure: the JNC 7 report. *JAMA* 2003;289:2560–2572.
198. Arauz-Pacheco C, Parrott MA, Raskin P. The treatment of hypertension in adult patients with diabetes. *Diabetes Care* 2002;25:134–147.
199. Efficacy of atenolol and captopril in reducing risk of macrovascular and microvascular complications in type 2 diabetes: UKPDS 39. *BMJ* 1998;317:713–720.
200. Tight blood pressure control and risk of macrovascular and microvascular complications in type 2 diabetes: UKPDS 38. *BMJ* 1998;317:703–713.
201. Brenner BM, Cooper ME, de Zeeuw D, et al. Effects of losartan on renal and cardiovascular outcomes in patients with type 2 diabetes and nephropathy. *N Engl J Med* 2001;345:861–869.
202. Tatti P, Pahor M, Byington RP, et al. Outcome results of the Fosinopril Versus Amlodipine Cardiovascular Events Randomized Trial (FACET) in patients with hypertension and NIDDM [see comments]. *Diabetes Care* 1998;21:597–603.

203. UK Prospective Diabetes Study (UKPDS) Group. Intensive blood-glucose control with sulphonylureas or insulin compared with conventional treatment and risk of complications in patients with type 2 diabetes (UKPDS 33). *Lancet* 1998;352:837–853.
204. Stratton IM, Adler AI, Neil HA, et al. Association of glycaemia with macrovascular and microvascular complications of type 2 diabetes (UKPDS 35): prospective observational study. *BMJ* 2000;321:405–412.
205. Langenfeld MR, Forst T, Hohberg C, et al. Pioglitazone decreases carotid intima-media thickness independently of glycemic control in patients with type 2 diabetes mellitus: results from a controlled randomized study. *Circulation* 2005;111:2525–2531.
206. Knowler WC, Barrett-Connor E, Fowler SE, et al. Reduction in the incidence of type 2 diabetes with lifestyle intervention or metformin. *N Engl J Med* 2002;346:393–403.
207. Tuomilehto J, Lindstrom J, Eriksson JG, et al. Prevention of type 2 diabetes mellitus by changes in lifestyle among subjects with impaired glucose tolerance. *N Engl J Med* 2001;344:1343–1350.
208. The prevention or delay of type 2 diabetes. *Diabetes Care* 2002;25:742–749.
209. Executive Summary of The Third Report of The National Cholesterol Education Program (NCEP) Expert Panel on Detection, Evaluation, and Treatment of High Blood Cholesterol in Adults (Adult Treatment Panel III). *JAMA* 2001;285:2486–2497.
210. Cerami A, Vlassara H, Brownlee M. Glucose and aging. *Sci Am* 1987; 256:90–96.

CHAPTER 5 ■ LIPID DISORDERS

DANIEL J. RADER

OVERVIEW

Lipoprotein disorders are common and are an important risk factor for coronary artery disease (CAD) and all types of atherosclerotic vascular disease (ASCVD). Intervention with diet and drugs to reduce low-density-lipoprotein (LDL) cholesterol has been proven to decrease the risk of subsequent cardiovascular events, including total mortality. In patients with established ASCVD or at high risk for developing it, treatment to reduce LDL-C is effective not only when the LDL-C level is elevated, but also when the cholesterol level is average. Based on the wealth of clinical trial data, it is widely agreed that virtually all patients with CAD should be treated aggressively with lipid-modifying drug therapy to reduce their risk of subsequent cardiovascular events. Unfortunately, sudden cardiac death at the time of the first myocardial infarction (MI) is common, and therefore waiting to initiate lipid-modifying therapy until symptoms of CAD have developed is not an acceptable strategy. Therefore, it is also generally agreed that patients who have a level of risk that is roughly equivalent to that of patients with established CAD should also be treated aggressively with lipid-modifying therapy. This category includes patients who have other forms of ASCVD (carotid disease, peripheral vascular disease), patients with diabetes mellitus, and patients who have an absolute risk of having a cardiovascular event over the next 10 years of greater than 20%. Finally, lipid-modifying drug therapy has been shown to reduce cardiovascular events even in less-high-risk patients. Therefore, a major challenge in the use of lipid-modifying drug therapy in the primary prevention setting is performing an accurate risk assessment so that patients can be treated with an appropriate level of lipid-modifying drug therapy. In addition to standard risk assessment based on traditional risk factors, the diagnosis of the metabolic syndrome may identify patients at higher risk. There may be a clinical role for additional tests to assess cardiovascular risk, such as laboratory tests and noninvasive imaging of subclinical atherosclerosis. LDL-C is not the only lipid parameter of interest, and triglycerides, non–high-density-lipoprotein (HDL) cholesterol, and HDL cholesterol are also of tremendous interest. Lipid-modifying therapy is a cornerstone of cardiovascular risk reduction. Strategies for achieving appropriate modification of plasma lipids and lipoproteins must include both broad-based public health measures oriented around diet and lifestyle and highly focused, aggressive intervention targeted toward those at highest risk for developing ASCVD.

GLOSSARY

Apolipoprotein: Major protein component of lipoproteins; there are multiple apolipoproteins with functions.

Cholesteryl ester transfer protein (CETP): Protein that transfers lipids among lipoproteins, especially cholesteryl ester from HDL to very low density lipoprotein (VLDL) in exchange for triglycerides.

Chylomicron: Intestinal triglyceride-rich lipoprotein; elevated when triglycerides are greater than 1,000 mg/dL.

Hepatic lipase (HL): Endothelial-anchored enzyme in liver primarily responsible for hydrolysis of triglycerides and phospholipids in intermediate-density lipoprotein (IDL) and HDL.

High-density lipoprotein (HDL): Small lipoprotein thought to participate in "reverse cholesterol transport;" levels are inversely associated with CAD risk.

Hydroxy-3-methylglutaryl coenzyme A (HMG-CoA) reductase: Rate-limiting enzyme in cholesterol biosynthesis; inhibition by "statins" results in reduction of plasma VLDL-cholesterol levels.

Intermediate-density lipoprotein (IDL): Lipoprotein formed by hydrolysis of triglycerides in VLDL; elevated in type III hyperlipoproteinemia.

Lecithin:cholesterol acyltransferase (LCAT): Enzyme that converts free cholesterol to cholesteryl ester on HDL.

Lipoprotein: Complex responsible for transporting lipids (cholesterol, triglyceride, phospholipids) within the blood.

Lipoprotein lipase (LPL): Endothelial-anchored enzyme primarily responsible for hydrolysis of chylomicron and VLDL triglycerides, especially in muscle and adipose tissue.

Low-density lipoprotein (LDL): Major cholesterol-containing lipoprotein and major atherogenic lipoprotein.

Primary prevention: Treatment for preventing atherosclerosis and CAD events in persons who do not have evidence of CAD.

Secondary prevention: Treatment for preventing recurrent CAD events in persons who have documented CAD.

Very low density lipoprotein (VLDL): Major triglyceride-containing lipoprotein when fasting triglycerides are less than 1,000 mg/dL; made by the liver.

HISTORICAL PERSPECTIVE

The association between elevated serum cholesterol and coronary heart disease (CHD) was first reported in the 1930s, and subsequent large epidemiologic studies confirmed the strong relationship between serum cholesterol and CHD. These studies formed the basis of the "cholesterol hypothesis" that the relationship between serum cholesterol and atherosclerosis is causal and that reduction of serum cholesterol would reduce atherosclerotic disease.

The Subfractionation of serum cholesterol into cholesterol contained within specific lipoproteins such as LDLs and HDLs was a major clinical advance. Cardiovascular risk was found to be positively associated with LDL-cholesterol (LDL-C) levels and inversely with HDL-C levels. The relationship between fasting serum triglycerides and cardiovascular risk has been confounded by the inverse association between triglycerides and HDL-C, as well as by the association of triglycerides with other risk factors such as diabetes mellitus and body mass. However, triglyceride levels are now considered an important independent predictor of cardiovascular risk.

LIPID-MODIFYING THERAPY AND EFFECTS ON ATHEROSCLEROTIC CARDIOVASCULAR EVENTS

Despite the wealth of epidemiologic and pathologic data linking serum cholesterol to atherosclerotic disease, proof of the cholesterol hypothesis required demonstration that reduction of cholesterol decreased atherosclerosis and clinical cardiovascular events. Over the last three decades, multiple trials have been reported that were designed to test this hypothesis.

Early Clinical Trials: Niacin, Bile Acid Sequestrants, and Partial Ileal Bypass

The early clinical trials used niacin, bile acid sequestrants, and even the surgical approach of partial ileal bypass to reduce serum cholesterol levels. The Coronary Drug Project demonstrated a modest benefit of niacin in reducing nonfatal MI after 6 years of treatment (1) and in reducing total mortality after 15 years of follow-up (2). The Program on the Surgical Control of Hyperlipidemias (POSCH) trial employed the surgical technique of partial ileal bypass surgery to reduce LDL-C levels and demonstrated a significant 35% relative reduction in fatal CHD and nonfatal MI, although not in total mortality (the primary endpoint of the trial) (3). In the Lipid Research Clinics Coronary Primary Prevention Trial (LRC-CPPT) with cholestyramine in hypercholesterolemic men (4,5), combined fatal CHD and nonfatal MI (the primary endpoint) was reduced by 19%.

3-Hydroxy-3-methylglutaryl Coenzyme A Reductase Inhibitor (Statin) Trials

The cholesterol hypothesis was finally definitively proven as a result of the clinical outcome trials with hydroxy-3-methylglutaryl-coenzyme A (HMG-CoA) reductase inhibitors (statins). In the Scandinavian Simvastatin Survival Study (4S) (6), 4,444 patients with CHD and elevated cholesterol were randomized to placebo or simvastatin 20 mg titrated to 40 mg as needed. Treatment with simvastatin was associated with a 30% relative risk reduction in total mortality and a 44% reduction in CHD death or MI. It is important that it was not only the subjects with the highest cholesterol levels who experienced a reduction in risk; the quartile with the lowest LDL-C levels at baseline had proportionately as much benefit from treatment as the highest quartile (7). This is important because least one third of persons with CHD have total cholesterol levels less than 200 mg/dL (8). In the Cholesterol and Recurrent Events (CARE) study (9), 4,159 patients who were post-MI and had total cholesterol levels less than 240 mg/dL were randomized to placebo or pravastatin 40 mg daily and followed for an average of 5 years. Treatment with pravastatin was associated with a significant 24% reduction in relative risk. In the Long-Term Intervention with Pravastatin in Ischemic Disease (LIPID) trial (10), 9,014 patients with CHD and a broad range of cholesterol levels were randomized to placebo or pravastatin 40 mg daily and followed for an average of 6 years. Treatment with pravastatin significantly reduced CHD mortality by 24% and total mortality by 22%. These three statin studies in patients with preexisting CHD reported in the 1990s definitively established the efficacy of statin therapy in reducing cardiovascular events and total mortality in patients with established CHD over a very wide range of baseline LDL-C levels.

Two additional large outcome studies with statins in the 1990s were carried out in patients without CHD. In the West of Scotland Coronary Prevention Study (WOSCOPS) (11), 6,595 healthy Scottish men with total cholesterol levels of less than 252 mg/dL were randomized to placebo or pravastatin 40 mg/day and followed for an average of 5 years. Treatment with pravastatin was associated with a significant 31% reduction in relative risk of nonfatal MI or CHD death. The Air Force/Texas Coronary Atherosclerosis Prevention Study (AFCAPS/ TexCAPS) (12) extended these findings into a population with modestly elevated to average cholesterol levels. A total of 6,608 men and women with LDL-C level 130 to 190 mg/dL and relatively low HDL-C levels were randomized to lovastatin 20 to 40 mg or placebo and followed for an average of 5.2 years. Treatment with lovastatin was associated with a 37% relative risk reduction in the primary endpoint of combined cardiovascular events in the lovastatin-treated group. These studies definitively confirmed that the benefits of cholesterol reduction extend to the primary prevention setting.

Subsequent studies have focused less on the issue of primary versus secondary prevention and instead have defined groups of patients based on their future risk of CHD events. The Heart Protection Study (HPS) was a more recent study in which 20,536 patients aged 40 to 80 years old with CHD, other atherosclerotic vascular disease, or diabetes were randomized to simvastatin 40 mg or placebo (13). For inclusion, total cholesterol needed only be greater than 135 mg/dL, ensuring that many subjects in this trial had average and even below-average cholesterol levels. Treatment with simvastatin was associated with a highly significant 24% reduction in major coronary events, 25% reduction in stroke, and 13% reduction in total mortality. Remarkably, the relative benefit of simvastatin therapy was similar across tertiles of baseline LDL-C, and even the group with LDL-C less than 100 mg/dL at baseline demonstrated benefit with simvastatin. The results of HPS led to the widespread concept that there are benefits of statin therapy in high-risk individuals regardless of baseline cholesterol levels.

In the Prospective Study of Pravastatin in the Elderly at Risk (PROSPER), 5,804 patients aged 70 to 80 years with vascular disease or risk factors were randomized to pravastatin 40 mg or placebo and followed for an average of 3.2 years (14). Pravastatin treatment was associated with a significant 15% reduction in a composite cardiovascular endpoint, demonstrating the benefit of statin therapy in the elderly. In the Antihypertensive and Lipid-Lowering Treatment to Prevent Heart Attack Trial (ALLHAT), 10,355 hypertensive patients were randomized to pravastatin 40 mg or usual care (in which up to about 30% of patients were receiving statin therapy prescribed by their physician by the end of the trial) (15). There was a trend but not a statistically significant reduction in coronary events associated with randomization to pravastatin in this trial, but the difference between the two groups in total cholesterol was only 9%. In the Anglo-Scandinavian Cardiac Outcomes Trial Lipid-lowering Arm (ASCOT-LLA), 19,342 hypertensive patients with at least three other risk factors and with total cholesterol levels less than 242 mg/dL were randomized to atorvastatin 10 mg or placebo (16). The study was stopped early after 3.3 years when a highly significant 36% relative risk reduction associated with atorvastatin was found. In the Collaborative Atorvastatin Diabetes Study (CARDS), 2,838 patients with type 2 diabetes were randomized to atorvastatin 10 mg or placebo (17). This study was also terminated early due to a significant 37% reduction in major cardiovascular events.

The first trial to directly compare two different doses of the same statin with regard to cardiovascular (CV) outcomes was the Treat to New Targets (TNT) trial (18). A total of 10,001 patients with CHD and LDL-C less than 130 mg/dL were randomized to atorvastatin 10 mg or 80 mg daily. The higher dose of atorvastatin resulted in a mean on-treatment LDL-C of 77 mg/dL (compared with 101 mg/dL for the lower dose) and a significant 22% reduction in major cardiovascular events. This trial conclusively proved that a higher dose of atorvastatin reduced CV events to a greater extent than a lower dose. The studies from HPS to TNT reviewed here substantially moved the field toward a "lower is better" approach to reducing LDL-C.

Statin trials have also been performed in patients presenting with acute coronary syndromes (ACS). In the Myocardial Ischemia Reduction with Aggressive Cholesterol Lowering (MIRACL) trial, patients presenting with ACS were randomized to immediate therapy with atorvastatin 80 mg or placebo and followed for 4 months (19). There was a 16% reduction in recurrent coronary events associated with immediate atorvastatin therapy that just achieved statistical significance (p = .48). Two more-recent ACS studies compared different statin regimens or doses and followed subjects for a longer period of time. In the Pravastatin or Atorvastatin Evaluation and Infection Therapy (PROVE-IT) study, ACS patients were randomized to atorvastatin 80 mg or pravastatin 40 mg and followed for a mean of 2 years (20). The more intensive regimen of atorvastatin 80 mg (mean on-treatment LDL-C of 62 mg/dL) was associated with a significant 16% relative risk reduction in major cardiovascular events compared with the less intensive pravastatin 40 mg regimen (mean on-treatment LDL-C of 95 mg/dL). In contrast, the Aggrastat to Zocor (A to Z) trial randomized ACS patients to simvastatin 40 mg versus placebo for 4 months, followed by titration to simvastatin 80 mg versus simvastatin 20 mg, and followed subjects for up to 2 years (21). This study failed to demonstrate a significant difference between the two arms with regard to the primary endpoint, but did demonstrate reduction in cardiovascular events during the follow-up period starting at 4 months. Overall the ACS studies have resulted in the standard practice of starting a statin in the hospital prior to discharge in patients admitted for ACS.

Fibrate Trials

There have been fewer clinical endpoint trials with fibrates than with statins. The Helsinki Heart Study (HHS) compared gemfibrozil 1,200 mg to placebo in men with elevated non-HDL-C greater than 200 mg/dL and demonstrated a significant 34% reduction in combined fatal and nonfatal MI (the primary endpoint) but no difference in total mortality (22). The Veteran Affairs High-Density Lipoprotein Cholesterol Intervention Trial (VA-HIT) tested the benefit of gemfibrozil 1,200 mg versus placebo in patients with CHD and average LDL-C levels (mean 112 mg/dL) but low HDL-C levels (mean 32 mg/dL) (23). Gemfibrozil therapy was associated with a significant 22% reduction in the primary endpoint (nonfatal myocardial infarction and coronary death) compared to placebo. In contrast, the Bezafibrate Infarction Prevention (BIP) trial in patients with established CHD, LDL-C less than 180 mg/dL and HDL-C less than 45 mg/dL randomized to either bezafibrate 400 mg daily or placebo (24) failed to demonstrate a significant reduction in the primary endpoint of fatal or nonfatal MI. A post hoc analysis in the subgroup with high baseline triglycerides (>200 mg/dL) suggested a reduction in events of 39%. These two latter trials differed in a number of important ways, including the fibrate used and the baseline LDL-C levels, which in BIP were 150 mg/dL compared with only 111 mg/dL in VA-HIT. A reasonable conclusion might be that fibrates are effective as monotherapy in reducing events in secondary prevention if the LDL-C is low, but not if it is elevated.

PHYSIOLOGY AND PATHOPHYSIOLOGY OF LIPOPROTEIN METABOLISM

Appropriate clinical management of patients with lipid disorders requires a general working knowledge of normal lipoprotein metabolism. Lipoproteins are large macromolecular complexes that transport cholesterol and triglycerides within the blood. They contain a hydrophobic neutral lipid core consisting of triglycerides and cholesteryl esters, which is surrounded by phospholipids and specialized proteins known as apolipoproteins. Apolipoproteins are required for the structural integrity of lipoproteins and direct their metabolic interactions with enzymes, lipid transport proteins, and cell surface receptors. The five major families of lipoproteins are chylomicrons, very low density lipoproteins, intermediate-density lipoproteins, low-density lipoproteins, and high-density lipoproteins Chylomicrons are the largest and most lipid-rich lipoproteins, whereas HDL are the smallest lipoproteins and contain the least amount of lipid. The major metabolic pathways of lipoproteins are shown in Figures 5.1 to 5.3 and are described in detail in the accompanying legends.

Disorders of lipoprotein metabolism involve perturbations that cause elevation of triglycerides and/or cholesterol, reduction of HDL-C, or alteration of properties of lipoproteins such as their size or composition. These perturbations can be genetic (primary) or occur as a result of other diseases, conditions, or drugs (secondary) (Table 5.4). Many (but not all) lipoprotein disorders have as their most important clinical consequence the increased risk of premature atherosclerotic cardiovascular disease. The next section of this chapter will focus specifically on the identification and diagnosis of specific lipid disorders, and the subsequent section will focus on the management of lipid disorders, especially regarding the prevention of atherosclerosis and its associated clinical events.

The mechanisms by which atherogenic lipoproteins promote atherosclerosis continue to be the subject of intensive research. In brief, LDL and other atherogenic lipoproteins probably must be aggregated, oxidized, or otherwise modified in order to be recognized by macrophage cell-surface receptors and be internalized, leading to foam cell formation (25). Atherogenic lipoproteins may influence macrophage function in ways that go beyond foam cell formation that also promote atherogenesis (26). On the other hand, HDL is believed to promote cholesterol efflux from macrophages and return it to the liver for excretion in the bile, a process known as reverse cholesterol transport (27). HDL may also have antioxidant and antiinflammatory effects that contribute to its antiatherogenic effects (28).

SECONDARY DISORDERS OF LIPOPROTEIN METABOLISM

Lipid disorders can be grouped into primary disorders (genetic or inherited) and secondary disorders (due to another disease or environmental factor). Clinically, it is useful to first consider and exclude secondary causes because they should be treated if found to be present. Some of the most important secondary causes of hyperlipidemia are reviewed briefly in what follows and are listed in Table 5.1.

Hypothyroidism

Hypothyroidism causes elevated LDL-C levels due primarily to downregulation of the LDL receptor. Because hypothyroidism can be subtle in its clinical presentation, patients presenting with hypercholesterolemia should be screened with a thyroid-stimulating hormone (TSH) test to rule out hypothyroidism. Thyroid replacement therapy usually results in resolution of the hypercholesterolemia. Hypothyroid patients who remain hypercholesterolemic after adequate replacement probably have an underlying lipoprotein disorder and may require lipid-lowering drug therapy.

TABLE 5.1

SELECTED DISORDERS ASSOCIATED WITH SECONDARY DYSLIPIDEMIA

	Cholesterol	Triglycerides	HDL-C
Metabolic/endocrine			
Hypothyroidism	++	N	N
Diabetes mellitus, type 2	+	++	−
Cushing syndrome	+	++	−
Renal			
Chronic kidney disease	+	+	−
Nephrotic syndrome	++	++	−
Hepatic			
Obstructive liver disease	++	N	−
Primary biliary cirrhosis	++	N	+
Drugs			
Alcohol	N	++	+
Thiazide diuretics	N	+	−
Beta blockers	N	+	−
Cyclosporine	++	N	N
Isotretinoin and etretinate		++	−
HIV-protease inhibitors	N	++	−

HDL-C, high-density-lipoprotein cholesterol.
++, Substantially increased; +, increased; N, not affected; −, decreased.

Diabetes Mellitus and Insulin Resistance

Patients with type II diabetes mellitus (and insulin resistance even in the absence of overt diabetes) frequently have associated dyslipidemia (29). Insulin resistance results in impaired capacity to catabolize chylomicrons and VLDL, as well as excess hepatic triglyceride and VLDL production. Type II diabetes mellitus, insulin resistance, and glucose intolerance are often associated with a constellation of lipid abnormalities including elevated triglycerides and VLDL-C, increased small, dense LDL, and decreased HDL-C. Occasionally, the triglycerides can be extremely elevated (>1,000 mg/dL) and predispose to acute pancreatitis. Significant elevation of LDL-C in the diabetic patient often suggests the presence of an additional lipoprotein abnormality. All patients presenting with hyperlipidemia should be screened for diabetes using a fasting glucose. Aggressive control of diabetes often results in improved control of hyperlipidemia. Furthermore, hyperlipidemia is a major risk factor for diabetic patients, and lipid disorders in diabetes should be aggressively treated in order to decrease the risk of cardiovascular disease.

Renal Diseases

Chronic renal insufficiency and especially end-stage renal disease are often associated with moderate hypertriglyceridemia due to a defect in triglyceride lipolysis and remnant clearance (30). Nephrotic syndrome is associated with a more pronounced hyperlipidemia involving both elevated triglycerides and cholesterol due to hepatic overproduction of VLDL. Both types of renal disease should be considered and excluded if suspected in patients presenting with hyperlipidemia. Resolution of the nephrotic syndrome improves the lipid profile, but patients with chronic nephrotic syndrome often require lipid-lowering drug therapy. Although the lipid abnormalities in end-stage renal disease are more modest, cardiovascular risk is high, and lipid-modifying drug therapy should be seriously considered. There has also been interest in the concept that atherogenic lipoproteins are nephrotoxic and lipid-lowering therapy might slow the progression of chronic renal insufficiency.

Alcohol

Alcohol intake often exacerbates hyperlipidemia, but its effects are highly variable. The greatest effects of alcohol are on triglyceride levels. Alcohol consumption inhibits oxidation of free fatty acids by the liver, which stimulates hepatic triglyceride synthesis and secretion of VLDL. The usual lipoprotein pattern associated with alcohol consumption is moderate hypertriglyceridemia, although it can raise total and LDL-C levels as well. Regular alcohol use also raises the HDL-C level by a mechanism that is not completely understood. Patients with hyperlipidemia who drink alcohol regularly should be advised to reduce their alcohol intake.

Drugs

Several drugs are known to influence plasma lipid levels and are listed in Table 5.1. Retinoids such as isotretinoin and etretinate used for acne are known to induce substantial hypertriglyceridemia in susceptible persons. Immunosuppressive therapy used in the posttransplantation setting is well known to cause both hypercholesterolemia and hypertriglyceridemia. Finally, since the introduction of the protease inhibitors for therapy for HIV, it has become recognized that many of these patients develop hyperlipidemia, which appears to result from a complex and poorly understood interaction between the disease and the effect of the drugs.

PRIMARY (GENETIC) DISORDERS OF APOLIPOPROTEIN B–CONTAINING LIPOPROTEINS CAUSING HYPERLIPOPROTEINEMIA

The classification of lipoprotein disorders is useful as a guide to accurate diagnosis and effective treatment. The Frederickson and Levy classification (Table 5.2) is based on the type of lipoprotein that is elevated and has been used for several decades. It is now gradually being replaced by a classification based on the understanding of the molecular etiology and pathophysiology of the lipoprotein disorders (Table 5.3). In this section, lipoprotein disorders are presented in a way intended to facilitate a practical clinical approach. This approach is based on classifying patients first according to triglyceride levels and can lead to a more rational approach to differential diagnosis and choice of appropriate therapy.

TABLE 5.2

FREDERICKSON AND LEVY CLASSIFICATION OF HYPERLIPOPROTEINEMIA PHENOTYPES

Phenotype	I	IIa	IIb	III	IV	V
Lipoprotein	CM	LDL	LDL and VLDL	Remnants	VLDL	CM and VLDL
Triglycerides	+++	N	+	+	++	+++
Cholesterol	+++	++	+	++	+	+++
Xanthomas	Eruptive	Tendon	None	Palmar and tuberoeruptive	None	Eruptive
Pancreatitis	+++	0	0	0	0	+++
Atherosclerosis	0	+++	+++	++	+/–	+/–
Molecular defect(s)	LPL, apoC-II	LDL receptor, apoB-100	Unknown	apoE	Unknown	Unknown

apoE, apolipoprotein E; CM, chylomicron; LDL, low-density lipoprotein; LPL, lipoprotein lipase; VLDL, very low density lipoprotein.

TABLE 5.3

PRIMARY (GENETIC) HYPERLIPOPROTEINEMIAS

Name	Molecular defect	Lipoproteins elevated	Lipoprotein phenotype	Clinical findings	Genetic transmission	Estimated incidence
Familial chylomicronemia syndrome	LPL deficiency, apoC-II deficiency	Chylomicrons	Type I	Eruptive xanthomas, hepatosplenomegaly	AR	1/1,000,000
Familial hypertriglyceridemia	Unknown	VLDL, occasionally chylomicrons	Type IV, occasionally V	Usually none	AD	1/500
Familial dysbetalipoproteinemia	Abnormal apoE (i.e., apoE-2/2)	Chylomicron and VLDL remnants	Type III	Palmar and tuberoeruptive xanthomas, premature atherosclerosis	AR or AC	1/5,000
Familial combined hyperlipidemia	Unknown	VLDL and LDL	Type IIb, sometimes IIa or IV, rarely V	Premature atherosclerosis	AD	1/200
Familial hepatic lipase deficiency	Hepatic lipase	VLDL remnants	Type III deficiency	Premature atherosclerosis	AR	Rare
Familial hypercholesterolemia	LDL-receptor	LDL	Type II	Tendon xanthomas, premature atherosclerosis	AC	
Familial defective apoB-100	Abnormal apoB-100 (i.e., $Arg_{3500} \rightarrow Gln$)	LDL	Type IIa	Tendon xanthomas, atherosclerosis	AC	1/600
Autosomal recessive hypercholesterolemia	ARH gene	LDL	Type IIa	Tendon xanthomas, premature atherosclerosis	AR	Rare
Autosomal dominant hypercholesterolemia	PCSK9 gene	LDL	Type IIa	Tendon xanthomas, premature atherosclerosis	AR	Rare

AC, autosomal codominant; AD, autosomal dominant; apo, apolipoprotein; AR, autosomal recessive; ARH, autosomal recessive hypercholesterolemia; LDL, low-density lipoprotein; LPL, lipoprotein lipase; PCSK9, proprotein convertase subtilisin/kexin type 9; VLDL, very low density lipoprotein.

Disorders Associated with Triglycerides Greater Than 1,000 mg/dL

Severe hypertriglyceridemia (fasting triglycerides >1,000 mg/dL) is virtually always an indication of hyperchylomicronemia in the fasting state and points to an underlying genetic predisposition, often exacerbated by another medical condition or a hormonal or environmental factor. The major clinical complication of severe hypertriglyceridemia is acute pancreatitis, and initial treatment is focused on decreasing the triglycerides below 1,000 mg/dL to prevent this serious complication. In addition, some but not all patients with severe hypertriglyceridemia are at risk for premature atherosclerotic CVD and require more aggressive therapy even once the triglycerides have been decreased below the 1,000-mg/dL threshold. The major disorders associated with severe hypertriglyceridemia are discussed in the following subsections.

Familial Chylomicronemia Syndrome: Lipoprotein Lipase Deficiency and Apolipoprotein C-II Deficiency

The familial hyperchylomicronemia syndrome is characterized by presentation in childhood with acute pancreatitis in the setting of triglyceride levels greater than 1,000 mg/dL. Recurrent abdominal pain is a common feature in children with this disorder. On physical exam, eruptive xanthomas (small papular lesions that occur in showers on the buttocks and back) are often seen. Lipemia retinalis (a pale appearance to the retinal veins) is a clue to the existence of severe hypertriglyceridemia, and hepatosplenomegaly due to ingestion of chylomicrons by the reticuloendothelial system is often found. Premature atherosclerotic cardiovascular disease is not a feature of this disease.

Two different genetic defects can cause the familial hyperchylomicronemia syndrome: lipoprotein lipase (LPL) deficiency and apolipoprotein C-II (apoC-II) deficiency. The hydrolysis of triglycerides in chylomicrons requires the action of LPL in tissue capillary beds, and apoC-II is a required cofactor for the activation of LPL (Fig. 5.1). Mutations in either the LPL gene or the apoC-II gene result in functional deficiency of LPL, inability to hydrolyze triglycerides in chylomicrons, and consequent massive hyperchylomicronemia. The disorder is autosomal recessive, meaning that both alleles of the LPL or apoC-II gene must be affected for the disorder to be present. Therefore, the parents of children with this disorder generally have normal or near-normal triglyceride levels. Both are rare disorders, but of the two, LPL deficiency is much more common (approximately 1 in 1 million persons) than apoC-II deficiency.

The diagnosis of the familial hyperchylomicronemia syndrome is usually made based on the clinical presentation and some key laboratory features. The plasma is often lactescent

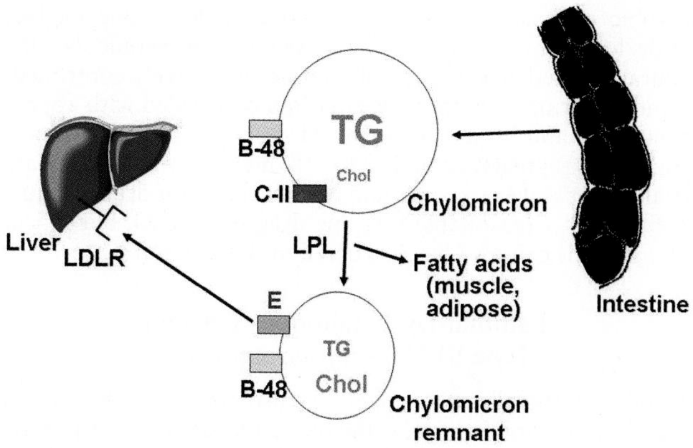

FIGURE 5.1. **Exogenous pathway of lipid transport.** Dietary fat is absorbed into chylomicrons, which contain the major structural apolipoprotein B-48. Chylomicrons bind to lipoprotein lipase (LPL) on the luminal surface of the capillary endothelium of tissues, especially muscle and adipose tissue. The LPL hydrolyzes the triglycerides (apolipoprotein C-II on the chylomicron surface is a required cofactor for LPL). The free fatty acids enter the tissue to be used for energy (muscle) or storage (adipose), and the triglyceride-depleted chylomicron remnant (CMR) is released. CMRs are taken up by the liver by binding of apolipoprotein E to the low-density-lipoprotein (LDL) receptor and the LDL-receptor–related protein (LRP). TG Chol, triglyceride cholesterol.

plasma, and after overnight refrigeration a cake of chylomicrons forms on the surface. Triglyceride levels are usually greater than 1,000 mg/dL and may be as high as 10,000 mg/dL or greater. Total cholesterol levels are also elevated due to the presence of cholesterol in chylomicrons. Lipoprotein electrophoresis demonstrates markedly elevated chylomicrons at the origin, but is not essential for making the diagnosis. The diagnosis of LPL deficiency can be confirmed at specialized centers by the measurement of LPL activity in the plasma after intravenous heparin injection (postheparin LPL activity). Patients with suspected familial hyperchylomicronemia syndrome should be referred to a specialized lipid center for diagnosis and management.

The mainstay of therapy for familial hyperchylomicronemia syndrome is restriction of total dietary fat. Consultation with a registered dietician familiar with this disorder is essential. Caloric supplementation with medium-chain triglycerides, which are absorbed directly into the portal vein and therefore do not promote chylomicron formation, can be useful if necessary. If dietary fat restriction alone is not successful, some patients may respond to a trial of fish oils or fibrates. For patients with apoC-II deficiency, an attack of acute pancreatitis can be treated with infusion of fresh-frozen plasma to provide apoC-II in an attempt to clear severe hypertriglyceridemia and promote resolution of the pancreatitis.

Familial Type V Hyperlipoproteinemia

Type V hyperlipoproteinemia (HLP) is a common diagnosis, which continues to use the nomenclature of the Frederickson classification system. The label of type V HLP is generally used for an adult with triglyceride levels greater than 1,000 mg/dL who does not have known familial chylomicronemia syndrome due to LPL or apoC-II deficiency (see prior discussion). Type V HLP is also associated with risk of acute pancreatitis, which can be the initial presentation of this syndrome and is the major rationale for aggressive treatment of this condition. Type V HLP can also be associated with increased risk of cardiovascular disease, although some patients with type V HLP do not appear to be at significantly increased risk.

Most but not all patients with type V HLP have a family history of hypertriglyceridemia, although specific genetic mutations causing type V HLP have not yet been identified. Type 2 diabetes mellitus or glucose intolerance frequently accompanies type V hyperlipidemia, but type V also occurs in people with normal glucose tolerance. Some patients with nephrotic syndrome can develop severe hypertriglyceridemia. Estrogen replacement therapy, oral contraceptives, isotretinoin or etretinate, and alcohol use can exacerbate moderate hypertriglyceridemia and lead to severe hypertriglyceridemia and even acute pancreatitis. Rarely, patients with familial dysbetalipoproteinemia (type III hyperlipidemia; see later discussion) can have triglycerides greater than 1,000 mg/dL, particularly if another factor is superimposed on the apoE mutation. The diagnostic evaluation of an adult patient presenting with triglycerides greater than 1,000 mg/dL should be focused on a search for underlying predisposing factors and an attempt to establish a history of complications (pancreatitis and cardiovascular disease). A comprehensive personal and family history should be obtained and all medications should be reviewed. On physical exam, lipemia retinalis and tiny eruptive xanthomas on the back or buttocks are the most specific findings for type V hyperlipidemia. Diabetes and renal disease should always be excluded as potential contributing factors. No specific laboratory tests are required for the diagnosis of type V except possibly lipoprotein centrifugation to exclude familial dysbetalipoproteinemia (see later discussion).

The management of type V hyperlipidemia is first targeted to decreasing triglycerides in order to reduce the risk of pancreatitis, followed by further lipid lowering depending on the presence of CAD or other risk factors for cardiovascular disease. Women taking estrogens and patients taking isotretinoin or etretinate should be encouraged to discontinue them if triglycerides are greater than 1,000 mg/dL. Diabetes mellitus should be controlled as optimally as possible. Patients should be referred to a registered dietician for dietary counseling. In general, dietary management includes restriction of total fat as well as simple sugars in the diet. Alcohol should be avoided. Regular aerobic exercise can have a significant effect on triglyceride levels and should be actively encouraged. If the patient is overweight, weight loss can help to decrease triglycerides as well.

When fasting triglyceride levels remain greater than 1,000 mg/dL despite institution of appropriate dietary and lifestyle measures and control of secondary causes, drug therapy must be considered in order to decrease the risk of acute pancreatitis. Drug therapy is usually straightforward, although a subset of patients is remarkably resistant to standard treatment. There are three major drug classes for consideration in treating very high triglycerides: fibrates, nicotinic acid, and fish oils (see later discussion). In practice, fibrates are generally recommended as the first-line agent. Nicotinic acid or fish oils should be considered for patients who fail to respond adequately to fibrates.

Frequently, once the triglycerides are adequately controlled, patients remain significantly hypercholesterolemic. This often raises the difficult issue of the need for a second medication to better control the LDL-C. The National Cholesterol Education Program (NCEP) guidelines represent a useful guide to the decision to institute further drug therapy in this setting (31). If the triglyceride levels are greater than 200 mg/dL, the non-HDL-C should be calculated by subtracting the HDL-C from the total cholesterol. Targets for non-HDL-C are 30 mg/dL higher than LDL-C targets. Many type V patients who have had their triglycerides managed are candidates for the addition of a statin to further reduce LDL-C and non-HDL-C levels. Although it is important to recognize that there is an increased risk of myopathy associated with the combination of fibrate and statin, the risk can be minimized as described later.

Lipid Disorders

Disorders Associated with Triglycerides 200 to 1,000 mg/dL

Fasting triglyceride levels less than 1,000 mg/dL are not generally associated with risk of acute pancreatitis, although patients with fasting TG greater than 500 mg/dL can often achieve TG levels greater than 1,000 mg/dL after a meal and therefore remain at some risk for pancreatitis. However, the importance of elevated triglyceride levels in the 200- to 1,000-mg/dL range is mostly related to their potential association with risk of atherosclerotic CVD. There has been increasing recognition of the importance of elevated fasting triglycerides in this range as an independent cardiovascular risk factor. The major primary causes of elevated triglycerides in the 200- to 1,000-mg/dL range are familial hypertriglyceridemia, familial dysbetalipoproteinemia (type III hyperlipidemia), and familial combined hyperlipidemia (FCHL). It is important to differentiate among them because familial dysbetalipoproteinemia and FCHL are both definitely associated with increased risk of premature atherosclerosis, whereas the risk associated with familial hypertriglyceridemia is variable. The clinical approach to a patient with triglycerides in the 200- to 1,000-mg/dL range is generally to rule out secondary causes (and treat them when present), differentiate among the major primary causes, assess the patient for the presence of ASCVD and other cardiovascular risk factors, and manage the lipid disorder based on the clinical assessment of cardiovascular risk. Because there are no clinical endpoint trials based on treatment of hypertriglyceridemia and no formal guidelines for the clinical management of patients with hypertriglyceridemia, the clinical approach to reducing cardiovascular risk remains focused on decreasing LDL-C. However, elevated triglycerides can make the determination of LDL-C difficult, can be associated with increased risk even in the presence of a normal LDL-C, and can complicate the therapeutic approach.

Familial Hypertriglyceridemia

Familial hypertriglyceridemia (FHTG) is a relatively common disorder characterized by moderately elevated triglycerides usually with average or only moderately elevated total cholesterol. FHTG occurs in approximately 1 in 500 persons. It is inherited as an autosomal dominant trait but is not usually expressed until adulthood. The molecular etiology is unknown. VLDL is elevated due either to increased production, impaired catabolism, or a combination of the two. LDL-C is generally not increased in this disorder. Increased intake of simple carbohydrates, a sedentary lifestyle, obesity, insulin resistance, alcohol use, and estrogens can all exacerbate the hypertriglyceridemia.

The diagnosis is suggested by elevated triglyceride levels (200 to 1,000 mg/dL) with normal or only mildly increased cholesterol levels (<240 mg/dL) and almost always a low HDL-C level. Hypertriglyceridemia in at least one first-degree relative is essential in making the diagnosis. It is important to consider and rule out secondary causes of the hypertriglyceridemia. In the differential diagnosis, both familial dysbetalipoproteinemia (type III hyperlipoproteinemia) and familial combined hyperlipidemia (FCHL) should be considered. This is not simply an academic exercise because these two conditions are associated with a significantly increased risk of atherosclerotic vascular disease, whereas FHTG often is not. The total cholesterol level relative to the triglyceride level is usually lower in FHTG compared with familial dysbetalipoproteinemia and FCHL, and the plasma apoB level is usually lower in FHTG than in the other two conditions.

Therapy for FHTG should begin with diet and lifestyle. Intake of simple carbohydrates should be reduced. Regular aerobic exercise can be very effective in decreasing triglyceride levels, as can weight loss. Alcohol use should be discouraged. Diabetes mellitus should be aggressively controlled. Lipid-lowering drug therapy can often be avoided with appropriate diet and lifestyle changes. However, patients who have triglycerides greater than 400 to 600 mg/dL after an adequate trial of diet and exercise should be considered for drug therapy. A fibrate is a reasonable first-line drug for FHTG, but niacin and fish oils can also be considered in this condition.

Familial Dysbetalipoproteinemia (Type III Hyperlipoproteinemia)

Familial dysbetalipoproteinemia is also commonly known as type III hyperlipidemia. It is the best understood of the genetic lipid disorders causing moderate triglyceride elevation and can usually be definitively diagnosed based on a combination of clinical and laboratory parameters. Patients with familial dysbetalipoproteinemia usually present in adulthood with distinctive xanthomas, premature atherosclerosis, or asymptomatic hyperlipidemia discovered on routine screening. Two types of xanthomas are seen in patients with familial dysbetalipoproteinemia. Tuberoeruptive xanthomas begin as clusters of small papules on the elbows, knees, or buttocks and can grow to the size of small grapes. Palmar xanthoma refers to orange-yellow discoloration to the creases of the palms and wrists. Either of these xanthomas is highly suggestive of familial dysbetalipoproteinemia. Premature atherosclerotic CVD is often seen in this disorder. Compared with other lipid disorders, peripheral vascular disease is particularly common in patients with familial dysbetalipoproteinemia.

The pattern of hyperlipidemia can be another clue to the diagnosis of familial dysbetalipoproteinemia. Patients generally have both hypertriglyceridemia and hypercholesterolemia, and in contrast to most other lipid disorders, the cholesterol and triglyceride are often elevated to a relatively similar degree. In addition, the HDL-C level is often relatively normal, in contrast to most hypertriglyceridemic conditions, in which the HDL-C level is usually reduced. The hyperlipidemia can be relatively mild or very severe, depending on the presence of other metabolic conditions and unknown factors.

Familial dysbetalipoproteinemia is caused by mutations in the gene for apolipoprotein E (apoE). ApoE is present on chylomicron and VLDL remnants and mediates their removal from the plasma by binding to receptors in the liver (Figs. 5.1 and 5.2). Defective apoE is impaired in its ability to bind to these receptors, resulting in accumulation of chylomicron and VLDL remnants in the plasma. The most common form of familial dysbetalipoproteinemia is related to a common polymorphism in the human apoE gene. The most common form of apoE is known as apoE3, but another form, called apoE2, has an allele frequency of about 7%. The apoE2 protein, which differs from apoE3 by a single amino acid, does not bind adequately to lipoprotein receptors, resulting in defective removal of chylomicron and VLDL remnants. Homozygosity for the E2 allele (the E2/E2 genotype) is the most common cause of familial dysbetalipoproteinemia. However, most persons with the apoE2/E2 genotype do not have familial dysbetalipoproteinemia; development of this disorder appears to require an additional factor or a "second hit." Some of these factors include obesity, diabetes mellitus, hypothyroidism, renal disease, and alcohol use, but many patients with familial dysbetalipoproteinemia do not have an obvious second hit in addition to the E2/E2 genotype. There is another common variant of apoE known as apoE4, which has an allele frequency of approximately 14%. Although associated with elevated LDL-C and increased risk of both CHD and Alzheimer disease, the common apoE4 allele is not associated with familial dysbetalipoproteinemia.

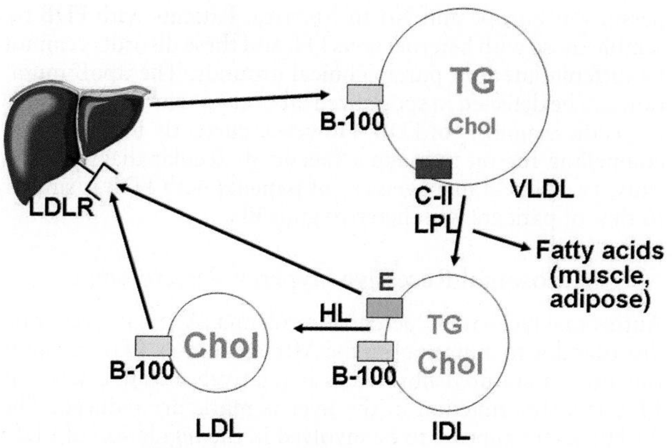

FIGURE 5.2. **Endogenous pathway of lipid transport.** The liver synthesizes triglycerides and cholesteryl esters and packages them into very low density lipoproteins (VLDL), which contain the major structural apolipoprotein B-100. VLDLs are hydrolyzed by lipoprotein lipase (LPL) to form intermediate-density lipoproteins (IDL). IDL can be taken up by the liver via binding of apolipoprotein E to the LDL receptor or the LDL-receptor–related protein (LRP). Alternatively, the triglyceride and phospholipid in IDL can be hydrolyzed by hepatic lipase (HL) within the hepatic sinusoids to form LDL. LDL can be taken up by peripheral cells or by the liver by the binding of apolipoprotein B-100 to the LDL receptor. TG Chol, triglyceride cholesterol.

Because familial dysbetalipoproteinemia is treated somewhat differently from other lipid disorders, it is important to consider the diagnosis and confirm it if suspected. The diagnosis can be made with reasonable confidence in several ways. The traditional approach is to use lipoprotein electrophoresis, which demonstrates a broad β band due to the presence of remnant lipoproteins. A second method is often referred to as a "beta quantification" in which plasma is subjected to ultracentrifugation and the cholesterol measured in the VLDL fraction. Because this disorder is associated with increased numbers of VLDL remnants that are enriched in cholesterol relative to triglycerides, an elevated ratio of VLDL-C to plasma triglycerides of greater than 0.3 is confirmatory of the diagnosis. A third approach is to perform advanced lipoprotein analysis, which reveals a substantial increase in IDL-sized particles. Finally, the apoE2/E2 pattern can be determined by using protein methods (apoE phenotype) or DNA-based methods (apoE genotype). The finding of an apoE2/E2 pattern by phenotyping or genotyping in a patient with suspected familial dysbetalipoproteinemia confirms the diagnosis. The absence of the apoE2/2 genotype decreases the likelihood but does not absolutely rule out the diagnosis of familial dysbetalipoproteinemia because other mutations in apoE other than E2 can also cause this condition.

Because familial dysbetalipoproteinemia is associated with increased risk of premature ASCVD, it should be aggressively treated. General therapeutic measures include decreased dietary fat, regular aerobic exercise, weight loss (if required), and discontinuance of alcohol. Statins, fibrates, and niacin are all effective in the treatment of familial dysbetalipoproteinemia and sometimes must be used in combination.

Familial Combined Hyperlipidemia

Familial combined hyperlipidemia (FCHL) is the most common primary lipid disorder, occurring in approximately 1 in 200 persons. Approximately 20% of patients with CHD younger than age 60 years have FCHL. FCHL is characterized by a mixed dyslipidemia usually associated with moderately elevated fasting triglycerides, moderately elevated cholesterol, and reduced HDL-C. In most cases, at least one first-degree relative also has hyperlipidemia, and there is often a family history of premature CHD as well. Xanthomas are not generally seen in patients with this disorder. Visceral obesity, glucose intolerance, insulin resistance, hypertension, and hyperuricemia are sometimes associated with FCHL. Patients with FCHL almost always have a significantly elevated plasma level of apolipoprotein B (apoB) that is disproportionate to the LDL-C level. This is indicative of the presence of small, dense LDL particles, which are characteristic of this syndrome and are considered to be highly atherogenic. FCHL is inherited as an autosomal dominant trait and can be expressed in childhood but is sometimes not fully expressed until adulthood.

The genetic basis of FCHL is not fully understood (32). Studies of lipoprotein metabolism in carefully selected individuals have indicated that hepatic overproduction of VLDL is a common metabolic basis of this condition. It has been suggested that a subset of patients with the familial combined hyperlipidemia phenotype may be heterozygous for lipoprotein lipase deficiency, but LPL mutations are probably not a common cause of FCHL. It is likely that more than one genetic etiology of the FCHL phenotype exists.

The diagnosis of FCHL is suggested by the presence of a mixed hyperlipidemia with fasting triglyceride levels from 200 to 800 mg/dL, cholesterol levels of 200 to 400 mg/dL, and decreased HDL-C levels in the absence of secondary causes of hyperlipidemia. A family history of hyperlipidemia and premature coronary disease is often present and supports the diagnosis. The finding of an elevated apoB level relative to the LDL-C level suggests increased levels of small, dense LDL. The LDL particle concentrations can be determined using nuclear magnetic resonance (NMR), which helps confirm the diagnosis and assists in decisions regarding therapy.

Because individuals with FCHL are at significantly increased risk of premature CHD, they should be treated aggressively. Decreased dietary intake of saturated fat and simple carbohydrates, regular aerobic exercise, and weight loss can all have beneficial effects on the lipid profile. However, many patients with FCHL require lipid-lowering drug therapy for adequate control. Statins are effective in lowering LDL-C and apoB, and the addition of ezetimibe may sometimes be required to achieve the LDL-C goal. Nicotinic acid decreases both LDL-C and triglycerides and raises HDL-C and is often used in combination with statins for this condition. Fibrates are also sometimes used in combination with statins in FCHL, particularly when the triglycerides are substantially elevated.

Disorders Associated with Triglycerides Less Than 200 mg/dL

Familial Hypercholesterolemia

Familial hypercholesterolemia (FH) is caused by mutations in the gene for the LDL receptor that prevent its appearance on the cell surface or impair its ability to bind and internalize LDL (33). FH is an autosomal codominant disorder, meaning that heterozygotes have hypercholesterolemia but homozygotes have even more severe hypercholesterolemia. One mutant LDL receptor allele results in the production of only about half of the normal number of LDL receptors, whereas the presence of two mutant alleles severely reduces or eliminates functional LDL receptors. The reduction in functional hepatic LDL receptors leads to reduced clearance of plasma LDL by the liver and substantial elevations in LDL-C. Elevated LDL-C levels lead directly to the major complication of this condition, premature atherosclerotic cardiovascular disease.

Heterozygous FH occurs in approximately 1 in 500 persons worldwide, making it one of the most common single-gene disorders. It is characterized by elevated LDL-C levels (usually 200 to 400 mg/dL) with normal triglycerides and a family history of hypercholesterolemia or premature cardiovascular disease. The finding of tendon xanthomas is virtually diagnostic of FH (although they can also been seen in related disorders, as discussed later). Tendon xanthomas are most easily recognized within the Achilles tendons, where they cause thickening and irregularity. Other common locations for tendon xanthomas are the digit extensor tendons of the metacarpophalangeal joints on the dorsum of the hands. Premature corneal arcus is frequently seen in patients with heterozygous FH. There is no definitive diagnostic test for heterozygous FH, which is diagnosed on clinical grounds.

Heterozygous FH is strongly associated with premature atherosclerotic cardiovascular disease, especially CHD. Therefore, patients should be aggressively treated to lower the LDL-C. Most heterozygous FH patients require lipid-lowering drug therapy. Statins are usually effective in heterozygous FH by inducing upregulation of the normal LDL receptor allele in the liver. If further LDL lowering is required, the addition of a cholesterol-absorption inhibitor (ezetimibe) to the statin can be used to achieve further LDL-C reduction. In some heterozygous FH patients, even high-dose statin plus ezetimibe fails to adequately reduce LDL-C levels. In this case, a bile acid sequestrant and/or niacin can also be added to the regimen. Even the combination of several drugs sometimes fails to adequately control the cholesterol, in which case LDL apheresis should be considered (see later discussion).

Homozygous FH is caused by the inheritance of two mutant LDL-receptor alleles, which results in the production of little or no LDL receptors and a severe defect in the catabolism of LDL. Homozygous FH occurs in approximately 1 in 1 million persons worldwide and is a much more severe clinical disorder than heterozygous FH. Patients with homozygous FH usually present in childhood with cutaneous xanthomas. Total cholesterol levels are usually greater than 500 mg/dL and can be as high as 1,200 mg/dL. The devastating complication of homozygous FH is accelerated atherosclerosis, which often develops first in the aortic root, causing aortic valvular or supravalvular stenosis, and extends into the coronary ostia. Untreated receptor-negative homozygous FH patients rarely survive beyond the second decade; receptor-defective patients have a better prognosis but invariably develop clinical atherosclerotic vascular disease by age 30 years and often much sooner. Patients with suspected homozygous FH should be referred to a specialized center. Statins and cholesterol-absorption inhibitors have either no or only modest effects in reducing cholesterol. Liver transplantation is effective in decreasing LDL-C levels but is associated with the substantial risks of surgery and long-term immunosuppression. The current treatment of choice for homozygous FH is LDL apheresis, which can promote regression of xanthomas and retard progression of atherosclerosis. Novel therapies, including gene therapy, are under development for homozygous FH.

Familial Defective Apolipoprotein B-100

Familial defective apoB-100 (FDB) resembles heterozygous FH clinically: it is characterized by elevated LDL-C with normal triglycerides, possible tendon xanthomas, and increased risk of premature atherosclerotic cardiovascular disease. In contrast to FH, FDB is caused by mutations in the receptor-binding region of apoB-100, the ligand for the LDL receptor, which impairs its binding and delays the clearance of LDL from the blood. The most common mutation causing FDB is a substitution of glutamine for arginine at position 3500 in apoB-100. However, other mutations have been reported that have a similar effect on apoB binding to the LDL receptor. FDB is a dominantly inherited disorder and occurs in approximately 1 in 700 persons in Europe and North America. Patients with FDB resemble those with heterozygous FH, and these disorders cannot be differentiated on purely clinical grounds. The apoB mutation can be detected in specialized laboratories in order to make a specific diagnosis of FDB. However, currently there is not a compelling reason to make a specific molecular diagnosis because the clinical management of patients with FDB is similar to that of patients with heterozygous FH.

Autosomal Recessive Hypercholesterolemia

Autosomal recessive hypercholesterolemia (ARH) is a very rare disorder due to mutations in the ARH gene (33). LDL-receptor function in cultured fibroblasts is relatively normal, whereas LDL-receptor function in the liver is markedly reduced. The ARH protein appears to be involved in the regulation of LDL-receptor–mediated endocytosis in the liver. ARH clinically resembles receptor-defective homozygous FH. Patients sometimes respond partially to treatment with statins, but they often require LDL apheresis for adequate control of their hypercholesterolemia.

Autosomal Dominant Hypercholesterolemia

Autosomal dominant hypercholesterolemia (ADH) is another rare disorder, and is due to gain-of-function mutations in the proprotein convertase subtilisin/kexin type 9 (PCSK9) gene (34). Patients have a phenotype very similar to heterozygous FH. The function of PCSK9 and its role in cholesterol metabolism is unclear. It is interesting that loss-of-function mutations in this gene appear to cause extremely low LDL-C levels (35).

Polygenic Hypercholesterolemia

Most forms of hypercholesterolemia are not single-gene disorders, but rather are due to a complex interaction of several genetic and environmental factors. For example, genetic differences in cholesterol absorption, cholesterol synthesis, or rates of bile acid synthesis may result in very different cholesterol levels in people challenged with a fat-rich diet. Polygenic hypercholesterolemia is characterized by a cholesterol level exceeding the 95th percentile for age and gender, with triglyceride levels that are usually relatively normal. In polygenic hypercholesterolemia, LDL-C levels are usually not as elevated as they are in heterozygous FH and FDB, and tendon xanthomas are not observed. In the differentiation of polygenic hypercholesterolemia from the single-gene disorders described previously, family studies are useful. Only about 7% of first-degree relatives of patients with polygenic hypercholesterolemia are hypercholesterolemic, whereas about half of relatives with FCHL, heterozygous FH, and FDB have dyslipidemia. Treatment of polygenic hypercholesterolemia follows the same guidelines as the approach to any patient with hypercholesterolemia as outlined previously.

PRIMARY DISORDERS OF HIGH-DENSITY-LIPOPROTEIN METABOLISM CAUSING LOW HIGH-DENSITY-LIPOPROTEIN–CHOLESTEROL LEVELS

HDL-C levels are inversely associated with CHD independent of LDL-C levels. Patients with low HDL-C levels are frequently identified. Many causes of low HDL-C are at least in part secondary to other factors. Cigarette smoking, obesity, and physical inactivity contribute to low HDL-C. Type II diabetes

TABLE 5.4

PRIMARY (GENETIC) DISORDERS ASSOCIATED WITH LOW HIGH-DENSITY-LIPOPROTEIN–CHOLESTEROL LEVELS

Genetic disorder	Molecular defect	Metabolic abnormalities	Lipoprotein findings	Clinical findings	Premature atherosclerosis	Genetic transmission
Familial apoA-I deficiency	ApoA-I absence	Absent apoA-I biosynthesis	HDL <5 mg/dL TG normal	Planar xanthomas, corneal opacities	++	Autosomal codominant
Familial apoA-I structural mutants	Mutant apoA-I	Rapid apoA-I catabolism	HDL 15–30 mg/dL TG normal to increased	Often none, sometimes corneal opacities	No	Autosomal dominant
Familial LCAT deficiency	LCAT deficiency (complete)	Rapid apoA-I catabolism	HDL <10 mg/dL TG increased	Corneal opacities, anemia, proteinuria, renal insufficiency	No	Autosomal recessive
Fish-eye disease	LCAT deficiency (partial)	Rapid apoA-I catabolism	HDL <10 mg/dL TG normal to increased	Corneal opacities	No	Autosomal recessive
Tangier disease	Mutant ABCA1	Very rapid apoA-I catabolism	HDL <5 mg/dL TG usually increased	Corneal opacities, enlarge orange tonsils, hepatosplenomegaly, peripheral neuropathy	+	Autosomal codominant
Familial hypoalphalipoproteinemia	Unknown	Usually rapid apoA-I catabolism	HDL 15–35 mg/dL TG normal	Often none, sometimes corneal opacities	No to ++	Autosomal dominant

apo, apolipoprotein; HDL, high-density lipoprotein; LCAT, lecithin:cholesterol acyltransferase; TG, triglycerides.

mellitus, end-stage renal disease, and hypertriglyceridemia from any cause are all associated with low HDL. Beta-blockers, thiazide diuretics, androgens, and progestins can all reduce HDL-C levels. It is important to note that a low-fat diet often results in a low level of HDL-C; for example, most vegetarians have low levels of HDL-C. In this case, the low HDL is not considered to be associated with an increased risk of CHD because persons who eat lo-fat diets are at substantially reduced risk of premature CHD. Many persons with low HDL-C levels have a genetic cause for the low HDL-C. However, only a few of the specific genes responsible for inherited low HDL syndromes have been identified, and these are reviewed in the following subsections (Table 5.4).

Primary Monogenic Disorders Causing Low High-Density-Lipoprotein–Cholesterol Levels

Familial Apoliporotein A-I Deficiency and Structural Apolipoprotein A-I Mutations

Complete genetic deficiency of apoA-I due to deletions of the apoA-I gene or nonsense mutations that prevent the biosynthesis of apoA-I protein result in virtually absent plasma HDL and increased risk of premature cardiovascular disease. Mutations in the apoA-I–coding sequence have been described in association with low levels of HDL-C (usually 15 to 30 mg/dL) but are a very rare cause of low HDL-C levels in the general population. The first of these mutants to be described was apoA-I Milano, which was not found to be associated with increased risk of premature CHD despite the low levels of HDL-C in persons bearing this mutation (36). It is of interest that a few apoA-I mutations have been described in association with systemic amyloidosis in addition to low HDL, and the mutant apoA-I has been found as a primary component of the amyloid plaque.

Familial Lecithin:Cholesterol Acyltransferase Deficiency and Fish-eye Disease

HDL cholesterol is esterified by the enzyme lecithin:cholesterol acyltransferase (LCAT) (Fig. 5.3). Two general types of genetic LCAT deficiency have been described in humans: complete deficiency (also called classic LCAT deficiency) and partial deficiency (also called fish-eye disease) (37). Progressive corneal opacification, very low plasma levels of HDL-C (usually <10 mg/dL), and variable hypertriglyceridemia are characteristic of both types. In partial LCAT deficiency, there are no other known clinical sequelae. In contrast, complete (classic) LCAT deficiency is characterized by anemia and progressive proteinuria and renal insufficiency. The diagnosis can be made in specialized laboratories by quantitation of LCAT activity in the plasma. It is remarkable that, despite the extremely low levels of HDL-C and apoA-I, there is no apparent increased risk of premature atherosclerotic cardiovascular disease in either complete or partial LCAT deficiency. This again demonstrates that the relationship between low HDL-C and increased risk of CHD is complex and in part depends on the specific cause of the low HDL.

Tangier Disease

Tangier disease is a very rare disorder associated with cholesterol accumulation in the reticuloendothelial system resulting in hepatosplenomegaly, intestinal mucosal abnormalities, pathognomonic enlarged orange tonsils, peripheral neuropathy, and extremely low levels of HDL-C and apoA-I (38). After several decades of investigation, Tangier disease was found to

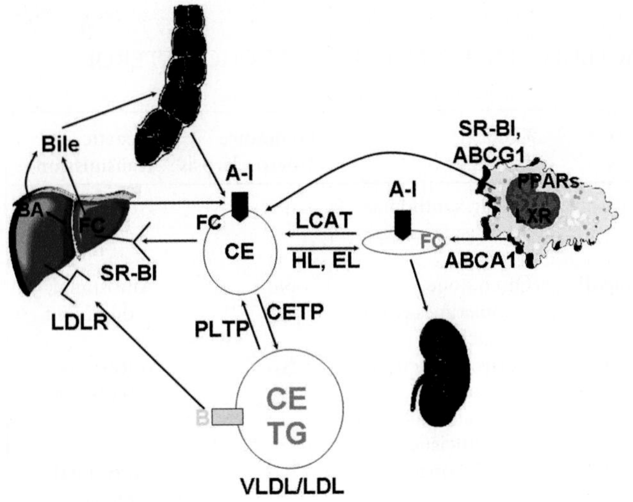

FIGURE 5.3. **High-density-lipid (HDL) metabolism and reverse cholesterol transport.** HDL and its major apolipoprotein, apoA-I, are synthesized by both the intestine and the liver. A second major HDL protein, apoA-II, is made only by the liver. Nascent HDL interacts with peripheral cells to facilitate the removal of excess free cholesterol through a process that is facilitated by the cellular protein ABCA1. Some of the acquired free cholesterol is esterified to cholesteryl ester on the HDL particle by the action of the enzyme lecithin:cholesterol acyltransferase (LCAT), and the nascent HDL particle becomes the larger HDL$_3$. HDL acquires further cholesteryl ester by continued LCAT action and eventually becomes the even larger HDL$_2$. HDL$_2$ can selectively transfer both cholesteryl ester and free cholesterol to the liver via an HDL receptor in the liver called scavenger receptor BI (SR-BI). Cholesteryl esters can also be transferred from HDL$_2$ to apoB-containing lipoproteins such as very low density lipoprotein (VLDL) and low-density lipoprotein (LDL) via the action of the cholesteryl ester transfer protein (CETP) and then returned to the liver by hepatic uptake of LDL. HDL$_2$ triglycerides and phospholipids can be hydrolyzed by hepatic lipase (HL) to remodel it to HDL$_3$. Cholesterol derived from HDL contributes to the hepatic cholesterol pool used for bile acid synthesis, and the cholesterol is eventually excreted into the bile and feces as bile acid or free cholesterol. The solid lines indicate the metabolism of the lipoprotein particles, and the broken lines indicate the flux of cholesterol independent of lipoprotein particle metabolism.

be caused by mutations in the gene encoding ABCA1, a cellular transporter that facilitates the efflux of unesterified cholesterol and phospholipids from cells to apoA-I as an acceptor (39). The absence of functional ABCA1 results in impaired cholesterol efflux from most tissues, increased cholesterol accumulation particularly in macrophages and certain other cell types, and impaired lipidation of nascent apoA-I, with subsequent rapid catabolism of apoA-I. Tangier disease is associated with some increased risk of premature atherosclerotic disease, but this risk does not seem to be proportional to the markedly decreased HDL-C and apoA-I levels and impaired cholesterol efflux. Heterozygotes for functional ABCA1 mutations have moderately reduced HDL-C levels (approximately 20 to 40 mg/dL) but have no evidence of cholesterol accumulation in tissues. However, the risk of premature atherosclerosis in heterozygotes appears to be moderately increased. Heterozygosity for rare mutations in ABCA1 may be a quantitatively important cause of low HDL-C levels in the general population (40).

Primary Hypoalphalipoproteinemia

The most common inherited form of low HDL is termed primary or familial hypoalphalipoproteinemia. It is defined as an HDL-C level below the 10th percentile in the setting of relatively normal cholesterol and triglyceride levels, no apparent secondary causes of low HDL-C, and no clinical signs of LCAT deficiency or Tangier disease. This syndrome is often referred to as "isolated low HDL." A family history of low HDL-C facilitates the diagnosis of an inherited condition, which usually follows the pattern of an autosomal dominant trait. The genetic etiology of this syndrome is unknown, although the metabolic etiology appears to be primarily accelerated catabolism of apoA-I. Although several kindreds with this syndrome have been described in association with an increased incidence of premature atherosclerotic cardiovascular disease, other families have been described in which there was no evidence of increased atherosclerosis. Therefore, the direct relationship of primary hypoalphalipoproteinemia to premature coronary disease is uncertain and may depend on the specific nature of the gene defect or metabolic cause of the low HDL-C level.

SCREENING AND MANAGEMENT OF PATIENTS WITH LIPID DISORDERS

Screening

A general approach to the screening and management of lipid disorders has been developed by an expert Adult Treatment Panel (ATP) convened by the National Cholesterol Education Program (NCEP) of the National Institutes of Health. The most recent full guidelines are the ATPIII guidelines from 2001 (31) with an update issued in 2004 based on new clinical trials that were reported since 2001 (41). The NCEP ATPIII guidelines recommend that all adults older than the age 20 years be screened for lipids by a fasting full-lipid panel, including triglycerides, total cholesterol, HDL-C, and calculated LDL-C levels. A detailed cardiovascular risk assessment should be performed at the same time. The LDL-C is usually calculated from the other lipid values using the following equation: LDL-C = total cholesterol – (triglycerides/5) – HDL-C (because VLDL usually contains triglyceride and cholesterol in a ratio of approximately 5 to 1, the fraction triglycerides/5 is an estimate of the VLDL-C). This formula is reasonably accurate if test results are obtained on fasting plasma and if the triglyceride level does not exceed 400 mg/dL. The determination of LDL-C levels in patients with triglyceride levels greater than 400 mg/dL usually requires application of ultracentrifuge techniques in specialized laboratories, although direct assays for LDL measurement have recently become available. The NCEP ATPIII guidelines recommended the clinical use of the non-HDL-C level as a secondary target of therapy in patients with fasting TG levels greater than 200 mg/dL. The non-HDL-C is calculated simply as follows: non-HDL-C = total cholesterol – HDL-C. Non-HDL-C targets are 30 mg/dL higher than the LDL-C targets.

Diagnosis and Classification of Lipid Disorders

Most patients with hyperlipidemia have a genetic factor contributing to their lipid disorder. However, the clinician should always consider whether a secondary medical disorder could be causing or contributing to the hyperlipidemia. Treatment of the underlying medical condition can often result in substantial improvement in the lipid profile and obviate the need for therapy directed at the lipids themselves. Once secondary causes have been considered, it is useful to use the fasting triglyceride level as an initial method of stratifying patients. This approach guides both the initial diagnostic evaluation and the choice of most effective therapy. It is important to consider the differential diagnosis of hyperlipidemia before treatment because the inherited disorders discussed previously are associated with different risks of developing CHD, differences in response to drug therapy, and differences with regard to family and genetic counseling.

Although extremely elevated triglyceride levels (>1,000 mg/dL) are associated with the risk of acute pancreatitis, the most important clinical consequence of lipid disorders is atherosclerotic cardiovascular disease (CVD), including coronary, cerebrovascular, and peripheral vascular disease. The clinical approach to a patient with a lipid disorder is significantly influenced by the presence of established CVD and/or other risk factors.

General Issues in the Nonpharmacologic Management of Lipid Disorders

Identify and Treat Secondary Causes of Hyperlipidemia

Secondary causes of hypercholesterolemia should be considered and excluded with appropriate laboratory testing. Because occult hypothyroidism can cause elevated LDL-C levels, patients with newly diagnosed elevated LDL-C should be screened with a TSH to exclude hypothyroidism. Treatment of hypothyroidism usually results in substantial improvement in hypercholesterolemia. A fasting glucose should always be obtained in the initial workup of hyperlipidemia. Diabetes mellitus should be controlled as effectively as possible, which often results in improvement in hyperlipidemia. Nephrotic syndrome and chronic renal insufficiency should be excluded if clinically suspected. Patients with hypertriglyceridemia who drink alcohol should be encouraged to decrease their intake. Sedentary lifestyle, obesity, and smoking are all associated with low HDL-C levels.

Counsel Patients on an Appropriate Diet

Dietary modification is an important component of the effective management of patients with lipid disorders. It is important for the physician to make a general assessment of the patient's diet, provide suggestions for improvement, and recognize whether a patient may benefit from referral to a dietician for more intensive counseling. If possible, the patient should receive specific instruction in the diet from a dietician or qualified professional. The dietary approach depends on the type of hyperlipidemia and the overall metabolic profile of the patient. Patients with primarily elevated LDL-C should focus on reducing their intake of saturated fats and cholesterol. On the other hand, patients with primary hypertriglyceridemia, particularly in the setting of obesity and/or insulin resistance, may need to primarily limit intake of simple carbohydrates and overall calories. Finally, patients with hyperchylomicronemia (generally fasting TG >1,000 mg/dL) should limit intake of total fat.

Certain types of "functional foods" can be used to modestly reduce cholesterol levels and in some cases avoid the need for drug therapy. Plant stanol and sterol esters reduce LDL-C levels in randomized, controlled trials when taken three times per day, are not absorbed, and are available in a variety of foods such as spreads, salad dressings, and snack bars. Chinese red yeast rice has been shown to reduce LDL-C levels and is known to contain small amounts of lovastatin, which accounts for its modest cholesterol-lowering properties. Addition of psyllium to the diet can reduce cholesterol levels. Soy protein has been shown to reduce cholesterol levels. Fish oils can reduce triglyceride levels at relatively high doses (see later discussion).

Encourage Regular Aerobic Exercise

Regular aerobic exercise can have a positive effect on plasma lipids. Elevated triglycerides are especially sensitive to aerobic exercise, and persons with hypertriglyceridemia can substantially lower their triglycerides by initiating an exercise program. The effect of exercise on LDL-C levels is more modest. Although widely believed to be a method for raising HDL-C, the effects of aerobic exercise on HDL-C are relatively modest in most individuals unless accompanied by weight loss.

Encourage Achieving and Maintaining Appropriate Weight

Obesity is often associated with dyslipidemia, especially with elevated triglycerides, low HDL-C, and small, dense LDL. In persons who are overweight, weight loss can have a significant favorable impact on the lipid profile and should be actively encouraged. Along with counseling on other dietary issues, a dietician should also advise patients on caloric restriction necessary for effective weight loss.

Lipid-Modifying Drug Therapy

The Decision to Initiate Lipid-Modifying Drug Therapy

The decision to initiate lipid-modifying drug therapy is highly dependent on the level of cardiovascular risk of the patient. The patient with known CHD has traditionally been considered in the class of highest-risk patient meriting the most aggressive lipid intervention. The NCEP ATPIII guidelines in 2001 established the concept of the "CHD-risk-equivalent" patient: the patient who does not have clinical CHD but whose risk is comparable and therefore who should be treated just as aggressively as patients with CHD (31). This includes those patients with other noncoronary atherosclerotic vascular disease, those with diabetes mellitus, and those with a global Framingham risk score of greater than 20% risk of a CHD event over 10 years. The ATPIII guidelines extended the goal of LDL-C less than 100 mg/dL to all CHD-risk-equivalent patients.

Studies such as HPS, ASCOT, CARDS, and PROVE-IT proved that statin therapy is beneficial in high-risk patients virtually regardless of the baseline LDL-C level and also suggested that the target of LDL-C less than 100 mg/dL may not be low enough in such patients. Therefore, in 2004 an NCEP white paper endorsed by the National Heart, Lung and Blood Institute (NHLBI), American College of Cardiologists (ACC), and American Heart Association (AHA) suggested that in "very high risk" patients an LDL-C goal of less than 70 mg/dL is a reasonable therapeutic option based on available clinical trial data (41). Many clinicians choose to treat all CHD and CHD-risk-equivalent patients to LDL-C less than 70 mg/dL when it is feasible to do so. Thus, the vast majority of CHD and CHD-risk-equivalent patients are candidates for lipid-modifying drug therapy, and many require high-dose statins or combination drug therapy to achieve LDL-C targets of less than 70 mg/dL.

The decision to initiate lipid-lowering drug therapy in patients who are not at as a high cardiovascular risk is often more difficult. Data certainly exist for the benefit of lipid-altering drug therapy even in the less-high-risk primary prevention setting. Absolute global 10-year cardiovascular risk should be quantitated using a simple approach based on the Framingham Heart Study database and used as a guide to the decision for initiating cholesterol-lowering drug therapy. In addition, persons with markedly elevated LDL-C levels (>190 mg/dL) have a high lifetime risk of developing ASCVD and should be seriously considered for drug therapy even if their 10-year absolute risk is not particularly elevated. However, it is often difficult to decide whether to initiate drug therapy in patients who have LDL-C levels in a gray zone. A high proportion of patients who eventually develop ASCVD have LDL-C levels that are in this range. Furthermore, many patients have average or below-average LDL-C levels but elevated triglycerides and/or low HDL-C, and the decision to initiate lipid-modifying drug therapy in these individuals is often difficult as well. Therefore, the use of certain blood and/or vascular imaging tests may be useful in helping to refine the risk assessment and therefore the decision about drug therapy (see later discussion). In persons with low 10-year absolute risk and considered to be at relatively low lifetime risk, the emphasis should remain primarily on dietary and lifestyle modification.

In certain patients, drug therapy should be targeted initially toward reduction of triglycerides rather than LDL-C. For example, when triglycerides are greater than 1,000 mg/dL the patient has a primary triglyceride disorder, usually hyperchylomicronemia, and should be treated to prevent the risk of acute pancreatitis. When triglycerides are 500 to 1,000 mg/dL, the decision to use drug therapy depends on the assessment of cardiovascular risk; however, if drug therapy is used, it should usually be first targeted to reducing the triglycerides because cholesterol reduction is difficult in the setting of substantially elevated triglycerides. It is important to note that the major clinical endpoint trials with statins have generally excluded persons with triglyceride levels greater than 400 to 600 mg/dL. Therefore, there are few data regarding the effectiveness of statins in reducing cardiovascular risk in persons with triglycerides above this range. If the triglycerides are less than 500 mg/dL, the initial emphasis in treatment should be on reduction of LDL-C, not the triglycerides. As mentioned previously, the NCEP ATPIII guidelines established the concept of non-HDL-C as a secondary target for therapy in patients with TG greater than 200 mg/dL (31). The non-HDL-C encompasses all atherogenic lipoproteins, including not just LDL but also VLDL and IDL. Thus, after focusing initially on lowering the LDL-C or if the LDL-C cannot be determined, one should use the non-HDL-C as a secondary target for therapy. The recommended targets for non-HDL-C are 30 mg/dL higher than the LDL-C targets, so the patient who should be targeted to LDL-C less than 100 mg/dL should also be targeted to non-HDL-C less than 130 mg/dL.

The Choice of a Lipid-Modifying Drug Therapy

Once the decision has been made to initiate drug therapy, the next decision involves the choice of drug. A summary of the major drugs for treating dyslipidemia is provided in Table 5.5 and the major classes of drugs are discussed in what follows.

3-Hydroxy-3-methylglutaryl Coenzyme A Reductase Inhibitors (Statins). HMG-CoA reductase is the rate-limiting step in cholesterol biosynthesis, and inhibition of this enzyme decreases cholesterol synthesis. There are six HMG-CoA reductase inhibitors currently available: lovastatin, pravastatin, simvastatin, fluvastatin, atorvastatin, and rosuvastatin. By inhibiting cholesterol biosynthesis, these drugs lead to increased hepatic LDL-receptor expression and in some situations to decreased hepatic production of VLDL as well. Their major effect is reduction of LDL-C, which they do in a dose-dependent fashion. There is wide interindividual variation in the initial response to a statin, but once a patient is on a statin, the doubling of the statin dose produces a very predictable 6% further reduction in LDL-C (42). Statins also reduce triglycerides in a dose-dependent fashion that is proportional to their LDL-C lowering effects. Statins have a modest HDL-C–raising effect by 5% to 10% that is not dose dependent. As reviewed earlier, there is now considerable evidence of efficacy for statins in reducing the risk of clinical cardiovascular events.

Statins are generally safe and well tolerated. However, a subgroup of patients develop muscle fatigue or pain on statin therapy, the mechanism of which is not well understood. Severe myopathy and rhabdomyolysis have been reported associated with statin therapy, and, although rare, represents the most important risk associated with statins. The risk of myopathy is dose dependent and more common at the highest doses of statins. Risk factors for statin myopathy include advanced age, female gender, frailty and low body weight, renal insufficiency, and occult hypothyroidism. The risk of statin-associated myopathy is increased by the administration of drugs that interfere with the cytochrome P450 (particularly 3A4) metabolism of statins, such as erythromycin-type antibiotics, antifungal agents, immunosuppressive drugs, amiodarone, gemfibrozil, and HIV-protease inhibitors. Statins that are not metabolized via P450 3A4 are less likely to be influenced by coadministration of these other drugs. Severe myopathy can usually be avoided by employing careful patient selection, avoiding interacting drugs, and informing the patient of its potential and advising immediate discontinuance of the drug in the event of new generalized muscle pain. Serum creatinine kinase (CK) levels need not be monitored on a routine basis. A CK level can be obtained in a patient taking a statin who complains of muscle pain; however, a normal level does not exclude the possibility that the symptoms are due to the drug. By convention and history, liver transaminases (alanine transaminase and aspartate transaminase) are monitored in patients taking statins (for example, 8 weeks after initiation of the drug and then every 6 months thereafter). However, substantial (greater than three times normal) elevation in transaminases is relatively rare, and mild to moderate (one to three times normal) elevation in transaminases in the absence of symptoms need not mandate discontinuing the medication. Severe clinical hepatitis associated with statins is exceedingly rare, if it occurs at all, and the trend is toward less frequent monitoring of transaminases in patients taking statins.

The overall interest in both the efficacy and safety of statins has increased in recently years (43,44). On one hand, as reviewed earlier, the data regarding the cardiovascular clinical benefits of statin therapy have increased dramatically in the last decade. On the other hand, the potential risks of statin therapy, particularly myopathy and rhabdomyolysis, were brought into sharper focus by the withdrawal of cerivastatin from the market. A joint statin advisory was issued by the ACC/AHA/NHLBI (45) and emphasized the overall safety of statins but the importance of understanding the risk factors for statin myopathy and the need to be careful in patients at risk, points reinforced by others (46). Finally, there has been growing interest in the concept that statins may exert their cardiovascular benefits at least in part through mechanisms that are independent of their cholesterol-lowering properties (so-called pleiotropic effects) (47). Although intriguing, this has not been definitively proven in humans, but is the subject of substantial ongoing research.

Cholesterol-Absorption Inhibitors. The small intestine mediates the active absorption of luminal cholesterol, which is derived from both the diet (about one third) and the liver via the bile (about two thirds). The first cholesterol absorption inhibitor, ezetimibe, was introduced onto the market in 2003 (48). Ezetimibe 10 mg was shown to inhibit cholesterol absorption in humans by almost 60% in a process that involves binding to and inhibiting the function of NPC1L1 (49). The inhibition of intestinal cholesterol absorption presumably reduces hepatic cholesterol stores and results in upregulation

TABLE 5.5

DRUGS AFFECTING LIPID METABOLISM AND USED FOR THE TREATMENT OF DYSLIPIDEMIA

Drug class and name	Major indication(s)	Starting daily dose	Maximal daily dose	Mechanism of class	Adverse events
HMG-CoA reductase inhibitors	Elevated LDL			Inhibit cholesterol synthesis and upregulate LDL receptors in liver	Myalgias, arthralgias, elevated LFTs
Lovastatin		20 mg	80 mg		
Pravastatin		20–40 mg	80 mg		
Simvastatin		20–40 mg	80 mg		
Fluvastatin		20 mg	80 mg		
Atorvastatin		10–20 mg	80 mg		
Rosuvastatin		5–10 mg	40 mg		
Cholesterol absorption inhibitors	Elevated LDL			Inhibit intestinal cholesterol absorption	Elevated LFTs when given with a statin
Ezetimibe		10 mg	10 mg		
Bile acid sequestrants	Elevated LDL			Inhibit intestinal bile acid reabsorption and upregulate LDL	Bloating, constipation, elevated triglycerides
Cholestyramine		1 g	4 g		
Colestipol		1 g	5 g		
Colesevalam		1.25–2.5 g	4.5 g		
Fibric acid derivatives	Elevated TG, low HDL			Stimulate lipoprotein lipase, reduce apoC-III, increase VLDL/LDL uptake	GI upset, myalgias, gallstones
Gemfibrozil		600 mg BID	1.2 mg		
Fenofibrate (micronized)		145 mg	145 mg		
Nicotinic acid	Low HDL, elevated TG and LDL-C			Inhibit adipocyte lipolysis, decrease VLDL synthesis, decrease HDL catabolism	Cutaneous flushing, GI upset, elevated LFTs, glucose, uric acid
Immediate-release		100 mg TID	3–4 g		
Sustained-release		250 mg BID	2–3 g		
Extended-release		500 mg QD	2 g		
Fish oils	Elevated TG			Decrease chylomicron and VLDL production, increase TG catabolism	GI upset, fishy taste and smell
Dietary supplement		2–3 g	6 g		
Prescription		2–4 g	4 g		

apo, apolipoprotein; BID, twice daily; HDL, high-density lipoprotein; GI, gastrointestinal; HMG-CoA, hydroxy-3-methylglutaryl coenzyme A; LDL, low-density lipoprotein; LDL-C, LDL cholesterol; LFTs, liver function tests; QD, daily; TG, triglycerides; TID, three times daily; VLDL, very low density lipoprotein.

of hepatic LDL-receptor expression, leading to reduction in LDL-C levels. The 10-mg dose of ezetimibe, the only dose marketed and used clinically, reduces LDL-C levels by about 18% on average as monotherapy (50) and to a similar extent when used in combination with a statin (51). Ezetimibe has very small but statistically significant effects in reducing TG and raising HDL-C levels. No cardiovascular outcome data have been reported with ezetimibe. The safety and tolerability of ezetimibe in placebo-controlled clinical trials were excellent, and in clinical practice it is generally well tolerated. When used in combination with a statin, monitoring of liver transaminases is recommended. Ezetimibe is used in combination with statins to further reduce LDL-C levels and in patients who are statin intolerant. A fixed-dose combination therapy product of ezetimibe plus simvastatin is available on the market.

Bile Acid Sequestrants (Resins). Cholesterol is used by the liver to actively synthesize bile acids, which are then excreted into the bile. Bile acids within the intestinal lumen are reabsorbed in the terminal ileum and returned to the liver, resulting in an enterohepatic circulation of bile acids. Bile acid sequestrants, which have been used clinically for several decades, bind bile acids in the intestine, prevent their reabsorption, and accelerate their loss in the feces. To maintain an adequate bile acid pool, the liver diverts cholesterol to bile acid synthesis, resulting in decreased hepatic cholesterol and upregulation of hepatic LDL-receptor expression. Bile acid sequestrants primarily reduce LDL-C and have very small effects on raising HDL-C levels. They tend to increase plasma triglyceride levels, probably through a mechanism that involves the bile acid nuclear receptor FXR (52). Bile acid sequestrants have been shown to reduce clinical cardiovascular events (4,5).

Bile acid sequestrants are very safe drugs that are not systemically absorbed and therefore are the cholesterol-lowering drug of choice in children and pregnant women. However, cholestyramine and colestipol are insoluble resins that must be suspended in liquid and are therefore often inconvenient and unpleasant to take. Colestipol is also available in large tablets but requires taking multiple tablets a day for substantial effect. Colesevalam was designed to combat the limitations of the traditional resins by making the molecule able to bind a larger number of bile acids. Colvesevalam is thus available as smaller tablets, but usually at least six tablets per day must be taken for effective reduction in LDL-C. Side effects of resins are generally limited to bloating and constipation. The older bile acid sequestrants interfere with the absorption of certain drugs (e.g., digoxin, warfarin) when taken around the same time, although this is less of an issue with colesevalam.

Fibric Acid Derivatives (Fibrates). Peroxisome proliferator-activated receptor-α(PPAR-α) is a nuclear hormone receptor expressed in multiple cells and tissues and involved in metabolic regulation. Fibric acid derivatives, or fibrates, are agonists of PPAR-α that have been used as lipid-modifying agents for several decades (53). This class includes clofibrate, gemfibrozil, fenofibrate, and bezafibrate. Fibrates have as their primary effect the lowering of triglycerides (up to 40%), with modest effects in raising HDL-C (up to 20% depending on the triglyceride levels) and minimal effects on LDL-C. Fibrates lower triglycerides by activating PPAR-α to stimulate lipoprotein lipase (enhancing triglyceride hydrolysis) and reduce hepatic apoC-III synthesis (enhancing clearance of TG-rich lipoproteins). Fibrates raise HDL-C indirectly by lowering triglycerides and possibly directly by promoting apoA-I and apoA-II production. Fibrates may also have direct antiinflammatory effects through PPAR-α activation (54). As noted earlier, fibrates have been demonstrated in several clinical trials to reduce cardiovascular events, particularly in patients with the phenotype of insulin resistance (55).

Fibrates are generally well tolerated, with the most common side effects being dyspepsia. They modestly increase the risk of gallstones. Elevated liver function tests can occur with fibrate therapy, but this is relatively uncommon and rarely presents a clinical issue. Myopathy has occurred with fibrate therapy, but in the absence of other drugs is rare.

The most clearly defined clinical role of fibrates is in the treatment of hypertriglyceridemia. After lifestyle intervention, fibrates are generally first-line agents in the setting of hyperchylomicronemia (generally TG >1,000 mg/dL) to prevent acute pancreatitis. Fibrates are also often considered first-line agents for persons with triglycerides greater than 500 mg/dL because statins are less effective and less proven to reduce cardiovascular risk in this setting. The issue of whether fibrates should be considered as first-line agents in some patients with TG levels in the 200- to 500-mg/dL range has not been resolved. Because fibrates raise HDL-C levels, they are sometimes also used in patients with isolated low HDL-C. Fibrates are effective in reducing cardiovascular events, particularly in patients with insulin resistance, metabolic syndrome, and/or type 2 diabetes (55). Increasingly, fibrates are being used in combination with statins (see later discussion). The ongoing ACCORD trial will determine the benefit of adding fenofibrate to a statin in patients with type 2 diabetes.

Nicotinic Acid (Niacin). Nicotinic acid, or niacin, is a B-complex vitamin that in high doses has been used clinically as a lipid-modifying drug for several decades (56,57). Niacin effectively reduces triglycerides and LDL-C and is the most effective of available lipid-modifying drugs in raising HDL-C levels. Niacin is also the only currently available lipid-lowering drug that decreases lipoprotein (a) levels. Its safety and efficacy were documented in the Coronary Drug Project, which showed that niacin reduced nonfatal MI after 6 years of treatment and total mortality after 15 years of follow-up.

Niacin has long been known to acutely reduce free fatty acid levels through inhibition of adipocyte triglyceride lipolysis, a mechanism believed to be at least partially responsible for its lipid-modifying effects (57). In 2003, a nicotinic acid receptor was reported, a G protein-coupled receptor primarily expressed on adipocytes that when activated results in inhibition of hormone-sensitive lipase and adipocyte TG lipolysis (58,59). Whether this mechanism accounts for all of the triglyceride and cholesterol lowering associated with niacin therapy is uncertain. Furthermore, the mechanism by which niacin increases HDL-C levels remains unclear; in vitro data suggest that niacin may have direct effects on the liver as well (56).

The clinical use of niacin has been limited by its major side effect, that of prostaglandin-mediated cutaneous flushing. This has resulted in many attempts to develop sustained-release and extended-release preparations of niacin that would reduce or eliminate the flushing response. Over-the-counter sustained-release niacin preparations, which are classically administered twice a day, have been used extensively but have been associated with several cases of severe hepatotoxicity (57). A Food and Drug Administration (FDA)-approved prescription extended-release niacin is administered once daily and has an excellent safety track record. Although flushing does often occur at the initiation of any form of niacin therapy, rapid tachyphylaxis to the flushing occurs within days or weeks, and a substantial number of patients who continue through the early flushing are able to tolerate niacin at therapeutic doses.

Use of niacin has been associated with elevation in uric acid and even precipitation of acute gout, and therefore niacin should be used with caution in patients with a history of gout. Niacin can also exacerbate peptic ulcer disease and symptoms of gastroesophageal reflux. Mild elevations in transaminases can occur with niacin therapy, but rarely does this require discontinuation. Niacin potentiates the effect of warfarin and should be used cautiously in this setting. Acanthosis nigricans, a dark-colored, coarse skin lesion, is a relatively rare side effect of niacin that is not dangerous but can be bothersome. Finally, niacin can modestly elevate fasting glucose in patients with type 2 diabetes or impaired fasting glucose. However, controlled trials have shown that this effect of niacin is generally of minimal clinical consequence (60).

The most common use of niacin clinically is in patients on a statin who have persistent elevated triglycerides and non-HDL-C levels and/or low HDL-C levels. In this situation, the addition of niacin generally reduces triglycerides and non-HDL-C and increases HDL-C (56,61,62). A fixed-dose combination product of extended-release niacin plus lovastatin is available on the market. The addition of niacin to chronic simvastatin was shown to reduce progression of carotid atherosclerosis compared with continuation of simvastatin alone (63). A clinical outcome trial of extended-release niacin plus simvastatin versus simvastatin alone called AIM-HIGH has been initiated and should definitively address the question of whether adding niacin to statin therapy further reduces cardiovascular events over statin monotherapy.

Omega-3 Fatty Acids (Fish Oils). Omega-3 fatty acids are useful tools in the management of hypertriglyceridemia (64,65). Omega-3 fatty acids are naturally found in high concentration in fish, and their use as concentrated fish oil capsules has been at the center of active investigation. Both epidemiologic and experimental studies have demonstrated the benefit of both dietary fish and concentrated fish oils in the reduction of CHD events. Most of the attention has been focused on the two active ω-3 fatty acids in fish oil, eicosapentanoic acid (EPA) and decohexanoic acid (DHA). Omega-3 fatty acids in doses of up to about 4 g/day decrease fasting and postprandial TGs. Omega-3 fatty acids are thus useful as therapy for patients with severe hypertriglyceridemia. Often they are used in patients who have not responded adequately to fibrates, but they can be used as first-line therapy as well. Fish oils should not be used for hypercholesterolemia in the absence of elevated triglycerides and have been reported to actually raise LDL-C levels in this setting. Omega-3 fatty acids come in various commercial forms with varying amounts of ω-3 fatty acids per capsule. Most commercially available fish oil preparations are sold as dietary supplements without a prescription. An FDA-approved prescription version of ω-3 fatty acids is the most highly concentrated of the preparations available, with 890 mg of DHA and EPA per 1-g capsule, and the recommended dose for severe hypertriglyceridemia is 4 g/day.

A second, potentially important clinical use of ω-3 fatty acids is in the reduction of cardiovascular risk (66). In addition to abundant data regarding dietary fish intake associated with reduced cardiovascular risk, a large randomized, controlled trial demonstrated that one fish oil capsule daily containing approximately 1 g of ω-3 fatty acids was associated with a significant reduction in cardiovascular events (67). Based on these data, many clinicians recommend lower-dose fish oils in patients with CHD or very high risk of CHD.

Combination Drug Therapy. Many patients with dyslipidemia require therapy with more than one lipid-modifying drug (68,69). There are several well-recognized situations in which more than one drug is required for effective management of lipid disorders and reduction of cardiovascular risk. These include inability to get LDL-C and/or non-HDL-C to goal, combined hyperlipidemia, severe hypertriglyceridemia, and low HDL-C.

As the LDL-C goals continue to be reduced for greater numbers of individuals, the number of individuals who cannot achieve their LDL-C goals on statin monotherapy continues to increase. Thus, the addition of a cholesterol-absorption inhibitor (ezetimibe) to a statin has become relatively common as a way to allow patients to achieve their LDL-C goals. Adding ezetimibe to a statin is safe and results in about a 20% further reduction in LDL-C (51). A fixed-dose combination product of simvastatin and ezetimibe is available. Bile acid sequestrants can also be used in combination with statins to achieve greater LDL-C reduction. In fact, ezetimibe and bile acid sequestrants are additive when used in combination (70), and therefore this combination has utility in combination with a statin in severely hypercholesterolemic patients as well as in statin-intolerant patients.

Patients with combined hyperlipidemia may achieve their LDL-C goal with a statin alone, but frequently have persistently elevated triglycerides and often do not achieve their non-HDL-C goal. In this situation, the addition of either niacin or a fibrate to the statin can be highly effective in reducing the triglycerides and non-HDL-C levels (61,62).

Many patients with severe hypertriglyceridemia (defined by NCEP ATPIII as >500 mg/dL) are treated with a fibrate as first-line therapy, but once the triglycerides are adequately reduced, the LDL-C and even non-HDL-C often remain above the appropriate goals for the patient. In this situation, the addition of a statin to the fibrate is often required to achieve LDL-C and non-HDL-C goals (71). Although the risk of myopathy with this combination is a concern, it can be minimized with appropriate patient selection and education (72). Some data suggest that combining statins with gemfibrozil is associated with considerably higher risk of myopathy than combining with fenofibrate (73). Although statin–fibrate combination therapy should be used with caution, it clearly has a role in the aggressive management of lipid disorders in high-risk patients.

Finally, low HDL-C is common, and many patients can be treated to LDL-C and even non-HDL-C goals and yet have persistent low HDL-C levels. Thus combination therapy, usually by adding niacin to the regimen, is commonly used in this setting in patients who are at higher-than-average cardiovascular risk. Issues in the management of low HDL-C are discussed later in the section on HDL.

Approaches to Reducing Low-Density-Lipoprotein Cholesterol When Maximally Tolerated Drug Therapy Is Not Adequately Effective

A fairly sizeable number of patients cannot achieve their LDL-C goal, even with maximally tolerated combination drug therapy. A subset of them are statin intolerant, and another subset simply cannot achieve the LDL-C goal, usually because of a genetic disorder making them less responsive to drug therapy. As a whole, these patients are at high risk for cardiovascular clinical events and should be referred to a specialized lipid center. The following approaches have been used in such patients. Because these approaches are not optimal, there continues to be interest in developing new small molecules that target molecular pathways involved in regulating LDL-C levels as new therapies to meet the unmet medical need associated with LDL-C reduction (74,75).

Partial Ileal Bypass

Partial ileal bypass was developed in the 1960s as a surgical procedure to decrease LDL-C levels. Similar to the mechanism of the bile acid sequestrants, partial ileal bypass interrupts the enterohepatic circulation of bile acids, resulting in upregulation of the hepatic LDL receptor. As discussed earlier, one controlled trial of partial ileal bypass in moderately hypercholesterolemic patients with established CHD demonstrated a 38% decrease in LDL-C and a 35% decrease in the combined endpoint of nonfatal MI and CHD death (3). Partial ileal bypass was developed in the pre-statin era and has not been proven to be effective in patients with severe hypercholesterolemia who do not respond adequately to statins with or without ezetimibe. Diarrhea is a common side effect of this procedure, and the incidence of kidney stones, gallstones, and intestinal obstruction is increased. The clinical utility of partial ileal bypass at this time is limited to hypercholesterolemic patients with established CHD who are unable to tolerate standard lipid-lowering medications and who do not wish to have LDL apheresis (see next subsection).

Low-Density-Lipoprotein Apheresis

The preferred option for management of patients with refractory or drug-resistant hypercholesterolemia is LDL apheresis. In this approach, the patient's plasma is passed over columns that selectively remove LDL, then the LDL-depleted plasma is returned to the patient (76,77). Most patients have it performed biweekly, although very severely hypercholesterolemic patients may have it weekly. Clinical trials have indicated that LDL apheresis can retard progression or cause regression of CAD in patients with severe drug-resistant hypercholesterolemia (78,79) and have even suggested a decrease in clinical cardiovascular events (79). LDL-apheresis is an FDA-approved procedure that is reimbursed by most insurance plans. Candidates for LDL apheresis are considered to be those patients who on maximally tolerated combination drug therapy have CHD and LDL-C greater than 200 mg/dL or no CHD and LDL-C greater than 300 mg/dL.

Approach to the Patient with Low High-Density-Lipoprotein Cholesterol

HDL-C is a strong independent negative risk factor for cardiovascular disease (80). Low HDL-C level is one of the most common findings in patients with premature CHD, and is also frequently found in healthy individuals as a result of routine lipid screening. Despite the importance of low HDL-C as a cardiovascular risk factor, there are no formal guidelines for the classification and management of patients with low HDL-C. Secondary causes of low HDL-C such as smoking, sedentary lifestyle, and obesity should be addressed with lifestyle intervention. Low HDL-C is particularly common in patients with other aspects of the "metabolic syndrome" that is usually associated with visceral obesity and some degree of insulin resistance.

The finding of a low HDL-C level often is used to support the use of statin therapy in settings where the LDL-C level is only modestly elevated. If the LDL-C level is optimally controlled, the difficult issue is whether pharmacologic intervention should be used to specifically raise an isolated HDL-C level. Statins raise HDL-C levels modestly by about 5% 10%, and whether this contributes to the benefits of statin therapy is unknown. Fibrates raise HDL-C by about 5% to 20% and are more effective at raising HDL-C the higher the baseline triglycerides. Niacin is the most effective HDL-C–raising therapy available, with increases in HDL-C of up to about 30% at the higher doses of greater than 1.5 g/day. In high-risk patients, the addition of niacin to existing statin therapy is often used to attempt to raise HDL-C levels in the hope of reducing cardiovascular risk. The therapy of low HDL-C is a major unmet medical need, and new therapies designed to raise HDL-C levels or promote HDL function are under active development (81,82).

CONTROVERSIES AND PERSONAL PERSPECTIVES

The case for aggressive reduction of LDL-C in the reduction of cardiovascular risk is now incontrovertible. In patients with CHD and other high-risk patients, the issue is no longer whether to treat aggressively, but only how low to reduce the LDL-C level. The "optional" goal of LDL less than 70 mg/dL in very high risk patients has been rapidly adopted by cardiologists and many primary care physicians, not only for the very highest risk patients, but also for many patients with CHD-risk-equivalent status. In turn, in many medical practices the goal of LDL less than 100 mg/dL has become almost standard for the majority of patients who have an indication for lipid-modifying drug therapy. Thus the controversies around LDL-C reduction have shifted from who and how aggressively to treat to several new and important topics. A key issue that is unresolved but promises to garner much attention in the coming years is whether statins have cardiovascular benefits that go beyond their ability to reduce LDL-C levels. This issue of the so-called "pleiotropic effects" of statins is supported by in vitro and animal studies but is extremely difficult to prove in humans. The issue is not purely academic because it raises a number of important questions that bear directly on clinical management of patients: (a) If pleiotropic effects of statins are clinically important, are they dose dependent? Should higher doses of statins therefore be used even if not required for further LDL-C reduction? (b) Are all methods of lowering LDL-C likely to result in similar cardiovascular event reductions, or if statins have additional properties, are they more beneficial even at a similar degree of LDL-C reduction? (c) What should be measured in clinical practice to monitor the "non-LDL" effects of statin therapy? This issue divides the experts into camps of those who believe that the overall body of evidence supports reduction of LDL (and other atherogenic lipoproteins) as the primary or even sole mechanism of statin benefit and those who believe that statins exert pleiotropic properties that contribute substantially to their beneficial effects. The only definitive resolution to this question would be to perform a clinical CV event trial of a statin compared with a nonstatin therapy producing similar LDL-C reductions, a trial that is highly unlikely to be performed. Thus, this debate is likely to rage for years with inadequate resolution. If adoption of aggressive LDL-C and non-HDL-C goals continues to be widespread (and the goals themselves may fall further), it may become a partially moot point because many patients will require relatively high dose statin therapy (often in combination with at least one other drug) to achieve aggressive LDL-C and non-HDL-C goals.

In many ways, the treatment of lipids in high-risk patients is fairly straightforward—few would disagree with aggressively targeting LDL-C and non-HDL-C goals in such patients by whatever means necessary. However, the approach to less-high-risk healthy individuals is much less clear in many cases. For example, a large number of healthy individuals have LDL-C levels that are not optimal but not all that elevated either. How can the clinician make rational decisions about which ones to treat with drug therapy? The issue of whether to use additional tests (beyond traditional risk factors) to further refine the risk assessment and guide the intensity of medical therapy remains controversial. On one side, many argue that traditional risk factors are quite good at predicting future cardiovascular risk and are adequate for making medical decisions such as whether to initiate a statin. On the other side, others argue that traditional risk factors miss many people who go on to develop premature (or "mature") CHD and that additional testing is indicated in order to guide the intensity of medical therapy. This debate will intensify as more interventions, such as inhibition of the RAS system and PPAR-α agonism, are shown to be effective in reducing cardiovascular risk independent of specific phenotype. Even if one concedes that additional tests may be useful, it is far from certain which tests should be employed on a routine basis and in what combination. For example, C-reactive protein (CRP) has gained a certain amount of favor in this regard, but as predictive as it is in observational studies, many clinicians remain unconvinced of its value in routine clinical practice. Lipoprotein-associated phospholipase A2 (Lp-PLA2) is independently predictive of CV risk in multiple studies and is clinically available as a test, but most clinicians are confused by it and unclear as to whether it offers improvements in addition to or in place of CRP. Lipoprotein (a) has a long history as a cardiovascular risk factor, but its clinical utility remains controversial. Even the issue of whether LDL-C is the best marker of atherogenic lipoproteins or whether apoB or LDL particle number gives a better prediction of future cardiovascular risk is one that continues to be actively debated. Furthermore, the number of new blood-based tests that purport to independently predict CV risk continues to grow annually, crowding the field and turning up the volume in this important area.

Beyond blood tests, the huge issue of noninvasive imaging of atherosclerosis as a way to predict future risk continues to gain momentum (83). B-mode carotid ultrasound can be used to quantitate carotid intimal-medial thickness (IMT) in asymptomatic persons, and this technique has been used to demonstrate that lipid lowering can retard the progression of intimal thickening compared with controls. Prospective studies in large population-based studies such as ARIC and CHS have shown that carotid IMT is predictive of future coronary events independent of known cardiovascular risk factors (84,85). Although carotid IMT testing has not traditionally been clinically available, this situation is changing, and many centers are setting up clinical IMT labs. Another marker for coronary atherosclerotic plaque is coronary calcification. Electron beam tomography and multidetector computed tomography can detect and quantitate coronary artery calcification as a specific marker for atherosclerotic plaque. Coronary calcification is highly correlated with extent of atherosclerotic disease on autopsy and with extent of angiographic coronary disease. Several prospective studies have indicated that the extent of coronary calcification is associated with the probability of a future coronary event (86). Therefore, both carotid IMT by ultrasound and coronary artery calcification scanning could potentially be used as noninvasive methods for stratifying selected asymptomatic persons according to cardiovascular risk as a guide to more informed decisions regarding drug therapy for cholesterol reduction. However, whether they should be used at all, and if so in which patients, which of the modalities should be used, and in combination with which blood-based tests as noted earlier, all remain to be resolved, and these issues will continue to generate much controversy.

The optimal approach to the healthy patient with hypertriglyceridemia, particularly in the 200- to 1,000-mg/dL range, continues to be controversial (87). Although all would agree that lifestyle management is the first line of therapy, many of these patients, most of whom have some degree of insulin resistance and the metabolic syndrome, will require drug therapy. Are statins the appropriate first-line drug for such patients? Or is there at least a subset of hypertriglyceridemic patients for whom fibrates, or even niacin, should be considered appropriate first-line therapy? All three classes of drugs have been shown to reduce cardiovascular risk, but they have never been compared head to head and probably never will be. Thus there will be continued debate about whether certain subsets of hypertriglyceridemic patients are better treated with a statin, a fibrate, or niacin or perhaps require no drug therapy at all.

The optimal approach to the healthy patient with isolated low HDL-C also is uncertain. It is far from clear that all such patients are necessarily at increased risk for cardiovascular disease, as the experience with apoA-I Milano taught the field several decades ago (36). Thus, which patients with isolated low HDL-C require drug therapy? Furthermore, even if the clinician decides that a patient with isolated low HDL-C is a candidate for lipid-modifying drug therapy, what approach is appropriate? Should it be a statin, based on the fact that statins reduce risk even when LDL-C is low? Should it be a fibrate, given that many of these patients are insulin resistant and fibrates appear to be most effective in reducing CV risk in insulin-resistant patients? Or should it be niacin, given that niacin is clearly the most effective HDL-raising drug on the market? This is yet another issue that is unlikely to be resolved with randomized clinical trials and thus will be subject to continued debate.

One of the most common clinical settings is the patient with CHD or diabetes who has been treated with a statin, is at or near LDL-C goal, but still has elevated TG and/or low HDL. Surprisingly, we still do not have any clinical trial data that speak to the issue of whether adding a second drug (such as a fibrate or niacin) will further reduce cardiovascular risk. This is one area of lipidology where practice has dramatically outpaced the evidence base, in that the majority of experts would probably add a second drug to the statin in this setting. Studies such as ACCORD (fenofibrate) and AIM-HIGH (extended-release niacin) are designed to address this lack of evidence, but will not be completed until after 2010. Even then, if both studies are positive, it will remain unclear whether adding a fibrate or niacin in this setting is optimal. Thus the issue of drug therapy for the HDL-TG axis in addition to statin therapy will continue to be a topic of substantial debate.

THE FUTURE

One can predict certain developments in the area of the clinical management of lipid disorders with some degree of confidence. First, it appears highly likely that the LDL-C and non-HDL-C goals will continue to fall for larger numbers of patients. Whether the LDL-C goal of less than 70 mg/dL in very high risk patients will fall even further is uncertain (but in my opinion likely); it seems almost certain that the goal of LDL-C less than 70 mg/dL will no longer be "optional" and will be formally extended to a larger number of patients, probably eventually to all CHD and CHD-risk-equivalent patients. Similarly, the goal of LDL-C less than 100 mg/dL will likely be formalized for all moderate-risk patients and may eventually be extended to all patients who are candidates for lipid-modifying drug therapy. The non-HDL-C goal will become more commonly used as clinical laboratories begin reporting it and as continued education around this issue takes place. The non-HDL-C goals will fall in parallel with the LDL-C goals, and a non-HDL-C of less than 100 mg/dL for patients with CHD/CHD-risk-equivalent status will become standard. The pressure to reduce LDL-C will drive the average dose of statin higher and result in substantial increases in the use of cholesterol-absorption inhibitors in combination with statins. There will be continued discussion of whether LDL-C and non-HDL-C should be replaced with a better marker of atherogenic particle number such as apoB or LDL particle number.

As there is greater appreciation of the "residual risk" associated with statin monotherapy, coupled to the observation that statin-treated patients who have subsequent events are more likely to have elevated triglycerides and/or reduced HDL-C levels, further increases in combination therapy, particularly statin–fibrate and statin–niacin combinations, will occur. This will be centered on higher-risk patients, but will not be exclusive to patients with existing CHD. If clinical trials designed to test the benefit of adding a fibrate or niacin to a statin demonstrate significant reduction in CV events, the use of combination therapy will become commonplace, much as it is now in the treatment of hypertension.

As the fact that traditional risk factors do not adequately predict who will develop premature CHD becomes increasingly recognized, the interest in using additional tests to predict risk and guide intensity of lipid-modifying drug therapy in healthy patients will increase dramatically. This will include increased use not only of additional blood tests, but also of noninvasive imaging tests. Much work is required to determine the optimal and most cost-effective combinations of blood and imaging tests to be used in clinical practice. Eventually, genetic profiling of cardiovascular risk will be used routinely in clinical practice to guide intensity of preventive therapies, including lipid-modification therapy.

As LDL-C and non-HDL-C targets fall and are broadened to more patients, the fact that millions of patients are unable to reach these aggressive targets will become more widely appreciated. This will lead to greater interest in novel therapies that address the unmet medical need in LDL-C and non-HDL-C reduction. Our basic scientific understanding of both the regulation of VLDL and LDL production by the liver, as well as the catabolism of apoB-containing lipoproteins by the liver, continues to expand, providing new targets for the development of novel therapeutics that will either reduce production or enhance catabolism of atherogenic lipoproteins. Finally, low HDL is clearly a major unmet medical need, and novel therapies that raise HDL or improve its function have the potential to produce major reductions in cardiovascular risk. The next several years will witness a variety of HDL-targeted therapeutics in early to late stage clinical development and probably the introduction of novel HDL-targeted therapies to the clinical marketplace.

References

1. The Coronary Drug Project Research Group. Clofibrate and niacin in coronary heart disease. *JAMA* 1975;231:360–381.
2. Canner PL, Berge KG, Wenger NK, et al. Fifteen year mortality in Coronary Drug Project patients: long-term benefit with niacin. *J Am Coll Cardiol* 1986;8:1245–1255.
3. Buchwald H, Varco RL, Matts JP, et al. Effect of partial ileal bypass surgery on mortality and morbidity from coronary heart disease in patients with hypercholesterolemia—report of the Program on the Surgical Control of the Hyperlipidemias (POSCH). *N Engl J Med* 1990;323:946–955.
4. Lipid Research Clinics Program. The Lipid Research Clinics Coronary Primary Prevention Trial results: II. The relationship of reduction in incidence of coronary heart disease to cholesterol lowering. *JAMA* 1984;251:365–374.
5. Lipid Research Clinics Program. The Lipid Research Clinics Coronary Primary Prevention Trial results. 1. Reduction in incidence of coronary heart disease. *JAMA* 1984;251:351–364.
6. Scandinavian Simvastatin Survival Study Group. Randomized trial of cholesterol lowering in 4444 patients with coronary heart disease: the Scandinavian Simvastatin Survival Study (4S). *Lancet* 1994;344:1383–11389.
7. Scandinavian Simvastatin Survival Study Group. Baseline serum cholesterol and treatment effect in the Scandinavian Simvastatin Survival Study (4S). *Lancet* 1995;345:1274–1275.

8. Kannel WB. Range of serum cholesterol values in the population developing coronary artery disease. *Am J Cardiol* 1995;76:69C–77C.
9. Sacks FM, Pfeffer MA, Moye L, et al. The effect of pravastatin on coronary events after myocardial infarction in patients with average cholesterol levels. *N Engl J Med* 1996;335:1001–1009.
10. Tonkin AM, Colquhoun D, Emberson J, et al. Effects of pravastatin in 3260 patients with unstable angina: results from the LIPID study. *Lancet* 2000;356:1871–1875.
11. Shepherd J, Cobbe SM, Ford I, et al. Prevention of coronary heart disease with pravastatin in men with hypercholesterolemia. *N Engl J Med.* 1995;333:1301–1307.
12. Downs JR, Clearfield M, Weis S, et al. Primary prevention of acute coronary events with lovastatin in men and women with average cholesterol levels. *JAMA* 1998;279:1615–1622.
13. MRC/BHF Heart Protection Study of cholesterol lowering with simvastatin in 20,536 high-risk individuals: a randomised placebo-controlled trial. *Lancet* 2002;360:7–22.
14. Shepherd J, Blauw GJ, Murphy MB, et al. Pravastatin in elderly individuals at risk of vascular disease (PROSPER): a randomised controlled trial. *Lancet* 2002;360:1623–1630.
15. Major outcomes in moderately hypercholesterolemic, hypertensive patients randomized to pravastatin vs usual care: the Antihypertensive and Lipid-Lowering Treatment to Prevent Heart Attack Trial (ALLHAT–LLT). *JAMA* 2002;288:2998–3007.
16. Sever PS, Dahlof B, Poulter NR, et al. Prevention of coronary and stroke events with atorvastatin in hypertensive patients who have average or lower-than-average cholesterol concentrations, in the Anglo-Scandinavian Cardiac Outcomes Trial–Lipid Lowering Arm (ASCOT–LLA): a multicentre randomised controlled trial. *Lancet* 2003;361:1149–1158.
17. Colhoun HM, Betteridge DJ, Durrington PN, et al. Primary prevention of cardiovascular disease with atorvastatin in type 2 diabetes in the Collaborative Atorvastatin Diabetes Study (CARDS): multicentre randomised placebo-controlled trial. *Lancet* 2004;364:685–696.
18. LaRosa JC, Grundy SM, Waters DD, et al. Intensive lipid lowering with atorvastatin in patients with stable coronary disease. *N Engl J Med* 2005;352: 1425–1435.
19. Schwartz GG, Olsson AG, Ezekowitz MD, et al. Effects of atorvastatin on early recurrent ischemic events in acute coronary syndromes: the MIRACL study: a randomized controlled trial. *JAMA* 2001;285:1711–1718.
20. Cannon CP, Braunwald E, McCabe CH, et al. Intensive versus moderate lipid lowering with statins after acute coronary syndromes. *N Engl J Med* 2004;350:1495–1504.
21. de Lemos JA, Blazing MA, Wiviott SD, et al. Early intensive vs a delayed conservative simvastatin strategy in patients with acute coronary syndromes: phase Z of the A to Z trial. *JAMA* 2004;292:1307–1316.
22. Frick MH, Elo O, Haapa K, Heinonen OP, et al. Helsinki Heart Study: primary-prevention trial with gemfibrozil in middle-aged men with dyslipidemia. Safety of treatment, changes in risk factors, and incidence of coronary heart disease. *N Engl J Med* 1987;317:1237–1245.
23. Rubins HB, Robins SJ, Collins D, et al. Gemfibrozil for the secondary prevention of coronary heart disease in men with low levels of high-density lipoprotein cholesterol. *N Engl J Med* 1999;341:410–418.
24. Secondary prevention by raising HDL cholesterol and reducing triglycerides in patients with coronary artery disease: the Bezafibrate Infarction Prevention (BIP) study. *Circulation* 2000;102:21–27.
25. Glass CK, Witztum JL. Atherosclerosis. the road ahead. *Cell* 2001;104:503–516.
26. Rader DJ, Pure E. Lipoproteins, macrophage function, and atherosclerosis: beyond the foam cell? *Cell Metab* 2005;1:223–230.
27. Lewis GF, Rader DJ. New insights into the regulation of HDL metabolism and reverse cholesterol transport. *Circ Res* 2005;96:1221–1232.
28. Barter PJ, Nicholls S, Rye KA, et al. Antiinflammatory properties of HDL. *Circ Res* 2004;95:764–772.
29. Brunzell JD, Ayyobi AF. Dyslipidemia in the metabolic syndrome and type 2 diabetes mellitus. *Am J Med.* 2003;115(Suppl 8A):24S–28S.
30. Quaschning T, Krane V, Metzger T, Wanner C. Abnormalities in uremic lipoprotein metabolism and its impact on cardiovascular disease. *Am J Kidney Dis* 2001;38:S14–S19.
31. Executive summary of the third report of the National Cholesterol Education Program (NCEP) Expert Panel on Detection, Evaluation, and Treatment of High Blood Cholesterol in Adults (Adult Treatment Panel III). *JAMA* 2001;285:2486–2497.
32. Shoulders CC, Jones EL, Naoumova RP. Genetics of familial combined hyperlipidemia and risk of coronary heart disease. *Hum Mol Genet* 2004;13(Spec No 1):R149–R160.
33. Rader DJ, Cohen J, Hobbs HH. Monogenic hypercholesterolemia: new insights in pathogenesis and treatment. *J Clin Invest* 2003;111:1795–1803.
34. Abifadel M, Varret M, Rabes JP, et al. Mutations in PCSK9 cause autosomal dominant hypercholesterolemia. *Nat Genet* 2003;34:154–156.
35. Cohen J, Pertsemlidis A, Kotowski IK, et al. Low LDL cholesterol in individuals of African descent resulting from frequent nonsense mutations in PCSK9. *Nat Genet* 2005;37:161–165.
36. Chiesa G, Sirtori CR. Apolipoprotein A-IMilano: current perspectives. *Curr Opin Lipidol* 2003;14:159–163.
37. Kuivenhoven JA, Pritchard H, Hill J, et al. The molecular pathology of lecithin:cholesterol acyltransferase (LCAT) deficiency syndromes. *J Lipid Res* 1997;38:191–205.
38. Hobbs HH, Rader DJ. ABC1: connecting yellow tonsils, neuropathy, and very low HDL. *J Clin Invest* 1999;104:1015–1017.
39. Tall AR. Role of ABCA1 in cellular cholesterol efflux and reverse cholesterol transport. *Arterioscler Thromb Vasc Biol* 2003;23:710–711.
40. Cohen JC, Kiss RS, Pertsemlidis A, et al. Multiple rare alleles contribute to low plasma levels of HDL cholesterol. *Science.* 2004;305:869–872.
41. Grundy SM, Cleeman JI, Merz CN, et al. Implications of recent clinical trials for the National Cholesterol Education Program Adult Treatment Panel III guidelines. *Circulation* 2004;110:227–239.
42. Gotto AM. Cholesterol management in theory and practice. *Circulation* 1997;96:4424–4430.
43. Gotto Jr AM. Risks and benefits of continued aggressive statin therapy. *Clin Cardiol* 2003;26:III3–III12.
44. Vaughan CJ, Gotto Jr AM. Update on statins: 2003. *Circulation* 2004; 110:886–892.
45. Pasternak RC, Smith Jr SC, Bairey-Merz CN, et al. ACC/AHA/NHLBI clinical advisory on the use and safety of statins. *J Am Coll Cardiol* 2002;40:567–572.
46. Grundy SM. The issue of statin safety: where do we stand? *Circulation* 2005;111:3016–3019.
47. Liao JK, Laufs U. Pleiotropic effects of statins. *Annu Rev Pharmacol Toxicol* 2005;45:89–118.
48. Lipka LJ. Ezetimibe: a first-in-class, novel cholesterol absorption inhibitor. *Cardiovasc Drug Rev* 2003;21:293–312.
49. Garcia-Calvo M, Lisnock J, Bull HG, et al. The target of ezetimibe is Niemann-Pick C1-Like 1 (NPC1L1). *Proc Natl Acad Sci USA* 2005;102: 8132–8137.
50. Bays HE, Moore PB, Drehobl MA, et al. Effectiveness and tolerability of ezetimibe in patients with primary hypercholesterolemia: pooled analysis of two phase II studies. *Clin Ther* 2001;23:1209–1230.
51. Davidson MH, Ballantyne CM, Kerzner B, et al. Efficacy and safety of ezetimibe coadministered with statins: randomised, placebo-controlled, blinded experience in 2382 patients with primary hypercholesterolemia. *Int J Clin Pract* 2004;58:746–755.
52. Claudel T, Staels B, Kuipers F. The farnesoid X receptor. A molecular link between bile acid and lipid and glucose metabolism. *Arterioscler Thromb Vasc Biol* 2005;25:2020–2030.
53. Despres JP, Lemieux I, Robins SJ. Role of fibric acid derivatives in the management of risk factors for coronary heart disease. *Drugs* 2004;64:2177–2198.
54. Tsimihodimos V, Miltiadous G, Daskalopoulou SS, et al. Fenofibrate: metabolic and pleiotropic effects. *Curr Vasc Pharmacol* 2005;3:87–98.
55. Steiner G. Fibrates in the metabolic syndrome and in diabetes. *Endocrinol Metab Clin North Am* 2004;33:545–555, vi–vii.
56. Meyers CD, Kamanna VS, Kashyap ML. Niacin therapy in atherosclerosis. *Curr Opin Lipidol* 2004;15:659–665.
57. Carlson LA. Nicotinic acid: the broad-spectrum lipid drug. A 50th anniversary review. *J Intern Med* 2005;258:94–114.
58. Pike NB, Wise A. Identification of a nicotinic acid receptor: is this the molecular target for the oldest lipid-lowering drug? *Curr Opin Investig Drugs* 2004;5:271–275.
59. Karpe F, Frayn KN. The nicotinic acid receptor—a new mechanism for an old drug. *Lancet* 2004;363:1892–1894.
60. Shepherd J, Betteridge J, Van Gaal L. Nicotinic acid in the management of dyslipidaemia associated with diabetes and metabolic syndrome: a position paper developed by a European Consensus Panel. *Curr Med Res Opin* 2005;21:665–682.
61. Levy DR, Pearson TA. Combination niacin and statin therapy in primary and secondary prevention of cardiovascular disease. *Clin Cardiol* 2005;28:317–320.
62. Koh KK, Quon MJ, Han SH, et al. Additive beneficial effects of fenofibrate combined with atorvastatin in the treatment of combined hyperlipidemia. *J Am Coll Cardiol* 2005;45:1649–1653.
63. Taylor AJ, Sullenberger LE, Lee HJ, et al. Arterial Biology for the Investigation of the Treatment Effects of Reducing Cholesterol (ARBITER) 2: a double-blind, placebo-controlled study of extended-release niacin on atherosclerosis progression in secondary prevention patients treated with statins. *Circulation* 2004;110:3512–3517.
64. Kris-Etherton PM, Harris WS, Appel LJ. Fish consumption, fish oil, omega-3 fatty acids, and cardiovascular disease. *Arterioscler Thromb Vasc Biol* 2003;23:e20–e30.
65. Hooper L, Thompson RL, Harrison RA, et al. Omega 3 fatty acids for prevention and treatment of cardiovascular disease. *Cochrane Database Syst Rev* 2004: CD003177.
66. Balk E, Chung M, Lichtenstein A, et al. Effects of omega-3 fatty acids on cardiovascular risk factors and intermediate markers of cardiovascular disease. *Evid Rep Technol Assess (Summ)* 2004:1–6.
67. Anonymous. Dietary supplementation with n-3 polyunsaturated fatty acids and vitamin E after myocardial infarction: results of the GISSI-Prevenzione trial. Gruppo Italiano per lo Studio della Sopravvivenza nell'Infarto miocardico. *Lancet* 1999;354:447–455.
68. Streja D. Combination therapy for the treatment of dyslipidemia. *Curr Opin Investig Drugs* 2004;5:306–312.

69. Ansell BJ. Rationale for combination therapy with statin drugs in the treatment of dyslipidemia. *Curr Atheroscler Rep* 2005;7:29–33.
70. Zema MJ. Colesevelam HCl and ezetimibe combination therapy provides effective lipid-lowering in difficult-to-treat patients with hypercholesterolemia. *Am J Ther* 2005;12:306–310.
71. Shek A, Ferrill MJ. Statin-fibrate combination therapy. *Ann Pharmacother* 2001;35:908–917.
72. Wierzbicki AS, Mikhailidis DP, Wray R, et al. Statin-fibrate combination: therapy for hyperlipidemia: a review. *Curr Med Res Opin* 2003;19:155–168.
73. Jones PH, Davidson MH. Reporting rate of rhabdomyolysis with fenofibrate + statin versus gemfibrozil + any statin. *Am J Cardiol* 2005;95:120–122.
74. Rader DJ. A new feature on the cholesterol-lowering landscape. *Nat Med* 2001;7:1282–1284.
75. Scharnagl H, Marz W. New lipid-lowering agents acting on LDL receptors. *Curr Top Med Chem* 2005;5:233–242.
76. Eder AF, Rader DJ. LDL-apheresis for severe refractory dyslipidemia. *Today's Therapeutic Trends* 1996;14:165–179.
77. Thompson GR. LDL apheresis. *Atherosclerosis.* 2003;167:1–13.
78. Tatami R, Inoue N, Itoh H, et al. Regression of coronary atherosclerosis by combined LDL-apheresis and lipid-lowering drug therapy in patients with familial hypercholesterolemia: a multicenter study. *Atherosclerosis* 1992;95:1–13.
79. Thompson GR, Maher V, Matthews S, et al. Familial hypercholesterolaemia regression study: a randomised trial of low-density lipoprotein apheresis. *Lancet* 1995;345:811–816.
80. Assmann G, Gotto Jr AM. HDL cholesterol and protective factors in atherosclerosis. *Circulation* 2004;109:III8–III14.
81. Linsel-Nitschke P, Tall AR. HDL as a target in the treatment of atherosclerotic cardiovascular disease. *Nat Rev Drug Discov* 2005;4:193–205.
82. Duffy D, Rader DJ. Drugs in development: targeting high-density lipoprotein metabolism and reverse cholesterol transport. *Curr Opin Cardiol* 2005; 20:301–306.
83. Grundy SM. Atherosclerosis imaging and the future of lipid management. *Circulation* 2004;110:3509–3511.
84. Chambless LE, Heiss G, Folsom AR, et al. Association of coronary heart disease incidence with carotid arterial wall thickness and major risk factors: the Atherosclerosis Risk in Communities (ARIC) Study, 1987–1993. *Am J Epidemiol* 1997;146:483–494.
85. Kuller LH, Shemanski L, Psaty BM, et al. Subclinical disease as an independent risk factor for cardiovascular disease. *Circulation* 1995;92:720–726.
86. Kondos GT, Hoff JA, Sevrukov A, et al. Electron–beam tomography coronary artery calcium and cardiac events: a 37-month follow-up of 5635 initially asymptomatic low- to intermediate-risk adults. *Circulation* 2003;107: 2571–2576.
87. Szapary PO, Rader DJ. The triglyceride–high-density lipoprotein axis: an important target of therapy? *Am Heart J* 2004;148:211–221.

CHAPTER 6 ■ EXERCISE AND PHYSICAL ACTIVITY

ERIC H. AWTRY AND GARY J. BALADY

PHYSICAL ACTIVITY AND PUBLIC HEALTH

Nearly 70 million (approximately 1 of every 4) persons in the United States have cardiovascular disease (CVD). Of these, 65 million suffer from hypertension, 13 million have coronary artery disease (CAD), 4.9 million have congestive heart failure, and 5.4 million have suffered a stroke (1). Despite the declining mortality rate from cardiovascular illness observed since 1950, 38% of all deaths in the United States are currently attributed to CVD. The morbidity and subsequent disability incurred from cardiovascular illness have far-reaching medical and socioeconomic implications, and accounted for an estimated total cost of $327 billion in 2000 (1).

Physical inactivity is a risk factor for the development of CVD (2) and is associated with a higher all-cause mortality rate (3,4). Conversely, regular exercise is associated with a lower incidence of cardiovascular symptoms and a reduction in cardiovascular mortality rates among asymptomatic persons (5,6) and patients with established CVD (7–9). Furthermore, a regular exercise program is a cost-effective intervention, with an estimated cost of less than $12,000 per year of life saved (10). Despite the clear benefits of physical activity, the proportion of Americans who are physically active is relatively small. The most recent report from the Centers for Disease Control and Prevention (CDC) indicates that only 25% of adult Americans engage in recommended levels of physical activity (11); 58% never participate in vigorous leisure-time activity (12), and 25% report no regular leisure time physical activity at all (13).

Many factors contribute to physical inactivity in adults; the most-cited reasons are a real or perceived risk of self-injury and lack of time. Other important barriers include physical limitations resulting from comorbid conditions, lack of companionship or encouragement, and the absence of an appropriate environment for exercise (e.g., no available paths for walking or biking, lack of exercise equipment, inclement weather, or unsafe neighborhoods). Although most Americans are aware of the health benefits of exercise, this awareness does not strongly correlate with engagement in physical activity. Rather, regular physical activity is more strongly associated with enjoyment of exercise, confidence in athletic ability, and participation in low to moderate levels of activity (14).

PHYSICAL ACTIVITY, EXERCISE, AND FITNESS

Physical activity, fitness, and exercise are related entities but have different definitions. The definitions described below are as defined in the Surgeon General's report on physical activity and health (15).

Physical activity refers to skeletal muscle contraction resulting in bodily movement that requires energy use, and can be further classified based on the specific mechanical and metabolic aspects of contraction. Mechanically, physical activities can be divided into those that produce muscle tension without limb movement (*isometric exercise*) and those that produce limb movement without a change in muscle tension (*isotonic exercise*). Metabolically physical activity can be classified as *aerobic* (energy derived in the presence of oxygen) or *anaerobic* (energy derived in the absence of oxygen). Most activity involves a combination of these forms of muscle contraction (15). The *intensity* of physical activity can be described as the energy required per unit of time for the performance of the activity and can be expressed in units of oxygen use, kilocalories (measure of heat), or kilojoules (measure of energy). This energy requirement can be most readily quantified by measuring the oxygen uptake required during the activity. Alternatively, activity intensity can be expressed as a measure of the force of muscle contraction required (in pounds or kilograms). The intensity of a physical activity can be related in relative terms by expressing it as a proportion of the individual's maximal capacity (e.g., the percentage of O_2max or the percentage of

TABLE 6.1

EFFORT INTENSITY FOR VARIOUS COMMONLY PERFORMED EXERCISE ACTIVITIES

Light (<0.3 METs[a] or <4 kcal/min)	Moderate (3.0–6.0 METs or 4–7 kcal/min)	Hard/Vigorous (>6.0 METs or >7 kcal/min^{-1})
Walking, slowly (strolling) (1–2 miles/h)	Walking, briskly (3–4 miles/h)	Walking, briskly uphill or with a load
Cycling, stationary (<50 W)	Cycling for pleasure or transportation (≤10 miles/h)	Cycling, fast or racing (>10 miles/h)
Swimming, slow treading	Swimming, moderate effort	Swimming, fast treading or crawl
Conditioning exercise, light stretching	Conditioning exercise, general calisthenics, racket sports, tennis	Conditioning exercise, stair ergometer, ski machine, racket sports, singles tennis, racquetball
Golf, power cart	Golf, pulling cart or carrying clubs	
Bowling		
Fishing, sitting	Fishing, standing/casting	Fishing in stream
Boating, power	Canoeing, leisurely (2.0–3.9 miles/h)	Canoeing, rapidly (≥4 miles/h)
Home care, carpet sweeping	Home care, general cleaning	Moving furniture
Mowing lawn, riding mower	Mowing lawn, power mower	Mowing lawn, hand mower
Home repair, carpentry	Home repairs, painting	

Abbreviation: MET, metabolic equivalent.
[a]1 MET = 3.5 kcal/kg/min.
Source: From Pate RR, Pratt M, Blair SN, et al. Physical activity and public health: a recommendation from the CDC and the American College of Sports Medicine. *JAMA* 1995;273:402–407, with permission.

maximum heart rate) or as a multiple of resting metabolic requirements (i.e., the number of metabolic equivalents [METs] required to perform the activity) (15) (Tables 6.1 and 6.2).

Physical exercise is a form of physical activity that is planned and performed with the goal of achieving or preserving physical fitness. *Exercise training* may be a more accurate term, because similar activity may be viewed as exercise by one person and not by others (15). *Physical fitness* is a set of attributes that enables an individual to perform physical activity (14). Physical fitness is best assessed by measures of O_2max, and is often estimated by measurement of the peak workrate or MET level achieved during graded exercise tests. Numerous exercise-training studies have evaluated the frequency, intensity, and duration of the training sessions required to achieve physical fitness. Based on these data, it appears that the most consistent benefit on O_2max is observed when exercise training is performed at an intensity of approximately 60% of the maximum heart rate or 50% of O_2max, for 20 to 60 minutes per session, for at least 3 to 5 sessions per week, for 12 or more weeks (16). Improvements in O_2max of 15% to 30% are usually achieved using the above guidelines. It also appears that intermittent activity at comparable exercise intensity and total duration can confer fitness benefits similar to those of continuous activity (17).

TABLE 6.2

CLASSIFICATION OF PHYSICAL ACTIVITY INTENSITY[a]

	Endurance-type activity					
	Relative intensity		Absolute intensity (METs) in healthy adults (age [y])			
Intensity	O_2max heart rate reserve (%)	Maximum heart rate (%)	Young (20–39)	Middle-aged (40–64)	Old (65–79)	Very old (80+)
Very light	<25	<30	<3.0	<2.5	<2.0	≤1.25
Light	25–39	30–49	3.0–4.7	2.5–4.4	2.0–3.5	1.26–2.20
Moderate	40–59	50–69	4.8–7.1	4.5–5.9	3.6–4.7	2.30–2.95
Hard	60–84	70–89	7.2–10.1	6.0–8.4	4.8–6.7	3.00–4.25
Very Hard	≥85	≥90	≥10.2	≥8.5	≥6.8	≥4.25
Maximum[b]	100	100	12.0	10.0	8.0	5.0

Abbreviations: MET, metabolic equivalent; O_2max, maximal oxygen uptake.
[a]Based on 8–12 repetitions for persons <50 years old and 10–15 repetitions for persons ≥50 years old.
[b]Maximum values are mean values achieved during maximum exercise by healthy adults. Absolute intensity (METs) values are approximate mean values for men. Mean values for women are approximately 1–2 METs lower than those for men.
Source: Adapted from U.S. Department of Health and Human Services. *Physical activity and health: a report of the surgeon general.* Atlanta: Center for Disease Control and Prevention, National Center for Chronic Disease Prevention and Promotion, 1996.

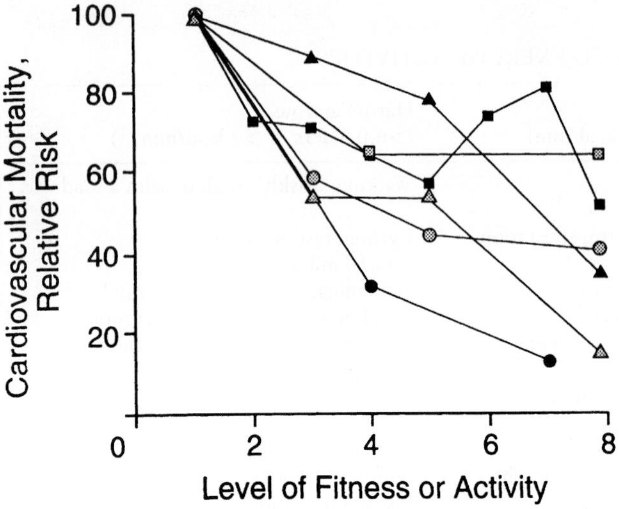

FIGURE 6.1. The relationship between physical activity or fitness and the relative risk for cardiovascular mortality. As fitness improves, the risk for cardiovascular death diminishes. ■, Paffenbarger et al. (26); ▲, Morris et al. (1990); ●, Blair et al. (2); ■, Leon et al. (1987); ▲, Ekelund et al. (1988); ● Sandvik et al. (1993). (*Source:* From Pate RR, Pratt M, Blair SN, et al. Physical activity and public health: a recommendation from the CDC and the American College of Sports Medicine. *JAMA* 1995;273:402–407, with permission.)

PHYSICAL ACTIVITY AND HEALTH: EPIDEMIOLOGIC OBSERVATIONS AND BIOLOGIC MECHANISMS

Effects on All-Cause Mortality

Data accumulated over the past 50 years confirm the health benefits of exercise; epidemiologic studies show that active individuals have a lower risk of developing many chronic illnesses, including CVD (14), and that as many as 12% of deaths in the United States are associated with inactivity (18) (Fig. 6.1). In addition, physical activity is associated with lower all-cause mortality rates in healthy individuals (2,19,20), individuals with chronic diseases (4), diabetic persons (21), and the elderly (22,23). A large-scale epidemiologic study involving 13,375 women and 17,265 men between the ages of 20 and 93 years reported a significant inverse association between leisure time physical activity and all-cause mortality, with active individuals enjoying a 30% to 50% reduction in mortality compared with their sedentary counterparts (24). Importantly, an evaluation of 5,209 men and women demonstrated that the performance of recent activity confers a reduction in all-cause mortality, whereas activity performed decades earlier without subsequent maintenance appears to have no long-term benefit (25). Nonetheless, the risk for all-cause mortality decreases among inactive men and women who subsequently become more physically active (26,27).

Effects on Cardiovascular Events

Multiple studies have demonstrated the efficacy of regular exercise and physical activity in the primary and secondary prevention of cardiovascular events (2,6,20,23). In the Harvard University alumni study, men without a history of CVD were assessed for their activity level and followed for 16 years (20). There was a 39% reduction in cardiovascular morbidity and a 24% reduction in cardiovascular mortality in subjects with exercise energy expenditures of more than 2,000 kcal/week. Additionally, the risk of death became progressively lower as weekly energy expenditures from physical activity increased from 500 to 3,500 kcal. Furthermore, alumni who were initially inactive and later increased their activity levels demonstrated significantly reduced cardiovascular risk compared with those who remained inactive (26). A similar graded effect of exercise was noted in the Honolulu Heart Program, which studied the effects of walking on 2,678 physically capable men aged 71 to 93 years who did not have known CVD (6). Participants who walked less than 0.25 mile daily had a twofold increased risk of developing coronary heart disease (CHD) compared with those who walked more than 1.5 mile/day (5.1% versus 2.5%, $P < 0.1$), whereas subjects who walked 0.5 to 1.5 mile daily had an intermediate risk (4.5%, $P < 0.5$). In the Nurses' Health Study of 73,029 women (aged 40 to 65 years), physical activity was inversely related to the risk of stroke and CAD (28,29). The largest benefit was seen between the lowest and second-lowest quintile groups for exercise, suggesting that the incremental value of exercise is greatest in the least-active subjects.

Exercise programs for patients with established CHD have been well studied (8,9,30–32). A meta-analysis of 48 randomizing trials encompassing 8,940 patients with CHD revealed that patients enrolled in cardiac rehabilitation programs had a 20% reduction in all-cause mortality and a 26% reduction in cardiac mortality, compared with subjects receiving usual care (9). Although individual trials have demonstrated a reduction in myocardial infarction (MI) in patients undergoing cardiac rehabilitation, there was no significant reduction in either MI or coronary revascularization noted in this meta-analysis. Among patients referred for or enrolled in cardiac rehabilitation programs, exercise capacity is a strong prognostic factor; incremental reductions in mortality risk are associated with progressively higher levels of fitness (31). Additionally, low exercise capacity predicts the need for future hospitalization (32). A recent meta-analysis regarding the use of exercise training in patients with heart failure has shown that exercise training in this population is safe, and is associated with a 35% reduction in mortality (8).

The specific mechanisms by which physical activity reduces CVD and CVD mortality have not been completely elucidated, but are likely multifactorial. In a cross-sectional analysis of a large cohort of men and women, higher levels of fitness were associated with lower levels of atherosclerotic risk factors in persons with and without CAD (33). However, modification of risk factors does not fully explain the benefits that have been observed. Other possible mechanisms—including effects on thrombosis, endothelial function, inflammation, and autonomic tone—may play an important role (Table 6.3).

TABLE 6.3

PHYSICAL ACTIVITY AND REDUCED CARDIOVASCULAR RISK: BIOLOGIC MECHANISMS

Lower blood pressure
Improved glucose tolerance
Reduced obesity
Improvement of lipid profile
Enhanced fibrinolysis
Reduced inflammation
Improved endothelial function
Enhanced parasympathetic autonomic tone

Atherosclerotic Risk Factors

Hypertension

Epidemiologic studies suggest that regular physical activity is associated with lower blood pressure in both normotensive and mildly hypertensive individuals (34–36), and that inactivity is associated with a significantly increased risk of developing hypertension (25). In mildly hypertensive men, short-term physical activity decreases blood pressure for 8 to 12 hours after exercise, and average resting blood pressure is lower on days during which exercise is performed (37). Furthermore, in severely hypertensive black men, moderate physical activity performed for 16 to 32 weeks results in a decrease in diastolic blood pressure that is sustained even after a reduction in antihypertensive medications, and is associated with a significant decrease in left ventricular (LV) hypertrophy as early as 16 weeks after the initiation of exercise (38). The magnitude of blood pressure reduction attained with exercise is modest, although significant (9,39,40). A meta-analysis of 54 randomized trials of aerobic exercise revealed significant reductions in both systolic (4 mm Hg) and diastolic (3 mm Hg) blood pressure (40). The blood pressure reduction was even greater in hypertensive patients (5 and 4 mm Hg, respectively), and was seen regardless of ethnicity, weight change, type of exercise, or exercise intensity.

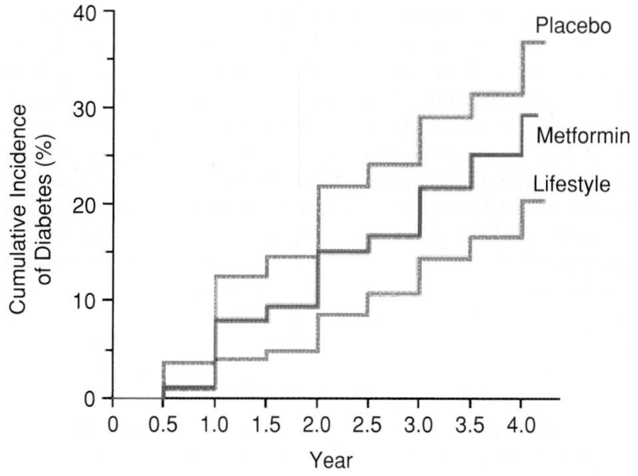

FIGURE 6.2. The effect of lifestyle intervention or metformin on the cumulative incidence of diabetes. The diagnosis of diabetes was based on the criteria of the American Diabetes Association. The incidence of diabetes differed significantly among the three groups ($P < .001$ for each comparison). (*Source:* Reproduced from Diabetes Prevention Program Research Group. Reduction in the incidence of type 2 diabetes with lifestyle intervention or metformin. *N Engl J Med* 2002;346:393–402, with permission.)

Diabetes Mellitus

Physical activity induces several beneficial effects on glucose metabolism, including increased insulin sensitivity, decreased hepatic glucose production, preferential use of glucose over fatty acids by exercising muscle, and reduced obesity (41). In addition, there is evidence that regular exercise may prevent the onset of diabetes mellitus. In a prospective study of 4,369 nondiabetic Finnish men and women, physical activity was inversely related to the future risk of developing type 2 diabetes, regardless of whether or not the subjects were obese or had impaired glucose tolerance at baseline (42). Furthermore, a randomized controlled trial found that in patients with impaired glucose tolerance, the risk of developing diabetes was significantly less in patients treated with a lifestyle intervention program (goal of 7% weight loss and >150 minutes of exercise per week) than with in patients treated with metformin (4.8% and 7.8%, respectively; Fig. 6.2) (43). In a population-based prospective study, men in the lowest fitness level had a 3.7-fold higher risk of developing diabetes compared with men in the highest fitness level (44). It appears that moderate exercise (e.g., walking) may have equal benefit to more vigorous exercise, providing that the total energy expenditure is similar (45), and, although relatively low levels of physical activity (40 minutes weekly) appear to have a beneficial effect on the risk of developing diabetes, there is a progressively greater effect seen at greater activity levels (46). Among patients with established type 2 diabetes, physical activity is associated with reductions in the risk of CVD (5) and of cardiovascular and total mortality (5,21), with greater reductions seen at higher levels of activity. Given these data, exercise should be strongly encouraged in patients with or at risk for type 2 diabetes; however, the role of physical activity in the prevention and treatment of type 1 diabetes has not been well studied.

Overweight and Obesity

The prevalence of being overweight (body mass index [BMI] ≥25) in the American adult population is 65% and the prevalence of obesity (BMI ≥30%) is 30%. The latter represents a 75% increase since 1991 (1). In addition, an estimated 9.2 million children aged 6 to 19 years are overweight or obese. The most likely explanation for this national trend is an increase in total caloric intake, along with a reduction in physical activity. Overweight and obesity are associated with significant increases in cardiovascular morbidity and mortality, effects that are mitigated by weight loss (47).

Exercise training appears to be an important component of weight loss programs, although most randomized controlled trials show only modest weight loss (average weight loss 2 to 3 kg) in the treated group versus the control group (48). Additionally, when compared to diet alone, exercise alone does not yield as great a loss of weight. When diet is added to an exercise regimen the average additional weight loss is 5.3 kg versus exercise alone (48), and the addition of an exercise regimen to dietary changes produces a 0.1 kg/week greater weight loss than diet alone (49). Despite the relatively modest effects of exercise on initial weight loss, studies suggests that exercise is necessary to maintain weight loss and prevent weight regain after diet-induced weight loss (50).

Body composition and fat distribution are also linked to cardiovascular mortality (51) and are favorably affected by exercise. On average, exercise training programs reduce body fat by approximately 2% (52) and, when added to a diet program, increase the percentage of weight lost as fat versus that lost as fat-free mass (53). In addition, physically active men and women have a more favorable waist–hip ratio than do sedentary individuals (54–56). Although significant, these changes are rather small, even after 1 year of diet and exercise (55). Importantly, physical activity appears to have favorable effects on lipoproteins, glucose metabolism, and blood pressure, even when weight loss is only modest (57). Furthermore, the results of several studies demonstrate that overweight individuals who are physically active have much lower cardiovascular and all-cause mortality rates than their obese, sedentary counterparts (58–60), although physical activity does not completely eliminate the higher mortality risk associated with obesity (61). This suggests that physical activity may reduce cardiovascular mortality in overweight individuals independent of weight loss.

Lipids

The effect of exercise on lipid levels has been an area of continued research. There is much variability in the results of exercise—lipid-lowering studies, at least in part owing to the heterogeneity of the study methods, populations, exercise interventions, and the use of adjunctive interventions such as diet or pharmacologic lipid-lowering agents. A meta-analysis of 31 randomized trials revealed small but statistically significant changes in lipoproteins in the aerobic exercise group, including a reduction in both total cholesterol and low-density lipoprotein (LDL) of 4 mg/dL, a reduction in triglycerides of 7 mg/dL, and an increase in high-density lipoprotein (HDL) cholesterol of 2 mg/dL (62). The effect of resistance exercise was inconclusive. The greatest changes in lipids during an exercise program appear to occur in patients who also lose weight, and, when body weight increases, lipid levels worsen (63). Moderate-intensity exercise (i.e., equivalent to briskly walking 10 miles per week), Step 2 American Heart Association (AHA) diet, and the combination of exercise plus diet were studied in a randomized controlled trial of postmenopausal women and middle-aged men (64). The most favorable changes in LDL (8% to 12% reduction) occurred among subjects in the diet and exercise group after 1 year. HDL levels decreased by 2% among women in the diet plus exercise groups, but among men there was a favorable 2% increase (64). In a study of 82 male and female patients with coronary disease, a 3-month exercise training program in conjunction with diet resulted in an 8% increase in HDL and a 22% decrease in triglycerides in subjects who had baseline triglyceride elevations. However, there was no significant improvement in body weight, LDL, glucose level, or insulin level (65).

It appears that the training intensities required to yield modest improvements in lipids are not as high as those required to improve fitness levels, although the magnitude of the effect may depend on the total amount of exercise performed (62,66,67). A meta-analysis of randomized controlled trials has shown that relatively modest amounts of exercise appeared to generate measurable effects on serum lipids, and that there was no incremental benefit of exercising more frequently than 3 times per week (68). Conversely, the results of a quantitative analysis of trials suggests that an exercise expenditure of 1,200 to 2,200 kcal/wk (~15–20 mi/week of brisk walking or jogging) is required to produce significant effects on lipoproteins, and that energy expenditures beyond this lead to even further benefits (66). It is noteworthy that long-term cessation of physical activity results in loss of much of this improvement in lipoproteins (69).

Other Factors

Thrombosis

Hemostasis reflects a balance between clot formation (thrombosis) and clot dissolution (fibrinolysis), and mounting evidence suggests that hemostatic parameters are important cardiovascular risk factors. In the Framingham Heart Study (70), elevated fibrinogen levels were associated with an increased risk of CHD in men and women between the ages of 47 and 59 years. In fact, patients in the upper tercile of fibrinogen levels had a two- to threefold higher incidence of CHD. Further evidence suggests that exercise training favorably affects the fibrinolytic system, which may help to explain the reduction in cardiac events observed in subjects who are more physically active. Strenuous endurance exercise for 6 months in healthy patients aged 60 to 82 years results in significant improvement in hemostatic parameters, including a reduction in plasma fibrinogen of 13%, an increase in mean tissue-plasminogen activator (t-PA) of 39%, an increase in active t-PA of 141%, and a reduction of plasminogen activator inhibitor-1 of 58% (71). Although patients aged 24 to 30 years in this trial did not show similar benefits, other studies have demonstrated favorable effects on fibrinolytic enzymes after exercise training in younger subjects (72) and in patients after MI (73). Furthermore, the reduction in hemostatic factors is inversely related to the amount and intensity of physical activity performed; patients with the highest levels of routine exercise have the most favorable hemostatic profiles (74).

Platelet activation is an important component of the pathophysiology of acute coronary syndromes, and may be affected by acute and chronic exercise. One study demonstrated that after acute strenuous treadmill exercise of similar duration and intensity, platelet activation and hyper-reactivity were increased in sedentary subjects but remained unchanged in physically fit individuals (75). Furthermore, a 12-week program of regular, moderate-intensity physical activity in middle-aged, overweight, mildly hypertensive men resulted in a 52% reduction in secondary platelet aggregation compared with a 17% decrease for the control group (76). Thus, it appears that, although acute exercise can lead to increased platelet activity, especially in sedentary individuals, regular exercise may abolish or improve this response.

Inflammation

Growing evidence suggests that inflammation plays a role in the pathogenesis of atherosclerosis and the pathophysiology of acute coronary syndromes. Although there are conflicting data (77,78), the weight of evidence suggests that regular exercise has a beneficial effect on the inflammatory process (74,79–82). Acute, prolonged, strenuous exercise (i.e., marathon running) is associated with a marked but transient increase in inflammatory markers (83,84) that appears to be proportional to the duration of the exercise performed (85). The relationship of chronic exercise to serum inflammatory markers such as C-reactive protein, tumor necrosis factor-α (TNF-α), various interleukins (IL-1, IL-6), and white blood cell count has been assessed in several studies. Most have found an inverse relationship between physical activity (74,79,80) or fitness (81) and the levels of these biomarkers (Fig. 6.3). Additionally, skeletal muscle biopsies of patients with heart failure have revealed local muscle levels of TNF-α, IL-6, IL-1, and inducible nitric oxide synthase to be significantly reduced by exercise training (82).

Endothelial Function

The vascular endothelium plays an important role in the regulation of arterial tone and local platelet aggregation, in part through the release of nitric oxide (NO) (82). Release of NO is stimulated by serotonin, thrombin, acetylcholine, and other receptor-dependent agonists (82), as well as by increased shear stress associated with acute and chronic increases in blood flow (86,87). NO, thus produced, results in vasodilation and inhibits platelet adhesion and aggregation by a guanylyl cyclase–dependent mechanism in vascular smooth muscle cells and platelets. This endothelium-dependent vasodilation is impaired in patients with CAD, peripheral arterial disease, or atherosclerotic risk factors, including hypercholesterolemia, diabetes mellitus, cigarette smoking, and hypertension (88–90). Convincing evidence exists that impaired NO action in atherosclerosis contributes to the pathophysiology of myocardial ischemia in patients with stable and unstable coronary syndromes (89,91).

A growing body of evidence supports the premise that exercise improves endothelial function (88–92). Animal studies suggest that an important consequence of chronic exercise is an improvement in vasomotor function, which is characterized by increased endothelium-dependent vasodilation in response to increased blood flow and clinically relevant NO agonists (93,94). Exercise training has been shown to improve endothelium-dependent, flow-mediated dilation in young,

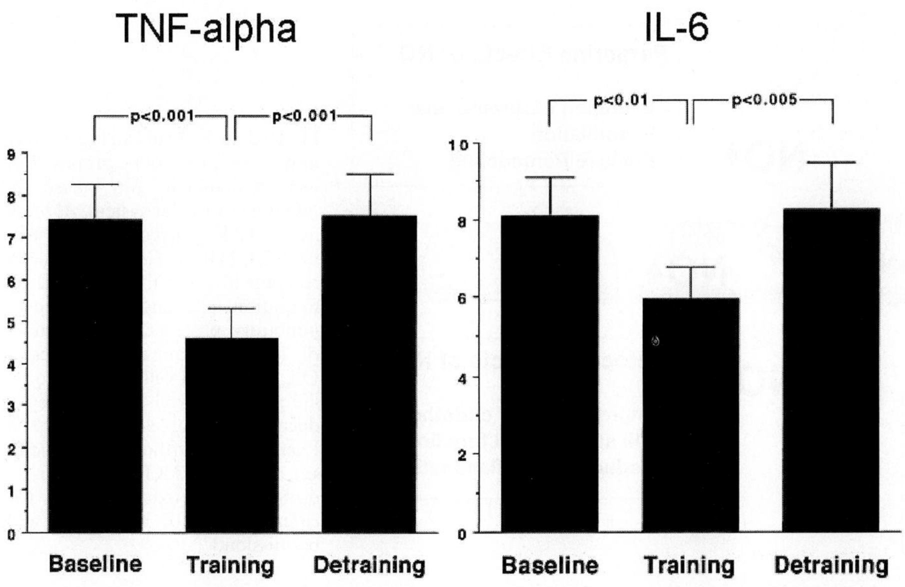

FIGURE 6.3. The effects of physical training and detraining on the proinflammatory cytokines TNF-α and IL-6 in patients with chronic heart failure. Training produced a significant reduction in TNF-α and IL-6 that was lost after detraining. (*Source:* Modified from Adamopoulos S, Parissis J, Karazas, et al. Physical training modulates proinflammatory cytokines and the soluble FAS/soluble FAS ligand system in patients with chronic heart failure. *J Am Coll Cardiol* 2002;39:653–663, with permission.)

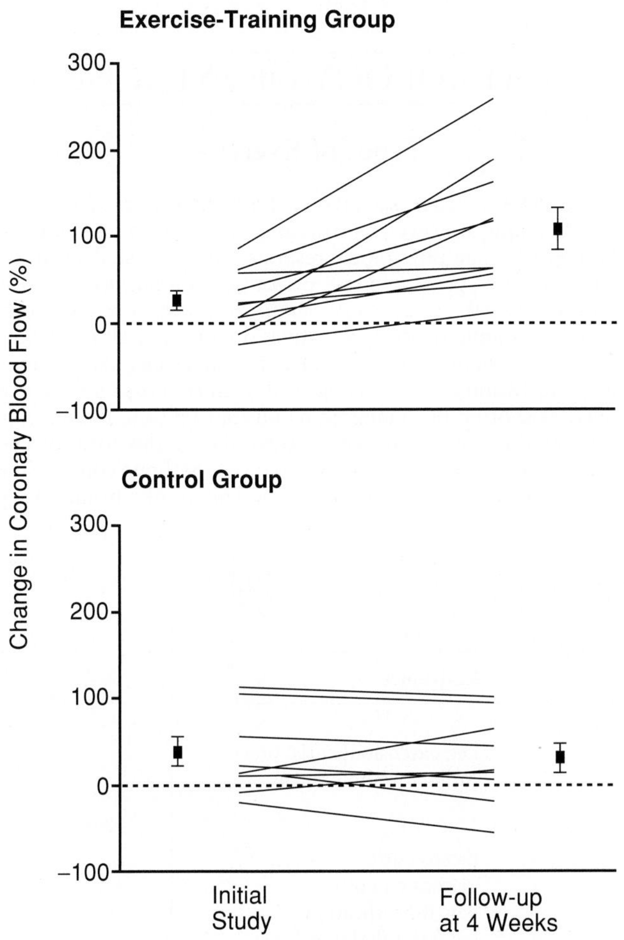

FIGURE 6.4. The effect of exercise on acetylcholine-induced changes in coronary blood flow. The mean percentage change in coronary blood flow differed significantly between the groups after 4 weeks of exercise ($P < .01$). Negative values indicate decreases in coronary blood flow. Each line represents the change in an individual subject, and the solid circles and bars represent the group means ± SE. (*Source:* Reproduced from Hambrecht R, Wolf A, Gielen S, et al. Effect of exercise on coronary endothelial function in patients with coronary artery disease. *N Engl J Med* 2000;342:454–460, with permission.)

healthy men (95). This effect was present in subjects with and without atherosclerotic risk factors and was not related to lipid levels. Similar effects have been demonstrated in patients with heart failure (88,90,96), as well as in the elderly (97), in whom regular aerobic exercise may prevent the age-associated decline in endothelial function, an effect that may be mediated by an exercise-induced increase in the availability of NO (98). In patients with CAD, a 4-week exercise regimen was associated with a 54% reduction in acetylcholine-induced coronary artery constriction and a 29% increase in coronary flow reserve, suggesting that exercise training improves endothelium-dependent vasoconstriction in both epicardial coronary arteries and in resistance vessels (Fig. 6.4) (91).

The improvement in endothelial function induced by exercise has the potential to positively impact outcomes in patients with CVD. For example, in patients with heart failure, the exercise-induced improvement in endothelial function correlates with a significant increase in exercise capacity (89). Several lifestyle modification and exercise training studies in patients with CAD have demonstrated a treatment-induced reduction in myocardial ischemia as measured by serial nuclear perfusion or positron emission tomography scans (87,99,100). This improvement in myocardial blood flow is associated with a significant reduction in coronary events (87) and is likely mediated, at least in part, by an improvement in endothelial function. The mechanisms whereby exercise improves endothelial function are not completely elucidated, but may involve a reduction in inflammatory factors that impair endothelial function (82,101) and an increase in endothelial NO synthesis (Fig. 6.5) (102). Additionally, there is a significant correlation between endothelial function and the levels of circulating endothelial progenitor cells in healthy men (103). Exercise appears to increase the production and circulating numbers of these cells (104).

Autonomic Function

Cardiovascular function is modulated, in part, by the balance between sympathetic and parasympathetic neural activity. Heart rate variability (HRV) is a well-accepted noninvasive technique for assessing this autonomic tone. Greater HRV implies augmentation of parasympathetic tone, which may protect against cardiovascular morbidity and mortality. Conversely, enhanced sympathetic activity is associated with decreased HRV and may be a risk factor for cardiac events.

In healthy subjects, HRV appears to be related to exercise training. The HRV of trained athletes is significantly greater

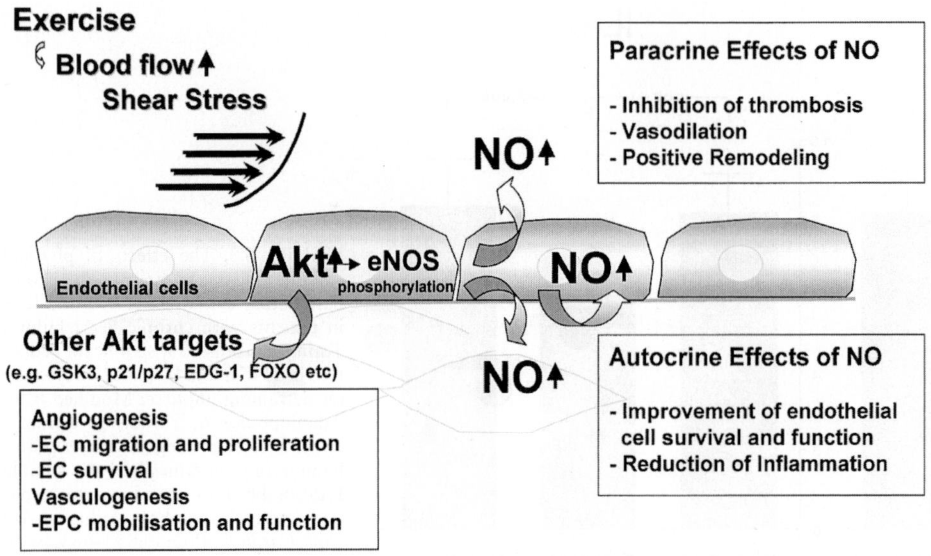

FIGURE 6.5. Transducing exercise into atheroprotection; proposed effects mediated by Akt kinase and NO in the vascular system. *Abbreviations:* GSK-3, glycogen synthase kinase 3β; EDG-1, G protein-coupled receptor involved in endothelial cell migration; p21 and p27, cell-cycle inhibitory proteins; FOXO, family of forkhead transcription factors; EC, endothelial cell; EPC, endothelial progenitor cell. (*Source:* Reproduced from Dimmeler S, Zeiher AM. Exercise and cardiovascular health: get active to "AKTivate" your endothelial nitric oxide synthase. *Circulation* 2003;107:3118–3120, with permission.)

than that of age-matched controls, suggesting that exercise training increases parasympathetic tone (105,106). Furthermore, the decrease in vagal tone associated with aging may be a manifestation of a decline in physical fitness rather than a result of the normal aging process (107). In patients with heart failure, exercise has been shown to significantly increase HRV while decreasing sympathetic activity as measured by radiolabeled norepinephrine techniques (96). Further evidence of the sympatholytic effect of exercise has been provided by performing direct recordings of the peroneal nerves in patients with heart failure (108). In this study, 4 months of supervised exercise training lead to a 37% reduction in muscle sympathetic nerve activity. This shift in the autonomic balance toward increased parasympathetic tone may have significant clinical benefit. In a study of 397 patients with advanced heart failure, those patients with the highest HRV at rest had the lowest mortality at follow-up, and HRV throughout the follow-up period was persistently lower in patients who died or were hospitalized for cardiovascular events (109). These findings offer the potential to identify high-risk patients and possibly alter their outcomes by intervening with exercise training. The effect of exercise on autonomic tone in patients with other forms of CVD is less well studied.

PHYSIOLOGY OF EXERCISE

Types of Exercise

Most types of exercise involve both endurance and resistance training; however, one training type usually predominates (Table 6.4). The physiologic responses to exercise depend, in part, on the type of exercise performed. *Endurance exercise* (also referred to as *aerobic, dynamic* or *isotonic exercise*) consists of dynamic or isotonic activity involving high-repetition movements against low resistance. Examples include walking, jogging, swimming, or cycling. Although *isotonic* implies that muscles shorten but maintain a constant tension, the tension actually does change to some degree during this form of exercise (16). Endurance exercise involves rhythmic contraction and relaxation of working muscles. This results in increased

TABLE 6.4

TYPES OF EXERCISE

	Endurance	Resistance
LOWER EXTREMITY		
	Walking Jogging/running Climbing stairs	Leg extension, curls, press Adductor/abductor
UPPER EXTREMITY		
	Arm ergometry	Biceps curls Triceps extension Bench/overhead press Lateral pull down/raises Bench-over/seated row
COMBINED UPPER AND LOWER EXTREMITY		
	Rowing Cross-country ski machines Combined arm/leg cycle Swimming Aerobics	

blood flow to active muscles during relaxation and increased venous return to the heart from the working muscles during contraction. Regular endurance exercise is referred to as *endurance training*, because it results in improved functional capacity, thereby enabling the individual to exercise for a longer duration or at a higher work rate.

Resistance exercise, also called *static exercise*, involves low-repetition movements against high resistance, such as weightlifting. This training may also be referred to as *isometric exercise*, because muscle tension develops predominantly without muscle shortening. The development of muscle tension during resistance training restricts blood flow during contraction. Regular resistance training leads to increased strength and is commonly referred to as *power* or *strength training*.

Responses to Exercise Training

Regular endurance or resistance training results in specific changes in the muscular, cardiovascular, and neurohumoral systems that lead to improvement in functional capacity and strength. These changes are referred to as the *training effect* and enable an individual to exercise to higher peak work rates with lower heart rates at each submaximal level of exercise.

Muscular Adaptations

Regular endurance training stimulates changes in skeletal muscle, including increases in mitochondria, myoglobin, capillary density, and metabolic enzymes (110). The increased mitochondrial number is specific to the muscle group exercised. For example, runners have more mitochondria in their lower extremity muscles than in their arm muscles. Additional capillaries in skeletal muscle serve to aid in the exchange of nutrients and metabolic byproducts during exercise. Increased metabolic enzymes enhance a muscle's capacity for converting fatty acids to adenosine 6-triphosphate so that more energy is derived from fatty acid metabolism, and glycogen stores are spared (110). As a result, less lactate is produced, and endurance is enhanced. The net effect of these changes in skeletal muscle is to promote aerobic metabolism, which, in turn, improves exercise capacity. In contrast to endurance training, regular resistance training leads to muscle cell hypertrophy owing to increased synthesis of contractile proteins and connective tissue (111).

Cardiovascular Adaptations

Endurance training results in increased venous return to the heart, leading to higher LV volumes and LV dilation. Conversely, resistance training exposes the patient to chronic increases in afterload owing to increased total peripheral resistance and elevated blood pressure, thereby stimulating an increase in LV wall thickness. These effects result in increased LV mass in both training groups (112). However, the increase in LV mass induced by resistance training is proportional to the increase in skeletal muscle mass, whereas there is a disproportionate increase in LV mass in endurance training. Thus, the LV mass–lean body mass ratio is elevated in the endurance trainer, whereas it is normal in the resistance trainer (113). The magnitude of these changes depends, in part, on the type of exercise performed; leg exercise yields greater increases in LV volume and mass than upper extremity exercise, compared with untrained control subjects (114).

Patients with CAD who undergo exercise training have less ischemia for a given rate–pressure product compared with that before training. Improvements in ischemic threshold manifest as less angina (115), less ST-segment depression (116), and greater myocardial perfusion (87,117) at the same levels of exercise. These findings suggest that exercise training improves myocardial oxygen supply in patients with CAD. Several studies have demonstrated a decline in maximal exercise capacity associated with aging in both men and women (118,119), which appears to be more marked with each successive decade of life (120). Habitual exercise may attenuate this loss of exercise capacity; however, it does not appear to prevent the progressively greater decline with advancing age. Nonetheless, habitual exercise does increase an individual's maximal exercise capacity at any given age (120).

Neurohumoral Adaptations

The neurohumoral response to exercise manifests as a lower resting heart rate and a reduced heart rate at any given level of submaximal exercise. This so-called *training bradycardia* relates to a shift in the balance of autonomic tone in favor of parasympathetic activity. The associated reduction in sympathetic activity is evidenced by lower levels of circulating catecholamines in trained versus untrained individuals (121). Exercise is also associated with changes in the neuroendocrine system. In patients with heart failure, exercise training is associated with significant reductions in resting levels of angiotensin, aldosterone, vasopressin, and atrial natriuretic peptide (122), potentially accounting, in part, for the clinical benefits of exercise seen in this population.

Detraining

Cessation of exercise training for as few as 3 weeks can lead to some loss of the training effect. This may be partially the result of a reduction in LV size and stroke volume induced by the loss of exercise-related augmentation of cardiac filling (123). Importantly, detraining may also reverse the beneficial effects of exercise on platelet aggregation (124), serum lipid levels (69,124), proinflammatory cytokines (see Figure 6.3) (101), and endothelium-dependent vasodilation (125).

PHYSICAL ACTIVITY AND EXERCISE: PRESCRIPTION FOR HEALTH AND FITNESS

Major public health statements have generated recommendations regarding the amount of exercise and physical activity that should be performed each week to generate health benefits. It is important to note that these recommendations are based on studies performed almost exclusively on men, although recent years have witnessed an increasing number of studies performed on women. The CDC, American College of Sports Medicine (14), AHA (126), Institute of Medicine (86), and the Surgeon General (15) all recommend that adults exercise for 30 to 60 minutes at moderate intensity levels on most, if not all, days of the week to achieve a weekly energy expenditure of at least 1,000 kcal. In addition, these recommendations stress that this physical activity can be accomplished in a single daily session or during multiple short intervals throughout the day. If exercise is of low intensity, it should be performed more frequently and for longer duration. The CDC recommendations rely on data that suggest that the benefits of exercise relate to the total energy expenditure or dose, measured in calories or duration of physical activity. Observational studies have shown that cardiovascular mortality decreases when duration of exercise increases from 15 to 47 minutes per day, and when caloric expenditure increases from 500 to 2,000 calories per week (20). The Harvard University alumni study demonstrated that brief durations of physical activity—as short as 15 minutes—conferred as great a reduction in CHD risk as longer sessions, as long as the total energy expenditure was equivalent (127).

RISKS

The inherent risks of physical activity must be considered to promote the health benefits of exercise while minimizing injury. Because nearly every activity carries some risk, the risk–benefit ratio must be examined for each individual. Major hazards involve the cardiovascular and musculoskeletal systems.

Cardiovascular Risks

The risks of cardiovascular morbidity and mortality during exercise depend on whether one studies the general population or individuals with CAD. Although the risk of death during exercise is low, death in individuals over 35 years of age is usually the result of atherosclerotic CAD, whereas younger individuals are more likely to suffer from genetic or congenital cardiac malformations (128). The incidence of sudden cardiac death during exercise for the population at large is one event per 565,000 hours of exercise (129), but is much lower for young individuals than for middle-aged and older adults. Among high school and college athletes, the sudden death rate is estimated to be 1 in 133,333 male athletes and 1 in 769,230 female athletes (130). The exertionally related sudden death rate in previously healthy middle-aged men is approximately 6 to 7 in 100,000 events per year (131,132).

For healthy sedentary men, the risk of cardiac arrest is 56 times higher during exercise compared with times of inactivity. In contrast, the risk for active men during exercise is 5 times the risk during times of inactivity. Despite this transient increased risk during strenuous exercise, regularly active men have a cumulative cardiac arrest risk that is 40% lower than the risk in inactive men (132). This and other studies (133,134) demonstrate that the risk of primary cardiac arrest during exertion is reduced among those who are physically active.

There is also evidence that heavy exertion may trigger acute MI. Two studies have found that the relative risk of MI within 1 hour after strenuous physical exertion is two- to sixfold higher than that of patients who are sedentary or less active during that hour (135,136). However, the risk is inversely related to the amount of leisure time physical activity performed by the subjects. Thus, the more active the individual, the lower the risk for developing acute MI during strenuous exertion.

In individuals with known CHD, exercise training is relatively safe. In a study of 167 cardiac rehabilitation programs involving 51,000 patients, the incidence of cardiac arrest was 1 in 112,000 person-hours, with a successful resuscitation rate of 86% (137). The incidence of MI was 1 in 294,000 person-hours, and the incidence of death was 1 in 784,000 person-hours. More recent data from a single cardiac rehabilitation center reports the incidence of major cardiovascular complications to be 1 in 60,000 participant-hours, with no deaths occurring (138).

CONTROVERSIES AND PERSONAL PERSPECTIVES

Promotion of Physical Activity

The message from America's leading scientists is clear, unequivocal, and unified: physical inactivity is a risk factor for CVD. It is highly prevalent and is a matter of public health. This unprecedented focus on physical activity and exercise is the product of copious research, including epidemiologic observational studies, cohort studies, randomized controlled trials, and basic research. It is clear that the promotion of physical activity has remained at the forefront of our national public health agenda since the publication of the 1996 Surgeon General's report on physical activity and health (15). Much work remains to promulgate this message and implement strategies to achieve the ambitious goals of the *Healthy People 2010* objectives (139) and beyond. Broad-based efforts that affect every level of our social infrastructure are needed ultimately to impact the health status of the United States. Although educational and media campaigns that directly target youth and adults are essential, these efforts must be supported by policy makers, legislators, educators, health care providers and insurers, employers, community leaders, and researchers.

THE FUTURE

Evidence regarding the health benefits of physical activity is overwhelming; however, there are many unanswered questions, and future research is needed. For example, further study of the specific mechanisms responsible for the decrease in cardiovascular events, as well as total mortality, is needed. In addition, whether specific physiologic and biochemical changes differ among the various types of exercise is undetermined. For instance, what are the effects of chronicity, intensity, and duration of activity on these parameters? Moreover, no prospective, randomized controlled trial has compared the effects that the high-dose versus low-dose range of these exercise recommendations has on fitness levels or modifiable cardiovascular risk factors (including weight, body composition, and lipid profile). Importantly, no study has evaluated the cardiovascular benefits of these recommendations on racial minorities.

The U.S. Department of Health and Human Services has published recommendations for the promotion of health and prevention of disease in Americans (139). A major objective is to enhance the physical activity of inactive individuals in an attempt to reduce chronic diseases and improve quality of life. Certain special populations have been targeted owing to their lack of participation in leisure time physical activity, including ethnic minorities such as blacks, Hispanics, Native Americans, low-income groups, the elderly, the disabled, and obese individuals. Methods that aid in promoting, implementing, and maintaining physical activity are needed.

References

1. American Heart Association. *Heart disease and stroke statistics—2005 update*. Dallas, TX: American Heart Association.
2. Blair SN, Kohl HW 3rd, Paffenbarger RS Jr, et al. Physical fitness and all-cause mortality. A prospective study of healthy men and women. *JAMA* 1989;262:2395–2401.
3. Powell KE, Thompson PD, Caspersen CJ, et al. Physical activity and the incidence of coronary heart disease. *Annu Rev Public Health* 1987;8:253–287.
4. Martinson BC, O'Connor PJ, Pronk NP. Physical inactivity and short-term all-cause mortality in adults with chronic disease. *Arch Intern Med* 2001;161:1173–1180.
5. Hu G, Eriksson J, Barengo NC, et al. Occupational, commuting, and leisure-time physical activity in relation to total and cardiovascular mortality among Finnish subjects with type 2 diabetes. *Circulation* 2004;110:666–673.
6. Hakim AA, Curb JD, Petrovitch H, et al. Effects of walking on coronary heart disease in elderly men—the Honolulu Heart Program. *Circulation* 1999;100:9–13.
7. Witt BJ, Jacobsen SJ, Weston SA, et al. Cardiac rehabilitation after myocardial infarction in the community. *J Am Coll Cardiol* 2004;44:988–996.
8. The ExTraMatch Collaborative. Exercise training meta-analysis of trials in patients with chronic heart failure. *BMJ Online* 2004;doi:10.1136/bmj.37938.645220.EE.

9. Taylor RS, Brown A, Ebrahim S, et al. Exercise-based rehabilitation for patients with coronary heart disease: systematic review and meta-analysis of randomized controlled trials. *Am J Med* 2004;116:682–692.
10. Lowensteyn I, Coupal L, Zowall H, et al. The cost-effectiveness of exercise training for the primary and secondary prevention of cardiovascular disease. *J Cardiopulm Rehabil* 2000;20:147–155.
11. Centers for Disease Control and Prevention. Physical activity trends—United States, 1990–1998. *MMWR* 2001;50:166–169.
12. Lucas JW, Schiller JS, Benson V. Summary health statistics for U.S. adults: National Health Interview Survey, 2001. *Vital Health Stat* 2004;10:1–134.
13. Centers for Disease Control and Prevention. Prevalence of no leisure-time physical activity—35 states and the District of Columbia, 1998–2002. *MMWR* 2004;53:82–86.
14. Pate RR, Pratt M, Blair SN, et al. Physical activity and public health: a recommendation from the Centers for Disease Control and Prevention and the American College of Sports Medicine. *JAMA* 1995;273:402–407.
15. U.S. Department of Health and Human Services. *Physical activity and health: a report of the surgeon general.* Atlanta: Centers for Disease Control and Prevention, 1996.
16. American College of Sports Medicine. Position stand on the recommended quantity and quality of exercise for developing and maintaining cardiorespiratory and muscular fitness and flexibility in healthy adults. *Med Sci Sports Exerc* 1998;30:975–991.
17. DeBusk RF, Stenestrand U, Sheehan M, et al. Training effects of long versus short bouts of exercise in healthy subjects. *Am J Cardiol* 1990;65:1010–1013.
18. McGinnis JM, Foege WH. Actual causes of death in the Unites States. *JAMA* 1993;270:2207–2212.
19. Gulati M, Pandey DK, Arnsdorf MF, et al. Exercise capacity and the risk of death in women—The St James Women Take Heart Project. *Circulation* 2003;108:1554–1559.
20. Paffenbarger RS, Hyde RT, Wing A, et al. Physical activity, all-cause mortality, and longevity of college alumni. *N Engl J Med* 1986;314:605–613.
21. Tanasescu M, Leitzmann MF, Rimm EB, et al. Physical activity in relation to cardiovascular disease and total mortality among men with type 2 diabetes. *Circulation* 2003;107:2435–2439.
22. Landi F, Cesari M, Lattanzio F, et al. Physical activity and mortality in frail, community-living, elderly patients. *J Gerontol A Biol Sci Med Sci* 2004;59:833–837.
23. Knoops KTB, de Groot LCPG, Kromhout D, et al. Mediterranean diet, lifestyle factors, and 10-year mortality in elderly European men and women. *JAMA* 2004;292:1433–1439.
24. Andersen LB, Schnohr P, Schroll M, et al. All-cause mortality associated with physical activity during leisure time, work, sports, and cycling to work. *Arch Intern Med* 2000;160:1621–1628.
25. Paffenbarger RS, Wing AL, Hyde RT: Physical activity and incidence of hypertension in college alumni. *Am J Epidemiol* 1983;117:245–257.
26. Paffenbarger RS, Hyde RT, Wing A, et al. The association of changes in physical activity level and other lifestyle characteristics with mortality among men. *N Engl J Med* 1993;328:538–545.
27. Gregg EW, Cauley JA, Stone K, et al. Relationship of changes in physical activity and mortality among older women. *JAMA* 2003;289:2379–2386.
28. Manson JE, Stampfer MJ, Colditz GA, et al. A prospective study of exercise and incidence of myocardial infarction in women. *Circulation* 1993;88:211–220.
29. Manson JE, Stampfer MJ, Willett WC, et al. Physical activity and the incidence of coronary heart disease and stroke in women. *Circulation* 1995; 92:927.
30. Wannamethee SG, Shaper AG, Walker MA. Physical activity and mortality in older men diagnosed with coronary heart disease. *Circulation* 2000; 102:1358–1363.
31. Kavanagh T, Mertens DJ, Hamm LF, et al. Prediction of long-term prognosis in 12,169 men referred for cardiac rehabilitation. *Circulation* 2002;106: 666–671.
32. Yu cm, Lau CP, Cheung BM, et al. Clinical predictors of morbidity and mortality in patients with myocardial infarction or revascularization who underwent cardiac rehabilitation, and importance of diabetes mellitus and exercise capacity. *Am J Cardiol* 2000;85:344–349.
33. LaMonte MJ, Eisenman PA, Adams TD, et al. Cardiorespiratory fitness and coronary heart disease risk factors. The LDS Hospital Fitness Institute Cohort. *Circulation* 2000;102:1623–1628.
34. Palatini P, Granier GR, Mormino P, et al. Relation between physical training and ambulatory blood pressure in stage I hypertensive subjects: results of the HARVEST trial. *Circulation* 1994;90:2870–2876.
35. Reaven PD, Barrett-Connor E, Edelstein S. Relation between leisure-time physical activity and blood pressure in older women. *Circulation* 1991;83:559–565.
36. Staessen J, Fagard R, Amery A. Lifestyle as a determinant of blood pressure in the general population. *Am J Hypertens* 1994;7:685–694.
37. Pescatello LS, Fargo AE, Leach CN, et al. Short term effect of dynamic exercise on arterial blood pressure. *Circulation* 1991;83:1557–1561.
38. Kokkinos PF, Narayan P, Colleran JA, et al. Effects of regular exercise on blood pressure and left ventricular hypertrophy in African-American men with severe hypertension. *N Engl J Med* 1995;333:1462–1467.
39. Appel LJ, Champagne CM, Harsha DW, et al. Effects of comprehensive lifestyle modification on blood pressure control: main results of the PREMIER clinical trial. *JAMA* 2003;289:2083–2093.
40. Whelton SP, Chin A, Xin X, et al. Effect of aerobic exercise on blood pressure: a meta-analysis of randomized, controlled trials. *Ann Intern Med* 2002;136:493–503.
41. Wasserman DH, Zinman B: Fuel homeostasis. In: Ruderman N, Devlin JT, eds. *The health professional's guide to diabetes and exercise.* Alexandria, VA: American Diabetes Association, 1995:29–47.
42. Hu G, Lindstrom J, Valle TT, et al. Physical activity, body mass index, and risk of type 2 diabetes in patients with normal and impaired glucose regulation. *Arch Intern Med* 2004;164:892–896.
43. Knowler WC, Barrett-Connor E, Fowler SE, et al. Reduction in the incidence of type 2 diabetes with lifestyle intervention or metformin. *N Engl J Med* 2002;346:393–403.
44. Wei M, Gibbons LW, Mitchell TD, et al. The association between cardiorespiratory fitness and impaired fasting glucose and type 2 diabetes mellitus in men. *Ann Intern Med* 1999;130:89–96.
45. Hu FB, Sigal RJ, Rich-Edwards JW, et al. Walking compared with vigorous physical activity and the risk of type 2 diabetes in women. *JAMA* 1999;282:1433–1439.
46. Lynch J, Helmrich SP, Lakka TA, et al. Moderately intense physical activities and high levels of cardiorespiratory fitness reduces the risk of non-insulin-dependent diabetes. *Ann Intern Med* 1996;156:1307–1314.
47. Klein S, Burke LE, Bray GA, et al. Clinical Implications of obesity with specific focus on cardiovascular disease. A statement for professionals from the American Heart Association Council on Nutrition, Physical Activity, and Metabolism. *Circulation* 2004;110:2952–2967.
48. National Institutes of Health. Clinical Guidelines on the identification, evaluation, and treatment of overweight and obesity in adults—the evidence report. *Obes Res* 1998;6[Suppl 2]:51S–209S.
49. Wing RR. Physical activity in the treatment of the adulthood overweight and obesity: current evidence and research issues. *Med Sci Sports Exerc* 1999;31:S547–S552.
50. Saris WH, Blair SN, van Baak MA, et al. How much physical activity is enough to prevent unhealthy weight gain? Outcome of the IASO 1st Stock Conference and consensus statement. *Obes Rev* 2003;4:101–114.
51. Blair SN. Evidence for success of exercise in weight loss and control. *Ann Intern Med* 1993;119:702–706.
52. Wilmore JH. Appetite and body composition consequent to physical activity. *Res Q Exerc Sport* 1983;54:415–425.
53. Garrow JS, Summerbell CD. Meta-analysis: effect of exercise, with or without dieting, on the body composition of overweight subjects. *J Clin Nutr* 1995;49:1–10.
54. Tremblay A, Despres JP, LeBlanc C, et al. Effect of intensity and physical activity on body fatness and fat distribution. *Am J Clin Nutr* 1990;51:153–157.
55. Seidell JC, Cigolini M, Deslypre JP, et al. Body fat distribution in relation to physical activity and smoking habits in 38-year old European men: the European Fat Distribution Study. *Am J Epidemiol* 1991;133:257–265.
56. Wing RR, Matthews KA, Kuller LH, et al. Waist to hip ratio in middle aged women: associations with behavioral and psychosocial factors and what changes in cardiovascular risk factors. *Arterioscler Thromb* 1991;11:1250–1257.
57. Krauss RM, Winston M, Fletcher BJ, et al. Obesity. Impact on cardiovascular disease. *Circulation* 1999;98:1472–1476.
58. Stevens J, Cai J, Evenson KR, et al. Fitness and fatness as predictors of mortality from all causes and from cardiovascular disease in men and women in the lipid research clinics study. *Am J Epidemiol* 2002;156:832–841.
59. Lee CD, Blair SN, Jackson AS. Cardiorespiratory fitness, body composition, and all-cause and cardiovascular disease mortality in men. *Am J Clin Nutr* 1999;69:373–380.
60. Wei M, Kampert JB, Barlow CE, et al. Relationship between low cardiorespiratory fitness and mortality in normal-weight, overweight, and obese men. *JAMA* 1999;282:1547–1553.
61. Hu FB, Willett WC, Li T, et al. Adiposity as compared with physical activity in predicting mortality among women. *N Engl J Med* 2004;351:2694–2703.
62. Halbert JA, Silagy CA, Finucane P, et al. Exercise training and blood lipids in hyperlipidemic and normolipidemic adults: a meta-analysis of randomized, controlled trials. *Eur J Clin Nutr* 1999;53:514–522.
63. Tran ZV, Weltman A. Differential effects of exercise on serum lipid and lipoprotein levels seen with changes in body weight. *JAMA* 1985;254:919–924.
64. Stafanick M, Mackey S, Sheehan M, et al. Effects of diet and exercise in men and postmenopausal women with low levels of HDL cholesterol and high levels of LDL cholesterol. *N Engl J Med* 1998;339:12–20.
65. Brochu M, Poehlman ET, Savage P, et al. Modest effects of exercise training alone on coronary risk factors and body composition in coronary patients. *J Cardiopulm Rehabil* 2000;20:180–188.
66. Durstine JL, Grandjean PW, Davis PG, et al. Blood lipid and lipoprotein adaptations to exercise: a quantitative analysis. *Sports Med* 2001;31:1033–1062.
67. Kraus WE, Houmard JA, Duscha BD, et al. Effects of the amount and intensity of exercise on plasma lipoproteins. *N Engl J Med* 2002;347:1483–1492.
68. Lawrence C. 'Definite and Material': coronary thrombosis and cardiologists in the 1920's. *Hosp Prac* 1992: 175–210.

69. Petibois C, Cassaigne A, Gin H, et al. Lipid profile disorders induced by long-term cessation of physical activity in previously high endurance-trained subjects. *J Clin Endocrinol Metab* 2004;89:3377–3384.
70. Kannel W, Wolf P, Castelli W, et al. Fibrinogen and risk of cardiovascular disease: the Framingham Heart Study. *JAMA* 1987;258:1183–1186.
71. Stratton JR, Chandler WL, Schwartz RS, et al. Effects of physical conditioning on fibrinolytic variables in young and old healthy adults. *Circulation* 1991;83:1692–1697.
72. de-Geus EJ, Kluft C, de-Bart AC, et al. Effects of exercise training on plasminogen activator inhibitor activity. *Med Sci Sports Exerc* 1992;24:1210–1219.
73. Suzuki T, Yamauchi K, Yamada Y, et al. Blood coagulability and fibrinolytic activity before and after physical training during the recovery phase of acute myocardial infarction. *Clin Cardiol* 1992;15:358–364.
74. Wannamethee SG, Lowe GDO, Whincup PH, et al. Physical activity and hemostatic and inflammatory variables in elderly men. *Circulation* 2002;105:1785–1790.
75. Kestin AS, Ellis PA, Barnard MR, et al. Effect of strenuous exercise on platelet activation state and reactivity. *Circulation* 1993;88:1502–1511.
76. Rauramaa R, Salonen JT, Seppanen K, et al. Inhibition of platelet aggregability by moderate-intensity physical exercise: a randomized clinical trial in overweight men. *Circulation* 1986;74:939–944.
77. Rauramaa R, Halonen P, Vaisanen SB, et al. Effects of aerobic exercise on inflammation and atherosclerosis in men: the DNASCO Study: a six-year randomized, controlled trial. *Ann Intern Med* 2004;140:1007–1014.
78. Nicklas BJ, Ambrosius W, Messier SP, et al. Diet-induced weight loss, exercise, and chronic inflammation in older, obese adults: a randomized controlled clinical trial. *Am J Clin Nutr* 2004;79:544–551.
79. Abramson JL, Vaccarino V. Relationship between physical activity and inflammation among apparently healthy middle-aged and older US adults. *Arch Intern Med* 2002;162:1286–1292.
80. Pitsavoss C, Chrysohoou C, Panagiotakos DB, et al. Association of leisure-time physical activity on inflammation markers (C-reactive protein, white cell blood count, serum amyloid A, and fibrinogen) in healthy subjects (from the ATTICA study). *Am J Cardiol* 2003;91:368–370.
81. Aronson D, Sella R, Sheikh-Ahman M, et al. The association between cardiorespiratory fitness and C-reactive protein in subjects with the metabolic syndrome. *J Am Coll Cardiol* 2004;44:2003–2007.
82. Gielen S, Adams V, Mobius-Winkler S, et al. Anti-inflammatory effects of exercise training in the skeletal muscle of patients with chronic heart failure. *J Am Coll Cardiol* 2003;42:861–868.
83. Weight LM, Alexander D, Jacobs P. Strenuous exercise: analogous to the acute-phase response? *Clin Sci* 1991;81:677–683.
84. Siegel AJ, Stec JJ, Lipinska I, et al. Effect of marathon running on inflammatory and hemostatic markers. *Am J Cardiol* 2001;88:918–920.
85. Strachan AF, Noakes TD, Kotzenberg G, et al. C reactive protein concentrations during long distance running. *Br Med J* 1984;289:1249–1251.
86. Brooks GA, Butte NF, Rand WM, et al. Chronicle of the Institute of Medicine physical activity recommendation: how a physical activity recommendation came to be among dietary recommendations. *Am J Clin Nutr* 2004;79[Suppl]:921S–930S.
87. Sdringola S, Nakagawa K, Nakagawa Y, et al. Combined intense lifestyle and pharmacologic lipid treatment further reduce coronary events and myocardial perfusion abnormalities compared with usual-care cholesterol-lowering drugs in coronary artery disease. *J Am Coll Cardiol* 2003;41:263–272.
88. Hornig B, Maier V, Drexler H. Physical training improves endothelial function in patients with chronic heart failure. *Circulation* 1996;93:210–214.
89. Hambrecht R, Fiehn E, Weigl C, et al. Regular physical exercise corrects endothelial dysfunction and improves exercise capacity in patients with chronic heart failure. *Circulation* 1998;98:2709–2715.
90. Linke A, Schoene N, Gielen S, et al. Endothelial dysfunction in patients with chronic heart failure: systemic effects of lower-limb exercise training. *J Am Coll Cardiol* 2001;37:392–397.
91. Hambrecht R, Wolf A, Geilen S, et al. Effect of exercise on coronary endothelial function in patients with coronary artery disease. *N Engl J Med* 2000;342:454–460.
92. Charo S, Gokce N, Vita JA. Endothelial dysfunction and coronary risk reduction. *J Cardiopulm Rehabil* 1998;18:60–67.
93. Sessa WC, Pitchard K, Seyedi N, et al. Chronic exercise in dogs increases coronary vascular nitric oxide production and endothelial cell nitric oxide synthase gene expression. *Circ Res* 1994;74:349–353.
94. Muller JM, Meyers PR, Laughlin H. Vasodilator responses of coronary resistance arteries of exercise-trained pigs. *Circulation* 1994;89:2308–2314.
95. Clarkson P, Montgomery HE, Muller MJ, et al. Exercise training enhances endothelial function in young men. *J Am Coll Cardiol* 1999;33:1379–1385.
96. Coats AJS, Adamopoulos S, Radaelli A, et al. Controlled trial of physical training in chronic heart failure: exercise performance, hemodynamics, ventilation, and autonomic function. *Circulation* 1992;85:2119–2131.
97. DeSouza CA, Shapiro LF, Clevenger CM, et al. Regular aerobic exercise prevents and restores age-related declines in endothelium-dependent vasodilation in healthy men. *Circulation* 2000;102:1351–1357.
98. Taddei S, Galetta F, Virdis A, et al. Physical activity prevents age-related impairment in nitric oxide availability in elderly athletes. *Circulation* 2000;101:2896–2901.
99. Gould KL, Ornish D, Scherwitz L, et al. Changes in myocardial perfusion abnormalities by positron emission tomography after long-term, intense risk factor modification. *JAMA* 1995;274:894–901.
100. Belardinelli R, Georgiou D, Ginzton L, et al. Effects of moderate exercise training on thallium uptake and contractile response to low-dose dobutamine of dysfunctional myocardium in patients with ischemic cardiomyopathy. *Circulation* 1998;97:553–561.
101. Adamopoulos S, Parissis J, Karatzas D, et al. Physical training modulates proinflammatory cytokines and the soluble Fas/soluble Fas ligand system in patients with chronic heart failure. *J Am Coll Cardiol* 2002;39:653–663.
102. Hambrecht R, Adams V, Erbs S, et al. Regular physical activity improves endothelial function in patients with coronary artery disease by increasing phosphorylation of endothelial nitric oxide synthase. *Circulation* 2003;107:3152–3158.
103. Hill JM, Zalos G, Halcox JP, et al. Circulating endothelial progenitor cells, vascular function, and cardiovascular risk. *N Engl J Med* 2003;348:593–600.
104. Laufs U, Werner N, Link A, et al. Physical training increases endothelial progenitor cells, inhibits neointima formation, and enhances angiogenesis. *Circulation* 2004;109:220–226.
105. Goldsmith RL, Bigger JT Jr, Steinman RC, et al. Comparison of 24-hour parasympathetic activity in endurance-trained and untrained young men. *J Am Coll Cardiol* 1992;20:552–558.
106. DeMeersman RE. Heart rate variability and aerobic fitness. *Am Heart J* 1993;125:726–731.
107. Goldsmith RL, Bigger JT Jr, Bloomfield DM, et al. Physical fitness as a determinant of vagal modulation. *Med Sci Sports Exerc* 1997;29:812–817.
108. Roveda F, Middlekauff HR, Rondon UPB, et al. The effects of exercise training on sympathetic neural activation in advanced heart failure. *J Am Coll Cardiol* 2003;42:854–860.
109. Adamson PB, Smith AL, Abraham WT, et al. Continuous autonomic assessment in patients with symptomatic heart failure: prognostic value of heart rate variability measured by implanted cardiac resynchronization device. *Circulation* 2004;110:2389–2394.
110. Holloszy JO, Coyle EF. Adaptations of skeletal muscle to endurance exercise and their metabolic consequences. *J Appl Physiol* 1984;56:831–838.
111. Sharkey B. Specificity of exercise. In Durstine JL, Pate RR, eds. *Resource manual for guidelines for exercise testing and prescription. American College of Sports Medicine*. Philadelphia: Lea & Febiger, 1988:55.
112. Pluim BM, Zwinderman AH, van der Laarse A, et al. The athlete's heart: a meta-analysis of cardiac structure and function. *Circulation* 1999;100:336–344.
113. Longhurst JC, Kelly AR, Gonyea WJ, et al. Echocardiographic left ventricular masses in distance runners and weightlifters. *J Appl Physiol* 1980;48:154–162.
114. Price DT, Davidoff R, Balady GJ. Comparison of cardiovascular adaptations to long term arm and leg exercise in wheelchair athletes vs. long distance runners. *Am J Cardiol* 2000;85:996–1001.
115. Ben-Ari E, Kelleman JJ, Rothbaum DA, et al. Effects of prolonged intensive versus moderate leg training on the untrained arm exercise response in angina pectoris. *Am J Cardiol* 1987;59:231–234.
116. Rogers MA, Yamamoto C, Hagberg JM, et al. The effects of seven years of intense exercise training on patients with coronary artery disease. *J Am Coll Cardiol* 1987;10:321–326.
117. Schuler G, Schierf G, Wirth A, et al. Low fat diet and regular supervised physical exercise in patients with symptomatic coronary artery disease: reduction of stress induced myocardial ischemia. *Circulation* 1988;77:172–188.
118. Fitzgerald MD, Tanaka H, Iran ZV, et al. Age-related declines in maximal aerobic exercise capacity in regular exercising vs. sedentary women: a meta-analysis. *J Appl Physiol* 1997;83:160–165.
119. Wilson TM, Tanaka H. Meta-analysis of the age-associated decline in maximal aerobic exercise capacity in men: relation to training status. *Am J Physiol Heart Circ Physiol* 2000;278:H829–H834.
120. Fleg JL, Morrell CH, Bos AG, et al. Accelerated longitudinal decline of aerobic capacity in healthy older adults. *Circulation* 2005;112:674–682.
121. Jennings G, Nelson L, Nestel P, et al. The effects of changes in physical activity on major cardiovascular risk factors, hemodynamics, sympathetic function, and glucose utilization in man: a controlled study of four levels of activity. *Circulation* 1986;73:30–40.
122. Braith RW, Welsh MA, Feigenbaum MS, et al. Neuroendocrine activation in heart failure is modified by endurance exercise training. *J Am Coll Cardiol* 1999;34:1170–1175.
123. Martin WH, Coyle EF, Bloomfield SA, et al. Effects of physical deconditioning after intense endurance training on left ventricular dimensions and stroke volume. *J Am Coll Cardiol* 1986;7:982–989.
124. Wang JS, Chow SE. Effects of exercise training and detraining on oxidized low-density lipoprotein-potentiated platelet function in men. *Arch Phys Med Rehabil* 2004;85:1531–1537.
125. Vona M, Rossi A, Capodaglio P, et al. Impact of physical training and detraining on endothelium-dependent vasodilation in patients with recent acute myocardial infarction. *Am Heart J* 2004;147:1039–1046.
126. Thompson PD, Buchner D, Pina IL, et al. AHA Scientific Statement: Exercise and physical activity in the prevention and treatment of atherosclerotic cardiovascular disease. *Circulation* 2003;107:3109–3116.

127. Fletcher GF, Balady GJ, Amsterdam EA, et al. Exercise standards for testing and training: a statement for health professionals from the American Heart Association. *Circulation* 2001;104:1694–1740.
128. Maron BJ, Shirani J, Poliac LC, et al. Sudden death in young competitive athletes: clinical, demographic and pathological profiles. *JAMA* 1996; 276:199–204.
129. Thompson PD, Buchner D, Pina IL, et al. Exercise and physical activity in the prevention and treatment of atherosclerotic cardiovascular disease: a statement from the Council on Clinical Cardiology (Subcommittee on Exercise, Rehabilitation, and Prevention) and the Council on Nutrition, Physical Activity, and Metabolism (Subcommittee on Physical Activity). *Circulation* 2003;107:3109–3116.
130. Van Camp SP, Bloor CM, Muelle FU, et al. Non-traumatic sports deaths in high school and college athletes. *Med Sci Sports Exerc* 1995;27:641–647.
131. Thompson PD, Funk EJ, Carlton RA, et al. Incidence of death during jogging in Rhode Island from 1975 through 1980. *JAMA* 1982;247:2535–2538.
132. Siscovick DS, Weiss NA, Fletcher RN, et al. The incidence of primary cardiac arrest during vigorous exercise. *N Engl J Med* 1984;311:874–877.
133. Albert CM, Mittelman MA, Chae CU, et al. Triggering of sudden death from cardiac causes by vigorous exertion. *N Engl J Med* 2000;343:1355–1361.
134. Lamaitre RN, Siscovick DS, Raghunathan TE, et al. Leisure-time physical activity and the risk of primary cardiac arrest. *Arch Intern Med* 1999; 59:686–690.
135. Mittleman MA, Maclure M, Tofler GH, et al. Triggering of acute myocardial infarction by heavy physical exertion: protection against triggering by regular exercise. *N Engl J Med* 1993;329:1677–1683.
136. Willich SN, Lewis M, Lowel H, et al. Physical exertion as a trigger of acute myocardial infarction. *N Engl J Med* 1993;329:1684–1690.
137. Van Camp SP, Peterson RA. Cardiovascular complications of out-patient cardiac rehabilitation programs. *JAMA* 1986;256:1160–1163.
138. Franklin BA, Bonzheim K, Gordon S, et al. Safety of medically supervised cardiac rehabilitation therapy: a 16 year followup. *Chest* 1998;114:902–906.
139. U.S. Department of Health and Human Services. *Healthy people 2010: Objectives for improving health.* Vol. 2. [Publication number (PHS) 017-001-00547-9].
140. Leon AS, Connett J, Jacobs DR Jr, et al. Leisure-time physical activity levels and risk of coronary heart disease and death: the Multiple Risk Factor Intervention Trial. *JAMA* 1987;258:2388–2395.
141. Morris JN, Clayton DG, Everett MG, et al. Exercise in leisure time: coronary attack and rats. *Br Heart J* 1990;63:325–334.
142. Sandvik L, Erikssen J, Thaulow E, et al. Physical fitness as a predictor of mortality among healthy middle-aged Norweigan men. *N Engl J Med* 1993; 328:533–537.

CHAPTER 7 ■ HYPERTENSION: CONTEXT AND MANAGEMENT

HEATHER COHEN HENRI AND PETER RUDD

Hypertension is a major cardiovascular risk factor that directly contributes to coronary artery disease, stroke, congestive heart failure (CHF), renal failure, and peripheral arterial disease (1). Optimal management of the condition depends on careful diagnosis, nonpharmacologic and pharmacologic treatment, parsimonious selection of tests, and practice efficiency.

Over the natural history of hypertension, early endothelial dysfunction and elevations of cardiac output usually evolve to increased peripheral vascular resistance, reflecting an array of genetic, environmental, and homeostatic factors. Early perturbations may be slight and reversible; subsequent chronic changes tend to be larger, slower, and irreversible.

Successful reduction in blood pressure (BP) and other cardiovascular risk factors can dramatically reduce the incidence of cerebrovascular and coronary morbidity and mortality, especially for individuals with the highest elevations of BP, those with multiple risk factors, and the elderly. Nonpharmacologic therapy may be sufficient for mild elevations in BP in patients without other risk factors. The large array of antihypertensive drug options necessitates individualization for particular patients and a thoughtful balance of antihypertensive efficacy, patient cost and convenience, and compelling indications and contraindications.

INTRODUCTION

During middle and older age, BP is strongly and directly related to vascular and overall mortality (2). Hypertension is the most common diagnosis cited in office visits to American physicians (3). BP-lowering agents are the most widely used prescription drugs among adults over age 65 (4). In 1998, Americans spent an estimated $109 billion in direct medical care costs attributable to hypertension and its complications (5).

Of the known cardiovascular risk factors, hypertension is the most prevalent. It occurs in 65% of the U.S. population over age 60. In 2000, there were about 58 million Americans who could benefit from antihypertensive intervention. Hypertension's prevalence increases with age, from 7% in individuals age 18 to 39 to 65% in individuals over age 59 (6). Most cases of uncontrolled hypertension occur in adults who do have access to health care and relatively frequent contact with physicians (7). Nevertheless, the percentage of hypertensives consistently controlled with medications has remained low: 25% (1988 to 1991) to 31% (1999 to 2000) (6). Figure 7.1 illustrates awareness, treatment and control of hypertension by gender and race/ethnicity from the NHANES 1999–2000 survey. Over the past decade, the prevalence of hypertension increased by about 10%. Nearly one third of respondents were unaware of their condition. Although two thirds were told to adopt lifestyle changes or take medications, only 31% achieved BP control of $\leq$140/90 mm Hg (8). Temporal trends show limited improvement in control over the past two decades.

Traditional definitions used systolic BP (SBP) >139 mm Hg and/or diastolic BP (DBP) >89 mm Hg to define hypertension. More recently, the recommendation shifted to defining normal BP as mean daytime SBP <120 mm Hg and DBP <80 mm Hg with pre- or established hypertension above these levels (9).

CLINICAL PROFILE

Natural History

Whether viewed as a distinct disease or as a cardiovascular risk factor, hypertension commonly produces structural changes in arteries and target organs in several patterns. During the prehypertension phase, repetitive perturbations of cardiovascular homeostasis occur, reflecting an array of hereditary and environmental factors. In time, these small changes accumulate and yield larger pathophysiologic changes that are recognizable as early hypertension. If the BP elevations are caught in time and reversed, normalization may occur. Reducing sodium intake, alcohol intake, and obesity lowered the incidence of hypertension from 19% to 9% in a 5-year trial of 201 individuals with high-normal BP (10). Patients with sustained elevations of

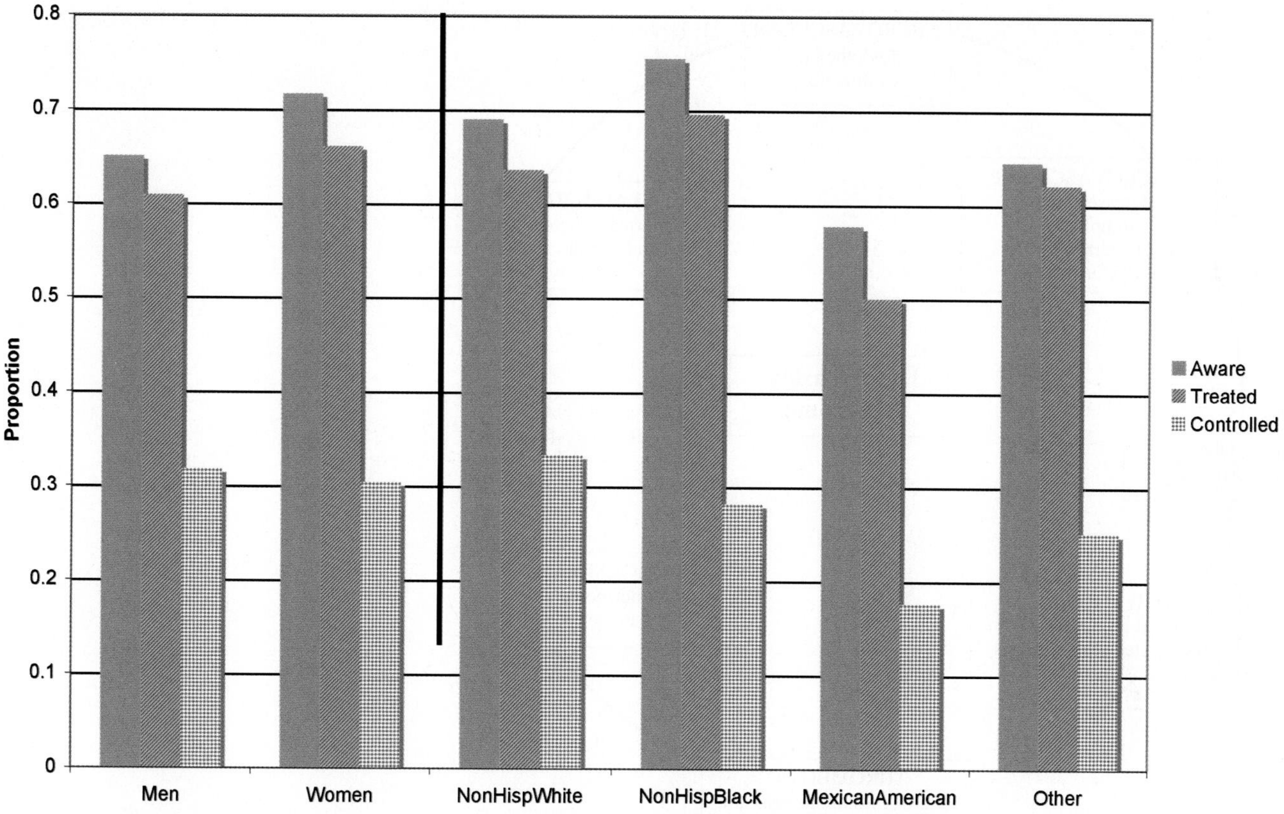

FIGURE 7.1. Awareness and management of hypertension by sociodemographic subgroups, NHAMES 1999–2000.

BP most often progress to established hypertension. A detailed discussion of the pathophysiology of hypertension appears in Chapter 100.

BP is only one factor among many that affects prognosis. Fewer than 5% of people with hypertension enter a fulminant course with rapid deterioration in cardiac, renal, and neurologic function. About half of hypertensives develop related end-organ damage if BP is left untreated over 7 to 10 years (11). The remaining patients exhibit a more indolent course with hypertensive complications occurring slowly, if at all (Fig. 7.2). The most common organ systems involved with destructive and remodeling processes include (a) the heart itself (diastolic

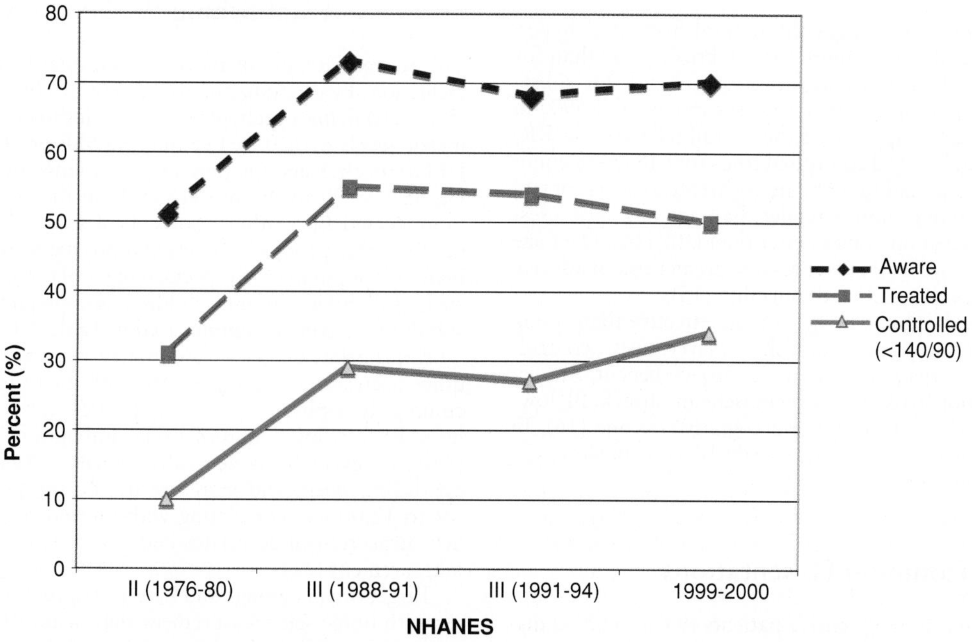

FIGURE 7.2. Awareness and management trends among hypertensives aged 18 to 74 years.

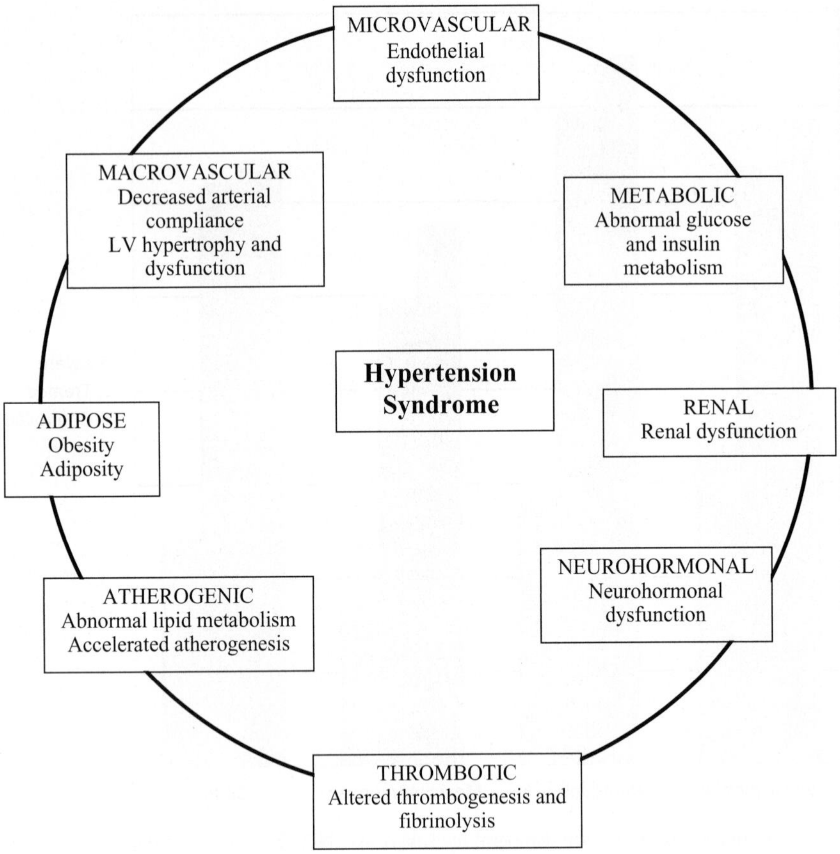

FIGURE 7.3. Hypertension syndrome.

dysfunction, left ventricular hypertrophy, endocardial scarring, CHF, and coronary insufficiency), (b) the large- and medium-sized arteries (accelerated atherosclerosis, aneurysm formation with or without dissection), (c) the brain and intracranial circulation (ischemia, both hemorrhagic and thrombotic infarction), and (d) renal circulation (nephrosclerosis, with and without renal failure). These target organ complications reflect a cluster of contributing factors termed the *hypertension syndrome* (12). Figure 7.3 displays the pathophysiologic derangements of the hypertension syndrome.

Effective treatment changes the natural history of hypertension-related end points, more for cerebrovascular than for coronary events. Hypertension carries a high risk for subsequent CHF, accounting for 39% of cases in men and 59% in women. Effective therapy lowers the overall relative risk (RR) of CHF in 12 randomized controlled trials to 0.48 (95% confidence interval [CI], 0.38 to 0.59) among treated versus control subjects (13). Among those younger than age 65, pulse pressure and SBP predict outcomes better than DBP (14). Over age 65, only elevated SBP and pulse pressure predict risk of adverse cardiovascular events and total mortality (15).

Preventing end-organ damage is more effective than trying to reverse the changes once established. Nevertheless, controlling BP after end-organ damage carries proven benefit. Among patients with prior stroke or transient ischemic attack, BP lowering reduces risk of dementia and cognitive decline (16). In patients with chronic renal failure, tight BP control slows decline in renal function (17).

Common Presentations

The vast majority of hypertensive patients (93% to 95%) display no demonstrable, curable abnormality of anatomy or physiology (18). Termed *primary hypertension,* the condition carries no consistent hallmark symptoms or signs, except for the elevated BP itself. Most cases are detected incidentally as part of routine examinations and generally in the absence of target organ damage at initial presentation. For the majority of hypertensives, specific symptoms and symptom levels do not correlate well with BP level, whether or not under medication treatment (19).

Establishing the Diagnosis

The Seventh Report of the Joint National Committee on the Detection, Evaluation, and Treatment of High Blood Pressure (JNC VII) defines prehypertension as indirect, sphygmomanometric levels of 120 to 139 mm Hg SBP or 80 to 89 mm Hg DBP, or both. Stage 1 hypertension is defined by 140 to 159 mm Hg SBP or 90 to 99 mm Hg DBP on the average of two or more seated BP readings on each of two or more office visits (9). Other groups have urged more stringent thresholds for high-risk populations in special danger of target organ damage, such as diabetics, infants, children, and pregnant women. The standard criteria are summarized in Table 7.1.

Appropriate diagnosis and management of hypertension require accurate and representative BP measurement. There is commonly a physiologic 15% to 20% variation in hour-to-hour BP readings. Studies using ambulatory BP monitoring (ABPM) reveal BP is generally highest during the day, lowest during sleep, and increases during the period from 4:00 AM to 12:00 PM, correlating with diurnal cortisol levels (20). Self-measurement correlates better with ABPM than office BP measurement (21).

Target organ damage and long-term prognosis correlate better with home self-measurement than with office BP measurements. In an 11-year cohort study of 1702 subjects with hypertension, the JNC VII classification had a stronger predictive

TABLE 7.1

BP CLASSIFICATION—ADULTS 18 YEARS OR OLDER[a]

Category	Systolic (mm Hg)	Diastolic (mm Hg)
Normal	<120	and <80
Prehypertension	120–139	or 80–89
Stage 1 hypertension	140–159	or 90–99
Stage 2 hypertension	>159	or >99

[a]When systolic and diastolic pressures fall into different categories, the higher category should guide classification (9).

power of first transient ischemic attack or stroke using home BP measurements compared to clinic BP readings (22).

No consensus currently exists about the optimal analysis for ABPM data, although the concept of BP load has gained special prominence. *Load* refers to the percentage of readings during which the SBP or DBP exceeds predefined limits (e.g., 140/90 mm Hg while awake and 120/80 mm Hg during sleep). Among patients with treated hypertension, a higher mean ABPM independently predicts cardiovascular events, even after adjustment for office measurements of BP and classic risk factors (23). Measuring BP outside the office helps to identify and address cases of apparent drug resistance, autonomic dysfunction, or when hypotensive symptoms are present (9,24).

Risk Assessment and Profile

When assessing a hypertensive patient, the clinician seeks to (a) confirm the existence and magnitude of hypertension, (b) assess the extent of end-organ damage, (c) evaluate for contributing comorbidities and risk factors, (d) screen for secondary causes of hypertension, (e) understand any special circumstances that may impact treatment over time, and (f) help to develop professional trust and the patient's ongoing commitment for reducing cardiovascular risk. The most important components of initial and follow-up visits in the ambulatory setting are enumerated in Table 7.2.

The physical examination should search for target organ damage and evidence of atherosclerotic disease, concentrating on evidence for cardiomegaly or heart failure, vascular insufficiency, bruits, and possible stigmata of secondary hypertension such as thyromegaly. Other priorities include identifying comorbidities that can complicate therapy, such as diabetes or renal dysfunction, and calculating body mass index for cardiac risk stratification. Thorough neurologic assessment provides a baseline for hypertensive complications including dementia (25). Routine fundoscopy usually shows only arteriolar narrowing with elevated BP, but hemorrhages or exudates as well as swelling of the optic discs indicate the need for urgent treatment (26).

TABLE 7.2

COMPONENTS OF AMBULATORY ANTIHYPERTENSIVE MANAGEMENT

INITIAL VISIT
- Role for home self BP measurement?
- Evidence for secondary hypertension?
- Evidence for current target organ damage?
- Clues for optimal future management?
- Opportunities to treat other cardiovascular risk factors?

FOLLOW-UP VISITS
- Interim symptoms/signs from hypertension-related pathology?
- Interim symptoms/signs attributable to antihypertensive treatment?
- Remediable obstacles to optimal medication/diet/exercise/other compliance?

Useful initial tests for patients with hypertension include (a) urinalysis (screen for proteinuria), (b) serum potassium, sodium, creatinine (calculate glomerular filtration rate and screen for secondary causes), (c) thyroid-stimulating hormone (screen for hyperthyroidism), and (d) total cholesterol, high-density lipoprotein, fasting glucose, and/or glycosylated hemoglobin (risk stratification) (27). A resting electrocardiogram (28) may show left ventricular hypertrophy, presence of coronary artery disease, and conduction blocks, important when using antihypertensive medications that have nodal blocking activity. Extensive laboratory and imaging evaluation for secondary causes of hypertension is not routinely indicated unless suggestive history or refractory BP control appears (9).

Hypertension often keeps close company with other cardiovascular risk factors, including diabetes mellitus, hyperinsulinemia, dyslipidemia, and exogenous obesity (29). In combination, these risk factors are synergistic rather than merely additive. Obesity brings a two- to six-fold increase in the probability of developing hypertension (30) and accounts for 65% to 78% of its attributable risk (31). Among patients with concomitant hypertension and dyslipidemia, coronary artery disease prevalence more than doubles compared with those with either condition alone (32). Aggressive multifactorial risk factor intervention reduces mortality by nearly 30% among hypertensive patients with hypercholesterolemia, diabetes, or a history of smoking (33).

Smoking and alcohol use also contribute to cardiovascular morbidity. Cigarette smoking leads to endothelial damage and atherosclerosis. Consuming three or more alcoholic drinks a day increases BP, even when controlling for body mass index, cigarette smoking, and age (34).

PRINCIPLES OF MANAGEMENT

Goal of Antihypertensive Therapy

Antihypertensive therapy seeks to prevent cardiovascular morbidity and mortality. Nonpharmacologic diet and lifestyle changes remain essential for all patients, especially those with only modestly elevated BP. Drug therapy offers value for those with hypertension and those with prehypertension who have compelling indications, such as chronic kidney disease or diabetes (9). The benefit of therapy rises for those with higher pretreatment BPs (35) or multiple risk factors (36). Benefit of treatment accrues to both genders (37) and continues throughout older age (15).

Nonpharmacologic Treatment

Diet and lifestyle approaches, including weight loss, exercise, and dietary adjustment, may prevent and control of hypertension (38). Combining nonpharmacologic and pharmacologic therapy controls BP better than nonpharmacologic treatment alone (39). Table 7.3 summarizes recommendations for nonpharmacologic therapy.

TABLE 7.3

RECOMMENDATIONS FOR NONPHARMACOLOGIC THERAPY

	Normotensive individuals	Prehypertensive and hypertensive patients	Health care professionals
Alcohol	Consume <2 drinks/d for men and no more than 1 drink/d for women (1 oz ethanol, 10 oz wine, 24 oz beer)	Consume <2 drinks/d for men and no more than 1 drink/d for women (1 oz ethanol, 10 oz wine, 24 oz beer)	Advise on effects of excess consumption, encourage reduction, refer as appropriate
Obesity	Reduce to goal body weight = BMI 18.5–24.9 kg/m^2 with diet and exercise	Reduce to goal body weight = BMI 18.5–24.9 kg/m^2 with diet and exercise	Inform patient, use proper BP cuff, refer as appropriate
Diet	Consume diet rich in fruits, vegetables, and low-fat dairy products with a reduced content of saturated and total fat (DASH diet)	Consume diet rich in fruits, vegetables, and low-fat dairy products with a reduced content of saturated and total fat (DASH diet)	Inform patient, refer as appropriate to community resources
Sodium/Salt	Minimize high-salt processed foods	Reduce intake to <100 mmol/d (<2.3 g sodium, <6.0 g salt/d)	Provide information on salt content of foods, counsel on methods to reduce salt intake
Smoking	Stop smoking	Stop smoking	Advise on effects of smoking, encourage quitting, refer as appropriate
Exercise	Regularly do exercise as beneficial for weight regulation and maintaining function throughout older age	Regularly do aerobic exercise for at least 30 minutes a day most days of the week	Encourage regular, appropriate physical activity; specify mode, intensity, duration, days per week
Calcium	Consume 1200 mg/d in dietary or nondietary supplement	Consume 1200 mg/d in dietary or nondietary supplement	Advise on calcium content in foods
Stress management	Insufficient evidence to recommendation stress reduction	Insufficient evidence to recommend stress reduction	Assess social situation as appropriate
Potassium and magnesium	No evidence to recommend supplementation beyond diet rich in fruits, vegetables, and low-fat dairy	No evidence to recommend supplementation beyond diet rich in fruits, vegetables, and low-fat dairy	Encourage diet rich in fruits, vegetables, and low-fat dairy products

Abbreviation: BMI, body mass index calculated as weight in kg divided by the square of height in meters.
(*Source:* Adapted from Touyz et al. [284] and Chobanian et al. [9].)

Weight Reduction

Losing excess weight reduces SBP and DBP. The Trials of Hypertension Prevention, phase II (40) studied 2382 prehypertensive patients and achieved an average of 4.4 kg weight loss at 6 months and reduction of SBP and DBP by 3.7 and 2.7 mm Hg, respectively. In a study of patients with established hypertension, weight management associated with an average 7.8 kg weight loss yielded 7 mm Hg SBP and 5 mm Hg DBP reductions in clinic BP (41).

Most trials confirm that BP reduction is directly related to the weight loss achieved. If weight gain recurs, hypertension may return, but the long-term benefits of BP reduction persist. After 7 years of following 181 participants, body weight was similar in the weight loss and control groups, but the odds of developing hypertension in the weight loss group were reduced by 77% ($P = .02$) (42). Caloric restriction and regular physical activity remain the two basic ingredients for successful weight loss.

Exercise

Adding physical activity to a weight-loss program accelerates the weight loss and augments BP reduction (43). An addition of even a 20-minute daily walk can reduce the risk of incident hypertension by 29% (44). The precise mechanism likely involves decreases in cardiac output and peripheral resistance as well as modifications in serum norepinephrine levels, insulin sensitivity, electrolyte balance, neural and baroreflex mechanisms, and vascular structure (41,45).

Cardiovascular exercise training is the most effective type of exercise for the prevention and treatment of hypertension. In a review of 39 studies using predominately walking or jogging exercise, lower intensity exercise resulted in greater BP reduction than did high-intensity exercise. Combined random and nonrandom trials showed average reductions in SBP of −13 mm Hg and in DBP of −18 mm Hg in hypertensive patients. Training more than three times per week or for more than 50 minutes per session did not confer added antihypertensive benefit (46). Current recommendations specify that exercise should occur for 20 to 60 minutes, 3 to 5 days per week, at low to moderate intensity (47).

Dietary Adjustment

Some of the most dramatic evidence supporting nonpharmacologic therapy has emerged from the Dietary Approaches to Stop Hypertension (DASH) trial (48). The study evaluated 459 adults with prehypertension or stage 1 hypertension (<160/80 to 95 mm Hg) randomized to usual diet or to a diet with increased fruits and vegetables with or without reduced total and saturated fat intake. During the trial, investigators kept patients' sodium intake and body weight at constant levels. After 8 weeks, the combined dietary intervention reduced BP by 11.4/5.5 mm Hg versus 7.2/2.8 mm Hg achieved by increasing fruits and vegetables alone ($P < .01$). Remarkably, 70% of subjects on combination diet—versus 23% on usual diet—were normotensive at the end of 8 weeks (49). Recent data establishes the combination diet as sustainable (50) and particularly effective in groups at highest risk of hypertension-related end-organ damage (African Americans, those with hypertension, and patients over age 50) (51).

The impact of reducing sodium on BP remains controversial, perhaps because salt sensitivity is heterogeneously distributed to a minority. In an unselected, normotensive population, there is insufficient evidence to recommend universal restriction of salt intake (52). In contrast, salt restriction may yield modest antihypertensive benefit among elderly hypertensives (53). Adding extra salt confers no medical value and possible harm. High sodium intake predicted mortality and risk of coronary disease among 2436 adults, independent of other cardiovascular risk factors including BP in a prospective trial (54) and cumulative mortality up to 27 years later (55).

There is consensus about the benefit of salt restriction among hypertensives (9). In the DASH-Sodium trial (56,57), subjects received the DASH diet or a typical U.S. diet and three levels of sodium (50, 100, and 150 mmol per 2100 kcal) for 30 days. Both the DASH diet group and the low-sodium groups had significant reductions in BP, but the greatest effect was seen in the combined groups (58). The benefit of BP reduction was greatest in the oldest subjects and in those with the lowest sodium intake. Moderate salt restriction with a target range of 90 to 130 mmol per day carries no associated adverse effects (52).

Importantly, sodium restriction often allows reduced need for antihypertensive medications, regardless of combination with weight loss (59). In one trial of sodium reduction with or without weight reduction among elderly hypertensives, over one third of patients were able to remain off their hypertensive medication, compared to only 16% who continued on their usual diet (60).

Adjustments in dietary and nondietary calcium supplementation may lower BP. In a meta-analysis of 42 randomized trials, calcium supplementation resulted in a small (about 1 mm Hg) but significant ($P < .001$) decrease in SBP and DBP (61). Recent data in elderly women demonstrate that adding vitamin D_3 supplementation to calcium may confer additional benefit in lowering BP versus supplementation with calcium alone. During an 8-week trial of 140 women with 25-hydroxycholecalciferol levels below 50 nmol/L, 81% of subjects in the combined vitamin D_3 and calcium group compared with 47% of subjects in the calcium alone group showed a decrease of at least 5 mm Hg SBP ($P = .04$) (62).

Most other dietary interventions appear to have trivial effects on BP. A randomized controlled intervention studying a low carbohydrate, high-protein, and high-fat diet (e.g., Atkins diet) did not significantly change SBP over 12 months (63). Reflecting a 1966–1996 Medline search, supplementing above the general dietary allowance of potassium and/or magnesium carries no demonstrable benefit in treating hypertension (64). More recently, isolated reports of mild benefit have appeared for potassium supplementation (65).

Alcohol Restriction and Smoking Cessation

Alcohol acts as a vasodilator at low doses (1 to 2 drinks per day) and as a pressor at high doses (66). Despite popular attention surrounding potential health benefits of red wine, there is insufficient rigorous evidence to recommend a "therapeutic" daily glass of wine (67). In contrast, among habitual drinkers there is ample evidence to recommend restriction of alcohol intake to two or fewer drinks. For individuals consuming four to six standard drinks a day, the pressor effect lasts throughout a 24-hour period (68). Alcohol may have a BP-lowering effect at 4 hours yet lead to BP elevations 10 hours later (69). Restricting habitual alcohol consumption can reduce BP in normotensive and hypertensive individuals (70). In a trial of hypertensive, alcohol-dependent patients, ethanol abstinence over a 24-hour period was associated with a decrease in mean BP of up to 12.5 mm Hg (71).

Among smokers, smoking cessation is commonly associated with a 3- to 4-kg weight gain and increased incidence of hypertension (72). Nevertheless, smoking cessation dramatically reduces overall cardiovascular risk.

Stress Reduction/Relaxation Training

For over 45 years, scientists have explored the relationship between mental stress and cardiovascular disease (73). Currently, insufficient evidence exists to support stress reduction as a principal or sufficient treatment for hypertension. Conflicting data exist as to whether high job stress alone is a predictor of subsequent hypertension or whether the methods used to cope with stress are more determinant (74). In a 5-year study of 292 healthy adult subjects, there was no increased risk among subjects with the highest perceived job stress, although 32% did progress to hypertension during the study period (75).

Although stress reduction programs have unclear impact on BP, device-assisted slow breathing shows promise. In a randomized study of 149 hypertensives, accumulated time spent in slow breathing resulted in significant decreases in BP. The greatest decreases in SBP (–15.0 mm Hg) were seen in subjects who spent more than 180 minutes over 8 weeks in device-assisted slow breathing. Postulated mechanisms involve effects on baroreceptor sensitivity, heart rate variability, and venous return (76). Additional studies of greater size and duration are needed before such BP-lowering techniques gain broad acceptance.

Pharmacologic Therapy

If 3 to 6 months of nonpharmacologic therapy fail to reduce BP to acceptable levels, the clinician should consider adding pharmacologic therapy or start it immediately along with nonpharmacologic therapy in patients with evidence of cardiovascular disease, target organ damage, or stage 2 hypertension (28).

The key goal is to lower BP to reduce adverse cardiovascular outcomes. In one study of 4736 hypertensive patients 60 years or older over a 5-year period, drug treatment lowered the RR of stroke by 36%, myocardial infarction by 27%, and total cardiovascular disease by 32% (77). BP lowering itself is of greater importance than the specific medication used (78). Thoughtful selection of appropriate single and combination drug therapy remains essential to maximize benefit and minimize adverse events.

Figure 7.4 displays the JNC VII recommended pathway for treating hypertensive patients. No single approach or drug is appropriate for every patient. An individualized approach helps to tailor therapy for maximal effectiveness. Initiation of monotherapy and combination therapy should take into account compelling indications for and adverse effects from each antihypertensive drug. A summary of antihypertensive drug therapy appears in Table 7.4.

Individualized Approach

The most comprehensive strategy for selecting antihypertensive therapy is the individualized approach. It takes into account

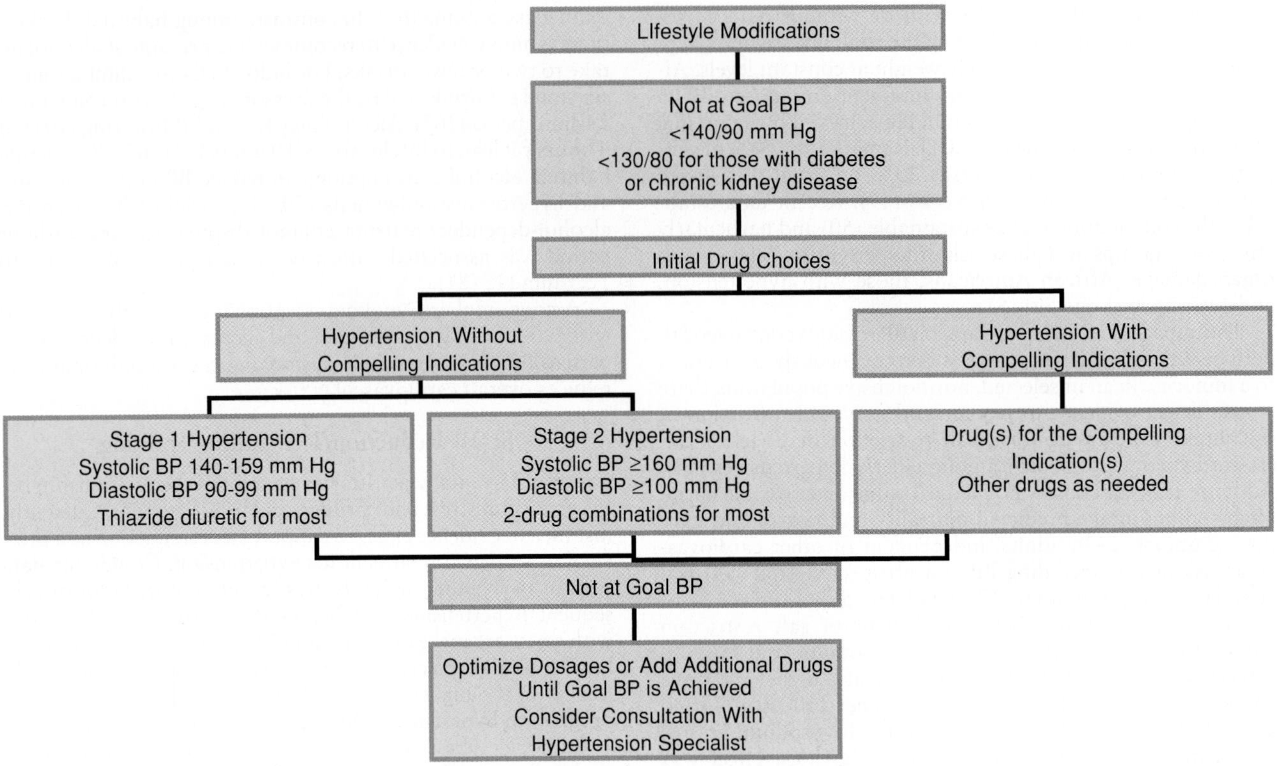

FIGURE 7.4. Algorithm for treating hypertension. (*Source:* Adapted from Chobanian et al. [9].)

several key components of each patient: profile of hemodynamics and pathophysiology, cardiovascular risk analysis, concurrent medical conditions and therapies, quality of life analysis, and cost. In essence, the customized approach corresponds to a type of "mosaic" model of treatment, incorporating a large number of variables that differ for each individual (79).

Responding to the projected *pathophysiology* and *hemodynamics,* the clinician chooses medications to reverse the underlying circulatory dysregulation, lowering the vascular resistance, if elevated, while preserving cardiac output and maintaining perfusion to critical target organs: at rest, with exercise, and over the entire 24 hours.

Reflecting *cardiovascular risk profile analysis,* the clinician should avoid medications that likely worsen the known risk profile, such as using high-dose thiazides in a patient with elevated low-density lipoprotein cholesterol (80,81). The clinician should prospectively monitor those regimen-affected factors that impact risk and adjust the regimen to minimize overall risk, whether related to atherosclerosis, arrhythmias, congestive failure, or sudden death (82).

Aware of *concurrent medical conditions and therapies,* the clinician prescribes the fewest antihypertensive drugs to treat the greatest number of concomitant conditions, such as using β-blockers when the need for coronary prophylaxis and hypertension are present in the absence of limiting bradycardia or bronchospasm. Such therapeutic parsimony facilitates medication adherence by simplifying the overall regimen and minimizes adverse drug reactions and drug–drug interactions.

For regimen adherence, the clinician seeks to optimize the patient's *quality of life* by considering physical and mental factors (83). For example, diuretic-based therapy may be more problematic in an older patient with incontinence (84). Similarly, β-blocker therapy has been associated with a small but significant increase in fatigue and sexual dysfunction (85). Such adjustments necessitate ongoing clinician–patient dialogue regarding disease- and treatment-mediated symptoms.

Rising health care expenditures, especially for medications, prompt both clinician and patient to consider cost. Key components include drug acquisition, concomitant treatment (e.g., potassium supplementation) and tests (e.g., monitoring serum potassium and renal function) (86), clinician visits, switching to a new agent after therapeutic failure or adverse event (87), and cost of not treating to goal BPs with attributable morbidity and mortality (88).

Best Options for Initial Monotherapy

The JNC VII recommends thiazide diuretics as the drug of choice for initial monotherapy in the absence of specific contraindications or compelling indications (9). In support, the Antihypertensive and Lipid-Lowering Treatment to Prevent Heart Attack Trial (ALLHAT) comprises the largest randomized trial comparing outcomes with antihypertensive monotherapy. The ALLHAT trial compared a calcium channel blocker, angiotensin-converting enzyme (ACE) inhibitor, and thiazide diuretic among 33,357 hypertensive adults over a mean of 5 years (89). All-cause mortality did not differ among the groups, but the rate of heart failure was lowest in the diuretic group. Similar results have been seen in both black and non-black patients (90,91). In a meta-analysis of 42 trials designed to compare several antihypertensive drugs, low-dose diuretics were the most effective initial treatment for prevention of cardiovascular morbidity and mortality (92). Whereas BP reductions were similar between comparison groups for every outcome studied (coronary heart disease, CHF, stroke, cardiovascular disease events, cardiovascular mortality, and total mortality), no drug was significantly better than low-dose diuretics. When analyzed from a financial perspective, thiazide therapy is the least expensive hypertensive agent available with the atypical exception of vasodilator therapy (86).

Despite concern about links between thiazide use and elevated blood glucose, recent data show that thiazides did not

TABLE 7.4

OVERVIEW OF ANTIHYPERTENSIVE MEDICATIONS

Class	Example(s)	Initial dose (mg/d)	Usual dose (mg/d)	Maximum dose (mg/d)	Mechanism(s)	Advantages	Disadvantages
DIURETICS							
Thiazides	Hydrochlorothiazide	12.5–25	25–50	100	Natriuresis	Potentiates other antihypertensives	↓K^+, ↓Na^+, ↑lipids
	Chlorothiazide	125–250	250–500	1000	Vasodilatation	Low cost	↑Glucose, ↑uric acid
Thiazide-like	Chlorthalidone	12.5–25	25–50	50		Lasts 24–48 hours	
	Indapamide	2.5	2.5–5	5	Natriuresis	Works even if GFR <50 mL/h	Same as thiazides
	Metolazone	0.5–2.5	0.5–5	5	Vasodilatation		
K^+-sparing	Spironolactone	25	25–50	100	Aldosterone	Spares potassium	Gynecomastia
	Triamterene	25–50	25–50	75	Antagonist	No effect on glucose, lipids	Limited hypotensive effect on its own
	Amiloride	5	5–10	10	Natriuresis		
	Eplerenone	25	25–50	100			
Loop	Furosemide	10–20	10–40	120	Natriuresis	More potent diuresis	↓K^+, ↓Na^+, ↑ lipids ↑ Glucose, ↑ uric acid
	Bumetanide	0.5	0.5–1.0	5			
	Ethacrynic acid	25	25–50	100			
ANTIADRENERGICS							
β-Blockers						Useful when CAD present or for agitation or tremor	Caution: bronchospasm
Lipophilic	Propranolol	20–40	40–160	320	Peripheral β-blocker		Caution: hepatic dysfunction
	Metoprolol	25–50	50–100	200			Decreases cardiac output
	Labetalol	100	100–200	1200	$[\alpha_1 + \beta]$		
	Carvedilol	12.5	12.5–50.0	50	$[\alpha_1 + \beta]$		
Hydrophilic	Atenolol	25–50	50–100	200			May worsen CHF
	Nadolol	20–40	40–120	320			
α_2-Agonists	Methyldopa	125–250	250–500	2000	↓CO, ↓HR	Useful when contraindications to β-blockers	May cause excess sedation, dry mouth, orthostasis, dermatitis from patch
	Clonidine	0.1–0.2	0.1–0.6	1.2	↓ Peripheral catecholamines		
	Clonidine patch	0.1	0.1–0.3	0.3			
	Guanabenz	2–4	2–8	64			
	Guanfacine	1	1–2	3			
α_1-Blockers	Prazosin	1	1–2	10	Peripheral postganglionic blocker	↑HDL, ↓LDL	Inadvisable as monotherapy
	Terazosin	1	1–2	10			
	Doxazosin	1	1–2	8			

(continued)

TABLE 7.4

(CONTINUED) OVERVIEW OF ANTIHYPERTENSIVE MEDICATIONS

Class	Example(s)	Initial dose (mg/d)	Usual dose (mg/d)	Maximum dose (mg/d)	Mechanism(s)	Advantages	Disadvantages
Peripheral antagonists	Reserpine	0.1	0.1–0.25	0.25	Peripheral ganglionic blocker	Long half-life	May cause sedation, depression, orthostasis
	Guanethidine	10	10–50	150			
	Guanadrel	10	10–50	100			
ACE INHIBITORS							
	Captopril	12.5	25–75	150	↓ Angiotensin II, ↓ aldosterone	Drugs of choice for diabetes mellitus	May cause ↑K^+, creatinine, proteinuria, dysgeusia, cough, rash
	Enalapril	2.5–5	10–20	40			
	Lisinopril	5	10–20	40	↓ Afterload	Useful for CHF	
	Benazepril	5–10	20–40	80			
	Ramipril	1.25–2.5	2.5–20	20			
ANGIOTENSIN RECEPTOR BLOCKERS							
	Losartan	25	25–100	100	Block, A-II, AT1 receptor ↓ Peripheral resistance	Less likely than ACE inhibitors to cause cough	May cause ↑K^+, creatinine
	Valsartan	80	160–320	320			
	Irbesartan	100	100–200	200			
CALCIUM ANTAGONISTS							
	Nifedipine	30	30–90	180	Vasodilatation	May aid natriuriesis	May cause edema, headache, flushing, weakness
	Amlodipine	2.5	2.5–10	15	↓ Afterload		
Dihydropyridines	Felodipine	2.5	2.5–10	20	Reflex sympathetic stimulation		
Negative inotropes	Diltiazem	60	90–240	360	↓HR, ↓CO	Control HR	May cause constipation, abdominal pain
	Verapamil	80–120	120–240	480			
DIRECT VASODILATORS							
	Hydralazine	25–50	50–200	300	Vasodilatation	Potent	May cause edema, ↑cardiac work, pericarditis
	Minoxidil	2.5–10	10–20	40		Rapid acting	

Abbreviations: ACE, angiotensin-converting enzyme; CAD, coronary artery disease; CHF, congestive heart failure; CO, cardiac output; GFR, glomerular filtration rate; HDL, high-density lipoprotein; HR, heart rate; LDL, low-density lipoprotein.

TABLE 7.5

COMPELLING INDICATIONS FOR INDIVIDUAL DRUG CLASSES

High-risk condition	Diuretic	β-Blocker	ACE inhibitor	A-II receptor antagonist	Calcium channel blocker	Aldosterone antagonist	Trial basis (reference)
Heart failure	•	•	•	•		•	(259–267)
Post-myocardial infarction		•	•			•	(268–272)
Coronary disease risk	•	•	•		•		(89,95,273–275)
Diabetes	•	•	•	•	•		(89,276–278)
Chronic kidney disease			•	•			(142,277,279–282)
Recurrent stroke prevention	•		•				(283)

(*Source:* Adapted from Chobanian et al. [9].)

increase risk of developing diabetes among 12,550 hypertensive adults. In contrast, use of β-blockers was associated with a 28% higher risk of subsequent diabetes (93). Similarly, over a mean 14-year follow-up in the Systolic Hypertension in the Elderly Program (94), diuretic treatment versus placebo or atenolol in diabetics was associated with the most improved long-term outcomes.

There are conflicting data regarding the superiority of diuretic therapy over ACE inhibitors as initial monotherapy for elderly patients. In a prospective, randomized, open-label study of 6083 hypertensive subjects followed over 4 years, use of ACE inhibitors and diuretics led to similar reductions of BP. Among older male hypertensives, ACE inhibitor therapy was associated with fewer cardiovascular events or deaths compared to diuretic therapy (hazard ratio 0.83; 95% CI, 0.71 to 0.97; $P = .02$) (95). The gender difference may result from the higher overall cardiovascular risk of men compared with women. Additional data show ACE inhibitor therapy is well tolerated in high-risk, elderly patients (96).

Angiotensin II receptor blockers may be used as alternative initial monotherapy. In the Losartan Intervention For Endpoint reduction in hypertension study, 9193 hypertensive patients treated with either losartan versus atenolol once daily were followed for 5 years. Despite similar BP reduction, losartan therapy displayed less risk of new onset atrial fibrillation (RR 0.67, 95% CI, 0.55 to 0.83; $P < .001$) and associated stroke (97).

In selecting initial monotherapy, compelling indications carry much weight. Randomized controlled trial data become compelling when outcomes show reduced condition-specific mortality. For example, β-blockers and ACE inhibitors confer mortality benefit to patients with coronary artery disease and should be utilized unless contraindicated in hypertensive patients with established coronary disease (83). Table 7.5 includes common high-risk conditions and guidelines for selecting individual drug classes based on comorbidities.

To balance compelling indications, the clinician seeks to minimize potential adverse effects, such as hyponatremia, hyperglycemia, hyperlipidemia, conduction blocks, bronchospasm, hyperkalemia, and fetal toxicity. Thiazide-induced hyponatremia occurs commonly and may produce mental status changes, seizures, or obtundation, especially with advanced patient age, low body weight, and low serum potassium. In contrast, duration of thiazide use and concomitant therapy with loop diuretics does not predict hyponatremic risk (98). High-dose thiazide diuretics may lead to adverse effects on lipid and carbohydrate metabolism, whereas low-dose diuretics yield side effect profiles similar to placebo (99). Both β-blockers and some calcium channel blockers are associated with nodal conduction delays, contraindicated in patients with bradycardia, sick sinus syndrome, and second- or third-degree atrioventricular block (100). Nonselective β-blockers can induce bronchospasm in patients with obstructive lung disease, but cardioselective β-blockers minimize this effect (101). Aldosterone antagonists may cause hyperkalemia with renal failure and should be avoided in patients with higher baseline serum potassium and/or creatinine levels (102). Lastly, pregnancy is an absolute contraindication for angiotensin II receptor antagonists and ACE inhibitors; these drugs have been associated with fetal toxicity (103).

Combination Drug Therapy

Up to 85% of hypertensive patients require combination drug therapy to reach goal BP (104). Combination therapy may reduce dose-related side effects and adverse events by avoiding higher doses of single drugs and utilizing two or more drugs with different mechanisms and side effect profiles (105). Low-dose combination therapy often provides greater BP control than titration upward of monotherapy in a patient without adequate response to initial monotherapy (106). In direct comparisons of three approaches to hypertension treatment (low-dose combination, sequential monotherapy, and stepped care), the low-dose combination groups had significantly greater success in achieving target BP (107,108) with fewer drug-related adverse events compared with the other two strategies (109). Successful drug combinations will likely reflect complementary mechanisms of antihypertensive therapy. Perhaps more subtly, some combinations of antihypertensive agents yield superior survival rates despite similar immediate BP-lowering effects. Women treated with a two-drug class regimen of calcium channel blocker and diuretic had an 85% greater risk of cardiovascular death when compared to women treated with a combination of diuretic and β-blocker. There was no significant difference in outcomes with ACE inhibitor plus diuretic therapy compared to β-blocker plus diuretic regimens (90).

SECONDARY FORMS OF HYPERTENSION

The vast majority of hypertensive patients exhibit no demonstrable, curable secondary cause. Only 4% to 9% of patients have identifiable underlying causes of hypertension, most commonly renal parenchymal disease with minimal reversibility. Most series from a variety of international settings indicate only 1% to 2% of hypertensives have a correctible secondary cause (110–112). Among older patients with atherosclerosis, the prevalence of secondary hypertension increases, especially for renovascular and primary hypothyroidism causes (110). Clues from history, physical examination, or baseline testing often provide the impetus to pursue causes of secondary hypertension. In the absence of specific indications, there is little justification for routine aggressive evaluation of every hypertensive patient for curable causes. The diagnostic process may resume if patients later exhibit new clues or refractoriness to treatment. In recent years, several isolated reports of higher prevalence of correctible secondary causes have emerged, especially for primary hyperaldosteronism (113). Table 7.6 summarizes several etiologies, diagnostic screening options and treatments for secondary hypertension.

Renal Parenchymal Disease

Renal parenchymal disease is both a cause and a consequence of hypertension. Accounting for up to 5% of all cases of hypertension, renal parenchymal damage is the most common cause of secondary hypertension (114). Hypertension and diabetes are the leading contributors to chronic renal failure (115,116). Parenchymal disease ultimately decreases the glomerular filtration rate and thereby increases BP by hindering the excretion of salt and excess fluid (117). Chronic renal parenchymal conditions are often irreversible and associated secondary hypertension may be related to several changes in the homeostatic balance.

The pathophysiology underlying hypertension-mediated glomerular disease is complex. Factors include activation of the sympathetic nervous system (118), the renin–angiotensin system, volume expansion, decreased synthesis of vasodilatory substances (119), and sodium retention. These processes ultimately result in nonfunctional connective tissue formation. Prominent histologic features consist of fibrosis, loss of native renal cells, and infiltration by monocytes and macrophages (120). Incremental increases in BP lead to elevated glomerular pressure once the kidney's ability to autoregulate pressure is disrupted (121). Left untreated, a vicious cycle of further renal parenchymal damage and hypertension ensues.

Many clinical conditions affect renal parenchyma and produce hypertension. Glomerular disease leading to nephrotic syndrome can be either primary or secondary. Among patients with primary nephrotic syndrome, minimal change disease is most commonly found among children; membranous nephropathy is more common in adults (122). Causes of secondary glomerular diseases include aforementioned diabetes, infections, connective tissue disorders, HIV-associated nephropathy (123) and, rarely, amyloidosis (124).

Glomerulonephritis comprises an important cause of acute and chronic kidney disease, characterized by hematuria, red cell casts, hypertension, and decreased glomerular filtration rate (125). Although many patients with acute nephritis may ultimately recover their renal function, histologic findings on renal biopsy such as tubular loss and interstitial fibrosis are predictive of hypertension (126) and correlate with development of end-stage renal disease (127).

Additional causes of acute renal failure include CHF, acute tubular necrosis, hypercalcemia (128), vasculitis, and analgesic use. Normally, nonsteroidal anti-inflammatory medications (NSAIDs) are well tolerated by the kidney. However, in the setting of underlying renal dysfunction or volume depletion, NSAIDs may cause acute tubulointerstitial nephritis, renal papillary necrosis (129), glomerulonephritis, and vasculitis (130).

Genetic disorders affecting renal parenchyma, such as polycystic kidney disease, may also lead to hypertension (131). Identifying polycystic kidney disease early allows aggressive BP treatment to improve prognosis (132).

Screening tests for parenchymal renal disease usually reveal azotemia, microalbuminuria (133), proteinuria, or abnormal urinary sediment. The most important management decisions usually revolve around the desirability and timing of dialysis or transplantation, optimal management of the volume component of the hypertension, and strictness of BP control. In a randomized trial of 840 patients with moderately to severely reduced glomerular filtration rate, low target BP (mean arterial pressure <92 mm Hg) versus usual target BP (mean arterial pressure <107 mm Hg) dramatically reduced end points of kidney failure and all cause mortality (134).

In addition to achieving control of elevated BP, reducing proteinuria is paramount in delaying progression of chronic renal disease. Microalbuminuria is a strong, continuous, and independent risk factor for renal dysfunction, cardiovascular disease, and death (135). The presence of both microalbuminuria and hypertension increases risk synergistically, exceeding the additive risk of either factor in isolation (136). In patients with at least 1.0 g/d of proteinuria, meta-analysis reveals benefit of reducing SBP to 110 to 129 mm Hg (137). Reducing proteinuria by half decreases risk of renal failure by half in patients with diabetic nephropathy (138).

Recent data demonstrate additional renoprotective effects of ACE inhibitors and angiotensin II receptor antagonists once BP is optimized (139). Combining these two agents does not improve BP control (140), but may provide superior renoprotection compared with monotherapy (141). These medications reduce proteinuria by strengthening the glomerular barrier, diminishing protein-mediated inflammatory cascades that lead to interstitial inflammation and disease progression (142). Close monitoring for hyperkalemia and worsening renal function remains essential with the use of these medications (143).

Vascular Causes

Hypertension may result from physiologically significant stenosis of the renal arteries, the aorta, and a variety of other vascular structures.

Renovascular Causes

Activation of the renin–angiotensin–aldosterone system can result from compromise of arterial flow to either or both kidneys. Depending on the status and participation of the contralateral kidney, the ischemic stimulus may elevate renin, promote fluid retention, or both.

Two clinical subgroups comprise the majority of patients with renovascular hypertension: fibromuscular dysplasia and atherosclerotic disease. Fibromuscular dysplasia of the renal arteries accounts for less than 10% of all renovascular hypertension and occurs mainly in younger women. Like atherosclerosis, the disease appears in arterial beds throughout the body. Lesions are classified as intimal, medial, or adventitial, with the vast majority of cases being medial and affecting the kidney—typically characterized by a "beaded" appearance on angiography (144). Patients with renal fibromuscular dysplasia typically have a renin-dependent hypertension, whereas patients with atherosclerotic renal disease usually have elevated BP that is not renin dependent (145). Among patients with fibromuscular dysplasia, percutaneous angioplasty cures up to 50% and improves 42% of patients (146).

Atherosclerotic renal artery stenosis is a progressive disease, accounting for about 90% of all renovascular hypertension (147). More prevalent with advanced age, it often coexists with other high-risk vascular diseases such as coronary artery

TABLE 7.6

SECONDARY HYPERTENSION: AN OVERVIEW

Condition	History	Physical exam	Initial tests	Screening	Definitive	Comments	Therapy
Renal parenchymal disease	Renal disease, hypertension, diabetes mellitus, glomerulonephritis, chronic analgesics	Flank/abdominal mass, volume overload, diabetic neuropathy/retinopathy	Elevated creatinine and GFR, anemia, active sediment, proteinuria	Spot and 24-hour urinary protein, renal ultrasound	Renal biopsy in selected cases	False reassurance with "normal" creatinine in elderly	Treat underlying condition, volume overload and electrolyte imbalances; aggressive BP control
Renovascular hypertension	Age <30 y, especially female; age >60, atherosclerosis; azotemia induced by ACE-I or ARB	Flank bruit; peripheral vascular insufficiency	Proteinuria, hyperlipidemia	Clinical prediction rules, ultrasound, CT, MRI, captopril renal scintigraphy	Renal arteriography	Angioplasty and surgery improve BP control but do not improve renal function, especially for elderly	ACE-I or ARB; close monitoring, BP and lipid control; surgery, angioplasty and stenting in selected cases
Coarctation of the aorta	Early onset hypertension, lower extremity claudication, mesenteric ischemia	Asymmetrical pulses and BP, systolic murmur or bruit	Bilateral ankle:brachial index, CXR	Ultrasound, MRI, CT	Transesophageal echo, aortography		Surgical repair
Cushing syndrome	Weight gain, acne, fluid retention, bruising, adrenal mass, steroid use	Abdominal mass, moon facies, truncal obesity, striae, hirsutism	Hyperglycemia, hyperlipidemia	24-h Urinary free cortisol, low-dose dexamethasone suppression test, midnight salivary cortisol	High dose dexamethasone suppression test; if ACTH dependent, pituitary MRI +/− inferior petrosal sampling	Screen for osteoporosis	Surgical excision versus drug suppression
Primary hyperaldosteronism	Onset at young age; weakness, fatigue, polyuria, polydipsia, muscle cramps		±Hypokalemia	PA/plasma renin activity, 24-h urinary aldosterone	Adrenal CT or MRI; scintigraphy +/- adrenal vein sampling		Excision for adenoma; anti-aldosterone therapy for adrenal hyperplasia
Pheochromocytoma	±Paroxysmal hypertension; palpitations, headache, sweating, autonomic instability	Tremor, orthostasis, cardiomyopathy, perspiration, incidentally discovered adrenal mass	Hyperglycemia	Plasma metanephrines; 24-h urinary metanephrines	Adrenal CT or MRI, scintigraphy, rarely PET scan		Surgical excision after pretreatment with a-blockers, fluid (phenoxybenzamine, labetalol)
Sleep apnea	Snoring, daytime somnolence or fatigue	Obesity, increased neck circumference, micrognathia			Polysomnography	Weight loss, avoidance of sedatives or alcohol	CPAP, surgery in selected refractory patients

Abbreviations: ACE-I, angiotensin converting enzyme inhibitor; ACTH, adrenocorticotropic hormone; ARB, angiotensin receptor blocker; BP, blood pressure; CPAP, continuous positive airway pressure; CT, computed tomography; CXR, chest radiograph; MRI, magnetic resonance imaging; PA, plasma aldosterone; PET, positron emission tomography.

disease (148). Atherosclerotic renal disease may extend for years without signaling its presence with hypertension or even elevated serum creatinine. Alternatively, it can cause progressive hypertension with pulmonary edema or need for dialysis (149). Clues predictive of significant renal artery stenosis include resistance to antihypertensive medication (150), abrupt onset or accelerated hypertension, unexplained azotemia, azotemia induced by ACE inhibitors or angiotensin II receptor blockers, asymmetric renal size, and CHF with normal ventricular function (145). Renal parenchymal damage plays an important role in prognosis: although renal artery anatomy does not correlate with baseline renal function or functional outcome, reduced renal function and proteinuria predict poor cardiovascular outcome and renal failure (151).

No simple and reliable screening test exists. When evaluated systematically, clinical prediction rules may have sensitivity of 65% and specificity of 87% in diagnosing renal artery stenosis (152). Although x-ray angiography is the gold standard for diagnosis, less invasive options include color Doppler sonography, computed tomographic (CT) angiography, magnetic resonance angiography (MRI), captopril renal scintigraphy, and the captopril test. Owing to lower cost and availability, sonography is often the first diagnostic modality utilized, with up to 95% sensitivity and 90% specificity achieved by highly trained operators (153). In direct comparison to captopril renography, ultrasound has equivalent if not better sensitivity, positive predictive value, specificity and negative predictive value (154). In a meta-analysis comparing several diagnostic tests utilizing angiography as the gold standard, CT angiography and three-dimensional MRI outperformed ultrasound, captopril renal scintigraphy, and the captopril test (155). Although promising, CT and MRI do remain less sensitive and reproducible than digital angiography (156).

Aggressively searching for renal stenosis in patients with hypertension remains a topic of debate, as only a small percentage may benefit from intervention. Tests that reliably predict which patients will respond to revascularization are not yet available (157). Methods such as angiography and noninvasive imaging currently assess the severity of stenosis but not the functional significance or associated differential pressure produced by stenosis. Developing techniques noninvasively to measure renal artery differential pressure may show promise (158).

Debate continues about whether surgical intervention or angioplasty and stenting in atherosclerotic renal disease help to preserve renal function and improve cardiovascular morbidity and mortality compared with medical therapy (147). Among patients with atherosclerotic renal stenosis, the best candidates for revascularization are those with bilateral disease (159), baseline serum creatinine <2.0 mg/dL, normal renal resistive indices, no proteinuria, and with evidence of end-organ injury (145). Balloon angioplasty and stenting are commonly the preferred revascularization techniques (160). Meta-analysis of three randomized studies comparing best medical therapy with balloon angioplasty shows angioplasty results in better BP control but not preservation of renal function (161). Fully 81% of patients who undergo angioplasty and stenting for renovascular hypertension will have lower BP at 1 year. However, renal function is stable or worse in about 75% of these patients (162). Surgical correction has similar effect on BP improvement. However, in one series of 500 patients with hypertension and atherosclerotic renal disease who underwent surgical correction, 5% died within 30 days of surgery. Fifty-seven percent of patients in this series had unchanged or worse renal function after surgery (163). Medical management for atherosclerotic renal stenosis includes ACE inhibitor or angiotensin II receptor blocker therapy (with careful monitoring of potassium and renal function), aggressive BP control, cholesterol lowering, and avoidance of nephrotoxic agents.

Aortic Coarctation

A variety of rare congenital, inflammatory, and infectious etiologies may produce malformations of the aorta (164). Although the majority of patients with congenital disease present during childhood, some may pass into adulthood before definitive diagnosis (165). Important clues include early onset hypertension, lower extremity claudication, and mesenteric ischemia (164). These conditions can be recognized on chest radiographs and confirmed by ultrasound, angiography, CT, or MRI. Other lesions of the aortic arch are characterized by aortic obstruction and include supraclavicular aortic stenosis, aortic arch interruption or atresia, and coarctation (166). Surgical repair with resection and anastomosis remains the treatment of choice in suitable operative candidates (167), with angioplasty available as an alternative (168).

Endocrinologic Causes

Cushing Syndrome

Chronic exposure to excess glucocorticoids results in Cushing syndrome. Although Cushing syndrome may be iatrogenic, endogenous disease is caused by excess adrenocorticotropic hormone (ACTH) production in 80% of cases (usually a pituitary adenoma, or rarely an extrapituitary ACTH-secreting tumor or corticotropin-releasing hormone-secreting tumor). About 20% of cases are ACTH independent (unilateral benign or malignant adrenocortical tumors or bilateral adrenal hyperplasia or dysplasia) (169).

Cushing syndrome with classic stigmata of hypercortisolism is a very rare disease, with an estimated incidence of 1 case per 100,000 persons. A much more common phenomenon, *subclinical Cushing syndrome,* has recently been described: without signs of frank cortisol excess but with hormonally active adrenal incidentilomas discovered by CT, MRI, or ultrasound. Affecting 5% to 20% of patients found to have adrenal incidentilomas, the estimated prevalence is 79 cases per 100,000 persons (170).

Both classic and subclinical Cushing syndrome carry associations with accelerated bone loss (171), truncal obesity, hyperglycemia, hyperlipidemia, hypertension, and increased cardiovascular risk (172). These features overlap with those of the metabolic syndrome (173). In contrast to the subclinical state, classic Cushing syndrome includes patients with frank signs of hypercortisolism such as moon facies, acne, striae, and buffalo hump.

Most patients with classic and subclinical Cushing syndrome display hypertension (174). Glucocorticoid-mediated hypertension is a low renin state (175). The precise mechanisms underlying elevated BP remain elusive. Increased pressor responsiveness has been reported, probably owing to local postsynaptic effector mechanisms in the resistance vessels (176). After cure of classic Cushing syndrome, rates of hypertension and mortality approximate those found in the general population (177). Among patients with subclinical Cushing syndrome treated with adrenalectomy, rates of hypertension and metabolic abnormalities also improve (174).

No screening test or diagnostic test for Cushing syndrome is 100% predictive (178). Three options for initial screening are available: 24-hour urinary free cortisol, low-dose dexamethasone suppression test, or late-night salivary cortisol (169). A 24-hour urinary free cortisol excretion greater than four times the normal level in a patient with typical clinical features can be diagnostic of cortisol excess (179). Although highly reliable, this test requires patient cooperation for completeness. Low-dose dexamethasone suppression test, utilizing either blood or urine samples, is another assay of excess autonomous cortisol production (180). However, the criterion for normal suppression of cortisol after dexamethasone is unclear, and the test may have a low sensitivity (181). Last, measuring midnight salivary cortisol is a noninvasive technique with comparable diagnostic accuracy to identify patients with cortisol excess (182).

After confirming excess cortisol in patients with classic Cushing syndrome, determination of plasma ACTH suppression guides further workup. Whereas ACTH levels alone rarely provide definitive diagnosis, the high-dose dexamethasone suppression test at least partially suppresses 80% to 90% of corticotroph adenomas, whereas ectopic and adrenal tumors are generally resistant to feedback. In patients with ACTH-dependent Cushing syndrome, further evaluation with pituitary MRI may provide definitive diagnosis. In patients with discordant or equivocal clinical, biochemical, and radiologic studies, bilateral inferior petrosal sampling may bring clarity (169). Such petrosal sampling measures sinus-to-peripheral ACTH ratio but has a 1% to 10% false-negative rate (183).

Both medical and surgical options exist for Cushing syndrome (184). Medical targets for therapy modulate signaling pathways and transcriptional regulation of ACTH biosynthesis, antagonize corticotrophin-releasing hormone, or glucocorticoid receptors, or inhibit glucocorticoid synthesis (185). Medical treatment applies occasionally as first-line treatment, and generally follows surgery. Surgical therapy involves a transsphenoidal approach in 99% of cases. Stereotactic gamma knife radiotherapy is utilized in selected cases (186).

Management of adrenal incidentilomas depends on two key factors: (a) hormonal activity (e.g., presence of subclinical Cushing disease) and (b) size. In cases of biochemical cortisol excess with clinical sequelae evident, adrenalectomy should follow (170,187). If malignancy is suspected (highest risk in masses >4 cm) for nonhormonally active adrenal incidentilomas, preferred management includes adrenalectomy or fine needle aspiration (187).

Primary Aldosteronism

Whereas Cushing syndrome reflects glucocorticoid excess, a variety of other conditions generate mineralocorticoid excess. These conditions include primary hyperaldosteronism (adenoma, carcinoma, or bilateral hyperplasia), enzymatic deficiencies (11-OH-hydroxylase deficiency, 17-OH-hydroxylase deficiency, and 11-OH-dehydrogenase deficiency syndromes), or chronic licorice ingestion containing glycyrrhetinic acid (188). Benign unilateral aldosterone-producing adenoma (APA) and bilateral idiopathic adrenal hyperplasia (IHA) are the leading causes of primary aldosteronism (189). These conditions yield inappropriately large and autonomous secretion of aldosterone with predictable metabolic and pathophysiologic consequences. Once secreted, aldosterone increases distal tubular sodium resorption and potassium secretion, increases intravascular volume, and suppresses renin secretion. When secreted in excess, aldosterone produces a volume-dependent hypertension. Additionally, downregulation of endothelial nitric oxide synthase is postulated to play a role in mineralocorticoid-mediated hypertension (190).

APAs, comprising about 80% of all primary aldosteronism, display response to corticotropin but not to renin. In normal individuals, the renin–angiotensin system regulates aldosterone secretion. However, even with volume expansion or increased sodium intake, a renin-unresponsive APA will continue to secrete plasma aldosterone (PA). In contrast to APA, IHA shows response to renin. Comprising about 20% of all primary aldosteronism, IHA exhibits responsiveness to increased plasma angiotensin II and a normal aldosterone response on postural testing (191).

Prevalence of primary aldosteronism is widely debated, reflecting a lack of diagnostic standardization (192,193). Difficulty establishing cutoffs for diagnosis relate to the continuum of elevated BP seen with elevation of aldosterone. Among a community-based sample of normotensive individuals, increased aldosterone levels within a physiologic range predispose to the development of hypertension. This phenomenon blurs the distinction between low renin essential hypertension and hyperaldosteronism (194). Although hypokalemia was originally considered a hallmark of primary aldosteronism, low potassium may be absent (195). In fact, most patients currently carrying the diagnosis are normokalemic (196). Patients may be asymptomatic or may display weakness, fatigue, polyuria, polydipsia, or muscle cramps (197).

Hypertensive patients who have hypokalemia, medication resistance, or onset at a young age should undergo screening for primary hyperaldosteronism (198). Ratio of PA concentration to plasma renin activity is a first-line screening test. Because the PA/renin ratio has limited sensitivity and specificity, it is not advocated as a routine screening test in the general hypertensive population (199). Concomitant antihypertensive medications may distort ratio results (200).

A positive screening test leads the clinician to confirmatory testing. Physiologic maneuvers that normally inhibit or stimulate aldosterone and renin secretion may assist definitive diagnosis (191). Radiocholesterol scintigraphy, CT, or MRI complements biochemical information. In a series of 49 patients with confirmed PA, the positive predictive value of adrenal imaging was 98% for scintigraphy, 85% for CT scan, and 83% for MRI, with a sensitivity of 85%, 85%, and 74% respectively (201).

Because management of APA and IHA differs, distinguishing between these two entities has clinical importance. Whereas laparoscopic adrenalectomy may cure APA, surgery offers no value in patients with IHA (195). Clinically, patients with APA have higher BP, lower serum potassium levels, higher serum and urinary aldosterone levels, and are younger compared with patients who have IHA. Adrenal venous sampling and imaging are also used to find asymmetry predictive of APA (202). Because CT or MRI may confound by demonstrating an unrelated adrenal nodule, performing adrenal venous sampling or scintigraphy distinguishes functional from structural asymmetry (203). Lateralization of aldosterone production is predictive of cure after adrenalectomy (204).

IHA warrants medical therapy with the nonselective aldosterone-receptor antagonist spironolactone as the mainstay of therapy. Spironolactone generates both anti-androgenic and progestational side effects. Alternatively, a more expensive, selective aldosterone receptor antagonist, eplerenone, has an improved side effect profile with similar safety and antihypertensive effect but higher cost (205).

Pheochromocytoma

Pheochromocytomas and other catecholamine-secreting tumors—termed *paragangliomas* when arising outside the adrenals—may prompt some of the most dramatic moments in hypertension. The clinical spectrum is wide, ranging from previously unsuspected tumors that first gain recognition from hypertensive crises after a procedure like anesthetic intubation, to incidentally discovered, slow-growing, sometimes large, metabolically almost inactive masses.

Nearly 80% of the tumors are limited to the adrenal glands, usually unilaterally. The tumors are more likely to be bilateral or multiple in pediatric presentations or in familial forms such as type 1 neurofibromatosis, von Hippel-Lindau disease, or multiple endocrine neoplasia type 2. An additional 10% to 20% arise in other intraabdominal sites, and less than 5% appear from intrathoracic sites along the neurosecretory crest or bladder. Fewer than 10% of all catecholamine-secreting tumors are malignant (206).

Recent advances in the fields of radiology, genetics, and immunohistochemistry shape our evolving understanding of this rare disorder. In one series of 41 consecutive patients undergoing surgery for pheochromocytoma between 1990 and 2002, almost half of the cases came to attention after abdominal imaging (ultrasound, CT, or MRI) performed for reasons unrelated to BP (207). Much as for subclinical Cushing disease, adrenal incidentilomas may lead to unexpected discovery. Whereas baseline prevalence of pheochromocytoma accounts for 0.5% of hypertensives tested, up to 4% of patients with adrenal incidentilomas may show the condition (208). Historically, only 10% of pheochromocytomas were thought hereditary. New data show 25% of patients with pheochromocytoma and no family history have germ-line mutations in one of four related susceptibility genes (209).

Disease manifestations reflect the direct and indirect effect of catecholamines, either hypersecreted at random intervals for variable durations or tonically released. The classic symptoms of pheochromocytoma (paroxysmal headache, sweating, palpitations, stress, and a sense of imminent death associated with a rise in BP) occur infrequently in combination (210). Only about one-quarter of patients report headaches, palpitations, and sweating. The majority do have hypertension, but rates of hypertension do not differ from those of the general adult population (207). Other findings that may suggest pheochromocytoma include nervousness and anxiety, tremor, nausea, abdominal or chest pain, glucose intolerance, orthostatic drop in BP, weight loss, and fatigue (206). Usually the most spectacular symptoms accompany the most dramatic BP elevations.

The diagnosis of pheochromocytoma should be considered in patients with refractory or paroxysmal hypertension, autonomic disturbances, panic attacks, adrenal incidentilomas, or relevant family history (211). Tumors that are metabolically active are often detected while still small. Those that are nearly silent metabolically may grow to larger size before detection.

Plasma metanephrines have gained special prominence as an initial screening test for pheochromocytoma, with negative predictive value of a normal test approaching 100% (212). Plasma metanephrines provide the best test for excluding the diagnosis when compared to plasma catecholamines, urinary catecholamines, urinary total and fractionated metanephrines, and urinary vanillylmandelic acid. Combining tests does not improve diagnostic yield above measuring plasma metanephrines alone (213). However, plasma metanephrines may have a false-positive rate up to 18% in low-risk patients. Adjusting for age (214) or eliminating confounding medications (215) may decrease the false-positive rate. Alternatively, 24-hour urinary total metanephrines and catecholamines yield fewer false-positive results (216).

Diagnosis and treatment of pheochromocytoma depend on localization of the tumor. CT is better than MRI at detecting adrenal pheochromocytoma, whereas MRI is optimal for detecting extra-adrenal tumors. CT and MRI have 93% to 100% sensitivity, with only 70% specificity. Scintigraphy provides superior specificity (95% to 100%) but lower sensitivity (77% to 90%) (217). In challenging cases, positron emission tomography may provide an additional diagnostic tool for localization (218).

In most situations, patients with catecholamine-secreting tumors undergo curative resection as definitive therapy. Perioperative management usually includes several weeks of α_1-blocker therapy, especially phenoxybenzamine, and rehydration to avoid abrupt hypotension from withdrawal of the elevated catecholamines once the tumor pedicle is clamped. β-Blockade can control arrhythmias during the perioperative period but should be administered only in conjunction with α_1-blockers to avoid unopposed α-agonist influence. Despite intraoperative hemodynamic lability, there were no perioperative deaths, myocardial infarctions or cerebrovascular accidents in one series of 143 patients who underwent surgical resection of pheochromocytomas and paragangliomas (219). Laparoscopic technique offers more stable hemodynamics and better postoperative results when compared with open adrenalectomy (220).

Sleep Apnea

Sleep-disordered breathing may contribute to hypertension. Among patients with obstructive sleep apnea (OSA), repetitive and partial or complete collapse of the pharynx occurs during sleep (221). The disorder affects up to 9% of women and 24% of men (222). The prospective Wisconsin Sleep Cohort Study demonstrated an independent dose–response relationship between sleep-disordered breathing and the development of hypertension (223). Because OSA is more prevalent in obese individuals, it may partially account for the strong association between obesity and hypertension. Postulated mechanisms mediating the relationship between OSA and hypertension include sympathetic activation, hyperleptinemia, insulin resistance, elevated angiotensin II and aldosterone levels, oxidative and inflammatory stress, endothelial dysfunction, and impaired baroreflex function (224). Sleep-disordered breathing may also contribute to the elevated cardiovascular disease risk in patients with the metabolic syndrome (225).

Common presentations include suggestive habitus, especially obese male patients (226). Patients may report loud snoring, disrupted sleep, and excessive daytime sleepiness. Neck circumference is the single best measure to predict OSA (227). The disorder may appear in patients with normal weight but a small, receding jaw (228). Measuring the cricomental space is helpful in excluding OSA, with greater than 1.5 cm giving a negative predictive value of 100% in one series of 75 patients referred to a tertiary sleep center (229).

The diagnostic gold standard is polysomnography in a sleep laboratory (230). Screening oximetry is less expensive, but has limited diagnostic accuracy (231). No standard exists for determination of the anatomic level of obstruction during pharyngeal collapse (232). Conservative treatment options for patients with mild disease include weight loss, abstaining from alcohol or sedative use, and avoiding the supine position. Continuous positive airway pressure (CPAP) is the most effective treatment for clinically significant disease (233). CPAP treatment in patients with moderate to severe OSA substantially reduces both daytime and nighttime BP. Among a series of patients treated effectively with CPAP, SBP and DBP decreased by about 10 mm Hg (234).

Some patients are unable to tolerate CPAP. They may experience nasal dryness and congestion, claustrophobia, facial skin abrasions, or air leaks. Measures to improve compliance include ensuring a comfortable fit, adding humidification, and providing close follow-up (235). For patients who are unable to tolerate CPAP or who are refractory to noninvasive therapy, surgical options include maxillomandibular advancement osteotomy or tonsillectomy (236). Localizing the level of anatomic obstruction appears to improve efficacy of surgical corrective procedures (237).

SPECIAL SITUATIONS

Hypertensive Crises

True hypertensive emergencies are unusual. Many reflect mismanagement and occur in patients with a background of poorly controlled BP (238), sometimes from patient nonadherence, medical system failures, or both factors. Rather than a search for secondary causes, the clinical priority should be the safe, prompt, and gradual lowering of BP without major side effects or complications.

Although SBP may exceed 180 to 200 mm Hg and DBP may exceed 110 to 120 mm Hg, the absolute level of BP is less important than the rate of rise and the absolute difference between the patient's usual BP and that observed during crises. Clinical decompensation rather than the BP level alone should define the situation as urgent (i.e., no target organ damage) or emergent (i.e., target organ damage present.) Others have emphasized the term *malignant hypertension* in reference to the association with encephalopathy or nephropathy (239). Although hypertensive urgency may successfully be treated with oral drugs to lower BP over a few hours, hypertensive emergency requires intensive monitoring and parenteral therapy (240).

Most patients offer few specific symptoms. Signs of target organ damage include cardiovascular decompensation such as palpitations, angina, or congestive failure. Neurologic manifestations include headache, nausea, seizure, or obtundation. Clinical examination may demonstrate retinopathy, CHF, arrhythmias, or focal neurologic deficits. Diagnostic workup includes laboratory evaluation (blood urea nitrogen, creatinine, electrolytes, a complete blood count), urinalysis, ECG, and chest radiography.

There is no single recipe for managing hypertensive crises. No large, randomized, controlled trials exist conclusively to determine relative mortality benefits of specific agents (241). Each situation should be assessed individually for critical organ involvement, desired time frame for lowering BP (minutes, hours, or days), and available options, including requisite personnel and equipment.

Refractory Hypertension

Resistant or *refractory hypertension* reflects failure to achieve target BP in a patient prescribed a regimen of at least three appropriate antihypertensive agents including a diuretic (9). Such a definition assumes that careful and appropriate measurement of BP has occurred on several occasions, including adequate patient preparation, elimination of interfering substances, and use of proper instruments and techniques. Although not common, refractory hypertension may lead to the diagnosis of secondary forms of hypertension. For example, increased BP after starting ACE inhibitor therapy may suggest occult, bilateral renovascular hypertension, especially in association with drug-induced renal insufficiency.

In clinical practice, inadequate BP control is more commonly due to factors related to the prescribing clinician and/or the patient. In one series of 800 hypertensive patients followed over 2 years, increases in hypertensive therapy occurred during only 7% of visits, despite 40% of the patients having stage II hypertension. Less intensive management by clinicians leads to significantly suboptimal BP control (242). Inappropriate or inadequate drug regimens are another important cause of poor BP control (243). Using more than one drug of the same drug class or creating adverse drug–drug interactions may blunt BP response.

A patient's failure to adhere to prescribed regimens frequently reflects suboptimal knowledge of the regimen or of the importance of consistent medication taking. Compliance-enhancing strategies for the clinician include (a) inquiring nonconfrontationally about compliance barriers, (b) encouraging the development and use of the patient's own medication-taking system, (c) providing simple and clear instructions, (d) monitoring progress to goal, (e) making explicit the value of the regimen and adherence to it, and (f) customizing the regimen to the patient's needs and preferences (244).

CONTROVERSIES AND PERSONAL PERSPECTIVES

In a field as vast and rapidly changing as hypertension, controversies thrive. Debate surrounding the significance of white coat hypertension deserves special attention.

White Coat Hypertension

In 1983, Mancia et al. (245) proposed *white coat syndrome* to define BP increases of ≤27 mm Hg SBP and ≤15 mm Hg DBP when a physician entered the patient's room during intra-arterial BP monitoring. Over time, the phrase *white coat effect* has come to describe the difference between clinic readings taken by a physician and the average daytime BP by other means. Patients have *white coat hypertension* when they display elevated BP as measured by a physician but have otherwise normal daytime mean pressure (246). The prevalence of such discrepant BP levels reaches up to 20% of men and 54% of women (247).

Patients with white coat hypertension show diversity in metabolic, neuroendocrine, and cardiac findings and display greater BP variability compared to those with sustained BP elevations (248). In general, white coat hypertension is associated with intermediate risk compared to sustained hypertension (249).

The most appropriate management of white coat hypertension remains debatable. Proponents of treatment argue that office BPs comprise the basis for most published clinical trials in which treating hypertension appears beneficial (250). Others advise treating patients with white coat hypertension only for demonstrable end-organ damage. All agree that patients with white coat hypertension should undergo BP checks to identify those who are misdiagnosed or those who develop sustained hypertension (251). Home self-measurement and ABPM shed light on an individual's BP load and pattern of hypertension. Although promising in their greater prognostic accuracy, their widespread routine application is not fully established.

THE FUTURE

Advances in the field of hypertension management predict exciting developments in several areas. First, basic scientific advances in molecular and genetic medicine will likely shed light on the initial and initiating events that cause the deranged physiology of hypertension (252). Genetic characterization may help to identify those at risk of target organ damage (253), as well as guide tailored therapy (254). Second, optimal use of antihypertensive drugs and goals of therapy continue to be reevaluated. Emerging evidence is shaping our definition of "normal" and optimal BP (255). Ongoing research will spur debate about the benefits of treating prehypertension (256,257) and challenge current guidelines (258). Last, hypertension has historically been an asymptomatic disease progressing silently until irreversible target organ damage develops. With recent emphasis on the prognostic benefit of home self-BP monitoring, patients increasingly seek a degree of self-management. Hopefully, in the near future, this patient participation will translate into improved levels of BP control and risk reduction.

References

1. Levy D, Larson MG, Vasan RS, et al. The progression from hypertension to congestive heart failure. *JAMA* 1996;275:1557–1562.

2. Lewington S, Clarke R, Qizilbash N, et al. Age-specific relevance of usual blood pressure to vascular mortality: a meta-analysis of individual data for one million adults in 61 prospective studies. *Lancet* 2002;360:1903–1913.
3. Woodwell DA, Cherry DK. National Ambulatory Medical Care Survey: 2002 summary. *Adv Data* 2004;26:1–44.
4. Moxey ED, O'Connor JP, Novielli KD, et al. Prescription drug use in the elderly: a descriptive analysis. *Health Care Financ Rev* 2003;24:127–141.
5. Hodgson TA, Cai L. Medical care expenditures for hypertension, its complications, and its comorbidities. *Med Care* 2001;39:599–615.
6. Hajjar I, Kotchen TA. Trends in prevalence, awareness, treatment, and control of hypertension in the United States, 1988–2000. *JAMA* 2003;290: 199–206.
7. Hyman DJ, Pavlik VN. Characteristics of patients with uncontrolled hypertension in the United States. *N Engl J Med* 2001;345:479–486.
8. Wang Y, Wang QJ. The prevalence of prehypertension and hypertension among US adults according to the new joint national committee guidelines: new challenges of the old problem. *Arch Intern Med* 2004;164:2126–2134.
9. Chobanian AV, Bakris GL, Black HR, et al. The Seventh Report of the Joint National Committee on Prevention, Detection, Evaluation, and Treatment of High Blood Pressure: the JNC 7 report. *JAMA* 2003;289:2560–2572.
10. Stamler R, Stamler J, Gosch FC, et al. Primary prevention of hypertension by nutritional-hygienic means. Final report of a randomized, controlled trial. *JAMA* 1989;262:1801–1807.
11. Fisher N, Williams G. Hypertensive vascular disease. In: Kasper DL, Braunwald E, Fauci A, et al., eds. *Harrison's Principles of Internal Medicine*. New York: McGraw-Hill, 2004.
12. Neutel JM, Smith DH, Weber MA. Is high blood pressure a late manifestation of the hypertension syndrome? *Am J Hypertens* 1999;12:215S–223S.
13. Moser M. Management of hypertension, Part I. *Am Fam Physician* 1996; 53:2295–2302.
14. Haider AW, Larson MG, Franklin SS, et al. Systolic blood pressure, diastolic blood pressure, and pulse pressure as predictors of risk for congestive heart failure in the Framingham Heart Study. *Ann Intern Med* 2003;138:10–16.
15. Cushman WC. The clinical significance of systolic hypertension. *Am J Hypertens* 1998;11:182S-185S.
16. Tzourio C, Anderson C, Chapman N, et al. Effects of blood pressure lowering with perindopril and indapamide therapy on dementia and cognitive decline in patients with cerebrovascular disease. *Arch Intern Med* 2003; 163:1069–1075.
17. Bakris GL, Weir MR, Shanifar S, et al. Effects of blood pressure level on progression of diabetic nephropathy: results from the RENAAL study. *Arch Intern Med* 2003;163:1555–1565.
18. Rudd P, Dzau V. Hypertension: evaluation and management. In: Loscalzo J, Creager M, Dzau V, eds. *Vascular Medicine*. Boston: Little, Brown; 1996: 609–638.
19. Pickering TG. Effects of stress and behavioral interventions in hypertension—headache and hypertension: something old, something new. *J Clin Hypertens (Greenwich)* 2000;2:345–347.
20. Neutel JM, Smith DH. The circadian pattern of blood pressure: cardiovascular risk and therapeutic opportunities. *Curr Opin Nephrol Hypertens* 1997;6:250–256.
21. Mengden T, Uen S, Baulmann J, et al. Significance of blood pressure self-measurement as compared with office blood pressure measurement and ambulatory 24-hour blood pressure measurement in pharmacological studies. *Blood Press Monit* 2003;8:169–172.
22. Asayama K, Ohkubo T, Kikuya M, et al. Prediction of stroke by self-measurement of blood pressure at home versus casual screening blood pressure measurement in relation to the Joint National Committee 7 classification: the Ohasama study. *Stroke* 2004;35:2356–2361.
23. Clement DL, De Buyzere ML, De Bacquer DA, et al. Prognostic value of ambulatory blood-pressure recordings in patients with treated hypertension. *N Engl J Med* 2003;348:2407–2415.
24. Pickering T. Recommendations for the use of home (self) and ambulatory blood pressure monitoring. American Society of Hypertension Ad Hoc Panel. *Am J Hypertens* 1996;9:1–11.
25. Skoog I, Lernfelt B, Landahl S, et al. 15-year longitudinal study of blood pressure and dementia. *Lancet* 1996;347:1141–1145.
26. Wong TY, Mitchell P. Hypertensive retinopathy. *N Engl J Med* 2004;351:2310–2317.
27. Khaw KT, Wareham N, Bingham S, et al. Association of hemoglobin A1c with cardiovascular disease and mortality in adults: the European prospective investigation into cancer in Norfolk. *Ann Intern Med* 2004;141:413–420.
28. August P. Initial treatment of hypertension. *N Engl J Med* 2003;348:610–617.
29. Haffner SM, Ferrannini E, Hazuda HP, et al. Clustering of cardiovascular risk factors in confirmed prehypertensive individuals. *Hypertension* 1992;20:38–45.
30. Van Itallie TB. Health implications of overweight and obesity in the United States. *Ann Intern Med* 1985;103:6:983–988.
31. Kannel WB. Framingham study insights into hypertensive risk of cardiovascular disease. *Hypertens Res* 1995;18:181–196.
32. Johnson ML, Pietz K, Battleman DS, et al. Prevalence of comorbid hypertension and dyslipidemia and associated cardiovascular disease. *Am J Manag Care* 2004;10:926–932.
33. Fagerberg B, Wikstrand J, Berglund G, et al. Mortality rates in treated hypertensive men with additional risk factors are high but can be reduced: a randomized intervention study. *Am J Hypertens* 1998;11:14–22.
34. Criqui MH, Mebane I, Wallace RB, et al. Multivariate correlates of adult blood pressures in nine North American populations: The Lipid Research Clinics Prevalence Study. *Prev Med* 1982;11:391–402.
35. Kawachi I, Malcolm LA. The cost-effectiveness of treating mild-to-moderate hypertension: a reappraisal. *J Hypertens* 1991;9:199–208.
36. Kannel WB. An epidemiological perspective in hypertension problem solving. *Cardiology* 1994;85[Suppl 1]:71–77.
37. Hayes SN, Taler SJ. Hypertension in women: current understanding of gender differences. *Mayo Clin Proc* 1998;73:157–165.
38. Labarthe D, Ayala C. Nondrug interventions in hypertension prevention and control. *Cardiol Clin* 2002;20:249–263.
39. Cutler JA. Combinations of lifestyle modification and drug treatment in management of mild-moderate hypertension: a review of randomized clinical trials. *Clin Exp Hypertens* 1993;15:1193–1204.
40. Effects of weight loss and sodium reduction intervention on blood pressure and hypertension incidence in overweight people with high-normal blood pressure. The Trials of Hypertension Prevention, phase II. The Trials of Hypertension Prevention Collaborative Research Group. *Arch Intern Med* 1997;157:657–667.
41. Blumenthal JA, Sherwood A, Gullette EC, et al. Exercise and weight loss reduce blood pressure in men and women with mild hypertension: effects on cardiovascular, metabolic, and hemodynamic functioning. *Arch Intern Med* 2000;160:1947–1958.
42. He J, Whelton PK, Appel LJ, et al. Long-term effects of weight loss and dietary sodium reduction on incidence of hypertension. *Hypertension* 2000;35:544–549.
43. Steffen PR, Sherwood A, Gullette EC, et al. Effects of exercise and weight loss on blood pressure during daily life. *Med Sci Sports Exerc* 2001;33:1635–1640.
44. Hayashi T, Tsumura K, Suematsu C, et al. Walking to work and the risk for hypertension in men: the Osaka Health Survey. *Ann Intern Med* 1999;131:21–26.
45. Watkins LL, Sherwood A, Feinglos M, et al. Effects of exercise and weight loss on cardiac risk factors associated with syndrome X. *Arch Intern Med* 2003;163:1889–1895.
46. Petrella RJ. How effective is exercise training for the treatment of hypertension? *Clin J Sport Med* 1998;8:224–231.
47. Wallace JP. Exercise in hypertension. A clinical review. *Sports Med* 2003;33:585–598.
48. Appel LJ, Moore TJ, Obarzanek E, et al. A clinical trial of the effects of dietary patterns on blood pressure. DASH Collaborative Research Group. *N Engl J Med* 1997;336:1117–1124.
49. Conlin PR, Chow D, Miller ER 3rd, et al. The effect of dietary patterns on blood pressure control in hypertensive patients: results from the Dietary Approaches to Stop Hypertension (DASH) trial. *Am J Hypertens* 2000;13:949–955.
50. Ard JD, Coffman CJ, Lin PH, et al. One-year follow-up study of blood pressure and dietary patterns in dietary approaches to stop hypertension (DASH)-sodium participants. *Am J Hypertens* 2004;17:1156–1162.
51. Svetkey LP, Erlinger TP, Vollmer WM, et al. Effect of lifestyle modifications on blood pressure by race, sex, hypertension status, and age. *J Hum Hypertens* 2005;19:21–31.
52. Fodor JG, Whitmore B, Leenen F, et al. Lifestyle modifications to prevent and control hypertension. 5. Recommendations on dietary salt. Canadian Hypertension Society, Canadian Coalition for High Blood Pressure Prevention and Control, Laboratory Centre for Disease Control at Health Canada, Heart and Stroke Foundation of Canada. *CMAJ* 1999;160[9 Suppl]:S29–34.
53. Midgley JP, Matthew AG, Greenwood CM, et al. Effect of reduced dietary sodium on blood pressure: a meta-analysis of randomized controlled trials. *JAMA* 1996;275:1590–1597.
54. Tuomilehto J, Jousilahti P, Rastenyte D, et al. Urinary sodium excretion and cardiovascular mortality in Finland: a prospective study. *Lancet* 2001;357:848–851.
55. Weinberger MH, Fineberg NS, Fineberg SE, et al. Salt sensitivity, pulse pressure, and death in normal and hypertensive humans. *Hypertension* 2001;37:429–432.
56. Bray GA, Vollmer WM, Sacks FM, et al. A further subgroup analysis of the effects of the DASH diet and three dietary sodium levels on blood pressure: results of the DASH-Sodium Trial. *Am J Cardiol* 2004;94:222–227.
57. Sacks FM, Svetkey LP, Vollmer WM, et al. Effects on blood pressure of reduced dietary sodium and the Dietary Approaches to Stop Hypertension (DASH) diet. DASH-Sodium Collaborative Research Group. *N Engl J Med* 2001;344:3–10.
58. Vollmer WM, Sacks FM, Ard J, et al. Effects of diet and sodium intake on blood pressure: subgroup analysis of the DASH-sodium trial. *Ann Intern Med* 2001;135:1019–1028.
59. Little P, Girling G, Hasler A, et al. A controlled trial of a low sodium, low fat, high fibre diet in treated hypertensive patients: effect on antihypertensive drug requirement in clinical practice. *J Hum Hypertens* 1991;5:175–181.
60. Whelton PK, Appel LJ, Espeland MA, et al. Sodium reduction and weight loss in the treatment of hypertension in older persons: a randomized

controlled trial of nonpharmacologic interventions in the elderly (TONE). TONE Collaborative Research Group. *JAMA* 1998;279:839–846.
61. Griffith LE, Guyatt GH, Cook RJ, et al. The influence of dietary and nondietary calcium supplementation on blood pressure: an updated metaanalysis of randomized controlled trials. *Am J Hypertens* 1999;12:84–92.
62. Pfeifer M, Begerow B, Minne HW, et al. Effects of a short-term vitamin D(3) and calcium supplementation on blood pressure and parathyroid hormone levels in elderly women. *J Clin Endocrinol Metab* 2001;86:1633–1637.
63. Foster GD, Wyatt HR, Hill JO, et al. A randomized trial of a low-carbohydrate diet for obesity. *N Engl J Med* 2003;348:2082–2090.
64. Burgess E, Lewanczuk R, Bolli P, et al. Lifestyle modifications to prevent and control hypertension. 6. Recommendations on potassium, magnesium and calcium. Canadian Hypertension Society, Canadian Coalition for High Blood Pressure Prevention and Control, Laboratory Centre for Disease Control at Health Canada, Heart and Stroke Foundation of Canada. *CMAJ* 1999;160[9 Suppl]:S35–45.
65. Naismith DJ, Braschi A. The effect of low-dose potassium supplementation on blood pressure in apparently healthy volunteers. *Br J Nutr* 2003;90:53–60.
66. Victor RG, Hansen J. Alcohol and blood pressure—a drink a day. *N Engl J Med* 1995;332:1782–1783.
67. Goldberg IJ. To drink or not to drink? *N Engl J Med* 2003;348:163–164.
68. Rakic V, Puddey IB, Burke V, et al. Influence of pattern of alcohol intake on blood pressure in regular drinkers: a controlled trial. *J Hypertens* 1998;16:165–174.
69. McFadden CB, Brensinger CM, Berlin JA, et al. Systematic review of the effect of daily alcohol intake on blood pressure. *Am J Hypertens* 2005; 18:276–286.
70. National High Blood Pressure Education Program Working Group. Report on primary prevention of hypertension. *Arch Intern Med* 1993;153:186–208.
71. Estruch R, Sacanella E, De la Sierra A, et al. Effects of alcohol withdrawal on 24 hour ambulatory blood pressure among alcohol-dependent patients. *Alcohol Clin Exp Res* 2003;27:2002–2008.
72. Janzon E, Hedblad B, Berglund G, et al. Changes in blood pressure and body weight following smoking cessation in women. *J Intern Med* 2004;255:266–272.
73. Kuchel O. Mental stress and hypertension, an evolutionary framework: some historical perspectives of the 1960 World Health Organization Prague Hypertension Meeting. *J Hypertens* 2003;21:639–641.
74. Beilin LJ, Puddey IB, Burke V. Lifestyle and hypertension. *Am J Hypertens* 1999;12:934–945.
75. Fauvel JP, M'Pio I, Quelin P, et al. Neither perceived job stress nor individual cardiovascular reactivity predict high blood pressure. *Hypertension* 2003;42:1112–1116.
76. Elliot WJ, Izzo JL Jr, White WB, et al. Graded blood pressure reduction in hypertensive outpatients associated with use of a device to assist with slow breathing. *J Clin Hypertens (Greenwich)* 2004;6:553–559; quiz 560–551.
77. Petrovitch H, Vogt TM, Berge KG. Isolated systolic hypertension: lowering the risk of stroke in older patients. SHEP Cooperative Research Group. *Geriatrics* 1992;47:30–32, 35–38.
78. Staessen JA, Wang JG, Thijs L. Cardiovascular prevention and blood pressure reduction: a quantitative overview updated until 1 March 2003. *J Hypertens* 2003;21:1055–1076.
79. Taylor RB. Patient profiling: individualization of hypertension therapy. *Am Fam Physician* 1990;42[5 Suppl]:29S–31S, 34S–36S.
80. Ashida T. [Treatment of hypertension with dyslipidemia]. *Nippon Rinsho* 2001;59:978–982.
81. Ott SM, LaCroix AZ, Ichikawa LE, et al. Effect of low-dose thiazide diuretics on plasma lipids: results from a double-blind, randomized clinical trial in older men and women. *J Am Geriatr Soc* 2003;51:340–347.
82. Materson BJ, Preston RA. Newer principles of patient profiling for antihypertensive therapy. *Circulation* 1989;80[6 Suppl]:IV128–135.
83. Erickson SR, Williams BC, Gruppen LD. Relationship between symptoms and health-related quality of life in patients treated for hypertension. *Pharmacotherapy* 2004;24:344–350.
84. Schneider T, Rubben H, Michel MC. [The medication-induced dysfunction of the urinary bladder]. *Urologe A* 2003;42:1588–1593.
85. Ko DT, Hebert PR, Coffey CS, et al. Beta-blocker therapy and symptoms of depression, fatigue, and sexual dysfunction. *JAMA* 2002;288:351–357.
86. Fischer MA, Avorn J. Economic implications of evidence-based prescribing for hypertension: can better care cost less? *JAMA* 2004;291:1850–1856.
87. Ramsey SD, Neil N, Sullivan SD, et al. An economic evaluation of the JNC hypertension guidelines using data from a randomized controlled trial. Joint National Committee. *J Am Board Fam Pract* 1999;12:105–114.
88. Moser M. The cost of treating hypertension: can we keep it under control without compromising the level of care? *Am J Hypertens* 1998;11:120S–127S; discussion 135S–137S.
89. Major outcomes in high-risk hypertensive patients randomized to angiotensin-converting enzyme inhibitor or calcium channel blocker vs diuretic: The Antihypertensive and Lipid-Lowering Treatment to Prevent Heart Attack Trial (ALLHAT). *JAMA* 2002;288:2981–2997.
90. Wassertheil-Smoller S, Psaty B, Greenland P, et al. Association between cardiovascular outcomes and antihypertensive drug treatment in older women. *JAMA* 2004;292:2849–2859.
91. Wright JT Jr, Dunn JK, Cutler JA, et al. Outcomes in hypertensive black and nonblack patients treated with chlorthalidone, amlodipine, and lisinopril. *JAMA* 2005;293:1595–1608.
92. Psaty BM, Lumley T, Furberg CD, et al. Health outcomes associated with various antihypertensive therapies used as first-line agents: a network meta-analysis. *JAMA* 2003;289:2534–2544.
93. Gress TW, Nieto FJ, Shahar E, et al. Hypertension and antihypertensive therapy as risk factors for type 2 diabetes mellitus. Atherosclerosis Risk in Communities Study. *N Engl J Med* 2000;342:905–912.
94. Kostis JB, Wilson AC, Freudenberger RS, et al. Long-term effect of diuretic-based therapy on fatal outcomes in subjects with isolated systolic hypertension with and without diabetes. *Am J Cardiol* 2005;95:29–35.
95. Wing LM, Reid CM, Ryan P, et al. A comparison of outcomes with angiotensin-converting-enzyme inhibitors and diuretics for hypertension in the elderly. *N Engl J Med* 2003;348:583–592.
96. Neutel JM, Weber MA, Julius S, et al. Clinical experience with perindopril in elderly hypertensive patients: a subgroup analysis of a large community trial. *Am J Cardiovasc Drugs* 2004;4:335–341.
97. Wachtell K, Lehto M, Gerdts E, et al. Angiotensin II receptor blockade reduces new-onset atrial fibrillation and subsequent stroke compared to atenolol: the Losartan Intervention For End Point Reduction in Hypertension (LIFE) study. *J Am Coll Cardiol* 2005;45:712–719.
98. Chow KM, Szeto CC, Wong TY, et al. Risk factors for thiazide-induced hyponatraemia. *QJM* 2003;96:911–917.
99. Neutel JM, Black HR, Weber MA. Combination therapy with diuretics: an evolution of understanding. *Am J Med* 1996;101:3A:61S–70S.
100. Edoute Y, Nagachandran P, Svirski B, et al. Cardiovascular adverse drug reaction associated with combined beta-adrenergic and calcium entry-blocking agents. *J Cardiovasc Pharmacol* 2000;35:556–559.
101. Everly MJ, Heaton PC, Cluxton RJ, Jr. Beta-blocker underuse in secondary prevention of myocardial infarction. *Ann Pharmacother* 2004;38:286–293.
102. Tamirisa KP, Aaronson KD, Koelling TM. Spironolactone-induced renal insufficiency and hyperkalemia in patients with heart failure. *Am Heart J* 2004;148:971–978.
103. Montan S. Drugs used in hypertensive diseases in pregnancy. *Curr Opin Obstet Gynecol* 2004;16:111–115.
104. Julius S, Kjeldsen SE, Brunner H, et al. VALUE trial: Long-term blood pressure trends in 13,449 patients with hypertension and high cardiovascular risk. *Am J Hypertens* 2003;16:544–548.
105. Rodgers PT. Combination drug therapy in hypertension: a rational approach for the pharmacist. *J Am Pharm Assoc (Wash)* 1998;38:469–479.
106. Neutel JM, Smith DH, Weber MA. Low dose combination therapy vs. high dose monotherapy in the management of hypertension. *J Clin Hypertens (Greenwich)* 1999;1:79–86.
107. Ruilope LM, de la Sierra A, Moreno E, et al. Prospective comparison of therapeutical attitudes in hypertensive type 2 diabetic patients uncontrolled on monotherapy. A randomized trial: the EDICTA study. *J Hypertens* 1999;17:1917–1923.
108. Kuschnir E, Bendersky M, Resk J, et al. Effects of the combination of low-dose nifedipine GITS 20 mg and losartan 50 mg in patients with mild to moderate hypertension. *J Cardiovasc Pharmacol* 2004;43:300–305.
109. Mourad JJ, Waeber B, Zannad F, et al. Comparison of different therapeutic strategies in hypertension: a low-dose combination of perindopril/indapamide versus a sequential monotherapy or a stepped-care approach. *J Hypertens* 2004;22:2379–2386.
110. Anderson GH Jr, Blakeman N, Streeten DH. The effect of age on prevalence of secondary forms of hypertension in 4429 consecutively referred patients. *J Hypertens* 1994;12:609–615.
111. Danielson M, Dammstrom B. The prevalence of secondary and curable hypertension. *Acta Med Scand* 1981;209:451–455.
112. Sinclair AM, Isles CG, Brown I, et al. Secondary hypertension in a blood pressure clinic. *Arch Intern Med* 1987;147:1289–1293.
113. Omura M, Saito J, Yamaguchi K, et al. Prospective study on the prevalence of secondary hypertension among hypertensive patients visiting a general outpatient clinic in Japan. *Hypertens Res* 2004;27:193–202.
114. Preston RA, Singer I, Epstein M. Renal parenchymal hypertension: current concepts of pathogenesis and management. *Arch Intern Med* 1996;156:602–611.
115. State-specific trends in chronic kidney failure—United States, 1990–2001. *MMWR Morb Mortal Wkly Rep* 2004;53:918–920.
116. Atkins RC. The epidemiology of chronic kidney disease. *Kidney Int Suppl* 2005:S14–18.
117. Oko A, Lochynska K, Idasiak-Piechocka I, et al. [Arterial hypertension in glomerulonephritis]. *Pol Merkuriusz Lek* 2003;15:344–346.
118. Klein IH, Ligtenberg G, Neumann J, et al. Sympathetic nerve activity is inappropriately increased in chronic renal disease. *J Am Soc Nephrol* 2003;14:3239–3244.
119. Soares-da-Silva P, Pestana M, Ferreira A, et al. Renal dopaminergic mechanisms in renal parenchymal diseases, hypertension, and heart failure. *Clin Exp Hypertens* 2000;22:251–268.
120. Yu HT. Progression of chronic renal failure. *Arch Intern Med* 2003;163:1417–1429.
121. Ljutic D, Kes P. The role of arterial hypertension in the progression of non-diabetic glomerular diseases. *Nephrol Dial Transplant* 2003;18[Suppl 5]: v28–30.
122. Rivera F, Lopez-Gomez JM, Perez-Garcia R. Clinicopathologic correlations of renal pathology in Spain. *Kidney Int* 2004;66:898–904.

123. Kimmel PL, Barisoni L, Kopp JB. Pathogenesis and treatment of HIV-associated renal diseases: lessons from clinical and animal studies, molecular pathologic correlations, and genetic investigations. *Ann Intern Med* 2003;139:214–226.
124. Kaaroud H, Boubaker K, Beji S, et al. Renal amyloidosis followed more than 5 years: report of 12 cases. *Transplant Proc* 2004;36:1796–1798.
125. Tumlin JA, Hennigar RA. Clinical presentation, natural history, and treatment of crescentic proliferative IgA nephropathy. *Semin Nephrol* 2004;24:256–268.
126. Szeto CC, Choi PC, To KF, et al. Grading of acute and chronic renal lesions in Henoch-Schonlein purpura. *Mod Pathol* 2001;14:635–640.
127. Kaplan-Pavlovcic S, Cerk K, Kveder R, et al. Clinical prognostic factors of renal outcome in anti-neutrophil cytoplasmic autoantibody (ANCA)-associated glomerulonephritis in elderly patients. *Nephrol Dial Transplant* 2003;18[Suppl 5]:v5–7.
128. Schmekal B, Pichler R, Biesenbach G. Causes and prognosis of nontraumatic acute renal failure requiring dialysis in adult patients with and without diabetes. *Ren Fail* 2004;26:39–43.
129. Elseviers MM, De Broe ME. Analgesic nephropathy: is it caused by multi-analgesic abuse or single substance use? *Drug Saf* 1999;20:15–24.
130. Wen SF. Nephrotoxicities of nonsteroidal anti-inflammatory drugs. *J Formos Med Assoc* 1997;96:157–171.
131. George AL Jr, Neilson EG. Genetics of kidney disease. *Am J Kidney Dis* 2000;35:4[Suppl 1]:S160–169.
132. Kelleher CL, McFann KK, Johnson AM, et al. Characteristics of hypertension in young adults with autosomal dominant polycystic kidney disease compared with the general U.S. population. *Am J Hypertens* 2004;17:1029–1034.
133. Derhaschnig U, Kittler H, Woisetschlager C, et al. Microalbumin measurement alone or calculation of the albumin/creatinine ratio for the screening of hypertension patients? *Nephrol Dial Transplant* 2002;17:81–85.
134. Sarnak MJ, Greene T, Wang X, et al. The effect of a lower target blood pressure on the progression of kidney disease: long-term follow-up of the modification of diet in renal disease study. *Ann Intern Med* 2005;142:342–351.
135. Mann JF, Yi QL, Gerstein HC. Albuminuria as a predictor of cardiovascular and renal outcomes in people with known atherosclerotic cardiovascular disease. *Kidney Int Suppl* 2004: S59–62.
136. Karalliedde J, Viberti G. Hypertension and microalbuminuria: risk factors for cardiovascular disease in diabetes. *Curr Hypertens Rep* 2005;7:1–2.
137. Jafar TH, Stark PC, Schmid CH, et al. Progression of chronic kidney disease: the role of blood pressure control, proteinuria, and angiotensin-converting enzyme inhibition: a patient-level meta-analysis. *Ann Intern Med* 2003;139:244–252.
138. Atkins RC, Briganti EM, Lewis JB, et al. Proteinuria reduction and progression to renal failure in patients with type 2 diabetes mellitus and overt nephropathy. *Am J Kidney Dis* 2005;45:281–287.
139. Campbell RC, Ruggenenti P, Remuzzi G. Proteinuria in diabetic nephropathy: treatment and evolution. *Curr Diab Rep* 2003;3:497–504.
140. Andersen N, Poulsen P, Knudsen S, et al. Long-term dual blockade with candesartan and lisinopril in hypertensive patients with diabetes: the CALM II study. *Diabetes Care* 2005: 273–277.
141. Nakao N, Yoshimura A, Morita H, et al. Combination treatment of angiotensin-II receptor blocker and angiotensin-converting-enzyme inhibitor in non-diabetic renal disease (COOPERATE): a randomised controlled trial. *Lancet* 2003;361:117–124.
142. Brenner BM, Cooper ME, de Zeeuw D, et al. Effects of losartan on renal and cardiovascular outcomes in patients with type 2 diabetes and nephropathy. *N Engl J Med* 2001;345:861–869.
143. Thurman JM, Schrier RW. Comparative effects of angiotensin-converting enzyme inhibitors and angiotensin receptor blockers on blood pressure and the kidney. *Am J Med* 2003;114:588–598.
144. Slovut DP, Olin JW. Fibromuscular dysplasia. *N Engl J Med* 2004;350:1862–1871.
145. Safian RD. Atherosclerotic Renal Artery Stenosis. *Curr Treat Options Cardiovasc Med* 2003;5:91–101.
146. Morganti A. Angioplasty of the renal artery: antihypertensive and renal effects. *J Nephrol* 2000;13[Suppl 3]:S28–33.
147. Zalunardo N, Tuttle KR. Atherosclerotic renal artery stenosis: current status and future directions. *Curr Opin Nephrol Hypertens* 2004;13:613–621.
148. Conlon PJ, O'Riordan E, Kalra PA. New insights into the epidemiologic and clinical manifestations of atherosclerotic renovascular disease. *Am J Kidney Dis* 2000;35:573–587.
149. Textor SC. Epidemiology and clinical presentation. *Semin Nephrol* 2000;20:426–431.
150. van Jaarsveld BC, Krijnen P, Derkx FH, et al. Resistance to antihypertensive medication as predictor of renal artery stenosis: comparison of two drug regimens. *J Hum Hypertens* 2001;15:669–676.
151. Wright JR, Shurrab AE, Cheung C, et al. A prospective study of the determinants of renal functional outcome and mortality in atherosclerotic renovascular disease. *Am J Kidney Dis* 2002;39:1153–1161.
152. Zoccali C, Mallamaci F, Finocchiaro P. Atherosclerotic renal artery stenosis: epidemiology, cardiovascular outcomes, and clinical prediction rules. *J Am Soc Nephrol* 2002;13[Suppl 3]:S179–183.
153. Rabbia C, Valpreda S. Duplex scan sonography of renal artery stenosis. *Int Angiol* 2003;22:101–115.
154. Johansson M, Jensen G, Aurell M, et al. Evaluation of duplex ultrasound and captopril renography for detection of renovascular hypertension. *Kidney Int* 2000;58:774–782.
155. Vasbinder GB, Nelemans PJ, Kessels AG, et al. Diagnostic tests for renal artery stenosis in patients suspected of having renovascular hypertension: a meta-analysis. *Ann Intern Med* 2001;135:401–411.
156. Vasbinder GB, Nelemans PJ, Kessels AG, et al. Accuracy of computed tomographic angiography and magnetic resonance angiography for diagnosing renal artery stenosis. *Ann Intern Med* 2004;141:674–682; discussion 682.
157. Textor SC, Wilcox CS. Renal artery stenosis: a common, treatable cause of renal failure? *Annu Rev Med* 2001;52:421–442.
158. Yim PJ, Cebral JR, Weaver A, et al. Estimation of the differential pressure at renal artery stenoses. *Magn Reson Med* 2004;51:969–977.
159. Krijnen P, van Jaarsveld BC, Deinum J, et al. Which patients with hypertension and atherosclerotic renal artery stenosis benefit from immediate intervention? *J Hum Hypertens* 2004;18:91–96.
160. Olin JW. Atherosclerotic renal artery disease. *Cardiol Clin* 2002;20:547–562, vi.
161. Zeller T. Percutaneous endovascular therapy of renal artery stenosis: technical and clinical developments in the past decade. *J Endovasc Ther* 2004;11[Suppl 2]:II96–106.
162. Nolan BW, Schermerhorn ML, Rowell E, et al. Outcomes of renal artery angioplasty and stenting using low-profile systems. *J Vasc Surg* 2005;41:46–52.
163. Cherr GS, Hansen KJ, Craven TE, et al. Surgical management of atherosclerotic renovascular disease. *J Vasc Surg* 2002;35:236–245.
164. Terramani TT, Salim A, Hood DB, et al. Hypoplasia of the descending thoracic and abdominal aorta: a report of two cases and review of the literature. *J Vasc Surg* 2002;36:844–848.
165. Jenkins NP, Ward C. Coarctation of the aorta: natural history and outcome after surgical treatment. *QJM* 1999;92:365–371.
166. Jaffe RB. Radiographic manifestations of congenital anomalies of the aortic arch. *Radiol Clin North Am* 1991;29:319–334.
167. Corno AF, Botta U, Hurni M, et al. Surgery for aortic coarctation: a 30 years experience. *Eur J Cardiothorac Surg* 2001;20:1202–1206.
168. Serfontein SJ, Kron IL. Complications of coarctation repair. *Semin Thorac Cardiovasc Surg Pediatr Card Surg Annu* 2002;5:206–211.
169. Arnaldi G, Angeli A, Atkinson AB, et al. Diagnosis and complications of Cushing's syndrome: a consensus statement. *J Clin Endocrinol Metab* 2003;88:5593–5602.
170. Reincke M. Subclinical Cushing's syndrome. *Endocrinol Metab Clin North Am* 2000;29:43–56.
171. Hadjidakis D, Tsagarakis S, Roboti C, et al. Does subclinical hypercortisolism adversely affect the bone mineral density of patients with adrenal incidentalomas? *Clin Endocrinol (Oxf)* 2003;58:72–77.
172. Tauchmanova L, Rossi R, Biondi B, et al. Patients with subclinical Cushing's syndrome due to adrenal adenoma have increased cardiovascular risk. *J Clin Endocrinol Metab* 2002;87:4872–4878.
173. Terzolo M, Pia A, Ali A, et al. Adrenal incidentaloma: a new cause of the metabolic syndrome? *J Clin Endocrinol Metab* 2002;87:998–1003.
174. Rossi R, Tauchmanova L, Luciano A, et al. Subclinical Cushing's syndrome in patients with adrenal incidentaloma: clinical and biochemical features. *J Clin Endocrinol Metab* 2000;85:1440–1448.
175. Chemaitilly W, Wilson RC, New MI. Hypertension and adrenal disorders. *Curr Hypertens Rep* 2003;5:498–504.
176. Whitworth JA, Mangos GJ, Kelly JJ. Cushing, cortisol, and cardiovascular disease. *Hypertension* 2000;36:912–916.
177. Baid S, Nieman LK. Glucocorticoid excess and hypertension. *Curr Hypertens Rep* 2004;6:493–499.
178. Morris DG, Grossman AB. Dynamic tests in the diagnosis and differential diagnosis of Cushing's syndrome. *J Endocrinol Invest* 2003;26:7[Suppl]:64–73.
179. Nieman LK. Diagnostic tests for Cushing's syndrome. *Ann NY Acad Sci* 2002;970:112–118.
180. Tsagarakis S, Kokkoris P, Roboti C, et al. The low-dose dexamethasone suppression test in patients with adrenal incidentalomas: comparisons with clinically euadrenal subjects and patients with Cushing's syndrome. *Clin Endocrinol (Oxf)* 1998;48:627–633.
181. Findling JW, Raff H, Aron DC. The low-dose dexamethasone suppression test: a reevaluation in patients with Cushing's syndrome. *J Clin Endocrinol Metab* 2004;89:1222–1226.
182. Yaneva M, Mosnier-Pudar H, Dugue MA, et al. Midnight salivary cortisol for the initial diagnosis of Cushing's syndrome of various causes. *J Clin Endocrinol Metab* 2004;89:3345–3351.
183. Findling JW, Kehoe ME, Raff H. Identification of patients with Cushing's disease with negative pituitary adrenocorticotropin gradients during inferior petrosal sinus sampling: prolactin as an index of pituitary venous effluent. *J Clin Endocrinol Metab* 2004;89:6005–6009.
184. Morris D, Grossman A. The medical management of Cushing's syndrome. *Ann NY Acad Sci* 2002;970:119–133.
185. Labeur M, Arzt E, Stalla GK, et al. New perspectives in the treatment of Cushing's syndrome. *Curr Drug Targets Immune Endocr Metabol Disord* 2004;4:335–342.

186. Chanson P, Salenave S. Diagnosis and treatment of pituitary adenomas. *Minerva Endocrinol* 2004;29:241–275.
187. Mantero F, Albiger N. A comprehensive approach to adrenal incidentalomas. *Arq Bras Endocrinol Metabol* 2004;48:583–591.
188. Stewart PM. Mineralocorticoid hypertension. *Lancet* 1999;353:1341–1347.
189. Veglio F, Morello F, Rabbia F, et al. Recent advances in diagnosis and treatment of primary aldosteronism. *Minerva Med* 2003;94:259–265.
190. Frey FJ, Odermatt A, Frey BM. Glucocorticoid-mediated mineralocorticoid receptor activation and hypertension. *Curr Opin Nephrol Hypertens* 2004;13:451–458.
191. Ganguly A. Primary aldosteronism. *N Engl J Med* 1998;339:1828–1834.
192. Plouin PF, Jeunemaitre X. Would wider screening for primary aldosteronism give any health benefits? *Eur J Endocrinol* 2004;151:305–308.
193. Failor RA, Capell PT. Hyperaldosteronism and pheochromocytoma: new tricks and tests. *Prim Care* 2003;30:801–820, viii.
194. Vasan RS, Evans JC, Larson MG, et al. Serum aldosterone and the incidence of hypertension in nonhypertensive persons. *N Engl J Med* 2004;351:33–41.
195. Al Fehaily M, Duh QY. Clinical manifestation of aldosteronoma. *Surg Clin North Am* 2004;84:887–905.
196. Stowasser M. Primary aldosteronism: rare bird or common cause of secondary hypertension? *Curr Hypertens Rep* 2001;3:230–239.
197. Nussberger J. Investigating mineralocorticoid hypertension. *J Hypertens Suppl* 2003;21[Suppl 2]:S25–30.
198. Nadar S, Lip GY, Beevers DG. Primary hyperaldosteronism. *Ann Clin Biochem* 2003;40:439–452.
199. Kaplan NM. The current epidemic of primary aldosteronism: causes and consequences. *J Hypertens* 2004;22:863–869.
200. Mulatero P, Rabbia F, Milan A, et al. Drug effects on aldosterone/plasma renin activity ratio in primary aldosteronism. *Hypertension* 2002;40:897–902.
201. Lumachi F, Marzola MC, Zucchetta P, et al. Non-invasive adrenal imaging in primary aldosteronism. Sensitivity and positive predictive value of radiocholesterol scintigraphy, CT scan and MRI. *Nucl Med Commun* 2003;24:683–688.
202. Young WF Jr. Minireview: primary aldosteronism—changing concepts in diagnosis and treatment. *Endocrinology* 2003;144:2208–2213.
203. Young WF, Stanson AW, Thompson GB, et al. Role for adrenal venous sampling in primary aldosteronism. *Surgery* 2004;136:1227–1235.
204. Blumenfeld JD, Vaughan ED Jr. Diagnosis and treatment of primary aldosteronism. *World J Urol* 1999;17:15–21.
205. Young WF, Jr. Primary aldosteronism—treatment options. *Growth Horm IGF Res* 2003;13[Suppl A]:S102–108.
206. Bravo EL, Gifford RW, Jr. Current concepts. Pheochromocytoma: diagnosis, localization and management. *N Engl J Med* 1984;311:1298–1303.
207. Baguet JP, Hammer L, Mazzuco TL, et al. Circumstances of discovery of phaeochromocytoma: a retrospective study of 41 consecutive patients. *Eur J Endocrinol* 2004;150:681–686.
208. Mantero F, Terzolo M, Arnaldi G, et al. A survey on adrenal incidentaloma in Italy. Study Group on Adrenal Tumors of the Italian Society of Endocrinology. *J Clin Endocrinol Metab* 2000;85:637–644.
209. Dluhy RG. Pheochromocytoma—death of an axiom. *N Engl J Med* 2002; 346:1486–1488.
210. Opocher G, Schiavi F, Conton P, et al. Clinical and genetic aspects of phaeochromocytoma. *Horm Res* 2003;59[Suppl 1]:56–61.
211. Langerman A, Schneider JA, Ward RP. Pheochromocytoma storm presenting as cardiovascular collapse at term pregnancy. *Rev Cardiovasc Med* 2004;5:226–230.
212. Lenders JW, Keiser HR, Goldstein DS, et al. Plasma metanephrines in the diagnosis of pheochromocytoma. *Ann Intern Med* 1995;123:101–109.
213. Lenders JW, Pacak K, Walther MM, et al. Biochemical diagnosis of pheochromocytoma: which test is best? *JAMA* 2002;287:1427–1434.
214. Sawka AM, Thabane L, Gafni A, et al. Measurement of fractionated plasma metanephrines for exclusion of pheochromocytoma: can specificity be improved by adjustment for age? *BMC Endocr Disord* 2005;5:1.
215. Eisenhofer G, Goldstein DS, Walther MM, et al. Biochemical diagnosis of pheochromocytoma: how to distinguish true- from false-positive test results. *J Clin Endocrinol Metab* 2003;88:2656–2666.
216. Sawka AM, Jaeschke R, Singh RJ, et al. A comparison of biochemical tests for pheochromocytoma: measurement of fractionated plasma metanephrines compared with the combination of 24-hour urinary metanephrines and catecholamines. *J Clin Endocrinol Metab* 2003;88:553–558.
217. Pacak K, Linehan WM, Eisenhofer G, et al. Recent advances in genetics, diagnosis, localization, and treatment of pheochromocytoma. *Ann Intern Med* 2001;134:315–329.
218. Goldstein DS, Eisenhofer G, Flynn JA, et al. Diagnosis and localization of pheochromocytoma. *Hypertension* 2004;43:907–910.
219. Kinney MA, Warner ME, vanHeerden JA, et al. Perianesthetic risks and outcomes of pheochromocytoma and paraganglioma resection. *Anesth Analg* 2000;91:1118–1123.
220. Kazaryan AM, Kuznetsov NS, Shulutko AM, et al. Evaluation of endoscopic and traditional open approaches to pheochromocytoma. *Surg Endosc* 2004;18:937–941.
221. August P. Hypertension in men. *J Clin Endocrinol Metab* 1999;84:3451–3454.
222. Young T, Palta M, Dempsey J, et al. The occurrence of sleep-disordered breathing among middle-aged adults. *N Engl J Med* 1993;328:1230–1235.
223. Peppard PE, Young T, Palta M, et al. Prospective study of the association between sleep-disordered breathing and hypertension. *N Engl J Med* 2000;342:1378–1384.
224. Wolk R, Shamsuzzaman AS, Somers VK. Obesity, sleep apnea, and hypertension. *Hypertension* 2003;42:1067–1074.
225. Svatikova A, Wolk R, Gami AS, et al. Interactions between obstructive sleep apnea and the metabolic syndrome. *Curr Diab Rep* 2005;5:53–58.
226. Sharma SK, Kurian S, Malik V, et al. A stepped approach for prediction of obstructive sleep apnea in overtly asymptomatic obese subjects: a hospital based study. *Sleep Med* 2004;5:351–357.
227. Dixon JB, Schachter LM, O'Brien PE. Predicting sleep apnea and excessive day sleepiness in the severely obese: indicators for polysomnography. *Chest* 2003;123:1134–1141.
228. Victor LD. Obstructive sleep apnea. *Am Fam Physician* 1999;60:2279–2286.
229. Tsai WH, Remmers JE, Brant R, et al. A decision rule for diagnostic testing in obstructive sleep apnea. *Am J Respir Crit Care Med* 2003;167:1427–1432.
230. Caples SM, Gami AS, Somers VK. Obstructive sleep apnea. *Ann Intern Med* 2005;142:187–197.
231. Epstein LJ, Dorlac GR. Cost-effectiveness analysis of nocturnal oximetry as a method of screening for sleep apnea-hypopnea syndrome. *Chest* 1998;113:97–103.
232. Faber CE, Grymer L. Available techniques for objective assessment of upper airway narrowing in snoring and sleep apnea. *Sleep Breath* 2003;7:77–86.
233. Malhotra A, White DP. Obstructive sleep apnoea. *Lancet* 2002;360:237–245.
234. Becker HF, Jerrentrup A, Ploch T, et al. Effect of nasal continuous positive airway pressure treatment on blood pressure in patients with obstructive sleep apnea. *Circulation* 2003;107:68–73.
235. Victor LD. Treatment of obstructive sleep apnea in primary care. *Am Fam Physician* 2004;69:561–568.
236. Pirsig W, Verse T. Long-term results in the treatment of obstructive sleep apnea. *Eur Arch Otorhinolaryngol* 2000;257:570–577.
237. Kao YH, Shnayder Y, Lee KC. The efficacy of anatomically based multilevel surgery for obstructive sleep apnea. *Otolaryngol Head Neck Surg* 2003;129:327–335.
238. Tisdale JE, Huang MB, Borzak S. Risk factors for hypertensive crisis: importance of out-patient blood pressure control. *Fam Pract* 2004;21:420–424.
239. Varon J, Marik PE. The diagnosis and management of hypertensive crises. *Chest* 2000;118:214–227.
240. Vaughan CJ, Delanty N. Hypertensive emergencies. *Lancet* 2000;356:411–417.
241. Cherney D, Straus S. Management of patients with hypertensive urgencies and emergencies: a systematic review of the literature. *J Gen Intern Med* 2002;17:937–945.
242. Berlowitz DR, Ash AS, Hickey EC, et al. Inadequate management of blood pressure in a hypertensive population. *N Engl J Med* 1998;339:1957–1963.
243. Setaro JF, Black HR. Refractory hypertension. *N Engl J Med* 1992;327:543–547.
244. Rudd P. The search for high-yield, low-risk antihypertensive treatment. *Am J Med* 2000;108:429–430.
245. Mancia G, Bertinieri G, Grassi G, et al. Effects of blood-pressure measurement by the doctor on patient's blood pressure and heart rate. *Lancet* 1983;2:695–698.
246. Pickering TG. Principles and techniques of blood pressure measurement. *Cardiol Clin* 2002;20:207–223.
247. MacDonald MB, Laing GP, Wilson MP, et al. Prevalence and predictors of white-coat response in patients with treated hypertension. *CMAJ* 1999;161:265–269.
248. Weber MA, Neutel JM, Smith DH, et al. Diagnosis of mild hypertension by ambulatory blood pressure monitoring. *Circulation* 1994;90:2291–2298.
249. Verdecchia P, Schillaci G, Borgioni C, et al. Prognostic significance of the white coat effect. *Hypertension* 1997;29:1218–1224.
250. Spence JD. Withholding treatment in white-coat hypertension: wishful thinking. *CMAJ* 1999;161:275–276.
251. Rao S, Liu CT, Wilder L, et al. Clinical inquiries. What is the best way to treat patients with white-coat hypertension? *J Fam Pract* 2004;53:408–412.
252. Staessen JA, Wang J, Bianchi G, et al. Essential hypertension. *Lancet* 2003;361:1629–1641.
253. Ho H, Pinto A, Hall SD, et al. Association Between the CYP3A5 Genotype and Blood Pressure. *Hypertension* 2005;45:294–298.
254. Turner ST, Schwartz GL. Gene markers and antihypertensive therapy. *Curr Hypertens Rep* 2005;7:21–30.
255. Freitag MH, Vasan RS. What is normal blood pressure? *Curr Opin Nephrol Hypertens* 2003;12:285–292.
256. Mainous AGr, Everett CJ, Liszka H, et al. Prehypertension and mortality in a nationally representative cohort. *Am J Cardiol* 2004;94:1496–1500.
257. Russell LB, Valiyeva E, Carson JL. Effects of prehypertension on admissions and deaths: a simulation. *Arch Intern Med* 2004;164:2119–2124.
258. Nissen SE, Tuzcu EM, Libby P, et al. Effect of antihypertensive agents on cardiovascular events in patients with coronary disease and normal

blood pressure: the CAMELOT study: a randomized controlled trial. *JAMA* 2004;292:2217–2225.
259. Pitt B, Zannad F, Remme WJ, et al. The effect of spironolactone on morbidity and mortality in patients with severe heart failure. Randomized Aldactone Evaluation Study Investigators. *N Engl J Med* 1999;341:709–717.
260. Hunt SA, Baker DW, Chin MH, et al. ACC/AHA guidelines for the evaluation and management of chronic heart failure in the adult: executive summary. A report of the American College of Cardiology/American Heart Association Task Force on Practice Guidelines (Committee to revise the 1995 Guidelines for the Evaluation and Management of Heart Failure). *J Am Coll Cardiol* 2001;38:2101–2113.
261. Tepper D. Frontiers in congestive heart failure: Effect of Metoprolol CR/XL in chronic heart failure: Metoprolol CR/XL Randomised Intervention Trial in Congestive Heart Failure (MERIT-HF). *Congest Heart Fail* 1999;5:184–185.
262. Packer M, Coats AJ, Fowler MB, et al. Effect of carvedilol on survival in severe chronic heart failure. *N Engl J Med* 2001;344:1651–1658.
263. A randomized trial of beta-blockade in heart failure. The Cardiac Insufficiency Bisoprolol Study (CIBIS). CIBIS Investigators and Committees. *Circulation* 1994;90:1765–1773.
264. Effect of enalapril on survival in patients with reduced left ventricular ejection fractions and congestive heart failure. The SOLVD Investigators. *N Engl J Med* 1991;325:293–302.
265. Effect of ramipril on mortality and morbidity of survivors of acute myocardial infarction with clinical evidence of heart failure. The Acute Infarction Ramipril Efficacy (AIRE) Study Investigators. *Lancet* 1993;342:821–828.
266. Kober L, Torp-Pedersen C, Carlsen JE, et al. A clinical trial of the angiotensin-converting-enzyme inhibitor trandolapril in patients with left ventricular dysfunction after myocardial infarction. Trandolapril Cardiac Evaluation (TRACE) Study Group. *N Engl J Med* 1995;333:1670–1676.
267. Cohn JN, Tognoni G. A randomized trial of the angiotensin-receptor blocker valsartan in chronic heart failure. *N Engl J Med* 2001;345:1667–1675.
268. Pitt B, Remme W, Zannad F, et al. Eplerenone, a selective aldosterone blocker, in patients with left ventricular dysfunction after myocardial infarction. *N Engl J Med* 2003;348:1309–1321.
269. Braunwald E, Antman EM, Beasley JW, et al. ACC/AHA 2002 guideline update for the management of patients with unstable angina and non-ST-segment elevation myocardial infarction—summary article: a report of the American College of Cardiology/American Heart Association task force on practice guidelines (Committee on the Management of Patients With Unstable Angina). *J Am Coll Cardiol* 2002;40:1366–1374.
270. A randomized trial of propranolol in patients with acute myocardial infarction. I. Mortality results. *JAMA* 1982;247:1707–1714.
271. Hager WD, Davis BR, Riba A, et al. Absence of a deleterious effect of calcium channel blockers in patients with left ventricular dysfunction after myocardial infarction: The SAVE Study Experience. SAVE Investigators. Survival and Ventricular Enlargement. *Am Heart J* 1998;135:406–413.
272. Dargie HJ. Effect of carvedilol on outcome after myocardial infarction in patients with left-ventricular dysfunction: the CAPRICORN randomised trial. *Lancet* 2001;357:1385–1390.
273. Black HR, Elliott WJ, Grandits G, et al. Principal results of the Controlled Onset Verapamil Investigation of Cardiovascular End Points (CONVINCE) trial. *JAMA* 2003;289:2073–2082.
274. Dahlof B, Devereux RB, Kjeldsen SE, et al. Cardiovascular morbidity and mortality in the Losartan Intervention For Endpoint reduction in hypertension study (LIFE): a randomised trial against atenolol. *Lancet* 2002;359:995–1003.
275. Yusuf S, Sleight P, Pogue J, et al. Effects of an angiotensin-converting-enzyme inhibitor, ramipril, on cardiovascular events in high-risk patients. The Heart Outcomes Prevention Evaluation Study Investigators. *N Engl J Med* 2000;342:145–153.
276. Arauz-Pacheco C, Parrott MA, Raskin P. Treatment of hypertension in adults with diabetes. *Diabetes Care* 2003;26[Suppl 1]:S80–82.
277. Guideline NKF. K/DOQI clinical practice guidelines for chronic kidney disease: Kidney Disease Outcome Quality Initiative. *Am J Kidney Dis* 2002;39[Suppl 2]:S1-S246.
278. Pacak K. Efficacy of atenolol and captopril in reducing risk of macrovascular and microvascular complications in type 2 diabetes: UKPDS 39. UK Prospective Diabetes Study Group. *BMJ* 1998;317:713–720.
279. Randomised placebo-controlled trial of effect of ramipril on decline in glomerular filtration rate and risk of terminal renal failure in proteinuric, non-diabetic nephropathy. The GISEN Group (Gruppo Italiano di Studi Epidemiologici in Nefrologia). *Lancet* 1997;349:1857–1863.
280. Lewis EJ, Hunsicker LG, Bain RP, et al. The effect of angiotensin-converting-enzyme inhibition on diabetic nephropathy. The Collaborative Study Group. *N Engl J Med* 1993;329:1456–1462.
281. Lewis EJ, Hunsicker LG, Clarke WR, et al. Renoprotective effect of the angiotensin-receptor antagonist irbesartan in patients with nephropathy due to type 2 diabetes. *N Engl J Med* 2001;345:851–860.
282. Wright JT Jr, Agodoa L, Contreras G, et al. Successful blood pressure control in the African American Study of Kidney Disease and Hypertension. *Arch Intern Med* 2002;162:1636–1643.
283. Randomised trial of a perindopril-based blood-pressure-lowering regimen among 6,105 individuals with previous stroke or transient ischaemic attack. *Lancet* 2001;358:1033–1041.
284. Touyz RM, Campbell N, Logan A, et al. The 2004 Canadian recommendations for the management of hypertension: part III—lifestyle modifications to prevent and control hypertension. *Can J Cardiol* 2004;20:55–59.

CHAPTER 8 ■ SMOKING

JOAQUIN BARNOYA AND STANTON A. GLANTZ

OVERVIEW

Tobacco smoke, either as active or passive smoking, is a leading cause of preventable cardiovascular diseases (CVD). In the United States, during 1997–2001, smoking was responsible for an annual average of 260,000 deaths among men and 178,000 deaths among women. One third (34.7%) of these deaths where from CVD (1). Ischemic heart disease (IHD) is the leading cause of death from secondhand smoke (SHS), accounting for more than 10 times the number of deaths from lung cancer (1). The effects of tobacco smoke on the cardiovascular system are multiple and reinforce each other. These effects include platelet activation, endothelial dysfunction, inflammation, altered lipid levels and metabolism, and hemodynamic effects. These effects occur rapidly, often within minutes of active or passive smoking.

Cessation of exposure to tobacco smoke leads to a fast decline in the risk associated with exposure. When someone stops smoking, exercise tolerance improves the next day. Half the excess risk of acute myocardial infarction (AMI) is gone in 1 year, most is gone in 3 years (2), and many of the acute effects on the cardiovascular system begin to disappear within hours after ending exposure.

Tobacco control should be viewed from both an individual and societal standpoint. From an individual standpoint, every smoker should be encouraged to quit or not to smoke around others and every nonsmoker should be encouraged to avoid exposure to SHS. Currently there are multiple pharmacologic treatments to help patients quit, and smoke-free environments have been shown to reduce smoking. Every cardiologist should become active in the societal fight against tobacco and SHS.

EPIDEMIOLOGY OF SMOKING AND EXPOSURE TO SECONDHAND SMOKE

Tobacco has been used for thousands of years. A Mayan stone carving more than 1,000 years ago displays the first record of tobacco use in human history. In 1884, James Bonsack developed the cigarette manufacturing machine, resulting in the mass production of cigarettes. In addition to this machine, the development in 1892 of the safety matches fueled an increase in cigarette consumption, along with the development of an aggressive increase in cigarette marketing (3). Since then, tobacco became a major public health problem; by 2020 smoking is expected to kill 10 million people per year, most of them (70%) in low- and middle-income countries (4).

Smoking prevalence in the United States has been declining. In 2003, approximately 21.6% (45.4 million) of U.S. adults were current smokers, half the rate in 1950 (44%) (Fig. 8.1) (5). Eighty-one percent of these smokers do so every day. More men than women smoke (24.1% and 19.2%, respectively) and more young than old people smoke (5). In addition, smoking is more prevalent among those living below the poverty level and in those with low educational level compared to those living above the poverty level and the highly educated (5).

The tobacco epidemic has spread worldwide. For example, in China, in 2001, 60% of men and 7% of women smoked, representing approximately 147 million men and 15 million women age 35 to 74 (6).

Most smokers want to quit smoking or cut down. In 2003, 41.1% (15.1 million) current smokers reported they had stopped smoking for at least 1 day during the past 12 months because they were trying to quit (5). Young adults have the highest spontaneous quit rates (7) and quitting before age 35 results in mortality patterns equal to that of nonsmokers (Fig. 8.2) (8). Regardless of age, every smoker should be encouraged to quit and at least be referred to a smoking cessation quit-line.

SHS exposure continues to be a major threat to most of the world's population. In the United States, only 43% of blue collar workers enjoy smoke-free environments compared to 75% of white collar workers (9). The 2000 National Youth Tobacco Survey found that 4 in 10 students (grades 6–12) live in homes where others smoke and 7 in 10 are exposed to smoke in public places (10). In China, a cross-sectional survey in 2000 and 2001, found that 27% of nonsmoking men and 26% of nonsmoking women were breathing SHS at the workplace (6). In Europe and Latin America, high concentrations of nicotine have been found in bars and restaurants, and in lower concentrations, in hospitals and high schools (11,12). Many

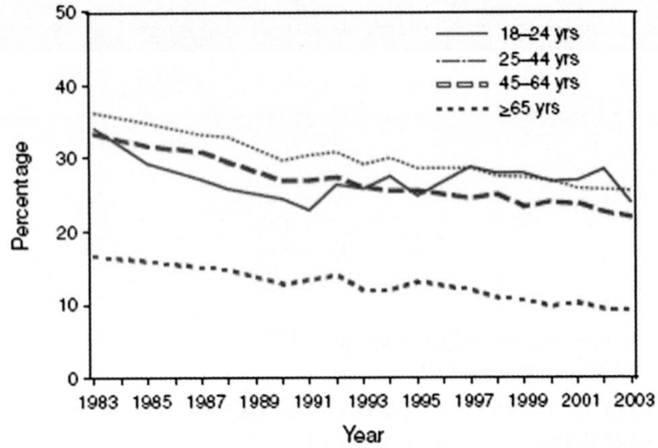

FIGURE 8.1. Smoking prevalence in the United States has declined over the last 20 years. The decline was faster in the first 10 years than in the last 10 years. In addition, most of the decline was among older age groups, the 18- to 24-year-old group has not experienced such an encouraging decline. (*Source:* Centers for Disease Control and Prevention. Cigarette Smoking Among Adults—United States, 2003. *MMWR* 2005;54:509–513.)

communities, some states in the United States, and several countries (Ireland, Norway, Sweden, New Zealand, Italy and Uruguay as of March 2006) have implemented smoke-free policies, setting an example to follow and protecting their citizens from the dangers of SHS.

SMOKING AND CARDIOVASCULAR DISEASE

Smoking is a leading risk factor for all CVD. Coronary heart disease (CHD), stroke, and peripheral artery disease are all increased in smokers compared to nonsmokers. IHD accounts for the largest number of deaths from CVD caused by smoking (64% in men and 60% in women) (1).

CHD, including AMI, IHD, and angina pectoris, risk increases continuously with daily cigarette smoking (13). The relative risk of nonfatal AMI in the 35- to 39-year age group is 4.9 (95% confidence interval [CI] 3.9–6.1) in men and 5.3 (95% CI 3.2–8.7) in women (13). The risk is dose dependent and declines with age (because the baseline risk of heart disease is greater at older age) (14). The fact that the risk is highest in young people highlights the particular relevance of smoking cessation among this group.

Compared to nonsmokers, smokers have a higher risk of sudden death (especially women taking oral contraceptives (15,16), recurrent ischemia after coronary artery bypass grafting (CABG), and reocclusion after an AMI (16). Smokers also have a higher incidence of abdominal aortic aneurysm, peripheral vascular disease, and renal artery stenosis (17,18). Erectile dysfunction has also been found to be associated with active and passive smoking (19) and is markedly improved by smoking cessation (20).

PASSIVE SMOKING AND CARDIOVASCULAR DISEASE

Passive smoking increases the risk of heart disease by about 30% (14,21,22). Despite the much lower dose of tobacco smoke inhaled by active smokers, the risk (using questionaires

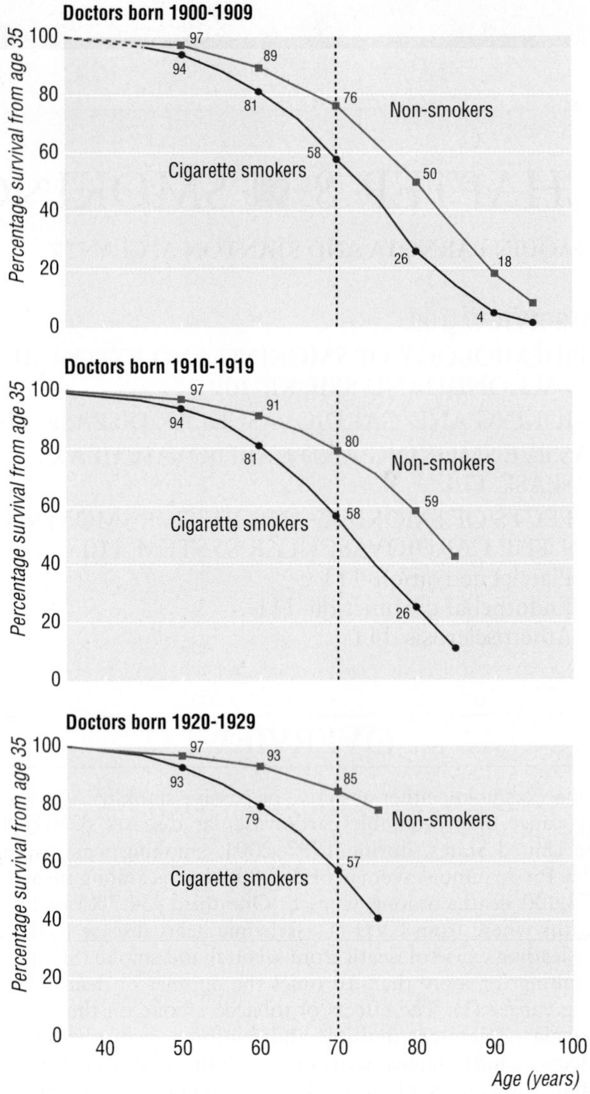

FIGURE 8.2. After smoking cessation there is an increase in survival, regardless of age at quitting. For those who quit before 40 years of age, survival improves almost to that of never smokers and for those who quit before age 35, survival is the same as survival in the never smokers group. (*Source:* From *BMJ*. 2004;328(7455):5 with permission from BMJ Publishing group.)

to assess exposure) is about one third the increase seen in active smokers (21). Cotinine, a stable metabolite of nicotine, has been used to assess exposure to SHS. Cotinine, unlike questionnaires, provides complete and objective measure of someone's total recent exposure to SHS. Using this better estimate of exposure based on cotinine, yields higher risk estimates for the effects of SHS than had been determined based on questionnaires; Whincup et al. (23) estimated the risk of CHD with exposure to SHS to be 1.57 (95% CI 1.08–2.28), similar to that found in light (1–9 cigarettes/d) active smokers (Fig. 8.3) (23).

EFFECTS OF SMOKING AND PASSIVE SMOKING ON THE CARDIOVASCULAR SYSTEM

Active and passive smoking affect the cardiovascular system through the same mechanisms. On average, the biological

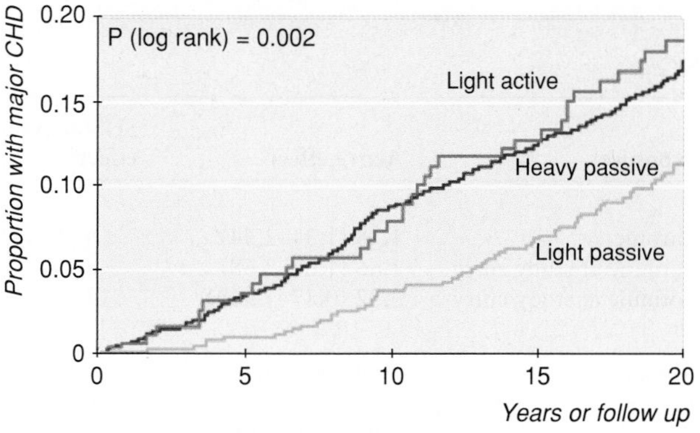

FIGURE 8.3. The risk of heart disease in heavy passive smokers is undistinguishable to the risk in light active smokers using cotinine levels at time zero as the measure of exposure. (*Source:* Reproduced from *BMJ*. 2004;329(7439):4 with permission from BMJ Publishing group.)

effects of passive smoking are nearly as large as the effects of active smoking (21). Table 8.1 summarizes the effects of SHS on the cardiovascular system and compares them to the effects of active smoking. These effects are synergistic and interact with other known cardiovascular risk factors (e.g., diabetes, obesity). In some cases, such as platelet activation and endothelial dysfunction, the effects occur within minutes of exposure to tobacco smoke (24,25).

Nicotine is the agent in tobacco that has been most widely researched. Even though it is responsible for the addiction, it is not the major agent acting on the cardiovascular system (26). Polycyclic aromatic hydrocarbons (27), oxidizing agents (16), particulate matter (28), and acrolein (29) are more likely the agents that affect the cardiovascular system.

Platelet Activation

Platelet activation leads to thrombosis, a key factor in AMI and sudden death. This prothrombotic state observed smokers partially explains the younger age, lower risk factor prevalence, and less underlying coronary disease observed in smokers compared to nonsmokers at the time of first MI. The immediate increase in the risk of IHD attributable to the increase in platelet aggregation is estimated to be 43% for active smoking and 34% for passive smoking (14).

Tobacco smoke activates platelets through several mechanisms. These mechanisms include endothelial dysfunction, oxidative stress, decrease platelet-derived nitric oxide (NO) production (16), and increased fibrinogen (17) and thromboxane (30). Platelet activation occurs soon after exposure. In active smokers (with established CHD) and passive smokers, platelet activation has been observed 5 minutes after smoking two cigarettes (31) and 20 minutes of breathing SHS (32). Despite the much lower dose of tobacco smoke inhaled by passive smokers, the effect on platelet activation is 96% of that observed in active smokers (21). In addition, side stream smoke (the main component of SHS) has been found to be 1.5 times more potent than mainstream smoke (the smoke inhaled by the smoker) in activating platelets under normal and shear stress conditions (30). "Light" and "mild" cigarette smoke extracts have also been found to be more potent activators than "full flavor" cigarette smoke (33).

The increased platelet aggregability resulting from smoking is ameliorated as early as 2 weeks after smoking cessation (34), suggesting that the effects of tobacco smoke on platelet aggregability are transient and partially reversible.

Endothelial Dysfunction

Endothelial dysfunction is strongly and independently associated with cardiovascular events (35). Endothelial dysfunction results in atherosclerosis, plaque rupture, and decreased blood flow owing to thrombosis and vasospasm. Tobacco smoke exposure (acute or chronic, active or passive) leads to endothelial dysfunction, which is manifest clinically in 15 to 30 minutes (21,25,36). Otsuka et al. (25) exposed healthy smokers and nonsmokers to 30 minutes of SHS at levels comparable to those in a bar. Before exposure, the coronary flow velocity reserve (CFVR, a surrogate marker of endothelial function) was better in nonsmokers than in smokers. After exposure, the CFVR of nonsmokers was undistinguishable from that of smokers. In contrast, smokers experienced no change in CFVR, suggesting that the effect of the smoke constituents was saturated in the smokers (25). Endothelial cell damage has been documented as early as 20 minutes of exposure to cigarette smoke (37,38). A dose–response relationship has also been documented between exposure to tobacco smoke and decreased endothelium-dependent vasodilation (24,39). Evidence suggests that the endothelium partially recovers after exposure has ended (1 year after exposure has ended) (39,40).

NO, secreted by the endothelium and responsible for vessel dilation, is decreased in active and passive smokers (41,42). In animal models with low levels of NO activity, the repair mechanism of the endothelium is impaired (35). Furthermore, the detrimental effects of tobacco smoke on endothelial function have been abolished by adding the NO precursor, L-arginine, to the diet of active and passive smokers (43–45).

Atherosclerosis

Lipid levels are altered in smokers and passive smokers (17,21). Tobacco smoke increases low-density lipoprotein (LDL) and decreases in high-density lipoprotein (HDL) (17). In addition to altering lipid levels, cigarette smoke renders LDL more prone to oxidation. Active and passive smokers have higher levels of products of lipid peroxidation and oxidized LDL (17,46). Oxidized LDL is rapidly ingested by macrophages which, in turn, form foam cells in atherosclerotic lesions. Insulin resistance, leading to an atherogenic lipid profile, is also increased by tobacco smoke (16,47).

Active and passive smokers also show evidence of increased inflammatory markers (17,48). Inflammation is now recognized as a key step in the atherosclerotic process (49). Inflammatory markers that have been found to be elevated with tobacco smoke exposure include leukocyte count, acute phase reactants (e.g., fibrinogen, C-reactive protein), interleukin-6, and tumor necrosis factor. The increase observed in passive smokers compared to that observed in active smokers is as or sometimes larger (see Table 8.1). This inflammatory state is reduced after smoking cessation (50).

Increased Oxidative Stress

Smokers and passive smokers have increased markers of oxidative stress (17,21). Under normal conditions, oxidative stress results from free radicals generated during the respiratory process. To protect blood vessels and LDL from oxidation, the body uses antioxidants such as folate, vitamin C, and β-carotene. Smokers and passive smokers have been found to

TABLE 8.1

COMPARATIVE EFFECTS OF PASSIVE AND ACTIVE SMOKING[a]

	SHS effect[b]	Exposure	Active effect[c]	SHS/active effect[d]
RISK OF HEART DISEASE (95% CI)				
OVERALL	1.31 (1.21–1.41)[k]	Chronic	1.78 (1.31–2.44)[e]	40%
Twenty years (23)	1.57 (1.08–2.28)[f]	Cotinine at study entry	1.66 (1.04–2.68)	86%
First 4 years (23)	3.73 (1.32–10.98)	Cotinine at study entry	3.32 (0.87–12.64)	122%
PLATELET FUNCTION				
Platelet activation (32) (SI PGI_2)[g]	0.550 ± 0.059	20 min	0.540 ± 0.069	96%
Platelet aggregate ratio (37,38) (change)	−.09	20 min	−.15	60%
Fibrinogen (48) (95% CI) (mg/dL)	5.2 (−1.2 to 12.0)	Chronic	6.9 (−0.9 to 14.0)	75%
Fibrinogen (119) (mg/dL) (SE)	11.2 ± 4.1	Chronic	18.1 ± 6.7	62%
Plasma thromboxane (30) (pg/mL)	3.30 ± 0.35	Acute	2.93 ± 0.07	113%
Plasma malondialdehyde (30) nmol/10^9 platelets	4.20 ± 0.17	Acute	3.90 ± 0.07	108%
ENDOTHELIUM AND ARTERIAL FUNCTION				
Endothelial cell count (change) (37,38) (mean number of anuclear cell carcasses on 0.9 μL chamber)	0.9	20 min	2.0	45%
CFVR (25) (cm/s)	68.8 ± 22.7	30 min	67.1 ± 15.0	91%
Flow-mediated dilation (24) (%)	3.1 ± 2.7	3 y	4.4 ± 3.1	134%
Aortic stiffness (60,61) (mm Hg/mm)	58	4 min	49	110%
HDL (120) (mg/dL)	48.26 ± 3.47	Chronic	45.59 ± 4.60	73%
Increase in intimal media thickness (121) (μm/3 y)	5.9	Chronic	14.3	41%
INFLAMMATORY MARKERS (48) (95% CI)				
White blood cells (×10^3/μL)	0.6 (0.3–0.8)	Chronic	0.6 (0.5–0.7)	100%
CRP (mg/dL)	0.08 (0.02–0.10)	Chronic	0.1 (0.08–0.20)	80%
Homocysteine (μmol/L)	0.4 (0.2–0.6)	Chronic	0.5 (0.1–0.9)	80%
Oxidized LDL (mg/dL)	3.3 (0.5–6.0)	Chronic	3.9 (1.4–7.0)	85%
ANTIOXIDANTS				
Vitamin C μmol/L (51), median (interquartile range)	53 (41–79)	Chronic	40 (25–58)	57%
Hypovitaminosis (51) (vitamin C <23 μmol/L)	12%	Chronic	24%	50%
Ratio of DHAA[i] to ascorbic acid (122)	10.3 ± 7.0	>6 mo	11.2 ± 6.9	78%
Vitamin C in children (123) mmol/L (mean ± SE)	−8.8 ± 1.5[h]	Chronic	−9.0 ± 2.3	98%
β-Carotene (124) (μmol/L) mean (SE)	0.129 ± 0.022	Chronic	0.155 ± 0.021	174%
β-Carotene (53) (μmol/L)	0.15	Chronic	0.17	128%
RBC folate mean decrease (52) nmol/L (95% CI)[j]	−50 (−69 to −31)	Chronic	−86 (−101 to −71)	58%

[a]Data are presented as mean values ± SD unless otherwise noted.
[b]Change in variable associated with passive smoking among nonsmokers (after minus before SHS exposure).
[c]Difference in variable between smokers and nonsmokers (smoker minus nonsmoker).
[d]Represents the difference between passive smoking effect divided by active smoking effect times 100%.
[e]Risk of death at age 65 smoking 20 cigarettes/d from Law et al. (14).
[f]Cotinine levels 2.8–14.0 ng/mL.
[g]Sensitivity index to prostacyclin.
[h]High-dose SHS group.
[i]Dehydroascorbic acid.
[j]High exposure to SHS.
[k]From Barnoya and Glantz (21).
Abbreviations: CFVR, coronary flow velocity reserve; CRP, C-reactive protein; HDL, high-density lipoprotein; SHS, second hand smoke.
Source: Barnoya J, Glantz SA. Cardiovascular effects of secondhand smoke: nearly as large as smoking. *Circulation* 2005;111:2684–2698.

have lower levels of antioxidants (51–53). Therefore, the harmful effects of tobacco smoke are twofold. First, tobacco smoke is a source of free radicals. Second, it leads to a decrease in antioxidant levels that normally would protect the body against oxidative damage.

Other Effects

Smoking leads to higher levels of epinephrine and norepinephrine, resulting in increased systemic arterial pressure, heart rate (up to 20 beats per minute), and myocardial contractility (17,54). These changes increase myocardial oxygen demand. This state is further complicated by a decrease in oxygen-carrying capacity owing to higher levels of carboxyhemoglobin observed in smokers. In addition, the heart's ability to transform oxygen into the energy molecule adenosine triphosphate is decreased with brief (30 minutes) exposure to SHS (55). The cell respiratory organ, the mitochondria, is also damaged with SHS exposure. This harmful effect is observed as early as 21 days of exposure to SHS and is worst if coupled with hypercholesterolemia (56).

Heart rate variability (HRV) is also reduced with SHS exposure. After 2 hours of exposure, the HRV was reduced 12% of the level before exposure (57). In addition, tobacco smoke has also been found to have arrhythmogenic potential (16). Arterial stiffness is also increased in smokers and passive smokers (58,59). The effect occurs in active smokers right after smoking one cigarette and in passive smokers within 4 minutes of breathing SHS (60,61).

TABLE 8.2

SOURCES OF INFORMATION ON TOBACCO CONTROL AND ADVOCACY

- Americans for Nonsmokers' Rights: www.no-smoke.org
- World Health Organization (Tobacco Free Initiative): www.who.int/tobacco/en
- Framework Convention Alliance on Tobacco Control: www.fctc.org
- Society for Nicotine and Tobacco Research (SRNT): www.srnt.org
- Tobacco Information and Prevention Sources (CDC): www.cdc.gov/tobacco/
- Smokefree.gov: http://smokefree.gov
- Action on Smoking and Health (ASH): www.ash.org.uk
- American Cancer Society: www.cancer.org
- American Heart Association: www.americanheart.org
- Tobacco Scam: www.tobaccoscam.ucsf.edu
- Legacy Tobacco Documents Library: http://legacy.library.ucsf.edu

PHYSICIANS AND TOBACCO CONTROL

Smoking prevalence among U.S. physicians is low (3.3%), yet it continues to be a problem in other countries (e.g., Guatemala 18%, Italy 31%) (62,63). Physicians can and should play several key roles in fighting against tobacco. They should be role models as nonsmokers and counsel every patient about the health dangers of active and passive smoking.

In 1996, the Agency for Health Care Policy and Research Tobacco Cessation Guideline suggested that even simple advice (taking 3 minutes) from a physician is effective in promoting cessation and gave counseling its highest recommendation (64). Results from the 2005 Global Health Professionals Survey found that almost all third-year medical students believe health professionals should give advice or information about smoking cessation to patients (65), yet few students receive any formal training in cessation counseling (65,66). In the United States, a 2000 survey among current smokers found that less than 50% reported receiving any cessation advice from a physician (67). Every patient should also receive advice to avoid exposure to SHS, because the adverse effects of SHS on the cardiovascular system are fast and nearly as large as active smoking (21).

From a societal standpoint, physicians and their organizations (e.g., American College of Cardiology and American Heart Association) should contribute to the implementation of effective public policies that reduce tobacco consumption. Table 8.2 provides a list of resources on tobacco control. These policies include smoke-free work and public places, increased taxation on tobacco products, and strong graphical health warning labels on cigarette packs (68).

A comprehensive tobacco control program has been shown to reduce heart disease mortality. In California, the Tobacco Control Program (which included a strong media campaign that exposed the tobacco industry tactics and promoted policies creating smoke-free environments) was associated with 59,000 fewer deaths from heart disease between 1989 and 1997 (69,70).

SMOKING CESSATION

Smoking cessation is a cost-effective intervention for reducing morbidity and mortality due to heart disease (Fig. 8.4) (71). Overall, 70% of smokers report wanting to quit, yet fewer than 5% are successful in doing so each year (72). In contrast, smokers who receive assistance—behavioral, pharmacologic, or both—achieve quit rates of around 20% at least 6 months after quitting (64,73,74). More than advice about diet, exercise, or alcohol use, advice about tobacco use and cessation is significantly associated with patient satisfaction with their physician (75). Furthermore, a clinician's failure to address tobacco use tacitly implies that "quitting is not important."

Smoking cessation can be considered as both primary and secondary prevention strategies for CVD; it not only prevents the development of CVD, but it also benefits smokers with manifest CVD (8,76). Compared to continuing smokers, former smokers who undergo a CABG have improved survival and decreased need for repeated revascularization (77). In smokers with heart failure, cessation reduces mortality 30% compared to continuing smokers (78), which is as much or more than that achieved with a β-blocker (34% mortality reduction [79]), an aldosterone inhibitor (30% mortality reduction [80]), or an angiotensin-converting enzyme (ACE) inhibitor (19% mortality reduction [81]). The cost of creating a long-term abstainer ranges from $400 (physician counseling only) to $1,100 (a 4- to 8-week course of nicotine replacement therapy [NRT]) (82); this one-time cost is comparable to the annual cost of an ACE inhibitor and β-blocker (range, $200–1,500 per year) (83–85).

There are a number of ways by which physicians can assist smokers with quitting. Even brief advice (<3 minutes) has been shown to increase quit rates by 70% (64). Clinicians can apply the "5 A's" strategy as a framework for smoking cessation counseling in providing advice to their patients (Table 8.3). Just as with other vital signs (e.g., blood pressure and heart rate), smoking status should be documented in every patients chart. If a patient smokes, a more detailed inquiry is warranted. Age at initiation, number of cigarettes smoked per day, and how soon the first cigarette is smoked after waking should be documented. This last question has been shown to be an acceptable proxy measure for the level of nicotine addiction; persons who smoke their first cigarette of the day within the first 30 minutes of waking are generally more dependent than are persons who smoke their first cigarette later in the day (86).

Even very brief advice can be effective. In the absence of time or expertise for providing comprehensive cessation counseling, clinicians should (at a minimum) ask each patient whether they smoke or use any form of tobacco, advise tobacco users to quit, and refer patients to local smoking cessation programs or a

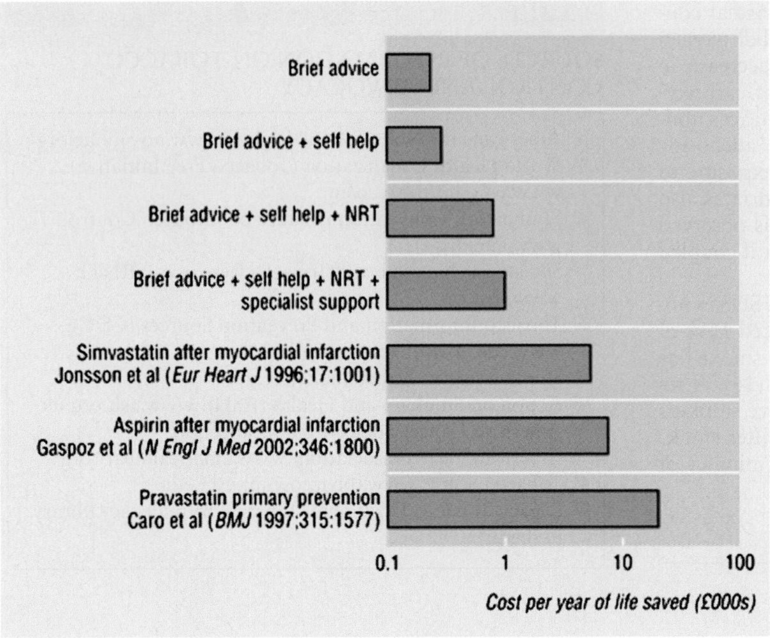

FIGURE 8.4. In addition to the benefits of smoking cessation, it is a cost-effective intervention when compared to other established treatments to reduce morality from heart disease. Even when compared to a relatively inexpensive drug as aspirin, smoking cessation is more cost effective. Despite this fact smoking cessation is rarely "prescribed" as a treatment to reduce heart disease mortality. (*Source:* From *BMJ*. 2004; 328(7445):948 with permission from BMJ Publishing group.)

toll-free quit-line (e.g., 1-800-QUIT NOW, accessible anywhere in the United States). Telephone quit-lines have proven to be a cost-effective strategy for smoking cessation (87–89). A randomized clinical trial comparing intensive telephone counseling against no counseling after quitting yielded almost a twofold higher abstinence rate for those receiving telephone counseling (87). Quit-lines are a viable cessation option for all smokers, but are especially useful for smokers who otherwise would have no access to treatment owing to lack of health insurance or geographic location.

In counseling patients, clinicians should focus not only on the harms of active smoking but also the effects of SHS on family and coworkers (7) and the benefits of cessation and the short time required for benefits to be incurred. It is also important to emphasize the fact that, although most patients "know" that smoking increases the risk of disease, the absolute risks are much higher than people believe (90,91). Patients should be particularly counseled about the immediate and large effects of both active and passive smoking on the heart and vascular system, because most people think of cancer rather than heart disease when they think about smoking, even though CVD accounts for more smoking-induced deaths than cancer.

TABLE 8.3

THE 5 A'S STRATEGY FOR BEHAVIORAL COUNSELING ON SMOKING CESSATION

Ask	Every cardiologist (or healthcare provider) should ask every patient "Do you smoke or use any tobacco product?"
Advise	All tobacco users, regardless of age or disease status, should be advised to quit.
Assess	Assess readiness to quit as (a) not ready to quit in the next month, (b) ready to quit in the next month, (c) recent quitter (<6 mo), (d) former smoker (>6 mo).
Assist	Behavioral counseling and pharmacotherapy should be offered to every smoker willing to quit.
Arrange	Follow-up counseling is important. Most relapse occurs within the first 3 months.

Source: From Fiore MC, Bailey WC, Cohen SJ, et al. *Treating tobacco use and dependence.* Clinical Practice Guideline. Rockville, MD: US Department of Health and Human Services, Public Health Service, 2000.

For patients who are not ready to quit, clinicians should apply the "5 R's" (64):

- *Relevance:* A personalized message should be delivered, emphasizing the effects of tobacco smoke on health, including the cardiovascular system.
- *Risks:* Short-term (e.g., bad breath, increased blood pressure), long-term (e.g., atherosclerosis, lipid abnormalities), and environmental (e.g., increase risk of disease in spouse, coworkers, and pets) effects should be highlighted.
- *Rewards:* Benefits of cessation should be explained, emphasizing the short-term benefits, regardless of age. The excess risk of AMI is reduced by 50% within 1 year of quitting (92).
- *Roadblocks:* Clinicians should assist patients in identifying barriers to quitting (e.g., weight gain or anxiety) and help to identify appropriate cognitive and behavioral coping strategies (e.g., emphasize that the benefits of quitting outweigh any possible weight gain and recommend pharmacotherapy as an option to decrease anxiety). Creating a smoke-free home and demanding smoke-free environments help to decrease the anxiety produced by the presence of other smokers, and this likely will increase the chance of success.
- *Repetition:* At each clinic visit, tobacco use should be addressed and appropriate interventions applied. Interventions should be documented in the medical record.

Pharmacotherapy

With the possible exception of light and occasional smokers (93), most smokers who are willing to quit should be offered pharmacotherapy (64). U.S. Food and Drug Administration (FDA)-approved agents for smoking cessation include five formulations of NRT and bupropion sustained release (SR). Light smokers (<10–15 cigarettes/d [93]), nondaily smokers (estimated to account for 19% of the smoking population [94]), and adolescents might not benefit from pharmacotherapy.

The presence of established CVD generally is not a contraindication to receiving pharmacotherapy for smoking cessation (95,96), although NRT is contraindicated in patients who have had a recent (in the preceding 2 weeks) MI, those with serious arrhythmias, and those with serious or worsening angina pectoris (64). All patients should receive behavioral counseling, either alone or in combination with pharmacotherapy.

Pregnant smokers deserve special attention. In addition to the obvious risks posed on the pregnant women by active smoking, the fetus will also be harmed by exposure to SHS. In utero exposure to SHS has been shown to be associated with an increased risk of spontaneous abortion and low birthweight (97), and as such, pregnant smokers should receive augmented intervention that exceeds minimal advice to quit. According to the Clinical Practice Guideline (64), despite potential risks and lack of an FDA indication for its use during pregnancy, NRT during pregnancy has been described as safer than smoking (98), and its use might be warranted in selected patients who are unable to quit using nonpharmacologic methods alone, or in cases for which the increased likelihood of quitting offsets the corresponding risks of NRT use (64). Given that postpartum relapse rates range from 70% to 80% among women who quit during pregnancy (99), relapse prevention is needed for those women who are able to quit successfully during pregnancy.

Pharmacotherapy is helpful in reducing withdrawal symptoms, although the nicotine levels achieved through smoking far exceed the levels received through pharmacotherapy (Fig. 8.5). Withdrawal symptoms, which generally peak within 24 to 48 hours after quitting and dissipate over the next 2 to 4 weeks (100), include anger/irritability, anxiety, cravings, difficulty concentrating, hunger/weight gain, impatience, restlessness, drowsiness, fatigue, impaired task performance, nervousness, and sleep disturbances (101).

Table 8.4 (from *Rx for Change*) presents the first-line medications currently approved by the FDA for smoking cessation. Each of these agents has been proven effective and approximately doubles patients' chances of quitting (Fig. 8.6). Product selection should be made according to patient preference. Product dosing for the NRT formulations should be determined based on either the time to first cigarette in the morning (nicotine lozenge) or the number of cigarettes smoked (all other NRT formulations; see Table 8.4). Nicotine gum reaches peak plasma concentrations approximately in 30 minutes (102). It should be chewed slowly until a "peppery" taste emerges, then "parked" between the cheek and gum for nicotine to be absorbed. Each piece lasts for about 30 minutes, and patients can use up to 24 pieces per day (102,103). The lozenge is similar to the gum in terms of nicotine content and peak concentrations. It is sucked and move from side to side of the mouth, like a hard candy, until fully dissolved (20–30 minutes). Acidic beverages (e.g., coffee and juice) should be avoided 15 minutes before and while using the gum or lozenge, because this alteration in pH can decrease the nicotine absorption through the buccal mucosa.

The nicotine oral inhaler, which is available only by prescription in the United States, delivers 4 mg of nicotine vapor from a porous plug that contains 10 mg of nicotine (103). Use of this formulation resembles the hand-to-mouth motion to which many smokers are accustomed (102). Peak plasma nicotine concentrations are reached within 30 to 45 minutes. The nicotine nasal spray, also available only by prescription, reaches peak plasma nicotine concentration more rapidly than any other NRT formulation (within 11–13 minutes [104]). Each dose provides 1 mg of nicotine, through two sprays, one (0.5-mg) spray in each nostril.

The nicotine transdermal patch delivers nicotine slowly but continuously for either 16 or 24 hours, depending on the formulation. The time to maximum concentration is 4 and

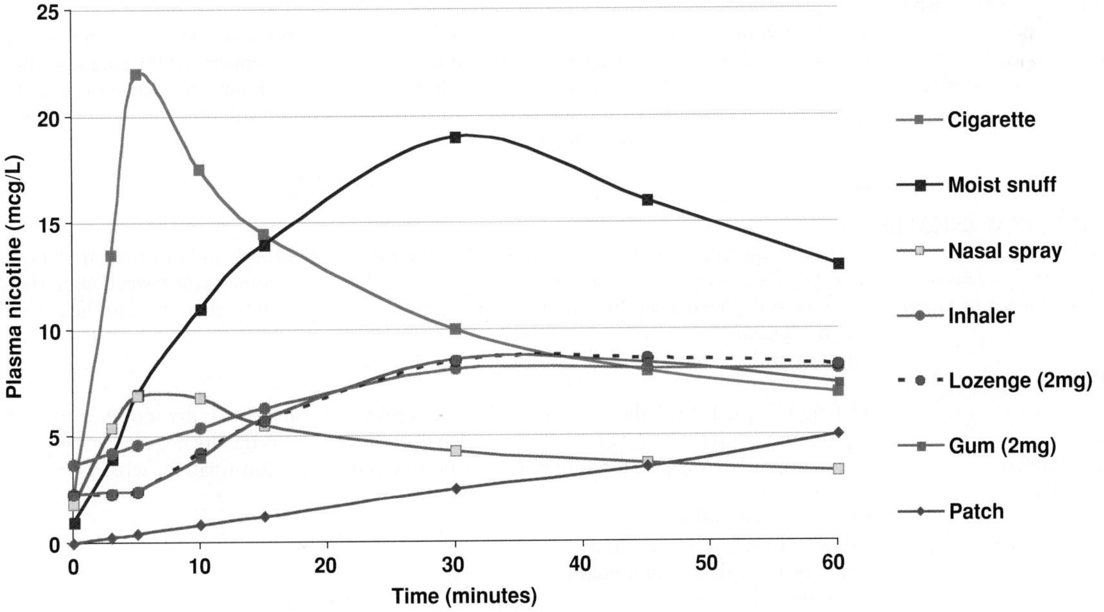

FIGURE 8.5. Plasma nicotine concentrations differ according to delivery system. The nicotine nasal spray is the one that most closely resembles the plasma nicotine concentrations achieved with smoking. Similar to smoking, plasma levels decline fast after reaching a peak level. The nicotine patch is the form of delivery that maintains a steady concentration for the longer period of time. Nicotine delivery choice is prescribed based on patient preference and number of cigarettes smoked per day. *Source:* Adapted with permission from *Rx for Change: Clinician-assisted tobacco cessation*. San Fransisco, CA: The Regents of the University of California, University of Southern California, and Western University of Health Sciences; 1999–2006. All rights reserved.

TABLE 8.4

PHARMACOTHERAPY OPTIONS: PRODUCTS, DOSING, RECOMMENDED DURATION OF TREATMENT, AND ADVERSE EFFECTS

Product	Dosing	Duration	Adverse effects
NICOTINE GUM			
Nicorette[a] generic gum 2 mg, 4 mg; regular, mint, orange, fresh mint[a]	≥25 cigarettes/d: 4 mg <25 cigarettes/d: 2 mg Week 1–6: 1 piece q1–2h Week 7–9: 1 piece q2–4h Week 10–12: 1 piece q4–8h	Up to 12 weeks	Mouth/jaw soreness, hiccups, dyspepsia, hypersalivation. Effects associated with incorrect chewing technique: lightheadedness, nausea and vomiting, throat, and mouth irritation.
NICOTINE LOZENGE			
Commit[a] 2 mg, 4 mg	First cigarette ≤30 min after waking: 4 mg First cigarette <30 min after waking: 2 mg Week 1–6: 1 lozenge q1–2h Week 7–9: 1 lozenge q2–4h Week 10–12: 1 lozenge q4–8h	Up to 12 weeks	Nausea, hiccups, cough, heartburn, headache, flatulence, insomnia.
NICOTINE TRANSDERMAL PATCH			
Nicoderm CQ[a] 7 mg, 14 mg, 21 mg 24-hour release	*>10 cigarettes/d:* 21 mg/d × 6 weeks 14 mg/d × 2 weeks 7 mg/d × 2 weeks *≤ 10 cigarettes/d:* 14 mg/d × 6 weeks 7 mg/d × 2 weeks	8–10 weeks	Local skin reactions (erythema, pruritus, burning), headache, sleep disturbances (insomnia) or abnormal/vivid dreams (associated with nocturnal nicotine absorption).
Generic patch[c,d] (formerly Habitrol) 7 mg, 14 mg, 21 mg 24-hour release	*>10 cigarettes/d:* 21 mg/d × 4 weeks 14 mg/d × 2 weeks 7 mg/d × 2 weeks *≤10 cigarettes/d:* 14 mg/d × 6 weeks 7 mg/d × 2 weeks	8 weeks	May wear patch for 16 h (remove at bedtime) if patient experiences sleep disturbances.
NICOTINE NASAL SPRAY			
Nicotrol NS[b] metered spray 0.5 mg nicotine in 50 μL aqueous nicotine solution	1–2 doses/h (8–40 doses/d) One dose = 2 sprays (1 in each nostril); each spray delivers 0.5 mg of nicotine to the nasal mucosa. For best results, initially use at least 8 doses/d. Do not exceed 5 doses/h or 40 doses/d.	3–6 mo Gradually decrease use over 3–6 mo	Nasal and/or throat irritation (hot, peppery, or burning sensation), rhinitis, tearing, sneezing, cough, headache.
NICOTINE ORAL INHALER			
Nicotrol inhaler[b] 10 mg cartridge delivers 4 mg inhaled nicotine vapor	6–16 cartridges/d; individualized dosing Initially, use at least 6 cartridges/d. Nicotine is depleted after 20 min of active puffing. Open cartridge retains potency for 24 h.	Up to 6 mo	Mouth and/or throat irritation, unpleasant taste, cough, rhinitis, dyspepsia, hiccups, headache.
BUPROPION SR			
Zyban Generics 150 mg sustained release tablet	150 mg PO qAM ×3 d, then increase to 150 mg PO BID Set quit date 1–2 weeks after initiation of therapy. Do not exceed 300 mg/d. Allow at least 8 h between doses. Avoid bedtime dosing to minimize insomnia.	7–12 weeks; maintenance up to 6 mo	Insomnia, dry mouth, nervousness, difficulty concentrating, rash, constipation, seizures (risk is 0.1%).

Source: Adapted with permission from *Rx for change: Clinician-assisted tobacco cessation.* San Francisco, CA: The Regents of the University of California, University of Southern California, and Western University of Health Sciences; 1999–2005. Copyright 1999–2006.
[a]Marketed by GlaxoSmithKline
[b]Marketed by Pfizer

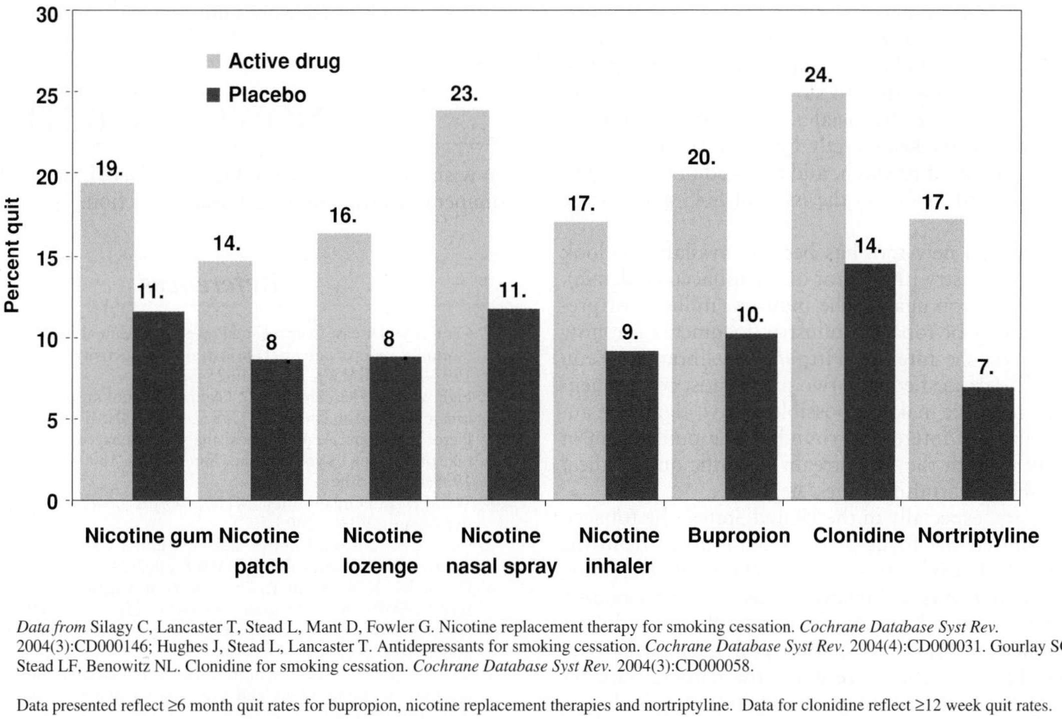

FIGURE 8.6. All available FDA-approved medications for smoking cessation have been shown to increase quitting rates at 6 months when compared to placebo. Even when receiving pharmacotherapy, all smokers trying to quit should receive behavioral counseling. *Source:* Adapted with permission from *Rx for Change: Clinician-assisted tobacco cessation.* San Fransisco, CA: The Regents of the University of California, University of Southern California, and Western University of Health Sciences; 1999–2006. All rights reserved.

9 hours (102). The patch should be worn in a dry, hairless skin area on the upper body or upper outer part of the arm, and to reduce skin irritation, the same area should not be used again for at least 1 week. Insomnia or vivid dreams can occur with the 24-hour patch, in which case the patch should be removed before bedtime or a 16-hour patch should be used.

Bupropion SR, also marketed in the United States as an oral antidepressant agent, is the only nonnicotine formulation with an FDA indication for smoking cessation. Similar to the NRT products, bupropion SR approximately doubles cessation rates compared to placebo (73). This oral tablet is contraindicated in patients with a previous history of seizures, current or prior diagnosis of bulimia or anorexia nervosa, use of monoamine oxidase inhibitors within the previous 14 days, or if taking other medications containing bupropion (64). A combination of nicotine patch and bupropion also can be used, although combination therapy generally is reserved for patients who have failed using monotherapy (64). For a complete list of all the precautions and contraindications of each of the drugs in Table 8.4, clinicians should refer to the manufacturer's complete prescribing information.

SMOKE-FREE ENVIRONMENTS AS A TOBACCO CONTROL TOOL

Smoke-free environments have a beneficial effect on smokers and nonsmokers. The tobacco industry itself recognizes the smokers' concern over SHS as a powerful motivator to quit smoking (7). Smoke-free workplaces have been associated with a 3.8% absolute reduction in smoking prevalence and three fewer cigarettes smoked per day for each continuing smoker (105,106). NRT has been proven successful in aiding smokers to quit, but when comparing a free NRT program against implementing smoke-free workplaces, the latter are nine times even more cost effective per new nonsmoker than the former (107).

Smoke-free environments also protect nonsmokers from the harmful and fast effects of SHS on the CVD. Tobacco control programs, stressing smoke-free environments, have been shown to quickly reduce the burden from heart disease (and lung cancer [108,109]) compared to trends if there is no program (69,110). Therefore, in addition to counseling smokers to quit, cardiologists are obligated to become active in the fight for smoke-free environments. There is little that a cardiologist can do that has the same rapid benefits for his or her patients and their families than help to liberate them from nicotine addiction and SHS exposure.

PERSONAL PERSPECTIVE AND CONTROVERSIES

Despite the overwhelming scientific and medical case that both smoking and passive smoking are leading preventable causes of death as well as the fact that there are established treatments and public policy interventions for reducing this toll, implementation of meaningful tobacco control strategies has moved forward very slowly. Even in 2006, few physicians aggressively intervene either at the level of individual patients or public policy to reduce the toll of smoking. Amazingly, given the strong scientific case, that passive smoking causes heart (and other) diseases, public acceptance of this link remains "controversial" (111).

This slow progress and continuing controversy is not surprising. The tobacco industry, in the last 50 years, has invested in a multimillion dollar campaign to confuse the public and keep this controversy alive to slow the rate of decline in cigarette consumption and the social acceptability of smoking. Worldwide, the industry has secretly hired consultants, sponsored symposia, financed research, and engaged in lobbying to get a more "balanced" view on the issue of SHS and disease (112–114).

In recent years, a new tool has become available to look into the tobacco industry (the vector of the tobacco epidemic). As a result of litigation against the industry, millions of previously secret pages of tobacco industry documents are now available to all via the Internet. Http://legacy.library.ucsf.edu and http://bat.library.ucsf.edu are two of the most comprehensive sites. This resource makes it possible to investigate the authors and conflicts of interest surrounding the publication of papers that differ with the mainstream scientific and medical opinion that SHS is harmful to ones' health.

In recent years, especially in the United States, the tobacco industry has shifted the focus of the debate away from the health effects of SHS over to economic claims that creating smoke-free environments will be disastrous for the hospitality industry. The tobacco industry has invested millions of dollars in the national restaurant association and its international counterparts (115), and, more recently, the gaming industry (116). Despite the fact that all of the high-quality, independently funded, peer-reviewed research in the area of the effects of smoke-free policies on the hospitality industry have consistently shown no effect or a positive effect (117,118), these claims continue to be pressed vigorously to oppose smoke-free public and workplaces. As with the industry's earlier efforts to create controversy about the evidence that smoking and passive smoking is dangerous or nicotine is addictive, these efforts to promote misinformation about the economic impacts of smoking restrictions continues to be widely accepted. It remains a challenge to educate restaurateurs and other people in the hospitality industry to prevent them from becoming the (often unknowing) foot soldiers for the tobacco industry in its effort to maintain sales.

If tobacco were to be introduced today as a new product, there is no doubt that regulatory authorities would simply forbid its introduction. Despite this fact, the tobacco industry remains a powerful political player because of its campaign contributions and generals to many other organizations in the arts, sciences, and elsewhere. Only as institutions concerned with health raise the political cost to other agencies of working with the tobacco industry (including universities, which continue to accept funding from the industry) will this power be attenuated. Although a difficult challenge, there is no question that progress has been made in recent decades. Much remains to be done.

THE FUTURE

The pathophysiology of smoking and passive smoking and CVD—the mechanism are already well known—and the depth of our understanding of the mechanisms for these effects continues to grow. Furthermore, the rapid and substantial benefits of smoking cessation should continue to be confirmed both on individual and societal levels. The fact that many cardiologists and hospitals still do not routinely screen for and treat tobacco use despite the overwhelming evidence of highly cost-effective clinical benefit is a serious shortcoming in current clinical practice. The real challenge remains integrating this knowledge into routine clinical practice at all levels of the medical care system, to make treatment of tobacco addiction as routine and expected as checking blood pressure and treating hypertension when it is identified.

ACKNOWLEDGMENT

We wish to thank Karen S. Hudmon DrPH, MS, RPh, for her comments on the smoking cessation section.

References

1. Centers for Disease Control and Prevention. Annual smoking—attributable mortality, years of potential life lost, and productivity losses—United States, 1997–2001. *MMWR* 2005;54:625–628.
2. Lightwood J, Fleischmann KE, Glantz SA. Smoking cessation in heart failure: it is never too late. *J Am Coll Cardiol* 2001;37:1683–1684.
3. Pierce JP, Gilpin EA. A historical analysis of tobacco marketing and the uptake of smoking by youth in the United States: 1890–1977. *Health Psychol* 1995;14:500–508.
4. World Health Organization (WHO). *Why is tobacco a public health priority?* Geneva: WHO, 2005.
5. Centers for Disease Control and Prevention. Cigarette Smoking Among Adults—United States, 2003. *MMWR* 2005;54:509–513.
6. Gu D, Wu X, Reynolds K, Duan X, et al. Cigarette smoking and exposure to environmental tobacco smoke in China: The International Collaborative Study of Cardiovascular Disease in Asia. *Am J Public Health* 2004;94:1972–1976.
7. Ling PM, Glantz SA. Tobacco industry research on smoking cessation recapturing young adults and other recent quitters. *J Gen Intern Med* 2004;19:419–426.
8. Doll R, Peto R, Boreham J, Sutherland I. Mortality in relation to smoking: 50 years' observations on male British doctors. *BMJ* 2004;328:1519.
9. Shopland DR, Anderson CM, Burns DM, Gerlach KK. Disparities in smoke-free workplace policies among food service workers. *J Occup Environ Med* 2004;46:347–356.
10. Centers for Disease Control and Prevention. *Global youth tobacco survey.* Atlanta: CDC, 2000.
11. Nebot M, Lopez MJ, Gorini G, et al. Environmental tobacco smoke exposure in public places of European cities. *Tob Control* 2005;14:60–63.
12. Navas-Acien A, Peruga A, Breysse P, et al. Secondhand tobacco smoke in public places in Latin America, 2002–2003. *JAMA* 2004;291:2741–2745.
13. Mahonen MS, McElduff P, Dobson AJ, et al. Current smoking and the risk of non-fatal myocardial infarction in the WHO MONICA Project populations. *Tob Control* 2004;13:244–250.
14. Law MR, Morris JK, Wald NJ. Environmental tobacco smoke exposure and ischaemic heart disease: an evaluation of the evidence. *BMJ* 1997;315: 973–980.
15. U.S. Department of Health and Human Services. *Women and smoking: a report of the Surgeon General.* Washington, DC: USDHHS, 2001.
16. Benowitz NL. Cigarette smoking and cardiovascular disease: pathophysiology and implications for treatment* 1. *Prog Cardiovasc Dis* 2003;46:91–111.
17. U.S. Department of Health and Human Services. *The health consequences of smoking. A report of the Surgeon General.* Washington, DC: Centers for Disease Control and Prevention, National Center for Chronic Disease Prevention and Health Promotion, Office on Smoking and Health, 2004.
18. Isselbacher EM. Thoracic and abdominal aortic aneurysms. *Circulation* 2005;111:816–828.
19. Gocmez SS, Utkan T, Duman C, et al. Secondhand tobacco smoke impairs neurogenic and endothelium-dependent relaxation of rabbit corpus cavernosum smooth muscle: improvement with chronic oral administration of L-arginine. *Int J Impot Res* 2005;17:437–444.
20. McVary KT, Carrier S, Wessells H. Smoking and erectile dysfunction: evidence based analysis. *J Urol* 2001;166:1624–1632.
21. Barnoya J, Glantz SA. Cardiovascular effects of secondhand smoke: nearly as large as smoking. *Circulation* 2005;111:2684–2698.
22. Thun M, Henley J, Apicella L. Epidemiologic studies of fatal and nonfatal cardiovascular disease and ETS exposure from spousal smoking. *Environ Health Perspect* 1999;107[Suppl 6]:841–846.
23. Whincup PH, Gilg JA, Emberson JR, et al. Passive smoking and risk of coronary heart disease and stroke: prospective study with cotinine measurement. *BMJ* doi:2004:bmj.38146.427188.55.
24. Celermajer DS, Adams MR, Clarkson P, et al. Passive smoking and impaired endothelium-dependent arterial dilatation in healthy young adults. *N Engl J Med* 1996;334:150–154.
25. Otsuka R, Watanabe H, Hirata K, et al. Acute effects of passive smoking on the coronary circulation in healthy young adults. *JAMA* 2001;286: 436–441.
26. Sun YP, Zhu BQ, Browne AE, et al. Nicotine does not influence arterial lipid deposits in rabbits exposed to second-hand smoke. *Circulation* 2001; 104:810–4.

27. Glantz S, Parmley W. Passive smoking and heart disease. Epidemiology, physiology, and biochemistry. *Circulation* 1991;83:1–12.
28. Brook RD, Franklin B, Cascio W, et al. Air pollution and cardiovascular disease: a statement for healthcare professionals from the Expert Panel on Population and Prevention Science of the American Heart Association. *Circulation* 2004;109:2655–2671.
29. Jaimes EA, DeMaster EG, Tian RX, Raij L. Stable compounds of cigarette smoke induce endothelial superoxide anion production via NADPH oxidase activation. *Arterioscler Thromb Vasc Biol* 2004;24:1031–1036.
30. Schmid P, Karanikas G, Kritz H, et al. Passive smoking and platelet thromboxane. *Thrombosis Res* 1996;81:451–460.
31. Hung J, Lam JY, Lacoste L, Letchacovski G. Cigarette smoking acutely increases platelet thrombus formation in patients with coronary artery disease taking aspirin. *Circulation* 1995;92:2432–2436.
32. Burghuber OC, Punzengruber C, Sinzinger H, et al. Platelet sensitivity to prostacyclin in smokers and non-smokers. *Chest* 1986;90:34–38.
33. Ramachandran J, Rubenstein D, Bluestein D, Jesty J. Activation of platelets exposed to shear stress in the presence of extracts of low-nicotine and zero-nicotine cigarettes: The protective effect of nicotine. *Nicotine Tob Res* 2004;6:835–841.
34. Morita H, Ikeda H, Haramaki N, et al. Only two-week smoking cessation improves platelet aggregability and intraplatelet redox imbalance of long-term smokers. *J Am Coll Cardiol* 2005;45:589–594.
35. Lerman A, Zeiher AM. Endothelial function: cardiac events. *Circulation* 2005;111:363–368.
36. Kato M, Roberts-Thomson P, Phillips BG, et al. The effects of short-term passive smoke exposure on endothelium-dependent and independent vasodilation. *J Hypertens* 1999;17:1395–1401.
37. Davis J, Shelton L, Watanabe I, Arnold J. Passive smoking affects endothelium and platelets. *Arch Intern Med* 1989;149:386–389.
38. Davis JW, Hartman CR, Lewis HD Jr, et al. Cigarette smoking-induced enhancement of platelet function: Lack of prevention by aspirin in men with coronary artery disease. *J Lab Clin Med* 1985;105:479–483.
39. Celermajer DS, Sorensen KE, Georgakopoulos D, et al. Cigarette smoking is associated with dose-related and potentially reversible impairment of endothelium-dependent dilation in healthy young adults. *Circulation* 1993;88:2149–2155.
40. Raitakari OT, Adams MR, McCredie RJ, et al. Arterial endothelial dysfunction related to passive smoking is potentially reversible in healthy young adults. *Ann Intern Med* 1999;130:578–581.
41. Barua RS, Ambrose JA, Eales-Reynolds LJ, et al. Dysfunctional endothelial nitric oxide biosynthesis in healthy smokers with impaired endothelium-dependent vasodilatation. *Circulation* 2001;104:1905–1910.
42. Barua RS, Ambrose JA, Eales-Reynolds L-J, et al. Heavy and light cigarette smokers have similar dysfunction of endothelial vasoregulatory activity: an in vivo and in vitro correlation. *J Am Coll Cardiol* 2002;39:1758–1763.
43. Hutchison SJ, Reitz MS, Sudhir K, et al. Chronic dietary L-arginine prevents endothelial dysfunction secondary to environmental tobacco smoke in normocholesterolemic rabbits. *Hypertension* 1997;29:1186–1191.
44. Hutchison SJ, Sudhir K, Sievers RE, et al. Effects of L-arginine on atherogenesis and endothelial dysfunction due to secondhand smoke. *Hypertension* 1999;34:44–50.
45. Campisi R, Czernin J, Schoder H, et al. L-Arginine normalizes coronary vasomotion in long-term smokers. *Circulation* 1999;99:491–497.
46. Valkonen M, Kuusi T. Passive smoking induces atherogenic changes in low-density lipoprotein. *Circulation* 1998;97:2012–2016.
47. Ambrose JA, Barua RS. The pathophysiology of cigarette smoking and cardiovascular disease: An update. *J Am Coll Cardiol* 2004;43:1731–1737.
48. Panagiotakos DB, Pitsavos C, Chrysohoou C, et al. Effect of exposure to secondhand smoke on markers of inflammation: the ATTICA study* 1. *Am J Med* 2004;116:145–150.
49. Libby P, Theroux P. Pathophysiology of coronary artery disease. *Circulation* 2005;111:3481–3488.
50. Ohsawa M, Okayama A, Nakamura M, et al. CRP levels are elevated in smokers but unrelated to the number of cigarettes and are decreased by long-term smoking cessation in male smokers. *Prev Med* 2005;41:651–656.
51. Tribble DL, Giuliano LJ, Fortmann SP. Reduced plasma ascorbic acid concentrations in nonsmokers regularly exposed to environmental tobacco smoke. *Am J Clin Nutr* 1993;58:886–890.
52. Mannino DM, Mulinare J, Ford ES, Schwartz J. Tobacco smoke exposure and decreased serum and red blood cell folate levels: data from the Third National Health and Nutrition Examination Survey. *Nicotine Tob Res* 2003;5:357–362.
53. Dietrich M, Block G, Norkus EP, et al. Smoking and exposure to environmental tobacco smoke decrease some plasma antioxidants and increase γ-tocopherol in vivo after adjustment for dietary antioxidant intakes. *Am J Clin Nutr* 2003;77:160–166.
54. Cryer PE, Haymond MW, Santiago JV, Shah SD. Norepinephrine and epinephrine release and adrenergic mediation of smoking-associated hemodynamic and metabolic events. *N Engl J Med* 1976;295:573–577.
55. Gvozdjakova A, Kucharska J, Gvozdjak J. Effect of smoking on the oxidative processes of cardiomyocytes. *Cardiology* 1992;1992:81–84.
56. Knight-Lozano CA, Young CG, Burow DL, et al. Cigarette smoke exposure and hypercholesterolemia increase mitochondrial damage in cardiovascular tissues. *Circulation* 2002;105:849–854.
57. Pope CA 3rd, Eatough DJ, Gold DR, et al. Acute exposure to environmental tobacco smoke and heart rate variability. *Environ Health Perspect* 2001;109:711–716.
58. Mahmud A, Feely J. Effect of Smoking on Arterial Stiffness and Pulse Pressure Amplification. *Hypertension* 2003;41:183–187.
59. Mahmud A, Feely J. Effects of passive smoking on blood pressure and aortic pressure waveform in healthy young adults—influence of gender. *Br J Clin Pharmacol* 2004;57:37–43.
60. Stefanadis C, Tsiamis E, Vlachopoulos C, et al. Unfavorable effect of smoking on the elastic properties of the human aorta. *Circulation* 1997;95:31–38.
61. Stefanadis C, Vlachopoulos C, Tsiamis E, et al. Unfavorable effects of passive smoking on aortic function in men. *Ann Intern Med* 1998;128: 426–434.
62. Nelson DE, Giovino GA, Emont SL, et al. Trends in cigarette smoking among US physicians and nurses. *JAMA* 1994;271:1273–1275.
63. Barnoya J, Glantz S. Knowledge and use of tobacco among Guatemalan physicians. *Cancer Causes Control* 2002;13:879–881.
64. Fiore MC, Bailey W, Cohen S, et al. *Treating tobacco use and dependence. Clinical practice guideline*. Rockville, MD: U.S. Department of Health and Human Services. Public Health Services, 2000.
65. Centers for Disease Control and Prevention. Tobacco use and cessation counseling—global health professionals survey pilot study, 10 countries, 2005. *MMWR* 2005;54:505–509.
66. Ferry LH, Grissino LM, Runfola PS. Tobacco dependence curricula in US undergraduate medical education. *JAMA* 1999;282:825–829.
67. Doescher MP, Saver BG. Physicians' advice to quit smoking. The glass remains half empty. *J Fam Pract* 2000;49:543–547.
68. Schroeder SA. Tobacco control in the wake of the 1998 master settlement agreement. *N Engl J Med* 2004;350:293–301.
69. Fichtenberg CM, Glantz SA. Association of the California Tobacco Control Program with declines in cigarette consumption and mortality from heart disease. *N Engl J Med* 2000;343:1772–1777.
70. Fichtenberg CM, Glantz SA. Controlling tobacco Use. *N Engl J Med* 2001; 344:1798–1799.
71. Parrott S, Godfrey C. Economics of smoking cessation. *BMJ* 2004;328: 947–949.
72. Centers for Disease Control and Prevention. Cigarette smoking among adults—United States, 2000. *MMWR* 2002;51:642–645.
73. Hughes J, Stead L, Lancaster T. Antidepressants for smoking cessation. *Cochrane Database Syst Rev* 2004:CD000031.
74. Silagy C, Lancaster T, Stead L, et al. Nicotine replacement therapy for smoking cessation. *Cochrane Database Syst Rev* 2004:CD000146.
75. Barzilai DA, Goodwin MA, Zyzanski SJ, Stange KC. Does health habit counseling affect patient satisfaction? *Prev Med* 2001;33:595–599.
76. Anthonisen NR, Skeans MA, Wise RA, et al. The effects of a smoking cessation intervention on 14.5-year mortality: a randomized clinical trial. *Ann Intern Med* 2005;142:233–239.
77. van Domburg RT, Meeter K, van Berkel DFM, et al. Smoking cessation reduces mortality after coronary artery bypass surgery: a 20-year follow-up study. *J Am Coll Cardiol* 2000;36:878–883.
78. Suskin N, Sheth T, Negassa A, Yusuf S. Relationship of current and past smoking to mortality and morbidity in patients with left ventricular dysfunction* 1. *J Am Coll Cardiol* 2001;37:1677–1682.
79. Effect of metoprolol CR/XL in chronic heart failure: Metoprolol CR/XL Randomised Intervention Trial in Congestive Heart Failure (MERIT-HF). *Lancet* 1999;353:2001–2007.
80. Pitt B, Zannad F, Remme WJ, et al. The effect of spironolactone on morbidity and mortality in patients with severe heart failure. Randomized Aldactone Evaluation Study Investigators. *N Engl J Med* 1999;341:709–717.
81. Effect of enalapril on survival in patients with reduced left ventricular ejection fractions and congestive heart failure. The SOLVD Investigators. *N Engl J Med* 1991;325:293–302.
82. Wasley MA, McNagny SE, Phillips VL, Ahluwalia JS. The cost-effectiveness of the nicotine transdermal patch for smoking cessation. *Prev Med* 1997;26:264–270.
83. Boyko WL Jr, Glick HA, Schulman KA. Economics and cost-effectiveness in evaluating the value of cardiovascular therapies. ACE inhibitors in the management of congestive heart failure: comparative economic data. *Am Heart J* 1999;137:S115–119.
84. Delea TE, Vera-Llonch M, Richner RE, et al. Cost effectiveness of carvedilol for heart failure. *Am J Cardiol* 1999;83:890–896.
85. Vanderhoff BT, Ruppel HM, Amsterdam PB. Carvedilol: the new role of beta blockers in congestive heart failure. *Am Fam Physician* 1998;58:1627–1634, 1641–1642.
86. Shiffman S, Dresler CM, Hajek P, et al. Efficacy of a nicotine lozenge for smoking cessation. *Arch Intern Med* 2002;162:1267–1276.
87. Zhu SH, Anderson CM, Tedeschi GJ, et al. Evidence of real-world effectiveness of a telephone quitline for smokers. *N Engl J Med* 2002;347: 1087–1093.
88. Tomson T, Helgason AR, Gilljam H. Quitline in smoking cessation: a cost-effectiveness analysis. *Int J Technol Assess Health Care* 2004;20:469–474.
89. Ossip-Klein DJ, McIntosh S. Quitlines in North America: evidence base and applications. *Am J Med Sci* 2003;326:201–205.
90. Ayanian JZ, Cleary PD. Perceived risks of heart disease and cancer among cigarette smokers. *JAMA* 1999;281:1019–1021.

91. Weinstein ND, Marcus SE, Moser RP. Smokers' unrealistic optimism about their risk. *Tob Control* 2005;14:55–59.
92. Lightwood JM, Glantz SA. Short-term economic and health benefits of smoking cessation: myocardial infarction and stroke. *Circulation* 1997;96:1089–1096.
93. Pierce JP, Gilpin EA. Impact of over-the-counter sales on effectiveness of pharmaceutical aids for smoking cessation. *JAMA* 2002;288:1260–1264.
94. Hassmiller KM, Warner KE, Mendez D, et al. Nondaily smokers: who are they? *Am J Public Health* 2003;93:1321–1327.
95. Meine TJ, Patel MR, Washam JB, et al. Safety and effectiveness of transdermal nicotine patch in smokers admitted with acute coronary syndromes. *Am J Cardiol* 2005;95:976–978.
96. Kimmel SE, Berlin JA, Miles C, et al. Risk of acute first myocardial infarction and use of nicotine patches in a general population. *J Am Coll Cardiol* 2001;37:1297–1302.
97. National Cancer Institute. *Health effects of exposure to environmental tobacco smoke: The report of the California Environmental Protection Agency, Smoking and Tobacco Control* [Monograph no. 10; Report No.: NIH Pub. No, 99-4645]. Bethesda, MD: Department of Health and Human Services, National Institutes of Health, National Cancer Institute, 1999.
98. Benowitz N, Dempsey D. Pharmacotherapy for smoking cessation during pregnancy. *Nicotine Tob Res* 2004;6[Suppl 2]:S189–S202.
99. Fang WL, Goldstein AO, Butzen AY, et al. Smoking cessation in pregnancy: a review of postpartum relapse prevention strategies. *J Am Board Fam Pract* 2004;17:264–275.
100. Benowitz NL. Cigarette smoking and nicotine addiction. *Med Clin North Am* 1992;76:415–437.
101. Hughes JR, Gust SW, Skoog K, et al. Symptoms of tobacco withdrawal. A replication and extension. *Arch Gen Psychiatry* 1991;48:52–59.
102. Fagerstrom KO. Nicotine-replacement therapies. In: Ferrence R, Slade J, Room R, Pope M, eds. *Nicotine and public health*. Washington, DC: American Public Health Association, 2000:199–207.
103. *Rx for change: Clinician-assisted tobacco cessation*. San Francisco, CA: The Regents of the University of California, University of Southern California, and Western University of Health Sciences; 1999–2005.
104. Schneider NG, Lunell E, Olmstead RE, Fagerstrom KO. Clinical pharmacokinetics of nasal nicotine delivery. A review and comparison to other nicotine systems. *Clin Pharmacokinet* 1996;31:65–80.
105. Fichtenberg CM, Glantz SA. Effect of smoke-free workplaces on smoking behaviour: systematic review. *BMJ* 2002;325:188.
106. Bauer JE, Hyland A, Li Q, et al. A longitudinal assessment of the impact of smoke-free worksite policies on tobacco use. *Am J Public Health* 2005; 95:1024–1029.
107. Ong MK, Glantz SA. Free nicotine replacement therapy programs vs implementing smoke-free workplaces: a cost-effectiveness comparison. *Am J Public Health* 2005;95:969–975.
108. Barnoya J, Glantz S. Association of the California tobacco control program with declines in lung cancer incidence. *Cancer Causes Control* 2004;15: 689–695.
109. Jemal A, Cokkinides VE, Shafey O, Thun MJ. Lung cancer trends in young adults: an early indicator of progress in tobacco control (United States). *Cancer Causes Control* 2003;14:579–585.
110. Sargent RP, Shepard RM, Glantz SA. Reduced incidence of admissions for myocardial infarction associated with public smoking ban: before and after study. *BMJ* 2004;328:977–980.
111. Kennedy GE, Bero LA. Print media coverage of research on passive smoking. *Tob Control* 1999;8:254–260.
112. Barnoya J, Glantz S. Tobacco industry success in preventing regulation of secondhand smoke in Latin America: the "Latin Project." *Tob Control* 2002;11:305–314.
113. Muggli ME, Hurt RD, Blanke DD. Science for hire: a tobacco industry strategy to influence public opinion on secondhand smoke. *Nicotine Tob Res* 2003;5:303–314.
114. Assunta M, Fields N, Knight J, Chapman S. "Care and feeding": the Asian environmental tobacco consultants programme. *Tob Control* 2004;13[Suppl 2]:4–12.
115. Dearlove JV, Bialous SA, Glantz SA. Tobacco industry manipulation of the hospitality industry to maintain smoking in public places. *Tob Control* 2002;11:94–104.
116. Mandel LL, Glantz SA. Hedging their bets: tobacco and gambling industries work against smoke-free policies. *Tob Control* 2004;13:268–276.
117. Scollo M, Lal A, Hyland A, Glantz S. Review of the quality of studies on the economic effects of smoke-free policies on the hospitality industry. *Tob Control* 2003;12:13–20.
118. Alamar BC, Glantz SA. Smoke-free ordinances increase restaurant profit and value. *Contemp Econ Policy* 2004;22:520–525.
119. Iso H, Shimamoto T, Sato S, et al. Passive smoking and plasma fibrinogen concentrations. *Am J Epidemiol* 1996;144:1151–1154.
120. Moffatt RJ, Stamford BA, Biggerstaff KD. Influence of worksite environmental tobacco smoke on serum lipoprotein profiles of female nonsmokers. *Metabolism* 1995;44:1536–1539.
121. Howard G, Wagenknecht LE, Burke GL, et al. Cigarette smoking and progression of atherosclerosis: The Atherosclerosis Risk in Communities (ARIC) Study. *JAMA* 1998;279:119–124.
122. Ayaori M, Hisada T, Suzukawa M, et al. Plasma levels and redox status of ascorbic acid and levels of lipid peroxidation products in active and passive smokers. *Environ Health Perspect* 2000;108:105–108.
123. Strauss RS. Environmental tobacco smoke and serum vitamin C levels in children. *Pediatrics* 2001;107:540–542.
124. Alberg AJ, Chen JC, Zhao H, et al. Household exposure to passive cigarette smoking and serum micronutrient concentrations. *Am J Clin Nutr* 2000;72:1576–1582.

CHAPTER 9 ■ ESTROGEN, FEMALE GENDER, AND HEART DISEASE

PATHMAJA PARAMSOTHY AND ROBERT H. KNOPP

OVERVIEW

Death from cardiovascular disease (CVD), meaning heart disease and stroke, is slightly more common in women than in men. CVD in women is a formidable problem because of difficulties in diagnosis and increased morbidity and mortality associated with CVD events at all ages. In the middle years, CVD is associated with multiple risk factors, generally more in women than in men of the same age. Among these, diabetes is a more severe risk factor in women than in men, raising CVD rates in women to those of men. Insulin resistance, obesity, and the metabolic syndrome also function in the same way. An example of this relationship is the greater risk of high triglyceride and low high-density lipoprotein (HDL) for CVD in women compared to men. In contrast, low-density lipoprotein (LDL) seems to be the more predominant CVD predictor in men. Smoking is also a very serious CVD risk factor in women. In the context of oral contraceptive use, smoking can multiply CVD risk many times. Postmenopausally, hormone replacement therapy (HRT) does not prevent CVD in women at mean ages of 64 and 67 years in two prospective trials. An increase in stroke incidence was observed in one of these trials. In contrast, estrogen may have CVD benefit if given before the development of advanced atherosclerosis, for instance at the time of menopause. On the other hand, women with advanced CVD at the time of menopause or combinations of risk factors may have increased risk from estrogen. Thus, complete risk factor assessment, including noninvasive vascular testing and careful clinical judgment are advisable in starting HRT at the time of menopause. The estrogen patch is an attractive modality of estrogen delivery, because it avoids the first-pass hepatic effect of oral estrogens on clotting factors. Potential distinctions among the vascular effects of the available progestins have not been ruled out.

GLOSSARY

Combined hyperlipidemia: The combined elevations of triglycerides above 200 mg/dL and LDL-C levels above National Cholesterol Education Program (NCEP) targets: 70, 100, 130, or 160 mg/dL.

Cholesterol ester transport protein (CETP): A protein that recycles cholesterol from HDL to LDL, thereby conserving the body's cholesterol.

Lipoprotein(a) [Lp(a)]: A protein on LDL that inhibits fibrinolysis in arterial clots, enhances LDL trapping in the arterial wall, and is risk factor for premature CVD, particularly in women.

Polycystic ovary syndrome (PCOS): A common manifestation of insulin resistance in young women, characterized by infertility, anovulation, hyperandrogenemia, irregular menses, and often obesity.

Remnant lipoprotein: An atherogenic particle, intermediate between very-low-density lipoprotein (VLDL) and LDL in size and metabolism having atherogenic potential.

Metabolic syndrome: A syndrome of insulin resistance in which at least three of the following five abnormalities are seen: abdominal obesity, hypertriglyceridemia, low HDL, hypertension, and increased fasting glucose.

The main points of this chapter are illustrated in the following true case. A 25-year-old woman who used oral contraceptives (OCs) and smoked one pack of cigarettes per day had vague chest pains for a year, initially diagnosed as anxiety and acid reflux. On July 4, 2000, she was seen at an emergency room (ER) for chest pain and sent away. Twelve hours later at the same ER, the possibility of a myocardial infarction (MI) was entertained as she went into shock. An emergency two-vessel angioplasty procedure was performed, saving the patient's life. Several other angioplasties and three-vessel bypass surgery have been done since, complicated by bilateral iliac vessel stenosis. She is now somewhat intellectually impaired. In clinic, her cholesterol was 182 mg/dL, triglyceride was 175 mg/dL, and HDL cholesterol (HDL-C) was 24 mg/dL on 40 mg atorvastatin. Her lipoprotein (a) [Lp(a)] level was 30 mg/dL, the seventy-fifth percentile.

Important questions are raised by this case. Why did this patient have an MI? Why was the MI not recognized during the ER room visit? Is this case really rare? Is the presentation and risk profile unique to this case or to women in general? What is the approach to managing this patient's lipid disorder? This chapter attempts to address these issues.

INCIDENCE OF CORONARY ARTERY DISEASE IN WOMEN VERSUS MEN

The perception persists that coronary artery disease (CAD) among women is uncommon, especially in the young, and that arteriosclerotic disease is less important overall. These perceptions are incorrect. CVD is an equal opportunity killer in men and women over their lifetimes. In Washington State, the incidence of CVD death was 42% in women and 39% in men in 1991 and 33% in women and 32% in men in 2003 (1,2). Nationwide, these numbers approach 50%. The slightly higher percentage of female cardiovascular deaths can be attributed to the greater longevity of women, age being an extremely powerful risk factor in its own right. Greater longevity allows female CVD mortality to "catch up" in old age, particularly with stroke, 9.4% in women versus 6.2% in men (2).

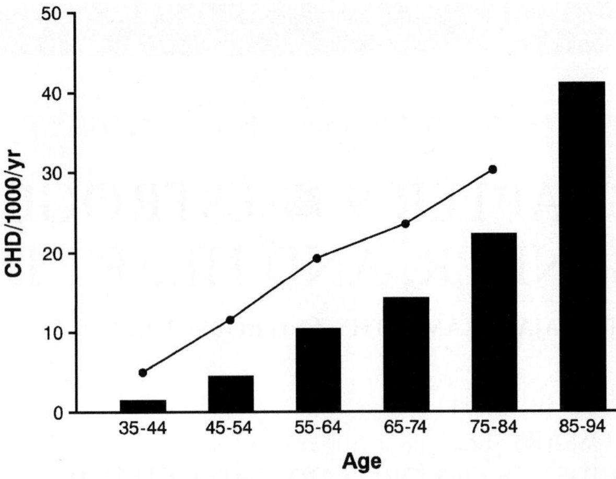

FIGURE 9.1. Annual rate of CHD in men (*line*) and women (*bars*), from the Framingham Heart Study. (*Source:* From Castelli WP. Cardiovascular disease in women. *Am J Obstet Gynecol* 1988;158:1553–1560, with permission.)

In youth, CVD rates are certainly lower in women than in men. However, the rate is not negligible and has defined relationships to cardiovascular risk factors. As shown in Figure 9.1, the increase in CVD with age in women in the Framingham study (3) is parallel to men but is delayed by 10 to 15 years. A similar delay in women is seen even in high-risk conditions such as heterozygous familial hypercholesterolemia. The delay in onset is attributed to the premenopausal exposure to endogenous ovarian estrogen, but is not immune to advancing age (Fig. 9.1). A slight increase in the female risk curve around the time of menopause may reflect the lack of estrogen (Fig. 9.1). Some women develop menopause early (especially smokers), and plasma estrogen levels decline in the 40s (a number of years before menopause), possibly contributing to an acceleration of atherogenesis prior to menopause.

The importance of CVD in young women can be appreciated by comparing CVD death rates in women to other causes of mortality. Since 1982, heart disease mortality has occurred at a rate of approximately 11 per 100,000 in women ages 25 to 45 years with little decline, reflecting the level rates for CVD in women overall in the last decade (4). The decline in Washington state since 1991 may be atypical (2). Among young women, approximately one third of heart disease deaths are coronary in etiology. In men ages 25 to 44 years, the CVD rate is approximately 30 per 100,000—almost 10 times more common than in women. As for other causes of mortality in women, cancer accounts for 29 per 100,000 and injuries for 14 per 100,000 (5). In a study of ER admissions among young persons (ages 18 to 45 years) for sudden death, 1 of 20 cases of coronary disease was in a young woman (6). In another study, one fourth of all MI survivors younger than 40 years at a major hospital were women (7). The main point is that CVD incidence in younger women is not negligible, ranging from one fourth to one twentieth the rate in men.

The early lesions of arteriosclerosis—fatty streaks and fibrous plaques—are seen in both young women and men. Half of the men and one fourth of the women in Bogalusa were so affected. Among blacks, men and women were affected equally. In both genders, the fatty streak lesions were proportional to the plasma LDL-C. However, the plasma very-low-density lipoprotein cholesterol (VLDL-C) level (8), was also associated with lesions, but only in women. When coronary lesions are examined, those in women are more lipid filled, rich in macrophages, and less densely fibrous (9). Thus, lesions in women could be more unstable under certain circumstances, as well as more readily reversed (10). Likewise, coronary calcification is half that of men on ultrafast computed tomography until age 60 years, when the difference between the genders narrows (11).

An excess of acute MI among young black women was observed in Bogalusa (8) and is confirmed nationally, where black women have a 50% to 75% greater risk of death from heart since 1950 (12) and into the 1990s (4). Age adjusted rates, per 100,000, were 190 for blacks and 110 for whites in 1988 (12). The reasons for this greater risk may reflect a greater CVD risk burden among African American women.

DIFFERENCES IN CARDIOVASCULAR DISEASE PRESENTATION, MANAGEMENT, AND OUTCOME IN WOMEN VERSUS MEN

The tendency to overlook CVD in women is compounded by a less classical presentation, which is more frequently angina in women compared to MI in men. Among women participating in the Framingham study, the annual incidence of angina pectoris exceeded that of MI by more than 2:1 in the age range of 45 to 64 years. In contrast, frank MI exceeded angina in men of all age groups, ranging from 1.5:1 between ages 45 and 64 years to 6.5:1 between ages 75 and 84 years (13,14). In a recent study, women presenting for stenting had fewer MIs than men (15).

Recognition of cardiac chest pain is difficult in women because it is unexpected, often atypical, and more often noncardiac than in men. Misdiagnosis as chronic fatigue or a psychiatric disorder is not uncommon. The greater incidence of silent MI in women (14) may also be related to the atypicality of presentation. For example, one of our patients complained of early fatigability with exercise but had no ST changes on treadmill testing. Eventually, she developed overt angina and had bypass surgery whereupon the fatigue resolved. Anatomic studies might have been done earlier if her severe combined hyperlipidemia, elevated Lp(a), and impaired fasting glucose (see the section Lipid Screening Guidelines for Hyperlipidemic Women) had been appreciated.

This case also illustrates the point that exercise tolerance testing in women is more susceptible to false-positive and false-negative results than in men. If doubt persists after a negative exercise test, radionuclide or echocardiographic imaging may be ordered after exercise (16,17). Furthermore, a normal or negative angiogram does not necessarily mean that early atherosclerosis or endothelial dysfunction is not present, especially in women with risk factors.

Frank MI in women has higher morbidity and mortality than in men. Sudden death is more frequent, and early post-MI mortality is greater in women than in men (18–20). Nearly all of the excess mortality in women is concentrated in the first 4 weeks post MI (Fig. 9.2). These data influence all subsequent statistics. After 1 year, a mortality rate of 32% in women versus 16% in men has been observed in the Framingham study (21,22). Thus, post-event, nonadjusted mortality is approximately 50% greater in women than in men for various intervals. These trends were confirmed recently and extended (23) with a higher risk for death relative to younger men (24).

Revascularization procedures including percutaneous intervention and bypass surgery also show greater short- and long-term morbidity and mortality in women than in men, although the probability of benefit remains high in both genders (25–27). Percutaneous interventions in women with coronary ischemia are associated with increased complications and decreased benefits (28,29). An analysis of stent experience from Germany found rates of death and MI greater in women at 30 days (3.1% versus 1.8% in men) but equal after 1 year (6.0 versus 5.8%) (15). Male–female differences in clinical presentation and prognosis are summarized in Table 9.1.

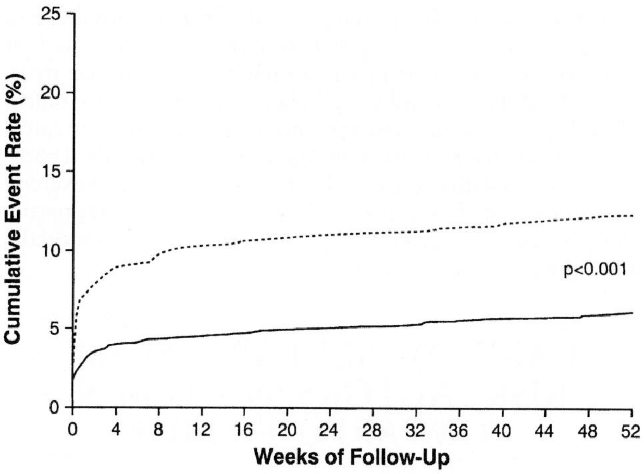

FIGURE 9.2. One-year Kaplan-Meier mortality curves for women and men. The solid line represents men; the dashed line represents women. (*Source:* From Becker RC, Terrin M, Ross R, et al. Comparison of clinical outcomes for women and men after acute myocardial infarction. *Ann Intern Med* 1994;120:635–645, with permission.)

As to whether a frank bias exists in physician management of coronary disease and cardiac catheterization between the genders, two investigations indicate that less aggressive decision making is appropriate in women at low risk for cardiac death and little probability of benefit (30,31), or with angina pectoris (32). A recent study found more orders for do not resuscitate, less aspirin prescription, and less thrombolytic therapy in women compared to men with acute MI (33). The gender difference persists in the latest reports, especially in African American women. Specifically, reperfusion therapy was done post MI in 86.5% of white men, 83.3% of white women, 80.4% of black men, and 77.8% of black women (34). Ultimately, a woman's care depends greatly on the interaction between patient and physician (35).

TABLE 9.1

DIFFERENCES IN CVD PRESENTATION AND OUTCOME IN WOMEN VERSUS MEN

	Comparison of women and men
PRESENTATION	
Angina	W > M
Atypical chest pain	W > M
Death from MI	W > M
Sudden death	W > M
False-positive exercise test	W > M
Angina prognosis for MI	W < M
CONSEQUENCES	
MI morbidity	W > M
MI morbidity (unadjusted)	W > M
MI mortality (adjusted)	W = to slightly > M
Coronary artery bypass graft mortality	W = to > M
Angioplasty mortality (adjusted and unadjusted)	W > M
Stenting death and MI	W ≥ M[a]

Abbreviations: M, men; MI, myocardial infarction; W, women.
[a]W > M at 30 days, W = M at 1 year.

The most important message from the greater morbidity and mortality associated with coronary disease in women is that high priority should be given to early recognition and treatment of risk factors and early ischemic symptoms in women. The other point is that obscure symptoms of fatigue or atypical chest pain should be worked up aggressively for potential coronary ischemia with exercise or vasodilator stress (when exercise is contraindicated) and myocardial perfusion imaging, particularly when risk factors for CAD are present and especially when present in combination.

CARDIOVASCULAR DISEASE RISK FACTORS IN WOMEN COMPARED TO MEN

Hypertension and smoking are risk factors for coronary disease in women as they are in men (13). Smoking was the worst of any single risk factor among male subjects (36), but seemed to have less impact among females. Nonetheless, in a study of 119,404 female nurses, the cardiovascular risk of smoking was clear (37) and appeared to be increasing in severity in recent birth cohorts (38). The interaction of smoking with OC use is also very strong (see the section Oral Contraceptive Use and Cardiovascular Disease Risk). Lp(a), fibrinogen, and homocysteine all function as risk factors in women, as well as in men (39–41). C-reactive protein (CRP), a marker of inflammation, is a strong and independent risk factor for CHD in women (41). Abdominal obesity, weight gain since age 18, and increments in body weight—even at body mass indexes less than 27—are associated with increased CVD incidence in women (42). Some of this association may be mediated by the strong CRP association with abdominal obesity (43). Two other risk factors in women are marital stress (44) and the initial days of the menstrual cycle (45).

Diabetes, elevated triglyceride, and low HDL levels are stronger risk factors for CVD in women than men. Diabetes confers a greater increment of susceptibility to atherosclerosis in women than men, resulting in diabetic women having an absolute coronary disease rate equaling or approaching that of men (46–48). Diabetes may confer a greater mortality risk than having a prior MI (without diabetes) in women (48). The exaggerated diabetic effect on CVD in women is most marked in middle-aged women and attenuates with age, as does the cholesterol effect owing to the increased incidence of coronary disease from other causes, especially age (49). The greater impact of diabetes on CVD in women compared to men is due to more greatly disturbed lipoprotein levels in women compared to men (50–52), as well as the other classical CVD risk factors (51). Whether female gender exaggerates additional atherogenic mechanisms in diabetes such as lipoprotein oxidation and glycoxidation requires further study.

Total plasma cholesterol relates to heart disease risk differently in women than in men. The increment in CVD in men from a low- to a high-cholesterol level is nearly 10-fold in men aged 35 years but attenuates with increasing age to only 1.2-fold by age 65 years. In women aged 65 years, the increase in CVD risk associated with high cholesterol is twofold, but at an absolute increment similar to men: 2.4% versus 1.9%. This trend persists to old age, where LDL has stronger relative risk in women than men (53). Again, the decline in relative risk of cholesterol is because of the dilution of this effect by the increased rate of CVD with age.

The cluster of risk factors associated with CVD in middle age also differs between men and women. Because women tend to be protected compared to men and have a 10- to 15-year delay in the curve describing the rise in CVD (see Fig. 9.1), it follows that for a woman to have coronary disease in middle age, she must have more risk factors or a greater risk burden than a man to experience CAD, as seen in many studies (15,54).

The leading condition embodying multiple risk factors is the metabolic syndrome, arising from obesity and insulin resistance (55). The metabolic syndrome is defined as having three of five criteria, namely, abdominal obesity; elevated blood pressure, glucose; and triglycerides; and decreased HDL-C (56). The two lipid criteria define combined hyperlipidemia (57,58). Clotting factor abnormalities are also associated, including elevated factor VII and plasminogen activator inhibitor-1 levels as are markers of inflammation such as CRP and serum amyloid A (SAA), which is associated with a dysfunctional, "inflammatory HDL" (59). Thus, a single entity, the metabolic syndrome, may embody three to eight risk factors or more and cause premature CAD in middle aged women.

Coronary disease in middle-aged women is highly associated with the metabolic syndrome. Diabetes and hypertension are overrepresented three- and five-fold, respectively, in women with coronary disease compared to women without. In addition, diabetes, hypertension, and hyperlipidemia are present in more women than men with acute MI in virtually every study (15,18–20,25,30,35,60–63). In the recent WISE study, the metabolic syndrome predicted coronary disease, whereas obesity alone did not (64).

Plasma triglyceride and HDL abnormalities are stronger risk predictors for CAD in women compared to men. Triglyceride elevations are associated with a 1.8-fold increase in CVD risk in women compared to a 1.2-fold increase in risk in men (65). Similarly, a reduction in HDL-C is more strongly associated with CVD risk in women than in men. A 1 mg/dL drop in HDL-C is associated with a 3% to 4% increase in CAD in women compared to a 2% increment in coronary disease in men (66).

The importance of triglyceride and HDL to CVD in women is confirmed when coronary arteriosclerosis is graded according to angiographic severity. Elevated total cholesterol, LDL-C, and apoprotein B are most strongly associated with severity in men. In contrast, elevated VLDL-C, intermediate-density lipoprotein cholesterol, LDL triglyceride, and low apoprotein A-I levels are most strongly associated with severity in women (67). Again, lipid abnormalities of the metabolic syndrome predominate over LDL as CVD risk factors in women.

In women, an early manifestation of the metabolic syndrome is polycystic ovary syndrome (PCOS), with the features of hyperandrogenemia, irregular periods, and male pattern baldness. Such individuals typically have the lipid profile of combined hyperlipidemia. Conversely, women with CAD more frequently have a history of PCOS (68). Treatments include metformin 500 mg BID for the first week and 1 g BID thereafter, if tolerated (diarrhea) and thiazolidinediones (e.g., pioglitazone), 15 or 30 mg QD if tolerated (fluid and subcutaneous weight gain). Both reduce hyperandrogenemia and dysmenorrhea (69,70). Weight loss by modifying diet and regular aerobic exercise is also very important.

A further argument that combined hyperlipidemia in the metabolic syndrome is a major cause of premature coronary disease in middle-aged women is made from the distribution of arteriosclerosis in the vascular tree in women versus men (1,71). The increase in arterial surface area affected by arteriosclerosis occurs later in women than in men by approximately 10 years, as does the clinical onset of coronary disease (3), but the distribution of arteriosclerosis in women is greater in the aorta and less in the coronary circulation than in men. The more peripheral distribution of arteriosclerotic vascular disease is typical of patients with diabetes, high triglycerides, and low HDL—all features of the metabolic syndrome.

In summary, the metabolic syndrome and its associated combined hyperlipidemia are more prevalent in women with arteriosclerosis in middle age than in men. Management should

TABLE 9.2

RISK FACTORS FOR CVD IN WOMEN

The metabolic syndrome (syndrome X)
Insulin resistance
Obesity
Hypertension[a]
Diabetes[a]
Combined hyperlipidemias
Low HDL cholesterol (<40 mg/dL)[a]
PCOS (amenorrhea, hirsutism, infertility)
Smoking[a]
Inactivity
Age ≥55 y[a]
Familial or polygenic hypercholesterolemia
Homocysteine elevations
Family history of premature coronary disease: younger than 55 y in men and 65 yr in women (first-degree relatives)[a]
Oral contraceptive use in the presence of other risk factors
Lp(a)

Abbreviations: HDL, high-density lipoprotein; Lp(a), lipoprotein (a); PCOS, polycystic ovary syndrome.
[a]Denotes official National Cholesterol Education Program risk factors. See Executive Summary of The Third Report of the National Cholesterol Education Program (NCEP) Expert Panel on Detection, Evaluation, and Treatment of High Blood Cholesterol in Adults (Adult Treatment Panel III). *JAMA* 2001;285:2486–2497.

be directed toward the entire metabolic disorder (e.g., insulin resistance, obesity, hypertension, hyperglycemia, dyslipidemia) (72) and not toward a single factor such as elevated LDL, as important as it is. Important risk factors in women are listed in Table 9.2.

DIETARY RESPONSE AND CARDIOVASCULAR DISEASE

Controlled feeding studies indicate that LDL in women is approximately 30% less responsive to diet and cholesterol feeding than men, though this is not seen in free-living dietary interventions (73,74). More consistent are greater HDL-C decreases in women on low fat-diet—5% to 6% as compared to 1% to 3% in men after 6 and 12 months of diet—with the greatest reduction in HDL_2-C, the estrogen-exercise–sensitive portion of HDL (74,75). Conversely, HDL is more sensitive to cholesterol and fat feeding in women.

There is no difference in dietary recommendation for men versus women in the current national guidelines (56). However, low-fat diets tend to raise triglycerides and lower HDL. Because these abnormalities are more important in women than in men, and higher fat intake lowers triglyceride levels (75,76), it follows that a diet more generous in allowable fats content may be more advisable. Currently, the NCEP allows 25% to 35% of dietary calories as fat, but as much as 40% of energy as fat may be beneficial (as polyunsaturated fat and monounsaturated fat) for the dyslipidemia of the metabolic syndrome and coronary disease prevention, especially in women (76,77).

EFFECTS OF GONADAL STEROIDS ON LIPOPROTEIN METABOLISM AND THEIR CLINICAL SIGNIFICANCE

The effects of sex hormones and gender on lipoprotein metabolism are shown in Figure 9.3. The main point from the illustration is that estrogen and female gender enhance the metabolic traffic of cholesterol transport in virtually every pathway, raising triglyceride, lowering LDL, and raising HDL, and favoring cholesterol recycling from LDL to HDL. Progestins, androgens, and male gender have the opposite effect (1,78,79).

Plasma Triglyceride Elevations

Probably the best-recognized effect of estrogen treatment is an increase in plasma triglycerides (80). This effect is greater when estrogen is given orally and less when given systemically by injection, patch, or natural ovarian secretion (1,78,79). The increase in plasma triglyceride concentrations is due to an increased hepatic triglyceride secretion in the form of increased entry of VLDL into the circulation. The most extreme, estrogen-dominant condition in nature is pregnancy (81,82).

Estrogen treatment can interact with diabetes or genetic lipoprotein lipase deficiency to cause a marked exaggeration of hypertriglyceridemia that can result in pancreatitis if levels

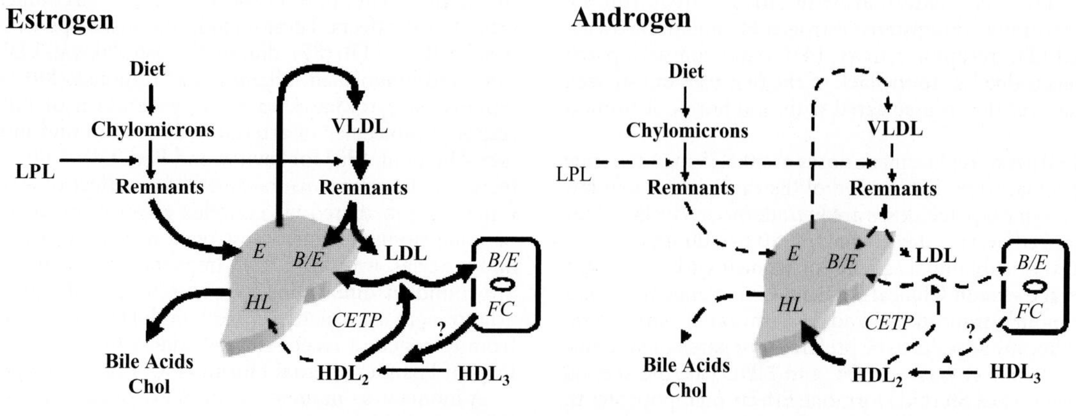

FIGURE 9.3. Effects of sex steroids on lipoprotein metabolism. Width of the lines indicates the rate of cholesterol traffic under the influence of estrogen or progestin/androgen. Question marks indicate effects for which documentation is uncertain or unclear. *Abbreviations:* B/E, low-density lipoprotein receptor; CETP, cholesterol ester transfer protein; Chol, cholesterol; E, LDL related protein or LRP which recognizes apo E; FC, free cholesterol; HDL, high-density lipoprotein; HL, hepatic lipase; LDL, low-density lipoprotein; LPL, lipoprotein lipase; VLDL, very-low-density lipoprotein.

exceed 2,000 mg/dL. The clinical significance is that women given estrogen, especially postmenopausal estrogen, should be checked first for triglyceride elevations. If plasma triglyceride levels are >300 mg/dL, oral estrogen should be withheld. Patch estrogen can be given postmenopausally in this situation because it has little triglyceride-raising effect in the absence of the hepatic first-pass effect (83). The selective estrogen receptor modulator raloxifene can raise triglyceride in such patients, although not in most postmenopausal women (83).

In contrast to estrogen, androgens and androgenic progestins antagonize the effect of estrogen and tend to lower plasma triglyceride levels. For example, an anabolic steroid such as stanozolol or oxandrolone can be used as a last resort in the management of severe hypertriglyceridemia (>2,000 mg/dL) and recurrent pancreatitis, although undesirable effects on LDL and HDL may result (84).

Remnant Lipoprotein Metabolism

Remnant lipoproteins are the product of the removal of triglyceride from chylomicrons and VLDL, as pictured in Figure 9.3. Hepatic LDL receptors recognize remnants by the presence of apoprotein E3 or E4 on the surface of the particle. Without this recognition, remnant removal disease, or type III hyperlipidemia, ensues. Because estrogen upregulates the LDL receptor, estrogen may correct remnant removal disease (1,80,85). Unfortunately, clinical experience indicates that estrogen-using hypertriglyceridemic women may present with remnant removal disease. This apparent discrepancy reflects the dual etiology of type III hyperlipidemia, which involves excessive entry of VLDL into the circulation and impaired remnant removal. Clinicians need to be alert to the possibility that estrogens may improve or aggravate type III hyperlipidemia.

A second step in the remnant removal process is the removal of triglyceride from the remnant by hepatic lipase (1). Hepatic lipase activity is reduced by estrogen, causing lipoproteins in pregnancy, oral contraception, and postmenopausal hormone replacement to increase in triglyceride content. Clinically, hepatic lipase deficiency looks like remnant removal disease, but estrogen makes it worse, not better. Progestins have the opposite effect of increasing hepatic lipase activity—an effect that is associated with increased CVD risk (86).

Low-Density Lipoprotein Metabolism

Decreased LDL-C concentrations with estrogen treatment are greatest with orally administered estrogen formulations owing to increased LDL receptor activity. LDL reduction with patch formulations is due less to the lack of the first pass of estrogen through the liver that is associated with oral hormone administration.

Typical estrogen replacement doses are 0.625 mg of equine estrogen (Premarin) or 17β -estradiol (Estrace) 1 or 2 mg/day, both orally. Typical patch doses are Estraderm or Vivelle, 50 or 100 μg changed every 3 days; Climara, 50 or 100 μg changed every 7 days; or sublingual estrace for women with patch sensitivity (see the section Clinical Advice). Costs range from $15 to $25 per month or more. Oral administration of estrogen replacement therapy appears to be preferable to patch or systemic administration for effects on LDL and HDL (see the section Postmenopausal Sex Steroid Hormone Effects on Lipoproteins, Carbohydrate Metabolism, and Clotting). However, oral estrogen can exaggerate hepatic synthesis of many other proteins, including VLDL and clotting factors. Thus, patch estrogen, which mimics the systemic entry of ovarian estrogen, appears to be preferable.

In contrast to estrogens, high-dose androgens increase LDL-C by diminishing LDL receptor activity. If the androgen is testosterone, which is partly converted to estradiol by tissue aromatases, no effect is seen on LDL levels (79).

Lipoprotein(a) Metabolism

Lp(a) is associated with LDL and exaggerates its inherent atherogenicity. Lp(a) is a nonfibrinolytic plasminogen homolog carried on LDL apoprotein B, thereby forming Lp(a) (36,39). Estrogen reduces Lp(a) levels in moderate to high doses (78,79). The selective estrogen receptor modulators raloxifene and tamoxifen also lower Lp(a) (78,79,83). Even more paradoxically, androgens lower Lp(a)(79).

High-Density Lipoprotein Metabolism

A well-known effect of estrogen is to increase plasma HDL cholesterol (HDL-C) concentrations. The HDL-C increase is confined to the more buoyant, lipid-rich HDL_2-C. HDL_3-C concentrations are unchanged. Because HDL_2-C is also selectively increased with hygienic measures such as exercise, it was originally thought that HDL_2-C was the only beneficial fraction of HDL-C. This conclusion no longer appears to be valid, but an increase in HDL_2-C is associated, nonetheless, with a reduction in CVD risk. The increase in HDL_2-C concentration is due to an increase in apoprotein A-I secretion from the liver and a reduction in hepatic lipase-mediated uptake of HDL_2-C and phospholipid—quantitatively the two most important HDL lipids.

Cholesterol from HDL can also be recycled back to LDL and VLDL, where it is made available again to cells by the plasma enzyme that accomplishes this process: cholesterol ester transfer protein (CETP), which is estrogen dependent. With estrogen also reducing hepatic cholesterol uptake by a decrease in hepatic lipase activity, the overall effect is to enhance cholesterol transport and recycling in the bloodstream (see references Knopp et al. [1, 78, 79] for reviews).

ENDOTHELIAL AND VASCULAR BIOLOGY EFFECTS OF ESTROGENS, PROGESTINS, AND ANDROGENS

In addition to lipoprotein effects, estrogen has numerous direct arterial wall effects. These include diminished penetration of arterial wall by LDL (87), diminished arterial wall LDL retention (88), and diminished inflammatory response (89), involving a diminished cytokine release and generation of inflammatory response molecules in arterial endothelium and intima media (see Zhu et al. [90] for review and Fig. 9.4). Some of these effects may be related to the antioxidant effect of estrogen (90). Others are mediated via complex receptor-mediated genomic or nongenomic effects on estrogen receptors or macrophages and arterial walls (91,92). Importantly, estrogen receptors are found in diminished amounts or are absent in areas of atherosclerosis, which may explain the lack of vascular benefit from estrogen in recent clinical trials (93) (see the section Effects of Postmenopausal Hormone Use on Coronary Disease).

A moment-to-moment effect of estrogen increases endothelial nitric oxide synthase activity, nitric oxide generation, and vasodilation. This effect can reverse the paradoxical vasoconstrictor response to acetylcholine in arteriosclerotic arteries (94) (Fig. 9.5). In fact, estrogen administration can reverse clinical vasospasm within minutes and may be a useful treatment in cardiologic syndrome X (95,96). In addition, estrogen is associated with lower plasma levels of the vasoconstrictor endothelin

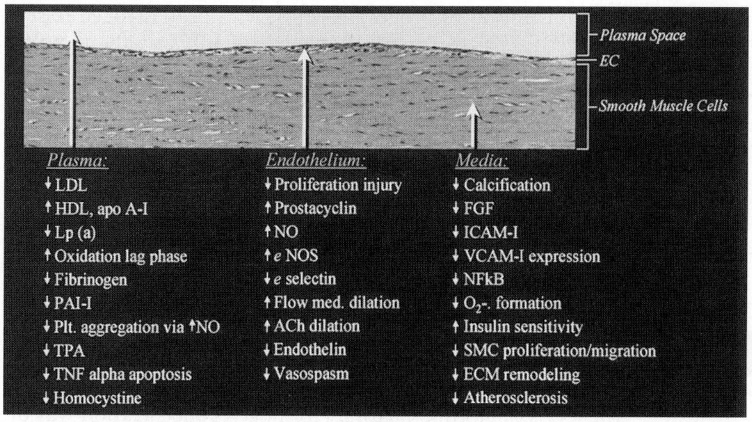

FIGURE 9.4. Beneficial effects of estrogen on arterial wall biology. In this scenario, estrogen-mediated events in plasma, endothelium, and intima media are beneficial to the arterial wall. *Abbreviations:* ACh, acetylcholine; apo, apoprotein; EC, epidermal cell; ECM, extracellular matrix; eNOS, endothelial nitric oxide synthase; FGF, fibroblast growth factor; HDL, high-density lipoprotein; ICAM-1, intercellular adhesion molecule-1; LDL, low-density lipoprotein; Lp(a), lipoprotein(a); NFκB, nuclear factor kappa B; NO, nitrous oxide; PAI-1, plasminogen activator inhibitor-1; Plt, platelet; SMC, smooth muscle cell; TNF, tumor necrosis factor; TPA, tissue plasminogen activator; VCAM-1, vascular cell adhesion molecule-1.

(97). Surprisingly, testosterone and other androgens may have a vasodilatory effect in healthy arteries (92,98,99).

Most recently, vasoconstrictive effects of progestins on arterial vasomotion have been reported (100), and medroxyprogesterone acetate (MPA) has been reported to abolish the antiatherosclerotic effect of estrogen in cholesterol-fed monkeys and rats (101,102). Testosterone and one androgenic progestin also promote atherogenesis in cholesterol-fed monkeys (103) as they are antiestrogens may also oppose the antioxidant effect of estrogen (104).

Another way in which sex hormones affect arterial wall physiology is through the arterial wall–prostaglandin system, which can favor vasoconstriction and platelet aggregation if thromboxane formation is dominant and vasodilation and diminished platelet aggregation if prostacyclin is dominant. Estrogen favors prostacyclin dominance, whereas testosterone favors thromboxane formation, diminishes prostacyclin formation, and enhances platelet thromboxane receptor binding on platelets (see Pratico and FitzGerald [99] for a review).

In summary, ample evidence exists for the presence of estrogen receptors in healthy arterial walls and direct, almost moment-to-moment regulation of endothelial nitric oxide generation and vasomotion, arterial wall LDL penetration and metabolism, and underlying inflammatory response.

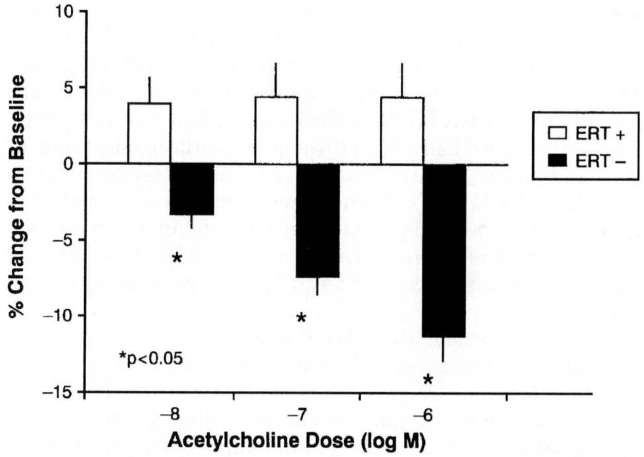

FIGURE 9.5. Mean percent change in coronary diameter after graded doses of acetylcholine. Vertical lines indicate standard error of the mean. Actual *P* values for comparison of estrogen replacement therapy (ERT)+ versus ERT− for each dose of acetylcholine are .03, .001, and .0004, respectively. (*Source:* From Herrington DM, Braden GA, Williams JK, et al. Endothelial-dependent coronary vasomotor responsiveness in postmenopausal women with and without estrogen replacement therapy. *Am J Cardiol* 1994; 73:951–952, with permission.)

ORAL CONTRACEPTIVE STEROID EFFECTS ON LIPOPROTEIN METABOLISM AND ATHEROGENESIS

The antagonism between estrogenic and progestogenic-androgenic effects on lipoproteins is played out in the three generations of OCs. The first generation contained high doses of estrogens and progestins, some estrogen dominant and some androgen dominant (105). Estrogen-dominant OCs were associated with high triglyceride, high HDL-C levels, and normal LDL-C levels, whereas progestin-androgen–dominant OCs had lower triglyceride, higher LDL-C levels, and lower HDL-C levels.

The second-generation formulations showed less marked effects on triglyceride, LDL-C levels, and HDL-C levels, although the estrogen– versus progestin-androgen–mediated differences could still be seen. The third-generation pills now in use are associated with normal LDL-C levels and increased HDL-C levels, and appear to be estrogen dominant. As a result, triglyceride elevations of 30% to 40% are still seen. As mentioned, a tendency to venous thrombosis persists (106,107). In addition, estrogen–progestin balance affects insulin sensitivity and clotting factor levels (108), with estrogen dominance favoring insulin sensitivity and a reduction in plasma fibrinogen levels (108).

The main point is that OC steroids, depending on their composition, can affect several arteriosclerotic risk factor axes. It makes good sense for women taking OCs to have their lipoprotein and glucose levels checked at least once after starting. Not all women respond the same and sometimes the hormone-induced changes in lipoproteins can be marked. It is also very important for women using OC steroids to manage heart disease risk factors aggressively.

ORAL CONTRACEPTIVE USE AND CARDIOVASCULAR DISEASE RISK

Shortly after the introduction of oral contraception in the 1960s, reports appeared of venous thrombosis and stroke with OC use. The occurrence of venous thrombosis is not surprising because the earliest OCs contained between 100 and 150 μg of ethinyl estradiol, 4 to 8 times current OC doses. Shortly after, reports of a threefold excess of CAD among OC users appeared, with combinations of risk factor increasing risk exponentially (109,110). These data demonstrate that the risk factor theory of arteriosclerosis applies to young women and that OC use exaggerates this risk.

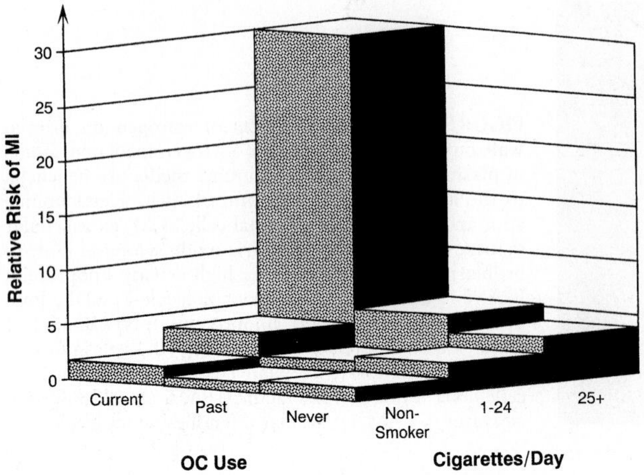

FIGURE 9.6. The effect of smoking and oral contraceptives (OCs) on the risk of MI in women younger than 50 years. (*Source:* Adapted from Rosenberg L, Kaufman DW, Helmrich S, et al. Myocardial infarction and cigarette smoking in women younger than 50 years of age. *JAMA* 1985;253:2965.)

Currently, daily OC estrogen doses are 20 to 35 μg of ethinyl-estradiol. Even at these doses, venous thrombosis still occurs (107) and may be promoted by procoagulant mutations such as factor V Leiden (106). The reduced androgenicity of some third-generation OCs appears to render the formulation more estrogenic, even though the estrogen dose is unchanged (108). Thus, heart disease appears to be two- to threefold increased, although at a low absolute rate (107,111). Again, interaction with CVD risk factors can greatly multiply this risk. Smoking is particularly notable. The risk of coronary disease in a cigarette-smoking OC user is increased approximately 20- to 30-fold from baseline and approximately six- to eightfold above the risk of cigarette smoking alone for coronary disease (112,113) (Fig. 9.6). The standard recommendation is that female smokers over 35 should not use OCs.

The mechanism for the increased CVD risk with OC use and smoking consists of arterial injury from smoking and thrombosis at the site of arterial injury from the estrogen component of the OC. Smoking-induced arterial injury includes acute endothelial erosion (114) as well as more chronic arteriosclerotic plaque formation (115).

The important message is that CVD risk must be considered when prescribing OCs and that every woman should have lipid profile, blood pressure, HbA1C, height, and weight checked when OC use is considered (116). CVD risk factors in women are summarized in Table 9.2.

POSTMENOPAUSAL SEX STEROID HORMONE EFFECTS ON LIPOPROTEINS, CARBOHYDRATE METABOLISM, AND CLOTTING

LDL-C levels are higher in postmenopausal women than in younger women, in part because of the absence of endogenous estrogen (1,78,79). When women have been studied through menopause and estrogen deficiency develops, the LDL-C level increases by 12.0 mg/dL (0.31 mmol) and HDL-C decreases by 3.5 mg/dL (0.09 mmol) (109). Insulin, glucose, and body weight also increase with menopause, indicating a broad effect of estrogen.

Oral estrogen raises HDL-C 6 to 8 mg/dL (0.15 to 0.2 mmol) (117). Lesser HDL increases occur with patch estrogen (117). Administration of progestin, MPA, with oral estrogen lessens the HDL-C increase to about 1.5 mg/dL (~0.04 mmol/L) above baseline. In contrast, the HDL-C rise with micronized natural progesterone and equine estrogen was almost entirely preserved (5 mg/dL or 0.13 mmol increase above baseline).

LDL-C reductions of approximately 14.5 to 17.5 mg/dL (0.37 to 0.45 mmol) were observed regardless of the amount or type of progestin in this study. Triglyceride elevations were minor, ranging from 11.4 to 13.7 mg/dL (0.13 to 0.15 mmol), and less than the triglyceride elevations associated with oral contraception. In the same study, plasma glucose and insulin levels were lowest with estrogen alone and highest with high-dose progestin plus estrogen (117).

The relative amounts of estrogen and progestin also affected the levels of clotting factors. Fibrinogen concentration was diminished among postmenopausal estrogen users, as with OC users (108). Addition of natural progesterone or increasing doses of MPA (Provera) had the opposite effect.

An increase in CRP levels with estrogen use has been seen in several studies (118). This increase may drive an increase in activity in the complement pathway and favor inflammatory processes (119). The effect is a result of the first pass of oral estrogen through the liver; patch estrogen is not associated with CRP elevation.

EFFECTS OF POSTMENOPAUSAL HORMONE USE ON CORONARY DISEASE

More than 50 case-controlled and prospective cohort studies compared arteriosclerotic vascular disease in estrogen users versus nonusers (1,78,79,120–122). These studies indicated that the incidence of CAD among estrogen users is approximately one half of that among nonusers. Even before the recent negative clinical trials of estrogen efficacy on heart disease, it was postulated that the putative estrogen benefit was due in part to a "healthy user effect" (i.e., healthier women use estrogen). Barrett-Connor (120) estimated that half of the CVD reduction from estrogen might be due this selection bias, for which there is no statistical adjustment.

This prediction was borne out and more-so by two randomized placebo controlled clinical trials. The combination of 0.625 mg/day of equine estrogen and 2.5 mg/day of MPA was without benefit in two studies, HERS (Heart and Estrogen/Progestin Replacement Study) (123,124) and WHI (Women's Health Initiative) (125). Both studies showed trends toward more heart disease, HERS in the first year in a post-hoc analysis (123) (Fig. 9.7) and WHI throughout, although not statistically significant (hazard ratio of 1.29 with confidence interval of 1.02 to 1.63) (125). Women given estrogen alone (without a uterus), had no cardiovascular benefit and an increased incidence of stroke (risk ratio 1.41 [1.07 to 1.85]) (126). Women in both of these studies were 14 to 17 years postmenopause on average.

A lack of benefit from HRT also was observed in coronary atherosclerosis quantified angiographically in the Estrogen Replacement Atherosclerosis (ERA) study (127). These were women with established coronary disease and an average age of 66 years. Decreases in minimum coronary diameter change and increases in percent stenosis were statistically indistinguishable in the three groups but with a worsening trend in the equine estrogen plus MPA group versus estrogen alone or placebo (Table 9.3).

The failure of these studies to demonstrate benefit has many explanations. The most plausible is that estrogen may be protective in healthy arteries with a normal compliment of

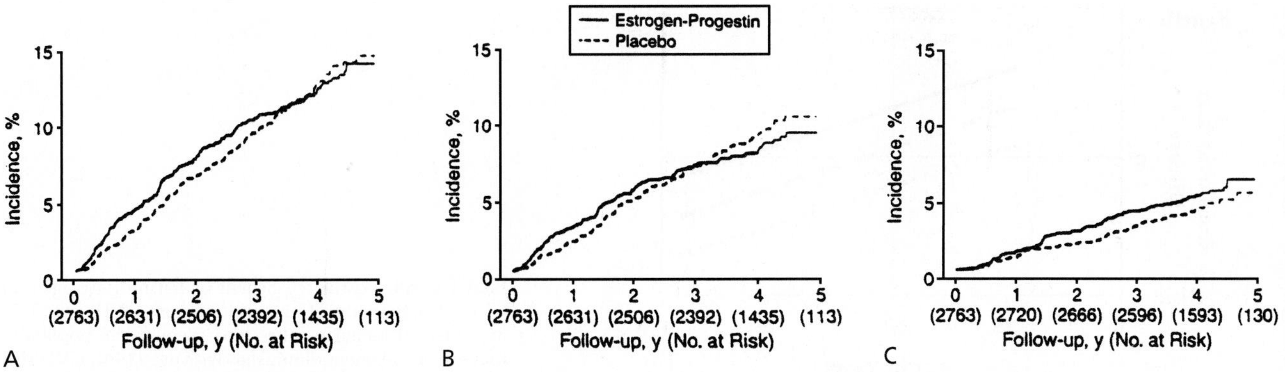

FIGURE 9.7. Heart and Estrogen/Progestin Replacement Study Kaplan-Meier curve estimates of the cumulative incidence of primary coronary heart disease and its constituents. **A:** All events. **B:** Nonfatal events. **C:** Fatal events. Numbers in parentheses are subjects followed to each time-point. Curves are fainter where the sample size falls to less than one half of the original cohort. (*Source:* From Hulley S, Grady D, Bush T, et al. Randomized trial of estrogen plus progesterone for secondary prevention of coronary heart disease in postmenopausal women. *JAMA* 1998;280:605–613, with permission.)

estrogen receptors. On the other hand, estrogen is less likely to be beneficial in a setting of established atherosclerosis with reduced arterial wall estrogen receptors typical of women in their mid-60s. This is the case in animal models of atherosclerosis (128,129). Increased risk could result from an enhanced thrombosis tendency from estrogen treatment in the presence of plaque rupture (123,124,130–133) (see Fig. 9.8). See reference Knopp et al. (134) for further discussion.

CLINICAL ADVICE

What should we tell patients? The results of HERS, HERS II, and WHI agree that oral HRT should not be used for either primary or secondary prevention of CHD in women in their mid-60s, well past menopause (135). However, the possibility of benefit has not been ruled out for hormone replacement begun at menopause, the typical time to start, and before the time when atherosclerosis accelerates postmenopausally. The potential additional benefit of patch estrogen is also unexamined. These points are discussed in recent reviews (92,134, 136,137).

Reasons remain to justify HRT, including skin flushing, as well as a sense of well-being, prevention of osteoporosis, preservation of skin turgor, preservation of vaginal mucosa, metabolic benefits (see below), and higher intellectual function (1,78,79). Most women come to this decision aware of at least some of the benefits and side effects and often have their own viewpoint about whether to take estrogen.

CHOLESTEROL-LOWERING INTERVENTIONS AND REDUCTIONS IN CORONARY ARTERY DISEASE IN WOMEN

Diet

As mentioned, some studies have found a diminished effect of diet on LDL-C and HDL-C levels in women compared to men. However, in a recent study of the largest group of free-living men and women studied to date, LDL-C lowering was equivalent in men and women, but the HDL-C lowering was greater in women (6% to 7%) than in men (1% to 3%)—even after 6 to 12 months, when the acute HDL-lowering effects of diet had worn off (73,74). These percentage differences are small in the aggregate but could be meaningful for atherosclerotic risk among individuals with marked HDL-C reductions. Higher fat intake is under investigation as a means to minimize this HDL-C decrease (75). The new NCEP guidelines favor a 25% to 35% fat diet, with only saturated fat restriction (56).

TABLE 9.3

EFFECTS OF POSTMENOPAUSAL HORMONE REPLACEMENT ON CORONARY LUMEN DIAMETER[a]

				P Values	
	Estrogen	Estrogen + MPA	Placebo	E vs Placebo	E + MPA vs Placebo
Minimal coronary diameters adjusted change (mm)	−0.09 ± 0.02	−0.12 ± 0.02	−0.09 ± 0.02	.97	.38
Stenosis adjusted change (%)	4.01 ± 0.92	4.75 ± 0.92	4.11 ± 4.93	.93	.56

Abbreviations: E, estrogen; MPA, medroxyprogesterone acetate.
[a]Data include all subjects with adjustments for baseline inequalities.
Source: From Herrington DM, Reboussin DM, Brosnihan KB, et al. Effects of estrogen replacement on the progression of coronary-artery atherosclerosis. *N Engl J Med* 2000;343:522–529, with permission.

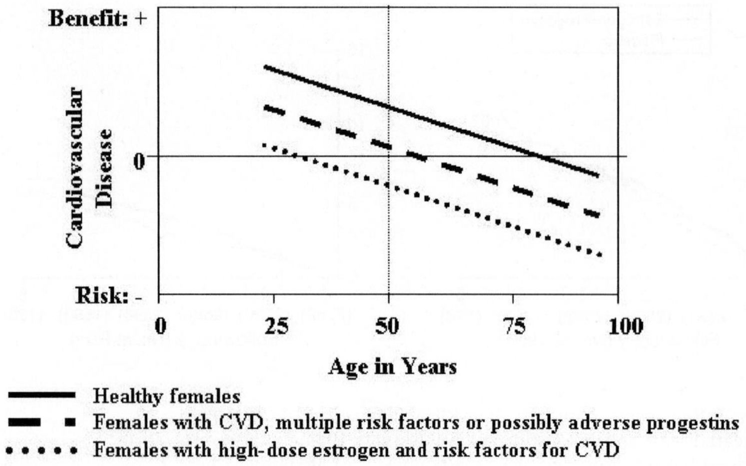

FIGURE 9.8. Postulated benefit or harm of estrogen on CVD as a function of age and inherent CVD risk. This hypothetical scenario takes into account the possibility that estrogen benefit diminishes with age (144), CVD risk (109,110), and estrogen dose (109,110,145). *Solid line*, healthy women; *dashed line*, women with CVD, multiple risk factors, or possibly adverse progestins; *dotted line*, women with high-dose estrogen and risk factors for CVD.

Drug Therapy Efficacy

LDL-C reductions are at least as good in women as in men with heterozygous familial hypercholesterolemia treated with reductase inhibitor, niacin, and bile acid–binding resin. In the authors' clinical experience, familial hypercholesterolemic women are more often successfully managed with single lipid-lowering agents (almost always reductase inhibitors) than are men, who often require combination therapy. The better response in women is not fully understood but could relate to lesser volume of distribution of standard drug doses.

Arteriosclerosis Prevention and Regression

Studies of angiographic regression and heart disease prevention tend to show better responses in women than in men. In the SCOR study, the mean percent coronary artery stenosis at baseline was approximately 48% in women and 55% in men at equivalent ages (40 to 43 years) (10). After several years of triple-drug therapy (reductase, resin, and niacin), angiographic improvement was greater in women (–2.1%) compared to men (–0.9%) (negative signs connote vessel enlargement).

The prevention of clinical manifestations of coronary disease in men and women in the CARE study confirm greater benefit in women (138). In this investigation, CAD reduction in women was 46% compared to 20% in men at equivalent doses (40 mg/day) of the reductase inhibitor pravastatin. The better preventive effect in women may be related to a less advanced stage of disease, to a greater LDL-C reduction, or to other inherent biologic differences. It is known that arteriosclerotic plaques in women are less fibrotic and contain more lipid-filled foam cells (139), implying greater potential for reversibility but also potentially greater vulnerability for plaque rupture and thrombosis. The main point is that impaired responsiveness to therapy cannot be used as a reason not to treat women at high risk for arteriosclerotic vascular disease.

Lipid Screening Guidelines for Hyperlipidemic Women

Based on low CVD mortality rates of women before the menopause (140), it was recommended that cholesterol screening not be done in premenopausal women unless a family history of CAD is present (141). Fortunately, current ATP-III guidelines recommend equivalent lipid profile screening in men and women, every 5 years from age 20 (56).

One needs to know whether plasma triglyceride levels are elevated in the context of using sex hormones—either for oral contraception in the reproductive years or for therapy as ovarian function wanes, even before the menopause. In addition, combined hyperlipidemia is a real threat for coronary disease in middle-aged women (see the section Cardiovascular Disease Risk Factors in Women Compared to Men). This condition is now more clearly addressed in the NCEP ATP-III guidelines (56).

LIPID-LOWERING TREATMENT GUIDELINES

The NCEP guidelines for lipid lowering specify that risk factors apply equally for men and women; except for family history of premature, CVD under age 65 in a female relative is considered to be premature and under age 55 in male relatives. Likewise, age as a risk factor is later in women (age 55 years) than in men (age 45 years). There is no gender distinction in the application of the HDL-C less than 40 mg/dL rule as a risk factor despite the fact that women have a mean HDL-C of approximately 55 mg/dL and men a mean HDL-C of 45 mg/dL. As a result, fewer women qualify for low HDL-C as a risk factor than men and more women qualify for subtracting one risk factor on the basis of HDL-C more than 60 mg/dL. Otherwise, the less than 160, 130, and 100 mg/dL LDL-C target values apply equally to men and women, with the gender differences in risk being embodied in the risk factor assessments.

GENDER DIFFERENCES IN PHARMACOLOGIC TREATMENT

Bile Acid–Binding Resin

Most patients object to the gustatory, upper gastrointestinal, and constipating side effects of bile acid–binding resin. Based on common sense, perhaps the most important point to keep in mind is that when resin is necessary, lower doses might be tried in women compared to men because of a woman's smaller size. Bile acid–binding resin tablets in the form of colestipol, although large, offer a somewhat more palatable alternative (1 capsule = 1 g, 4 capsules = one scoop or packet). Recently, colesevelam (WelChol) has become available, which is the first well-tolerated, high-affinity bile acid–binding resin in both sexes.

Niacin

In addition to the usual flushing, side effects of niacin include acanthosis nigricans, ichthyosis, thickening of the skin, and, more subtly, winter dryness. These skin symptoms are less well tolerated in women than in men. Apart from scrubbing with pumice to remove acanthosis, there is no good solution except to tailor the dose to the level of tolerable side effects. Clinical experience indicates that lower doses of 1 to 2 g/day are worthwhile because a beneficial effect on HDL and triglyceride levels can still be obtained at these doses (85), whereas the need for LDL-C lowering can be met by adding reductase inhibitor agents in combination. The tendency for plasma glucose levels to rise with niacin therapy does not have a known gender specificity (85).

Fibric Acid Derivatives

Fibric acid derivatives are almost essential in the management of hypertriglyceridemia associated pancreatitis (>1,000 to 2,000 mg/dL). Whether these agents cause cancer in humans is moot in male subjects, and studies in women are lacking. More clear is the tendency of all fibrates to increase gallbladder bile saturation with cholesterol and cause gallstones (85). Because overweight, middle-aged women are more prone to this condition, gallstone disease from fibrate use adds to the reasons to try to find other approaches to high-triglyceride management, which includes weight loss agents, insulin-sensitivity improvers such as metformin, and weak triglyceride lowerers such as fish oil and a low-fat diet.

Reductase Inhibitors

The largest available study of a reductase inhibitor is the Excel study of lovastatin. Results show a greater degree of lipid lowering in older women (142). As higher doses of reductases are being recommended (85), it may be anticipated that more hepatotoxicity and myotoxicity may occur in women because of their smaller body mass relative to dose than that of men. However, high-dose therapy may not be as necessary in women compared with men (142).

Reductase and Fibrate Combination Therapy

Myotoxicity is more common among women with impaired renal function who take the combination of gemfibrozil and lovastatin than among men (143). Clofibrate alone is highly myotoxic in renal failure because of its renal elimination. It is no longer manufactured. Gemfibrozil seems less so, but it can also produce myotoxicity under the conditions described above and with the additional potential for rhabdomyolysis and acute renal failure (143). Fenofibrate has the best compatibility with statins.

CONTROVERSIES AND PERSONAL PERSPECTIVES

Postmenopausal Hormone Replacement Therapy

The take home message is that estrogen and progestin currently cannot be prescribed for CVD prevention with any assurance for benefit in women past menopause. On the other hand, if a woman has been taking HRT since menopause, and is now in her mid-60s, there may be no justification for hormones being stopped, because CVD benefit may have been maintained from menopause. The only clear-cut justification for stopping postmenopausal estrogen is if a woman already has developed CAD. Patch estrogen treatment is an excellent alternative to oral therapy because it minimizes the clotting factor effects of oral therapy and the increase in CRP secretion.

When counseling patients, we tell them what we know, but we also listen to their concerns. If HRT is initiated, it must be in conjunction with annual lipid evaluation, CHD symptom and risk factor screening, gynecologic evaluation, breast examination, and mammography.

CONCLUSIONS

CVD can occur in women of all ages, depending on risk factor burden. The metabolic syndrome is a more important CVD risk factor in women than in men. The global burden of CHD is rising along with the industrialization of the Third World and the lack of exercise in the modern lifestyle. It is also important to recognize the increased propensity for insulin resistance and metabolic syndrome in certain groups such as Asian and Hispanic ethnicities. Triglyceride and HDL levels are more important in women than in men. Because almost every category of overt CVD and its operative management carries worse morbidity and mortality in women compared to men, it is important to use every means to prevent its occurrence. The interplay of estrogen and progestin bears on this issue in all stages of life and has to be considered, along with all other cardiovascular therapies.

In general, estrogen at replacement hormone–dose levels is associated with a favorable effect on lipoprotein metabolism, arterial wall penetration of LDL, insulin sensitivity, and plasma glucose concentrations. The best available information from clinical trials in older postmenopausal in women is that HRT is without cardiovascular benefit. It remains to be seen if SERMS will have benefit in a primary prevention setting or HRT especially as a patch in women at the time of menopause.

Caution is also advised for clinicians giving estrogen in any case in which the patient has underlying hypertriglyceridemia or a history of thrombosis. Should hypertriglyceridemia result from estrogen administration or if the patient has a baseline plasma triglyceride level above 300 mg/dL (3.38 mmol), an estrogen patch regimen should be used as an alte1ative.

With the recent growth in understanding of the effects of sex steroid hormones on many body functions and of the many differences between the genders in arterial physiology and pathophysiology, the prospect remains that this knowledge can be used to minimize coronary disease in both men and women if the undesirable side effects can be avoided.

THE FUTURE

The following statements are as much hopes as predictions. First, physicians and caregivers will remember that coronary disease and arteriosclerotic vascular disease are equivalent causes of death in women as well as in men, but that symptomatologies and presentations differ often. Second, physicians and caregivers will have the patience to let patients tell us the story as they see it, so that we can better appreciate and describe the male–female difference and treat appropriately. The third expectation is that ongoing clinical trials will further refine the nature and extent of the heightened vulnerability of women for certain morbidities associated with coronary disease. The fourth expectation is that we will learn the reasons for these excessive morbidities and find better ways to prevent and treat them. The fifth hope is that caregivers will recognize that treatable CVD risk factors—especially hypertension, diabetes, and the metabolic syndrome with its associated dyslipidemia—are consistently more common among women with CVD than among men. The sixth expectation is that we will learn to use metabolic treatments more effectively and in combination to treat these risk factors. These treatments will include use of antihypertensives without adverse metabolic effect, agents to minimize insulin resistance, cautious use of existing and forthcoming appetite suppressants, and more informed, target-oriented treatment of diabetes and dyslipidemia. Treatments will also include management of female hyperandrogenic states premenopausally and hormone replacement postmenopausally in those settings where patient symptoms dictate at the time of menopause. Seventh, women and men should be treated aggressively with lipid-lowering agents to target. The eighth expectation is that good nutrition and physical activity will become a nationwide effort for all women, men, and children to minimize the risk of developing metabolic syndrome, diabetes, and CVD. The ninth expectation is that we will recognize the global epidemic of CVD and that future research and therapies will reflect this.

Clinical trials are beginning to evaluate the effect of postmenopausal HRT on cardiovascular health in healthy postmenopausal women at the time of menopause. We can also expect development of estrogenic compounds with hybrid or chimeric estrogen and progestin effects or that only act on certain estrogen-sensitive systems (e.g., the selective estrogen receptor modulators [SERMS]). One of these agents, raloxifene, has had no deleterious effect on CVD to date. These specific therapies may eventually be directed to the arterial wall or bone, for instance, without effects on clotting, hepatic lipoprotein production, or breast metaplasia. Knowledge is also developing rapidly in understanding the postreceptor signaling system of the estrogen receptor (92) and the specificities it entails that may eventually be used for pharmacologic benefit.

Female–Male Cardiovascular Disease Issues

The epidemiology, management, risk predictors, and subsequent morbidities of CVD are incompletely distinguished in women compared to men. Although better descriptions are constantly appearing (18,25,26,61), we will never discover a better way to treat CVD in women without listening to and looking for the ways that early CVD presents differently in women than in men. In this regard, the basic skills of the practitioner must be joined with those of the epidemiologist, clinical trialist, and clinical and basic researchers to carry this field forward.

References

1. Knopp RH, Zhu X, Bonet B. Effects of estrogens on lipoprotein metabolism and cardiovascular disease in women. *Atherosclerosis* 1994;110[Suppl]: S83–91.
2. Washington State Vital Statistics, 2003. In: *Statistics*. Center for Health Statistics. Olympia: Washington State Department of Health, 2005:183.
3. Castelli WP. Cardiovascular disease in women. *Am J Obstet Gynecol* 1988;158:1553–1560, 1566–1557.
4. Rosamond WD, Chambless LE, Folsom AR, et al. Trends in the incidence of myocardial infarction and in mortality due to coronary heart disease, 1987 to 1994. *N Engl J Med* Sep 24 1998;339:861–867.
5. Centers for Disease Control and Prevention. Update: mortality attributable to HIV infection among persons aged 25–44 years in the United States, 1994. *MMWR Morb Mortal Wkly Rep* 1996;45:121–125.
6. Raymond JR, van den Berg EK Jr, Knapp MJ. Nontraumatic prehospital sudden death in young adults. *Arch Intern Med* Feb 1988;148:303–308.
7. Negus BH, Willard JE, Glamann DB, et al. Coronary anatomy and prognosis of young, asymptomatic survivors of myocardial infarction. *Am J Med* 1994;96:354–358.
8. Berenson GS, Wattigney WA, Tracy RE, et al. Atherosclerosis of the aorta and coronary arteries and cardiovascular risk factors in persons aged 6 to 30 years and studied at necropsy (The Bogalusa Heart Study). *Am J Cardiol* 1992;70:851–858.
9. Mautner SL, Lin F, Mautner GC, et al. Comparison in women versus men of composition of atherosclerotic plaques in native coronary arteries and in saphenous veins used as aortocoronary conduits. *J Am Coll Cardiol* May 1993;21:1312–1318.
10. Kane JP, Malloy MJ, Ports TA, et al. Regression of coronary atherosclerosis during treatment of familial hypercholesterolemia with combined drug regimens. *JAMA* 1990;264:3007–3012.
11. Janowitz WR, Agatston AS, Kaplan G, et al. Differences in prevalence and extent of coronary artery calcium detected by ultrafast computed tomography in asymptomatic men and women. *Am J Cardiol* 1993;72:247–254.
12. U.S. Public Health Service, National Center for Health Statistics. *Health, United States, 1988* [publication P]. Washington, DC: U.S. Government Printing Office, 1988:89–1232.
13. Dustan HP. Coronary artery disease in women. *Can J Cardiol* 1990;6[Suppl B]:19B–21B.
14. Lerner DJ, Kannel WB. Patterns of coronary heart disease morbidity and mortality in the sexes: a 26-year follow-up of the Framingham population. *Am Heart J* 1986;111:383–390.
15. Mehilli J, Kastrati A, Dirschinger J, et al. Differences in prognostic factors and outcomes between women and men undergoing coronary artery stenting. *JAMA* 2000;284:1799–1805.
16. Wenger NK, Speroff L, Packard B. Cardiovascular health and disease in women. *N Engl J Med* 1993;329:247–256.
17. Wenger NK. Coronary heart disease in women: an overview (myths, misperceptions and missed opportunities). In: Wenger NK, Speroff L, Packard B, eds. *Cardiovascular disease and health in women*. Greenwich, CT: LeJacq Communications, 1993:21–29.
18. Becker RC, Terrin M, Ross R, et al. Comparison of clinical outcomes for women and men after acute myocardial infarction. The Thrombolysis in Myocardial Infarction Investigators. *Ann Intern Med* 1994;120:638–645.
19. Moen EK, Asher CR, Miller DP, et al. Long-term follow-up of gender-specific outcomes after thrombolytic therapy for acute myocardial infarction from the GUSTO-I trial. Global Utilization of Streptokinase and Tissue Plasminogen Activator for Occluded Coronary Arteries. *J Womens Health* 1997;6:285–293.
20. Kober L, Torp-Pedersen C, Ottesen M, et al. Influence of gender on short- and long-term mortality after acute myocardial infarction. TRACE study group. *Am J Cardiol* 1996;77:1052–1056.
21. Cupples L, D'Agostino R. Some risk factors related to the annual incidence of cardiovascular disease and death using pooled repeated biennial measurements: Framingham Heart Study, 30-year follow-up. In: Kannel WB, Wolf P, Garrison R, eds. *The Framingham Heart Study, an epidemiological investigation of heart disease* [Vol. NIH Publication 87-2703, Section 34]. Rockville, MD: National Heart, Lung and Blood Institute, 1987.
22. Higgins M, Thom T. Cardiovascular disease in women as a public health problem. In: Wenger NK, Speroff L, Packard B, eds. *Cardiovascular disease and health in women*. Greenwich, CT: LeJacq Communications, 1993: 15–19.
23. Hochman JS, Tamis JE, Thompson TD, et al. Sex, clinical presentation, and outcome in patients with acute coronary syndromes. Global Use of Strategies to Open Occluded Coronary Arteries in Acute Coronary Syndromes IIb Investigators. *N Engl J Med* 1999;341:226–232.
24. Vaccarino V, Parsons L, Every NR, et al. Sex-based differences in early mortality after myocardial infarction. National Registry of Myocardial Infarction 2 Participants. *N Engl J Med* 1999;341:217–225.
25. Lincoff AM, Califf RM, Ellis SG, et al. Thrombolytic therapy for women with myocardial infarction: is there a gender gap? Thrombolysis and Angioplasty in Myocardial Infarction Study Group. *J Am Coll Cardiol* 1993; 22:1780–1787.
26. Bell MR, Holmes DR Jr, Berger PB, et al. The changing in-hospital mortality of women undergoing percutaneous transluminal coronary angioplasty. *JAMA* 1993;269:2091–2095.
27. Khan SS, Nessim S, Gray R, et al. Increased mortality of women in coronary artery bypass surgery: evidence for referral bias. *Ann Intern Med* 1990;112:561–567.
28. Nabel EG, Selker HP, Califf RM, et al. Women's Ischemic Syndrome Evaluation: current status and future research directions: report of the National Heart, Lung and Blood Institute workshop: October 2–4, 2002: Section 3: diagnosis and treatment of acute cardiac ischemia: gender issues. *Circulation* 2004;109:e50–52.
29. Lagerqvist B, Safstrom K, Stahle E, et al. Is early invasive treatment of unstable coronary artery disease equally effective for both women and men? FRISC II Study Group Investigators. *J Am Coll Cardiol* 2001;38:41–48.
30. Bickell NA, Pieper KS, Lee KL, et al. Referral patterns for coronary artery disease treatment: gender bias or good clinical judgment? *Ann Intern Med* 1992;116:791–797.
31. Mark DB, Shaw LK, DeLong ER, et al. Absence of sex bias in the referral of patients for cardiac catheterization. *N Engl J Med* 1994;330:1101–1106.

32. Maynard C, Beshansky JR, Griffith JL, et al. Influence of sex on the use of cardiac procedures in patients presenting to the emergency department. A prospective multicenter study. *Circulation* 1996;94[9 Suppl]:II93–98.
33. Gan SC, Beaver SK, Houck PM, et al. Treatment of acute myocardial infarction and 30-day mortality among women and men. *N Engl J Med* 2000;343:8–15.
34. Vaccarino V, Rathore SS, Wenger NK, et al. Sex and racial differences in the management of acute myocardial infarction, 1994 through 2002. *N Engl J Med* 2005;353:671–682.
35. Healy B. The Yentl syndrome. *N Engl J Med* 1991;325:274–276.
36. Bostom AG, Cupples LA, Jenner JL, et al. Elevated plasma lipoprotein(a) and coronary heart disease in men aged 55 years and younger. A prospective study. *JAMA* 1996;276:544–548.
37. Willett WC, Green A, Stampfer MJ, et al. Relative and absolute excess risks of coronary heart disease among women who smoke cigarettes. *N Engl J Med* 1987;317:1303–1309.
38. Thun MJ, Day-Lally CA, Calle EE, et al. Excess mortality among cigarette smokers: changes in a 20-year interval. *Am J Public Health* 1995;85:1223–1230.
39. Guyton JR, Dahlen GH, Patsch W, et al. Relationship of plasma lipoprotein Lp(a) levels to race and to apolipoprotein B. *Arteriosclerosis* 1985;5:265–272.
40. Kannel WB, Wolf PA, Castelli WP, et al. Fibrinogen and risk of cardiovascular disease. The Framingham Study. *JAMA* 1987;258:1183–1186.
41. Pai JK, Pischon T, Ma J, et al. Inflammatory markers and the risk of coronary heart disease in men and women. *N Engl J Med* 2004;351:2599–2610.
42. Willett WC, Manson JE, Stampfer MJ, et al. Weight, weight change, and coronary heart disease in women. Risk within the 'normal' weight range. *JAMA* 1995;273:461–465.
43. Lambert M, Delvin EE, Paradis G, et al. C-reactive protein and features of the metabolic syndrome in a population-based sample of children and adolescents. *Clin Chem* 2004;50:1762–1768.
44. Orth-Gomer K, Wamala SP, Horsten M, et al. Marital stress worsens prognosis in women with coronary heart disease: The Stockholm Female Coronary Risk Study. *JAMA* 2000;284:3008–3014.
45. Methot J, Bogaty P, Poirier P, et al. The relationship of the occurrence of acute coronary events in women to the timing of their menstrual cycle. *Circulation* 2000;102[Suppl II]:II–613.
46. Knopp R, Broyles F, Bonet B. Exaggerated lipoprotein abnormalities in diabetic women as compared with diabetic men: possible significance for atherosclerosis. In: Wenger NK, Speroff L, Packard B, eds. *Cardiovascular disease and health in women.* Greenwich, CT: LeJacq Communications, 1993:131–138.
47. Kannel W. Cardiovascular sequelae in diabetes. In: Moskowitz J, ed. *Diabetes and atherosclerosis connection.* Rockville, MD: National Heart, Lung and Blood Institution, 1981:5–15.
48. Hu G, Jousilahti P, Qiao Q, et al. The gender-specific impact of diabetes and myocardial infarction at baseline and during follow-up on mortality from all causes and coronary heart disease. *J Am Coll Cardiol* 2005;45:1413–1418.
49. Bueno H, Vidan MT, Almazan A, et al. Influence of sex on the short-term outcome of elderly patients with a first acute myocardial infarction. *Circulation* 1995;92:1133–1140.
50. Walden CE, Knopp RH, Wahl PW, et al. Sex differences in the effect of diabetes mellitus on lipoprotein triglyceride and cholesterol concentrations. *N Engl J Med* 1984;311:953–959.
51. Barrett-Connor E, Giardina EG, Gitt AK, et al. Women and heart disease: the role of diabetes and hyperglycemia. *Arch Intern Med* 2004;164:934–942.
52. Siegel RD, Cupples A, Schaefer EJ, et al. Lipoproteins, apolipoproteins, and low-density lipoprotein size among diabetics in the Framingham offspring study. *Metabolism* 1996;45:1267–1272.
53. Corti MC, Guralnik JM, Salive ME, et al. HDL cholesterol predicts coronary heart disease mortality in older persons. *JAMA* 1995;274:539–544.
54. Arnold AM, Mick MJ, Piedmonte MR, et al. Gender differences for coronary angioplasty. *Am J Cardiol* 1994;74:18–21.
55. Reaven GM. Banting lecture 1988. Role of insulin resistance in human disease. *Diabetes* 1988;37:1595–1607.
56. Executive Summary of The Third Report of The National Cholesterol Education Program (NCEP) Expert Panel on Detection, Evaluation, and Treatment of High Blood Cholesterol In Adults (Adult Treatment Panel III). *JAMA* 2001;285:2486–2497.
57. Kwiterovich PO Jr, Motevalli M, Miller M, et al. Further insights into the pathophysiology of hyperapobetalipoproteinemia: role of basic proteins I, II, III. *Clin Chem* 1991;37:317–326.
58. Brunzell JD, Albers JJ, Chait A, et al. Plasma lipoproteins in familial combined hyperlipidemia and monogenic familial hypertriglyceridemia. *J Lipid Res* 1983;24:147–155.
59. Tannock LR, O'Brien KD, Knopp RH, et al. Cholesterol feeding increases C-reactive protein and serum amyloid A levels in lean insulin-sensitive subjects. *Circulation* 2005;111:3058–3062.
60. Maynard C, Litwin PE, Martin JS, et al. Gender differences in the treatment and outcome of acute myocardial infarction. Results from the Myocardial Infarction Triage and Intervention Registry. *Arch Intern Med* 1992;152:972–976.
61. Weaver WD, White HD, Wilcox RG, et al. Comparisons of characteristics and outcomes among women and men with acute myocardial infarction treated with thrombolytic therapy. GUSTO-I investigators. *JAMA* 1996;275:777–782.
62. Kostis JB, Wilson AC, O'Dowd K, et al. Sex differences in the management and long-term outcome of acute myocardial infarction. A statewide study. MIDAS Study Group. Myocardial Infarction Data Acquisition System. *Circulation* 1994;90:1715–1730.
63. Yarzebski J, Col N, Pagley P, Savageau J, et al. Gender differences and factors associated with the receipt of thrombolytic therapy in patients with acute myocardial infarction: a community-wide perspective. *Am Heart J* 1996;131:43–50.
64. Kip KE, Marroquin OC, Kelley DE, et al. Clinical importance of obesity versus the metabolic syndrome in cardiovascular risk in women: a report from the Women's Ischemia Syndrome Evaluation (WISE) study. *Circulation* 2004;109:706–713.
65. Hokanson JE, Austin MA. Plasma triglyceride level is a risk factor for cardiovascular disease independent of high-density lipoprotein cholesterol level: a meta-analysis of population-based prospective studies. *J Cardiovasc Risk* 1996;3:213–219.
66. Gordon DJ, Probstfield JL, Garrison RJ, et al. High-density lipoprotein cholesterol and cardiovascular disease. Four prospective American studies. *Circulation* 1989;79:8–15.
67. Reardon MF, Nestel PJ, Craig IH, et al. Lipoprotein predictors of the severity of coronary artery disease in men and women. *Circulation* 1985;71:881–888.
68. Birdsall MA, Farquhar CM, White HD. Association between polycystic ovaries and extent of coronary artery disease in women having cardiac catheterization. *Ann Intern Med* 1997;126:32–35.
69. Nestler JE, Jakubowicz DJ. Decreases in ovarian cytochrome P450c17 alpha activity and serum free testosterone after reduction of insulin secretion in polycystic ovary syndrome. *N Engl J Med* 1996;335:617–623.
70. Gasic S, Bodenburg Y, Nagamani M, et al. Troglitazone inhibits progesterone production in porcine granulosa cells. *Endocrinology* 1998;139: 4962–4966.
71. Blankenhorn DH, Hodis HN. George Lyman Duff Memorial Lecture. Arterial imaging and atherosclerosis reversal. *Arterioscler Thromb* 1994;14: 177–192.
72. Kannel WB, Wilson PW. Risk factors that attenuate the female coronary disease advantage. *Arch Intern Med* 1995;155:57–61.
73. Walden CE, Retzlaff BM, Buck BL, et al. Lipoprotein lipid response to the National Cholesterol Education Program step II diet by hypercholesterolemic and combined hyperlipidemic women and men. *Arterioscler Thromb Vasc Biol* 1997;17:375–382.
74. Walden CE, Retzlaff BM, Buck BL, et al. Differential effect of National Cholesterol Education Program (NCEP) Step II diet on HDL cholesterol, its subfractions, and apoprotein A-I levels in hypercholesterolemic women and men after 1 year: the beFIT Study. *Arterioscler Thromb Vasc Biol* 2000;20:1580–1587.
75. Knopp RH, Paramsothy P, Retzlaff BM, et al. Gender differences in lipoprotein metabolism and dietary response: basis in hormonal differences and implications for cardiovascular disease. *Current Atheroscl Rep* 2005;7:472–749.
76. Knopp RH, Retzlaff BM. Saturated fat prevents coronary artery disease? An American paradox. *Am J Clin Nutr* 2004;80:1102–1103.
77. Mozaffarian D, Rimm EB, Herrington DM. Dietary fats, carbohydrate, and progression of coronary atherosclerosis in postmenopausal women. *Am J Clin Nutr* 2004;80:1175–1184.
78. Knopp R, Zhu X-D, Lau J, Walden C. Sex hormones and lipid interactions: Implications for cardiovascular disease in women. *The Endocrinologist* 1994;4:286–301.
79. Knopp RH, Zhu X, Bonet B, et al. Effects of sex steroid hormones on lipoproteins, clotting, and the arterial wall. *Semin Reprod Endocrinol* 1996;14:15–27.
80. Applebaum-Bowden D, McLean P, Steinmetz A, et al. Lipoprotein, apolipoprotein, and lipolytic enzyme changes following estrogen administration in postmenopausal women. *J Lipid Res* 1989;30:1895–1906.
81. Knopp RH, Bergelin RO, Wahl PW, et al. Population-based lipoprotein lipid reference values for pregnant women compared to nonpregnant women classified by sex hormone usage. *Am J Obstet Gynecol* 1982;143:626–637.
82. Knopp RH BB, Zhu X-D. Lipid metabolism in pregnancy. In: Cowett RM, ed. *Principles of perinatal-neonatal metabolism.* 2nd ed. New York: Springer-Verlag, 1998:221–258.
83. Carr MC, Knopp RH, Brunzell JD, et al. Effect of raloxifene on serum triglycerides in women with a history of hypertriglyceridemia while on oral estrogen therapy. *Diabetes Care* 2005;28:1555–1561.
84. Olsson AG, Oro L, Rossner S. Effects of oxandrolone on plasma lipoproteins and the intravenous fat tolerance in man. *Atherosclerosis* 1974;19:337–346.
85. Knopp RH. Drug treatment of lipid disorders. *N Engl J Med* 1999;341: 498–511.
86. Zambon A, Brown BG, Deeb SS, et al. Hepatic lipase as a focal point for the development and treatment of coronary artery disease. *J Investig Med* 2001;49:112–118.
87. Wagner JD, Clarkson TB, St Clair RW, et al. Estrogen and progesterone

replacement therapy reduces low density lipoprotein accumulation in the coronary arteries of surgically postmenopausal cynomolgus monkeys. *J Clin Invest* 1991;88:1995–2002.
88. Haarbo J, Nielsen LB, Stender S, et al. Aortic permeability to LDL during estrogen therapy. A study in normocholesterolemic rabbits. *Arterioscler Thromb* 1994;14:243–247.
89. Chen SJ, Li H, Durand J, Oparil S, et al. Estrogen reduces myointimal proliferation after balloon injury of rat carotid artery. *Circulation* 1996; 93:577–584.
90. Zhu X, Bonet B, Gillenwater H, et al. Opposing effects of estrogen and progestins on LDL oxidation and vascular wall cytotoxicity: implications for atherogenesis. *Proc Soc Exp Biol Med* 1999;222:214–221.
91. Mendelsohn ME, Karas RH. The protective effects of estrogen on the cardiovascular system. *N Engl J Med* 1999;340:1801–1811.
92. Mendelsohn ME, Karas RH. Molecular and cellular basis of cardiovascular gender differences. *Science* 2005;308:1583–1587.
93. Losordo DW, Kearney M, Kim EA, et al. Variable expression of the estrogen receptor in normal and atherosclerotic coronary arteries of premenopausal women. *Circulation* 1994;89:1501–1510.
94. Herrington DM, Braden GA, Williams JK, et al. Endothelial-dependent coronary vasomotor responsiveness in postmenopausal women with and without estrogen replacement therapy. *Am J Cardiol* 1994;73:951–952.
95. Gerhard M, Ganz P. How do we explain the clinical benefits of estrogen? From bedside to bench. *Circulation* 1995;92:5–8.
96. Guetta V, Cannon RO 3rd. Cardiovascular effects of estrogen and lipid-lowering therapies in postmenopausal women. *Circulation* 1996;93:1928–1937.
97. Polderman KH, Stehouwer CD, van Kamp GJ, et al. Influence of sex hormones on plasma endothelin levels. *Ann Intern Med* 1993;118:429–432.
98. Yue P, Chatterjee K, Beale C, et al. Testosterone relaxes rabbit coronary arteries and aorta. *Circulation* 1995;91:1154–1160.
99. Pratico D, FitzGerald GA. Testosterone and thromboxane. Of muscles, mice, and men. *Circulation* 1995;91:2694–2698.
100. Miller VM, Vanhoutte PM. Progesterone and modulation of endothelium-dependent responses in canine coronary arteries. *Am J Physiol* 1991;261: R1022–1027.
101. Adams MR, Register TC, Golden DL, et al. Medroxyprogesterone acetate antagonizes inhibitory effects of conjugated equine estrogens on coronary artery atherosclerosis. *Arterioscler Thromb Vasc Biol* 1997;17:217–221.
102. Levine RL, Chen SJ, Durand J, et al. Medroxyprogesterone attenuates estrogen-mediated inhibition of neointima formation after balloon injury of the rat carotid artery. *Circulation* 1996;94:2221–2227.
103. Adams MR, Williams JK, Kaplan JR. Effects of androgens on coronary artery atherosclerosis and atherosclerosis-related impairment of vascular responsiveness. *Arterioscler Thromb Vasc Biol* 1995;15:562–570.
104. Zhu X, Bonet B, Knopp RH. Estradiol 17beta inhibition of LDL oxidation and endothelial cell cytotoxicity is opposed by progestins to different degrees. *Atherosclerosis* 2000;148:31–41.
105. Wahl P, Walden C, Knopp R, et al. Effect of estrogen/progestin potency on lipid/lipoprotein cholesterol. *N Engl J Med* 1983;308:862–867.
106. Bloemenkamp KW, Rosendaal FR, Helmerhorst FM, et al. Enhancement by factor V Leiden mutation of risk of deep-vein thrombosis associated with oral contraceptives containing a third-generation progestagen. *Lancet* 1995;346:1593–1596.
107. Lewis MA, Spitzer WO, Heinemann LA, et al. Third generation oral contraceptives and risk of myocardial infarction: an international case-control study. Transnational Research Group on Oral Contraceptives and the Health of Young Women. *BMJ* 1996;312:88–90.
108. Knopp RH, Broyles FE, Cheung M, et al. Comparison of the lipoprotein, carbohydrate, and hemostatic effects of phasic oral contraceptives containing desogestrel or levonorgestrel. *Contraception* 2001;63:1–11.
109. Mann JI, Vessey MP, Thorogood M, et al. Myocardial infarction in young women with special reference to oral contraceptive practice. *Br Med J* 1975;2:241–245.
110. Mann JI, Inman WH. Oral contraceptives and death from myocardial infarction. *Br Med J* 1975;2:245–248.
111. Baillargeon JP, McClish DK, Essah PA, et al. Association between the current use of low-dose oral contraceptives and cardiovascular arterial disease: a meta-analysis. *J Clin Endocrinol Metab* 2005;90:3863–3870.
112. Croft P, Hannaford PC. Risk factors for acute myocardial infarction in women: evidence from the Royal College of General Practitioners' oral contraception study. *BMJ* 1989;298:165–168.
113. Rosenberg L, Kaufman DW, Helmrich SP, et al. Myocardial infarction and cigarette smoking in women younger than 50 years of age. *JAMA* 1985;253:2965–2969.
114. Spain D. Concerning the pathology of acute coronary heart disease in young women. In: Olver M, ed. *Coronary heart disease in young women*. Edinburgh: Churchill Livingstone, 1978:61–70.
115. Holden J Sudden death in a 29-year old woman [clinical conference]. *Am J Med* 1988;84:265–272.
116. Knopp RH, LaRosa JC, Burkman RT Jr. Contraception and dyslipidemia. *Am J Obstet Gynecol* 1993;168:1994–2005.
117. The Writing Group for the PEPI Trial. Effects of estrogen or estrogen/progestin regimens on heart disease risk factors in postmenopausal women. The Postmenopausal Estrogen/Progestin Interventions (PEPI) Trial. *JAMA* 1995;273:199–208.
118. Cushman M, Legault C, Barrett-Connor E, et al. Effect of postmenopausal hormones on inflammation-sensitive proteins: the Postmenopausal Estrogen/Progestin Interventions (PEPI) Study. *Circulation* 1999;100:717–722.
119. Pasceri V, Willerson JT, Yeh ET. Direct proinflammatory effect of C-reactive protein on human endothelial cells. *Circulation* 2000;102:2165–2168.
120. Barrett-Connor E. Postmenopausal estrogen and prevention bias. *Ann Intern Med* 1991;115:455–456.
121. Grodstein F, Stampfer MJ, Manson JE, et al. Postmenopausal estrogen and progestin use and the risk of cardiovascular disease. *N Engl J Med* 1996;335:453–461.
122. Psaty BM, Heckbert SR, Atkins D, et al. The risk of myocardial infarction associated with the combined use of estrogens and progestins in postmenopausal women. *Arch Intern Med* 1994;154:1333–1339.
123. Hulley S, Grady D, Bush T, et al. Randomized trial of estrogen plus progestin for secondary prevention of coronary heart disease in postmenopausal women. Heart and Estrogen/progestin Replacement Study (HERS) Research Group. *JAMA* 1998;280:605–613.
124. Grady D, Herrington D, Bittner V, et al. Cardiovascular disease outcomes during 6.8 years of hormone therapy: Heart and Estrogen/progestin Replacement Study follow-up (HERS II). *JAMA* 2002;288:49–57.
125. Rossouw JE, Anderson GL, Prentice RL, et al. Risks and benefits of estrogen plus progestin in healthy postmenopausal women: principal results From the Women's Health Initiative randomized controlled trial. *JAMA* 2002;288:321–333.
126. Anderson GL, Limacher M, Assaf AR, et al. Effects of conjugated equine estrogen in postmenopausal women with hysterectomy: the Women's Health Initiative randomized controlled trial. *JAMA* 2004;291:1701–1712.
127. Herrington DM, Reboussin DM, Brosnihan KB, et al. Effects of estrogen replacement on the progression of coronary-artery atherosclerosis. *N Engl J Med* 2000;343:522–529.
128. Hanke H, Kamenz J, Hanke S, et al. Effect of 17-beta estradiol on pre-existing atherosclerotic lesions: role of the endothelium. *Atherosclerosis* 1999;147:123–132.
129. Williams JK, Anthony MS, Honore EK, et al. Regression of atherosclerosis in female monkeys. *Arterioscler Thromb Vasc Biol* 1995;15:827–836.
130. Daly E, Vessey MP, Hawkins MM, et al. Risk of venous thromboembolism in users of hormone replacement therapy. *Lancet* 1996;348:977–980.
131. Jick H, Derby LE, Myers MW, et al. Risk of hospital admission for idiopathic venous thromboembolism among users of postmenopausal oestrogens. *Lancet* 1996;348:981–983.
132. Grodstein F, Stampfer MJ, Goldhaber SZ, et al. Prospective study of exogenous hormones and risk of pulmonary embolism in women. *Lancet* 1996;348:983–987.
133. Grady D, Wenger NK, Herrington D, et al. Postmenopausal hormone therapy increases risk for venous thromboembolic disease. The Heart and Estrogen/progestin Replacement Study. *Ann Intern Med* 2000;132:689–696.
134. Knopp RH, Aikawa K, Knopp EA. Estrogen therapies, lipids, and the heart disease prevention controversy. *Curr Cardiol Rep* 2003;5:477–482.
135. Mosca L, Appel LJ, Benjamin EJ, et al. Evidence-based guidelines for cardiovascular disease prevention in women. *Circulation* 2004;109:672–693.
136. Turgeon JL, McDonnell DP, Martin KA, et al. Hormone therapy: physiological complexity belies therapeutic simplicity. *Science* 2004;304:1269–1273.
137. Seed M, Knopp RH. Estrogens, lipoproteins, and cardiovascular risk factors: an update following the randomized placebo-controlled trials of hormone-replacement therapy. *Curr Opin Lipidol* 2004;15:459–467.
138. Sacks FM, Pfeffer MA, Moye LA, et al. The effect of pravastatin on coronary events after myocardial infarction in patients with average cholesterol levels. Cholesterol and Recurrent Events Trial investigators. *N Engl J Med* 1996;335:1001–1009.
139. Dollar AL, Kragel AH, Fernicola DJ, et al. Composition of atherosclerotic plaques in coronary arteries in women less than 40 years of age with fatal coronary artery disease and implications for plaque reversibility. *Am J Cardiol* 1991;67:1223–1227.
140. Jacobs D, Blackburn H, Higgins M, et al. Report of the Conference on Low Blood Cholesterol: Mortality Associations. *Circulation* 1992;86:1046–1060.
141. Hulley SB, Walsh JM, Newman TB. Health policy on blood cholesterol. Time to change directions. *Circulation* 1992;86:1026–1029.
142. Shear CL, Franklin FA, Stinnett S, et al. Expanded Clinical Evaluation of Lovastatin (EXCEL) study results. Effect of patient characteristics on lovastatin-induced changes in plasma concentrations of lipids and lipoproteins. *Circulation* 1992;85:1293–1303.
143. Pierce LR, Wysowski DK, Gross TP. Myopathy and rhabdomyolysis associated with lovastatin-gemfibrozil combination therapy. *JAMA* 1990; 264:71–75.
144. Rosenfeld ME, Polinsky P, Virmani R, et al. Advanced atherosclerotic lesions in the innominate artery of the ApoE knockout mouse. *Arterioscler Thromb Vasc Biol* 2000;20:2587–2592.
145. Wilson PW, Garrison RJ, Castelli WP. Postmenopausal estrogen use, cigarette smoking, and cardiovascular morbidity in women over 50. The Framingham Study. *N Engl J Med* 1985;313:1038–1043.

CHAPTER 10 ■ ETHANOL AND THE HEART

MICHAEL H. CRIQUI AND LORI B. DANIELS

OVERVIEW

Epidemiologic studies have consistently shown that light to moderate alcohol consumption is associated with reduced morbidity and mortality from coronary heart disease (CHD) (1). However, higher levels of alcohol use can be cardiotoxic and contribute to hypertension, arrhythmias, and cardiomyopathy and ultimately lead to increased cardiovascular disease (CVD). In addition, other disease endpoints, including cancer, cirrhosis, and accidental and violent death, are increased at higher levels of alcohol consumption. This J-shaped relationship between alcohol intake and survival has been extensively described (2).

EPIDEMIOLOGY

Approximately 63% of the U.S. population consumes alcohol, and approximately one tenth of these are considered heavy drinkers. The prevalence of alcohol consumption differs by gender and by age, and is higher in men and in younger individuals (3). Among the identifiable etiologies of nonischemic dilated cardiomyopathy (DCM) in the United States, alcohol is the most common in both sexes and all races, accounting for almost half of all cases (4). Furthermore, excessive alcohol intake is reported in 3% to 40% of patients with otherwise unexplained idiopathic DCM (5). With early detection and abstinence from further alcohol, cardiac function can recover in some cases (6,7).

ANATOMY AND PATHOLOGY

Specimens from autopsies and biopsies of alcoholic hearts have shown varying degrees of morphologic abnormalities, depending on the stage and progression of the disease. During the preclinical phase, left ventricular (LV) dilation and a normal or moderately increased LV mass may be seen. Some patients may also have wall thickening, which may offset the LV dilation and lead to a compensated, asymptomatic state. With progression of the disease, varying degrees of cardiomegaly reflecting chamber dilation are seen, particularly when there is concomitant mitral insufficiency. On gross observation, the heart appears flabby, large, and pale (4).

The exact pathogenesis of alcoholic cardiomyopathy is incompletely understood. At a microscopic level, alcohol affects mitochondrial structure and function, which can be observed on biopsy (8). Changes in the sarcoplasmic reticulum, contractile proteins, and calcium homeostasis also contribute to myocardial cell dysfunction (4).

PATHOPHYSIOLOGY

Acutely, ethanol ingestion exerts a transient direct toxic effect on cardiac performance, acting as a negative inotrope (9–11). Increased autonomic activity may lead to a modest increase in heart rate (10). Because these actions of alcohol tend to have opposing effects, overt evidence of hemodynamic derangements from alcohol can be minimal in healthy individuals. Still, asymptomatic cardiac dysfunction may be present even in healthy "social drinkers" who consume smaller quantities of alcohol (12).

The transient negative inotropic effect on myocardial function can become permanent with chronic consumption. In addition, chronic users often exhibit greater hemodynamic derangements from alcohol, especially in the setting of underlying cardiac disease. Increased diastolic stiffness, possibly due to accumulation of myocardial collagen in the extracellular matrix, may contribute to clinical presentations of the alcoholic heart. The role of ethanol in the accumulation of collagen can be enhanced by the use of tobacco (13), which is a common coaddiction. With both acute and chronic ingestion, abnormalities in myofibrillar protein turnover can contribute to myocardial damage, perhaps with involvement of oxidative stress (14). Reactive oxygen species may impair myocyte function by interfering with calcium handling (4). Toxic effects of acetaldehyde and fatty acid ethyl esters, metabolites and byproducts of alcohol, may also potentiate myocardial damage via impairment of mitochondrial oxidative phosphorylation (9).

Alcohol-induced hypertension also contributes to chronic myocardial dysfunction in chronic drinkers, in a dose-related fashion (15–18). Individuals who drink more than two alcoholic beverages per day have twice the incidence of hypertension compared with nondrinkers (19).

Thiamine deficiency is another factor contributing to alcoholic cardiomyopathy in many instances. Approximately 15% of asymptomatic alcoholics are moderately deficient in thiamine (20). The physiologic derangements seen in beriberi heart disease, however, are different from those seen in alcoholic cardiomyopathy, and include a hyperdynamic state with decreased peripheral vascular resistance, increased cardiac output, tachycardia, and biventricular failure (21).

Finally, some alcoholic beverages contain additives such as cobalt that may be directly cardiotoxic (22).

CLINICAL PRESENTATIONS

Hypertension

Heavy alcohol consumption is an independent risk factor for hypertension, with up to a twofold increased incidence of hypertension in drinkers compared with nondrinkers (15,17,19,23,24). Some studies have shown an association with increased incidence of hypertension from even low to moderate alcohol consumption (17,24), although the risk appears to be dose dependent (15–17). At three or more drinks per day, there is a relatively linear relationship between alcohol intake and blood pressure in a variety of populations, irrespective of race and gender (25) (Fig. 10.1).

Cardiomyopathy and Heart Failure

Chronic ethanol abuse induces a marked decrease in left ventricular function compared to normal individuals. In fact, alcohol has been implicated as a major cause of up to 30% of all dilated cardiomyopathies (26). The risk of developing alcoholic cardiomyopathy is related to both the mean daily alcohol intake and the duration of drinking, although there is significant individual susceptibility to the toxic effects of alcohol (26–28). Most patients in whom alcoholic cardiomyopathy develops have been drinking greater than 80 grams per day for more than 5 years (27,29). Early changes in LV function in chronic asymptomatic alcoholics demonstrate dilation with preserved ejection fraction and impaired relaxation. With increased duration of alcoholism, the LV diastolic filling abnormalities progress (30) and there is progressive decline in LV systolic function (26).

As previously mentioned, thiamine deficiency should also be considered as a potential factor contributing to alcoholic cardiomyopathy because 15% of asymptomatic alcoholics are moderately deficient in thiamine as determined by dietary history and excretion of vitamin metabolites (20). For the diagnosis of beriberi heart disease, several criteria are required, including a history of thiamine deficiency for more than 3 months, absence of another etiology of heart failure, evidence of peripheral neuropathy, and a therapeutic response to thiamine (21).

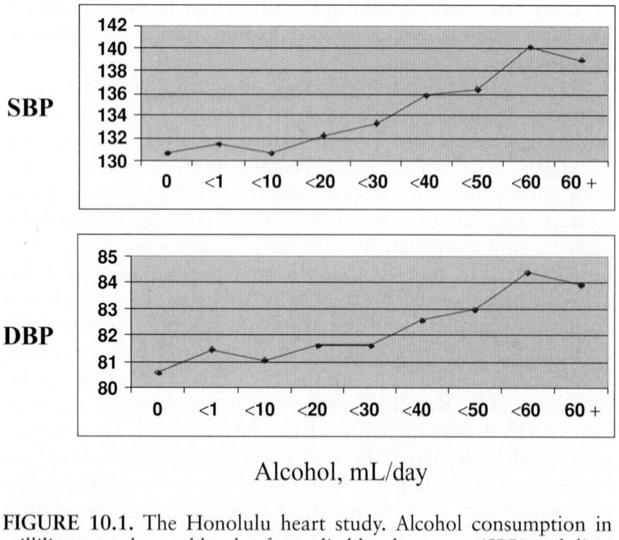

FIGURE 10.1. The Honolulu heart study. Alcohol consumption in milliliters per day and levels of systolic blood pressure (SBP) and diastolic blood pressure (DBP). (Modified from Criqui MH, Langer RD, Reed DM. Dietary alcohol, calcium, and potassium. Independent and combined effects on blood pressure. *Circulation* 1989;80:609–614.)

Dysrhythmias

Dysrhythmias are associated with underlying changes in myocardial composition and electrophysiology as a consequence of chronic alcohol ingestion, although they may occur in up to 60% of binge drinkers even in the absence of underlying myocardial damage (31,32). Electrolyte abnormalities such as hypokalemia and hypomagnesemia, which occur more frequently in chronic alcoholics, may also contribute (33–35).

The most common alcohol-related arrhythmias are paroxysmal atrial arrhythmias, especially atrial fibrillation, although ventricular dysrhythmias can also occur (31,36). *Holiday heart* describes the development of an acute arrhythmic process, generally atrial fibrillation, after an episode of heavy alcohol consumption. These episodes frequently occur over long weekends or holidays, thus the name *holiday heart* (31).

Sudden Cardiac Death

An increased incidence of sudden cardiac death (SCD) has been found among the alcoholic population (37,38), with one study showing heavy drinkers with a 60% increased risk compared with occasional or light drinkers (39).

Dose is an important factor in determining the relationship of alcohol to the development of sudden death. In contrast to the increased risk of sudden death with heavy drinking, moderate or light alcohol intake (two to six drinks per week) reduced sudden death in a prospective study of more than 21,000 male physicians compared with those who rarely or never consumed alcohol (40). This dose-dependent relationship was also seen in an analysis of the Framingham population, in which individuals who consumed more than 2,500 grams of alcohol per month had an increased risk of sudden death (41).

Possible mechanisms for the observed association between alcohol and SCD include prolongation of the QT interval leading to ventricular tachyarrhythmias, rapid degeneration of ventricular tachycardias into ventricular fibrillation, electrolyte abnormalities, sympathoadrenal stimulation, and decreased vagal input (25).

DIAGNOSIS, MANAGEMENT, AND PROGNOSIS

The diagnosis of alcoholic cardiomyopathy can be suspected when congestive heart failure is present along with cardiomegaly and a history of heavy and prolonged alcohol consumption. Laboratory data have a low sensitivity and specificity for the diagnosis of alcoholic cardiomyopathy, but findings such as an elevated red cell mean corpuscular volume, aspartate aminotransferase, γ-glutamyl transferase, serum uric acid, and high-density lipoprotein or mild thrombocytopenia may suggest alcohol abuse (42,43). Carbohydrate-deficient transferrin, a more recently developed biologic marker of heavy alcohol abuse, may be a superior test to use especially in men younger than 40 years old and in smokers (44–46). Endomyocardial biopsy is not generally necessary for the diagnosis of alcoholic cardiomyopathy, but it may help to distinguish among various etiologies when the diagnosis is in question.

The therapy of heart failure in alcoholic patients is guided by the same principles as in other forms of cardiomyopathy, with diuretics, β blockers, angiotensin-converting enzymes, and digoxin used according to standard guidelines. However, abstinence from alcohol is crucial and can lead to improved LV function, especially if the myocardium has not yet fibrosed (47,48). Treatment of dysrhythmias secondary to ethanol should also follow standard arrhythmia management practices but also involves alcohol cessation and correction of electrolyte abnormalities, especially potassium and magnesium.

Prognosis in alcoholic cardiomyopathy may be significantly better than in idiopathic cardiomyopathy (49), but some studies suggest that this is only true in patients who are able to abstain from further alcohol (49,50). One study of 55 men with alcoholic cardiomyopathy showed that left ventricular function can improve with even limited "controlled" drinking of up to 60 grams of ethanol per day (four drinks), whereas consuming more than 80 grams per day was associated with further deterioration in function (51).

BENEFITS OF LIGHT TO MODERATE ALCOHOL CONSUMPTION

A series of epidemiologic studies have suggested that light to moderate alcohol consumption, defined as one to two drinks a day of any alcoholic beverage, helps to protect against coronary artery disease (1,52–60) and reduces cardiovascular mortality (2,53,61–63) as well as all-cause mortality (64,65).

The beneficial effects of light to moderate drinking on CVD have been shown in multiple populations, including various ethnic groups, both genders (66), young and old (67), patients with known heart disease (62,63,68) and without underlying CVD (40), and type 2 diabetics (69,70). Recent studies have also suggested that light to moderate alcohol consumption is associated with a reduced risk of ischemic stroke (71) and peripheral vascular disease (72,73).

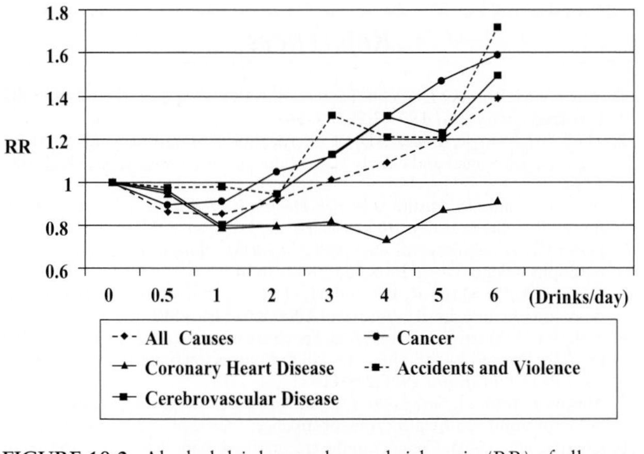

FIGURE 10.2. Alcohol drinks per day and risk ratio (RR) of all-cause and cause-specific mortality over 12 years in the American Cancer Society prospective study of 276,802 men aged 40 to 59 years. Risk ratios are adjusted for age and smoking habits.

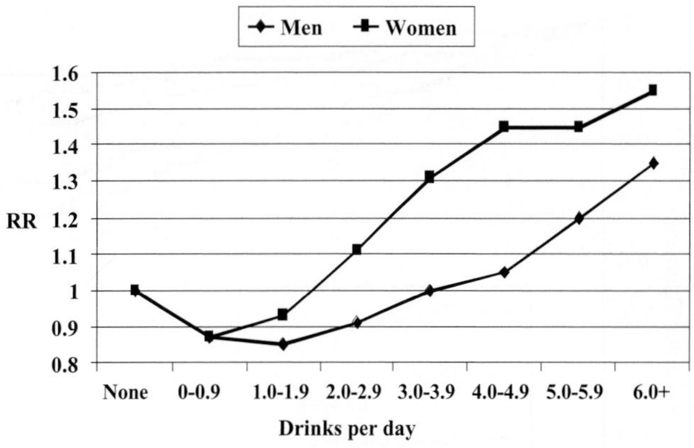

FIGURE 10.3. Relationship of usual alcohol intake to all-cause mortality, derived from a pooled analysis of 14 cohort studies. RR, risk ratio.

Total morbidity and mortality seem to be minimized at about one drink per day. A J-shaped pattern with a lower risk among light to moderate drinkers and an increased incidence of cardiac mortality in heavy drinkers may be secondary to alcohol-related arrhythmias, hypertension, or cardiomyopathy (Figs. 10.2 and 10.3). Despite widespread opinion to the contrary, the beneficial effects of moderate alcohol consumption are unrelated to the type of beverage consumed per se (55), but they may reflect the manner in which different alcoholic beverages are consumed (59,74,75).

A biologically plausible basis for these beneficial effects of light to moderate drinking is the approximately 30% rise in high-density-lipoprotein (HDL) cholesterol levels, which are inversely related to CHD risk (76–78). In addition, ethanol ingestion induces increased thrombolytic activity via enhanced endogenous tissue plasminogen activator (79,80), downregulation of plasminogen activator inhibitor-I (81), decreased platelet activity (82,83), and reduced fibrinogen levels (84). Alcohol also may favorably affect insulin resistance (85,86), and may have antioxidant activity (87–89) and antiinflammatory activity (90,91). Several studies have also raised the possibility that some of the cardioprotective benefit from low to moderate consumption results from alcohol acting as a preconditioning agent (92).

SPECIAL GROUPS

Women

For any given amount of alcohol consumed, women on average achieve a higher blood alcohol level than men. The likelihood of developing alcoholic cardiomyopathy correlates with total lifetime alcohol consumption in both sexes; however, women may be more sensitive to the cardiotoxic effects of alcohol and develop similar degrees of left ventricular dysfunction with a lower total lifetime dose and a lower daily dose of alcohol than men (93). In addition, alcohol is a dose-dependent risk factor for breast cancer (94). At the same time, the overall risk of CVD is somewhat lower in women than in men. As shown in Figure 10.3, which depicts the association between number of drinks consumed per day and all-cause mortality in a meta-analysis of 14 studies, there is a less favorable risk–benefit ratio for alcohol in women than in men (95).

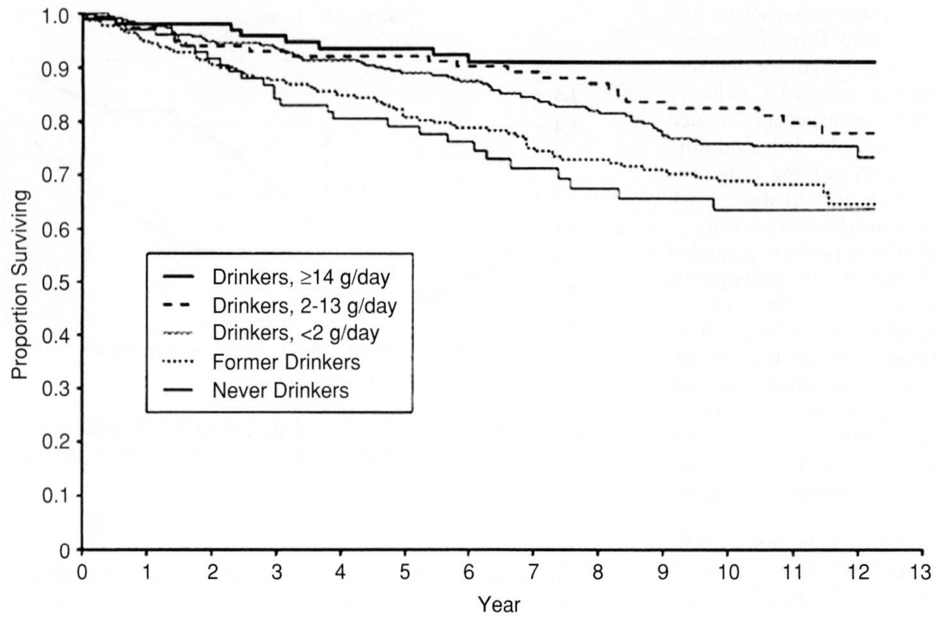

FIGURE 10.4. Survival curves for coronary heart disease mortality according to alcohol intake in 983 older-onset diabetic persons in the Wisconsin Epidemiologic Study of Diabetic Retinopathy, 1984 to 1996. (From Valmadrid CT, Klein R, Moss SE, et al. Alcohol intake and the risk of coronary heart disease mortality in persons with older-onset diabetes mellitus. *JAMA* 1999;282:239–246.)

Diabetics

As in other patients at high risk for CHD, mild to moderate alcohol consumption appears to reduce CHD and all-cause mortality in diabetics (70,96–98) (Fig. 10.4). However, the highest consumption category in this study was one or more drinks per day, so heavy drinkers were not represented. In addition, any potential benefits must be carefully weighed against the possible risks, some of which are unique to diabetics. Alcohol may both induce and mask potentially severe hypoglycemia by exaggerating hypoglycemic effects caused by other factors, such as exercise, insulin, sulfonylureas, and β blockers. Finally, heavy alcohol may worsen diabetic neuropathy (69).

CONTROVERSIES AND PERSONAL PERSPECTIVES

Although light to moderate alcohol consumption clearly affords some protection against CVD, a general public health recommendation endorsing drinking is contraindicated. The American Heart Association/American College of Cardiology science advisories have concluded that, in the absence of proof of causality, the use of alcohol as a cardioprotective strategy is not recommended (25). Although the evidence supporting the cardiovascular benefits of moderate alcohol ingestion is reassuring, as an intoxicating substance with a high addiction potential, alcohol is nonetheless a leading cause of morbidity and mortality. Any recommendation that nondrinkers start drinking alcohol or that light drinkers drink more is likely to increase alcohol abuse, which appears to correlate with overall alcohol consumption in the general population. Such an increase would be differentially greater in the young, who are at low risk for CVD but are at high risk for alcohol-related adverse outcomes including vehicular accidents. Except in highly selected situations, alcohol is too dangerous to be employed as a pharmacologic agent (99).

If alcohol were a new drug undergoing regulatory review for approval as a therapeutic agent to treat those at risk for CVD, the Food and Drug Administration would be presented with clinical trials showing a dose-related impairment in coordination and cognition in all subjects leading to significant morbidity and mortality, severe psychosocial dysfunction in some, and a profound dependency in about 10% of those receiving the drug. There is virtually no chance that alcohol would receive Food and Drug Administration approval as a pharmacologic agent, regardless of any cardioprotective effects.

THE FUTURE

Future studies of alcohol and the cardiovascular system have much to uncover. Recently, a panel of experts was convened and identified several key areas for future studies, including elucidation of the role that genetic susceptibility plays in alcohol's cardiotoxic and cardioprotective effects and determination of the mechanisms underlying alcohol-induced CVD as well as alcohol-induced cardioprotection. Another exciting area of focus for future research is the potential for stem cells to assist with myocardial regeneration and repair in hearts damaged by alcohol (25).

References

1. Marmot M, Brunner E. Alcohol and cardiovascular disease: the status of the U shaped curve. *BMJ* 1991;303:565–568.
2. Thun MJ, Peto R, Lopez AD, et al. Alcohol consumption and mortality among middle-aged and elderly U.S. adults. *N Engl J Med* 1997;337:1705–1714.
3. National Center for Health Statistics. *Health, United States, 2004 with chartbook on trends in the health of Americans.* Hyattsville, MD: 2004.
4. Piano MR. Alcoholic cardiomyopathy: incidence, clinical characteristics, and pathophysiology. *Chest* 2002;121:1638–1650.
5. Gavazzi A, De Maria R, Parolini M, et al. Alcohol abuse and dilated cardiomyopathy in men. *Am J Cardiol* 2000;85:1114–1118.
6. Ballester M, Marti V, Carrio I, et al. Spectrum of alcohol-induced myocardial damage detected by indium-111—labeled monoclonal antimyosin antibodies. *J Am Coll Cardiol* 1997;29:160–167.
7. Masani F, Kato H, Sasagawa Y, et al. An echocardiographic study of alcoholic cardiomyopathy after total abstinence. *J Cardiol* 1990;20:627–634.
8. Cherpachenko NM. Changes in the enzymatic activity in the myocardium of patients with idiopathic and secondary dilated cardiomyopathy. *Arkh Patol* 1993;55:69–73.
9. Patel VB, Why HJ, Richardson PJ, et al. The effects of alcohol on the heart. *Adverse Drug React Toxicol Rev* 1997;16:15–43.

10. Thomas AP, Rozanski DJ, Renard DC, et al. Effects of ethanol on the contractile function of the heart: a review. *Alcohol Clin Exp Res* 1994;18:121–131.
11. Lange LG, Sobel BE. Mitochondrial dysfunction induced by fatty acid ethyl esters, myocardial metabolites of ethanol. *J Clin Invest* 1983;72:724–731.
12. Kelbaek H, Gjorup T, Brynjolf I, et al. Acute effects of alcohol on left ventricular function in healthy subjects at rest and during upright exercise. *Am J Cardiol* 1985;55:164–167.
13. Rajiyah G, Agarwal R, Avendano G, et al. Influence of nicotine on myocardial stiffness and fibrosis during chronic ethanol use. *Alcohol Clin Exp Res* 1996;20:985–989.
14. Preedy VR, Atkinson LM, Richardson PJ, et al. Mechanisms of ethanol-induced cardiac damage. *Br Heart J* 1993;69:197–200.
15. Thadhani R, Camargo Jr CA, Stampfer MJ, et al. Prospective study of moderate alcohol consumption and risk of hypertension in young women. *Arch Intern Med* 2002;162:569–574.
16. Kaplan NM. Alcohol and hypertension. *Lancet* 1995;345:1588–1589.
17. Fuchs FD, Chambless LE, Whelton PK, et al. Alcohol consumption and the incidence of hypertension: The Atherosclerosis Risk in Communities Study. *Hypertension* 2001;37:1242–1250.
18. Criqui MH, Langer RD, Reed DM. Dietary alcohol, calcium, and potassium. Independent and combined effects on blood pressure. *Circulation* 1989;80:609–614.
19. Klatsky AL, Friedman GD, Siegelaub AB, et al. Alcohol consumption and blood pressure Kaiser-Permanente Multiphasic Health Examination data. *N Engl J Med* 1977;296:1194–1200.
20. Neville JN, Eagles JA, Samson G, et al. Nutritional status of alcoholics. *Am J Clin Nutr* 1968;21:1329–1340.
21. Blakenhorn MA. Effects of vitamin deficiency on the heart and circulation. *Circulation* 1955;11:288–291.
22. Alexander CS. Cobalt-beer cardiomyopathy. A clinical and pathologic study of twenty-eight cases. *Am J Med* 1972;53:395–417.
23. Nakanishi N, Yoshida H, Nakamura K, et al. Alcohol consumption and risk for hypertension in middle-aged Japanese men. *J Hypertens* 2001;19:851–855.
24. Stranges S, Wu T, Dorn JM, et al. Relationship of alcohol drinking pattern to risk of hypertension: a population-based study. *Hypertension* 2004;44:813–819.
25. Lucas DL, Brown RA, Wassef M, et al. Alcohol and the cardiovascular system research challenges and opportunities. *J Am Coll Cardiol* 2005;45:1916–1924.
26. Lee WK, Regan TJ. Alcoholic cardiomyopathy: is it dose-dependent? *Congest Heart Fail* 2002;8:303–306.
27. Wilke A, Kaiser A, Ferency I, et al. Alcohol and myocarditis. *Herz* 1996; 21:248–257.
28. Kajander OA, Kupari M, Laippala P, et al. Dose dependent but non-linear effects of alcohol on the left and right ventricle. *Heart* 2001;86:417–423.
29. Regan TJ. Alcohol and the cardiovascular system. *JAMA* 1990;264:377–381.
30. Lazarevic AM, Nakatani S, Neskovic AN, et al. Early changes in left ventricular function in chronic asymptomatic alcoholics: relation to the duration of heavy drinking. *J Am Coll Cardiol* 2000;35:1599–1606.
31. Ettinger PO. Holiday heart arrhythmias. *Int J Cardiol* 1984;5:540–542.
32. Ettinger PO, Wu CF, De La Cruz Jr C, et al. Arrhythmias and the "holiday heart": alcohol-associated cardiac rhythm disorders. *Am Heart J* 1978;95:555–562.
33. Elisaf M, Liberopoulos E, Bairaktari E, et al. Hypokalaemia in alcoholic patients. *Drug Alcohol Rev* 2002;21:73–76.
34. Fauchier L. Alcoholic cardiomyopathy and ventricular arrhythmias. *Chest* 2003;123:1320.
35. Elisaf M, Bairaktari E, Kalaitzidis R, et al. Hypomagnesemia in alcoholic patients. *Alcohol Clin Exp Res* 1998;22:134.
36. Buckingham TA, Kennedy HL, Goenjian AK, et al. Cardiac arrhythmias in a population admitted to an acute alcoholic detoxification center. *Am Heart J* 1985;110:961–965.
37. Vikhert AM, Tsiplenkova VG, Cherpachenko NM. Alcoholic cardiomyopathy and sudden cardiac death. *J Am Coll Cardiol* 1986;8:3A–11A.
38. Rosengren A, Wilhelmsen L, Wedel H. Separate and combined effects of smoking and alcohol abuse in middle-aged men. *Acta Med Scand* 1988;223: 111–118.
39. Wannamethee G, Shaper AG. Alcohol and sudden cardiac death. *Br Heart J* 1992;68:443–448.
40. Albert CM, Manson JE, Cook NR, et al. Moderate alcohol consumption and the risk of sudden cardiac death among US male physicians. *Circulation* 1999;100:944–950.
41. Gordon T, Kannel WB. Drinking habits and cardiovascular disease: the Framingham Study. *Am Heart J* 1983;105:667–673.
42. Afzal A, Ananthasubramaniam K, Sharma N, et al. Racial differences in patients with heart failure. *Clin Cardiol* 1999;22:791–794.
43. Wang RY, Alterman AI, Searles JS, et al. Alcohol abuse in patients with dilated cardiomyopathy. Laboratory vs clinical detection. *Arch Intern Med* 1990;150:1079–1082.
44. Yersin B, Nicolet JF, Dercrey H, et al. Screening for excessive alcohol drinking. Comparative value of carbohydrate-deficient transferrin, gamma-glutamyltransferase, and mean corpuscular volume. *Arch Intern Med* 1995; 155:1907–1911.
45. Anton RF, Lieber C, Tabakoff B. Carbohydrate-deficient transferrin and gamma-glutamyltransferase for the detection and monitoring of alcohol use: results from a multisite study. *Alcohol Clin Exp Res* 2002;26:1215–1222.
46. Bell H, Tallaksen CM, Try K, et al. Carbohydrate-deficient transferrin and other markers of high alcohol consumption: a study of 502 patients admitted consecutively to a medical department. *Alcohol Clin Exp Res* 1994;18:1103–1108.
47. Demakis JG, Proskey A, Rahimtoola SH, et al. The natural course of alcoholic cardiomyopathy. *Ann Intern Med* 1974;80:293–297.
48. Guillo P, Mansourati J, Maheu B, et al. Long-term prognosis in patients with alcoholic cardiomyopathy and severe heart failure after total abstinence. *Am J Cardiol* 1997;79:1276–1278.
49. Prazak P, Pfisterer M, Osswald S, et al. Differences of disease progression in congestive heart failure due to alcoholic as compared to idiopathic dilated cardiomyopathy. *Eur Heart J* 1996;17:251–257.
50. Fauchier L, Babuty D, Poret P, et al. Comparison of long-term outcome of alcoholic and idiopathic dilated cardiomyopathy. *Eur Heart J* 2000;21:306–314.
51. Nicolas JM, Fernandez-Sola J, Estruch R, et al. The effect of controlled drinking in alcoholic cardiomyopathy. *Ann Intern Med* 2002;136:192–200.
52. Jackson R, Scragg R, Beaglehole R. Alcohol consumption and risk of coronary heart disease. *BMJ* 1991;303:211–216.
53. Stampfer MJ, Colditz GA, Willett WC, et al. A prospective study of moderate alcohol consumption and the risk of coronary disease and stroke in women. *N Engl J Med* 1988;319:267–273.
54. Mukamal KJ, Conigrave KM, Mittleman MA, et al. Roles of drinking pattern and type of alcohol consumed in coronary heart disease in men. *N Engl J Med* 2003;348:109–118.
55. Rimm EB, Klatsky A, Grobbee D, et al. Review of moderate alcohol consumption and reduced risk of coronary heart disease: is the effect due to beer, wine, or spirits. *BMJ* 1996;312:731–736.
56. Fuchs CS, Stampfer MJ, Colditz GA, et al. Alcohol consumption and mortality among women. *N Engl J Med* 1995;332:1245–1250.
57. Gaziano JM, Gaziano TA, Glynn RJ, et al. Light-to-moderate alcohol consumption and mortality in the Physicians' Health Study enrollment cohort. *J Am Coll Cardiol* 2000;35:96–105.
58. Klatsky AL, Armstrong MA, Friedman GD. Alcohol and mortality. *Ann Intern Med* 1992;117:646–654.
59. Criqui MH, Ringel BL. Does diet or alcohol explain the French paradox? *Lancet* 1994;344:1719–1723.
60. Janszky I, Mukamal KJ, Orth-Gomer K, et al. Alcohol consumption and coronary atherosclerosis progression—the Stockholm Female Coronary Risk Angiographic Study. *Atherosclerosis* 2004;176:311–319.
61. Hein HO, Suadicani P, Gyntelberg F. Alcohol consumption, serum low density lipoprotein cholesterol concentration, and risk of ischaemic heart disease: six year follow up in the Copenhagen male study. *BMJ* 1996;312:736–741.
62. Muntwyler J, Hennekens CH, Buring JE, et al. Mortality and light to moderate alcohol consumption after myocardial infarction. *Lancet* 1998;352: 1882–1885.
63. Mukamal KJ, Maclure M, Muller JE, et al. Prior alcohol consumption and mortality following acute myocardial infarction. *JAMA* 2001;285:1965–1970.
64. Gmel G, Gutjahr E, Rehm J. How stable is the risk curve between alcohol and all-cause mortality and what factors influence the shape? A precision-weighted hierarchical meta-analysis. *Eur J Epidemiol* 2003;18:631–642.
65. Boffetta P, Garfinkel L. Alcohol drinking and mortality among men enrolled in an American Cancer Society prospective study. *Epidemiology* 1990;1: 342–348.
66. Klatsky AL, Armstrong MA, Friedman GD. Relations of alcoholic beverage use to subsequent coronary artery disease hospitalization. *Am J Cardiol* 1986;58:710–714.
67. Abramson JL, Williams SA, Krumholz HM, et al. Moderate alcohol consumption and risk of heart failure among older persons. *JAMA* 2001; 285:1971–1977.
68. Criqui M. Alcohol in the myocardial infarction patient. *Lancet* 1998; 352:1873.
69. Criqui MH, Golomb BA. Should patients with diabetes drink to their health? *JAMA* 1999;282:279–280.
70. Valmadrid CT, Klein R, Moss SE, et al. Alcohol intake and the risk of coronary heart disease mortality in persons with older-onset diabetes mellitus. *JAMA* 1999;282:239–246.
71. Djousse L, Ellison RC, Beiser A, et al. Alcohol consumption and risk of ischemic stroke: the Framingham Study. *Stroke* 2002;33:907–912.
72. Djousse L, Levy D, Murabito JM, et al. Alcohol consumption and risk of intermittent claudication in the Framingham Heart Study. *Circulation* 2000;102:3092–3097.
73. Camargo Jr CA, Stampfer MJ, Glynn RJ, et al. Prospective study of moderate alcohol consumption and risk of peripheral arterial disease in US male physicians. *Circulation* 1997;95:577–580.
74. Gronbaek M, Becker U, Johansen D, et al. Type of alcohol consumed and mortality from all causes, coronary heart disease, and cancer. *Ann Intern Med* 2000;133:411–419.
75. Di Castelnuovo A, Rotondo S, Iacoviello L, et al. Meta-analysis of wine and beer consumption in relation to vascular risk. *Circulation* 2002;105:2836–2844.
76. Gardner CD, Tribble DL, Young DR, et al. Associations of HDL, HDL(2), and HDL(3) cholesterol and apolipoproteins A-I and B with lifestyle factors

in healthy women and men: the Stanford Five City Project. *Prev Med* 2000; 31:346–356.
77. Criqui MH. The reduction of coronary heart disease with light to moderate alcohol consumption: effect or artifact? *Br J Addict Alcohol Other Drugs* 1990;85:854–857.
78. Gaziano JM, Buring JE, Breslow JL, et al. Moderate alcohol intake, increased levels of high-density lipoprotein and its subfractions, and decreased risk of myocardial infarction. *N Engl J Med* 1993;329:1829–1834.
79. Ridker PM, Vaughan DE, Stampfer MJ, et al. Association of moderate alcohol consumption and plasma concentration of endogenous tissue-type plasminogen activator. *JAMA* 1994;272:929–933.
80. Margaglione M, Cappucci G, Colaizzo D, et al. Fibrinogen plasma levels in an apparently healthy general population–relation to environmental and genetic determinants. *Thromb Haemost* 1998;80:805–810.
81. Grenett HE, Aikens ML, Tabengwa EM, et al. Ethanol downregulates transcription of the PAI-1 gene in cultured human endothelial cells. *Thromb Res* 2000;97:247–255.
82. Haut MJ, Cowan DH. The effect of ethanol on hemostatic properties of human blood platelets. *Am J Med* 1974;56:22–33.
83. Mikhailidis DP, Jeremy JY, Barradas MA, et al. Effect of ethanol on vascular prostacyclin (prostaglandin I2) synthesis, platelet aggregation, and platelet thromboxane release. *Br Med J (Clin Res Ed)* 1983;287:1495–1498.
84. McConnell MV, Vavouranakis I, Wu LL, et al. Effects of a single, daily alcoholic beverage on lipid and hemostatic markers of cardiovascular risk. *Am J Cardiol* 1997;80:1226–1228.
85. Razay G, Heaton KW, Bolton CH, et al. Alcohol consumption and its relation to cardiovascular risk factors in British women. *BMJ* 1992;304:80–83.
86. Kiechl S, Willeit J, Poewe W, et al. Insulin sensitivity and regular alcohol consumption: large, prospective, cross sectional population study (Bruneck study). *BMJ* 1996;313:1040–1044.
87. Frankel EN, Kanner J, German JB, et al. Inhibition of oxidation of human low-density lipoprotein by phenolic substances in red wine. *Lancet* 1993; 341:454–457.
88. Miyagi Y, Miwa K, Inoue H. Inhibition of human low-density lipoprotein oxidation by flavonoids in red wine and grape juice. *Am J Cardiol* 1997;80:1627–1631.
89. Kerry NL, Abbey M. Red wine and fractionated phenolic compounds prepared from red wine inhibit low density lipoprotein oxidation in vitro. *Atherosclerosis* 1997;135:93–102.
90. Albert MA, Glynn RJ, Ridker PM. Alcohol consumption and plasma concentration of C-reactive protein. *Circulation* 2003;107:443–447.
91. Volpato S, Pahor M, Ferrucci L, et al. Relationship of alcohol intake with inflammatory markers and plasminogen activator inhibitor-1 in well-functioning older adults: the Health, Aging, and Body Composition study. *Circulation* 2004;109:607–612.
92. Zhou HZ, Karliner JS, Gray MO. Moderate alcohol consumption induces sustained cardiac protection by activating PKC-epsilon and Akt. *Am J Physiol Heart Circ Physiol* 2002;283:H165–H174.
93. Urbano-Marquez A, Estruch R, Fernandez-Sola J, et al. The greater risk of alcoholic cardiomyopathy and myopathy in women compared with men. *JAMA* 1995;274:149–154.
94. Longnecker MP, Berlin JA, Orza MJ, et al. A meta-analysis of alcohol consumption in relation to risk of breast cancer. *JAMA* 1988;260:652–656.
95. Holman CD, English DR, Milne E, et al. Meta-analysis of alcohol and all-cause mortality: a validation of NHMRC recommendations. *Med J Aust* 1996;164:141–145.
96. Ajani UA, Gaziano JM, Lotufo PA, et al. Alcohol consumption and risk of coronary heart disease by diabetes status. *Circulation* 2000;102:500–505.
97. Tanasescu M, Hu FB, Willett WC, et al. Alcohol consumption and risk of coronary heart disease among men with type 2 diabetes mellitus. *J Am Coll Cardiol* 2001;38:1836–1842.
98. Solomon CG, Hu FB, Stampfer MJ, et al. Moderate alcohol consumption and risk of coronary heart disease among women with type 2 diabetes mellitus. *Circulation* 2000;102:494–499.
99. Criqui MH. Alcohol and coronary heart disease risk: implications for public policy. *J Stud Alcohol* 1997;58:453–454.

CHAPTER 11 ■ OTHER RISK FACTORS FOR CORONARY ARTERY DISEASE

LIVIU KLEIN AND PHILIP GREENLAND

OVERVIEW

More than 80% of patients who develop clinically significant coronary artery disease (CAD), and more than 95% of those who will experience a fatal CAD event, have at least one major cardiac risk factor (1,2). Nonetheless, the prevalence of traditional risk factors is almost as high in those without disease as in subsequently affected individuals (1–6). As a consequence, the predictive models for risk assessment (7,8), the cornerstone of primary prevention, have a lower than desired accuracy in predicting CAD risk in any individual patient. The search for new risk factors that could refine risk assessment combined with advances in vascular biology in recent years have led to the discovery of a plethora of circulating biomarkers implicated in the pathology of atherosclerosis (Table 11.1). This chapter outlines the relationship between the leading candidate biomarkers and novel risk factors for CAD.

C-REACTIVE PROTEIN

Historical Considerations and Chemical Structure

C-reactive protein (CRP) was first detected in 1930 by Tillet and Frances, who identified a substance in the sera of patients acutely infected with pneumococcal pneumonia that formed a precipitate when combined with polysaccharide C of *Streptococcus pneumoniae* (9). It was found subsequently that this reaction was not unique to pneumococcal pneumonia but could be observed with a large variety of other acute infections and inflammatory states.

CRP is a calcium-binding pentameric protein consisting of five identical, noncovalently linked, 23-kDa subunits (10). It is present in trace amounts in humans and appears to have

TABLE 11.1

SELECTED NOVEL RISK FACTORS FOR CAD

INFLAMMATORY MARKERS
C-reactive protein
Interleukins (e.g., IL-6)
Vascular and cellular adhesion molecules (e.g., VCAM, ICAM)
Serum amyloid A
Soluble CD 40-ligand
Leukocyte count
HEMOSTASIS/THROMBOSIS MARKERS
Fibrinogen
von Willebrand factor antigen
PAI-1
Tissue-plasminogen activator
Fibrinopeptide A
Prothrombin fragment 1 + 2
Factors V, VII, and VIII
D-Dimer
LIPID-RELATED FACTORS
Lipoprotein(a)
Small dense LDL
HDL subtypes
Remnant lipoproteins
Apolipoproteins A1 and B
Oxidized LDL
PLATELET-RELATED FACTORS
Platelet aggregation
Platelet activity
Platelet size and volume
OTHER FACTORS
Homocysteine
Lipoprotein-associated phospholipase A_2
Microalbuminuria
PAI-1 genotype
ApoE genotype
Angiotensin-converting enzyme genotype
Infectious agents (e.g., *Chlamydia pneumonia*, cytomegalovirus, Herpes simplex virus, *Helicobacter pylori*)

Abbreviations: ApoE, apolipoprotein E; HDL, high-density lipoprotein; ICAM, intercellular adhesion molecule; LDL, low-density lipoprotein; PAI-1 plasminogen activator inhibitor 1; VCAM, vascular cell adhesion molecule.

been highly conserved over hundreds of millions of years (11). CRP is synthesized primarily by hepatocytes in response to activation of several cytokines, such as interleukins 1 and 6, and tumor necrosis factor-α (TNF-α). Because the clearance rate of CRP remains constant, its serum level is determined only by its rate of production.

Measurement and Plasma Concentration

When monitoring states of extremely active inflammation such as sepsis or arthritis that yield CRP levels above 20 to 30 mg/L, qualitative or semiquantitative laboratory techniques, most commonly latex agglutination, have been used. The development of high-sensitivity methods with lower detection limits of 0.2 mg/L allow differentiation of low-level states of inflammation that are required for use in CAD risk assessment. Accurate and rapid quantitative measures of high-sensitivity CRP are obtained using laser nephelometry, rate immunonephelometry or turbidimetry, and enzyme immunoassay (12). Taking into account the day-to-day variability of CRP measurements over time, its predictive value can be improved by using the average of several serial measurements (13).

In healthy persons in the absence of active inflammatory states, CRP levels are usually below 1 mg/L (14). There is no apparent circadian variability, as is observed with cytokines (15), and there is no evidence for seasonal variations as has been reported for fibrinogen (16). CRP has a long half-life, and concentrations appear to be fairly stable over long periods of time in most individuals (17). Heritability studies suggest that 35% to 40% of the variance in CRP levels is genetically determined (18).

CRP serum concentration is physiologically elevated in the third trimester of pregnancy as well as in patients taking oral contraceptives or hormone replacement therapy (19). Levels of CRP are higher in women than in men (20) and are markedly different among different ethnicities: African-American women have higher levels than Caucasians or Hispanics, whereas Chinese women have the lowest CRP levels (20–22). Obesity has been associated with high levels of CRP (23) and weight loss leads to a prompt reduction in serum CRP (24).

C-Reactive Protein and Atherosclerosis

Evidence accumulated over the past decade supports a central role for inflammation in all phases of the atherosclerotic process, from lesion initiation through progression and, ultimately, plaque rupture (25). Recruitment of mononuclear leukocytes to the intima is one of the earliest events in the formation of an atherosclerotic lesion and is followed shortly by their adhesion, transmigration into the subendothelial space and transformation into foam cells (26). T lymphocytes are also attracted to the site of early lesion development (27) and along with the endothelial cells secrete cytokines and growth factors, further amplifying the proinflammatory state and promoting migration and proliferation of smooth muscle cells (27). The cells of the atheromatous plaque produce TNF-α, which together with interferon-γ and interleukin-1, increase interleukin-6 and CRP production (27). CRP is expressed in atherosclerotic plaque (28) and may enhance expression of local adhesion molecules (29), increase expression of endothelial plasminogen activator inhibitor 1 (30), reduce endothelial nitric oxide bioactivity (31), and alter low-density lipoprotein (LDL) cholesterol uptake by macrophages (32). The expression of human CRP in CRP-transgenic mice directly enhances intravascular thrombosis (33) and accelerates atherogenesis (34). CRP has been found within thin cap atheromas and immunohistochemical deposition of CRP within plaques corroborates the concept that inflammation is an important component to plaque instability reflected by serum CRP (35).

C-Reactive Protein and Prediction of Cardiovascular Events in Asymptomatic Individuals

The first association of CRP with CAD events in asymptomatic individuals derives from a nested case control study of the observational component of the Multiple Risk Factor Intervention Trial (MRFIT). The study showed that over 17 years of follow-up, CAD deaths among smokers were 4.3-fold greater among those in the highest versus the lowest quartile of CRP (36). These findings were later confirmed in the Physicians' Health Study, where baseline CRP values were compared for

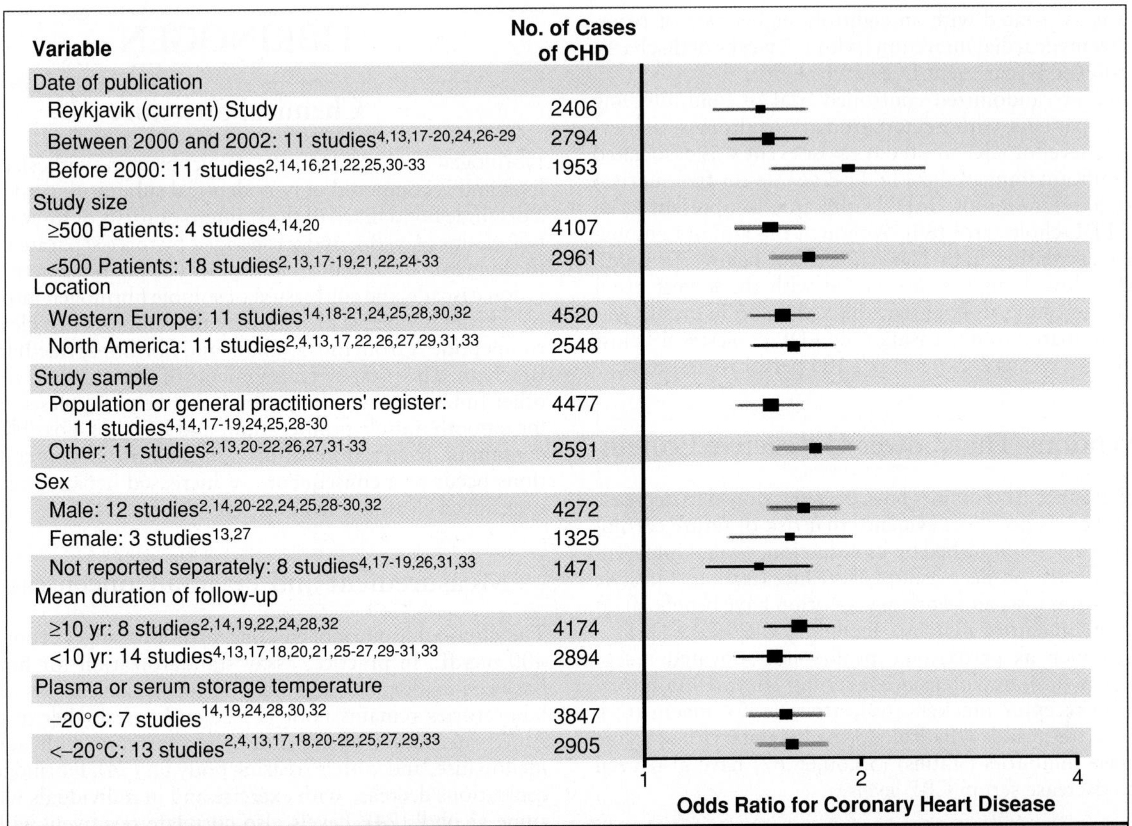

Figure 2. **Twenty-Two Prospective Studies of the Association of C-Reactive Protein Concentrations with the Risk of Coronary Heart Disease (CHD) in Essentially General Populations, Grouped According to Several Study Characteristics.**

One of the 11 studies published before 2000 was updated in 2002[13,16]; hence, data on 85 cases from this study contributed to two subtotals, but we did not double-count these cases in estimating the overall odds ratio. Two studies[17,18] published in 1999 (comprising a total of 98 cases) were not included in a previous meta-analysis of studies published before March 2000[14]; they have been included in the 11 studies published between 2000 and 2002. Although three studies published after 2000,[17-19] involving a total of 245 cases of coronary heart disease, reported results for deaths from cardiovascular causes rather than specifically from coronary heart disease, the majority of these deaths were likely to have been due to coronary heart disease. It was not possible to separate results for 77 cases of coronary revascularization from results for nonfatal myocardial infarction and death from coronary heart disease in another study.[20] The odds ratios used were those reported in studies that had adjusted for age, sex, smoking status, and other established risk factors for coronary heart disease (such as blood lipid levels, blood pressure, body-mass index, and diabetes status). The "Other" category in "Sample" includes participants selected according to various criteria (e.g., the absence of a history of coronary disease in randomized trials). The Reykjavik Study provided separate estimates for men (732 cases with C-reactive protein values) and women (674 cases with C-reactive protein values). Information on the storage temperature used for samples was unavailable for two studies involving a total of 316 cases.[26,31] Odds ratios involve comparisons of patients in the top third versus those in the bottom third of C-reactive protein concentrations. The horizontal lines represent 99 percent confidence intervals.

FIGURE 11.1. Prospective studies of CRP and CAD. (*Source:* Reproduced with permission from Danesh et al. [39]).

543 subjects without cardiovascular disease and for 543 who developed such vascular disease over 8 years of follow-up. Men in the highest quartile had a relative risk for myocardial infarction of 2.9 compared with men in the lowest quartile, independent of many of the usual cardiovascular risk factors (37). The same investigators have demonstrated subsequently that women who developed cardiovascular events had higher baseline CRP levels than control subjects and those with the highest levels at baseline had a sevenfold increase in the risk of myocardial infarction or stroke over 3 years of follow-up (38).

Since the publication of these initial reports, there have been a plethora of studies supporting a role for CRP in cardiovascular event prediction among apparently healthy individuals (39–56). These data are robust and remarkably consistent across over 20 European and American cohorts that included men, women, and middle-aged and older individuals (39–56) (Fig. 11.1). Although the initial studies have suggested an odds ratio for CAD events of about 2.0 (57), more recent data indicate an odds ratio in the range of 1.4 to 1.6 in comparing individuals with baseline values in the top third with those in the bottom third of CRP distribution (39).

C-Reactive Protein and Prediction of Cardiovascular Events in Individuals With Preexisting Cardiovascular Disease

Several studies examined the role of CRP in predicting recurrent events in patients with acute coronary syndromes. One such study found that elevated CRP on admission for ST-elevation myocardial infarction was associated with a sixfold higher rate of ischemic events (recurrent angina, myocardial infarction) and a lower 1-year event-free survival rate (58). In another study, predischarge CRP in the setting of unstable angina was associated with an eightfold higher rate of recurrent or new myocardial infarctions within 2 weeks of discharge and with lower 1-year event-free survival (59).

In a recent randomized controlled trial of lipid-lowering strategy in patients with acute coronary syndromes, achieving a lower level of CRP at 30 days post event was associated with a significant improvement in the 2-year event-free survival (myocardial infarction or CAD death), an effect present at all levels of LDL-cholesterol (60). Although the authors emphasized that decreasing both LDL cholesterol below 70 mg/dL and CRP below 1 mg/L is associated with the lowest event rate, it is interesting to note that this reduction in events was minimal compared to decreasing only LDL cholesterol below 70 mg/dL (1.9 versus 2.7 events per 100 person-years) (60).

Interventions That Lower C-Reactive Protein

Although no specific therapies have been developed to decrease CRP and there is no direct evidence that risk of future cardiovascular events is diminished by its reduction, several interventions are effective in decreasing CRP concentration. Lifestyle changes, weight loss, and smoking cessation have beneficial effects on inflammatory markers, including CRP (24,61). Several drugs such as peroxisome proliferator-activated receptors agonists (62), angiotensin converting enzyme inhibitors/angiotensin receptor blockers (63), aspirin (37), niacin (64), clopidogrel (65), and 3 hydroxy-3-methylglutaryl coenzyme A reductase inhibitors (statins) (55,60,66,67) have also been shown to decrease serum CRP levels.

Clinical Implications

Although CRP has been found to be an independent predictor for future cardiovascular events in asymptomatic individuals, most of the epidemiologic studies report only the relative risk and fail to show the absolute risk associated with increased CRP or the receiver operating curve comparing CRP to other risk factors, making it difficult to gauge the true incremental value of using CRP for cardiovascular risk prediction. Recent studies have shown that CRP may have a role in refining the Framingham risk prediction model in middle-aged and older individuals at intermediate risk of CAD events (10-year risk of 10% to 20%) (56,68–70) and therefore the most logical use of CRP is in these individuals.

The American Heart Association and the Centers for Disease Control and Prevention issued recommendations on using CRP for risk stratification in primary prevention (71). These recommendations advocate obtaining at least two CRP measurements, preferably 2 weeks apart, and categorizing CRP levels according to approximate tertiles in adult populations: low risk (<1 mg/L), average risk (1.0 to 3.0 mg/L), and high risk (>3.0 mg/L). CRP levels above 10 mg/L generally indicates presence of a significant acute phase response, and further assessment is required to determine the cause. Individuals reclassified as high risk (10-year risk of >20%) based on CRP should have the traditional risk factors treated intensively, and those reclassified as low risk (10-year risk of <10%) may follow a more conservative approach.

Further data from prospective clinical trials are needed to determine if patients should be treated on the basis of elevated CRP alone. One such trial, currently in progress in the United States, is the Justification for the Use of statins in Primary prevention: an Intervention Trial Evaluating Rosuvastatin (JUPITER) (72). This study is investigating whether long-term treatment with rosuvastatin decreases the rate of major cardiovascular events in patients with lower LDL cholesterol and high CRP.

FIBRINOGEN

Chemical Structure

Fibrinogen is a large (340-kDa) glycoprotein synthesized in the liver and is composed of two identical subunits linked through a disulfide bond. Each of the subunits consists of three polypeptide chains (Aα, Bβ, and γ) encoded by three separate genes on the long arm of chromosome 4 (73). The final step in the coagulation cascade, the conversion of soluble fibrinogen into insoluble fibrin polymer, is mediated by thrombin, which cleaves fibrinopeptide A from the Aα chain and fibrinopeptide B from the Bβ chain. The proteolytic fragments of fibrinogen have several other functions, including stimulating hematopoiesis, promoting smooth muscle proliferation, and having a possible role in containing bacterial infection. Elevated fibrinogen concentrations occur as a consequence of increased hepatic production or reduced clearance from the circulation (74).

Measurement and Plasma Concentration

The circulating fibrinogen concentration ranges from 200 to 400 mg/dL. In practice, assay standardization for fibrinogen has been inadequate, and analytic consistency across reference laboratories remains poor (74). Levels are higher in African Americans and women, and levels increase with age, after menopause, and with increasing body fat (74). Fibrinogen concentrations decrease with exercise and in individuals who consume alcohol (74). Levels also correlate positively with other risk factors for vascular disease, increasing with concentrations of LDL cholesterol and lipoprotein (a) and decreasing with increasing high density lipoprotein (HDL) cholesterol (74). Fibrinogen levels are also higher in patients with hypertension (75) and diabetes mellitus (76). Smoking also increases fibrinogen concentration (77), which may decrease upon smoking cessation (74,78). Higher concentrations of plasma fibrinogen have been observed in smokers with the T148-A455 allele compared with homozygotes for the common C148-G455 allele (79). In addition, fibrinogen is an acute phase reactant that increases in a variety of disorders, including infections, neoplasms, and hepatitis (74).

Fibrinogen and Atherosclerosis

Plasma fibrinogen regulates cell adhesion, chemotaxis, and proliferation, influences platelet aggregation and blood viscosity, interacts with plasminogen binding, and, in combination with thrombin, mediates the final step in clot formation and the response to vascular injury (80–82). Recent data also suggest that the association of fibrinogen with CAD may relate to its role in inflammation (83).

Fibrinogen and Prediction of Cardiovascular Events in Asymptomatic Individuals

Many studies demonstrate a link between fibrinogen and cardiovascular disease (84). Among the largest to report an association between fibrinogen and CAD, the Atherosclerosis Risk in Communities (ARIC) study showed that in over 14,000 middle-aged adults elevated levels of fibrinogen were associated with 1.5-fold increased risk of developing myocardial infarction or coronary death over 5 years of follow-up (85). Two recent meta-analyses of 12 prospective, long-term studies found an odds ratio of 1.8 for CAD events for asymptomatic individuals in the upper tertile of baseline fibrinogen (350 mg/dL)

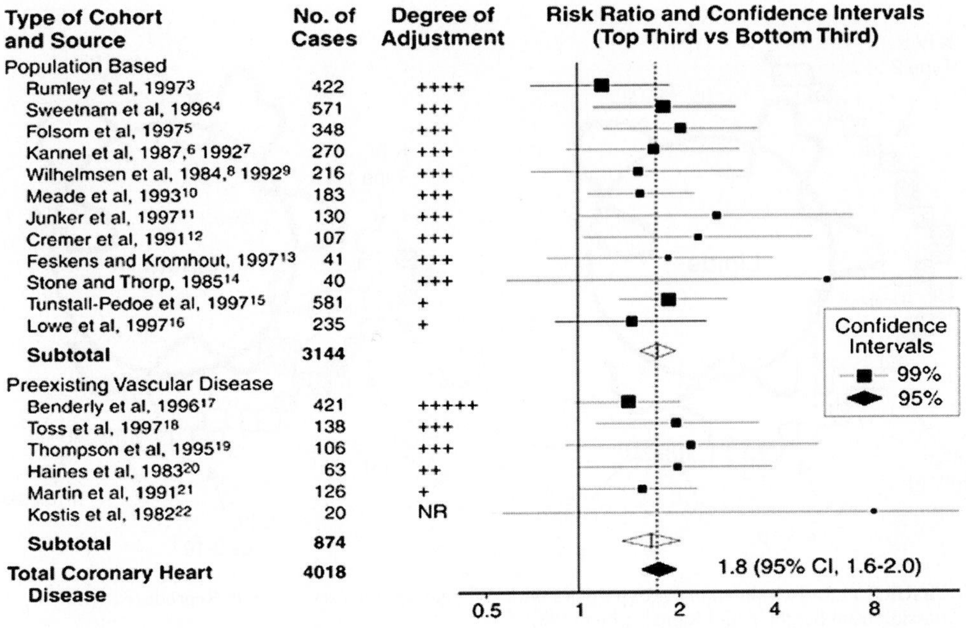

FIGURE 11.2. Prospective studies of fibrinogen and CAD. (*Source:* Reproduced with permission from Danesh et al. [86]).

compared to those in the lowest tertile (250 mg/dL) (86,87) (Fig. 11.2).

Fibrinogen and Prediction of Cardiovascular Events in Individuals With Preexisting Cardiovascular Disease

The same two meta-analyses also reviewed studies conducted in individuals with preexisting coronary, peripheral vascular, or cerebrovascular disease, and found an odds ratio of 1.7 for recurrent CAD events for individuals in the upper tertile of baseline fibrinogen compared to those in the lowest tertile (86,87). Fibrinogen is, thus, a moderate predictor of future events, independent of traditional risk factors in individuals with and without previous cardiovascular disease.

Interventions That Lower Fibrinogen

Exercise, moderate alcohol consumption, and smoking cessation lower fibrinogen levels (74,78,88). Although a specific fibrinogen-lowering agent is not yet available, niacin (88), fibrates (89,90), and hormone replacement therapy (91) lower fibrinogen concentration; statin and aspirin do not (88). Even in the clinical trials in which fibrinogen levels were decreased, there was no reduction in cardiovascular events.

Clinical Implications

Only one study evaluated the role of fibrinogen in refining risk prediction models in primary prevention and found only modest incremental effects, with an odds ratio of 1.18 for future coronary events for individuals in the upper versus lower quartile of fibrinogen, after adjustment for Framingham risk score (92). Owing to its limited additive effect on top of the Framingham risk score, the fact that assay standardization has been inadequate, and that levels are elevated in certain groups, fibrinogen measurement has a limited use in clinical practice.

LIPOPROTEIN(a)

Historical Considerations and Chemical Structure

Lipoprotein(a) was discovered in 1963 by Berg (93) and consists of two major components: an LDL particle containing the apoprotein B-100 molecule and an apoprotein(a) [apo(a)] molecule linked by a single disulfide bond (94). Apo(a) is a large protein with an amino acid sequence similar to that of plasminogen. Both the apo(a) and plasminogen genes consist of specific coding sequences for loop structures stabilized by intrachain disulfide bonds, referred to as *kringle domains.* Five different kringle domains (K1 to K5) are found in the plasminogen gene, and only K4 and K5 are present in apo(a) gene (94,95). The K4 sequence is repeated many-fold in the apo(a) gene; the multiple copies are similar but not identical to each other (96) (Fig. 11.3). This variation of apo(a) gene size leads to the heterogeneity of apo(a) protein size that also impacts on plasma Lp(a) level (97,98). In general, it is widely believed that smaller apo(a) sizes leads to higher plasma Lp(a) levels, although the relationship is complex (99,100).

Lp(a) is synthesized in the liver, and its molecular weight varies from 400 to 700 kDa. Although the plasma LDL concentration is primarily determined by the rate of removal, the Lp(a) level is controlled by the rate of synthesis at the level of the gene that encodes apo(a) (101).

Measurement and Plasma Concentration

Lp(a) concentration in plasma ranges from 1 mg to 100 mg/dL. Most values lie below 20 mg/dL, and the concentration distribution is, therefore, markedly skewed in most populations (96). Plasma levels vary widely among individuals and appear to be highly heritable (102). Nongenetic mechanisms that regulate Lp(a) levels are largely unknown, although Lp(a) levels are increased in patients with renal failure, nephrotic syndrome, and diabetes as well as in menopausal women (96). African

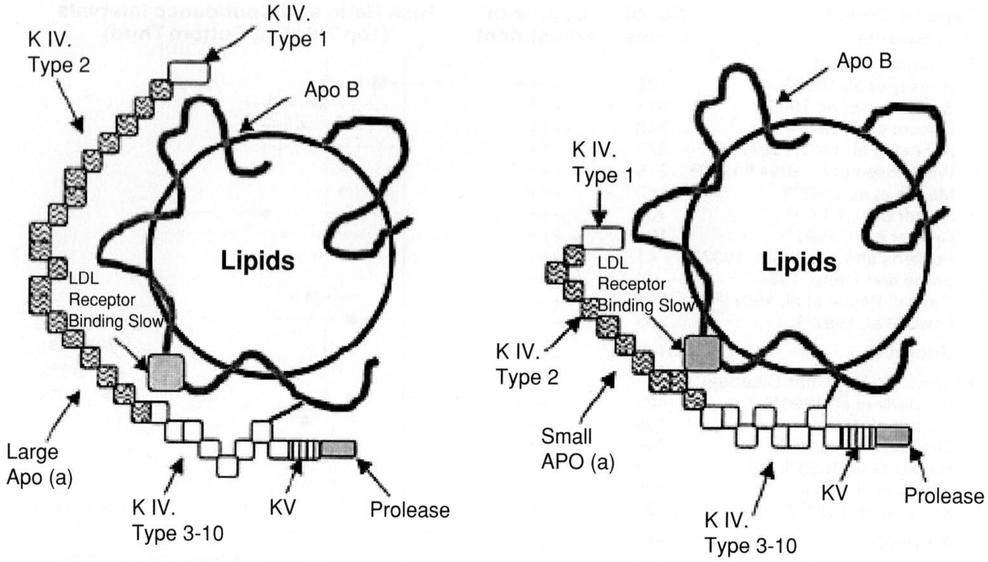

FIGURE 11.3. Two different Lp(a) particles with different apo(a) sizes. (*Source:* Reproduced with permission from Berglund and Ramakrishnan [96]).

Americans have substantially higher Lp(a) levels than do Caucasians or Asians, and this difference is not explained by differences in apo(a) size distribution or other genetic factors (103).

Lp(a) level measurements reflect particle concentrations, including both lipid and protein components. Older studies have expressed Lp(a) levels in mass units (mg/dL) and this requires an assumption of a particular apo(a) mass and ignores apo(a) size variation. The use of molar units (nmol/L) is therefore preferable and has been advocated for standardization of Lp(a) measurements (104).

Lipoprotein(a) and Atherosclerosis

When present at low levels, Lp(a) may serve a protective function by binding and possibly degrading of oxidized phospholipids formed during normal homeostasis or in acutely stressful situations (105). Lp(a) has also been shown to be involved in wound healing (106), and elevated levels have been noted in centenarians (107). When levels are chronically elevated, Lp(a) may be proatherogenic particularly because it has enhanced binding to the extracellular matrix of the artery wall (108). The close homology between Lp(a) and plasminogen has raised the possibility that it may inhibit endogenous fibrinolysis by competing with plasminogen binding on the endothelium. Lp(a) may bind and inactivate tissue factor pathway inhibitor and may upregulate the expression of plasminogen activator inhibitor (109,110).

Lipoprotein(a) and Prediction of Cardiovascular Events in Asymptomatic Individuals

Data from prospective studies are conflicting regarding the risk for CAD events associated with increased levels of Lp(a). A recent meta-analysis of 18 studies with a mean follow-up period of 10 years found that asymptomatic individuals with Lp(a) levels in the top tertile of the distribution had a risk of CAD events 1.7 times higher compared to those with Lp(a) levels in the lower tertile (111). Although one of those studies accounted for almost half the cases, the risk ratio in that study was almost identical to the risk ratio of in the aggregated results of the others (1.66 versus 1.69) (111,112) (Fig. 11.4).

The conflicting data from other studies may be a result of the variability in the methods used to determine Lp(a) levels and the fact that different isoforms of apo(a) may differ in their atherogenic potential (96,113). The risk associated with increased Lp(a) may also be dependent on age, gender (114), or interaction with other factors such as fibrinogen and CRP (115). One study evaluating the role of Lp(a) in refining the risk prediction models in primary prevention found that the risk was confined only to the high-risk men (as identified by the PROCAM score), in which 83% of all coronary events occurred (116). These observations may explain why Lp(a) was found to be a risk factor of coronary events only in those studies where participants were at high risk for coronary events (117), and not in others (118).

Lipoprotein(a) and Prediction of Cardiovascular Events in Individuals With Preexisting Cardiovascular Disease

A recent meta-analysis found that in the nine studies of patients who already had cardiovascular disease at baseline, the combined risk ratio for future cardiovascular events was 1.3, which was significantly smaller than that for the studies conducted in healthy populations (111). This result for studies in patients with preexisting disease was dominated by one large study of patients with a history of myocardial infarction, which accounted for three fourths of the evidence (116).

Interventions That Lower Lipoprotein(a)

Niacin (119,120), neomycin (119), stanozolol (121), *N*-acetylcysteine (122), and hormone replacement therapy (123) may lower Lp(a) levels; statins do not (124). Lp(a) levels can also be dramatically lowered by LDL apheresis (125). In patients with a borderline LDL cholesterol level, an elevated Lp(a) level may provide a rationale for more aggressive LDL-lowering therapy. In one study, higher levels of Lp(a) did not confer greater cardiovascular risk if LDL had been lowered (126).

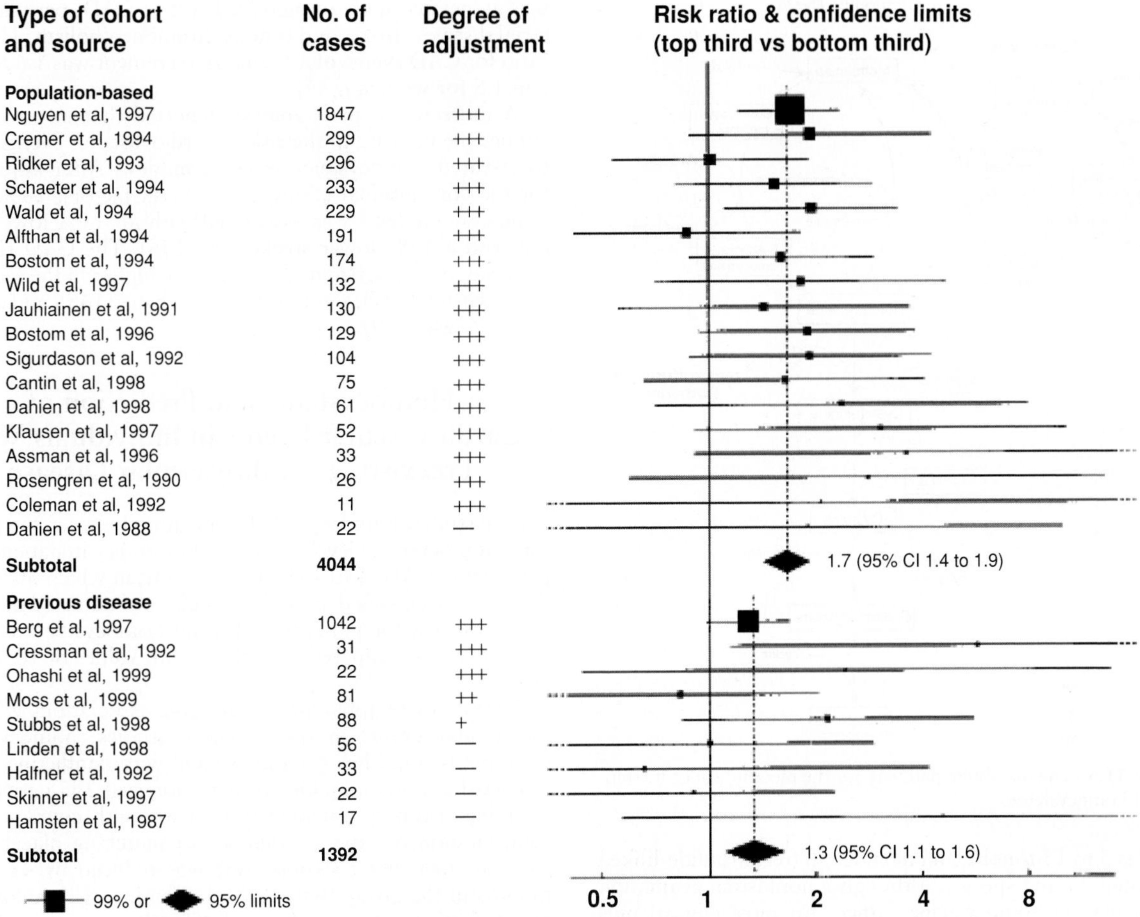
Type of cohort and source
No. of cases
Degree of adjustment
Risk ratio & confidence limits (top third vs bottom third)
Population-based
Nguyen et al, 1997 1847 +++
Cremer et al, 1994 299 +++
Ridker et al, 1993 296 +++
Schaeter et al, 1994 233 +++
Wald et al, 1994 229 +++
Alfthan et al, 1994 191 +++
Bostom et al, 1994 174 +++
Wild et al, 1997 132 +++
Jauhiainen et al, 1991 130 +++
Bostom et al, 1996 129 +++
Sigurdason et al, 1992 104 +++
Cantin et al, 1998 75 +++
Dahien et al, 1998 61 +++
Klausen et al, 1997 52 +++
Assman et al, 1996 33 +++
Rosengren et al, 1990 26 +++
Coleman et al, 1992 11 +++
Dahien et al, 1988 22 —
Subtotal 4044
1.7 (95% CI 1.4 to 1.9)
Previous disease
Berg et al, 1997 1042 +++
Cressman et al, 1992 31 +++
Ohashi et al, 1999 22 +++
Moss et al, 1999 81 ++
Stubbs et al, 1998 88 +
Linden et al, 1998 56 —
Halfner et al, 1992 33 —
Skinner et al, 1997 22 —
Hamsten et al, 1987 17 —
Subtotal 1392
1.3 (95% CI 1.1 to 1.6)
99% or 95% limits
0.5
1
2
4
8

FIGURE 11.4. Prospective studies of lipoprotein(a) and CAD. Prospective studies of lipoprotein(a) and CAD. Risk ratios compare top and bottom thirds of baseline measurements. Black squares indicate risk ratio in each study, with square size proportional to number of cases and horizontal lines representing 99% confidence intervals (CI). The combined risk ratios and their 95% CI are indicated by shaded diamonds. Degree of adjustment for possible confounders is denoted as follows: +, adjustment for age and gender only; ++, adjustment for the preceding plus smoking; and +++, adjustment for the preceding plus some other classical vascular risk factors. (*Source:* Reproduced with permission from Danesh et al. [111]).

Clinical Implications

Lack of a standardized assay and limited therapeutic options in the treatment of elevated levels have hindered widespread use of Lp(a) in risk assessment. In addition, whether the assessment of Lp(a) truly adds prognostic information to standard global risk prediction in primary prevention remains uncertain, because in most studies Lp(a) has been predictive only among those already known to be at high risk. Thus, in terms of general population screening, lp(a) evaluation has limited utility.

HOMOCYSTEINE

Historical Considerations and Chemical Structure

Homocysteine is a sulfur-containing amino acid formed as a byproduct of the metabolism of the essential amino acid methionine (127). Following ingestion, methionine is converted to *S*-adenosylmethionine and then to *S*-adenosylhomocysteine, from which homocysteine is formed. Cells remetabolize homocysteine by a number of possible pathways involving several different enzymes that variously use B vitamins as substrates or cofactors (i.e., folate, cobalamin, and pyridoxine) (127). Homocysteine enters the transsulfuration pathway, where it is converted to cystathionine by pyridoxine-dependent cystathionine β-synthase (Fig. 11.5). Plasma homocysteine concentrations may increase, owing to decreased activity of certain enzymes, reduced vitamin cofactor availability, or both.

In the early 1970s, three different inborn errors of homocysteine metabolism involving these enzymes were described (*homozygous homocystinurias*) that lead to extremely high levels of homocysteine in the blood (>100 μmol/L) and urine of individuals homozygous for these mutations; half of affected individuals developed arterial or venous thrombosis by 30 years of age (127–130). From these initial observations, a link has been established between more moderate elevations of plasma homocysteine concentrations and atherosclerosis (131–133).

Measurement and Plasma Concentration

Until recently, total plasma homocysteine was measured predominantly by high-performance liquid chromatography. Reliable and less expensive immunoassays have become available, making wider screening for hyperhomocysteinemia possible (127). The range of fasting homocysteine currently reported as

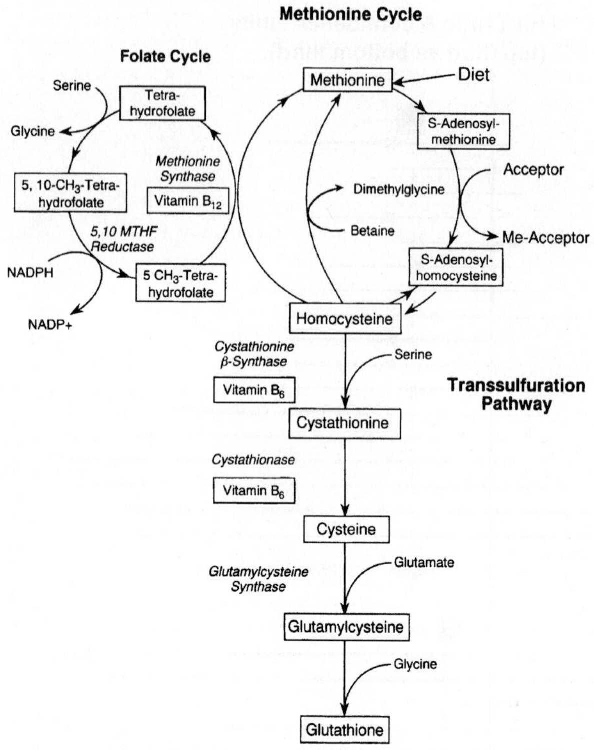

FIGURE 11.5. The metabolic pathway for the metabolism of methionine and homocysteine.

normal is 5 to 15 μmol/L and includes all free, disulfide-linked and protein-bound species. Although a nonfasting evaluation of total plasma homocysteine suffices for most clinical purposes, measurement of homocysteine levels 2 to 6 hours after ingestion of an oral methionine load (0.1 g/kg body mass) can identify individuals with impaired homocysteine metabolism despite normal fasting levels (127).

Increases in homocysteine levels can occur with aging (134), menopause (135), hypothyroidism (136), vitamin B_6, B_{12}, and folate deficiencies (137) and chronic renal failure (138). Genetic variation in enzymes involved in homocysteine metabolism (such as methylene tetrahydrofolate reductase 677C $\rightarrow$ T) contributes to interindividual differences in plasma homocysteine levels (139).

Homocysteine and Atherosclerosis

Although a high circulating level of homocysteine is associated with atherosclerosis and thromboembolic disorders, the underlying mechanisms of vascular damage remain obscure. These may include endothelial dysfunction, accelerated oxidation of LDL cholesterol, impairment of flow-mediated endothelial-derived relaxing factor with subsequent reduction in arterial vasodilation, platelet activation, increased expression of monocyte chemoattractant protein, and interleukin-8 leading to a proinflammatory response, and oxidative stress (140–144).

Homocysteine and Prediction of Cardiovascular Events in Asymptomatic Individuals

Many, but not all, prospective studies of homocysteine and cardiovascular disease show homocysteine to be associated with cardiovascular events. An older meta-analysis of 27 studies indicated that an elevation in homocysteine levels (>15 μmol/L) was associated with an increased risk of CAD, peripheral arterial disease, stroke, and venous thromboembolism. The odds ratio for CAD events of a 5 μmol/L increment was 1.6 for men and 1.8 for women (145).

A more recent meta-analysis reported that in prospective studies the increase in the risk of cardiovascular events owing to elevated homocysteine levels is modest. After adjustment for the conventional cardiovascular risk factors, 25% lower homocysteine level was associated with an 11% lower CAD risk and a 19% lower stroke risk (146). The CAD risk due to elevated homocysteine levels may be higher in the setting of hypertension (147), smoking (147), diabetes (148), and chronic renal disease (149).

Homocysteine and Prediction of Cardiovascular Events in Individuals With Preexisting Cardiovascular Disease

Several studies found a graded association between the plasma total homocysteine level and overall mortality in patients with preexisting CAD (150,151). In one study, in which 80% of all deaths were classified as cardiovascular, the adjusted mortality ratio was 1.6 for patients with total homocysteine levels of 15 μmol/L as compared with those with values of 10 μmol/L (150).

Despite these apparently convincing associations with cardiovascular events in observational studies, homocysteine-lowering therapy has been associated with conflicting results in regard to outcomes. One trial randomized 205 patients undergoing coronary angioplasty to a 6-month course of folic acid, vitamin B_6, and vitamin B_{12} or matching placebo. Despite the fact that restenosis rate was reduced by 48% at 6 months in the group that received vitamins, with a concomitant reduction in homocysteine of 35%, there was no reduction in myocardial infarction or death (152). Furthermore, recent data from another randomized controlled study of 626 patients treated with B-vitamin therapy following percutaneous coronary intervention found increased rates of restenosis and major adverse cardiac events in the vitamin treatment group after 6 months of follow-up (153).

Interventions That Lower Homocysteine

In healthy subjects and in patients with atherosclerotic vascular disease, homocysteine concentrations may be reduced by folic acid alone or in combination with vitamins B_6 or B_{12}. The effect is greatest with folic acid, which, in doses of only 0.4 mg/day, may reduce homocysteine concentrations by approximately 25%. Addition of vitamin B_{12} may produce another modest 7% reduction (154,155).

In the Vitamin Intervention for Stroke Prevention trial patients with ischemic stroke and a homocysteine level at the 25th percentile or greater of the North American stroke population were randomized to a high-dose multivitamin formulation that included 2.5 mg of folic acid and a low-dose formulation that included 0.2 mg of folic acid. The mean reduction in homocysteine levels was 2 μmol/L greater in the high-dose group than in the low-dose group, but there was no effect on recurrent strokes, CAD events, or death after a mean follow-up of 2 years (156). Several other trials are near completion and should provide a definite answer to this issue (157–159).

Clinical Implications

Despite availability of newer assays, measurement of homocysteine remains controversial and recent guidelines do not advocate their use. Many of the prospective studies showing increased risk with higher homocysteine concentrations began well before fortification of the food supply with folic acid. Food fortification has greatly reduced the frequency of low folate and elevated homocysteine levels, particularly for persons initially in the moderately elevated range (160). Thus, the number of individuals potentially identifiable by general screening for homocysteine has decreased considerably. In addition, because vitamin supplementation is inexpensive and has low toxicity, it may be a more cost-effective approach for high-risk groups than screening.

Last, there is no evidence demonstrating that homocysteine screening adds to standard lipid evaluation or to the Framingham risk score. Perhaps homocysteine evaluation may be appropriate in those lacking traditional risk factors, in the setting of renal failure, or among those with premature atherosclerosis or a family history of myocardial infarction and stroke at a young age.

CONTROVERSIES AND PERSONAL PERSPECTIVE

The discovery of novel risk markers provides exciting clues to the pathophysiology of atherosclerosis, improved diagnostic capabilities, and ultimately, better patient care. Crossing the boundary from research to clinical practice, however, requires a number of questions to be answered. First, there must be an available, standardized, reproducible, and accurate laboratory test that has been prospectively validated in the population to which it will be applied. For now, this is the case only for CRP and homocysteine.

Second, it must be demonstrated that measurement of the novel risk factor adds to the information obtained from existing standard approaches to cardiovascular risk stratification (global risk assessment). As described in the text, CRP is the only biomarker that possibly adds information to that obtained from the one such risk model (Framingham risk score). Accordingly, its best use is in individuals at intermediate risk for coronary events (71).

Third, there must be prospective controlled trials demonstrating that targeting individuals with elevated levels of these novel risk factors and reducing them decreases important clinical end points, such as mortality, nonfatal myocardial infarction, and stroke. As of 2005, there is no evidence that reducing any of the novel risk factors is associated with improvement in clinically important outcomes, although a number of studies are still ongoing, particularly with respect to CRP and homocysteine (72,157–159).

Until additional supportive data are forthcoming, specific interventions to modify novel markers should be reserved for investigative purposes and perhaps for selected cases such as (a) asymptomatic individuals with strong family histories of vascular disease in whom traditional risk factors are not apparent; (b) patients with premature vascular disease with no apparent explanatory factors; and (c) individuals with recurrent disease despite intensive and optimal management of all traditional risk factors.

THE FUTURE

At present, approximately 40% of the adult U.S. population is at intermediate risk for CAD events (10-year estimated risk of 10% to 20%) (161,162), and current practice guidelines do not advocate intensive risk factor management (e.g., lipid lowering) in these individuals (163). Although several novel biomarkers have been identified that may help in the detection of persons at higher risk for future vascular events, CRP is the only one that has been given serious consideration for its potential role in refining risk estimation. CRP has a standardized, accurate assay and it has been shown to add modest prognostic information to the Framingham risk estimation in Caucasian populations, particularly in the individuals at intermediate risk for CAD events (56,69). One large population study is addressing the role of CRP for risk prediction in African-American, Chinese, and Hispanic middle-aged adults (164); a larger clinical trial is exploring whether lowering CRP in individuals without known cardiovascular disease will translate into a reduction of cardiovascular events (72). The results of these studies, which should be available in the next 5 years, will further define the role of CRP for risk prediction in everyday clinical practice.

As to the possibility of other newer markers being strong enough to add substantially to the discrimination of current risk prediction methods, that seems rather unlikely at this point given the requirements that such a new marker be largely independent of existing predictors, that the assay be repeatable and stable, and that the intensity of the contribution to relative risk be much stronger than the typical 1.5- to 2.0-fold increase seen with nearly every new marker. However, it remains possible than one or more new markers may become a target of therapy to improve outcomes, even if the marker does not strongly add to risk prediction. Several current markers (CRP, lipoprotein-associated phospholipase A_2, and others) are being evaluated for this possibility, and future work may confirm one or more of these as a new strategy for intervention.

KEY CONCEPTS

- **The risk predictive models (e.g., Framingham risk score, PROCAM, SCORE) have a lower than desired accuracy in predicting coronary artery disease events in an individual patient.**
- **Novel risk factors implicated in the pathophysiology of atherosclerosis (e.g., C-reactive protein, fibrinogen, lp[a]) may refine the risk assessment.**
- **CRP, an acute phase reactant linking inflammation and atherosclerosis, is probably the only available novel risk factor that will play a role in refining the cardiovascular risk. Its use in individuals at intermediate risk for coronary artery disease events may alter the intensity of traditional risk factor management (e.g., cholesterol lowering).**
- **Fibrinogen and other prothrombotic risk factors are involved in atherogenesis and may increase the risk for coronary artery disease events.**
- **Lp(a) confers an independent risk for coronary artery disease events in selected populations and may do so by impairing fibrinolysis, promoting thrombosis, or stimulating vascular smooth muscle cell proliferation.**
- **Hyperhomocysteinemia confers a modest increase risk for coronary artery disease events, by imparting oxidative stress-induced endothelial dysfunction and inducing atherothrombosis.**

References

1. Greenland P, Knoll MD, Stamler J, et al. Major risk factors as antecedents of fatal and nonfatal coronary heart disease events. *JAMA* 2003;290:891–897.
2. Khot UN, Khot MB, Bajzer CT, et al. Prevalence of conventional risk factors in patients with coronary heart disease. *JAMA* 2003;290:898–904.
3. Keys A. Coronary artery disease in seven countries. *Circulation* 1970;41:1–211.
4. American Heart Association. *Heart disease and stroke statistics—2005 update*. Dallas, TX: American Heart Association, 2004.
5. Wilson PW, D'Agostino RB, Levy D, et al. Prediction of coronary heart disease using risk factor categories. *Circulation* 1998;97:1837–1847.
6. Reddy KS, Yusuf S. Emerging epidemic of cardiovascular disease in developing countries. *Circulation* 1998;97:596–601.

7. Grundy SM, Pasternak R, Greenland P, et al. Assessment of cardiovascular risk by use of multiple-risk-factor assessment equations; a statement for healthcare professionals from the American Heart Association and the American College of Cardiology. *Circulation* 1999;100:1481–1492.
8. Conroy RM, Pyorala K, Fitzgerald AP, et al. SCORE project group. Estimation of ten-year risk of fatal cardiovascular disease in Europe: the SCORE project. *Eur Heart J* 2003;24:987–1003.
9. Tillett WS, Francis T. Serological reactions in pneumonia with a non-protein somatic fraction of the pneumococcus. *J Exp Med* 1930;52:561–571.
10. Macintyre SS. C-reactive protein. *Methods Enzymol* 1988;163:383–399.
11. Shrive AK, Metcalfe AM, Cartwright JR, et al. C-reactive protein and SAP-like pentraxin are both present in Limulus polyphemus haemolymph: crystal structure of Limulus SAP. *J Mol Biol* 1999;290:997–1008.
12. Ledue TB, Rifai N. Preanalytic and analytic sources of variations in C-reactive protein measurement: implications for cardiovascular disease risk assessment. *Clin Chem* 2003;49:1258–1271.
13. Koenig W, Sund M, Frfhlich M, et al. Refinement of the association of serum C-reactive protein concentration and coronary heart disease risk by correction for within subject variation over time. Results from the MONICA-Augsburg studies 1984 and 1987. *Am J Epidemiol* 2003;158:357–364.
14. Ridker PM. Clinical application of C-reactive protein for cardiovascular disease detection and prevention. *Circulation* 2003;107:363–369.
15. Meier-Ewert HK, Ridker PM, Rifai N, et al. Absence of diurnal variation of C-reactive protein concentrations in healthy subjects. *Clin Chem* 2001;47:426–430.
16. Frohlich M, Sund M, Thorand B, et al. Lack of seasonal variation in C-reactive protein. *Clin Chem* 2002;48:575–577.
17. Ockene IS, Matthews CE, Rifai N, et al. Variability and classification accuracy of serial high sensitivity C-reactive protein measurements in healthy adults. *Clin Chem* 2001;47:444–450.
18. Pankow JS, Folsom AR, Cushman M, et al. Familial and genetic determinants of systemic markers of inflammation: the NHLBI family heart study. *Atherosclerosis* 2001;154:681–689.
19. Ridker PM, Hennekens CH, Rifai N, et al. Hormone replacement therapy and increased plasma concentration of C-reactive protein. *Circulation* 1999;100:713–716.
20. Woloshin S, Schwartz LM. Distribution of C-reactive protein values in the United States. *N Engl J Med* 2005;352:1611–1613.
21. Albert MA, Glynn RJ, Buring J, et al. C-reactive protein levels among women of various ethnic groups living in the United States (from the Women's Health Study). *Am J Cardiol* 2004;93:1238–1242.
22. Khera A, McGuire DK, Murphy SA, et al. Race and gender differences in C-reactive protein levels. *J Am Coll Cardiol* 2005;46:464–469.
23. Visser M, Bouter LM, McQuillan GM, et al. Elevated C-reactive protein levels in overweight and obese adults. *JAMA* 1999;282:2131–2135.
24. Tchernof A, Nolan A, Sites CK, et al. Weight loss reduces C–reactive protein levels in obese postmenopausal women. *Circulation* 2002;105:564–569.
25. Ross R. Atherosclerosis—an inflammatory disease. *N Engl J Med* 1999; 340:115–126.
26. Skalen K, Gustafsson M, Rydberg EK, et al. Subendothelial retention of atherogenic lipoproteins in early atherosclerosis. *Nature* 2002;417:750–754.
27. Hansson GK. Inflammation, atherosclerosis and coronary artery disease. *N Engl J Med* 2005;352:1685–1692.
28. Torzewski J, Torzewski M, Bowyer DE, et al. C-reactive protein frequently co-localizes with the terminal complement complex in the intima of early atherosclerotic lesions of human coronary arteries. *Arterioscler Thromb Vasc Biol* 1998;18:1386–1392.
29. Pasceri V, Willerson JT, Yeh ET. Direct pro-inflammatory effect of C-reactive protein on human endothelial cells. *Circulation* 2000;102:2165–2168.
30. Devaraj S, Xu DY, Jialal I. C-reactive protein increases plasminogen activator inhibitor-1 expression and activity in human aortic endothelial cells: implications for the metabolic syndrome and atherothrombosis. *Circulation* 2003;107:398–404.
31. Venugopal SK, Devaraj S, Yuhanna I, et al. Demonstration that C-reactive protein decreases eNOS expression and bioactivity in human aortic endothelial cells. *Circulation* 2002;106:1439–1441.
32. Zwaka TP, Hombach V, Torzewski J. C-reactive protein-mediated low density lipoprotein uptake by macrophages: implications for atherosclerosis. *Circulation* 2001;103:1194–1197.
33. Danenberg HD, Szalai AJ, Swaminathan RV, et al. Increased thrombosis after arterial injury in human C-reactive protein-transgenic mice. *Circulation* 2003;108:512–515.
34. Paul A, Ko KW, Yechoor V, et al. C-reactive protein accelerates the progression of atherosclerosis in apolipoprotein E-deficient mice. *Circulation* 2004;109:647–655.
35. Burke AP, Tracy RP, Kolodgie F, et al. Elevated C-reactive protein values and atherosclerosis in sudden coronary death: association with different pathologies. *Circulation* 2002;105:2019–2023.
36. Kuller LH, Tracy RP, Shaten J, et al. Relation of C-reactive protein and coronary heart disease in the MRFIT nested case-control study. Multiple Risk Factor Intervention Trial. *Am J Epidemiol* 1996;144:537–547.
37. Ridker PM, Cushman M, Stampfer MJ, et al. Inflammation, aspirin, and the risk of cardiovascular disease in apparently healthy men. *N Engl J Med* 1997;336:973–979.
38. Ridker PM, Buring JE, Shih J, et al. Prospective study of C-reactive protein and the risk of future cardiovascular events among apparently healthy women. *Circulation* 1998;98:731–733.
39. Danesh J, Wheeler JG, Hirschfield GM, et al. C-reactive protein and other circulating markers of inflammation in the prediction of coronary heart disease. *N Engl J Med* 2004;350:1387–1397.
40. Folsom AR, Aleksic N, Catellier D, et al. C-reactive protein and incident coronary heart disease in the Atherosclerosis Risk In Communities (ARIC) study. *Am Heart J* 2002;144:233–238.
41. Gram J, Bladbjerg EM, Møller L, et al. Tissue-type plasminogen activator and C-reactive protein in acute coronary heart disease: a nested case-control study. *J Intern Med* 2000;247:205–212.
42. Harris TB, Ferrucci L, Tracy RP, et al. Associations of elevated interleukin-6 and C-reactive protein levels with mortality in the elderly. *Am J Med* 1999;106:506–512.
43. Jager A, van Hinsbergh VWM, Kostense PJ, et al. von Willebrand factor, C-reactive protein, and 5-year mortality in diabetic and non diabetic subjects: the Hoorn Study. *Arterioscler Thromb Vasc Biol* 1999;19:3071–3078.
44. Koenig W, Sund M, Fröhlich M, et al. C-reactive protein, a sensitive marker of inflammation, predicts future risk of coronary heart disease in initially healthy middleaged men: results from the MONICA (Monitoring Trends and Determinants in Cardiovascular Disease) Augsburg Cohort Study, 1984 to 1992. *Circulation* 1999;99:237–242.
45. Lowe GDO, Rumley A, Sweetnam PM, et al. Fibrin D-dimer, C-reactive protein and risk of ischaemic heart disease: the Speedwell study. *Blood Coagul Fibrinolysis* 1999;10:S92-S93.
46. Mendall MA, Strachan DP, Butland BK, et al. C-reactive protein: relation to total mortality, cardiovascular mortality and cardiovascular risk factors in men. *Eur Heart* 2000;21:1584–1590.
47. Packard CJ, O'Reilly DSJ, Caslake MJ, et al. Lipoprotein-associated phospholipase A2 as an independent predictor of coronary heart disease. *N Engl J Med* 2000;343:1148–1155.
48. Pirro M, Bergeron J, Dagenais GR, et al. Age and duration of follow-up as modulators of the risk for ischemic heart disease associated with high plasma C-reactive protein levels in men. *Arch Intern Med* 2001;161:2474–2480.
49. Pradhan AD, Manson JE, Rossouw JE, et al. Inflammatory biomarkers, hormone replacement therapy, and incident coronary heart disease: prospective analysis from the Women's Health Initiative observational study. *JAMA* 2002;288:980–987.
50. Roivainen M, Viik-Kajander M, Palosuo T, et al. Infections, inflammation, and the risk of coronary heart disease. *Circulation* 2000;101:252–257.
51. Strandberg TE, Tilvis RS. C-reactive protein, cardiovascular risk factors, and mortality in a prospective study in the elderly. *Arterioscler Thromb Vasc Biol* 2000;20:1057–1060.
52. Tracy RP, Lemaitre RN, Psaty BM, et al. Relationship of C-reactive protein to risk of cardiovascular disease in the elderly: results from the Cardiovascular Health Study and the Rural Health Promotion Project. *Arterioscler Thromb Vasc Biol* 1997;17:1121–1127.
53. Ridker PM, Rifai N, Clearfield M, et al. Measurement of C-reactive protein for the targeting of statin therapy in the primary prevention of acute coronary events. *N Engl J Med* 2001;344:1959–1965.
54. Ridker PM, Rifai N, Rose L, et al. Comparison of C-reactive protein and low-density lipoprotein cholesterol levels in the prediction of first cardiovascular events. *N Engl J Med* 2002;347:1557–1565.
55. Ridker PM, Rifai N, Pfeffer MA, et al, for the Cholesterol And Recurrent Events (CARE) Investigators. Long-term effects of pravastatin on plasma concentration of C-reactive protein. *Circulation* 1999;100:230–235.
56. Cushman M, Arnold AM, Psaty BM, et al. C-reactive protein and the 10-year incidence of coronary heart disease in older men and women: the Cardiovascular Health Study. *Circulation* 2005;112:25–31.
57. Danesh J, Whincup P, Walker M, et al. Low-grade inflammation and coronary heart disease: prospective study and updated meta-analyses. *BMJ* 2000;321:199–204.
58. Tommasi S, Carluccio E, Bentivoglio M, et al. C-reactive protein as a marker for cardiac ischemic events in the year after a first, uncomplicated myocardial infarction. *Am J Cardiol* 1999;83:1595–1599.
59. Biasucci LM, Liuzzo G, Grillo KL, et al. Elevated levels of c-reactive protein at discharge in patients with unstable angina predict recurrent instability. *Circulation* 1999;99:855–860.
60. Ridker PM, Cannon CP, Morrow D, et al. Pravastatin or Atorvastatin Evaluation and Infection Therapy-Thrombolysis in Myocardial Infarction 22 (PROVE IT-TIMI 22) Investigators. C-reactive protein levels and outcomes after statin therapy. *N Engl J Med* 2005;352:20–28.
61. Esposito K, Pontillo A, Di Palo C, et al. Effect of weight loss and lifestyle changes on vascular inflammatory markers in obese women: a randomized trial. *JAMA* 2003;289:1799–1804.
62. Haffner SM, Greenberg AS, Weston WM, et al. Effect of rosiglitazone treatment on nontraditional markers of cardiovascular disease in patients with type 2 diabetes mellitus. *Circulation* 2002;106:679–684.
63. Lauten WB, Khan QA, Rajagopalan S, et al. Usefulness of quinapril and irbesartan to improve the anti-inflammatory response of atorvastatin and aspirin in patients with coronary heart disease. *Am J Cardiol* 2003;91:1116–1119.
64. Grundy SM, Vega GL, McGovern ME, et al. Efficacy, safety and tolerability

of once-daily niacin for the treatment of dyslipidemia associated with type 2 diabetes. *Arch Intern Med* 2002;162:1568–1576.
65. Chew DP, Bhatt DL, Robbins MA, et al. Effect of clopidogrel added to aspirin before percutaneous coronary intervention on the risk associated with C-reactive protein. *Am J Cardiol* 2001;88:672–674.
66. Albert MA, Danielson E, Rifai N, et al., for the PRINCE Investigators. Effect of statin therapy on C-reactive protein levels: the pravastatin inflammation/CRP evaluation (PRINCE): a randomized trial and cohort study. *JAMA* 2001;286:64–70.
67. Ridker PM, Rifai N, Clearfield M, et al., for the Air Force/Texas Coronary Atherosclerosis Prevention Study Investigators. Measurement of C-reactive protein for the targeting of statin therapy in the primary prevention of acute coronary events. *N Engl J Med* 2001;344:1959–1965.
68. Albert MA, Glynn RJ, Ridker PM. Plasma concentration of C-reactive protein and the calculated Framingham coronary heart disease risk score. *Circulation* 2003;108:161–165.
69. Koenig W, Lowel H, Baumert J, et al., C-reactive protein modulates risk prediction based on the Framingham Score: implications for future risk assessment: results from a large cohort study in southern Germany. *Circulation* 2004;109:1349–1353.
70. Ridker PM, Cook N. Clinical usefulness of very high and very low levels of C-reactive protein across the full range of Framingham Risk Scores. *Circulation* 2004;109:1955–1959.
71. Smith SC Jr, Anderson JL, Cannon RO 3rd, et al., CDC; AHA. CDC/AHA Workshop on Markers of Inflammation and Cardiovascular Disease: application to clinical and public health practice: report from the clinical practice discussion group. *Circulation* 2004;110:e550–553.
72. Ridker PM. Rosuvastatin in the primary prevention of cardiovascular disease among patients with low levels of low-density lipoprotein cholesterol and elevated high-sensitivity C-reactive protein: rationale and design of the JUPITER trial. *Circulation* 2003;108:2292–2297.
73. Kant JA, Fornace AJ, Saxe D, et al. Evolution and organization of the fibrinogen locus on chromosome 4: gene duplication accompanied by transposition and inversion. *Proc Natl Acad Sci U S A* 1985;82:2344–2348.
74. Folsom AR. Epidemiology of fibrinogen. *Eur Heart J* 1995;16:21–24.
75. Letcher RI, Chien S, Pickering TG, et al. Direct relationship between blood pressure and blood viscosity in normal and hypertensive subjects. Role of fibrinogen concentration. *Am J Med* 1981;70:1195–1202.
76. Kannel WB, D'Agostino RB, Wilson PW, et al. Diabetes, fibrinogen, and risk of cardiovascular disease: the Framingham experience. *Am Heart J* 1990;120:672–676.
77. Ernst E, Matrai A, Scholzl C, et al. Dose-effect relationship between smoking and blood rheology. *Br J Haematol* 1987;65:485–487.
78. Yarnell JW, Sweetnam PM, Rogers S, et al. Some long-term effects of smoking on the haemostatic system: a report from the Caerphilly and Speedwell Collaborative Surveys. *J Clin Pathol* 1987;40:909–913.
79. Kannel WB, Wolf PA, Castelli WP, et al. Fibrinogen and risk of cardiovascular disease. The Framingham Study. *JAMA* 1987;258:1183–1186.
80. Herrick S, Blanc-Brude O, Gray A, Laurent G. Fibrinogen. *Int J Biochem Cell Biol* 1999;31:741–746.
81. Smith EB, Keen GA, Grant A, et al. Fate of fibrinogen in human arterial intima. *Arteriosclerosis* 1990;10:263–275.
82. Rabbani LE, Loscalzo J. Recent observations on the role of hemostatic determinants in the development of atherothrombotic plaque. *Atherosclerosis* 1994;105:1–7.
83. Andreotti F, Burzotta F, Maseri A. Fibrinogen as a marker of inflammation: a clinical view. *Blood Coagul Fibrinolysis* 1999;10:S3-S4.
84. Ernst E, Resch KL. Fibrinogen as a cardiovascular risk factor: a meta-analysis and review of the literature. *Ann Intern Med* 1993;118:956–963.
85. Folsom AR, Wu KK, Rosamond WD, et al. Prospective study of hemostatic factors and incidence of coronary heart disease: the Atherosclerosis Risk in Communities (ARIC) Study. *Circulation* 1997;96:1102–1108.
86. Danesh J, Collins R, Appleby P, et al. Association of fibrinogen, C-reactive protein, albumin, or leukocyte count with coronary heart disease: meta-analyses of prospective studies. *JAMA* 1998;279:1477–1482.
87. Maresca G, Di Blasio A, Marchioli R, et al. Measuring plasma fibrinogen to predict stroke and myocardial infarction: an update. *Arterioscler Thromb Vasc Biol* 1999;19:1368–1377.
88. Ernst E, Resch KL. Therapeutic interventions to lower fibrinogen concentration. *Eur Heart J* 1995;16:47–53.
89. Secondary prevention by raising HDL cholesterol and reducing triglycerides in patients with coronary artery disease: the Bezafibrate Infarction Prevention (BIP) study. *Circulation* 2000;102:21–27.
90. Meade T, Zuhrie R, Cook C, et al. Bezafibrate in men with lower extremity arterial disease: randomised controlled trial. *BMJ* 2000;325:1139–1143.
91. Hulley S, Grady D, Bush T, et al. Randomized trial of estrogen plus progestin for secondary prevention of coronary heart disease in postmenopausal women. Heart and Estrogen/progestin Replacement Study (HERS) Research Group. *JAMA* 1998;280:605–613.
92. Acevedo M, Pearce GL, Kottke-Marchant K, et al. Elevated fibrinogen and homocysteine levels enhance the risk of mortality in patients from a high-risk preventive cardiology clinic. *Arterioscler Thromb Vasc Biol* 2002;22:1042–1045.
93. Berg K. A new serum system type in man-the Lp system. *Acta Pathol Microbiol Scand* 1963;59:369–382.
94. Utermann G. The mysteries of lipoprotein(a). *Science* 1989;246:904–910.
95. McLean JW, Tomlinson JE, Kuang W-J, et al. cDNA sequence of human apolipoprotein (a) is homologous to plasminogen. *Nature* 1987;330:132–137.
96. Berglund L, Ramakrishnan R. Lipoprotein(a): an elusive cardiovascular risk factor. *Arterioscler Thromb Vasc Biol* 2004;24:2219–2226.
97. van der Hoek YY, Wittekoek ME, Beisiegel U, et al. The apolipoprotein kringle IV repeats which differ from the major repeat kringle are present in variably-sized isoforms. *Hum Mol Genet* 1993;2:361–366.
98. Koschinsky ML, Beisiegel U, Henne-Bruns D, et al. Apolipoprotein (a) size heterogeneity is related to variable number of repeat sequences in its mRNA. *Biochemistry* 1990;29:640–644.
99. Gavish D, Azrolan N, Breslow J. Plasma Lp(a) concentration is inversely correlated with the ratio of Kringle IV/Kringle V encoding domains in the apo(a) gene. *J Clin Invest* 1989;84:2021–2027.
100. Kraft HG, Kochl S, Menzel HJ, et al. The apolipoprotein[a] gene-a transcribed hypervariable locus controlling plasma lipoprotein[a] concentration. *Hum Genet* 1992;90:220–230.
101. Rader DJ, Cain W, Ikewaki K, et al. The inverse association of plasma lipoprotein(a) concentrations with apolipoprotein(a) isoform size is not due to differences in Lp(a) catabolism but to differences in production rate. *J Clin Invest* 1994;93:2758–2763.
102. Boerwinkle E, Leffert CC, Lin J, et al. Apolipoprotein(a) gene accounts for greater than 90% of the variation in plasma lipoprotein(a) concentrations. *J Clin Invest* 1992;90:52–60.
103. Marcovina SM, Albers JJ, Wijsman E, et al. Differences in Lp(a) concentrations and apo(a) polymorphs between black and white Americans. *J Lipid Res* 1996;37:2569–2585.
104. Marcovina SM, Koschinsky ML, Albers JJ, et al. Report of the National Heart, Lung, and Blood Institute Workshop on lipoprotein(a) and cardiovascular disease: recent advances and future directions. *Clin Chem* 2003;49:1785–1796.
105. Tsimikas S, Lau HK, Han KR, et al. Percutaneous coronary intervention results in acute increases in oxidized phospholipids and lipoprotein(a): short-term and long-term immunologic responses to oxidized low-density lipoprotein. *Circulation* 2004;109:3164–3170.
106. Yano Y, Shimokawa K, Okada Y, et al. Immunolocalization of lipoprotein(a) in wounded tissues. *J Histochem Cytochem* 1997;45:559–568.
107. Thillet J, Doucet C, Chapman J, et al. Elevated lipoprotein(a) levels and small apo(a) isoforms are compatible with longevity: evidence from a large population of French centenarians. *Atherosclerosis* 1998;136:389–394.
108. Dangas G, Mehran R, Harpel PC, et al. Lipoprotein(a) and inflammation in human coronary atheroma: association with the severity of clinical presentation. *J Am Coll Cardiol* 1998;32:2035–2042.
109. Caplice NM, Panetta C, Peterson TE, et al. Lipoprotein(a) binds and inactivates tissue factor pathway inhibitor: a novel link between lipoproteins and thrombosis. *Blood* 2001;98:2980–2987.
110. Buechler C, Ullrich H, Ritter M, et al. Lipoprotein(a) up-regulates the expression of the plasminogen activator inhibitor 2 in human blood monocytes. *Blood* 2001;97:981–986.
111. Danesh J, Collins R, Peto R. Lipoprotein(a) and coronary heart disease: meta-analysis of prospective studies. *Circulation* 2000;102:1082–1085.
112. Nguyen TT, Ellefson RD, Hodge DO, et al. Predictive value of electrophoretically detected lipoprotein(a) for coronary heart disease and cerebrovascular disease in a community-based cohort of 9936 men and women. *Circulation* 1997;96:1390–1397.
113. Tsimikas S, Brilakis ES, Miller ER, et al. Oxidized phospholipids, Lp(a) lipoprotein, and coronary artery disease. *N Engl J Med* 2005;353:46–57.
114. Ariyo AA, Thach C, Tracy R. Cardiovascular Health Study Investigators. Lp(a) lipoprotein, vascular disease, and mortality in the elderly. *N Engl J Med* 2003;349:2108–2115.
115. Shai I, Rimm EB, Hankinson SE, et al. Lipoprotein (a) and coronary heart disease among women: beyond a cholesterol carrier? *Eur Heart J* 2005;26:1633–1639.
116. von Eckardstein A, Schulte H, Cullen P, et al. Lipoprotein(a) further increases the risk of coronary events in men with high global cardiovascular risk. *J Am Coll Cardiol* 2001;37:434–439.
117. Berg K, Dahlen G, Christopherson B, et al. Lp(a) lipoprotein level predicts survival and major coronary events in the Scandinavian Simvastatin Survival Study. *Clin Genet* 1997;52:254–261.
118. Ridker PM, Hennekens CH, Stampfer MJ. A prospective study of lipoprotein(a) and the risk of myocardial infarction. *JAMA* 1993;270:2195–2199.
119. Gurakar A, Hoeg JM, Kostner G, et al. Levels of lipoprotein Lp(a) decline with neomycin and niacin treatment. *Atherosclerosis* 1985;57:293–301.
120. Carlson LA, Hamsten A, Asplund A. Pronounced lowering of serum levels of lipoprotein Lp(a) in hyperlipidaemic subjects treated with nicotinic acid. *J Intern Med* 1989;226:271–276.
121. Glueck CJ, Freiberg R, Glueck HI, et al. Idiopathic osteonecrosis, hypofibrinolysis, high plasminogen activator inhibitor, high lipoprotein(a), and therapy with stanozolol. *Am J Hematol* 1995;48:213–220.
122. Gavish D, Breslow JL. Lipoprotein(a) reduction by (N)-acetylcysteine. *Lancet* 1991;337:203–204.
123. Sachs FM, McPherson R, Walsh BW. Effects of postmenopausal estrogen replacement on plasma Lp(a) lipoprotein concentrations. *Arch Intern Med* 1994;154:1106–1110.

124. Kostner GM, Gavish D, Leopold B, et al. HMG CoA reductase inhibitors lower LDL cholesterol without reducing Lp(a) levels. *Circulation* 1989;80:1313–1319.
125. Bambauer R. Is lipoprotein (a)-apheresis useful? *Ther Apher Dial* 2005; 9:142–147.
126. Maher V, Brown BG, Marcovina SM, et al. Effects of lowering LDL cholesterol on the cardiovascular risk of lipoprotein(a). *JAMA* 1995;274;1771–1774.
127. Mangoni AA, Jackson SH. Homocysteine and cardiovascular disease: current evidence and future prospects. *Am J Med* 2002;112:556–565.
128. Mudd SH, Skovby F, Levy HL, et al. The natural history of homocystinuria due to cystathionine beta-synthase deficiency. *Am J Hum Genet* 1985;37:1–31.
129. McCully KS. Homocystinuria, arteriosclerosis, methylmalonic aciduria, and methyltransferase deficiency: a key case revisited. *Nutr Rev* 1992;50:7–12.
130. Yap S, Naughten ER, Wilcken B, et al. Vascular complications of severe hyperhomocysteinemia in patients with homocystinuria due to cystathionine beta-synthase deficiency: effects of homocysteine-lowering therapy. *Semin Thromb Hemost* 2000;26:335–340.
131. Boers GH, Smals AG, Trijbels FJ, et al. Heterozygosity for homocystinuria in premature peripheral and cerebral occlusive arterial disease. *N Engl J Med* 1985;313:709–715.
132. Malinow MR, Kang SS, Taylor LM, et al. Prevalence of hyperhomocyst(e)inemia in patients with peripheral arterial occlusive disease. *Circulation* 1989;79:1180–1188.
133. Clarke R, Daly L, Robinson K, et al. Hyperhomocysteinemia: an independent risk factor for vascular disease. *N Engl J Med* 1991;324:1149–1155.
134. Kang SS, Wong PW, Cook HY, et al. Protein-bound homocyst(e)ine: a possible risk factor for coronary artery disease. *J Clin Invest* 1986;77:1482–1486.
135. Jacobsen DW, Gatautis VJ, Green R, et al. Rapid HPLC determination of total homocysteine and other thiols in serum and plasma; sex differences and correlation with cobalamin and folate concentrations in healthy subjects. *Clin Chem* 1994;40:873–881.
136. Nedrebo BG, Ericsson UB, Nygard O, et al. Plasma total homocysteine levels in hyperthyroid and hypothyroid patients. *Metabolism* 1998;47:89–93.
137. Ubbink JB, Vemiaak WJ, van der Merwe A, et al. Vitamin B-12, vitamin B-6, and folate nutritional status in men with hyperhomocysteinemia. *Am J Clin Nutr* 1993;57:47–53.
138. Bostom AG, Culleton BF. Hyperhomocysteinemia in chronic renal disease. *J Am Soc Nephrol* 1999;10:891–900.
139. Jacques PF, Bostom AG, Williams RR, et al. Relation between folate status, a common mutation in methylenetetrahydrofolate reductase, and plasma homocysteine concentrations. *Circulation* 1996;93:7–9.
140. Welch GN, Loscalzo J. Homocysteine and atherothrombosis. *N Engl J Med* 1998;338:1042–1050.
141. Chambers JC, Ueland PM, Obeid OA, et al. Improved vascular endothelial function after oral B vitamins: an effect mediated through reduced concentrations of free plasma homocysteine. *Circulation* 2000;102:2479–2483.
142. Bellamy MF, McDowell IF, Ramsey MW, et al. Hyperhomocysteinemia after an oral methionine load acutely impairs endothelial function in healthy adults. *Circulation* 1998;98:1848–1852.
143. Poddar R, Sivasubramanian N, DiBello PM, et al. Homocysteine induces expression and secretion of monocyte chemoattractant protein-1 and interleukin-8 in human aortic endothelial cells: implications for vascular disease. *Circulation* 2001;103:2717–2723.
144. Werstuck GH, Lentz SR, Dayal S, et al. Homocysteine-induced endoplasmic reticulum stress causes dysregulation of the cholesterol and triglyceride biosynthetic pathways. *J Clin Invest* 2001;107:1263–1273.
145. Boushey CJ, Beresford SA, Omenn GS, et al. A quantitative assessment of plasma homocysteine as a risk factor for vascular disease. Probable benefits of increasing folic acid intakes. *JAMA* 1995;274:1049–1057.
146. Homocysteine Studies Collaboration. Homocysteine and risk of ischemic heart disease and stroke: a meta-analysis. *JAMA* 2002;288:2015–2022.
147. Graham IM, Daly LE, Refsum HM, et al. Plasma homocysteine as a risk factor for vascular disease: the European Concerted Action Project. *JAMA* 1997;277:1775–1781.
148. Soinio M, Mamiemi J, Laakso M, et al. Elevated plasma homocysteine level is an independent predictor of coronary heart disease events in patients with type 2 diabetes mellitus. *Ann Intern Med* 2004;140:94–100.
149. Moustapha A, Naso A, Nahlawi M, et al. Prospective study of hyperhomocysteinemia as an adverse cardiovascular risk factor in end-stage renal disease. *Circulation* 1998;97:138–141.
150. Nygard O, Nordrehaug JE, Refsum H, et al. Plasma homocysteine levels and mortality in patients with coronary artery disease. *N Engl J Med* 1997;337:230–236.
151. Al-Obaidi MK, Stubbs PJ, Collinson P, et al. Elevated homocysteine levels are associated with increased ischemic myocardial injury in acute coronary syndromes. *J Am Coll Cardiol* 2000;36:1217–1222.
152. Schnyder G, Roffi M, Flammer Y, et al. Effect of homocysteine-lowering therapy with folic acid, vitamin B(12), and vitamin B(6) on clinical outcome after percutaneous coronary intervention: the Swiss Heart study: a randomized controlled trial. *JAMA* 2002;288:973–979.
153. Lange H, Suryapranata H, De Luca G, et al. Folate therapy and in-stent restenosis after coronary stenting. *N Engl J Med* 2004;350:2673–2681.
154. Homocysteine Lowering Trialists' Collaboration. Lowering blood homocysteine with folic acid based supplements: meta-analysis of randomised trials. *BMJ* 1998;316:894–898.
155. Wald DS, Bishop L, Wald NJ, et al. Randomized trial of folic acid supplementation and serum homocysteine levels. *Arch Intern Med* 2001; 161:695–700.
156. Toole JF, Malinow MR, Chambless LE, et al. Lowering homocysteine in patients with ischemic stroke to prevent recurrent stroke, myocardial infarction, and death: the Vitamin Intervention for Stroke Prevention (VISP) randomized controlled trial. *JAMA* 2004;291:565–575.
157. The VITATOPS (Vitamins to Prevent Stroke) Trial. Rationale and design of an international, large, simple, randomised trial of homocysteine-lowering multivitamin therapy in patients with recent transient ischaemic attack or stroke. *Cerebrovasc Dis* 2002;13:120–126.
158. MacMahon M, Kirkpatrick C, Cummings CE, et al. A pilot study with simvastatin and folic acid/vitamin B12 in preparation for the Study of the Effectiveness of Additional Reductions in Cholesterol and Homocysteine (SEARCH). *Nutr Metab Cardiovasc Dis* 2000;10:195–203.
159. Manson JE, Gaziano JM, Spelsberg A, et al. A secondary prevention trial of antioxidant vitamins and cardiovascular disease in women: rationale, design, and methods. The WACS Research Group. *Ann Epidemiol* 1995;5:261–269.
160. Jacques PF, Selhub J, Bostom AG, et al. The effect of folic acid fortification on plasma folate and total homocysteine concentrations. *N Engl J Med* 1999;340:1449–1454.
161. Ford ES, Giles WH, Mokdad AH. The distribution of 10-Year risk for coronary heart disease among US adults: findings from the National Health and Nutrition Examination Survey III. *J Am Coll Cardiol* 2004;43:1791–1796.
162. Jacobson TA, Griffiths GG, Varas C, et al. Impact of evidence-based "clinical judgment" on the number of American adults requiring lipid-lowering therapy based on updated NHANES III data. National Health and Nutrition Examination Survey. *Arch Intern Med* 2000;160:1361–1369.
163. Greenland P, Smith SC Jr, Grundy SM. Improving coronary heart disease risk assessment in asymptomatic people: role of traditional risk factors and noninvasive cardiovascular tests. *Circulation* 2001;104:1863–1867.
164. Bild DE, Bluemke DA, Burke GL, et al. Multi-ethnic study of atherosclerosis: objectives and design. *Am J Epidemiol* 2002;156:871–881.

CHAPTER 12 ■ BEHAVIORAL CARDIOLOGY AND HEART DISEASE

ELLEN A. DORNELAS AND MATTHEW M. BURG

HISTORICAL PERSPECTIVE AND OVERVIEW

The earliest appreciation that psychological factors contribute to diseases of the heart can be attributed to Celsus, who is reported to have said, "Fear and anger and any other state of mind may often be apt to excite the pulse." John Hunter, a leading pioneer of cardiovascular medicine and pathology, acknowledged the links between his outbursts of anger and his anginal attacks, proclaiming, "My life is in the hands of any rascal who chooses to put me in a passion." He died suddenly in 1793 after participating in a violent argument at a faculty meeting. Sir William Osler later described the circumstances of Hunter's death: "In silent rage and in the next room he gave a deep groan and fell down dead" (1). Although these reports are anecdotal indications that physicians understood the importance of psychological factors for their cardiac patients, it was two cardiologists, Meyer Friedman and Ray Rosenman, who in 1959 were the first to conduct rigorous scientific studies of these factors and their relationship to CHD. The results of their work drew widespread attention to a clustering of behaviors, including a highly competitive, goal-driven approach to daily activities, aggressive behaviors, a need to perform activities at an unusually high rate of speed, hyperarousal of emotional and physical alertness, and hostile affect, that came to be called the "Type A Behavior Pattern" (2). Although their early studies found an association between this behavior pattern and onset of coronary heart disease (CHD), later studies were unable to replicate this finding. The work of Friedman and Rosenman, however, led to the development of a field, now called *Behavioral Cardiology,* which applies the theories and principles of the behavioral sciences to the practice of medicine with cardiac patients. The past four decades have seen exponential growth in the understanding that psychological factors are important, both as precipitants and sequelae of cardiac events. Psychosocial factors associated with risk for CHD include stress and emotional elements (e.g., anger, depression), personality traits (e.g., cynicism), social factors (e.g., social support), and lifestyle choices (e.g., tobacco use). This chapter focuses on the role that these factors can play in promoting risk for an acute cardiac event and on recovery from these events.

PSYCHOLOGICAL FACTORS AND HEART DISEASE

Stress

Stress has been used ubiquitously to describe both external precipitants and internal reactions that can include emotional, behavioral, cognitive, and physiological responses to environmental triggers. In the section that follows, a heuristic definition is used that defines stress as an external or environmental situation that may tax a person's coping abilities. In the following section, the relationship between acute and chronic external stressors to CHD is described. Following this section, known psychosocial risk factors (hostility, depression, anxiety, and social support) are described as precipitants and sequelae of cardiac disease.

Acute Stress

Early case series (3,4) describe cardiac arrest or sudden death in response to acute stress such as grief or fear. A recent observational study receiving a great deal of attention in the media reported that sudden emotional stress (e.g., tragic news or news of a close relative or friend's death) can precipitate severe but reversible left ventricular dysfunction in patients without cardiac disease (5). Epidemiologic studies have shown that sudden death increases in populations suffering emotionally devastating disasters such as earthquake or war (6,7). Toivonen et al. (8) observed proarrhythmic repolarization changes in the ECG of healthy house officers exposed to the sudden stress of an on-call alarm, and an increase in implantable cardioverter devices shock-treated ventricular arrhythmias was seen in the weeks following the terrorist attacks of 9/11, in both New York City (9) and distant locales (10). In working patients with implantable cardioverter devices, ventricular tachycardia occurs more frequently on the first day of the work week (11).

Acute stress is also a potent trigger of myocardial ischemia in patients with coronary artery disease (CAD). Holter monitoring studies have found ischemia to be common during periods of low physical exertion but moderate to high mental and emotional stress, with the incidence and duration of these episodes directly related to the intensity of the stress experienced (12,13). Studies in the laboratory with measures of ischemia (left ventricular dysfunction, new regional wall motion abnormality by stress echo, myocardial perfusion defects) have shown that acute mental stress can provoke myocardial ischemia in up to 50% of patients with CAD and the prognostic significance of this "mental stress ischemia" has been demonstrated in several studies (14–16). In these studies, patients with ischemia during acute laboratory stress demonstrate 2.4 to 3.0 times increased risk of myocardial infarction (MI) or unstable angina 1 to 4 years later (17–19). In addition, the Psychophysiological Investigations of Myocardial Ischemia (PIMI) study investigators (20) reported a 3.0 rate ratio for death over a 5-year follow-up among CAD patients with mental stress ischemia. This was the first study powered to demonstrate an effect for death tied to mental stress ischemia in the lab. Overall, there is consistent evidence that emotional distress, anger, and extreme excitement can trigger acute coronary syndrome (ACS) and sudden cardiac death in susceptible individuals with both immediate (21) and long-lasting impact (20).

Chronic Stress

Chronic stress, assessed as a function of events such as divorce, loss of job, death of a loved one, or catastrophic illness, can play a role in first occurrence of cardiac events. For example, one case control study showed that the cardiac patients reported greater numbers of recent stressful life events than controls (22). In addition, the world-wide INTERHEART study comparing 11,119 first MI patients to 13,648 matched on age and gender controls also showed that stressful life events in the year preceding the index MI were more common in cardiac patients compared to the control group (23).

The work environment has most often been used to study chronic stress as it relates to CAD (24). In this research, *job strain,* defined as the confluence of high job demands and low job control, has been associated with increased CVD prevalence (25). Greater numbers of work-related stressors are also associated with increased risk for cardiac mortality (26). Overall, the data suggest that chronic stressors influence the development and progression of CAD. Job strain has been the most often studied model of chronic stress and lack of control (e.g., the perception of little power to impact on decision making) is thought to be the most pathogenic component of work-related stress (27). Although environmental stressors have an independent effect on CHD, it is the combination of external stressors and internal psychological factors, such as those described below, that exert the greatest degree of influence on the development and course of CHD.

Hostility and Anger

Hostility is a multidimensional psychological construct that involves three primary factors: cynicism/mistrust (cognitions), anger/contempt (emotions), and verbal/physical aggression (behaviors) (28). *Anger* is an affective experience, ranging from mild irritation or annoyance, to full-blown rage (29). As described, a relationship between anger/hostility and CHD has been proposed throughout the centuries, with Rosenman and Friedman in the 1950s launching scientific investigations into the Type A Behavior Pattern. They found this behavior pattern to incur a greater than twofold increased risk of developing ischemic heart disease, controlling for traditional risk factors, in an initially healthy sample (30). A detailed analysis of this data (31) revealed the relative importance of the hostility and anger components as predictors of CHD onset. Hostility is also associated with a 1.9-fold increased risk of death (32), up to a 14.6-fold increased risk of cardiac events among patients with CAD (33), and a 2.5-fold increased risk of restenosis after percutaneous transluminal coronary angioplasty (PTCA) (34). Highly hostile patients also demonstrate more rapid progression of carotid atherosclerosis (35) and are more likely to evidence myocardial ischemia during mental stress testing (36,37). The experience of moderate to extreme anger is associated with a 2.5-fold increased risk of MI for up to 2 hours after anger provocation (38); the induction of anger in the laboratory, either by structured interview (36) or by recall of a previous anger-provoking incident (39,40), can provoke myocardial ischemia in patients with CHD. Thus, hostility has come to be thought of as the most pathogenic aspect of the type A behavior pattern. This line of research has led to new developments in the understanding of how other negative emotions, particularly depression, are related to CHD.

Depression

Depression refers to both a diagnostic entity (e.g., major depressive disorder) and a clustering of symptoms with psychological (e.g., feelings of sadness), behavioral (e.g., difficulty functioning in ordinary role activities), and somatic (e.g., sleep problems) characteristics. Symptoms of depression are seen in up to 65% of patients after MI, with between 16% and 22% evidencing major depression (41–43) and up to one third developing depression over 12 months (44). For these patients, depression follows a chronic relapsing course, particularly if a full remission is not realized (44). Life-time history of depression increases risk for cardiac-related morbidity and mortality (45–47). In patients with chronic CAD, a diagnosis of major depression incurs a twofold risk of ACS (41), and depression after acute MI incurs a greater than fourfold risk of 6-month mortality, and ongoing mortality risk for 5 years (44,48,49). Depression after MI also increases the risk for reinfarction, particularly for patients with post-MI ventricular arrhythmias (50). This effect of depression is independent of CAD severity, left ventricular dysfunction, or history of MI. In addition, this effect is seen for both diagnostic depression (41) and subsyndromal depression (e.g., score $\geq$10 on the Beck Depression Inventory) (42,44,49). Depression prior to or after coronary artery bypass grafting (50) also incurs a threefold risk for CAD progression over 6 months (51) and a fourfold risk of cardiovascular death over 2 years (51), independent of a range of medical comorbidities, behavioral health risks, or surgical complications.

Anxiety

Anxiety is a clustering of symptoms that include psychological (uncontrollable worry) and somatic (acute physiologic arousal) features. Between 15% and 30% of post-ACS patients experience symptoms of anxiety (52). Although normative, higher symptom levels at the time of hospitalization for ACS are related to poorer subsequent psychological and psychiatric outcomes (53,54). Panic attacks, characterized by palpitations, sweating, dyspnea, chest pain, and feelings of losing control or going crazy, are common manifestations of anxiety disorders.

The prevalence of panic disorder in cardiac populations ranges from 10% to 15% (55) and 30% to 50% of patients with recurrent chest pain and normal coronary arteries meet criteria for panic disorder (56).

Studies of initially healthy populations have linked anxiety to ACS incidence (57,58). In addition, the few studies concerning post-ACS anxiety and prognosis demonstrate almost fivefold independent risk of in-hospital cardiac complications or death (59), 2.5-fold independent risk for 1-year recurrent MI (60), and 8-year, 4.7-fold independent risk of a cardiac event for patients with both high anxiety and social inhibition (61). Although these studies are clearly suggestive, they rely mostly on self-report of symptoms and have been accomplished with small numbers of post-MI patients. There is a well-established relationship between depression, hostility, and heart disease, but there is a need for additional research to determine the impact of anxiety on CHD prognosis.

Social Support

Social support is an important predictor of initial ACS incidence and subsequent mortality. In addition, high levels of support can buffer the impact of the ACS event. Lack of social support in combination with high levels of stress was associated with a more than fourfold increased mortality risk among patients in the Beta Blocker Trial (62). Subsequent studies have linked the presence, degree, and quality of intimate social ties—including marital status, whether the person lives alone or with others, and the availability of various sources of emotional support—to mortality in patients after ACS (63–66). Indices of social network size, frequency of social activity, group membership, and perceived support have also been found to predict survival (67–70) controlling for sociodemographic and disease severity indices.

A number of explanations have been offered for the beneficial effects of social support on cardiovascular disease (71). For example, social contacts may foster better health habits, treatment adherence, and proper use of health care resources, whereas social isolation may be accompanied by potentially deleterious physiologic activity involving the autonomic nervous system and immune function. Finally, social support has been shown to reduce psychological distress, which is high in cardiac patients and associated with elevated mortality risk.

Pathophysiologic Mechanisms by Which Emotions May Affect the Heart

Biological and behavioral pathways have been examined as potential mechanisms tying psychological and emotional factors to CHD development and prognosis. Promising findings in the biological domain focus on autonomic balance, cardiovascular and neuroendocrine reactivity, inflammation, and endothelial function, with an emerging picture in which dysregulation of autonomic nervous system function in general, and of hypothalamic–pituitary–adrenal axis function specifically, links emotions and CHD.

Depression-related dysregulation of the autonomic nervous system and hypothalamic–pituitary–adrenal axis has been linked to hypercortisolemia, elevated plasma and urinary catecholamines, impairments in platelet functioning, elevated heart rate, reduced heart rate variability, and impaired vagal control, all of which may negatively impact CHD prognosis (72–78). Recent studies have also linked depression to markers of inflammation, including activity of adhesion molecules, leukocyte adhesiveness/aggregation, phagocytic activity, T-cell activation markers, and proinflammatory cytokines (79–81), processes known to promote CAD progression by increasing macrophage and lipid deposition within coronary arteries, and instability and rupture of existing atherosclerotic lesions (82,83). Similarly, anxiety has been linked to abnormal cardiac autonomic control, which can increase the risk of potentially fatal ventricular arrhythmias. Acute anxiety states are also believed to be capable of triggering coronary vasospasm, which can lead to rupture of atherosclerotic plaques (57,58). Acute and chronic stress can also provoke a hypercoagulable state that can be particularly harmful for patients with CHD who already have impaired endothelial and anticoagulant functioning (84).

The anger/hostility constellation has also been linked to chronic over stimulation of the sympathetic nervous system (85), which can lead to arterial constriction, increased blood pressure and heart rate, impaired ventricular function, elevated circulating catecholamines and corticosteroids, release of free fatty acids into the blood stream, and increased platelet aggregation (58,86).

In addition to direct physiologic pathways, negative emotions can influence key health risk behaviors. CHD patients with depression, anxiety, and higher levels of hostility/anger are more likely to engage in CHD risk behaviors such as smoking, overeating, decreased physical activity, decreased sleep, and increased use of alcohol and drugs (28,87). Depressed patients in particular are prone to nonadherence with treatment regimens, making them less likely to take proper medications and make appropriate lifestyle changes. Such health behaviors may mediate the relationship between negative emotions and CHD (58,88,89). Thus, it appears that not only are there direct physiologic pathways by which depression, anger/hostility, and anxiety can lead to poorer health outcomes in patients with CHD, but also various risk behaviors associated with these negative affect states may have physical consequences that serve as additional health risk factors.

Summary

In summary, the importance of psychological and emotional factors as contributors to CHD incidence and prognosis has been appreciated since the time of the ancient Greeks. Research conducted over the past 35 years has demonstrated that factors such as acute and chronic stress, anger and hostility, depression and anxiety, and lack of social support are associated with independent and significant risk for ACS onset and subsequent event-free survival, with the size of the effect equal to or greater than that associated with such accepted risk factors as hypertension and hypercholesterolemia. Plausible mechanisms to account for this risk have been proposed and tested, and these mechanisms include both physiologic and behavioral pathways, possibly working in concert. Further, as suggested by Williams et al. (90), psychosocial risk factors tend to cluster together and often co-occur in the same subgroups (e.g., cigarette smokers), perhaps imparting synergistic effects on cardiovascular disease. In the remainder of this chapter, we review the literature concerning behavioral interventions for patients with CHD, and use a discussion of current controversies to articulate directions for future research.

BEHAVIORAL INTERVENTIONS FOR CARDIAC PATIENTS

Cardiac Rehabilitation

There is ample evidence that multifactorial cardiac rehabilitation can improve psychological functioning and quality of life.

The exercise and social support components have particular benefit for depressed and anxious cardiac patients, even when there is no demonstrable effect on aerobic fitness (91). Not all cardiac rehabilitation programs include a psychosocial component, but adding psychosocial treatment to standard cardiac rehabilitation is associated with improvement in psychological distress and medical outcomes (92).

Cardiac rehabilitation can also provide an ideal context for targeting behavioral problems that often go unaddressed, such as sexual functioning. Between 25% and 40% of cardiac patients report sexual performance problems (93), which have significant anxiety and relational components. Patients' fears about cardiac exertion during sex can be addressed with education and information. In addition, the goals of cardiac rehabilitation include the initiation and maintenance of long-term health risk behavioral change. The integration into cardiac rehabilitation of behavioral treatments for such things as tobacco cessation, proper diet, and medication adherence demonstrate the role that behavioral cardiology can play in the success of multifactorial rehabilitation efforts.

Despite the positive outcomes associated with rehabilitation, it is greatly underutilized. Although part of this problem is a function of referral and reimbursement patterns, psychological factors can play a key role in determining whether patients attend and adhere to cardiac rehabilitation. Factors associated with nonattendance include denial of illness severity, perceived lack of control over illness (94), depression, anxiety, living alone, substance abuse, and impaired cognitive functioning (93). Attention to these factors may improve acceptance of, and adherence with referral to cardiac rehabilitation programs.

Stress Management

Lifestyle interventions and cardiac rehabilitation programs tend to have multiple components that often incorporate stress management, which can include relaxation training (e.g., diaphragmatic breathing, progressive muscle relaxation, visual imagery) and use of cognitive strategies (e.g., coping skills training, problem solving, self-observation) to reduce distress, promote psychological well-being, and facilitate return to normal psychological functioning after a cardiac event. Stress management interventions are most often provided in groups, although they can be offered individually and can range in intensity from one to multiple sessions. For example, the Recurrent Coronary Prevention Project utilized a group-based cognitive-behavioral stress reduction treatment to modify the type A behavior pattern in patients after acute MI demonstrating a fourfold decrease in type A behavior that translated into 44% fewer recurrent cardiac events (95). Smaller studies have also demonstrated the effectiveness of stress reduction treatment for decreasing anger and hostility (96) or general distress-related risk (97,98) in CHD patients. Recently Blumenthal et al. (99,100) have shown that stress management treatment reduced myocardial ischemia, both during a laboratory mental stress protocol and during 48-hour holter monitoring. Compared to a usual care control condition, stress management was associated with better 5-year event-free survival, significant reductions in hostility and improvements in quality of life, and improvement in baroreflex sensitivity and heart rate variability. Similar treatment approaches have been used in small studies of patients with implantable cardioverter devices, with modest effects on indices of anxiety (101,102), and improvements in quality of life, depression, activity level, and sexual functioning (103,104).

The impact of stress management on anxiety and depression is less clear; one large trial (105) showed no effect on anxiety or depression. However, all patients were randomized, whether or not there was evidence of elevated distress levels and when reviewed by Linden (106), it was noted that this null finding reflected a floor effect, in that patients who are not depressed or anxious have little room for improvement. A recent Cochrane review (107) evaluating 18 trials of 5,242 patients randomized to stress management compared to some form of control group demonstrated a beneficial effect on composite measures of psychological well-being and quality-of-life indices.

Psychotherapy

Two recent randomized clinical trials directly examined treatment of distress and/or depression in post-MI patients, and the resulting impact on death and reinfarction. The Montreal Heart Attack Readjustment Trial (M-HART) regularly assessed distressed, post-MI patients and provided supportive home visits from a nurse to those randomized to the treatment condition when distress reached at least moderate levels (108). No overall survival benefit was demonstrated for the treatment; however, increased mortality was seen for older women in the treatment condition. Post hoc analyses (109) revealed enhanced survival for those who benefited psychologically from the nurse visits, highlighting the importance of offering depression/distress treatments of known efficacy when working with cardiac patients.

The Enhancing Recovery in Coronary Heart Disease (ENRICHD) Trial (110,111) was a multicenter, randomized controlled clinical trial funded by the National Heart, Lung and Blood Institute that was designed to determine the effect on medical prognosis (death, reinfarction) of a psychotherapy treatment for acute MI patients with depression and/or low social support. ENRICHD demonstrated a modest treatment effect for depression that did not translate into improved survival, except for patients with the most severe depression (111). A subgroup of the 1,165 patients enrolled into the treatment arm whose depression did not improve, had higher late (≥6 months post-MI) cardiac mortality rates than intervention patients whose depression responded to treatment (112). Of note, patients randomized to the usual care condition also demonstrated improvement in depression symptoms, and by 30 months of follow-up, no group differences in these symptoms remained. Cumulatively, the data from the ENRICHD trial suggest that early identification of cardiac patients with treatment refractory depression is important, so that such patients can be treated more aggressively. Further, these findings demonstrate the need for research to determine (a) the threshold treatment effects on depression for improved event-free survival after ACS, (b) the treatment dose necessary to affect the mechanism(s) that link depression to post-ACS prognosis, and (c) the ideal time to intervene on depression after ACS (111).

Pharmacotherapy for Depression in Cardiac Patients

Pharmacologic treatment of depression in CHD patients is complex and entails certain limitations and contraindications. For example, tricyclic and monoamine oxidase inhibitor medications affect cardiac conduction, contractility, and rhythm, and are associated with orthostatic hypotension (113,114). The more benign side effect profile of the newer selective serotonin reuptake inhibitor (SSRI) medications makes them the class of choice for cardiac patients. The recently completed SADHART trial demonstrated their safety, with data analyses indicating a trend to improved event-free survival (115). Post hoc analyses from ENRICHD also demonstrated a survival benefit for patients in both usual care and treatment conditions who received

SSRIs during the study (116). This effect is likely due to the impact of SSRIs on serotonergic platelet receptor function.

CONTROVERSIES AND PERSONAL PERSPECTIVES

Given the amount of data reviewed in this chapter and the strength of association between psychological/emotional factors and CHD incidence and prognosis that these data demonstrate, perhaps the greatest controversy concerns the general absence of these factors from the clinical pathways that guide the diagnosis and treatment of patients with CHD. There are likely many reasons for this. For example, in the past, emotional distress in CHD patients was thought to be part of a "normal reaction" to a new diagnosis of CAD or to an ACS event, a reaction that quickly dissipated with return to a person's normal routine. It is now known that a significant number of cardiac patients experience symptoms of depression and anxiety that are more severe than normal adjustment reactions. Many cardiologists feel themselves ill equipped to identify, let alone treat the problems discussed in this chapter. Yet, clinical cardiologists are arguably in an ideal position to recognize the psychological issues faced by their patients—because of the close and regular contact they have with them and the life-threatening nature of the disease(s) for which they are treating them. Rozanski et al. (117) have suggested that open-ended items to screen for symptomatic distress (e.g., depression), chronic stress (e.g., work-related problems), and somatic problems with possible psychological causes (e.g., sleep problems) be included in the review of systems during routine office visits. Cardiologists who start with open-ended questions about a patient's mood, stress at work or home, sleep problems, and energy level (117) can quickly determine whether patients perceive themselves to be in distress. Table 12.1 provides examples of questions that assess known psychosocial risk factors for heart disease.

Even patients who appear distressed but deny it can benefit when their physician normalizes and acknowledges their distress. Simple principles of motivational interviewing can be invaluable in this regard (118). *Motivational interviewing* is a style of communicating with patients designed to increase their belief that it is worthwhile to change a behavior or in this case, to seek help for psychosocial distress. If motivation is a problem, it must be dealt with first, before any behavior change programs can be effectively initiated (119). The physician is in the ideal position to build motivation to seek help for psychosocial problems. Questions that can also increase desire in patients to get relief from their distress include:

- Is it getting better on its own?
- Is this affecting other parts of your life?
- Have other people commented that you seem distressed?

TABLE 12.1

PSYCHOLOGICAL ASSESSMENT OF THE CARDIAC PATIENT

I. Chronic stressors
  A. Current employment: How stressful is your work?
  B. Social support
    1. Who lives at home?
    2. How is your relationship with (the relatives) at home?
    3. Sexual functioning: Are you happy with your sexual relationship?
    4. Do you have close friends or relatives who help you when you need it?
II. Symptoms of psychological distress
  a. Current treatment: Do you see a counselor or go to any support groups?
  b. Depression: How often do you feel sad or blue?
  c. Anxiety: How often do you feel nervous or uptight?
  d. Anger: How often do you feel frustrated or irritated?
III. Risk factors for cardiovascular disease
  A. Cigarette smoking/tobacco use
  B. Sedentary lifestyle
  C. Poor diet
  D. Nonadherence to medical regimen
  E. Drinking/drug use

Mood disturbances that worsen over time should be evaluated by a mental health professional. Cardiologists who encounter distressed patients should avoid offering too many solutions at once. Prioritizing the psychosocial needs and addressing the most important one first will avoid overwhelming the patient. Given the complexity of behavioral change, enlisting a multidisciplinary team is important for successful treatment, and the clinician is encouraged to either develop a structure of collaboration with mental health providers, or to rely on interdisciplinary cardiac rehabilitation programs for this effort. Figure 12.1 provides a simple algorithm to guide the clinician in determining what types of treatment might meet the psychosocial needs of their cardiac patients. Given the wide array of potential behavioral treatments that exist, the referral process can seem complex, but developing a relationship with at least one behavioral health specialist (e.g., psychologist or psychiatrist) can help in guiding the patient to the appropriate behavioral treatment.

Perhaps a second major controversy concerns the establishment of an evidence base for treating the psychosocial factors described in this chapter. Our review of the few trials conducted over the past 30 years shows their promise, particularly for stress (99,100) and hostility/anger reduction (95) treatments, while also revealing many of the treatment issues that factors such as depression give rise to (110,111). Phase III clinical trials can support this effort, testing stress management treatment with larger patient groups, and expanding the target populations to include those with arrhythmia (e.g., implantable cardioverter device) and congestive heart disease (congestive heart failure). These trials should also include ancillary studies designed to address questions concerning the pathways by which stress-related factors contribute to event-free survival. In addition to Phase III trials, smaller trials, perhaps with surrogate endpoints involving proposed pathophysiologic pathways, could help to disentangle issues concerning the treatment of depression in ACS patients, particularly with regard to the better identification of at-risk groups, the determination of treatment dose necessary to affect ACS-related endpoints, and the design and delivery of treatments acceptable to the patient group that does not self-identify as depressed. These factors will also be important for patients with congestive heart failure where depression can profoundly influence the disease trajectory (120). This research, although costly, must move forward, given the strength of factors such as depression in the prognostic equation. Cardiologists will play a crucial role in this effort, given their involvement in the care of the patient population and their experience in the conduct of clinical trials.

THE FUTURE

The integration of psychosocial risk identification and reduction into clinical pathways, the conduct of clinical trials to establish an evidence base for treatment, and the use of these trials to address questions concerning questions of pathophysiology

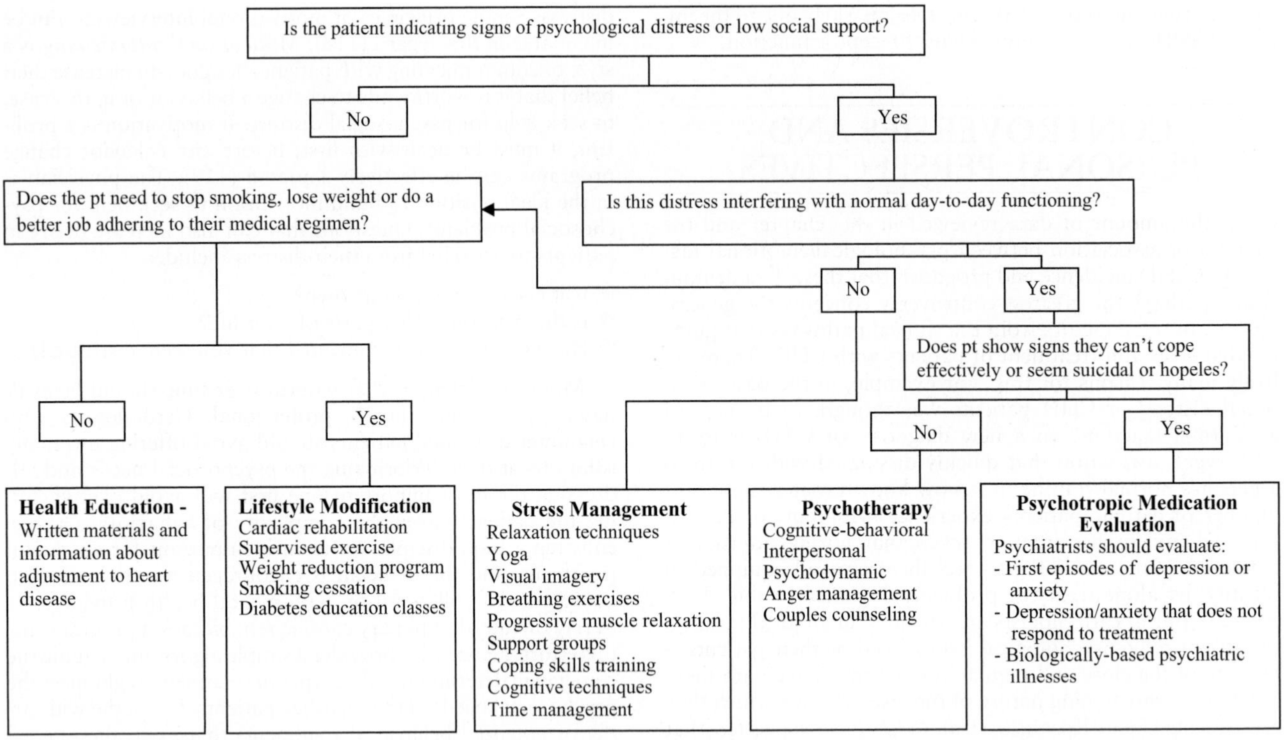

FIGURE 12.1. Screening and referral for psychosocial distress.

will all be part of the future research agenda. Research is also needed, however, to promote a greater understanding of the risk equation. For example, anecdotal evidence is rich with accounts of those who appear immune to the health effects of tobacco use. Similarly, not all people suffer the negative health consequences of stress, although many who appear depressed in the days after ACS quickly rebound to the previous level of functioning, and others experience personal growth as a function of their potentially catastrophic ACS experience.

Genetic susceptibility may play a role in these issues, lowering the threshold for the stress and associated factors to affect the cardiovascular system. For example, functional polymorphism (5-HTTLPR) of the serotonin transporter gene (*SLC6A4*) in cardiac patients has been examined (121) in a Japanese sample of 2,509 ACS patients, revealing that depressive symptoms were more common in carriers of the low-activity transporter polymorphism compared to noncarriers (48.3% versus 35%). Of note, 2-year cardiac events were also more common in carriers than noncarriers (31.3% versus 22.3%), but the effect became nonsignificant when depression was statistically controlled. Overall, these data suggest that the polymorphism 5-HTTLPR is associated with an increased risk for recurrent cardiac events that is mediated in part by depressive symptoms following AMI, demonstrating the complex interplay of genetic factors with susceptibility and risk.

Although much of this chapter has been devoted to the risks incurred by psychological distress, a new diagnosis of heart disease can also have a positive impact for some. Cardiac disease can precipitate emotional maturation by leading to a heightened awareness of mortality, greater clarity of personal values, and increased appreciation for important interpersonal relationships (122). An emerging research focus is on *resilience,* the ability of an individual to ostensibly "bounce back" and/or experience growth from difficult circumstances (123). A comparable emerging research focus is on positive psychology or those factors that contribute to enhanced survival and outcomes (124). These areas represent a potentially critical research focus for patients with CHD, because they will help to identify those intrapersonal factors that can be enhanced to improve medical outcomes, rather than only identifying those areas in need of remedy to forestall poorer outcomes.

References

1. DeBakey M, Gotto A. *The living heart.* New York: Charter Books, 1977.
2. Friedman M, Rosenman RH. Association of specific overt behavior pattern with blood and cardiovascular findings: blood cholesterol level, blood clotting time, incidence of arcus senilis, and clinical coronary artery disease. *JAMA* 1959;169:1286–1296.
3. Engel GL. Sudden and rapid death during psychological stress. *Ann Intern Med* 1971;74:771–782.
4. Reich P, DeSilva RA, Lown B, et al. Acute psychological disturbances preceding life-threatening ventricular arrhythmias. *JAMA* 1981;246:233–235.
5. Wittstein IS, Thiemann DR, Lima JA, et al. Neurohumoral features of myocardial stunning due to sudden emotional stress. *N Engl J Med* 2005; 352:539–548.
6. Leor J, Poole WK, Kloner RA. Sudden cardiac death triggered by an earthquake. *N Engl J Med* 1996;334:413–419.
7. Meisel SR, Kutz I, Dayan KI, et al. Effect of Iraqi missile war on incidence of acute myocardial infarction and sudden death in Israeli civilians. *Lancet* 1991;338:660–661.
8. Toivonen L, Helenius K, Viitasalo M. Electrocardiographic repolarization during stress from awakening on alarm call. *J Am Coll Cardiol* 1997; 30:774–779.
9. Steinberg JS, Arshad A, Kowalski M, et al. Increased incidence of life-threatening ventricular arrhythmias in implantable defibrillator patients after the World Trade Center attack. *J Am Coll Cardiol* 2004;44:1261–1264.
10. Shedd OL, Sears SF, Harvill JL, et al. The World Trade Center attack: increased frequency of defibrillator shocks for ventricular arrhythmias in patients living remotely from New York City. *J Am Coll Cardiol* 2004; 44:1265–1267.
11. Peters RW, McQuillan S, Resnick SK, et al. Increased Monday incidence of life-threatening ventricular arrhythmias. *Circulation* 1996;94:1346–1349.
12. Gabbay FH, Krantz DS, Kop WJ, et al. Triggers of myocardial ischemia during daily life in patients with coronary artery disease: physical and mental activities, anger and smoking. *J Am Coll Cardiol* 1996;27:585–592.

13. Gullette EC, Blumenthal JA, Babyak M, et al. Effects of mental stress on myocardial ischemia during daily life. *JAMA* 1997;277:1521–1526.
14. Burg MM, Jain D, Soufer R, et al. Role of behavioral and psychological factors in mental stress-induced silent left ventricular dysfunction in coronary artery disease. *J Am Coll Cardiol* 1993;22:440–448.
15. Jain D, Shaker SM, Burg M, et al. Effects of mental stress on left ventricular and peripheral vascular performance in patients with coronary artery disease. *J Am Coll Cardiol* 1998;31:1314–1322.
16. Rozanski A, Bairey CN, Krantz DS, et al. Mental stress and the induction of silent myocardial ischemia in patients with coronary artery disease. *N Engl J Med* 1988;318:1005–1012.
17. Jain D, Burg M, Soufer R, et al. Prognostic implications of mental stress-induced silent left ventricular dysfunction in patients with stable angina pectoris. *Am J Cardiol* 1995;76:31–35.
18. Jiang W, Babyak M, Krantz DS, et al. Mental stress—induced myocardial ischemia and cardiac events. *JAMA* 1996;275:1651–1656.
19. Krantz DS, Santiago HT, Kop WJ, et al. Prognostic value of mental stress testing in coronary artery disease. *Am J Cardiol* 1999;84:1292–1297.
20. Sheps DS, McMahon RP, Becker L, et al. Mental stress-induced ischemia and all-cause mortality in patients with coronary artery disease: results from the Psychophysiological Investigations of Myocardial Ischemia study. *Circulation* 2002;105:1780–1784.
21. Strike PC, Steptoe A. Behavioral and emotional triggers of acute coronary syndromes: a systematic review and critique. *Psychosom Med* 2005;67: 179–186.
22. Rafanelli C, Pancaldi LG, Ferranti G, et al. Stressful Life Events and Depressive Disorders as Risk Factors for Acute Coronary Heart Disease. *Ital Heart J Suppl* 2005;6:105–110.
23. Rosengren A, Hawken S, Ounpuu S, et al. Association of psychosocial risk factors with risk of acute myocardial infarction in 11,119 cases and 13,648 controls from 52 countries (the INTERHEART study): case-control study. *Lancet* 2004;364:953–962.
24. Peter R, Siegrist J. Psychosocial work environment and the risk of coronary heart disuse. *Int Arch Occup Environ Health* 2000;73:S41–S45.
25. Theorell T, Karasek RA. Current issues relating to psychosocial job strain and cardiovascular disease research. *J Occup Health Psychol* 1996;1:9–26.
26. Matthews KA, Gump BB. Chronic work stress and marital dissolution increase risk of posttrial mortality in men from the Multiple Risk Factor Intervention Trial. *Arch Intern Med* 2002;162:309–315.
27. Hammer N, Alfredsson L, Johnson JV. Job strain, social support at work, and incidence of myocardial infarction. *Occup Environ Med* 1998;55:548–553.
28. Smith TW, Ruiz JM. Psychosocial influences on the development and course of coronary heart disease: current status and implication for research and practice. *J Consult Clin Psychol* 2002;70:548–568.
29. Spielberger CD, Johnson EH, Russell SF, et al. The experience and expression of anger: construction and validation of an anger expression scale. In: Chesney MS, Rosenman RH, eds. *Anger and hostility in cardiovascular and behavioral disorders*. New York: McGraw-Hill,1985:5–30.
30. Rosenman RH, Brand RJ, Jenkins et al. Coronary heart disease in the Western Collaborative Group Study: final follow-up experience of 8 1/2 years. *JAMA* 1975;223:872–877.
31. Matthews KA, Glass DC, Rosenman RH, et al. Competitive drive, pattern A, and coronary heart disease: a further analysis of some data from the Western Collaborative Group Study. *J Chronic Dis* 1977;30:489–498.
32. Hecker MH, Chesney MA, Black GW, et al. Coronary-prone behaviors in the Western Collaborative Group Study. *Psychosom Med* 1988;50:153–164.
33. Koskenvuo M, Kaprio J, Rose RJ, et al. Hostility as a risk factor for mortality and ischemic heart disease in men. *Psychosom Med* 1988;50:330–340.
34. Goodman M, Quigley J, Moran G, et al. Hostility predicts restenosis after percutaneous transluminal coronary angioplasty. *Mayo Clinic Proc* 1996; 71:729–734.
35. Julkunen J, Salonen R, Kaplan GA, et al. Hostility and the progression of carotid atherosclerosis. *Psychosom Med* 1994;56:519–525.
36. Burg MM, Jain D, Soufer R, et al. Role of behavioral and psychological factors in mental stress induced silent left ventricular dysfunction in coronary artery disease. *J Am Coll Cardiol* 1993;22:440–448.
37. Helmers KF, Krant DS, Howell RH, et al. Hostility and myocardial ischemia in coronary artery disease patients: evaluation by gender and ischemic index. *Psychosom Med* 1993;55:29–36.
38. Mittleman MA, Maclure M, et al. Triggering of acute myocardial infarction onset by episodes of anger. *Circulation* 1995;92:1720–1725.
39. Ironson G, Taylor CB, Boltwood M, et al. Effects of anger on left ventricular ejection fraction in coronary artery disease. *Am J Cardiol* 1992;70:281–285.
40. Boltwood MD, Taylor CB, Burke MB, et al. Anger report predicts coronary artery vasomotor response to mental stress in atherosclerotic segments. *Am J Cardiol* 1993;72:1361–1365.
41. Carney RM, Rich MW, Freedland KE, et al. Major depressive disorder predicts cardiac events in patients with coronary artery disease. *Psychosom Med* 1988;50:627–633.
42. Frasure-Smith N, Lesperance F, Talajic M. Depression following myocardial infarction. Impact on 6-month survival. *JAMA* 1993;270:1819–1825.
43. Schleifer SJ, Macari-Hinson MM, Coyle DA, et al. The nature and course of depression following myocardial infarction. *Arch Intern Med* 1989;149:1785–1789.
44. Lesperance F, Frasure-Smith N, Talajic M. Major depression before and after myocardial infarction: its nature and consequences. *Psychosom Med* 1996;58:99–110.
45. Ford DE, Mead LA, Chang PP, et al. Depression is a risk factor for coronary artery disease in men: the precursors study. *Arch Intern Med* 1998; 158:1422–1426.
46. Barefoot JC, Schroll M. Symptoms of depression, acute myocardial infarction, and total mortality in a community sample. *Circulation* 1996;93:1976–1980.
47. Kawachi I, Sparrow D, Spiro IIIA, et al. A prospective study of anger and coronary artery disease. *Circulation* 1996;94:2090–2095.
48. Lesperance F, Frasure-Smith N, Talajic M, et al. Five-year risk of cardiac mortality in relation to initial severity and one-year changes in depression symptoms after myocardial infarction. *Circulation* 2002;105:1049–1033.
49. Frasure-Smith N, Lesperance F, Gravel G, et al. Social support, depression, and mortality during the first year after myocardial infarction. *Circulation* 2000;101:1919–1924.
50. Connerney I, Shapiro PA, McLaughlin JS, et al. In-hospital depression after CABG surgery predicts 12-month outcome. *Psychosom Med* 1999;62:106.
51. Burg MM, Benedetto CM, Rosenberg R, et al. Depression prior to CABG predicts 6-month and 2-year morbidity and mortality. *Psychosom Med* 2001;63:103.
52. Dusseldorp E, van Elderen T, Maes S, et al. A meta-analysis of psychoeducational programs for coronary heart disease patients. *Health Psychol* 1999;18:506–519.
53. Terry DJ. Stress, coping and coping resources as correlates of adaptation in myocardial infarction patients. *Br J Clin Psychol* 1992;31:215–225.
54. Mayou RA, Gill D, Thompson R, et al. Depression and anxiety as predictors of outcomes after myocardial infarction. *Psychosom Med* 2000; 62:212–219.
55. Fleet R, Lavoie K, Beitman BD. Is panic disorder associated with coronary artery disease? A critical review of the literature. *J Psychosom Res* 2000;48:347–356.
56. Carter CS, Servan-Schreiber D, Perlstein WM. Anxiety disorders and the syndrome of chest pain with normal coronary arteries: prevalence and pathophysiology. *J Clin Psychiatry* 1997;58[Suppl]:70–73.
57. Kubzansky LD, Kawachi I, Weiss ST, et al. Anxiety and coronary heart disease: a synthesis of epidemiological, psychological and experimental evidence. *Ann Behav Med* 1998;20:47–58.
58. Rozanzki A, Blumenthal JA, Kaplan J. Impact of psychological factors on the pathogenesis of cardiovascular disease and implications for therapy. *Circulation* 1999;99:2192–2217.
59. Moser DK, Dracup K. Is anxiety early after myocardial infarction associated with subsequent ischemic and arrhythmic events? *Psychosom Med* 1996;58:395–401.
60. Frasure-Smith N, Lesperance F, Talajic M. The impact of negative emotions on prognosis following myocardial infarction: is it more than just depression? *Health Psychol* 1995;14:388–398.
61. Denollet J, Sys SU, Brutsaert DL. Personality and mortality after myocardial infarction. *Psychosom Med* 1995;57:582–591.
62. Ruberman W, Weinblatt E, Goldberg JD, et al. Psychosocial influences on mortality after myocardial infarction. *N Engl J Med* 1984;311:552–559.
63. Berkman LF, Leo-Summers L, Horwitz RI. Emotional support and survival following myocardial infarction: a prospective population-based study of the elderly. *Ann Intern Med* 1992;117:1003–1009.
64. Case RB, Moss AJ, Case N, et al. Living alone after myocardial infarction. *JAMA* 1992;267:520–524.
65. Farmer I, Meyer PS, Ramsey DJ, et al. Higher levels of social support predict greater survival following acute myocardial infarction: the Corpus Christi Heart Project. *Behav Med* 1996;22:59–66.
66. Williams RB, Barefoot JC, Califf RM, et al. Prognostic importance of social and economic resources among medically treated patients with angiographically documented coronary artery disease. *JAMA* 1992;267:520–524.
67. Brummett BH, Barefoot JC, Siegler IC, et al. Characteristics of socially isolated patients with coronary artery disease who are at elevated risk for mortality. *Psychosom Med* 2001;63:267–272.
68. Oxman TE, Freeman DH, Manheimer ED. Lack of social participation or religious strength and comfort as risk factors for death after cardiac surgery in the elderly. *Psychosom Med* 1995;57:5–15.
69. Orth-Gomér K, Undén AL, Edwards ME. Social isolation and mortality in ischemic heart disease: a 10-year follow-up study of 150 middle-aged men. *Acta Med Scand* 1988;224:205–215.
70. Welin C, Lappas G, Wilhelmsen L. Independent importance of psychosocial factors for prognosis after myocardial infarction. *J Intern Med* 2000;247:629–639.
71. House JS. Social isolation kills, but how and why? *Psychosom Med* 2001;63:273–274.
72. Carney RM, Freedland KE, Stein PK, et al. Change in heart rate and heart rate variability during treatment for depression in patients with coronary heart disease. *Psychosom Med* 2000;62:639–647.
73. Carney RM, Rich MW, TeVelde A, et al. The relationship between heart rate, heart rate variability and depression in patients with coronary artery disease. *J Psychosom Res* 1988;32:159–164.

74. Dallack GW Roose SP. Perspectives of the relationship between cardiovascular disease and affective disorder. *J Clin Psychiatry* 1990;51:4–9.
75. Lahmeyer HW, Bellier SN. Cardiac regulation and depression. *J Psychiatr Res* 1987;21:1–6.
76. Rechlin T. Are affective disorders associated with alterations of heart rate variability? *J Affect Disord* 1994;32:271–275.
77. Roy A, Pickar D, De Jong J, et al. Norepinephrine and its metabolites in cerebrospinal fluid, plasma, and urine. Relationship to hypothalamic-pituitary-adrenal axis function in depression. *Arch Gen Psychiatry* 1988; 45:849–857.
78. Siever L, Davis K. Overview: toward a dysregulation hypothesis of depression. *Am J Psychiatry* 1985;142:1017–1031.
79. Lerman Y, Melamed S, Shragin Y, et al. Association between burnout at work and leukocyte adhesiveness/aggregation. *Psychosom Med* 1999; 61:828–833.
80. Maes M, Stevens WJ, Declerck LS, et al. Significantly increased expression of T-cell activation markers in depression: further evidence for an inflammatory process during that illness. *Prog Neuropsychopharmacol Biol Psychiatry* 1993;17:241–255.
81. Maes M, Van der Planken M, Stevens WJ, et al. Leukocytosis, monocytosis, and neutrophilia: hallmarks of severe depression. *J Psychiatr Res* 1992; 26:125–134.
82. Kop W, Cohen N. Psychological risk factors and immune system involvement in cardiovascular disease. In: Ader R, Felton DL, Cohen N, eds. *Psychoneuroimmunology*, 3rd ed. San Diego: Academic Press, 2000.
83. Ross R. Atherosclerosis—an inflammatory disease. *N Engl J Med* 1999; 340:115–126.
84. von Kanel R, Mills PJ, Fainman C, et al. Effects of psychological stress and psychiatric disorders on blood coagulation and fibrinolysis: a biobehavioral pathway to coronary artery disease? *Psychosom Med* 2001;63:531–544.
85. Keefe FJ, Castell PJ, Blumenthal JA. Angina pectoris in type A and type B cardiac patients. *Pain* 1986;27:211–218.
86. Thoresen CE, Powell LH. Type A behavior pattern: new perspectives on theory, assessment, and intervention. *J Consult Clin Psychol* 1992;60:595–604.
87. Ziegelstein RC, Fauerbach JA, Stevens SS, et al. Patients with depression are less likely to follow recommendations to reduce cardiac risk during recovery from a myocardial infarction. *Arch Intern Med* 2000;160:1818–1823.
88. Carney RM, Freedland KE, Rich MW, et al. Depression as a risk factor for cardiac events in established coronary heart disease: a review of possible mechanisms. *Annals of Behav Med* 1995;17:2–149.
89. Katon W, Berg AO, Robins AJ, et al. Depression-medical utilization and somatization. *West J Med* 1986: 564–568.
90. Williams RB, Barefoot JC, Schneiderman N. Psychosocial risk factors for cardiovascular disease: more than one culprit at work. *JAMA* 2003; 290:2190–2192.
91. Lane D, Carroll D, Lip GY. Psychology in coronary care. *QJM* 1999; 92:425–431.
92. Linden W, Stossel C, Maurice J. Psychosocial interventions for patients with coronary artery disease: a meta analysis. *Arch Intern Med* 1996;156: 745–752.
93. Sotile Wm. *Psychosocial interventions for cardiopulmonary patients.* Champaign, IL: Human Kinetics Press, 1996.
94. Cooper AF, Jackson G, Weinman J, et al. Factors associated with cardiac rehabilitation attendance: a systematic review of the literature. *Clin Rehabil* 2002;16:541–552.
95. Friedman M, Thoresen CE, Gill J, et al. Alteration of type A behavior and its effect on cardiac recurrences in post-myocardial infarction patients: summary results of the recurrent coronary prevention project. *Am Heart J* 1986;112:653–665.
96. Gidron Y, Davidson K, Bata I. The short-term effects of a hostility-reduction intervention on male coronary artery disease patients. *Health Psychol* 1999;18:416–420.
97. Frasure-Smith N, Prince R. The ischemic heart disease life stress monitoring program: impact on mortality. *Psychsom Med* 1985;47:431–445.
98. Frasure-Smith N, Prince R. Long-term follow-up of the ischemic heart disease life stress monitoring program. *Psychosom Med* 1989;51:485–513.
99. Blumenthal JA, Sherwood A, Babyak MA, et al. Effects of exercise and stress management training on markers of cardiovascular risk in patients with ischemic heart disease: a randomized controlled trial. *JAMA* 2005;293:1626–1634.
100. Blumenthal JA, Wei J, Babyak MA, et al. Stress management and exercise training in cardiac patients with myocardial ischemia. *Arch Intern Med* 1997;157:2213–2223.
101. Dougherty CM, Pyper GP, Frasz HA. Description of a nursing intervention program after an implantable cardioverter defibrillator. *Heart Lung* 2004;33:183–190.
102. Dougherty CM, Lewis FM, Thompson EA, et al. Short-term efficacy of a telephone intervention by expert nurses after an implantable cardioverter defibrillator. *Pacing Clin Electrophysiol* 2004;27:1594–1602.
103. Frizelle DJ, Lewin RJP, Kaye G, et al. Cognitive-behavioural rehabilitation programme for patients with an implanted cardioverter-defibrillator: a pilot study. *Br J Health Psychol* 2004;9:381–392.
104. Kohn CS, Petrucci RJ, Baessler C, et al. The effect of psychological intervention on patients' long-term adjustment to the ICD: a prospective study. *Pacing Clin Electrophysiol* 2000;23:450–456.
105. Jones DA, West RR. Psychological rehabilitation after myocardial infarction: multicentre randomized controlled trial. *BMJ* 1996;314:1517–1521.
106. Linden W. Psychological treatments in cardiac rehabilitation: a review of rationales and outcomes. *J Psychosom Res* 2000: 48;443–454.
107. Rees K, Bennett P, West R, et al. Psychological interventions for coronary heart disease. *Cochrane Database Syst Rev* 2004;2:CD002902. DOI:10.1002/14651858.CD002902.pub2
108. Fraser-Smith N, Lesperance F, Prince RH, et al. Randomised trial of home-based psychosocial nursing intervention for patients recovering from myocardial infarction. *Lancet* 1997;350:473–479.
109. Cossette S, Fraser-Smith N, Lesperance F. Impact of improving psychological distress in post-MI patients. *Psychosom Med* 1990: 61:93.
110. ENRICHD Investigators. Enhancing Recovery in Coronary Heart Disease (ENRICHD) study intervention: rationale and design. *Psychosom Med* 2001;63:747–755.
111. ENRICHD Investigators. Effects of treating depression and low perceived social support on clinical events after myocardial infarction: the Enhancing Recovery in Coronary Heart Disease Patients (ENRICHD) Randomized Trial. *JAMA* 2003;28:3106–3116.
112. Carney R, Blumentahl J, Freedland KE, et al. Depression and late mortality after myocardial infarction in the Enhancing Recovery in Coronary Heart Disease (ENRICHD) Study. *Psychosom Med* 2004;66:466–474.
113. Glassman AH, Roose SP, Bigger JT. The safety of tricyclic antidepressants in cardiac patients. Risk-benefit reconsidered. *JAMA* 1993;269:2673–2675.
114. Cohen HW, Gibson G, Alderman MH. Excess risk of myocardial infarction in patients treated with antidepressant medications: association with use of tricyclic agents. *Am J Med* 2000;108:87–88.
115. Glassman AH, O'Connor CM, Califf RM, et al. Sertraline Antidepressant Heart Attack Randomized Trial (SADHART) Group. Sertraline treatment of major depression in patients with acute MI or unstable angina. *JAMA* 2002;288:701–709.
116. Taylor CB, Youngblood ME, Catellier D, et al., for the ENRICHD Investigators. Effects of antidepressant medication on morbidity and mortality in depressed post-MI patients. *Arch Gen Psychiatry* 2005;62:792–798.
117. Rozanski A, Blumenthal JA, Davidson KW, et al. The epidemiology, pathophysiology, and management of psychosocial risk factors in cardiac practice: the emerging field of behavioral cardiology. *J Am Coll Cardiol* 2005;45:637–651.
118. Miller WR, Rollnick S. *Motivational Interviewing: preparing people to change addictive behavior*. New York: The Guilford Press, 1991.
119. Rollnick S, Heather N, Bell A. Negotiating behaviour change in medical settings: the development of brief motivational interviewing. *J Mental Health* 1992;1:25–37.
120. Parissis JT, Fountoulaki K, Paraskevaidis I, et al. Depression in chronic heart failure: novel pathophysiological mechanisms and therapeutic approaches. *Expert Opin Investig Drugs* 2005;14:567–577.
121. Nakatani D, Sato H, Sakata Y, et al. Influence of serotonin transporter gene polymorphism on depressive symptoms and new cardiac events after acute myocardial infarction. *Am Heart J* 2004;150:652–658.
122. Dornelas EA, Thompson PD. Perspectives from health psychology: psychodynamic treatment for cardiac patients. In: Magnavita JJ, ed. *Comprehensive handbook of psychotherapy.* Vol. 1 : *Psychodynamic/object relations.* New York: John Wiley & Sons, Inc., 2002: 549–564.
123. Kelley TM. Natural resilience and innate mental health. *Am Psychol* 2005;60;265–267.
124. Seligman ME, Steen TA, Park N, et al. Positive psychology progress: empirical validation of interventions. *Am Psychol* 2005;60:410–421.

CHAPTER 13 ■ CARDIAC REHABILITATION AND SECONDARY PREVENTION

PHILIP A. ADES AND RAINER HAMBRECHT

BACKGROUND

> Cardiac rehabilitation is a multifactorial process that includes exercise training, education and behavioral counseling regarding risk reduction and lifestyle changes. These services should be integrated into the comprehensive care of cardiac patients. (1)

Cardiac rehabilitation–lifestyle therapy for coronary heart disease (CHD) is fundamentally different from other well-established pharmacologic, interventional, or surgical therapies: It does not rely on a single pathogenic mechanism for intervention, it is not a "single-bullet" treatment, and requires the ongoing cooperation and participation of the patient. These characteristics are not signs of an ill-defined polypragmatic approach without a sound scientific basis, but rather are deeply rooted in the chronic multifactorial disease process that drives the progression of atherosclerosis. The risk factor concept of atherogenesis derived from population-based studies such as The Framingham Study (2) has greatly advanced our understanding of the determining environmental and behavioral factors. Many of the mechanisms that mediate the adverse cardiovascular effects of physical inactivity are still unknown. Nonetheless, the epidemiologic link between lack of physical activity and/or diminished fitness and increased risk for CHD is clear and well proven (3).

Cardiac rehabilitation is a therapeutic approach based on epidemiologic and pathophysiologic mechanisms, which is aimed at modifying the atherogenic disease process on the individual level. Although some approach the area of cardiac rehabilitation with skepticism and consider it inferior to "high-tech" interventions, the ultimate goal of medical care continues to be to prolong and improve quality of life. Using prognostic impact as a measure of therapeutic efficacy, cardiac rehabilitation is by no means inferior to conventional pharmacologic or interventional care. For example, it was recently demonstrated that cardiac rehabilitation with a 12-month outpatient exercise training program is superior to percutaneous coronary interventions regarding the prevention of subsequent cardiovascular events and improvement of exercise tolerance (4). The mortality reduction in stable CHD achieved by exercise-based rehabilitation is 27%, which is comparable to the effects of our most potent drugs such as β-blocking agents, lipid-lowering drugs, and angiotensin converting enzyme inhibitors (5). Furthermore, an invasive interventional approach in the nonacute setting is severely handicapped by the fact that you only treat the most advanced coronary lesions but are unable to modify overall disease progression of what is, in essence, a diffuse metabolic disease. Exercise-based rehabilitation, on the other hand, embraces the concept that it is most often not the highest grade stenoses that initiate an acute coronary event but rather a ruptured plaque in a less severe obstruction that is the culprit. Comprehensive cardiac rehabilitation aims at influencing all determinants of the atherosclerotic disease process.

Comprehensive cardiac rehabilitation services include medical evaluation, prescribed exercise, cardiac risk factor modification, and lifestyle counseling. The clinical implementation of cardiac rehabilitation is frequently linked to a structured "secondary prevention center," with on-site and home-based exercise programs, lipid clinics, weight loss programs, and other risk factor modification components aimed at preventing second coronary events, cardiac rehospitalizations, and cardiac disability in patients with established CHD (6,7). Services are tied to a series of short-term and longer term outcomes, which include return to work and measures of physical functioning, cardiac symptoms, psychological well-being, risk factors, progression of coronary atherosclerosis, recurrence of cardiac events, and number of rehospitalizations. Cardiac rehabilitation is prescribed for patients after myocardial infarction (MI), coronary bypass surgery, or after percutaneous coronary interventions, in addition to patients with chronic angina pectoris, chronic heart failure, or heart transplantation and finally for selected patients after valvular heart surgery or exertional arrhythmias (1,8). Debate is ongoing as to whether early outpatient exercise training requires direct supervision or whether it could effectively be more widely applied, for low- and moderate-risk patients, in the home setting (9–12). The clinical application of training therapy in coronary artery disease (CAD) and chronic heart failure patients is detailed in Table 13.1.

Cardiac rehabilitation is highly cost effective and is associated with a decrease in cardiac hospitalizations (13–16). The cardiac rehabilitation facility should be viewed as the clinical site at which systematic secondary prevention services are delivered in an outpatient setting in collaboration with the primary physician. Maintaining physical functioning, preventing coronary disability, and preventing recurrent coronary events are the primary outcome goals.

THE EVOLUTION OF MODERN CARDIAC REHABILITATION AND SECONDARY PREVENTION

Historical Background: Evolution From Symptomatic to Prognostic Intervention

Cardiac rehabilitation was conceived in an era when post-MI activity prescriptions were evolving from 6 weeks of bed rest in the 1930s, to "chair" therapy in the 1940s, to 3 to 5 minutes of walking per day at 4 weeks in the 1950s (17–19). By the early 1960s, clinicians recognized that early ambulation helped patients to avoid many of the complications of bed rest, such as pulmonary embolism and deconditioning, and in-hospital ambulation gradually displaced long-term bed rest as the standard of care (20–22). As the ambulation process extended beyond hospital discharge, concerns about the safety of unsupervised exercise resulted in the development of highly structured, physician-supervised, electrocardiographically monitored exercise programs in the 1970s. The focus was almost exclusively on exercise and on the physical recovery process. By the 1990s, hospitalizations for acute MI shortened and are now as brief as 3 to 4 days (23), such that deconditioning is minimal. However, also minimized is the ability to counsel patients about risk factor modification. Smoking relapse prevention programs, initiated in hospital, have proven effective (24), but therapy and education for other modifiable risk factors are largely left for the postdischarge period.

With the development of a body of literature supporting the benefits of risk factor modification in coronary patients (called *secondary prevention*), the cardiac rehabilitation center has evolved to become a clinical site for the systematic delivery of secondary prevention services. Recently demonstrated benefits of cardiac rehabilitation and secondary prevention in coronary patients are broad and compelling. A recent meta-analysis of patients participating in exercise-based rehabilitation programs following an acute MI documented a significant 27% reduction of total mortality among training patients and a 31% reduction in cardiac mortality, confirming earlier work (5,25,26). A recent report from Olmstead county in Minnesota provides encouraging and interesting observations in a "real world" setting (27). These investigators identified 1821 patients with MI discharged from the hospital alive between 1982 and 1998 and 55% of patients participated in cardiac rehabilitation, defined conservatively as attendance at a single visit. Three-year survival was 95% in participants and 64% in nonparticipants. This survival benefit was maintained after adjusting for propensity to participate in cardiac rehabilitation with an overall 56% reduction in mortality, which was similar across age and gender subgroups. Participation in cardiac rehabilitation was further associated with a 28% reduction

TABLE 13.1

INDICATIONS, EXERCISE PRESCRIPTION, AND EXPECTED OUTCOMES FOR EXERCISE-BASED CARDIAC REHABILITATION IN SELECTED PATIENT POPULATIONS

CORONARY HEART DISEASE

Indications
- Stable CHD
- Post-MI
- Post-cardiac revascularization procedure (surgical or percutaneous)

Contraindications
- Acute MI <7 days
- Unstable angina or arrhythmias
- Decompensated congestive heart failure
- Uncontrolled hypertension
- Acute myocarditis or pericarditis
- Symptomatic aortic stenosis or hypertrophic cardiomyopathy
- Acute systemic illness

Suggested Exercise Program
- Endurance exercise training at 60–70% of maximal exercise capacity or 70–85% maximal heart rate
- Resistance training, particularly for older patients, women, physical occupations

Expected Clinical Outcome
- 27% reduction in total mortality
- 31% reduction in cardiac mortality
- Increases in symptom-free exercise tolerance

Adverse Event Risk
- 1 cardiac arrest per 112.000 patient training hours
- 1 MI per 294.000 patient training hours
- 1 cardiac death per 784.000 patient training hours

CHRONIC HEART FAILURE

Indications
- Stable chronic heart failure (NYHA I-III)

Contraindications
- Decompensated congestive heart failure within the last 3 months
- Acute MI <7 days
- Unstable angina or high-risk arrhythmias
- Uncontrolled hypertension
- Acute myocarditis or pericarditis
- Symptomatic aortic stenosis or hypertrophic cardiomyopathy
- Acute systemic illness
- (N.B. Implantable Cardioverter Defibrillators are not a contraindication for exercise training)

Suggested Exercise Program
- Endurance exercise training at 50%–70% of maximal exercise capacity or 70–85% maximal heart rate
- Start low (40%–50% of V_{O_2} max) for short training intervals (10 minutes)
- Increase first training duration, then workload.
- Consider resistance training

Expected Clinical Outcome
- Reduction of total mortality by 35% (odds ratio 0.65; CI 0.46–0.92, $P = .015$)
- Reduction of hospitalization by 28% (odds ratio 0.72; CI 0.56–0.93, $P = .018$)
- Increase in symptom-free exercise tolerance by 12%–31%

Adverse Event Risk
- Minimal risk of cardiac decompensation
- Cardiac arrhythmias
- Increased risk of cardiac death among chronic heart failure training patients is not established

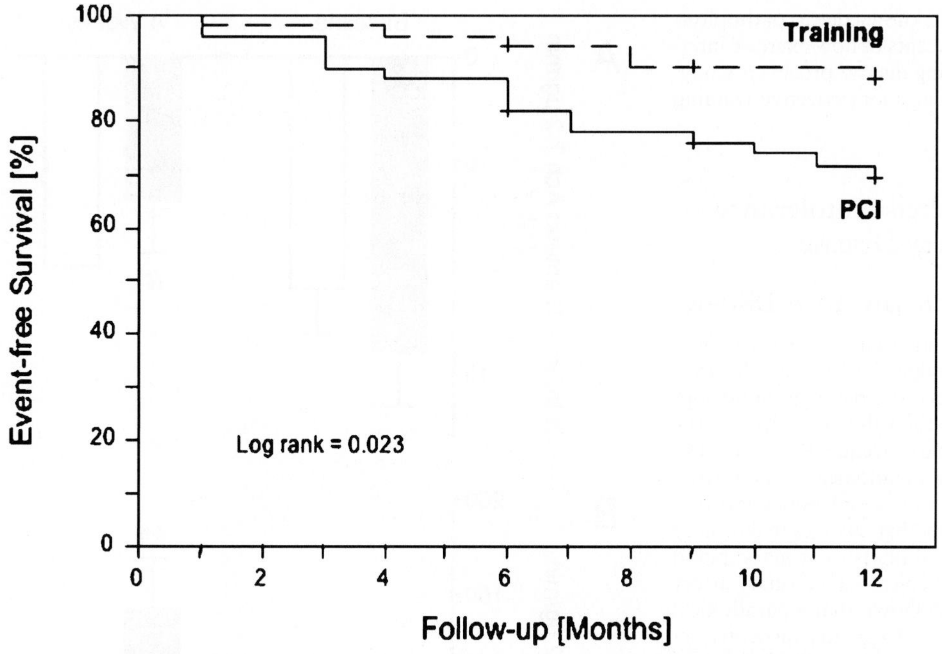

FIGURE 13.1. Kaplan-Meier survival curve of patients with stable coronary artery disease randomized to either interventional treatment (PCI) or aerobic endurance exercise training (Training) over 12 months. Training was associated with a significantly lower rate of major cardiovascular events (death, MI, stroke, hospitalization for worsening angina, need for revascularization) as compared to conventional PCI. Reprinted with permission (4).

in recurrent MI. Interestingly, the benefits of cardiac rehabilitation were more pronounced in recent years, coincident with greater participation of elderly, women, and patients with more medical comorbidities.

The therapeutic benefit of regular physical exercise has also been confirmed in direct comparison with an interventional strategy: 12 months of exercise therapy in stable CAD patients was associated with a higher event-free survival and an increased exercise capacity than a percutaneous coronary intervention (Fig. 13.1) (4). Furthermore, the combination of exercise and low-fat diets has been documented to slow the atherogenic process (28,29), and studies that incorporated multiple risk factor interventions (9), pharmacologic lipid lowering, or both, demonstrated a decrease in coronary events and a retardation of atherosclerosis (30).

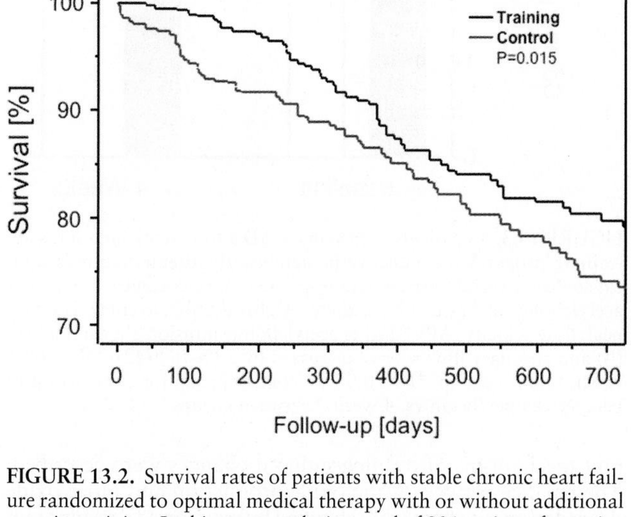

FIGURE 13.2. Survival rates of patients with stable chronic heart failure randomized to optimal medical therapy with or without additional exercise training. In this meta-analysis a total of 801 patients from nine independent prospective randomized clinical trials were included. Over a follow-up period of 705 days training was associated with a 35% reduction of all-cause mortality. Reprinted with permission (31).

Over the past two decades, rehabilitation programs have been extended into new diagnostic categories beyond standard post-MI treatment. In stable chronic heart failure, physical activity was traditionally discouraged, with negative physiologic consequences for the patients. Exercise intolerance worsened and the progression of disease-related muscular atrophy accelerated. However, carefully designed exercise programs with an intensity of 50% to 70% of maximal oxygen uptake or 70% to 85% of maximal heart rate, have proven to be effective in increasing exercise capacity by approximately 20%. As confirmed by a recent meta-analysis, exercise therapy reduces the relative risk of chronic heart failure mortality by 35% and chronic heart failure–related hospitalizations by 28% (Fig. 13.2) (31).

The general focus of cardiac rehabilitation today is no longer just to limit the devastating physical and mental consequences of a serious cardiovascular event, but to prevent future cardiac events by combining individually tailored exercise programs with chronic disease management skills as a long-term intervention. In the context of this process, exercise training is offered to most patients with chronic stable cardiovascular diseases including CHD, chronic heart failure, valvular heart disease, congenital heart disease, peripheral vascular occlusive disease, and after cardiac transplantation. Despite well-described benefits, fewer than 15% of patients who might benefit currently participate in formal cardiac rehabilitation, due in part to a lack of geographically available programs (32,33).

SCIENTIFIC FOUNDATION OF CARDIAC REHABILITATION AND SECONDARY PREVENTION

As the primary goal of cardiac rehabilitation interventions has changed from regaining muscle strength to modification of atherosclerotic progression and improving prognosis, studies of exercise or comprehensive interventions have focused on mechanistic as well as symptomatic outcomes. This development shifted the scientific basis of rehabilitation interventions in many patient groups, most notably in CHD and chronic heart failure patients, from empirical knowledge to pathophysiologic evidence. The molecular concepts of how exercise interventions interfere with the underlying disease process are now providing a new basis for developing more effective training programs.

Pathophysiology of Exercise Intolerance in Coronary Artery Disease

The Exercise Limitation in Coronary Artery Disease

Traditionally, coronary stenoses were regarded as static flow obstructions leading to exercise-induced ischemia whenever myocardial oxygen demand exceeded the regional blood supply. Although this mechanism is still valid to a degree, the pathogenesis of myocardial ischemia is frequently more complex. From the first description of a paradoxical vasoconstriction of atherosclerotic segments during acetylcholine infusion into coronary arteries (34), we know that changes in coronary endothelial function can critically diminish coronary blood flow even in patients with moderate epicardial coronary artery stenoses (50% to 70%). It has been shown that a paradoxical response to acetylcholine is indicative of a greater vasoconstrictive effect to both endogenous and exogenous catecholamines (35). Sympathetic activation and consecutive release of catecholamines occurs during physical activity, exposure to cold, or mental stress. In all these contexts, paradoxical epicardial coronary vasoconstriction has been described (36–38), which makes endothelial dysfunction a likely pathomechanism to explain stress- or exercise-induced angina pectoris in stable CAD (39).

Cardiovascular Effects of Exercise in Coronary Artery Disease

The first era of mechanistic rehabilitation research started in the late 1980s and assessed the effects of aggressive lifestyle interventions including exercise on the progression of coronary atherosclerosis. Studies evaluating the *regression hypothesis* used quantitative coronary angiography to quantify changes in target lesion diameter.

Three major studies—the *Lifestyle Heart Trial* (29), the *Stanford Coronary Risk Intervention Project* (SCRIP) (9), and the *Heidelberg Regression Study* (28)—confirmed that comprehensive lifestyle changes including a low-fat diet and/or lipid-lowering medication and exercise training were effective in slowing or slightly reversing the progression of coronary atherosclerosis and in reducing the cardiac adverse event rate. However, only a minority of trained patients actually had a significant regression in minimal stenosis diameter, those who exercised more than 5 to 6 hours of per week (>2500 kcal/week) (40). In contrast, myocardial perfusion was improved and coronary event rate was reduced out of proportion to the minimal angiographic regression noted (41).

With the observation of the importance of endothelial function came an awareness that the luminal diameter of epicardial vessels is highly dynamic in response to mechanical (flow-related) or agonist-mediated (endogenous or pharmacologic) stimuli. Hence, a new era of research assessed the effects of endurance training on coronary endothelial function. Hambrecht and colleagues (42) documented a significant improvement in coronary endothelial function in patients with stable CAD after only 4 weeks of high-intensity exercise training (60 minutes at 70% of Vo_2 max/d) (Fig. 13.3). In two consecutive studies of moderate exercise training in patients awaiting coronary bypass grafting surgery, where intraoperative harvesting of left internal mammary artery samples was possible, two important mechanisms of training-induced changes were described: The balance between nitric oxide production and nitric oxide degradation was favorably changed by training as a result of increased vascular extracellular nitric oxide synthase expression and activity and reduced generation of reactive oxygen species

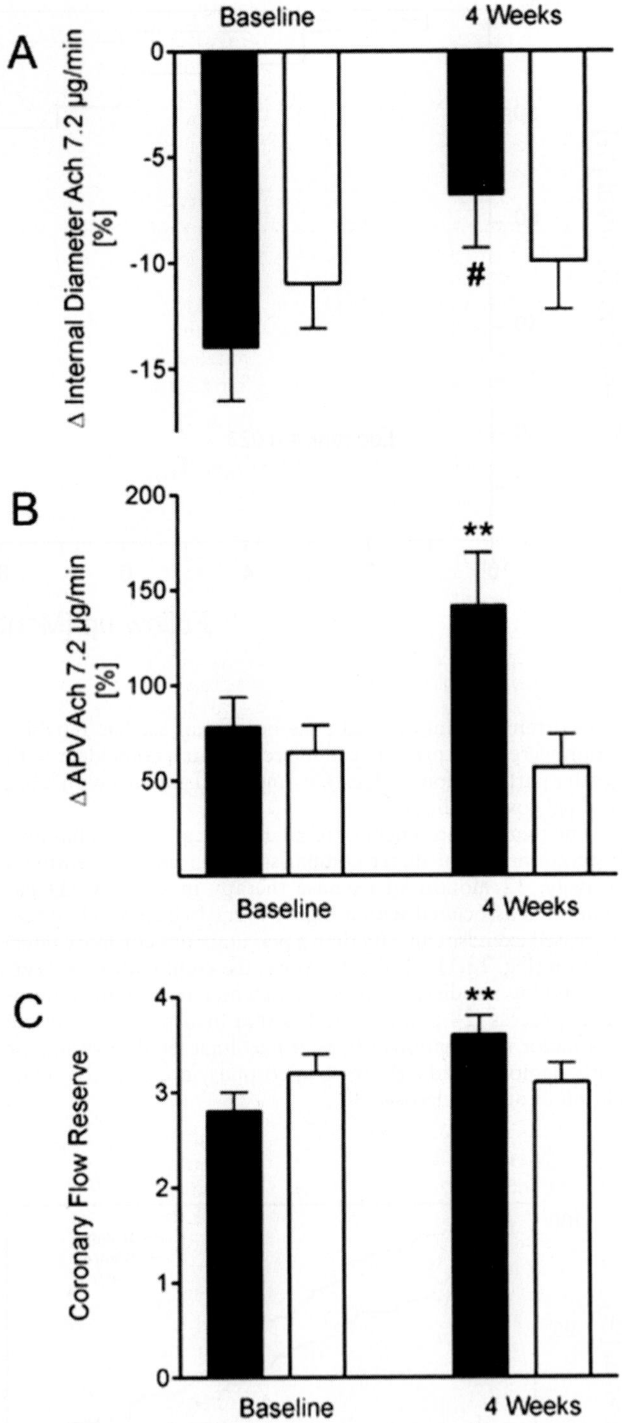

FIGURE 13.3. In patients with stable CAD a four-week high-intensity training program was effective in significantly attenuating paradoxical coronary vasoconstriction in response to intracoronary infusion of acetylcholine at a rate of 7.2 μg/min (A). In addition, average coronary peak flow velocity (APV) during acetylcholine infusion almost doubled (B) and coronary flow reserve increased by 29% (C) (42). $^{**}P < 0.01$ versus control group. $^{\#}P < 0.05$ vs. control group for comparison of percent change (begin vs. 4 weeks) between groups.

produced by vascular NAD(P)H oxidases (43,44). In addition, animal experiments indicate improved vascular antioxidative protection by elevated extracellular superoxide dismutase activity after training (45). The significance of these data is underscored by long-term follow-up studies, which confirmed the predictive value of endothelial dysfunction for future cardiovascular events (46,47).

Recently, yet another potential mechanism of training-induced improvement of myocardial perfusion has been identified: Contrary to previous concepts, postnatal vasculogenesis has been confirmed in humans, which is initiated by pluripotent bone marrow–derived circulating endothelial progenitor cells (EPCs) (48). Training increases the number of circulating EPCs and may thereby improve endothelial regeneration and collateral formation into ischemic tissue areas (49,50).

Pathophysiology of Exercise Intolerance in Chronic Heart Failure

Exercise Intolerance in Chronic Heart Failure

It was originally hypothesized that exercise intolerance in chronic heart failure occurred as a direct consequence of insufficient adaptation of cardiac output to the increased demands during physical exertion and that any extra workload placed on the diseased myocardium would inevitably lead to further deterioration of left ventricular function. However, exercise studies in chronic heart failure patients documented a complete lack of correlation between the left ventricular ejection fraction and exercise capacity (51).

If central hemodynamics are not the principal determining factor of exercise capacity, what other factors should be considered? The first focus of interest was on systemic neurohumeral alterations—a concept of chronic heart failure evolving as a clinical process that was initiated by myocardial dysfunction but which then affected virtually any organ system as a consequence of neurohormonal activation (52,53). This pathophysiologic model of chronic heart failure is still valid today and has been extended by demonstration of significant immune activation and inflammation in chronic heart failure (54,55).

Building on this model, peripheral changes associated with neurohumoral and inflammatory activation have been systematically analyzed in the last decade. Characteristic changes of endothelial function, respiration, and skeletal muscle function have been found. Today it is well-established that chronic heart failure causes a peripheral hypoperfusion owing to impaired endothelium-dependent vasodilation (56) leading to cytokine activation (57), a reduction in the strength of respiratory muscles (58), and profound morphologic (59,60), metabolic (61,62), and functional alterations in skeletal muscle (63). In the course of these scientific advances, peripheral changes have become a new therapeutic target (Fig. 13.4).

Effects of Exercise

With regard to symptomatic benefit after exercise training in chronic heart failure, a recent meta-analysis of randomized controlled trials by the European Heart Failure Training Group revealed an improvement of peak Vo_2 by up to 2 mL/kg·min^{-1} with a range of +14% to +31% increase versus control patients (64). Although modest in absolute terms this increase of about 20% translates into a considerably better quality of life for most patients. Cardiac function is not worsened by exercise training; rather, there was a small but significant improvement of ejection fraction and a reduction in cardiomegaly (65). Exercise training is a nonspecific intervention that affects several functional systems in chronic heart failure patients, namely, vascular endothelial function, central hemodynamics, neurohumoral activation, the respiratory system, and skeletal muscle metabolism and function.

Endothelium-dependent vasodilation, especially during exercise, is significantly improved by endurance training in chronic heart failure patients (66,67), which contributes to a reduced cardiac afterload and enhanced skeletal muscle perfusion. *Cardiac function* is enhanced, most likely as a consequence of afterload reduction after a 6-month training program (Fig. 13.5) (65). Apart from systolic function, clinical studies indicate an improved left ventricular early diastolic filling following exercise interventions in chronic heart failure subgroups with relaxation abnormalities (68).

Neurohumoral activation as indicated by circulating levels of angiotensin II, aldosterone, and atrial natriuretic peptide was reduced by 25% to 32% after long-term exercise training (69). The activity and strength of *inspiratory muscles* is decreased in chronic heart failure patients contributing to a reduction of the key clinical symptom of exercise-induced dyspnea. Both systemic exercise training and selective respiratory muscle training improve ventilation dynamics and exercise performance (58).

Skeletal muscle morphology, metabolism, and function are significantly altered in chronic heart failure. These changes are not just a consequence of deconditioning but represent intrinsic changes induced by systemic neurohumoral and inflammatory responses in chronic heart failure. All aspects of skeletal muscle characteristics can be positively influenced by training: On the ultrastructural level, the volume density of cytochrome C–positive mitochondria is increased permitting an enhanced oxidative phosphorylation. In addition to metabolic improvements, recent studies indicate that training has the potential to reverse the inflammatory activation with increased expression of cytokines like tumor necrosis factor-α (TNF-α), interleukin (IL)-1β, and IL-6 in the skeletal muscle (57). It is hoped that these changes might also attenuate the proapoptotic environment with reduced IGF-I in the skeletal muscle (70,71).

Clinical Application of Exercise Training

In light of the multiple beneficial effects of exercise in chronic heart failure, training programs are recommended by current guidelines on chronic heart failure treatment. Both the American Heart Association and the European Society of Cardiology agree that exercise programs should be encouraged in stable NYHA class II and III patients (72–74). Clinical stability is defined by stable symptoms, absence of resting symptoms and postural hypotension, stable fluid balance (need of an increase in diuretic dosage no more than once a week), freedom from evidence of congestion, stable renal function (creatinine level), and normal or near-normal electrolyte values (75). With respect to the 15% to 25% functional improvement of exercise tolerance, the reduction of symptoms, and the improved quality of life, exercise training is therefore recommended in stable chronic heart failure (73).

Exercise training is usually performed as a steady-state or interval program of 50% to 80% of the maximal heart rate or at an exercise intensity (in Watts (W)) equivalent to 50% to 70% of the maximal exercise capacity reached during exercise testing. Exercise sessions should start at a low level (e.g., 50% of maximal heart rate for 10 minutes) and individual titration of exercise training should be performed in the following order: duration (up to 20 minutes per unit), then frequency (up to three times a day and/or three to five times per week), and then intensity (up to 70% to 80% of peak heart rate) (73).

In chronic heart failure patients, aerobic training should be combined with resistance exercise to antagonize the muscle

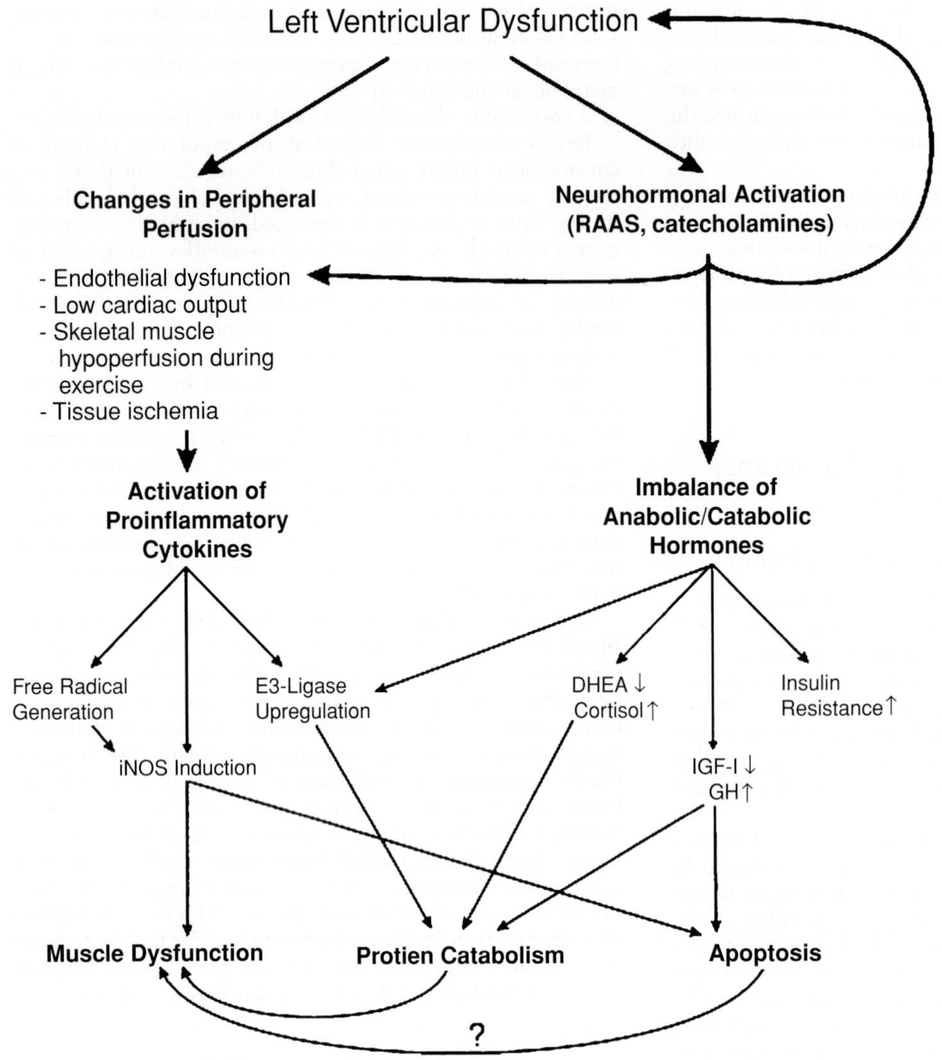

FIGURE 13.4. The pathogenesis of skeletal muscle dysfunction in chronic heart failure has been elucidated in recent years: It is believed that skeletal muscle hypoperfusion—especially during exercise—leads to cytokine activation and increased local generation of reactive oxygen species (ROS). Both ROS and cytokines promote the induction of inducible nitric oxide synthase (iNOS) which inhibits muscle oxidative metabolism by production of excess NO. Cytokine-induced expression of E3-ligases (Murf1, MafBx) accelerate proteasome-mediated protein degradation and catabolism. The catabolic–anabolic imbalance is further aggravated by reduced local IGF-I concentrations and an elevated cortisol/dehydroepiandrosterone (DHEA) ratio. Free radicals, NO, and IGF-I deficiency may also increase apoptosis of skeletal muscle myonuclei, although the functional relevance of apoptosis in multinucleated cells is still under debate.

catabolism seen in more advanced stages of heart failure, although this has been a topic of some controversy. The reluctance to include resistance exercise in training programs for chronic heart failure patients is based on older studies that found a rise in afterload along with an acute reduction in cardiac output and an increase in the severity of mitral regurgitation with prolonged isometric exercise (74,75). More recent studies with a maximum of 2 × 10 repetition exercises at 70% of maximal capacity, however, show no significant decrease in ejection fraction or an increase in systolic BP (78–80).

In a study of resistance training in older women with chronic heart failure, strength was increased by 43%, muscle endurance by 299%, and 6-minute walk by 49%, all associated with favorable ultrastructural adaptations in skeletal muscle (81). Although pure resistance training in chronic heart failure patients leads to an increase in muscular strength, it does not affect maximal oxygen uptake. There is, on the other hand, good reason to believe that combining resistance with endurance training might enhance the gain in muscle mass derived from the training intervention (82). When initiating resistance exercise in chronic heart failure patients short stress phases (10 repetitions maximum) at 30% to 50% of the maximal voluntary contraction, interrupted by phases of muscle relaxation are unlikely to cause hemodynamic deterioration. As a supplementary training modality, resistance training can complement, but not replace, the well-established aerobic endurance training.

Risk Factor Modifying Effects of Comprehensive Exercise Rehabilitation Interventions

Effects on Lipid Levels and Obesity

It is now very well established that lowering blood lipid levels reduces clinical events and mortality rates in patients known to have CHD. Numerous controlled clinical trials, most with quantitative coronary angiography, have demonstrated the efficacy of pharmacologic and diet-induced lipid lowering on slowing the progression of angiographic measures of atherosclerosis and on reducing clinical coronary events (9,28, 29,83–86). Low-fat diets, without accompanying drug treatment, have been effective in reducing the prevalence of angiographic progression of CAD when combined with exercise (28,29) and stress management (29), which strengthens the case for widespread institution of lipid-lowering dietary therapy. The reduction in clinical coronary events was conclusively demonstrated in the Scandinavian Simvastatin Survival Study, which reported a 30% to 35% reduction in deaths and major coronary events (83). The National Cholesterol Education Program now recommends setting an LDL cholesterol level of <70 mg/dL as a goal of therapy for all coronary patients based on newer studies (87).

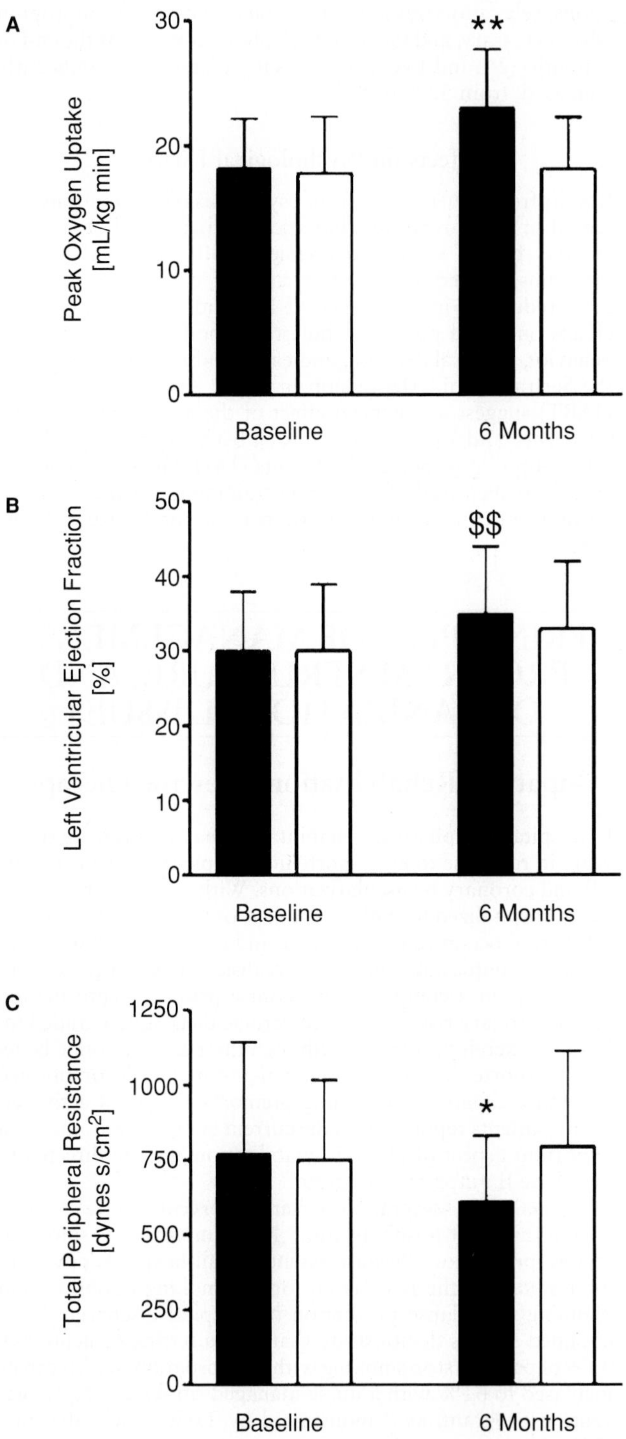

FIGURE 13.5. In patients with stable chronic heart failure a 6 months training program succeeded in increasing maximal oxygen uptake (A), and improving left ventricular ejection fraction (EF, B). However, the improved increased EF is most likely not related to direct training effects on the myocardium, but rather the result of the afterload reduction (decline in total peripheral resistance at rest and during peak exercise) (C) (64). $^{*}P < .05$ versus control group. $^{**}P < .01$ versus control group. $^{\$\$}P < .01$ versus baseline.

The cardiac rehabilitation program is an optimal site for systematic screening and treatment of hyperlipidemia. This includes dietary counseling and active participation by the patient in pharmacologic therapy. A rehabilitation-based screening and treatment program has been documented to triple the likelihood that patients for whom such treatment is appropriate receive lipid-lowering therapy (88). Affiliation with a clinician expert in lipid management is advantageous, and in many cases a lipid clinic can be organized at the rehabilitation facility itself.

Although exercise training has no consistent effect on low-density lipoprotein (LDL) cholesterol levels, a consistent favorable increase of high-density lipoprotein (HDL) cholesterol of 8% to 23% has been demonstrated (89–91). Decreases of 3% to 21% in serum triglyceride levels after 1 to 2 years of exercise have also been demonstrated (92–94). Numerous studies that combined exercise with behavioral counseling and dietary instruction have documented consistent beneficial effects on serum lipid levels that include decreases in LDL cholesterol and serum triglyceride levels and maintenance or slight increase in HDL cholesterol (9,28,29). For example, in the diet-exercise studies of Schuler and associates (28) and Ornish and co-workers (29), reductions in LDL cholesterol of 11% and 37%, respectively, were attained. In some patients, lipid-lowering medications are required to meet treatment goals (87), and the benefits of aggressive therapy include a retardation of the atherosclerotic process and a decrease in long-term coronary events (9,30).

Over 80% of patients starting cardiac rehabilitation in the United States are overweight and 51% to 58% have full-blown metabolic syndrome (95,96). Studies on the effect of cardiac rehabilitation exercise without intensive nutritional counseling on measures of obesity have documented only modest benefits (97–99). This may be because of the surprisingly low exercise-related caloric expenditure noted with cardiac rehabilitation exercise programs, particularly in female and older participants (100,101). A promising intervention that merits further study is the modification of cardiac rehabilitation exercise protocols to maximize caloric expenditure (102,103). This involves increasing the frequency and duration of exercise, at slightly lower intensities, and using non–weight-supported exercise such as walking (102,103). In studies that incorporated a very low-fat dietary intervention in addition to the exercise intervention, consistent improvements in body mass index [(weight in kg)/(height in m)^2] have been demonstrated (9,28,29). Although obesity is an independent risk factor for the development of CAD (104,105), in the setting of established CAD, reduction of obesity, particularly abdominal obesity, acts as a multifactorial intervention with associated improvements in lipid profiles, measures of insulin resistance, and lowering of blood pressure (98,106–108) and systemic inflammation (109). Aerobic exercise training alone is associated with a reduction in abdominal obesity, even in the absence of major changes of weight in healthy elderly individuals and in CHD patients (90,110).

Although no study has yet addressed the effect of weight reduction on second coronary events, the presence of the metabolic syndrome clearly portends a worsened long-term prognosis after MI (111). Nutrition education combined with behavioral interventions and prescribed exercise can achieve modest and sustained weight loss in the rehabilitation setting (112). However, the accomplishment of weight loss in cardiac rehabilitation is not a passive process, and it requires the development of a weight loss module for selected patients, staffed by appropriately trained professionals, with clear definitions of goals and desired outcomes and long-term follow-up. A well-established and effective behavior-based weight reduction program has been adapted to the cardiac rehabilitation setting (113,114). The intervention includes behavioral concepts of stimulus control, self-monitoring, problem solving, and social support; a daily caloric goal; and a daily calorie count. In many cases, a relatively modest but sustained weight loss of 5% to 10% of body weight significantly improves risk factors such as lipid measures and insulin resistance. An advantage of cardiac rehabilitation–based weight reduction programs is that patients are already performing the requisite exercise component needed to prevent them from regaining lost weight (115).

Effects on Glycemic Control and Diabetes Mellitus

Together with a high-caloric, low-fiber diet, a sedentary lifestyle is a key risk factor for the development of pathologic glucose tolerance and type 2 diabetes mellitus. Several follow-up studies documented a clear risk reduction for the development of type 2 diabetes among physically active individuals as compared with their inactive counterparts, a relationship that was evident across all body mass index groups (116,117). Exercise continues to be effective for preventing the development of overt type 2 diabetes mellitus among patients with impaired glucose tolerance (118,119).

No clinical trials involving patients with established CAD have been carried out to determine whether tight control of diabetes in patients with either type 1 or type 2 diabetes prevents cardiac complications or slows the course of macrovascular disease. Results of a multicenter clinical trial of tight glucose control in patients with type 1 (insulin-dependent) diabetes who did not have CAD demonstrated improved lipid profiles, an increase in body weight, a decrease in microvascular complications (retinal and renal), and a trend toward decreased macrovascular events, with such events (cardiac and cerebrovascular) reduced by almost 50% (120). In patients with type 2 diabetes, exercise, and weight reduction resulted in improved measures of insulin resistance and associated coronary risk factors, such as lipid abnormalities and hypertension (121,122). Poor glycemic control predicts an increased likelihood of cardiac events in type 2 diabetes (123,124). An important role of the cardiac rehabilitation program, beyond encouraging exercise and proper nutrition, is to assist primary physicians with monitoring and treatment of diabetes. Patients are taught self-monitoring techniques and medications are adjusted as needed (6,125).

Effects on Blood Pressure Control and Hypertension

Rehabilitation programs assist primary physicians with the treatment and follow-up of coronary patients with hypertension. Although weight reduction, exercise, and salt restriction have all been associated with modest reductions in systemic blood pressure, definite benefits in the cardiac rehabilitation setting have not been demonstrated. Frequent surveillance of blood pressure, teaching of self-monitoring techniques, nutritional instruction, and adjustment of medications are all useful (6,126).

Effects on Smoking Cessation

Cigarette smoking cessation is associated with a marked decrease in coronary event rates in coronary patients (127,128). In the study of Wilhelmsson and associates (128), patients who quit smoking after experiencing MI reduced their 1-year mortality rate from 10% to 5% and their 1-year reinfarction rate from 18% to 9%. Exercise training in and of itself has minimal, if any, effect on smoking cessation rates in coronary patients (129). The best results with smoking cessation after a coronary event have been obtained using a physician-recommended, nurse-managed intervention that takes place during hospitalization for an acute coronary event (while patients are unable to smoke) and is aimed at relapse prevention (10,24). These interventions include teaching skills to deal with high-risk situations, relaxation training, provision of nicotine or bupropion when necessary, and long-term telephone contact. At the end of 6 months (24) and 1 year (10), cessation rates were significantly increased, from 32% to 61%.

Effects on Psychological Factors

Results from a meta-analysis of psychosocial interventions presented in the cardiac rehabilitation setting aimed at modifying risk factors such as depression (130) suggest that these programs yielded a 37% reduction in cardiac mortality, a 29% reduction in recurrence of MI, and significant positive effects on blood pressure, cholesterol, body weight, smoking behavior, physical exercise, and eating habits. Initial results of the Sertraline and Depression in Heart Attack Study (SADHART) suggest a beneficial effect of the antidepressant drug on events and overall clinical well-being over 6 months of follow-up in post-acute MI patients (131). Finally, a randomized controlled trial of relaxation training in cardiac rehabilitation resulted in a significant decrease in total cardiac events (132).

PRINCIPLES OF MANAGEMENT, PROGRAM STRUCTURE, AND ORGANIZATIONAL ISSUES

Inpatient Rehabilitation/Exercise Therapy

In-hospital, or phase I, rehabilitation has evolved in recent years in response to ever-shortening hospitalizations for acute MI and coronary revascularizations. With many infarction patients hospitalized for only 4 to 6 days or less (23), and much of this period occupied by acute care and recovery from interventional techniques, it is no longer realistic to expect patients to participate in a comprehensive course providing information about coronary risk factors and cardiac diets, and a graded in-hospital exercise program. Although there are economic benefits of a shorter hospitalization, patients are less deconditioned and more capable of resuming premorbid physical activities. Many patients report that in the current environment, the most important aspect of phase I rehabilitation is to be directed to the phase II outpatient program.

Nonetheless, several important interventions take place during this brief hospitalization. Most important is smoking-relapse prevention. Because essentially all hospitals now prohibit smoking, the issue is no longer smoking cessation, but planning for relapse prevention on hospital discharge. Well-designed studies demonstrate that in the setting of acute MI, 32% of patients stop smoking without a program, which can be increased to 61% with a nurse-managed smoking-relapse prevention program, as demonstrated by Taylor and colleagues (24).

It is also important during this brief index admission to define coronary risk factors and set up an outpatient plan for long-term therapy. Defining the lipid profile is of particular importance; studies of aggressive lipid lowering in coronary patients document decreasing secondary event rates beginning 6 months after therapy is begun (83,86). Serum lipid values are accurate when measured within 24 hours of MI. When they are measured later in a hospitalization for MI, they are inaccurate, with total, LDL, and HDL cholesterol levels lower and triglyceride levels higher (133–136). For 1 month after coronary bypass surgery, serum cholesterol levels measure falsely low, and therefore baseline measures should be determined preoperatively, with follow-up measures performed after 1 month (137).

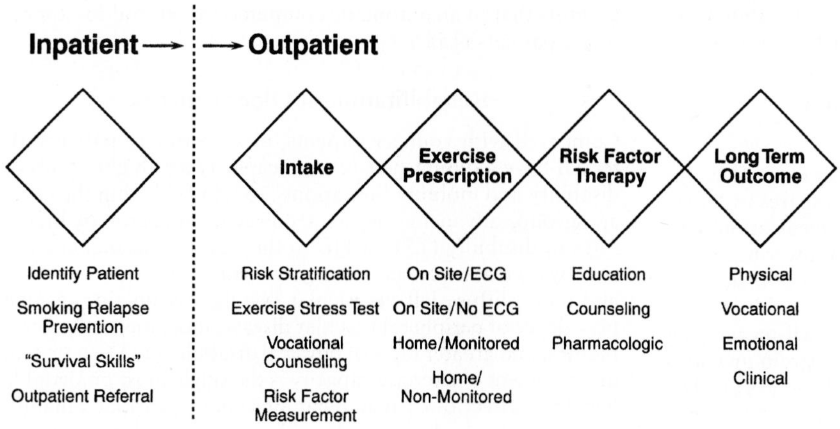

FIGURE 13.6. Elements of cardiac rehabilitation. *Abbreviation:* ECG = electrocardiographic monitoring.

Outpatient Rehabilitation/Exercise Therapy

Intake Evaluation

The cardiac rehabilitation intake evaluation is an optimal opportunity to systematically define secondary risk factors for the progression of CAD (Fig. 13.6). Therefore, as part of this evaluation, a fasting lipid profile and a glucose measure should be obtained for all patients. Other risk factors, such as smoking status, blood pressure, obesity, and diabetes-related measures, should also be assessed.

An exercise tolerance test needs to be performed so that an exercise prescription can be developed and the risk associated with exercise can be assessed. Patients in whom high-risk characteristics are identified at risk stratification (Table 13.2) should participate in a supervised program in which electrocardiographic (ECG) monitoring is available. Patients who are stratified to low- or intermediate-risk groups can be considered for a non-ECG monitored or a home-based exercise program. Although the requirements for ECG monitoring remain poorly defined, the American College of Cardiology, in its "Report on Cardiac Rehabilitation," recommends ECG monitoring for high-risk patients (138).

Only 15% of eligible patients in the United States receive cardiac rehabilitation services (1). In many cases, cardiac rehabilitation programs are not geographically available, whereas in other cases, formal rehabilitation is not recommended by the primary physician (139,140). For some patients, insurance coverage is incomplete or unavailable. Whereas cardiac rehabilitation services have classically been delivered on site at a well-defined exercise training facility, the need to expand preventive cardiology services to include the majority of eligible patients necessitates a redefinition of this model.

The development of alternate approaches to delivery of cardiac rehabilitation services is an ongoing process, aimed at a goal of expanding the base of patients who receive services, at the lowest possible health care cost. Numerous investigators have documented the safety of home-based exercise programs for individuals who are at low to medium risk by use of varying degrees of transtelephonic monitoring (11,12,141). Case management (evaluation and management of risk factors for the individual patient) complements exercise conditioning and allows the individualization of preventive care in health care delivery systems that focus on efficiency and outcomes. Case management, whether delivered in an office practice or in a structured rehabilitation program, should focus on attainment of risk factor goals and identification of highest risk patients (see Table 13.2) (9,10). Exercise programs can be individualized for moderate- and high-risk patients, and patients at

TABLE 13.2

GUIDELINES FOR RISK-STRATIFICATION

Risk level	Characteristics
Low	No significant left ventricular dysfunction (i.e., ejection fraction, ≥50%) No resting or exercise-induced myocardial ischemia manifested as angina and/or ST segment displacement No resting or exercise-induced complex arrhythmias Uncomplicated myocardial infarction, coronary artery bypass surgery, angioplasty, or atherectomy Functional capacity ≥6 METs on graded exercise test ≥3 weeks after clinical event
Intermediate	Mildly to moderately depressed left ventricular function (ejection fraction, 31–49%) Functional capacity <5–6 METs on graded exercise test ≥3 wk after clinical event Failure to comply with exercise intensity prescription Exercise-induced myocardial ischemia (1–2 mm ST segment depression) or reversible ischemic defects (seen on echocardiography or nuclear radiography)
High	Severely depressed left ventricular function (ejection fraction, ≤30%) Complex ventricular arrhythmias while patient is at rest or appearing or increasing with exercise Decrease in systolic blood pressure of >15 mm Hg during exercise or failure to rise with increasing exercise workloads Patient is survivor of sudden cardiac death Myocardial infarction complicated by congestive heart failure, cardiogenic shock, and/or complex ventricular arrhythmias Severe coronary artery disease and marked exercise-induced myocardial ischemia (>2 mm ST segment depression)

METs, multiple of resting energy expenditure.
From American Association of Cardiovascular and Pulmonary Rehabilitation. *Guidelines for cardiac rehabilitation programs.* Champaign, IL: Human Kinetics Books, 1995, with permission.

highest risk of disability should be referred to a rehabilitation program for closer supervision and monitoring.

Compliance With Exercise and Long-Term Follow-Up

Long-term adherence to cardiac rehabilitation exercise is approximately 50% at 1 year (142,143). This compares to 1-year adherence rates of 64% for antihypertensive medication regimens (144) and 82% for treatment with lipid-lowering agents (145). Several interventions have been shown to optimize compliance with cardiac rehabilitation exercises. A gradual transition to home-based exercise sessions with self-monitoring while the patient is still in the rehabilitation program increases 6-month compliance rates from 76% to 92% (146). The use of lower intensity exercise (147), participation of nurse case-managers (9,10), and the signing of a written agreement (148) have all been associated with increased long-term compliance with the exercise component of cardiac rehabilitation.

Provisions for the long-term continuation of risk factor modification also need to be specified. The long-term surveillance and treatment of coronary risk factors is generally transferred to the primary physician, in a case management format, whereas the long-term surveillance and maintenance of the exercise component is often delegated to the rehabilitation program. Long-term, institutional phase III cardiac rehabilitation programs successfully maintain patients in a supervised exercise program and are particularly useful for older patients because they provide supervision and social interactions.

Strategies to improve participation in cardiac rehabilitation programs are of major importance in view of the relationship between adherence with preventive cardiology recommendations and better clinical outcomes (149–151). The most important determinant of early post–coronary event cardiac rehabilitation participation, studied in a population of patients 62 years old or older, is the strength of the primary physician's recommendation for participation (140). When the recommendation was graded as moderate to strong (4 to 5, on a scale of 1 to 5), participation was 70%; when the recommendation was weak (1 to 3), participation rate was 2% (Fig. 13.7). Other predictors of poor participation rates included older age; presence of comorbidities, especially arthritis; and the presence of mental depression (140). A recent intervention that may be of promise in increasing referral to cardiac rehabilitation programs is that of an automatic computerized referral for appropriate patients (152).

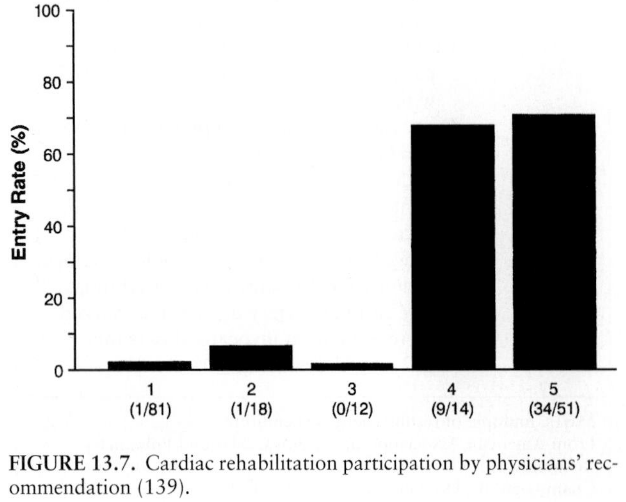

FIGURE 13.7. Cardiac rehabilitation participation by physicians' recommendation (139).

Rehabilitation of Older Patients

Compared with younger patients, older coronary patients after MI have a diminished exercise capacity and higher rates of disability and mobility limitations (153,154). Within the older age group, advancing age is a powerful predictor of higher rates of disability (154). CHD in the elderly is also characterized by a greater severity of angiographic disease, more severe and more diffuse left ventricular systolic dysfunction, a high prevalence of peripheral vascular disease, more medical comorbidities, and greater rates of physical disability (155). In that an improvement of exercise capacity is the single most predictable beneficial effect of cardiac rehabilitation (1), cardiac rehabilitation effectively distances the older participant from physical disability, particularly with long-term participation (155). For clinicians in the field, this is by far the most evident clinical benefit of cardiac rehabilitation in older patients after MI. It should be noted that cardiac rehabilitation exercise training includes both aerobic and resistance training. A randomized controlled trial of resistance training in disabled older women with CHD (post-MI and postrevascularization) documented improvements in directly measured physical functional performance, which included both household activities and measures of endurance activities such as stair climbing, grocery carrying, and 6-minute walk distance (156,157).

Rehabilitation of Women

The current model of cardiac rehabilitation was developed primarily in middle-aged male coronary patients in the 1960s and 1970s. Women continue to form a minority of cardiac rehabilitation participants (158). The primary reason for this appears to be lower referral rates by primary physicians rather than clinical differences between male and female patients (158). Early after MI, women have a lower functional capacity than men, are older, are more likely to have residual angina, and have more prominent risk factor profiles, and are therefore are excellent candidates for rehabilitation (158–161). There has been relatively little study of the relative benefits and special needs of women in cardiac rehabilitation, although women improve their exercise capacity with training to a similar degree as men (158,162). Women, however, appear to experience less weight loss and improve risk factors to a lesser degree, probably due to a significantly lower exercise-related energy expenditure during cardiac rehabilitation sessions (101).

CONTROVERSIES, PERSONAL PERSPECTIVES, AND THE FUTURE

The evolution of cardiac rehabilitation has reached a critical phase where it may soon become necessary to redefine its place in clinical medicine. Forces from four major directions push cardiac rehabilitation to a new frontier:

1. Growing economic limitations of clinical medicine force us to place more and more responsibility on the patients' lifestyle as a predictor of health outcomes. It becomes increasingly difficult for society to accept that some individuals will place an extra burden on public health expenditures by continuing unhealthy habits and/or refusing to participate in preventive programs that emphasize lifestyle modifications.
2. The prevalence of a complete absence of leisure-time physical activity is estimated to be 40% for the entire population,

but may reach over 55% in ethnic subgroups. It is estimated that adult obesity rates (body mass index >30) will reach 30% in 2015 and >40% in 2025 in the United States. Concurrently, the prevalence of diseases and conditions caused by lack of physical activity and a hypercaloric diet, such as type 2 diabetes and the metabolic syndrome, is accelerating.

3. The scientific evidence base for exercise-based and comprehensive rehabilitation has never been better: An increasing number of clinical trials confirm multiple clinical benefits and basic science experiments have greatly enhanced insight into the molecular mechanisms involved in mediating training-induced changes in endothelial function. For many rehabilitation interventions a clear prognostic benefit has been documented.
4. The gap between increasing rates of obesity and inactivity-related diseases and shrinking health budgets can only be closed by a paradigm shift from reparative to preventive clinical interventions.

We must make promotion of physical activity and healthy nutritional habits a number one priority of our public health system. Interventions need to start early in childhood, when unhealthy eating habits are developed and sedentary lifestyles are copied from adults. The degree to which unhealthy behaviors are regarded as a "private issue" must be publicly discussed. A balance needs to be struck between a reasonable minimum effort of the individual to reduce healthcare costs and the intrusion of an investigative healthcare system into personal lifestyle. As is true of other prevention interventions, we need not await a "magic bullet." If cardiac rehabilitation and secondary preventive therapies can be systematically applied to targeted populations, recurrent coronary event rates will plummet and coronary disability will be minimized.

References

1. Wenger NK, Froehlicher ES, Smith LK, et al. *Cardiac rehabilitation: clinical practice guidelines.* AHCPR publication no. 96-0672. Rockville, MD:U.S. Department of Health and Human Services, Public Health Service, Agency for Health Care Policy and Research, and the National Heart, Lung, and Blood Institute, 1995.
2. Dawber TR, Kannel WB, Revotskie N, et al. Some factors associated with the development of coronary heart disease: six years' follow-up experience in the Framingham Study. *Am J Publ Health* 1959;49:1349–1356.
3. Pate RR, Pratt M, Blair SN, et al. Physical activity and public health: a recommendation from the Centers for Disease Control and Prevention and the American College of Sports Medicine. *JAMA* 1995;273:402–407.
4. Hambrecht R, Walther C, Mobius-Winkler S, et al. Percutaneous coronary angioplasty compared with exercise training in patients with stable coronary artery disease: a randomized trial. *Circulation* 2004;109:1371–1378.
5. Joliffe JA, Rees K, Taylor RS, et al. *Exercise-based rehabilitation for coronary heart disease* . Oxford: Update Software, 2002.
6. Balady GJ, Ades PA, Comoss P, et al. Core components of cardiac rehabilitation/secondary prevention programs: a statement for healthcare professionals from the American Heart Association and the American Association of Cardiovascular and Pulmonary Rehabilitation Writing Group. *Circulation* 2000;102:1069–1073.
7. Ades PA. Cardiac rehabilitation and the secondary prevention of coronary heart disease. *N Engl J Med* 2001;345:892–902.
8. Feigenbaum E, Carter E. *Health technology assessment report*, 1987, no. 6. Rockville, MD: U.S. Department of Health and Human Services, Public Health Service, National Center for Health Services Research and Health-Care Technology Assessment, 1988.
9. Haskell WL, Alderman EL, Fair JM, et al. Effects of intensive multiple risk factor reduction on coronary atherosclerosis and clinical cardiac events in men and women with coronary artery disease: the Stanford Coronary Risk Intervention Project (SCRIP). *Circulation* 1994;89:975–990.
10. DeBusk RF, Houston-Miller N, Superko HR, et al. A case-management system for coronary risk factor modification after acute myocardial infarction. *Ann Intern Med* 1994;120:721–729.
11. DeBusk RF, Haskell WL, Miller NH, et al. Medically directed at-home rehabilitation soon after uncomplicated acute myocardial infarction: a new model for patient care. *Am J Cardiol* 1985;55:251–257.
12. Ades PA, Pashkow F, Fletcher G, et al. A controlled trial of cardiac rehabilitation in the home setting using electrocardiographic and voice transtelephonic monitoring. *Am Heart J* 2000;139:543–548.
13. Ades PA, Pashkow F, Nestor J. Cost-effectiveness of cardiac rehabilitation after myocardial infarction. *J Cardiopulm Rehabil* 1997;17:222–231.
14. Ades P, Huang D, Weaver S. Cardiac rehabilitation participation predicts lower rehospitalization costs. *Am Heart J* 1992;123:916–921.
15. Levin LA, Perk J, Hedback B. Cardiac rehabilitation: a cost analysis. *J Intern Med* 1991;230:427–434.
16. Bondestam E, Breikss A, Hartford M. Effects of early rehabilitation on consumption of medical care during the first year after acute myocardial infarction in patients >65 years of age. *Am J Cardiol* 1995;75:767–771.
17. Mallory G, Shite P, Salcedo-Salgar J. The speed of healing of myocardial infarction: a study of the pathological anatomy in seventy-two cases. *Am Heart J* 1939;18:647–671.
18. Levine S, Lown B. "Armchair" treatment of acute coronary thrombosis. *JAMA* 1952;148:1365–1369.
19. Newman L, Andrews M, Koblish M. Physical medicine and rehabilitation in acute myocardial infarction. *Arch Intern Med* 1952;89:552–561.
20. Cain HD, Frasher WG, Stivelman R. Graded activity program for safe return to self-care after myocardial infarction. *JAMA* 1961;177:111–115.
21. Berra K. Cardiac and pulmonary rehabilitation: historical perspectives and future needs. *J Cardiopulm Rehabil* 1991;11:8–15.
22. Pashkow FJ. Issues in contemporary cardiac rehabilitation: a historical perspective. *J Am Coll Cardiol* 1993;21:822–834.
23. Newby LK, Eisenstein EL, Califf RM, et al. Cost effectiveness of early discharge after uncomplicated acute myocardial infarction. *N Engl J Med* 2000;342:749–755.
24. Taylor CB, Houston-Miller N, Killen JD, et al. Smoking cessation after acute myocardial infarction: effects of a nurse-managed intervention. *Ann Intern Med* 1990;113:118–123.
25. Oldridge NB, Guyatt GH, Fischer ME, et al. Cardiac rehabilitation after myocardial infarction: combined experience of randomized clinical trials. *JAMA* 1988;260:945–950.
26. O'Connor GT, Buring JE, Yusuf S, et al. An overview of randomized trials of rehabilitation with exercise after myocardial infarction. *Circulation* 1989;80:234–244.
27. Witt BJ, Jacobsen SJ, Weston SA et al. Cardiac rehabilitation after myocardial infarction in the community. *J Am Coll Cardiol* 2004;44:988–996.
28. Schuler G, Hambrecht R, Schlierf G, et al. Regular physical exercise and low-fat diets: effects on progression of coronary artery disease. *Circulation* 1992;86:1–11.
29. Ornish D, Brown SE, Scherwitz LW, et al. Can lifestyle changes reverse coronary heart disease? The Lifestyle Heart Trial. *Lancet* 1990;336: 129–133.
30. Brown BG, Zhao XQ, Sacco DE, et al. Lipid lowering and plaque regression: new insights into prevention of plaque disruption and clinical events in coronary disease. *Circulation* 1993;87:1781–1791.
31. Piepoli MF, Davos C, Francis DP, et al. Exercise training meta-analysis of trials in patients with chronic heart failure (ExTraMATCH). *BMJ* 2004; 328:189.
32. Leon AS, Certo C, Comoss P, et al. Scientific evidence of the value of cardiac rehabilitation services with emphasis on patients following myocardial infarction. Section I: exercise conditioning component. *J Cardiopulm Rehabil* 1990;10:79–87.
33. Curnier D, Savage PD, Ades PA. Geographic distribution of cardiac rehabilitation programs in the U.S. *J Cardiopulm Rehabil.* 2005:25:80–84.
34. Ludmer PL, Selwyn AP, Shook TL, et al. Paradoxical vasoconstriction induced by acetylcholine in atherosclerotic coronary arteries. *N Engl J Med* 1986;315:1046–1051.
35. Vita JA, Treasure CB, Yeung AC, et al. Patients with evidence of coronary endothelial dysfunction as assessed by acetylcholine infusion demonstrate marked increase in sensitivity to constrictor effects of catecholamines. *Circulation* 1992;85:1390–1397.
36. Gordon JB, Ganz P, Nabel EG, et al. Atherosclerosis influences the vasomotor response of epicardial coronary arteries to exercise. *J Clin Invest* 1989;83:1946–1952.
37. Zeiher AM, Drexler H, Wollschlaeger H, et al. Coronary vasomotion in response to sympathetic stimulation in humans: importance of the functional integrity of the endothelium. *J Am Coll Cardiol* 1989;14:1181–1190.
38. Yeung AC, Vekshtein VI, Krantz DS, et al. The effect of atherosclerosis on the vasomotor response of coronary arteries to mental stress. *N Engl J Med* 1991;325:1551–1556.
39. Hasdai D, Gibbons RJ, Holmes DR, et al. Coronary endothelial dysfunction in humans is associated with myocardial perfusion defects. *Circulation* 1997;96:3390–3395.
40. Hambrecht R, Niebauer J, Marburger Ch, et al. Various intensities of leisure time physical activity in patients with coronary artery disease: effects on cardiorespiratory fitness and progression of coronary atherosclerotic lesions. *J Am Coll Cardiol* 1993;22:468–477.

41. Schuler G, Hambrecht R, Schlierf G, et al. Myocardial perfusion and regression of coronary artery disease in patients on a regimen of intensive physical exercise and low fat diet. *J Am Coll Cardiol* 1992;19:34–42.
42. Hambrecht R, Wolf A, Gielen S, et al. Effect of exercise on coronary endothelial function in patients with coronary artery disease. *N Engl J Med* 2000;342:454–460.
43. Hambrecht R, Adams V, Erbs S, et al. Regular physical activity improves endothelial function in patients with coronary artery disease by increasing phosphorylation of endothelial nitric oxide synthase. *Circulation* 2003;107:3152–3158.
44. Adams V, Linke A, Kränkell N, et al. Impact of regular physical activity on the NAD(P)H oxidase and angiotensin receptor system in patients with coronary artery disease. *Circulation* 2005;111:555–562.
45. Fukai T, Siefried MR, Fukai M, et al. Regulation of the vascular extracellular superoxide dismutase by nitric oxide and exercise training. *J Clin Invest* 2000;105:1631–1639.
46. Schächinger V, Britten MB, Zeiher A. Prognostic impact of coronary vasodilator dysfunction on adverse long-term outcome of coronary heart disease. *Circulation* 2000;101:1899–1906.
47. Suwaidi JA, Hamasaki S, Higano ST, et al. Long-term follow-up of patients with mild coronary artery disease and endothelial dysfunction. *Circulation* 2000;101:948–954.
48. Asahara T, Masuda H, Takahashi T, et al. Bone marrow origin of endothelial progenitor cells responsible for postnatal vasculogenesis in physiological and pathological neovascularization. *Circ Res* 1999;85:221–228.
49. Adams V, Lenk K, Linke A, et al. Increase of circulating endothelial progenitor cells in patients with coronary artery disease after exercise-induced ischemia. *Arterioscler Thromb Vasc Biol* 2004;24:684–690.
50. Laufs U, Werner N, Link A, et al. Physical training increases endothelial progenitor cells, inhibits neointima formation, and enhances angiogenesis. *Circulation* 2004;109:220–226.
51. Franciosa JA, Park M, Levine TB. Lack of correlation between exercise capacity and indexes of resting left ventricular performance in heart failure. *Am J Cardiol* 1981;47:33–39.
52. Cohn JN, Levine TB, Francis GS, et al. Neurohumoral control mechanisms in congestive heart failure. *Am Heart J* 1981;102:509–514.
53. Levine TB, Francis GS, Goldsmith SR, et al. Activity of the sympathetic nervous system and renin-angiotensin system assessed by plasma hormone levels and their relation to hemodynamic abnormalities in congestive heart failure. *Am J Cardiol* 1982;49:1659–1666.
54. Levine B, Kalman J, Mayer L, et al. Elevated circulating levels of tumor necrosis factor in severe chronic heart failure. *N Engl J Med* 1990;323:236–241.
55. Seta Y, Shan K, Bozkurt B, et al. Basic mechanisms in heart failure: the cytokine hypothesis. *J Card Fail* 1996;2:243–249.
56. Kubo SH, Rector TC, Williams RE, et al. Endothelium dependent vasodilation is attenuated in patients with heart failure. *Circulation* 1991;84:1589–1596.
57. Gielen S, Adams V, Möbius-Winkler S, et al. Anti-inflammatory effects of exercise training in the skeletal muscle of patients with chronic heart failure. *J Am Coll Cardiol* 2003;42:861–868.
58. Mancini DM, Henson D, LaMacna J, et al. Respiratory muscle function and dyspnea in patients with chronic congestive heart failure. *Circulation* 1992;86:909–918.
59. Sullivan MJ, Green HJ, Cobb FR. Skeletal muscle biochemistry and histology in ambulatory patients with long-term heart failure. *Circulation* 1990;81:518–527.
60. Simonini A, Long CS, Dudley GA, et al. Heart failure in rats causes changes in skeletal muscle morphology and gene expression that are not explained by reduced activity. *Circ Res* 1996;79:128–136.
61. Mancini DM, Coyle E, Coggan A, et al. Contribution of intrinsic skeletal muscle changes to 31-P NMR skeletal muscle metabolic abnormalities in patients with chronic heart failure. *Circulation* 1989;80:1338–1346.
62. Okita K, Yonezawa K, Nishijima H, et al. Skeletal muscle metabolism limits exercise capacity in patients with chronic heart failure. *Circulation* 1998;98:1886–1891.
63. Opasich C, Ambrosino N, Felicetti G, et al. Skeletal and respiratory muscle strength in chronic heart failure. *G Ital Cardiol* 1993;23:759–766.
64. European Heart Failure Training Group. Experience from controlled trials of physical training in chronic heart failure. Protocol and patient factors in effectiveness in the improvement in exercise tolerance. *Eur Heart J* 1998;19:466–475.
65. Hambrecht R, Gielen S, Linke A, et al. Effects of exercise training on left ventricular function and peripheral resistance in patients with chronic heart failure. A randomised trial. *JAMA* 2000;283:3095–3101.
66. Hambrecht R, Fiehn E, Weigl C, et al. Regular physical exercise corrects endothelial dysfunction and improves exercise capacity in patients with chronic heart failure. *Circulation* 1998;98:2709–2715.
67. Linke A, Schoene N, Gielen S, et al. Endothelial dysfunction in patients with chronic heart failure: systemic effects of lower-limb exercise training. *J Am Coll Cardiol* 2001;37:392–397.
68. Belardinelli R, Georgiou D, Cianci G, et al. Effects of exercise training on left ventricular filling at rest and during exercise in patients with ischemic cardiomyopathy and severe left ventricular systolic dysfunction. *Am Heart J* 1996;132:61–70.
69. Braith R, Welsch M, Feigenbaum M, et al. Neuroendocrine activation in heart failure is modified by endurance training. *J Am Coll Cardiol* 1999;34:1170–1175.
70. Hambrecht R, Schulze PC, Gielen S, et al. Reduction of insulin-like growth factor-I expression in the skeletal muscle of noncachectic patients with chronic heart failure. *J Am Coll Cardiol* 2002;39:1175–1181.
71. Adams V, Jiang H, Yu J, et al. Apoptosis in skeletal myocytes of patients with chronic heart failure is associated with exercise intolerance. *J Am Coll Cardiol* 1999;33:959–965.
72. Pina I, Apstein CS, Balady GJ, et al. Exercise and heart failure: a statement from the American Heart Association Committee on exercise, rehabilitation, and prevention. *Circulation* 2003;107:1210–1225.
73. Swedberg K, Cleland J, Dargie H, et al. Guidelines for the diagnosis and treatment of chronic heart failure: executive summary (update 2005): The Task Force for the Diagnosis and Treatment of Chronic Heart Failure of the European Society of Cardiology. *Eur Heart J* 2005;26:1115–1140.
74. Working Group on Cardiac Rehabilitation & Exercise Physiology and Working Group on Heart Failure of the European Society of Cardiology. Recommendations on exercise testing in chronic heart failure patients. *Eur Heart J* 2001;22:37–45.
75. Stevenson LW, Massie BM, Francis G. Optimizing therapy for complex or refractory heart failure: a management algorithm. *Am Heart J* 1998;135:S293-S309.
76. Elkayam U, Roth A, Weber L, et al. Isometric exercise in patients with chronic advanced heart failure: hemodynamic and neurohumoral evaluation. *Circulation* 1985;72:975–981.
77. Reddy HK, Weber KT, Janicki JS, et al. Hemodynamic, ventilatory and metabolic effects of light isometric exercise in patients with chronic heart failure. *J Am Coll Cardiol* 1988;12:353–358.
78. Karlsdottir AE, Foster C, Porcari JP, et al. Hemodynamic responses during aerobic and resistance exercise. *J Cardiopulm Rehabil* 2002;22:170–177.
79. McKelvie RS, McCartney N, Tomlinson C, et al. Comparison of hemodynamic responses to cycling and resistance exercise in congestive heart failure secondary to ischemic cardiomyopathy. *Am J Cardiol* 1995;76:977–979.
80. Meyer K, Hajric R, Westbrook S, et al. Hemodynamic responses during leg press exercise in patients with chronic congestive heart failure. *Am J Cardiol* 1999;83:1537–1543.
81. Pu CT, Johnson MT, Forman DE, et al. Randomized trial of progressive resistance training to counteract the myopathy of chronic heart failure. *J Appl Physiol* 2001;90:2341–2350.
82. McKoy G, Ashley W, Mander J, et al. Expression of insulin growth factor-1 splice variants and structural genes in rabbit skeletal muscle induced by stretch and stimulation. *J Physiol* 1999;516:583–592.
83. Scandinavian Simvastatin Survival Study Group. Randomized trial of cholesterol lowering in 4444 patients with coronary heart disease. *Lancet* 1994;345:1383–1389.
84. Blankenhorn DH, Nessim SA, Johnson RL, et al. Beneficial effects of combined colestipol-niacin therapy on coronary atherosclerosis and coronary venous bypass grafts. *JAMA* 1987;257:3233–3240.
85. Brown G, Alvers JJ, Fisher LD, et al. Regression of coronary artery disease as a result of intensive lipid-lowering therapy in men with high levels of apolipoprotein B. *N Engl J Med* 1990;323:1289–1298.
86. Sacks FM, Pfeffer MA, Moye LA, et al. The effect of pravastatin on coronary events after myocardial infarction in patients with average cholesterol levels. Cholesterol and Recurrent Events Trial investigators. *N Engl J Med* 1996;335:1001–1009.
87. Grundy SM, Cleeman JI, Merz CN, et al. Implications of recent clinical trials for the National Cholesterol Education Program Adult Treatment Panel III guidelines. *Circulation* 2004;110:227–239.
88. Ades PA, Savage PD, Poehlman ET, et al. Lipid lowering in the cardiac rehabilitation setting. *J Cardiopulm Rehabil* 1999;19:255–260.
89. Warner JG Jr, Brubaker PH, Zhu Y, et al. Long-term (5-year) changes in HDL cholesterol in cardiac rehabilitation patients: do sex differences exist? *Circulation* 1995;92:772–777.
90. Brochu M, Poehlman ET, Savage P, et al. Modest effects of exercise training alone on coronary risk factors and body composition in coronary patients. *J Cardiopulm Rehabil* 2000;20:180–188.
91. Mendoza SG, Carrasco H, Zerpa A, et al. Effect of physical training on lipids, lipoproteins, apolipoproteins, lipases, and endogenous sex hormones in men with premature myocardial infarction. *Metabolism* 1991;40:368–377.
92. Wilhelmsen L, Sanne H, Elmfeldt D, et al. A controlled trial of physical training after myocardial infarction: effects of risk factors, nonfatal reinfarction, and death. *Prev Med* 1975;4:491–508.
93. Oberman A, Cleary P, Larosa JC, et al. Changes in risk factors among participants in a long-term exercise rehabilitation program. *Adv Cardiol* 1982;31:168–175.
94. Engblom E, Hietanen EK, Hamalainen H, et al. Exercise habits and physical performance during comprehensive rehabilitation after coronary bypass surgery. *Eur Heart J* 1992;13:1053–1059.
95. Savage PD, Banzer JA, Balady GJ, et al. Prevalence of metabolic syndrome in cardiac rehabilitation/secondary prevention programs. *Am Heart J* 2005;149:627–631.

96. Milani RV, Lavie CJ. Prevalence and profile of metabolic syndrome in patients following acute coronary events and effects of therapeutic lifestyle change with cardiac rehabilitation. *Am J Cardiol* 2003;92:50–54.
97. Brochu M, Poehlman EP, Savage PD, et al. Coronary risk profiles in male coronary patients: effects of body composition, fat distribution, age and fitness. *Coron Artery Dis* 2000;11:137–144.
98. Lavie CJ, Milani RV. Effects of cardiac rehabilitation and exercise training in obese patients with coronary artery disease. *Chest* 1996;109:52–56.
99. Brochu M, Poehlman ET, Ades PA. Obesity, body fat distribution and coronary artery disease. *J Cardiopulm Rehabil* 2000;20:96–108.
100. Schairer JR, Kostelnik T, Proffitt SM, et al. Caloric expenditure during cardiac rehabilitation. *J Cardiopulm Rehabil* 1998;18:290–294.
101. Savage PD, Brochu M, Scott P, et al. Low caloric expenditure in cardiac rehabilitation. *Am Heart J* 2000;140:527–533.
102. Savage P, Brochu M, Poehlman E, et al. Reduction in obesity and coronary risk factors after high caloric exercise training in overweight coronary patients. *Am Heart J* 2003;146:317–323.
103. Mertens DJ, Kavanagh T, Campbell RB, et al. Exercise without dietary restriction as a means to long-term fat loss in the obese cardiac patient. *J Sports Med Phys Fitness* 1998;38:310–316.
104. Hubert HB, Feinleib M, McNamara PM, et al. Obesity as an independent risk factor for cardiovascular disease: a 26-year follow-up of participants in the Framingham Heart Study. *Circulation* 1983;67:968–977.
105. Manson SE, Colditz GA, Stampfer MJ, et al. A prospective study of obesity and risk of coronary heart disease in women. *N Engl J Med* 1990;322: 882–889.
106. Wood PD, Stephanick ML, Dreon D, et al. Changes in plasma lipids and lipoproteins in overweight men during weight loss through dieting as compared with exercise. *N Engl J Med* 1988;319:1173–1179.
107. Schotte DE, Stunkard AJ. The effects of weight reduction on blood pressure in 201 obese patients. *Arch Intern Med* 1990;150:1701–1704.
108. Consensus development conference. Diet and exercise in non-insulin dependent diabetes mellitus. *Diabetes Care* 1987;10:639–644.
109. Tchernof A, Nolan A, Sites CK, et al. Weight loss reduces C-reactive protein levels in obese postmenopausal women. *Circulation* 2002;105:564–569.
110. Kohrt WM, Obert KA, Holloszy JO. Exercise training improves fat distribution patterns in 60–70-year old men and women. *J Gerontol* 1992;47:M99–M105.
111. Levantesi G, Macchia A, Marfisi R, et al. Metabolic syndrome and risk of cardiovascular events after myocardial infarction. *J Am Coll Cardiol* 2005;46:277–283.
112. Dracup K, Meleis AI, Clark S, et al. Group counseling in cardiac rehabilitation: effect on patient compliance. *Patient Educ Couns* 1984;6:169–177.
113. Brownell KD. *The LEARN program for weight control,* 6th ed. Dallas: American Health Publishing Company, 1994.
114. Harvey-Berino J. Weight loss in the clinical setting: applications for cardiac rehabilitation. *Coron Artery Dis* 1998;9:795–798.
115. Savage P, Lee M, James S, et al. Weight reduction in the cardiac rehabilitation setting. *J Cardiopulm Rehabil* 2002;22:154–160.
116. Helmrich SP, Ragland DR, Leung RW, et al. Physical activity and reduced occurrence of non-insulin-dependent diabetes mellitus. *N Engl J Med* 1991;325:147–152.
117. Manson JE, Rimm EB, Stampfer MJ, et al. Physical activity and incidence of non-insulin-dependent diabetes mellitus in women. *Lancet* 1991;338: 774–778.
118. Pan XR, Li GW, Hu YH, et al. Effects of diet and exercise in preventing NIDDM in people with impaired glucose tolerance. The Da Qing IGT and Diabetes Study. *Diabetes Care* 1997;20:537–544.
119. Tuomilehto J, Lindstrom J, Eriksson JG, et al. Prevention of type 2 diabetes mellitus by changes in lifestyle among subjects with impaired glucose tolerance. *N Engl J Med* 2001;344:1343–1350.
120. Diabetes Control and Complications Trial (DCCT) Research Group. Effect of intensive diabetes management on macrovascular events and risk factors in the Diabetes Control and Complications Trial. *Am J Cardiol* 1995;75: 894–903.
121. Horton ES. Role and management of exercise in diabetes mellitus. *Diabetes Care* 1988;11:201–211.
122. Dylewicz P, Bienkowska S, Szczesniak L, et al. Beneficial effect of short-term endurance training on glucose metabolism during rehabilitation after coronary bypass surgery. *Chest* 2000;117:47–51.
123. Lehto S, Ronnemaa T, Haffner SM, et al. Dyslipidemia and hyperglycemia predict coronary heart disease events in middle-aged patients with NIDDM. *Diabetes* 1997;46:1354–1359.
124. Haffner SM. Epidemiological studies on the effects of hyperglycemia and improvement of glycemic control on macrovascular events in type 2 diabetes. *Diabetes Care* 1999;22[Suppl 3]:C54–C56.
125. Ruderman N, Devlin JT, eds. *The health professional's guide to diabetes and exercise.* Alexandria, VA: American Diabetes Association, 1995.
126. Vongvanich P, Bairey Merz CN. Supervised exercise and electrocardiographic monitoring during cardiac rehabilitation: impact on patient care. *J Cardiopulm Rehabil* 1996;16:233–238.
127. Hermanson B, Omenn GS, Kronmal RA, et al. Beneficial six-year outcome of smoking cessation in older men and women with coronary artery disease. *N Engl J Med* 1988;319:1365–1369.
128. Wilhelmsson C, Vedin JA, Elmfeldt D, et al. Smoking and myocardial infarction. *Lancet* 1975;1:415–419.
129. Carson P, Phillips R, Lloyd M, et al. Exercise after myocardial infarction: a controlled trial. *J R Coll Physicians Lond* 1982;16:147–151.
130. Linden W, Stossel C, Maurice J. Psychosocial interventions for patients with coronary artery disease: a meta-analysis. *Arch Intern Med* 1996;156: 745–752.
131. Glassman AH, O'Connor CM, Califf RM, et al. Sertraline treatment of major depression in patients with acute MI or unstable angina. *JAMA* 2002;288:701–709.
132. van Dixhoorn J, Duivenvoorden HJ. Effect of relaxation therapy on cardiac events after myocardial infarction: a five-year follow-up study. *J Cardiopulm Rehabil* 1999;19:178–185.
133. Watson WC, Buchanan KD, Dickson C. Serum cholesterol levels after myocardial infarction. *Br Med J* 1963;2:709–712.
134. Ronnemaa T, Viikari J, Irjala K, et al. Marked decrease in serum HDL cholesterol level during acute myocardial infarction. *Acta Med Scand* 1980;207:161–166.
135. Ryder REJ, Hayes TM, Mulligan IP, et al. How soon after myocardial infarction should plasma lipid values be assessed? *Br Med J* 1984;289: 1651–1653.
136. Rosenson R. Myocardial injury: the acute phase response and lipoprotein metabolism. *J Am Coll Cardiol* 1993;22:933–940.
137. Cunningham MJ, Boucher TM, McCabe CH, et al. Changes in total cholesterol and high-density lipoprotein cholesterol in men after coronary bypass grafting. *Am J Cardiol* 1987;60:1393–1394.
138. Parmley WW. Position report on cardiac rehabilitation: recommendations of the American College of Cardiology on cardiovascular rehabilitation. *J Am Coll Cardiol* 1986;7:451–453.
139. Curnier D, Savage PD, Ades PA. Geographic distribution of cardiac rehabilitation programs in the U.S. *J Cardiopulm Rehabil* 2005:25:80–84.
140. Ades PA, Waldmann ML, McCann W, et al. Predictors of cardiac rehabilitation participation in older coronary patients. *Arch Intern Med* 1992; 152:1033–1035.
141. Fletcher GF, Chiaramida AJ, LeMay MR, et al. Telephonically-monitored home exercise early after coronary bypass surgery. *Chest* 1984;86: 198–202.
142. Oldridge NB. Compliance and dropout in cardiac rehabilitation. *J Cardiac Rehabil* 1984;4:166–177.
143. Burke L, Dunbar-Jacob J, Hill M. Compliance with cardiovascular disease prevention strategies: a review of the research. *Ann Behav Med* 1997;19: 239–263.
144. Dunbar-Jacob J, Dwyer K, Dunning E. Compliance with antihypertensive regimen: a review of the research in the 1980's. *Ann Behav Med* 1991; 13:31–39.
145. Kruse W. Compliance with treatment of hyperlipoproteinemia in medical practice and clinical trials. In: Kramer J, Spilker B, eds. *Patient compliance in medical practice and clinical trials.* New York: Raven Press, 1991: 175–186.
146. Carlson JJ, Johnson JA, Franklin BA, et al. Program participation, exercise adherence, cardiovascular outcomes, and program cost of traditional versus modified cardiac rehabilitation. *Am J Cardiol* 2000;86:17–23.
147. Lee JY, Jensen BE, Oberman A, et al. Adherence in the training levels comparison trial. *Med Sci Sports Exerc* 1996;28:47–52.
148. Oldridge N, Jones N. Improving patient compliance in cardiac exercise rehabilitation: effects of a written agreement and self-monitoring. *J Cardiopulm Rehabil* 1983;3:257–262.
149. Mulcahy R. Influence of cigarette smoking on morbidity and mortality after myocardial infarction. *Br Heart J* 1983;49:410–415.
150. Singh RB, Rostogi S, Verma R, et al. Randomized controlled trial of cardioprotective diet in patients with recent acute myocardial infarction: results of one year follow up. *Br Med J* 1992;304:1015–1019.
151. Hypertension Detection and Follow-up Program Cooperative Group. Persistence of reduction in blood pressure and mortality of participants in the Hypertension Detection and Follow-up Program. *JAMA* 1988;259: 2113–2122.
152. Grace SL, Evindar A, Kung T, et al. Increasing access to cardiac rehabilitation: automatic referral to the program nearest home. *J Cardiopulm Rehabil* 2004;24:171–174.
153. Nickel JT, Chirikos TN. Functional disability of elderly patients with long-term coronary heart disease: a sex-stratified analysis. *J Gerontol* 1990;45: S60–68.
154. Pinsky JL, Jette AM, Branch LG, et al. The Framingham Disability Study: relationship of various coronary heart disease manifestations to disability in older persons living in the community. *Am J Public Health* 1990;80:1363–1368.
155. Ades PA. Cardiac rehabilitation in older coronary patients. *J Am Geriatr Soc* 1999;47:98–105.
156. Brochu M, Savage P, Lee M, et al. Effects of resistance training on physical function in older disabled women with coronary heart disease. *J Appl Physiol* 2002;92:672–678.
157. Ades PA, Savage PD, Cress ME, et al. Resistance training improves performance of daily activities in disabled older women with coronary heart disease. *Med Sci Sports Exerc* 2003;35:1265–1270.
158. Ades PA, Waldmann ML, Polk D, et al. Referral patterns and exercise response in the rehabilitation of female coronary patients aged ≥62 years. *Am J Cardiol* 1992;69:1422–1425.

159. Bueno H. Influence of sex on the short-term outcome of elderly patients with a first acute myocardial infarction. *Circulation* 1995;92:1133–1140.
160. Cannistra LB, Balady GJ, O'Malley CJ, et al. Comparison of the clinical profile and outcome of women and men in cardiac rehabilitation. *Am J Cardiol* 1992;69:1274–1279.
161. Rich MW, Bosner MS, Chung MK, et al. Is age an independent predictor of early and late mortality in patients with acute myocardial infarction? *Am J Med* 1992;92:7–13.
162. Balady GJ, Jette D, Scheer J, et al. Changes in exercise capacity following cardiac rehabilitation in patients stratified according to age and gender. *J Cardiopulm Rehabil* 1996;16:38–46.

CHAPTER 14 ■ AN INTEGRATED APPROACH TO RISK FACTOR MODIFICATION

ROBERT C. BLOCK AND THOMAS A. PEARSON

NEED FOR A SYSTEMATIC APPROACH TO PREVENTIVE CARDIOLOGY

An extensive base of scientific evidence supporting the practice of preventive cardiology grows significantly each year. The role of various risk factors in the atherosclerotic process and the effects of their reduction on clinical course have been clearly outlined in studies of vascular biology, natural history, and clinical trials. The development of consensus statements regarding clinical recommendations is helping to transform the practice of cardiovascular disease (CVD) prevention, but the translation of knowledge into effective clinical practice has been shown to be consistently inadequate (1–4). The time has come to "use what we know" (3). Said another way, by Claude Lenfant, former director of the National Heart, Lung and Blood Institute, "the real challenge of this new millennium may indeed be to strike an appropriate balance between the pursuit of exciting new knowledge and the full application of strategies known to be extremely effective, but considered underused" (5).

Rationale for a Comprehensive Prevention Strategy

The practice of cardiology has become increasingly specialized, with the creation of clinical subdisciplines limited to invasive cardiology, heart failure, hypertension, lipidology, and so on. The central thesis of this chapter emphasizes one characteristic shared by all patients with CVD, namely the need for both short-term and long-term reductions in risk of myocardial infarction and cardiac death. The rationale for a comprehensive approach to CVD risk management is therefore shared by a wide spectrum of patients (Table 14.1).

First, atherosclerosis is a diffuse disease involving multiple arterial beds and target organs, potentially leading to a host of life-threatening complications other than coronary artery disease. Once acute manifestations of ischemia are controlled, the focus of attention must be on the pathophysiology of the atherosclerotic process. Although revascularization is highly effective in relieving symptoms caused by severe atherosclerotic lesions in the short term, it cannot address the underlying diffuse nature of the atherosclerotic process. Many interventions such as the use of antiplatelet drugs, angiotensin-converting-enzyme (ACE) inhibitors, and β blockers, show sustained benefits compared to placebo over the long term. Clinical trials of lifestyle change and drugs that lower low-density-lipoprotein (LDL) cholesterol, such as hydroxymethylglutaryl coenzyme A (HMG-CoA) reductase inhibitors, show progressive gains in benefit over the course of the trials, suggesting enhanced survival benefit after several years of therapy, across a range of cardiac outcomes, such as angina, the need for revascularization, congestive heart failure, cardiac mortality, and total mortality.

Second, because atherosclerosis is a diffuse disease, it involves the renal, peripheral, and cerebrovascular beds. To focus on disease in one vascular bed without attention to inevitable multiorgan complications would detract from a cohesive preventive strategy. For many chronic vascular diseases such as peripheral arterial disease, aortic aneurysm, and cerebrovascular disease, the main cause of death is myocardial infarction and sudden cardiac death. Indeed, the control of hyperlipidemia, hypertension, smoking, and other CVD risk factors demonstrates reduction in clinical events in all vascular beds, and trials frequently use a composite endpoint to provide a more comprehensive view of the intervention's benefits.

Third, a number of randomized trials have better defined the role of risk factor management in the overall treatment of the patient with an acute coronary syndrome (ACS). One observation is that reductions in clinical events in ACS can occur rapidly after initiation of aggressive risk factor management. For example, the PROVE-IT Study (6), a randomized trial of atorvastatin 80 mg/day versus pravastatin 40 mg/day in ACS patients, gave evidence for a benefit for atorvastatin after only a few weeks of therapy, and significant benefits in the

TABLE 14.1

RATIONALE FOR COMPREHENSIVE RISK FACTOR MODIFICATION INTEGRATED INTO THE OVERALL MANAGEMENT OF THE PATIENT WITH CORONARY ARTERY DISEASE

- Address the underlying atherosclerotic disease rather than its symptomatic presentation
  - Cumulative reduction in events over a long period
  - Reduced risk of disease and symptoms in other vascular beds (e.g., renal, peripheral, and cerebrovascular)
- Improve effectiveness of acute cardiac care
  - Risk factor modifications improve outcomes when instituted early
  - Risk factor modifications complement acute interventions
  - Benefits are additive to those of other cardiologic procedures
- Improve safety of interventions
  - Reduce adverse interactions among risk factor modifications
  - Improve monitoring of adverse events in the setting of acute intervention
- Improve continuing care and adherence by making risk factor modification the primary treatment paradigm in both acute and chronic stages of cardiologic care

atorvastatin arm were observed in both the 0- to 6-month and 6- to18-month periods of the study. PROVE-IT and other studies support recommendations that risk factor interventions be implemented immediately rather than put off to a follow-up visit or cardiac rehabilitation program (7).

Fourth, there is strong evidence that risk factor management complements cardiologic interventions targeting ischemia, arrhythmias, and congestive heart failure. Analyses of randomized trials of antiplatelet and lipid-lowering drugs routinely identify benefits independent of β blockers, ACE inhibitors, revascularization, and so on. Indeed, certain interventions may synergize to multiply the benefits. An analysis of placebo-controlled trials of pravastatin suggests such a synergistic interaction with aspirin, in which combined aspirin and pravastatin provides greater risk reduction than that expected for the sum of risk reductions of either intervention alone (8). One consequence of these additive benefits is the striking reduction in case-fatality rates in patients in contemporary randomized trials. For example, the TNT Study suggested that, even in the atorvastatin 10-mg/day arm, the coronary death rate among patients with stable coronary disease was as low at 2.5% over the 4.9-year course of the study as compared to the threefold- to fourfold-greater coronary mortality rates in historic cohorts of patients with chronic coronary disease (9).

Fifth, the long-term medical management of CVD with drugs and devices will likely expand significantly. An increasing array of prescription medications is being added to our armamentarium, with potential for benefit as well as adverse drug–drug and drug–device interactions. Strong evidence supports the notion that statin treatment benefits everyone at high risk of CVD, regardless of their LDL, shifting the paradigm from LDL-goal attainment to one focused on universal and aggressive lipid reduction. Results of the Heart Protection Study, PROVE-IT (6), TNT (9), IDEAL (10), and others support revision of the recommendations of the Adult Treatment Panel III (ATP III) of the National Cholesterol Education Program toward more aggressive lipid reduction, particularly for those at very high risk (7). Therefore, more patients treated with aggressive interventions require diligent monitoring for adverse side effects of single agents as well as drug interactions. The ASCOT Study may provide a good example (11). One arm of the study compared two antihypertensive regimens: β blocker (atenolol) with thiazide diuretic, as needed, versus calcium channel blocker (amlodipine) plus ACE inhibitor (perindopril), as needed. The calcium channel blocker/ACE arm led to a small (1.9 to 2.7 mm Hg) blood pressure reduction but an impressive reduction (16%) in total cardiovascular events. The β blocker/thiazide arm demonstrated an 11% reduction in high-density-lipoprotein (HDL) cholesterol and a 23% increase in serum triglyceride levels. HDL-cholesterol change was the largest contributor to the endpoint differences. This suggests that blood pressure management that has a detrimental effect on the lipid profile may be inferior to one that does not. If reduction in the overall risk of a cardiac event is the goal of therapy, these unforeseen effects of risk factor interventions need to be considered in selecting the "best" regimen.

Finally, a number of psychosocial benefits to the patient accrue from an integrated approach to risk factor modification. The amelioration of the effects of depression, enhanced social support, and improved compliance/adherence with lifestyle and pharmacologic interventions are all positive consequences of a comprehensive risk factor management program. An acute coronary syndrome or a revascularization procedure provides the "teachable moment" in which the patient might adopt fundamental changes in lifestyle and commitment to long-term drug therapy. The delay in instituting preventive interventions for weeks or months sends the message that these interventions are of secondary importance and mere adjuncts to more effective cardiologic procedures. As previously discussed, the evidence from randomized trials overwhelmingly supports at least as powerful a role for lifestyle and pharmacologic interventions over the short and long term as any others in modern cardiology. The message to the patient should be that the acute management of symptomatic disease must be followed up by treatment of the underlying disease process over the remainder of the patient's life.

Evidence for the Underutilization of Interventions to Reduce Risk

The American College of Cardiology (ACC), American Heart Association (AHA), and other organizations have developed a number of preventive cardiology guideline statementsbased on basic science, epidemiologic, and randomized, controlled trial evidence. Despite this body of evidence and a consensus on effectiveness, use of risk reduction interventions is disappointing when seen from a variety of viewpoints.

From a population perspective, blood pressure control improved in the 1990s, yet only an estimated 49% of individuals aged 65 and older with hypertension have a blood pressure of less than 140/90 mm Hg (12). Data for all age groups from the 1999–2000 National Health and Nutrition Examination Survey demonstrated that 68.9% of individuals with hypertension were aware of their diagnosis, 58.4% were treated, and only 31% had their blood pressure controlled (13). Mexican Americans, women, and those aged 60 years and older had significantly lower rates of control than men, non-Hispanic whites, and younger individuals (Fig. 14.1).

The evidence also demonstrates low success in achieving lipid-lowering treatment goals, particularly in coronary heart disease and high-risk noncoronary disease groups (2). In the Lipid Treatment Assessment Project study performed in 1997 in 618 physicians who were frequent prescribers of lipid-lowering drugs, only 18% of their patients with known coronary heart disease achieved the National Cholesterol Education Program's goal for LDL cholesterol, along with 37% of high-risk and 68% of low-risk patients. The reasons for the low success rate were

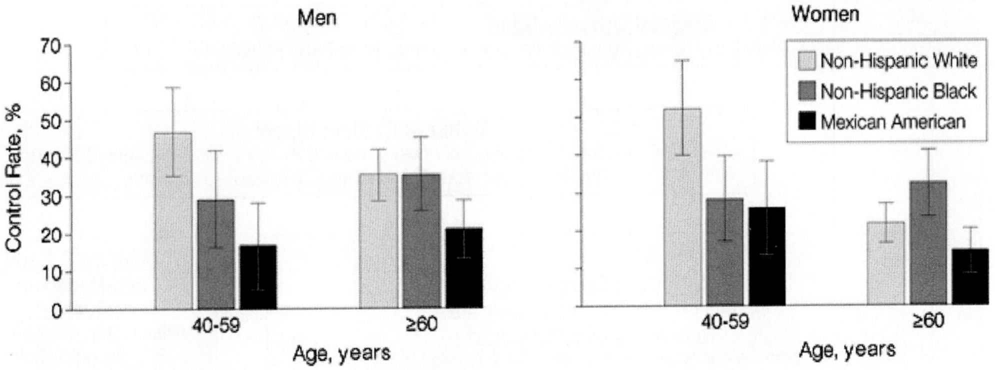

FIGURE 14.1. Overall hypertension control rates in 1999 to 2000 by age and race/ethnicity in men and women. Error bars indicate 95% confidence intervals. Data are weighted to the U.S. population. For comparisons between racial/ethnic groups (with non-Hispanic whites as the referent), p values are as follows: For Mexican Americans, men aged 40 to 59 years, $p < .001$; men aged at least 60 years, $p = .003$; women aged 40 to 59 years, $p = .002$; and women aged at least 60 years, $p = .04$. For non-Hispanic blacks, men aged 40 to 59 years, $p = .02$; men aged at least 60 years, $p = .51$; women aged 40 to 59 years, $p = .003$; and women aged at least 60 years, $p = .98$. (From Hajjar I, Kotchen TA. Trends in prevalence, awareness, treatment, and control of hypertension in the United States, 1988–2000. *JAMA* 2003;290(2): 199–206.)

identified as a lack of the use of medications, inappropriate choices or doses of medication, and infrequent use of medicine combinations. Eighty percent of patients did not receive dietary advice. The NEPTUNE II Study (14), performed in 2004, used a protocol similar to that of the L-TAP Study. A significant improvement in achievement of LDL-cholesterol goals was found, but only 57% of CHD patients attained their LDL-cholesterol goals. Physicians in the United States also do not appear to follow national recommendations pertaining to the screening of family members of their high-risk CVD patients. In one study, the documentation of a discharge plan recommending the screening of family members of patients younger than age 55 years was made in less than 1% of inpatient medical records (15). More optimistic data reveal that hospital compliance with smoking cessation guidelines for patients with an acute myocardial infarction has improved, with an estimated 84% receiving counseling (16). The data reveal that what is achievable in clinical trials does not generally translate into everyday practice, a phenomenon otherwise known as the "treatment gap."

STRATEGIES FOR INTEGRATION OF COMPREHENSIVE RISK REDUCTION INTO CARDIOLOGIC PRACTICE

The treatment gaps observed in cardiovascular risk reduction are also seen in the management of a variety of other chronic diseases. Cardiovascular risk factor modification is a long-term process that requires patient and physician to assume a chronic disease management paradigm that demands significant modification in lifestyle and adherence to pharmacologic interventions. For such regimens to be successful, a multidimensional and comprehensive approach requires careful and proactive consideration. The Chronic Care Model (17) described by Wagner for primary care practices can also be applied to cardiovascular disease risk management, given the inherent challenges of any long-term therapy that often involves multiple interventions. The Chronic Care Model has six elements (Table 14.2), which can be applied to cardiovascular disease, with risk factor modification the cornerstone for successful management of the chronic disease (Fig. 14.2).

Role of Societal Organizations

Health care organizations do not function in a vacuum, but are influenced philosophically, intellectually, economically, and legally by a variety of societal organizations, including professional societies (e.g., the American College of Cardiology), voluntary health organizations (e.g., the American Heart Association), governments at the local, state or province, and national levels, and third-party payers, either private or public. One such influence is the development of standards or guidelines on what constitutes good care. A large number of clinical practice guidelines to address the spectrum of issues related to CVD have been published by professional groups, most notably the American Heart Association, the American College of Cardiology, and the U.S. Preventive Services Task Force. These guidelines are comprehensive and designed to be useful in practice settings while incorporating the most recent evidence from the research arena. Included in these guidelines are the evaluation and treatment of patients with (18–20) and without diagnosed CVD (19,20); CVD and its risk factors in minorities (21), women (22), and patients with the metabolic syndrome (23), diabetes (24), hyperlipidemia (7), and hypertension (25); individuals who smoke (26); persons older than the age of 75 years (27); and children and adolescents (28,29). A comprehensive guide to improving cardiovascular health at the community level is also available targeted at health care providers, public health practitioners, and health policy

TABLE 14.2

SIX ELEMENTS OF THE CHRONIC CARE MODEL

Health care organization
Delivery system redesign
Decision support
Clinical information systems
Self-management support
Community resources

Adapted from Bodenheimer T, Wagner EH, Grumbach K. Improving primary care for patients with chronic disease. *JAMA* 2002;288: 1775–1779.

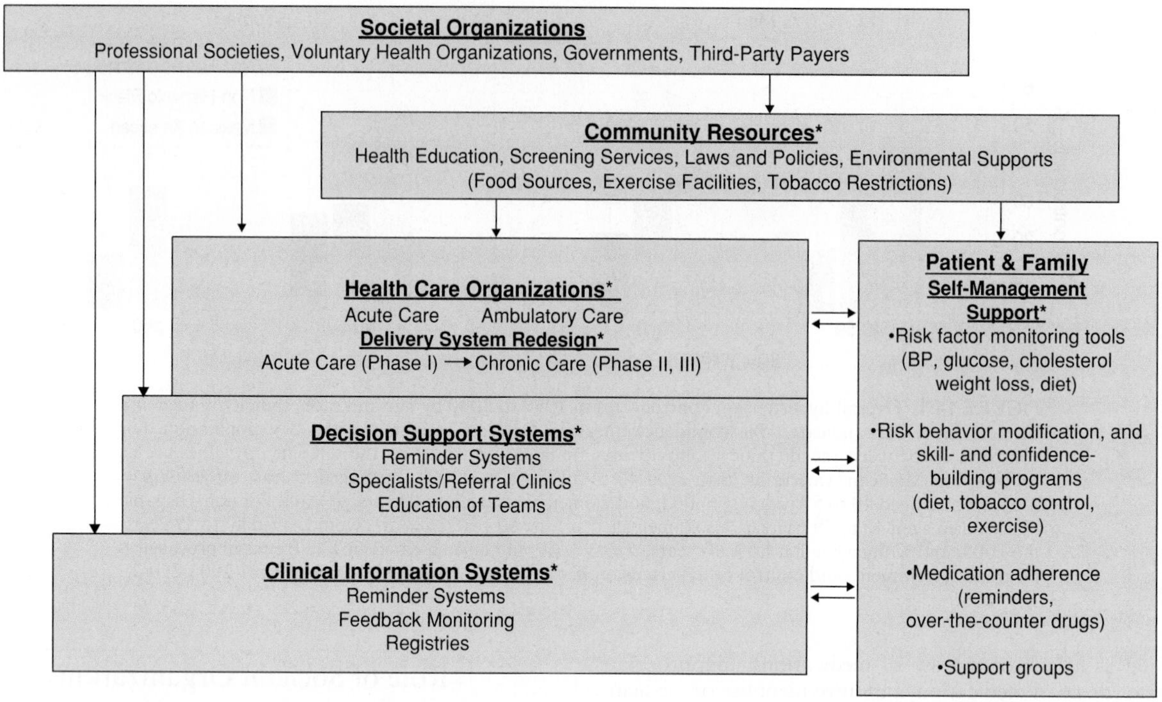

FIGURE 14.2. The Chronic Care Model applied to cardiovascular disease. Asterisks indicate elements of the Chronic Care Model. BP, blood pressure.

makers (30). These guidelines provide a wealth of evidence-based information and are invaluable resources for health care organizations, practicing clinicians, and other stakeholders in the areas of CVD treatment and prevention.

Community Resources

The Chronic Care Model recognizes the need for patients and family to be care providers in a system of self-management. Aiding in this is a community environment that assists both patients and care providers to enable patients to modify lifestyles, access acute and ambulatory health care services, and adhere to complex treatment regimens. The American Heart Association Guide to Improving Cardiovascular Health at the Community Level (30) provides evidence-based recommendations for community-based strategies for CVD reduction (Fig. 14.3). These guidelines specifically address population-based changes in diet, sedentary lifestyle, and tobacco use, diagnosis and treatment of hyperlipidemia and hypertension, and early recognition of symptoms of myocardial infarction and stroke. Although they are applicable to low-risk children and adults, the guidelines have general relevance to patients and providers who would benefit from an environment conducive and supportive

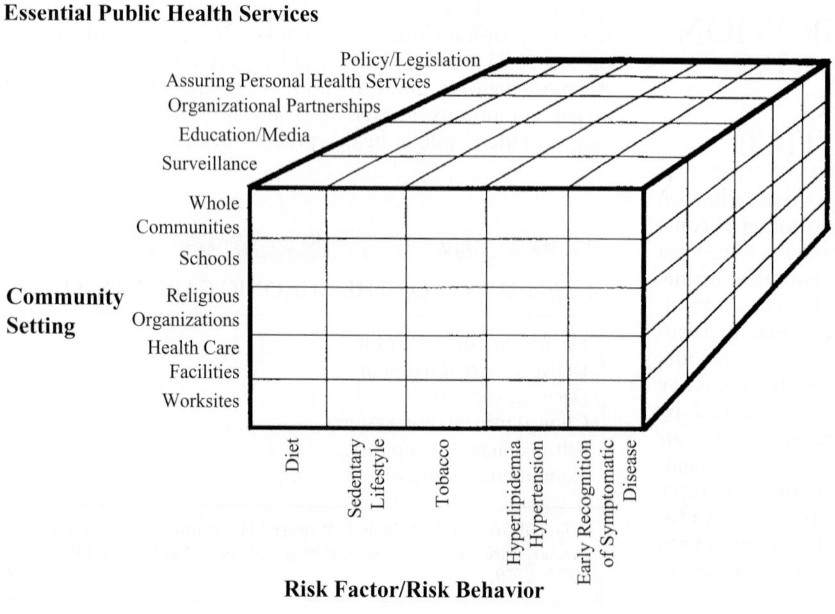

FIGURE 14.3. A conceptual framework for public health practice in cardiovascular disease prevention. (From Pearson TA, Bazzarre TL, Daniels SR, et al. AHA scientific statement. American Heart Association guide for improving cardiovascular health at the community level. A statement for public health practitioners, healthcare providers, and health policy makers from the American Heart Association Expert Panel on Population and Prevention Science. *Circulation* 2003;107;645–651.)

TABLE 14.3

TREATMENT RATES AT DISCHARGE AND AT ONE-YEAR FOLLOW-UP

	Pre-CHAMP (%)		Post-CHAMP (%)	
Therapy	Discharge	One year	Discharge	One year
Aspirin	78	68	92*	94*
β Blocker	12	18	61*	57*
Nitrates	62	42	34*	18*
Calcium blocker	68	58	12*	6*
ACE inhibitor	4	16	56*	48*
Statin	6	10	86*	91*

*$P < 0.01$ pre vs. post-CHAMP at discharge and at one year.
ACE, angiotensin-converting enzyme; CHAMP, Cardiac Hospitalization Atherosclerosis Management Program.

of efforts to control risk factors. Such an environment may include surveillance of the heart disease burden, health education programs, screening services, and government policies supporting healthier foods, exercise facilities, tobacco-free air, and so on. These resources are found in whole communities, but also in places where people work, study, worship, and receive health care.

The Chronic Care Model (17) also incorporates other community resources, including self-help groups, senior centers, and home agencies. Such support for those with cardiovascular disease can help patients by providing rehabilitation after hospitalization, social support, and assistance in chronic disease self-management. Home care agencies, in particular, provide crucial monitoring of carefully designed multidrug regimens that might be life threatening and less effective when patients attempt to manage these issues independently.

Role of Health Care Organizations

The Chronic Care Model alludes to the "Tyranny of the Urgent" (17) as a barrier to the implementation of chronic disease management programs. Health care organizations must identify chronic disease as a priority and provide resources, facilities, systems, and staff, as well as commitment to implement guidelines and standards of chronic disease care. The rationale to do this, even in acute care facilities, is strong (Table 14.1).

Delivery System Redesign

Opportunities for Hospital Services

An inpatient hospital service can reliably and efficiently assess the levels of risk factors present in those patients admitted for revascularization procedures or acute coronary syndromes. The AHA has developed the "Get with the Guidelines" program, a Web-based interactive care coordination and guideline adherence improvement tool that is being used in acute care settings. This tool is designed to be user-friendly for health providers and patients and includes straightforward data tracking that can be provided as feedback to hospitals. The program has been shown to enhance adherence to current guidelines, including lipid treatment and measurement, smoking cessation counseling, and cardiac rehabilitation referral patterns (31). The American College of Cardiology's tool for improving acute myocardial infarction care, Guidelines Applied in Practice (GAP), has also been shown to improve quality when applied to a range of patients, health care providers, and institutions (32). Critical pathway advances, such as the AHA/ACC guidelines for the management of individuals with acute myocardial infarction (33), comprehensively define the care of specific clinical conditions and incorporate secondary prevention guidelines. The Cardiac Hospitalization Atherosclerosis Management Program (CHAMP) at the University of California-Los Angeles has developed and implemented a case-management program that integrates early risk factor intervention in acute care settings with outpatient exercise, smoking cessation, and nutrition programs. This program translated into increasing rates of use of interventions of proven effectiveness during long-term follow-up (34) (Table 14.3) and improved levels of risk factors such as LDL-cholesterol levels (Table 14.4).

The hospital setting represents an opportunity for the inclusion of cardiologists and hospitalists in the assessment and management of cardiovascular disease and the continuation of those recommendations to the primary care setting. An acute coronary syndrome does not occur in a vacuum of other chronic diseases and risk factors. The treatment plans for these patients frequently require revision to be concordant with current guidelines. Primary care involvement while the patient is hospitalized can add credence to specialist recommendations, taking advantage of the "teachable moment" phenomenon, and thus improve long-term care.

TABLE 14.4

LOW-DENSITY-LIPOPROTEIN (LDL) CHOLESTEROL LEVELS DURING FOLLOW-UP

LDL (mg/dL)	Pre-CHAMP 1992/1993 (%) ($n = 256$)	Post-CHAMP 1994/1995 (%) ($n = 301$)
$\leq$100	6	58
101–130	15	16
131–160	18	4
>160	14	0
Not documented	48	22

CHAMP, Cardiac Hospitalization Atherosclerosis Management Program.
From Fonarow GC, Gawlinski A, Moughrabi A, et al. Improved treatment of coronary heart disease by implementation of a Cardiac Hospitalization Atherosclerosis Management Program (CHAMP). *Am J Cardiol* 2001;87:819–822.

Optimal use of the hospital laboratory illustrates the potential for improving risk factor identification. A baseline lipid assessment performed per protocol at the time of hospital admission for acute myocardial infarction is useful because it obtains serum prior to the well-documented reduction of cholesterol levels 24 hours after a myocardial infarction, complies with the AHA/ACC guideline for management of this illness, and ensures the availability of these useful data by clinicians. The process of highlighting abnormal lipid levels aids in their integration into decision-making, promotes guideline adherence, and subsequently improves patient outcomes.

Opportunities for the Cardiovascular Specialist

The physician admitting patients acutely ill with vascular disease, or the cardiovascular specialist who is consulted for advice, diagnoses the condition and outlines a treatment strategy. As this role is defined for the acute illness, it should also incorporate the first phases of risk factor modification. The American College of Cardiology stated that the duties and responsibilities of cardiologists should include service as champions of prevention with "a clear mandate for addressing primary prevention and risk factor control in all settings of patient encounters" (33). The inpatient team provides these high-risk patients with the opportunity to optimize risk factors, with the physician assuming the responsibility to provide a management plan with regard to medical and lifestyle interventions implemented by a multidisciplinary team (nurses, nutritionists, rehabilitation specialists, etc).

Through effective communication to the outpatient team, the plan to modify risk factors initiated in the hospital can be continued on an outpatient basis indefinitely. Effective communication via a discharge summary should emphasize specific risk factor identification and a comprehensive risk management strategy. This, along with the cardiovascular specialist's initiation of an optimal medication regimen at the time of discharge, will help to ensure a focus on preventive measures in which patient and primary care providers alike will receive a consistent message from the specialist (33).

Opportunities for the Primary Care Provider

Primary care providers play a vital role in the prevention of cardiovascular disease. The American Heart Association's 2002 guideline for the primary prevention of cardiovascular disease and stroke recommends a global risk assessment and management strategy for primary care providers with an initial assessment of risk factors at age 20 years (20). This consensus panel stressed the importance of expanding the scope of preventive practice to include a larger number of patients at earlier stages in the disease process, using an environment conducive to long-term relationship building and risk factor modification.

The task of maintaining current knowledge regarding the multitude of diseases addressed by primary care providers is challenging. In addition to the efforts of other organizations, however, the American College of Physicians (ACP) has assisted in this process by outlining primary care guidelines for the management of risk factors and other conditions common in primary care practice (35–39).

Redesign of the ambulatory care protocol should focus on guidelines, involve a multidisciplinary team with defined roles for its members, and use reminder systems or clinical provider education (40,41). Case-management efforts have frequently improved outcomes for individuals with diabetes, mixed comorbidities, and congestive heart failure (42). Clinical care interactive workshop sessions have also been shown to improve physician practice (43). Regular contact of patients with health professionals, nurse case-management programs, and immediate postinterventional prescription of therapy can also improve compliance (44). Data from the Practice Partner Research Network (PPRNet) demonstrated that increased medical system decision support of medical providers can improve chronic disease outcomes and that such enhanced support has the potential to be the most important predictor of these outcomes (45).

Role of Specialty Clinics and Cardiac Rehabilitation Units

A subgroup of patients may benefit from the resources of a preventive cardiology specialty practice. These patients tend to have issues that fall into the categories of rare, risky, recalcitrant, or resistant (the four R's) or a combination of these (5). Some individuals are not responsive to standard treatment and thus would benefit from consultation with a clinician who has extensive experience with more challenging clinical issues. Recalcitrant individuals, for example, may benefit from a team of health care professionals skilled in counseling and behavior modification. A comprehensive preventive cardiology approach may also instill a sense of urgency in patients regarding the need for significant lifestyle change and adherence to medical therapy.

Preventive cardiology programs vary in their structure and expertise, but generally they are more likely to be successful by approaching each patient with a global atherosclerotic disease prevention focus rather than treatment of only one risk factor (46). Programs generally include the services of one or more physicians, as well as nurses, nutritionists, exercise physiologists, ad behavioral scientists, all of whom should have experience with comprehensive risk factor management. Cardiac rehabilitation programs have proven to be beneficial as part of a secondary prevention strategy (47), but, unfortunately, they have been underutilized for a variety of reasons (47,48), with only an estimated 10% to 47% of eligible individuals participating (49). The need exists to extend the benefits of cardiac rehabilitation to groups underrepresented in their use of these programs, such as women, minority groups, and indigent patients, all of whom can also derive significant benefit from such comprehensive and aggressive treatment (50,51). When used, these programs are most effective if they entail a comprehensive, active, and participatory approach to CVD risk reduction (47,48,52) rather than a simple focus on physical training.

To take advantage of the potential social, psychological, and medical benefits inherent within programs, the AHA recommends that programs that consist of exercise training alone do not meet the definition of cardiac rehabilitation (53,54) (Table 14.5).

TABLE 14.5

COMPONENTS OF CARDIAC REHABILITATION FOR COMPREHENSIVE RISK MANAGEMENT

Initial evaluation
Management of lipid levels
Management of hypertension
Cessation of smoking
Weight reduction
Management of diabetes
Psychosocial management
Physical activity counseling and exercise training

Adapted from Balady GJ, Ades PA, Comoss P, et al. Core components of cardiac rehabilitation/secondary prevention programs. A statement for healthcare professionals from the American Heart Association and the American Association of Cardiovascular and Pulmonary Rehabilitation. *Circulation* 2000; 102:1069–1073.

Clinical Information Systems and Decision Support

The Institute of Medicine (IOM) recommends formal incentives for providers to create organized processes of care to improve quality and calls for governmental economic assistance for provider organizations to improve their clinical information technology (IT) (55,56). Such IT is felt by many to be fundamental to the process of improving health care (41), and the U.S. Department of Health and Human Services has outlined a goal to achieve a nationally relevant electronic medical record by the year 2014.

Computer-based clinical decision support systems have been shown to improve clinical performance for preventive care, drug dosing, and other aspects of medical care (57). This enhanced performance is consistent with data that suggest that most clinical errors are probably related to human limitations in data processing, and that prospective physician reminders can reduce these mistakes (58,59). Data from the Practice Partner Research Network has demonstrated that increasing the medical system decision support of medical providers has the potential to be the most important predictor of improved chronic disease outcomes while achieving lower care costs when compared with older record systems (45,60,61). Physician reminders have the potential to improve cholesterol and hypertension management of cardiovascular disease patients through the use of real-time feedback (62–65). Although clinician resistance to the use of an electronic medical record (EMR) needs to be considered, evidence has shown that preexisting concerns are generally outweighed by positive experiences (66). Attention to organizational culture throughout the process of EMR design and implementation is also associated with improved clinician enthusiasm (67).

Self-Management Support for Patients and Their Families

Patients with chronic conditions often become their own caregivers, with assumption of self-control over a range of lifestyle and pharmacologic interventions (17). Self-management support is the process of empowering patients to have confidence in the treatment regimen as well as their ability to fully implement it. Adherence to recommended therapies is one measure of the ability of an individual to understand the rationale for a regimen as well as the need to implement it chronically. Deficiencies in optimal treatment as a result of poor adherence to recommendations represent a huge issue, with an estimated 50% of patients following instructions for prescribed therapies and poor compliance with prescribed medication or placebo associated with increased mortality (65–67). Noncompliance includes patients keeping about 75% of the appointments that they make and 50% of those made for them and approximately 50% of medications prescribed in the United States each year being taken improperly (68,69).

Barriers identified as important in predicting poor adherence to recommended therapies include limited patient motivation and poor habit reinforcement, prompt and intolerable medication side effects, and complex or confusing regimens (69). In dietary approaches to controlling hypertension, the number of complaints about the diets, attendance at treatment sessions, household composition, and baseline physiologic levels are predictive of compliance (70). Other issues that correlate with compliance include patient knowledge, confidence in his or her ability to follow recommended behaviors, perceptions of health, availability of social support, the physician–patient relationship (71), and prior levels of compliance (72–74) (Table 14.6).

TABLE 14.6

STRATEGIES DEMONSTRATED TO BE SUCCESSFUL IN IMPROVING COMPLIANCE WITH CARDIOVASCULAR DISEASE PREVENTION REGIMENS

Signed agreements
Behavioral skill training
Self-monitoring
Telephone/mail contact
Spouse support
Self-efficacy enhancement
Contingency contracting
Exercise prescription: frequent short periods
External cognitive aids: appointment reminder letter, follow-up letter for missed appointments, medication refill reminder, unit-of-use packaging, medication reminder chart
Persuasive communication
Convenience: work-site clinic (nurse managed)
Nurse-managed intervention
School-based food service program plus education

Adapted from Burke LE, Dunbar-Jacob GM, Hill MN. Compliance with cardiovascular disease prevention strategies: a review of the research. *Ann Behav Med* 1997;19:239–263.

A variety of methods to improve adherence has been investigated. Reducing the need for multiple daily doses has been documented to improve compliance, particularly for medications that are required chronically (75,76). An increase in patient-centeredness that incorporates shared decision-making may lead to improved adherence to these therapies (77). A variety of devices to monitor risk factor change is available for personal use, including home blood pressure and glucose monitors, accurate scales for body weight, and a number of nutritional assessment programs for tracking dietary change. Patient education by members of the preventive cardiology team should focus on building skills and confidence in lifestyle modification such as exercise regimens, dietary change, and tobacco cessation. Other steps found to be effective involve information and reminders, self-monitoring, more convenient care, reinforcement, family therapy, counseling, and other measures that focus the attention of, or provide more supervision by, health care providers (78).

CONTROVERSIES AND PERSONAL PERSPECTIVES

The total burden of CVD and its risk factors will continue to increase. First, on the basis of the aging of the population and falling case-fatality rates, one can predict that the prevalence of CVD and other vascular diseases will continue to increase for at least the next 30 years. Second, current guidelines greatly expand the indications for aggressive treatment of risk factors, identifying an increasing number of individuals who are at levels of risk requiring intervention. Third, the earlier identification of CVD through improved technologies will expand the number of high risk individuals, thus providing additional patients requiring clinical care in this population. These worrisome and highly likely scenarios will force us to expend our resources prudently, based on efficiency and cost-effectiveness proven in randomized trials. The use of new interventions can be accepted only if they can be proven to enhance or replace older ones (4).

Only through shared responsibilities can efforts truly succeed. More and more, medicine is becoming collaborative and less authoritarian, as emphasized in the Chronic Care Model. These tenets should be applied throughout the stages of care of those with CVD, translating into cooperation among nurses, pharmacists, primary care providers, and cardiovascular specialists, using comprehensive, evidence-based care. Cardiovascular specialists cannot avoid managing risk factors, nor can they relieve primary care providers of their responsibility to perform chronic risk factor management.

THE FUTURE

The myriad of preventive options has demonstrated huge potential benefits in the management of CVD. The cardiovascular specialist's role needs to include mastery of these skills that show such benefits. At the same time, primary care providers also need to practice risk factor management, given their central role in primary prevention as well as their commitment to treating patients globally. Finally, patients and their families need to be supported in their efforts to self-manage their cardiovascular risk, which may include assessments (e.g., blood pressure and glucose measurements) as well as interventions (e.g., over-the-counter drugs such as aspirin and cholesterol-lowering agents) that previously had been under the exclusive control of the physician. The persistent treatment gap suggests that old models of specialist–patient care require revision into fundamentally different systems of care, such as that proposed by the Chronic Care Model.

ACKNOWLEDGMENT

We acknowledge an Institutional National Research Service Award (T32 HL07937) from the National Heart, Lung, and Blood Institute, National Institutes of Health, supporting Dr. Block's Preventive Cardiology Research Fellowship.

References

1. Benjamin IJ, Smith SC, Cooper RS, et al. 33rd Bethesda Conference: Task Force #1. Magnitude of the prevention problem: opportunities and challenges. *J Am Coll Cardiol* 2002: 40(4):588–603.
2. Pearson TA, Laurora I, Chu H, et al. The Lipid Treatment Assessment Project (L-TAP): a multicenter survey to evaluate the percentages of dyslipidemic patients receiving lipid-lowering therapy and achieving low-density lipoprotein goals. *Arch Intern Med* 2000: 160(4):459–467.
3. World Health Organization. *Integrated management of cardiovascular risk. Report of a WHO meeting. Geneva, 9-12, July 2002.* Geneva: World Health Organization, 2002.
4. Ockene IS, Hayman LL, Pasternak RC, et al. 33rd Bethesda Conference: Task Force #4. Adherence issues and behavior changes: achieving a long-term solution. *J Am Coll Cardiol* 2002: 40(4):630–640.
5. Lenfant C. Conquering cardiovascular disease: progress and promise. *JAMA* 1999;282:2068–2070.
6. Cannon CP, Braunwald E, McCabe CH, et al. Pravastatin or Atorvastatin Evaluation and Infection Therapy-Thrombolysis in Myocardial Infarction 22 Investigators. Intensive versus moderate lipid lowering with statins after acute coronary syndromes. *N Engl J Med* 2004;350:1495–1504.
7. Grundy SM, Cleeman JI, Merz NB, et al. Implications of recent clinical trials for the National Cholesterol Education Program Adult Treatment Panel III Guidelines. *Circulation* 2004;110:227–239.
8. Hennekens CH, Sacks FM, Tonkin A, et al Additive benefits of pravastatin and aspirin to decrease risks of cardiovascular disease: randomized and observational comparisons of secondary prevention trials and their meta-analyses. *Arch Intern Med* 2004;164(1):40–44.
9. LaRosa JC, Grundy SM, Waters DD, et al. Intensive lipid lowering with atorvastatin in patients with stable coronary disease. *N Engl J Med* 2005; 352:1425–1435.
10. Pedersen TR, Faergeman O, Kastelein JJP, et al. High-dose atorvastatin versus usual-dose simvastatin for secondary prevention after myocardial infarction: the IDEAL study: a randomized controlled trial. *JAMA* 2005; 294:2437–2445.
11. Sever PS, Dahlof B, Poulter NR, et al; ASCOT investigators. Prevention of coronary and stroke events with atorvastatin in hypertensive patients who have average or lower-than-average cholesterol concentrations, in the Anglo-Scandinavian Cardiac Outcomes Trial-Lipid Lowering Arm (ASCOT-LLA): a multicentre randomised controlled trial. *Lancet* 2003;361:1149–1158.
12. Psaty BM, Manolio TA, Smith NL, et al. Time trends in high blood pressure control and the use of antihypertensive medications in older adults. The Cardiovascular Health Study. *Arch Intern Med* 2002;162:2325–2332.
13. Hajjar I, Kotchen TA. Trends in prevalence, awareness, treatment, and control of hypertension in the United States, 1988–2000. *JAMA* 2003; 290(2):199–206.
14. Davidson MH, Maki KC, Pearson TA, et al. Results of the National Cholesterol Education (NCEP) Program Evaluation Project Utilizing Novel E-Technology (NEPTUNE) II survey and implications for treatment under the recent NCEP Writing Group recommendations. *Am J Cardiol* 2005;96(4): 556–563.
15. Swanson JR, Pearson, TA. Screening family members at high risk for coronary artery disease, why isn't it done? *Am J. Prev Med* 2001;20:50–55(6).
16. Williams SC, Schmaltz SP, Morton DJ, et al. Quality of care in US hospitals as reflected by standardized measures, 2002–2004. *N Eng J Med* 2005;353(3):255–264.
17. Bodenheimer T, Wagner EH, Grumbach K. Improving primary care for patients with chronic disease. *JAMA* 2002;288:1775–1779.
18. Smith Jr SC, Blair SN, Bonow RO, et al. AHA/ACC guidelines for preventing heart attack and death in patients with atherosclerotic disease: 2001 update. *Circulation* 2001;104:1577–1579.
19. Smith S, Jackson R, Pearson TA, et al. Principles for national and regional guidelines on cardiovascular disease prevention. A scientific statement from the World Heart and Stroke Forum. *Circulation* 2004;109:3112–3121.
20. Pearson TA, Blair SN, Daniels SR, et al. AHA guidelines for primary prevention of cardiovascular disease and stroke: 2002 Update. Consensus panel guide to comprehensive risk reduction for adult patients without coronary or other atherosclerotic diseases. *Circulation* 2002;106:388–391.
21. Yancey AK, Robinson RG, Ross RK, et al. Discovering the full spectrum of cardiovascular disease. Minority Health Summit 2003. Report of the Advocacy Writing Group. *Circulation* 2005;111:e140–e149.
22. Mosca L, Appel LJ, Benjamin EJ, et al. Evidence-based guidelines for cardiovascular disease prevention in women. *Circulation* 2004;109:672–693.
23. Grundy SM, Hansen B, Smith S, et al. Clinical management of metabolic syndrome. Report of the American Heart Association/National Heart, Lung, and Blood Institute/American Diabetes Association Conference on Scientific Issues Related to Management. *Circulation* 2004;109:551–556.
24. Grundy SM, Howard B, Smith S, et al. Prevention Conference VI: diabetes and cardiovascular disease. Executive summary. Conference proceeding for healthcare professionals from a special writing group of the American Heart Association. *Circulation* 2002: 105:2231–2239.
25. Chobanian AV, Bakris GL, Black HR, et al. Seventh report of the Joint National Committee on Prevention, Detection, Evaluation, and Treatment of High Blood Pressure. *Hypertension* 2003;42:1206–1252.
26. Ockene IS, Miller NH. Cigarette smoking, cardiovascular disease, and stroke. *Circulation* 1997;96:3243–3247.
27. Williams MA, Fleg JL, Ades PA, et al. Secondary prevention of coronary artery disease in the elderly (with emphasis on patients >or=75 years of age). An American Heart Association scientific statement from the Council on Clinical Cardiology Subcommittee on Exercise, Cardiac Rehabilitation, and Prevention. *Circulation* 2002;105:1735–1743.
28. Daniels SR, Arnett DK, Eckel RH, et al. Overweight in children and adolescents. Pathophysiology, consequences, prevention, and treatment. *Circulation* 2005;111:1999–2012.
29. Kavey RW, Daniels SR, Lauer RM, et al. American Heart Association guidelines for primary prevention of atherosclerotic cardiovascular disease beginning in childhood. *Circulation* 2003;107:1562–1566.
30. Pearson TA, Bazzarre TL, Daniels SR, et al. American Heart Association guide for improving cardiovascular health at the community level. A statement for public health practitioners, healthcare providers, and health policy makers from the American Heart Association Expert Panel on Population and Prevention Science. *Circulation* 2003;107:645–651.
31. LaBresh KA, Ellrodt AG, Gliklich R, et al. Get with the guidelines for cardiovascular secondary prevention. *Arch Intern Med* 2004;164:203–209.
32. Mehta RH, Montoye CK, Gallogly M, et al, for the GAP Steering Committee of the American College of Cardiology. Improving quality of care for acute myocardial infarction: the Guidelines Applied in Practice (GAP) initiative. *JAMA* 2002;287:1269–1276.
33. Merz CNB, Mensah GA, Fuster V, et al. Task Force #5. The role of cardiovascular specialists as leaders in prevention: From training to champion. 33rd Bethesda Conference: preventive cardiology: how can we do better? *J Am Coll Cardiol* 2002;40:641–649.
34. Fonarow GC, Gawlinski A, Moughrabi S, et al. Improved treatment of coronary heart disease by implementation of a Cardiac Hospitalization Atherosclerosis Management Program (CHAMP). *Am J Cardiol* 2001; 87(7):819–822.
35. Snow V, Barry P, Fihn SD, et al., for the American College of Physicians/American College of Cardiology Chronic Stable Angina Panel. Primary

care management of chronic stable angina and asymptomatic suspected or known coronary artery disease: a clinical practice guideline from the American College of Physicians. *Ann Intern Med* 2004;141:562–567.

36. Snow V, Barry P, Fihn SD, et al. (the ACP/ACC Chronic Stable Angina Panel). Evaluation of primary care patients with chronic stable angina: guidelines from the American College of Physicians. *Ann Intern Med* 2004;141:57–64.
37. Snow V, Aronson MD, Hornbake R, et al., for the Clinical Efficacy Assessment Subcommittee of the American College of Physicians. Lipid control in the management of type 2 diabetes mellitus: a clinical practice guideline from the American College of Physicians. *Ann Intern Med* 2004;140:644–649.
38. Vijan, S, Hayward, RA. Pharmacologic lipid-lowering therapy in type 2 diabetes mellitus: background paper for the American College of Physicians. *Ann Intern Med* 2004;140:650–658.
39. Snow V, Weiss KB, Mottur-Pilson C, for the Clinical Efficacy Assessment Subcommittee of the American College of Physicians. The evidence base for tight blood pressure control in the management of type 2 diabetes mellitus. *Ann Intern Med* 2003;138:587–592.
40. Vijan, S, Hayward RA. Treatment of hypertension in type 2 diabetes mellitus: Blood pressure goals, choice of agents, and setting priorities in diabetes care. *Ann Intern Med* 2003;138:593–602.
41. Casalino L, Gillies RR, Shortell SM, et al. External incentives, information technology, and organized processes to improve health care quality for patients with chronic diseases. *JAMA* 2003;289:434–441.
42. Ornstein S, Jenkins RG, Nietert PJ, et al. A multimethod quality improvement intervention to improve preventive cardiovascular care. *Ann Intern Med* 2004;141:523–532.
43. Thomson O, Freemantle N, Oxman AD, et al. Continuing education meetings and workshops. *Cochrane Database Syst Rev* 2005: 4.
44. Smith SC. Clinical treatment of dyslipidemia: practice patterns and missed opportunities. *Am J Cardiol* 2000;86(12A):62L–65L.
45. Fiefer C, Ornstein SM, Niebert PJ, et al. System supports for chronic illness care and their relationship to clinical outcomes. *Top Health Inf Manage* 2001;22(2):65–72.
46. Genest J. Prevalence of risk factors in men with premature coronary artery disease. *Am J Cardiol* 1991;67:1185–1190.
47. Ades PA. Transforming exercise-based cardiac rehabilitation programs into secondary prevention centers: A national imperative. *J Cardiopulm Rehabil* 2001;21:263–272.
48. Haskell WL, Alderman EL, Fair JM, et al. Effects of intensive multiple risk factor reduction on coronary atherosclerosis and clinical cardiac events in men and women with coronary artery disease. The Stanford Coronary Risk Intervention Project (SCRIP). *Circulation* 1994;89:975–990.
49. Wenger NK, Froelicher ES, Ades PA, et al. *Cardiac rehabilitation: clinical practice guidelines.* (AHCPR publication no. 96-0672) Rockville, MD: Agency for Health Care Policy and Research and the National Heart, Lung, and Blood Institute, 1995.
50. Friedman DB, Williams AN, Levine BD. Compliance and efficacy of cardiac rehabilitation and risk factor modification in the medically indigent. *Am J Cardiol* 1997;79:281–285.
51. Cannistra LB, O'Malley CJ, Balady GJ. Comparison of outcome of cardiac rehabilitation in black women and white women. *Am J Cardiol* 1995;75:890–893.
52. DeBusk RF, Miller NH, Superko HR, et al. A case-management system for coronary risk factor modification after acute myocardial infarction. *Ann Intern Med* 1994;120(9):721–729.
53. Balady GJ, Ades PA, Comoss P, et al. Core components of cardiac rehabilitation/secondary prevention programs. A statement for healthcare professionals from the American Heart Association and the American Association of Cardiovascular and Pulmonary Rehabilitation. *Circulation* 2000; 102:1069–1073.
54. Ades PA. Cardiac rehabilitation and secondary prevention of coronary heart disease. *N Engl J Med* 2001;345(12):892–902.
55. Institute of Medicine. *Crossing the quality chasm: a new health system for the 21st century.* Washington, DC: National Academy Press, 2001.
56. Institute of Medicine. *Leadership by example: coordinating government roles in improving health care policy.* Washington, DC: National Academy Press, 2002.
57. Hunt DL, Haynes RB, Hanna SE, et al. Effects of computer-based clinical decision support systems on physician performance and patient outcomes. *JAMA* 1998;280:1339–1346.
58. Kaushal R, Shojania KG, Bates DW. Effects of computerized physician order entry and clinical decision support systems on medication safety. A systematic review. *Arch Intern Med* 2003;163:1409–1416.
59. McDonald CJ. Protocol-based computer reminders, the quality of care and the non-perfectability of man. *N Engl J Med* 1976;295:1351–1355.
60. Litvin CB, Ornstein SM, Anthony WE, et al. Quality improvement using electronic medical records: a case study of a high-performing practice. *Top Health Inf Manage* 2001;22(2):59–64.
61. Hunt J, Siemienczuk J, Erstgaard P, et al. Use of an electronic medical record in disease management programs: a case study in hyperlipidemia. *Medinfo* 2001;10(Pt 1):825–829.
62. Kinn JW, Marek JC, O'Toole MF, et al. Effectiveness of the electronic medical record in improving the management of hypertension. *J Clin Hypertens* 2002;4(6):415–419.
63. Earnest MA, Ross SE, Wittevrongel L, et al. Use of a patient-accessible electronic medical record in a practice for congestive heart failure: patient and physician experiences. *J Am Med Inf Assoc* 2004;11(5):410–417.
64. Goldstein MK, Coleman RW, Tu SW, et al. Translating research into practice: organization issues in implementing automated decision support for hypertension in three medical centers. *J Am Med Inf Assoc* 2004;11(5);368–376.
65. Irvine J, Baker B, Smith J, et al. Poor adherence to placebo or amiodarone therapy predicts mortality: results from the CAMIAT study. *Psychosom Med* 1999;61(4):566–575.
66. Coronary Drug Project Research Group. Influence of adherence to treatment and response of cholesterol on mortality in the Coronary Drug Project Group. *N Engl J Med* 1980;303:1038–1041.
67. Horwitz R, Viscoli CM, Berkman L, et al. Treatment adherence and risk of death after a myocardial infarction. *Lancet* 1990;336:542–545.
68. Berg JS, Dischler J, Wagner DJ, et al. Medication compliance: a health care problem. *Ann Pharmacother* 1993;27(Suppl):S2–S22.
69. Levine DM. Behavioral and psychosocial factors, processes and strategies. In: Pearson TA, Criqui MH, Luepker RV, et al., eds. *Primer in preventive cardiology*. Dallas, TX: American Heart Association, 1994:217–226.
70. Rudd P. Clinicians and patients with hypertension: unsettled issues about compliance. *Am Heart J* 1995;130(3):572–579.
71. Ciechanowski P, Russo J, Katon W, et al. Influence of patient attachment style on self-care and outcomes in diabetes. *Psychosom Med* 2004;66(5): 720–728.
72. Schmid TL, Jeffrey RW, Onstad L, et al. Demographic, knowledge, physiological, and behavioral variables as predictors of compliance with dietary treatment goals in hypertension. *Addict Behav* 1991;16:151–160.
73. Burke LE, Dunbar-Jacob JM, Hill MN. Compliance with cardiovascular disease prevention strategies: a review of the research. *Ann Behav Med* 1997;19:239–263.
74. Miller NH, Hill M, Kottke T, et al. The multilevel compliance challenge: recommendations for a call to action. *Circulation* 1997;95:1085–1090.
75. Haynes RB, Sackett DL, Taylor DW, et al. Manipulation of the therapeutic regimen to improve compliance: conceptions and misconceptions. *Clin Pharmacol Ther* 1977;22:125–130.
76. Greenberg RN. Overview of patient compliance with medication dosing: a literature review. *Clin Ther* 1984;6:592–599.
77. Schedlbauer A, Schroeder K, Peters TJ, et al. Interventions to improve adherence to lipid lowering medication. *Cochrane Database Syst Rev* 2005;1.
78. Haynes RB, McDonald H, Garg AX, et al. Interventions for helping patients to follow prescriptions for medications. *Cochrane Database Syst Rev* 2005;1.

SECTION TWO
CLINICAL CARDIOLOGY

ROBERT M. CALIFF, M.D.

CHAPTER 15 ■ THE HISTORY

ERIC J. TOPOL

OVERVIEW

The history is the most essential part of the diagnostic evaluation. With the advances in cardiovascular genetics, a detailed family history is more important than ever before. A careful interview with the patient not only lays the foundation for an appropriate further workup, but it also serves as the framework for a bond between patient and physician, thereby promoting mutual respect, trust, and understanding. The need to listen to the patient cannot be adequately emphasized, and this goes beyond what is verbally communicated through gestures and nonverbal language. The major symptoms to review with each patient include chest discomfort or pain, dyspnea or cough, and syncope or palpitations—each of which is discussed in more depth. It is hoped that directly obtaining a meticulous history will become more routine and prioritized in the years ahead.

GENERAL PERSPECTIVE

Obtaining a careful, detailed history is fundamental to the proper evaluation of the patient. This takes time because it requires listening to the patient and, ideally, his or her family members without interruption. Beyond listening, it is vital to cue in to the patient's nonverbal communication, such as affect and gestures. The time spent with the patient and the attitude displayed set the tone for the whole relationship and therefore represent a critical investment for the long-term bond and mutual trust that need to be nurtured. It is important for the patient to understand that the physician is a compassionate person who cares about his or her condition and genuinely wants to help. The relationship that is built on strong communication with attention to details during the interview leads to a "full disclosure" history that often preempts the need for expensive, potentially hazardous, and certainly inconvenient diagnostic testing (1,2). History taking is a true art that yields unique and valuable information.

Before zooming in on the chief complaint, it is helpful to establish the patient's noncardiovascular history and medications and to query the risk factors for atherosclerosis. Pertinent conditions such as thyroid disease, anemia or gastrointestinal bleeding, asthma or chronic bronchitis, recent upper respiratory or viral illness, prostatitis, or arthritis are frequently related to the chief complaint and need to be fully characterized. Similarly, trauma or recent procedures such as oral surgery need to be surveyed. The entire list of medications with corresponding dosages must be known, given the preponderance of symptoms that can arise from side effects of drug therapy. Furthermore, the list of medications often serves as a checkpoint that all relevant medical conditions have been reviewed. With the very common use of supplements, vitamins, and other nontraditional remedies, it is imperative to collect this information. Known allergies should be ascertained, and if coronary angiography is even a remote possibility, direct questioning about exposure to contrast dye or shellfish is imperative.

The risk factors for atherosclerosis must be carefully examined. As reviewed in detail in the first section of this book, each of the "big five"—hypertension, smoking, diabetes, hypercholesterolemia, and family history—is discussed. In this era of recognition of the primacy of genetics for influencing diseases, it is especially essential to obtain a detailed family history to consider for precocious atherosclerotic coronary disease (presenting at younger than 40 years for men or 45 years for women), any history of coronary artery disease, and other heart disease such as hypertrophic cardiomyopathy, arrhythmias, or other conditions (see Chapters 93 and 95). Although a family history of myocardial infarction may not be accurate (3,4), the prognostic value of family history of cardiovascular disease in siblings has been recently emphasized (5).

The patient's weight at the time of graduation from high school and over the next few years (with any significant fluctuations) is helpful information. For a woman, determination of menstrual status and, if she is postmenopausal, of whether hormone replacement therapy has been recommended are important to resolve but are too frequently overlooked. The patient's diet and nutritional status are worthy of full review, and provide some insight into a patient's level of commitment to a healthy lifestyle. Similarly, the level of physical activity and whether regular exercise is part of the patient's weekly routine frame the symptomatic assessment and corroborate the previous commitment to cardiovascular health. The pattern of alcohol use is a particularly worthwhile item about which to question the patient. Similarly, the potential for drug abuse should be explored in particular circumstances. Considerable insight into the psychosocial makeup of the patient is possible if the physician attends to the intensity level and manner in which the patient's words and responses are conveyed.

TABLE 15.1

ASSESSING CARDIOVASCULAR DISABILITY

Canadian cardiovascular society functional classification	Specific activity scale
Ordinary physical activity, such as walking and climbing stairs, does not cause angina. Angina with strenuous, rapid, or prolonged exertion at work or recreation.	Patients can perform to completion any activity requiring ≤7 metabolic equivalents [e.g., can carry 24 lb up eight steps, carry objects that weigh 80 lb, do outdoor work (shovel snow, spade soil), and do recreational activities (skiing, basketball, squash, handball, jog/walk 5 mph)].
Slight limitation of ordinary activity. Walking or climbing stairs rapidly, walking uphill, walking or stair climbing after meals, in cold, in wind, or when under emotional stress, or only during the few hours after awakening. Walking more than two blocks on the level and climbing more than one flight of ordinary stairs at a normal pace and in normal conditions.	Patients can perform to completion any activity requiring ≤5 metabolic equivalents (e.g., have sexual intercourse without stopping, garden, rake, weed, roller skate, dance fox trot, walk at 4 mph on level ground), but cannot and do not perform to completion activities requiring ≥6 metabolic equivalents.
Marked limitation of ordinary physical activity. Walking one to two blocks on the level and climbing more than one flight in normal conditions.	Patients can perform to completion any activity requiring ≤2 metabolic equivalents (e.g., shower without stopping, strip and make bed, clean windows, walk 2.5 mph, bowl, play golf, dress without stopping), but cannot and do not perform to completion any activities requiring ≥3 metabolic equivalents.
Inability to perform any physical activity without discomfort—anginal syndrome may be present at rest.	Patients cannot or do not perform to completion activities requiring ≤2 metabolic equivalents.

Adapted from Criteria Committee, New York Heart Association. *Diseases of the heart and blood vessels: nomenclature and criteria for diagnosis,* 6th ed. Boston: Little, Brown, 1964:114; and Goldman L, Hashimoto B, Cook EF, et al. Comparative reproducibility and validity of systems for assessing cardiovascular functional class: advantages of a new specific activity scale. *Circulation* 1981;64:1227–1234.

EVALUATION OF CARDIOVASCULAR SYMPTOMS

For each patient, a review of cardiovascular symptoms beyond the primary symptom is useful. The major symptoms are chest discomfort, dyspnea, syncope, edema, and fatigue. Other symptoms such as cough, palpitations, orthopnea, and dizziness or light-headedness are supportive and need to be ascertained in relation to the primary complaint. Often, a patient is not in touch with the symptoms or is in such fear or denial that he or she is unlikely to volunteer the information. For this reason, it is imperative to perform detailed questioning about chest discomfort or dyspnea in patients with a clustering of risk factors for atherosclerosis even in the absence of a complaint. Symptoms of atherosclerosis of other arterial beds are systematically surveyed. For the cerebrovasculature, a check on symptoms such as transient loss of speech or motor function (suggesting a transient ischemic attack) or, for the peripheral blood vessels, calf discomfort on exertion that is promptly relieved by rest (suggesting intermittent claudication) helps to resolve the diffuseness of the atherosclerotic process, if present.

A functional classification of the patient's symptoms should be obtained (6,7). For angina, the Canadian Cardiovascular Society Functional Classification System is usually used (Table 15.1), whereas for dyspnea and other symptoms of heart failure, the New York Heart Association Functional Classification is relied on (Table 15.2).

Chest Discomfort, Pain, and Related Symptoms

One of the most frequent yet difficult symptoms to assess is chest discomfort or pain (8–24). Because this can be so frightening to patients, these symptoms may precipitate emergency evaluation. A variety of cardiac and noncardiac conditions can produce chest discomfort or pain, as summarized in Table 15.3. The key to determining whether the discomfort is cardiac is to review its character, location, and precipitating factors. Because conditions such as esophageal reflux and musculoskeletal abnormalities are quite common, it is not unusual for a given

TABLE 15.2

FUNCTIONAL CLASSIFICATION

Class	New York Heart Association functional classification
I	Patients with cardiac disease but without resulting limitations of physical activity. Ordinary physical activity does not cause undue fatigue, palpitations, dyspnea, or anginal pain.
II	Patients with cardiac disease resulting in slight limitation of physical activity. They are comfortable at rest. Ordinary physical activity results in fatigue, palpitation, dyspnea, or anginal pain.
III	Patients with cardiac disease resulting in marked limitation of physical activities. They are comfortable at rest. Less-than-ordinary physical activity causes fatigue, palpitation, dyspnea, or anginal pain.
IV	Patients with cardiac disease resulting in inability to perform any physical activity without discomfort.

Goldman L, Hashimoto B, Cook EF, et al. Comparative reproducibility and validity of systems for assessing cardiovascular functional class: advantages of a new specific activity scale. *Circulation* 1981;64:1227–1234.

TABLE 15.3

CAUSES OF CHEST DISCOMFORT AND PAIN

Cardiac	Noncardiac
Angina	Esophagitis, esophageal spasm, or reflex
Acute myocardial infarction	Peptic ulcer
Aortic dissection	Gallbladder disease
Pericarditis	Musculoskeletal causes, including osteochondritis or cervical disk, thoracic outlet syndrome
Myocarditis	Hyperventilation
	Anxiety
	Psychogenic causes
Mitral valve prolapse	Pneumonia
	Pulmonary embolus
	Pneumothorax
	Pulmonary hypertension

patient to have two or more different types of chest discomfort (23,24). In such instances, a careful assessment of each of the symptom complexes is necessary to determine the underlying condition(s).

Character and Location

Although *angina* literally means "choking," most patients with true angina do not use this term to describe their sensation. Despite Herberden's early description in 1768 of a "painful and most disagreeable sensation in the breast" (25), the unpleasant sensation is more typically characterized as a pressure, tightness, heaviness, or burning. The pressure is not perceived by the patient as "pain," such that the interviewer who specifically asks about pain may be misled. On the other hand, "pain" is much more apt to be used by the patient to describe a heart attack; on occasion, the patient may clench the fist while describing the discomfort—the so-called Levine sign. The discomfort of angina is usually easy to differentiate from the pain of acute myocardial infarction by the duration, radiation, and lack of precipitating or alleviating factors. As opposed to angina, which usually lasts for 1 to 3 minutes, heart attack pain lasts for longer than 10 minutes; rather than having one focus (usually the retrosternal region), there is commonly radiation of the pain, such as down the arm. Heart attack pain is described in more depth in Chapter 19. Angina most commonly is felt in the midline of the chest, but it can manifest exclusively in the jaw or neck, the left shoulder or arm, and, when present in the arm, particularly on the ulnar aspect of the forearm and hand (Table 15.4). Rather than in the chest, the principal pressure or burning can be perceived in the epigastrium, causing the patient to believe the problem is simple indigestion. More rarely, the back interscapular region or the right side of the chest, shoulder, arm, or forearm is involved. Unlike the chest discomfort of angina, severe pain that radiates to the back is a classic indication of aortic dissection. However, patients with aortic dissection or expanding aortic aneurysm can have predominant anterior chest pain that may be mistaken for acute myocardial infarction. In the course of evaluating patients with chest pain, it is helpful to adopt the philosophy of "aortic dissection until proven otherwise" so that this diagnosis is never missed, even though it is a relatively uncommon entity in the current era of improved control of hypertension.

TABLE 15.4

ANGINAL "EQUIVALENTS"

Dyspnea
Jaw or neck discomfort
Shoulder, elbow, or arm discomfort, particularly along the side of the left forearm and hand
Epigastric discomfort
Back (interscapular) discomfort

Chest pain or discomfort in women is more difficult to assess, and there have been studies to address the issue of whether there is gender bias resulting in inappropriate underinvestigation or undertreatment in women (26,27). A careful history and assessment of risk is especially critical among women because the correct diagnosis is more elusive—even with noninvasive testing—and pivotal.

Acute pericarditis is a precordial pain that is typically left sided; it is usually worse with inspiration and described as sharp, often referred to the neck. Unlike angina or myocardial infarction pain, this pain is often positional in character such that if the patient sits up and leans forward, the pain may be relieved. Congenital absence of the pericardium is exceedingly rare, but the telltale symptom is chest pain produced by lying on the left side lasting only a few seconds or minutes (28). On occasion, patients with acute myocarditis may present with chest pain, which may be attributed to pericardial involvement or the actual inflammation of cardiac muscle. Mitral valve prolapse often is accompanied by atypical chest discomfort because it is sharp, stabbing, protracted in duration, and associated with a constellation of symptoms (see Chapter 22).

A long list of noncardiac causes of chest pain or discomfort (Table 15.3) is capped by the esophageal disorders of reflux, esophagitis, or spasm, all of which may coexist in certain patients with myocardial ischemia. Esophageal discomfort can fully mimic the character and location of myocardial ischemic symptoms, but, more commonly, the retrosternal burning or epigastric heaviness is brought on by food ingestion and recumbency, with relief by antacids and H_2-blockers. When there is a sour taste in the mouth (so-called water brash) as a result of the acid reflux, this is helpful in differentiating esophageal-induced symptoms from other etiologies. Other gastrointestinal disorders such as peptic ulcer disease, gall bladder disease, and pancreatitis can produce epigastric discomfort and need to be considered in the differential diagnosis.

The symptoms of chest discomfort may be the presenting feature for a host of musculoskeletal conditions. Costal chondritis, or Tietze syndrome (12), is characterized by a chest wall pain that includes point tenderness and frequently is exacerbated by movement or coughing. Chest wall syndromes are particularly common among cigarette smokers and seem to be responsive to cessation of smoking; the etiology is unclear. A thoracic outlet syndrome is associated with ulnar distribution paresthesias in the arm and forearm that are worsened by arm abduction or lifting. Herpes zoster of the chest wall displays a specific dermatome pattern of the pain with exquisite sensitivity of the skin to touch and ultimately the development of characteristic skin vesicles.

In the continuum of musculoskeletal chest discomfort, terms frequently used for discharge diagnosis in emergency departments when the cause is uncertain are *hyperventilation*, *anxiety*, and the *Da Costa syndromes* (also known as *neurocirculatory asthenia*) (11). Emotional stress precipitates pain characterized by a dull, persistent ache and may be accompanied by point or even diffuse chest wall tenderness (29–33). This pain may last for hours or even days and may be quite localized (e.g., below the left nipple) with a "stabbing" quality. A component of hyperventilation may be diagnosed by eliciting the symptoms of circumoral or fingertip paresthesias with occasional carpal-pedal spasm and the response of the symptoms to breathing into a paper bag. Pulmonary causes of chest discomfort include pneumonia, pneumothorax, pulmonary hypertension, and pulmonary embolus. On occasion, pneumonia can present simultaneously with acute myocardial infarction such that the "either/or" process of ruling out one diagnosis should be considered carefully. Pulmonary hypertension may simulate angina, likely due to right ventricular ischemia. A pneumothorax presents with sudden onset of chest pain in the lateral chest with acute shortness of breath. Pulmonary embolism is also sudden, occurring at rest, and is usually associated with pleuritic chest pain exacerbated by coughing.

Exacerbating and Alleviating Factors

The most helpful aspect of angina is the classic precipitation by exercise or emotional stress. Interestingly, some patients never have angina with peak levels of robust exercise but rather experience the tightness or burning during a high-pressure business meeting or a stressful emotional incident. Cold weather, rushing to do an activity, and heavy meals are all common precipitants of angina. When angina occurs nocturnally or in the early morning hours on a cyclic basis or when it occurs at rest, the possibility of coronary artery spasm or Prinzmetal angina should be considered. This "variant" angina may be associated with a history of migraine headaches, Raynaud phenomenon, or both, signifying a vasospastic tendency of multiple arterial beds. Coronary artery spasm, expressed as rest pain or discomfort, can occur concomitantly with classic exertional angina.

Alleviating factors that help in the diagnosis are relief by cessation of the activity or by sublingual nitroglycerin. Getting out of the cold or completing the uphill walk are excellent examples of ways that angina is usually relieved. Of interesting, lying down may not relieve angina and at times may precipitate it by the increase in venous return. The response to nitroglycerin is not specific because esophageal spasm also is alleviated by nitroglycerin. However, the rapidity of relief for angina is quite impressive. The freshness of the nitroglycerin tablets needs to be ascertained in the context of whether the discomfort was responsive; if the tablets are old and did not induce mucosal tingling or a headache, it remains unclear whether a true effect was tested.

Precipitating Factors

There are several key subgroups of patients that deserve particular emphasis. Diabetes mellitus frequently leads to significant atherosclerotic coronary disease, but the symptoms are much less apt to be present and probably are related to a sensory neuropathy (14). Silent ischemia must, therefore, be considered in these patients, but careful interrogation for anginal equivalent symptoms (Table 15.4) is especially worthwhile. Of course, many diabetics have classic angina, but missing the underlying coronary disease in patients who are not fortunate enough to have an intact "alarm system" can have serious or even fatal consequences. Compared with men, women with documented coronary artery disease more often do not have the characteristic symptoms of angina, for unclear reasons. Whereas an exertional or emotional stress component is frequently elicited, the quality of the discomfort can be misleading and seem atypical. A full diagnostic evaluation and extra time to delineate fully the symptoms, precipitants, and risk factors are imperative.

After cardiac transplantation, patients cannot expect to experience chest pain or discomfort due to denervation, except in rare situations in which apparent reinnervation occurs (34,35). Systematic screening for coronary atherosclerosis has to be set up (see Chapter 89). For patients presenting with the chest pain of acute myocardial infarction, women, the elderly, and minority patients (particularly African Americans and Hispanics) tend to present later in the course of the event and are more apt to have atypical or nonclassic features (16–18).

Dyspnea and Cough

Difficulty breathing is one of the cardinal symptoms of cardiac and pulmonary disease. Strictly, *dyspnea* denotes an abnormally uncomfortable awareness of breathing that is easily differentiated from normal, quiet, unnoticed breathing. The history can be particularly important in pinpointing the cause of dyspnea because there are a number of potential etiologies (36,37), including heart failure, pulmonary edema, obstructive airway disease, and pulmonary embolism.

Sudden dyspnea occurs not only with acute pulmonary edema, but also with a pneumothorax, pulmonary embolism, or airway obstruction. In congestive heart failure, the onset of dyspnea is insidious and frequently precipitated by exertion. Conditions that simulate the chronic development of dyspnea are chronic obstructive pulmonary disease, pleural effusions, pregnancy, and obesity. Asthma or obstructive airway disease is suggested by inspiratory dyspnea, wheezing, and prior episodes responsive to bronchodilators. Although it is a rare symptom, sudden dyspnea while sitting rather than recumbent suggests the possibility of atrial myxoma, whereas dyspnea relieved by squatting is a classic indication for the congenital lesion of tetralogy of Fallot.

Paroxysmal nocturnal dyspnea is a classic sign of interstitial pulmonary edema and is most commonly due to heart failure. It usually begins 2 to 4 hours after going to sleep; is associated with sweating, cough, and, at times, wheezing; and can gradually improve (over 10 to 20 minutes) by getting out of bed or sitting on the side of the bed. The cough follows the dyspnea in heart failure but occurs in the opposite order in patients with chronic obstructive pulmonary disease. Of lesser severity is orthopnea due to pulmonary venous hypertension, which occurs in the recumbent position with relief by sitting upright or standing. The number of pillows used by the patient is a good way to semiquantify orthopnea because patients learn to use one or more extra pillows to combat their sense of breathlessness. Symptoms of heart failure that also cluster with dyspnea and orthopnea are nocturia, edema, and, more rarely, upper abdominal discomfort due to hepatosplenomegaly.

Dyspnea on exertion as a sole symptom may signify an anginal equivalent (Table 15.4); if it occurs with angina, there is an increased likelihood of a large myocardium in jeopardy, compared with angina and no symptoms of breathlessness.

Two alterations of breathing, both with a component of apnea, deserve mention. *Cheyne-Stokes respiration* refers to periods of hyperpnea followed by apnea. The pattern is a feature of the elderly who have heart failure, often with concomitant cerebrovascular disease. Sleep apnea has emerged as an important trigger of pulmonary hypertension and is characterized by episodes of snoring with prolonged periods of apnea due to upper airway obstruction. It typically occurs in patients who are overweight or mildly obese and can be responsive to measures that counter the upper airway obstruction. The diagnosis, however, can only be supported by obtaining a history from the patient's spouse or significant other.

Cough as a symptom is considerably more frequent but equally less specific (38). Perhaps the most common cause of cough today results from the side effect of angiotensin-converting-enzyme inhibitors—popularly used for the treatment of hypertension and heart failure—that occurs as a result of activating bradykinin. The dry cough from this class of medications can be difficult to differentiate from that of pulmonary hypertension or mitral stenosis. Both types of cough are irritating and spasmodic, although the heart failure or mitral stenosis cough is more likely to be nocturnal, despite considerable overlap. Cough associated with hoarseness in the absence of upper respiratory disease may suggest a very enlarged left atrium with compression of the recurrent laryngeal nerve. Hoarseness without obvious upper respiratory infection in such patients is known as *Ortner syndrome*, in which the large left atrium exerts pressure on an enlarged pulmonary artery and peribronchial lymph nodes to compress the recurrent laryngeal nerve. Dysphagia and right posterior chest pain occur only if left atrial enlargement is extreme due to severe chronic mitral regurgitation.

Sputum production and, particularly, hemoptysis are symptoms that tend to localize the disorder in the lungs, except for hemoptysis that is associated with severe mitral stenosis and is characterized by sudden increases in left atrial pressure and rupture of small bronchopulmonary veins. Frank hemoptysis that occurs with pulmonary arterial hypertension due to congenital left-to-right shunts may not share this pathophysiology because bronchial arterioles rupture, in this case, to cause massive hemorrhage.

In patients with dyspnea and suspect valvular disease, determining whether there is a history of rheumatic fever is customary but can be misleading. Determination of whether there was scarlet fever with a rash, joint pains, chorea (St. Vitus' dance) with twitches or clumsiness, frequent sore throats, prolonged bed rest, or a family history of rheumatic fever are all in this line of questioning. However, frequently, the absence of these symptoms does not rule out rheumatic fever; a positive history can also be inaccurate (39).

Syncope and Palpitations

Syncope is a loss of consciousness due to inadequate perfusion of the brain. The history is fundamental for narrowing down a wide differential diagnosis (see Chapter 70). Sudden loss of consciousness without an aura or warning characterizes cardiac syncope. This condition can result from an arrhythmia such as ventricular fibrillation, ventricular tachycardia, advanced atrioventricular block, or asystole (39,40). A family history of syncope raises the possibility of a long-QT syndrome (see Chapter 93). Beyond arrhythmic causes of syncope, the hemodynamically significant lesions of aortic stenosis, hypertrophic cardiomyopathy, and primary pulmonary hypertension are important causes of cardiac syncope. With these disorders, syncope classically occurs just after exertion, and although hemodynamic lesions are present that can account for the loss of consciousness, serious arrhythmias should not be discounted as the primary trigger. Hypertrophic cardiomyopathy is usually familial, and so the family history is important to raise or support this possibility. Besides the postexertional syncope, fainting during prolonged standing, posttussive, or even during exertion can occur with this condition.

The most common cause of cardiac syncope is known as *vasodepressor* and is mediated through the autonomic nervous system, with unconsciousness developing a bit more gradually and lasting for a few seconds; this condition can be induced by emotional stress or pain. It can be preceded by dim vision, sweating, nausea, light-headedness, giddiness, or yawning, reflecting autonomic nervous system hyperactivity, and can be fully alleviated by lying down. After the spell, it is common for the patient to be quite pale and to have a slow heart rate. Closely related in underlying pathophysiology is the syncope due to direct stimulation of the carotid sinus in patients who are "hypersensitive;" this syncope is manifested by fainting spells after sudden head motion or wearing of a tight collar. Hypovolemia in patients experiencing fainting while standing and orthostatic hypotension-related syncope are other possible and related etiologies of cardiac syncope.

Compared with cardiac syncope, neurologic causes often have an aura, as in the case of epilepsy (which is familial in some cases and posttraumatic in others) or associated neurologic deficits of transient cerebrovascular ischemia (e.g., vision loss, speech impairment, or motor weakness). Furthermore, after some neurologic causes of syncope such as a grand mal seizure, there is postictal confusion. It is important to note that vasodepressor syncope is not typically linked with trauma, but patients with seizures or other forms of sudden cardiac syncope can sustain physical injury with a fainting spell. Near-syncope, which is described by patients as "nearly" losing consciousness or "graying" out, is similar in its differential to actual syncope, but overall it is less likely to be associated with serious pathologic conditions compared with true loss of consciousness.

Calkins and colleagues (40) studied the differentiating symptoms of the history to resolve the etiology of syncope. Features of the history predictive of syncope not due to ventricular tachycardia or atrioventricular block were palpitation, blurred vision, nausea, warmth, diaphoresis, and lightheadedness before syncope and nausea, warmth, diaphoresis, and fatigue after the syncopal event (41).

Palpitations represent an unpleasant awareness of the heartbeat and frequently are described as "skipping," "jumping," "pounding," or "racing." The skipping is often attributed to the postextrasystolic pause, whereas the pounding or forceful beat is accounted for by the postextrasystolic potentiation of contractility. A variety of rhythm disturbances may be considered, with the full spectrum from bradyarrhythmias to supraventricular or ventricular tachycardias being potential triggers. Palpitations are remarkably common and can simply occur with anxiety (e.g., palpitations occurring with the syndrome of hyperventilation previously described), with tingling around the mouth and in the hands, although the underlying rhythm is sinus tachycardia. Similarly, other benign forms occur with postural hypotension due to the reflex heart acceleration or in response to medications (e.g., amphetamines), cocaine, alcohol, tobacco, and caffeine. With physical exertion, a sense of the heart "pounding" may certainly be anticipated.

When the complaint occurs despite lack of exertion or with only minimal effort, other causes need to be surveyed, such as heart failure, anemia, thyrotoxicosis, and atrial fibrillation. A pulse rate of approximately 150 beats per minute suggests atrial flutter, whereas faster rates suggest paroxysmal supraventricular tachycardia. Rates slower than 140 beats per minute (as low as 100 beats per minute) are more suggestive of sinus tachycardia and therefore are more likely to be benign.

Edema, Fatigue, and Other Symptoms

Swollen legs manifesting at the end of the day are characteristic of heart failure or chronic venous insufficiency. Early on, this can sometimes be associated only with difficulty in getting one's shoes on, but it can also be linked to appreciable weight gain due to fluid retention. Usually, the edema is symmetric and progresses "from the ground up." In patients with prior bypass surgery who have had saphenous vein grafts harvested, the edema may begin unilaterally on the side of decreased venous competence. In patients confined to bed with heart failure, presacral edema is common. In the presence of hyperpigmentation of the legs, ulcers, and other changes suggesting venous stasis, chronic venous insufficiency may be the likely explanation, but frequently the coincident finding of heart failure and chronic venous insufficiency is present. This is especially true in patients who have had long-standing heart failure and other reasons for venous insufficiency (e.g., marked obesity). Generalized edema, known as *anasarca*, can occur with severe heart failure but also with cirrhosis and the nephrotic syndrome. Periorbital edema occurs with hypoproteinemia, myxedema, hereditary angioneurotic edema, and acute glomerulonephritis. Edema localized to the upper body, involving the face, arms, and neck, raises the possibility of a superior vena cava syndrome, which may herald carcinoma of the lung. Edema of cardiac origin that is not associated with dyspnea or orthopnea suggests a right-sided heart lesion such as constrictive pericarditis, tricuspid stenosis, or, for example, a tumor that has invaded the inferior vena cava or right atrium.

Fatigue is a nonspecific and common symptom that may not have cardiovascular basis. However, it may signal poor cardiac output or result from overdiuresis or from the use of β-blocker drugs. In some cases, episodic fatigue from physical exertion or emotional stress disproportionate to the amount of effort expended may represent an anginal equivalent.

Nausea and vomiting can occur with acute myocardial infarction (see Chapter 19). Fever and chills, along with other constitutional signs, may be associated with infectious endocarditis (see Chapter 26).

CONTROVERSIES AND PERSONAL PERSPECTIVES

It is clear that taking a thorough history has become less of a priority for a few pivotal reasons. First, there is less time available for physician–patient direct contact as a result of the demands placed on a physician's time. Frequently, a physician extender or nurse obtains part or all of the history to reduce the time burden on the doctor. Under the putative heading of "efficiency," the priority of the detailed, thorough interview has been markedly reduced. Second, with advances in technology, the history and physical examination have been partially supplanted by rapid use of bedside tools such as the two-dimensional echocardiogram, a treadmill or dobutamine thallium test, a Holter recording, or even diagnostic angiography or electrophysiologic study—all instead of the meticulous history.

These two forces are unfortunate. The history is the most important way to create a physician–patient bond and is precious and irreplaceable. Ideally, the task should not be delegated to a physician extender, except for such perfunctory aspects as the medications and doses, risk factors, and minor details. It is absolutely essential to query the patient directly and in depth for the principal symptoms (e.g., chest discomfort, loss of consciousness, or dyspnea). Only in this way can there be the optimal accuracy and relationship building that are critical. In addition, the use of advanced diagnostic technology easily can be imprudent with respect to cost and can uncover findings that, although accurate, have no bearing on the patient's symptoms. The detailed history preempts or properly guides the use of more refined diagnostic tests. Intuitively, the history is the most cost-effective tool that one can use to lay a sound foundation for the patient's evaluation.

THE FUTURE

Although the history has been deemphasized in the last decade, it will become increasingly relied on in the future because of its relatively low cost and pivotal importance in guiding more diagnostic and therapeutic decision making. To counter the reduced sense of patient satisfaction and bonding with the physician, spending more time with the patient to relay information and develop mutual understanding and trust can override the forces that have deprioritized such a core component of high-quality cardiovascular care.

References

1. Belkin BM, Neelon FA. The art of observation: William Osler and the method of Zadig. *Ann Intern Med* 1992;116:863–866.
2. Sandler G. The importance of the history in the medical clinic and the cost of unnecessary tests. *Am Heart J* 1980;100:928.
3. Kee F, Tiret L, Robo JY, et al. Reliability of reported family history of myocardial infarction. *BMJ* 1993;307:1528–1530.
4. Hunt K, Emslie C, Watt G. Lay constructions of a family history of heart disease: potential for misunderstandings in the clinical encounter? *Lancet* 2001;357:1168–1171.
5. Murabito J, Pencina M, Nam BH, et al. Sibling cardiovascular disease as a risk factor for cardiovascular disease in middle-aged adults. *JAMA* 2005; 294:3117–3123.
6. Goldman L, Hashimoto B, Cook EF, et al. Comparative reproducibility and validity of systems for assessing cardiovascular functional class: advantages of a new specific activity scale. *Circulation* 1981;64:1227–1234.
7. Criteria Committee, New York Heart Association. *Diseases of the heart and blood vessels: nomenclature and criteria for diagnosis,* 6th ed. Boston: Little, Brown, 1964: 114.
8. Serlie AW, Erdman RA, Passchier J, et al. Psychological aspects of non-cardiac chest pain [review]. *Psychother Psychosom* 1995;64:62–73.
9. Pryor DB, Shaw L, McCants CB, et al. Value of the history and physical in identifying patients at increased risk for coronary artery disease. *Ann Intern Med* 1993;118:81–90.
10. Tatum JL, Jesse RL, Kontos MC, et al. Comprehensive strategy for the evaluation and triage of the chest pain patient. *Ann Emerg Med* 1997;29:116–125.
11. Jarcho S. Functional heart disease in the Civil War (Da Costa, 1871). *Am J Cardiol* 1959;4:809–817.
12. Levey GS, Calabro JJ. Tietze's syndrome: report of two cases and review of the literature. *Arthritis Rheum* 1962;5:261.
13. Epstein SE, Gerber LN, Boren JS. Chest wall syndrome: a common cause of unexpected pain. *JAMA* 1979;241:279.
14. Chiariello M, Indolfi C. Silent myocardial ischemia in patients with diabetes mellitus. *Circulation* 1996;93:2089–2091.
15. Gregor RD, Bata IR, Eastwood BJ, et al. Gender differences in the presentation, treatment, and short-term mortality of acute chest pain. *Clin Invest Med* 1994;17:551–562.
16. Ell K, Haywood LJ, Sobel E, et al. Acute chest pain in African Americans: factors in the delay in seeking emergency care. *Am J Public Health* 1994;84:965–970.
17. Haywood LJ, Ell K, deGuman M, et al. Chest pain admissions: characteristics of black, Latino, and white patients in low- and mid-socioeconomic strata. *J Natl Med Assoc* 1993;85:749–757.
18. Johnson PA, Goldman L, Orav EJ, et al. Comparison of the Medical Outcomes Study short-form 36-item health survey in black patients and white patients with acute chest pain. *Med Care* 1995;33:145–160.
19. Lehmann JB, Wehner PS, Lehmann CU, et al. Gender bias in the evaluation of chest pain in the emergency department. *Am J Cardiol* 1996;77:641–644.
20. Chang RA, Rossi NF. Intermittent cocaine use associated with recurrent dissection of the thoracic and abdominal aorta. *Chest* 1995;108:1758–1762.
21. Hollander JE, Todd KH, Green G, et al. Chest pain associated with cocaine: an assessment of prevalence in suburban and urban emergency departments. *Ann Emerg Med* 1995;26:671–676.
22. Hollander JE. The management of cocaine-associated myocardial ischemia. *N Engl J Med* 1995;333:1267–1272.
23. Chauhan A, Petch MC, Schofield PM. Cardioesophageal reflex in humans as a mechanism for "linked angina." *Eur Heart J* 1996;17:407–413.
24. Saltissi S. Cardio-esophageal reflex and "linked angina"—is the way to a man's (or woman's) heart through the stomach? *Eur Heart J* 1996;17:329–331.
25. Eslick GD. Chest pain: a historical perspective. *Int J Cardiol* 2001;77:5–11.
26. Wong Y, Rodwell A, Livesey SA, et al. Sex differences in investigation results and treatment in subjects referred for investigation of chest pain. *Heart* 2001;85:149–152.
27. Sharaf BL, Pepine CJ, Kerensky RA, et al. Detailed angiographic analysis of women with suspected ischemic chest pain (pilot phase data from the NHLBI-sponsored Women's Ischemia Syndrome Evaluation [WISE] study angiographic core laboratory). *Am J Cardiol* 2001;87:937–941.
28. Constant J, ed. *Bedside cardiology,* 2nd ed. Boston: Little, Brown, 1976.
29. Bradley LA, Richter JE, Scarinci IC, et al. Psychosocial and psychophysical assessments of patients with unexplained chest pain. *Am J Med* 1992;92:65S–73S.
30. Yingling KW, Wulsin LR, Arnold LM, et al. Estimated prevalences of panic disorder and depression among consecutive patients seen in an emergency department with acute chest pain. *J Gen Intern Med* 1993;8:231–235.
31. Tew R, Guthrie EA, Creed FH, et al. A long-term follow-up study of patients with ischemic heart disease versus patients with nonspecific chest pain. *J Psychosom Res* 1995;39:977–985.
32. Mayou R, Bryant B, Forfar C, et al. Non-cardiac chest pain and benign palpitations in the cardiac clinic. *Br Heart J* 1994;72:548–553.
33. Cannon RO III, Quyyumi AA, Mincemoyer R, et al. Imipramine in patients

with chest pain despite normal coronary angiograms. *N Engl J Med* 1994;330:1411–1417.
34. Schroeder JS, Hunt SA. Chest pain in heart-transplant recipients. *N Engl J Med* 1986;324:1805–1807.
35. Stark RP, McGinn AL, Wilson RF. Chest pain in cardiac-transplant recipients: Evidence of sensory reinnervation after cardiac transplantation. *N Engl J Med* 1991;324:1791–1794.
36. Duncan AK, Vittone J, Fleming KC, et al. Cardiovascular disease in elderly patients. *Mayo Clin Proc* 1996;71:184–196.
37. Valacio R, Lye M. Heart failure in the elderly patient. *Br J Clin Pract* 1995; 49:200–204.
38. Irwin RS, Curley FJ, French CL, et al. Chronic cough: the spectrum and frequency of causes, key components of the diagnostic evaluation, and outcome of specific therapy. *Am Rev Respir Dis* 1990;141:640–647.
39. Reichek N, Shelburne JC, Perloff JK. Clinical aspects of rheumatic valvular disease. *Prog Cardiovasc Dis* 1973;15:491–537.
40. Calkins H, Shyr Y, Frumin H, et al. The value of the clinical history in the differentiation of syncope due to ventricular tachycardia, atrioventricular block, and neurocardiogenic syncope. *Am J Med* 1995;98:365–373.
41. Sutton R, Nathan A, Perrins J, et al. Syncope: a good history is not enough. *BMJ* 1994;309:474.

CHAPTER 16 ■ PHYSICAL EXAMINATION

KANU CHATTERJEE

OVERVIEW

A systematic approach to the bedside examination of a patient is essential in determining the significance of an abnormal physical finding, such as decreased or increased intensity of the first heart sound (S_1), a pathologic third heart sound (S_3), or a systolic or diastolic murmur. Assessment of the abnormalities of the systemic venous pressure and pulse, arterial pulse, precordial impulse, heart sound, and murmurs provides clues not only for the diagnosis of the anatomic abnormalities, but also for the determination of the severity of the hemodynamic abnormalities.

Furthermore, a careful, systematic, and methodical bedside clinical evaluation—including analysis of clinical history—can provide enough information to decide on appropriate further investigations to establish the diagnosis.

INSPECTION

General

During general inspection (1,2), the stature, body habitus, and presence or absence of obesity are noted. An unusually short stature is seen in patients with osteogenesis imperfecta, which is associated with aortic and mitral regurgitation and calcification of the arterial system. Congenital heart disease, such as Noonan syndrome, occurs in association with short stature, web neck, dental malocclusion, antimongoloid slanting of the eyes, mental retardation, and hypogonadism. Pulmonary valve stenosis and obstructive and nonobstructive cardiomyopathy are also observed. Dwarfism is an essential phenotypic feature of the various types of mucopolysaccharidosis, which can be associated with various valvular and myocardial dysfunctions. An unusually tall stature is seen in patients with Marfan syndrome, which is associated with aortic aneurysm, aortic regurgitation, and mitral regurgitation. When severe chest or back pain is the presenting symptom in a patient with Marfan syndrome, acute aortic dissection should be suspected. A tall stature, long extremities, and eunuchoid appearance is observed in patients with Klinefelter syndrome, which can be associated with congenital heart diseases such as ventricular septal defects, patent ductus arteriosus, and tetralogy of Fallot. During initial cardiac evaluation, it is customary to notice any obvious musculoskeletal deformity, such as kyphoscoliosis, straight back, and pectus deformity. A higher incidence of mitral valve prolapse is observed in the presence of such musculoskeletal deformities. An increased incidence of mitral valve prolapse is also observed in females with smaller breasts. Muscular dystrophies such as pseudohypertrophic, fascioscapular humoral, or limb girdle varieties can be suspected during general inspection. These muscular dystrophies may be associated with various cardiovascular abnormalities, including myocardial disease, mitral valve prolapse, ventricular septal defect, and dysrhythmias.

Gait

Neurologic deficits resulting from cardioembolic strokes or hypertensive cerebrovascular disease may be associated with abnormalities of gait. A parkinsonian gait may indicate Shy-Drager syndrome, which may be associated with orthostatic hypotension and supine hypertension (3). Certain metabolic disorders (e.g., hyperthyroidism, hypothyroidism, Cushing syndrome, and acromegaly) can be suspected during inspection, and these metabolic diseases may be associated with various cardiovascular abnormalities, including systemic and pulmonary hypertension and myocardial and pericardial diseases.

Body Habitus

Marked weight loss, wasting, and cachexia are manifestations of severe, chronic congestive heart failure (CHF). Cardiac cachexia (4) does not correlate with cardiac output as usually perceived, but to a marked neuroendocrine abnormality characterized by an activated renin–angiotensin system and increased levels of cytokines, including tumor necrosis factor and interleukins. Furthermore, cardiac cachexia is associated with poor prognosis. The presence and severity of obesity should be noted; various cardiovascular abnormalities can be associated with obesity. Obesity, particularly abdominal and truncal types, is one of the components of the metabolic syndrome X, which comprises hypertension, hyperlipidemia, and insulin resistance (5,6). In patients with metabolic syndrome, there is increased risk of atherosclerotic macrovascular disease, including coronary artery disease. In markedly obese patients, there is increased incidence of sleep apnea, hypertension, and dilated cardiomyopathy. Truncal obesity, if associated with buffalo hump or moon facies, should raise the suspicion of Cushing syndrome, which may be complicated by hypertension and hypertensive heart disease. In African Americans, severe obesity and marked increase in body mass index and diabetes are more important predictors of primary diastolic heart failure than hypertension or coronary artery disease.

Respiration

During inspection, presence of respiratory distress and types of altered respiration should be observed. Inability to lie down or a dry, irritating cough with dyspnea in the supine position usually indicates pulmonary venous congestion. Sleep-disordered breathing is common in chronic CHF (7). Typical Cheyne-Stokes respiration with central sleep apnea is observed in 20% to 30% of patients with moderate or severe systolic CHF. Cheyne-Stokes respiration with central sleep apnea is a risk factor for increased mortality (8). Also, patients with central sleep apnea are likely to benefit from continuous positive airway pressure therapy (9). Frequent sighing respirations and a restless, anxious look are more frequently encountered in patients with anxiety and neurocirculatory asthenia. The "blue bloater" and "pink puffer" appearances, which can be detected during inspection, usually indicate chronic obstructive pulmonary disease (COPD). During inspection, it is desirable to note any changes in the color of the skin. A bluish discoloration of the skin may indicate cyanosis, which can be either peripheral or central. Peripheral cyanosis is detected in exposed skin (e.g., lips, nose, and earlobes, and extremities) and indicates impaired peripheral perfusion. A bluish discoloration of the tongue, uvula, and buccal mucus membrane suggests central cyanosis, which results from intrapulmonary or intracardiac right-to-left shunt. When differential cyanosis (i.e., cyanosis in the inferior extremities without cyanosis in the superior extremity) is observed along with differential clubbing, Eisenmenger syndrome associated with patent ductus arteriosus should be suspected.

Edema

Generalized edema can be detected during inspection, which usually results from nephrotic syndrome and sepsis, and rarely from severe heart failure. Dependent edema, on the other hand, is associated with right heart failure. The presence of ascites, which also may be a manifestation of right heart failure, can be suspected from the protuberant abdomen. Ascites in the absence of edema of the lower extremities is more frequently a manifestation of liver disease, such as cirrhosis, rather than of heart failure. However, in patients with constrictive pericarditis and restrictive cardiomyopathy, disproportionately large ascites with little or no edema of the lower extremities can be observed (10).

Skin

Slate or bronze pigmentation of the skin may suggest hemochromatosis, which may be associated with various cardiac complications (e.g., restrictive or dilated cardiomyopathy, arrhythmias, and conduction disturbances). It should be appreciated that patients on chronic amiodarone therapy develop similar discoloration of the skin with exposure to sunlight (11). Discoloration of the skin similar to marked suntan is also seen in patients with carcinoid syndrome. Mild jaundice may be observed in patients with heart failure with congestive hepatopathy. Prosthetic valve malfunction should be suspected if jaundice is obvious in a patient with artificial heart valves. The livido reticulares with cyanosis of the toes and preserved peripheral pulses (blue toes syndrome) suggest cholesterol emboli (12). Acrosclerosis with taut, thickened, or edematous skin bound tightly to subcutaneous tissue in the hands and fingers suggests systemic sclerosis, which may be associated with pulmonary hypertension, pericarditis, right heart failure, systemic hypertension, restrictive cardiomyopathy, and dilated cardiomyopathy. If malar flush is detected, mitral stenosis with pulmonary hypertension should be suspected. Malar flush, however, can also occur in patients with severe precapillary pulmonary hypertension and may be confused with butterfly rash of lupus erythematosus. Transverse or diagonal earlobe creases in a relatively young person (<45 years of age), along with corneal arcus—a circumferential light ream around the iris that begins inferiorly—is associated with increased risk of atherosclerotic coronary artery disease. Arcus is also frequently associated with hypercholesterolemia and xanthelasma (deposits of cholesterol on the eyelids). When telangiectasia of the lips, tongue, and buccal mucosa are detected, Osler-Weber-Rendu disease, which is associated with pulmonary arteriovenous fistulae, should be suspected. Exfoliative dermatitis, purpura, and petechial rashes may indicate drug reactions. Although an erythema marginatum is characteristic of acute rheumatic fever, erythema nodosum is a nonspecific finding and occurs in many systemic diseases. In patients with suspected bacterial endocarditis, searches should be made for conjunctival hemorrhages, skin purpuric, and petechial lesions, as well as for splinter hemorrhages. It should be realized that splinter hemorrhages in the nail beds may occur in normal patients after mild trauma and in patients with trichinosis or hemorrhagic disorders.

During examination of the skin, it is customary to check for the presence of cutaneous and subcutaneous nodular lesions, which may suggest some systemic and metabolic diseases. The rheumatic nodules associated with acute rheumatic fever are small, nontender, and most frequently are present on the knuckles, extensor surface of the elbows, and suboccipital regions. Rheumatoid nodules, on the other hand, are large, nontender, and characteristically localized over points of pressure or friction—most commonly the extensor surfaces of the proximal forearms. If rheumatoid nodules are detected, attention should be directed to detect the cardiovascular complications of rheumatoid arthritis (e.g., pericarditis, aortic and mitral valvular disease, conduction disturbances, and, rarely, cardiomyopathy). Xanthomas—cholesterol-filled nodules—occur in different types of abnormalities of lipoprotein metabolism, and recognition of the distribution of xanthomas aids in the diagnosis of these disorders. Tendon xanthomas, xanthomas occurring on digital extensors, and tuberous xanthomas occur in familial hypercholesterolemia (13). Eruptive xanthomas are small, yellow papules in the skin surrounded by an erythematous halo. They occur in patients with primary familial hypertriglyceridemia that results from lipoprotein lipase deficiency and is associated with recurrent episodes of pancreatitis, but not with premature coronary artery disease. Eruptive xanthomas also occur in patients with endogenous and mixed hypertriglyceridemia, which can be associated with ischemic vascular disease. In patients with suspected bacterial endocarditis, it is desirable to search for Osler nodes and Janeway lesions. Osler nodes are most frequently observed on the palms, soles of the feet, and pads of the fingers or toes. These nodes are tender, nodular, erythematous skin lesions and result from emboli. Janeway lesions are nontender, raised, hemorrhagic nodules that usually occur on the palms of the hands and soles of the feet. These lesions were initially thought to be due to vasculitis, but they also appear to be of embolic origin. Café-au-lait spots—sometimes detected only in the axilla—occur in neurofibromatosis, which occasionally is associated with hypertrophic cardiomyopathy.

Funduscopy

In patients with established or suspected systemic hypertension, funduscopic examination should be performed. Several grades of changes may be observed (14). Grade 1 consists of minimal irregularity of the arterial lumen and narrowing with increased light reflex. Grade 2 changes consist of arteriovenous nicking, more marked narrowing and irregularity of the arterioles, and distention of the veins. Grade 3 changes are characterized by the presence of flame-shaped hemorrhages and fluffy "cotton wool" exudates in addition to arterial changes. Hard exudates may also be present. Grade 4 funduscopic changes are characterized by the presence of papilledema and any other changes in grades 1 through 3. Generally, grade 1 and 2 changes are present in benign hypertension, whereas grade 3 or 4 changes are seen in accelerated or malignant hypertension. Funduscopic examination should also be performed in patients with suspected bacterial endocarditis and may reveal vascular occlusions and hemorrhagic areas with white centers (Roth spots), which result from emboli in the nerve fiber retinal layer. Roth spots, however, are not diagnostic of bacterial endocarditis and can be seen in hemorrhagic disorders, including leukemia. Mycotic aneurysms resulting from large emboli occasionally may be discovered in retinal vessels during funduscopic examination. Identification of such lesions should lead to further evaluation for the source of emboli, and appropriate investigations—including transthoracic and, occasionally, transesophageal echocardiography—must be undertaken. Occasionally, funduscopic examination may reveal unusual findings such as beading of the retinal artery (hypercholesterolemia), microinfarction in the peripheral retina (sickle cell disease), or angioid streaks (pseudoxanthoma elasticum). These disorders may be associated with cardiovascular complications. A wreath-like arteriovenous anastomosis around the optic disk is a characteristic of Takayasu syndrome. In adult cardiology practice, the abnormal findings that are often detected during inspection, along with their significance, are summarized in Table 16.1.

TABLE 16.1

INSPECTION

CYANOSIS
- *Peripheral cyanosis only*—suspect low cardiac output and impaired peripheral perfusion
- *Central cyanosis*—suspect intrapulmonary or intracardiac right-to-left shunt
- *Differential cyanosis*—suspect Eisenmenger syndrome with patent ductus arteriosus

RESPIRATORY DISTRESS
- *Cheyne-Stokes respiration with central sleep apnea*—suspect heart failure
- *Blue bloater and pink puffer*—suspect pulmonary disease
- *Frequent sighing respiration*—suspect anxiety syndromes

NUTRITIONAL STATUS
- *Cachexia*—suspect severe heart failure with abnormal neuroendocrine profile
- *Obesity*—suspect metabolic syndrome X, sleep apnea, cardiomyopathy
- *Ascites and peripheral edema*—suspect severe heart failure, constrictive pericarditis

MUSCULOSKELETAL DEFORMITY, KYPHOSCOLIOSIS, STRAIGHT BACK, PECTUS EXCAVATUM
- Suspect mitral valve prolapse, aortic and mitral valve regurgitation, congenital heart disease such as atrial septal defect

ABNORMAL MOVEMENT OF THE HEAD AND NECK
- *Bobbing of the head,* coincident with each heart beat—suspect severe aortic regurgitation
- *Lateral movements of the earlobes* with each cardiac cycle—suspect severe tricuspid regurgitation

SLATE OR BRONZE DISCOLORATION OF THE SKIN
- Suspect chronic amiodarone therapy, hemochromatosis, carcinoid syndrome

Examination of the Arterial Pulse

During initial evaluation, all accessible arterial pulses should be examined; in the inferior extremities, dorsales pedes, posterior tibials, and femoral pulses should be examined bilaterally. In the upper extremities, both brachial and radial pulses should be examined, and, in special circumstances, the ulnar pulses and axillary arterial pulses should also be examined. Temporal arteries are examined when temporal arteritis is suspected in patients with headache and jaw claudication. Carotid arteries should be examined sequentially in all patients. Diminished or absent dorsalis pedis pulses is associated with increased incidence of atherosclerotic coronary artery disease. Loss of or decreased femoral pulse unilaterally or bilaterally most frequently suggests local obstructive lesions due to atherosclerotic disease. However, diminished amplitudes of the lower extremity pulses, including femoral, popliteals, posterior tibials, and dorsales pedes arterial pulsations, also occur from isolated aortoiliac diseases, such as Leriche syndrome (15), postsubclavian coarctation of the aorta, aortic dissection, descending thoracic and abdominal aortic aneurysms, and abdominal aortic disease such as giant cell arteritis. When coarctation of the aorta is suspected, the radial and femoral pulses should be examined simultaneously to assess radial/femoral delay.

In a normal adult, the pulse transmission time from aorta to the radial artery is approximately 75 ms and to the femoral artery is approximately 70 ms. Thus, in the presence of coarctation, delay in the onset of femoral pulse compared to that of radial pulse can be detected. The radial/femoral delay is rarely observed in patients with Leriche syndrome and abdominal coarctation. Also in pseudocoarctation, the degree of obstruction is not severe enough to decrease the amplitude of the femoral pulse or to cause delay in the onset of femoral pulse compared with that of radial pulse (16). In patients with radial/femoral delay and suspected coarctation, blood pressure should be recorded in the upper and lower extremities. In the supine position, the inferior extremity pressure is normally slightly higher than that of the upper extremity arterial pressure. In coarctation, inferior extremity pressure is lower than upper extremity pressure.

While examining the peripheral arterial pulses, it is desirable to assess the rigidity and elasticity of the arteries. The rigidity of the arterial pulses are best appreciated by examining the femoral, radial, brachial, and carotid pulses. In clinical practice, the thickness and firmness of the arterial walls are examined by rolling the vessel, usually the radial artery, against underlying tissue. The more rigid the artery, the less it is compressible. The appreciation of nonelastic, rigid peripheral arteries may indicate the presence of systolic hypertension. If the significant rigidity of the peripheral arteries is observed, it is desirable to perform Osler maneuver. Osler maneuver is performed by elevating the cuff pressure to obliterate the radial pulse; if, after obliteration of the pulse, the radial artery is easily palpable and appears rigid (positive Osler sign), then there might be a significant difference between indirect measurement of arterial pressure by cuff method and directly determined intraarterial pressure.

The peripheral arterial pulses are also examined at the bedside for detection of arrhythmias. If the pulse rate is regular but slow, sinus bradycardia, junctional rhythm, or complete atrioventricular block is suspected. Occasionally, bigeminy may produce an irregular slow pulse because of the nonconducted pulse associated with the ectopic beat. Careful examination of the venous pulse and simultaneous auscultation may be helpful for the differential diagnosis of slow regular pulse. If regular cannon waves with each cardiac cycle are recognized, junctional rhythm is suspected. In the presence of a slow regular pulse, if irregular cannon waves and changing intensity of the S_1 are observed, atrioventricular dissociation owing to complete atrioventricular block is the most likely diagnosis. Bigeminy can be diagnosed easily by auscultation, which demonstrates the postectopic compensatory pause. Atrial fibrillation can be suspected if irregularly irregular pulses are appreciated. However, frequent premature beats or multifocal atrial tachycardia can also produce an irregularly irregular pulse. If atrial fibrillation is suspected, it is desirable to determine the ventricular rate by simultaneous auscultation to assess the degree of pulse deficit. The difference between the heart rate by auscultation and the pulse rate is the pulse deficit. The rapid ventricular responses are the cause of the hemodynamic abnormalities of atrial fibrillation. A fast and regular pulse rate ($\geq$150 beats) should raise the possibility of supraventricular or ventricular tachycardia. It is mandatory to do electrocardiographic evaluation of every patient with suspected arrhythmia.

Peripheral arterial pulses are also examined to detect any alteration of the character of the pulse, which can provide important diagnostic clues. Pulsus alternans is suspected when strong and weak amplitude pulses are appreciated with alternate beats in the presence of a regular pulse. Pulsus alternans can be confirmed by measuring blood pressure by sphygmomanometer. When the cuff pressure is slowly released, phase I Korotkoff sound is heard initially only during the alternate strong beats; with further release of cuff pressure, the softer sounds of the weak beat also appear. The most important cause of pulsus alternans is left ventricular systolic failure. Pulsus alternans is rarely encountered in patients with cardiac tamponade with pulsus paradoxus, if the respiratory rate is half of the heart rate. However, in these patients, when respiration is held transiently, the pulsus alternans is resolved. Pulsus alternans (mechanical alternans) can also occur occasionally in aortic stenosis, in hypertrophic obstructive cardiomyopathy, with sudden increase of afterload, with ischemia, with abrupt fall of preload, and with the onset of a tachyarrhythmia. Rapid atrial pacing may induce pulsus alternans in the presence of normal left ventricular systolic function. However, clinically detectable sustained pulsus alternans almost always indicates left ventricular systolic dysfunction.

In experimental and clinical studies, alternating changes in preload, afterload, and contractility have been suggested as potential mechanisms for mechanical alternans (17); ventricular dyssynchrony with alternating contraction of the interventricular septum, incomplete relaxation in the alternate beats, partial asystole of the left ventricle, alternating changes in action potential duration, and alternating amounts of Ca^{2+} sparks from the sarcoplasmic reticulum are the other proposed mechanisms (18). The failing heart is sensitive to altered afterload and resistance to left ventricular ejection. The increased arterial pressure associated with a strong beat increases the resistance to left ventricular ejection for the following beat, which is thus associated with decreased forward stroke volume and decreased arterial pressure. This reduction in arterial pressure lowers the resistance to left ventricular ejection, which allows increase in forward stroke volume and, therefore, increase in arterial pressure. These changes in arterial pressure, reflecting changes in the ejection impedance with alternate beats, can perpetuate pulsus alternans (Fig. 16.1).

A substantial reduction in the amplitude of the arterial pulse during inspiration may suggest pulsus paradoxus. Determination of arterial pressure by sphygmomanometry during inspiration and expiration should be performed to confirm. Systolic arterial pressure normally falls during inspiration; however, the

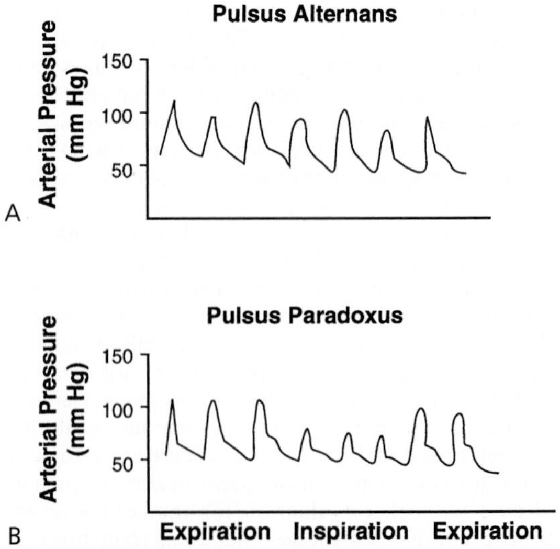

FIGURE 16.1. Schematic illustrations of pulsus alternans (A) and pulsus paradoxus (B). In clinical practice, pulsus alternans usually indicates systolic ventricular failure and occurs in patients with chronic ischemic or nonischemic dilated cardiomyopathy, aortic stenosis, and acute myocardial infarction. Pulsus paradoxus, however, is observed in pericardial tamponade, constrictive pericarditis (rare), emphysema, asthma, marked obesity, and severe CHF (rare).

magnitude of fall in arterial pressure during inspiration usually does not exceed 8 to 12 mm Hg. A more marked inspiratory decrease in arterial pressure exceeding 12 to 15 mm Hg is regarded as pulsus paradoxus. When the cuff pressure is slowly released, the systolic pressure at expiration is noted. With further slow deflation of the cuff, the systolic pressure during inspiration can also be detected. The difference between the pressure during expiration and inspiration is the magnitude of the pulsus paradoxus. The abnormal pulsus paradoxus is an important physical finding of cardiac tamponade (19). The marked inspiratory decrease in arterial pressure in tamponade results from the marked inspiratory decline of left ventricular stroke volume due to a decreased end-diastolic volume. In cardiac tamponade during inspiration, there is an increase in venous return to the right atrium and the right ventricle. Because of increased intrapericardial pressure, the intraventricular septum shifts toward the left ventricle during inspiration, which decreases left ventricular preload. There is also an expected decrease in venous return to the left ventricle during inspiration because of increased pulmonary venous reservoir capacity during inspiration. In clinical practice, besides cardiac tamponade, pulsus paradoxus is observed in patients with COPD. It should be emphasized that pulsus paradoxus is a rare finding in patients with constrictive pericarditis. Pulsus paradoxus is rarely observed in pulmonary embolism, pregnancy, marked obesity, and partial obstruction of the superior vena cava. In patients with significant aortic regurgitation and atrial septal defect, pulsus paradoxus may not occur despite cardiac tamponade. In hypertrophic obstructive cardiomyopathy, arterial pressure occasionally increases during inspiration (reversed pulsus paradoxus) (20). The precise mechanism for this phenomenon is not clear.

The amplitude of the peripheral arterial pulse may provide some information about stroke volume, systemic vascular resistance, and compliance of the arteries. A small-amplitude, rapid pulse usually indicates hypotension, reduced stroke volume, and increased systemic vascular resistance. A large-amplitude, arterial pulse suggests large stroke volume or decreased compliance. A large-volume, bounding pulse is noted after exercise; in high-output states such as chronic anemia, hyperthyroidism, and aortic regurgitation; and in patients with bradycardia (e.g., complete heart block). Decreased compliance and increased rigidity of the peripheral arteries may also increase the amplitude of the arterial pulse, as seen in elderly patients with systolic hypertension. In elderly patients, when the carotid pulse amplitude is decreased, local carotid disease or aortic stenosis should be suspected.

Changes in the contour of the arterial pulses (Fig. 16.2) should also be noted. In patients with significant aortic valve stenosis, a delayed upstroke of the ascending limb of the carotid pulse (so-called pulsus tardus), an anacrotic character of the carotid pulse, delayed peak, and small amplitude (pulsus parvus) of the carotid pulse are frequently appreciated. In patients with aortic stenosis, a thrill over the carotid pulse may also be detected. These abnormalities are best appreciated in the central pulse. In the central aortic ascending pressure pulse, normally there is a notch on the ascending limb: the anacrotic notch. On the upstroke of the carotid pulse, however, the anacrotic notch is not normally appreciated. An anacrotic carotid pulse gives the impression of interruption of the ascending limb or the upstroke of the carotid pulse. When the anacrotic notch is felt immediately after the onset of the upstroke, aortic stenosis is likely to be hemodynamically significant. An anacrotic radial pulse also suggests moderate to severe aortic stenosis. At the bedside, the delayed peak of the carotid pulse is appreciated by simultaneous auscultation of the duration of the systole. Normally, the peak of the carotid pulse is closer to the S_1. In the presence of significant aortic stenosis, the peak of the carotid pulse is delayed and is closer to the second heart sound (S_2). With increasing severity of aortic stenosis, the peak of the carotid pulse is not only further delayed and closer to the S_2, but the amplitude of the carotid pulse is also substantially reduced. It needs to be emphasized, however, that these changes in the contour of the carotid pulse may not be present in elderly patients with aortic stenosis with decreased and noncompliant carotid arteries. When aortic stenosis is suspected, whether in young or older patients, an echocardiographic evaluation is highly desirable.

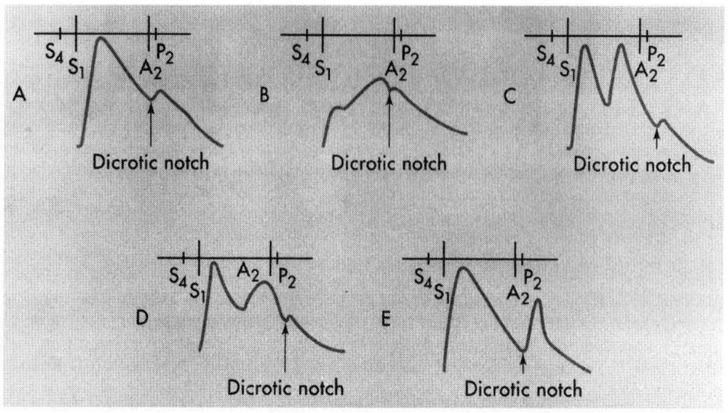

FIGURE 16.2. Schematic illustration of the configurational changes in the carotid pulse and their differential diagnoses. Heart sounds are also illustrated. **A:** Normal. **B:** Anacrotic pulse with slow initial upstroke and delayed peak, which is close to the aortic component of the second heart sound (A_2), indicate fixed aortic stenosis. **C:** Pulsus bisferiens with increased amplitude of percussion and tidal waves occurs during systole. This type of pulsus bisferiens carotid pulse is most frequently observed in patients with significant aortic regurgitation. **D:** Pulsus bisferiens in hypertrophic obstructive cardiomyopathy is rarely appreciated at the bedside. **E:** Dicrotic pulse results from an accentuated dicrotic wave and tends to occur in severe heart failure, hypovolemic shock, cardiac tamponade, sepsis, and after aortic valve replacement. *Abbreviations:* P_2, pulmonary component of the second heart sound; S_1, first heart sound; S_4, atrial sound. (*Source:* From Chatterjee K. Bedside evaluation of the heart: the physical examination. In: Parmley W, Chatterjee K, eds. *Cardiology*. Philadelphia: JB Lippincott Co, 1997;1:13, with permission.)

Pulsus bisferiens is appreciated by the presence of two positive impulses near the peak of the arterial pulse. These two positive impulses represent accentuated percussion and tidal waves, which can be recorded in the carotid arterial pulse tracing and the central aortic pulse waveform, even in normal subjects. The percussion wave results from the rapid left ventricular ejection, and a second, usually smaller, peak represents the tidal wave that results from a reflected wave from the periphery. Normally, radial and femoral pulse tracings demonstrate a single sharp peak. In pulsus bisferiens, percussion and tidal waves are accentuated. At the bedside, it is often difficult to distinguish between anacrotic, pulsus bisferiens, and dicrotic pulse. The anacrotic pulse, however, is characterized by a positive palpable wave during the ascending limb of the arterial pulse. Thus, it should be easily distinguished from pulsus bisferiens or the dicrotic pulse. However, if the two positive waves are felt near where the maximum amplitude of the pulse wave occurs, it is difficult to distinguish between pulsus bisferiens and dicrotic pulse. In these circumstances, one has to rely on detection of the etiologic conditions that can be associated with pulsus bisferiens or dicrotic pulse (21). The conditions most frequently associated with pulsus bisferiens are isolated hemodynamically significant aortic regurgitation, mixed aortic stenosis and regurgitation with predominant aortic regurgitation, and obstructive hypertrophic cardiomyopathy. Pulsus bisferiens is rarely appreciated in patients with large patent ductus arteriosus with large left-to-right shunt, multiple arteriovenous fistulas, and complete heart block. If these etiologies are excluded at the bedside, then one

TABLE 16.2

ALTERED CHARACTERS OF THE ARTERIAL PULSE AND THEIR CLINICAL SIGNIFICANCE

- *Pulsus alternans*—suspect acute or chronic reduction in left ventricular ejection fraction
- *Anacrotic pulse, delayed upstroke, palpable thrill, delayed peak*—suspect fixed left ventricular outflow tract obstruction such as aortic valve stenosis
- *Pulsus biferiens*—suspect aortic regurgitation, aortic stenosis with dominant aortic regurgitation, dynamic left ventricular outflow tract obstruction (obstructive hypertrophic cardiomyopathy), large patent ductus arteriosus with left-to-right shunt, complete heart block, hyperkinetic heart syndrome (e.g., in hyperthyroidism)
- *Dicrotic pulse*—suspect low-output syndrome with increased systemic vascular resistance, high output with low systemic resistance (e.g., in septic shock), postaortic valve replacement with depressed left ventricular ejection fraction
- *Pulsus paradoxus*—suspect tamponade, emphysema

should consider dicrotic pulse if double-picked arterial pulse is appreciated. The arterial pressure waveform, when recorded, reveals a single percussion wave and a prominent, accentuated dicrotic wave. At the bedside, however, it is difficult to differentiate between dicrotic pulse and pulsus bisferiens. The dicrotic pulse is appreciated in some patients with severe heart failure, for example, due to dilated cardiomyopathy, low cardiac output, and increased systemic vascular resistance. On the other hand, dicrotic pulse is also appreciated in patients with septic shock with high cardiac output and low systemic vascular resistance. However, a dicrotic pulse is also appreciated in patients after aortic valve replacement and usually indicates impaired left ventricular systolic function. In patients with aortic valve replacement, if a double-picked carotid pulse with sharp initial upstroke is appreciated, it is desirable to evaluate prosthetic valve and left ventricular function by echocardiography to exclude paraprosthetic leak.

Corrigan pulse, or water-hammer pulse, is typically observed in patients with significant chronic aortic regurgitation and is characterized by an abrupt, very rapid upstroke of the peripheral pulse followed by rapid collapse. It is best appreciated by raising the arm abruptly and feeling the changes in the radial pulse. The significance of altered character of the arterial pulse in adult patients is summarized in Table 16.2.

Examination of Jugular Venous Pulse and Pressure

Examination of jugular venous pulse and pressure (1,2) is essential to assess hemodynamic changes in the right side of the heart. Jugular venous pressure and pulses usually are examined with the patient in a 45-degree, semirecumbent position. However, if, in this position, the venous pulsations are not recognized, the examination of venous pressure and pulse should be done with the patient in a supine position or even with the head and neck tilted below the level of the chest. Occasionally, if the venous pressure is normal or low, the legs need to be raised to increase the venous return and increase right-sided venous pressure. When the venous pressure is extremely elevated and the veins appear to be distended, it is preferable to examine the jugular venous pulses with the patient in an upright position or even in a standing position. It is preferable to examine the internal jugular venous pressure and pulse. In adults, particularly in elderly patients, the external jugular venous pressure may be elevated because of partial obstruction at the level of the external jugular venous bulb owing to partial thrombosis or even obstruction by the platysma muscle. The internal jugular venous pulse is located medial to the mandibular portion of the sternomastoid muscle. The proximal internal jugular venous pulse is located in the supraclavicular area between the two proximal heads of the sternomastoid muscle. Both right and left jugular venous pulsations need to be examined, because sometimes disparity between left and right internal jugular venous pressures can be recognized. Occasionally in elderly patients, the left internal jugular venous pressure is higher than the right internal jugular venous pressure because of the partial obstruction of the left innominate vein by unfolded aorta. In these circumstances, with inspiration and descent of the diaphragm, partial obstruction of the left innominate vein is relieved, and the pressures in the right and left internal jugular veins become equal.

At the bedside, venous pulsation needs to be differentiated from carotid artery pulsation. By inspection, the venous pulse is characterized by a sharp inward movement, whereas the arterial pulse is characterized by a sharp outward movement. During inspection, the venous pulse is also recognized by its double undulation character in sinus rhythm. In the presence of atrial fibrillation, the double undulation character of the venous pulse is lost because of the absence of an 'a' wave associated with atrial systole. The venous pressure and the amplitude of the venous pulse can be decreased or increased by appropriate maneuvers. The pressure and amplitude can be decreased by raising the level of the head and trunk above the level of the right atrium (in a sitting or standing position), or they can be increased by enhancing the venous return to the right side of the heart by raising the legs or by abdominal compression. In the presence of low systemic venous pressure, when a patient is examined in a head-down position, it is possible to recognize the venous pulsation in the neck. When a pulsation in the neck is recognized, a gentle to moderate compression—by the fingers or stethoscope tubes—at the root of the neck obliterates the venous pulse, but the arterial pulse remains visible. This maneuver is extremely useful for differentiating between arterial and venous pulsations. Normally during inspection, the jugular venous pulse amplitude decreases during inspiration, whereas the arterial pulse amplitude does not change during respiration.

After recognizing the venous pulse, the venous pressure is estimated by noting the height of the oscillating top of the venous pulse above the sternal angle. Right atrial pressure is approximated by adding 5 cm to the height of the venous column, because it is assumed that the right atrium is located about 5 cm below the sternal angle. The normal right atrial pressure is less than 9 cm of water. If the jugular venous pressure is increased in the absence of obvious pulsation, it is desirable to exclude superior vena cava obstruction, which does not permit transmission of right atrial pulsation to the internal jugular veins. If pulsation of the neck veins can be recognized, the estimated venous pressure can be used to estimate right atrial pressure. The character of the venous pulse and other physical findings need to be incorporated to assess the cause of elevation of systemic venous and right atrial pressures. The normal jugular venous pulse wave or right atrial pressure wave recordings usually consist of three positive waves ('a,' 'c,' and 'v') and two negative waves ('x' and 'y' descents) (Fig. 16.3). The 'a' wave is caused by transmitted right atrial pressure to the jugular veins during right atrial systole. The 'a' wave in the jugular venous pulse is appreciated by its occurrence just prior to the left ventricular ejection, which is recognized by simultaneous palpation of the carotid pulse upstroke. At the bedside, simultaneous palpation of the carotid pulse upstroke and inspection of the venous pulse give the impression that the 'a' wave of the venous pulse and the carotid pulse upstroke occur out of phase. On the other hand, the prominent

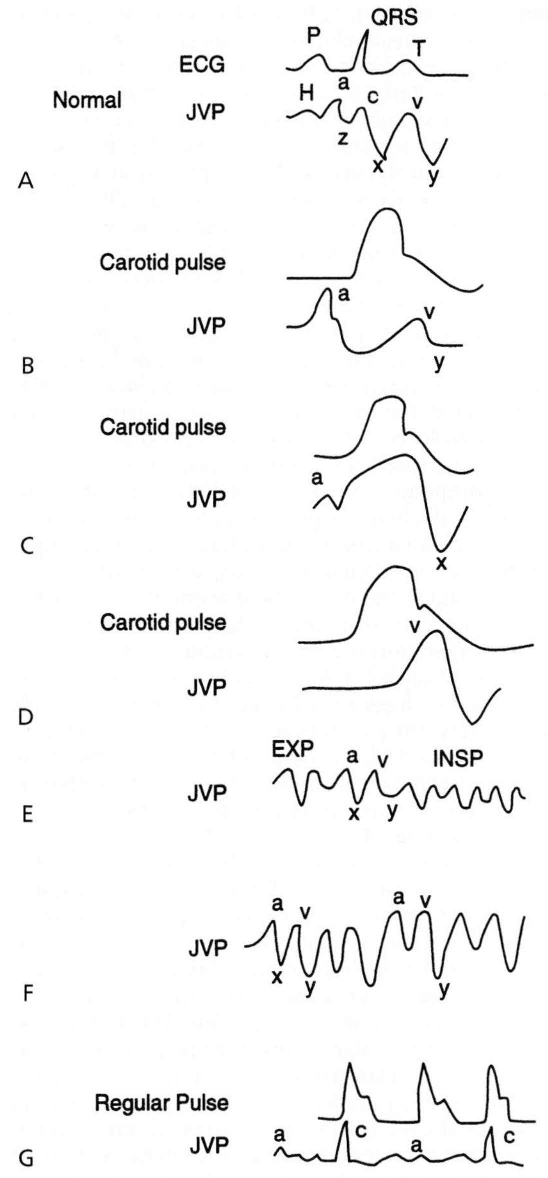

FIGURE 16.3. Schematic illustrations of a normal jugular venous pulse (JVP) and a few commonly encountered abnormalities of the JVP. **A:** Normal venous pulse along with electrocardiogram (ECG). The 'a' wave associated with right atrial systole occurs after the P wave and just before the upstroke of the carotid pulse. Normally, 'a' wave is dominant and appears more obvious during inspiration. During simultaneous palpitation of the carotid pulse at the bedside, an impression of "out of phase" between the 'a' wave and the carotid pulse upstroke is appreciated. During right atrial relaxation, the venous pulse descends and may continue up to a plateau interval (z) or can be interrupted by the 'c' wave, which is produced by the bulging of the tricuspid valve into the right atrium at the onset of the isovolumic systole and also transmitted from the carotid pulse when observed in the neck. After the 'c' wave, the venous pulse descends (x), which results from atrial relaxation. The 'v' wave occurs during right atrial filling with closed tricuspid valve and during right ventricular ejection. After the peak of the 'v' wave, which corresponds to the T wave of the ECG, right atrial pressure exceeds right ventricular diastolic pressure, which causes opening of the tricuspid valve, rapid filling of the right ventricle, and subsequent 'y' descent. When diastole is long (e.g., with a slow heart rate), the 'y' descent may be followed by a brief positive wave (H) or a plateau. It should be recognized that, at the bedside, it is difficult to appreciate the 'x' descent, H wave, and 'z' wave; usually only 'a' and 'v' waves and 'y' descents are appreciated. **B:** A prominent 'a' wave precedes the carotid pulse upstroke; when jugular venous pulse is inspected during simultaneous palpitation of the carotid pulse upstroke, an impression of "out of phase" between pulses is appreciated at the bedside. **C:** Prominent 'v' wave (regurgitant wave) followed by a sharp 'y' descent and coincident with the carotid pulse. At the bedside, venous pulse appears in phase with carotid pulse, and tricuspid regurgitation is the most common cause. **D:** In atrial fibrillation, a prominent 'v' in the JVP in the absence of tricuspid regurgitation can be recognized. **E:** In cardiac tamponade, mean JVP is elevated, and a lack of a sharp 'x' or 'y' descent is appreciated at the bedside. *Abbreviations:* EXP, expiration; INSP, inspiration. **F:** Jugular venous pulsation in constrictive pericarditis usually reveals a marked elevation of the mean venous pressure and sharp 'y' descent. During inspiration, the venous pressure may not decrease and may even increase (Kussmaul sign). These altered characteristics of the JVP, however, are nondiagnostic of constrictive pericarditis and can be present in patients with right ventricular infarction, pulmonary embolism, restrictive cardiomyopathy, and severe tricuspid regurgitation. **G:** In a patient with a slow regular pulse, appreciation of irregular cannon waves ('c') in the jugular venous pulse suggests complete atrioventricular block.

'v' wave in the venous pulse occurs more or less simultaneously with the carotid pulse upstroke. Atrial relaxation initiates the descent of the 'a' wave. Rarely, when the PR interval is markedly prolonged, the descent may continue until a plateau is reached, the 'z' point, which occurs just prior to the ventricular systole. The descent after atrial systole usually is interrupted by the 'c' wave. In the right atrial pressure pulse, the 'c' wave is recognized with the onset of right ventricular systole and occurs from bulging of the tricuspid valve into the right atrium. It should be emphasized, however, that the 'c' wave in the jugular venous pulse probably results from transmission of the carotid artery pulsation and not from the transmission of the right atrial 'c' wave. The 'v' wave is caused by the rise in right atrial and jugular venous pressure due to continued inflow of blood to the venous system during right ventricular systole when the tricuspid valve is still closed. Although in right atrial and jugular venous pressure tracings, the peak of the normal 'v' wave occurs immediately after ventricular systole; at the bedside, the normal or abnormal 'v' wave coincides with the carotid pulse upstroke and downstroke. Although the regurgitant wave of tricuspid regurgitation (a prominent 'v' wave) occurs earlier and coincides with the beginning of left ventricular ejection, at the bedside the tricuspid regurgitant wave is appreciated simultaneously with the carotid pulse upstroke (see Fig. 16.3).

The descending limb of the 'v' wave—the 'y' descent—is caused by the opening of the tricuspid valve and the rapid inflow of blood to the right ventricle from the right atrium. The 'y' descent is almost always recognized in the jugular venous pulse, and it follows the 'v' wave.

During examination of the jugular venous pulse at the bedside, if a prominent 'a' wave is appreciated, conditions associated with increased resistance to right atrial emptying during atrial systole should be considered. The 'a' waves need to be distinguished from regular cannon waves, which occur in junctional rhythm or ventricular tachycardia with retrograde ventriculoatrial conduction. Cannon waves occur during atrial systole with closed tricuspid valve. Cannon waves, therefore, occur concurrently with the onset of ventricular systole (i.e., concurrently with carotid pulse upstroke). Cannon waves are distinguished from 'v' waves by lack of obvious 'y' descents that follow 'v' waves or regurgitant waves. In the presence of a regular pulse, if irregular cannon waves are recognized by a sudden appearance of a large positive wave coincident with ventricular systole (with carotid upstroke), atrioventricular dissociation should be suspected. Regular cannon waves also occur in patients with a prolonged PR interval when atrial systole occurs during the preceding ventricular systole. When a prominent 'a' wave with large amplitude is appreciated, it is desirable to exclude tricuspid valve obstruction; this can be done by noting absence of a mid-diastolic rumble along the lower left sternal border, which increases in intensity during inspiration. Although in severe tricuspid stenosis the 'y' descent is abbreviated and presystolic hepatic pulsations can be observed, such a degree of tricuspid stenosis is rarely encountered. It should also be emphasized that isolated tricuspid stenosis is almost never encountered in rheumatic heart disease, and rheumatic tricuspid stenosis occurs almost always in the presence of mitral or aortic valve disease and in patients who are usually in atrial fibrillation. In adult cardiac patients, if isolated tricuspid stenosis is recognized with a prominent 'a' wave with a mid-diastolic rumble along the lower left sternal border that increases in intensity during inspiration (Carvello sign), right atrial myxoma or carcinoid heart disease should be considered in the differential diagnosis. However, the most common cause of a prominent 'a' wave in adults is right ventricular hypertrophy, which offers increased resistance to right atrial emptying during right atrial systole. Right ventricular hypertrophy may result from a right ventricular outflow tract obstruction, such as pulmonary valve stenosis or precapillary or postcapillary pulmonary hypertension. Significant pulmonary valve stenosis can be easily diagnosed by noting a long ejection systolic murmur, which is heard best over the left second intercostal space, a pulmonary ejection sound, and a widely split S_2 with reduced intensity of the pulmonary component of the S_2. Pulmonary hypertension is also easily recognized at the bedside by noting the increased intensity of the pulmonic component of the S_2 and its transmission to the cardiac apex (mitral area).

If a prominent 'v' wave in the jugular venous pulse is recognized at the bedside, tricuspid regurgitation should be suspected, and physical findings to confirm the diagnosis should be sought. In tricuspid regurgitation, jugular venous pulse reveals a sharp 'y' descent after a prominent 'v' wave. In severe tricuspid regurgitation, lateral pulsatile motions of the earlobes coincident with each cardiac cycle are observed in many patients. There usually is a systolic murmur either early or pansystolic in duration, which is heard best over the left third and fourth intercostal spaces, along the left sternal border. Tricuspid regurgitation murmur frequently radiates to the epigastrium and the right side of the sternum. It may be heard even over the jugular venous pulse. The tricuspid regurgitation murmur also increases in intensity after inspiration. When the diagnosis of tricuspid regurgitation is confirmed, it is desirable to assess carefully the intensity of the pulmonic component of the S_2 to distinguish between primary and secondary tricuspid regurgitation. Secondary tricuspid regurgitation is defined when tricuspid regurgitation occurs owing to right ventricular dilatation and failure secondary to pulmonary hypertension.

Occasionally, a prominent 'v' wave is detected in patients with atrial septal defect in the absence of pulmonary arterial hypertension and tricuspid regurgitation (22). The mechanism of the prominent 'v' wave in atrial septal defect is not clear; however, a concomitant increase in systemic venous return and left-to-right shunt during ventricular systole may cause a rapid increase in right atrial pressure—hence, a prominent 'v' wave. It should be emphasized that a prominent 'v' wave in patients with atrial septal defect is not followed by a sharp 'y' descent.

Although a sharp 'y' descent most frequently occurs in tricuspid regurgitation, it can be observed in constrictive pericarditis and restrictive cardiomyopathy. In constrictive pericarditis and restrictive cardiomyopathy, systemic venous pressure is elevated, and inspection of the jugular venous pulse may reveal a sharp 'y' descent of brief duration. In constrictive pericarditis or restrictive cardiomyopathy, the jugular venous pressure does not fall appropriately or even increase during inspiration (Kussmaul sign) (23) (see Fig. 16.3). It should be recognized that the Kussmaul sign is not diagnostic of constrictive pericarditis or restrictive cardiomyopathy. Kussmaul sign can be observed in patients with right ventricular infarction (24), primary severe right ventricular failure resulting from any cause, primary or secondary severe tricuspid regurgitation, partial obstruction of the vena cava, or right atrial and right ventricular tumors; in some patients with severe CHF without tricuspid regurgitation; and, occasionally, in patients with tricuspid stenosis. The Kussmaul sign is observed in some elderly patients without any obvious pathology (personal observation). The Kussmaul sign is uncommon and seldom noted in cardiac tamponade. The mechanism of the Kussmaul sign has not been adequately studied; however, increased resistance to right atrial filling during inspiration seems to be a common contributory factor. For practical purposes, in patients with chronic CHF, a presence of the Kussmaul sign should raise the possibility of constrictive pericarditis or restrictive cardiomyopathy, and appropriate evaluations should be considered. The presence of physical findings of pulmonary hypertension (e.g., a sustained systolic left parasternal lift, a loud pulmonic component of the S_2, and severe tricuspid regurgitation with pulsatile hepatic impulse) favor the diagnosis of restrictive cardiomyopathy. In contrast, lack of findings suggestive of pulmonary hypertension, a quiet precordium or presence of a prominent diastolic left parasternal impulse, and absence of hepatic pulsation favor the diagnosis of constrictive pericarditis. In constrictive pericarditis, a pericardial "knock" (similar to right-sided S_3 gallop) and, rarely, a mid-diastolic murmur are heard. Once constrictive pericarditis or restrictive cardiomyopathy are suspected, appropriate investigations should be performed (see Chapter 54).

In patients with suspected CHF, it is desirable to perform the hepatojugular reflux test (25,26). With the patient breathing normally and in the semirecumbent position, firm pressure is applied with the palm of the hand to the upper right quadrant of the abdomen for at least 10 seconds. In normal patients, there may be a transient increase in jugular venous pressure with rapid return to or near baseline in less than 10 seconds. The abnormal hepatojugular reflux is defined when there is a rapid increase in jugular venous pressure that remains elevated by 4 cm or more until abdominal compression is released. During abdominal compression with increased intraabdominal pressure, there is an increase in venous return to the right atrium and right ventricle. Concurrently, there is an increase in right ventricular afterload owing to upward movement of the diaphragm, which reduces the intrathoracic volume capacity. The normally functioning right ventricle handles this increase in preload and afterload, and systemic venous pressure remains normal. The dysfunctioning right ventricle, however, fails to accept this increase in preload and afterload; therefore, there is a persistent elevation of systemic venous pressure. A positive hepatojugular reflux is most frequently associated with CHF resulting from left heart failure (27). In these circumstances, an abnormal sustained elevation of right atrial pressure during hepatojugular reflux indicates incipient right heart failure or abnormal compliance of the right ventricle in the presence of intact pericardium (Fig. 16.4). It should be emphasized that a positive hepatojugular reflux is noted in patients with isolated right heart failure due to precapillary pulmonary hypertension or right ventricular infarction. The abnormalities of the venous pressure and pulse and associated suspected cardiovascular disorders are summarized in Table 16.3.

Examination of the Precordial Pulsations

Inspection and palpation of precordial pulsation is best performed in patients in supine position with head and trunk

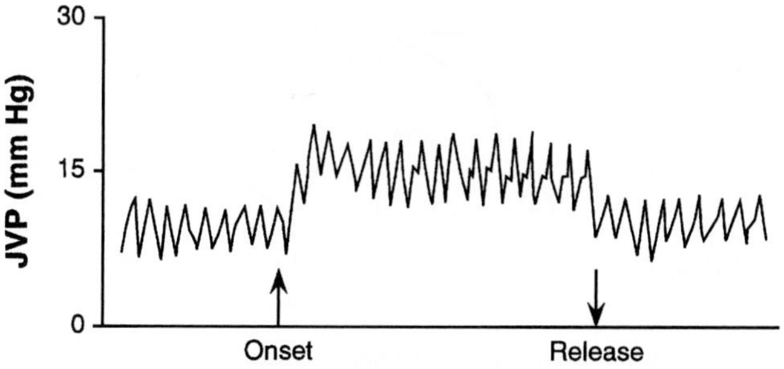

FIGURE 16.4. An example of a positive hepatojugular reflux (abdominojugular maneuver). Jugular venous pressure (JVP) increases with the onset of abdominal compression (≠) and remains elevated until it is released (□). In adults, the most common cause of positive hepatojugular reflux is left heart failure due to dilated cardiomyopathy. However, positive hepatojugular reflux also is observed in tricuspid stenosis and isolated right ventricular failure due to pulmonary hypertension and right ventricular infarction.

elevated (45degrees) (1,2). Normally, a slight, abrupt, inward pulsation can be seen occasionally over the lower left parasternal area, particularly in children and thin-chested patients. Epigastric and subxyphoid pulsations are usually abnormal, although they can be seen in patients with COPD. A pronounced epigastric or subxyphoid pulsation should raise the possibility of right ventricular failure or abdominal aortic aneurysm. A visible pulsation over the right second intercostal space or right sternoclavicular joint may indicate aneurysm of the ascending aorta. Aneurysm of the arch of the aorta may also cause suprasternal pulsation. The most common cause of right supraclavicular pulsation is a kinked, tortuous right carotid artery. A visible pulsation over the left second or third interspace may be due to dilated pulmonary artery, which may result from increased flow, such as with atrial septal defect or increased pressure, as in patients with precapillary or postcapillary pulmonary hypertension. Systolic outward parasternal and left ventricular outward movements are better appreciated by palpation. However, in many patients, an abnormal left ventricular apical impulse is visible and may result from a pronounced, sustained, outward movement or hyperdynamic left ventricular apical impulse. When cardiac pulsations are visible lateral to the left midclavicular line, cardiac enlargement should be suspected. Leftward displacement of the cardiac apex may occur due to fibrosis of the left lung, right-sided tension pneumothorax, or massive left pleural effusion. Absent left pericardium (a congenital anomaly) and thoracic deformity may also cause visible pulsations beyond the midclavicular line. Occasionally in patients with adhesive pericarditis, retraction of the ribs in the left axilla (Broadbent sign) are recognized. In patients with severe dilated congestive cardiomyopathy, a double or triple impulse over the left ventricular apex can be recognized and represents a sustained left ventricular outward movement, a prominent atrial filling wave, and early diastolic filling impulse.

Palpation of left ventricular impulse and left parasternal impulse provide useful information to assess changes in cardiac dynamics and function. The left ventricular apical impulse is best palpated when the patient lies in a partial left lateral decubitus position. The outward movement of the left ventricular apical impulse is normally brief and localized and does not extend significantly into the left ventricular ejection phase (Fig. 16.5). The beginning of left ventricular ejection at the bedside is appreciated by the onset of the carotid pulse upstroke. The normal outward movement of the left ventricular apical impulse recedes from the chest wall and becomes impalpable with the onset of ejection after the upstroke of the carotid pulse and during the downstroke of the carotid pulse (28). Thus, at the bedside, when carotid pulse and left ventricular apical impulse are examined concurrently, these two impulses appear out of phase or asynchronous. The sustained apical impulse is characterized by a prolonged duration of the outward movement extending into the ejection phase of the left ventricle. Usually, this outward movement is diffuse and occupies more than one intercostal space. When the carotid pulse upstroke and duration are evaluated simultaneously with the left ventricular outward movement, the sustained apical impulse appears in phase with the carotid pulse upstroke and remains palpable during the downstroke of the carotid pulse.

With a hyperdynamic apical impulse, the amplitude of the outward movement is increased, but the sequence between the onset of the carotid pulse and the outward movement remains normal. The hyperdynamic apical impulse is appreciated as a thrust of large amplitude that immediately disappears from the palpating fingers. When the duration of the ejection phase is estimated from the carotid pulse upstroke and downstroke or from the interval between the S_1 and S_2, the hyperdynamic apical impulse does not extend throughout systole. The sustained outward movement usually is felt as a heave. The duration of the outward movement of the apical impulse when it is sustained extends throughout the ejection phase. A sustained apical impulse usually is found when there is significant impairment of left ventricular systolic function (i.e., reduced ejection fraction) (29,30). Another cause of sustained apical impulse is marked left ventricular hypertrophy resulting from systemic hypertension or left ventricular outflow tract obstruction. In patients with known coronary artery disease or previous myocardial infarction and dilated cardiomyopathy, a sustained apical impulse almost invariably indicates reduced left ventricular ejection fraction. Systolic bulges occasionally may be appreciated in the absence of previous myocardial infarction and probably result from myocardial ischemia. At the bedside, however, these transient abnormal systolic motions are difficult to appreciate. Occasionally in patients with mitral valve prolapse, a deep notch in the systolic portion of the left ventricular apical impulse, which coincides with the midsystolic click, is recorded in the apex cardiogram, but it is difficult to recognize at the bedside. The hyperdynamic apical impulse occurs in conditions associated with an increased stroke volume or volume overload. Hyperdynamic impulse is found in patients with hypermetabolic state, such as hyperthyroidism, anemia, primary mitral regurgitation, and aortic regurgitation, and in some patients

TABLE 16.3

ABNORMALITIES OF THE VENOUS PRESSURE AND PULSE AND THEIR CLINICAL SIGNIFICANCE

- *Positive hepatojugular reflux*—suspect CHF, particularly left ventricular systolic dysfunction
- *Elevated systemic venous pressure without obvious 'x' or 'y' descent and quiet precordium and pulsus paradoxus*—suspect cardiac tamponade
- *Elevated systemic venous pressure with sharp 'y' descent, Kussmaul sign, and quiet precordium*—suspect constrictive pericarditis
- *Elevated systemic venous pressure with a sharp, brief 'y' descent, Kussmaul sign, and evidence of pulmonary hypertension and tricuspid regurgitation*—suspect restrictive cardiomyopathy
- *A prominent 'a' wave with or without elevation of mean systemic venous pressure*—exclude tricuspid stenosis, right ventricular hypertrophy due to pulmonary stenosis, and pulmonary hypertension
- *A prominent 'v' wave with a sharp 'y' descent*—suspect tricuspid regurgitation

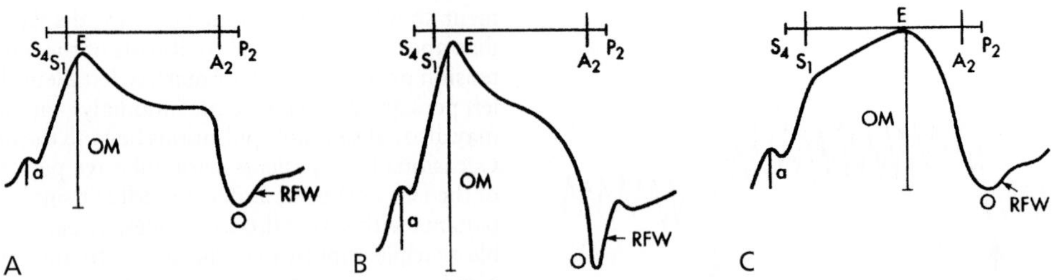

FIGURE 16.5. Schematic diagrams of normal, hyperdynamic, and sustained left ventricular impulse. Heart sounds are also illustrated. **A:** Normal apical impulse. The 'a' wave related to ventricular filling during atrial systole usually is not palpable. Similarly, the rapid filling wave (RFW) in early diastole is also not palpable. The E point, which coincides with the beginning of the left ventricular ejection, is brief in normal individuals. Normal apical impulse usually is associated with normal left ventricular ejection fraction. **B:** Hyperdynamic left ventricular impulse usually is seen in left ventricular volume overloaded conditions such as primary mitral regurgitation and aortic regurgitation. Left ventricular ejection fraction usually is normal. A palpable 'a' wave or presystolic wave indicates increased left ventricular end-diastolic pressure. **C:** Sustained left ventricular impulse, which extends into the ejection phase, usually is seen in the presence of decreased left ventricular ejection fraction or when there is marked left ventricular hypertrophy. A palpable 'a' wave or early rapid filling spike is associated with increased diastolic pressure. *Abbreviations:* A_2, aortic component of the second heart sound; P_2, pulmonary component of the second heart sound; S_1, first heart sound; S_4, fourth heart sound.

with a patent ductus arteriosus and ventricular septal defect with a large left-to-right shunt. A hyperdynamic impulse, in general, suggests preserved left ventricular ejection fraction.

While examining the left ventricular apical impulse, particularly with the patient in the left lateral decubitus position, a double impulse is felt and almost always represents a palpable 'a' wave (presystolic wave) and a prominent outward movement. The palpable 'a' wave is related to an accentuated atrial filling wave and is most frequently observed in patients with noncompliant left ventricle, such as in patients with aortic stenosis, hypertensive heart disease, or ischemic heart disease. The hemodynamic correlate of palpable 'a' wave is increased left ventricular end-diastolic pressure. Occasionally, a palpable, rapid filling spike, which coincides with a prominent S_3 gallop, is appreciated during palpation of left ventricular apical impulse. At the bedside, this palpable early diastolic rapid filling spike is appreciated after the outward movement. The hemodynamic correlate of palpable S_3 gallop is also increased left ventricular diastolic pressure. In occasional patients with obstructive hypertrophic cardiomyopathy, the apical impulse may have a bifid outward movement and if there is a prominent 'a' wave, a triple impulse may be felt (31,32). The characteristics of the left ventricular outward movement, along with changes in the filling waves, are illustrated in Fig. 16.5.

Right ventricular impulse is appreciated by palpation of the lower left parasternal area. In children and in some adults with thin chest walls, a brief, gentle impulse may be palpable over the left third and fourth interspaces. This impulse usually is in diastole. A prolonged left parasternal impulse extending during the ejection phase (i.e., throughout the carotid pulse upstroke and downstroke or between S_1 and S_2) is distinctly abnormal and reflects right ventricular failure or right ventricular hypertrophy. In the presence of significant mitral regurgitation, left atrial expansion during left ventricular systole may also produce a sustained systolic left parasternal impulse. In patients with right ventricular hypertrophy and failure, a sustained epigastric impulse is also appreciated. An inward systolic movement and an outward diastolic movement are sometimes appreciated in some patients with constrictive pericarditis (33). The diastolic movement usually coincides in timing with the pericardial knock. The precise explanation for these unusual precordial impulses in constrictive pericarditis has not been clarified. It has been suggested that this unusual outward movement during isovolumic systole is inhibited by the constriction, and the outward movement during early diastole becomes accentuated. In patients with severe chronic constrictive pericarditis, however, the precordium usually is quiet, and no obvious precordial impulses are appreciated at the bedside. In patients with Ebstein anomaly, the precordium may also be quiet. In some patients with Ebstein anomaly, a right parasternal systolic outward movement resulting from a large, ventricularized right atrium is appreciated. A hyperdynamic left parasternal impulse may be palpable in volume overloaded right ventricle as with an atrial septal defect or tricuspid regurgitation (34).

A left ventricular aneurysm can be associated with a systolic impulse in unusual locations, such as over the midprecordium. Pulsation in the left second interspace usually reflects an enlarged pulmonary artery resulting from chronic severe pulmonary arterial hypertension or from increased pulmonary flow, as in atrial septal defect. Occasionally, a higher frequency impulse is appreciated coincident with the downstroke of the carotid pulse in the left second interspace and usually reflects an accentuated pulmonary component of the S_2, as in patients with severe chronic pulmonary hypertension. A pulsatile mass in the suprasternal notch may indicate aneurysm of the ascending aorta. Aneurysm of the ascending aorta is sometimes associated with the tracheal tug, which is appreciated when the trachea is slightly pulled upward and the pulsation in the trachea is recognized with each cardiac cycle. A pulsatile mass in the right supraclavicular area is most frequently caused by a kinked right carotid artery. Such an abnormal impulse may indicate the presence of atherosclerotic peripheral vascular disease.

Auscultation

A systematic and careful cardiac auscultation (1,35) is essential for the diagnosis of a cardiovascular abnormality. Auscultation should be performed whenever possible with the patient in the left lateral decubitus, supine, and sitting positions. Auscultation can begin over the cardiac apex—the so-called mitral area—and one can proceed counterclockwise to the left fourth interspace (tricuspid area), left third interspace, left second interspace (pulmonic area), and right second interspace (aortic area), sometimes, over the right fourth interspace adjacent to the sternal borders, and, finally, over the epigastrium. It is customary to assess the intensity and splitting of the S_1 and S_2 and the presence of S_3 and the fourth heart sound (S_4). It is also desirable to listen for the presence of abnormal early systolic, midsystolic, early diastolic, and late diastolic heart sounds.

After the analysis of the normal and abnormal heart sounds, heart murmurs, if present, are analyzed. When certain diagnoses are suspected, areas of auscultation should include the left axilla, thoracic and lumber spine, vortex (mitral regurgitation), axilla and back (pulmonary artery branch stenosis), posterior chest (coarctation of the aorta), left infraclavicular area (patent ductus arteriosus), and sternoclavicular joints (venous hum).

FIRST HEART SOUND

Intensity

For the analysis of the S_1, the diaphragm is used, and auscultation is performed over the mitral and tricuspid areas. The intensity of the S_1 is determined primarily by the intensity of mitral component (M_1) of the S_1. Several factors contribute to the intensity of M_1 (36,37). The position of the mitral valve at the onset of systole, the rate of mitral valve closure, the mobility of the mitral valve, the PR interval, and the dP/dT of the left ventricle—all are important factors that influence the intensity of M_1. The position of the atrioventricular valves at the beginning of the ventricular systole, and the velocity of closure seem to be the major determinants of the intensity of the S_1. When the mitral valve remains fully open until the very end of diastole and then closes rapidly, the intensity of M_1 is increased. The greater the distance that the mitral valve leaflets have to travel from the open to closed positions and the greater the velocity of closure of the mitral valve, the louder the S_1. If a substantial increase in the intensity of the S_1 is recognized, an increase in transmitral valvular pressure gradient (e.g., in mitral stenosis), increased transvalvular flow (e.g., in the presence of large left-to-right shunt owing to ventricular septal defect or a patent ductus arteriosus), a very short PR interval (e.g., in preexcitation syndrome), or markedly shortened left ventricular diastole (e.g., in tachycardia) should be suspected. When mitral valve obstruction and short PR interval are excluded, increased intensity of the S_1 may reflect an increased left ventricular dP/dT, as during adrenergic stimulation. The increased intensity of the tricuspid valve closure sound (T_1), which is appreciated over the left third and fourth interspaces along the lower sternal border, usually occurs when the transtricuspid valve pressure gradient is increased, as in patients with tricuspid stenosis or right atrial myxoma. A substantial increase in diastolic flow across the tricuspid valve, as in large atrial septal defect, may also increase the intensity of the T_1. Intermittent increased intensity of the S_1 in the presence of regular pulse and heart rhythms indicates atrioventricular dissociation, results from varying PR intervals, and is associated with variable rates of closure of atrioventricular valves. An increase in intensity of the S_1 has been observed in some patients with mitral valve prolapse, despite mitral regurgitation, and probably reflects increased adrenergic activity (38).

A decrease in intensity of the S_1 can result from a substantial loss of the tissue mass of the atrioventricular valves, as occurs in severe rheumatic tricuspid and mitral valve diseases and bacterial endocarditis. This decrease can also result from the marked restriction of the movement of the atrioventricular valves because of calcification or sclerosis of the valve leaflets, which occasionally occurs in patients with rheumatic mitral valve stenosis and may be associated with decreased—rather than increased—intensity of the S_1. When the PR interval is prolonged (>200 ms), the intensity of the S_1 decreases because semiclosure of the mitral valve occurs after atrial systole and before ventricular systole begins. In severe aortic regurgitation, premature closure of the mitral valve may occur owing to a rapid rise in left ventricular diastolic pressure, and the mitral valve may be virtually closed at the onset of ventricular systole, resulting in a markedly decreased intensity of the S_1. In patients with acute severe aortic regurgitation associated with marked increase in left ventricular diastolic pressure, the S_1 may be inaudible and should be regarded as an indication for surgical intervention (39). A substantial increase in left ventricular diastolic pressure is an important mechanism for decreased intensity of the S_1 in the absence of prolonged PR interval and restricted mitral valve mobility. Impaired contractile function, as in dilated cardiomyopathy, is contributory to reduced intensity of the S_1. In these patients, left ventricular diastolic pressure is also frequently elevated. Occasionally, decreased intensity of S_1 is observed in isolated left bundle branch block, probably reflecting impaired left ventricular function (40).

A variable intensity of the S_1 is common in atrial fibrillation. Auscultatory alternans—in which the S_1 is soft and loud in intensity with alternate beats—is a rare finding of severe cardiac tamponade and is almost always associated with electrical alternans and pulsus paradoxus. Auscultatory alternans also has been observed in patients with pulsus alternans, in whom beat-to-beat alteration in the left ventricular dP/dT occurs (41).

Decreased conduction of sounds through the chest wall reduces the intensity of the S_1 in patients with COPD, obesity, and pericardial effusion. In these circumstances, all heart sounds appear soft and distant. One of the practical difficulties in assessing the intensity of the S_1 at the bedside is the lack of any objective method to standardize its intensity. The S_1 normally is loudest at the apex and along the lower left sternal border.

Splitting

The splitting of the S_1 (42) is best appreciated along the left parasternal areas and is most frequently observed in the presence of complete or incomplete right bundle branch block. In right bundle branch block, the S_2 is also widely split, and the A_2–P_2 interval widens during inspiration. Delayed closure of T_1 because of increased flow across the tricuspid valve (atrial septal defect) or increased transtricuspid valve pressure gradient (tricuspid stenosis) causes wide splitting of S_1 without splitting of the S_2. The widely split S_1 is recognized in patients with the Ebstein anomaly, not only because of right ventricular conduction disturbances but also from the delayed closure of the tricuspid valve owing to atrialization of the right ventricle. In Ebstein anomaly, the S_2 is also widely split, and, frequently, systolic and diastolic, scratchy, superficial sounds—so-called sail sounds—are present (43). The reversed splitting of the S_1 is extremely rare and difficult to recognize at the bedside. Reversed splitting of the S_1 can result from severe mitral stenosis and is rarely caused by left bundle branch block. In patients with severe mitral stenosis, delayed closure of the mitral valve contributes to the reversed splitting of the S_1. However, earlier closure of the tricuspid valve resulting from secondary tricuspid regurgitation is also necessary for the reversed splitting of the S_1 in mitral stenosis.

Sounds Mimicking the First Heart Sound

At the bedside, it is necessary to distinguish between splitting of the S_1 and the presence of a loud atrial sound preceding the S_1 (Fig. 16.6). The left ventricular atrial sound (S_4) usually is localized over the cardiac apex and is heard best with the bell of the stethoscope. When auscultation is started with the use of the bell over the cardiac apex, S_1 and S_4 are heard easily. When the bell is converted to the diaphragm by applying firm pressure over the underlying skin, the S_4 decreases in intensity or disappears, whereas the splitting of the S_1 becomes more obvious.

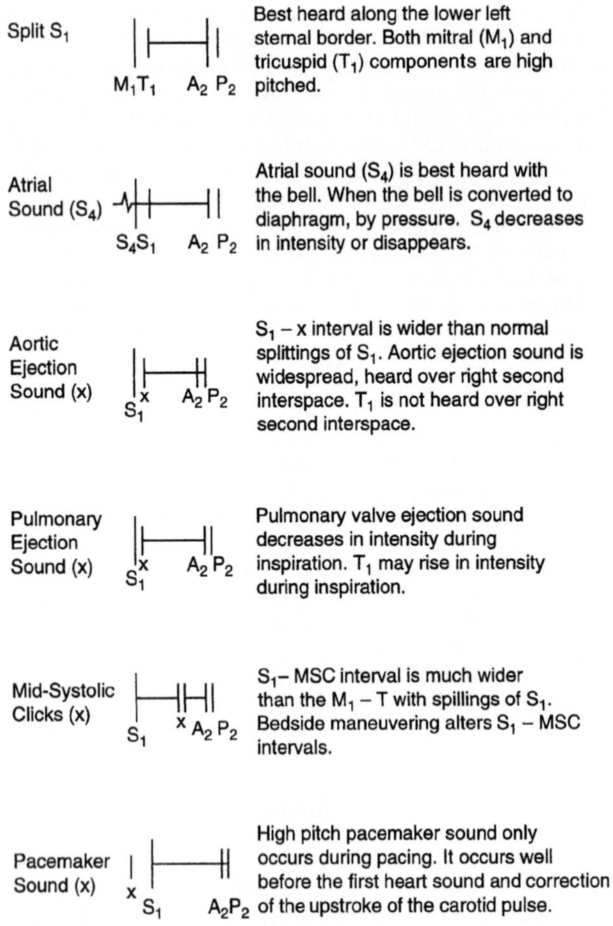

Split S_1
M_1T_1 A_2 P_2
Best heard along the lower left sternal border. Both mitral (M_1) and tricuspid (T_1) components are high pitched.
Atrial Sound (S_4)
S_4S_1 A_2 P_2
Atrial sound (S_4) is best heard with the bell. When the bell is converted to diaphragm, by pressure. S_4 decreases in intensity or disappears.
Aortic Ejection Sound (x)
S_1 x A_2 P_2
S_1 – x interval is wider than normal splittings of S_1. Aortic ejection sound is widespread, heard over right second interspace. T_1 is not heard over right second interspace.
Pulmonary Ejection Sound (x)
S_1 x A_2 P_2
Pulmonary valve ejection sound decreases in intensity during inspiration. T_1 may rise in intensity during inspiration.
Mid-Systolic Clicks (x)
S_1 x A_2 P_2
S_1– MSC interval is much wider than the M_1 – T with spillings of S_1. Bedside maneuvering alters S_1 – MSC intervals.
Pacemaker Sound (x)
x S_1 A_2P_2
High pitch pacemaker sound only occurs during pacing. It occurs well before the first heart sound and correction of the upstroke of the carotid pulse.

FIGURE 16.6. The causes and differential diagnosis of the first heart sound (S_1). *Abbreviations:* A_2, aortic component of the second heart sound; P_2, pulmonary component of the second heart sound.

The combination of a systolic ejection sound and S_1 may also appear as split S_1. The S_1 and the ejection sound interval usually is greater than the normal M_1–T_1 interval. The aortic ejection sound is widely transmitted and, therefore, can be heard easily over the aortic area, along the left sternal border, and over the cardiac apex. On the other hand, the split S_1 is best appreciated along the lower left sternal border, over the left third and fourth interspaces. Pulmonary valvular ejection sounds can be easily distinguished from T_1. Pulmonary ejection sounds are usually localized and heard best over the left second interspace. Pulmonary valvular ejection sounds decrease in intensity during inspiration, whereas the intensity of T_1 remains unchanged or increases after inspiration.

A combination of S_1 and a midsystolic click owing to mitral valve prolapse is rarely confused with a split S_1. The interval between S_1 and a midsystolic click is much greater than the interval between M_1 and T_1. Furthermore, the S_1 to midsystolic click interval can be changed by maneuvers such as standing and squatting. These maneuvers, however, usually do not alter the interval between M_1 and T_1 significantly enough to be appreciated at the bedside. The presence of a pacemaker sound preceding S_1 may seem like a widely split S_1. The pacemaker sound results from the stimulation of the intercostal muscles during pacing, precedes S_1, and occurs well before the upstroke of the carotid pulse (44). Furthermore, the pacemaker sound disappears with discontinuation of pacing. The causes and the differential diagnosis of the abnormalities of the S_1 are summarized in Table 16.4.

TABLE 16.4

USUAL CAUSES OF THE ABNORMALITIES OF THE FIRST HEART SOUND

INCREASED INTENSITY

- *Mitral or tricuspid valve obstruction*—mitral stenosis, left atrial myxoma, tricuspid stenosis, and right atrial myxoma; associated with other findings of atrioventricular valvular obstruction such as mid-diastolic rumble
- *Increased transatrioventricular valve flow*—patent ductus arteriosus, ventricular septal defect, atrial septal defect; associated with characteristic findings such as continuous murmur, pansystolic murmur, or widely split second heart sound, respectively
- *Increased dP/dT*—hyperkinetic heart syndrome, tachycardia, mitral valve prolapse; also associated with additional physical findings such as midsystolic click in mitral valve prolapse
- *Short PR interval*—preexcitation syndrome confirmed by electrocardiographic findings

DECREASED INTENSITY

- *Restrictive mitral valve movement*—calcific mitral stenosis; also associated with other auscultatory findings such as mid-diastolic rumble and findings suggestive of pulmonary hypertension
- *Lack of apposition of the mitral valve leaflets*—rheumatic mitral regurgitation, which is associated with a pansystolic murmur over the cardiac apex
- *Presystolic semiclosure of the mitral valves owing to increase in left ventricular diastolic pressure*—noncompliant left ventricle, acute aortic regurgitation, dilated cardiomyopathy
- *Conduction anomaly, left bundle branch block, prolonged PR interval*—confirmed by electrocardiography

WIDE SPLITTING OF THE FIRST HEART SOUND

- *Conduction abnormalities*—complete right bundle branch block, left ventricular pacing, preexcitation syndrome with left ventricular connection; confirmed by other associated findings, as well as by electrocardiography
- *Ebstein anomaly*—also associated with widely split second heart sound, sail sounds, and tricuspid regurgitation murmur
- *Mechanical*—tricuspid stenosis, atrial septal defect; also associated with characteristic physical findings such as mid-diastolic rumble and wide fixed splitting of the second heart sound, respectively

REVERSED SPLITTING OF THE FIRST HEART SOUND

- *Arrhythmias*—premature beats of right ventricular origin
- *Conduction disturbances*—left bundle branch block, right ventricular pacing; confirmed by electrocardiography
- *Mechanical*—severe mitral stenosis and left atrial myxoma

Abbreviation: dP/dT, upstroke pattern.

SECOND HEART SOUND

The genesis of the S_2 appears to be related to closure of the aortic and pulmonary valves; thus, the S_2 traditionally is regarded to consist of two components designated as A_2 (associated with aortic valve closure) and P_2 (associated with pulmonary valve closure). The first high-frequency component of A_2 and P_2 is coincident with completion of closure of these semilunar valves (45). It should be appreciated that A_2 and P_2 are not produced by the clapping together of the valve leaflets but by the sudden deceleration of retrograde flow of the blood column in the aorta and pulmonary artery when the maximum tensing of these valve leaflets occurs. The abrupt deceleration of flow produces the vibration of the cardiohemic system, and the lower frequency vibrations are coincident with the incisura of the great vessels, whereas the higher frequency components cause A_2 and P_2.

Intensity

Aortic Component

The amplitude and intensity of A_2 and P_2 are directly proportional to the rate of change of the diastolic pressure gradient that develops across the semilunar valves—that is, the driving force that accelerates the blood mass retrograde into the base of the great vessels (46). The rate of pressure decline in the ventricle and the level of the diastolic pressure in the great vessels determine the pressure gradient in the root of the great vessels. Normally, the diastolic pressure gradient in the aorta is significantly greater than that in the pulmonary artery, which explains the normal increased intensity of A_2 compared with that of P_2. The most common cause of the increased intensity of A_2 is systemic hypertension. Occasionally, in addition to the increased intensity, a tambour quality of A_2 is recognized in systemic hypertension. Such altered quality of A_2 also is appreciated in some patients with aneurysm of the ascending aorta. The decreased intensity of A_2 most frequently occurs from immobility of calcified, sclerosed aortic valves in calcific aortic stenosis. In aortic regurgitation resulting from fibrosed and retracted aortic valve leaflets, as in syphilitic aortic regurgitation, the aortic component of the S_2 also is decreased in intensity. Normally, A_2 is widely transmitted and well heard at the cardiac apex. However, in patients with significant primary mitral regurgitation, A_2 may be drowned at the cardiac apex by the regurgitant murmur that frequently extends beyond the aortic valve closure.

Pulmonic Component

The pulmonic component of the S_2—that is, P_2—is softer than A_2 and is rarely audible at the apex. Increase in the intensity of P_2 indicates pulmonary hypertension, irrespective of its etiology. When there is a substantial increase in its intensity, P_2 is also heard at the cardiac apex. Without pulmonary hypertension, it is uncommon for the P_2 to be transmitted to the cardiac apex. In only approximately 5% of healthy subjects, and only when they are young (<20 years old), can P_2 be recorded by phonocardiography over the cardiac apex (47). A palpable P_2 over the left second interspace indicates severe pulmonary hypertension.

When the cardiac apex is occupied by the right ventricle—as in patients with large atrial septal defects—P_2 can be heard at the apex, even when the pulmonary artery pressure is not increased. Similarly, in patients with primary tricuspid regurgitation without pulmonary hypertension, P_2 occasionally is heard at the apex. In patients with a widely split S_2 secondary to right bundle branch block, P_2 rarely can be heard at the apex in the absence of pulmonary hypertension.

Decreased intensity of P_2 results from a reduction in the pulmonary artery diastolic pressure, as in patients with pulmonary valve stenosis. Decreased intensity of P_2 or absence of P_2 may also occur from the loss of the pulmonary valve leaflets or from the congenital absence of the pulmonary valves.

Splitting

The sequence of closure of the aortic and pulmonary valves during respiratory phases should be analyzed whenever feasible.

In adults, the splitting of the S_2 during the expiratory phase of respiration usually is not appreciated at the bedside, because the degree of splitting usually does not exceed 30 ms. However, during inspiration, the splitting is easily appreciated, particularly in the semirecumbent position and even in elderly patients. The splitting of the S_2 should be assessed during normal respiration with the diaphragm of the stethoscope over the left second and third interspaces close to the sternal border. Normally, the aortic component of the S_2 (A_2) precedes the pulmonic component (P_2). The normal splitting of the S_2 primarily results from the differences between pulmonary artery and aortic "hangout" times (48). The left ventricular ejection starts a few milliseconds before the onset of right ventricular ejection because of the earlier onset of left ventricular depolarization. The earlier onset of left ventricular ejection certainly contributes to the earlier completion of left ventricular ejection. However, this earlier completion of left ventricular ejection only accounts for 10 to 15 ms of the degree of splitting of the S_2. The hangout time is the interval between the end of ventricular ejection and the closure of the semilunar valves. The hangout time in the aorta is considerably shorter than that of the pulmonary artery. The hangout time in the pulmonary artery may be as long as 60 to 70 ms; the hangout time in the aorta may be as short as 15 to 30 ms. The difference between the pulmonary artery and aortic hangout times primarily determines the degree of splitting of the S_2, both in physiologic situations and in many pathologic conditions (Fig. 16.7). The hangout time also is determined by the compliance of the aorta and the pulmonary artery. Normally, the aorta is much stiffer than the pulmonary artery—a characteristic that accounts for the shorter hangout time in the aorta than in the pulmonary artery. When pulmonary artery compliance decreases, as in chronic pulmonary hypertension, hangout time also decreases; thus, the degree of splitting of the S_2 may actually be shorter in the presence of significant chronic pulmonary arterial hypertension. The A_2–P_2 interval increases during inspiration. The normal inspiratory splitting of the S_2 is

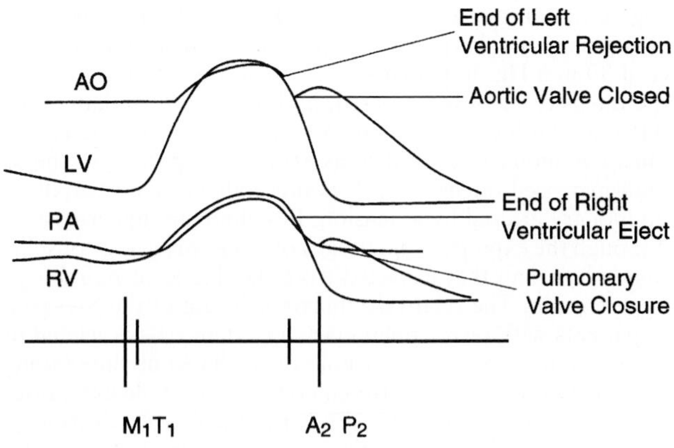

FIGURE 16.7. Schematic illustrations of hangout times, which are the time intervals between the end of ventricular ejection and closure of the aortic valve (A_2) and closure of the pulmonary valve (P_2). Hangout time is primarily determined by the compliance of the great vessels and the stroke volume ejected into the great vessels. The aortic hangout time is much shorter (the aorta is less compliant than the pulmonary artery) than that of the pulmonary artery. The differences between the pulmonary and aortic hangout time may explain physiologic or pathologic splitting of the second heart sound. The mitral component (M_1) and the tricuspid component (T_1) of the first heart sound and left ventricular (LV), right ventricular (RV), aortic (AO), and pulmonary artery (PA) pressure waveforms are also illustrated.

explained by an increase in the pulmonary hangout time during inspiration that results from an increase in right ventricular stroke volume. An increase in the right ventricular ejection time after inspiration also contributes to the inspiratory splitting of the S_2. More negative intrathoracic pressure during inspiration is associated with an increased venous return to the right ventricle and an increased right ventricular stroke volume. During inspiration, A_2 occurs slightly earlier because of the slight reduction of left ventricular ejection time associated with a transient, slight reduction of left ventricular stroke volume. During normal respiration, prolongation of left ventricular ejection time and a delayed A_2 usually occur during the expiratory phase, whereas lengthening of the right ventricular ejection time and delay in P_2 coincide with the inspiratory phase.

Wide Splitting

In adults, when splitting of the S_2 is appreciated during expiration, abnormal wide splitting of the S_2 should be suspected. The inspiratory increase in the degree of splitting of the S_2 indicates the presence of physiologic delay in the pulmonary valve closure sound. The widely split S_2 during expiration (with further increase in splitting during inspiration) most frequently occurs in right bundle branch block. A widely split S_2 may be present in Wolff-Parkinson-White syndrome with left ventricular preexcitation. Left ventricular pacing also produces right bundle branch block–types of conduction disturbances and is associated with widely split S_2. The wide splitting of the S_2 in conduction disturbances occurs from delayed activation of the right ventricle and consequently delayed completion of right ventricular ejection.

The wide splitting of the S_2 may also result from increased resistance of right ventricular ejection, as in patients with pulmonary valve stenosis, infundibular stenosis, supravalvular stenosis, and pulmonary branch stenosis. In pulmonary valve stenosis, the intensity of the P_2 is substantially decreased. In pulmonary valve stenosis, the degree of expiratory splitting of the S_2 is directly related to the severity of stenosis and right ventricular systolic hypertension (49). If the expiratory splitting of the S_2 is approximately 40 to 50 ms, right ventricular systolic pressure is also 40 to 50 mm Hg. When the degree of splitting of the S_2 exceeds 70 to 80 ms, the right ventricular systolic pressure is extremely high and may exceed 80 mm Hg. In patients with pulmonary branch stenosis, the intensity of P_2 is increased, and, frequently, unilateral or bilateral continuous murmurs are appreciated. In adults, the most common cause of obvious expiratory splitting of the S_2 with increased intensity of P_2 is precapillary or postcapillary pulmonary arterial hypertension. In pulmonary hypertension, although the expiratory splitting is obvious, the degree of splitting is less than that expected from the degree of pulmonary hypertension. The relatively shorter splitting of the S_2—even in patients with severe pulmonary hypertension—is related to the substantial reduction in pulmonary hangout time owing to decreased pulmonary arterial compliance. Wide expiratory splitting of the S_2 may also result from isolated reduction of the left ventricular ejection time, as in patients with hemodynamically significant mitral regurgitation (50). In patients with severe mitral regurgitation with relatively preserved left ventricular ejection fraction, as in patients with primary mitral regurgitation, left ventricular forward stroke volume may decrease with a substantial shortening of left ventricular ejection time and an earlier occurrence of A_2 (51). In patients with unrestricted ventricular septal defect with increased pulmonary flow and decreased pulmonary vascular resistance, a widely split S_2 is appreciated because of a decrease in left ventricular ejection time and aortic hangout time and an increase in pulmonary artery hangout time (52). In constrictive pericarditis, a wide inspiratory splitting of the S_2 occasionally is observed, and it results from marked reduction in left ventricular ejection time during inspiration (53). Decreased impedance of the pulmonary vascular bed resulting in an increase in pulmonary hangout time may also cause a wide splitting of the S_2 (35). In patients with idiopathic dilatation of the pulmonary artery, mild pulmonary valve stenosis, and atrial septal defect with normal pulmonary artery pressure, the increase in pulmonary hangout time is the principal mechanism for the wide splitting of the S_2. In patients with a primum or secundum type of atrial septal defect and also with common atrium, the interval between A_2 and P_2 during expiration and inspiration may not change significantly (widely split fixed S_2). The mechanism of wide expiratory splitting of the S_2 appears to be due to isolated shortening of the ejection time of the left ventricle, whereas the right ventricular ejection time remains normal. There is also an increase in the pulmonary hangout time, which results from the decreased pulmonary vascular impedance. During inspiration, P_2 is delayed, as in healthy patients, owing to prolongation of the right ventricular ejection time. However, in atrial septal defect, A_2 does not occur earlier, suggesting the absence of inspiratory shortening of left ventricular ejection time (54). This lack of shortening of left ventricular ejection time may result from the transient increase in the venous return to the left ventricle due to a reduction in the magnitude in the left-to-right shunt. Thus, the A_2–P_2 interval may remain relatively constant during normal expiration and inspiration.

In adults, the most frequent cause of fixed splitting of the S_2 is the occurrence of severe right ventricular failure when there is little or no increase in right ventricular stroke volume after inspiration. The degree of splitting of the S_2 during expiration, however, usually is normal in the absence of right bundle branch block. In patients with severe right ventricular failure and right bundle branch block, a wide fixed splitting of the S_2 frequently is appreciated at the bedside.

Widely Split Second Heart Sound

A marked increase in the intensity of the pulmonic component of the S_2 (P_2) with narrow expiratory splitting of the S_2 is a common and almost universally present physical finding in severe pulmonary hypertension. The degree of expiratory splitting (the A_2–P_2 interval) may even be more than 30 ms in patients with pulmonary hypertension, but the splitting is still clearly appreciated because of the marked increase in the intensity of P_2 (55). In some patients with pulmonary hypertension, a wide splitting with an increased amplitude of P_2 is present in the absence of right bundle branch block (56). It has been suggested that, in these circumstances, wide splitting may represent impairment of right ventricular systolic function. In some patients with severe pulmonary hypertension, fixed splitting of the S_2 has been observed, and it has been suggested that this fixed splitting occurs because of concomitant right ventricular failure secondary to pulmonary hypertension.

At the bedside, when pulmonary hypertension is suspected, it is desirable to search for other findings that may be associated with or result from chronic severe pulmonary hypertension. These findings include the pulmonary ejection sound, left parasternal systolic lift, pulmonary insufficiency murmur, right ventricular S_4, S_3 gallops, and tricuspid regurgitation. It is also desirable to investigate at the bedside the potential etiology of pulmonary hypertension. In adult patients, Eisenmenger syndrome is suspected from the presence of cyanosis and clubbing and the characteristic changes in the S_2. In Eisenmenger syndrome, central cyanosis occurs because of intracardiac right-to-left shunt. In Eisenmenger syndrome associated with atrial and ventricular septal defects, peripheral cyanosis and clubbing involve fingers and toes bilaterally. In Eisenmenger syndrome associated with patent ductus arteriosus, however, the cyanosis and clubbing are usually recognized in the toes, and the fingers are spared. Differential cyanosis and clubbing in adult patients almost always indicate patent ductus arteriosus and reversal of shunt, and preferential reverse shunting to the descending thoracic aorta. The S_2 in Eisenmenger syndrome associated with atrial septal defect remains widely split, and the degree of splitting during expiration and inspiration usually does not change significantly (wide fixed splitting of S_2). In Eisenmenger syndrome associated with a ventricular septal defect, the duration of right and left ventricular systole is essentially equal; therefore, a loud, single S_2 is appreciated because of simultaneous closure of the aortic and pulmonary valves (47). In Eisenmenger syndrome associated with patent ductus arteriosus, the S_2 behaves like that in precapillary primary pulmonary hypertension. It should be appreciated that pulmonary hypertension and central and peripheral cyanosis and clubbing can also occur from primary pulmonary disease, such as severe pulmonary fibrosis.

In adults, postcapillary pulmonary hypertension is much more frequent than precapillary pulmonary hypertension. Postcapillary pulmonary hypertension can be caused by mitral valve obstruction, such as rheumatic mitral stenosis, mitral regurgitation, aortic stenosis, and aortic regurgitation. These valvular abnormalities can be suspected at the bedside. If valvular heart disease is excluded, an increase in left ventricular diastolic pressure resulting from left ventricular myocardial dysfunction should be suspected. If a left ventricular S_3 gallop is appreciated in patients with suspected dilated cardiomyopathy or aortic valve disease, an abnormally elevated left ventricular diastolic pressure and, thus, postcapillary pulmonary hypertension, should be suspected. The causes of precapillary pulmonary hypertension in adults include primary pulmonary diseases, such as COPD, chronic thromboembolic pulmonary hypertension, and primary pulmonary hypertension. When precapillary pulmonary hypertension is suspected, it is desirable to look for conditions such as systemic lupus erythematosus, scleroderma, or CREST syndrome (calcinosis, Raynaud phenomenon, esophageal dysmotility, sclerodactyly, and telangiectasia), which can also be associated with precapillary pulmonary hypertension.

Paradoxical Split

Reversed or paradoxical splitting of the S_2 is recognized when splitting of the S_2 during expiration is appreciated. And, during inspiration, the A_2–P_2 interval shortens, and the S_2 may appear single (54). The sequence of these closure sounds is reversed, with P_2 preceding A_2 during expiration. During inspiration, P_2 moves toward A_2, and the splitting of the interval narrows. The reversed splitting of the S_2 may occur because of a delay in the electrical activation of the left ventricle, which results in a delay in the onset and completion of left ventricular ejection. The most common cause of reversed splitting of the S_2 is left bundle branch block, which is associated with a prolonged electromechanical interval. Right ventricular ectopic beats and right ventricular pacing produce a delay in the onset of left ventricular contraction and result in reversed splitting of the S_2. The Wolff-Parkinson-White syndrome with right ventricular preexcitation is associated with reversed splitting of the S_2. It should be appreciated that left ventricular systolic function may also be impaired and can accompany conduction disturbances (57). In these circumstances, the degree of expiratory reversed splitting may be significantly greater than when the conduction disturbances are present without myocardial dysfunction.

Reversed splitting of the S_2 may occur owing to prolongation of the left ventricular ejection time, resulting from selective increase in the left ventricular forward stroke volume or a marked increase in resistance to left ventricular ejection. A selective increase in left ventricular forward stroke volume can occur in patients with significant aortic regurgitation or with patent ductus arteriosus with a large left-to-right shunt. Increased resistance to left ventricular ejection occurs in patients with significant aortic stenosis and obstructive hypertrophic cardiomyopathy. In patients with aortic stenosis, reversed splitting in the absence of left bundle branch block indicates hemodynamically significant aortic stenosis. In patients with hypertrophic cardiomyopathy with left ventricular outflow tract obstruction, reversed splitting occurs despite significant mitral regurgitation (58). The systolic murmur associated with primary mitral regurgitation, ventricular septal defect, and hypertrophic obstructive cardiomyopathy may appear similar in character and duration at the bedside. The behavior of the S_2 may be useful in the differential diagnosis of these conditions. If the S_2 is paradoxically split in the absence of left bundle branch block, the diagnosis of hypertrophic cardiomyopathy is most likely. The presence of widely split S_2 favors the diagnosis of primary mitral regurgitation or ventricular septal defect. Reversed splitting also occurs occasionally in patients with severe chronic systemic hypertension. However, a compensatory increase in adrenergic activity and left ventricular wall thickness, which reduces left ventricular wall stress, may normalize left ventricular ejection time; therefore, S_2 may be normal. In systemic hypertension, the intensity of A_2 is always increased. Acute elevation of systemic arterial pressure (e.g., during administration of methoxamine) has been shown to produce reversed splitting of the S_2, even in normal subjects, suggesting that acute increase in left ventricular afterload may cause a substantial prolongation of the left ventricular ejection time (59). Reversed splitting of the S_2 also has been recognized in patients with ischemic heart disease and during episodes of angina. These findings, however, are rarely encountered. Poststenotic aortic root dilatation is associated with a decrease in the impedance in the systemic vascular bed; delayed A_2 can occur, which may contribute to the reversed splitting of the S_2 (60). Such mechanisms have also been entertained in explaining the reversed splitting of the S_2 in patients with chronic aortic regurgitation and patent ductus arteriosus.

Single Second Heart Sound

Single S_2 may result from the absence of either of the two components of the S_2 or from the fusion of A_2 and P_2 without the inspiratory splitting. The most common cause of an apparently single S_2 is the inability to hear the faint pulmonic component because of chronic obstructive lung disease, obesity, or even normal but accentuated respiratory noise. Another common cause of single S_2 is advanced age and most likely occurs because of a decreased inspiratory delay in P_2, rather than a delayed A_2. Decreased inspiratory delay of P_2 probably results from a decreased right-sided hangout interval related to aging changes in the pulmonary artery compliance. However, all conditions that can delay A_2 may produce a single S_2 when the splitting interval becomes greater than 30 ms. In conditions in which one component of the S_2 is absent or inaudible (e.g., in patients with severe tetralogy of Fallot, severe pulmonary valve stenosis, severe aortic stenosis, pulmonary atresia, and most cases of tricuspid atresia), S_2 is single. The abnormalities of the S_2 and their potential mechanisms and associated causes are summarized in Table 16.5.

EJECTION SOUNDS

The ejection sounds are relatively high-pitched sounds occurring with the onset or soon after ventricular ejection starts.

TABLE 16.5

ABNORMALITIES OF THE SECOND HEART SOUND

SINGLE S_2

- If there is no evidence of left ventricular outflow tract obstruction, hypertensive heart disease, Eisenmenger syndrome with ventricular septal defect, and right ventricular outflow obstruction (e.g., tetralogy of Fallot), a clinically relevant pathology can be excluded.

WIDE SPLITTING OF S_2 WITH INSPIRATORY DELAY OF P_2

- *No other abnormal finding except widely split S_2*—suspect right ventricular conduction delay such as right bundle branch block.
- *Pulmonary ejection sound, ejection systolic murmur, a short early diastolic murmur in the left second interspace*—suspect idiopathic dilatation of the pulmonary artery or mild pulmonary valve stenosis.
- *Longer ejection systolic murmur with or without pulmonary ejection sound and decreased intensity of the P_2*—suspect pulmonary valve stenosis or right ventricular infundibular stenosis.
- *Increased intensity of P_2 with or without a short ejection systolic murmur along left sternal border; with or without evidence of right ventricular hypertrophy, tricuspid regurgitation, and right heart failure; and unilateral or bilateral continuous murmur*—suspect peripheral pulmonary artery branch stenosis.
- *Increased intensity of the P_2 with or without ejection systolic murmur and evidence of right ventricular hypertrophy or failure*—suspect precapillary pulmonary hypertension.

WIDELY SPLIT FIXED S_2—SUSPECT PRIMUM OR SECUNDUM ATRIAL SEPTAL DEFECT

- *In the presence of cyanosis or pulmonary hypertension*—suspect Eisenmenger syndrome with atrial septal defect or complete atrioventricular canal or common atrium.

INCREASED INTENSITY OF P_2 WITH P_2 TRANSMITTED TO THE CARDIAC APEX SUGGESTING PULMONARY HYPERTENSION

- Search for evidence for right ventricular hypertrophy, right ventricular failure, and secondary tricuspid regurgitation.
- *Cyanosis and clubbing*—suspect Eisenmenger syndrome.
- *Differential cyanosis and clubbing*—suspect patent ductus arteriosus.
- *Widely split S_2*—suspect atrial septal defect.
- *Single S_2*—suspect ventricular septal defect.
- *In the absence of Eisenmenger syndrome*—suspect primary pulmonary disease.
- *Mid-diastolic rumble in left lateral decubitus*—suspect mitral valve obstruction.
- *Early systolic or pansystolic regurgitant murmur over the cardiac apex*—suspect mitral regurgitation.
- *Ejection systolic murmur with a small-volume, delayed upstroke and peaked carotid pulse*—suspect aortic stenosis.
- *Ejection systolic murmur along the left sternal border with or without a regurgitant murmur and a normal carotid pulse upstroke*—suspect obstructive hypertrophic cardiomyopathy.
- *Early diastolic murmur with displaced hyperdynamic or sustained left ventricular apical impulse*—suspect aortic regurgitation.
- *In the absence of evidence for valvular heart disease, a sustained left ventricular apical impulse with a left ventricular S_3 gallop*—suspect nonischemic or ischemic dilated cardiomyopathy.
- *Elevated systemic venous pressure with sharp 'y' descent and positive Kussmaul sign*—suspect restrictive cardiomyopathy.
- *After exclusion of the causes of postcapillary pulmonary hypertension*—suspect precapillary pulmonary hypertension such as thromboembolic pulmonary hypertension, collagen vascular disease, primary pulmonary disease, and primary pulmonary hypertension.

PARADOXICAL SPLITTING OF THE S_2

- Suspect conduction disturbances such as left bundle branch block, preexcitation syndrome, arrhythmias, right ventricular pacing.
- *Ejection systolic murmur*—suspect aortic stenosis, obstructive hypertrophic cardiomyopathy.
- *Early diastolic murmur*—suspect aortic regurgitation.
- *Loud A_2*—suspect hypertension.

Abbreviations: A_2, aortic component of the second heart sound; MRI, magnetic resonance imaging; P_2, pulmonary component of the second heart sound; S_1, first heart sound; S_2, second heart sound; S_3, third heart sound.

The ejection sounds are classified as valvular (arising from deformed aortic or pulmonic valves) or vascular (caused by a forceful ejection of blood into the great vessels).

Aortic Ejection Sound

Aortic valvular ejection sounds are recognized in bicuspid aortic valve and valvular aortic stenosis. The aortic ejection sounds occur 20 to 40 ms after the onset of pressure rises in the central aorta, and they coincide with the sharp anacrotic notch on the upstroke of the aortic pressure curve. The aortic ejection sounds also coincide with the maximal excursion of the domed valve. When the aortic valve is immobile because of severe calcification, no excursion or pistol-like ascent of the deformed valve is present; therefore, in severe calcific aortic stenosis, ejection sound is frequently absent. The intensity of the aortic valvular ejection sound also correlates directly with the mobility of the valve. Thus, if the ejection sound is present in patients with aortic valvular stenosis, it indicates the presence of a mobile stenotic valve. In bicuspid aortic valve, the ejection sound usually is loud and is followed by a short ejection systolic murmur, normal S_2, and trivial aortic regurgitation. The aortic valvular ejection sound is widely transmitted and often heard best at the apex. Aortic vascular ejection sounds originate from the aortic root and are common in systemic hypertension, aortic aneurysm, and, sometimes, with aortic root dilatation owing to aortic regurgitation. Aortic vascular ejection sounds occur later than aortic valvular ejection sounds and frequently are localized and poorly transmitted. Aortic vascular ejection sounds are sometimes confused with tricuspid valve closure sounds. The differential diagnosis between tricuspid valve closure sounds and aortic vascular ejection sounds depends on the clinical circumstances when these sounds are expected to be present.

Pulmonic Ejection Sound

Pulmonary valvular ejection sounds are observed in mild to moderate pulmonary valve stenosis and idiopathic dilatation of the pulmonary artery. Pulmonary valvular ejection sounds occur at the maximal excursion of the stenotic pulmonary valve. In contrast to the aortic valvular ejection sounds and to most right-sided sounds and murmurs, a pulmonary ejection sound or click decreases in intensity—or even disappears—with inspiration (61). The pulmonary valvular ejection sounds coincide with the movement of the domed pulmonary valve. During expiration, a pressure gradient between the pulmonary artery end-diastolic pressure and right ventricular end-diastolic pressure exists, allowing the deformed domed pulmonary valve excursion and, therefore, the presence of the ejection sounds. During inspiration, the pressure gradient between the pulmonary artery and the right ventricle in end diastole substantially decreases, and there is preopening of the pulmonary valve; there is no further excursion of the domed pulmonary valve, which explains the absence of pulmonary ejection sounds during inspiration. In severe pulmonary stenosis, the pulmonary valvular ejection sounds appear fused with the S_1, which may explain the lack of pulmonary valvular ejection sounds in these patients. Pulmonary vascular ejection sounds arise from the pulmonary artery and are associated with dilatation of the pulmonary artery. The dilated pulmonary artery can be seen in patients with idiopathic dilatation of the pulmonary artery or secondary to severe pulmonary hypertension. Vascular pulmonary ejection sounds are louder in the second and third left intercostal spaces. Echocardiographic studies have suggested that pulmonary vascular ejection sounds coincide with the complete opening of the pulmonary valve and occur during the upstroke of the pulmonary artery pressure recordings (62). It should be recognized that the intensity of pulmonary vascular ejection sounds may not vary substantially during the phases of respiration. In patients with pulmonary hypertension with vascular pulmonary ejection sounds, the intensity of P_2 is markedly accentuated. In idiopathic dilatation of the pulmonary artery, the S_2 intensity is normal and may or may not be associated with an ejection systolic murmur or an early diastolic murmur. In pulmonary valve stenosis with pulmonary valvular ejection sounds, there is a long ejection systolic murmur. The S_2 is widely split, and the intensity of P_2 is decreased.

NONEJECTION SOUNDS

Clicks

Systolic nonejection sounds (midsystolic clicks) occur most frequently in mitral valve prolapse syndrome. Midsystolic clicks also occur with prolapse of the tricuspid valve. The mechanism of the midsystolic click is the tensing of the atrioventricular valves during systole.

The click sound has a sharp, high-frequency, clicking quality, and, although it is heard best over the cardiac apex, it can be transmitted widely. It may be an isolated finding occurring in middle to late systole, or there may be multiple clicks resulting from prolapsing of the different areas of the large, redundant, scalloped mitral leaflets at different times. Echocardiographic studies have shown the presence of the middle to late systolic prolapse, as well as pansystolic prolapse, in patients with midsystolic clicks. All of these different types of prolapse of the mitral valve can occur in patients with only systolic clicks, with clicks and late systolic murmur, or with late systolic murmur alone (63–65). Midsystolic clicks usually occur at the time of maximum prolapse. Valvuloventricular disproportion (a valve too big for the ventricle) has been thought to be the principal cause of mitral valve prolapse. It has been suggested that the ventricular volume or dimension associated with prolapse of the mitral valve (click dimension) is relatively fixed in a given patient. After the onset of ejection, the mitral valve prolapse occurs whenever this click dimension is reached (66). Thus, the S_1–click interval and the relative proportion of systole occupied by the regurgitant murmur vary with maneuvers (Fig. 16.8). When the patient maintains an upright posture and the ventricular volume is reduced, the S_1–click interval is shorter, and the duration of the murmur is longer. When the patient is supine and the ventricular volume is increased, the S_1–click interval is longer, and the duration of the murmur is shorter. With the postectopic beat—even though the ventricular volume is increased—the postectopic potentiation causes a

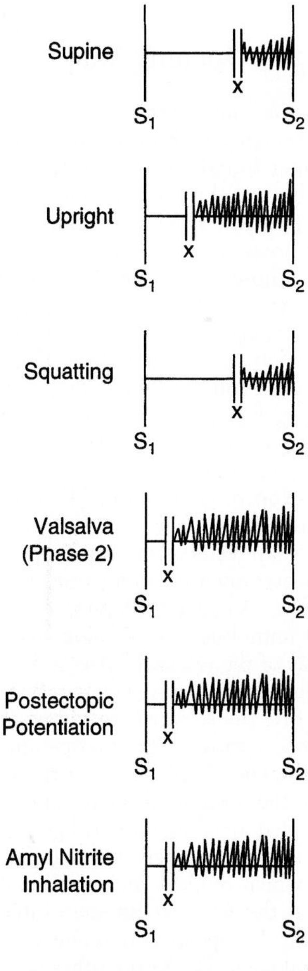

FIGURE 16.8. The influences of various bedside maneuvers on the first heart sound (S_1) and midsystolic click (x) intervals and the duration of the late systolic murmur, which usually extends to the second heart sound (S_2). With an increase in left ventricular volumes (supine and squatting), S_1–x intervals are longer and the duration of the late systolic murmur is shorter. With a smaller left ventricular diastolic volume (upright, Valsalva phase 2, amyl nitrite inhalation), S_1–x intervals are shorter and the duration of the late systolic murmur is relatively longer.

rapid ejection; therefore, the S_1–click interval gets shorter, and the duration of the murmur gets longer (66). These bedside maneuvers are helpful for the differential diagnosis between nonejection click and early ejection sound, a split S_2, and an S_3.

Although mitral and tricuspid valve prolapse are the most frequent causes of midsystolic clicks, nonejection sounds also have been observed in patients with left-sided pneumothorax, adhesive pericarditis, atrial myxomas, left ventricular aneurysm, and aneurysm associated with ventricular septal defects (67–70). These nonejection clicks vary in their timing, and the maneuvers that influence the midsystolic click associated with mitral valve prolapse and the S_1 interval are not recognized in these patients. In some patients with hypertrophic cardiomyopathy, a nonejection sound has been observed to occur with systolic anterior motion of the anterior mitral leaflet. This sound, termed *pseudoejection sound*, begins considerably after the upstroke of the carotid pulse (71). The precise mechanism of this pseudoejection sound in hypertrophic cardiomyopathy remains unclear. It may result from the contact of the anterior leaflet with the septum or from the deceleration of blood flow in the left ventricular outflow tract. The S_1–pseudoejection sound interval also does not change with maneuvers. The effects of different maneuvers on the S_1–midsystolic click interval and mitral regurgitation murmur associated with mitral valve prolapse are summarized in Fig. 16.8.

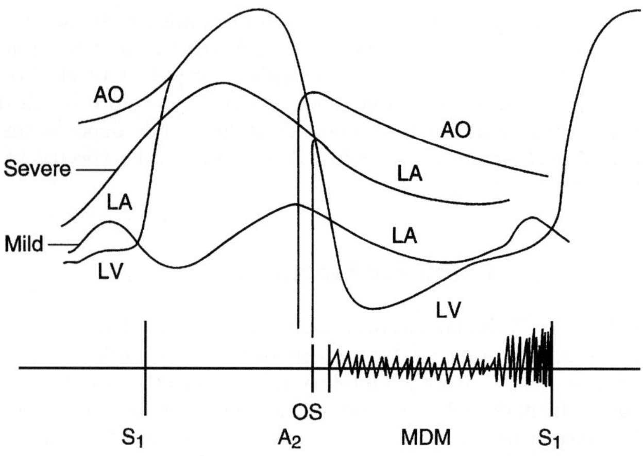

FIGURE 16.9. Schematic illustrations of left ventricular (LV), aortic (AO), and left atrial (LA) pressures to explain the relationship between the severity of mitral stenosis and the interval between the closure of the aortic valve sound (A_2) and the opening snap (OS). Compared to mild mitral stenosis, left atrial pressure is higher in severe mitral stenosis; thus, LA–LV pressures cross over at the end of isovolumic relaxation phase occur closer to A_2; thus, the A_2–OS interval is shorter with more severe mitral stenosis. The mid-diastolic murmur (MDM) is longer in more severe mitral stenosis and may extend to a loud first heart sound (S_1). The A_2–OS interval, however, is related to aortic pressure at the time of aortic valve closure; the interval is related to left ventricular pressure at the time of the opening of the mitral valve, which is also related to arterial pressure, ventricular relaxation, associated mitral regurgitation, aortic stenosis, and aortic regurgitation, as well as heart rate, which influences the duration of diastole.

Opening Snap

The opening snap is a high-pitched (high-frequency), early diastolic sound associated with mitral or tricuspid valve opening. These opening sounds of the atrioventricular valves are normally silent, but they become audible in the presence of mitral or tricuspid stenosis. The most common cause of opening snap is mitral stenosis, and the snap is heard best with the diaphragm of the stethoscope just medial to the cardiac apex. The opening snap associated with mitral stenosis usually is widely transmitted and frequently heard along the left sternal border and even over the left second interspace. Thus, the transmitted opening snap can be confused with the pulmonic component of the S_2. However, during the inspiratory phase of respiration, three high-frequency sounds can be recognized: The initial two sounds are the two components of the S_2, and the third is the opening snap. The opening snap coincides with the full opening of the mitral valve and usually occurs 40 to 100 ms after the S_2. The opening snap results from rapid opening of the mitral valve to its maximal open position; thus, the mobility of the valve contributes to its genesis. When the mitral valve is heavily calcified and immobile, the opening snap may be absent. A careful analysis of the interval between A_2 and the opening snap can provide information regarding the severity of mitral stenosis. The shorter the A_2–opening snap interval is, the more severe is the mitral stenosis. The A_2–opening snap interval is related to the difference in pressures at the time of the aortic valve closure and the opening of the mitral valve. When mitral stenosis is severe, left atrial pressure is higher, and the pressure crossover point between the left ventricle and the left atrium is closer to A_2, which reduces the A_2–opening snap interval. At the bedside, if the A_2–opening snap interval appears like widely split S_2, the A_2–opening snap interval is short and suggests severe mitral stenosis. On the other hand, if the opening snap seems to occur at the time when the S_3 gallop is expected, the A_2–opening snap interval is wide and indicates mild mitral stenosis. It needs to be emphasized that the A_2–opening snap interval should be assessed when the heart rate is relatively normal. When the heart rate is fast, the A_2–opening snap interval is shorter, even when the mitral stenosis is not severe. Similarly, in the presence of aortic stenosis, mitral regurgitation, or aortic regurgitation, it is difficult to assess the severity of mitral stenosis based on the A_2–opening snap interval (72) (Fig. 16.9).

Although an opening snap is most frequently encountered in mitral stenosis, it also can occur in patients with tricuspid stenosis. Left atrial and right atrial myxomas may cause an early diastolic sound (tumor plop) and seem to occur when tumors move into the ventricle and come to a sudden halt. In some patients with hypertrophic cardiomyopathy with a decreased left ventricular cavity, high-frequency, early diastolic sounds are heard; these sounds coincide with the time of contact of the anterior leaflet of the mitral valve to the interventricular septum (73). The tricuspid opening snap also can be heard in patients with atrial septal defect with a large left-to-right shunt. Rarely, a high-pitched diastolic sound can be heard in patients with mitral valve prolapse. This high-frequency sound seems to be related to the rapid, inward movement of the prolapsed mitral valve toward the left ventricular cavity before the opening of the mitral valve. Also, rarely in patients with severe mitral regurgitation secondary to ruptured chordae, a high-pitched, early diastolic sound similar to the opening snap can be heard (50). If a high-frequency, early diastolic sound is heard in clinical practice, one should exclude mitral valve stenosis by echocardiography.

Bioprosthesis and mechanical prosthesis also produce systolic and diastolic high-pitched sounds. The relative intensity of the opening and closing sounds vary according to the type and design of the prosthetic valve. With the ball-and-cage type of valve, the opening and closing sounds are loud and clicking in character. With the disc valve, however, the closing sound is louder and clickier than the opening sound. Artificial valve sounds are of high frequency and are much louder than normal valve sounds. The opening or closing sounds may consist of multiple clicks, which do not necessarily indicate valve malfunction. The absence of an opening click has been observed with normally functioning mitral valve prosthesis. Obstruction of a prosthetic valve in the mitral position may be associated with a markedly decreased A_2–opening click interval. For the diagnosis of the malfunction of prosthetic valve, however, one should not rely on the physical findings.

THIRD AND FOURTH HEART SOUNDS

S_3 and S_4 are of relatively low frequency, lower pitched sounds, and are related to early and late diastole filling of the ventricles (74). When these sounds are recognized in the pathologic states, they are termed *gallop sounds*. The S_3 is commonly heard in children, adolescents, and young adults in the absence of any pathologic condition or hemodynamic abnormality and is termed *physiologic* S_3. The physiologic or pathologic S_3 is a low-frequency sound that follows A_2 by 120 to 200 ms and occurs during the ventricular early rapid filling phase.

The mechanisms for the production of physiologic and pathologic S_3 have not been precisely determined. The opening and tensing of the atrioventricular valves in early diastole, the tensing of the ventricular wall, and the impact of the ventricular wall with the chest wall at the end of the rapid filling phase had been proposed as the mechanisms. Fast cineangiographic, echocardiographic, and Doppler studies have indicated that the S_3 is most likely related to the rapid deceleration of flow in early diastole. During the early filling phase—when there is an abrupt deceleration of the column of blood entering the ventricle after the opening of the atrioventricular valves—the cardiohemic system is set into vibration, which contributes to the genesis of the S_3 (75). It also has been suggested that the dynamic impact of the heart with the chest wall at the end of the rapid filling phase may contribute to the genesis of the S_3 that is recognized at the bedside (76).

At the bedside, S_3 is best recognized when the bell of the stethoscope is pressed very lightly over the skin in the left lateral decubitus position. When the bell of the stethoscope is pressed harder and converted to a diaphragm, the intensity of the S_3 decreases and may even disappear. However, the accuracy and interobserver agreement in detecting gallop sounds by auscultation is poor (77). In a number of pathologic conditions, an S_3 gallop indicates an increase in left ventricular diastolic pressure (78,79). In patients with chronic aortic regurgitation, the presence of an S_3 gallop has been reported to reflect reduced left ventricular ejection fraction (80). An S_3 gallop is very common in aortic regurgitation and usually is followed by a mid-diastolic rumble of the Austin Flint murmur.

An S_3 is frequently appreciated in patients with hemodynamically significant mitral and tricuspid regurgitation. An S_3 gallop also is heard in patients with a large left-to-right shunt owing to high flow across the mitral valve with ventricular septal defect or patent ductus arteriosus and to high flow across the tricuspid valve with atrial septal defects. The presence of S_3 in these conditions does not imply abnormal ventricular function or CHF. An S_3 gallop may be present in systolic and diastolic heart failure, aortic valve disease, and coronary artery disease (81). In such patients, S_3 gallop is usually associated with increased left ventricular end-diastolic pressure (>15 mm Hg) and elevated B-type natriuretic peptide levels (82). However, it should be emphasized that even phonocardiographic S_3 and S_4 is not a sensitive marker of left ventricular dysfunction, although specific for an elevated left ventricular end-diastolic pressure, reduced left ventricular ejection fraction, and elevated B-type natriuretic (83). An S_3 is often present in high-output states such as thyrotoxicosis and pregnancy and does not indicate left ventricular dysfunction (84).

An S_3 is almost invariably recognized in patients with restrictive cardiomyopathy. The S_3 in constrictive pericarditis is termed the *pericardial knock*. The frequency of the pericardial knock is somewhat higher than the physiologic or other pathologic S_3. The pericardial knock or S_3 associated with restrictive cardiomyopathy may occur earlier and soon after A_2 and may be confused with opening snap; it usually increases in intensity with inspiration and occurs coincident with the 'y' descent of the jugular venous pulse. An audible gallop sound is associated with worse prognosis in patients undergoing noncardiac surgery, in patients with asymptomatic left ventricular dysfunction, and in those with overt heart failure (85–88).

The S_4 is related to ventricular filling during atrial systole and, therefore, is absent in patients with atrial fibrillation. The S_4 precedes the S_1; thus, it is frequently termed the *atrial diastolic gallop* or the *presystolic gallop*. The S_4 is heard best at the cardiac apex with the patient in the left lateral decubitus position. The right ventricular S_4 gallop, however, is heard best along the lower left sternal border over the third or fourth intercostal space. The intensity of the right-sided S_4 increases after inspiration. In contrast, the left-sided S_4 is heard best during expiration. Occasionally, a loud, audible S_4 is accompanied by a palpable presystolic apical impulse—the so-called palpable S_4. The precise mechanism for the genesis of the S_4 has not been identified; however, both the ventricular origin owing to the abrupt deceleration of the incoming blood column during atrial contraction and the impact theory have been proposed (76,89). The common pathologic conditions in which a prominent left-sided S_4 is recognized are systemic hypertension, aortic valvular stenosis, and hypertrophic cardiomyopathy associated with left ventricular hypertrophy. Similarly, pulmonary hypertension and pulmonary valvular stenosis, which produce right ventricular hypertrophy, are associated with right-sided S_4. Although it initially was thought that the presence of S_4 in a patient with aortic stenosis indicated hemodynamically significant aortic valvular stenosis with a gradient of 70 mm Hg or greater and a left ventricular end-diastolic pressure of 13 mm Hg or greater (90), other studies have suggested that S_4 is good evidence of significant aortic stenosis only in patients younger than age 40 (91).

An audible S_4 with or without a palpable presystolic impulse is common in patients during angina and acute myocardial infarction (92). In the absence of acute ischemia, S_4 is uncommon, except in patients with ischemic dilated cardiomyopathy with elevated left ventricular diastolic pressure. In patients with left ventricular aneurysm or idiopathic or ischemic cardiomyopathy, the S_4 is often associated with a pathologic S_3, producing a quadruple rhythm. If there is also tachycardia or a markedly prolonged PR interval, S_3 and S_4 can be fused and give rise to a loud summation gallop. In acute atrioventricular valve regurgitation, as in patients with mitral regurgitation owing to ruptured chordae, an S_4 associated with a presystolic apical impulse is frequently present (93). In chronic mitral regurgitation an S_4 is uncommon, whereas an S_3 is frequently present. In patients with first degree atrioventricular block, S_4 is more easily heard because of its separation of the S_1. In complete atrioventricular block, intermittent S_4 is recognized frequently. The clinical significance of the gallop sounds are summarized in Table 16.6.

PERICARDIAL FRICTION RUB

Pericardial friction sounds are high pitched, leathery, and scratchy in quality and heard best with the patient leaning

TABLE 16.6

CLINICAL SIGNIFICANCE OF GALLOP SOUNDS

- S_3 is common in children and young adults (physiologic), but it is uncommon in normal subjects >40 years.
- S_3 usually indicates an increase in left or right ventricular diastolic pressure in the presence of impaired ejection fraction.
- *Chronic aortic regurgitation*—the presence of S_3 indicates impaired left ventricular ejection fraction.
- *Right ventricular failure resulting from congenital heart disease and pulmonary hypertension or primary right ventricular failure*—S_3 gallop indicates an increase in right ventricular diastolic pressure and reduced right ventricular ejection fraction.
- In hyperkinetic states, hyperthyroidism, anemia, arteriovenous fistulae, left-to-right shunts, and chronic tricuspid or mitral regurgitation, S_3 does not indicate hemodynamic abnormalities.
- *Primary myocardial or pericardial disease* (constrictive pericarditis)—S_3 and S_4 gallops indicate increased ventricular diastolic pressures.
- In the presence of first-degree atrioventricular block, S_4 can be audible without any associated hemodynamic abnormality.

Abbreviations: S_3, third heart sound; S_4, fourth heart sound.

forward or in the knee/chest position during held, forced expiration. The pericardial rub may have three components: (a) during atrial systole, (b) during ventricular systole, and (c) during rapid ventricular filling. Three-component pericardial rubs are more frequently observed in patients with acute primary pericarditis, uremic pericarditis, postoperative pericarditis, and traumatic pericarditis. In episternal pericarditis after acute myocardial infarction, it is more common to recognize one or two components of the pericardial rub.

A one-component pericardial rub occurring during ventricular systole can be confused with certain midsystolic ejection murmurs with a scratchy quality, as recognized in some patients with hyperthyroidism (Means-Lerman sign) (94). Superficial, scratchy ejection systolic murmurs also are recognized in patients with Ebstein anomaly.

Mediastinal crunch (Hamman sign) is a series of scratchy sounds that occur with cardiac cycles and result from the presence of air in the pericardium and mediastinum (95). The pleuropericardial rubs are accentuated during inspiration. The character of the pleuropericardial rub is different from that of the mediastinal crunch. Mediastinal crunch is observed in patients with mediastinal emphysema, which may also be associated with chest pain syndrome similar to angina. Mediastinal emphysema is associated with crepitations in the neck, secondary to subcutaneous air. The most common cause of mediastinal crunch is the presence of air and blood in the open pericardial sac after cardiac surgery, and does not indicate any significant hemodynamic abnormality.

Pacemaker sounds are also high-frequency sounds of brief duration and are produced by the contraction of the intercostal muscles resulting from stimulation of the intercostal nerves by the transvenous pacemakers located in the right ventricular apex (44). The pacemaker sounds coincide with the pacemaker stimuli and are abolished when the pacing is discontinued. The stimulation of pectoral muscles and the diaphragm during epicardial or endocardial pacing may also produce extracardiac sounds.

EVALUATION OF HEART MURMURS

During bedside evaluation of a cardiovascular murmur, it is customary to assess the location of the maximum intensity, radiation, timing (systolic, diastolic, or continuous), intensity (loudness), and frequency (pitch) of the murmur, as well as its configuration (shape, quality, and duration). It is generally agreed that turbulence is the principle determinant for the genesis of most murmurs. In clinical practice, six grades are used to assess the intensity of a murmur. Grade 1 is the faintest murmur and can be heard only with special effort or maneuvers. A grade 2 murmur is faint but can be heard easily. A grade 3 murmur is moderately loud. A grade 4 murmur is very loud, and a grade 5 murmur is extremely loud and can be heard with a light touch of the stethoscope. A grade 6 murmur is exceptionally loud and can be heard with the stethoscope just removed from contact with the chest. Systolic murmurs of grade 4 or higher usually are associated with a palpable thrill. The frequency of the murmur determines its pitch, which may be high or low. Several shapes or configurations of a murmur can be recognized: a crescendo (increasing); a decrescendo (diminishing); crescendo/decrescendo (increasing and decreasing or diamond shaped); and a plateau (no change in intensity of the murmur). The quality of a murmur can be harsh, rumbling, scratchy, grunting, blowing, squeaky, or musical. The duration of a murmur is assessed by determining the length of systole or diastole that the murmur occupies. The murmur can be long or brief. The direction of radiation of a murmur follows the direction of blood flow and can provide information regarding the origin of the murmur. It is essential to determine the timing of the murmur in relation to the cardiac cycle. A murmur can be systolic, diastolic, or continuous. Systolic and diastolic murmurs can be left sided or right sided. At normal heart rate, systole is much shorter in duration than diastole. Whenever there is any doubt about the timing of a given murmur, it is desirable to auscultate and identify S_1 and S_2 with simultaneous palpation of the carotid pulse. After recognizing a systolic murmur, it is necessary to determine whether the systolic murmur is of ejection type (midsystolic) or regurgitant type (Fig. 16.10). The ejection systolic murmur starts after the S_1 and does not extend to the S_2. A left-sided ejection systolic murmur ends before A_2, and a right-sided ejection systolic murmur ends before P_2. The ejection murmur is related to flow across the semilunar valves. Onset of the murmur coincides with the beginning of the ejection, and termination of the murmur coincides with the cessation of forward flow. The S_1 occurs at the onset of isovolumic systole, and the beginning of ejection occurs at the end of the isovolumic systole, explaining why ejection systolic murmur starts after the S_1. The ventricular ejection ends before closure of the semilunar valves; thus, an ejection systolic murmur cannot extend to the semilunar valve closure sounds. The configuration or shape of most ejection systolic murmurs is crescendo/decrescendo. The crescendo part of the ejection systolic murmur is related to the initial rapid ejection phase, and the decrescendo part of the ejection systolic murmur is related to the slower ejection phase. A regurgitant murmur can be pan- or holosystolic (murmur starts with S_1 and extends up to or beyond A_2 [left sided] or P_2 [right sided]), an early systolic (murmur starts with S_1 but does not extend to A_2) and late systolic (murmur starts after S_1 and extends to S_2).

Ejection Systolic Versus Regurgitant Murmur

When the S_1 and S_2 are decreased in intensity, it is often difficult to distinguish between an ejection systolic murmur and

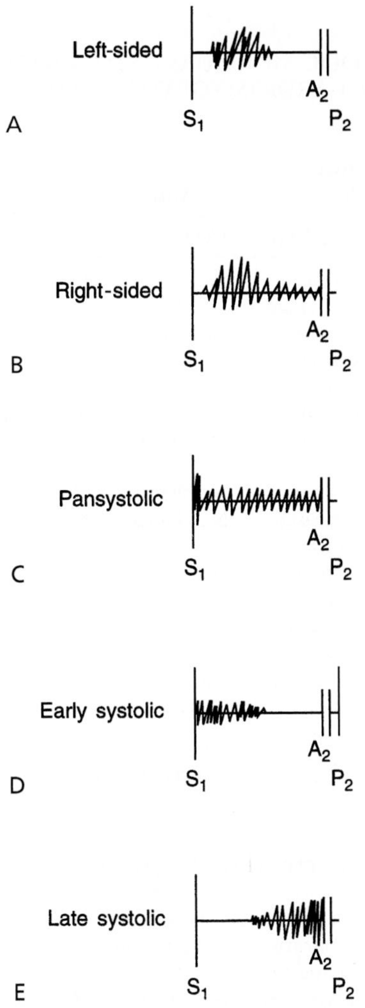

FIGURE 16.10. A left-sided ejection systolic murmur starts after the first heart sound (S_1) and terminates before the aortic component of the second heart sound (A_2). A right-sided ejection systolic murmur starts after S_1 and terminates before the pulmonary component of the second heart sound (P_2). A pansystolic murmur starts with S_1 and extends to the second heart sound. An early systolic murmur starts with the S_1 and terminates before the second heart sound. A late systolic murmur starts after the S_1 and extends up to second heart sound. **A:** Aortic stenosis, aortic sclerosis, flow murmur, innocent murmur, hypertrophic cardiomyopathy, and bicuspid aortic valve. **B:** Pulmonary stenosis, infundibular stenosis, flow murmur (atrial septal defect), idiopathic dilatation of the pulmonary artery, and innocent murmurs. **C:** Mitral regurgitation, tricuspid regurgitation, and ventricular septal defect. **D:** Mitral regurgitation, tricuspid regurgitation, and ventricular septal defect. **E:** Mitral regurgitation and tricuspid regurgitation.

a regurgitant murmur. There are a number of distinguishing features, however, that can be appreciated at the bedside (95). If A_2 is clearly audible over the cardiac apex, the murmur is likely to be ejection type (96). If A_2 is heard over the right and left second interspaces but not over the apex, it is likely that A_2 is drowned out by the holosystolic murmur of mitral regurgitation. If the patient is in atrial fibrillation, and if the intensity of the murmur substantially increases with longer RR cycle length, the murmur is likely to be an ejection murmur. Similarly, if the intensity of the murmur increases during the postectopic beat after a postectopic pause, the murmur is likely to be of ejection variety. A response to hand grip can be used to distinguish between left-sided ejection and regurgitant murmurs. In response to sustained hand grip, the intensity of a mitral regurgitation murmur increases, whereas the intensity of murmur associated with aortic stenosis usually decreases. The physiologic responses to hand grip are complex. In addition to an increase in systemic vascular resistance and arterial pressure, a reflex increase in contractility may also occur, which can increase the intensity of the stenotic murmur. Amyl nitrite inhalation is also a helpful bedside pharmacologic maneuver to distinguish between an ejection systolic murmur and a holosystolic regurgitant murmur of left ventricular origin. The intensity of the ejection systolic murmur increases, whereas the intensity of the regurgitant holosystolic murmur decreases. Amyl nitrite inhalation is associated with decreased systemic vascular resistance and arterial pressure, which decreases the severity of the regurgitation—hence, the intensity of the regurgitation murmur. In aortic stenosis, the intensity of the systolic murmur increases because of the increased flow across the stenotic aortic valve. In obstructive hypertrophic cardiomyopathy, the intensity of the murmur in response to amyl nitrite inhalation increases because of accentuated left ventricular outflow obstruction. The intensity of an ejection systolic murmur is markedly influenced by the changes in stroke volume. With increased stroke volume—such as during exercise, anxiety, or fever; after volume loading or passive leg elevation; or with a long diastolic filling period—the intensity of the ejection systolic murmur increases. Likewise, conditions that decrease cardiac output and stroke volume (e.g., CHF, β-blockade, or other negative inotropic agents) decrease the intensity of the ejection murmur. The effects of different pharmacologic and nonpharmacologic interventions on systolic murmurs of fixed and dynamic left ventricular outflow obstruction and of mitral regurgitation are summarized in Table 16.7.

Once the presence of an ejection systolic murmur is established, a systematic evaluation to establish its etiology should be undertaken (Table 16.8). Congenital aortic, valvular, subvalvular, or supravalvular stenosis, acquired aortic stenosis, and hypertrophic obstructive cardiomyopathy are all associated with an ejection systolic murmur. The murmur of fixed stenosis of the left ventricular outflow tract is crescendo/decrescendo in configuration and usually is heard best at the right second and left second and third interspaces near the sternal border. This murmur usually radiates widely into the neck and along the great vessels. The murmur of aortic stenosis is of lower pitch and has a harsh quality. With calcific aortic stenosis, particularly in the elderly, the murmur may radiate to the apex. Also in calcific aortic stenosis in the elderly, the high-frequency components of the murmur may predominate, and the apical murmur may have a high pitch and, often, a musical quality (Gallavardin sign) (97). This murmur is frequently confused with the mitral regurgitation murmur. An aortic ejection sound is frequently appreciated in congenital and acquired valvular aortic stenosis. With increasing severity of aortic stenosis and with calcification of the aortic valves, however, the aortic ejection sound may not occur. In congenital aortic stenosis—whether valvular, subvalvular, or supravalvular—the S_2 splitting usually is normal or single. In acquired aortic stenosis, the S_2 usually is single, or it may be reversed with severe outflow obstruction. The intensity of A_2 in congenital valvular aortic stenosis usually is normal but may decrease with calcification. The intensity of A_2 in subvalvular and supravalvular aortic stenosis is normal or decreased. In acquired aortic stenosis, the intensity of A_2 is decreased, or it may be absent with calcification of the aortic valve. The murmur of aortic regurgitation frequently is present in congenital valvular and subvalvular aortic stenosis, as well as in acquired aortic valvular stenosis. A murmur of aortic regurgitation is uncommon in supravalvular congenital aortic stenosis. In supravalvular congenital aortic stenosis (William syndrome), elf-like facial appearance, mental retardation, and hypercalcemia are common (98). The carotid artery upstroke is slow rising, the peak is delayed, and the amplitude is decreased in congenital valvular

TABLE 16.7

EFFECTS OF MANEUVERS ON THE INTENSITY OF THE SYSTOLIC MURMURS AND CAROTID PULSE IN AORTIC STENOSIS, HYPERTROPHIC OBSTRUCTIVE CARDIOMYOPATHY, AND MITRAL REGURGITATION

	Aortic stenosis		Hypertrophic obstructive cardiomyopathy		Mitral regurgitation	
Maneuvers	ESM	CAR AMP	ESM	CAR AMP	PSM	CAR AMP
Leg raising	Increased	Increased	Decreased	Increased No change	Increased	Decreased No change
Standing	Decreased	Decreased No change	Increased	Decreased No change	Decreased	Increased No change
Squatting	Decreased No change	No change	Decreased	Increased No change	Increased	Decreased No change
Hand grip	Decreased Increased	Increased No change	Decreased	No change	Increased	No change
Supine position	No change	No change	Decreased	No change	No change	No change
Postectopic beat	Increased	Increased	Increased	Decreased No change	No change	No change
Valsalva (phase 2)	Decreased	Decreased	Increased	Decreased	Decreased	Decreased
Amyl nitrite	Increased	Increased	Increased	Decreased No change	Decreased	Increased No change

Abbreviations: CAR AMP, carotid pulse amplitude; ESM, ejection systolic murmur; PSM, pansystolic murmur.

and subvalvular aortic stenosis, as well as in acquired aortic stenosis. In congenital supravalvular aortic stenosis, the right brachial and carotid pulsations have greater amplitudes than those of left brachial and left carotid pulsations. Left ventricular hypertrophy can occur in response to valvular, subvalvular, supravalvular, and acquired aortic stenosis; thus, it can be associated with a sustained left ventricular apical impulse. A significant hypertrophy and noncompliant ventricle may also be associated with a palpable presystolic impulse (S_4).

Severity of Aortic Stenosis

After establishing the diagnosis of aortic stenosis, attempts should be made to assess its severity (Fig. 16.11). A palpable anacrotic character of radial pulse, slow-rising carotid pulse, and reduced amplitude and delayed peak of the carotid pulse indicate significant aortic stenosis. The decrease in intensity of the S_1 in the absence of prolonged PR interval (first-degree atrioventricular block) indicates an increase in left ventricular end-diastolic pressure, which indirectly suggests hemodynamically significant aortic stenosis. The intensity of the aortic valve closure sound (A_2) does not correlate with the severity of aortic stenosis. A longer and delayed peaking ejection systolic murmur suggests significant aortic stenosis. However, in the presence of heart failure and reduced stroke volume, the duration and intensity of the ejection murmur is decreased, and it may even be absent (silent aortic stenosis). Hemodynamically significant aortic stenosis usually is associated with left ventricular hypertrophy, which can be appreciated at the bedside by the presence of a sustained left ventricular apical impulse. In elderly patients, diagnosis of hemodynamically significant aortic valve stenosis may be difficult (99). The ejection murmur is often of low intensity due to decreased stroke volume associated with impaired left ventricular ejection fraction. The murmur is often loudest at the apex, may have a high-frequency component, and may be difficult to define as ejection in nature because of decreased S_1 and S_2. In the elderly, the carotid pulse upstroke and amplitude may be normal or near normal because of the sclerotic changes in the carotid arteries. In elderly patients with aortic stenosis, hypertension may coexist and cause further difficulties in the diagnosis.

Hypertrophic Cardiomyopathy

It is generally believed that the systolic anterior motion of the mitral valve apparatus, impinging on the thickened interventricular septum and producing high-velocity flow and obstruction during midsystole, causes the midsystolic ejection murmur in hypertrophic cardiomyopathy. The maximum intensity of this ejection murmur is appreciated over the left second or third interspace along the sternal edge. In many patients with obstructive hypertrophic cardiomyopathy, the systolic murmur along the left sternal edge is longer in duration and may appear regurgitant in nature. In many patients with obstructive hypertrophic cardiomyopathy, mitral regurgitation occurs after the onset of left ventricular outflow tract obstruction. The sequence of dynamic events in these patients is rapid, high-velocity ejection in midsystole followed by obstruction in the left ventricular outflow tract due to systolic anterior motion, which also produces incompetence of the mitral valve associated with mitral regurgitation (ejection, obstruction, regurgitation). The initial part of the systolic murmur seems to be related to left ventricular outflow tract obstruction, and the latter part is related to mitral regurgitation (100). The ejection murmur that is appreciated at the bedside is the summation of both murmurs. In patients with obstructive hypertrophic cardiomyopathy, the intensity of the systolic murmur varies directly with the degree of left ventricular outflow tract obstruction and pressure gradient and, therefore, the orifice size of the left ventricular outflow tract (101). The size of the left ventricular outflow tract is directly related to left ventricular volume and intraventricular pressure during systole and inversely related to muscle tension and contractile state. The higher the distending pressure (the arterial pressure), the larger the left ventricular outflow tract and, therefore, the softer the murmur. Similarly, the larger the left ventricular volume, the larger the size of the left ventricular outflow tract and the softer the murmur. With increased inotropic state, such as during postectopic potentiation or during the challenge with positive inotropic drugs, the size of the

TABLE 16.8

DIFFERENTIAL DIAGNOSIS OF SYSTOLIC MURMURS—BEDSIDE EVALUATION

DETERMINE THE TIMING OF THE SYSTOLIC MURMUR; THE MURMUR STARTS AFTER THE S_1 AND DOES NOT EXTEND UP TO THE S_2—EJECTION SYSTOLIC MURMUR

- Consider conditions associated with left or right ventricular outflow tract obstruction such as aortic stenosis, pulmonary stenosis, or hypertrophic cardiomyopathy.
- The flow murmurs in systole are ejection systolic murmurs and can be observed in hyperkinetic states such as hyperthyroidism and after exercise.
- The flow murmurs in systole are ejection systolic murmurs and can be observed in hyperkinetic states such as hyperthyroidism and after exercise.
- The murmur associated with aortic sclerosis (grunting quality) is an ejection systolic murmur.
- The innocent murmur in children (Still murmur) is an ejection systolic murmur.
- In patients with suspected aortic stenosis, careful analysis of the changes in the carotid pulse upstroke, volume, and presence or absence of left ventricular hypertrophy, behavior of the S_2, and intensity of the S_1 to assess the severity of aortic stenosis.
- Hypertrophic cardiomyopathy is suspected from the presence of an ejection systolic murmur and normal or sharp carotid pulse upstroke. Auscultation and simultaneous palpations of the carotid pulse volume during Valsalva maneuvers. Standing and squatting and amyl nitrate inhalation are used to confirm the diagnosis.
- Bicuspid aortic valve suspected from the presence of an aortic ejection sound, normal S_2, and a brief, early diastolic murmur of aortic regurgitation.
- *Superficial, scratchy ejection systolic murmur*—suspect Means-Lerman scratch of hyperthyroidism, Ebstein anomaly, one-component pericardial friction rub.
- *Long ejection systolic murmur with widely split S_2 and reduced intensity of P_2*—suspect pulmonary stenosis. Presence of a pulmonary valve ejection sound suggests pulmonary valve stenosis; absence of a pulmonary valve ejection sound suggests infundibular stenosis.
- *Presence of a pulmonary valve ejection sound short ejection systolic murmur, normal physiologic splitting of the S_2 with or without short early diastolic murmur*—suspect idiopathic dilatation of the pulmonary artery.
- *Pulmonary vascular ejection sound, a short ejection systolic murmur, and increased intensity of the P_2*—suspect pulmonary hypertension; the presence of a left parasternal systolic lift, secondary tricuspid, and pulmonary regurgitation suggests severe pulmonary hypertension. Once pulmonary hypertension is suspected, causes for postcapillary pulmonary hypertension should be excluded before the diagnosis of precapillary pulmonary hypertension is entertained.
- When an ejection systolic murmur is recognized without any evidence of left or right ventricular outflow obstruction, hyperkinetic states and innocent ejection systolic murmur are diagnosed.

MURMURS START WITH THE S_1 AND EXTEND UP TO THE S_2 OR BEYOND—PANSYSTOLIC OR HOLOSYSTOLIC MURMUR

- These murmurs can be associated with mitral regurgitation, tricuspid regurgitation, or VSD. Mitral regurgitation is suspected from the radiation of murmur to the axilla or to the base and changes in the intensity and duration with maneuvers such as hand grip and amyl nitrite inhalation.
- Tricuspid regurgitation murmur is suspected when there is an increase in intensity of the murmur during inspiration. Associated findings of tricuspid regurgitation are a prominent 'v' wave and 'y' descent in jugular venous pulse and hepatic pulsation. Secondary tricuspid regurgitation is associated with increased intensity of P_2.
- The pansystolic murmur of VSD is associated with a palpable thrill and does not change in intensity with inspiration and does not radiate to the axilla.

MURMURS START WITH THE S_1 AND DO NOT EXTEND UP TO THE S_2—EARLY SYSTOLIC MURMUR

- The early systolic murmur can be due to either mild or severe mitral regurgitation. Acute severe mitral regurgitation is associated with a crescendo/decrescendo, early systolic murmur and pulmonary hypertension. If left ventricular ejection fraction is normal, suspect primary acute severe mitral regurgitation such as ruptured chordae. If left ventricular ejection fraction is depressed, suspect papillary muscle dysfunction and coronary artery disease.
- Early systolic murmur can also result from mild mitral regurgitation associated with ventricular dilatation, as in patients with ischemic or nonischemic dilated cardiomyopathy or annular calcification of the mitral valve.
- Early systolic murmur may also result from tricuspid regurgitation. If the murmur increases in intensity during inspiration, tricuspid regurgitation should be considered. Early systolic murmur associated with tricuspid regurgitation most frequently results from secondary severe tricuspid regurgitation associated with pulmonary hypertension. A prominent 'v' wave with a sharp 'y' descent and systolic hepatic pulsation confirm the diagnosis of severe tricuspid regurgitation. If the intensity of P_2 is increased, it suggests that tricuspid regurgitation is secondary. Primary tricuspid regurgitation in the absence of evidence of pulmonary hypertension occurs in patients with carcinoid heart disease, right ventricular infarct, and traumatic rupture of the chordae of the tricuspid valve.

MURMURS START AFTER THE S_1 AND EXTEND UP TO THE S_2—LATE SYSTOLIC MURMUR

- The most common cause of late systolic murmurs is mitral valve prolapse, which is frequently associated with midsystolic clicks. The S_1–midsystolic click interval and the onset of late systolic murmur in mitral valve prolapse are influenced by left ventricular volume and inotropic state. Maneuvers such as sitting, the supine, squatting, and standing positions, and amyl nitrite inhalation can confirm the diagnosis of mitral valve prolapse at the bedside.
- Tricuspid regurgitation secondary to tricuspid valve prolapse can also produce a late systolic murmur and midsystolic clicks. The late systolic murmur associated with tricuspid valve prolapse increases in intensity during inspiration.

Abbreviations: P_2, pulmonary component of the second heart sound; S_1, first heart sound; S_2, second heart sound; VSD, ventral septal defect.

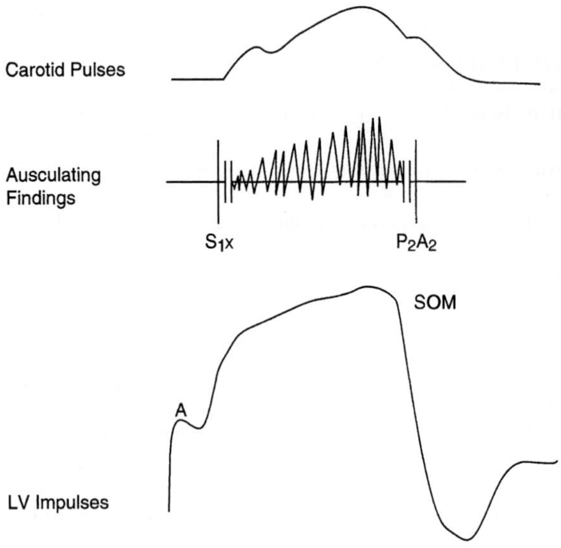

FIGURE 16.11. Schematic illustration of the physical findings of aortic stenosis, which suggest hemodynamically significant aortic stenosis, are slow-rising, delayed-peaking anacrotic pulse (carotid pulse), palpable presystolic (A) and sustained outward movement (SOM) in left ventricular (LV) impulse and delayed-peaking ejection systolic murmur, reversed splitting of the second heart sound in the absence of left bundle branch block, and reduced intensity of the first heart sound (S_1) (see text). *Abbreviations:* A_2, aortic component of the second heart sound; P_2, pulmonary component of the second heart sound; x, aortic ejection sound.

left ventricular outflow tract decreases with an increase in the pressure gradient and intensity of the ejection systolic murmur. Certain maneuvers that change the intensity of the murmur may confirm the diagnosis (Table 16.9). The systolic murmur in obstructive hypertrophic cardiomyopathy increases in intensity while standing and decreases in intensity in the supine and squatting positions. The Valsalva maneuver is another intervention that can be applied at the bedside to establish the diagnosis of obstructive hypertrophic cardiomyopathy. During phase 2 of the Valsalva maneuver, there is a decrease in venous return, which reduces left ventricular volume; a decrease in arterial pressure, which results from decreased stroke volume; and a reflex increase in heart rate. All of these hemodynamic changes enhance left ventricular outflow obstruction and increase the intensity of the murmur and decrease carotid pulse amplitude. In patients with aortic stenosis during phase 2 of the Valsalva maneuver, the carotid pulse volume decreases, but there is also a reduction in the intensity of the ejection systolic murmur. Similarly, during phase 2 of a Valsalva maneuver in patients with primary mitral regurgitation, there is a reduction in the carotid pulse volume and the intensity of the regurgitant murmur (see Table 16.7).

In obstructive hypertrophic cardiomyopathy, following a premature beat, postectopic potentiation increases the left ventricular outflow pressure gradient; therefore, the intensity of the murmur is increased. However, the carotid pulse volume is either decreased or remains unchanged. In patients with aortic stenosis, the intensity of the murmur increases during the postectopic beat, but there is also a substantial increase in the carotid pulse volume. The most useful pharmacologic intervention that can be applied easily at the bedside is the use of amyl nitrite inhalation. After inhalation of amyl nitrite, the intensity of the ejection systolic murmur in obstructive hypertrophic cardiomyopathy increases along with decreased or unchanged carotid pulse volume. The murmur of mitral regurgitation decreases with amyl nitrite inhalation as a decrease in systemic vascular resistance and arterial pressure decreases the severity of mitral regurgitation. In aortic stenosis, the intensity of the murmur tends to increase after amyl nitrite inhalation. The pharmacologic agents that increase the contractile state (e.g., isoprenaline, dobutamine, or dopamine) increase the intensity of the murmur; agents that decrease the inotropic state (e.g., intravenous β-blocker or disopyramide) decrease the intensity of the murmur. Similarly, pharmacologic agents that increase left ventricular outflow resistance (e.g., methoxamine or phenylephrine) decrease the intensity of the murmur as the left ventricular outflow tract obstruction decreases (102). In clinical practice, however, these pharmacologic agents are rarely used or necessary for the differential diagnosis of obstructive hypertrophic cardiomyopathy, aortic stenosis, or mitral regurgitation. In patients with significant left ventricular outflow tract obstruction, the carotid pulse usually has a sharp initial upstroke, a large volume, and, occasionally, a bisferiens quality. The left ventricular apical impulse frequently is sustained because of a significant increase in left ventricular mass. A presystolic wave (a palpable S_4) also is frequently appreciated. The

TABLE 16.9

DIAGNOSIS OF OBSTRUCTIVE HYPERTROPHIC CARDIOMYOPATHY

Maneuvers	Hemodynamic changes	LV outflow tract size	LV outflow pressure gradient	Intensity of the murmur
Standing	↑ LV volume ≠ Heart rate	↑	≠	≠
Squatting	≠ LV volume ≠ SVR, ART pressure	≠	↑	↑
Valsalva phase 2	≠ Heart rate ↑↑ LV volume	↑↑	#	#
Hand grip	↑ Heart rate ≠ ART pressure	≠	↑	↑
Post-PVC	# Contractility ≠ LV volume	↑↑	#	#
Amyl nitrite inhalation	≠ Heart rate ↑ LV volume ↑ ART pressure	↑↑	#	#

Abbreviations: ART, arterial; LV, left ventricular; PVC, premature ventricular contraction; SVR, systemic vascular resistance; ≠, mild increase; ↑, mild decrease; #, marked increase; ↑↑, marked decrease.

outward movement of the left ventricular apical impulse may occasionally have bifid character. If the left ventricular outward movement is associated with a presystolic wave, three distinct impulses can be appreciated in rare patients (triple ripple). It should also be realized that in patients with hypertrophic nonobstructive cardiomyopathy, the carotid pulse character may be normal and ejection systolic murmur may be absent. The only indication of hypertrophic cardiomyopathy may be an S_4 or a sustained left ventricular apical impulse. In apical hypertrophic cardiomyopathy, the electrocardiogram may provide some clues for the diagnosis. The electrocardiogram in apical hypertrophic cardiomyopathy frequently reveals a giant T-wave inversion in the lateral precordial leads, along with large QRS voltages owing to left ventricular hypertrophy (103). Absence of electrocardiographic changes, however, does not exclude nonobstructive hypertrophic cardiomyopathy. In all patients with suspected hypertrophic cardiomyopathy, echocardiographic evaluation is essential.

Other Left-Sided Ejection Systolic Murmurs

Hemodynamically significant isolated aortic regurgitation can also be associated with an ejection systolic murmur, which usually reflects increased flow during systole. A bicuspid aortic valve may be associated with an ejection systolic murmur. The bicuspid aortic valve at the bedside is suspected from the presence of an aortic ejection sound, normal carotid pulse upstroke, a short early diastolic murmur, and no evidence of hemodynamically significant aortic stenosis. A left-sided ejection systolic murmur is also recognized in the presence of normal valves when the flow across the aortic valve is significantly increased, as in anemia in pregnancy or thyrotoxicosis. The murmur of so-called aortic sclerosis is also a midsystolic ejection murmur. In aortic sclerosis, the physical findings of left ventricular outflow tract obstruction are absent. It results from the stiffening and degenerative fibrous thickening of the roots of the aortic cusps at the site of their insertions. The murmur of aortic sclerosis usually is heard best over the right second interspace, and the murmur usually does not radiate to the carotid arteries. In some patients, a musical, high-frequency murmur of brief duration can be heard along the lower left sternal border and cardiac apex. The S_1 and S_2 are normal, and there is no evidence of aortic regurgitation. Clinical recognition of aortic sclerosis is relevant; it is an adverse risk factor for long-term prognosis probably because of increased atherothrombotic complications. An ejection systolic murmur similar to that of hypertrophic obstructive cardiomyopathy has been observed in patients who develop transiently left ventricular outflow obstruction during acute myocardial infarction, or in patients with apical ballooning syndrome (104). Aortic root dilation associated with bicuspid aortic valve, ascending aortic aneurysm or aortitis, and hypertension, can be associated with ejection systolic murmur.

Right-Sided Ejection Systolic Murmurs

Right-sided ejection systolic murmurs can result from obstructions to right ventricular outflow, such as pulmonary valvular stenosis, subvalvular right ventricular outflow obstruction, or supravalvular pulmonary stenosis. Isolated infundibular pulmonary stenosis without ventricular septal defect is rare. Infundibular pulmonary stenosis usually is associated with ventricular septal defect, as in patients with tetralogy of Fallot. One finding at the bedside that suggests the presence of pulmonary valvular stenosis is a long ejection systolic murmur that starts after the S_1 and terminates before the P_2 and that can be markedly decreased in intensity. Frequently, a pulmonic valvular ejection sound is also present. There may or may not be an associated early diastolic murmur owing to pulmonary insufficiency. Depending on the severity of pulmonary valvular stenosis, evidence of right ventricular hypertrophy may be recognized. Significant pulmonary valvular stenosis causing right ventricular hypertrophy is associated with a prominent 'a' wave in the jugular venous pulse, which reflects increased resistance to right ventricular filling during right atrial systole. Typically, in pulmonary valvular stenosis and isolated subvalvular right ventricular outflow obstruction, the S_2 is widely split. The degree of splitting of the S_2 roughly correlates to the severity of the pressure gradient across the right ventricular outflow tract. The intensity of P_2 is decreased. In patients with supravalvular pulmonary stenosis, however, the intensity of P_2 is not decreased. Supravalvular pulmonary stenosis, or pulmonary artery branch stenosis, is frequently associated with a continuous murmur. Pulmonary valve stenosis, or obstruction in the right ventricular outflow tract, and supravalvular pulmonary stenosis can be associated with significant right ventricular hypertrophy.

The idiopathic dilatation of the pulmonary artery may be associated with a right-sided ejection systolic murmur. The usual findings of idiopathic dilatation of the pulmonary artery are a pulmonary ejection sound, short ejection systolic murmur, relatively widely split S_2 with normal intensity of P_2, and, occasionally, short pulmonary insufficiency murmur. There is no hemodynamic abnormality. In patients with precapillary or postcapillary pulmonary hypertension, an ejection systolic murmur may be present. The S_2 is narrowly split, with P_2 markedly accentuated in intensity, and the pulmonary ejection sound is late because of its vascular origin. Evidence of pulmonary insufficiency, right ventricular hypertrophy, and tricuspid regurgitation may be present. A right-sided ejection systolic murmur also is heard in atrial septal defect with relatively large left-to-right shunt. This ejection murmur occurs because of increased flow across the pulmonary valve, and it is not related to any pulmonary valve stenosis. Atrial septal defect can be suspected from the presence of wide fixed splitting of the S_2 and the evidence for right ventricular volume overload. Increased flow across the pulmonary valve associated with increased flow due to hyperthyroidism may also be associated with an ejection systolic murmur. The ejection systolic murmur owing to hyperthyroidism may have a scratchy quality (Means-Lerman scratch), and, frequently, the intensity of P_2 is increased because of mild to moderate pulmonary hypertension (94). The right-sided flow murmurs, however, usually are not associated with evidence of any hemodynamic compromise, such as right ventricular hypertrophy or right heart failure.

Innocent Murmurs

Innocent murmurs are, by and large, ejection in type and midsystolic in timing. In adults, innocent ejection systolic murmurs are diagnosed when there is no evidence for right or left ventricular outflow tract obstruction. The short ejection systolic murmur associated with aortic sclerosis is often regarded as an innocent murmur. In children, a short, vibrating murmur can be heard over the midprecordium and it is not accompanied by any other abnormality. The precise mechanism of this murmur, termed *Still murmur*, is not known (105,106). Another type of innocent systolic ejection murmur most frequently heard in children has a blowing quality and is heard best over the left second interspace. This murmur is thought to originate from the flow across the pulmonary artery. With increasing age, these innocent murmurs tend to decrease in intensity and, ultimately, disappear. In patients with straight back syndrome with a decreased anteroposterior diameter of the chest, a superficial ejection systolic murmur is heard over the left second interspace. The mechanism of this murmur remains unclear. It should be emphasized that whether an ejection systolic murmur is innocent should not depend on the duration or intensity of the murmur, but rather on whether any other abnormal finding is present. If any abnormal finding coexists, such as an abnormality of S_2, even a short and sharp ejection systolic murmur should not be considered benign or innocent.

Regurgitant Systolic Murmurs

In clinical practice, when a pansystolic or holosystolic murmur is recognized, mitral regurgitation, tricuspid regurgitation, or ventricular septal defect should be considered in the differential diagnosis. The pansystolic mitral regurgitation murmur usually is of higher pitch and has a blowing character. The murmur frequently extends beyond the left ventricular systole, and A_2 is frequently drowned by the murmur. In patients with hemodynamically significant primary mitral regurgitation, the left ventricular pressure remains higher than the left atrial pressure throughout the systole and during the isovolumic relaxation phase. This hemodynamic abnormality explains the onset of pansystolic murmur with S_1 and extension of the murmur beyond A_2. Primary mitral regurgitation is defined when mitral regurgitation occurs because of the abnormalities of the components of the mitral valve apparatus, particularly of the mitral valve leaflets. Rheumatic mitral valve disease, bacterial endocarditis, and ruptured chordae that produce pansystolic mitral valve prolapse are examples of primary mitral regurgitation. Hemodynamically significant mitral regurgitation usually is associated with an S_3 gallop and left ventricular dilatation with preserved left ventricular ejection fraction. When mitral regurgitation results from mitral valve prolapse, particularly of the posterior leaflet, the radiation of the murmur occurs toward the base and occasionally radiates to the neck. Thus, this murmur can be confused with an ejection systolic murmur owing to aortic stenosis. The pansystolic murmur due to mitral valve prolapse occasionally can be confused with the ejection systolic murmur resulting from left ventricular outflow obstruction in hypertrophic cardiomyopathy. Bedside maneuvers (e.g., Valsalva, hand grip, squatting, and standing) usually can differentiate between obstructive hypertrophic cardiomyopathy and primary mitral regurgitation. Posterior radiation of the mitral regurgitation murmur can be detected when auscultation is done over the thoracic spine or on the vortex. When the regurgitant murmur is heard over the lower back (on the lumbar spine), a substantial increase in left atrial size should be suspected. The S_2 in hemodynamically significant primary mitral regurgitation usually is widely split—a condition that results from decreased left ventricular ejection time. The intensity of P_2 remains normal until pulmonary hypertension develops, when its intensity is increased.

Tricuspid Regurgitation

The pansystolic murmur of tricuspid regurgitation usually is heard best at the lower left sternal border. The tricuspid regurgitation murmur does not radiate to the left axilla. The murmur of tricuspid regurgitation may be heard along the right sternal border, over the epigastrium, and over the right subcostal region. The intensity of the murmur, as expected, increases during inspiration owing to the increased venous return and right ventricular filling. Occasionally, severe tricuspid regurgitation is associated with a diastolic flow murmur that is characterized as a short diastolic rumble along the lower left sternal border. When present, this murmur also increases in intensity during inspiration. Hemodynamically significant tricuspid regurgitation frequently is associated with right ventricular S_3 gallop, which also increases in intensity during inspiration. Tricuspid regurgitation is diagnosed at the bedside from the presence of a prominent 'v' wave followed by a sharp 'y' descent in the jugular venous pulse and systolic hepatic pulsation. Tricuspid regurgitation is most often secondary to pulmonary arterial hypertension; thus, a prominent left parasternal impulse and narrow splitting of S_2 with an accentuated P_2 suggest secondary tricuspid regurgitation. Although severe tricuspid regurgitation can be associated with reversed splitting of the S_2 owing to a marked reduction in right ventricular ejection time, this finding is rarely observed. Tricuspid regurgitation not accompanied by pulmonary hypertension (primary tricuspid regurgitation) can occur after right-sided bacterial endocarditis, right ventricular infarction, Ebstein anomaly, carcinoid heart disease, right ventricular papillary muscle dysfunction or infarction, or traumatic rupture of the chordae of the tricuspid valve. Predominant tricuspid regurgitation also can occur in rheumatic heart disease; however, rheumatic tricuspid regurgitation is almost always accompanied by aortic or mitral valvular disease.

Ventricular Septal Defect

Ventricular septal defect is associated with a pansystolic murmur, because the pressure in the right ventricle is lower than the pressure in the left ventricle throughout systole (107). This hemodynamic profile is observed in unrestricted ventricular septal defect with normal pulmonary vascular resistance. Thus, the S_2 in these patients usually is normal. The murmur is loud and may be accompanied by a thrill (52). The murmur is heard best over the left third or fourth interspace along the left sternal border. In supracristal ventricular septal defect, the maximum intensity of the murmur may be located over the left second interspace, and it can be confused with the murmur of pulmonary valve stenosis. A wide splitting of the S_2 with reduced intensity of P_2 is present in pulmonary stenosis, and a normal S_2 favors ventricular septal defect. The murmur of ventricular septal defect does not radiate to the axilla, as with mitral regurgitation, and does not increase in intensity with inspiration, as with tricuspid regurgitation. When the magnitude of the left-to-right shunt is large, wide physiologic splitting of the S_2 with normal intensity of P_2 is recognized. Furthermore, left ventricular S_3 gallop with or without a mid-diastolic rumble suggesting increased flow across the mitral valve can be heard at the cardiac apex. It should be appreciated that the intensity of the murmur correlates poorly with the degree of left-to-right shunt. A grade 5 murmur usually is associated with a high-velocity flow through a small hemodynamically insignificant ventricular septal defect (108). When the septal defect is large and the right and left ventricular pressures are equal, no murmur may be produced across the defect (109). Pansystolic murmur of mitral regurgitation and the murmur of ventricular septal defect decrease in intensity in response to amyl nitrite. Amyl nitrite inhalation reduces systemic vascular resistance and left ventricular/right ventricular pressure gradient associated with decreased left-to-right shunt.

Early systolic regurgitant murmurs can occur in mitral and tricuspid valvular regurgitation and in certain types of ventricular septal defects. Early systolic regurgitant murmurs begin with the S_1 but do not extend to S_2 and generally have a decrescendo configuration. The early systolic murmur associated with mitral regurgitation is heard best at the cardiac apex, but it may have limited radiation. The early systolic murmur usually suggests relatively mild mitral regurgitation and results most frequently from left ventricular dilatation with or without annular dilatation. In some patients with mitral stenosis, an early systolic murmur is heard and probably represents mild mitral regurgitation. Mitral annular calcification may also be associated with an early systolic murmur, indicating mild mitral regurgitation. Mitral annular calcification is associated with

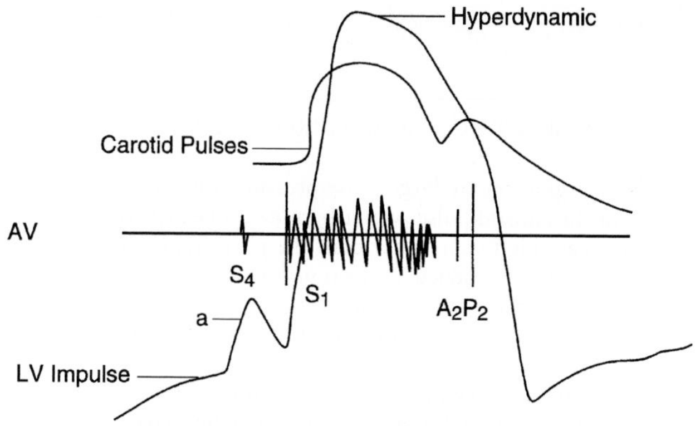

FIGURE 16.12. Schematic illustrations of the physical findings suggestive of acute or subacute severe primary mitral regurgitation (e.g., due to ruptured chordae). Examination of the carotid pulse reveals a sharp upstroke, but the amplitude is small. Palpation of the left ventricular (LV) impulse usually reveals a palpable 'a' wave and a hyperdynamic outward movement, indicating increased LV diastolic pressure and normal LV ejection fraction, respectively. Auscultation usually reveals a fourth heart sound (S_4), an early systolic murmur, and a relatively widely split second heart sound. The pulmonary component of the second heart sound (P_2) usually is accentuated, indicating pulmonary hypertension. *Abbreviations:* A_2, aortic component of the second heart sound; AV, atrioventricular; S_1, first heart sound.

lack of a reduction of the circumference of the annulus at the beginning of the systole, thus inducing mild mitral regurgitation.

Early systolic murmur may also be associated with acute severe mitral regurgitation (110). The conditions producing acute severe mitral regurgitation include spontaneous rupture of the chordae, bacterial endocarditis of the mitral valve, papillary muscle rupture or infarction secondary to acute myocardial infarction, and disruption of the mitral valve apparatus owing to chest trauma. In acute severe mitral regurgitation, there is regurgitation of a relatively large volume of blood into a normal-sized left atrium. As a result, there is a rapid increase in the magnitude of 'v' wave, and, during middle or late systole, 'v' wave pressure may be similar to that of left ventricular systolic pressure; this loss of the pressure gradient between the left ventricle and left atrium during midsystole stops the regurgitation, and, therefore, the murmur terminates before the A_2 (Fig. 16.12). In patients with ruptured chordae, left ventricular apical impulse usually is normal in character, indicating normal ejection fraction. In contrast, when mitral regurgitation occurs after acute myocardial infarction, left ventricular ejection fraction usually is depressed. In acute mitral regurgitation, a palpable S_4 and audible S_4 are commonly recognized. In contrast to chronic mitral regurgitation, an S_3 gallop may be absent. Acute severe mitral regurgitation almost always is associated with a substantial increase in the left atrial and pulmonary capillary wedge pressure and with postcapillary pulmonary hypertension. The S_2 is widely split, and the intensity of P_2 is increased (see Fig. 16.12). The systolic murmur of acute mitral regurgitation may radiate to the axilla and back, especially if it is due to prolapse of the anterior leaflet of the mitral valve. When the murmur is loud, it may be conducted to the top of the head and to the lower back along the spinal column. Occasionally, the murmur is conducted to the base of the heart and over the neck vessels and can be confused with the murmur of aortic stenosis. The systolic murmur associated with primary tricuspid regurgitation is often early systolic and ends well before the S_2 (111). Early systolic murmur may also represent severe tricuspid regurgitation. When the right ventricular pressure is near normal and there is minimal gradient between right ventricular systolic pressure and right atrial pressure, the flow velocity is low and there is minimal turbulence, producing an abbreviated systolic murmur. In these patients, a large 'v' wave with a sharp 'y' descent frequently is encountered, indicating severe tricuspid regurgitation. There may also be a short mid-diastolic rumble (flow murmur) along the left sternal border, which increases in intensity during inspiration. Frequently, a right-sided S_3 gallop is appreciated. The early systolic murmur associated with severe tricuspid regurgitation also increases in intensity during inspiration. A right-sided S_4 with a prominent diastolic tricuspid flow rumble is appreciated when the tricuspid regurgitation is acute and severe, as occurs in endocarditis of the tricuspid valve. After total excision of the tricuspid valve, severe tricuspid regurgitation may not be associated with any systolic murmur, although there is a prominent 'v' wave in the jugular venous pulse, and systolic hepatic pulsations are easily appreciated. Palpable venous thrills and a murmur at the base of the neck are a result rapid retrograde flow to the jugular venous system (112).

An early systolic murmur may occur in certain types of ventricular septal defects. The ventricular septal defects causing early systolic murmur usually are small and located in the muscular septa, which are sealed because of systolic thickening of the ventricular septa (113). This early systolic murmur associated with ventricular septal defect may indicate that the defect may eventually close spontaneously.

Late Systolic Murmurs

Late systolic murmurs are most frequently recognized in mitral regurgitation owing to papillary muscle dysfunction or mitral valve prolapse. The late systolic murmur resulting from papillary muscle dysfunction may or may not be associated with midsystolic clicks. The late systolic murmur due to papillary muscle dysfunction can be intermittent or constant and may occur only during myocardial ischemia. Late systolic murmur with or without midsystolic clicks may occur due to fibrosis of the posterior left ventricular wall, as seen in patients with pseudohypertrophic muscular dystrophy. In these patients, the electrocardiogram always reveals evidence of posterior wall infarction (a tall R wave in leads V_1 and V_2). Mitral valve prolapse associated with myxomatous disease of the mitral valve is the most common cause of late systolic murmur. The murmur is heard best at the apex and often has a late systolic crescendo character. Single or multiple midsystolic clicks frequently accompany late systolic murmur.

Precordial whoop or honk is also associated with mitral valve prolapse. These murmurs are loud, high pitched, musical, sonorous, and vibratory. These murmurs are heard best at the apex in late systole and can be intermittent. The unusual quality of this precordial whoop or honk is secondary to the high-frequency vibrations of the mitral apparatus.

Late systolic murmur with or without midsystolic clicks can be observed in tricuspid regurgitation due to prolapse of the tricuspid valve. Isolated prolapse of the tricuspid valve is extremely unusual and almost always accompanies mitral valve prolapse. However, isolated tricuspid valve prolapse can be observed in patients with the Ebstein anomaly. Tricuspid valve prolapse may also produce precordial whoop or honk, as with mitral valve prolapse.

DIASTOLIC MURMURS

Early Diastolic Murmurs (Aortic Regurgitation)

Early diastolic murmurs typically start at the time of closure of the semilunar valves, and their onset coincides with S_2

TABLE 16.10

DIFFERENTIAL DIAGNOSIS OF THE DIASTOLIC MURMUR

MURMURS START WITH S_2 AND HAVE A DECRESCENDO QUALITY—SUSPECT AORTIC REGURGITATION OR PULMONARY REGURGITATION

- Chronic aortic regurgitation signs of hemodynamically significant aortic regurgitation are large pulse pressure, low arterial diastolic pressure, sharp carotid pulse upstroke, pulsus bisferiens quality of the carotid pulse, water-hammer pulse, Corrigan sign, and left ventricular enlargement. Reduced intensity of S_1 indicates increased left ventricular diastolic pressure. Presence of S_3 gallop indicates increased left ventricular end-diastolic pressures and reduced left ventricular ejection fraction.
- If aortic regurgitation is associated with increased intensity of A_2, suspect hypertensive aortic regurgitation.
- Aortic regurgitation due to bicuspid aortic valve is associated with an aortic ejection sound, short ejection systolic murmur, and normal S_2.
- If early diastolic murmur increases in intensity during inspiration, suspect pulmonary insufficiency. Once pulmonary insufficiency is suspected, a careful analysis of the intensity of the P_2 should be performed to assess whether pulmonary insufficiency is secondary to pulmonary hypertension. If the intensity of P_2 is increased, one should suspect secondary pulmonary insufficiency. This can occur in patients with precapillary or postcapillary pulmonary hypertension. Once secondary pulmonary hypertension is suspected, conditions that can be associated with postcapillary pulmonary hypertension—such as mitral stenosis and mitral regurgitation, aortic stenosis and aortic regurgitation, and primary left ventricular myocardial dysfunction (dilated, hypertrophic, and restrictive cardiomyopathy)—should be excluded before the diagnosis of precapillary pulmonary hypertension causing pulmonary regurgitation can be entertained.
- When the intensity of P_2 is normal or decreased, consider primary pulmonary regurgitation. Primary pulmonary regurgitation can occur from bacterial endocarditis, congenital absence of the pulmonary valve, or after pulmonary valvulotomy.

THE MURMUR STARTS AFTER S_2 AND EXTENDS TO S_1 (MID-DIASTOLIC RUMBLE WITH OR WITHOUT PRESYSTOLIC ACCENTUATION); CONSIDER ORGANIC OR FUNCTIONAL MITRAL OR TRICUSPID VALVE STENOSIS

- The presence of an opening snap indicates organic mitral or tricuspid stenosis.
- Left or right atrial myxomas are associated with similar auscultatory findings of mitral and tricuspid stenosis of rheumatic origin.
- Once organic mitral and tricuspid valve obstruction are excluded, increased flow across the atrioventricular valves should be suspected as the cause of the mid-diastolic flow murmur. Under these circumstances, one is obliged to exclude atrial septal defect, ventricular septal defect, hyperkinetic heart syndromes, and aortic regurgitation.

Abbreviations: A_2, aortic component of the second heart sound; P_2, pulmonary component of the second heart sound; S_1, first heart sound; S_2, second heart sound; S_3, third heart sound.

(Table 16.10; Fig. 16.13). The aortic regurgitation murmur begins with the A_2, whereas the pulmonary regurgitation murmur begins with the P_2. The configuration of the aortic regurgitation murmur usually is decrescendo. The aortic regurgitation diastolic murmurs are high pitched and have a blowing character. Occasionally, these murmurs have a musical quality (diastolic whoop) and can be heard best with the diaphragm of the stethoscope. The musical quality of the aortic regurgitation murmur has been attributed to everted aortic cusps or perforated aortic cusps (114). The duration of the murmur is variable but usually terminates before the S_1. The low-intensity, high-pitched murmur of aortic regurgitation may not be heard easily until the patient sits and leans forward with the breath held during expiration and firm pressure with the diaphragm of the stethoscope is applied along the left sternal border or over the right second interspace. The radiation of an aortic regurgitation murmur is toward the cardiac apex. In some patients, the murmur can be heard best over the midprecordium, along the lower left sternal border, or even over the cardiac apex. Radiation of the murmur along the right sternal border is more frequent in aortic regurgitation caused by aortic root abnormalities (115). The presence of an early diastolic murmur appears to be the most useful finding for establishing the diagnosis of aortic regurgitation (positive likelihood ratio 8.8) and its absence to exclude aortic regurgitation (negative likelihood ratio –0.2) (116). After the diagnosis of aortic regurgitation is suspected, it is desirable to assess the severity of aortic regurgitation (Fig. 16.14). In hemodynamically significant chronic aortic regurgitation, the carotid pulse upstroke is sharp, and the volume is increased. Frequently, a pulsus bisferiens quality of the carotid arterial pulse is appreciated. Arterial diastolic pressure usually is below 60 mm Hg. The pulse pressure is increased substantially. The presence of water-hammer pulse or Corrigan pulse is also suggestive of hemodynamically significant chronic aortic regurgitation. The various peripheral signs of chronic aortic regurgitation are also present. Hemodynamically significant chronic aortic regurgitation is associated with a considerable increase in left ventricular size, which can be determined at the bedside and by chest x-ray. In severe aortic regurgitation,

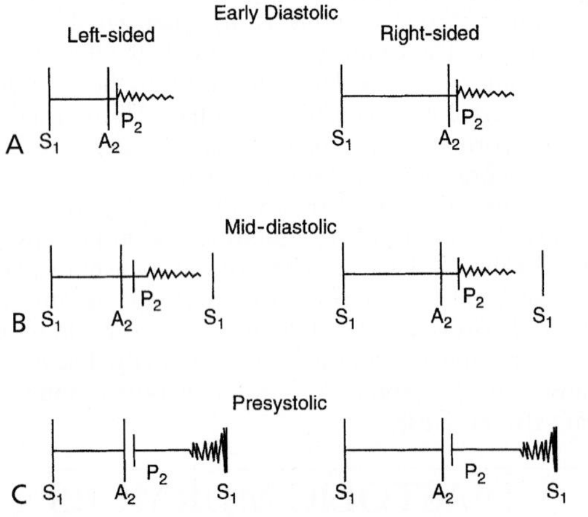

FIGURE 16.13. **A:** An early diastolic murmur, when the left-sided murmur starts with the aortic component of the second heart sound (A_2) and when the right-sided murmur starts with the pulmonary component of the second heart sound (P_2) or soon after P_2. **B:** A mid-diastolic murmur starts after A_2 when left sided and after P_2 when right sided and does not extend up to the first heart sound (S_1). **C:** A presystolic murmur starts before S_1 and terminates at S_1.

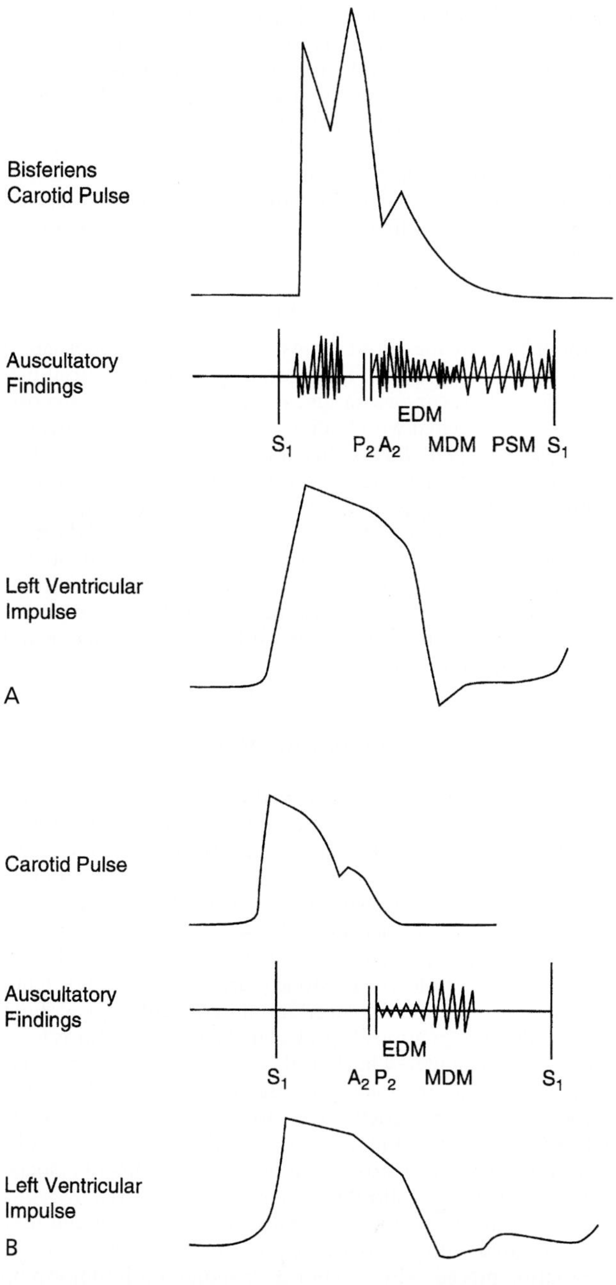

FIGURE 16.14. **A:** Schematic illustrations of the physical findings that can indicate hemodynamically significant chronic aortic regurgitation and can be appreciated at the bedside. The carotid pulse upstroke is sharp or may have bisferiens quality. The amplitude is increased. Left ventricular apical impulse reveals a hyperdynamic quality that suggests increased left ventricular volume with normal ejection fraction. Auscultation usually reveals an early diastolic murmur (EDM), and an Austin Flint murmur with both mid-diastolic (MDM) and presystolic (PSM) components are usually appreciated. The second heart sound can be paradoxically split (P_2–A_2), and the first heart sound (S_1) may be soft if left ventricular diastolic pressure is elevated. **B:** Schematic illustrations of the physical findings that may indicate hemodynamically significant acute aortic regurgitation. The carotid pulse usually is normal. Left ventricular apical impulse is also normal. The EDM of aortic regurgitation usually is brief. Austin Flint murmur only consists of an MDM component. The S_1 is soft or absent as the second heart sound is physiologically split (A_2–P_2), but the pulmonary component of the second heart sound (P_2) may be increased in intensity, indicating pulmonary hypertension. *Abbreviation:* A_2, aortic component of the second heart sound.

ejection systolic murmur along the left sternal border and over the aortic area indicates increased stroke volume rather than aortic stenosis. S_2 can be paradoxically split owing to selective increase in the left ventricular stroke volume, which increases its ejection time. Frequently, it is difficult to appreciate A_2, which may be decreased in intensity or absent because of the lack of coaptation of the valve cusp (117). Left ventricular apical impulse usually is displaced downward and laterally and maintains the normal asynchronous sequence with the carotid pulse upstroke, indicating normal left ventricular ejection fraction. In severe chronic aortic regurgitation, there may be a substantial increase in left ventricular mass due to eccentric hypertrophy that may be associated with a sustained left ventricular apical impulse. The presence of S_3 gallop usually indicates reduced left ventricular ejection fraction. The presence of S_3 may also indicate increased left ventricular diastolic pressure. A soft S_1 in the absence of a prolonged PR interval indicates elevated left ventricular diastolic pressure. The Austin Flint murmur is a mid-diastolic rumble with late systolic accentuation; it is heard best at the cardiac apex and results from relative functional mitral stenosis. Evidence of pulmonary venous congestion and pulmonary hypertension should also be considered indicative of hemodynamically significant aortic regurgitation.

The hemodynamic consequences of acute severe aortic regurgitation are characterized by a sudden, severe volume overload to a nondilated left ventricle, which is associated with a rapid increase in left ventricular diastolic pressure and, often, equalization of left ventricular and aortic pressures in mid-diastole. The regurgitant murmur, therefore, can be brief (118). Because of a noncompliant ventricle and a substantial increase in left ventricular diastolic pressure, pulmonary venous pressure and pulmonary artery pressure may increase considerably—a condition that can be suspected from the increased intensity of P_2. The apical impulse maintains the normal character, indicating normal ejection fraction. Decreased intensity of the S_1 or absent S_1 indicates acute severe aortic regurgitation and results from premature closure of the mitral valve owing to a marked and rapid increase in left ventricular diastolic pressure (see Fig. 16.14). A marked increase in left ventricular end-diastolic pressure may also prevent effective left ventricular filling during left atrial systole; thus, an S_4 gallop may be absent in acute aortic regurgitation.

Mild aortic regurgitation without any hemodynamic compromise can occur in association with bicuspid aortic valve or systemic hypertension. Aortic regurgitation resulting from systemic hypertension usually is associated with an accentuated A_2, and the duration of the regurgitation is brief.

Dock Murmur

Diastolic murmur similar to murmurs of aortic regurgitation can be heard in some patients with stenosis of the left anterior descending coronary artery (Dock murmur) (119). The murmur of left anterior descending coronary artery stenosis, however, is not transmitted widely and usually is heard best over the left second or third interspace, a little lateral to the left sternal border. This murmur is caused by turbulent flow across the coronary artery stenosis, and its duration may be short or long. After successful angioplasty or coronary artery bypass surgery, this murmur is abolished.

Pulmonary Regurgitation (Graham Steell Murmur)

An early diastolic murmur also results from pulmonary regurgitation. In adult patients, pulmonary regurgitation occurs most frequently due to pulmonary artery hypertension (Graham Steell murmur) (120,121). The early diastolic murmur associated with pulmonary hypertension is a high-pitched, blowing murmur that starts with an accentuated P_2 and can be of variable duration. In Eisenmenger syndromes associated with atrial septal defect or patent ductus arteriosus, when right ventricular diastolic pressure may remain normal, the pulmonary regurgitant murmur may be pandiastolic. On the other hand, in the presence of modest precapillary or postcapillary pulmonary hypertension, the duration of the murmur may be brief. The pulmonary regurgitant murmur has a decrescendo configuration like that of aortic regurgitation. The murmur may increase in intensity during inspiration and may be very localized. It is heard best over the left second and third interspaces.

Pulmonary regurgitation can occur in the absence of pulmonary hypertension, as in patients with idiopathic dilatation of the pulmonary artery. Pulmonary regurgitation is also frequently observed after pulmonary valvulotomy. It may occur as a complication of right-sided endocarditis and with the congenital absence of the pulmonary valve. In these conditions, the pulmonary artery diastolic pressure is normal or low, and the pulmonary regurgitant murmur is of lower pitch. The murmur usually begins after the onset of P_2 (122). Congenital absence of the pulmonary valve may be associated with severe pulmonary regurgitation, and a loud "to and fro" murmur and absent pulmonary component of the S_2 should raise the suspicion of absent pulmonary valve.

Mid-Diastolic Murmurs

The mid-diastolic murmurs result from turbulent flow across the atrioventricular valves during ventricular diastole. These murmurs result from either functional or organic mitral or tricuspid valve stenosis.

Mitral Stenosis

The mid-diastolic murmur of mitral stenosis has a rumbling character and is heard best with the bell of the stethoscope and over the left ventricular impulse and with the patient in the left lateral decubitus position. If the stenotic mitral valve is mobile, an opening snap and a loud S_1 are present. The mid-diastolic rumble starts with the opening snap and may extend to the S_1 with presystolic accentuation (see Fig. 16.9). The presystolic component of the mid-diastolic murmur of mitral stenosis may be present in sinus rhythm and atrial fibrillation (123). The mechanism of the presystolic accentuation of the mid-diastolic murmur is not entirely clear. It was initially thought to be related to atrial systole. However, it may occur in the presence of atrial fibrillation. Doppler echocardiographic studies have suggested that the presystolic murmur is related to antegrade flow through a progressively narrowing mitral orifice during the end of the ventricular diastole. It should be recognized that the onset of mitral valve closure starts approximately 60 ms before the valves close and produce S_1. With an obstructed mitral valve, the presence of a pressure gradient at end diastole allows antegrade flow across the closing mitral valve before the mitral valves close completely, explaining the presystolic murmur—even in patients with atrial fibrillation. The duration of the murmur correlates well with the severity of mitral stenosis. The longer the mid-diastolic murmur, the more severe the mitral stenosis. The intensity of the murmur is related not only to the severity of the mitral valve obstruction but also to the flow across the valve. When there is a marked reduction in cardiac output resulting from severe mitral valve obstruction, the flow across the valve also is markedly reduced and may be associated with a soft murmur or absent murmur (silent mitral stenosis). The severity of mitral stenosis also can be assessed by noting the A_2–opening snap interval. The shorter the A_2–opening snap interval, the higher the left atrial pressure and the higher the pressure gradient across the mitral valve. In patients with severe postcapillary pulmonary hypertension associated with low cardiac output and calcified immobile mitral valve, the auscultatory findings of mitral stenosis may not be recognized. The severity of mitral stenosis also should be suspected from the associated findings, such as evidence of pulmonary hypertension.

Left Atrial Myxoma and Tumor Plop

Although rheumatic mitral stenosis is the most common cause of mitral valve obstruction, left atrial myxoma, left atrial ball valve thrombus, cor triatriatum, and congenital mitral stenosis all can be associated with findings of mitral valve obstruction. The auscultatory findings with left atrial myxoma may be identical to those of rheumatic mitral stenosis (124). A loud tumor plop sound at the beginning of the mid-diastolic rumble may be similar to opening snap. The presystolic component of the mid-diastolic murmur may occur when the tumor is ejected into the left atrium at the beginning of the systole. A systolic murmur of mitral regurgitation may also be present. Patients with left atrial myxoma may also present with positional syncope and intermittent pulmonary edema.

Other Diastolic Murmurs

Tricuspid valve stenosis is associated with a mid-diastolic rumbling murmur, which usually is heard best or over the lower left third and fourth interspaces along the sternal border. The diastolic murmur resulting from tricuspid valve obstruction increases in intensity during inspiration (Carvello sign). The mid-diastolic murmur of tricuspid valve stenosis may be preceded by tricuspid opening snap. As right atrial systole occurs before the left atrial systole, the diastolic murmur of tricuspid stenosis may have a crescendo/decrescendo configuration without presystolic accentuation (125). Isolated tricuspid stenosis is infrequently encountered in clinical practice. Systemic lupus erythematosus and carcinoid heart disease may produce tricuspid stenosis. Rarely, constrictive pericarditis may cause functional tricuspid stenosis and may be associated with a mid-diastolic murmur. Tricuspid stenosis most frequently occurs in association with rheumatic mitral valve disease. Right atrial myxoma is an infrequent cause of tricuspid valve obstruction and may be associated with mid-diastolic murmur with presystolic accentuation preceded by a tumor plop sound. Both tumor plop sound and mid-diastolic murmur resulting from tricuspid valve obstruction owing to right atrial myxoma increase in intensity during inspiration.

Diastolic rumbles may occur because of high flow across the atrioventricular valves. Diastolic murmurs at the cardiac apex are appreciated in patients with severe isolated mitral regurgitation or ventricular septal defect and patent ductus arteriosus with a large left-to-right shunt. Similarly, a large left-to-right shunt associated with atrial septal defect may cause a mid-diastolic murmur along the left sternal border owing to increased flow across the tricuspid valve. Similar low-pitched, rumbling murmurs may be present in hyperkinetic states such as hyperthyroidism, chronic severe anemia, and arteriovenous fistulae.

Carey-Coombs Murmur

Mitral valvulitis associated with acute rheumatic fever may cause a short diastolic rumble (Carey-Coombs murmur) (126). This rumble usually is preceded by an S_3 gallop and most often is recognized in children in the presence of fever and anemia.

These physical findings do not indicate mitral valve obstruction, but they do indicate rheumatic carditis.

Austin Flint Murmur

The mid-diastolic murmur associated with aortic regurgitation is called the *Austin Flint murmur*, after the man who first described this murmur in 1862 (127). It is heard best at the apex and can be mid-diastolic or presystolic in timing. In some patients, however, a long mid-diastolic rumble with presystolic accentuation is appreciated. Unlike organic mitral stenosis, the Austin Flint murmur is preceded by an S_3 gallop rather than opening snap. The S_1 in patients with aortic regurgitation and the Austin Flint murmur is normal or decreased in amplitude, but in mitral stenosis, S_1 usually is increased in amplitude. With amyl nitrite inhalation and when aortic regurgitation is decreased, the Austin Flint murmur is decreased in duration and intensity. The mid-diastolic murmur of organic mitral stenosis, however, increases in intensity and duration after amyl nitrite inhalation. The mechanisms of the genesis of the Austin Flint murmur are incompletely understood and likely to be multifactorial (128). Although late diastolic mitral regurgitation has been excluded as one of the mechanisms, antegrade flow across the mitral valve with closing mitral orifice and incomplete mitral valve opening may be contributory to the genesis of the Austin Flint murmur. Echo Doppler and magnetic resonance imaging suggest that the murmur arises from the regurgitant jets that are directed at the left ventricular free wall (129).

Rytand Murmur

Occasionally in patients with complete atrioventricular heart block, a mid-diastolic murmur is heard at the apex (Rytand's murmur) and may be confused with mitral stenosis. The slow heart rate, variable duration of the murmur, changing intensity of the S_1, and lack of opening snap are helpful findings for the differential diagnosis. The mechanism of Rytand's murmur is not clear, but increased flow owing to slow heart rate and increased antegrade flow with atrial contraction, which occurs randomly, may be contributory (130).

Continuous Murmurs

Continuous murmurs (131) begin in systole and extend up to diastole without interruption. Continuous murmurs do not necessarily occupy the total duration of systole and diastole. These murmurs may result from blood flow from a higher pressure chamber or vessel to a lower pressure system associated with the persistent pressure gradient between the structures during systole and diastole. Patent ductus arteriosus is one relatively common cause of a continuous murmur. Descending thoracic, aortic pressure is higher than pulmonary artery pressure during both systole and diastole, and the blood flow from the high-pressure descending thoracic aorta to the low-pressure pulmonary artery causes the continuous machinery murmur (Gibson murmur) (132). The maximum intensity of the murmur usually occurs at the S_2; the duration of the murmur varies and depends on the pressure difference between aorta and the pulmonary artery. When pulmonary hypertension develops, pulmonary diastolic pressure increases, and the diastolic portion of the continuous murmur becomes shorter. When the diastolic pressure in the pulmonary artery is equal to the aortic pressure, the diastolic component of the continuous murmur is absent. With more severe pulmonary hypertension, the pulmonary artery systolic pressure may be similar to the aortic systolic pressure, and the systolic component of the murmur may be absent (silent patent ductus arteriosus). In patients with severe pulmonary hypertension with reversal of shunt across the patent ductus arteriosus (Eisenmenger syndrome), differential cyanosis and clubbing may provide clues for diagnosis.

Continuous murmurs may be present in patients with aorticopulmonary window or Lutembacher syndrome, which consists of a small atrial septal defect and mitral valve obstruction (133), total anomalous pulmonary venous drainage, and mitral stenosis with a persistent left superior vena cava. A communication between the sinus of Valsalva and the right atrium or right ventricle is associated with a continuous murmur. Systemic and pulmonary arteriovenous fistulae also produce continuous murmurs. Systemic arteriovenous communications usually produce loud continuous murmurs. The murmurs of pulmonary arteriovenous fistulae are softer and may be primarily systolic. Coronary arteriovenous fistulae are occasionally encountered in adult cardiac patients. The location, duration, and character of the continuous murmur due to a coronary atriovenous communication depend on the anatomic type of coronary arteriovenous fistulae. The right coronary and right atrial or coronary sinus communication produce continuous murmurs that usually are located along the parasternal areas. The circumflex coronary artery–coronary sinus communication, however, produces continuous murmurs in the left axilla (134).

Constriction in the systemic or pulmonary arteries can be associated with a continuous murmur owing to a pressure gradient across the narrow segment during both systole and diastole. In coarctation of the aorta, a continuous murmur can be heard in the back overlying the areas of constriction. Continuous murmurs in coarctation of the aorta may also originate from the tortuous collateral arteries, which are heard in the back over the interscapular regions. Sometimes, large, tortuous intercostal vessels are visible when the shoulders are rotated and separated (Suzman sign) (135). Pulmonary artery branch stenosis may also be associated with continuous murmur. Chronic obstruction of the pulmonary artery from pulmonary embolism has been shown to produce continuous murmur on rare occasions. Bronchial arterial collateral vessels develop in certain types of cyanotic congenital heart disease, as in tricuspid atresia and pulmonary atresia with ventricular septal defect; these collateral vessels can produce continuous murmur. An example of innocent continuous murmur is venous hum (136). The venous hum is heard with the patient in the sitting position and usually in the supraclavicular areas; it disappears when the patient is in the supine position. A loud, left-sided venous hum transmitted below the clavicle should not be mistaken for the patent ductus arteriosus. A venous hum is not heard in the supine position, and pressure on the internal jugular vein abolishes the venous hum. The mammary shuffle associated with pregnancy is another example of an innocent continuous murmur. These innocent murmurs are usually of higher frequency (high pitched) and louder in systole. Fistulous connection between internal mammary graft and left anterior descending vein or pulmonary vasculature may also case continuous murmur (137). The causes of continuous murmurs and the mechanisms of their geneses are summarized in Table 16.11.

CONTROVERSIES AND PERSONAL PERSPECTIVES

Often in today's clinical practice, bedside examination is considered unnecessary and a waste of time. Indeed, the investigative tools available today are far superior to the bedside examination in establishing the diagnosis of the anatomic abnormality and severity of the pathophysiologic consequences. However, only bedside examination allows you to know the patient, understand the patient's sufferings and expectations, and establish rapport with the patient. Furthermore, repeated and frequent echocardiographic evaluations during follow up

TABLE 16.11

CAUSES OF CONTINUOUS MURMUR

CONTINUOUS MURMUR DUE TO FLOW FROM HIGH- TO LOW-PRESSURE SYSTEMS

- *Systemic artery to pulmonary artery connection*—patent ductus arteriosus, aortopulmonary window, truncus arteriosus, pulmonary atresia, and coronary arteriovenous fistulae
- *Systemic artery to right heart connection*—rupture of sinus of Valsalva coronary artery fistulae
- *Left-to-right atrial shunting*—Lutembacher syndrome
- *Venovenous shunts*—anomalous pulmonary veins, portosystemic shunts
- *Arteriovenous fistulae*—systemic or pulmonic

CONTINUOUS MURMUR SECONDARY TO LOCALIZED ARTERIAL OBSTRUCTION

- Coarctation of the aorta
- Pulmonary artery branch stenosis
- Carotid stenosis

CONTINUOUS MURMUR DUE TO RAPID BLOOD FLOW

- Venous hum
- Mammary shuffle

evaluation is clearly expensive and not cost effective. With better teaching and practice it is possible to use bedside examination as a more effective tool. Thus, I believe that we should practice more—not less—bedside physical examination.

CONCLUSIONS

Bedside clinical examination of the cardiovascular system provides useful information about the potential etiology of valvular, myocardial, and pericardial diseases, which can be confirmed by further noninvasive and invasive investigations. Physical examination also is helpful in deciding the appropriate investigations to establish the diagnosis. Furthermore, appropriate clinical evaluations are helpful to assess the therapeutic response and prognosis of patients with cardiovascular disorders. There is no cost-effective substitute for the information and insight derived from a careful bedside examination.

THE FUTURE

The future of the physical examination as an investigation tool is likely to be compromised with the increasing availability of sonocardiographic and other allied imaging techniques. It should be remembered, however, that the bedside physical examination is still the least expensive and, in certain circumstances, most informative investigation.

References

1. Chatterjee K. Bedside evaluation of the heart: the physical examination. In: Parmley W, Chatterjee K, eds. *Cardiology*. Philadelphia: JB Lippincott Co, 1997.
2. O'Rourke RA, Silverman ME, Schlant RC. General examination of the patient. In: Schlant RC, Alexander RW, eds. *Hurst's the heart,* 8th ed. New York: McGraw-Hill, 1994:10217.
3. Shy GM, Drager GA. A neurologic syndrome associated with orthostatic hypotension: a clinical-pathologic study. *Arch Neurol* 1960;2:511.
4. Anker SD, Coats AJS. Syndrome of cardiac cachexia. In: Poole-Wilson PA, Colucci WS, Massie BM, et al., eds. *Heart failure*. New York: Churchill Livingstone, 1997:18261.
5. Kaplan NM. The deadly quartet. Upper-body obesity, glucose intolerance, hypertriglyceridemia, and hypertension. *Arch Intern Med* 1989;149: 1514.
6. Solymoss BC, Marcil M, Chadur M, et al. Fasting hyperinsulinism, insulin resistance syndrome, and coronary artery disease in men and women. *Am J Cardiol* 1995;76:1152.
7. Javaheri S, Parker TJ, Liming JD, et al. Sleep apnea in 81 ambulatory male patients with stable heart failure: types and their prevalences. *Circulation* 1998;97:1254.
8. Lanfranchi PA, Braghiroli A, Bosmini E, et al. Prognostic value of nocturnal Cheyne-Stokes respiration in chronic heart failure. *Circulation* 1999;99: 1435.
9. Sin D, Logan A, Fitzgerald F, et al. Effects of continuous positive airway pressure on cardiovascular outcomes in heart failure patients with and without Cheyne-Stokes respiration. *Circulation* 2000;102:61.
10. Benotti JR, Grossman W, Cohn EF. Clinical profile of restrictive cardiomyopathy. *Circulation* 1980;61:1206.
11. Zachary CB, Slater DN, Holt DW, et al. The pathogenesis of amiodarone-induced pigmentation and photosensitivity. *Br J Dermatol* 1984;110:451.
12. Richards AM, Eliot RS, Kanjuh VI, et al. Cholesterol embolism: a multiple-system disease masquerading as polyarteritis nodosa. *Am J Cardiol* 1965; 15:696.
13. Malloy MJ, Kane JP, Kunitake ST, et al. Complementarity of colestipol, niacin, and lovastatin in treatment of severe familial hypercholesterolemia. *Ann Intern Med* 1987;107:616.
14. Keith NM, Wagener HP, Barker ND. Some different types of essential hypertension: their course and prognosis. *Am J Med Sci* 1939;197:332.
15. Leriche R, Morel A. The syndrome of thrombotic obliteration of the aortic bifurcation. *Ann Surg* 1948;127:193.
16. Smyth PT, Edwards JE. Pseudocoarctation, kinking, or buckling of the aorta. *Circulation* 1972;46:1027.
17. McGaughey MD, Maughan L, Sunagawa K, et al. Alternating contractility in pulsus alternans studied in the isolated canine heart. *Circulation* 1985; 71:357.
18. Narayan P, McCune SA, Robitaille PML, et al. Mechanical alternans and the force-frequency relationship in failing rat hearts. *J Moll Cell Cardiol* 1995;27:523.
19. Chabetai R, Fowler NO, Guntheroth WG. The hemodynamics of cardiac tamponade and constrictive pericarditis. *Am J Cardiol* 1970;26:480.
20. Massumi RA, Mason DT, Zakuddin V, et al. Reserved pulsus paradoxus. *N Engl J Med* 1973;289:1272.
21. Robinson B. The carotid pulse: 1. Diagnosis of aortic stenosis by external recordings. *Br Heart J* 1963;25:51.
22. Dexter L. Atrial septal defect. *Br Heart J* 1956;18:209.
23. Kussmaul A. User schwielige Mediastino-pericarditis und den parodoxen pulse. *Berl Klin Wochenschr* 1873;10:433.
24. Dell'Italia L, Starling MR, O'Rourke RA. Physical examination for exclusion of hemodynamically important right ventricular infarction. *Ann Intern Med* 1983;99:608.
25. Ducas J, Magder S, McGregor M. Validity of the hepatojugular reflux as a clinical test for congestive heart failure. *Am J Cardiol* 1983;52:1299.
26. Ewy GA. The abdominojugular test: technique and hemodynamic correlates. *Ann Intern Med* 1989;108:456.
27. Cohn J, Hamosh P. Experimental observations on pulsus paradoxus and hepatojugular reflux. In: Reddy PS, ed. *Pericardial disease*. New York: Raven, 1982:249.
28. Sutton GC, Craige E. Quantitation of precordial movement: I. Normal subjects. *Circulation* 1967;35:476.
29. Sutton GC, Prewitt TA, Craige E. Relationship between quantitated precordial movement and left ventricular function. *Circulation* 1970;31:179.
30. Manttleman SJ, Hakki AH, Iskandrian AS, et al. Reliability of bedside evaluation in determining left ventricular function: correlation with left ventricular ejection fraction determined by radionuclide ventriculography. *J Am Coll Cardiol* 1983;1:417.
31. Braunwald E, Lambrew CT, Rockoff SD, et al. Idiopathic hypertrophic subaortic stenosis: 1. A description of the disease based upon an analysis of 64 patients. *Circulation* 1964;30:3.
32. Tafur E, Cohen LS, Levine HD. The apex cardiogram in left ventricular outflow obstruction. *Circulation* 1964;30:392.
33. El-Sherif A, El-said G. Jugular, hepatic and precordial pulsations in constrictive pericarditis. *Br Heart J* 1971;33:305.
34. Armstrong TG, Gotsman MS. The left parasternal lift in tricuspid incompetence. *Am Heart J* 1974;88:183.
35. Shaver JA, Salerni R. Auscultation of the heart. In: Schlant RC, Alexander RW, eds. *Hurst's the heart,* 8th ed. New York: McGraw-Hill, 1994:253.
36. Leech G, Brooks N, Green-Wilkinson A, Leatham A. Mechanisms of influence of P-R interval on loudness of first heart sound. *Br Heart J* 1980;43:138.
37. Shah PM. Hemodynamic determinants of the first heart sound. In: Leon DF, Shaver JA, eds. *Physiologic principles of heart sounds and murmurs. Monograph 46*. New York: American Heart Association, 1975:2.
38. Tei C, Shah PM, Cherian G, et al. The correlates of an abnormal first heart sound in mitral valve prolapse syndromes. *N Engl J Med* 1982;307:334.

39. Mann T, McLaurin L, Grossman W, et al. Acute aortic regurgitation due to infective endocarditis. *N Engl J Med* 1975;293:108.
40. Shaver JA, Rahko PS, Grines CL, et al. Effect of left bundle branch block on the events of the cardiac cycle. *Acta Cardiol* 1988;4:459.
41. Sakamoto T, Kusukawa R, MacCanon DM, Luisada AA. First heart sound amplitude in experimentally induced alternans. *Dis Chest* 1966;50:470.
42. Leatham A. Splitting of the first and second heart sounds. *Lancet* 1954; 267:607.
43. Crews TL, Pridie RB, Benham R, et al. Auscultatory and phonocardiographic findings in Ebstein's anomaly: correlation of first heart sound with ultrasonic records of tricuspid valve movement. *Br Heart J* 1972;34: 681.
44. Harris A. Pacemaker "heart sound." *Br Heart J* 1967;29:608.
45. Hirschfeld S, Liebman J, Borkat G, Bormuth C. Intracardiac pressure-sound correlates of echocardiographic aortic valve closure. *Circulation* 1977;55:602.
46. Stein PD, Sabbah HN, Anbe DT, Khaja F. Hemodynamic and anatomic determinants of relative differences in amplitude of the aortic and pulmonary components of the second heart sound. *Am J Cardiol* 1978;42:539.
47. Harris A, Leatham A, Sutton G. The second heart sound in pulmonary hypertension. *Br Heart J* 1968;30:743.
48. Shaver JA, Nadolny RA, O'Toole JD, et al. Sound pressure correlates of the second heart sound: an intracardiac sound study. *Circulation* 1974;49:316.
49. Leatham A, Weitzman DW. Auscultatory and phonocardiographic signs of pulmonary stenosis. *Br Heart J* 1957;19:303.
50. Sutton GC, Chatterjee K, Caves PK. Diagnosis of severe mitral regurgitation due to nonrheumatic chordal abnormalities. *Br Heart J* 1973;35:877.
51. Adolph RJ. Second heart sound: role of altered electromechanical events. In: Leon DF, Shaver JA, eds. *Physiologic principles of heart sounds and murmurs. Monograph 46*. New York: American Heart Association, 1975:45.
52. Leatham, Segal B. Auscultatory and phonocardiographic signs of ventricular septal defect with left to right shunt. *Circulation* 1962;25:318.
53. Beck W, Schrire V, Vogelpoel L. Splitting of the second heart sound in constrictive pericarditis with observations on the mechanism of pulsus paradoxus. *Am Heart J* 1962;64:765.
54. Gray I. Paradoxical splitting of the second heart sound. *Br Heart J* 1956; 18:21.
55. Perloff JK. Auscultatory and phonocardiographic manifestations of pulmonary hypertension. *Prog Cardiovasc Dis* 1967;9:303.
56. Shapiro S, Clark TJH, Goodwin JF. Delayed closure of the pulmonary valve in obliterative pulmonary hypertension. *Lancet* 1965;2:1207.
57. Luisada AA, Kumar S, Pouget MJ. On the causes of the changes of the second heart sound in left bundle branch block. *Jpn Heart J* 1972;13: 281.
58. Alvares RF, Shaver JA, Gamble WH, Goodwin JF. The isovolumic relaxation period in hypertrophic cardiomyopathy. *J Am Coll Cardiol* 1984;3:71.
59. Shaver JA, Kroetz FW, Leonard JJ, Paley HW. Effect of study state increase in systemic arterial pressure on the duration of left ventricular ejection time. *J Clin Invest* 1968;47:217.
60. Shaver JA, O'Toole JD. The second heart sound: newer concepts, part 2. Paradoxical splitting and narrow physiologic splitting. *Mod Concepts Cardiovasc Dis* 1977;46:13.
61. Hultgren HN, Reeve R, Cohn K, McLeod R. The ejection click of valvular pulmonic stenosis. *Circulation* 1969;40:631.
62. Sakamoto T, Matsuhisa M, Hayashi T, Ichiyasu H. Echocardiogram and phonocardiogram related to the movement of the pulmonary valve. *Jpn Heart J* 1975;16:107.
63. Barlow JB, Pocock WA, Marchand P, Denny M. The significance of late systolic murmurs. *Am Heart J* 1963;66:443.
64. Criley JM, Lewis KB, Humphries JO, Ross RS. Prolapse of the mitral valve: clinical and cine-angiographic findings. *Br Heart J* 1966;28:488.
65. Popp RL, Brown OR, Silverman JF, Harrison D. Echocardiographic abnormalities in the mitral valve prolapse syndrome. *Circulation* 1974;49: 428.
66. Mathey DG, Decodt PR, Allen HN, Swan HJC. The determinants of onset of mitral valve prolapse in the systolic click-late systolic murmur syndrome. *Circulation* 1976;53:872.
67. Roelandt J, Willems J, Van der Hauwaert LG, deGreest H. Clicks and sounds (whoops) in left-sided pneumothorax: clinical and phonocardiographic study. *Dis Chest* 1969;56:31.
68. Martin CE, Hufnagel CA, deLeon AC Jr. Calcified atrial myxoma: diagnostic significance of the "systolic tumor sound" in a case presenting as tricuspid insufficiency. *Am Heart J* 1969;78:245.
69. Pickering D, Keith JD. Systolic clicks, with ventricular septal defects: a sign of aneurysm of ventricular septum? *Br Heart J* 1971;22:538.
70. Killebrew E, Cohn K. Observations on murmurs originating from incompetent heterograft mitral valves. *Am Heart J* 1971;81:490.
71. Sze KC, Shah PM. Pseudoejection sound in hypertrophic subaortic stenosis: an echocardiographic correlative study. *Circulation* 1976;54:504.
72. Ranko PS, Shaver JA, Salerni R, et al. Echo-phonocardiographic estimates of pulmonary artery wedge pressure in mitral stenosis. *Am J Cardiol* 1985; 55:462.
73. Spodick DH. Hypertrophic obstructive cardiomyopathy of the left ventricular (idiopathic hypertrophic subaortic stenosis). In: Burch GE, Brest AN, eds. *Cardiovascular clinics*. Philadelphia: FA Davis, 1972:156.
74. Abrams J. The third and fourth heart sounds. *Primary Cardiol* 1982;8:47.
75. Vancheri F, Gibson D. Relation of third and fourth heart sounds to blood velocity during left ventricular filling. *Br Heart J* 1989;61:144.
76. Reddy PS, Salerni R, Shaver JA. Normal and abnormal heart sounds in cardiac diagnosis: part II. Diastolic sounds. *Current Probl Cardiol* 1985; April:10.
77. Lok CE, Morgan CD, Ranganathan N. The accuracy and interobserver agreement in detecting the "gallop sounds" by cardiac auscultation. *Chest* 1998;114:1283.
78. Shah PM, Jackson D. Third heart sound and summation gallop. In: Leon DF, Shaver JA, eds. *Physiologic principles of heart sounds and murmurs. Monograph 46*. New York: American Heart Association, 1975:79.
79. Patel R, Bushnell DL, Sobotka PA. Implications of an audible third heart sound in evaluating cardiac function. *West J Med* 1993;158:606.
80. Abdulla AM, Frank MJ, Erdin RA Jr, et al. Clinical significance and hemodynamic correlates of the third heart sound gallop in aortic regurgitation: a guide to optimal timing of cardiac catheterization. *Circulation* 1981;64:463.
81. Zile MR, Brutsaert DL. New concepts in diastolic function and diastolic heart failure. Part I: Diagnosis, prognosis and measurements of diastolic function. *Circulation* 2002;105:1387.
82. Marcus GM, Michaels AD, DeMarco T, et al. Usefulness of the third heart sound in predicting an elevated level of B-type natriuretic peptide. *Am J Cardiol* 2004;93:1312.
83. Marcus GM, Gerber IL, McKeown BH, et al. Association between third and fourth heart sounds and objective measures of left ventricular function. *JAMA* 2005;293:2238.
84. Nixon PG. The genesis of the third heart sound. *Am Heart J* 1963;65:712.
85. Maisel AS, Gilpin E, Hoit B, et al. Survival after hospital discharge in matched populations with inferior or anterior myocardial infarction. *J Am Coll Cardiol* 1985;6:731.
86. Goldman L, Caldera DL, Nussbaum SR, et al. Multifactorial index of cardiac risk in noncardiac surgical procedures. *N Engl J Med* 1977;297:845.
87. Drazner MH, Rame JE, Dries DL. Third heart sound and elevated jugular venous pressure as markers of the subsequent development of heart failure in patients with asymptomatic left ventricular dysfunction. *Am J Med* 2003;114:431.
88. Drazner MH, Rame JE, Stevenson LW, Dries DL. Prognostic importance of elevated jugular venous pressure and a third heart sound in patients with heart failure. *N Engl J Med* 2001;345:574.
89. Vandewerf F, Minten J, Carmeliet P, et al. The genesis of the third and fourth heart sounds: a pressure-flow study in dogs. *J Clin Invest* 1984;73:1400.
90. Goldblatt A, Aygen MM, Braunwald E. Hemodynamic-phonocardiographic correlations of the fourth heart sound in aortic stenosis. *Circulation* 1962;26:92.
91. Caulfield WH, deLeon AC, Perloff JK, Steelman RB. The clinical significance of the fourth heart sound in aortic stenosis. *Am J Cardiol* 1971; 28:179.
92. Hill JC, O'Rourke RA, Lewis RP, McGranahan GM. The diagnostic value of the atrial gallop in acute myocardial infarction. *Am Heart J* 1969;78:194.
93. Sutton GC, Chatterjee K, Caves PK. Diagnosis of severe mitral regurgitation due to non-rheumatic chordal abnormalities. *Br Heart J* 1973;35:877.
94. Lerman J, Means JH. Cardiovascular symptomatology in exophthalmic goiter. *Am Heart J* 1932;8:55.
95. Hamman L. Spontaneous mediastinal emphysema. *Bull Johns Hopkins Hosp* 1939;64:1.
96. Lembo NJ, Dell'Italia LJ, Crawford MH, O'Rourke RA. Bedside diagnosis of systolic murmurs. *N Engl J Med* 1988;318:1572.
97. Gallavardin L, Ravault P. Le souffle du retre'cissem-ent aortique puce changer de timbre et devenir musical dans sa propagation apexienne. *Lyon Med* 1925;135:523.
98. Pagon RA, Bennett FC, La Veek B, et al. Williams syndrome. *J Pediatr* 1987;80:85.
99. Thompson ME, Shaver JA. Aortic stenosis in the elderly. *Geriatrics* 1983; 38:50.
100. Shaver JA, Alvares RF, Reddy PS, Salerni R. Phonoechocardiography and intracardiac phonocardiography in hypertrophic cardiomyopathy. *Postgrad Med J* 1986;62:527.
101. Shah PM. Controversies in hypertrophic cardiomyopathy. *Curr Probl Cardiol* 1986;11:563.
102. Braunwald E, Lambrew CT, Rockoff SD, et al. Idiopathic hypertrophic subaortic stenosis: I. A description of the disease based upon analysis of 64 patients. *Circulation* 1964;30[Suppl 4]:3.
103. Yamaguchi H, Ishimura T, Nishiyama S, et al. Hypertrophic nonobstructive cardiomyopathy with giant negative T-waves (apical hypertrophy): ventriculographic and echocardiographic features in 30 patients. *Am J Cardiol* 1979;44:401.
104. Mineo K, Cummings J, Josephson R, Nanda NC. Acquired left ventricular outflow tract obstruction during acute myocardial infarction. Diagnosis of a new cardiac murmur. *Am J Geriatric Cardiol* 2001;10:283.
105. Darazs B, Hesdorfer CS, Butterworth AM, Ziady F. The possible etiology of the vibratory systolic murmur. *Clin Cardiol* 1987;10:341.
106. Schwartz ML, Goldberg SJ, Wilson N, et al. Relation of Still's murmur, small aortic diameter, and high aortic velocity. *Am J Cardiol* 1986;57:1344.
107. Craig E. Phonocardiography in interventricular septal defects. *Am Heart J* 1960;60:51.

108. Roger H. Recherches cliniques sur la communication congenitale. Des deux coeurs par inocclusion du septum interventriculaire. *Bull Acad Med (Paris)* 1879;8:1074.
109. Wood P. The Eisenmenger syndrome or pulmonary hypertension with reversed central shunt. *BMJ* 1958;Sept:701.
110. Sutton GC, Craig E. Clinical signs of severe acute mitral regurgitation. *Am J Cardiol* 1967;20:141.
111. Rios JC, Massumi RA, Breesmen WT, Sarin RK. Auscultatory features of acute tricuspid regurgitation. *Am J Cardiol* 1969;23:4.
112. Amidi M, Irwin JM, Salerni R, et al. Venous systolic thrill and murmur in the neck: a consequence of severe tricuspid insufficiency. *J Am Coll Cardiol* 1986;7:942.
113. Vogelpoel L, Schrire V, Beck W, et al. A typical systolic murmur of minute ventricular septal defect and its recognition by amyl nitrite and phenylephrine. *Am Heart J* 1961;62:101.
114. Gelfand D, Bellet S. The musical murmur of aortic insufficiency: clinical manifestations based on study of 18 cases. *Am J Med Sci* 1951;221:644.
115. Harvey WP, Corrado MA, Perloff JK. Right sided murmurs of aortic insufficiency. *Am J Med Sci* 1963;245:533.
116. Choudhry NK, Etchells EE. Does this patient have aortic regurgitation? *JAMA* 1999;281:2231.
117. Sabbah HN, Khaja F, Anbe DT, Stein PD. The aortic closure sound in pure aortic insufficiency. *Circulation* 1977;56:859.
118. Reddy PS, Leon DF, Krishnaswami V, et al. Syndrome of acute regurgitation. In: Leon DF, Shaver JA, eds. *Physiologic principles of heart sounds and murmurs. Monograph 46*. New York: American Heart Association, 1975: 166.
119. Dock W, Zoneraich S. A diastolic murmur arising in a stenosed coronary artery. *Am J Med* 1967;742:617.
120. Steell G. The murmur of high pressure in the pulmonary artery. *Med Chron* 1888;9:182.
121. Runco V, Molnar W, Meckstroth CV, Ryan JM. The Graham Steell murmur versus aortic regurgitation in rheumatic heart disease. *Am J Med* 1961;31:71.
122. Runco V, Levin HS. The spectrum of pulmonic regurgitation. In: Leon DF, Shaver JA, eds. *Physiologic principles and heart sounds and murmurs. Monograph 46*. New York: American Heart Association, 1975:175.
123. Criley JM, Hermer AJ. The crescendo presystolic murmur of mitral stenosis with atrial fibrillation. *N Engl J Med* 1971;285:1284.
124. Nasser WK, Davis RH, Dillon JC, et al. Atrial myxoma: II. Phonocardiographic, echocardiographic, hemodynamic and angiographic features in nine cases. *Am Heart J* 1972;83:810.
125. Wooley CF, Fontana ME, Kilman JW, Ryan JM. Tricuspid sounds: atrial systolic murmur, tricuspid opening snap, and right atrial pressure pulse. *Am J Med* 1985;78:375.
126. Coombs CF. *Rheumatic Heart Disease*. New York: William Wood, 1924: 190.
127. Flint A. On cardiac murmurs. *Am J Med Sci* 1862;44:29.
128. Reddy PS, Curtiss EI, Salerni R, et al. Sound pressure correlates of the Austin Flint murmur: An intracardiac sound study. *Circulation* 1976;53:210.
129. Landzberg JS, Pflugfelder PW, Cassidy MM, et al. Etiology of the Austin Flint Murmur. *J Am Coll Cardiol* 1992;20:408.
130. Panidis IP, Ross J, Munley B, et al. Diastolic mitral regurgitation in patients with atrioventricular conduction abnormalities: a common finding by Doppler echocardiography. *J Am Coll Cardiol* 1986;7:768.
131. Craige E, Milward DK. Diastolic and continuous murmurs. *Prog Cardiovasc Dis* 1971;14:38.
132. Gibson GA. Lecture on patent ductus arteriosus. *Edinburgh Med J* 1900; 8:1.
133. Steinbrunn W, Cohn KE, Selzer A. Atrial septal defect associated with mitral stenosis: the Lutembacher syndrome revisited. *Am J Med* 1970;48:295.
134. Harris A, Jefferson K, Chatterjee K. Coronary arteriovenous fistula with aneurysm of coronary sinus. *Br Heart J* 1969;31:400.
135. Campbell M, Suzman SS. Coarctation of the aorta. *Br Heart J* 1947;9: 185.
136. Fowler NO, Gause R. The cervical venous hum. *Am Heart J* 1964;67:135.
137. Guray U, Guray Y, Ozbakir C, et al. Fistulous connection between internal mammary graft and pulmonary vasculature after coronary bypass grafting: A rare cause of continuous murmur. *Int J Cardiol* 2004;96:489.

CHAPTER 17 ■ CHRONIC STABLE CORONARY DISEASE

KEITH A. A. FOX

INTRODUCTION

The prevalence of occult atheromatous coronary disease among industrialized communities is so high that the incidental finding of coronary disease on pathologic examination is the norm rather than the exception (see Atherosclerotic Biology and Epidemiology of Disease). Thus, most individuals with nonobstructive coronary arterial disease are asymptomatic and manifest no clinical signs nor symptoms of the disease process. Managing the preclinical phase of the disease, including risk factors modification is considered in Preventive Cardiology. This chapter focuses on chronic stable coronary disease manifest through symptoms, clinical signs, or cardiac complications.

Chronic stable angina is the most common symptomatic manifestation of obstructive coronary artery disease. Although myocardial oxygen supply–demand imbalance may result in angina in the absence of detectable atheromatous coronary artery disease, the vast majority of angina occurs in the presence of obstructive coronary artery plaques. However, the threshold for provoking angina and the severity of symptoms depend on a variety of factors that influence loading conditions, oxygen demand, and cellular cytoprotective pathways because myocardial ischemia is more prevalent than symptomatic angina and the threshold for provoking symptoms varies within and between patients. Rather than an isolated condition, chronic stable angina should be regarded as a symptomatic manifestation of predominantly obstructive coronary artery disease and a relatively stable interlude in the pathophysiology of progression of atheromatous coronary artery disease.

Despite the absence of symptoms and clinical manifestations early in the progression of coronary disease, markers of the disease process "intermediate phenotypes" may be detectable biochemically and by noninvasive and invasive testing and prognosis may be altered by interventions that aim to mitigate the progression of atheroma.

PREVALENCE AND INCIDENCE OF ANGINA

The elegant description by William Heberden in 1768 captures the key features of angina:

> a disorder of the breast marked with strong and peculiar symptoms, considerable for the kind of danger belonging to it, and not extremely rare, the sense of strangling and anxiety with which it is attended, may make it not improperly be called angina pectoris. Those who are afflicted with it are seized while they are walking (more especially if it be uphill, and soon after eating), with a painful and most disagreeable sensation in the breast, which seems as if it

would extinguish life, if it were to increase or to continue; but the moment they stand still, all this uneasiness vanishes.

As observed by William Heberden, angina is "not extremely rare": it affects approximately 3.1 million men and 3.3 million women in the United States (overall, 3.8% of the population) and there are an additional 400,000 new cases each year (1). The prevalence of angina rises markedly with age (21.1% in men, 13.7% in women 65 to 69 and 27.3% and 24.7%, respectively, for men and women 80 to 84 years of age) (2). Thus, angina is highly prevalent especially in the elderly, has a major impact on lifestyle and quality of life, and imposes a major financial burden on the individual and a huge socioeconomic impact on the community.

PATHOPHYSIOLOGY OF ANGINA

Cardiac ischemic pain is transmitted via sensory afferents located in the coronary vessels and myocardium (3). These afferents are sensitive to both stretch and by local expression of specific chemical stimuli (4). Maseri and colleagues (3) categorized cardiac ischemic pain into three components: (a) a diffuse visceral component, (b) a better defined somatic component conforming to a distribution by dermatomes, and (c) an interpretive component modulated by psychological factors. Pain-producing stimuli traveling through afferent nerve endings converge with others from the same dermatome on the same dorsal horn spinal neurons. Cardiac afferents distributed from the first to the fourth thoracic spinal neurons interact with other afferents and descending signals from supraspinal sources, then ascend to the thalamus and from thence to the cortex, where the decoding is processed by a complex collage of physical, emotional, and other factors.

The symptomatic discomfort that represents angina pectoris usually reflects underlying coronary atherosclerosis sufficient to reduce maximal blood flow during exercise (5) (Table 17.1). Whereas fixed segmental coronary stenosis (e.g., >50% diameter stenosis) may prevent sufficient myocardial blood flow to meet the increased oxygen requirements imposed by physical exercise; changes in vascular tone also modulate the threshold for ischemia. Failure of flow mediated dilation is due to deficient endothelial-dependent relaxation (6–8) and is associated with the diffuse nature of coronary artery disease, even in the absence of stenotic atheromatous lesions. Thus, angina may result from exercise-induced coronary vasoconstriction of noncritically narrowed coronary arteries and imbalance between oxygen supply and demand.

Mental or physical stress can precipitate angina pectoris and ischemia; mental stress is mediated by sympathetic activation, with a commensurate increase in myocardial oxygen requirements resulting from tachycardia, hypertension, and increased contractility (9). This exerts a double jeopardy on the ischemic myocardium by also reducing regional coronary flow (10). Failure of endothelial-dependent epicardial coronary vasodilatation is evident during mental stress in patients with stable angina (10), and, vasoconstriction of coronary resistance vessels may be present. Several neurohumoral factors contribute including serotonin, neuropeptide Y, norepinephrine, angiotensin II, thromboxane A_2, endothelin, and arginine vasopressin (11,12). As many as one of five stable angina patients have features of recent injury and/or repair in their culprit coronary lesions. Aggregation and activation of platelets can contribute to the alterations in vascular tone (13).

STABLE ANGINA: A SYMPTOM COMPLEX

Most patients with stable angina describe retrosternal chest discomfort or distress, rather than "pain." Anginal discomfort is sometimes characterized as heaviness, burning, tightness, or a choking sensation. It is commonly felt in the center of the chest, characteristically gestured with a clenched-fist or the flat of the hand across the sternum (14). In some patients, it is exclusively located outside the chest, in the arms, shoulders, back, jaw, or epigastrium. Patterns of anginal radiation are associated with severe ischemia and can spread from the chest to the neck, shoulders, arms (usually left), and jaw. Anginal equivalents characterized by dyspnea, profound fatigue, weakness, or syncope may occur in the absence of any discomfort. Ischemic symptoms during stable angina are usually of brief duration, persisting for 3 to 5 minutes, and are typically relieved by rest, dissipation of emotional distress, or the administration of nitroglycerin. Typically, the symptoms are produced by vigorous physical activity or emotional distress, and the threshold at which they occur may be lowered by exposure to cold weather, by smoking a cigarette, or after ingestion of a meal. Some patients experience warm-up angina (possibly a form of ischemic preconditioning) such that they experience angina much more readily on initiating exercise, than after the episode of angina. After pausing for the initial episode of angina to dissipate, they are able to continue for a sustained time at the same or even an accelerated pace. Warm-up angina is evident in approximately 20% of patients; hence, the second exertional effort is predictably better than the first if there is separation of at least

TABLE 17.1

CAUSES OF ANGINAL CHEST PAIN

CORONARY ARTERIAL DISEASE	**VASCULAR DISORDERS**
Fixed obstructive coronary disease	Variant angina
Coronary disease with dynamic flow limitation	Coronary vasospasm (see Printzmetal angina)
Microvascular angina (Syndrome X)	Syndrome X (without obstructive vascular disease)
OTHER CARDIAC DISORDERS	**SYSTEMIC DISORDERS PRECIPITATING ANGINA**
Aortic stenosis	Anaemia
Hypertrophic cardiomyopathy	Thyrotoxicosis
Hypertensive heart disease and left ventricular hypertrophy	High-output states (e.g., arterio-venous shunts)
Mitral valve prolapse	
Severe pulmonary hypertension and right ventricular hypertrophy	

2 to 5 minutes between them (15). However, if the second effort is initiated later than 30 to 60 minutes after the first, the improvement disappears. Marber and colleagues (15), along with others (16–18), have suggested a pathophysiologic link triggered by favorable adaptive myocardial metabolic changes that result in less of a decline in high-energy phosphate and less lactate production despite recurrent ischemia. Experimental insights into the phenomenon of ischemic preconditioning have demonstrated changes in mitochondrial K_{ATP} channel function, leading to reduced requirement for oxygenated substrate and attendant reduction in myocardial oxygen consumption (18,19).

Angina is traditionally categorized into four grades based on the Canadian Cardiovascular Society grading scale (20). In class I, patients experience angina only with strenuous or protracted physical activity; those in class II experience only slight limitation with vigorous physical activity such as walking up a hill briskly. Patients in class III have marked limitation, with symptoms during the activities of everyday living, and those in class IV have the inability to perform the activities of daily living because of symptoms as well as angina that may occur at rest. This classification does not address changes in the pattern or frequency of angina (including the development of unstable angina) or take into account the warm-up effect or the self-imposed alteration in activities of daily living that may subtly modify symptomatic status (21).

SILENT ISCHEMIA

The chronologic sequence of events during ischemia begins with diminished myocardial perfusion and is followed by diminished diastolic and systolic left ventricular function, abnormal myocardial lactate metabolism, electrocardiographic (ECG) changes, and then finally symptoms of angina pectoris (22,23). Most ischemic episodes in patients with stable angina (>75%) are clinically silent, and despite symptomatic control of angina, a substantial proportion (40% of patients with stable angina) continue to demonstrate ischemia on ambulatory monitoring (22).

Impairment of contractile function may persist for an extended period of time (60–120 minutes after exercise-induced angina) despite abrupt normalization of hemodynamic and ECG parameters. Ambrosio and colleagues (24) demonstrated the delay in return of contractile performance despite normal perfusion after the development and relief of exertional angina (myocardial stunning), in the context of severely obstructive coronary artery disease.

SYNDROME X

Cardiac syndrome X represents a heterogeneous group of disorders best characterized by a reduced capacity of the coronary circulation to augment flow in the face of an increase in oxygen demand. Abnormalities of coronary vasomotor tone and angina, or angina-like chest pain may occur in the presence of angiographically normal coronary arteries (25). In addition, about 25% of patients with stable angina have coronary lesions on angiography that do not alter exercise-induced coronary flow (26,27). Evidence for myocardial ischemia in such patients has been demonstrated by reversible perfusion defects with thallium scintigraphy and transient impairment of global and regional left ventricular function by radionuclide ventriculography (28). Survival in patients with syndrome X is not significantly impaired in comparison with age- and gender-matched controls (29).

PRINZMETAL'S VARIANT ANGINA

Focal coronary spasm has been demonstrated as a mechanism for variant angina based on the association of transient ST elevation concurrent with symptoms and localized myocardial perfusion and functional abnormalities (30,31). This uncommon but well-recognized syndrome (30) is evident in up to 2% of patients presenting with chest pain undergoing invasive study. It is usually associated with underlying fixed coronary obstruction, but a substantial cohort may have angiographically normal coronary arteries or minimally evident disease (32).

DEMOGRAPHICS AND OUTCOME OF PATIENTS WITH ANGINA

Evaluation of a general outpatient population of 5,125 patients with stable angina enrolled by 1,266 primary care physicians in the United States demonstrates approximately equal gender distribution (mean age of women of 71 years and that of men of 67 years) (33). In the Coronary Artery Surgery Study, 62% of women with definite angina had coronary disease compared with a much higher proportion (89%) of men (34). Most patients had more than one cardiovascular-related illness, usually systemic hypertension, hypercholesterolemia, prior infarction, heart failure, or diabetes. The majority perceived their health to be either poor or fair and had experienced at least two episodes of angina per week, and although more than 90% had angina with activity, nearly half also experienced angina at rest, highlighting the commonality of mixed angina. Recently, the 5-year outcome and risk characteristics of a trial population of patients with chronic ischemic heart disease was defined (35). The rate of death, nonfatal myocardial infarction (MI), or stroke varied almost 10-fold according to baseline risk characteristics (from 1% to 9%) (Table 17.2). Thus, estimating baseline risk is critically important in weighing up the balance between risk and benefit of therapeutic interventions.

New-onset angina, defined as occurring within 2 to 3 months of presentation, is associated with at least a doubling of the risk of nonfatal MI within the first year after onset (36). This accentuated risk over patients with chronic coronary disease appears in spite of a lesser extent of triple-vessel disease and a greater frequency of single-vessel disease than in patients with chronic stable angina (37).

African Americans, especially those born in the southern United States, have an excess of cardiovascular mortality compared with American whites (38). Less aggressive use of diagnostic procedures has been recorded in African Americans (39,40). Asian Indians living outside of India have an excess risk of MI (range, 2.5 to 5.0) and mortality for coronary artery disease (range, 1.5 to 3.0) compared with indigenous populations (41). Their disease is characterized by premature onset and a severe and diffuse nature such that it is less amenable to coronary artery bypass grafting (CABG) and more likely to lead to permanent disability. Factors promoting this more malignant course include increased triglycerides and lipoprotein(a) levels, low high-density lipoprotein (HDL) cholesterol levels, insulin resistance, and more prevalent diabetes occurring earlier in life (42). A consistent inverse relationship exists between indicators of socioeconomic status and coronary artery disease (43). Although socioeconomic status is strongly and inversely linked to conventional risk factors such as cigarette smoking, hypertension, cholesterol, and obesity, it is likely to be an independent risk factor for cardiovascular disease.

TABLE 17.2

RISK FACTORS FOR ADVERSE PROGNOSIS IN PATIENTS WITH CHRONIC CORONARY ARTERY DISEASE (38)

- Age: the likelihood of death or nonfatal ischemic event increases with age
- Smoking status
- Diabetes/glucose intolerance
- Previous myocardial infarction or stroke
- Recent episode of unstable angina or new-onset stable angina
- Coexisting heart failure or evidence of left ventricular dysfunction
- Coexisting risk factors for coronary artery disease, such as hypertension
- Frequent anginal symptoms: quiescent angina is associated with a reduced risk of death and cardiac ischemic events
- Renal dysfunction/creatinine elevation
- Elevated white cell count
- Male gender

PRINCIPLES OF MANAGEMENT

The clinical assessment of patients with angina pectoris should involve a systematic review of cardiac and extracardiac factors that might contribute to the genesis of symptoms. Hence, cardiovascular factors such as hypertension, left ventricular hypertrophy, aortic and other valvular disease, and arteritis must be considered. Important contributory systemic illnesses such as anemia, thyrotoxicosis, renal disease, chronic volume overload, and high-output states need identification. Homocysteinuria (estimated prevalence of 1% to 2% of the population in a heterozygous state) has been found to be associated with symptomatic coronary artery disease (43). In the U.S. Physician Health Study, the adjusted relative risk for disease in the highest 5% versus the lowest 90% of homocysteine levels was 3.4 (95% confidence interval, 1.3–8.8%, $P = .01$) compared with matched-paired controls (44). However, correction of elevated homocysteine with folic acid does not appear to improve outcome (NORVIT, ESC 2005 Hotline Presentation) (44a).

Identification is required of cardiac and systemic factors that support the clinical suspicion of coronary disease (lipid profiles; hypertension with signs of target organ damage; microalbuminuria; concomitant vascular disease in extracranial neck vessels, abdominal aorta, or peripheral arteries). Left ventricular dysfunction and elevated left ventricular filling pressure may, uncommonly, be accompanied by a presystolic fourth heart sound, cardiomegaly, mitral regurgitation, or paradoxical splitting of the second sound. However, most commonly findings on physical examination of a patient with chronic stable angina are normal unless signs of the contributory illnesses or cardiac complications are present.

DIAGNOSTIC TESTS

The ECG at rest is commonly normal in patients with angina pectoris, but it can demonstrate evidence of prior infarction or with persisting ST-segment elevation, aneurysm, T-wave change, intraventricular conduction defects, and atrial abnormalities may also be evident. ECG observations captured during an episode of angina permit evaluation of the location and extent of ECG changes. When the total amount of ST-segment change is extensive (>12 mm), there is a high positive predictive accuracy for the detection of three-vessel or left main coronary disease (45). Frequency of angina, especially with dysfunction, predicts three-vessel coronary disease (Fig. 17.1).

The graded exercise stress test forms the cornerstone of diagnostic testing in patients with known or suspected stable angina pectoris. It should be performed in all such patients before undertaking more detailed or invasive procedures. At least four

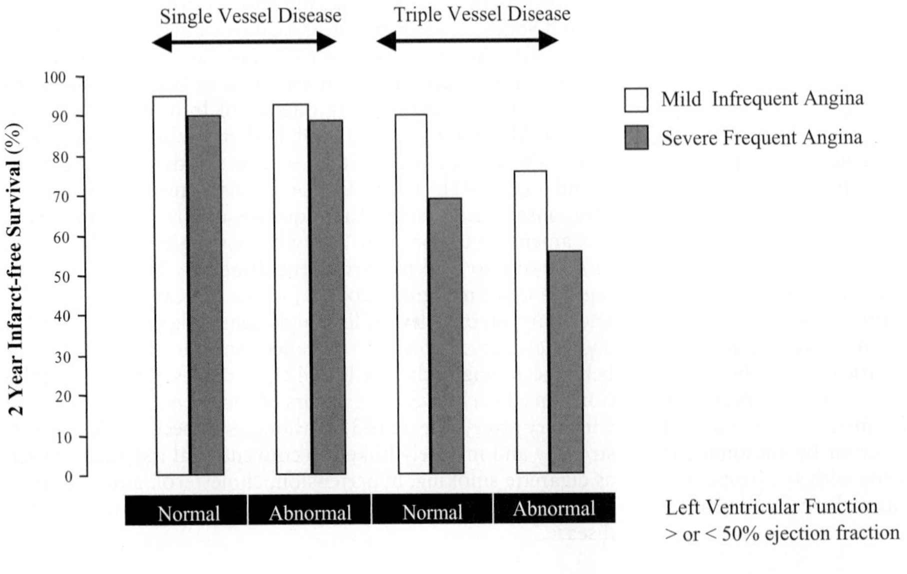

FIGURE 17.1. Infarction-free survival (2 year) of patients with angina pectoris according to angina frequency, extent of coronary artery disease, and left ventricular function (ejection fraction: normal, ≥50%; abnormal, <50%). (*Source:* Data from Califf RM, Mark DB, Harrell FE, et al: Importance of clinical measures of ischemia in the prognosis of patients with documented coronary artery disease. *J Am Coll Cardiol* 1988;11:20.)

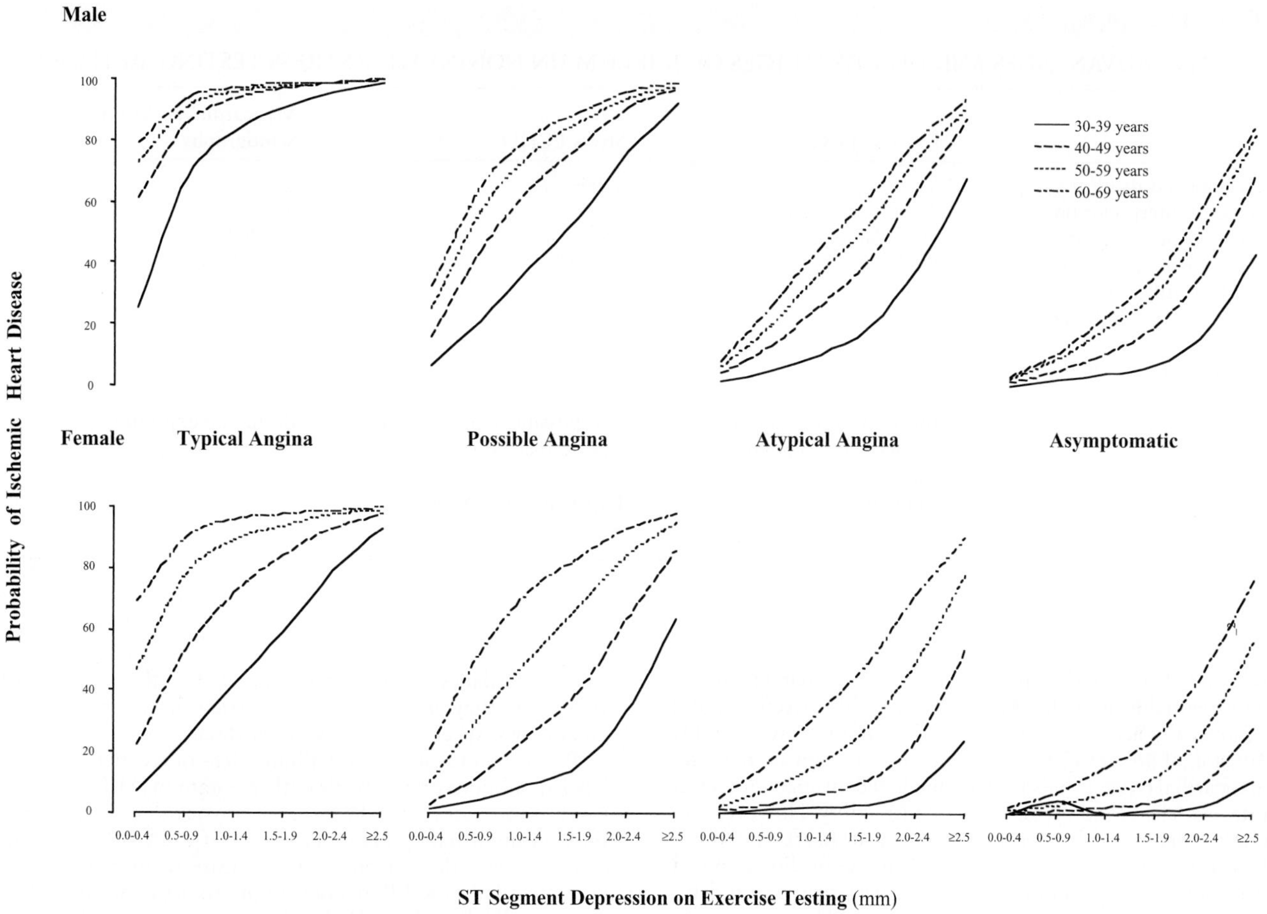

FIGURE 17.2. Exercise stress testing. Coronary heart disease probability according to age, sex, clinical history, and ST-segment depression. (*Source:* Data from European Society of Cardiology Working Group on Exercise Physiology, Physiopathology and Electrocardiography. Guidelines for cardiac exercise testing. *Eur Heart J* 1993;14:969.)

important potential objectives may be achieved by conducting this test:

1. Correlation of patient symptoms with the presence of ischemia. When angina occurs with ischemic ECG changes, the prediction of coronary disease is more reliable (46) but the predictive accuracy is lower in women (Fig. 17.2).
2. Definition of risk of future events. Those patients who are unable to exercise for more than 6 minutes on the Bruce protocol or demonstrate significant ischemia within this temporal window are at increased risk and merit further investigation (47). A summary of high-risk variables associated with unfavorable prognosis during exercise testing is shown in Table 17.3. A recent addition to this profile is the observation that a delay in the decrease in heart rate during the first minute after a graded exercise test was strongly predictive of mortality at 6 years (19% versus 5%; relative risk of 4.0).
3. To assess the level of activity and heart rate–blood pressure product at which ischemia develops.
4. To evaluate the efficacy of pharmacologic and/or revascularization therapy by assessing subjective and objective manifestations of ischemia.

Deriving an index or score from information relating to the duration of exercise, the extent of ST-segment deviation, and the reproduction of limiting or nonlimiting angina can provide a more precise estimation of prognosis.

In various circumstances, more specialized noninvasive assessment is warranted. When an adequate exercise test

TABLE 17.3

FEATURES ASSOCIATED WITH A POOR PROGNOSIS AND INDICATIVE OF SEVERE DISEASE

a) **Exercise ECG:**
- Inability to perform exercise ECG on account of limiting symptoms
- Poor maximal exercise capacity (less than stage 3 of the Bruce protocol)
- Early positive test (<3 min) or strongly positive test:
  - ≥1-mm ST-segment depression during stage 2 or less (Bruce protocol)
  - ≥2-mm ST-segment depression at any time
  - Downsloping ST depression
- Flat or lowered blood pressure response (fall or no rise from baseline)
- Delayed recovery or delayed decrease in heart rate on cessation of exercise
- Ventricular arrhythmia on exercise (rate >120/min)

b) **Radionuclide imaging:**
- Reversible radionuclide perfusion defect in more than one territory
- Large perfusion defect (>15% of ventricle)
- Presence of fixed and reversible perfusion defects
- Reduced radionuclide ejection fraction with exercise
- Increased lung uptake of radionuclide after exercise

TABLE 17.4

RELATIVE ADVANTAGES AND DISADVANTAGES OF THREE MAIN NONINVASIVE STRESS TESTING METHODS

	Exercise ECG	Stress ECHO	Myocardial Perfusion Scintigraphy
Technical difficulty	+	+++	++
Ease of interpretation	+	+++	++
Diagnostic sensitivity	50–80%	65–90%	65–90%
Diagnostic specificity	80–95%	90–95%	90–95%
Risk stratification	++	++	++
Identification of hibernating myocardium	–	+++	++
Identification of ischemic territory	+	++	++
Limitations	Intraventricular conduction defects and repolarization abnormalities	Not possible in patients with poor image quality	Radiation exposure
	Limited sensitivity	Expert interpretation	
Cost	+	++	+++

is coupled with either myocardial nuclear imaging or two-dimensional echocardiography, it is a highly effective and diagnostically accurate test (Table 17.4). Both exercise and the infusion of dobutamine induce ischemia through an increase in myocardial oxygen consumption mediated by augmented heart rate, systolic blood pressure, and contractility. However, exercise results in a 50% greater increment in heart rate systolic blood pressure product versus dobutamine in direct comparisons, probably accounting for its greater sensitivity in detecting coronary artery disease in some series (48).

Given that a high proportion of patients with stable angina have prior infarction and/or wall motion abnormalities at rest detected by two-dimensional echocardiography or resting perfusion defects, the question of whether such wall motion abnormalities possess residual myocardial perfusion and viability becomes highly relevant in therapeutic planning. Dobutamine enhancement of left ventricular dysfunction or inotropic stimulation evident after a ventricular premature beat is predictive of improvement in function with revascularization of the affected segment (49). Delayed imaging, 18 to 24 hours after thallium exercise scintigraphy, reveals that 50% or more of segments with apparently irreversible thallium defects on delayed imaging (at 3–4 hours) demonstrate isotope redistribution thought to be indicative of severe ischemia and predictive of favorable response to revascularization (50). Thallium reinjection at rest, 3 to 4 hours after stress imaging, has been demonstrated to provide similar information to delayed imaging in a more time-efficient and practical fashion (51). The use of thallium in this fashion to detect myocardial viability has been validated by concomitant metabolic imaging using positron emission tomography with oxygen-15–labeled water and exogenous glucose use with fluorine-18–labeled fluorodeoxyglucose (51).

By contrast, dipyridamole- and adenosine-induced hyperemia results in maldistribution of coronary flow by maximally dilating normal vascular segments, whereas those with fixed coronary stenosis already have near-maximal dilatation, resulting in image defects. Adenosine's rapid onset of action and extremely short half-life, as opposed to that of dipyramidole, circumvents the need for theophylline reversal of troublesome side effects such as bronchial constriction (52). Two-dimensional echocardiography performed before and immediately after exercise testing and continuously before, during, and after dobutamine infusion is used to detect new or worsening preexisting wall motion abnormalities (53,54). These findings show excellent concordance with the territory of the affected coronary vessel (48); they demonstrate prognostic value in patients with known or suspected coronary artery disease (55–57).

Perfusion imaging with thallium-201– or technetium-99m–labeled radiopharmaceuticals (either sestamibi [MIBI] or tetrofosmin) provides visualization of myocardial blood flow. Injected immediately before cessation of exercise or pharmacologic stress, these agents can delineate relative differences in myocardial blood flow conforming to areas of myocardial ischemia. With thallium-201, a late image associated with redistribution of blood flow 3 to 4 hours after exercise can be obtained to assess reversibility of defects observed during exercise (58). By contrast, with the technetium-99m–labeled MIBI, myocardial distribution is relatively fixed without significant redistribution; hence, imaging can be conducted for a few hours after the time of injection during pharmacologic or exercise stress (59). A second injection is necessary to characterize blood flow at rest. Perfusion is also useful in assessing ischemia in specific vascular segments when coronary disease has been established (28). Substantial data are available to support the role of myocardial perfusion imaging in more precisely defining prognosis; in this regard, a high-risk scan may be especially useful, and the characteristics of this finding are depicted in Table 17.3 (60–64).

Although coronary calcification has long been recognized as a marker of atherosclerosis, its clinical utility has been limited. The availability of electron beam (ultrafast) tomography has dramatically increased the sensitivity of coronary calcium detection (65). However, there may be marked intrapatient variability on repeat testing and its role remains controversial (66). An American College of Cardiology/American Heart Association consensus document concluded that "the test has proven to have a predictive accuracy approximately equivalent to alternative methods for diagnosing coronary artery disease but has not been found to be superior to alternative non-invasive tests" (67).

Intravascular Imaging

Fiber-Optic Imaging (Angioscopy)

Visualization of the physical appearance of atheromatous lesions, and in particular the detection of unsuspected plaque

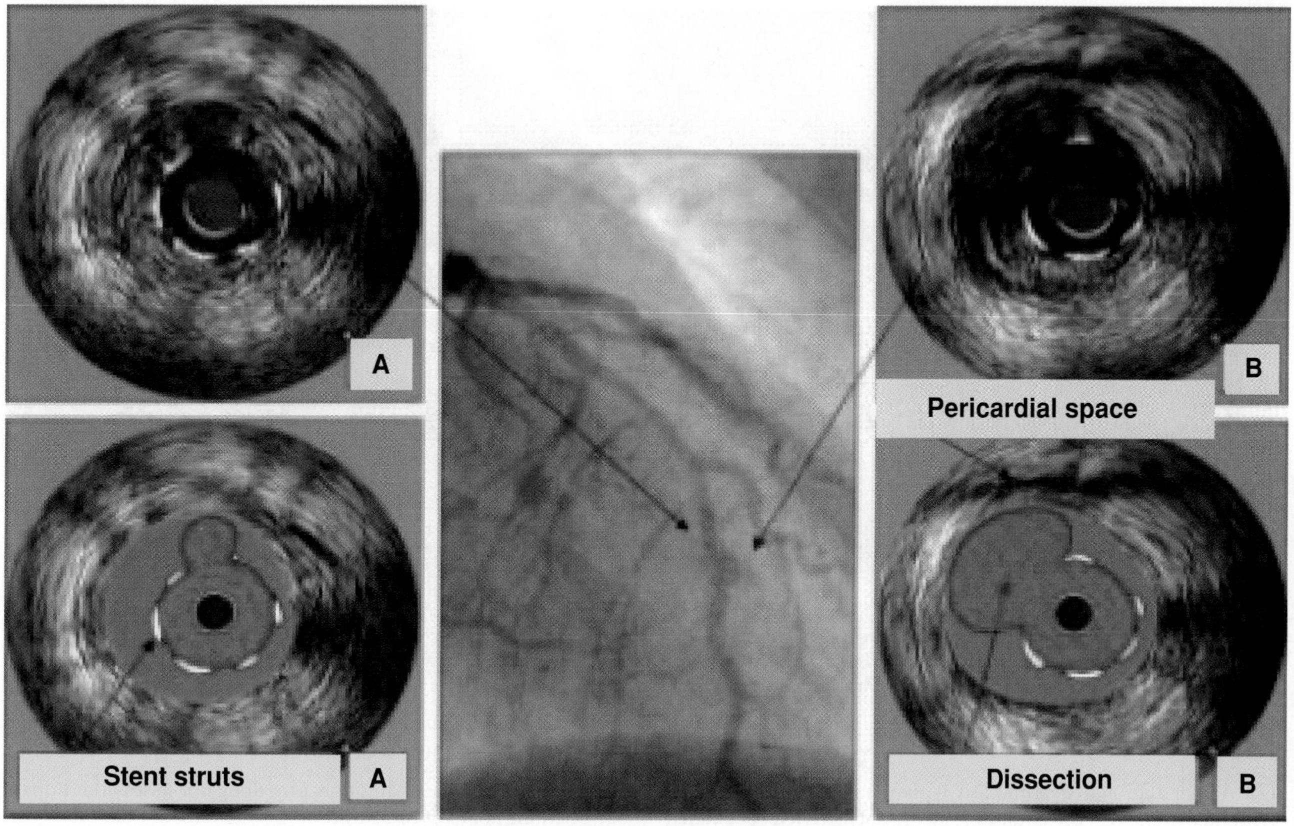

FIGURE 17.3. Coronary angiography and IVUS: segment of vessel with dissection (see arrows on angiogram) and flow within the dissection cavity. IVUS showing stent struts (**A**) and dissection (**B**). (*Source:* Data from Schoenhagen P, Nissen S. Understanding coronary artery disease: tomographic imaging with intravascular ultrasound. *Heart* 2002;88:91–96).

rupture events, has provided new information on the diffuse nature of coronary arterial disease. In particular, the detection of multiple "vulnerable" plaques in segments of coronary artery without detectable abnormality on angiography has led to key insights into the mechanisms of progression of acute coronary arterial disease (68). In support, Buffon and colleagues measured myeloperoxidase proximal and distal to suspected unstable plaques (69). These findings suggest multiple sites of plaque disruption with associated platelet aggregation and thrombosis. However, angioscopy remains a research tool and its focus is mainly in the field of acute coronary artery disease rather than stable ischemic syndromes.

Intravascular Ultrasound

High-resolution intravascular ultrasound (IVUS) has provided critically important observations that demonstrate the extent and distribution coronary artery disease and reveal the severity and eccentric nature of plaque lesions. These may be underestimated on angiography (Fig. 17.3). Vascular remodeling (as originally described by Glagov, 73) results in extensive atheroma but relative preservation of the coronary arterial lumen until late in the disease process.

IVUS has also provided insights into plaque composition, including the distribution and extent of lipid-rich plaques, extent of calcification, and thickness of the fibrous cap (70). All of these features provide evidence of susceptibility of atheromatous plaques to rupture, but validated outcome studies are required to demonstrate that interventions on such nonstenotic lesions alter clinical outcome.

Optical Coherence Tomography

Using light from an intravascular device, and having cleared red cells from the field of view, it is possible to obtain exquisite resolution of structures in the vascular wall (71) (Fig. 17.4). This technique has great potential as an experimental tool, but it may have limited clinical application on account of the need for a blood-free field and the fact that only limited segments of the coronary arterial tree are currently accessible with this device.

Magnetic Resonance Imaging

Magnetic resonance imaging (MRI) is emerging as the reference standard for clinical assessment of ischemia and for evaluation of myocardial viability. The exquisite structural information provided by either MRI (72) (Fig. 17.5A) or multislice CT (73,74). In addition to such structural information, MRI in conjunction with administration of a contrast agent (e.g., gadolinium chelate) can be used to detect perfusion abnormalities and viability (75) (Fig. 17.5B). Perfusion measurements were first investigated based on tissue water content detected by MRI and evaluation of T_1 and T_2 signals. However, such assessment is not sufficiently reliable without the administration of MRI contrast material (75–79). First-pass imaging in the presence of a contrast agent allows the detection of impaired perfusion and can provide assessment of the physiologic significance of stenoses in different vascular beds.

An alternative approach involves the detection of reversible left ventricular contractile dysfunction using multiphasic MRI

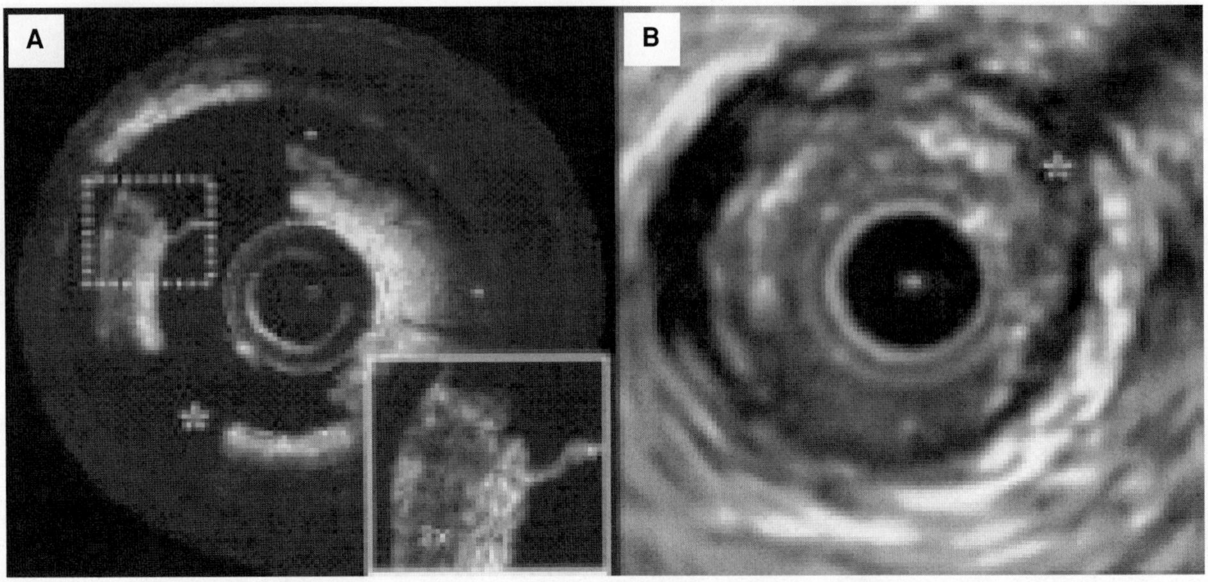

FIGURE 17.4. Coronary dissection demonstrated with optical coherence tomography (**A**) and IVUS (**B**), following balloon angioplasty. The dissection flap is more readily distinguished in the optical coherence image. (*Source:* Data from Bouma BE, Tearney GJ, Yabushita H, et al. Evaluation of intracoronary stenting by intravascular optical coherence tomography. *Heart* 2003;89:317–321.)

(75). Such regional dysfunction is associated with reversible ischemia (e.g., with dipyridamole stress). Sensitivity, specificity, and accuracy of 91%, 80%, and 90%, respectively, have been reported, and dobutamine stress MRI avoids the problems of poor acoustic windows in patients assessed with dobutamine stress echo.

In addition to assessing the volume of myocardial flow affected by decreased perfusion, late enhancement of gadolinium chelate allows the detection of reperfused but viable myocardium and the potential for distinguishing such zones from myocardium with impaired perfusion but without the potential for function recovery (79). Thus, MRI imaging with the aid of MRI contrast agents can detect abnormalities in structure and function of the ventricle, estimate the volume of myocardium with reduced perfusion, and demonstrate potentially viable segments. For these reasons, MRI is emerging as the reference standard for the assessment of the impact of functional stenoses in coronary arteries.

Coronary Angiography

Selective coronary angiography is the most widely used diagnostic investigation to define the extent and severity of intrinsic coronary narrowing. In general, it should be performed in patients (a) when the diagnosis of coronary disease is important to establish yet remains in doubt after noninvasive assessment, (b) when high-risk coronary disease is suspected based on the results of clinical and noninvasive evaluation, and (c) in non–high-risk patients when significant symptoms persist despite adequate medical therapy or medical therapy is poorly tolerated.

Coronary angiography is widely applied, but significant limitations need to be considered:

- Angiographically apparently "normal" vessels may have extensive nonstenotic coronary disease, as demonstrated histopathologically or with high-resolution IVUS.
- The physiologic importance of moderate and apparently similar stenoses may differ markedly (as demonstrated by measurements of coronary flow reserve) (80,81).
- Standard coronary angiography does not assess the impact of changes in vascular tone.
- As a result of collateral development, angiographic appearances may underestimate or overestimate the impact of stenosis on myocardial perfusion.
- The angiogram does not provide insights into the histologic structure of stenotic lesions or the likelihood of plaque rupture.
- Disrupted endothelium or minor plaque fissures may precipitate signs and symptoms of non–ST-elevation acute coronary syndrome and yet may be difficult to detect on coronary angiography.

Despite these limitations, coronary angiography provides key information on the extent and distribution of coronary stenoses and long-term survival (Fig. 17.6). It may be combined with provocative testing with ergonovine maleate in patients with known or suspected Prinzmetal variant angina and may identify the location and extent of provokable coronary spasm (82). In patients without major anatomic narrowing and in the absence of Prinzmetal variant angina, vasoreactivity of lesions may be provoked by intravenous ergonovine in almost 20% of patients. Combined with IVUS to provide precise definition of not only the extent of coronary narrowing and the thickness and extent of atheroma in the coronary arterial wall (83,84).

Multislice CT (64 slice) can provide accurate detection of coronary stenosis with high negative predictive accuracy (74). It may facilitate rapid triage of patients with suspected cardiac pain (74).

THERAPEUTIC INTERVENTIONS

In chronic stable coronary disease, the goals of treatment are to relieve symptoms and reduce the risk of future cardiac events (including acute coronary syndrome, heart failure, and death) (Fig. 17.7). Simultaneous rather than alternative approaches are required: these include lifestyle modification, management

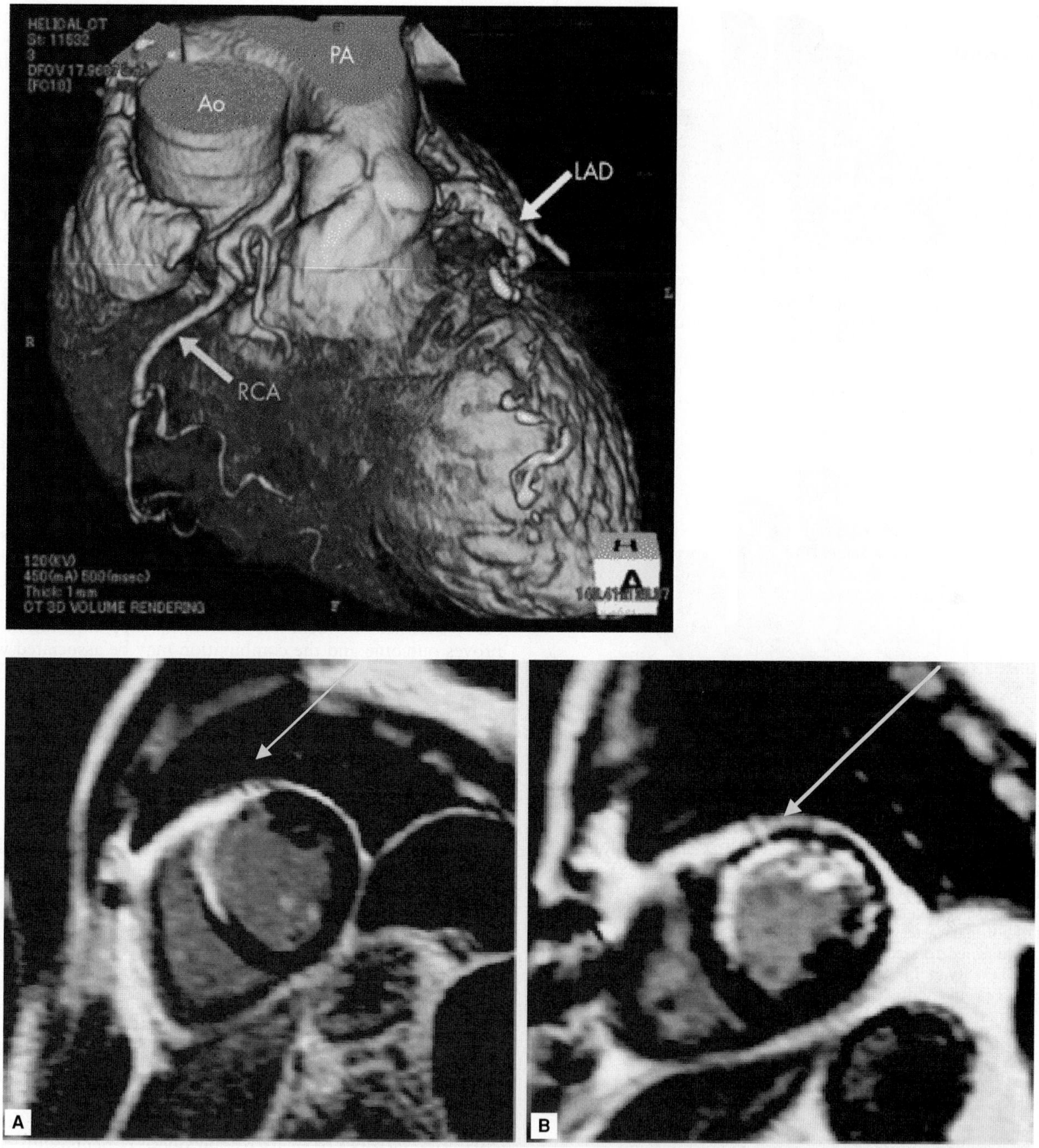

FIGURE 17.5. (*upper panel*) Imaging to define anatomy: contrast-enhanced multidetector computed tomography. (*Source:* Kobayashi K, Tokunaga T, Isobe M. A case of anomalous of the right coronary artery from the pulmonary artery complicated by acute myocardial infarction. *Heart* 2005;91:1130). (*lower panels A, B*) Imaging to detect MI. Contrast enhanced magnetic resonance imaging. (**A**) Transmural anteroseptal infarction with hyperenhancement shown in white. (**B**) Nontransmural infarction extending from septum to lateral wall (*arrows*) (79).

of risk factors, pharmacologic therapy, and coronary revascularization. All forms of intervention present some hazard and hence they should be instituted when the perceived benefits, in terms of improved symptoms and prognosis, outweigh the associated risks. The clinician, and the informed patient, need to institute an overall treatment strategy to minimize the impact of the disease throughout the remainder of the patient's life. Accurate assessment of prognostic risk is critically important in this regard.

LIFESTYLE AND RISK FACTOR MODIFICATION

Lifestyle and risk factor modifications are integral to treatment of patients with chronic stable coronary disease. They may provide both symptomatic and prognostic benefits and their impact may enhance mechanical or pharmacologic treatment

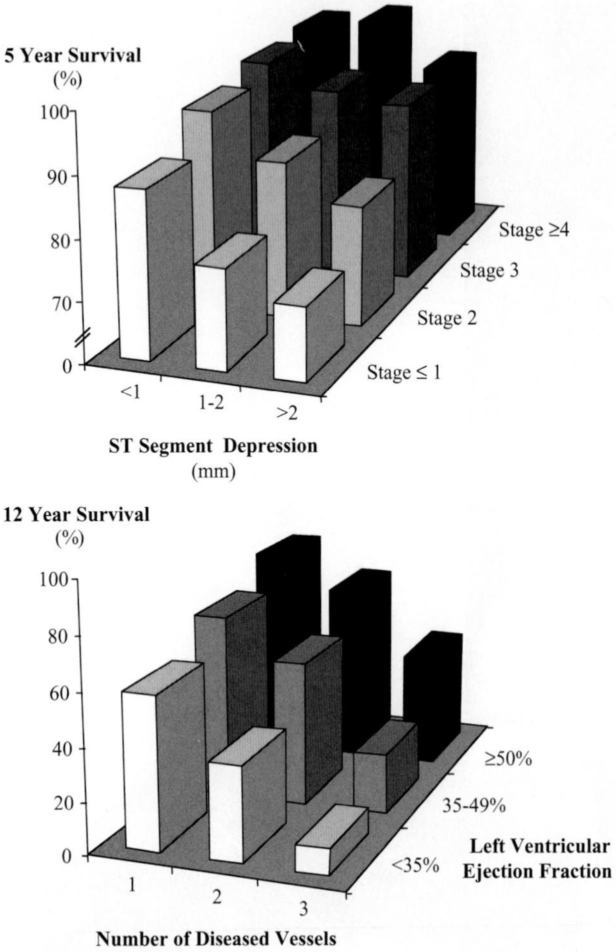

FIGURE 17.6. Five- and 12-year survival rates of medically treated patients according to exercise tolerance, exercise-induced ST-segment depression, number of diseased vessels, and left ventricular function. (*Source:* The Coronary Artery Surgery Study [CASS]. A randomized trial of coronary artery bypass surgery: quality of life in patients randomly assigned to treatment groups. *Circulation* 1983;68:951 and Weiner DA, Ryan TJ, McCabe CH, et al: Prognostic importance of a clinical profile and exercise test in medically treated patients with coronary artery disease. *J Am Coll Cardiol* 1984;3:772.)

and their lack of impact may substantially diminish potential benefits.

Smoking

Based on data from the INTERHEART study (85), smoking accounts for about one third of the excess risk of MI, and this is observed consistently across all geographic regions. Cessation of smoking is associated with major benefits (86) and repeated brief and supportive advice should be given to all patients (87). Short-term nicotine replacement therapy should be offered to those individuals with a heavy consumption of tobacco (>10 cigarettes/d), because it is associated with up to a ninefold increased likelihood of success (82,88). The antidepressants bupropion and nortriptyline may aid long-term smoking cessation, but selective serotonin reuptake inhibitors such as fluoxetine do not (89). This suggests that these agents produce their beneficial effects independent of an antidepressant effect. Recent studies of a CB_1 cannabinoid receptor antagonist (rimonabant) suggest that smoking cessation may be enhanced by this approach. Challenges remain to avoid relapse in smokers who have successfully quit for a short time; supportive groups and counseling may enhance longer term abstention (90).

Dietary Interventions

Dietary intervention complements the use of lipid-lowering therapy, but on average a low-fat diet reduces serum cholesterol concentrations by only 5% (91), even in motivated individuals (92). Nevertheless, dietary modification may provide additional preventative benefits, such as those obtained from a Mediterranean-type diet (93) or those high in (*n*-3) polyunsaturated fatty acids of fish oils (94,95). Observational studies (96,97) and randomized trials (98) have suggested that the consumption of fruits and vegetables containing high levels of antioxidant vitamins or supplementation with vitamin E (99,100) is protective against the development of coronary events. However, three large-scale ($n = 6{,}000$–$30{,}000$) multicenter randomized controlled trials (95,101,102) demonstrated that low- or high-dose vitamin E supplementation has no effect on cardiovascular outcomes. Finally, modest alcohol consumption is associated with a reduced risk of coronary heart disease and should be limited to 21 to 28 units per week (1 U = 8 g of absolute alcohol) for a man and 14 to 21 units a week for a woman (103). Neither folic acid nor vitamin B_6 supplementation improves outcome and the combination may be associated with increased hazards of fatal or nonfatal stroke or MI (NORVIT study ESC Hotline 2005) (44a).

Obesity

There are escalating levels of obesity, not only in Western societies, but also in other societies undergoing industrialization. These demographic changes have the potential for a major adverse impact on the incidence and prevalence of cardiovascular disease in the future (104). Obesity, and particularly abdominal obesity (increased waist-to-hip ratio), is associated with increased risk of MI (85). Abdominal obesity, and to a lesser extent increased BMI, is associated with the development of the "metabolic syndrome" characterized by obesity, insulin resistance, hypertension, and dyslipidemia. Novel therapeutic strategies may be able to reduce obesity and the metabolic syndrome. For example, cannabinoid type-1 receptor antagonism, when combined with a low-calorie diet, markedly enhances weight loss and improves many of the associated cardiovascular risk factors (105). Its role in obese patients with coronary heart disease has yet to be established. Despite the high prevalence of obesity, there have been no interventional trials to show that weight reduction in obese patients with chronic stable angina or coronary artery disease improves symptoms or outcome. However, it is reasonable to assume that weight reduction would reduce the frequency of anginal episodes and potentially improve prognosis.

Diabetes Mellitus

Good glycemic control is essential in all patients with diabetes mellitus because of the reduced risk of long-term complications, including coronary artery disease. Although there are no specific trials of diabetic control in patients with chronic stable angina, primary prevention trials (106,107) and secondary prevention trials in patients after MI (108) indicate that cardiovascular morbidity and mortality rates are reduced

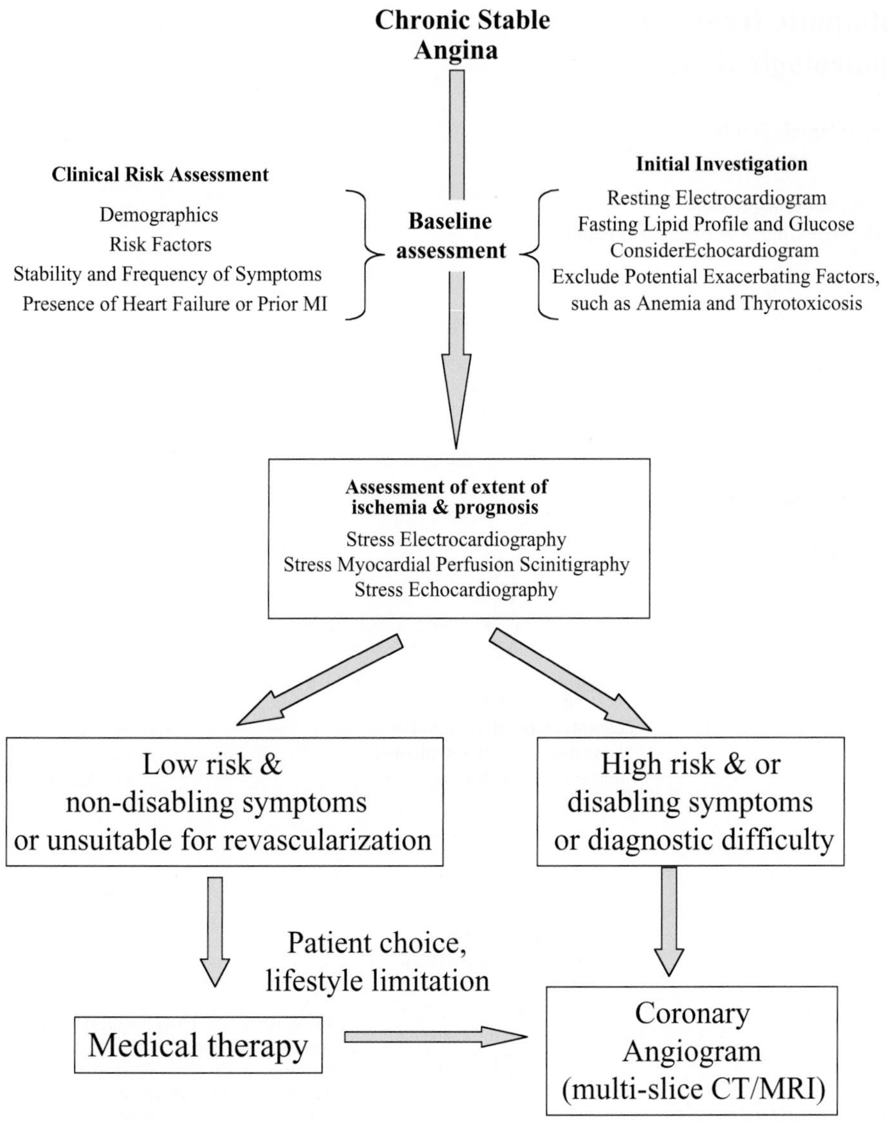

FIGURE 17.7. Flow diagram for the initial assessment and investigation of patients with chronic stable angina: differentiation of lower and higher risk.

with intensive hypoglycemic therapy regimens. Moreover, poor glycemic control at the time of presentation with MI is a poor prognostic sign (109). Although previous studies (110) suggested that sulfonylureas, in particular, tolbutamide, are associated with an increased risk of cardiovascular death, this was not confirmed in the UK Prospective Diabetes Study (UKPDS) trial (111). The latter trial did, however, suggest that metformin should be the first-line agent of choice in overweight patients with diabetes mellitus because it is associated with a decreased risk of diabetes-related end points, less weight gain, and fewer hypoglycemic episodes.

SYMPTOMATIC THERAPY

Pharmacologic Therapy

No single class of antianginal drug has been shown to be superior to another in the reduction of anginal episodes, nor in reducing outcome events. However, because of the inferred secondary preventative benefits of ß-blockers, they should be the first-line agents (Figs. 17.8 and 17.9). A meta-analysis suggests that ß-blockers are better tolerated and may be more efficacious than calcium antagonists in the treatment of chronic stable angina (112).

If monotherapy does not control anginal symptoms, the introduction of a second antianginal agent provides significant but modest additional benefits. The combination of ß-blockade and rate-limiting calcium antagonism may cause excessive bradycardia or heart block. However, this interaction is uncommon, and if there is concern, a long-acting dihydropyridine-type calcium antagonist should be coprescribed. There is no definitive evidence that triple or quadruple antianginal therapy produces further benefit beyond dual therapy.

ß-Blockers

Randomized controlled trials (113,114) have demonstrated that ß-blocker therapy is efficacious in reducing symptoms of angina and episodes of ischemia and in improving exercise capacity. ß-Blockers inhibit the ß-adrenergic receptors of the myocardium to produce negative chronotropism and negative inotropism of the heart. The attenuation of the heart rate response to exercise and stress reduces the myocardial oxygen

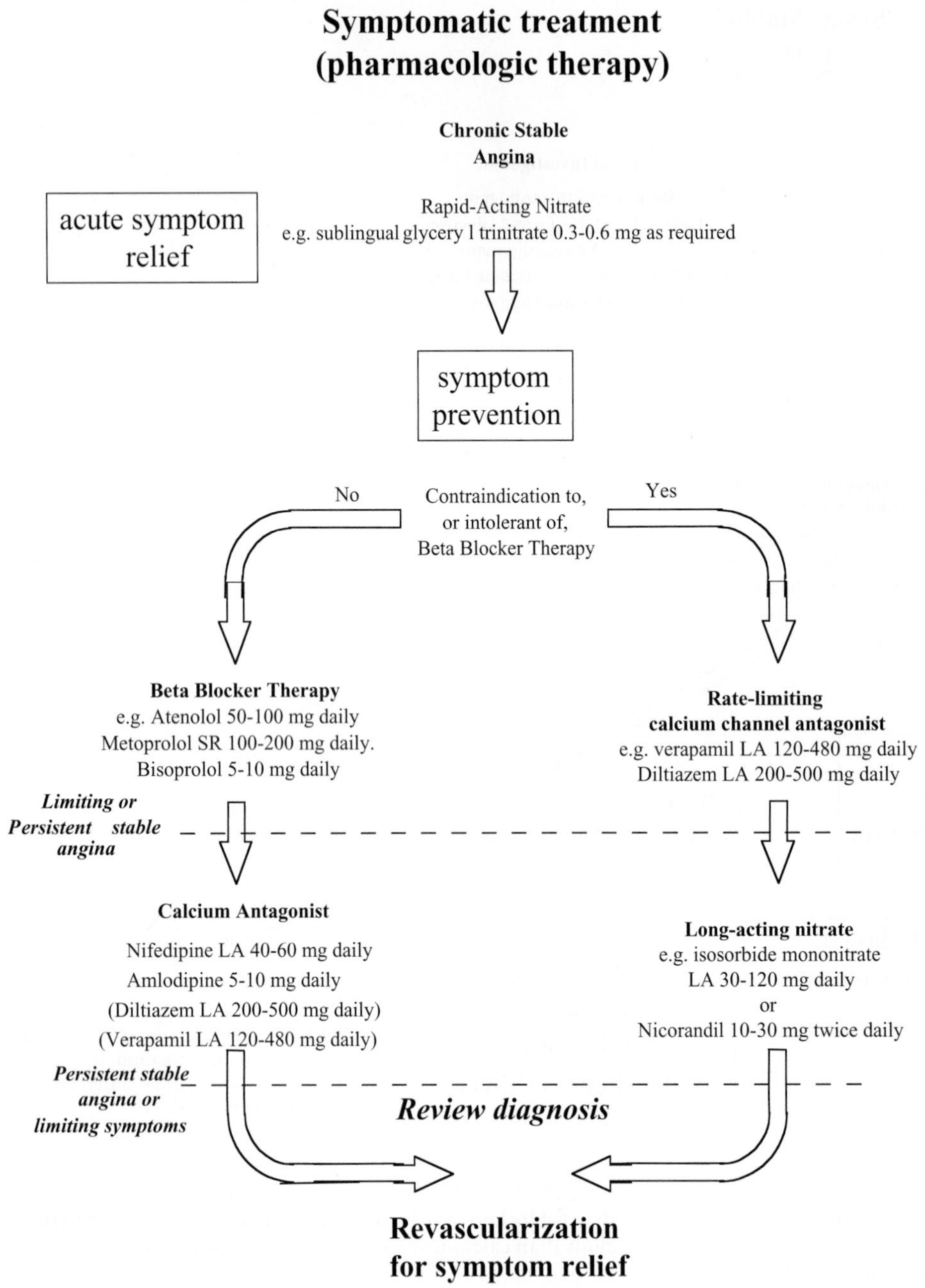

FIGURE 17.8. Flow diagram for symptomatic pharmacologic therapy of patients with chronic stable angina. Treatment for symptom relief and symptom prevention. *Note:* The specific drugs and dosages are illustrations rather than preferred sequences based on clinical trials. They do not exclude other drugs within the same class. Caution is required in combining ß-blockers and heart rate limiting calcium antagonists.

demand and severity of ischemia. They also prolong diastole, a major determinant of myocardial perfusion time.

There is no evidence to support the suggestion that one type of ß-blocker is superior to another. However, the secondary preventive benefits of ß-blockers may be lost where agents have intrinsic sympathomimetic action (115) and the use of such agents should therefore be avoided.

True side effects from ß-blocker therapy are not common (<10%), but include symptoms such as fatigue and lethargy. Because such symptoms are encountered in patients with stable coronary disease, a causative association should be established before permanent discontinuation of ß-blocker therapy. Because of ß-adrenergic receptor upregulation in the presence of ß-blockade, patients should not be rapidly withdrawn from therapy. This can cause an acute withdrawal syndrome and may even precipitate acute MI (116,117).

Calcium Antagonists

Patients who are intolerant of a ß-blocker should be prescribed a rate-limiting calcium channel antagonist such as diltiazem or verapamil. In the Danish Verapamil Infarction Trial (DAVIT) II trial, a post hoc analysis suggested that verapamil may be beneficial after MI in the absence of heart failure (118). However, other calcium channel antagonists (119,120) and classes of antianginal agents (121–123) are equally effective in relieving symptoms. The ACTION trial (3,825 patients with stable coronary disease treated over 5 years) suggests that long-acting nifedipine has a neutral effect on survival, MI, and stroke, but it reduces angina and the need for coronary angiography and revascularization (124).

There is controversy as to whether calcium channel blockers can be used safely in patients with heart failure (125), but

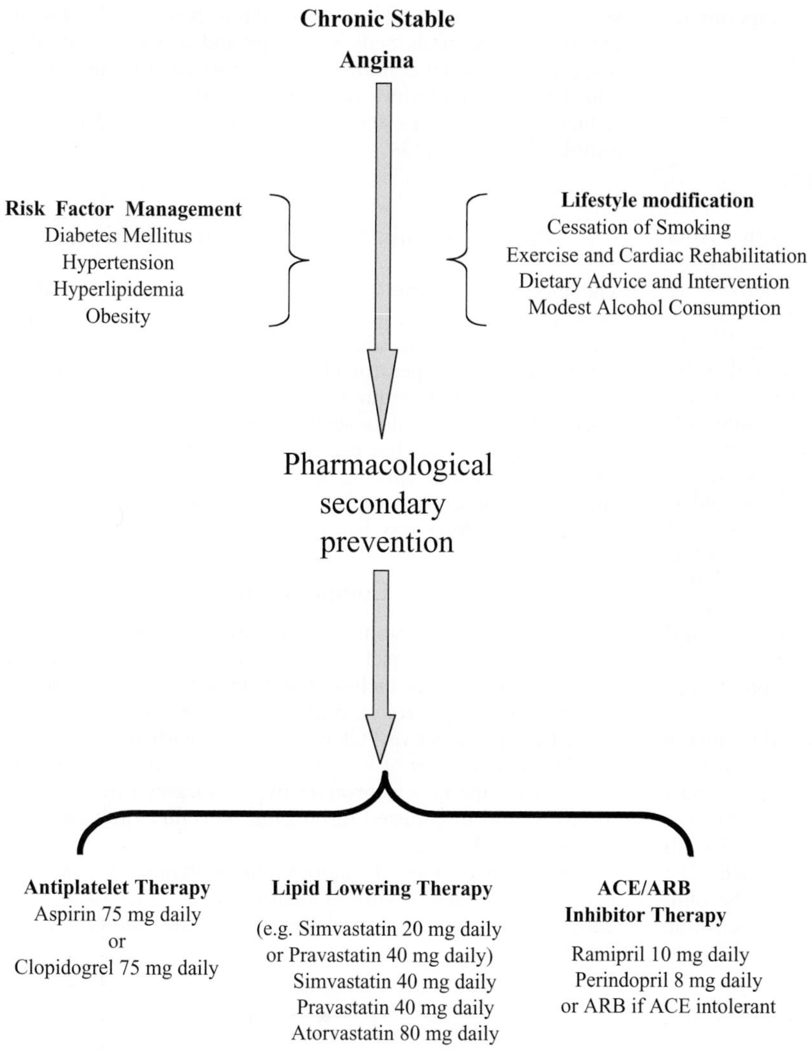

FIGURE 17.9. Flow diagram for secondary prevention in patients with chronic stable angina. For higher risk patients, consider coronary angiography provided the patient is suitable for revascularization. *Note:* The specific drug and dosage are illustrations and are not arranged in preferred sequence based on clinical trials and do not exclude other drugs within the same class.

amlodipine has been shown to have a neutral effect on mortality rates in patients with heart failure (126).

Nitrates

Nitrates were the first form of antianginal drug and their mechanism of action is through the release of nitric oxide either indirectly (glyceryl trinitrate) by reactions with sulfhydryl groups, such as methionine or cysteine, or by interaction with plasma or cell membranes. The liberated nitric oxide causes endothelium-independent relaxation of vascular smooth muscle by increasing intracellular cyclic guanidine monophosphate.

Randomized controlled trials (121,127) have demonstrated that nitrates are effective in reducing the frequency of anginal symptoms and in improving exercise capacity. However, as with calcium antagonists, their use in severe aortic stenosis and hypertrophic obstructive cardiomyopathy should be avoided because of the potential to compromise coronary perfusion through peripheral vasodilatation and systemic arterial hypotension.

Acute Relief of Angina

Sublingual or buccal nitrates produce rapid and effective relief of acute anginal episodes. All patients should be provided with a sublingual nitrate preparation. Buccal preparations provide a more protracted release of nitrate, which is appropriate for prolonged activities that may provoke episodes of angina.

Prevention of Anginal Episodes

Long-acting nitrates, either oral or transdermal, provide effective relief of angina. Nitrates undergo extensive first-pass metabolism through hepatic glutathione reductases. Topical and transdermal nitrate preparations are able to bypass such metabolism, and some nitrate preparations, such as isosorbide mononitrate, undergo less extensive hepatic metabolism and have better bioavailability and more prolonged action. One of the main limitations of prophylactic nitrate use is the development of tolerance (128) and this phenomenon requires a daily nitrate-free period (129,130).

Potassium Channel Agonists

This class of antianginal agents has nitrate like vasodilatory propetics and potential cardioprotective actions. Potassium channel openers act on the ion channels of vascular smooth muscle cells and cardiac myocytes. Consequently, they may enhance ischemic preconditioning (131) and improve the myocardial response to an ischemic insult (132).

Nicorandil is the only preparation of this class in clinical use. It is effective in the treatment of angina and has both nitrate and potassium channel-opening properties. However, there is no evidence that potassium channel openers are superior to other classes of antianginal agents.

CORONARY REVASCULARIZATION

Although periprocedural risks have diminished, both CABG and percutaneous coronary intervention (PCI) carry a measurable early morbidity and mortality risk that exceeds the early risks of medical therapy in patients with chronic stable ischemic disease. These risks have diminished over time (Fig. 17.10). Revascularization should be instituted if the perceived benefits, in terms of improved symptoms and prognosis, are likely to outweigh the associated risks. This is particularly important when the therapy is for symptomatic rather than prognostic benefits, such as with PCI or CABG for one-vessel disease.

Selection of the appropriateness and the type of revascularization procedure is heavily influenced by technical aspects of the coronary anatomy, as well as by factors such as comorbidity and patient preference. Patients vary greatly in what is considered an acceptable level of symptoms, optimal medical therapy, and tolerable drug side effects. Thus, the need for, and type of, coronary revascularization should take into account both objective clinical criteria and the patient's symptoms and informed choices.

Several factors must also be considered when evaluating the applicability and evidence of the clinical usefulness of coronary revascularization strategies. First, the major randomized trials are based on highly selected patient groups and may not reflect the broad mix of patients who present to the clinic (133). In the Angioplasty Compared with Medicine trial (ACME) 212 out of almost 5,000 screened patients were included. Second, most trials have not exclusively selected patients with chronic stable angina pectoris. Third, many datasets reported in the literature are outdated; medical therapy and surgical techniques (e.g., use of arterial conduits) have improved substantially. In addition, the early failure and restenosis rates in PCI have been reduced with coronary stents, drug-eluting stents, and adjuvant antiplatelet agents (134).

Percutaneous Coronary Intervention

The success and complication rates of PCI are influenced by factors including age, gender, clinical presentation, left ventricular function, comorbidity (e.g., diabetes mellitus), and the experience of the operator (135,136). The nature of the target lesion is a key determinant of outcome. For example, short discrete lesions on straight segments of artery that do not compromise major branches are ideal for PCI. Lesions that are less suitable include chronic total occlusions, long lesions, calcifications, those on complex tortuous segments, flexures, or complex branching vessels.

Complications

The most common serious complication of PCI is acute occlusion of the dilated vessel owing to dissection or thrombosis. Other complications include vascular damage, thromboembolism (including stroke), and hemorrhage due to anticoagulant therapy. Elective PCI is associated with overall angiographic success rates of 96% to 99%; transmural MI rates of 1% to 3%, emergency coronary bypass surgery rates of 0.2% to 3.0%, and unadjusted in-hospital mortality rates of 0.5% to 1.4% (136).

The reported risk of angiographic restenosis for isolated balloon angioplasty (without stenting) is 25% to 40% (137–140). Restenosis occurs predominantly within the first 3 to 6

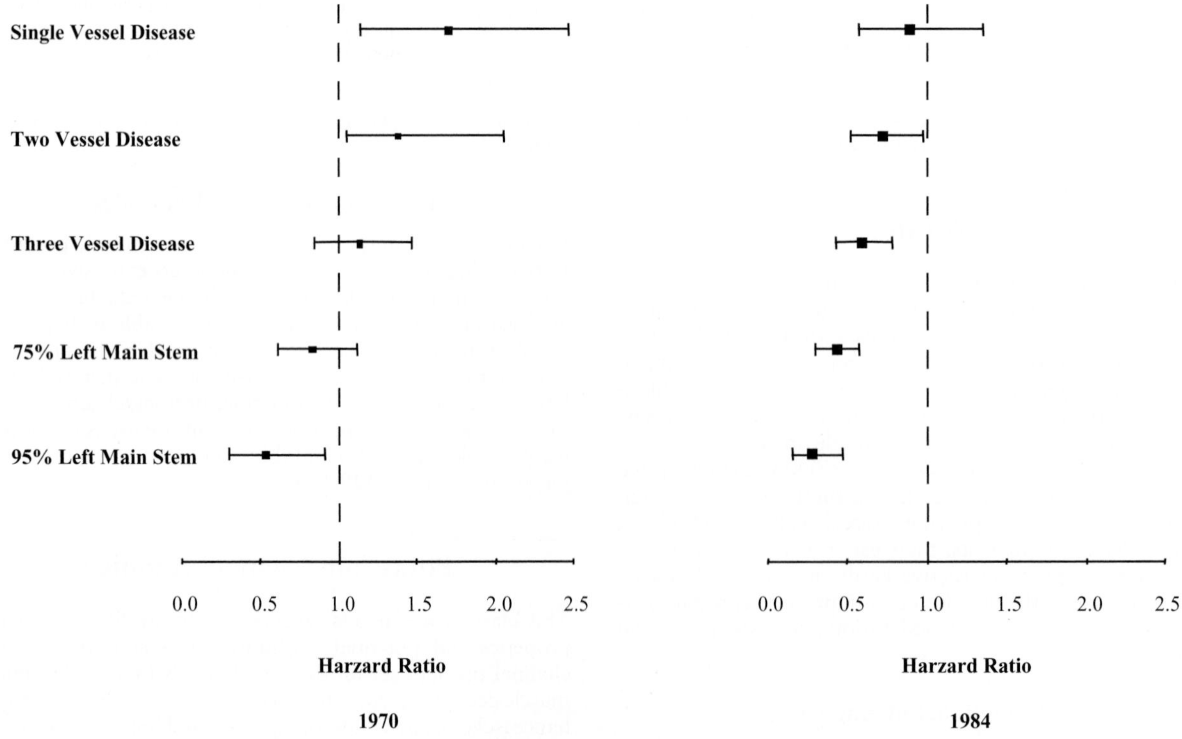

FIGURE 17.10. Improvements in survival with coronary artery bypass graft surgery (to left of vertical dashed lines) during a 14-year period. (*Source:* Data from Califf RM, Harrell FE, Lee KL, et al: The evolution of medical and surgical therapy for coronary artery disease; a 15-year perspective. *JAMA* 1989;261:2077.)

months (138,139) does not always lead to recurrent symptoms, and has been dramatically reduced by the widespread use of intracoronary stents (137,141–145), particularly drug-eluting stents. Current rates of restenosis with drug-eluting stents are 5% to 10% (146).

Percutaneous Coronary Intervention Versus Medical Treatment. ACME was the first randomized controlled trial to assess PCI in comparison with medical therapy (133) (one-vessel disease, >90% stable angina pectoris). PCI subjectively and objectively improved anginal symptoms at 6 months (133,147) at the cost of some complications and recurrent revascularization procedures.

The Randomised Intervention Treatment of Angina (RITA-2) trial (148) was a more powerful (n = 1018) randomized controlled trial and was designed to compare the effects of PCI with medical therapy in patients with angina and one-vessel (60%) or multivessel (40%) disease. The study population included patients with quiescent angina (no symptoms in 20%) or recent unstable angina (10%). Consistent with the ACME trial (133), an initial strategy of PCI was associated with significantly less angina for at least 2 years after the procedure compared with medical treatment. Anginal symptoms and antianginal drug therapy were reduced, exercise capacity increased, and quality of life improved (148,149). Nevertheless PCI was associated with nearly twice the risk of death or nonfatal MI (6.3% versus 3.3% at 2.7 years; $P = .02$), which occurred predominantly in the first 3 months after randomization.

The symptomatic benefits of PCI in the RITA-2 trial (148) appeared to be most marked in the patients with severe symptoms or limited exercise tolerance. It may therefore be necessary to accept a small initial procedure-related hazard from PCI to gain relief from severe or limiting anginal symptoms. However, improved imaging and stent technologies combined with better antiplatelet therapies, such as the thienopyridines and glycoprotein IIb/IIIa receptor antagonists, mean that the hazards identified in RITA-2 (148) have been overestimated in the current era. PCI is an appropriate intervention in patients with suitable coronary anatomy who have chronic stable angina with limiting symptoms despite medical treatment.

Percutaneous Coronary Intervention Versus Coronary Artery Bypass Grafting. A meta-analysis (150) of eight large randomized controlled trials that compared PCI (n = 1,710) with CABG (n = 1,661) in patients with predominantly stable angina (80%) has shown no significant difference in survival between the two revascularization strategies during a mean follow-up of 2.7 years. There is, however, a significant difference in the subsequent need for additional revascularization, with 17.8% of patients randomized to PCI requiring CABG within 1 year and about 2% requiring CABG per year in subsequent years. The prevalence of angina at 1 year was considerably higher in the PCI group (1.5- to 2-fold), but at 3 years, this difference was no longer significant (150).

The Bypass Angioplasty Revascularization Investigation trial (151) was published after the meta-analysis by Pocock and colleagues (150) and is the largest study to compare PCI with CABG (40% of patients had stable angina). There was no significant difference in survival or risk of MI between PCI and CABG patients, but PCI was associated with a higher rate of subsequent revascularization (8% for CABG versus 54% for PCI at 5 years). In the Arterial Revascularisation Therapy Study (ARTS) (152) and Stent or Surgery (SOS) trials (153), elective coronary artery stenting was associated with reduced need for recurrent revascularization in patients with multivessel disease (4–6% for CABG versus 17–21% for PCI at 1–2 years). The additional impact of drug-eluting stents on recurrent revascularization procedures following PCI has not yet been assessed in comparison to a strategy of CABG.

The Duke University database (n = 9,263) is a single-center prospective experience of patients with ischemic heart disease (20% of patients had stable angina) who were managed with medical therapy, PCI, or CABG. It suggests that patients with one- or two-vessel disease without involvement of the proximal left anterior descending coronary artery (LAD) experience better clinical outcomes with PCI than with CABG (154–156). Trial data are awaited for definitive evidence in the era of drug-eluting stents and modern surgery.

Feasibility of PCI has been established in multivessel angioplasty (>2 vessels), but no definitive outcome data are available comparing PCI and CABG with current technology in multivessel disease. The absence of definitive outcome data for multivessel PCI versus surgery leads to the following recommendation: PCI is an appropriate alternative to CABG in patients with symptom-limiting angina despite medical treatment who have suitable one- or two-vessel disease without a significant proximal LAD stenosis.

Culprit Lesion Percutaneous Coronary Intervention. When the purpose of revascularization is relief of angina, PCI of the lesion that is thought to be responsible for the patient's symptoms may be undertaken, even with multivessel disease. This strategy, "culprit lesion PCI," may be appropriate in symptomatic patients with multivessel coronary artery disease who have an exceptionally severe stenosis and many minor lesions or in patients unsuitable for CABG because of comorbid conditions (157). Culprit lesion PCI is also a reasonable option if surgical revascularization with CABG would be incomplete and therefore may not confer prognostic benefit.

Percutaneous Coronary Intervention After Coronary Artery Bypass Grafting. Five years after undergoing CABG, 50% of patients will have redeveloped angina, and by 12 years, 30% will have undergone repeat revascularization (158). However, these data do not reflect the current high use and improved patency of arterial conduits. Repeat CABG is associated with a higher risk and a lower likelihood of benefit than the initial intervention. In an analysis of 632 nonrandomized patients with previous CABG who required either elective repeat CABG or PCI, complete revascularization was achieved in 38% of patients who underwent PCI compared with 92% of patients who underwent CABG. However, complications were significantly lower with PCI (0.3% versus 7.3%), and survival was similar at 1 and 6 years of follow-up (159,160). In patients with limiting angina despite previous CABG and medical therapy when technically feasible, an initial strategy of PCI may be preferred to repeat CABG.

Stents

Intracoronary stents were employed initially to minimize the risk of acute or threatened vessel occlusion. They enhanced vessel patency and led to a reduction in the need for emergency CABG after PCI (145,161–165).

Randomized controlled trials have demonstrated the efficacy of elective intracoronary stenting. Some studies have methodologic limitations such as control patients who did not receive matched anticoagulation regimens (the STent REStenosis Study [STRESS] trial) (137) or investigators who were not fully blinded (the BElgian NEtherlands STENT [BENESTENT] and Stenting In Chronic Coronary Occlusion [SICCO] trials) (141,166,167). Nevertheless, all trials reported consistent findings, with elective stenting being associated with improved procedural and clinical outcomes and a reduction in the need for subsequent revascularization procedures. The clearest evidence has come from PCI procedures for higher risk lesions, namely chronically occluded arteries (167–169), saphenous vein grafts

(170), proximal LAD stenosis (144), and restenosis after prior PCI (171,172), and when conventional PCI has produced a suboptimal result (142).

The effect of elective stenting of all lesions was compared in the BENESTENT study (141) with the use of PCI alone in patients with stable angina and a single new lesion. There were no procedure-related deaths in this trial, and stenting was associated with improved clinical and angiographic outcomes. The BENESTENT II study (173) included patients with unstable angina (40%) and confirmed the benefits of elective stent implantation using heparin-coated stents. It has been proposed that, a more selective approach of stent implantation for high-risk lesions or suboptimal angiographic results may confer similar benefits (174). Importantly, after stent implantation, patients have less restenosis and greater MI-free survival and reduced needs for repeated coronary intervention (137,141,145, 161,166,175,176).

To reduce the incidence of stent thrombosis and restenosis, coated stents have been developed (e.g., with heparin), but these stents had limited benefits over bare metal stents. In contrast, a major development involves drug-eluting stents that contain antiproliferative agents. Sirolimus is a macrolide antibiotic with antifungal, immunosuppressive, and antimitotic properties that has been used in the prevention of renal transplant rejection. Sirolimus-coated stents were associated with a dramatic reduction in the incidence of in-stent restenosis, with failure of target vessel revascularization falling from 21.0% to 8.6% in the SIRUS study (146). Paclitaxel is a microtubule-stabilizing agent with potent antitumor activity that has also been successfully used in stent coatings with similar reductions in in-stent restenosis.

Antiplatelet Therapy for Percutaneous Coronary Intervention

Aspirin therapy is associated with a 50% reduction in the rate of vascular occlusion after PCI (4% versus 8%) (Fig. 17.11) (177,178) and compared with conventional anticoagulant therapy, the combination of ticlopidine (250 mg BID) and aspirin (100 mg BID) was superior to aspirin alone or aspirin in combination with warfarin (179,180). Clopidogrel avoids the adverse hematologic risks of ticlopidine and observational data indicate that it is as efficacious as ticlopidine in the prevention of stent thrombosis; it is currently the thienopyridine of choice in this setting (181,182).

More potent platelet antagonists have been tested in the peri-PCI setting. Several large-scale randomized controlled trials (134,183–186) assessed the short-term use of IV platelet glycoprotein IIb/IIIa antagonists in PCI. Most studies focused on high-risk PCI procedures in patients with recent MI, unstable angina, or complex lesions and they demonstrated significant reductions in the combined rate of death, MI, and revascularization. The major impact was on markers indicative of myocyte necrosis (troponins). Most benefit is seen in the first 30 days, but a small benefit was still demonstrable at 3-year follow-up (134,184,187). The benefit was at the expense of an increased risk of minor bleeding complications.

Subgroup analysis is not available for elective patients in the three trials included patients undergoing PCI: Evaluation in PCI to Improve Long-term Outcome with abciximab GP IIb/IIIa blockade (EPILOG) (30% of the study population) (184), Evaluation of Platelet IIb/IIIa Inhibitor for Stenting (EPISTENT) (40%) (138), and Integrilin to Minimise Platelet Aggregation and Coronary Thrombosis (IMPACT-II) (60%) (185). In contrast to the other studies, the IMPACT-II trial (185) failed to demonstrate a consistent and prolonged benefit with IIb/IIIa antagonism, although the dosage regimen may have been inadequate. The EPISTENT trial (134) suggests that IIb/IIIa receptor antagonism is beneficial, particularly in the presence of stent implantation, and confers long-term and economic benefits (187).

A meta-analysis (188) of 16 randomized controlled trials incorporating 32,135 patients confirms the modest beneficial effects of platelet glycoprotein IIb/IIIa antagonists in patients during PCI or acute coronary syndromes. The recent ISAR-REACT trial has questioned the role of glycoprotein IIb/IIIa receptor antagonists in elective PCI (189) when all patients (low risk) were pretreated with clopidogrel (600-mg loading dose). No additional benefit of a glycoprotein IIb/IIIa receptor antagonist was demonstrated. Glycoprotein IIb/IIIa inhibitors reduce cardiac complications in high risk patients undergoing PCI. All patients with chronic stable angina should be pretreated with clopidogrel before elective PCI.

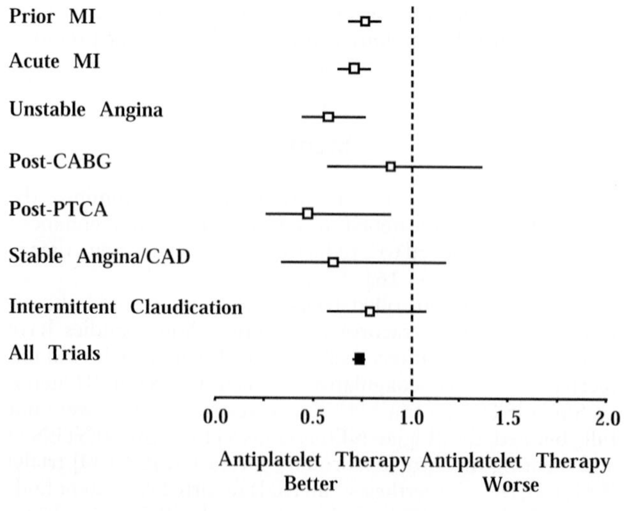

FIGURE 17.11. Proportionate benefits of antiplatelet therapy in patients with ischemic heart disease. $n = \sim 100{,}000$, $P < .00001$. *Abbreviations:* MI, myocardial infarction; CABG, coronary artery bypass graft surgery; PCI, percutaneous coronary intervention; CAD, coronary artery disease (181).

Coronary Artery Bypass Graft Surgery

Choice of Coronary Artery Bypass Grafting Versus Medical Treatment

The three major randomized controlled trials compared CABG with medical therapy: the Coronary Artery Surgery Study (CASS) (190), the Veterans Administration Cooperative Study (191), and the European Coronary Surgery Study [ECSS] (192). These studies form the basis of the meta-analysis by Yusuf and colleagues (193) that compares CABG with medical therapy in patients with chronic stable angina. All of these trials predate modern surgical techniques, the widespread use of arterial conduits, and modern medical therapy. Nevertheless, in comparison with medical therapy, CABG significantly improves symptoms of angina and exercise capacity and reduces the need for antianginal therapy (190). After CABG, more than 70% of patients are free of angina at 1 year and 50% are free at 5 years (190,193). Patients experience a better quality of life after CABG (190,194,195) and report less limitation in physical activity (190). Moreover, 73% of patients are working 1 year after CABG (195). CABG is an appropriate intervention in patients who have suitable coronary anatomy with chronic stable and symptom-limiting angina despite medical treatment.

Arterial Conduits

Saphenous vein bypass grafts undergo progressive obstruction and occlusion (graft vasculopathy) and have an accelerated failure rate that is particularly evident beyond the fifth year. Arterial conduits are increasingly used to improve graft survival and reduce the need for reoperation (196–198). The internal mammary arteries are the principal conduits to have been assessed, although other conduits, such as the radial and gastroepiploic arteries, may also be used.

Ten years after CABG, 83% of internal mammary artery grafts remain patent compared with only 41% of saphenous vein grafts (199). Observational studies suggest that this improved patency rate is associated with better long-term survival rates and a reduction in the risk of angina, hospitalization, MI, and repeat operation (196–198). Overall, patients who undergo CABG with saphenous vein grafts have a 1.6-fold greater risk of death over 10 years compared with those who receive an internal mammary artery graft (196).

In patients with chronic stable angina, elective surgical mortality rate is in the range of 2% to 4%, depending on the case mix (200). Various factors influence surgical mortality rates, including age, gender, degree of left ventricular impairment, and the presence of other comorbid conditions (200). If technically feasible, CABG surgery should incorporate the use of arterial conduits such as one or both of the internal mammary arteries.

SECONDARY PREVENTION

Certain lifestyle interventions (e.g., smoking cessation) and risk factor modifications have been shown to improve the prognosis of patients with ischemic heart disease, but others remain unproven or have neutral effects. The major secondary prevention therapies are associated with very modest rates for hazard (e.g., bleeding risk with aspirin) and side effects, (e.g., with statin therapy) and the hazards are outweighed by benefits in outcome (Fig. 17.12).

Antiplatelet Therapy

Aspirin has been described as a weak inhibitor of platelet aggregation, based on in vitro responses to specific agonists. However, it substantially reduces cardiovascular events across the spectrum of vascular risk. It is a simple and effective treatment in patients with chronic stable angina. In a landmark meta-analysis the Antiplatelet Trialists' Collaboration demonstrated a significant morbidity and mortality benefit with long-term aspirin therapy in patients with ischemic heart disease (177), especially in those who have undergone coronary revascularization (178).

Although the proportionate reductions in events for patients with chronic stable angina as an isolated group (37%) were comparable to the overall reduction in all patients with ischemic heart disease (27%), the confidence intervals were wide and included unity. Long-term aspirin (<100 mg/d) is recommended to reduce the risk of death and MI in all patients with chronic ischemic heart disease.

The frequency of cardiovascular events despite aspirin therapy has led to the search for other, more potent antiplatelet agents. In the CAPRIE trial (201), long-term clopidogrel treatment (75 mg/d) was at least as efficacious as aspirin in the prevention of ischemic stroke, MI, or vascular death in patients with atherosclerotic vascular disease. The overall secondary

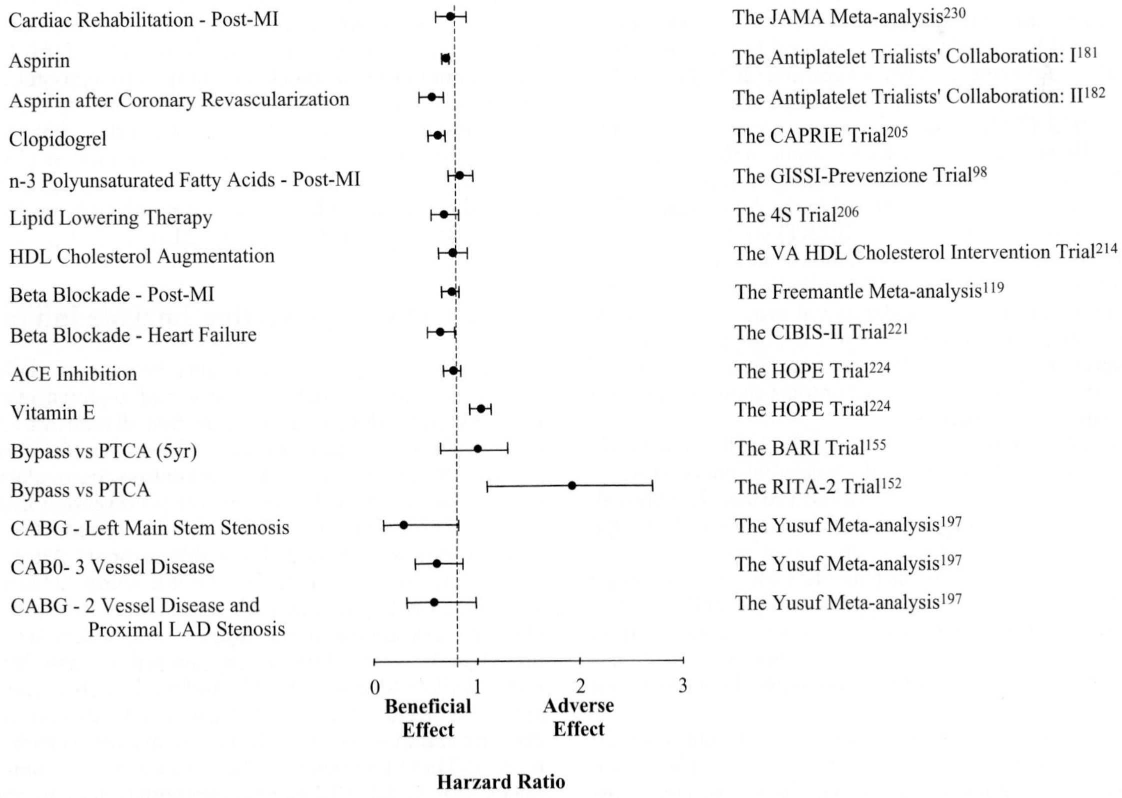

FIGURE 17.12. Proportionate benefits of a range of potential secondary preventive therapies. *The RITA-2 trial predominantly recruited patients with a low cardiovascular risk (152).

preventive benefits of clopidogrel statistically exceeded those of aspirin, but the relative benefits were modest (relative risk reduction, 8.7%; $P = .04$) (201). Clopidogrel is indicated as an alternative to aspirin in patients with aspirin intolerance. There is no outcome evidence to support the practice of clopidogrel treatment when administered at the time of PCI.

Clopidogrel is beneficial when used in combination with aspirin, in patients with acute non–ST-elevation ACS (see discussion of CURE study). Combination aspirin and clopidogrel did not show significant improvement in the risk of death or MI or stroke (N Eng J Med 2006), although there were trends for better outcome in those with pre-existing vascular disease.

Lipid-Lowering Therapy

Serum cholesterol concentrations should be assessed in all patients with chronic stable angina, but the summation of evidence suggests that cholesterol-lowering therapy confers benefit to almost all patients (at least for total cholesterol >136 mg/dL; see below). Thus, all patients with chronic ischemic heart disease should be treated with an hydroxy-3-methyl glutaryl coenzyme A reductase inhibitor or statin, irrespective of the serum cholesterol concentration. Several large-scale randomized controlled trials addressed lipid-lowering therapy in patients with ischemic heart disease and the Scandinavian Simvastatin Survival Study (4S) trial (202) was the first to demonstrate a significant improvement in mortality in patients with a serum cholesterol concentration of more than 210 mg/dL (>5.5 mmol/L) (relative risk reduction, 30%). Mortality benefits have been demonstrated with simvastatin (202) or pravastatin (203,204). The Cholesterol and Recurrent Events (CARE) study (203) demonstrated that patients with average cholesterol concentrations (low-density lipoprotein [LDL] cholesterol, 120–150 mg/dL; 3.2–3.9 mmol/L) benefit from lipid-lowering therapy. However, the absolute risk of subsequent cardiac events is proportionately lower in patients with "average" concentrations of cholesterol. In contrast, more aggressive lipid-lowering appears to have additional benefits in patients after saphenous vein bypass grafting (205) (target LDL cholesterol <100 mg/dL or <2.6 mmol/L).

The 4S trial (202) is the only large-scale mortality study to specifically recruit patients with chronic stable angina (or prior MI), but the benefits of lipid-lowering therapy in chronic stable angina were also demonstrated in the Atorvastatin VErsus Revascularization Treatment (AVERT) study (206). Over 18 months of treatment, AVERT demonstrated a reduced the number of acute ischemic events—hospitalization for worsening angina or coronary revascularization procedures with the statin in comparison with intervention with PCI (13% versus 21%, respectively). However, PCI was associated with a greater improvement in chronic anginal symptoms than atorvastatin (54% versus 41%, respectively).

The initial secondary prevention trials predominantly recruited patients with serum total cholesterol concentrations above a certain threshold, usually around 190 mg/dL. Although a threshold effect was suggested based on data from the CARE trial (203) the subsequent Heart Protection Study (207) has definitively established that all patients with coronary heart disease should receive statin therapy. It is the overall absolute risk that is important rather than the cholesterol concentration per se. If a patient is at high risk, they will benefit from cholesterol reduction irrespective of their cholesterol concentration (207).

How low should the serum cholesterol concentration be reduced in patients with chronic stable angina? The recent PROVE-IT (208) and TNT (209) trials have respectively assessed whether more intensive lipid-lowering therapy is associated with better outcomes in patients with recent unstable or chronic stable coronary heart disease. Both trials show a consistent benefit in reducing serum LDL cholesterol concentrations below current guidelines (to a mean of 62–77 mg/dL).

Other classes of drugs, such as fibrates, also lower serum lipid concentrations, but the benefits on mortality are inferred rather than demonstrated directly. An exception is the Veterans Affairs trial of gemfibrozil, which demonstrated significant secondary preventive benefits of elevating reduced HDL cholesterol concentrations (210). Fibrates should therefore be considered in patients with normal LDL but low HDL cholesterol concentrations.

ß-Blockers for Secondary Prevention

There have been no randomized controlled trials to demonstrate that ß-blocker therapy improves survival in patients with chronic stable angina. However, post-MI (211), in hypertension (212), and in case-control (213) studies patients maintained on ß-blockers are less likely to have a vascular event and have a reduced mortality rate if they subsequently experience an MI. For these reasons, it is reasonable that ß-blockers should be the first-line agents of choice for patients with chronic stable angina. Concerns that ß-blocker therapy is associated with reduced peripheral perfusion owing to unopposed α-adrenergic vasoconstriction and blockade of $ß_2$ vascular receptors, are unfounded (214), even in patients with peripheral vascular disease (215). Because of the common risk factor of smoking, many patients with angina have chronic obstructive pulmonary disease and are denied ß-blocker therapy because of the concern of provoking bronchospasm. However, there is a large body of observational data demonstrating that patients with obstructive pulmonary disease derive similar mortality benefits (40% relative risk reduction) after MI with ß-blocker therapy (211).

Patients with chronic stable angina and coexistent heart failure are particularly at risk and should be given ß-blocker therapy as the agent of choice. Several large randomized controlled trials have demonstrated major mortality and morbidity benefits in patients with mild to severe heart failure (212,213) who were maintained on ß-blocker therapy. Although cautious dose uptitration and close clinical observation for cardiac decompensation are necessary, the withdrawal rates of patients with heart failure from ß-blocker therapy are modest (15%) and equivalent to those for placebo (213). Moreover, rates of rehospitalization are reduced and symptoms of heart failure are improved with ß-blocker therapy (213).

Angiotensin-Converting Enzyme Inhibition

The major morbidity and mortality benefits of angiotensin-converting enzyme (ACE) inhibitor and angiotensin receptor blockers (and ARB) therapy were first demonstrated in patients with heart failure (214,215). These benefits may reflect an antiischemic action of ACE inhibition, particularly given the evidence from the Heart Outcomes Prevention Evaluation (HOPE) (216) and the EURopean trial On reduction of cardiac events with Perindopril in stable coronary Artery disease (EUROPA) studies (217). The HOPE study (216) assessed 9,297 high-risk patients with vascular disease (55% with chronic stable angina) in the absence of documented heart failure. Over 4.5 years of treatment, ramipril was associated with reduced all-cause mortality, MI, and stroke (216). The benefits appear to be independent of the associated reductions in blood pressure and were particularly marked in patients with diabetes mellitus.These findings have been subsequently confirmed in the EUROPA trial of 13,655 patients with stable coronary heart disease (217). Perindopril 8 mg/d was associated with a 20% relative risk reduction in the likelihood of cardiovascular death,

MI or cardiac arrest (50 patients treated for 4 years to avoid one event). The recent Prevention of Events with Angiotensin Converting Enzyme inhibition (PEACE) trial (218) contrasts to the HOPE (216) and EUROPA (217) trials because it failed to demonstrate a benefit of trandolipril in 8,290 patients with stable coronary heart disease. However, very low-risk patients were recruited and the event rate was below the rate in the treatment arms of either HOPE or EUROPA (216,217). Patients with chronic stable angina and a predicted 10-year event rate below 15% should receive ACE inhibitor therapy on account of the major secondary preventive benefits.

Coronary Revascularization

There have been no randomized controlled trials to test whether PCI improves long-term survival in patients with chronic stable angina. In the short to medium term, the hazards of PCI exceed those of medical therapy (147,206). In contrast, in selected groups, CABG is associated with significant reductions in mortality rates compared with medical therapy. Comparisons of the prognostic benefits of PCI and CABG demonstrated no statistically significant differences between the two approaches (150,151), but this does not establish equivalence. Thus, in patients with chronic stable angina, PCI is an important treatment to relieve symptoms, but is associated with a small excess early risk.

In comparison with medical therapy, CABG improves long-term (10-year) survival in patients with stable angina. Subgroup analysis demonstrates that patients with greater than 50% left main stem stenosis had the greatest survival benefit with CABG (193,219,220). Survival benefits are also seen in patients with three-vessel disease or two-vessel disease that includes proximal LAD stenosis, especially in the context of LV dysfunction (193,220). However, for patients with two-vessel disease without proximal LAD stenosis or one-vessel disease, there is no evidence of a survival advantage from CABG. It has not yet been established in these patient populations whether PCI with current stent technology has a similar impact on survival. Patients with abnormal left ventricular function, high-risk anatomy (e.g., left main or proximal LAD stenosis), or strongly positive exercise tests derive greater absolute survival benefit from CABG than from medical therapy.

It is important to note that in the trials a significant number of patients with three-vessel disease who were initially randomized to medical therapy crossed over to surgery (41% at 10 years). These studies compared strategies rather than surgery per se, and may underestimate the benefits of surgery. Thus, randomized controlled trials may underestimate the benefits of modern CABG techniques with arterial conduits and do not take into account improvements in secondary preventive therapy (220).

Cardiac Rehabilitation

Cardiac rehabilitation involves a multidisciplinary approach addressing medical and psychosocial care, exercise, education, secondary prevention, and vocational advice (221). Although predominantly applied to the immediate post-MI or post-CABG period, it is also applicable to patients with chronic stable angina. The rehabilitation process encompasses three main components:

1. Explanation and understanding.
2. Specific interventions: secondary prevention, exercise training, and psychological support.
3. Long-term adaptation and education.

Patients with stable angina who attend a regular exercise and rehabilitation program have less angina and may have fewer recurrent MIs, as well as better cardiorespiratory fitness and vocational status (222,223). Exercise programs improve patient confidence and functional capacity, and although they are labor intensive, are potentially cost effective (224–226).

Benefits appear to be most prominent in the first 2 years (225,226); secondary preventive effects appear to be sustained over 10 years (226). Although these benefits have not been definitively demonstrated in populations of patients with chronic stable angina in the absence of MI, the referral of such patients to a cardiac rehabilitation program can improve symptoms and enhance measures of quality of life.

CONTROVERSIES AND PERSONAL PERSPECTIVES

The vast majority of individuals with chronic stable coronary disease are asymptomatic and exhibit no clinical manifestations of the disease process. Individuals only become patients relatively late in the time course of coronary atherogenesis. Our current diagnostic and therapeutic interventions are targeted at those who develop complications of the disease (angina, MI, heart failure) rather than individuals at particular risk of atheroma progression and plaque rupture. Smarter primary prevention strategies would allow higher risk individuals to be targeted. Based on clinical risk factors, family history, and phenotypic and genetic markers of susceptibility, such approaches have greater potential for benefit, and greater cost effectiveness, than blanket strategies in primary prevention.

In patients with symptomatic chronic stable coronary disease, the syndrome describes a relatively quiescent interval between symptomatic episodes of plaque rupture or between cardiac complications. Nevertheless, the disease process involves atheroma progression and thrombotic complications and is potentially amenable to intervention. Novel approaches may allow identification of vulnerable plaques and both mechanical interventions and pharmacologic interventions may modify the balance between inflammation and plaque rupture versus stabilization and repair.

Until such approaches are developed, the main focus in patients with chronic stable coronary disease is the control of symptoms and improvement in prognosis with current therapeutic interventions. These approaches would be enhanced by systematic and careful risk stratification, not only to provide insights into prognosis, but also to guide therapeutic decisions. Currently, a major "gap" exists between evidence of benefit and the systematic application of evidence-based therapy. Redressing this gap is an urgent clinical imperative.

THE FUTURE

Diagnostic Tools

Developments in several imaging modalities now provide insights into the extent, and limited information on the structure of coronary atheromatous plaque (e.g., high-resolution IVUS, positron emission tomography with labeling of plaque metabolic activity, optical coherence tomography). As yet, none of the these techniques has demonstrated that the enhanced anatomic and biological information translates into therapeutic decisions and altered patient outcome. However, such techniques provide major advances over the current reference standard in chronic ischemic heart disease, coronary angiography. Although angiography provides critical information to guide revascularization, it is limited to assessing the extent of encroachment of plaque into the arterial lumen (stenosis severity).

A critical goal for novel diagnostic techniques is to distinguish biologically active plaques, with enhanced risks of rupture and thrombotic events, from quiescent plaques with stable anatomic and biological features. Such differentiation would allow targeted therapy of nonstenotic but vulnerable plaques and avoid unnecessary treatment of stable quiescent and nonobstructive lesions. This goal is yet to be realized.

Risk Assessment in Chronic Stable Angina

In contrast to the settings of acute coronary syndrome or heart failure, limited risk stratification information has been available to guide therapeutic choices in chronic stable angina. Indeed, recent long-term trials have demonstrated the relatively low risk of cardiovascular events in patients with chronic stable ischemic heart disease annual mortality in the range of 1.5%, (124,216,217). However, these overall figures obscure a substantial range of almost 10-fold in risk depending on baseline characteristics (35). Such risk stratification is based on clinical characteristics (many of which are nonmodifiable, like age or prior myocardial injury) and includes commonly available biochemical or hematologic, measurements (e.g., creatinine, glucose, white blood cell count). It is critically important to determine whether markers of upregulation of the inflammatory and coagulation systems may provide additional and more accurate prognostic information (e.g., hsCRP, CD40, IL1, serum amyloid A, markers of platelet activation).

A longer term goal is to establish the extent to which environmental factors modify the expression and the impact of specific genetic characteristics (rather than single gene polymorphisms). Unraveling the influence of many different genetic influences on phenotype expression may provide more accurate prognostic information, guide therapeutic choices, and avoid adverse drug effects in specific individuals.

Therapeutic Interventions

The role of percutaneous revascularization has evolved remarkably rapidly and it is critical that PCI with modern technology be tested against best currently available surgical revascularization in the context with secondary prevention. Until this is done, it is uncertain whether the current displacement of CABG surgery by PCI procedures in patients with multivessel lesions is appropriate in terms of outcome complications and cost effectiveness.

Smart technologies have already altered proliferative responses to stent implantation with cell-cycle inhibitors. Whether more sophisticated drug-eluting stents may alter the behavior and susceptibility of other plaques to rupture (by achieving higher local concentrations of agents to modify plaque inflammation) remains to be determined.

Angiogenesis has great potential and promised much as a method of improving coronary revascularization. Much of this promise is yet to be fulfilled and the clinical importance of blood flow changes induced by angiogenesis requires further development. Nevertheless, in conjunction with major developments in gene transfer therapy (203,204), it may provide highly innovative future methods of improving myocardial perfusion.

Cytoprotection mechanisms, including pre- and postconditioning, have been demonstrated in experimental studies to have a major impact on cell survival in tissues subject to ischemia and reperfusion. As yet, these approaches have not translated into therapeutic interventions, but they have the potential to do so.

Thus, a series of approaches will allow more accurate diagnostic, risk prediction, and therapeutic interventions and a move from "blanket" approaches to treatment to smarter and more individualized therapies.

References

1. *2005 Heart and stroke statistical update [report]*. Dallas, TX: American Heart Association, 2005.
2. *Heart and stroke facts: 1996 statistical supplement [report]*. Dallas, TX: American Heart Association, 1997.
3. Maseri A, Crea F, Kaski JC, et al. Mechanisms and significance of cardiac ischemic pain. *Prog Cardiovasc Dis* 1992;35:1–18.
4. Crea F, Pupita G, Galassi AR, et al. Role of adenosine in pathogenesis of anginal pain. *Circulation* 1990;81:164–172.
5. Gould KL, Lipscomb K, Hamilton GW. Physiologic basis for assessing critical coronary stenosis: instantaneous flow response and regional distribution during coronary hyperemia as measures of coronary flow reserve. *Am J Cardiol* 1974;33:87–94.
6. Treasure CB, Klein JL, Weintraub WS, et al. Beneficial effects of cholesterol-lowering therapy on the coronary endothelium in patients with coronary artery disease. *N Engl J Med* 1995;332:481–487.
7. Uren NG, Crake T, Lefroy DC, et al. Reduced coronary vasodilator function in infarcted and normal myocardium after myocardial infarction. *N Engl J Med* 1994;331:222–227.
8. Uren NG, Marraccini P, Gistri R, et al. Altered coronary vasodilator reserve and metabolism in myocardium subtended by normal arteries in patients with coronary artery disease. *J Am Coll Cardiol* 1993;22:650–658.
9. Deanfield JE, Selwyn AP, Chierchia S, et al. Myocardial ischaemia during daily life in patients with stable angina: its relation to symptoms and heart rate changes. *Lancet* 1983;2:753–758.
10. Yeung AC, Vekshtein VI, Krantz DS, et al. The effect of atherosclerosis on the vasomotor response of coronary arteries to mental stress. *N Engl J Med* 1991;325:1551–1556.
11. Rubanyi GM, Frye R, Holmes DR, et al. Vasoconstrictor activity of coronary sinus plasma from patients with coronary artery disease. *J Am Coll Cardiol* 1987;9:1243–1249.
12. Golino P, Piscione F, Benedict CR, et al. Local effect of serotonin released during coronary angioplasty. *N Engl J Med* 1994;330:523–528.
13. van der Wal AC, Becker AE, Koch KT, et al. Clinically stable angina pectoris is not necessarily associated with histologically stable atherosclerotic plaques. *Heart* 1996;76:312–316.
14. Edmonstone WM. Cardiac chest pain: does body language help the diagnosis? *BMJ* 1995;311:1660–1661.
15. Marber MS, Joy MD, Yellon DM. Is warm-up in angina ischaemic preconditioning? *Br Heart J* 1994;72:213–215.
16. Rinaldi CA, Masani ND, Linka AZ, et al. Effect of repetitive episodes of exercise induced myocardial ischaemia on left ventricular function in patients with chronic stable angina: evidence for cumulative stunning or ischaemic preconditioning? *Heart* 1999;81:404–411.
17. Stewart RAH, Simmonds MB, Williams MJA. Time course of "warm up" in stable angina. *Am J Cardiol* 1995;76:70–73.
18. Williams DO, Bass TA, Gewirtz H, et al. Adaptation to the stress of tachycardia in patients with coronary artery disease: insight into the mechanism of the warm-up phenomenon. *Circulation* 1985;71:687–692.
19. Okazaki Y, Kodama K, Sato H, et al. Attenuation of increased regional myocardial oxygen consumption during exercise as a major cause of warm-up phenomenon. *J Am Coll Cardiol* 1993;21:1597–1604.
20. Campeau L. Grading of angina pectoris. *Circulation* 1976;54:522–523.
21. Cox J, Naylor CD. The Canadian Cardiovascular Society grading scale for angina pectoris: is it time for refinements? *Ann Intern Med* 1992;117:677–683.
22. Parker JO, Chiong MA, West RO, et al. Sequential alterations in myocardial lactate metabolism, S-T segments, and left ventricular function during angina induced by atrial pacing. *Circulation* 1969;XL:113–131.
23. Upton MT, Rerych SK, Newman GE, et al. Detecting abnormalities in left ventricular function during exercise before angina and ST-segment depression. *Circulation* 1980;62:341–349.
24. Ambrosio G, Betocchi S, Pace L, et al. Prolonged impairment of regional contractile function after resolution of exercise-induced angina. *Circulation* 1996;94:2455–2464.
25. Kemp HG, Vokonas PS, Cohn PF, et al. The anginal syndrome associated with normal coronary arteriograms: report of a six year experience. *Am J Med* 1973;54:735–742.
26. Likoff W, Segal BL, Kasparian H. Paradox of normal selective coronary arteriograms in patients considered to have unmistakable coronary heart disease. *N Engl J Med* 1967;276:1063–1066.
27. Kemp HG, Elliott WC, Gorlin R. The anginal syndrome with normal coronary arteriography. *Trans Assoc Am Physicians* 1967;80:59–70.
28. Ladenheim ML, Pollock BH, Rozanski A, et al. Extent and severity of myocardial hypoperfusion as predictors of prognosis in patients with suspected coronary artery disease. *J Am Coll Cardiol* 1986;7:464–471.

29. Kaski JE, Rosano GMC, Collins P, et al. Cardiac syndrome x: clinical characteristics and left ventricular function. Long term follow-up. *J Am Coll Cardiol* 1995;25:807–814.
30. Prinzmetal M, Kennamer R, Merliss R, et al. Angina pectoris: I. A variant form of angina pectoris. *Am J Med* 1959;27:375–388.
31. Maseri A, Parodi O, Severi S, et al. Transient transmural reduction of myocardial blood flow, demonstrated by thallium-201 scintigraphy, as a cause of variant angina. *Circulation* 1976;54:280–288.
32. Mark DB, Califf RM, Morris KG, et al. Clinical characteristics and long-term survival of patients with variant angina. *Circulation* 1984;69:880–888.
33. Pepine CJ, Abrams J, Mark RG, et al. Characteristics of a contemporary population with angina pectoris. *Am J Cardiol* 1994;74:226–231.
34. Weiner DA, Ryan TJ, McCabe CH, et al. Exercise stress testing: correlations among history of angina, ST-segment response and prevalence of coronary-artery disease in the Coronary Artery Surgery Study (CASS). *N Engl J Med* 1979;301:230–235.
35. Clayton T, Lubsen J, Pocock SJ, et al. A risk score for predicting death, myocardial infarction and stroke in patients with stable angina, based on a large randomized trial cohort of patients. *BMJ* 2005;331:869.
36. Roberts KB, Califf RM, Harrell FE Jr, et al. The prognosis for patients with new-onset angina who have undergone cardiac catheterization. *Circulation* 1983;68:970–978.
37. Castaner A, Roig E, Serra A, et al. Risk stratification and prognosis of patients with recent onset angina. *Eur Heart J* 1990;11:868–875.
38. Fang J, Madhavan S, Alderman MH. The association between birthplace and mortality from cardiovascular causes among black and white residents of New York City. *N Engl J Med* 1996;335:1545–1551.
39. Peterson ED, Shaw LK, DeLong ER, et al. Racial variation in the use of coronary-revascularization procedures. *N Engl J Med* 1997;336:480–486.
40. Whittle J, Conigliaro J, Good CB, et al. Racial differences in the use of invasive cardiovascular procedures in the Department of Veterans Affairs medical system. *N Engl J Med* 1993;329:621–627.
41. Enas EA, Yusuf S, Mehta JL. Prevalence of coronary artery disease in Asian Indians. *Am J Cardiol* 1992;70:945–949.
42. Kaplan GA, Keil JE. Socioeconomic factors and cardiovascular disease: a review of the literature [AHA Medical/Scientific Statement-Special Report]. *Circulation* 1993;88:1973–1998.
43. Clarke R, Daly L, Robinson K, et al. Hyperhomocysteinemia: an independent risk factor for vascular disease. *N Engl J Med* 1991;324:1149–1155.
44. Stampfer MJ, Malinow MR, Willett WC, et al. A prospective study of plasma homocyst(e)ine and risk of myocardial infarction in US physicians. *JAMA* 1992;268:877–881.
44a. Bønaa KH, Njølstad I, Ueland PM, et al., for the NORVIT Trial Investigators. Homocysteine lowering and cardiovascular events after acute myocardial infarction. *N Engl J Med* 2006; DOI 10.1056/NEJMoa055227.
45. Gorgels APM, Vos MA, Mulleneers R, et al. Value of the electrocardiogram in diagnosing the number of severely narrowed coronary arteries in rest angina pectoris. *Am J Cardiol* 1993;72:999–1003.
46. Weiner DA, McCabe C, Hueter DC, et al. The predictive value of anginal chest pain as an indicator of coronary disease during exercise testing. *Am Heart J* 1978;96:458–462.
47. Goldschlager N, Sox HC Jr. The diagnostic and prognostic value of the treadmill exercise test in the evaluation of chest pain, in patients with recent myocardial infarction, and in asymptomatic individuals. *Am Heart J* 1988;116:523–535.
48. Dagianti A, Penco M, Agati L, et al. Stress echocardiography: comparison of exercise, dipyridamole and dobutamine in detecting and predicting the extent of coronary artery disease. *J Am Coll Cardiol* 1995;26:18–25.
49. Nesto RW, Cohn LH, Collins JJ Jr, et al. Inotropic contractile reserve: a useful predictor of increased 5 year survival and improved postoperative left ventricular function in patients with coronary artery disease and reduced ejection fraction. *Am J Cardiol* 1982;50:39–44.
50. Bonow RO, Dilsizian V, Cuocolo A, et al. Identification of viable myocardium in patients with chronic coronary artery disease and left ventricular dysfunction. *Circulation* 1991;83:26–37.
51. Dilsizian V, Smeltzer WR, Freedman NMT, et al. Thallium reinjection after stress re-distribution imaging. Does 24-hour delayed imaging after reinjection enhance detection of viable myocardium? *Circulation* 1991;83:1247–1255.
52. Marwick T, Willemart B, D'Hondt AM, et al. Selection of the optimal nonexercise stress for the evaluation of ischemic regional myocardial dysfunction and malperfusion. *Circulation* 1993;87:345–354.
53. Ling LH, Pellikka PA, Mahoney DW, et al. Atropine augmentation in dobutamine stress echocardiography: role and incremental value in a clinical practice setting. *J Am Coll Cardiol* 1996;28:551–557.
54. Beleslin BD, Ostojic M, Stepanovic J, et al. Stress echocardiography in the detection of myocardial ischemia. *Circulation* 1994;90:1168–1176.
55. Kamaran M, Teague SM, Finkelhor RS, et al. Prognostic value of dobutamine stress echocardiography in patients referred because of suspected coronary artery disease. *Am J Cardiol* 1995;76:887–889.
56. Williams MJ, Odabashian J, Lauer MS, et al. Prognostic value of dobutamine echocardiography in patients with left ventricular dysfunction. *J Am Coll Cardiol* 1996;27:132–139.
57. Marcovitz PA, Shayna V, Horn RA, et al. Value of dobutamine stress echocardiography in determining the prognosis of patients with known or suspected coronary artery disease. *Am J Cardiol* 1996;78:404–408.
58. Kaul S, Lilly DR, Gascho JA, et al. Prognostic utility of the exercise thallium-201 test in ambulatory patients with chest pain: comparison with cardiac catheterization. *Circulation* 1988;77:745–758.
59. Berman DS, Hachamovitch R, Kiat H, et al. Incremental value of prognostic testing in patients with known or suspected ischemic heart disease: a basis for optimal utilization of exercise technetium-99m sestamibi myocardial perfusion single-photon emission computed tomography. *J Am Coll Cardiol* 1995;26:639–647.
60. Brown KA. Prognostic value of thallium-201 myocardial perfusion imaging: a diagnostic tool comes of age. *Circulation* 1991;83:363–381.
61. Shaw L, Chaitman BR, Hilton TC, et al. Prognostic value of dipyridamole thallium-201 imaging in elderly patients. *J Am Coll Cardiol* 1992;19:1390–1398.
62. Zabel KM, Califf RM. The value of exercise thallium imaging [editorial]. *Ann Intern Med* 1994;121:891–893.
63. Nygaard TW, Gibson RS, Ryan JM, et al. Prevalence of high-risk thallium-201 scintigraphic findings in left main coronary artery stenosis: Comparison with patients with multiple- and single-vessel coronary artery disease. *Am J Cardiol* 1984;53:462–469.
64. Dash H, Massie BM, Botvinick EH, et al. The noninvasive identification of left main and three vessel coronary artery disease by myocardial stress perfusion scintigraphy and treadmill exercise electrocardiography. *Circulation* 1979;60:276–284.
65. Taylor AJ, Bindeman J, Feuerstein I, et al. Coronary calcium independently predicts incident premature coronary heart disease over measured cardiovascular risk factors mean three-year outcomes in the Prospective Army Coronary Calcium (PACC) Project. *J Am Coll Cardiol* 2005;46:807–814.
66. Gibbons RJ, Chatterjee K, Daley J, et al. ACC/AHA/ACP-ASIM guidelines for the management of patients with chronic stable angina: a report of the American College of Cardiology/American Heart Association Task Force on Practice Guidelines (Committee on the Management of Patients with Chronic Stable Angina). *J Am Coll Cardiol* 1999;33:2092–2197.
67. O'Rourke RA, Brundage BH, Froelicher VF, et al. American College of Cardiology/American Heart Association Expert Consensus document on electron-beam computed tomography for the diagnosis and prognosis of coronary artery disease. *Circulation* 2000;102:126–140.
68. Asakura M, Ueda Y, Yamaguchi O, et al. Extensive development of vulnerable plaques as a pan-coronary process in patients with myocardial infarction: an angioscopic study. *J Am Coll Cardiol* 2001;37:1284–1288.
69. Buffon A, Biasuci LM, Liuzzo G, et al. Widespread coronary inflammation in unstable angina. *N Engl J Med* 2002;347:5–12.
70. Okazaki S, YokoyamaT, Miyauchi K, et al. Early statin treatment in patients with acute coronary syndrome: demonstration of the beneficial effect on atherosclerotic lesions by serial volumetric intravascular ultrasound analysis during half a year after coronary event: the ESTABLISH study. *Circulation* 2004;110:1061–1068.
71. Jan IK, Bouma BE, Kang DH, et al. Visualization of Coronary atherosclerotic plaques in patients using optical coherence tomography: comparison with intravascular ultrasound. *J Am Coll Cardiol* 2002;39:604–609.
72. Defer J, Coche E, Legros G, et al. Head-to-head comparison of three-dimensional navigator-gated magnetic resonance imaging and 16-slice computed tomography to detect coronary artery stenosis in patients. *J Am Coll Cardiol* 2005;46:92–100.
73. Leber AW, Knez A, von Ziegler F, et al. Quantification of obstructive and nonobstructive coronary lesions by 64-slice computed tomography: a comparative study with quantitative coronary angiography and intravascular ultrasound. *J Am Coll Cardiol* 2005;46:147.
74. Raff GL, Gallagher MJ, O'Neill WW, et al. Diagnostic accuracy of noninvasive coronary angiography using 64-slice spiral computed tomography. *J Am Coll Cardiol* 2005;46:552–557.
75. Kaandorp TA, Lamb HJ, Van der Wall EE, et al. Cardiovascular MR to access myocardial viability in chronic ischaemic LV dysfunction. *Heart* 2005;91:1359–1365.
76. Bax JJ, Van Der Wall EE, Harbinson M. Radionuclide techniques for the assessment of myocardial viability and hibernation. *Heart* 2004;90[Suppl 5]: v26–33.
77. Baer FM, Thissen P, Schneider CA, et al. Dobutamine magnetic resonance imaging predicts contractile recovery of chronically dysfunctional myocardium after successful revascularization. *J Am Coll Cardiol* 1998;31: 1040–1048.
78. John AS, Dreyfus GD, Pennell DJ. Images in cardiovascular medicine. Reversible wall thinning in hibernation predicted by cardiovascular magnetic resonance. *Circulation* 2005;111:e24–25.
79. Kim RJ, Wu E, Rafael A, et al. The use of contrast-enhanced magnetic resonance imaging to identify reversible myocardial dysfunction. *N Engl J Med* 2000;343:1445–1453.
80. Wilson RF. Assessing the severity of coronary-artery stenoses [editorial]. *N Engl J Med* 1996;334:1735–1737.
81. Pijls NHJ, De Bruyne B, Peels K, et al. Measurement of fractional flow reserve to assess the functional severity of coronary-artery stenoses. *N Engl J Med* 1996;334:1703–1708.
82. Silagy C, Mant D, Fowler G, et al. *Nicotine replacement therapy for smoking cessation* (Cochrane review) [The Cochrane Library, Issue 2]. Oxford: Update Software, 1997.

83. Forrester JS, Litvack F, Grundfest W, et al. A perspective of coronary disease seen through the arteries of living man. *Circulation* 1987;75:505–513.
84. Nissen SE, Yock P. Intravascular ultrasound: novel pathophysiologic insights and current clinical applications. *Circulation* 2001;103:604–616.
85. Yusuf S, Hawken S, Oupuu S, et al. Effect of potentially modifiable risk factors associated with myocardial infarction in 52 countries (the INTERHEART study): case-control study. *Lancet* 2004;364:937–952.
86. Wilhelmsson C. Coronary heart disease: epidemiology of smoking and intervention studies of smoking. *Am Heart J* 1988;115:242.
87. Kottke TE, Battista RN, DeFriese GH, et al. Attributes of successful smoking cessation interventions in medical practice: a meta-analysis of 39 controlled trials. *JAMA* 1988;259:2883.
88. Miller N, Frieden TR, Liu SY, et al. Effectiveness of a large-scale distribution programme of free nicotine patches: a prospective evaluation. *Lancet* 2005;365:1849.
89. Hughes J, Stead L, Lancaster T. Antidepressants for smoking cessation. *Cochrane Database Syst Rev* 2004;CD000031.
90. Hajek P, Stead LF, West R, Jarvis M. Relapse prevention interventions for smoking cessation. *Cochrane Database Syst Rev* 2005: CD003999.
91. Tang JL, Armitage JM, Lancaster T, et al. Systematic review of dietary intervention trials to lower blood total cholesterol in free-living subjects. *Br Med J* 1998;316:1213.
92. Acquilani R, Tramarin R, Pedretti RFE, et al. Despite good compliance, very low fat diet alone does not achieve recommended cholesterol goals in outpatients with coronary heart disease. *Eur Heart J* 1999;20:1020.
93. de Lorgeril M, Renaud S, Mamelle N, et al. Mediterranean alpha-linoleic acid-rich diet in the secondary prevention of coronary heart disease. *Lancet* 1994;343:1454.
94. Burr ML, Fehily AM, Gilbert JF, et al. Effects of changes in fat, fish and fibre intakes on death and myocardial reinfarction: diet and reinfarction trial. *Lancet* 1994;343:1454.
95. The GISSI-Prevenzione Trial. Dietary supplementation with n-3 polyunsaturated fatty acids and vitamin E after myocardial infarction: results of the GISSI-Prevenzione Trial. *Lancet* 1999;354:447.
96. Knekt P, Reunanen A, Jarvinen R, et al. Antioxidant vitamin intake and coronary mortality in a longitudinal population study. *Am J Epidemiol* 1994;139:1180.
97. Kushi LH, Folsom AR, Prineas RJ, et al. Dietary antioxidant vitamins and death from coronary heart disease in post-menopausal women. *N Engl J Med* 1996;334:1156.
98. Singh RB, Rastogi SS, Verma R, et al. Randomised controlled trial of cardioprotective diet in patients with recent acute myocardial infarction: results of one year follow up. *Br Med J* 1992;304:1015.
99. Stampfer MJ, Hennekens CH, Manson JE, et al. Vitamin E consumption and the risk of coronary heart disease in women. *N Engl J Med* 1993;328:1444.
100. Rimm EB, Stampfer MJ, Ascherio A, et al. Vitamin E consumption and the risk of coronary heart disease in men. *N Engl J Med* 1993;328:1450.
101. The Alpha-Tocopherol, Beta Carotene Cancer Prevention Study Group. The effect of vitamin E and beta carotene on the incidence of lung cancer and other cancers in male smokers. *N Engl J Med* 1994;330:1029.
102. The Heart Outcomes Prevention Evaluation Study Investigators. Vitamin E supplementation and cardiovascular events in high-risk patients. *N Engl J Med* 2000;342:154.
103. Gaziano JM, Buring JE, Breslow JL, et al. Moderate alcohol intake increased levels of high-density lipoprotein and its subfractions, and decreased risk of myocardial infarction. *N Engl J Med* 1993;329:1829.
104. Calle EE, Thun MJ, Petrelli JM, et al. Body-mass index and mortality in a prospective cohort of U.S. adults. *N Engl J Med* 1999;341:1097.
105. Van Gaal LF, Rissanen AM, Scheen AJ, et al., RIO-Europe Study Group. Effects of the cannabinoid-1 receptor blocker rimonabant on weight reduction and cardiovascular risk factors in overweight patients: 1-year experience from the RIO-Europe study. *Lancet* 2005;365:1389.
106. The UK Prospective Diabetes Study (UKPDS) Group. Effect of intensive blood-glucose control with metformin on complications in overweight patients with type 2 diabetes (UKPDS 34). *Lancet* 1998;352:854.
107. The Diabetes Control and Complications Trial Research Group. The effect of intensive treatment of diabetes on the development and progression of long-term complications in insulin-dependent diabetes mellitus. *N Engl J Med* 1993;329:977.
108. Malmberg K. Prospective randomised study of intensive insulin treatment on long term survival after acute myocardial infarction in patients with diabetes mellitus. DIGAMI (Diabetes Mellitus, Insulin Glucose Infusion in Acute Myocardial Infarction) Study Group. *Br Med J* 1997;314:1512.
109. Malmberg K, Norhammar A, Wedel H, et al. Glycometabolic state at admission: important risk marker of mortality in conventionally treated patients with diabetes mellitus and acute myocardial infarction: long-term results from the Diabetes and Insulin-Glucose Infusion in Acute Myocardial Infarction (DIGAMI) study. *Circulation* 1999;99:2626.
110. The University Group Diabetes Program. A study of the effects of hypoglycemic agents on vascular complications in patients with adult-onset diabetes. *Diabetes* 1976;egression analysis. *Br Med J* 1999;318:1730.
111. The UK Prospective Diabetes Study (UKPDS) Group. Intensive blood-glucose control with sulphonylureas or insulin compared with conventional treatment and risk of complications in patients with type 2 diabetes (UKPDS 33). *Lancet* 1998;352:837.
112. Heidenreich PA, McDonald KM, Hastie T, et al. Meta-analysis of trials comparing beta-blockers, calcium antagonists and nitrates for stable angina. *J Am Coll Cardiol* 1999;281:1927.
113. Stone PH, Gibson RS, Glasser SP, et al. Comparison of propranolol, diltiazem and nifedipine in the treatment of ambulatory ischemia in patients with stable angina. *Circulation* 1990;82:1962.
114. Dargie HJ, Ford I, Fox KM. Total Ischaemic Burden European Trial (TIBET). Effects of ischaemia and treatment with atenolol, nifedipine SR and their combination on outcome in patients with chronic stable angina. *Eur Heart J* 1996;7:104.
115. Freemantle N, Cleland J, Young P, et al. ß-blockade after myocardial infarction: systematic review and meta regression analysis. *Br Med J* 1999;318:1730.
116. Miller RR, Olson HG, Amsterdam EA, et al. Propranolol withdrawal rebound phenomenon: exacerbation of coronary events after abrupt cessation of antianginal therapy. *N Engl J Med* 1975;293:416.
117. Psaty BM, Koepsell TD, Wagner EH, et al. The relative risk of incident coronary heart disease associated with recently stopping the use of ß-blockers. *JAMA* 1990;263:1653.
118. The Danish Study Group on Verapamil in Myocardial Infarction. Effect of verapamil on mortality and major events after acute myocardial infarction (The Danish Verapamil Infarction Trial—DAVIT II). *Am J Cardiol* 1990;66:779.
119. Rodrigues EA, Kohli RS, Hains ADB, et al. Comparison of nicardipine and verapamil in the management of chronic stable angina. *Int J Cardiol* 1988;18:357.
120. Bowles MJ, Khurmi NS, O'Hara MJ, et al. Randomised double-blind placebo-controlled comparison of nicardipine and nifedipine in patients with chronic stable angina pectoris. *Chest* 1986;89:260.
121. Friedensohn A, Meshulam R, Schlesinger Z. Randomised double-blind comparison of the effects of isosorbide dinitrate retard, verapamil sustained-release, and their combination on myocardial ischaemic episodes. *Cardiology* 1991;79[Suppl 2]:31.
122. Steffensen R, Grande P, Pedersen F, et al. Effects of atenolol and diltiazem on exercise tolerance and ambulatory ischaemia. *Int J Cardiol* 1993;40:143.
123. van der Does R, Eberhardt R, Derr I, et al. Treatment of chronic stable angina with carvedilol in comparison with nifedipine slow release. *Eur Heart J* 1991;12:60.
124. Poole-Wilson PA, Lubsen J, Kirwen BA, et al. Effect of long-acting nifedipine on mortality and cardiovascular morbidity in patients with stable angina requiring treatment (ACTION trial): randomised controlled trial. *Lancet* 2004;364:849–857.
125. Elkayam U, Amin J, Mehra A, et al. A prospective, randomised, double blind, cross-over study to compare the efficacy and safety of chronic nifedipine therapy with that of isosorbide dinitrate and their combination in the treatment of chronic congestive heart failure. *Circulation* 1990;82:1954.
126. Packer M, O'Connor CM, Ghali JK, et al, for the Prospective Randomized Amlodipine Survival Evaluation Study Group. Effect of amlodipine on mortality and morbidity in severe chronic heart failure. *N Engl J Med* 1996;335:1107.
127. Chrysant SG, Glasser SP, Bittar N, et al. Efficacy and safety of extended release isosorbide mononitrate for stable effort angina pectoris. *Am J Cardiol* 1993;72:1249.
128. Reichek N, Goldstein RE, Redwood DR, et al. Sustained effects of nitroglycerin ointment in patients with angina pectoris. *Circulation* 1974;50:348.
129. Parker JO, Farrell B, Lahey KA, et al. Effect of intervals between doses on the development of tolerance to isosorbide dinitrate. *N Engl J Med* 1987;316:1440.
130. DeMots H, Glasser SP. Intermittent transdermal nitroglycerin therapy in the treatment of chronic stable angina. *J Am Coll Cardiol* 1989;13:786.
131. Matsubara T, Minatoguchi S, Matsuo H, et al. Three minute, but not one minute, ischemia and nicorandil have a preconditioning effect in patients with coronary artery disease. *J Am Coll Cardiol* 2000;35:345.
132. Patel DJ, Purcell HJ, Fox KM. Cardioprotection by opening of the K(ATP) channel in unstable angina. *Eur Heart J* 1999;20:51.
133. Parisi AF, Folland ED, Hartigan P, for the Veterans Affairs ACME Investigators. A comparison of angioplasty with medical therapy in the treatment of single-vessel coronary artery disease. *N Engl J Med* 1992;326:10.
134. The EPISTENT Investigators. Randomised placebo-controlled and balloon-angioplasty-controlled trial to assess safety of coronary stenting with the use of platelet glycoprotein-IIb/IIIa blockade. *Lancet* 1998;352:87.
135. Ellis SG, Weintraub W, Holmes D, et al. Relation of operator volume and experience to procedural outcome of percutaneous coronary revascularization at hospitals with high interventional volumes. *Circulation* 1997;95:2479.
136. Smith SC Jr, Dove JT, Jacobs AK, et al. American College of Cardiology/American Heart Association task force on practice guidelines (Committee to revise the 1993 guidelines for percutaneous transluminal coronary angioplasty); Society for Cardiac Angiography and Interventions. ACC/AHA guidelines for percutaneous coronary intervention (revision of the 1993 PTCA guidelines)-executive summary: a report of the American College of Cardiology/American Heart Association task force on practice guidelines (Committee to revise the 1993 guidelines for percutaneous transluminal coronary angioplasty) endorsed by the Society for Cardiac Angiography and Interventions. *Circulation* 2001;103:3019.

137. Fischman DL, Leon MB, Baim DS, et al, for the STent REStenosis Study Investigators. A randomized comparison of coronary-stent placement and balloon angioplasty in the treatment of coronary artery disease. *N Engl J Med* 1994;331:496.
138. Gruentzig AR, King SB, Schlumpf M, et al. Long-term follow-up after percutaneous transluminal coronary angioplasty: the early Zurich experience. *N Engl J Med* 1987;316:1127.
139. Nobuyoshi M, Kimura T, Nosaka H, et al. Restenosis after successful percutaneous transluminal coronary angioplasty: serial angiographic follow-up of 229 patients. *J Am Coll Cardiol* 1988;12:616.
140. Topol EJ, Califf RM, Weisman HF, et al. Randomised trial of coronary intervention with antibody against platelet IIb/IIIa integrin for reduction of clinical restenosis: results at six months: the EPIC Investigators. *Lancet* 1994;343:881.
141. Serruys PW, de Jaegere P, Kiemeneij F, et al., for the Benestent Study Group. A comparison of balloon-expandable-stent implantation with balloon angioplasty in patients with coronary artery disease. *N Engl J Med* 1994; 331:489.
142. Knight CJ, Curzen NP, Groves PH, et al. Stenting implantation reduces restenosis in patients with suboptimal results following coronary angioplasty. *Eur Heart J* 1999;20:1783.
143. Serruys PW, Emannuelsson H, van der Giessen W, et al. Heparin-coated Palmaz-Schatz stents in human coronary arteries: early outcome of the Benestent-II Pilot Study. *Circulation* 1996;93:412.
144. Versaci F, Gaspardone A, Tomai F, et al. A comparison of coronary-artery stenting with angioplasty for isolated stenosis of the proximal left anterior descending coronary artery. *N Engl J Med* 1997;336:817.
145. Rankin JM, Spinelli JJ, Carere RG, et al. Improved clinical outcome after widespread use of coronary artery stenting in Canada. *N Engl J Med* 1999; 341:1957.
146. Moses JW, Leon MB, Popma JJ, et al. SIRIUS Investigators. Sirolimus-eluting stents versus standard stents in patients with stenosis in a native coronary artery. *N Engl J Med* 2003;349:1315.
147. Strauss WE, Fortin T, Hartigan P, et al, for the Veterans Affairs Study of Angioplasty Compared to Medical Therapy Investigators. A comparison of quality of life scores in patients with angina pectoris after angioplasty compared with after medical therapy: outcomes of a randomized clinical trial. *Circulation* 1995;92:1710.
148. The RITA-2 Trial Participants. Coronary angioplasty versus medical therapy for angina: the second Randomised Intervention Treatment of Angina (RITA-2) trial. *Lancet* 1997;350:461.
149. Pocock SJ, Henderson RA, Clayton T, et al. Quality of life after coronary angioplasty or continued medical treatment for angina: three-year follow-up in the RITA-2 trial. Randomized Intervention Treatment of Angina. *J Am Coll Cardiol* 2000;35:907.
150. Pocock SJ, Henderson RA, Rickards AF, et al. Meta-analysis of randomised trials comparing coronary angioplasty with bypass surgery. *Lancet* 1995;346:1184.
151. The Bypass Angioplasty Revascularization Investigation (BARI) Investigators. Comparison of coronary bypass surgery with angioplasty in patients with multivessel disease. *N Engl J Med* 1996;335:217.
152. Serruys PW, Unger F, Sousa JE, et al. Comparison of coronary-artery bypass surgery and stenting for the treatment of multivessel disease. *N Engl J Med* 2001;344:1117.
153. Stent or Surgery Investigators. Coronary artery bypass surgery versus percutaneous coronary intervention with stent implantation in patients with multivessel coronary artery disease (the Stent or Surgery trial): a randomised controlled trial. *Lancet* 2002;360:965.
154. Mark DB, Nelson CL, Califf RM, et al. Continuing evolution of therapy for coronary artery disease: initial results from the era of coronary angioplasty. *Circulation* 1994;89:2015.
155. Jones RH, Kesler K, Phillips HR, et al. Long-term survival benefits of coronary artery bypass grafting and percutaneous transluminal angioplasty in patients with coronary artery disease. *J Thorac Cardiovasc Surg* 1996;111: 1013.
156. The RITA Trial Participants. Coronary angioplasty versus coronary artery bypass surgery: the Randomized Intervention Treatment of Angina (RITA) trial. *Lancet* 1993;341:573.
157. Ryan TJ, Bauman WB, Kennedy JW, et al. Guidelines for percutaneous transluminal coronary angioplasty: a report of the American College of Cardiology/American Heart Association Task Force on Assessment of Diagnostic and Therapeutic Cardiovascular Procedures (Committee on Percutaneous Transluminal Coronary Angioplasty). *J Am Coll Cardiol* 1993; 22:2033.
158. Weintraub WS, Jones EL, Craver JM, et al. Frequency of repeat coronary bypass or coronary angioplasty after coronary artery bypass surgery using saphenous vein grafts. *Am J Cardiol* 1994;73:103.
159. Stephan WJ, O'Keefe JH, Piehler JM, et al. Coronary angioplasty versus repeat coronary bypass grafting for patients with previous bypass surgery. *J Am Coll Cardiol* 1996;28:1140.
160. Weintraub WS, Jones EL, Morris DC, et al. Outcome of reoperative coronary bypass surgery versus coronary angioplasty after previous bypass surgery. *Circulation* 1997;95:868.
161. Altmann DB, Racz M, Battleman DS, et al. Reduction in angioplasty complications after the introduction of coronary stents: results from a consecutive series of 2242 patients. *Am Heart J* 1996;132:503.
162. Sigwart U, Puel J, Mirkovitch V, et al. Intravascular stents to prevent occlusion and restenosis after transluminal angioplasty. *N Engl J Med* 1987; 316:701.
163. Roubin GS, Cannon AD, Agrawal SK, et al. Intracoronary stenting for acute and threatened closure complicating percutaneous transluminal coronary angioplasty. *Circulation* 1992;85:916.
164. Haude M, Erbel R, Hopp HW, et al. STENT-BY Study: a prospective randomised trial comparing immediate stenting versus conservative treatment strategies in abrupt vessel closure or symptomatic dissections during coronary balloon angioplasty. *Eur Heart J* 1996;17:172. Abstract.
165. Ray SG, Penn IM, Ricci DR, et al. Mechanisms of benefit of stenting in failed angioplasty: final results from the Trial of Angioplasty and Stents in Canada (TASC II). *J Am Coll Cardiol* 1995;25:935–936. Abstract.
166. Macaya C, Serruys PW, Ruygrok P, et al, for the Benestent Study Group. Continued benefit of coronary stenting versus balloon angioplasty: one-year clinical follow-up of Benestent trial. *J Am Coll Cardiol* 1996;27:255.
167. Sirnes PA, Golf S, Myreng Y, et al. Stenting In Chronic Coronary Occlusion (SICCO): a randomised controlled trial of adding stent implantation after successful angioplasty. *J Am Coll Cardiol* 1996;28:1444.
168. Rubartelli P, Niccoli L, Verna E, et al. Stent implantation versus balloon angioplasty in chronic coronary occlusion: results for the GISSOC trial. *J Am Coll Cardiol* 1998;32:90.
169. Hoher M, Wohrle J, Grebe OC, et al. A randomized trial of elective stenting after balloon recanalization of chronic total occlusions. *J Am Coll Cardiol* 1999;34:722.
170. Savage MP, Douglas JS, Fischman DL, et al. Stent placement compared with balloon angioplasty for obstructed coronary bypass grafts: Saphenous Vein De Novo Trial Investigators. *N Engl J Med* 1997;337:740.
171. Colombo A, Ferraro M, Itoh A, et al. Results of coronary stenting for restenosis. *J Am Coll Cardiol* 1996;28:830.
172. Erbel R, Haude M, Hopp HW, et al, for the REstenosis STent (REST) Study. Coronary-artery stenting compared with balloon angioplasty for restenosis after initial balloon angioplasty. *N Engl J Med* 1998;339:1672.
173. Serruys PW, van Hout B, Bonnier H, et al. Randomised comparison of implantation of heparin-coated stents with balloon angioplasty in selected patients with coronary artery disease. *Lancet* 1998;352:673.
174. Rodriguez A, Ayala F, Bernardi V, et al. Optimal coronary balloon angioplasty with provisional stenting versus primary stent (OCBAS): immediate and long-term follow-up results. *J Am Coll Cardiol* 1998;32:1351.
175. Kimura T, Yokoi H, Nakagawa Y, et al. Three-year follow-up after implantation of metallic coronary-artery stents. *N Engl J Med* 1996;334: 561.
176. Betriu A, Masotti M, Serra A, et al. Randomized comparison of coronary stent implantation and balloon angioplasty in the treatment of de novo coronary artery lesions (START): a four year follow-up. *J Am Coll Cardiol* 1999;34:1498.
177. The Antiplatelet Trialists' Collaboration. Collaborative overview of randomised trials of antiplatelet therapy, I: prevention of death, myocardial infarction, and stroke by prolonged antiplatelet therapy in various categories of patients. *Br Med J* 1994;308:81.
178. The Antiplatelet Trialists' Collaboration. Collaborative overview of randomised trials of antiplatelet therapy, II: maintenance of vascular graft or arterial patency by antiplatelet therapy. *Br Med J* 1994;308:159.
179. Schömig A, Neumann FJ, Kastrati A, et al. A randomized comparison of antiplatelet and anticoagulant therapy after the placement of coronary-artery stents. *N Engl J Med* 1996;334:1084.
180. Leon MB, Baim DS, Popma JJ, et al, for the STent Anticoagulation Restenosis Study Investigators. A clinical trial comparing three antithrombotic-drug regimens after coronary-artery stenting. *N Engl J Med* 1998;339:1665.
181. Berger PB, Bell MR, Rihal CS, et al. Clopidogrel versus ticlopidine after intracoronary stent placement. *J Am Coll Cardiol* 1999;34:1891.
182. Brookes CIO, Sigwart U. Taming platelets in coronary stenting: ticlopidine out, clopidogrel in? Heart 1999;82:651.
183. The EPIC Investigators. Use of a monoclonal antibody directed against the platelet glycoprotein IIb/IIIa receptor in high-risk coronary angioplasty. *N Engl J Med* 1994;330:956.
184. The EPILOG Investigators. Platelet glycoprotein IIb/IIIa receptor blockade and low-dose heparin during percutaneous coronary revascularization. *N Engl J Med* 1997;336:1689.
185. The IMPACT Study Investigators. Randomised placebo-controlled trial of effect of eptifibatide on complications of percutaneous coronary intervention: IMPACT-II. Integrilin to Minimise Platelet Aggregation and Coronary Thrombosis-II. *Lancet* 1997;349:1422.
186. The CAPTURE Study Investigators. Randomised placebo-controlled trial of abciximab before and during coronary intervention in refractory unstable angina: the CAPTURE Study. *Lancet* 1997;349:1429.
187. Topol EJ, Mark DB, Lincoff AM, et al. Outcomes at 1 year and economic implications of platelet glycoprotein IIb/IIIa blockade in patients undergoing coronary stenting: results from a multicentre randomised trial. *Lancet* 1999;354:2019.
188. Kong DF, Califf RM, Miller DP, et al. Clinical outcomes of therapeutic agents that block the glycoprotein IIb/IIIa integrin in ischemic heart disease. *Circulation* 1998;98:2829.
189. Kastrati A, Mehilli J, Schuhlen H, et al. Intracoronary Stenting and Antithrombotic Regimen-Rapid Early Action for Coronary Treatment Study Investigators. A clinical trial of abciximab in elective percutaneous coronary

intervention after pretreatment with clopidogrel. *N Engl J Med* 2004;350:232.
190. The Coronary Artery Surgery Study (CASS). A randomized trial of coronary artery bypass surgery: quality of life in patients randomly assigned to treatment groups. *Circulation* 1983;68:951.
191. The Veterans Affairs Coronary Artery Bypass Surgery Cooperative Study Group. Eighteen-year follow-up in the Veterans Affairs Cooperative Study of Coronary Artery Bypass Surgery for stable angina. *Circulation* 1992;86:121.
192. The European Coronary Surgery Study Group. Prospective randomised study of coronary artery bypass surgery in stable angina pectoris: second interim report by the European Coronary Surgery Study Group. *Lancet* 1980;ii:491.
193. Yusuf S, Zucker D, Peduzzi P, et al. Effect of coronary artery bypass graft surgery on survival: overview of 10-year results from randomised trials by the Coronary Artery Bypass Graft Surgery Trialists Collaboration. *Lancet* 1994;344:563.
194. Sjoland H, Wiklund I, Caidahl K, et al. Improvement in quality of life and exercise capacity after coronary bypass surgery. *Arch Intern Med* 1996;156:265.
195. Caine N, Harrison SCW, Sharples LD, et al. Prospective study of quality of life before and after coronary artery bypass grafting. *Br Med J* 1991;302:511.
196. Loop FD, Lytle BW, Cosgrove DM, et al. Influence of the internal-mammary-artery graft on 10-year survival and other cardiac events. *N Engl J Med* 1986;314:1.
197. Azariades M, Fessler CL, Floten HS, et al. Five-year results of coronary bypass grafting for patients older than 70 years: role of internal mammary artery. *Ann Thorac Surg* 1990;50:940.
198. Boylan MJ, Lytle BW, Loop FD, et al. Surgical treatment of isolated left anterior descending coronary stenosis: comparison of left internal mammary artery and venous autograft at 18 to 20 years of follow-up. *J Thorac Cardiovasc Surg* 1994;107:657.
199. Barner HB, Standeven JW, Reese J. Twelve-year experience with internal mammary artery for coronary artery bypass. *J Thorac Cardiovasc Surg* 1985;90:668.
200. O'Connor GT, Morton JR, Diehl MJ, et al, for the Northern New England Cardiovascular Disease Study Group. Differences between men and women in hospital mortality associated with coronary artery bypass graft surgery. *Circulation* 1993;88:2104.
201. The CAPRIE Steering Committee. A randomised, blinded, trial of clopidogrel versus aspirin in patients at risk of ischaemic events. *Lancet* 1996;348:1329.
202. The Scandinavian Simvastatin Survival Study Group. Randomised trial of cholesterol lowering in 4444 patients with coronary heart disease: the Scandinavian Simvastatin Survival Study (4S). *Lancet* 1994;344:1383.
203. Sacks FM, Pfeffer MA, Moye LA, et al. The effect of pravastatin on coronary events after myocardial infarction in patients with average cholesterol levels. *N Engl J Med* 1996;335:1001.
204. The LIPID Study Group. Prevention of cardiovascular events and death with pravastatin in patients with coronary heart disease and a broad range of initial cholesterol levels. *N Engl J Med* 1998;339:1349.
205. The Post Coronary Artery Bypass Graft Trial Investigators. The effect of aggressive lowering of low-density lipoprotein cholesterol levels and low-dose anticoagulation on obstructive changes in saphenous-vein coronary-artery bypass grafts. *N Engl J Med* 1997;336:153.
206. Pitt B, Waters D, Brown WV, et al., for the Atorvastatin VErsus Revascularization Treatment Investigators. Aggressive lipid-lowering therapy compared with angioplasty in stable coronary artery disease. *N Engl J Med* 1999;341:70.
207. MRC/BHF Heart Protection Study of cholesterol lowering with simvastatin in 20,536 high-risk individuals: a randomised placebo-controlled trial. *Lancet*. 2002;360:7.
208. Cannon CP, Braunwald E, McCabe CH, et al. Pravastatin or atorvastatin evaluation and infection therapy—thrombolysis in myocardial infarction 22 investigators. Intensive versus moderate lipid lowering with statins after acute coronary syndromes. *N Engl J Med* 2004;350:1495.
209. LaRosa JC, Grundy SM, Waters DD, et al. Treating to New Targets (TNT) Investigators. Intensive lipid lowering with atorvastatin in patients with stable coronary disease. *N Engl J Med* 2005;352:1425.
210. Bloomfield Rubins H, Robins SJ, Collins D, et al, for the Veterans Affairs High-Density Lipoprotein Cholesterol Intervention Trial Study Group. Gemfibrozil for the secondary prevention of coronary heart disease in men with low levels of high-density lipoprotein cholesterol. *N Engl J Med* 1999;341:410.
211. Gottlieb SS, McCarter RJ, Vogel RA. Effect of ß-blockade on mortality among high risk and low risk patients after myocardial infarction. *N Engl J Med* 1998;339:489.
212. Beevers DG, Johnston JH, Larkin H, et al. Clinical evidence that ß-adrenoreceptor blockers prevent more cardiovascular complications than other antihypertensive drugs. *Drugs* 1983;25[Suppl 2]:326.
213. Nidorf SM, Thompson PL, Jamrozik KD, Hobbs MST. Reduced risk of death at 28 days in patients taking ß-blocker before admission to hospital with myocardial infarction. *Br Med J* 1990;300:71.
214. Mimran A, Ducailar G. Systemic and regional haemodynamic profile of diuretics and alpha- and beta-blockers. Drugs 1988;35[Suppl 6]:60.
215. Hiatt WR, Stoll S, Nies AS. Effect of ß-adrenergic blockers on the peripheral circulation in patients with peripheral vascular disease. *Circulation* 1985;72:1226.
216. Packer M, Bristow MR, Cohn JN, et al., for the U.S. Carvedilol Heart Failure Study Group. The effect of carvedilol on morbidity and mortality in patients with chronic heart failure. *N Engl J Med* 1996;334:1349.
217. The CIBIS II Investigators and Committees. The Cardiac Insufficiency Bisoprolol Study II (CIBIS II): a randomised trial. *Lancet* 1999;353:9.
218. The CONSENSUS Trial Study Group. Effects of enalapril on mortality in severe congestive heart failure: results of the Cooperative North Scandinavian Enalapril Survival Study (CONSENSUS). *N Engl J Med* 1987;316:1429.
219. The SOLVD Investigators. Effect of enalapril on survival in patients with reduced left ventricular ejection fractions and congestive heart failure. *N Engl J Med* 1991;325:293.
220. The Heart Outcomes Prevention Evaluation Study Investigators. Effects of an angiotensin-converting enzyme inhibitor, ramipril, on cardiovascular events in high-risk patients. *N Engl J Med* 2000;342:145.
221. Angiotensin-converting-enzyme inhibition in stable coronary artery disease. *N Engl J Med* 2004;351:2058.
222. Cox J, Naylor CD. The Canadian Cardiovascular Society grading scale for angina pectoris: is it time for refinements? *Ann Intern Med* 1992;117:677.
223. Califf RM, Harrell FE, Lee KL, et al. The evolution of medical and surgical therapy for coronary artery disease: a 15 year perspective. *JAMA* 1989;261:2077.
224. Linden W, Stossel C, Maurice J. Psychosocial interventions for patients with coronary artery disease: a meta-analysis. *Arch Intern Med* 1996;156:745.
225. Oldridge NB, Guyatt GH, Fischer ME, Rimm AA. Cardiac rehabilitation after myocardial infarction: combined experience of randomised controlled trials. *JAMA* 1988;260:945.
226. Hedbäck B, Perk J, Wodlin P. Long-term reduction of cardiac mortality after myocardial infarction: 10-year results of a comprehensive rehabilitation programme. *Eur Heart J* 1993;14:831.

CHAPTER 18 ■ UNSTABLE ANGINA: ISCHEMIC SYNDROMES

HARVEY D. WHITE

OVERVIEW

The prevalence of non–ST-elevation acute coronary syndromes (NSTEACS) is increasing. The major pathophysiologic mechanism is plaque rupture or fissuring with superimposed thrombus. Risk profiling should be performed at admission and repeated on several subsequent occasions to incorporate new information regarding the patient's response to therapy and risk factors. Treatment should be tailored according to individual patient characteristics and risk.

Patients should initially receive intensive antithrombotic therapy to passivate the thrombotic activity of the culprit unstable plaque. The optimal antithrombotic regimen has not yet been defined. Aspirin reduces the risk of cardiac events by 20%. In comparison with unfractionated heparin (UFH), enoxaparin has been shown to reduce the combined incidence of death and myocardial infarction (MI) by 9% at 30 days, and may be favored for patients being managed conservatively because of its ease of use. In patients managed invasively, enoxaparin and UFH produce similar outcomes, although enoxaparin is associated with a modest increase in bleeding. In patients not selected for early percutaneous coronary intervention (PCI), glycoprotein (GP) IIb/IIIa antagonists have been shown to reduce 30-day death/MI rates by 9% overall and by 18% in patients with elevated troponin levels, although there was no benefit in patients without elevated troponin levels. Adjunctive use of clopidogrel with aspirin has a synergistic effect, reducing cardiovascular death/MI/stroke by 20% in patients with and patients without elevated troponin levels.

β-Blockers, nitrates, and calcium channel antagonists relieve angina, but have no significant effect on intracoronary thrombus and do not necessarily reduce the risk of death/MI. The risk of cardiac events is decreased by reduction of low-density lipoprotein cholesterol (LDL-C) levels to below 62 mg/dL (1.6 mmol/L) using early aggressive statin therapy.

Early angiography and revascularization are integral to the management of NSTEACS. When compared with conservative medical treatment, early revascularization reduces the risk of death/MI in high-risk patients, decreases the need for antianginal medications, allows a shorter hospital stay, and results in fewer readmissions. This approach is cost effective in many healthcare settings. Patients selected for early revascularization should have the procedure within 48 hours of admission; the optimal timing of intervention has not yet been established. Intermediate-risk patients should be admitted to a coronary care or chest pain unit, monitored closely, and given intensive antithrombotic therapy. If patients become high-risk (i.e., they have recent ischemia or their troponin levels rise), they should have early angiography and revascularization if appropriate. If symptoms settle and troponin levels are not elevated, patients should be managed according to whether or not they have inducible ischemia. Low-risk patients should be discharged early with appropriate arrangements for follow-up and review.

The risk of ischemic events remains high in patients with NSTEACS, and management continues to pose a major clinical challenge. Better treatments and new therapeutic strategies are needed. It is important that evidence-based therapies be used and that primary and secondary preventative measures be instituted to reduce the community burden of acute coronary syndromes (ACS).

GLOSSARY

Conservative management: Risk profiling and medical therapy with selective use of angiography and revascularization procedures depending on symptoms, response to therapy, and the presence of inducible ischemia at low workloads or low doses of pharmacologic agents.

Invasive management: Medical therapy plus early coronary angiography and revascularization.

Plaque instability: Propensity for atheromatous plaque to rupture or fissure.

Plaque passivation: Inactivation of the platelet-active surface of a ruptured or fissured plaque.

Rebound ischemia: Increase in ischemic events when heparin therapy is stopped.

Risk profiling: Estimation of the risk of coronary events (usually death or MI) by assessment of patient characteristics and investigative findings.

INTRODUCTION

The first documented description of a patient with an acute ischemic syndrome is in the Ebers papyrus from 2,600 BCE, which states, "If you find a man with heart discomfort, with pain in his arms, at the side of his heart, death is near." This description remains apt, but the prognosis has changed over the centuries. Today, unstable angina is one of the commonest causes of hospitalization (1). Each year, more than 1.4 million patients in the United States (2) and more than 4 million worldwide (3) are hospitalized with NSTEACS. These numbers will continue to rise as the prevalence of patients with obesity and diabetes increases (3).

The syndromes of unstable angina, non–ST-elevation MI (NSTEMI) and ST-elevation MI (STEMI) are a continuum, and the pathophysiology is heterogeneous and dynamic. Clinical presentation depends on the severity of the arterial injury, the size and type of thrombus formed, the extent and duration of ischemia, and the amount of previous myocardial necrosis. The extent of ischemia depends on the myocardial distribution of the ischemia-producing artery, the severity of the ischemia-producing stenosis, the absence or presence of collateral circulation, and factors that affect the supply of oxygenated blood or that increase myocardial demands, such as the heart rate, blood pressure, and contractility. Patients may die or may develop MI, recurrent ischemia, heart failure, arrhythmia, or a stroke.

DEFINITIONS

Acute coronary syndromes describes a spectrum of clinical syndromes ranging from unstable angina to NSTEMI and STEMI. Patients presenting with ACS are divided into those with ST elevation (lasting $\geq$20 minutes) or new left bundle branch block, and those with NSTEACS which includes transient ST elevation (lasting <20 minutes), unstable angina, and NSTEMI (4).

Unstable angina is a syndrome intermediate between chronic stable angina and MI. It is a clinical diagnosis based on a history of chest pain and exclusion of the diagnosis of MI by electrocardiography (ECG) and biomarker testing for myocardial necrosis. The chest pain may be prolonged at rest or of new onset, may represent accelerating symptoms of previously stable angina, or may occur after MI. Patients presenting without ST elevation on the ECG are diagnosed as having either NSTEMI or unstable angina based on whether or not their troponin or creatine kinase (CK)-MB levels are elevated (5). Between 2% and 15% of patients diagnosed with unstable angina subsequently develop Q-wave MI.

The unstable angina classification developed by Braunwald (6) is based on the severity of symptoms, their clinical context, and the intensity of medical treatment. The classification has been validated clinically (7), has been shown to correlate with coronary angiographic findings (8), and has now been updated to include troponin levels (Table 18.1) (9). Prinzmetal angina (recurrent rest angina accompanied by ST elevation on the ECG owing to coronary artery spasm) is considered a separate entity (10).

PATHOPHYSIOLOGY

The five major causes of ACS are thrombus, mechanical obstruction, dynamic obstruction, inflammation, and increased oxygen demand (11). The major pathophysiologic mechanism is rupture or fissuring of an atheromatous plaque with superimposed thrombus (12–15). Other mechanisms include superficial erosion (which is more common in women), intraplaque hemorrhage, and erosion of a calcified nodule (16). Patients with ACS often have more than one ulcerated plaque, as shown by angiography (17), intravascular ultrasound (18), angioscopy (19), and release of inflammatory markers such as myeloperoxidase across nonculprit coronary vascular beds (20). Multiple plaque ruptures are more common in patients with increased C-reactive protein (CRP) levels (21).

In some patients, thrombogenicity of the blood (sometimes referred to as "vulnerable blood" leading to the concept of "vulnerable patients") is implicated, with alterations in circulatory prothrombotic or antifibrinolytic mechanisms. Levels of

TABLE 18.1

CLASSIFICATION OF UNSTABLE ANGINA (9)[a]

Severity	Clinical circumstances: (A) Develops in presence of extracardiac condition that intensifies myocardial ischemia (secondary unstable angina)	(B) Develops in absence of extracardiac condition (primary unstable angina)	(C) Develops within 2 weeks after acute MI (postinfarction unstable angina)
(I) New onset of severe angina or accelerated angina; no rest pain	IA	IB	IC
(II) Angina at rest within past month but not within preceding 48 hours (angina at rest, subacute)	IIA	IIB	IIC
(III) Angina at rest within 48 hours (angina at rest, acute)	IIIA	IIIB (troponin negative) IIIB (troponin positive)	IIIC

[a]Patients with unstable angina can also be divided into three groups, depending on whether unstable angina occurs: (a) in the absence of treatment for chronic stable angina; (b) during treatment for chronic stable angina; or (c) despite maximal antiischemic drug therapy. These three groups can be designated by subscripts 1, 2, or 3, respectively. Patients with unstable angina can be further divided into those with and those without transient ST-T-wave changes during chest pain.

(*Source:* Adapted from Hamm CW, Braunwald E. A classification of unstable angina revisited. *Circulation* 2000;102:118–122, with permission.)

plasminogen activator inhibitor-1 are increased in patients with obesity or diabetes (22).

Superficial fissuring of a plaque usually results in platelet deposition. There is less superimposed thrombus formation in patients with NSTEACS than in those with STEMI, which is usually associated with deep arterial injury and occlusive thrombus (Fig. 18.1) (14,15). Angioscopic findings show that the thrombus associated with unstable angina is white or gray and consists mostly of platelets, whereas the thrombus associated with STEMI consists mostly of red blood cells (23).

Inflammation plays a major role in atherosclerosis (24,25), and activation of macrophages triggers inflammatory processes that lead to plaque instability, procoagulation, and clinical events. Plaque rupture or fissuring can be triggered by increased shear forces with sudden changes in pressure or tone. Rupture most often occurs on minor plaques (26–31) that are eccentric (32) and have a large lipid core with a thin fibrous cap (33), increased concentrations of macrophages (34), and local expression of tissue factor. Macrophages produce metalloproteases such as collagenase, elastases, and stromelysins, which digest extracellular matrix (25). Macrophage-rich areas are more commonly found in atherectomy specimens from patients with unstable angina than from those with stable angina (35). Activated T lymphocytes are present at sites of plaque rupture (36) and they release various cytokines which activate macrophages and promote smooth muscle cell proliferation (25). Mast cells are found on plaque edges at sites that are likely to rupture (37). Increased levels of CRP (38) and its major inducer, interleukin-6 (39), have been found in patients with unstable angina, and are associated with higher rates of death/MI at hospital discharge and at 1 year (40–42).

The inflammatory stimulus for triggering expression of soluble cell adhesion molecules has been shown to persist for 6 months after presentation with NSTEACS (43). The inflammatory nature of the cells at the site of plaque rupture and shared T-cell receptor sequences in clonotypes from different patients (43,44) have led to speculation that chronic stimulation by a common antigen or certain bacterial infections, such as *Chlamydia pneumoniae* or *Helicobacter pylori*, may be associated with an increased risk of plaque rupture (45–47).

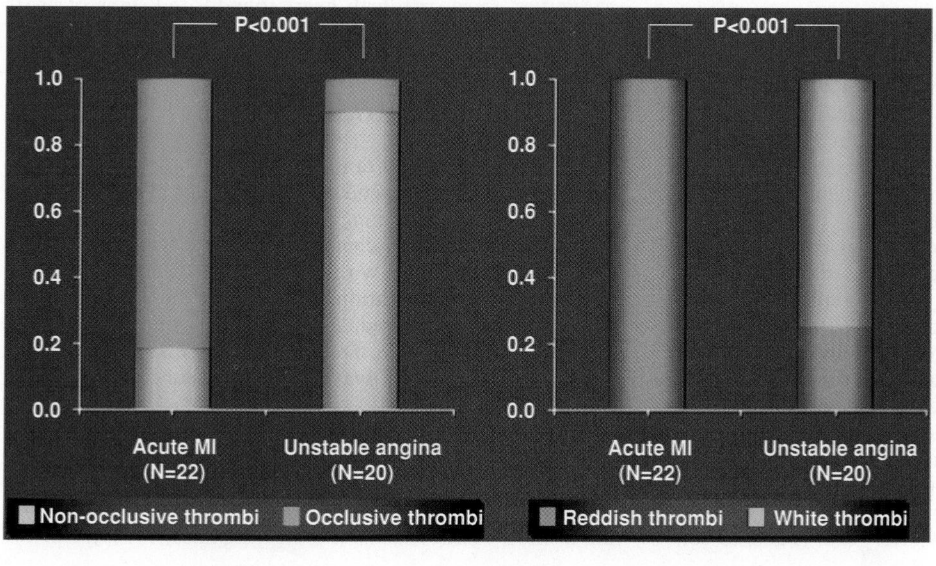

FIGURE 18.1. Angioscopic findings in acute ischemic syndromes showing (*left*) the proportions of occlusive and nonocclusive thrombi and (*right*) the differing character of thrombi in acute MI and unstable angina (23). (*Source:* Redrawn from Mizuno K. Angioscopy in acute coronary syndromes. *Cardiology Today* 1992;20:1, with permission.)

The T-cell response in patients with unstable angina is antigen-driven and directed toward antigens carried in culprit coronary atherosclerotic plaques (48). Cytomegalovirus has been found in atheromatous plaque specimens, but active replication of the virus is not thought to be a major cause of plaque instability (49).

After plaque rupture or fissuring, subendothelial adhesive proteins, collagen tissue factor, and von Willebrand factor are exposed, and tissue factor is released. Platelets adhere to GP Ia and Ib, change their shape, and release serotonin, thromboxane A_2, and adenosine diphosphate (ADP). In animal models, episodic platelet aggregation at sites of coronary stenosis has been shown to cause cyclic coronary blood flow (50). Platelet emboli have been found downstream from atheromatous plaques in small intramyocardial vessels from patients who have died suddenly (51). Platelet activation may manifest in anginal episodes associated with increased urinary levels of thromboxane B_2 (52).

Released tissue factor combines with factor VII, stimulating the extrinsic coagulation cascade to form thrombin, a very potent stimulus of platelet aggregation. At the platelet surface, factors V and X are activated to form the prothrombinase complex, which generates more thrombin. Damage to endothelium without plaque rupture may also result in thrombus formation (53). Evidence of a hypercoagulable state has been found in patients with unstable angina (54). During anginal episodes, increases occur in the plasma concentrations of prothrombin fragments 1 and 2 (signifying increased activity of factor X_a and thrombin formation) and fibrinopeptide A (a sign of increased thrombin activity and fibrin formation). These markers remain elevated for at least 6 months after ACS (55), and platelets remain activated for at least 28 days (56). Intracoronary thrombus is visualized in 35% to 52% of patients having coronary angiography for unstable angina (8,57–59); the detection rate rises to 70% to 93% when angioscopy is performed (23,58,60–62). The presence of thrombus at angiography denotes an increased risk of recurrent ischemia and MI (57). Another potential mechanism of ACS is increased narrowing of a coronary artery due to progression of atherosclerosis or plaque rupture (63).

Cocaine is toxic to the heart, and its use may be associated with ACS, even in patients with angiographically normal coronary arteries (64). There is a circadian variation in the onset of ACS (65). Platelet aggregation increases in the morning, elevating the risk of MI or sudden death (66). Activities such as heavy exertion, which produces acute physiologic effects, may also trigger ischemic events (67).

Coronary Artery Spasm

In 1959, Prinzmetal et al. (10) described a variant form of angina characterized by chest pain predominantly at rest and usually associated with ST elevation on the ECG. Rarely, variant angina is associated with other vasospastic disorders (such as migraine or Raynaud syndrome) in patients with angiographically normal coronary arteries.

Physiologic contraction of an epicardial coronary artery may be triggered by stimuli such as increased adrenergic activity (68), increased vagal activity (69), secretion of vasoconstrictor substances such as thromboxane A_2 (70), and increased production of endothelin-1 by endothelial cells (71). Increased vasomotor hyperreactivity may be localized to regions of coronary atheroma or may occur in angiographically normal arterial segments (72). In the presence of endothelial dysfunction, stimuli such as acetylcholine that normally cause vasodilation may instead cause vasoconstriction (73). In the presence of a severe atherosclerotic stenosis (particularly one that is eccentric with an arc of normal coronary artery that is able to contract), increased coronary tone can cause a critical reduction in coronary blood flow. Cold-pressor testing has demonstrated excessive vasoreactivity in unstable angina patients compared with stable angina patients (74).

Pathophysiologic Implications for Clinical Management

The management of patients with NSTEACS should focus on the pathophysiology (11). The primary aims of treatment are to reduce initial symptoms and ischemia, prevent MI, minimize necrosis in the event of MI, and reduce mortality. In individual patients, the mechanisms of plaque rupture or fissuring, platelet aggregation, thrombus formation, and increased vasomotor tone may play different roles at different times. A variety of therapeutic approaches are needed to modify these processes.

The mainstays of medical management are intensive antithrombotic therapy with aspirin and heparin (75) (either UFH [75] or low-molecular-weight heparin [LMWH] [76]), and antiplatelet therapy with clopidogrel (77) and/or GP IIb/IIIa antagonists (78). β-Blockers, nitrates, and calcium channel antagonists should be used for relief of symptoms. Early angiography and revascularization are recommended for patients at high risk or with recurrent symptoms. Risk profiling is pivotal to triage, and the results determine whether patients should be discharged early, admitted and monitored closely, or have early angiography and revascularization (Fig. 18.2).

Patients with an increased oxygen demand or a decreased oxygen supply (e.g., those with anemia or thyrotoxicosis) need to be managed appropriately. Patients with vasospasm require therapies such as nitrates and calcium channel antagonists. It has not yet been established how patients with evidence of inflammation should be managed, although falls in CRP levels have been noted with aspirin (79) and with statins, which improve outcomes independently of their effect on LDL-C (80,81).

CLINICAL PROFILE

History and Physical Examination

The physical findings and the site, character, and radiation of the discomfort are similar to those seen in patients with MI. The physical examination is usually normal unless ischemia causes signs of poor tissue perfusion, with sweating, tachycardia, cool extremities, third or fourth heart sounds, and signs of heart failure or cardiogenic shock.

Electrocardiography

The ECG is a very important investigative tool; prognosis and management critical depend on ECG findings. An ECG should be performed at admission, daily throughout hospitalization, and during episodes of ischemia. If there are symptoms lasting longer than 20 minutes with ST elevation or new left bundle branch block, administration of fibrinolytic therapy or primary PCI should be considered. A normal ECG does not exclude the possibility of an ACS. Transient ST depression (or, less frequently, elevation) and T-wave inversion occur commonly only during ischemia (82–85).

In the Global Use of Strategies to Open Occluded Coronary Arteries (GUSTO)-IIB trial, patients with 2 mm of ST depression in two ECG leads had 6 to 10 times the mortality rate of patients with normal ECGs (86). ST depression of 0.5 mm or more has been shown to be a significant risk factor for

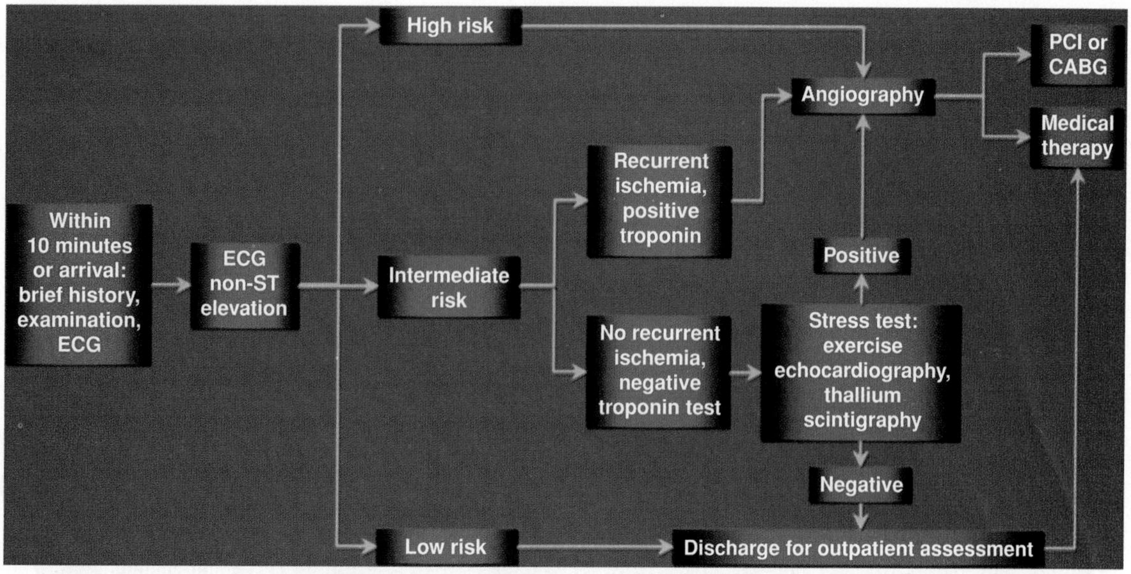

FIGURE 18.2. Algorithm for management of NSTEACS.

death/MI at 1 (84) and 4 years (85). In GUSTO-IIB, patients with ST depression were more likely to have triple-vessel disease (36%), whereas those with T-wave inversion were more likely to have normal coronary arteries (19%). Thirty-day mortality was 5.1% in those with ST depression and 1.7% in those with isolated T-wave inversion (83). Patients with inverted T waves in 5 leads or more are at higher risk (87) and have better outcomes with revascularization than with conservative therapy (88). Little information is available regarding the outcome of patients with deep T-wave inversion (>0.2 mV), who are usually classified as being at intermediate risk.

In the Fragmin During Instability in Coronary Artery Disease (FRISC) trial, the benefit of early revascularization was proportional to the depth of ST depression (89), and this association was independent of age, gender, and troponin levels. Revascularization was most beneficial in patients who had both ST depression and elevated troponin levels (90). However, the Treat Angina With Aggrastat and Determine Cost of Therapy with an Invasive or Conservative Strategy–Thrombolysis in Myocardial Infarction-18 (TACTICS–TIMI-18) trial (91) and the Randomised Intervention Trial of Unstable Angina (RITA-3) trial (92) found no association between ST-segment changes and the benefits of revascularization.

Continuous Electrocardiographic Monitoring

Ischemic ST-segment changes are detected on continuous ECG monitoring in 85% to 90% of patients with unstable angina, but the changes are often silent (93,94). Silent ischemia during Holter monitoring has been shown to correlate with reduced myocardial perfusion and impaired ventricular function (94), and patients with silent ischemia are more likely to die, develop MI, or require revascularization (94–96). The European Society of Cardiology (ESC) guidelines for the management of NSTEACS (97) recommend that patients should have multilead continuous ST-segment monitoring if it is available or, failing that, frequent ECGs.

Chest X-Ray

Unless MI has occurred previously, heart size is usually normal. Transient pulmonary edema may occur with global ischemia, and suggests the possibility of a left main coronary stenosis.

Troponins

The cardiac troponins are sensitive and specific markers of myocyte necrosis (98) and are the markers of choice for the diagnosis of MI (5). Short- and long-term studies have shown that troponin levels correlate with the risk of death and the combined risk of death/MI (99–103), with a clear gradient of risk as troponin levels increase (100,104). Troponin levels have been shown to be more powerful prognosticators than CK-MB levels (105). Thirty percent of patients who present with NSTEACS and normal CK-MB levels have elevated troponin levels (100,102,106), and these patients have poor outcomes. The combination of troponin T testing and exercise testing further defines patients at low, intermediate, and high risk (107).

Elevated troponin levels correlate with the pathophysiology of ACS (the presence of thrombus in the coronary artery) (108), and reflect the thrombogenic activity of ruptured or fissured plaques with embolism downstream and resultant myocyte necrosis (90,108). The prognostic value of troponins is greater than would be expected from the extent of myocyte necrosis and left ventricular impairment, perhaps reflecting preceding episodes of embolic episodes (Fig. 18.3) (109). Angiographic studies have shown that evidence of thrombus, complex lesions, and a reduced TIMI flow grade (110) were more common in patients with elevated troponin levels than in those with normal levels (90,108).

Troponin levels identify patients who are most likely to benefit from LMWH (106), GP IIb/IIIa antagonists (104,111,112), and revascularization (91,113). Troponin testing may be the only biomarker assay needed if utilized in a chest pain pathway (114). Point-of-care testing is recommended in institutions that cannot consistently deliver laboratory results within 1 hour for logistical reasons (115). Baseline point-of-care use of a multimarker assay including myoglobin (which is released earlier than troponins) has been shown to be a more effective means of risk profiling than single-marker, laboratory-based testing (116).

Troponins are very sensitive markers of myocyte necrosis, and elevated levels may be detected in contexts other than spontaneous myocardial ischemia or PCI (117). Apart from ACS, the most common causes of elevated troponin levels are atrial or ventricular tachycardia (often with hypotension and an increased myocardial oxygen demand), pulmonary emboli with right ventricular MI, cardiac failure (118), cardiac surgery,

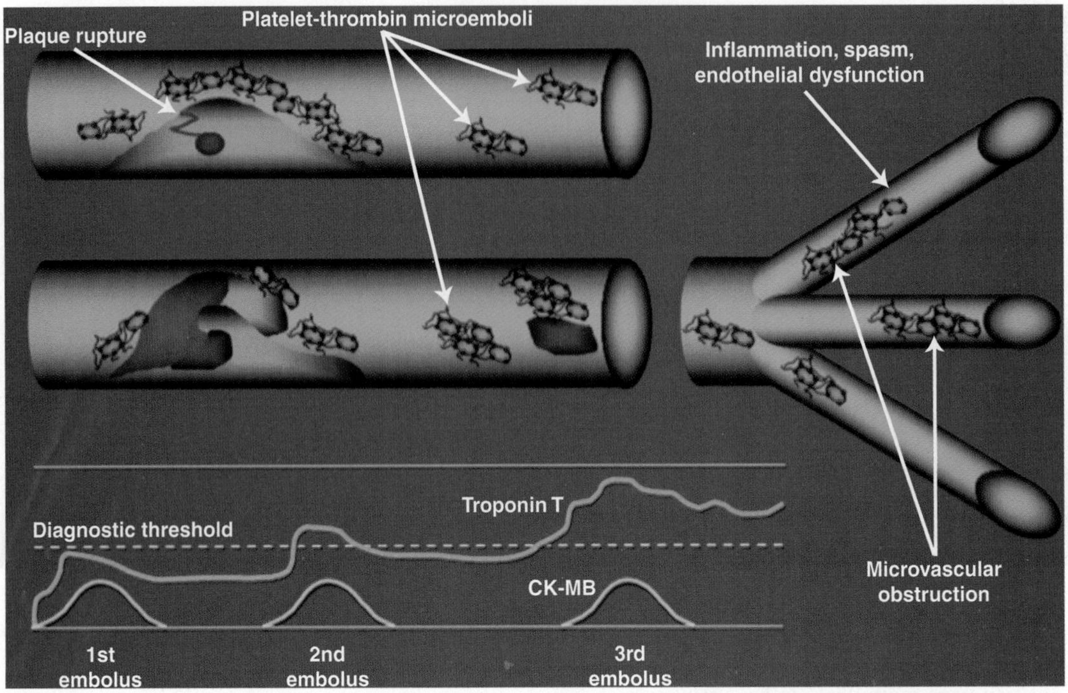

FIGURE 18.3. Microvascular obstruction after plaque rupture (109). (*Source:* Adapted from Goldmann BU, Christenson RH, Hamm CW, et al. Implications of troponin testing in clinical medicine. Curr Control Trials Cardiovasc Med 2001;2:75–84, with permission.)

myocarditis, and renal failure. Other tests such as myosin light-chain assays (119) are not currently recommended as standard practice.

White Blood Cell Count

The white blood cell count is usually normal. An elevated count is associated with higher risks of mortality and MI (120–122).

Renal Function

Impaired renal function is associated with a poor prognosis (123–126) and requires modification of the dosing regimen if LMWH is used (127).

Inflammatory Markers

There has been extensive research into the roles of inflammation and inflammatory markers in NSTEACS. The levels of high-sensitivity CRP, interleukin-6 and, more recently, CD-40 ligand (which has prothrombotic effects) have been shown to provide independent prognostic information (128). Elevated levels of other inflammatory markers such as adhesion molecules (129), interleukin-7 (130), and matrix-metalloproteinases (including pregnancy-associated plasma protein A) (131) have also been observed in patients with NSTEACS.

C-Reactive Protein

CRP is an acute-phase protein produced by the liver when there is tissue injury, infection, or inflammation. High-sensitivity CRP levels are elevated in 50% to 70% of patients with Braunwald class IIIB angina (40). Patients with elevated CRP levels at admission have been shown to have worse in-hospital and 1-year outcomes, and elevated levels at discharge have been associated with recurrent instability in the long term (41). In the TIMI-11A study, mortality at 14 days was 9.1% when both CRP and troponin levels were elevated compared with 4.7% if either was elevated and 0.4% if neither was elevated (132). The major application of CRP testing appears to be in determining the long-term prognosis after hospital discharge. Low CRP levels have been observed with aspirin (79) and statin therapy (133).

CD40 Ligand

CD40 ligand is expressed on activated platelets, and is prothrombotic and proinflammatory (134,135). Elevated levels are associated with increased rates of death, MI, and recurrent ischemia (136,137).

Amyloid A

Amyloid A is an acute-phase protein produced by the liver. Its predictive value appears to be similar to that of CRP (40).

Fibrinopeptide A

Fibrinopeptide A is a polypeptide cleaved from fibrinogen by thrombin. It is a sensitive marker of thrombin activity and fibrin generation. Elevated urinary fibrinopeptide A levels are associated with the presence of intracoronary thrombus (138) and signify an increased risk of death, MI, or revascularization. Persistently elevated levels denote an increased risk of coronary events (55).

B-Type Natriuretic Peptide

B-type natriuretic peptide (BNP) and the *N*-terminal fragment of the BNP prohormone (NT-proBNP) are synthesized in the

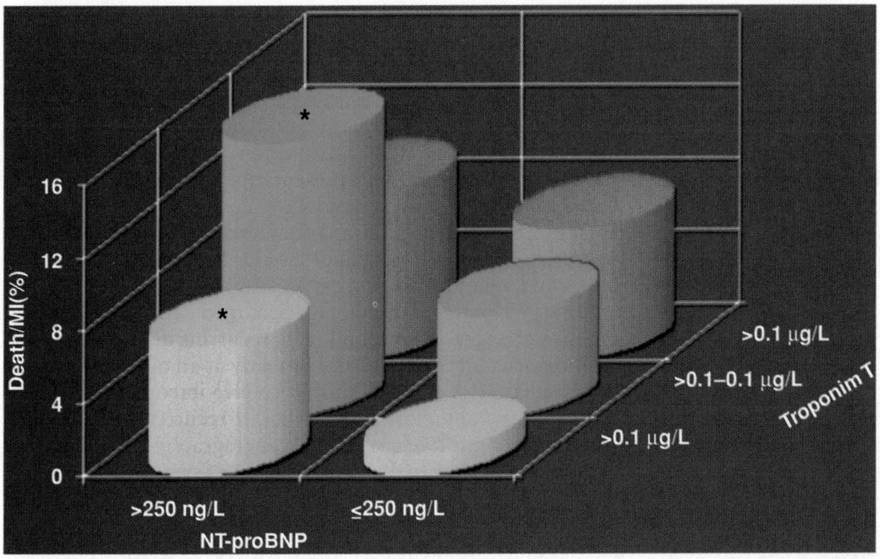

FIGURE 18.4. Predictive value of baseline NT-proBNP in relation to presence and absence of myocardial necrosis as evidenced by elevated levels of TnT ($n = 1791$) (141). *$P < .01$ versus NT-proBNP ≤250 ng/L. (*Source:* Redrawn from Heeschen C, Hamm CW, Mitrovic V, et al. N-terminal pro-B-type natriuretic peptide levels for dynamic risk stratification of patients with acute coronary syndromes. *Circulation* 2004;110:3206–3212, with permission.)

ventricles, and are important markers of neurohormonal activity. BNP levels correlate with left ventricular pressure, and increase in response to myocardial stretching in the event of myocardial ischemia (139). Several studies have shown that BNP and NT-proBNP levels have powerful prognostic value for death and MI in patients with NSTEACS (140–143), independent of markers of myocardial necrosis or inflammation. The FRISC-II trial (144) found that BNP levels predicted the benefit of revascularization, but there was no such association in TACTICS–TIMI-18 (142,145). Serial BNP measurements can be used for dynamic risk profiling (Fig. 18.4) (141). Patients with normal troponin levels and low BNP levels are at very low risk of cardiovascular events (Fig. 18.5) (141).

Other Markers

A number of other markers are currently under investigation, including interleukin-6, intercellular adhesion molecule-1, lipoprotein-associated phospholipase A_2, and various tissue

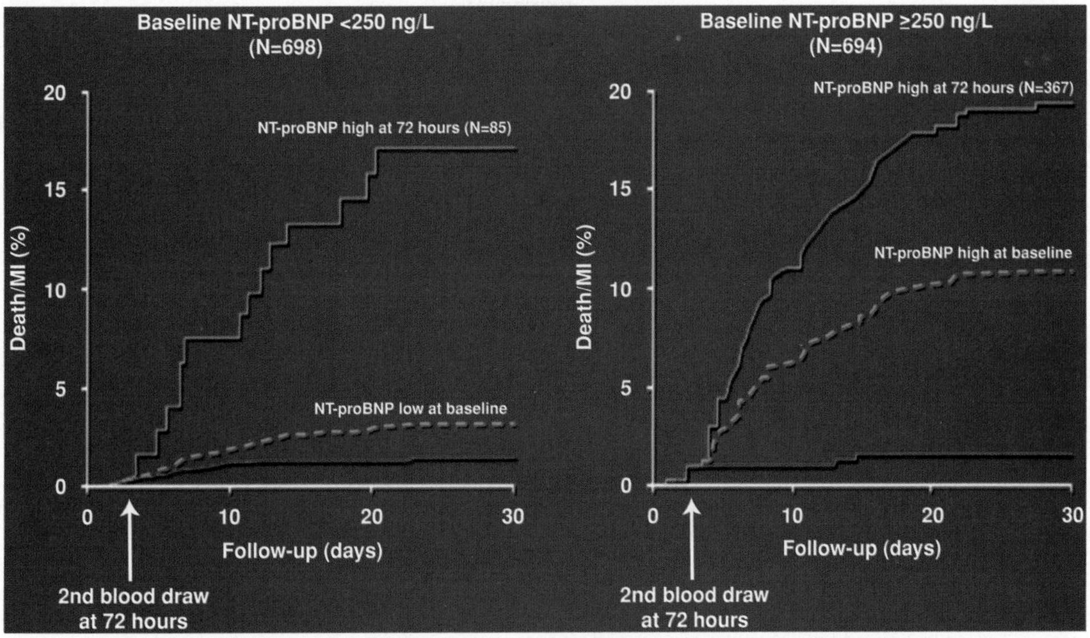

FIGURE 18.5. Dynamic risk profiling in patients with ACS using serial NT-proBNP measurements ($n =$ 1392 patients without death/MI during the first 72 hours) (141). Despite NT-proBNP levels of <250 ng/L at baseline, an increase in NT-proBNP levels during the following 72 hours indicated an adverse clinical course for these patients (*left*). In contrast, in patients with NT-proBNP levels >250 ng/L at baseline, rapid decline over the following 72 hours indicated low cardiac risk during the subsequent 27 days, whereas patients with consistently high NT-proBNP levels continued to be at increased cardiac risk (*right*). The *dashed lines* indicate event rate curves based on baseline NT-proBNP levels. (*Source:* Redrawn from Heeschen C, Hamm CW, Mitrovic V, et al. N-terminal pro-B-type natriuretic peptide levels for dynamic risk stratification of patients with acute coronary syndromes. *Circulation* 2004;110:3206–3212, with permission.)

inhibitors of metalloproteinases. Current guidelines do not recommend routine assessment of inflammatory markers.

Other Laboratory Tests

Primary risk factors, such as cholesterol and glucose levels, should be assessed at admission. Possible secondary causes of unstable angina should be investigated depending on the clinical circumstances, namely anemia, thyrotoxicosis, pulmonary embolism, and aortic dissection.

RISK PROFILING

Risk profiling is critical because it determines the choice of treatment strategy and provides prognostic information for the patient and relatives. It also enhances the cost effectiveness of patient care by allowing evidence-based treatments to be targeted at patients most likely to benefit from them. Risk profiling should take into account clinical factors, ECG features, cardiac marker levels, evidence of spontaneous or inducible ischemia, measures of left ventricular function, and coronary anatomy (Table 18.2) (1,146,147). Certain clinical features are not included in risk profiling models, and the clinical assessment should always be regarded as paramount. For instance, a patient who is gray, sweating, and anxious is likely to be at higher risk than one who is relaxed and appears well. Patients should be assessed fully at presentation and then reviewed at 6 to 8 hours for recurrence of ischemia, response to treatment, and the results of cardiac marker tests, particularly the troponins. Further risk profiling should be done at 12 and 24 hours and again before discharge.

Low-risk patients should be discharged early, advised to report any changes in symptoms (e.g., recurring discomfort at rest or at night), and reviewed subsequently at an outpatient clinic. Intermediate-risk patients should receive intensive antithrombotic therapy and close monitoring. If recurrent ischemia occurs or troponin levels rise, early angiography should be performed with a view to revascularization. If symptoms settle and troponin levels do not rise, tests for inducible ischemia should be performed. If the tests show ischemia at a low workload, angiography should be performed with revascularization as appropriate; otherwise, the patient can be managed medically.

TABLE 18.2

SHORT-TERM RISK OF DEATH/MI IN PATIENTS WITH UNSTABLE ANGINA[a] (1,146,147)

	High-risk: At least one of the following features must be present	Intermediate risk: No high-risk feature but must have one of the following features	Low risk: No high- or intermediate-risk feature but may have any of the following features
History	Accelerating tempo of ischemic symptoms in the preceding 48 hours	Previous MI, previous peripheral or cerebrovascular disease, previous CABG, previous aspirin use	
Character of pain	Prolonged ongoing (>20 min) rest pain	Prolonged (>20 min) rest angina, now resolved, with moderate or high likelihood of CAD Rest angina (<20 min) or angina relieved by rest or sublingual nitroglycerin	New-onset CCS class III or IV angina in the preceding 2 weeks without prolonged (>20 min) rest pain but with moderate or high likelihood of CAD
Clinical findings	Pulmonary edema, most likely due to ischemia New or worsening murmur of mitral regurgitation Third heart sound or new/worsening rales Hypotension, bradycardia, tachycardia Age >75 years	Age >70 y	
ECG findings	Rest angina with transient ST-segment changes ≥0.05 mV New or presumed-new bundle branch block Sustained ventricular tachycardia	T-wave inversion >0.2 mV Pathologic Q waves	Normal or unchanged ECG during an episode of chest discomfort
Cardiac markers	Elevated levels (e.g., troponin T or troponin I)		Normal

[a]Estimation of the short-term risks of death and nonfatal cardiac ischemic events in unstable angina is a complex multivariable problem that cannot be fully specified in a table such as this; therefore, this table is meant to offer general guidance and illustration rather than rigid algorithms.
Abbreviations: CABG, coronary artery bypass graft; CAD, coronary artery disease; CCS, Canadian Cardiovascular Society; ECG, electrocardiography; MI, myocardial infarction.
(*Source:* Adapted from AHCPR Clinical Practice Guideline No. 10, Unstable Angina: Diagnosis and Management, May 1994. Braunwald E, Mark DB, Jones RH, et al. Unstable angina: diagnosis and management. Rockville, MD: Agency for Health Care Policy and Research and the National Heart, Lung, and Blood Institute. US Public Health Service, US Department of Health and Human Services, 1994; AHCPR Publication No. 94-0602, with permission.)

TABLE 18.3

FACTORS INCLUDED IN RISK PROFILING MODELS FOR PATIENTS WITH NSTEACS

	GUSTO-IIB (148)	PURSUIT (149)	TIMI-11B (150)	GRACE (151)	FRISC (152)
Age	*	*	*	*	*
Male gender					*
Cardiac biomarkers	*	*	*	*	*
ST-segment deviation	*	*	*	*	*
≥2 Episodes of angina within 24 hours			*		
Higher angina classification		*			
Congestive heart failure	*	*			
Previous CAD or MI	*	*	*		*
Risk factors	*	*	*		*
Diabetes					*
Previous β-blocker therapy		*			
Previous aspirin therapy		*	*		
Previous CABG		*			
Renal insufficiency	*			*	
Severe chronic obstructive respiratory disease	*				
Inflammatory markers				*	*
Heart rate				*	
Blood pressure				*	
Killip class				*	
Cardiac arrest				*	

Abbreviations: AMI, acute myocardial infarction; CABG, coronary artery bypass graft; CAD, coronary artery disease.

High-risk patients should receive intensive antithrombotic therapy and have early angiography and revascularization if their coronary anatomy is suitable.

Various risk models have been developed for NSTEACS (Table 18.3) (148–152). The Platelet Glycoprotein IIb/IIIa in Unstable Angina: Receptor Suppression Using Integrilin Therapy (PURSUIT) investigators (149) found that most of the prognostic information was provided by seven variables: age, gender, Canadian Cardiovascular Society angina classification, heart rate, blood pressure, presence of rales, and presence of ST depression. Different models were developed for the endpoints of death and death/MI, and for NSTEMI and NSTEACS without MI.

The TIMI-11B risk model is based on seven readily quantifiable variables: age 65 years or older, three or more risk factors for coronary artery disease (CAD), prior coronary stenosis of 50% or more, ST-segment changes at presentation, two or more anginal events within the previous 24 hours, use of aspirin within the previous 7 days, and elevated serum cardiac marker levels (150). The advantage of this model is its simplicity. An electronic version of the model is available for palmtop computers (153).

The FRISC risk score includes seven risk factors: age over 70 years, male gender, diabetes, previous MI, ST depression, increased troponin levels, and inflammatory markers (CRP or interleukin-6) (152). In FRISC-II (113), invasive treatment was most beneficial in patients with five or more of these factors who had a 12-month relative risk (RR) for death/MI of 0.34 (95% confidence interval [CI] 0.15–0.78) versus 0.69 (95% CI 0.50–0.94) in patients with three or four risk factors (152). Invasive treatment had no benefit in patients with two or more risk factors. The Global Registry of Acute Coronary Events (GRACE) risk algorithm (151) was developed from an international registry. It includes renal function, and may perform slightly better than trial-based risk scores (154,155).

NONINVASIVE INVESTIGATIONS

Stress Testing

Exercise or pharmacologic testing (with or without imaging) can be performed as part of a chest pain unit assessment or when patients have been asymptomatic on antithrombotic therapy for 24 to 48 hours. Ischemia occurring at a low workload (<6 metabolic equivalents) is associated with a poor prognosis (156). When exercise testing for ischemia is negative in patients with a normal baseline ECG, the 5-year survival rate is 95% (156). Exercise thallium imaging can be used to assess the severity of CAD and the risk of subsequent cardiac events in patients with unstable angina (157,158).

Some patients have physical limitations that preclude exercise testing and others have ECG changes that are difficult to interpret because of baseline abnormalities such as left ventricular hypertrophy, left bundle branch block, preexcitation, or the effects of digoxin. Pharmacologic stress testing is of particular value in these patients (159). Although stress testing can indicate the presence of severe coronary stenoses (160) and the likelihood of multivessel disease, it cannot detect instability of coronary artery plaques.

Echocardiography

Two-dimensional echocardiography can provide anatomic and functional information, which is helpful in determining the diagnosis and prognosis. Transient wall motion abnormalities and changes in ventricular volumes can be detected during ischemia (161). These findings may be helpful if symptoms are atypical or if ECG findings are nondiagnostic. Echocardiographic changes may precede chest pain or ischemic ST-segment changes. Transesophageal echocardiography is particularly

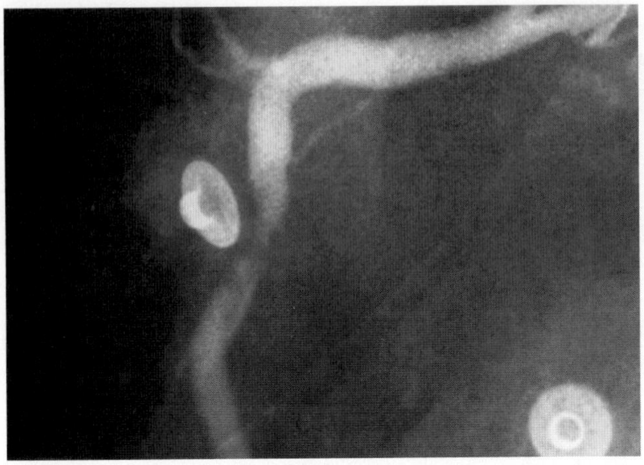

FIGURE 18.6. Right coronary angiogram showing a complex mid-coronary stenosis and protruding thrombus downstream.

valuable for evaluating the possibility of aortic dissection and structural abnormalities of the mitral valve. Dobutamine stress echocardiography is very useful for assessing ischemia and the viability of myocardium.

Cardiac Magnetic Resonance Imaging

Cardiac magnetic resonance imaging (MRI) has been shown to accurately predict the presence of significant CAD in patients with NSTEACS (162,163). It can also be used to assess global and regional cardiac function, myocardial perfusion, and myocardial viability (164,165).

CORONARY ANGIOGRAPHY

The findings at coronary angiography depend on the population studied. Angiography outlines only the arterial lumen, and may not detect large plaques within the arterial wall (163). In the TIMI-IIIB trial (166), 19% of patients had no coronary stenoses of more than 60% narrowing, and 4% had a left main coronary stenosis of more than 50%. Single-vessel disease was found in 38%, double-vessel disease in 29%, and triple-vessel disease in 15%. Eccentric plaques and complex plaques (Fig. 18.6) are more common in patients with unstable angina than in those with chronic stable angina (8). Coronary artery thrombi may be detected in 40% of patients having angiography soon after an episode of rest pain (57). Impaired coronary flow is common (167,168).

LEFT VENTRICULOGRAPHY

Left ventriculography may detect abnormalities of regional wall motion caused by previous MI or "hibernation" owing to prolonged or recurrent ischemia. Wall motion abnormalities and changes in ventricular volumes may occur during episodes of acute ischemia (169). The presence of mitral regurgitation can be detected and its severity assessed.

PROGNOSIS

The prognosis is worse in patients with NSTEACS than in patients with STEMI (83). Within 1 month, 2% to 5% die and 5% to 16% have an MI (91,170,171). Within 1 year, 26% to 35% require readmission to hospital for recurrent symptoms (172) and 4% to 15% die (166,172–176). Patients with unstable angina and a normal coronary angiogram have good short- (177) and long-term prognoses (178).

In a TACTICS–TIMI-18 substudy of patients without stenoses of 50% or more (179), the 6-month death/MI rate was 3.1% in those with elevated troponin I levels versus 0% in those without elevated troponin I levels. These patients may have had elevated troponin levels for another reason, or they may have had coronary atherothrombosis undetected by angiography. Coronary artery spasm may also have played a role (117).

Clinical Variables

The most important prognostic variables are age (149), left ventricular function (149), coronary anatomy (180), diabetes (91,170,171,181), and comorbid conditions such as chronic obstructive pulmonary disease, renal failure, cerebrovascular disease, peripheral vascular disease (182), and malignancy.

Rest pain at admission and recurrent ischemic episodes are high-risk features (82,166,183–185). Patients who have recurrent rest pain within 48 hours after admission have a 20% lower survival rate (184). MI occurs in approximately 3% of patients who have accelerating angina without ECG changes and in approximately 18% of those who have rest pain with ECG changes (185). Ischemic ST-segment changes on the admission ECG are high-risk features (82,148,184). Patients who have myocardial ischemia on continuous ST-segment monitoring have a significantly increased risk of death/MI (96). Mortality at 1 year can be predicted by the depth of ST depression on the admission ECG. ST depression of more than 1 mm after admission has 89% sensitivity for predicting MI, further angina, or the need for revascularization (82). The number of ischemic episodes correlates with outcomes (148). ST-segment shifts increase the risk of death or MI (82). Patients with ischemia during continuous ST-segment monitoring have an increased risk of death/MI at 1 year (18.4% versus 8.3%, $P = .02$) (186).

The medicines that patients are receiving at the time of presentation can be an important indicator of risk. In the TIMI-IIIB trial, patients who developed unstable angina while on β-blockers did worse, whereas those who had unstable angina while on angiotensin-converting enzyme (ACE) inhibitors did better (166). Patients who develop an ACS while on aspirin are at high risk, and thus current aspirin therapy is listed as a risk factor in the TIMI risk score (see Table 18.3) (150).

PRINCIPLES OF MANAGEMENT

Aims of Treatment

The immediate aims of treatment are to relieve pain with morphine and antianginal therapy, and to prevent MI and death by stabilizing the thrombotic process with antithrombotic therapy. If MI develops, treatments to preserve myocardium should be used, such as fibrinolytic therapy or primary PCI in the event of ST elevation or new-onset left bundle branch block.

Longer term goals include identification and treatment of cardiac risk factors such as hypertension, dyslipidemia, smoking, obesity, and lack of exercise. Patients should be assessed for anxiety and depression, and treated appropriately (187,188). They should also be enrolled in a cardiac rehabilitation program. It is incumbent upon physicians to use the most cost-effective strategy available.

General Measures

Patients with rest pain and ECG changes within the previous 48 hours should be admitted to hospital. Antithrombotic and antiischemic therapy should be commenced without delay when the patient is first seen in the emergency department, chest pain unit (189), or coronary care unit. Patients should be placed on bed rest, ideally with continuous ECG monitoring for arrhythmias and ischemia. Failing that, 12-lead ECGs should be performed at baseline, at 30 minutes, and at 1 hour, and repeated if further pain occurs.

Oxygen

Oxygen is commonly administered to all patients with acute chest pain. The Agency for Health Care Policy and Research guidelines recommend more selective use of oxygen in patients with obvious cyanosis, respiratory distress, or high-risk features (1).

Morphine

Morphine is effective for relieving pain and anxiety. It may also reduce cardiac workload and oxygen consumption by causing venodilation and slightly decreasing the heart rate and blood pressure. Morphine should be administered in IV doses of 2 to 5 mg if angina has not been relieved by nitroglycerin tablets or spray (see Nitrates), provided there are no contraindications. The dose can be repeated every 5 to 30 minutes.

Antiplatelet Agents

Aspirin

Aspirin potently inhibits thromboxane A_2-dependent platelet aggregation by irreversibly inhibiting the platelet enzyme, cyclooxygenase, and consequently reducing platelet synthesis of thromboxane A_2. Platelet adhesion to damaged endothelium is not affected (190). Aspirin does not prevent platelet degranulation (190) and does not inhibit platelet aggregation in response to stimuli such as thrombin, ADP, collagen, catecholamines, and shear-induced platelet aggregation (191). Aspirin resistance occurs in up to 40% of patients and is more common in women and the elderly (192,193). However, patients with PIA2 polymorphism of the GP IIb/IIIa receptor have been shown to be more responsive to aspirin (194). Some patients cannot tolerate aspirin because of gastrointestinal side effects, bleeding, or allergy (195–197), and these patients should receive clopidogrel instead (195–198).

Aspirin has a number of nonplatelet effects. It inhibits prostaglandin, interleukin-6 synthesis in leukocytes (199), and the activity of endothelial nitric oxide inhibitors (200). These features may explain why aspirin appears to have greater effects than would be expected from inhibition of thromboxane A_2-dependent platelet aggregation alone (201). At high doses, aspirin reduces endothelial production of the vasodilating prostaglandin, prostacyclin (202).

Despite these limitations, aspirin has been shown to reduce the risk of death or MI by approximately 50% in patients with NSTEACS (113,173,174,203). The doses used in these studies varied from 75 mg/d (203) to 325 mg four times daily (174). The effect of aspirin is rapid. In a study of normal volunteers, 162.5 mg of aspirin inhibited 91% of arachidonic acid–induced platelet aggregation ex vivo within 15 minutes (204).

All patients with NSTEACS should receive aspirin as soon as possible unless there is active bleeding or documented hypersensitivity. The initial dose should be 150 to 325 mg to allow for the possibility of reduced intestinal blood flow during ischemia and ensure complete inhibition of thromboxane A_2 production. In the long term, a dose of 75 to 162 mg should be used (205,206).

Ticlopidine and Clopidogrel

Ticlopidine and clopidogrel are thienopyridine derivatives, and both are prodrugs. They are selective antagonists of ADP-induced aggregation and reduce responses to other agonists that require ADP. Because of its side effects and delayed onset of action (2–3 days for maximal antiplatelet effect), ticlopidine is not recommended as initial therapy for patients with unstable angina.

The Clopidogrel in Unstable Angina to Prevent Recurrent Events (CURE) trial randomized 12,562 patients with ACS to receive either aspirin alone (75–325 mg/d) or aspirin plus clopidogrel, given as a 300 mg loading dose followed by 75 mg/d (77). At 12 months, the combined incidence of cardiovascular death/MI/stroke was reduced by 23% (from 11.47–9.28%) in patients treated with aspirin plus clopidogrel ($P < .001$) (Fig. 18.7). The major component of the reduction was a 23% decrease in MI, and most of the benefit was observed in the first 3 months. The benefits of clopidogrel were consistent in patients with and patients without elevated troponin or CK levels (207), and in low-, intermediate- and high-risk subgroups stratified by the TIMI risk score (207). The number of patients needed to treat for 9 months was 63 in the low-risk group (TIMI score 0–2), 63 in the intermediate-risk group (TIMI score 3–4), and 21 in the high-risk group (TIMI score >4). There was a 1% absolute increase in major bleeding in patients receiving aspirin plus clopidogrel (3.6% versus 2.7% in patients given aspirin alone, $P < .01$) (77).

The Percutaneous Coronary Intervention-Clopidogrel in Unstable Angina to Prevent Recurrent Events (PCI-CURE) investigators (208) studied the outcome of CURE trial patients who had PCI, mostly for refractory ischemia. The median period of clopidogrel pretreatment was 6 days. At 30 days the combined incidence of cardiovascular death/MI/stroke was reduced from 6.4% to 4.5% ($P < .05$).

The Clopidogrel for the Reduction of Events During Observation (CREDO) trial (209) compared clopidogrel 300 mg with a placebo administered 3 to 24 hours before PCI in patients with chronic stable angina. Both groups received a maintenance dose of clopidogrel (75 mg/d) for 30 days. There was a trend for death/MI/urgent target vessel revascularization to be reduced at 30 days in patients receiving clopidogrel more than 6 hours before PCI (RR 0.614, $P = .051$).

There has been controversy over the optimal timing and size of the loading dose of clopidrogrel (210). The American College of Cardiology/American Heart Association (ACC/AHA) and ESC guidelines recommend that a loading dose of 300 mg of clopidogrel be given at the time of PCI (1,211).

In the CURE trial, approximately 1,000 patients had coronary artery bypass grafting (CABG) during the initial hospitalization. Their combined incidence of cardiovascular death/MI/stroke was reduced from 4.7% to 2.9% (RR 0.56, 95% CI 0.29–1.08) (212). Life-threatening bleeding occurred in 5.6% of patients randomized to aspirin plus clopidogrel versus 4.2% of those randomized to aspirin alone (RR 1.30, 95% CI 0.91–1.95). There was no excess bleeding in patients who stopped clopidogrel more than 5 days before surgery, but those who continued to receive clopidogrel within 5 days prior to surgery had a nonsignificant excess of major bleeding and a trend toward a higher reoperation rate (RR 1.79, 95% CI 0.85–3.74).

A prospective registry of patients receiving clopidogrel within 7 days prior to CABG reported greater chest tube

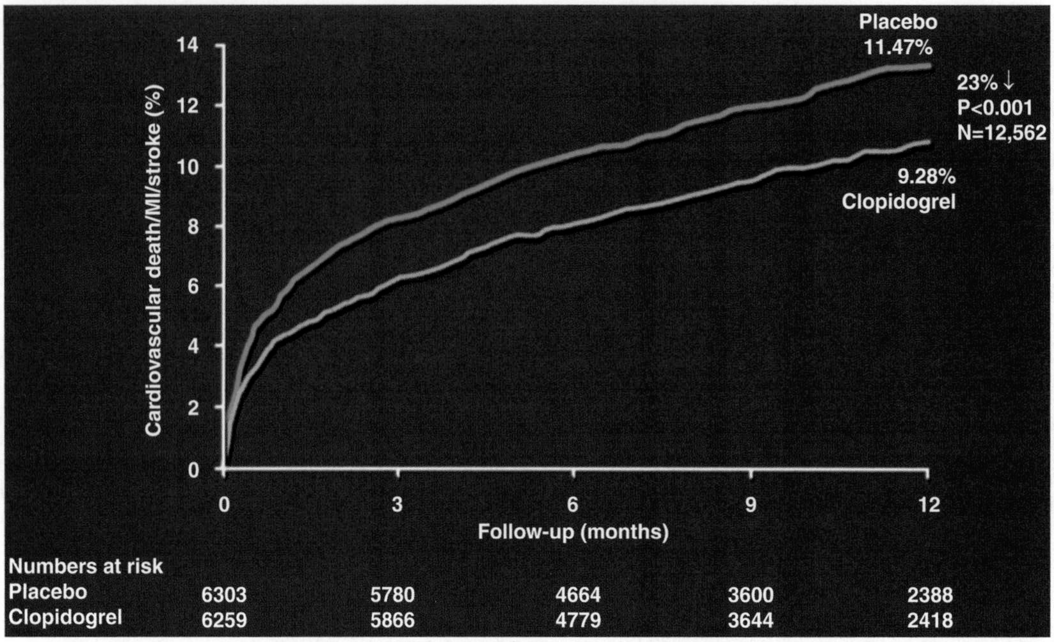

FIGURE 18.7. Cumulative hazard rates of cardiovascular death/MI/stroke within 12 months in the CURE trial evaluating aspirin plus clopidogrel versus aspirin alone (77). (*Source:* Redrawn from The Clopidogrel in Unstable Angina to Prevent Recurrent Events Trial Investigators. Effects of clopidogrel in addition to aspirin in patients with acute coronary syndromes without ST-segment elevation. *N Engl J Med* 2001;345:494–502, with permission.)

drainage, greater need for transfusion, and a 10-fold higher need for reoperation due to bleeding when compared with matched patients not receiving preoperative clopidogrel (6.8% versus 0.6%, $P = .018$) (213).

There is marked interpatient variability in the antiplatelet effects of clopidogrel, and 30% of patients receiving a 600-mg loading dose achieve suboptimal levels of platelet inhibition (210). Individualized measurement of platelet aggregation responses, receptor polymorphisms and cytochrome P450 3A4 activity levels allows titration of the dose to maximize efficacy and safety (210).

There are a number of different approaches to prescribing clopidogrel in patients with NSTEACS. One approach is to treat all patients except those likely to have CABG (patients with ECG changes suggestive of left main CAD, multiple regional wall motion abnormalities on echocardiography, hemodynamic instability, or left ventricular failure). An alternative approach is to use clopidogrel at the time of angiography after the coronary anatomy is known.

Clopidogrel is indicated for acute and long-term treatment (for $\geq$1 month and ideally for $\geq$9 months) in addition to aspirin in all patients with NSTEACS. It is particularly useful for patients who cannot tolerate aspirin. In high-risk patients, use of clopidogrel should be considered in addition to GP IIb/IIIa antagonists (214,215).

Platelet Glycoprotein IIb/IIIa Antagonists

The final common pathway to platelet aggregation is the binding of fibrinogen to GP IIb/IIIa receptors on platelet surfaces, with cross-linking and formation of a platelet thrombus. The surface of each platelet has 50,000 to 80,000 of these receptors, but they are usually unactivated unless conformational changes are induced by disruption of endothelium. Inhibition of these receptors blocks the final common pathway to platelet aggregation (Fig. 18.8). The effects of multiple antagonists inducing thrombin, thromboxane A_2, collagen, ADP, catecholamine, and shear-induced platelet aggregation can be prevented by blocking these receptors.

In a pooled analysis of trials totaling 31,402 patients with NSTEACS who were not selected for early revascularization (78), use of GP IIb/IIIa antagonists reduced the combined incidence of death/MI by 9% at 30 days ($P = .015$; Fig. 18.9) (216,217). Major bleeding occurred in 2.4% of patients receiving GP IIb/IIIa antagonists versus 1.4% of those receiving control treatment ($P < .0001$). In a systematic overview of trials in patients having PCI, GP IIb/IIIa antagonists were found to reduce death/MI by approximately 35% at 30 days (218).

Abciximab. Abciximab is a monoclonal antibody to the GP IIb/IIIa receptor, and binds for the life of the platelet. It can cause thrombocytopenia in approximately 1% of patients. The GUSTO IV trial has specifically tested abciximab in patients with NSTEACS.

In GUSTO-IV (219), 7,800 patients presenting within 24 hours of the onset of chest pain lasting 5 minutes or longer and either 0.5 mm or more of ST depression or elevated troponin I or T levels were randomized to receive either a placebo infusion, an abciximab infusion for 24 hours, or an abciximab infusion for 48 hours. The aim of the trial was to test an intensive medical regimen, and PCI was discouraged. Only 1.6% of patients had PCI in the first 48 hours. Abciximab had no effect on death/MI at 30 days, which occurred in 8.0% of patients given the placebo, 8.2% of those given abciximab for 24 hours, and 9.1% of those given abciximab for 48 hours. These results are markedly inconsistent with those of previous trials, and several explanations have been proposed including the possibility that abciximab might be a procoagulant as the effect of the bolus attenuates during the course of the infusion (220–222).

Based on the CAPTURE trial which slowed benefit of abciximab, abciximab (0.25 mg/kg IV bolus and 0.125 μg/kg/min infusion) should be administered for 24 hours prior to PCI in high-risk patients with known coronary anatomy (223) or for 12 hours starting at the time of PCI.

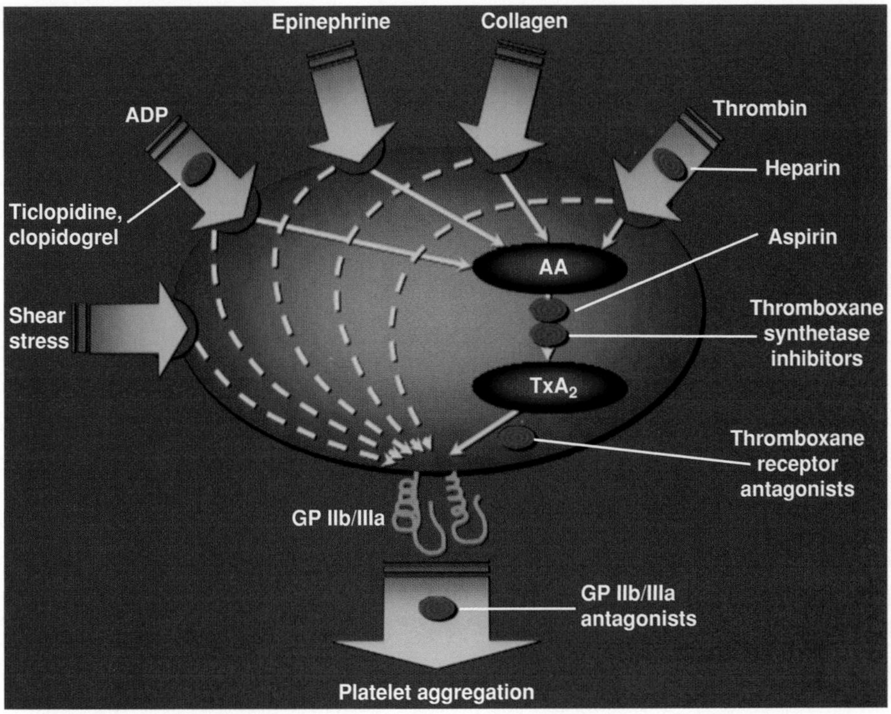

FIGURE 18.8. Stimuli that increase the affinity of the GP IIb/IIIa receptor for fibrinogen. *Abbreviations:* AA, arachidonic acid; TxA_2, thromboxane A_2.

Tirofiban. Tirofiban is a small nonpeptide antagonist of the GP IIb/IIIa receptor, and mimics the tripeptide arginine–glycine–aspartate sequence in fibrinogen. It is nonimmunogenic and highly selective for the platelet fibrinogen receptor, producing an acute effect within 5 minutes of administration. The effects are reversible in 4 to 6 hours. Two trials have tested tirofiban in NSTEACS (170,224).

The Platelet Receptor Inhibition in Ischemic Syndrome Management (PRISM) study (224) compared tirofiban with heparin in 3231 patients. Tirofiban reduced all components of the composite primary endpoint (death/MI/refractory ischemia) by approximately 33% during the 48-hour infusion period ($P = .007$).

The Platelet Receptor Inhibition in Ischemic Syndrome Management in Patients Limited by Unstable Signs and Symptoms (PRISM-Plus) study of 1,560 high-risk patients (170) compared tirofiban, heparin, and combination treatment with both agents. The tirofiban-alone limb of the trial was stopped early because of a trend toward higher mortality. Combination treatment reduced death/MI by 30% at 30 days (8.7% versus 11.9%, $P = .03$). Neither PRISM nor PRISM-Plus observed any increase in bleeding with tirofiban.

Tirofiban is indicated for "upstream" treatment prior to PCI. The recommended treatment regimen is 0.4 μg/kg per minute for 30 minutes followed by 0.10 μg/kg per minute. The infusion should be continued for 12 to 24 hours after PCI.

Trials	N	Placebo (%)	GP IIb/IIa antagonists (%)	RP for death/MI
All PCI trials	17,393	8.5	5.6	0.65
All ACS trials	31,402	11.8	10.8	0.91
Troponin negative	3458	11.3	9.3	0.82
Troponin positive	4144	6.9	6.5	1.10
PCI	4378	14.5	11.8	0.77
No PCI	12,685	14.3	13.3	0.93
All oral trials	33,340	6.5	7.2	1.11

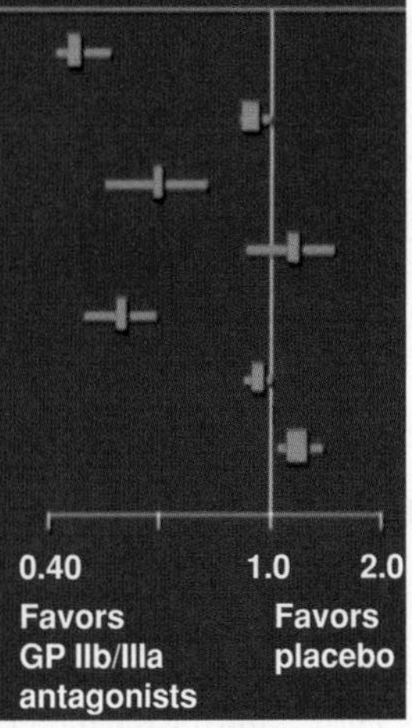

FIGURE 18.9. Relative risks of death/MI in trials evaluating GP IIb/IIIa antagonists in patients treated with PCI (216), patients managed conservatively (78), and patients receiving oral GP IIb/IIIa antagonists (217). (*Source:* Adapted from Chew DP, Moliterno DJ. A critical appraisal of platelet glycoprotein IIb/IIIa inhibition. *J Am Coll Cardiol* 2000;36:2028–2035.)

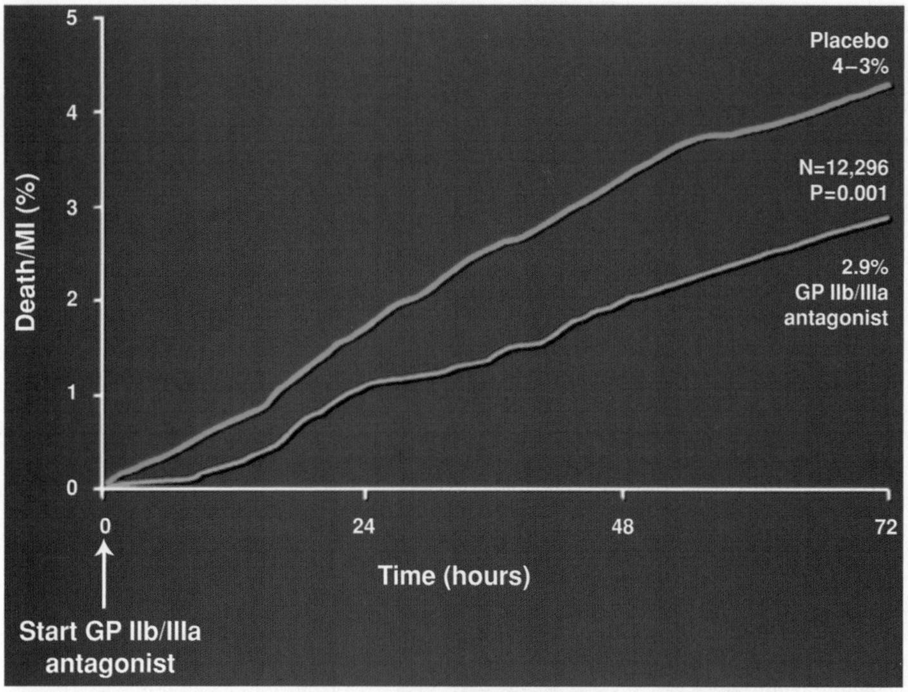

FIGURE 18.10. Event rates before intervention in the CAPTURE (223), PRISM-Plus (170), and PURSUIT (171) trials of GP IIb/IIIa antagonists in patients with NSTEACS (226). (*Source:* Redrawn from Boersma E, Akkerhuis M, Théroux P, et al. Platelet glycoprotein IIb/IIIa receptor inhibition in non–ST-elevation acute coronary syndromes: early benefit during medical treatment only, with additional protection during percutaneous coronary intervention. *Circulation* 1999;100: 2045–2048, with permission.)

Eptifibatide. Eptifibatide is a cyclic peptide inhibitor of the GP IIb/IIIa receptor that exerts rapid platelet inhibition. It has a short half-life, and platelet aggregation returns to baseline within 2 to 4 hours. It has been tested in three trials of patients with NSTEACS (171,214,225).

The Integrilin (Eptifibatide) to Minimize Platelet Aggregation and Coronary Thrombosis II study compared eptifibatide with a placebo in 4,010 patients. There was no significant difference in death/MI/revascularization at 30 days (9.9% with eptifibatide versus 11.4% with the placebo, $P = 0.18$) (225). In the PURSUIT trial, eptifibatide was compared with a placebo in 9,461 patients, and reduced death/MI from 15.7% to 14.2% at 30 days ($P = .03$) (171).

The Enhanced Suppression of the Platelet IIb/IIIa Receptor with Integrilin Therapy trial (214) compared eptifibatide (two 180-mg/kg boluses followed by 2.0 mg/kg/h for 18–24 h) with a placebo in 2,064 patients who also received stents, aspirin, low-dose heparin, and loading doses of ticlopidine or clopidogrel. The trial was stopped early after an interim analysis showed that the combined 48-hour incidence of death/MI/urgent revascularization/thrombotic bailout/use of GP IIb/IIIa antagonists was significantly lower among patients receiving eptifibatide (6.6% versus 10.5%, $P = .0015$). Fourteen percent of the trial cohort had presented within 2 days of an ACS, and in these patients there was a trend toward a reduction in event rates from 20.4% to 11.4% ($P = .24$).

Eptifibatide is indicated for both upstream use prior to PCI and/or a 24-hour infusion starting at the time of PCI. The recommended dosing regimen is two 180-μg/kg boluses followed by 2.0 μg/kg per hour.

Upstream Treatment With Glycoprotein IIb/IIIa Antagonists. GP IIb/IIIa antagonists may be beneficial before CABG, before PCI, during PCI, and in patients receiving medical therapy alone. Upstream treatment with GP IIb/IIIa antagonists prior to revascularization was assessed in the CAPTURE (223), PRISM-Plus (170), and PURSUIT (171) trials totaling more than 12,000 patients. Overall, there was a substantial reduction in death/MI in the period before intervention (from 4.3% to 2.9%, equating to 14 fewer events per 1,000 patients treated) (Fig. 18.10) (226). Most of this reduction was in MI rather than death.

Upstream treatment with a GP IIb/IIIa antagonist also reduces the risk of MI before CABG (170), and may reduce the risk of perioperative events. In the PURSUIT trial, the reduction in events was greatest among patients who received eptifibatide within 72 hours of CABG (23.8% versus 33.6% with placebo, $P = .002$). There was no increase in major bleeding with eptifibatide (58.2% versus 56.6% with the placebo, $P = .7$) (227).

Use of Glycoprotein IIb/IIIa Antagonists in Patients Managed Without Interventions. In the PARAGON-A (228), PRISM (224), PRISM-Plus (170), PURSUIT (171) PARAGON-B (229), and GUSTO-IV (219) trials, intervention was not recommended routinely, and only about 6% of patients had revascularization procedures while on GP IIb/IIIa antagonists. Overall, GP IIb/IIIa antagonists reduced the incidence of death/MI by 9% at 30 days (see Fig. 18.9). In the PURSUIT trial, PCI was performed at the discretion of the treating physician, and an analysis with censoring for PCI across the 30-day follow-up period showed that eptifibatide reduced the incidence of death/MI by 31% (from 16.8% to 15.1%, $P = .035$) (230).

Which Patients Should Receive Glycoprotein IIb/IIIa Antagonists? GP IIb/IIIa antagonists should be used in patients with elevated troponin levels, ST depression, a TIMI risk score above 3, or diabetes (1,211,231). A few studies have evaluated the cost effectiveness of GP IIb/IIIa antagonists, and found them to be in the same cost range as other accepted therapies (232).

Combination Treatment With Glycoprotein IIb/IIIa Antagonists and Clopidogrel. There is in vitro evidence that this combination enhances inhibition of platelet function (233), and nonrandomized retrospective analysis has suggested that combination treatment is both beneficial and safe in patients with NSTEACS (77) and those having elective PCI (215).

The ISAR-REACT 2 trial randomized patients in the catheterization laboratory to 600 mg clopidrogrel vs 600 mg clopidrogrel plus abciximab (A. Kastrati. HOTLINE Sessions, ACC, March 2006, Atlanta). Event rates (death, MI, urgent revascularization at 30 days) were reduced with abciximab but only in those with raised troponins (13.1% vs 18.3%, $P = 0.02$). Upstream use of clopidogrel and a GP IIb/IIIa antagonist prior to PCI should be considered in high-risk patients, particularly in those with elevated troponins but avoided in those likely to require urgent CABG.

Heparin

A number of trials have compared UFH with a placebo or control aspirin therapy in patients with unstable angina (75,96, 203,234–236). A pooled analysis showed that there was a trend for UFH to reduce death/MI at 30 days (237).

Low-Molecular-Weight Heparins. Although LMWHs lack the minimum 18 saccharides that are required for simultaneous binding of thrombin and antithrombin III, and bind to and inhibit factor X_a more effectively than UFH does. Because the different LMWHs have different chemical structures and different molecular weights, they have different biological properties, different antifactor X_a to antifactor II_a ratios, and different effects on the release of tissue factor pathway inhibitor. The antifactor X_a effects of LMWHs can be partially reversed (by approximately 60%) by administration of protamine sulfate (238).

LMWHs have a number of advantages over UFH, including greater bioavailability, a more predictable dose response owing to minimal protein binding, higher antifactor X_a to antifactor II_a ratios, greater ability to inhibit thrombin generation, inhibition of von Willebrand factor release, resistance to inactivation by platelet factor 4, lack of heparin resistance, and lack of platelet activation. LMWHs are more convenient to use than UFH because they require no monitoring of the activated partial thromboplastin time (APTT) and no IV lines. Use of LMWHs has been shown to save money in some healthcare systems (239). Thrombocytopenia and osteoporosis are less common with LMWHs than with UFH (240), and rebound ischemia may be less common after cessation of LMWHs (186). When used for prolonged treatment, however, LMWHs have not been shown to be superior to UFH (241–245).

In a systematic overview of six trials comparing enoxaparin with UFH in a total of 21,946 patients, there were no differences in mortality, major bleeding, or need for transfusion (76). However, enoxaparin was associated with a significant reduction in death/MI at 30 days (10.1% versus 11.0%, odds ratio [OR] 0.91, 95% CI 0.83–0.99; Fig. 18.11).

These trials covered the full spectrum of NSTEACS management, from conservative treatment with angiography in approximately 50% of cases (241,246), to a more invasive approach with angiography in 60% to 65% (247–249), to a very invasive strategy with angiography in 92% of patients (250). In the trials that used a conservative approach, enoxaparin reduced event rates more effectively than UFH without increasing bleeding (241,247). In the trials with higher rates of revascularization, both agents had similar efficacy, but bleeding was more common with enoxaparin (248–251).

Three trials have examined the safety and efficacy of combination treatment with enoxaparin and a GP IIb/IIIa antagonist (248–251). In the Aggrastat to Zocor (A to Z) trial, 3,987 patients with NSTEACS were given aspirin and tirofiban and randomized to receive either enoxaparin or UFH (249). The aim of the trial was to show that enoxaparin was noninferior to UFH. The primary composite endpoint of the trial was death/MI/refractory ischemia at 7 days. The results fell within the prespecified noninferiority boundaries, with primary endpoint events occurring in 8.4% of the enoxaparin treatment group and 9.4% of the UFH treatment group (hazard ratio 0.88, 95% CI 0.71–1.08) (249). Enoxaparin had no significant advantage over UFH in patients selected for early revascularization. Among patients selected for early conservative treatment, however, those receiving enoxaparin had fewer primary endpoint events than those receiving UFH (7.7% versus 10.6%, hazard ratio 0.72, 95% CI 0.53–0.99, $P = .04$) (251).

In the Integrilin and Enoxaparin Randomized Assessment of Acute Coronary Syndrome Treatment (INTERACT) trial, 746 NSTEACS patients were given eptifibatide and aspirin and randomized to receive either UFH or enoxaparin. Approximately 15% of patients had angiography in the first 48 hours. Enoxaparin was associated with a lower rate of major bleeding unrelated to CABG at 96 hours (1.8% versus 4.6% with UFH, $P = .03$) and a lower rate of death/MI at 30 days (5% versus 9% with UFH, $P = .03$) (248).

In the Superior Yield of the New Strategy of Enoxaparin, Revascularization and Glycoprotein IIb/IIIa Inhibitors (SYNERGY) trial, 10,027 patients were randomized to receive either enoxaparin or UFH; 57% also received a GP IIb/IIIa antagonist. Angiography was performed in 92% of patients at a

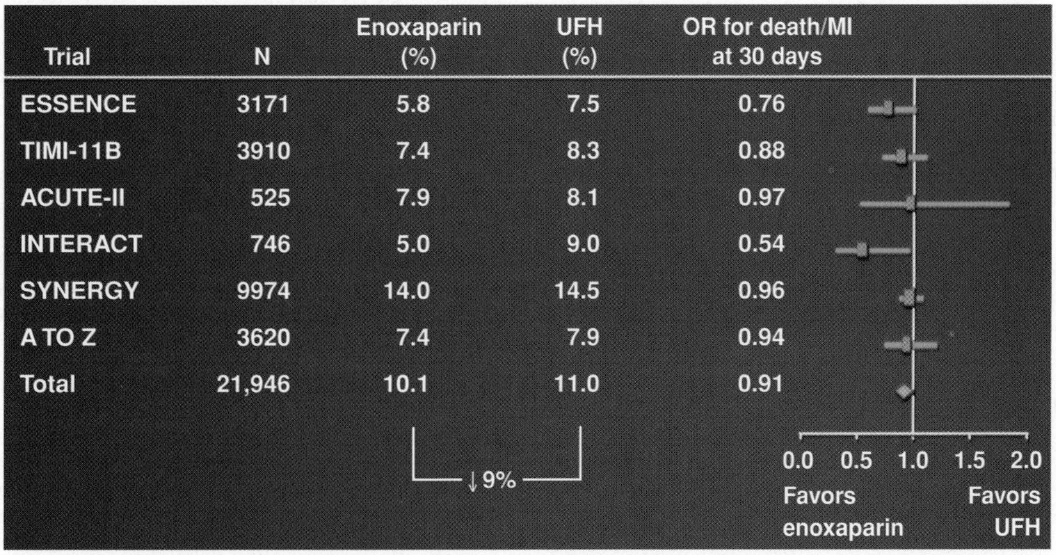
Trial
N
Enoxaparin (%)
UFH (%)
OR for death/MI at 30 days
ESSENCE 3171 5.8 7.5 0.76
TIMI-11B 3910 7.4 8.3 0.88
ACUTE-II 525 7.9 8.1 0.97
INTERACT 746 5.0 9.0 0.54
SYNERGY 9974 14.0 14.5 0.96
A TO Z 3620 7.4 7.9 0.94
Total 21,946 10.1 11.0 0.91
↓9%
0.0 0.5 1.0 1.5 2.0
Favors enoxaparin
Favors UFH

FIGURE 18.11. Systematic overview of death/MI at 30 days in trials comparing enoxaparin with UFH (76). *Abbreviations:* ESSENCE, Efficacy and Safety of Subcutaneous Enoxaparin in Non-Q-Wave Coronary Events; ACUTE-II, Antithrombotic Combination Using Tirofiban and Enoxaparin-II. (*Source:* Redrawn from Petersen JL, Mahaffey KW, Hasselblad V, et al. Efficacy and bleeding complications among patients randomized to enoxaparin or unfractionated heparin for antithrombin therapy in non–ST-segment elevation acute coronary syndromes: a systematic overview. *JAMA* 2004;292:89–96, with permission.)

median time of 21.6 hours (250). There was no difference in death/MI at 30 days (14.0% with enoxaparin versus 14.5% with UFH), but TIMI major bleeding (252) was more common with enoxaparin (9.1% versus 7.6%, $P = .008$). Patients who crossed over between the different antithrombotic treatment groups had increased bleeding and death/MI rates.

Recommendations for Heparin Use. Patients with intermediate- or high-risk NSTEACS should receive either enoxaparin (1 mg/kg twice daily) or weight-adjusted IV UFH immediately, provided they have no contraindications (1). The initial dose of UFH should be a weight-adjusted bolus (60 IU/kg) followed by an infusion of 12 IU/kg per hour to maintain the APTT at 50 to 70 seconds (253). The infusion should be continued for 2 days or until revascularization (1).

Enoxaparin is the preferred antithrombotic agent in low-risk patients and in intermediate- or high-risk patients who are being managed conservatively for reasons such as multiple comorbidities. For other intermediate- and high-risk patients, UFH and enoxaparin offer similar benefits, although enoxaparin is associated with increased bleeding. Patients should not be switched from one antithrombotic therapy to another.

Direct Antithrombins

Heparin has a number of limitations. It requires monitoring, has a limited effect on fibrin and platelet-bound thrombin (254), requires antithrombin III as a cofactor, is inactivated by platelet secretion products such as platelet factor 4 and thrombospondin, and carries a risk of thrombocytopenia. Conversely, direct antithrombins have a more predictable and consistent effect on the APTT, are able to inactivate clot-bound thrombin, do not require antithrombin III, and are only minimally affected by plasma proteins or platelet factor 4 (255). A meta-analysis of trials in patients with NSTEACS showed that hirudin reduced the incidence of death/MI by 20% during the treatment period (from 4.6% to 3.7%, OR 0.80, 95% CI 0.70–0.92) (256).

Bivalirudin. Bivalirudin (formerly known as Hirulog) is a synthetic 20–amino-acid peptide. Its half-life is shorter than that of hirudin (25 minutes versus 2.3 hours) and its action is reversible (257). By inhibiting both fibrin-bound and circulating thrombin directly, bivalirudin blocks the powerful effect of thrombin on platelet aggregation. In the Hirulog Angioplasty study, 4,098 patients undergoing PCI for unstable or postinfarction angina were randomized to receive either heparin or bivalirudin (258). Bivalirudin reduced the combined incidence of death/MI/abrupt vessel closure/CABG/intraaortic balloon pumping [IABP]/repeat PCI from 14.2% to 9.1% ($P < .05$) in patients with postinfarction angina, and overall was associated with lower bleeding rates than heparin. Transfusions were required in 3.7% of patients receiving bivalirudin versus 8.6% of those receiving heparin ($P < .001$).

In the Randomized Evaluation in PCI Linking Angiomax to Reduced Clinical Events-2 (REPLACE-2) trial, 6,002 patients undergoing urgent or elective PCI (40% of whom had NSTEACS) were randomized to receive either heparin plus routine abciximab or eptifibatide, or bivalirudin with bailout use of a GP IIb/IIIa antagonist (7.2%). There was no difference in the combined incidence of death/MI/urgent revascularization (9.2% with bivalirudin versus 10.0% with heparin plus GP IIb/IIIa antagonism), but major bleeding was less common with bivalirudin (2.4% versus 4.1%, $P < .0001$) (259).

The Acute Catheterization and Urgent Intervention Triage Strategy (ACUITY) trial randomized 9207 patients to receive one of five different treatment regimens: UFH or enoxaparin with upstream administration of a GP IIb/IIIa antagonist, bivalirudin plus a GP IIb/IIIa antagonist upstream or with PCI, or bivalirudin plus selective use of a GP IIb/IIIa antagonist if bailout is required (260). Clopidogrel therapy was used in all treatment groups according to local practice. The primary endpoint was a composite of death, MI or unplanned revascularization for ischemia plus major bleeding. The primary endpoint showed non-inferiority for the net clinical outcome; 11.7% heparin + IIb/IIIa groups vs. 11.8% bivalirudin + IIb/IIIa groups, $p < 0.001$. The ischemic composite was 7.3% vs. 7.7%, $p = 0.015$, for non-inferiority and major bleeding was 5.7% vs. 5.3%, $p < 0.001$ for non-inferiority. The results for bivalirudin group alone was 10.1% for the composite endpoint, $p < 0.0001$; 7.8% for the ischemic endpoint, $p = 0.32$ and 3.0% for major bleeding $p < .001$, (all p values for superiority). All causes of major bleeding were numerically lower with bivalirudin, except for intracranial hemorrhage, 0.07% vs. 0.07%. Notably transfusions were less frequent with bivalirudin; 2.7% heparin + GP IIb/IIIa vs. 1.6%, $p < .001$. Thus the simpler regimen of bivalirudin alone resulted in significantly greater net clinical benefit (G. Stone, HOTLINE Sessions, ACC, March 2006, Atlanta).

β-Adrenoreceptor Blockers

β-Blockers are effective when used singly in unstable angina (175,176,261,262) and in combination with nitrates (263) to reduce recurrent ischemia. In a review of 4,700 randomized patients, β-blockers reduced the percentage of those developing MI by 13% (from 32% to 29%, $P < .05$) (262).

Patients should be started on a β-blocker or have their existing dose adjusted to maintain the resting heart rate at 50 to 60 beats per minute. IV β-blockers should be considered in high-risk patients with rest pain and widespread ST-segment changes or tachycardia. Standard contraindications include marked first- (>0.24 s), second-, or third-degree atrioventricular block, asthma, and severe left ventricular dysfunction. Therapy should be continued in the long term.

Nitrates

No large randomized trials of nitrates in unstable angina have been performed, and there is no compelling evidence that they reduce the risk of death/MI. They do, however, relieve angina. Nitrates are of particular value in patients with vasospasm or a physiologic increase in coronary artery tone. Although they reduce ischemia very effectively, tolerance can develop within 24 hours. Small doses or concomitant administration of the sulfhydryl donor, *N*-acetylcysteine, may augment the effect of nitroglycerin and decrease tolerance (264). Nitrates should not be used within 24 hours of sildenafil (Viagra) because of the risk of severe hypotension (265).

Nitroglycerin should be given immediately, either as a sublingual tablet or spray, to relieve angina. If this does not relieve the symptoms, IV nitroglycerin can be infused to relieve pain and to optimize hemodynamics, starting at an infusion rate of 5 to 10 μg/min, with increases every 5 to 10 minutes depending on symptoms and side effects such as headache or hypotension.

Calcium Channel Antagonists

Calcium channel antagonists dilate coronary arteries by reducing the cellular membrane influx of calcium. They have variable vasodilatory effects in peripheral arteries and have negative inotropic, chronotropic, and atrioventricular conduction-slowing effects. They may enhance diastolic relaxation and left ventricular compliance. When used without a β-blocker, agents that increase the heart rate (e.g., short-acting nifedipine) may result in worse outcomes than agents that reduce the heart rate (e.g., verapamil or diltiazem) (266,267).

Calcium channel antagonists should be used in patients who have refractory ischemia in the presence of β-blocker and nitrate therapy, or in combination with a β-blocker if hypertension is present. Calcium channel antagonists should be avoided in patients with pulmonary edema or left ventricular dysfunction, but are the agents of choice in individuals with variant angina.

Other Agents

Nicorandil has nitrate and potassium channel-opening effects. When compared with a placebo in 188 patients with unstable angina, nicorandil was found to reduce the incidence of recurrent ischemia but not death or MI (268). Ranolazine increases the efficacy of energy production by decreasing fatty acid oxidation and promoting glucose utilization. It is currently being tested in large clinical trials (269).

Oral Anticoagulants

Because of their delayed onset of action, oral anticoagulants are not appropriate for acute treatment, but can be considered for long-term use if aspirin is contraindicated.

New Agents

There are a number of new antiplatelet drugs in development. Some block the $P2Y_{12}$ ADP receptor inhibiting platelet secretion and sustained aggregation; others block the $P2Y_1$ ADP receptor on platelets inhibiting shape change and transient aggregation (270).

Tissue factor is an integral protein of vascular endothelium, and an essential cofactor for the proteolytic activity of factor VII toward its substrates, factors IX and X. Human plasma contains a tissue factor inhibitor that inhibits coagulation. A recombinant tissue factor pathway inhibitor, targeted at exposed subendothelium, is currently in development (271).

Ximelagatran is an oral direct thrombin inhibitor that requires no coagulation monitoring and can be given in a fixed dose. In a pilot trial of patients with NSTEACS, it reduced the combined incidence of death/MI/severe recurrent ischemia from 11.2% to 7.4% ($P = .01$) (272). Pentasaccharides, which are indirect inhibitors of factor Xa, are currently being tested in clinical trials (273).

Thrombolytic Therapy

Thrombolytic therapy is not recommended for routine use in patients with unstable angina because it has been shown to increase the risk of MI (274).

Intraaortic Balloon Pumping

IABP stabilizes patients and relieves symptoms very effectively (275). By increasing aortic diastolic pressure, coronary blood flow is improved distal to critical stenoses, and there is a decrease in myocardial oxygen demands owing to reduction of afterload. No randomized trials of IABP have been done in patients with unstable angina. IABP should be considered in patients with refractory symptoms or hemodynamic instability to stabilize patients during angiography or prior to CABG.

Indications for Angiography

Coronary angiography determines the extent and severity of CAD, and may detect thrombus. Assessment of valvular and left ventricular function can be performed at the same time. Indications for angiography (other than as part of an invasive treatment strategy) are listed in Table 18.4.

TABLE 18.4

INDICATIONS FOR ANGIOGRAPHY WITH A CONSERVATIVE STRATEGY

Suspicion of left main CAD
Two ischemic episodes lasting ≥5 min
Chest pain lasting ≥20 min
≥1 mm of ST depression or T-wave inversion while on heparin with a therapeutic APTT
≥2 mm of ST depression or T-wave inversion with or without pain
Ischemia with development of pulmonary edema, mitral regurgitation, or hypotension
PCI within previous 6 months
Previous CABG
Significant ventricular arrhythmias
Impaired left ventricular function
Abnormal stress testing at the nonacute stage
Diagnosis of CAD in a patient with atypical symptoms

Abbreviations: APTT, activated partial thromboplastin time; CABG, coronary artery bypass grafting; CAD, coronary artery disease; PCI, percutaneous coronary intervention.

Revascularization

A number of trials have compared conservative therapy with revascularization (91,92,113,166,276–280). FRISC-II (113), TACTICS–TIMI-18 (91), and RITA-3 (92) concluded that high-risk patients should be revascularized.

The proportions of patients in these trials who had revascularization procedures after being randomized to receive conservative treatment varied from 2% (281) to 47% (276). In some trials, there was little difference in revascularization rates between the invasive and conservative treatment groups, for example, in the Veterans Affairs Non–Q-Wave Infarction Strategies in Hospital (VANQWISH) trial, revascularization was performed in 33% of the conservative treatment group versus 44% of the invasive treatment group (277). In contrast, only 9% of the conservative treatment group in FRISC-II were revascularized, as opposed to 71% of the invasive treatment group (113).

In VANQWISH, mortality was higher in patients who had revascularization procedures. Most of these deaths occurred in patients treated acutely with CABG (11.6%) (277), and acuity is known to be one of the most powerful adverse prognosticators after CABG (282). At 23-month follow-up, however, there was no difference in death/MI between the invasive and conservative treatment groups.

FRISC-II (113) found that patients benefited from revascularization preceded by dalteparin treatment for 4 days before PCI and for 7 days before CABG. Owing to periprocedural events, the invasive treatment group had a higher rate of MI than the conservative treatment group at 1 month, but a lower rate of MI from then on. At 1 year, the invasive treatment group had lower rates of mortality (2.2% versus 3.9%, $P < .02$), MI (8.6% versus 11.6%, $P = .02$), and readmissions (37% versus 57%, $P < .001$) (283). The patients who benefited most from revascularization were those with ST depression and elevated troponin T levels (90).

TACTICS–TIMI-18 (91) randomized 2,220 intermediate- to high-risk patients to receive either conservative treatment or revascularization (performed between 4 and 48 hours). The

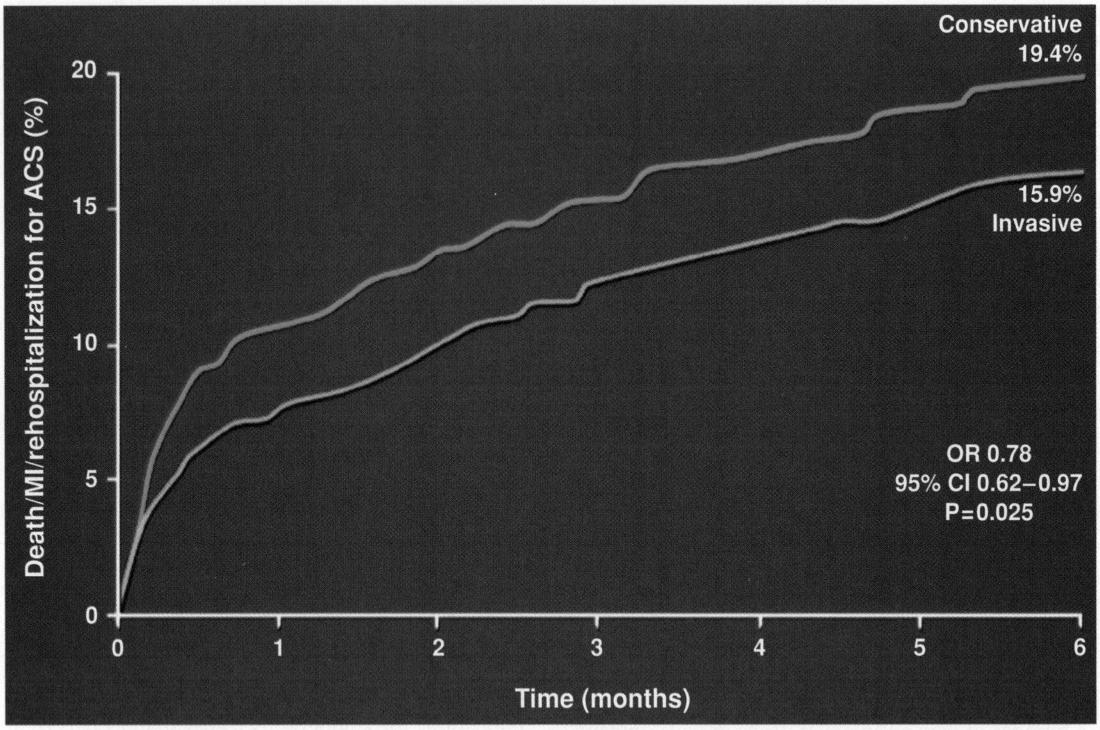

FIGURE 18.12. Cumulative incidence of death/MI/rehospitalization for ACS within 6 months in patients managed either conservatively or invasively in the TACTICS–TIMI-18 trial (91). (*Source:* Redrawn from Cannon CP, Weintraub WS, Demopoulos LA, et al. Comparison of early invasive and conservative strategies in patients with unstable coronary syndromes treated with the glycoprotein IIb/IIIa inhibitor tirofiban. *N Engl J Med* 2001;344:1879–1887, with permission.)

conservative treatment group received heparin, aspirin, and tirofiban for 48 to 108 hours. In the invasive treatment group, the mean duration of the tirofiban infusion before catheterization was 24 hours, and 41% of patients had PCI, 19% had CABG, and 40% had no intervention. The combined incidence of death/MI/rehospitalization was reduced from 19.4% in the conservative treatment group to 15.9% in the invasive treatment group (OR 0.78, P = .025) (Fig. 18.12). Patients pretreated with tirofiban did not have an increased rate of periprocedural MI. Revascularization was beneficial in patients with elevated troponin levels and in those with ST depression, but not in patients with a low TIMI risk score of 0 to 2, who constituted 25% of the study cohort. The ORs for death/MI/rehospitalization were 0.76 (95% CI 0.57–1.00) in intermediate-risk patients and 0.56 (95% CI 0.33–0.95) in high-risk patients.

In RITA-3, 1,810 patients with NSTEACS were given aspirin and enoxaparin and randomized to receive either early invasive or conservative treatment (92). The combined incidence of death/MI/refractory angina at 12 months was reduced by early revascularization from 14.5% to 9.6% (RR 0.66, 95% CI 0.51–0.85). Most of this reduction was in refractory ischemia, and there were no differences in the endpoints of death and death/MI. The protocol definition of MI required a CK rise to three times normal in patients treated with revascularization and to twice normal in patients treated conservatively. When the ESC/AHA definition of MI (5) was applied (2× increase in CK for revascularization), revascularization was associated with a significant reduction in MI from 13.3% to 8.9% at 4 months (P = .005). Quality of life was also improved by early revascularization.

The recent Invasive Versus Conservative Treatment in Unstable Coronary Syndromes (ICTUS) trial (276) randomized 1,200 patients with elevated troponin levels to receive either early revascularization (performed at a median of 23 [95% CI 14–42] hours) or selective revascularization (performed at a median of 142 [95% CI 37–243] hours). All patients received aspirin, enoxaparin, and clopidogrel upstream, and abciximab was used during PCI. Angiography was performed in 97% of the early revascularization treatment group and in 67% of the selective revascularization treatment group, with 47% having revascularization procedures within 1 year. There were no differences in the combined incidence of death/MI/rehospitalization for ACS at 1 year (21.7% with early revascularization versus 20.4% with selective revascularization, P = .59), although the rate of MI was reduced by early revascularization from 14.6% to 9.4% (P = .006). The GRACE registry (284) found no evidence that patients treated in hospitals with catheterization facilities achieved better clinical outcomes.

A meta-analysis of seven trials comparing invasive treatment with conservative treatment in a total of 9,212 patients found that patients managed invasively had reduced rates of MI (7.3% versus 9.4%, OR 0.75, 95% CI 0.65–0.87, P = .0002), rehospitalization (32.5% versus 41.3%, OR 0.66, P <.000001), and severe angina (11.2% versus 14.0%, OR 0.77, P = .00006) (285). Although mortality was not significantly reduced by invasive treatment (5.5% versus 6.0%, OR 0.92, 95% CI 0.77–1.09), the combined incidence of death/MI was reduced from 14.4% to 12.2% (OR 0.82, 95% CI 0.72–0.93, P = .001). The major benefit of invasive treatment was seen in higher risk patients with elevated cardiac marker levels at randomization; there was no significant benefit in lower risk patients. Addition of the ICTUS trial results (276) to this meta-analysis shows a nonsignificant 8% reduction in mortality (OR 0.92, 95% CI 0.78–1.10; Fig. 18.13) and a 15% reduction in MI (OR 0.85, 95% CI 0.74–0.97; Fig. 18.14).

There are few published data regarding treatment in the elderly. In TACTICS–TIMI-18 (286), patients older than 75 years had an absolute reduction in death/MI of 10.8% at

Trial	N	Routine invasive (%)	Selective invasive (%)	OR for mortality
TIMI-IIB	1473	4.9	5.2	0.94
VANQWISH	920	17.3	12.9	1.42
MATE	201	10.8	10.0	1.09
FRISC-II	2457	2.2	3.9	0.56
TACTICS–TIMI-18	2220	3.3	3.5	0.94
VINO	131	0.1	13.4	0.21
RITA-3	1810	6.7	7.9	0.84
ICTUS	1201	2.2	2.0	1.07
Combined	10,413	5.1	5.5	0.92

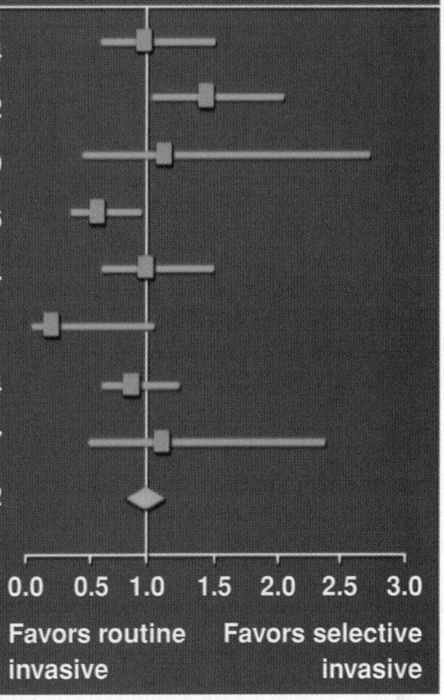

Test for homogeneity of ORs: P=0.0602

FIGURE 18.13. Meta-analysis of mortality from randomization to end of follow-up in trials of routine versus selective invasive management of ACS (276,285). (*Source:* Adapted from Mehta SR, Cannon CP, Fox KA, et al. Routine vs selective invasive strategies in patients with acute coronary syndromes: a collaborative meta-analysis of randomized trials. *JAMA* 2005;293:2908–2917, with permission.)

Trial	N	Routine invasive (%)	Selective invasive (%)	OR for MI
TIMI-IIIB	1473	8.4	10.1	0.81
VANQWISH	920	15.6	17.5	0.87
MATE	201	3.6	2.2	1.64
FRISC-II	2457	8.6	11.6	0.72
TACTICS–TIMI-18	2220	4.8	6.9	0.68
VINO	131	3.1	14.9	0.18
RITA-3	1810	4.1	5.2	0.78
ICTUS	1201	14.6	9.4	1.65
Combined	10,413	8.1	9.4	0.85

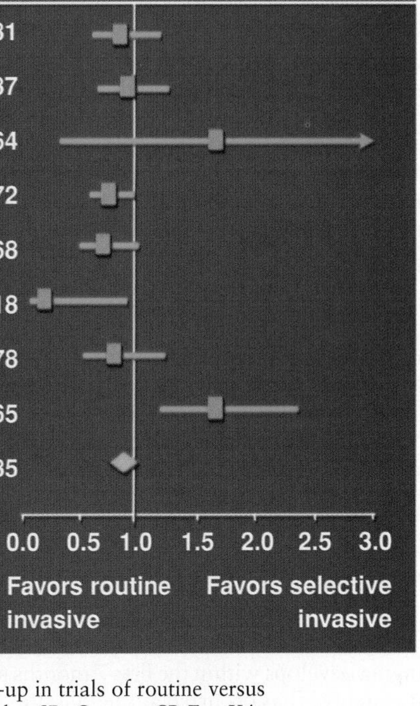

Test for homogeneity of ORs: P=0.004

FIGURE 18.14. Meta-analysis of MI from randomization to end of follow-up in trials of routine versus selective invasive management of ACS (276,285). (*Source:* Adapted from Mehta SR, Cannon CP, Fox KA, et al. Routine vs selective invasive strategies in patients with acute coronary syndromes: a collaborative meta-analysis of randomized trials. *JAMA* 2005;293:2908–2917, with permission.)

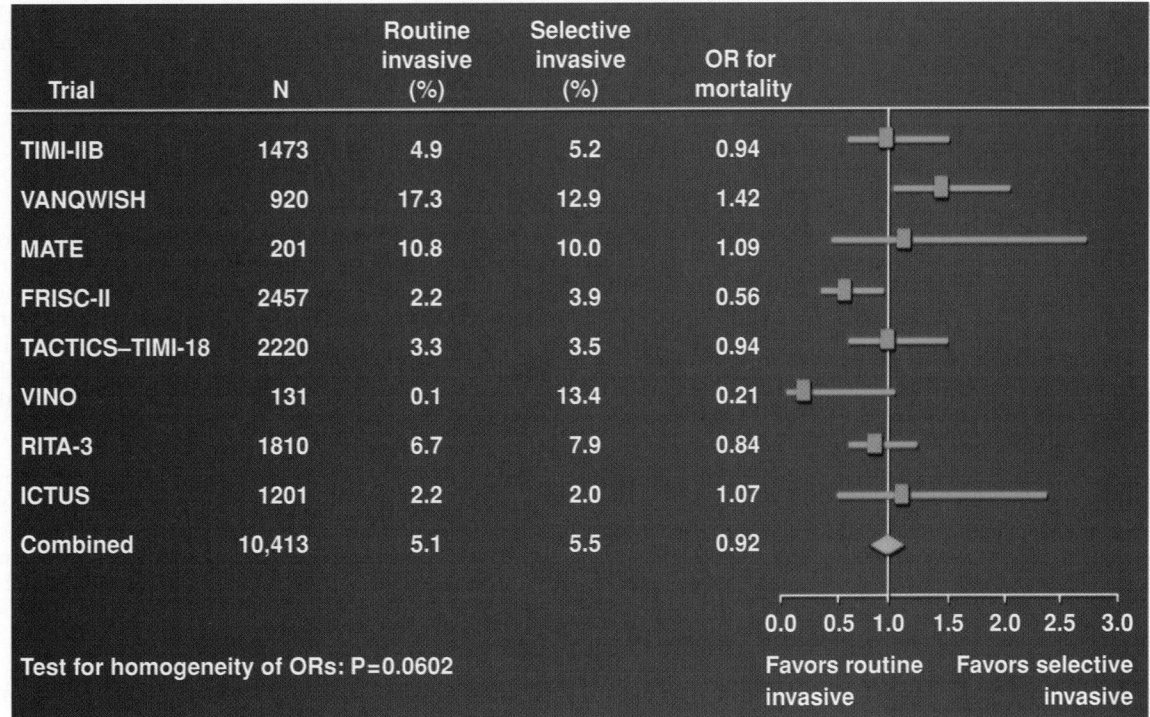

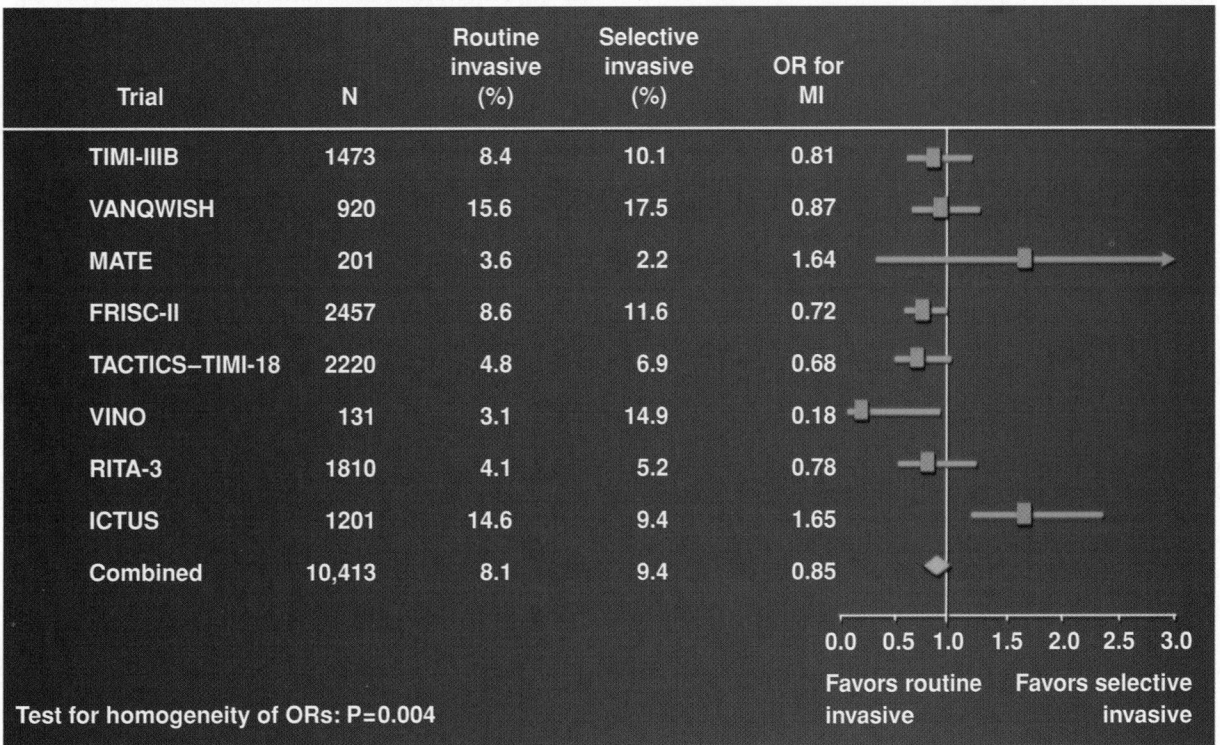

6 months with revascularization (10.8% versus 21.6%, $P = .016$). However, transfusions were required in 20.9% of elderly patients having revascularization procedures versus 7.9% of those managed conservatively ($P = .002$). There are higher initial costs with revascularization, but shorter hospital stays and fewer readmissions translate into lower postprocedural costs. In TACTICS–TIMI-18 there was no difference in 6-month costs between invasive and conservative treatment (287). Invasive treatment was found to be cost effective in an analysis of the FRISC-II trial (288).

It is recommended that high-risk patients have early revascularization accompanied by aspirin, clopidogrel, UFH or enoxaparin, and a small-molecule GP IIb/IIIa antagonist for 4 to 48 hours prior to angiography. An alternative approach is to withhold GP IIb/IIIa antagonists, clopidogrel, or both until the coronary anatomy has been defined. The superiority of either approach is yet to be determined in clinical trials.

Timing of Intervention

The Intracoronary Stenting with Antithrombotic Regimen Cooling-Off (ISAR-COOL) study (289) randomized 410 patients to be managed either with early revascularization or with a "cooling off" period (median time to catheterization 86 hours) during which patients received aspirin, clopidogrel, tirofiban, and UFH. Early revascularization (performed at a median time of 2.4 hours) reduced death/MI from 11.6% to 5.9% ($P = .04$). Most of the events in the conservative treatment group were MIs occurring in the period before PCI. In the context of current medical management and current PCI techniques, delaying of PCI to allow time for "passivation" of the culprit lesion results in increased event rates prior to PCI. Although early angiography appears preferable to delayed angiography, the optimal timing of angiography has not yet been defined (see Controversies and Personal Perspectives).

Percutaneous Coronary Intervention

PCI techniques have evolved rapidly over the past several years with the advent of drug-eluting stents. Although PCI improves coronary flow, it may be associated with periprocedural MI owing to obstruction of branch vessels or distal embolization of thrombus or plaque material. In the past, acute thrombotic closure and MI associated with PCI were more common in patients with NSTEACS than in those having elective interventions (290,291). PCI is aimed at treating the culprit lesion rather than non–flow-limiting plaques, although the latter are more likely to cause NSTEACS (17,292). Revascularization is not recommended unless the benefits are likely to outweigh the risks.

Coronary Artery Bypass Grafting

CABG is an excellent treatment for relieving angina, and grafts protect against proximal minor plaque instability (293). CABG was an important component of the FRISC-II and TACTICS–TIMI-18 trials, being performed in 35% of the FRISC-II invasive treatment group (113) and in 20% of the TACTICS–TIMI-18 invasive treatment group (91).

Unstable Angina after Percutaneous Coronary Intervention

If angina develops within the first 7 months after PCI, it is likely that restenosis has occurred at the PCI site. Another possibility is acute thrombotic closure, which may occur late after implantation of a drug-eluting stent (294). In the event of angina occurring after revascularization, angiography should be performed expeditiously with repeat revascularization if indicated. IV nitroglycerin has been shown to be superior to antithrombotic therapy in preventing recurrent or refractory angina after balloon angioplasty (295).

Unstable Angina after Coronary Artery Bypass Grafting

Within the first 12 months after CABG using venous conduits, 10% to 15% of grafts occlude owing to technical reasons and fibroproliferation with or without superimposed thrombus formation (296). Internal mammary artery grafts have better long-term patency rates (approximately 92%) (297), but are vulnerable to early stenosis. In the long term, late graft disease occurs as a result of atherosclerosis and superimposed thrombosis (298). Progression of atherosclerosis also occurs in the native coronary arteries.

Patients with NSTEACS after CABG should have expeditious angiography. Stenting may prevent occlusion of a severely stenosed vein graft, thereby avoiding reoperation and its associated risks. Unfortunately, disease progression commonly occurs in nonstented segments of the vein graft within 2 years (299).

The Case for Conservative Management in Intermediate- and Low-Risk Patients

The favorable prognosis of low-risk patients justifies a conservative approach because they are unlikely to require revascularization. These patients can be managed initially with antithrombotic and antianginal therapy to passivate the ruptured or fissured plaque. Subsequent management depends on the severity of recurrent or inducible ischemia. Stress testing can be performed to assess the hemodynamic significance of CAD, and should be delayed until 24 to 48 hours after the last episode of angina. It should be noted, however, that noninvasive stress testing does not predict plaque instability or the risk of future MI; thus, it is important that these patients be reviewed and instructed to report any continuing symptoms.

Early Lipid Lowering

The concept that lipid lowering may stabilize plaques is supported by numerous trials showing that statin therapy reduces the risk of clinical events despite only modest angiographic reductions in the severity of coronary stenoses (300,301). The pleiotrophic effects of statins may improve clinical outcomes independently of lipid changes in patients with ACS. Statins may also suppress inflammatory cell activity (302) and reduce thrombus formation (303). Statin trials have reported rapid improvements in endothelial function (304–307) and reduced levels of inflammatory markers such as CRP (80).

In the Long-Term Intervention With Pravastatin in Ischemic Disease (LIPID) trial, 3,260 patients were randomized to receive either pravastatin or a placebo starting 3 to 36 months after hospitalization for unstable angina. Mortality at 6 years was reduced from 13% to 9.7% with pravastatin ($P = .004$) (308).

In the Myocardial Ischemia Reduction with Aggressive Cholesterol Lowering (MIRACL) trial (309), 3,086 patients were randomized to receive either 80 mg of atorvastatin daily or a placebo 1 to 4 days after presenting with ACS. On average, atorvastatin increased high-density lipoprotein cholesterol levels by 4%, and reduced total cholesterol by 27%, LDL-C by 40% and triglycerides by 16%. At 16 weeks the combined incidence of death/MI/resuscitated cardiac arrest/worsening angina/urgent rehospitalization was reduced from 17.4% to 14.8% ($P = .048$).

In phase 2 of the A to Z trial, 4,487 patients with ACS received either 40 mg of simvastatin for 1 month followed by 80 mg of simvastatin daily, or a placebo for 4 months followed by 20 mg of simvastatin daily (310). The median follow-up period was 721 days. In patients receiving the more intensive regimen, there was a trend toward a reduction in cardiovascular death/MI/stroke/readmission with ACS (14.4% versus 16.7%, $P = .14$).

In the Pravastatin or Atorvastatin Evaluation and Infection Therapy–Thrombolysis in Myocardial Infarction-22 (PROVE-IT) trial, 4,162 patients developing an ACS within the preceding 10 days were randomized to receive either 40 mg of pravastatin or 80 mg of atorvastatin daily (80). LDL-C levels were lowered to 95 mg/dL (2.46 mmol/L) in the pravastatin treatment group and to 62 mg/dL (1.60 mmol/L) in the atorvastatin treatment group. Atorvastatin reduced the combined incidence of death/ MI/admission for ACS/revascularization (after 30 days)/stroke by 16%, from 26.3% to 22.4% ($P < .001$). The benefit of atorvastatin was apparent within 30 days, and mortality at 2 years was reduced from 3.2% to 2.2% ($P = .07$).

A major rationale for early commencement of lipid lowering therapy is that it emphasizes to patients that this treatment is important and needs to be continued in the long term. Also patients may be more likely to comply with therapy and achieve their target lipid levels if therapy is commenced and dietary advice is provided during hospitalization (311).

Antiinflammatory Agents

A small randomized trial compared 48 hours of methylprednisolone therapy with a placebo in 166 patients with unstable angina, and reported a reduction in CRP levels, but no effect on short-term outcomes (312). A study of long-term therapy with antichlamydial antibiotics found that there was no reduction in the risk of ischemic events after ACS (313).

Secondary Prevention

Smoking cessation and treatment of dyslipidemia and hypertension are important secondary preventative measures in all patients with CAD. Other measures that should be instituted include achievement of ideal weight, a regular exercise program, an appropriate low–cardiovascular-risk diet, and achievement of optimal diabetic control where necessary. If facilities are available, patients should be referred to a cardiac rehabilitation program (314). Aspirin, β-blockers, statins, and ACE inhibitors should be prescribed in all patients without contraindications (315–317).

GUIDELINES

There is strong evidence that better outcomes are achieved by institutions with higher usage rates of evidence-based therapies (318,319). The uptake of treatment guidelines has been variable (320). The Can Rapid Risk Stratification of Unstable Angina Patients Suppress Adverse Outcomes With Early Implementation of the ACC/AHA Guidelines investigators (CRUSADE) (321) reported that an early invasive strategy was utilized in only 44.89% of high-risk patients with NSTEACS. Predictors of early invasive treatment included younger age, male gender, lack of comorbidities, and management by cardiologists. When an early invasive strategy was used, there was a lower risk of in-hospital mortality after adjustment for differences in clinical characteristics (2.5% versus 3.7%, $P < .001$).

CONTROVERSIES AND PERSONAL PERSPECTIVES

Optimal Timing of Revascularization

The optimal timing of revascularization has not been defined. There is increasing evidence that the earlier intervention is undertaken, the better the outcomes are (322). However, this is balanced by evidence from TACTICS–TIMI-18, where the TIMI flow grade (110) and myocardial perfusion were found to correlate with the length of tirofiban treatment before PCI (323). Moreover, at 6 months there was no significant difference in death/MI/rehospitalization between patients having angiography within 48 hours and those having angiography after 48 hours (15.4% versus 19.5%, $P = .34$) (324), although there was a trend for MI rates to be lower in those having angiography within 48 hours (2.9% versus 6.5%, $P = .08$).

In the GRACE registry (325), patients having angiography within 24 hours had higher in-hospital mortality (3.5%) than those having angiography between 24 and 48 hours (1.4%) or after 48 hours (2.0%; $P < .0001$). The mortality difference persisted at 6 months (7.0% versus 3.9% and 5.9%, respectively). It should be noted that the timing of angiography in the GRACE registry was not randomized, and it is very likely that patients having earlier angiography were at higher risk and more unstable. Furthermore, it is not known how many patients in each group received upstream GP IIb/IIIa antagonists, which reduce the risk of events prior to angiography (226).

The optimal timing of intervention may depend on the patient's risk status. Very high-risk patients, such as those with hemodynamic instability or important ventricular arrhythmias, should have angiography as soon as possible. Patients with dynamic ST-segment changes are also likely to benefit from very early intervention, whereas patients with elevated troponin levels may benefit from upstream treatment with GP IIb/IIIa antagonists before angiography within the first 24 to 48 hours. The only way to determine whether early angiography (e.g., within 4 hours) is preferable to delayed angiography (e.g., at 12–24 hours) is to conduct prospective trials in which the timing of planned angiography is randomized.

Upstream Versus In-Laboratory Administration of Glycoprotein IIb/IIIa Antagonists

A distinct advantage of starting a GP IIb/IIIa antagonist prior to intervention is that it extends the benefit of this therapy to patients not having PCI (i.e., those having CABG or no intervention) (226). Conversely, if GP IIb/IIIa antagonist use is limited to the catheterization laboratory, only 40% to 60% of all patients presenting with NSTEACS receive its benefits, and overall the treatment is less beneficial than if it had been administered upstream. In the ACUITY trial deferred use of GP IIb/IIIa antagonists resulted in a 12% (−3 to 29%) increase in ischemic events (death, MI, unplanned revascularization), but increased major bleeding (4.9% vs. 6.1%, $p = 0.009$). The median time of upstream treatment was only $4^{1}/_{2}$ hours.

Benefits of Upstream Combination Antithrombotic Therapy

The concept of upstream treatment can also be applied to clopidogrel and enoxaparin. When administered upstream, clopidogrel reduces event rates prior to intervention. In the CURE trial, the combined incidence of cardiovascular death/MI/stroke was reduced from 2.1% to 1.4% at 24 hours ($P < .05$), translating into 7 fewer events per 1,000 patients randomized (77).

In a systematic overview of five trials comparing enoxaparin with UFH in a total of 9,835 patients receiving no antithrombotic therapy prior to randomization, enoxaparin reduced death/MI by 19% at 30 days (76). This benefit may be applicable to patients receiving upstream enoxaparin prior to revascularization. For every 1,000 patients with elevated troponin levels who receive clopidregrel, enoxaparin and IIb/IIIa antagonists upstream, there may be a 60% relative reduction in event rates and 12 fewer cardiovascular events based on the following calculations: if the event rate is 2% in the first 24 hours, clopidogrel may prevent four cardiovascular deaths, MIs, or strokes (based on a 20% overall reduction in the CURE trial) (77); GP IIb/IIIa antagonists may prevent four deaths or MIs (based on an 18% reduction in patients with elevated troponin levels in the Boersma meta-analysis) (78); and enoxaparin may prevent four deaths or MIs (based on a 19% reduction in Petersen's systematic overview) (76). If these benefits are additive, 12 major cardiovascular events per 1,000 patients treated may be prevented by upstream administration of intensive antithrombotic therapy. These benefits will need to be balanced with increased bleeding rates.

THE FUTURE

Despite considerable advances in treatment, patients with NSTEACS continue to have high morbidity and mortality rates. The number of patients with NSTEACS is likely to increase as the current epidemic of obesity and the metabolic syndrome impact on the prevalence of CAD (3). There are now six evidence-based treatments available for the treatment of NSTEACS (aspirin, clopidogrel, GP IIb/IIa antagonists, enoxaparin, bivalirudin, and revascularization) and the challenge now facing clinicians is to use them in suitable combinations (78,242,326). New biomarkers such as BNP and inflammatory markers such as interleukin-6 and CRP need to be integrated into risk algorithms.

Dynamic multimarker risk profiling needs to be integrated into routine clinical management, perhaps with the use of computer algorithms. New biomarkers for risk profiling—including markers of ischemia, inflammation, thrombosis, myocyte necrosis, and plaque instability—will enable targeting of therapies for efficacy and safety.

High-resolution, three-dimensional MRI can distinguish intact thick and fibrous plaque caps from intact thin and disrupted caps in human carotid arteries (327). This technology may allow examination of the association between fibrous cap changes and clinical outcomes, enabling the development of therapies to stabilize plaques. Innovative research is currently being done on noninvasive assessment of plaque temperature (328,329). Warmer plaques have increased numbers of macrophages and a greater propensity for rupture (329).

Further developments in noninvasive imaging may enable detection of coronary thrombi composed mostly of platelets, at which agents such as GP IIb/IIIa antagonists could be targeted. If imaging showed that a thrombus consisted mostly of red blood cells, a direct antithrombin might be more effective, whereas if the thrombus was a mixture of platelets and red blood cells, combination therapy might be more suitable. If an elevated plaque with little thrombus was detected, PCI without adjunctive drug therapy might be the most appropriate first-line treatment.

Our knowledge of the mechanisms that lead to plaque instability will continue to expand. Predictors of plaque instability need to be identified so that high-risk patients can be targeted with specific therapies. Apoptotic macrophages can be detected in recently disrupted plaques by scintigraphy using radiolabeled antiannexin antibodies (330–332). Treatments that may reduce the vulnerability of plaques to rupture include matrix metalloproteinase inhibitors and locally delivered growth factor inhibitors. Modulation of the ability of the myocardium to survive ischemia, including angiogenesis and metabolic manipulation, will be the focus of active research. Diagnostic modalities such as single-photon emission with radiolabeled B-methyl iodophenyl pentadecanoic acid can detect myocardium that has been ischemic in the last 24 to 36 hours. It may be possible to combine this technology with high-resolution computed tomography for noninvasive detection of thrombogenic coronary plaques. Rapid genomic profiling tests may be developed for bedside use so that therapies can be targeted at patients who are most likely to benefit and least likely to experience side effects. Clinical outcomes may be improved by combinations of current therapies with different dosing regimens. Nevertheless, there is still a need for safer, more effective, cost-effective, and easily administered treatments, including oral medications. In the long term, greater emphasis must be placed on primary prevention.

ACKNOWLEDGMENTS

The author gratefully acknowledges the assistance of Charlene Nell, who provided secretarial assistance, and Anna Breckon, ELS, who edited the manuscript and prepared the artwork.

References

1. Braunwald E, Antman EM, Beasley JW, et al. ACC/AHA 2002 guideline update for the management of patients with unstable angina and non-ST-segment elevation myocardial infarction—summary article: a report of the American College of Cardiology/American Heart Association Task Force on Practice Guidelines (Committee on the Management of Patients With Unstable Angina). *J Am Coll Cardiol* 2002;40:1366–1374.
2. Gibler WB, Cannon CP, Blomkalns AL, et al. Practical implementation of the guidelines for unstable angina/non-ST-segment elevation myocardial infarction in the emergency department: a scientific statement from the American Heart Association Council on Clinical Cardiology (Subcommittee on Acute Cardiac Care), Council on Cardiovascular Nursing, and Quality of Care and Outcomes Research Interdisciplinary Working Group, in Collaboration With the Society of Chest Pain Centers. *Circulation* 2005; 111:2699–2710.
3. Kleiman NS, White HD. The declining prevalence of ST elevation myocardial infarction in patients presenting with acute coronary syndromes [editorial]. *Heart* 2005;91:1121–1123.
4. Aroney C, Boyden AN, Jelinek MV, et al. Management of unstable angina: guidelines—2000. *Med J Aust* 2000;173[Suppl]:S65–S88.
5. The Joint European Society of Cardiology/American College of Cardiology Committee. Myocardial infarction redefined—a consensus document of the Joint European Society of Cardiology/American College of Cardiology Committee for the Redefinition of Myocardial Infarction. *J Am Coll Cardiol* 2000;36:959–969.
6. Braunwald E. Unstable angina: a classification. *Circulation* 1989;80:410–414.
7. Scirica BM, Cannon CP, McCabe CH, et al. Prognosis in the Thrombolysis in Myocardial Ischemia III registry according to the Braunwald unstable angina pectoris classification. *Am J Cardiol* 2002;90:821–826.
8. Ahmed WH, Bittl JA, Braunwald E. Relation between clinical presentation and angiographic findings in unstable angina pectoris, and comparison with that in stable angina. *Am J Cardiol* 1993;72:544–550.
9. Hamm CW, Braunwald E. A classification of unstable angina revisited. *Circulation* 2000;102:118–122.
10. Prinzmetal M, Kennamer R, Merliss R, et al. A variant form of angina pectoris. *Am J Med* 1959;27:375–388.
11. Braunwald E. Unstable angina: an etiologic approach to management [editorial]. *Circulation* 1998;98:2219–2222.
12. Falk E. Plaque rupture with severe pre-existing stenosis precipitating coronary thrombosis: characteristics of coronary atherosclerotic plaques underlying fatal occlusive thrombi. *Br Heart J* 1983;50:127–134.
13. Davies MJ, Thomas AC. Plaque fissuring: the cause of acute myocardial infarction, sudden ischemic death, and crescendo angina. *Br Heart J* 1985;53:363–373.
14. Fuster V, Badimon L, Badimon JJ, et al. The pathogenesis of coronary artery disease and the acute coronary syndromes (1). *N Engl J Med* 1992; 326:242–250.

15. Fuster V, Badimon L, Badimon JJ, et al. The pathogenesis of coronary artery disease and the acute coronary syndromes (2). *N Engl J Med* 1992;326:310–318.
16. Virmani R, Burke AP, Farb A, et al. Pathology of the unstable plaque. *Prog Cardiovasc Dis* 2002;44:349–356.
17. Goldstein JA, Demetriou D, Grines CL, et al. Multiple complex coronary plaques in patients with acute myocardial infarction. *N Engl J Med* 2000;343:915–922.
18. Rioufol G, Finet G, Ginon I, et al. Multiple atherosclerotic plaque rupture in acute coronary syndrome: a three-vessel intravascular ultrasound study. *Circulation* 2002;106:804–808.
19. Asakura M, Ueda Y, Yamaguchi O, et al. Extensive development of vulnerable plaques as a pan-coronary process in patients with myocardial infarction: an angioscopic study. *J Am Coll Cardiol* 2001;37:1284–1288.
20. Buffon A, Biasucci LM, Liuzzo G, et al. Widespread coronary inflammation in unstable angina. *N Engl J Med* 2002;347:5–12.
21. Zairis MN, Papadaki OA, Manousakis SJ, et al. C-reactive protein and multiple complex coronary artery plaques in patients with primary unstable angina. *Atherosclerosis* 2002;164:355–359.
22. Vaughan DE. Plasminogen activator inhibitor-1 and the calculus of mortality after myocardial infarction. *Circulation* 2003;108:376–377.
23. Mizuno K, Satomura K, Miyamoto A, et al. Angioscopic evaluation of coronary-artery thrombi in acute coronary syndromes. *N Engl J Med* 1992;326:287–291.
24. Ross R. Atherosclerosis—an inflammatory disease. *N Engl J Med* 1999;340:115–126.
25. Libby P. Molecular bases of the acute coronary syndromes. *Circulation* 1995;91:2844–2850.
26. Little WC, Constantinescu M, Applegate RJ, et al. Can coronary angiography predict the site of a subsequent myocardial infarction in patients with mild-to-moderate coronary artery disease? *Circulation* 1988;78:1157–1166.
27. Haft JI, Haik BJ, Goldstein JE, et al. Development of significant coronary artery lesions in areas of minimal disease: a common mechanism for coronary disease progression. *Chest* 1988;94:731–736.
28. Ambrose JA, Tannenbaum MA, Alexopoulos D, et al. Angiographic progression of coronary artery disease and the development of myocardial infarction. *J Am Coll Cardiol* 1988;12:56–62.
29. Hackett D, Verwilghen J, Davies G, et al. Coronary stenoses before and after acute myocardial infarction. *Am J Cardiol* 1989;63:1517–1518.
30. Giroud D, Li JM, Urban P, et al. Relation of the site of acute myocardial infarction to the most severe coronary arterial stenosis at prior angiography. *Am J Cardiol* 1992;69:729–732.
31. Pétursson MK, Jónmundsson EH, Brekkan A, et al. Angiographic predictors of new coronary occlusions. *Am Heart J* 1995;129:515–520.
32. Yamagishi M, Terashima M, Awano K, et al. Morphology of vulnerable coronary plaque: insights from follow-up of patients examined by intravascular ultrasound before an acute coronary syndrome. *J Am Coll Cardiol* 2000;35:106–111.
33. Davies MJ, Richardson PD, Woolf N, et al. Risk of thrombosis in human atherosclerotic plaques: role of extracellular lipid, macrophage, and smooth muscle cell content. *Br Heart J* 1993;69:377–381.
34. Moreno PR, Falk E, Palacios IF, et al. Macrophage infiltration in acute coronary syndromes. Implications for plaque rupture. *Circulation* 1994;90:775–778.
35. van der Wal AC, Becker AE, van der Loos CM, et al. Site of intimal rupture or erosion of thrombosed coronary atherosclerotic plaques is characterized by an inflammatory process irrespective of the dominant plaque morphology. *Circulation* 1994;89:36–44.
36. van der Wal AC, Piek JJ, de Boer OJ, et al. Recent activation of the plaque immune response in coronary lesions underlying acute coronary syndromes. *Heart* 1998;80:14–18.
37. Kaartinen M, Penttila A, Kovanen PT. Accumulation of activated mast cells in the shoulder region of human coronary atheroma, the predilection site of atheromatous rupture. *Circulation* 1994;90:1669–1678.
38. Adams JEI, Sicard GA, Allen BT, et al. Diagnosis of perioperative myocardial infarction with measurement of cardiac troponin I. *N Engl J Med* 1994;330:670–674.
39. Biasucci LM, Liuzzo G, Fantuzzi G, et al. Increasing levels of interleukin (IL)-1Ra and IL-6 during the first 2 days of hospitalization in unstable angina are associated with increased risk of in-hospital coronary events. *Circulation* 1999;99:2079–2084.
40. Liuzzo G, Biasucci LM, Gallimore JR, et al. The prognostic value of C-reactive protein and serum amyloid A protein in severe unstable angina. *N Engl J Med* 1994;331:417–424.
41. Biasucci LM, Liuzzo G, Grillo RL, et al. Elevated levels of C-reactive protein at discharge in patients with unstable angina predict recurrent instability. *Circulation* 1999;99:855–860.
42. Milazzo D, Biasucci LM, Luciani N, et al. Elevated levels of C-reactive protein before coronary artery bypass grafting predict recurrence of ischemic events. *Am J Cardiol* 1999;84:459–461.
43. Mulvihill NT, Foley JB, Murphy R, et al. Evidence of prolonged inflammation in unstable angina and non-Q wave myocardial infarction. *J Am Coll Cardiol* 2000;36:1210–1216.
44. Liuzzo G, Kopecky SL, Frye RL, et al. Perturbation of the T-cell repertoire in patients with unstable angina. *Circulation* 1999;100:2135–2139.
45. Kuo CC, Shor A, Campbell LA, et al. Demonstration of *Chlamydia pneumoniae* in atherosclerotic lesions of coronary arteries. *J Infect Dis* 1993;167:841–849.
46. Mendall MA, Goggin PM, Molineaux N, et al. Relation of *Helicobacter pylori* infection and coronary heart disease. *Br Heart J* 1994;71:437–439.
47. Mendall MA, Patel P, Ballam L, et al. C-reactive protein and its relation to cardiovascular risk factors; a population based cross-sectional study. *Br Med J* 1996;312:1061–1065.
48. Caligiuri G, Paulsson G, Nicoletti A, et al. Evidence for antigen-driven T-cell response in unstable angina. *Circulation* 2000;102:1114–1119.
49. Kol A, Sperti G, Shani J, et al. Cytomegalovirus replication is not a cause of instability in unstable angina. *Circulation* 1995;91:1910–1913.
50. Folts JD, Crowell EB, Rowe GG. Platelet aggregation in partially obstructed vessels and its elimination with aspirin. *Circulation* 1976;54:365–370.
51. Davies MJ, Thomas AC, Knapman PA, et al. Intramyocardial platelet aggregation in patients with unstable angina suffering sudden ischemic cardiac death. *Circulation* 1986;73:418–427.
52. Fitzgerald DJ, Roy L, Catella F, et al. Platelet activation in unstable coronary disease. *N Engl J Med* 1986;315:983–989.
53. Buja LM, Willerson JT. Role of inflammation in coronary plaque disruption [editorial]. *Circulation* 1994;89:503–505.
54. Hoffmeister HM, Jur M, Wendel HP, et al. Alterations of coagulation and fibrinolytic and kallikrein-kinin systems in the acute and postacute phases in patients with unstable angina pectoris. *Circulation* 1995;91:2520–2527.
55. Merlini PA, Bauer KA, Oltrona L, et al. Persistent activation of coagulation mechanism in unstable angina and myocardial infarction. *Circulation* 1994;90:61–68.
56. Ault KA, Cannon CP, Mitchell J, et al. Platelet activation in patients after an acute coronary syndrome: results from the TIMI-12 trial. *J Am Coll Cardiol* 1999;33:634–639.
57. Freeman MR, Williams AE, Chisholm RJ, et al. Intracoronary thrombus and complex morphology in unstable angina: relation to timing of angiography and in-hospital cardiac events. *Circulation* 1989;80:17–23.
58. Ambrose JA, Winters SL, Stern A, et al. Angiographic morphology and the pathogenesis of unstable angina pectoris. *J Am Coll Cardiol* 1985;5:609–616.
59. Gotoh K, Minamino T, Katoh O, et al. The role of intracoronary thrombus in unstable angina: angiographic assessment and thrombolytic therapy during ongoing angina attacks. *Circulation* 1988;77:526–534.
60. Sherman CT, Litvak F, Grundfest W, et al. Coronary angioscopy in patients with unstable angina pectoris. *N Engl J Med* 1986;315:913–919.
61. Mizuno K. Angioscopy in acute coronary syndromes. *Cardiology Today* 1992;20:1–2.
62. De Feyter PJ, Ozaki Y, Baptista J, et al. Ischemia-related lesion characteristics in patients with stable or unstable angina: a study with intracoronary angioscopy and ultrasound. *Circulation* 1995;92:1408–1413.
63. Moise A, Theroux P, Taeymans Y, et al. Unstable angina and progression of coronary atherosclerosis. *N Engl J Med* 1983;309:685–689.
64. Kloner RA, Hale S, Alker K, et al. The effects of acute and chronic cocaine use on the heart. *Circulation* 1992;85:407–419.
65. Muller JE, Stone PH, Turi ZG, et al. Circadian variation in the frequency of onset of acute myocardial infarction. *N Engl J Med* 1985;313:1315–1322.
66. Tofler GH, Brezinski D, Schafer AI, et al. Concurrent morning increase in platelet aggregability and the risk of myocardial infarction and sudden cardiac death. *N Engl J Med* 1987;316:1514–1518.
67. Mittleman MA, Maclure M, Tofler GH, et al. Triggering of acute myocardial infarction by heavy physical exertion: protection against triggering by regular exertion. *N Engl J Med* 1993;329:1677–1683.
68. Baroldi G. Coronary thrombosis: facts and beliefs. *Am Heart J* 1976;91:683–688.
69. Yasue H, Horio Y, Nakamura N, et al. Induction of coronary artery spasm by acetylcholine in patients with variant angina: possible role of the parasympathetic nervous system in the pathogenesis of coronary artery spasm. *Circulation* 1986;74:955–963.
70. McFadden EP, Clarke JG, Davies GJ, et al. Effect of intracoronary serotonin on coronary vessels in patients with stable angina and patients with variant angina. *N Engl J Med* 1991;324:648–654.
71. Toyo-Oka T, Aizawa T, Suzuki N, et al. Increased plasma level of endothelin-1 and coronary spasm induction in patients with vasospastic angina pectoris. *Circulation* 1991;83:476–483.
72. Brown BG, Bolson EL, Dodge HT. Dynamic mechanisms in human coronary stenosis. *Circulation* 1984;70:917–922.
73. Ludmer PL, Selwyn AP, Shook TL, et al. Paradoxical vasoconstriction induced by acetylcholine in atherosclerotic coronary arteries. *N Engl J Med* 1986;315:1046–1051.
74. Bogaty P, Hackett D, Davies G, et al. Vasoreactivity of the culprit lesion in unstable angina. *Circulation* 1994;90:5–11.
75. Theroux P, Ouimet H, McCans J, et al. Aspirin, heparin, or both to treat acute unstable angina. *N Engl J Med* 1988;319:1105–1111.
76. Petersen JL, Mahaffey KW, Hasselblad V, et al. Efficacy and bleeding complications among patients randomized to enoxaparin or unfractionated heparin for antithrombin therapy in non-ST-segment elevation acute coronary syndromes: a systematic overview. *JAMA* 2004;292:89–96.
77. Yusuf S, Zhao F, Mehta SR, et al. Effects of clopidogrel in addition to aspirin in patients with acute coronary syndromes without ST-segment elevation. *N Engl J Med* 2001;345:494–502.

78. Boersma E, Harrington RA, Moliterno DJ, et al. Platelet glycoprotein IIb/IIIa inhibitors in acute coronary syndromes: a meta-analysis of all major randomised clinical trials. *Lancet* 2002;359:189–198.
79. Ikonomidis I, Andreotti F, Economou E, et al. Increased proinflammatory cytokines in patients with chronic stable angina and their reduction by aspirin. *Circulation* 1999;100:793–798.
80. Cannon CP, Braunwald E, McCabe CH, et al. Intensive versus moderate lipid lowering with statins after acute coronary syndromes. *N Engl J Med* 2004;350:1495–1504.
81. Ridker PM, Cannon CP, Morrow D, et al. C-reactive protein levels and outcomes after statin therapy. *N Engl J Med* 2005;352:20–28.
82. Langer A, Freeman MR, Armstrong PW. ST segment shift in unstable angina: pathophysiology and association with coronary anatomy and hospital outcome. *J Am Coll Cardiol* 1989;13:1495–1502.
83. Savonitto S, Ardissino D, Granger CB, et al. Prognostic value of the admission electrocardiogram in acute coronary syndromes. *JAMA* 1999; 281:707–713.
84. Cannon CP, McCabe CH, Stone PH, et al. The electrocardiogram predicts one-year outcome of patients with unstable angina and non-Q wave myocardial infarction: results of the TIMI III registry ECG ancillary study. *J Am Coll Cardiol* 1997;30:133–140.
85. Hyde TA, French JK, Wong CK, et al. Four-year survival of patients with acute coronary syndromes without ST-segment elevation and prognostic significance of 0.5-mm ST-segment depression. *Am J Cardiol* 1999;84:379–385.
86. Kaul P, Newby LK, Fu Y, et al. Relation between baseline risk and treatment decisions in non-ST elevation acute coronary syndromes: an examination of international practice patterns. *Heart* 2005;91:876–881.
87. Holmvang L, Luscher MS, Clemmensen P, et al. Very early risk stratification using combined ECG and biochemical assessment in patients with unstable coronary artery disease (a Thrombin Inhibition in Myocardial Ischemia [TRIM] Substudy). *Circulation* 1998;98:2004–2009.
88. Jacobsen MD, Wagner GS, Holmvang L, et al. Quantitative T-wave analysis predicts 1 year prognosis and benefit from early invasive treatment in the FRISC II study population. *Eur Heart J* 2005;26:112–118.
89. Holmvang L, Clemmensen P, Lindahl B, et al. Quantitative analysis of the admission electrocardiogram identifies patients with unstable coronary artery disease who benefit the most from early invasive treatment. *J Am Coll Cardiol* 2003;41:905–915.
90. Diderholm E, Andrén B, Frostfeldt G, et al. The prognostic and therapeutic implications of increased troponin T levels and ST depression in unstable coronary artery disease: the FRISC II invasive troponin T electrocardiogram substudy. *Am Heart J* 2002;143:760–767.
91. Cannon CP, Weintraub WS, Demopoulos LA, et al. Comparison of early invasive and conservative strategies in patients with unstable coronary syndromes treated with the glycoprotein IIb/IIIa inhibitor tirofiban. *N Engl J Med* 2001;344:1879–1887.
92. Fox K, Poole-Wilson P, Henderson R, et al. Interventional versus conservative treatment for patients with unstable angina or non-ST-elevation myocardial infarction: the British Heart Foundation RITA 3 randomised trial. *Lancet* 2002;360:743–751.
93. Deanfield JE, Maseri A, Selwyn AP, et al. Myocardial ischaemia during daily life in patients with stable angina: its relation to symptoms and heart rate changes. *Lancet* 1983;ii:753–758.
94. Chierchia S, Lazzari M, Freedman B, et al. Impairment of myocardial perfusion and function during painless myocardial ischemia. *J Am Coll Cardiol* 1983;1:924–930.
95. Gottlieb SO, Weisfeldt ML, Ouyang P, et al. Silent ischemia as a marker for early unfavorable outcomes in patients with unstable angina. *N Engl J Med* 1986;314:1214–1219.
96. Holdright D, Patel D, Cunningham D, et al. Comparison of the effect of heparin and aspirin versus aspirin alone on transient myocardial ischemia and in-hospital prognosis in patients with unstable angina. *J Am Coll Cardiol* 1994;24:39–45.
97. Bertrand ME, Simoons ML, Fox KAA, et al. Management of acute coronary syndromes: acute coronary syndromes *without* persistent ST segment elevation: recommendations of the Task Force of the European Society of Cardiology. *Eur Heart J* 2000;21:1406–1432.
98. Jaffe AS, Ravkilde J, Roberts R, et al. It's time for a change to a troponin standard. *Circulation* 2000;102:1216–1220.
99. Hamm CW, Goldmann BU, Heeschen C, et al. Emergency room triage of patients with acute chest pain by means of rapid testing for cardiac troponin T or troponin I. *N Engl J Med* 1997;337:1648–1653.
100. Antman EM, Tanasijevic MJ, Thompson B, et al. Cardiac-specific troponin I levels to predict the risk of mortality in patients with acute coronary syndromes. *N Engl J Med* 1996;335:1342–1349.
101. Hamm CW, Ravkilde J, Gerhardt W, et al. The prognostic value of serum troponin T in unstable angina. *N Engl J Med* 1992;327:146–150.
102. Ohman EM, Armstrong PW, Christenson RH, et al. Cardiac troponin T levels for risk stratification in acute myocardial ischemia. *N Engl J Med* 1996;335:1333–1341.
103. Ottani F, Galvani M, Nicolini FA, et al. Elevated cardiac troponin levels predict the risk of adverse outcome in patients with acute coronary syndromes. *Am Heart J* 2000;140:917–927.
104. Heeschen C, Hamm CW, Goldmann B, et al. Troponin concentrations for stratification of patients with acute coronary syndromes in relation to therapeutic efficacy of tirofiban. PRISM Study Investigators. Platelet Receptor Inhibition in Ischemic Syndrome Management. *Lancet* 1999;354:1757–1762.
105. Newby LK, Kaplan AL, Granger BB, et al. Comparison of cardiac troponin I versus creatine kinase-MB for risk stratification in a chest pain evaluation unit. *Am J Cardiol* 2000;85:801–805.
106. Lindahl B, Venge P, Wallentin L, et al. Relation between troponin T and the risk of subsequent cardiac events in unstable coronary artery disease. *Circulation* 1996;93:1651–1657.
107. Lindahl B, Andrén B, Ohlsson J, et al. Risk stratification in unstable coronary artery disease: additive value of troponin T determinations and predischarge exercise tests. *Eur Heart J* 1997;18:762–770.
108. Heeschen C, van den Brand MJ, Hamm CW, et al. Angiographic findings in patients with refractory unstable angina according to troponin T status. *Circulation* 1999;104:1509–1514.
109. Goldmann BU, Christenson RH, Hamm CW, et al. Implications of troponin testing in clinical medicine. *Curr Control Trials Cardiovasc Med* 2001;2:75–84.
110. Chesebro JH, Knatterud G, Roberts R, et al. Thrombolysis in Myocardial Infarction (TIMI) trial, phase I: a comparison between intravenous tissue plasminogen activator and intravenous streptokinase: clinical findings through hospital discharge. *Circulation* 1987;76:142–154.
111. Hamm CW, Heeschen C, Goldmann B, et al. Benefit of abciximab in patients with refractory unstable angina in relation to serum troponin T levels. *N Engl J Med* 1999;340:1623–1629.
112. Newby LK, Ohman EM, Christenson RH, et al. Benefit of glycoprotein IIb/IIIa inhibition in patients with acute coronary syndromes and troponin T-positive status: the PARAGON-B troponin T substudy. *Circulation* 2001;103:2891–2896.
113. Fragmin and Fast Revascularisation During Instability in Coronary Artery Disease (FRISC II) Investigators. Invasive compared with non-invasive treatment in unstable coronary-artery disease: FRISC II prospective randomised multicentre study. *Lancet* 1999;354:708–715.
114. Hamm CW. Cardiac biomarkers for rapid evaluation of chest pain. *Circulation* 2001;104:1454–1456.
115. Wu AH, Apple FS, Gibler WB, et al. National Academy of Clinical Biochemistry Standards of Laboratory Practice: recommendations for the use of cardiac markers in coronary artery diseases. *Clin Chem* 1999;45:1104–1121.
116. Newby LK, Storrow AB, Gibler WB, et al. Bedside multimarker testing for risk stratification in chest pain units: the Chest Pain Evaluation by Creatine Kinase-MB, Myoglobin, and Troponin I (CHECKMATE) study. *Circulation* 2001;103:1832–1837.
117. French JK, White HD. Clinical implications of the new definition of myocardial infarction. *Heart* 2004;90:99–106.
118. Perna ER, Macin SM, Parras JI, et al. Cardiac troponin T levels are associated with poor short- and long-term prognosis in patients with acute cardiogenic pulmonary edema. *Am Heart J* 2002;143:814–820.
119. Sonel A, Sasseen BM, Fineberg N, et al. Prospective study correlating fibrinopeptide A, troponin I, myoglobin, and myosin light chain levels with early and late ischemic events in consecutive patients presenting to the emergency department with chest pain. *Circulation* 2000;102:1107–1113.
120. Cannon CP, McCabe CH, Wilcox RG, et al. Association of white blood cell count with increased mortality in acute myocardial infarction and unstable angina pectoris. *Am J Cardiol* 2001;87:636–639.
121. Mueller C, Neumann FJ, Roskamm H, et al. Women do have an improved long-term outcome after non-ST-elevation acute coronary syndromes treated very early and predominantly with percutaneous coronary intervention: a prospective study in 1,450 consecutive patients. *J Am Coll Cardiol* 2002;40:245–250.
122. Sabatine MS, Morrow DA, Cannon CP, et al. Relationship between baseline white blood cell count and degree of coronary artery disease and mortality in patients with acute coronary syndromes: a TACTICS-TIMI 18 substudy. *J Am Coll Cardiol* 2002;40:1761–1768.
123. Aviles RJ, Askari AT, Lindahl B, et al. Troponin T levels in patients with acute coronary syndromes, with or without renal dysfunction. *N Engl J Med* 2002;346:2047–2052.
124. Gibson CM, Pinto DS, Murphy SA, et al. Association of creatinine and creatinine clearance on presentation in acute myocardial infarction with subsequent mortality. *J Am Coll Cardiol* 2003;42:1535–1543.
125. Januzzi JL, Cannon CP, DiBattiste PM, et al. Effects of renal insufficiency on early invasive management in patients with acute coronary syndromes (the TACTICS-TIMI 18 trial). *Am J Cardiol* 2002;90:1246–1249.
126. Januzzi JL Jr, Snapinn SM, DiBattiste PM, et al. Benefits and safety of tirofiban among acute coronary syndrome patients with mild to moderate renal insufficiency: results from the Platelet Receptor Inhibition in Ischemic Syndrome Management in Patients Limited by Unstable Signs and Symptoms (PRISM-PLUS) trial. *Circulation* 2002;105:2361–2366.
127. Becker RC, Spencer FA, Gibson M, et al. Influence of patient characteristics and renal function on factor Xa inhibition pharmacokinetics and pharmacodynamics after enoxaparin administration in non-ST-segment elevation acute coronary syndromes. *Am Heart J* 2002;143:753–759.
128. Libby P, Ridker PM, Maseri A. Inflammation and atherosclerosis. *Circulation* 2002;105:1135–1143.
129. Mazzone A, De Servi S, Ricevuti G, et al. Increased expression of neutrophil and monocyte adhesion molecules in unstable coronary artery disease. *Circulation* 1993;88:358–363.

130. Damas JK, Waehre T, Yndestad A, et al. Interleukin-7-mediated inflammation in unstable angina: possible role of chemokines and platelets. *Circulation* 2003;107:2670–2676.
131. Bayes-Genis A, Conover CA, Overgaard MT, et al. Pregnancy-associated plasma protein A as a marker of acute coronary syndromes. *N Engl J Med* 2001;345:1022–1029.
132. Morrow DA, Rifai N, Antman EM, et al. C-reactive protein is a potent predictor of mortality independently of and in combination with troponin T in acute coronary syndromes: a TIMI 11A substudy. *J Am Coll Cardiol* 1998;31:1460–1465.
133. Ridker PM, Rifai N, Pfeffer MA, et al. Long-term effects of pravastatin on plasma concentration of C-reactive protein. The Cholesterol and Recurrent Events (CARE) Investigators. *Circulation* 1999;100:230–235.
134. Andre P, Prasad KS, Denis CV, et al. CD40L stabilizes arterial thrombi by a beta$_3$ integrin-dependent mechanism. *Nat Med* 2002;8:247–252.
135. Schonbeck U, Sukhova GK, Shimizu K, et al. Inhibition of CD40 signaling limits evolution of established atherosclerosis in mice. *Proc Natl Acad Sci U S A* 2000;97:7458–7463.
136. Heeschen C, Dimmeler S, Hamm CW, et al. Soluble CD40 ligand in acute coronary syndromes. *N Engl J Med* 2003;348:1104–1111.
137. Varo N, de Lemos JA, Libby P, et al. Soluble CD40L: risk prediction after acute coronary syndromes. *Circulation* 2003;108:1049–1052.
138. Wilensky RL, Bourdillon PD, Vix VA, et al. Intracoronary artery thrombus formation in unstable angina: a clinical, biochemical and angiographic correlation. *J Am Coll Cardiol* 1993;21:692–699.
139. Wiese S, Breyer T, Dragu A, et al. Gene expression of brain natriuretic peptide in isolated atrial and ventricular human myocardium: influence of angiotensin II and diastolic fiber length. *Circulation* 2000;102:3074–3079.
140. de Lemos JA, Morrow DA, Bentley JH, et al. The prognostic value of B-type natriuretic peptide in patients with acute coronary syndromes. *N Engl J Med* 2001;345:1014–1021.
141. Heeschen C, Hamm CW, Mitrovic V, et al. N-terminal pro-B-type natriuretic peptide levels for dynamic risk stratification of patients with acute coronary syndromes. *Circulation* 2004;110:3206–3212.
142. Morrow DA, de Lemos JA, Sabatine MS, et al. Evaluation of B-type natriuretic peptide for risk assessment in unstable angina/non-ST-elevation myocardial infarction: B-type natriuretic peptide and prognosis in TACTICS-TIMI 18. *J Am Coll Cardiol* 2003;41:1264–1272.
143. Omland T, de Lemos JA, Morrow DA, et al. Prognostic value of N-terminal pro-atrial and pro-brain natriuretic peptide in patients with acute coronary syndromes. *Am J Cardiol* 2002;89:463–465.
144. Jernberg T, Lindahl B, Siegbahn A, et al. N-terminal pro brain natriuretic peptide in relation to inflammation, myocardial necrosis, and the effect of an invasive strategy in unstable coronary artery disease. *J Am Coll Cardiol* 2003;42:1909–1916.
145. White HD, French JK. Use of brain natriuretic peptide levels for risk assessment in non-ST-elevation acute coronary syndromes [editorial]. *J Am Coll Cardiol* 2003;42:1917–1920.
146. Braunwald E, Jones RH, Mark DB, et al. *Unstable angina: diagnosis and management* [AHCPR Publication No. 940602]. Rockville, MD: Agency for Health Care Policy and Research and the National Heart, Lung, and Blood Institute. US Public Health Service, US Department of Health and Human Services,1994.
147. Braunwald E, Antman EM, Beasley JW, et al. ACC/AHA guidelines for the management of patients with unstable angina and non-ST-segment elevation myocardial infarction. A report of the American College of Cardiology/American Heart Association Task Force on Practice Guidelines (Committee on the Management of Patients With Unstable Angina). *J Am Coll Cardiol* 2000;36:970–1062. Erratum in *J Am Coll Cardiol* 2001;38:294–295.
148. Armstrong PW, Fu Y, Chang W-C, et al. Acute coronary syndromes in the GUSTO-IIb trial: prognostic insights and impact of recurrent ischemia. *Circulation* 1998;98:1860–1868.
149. Boersma E, Pieper KS, Steyerberg EW, et al. Predictors of outcome in patients with acute coronary syndromes without persistent ST-segment elevation: results from an international trial of 9461 patients. *Circulation* 2000;101:2557–2567.
150. Antman EM, Cohen M, Bernink PJLM, et al. The TIMI risk score for unstable angina/non-ST elevation MI: a method for prognostication and therapeutic decision making. *JAMA* 2000;284:835–842.
151. Granger CB, Goldberg RJ, Dabbous O, et al. Predictors of hospital mortality in the Global Registry of Acute Coronary Events. *Arch Intern Med* 2003;163:2345–2353.
152. Lagerqvist B, Diderholm E, Lindahl B, et al. FRISC score for selection of patients for an early invasive treatment strategy in unstable coronary artery disease. *Heart* 2005;91:1047–1052.
153. The TIMI Study Group [homepage on the internet] Boston: The TIMI Study Group [updated November 2003]. Palm Pilot software [about 1 screen]. Available: www.timi.org/files/palmsoftware/palmsoftware.htm. Accessed August 1, 2005.
154. de Araujo Goncalves P, Ferreira J, Aguiar C, et al. TIMI, PURSUIT, and GRACE risk scores: sustained prognostic value and interaction with revascularization in NSTE-ACS. *Eur Heart J* 2005;26:865–872.
155. Wong CK, White HD. Value of community-derived risk models for stratifying patients with non-ST elevation acute coronary syndromes [editorial]. *Eur Heart J* 2005;26:851–852.
156. Severi S, Orsini E, Marraccini P, et al. The basal electrocardiogram and the exercise stress test in assessing prognosis in patients with unstable angina. *Eur Heart J* 1988;9:441–446.
157. Brown KA. Prognostic value of thallium-201 myocardial perfusion imaging in patients with unstable angina who respond to medical treatment. *J Am Coll Cardiol* 1991;17:1053–1057. Erratum in: *J Am Coll Cardiol* 1991;18:889.
158. Hilton TC, Thompson RC, Williams HJ, et al. Technetium-99m sestamibi myocardial perfusion imaging in the emergency room evaluation of chest pain. *J Am Coll Cardiol* 1994;23:1016–1022.
159. Zhu YY, Chung WS, Botvinick EH, et al. Dipyridamole perfusion scintigraphy: the experience with its application in one hundred seventy patients with known or suspected unstable angina. *Am Heart J* 1991;121:33–43.
160. Wilson RF, Marcus ML, Christensen BV, et al. Accuracy of exercise electrocardiography in detecting physiologically significant coronary arterial lesions. *Circulation* 1991;83:412–421.
161. Nixon JV, Brown CN, Smitherman TC. Identification of transient and persistent segmental wall motion abnormalities in patients with unstable angina by two-dimensional echocardiography. *Circulation* 1982;65:1497–1503.
162. Plein S, Greenwood JP, Ridgway JP, et al. Assessment of non-ST-segment elevation acute coronary syndromes with cardiac magnetic resonance imaging. *J Am Coll Cardiol* 2004;44:2173–2181.
163. Kim WY, Danias PG, Stuber M, et al. Coronary magnetic resonance angiography for the detection of coronary stenoses. *N Engl J Med* 2001;345:1863–1869.
164. Schwitter J, Nanz D, Kneifel S, et al. Assessment of myocardial perfusion in coronary artery disease by magnetic resonance: a comparison with positron emission tomography and coronary angiography. *Circulation* 2001;103:2230–2235.
165. Kim RJ, Wu E, Rafael A, et al. The use of contrast-enhanced magnetic resonance imaging to identify reversible myocardial dysfunction. *N Engl J Med* 2000;343:1445–1453.
166. The TIMI IIIB Investigators. Effects of tissue plasminogen activator and a comparison of early invasive and conservative strategies in unstable angina and non-Q-wave myocardial infarction: results of the TIMI IIIB trial. *Circulation* 1994;89:1545–1556.
167. Wong GC, Morrow DA, Murphy S, et al. Elevations in troponin T and I are associated with abnormal tissue level perfusion: a TACTICS-TIMI 18 substudy. Treat Angina with Aggrastat and Determine Cost of Therapy with an Invasive or Conservative Strategy—Thrombolysis in Myocardial Infarction. *Circulation* 2002;106:202–207.
168. Zhao XQ, Théroux P, Snapinn SM, et al. Intracoronary thrombus and platelet glycoprotein IIb/IIIa receptor blockade with tirofiban in unstable angina or non-Q-wave myocardial infarction: angiographic results from the PRISM-PLUS trial (Platelet Receptor Inhibition for Ischemic Syndrome Management in Patients Limited by Unstable Signs and Symptoms). *Circulation* 1999;100:1609–1615.
169. Davies GJ, Bencivelli W, Fragasso G, et al. Sequence and magnitude of ventricular volume changes in painful and painless myocardial ischemia. *Circulation* 1988;78:310–319.
170. The Platelet Receptor Inhibition in Ischemic Syndrome Management in Patients Limited by Unstable Signs and Symptoms (PRISM-Plus) Study Investigators. Inhibition of the platelet glycoprotein IIb/IIIa receptor with tirofiban in unstable angina and non-Q-wave myocardial infarction. *N Engl J Med* 1998;338:1488–1497.
171. The PURSUIT Trial Investigators. Inhibition of platelet glycoprotein IIb/IIIa with eptifibatide in patients with acute coronary syndromes. *N Engl J Med* 1998;339:436–443.
172. Anderson HV, Cannon CP, Stone PH, et al. One-year results of the Thrombolysis In Myocardial Infarction (TIMI) IIIB clinical trial: a randomized comparison of tissue-type plasminogen activator versus placebo and early invasive versus early conservative strategies in unstable angina and non-Q wave myocardial infarction. *J Am Coll Cardiol* 1995;26:1643–1650.
173. Lewis HD, Davis JW, Archibald DG, et al. Protective effects of aspirin against acute myocardial infarction and death in men with unstable angina: results of a Veterans Administration cooperative study. *N Engl J Med* 1983;309:396–403.
174. Cairns JA, Gent M, Singer J, et al. Aspirin, sulfinpyrazone, or both in unstable angina: results of a Canadian multicenter trial. *N Engl J Med* 1985;313:1369–1375.
175. Lubsen J, Tijssen JGP, Kerkkamp HJJ. Early treatment of unstable angina in the coronary care unit: a randomised, double blind, placebo controlled comparison of recurrent ischaemia in patients treated with nifedipine or metoprolol or both: report of the Holland Interuniversity Nifedipine/Metoprolol Trial (HINT) Research Group. *Br Heart J* 1986;56:400–413.
176. Gottlieb SO, Weisfeldt ML, Ouyang P, et al. Effect of the addition of propranolol to therapy with nifedipine for unstable angina pectoris: a randomized, double-blind, placebo-controlled trial. *Circulation* 1986;73:331–337.
177. Diver DJ, Bier JD, Ferreira PE, et al. Clinical and arteriographic characterization of patients with unstable angina without critical coronary arterial narrowing (from the TIMI-IIIA trial). *Am J Cardiol* 1994;74:531–537.
178. Yasue H, Takizawa A, Nagao M, et al. Long-term prognosis for patients with variant angina and influential factors. *Circulation* 1988;78:1–9.
179. Dokainish H, Pillai M, Murphy SA, et al. Prognostic implications of elevated troponin in patients with suspected acute coronary syndrome but no

critical epicardial coronary disease: a TACTICS-TIMI-18 substudy. *J Am Coll Cardiol* 2005;45:19–24.
180. McCormick JR, Schick EC Jr, McCabe CH, et al. Determinants of operative mortality and long-term survival in patients with unstable angina: the CASS experience. *J Thorac Cardiovasc Surg* 1985;89:683–688.
181. Roffi M, Chew DP, Mukherjee D, et al. Platelet glycoprotein IIb/IIIa inhibitors reduce mortality in diabetic patients with non-ST-segment elevation acute coronary syndromes. *Circulation* 2001;104:2767–2771.
182. Cotter G, Cannon CP, McCabe CH, et al. Prior peripheral arterial disease and cerebrovascular disease are independent predictors of adverse outcome in patients with acute coronary syndromes: are we doing enough? Results from the Orbofiban in Patients with Unstable Coronary Syndromes-Thrombolysis In Myocardial Infarction (OPUS-TIMI) 16 study. *Am Heart J* 2003;145:622–627.
183. Bazzino O, Díaz R, Tajer C, et al. Clinical predictors of in-hospital prognosis in unstable angina: ECLA 3. *Am Heart J* 1999;137:322–331.
184. Betriu A, Heras M, Cohen M, et al. Unstable angina: outcome according to clinical presentation. *J Am Coll Cardiol* 1992;19:1659–1663.
185. Rizik DG, Healy S, Margulis A, et al. A new clinical classification for hospital prognosis of unstable angina pectoris. *Am J Cardiol* 1995;75:993–997.
186. Goodman SG, Barr A, Sobtchouk A, et al. Low molecular weight heparin decreases rebound ischemia in unstable angina or non-Q-wave myocardial infarction: the Canadian ESSENCE ST segment monitoring substudy. *J Am Coll Cardiol* 2000;36:1507–1513.
187. Glassman AH, O'Connor CM, Califf RM, et al. Sertraline treatment of major depression in patients with acute MI or unstable angina. *JAMA* 2002;288:701–709. Erratum in *JAMA* 2002;14:1720.
188. Swenson JR, O'Connor CM, Barton D, et al. Influence of depression and effect of treatment with sertraline on quality of life after hospitalization for acute coronary syndrome. *Am J Cardiol* 2003;92:1271–1276.
189. Farkouh ME, Smars PA, Reeder GS, et al. A clinical trial of a chest-pain observation unit for patients with unstable angina. *N Engl J Med* 1998; 339:1882–1888.
190. Tschopp TB. Aspirin inhibits platelet aggregation on, but not adhesion to, collagen fibrils: an assessment of platelet adhesion and deposited platelet mass by morphometry and ^{51}Cr-labeling. *Thromb Res* 1977;11:619–632.
191. Oates JA, Fitzgerald GA, Branch RA, et al. Clinical implications of prostaglandin and thromboxane A2 formation (1). *N Engl J Med* 1988;319: 689–698.
192. Buchanan MR, Brister SJ. Individual variation in the effects of ASA on platelet function: implications for the use of ASA clinically. *Can J Cardiol* 1995;11:221–227.
193. Pappas JM, Westengard JC, Bull BS. Population variability in the effect of aspirin on platelet function: implications for clinical trials and therapy. *Arch Pathol Lab Med* 1994;118:801–804.
194. Cooke GE, Bray PF, Hamlington JD, et al. PIA2 polymorphism and efficacy of aspirin [letter]. *Lancet* 1998;351:1253.
195. Derry S, Loke YK. Risk of gastrointestinal haemorrhage with long term use of aspirin: meta-analysis. *Br Med J* 2000;321:1183–1187.
196. Patrono C, Coller B, Dalen JE, et al. Platelet-active drugs: the relationships among dose, effectiveness, and side effects. *Chest* 1998;114:470S–488S.
197. Roderick PJ, Wilkes HC, Meade TW. The gastrointestinal toxicity of aspirin: an overview of randomised controlled trials. *Br J Clin Pharmacol* 1993;35:219–226.
198. CAPRIE Steering Committee. A randomised, blinded, trial of clopidogrel versus aspirin in patients at risk of ischaemic events (CAPRIE). *Lancet* 1996;348:1329–1339.
199. Komatsu H, Yaju H, Chiba K, et al. Inhibition by cyclo-oxygenase inhibitors of interleukin-6 production by human peripheral blood mononuclear cells. *Int J Immunopharmacol* 1991;13:1137–1146.
200. Rosenblum WI, Nishimura H, Nelson GH. L-NMMA in brain microcirculation of mice is inhibited by blockade of cyclooxygenase and by superoxide dismutase. *Am J Physiol* 1992;262:H1343–H1349.
201. Mehta P, Mehta JL. Effects of aspirin in arterial thrombosis: why don't animals behave the way humans do? [editorial]. *J Am Coll Cardiol* 1993; 21:511–513.
202. Kyrle PA, Eichler HG, Jager U, et al. Inhibition of prostacyclin and thromboxane A2 generation by low-dose aspirin at the site of plug formation in man in vivo. *Circulation* 1987;75:1025–1029.
203. The RISC Group. Risk of myocardial infarction and death during treatment with low dose aspirin and intravenous heparin in men with unstable coronary artery disease. *Lancet* 1990;336:827–830.
204. Dabaghi SF, Kamat SG, Payne J, et al. Effects of low-dose aspirin on in vitro platelet aggregation in the early minutes after ingestion in normal subjects. *Am J Cardiol* 1994;74:720–723.
205. Antiplatelet Trialists' Collaboration. Collaborative overview of randomised trials of antiplatelet therapy - I: prevention of death, myocardial infarction, and stroke by prolonged antiplatelet therapy in various categories of patients. *Br Med J* 1994;308:81–106.
206. Peters RJ, Mehta SR, Fox KA, et al. Effects of aspirin dose when used alone or in combination with clopidogrel in patients with acute coronary syndromes: observations from the Clopidogrel in Unstable Angina to Prevent Recurrent Events (CURE) study. *Circulation* 2003;108:1682–1687.
207. Budaj A, Yusuf S, Mehta SR, et al. Benefit of clopidogrel in patients with acute coronary syndromes without ST-segment elevation in various risk groups. *Circulation* 2002;106:1622–1626.
208. Mehta SR, Yusuf S, Peters RJ, et al. Effects of pretreatment with clopidogrel and aspirin followed by long-term therapy in patients undergoing percutaneous coronary intervention: the PCI-CURE study. *Lancet* 2001;358:527–533.
209. Steinhubl SR, Berger PB, Mann JT, et al. Early and sustained dual oral antiplatelet therapy following percutaneous coronary intervention: A randomized Controlled Trial. *JAMA* 2002;288:2411–2420.
210. Bates ER, Lau WC, Bleske BE. Loading, pretreatment, and interindividual variability issues with clopidogrel dosing. *Circulation* 2005;111:2557–2559.
211. Bertrand ME, Simoons ML, Fox KAA, et al. Management of acute coronary syndromes in patients presenting *without* persistent ST-segment elevation: the Task Force on the Management of Acute Coronary Syndromes of the European Society of Cardiology. *Eur Heart J* 2002;23:1809–1840.
212. Fox KA, Mehta SR, Peters R, et al. Benefits and risks of the combination of clopidogrel and aspirin in patients undergoing surgical revascularization for non-ST-elevation acute coronary syndrome: the Clopidogrel in Unstable Angina to Prevent Recurrent Ischemic Events (CURE) trial. *Circulation* 2004;110:1202–1208.
213. Hongo RH, Ley J, Dick SE, et al. The effect of clopidogrel in combination with aspirin when given before coronary artery bypass grafting. *J Am Coll Cardiol* 2002;40:231–237.
214. The ESPRIT Investigators. Novel dosing regimen of eptifibatide in planned coronary stent implantation (ESPRIT): a randomised, placebo-controlled trial. *Lancet* 2000;356:2037–2044.
215. Topol EJ, Moliterno DJ, Herrmann HC, et al. Comparison of two platelet glycoprotein IIb/IIIa inhibitors, tirofiban and abciximab, for the prevention of ischemic events with percutaneous coronary revascularization. *N Engl J Med* 2001;344:1888–1894.
216. Chew DP, Moliterno DJ. A critical appraisal of platelet glycoprotein IIb/IIIa inhibition. *J Am Coll Cardiol* 2000;36:2028–2035.
217. Chew DP, Bhatt DL, Sapp S, et al. Increased mortality with oral platelet glycoprotein IIb/IIIa antagonists: a meta-analysis of phase III multicenter randomized trials. *Circulation* 2001;103:201–206.
218. Kong DF, Califf RM, Miller DP, et al. Clinical outcomes of therapeutic agents that block the platelet glycoprotein IIb/IIIa integrin in ischemic heart disease. *Circulation* 1998;98:2829–2835.
219. The GUSTO IV-ACS Investigators. Effects of glycoprotein IIb/IIIa receptor blocker abciximab on outcome in patients with acute coronary syndromes without early coronary revascularisation: the GUSTO IV-ACS randomized trial. *Lancet* 2001;357:1915–1924.
220. Mascelli MA, Lance ET, Damaraju L, et al. Pharmacodynamic profile of short-term abciximab treatment demonstrates prolonged platelet inhibition with gradual recovery from GP IIb/IIIa receptor blockade. *Circulation* 1998;97:1680–1688.
221. Kereiakes DJ, Broderick TM, Roth EM, et al. Time course, magnitude, and consistency of platelet inhibition by abciximab, tirofiban, or eptifibatide in patients with unstable angina pectoris undergoing percutaneous coronary intervention. *Am J Cardiol* 1999;84:391–395.
222. Quinn MJ, Murphy RT, Dooley M, et al. Occupancy of the internal and external pools of glycoprotein IIb/IIIa following abciximab bolus and infusion. *J Pharmacol Exp Ther* 2001;297:496–500.
223. The CAPTURE Investigators. Randomised placebo-controlled trial of abciximab before and during coronary intervention in refractory unstable angina: the CAPTURE study. *Lancet* 1997;349:1429–1435.
224. The Platelet Receptor Inhibition in Ischemic Syndrome Management (PRISM) Study Investigators. A comparison of aspirin plus tirofiban with aspirin plus heparin for unstable angina. Platelet Receptor Inhibition in Ischemic Syndrome Management (PRISM) Study Investigators. *N Engl J Med* 1998;338:1498–1505.
225. Randomised placebo-controlled trial of effect of eptifibatide on complications of percutaneous coronary intervention: IMPACT-II. Integrilin to Minimise Platelet Aggregation and Coronary Thrombosis-II. *Lancet* 1997; 349:1422–1428.
226. Boersma E, Akkerhuis KM, Theroux P, et al. Platelet glycoprotein IIb/IIIa receptor inhibition in non-ST-elevation acute coronary syndromes: early benefit during medical treatment only, with additional protection during percutaneous coronary intervention. *Circulation* 1999;100:2045–2048.
227. Marso SP, Bhatt DL, Roe MT, et al. Enhanced efficacy of eptifibatide administration in patients with acute coronary syndrome requiring in-hospital coronary artery bypass grafting. PURSUIT Investigators. *Circulation* 2000; 102:2952–2958.
228. The PARAGON Investigators. International, randomized, controlled trial of lamifiban (a platelet glycoprotein IIb/IIIa inhibitor), heparin, or both in unstable angina. The PARAGON Investigators. Platelet IIb/IIIa Antagonism for the Reduction of Acute Coronary Syndrome Events in a Global Organization Network. *Circulation* 1998;97:2386–2395.
229. The Platelet IIb/IIIa Antagonist for the Reduction of Acute Coronary Syndrome Events in a Global Organization Network (PARAGON)-B Investigators. Randomized, placebo-controlled trial of titrated intravenous lamifiban for acute coronary syndromes. *Circulation* 2002;105:316–321.
230. Kleiman NS, Lincoff AM, Flaker GC, et al. Early percutaneous coronary intervention, platelet inhibition with eptifibatide, and clinical outcomes in patients with acute coronary syndromes. *Circulation* 2000;101:751–757.
231. Morrow DA, Antman EM, Snapinn SM, et al. An integrated clinical approach to predicting the benefit of tirofiban in non-ST elevation acute

coronary syndromes: application of the TIMI risk score for UA/NSTEMI in PRISM-Plus. *Eur Heart J* 2002;23:223–229.
232. Szucs TD, Meyer BJ, Kiowski W. Economic assessment of tirofiban in the management of acute coronary syndromes in the hospital setting: an analysis based on the PRISM PLUS Trial. *Eur Heart J* 1999;20:1253–1260.
233. Dalby M, Montalescot G, Bal dit Sollier C, et al. Eptifibatide provides additional platelet inhibition in non-ST-elevation myocardial infarction patients already treated with aspirin and clopidogrel: results of the Platelet Activity Extinction in Non-Q-Wave Myocardial Infarction With Aspirin, Clopidogrel, and Eptifibatide (PEACE) study. *J Am Coll Cardiol* 2004;43:162–168.
234. Cohen M, Adams PC, Hawkins L, et al. Usefulness of antithrombotic therapy in resting angina pectoris or non-Q-wave myocardial infarction in preventing death and myocardial infarction (a pilot study from the Antithrombotic Therapy in Acute Coronary Syndromes Study Group). *Am J Cardiol* 1990;66:1287–1292.
235. Cohen M, Adams PC, Parry G, et al. Combination antithrombotic therapy in unstable rest angina and non-Q-wave infarction in nonprior aspirin users. Primary end points analysis from the ATACS trial. Antithrombotic Therapy in Acute Coronary Syndromes Research Group. *Circulation* 1994;89:81–88.
236. Gurfinkel EP, Manos EJ, Mejail RI, et al. Low molecular weight heparin versus regular heparin or aspirin in the treatment of unstable angina and silent ischemia. *J Am Coll Cardiol* 1995;26:313–318.
237. Oler A, Whooley MA, Oler J, et al. Adding heparin to aspirin reduces the incidence of myocardial infarction and death in patients with unstable angina: a meta-analysis. *JAMA* 1996;276:811–815.
238. Massonnet-Castel S, Pelissier E, Bara L, et al. Partial reversal of low molecular weight heparin (PK 10169) anti-Xa activity by protamine sulfate: in vitro and in vivo study during cardiac surgery with extracorporeal circulation. *Haemostasis* 1986;16:139–146.
239. Mark DB, Cowper PA, Berkowitz SD, et al. Economic assessment of low-molecular-weight heparin (enoxaparin) versus unfractionated heparin in acute coronary syndrome patients: results from the ESSENCE randomized trial. Efficacy and Safety of Subcutaneous Enoxaparin in Non-Q Wave Coronary Events [unstable angina or non-Q-wave myocardial infarction]. *Circulation* 1998;97:1702–1707.
240. Warkentin TE, Levine MN, Hirsh J, et al. Heparin-induced thrombocytopenia in patients treated with low-molecular-weight heparin or unfractionated heparin. *N Engl J Med* 1995;332:1330–1335.
241. Antman EM, McCabe CH, Gurfinkel EP, et al. Enoxaparin prevents death and cardiac ischemic events in unstable angina/non-Q-wave myocardial infarction: results of the Thrombolysis in Myocardial Infarction (TIMI) 11B trial. *Circulation* 1999;100:1593–1601.
242. Fragmin and Fast Revascularisation During Instability in Coronary Artery Disease (FRISC II) Investigators. Long-term low-molecular-mass heparin in unstable coronary-artery disease: FRISC II prospective randomised multicentre study. *Lancet* 1999;354:701–707. Erratum in *Lancet* 1999;354:1478.
243. Fragmin During Instability in Coronary Artery Disease (FRISC) Study Group. Low-molecular-weight heparin during instability in coronary artery disease. *Lancet* 1996;347:561–568.
244. Klein W, Buchwald A, Hillis SE, et al. Comparison of low-molecular-weight heparin with unfractionated heparin acutely and with placebo for 6 weeks in the management of unstable coronary artery disease: Fragmin in Unstable Coronary Artery Disease Study (FRIC). *Circulation* 1997;96:61–68.
245. The FRAXIS Study Group. Comparison of two treatment durations (6 days and 14 days) of a low molecular weight heparin with a 6-day treatment of unfractionated heparin in the initial management of unstable angina or non-Q wave myocardial infarction: FRAXIS (Fraxiparine in Ischaemic Syndrome). *Eur Heart J* 1999;20:1553–1562.
246. Cohen M, Demers C, Gurfinkel EP, et al. A comparison of low-molecular-weight heparin with unfractionated heparin for unstable coronary artery disease. *N Engl J Med* 1997;337:447–452.
247. Cohen M, Théroux P, Borzak S, et al. Randomized double-blind safety study of enoxaparin versus unfractionated heparin in patients with non-ST-segment elevation acute coronary syndromes treated with tirofiban and aspirin: the ACUTE II study. *Am Heart J* 2002;144:470–477.
248. Goodman SG, Fitchett D, Armstrong PW, et al. Randomized evaluation of the safety and efficacy of enoxaparin versus unfractionated heparin in high-risk patients with non-ST-segment elevation acute coronary syndromes receiving the glycoprotein IIb/IIIa inhibitor eptifibatide. *Circulation* 2003;107:238–244.
249. Blazing MA, de Lemos JA, White HD, et al. Safety and efficacy of enoxaparin vs unfractionated heparin in patients with non-ST-segment elevation acute coronary syndromes who receive tirofiban and aspirin: a randomized controlled trial. *JAMA* 2004;292:55–64. Erratum in: *JAMA* 2004;292:1178.
250. Ferguson JJ, Califf RM, Antman EM, et al. Enoxaparin vs unfractionated heparin in high-risk patients with non-ST-segment elevation acute coronary syndromes managed with an intended early invasive strategy: primary results of the SYNERGY randomized trial. *JAMA* 2004;292:45–54.
251. de Lemos JA, Blazing MA, Wiviott SD, et al. Enoxaparin versus unfractionated heparin in patients treated with tirofiban, aspirin and an early conservative initial management strategy: results from the A phase of the A-to-Z trial. *Eur Heart J* 2004;25:1688–1694.
252. Rao AK, Pratt C, Berke A, et al. Thrombolysis in Myocardial Infarction (TIMI) trial—phase I: hemorrhagic manifestations and changes in plasma fibrinogen and the fibrinolytic system in patients treated with recombinant tissue plasminogen activator and streptokinase. *J Am Coll Cardiol* 1988;11:1–11.
253. Lee MS, Wali AU, Menon V, et al. The determinants of activated partial thromboplastin time, relation of activated partial thromboplastin time to clinical outcomes, and optimal dosing regimens for heparin treated patients with acute coronary syndromes: a review of GUSTO-IIb. *J Thromb Thrombolysis* 2002;14:91–101.
254. Weitz JI, Hudoba M, Massel D, et al. Clot-bound thrombin is protected from inhibition by heparin-antithrombin III but is susceptible to inactivation by antithrombin III-independent inhibitors. *J Clin Invest* 1990;86:385–391.
255. Lefkovits J, Topol EJ. Direct thrombin inhibitors in cardiovascular medicine. *Circulation* 1994;90:1522–1536.
256. The Direct Thrombin Inhibitor Trialists' Collaborative Group. Direct thrombin inhibitors in acute coronary syndromes: principal results of a meta-analysis based on individual patients' data. *Lancet* 2002;359:294–302.
257. Bates SM, Weitz JI. Direct thrombin inhibitors for treatment of arterial thrombosis: potential differences between bivalirudin and hirudin. *Am J Cardiol* 1998;82:12P–18P.
258. Bittl JA, Strony J, Brinker JA, et al. Treatment with bivalirudin (hirulog) as compared with heparin during coronary angioplasty for unstable or postinfarction angina. *N Engl J Med* 1995;333:764–769.
259. Lincoff AM, Kleiman NS, Kereiakes DJ, et al. Long-term efficacy of bivalirudin and provisional glycoprotein IIb/IIIa blockade vs heparin and planned glycoprotein IIb/IIIa blockade during percutaneous coronary revascularization: REPLACE-2 randomized trial. *JAMA* 2004;292:696–703.
260. Stone GW, Bertrand M, Colombo A, et al. Acute Catheterization and Urgent Intervention Triage Strategy (ACUITY) trial: study design and rationale. *Am Heart J* 2004;148:764–775.
261. Telford AM, Wilson C. Trial of heparin versus atenolol in prevention of myocardial infarction in intermediate coronary syndrome. *Lancet* 1981;i:1225–1228.
262. Yusuf S, Wittes J, Friedman L. Overview of results of randomized clinical trials in heart disease. II. Unstable angina, heart failure, primary prevention with aspirin, and risk factor modification. *JAMA* 1988;260:2259–2263.
263. Muller JE, Turi ZG, Pearle DL, et al. Nifedipine and conventional therapy for unstable angina pectoris: a randomized, double-blind comparison. *Circulation* 1984;69:728–739.
264. Horowitz JD, Henry CA, Syrjanen ML, et al. Combined use of nitroglycerin and N-acetylcysteine in the management of unstable angina pectoris. *Circulation* 1988;77:787–794.
265. Cheitlin MD, Hutter AM Jr, Brindis RG, et al. ACC/AHA expert consensus document. Use of sildenafil (Viagra) in patients with cardiovascular disease. American College of Cardiology/American Heart Association. *J Am Coll Cardiol* 1999;33:273–282.
266. Gibson RS, Boden WE, Theroux P, et al. Diltiazem and reinfarction in patients with non-Q-wave myocardial infarction. Results of a double-blind, randomized, multicenter trial. *N Engl J Med* 1986;315:423–429.
267. Hansen JF, Hagerup L, Sigurd B, et al. Cardiac event rates after acute myocardial infarction in patients treated with verapamil and trandolapril versus trandolapril alone. Danish Verapamil Infarction Trial (DAVIT) Study Group. *Am J Cardiol* 1997;79:738–741.
268. Patel DJ, Purcell HJ, Fox KM, et al. Cardioprotection by opening of the K_{ATP} channel in unstable angina: is this a clinical manifestation of myocardial preconditioning? Results of a randomized study with nicorandil. *Eur Heart J* 1999;20:51–57.
269. Chaitman BR, Skettino SL, Parker JO, et al. Anti-ischemic effects and long-term survival during ranolazine monotherapy in patients with chronic severe angina. *J Am Coll Cardiol* 2004;43:1375–1382.
270. Storey RF, Newby LJ, Heptinstall S. Effects of P2Y1 and P2Y12 receptor antagonists on platelet aggregation induced by different agonists in human whole blood. *Platelets* 2001;12:443–447.
271. Abendschein DR, Meng YY, Torr-Brown S, et al. Maintenance of coronary patency after fibrinolysis with tissue factor pathway inhibitor. *Circulation* 1995;92:944–949.
272. Wallentin L, Wilcox RG, Weaver WD, et al. Oral ximelagatran for secondary prophylaxis after myocardial infarction: the ESTEEM randomised controlled trial. *Lancet* 2003;362:789–797.
273. Turpie AG, Gallus AS, Hoek JA. A synthetic pentasaccharide for the prevention of deep-vein thrombosis after total hip replacement. *N Engl J Med* 2001;344:619–625.
274. Waters D, Lam JYT. Is thrombolytic therapy striking out in unstable angina? *Circulation* 1992;86:1642–1644.
275. Szatmary LJ, Marco J, Fajadet J, et al. The combined use of diastolic counterpulsation and coronary dilation in unstable angina due to multivessel disease under unstable hemodynamic conditions. *Int J Cardiol* 1988;19:59–66.
276. de Winter RJ, Windhausen F, Cornel JH, et al. Early invasive versus selectively invasive management for acute coronary syndromes. *N Engl J Med* 2005;353:1095–1104.
277. Boden WE, O'Rourke RA, Crawford MH, et al. Outcomes in patients with

acute non-Q-wave myocardial infarction randomly assigned to an invasive as compared with a conservative management strategy. Veterans Affairs Non-Q-Wave Infarction Strategies in Hospital (VANQWISH) Trial Investigators. *N Engl J Med* 1998;338:1785–1792.

278. McCullough PA, O'Neill WW, Graham M, et al. A prospective randomized trial of triage angiography in acute coronary syndromes ineligible for thrombolytic therapy: results of the Medicine Versus Angiography in Thrombolytic Exclusion (MATE) Trial. *J Am Coll Cardiol* 1998;32:596–605.
279. Michalis LK, Stroumbis CS, Pappas K, et al. Treatment of refractory unstable angina in geographically isolated areas without cardiac surgery: invasive versus conservative strategy (TRUCS study). *Eur Heart J* 2000;21:1954–1959.
280. Spacek R, Widimsky P, Straka Z, et al. Value of first day angiography/angioplasty in evolving non-ST segment elevation myocardial infarction: an open multicenter randomized trial. The VINO study. *Eur Heart J* 2002;23:230–238.
281. Madsen JK, Grande P, Saunamäki K, et al. Danish multicenter randomized study of invasive versus conservative treatment in patients with inducible ischemia after thrombolysis in acute myocardial infarction (DANAMI). *Circulation* 1997;96:748–755.
282. Jones RH, Hannan EL, Hammermeister KE, et al. Identification of preoperative variables needed for risk adjustment of short-term mortality after coronary artery bypass graft surgery. The Working Group Panel on the Cooperative CABG Database Project. *J Am Coll Cardiol* 1996;28:1478–1487.
283. Wallentin L, Lagerqvist B, Husted S, et al. Outcome at 1 year after an invasive compared with a non-invasive strategy in unstable coronary-artery disease: the FRISC II invasive randomised trial. *Lancet* 2000;356:9–16.
284. Van de Werf F, Gore JM, Avezum A, et al. Access to catheterisation facilities in patients admitted with acute coronary syndrome: multinational registry study. *Br Med J* 2005;330:441.
285. Mehta SR, Cannon CP, Fox KA, et al. Routine vs selective invasive strategies in patients with acute coronary syndromes: a collaborative meta-analysis of randomized trials. *JAMA* 2005;293:2908–2917.
286. Bach RG, Cannon CP, Weintraub WS, et al. The effect of routine, early invasive management on outcome for elderly patients with non-ST-segment elevation acute coronary syndromes. *Ann Intern Med* 2004;141:186–195.
287. Mahoney EM, Jurkovitz CT, Chu H, et al. Cost and cost-effectiveness of an early invasive vs conservative strategy for the treatment of unstable angina and non-ST-segment elevation myocardial infarction. *JAMA* 2002;288:1851–1858.
288. Janzon M, Levin LA, Swahn E, et al. Cost-effectiveness of an invasive strategy in unstable coronary artery disease: results from the FRISC II invasive trial. *Eur Heart J* 2002;23:31–40.
289. Neumann FJ, Kastrati A, Pogatsa-Murray G, et al. Evaluation of prolonged antithrombotic pretreatment ("cooling-off" strategy) before intervention in patients with unstable coronary syndromes: a randomized controlled trial. *JAMA* 2003;290:1593–1599.
290. De Feyter PJ, Suryapranata H, Serruys PW, et al. Coronary angioplasty for unstable angina: immediate and late results in 200 consecutive patients with identification of risk factors for unfavorable early and late outcome. *J Am Coll Cardiol* 1988;12:324–333.
291. Ellis SG, Roubin GS, King SBI, et al. Angiographic and clinical predictors of acute closure after native vessel coronary angioplasty. *Circulation* 1988;77:372–379.
292. Little WC, Applegate RJ. Role of plaque size and degree of stenosis in acute myocardial infarction. *Cardiol Clin* 1996;14:221–228.
293. White HD. Angioplasty versus bypass surgery [commentary]. *Lancet* 1995;346:1174–1175.
294. McFadden EP, Stabile E, Regar E, et al. Late thrombosis in drug-eluting coronary stents after discontinuation of antiplatelet therapy. *Lancet* 2004;364:1519–1521.
295. Doucet S, Malekianpour M, Theroux P, et al. Randomized trial comparing intravenous nitroglycerin and heparin for treatment of unstable angina secondary to restenosis after coronary artery angioplasty. *Circulation* 2000;101:955–961.
296. FitzGibbon GM, Leach AJ, Keon WJ, et al. Coronary bypass graft fate. Angiographic study of 1,179 vein grafts early, one year, and five years after operation. *J Thorac Cardiovasc Surg* 1986;91:773–778.
297. Galbut DL, Traad EA, Dorman MJ, et al. Seventeen-year experience with bilateral internal mammary artery grafts. *Ann Thorac Surg* 1990;49:195–201.
298. Campeau L, Enjalbert M, Lesperance J, et al. Atherosclerosis and late closure of aortocoronary saphenous vein grafts: sequential angiographic studies at 2 weeks, 1 year, 5 to 7 years, and 10 to 12 years after surgery. *Circulation* 1983;68[Suppl II]:II-1–II-7.
299. Piana RN, Moscucci M, Cohen DJ, et al. Palmaz-Schatz stenting for treatment of focal vein graft stenosis: immediate results and long-term outcome. *J Am Coll Cardiol* 1994;23:1296–1304.
300. Brown G, Albers JJ, Fisher LD, et al. Regression of coronary artery disease as a result of intensive lipid-lowering therapy in men with high levels of apolipoprotein B. *N Engl J Med* 1990;323:1289–1298.
301. Loscalzo J. Regression of coronary atherosclerosis [editorial]. *N Engl J Med* 1990;323:1337–1339.
302. Weber C, Erl W, Weber KS, et al. HMG-CoA reductase inhibitors decrease CD11b expression and CD11b-dependent adhesion of monocytes to endothelium and reduce increased adhesiveness of monocytes isolated from patients with hypercholesterolemia. *J Am Coll Cardiol* 1997;30:1212–1217.
303. Lacoste L, Lam JY, Hung J, et al. Hyperlipidemia and coronary disease. Correction of the increased thrombogenic potential with cholesterol reduction. *Circulation* 1995;92:3172–3177.
304. Anderson TJ, Meredith IT, Yeung AC, et al. The effect of cholesterol-lowering and antioxidant therapy on endothelium-dependent coronary vasomotion. *N Engl J Med* 1995;332:488–493.
305. Andrews TC, Raby K, Barry J, et al. Effect of cholesterol reduction on myocardial ischemia in patients with coronary disease. *Circulation* 1997;95:324–328.
306. Dupuis J, Tardif JC, Cernacek P, et al. Cholesterol reduction rapidly improves endothelial function after acute coronary syndromes: the RECIFE (Reduction of Cholesterol in Ischemia and Function of the Endothelium) trial. *Circulation* 1999;99:3227–3233.
307. Treasure CB, Klein JL, Weintraub WS, et al. Beneficial effects of cholesterol-lowering therapy on the coronary endothelium in patients with coronary artery disease. *N Engl J Med* 1995;332:481–487.
308. Tonkin AM, Colquhoun D, Emberson J, et al. Effect of pravastatin in 3260 patients with unstable angina: results from the LIPID Study. *Lancet* 2000;356:1871–1875.
309. Schwartz GG, Olsson AG, Ezekowitz MD, et al. Effects of atorvastatin on early recurrent ischemic events in acute coronary syndromes: the MIRACL study: a randomized controlled trial. *JAMA* 2001;285:1711–1718.
310. de Lemos JA, Blazing MA, Wiviott SD, et al. Early intensive vs a delayed conservative simvastatin strategy in patients with acute coronary syndromes: phase Z of the A to Z trial. *JAMA* 2004;292:1307–1316.
311. Fonarow GC, Gawlinski A, Moughrabi S, et al. Improved treatment of coronary heart disease by implementation of a Cardiac Hospitalization Atherosclerosis Management Program (CHAMP). *Am J Cardiol* 2001;87:819–822.
312. Azar RR, Rinfret S, Theroux P, et al. A randomized placebo-controlled trial to assess the efficacy of antiinflammatory therapy with methylprednisolone in unstable angina (MUNA trial). *Eur Heart J* 2000;21:2026–2032.
313. Cannon CP, Braunwald E, McCabe CH, et al. Antibiotic treatment of *Chlamydia pneumoniae* after acute coronary syndrome. *N Engl J Med* 2005;352:1646–1654.
314. O'Connor GT, Buring JE, Yusuf S, et al. An overview of randomized trials of rehabilitation with exercise after myocardial infarction. *Circulation* 1989;80:234–244.
315. Heart Outcome Prevention Evaluation Study Investigators. Effects of ramipril on cardiovascular and microvascular outcomes in people with diabetes mellitus: results of the HOPE study and MICRO-HOPE substudy. *Lancet* 2000;355:253–259.
316. The European Trial on Reduction of Cardiac Events With Perindopril in Stable Coronary Artery Disease Investigators. Efficacy of perindopril in reduction of cardiovascular events among patients with stable coronary artery disease: randomised, double-blind, placebo-controlled, multicentre trial (the EUROPA study). *Lancet* 2003;362:782–788.
317. White HD. Should all patients with coronary disease receive angiotensin-converting-enzyme inhibitors? [commentary]. *Lancet* 2003;362:755–757.
318. Thiemann DR, Coresh J, Oetgen WJ, et al. The association between hospital volume and survival after acute myocardial infarction in elderly patients. *N Engl J Med* 1999;340:1640–1648.
319. White HD, Willerson JT. We must use the knowledge that we have to treat patients with acute coronary syndromes [editorial]. *Circulation* 2004;109:698–700.
320. McGlynn EA, Asch SM, Adams J, et al. The quality of health care delivered to adults in the United States. *N Engl J Med* 2003;348:2635–2645.
321. Bhatt DL, Roe MT, Peterson ED, et al. Utilization of early invasive management strategies for high-risk patients with non-ST-segment elevation acute coronary syndromes: results from the CRUSADE quality improvement initiative. *JAMA* 2004;292:2096–2104.
322. Kastrati A, Mehilli J, Schühlen H, et al. A clinical trial of abciximab in elective percutaneous coronary intervention after pretreatment with clopidogrel. *N Engl J Med* 2004;350:232–238.
323. Gibson CM, Singh KP, Murphy SA, et al. Association between duration of tirofiban therapy before percutaneous intervention and tissue level perfusion (a TACTICS-TIMI 18 substudy). *Am J Cardiol* 2004;94:492–494.
324. McCullough PA, Gibson CM, DiBattiste PM, et al. Timing of angiography and revascularization in acute coronary syndromes: an analysis of the TACTICS-TIMI-18 trial. *J Interv Cardiol* 2004;17:81–86.
325. Montalescot G, Dabbous OH, Lim MJ, et al. Relation of timing of cardiac catheterization to outcomes in patients with non-ST-segment elevation myocardial infarction or unstable angina pectoris enrolled in the multinational Global Registry of Acute Coronary Events. *Am J Cardiol* 2005;95:1397–1403.
326. Antman EM, Cohen M, Radley D, et al. Assessment of the treatment effect of enoxaparin for unstable angina/non-Q-wave myocardial infarction: TIMI 11B-ESSENCE meta-analysis. *Circulation* 1999;100:1602–1608.
327. Hatsukami TS, Ross R, Polissar NL, et al. Visualization of fibrous cap thickness and rupture in human atherosclerotic carotid plaque in vivo with high-resolution magnetic resonance imaging. *Circulation* 2000;102:959–964.

328. Casscells W, Hathorn B, David M, et al. Thermal detection of cellular infiltrates in living atherosclerotic plaques: possible implications for plaque rupture and thrombosis. *Lancet* 1996;347:1447–1451.
329. Stefanadis C, Diamantopoulos L, Vlachopoulos C, et al. Thermal heterogeneity within human atherosclerotic coronary arteries detected in vivo: a new method of detection by application of a special thermography catheter. *Circulation* 1999;99:1965–1971.
330. Kolodgie FD, Petrov A, Virmani R, et al. Targeting of apoptotic macrophages and experimental atheroma with radiolabeled annexin V: a technique with potential for noninvasive imaging of vulnerable plaque. *Circulation* 2003;108:3134–3139.
331. Taki J, Higuchi T, Kawashima A, et al. Detection of cardiomyocyte death in a rat model of ischemia and reperfusion using 99mTc-labeled annexin V. *J Nucl Med* 2004;45:1536–1541.
332. Hosokawa R, Nohara R, Hirai T, et al. Myocardial metabolism of (123)I-BMIPP under low-dose dobutamine infusion: implications for clinical SPECT imaging of ischemic heart disease. *Eur J Nucl Med Mol Imaging* 2005;32:75–83.

CHAPTER 19 ■ ACUTE MYOCARDIAL INFARCTION: EARLY DIAGNOSIS AND MANAGEMENT

ERIC J. TOPOL AND FRANS J. VAN DE WERF

OVERVIEW

The aggressive approach to reperfusion for acute myocardial infarction (MI) continues to be refined. For suitable patients, the cardinal goal is to achieve rapid, complete, and durable restoration of myocardial blood flow. This requires immediate use of either fibrinolytic or catheter-based therapy, and much new data support the latter as the preferred approach when this can be made available. The admission electrocardiogram (ECG), which provides the location and approximate size of the infarct, is remarkably important for prognosis, and combined with the main clinical parameters of age (the single most important parameter), heart rate, blood pressure, and Killip class, more than 90% of prognostic information is quickly assembled.

Patients without ST-segment elevation have non–Q-wave MI or unstable angina and are generally treated the same way, except without the use of fibrinolytic agents. Therapy with aspirin, anticoagulation, and β-blockade is appropriate in most patients. If primary coronary intervention is not used, consideration for coronary angiography, either on an urgent or elective basis, and coronary revascularization, are key decisions that need to be made as a function of the patient's risk profile, the occurrence of recurrent ischemia, and resource availability.

Although there has been considerable progress in recent years, our current armamentarium leaves many patients with suboptimal reperfusion at the tissue level. This problem has not yet been adequately addressed despite attempts with platelet glycoprotein IIb/IIIa inhibitors and other antiplatelet agents, better anticoagulants, antiinflammatory agents, and emboli capture devices for catheter-based reperfusion. Undoubtedly, we need to more effective restoration of epicardial and tissue-level perfusion.

GLOSSARY

Myocardial reperfusion: Restoration of coronary blood flow through the infarct-related artery.
Primary angioplasty: Use of balloon angioplasty to achieve myocardial reperfusion.
Rescue angioplasty: For patients who fail fibrinolytic therapy, the use of catheter-based reperfusion as a fallback approach in the early hours of the event.
Facilitated reperfusion: The use of a pharmacologic approach as a bridge to catheter-based reperfusion.
TIMI-3 flow: Brisk, complete flow as assessed by the Thrombolysis in Myocardial Infarction semiquantitative scoring system.

PATHOPHYSIOLOGY

Coronary atherosclerotic disease is the underlying substrate in nearly all patients with acute MI. The initiating event is a crack or fissure in the diseased arterial wall, which occurs as a result of loss of integrity of the plaque cap (the fibrous tissue overlying the plaque and partitioning the atheroma from the arterial lumen). The fissure or even frank plaque rupture leads to exposure of subendothelial matrix elements such as collagen, stimulating platelet activation and thrombus formation. Furthermore, tissue factor is released with the arterial injury, which directly activates the extrinsic coagulation cascade and promotes the formation of fibrin. If an occlusive thrombus forms, patients may develop an acute ST-segment elevation MI unless the subtended myocardium is richly collateralized. On the other hand, the thrombus formed may not be occlusive, but rather mural, and the patient may develop unstable angina or non–ST-segment elevation changes on the ECG (ST-depression or T-wave changes), which denote the lack of a "current of injury" or full-thickness (subendocardial to epicardial) myocardial ischemia.

Understanding the reasons why plaques crack may provide a better means of preventing acute MI, rather than intervening at the late phase after the event has been initiated. Plaques that rupture or fissure tend to have a thin fibrous cap, a high lipid content, few smooth muscle cells, and a high proportion of macrophages and monocytes (1). These mononuclear cells are conceived as a major trigger in plaque rupture by their release of such proteases as monocyte chemotactic protein and matrix metalloproteinases (e.g., collagenases, stromelysin, elastases), which chemically digest the plaque cap. Of note, the 3-hydroxy-3-methylglutaryl coenzyme A (HMG-CoA) reductase inhibitors have been shown to reduce the incidence of MI, and this is likely related to reduction in lipid content, as well as a favorable antiinflammatory effect on the cellular plaque constituents and chemokines (2). Loss of integrity of the arterial wall and platelet thrombus, with cessation of coronary blood flow through the infarct-related artery, thus drives myocardial ischemia and injury. As elegantly described by Reimer and Jennings, the *wavefront* of necrosis extends from the subendocardium to the subepicardium (3), and the extent of necrosis varies as a function of collateral flow, the length of time that coronary blood flow has halted, and the extent of diminution of coronary blood flow. In many patients, there is a stuttering quality of MI with severe pain often denoting the cutoff of blood supply, and less chest pain with partial, albeit insufficient, reflow. This dynamic quality of the infarct vessel blood flow pattern in acute MI (altered vasomotor tone or spasm) is likely related to the release of vasoactive amines from the activated platelets and loss of endothelial function.

The thrombus that occludes the coronary artery is a mixture of white (platelet-rich) and red (fibrin- and erythrocyte-rich) clots. In some patients, there is a more dominant role of platelets, whereas in others predominantly fibrin-rich thrombus at the arterial injury site is found. Stagnation thrombosis results from the lack of blood flow through the infarct vessel, leading to calumniation of red thrombus proximal to the original occlusion site (4). There is rarely frank herniation of the plaque occluding the lumen, which is known as *plaque disaster* (4).

On the other hand, the mural thrombus in patients without ST-segment elevation MI is apt to be platelet rich and not accompanied by stagnation; there is not sustained cutoff of coronary blood flow. Depending on the extent and duration of ischemia, the patient may not experience any myocardial necrosis (unstable angina) or develop myocardial damage (non–ST-elevation or non–Q-wave infarction). Beyond what is occurring at the arterial injury site and proximal to it, there is the potential for embolization of atheroma constituents or platelet thrombus distally. This is not typically found at routine postmortem but requires careful histologic inspection (5). When this occurs, a further explanation to cessation of myocardial blood flow is provided.

INCIDENCE AND SIGNIFICANCE

The true incidence of acute MI is unknown. Beyond the significant proportion of patients who die before reaching the hospital, estimated at 300,000 to 400,000 patients annually in the United States (6), it is estimated that approximately 1 million patients present to a hospital each year with some type of MI as the principal diagnosis (7). Of these, we know that roughly 200,000 patients receive reperfusion therapy in the United States per year, and that this represents only 20% to 30% of the patients who are assessed for eligibility for aggressive management (8,9). The breakdown of infarctions is also unclear, with a split between the classic ST-segment elevation and the non–ST-segment elevation. The latter group is increasingly common but difficult to differentiate from unstable angina on presentation. It is estimated that the majority of patients with acute coronary syndromes now present with no definitive ECG changes, or have abnormal ST-segment depression or T-wave inversion.

The incidence and mortality resulting from MI is on the decline. Not only has the fatality rate been reduced as better therapies have evolved, but the absolute number of MI events has continued to decrease since the 1970s. This is likely attributable to the many advances in preventive cardiology, including treatment of hypertension, avoidance of smoking, management of hypercholesterolemia, improved diet and exercise, and the prophylactic use of aspirin. It may also be an outgrowth of the high rates of surgical and percutaneous coronary revascularization in the United States, where the treatment of angina is more apt to be bypass surgery or stenting, rather than medical management. Although prevention of MI is not a prominent effect of coronary revascularization, intervening early in the course of atherosclerotic coronary disease may change its long-term natural history. A pronounced effect on reducing the incidence of MI appears to have resulted from the use of HMG-CoA reductase inhibitors (2), which has led to the concept that acute MI may even be "extinct" someday (10). Clearly, the most important initiatives for the condition of MI are in its prevention, because once the process of plaque rupture is unleashed, it is much more difficult to interrupt.

Although the incidence is declining, acute MI remains the principal cause of death in Western society and it is projected by 2020 for this to be the case worldwide (11). With the many rapid advances that have occurred in this field, the serious and potentially catastrophic outcome of an MI event has been underestimated in more recent years. Although reperfusion has made important progress in lowering mortality, most patients with acute MI are not eligible for this therapy and face in-hospital death rates of 10% to 20% (8). With the increasing proportion of our population being represented by the elderly, who have a high incidence of fatality even with reperfusion therapy, MI remains as the most critical single event in medicine.

DIAGNOSIS

Acute MI is a clinical syndrome for which a constellation of subjective and objective parameters need to be assessed. The diagnosis must be obtained rapidly and accurately, and misdiagnosis can have catastrophic sequelae. The individual components of making the diagnosis are discussed separately, but it is their integration that facilitates the accuracy and speed of the clinical syndrome recognition.

History

The classic symptoms of MI are intense, oppressive, durable, excruciating chest pressure, with an impending sense of doom and radiation of the pain to the left arm. However, the other symptoms of chest heaviness or burning, radiation to the jaw, neck, shoulder, back, or both arms may be encountered. Indigestion is common, especially with inferior wall MI. Nausea (particularly) and vomiting are typical. Profuse diaphoresis is also a frequent characteristic. Taken together, the patient with a clear-cut presentation is experiencing a unique, discrete, painful event that has induced fear. However, the subtleties of the history are more common and challenging. It is important to ask whether there were premonitory signs of chest discomfort (not necessarily pain) in the preceding week or two. Pain or discomfort may be completely localized to the arm or shoulder. Quite commonly, only the symptoms of indigestion and nausea prevail, such that the patient attributes the episode to heartburn and resorts to taking antacids.

The identification of risk factors, such as smoking, known cholesterol elevation, diabetes, hypertension, and family history, is a supportive piece that helps to put the acute history into context. The chest discomfort that causes the patient to seek medical attention is usually sustained (>20 minutes), but can be stuttering.

Other accompanying symptoms include dyspnea, which is of concern because it may denote incipient congestive heart failure or, alternatively, is an outgrowth of the patient's anxiety. Palpitations or syncope are unusual, but a history of lightheadedness or dizziness and presyncope often reflects the underlying vagotonia or bradyarrhythmias. When syncope, or an out-of-hospital arrest, has occurred there is a high likelihood of ventricular tachycardia as an explanation.

The differential diagnosis is quite broad (because many conditions can masquerade as acute MI) including aortic dissection, pericarditis, esophagitis, myocarditis, pneumonia, cholecystitis, and pancreatitis. Of these conditions, it is always worth considering that the patient has aortic dissection until proven otherwise, so that this diagnosis is not missed. Although considerably less common than acute MI, the therapies for the two conditions are entirely different and, for example, the use of fibrinolytic therapy for aortic dissection could be disastrous.

Physical Examination

The patient appears to be in distress and may even be writhing in pain. Pallor is common. The pulse is usually regular, although ventricular extrasystoles may be present. Bradycardia or tachycardia is helpful in understanding the infarct location, the effect on the conduction system, the vagal tone, and the extent of myocardium at jeopardy. Significant tachycardia (pulse >120) is worrisome and usually denotes an extensive MI, although a "hyperdynamic" subset of patients who have relatively small infarcts, but are hyperadrenergic, may be encountered. The blood pressure is typically elevated owing to the body's response to pain. Hypotension is either due to vagotonia, dehydration, a right ventricular infarction, or impending power failure.

Major examination findings to be aware of include whether there is elevation of jugular venous pressure, the character and location of the apical impulse, the splitting of the second heart sound, the presence of a third or fourth heart sound, a mitral regurgitant murmur, and whether there are rales. Examination of the peripheral pulses and the extremities is important. Collectively, this information provides a sense of the size of the myocardial infarct. If a third heart sound is present, along with rales halfway up the posterior chest fields (Killip class II), a large anterior wall MI is likely present. On the other hand, a normal examination suggests either a small infarction or that more extensive myocardial damage has not yet occurred.

Electrocardiography

It is imperative to obtain a 12-lead ECG as quickly as possible to secure the diagnosis. The presence of a true normal ECG rules out the occlusion of a major epicardial vessel at the moment the tracing was obtained. Hyperacute, tall T-wave changes are the first manifestations of acute coronary occlusion, but are frequently not present when the patient reaches the hospital for medical attention. The presence of ST-segment elevation is the principal feature that denotes "current of injury" and should be associated with reciprocal depression in contralateral leads. If only minimal (1–2 mm) ST elevation is present, then either the patient has collaterals to the infarct territory, the vessel is not fully occluded, or there has already been evolution of the ECG changes. If only ST-segment depression or T-wave inversion or both are manifest, this may denote either unstable angina or a non–ST-elevation (non–Q-wave) MI. This usually is not associated with an occluded infarct vessel, but rather one that is stenotic with myocardial ischemia. If a patient has a normal ECG, but the history is suggestive or even compelling, it is vital to observe the patient over an extended period (6–24 hours) to obtain additional ECG tracings and to determine if the chest discomfort or other symptoms recur. Certainly transient but marked ischemia can resolve before the patient has an ECG and a normal ECG can be recorded. It is worthwhile to give sublingual nitroglycerin (0.4 mg) to a patient with marked ST-segment elevation to see if this represents coronary artery spasm while more definitive therapy (vide infra) is being initiated. If the patient's chest pain and ECG quickly revert to normal after nitroglycerin, this strongly suggests vasospasm as the principal trigger.

In patients with ST-segment elevation largely confined to the right precordial leads (V_1–V_2), it is important to differentiate ST-segment elevation owing to current of injury and fast (early) repolarization, which is a normal variant and especially common in young African-American men. Early repolarization is diminished or undetectable when the heart rate is increased, so that if the ECG remains equivocal it may be helpful to have the patient do some sit-ups to increase the heart rate, and then repeat the ECG.

Creatine Phosphokinase

Plasma levels of creatine phosphokinase (CK), or of the isoenzyme CK-MB, which is primarily localized in the heart, are unhelpful in making the initial diagnosis. It takes at least 6 hours for there to be an enzyme "leak," which denotes myocardial cell necrosis. Enzymes should be assessed every 8 hours for the first 24 hours, and longer if the peak is not firmly established. Peak CPK occurs earlier when there has been successful reperfusion (12,13). This enzyme is much more helpful in gauging the size of the MI than in making the diagnosis.

Troponin T and I

More sensitive measures of myocardial necrosis have become available, which have a similar or even greater obligatory lag in appearing in the blood (as CK or CK-MB) but appear to detect cell damage more readily (14). The troponins are part of the tropomyosin-binding protein of the contractile apparatus of cardiac myocytes and therefore are highly specific for cardiac origin. A rapid bedside assay for troponin is available and is a practical, rapid way to assess patients with ischemic symptoms and non–ST-segment elevation. The off-line quantitative assays of both troponin T and I have been particularly helpful in differentiating risk, better than CK, in patients with unstable angina and non–ST-elevation MI. Both offer a more sensitive means of not only diagnosing whether infarction has occurred, but also discriminating the risk. However, the real utility of tests such as troponin goes beyond the determination of risk level to favorably alter the prognosis of the patient by knowledge of whether the test result is abnormal or not. Indeed, responses of patients to either IIb/IIIa inhibitors or low-molecular-weight heparins are predicted by abnormal troponin. These sensitive markers should be applied routinely for patients without ST-segment elevation. Troponins offer little incremental value in classic ST-elevation MI.

Echocardiography

The diagnosis of acute MI cannot be made by echocardiography because diagnosis is based on the combination of symptoms, the ECG findings, and the enzyme abnormalities. However, there are several findings that may be considered ancillary from a two-dimensional echocardiography, including a segmental wall abnormality and hyperkinesis of the contralateral wall. If a segment is akinetic, dyskinetic, or severely hypokinetic, it is not possible to know whether there was ischemia, with attendant dysfunction or stunning, or irrevocable damage due to necrosis. This can only be differentiated by serial echocardiographic examination. However, the finding of lack of hyperkinesis of the contralateral territory (e.g., the anterolateral wall in an inferior MI) in the acute setting suggests that the infarct vessel has recanalized or that there is multivessel coronary disease. This finding may be especially valuable in assessing a patient with congestive heart failure or cardiogenic shock; the main compensation of the ventricle to preserve its global ejection fraction is preempted if there is a significant stenosis of a major epicardial vessel supplying the noninfarcted territory. In patients with inferior MI, an echocardiogram of the right ventricle is helpful in demonstrating dilation or hypocontractility and is more sensitive than the right precordial ECG lead ST-segment elevation. A significant prior MI is also diagnosed by scarring and thinning of a specific territory and can easily be differentiated from an acute MI by its echocardiographic appearance.

Angiography

On occasion, even with all of the tools outlined, the diagnosis is uncertain. This may be the result of atypical symptoms and an ECG that is difficult to interpret. In a patient in whom reperfusion therapy is contemplated, an approach that can rapidly establish the diagnosis is emergency coronary angiography. By demonstrating an acutely occluded infarct vessel, with the characteristic appearance of thrombus or a cutoff sign at the point of occlusion, coupled with left ventriculography to ascertain the segmental wall motion profile, angiography can at times be helpful in a difficult diagnosis. Examples of patients who may present with ambiguity are those with an acute myocarditis with diffuse ECG changes, or patients with prior bypass surgery and previous MI, or those without a characteristic pattern on ECG. Furthermore, angiography can serve as the foundation for primary angioplasty to achieve reperfusion.

MAJOR SUBGROUPS AT PRESENTATION

By Electrocardiography

In Table 19.1, the five types of ST-segment elevation MI are presented. These represent specific patterns of ECG abnormalities that correlate with a clinical presentation, the underlying coronary anatomy, and prognosis. The most worrisome type is the proximal left anterior descending (LAD) MI, often referred to as the *widow-maker* infarction, which carries a high mortality and is attributed to an occlusion of the LAD before or at the first septal perforator. All of the precordial leads and I and aVL show ST-segment elevation. The proximal location of occlusion is associated with compromised perfusion to the His-Purkinje conduction tissue owing to loss of septal supply and often accompanied by a new bundle branch block. Usually, left anterior hemiblock or right bundle branch block is present, but bifascicular blocks, left bundle branch block, or Mobitz II atrioventricular block are all possible. Cardiogenic shock or power failure is not unexpected in this subgroup, unless there has been effective reperfusion established.

In contrast, occlusion of the LAD just distal to the first septal perforator is an anterior MI, which is less serious and called the *mid-LAD infarction.* Although the ECG may be indistinguishable from that of the proximal anterior MI patient with respect to the leads with ST elevation, there is no conduction disturbance. Cardiogenic shock in these patients is considerably less frequent, as restriction of the damage to the anterolateral and anteroapical segments spares the proximal interventricular septum. If shock is present, one should be concerned about prior myocardial damage or other noncardiac causes such as massive hemorrhage. Heart failure can occur, and the complications of ventricular aneurysm with potential of apical thrombus are common, especially if reperfusion has been delayed or is unsuccessful.

One segment distal in the LAD, sparing a large diagonal, represents the distal LAD infarction, which is less common. Only leads V_1 to V_4 are affected, but still there is the potential for apical hypokinesis, thrombus formation, and a milder form of the mid-LAD infarct clinical syndrome. Importantly, cardiogenic shock cannot result from this type of infarction per se.

Two types of infarcts that are relatively small are due to less significant territory affected. These are the LAD diagonal branch "lateral" MI, involving only leads I, aVL, V_5, and V_6,

TABLE 19.1

A CLASSIFICATION OF ACUTE MI BASED ON ELECTROCARDIOGRAPHIC ENTRY CRITERIA WITH ANGIOGRAPHIC CORRELATION

Categories	Anatomy of occlusion	Electrocardiographic entry	30-day mortality (%)[a]	1-year mortality (%)[a]
1. Proximal LAD	Proximal to first septal perforator	ST ↑ V_{1-6}, I, aVL, and fascicular or bundle branch block	19.6	25.6
2. Mid-LAD	Proximal to large diagonal, but distal to first septal perforator	ST ↑ V_{1-6}, I, aVL	9.2	12.4
3. Distal LAD or diagonal	Distal to large diagonal or of diagonal itself	ST ↑ V_{1-4} or ST ↑ I, aVL, V_{5-6}	6.8	10.2
4. Moderate to large inferior (posterior, lateral, right ventricular)	Proximal RCA or left circumflex	ST ↑ II, III, aVF and any or all of the following: a. V_1, V_3R, V_4R *or* b. V_5V_6 *or* c. R > S in V_1, V_2	6.4	8.4
5. Small inferior	Distal RCA or left circumflex, branch occlusion	ST ↑ II, III, aVF only	4.5	6.7

Abbreviations: LAD, left anterior descending; RCA, right coronary artery.
[a]Based on Global Use of Streptokinase and t-PA for Occluded Coronary Arteries (GUSTO-I) cohort population in each of the 5-year categories, all receiving reperfusion therapy.

also classified in the distal LAD territory MI, and the small inferior MI, with ECG ST elevation confined to leads II, III, and aVF. The latter is usually attributed to a distal right coronary artery lesion or branch (posterolateral or posterior descending), but in patients with a dominant left circumflex, it may be a branch from this vessel. Both of these types of MIs are usually uncomplicated and rarely associated with serious outcomes such as congestive heart failure or significant arrhythmias.

Patients with moderate or large inferior MIs are a key subgroup, which is heterogeneous, representing a spectrum of involvement of the inferior, posterior, lateral, and right ventricular myocardial involvement. The proximal, dominant right coronary artery is responsible for supplying all of these territories and can result in a large and potentially catastrophic event. The ECG leads involved include II, III, and aVF, and additional changes in the V_5, V_6 lateral leads, right ventricular leads (V_1 or V_{3R}, V_{4R}), or posterior leads (R/S ratio >1 in V_1, V_2, with or without ST depression, ST elevation in aVR). The largest inferior MI involves the composite of all of these territories. Dreaded complications, such as power failure or cardiogenic shock due to a large right ventricular infarct, or the development of a ventricular septal defect due to extensive distal septal necrosis, are possible. In all patients with inferior MI, a systematic approach to obtaining the right precordial ECG must be incorporated. Although right ventricular lead ST elevation of 1 to 2 mm in V_{3R} or V_{4R} is highly specific for right ventricular infarct, the sensitivity is suboptimal, and one should carefully examine the patient for elevated jugular venous pressure, a right-sided S_3 gallop, and, in cases in which there is uncertainty, perform either or both echocardiography or right-sided heart catheterization. Inferior MI is characterized by hypervagotonia, with bradycardia and hypotension that is responsive to atropine (0.6–1.0 mg intravenously). Type I atrioventricular block (Wenckebach) is exceedingly common with inferior MI, particularly if continuous ECG monitoring is reviewed. The conduction disturbances and bradyarrhythmias of inferior MI are usually benign, most often not requiring specific therapy other than occasional atropine.

Diagnosis of a true posterior infarction is rare, but the posterior wall is the least well expressed on the 12-lead ECG, such that occlusion of the left circumflex branches, which are usually responsible for the true posterior myocardial territory, can be missed. When the findings of ST depression in V_1 to V_4 are present, especially when accompanied by an R greater than S wave in V_1 or V_2 (or both), the ECG is highly supportive of a posterior MI. The ST depression follows the "mirror rule" as the reflection of the tracing would fit the conventional ST-elevation pattern that one would expect in other MI locations. Posterior wall MIs are usually well tolerated, but it is imperative to interrogate the possibility of concomitant involvement of the right ventricle and free wall of the left ventricle.

All of the patterns described have associated reciprocal ECG changes, which are important to confirm the diagnosis. For example, most patients with inferior MI have ST depression in either leads I, aVL, or precordial leads V_1 to V_4, and the prognostic significance of this latter finding has been debated for many years. The extent of reciprocal changes is usually similar to the primary current of injury, such that if there is 5 mm of ST elevation, there is more pronounced evidence of contralateral, reciprocal ECG changes. For the most part, this finding is useful for confirming the diagnosis and represents an ECG contrecoup expression, which does not carry vital clinical prognostic information. In most series, however, there is some incremental risk of adverse outcomes as a function of the extent and severity of reciprocal ST-segment depression (15).

Repeat 12-lead ECGs are vital 60 to 90 minutes after administration of fibrinolytic therapy to detect whether tissue-level reperfusion has occurred. As shown in Table 19.2, with the early repeat ECG in many large-scale trials (16–21) the prognosis of patients is greatly differentiated by whether there has been greater than or equal to 70% resolution of ST-segment elevation. This has come to serve as the "lie detector" or "truth serum" as an inexpensive, readily available means of assessing

TABLE 19.2

MYOCARDIAL REPERFUSION: ST RESOLUTION VERSUS MORTALITY (30 DAY)

Study (reference)	Time (min)	Complete	Partial	No
ISAM (20)	180	2.8	4.3	9.2
INJECT (16)	180	2.5	4.3	17.5
HIT 4 (17)	180	2.8	6.0	14.3
GUSTO-III (21)	90	4.0	5.4	10.7
TIMI 14 (18)	90	1.0	4.2	5.9
InTIME (19)	60	1.7	4.5	7.7

tissue-level reperfusion. It is also worthwhile to recheck the ECG after catheter-based reperfusion because approximately 20% to 30% of patients do not achieve ST-segment resolution, even in the presence of TIMI flow grade 3, and carry an unfavorable prognosis (22). This criterion of incomplete ST-segment resolution has served as the basis for rescue catheter-based reperfusion trials, the results of which will be reviewed.

Non–ST-Segment Elevation

Patients with acute ECG changes but without ST-segment elevation fit into the non–ST-elevation category. This was formerly known as *subendocardial, non–Q-wave MI,* but the reperfusion era has provided ample evidence that many patients with initial ST elevation do not go on to evolve a Q-wave MI (23). Giant T-wave inversion, characteristic of a proximal LAD lesion if occurring throughout the precordial leads, is an example of a non–ST-elevation MI with a discrete ECG pattern. However, many of the ECGs in this patient group do not fit a particular pattern of myocardial necrosis or ischemia, and at the time of evaluation, one is uncertain whether the changes are fixed or transient. Clearly, ST-segment depression is more ominous than T-wave inversion for 30-day mortality or nonfatal reinfarction. In a large-scale trial, the death rates were 6.8% versus 1.4%, and the composite event rates were 12.4% and 6.8%, respectively (24). Especially worrisome is the finding of global ischemia, when there is an ST depression in virtually every lead except aVR (where there is elevation); this frequently denotes a left main or equivalent non–ST-elevation MI.

By Hemodynamic (Killip) Class

Beside the ECG, which establishes the location of the infarct and often the precise location of the affected coronary artery, it is important to establish the patient's hemodynamic class. The Killip categories are most useful and validated for this purpose (25). Killip class I is the most common presenting class, occurring in 85% of patients with MI, and, by definition, with no evidence of heart failure. Early heart failure, as manifested by bibasilar rales and at times an S_3 gallop, is present in Killip II, the category that approximately 10% of patients present with. Pulmonary edema, as denoted by Killip III, and cardiogenic shock, classified as Killip IV, are uncommon, collectively accounting for 5% of patients in large-scale trials. In evaluating the patient's risk, five simple baseline parameters have been demonstrated, explaining more than 90% of the prognostic information for 30-day mortality. As shown in the pyramid (Fig. 19.1), the key five characteristics are age, systolic blood pressure, Killip class, heart rate, and location of the MI (26). Thus, evaluation of the patient's age, ECG, and hemodynamics provides crucial information that stratifies risk and may be helpful in guiding therapy. More recently, the prognostic value of the baseline serum creatinine has been highlighted (27).

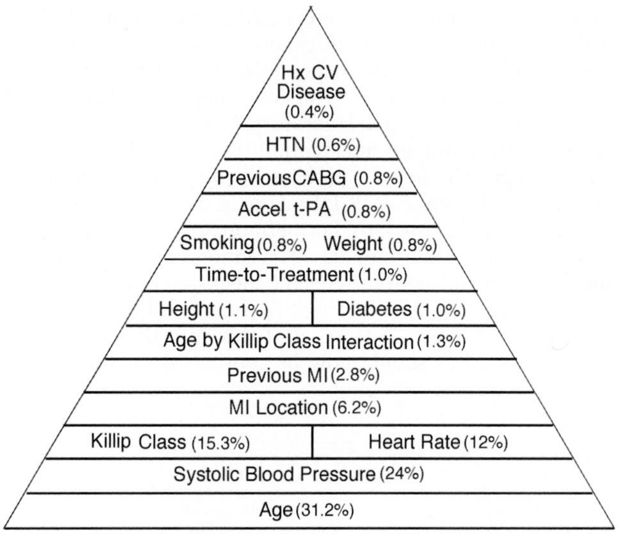

FIGURE 19.1. A multivariate model of mortality at 30 days in the Global Utilization of Streptokinase and t-PA for Occluded Coronary Arteries (GUSTO-I) trial. The factors in the pyramid provide the relative importance in affecting mortality among the 41,021 patients studied. *Abbreviations:* CABG, coronary artery bypass grafting; HTN, hypertension; Hx CV, history of cardiovascular disease; MI, myocardial infarction; t-PA, tissue plasminogen activator. (*Source:* Data adapted from Lee KL, Woodlief L, Topol EJ, et al. Predictors of 30-day mortality in the era of reperfusion for acute myocardial infarction: results from an international trial of 41,021 patients. *Circulation* 1995;91:1659–1668.)

PATIENT SELECTION FOR REPERFUSION THERAPY

All patients with ST-segment elevation MI who present within 12 hours from the onset of symptoms should be considered for myocardial reperfusion therapy. The only definite contraindications for fibrinolytic therapy are any previous intracranial hemorrhage, active bleeding, and recent stroke, trauma, or major surgery. Relative contraindications include severe or uncontrolled hypertension (systolic blood pressure >180/110 mm Hg), any previous cerebrovascular history, prior gastrointestinal hemorrhage, active menstruation, pregnancy, prolonged cardiopulmonary resuscitation (>10 minutes), noncompressible vascular punctures, and coumadin therapy with an international normalized ratio of greater than 2. For patients with relative contraindications to fibrinolytic therapy, primary angioplasty is the preferred reperfusion therapy.

Patients with new bundle branch block are also considered suitable candidates for reperfusion on the basis of the collaborative overview of the large-scale controlled trials of fibrinolytic therapy (28). Furthermore, right bundle branch block does not obscure ST elevation, and ST-segment elevation MI can frequently be diagnosed in the presence of left bundle branch block (29). Thus, for the most part, ST-segment elevation is the hallmark ECG feature guiding the use of reperfusion therapy along with symptoms, appropriate timing, and consideration of the clinical profile.

The benefit of reperfusion therapy generally appears to be independent of age, gender, and most baseline characteristics. However, the patients who derive the most benefit are patients treated earliest, those with anterior MI, and, in general, those with the highest risk. The critical dogma is to restore myocardial perfusion as quickly as possible. Accordingly, in a hospital with an experienced team for acute MI catheter-based intervention with an open laboratory, there is no question that percutaneous coronary intervention (PCI) would be the optimal strategy. The field of patients eligible for reperfusion is extended with the use of PCI, because of the contraindications to fibrinolytic therapy (30). Furthermore, owing to the relative lack of efficacy of fibrinolytic intervention in specific settings, such as in patients with cardiogenic shock and those with prior bypass surgery, PCI is preferred. As reviewed here, whenever available on a timely basis, even if this necessitates interhospital transfer, PCI should now be considered the reperfusion strategy of choice.

TREATMENT

Fibrinolytics or Catheter-Based Reperfusion

For many years there has been an active debate as to which reperfusion therapy is preferred—fibrinolytics or catheter-based reperfusion. Cumulatively, 23 randomized trials in 7,739 patients, show an advantage for primary angioplasty (31). The advantages, shown in Figure 19.2, are manifest in short-term reduction in mortality, reinfarction, and stroke. The vast majority of patients in these 23 trials underwent balloon angioplasty, but in recent years the use of stenting has largely replaced balloon angioplasty for catheter-based reperfusion. This change in practice was solidified with the results of randomized trials comparing balloon angioplasty with stenting for acute MI (31–41). As summarized in pooled analysis of the nine trials, primary stenting offered significant advantages compared with balloon angioplasty for the reduction of reinfarction (Fig. 19.3) and repeat target vessel revascularization. However, in this combined study of 4,433 patients, there was actually a 17%, increase in mortality at 30 days, albeit not statistically significant, for stenting compared with balloon angioplasty (31).

The advantages of catheter-based reperfusion over intravenous fibrinolytics was greatly extended by randomized trials that incorporated transfer of patients to a facility in which the PCI could be performed. The largest trial, the Danish Multicenter Randomized Study on Fibrinolytic Therapy Versus Acute Coronary Angioplasty in Acute Myocardial Infarction (DANAMI-2), showed a striking advantage for reduction of the composite of death, disabling stroke, or reinfarction, both for referral hospitals (requiring interhospital transfer) and invasive treatment centers (Fig. 19.4) (42). In this trial, the catheter-based reperfusion consisted of stents in 93% of the patients.

Other trials comparing fibrinolytics and interhospital transfer for catheter-based reperfusion have confirmed and extended the DANAMI-2 results (43–45). Interestingly, for the three trials summarized in Figure 19.5, there is remarkable similarity of the event rates among the transported patients, and the magnitude of reduction of events of death, reinfarction, and stroke (43). In the CAPTIM trial, prehospital administration of a lytic agent followed by rescue PCI, if needed, was associated with a lower mortality when compared with primary PCI, especially when the lytic was given very early(<2 hours) after onset of symptoms (46). Similar results were found in registries in Europe. These results should be viewed in the light of the negative outcomes after facilitated PCI with lytic agents (see below).

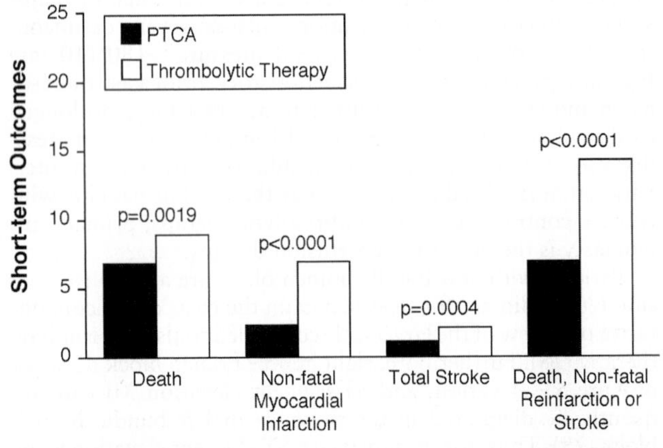

FIGURE 19.2. Short- and long-term clinical outcomes in individuals treated with primary PTCA or thrombolytic therapy. *Abbreviation:* PTCA, percutaneous transluminal coronary angioplasty. (*Source:* From Keeley EC, Boura JA, Grines CL. Primary angioplasty versus intravenous thrombolytic therapy for acute myocardial infarction: a quantitative review of 23 randomised trials. *Lancet* 2003;361:13–20, with permission.)

Analgesia and Supportive Measures

The first step in treating the patient, while more definitive therapy is being prepared (such as fibrinolytics or transfer to a cardiac catheterization laboratory), is to make the patient comfortable via supplemental oxygen (usually nasal cannula at 2 L/min) and morphine (2–4 mg intravenously and repeat as necessary). Before using morphine, it is helpful to have quickly tried sublingual nitroglycerin to determine whether there is a reversible component of the ischemia, pain, and ECG changes.

Aspirin

The use of aspirin is a cornerstone of therapy for patients with acute coronary syndromes. It should be initiated as quickly as possible when the diagnosis is made, at a dose of 160 mg by chewable administration (two 80-mg "baby" aspirin) or a 325-mg orally administered tablet. No enteric coated formulation of aspirin should be used. The validation for the importance of aspirin in this setting is derived from the landmark International Studies of Infarct Survival (ISIS-2) trial (Fig. 19.6), which showed it is lifesaving (47). Since this trial, aspirin has been used in virtually all patients with acute MI, and other trials have provided strong evidence for its use in unstable angina and non–ST-elevation MI . The dose that has been routinely recommended is 325 mg/day. For long-term use, a daily dose of 75 to 81 mg may represent the best balance of efficacy and safety, but no definitive randomized trials of aspirin dosing are available.

Clopidogrel

Recent trials have addressed the addition of clopidogrel to aspirin, as compared to aspirin alone, in the setting of ST-segment elevation MI. In the CLARITY trial of 3,491 patients (48) with a hybrid angiographic and clinical composite endpoint (Fig. 19.7A), there was a 36% reduction of an occluded infarct artery at early angiography, death, or recurrent MI. This trial focused on patients younger than 76 years, such that the potential for bleeding complications, chiefly occurring in the elderly when angiography is performed early, was not directly assessed. In the COMMIT trial conducted in China with 45,852 patients (49), there was a 9%, statistically significant reduction

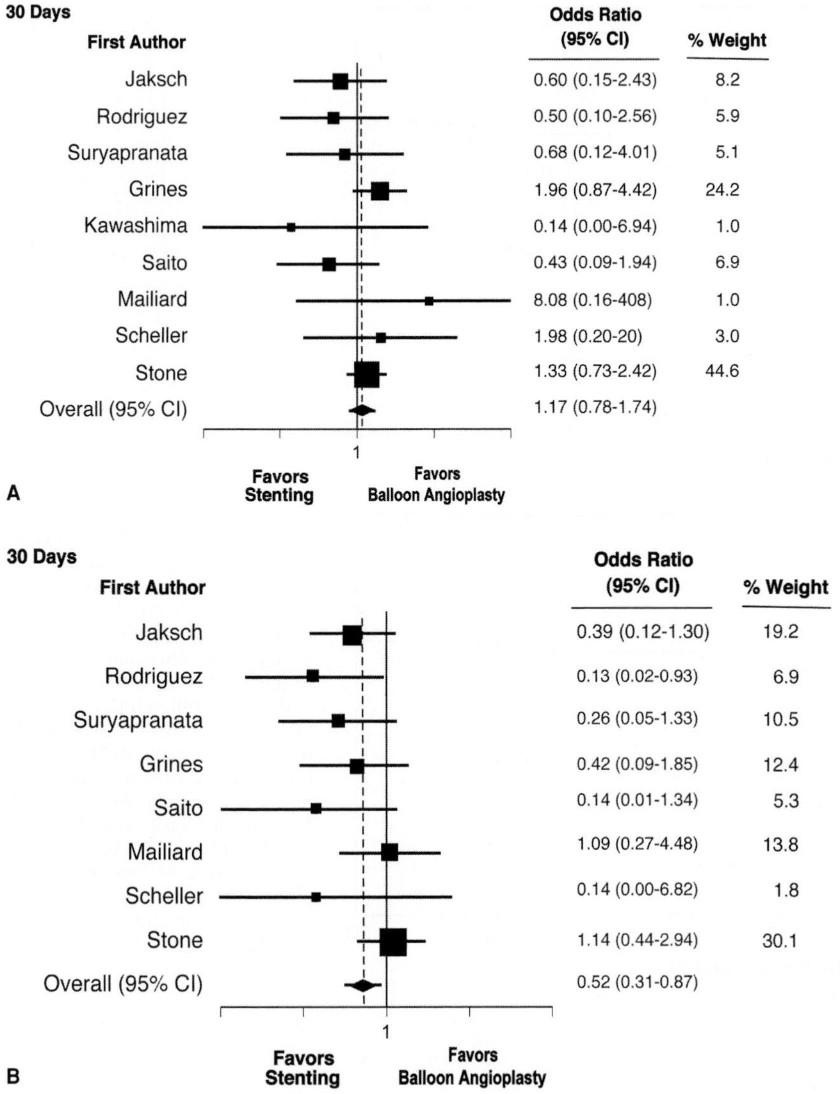

FIGURE 19.3. (**A**) Odds ratios for mortality in patients with myocardial infarction who were treated with primary stenting versus balloon angioplasty. *Abbreviation:* CI, confidence interval. (**B**) Odds ratio for reinfarction in patients with myocardial infarction who were treated with primary stenting versus balloon angioplasty. (*Source:* From Nordmann AJ, Hengstler P, Harr T, et al. Clinical outcomes of primary stenting versus balloon angioplasty in patients with myocardial infarction: a meta-analysis of randomized controlled trials. *Am J Med* 2004; 116:253–262, with permission).

of death, reinfarction, or stroke with the addition of clopidogrel on top of aspirin (Fig. 19.7B). These two trials taken together suggest strong consideration should be given that in patients for whom reperfusion therapy is appropriate, that early clopidogrel is added to aspirin. A loading dose of 300 to 600 mg may be optimal, but no loading was used in COMMIT and likely an insufficient loading (300 mg) was used in CLARITY. The desired rapid antiplatelet action would support the higher loading dose for this orally administered medicine.

Time to Treatment

The time to treatment is a pivotal parameter in reperfusion. Patients treated in the first hour have the highest absolute and relative mortality benefit (50). This observation has led to the first 60 minutes to be referred to as the *golden hour* of reperfusion. The dominant explanation for the exaggerated benefit appears to be related to prevention of myocardial damage, as thallium studies have indicated the ability to prevent an MI in up to 40% of such patients (51). However, as judged from the high placebo group mortality of patients treated in the first hour, it may be that patients who present early (e.g., within 30 minutes of onset of symptoms) have a larger MI and are therefore preselected to derive pronounced benefit. Certainly all of the trials convey an inverse relationship between treatment onset and survival benefit with little to no beneficial effect for patients treated at 12 hours or beyond. Two large-scale trials have been dedicated to the issue of late therapy (52,53), and both suggest that treatment benefit is restricted to the first 12 hours. The benefit of prehospital initiation of fibrinolysis (17% reduction in hospital mortality when compared with in-hospital initiation in a metaanalysis by Morrison et al. [54]) underlines the importance time to treatment.

With PCI there has been recent debate as to whether there is a similar gradient of benefit over time to reperfusion as seen with fibrinolytics, or that the strategy is time insensitive. Brodie et al. (55) reviewed their extensive data on primary PCI and showed that in higher risk patients, there was indeed a gradient of benefit as a function of time (Fig. 19.8).

The use of emboli protection devices was thought to be particularly useful in MI, with the extensive clot burden and atheromatous debris that might be embolized at the time of catheter-based reperfusion. Surprisingly, the data to validate the use of such devices has not panned out. The EMERALD trial testing one such device in 501 patients without improvement in microvascular flow, reduced infarct size, or enhanced event-free survival (56). More studies are underway and the possibility of improved technology to avoid embolization at the time of the initial device deployment in the infarct vessel may occur. But no evidence currently exists to support the use of such devices at this time.

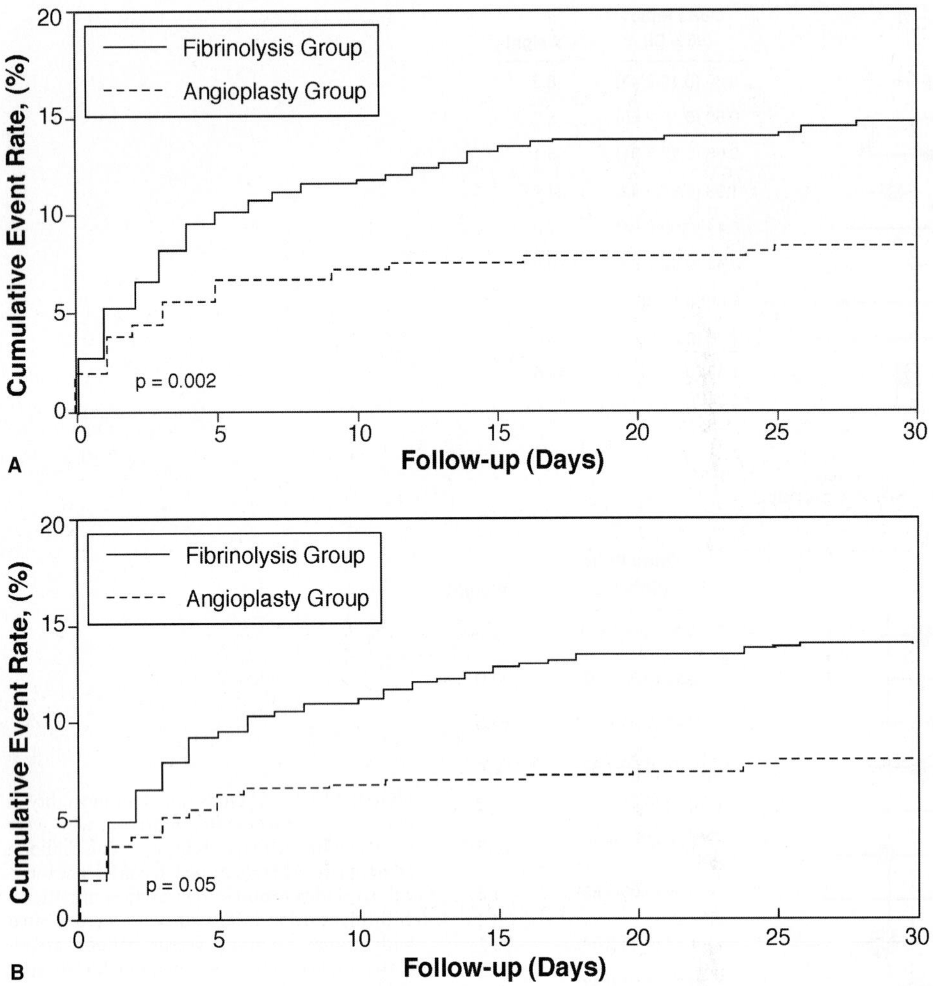

FIGURE 19.4. (A) Kaplan-Meier curves showing cumulative event rates for the primary composite end point of death, clinical reinfarction, or disabling stroke during 30 days of follow-up. This panel shows the results for the 1,129 patients who underwent randomization at referral hospitals. (B) Results for 443 patients who underwent randomization at invasive treatment centers. (*Source:* From Anderson HR, Nielson TT, Rasmussen K, et al., for the DANAMI-2 Investigators. A comparison of coronary angioplasty with fibrinolytic therapy in acute myocardial infarction. *N Eng J Med* 2003;349:733–742, with permission.)

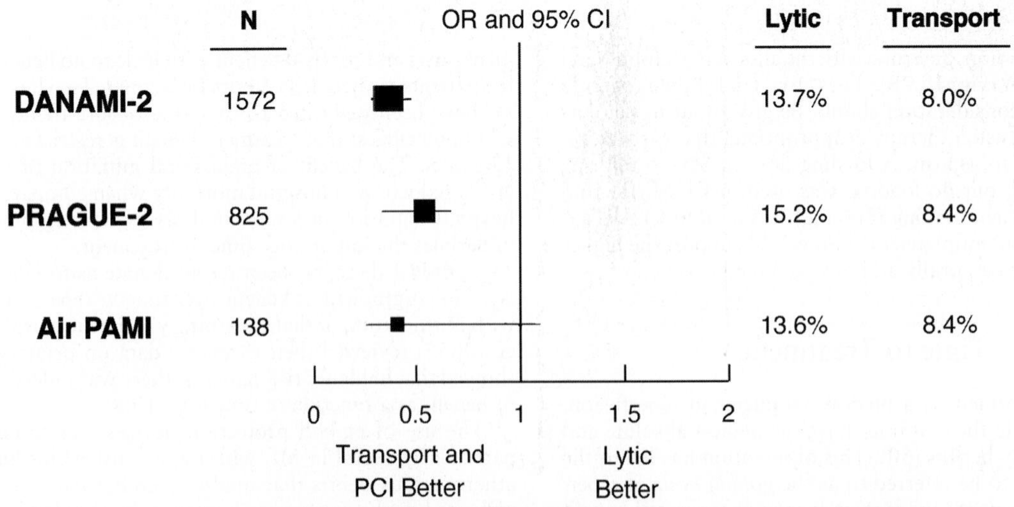

FIGURE 19.5. Odds ratio and 95% confidence intervals for the composite endpoint of death, reinfarction, and stroke at 30 days for the fibrinolytic (lytic) and transport plus coronary intervention arms in 3 randomized trials. *Abbreviations:* DANAMI, DANish multicenter randomized study on thrombolytic therapy versus coronary angioplasty in Acute Myocardial Infarction-2; PCI, percutaneous coronary intervention; PRAGUE-2, PRimary Angioplasty in AMI patients from General community hospitals transported to PTCA Units vs Emergency thrombolysis; Air PAMI, A randomlzed trial of transfer for Primary Angioplasty versus on-site thrombolysis in patients with high-risk Myocardial Infarction. (*Source:* From Topol EJ, Kereiakes DJ. Regionalization of care for acute ischemic heart disease: a call for specialized centers. *Circulation* 2003;107:1463–1466.)

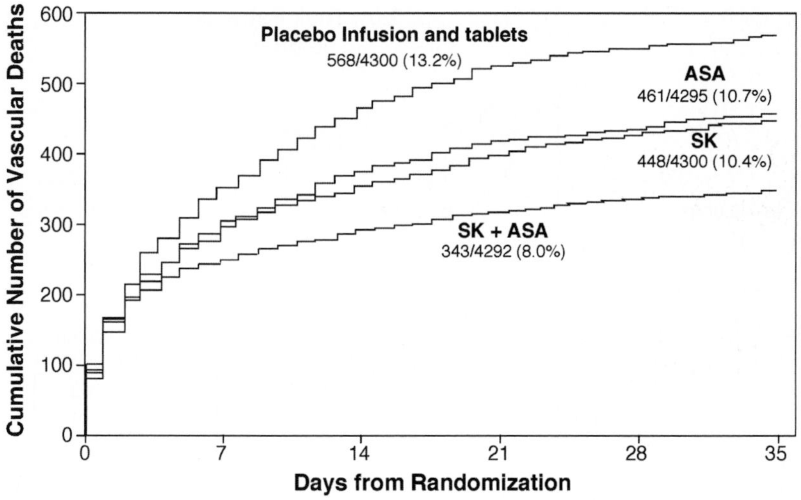

FIGURE 19.6. Second International Study of Infarct Survival (ISIS-2) showing significant reduction of mortality at 35 days for aspirin or streptokinase, and an additive effect for the two combined. *Abbreviations:* ASA, aspirin; SK, streptokinase. (*Source:* From ISIS-2 [Second international study of infarct survival] Collaborative Group. Randomized trial of intravenous streptokinase, oral aspirin, both, or neither among 17,187 cases of suspected acute myocardial infarction. *Lancet* 1988;11:349–360, with permission.)

Selection of Fibrinolytic Agents

There have been three large trials that studied the differences in effects on mortality for tissue plasminogen activator (t-PA) and streptokinase (SK) (57–60). In the GISSI-2/International trial (56), 20,891 patients were randomly assigned to t-PA or SK, with a factorial design also randomized to subcutaneous heparin started after 12 hours or no heparin. The t-PA was alteplase given over 3 hours. Mortality at 30 days was 8.9%

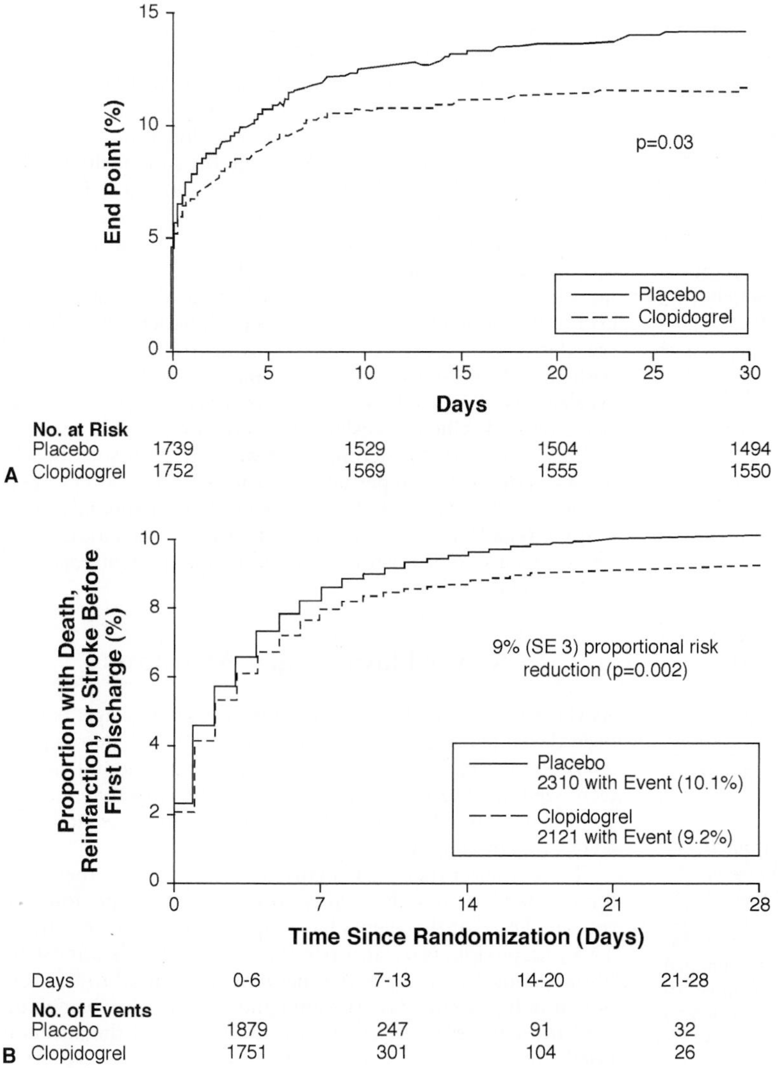

FIGURE 19.7. (A) Cumulative incidence of the end point of death from cardiovascular causes, recurrent myocardial infarction, or recurrent ischemia leading to the need for urgent revascularization. The odds ratio for this end point was significantly lower in the clopidogrel group than in the placebo group at 30 days 911.6% versus 14.1%; odds ratio, 0.80 (95% confidence interval, 0.65–0.97); $P = .030$. (*Source:* From Sabatine MS, Cannon CP, Gibson CM, et al. Addition of clopidogrel to aspirin and fibrinolytic therapy for myocardial infarction with ST-segment elevation. *N Eng J Med* 2005;352:1179–1189, with permission.) (B) Effects of clopidogrel allocation on death, reinfarction, or stroke before first discharge from hospital. Time-to-event analyses based on first relevant event during scheduled treatment period. Mean treatment duration in survivors was 14.9 days. Flatness of right-hand ends of graph is because events after discharge were not included. (*Source:* From COMMIT [Clopidrogrel and Metoprolol in Myocardial Infarction Trial] collaborative group. Addition of clopidogrel to aspirin in 45,852 patients with acute myocardial infarction: randomized placebo-controlled trial. *Lancet* 2005;366:1607–1621, with permission.)

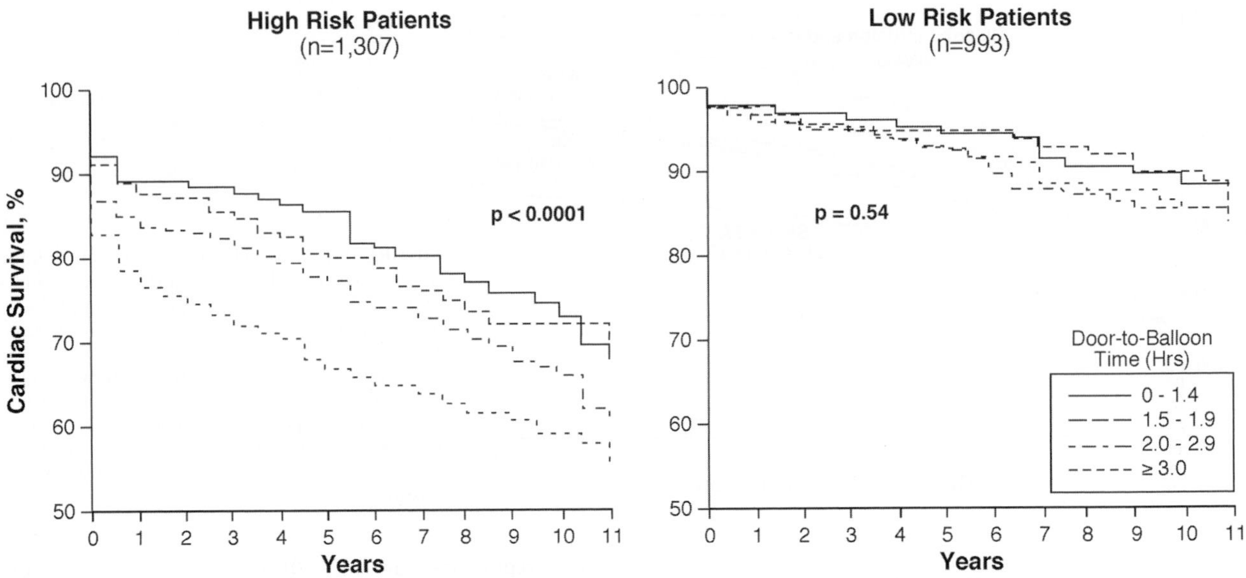

FIGURE 19.8. Kaplan-Meier estimates of late cardiac survival in patients treated with primary PCI for ST-segment elevation MI according to door-to-balloon times. (A) High-risk patients (Killip class 3–4, age >70 years, or anterior infarction). (B) Low-risk patients. (*Source:* From Brodie BR, Hansen C, Stuckey TD, et al. Door-to-balloon time with primary PCI for acute myocardial infarction impacts late cardiac mortality in high-risk patients and patients presenting early after the onset of symptoms. *J Am Coll Cardiol* 2006;47:289–295, with permission.)

and 8.5%, respectively (58). The ISIS-3 trial evaluated 41,299 patients with three different fibrinolytic agents: the duteplase form of t-PA, which has not been commercially developed; SK; and anistreplase. A factorial design for evaluating subcutaneous heparin started after 4 hours versus placebo was also used. There were no differences in mortality (10.3%, 10.5%, and 10.6%, respectively) (59). Subsequently, the Global Use of Streptokinase and t-PA for Occluded Coronary Arteries (GUSTO-I) trial evaluated 41,021 patients randomly assigned to one of four fibrinolytic strategies (60). Accelerated alteplase t-PA over 90 minutes, administered with intravenous heparin, was shown to significantly reduce 30-day mortality by 15% as compared with SK with intravenous or with subcutaneous heparin, or the combination of t-PA and SK with intravenous heparin (Fig. 19.9). The benefit was highly consistent across virtually all subcategories, including age, location of MI, and the time from symptom onset Although the superiority of t-PA was contested because of the 8- to 10-fold increase in its cost compared with SK ($2,200 versus $300), the differences were highly significant, consistent, and durable at 1 year of follow-up (61). The mechanism for the benefit, with earlier complete infarct vessel patency, as discussed later in this chapter, was also fully characterized (62). As expected, patients with higher risk derived the most substantial benefit from t-PA compared with SK (62). Formal cost-effectiveness analysis has shown that accelerated t-PA saved 14 additional years of life per 1,000 patients treated, which translates to a cost of $32,678 per year of life saved (63). This compares favorably with such benchmarks as the cost of hypertension treatment ($20,000 per year of life saved) or the cost-effectiveness ratio of hemodialysis for chronic renal failure ($35,000 per year of life saved), but still represents a significant toll on an individual patient basis and on a societal level (63).

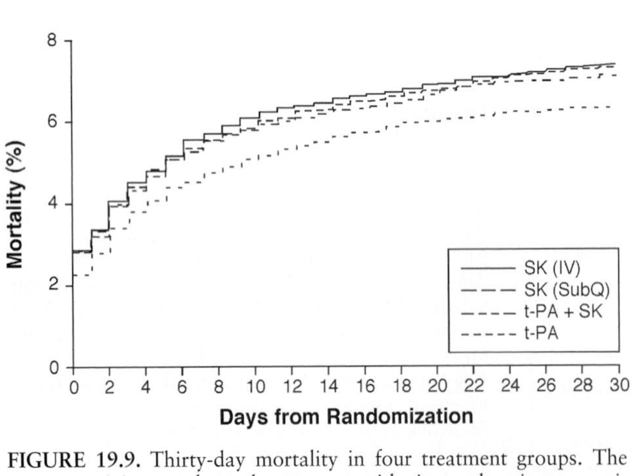

FIGURE 19.9. Thirty-day mortality in four treatment groups. The group receiving accelerated treatment with tissue plasminogen activator (t-PA) had lower mortality than both the two streptokinase (SK) groups ($P = .001$) and each individual treatment group: streptokinase and subcutaneous (SubQ) heparin ($p = .009$), streptokinase and intravenous (IV) heparin ($P = .003$), and t-PA and streptokinase combined with IV heparin ($P = .04$). (*Source:* From The GUSTO Investigators. An international randomized trial comparing four fibrinolytic strategies for acute myocardial infarction. *N Engl J Med* 1993;329:1615–1622, with permission.)

Newer Plasminogen Activators

As shown in Figure 19.10, many new fibrinolytic agents have been developed. The mutants of native t-PA include reteplase (r-PA, Retavase), and TNK tenecteplase (a triple mutant Genentech; see Fig. 19.10). Other agents being developed include recombinant staphylokinase, vampire bat plasminogen activator (PA), and amediplase.

The common theme for many of these agents is their prolonged half-life and the ability to use a bolus-type administration. Three of the agents have remarkable fibrin specificity: TNK, staphylokinase, and bat PA, which affords almost no fibrinogenolysis. All have the theoretical potential to be more potent in lysing coronary thrombi and therefore are being pursued for acute MI as a chief indication. Each of the agents is briefly addressed.

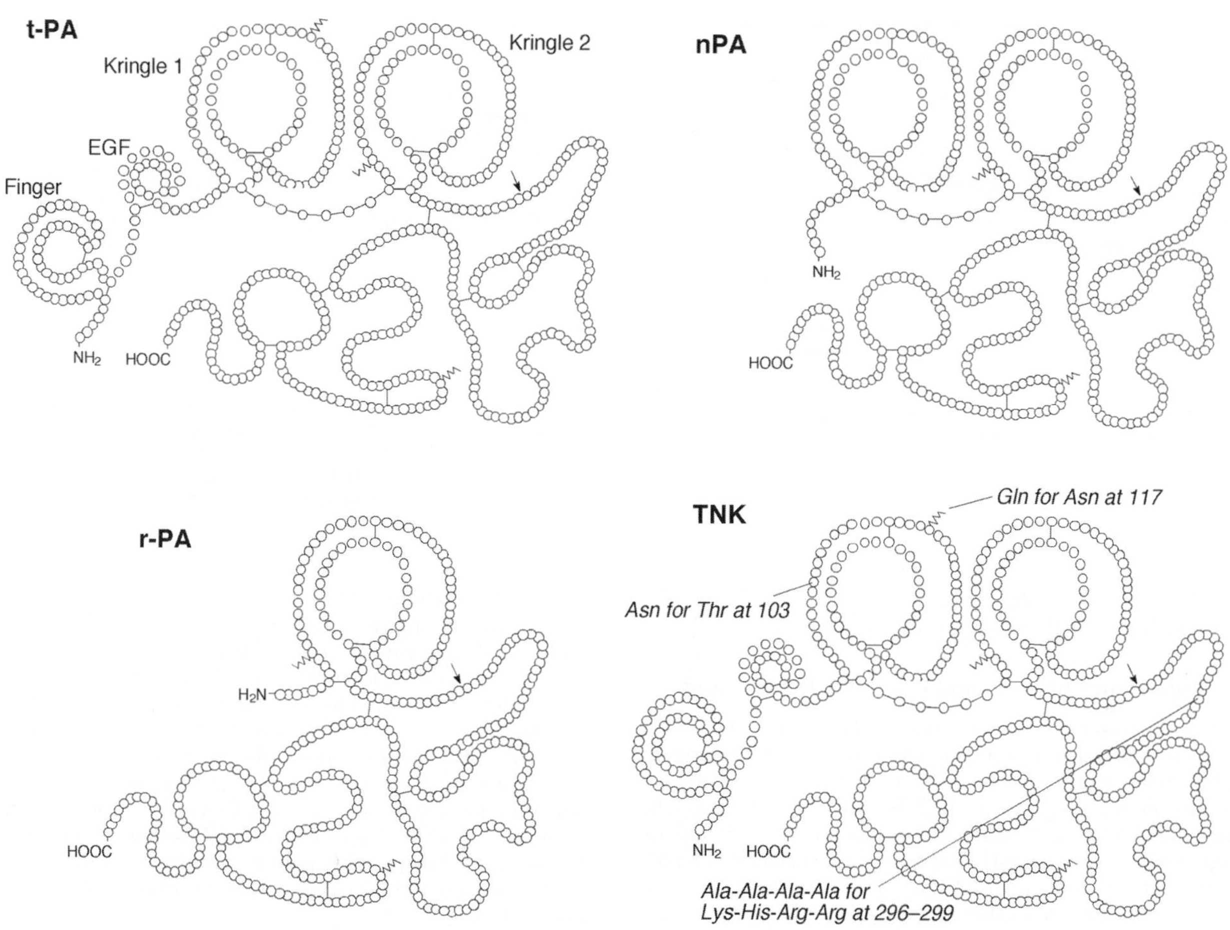

FIGURE 19.10. Structure of wild-type tissue plasminogen activator (t-PA) and three mutants. Reteplase (r-PA) is missing the finger, epidermal growth factor, and Kringle-1 domain. Lanoteplase (nPA) is similar to r-PA but maintains the Kringle-1. TNK is a triple site-directed mutagenic plasminogen activator with changes at three sites, as shown.

Acute Myocardial Infarction

Reteplase

r-PA was approved for use in the United States in 1996 and represents the first of the third-generation fibrinolytics to become commercially available. As shown in Fig. 19.10, it is a deletion mutant of t-PA and is given as two 10-MU boluses, 30 minutes apart. Like t-PA, intravenous heparin is used in conjunction with r-PA, and the results of two angiographic trials (64,65) indicate the potential of superiority for speed and extent of coronary thrombolysis for r-PA compared with conventional or accelerated t-PA. The International Joint Evaluation of Coronary Thrombolysis trial compared r-PA with SK in over 6,000 patients and demonstrated a small, but not statistically meaningful, benefit for r-PA (66). The GUSTO-III trial compared r-PA and accelerated t-PA in 15,072 patients. No benefit for r-PA over t-PA was demonstrated (21). There was a higher mortality and hemorrhagic stroke rate in GUSTO-III compared with previous trials, probably owing to a more aged population enrolled. Both t-PA and r-PA cost approximately $2,200 per dose. The major benefit of r-PA over t-PA is the ease of use. Equivalence or "noninferiority" of r-PA to t-PA has not been established at 30 days or 1 year with respect to mortality point estimates.

Tenecteplase

An outgrowth of the Assessment of the Safety and Efficacy of a New Fibrinolytic (ASSENT-2) trial (67) was the validation of TNK as equivalent (or not inferior) to accelerated t-PA. As shown in Figure 19.11, mortality at 30 days was remarkably similar with this single-bolus agent compared with the more complicated accelerated t-PA regimen. Furthermore, there was superiority established for patients presenting late (receiving therapy after 4 hours) and a significant reduction in noncerebral bleeding complications. Taken together, the profile of TNK is particularly favorable, and this is the most fibrin-specific agent currently available. Its cost, however, is similar to alteplase and r-PA.

Other Agents

n-PA was studied in the Intravenous nPA for Treatment of Infracting Myocardium Early (InTIME)-2 trial and did not fare particularly well against accelerated t-PA (19). Although the mortality at 30 days was within 0.3% absolute, possibly fulfilling noninferiority criteria, there was a significant excess in intracerebral hemorrhage with this single-bolus mutant t-PA. Likely related to this finding, n-PA has not become commercially available. Amediplase is a chimeric molecule consisting of the Kringle-2 domain of alteplase and the catalytic part of pro-urokinase. It can be given as a single bolus, is nonimmunogenic and induces a patency rate of the infarct vessel similar to alteplase. A large phase III mortality study with this agent is being considered.

Rescue Angioplasty

The strategy of using catheter-based reperfusion as a fallback when fibrinolytics have been deemed to fail has been studied

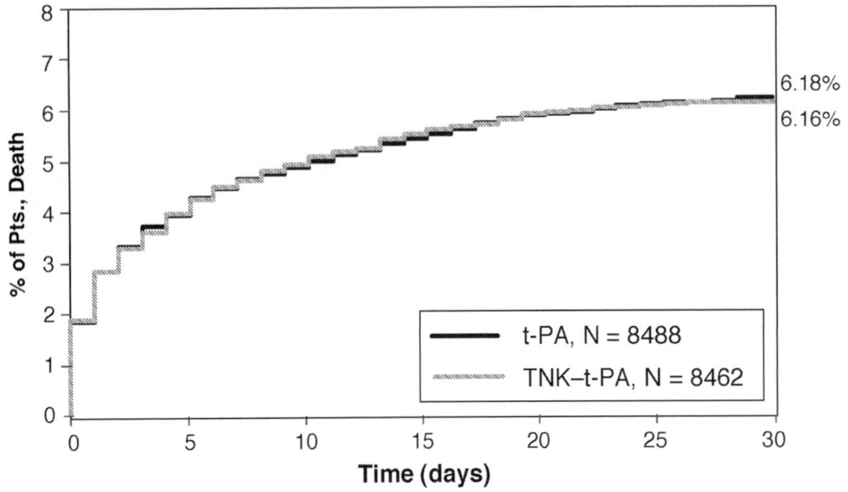

FIGURE 19.11. Primary results of Global Utilization of Streptokinase and t-PA for Occluded Coronary Arteries (GUSTO-III) trial for 30-day mortality. *Abbreviations:* r-PA, reteplase; t-PA, tissue plasminogen activator.

over the past two decades. Before reviewing recent data for this strategy, the rationale will be presented.

Importance of Early and Complete Reperfusion

The mechanism of benefit of accelerated t-PA in the GUSTO-I trial was clearly demonstrated to be the improvement in timely and complete restoration of coronary blood flow (62,68). The proportion of patients in the GUSTO angiographic trial who had TIMI-3 flow at 90 minutes after therapy was initiated, reflecting brisk infarct vessel blood flow, was considerably higher for the patients receiving t-PA compared with the other three strategies assessed. Nonetheless, even for accelerated t-PA, the rate of TIMI-3 flow was only 54%, leaving room for improvement in future pharmacologic reperfusion strategies (62,68). The patency status at 90 minutes was a critical index of outcomes, including survival at 24 hours, 30 days, and 1 and 2 years (62,68). Beside the salutary effects on improving survival, the TIMI-3 flow status was closely associated with global left ventricular function, cavity dilatation, and regional wall motion of the infarct zone (62,68). Two groups of patients known to have a high failure rate of fibrinolytics are those presenting with cardiogenic shock, due to poor perfusion, and occlusion of saphenous vein grafts, in which there is extensive clot burden.

Clinical Detection of Reperfusion

Apart from administering fibrinolytic therapy or performing PCI as rapidly as possible after the diagnosis is established, it is important to emphasize that in most patients one cannot rely on bedside signs to reliably detect whether pharmacologic reperfusion has been successful (69). First, it is not possible to use the patient's chest pain as a guide to whether the therapy is effective. The reasons for this are multiple, including the confounding effects of narcotic analgesics, the partial denervation that occurs at some point after coronary thrombosis in some patients with MI, the stuttering pattern of infarct vessel blood flow in the early hours of infarction, and the natural evolution of the necrosis with eventual attenuation or relief from chest pain. Second, so-called reperfusion arrhythmias are a misnomer, such as ventricular tachycardia; they more commonly occur in patients who either do not receive reperfusion therapy or fail to achieve successful reperfusion. One arrhythmia that has been correlated with restoration of infarct vessel patency is accelerated idioventricular rhythm. Third, resolution of the ST-segment elevation is an unreliable means of establishing reperfusion success. There may be partial resolution from natural, evolutionary features of the event or the dynamic blood flow pattern so characteristic of the first 12 hours of acute MI. If a patient develops sudden and near-complete relief of chest pain, full resolution of the ECG abnormalities, and has a run of accelerated idioventricular rhythm, this is highly specific for successful reperfusion, but this only occurs in less than 10% of patients receiving fibrinolytic therapy. Nevertheless, the accepted convention for diagnosing failure or reperfusion after fibrinolytics has been the ECG criteria of not achieving more than 50% resolution of the ST segment elevation 60 minutes into therapy. This failure parameter has indeed been correlated with an adverse prognosis of 30 day mortality (see Table 19.2).

Two recent trials of rescue PCI are helpful to validate the continued use of this strategy. Schomig et al. (70) performed a trial of 181 patients comparing balloon angioplasty and stenting. The stent group of patients had significantly greater myocardial salvage (70). In the best trial that has been done to date, Gershlick et al. for the REACT study group (71) randomized 427 patients to repeat fibrinolytics, conservative treatment, or rescue PCI. As shown in Figure 19.12, there was a significantly better outcome for rescue PCI compared with the other strategies. The end point utilized was a composite of reduction of death, reinfarction, stroke, or severe heart failure (71).

Platelet Glycoprotein IIb/IIIa Inhibitors and Facilitated Reperfusion

Beyond aspirin and clopidogrel, there has been intensive study of the use of intravenous IIb/IIIa inhibitors in the setting of reperfusion therapy. With primary PCI, there is clear evidence from five randomized trials that adding IIb/IIIa inhibitors will reduce the composite of death, reinfarction, and repeat target vessel revascularization (72–77) (Fig. 19.13). The benefits are sustained at 6 months for reduction of death or reinfarction (70). Montalescot et al. (78) pooled data from 6 placebo-controlled trials of IIb/IIIa inhibitors and PCI to determine the value of early versus late administration. This is comparing giving the drug in the emergency room at the earliest time after presentation or giving the drug at the time of PCI. A much higher rate of infarct vessel patency was consistently noted for use of early IIb/IIIa inhibition, and even among only 933 patients analyzed there was a 28%, nonstatistically significant reduction in mortality. In reviewing all these data, it appears that early IIb/III inhibition with PCI may be considered the

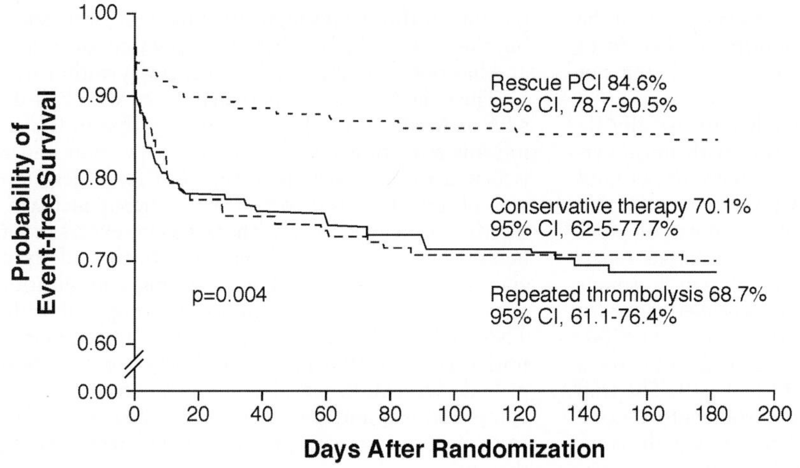

No. of Events

Rescue PCI	110	106	105	101	99	99	96	95	93
Conservative therapy	109	104	102	99	98	97	96	95	93
Repeat thrombolysis	129	127	124	122	120	117	117	116	115

FIGURE 19.12. Kaplan-Meier estimates of the cumulative rate of the composite primary endpoint (death, recurrent myocardial infarction, severe heart failure, or cerebrovascular event) within 6 months. *Abbreviations:* PCI, percutaneous coronary intervention; CI, confidence interval. (*Source:* From Gershlick AH, Stephens-Lloyd A, Hughes S, et al. Rescue angioplasty after failed thrombolytic therapy for acute myocardial infarction. *N Engl J Med* 2005;353:2758–2768, with permission.)

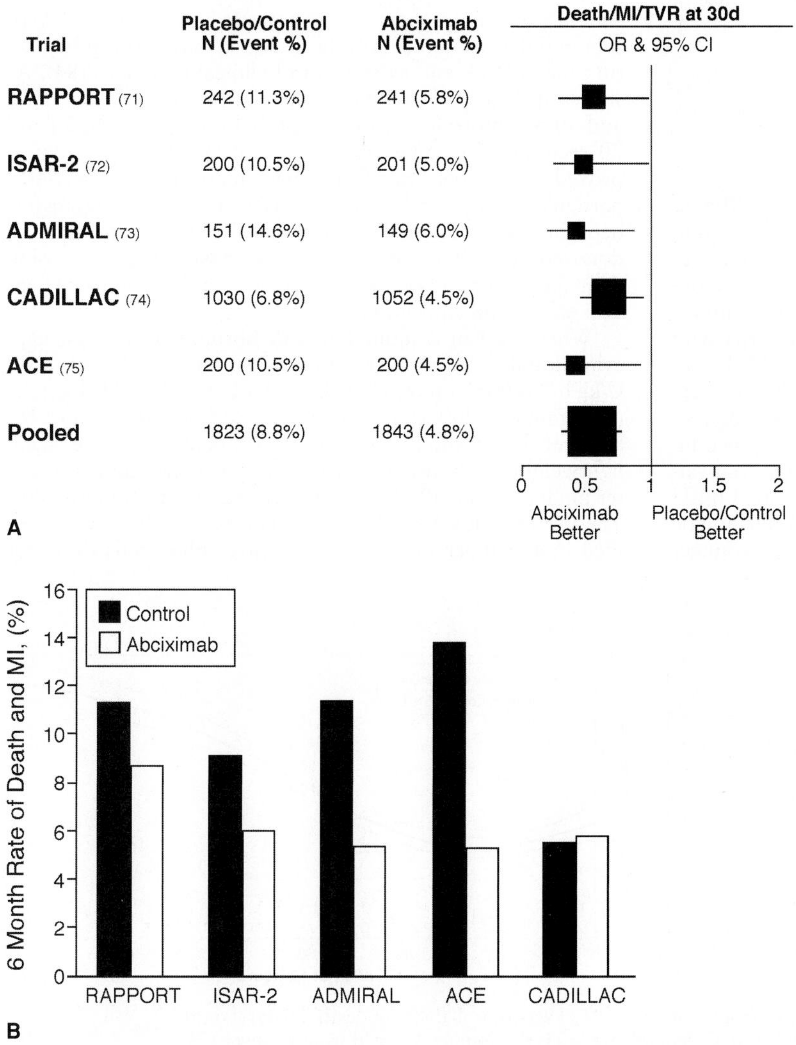

FIGURE 19.13. (**A**) Death, reinfarction, target vessel revascularization at 30 days. Two trials included stroke in the composite endpoint (ACE, CADILLAC) but the incidence was quite low. (**B**) Rate of death and MI at 6 months for 5 clinical trials of percutaneous coronary revascularization with and without abciximab. *Abbreviations:* ACE, Abciximab and Carbostent Evaluation; ADMIRAL, Abciximab before Direct angioplasty and stenting in Myocardial Infarction Regarding Acute and Long-term follow-up; CADILLAC, Controlled Abciximab and Device Investigation to Lower Late Angioplasty Complications; ISAR-2, Intracoronary tenting and Antithrombotic Regimen-2; RAPPORT, ReoPro and Primary PTCA Organization and Randomized Trial. (*Source:* From Topol EJ, Neumann F-J, Montalescot G. A preferred reperfusion strategy for acute myocardial infarction. *J Am Coll Cardiol* 2003;42:1886–1889.)

optimal reperfusion strategy (78). A recent metaanalysis of the use of abciximab in ST-elevation MI confirms the benefit of IIb/IIIa inhibition in conjunction with primary PCI (but not with thrombolysis) (79).

These trials addressed when and whether to use IIb/IIIa inhibitors for PCI alone, not in conjunction with fibrinolytics. But the data for use of fibrinolytics, with or without IIb/IIIa inhibitors, in conjunction with PCI has frequently been referred to as *facilitated PCI*. This conveys the use of pharmacologic therapy as a bridge to the catheter-based reperfusion strategy, which even in the most efficient hospitals carries a typical 60-minute delay of the so-called door-to-balloon time. The most recent completed trial is ASSENT-4, in which 1,667 patients were randomly assigned to PCI or a combination of full-dose tenecteplase and PCI (80). The trial had to be stopped prematurely (planned enrollment of 4,000 patients) because of increased in-hospital mortality in the combination arm (6.0% versus 3.0%, $P = .0105$) (80). As these patients were followed at 90 days, there was a significant excess of all major adverse events. A quantitative overview by Keeley et al. (81) of all randomized trials, including ASSENT-4 PCI, confirms the lack of benefit of facilitated PCI as compared with primary PCI. Taking all available data together, it appears that facilitated PCI should not incorporate fibrinolytics unless new data emerge that document their advantage. One such trial, FINESSE, is ongoing and directly compares half-dose reteplase plus abciximab, abciximab alone, or primary PCI with use of abciximab in the catheterization laboratory.

Combination Low-Dose Fibrinolytic and IIb/IIIa Inhibition

The GUSTO-V trial tested low-dose fibrinolytic and IIb/IIIa inhibition. With enrollment of more than 16,000 patients comparing r-PA with r-PA at half-dose and abciximab, there was little difference in mortality (5.9% versus 5.6%) (82). Noninferiority was established for the new strategy of combined therapy with respect to 30-day mortality, and superiority with respect to significantly less reinfarction and almost all MI complications (82) was demonstrated. On the other hand, there was an excess of bleeding complications (5.6% versus 3.9%). Of note, no increase in intracerebral hemorrhage was encountered (0.6% in both groups). Overall, the GUSTO-V trial validated combined fibrinolytics (at reduced doses) with IIb/IIIa inhibition as an alternative therapy to traditional fibrinolytic monotherapy. This may be particularly well suited for younger patients or those with high-risk MIs such as anterior location, but this strategy has not been incorporated for routine practice and has not been approved by regulatory authorities.

The overall effect of abciximab given with half-dose TNK–t-PA in ASSENT-3 (83) was similar to that in GUSTO-V. Significant reduction for in-hospital reinfarction and refractory ischemia rates as well as in the need for urgent intervention was observed, at the cost of a significant increase in major bleedings. Like GUSTO-V, there was no excess in intracranial hemorrhage with this combination. In the elderly no beneficial effects were seen. Major bleeding complications in this age category more than doubled as compared with full-dose TNK and unfractionated heparin (83). In summary, low-dose fibrinolytic and IIb/IIIa inhibition has not been borne out to provide survival benefit, has been shown to increase bleeding complications, and should not be considered a viable strategy for the vast majority of patients receiving reperfusion therapy.

Anticoagulation: Unfractionated or Low-Molecular-Weight Heparin and Direct Thrombin Inhibitors

A critical advance came with the analysis of the GUSTO-I trial in which more than 30,000 patients had intravenous heparin, serial measurements of the activated partial thromboplastin time (aPTT), and assessment of clinical outcomes (84). As shown in Figure 19.14, there is a relationship between aPTT and 30-day mortality, with the optimal range between 50 and 70 seconds. The same preferred range of 50 to 70 seconds proved to be associated with fewer bleeding complications, particularly intracerebral hemorrhage, than more aggressive heparin effects. These data, importantly, are not from a randomized trial of conservative or aggressive heparin dosing strategies, but represent the largest data set that compares heparin effects and clinical outcomes.

When used in conjunction with fibrinolytic therapy, heparin should be administered on a weight-adjusted basis at 60 U/kg bolus (maximum, 4,000 U) and followed by 12 U/kg/hour (maximum, 1,000 U/h initially) (85–90). Consideration for a lower bolus should be given in patients who are aged, lightweight (<50 kg), and female, as these are the major determinants of the aPTT after heparin administration (85–90). The use of intravenous heparin is essential with t-PA, as verified in a number of controlled angiographic trials (85), but

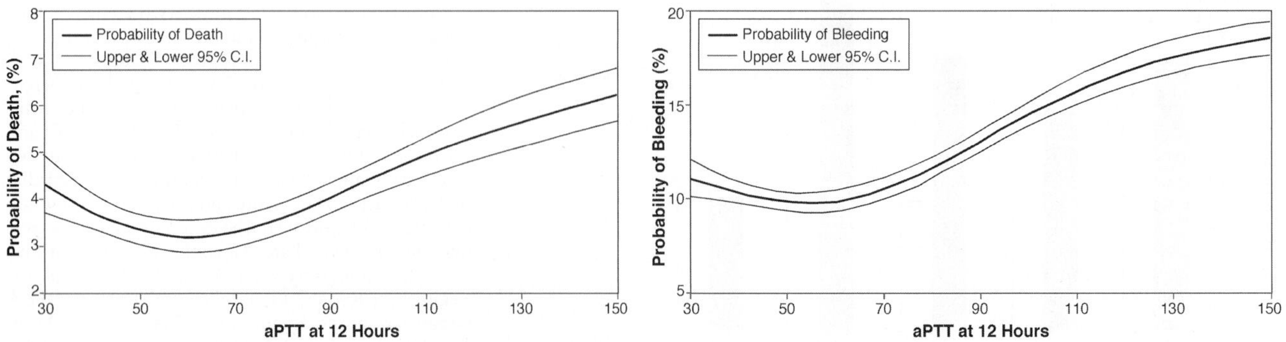

FIGURE 19.14. Activated partial thromboplastin time (aPTT) versus probability of death (30 days) or of severe or moderate bleeding. *Abbreviation:* CI, confidence interval. (*Source:* Adapted from Granger CB, Hirsh J, Califf RM, et al. Activated partial thromboplastin time and outcome after fibrinolytic therapy for acute myocardial infarction. *Circulation* 1996;93:870–878.)

less documented with SK (85–90). SK has considerably more fibrinogenolytic action, such that it will intrinsically elevate the aPTT to a higher extent than t-PA. In the GISSI-2/International and ISIS-3 controlled trials of high-dose subcutaneous heparin after SK, there was little evidence of mortality reduction and more bleeding complications (57,58). In GUSTO-I, comparing SK with intravenous versus subcutaneous heparin, there were no significant differences for mortality even though predischarge infarct vessel patency favored intravenous heparin in the angiographic trial (62). There is considerable debate as to whether any heparin should be routinely conjunctively administered with SK (91), but more recent trials of direct thrombin inhibitors strongly suggest the potential for better adjunctive therapy with this plasminogen activator (92). When selected, unfractionated heparin is used for the first 48 hours, with serial assessment of the aPTT at 6, 12, and 24 hours and active titration of the aPTT to the 50- to 70-second value. After 24 hours, in the uncomplicated patient, heparin can be discontinued. In patients with recurrent ischemia, however, atrial fibrillation, or those with an anteroapical MI who may require oral anticoagulation to prevent stroke (see Chapters 20 and 21), heparin should be continued until hospital discharge or the oral anticoagulation effect is fully established.

The use of low-molecular-weight heparin in ST-segment elevation MI has been studied in five trials, as reviewed by Eikelboom et al. (91) (Fig. 19.15). This pooled analysis of over 5,400 patients in five trials suggests a reduction in reinfarction without excess of bleeding for low-molecular-weight heparins in ST-segment elevation MI (91) Considerably more data became available with the EXTRACT data trial. In this trial enoxaparin was compared with unfractionated heparin in 20,506 patients (93). This trial provided definite evidence for superiority of enoxaparin compared with unfractionated heparin, albeit with an increase in major bleeding episodes.

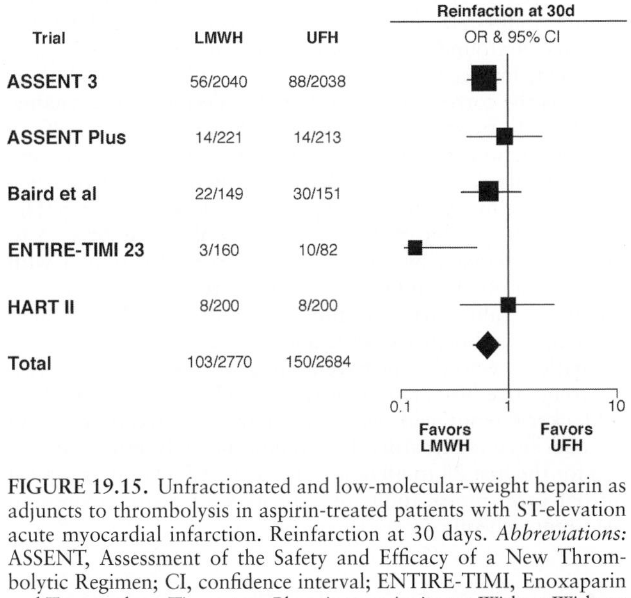

FIGURE 19.15. Unfractionated and low-molecular-weight heparin as adjuncts to thrombolysis in aspirin-treated patients with ST-elevation acute myocardial infarction. Reinfarction at 30 days. *Abbreviations:* ASSENT, Assessment of the Safety and Efficacy of a New Thrombolytic Regimen; CI, confidence interval; ENTIRE-TIMI, Enoxaparin and Tenecteplase–Tissue-type Plasminogen Activator With or Without Glycoprotein IIb/IIIa Inhibitor as Reperfusion Strategy in ST-Segment Elevation Myocardial Infarction–Thrombolysis in Myocardial Infarction; HART, Heparin-Aspirin Reperfusion Therapy; LMWH, low-molecular-weight heparin; OR, odds ratio; UFH, unfractionated heparin. *Outcome for Baird et al., *EHJ* 2002;8:627–632, is at 90 days. (*Source:* From Eikelboom JW, Quinlan DJ, Mehta SR, et al. Unfractionated and low-molecular-weight heparin as adjuncts to thrombolysis in aspirin-treated patients with ST-elevation acute myocardial infarction: a meta-analysis of the randomized trials. *Circulation* 2005;20:3855–3867, with permission.)

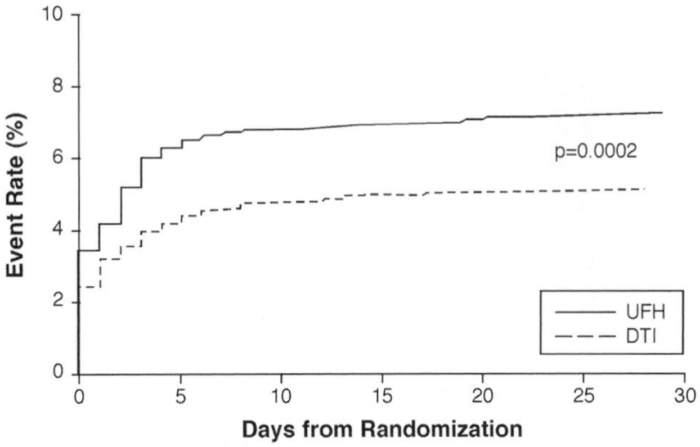

FIGURE 19.16. Kaplan-Meier event curves for death or myocardial infarction through 30 days in all patients undergoing early PCI. *Abbreviations:* DTI, direct thrombin inhibitor; UFH, unfractionated heparin. (*Source:* From Sinnaeve PR, Simes J, Yusuf S, et al. Direct thrombin inhibitors in acute coronary syndromes: effect in patients undergoing early percutaneous coronary intervention. *Eur Heart J* 2005;26:2396–2403, with permission.)

Direct thrombin inhibitors are the other anticoagulant class that has been tested in ST-segment elevation MI. Considerable benefit is evident in the catheter-based reperfusion trials of patients with acute coronary syndromes (94) (Fig. 19.16). An exhaustive review of 35,970 patients of direct thrombin inhibitors in 11 trials showed a 15% reduction in death or reinfarction, particularly with hirudin or bivalirudin, and less bleeding with bivalirudin compared with unfractionated heparin (92) (Fig. 19.17). There have not been head-to-head trials of direct thrombin inhibitors with low-molecular-weight heparin in this setting, and it appears that both classes of agents offer reinfarction protection compared with unfractionated heparin.

Bleeding Complications of Fibrinolytics and Anticoagulation

With the judicious use of heparin, the potential for bleeding complications of fibrinolytics is reduced. Nevertheless, the most feared complication of intracerebral hemorrhage occurs in approximately 1 of 200 patients (0.5%) treated with fibrinolytic therapy. The incidence is definitely higher with t-PA (0.7%) than SK (0.4%) (95,96). Prompt recognition of this catastrophe can be helpful because there are case reports of successful neurosurgical evacuation of the hemorrhage or hematoma, and in many patients, the location of the event is one that will not incur long-term disability (95,96). Presentation can be heralded by the complaint of a headache, an acute confusional state, a seizure, visual disturbance, or any new, focal neurologic sign. Still, even with rapid recognition and immediate computed tomography or magnetic resonance brain imaging, approximately two thirds of patients with an intracerebral hemorrhage will die or sustain fixed neurologic disability (95,96). In patients older than 75 years of age, the rate of fatality exceeds 90% (95–97). In the clinical trials that have evaluated fibrinolytics, the mortality incorporates all causes, and the end point of death plus nonfatal, disabling stroke is important to consider (98) to understand the net clinical benefit of a particular reperfusion strategy. Other sites of serious bleeding, such as gastrointestinal or retroperitoneal, are unusual (<5%), but can be life threatening if not quickly diagnosed and treated. The most common cause of bleeding—periaccess site—is usually self-limiting (99).

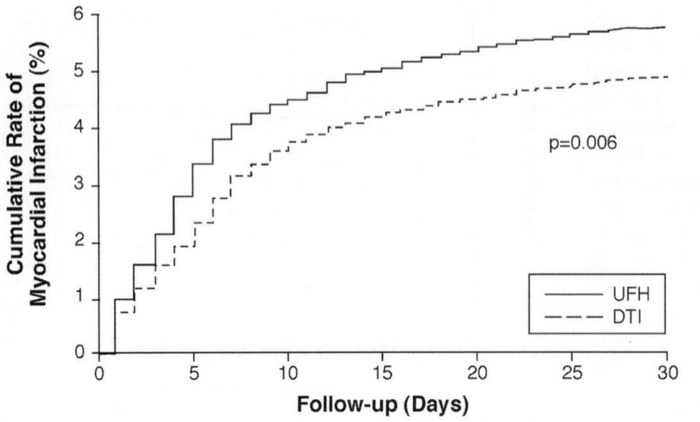

No. at Risk							
Unfractioned Heparin	17,184	16,211	15,930	15,764	15,680	15,602	15,500
Direct Thrombin Inhibitor	18,786	17,799	17,427	17,284	17,187	17,104	16,991

FIGURE 19.17. Death or myocardial infarction at 30 days. *Abbreviations:* DTI, direct thrombin inhibitor; UFH, unfractionated heparin. (*Source:* From The Direct Thrombin Inhibitor Trialists' Collaborative Group. Direct thrombin inhibitors in acute coronary syndromes: principal results of a meta-analysis based on individual patients' data. *Lancet* 2002;359:294–302, with permission.)

β-Blockade

Most of the data available on the use of β-blockers in acute MI are derived from the prereperfusion era. There is extensive support for the usefulness of β-blockade to reduce recurrent ischemia and arrhythmias and improve survival in the absence of reperfusion therapy (100,101). The largest trial of intravenous β-blockade, ISIS-1, suggested that the predominant benefit was mediated via the reduction of cardiac rupture events (101). Two relatively small placebo-controlled trials of intravenous β-blockade in conjunction with reperfusion therapy have been conducted some years ago; one (102) showed a reduction in recurrent ischemia with the use of early intravenous followed by oral metoprolol. The trial was relatively small, however, and the primary end point of preserving cardiac function was not significantly affected. The second trial with atenolol conducted by Van de Werf et al. (102,103) was negative and even suggested an increase in the risk of pulmonary edema in the β-blocker arm. The most recent and very large COMMIT trial in 45,852 patients (93% with ST-segment elevations or bundle branch block) failed to show a mortality reduction with intravenous metoprolol (104). In this trial, intravenous metoprolol was associated with an increase in the risk of cardiogenic shock. In a retrospective analysis of the GUSTO-I trial, the use of intravenous β-blockade (in 44% of the patients) was also associated with an adverse profile of clinical outcomes including worse mortality and congestive heart failure (105). Current recommendations therefore are to start the use of β-blockers with a low oral dose on the first or second day after presentation. Intravenous β-blockade should be restricted to patients who are hyperdynamic and hyperadrenergic, representing the unusual subset of relatively young patients who have tachycardia and hypertension disproportionate to the smallness of their MI territory. The potential for reducing intracerebral hemorrhage, as suggested in the TIMI-2 trial, has not yet been confirmed in subsequent large-scale efforts.

The CAPRICORN trial enrolled 1,959 patients 3 to 21 days after MI presentation, many of who received reperfusion therapy (101). The use of the β-blocker carvedilol in patients with ejection fraction lower than 40% was associated with a 23% reduction of mortality during extended 2-year follow-up. Accordingly, for patients who have diminished ejection fraction post-MI, use of β-blockade should be contemplated. Importantly, this does not refer to acute-phase management (106).

Nitrates

Intravenous nitroglycerin is frequently used (60), but the data to support its use do not originate from trials conducted in the era of myocardial reperfusion. A review of trials conducted with nitrates in the period that antedated fibrinolytic therapy suggested a significant 35% mortality benefit (107,108). The benefit is believed to be related to reduction of infarct size and improvement of regional myocardial function, along with reduction in right and left ventricular preload. More recent large-scale trials that have assessed either intravenous nitrates or long-acting oral nitrate preparations have failed to demonstrate benefit (109,110). However, in these trials there was extensive use of nitrates in the first few hospital days in the control group patients, confounding the assessment of the effect.

Often, intravenous nitroglycerin is inadequately administered, as the correct dose to achieve the desired hemodynamic benefit is to titrate the infusion to achieve at least a 10% to 15% reduction in the systolic blood pressure for normotensive patients and a 30% reduction in hypertensive patients, not to lower the systolic blood pressure to less than 90 mm Hg. Appropriate administration is to use a bolus dose of 12.5 to 20.0 μg, followed by an infusion of 10 to 20 μg/min with an increase in this infusion level by 5 to 10 μg every 5 to 10 minutes, along with careful surveillance of blood pressure, heart rate, and hemodynamic and clinical signs. In appropriate patients who do not have a large MI and are not at risk for congestive heart failure, it is especially helpful to combine β-blocker therapy with the intravenous nitroglycerin to avoid the undesired tachycardia. Intravenous nitroglycerin is continued for the first 24 to 48 hours and replaced by oral or topical nitroglycerin preparations in patients with heart failure and recurrent ischemia.

Angiotensin-Converting Enzyme Inhibitors

One of the most important advances in cardiovascular medicine in the last decade has been the demonstration of survival benefit for angiotensin-converting enzyme (ACE) inhibitors in patients with left ventricular dysfunction. In several trials of acute MI (109,110) various ACE inhibitors have been tested and shown, in aggregate, to promote survival, reduce the incidence of heart failure, and, in selected trials, reduce the incidence of reinfarction and the need for revascularization. The details of these trials and the rationale are reviewed in Chapters 20 and 21. ACE inhibitors can be recommended in the first 24 hours of an anterior MI (proximal or mid-LAD; see Table 19.1) or an MI complicated by either heart failure or ejection fraction less than 40%, or both. A graded dose schedule is used to avoid hypotension, especially with the first dose, with initiation of therapy on the first hospital day once the blood pressure is stabilized. The Heart Outcomes Preventions Evaluation trial findings of ramipril compared with placebo in a broad population of patients with coronary disease supports a greater than or equal to 20% reduction of death, recurrent MI, stroke, or need for revascularization (111). The combination of ACE inhibitors and β-blockers with asymptomatic left ventricular dysfunction was studied in post-MI patients and appears to provide additive benefit (112). Most recently, the use of valsartan or captopril or both was studied in patients with MI complicated by heart failure or documented left ventricular dysfunction (ejection fraction <40%) (108). In the VALIANT trial, 14,703 patients were assessed with mortality as the primary end point. There were no differences in mortality among the three treatment arms and no other clinical advantage of valsartan or the combination was found besides a lower rate of cough or angioedema with valsartan alone (113). In MI patients who cannot tolerate an ACE inhibitor, valsartan is a valid alternative.

Calcium Channel Blockade

Unlike ACE inhibitors, which have almost uniformly been shown to have salutary effects, the calcium channel blockers have limited data to support their use in this setting and, more recently, there has been heightened awareness of their potential for toxicity and risk of mortality (114). Nifedipine is contraindicated because of its intrinsic negative inotropic effects, reflex sympathetic activation, tachycardia, and hypotension. The excess of adverse outcomes in four placebo-controlled post-MI trials of nifedipine (none with reperfusion) (114–117) raised the possibility that coronary steal was occurring, referring to an imbalance in vasodilatation and reduction in coronary perfusion pressure. Other calcium channel β-blockers, such as verapamil or diltiazem, may be used for specific indications, such as treatment of supraventricular tachyarrhythmia or relief of postinfarction angina, if nitrates and β-blockers are ineffective or not adequately tolerated. All calcium channel blockers should otherwise be avoided, especially in patients who develop heart failure.

Statins and Management of Lipids

With the marked salutary effects on long-term survival, prevention of reinfarction, and subsequent coronary revascularization of HMG-CoA reductase drugs (85), it is important that a cholesterol panel (total, low-density lipoprotein, and high-density lipoprotein) be obtained on admission and no later than the first 24 hours. Trials of patients with acute coronary syndromes have reinforced the benefit of early initiation of statins, and this is discussed more fully in Chapter 21.

Management of Blood Sugar and Diabetes

There is mounting evidence of the importance of hyperglycemia in the setting of acute MI, both with respect for its unfavorable prognosis and the benefit of restoring normal glucose levels in the setting of catheter-based reperfusion (118).

Implantable Defibrillators

In the past, it was accepted that the decision to recommend an implantable defibrillator should be assessed at least 4 to 6 weeks after acute MI. But this notion was challenged by a report from the VALIANT investigators who studied 14,409 patients with reduced ejection fraction after MI (119). Of note, 19% of the sudden death or cardiac arrest events occurred in the first 30 days following MI. Although the custom of waiting to reassess left ventricular function needs to be revisited, it is important to acknowledge that there is appreciable risk in the first month, especially in patients with ejection fraction of less than 30% (119).

Non–ST-Elevation Myocardial Infarction

A considerable part of this chapter has been dedicated to ST elevation because of the pressing need to establish reperfusion therapy. Patients without ST elevation, unless they have true posterior MI, do not usually have an occluded infarct-related artery and have not been shown to benefit from fibrinolytic therapy. In fact, the aggregate data suggest that these patients may be put at risk of reinfarction if fibrinolytic therapy is used. The reasons for this include the presence of a mural thrombus rather than an occlusive one with the potential for a plasminogen activator to engender free thrombin and facilitate platelet aggregation and the autocatalytic formation of thrombin. Essentially, the prothrombotic effects of fibrinolytic therapy pose a risk in this setting, and this class of agents should be avoided. As we learned from the GUSTO-IIb trial (120), which enrolled more than 12,140 patients without ST elevation, they are clearly older and more frequently female, diabetic, and hypertensive than their ST-elevation counterparts. In many respects, their characteristics pull together the features of the three previous subgroups of the aged, women, and prior MI. They are twice as likely to have had a prior MI (32% versus 17%) and have more than twice the frequency of prior coronary artery bypass grafting (CABG) (12% versus 5%). The outcomes for these patients are still indicative of the need for improved therapies, as the incidence of death and nonfatal MI in the first 30 days was 9.4% and quite similar to the patients with ST-segment elevation. Of this composite, the non–ST-elevation patients have more reinfarction than death as compared with the ST-elevation patients (120). The therapy for non–ST-elevation MI is the same as that delineated for the ST-elevation MI patients, with emphasis on the use of aspirin, heparin, nitrates, and β-blockade. The use of low-molecular-weight heparin or direct thrombin inhibitors as preferred anticoagulation agents instead of unfractionated heparin has been the subject of intensive clinical trial evaluation. Similarly, platelet glycoprotein IIb/IIIa blockade (eptifibatide or tirofiban) has been shown to have a modest reduction of events as a medical management strategy for patients with non–ST-segment elevation MI (121,122). Interestingly, the use of the newer anticoagulants or IIb/IIIa blockers can be better justified in patients with abnormal troponin, likely reflecting their heightened risk and perhaps microvascular thrombotic obstruction (123). It remains unclear whether the use of enoxaparin instead of heparin is warranted in patients who are having early invasive procedures, because the efficacy differences between low-molecular-weight and unfractionated heparin are small, and not statistically significant, but the bleeding complications are clearly exacerbated with low-molecular-weight heparin in this setting (123). The use of calcium channel blockers in this setting is supported by the results of one trial, albeit with marginal statistical significance (124).

Regional Centers of Excellence for Acute Myocardial Infarction

With the new body of data strongly favoring catheter-based reperfusion, along with evidence supporting early angiography and intervention for patients with non–ST-segment elevation, the idea of establishing specialized centers has been fostered (5). The committed and experienced centers have higher volume and shorter door-to-balloon times along with better outcomes for patients with respect to risk-adjusted mortality (125).

Emergency Bypass Surgery

Still an essential part of reperfusion strategies today, although infrequently reported on, is the use of emergency bypass surgery for patients who undergo early coronary angiography, with or without fibrinolytic therapy. In patients who are intended to undergo primary mechanical reperfusion, but an unsuspected critical left main stem lesion is detected, or there is the equivalent scenario with advanced, diffuse, three-vessel coronary artery disease that is not approachable by percutaneous revascularization, emergency bypass surgery should be contemplated. In 1% to 2% of primary PCI cases, emergency surgery proves to be necessary (126) and for this reason having a facility with rapid, in-house surgical capabilities is quite important. The results for emergency bypass surgery as a reperfusion treatment for acute MI are particularly encouraging, despite the lack of a randomized controlled design and the fact that these studies were reported in the 1980s before pharmacologic and catheter-based reperfusion was popularized (127–130).

PREDISCHARGE ASSESSMENT AND ELECTIVE REVASCULARIZATION

Elective Coronary Angiography and Revascularization

In the GUSTO-I trial of 21,722 patients in the United States with acute MI, 71% underwent coronary angiography (131), and most of this was elective, predischarge. The major determinants of angiography were patient age, hospital availability, and recurrent ischemia. The age characteristic is particularly troubling; there was a pronounced reduction for use of angiography patients older than 73 years, and it is precisely these patients who have the highest risk of major events (131). Other studies have confirmed that hospital availability of the procedure is a key predictive factor of its use (132), which is also a sobering realization. Of note, recurrent ischemia, which could have been conceived as the most salient driving feature for performing coronary angiography, was third in importance (131). There is marked variability in the use of coronary angiography in the eight different regions of the United States, ranging from 52% to 81%, and reflective of the uncertainty of how this procedure should be applied (133).

When angiography is performed, patients can be categorized into five groups. An interesting group is the 15% of patients who have "minimal lesion syndrome" (134). These patients are usually young, quite often smokers, and male, who at the time of predischarge angiography have less than 30% residual stenosis. The underlying pathophysiology is likely to involve coronary vasospasm, or fissure, with subsequent thrombus formation overlying a minimally encroaching atherosclerotic plaque. Of course, revascularization is not necessary, but it is vital for smoking cessation to be achieved. The prognosis for these patients is excellent, but in 2% despite the use of nitrates, calcium channel blockers, or both, there is recurrence. The other angiographic subsets include patients with occluded infarct vessels and single-vessel disease, patients with single-vessel disease of the infarct-related artery, those with two- or three-vessel disease, and the small subgroup of patients with left main stem lesions.

Coronary angiography is advocated for all patients who have recurrent ischemia. For the reasons discussed for using emergency angiography, as far as establishing infarct vessel patency, extent of multivessel disease, and suitability for revascularization, angiography can be considered an integral part of the early post-MI assessment. Of note, if a patient has provocable ischemia, angiography is fully justified with the results of the Danish Multicenter Study of Acute MI trial (135).

A major question remains as to patients who do not have provocable ischemia or do not undergo functional testing but, by clinical criteria, have evidence of viable myocardium of the infarct zone. These criteria may include a lower peak CK or peak CK-MB than expected, hypokinesia but not akinesia of the infarct zone by echocardiography, early fibrinolytic therapy in the first 2 hours of symptom onset with rapid relief of chest pain and ECG findings, or the lack of development of Q waves on the ECG. These patients, on an empiric basis, may be suitable for coronary angiography because of the clinical judgment that they have sustained an "incomplete" infarct and will likely have a significant residual stenosis of the infarct vessel. On the other hand, patients with complicated MI, with such features as congestive heart failure or ventricular tachycardia, are at high risk for subsequent events and deserve consideration for angiography. The groups of patients who do not need angiography are those in whom revascularization, be it percutaneous or surgical, could not be considered or those patients with a small inferior or lateral infarct who do not have provocable ischemia. This analysis suggests that a substantial portion of patients probably deserve consideration for predischarge angiography, but this must be considered an unsettled controversy; there has not been a clinical trial to address this issue per se.

Coronary Angioplasty or Bypass Surgery

Revascularization is used commonly in hospitals in the United States, as evidenced by the GUSTO-I data of 30% use of percutaneous transluminal coronary angioplasty (PTCA) and 13% use of CABG (131). The coronary anatomy strongly predicts which procedure is performed, with single-vessel disease resulting in PTCA for 86% of patients undergoing any revascularization, whereas CABG was used in 79% of patients with three-vessel disease who had some form of revascularization (131). Even though the use of coronary angiography and revascularization was much lower outside the United States in this large trial, the proportionate use of angioplasty and bypass surgery among patients undergoing angioplasty was similar (136). Bypass surgery carries a risk of mortality that is independent of the acute MI event and, even risk adjusted, in the first year after surgery there is a small excess of deaths (not statistically meaningful) compared with patients not undergoing surgery (137). However, the benefit of complete revascularization in these patients with advanced, multivessel disease is much more likely to be manifest over a more prolonged follow-up (137). One of the controversies in surgical revascularization in this setting is whether bypass surgery to the infarct-related vessel, especially if it was not successfully rendered patent from reperfusion therapy, is worthwhile. This dilemma is usually resolved by grafting the infarct-related territory, but determination of viability (see Chapter 54) may be helpful. In patients with spontaneous or provocable ischemia who have extensive and diffuse atherosclerotic involvement, bypass surgery should be strongly considered as the revascularization procedure of choice, provided that the distal vessels are suitable for grafting. It would be anticipated that the patients with compromised left ventricular function would stand the most to benefit from the standpoint of survival.

CONTROVERSIES AND PERSONAL PERSPECTIVES

Over time, the controversy of fibrinolytic therapy compared with catheter-based reperfusion has largely been settled. Nonetheless, the advantage of the latter will only be fully realized with a regional approach of care, such as has been established in Denmark or the Czech Republic. The question as to whether sites who perform primary PCI should have emergency CABG backup remains controversial, even though such a small proportion of patients (approximately 1%–2%) require urgent bypass surgery. The differences between sites with respect to hospital and operator volume, door-to-balloon time, and risk-adjusted outcomes is concerning and suggests marked heterogeneity in quality of care. The use of drug-coated stents in MI, instead of their less expensive bare metal stent predecessor, has been commonplace despite the lack of any meaningful randomized comparative data in this setting. Because of the liability of drug-coated stents, which carry a somewhat higher risk of late thrombosis than bare metal stents, it is a concern that there might be an increased risk in MI patients who already have manifest prothrombotic potential. Whether pharmacologic reperfusion therapy provides any benefit in patients with a long transport time to the PCI center remains unclear.

THE FUTURE

There is little evidence for a major reduction of mortality in the past decade of fibrinolytic trials, and no evidence that patients are presenting any earlier with ST-segment elevation MI. Therefore, for many patients the "damage is done" largely before they reach the hospital or before myocardial reperfusion at the tissue level is achieved. Although it will be worthwhile to continue to refine strategies to optimize reperfusion, it appears that even more emphasis should be placed on preventing these events. This has been the beginning of defining the genes responsible for acute MI, such that at some point the risk could be ascertained very early in life. This could allow for appropriate lifestyle and, if necessary, drug therapy, to prevent the MI.

The other major area not covered in the chapter is the potential for stem cell therapy. Although there are experimental and small clinical studies to suggest feasibility, it remains to be seen whether a practical strategy can be developed that improves cardiac function and prognosis for patients who have sustained extensive damage. Moreover, the mechanism by which stem cells can achieve salutary effects remains unclear; actual proof of myocardial regeneration has been elusive. Notwithstanding these concerns, should stem cell therapy be proven successful for preventing death or heart failure, this would be considered an extraordinary step forward in the management of acute MI.

References

1. Libby P. Molecular basis of the acute coronary syndromes. *Circulation* 1995;91:2844–2850.
2. Vaughan CJ, Murphy MB, Buckley BM. Statins do more than just lower cholesterol. *Lancet* 1996;348:1079–1082.
3. Reimer KA, Jennings RB. The "wavefront phenomenon" of myocardial ischemic cell death. II. Transmural progression of necrosis within the framework of ischemic bed size (myocardium at risk) and collateral flow. *Lab Invest* 1979;40:633–644.
4. Falk E. Morphologic features of unstable atherothrombotic plaques underlying acute coronary syndromes. *Am J Cardiol* 1989;63:114E–120E.
5. Topol EJ, Yadav J. Recognition of the importance of embolization in atherosclerotic vascular disease. *Circulation* 2000;101:570–580.
6. Zipes DP, Wellens HJJ. Sudden cardiac death. *Circulation* 1998;98:2334–2351.
7. American Heart Association. Heart and stroke facts. Available: www.americanheart.org/presenter.jhtml?identifier=3000333. Accessed 4/13/06.
8. Cragg DR, Friedman HZ, Bonema JD, et al. Outcome of patients with acute myocardial infarction who are ineligible for fibrinolytic therapy. *Ann Intern Med* 1991;115:173–177.
9. Pfeffer MA, Moye LA, Braunwald E, et al. Selection bias in the use of fibrinolytic therapy in acute myocardial infarction. *JAMA* 1991;266:528–532.
10. Brown MS, Goldstein JL. Heart attacks: gone with the century. *Science* 1996;272:629.
11. Murray CL, Lopez AD. Evidence-based health policy—lessons from the Global Burden of Disease Study. *Science* 1996;274:740–743.
12. Puleo PR, Meyer D, Wathen C, et al. Use of a rapid assay of subforms of creatine kinase MB to diagnose or rule out acute myocardial infarction. *N Engl J Med* 1994;331:561–566.
13. Christensen RH, Ohman EM, Topol EJ, et al. Assessment of coronary reperfusion after thrombolysis with a model containing myoglobin, creatine kinase-MB, and clinical variables. *Circulation* 1997;96:1776–1782.
14. Ohman EM, Armstrong PW, Christenson RH, et al. for the GUSTO-IIa Investigators. Risk stratification with admission cardiac troponin T levels in acute myocardial ischemia. *N Engl J Med* 1996;335:1333–1341.
15. Peterson ED, Hathaway WR, Zabel KM, et al. Prognostic significance of precordial ST segment depression during inferior myocardial infarction in the fibrinolytic era: results in 16,521 patients. *J Am Coll Cardiol* 1996;28:305–312.
16. Schroder R, Wegscheider K, Schroeder K, et al. , for the INJECT Trial Group. Extent of early ST-segment elevation resolution: a simple but strong predictor of outcome in patients with acute myocardial infarction and a sensitive measure to compare fibrinolytic regimens. A substudy of the International Joint Efficacy Comparison of Fibrinolytics (INJECT) Trial. *J Am Coll Cardiol* 1995;26:1657–1664.
17. Zeymer U, Schroder R, Tebbe U, et al. Non-invasive detection of early infarct vessel patency by resolution of ST-segment elevation in patients with thrombolysis for acute myocardial infarction. *Eur Heart J* 2001;22:769–775.
18. de Lemos JA, Antman EM, Giugliana RP, et al. for the TIMI 14 Investigators. ST segment resolution and infarct-related artery patency and flow after fibrinolytic therapy. *Am J Cardiol* 2000;85:299–304.
19. de Lemos JA, Antman EM, Giugliano RP, et al. , for the InTIME-II Investigators. Very early risk stratification after fibrinolytic therapy with a bedside myoglobin assay and the 12-lead electrocardiogram. *Am Heart J* 2000;140:373–378.
20. Schroder R, Dissmann R, Bruggemann T, et al. Extent of early ST segment elevation resolution: a simple but strong predictor of outcome in patients with acute myocardial infarction. *J Am Coll Cardiol* 1994;24:384–391.
21. The GUSTO-III Investigators. An international, multicenter, randomized comparison of reteplase with alteplase for acute myocardial infarction. *N Engl J Med* 1997;337:1118–1123.
22. Claeys MJ, Bosmans J, Veenstra L, et al. Determinants and prognostic implications of persistent ST-segment elevation after primary angioplasty for acute myocardial infarction: importance of microvascular reperfusion injury on clinical outcome. *Circulation* 1999;99:1972–1977.
23. Schechtman KB, Capone RJ, Kleiger RE, et al. Risk stratification of patients with non-Q wave myocardial infarction. *Circulation* 1989;80:1148–1158.
24. Savonitto S, Cohen MG, Politi A, et al. The extent of ST-segment depression on the admission electrocardiogram is a powerful predictor of mortality in the non-ST elevation acute coronary syndromes. *Eur Heart J* 2005;26:2106–2113.
25. Killip T, Kimball JT. Treatment of myocardial infarction in a coronary unit: a two-year experience with 250 patients. *Am J Cardiol* 1967;20:457–464.
26. Lee KL, Woodlief L, Topol EJ, et al. Predictors of 30-day mortality in the era of reperfusion for acute myocardial infarction: results from an international trial of 41,021 patients. *Circulation* 1995;91:1659–1668.
27. Anavekar NS, McMurray JJV, Velazquez EJ, et al. Relation between renal dysfunction and cardiovascular outcomes after myocardial infarction. *N Engl J Med* 2004;351:1285–1295.
28. Fibrinolytic therapy trialists' (FTT) collaborative group. Indications for fibrinolytic therapy in suspected acute myocardial infarction: collaborative overview of early mortality and major morbidity results from all randomized trials of more than 1000 patients. *Lancet* 1994;343:311–322.
29. Sgarbossa E, Pinski SL, Barbagelata A, et al. Electrocardiographic diagnosis of acute myocardial infarction in the presence of left bundle branch block. *N Engl J Med* 1996;334:481–487.
30. Muller DWM, Topol EJ. Selection of patients with acute myocardial infarction for fibrinolytic therapy. *Ann Intern Med* 1990;113:949–960.

31. Keeley EC, Boura JA, Grines CL. Primary angioplasty versus intravenous thrombolytic therapy for acute myocardial infarction: a quantitative review of 23 randomised trials. *Lancet* 2003;361:13–20.
32. Nordmann AJ, Hengstler P, Harr T, et al. Clinical outcomes of primary stenting versus balloon angioplasty in patients with myocardial infarction: a meta-analysis of randomized controlled trials. *Am J Med* 2004;116:253–262.
33. Jaksch R, Niehus R, Knobloch W, Schiele T. PTCA versus stenting in acute myocardial infarction. *Eur Heart J* 1998;19:1341.
34. Rodriguez A, Bernardi V, Fernandez M, et al. In-hospital and late results of coronary stents versus conventional balloon angioplasty in acute myocardial infarction (GRAMI trial). Gianturco-Roubin in Acute Myocardial Infarction. *Am J Cardiol* 1998;81:1286–1291.
35. Suryapranata H, van't Hof AW, Hoorntje JC, et al. Randomized comparison of coronary stenting with balloon angioplasty in selected patients with acute myocardial infarction. *Circulation* 1998;97:2502–2505.
36. Grines CL, Cox DA, Stone GW, et al. Coronary angioplasty with or without stent implantation for acute myocardial infarction. Stent Primary Angioplasty in Myocardial Infarction Study Group. *N Engl J Med* 1999;341: 1949–1956.
37. Kawashima A, Ueda K, Nishida Y, et al. Quantitative angiographic analysis of restenosis of primary stenting using Wiktor stent for acute myocardial infarction—results from a multicenter randomized PRISAM study. *Circulation* 1999;100[Suppl 1]:I–856.
38. Saito S, Hosokawa G, Tanaka S, et al. Primary stent implantation is superior to balloon angioplasty in acute myocardial infarction—final results of the primary angioplasty versus stent implantation in acute myocardial infarction (PASTA) trial. PASTA Trial Investigators. *Catheter Cardiovasc Interv* 1999;48:262–268.
39. Maillard L, Hamon M, Khalife K, et al. A comparison of systematic stenting and conventional balloon angioplasty during primary percutaneous transluminal coronary angioplasty for acute myocardial infarction. STENTIM-2 Investigators. *J Am Coll Cardiol* 2000;35:1729–1736.
40. Scheller B, Hennen B, Severin-Kneib S, et al. Long-term follow-up of a randomized study of primary stenting versus angioplasty in acute myocardial infarction. *Am J Med* 2001;110:1–6.
41. Stone GW, Grines CL, Cox DA, et al. Comparison of angioplasty with stenting, with or without abciximab, in acute myocardial infarction. *N Engl J Med* 2002;346:957–966.
42. Anderson HR, Nielson TT, Rasmussen K, et al., for the DANAMI-2 Investigators. A comparison of coronary angioplasty with fibrinolytic therapy in acute myocardial infarction. *N Engl J Med* 2003;349:733–742.
43. Topol EJ, Kereiakes DJ. Regionalization of care for acute ischemic heart disease: a call for specialized centers. *Circulation* 2003;107:1463–1466.
44. Widimsky P, Budesinsky T, Vorac D, et al. Long distance transport for primary angioplasty vs immediate thrombolysis in acute myocardial infarction. Final results of the randomized national multicenter trial—PRAGUE-2. *Eur Heart J* 2003;24:94–104.
45. Grines CL, Westerhausen DR, Grines LL, et al. for the Air PAMI Study Group. A randomized trial of transfer for primary angioplasty versus onsite thrombolysis in patients with high-risk myocardial infarction: the Air Primary Angioplasty in Myocardial Infarction Study. *J Am Coll Cardiol* 2002;39:1713–1719.
46. Steg PG, Bonnefoy E, Chabaud S, et al. Impact of time to treatment on mortality after prehospital fibrinolysis or primary angioplasty: data from the CAPTIM randomized clinical trial. *Circulation* 2003;108:2851–2856.
47. ISIS-2 (Second international study of infarct survival) Collaborative Group. Randomized trial of intravenous streptokinase, oral aspirin, both, or neither among 17,187 cases of suspected acute myocardial infarction. *Lancet* 1988;11:349–360.
48. Sabatine MS, Cannon CP, Gibson CM, et al. Addition of clopidogrel to aspirin and fibrinolytic therapy for myocardial infarction with ST-segment elevation. *N Engl J Med* 2005;352:1179–1189.
49. COMMIT (ClOpidogrel and Metoprolol in Myocardial Infarction Trial) collaborative group. Addition of clopidogrel to aspirin in 45,852 patients with acute myocardial infarction: randomized placebo-controlled trial. *Lancet* 2005;366:1607–1621.
50. Lincoff AM, Topol EJ. The illusion of reperfusion. Does anyone achieve optimal myocardial reperfusion? *Circulation* 1993;87:1792–1805, and 88: 1361–1374.
51. Weaver WD, Cerqueira M, Hallstrom AP, et al. Prehospital-initiated vs hospital-initiated fibrinolytic therapy. *JAMA* 1993;270:1211–1216.
52. LATE Study Group. Late assessment of fibrinolytic efficacy (LATE) study with alteplase 6–24 hours after onset of acute myocardial infarction. *Lancet* 1993;342:759–766.
53. Estudio Multicentrico Estreptoquinasa Republicas de Americas del Sur (EMERAS). Randomized trial of late thrombolysis in patients with suspected acute myocardial infarction. *Lancet* 1993;342:767–772.
54. Morrison LJ, Verbeek RP, McDonald AC, et al. Mortality and prehospital thrombolysis for acute myocardial infarction: A meta-analysis. *JAMA* 2000;283:2686–2692.
55. Brodie BR, Hansen C, Stuckey TD, et al. Door-to-balloon time with primary percutaneous coronary intervention for acute myocardial infarction impacts late cardiac mortality in high-risk patients and patients presenting early after the onset of symptoms. *J Am Coll Cardiol* 2006;47:289–295.
56. Stone GW, Webb J, Cox DA, et al. Distal microcirculatory protection during percutaneous coronary intervention in acute ST-segment elevation myocardial infarction. *JAMA* 2005;293:1063–1072.
57. Gruppo Italiano Per Lo Studio Della Sopravvivenza Nell'Infarto Miocardico. GISSI-2: a factorial randomized trial of alteplase versus streptokinase and heparin versus no heparin among 12,490 patients with acute myocardial infarction. *Lancet* 1990;336:65–71.
58. The International Study Group. In-hospital mortality and clinical course of 20,891 patients with suspected acute myocardial infarction randomized between alteplase and streptokinase with or without heparin. *Lancet* 1990;336:71–75.
59. ISIS-3 (Third International Study of Infarct Survival) Collaborative Group. ISIS-3: a randomized comparison of streptokinase vs tissue plasminogen activator vs anistreplase and of aspirin plus heparin vs aspirin among 41,299 cases of suspected acute myocardial infarction. *Lancet* 1992;339:753–770.
60. The GUSTO Investigators. An international randomized trial comparing four fibrinolytic strategies for acute myocardial infarction. *N Engl J Med* 1993;329:1615–1622.
61. Califf RM, White HD, Van de Werf F, et al. One-year results from the Global Utilization of Streptokinase and TPA for Occluded Coronary Arteries (GUSTO-I) Trial. *Circulation* 1996;94:1233–1238.
62. The GUSTO Angiographic Investigators. The effects of tissue plasminogen activator, streptokinase, or both on coronary-artery patency, ventricular function, and survival after acute myocardial infarction. *N Engl J Med* 1993;329:1615–1622.
63. Mark DB, Hlatky MA, Califf RM, et al. Cost effectiveness of fibrinolytic therapy with tissue plasminogen activator as compared with streptokinase for acute myocardial infarction. *N Engl J Med* 1995;332:1418–1424.
64. Smalling RW, Bode C, Kalbfleisch J, et al. More rapid, complete, and stable coronary thrombolysis with bolus administration of reteplase compared with alteplase infusion in acute myocardial infarction. *Circulation* 1995;91:2725–2732.
65. Bode C, Smalling RW, Berg G, et al. Randomized comparison of coronary thrombolysis achieved with double-bolus reteplase (recombinant plasminogen activator) and front-loaded, accelerated alteplase (recombinant tissue plasminogen activator) in patients with acute myocardial infarction. *Circulation* 1996;94:891–898.
66. International Joint Efficacy Comparison of Fibrinolytics. Randomised, double-blind comparison of reteplase double-bolus administration with streptokinase in acute myocardial infarction (INJECT): trial to investigate equivalence. *Lancet* 1995;346:329–336.
67. ASSENT-2 Investigators (Assessment of the Safety and Efficacy of a New Fibrinolytic). Single-bolus tenecteplase compared with front-loaded alteplase in acute myocardial infarction: the ASSENT-2 double-blind randomized trial. *Lancet* 1999;354:716–722.
68. Simes RJ, Topol EJ, Holmes DR, et al. The link between the angiographic substudy and mortality outcomes in a large randomized trial of myocardial reperfusion: the importance of early and complete infarct artery reperfusion. *Circulation* 1995;91:1923–1928.
69. Kleiman NS, White, Ohman EM, et al. Mortality within 24 hours of thrombolysis for myocardial infarction: the importance of early reperfusion. *Circulation* 1994;90:2658–2666.
70. Schomig A, Ndrepepa G, Mehilli J, et al. A randomized trial of coronary stenting versus balloon angioplasty as a rescue intervention after failed thrombolysis in patients with acute myocardial infarction. *J Am Coll Cardiol* 2004;44:2073–2079.
71. Gershlick AH, Stephens-Lloyd A, Hughes S, et al. Rescue angioplasty after failed thrombolytic therapy for acute myocardial infarction. *N Engl J Med* 2005;353:2758–2768.
72. Topol EJ, Neumann F-J, Montalescot G. A preferred reperfusion strategy for acute myocardial infarction. *J Am Coll Cardiol* 2003;42:1886–1889.
73. Brener SJ, Barr LA, Burchenal JE, et al. Randomized, placebo-controlled trial of platelet glycoprotein IIb/IIIa blockade with primary angioplasty for acute myocardial infarction. ReoPro and Primary PTCA Organization and Randomized Trial (RAPPORT) Investigators. *Circulation* 1998;98:734–741.
74. Neumann FJ, Kastrani A, Schmitt C, et al. Effect of glycoprotein IIb/IIIa receptor blockade with abciximab on clinical and angiographic restenosis rate after the placement of coronary stents following acute myocardial infarction. *J Am Coll Cardiol* 2000;35:915–921.
75. Montalescot G, Barragan P, Wittenberg O, et al., for the ADMIRAL Investigators. Platelet glycoprotein IIb/IIIa inhibition with coronary stenting for acute myocardial infarction. *N Engl J Med* 2001;344:1895–1903.
76. Stone GW, Grines CL, Cox DA, et al., for the CADILLAC Investigators. Comparison of angioplasty with stenting, with or without abciximab, in acute myocardial infarction. *N Engl J Med* 2002;346:957–966.
77. Antoniucci D, Rodriguez A, Hempel A, et al. A randomized trial comparing primary infarct artery stenting with or without abciximab in acute myocardial infarction. *J Am Coll Cardiol* 2003;42:1879–1885.
78. Montalescot G, Borentain M, Payot L. Early vs late administration of glycoprotein IIb/IIIa inhibitors in primary percutaneous coronary intervention of acute ST-segment elevation myocardial infarction. A meta-analysis. *JAMA* 2004;292:362–366.

79. DeLuca G, Suryapranata H, Stonw GW, et al. Abciximab as adjunctive therapy to reperfusion in acute ST-segment elevation myocardial infarction. A meta-analysis of randomized trials. *JAMA* 2005;293:1759–1765.
80. ASSENT-4 Investigators. Primary versus tenecteplase-facilitated percutaneous coronary intervention in patients with ST-segment elevation acute myocardial infarction (ASSENT-4 PCI): randomised trial. *Lancet* 2006; 367:569–578.
81. Keeley EC, Boura JA, Grines CL. Comparison of primary and facilitated percutaneous coronary interventions for ST-elevation myocardial infarction: quantitative review of randomised trials. *Lancet* 2006;367:579–588.
82. The GUSTO V Investigators. Reperfusion therapy for acute myocardial infarction with fibrinolytic therapy or combination low dose fibrinolytic therapy and platelet glycoprotein IIb/IIIa inhibition: the GUSTO 5 trial. *Lancet* 2001;357:1905–1914.
83. Ambrosioni E, Borghi C, Magnani B. The effect of the angiotensin-converting enzyme inhibitor zofenopril on mortality and morbidity after anterior myocardial infarction. *N Engl J Med* 1995;332:80–85.
84. Granger CB, Hirsh J, Califf RM, et al. Activated partial thromboplastin time and outcome after fibrinolytic therapy for acute myocardial infarction. *Circulation* 1996;93:870–878.
85. Antman EM, Anbe DT, Armstrong PW, et al. ACC/AHA guidelines for the management of patients with ST-elevation myocardial infarction—Executive Summary: A report of the American College of Cardiology/American Heart Association Task Force on Practice Guidelines (Writing Committee to revise the 1999 Guidelines for the Management of Patients with Acute Myocardial Infarction) *Circulation* 2004;110:588–636.
86. Hsia J, Hamilton WP, Kleiman N, et al. A comparison between heparin and low-dose aspirin as adjunctive therapy with tissue plasminogen activator for acute myocardial infarction. *N Engl J Med* 1990;323:1433–1437.
87. Thompson PL, Aylward PE, Federman J, et al. A randomized comparison of intravenous heparin with oral aspirin and dipyridamole 24 hours after recombinant tissue-type plasminogen activator for acute myocardial infarction. *Circulation* 1991;83:1534–1542.
88. de Bono DP, Simoons JL, Tijssen J, et al. Effect of early intravenous heparin on coronary patency, infarct size, and bleeding complications after alteplase thrombolysis: results of a randomized double blind European Cooperative Study Group trial. *Br Heart J* 1992;67:122–128.
89. Bleich SD, Nichols TC, Schumacher RR, et al. Effect of heparin on coronary arterial patency after thrombolysis with tissue plasminogen activator in acute myocardial infarction. *Am J Cardiol* 1990;66:1412–1417.
90. White HD, Yusuf S. Issues regarding the use of heparin following streptokinase therapy. *J Thromb Thrombol* 1995;2:5–10.
91. Eikelboom JW, Quinlan DJ, Mehta SR, et al. Unfractionated and low-molecular-weight heparin as adjuncts to thrombolysis in aspirin-treated patients with ST-elevation acute myocardial infarction: a meta-analysis of the randomized trials. *Circulation* 2005;20:3855–3867.
92. The Direct Thrombin Inhibitor Trialists' Collaborative Group. Direct thrombin inhibitors in acute coronary syndromes: principal results of a meta-analysis based on individual patients' data. *Lancet* 2002;359:294–302.
93. Antman EM, Morrow DA, McCabe CH, et al. Enoxaparin versus unfractionated heparin with fibrinolysis for ST-elevation myocardial infarction. *N Engl J Med* 2006;354:1477–1488.
94. Sinnaeve PR, Simes J, Yusuf S, et al. Direct thrombin inhibitors in acute coronary syndromes: effect in patients undergoing early percutaneous coronary intervention. *Eur Heart J* 2005;26:2396–2403.
95. Gore JM, Granger CB, Simoons ML, et al. Stroke after thrombolysis: mortality and functional outcomes in the GUSTO-I trial. *Circulation* 1995;92:2811–2818.
96. Neuhaus KL. More on thrombolysis and hemorrhagic stroke. *Circulation* 1995;92:2794–2795.
97. White H, Barbash GI, Califf RM, et al. Age and outcome with contemporary fibrinolytic therapy: results from the GUSTO trial. *Circulation* 1996;94:1826–1833.
98. Topol EJ, Califf RM. Fibrinolytic therapy for elderly patients. *N Engl J Med* 1992;327:45–46.
99. Califf RM, Topol EJ, George BS, et al. Hemorrhagic complications associated with the use of intravenous tissue plasminogen activator in treatment of acute myocardial infarction. *Am J Med* 1988;85:353–359.
100. ISIS-1 (First International Study of Infarct Survival) Collaborative Study. Randomized trial of intravenous atenolol among 16,027 cases of suspected acute myocardial infarction: ISIS-1. *Lancet* 1986;2:57–65.
101. ISIS-1 (First International Study of Infarct Survival) Collaborative Group. Mechanisms for the early mortality reduction produced by beta-blockade started early in acute myocardial infarction: ISIS-1. *Lancet* 1988;1:823–921.
102. The TIMI Study Group. Comparison of invasive and conservative strategies after treatment with intravenous tissue plasminogen activator in acute myocardial infarction. Results of the thrombolysis in myocardial infarction (TIMI) phase II trial. The TIMI Study Group. *N Engl J Med* 1989;320:618–627.
103. Van de Werf F, Janssens L, Brzostek T, et al. Short-term effects of early intravenous treatment with a beta-adrenergic blocking agent or a specific bradycardiac agent in patients with acute myocardial infarction receiving fibrinolytic therapy. *J Am Coll Cardiol* 1993;22:407–416.
104. The COMMIT Collaborative Group. Early intravenous then oral metoprolol in 45,852 patients with acute myocardial infarction: randomised placebo-controlled trial. *Lancet* 2005;366:1622–1632.
105. Pfisterer M, Cox JL, Granger CB, et al., for the GUSTO-I Investigators. Atenolol use and clinical outcomes after thrombolysis for acute myocardial infarction: The GUSTO-I Experience. *J Am Coll Cardiol* 1998;32:634–640.
106. Dargie HJ. Effect of carvedilol on outcome after myocardial infarction in patients with left-ventricular dysfunction: the CAPRICORN randomized trial. *Lancet* 2001;357:1385–1390.
107. Yusuf S, Collins R, MacMahon S, et al. Effect of intravenous nitrates on mortality in acute myocardial infarction: an overview of the randomized trials. *Lancet* 1988;1:1088–1092.
108. Yusuf S, Wittes J, Friedman L. Overview of results of randomized clinical trials in heart disease. Treatments following myocardial infarction. *JAMA* 1988;260:2088–2093.
109. ISIS-4 (Fourth International Study of Infarct Survival) Collaborative Group. ISIS-4: a randomised factorial trial assessing early oral captopril, oral mononitrate, and intravenous magnesium sulphate in 58,050 patients with suspected acute myocardial infarction. *Lancet* 1995;345:669–685.
110. Gruppo Italiano per lo Studio della Sopravvivenza nell'Infarto Miocardico. GISSI-3: effects of lisinopril and transdermal glyceryl trinitrate singly and together on 6-week mortality and ventricular function after acute myocardial infarction. *Lancet* 1994;343:1115–1122.
111. Chinese cardiac study collaborative group. Oral captopril versus placebo among 13,634 patients with suspected acute myocardial infarction: interim report from the Chinese Cardiac Study (CCS-1). *Lancet* 1995;345:686–687.
112. Vantrimpont P, Rouleau JL, Chuan-Chuan W, et al. Additive beneficial effects of beta-blockers to angiotensin-converting enzyme inhibitors in the survival and ventricular enlargement (SAVE) study. *J Am Coll Cardiol* 1997;29:229–236.
113. Pfeffer MA, McMurray JJV, Velazquez EJ, et al. for the Valsartan in Acute Myocardial Infarction Trial (VALIANT) Investigators. Valsartan, Captopril, or both in myocardial infarction complicated by heart failure, left ventricular dysfunction, or both. *N Engl J Med* 2003;349:1893–1906.
114. Furberg CD, Psaty BM, Mayer JV. Nifedipine: dose-related increase in mortality in patients with coronary heart disease. *Circulation* 1995;92:1326–1331.
115. The Israeli Sprint Study Group. Secondary Prevention Reinfarction Israeli Nifedipine Trial (SPRINT): a randomized intervention trial of nifedipine in patients with acute myocardial infarction. *Eur Heart J* 1988;9:354–364.
116. Muller JE, Morrison J, Stone PH, et al. Nifedipine therapy for patients with threatened and acute myocardial infarction: a randomized, double-blind, placebo-controlled comparison. *Circulation* 1984;69:740–747.
117. Sirnes PA, Overskeid K, Pedersen TR, et al. Evolution of infarct size during the early use of nifedipine in patients with acute myocardial infarction: the Norwegian Nifedipine Multicenter Trial. *Circulation* 1984;70:638–644.
118. Kosiborod M, Rathore SS, Inzucchi SE, et al. Admission glucose and mortality in elderly patients hospitalized with acute myocardial infarction. *Circulation* 2005;111:3078–3086.
119. Solomon SD, Zelenkofske S, McMurray JJV, et al., for the Valsartan in Acute Myocardial Infarction Trial (VALIANT) Investigators. Sudden death in patients with myocardial infarction and left ventricular dysfunction, heart failure, or both. *N Engl J Med* 2005;352:2581–2588.
120. The Global Use of Strategies to Open Occluded Coronary Arteries (GUSTO) IIb Investigators. A comparison of recombinant hirudin with heparin for the treatment of acute coronary syndromes. *N Engl J Med* 1996;335:775–782.
121. Roffi M, Topol EJ. Percutaneous coronary intervention in diabetic patients with non-ST-segment elevation acute coronary syndromes. *Eur Heart J* 2004;25:190–198.
122. Boersma E, Mercado N, Poldermans D, et al. Acute myocardial infarction. *Lancet* 2003;361:847–858.
123. Topol EJ. A contemporary assessment of low-molecular-weight heparin for the treatment of acute coronary syndromes: Factoring in new trials and meta-analysis data. *Am Heart J* 2005;149:S100–S106.
124. Gibson RS, Boden WE, Theroux P, et al. Diltiazem and reinfarction in patients with non-Q-wave myocardial infarction: results of a double-blind, randomized, multicenter trial. *N Engl J Med* 1986;315:423–429.
125. Nallamothu BK, Wang Y, Magid DJ, et al. For the National Registry of Myocardial Infarction (NRMI) Investigators. Relation between hospital specialization with primary percutaneous coronary intervention and clinical outcomes in ST-segment elevation myocardial infarction. National Registry of Myocardial Infarction-4 Analysis. *Circulation* 2006;113:222–229.
126. GUSTO II Angioplasty Substudy Investigators. An international randomized trial of 1138 patients comparing primary coronary angioplasty versus tissue plasminogen activator for acute myocardial infarction. *N Engl J Med* 1997;336:1621–1628.
127. Phillips SJ, Zeff RH, Skinner JR, et al. Reperfusion protocol and results in 738 patients with evolving myocardial infarction. *Ann Thorac Surg* 1986;41:119–125.
128. Flameng W, Sargeant P, Vanhaecke J, et al. Emergency coronary bypass grafting for evolving myocardial infarction. *Cardiovasc Surg* 1987;94:124–131.

129. DeWood MA, Notske RN, Berg RJ, et al. Medical and surgical management of early Q wave myocardial infarction. I. Effects of surgical reperfusion on survival, recurrent myocardial infarction, sudden death and functional class at 10 or more years of follow-up. *J Am Coll Cardiol* 1989;14:65–77.
130. Kennedy JW, Ivey TD, Misbach G, et al. Coronary artery bypass graft surgery early after acute myocardial infarction. *Circulation* 1989;79:173–178.
131. Pilote L, Miller DP, Califf RM, et al. Determinants of the use of coronary angiography and revascularization after thrombolysis for acute myocardial infarction in the United States. *N Engl J Med* 1996;335:1198–1205.
132. Every NR, Larson EB, Litwin PE, et al. The association between onsite cardiac catheterization facilities and the use of coronary angiography after acute myocardial infarction. *N Engl J Med* 1993;329:546–551.
133. Pilote L, Califf RM, Sapp S, et al. Regional variability in the United States for the management of acute myocardial infarction: insights from the GUSTO trial. *N Engl J Med* 1995;333:565–572.
134. Kereiakes DJ, Topol EJ, George BS, et al. The Thrombolysis and Angioplasty in Myocardial Infarction (TAMI) Study Group: myocardial infarction with minimal coronary atherosclerosis in the era of myocardial reperfusion. *J Am Coll Cardiol* 1991;17:304–312.
135. Madsen JK, Grand P, Saunamaki K, et al. The Danish multicentre randomized study of invasive vs conservative treatment in patients with inducible ischemia following thrombolysis in acute myocardial infarction (DANAMI). *Circulation* 1997;96:748–755.
136. Van de Werf F, Topol EJ, Lee KL, et al. Variations in patient management and outcomes for acute myocardial infarction in the United States and other countries. *JAMA* 1995;273:1586–1591.
137. Tardiff BE, Califf RM, Morris D, et al. Coronary revascularization surgery following myocardial infarction: the effect of bypass surgery on survival following thrombolysis. *J Am Coll Cardiol* 1997;29:240–249.

CHAPTER 20 ■ ACUTE MYOCARDIAL INFARCTION: COMPLICATIONS

JUDITH S. HOCHMAN

OVERVIEW

Complications of myocardial infarction (MI) include (a) pump failure [left ventricular [LV] or right ventricular (RV)], which is the leading cause of death in hospitalized MI patients; (b) LV aneurysm; (c) systemic emboli; (d) reinfarction (infarct extension); (e) ischemia; (f) myocardial rupture (free wall, ventricular septal, and papillary muscle); (g) pericardial effusion; and (h) pericarditis. Except for reinfarction and hemorrhagic complications, reperfusion therapy reduces the incidence of most complications.

Echocardiography with color flow Doppler is an excellent tool for rapidly assessing all complications and for evaluating hypotension, congestive heart failure (CHF), and cardiogenic shock. Conditions that mimic shock complicating acute MI, such as aortic dissection, can be readily detected. Management of each complication must be related to its pathophysiology. Mechanical problems, such as ventricular septal rupture (VSR) and mitral regurgitation (MR), should be surgically corrected. Increasing use of early revascularization for cardiogenic shock, based on randomized trial evidence demonstrating improved survival, has resulted in decreasing mortality rates over time in large, community-based studies of patients in cardiogenic shock. Nevertheless, the mortality rate remains high. Early reinfarction, which is associated with increased mortality, may be managed preferentially with percutaneous coronary intervention (PCI) or thrombolysis when ST elevations occur. Future efforts must focus on preventing complications, because mortality rates are high once complications develop.

GENERAL PATHOPHYSIOLOGY

The spectrum of complications of myocardial necrosis, from CHF to arrhythmias to post-MI angina, is illustrated in Figure 20.1 (1). Complications of MI tend to occur when infarcts are large and extensively transmural, in the absence of tissue perfusion due to microvasculature obstruction (2–4). A large, transmural infarct is more prone to expansion (i.e., thinning and dilation) with its attendant increased risk for myocardial

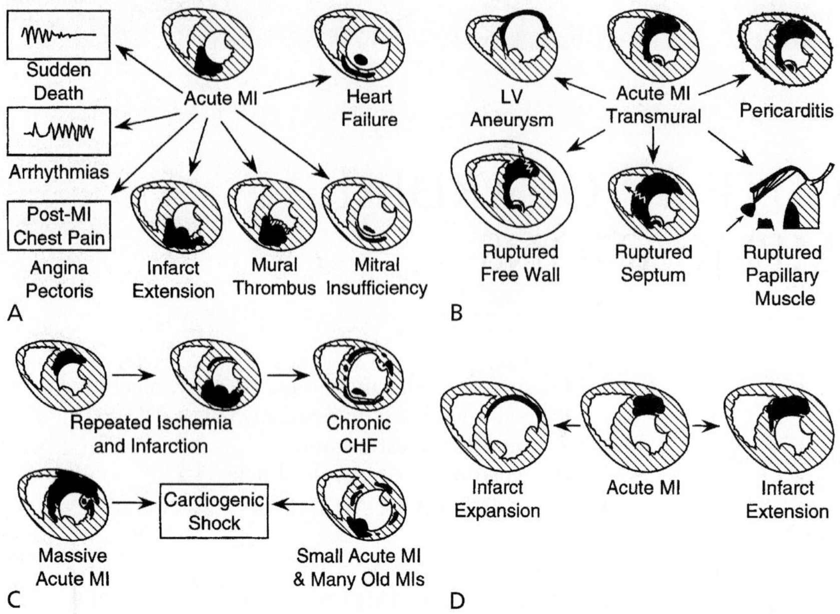

FIGURE 20.1. Complications of MI (schematic). (**A**) General complications. (**B**) Complications of transmural infarctions. (**C**) Cardiogenic shock as a result of either a massive acute infarction or a small acute process in a heart already involved by multiple old infarctions. (**D**) Comparison of infarct expansion (aneurysm formation) and infarct extension (reinfarction). *Abbreviations:* CHF, congestive heart failure; LV, left ventricle. (*Source:* From Edwards WD. Pathology of myocardial infarction and reperfusion. In: Gersh BJ, Rahimtoola SH, eds. *Acute myocardial infarction.* Boston: Chapman & Hall, 1996:16–50, with permission.)

rupture, LV aneurysm, LV thrombus, pump failure, and pericarditis (see Fig. 20.1) (1). Refractory, sustained ventricular tachycardia develops after MI most frequently in relation to large transmural infarcts that result in LV dilation. Although infarct size is a major determinant of complications, certain strategic locations of small, extensively transmural infarcts can result in devastating complications, such as LV free-wall rupture or rupture of the posteromedial papillary muscle, even when expansion does not occur (Fig. 20.1) (1). Indeed, in an autopsy study of patients dying of acute MI, infarct size was substantially smaller in patients with cardiac rupture than in patients dying of primary pump function or arrhythmias. An anteroapical location of MI increases the likelihood of acute infarct expansion and mural thrombosis. Massive acute myocardial necrosis, multiple small infarcts (acute and prior), and recurrent ischemia or reinfarction may each lead to cardiogenic shock (Fig. 30.1) (1). New myocardial necrosis or infarct extension (i.e., reinfarction) may occur after the initial MI and result in a larger total area of infarction. In contrast, infarct expansion involves no additional myocardial necrosis, but results in a larger functional infarct size with a greater percentage of the LV being composed of necrotic myocardium or scar (5). These two complications are compared in Fig. 20.1 (1). Extent and severity of disease in non–infarct-related coronary arteries and important characteristics of the patient—including age, gender, and comorbidities (e.g., diabetes mellitus and prior hypertension)—also contribute significantly to the development of acute MI complications. These complications are not entirely independent, and each can lead to other complications.

INFARCT EXPANSION, LEFT VENTRICULAR REMODELING, AND LEFT VENTRICULAR ANEURYSM

Pathophysiology

LV remodeling after MI refers to structural and functional changes in the infarct zone and in remote, uninfarcted myocardium that begin minutes after MI and may continue for months or years. These changes include (a) infarct expansion (thinning and dilation of the infarct zone); (b) subsequent dilation of the remote, uninfarcted myocardium with hypertrophy; (c) interstitial fibrosis and impairment of contraction; and (d) global change from a normal LV, elongated ellipse to a more spherical shape (6–10). Neurohormonal mediators and matrix metalloproteinases play an important role in this process (11). LV aneurysm, a discrete bulge of the LV composed of fibrotic tissue, results when severe infarct expansion persists and scar is laid down on the topographic substrate.

Infarct Expansion and Left Ventricular Remodeling

Infarct expansion occurs soon after onset of coronary occlusion (6,12). It is reversible if coronary flow is reestablished rapidly; however, it may progress in a time-dependent manner if flow is not reestablished or is reestablished late (13). Absence of myocardial perfusion at the microvascular level, even in the presence of Thrombolysis in Myocardial Infarction (TIMI) III flow, is associated with progressive LV dilation (2,3). Infarct size is a major determinant, with large infarcts expanding more frequently and more severely than small ones (7,9). Anterior infarcts and those involving the apex are at greatest risk for infarct expansion (5,6), probably as a result of a thinner LV wall and greater radius of curvature at the apex, which increase stress on the LV wall per Laplace's equation. Transmural infarcts are more likely to expand; nontransmural infarcts are largely protected from expansion (7,13). Infarct expansion is the pathologic substrate for type III cardiac rupture. Disruption of the intercellular collagen matrix may lead to slippage of sheets of myofibrils and expansion of the affected area (10,15).

Infarct expansion results in early LV dilation (6,7) and MR (see Mitral Regurgitation). It is associated with CHF and LV intracavitary thrombosis (8,15,16). Long-term global remodeling with dilation and impairment of uninfarcted myocardial segment contraction begins soon after a large infarction and progresses for months to years (9,10). LV volume strongly correlates with long-term mortality (17,18).

Left Ventricular Aneurysm

Regional expansion of the infarct zone that results in a discrete diastolic and systolic bulge and that is not reversed by reperfusion or other measures produces chronic, true LV aneurysm. Early LV aneurysms may be referred to as functional aneurysms (20) because they may be reversible. In time, scar tissue is laid down on the already spatially deformed infarct zone. Pathologic examination of LV aneurysm reveals primary scar tissue (19,22); however, LV aneurysms resected years after MI sometimes contain viable and presumably hibernating myocardium (21). In contrast to true LV aneurysm, pseudoaneurysm or false LV aneurysm represents localized rupture of the myocardium and is discussed later in this chapter (22).

Left Ventricular Thrombus

Inflammation of the endocardium resulting from myocardial necrosis in any location may produce layered, mural thrombus; however, thrombus most frequently develops in anterior infarcts (16,23) with expansion or aneurysmal dilation that involves the apex, caused by the combination of endocardial inflammation and stasis. More extensive thrombi with a protruding appearance are at increased risk for systemic embolization (16), and they typically occur in the apex.

Clinical Profile

Risk Factors

Patients with myocardial infarcts that involve the apex of the left ventricle, particularly those with anteroapical, Q-wave infarcts are at greatest risk for infarct expansion and aneurysm formation (5,6). A discrete, posterobasal aneurysm may less frequently develop following inferoposterior MI. Patients who do not receive reperfusion therapy or in whom reperfusion therapy fails to reestablish myocardial perfusion are at greater risk for aneurysm formation.

High ventricular afterload states, such as hypertension during acute MI and elevated plasma angiotensin-converting enzyme (ACE) activity levels, are associated with infarct expansion (15,24,25). Administration of corticosteroids after acute MI is associated with delayed infarct healing and development of LV aneurysms (26). Both corticosteroids and nonsteroidal antiinflammatory drugs have been demonstrated experimentally to induce infarct expansion when administered acutely after coronary occlusion (27–29).

Diagnosis

Clinical Findings

The classic physical finding of LV aneurysm is a dyskinetic apical impulse on palpation. The electrogradiogram (ECG) typically shows an extensive, anteroapical Q-wave MI with persistent ST-segment elevation. Persistent T-wave inversion is also a marker of progressive LV dilation (30). Chest roentgenography is insensitive but typically demonstrates a bulge in the LV silhouette.

Imaging

On imaging, LV aneurysm is defined as a discrete bulge in the LV contour during both diastole and systole, which typically exhibits dyskinetic (i.e., paradoxical) expansion during systole. Echocardiography with color flow Doppler is the imaging modality of choice and can be used to distinguish discrete LV aneurysms from false aneurysms. Other techniques to assess an aneurysm include biplane left ventriculography, radionuclide ventriculography, computed tomography, and magnetic resonance imaging (MRI).

Clinical Consequences

Cardiac Rupture, Congestive Heart Failure, and Arrhythmias

Rupture of the myocardium may result from acute infarct expansion, but it does not occur in chronic LV aneurysms with scar. Acute CHF complicating MI more frequently occurs when infarct expansion is demonstrated (8,15). Infarct expansion and acute aneurysmal dilation may result in CHF caused by paradoxic systolic bulging with reduced mechanical efficiency of the left ventricle (i.e., wasted work) (21) and elevated wall stress in the remote, uninfarcted myocardium, causing global ischemia. Chronic LV aneurysms are associated with chronic CHF. In this context, the extent of systolic bulging with chronic scar is minimal and wasted work only plays a significant role when the aneurysm is composed of viable myocardium interspersed with scar tissue or of thin scar that expands with each systole (22).

Recurrent and sustained monomorphic ventricular tachycardia may occur in acute infarct expansion or in chronic LV aneurysm and may be refractory to antiarrhythmic therapy (see Chapter 66). LV volume correlates strongly with short- and long-term mortality (17,18), with sudden cardiac death occurring at least as frequently as death from progressive pump failure. Early LV dilation results in late progressive LV enlargement with associated CHF and malignant ventricular arrhythmias late post-MI (31).

Left Ventricular Thrombi, Systemic Emboli, and Stroke

Layered mural and protruding thrombi typically develop within the first week following acute MIs with expanded or aneurysmal akinetic or dyskinetic segments, especially those involving the LV anterior wall and apex. Because LV thrombi more frequently occur with large infarctions they have become less common in the reperfusion era. Recent data suggest that 4% to 8% of all MI patients develop LV thrombus (32–34). Risk factors for LV thrombus are Killip class greater than I, ejection fraction (EF) less than 40%, anterior infarction, no reperfusion, and early intravenous β-blocker use (23). LV thrombi are associated with increased risk for systemic embolization, particularly when they have a protruding appearance (16). Stroke is the primary manifestation of cardiac emboli (occurring in 85% of cases); however, the overall incidence of arterial embolism is low (35–38), whether LV thrombus is visualized or not. The reported incidence (38) of systemic emboli associated with anterior MI in the prereperfusion era was 2% to 6%. Patients with atrial fibrillation (AF) after MI are at increased risk for systemic emboli from left atrial thrombi. Patients with chronic LV aneurysm are at low risk for systemic embolization (39), perhaps because the aneurysmal area containing thrombus is noncontractile and there is no longer endocardial inflammation. However, when global LVEF is reduced after MI (<40%), the rate of stroke is 1.5% per year even when CHF is not present. The risk increases with decreasing EF and older age (40). Patients with LVEF less than 28% have a 5-year stroke rate of 8.9%. However, many of these strokes are likely caused by cerebrovascular ulcerated plaques (as opposed to cardiac emboli) given the evidence that multiple ulcerated plaques occur throughout the vasculature.

Management

Medical Therapy

Inhibition of the Renin/Angiotensin/Aldosterone Axis. ACE inhibitors have been shown in experimental models and in clinical investigations (31,41,42) to reduce acute infarct expansion and progressive LV remodeling. When successful reperfusion has inhibited infarct expansion and aneurysm formation, ACE inhibitors have not been clearly shown to limit expansion further (43). A detailed discussion of the use of ACE inhibitors in MI can be found elsewhere in this textbook (see Chapters 19 and 21). Because infarct expansion begins early, therapy should be instituted within the first 24 hours of onset of MI in patients at risk for expansion and aneurysms (i.e., those with nonreperfused or large anteroapical Q-wave MIs, particularly with associated hypertension). A short-acting ACE inhibitor is recommended for initial therapy (e.g., captopril), so that it can be discontinued if hypotension develops. The initial dose should be 6.25 mg followed by 12.5 mg, then 25 to 50 mg every 8 hours as tolerated. After several days, the patient may be switched to a long-acting ACE inhibitor. Aldosterone antagonists and angiotensin receptor blockers also reduce adverse LV remodeling in experimental models, but have not been extensively clinically tested within 24 hours of acute MI (44,45). The use of these agents in patients with pulmonary congestion is discussed in the section on Acute Left Ventricular Failure.

Anticoagulation: Therapy for Left Ventricular Thrombus. Full oral anticoagulation for 3 months significantly accelerated the resolution of LV thrombus in a small randomized trial (46) of acenocoumarol versus sulfinpyrazone versus placebo. Full-dose warfarin is recommended when LV thrombus is visualized, although there are no data for this subset from randomized trials.

Anticoagulation: Prevention of Systemic Emboli. In the prereperfusion era, when patients were hospitalized for weeks, anticoagulant therapy reduced the occurrence of systemic and pulmonary embolism (PE) (47,48). The 30-day rate of stroke in a largely reperfused ST-elevation MI population was not reduced by heparin (reviparin) compared to placebo in the context of therapy with aspirin (ASA) in 97% and thienopyridines in 50% (49).

The Survival and Ventricular Enlargement investigators (40) reported that long-term use of warfarin in patients with EF less than 40% after MI was strongly associated with a reduced 5-year stroke rate. Of note, ASA was less strongly associated with a reduced risk (40). In the Anticoagulants in the Secondary Prevention of Events in Coronary Thrombosis-2 (51) and Warfarin-Aspirin Reinfarction Study-2 (52) randomized trials, warfarin alone or in combination with ASA was superior to ASA alone post-MI in preventing stroke as well as MI and death (52). However, stroke, MI, and death were not reduced by lower intensity warfarin (Coumadin) plus ASA compared with ASA alone in the Combined Hemotherapy and Mortality Prevention (53), the Low-dose Warfarin and Aspirin Study (54), or the Coumadin Aspirin Reinfarction Study (54,55).

Anticoagulant Regimens

Warfarin dosing. Warfarin therapy (full dosing or moderate intensity when combined with ASA) is recommended following infarction in patients with documented LV thrombus, systemic emboli and in those with AF (56,57). It is recommended that patients with these high-risk characteristics be treated with warfarin indefinitely if they are not at increased risk of bleeding. It is also reasonable to use warfarin for patients with extensive wall motion abnormalities, particularly those with large anterior MI or apical akinesis or dyskinesis, for 3 months or indefinitely in those who are not at increased risk of bleeding. This approach is supported by the Antithrombotics in the Secondary Prevention of Events in Coronary Thrombosis 2 and Warfarin Reinfarction Study (WARIS) II studies, which demonstrated reduction of vascular events, stroke, death, and MI with high-intensity warfarin (international normalized ratio [INR] 2.8–4.0) or moderate-intensity warfarin (INR 2.0–2.5) plus ASA compared to ASA alone, albeit at the expense of excess bleeding (51,52). However, lower intensity warfarin plus ASA compared with ASA alone resulted in similar event rates in three trials (53–55).

REINFARCTION AND ISCHEMIA

Pathophysiology

Importance of Coronary Perfusion Pressure

It is critical to maintain coronary perfusion pressure during acute MI to facilitate reperfusion and sustain patency of the Infarct related artery (IRA) postfibrinolysis or post-PCI (58,59). There is evidence of worse outcomes and larger MIs when hypotension occurs with use of nitrates and ACE inhibitors early in acute MI (60,61).

Clinical Profile

Diagnosis

The incidence of reinfarction or infarct extension varies widely, depending on the clinical definition and the diligence with which it is sought. ECG changes alone are the least specific method of diagnosing infarct extension, and they markedly overestimate its occurrence (5). ST-segment elevation that progresses days after MI may represent pericarditis or infarct expansion. Evolution of deepening T waves is typical after MI and does not usually represent ischemia or infarct extension. Recurrent chest pain is also nonspecific, with angina or pericarditis as other causes of post-MI chest pain. Recurrent elevations in creatine kinase with muscle and brain subunits (CK-MB) after its disappearance or to higher than 50% of the prior value are regarded as the standard for reinfarction. Because troponin I and T may remain elevated for up to 2 weeks, they are not used to diagnose reinfarction (56). The full constellation of recurrent chest discomfort and recurrent elevation in ST segments followed by recurrent elevation in CK-MB infrequently occurs but constitutes the typical diagnosis, both in large clinical trials and in clinical practice. We recommend obtaining daily CK-MB measurements for 2 days after MI as well as 8-hour samplings for 24 hours if a recurrent event develops (e.g., chest pain, worsening ST elevations or depressions).

Incidence, Risk Factors, and Prognosis

The incidence of early reinfarction varies depending on the initial therapy and ranges from 16% in observational studies of nonreperfused patients to less than 5% in randomized clinical trials (see Chapter 19).

Independent risk factors for recurrent MI in both reperfused and nonreperfused patients include previous MI, female gender, and diagnostic first ECG (62). Recurrent ischemia is a risk factor for reinfarction and reinfarction substantially increases the risk of death after MI (62–64).

Prevention

Recurrent MI is, in part, related to the early therapy used in treating the initial MI; this is discussed in Chapter 19.

Management

Reinfarction is managed using the same medications as those used for the initial ST-elevation or non–ST-elevation MI (see Chapters 18 and 19), including ASA, heparin (low-molecular-weight or unfractionated heparin), clopidogrel, GP IIb/IIIa antagonists, and β-blockers, but with the caveat that patients with recurrent ischemia are a high-risk group who merit early cardiac catheterization. Readministration of thrombolytics for recurrent MI with recurrent ST-segment elevations on ECG has been used (65), with high successful response rates. Direct PCI should be performed, if available, for recurrent coronary artery occlusion.

Calcium channel blockers may be added if recurrent angina occurs on maximal doses of β-blockers and nitrates. Intraaortic balloon pump (IABP) counterpulsation should be used for patients with ischemia and hemodynamic instability (i.e., hypotension, hypoperfusion, or low cardiac output) and for refractory ischemia if revascularization facilities are not immediately available.

Reinfarction and postinfarction ischemia identify a high-risk subgroup of patients in whom urgent cardiac catheterization is indicated with prompt revascularization with PCI or coronary artery bypass grafting (CABG) to reduce the risk of long-term events, depending on the coronary anatomy, LV function, and the extent of myocardial jeopardy.

ACUTE LEFT VENTRICULAR FAILURE

Pathophysiologic Principles

General

LV failure in acute MI varies widely in terms of pathophysiology and severity. Mild-to-severe pulmonary congestion may occur alone or in association with depressed stroke volume (SV) and cardiac output (66,67). Diastolic or systolic dysfunction may predominate. At the severe end of the spectrum of pump failure, cardiogenic shock is a state of severe tissue hypoperfusion caused by cardiac dysfunction.

Congestive Heart Failure

After acute coronary occlusion, LV systolic and diastolic function changes over minutes, hours, and weeks. Superimposed fixed or transient MR, recurrent ischemia, or reinfarction may have a major effect. Compliance of the infarct zone evolves over time (68), and stunned myocardium may recover function (69,70). Elevations in LV filling pressures resulting from systolic or diastolic dysfunction may reduce the pressure gradient that maintains coronary blood flow and thereby initiate a cycle of hypoperfusion and worsening LV dysfunction (Fig. 20.2) (71).

Systolic Dysfunction

The composite effect of dysfunctional myocardial segments, as well as the hyperkinetic or normokinetic motion of the uninfarcted myocardium, determines global LV function. These abnormalities may be old (e.g., caused by prior infarctions) or new and may be reversible or irreversible. Global LV function is the strongest determinant of pump failure and death caused by MI (72–74). Lack of compensatory hyperkinesis of uninfarcted zones correlates with the development of pump failure. The LV typically dilates when significant systolic dysfunction is present, caused by early infarct expansion and the effect of the resultant increased wall stress on the remote myocardium. LV dilation plays an acute compensatory role by allowing the high end-diastolic volume (EDV) to maintain SV when EF is significantly depressed. This acute adaptive effect is counterbalanced by deleterious long-term effects of LV dilation including increased wall stress, hypertrophy, and further dilation, followed by failure of the remote myocardium.

The clinical manifestations of CHF when LV systolic function is depressed vary. Neurohormonal (75–77) (see Fig. 20.2) and hydration status may explain why some patients with low EFs have pulmonary congestion and others do not (78). Diastolic dysfunction owing to infarction contributes substantially to increased filling pressure. Furthermore, changes in peripheral circulation and in end organs, particularly in patients with prior LV damage, may influence the symptomatic response to the acute insult.

Recovery of contractile function in akinetic and even dyskinetic segments following acute MI is well documented and is caused by resolution of myocardial stunning and hibernation. Stunning may take weeks to months to resolve, and function of hibernating myocardium is only restored when coronary flow is normalized. Even late reperfusion may improve wall motion and global EF.

Diastolic Dysfunction

Diastolic dysfunction with reduced LV compliance is a relatively common cause of pulmonary congestion in acute MI. Ischemia causes impaired myocardial relaxation (79). Severe pulmonary edema may result from global subendocardial ischemia caused by three-vessel or left main coronary artery disease (CAD) with a normal heart size. Additionally, the infarct zone undergoes alterations in compliance that result in varying LV distensibility over time following coronary occlusion (68). Reperfusion into areas of irreversible necrosis leads to contraction band necrosis, hemorrhage, and edema, resulting in acutely stiff infarcts zones (80) and, therefore, reduced LV compliance.

Diastolic abnormalities of the LV that impede LV filling may result in both an increase in LV filling pressures and a decrease in SV in the absence of global LV systolic dysfunction. Preexisting conditions that may cause reductions in ventricular compliance, such as hypertension and diabetes, result in an even greater shift of the pressure–volume curve when ischemia or infarction is superimposed.

Cardiogenic Shock Caused by Primary Left Ventricular Failure

LV failure is the most common cause of cardiogenic shock complicating acute MI. The prospective SHOCK Trial Registry identified LV failure as the etiology of shock in 79% of patients (81).

Patients with acute MI who develop cardiogenic shock typically have severe atherosclerotic disease involving all three major coronary arteries and often a severe stenosis in the Left anterior descending (LAD) coronary artery. Significant stenosis in the left main coronary artery is seen in 16% to 21% of patients (82–84). Prior MI is present in approximately 40% of patients; when an old infarct is extensive, even a small, new infarction may lead to shock. Although autopsy studies traditionally have demonstrated that at least 40% of the LV mass is affected in patients dying from cardiogenic shock complicating MI (83,85), recent evidence demonstrates that shock can

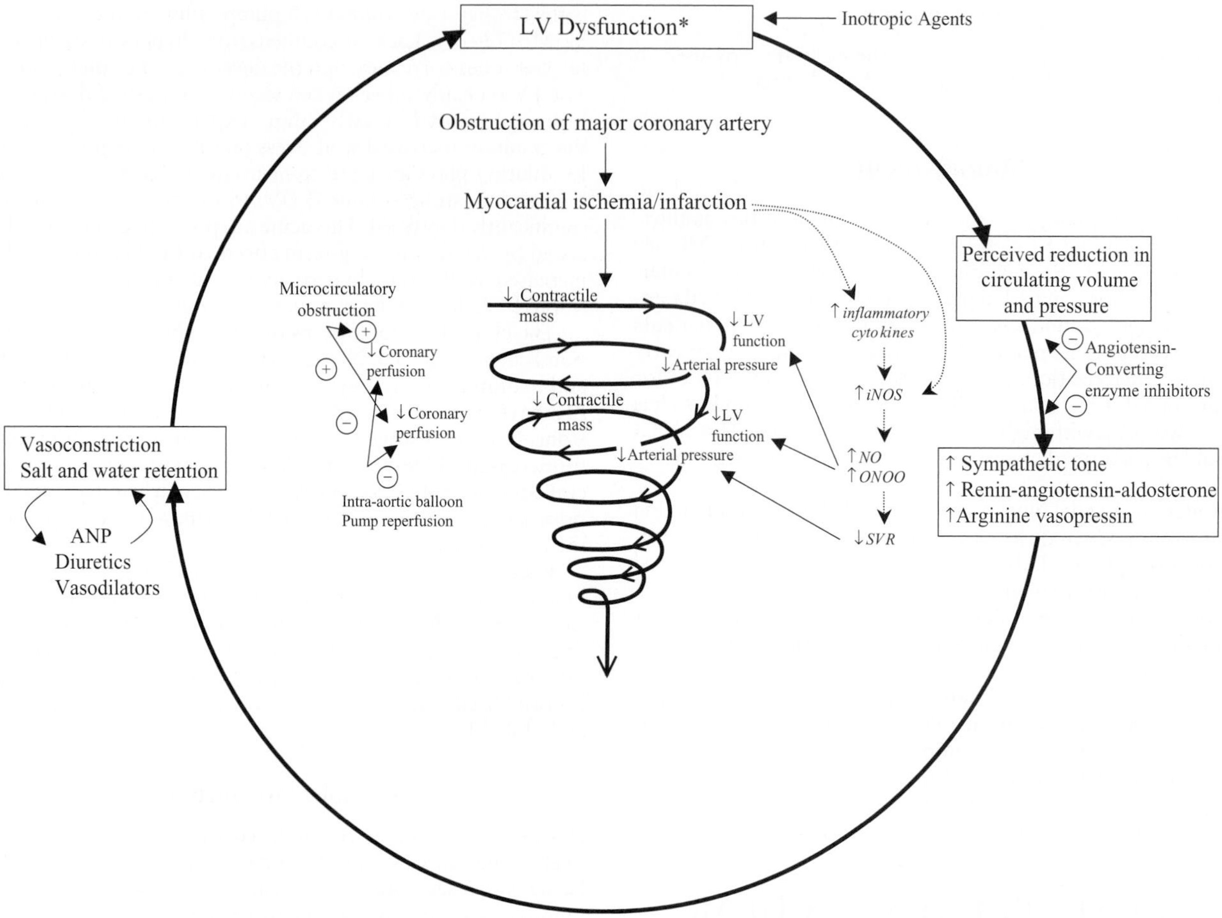

FIGURE 20.2. Pathophysiology of cardiogenic shock caused by primary LV failure. The complex interplay of LV dysfunction, neurohormonal activation, inflammatory mediators, and the vicious cycle of progressively worsening ventricular function that characterizes cardiogenic shock is illustrated. At the onset of shock, SVR is often not elevated, probably because a systemic inflammatory response blunts the expected vasoconstrictor response to hypotension. Later, a neurohumoral response usually increases SVR, as illustrated in the outer circle above. The italicized print represents the newly hypothesized role of the systemic inflammatory response in the genesis and maintenance of shock. For discussion, see text. *Abbreviations:* ANP, atrial natriuretic peptide; iNOS, inducible nitric oxide synthase; LV, left ventricular; NO, nitric oxide; ONOO, peroxynitrite. (*Source:* Adapted from Califf RM, Bengtson JR. Cardiogenic shock. *N Engl J Med* 1994;330:1724–1730; and Hochman JS. Cardiogenic shock complicating acute myocardial infarction: expanding the paradigm. *Circulation* 2003;107:2998–3002.)

occur because of reversible ischemia or because of a mismatch between inappropriate systemic vasodilation and reduced cardiac output due to LV dysfunction. Evidence for elevated levels of inflammatory markers and adverse effects of inducible nitric oxide synthase suggest that a systemic inflammatory response syndrome and high levels of nitric oxide seen in other etiologies of shock, play a role in the genesis and persistence of cardiogenic shock (87–91) (see Fig. 20.2). There is a wide range of EFs demonstrated on patients with cardiogenic shock due to LV failure (average LVEF ~30%, range <10% to >50%) (92–94).

Other Conditions

Conditions that result in high-output failure, including fever and anemia, may occur in acute MI (Table 20.1). Use of negative inotropic agents, such as β-blockers and calcium channel antagonists, particularly in patients with large infarctions, may result in CHF, hypotension, and shock (95). When hypotension is present, noncardiogenic causes of shock, including volume depletion, with or without hemorrhage, sepsis, and PE must be excluded. Even when shock results from primary LV failure, MR caused by papillary muscle dysfunction (96,97) often contributes to shock. Each of the mechanical causes of cardiogenic shock discussed later in this chapter must be excluded. CHF or shock may develop in response to severe emotional stress in the absence of obstructive CAD, as seen in LV Apical Ballooning/Takotsubo Cardiomyopathy (98,99). Aortic dissection with acute aortic regurgitation, tamponade, or both may mimic acute MI with cardiogenic shock (see Table 20.1). An acute MI may occur in association with another catastrophic event (e.g., ruptured aortic aneurysm, ischemic bowel), and the diagnosis may be difficult in an obtunded patient in shock.

Clinical Profile: Congestive Heart Failure and Cardiogenic Shock

The Killip clinical classification system (100) stratifies patients based on clinical evidence of LV failure:

1. Killip class I is defined as no evidence of CHF.
2. Killip class II is defined as presence of a third heart sound gallop, basilar rales, or both.
3. Killip class III is defined as pulmonary edema.
4. Killip class IV is defined as cardiogenic shock.

TABLE 20.1

CARDIOGENIC SHOCK: DIFFERENTIAL DIAGNOSIS

Complications of acute MI
Extensive LV infarction and ischemia
Extensive RV infarction and ischemia
VSR
Acute, severe MR
Tamponade
With free wall rupture
Without free wall rupture
Other conditions
Aortic dissection
Myocarditis
PE
Critical aortic or mitral stenosis
Hypertrophic cardiomyopathy with outflow obstruction
Acute aortic or MR
Pericarditis with tamponade
LV apical ballooning/Takostubo cardiomyopathy
Metabolic/toxic
Calcium channel or β-blocker overdose
Acidosis, hyperkalemia, hypoxemia
Thyroid storm, myxedema coma
Acute MI with
Ischemic/infarcted bowel
Ruptured abdominal aortic aneurysm
Sepsis
Hemorrhage
Anaphylaxis
Excessive β- or calcium channel blockade

Abbreviations: LV, left ventricular; MI, myocardial infarction; MR, mitral regurgitation; PE, pulmonary embolism; RV, right ventricular; SVR, systemic vascular resistance; VSR, ventricular septal rupture.

The worst Killip class may be present on hospital admission or may develop at any point during hospitalization. This clinical classification system provides a useful approach with continued applicability in the reperfusion era.

Incidence of Congestive Heart Failure and Cardiogenic Shock

The incidence of CHF complicating MI appears to have decreased over the past 30 years from 48% to 36%, with half that rate reported in randomized trials (Tables 20.2 and 20.3) (101,102). Placebo-controlled, randomized trials assessing the effect of thrombolysis on the occurrence of CHF after hospital admission demonstrate variable results (103–107), but overall the incidence of CHF is slightly lower in the thrombolytic than in the placebo group. Primary PCI appears to be associated with lower rates of CHF than thrombolytic therapy (see Tables 20.2 and 20.3) (108–116). In one study, prehospital thrombolysis resulted in a lower incidence of early cardiogenic shock compared to primary PCI, particularly in those who presented within 2 hours of MI onset (117).

Despite the efficacy of early reperfusion for preventing shock there has been no change in the nearly 8% incidence of cardiogenic shock in larger registries (118,119) and pump failure remains the leading cause of death in patients hospitalized with acute MI in the reperfusion era (120).

Congestive Heart Failure and Cardiogenic Shock: Risk Factors

Patient Profile. Age, female gender, prior MI, and diabetes are associated with risk of pump failure, as is anterior MI location (86,121,122). The characteristics of 1,190 patients with suspected cardiogenic shock in the prospective SHOCK Trial Registry, which includes all etiologies, infarct types, and therapies, were age 68.7, 40% women, history of MI in 37%, hypertension in 53%, and diabetes in 33% (81). Lower systolic blood pressure, higher hear rate, and Killip class II or III on admission provide clinical evidence of pump dysfunction and predict the development of shock. Other risk factors include EF of 35% or less, persistent occlusion of the IRA, and the absence of hyperkinesis of the uninfarcted LV segments (72).

Non–ST-Elevation Myocardial Infarction. Cardiogenic shock complicates non–ST-elevation MI approximately half as often as it does ST-elevation MI (123). In the SHOCK Trial Registry, 17% of patients with predominant LV failure had non–ST-elevation MI (124) and 2.6% of CRUSADE non–ST-elevation acute coronary syndrome patients developed cardiogenic shock (125). These patients are older and have more prior MI, CHF, CABG, peripheral vascular disease, severe three-vessel, and left main CAD than patients with ST-elevation MI. Importantly, in 35% the circumflex artery was the culprit vessel (124).

Congestive Heart Failure and Cardiogenic Shock: Timing

Patients often develop CHF and cardiogenic shock after hospital admission. In the SHOCK Trial Registry, patients with cardiogenic shock caused by primary LV failure demonstrated a predominance of early shock: 47% within the first 6 hours and 72% within 24 hours of MI onset (126). Nevertheless, only 27% of those with cardiogenic shock presented to the hospital in shock. Similarly the large NRMI Registry reported that 29% of all cardiogenic shock patients presented to hospital already in shock (118).

Clinical Assessment

Overview. Patients who develop pump failure must be assessed for other complicating conditions (see Table 20.1) (see also Pathophysiologic Principles). A targeted history should be obtained and a physical examination should be performed rapidly as well as ECG, arterial blood gas analysis, and hematology and chemistry profiles. Chest roentgenography should be promptly performed.

Clinical Findings: Congestive Heart Failure

Pump failure most frequently manifests as pulmonary congestion with pulmonary rales on examination, and pulmonary vascular redistribution with interstitial edema on chest roentgenography, initially with a normal heart size. Patients with mild CHF (Killip class II) may or may not report dyspnea. Tachypnea is usually present, but the respiratory rate may be only mildly elevated. Tachycardia and hypertension may or may not be present. Pulmonary edema (Killip class III) with acute interstitial and alveolar edema is associated with tachypnea, tachycardia, and hypertension caused by sympathetic stimulation. Lack of hypertension suggests profound LV failure and impending cardiogenic shock.

Electrocardiographic Findings: Congestive Heart Failure

There are large variations in the ECG findings in patients with pulmonary congestion, although most patients have changes consistent with a large infarction. Extensive ST-segment depressions are not uncommon and may represent extensive subendocardial infarction or small infarcts with extensive ischemia.

TABLE 20.2

INCIDENCE OF HEART FAILURE AFTER MI AND ITS INFLUENCE ON IN-HOSPITAL, 30-DAY, AND 1-YEAR MORTALITY

Study/Reference	Total number of patients	Incidence (%)	Mortality (%)	
			No CHF	CHF
Killip and Kimball, 1967 (100)	250	48.8	6.0	21.3
COMMUNITY STUDIES				
Worcester, MA (101)				
1975–1978	1402	38.3	7.0	32.6
1981–1984	1439	43.6		
1986–1988	1231	37.5		
1990–1991	1259	35.6		
1993–1995	1467	33.1	9.0	17.7
Olmsted, MN (102)				
1979–1984	501	27.0		
1985–1989	466	24.0		
1990–1994	570	23.0		
REGISTRIES				
VALIANT,[a] 2004 (239)	5566	42.0	2.3	13.0
BEAT,[b] 2003 (240)	3326	46.0	6.0	22.0/35.0
NRMI, 2002 (108)	190,518	19.1	7.2	21.4
RCTs				
Thrombolytic				
ASSENT-II, 2003 (109)	16,949		5.0	13.4
GUSTO, ASSENT-II (Pooled),[c] 2003 (110)	61,041	29.4	2.0	8.0
Primary PCI				
PAMI (Pooled),[d] 2001 (111)	2654	13.1	2.4	8.6

[a]Rates include heart failure and/or LV systolic dysfunction.
[b]Mortality rates at 1 year in patients with heart failure with preserved systolic LV function (22%) and heart failure with systolic dysfunction (35%).
[c]Patients enrolled in GUSTO-I, GUSTO-IIb, GUSTO-III, and ASSENT-II.
[d]Patients enrolled in PAMI-2, PAMI-Stent, and PAMI No SOS.
Rates presented do not include patients with cardiogenic shock for Killip, Pooled PAMI, NRMI, Pooled GUSTO ASSENT II studies.

Mortality rates for patients with heart failure on admission in Killip, NRMI, ASSENT-II, and Pooled PAMI studies and for patients with CHF at any time during hospitalization in Worcester, VALIANT, BEAT, and Pooled GUSTO ASSENT II studies.

Mortality rates for patients with CHF significantly higher than patients without CHF. (No *P*-values were reported in ASSENT-2).

Abbreviations: CHF, congestive heart failure; VALIANT, Valsartan in Acute Myocardial Infarction Trial; BEAT, Bucindolol Evaluation in Acute Myocardial Infarction Trial; NRMI, National Registry of Myocardial Infarction; ASSENT, Assessment of the Safety and Efficacy of a New Thrombolytic; GUSTO, Global Utilization of Strategies to Open Occluded Coronary Arteries in Acute Coronary Syndromes; PAMI, Primary Angioplasty in Myocardial Infarction; PAMI No SOS, PAMI No Surgery on Site: RCT, randomized controlled trials.

Clinical Findings: Cardiogenic Shock

The patient with classic cardiogenic shock complicating acute MI has severe systemic hypotension, end-organ hypoperfusion with cool extremities and oliguria, and respiratory distress caused by pulmonary congestion. This syndrome may develop either as a sudden event or slowly after hospital admission. There is a wide range in the clinical manifestations and severity of cardiogenic shock, and all components for classic cardiogenic shock may not be present. Clinical pulmonary edema need not be present to diagnose or suspect cardiogenic shock. An adequate or elevated pulmonary capillary wedge pressure (PCWP) should be documented by right-sided heart catheterization in the setting of systemic hypotension to confirm the diagnosis when pulmonary edema is not present (unless RV cardiogenic shock is diagnosed) (see Right Ventricular Infarction). A short mitral deceleration time by echo Doppler confirms elevated LV filling pressures, but a normal deceleration time does not exclude it (127). In the SHOCK Trial Registry, 29% of patients diagnosed with cardiogenic shock caused by predominant LV failure had no pulmonary congestion on physical or radiographic examination, despite having mean PCWP of 22 mm Hg and LVEF of 30% (128).

Preshock

Categorization of patients is not absolute, and gray zones exist. Patients who develop delayed cardiogenic shock following MI often slowly slip into shock, with evidence of a low cardiac output clinically before the onset of hypotension. Sympathetic stimulation may result in maintenance of normal BP in patients with high systemic vascular resistance (SVR) and low cardiac

TABLE 20.3

INCIDENCE OF HEART FAILURE BY INITIAL REPERFUSION THERAPY AND MORTALITY AT 30 DAYS OR 6 MONTH FOR PATIENTS WHO PRESENT WITH HEART FAILURE

		Thrombolysis			PCI		
			Mortality (%)			Mortality (%)	
Study/reference	Total patients (*n*)	Incidence (%)	No CHF	CHF	Incidence (%)	No CHF	CHF
REGISTRIES							
ESCAMI,[a] 2003 (112)	1,379	17.6			11.2		
IWGICC, 2001 (241)	3,113		3.2	15.6		1.6	7.6
RCTs							
Thrombolytic							
ASSET,[b] 1988 (103)	5,005	17.7					
Primary PCI							
GUSTO IIb,[c] 1997 (113,114)	1138	4.9	12.8	21.7	4.3	8.9	10.2
Rescue PCI							
MERLIN, 2004 (115)	307	29.9			24.2		
REACT,[d] 2004 (116)	427	14.8			9.0		

[a]Retrospective comparison of patients enrolled in ESCAMI trial. Incidence of CHF was significantly lower in PCI versus fibrinolytic treated patients.
[b]ASSET: Incidence of CHF in placebo group was18.4% (*P* not significant versus thrombolysis).
[c]Six-month mortality.
[d]REACT: Incidence of severe CHF at 6 months; conservative therapy group (heparin)—15.6%. (Rescue PCI significantly reduced the composite endpoint of death, reinfarction, cerebrovascular accident and severe CHF, but not severe CHF alone.)
Mortality rate for patients with CHF was significantly lower in PCI versus fibrinolytic treated patients in Rott and GUSTO-IIb studies.
Rates presented do not include patients with cardiogenic shock for ESCAMI, IWGICC, and MERLIN studies.
Abbreviations: PCI, percutaneous coronary intervention; ESCAMI, Evaluation of the Safety and Cardioprotective effects of eniporide in Acute Myocardial Infarction; IWGICC, Israeli Working Group on Intensive Cardiac Care, Israel Heart Society; ASSET, Anglo-Scandinavian Study of Early Thrombolysis; GUSTO, Global Utilization of Strategies to Open Occluded Coronary Arteries in Acute Coronary Syndromes; MERLIN, Middlesbrough Early Revascularization to Limit Infarction Trial; REACT, Rescue Angioplasty versus Conservative Treatment or Repeat Thrombolysis Trial.

output. This preshock or nonhypotensive shock state is associated with predominantly anterior MI and a 46% in-hospital mortality in the SHOCK Trial Registry (129). Sinus tachycardia and low urine output are clinical findings of reduced SV and cardiac output. It must be appreciated that these signs reflect severe depression of cardiac output and necessitate rapid evaluation of patients before the onset of frank hypotension.

Electrocardiographic Findings: Cardiogenic Shock

Most patients have ECG findings consistent with an ST-elevation MI; however, 15% to 30% of patients who develop cardiogenic shock may have nonspecific ECG findings (81,123,124), including widespread ST-segment depression. Anterior ST depression with upright T waves that improve across the precordium suggests acute posterior MI. Most infarcts (81) are anterior. Patients often have multiple infarct locations on ECG that are a composite of old and new MIs.

Patients with cardiogenic shock caused by LV failure should have extensive ECG abnormalities consistent with massive, acute infarct, severe and diffuse acute ischemia, or evidence of prior substantial damage (e.g., extensive pathologic Q waves or left bundle branch block). A relative lack of ECG abnormalities in contrast to the severity of the hemodynamic status should alert one to another cause of cardiogenic shock such as aortic dissection or rupture of the myocardium (i.e., free wall, ventricular septum, papillary muscle, or chordae) or hemorrhage (see Table 20.1). Patients with first inferior or posterior or lateral MI do not develop cardiogenic shock caused by LV failure, and one should suspect acute severe MR. In patients with cardiogenic shock and mild ECG abnormalities, such as only limited ST-segment elevations, aortic dissection should be ruled out (see Table 20.1).

Echocardiography With Color Flow Doppler

Echocardiography with color flow Doppler is an extremely valuable diagnostic tool and should be obtained as rapidly as possible once CHF or cardiogenic shock is suspected. LV and RV function can be visualized, left atrial pressure and cardiac output estimated, and tamponade can be diagnosed (130–132). Color flow Doppler mapping can diagnose severe MR and VSR (132). Proximal aortic dissection with aortic insufficiency, pericardial tamponade, or both can also be visualized. In critically ill patients, who are often supported by mechanical ventilation, it may be difficult to obtain adequate images with transthoracic echocardiography, and transesophageal echocardiography may reveal a mechanical complication (133). Even adequate transthoracic echocardiography may miss localized MR caused by a flail mitral leaflet (130).

Management: Pharmacologic Therapy, Mechanical Support, and Revascularization

General Measures

Hypoxemia caused by pulmonary congestion must be corrected rapidly with mechanical ventilatory support to reduce the work of breathing and improve oxygenation, as necessary. Lactic acidosis, which is common in cardiogenic shock, leads to further myocardial depression and resistance to the vasopressor effects of catecholamines. Rapid correction of acidosis is extremely important and empiric hyperventilation is appropriate until arterial blood gas results can be obtained. Ventilator settings can then be guided by arterial blood gas values. Hyperventilation is preferred to administration of sodium bicarbonate for correction of acidosis because the buffering capacity of sodium bicarbonate is limited and short lived, requiring a large sodium load.

Bradycardia and atrioventricular (AV) block must be corrected. If pacing is indicated, dual chamber pacing is preferred to preserve atrial contraction. New-onset AF should be rapidly cardioverted. An antiarrhythmic agent, such as amiodarone, may be required to maintain sinus rhythm. When severe LV dysfunction leads to reduction in SV, high heart rates are necessary to maintain cardiac output. This needs to be taken into account when setting the heart rate for patients with hemodynamically significant bradycardia who require pacing. In general, heart rates of approximately 90 to 100 beats per minute are advisable.

Volume Status

Pulmonary Congestion. Pulmonary congestion with acute MI is caused by a transient or sustained increase in the PCWP. Patients who present with pulmonary edema who have no prior history of myocardial dysfunction and have not received fluid administration have a normal total body sodium and fluid status. There is acute redistribution of fluid into the lungs, and with diaphoresis and no oral intake, there is relative intravascular depletion in the early phase. Diuretics can cause further intravascular depletion and hypotension and can precipitate cardiogenic shock. It must also be appreciated that there is a lag between normalization of the PCWP and resolution of interstitial and alveolar edema (134). Patients with findings on examination or on chest roentgenography suggesting congestion (e.g., basilar rales or interstitial fluid) for 24 hours do not necessarily require continued diuretic therapy provided dyspnea is resolving and respiratory status is improving. Excessive diuresis may result in severe intravascular depletion in patients who present with pulmonary edema, which initiates a vicious cycle of hypotension, hypoperfusion, infarct extension, ischemia, additional LV dysfunction, and so forth (see Fig. 20.2). The best means of assessing volume status is careful measurement of the intake and output record, including the prehospital and emergency department phases as well as patient weight. Measurement of PCWP is useful but reflects ventricular compliance as well as volume status. An elevated blood urea nitrogen to creatinine ratio may reflect intravascular depletion or poor renal perfusion caused by a low cardiac index (CI). However, a low blood urea nitrogen level in a patient with severely depressed LVEF and persistent pulmonary congestion reflects underdiuresis.

The volume status of patients with prior myocardial dysfunction and prior use of diuretics is more variable. These patients may be volume overloaded because of chronic CHF, or those on chronic diuretics may be intravascularly depleted at the time of onset of their acute MI, with a sudden increase in PCWP caused by acute infarction.

Hypotension. Hypotension complicating acute MI may be caused by hypovolemia as a result of vomiting, diaphoresis, use of diuretics, or associated hemorrhage. In addition, many of the medications (e.g., nitrates, morphine) administered during acute MI cause venodilation and preload reduction, which, in turn, causes hypotension. Placing the patient in Trendelenburg position is appropriate for treatment of these causes of hypotension. For patients who do not have evidence on examination or on chest roentgenography of pulmonary congestion and who are not in respiratory distress, an empiric intravenous volume challenge of 250 mL of normal saline can be given. Repeated empiric fluid challenges may be used before pulmonary artery catheterization or echo Doppler assessment, but caution must be exercised for those at increased risk for precipitation of CHF with volume infusion (e.g., older patients, patients with prior MI, prior CHF or impaired LV function, hypertensive heart disease, diabetes, and a small body size). Transcutaneous continuous oximetric monitoring of systemic oxygen saturation is advised. In some patients, hypotension and bradycardia are manifestations of Bezold–Jarisch reflex or a vasovagal response to volume depletion. Although atropine may be helpful, the key to management is fluid administration. This is particularly true in patients with a first inferior MI and in association with the administration of nitrates, which accentuates preload reduction in an already volume-depleted patient. Pulmonary artery catheterization is needed only in refractory patients. Overly vigorous fluid challenges in patients with extensive LV infarction result in pulmonary edema and should be avoided. Elderly patients, in particular, have reduced LV compliance and are sensitive to excessive administration of fluids.

Pulmonary Congestion and Hypotension—Cardiogenic Shock

When pulmonary congestion and hypotension are both present, and cardiogenic shock is diagnosed, and a fluid challenge is contraindicated. Diuretics have a limited role in the acute management of these patients because they can cause further hypotension and are ineffective because of marked reduction in renal blood flow and glomerular filtration. The circulation must be first supported by pharmacologic and mechanical interventions discussed in the following sections, followed by intravenous diuretics.

Medications

General. Negative inotropic agents such as β-blockers and calcium channel antagonists should be avoided in patients with acute large infarctions and pump failure. This does not preclude the use of β-blockers as secondary prevention at a later time in the clinical course once hemodynamics are stabilized. β-Blockers, initiated in low doses, are indicated in these patients before hospital discharge (56). Amiodarone is the agent of choice for ventricular tachycardia or fibrillation that occurs in patients with severe pump failure. Medications cleared primarily by the kidneys or liver must be used in reduced doses in patients with hepatic or renal dysfunction and end-organ hypoperfusion. In particular, lidocaine doses must be reduced when this agent is used to treat ventricular arrhythmias.

Morphine sulfate reduces preload and therefore improves pulmonary congestion. It also provides analgesia and lessens anxiety. To avoid hypotension, small incremental doses (2 to 4 mg) should be administered.

Medications that are used in acute MI patients with or without pump failure are discussed in Chapter 19.

Specific Medications

Diuretics. Furosemide, 20 mg intravenously, should be the initial dose for patients who have not been given diuretics and who have normal creatinine levels; higher and repeated doses should be given as needed. Other loop diuretics, such as torsemide, bumetanide, or ethacrynic acid, are alternatives. After the early phase of acute MI with pulmonary congestion, continued doses of diuretics are necessary for patients with significantly impaired LV systolic function and persistent CHF. Potent loop diuretics also activate the renin–angiotensin–aldosterone system, thereby leading to an increase in cardiac afterload and promoting sodium retention once their short-term effects resolve. For refractory patients, a combination of a loop and a thiazide diuretic, such as hydrochlorothiazide or metolazone, produces additive effects. Diuretics should be withheld or the dosage reduced when ACE inhibitors are initiated to avoid hypotension and transient renal insufficiency.

Nitrates. Sublingual followed by intravenous nitroglycerin is the ideal medication for patients with elevated LV pressures, moderate or no reduction in cardiac output, and normal or elevated systemic arterial pressure. Its acute use is preferred over intravenous loop diuretics for the treatment of pulmonary congestion for the reasons discussed (135,136). At low doses (<10 μg/minute), the dominant effect of nitroglycerin is on the venous circulation. At higher doses, intravenous nitroglycerin dilates the arteriolar circulation as well, and therefore may significantly decrease systemic arterial pressure (61). PCWP falls promptly, which rapidly improves symptoms of dyspnea. Myocardial ischemia is decreased by a reduction in myocardial diastolic wall tension, which decreases myocardial oxygen requirements. Nitroglycerin also may improve oxygen delivery by dilating coronary vessels and decreasing resistance in the coronary collateral circulation (135). Nitroglycerin reduces ischemic MR due to LV dilatation by reducing the LVEDV (137).

Renin–angiotensin–aldosterone system inhibitors. ACE inhibitors improve LV performance by reducing cardiac preload and afterload in patients with heart failure and acute MI. The renin–angiotensin–aldosterone system is frequently activated in patients with acute MI (76) and further activated in patients with CHF. In addition to directly blocking the renin–angiotensin–aldosterone system, ACE inhibitors vasodilate by increasing circulating bradykinins (138). Other beneficial effects on atherogenesis and plaque rupture may occur at a cellular level and the long-term vascular event rate is reduced. ACE inhibitors produce a dilating effect on the cerebral, coronary, and renal circulation, decreasing blood flow in the hepatic and splanchnic circulations (139,140). ACE inhibitors should be instituted early in patients with pulmonary congestion and particularly in those with hypertension. They should be administered orally and initiated in low doses with rapid upward titration, provided hypotension is not induced. ACE inhibitors should not be used acutely in patients who are hypotensive.

Ramipril instituted between days 3 and 10 significantly reduced 30-day mortality (relative hazard, 0.73; 95% confidence interval: 0.602–0.89; $P < .002$) in patients presenting with acute CHF complicating MI (141). Patients with pump failure complicating acute MI, including those whose cardiogenic shock has resolved, should be treated with ACE inhibitors. The timing of initiation depends on blood pressure stability, with hypertensive or normotensive patients tolerating early initiation. Early (≤ 12 hours) oral initiation of captopril, 6.25 mg, is recommended for patients presenting with pulmonary congestion. The dosage may be doubled with each subsequent dose, as tolerated up to 25 to 50 mg every 8 hours. Hypotension should be avoided, particularly during reperfusion; we therefore recommend initiating oral ACE inhibitors after direct PCI or thrombolysis has established reperfusion. If reperfusion fails or is not attempted, early administration of ACE inhibitors plays an important role. Long-acting ACE inhibitors (e.g., enalapril, lisinopril, ramipril, trandolapril) can be given after the acute phase.

Angiotensin receptor blockers are an acceptable alternative to ACE inhibitors for patients with LV dysfunction or heart failure following MI based on their similar efficacy in the Valsartan in Acute Myocardial Infarction Trial study (142). An aldosterone antagonist, eplerenone reduced all-cause mortality at 1 year by 15% when added to optimal management in patients with EF <40% and heart failure or diabetes. An aldosterone antagonist (eplerenone or aldactone) is recommended for these patients who do not have hyperkalemia or creatinine of at least 2.5 (143).

Pharmacologic Circulatory Support

General. The choice of a sympathomimetic agent for patients with pump failure depends on the patient's hemodynamics and, specifically, whether hypotension is present. Patients with pulmonary congestion without significantly depressed cardiac output should be treated with vasodilators alone. Patients with an elevated PCWP and a CI of 2.5 L/min/m^2 or less and with systolic blood pressure of at least 100 mm Hg can be treated with combined inotropic and vasodilating agents, such as dobutamine or milrinone if needed for hypoperfusion. Patients with cardiogenic shock and profound hypoperfusion need initial vasopressor support with alpha-dose dopamine or norepinephrine.

The lowest doses of sympathomimetic amines needed to maintain adequate cardiac output and adequate systemic perfusion should be used. For patients in cardiogenic shock, pulmonary artery catheter measurements are useful to guide therapy, but the targets for medication titration are clinical measures of systemic perfusion and oxygenation, not hemodynamic values. All sympathomimetic agents may cause atrial and ventricular tachyarrhythmias.

Dobutamine. This synthetic catecholamine increases myocardial contractility through preferential stimulation of myocardial β_1-adrenergic receptors. β_2-Peripheral vasodilator receptors and myocardial α_1-adrenergic receptors are also stimulated, but to a lesser extent. Dobutamine has less chronotropic effect than does dopamine and typically does not cause significant changes in heart rate when the dose is less than 15 μg/kg/min. The initial dose of dobutamine is 2 μg/kg/min followed by a gradual increase in dose to 15 μg/kg/min as needed. The lowest dosage required should be used for maintenance. Cardiac output should increase, and PCWP should decrease. SVR decreases somewhat, and the balance of the increase in cardiac output and the decrease in SVR results in unchanged blood pressure. Dobutamine therefore is not the drug of choice for hypotension. Its short half life—approximately 2 minutes—is highly desirable because it can be discontinued if ventricular tachycardia develops or it can be titrated down for excess increases in heart rate.

A concern with use of any inotropic agent is the risk for increase in myocardial oxygen requirements by increased myocardial contractility, tachycardia, and exacerbation of myocardial ischemia. However, when LV dilation and elevated diastolic filling pressures are present, wall tension decreases because dobutamine reduces EDV and pressure (144,145). Although dobutamine improves the patient's immediate hemodynamic status, there are no randomized trials assessing its effect on outcome.

Dopamine. The hemodynamic effects of dopamine are dose dependent and vary from patient to patient. Low doses (1–3 μg/kg/min) result in renal vasodilation caused by dopamine receptor stimulation. Intermediate doses of 5 to 10 μg/kg/min result in β_1-adrenergic stimulation and increased myocardial contractility. High doses (≥ 15 μg/kg/min) result in α_1-receptor stimulation and arterial vasoconstriction. High-dose dopamine increases pulmonary vascular pressures, including PCWP, as well as systemic arterial pressure. High-dose dopamine is required for cardiogenic shock with profound hypotension to support perfusion of the vital organs. As other support measures are instituted (e.g., IABP), dopamine should be titrated down to the minimum dosage required.

Norepinephrine and Epinephrine. Norepinephrine is a powerful α_1 stimulant that results in arterial vasoconstriction and is a β_1-stimulant that increases inotropy. It is used primarily for profound hypotension—for example, systolic blood pressure less than 70 mmHg—to maintain systemic and coronary perfusion pressures. Epinephrine also acts on the β_1 myocardial receptors and on both α_2- and β_2-receptors in peripheral blood vessels. Small amounts may constrict renal as well as cutaneous vessels while dilating skeletal and mesenteric vessels, which may result in a decrease in blood pressure. At higher doses, epinephrine acts primarily as a vasoconstrictor. It causes tachycardia and arrhythmias, which limit its use in acute MI with cardiogenic shock, except in resuscitating patients in cardiac arrest.

When dynamic outflow obstruction contributes to hemodynamic instability, as in hypertrophic or Takotsubo cardiomyopathy, predominant α_1 stimulants are preferred.

Other Medications. Digoxin increases myocardial contractility to a lesser extent than dobutamine or phosphodiesterase inhibitors, and is associated with an increased risk of ventricular arrhythmias during the first 24 hours of acute MI. Therefore, digoxin has no clear role in acute pulmonary congestion or cardiogenic shock complicating MI. Digoxin may be useful for patients with pump failure and AF with a rapid ventricular response, because it does not have the negative inotropic properties of β-blockers or verapamil and diltiazem.

Phosphodiesterase inhibitors, such as milrinone and amrinone, are positive inotropic and vasodilating agents. When cardiac output is severely reduced, the combination of lower doses of phosphodiesterase inhibitors and dobutamine may produce additive effects. Phosphodiesterase inhibitors have been studied in a limited number of patients with acute MI (146).

Levosimendan, a calcium-sensitizing drug with positive inotropic and vasodilating properties, reduced the rate of death or worsening heart failure in a placebo-controlled dose-ranging study of 504 patients with LV failure complicating acute MI (147). In a small case study, levosimendan administration resulted in an increase in CI and a decrease in SVR in cardiogenic shock patients supported with vasopressors and IABP (148).

Arginine vasopressin (AVP) a potent vasopressor hormone, is effective at raising blood pressure in vasodilatory shock states. In preliminary results of a small study of AVP versus dopamine for cardiogenic shock, AVP resulted in beneficial hemodynamic effects (149).

Nitric oxide synthase inhibitors (LNNMA and LNAME) block the synthesis of nitric oxide. These agents appeared to result in improved hemodynamics and survival in two small single center studies (89,150). A phase II dose-ranging trial demonstrated dose-related early rise in blood pressure; a phase III trial is in progress.

Nesiritide has not been investigated in patients with recent MI and should not be used in this setting.

Mechanical Circulatory Support

Mechanical circulatory support plays an extremely important role in providing temporary support for patients in cardiogenic shock. Support devices are superior to pharmacologic support for cardiogenic shock in that perfusion is improved without increasing myocardial work or O_2 consumption. It must be noted, however, that mechanical circulatory support alone has never been demonstrated in randomized trials to improve outcome in patients with cardiogenic shock.

Intraaortic Balloon Counterpulsation. The IABP is placed through the femoral artery into the descending thoracic aorta distal to the left subclavian artery and above the renal arteries, with balloon inflations and deflations synchronized with the cardiac cycle. This augments diastolic blood flow in the coronary and systemic circulation, and reduces afterload and aortic impedance. Both mechanisms increase CI and systemic and coronary diastolic pressures and improve myocardial metabolism (152). There are conflicting data on whether coronary flow distal to a critical stenosis increases with IABP. However, in hypotensive states an increase in aortic pressure by IABP should improve coronary blood flow (153), particularly when combined with PCI.

IABP remains extremely effective in supporting patients undergoing coronary angiography, PCI, and CABG in cardiogenic shock. It also provides bridging support until an LV assistance device can be implanted or cardiac transplantation can be performed.

IABP use in cardiogenic shock was independently associated with improved survival when combined with fibrinolytic therapy, PCI, or no reperfusion therapy only in centers that insert several devices per month (154). Rapid IABP insertion and transfer of patients from primary to tertiary care hospitals is associated with improved survival. American College of Cardiology/American Heart Association guideline indications for use of IABP include preparation for angiography and revascularization in cardiogenic shock that has not quickly reversed, acute MR or VSR, refractory post-MI angina (56), and refractory ventricular arrhythmias with hemodynamic instability. Less firm indications include hemodynamic instability without shock, poor LV function, or persistent ischemia with large regions at risk (56). Risks associated with IABP include (a) leg ischemia possibly necessitating thrombectomy, vascular surgery, or amputation; (b) dissection, perforation, or damage to the aorta with insertion; (c) hemorrhage; and (d) infection and thrombocytopenia. Full-dose intravenous heparin is required. IABP is contraindicated when significant aortic insufficiency is present or when peripheral vascular disease is severe or aortic pathology (e.g., aortic aneurysm) precludes it. IABP is not effective when there is no spontaneous circulation, and the timing of IABP inflation is difficult when there are uncontrolled tachyarrhythmias.

Other Percutaneous Left Ventricular Support Devices. The Tandem Heart provides nonpulsatile flow of oxygenated blood, extracted from the left atrium through septal puncture, into the femoral artery. Hemodynamics are improved compared to IABP but survival appears to be similar with increased complications in patients supported with the Tandem Heart (155, 156). A motor-driven turbine catheter (Impella device), advanced retrograde into the LV, increases CI and reduces PCWP (157). Surgically implanted ventricular assist devices may be used as a bridge to cardiac transplantation for suitable candidates.

Coronary Artery Reperfusion and Revascularization

Rapid reestablishment of blood flow in a totally occluded IRA is the single most important treatment of acute MI. This is true for patients with pump failure, in whom the absolute gain is large based on the high event rates (158–163). Randomized trial results confirm that early revascularization with either PCI or CABG improves 1-year survival compared with initial aggressive medical stabilization, including thrombolysis and IABP (163).

Congestive Heart Failure

Mortality among patients with CHF complicating acute MI (Killip classes II and III) has been modestly reduced by reperfusion therapy (see Table 20.3) (50,107). Limited trial and large registry data show superiority of primary PCI over fibrinolysis for patients with CHF complicating acute MI. Absolute reduction in events with direct PCI is larger than for Killip class I patients based on higher risk. Unfortunately, mortality remains high even with direct PCI. It is likely that prior and acute irreversible myocardial damage in many of these patients results in mortality that is significantly higher than among patients who present without CHF. Nevertheless, early successful reperfusion is the goal. We recommend direct PCI when available; if direct PCI is not available, thrombolytic therapy should be administered with rescue PCI for failure of reperfusion. Based on the high event rate among patients with CHF complicating MI if early PCI was not performed, subsequent revascularization is indicated based on the anatomy. If CABG is indicated for multivessel disease, its timing must be individualized based on whether the IRA is patent and on the patient's degree of pulmonary congestion and clinical stability.

Cardiogenic Shock

Thrombolysis. There is limited efficacy of thrombolysis in patients who present in shock, but if blood pressure is augmented by aggressive use of vasopressors or by IABP (58) during reperfusion, the rate of thrombus dissolution can be improved. If mechanical revascularization is not feasible, firbinolytic therapy is indicated and results in improved survival (7 lives saved per 100 patients treated) (164).

Mechanical Revascularization

Percutaneous transluminal coronary angioplasty. The in-hospital mortality ranges from 30% to 60% in patients undergoing PCI for cardiogenic shock (94,118,159,160). The overall success rate for PCI in shock is lower (~75%) than for primary PCI for acute MI and failure to achieve TIMI 2 or 3 flow is highly associated with in-hospital death.

The randomized SHOCK Trial Registry compared a direct invasive strategy of emergency early revascularization to initial medical stabilization including thrombolysis and IABP, followed by delayed revascularization as clinically determined. At 6 and 12 months, 13 lives were saved for every 100 patients treated with early revascularization compared with intensive medical therapy, thrombolysis, and delayed revascularization if warranted (163). This benefit is comparable with that seen at 1 year with CABG surgery for left main disease in stable patients and is sustained at up to 8 years of follow-up (Fig. 20.3). The improved survival was seen for patients with early

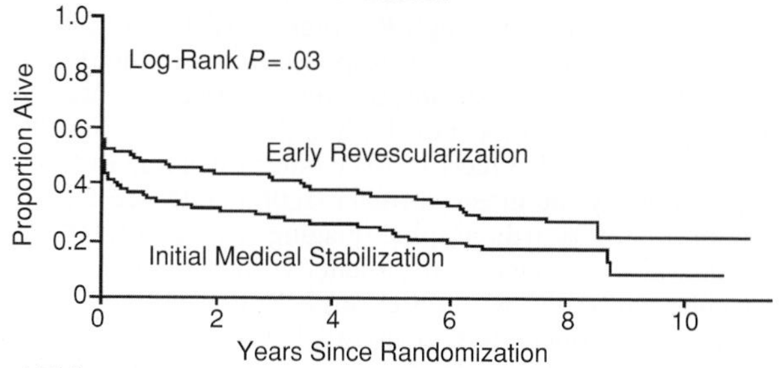

No. of Risk						
ERV	152	56	42	33	16	3
IMS	150	38	20	19	9	2

FIGURE 20.3. Kaplan-Meier survival curve up to 11 years postrandomization for patients with acute myocardial infarction complicated by cardiogenic shock caused by predominant left ventricular failure. Among all patients, the survival rates in the early revascularization (ERV) and initial medical stabilization (IMS) groups, respectively, were 41.4% vs. 28.3% at 3 years and 32.8% vs. 19.6% at 6 years. Among hospital survivors, the survival rates in the ERV and IMS groups, respectively, were 78.8% vs. 64.3% at 3 years and 62.4% vs. 44.4% at 6 years. *JAMA* 2006;295:2511–2515.

and late shock and regardless of infarct location or the presence of comorbidities (e.g., diabetes, prior hypertension, or MI). Although the small subgroup of those older than 75 years ($n = 56$) did not appear to benefit, there were imbalances between the groups and larger registries demonstrate a markedly lower in-hospital mortality for elderly patients who were clinically selected for early revascularization, even after adjustment for their lower risk profile (165–167). More than 80% of trial survivors were in New York Heart Association CHF class I to II at 1 year postinfarct (168).

PCI should be performed with IABP support. Use of stents and GP IIb/IIIa antagonists are independently associated with improved survival (94). The outcome of patients who underwent rescue PCI after thrombolysis was similar to those who underwent direct PCI in the SHOCK Trial (169). Most patients have triple-vessel disease (65%) and the options for revascularization include (a) PCI of the IRA followed by complete revascularization by multivessel PCI; (b) initial multivessel PCI; (c) initial CABG; and (d) PCI of the IRA followed by CABG. These strategies have not been directly compared. We recommend PCI for patients with one-, two-, or moderate three-vessel disease and CABG for those with severe three-vessel or left main disease. (87). Continuous noninvasive monitoring of the systemic oxygen saturation is required. Most patients with cardiogenic shock have required prior intubation; for others, intubation is recommended before injecting angiographic dye. Low osmolality ionic contrast dye is recommended. Despite these measures, relatively low PCI success rates and no reflow remain challenges. Approximately one third of patients improve rapidly and dramatically after PCI, whereas most show no immediate hemodynamic improvement. Patients may deteriorate hemodynamically after reperfusion is established, particularly if they are reperfused late. It is not uncommon for significant arrhythmias, including profound bradycardia and ventricular fibrillation, to develop during reperfusion in these patients. Immediate therapy must be available.

Coronary artery bypass surgery. In patients with shock, severe triple-vessel disease is present in most, and left main disease is present in 20% (159,170). Such patients are often unsuitable for PCI; hence, CABG is the preferred alternative. The in-hospital mortality among patients who underwent CABG at some time during their hospitalization for cardiogenic shock complicating acute MI was 35%. This constitutes the lowest mortality reported for cardiogenic shock in acute MI (81,161,170). Despite significantly higher rates of left main and triple-vessel CAD the 30-day and 1-year mortality for those who underwent emergency CABG was the same as for those who underwent emergency PCI (159,171).

We recommend emergency early CABG with IABP support for patients with cardiogenic shock and severe triple-vessel or left main disease, or with associated severe MR. Although some surgeons prefer a period of medical stabilization, there is a high risk of death on the first day (almost 50% of all deaths). The SHOCK Trial demonstrated that an initial intensive medical stabilization approach was associated with poorer 1-year survival than early revascularization (163).

Optimization of cardioprotection is most critical in patients with severe LV dysfunction and shock, and cardioprotective techniques including antegrade and retrograde cardioplegia, warm induction, prolonged vented bypass, and use of substrate-enriched blood have been advocated (170).

Summary

Rapid support of the circulation and restoration of IRA blood flow is the goal for managing patients with acute LV failure complicating MI. We strongly recommend rapid IABP support, coronary angiography, and revascularization. The choice of PCI or CABG is based on the coronary anatomy and the experience of the personnel. For hospitals without the facilities for PCI or CABG, thrombolytic agents should be administered for patients within 3 hours of MI onset with aggressive measures to augment blood pressure, including IABP, followed rapidly by transfer to tertiary care facilities. For young patients who do not respond to available measures, LV assistance devices should be considered as a bridge to urgent cardiac transplantation. Despite the marked reduction in mortality and the good functional class of survivors, overall 30-day survival is only 50% with aggressive care. Patients, especially the elderly, and their families must be involved in the decisions regarding their care, which should be individualized.

RIGHT VENTRICULAR INFARCTION

Pathology

RV infarction is typically associated with an inferior MI involving the interventricular septum and with occlusion of the proximal right coronary artery. Because the right ventricle is a thin-walled chamber that functions at low oxygen demands and low pressure with coronary perfusion throughout systole and diastole, extensive irreversible infarction is unusual with long-term recovery of function being the rule (172,173). RV infarction is typically seen in association with LV infarction (174).

Clinical Profile

Incidence

Depending on the diagnostic criteria used, the incidence of RV infarction in patients with inferior MI ranges from 10% to 50%. Most of these patients do not develop hypotension or cardiogenic shock. In the SHOCK Trial Registry, 2.8% of patients with suspected cardiogenic shock had shock caused by isolated RV failure (175).

Clinical Findings

The clinical manifestations of RV infarction include marked sensitivity to preload reduction (nitrates, morphine sulphate, diuretics), hypotension, and, infrequently, cardiogenic shock (176–178). High-grade AV block and bradyarrhythmias are common (179,180) because they are both consequences of proximal right coronary artery occlusion. Right atrial (RA) to left atrial shunting resulting in hypoxemia occurs infrequently in patients with RV failure and patent foramen ovale or atrial septal defect (181). RV free wall rupture and tamponade are rare, but patients with extensive RV necrosis are at risk for RV catheter-related perforation.

Diagnosis

The classic, clinical constellation of hypotension, elevated jugular venous pressure with clear lung fields, and no dyspnea is specific but insensitive for RV infarction (182). When performed early after onset of symptoms, ECG can be highly sensitive and specific. Right precordial (RV) leads should be obtained in patients with inferior MI. An ST elevation of 0.5 mm or more in lead V_{4R} is highly sensitive (183) and correlates with major clinical complications (184). Echocardiography and gated blood pool scintigraphy are effective (185) in diagnosing clinically significant RV infarction by assessing RV size and wall motion. Echocardiography is typically preferred because it can be performed at the bedside and simultaneously offers assessment of pericardial effusion and tamponade and acute PE, which are the chief differential diagnoses when predominant RV infarction and hypotension are present.

Accepted hemodynamic criteria for dominant RV infarction include a RA pressure greater than 10 mm Hg, an RA/PCWP ratio of 0.8 or more, or an RA pressure that is no less than 5 mm Hg below the PCWP. These values may only be demonstrated after volume infusion (186). Equalization of RA pressure and PCWP is often seen, necessitating exclusion of cardiac tamponade. The CI will be no more than 2.2 L/min/m^2 in patients with severe RV dysfunction.

Prognosis

The prognosis for RV infarction is largely determined by the degree of associated LV infarction (187). Overall, RV infarction is an independent risk factor for death in patients with inferior MI, and this risk increases substantially with increasing age (188,189). For the small subset with shock, the in-hospital mortality is 53% (175). This poor prognosis is despite the predominance of single-vessel disease (65%). For survivors of acute RV infarction, the long-term prognosis is excellent, with improved RVEF seen over time (172,190).

Hemodynamics and Management

Although RV cauterization in animal models with normal pulmonary vascular resistance and an open pericardium has not resulted in significant hemodynamic abnormalities, the clinical syndrome of hemodynamic compromise with RV infarction has been well described (191,192). The difference between the animal model of isolated RV infarction and clinical isolated RV infarction is that in the latter, the associated infarction of the LV and the interventricular septum result in relatively elevated LV filling pressures and RV afterload as well as loss of the interventricular septal contribution to normal RV function (193). The role of the pericardium and ventricular interdependence is important to the understanding of the pathophysiology of RV failure. As the size of the RV cavity increases because of extensive infarction and volume administration, flattening of the interventricular septum or bowing of the septum into the left ventricle develops, resulting in restriction of LV filling (194,195) (Fig. 20.4). This resolves when the pericardium is removed (194).

Volume infusion became standard treatment for hypotension and low cardiac output in RV infarction based on the experimental data and early clinical series (176). However, CI rises in response to volume only in patients with low RA pressures. In patients with high RA pressures, the thin, infarcted RV wall markedly dilates in response to excess fluid and, because of pericardial restraint, the interventricular septum shifts into the LV. This important finding demonstrates that PCWP may not accurately reflect LVEDV but, rather, impaired LV filling caused by the interventricular septal shift (see Fig. 20.4). Therefore, echocardiographic imaging is critical for the diagnosis and management of patients with hemodynamic compromise caused by RV infarction, because the PCWP may be misleading. Nonetheless, an elevated PCWP is detrimental as a component of RV afterload. Hemodynamic monitoring is advisable. In patients with low output caused by dominant RV infarction, the RA should be maintained at 10 to 15 mm Hg and the PCWP should be maintained at less than or equal to 15 mm Hg. Ventricular interaction with limitation of LV filling by RV dilation may cause patients to deteriorate with excess volume administration. In addition, excess volume administration precipitates pulmonary edema when LV infarction is present in association with RV infarction.

If the jugular venous pressure is elevated in a patient with an inferior MI without hypotension, all that is necessary is to avoid preload reduction. For patients with hypotension and RV

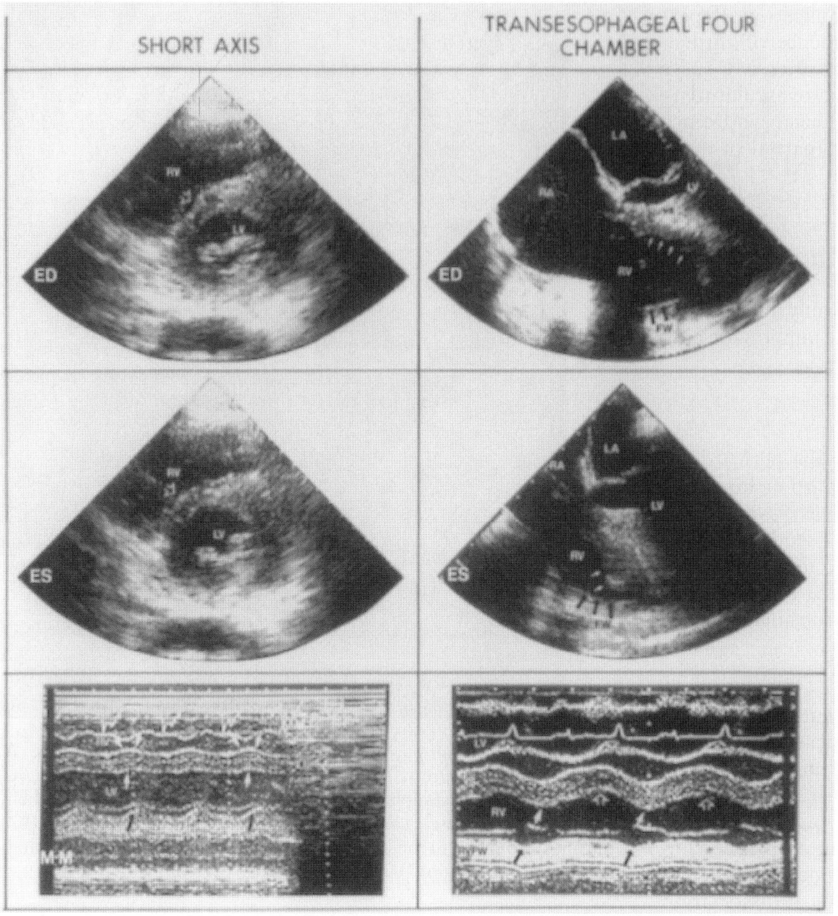

FIGURE 20.4. Transthoracic, transesophageal, and M-mode echocardiograms from a patient with RV infarction, refractory shock, and RA infarction. In short axis at end diastole (ED), the right ventricle (RV) is markedly dilatated, and the interventricular septal curvature is reversed (*open arrow*) with a shift into the left ventricle (LV). The four-chamber view demonstrates marked RA enlargement as well as severe RV dilation and bowing of the septum into the LV (*white arrows*). At end systole (ES), the septum bulges paradoxically into the RV in both short-axis (*open arrow*) and four-chamber views (*white arrows*). RV free wall (FW, *dark arrows*) was dyskinetic in four-chamber view. These findings are confirmed in the M-mode views from the transthoracic and transesophageal images. Excess volume administration can cause RV dilatation, septal shift into the LV with impairment of LV filling, and paradoxic decrease in cardiac output despite an increase of pulmonary capillary wedge pressure. (*Source:* From Goldstein JA, Barzilai B, Rosamound TL, et al. Determinants of hemodynamic compromise with severe right ventricular infarction. *Circulation* 1990;82:359–368, with permission. Original figure courtesy of Dr. J. Goldstein.)

and first inferior MI, emergency empiric volume administration is indicated. These patients require variable amounts of fluid (200 mL to 1 L of fluid over the first several hours) depending on the estimated or measured RA pressure. If hypotension or evidence of low cardiac output persists, an emergency echocardiogram should be obtained, and subsequent management should be guided by pulmonary artery catheter monitoring of cardiac output. As noted, additional fluid administration may be detrimental. Patients who are at risk for pulmonary edema should not receive this degree of rapid volume administration. These patients include those with (a) prior MIs; (b) acute, extensive LV infarction; (c) associated MR or other valvular lesions; (d) acute anterior MI; and (e) advanced age. If pulmonary congestion is not present, these patients may receive 200 to 250 mL of fluid, and an emergency echocardiogram should be obtained.

The positive inotropic effects of dobutamine play an important role in managing patients with RV infarction and low CI. Dobutamine significantly increases the CI and RVEF and is superior to afterload reduction therapy with nitroprusside (196). Patients in whom the initial central venous pressure or RA pressure are greater than 10 mm Hg or in whom an initial volume infusion fails and leads to an increase in RA and PCWP but a persistently low CI should be treated with dobutamine. When pacing is indicated for sinus bradycardia or complete heart block, it should be dual-chamber pacing. Of note, there is an increased incidence of ventricular fibrillation with RV pacing caused by RV ischemia (197). IABP and pulmonary artery counterpulsation have been used for RV shock (198,199). In rare cases of refractory shock caused by RV infarction, pericardiectomy should be considered (194).

Reperfusion Therapy

Rapid reperfusion with either thrombolytics or direct PCI should be the initial treatment for RV infarction (200). RV infarction is associated with low rates of reperfusion by thrombolysis, possibly because of prolonged hypotension (59). Systemic arterial pressure should be augmented during thrombolytic administration for RV infarction with hypotension (58). We recommend direct (or rescue) PCI for those with hypotension.

MECHANICAL COMPLICATIONS OF ACUTE MYOCARDIAL INFARCTION

Cardiac Rupture: Overview

Rupture may occur through a zone of necrosis in the LV free wall, interventricular septum, papillary muscle, or the contiguous chordae tendineae (201,202). Spontaneous RV free wall rupture rarely occurs. When one of these types of rupture occurs, it is typically referred to as a *mechanical complication* of acute MI; when shock results, this is termed a *mechanical cause* of shock. The relative infrequency of the often lethal mechanical complications of acute MI should not detract from their importance because they are amenable to surgical repair and compatible with an excellent long-term prognosis among perioperative survivors. Acute MR without papillary muscle rupture can cause severe hemodynamic compromise and is discussed in this section as a mechanical complication. Reperfusion therapy has reduced the overall incidence of cardiac rupture and shifted its occurrence to earlier after MI onset (203,204). Failure to establish flow in the microvasculature is a risk factor for rupture (2,3,205). Distinct clinical syndromes result, depending on the location and extent (partial or complete) of the rupture.

Left Ventricular Free Wall Rupture

Rupture of the LV free wall is not a uniformly fatal event, and early recognition of rupture with subacute tamponade may result in successful intervention.

Pathology

Pseudoaneurysm. Rupture that is sealed by the pericardium and then develops into a discrete aneurysmal outpouching with a narrow neck is referred to as a *pseudoaneurysm* or false aneurysm (see Fig. 20.3) (22). The wall of a pseudoaneurysm is composed of pericardium and not infarcted myocardium or scar tissue, in contrast to a true LV aneurysm. The neck of a pseudoaneurysm is narrower than that of a true aneurysm.

Clinical Profile

Subacute Ventricular Wall Rupture and Subacute Tamponade. Rupture with a period of temporary pericardial sealing (less stable than pseudoaneurysm) and subacute tamponade has been characterized in a (206) series of 1,457 consecutive patients with acute MI; approximately one third of 6.2% diagnosed with free wall rupture had a subacute presentation. The clinical constellation in these patients may include transient hypotension, syncope, transient electro-mechanical dissociation (EMD), chest pain (206), and transient bradycardia, repetitive emesis, and restlessness. These clinical findings are sensitive but nonspecific. The ECG findings of pericarditis may be seen and include persistent or new ST-segment elevations, persistently positive T waves, or inverted T waves becoming positive. However, these findings are insensitive and nonspecific (206). Subacute rupture can often be identified on echocardiography and successfully repaired (206,207). This is in contrast to the classic constellation of sudden chest pain and cardiovascular collapse with EMD seen in uncontained free wall rupture with tamponade. A right-sided heart catheterization can be performed to confirm tamponade hemodynamics with equalization of diastolic pressures, or MRI may show a rupture site (205) if the echocardiogram is not diagnostic.

Management

Early recognition of subacute rupture with echocardiography is critical for early intervention before uncontained intrapericardial hemorrhage and acute tamponade. Pericardiocentesis has been used to confirm that effusion is hemorrhagic and to relieve tamponade. However, we recommend emergency open drainage and repair, when possible, for subacute rupture with subacute tamponade. A stabilized patient with temporary sealing of the rupture site by thrombus on the epicardial surface is at risk for dislocation of the thrombus and precipitation of acute tamponade. Surgical repair is often successful and is accepted therapy (206,207). Unfortunately, the diagnostic criteria are not specific, and the decision to undergo surgical exploration frequently has to be made on the basis of a high index of clinical suspicion without definitive documentation of a site of rupture. Echocardiography may be helpful with the demonstration of an effusion, RV and RA compression, and shaggy, intrapericardial echo densities consistent with thrombus, at times visualized as a thrombus on the epicardial surface of the heart.

A,B

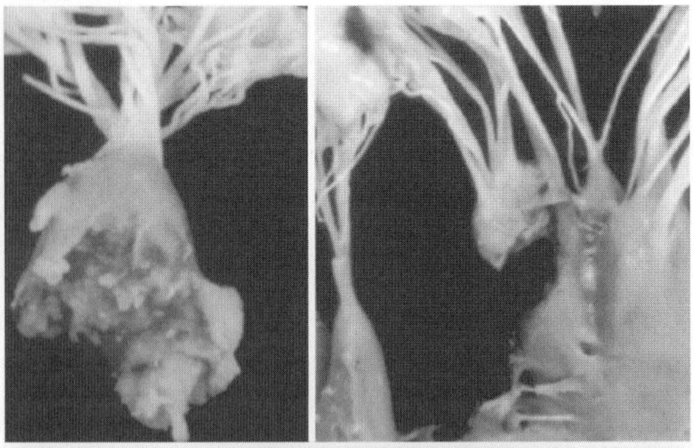

C

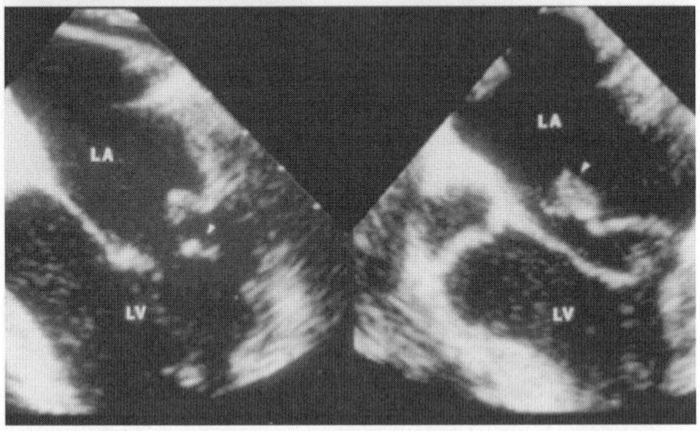

FIGURE 20.5. Examples of a ruptured belly of a papillary muscle (A) and a partial rupture (B) following acute myocardial infarction. (C) The utility of transesophageal echocardiography. The ruptured belly of the papillary muscle can be seen prolapsing into the left atrium (LA) during systole and in the left ventricle (LV) during diastole. (Pathology specimens courtesy of Dr. W. D. Edwards.)

Post–Myocardial Infarction Mitral Regurgitation

Pathophysiology

Post-MI MR may be due to papillary muscle rupture or, more commonly, LV remodeling. Dilation of the LV, which may be acute, alters the geometry of the mitral apparatus. The resultant tethering of the leaflets results in MR (208,209). Rupture of the papillary muscle may be partial or complete, but either condition results in severe MR (Fig. 20.5). The striking predominance of inferior infarcts in multiple studies of papillary muscle rupture (210,211) underscores the vulnerability of the posteromedial papillary muscle, which has blood supply from the posterior descending coronary artery alone, in contrast to the dual blood supply of the anterolateral papillary muscle from the LAD and circumflex arteries. Excellent long-term results from surgical correction may be obtained, largely because of the limited extent of LV necrosis (212). Medical therapy is ineffective in papillary muscle rupture.

Clinical Profile

Incidence, Patient Characteristics, and Prognosis. Acute MR often is common during the early phase of MI. It may be transient and is not usually the cause of hemodynamic compromise. The frequency of a murmur during MI has been reported to be 20% to 55% (213), but significant MR can often be silent. Angiographic studies (214,215) reported incidences of MR of 13% to 18% within hours of MI, while echocardiographic studies report 39% (213). The degree of MR after MI both early and later (216) in the course of MI is associated with mortality.

Acute severe MR was the cause of shock in 7% of patients with cardiogenic shock complicating MI in the SHOCK Trial Registry (81,217). Compared with those with LV failure, MR patients were more often female and had inferior and posterior infarcts. Although the EF was higher in patients with MR, the mean EF for those in shock was only 37%. The in-hospital mortality (55%) was similar to those with shock caused by LV failure (59%) (81).

Clinical Presentation and Diagnosis

The clinical picture of acute papillary muscle rupture is characterized by the sudden onset of pulmonary edema, hypotension, or both. Although older studies reported the onset approximately 2 to 7 days post-MI (210), the median time in the SHOCK Trial Registry was 22 hours (25%, 75%: 2, 36 hours) (217). As with other locations of myocardial rupture, thrombolytic therapy is associated with earlier occurrence and a reduced incidence of papillary muscle rupture. Other findings and physical examination are nonspecific. The apex beat may be dyskinetic, and heart sounds are usually soft, muffled, or masked by the auscultatory features of severe pulmonary edema. Accentuated pulmonary component of the second heart sound caused by pulmonary hypertension is often not appreciable. A harsh, but relatively short, systolic murmur typically is heard at the apex and left sternal edge; a thrill is uncommon. It should be strongly emphasized that the murmur may be soft or even absent as a result of the early pressure equalization between the left ventricle and left atrium caused by severe regurgitation into a nondilated atrial chamber and low-flow state. The key to the diagnosis is a high index of clinical suspicion, which should always be entertained in any patient with an inferior MI, particularly a first MI, who is hemodynamically compromised, particularly in the absence of any identifiable cause (e.g., large area of injury, an arrhythmia, PE, or tamponade) (Table 20.4).

Two-dimensional, and often transesophageal, echocardiography is a pivotal noninvasive diagnostic tool (218,219) (see Fig. 20.5). Identification of the freely mobile head of the papillary muscle either in the left atrium or the left ventricle or of a flail mitral leaflet is diagnostic (219). The addition of color flow imaging, with the aim of semiquantitation of the severity of MR, is very helpful. Transesophageal echocardiography may be particularly advantageous in patients on mechanical ventilation because transthoracic echocardiography may not provide adequate images. An extremely helpful clinical feature, particularly when the mitral valve apparatus is not well visualized, is the demonstration of reasonably well-preserved or even hyperdynamic LV function in the face of pulmonary edema, cardiogenic shock, or both. This constellation of clinical and echocardiographic features should point toward a mechanical complication as the cause of pulmonary edema or shock. Those in shock often may have depressed LV function (217). Documentation of tall V waves on PCWP tracing catheterization is a helpful finding but has limitations (220), and the role of pulmonary artery catheterization as a diagnostic modality has been superseded by advances in echocardiography. Nonetheless, pulmonary artery catheterization may be useful in monitoring the effects of pharmacologic therapy. Ventriculography may be required to confirm the severity of the MR in patients for whom surgery is being considered.

Management

The cornerstone of management is prompt diagnosis and aggressive medical therapy with a view to emergency cardiac surgery. Rapid IABP support is recommended for those in severe CHF or cardiogenic shock. The natural history of medically treated chordal or papillary muscle rupture, whether partial or complete, is poor and characterized by a volatile, unpredictable clinical course even when medical therapy results in initial stabilization (210). Sudden hemodynamic deterioration is frequent, and the consequences are usually catastrophic.

Papillary muscle rupture remains a potentially catastrophic and fatal complication of acute MI; however, there is a window of opportunity for emergency surgical correction with the encouraging prospect of excellent long-term survival and a return to an active life.

In contrast, patients with moderate or severe MR in the face of severely compromised LV function (i.e., EF <30%–35%), in whom clear evidence of papillary muscle or chordal rupture is not documented by echocardiography, pose a particularly difficult problem in diagnosis and management. The mechanism of MR in these patients may be underlying LV failure with dilation of the annulus or malalignment of the mitral valve apparatus caused by a severe regional wall motion abnormality adjacent to a papillary muscle or multiple areas by dyssynergy (209). A more prudent approach in these patients is aggressive medical therapy, including high-dose vasodilators and perhaps IABP. This may give time for LV function to improve and for additional diagnostic testing to help avoid the dilemma of a surgical procedure in the absence of a clearly delineated correctable cause of CHF. Factors to be addressed before performing surgery are the extent and reversibility of LV dysfunction, the potential for revascularization to improve LV size and function, the degree of MR, and the extent of structural abnormalities of the mitral valve apparatus.

TABLE 20.4

DIAGNOSTIC CONSIDERATIONS IN PATIENTS WITH INFERIOR MI AND CHF OR CARDIOGENIC SHOCK

Prior MI
High-grade AV block/bradyarrhythmias
Acute severe MR
RV infarction (characterized by an absence of pulmonary edema)
LV pseudorupture/subacute rupture
PE
Acute interventricular septal rupture

Abbreviations: AV, atrioventricular; CHF, congestive heart failure; LV, left ventricular; MI, myocardial infarction; MR, mitral regurgitation; PE, pulmonary embolism; RV right ventricular.

Acute Interventricular Septal Rupture

Incidence, Timing, Clinical Profile, and Prognosis

Acute rupture of the interventricular septum occurs in approximately 1% to 3% of all infarcts (221). In the SHOCK Trial Registry, VSR was the etiology of shock in 3.9% of those with shock complicating MI. Patients with VSR are more often older, female, with less prior MI and comorbidity compared with those without mechanical complications of MI (222) and with those with shock caused by LV failure. Older reports suggested that rupture occurred several days post-MI. However, in GUSTO 1 the median time to rupture was 1 day (223). When VSR causes shock, it occurs early after MI onset, with a median time of 16 hours for patients in the SHOCK Trial Registry. Once shock has developed, the prognosis is grim (87% mortality) (222).

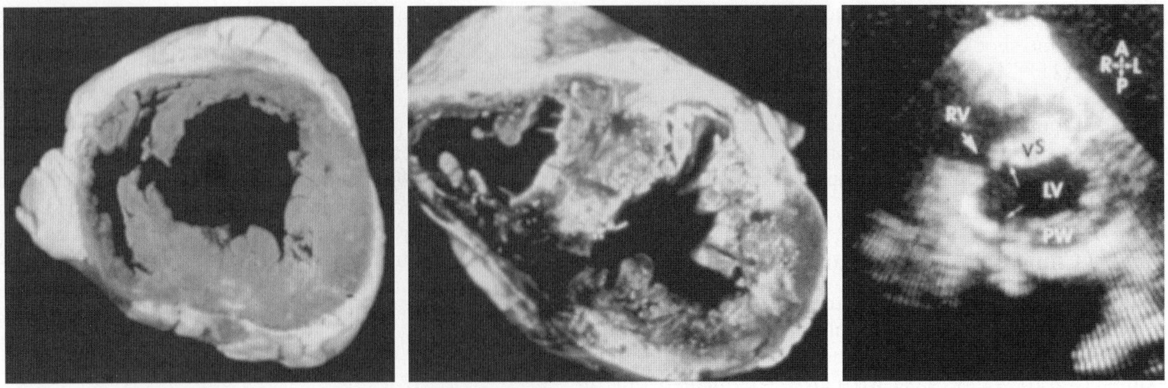

A–C

FIGURE 20.6. VSR complicating acute myocardial infarction. This illustrates two types of rupture of the ventricular septum, which in 53 autopsied hearts were simple (in 28 patients) or complex (in 25 patients). (**A**) Simple rupture is a direct through-and-through defect. (**B**) Complex ruptures are associated with serpiginous dissection tracts, which are remote from the primary site of tear of the ventricular septum. Complex ruptures are more frequent with inferior infarcts involving the inferobasal portion of the septum and may be associated with rupture of a second structure, such as the free wall of the right ventricle (RV) in this patient. (**C**) The marked utility of two-dimensional echocardiography in the diagnosis, illustrating a parasternal short-access view using transthoracic echocardiography. The echocardiogram illustrates a complex ventricular septal rupture. *Abbreviations:* LV, left ventricle; PW, posterior wall; VS, ventricular septum. (*Source:* From Edwards BS, Edwards WD, Edwards JE. Ventricular septal rupture complicating acute myocardial infarction: identification of simple and complex types in 53 autopsied hearts. *Am J Cardiol* 1984;54:1201–1205, with permission.)

Pathophysiology

Interventricular septal rupture is nearly always a complication of a transmural MI, particularly a first MI; however, in contrast to papillary muscle rupture, anterior or anterolateral infarcts are slightly more frequent than are inferior infarcts (223–225). A history of prior angina is uncommon, and hypertension may be a predisposing factor (223,225). Concomitant involvement of other structures including the papillary muscles and free wall of the left and right ventricles has been well described (224). Septal rupture may occur in patients with single-vessel disease, but multivessel disease is common. Two- or three-vessel CAD was present in 43% and 31%, respectively, in the SHOCK Trial Registry (222) and in 51% in GUSTO (223).

Interventricular septal rupture has been categorized morphologically into simple and complex forms (Fig. 20.6). The former is a discrete defect with a direct through-and-through communication across the septum, usually the apical septum. The ventricular openings are therefore at the same level on both sides of the septum. Complex ruptures are characterized by extensive hemorrhage around irregular, serpiginous tracts that extend in different directions within extensive necrotic tissue; they more frequently involve the inferobasal septum as a complication of inferior MIs. Complex ruptures are more likely to involve associated structures including extensive areas of the right ventricle (224).

Clinical Presentation and Diagnosis

The typical presentation is the acute development of shock and pulmonary edema in the face of severe right-sided heart failure and a new systolic murmur. The murmur is usually loud, pansystolic, and accompanied by a thrill in 50% of patients. The distinction between papillary muscle rupture and acute interventricular septal rupture can be made clinically on the basis of the intensity and characteristics of the murmur and the presence of a thrill and right-sided heart failure in most patients with septal rupture. Nonetheless, physical findings may be unreliable, particularly in a low-output state. Echocardiography with color flow Doppler demonstrates the interventricular shunt and may visualize the rupture site when adequate views are obtained.

If echocardiographic findings are not diagnostic, right heart catheterization can confirm the diagnosis by demonstration of a step-up in oxygen saturation in blood obtained from right ventricle compared to the right atrium. Left ventriculography can also confirm the diagnosis, but the decision to employ this diagnostic modality depends on the patient's hemodynamic stability and the need to identify the coronary anatomy in the event that concomitant coronary artery bypass surgery is being considered.

Management

The key to management is prompt diagnosis, an aggressive approach to stabilization, rapid angiography, and surgery (226). Medical therapy consists of diuretics, vasodilators, and frequently inotropes in addition to intermittent positive-pressure ventilation and IABP in patients with severe CHF or cardiogenic shock. As with papillary muscle rupture, initial stabilization via medical therapy may provide only a temporary respite.

A small, asymptomatic VSR may be managed without surgery. For most patients with VSR who are severely symptomatic, the need for surgical repair has never been questioned, but its timing has been an issue of debate. The current approach is to advocate early or emergency surgery in all patients, preferably before decompensation. It must be accepted that an aggressive approach may be associated with high perioperative mortality but may have the potential for an overall reduction in mortality (222,225). This is particularly relevant in patients with cardiogenic shock (as opposed to pulmonary edema alone); in patients with shock, short-term survival with medical therapy is extremely poor and apparent stabilization is usually transient (227–230). Percutaneous closure devices may play a role in very high-risk patients (231).

There is little consensus in the literature regarding the need for concomitant coronary revascularization during surgical repair of postinfarction VSR. Theoretically, revascularization of residual and viable but ischemic myocardium should facilitate weaning the patient off cardiopulmonary bypass and should accelerate recovery during the perioperative period as well as provide a beneficial effect on long-term outcome. There are, however, no prospective studies documenting the merits of such an approach. On balance, preoperative coronary angiography with a view to concomitant CABG appears reasonable and may be indicated, provided the patient is sufficiently stable as to tolerate the procedure (232).

In summary, the approach to patients with acute septal rupture and hemodynamic decompensation is rapid stabilization with IABP and prompt surgery. Rarely, patients with small shunts and without CHF who remain hemodynamically stable may be managed medically over the long term.

MISCELLANEOUS COMPLICATIONS OF ACUTE MYOCARDIAL INFARCTION

Pericarditis

Inflammation of the pericardium may occur acutely during MI and may be largely localized to the pericardium adjacent to the infarction, or it may occur as a delayed, more generalized inflammatory syndrome (Dressler syndrome). Pericarditis associated with acute infarction results from the infarction extending to the epicardial surface of the heart, with an associated inflammatory response.

Diagnosis

The diagnosis is made clinically by history, physical examination, and ECG. Pericarditic chest pain is typically sharp, severe, substernal pain that may radiate to the neck, shoulders, and back, increasing with inspiration and on reclining. Patients with pericarditis are often severely distressed and uncomfortable. A typical three-component pericardial friction rub may be heard, but may be absent when effusion develops. The typical ECG changes of pericarditis are uncommon when the pericarditis is localized to the infarct zone (233). Nonetheless, persistent or new ST-segment elevations in multiple leads may be seen when pericarditis is more generalized. Pericarditis should heighten the index of suspicion for subacute rupture and warrants echocardiography. Atypical T-wave evolution, either with T waves remaining consistently positive for 48 hours or longer after onset of acute MI or with initially inverted T waves gradually becoming positive deflections, has been described in postinfarction pericarditis (234). An effusion may or may not be present on echocardiography; presence of effusion is more common than clinical pericarditis (235). Most cases of acute pericarditis are diagnosed within 3 days of acute MI (236) but may occur as early as day 1.

Incidence

Clinical studies (236) report a higher incidence of pericarditis in patients with Q-wave MI than in patients with non–Q-wave MI; it is more common with large infarcts. Its clinical incidence varies depending on the diagnostic criteria. Most studies require a pericardial friction rub to be present. Large clinical trials such as GISSI-1 (50) define pericarditis as either a friction rub or as typical pericarditic chest pain. The incidence of postinfarction pericarditis has decreased by approximately 50% in patients treated with reperfusion therapy (50,233,236,237). Reperfusion therapy results in smaller infarcts that less often extend to the epicardial surface, resulting in less localized pericarditis.

Pericardial Effusion

Pericardial effusions occur relatively frequently after acute MI (incidence up to 45%) (235). They are more common with large, anterior infarcts and when CHF is present. They are typically asymptomatic. If tamponade develops, it is usually caused by free wall rupture or hemorrhage into the pericardium. Effusions most frequently occur without clinical pericarditis. Conversely, patients with clinical pericarditis frequently do not have associated effusion.

CONTROVERSIES AND PERSONAL PERSPECTIVES

Pump Failure

Randomized trial and large observational studies demonstrate that a direct invasive strategy, with IABP-supported rapid angiography, PCI, or CABG, markedly improves 1-year and long-term survival when post-MI shock develops caused by predominant LV failure. The treatment benefit is derived despite comorbidities such as diabetes and despite profound hemodynamic abnormalities. Regional care centers should be developed and patients directly transported to these centers to optimize outcomes in these critically ill patients who require expert specialized care. Although long-term survival is improved by intervention, even successful procedures are associated with high in-hospital mortality, and operators may be reluctant to intervene, particularly in states with "scorecard" public reporting of procedural complications (238). There is a wide range of mortality rates for those with shock and models currently used for risk prediction are inadequate because the hemodynamic parameters that have the best prognostic value, such as stroke work, may not be routinely assessed. State databases should separately analyze shock patients. Quality improvement measures must track not only procedural death rates but the rate of refusals for interventions based on the high-risk profile. However, when the outcome is grim even with intervention, such as surgery for VSR with inferior and RV MI once shock is present, treatment may be deemed futile.

Reperfusing Occluded Infarct-Related Arteries in Asymptomatic Patients: Any Benefits?

Despite the wealth of data implicating a beneficial effect of an open artery independent of myocardial salvage, the late open artery concept remains a tantalizing but unproven hypothesis. The implications for clinical practice, however, are far reaching. If it could be demonstrated that reperfusion of a closed IRA in asymptomatic patients without stress-induced ischemia reduces mortality or improves LV function, routine angiography in all MI survivors might then be recommended to identify those with an occluded IRA. To accomplish this, a randomized trial is ongoing.

THE FUTURE

Pump Failure

Prevention

Very early successful reperfusion is the most effective strategy to prevent pump failure. Effective public education and EMS systems are needed to reduce time to reperfusion. Strategies to prevent pump failure in patients at high risk need to be further investigated. Such studies should include (a) agents that inhibit the inflammatory response (e.g., complement inhibitors); (b) agents that inhibit production of high levels of nitric oxide and peroxynitrites; (c) therapies to limit myocardial necrosis such as cooling of ischemic myocardium or reperfusion with aqueous oxygenated blood.

Treatment

Agents that inhibit ongoing production of high levels of nitric oxide and alternative vasopressors and inotropes such as vasopressin and levosimendan should be investigated further. The role of newer LV support devices compared with IABP and criteria for selecting appropriate patients for LV support devices need to be defined.

Cardiac Rupture and Left Ventricular Remodeling: Basic Mechanisms

Measures to prevent cardiac rupture in patients at increased risk need to be evaluated. The role of interstitial matrix degradation by metalloproteinases in myocardial rupture should be explored further and metalloproteinase inhibitor evaluated in high-risk patients. Similarly, the effects of disruption of the intercellular collagen struts that link myofibrils with potential slippage of myocytes, infarct expansion, and LV remodeling and the role metalloproteinase inhibitors for patients at risk need to be investigated.

In summary, despite the dramatic advances in the treatment of acute MI, pump failure and myocardial rupture remain major challenges for the future and their basic mechanisms, prevention, and management must be explored and elucidated.

ACKNOWLEDGMENTS

We gratefully acknowledge the following persons for their help in the preparation of this chapter: Vinod Jorapur, MD, for his assistance with review of the literature and preparation of tables and references; Richard M. Fuchs, MD, and Harmony Reynolds, MD, for review and editing of the manuscript; Bernard Gersh, MD, for his contribution to prior editions; and Rachel Mansingh for assistance with all aspects of the manuscript preparation.

References

1. Edwards WD. Pathology of myocardial infarction and reperfusion. In: Gersh BJ, Rahimtoola SH, eds. *Acute myocardial infarction*. Boston: Chapman & Hall, 1996:16–50.
2. Ito H, Maruyama A, Iwakura K, et al. Clinical implications of the "no reflow" phenomenon: a predictor of complications and left ventricular remodeling in reperfused anterior wall myocardial infarction. *Circulation* 1996;93:223–228.
3. Bolognese L, Carrabba N, Parodi G, et al. Impact of microvascular dysfunction on left ventricular remodeling and long-term clinical outcome after primary coronary angioplasty for acute myocardial infarction. *Circulation* 2004;109:1121–1126.
4. Taylor AJ, Al-Saadi N, Abdel-Aty H, et al. Detection of acutely impaired microvascular reperfusion after infarct angioplasty with magnetic resonance imaging. *Circulation* 2004;109:2080–2085.
5. Hutchins GM, Bulkley BH. Infarct expansion versus extension: two different complications of acute myocardial infarction. *Am J Cardiol* 1978;41:1127.
6. Picard MH, Wilkins GT, Gillam LD, et al. Immediate regional endocardial surface expansion following coronary occlusion in the canine left ventricle: disproportionate effects of anterior versus inferior ischemia. *Am Heart J* 1991;121:753–762.
7. Hochman JS, Bulkley BH. Expansion of acute myocardial infarction: an experimental study. *Circulation* 1982;65:1446–1450.
8. Eaton LW, Weiss JL, Bulkley BH, et al. Regional cardiac dilatation after acute myocardial infarction: recognition by two-dimensional echocardiography. *N Engl J Med* 1979;300:57–62.
9. Pfeffer JM, Pfeffer MA, Fletcher PJ, et al. Progressive ventricular remodeling in rats with myocardial infarction. *Am J Physiol* 1991;260:H1406–H1414.
10. Olivetti G, Capasso JM, Sonnenblick EH, et al. Side-to-side slippage of myocytes participates in ventricular wall remodeling acutely after myocardial infarction in rats. *Circ Res* 1990;67:23–34.
11. Tziakas DN, Chalikias GK, Hatzinikolaou EI, et al. N-terminal pro-B-type natriuretic peptide and matrix metalloproteinases in early and late left ventricular remodeling after acute myocardial infarction. *Am J Cardiol* 2005;96:31–34.
12. Tennant R, Wiggers CJ. The effect of coronary occlusion on myocardial contraction. *Am J Physiol* 1935;112:351–361.
13. Hochman JS, Choo H. Limitation of myocardial infarct expansion by reperfusion independent of myocardial salvage. *Circulation* 1987;75:299–306.
14. Herzog E, Gu A, Kohmoto T, et al. Early activation of metalloproteinases after experimental myocardial infarction occurs in infarct and non-infarct zones. *Cardiovasc Pathol* 1998;7:307–312.
15. Pierard LA, Albert A, Gilis F, et al. Hemodynamic profile of patients with acute myocardial infarction at risk of infarct expansion. *Am J Cardiol* 1987;60:5–9.
16. Meltzer RS, Visser CA, Kan G, et al. Two-dimensional echocardiographic appearance of left ventricular thrombi with systemic emboli after myocardial infarction. *Am J Cardiol* 1984;53:1511–1513.
17. White HD, Norris RM, Brown MA, et al. Left ventricular end-systolic volume as the major determinant of survival after recovery from myocardial infarction. *Circulation* 1987;76:44–51.
18. Migrino RQ, Young JB, Ellis SG, et al. End-systolic volume index at 90 to 180 minutes into reperfusion therapy for acute myocardial infarction is a strong predictor of early and late mortality. The Global Utilization of Streptokinase and t-PA for Occluded Coronary Arteries (GUSTO)-I Angiographic Investigators. *Circulation* 1997;96:116–121.
19. Hochman JS, Bulkley BH. Pathogenesis of left ventricular aneurysms: an experimental study in the rat model. *Am J Cardiol* 1982;50:83–88.
20. Visser CA, Kan G, Meltzer RS, et al. Incidence, timing, and prognostic value of left ventricular aneurysm formation after myocardial infarction: a prospective serial echocardiographic study of 158 patients. *Am J Cardiol* 1986;57:729.
21. Gorlin R, Klein MD, Sullivan JM. Prospective correlative study of ventricular aneurysm: mechanistic concept and clinical recognition. *Am J Med* 1967;42:512–531.
22. Cabin HS, Roberts WC. Left ventricular aneurysm, intraaneurysmal thrombus, and systemic embolus in coronary heart disease. *Chest* 1980;77:586.
23. Chiarella F, Santoro E, Domenicucci S, et al. Predischarge two-dimensional echocardiographic evaluation of left ventricular thrombosis after acute myocardial infarction in the GISSI-3 study. *Am J Cardiol* 1998;8:822–827.
24. Nolan SE, Mannisi JA, Bush DE, et al. Increased afterload aggravates infarct expansion after acute myocardial infarction. *J Am Coll Cardiol* 1988;12:1318–1325.
25. Oosterga M, Voors AA, de Kam PJ, et al. Plasma angiotensin-converting enzyme activity and left ventricular dilation after myocardial infarction. *Circulation* 1997;95:2607–2609.
26. Bulkley BH, Roberts WC. Steroid therapy during acute myocardial infarction: a cause of delayed healing and of ventricular aneurysm. *Am J Med* 1974;56:244–250.
27. Jugdutt BI, Basualdo CA. Myocardial infarct expansion during indomethacin or ibuprofen therapy for symptomatic post infarction pericarditis: influence of other pharmacologic agents during remodeling. *Can J Cardiol* 1989;5:211–221.
28. Hammerman H, Kloner RA, Schoen FJ, et al. Indomethacin-induced scar thinning after experimental myocardial infarction. *Circulation* 1983;67:1290–1295.
29. Hammerman H, Kloner RA, Hale S, et al. Dose-dependent effects of short-term methylprednisolone on myocardial infarct extent, scar formation, and ventricular function. *Circulation* 1983;68:446–452.
30. Bosimini E, Giannuzzi P, Temporelli PL, et al. Electrocardiographic evolutionary changes and left ventricular remodeling after acute myocardial infarction: results of the GISSI-3 Echo substudy. *J Am Coll Cardiol* 2000;35:135–137.
31. St. John Sutton M, Pfeffer MA, Plappert T, et al. Quantitative two-dimensional echocardiographic measurements are major predictors of adverse cardiovascular events after acute myocardial infarction. The protective effects of captopril. *Circulation* 1994;89:68–75.
32. Ascione L, Antonini-Canterin F, Macor F, et al. Relation between early mitral regurgitation and left ventricular thrombus formation after acute myocardial infarction: results of the GISSI-3 echo substudy. *Heart* 2002;88:131–136.
33. Kalra A, Jang IK. Prevalence of early left ventricular thrombus after primary coronary intervention for acute myocardial infarction. *J Thromb Thrombolysis* 2000;10:133–136.
34. Toth C, Ujhelyi E, Fulop T, Istvan E. Clinical predictors of early left ventricular thrombus formation in acute myocardial infarction. *Acta Cardiol* 2002;57:205–211.
35. Meltzer RS, Visser CA, Fuster V. Intracardiac thrombi and systemic embolization. *Ann Intern Med* 1986;104:689–698.
36. Kontny F, Dale J, Hegrerves L, et al. Left ventricular thrombosis and arterial embolism after thrombolysis in acute anterior myocardial infarction: predictors and effects of adjunctive antithrombotic therapy. *Eur Heart J* 1993;14:1489–1492.

37. Mooe T, Teien D, Karp K, et al. Left ventricular thrombosis after anterior myocardial infarction with and without thrombolytic treatment. *J Intern Med* 1995;237:563–569.
38. Hirsh J, Fuster V. Guide to anticoagulant therapy. Part 2: oral anticoagulants. *Circulation* 1994;89:1469–1480.
39. Lapeyre AC III, Steele PM, Kazmier FJ, et al. Systemic embolism in chronic left ventricular aneurysm: incidence and the role of anticoagulation. *J Am Coll Cardiol* 1985;6:534–538.
40. Loh E, St. John Sutton M, Wun CCC, et al. Ventricular dysfunction and the risk of stroke after myocardial infarction. *N Engl J Med* 1997;336:251–257.
41. Pfeffer MA, Lamas GA, Vaughan DE, et al. Effect of captopril on progressive ventricular dilatation after anterior myocardial infarction. *N Engl J Med* 1988;319:80–86.
42. Carstensen S, Bonarjee VVS, Berning J, et al. Effects of early enalapril treatment on global and regional wall motion in acute myocardial infarction. *Am Heart J* 1995;129:1101–1107.
43. de Kam PJ, Voors AA, van der Berg MP, et al. Effect of very early angiotensin-converting enzyme inhibition on left ventricular dilation after myocardial infarction in patients receiving thrombolysis: results of a meta-analysis of 845 patients. *J Am Coll Cardiol* 2000;36:2047–2053.
44. Nakamura Y, Yoshiyama M, Omura T, et al. Beneficial effects of combination of ACE inhibitor and angiotensin II type 1 receptor blocker on cardiac remodeling in rat myocardial infarction. *Cardiovasc Res* 2003;57:48–54.
45. Hayashi M, Tsutamoto T, Wada A, et al. Immediate administration of mineralocorticoid receptor antagonist spironolactone prevents post-infarct left ventricular remodeling associated with suppression of a marker of myocardial collagen synthesis in patients with first anterior acute myocardial infarction. *Circulation* 2003;107:2559–2565.
46. Tramarin R, Pozzoli M, Febo O, et al. Echocardiographic assessment of therapy efficacy in left ventricular thrombosis post myocardial infarction. *Eur Heart J* 1986;7:482–492.
47. Medical Research Council. Assessment of short-anticoagulant administration after cardiac infarction: report of the Working Party on Anticoagulant Therapy in Coronary Thrombosis to the Medical Research Council. *BMJ* 1969;1:335–342.
48. Veterans Administration Hospital Investigators. Anticoagulants in acute myocardial infarction: results of a cooperative clinical trial. *JAMA* 1973; 225:724–729.
49. Yusuf S, Mehta SR, Xie C, et al., for the CREATE Trial Group Investigators. Effects of reviparin, a low-molecular-weight heparin, on mortality, reinfarction, and strokes in patients with acute myocardial infarction presenting with ST-segment elevation. *JAMA* 2005;293:427–435.
50. Gruppo Italiano Per Lo Studio Della Streptochinasi nell'Infarto Miocardico (GISSI). Effectiveness of intravenous thrombolytic treatment in acute myocardial infarction. *Lancet* 1986;2:397–401.
51. van Es RF, Jonker JJ, Verheugt FW, et al., for the Antithrombotics in the Secondary Prevention of Events in Coronary Thrombosis-2 (ASPECT-2) Research Group. Aspirin and Coumadin after acute coronary syndromes (the ASPECT-2 study): a randomised controlled trial. *Lancet* 2002;360: 109–113.
52. Hurlen M, Abdelnoor M, Smith P, et al. Warfarin, aspirin, or both after myocardial infarction. *N Engl J Med* 2002;347:969–974.
53. Fiore LD, Ezekowitz MD, Brophy MT, et al., for the Combination Hemotherapy and Mortality Prevention (CHAMP) Study Group. Department of Veterans Affairs Cooperative Studies Program Clinical Trial comparing combined warfarin and aspirin with aspirin alone in survivors of acute myocardial infarction: primary results of the CHAMP study. *Circulation* 2002;105:557–563.
54. Herlitz J, Holm J, Peterson M, et al., for the LoWASA study group. Effect of fixed low-dose warfarin added to aspirin in the long term after acute myocardial infarction; the LoWASA Study. *Eur Heart J* 2004;25:232–239.
55. Coumadin Aspirin Reinfarction Study (CARS) Investigators. Randomized double-blind trial of fixed low-dose warfarin with aspirin after myocardial infarction. *Lancet* 1997;350:389–396.
56. Antman EM, Anbe DT, Armstrong PW, et al., for the American College of Cardiology; American Heart Association; Canadian Cardiovascular Society. ACC/AHA guidelines for the management of patients with ST-elevation myocardial infarction—executive summary. A report of the American College of Cardiology/American Heart Association Task Force on Practice Guidelines (Writing Committee to revise the 1999 guidelines for the management of patients with acute myocardial infarction). *J Am Coll Cardiol* 2004;44:671–719.
57. Harrington RA, Becker RC, Ezekowitz M, et al. Antithrombotic therapy for coronary artery disease. The Seventh ACCP Conference on Antithrombotic and Thrombolytic Therapy. *Chest* 2004;216:513S–548S.
58. Prewitt RM, Gu S, Schick U, et al. Intraaortic balloon counterpulsation enhances coronary thrombolysis induced by intravenous administration of a thrombolytic agent. *J Am Coll Cardiol* 1994;23:794–798.
59. Giannitsis E, Potratz J, Schmuecker G, et al. Impact of right ventricular infarction on in-hospital patency after early thrombolysis with an accelerated dose regimen of 100 mg tPA. *Circulation* 1996;94[Suppl]:I-733.
60. Swedberg K, Held P, Kjekshus J, et al. Effects of the early administration of enalapril on mortality in patients with acute myocardial infarction: results of the Cooperative New Scandinavian Enalapril Survival Study II (CONSENSUS II). *N Engl J Med* 1992;327:678–684.
61. Jugdutt BI, Warnica JW. Intravenous nitroglycerin therapy to limit myocardial infarct size, expansion, and complications: effect of timing, dosage, and infarct location. *Circulation* 1988;78:906–919.
62. Donges K, Schiele R, Gitt A, et al. , for the Maximal Individual Therapy in Acute Myocardial Infarction (MITRA) and Myocardial Infarction Registry (MIR) Study Groups. Incidence, determinants, and clinical course of reinfarction in-hospital after index acute myocardial infarction (results from the pooled data of the maximal individual therapy in acute myocardial infarction [MITRA], and the myocardial infarction registry [MIR]). *Am J Cardiol* 2001;87:1039–1044.
63. Armstrong PW, Fu Y, Chang WC, et al. Acute coronary syndromes in the GUSTO-IIb trial: prognostic insights and impact of recurrent ischemia. The GUSTO-IIb Investigators. *Circulation* 1998;98:1860–1868.
64. Mueller HS, Forman SA, Menegus MA, et al. Prognostic significance of nonfatal reinfarction during 3-year follow-up: results of the Thrombolysis in Myocardial Infarction (TIMI) phase II clinical trial. *J Am Coll Cardiol* 1995;26:900–907.
65. Hudson MP, Barbash GI, Granger CB, et al. Temporal and regional differences in therapy for reinfarction following thrombolysis: results from GUSTO I and ASSENT II. *J Am Coll Cardiol* 2000;76:386A.
66. Forrester JS, Diamond G, Chatterjee K, et al. Medical therapy of acute myocardial infarction by application of hemodynamic subsets (first of two parts). *N Engl J Med* 1976;295:1356–1362.
67. Forrester JS, Diamond GC, Chatterjee K, et al. Medical therapy of acute myocardial infarction by application of hemodynamic subsets (second of two parts). *N Engl J Med* 1976;295:1404–1413.
68. Vokonas PS, Pirzada F, Hood WB Jr. Experimental myocardial infarction. XII. Dynamic changes in segmental mechanical behavior of infarcted and noninfarcted myocardium. *Am J Cardiol* 1976;37:853–859.
69. Becker LC, Levine JH, DiPaula AF, et al. Reversal of dysfunction in postischemic stunned myocardium by epinephrine and postextrasystolic potentiation. *J Am Coll Cardiol* 1986;7:580–589.
70. Ross J Jr. Myocardial perfusion-contraction matching: implications for coronary heart disease and hibernation. *Circulation* 1991;83:1076–1083.
71. Califf RM, Bengtson JR. Cardiogenic shock. *N Engl J Med* 1994;330: 1724–1730.
72. Berning J, Steensgaard-Hansen F. Early estimation of risk by echocardiographic determination of wall motion index in an unselected population with acute myocardial infarction. *Am J Cardiol* 1990;65:567–576.
73. Nishimura RA, Tajik AJ, Shub C, et al. Role of two-dimensional echocardiography in the prediction of in-hospital complications after acute myocardial infarction. *J Am Coll Cardiol* 1984;4:1080–1087.
74. Volpi A, De Vita C, Franzosi MG, et al. Determinants of 6-month mortality in survivors of myocardial infarction after thrombolysis: results of the GISSI-2 data base. *Circulation* 1993;88:416–429.
75. Remme WJ, Look MP, Bootsma M, et al. Neurohumoral activation during acute myocardial ischaemia: effects of ACE inhibition. *Eur Heart J* 1990;[Suppl B]:162–171.
76. Dargie HJ, McAlpine HM, Morton JJ. Neuroendocrine activation in acute myocardial infarction. *J Cardiovasc Pharmacol* 1987;9[Suppl 2]:21S–24S.
77. Omland T. Natriuretic peptides as markers of ventricular dysfunction. *Hypertension* 1997;30:305–306.
78. Sanford CF, Corbett J, Nicod P, et al. Value of radionuclide ventriculography in the immediate characterization of patients with acute myocardial infarction. *Am J Cardiol* 1982;49:637–644.
79. Oh JK, Ding ZP, Gersh BJ, et al. Restrictive left ventricular diastolic filling identifies the patients with heart failure after acute myocardial infarction. *J Am Soc Echocardiol* 1992;5:497–503.
80. Brown EJ, Swinford RD, Gadde P, et al. Acute effects of delayed reperfusion on myocardial infarct shape and left ventricular volume: a potential mechanism of additional benefits from thrombolytic therapy. *J Am Coll Cardiol* 1991;17:1641–1650.
81. Hochman JS, Buller CE, Sleeper LA, et al. Cardiogenic shock complicating acute myocardial infarction—etiologies, management and outcome; overall findings of the SHOCK Trial Registry. *J Am Coll Cardiol* 2000;36:1063–1070.
82. Himbert D, Juliard JM, Steg PG, et al. Limits of reperfusion therapy for immediate cardiogenic shock complicating acute myocardial infarction. *Am J Cardiol* 1994;74:492–494.
83. Alonso DR, Scheidt S, Post M, et al. Pathophysiology of cardiogenic shock: quantification of myocardial necrosis, clinical, pathologic, and electrocardiographic correlations. *Circulation* 1973;48:588–596.
84. Wong SC, Antonelli T, Sleeper LA, et al. Angiographic findings and clinical correlates in patients with cardiogenic shock complicating acute myocardial infarction in the SHOCK Registry. *J Am Coll Cardiol* 2000;36:1077–1083.
85. Page DL, Caulfield JB, Kastor JA, et al. Myocardial changes associated with cardiogenic shock. *N Engl J Med* 1971;285:133–137.
86. Holmes DR Jr, Bates ER, Kleiman NS, et al. for the GUSTO-I Investigators. Contemporary reperfusion therapy for cardiogenic shock: the GUSTO-I trial experience. Global utilization of streptokinase and tissue plasminogen activator for occluded coronary arteries. *J Am Coll Cardiol* 1995;26:668–674.
87. Hochman JS. Cardiogenic shock complicating acute myocardial infarction: expanding the paradigm. *Circulation* 2003;107:2998–3002.

88. Kohsaka S, Menon V, Lowe AM, et al. , for the SHOCK Investigators. Systemic inflammatory response syndrome after acute myocardial infarction complicated by cardiogenic shock. *Arch Intern Med* 2005;165:1643–1650.
89. Cotter G, Kaluski E, Milo O, et al. LINCS: L-NAME (a NO synthase inhibitor) in the treatment of refractory cardiogenic shock: a prospective randomized study. *Eur Heart J* 2003;24:1287–1295.
90. Theroux P, Armstrong PW, Mahaffey KW, et al. Prognostic significance of blood markers of inflammation in patients with ST-segment elevation myocardial infarction undergoing primary angioplasty and effects of pexelizumab, a C5 inhibitor: a substudy of the COMMA trial. *Eur Heart J* 2005;26:1964–1970.
91. Valencia R, Theroux P, Granger CB, et al. Congestive heart failure and cardiogenic shock complicating AMI have high mortality and are associated with intense inflammatory response: results from the CARDINAL trials. *J Am Coll Cardiol* 2004;43[Suppl 2]:A291.
92. Picard MH, Davidoff R, Sleeper LA, et al., for the SHOCK Trial. SHould we emergently revascularize Occluded Coronaries for cardiogenic shocK. Echocardiographic predictors of survival and response to early revascularization in cardiogenic shock. *Circulation* 2003;107:279–284.
93. Sanborn TA, Sleeper LA, Webb JG, et al., for the SHOCK Investigators. Correlates of one-year survival inpatients with cardiogenic shock complicating acute myocardial infarction: angiographic findings from the SHOCK trial. *J Am Coll Cardiol* 2003;42:1373–1379.
94. Klein LW, Shaw RE, Krone RJ, et al. , for the American College of Cardiology National Cardiovascular Data Registry. Mortality after emergent percutaneous coronary intervention in cardiogenic shock secondary to acute myocardial infarction and usefulness of a mortality prediction model. *Am J Cardiol* 2005;96:35–41.
95. Chen ZM, Pan HC, Chen YP, et al. COMMIT (Clopidrogrel and Metoprolol in Myocardial Infarction Trial) collaborative group. Early intravenous then oral metroprolol in 45,852 patients with acute myocardial infarction: randomised placebo-controlled trial. *Lancet* 2005;366(9497):1622–1632.
96. Ballester M, Tasca R, Marin L. Different mechanisms of mitral regurgitation in acute and chronic forms of coronary heart disease. *Eur Heart J* 1983;4:557–565.
97. Forrester JS, Diamond G, Freedman S, et al. Silent mitral insufficiency in acute myocardial infarction. *Circulation* 1971;44:877–883.
98. Tsuchihashi K, Ueshima K, Uchida T, et al., for the Angina Pectoris-Myocardial Infarction Investigations in Japan. Transient left ventricular apical ballooning without coronary artery stenosis: a novel heart syndrome mimicking acute myocardial infarction. *J Am Coll Cardiol* 2001;38:11–18.
99. Desmet WJR, Adriaenssens BFM, Dens JAY. Apical ballooning of the left ventricle: first series in white patients. *Heart* 2003;89:1027–1031.
100. Killip T, Kimball JT. Treatment of myocardial infarction in a coronary care unit: a two-year experience with 250 patients. *Am J Cardiol* 1967;20:457–464.
101. Spencer FA, Meyer TE, Goldberg RJ, et al. Twenty year trends (1975–1995) in the incidence, in-hospital and long-term death rates associated with heart failure complicating acute myocardial infarction: a community-wide perspective. *J Am Coll Cardiol* 1999;34:1378–1387.
102. Hellermann JP, Goraya TY, Jacobsen SJ, et al. Incidence of heart failure after myocardial infarction: is it changing over time? *Am J Epidemiol* 2003;157:1101–1107.
103. Wilcox RG, Von der Lippe G, Olsson CG, et al. Trial of tissue plasminogen activator for mortality reduction in acute myocardial infarction. Anglo-Scandinavian study of early thrombolysis (ASSET). *Lancet* 1988;2:525–530.
104. National Heart Foundation of Australia Coronary Thrombolysis Group. Coronary thrombolysis and myocardial salvage by tissue plasminogen activator given up to 4 hours after onset of myocardial infarction. *Lancet* 1988;1:203–208.
105. Meinertz T, Kasper W, Schumacher M, et al., for the APSAC Multicenter Trial Group. The German multicenter trial of anisoylated plasminogen streptokinase activator complex versus heparin for acute myocardial infarction. *Am J Cardiol* 1988;62:347–351.
106. Bassand JP, Machecourt J, Cassagnes J, et al. Multicenter trial of intravenous anisoylated plasminogen streptokinase activator complex (APSAC) in acute myocardial infarction: effects on infarct size and left ventricular function. *J Am Coll Cardiol* 1989;13:988–997.
107. Bates ER, Topol EJ. Limitations of thrombolytic therapy for acute myocardial infarction complicated by congestive heart failure and cardiogenic shock. *J Am Coll Cardiol* 1991;18:1077–1084.
108. Wu AH, Parsons L, Every NR, Bates ER, for the Second National Registry of Myocardial Infarction. Hospital outcomes in patients presenting with congestive heart failure complicating acute myocardial infarction: a report from the Second National Registry of Myocardial Infarction (NRMI-2). *J Am Coll Cardiol* 2002;40:1389–1394.
109. Single-bolus tenecteplase compared with front-loaded alteplase in acute myocardial infarction: the ASSENT-2 double-blind randomized trial. *Lancet* 1999;354:716–722.
110. Hasdai D, Topol EJ, Kilaru R, et al. Frequency, patient characteristics, and outcomes of mild-to-moderate heart failure complicating ST-segment elevation acute myocardial infarction: lessons from 4 international fibrinolytic therapy trials. *Am Heart J* 2003;145:73–79.
111. DeGeare VS, Boura JA, Grines LL, et al. Predictive value of the Killip classification in patients undergoing primary percutaneous coronary intervention for acute myocardial infarction. *Am J Cardiol* 2001;87:1035–1038.
112. Zeymer U, Schroder R, Machnig T, Neuhaus KL. Primary percutaneous transluminal coronary angioplasty accelerates early myocardial reperfusion compared to thrombolytic therapy in patients with acute myocardial infarction. *Am Heart J* 2003;146:686–691.
113. The GUSTO IIb Angioplasty Substudy Investigators. A clinical trial comparing primary coronary angioplasty with tissue plasminogen activator for acute myocardial infarction. *N Engl J Med* 1997;23:1621–1628.
114. Hochman JS, Jaber W, Bates ER, et al. Angioplasty versus thrombolytics for patients presenting with congestive heart failure: GUSTO IIb substudy findings. *J Am Coll Cardiol* 1998;31:856–864.
115. Sutton AG, Campbell PG, Graham R, et al. A randomized trial of rescue angioplasty versus a conservative approach for failed fibrinolysis in ST-segment elevation myocardial infarction: the Middlesbrough Early Revascularization to Limit INfarction (MERLIN) trial. *J Am Coll Cardiol* 2004; 44:287–296.
116. Gershlick AH. Rescue Angioplasty versus conservative treatment or repeat thrombolysis (REACT). American Heart Association Scientific Sessions, New Orleans, LA, November, 2004.
117. Steg PG, Bonnefoy E, Chabaud S, et al. Comparison of Angioplasty and Prehospital Thrombolysis In acute Myocardial infarction (CAPTIM) Investigators. Impact of time to treatment on mortality after prehospital fibrinolysis or primary angioplasty: data from the CAPTIM randomized clinical trial. *Circulation* 2003;108:2851–2856.
118. Babaev A, Frederick PD, Pasta DJ, et al. NRMI Investigators. Trends in management and outcomes of patients with acute myocardial infarction complicated by cardiogenic shock. *JAMA* 2005;294:448–454.
119. Dauerman HL, Goldberg RJ, White K, et al. Global Registry of Acute Coronary Events. GRACE Investigators. Revascularization, stenting, and outcomes of patients with acute myocardial infarction complicated by cardiogenic shock. *Am J Cardiol* 2002;90:838–842.
120. Rogers WJ, Bowlby LJ, Chandra NC, et al. Treatment of myocardial infarction in the United States (1990 to 1993). Observations from the national registry of myocardial infarction. *Circulation* 1994;90:2103–2114.
121. Goldberg RJ, Samad NA, Yarzebski J, et al. Temporal trends in cardiogenic shock complicating acute myocardial infarction. *N Engl J Med* 1999; 340:1162–1168.
122. Hasdai D, Califf RM, Thompson TD, et al. Predictors of cardiogenic shock after thrombolytic therapy for acute myocardial infarction. *J Am Coll Cardiol* 1999;35:136–143.
123. Holmes DR Jr, Berger PB, Granger CB, et al. Cardiogenic shock in patients with acute ischemic syndromes with and without ST-segment elevation. *Circulation* 1999;100:2067–2073.
124. Jacobs AK, French J, Col J, et al. Cardiogenic shock without ST segment elevation myocardial infarction. A report from the SHOCK Registry. *J Am Coll Cardiol* 2000;36:1091–1096.
125. Ohman EM, Kandzari D, Menon V, et al. Underutilization of revascularization in early cardiogenic shock among patients with non-ST-segment elevation acute coronary syndromes: observations from the CRUSADE initiative [Abstract 1938]. *Circulation* 2004;110[Suppl III]:410.
126. Webb JG, Buller CE, Thompson CR, et al. Implications of the timing of onset of cardiogenic shock after acute myocardial infarction: a report from the SHOCK Registry. *J Am Coll Cardiol* 2000;36:1084–1090.
127. Reynolds HR, Anand SK, Fox JM, et al. Restrictive physiology in cardiogenic shock: observations from Echocardiography. *Am Heart J* 2006;154: e9–e15.
128. Menon V, White H, LeJemtel T, et al. The clinical profile of patients with suspected cardiogenic shock due to predominant left ventricular failure. *J Am Coll Cardiol* 2000;36:1071–1076.
129. Menon V, Slater JN, White HD, et al. Acute myocardial infarction complicated by systemic hypoperfusion: report of the SHOCK Registry. *Am J Med* 2000;108:374–380.
130. Chirillo F, Cavarzerani A, Ius P, et al. Role of transthoracic, transesophageal, and transgastric two-dimensional and color Doppler echocardiography in the evaluation of mechanical complications of acute myocardial infarction. *Am J Cardiol* 1995;76:833–836.
131. Heidenreich PA, Stainback RF, Redberg RF, et al. Transesophageal echocardiography predicts mortality in critically ill patients with unexplained hypotension. *J Am Coll Cardiol* 1995;26:152–158.
132. Smyllie JH, Sutherland GR, Geuskens R, et al. Doppler color flow mapping in the diagnosis of ventricular septal rupture and acute mitral regurgitation after myocardial infarction. *J Am Coll Cardiol* 1990;15:1449–1455.
133. Oh JK, Seward JB, Khandheria BK, et al. Transesophageal echocardiography in critically ill patients. *Am J Cardiol* 1990;66:1492–1495.
134. Biddle TL, Yu PN. Effect of furosemide on hemodynamics and lung water in acute pulmonary edema secondary to myocardial infarction. *Am J Cardiol* 1979;43:86–90.
135. Armstrong PW, Walker DC, Burton JR, Parker JO. Vasodilator therapy in acute myocardial infarction. A comparison of sodium nitroprusside and nitroglycerin. *Circulation* 1975;52:1118.
136. Cotter G, Metzkor E, Kaluski E, et al. Randomised trial of high-dose isosorbide dinitrate plus low-dose furosemide versus high-dose furosemide plus low-dose isosorbide dinitrate in severe pulmonary oedema. *Lancet* 1998; 351:389–393.
137. Keren G, Bier A, LeJemtel TH. Improvement in forward cardiac output without a change in ejection fraction during nitroglycerin therapy in patients with functional mitral regurgitation. *Can J Cardiol* 1986;2:206–211.

138. Cody RJ. Renin system inhibition: beginning the fourth epoch [editorial]. *Circulation* 1992;85:362–364.
139. Kugler J, Maskin C, Frishman WH, et al. Regional and systemic metabolic effects of angiotensin converting enzyme inhibition during exercise in patients with severe heart failure. *Circulation* 1982;66:1256–1261.
140. Foult JM, Tavolaro O, Antony I, et al. Direct myocardial and coronary effects of enalaprilat in patients with dilated cardiomyopathy: assessment by a bilateral intracoronary infusion technique. *Circulation* 1988;77:337–344.
141. The Acute Infarction Ramipril Efficacy (AIRE) Study Investigators. Effect of ramipril on mortality and morbidity of survivors of acute myocardial infarction with clinical evidence of heart failure. *Lancet* 1993;342:821–828.
142. Pfeffer MA, McMurray JJ, Velazquez EJ, et al. Valsartan in Acute Myocardial Infarction Trial Investigators. Valsartan, captopril, or both in myocardial infarction complicated by heart failure, left ventricular dysfunction, or both. *N Engl J Med* 2003;349:1893–1906.
143. Pitt B, Remme W, Zannad F, et al. Eplerenone Post-Acute Myocardial Infarction Heart Failure Efficacy and Survival Study Investigators. Eplerenone, a selective aldosterone blocker, in patients with left ventricular dysfunction after myocardial infarction. *N Engl J Med* 2003;348:1309–1321.
144. Kirk ES, LeJemtel TH, Nelson GR, et al. Mechanisms of beneficial effects of vasodilators and inotropic stimulation in the experimental failing ischemic heart. *Am J Med* 1978;65:189–196.
145. Tuttle RR, Pollock GD, Todd G, et al. The effect of dobutamine on cardiac oxygen balance, regional blood flow, and infarction severity after coronary artery narrowing in dogs. *Circ Res* 1977;41:357–364.
146. Karlsberg RP, DeWood MA, DeMaria AN, et al. Comparative efficacy of short-term intravenous infusions of milrinone and dobutamine in acute congestive heart failure following acute myocardial infarction. Milrinone-Dobutamine Study Group. *Clin Cardiol* 1996;19:21–30.
147. Moiseyev VS, Poder P, Andrejevs N, et al. RUSSLAN Study Investigators. Safety and efficacy of a novel calcium sensitizer, levosimendan, in patients with left ventricular failure due to an acute myocardial infarction. A randomized, placebo-controlled, double-blind study (RUSSLAN). *Eur Heart J* 2002;23:1422–1432.
148. Lehmann A, Lang J, Boldt J, et al. Levosimendan in patients with cardiogenic shock undergoing surgical revascularization: a case series. *Med Sci Monit* 2004;10:MT89–93.
149. Yamane M, Kinebuchi O, Yamane A, et al. A comparison of continuous intravenous infusion of arginine vasopressin to dopamine in the treatment of cardiogenic shock. *J Am Coll Cardiol* 2005;45:78A.
150. Cotter G, Kaluski E, Blatt A, et al. L-NMMA (a nitric oxide synthase inhibitor) is effective in the treatment of cardiogenic shock. *Circulation* 2000;101:1358–1361.
151. Dzavik V. The effect of nitric oxide synthase inhibition on hemodynamics and outcome in patients with acute myocardial infarction complicated by cardiogenic shock—a dose ranging study. *Circulation* 2004;III-413:1949.
152. Nanas JN, Moulopoulos SD. Counterpulsation: historical background, technical improvements, hemodynamic and metabolic effects. *Cardiology* 1994;84:156–167.
153. Williams DO. Intra-aortic balloon counterpulsation: deciphering its effects on coronary flow. *J Am Coll Cardiol* 1996;27:817–818.
154. Chen EW, Canto JG, Parsons LS, et al. Investigators in the National Registry of Myocardial Infarction 2. Relation between hospital intra-aortic balloon counterpulsation volume and mortality in acute myocardial infarction complicated by cardiogenic shock. *Circulation* 2003;108:951–957.
155. Thiele H, Sick P, Boudriot E, et al. Randomized comparison of intra-aortic balloon support with a percutaneous left ventricular assist device in patients with revascularized acute myocardial infarction complicated by cardiogenic shock. *Eur Heart J* 2005;26:1276–1283.
156. Burkaff D, Cohen H, Brunckherst C, et al. For the Tandem Heart Investigators Group. A Randomized Multicenter Clinical Study to Evaluate the Safety and Efficacy of the Tandem Heart Percutaneous Ventricular Assist Device versus Conventional Therapy with Intra-Aortic Balloon Pumping for Treatment of Cardiogenic Shock. *Am Heart J* (in press).
157. Meyns B, Dens J, Sergeant P, et al. Initial experiences with the Impella device in patients with cardiogenic shock—Impella support for cardiogenic shock. *Thorac Cardiovasc Surg* 2003;51:312–317.
158. Holmes DR, Califf RM, Van de Werf F, et al. Difference in countries' use of resources and clinical outcome for patients with cardiogenic shock after myocardial infarction: results from the GUSTO trial. *Lancet* 1997;349:75–78.
159. Hochman JS, Sleeper LA, White HD, et al. Early revascularization in acute myocardial infarction complicated by cardiogenic shock. *N Engl J Med* 1999;341:625–634.
160. Zeymer U, Vogt A, Zahn R, et al. The Arbeitsgemeinschaft Leitende Kardiologische Krankenhausarzte (ALKK). Predictors of in-hospital mortality in 1333 patients with acute myocardial infarction complicated by cardiogenic shock treated with primary percutaneous coronary intervention (PCI); Results of the primary PCI registry of the Arbeitsgemeinschaft Leitende Kardiologische Krankenhausarzte (ALKK). *Eur Heart J* 2004 Feb;25:322–328.
161. Bengtson JR, Kaplan AJ, Pieper KS, et al. Prognosis in cardiogenic shock after acute myocardial infarction in the interventional era. *J Am Coll Cardiol* 1992;20:1482–1489.
162. Lee L, Erbel R, Brown TM, et al. Multicenter registry of angioplasty therapy of cardiogenic shock: initial and long-term survival. *J Am Coll Cardiol* 1991;17:599–603.
163. Hochman JS, Sleeper LA, White HD, et al. One year survival following early revascularization for acute myocardial infarction complicated by cardiogenic shock. *JAMA* 2001;285:190–192.
164. Fibrinolytic Therapy Trialists' (FTT) Collaborative Group. Indications for fibrinolytic therapy in suspected acute myocardial infarction: collaborative overview of early mortality and major morbidity results from all randomised trials of more than 1000 patients. *Lancet* 1994;343:311–322.
165. Dauerman HL, Ryan TJ Jr, Piper WD, et al. Outcomes of percutaneous coronary intervention among elderly patients in cardiogenic shock: a multicenter, decade-long experience. *J Invasive Cardiol* 2003;15:380–384.
166. Dzavik V, Sleeper LA, Cocke TP, et al. SHOCK Investigators. Early revascularization is associated with improved survival in elderly patients with acute myocardial infarction complicated by cardiogenic shock: a report from the SHOCK Trial Registry. *Eur Heart J* 2003;24:828–837.
167. Dzavik V, Sleeper LA, Picard MH, et al. SHould we emergently revascularize Occluded Coronaries in cardiogenic shocK Investigators. Outcome of patients aged ≥75 years in the SHould we emergently revascularize Occluded Coronaries in cardiogenic shocK (SHOCK) trial: do elderly patients with acute myocardial infarction complicated by cardiogenic shock respond differently to emergent revascularization? *Am Heart J* 2005;149:1128–1134.
168. Sleeper LA, Ramanathan K, Picard MH, et al. SHOCK Investigators. Functional status and quality of life after emergency revascularization for cardiogenic shock complicating acute myocardial infarction. *J Am Coll Cardiol* 2005;46:266–273.
169. Webb JG, Lowe AM, Sanborn TA, et al. SHOCK Investigators. Percutaneous coronary intervention for cardiogenic shock in the SHOCK trial. *J Am Coll Cardiol* 2003;42:1380–1386.
170. Allen BS, Buckberg GD, Fontan FM, et al. Superiority of controlled surgical reperfusion versus percutaneous transluminal coronary angioplasty in acute coronary occlusion. *J Thorac Cardiovasc Surg* 1993;105:864.
171. White HD, Assmann SF, Sanborn TA, et al. Comparison of percutaneous coronary intervention and coronary artery bypass grafting after acute myocardial infarction complicated by cardiogenic shock: results from the SHould We Emergently Revascularize Occluded Coronaries for Cardiogenic ShocK (SHOCK) trial. *Circulation* 2005;112:1992–2001.
172. Dell'Italia LJ, Lembo NJ, Starling MR, et al. Hemodynamically important right ventricular infarction: follow-up evaluation of right ventricular systolic function at rest and during exercise with radionuclide ventriculography and respiratory gas exchange. *Circulation* 1987;75:996.
173. Steele P, Kirch D, Ellis J, et al. Prompt return to normal of depressed right ventricular ejection fraction in acute inferior infarction. *Br Heart J* 1977;39:1319.
174. Setaro JF, Cabin HS. Right ventricular infarction. *Cardiol Clin* 1992;10:69–90.
175. Jacobs AK, Leopold JA, Modur S, et al. Right ventricular infarction complicated by cardiogenic shock: observations and implications. The NHLBI SHOCK Registry. *J Am Coll Cardiol* 2000;873:385A.
176. Cohn JN, Guiha NH, Broder MI, et al. Right ventricular infarction. Clinical and hemodynamic features. *Am J Cardiol* 1974;33:209.
177. Cintron GB, Hernandez E, Linares E, et al. Bedside recognition, incidence, and clinical course of right ventricular infarction. *Am J Cardiol* 1981;47:224.
178. Baigre RS, Hag A, Morgan CD, et al. The spectrum of right ventricular involvement in inferior wall myocardial infarction: a clinical, hemodynamic, and noninvasive study. *J Am Coll Cardiol* 1983;1:1396.
179. Braat SH, de Zwann C, Brugada P, et al. Right ventricular involvement with acute inferior wall myocardial infarction identifies high risk of developing atrioventricular nodal conduction disturbances. *Am Heart J* 1984;107:1183–1187.
180. Love JC, Haffajee CI, Gore JM, et al. Reversibility of hypotension and shock by atrial or atrioventricular sequential pacing in patients with right ventricular infarction. *Am Heart J* 1984;108:5–13.
181. Rietveld AP, Merrman L, Essed CE, et al. Right-to-left shunt with severe hypoxemia at the atrial level in a patient with hemodynamically important right ventricular infarction. *J Am Coll Cardiol* 1983;2:776.
182. Dell'Italia LJ, Starling MR, O'Rourke RA. Physical examination for exclusion of hemodynamically important right ventricular infarction. *Ann Intern Med* 1983;99:608.
183. Lopez-Sendon J, Coma-Canella I, Alcasena S, et al. Electrocardiographic findings in acute right ventricular infarction: sensitivity and specificity of electrocardiographic alterations in right precordial leads V4R, V3R, V1, V2 and V3. *J Am Coll Cardiol* 1984;6:1273.
184. Zehender M, Kasper W, Kauder E, et al. Right ventricular infarction as an independent predictor of prognosis after acute inferior myocardial infarction. *N Engl J Med* 1993;328:981–988.
185. Sharpe DN, Botvinick EH, Shames DM, et al. The noninvasive diagnosis of right ventricular infarction. *Circulation* 1978;57:483.
186. Dell'Italia LJ, Starling MR, Crawford MH, et al. Right ventricular infarction: Identification by hemodynamic measurements before and after volume loading and correlation with noninvasive techniques. *J Am Coll Cardiol* 1984;4:931–939.
187. Lloyd EA, Gersh BJ, Kennelly BM. Hemodynamic spectrum of "dominant" right ventricular infarction in 19 patients. *Am J Cardiol* 1981;48:1016.
188. Mehta SR, Eikelboom JW, Natarajan MK, et al. Impact of right ventricular involvement on mortality and morbidity in patients with inferior myocardial infarction. *J Am Coll Cardiol* 2001;27:37–43.

189. Bueno H, Lopez-Palop R, Perez-David E, et al. Combined effect of age and right ventricular involvement on acute inferior myocardial infarction prognosis. *Circulation* 1998;27:1714–1720.
190. Haines DE, Beller GA, Watson DD, et al. A prospective clinical, scintigraphic, angiographic, and functional evaluation of patients after inferior myocardial infarction with and without right ventricular dysfunction. *J Am Coll Cardiol* 1985;6:995.
191. Kagan A. Dynamic responses of the right ventricle following extensive damage by cauterization. *Circulation* 1952;5:816.
192. Donald DE, Essex HE. Pressure studies after inactivation of the major portion of the canine right ventricle. *Am J Physiol* 1954;176:155.
193. Goldstein JA, Tweddell JS, Barzilai B, et al. Importance of left ventricular function and systolic ventricular interaction to right ventricular performance during acute right heart ischemia. *J Am Coll Cardiol* 1992;19:704–711.
194. Goldstein JA, Vlahakes GJ, Verrier ED, et al. The role of right ventricular systolic dysfunction and elevated intrapericardiac pressure in the genesis of low output in experimental right ventricular infarction. *Circulation* 1982; 65:513.
195. Sharkey SW, Shelley W, Carlyle PF, et al. M-mode and two-dimensional echocardiographic analysis of the septum in experimental right ventricular infarction: correlation with hemodynamic alterations. *Am Heart J* 1985; 110:1210.
196. Dell'Italia LJ, Starling MR, Blumhardt R, et al. Comparative effects of volume loading, dobutamine, and nitroprusside in patients with predominant right ventricular infarction. *Circulation* 1985;72:1327.
197. Sclarovsky S, Zafrir N, Strasberg B, et al. Ventricular fibrillation complicating temporary ventricular pacing in acute myocardial infarction: significance of right ventricular infarction. *Am J Cardiol* 1981;48:1160–1166.
198. Iqbal MZ, Liebson PR. Counterpulsation and dobutamine: their use in treatment of cardiogenic shock due to right ventricular infarct. *Arch Intern Med* 1981;141:247–249.
199. Moran JM, Opravil M, Gorman AF. Pulmonary artery balloon counterpulsation for right ventricular failure. II. Clinical experience. *Ann Thorac Surg* 1984;38:254.
200. Bowers TR, O'Neill WW, Grene C, et al. Effect of reperfusion on ventricular function and survival after right ventricular infarction. *N Engl J Med* 1998;338:933–940.
201. Saffitz JE, Fredrickson RC, Roberts WC. Relation of size of transmural acute myocardial infarct to mode of death: interval between infarction and death in frequency of coronary arterial thrombus. *Am J Cardiol* 1986;112:1088–1090.
202. Becker AE, van Mantgem JP. Cardiac tamponade: a study of 50 hearts. *Eur J Cardiol* 1975;15:349–358.
203. Becker R, Charlesworth A, Wilcox R, et al. Cardiac rupture associated with thrombolytic therapy: impact of time to treatment in the Late Assessment of Thrombolytic Efficacy (LATE) study. *J Am Coll Cardiol* 1995;25:1063–1068.
204. Becker RC, Gore JM, Lambrew C, et al. A composite view of cardiac rupture in the United States National Registry of Myocardial Infarction. *J Am Coll Cardiol* 1996;27:1321–1326.
205. Lesser JR, Johnson K, Lindberg JL, et al. Images in cardiovascular medicine. Myocardial rupture, microvascular obstruction, and infarct expansion: elucidation by cardiac magnetic resonance. *Circulation* 2003;108:116–117.
206. Lopez-Sendon J, Gonzales A, Lopez de Sa E, et al. Diagnosis of subacute ventricular wall rupture after acute myocardial infarction: sensitivity and specificity of clinical, hemodynamic, and echocardiographic criteria. *J Am Coll Cardiol* 1992;19:1145–1153.
207. Park WM, Connery CP, Hochman JS, et al. Successful repair of myocardial free wall rupture after thrombolytic therapy for acute infarction. *Ann Thorac Surg* 2000;70:1345–1349.
208. Nesta F, Otsuji Y, Handschumacher MD, et al. Leaflet concavity: a rapid visual clue to the presence and mechanism of functional mitral regurgitation. *J Am Soc Echocardiogr* 2003;16:1301–1308.
209. Kono T, Sabbah HN, Stein PD, et al. Left ventricular shape as a determinant of functional mitral regurgitation in patients with severe heart failure secondary to either coronary artery disease or idiopathic dilated cardiomyopathy. *Am J Cardiol* 1991;68:355–359.
210. Wei JY, Hutchins GM, Bulkley BH. Papillary muscle rupture in fatal acute myocardial infarction: a potentially treatable form of cardiogenic shock. *Ann Intern Med* 1979;90:149–152.
211. Voci P, Bilotta F, Caretta Q, et al. Papillary muscle perfusion pattern: a hypothesis for ischemic papillary muscle dysfunction. *Circulation* 1995;91: 1714–1718.
212. Nishimura RA, Scaff HV, Gersh BJ, et al. Early repair of mechanical complications after acute myocardial infarction. *JAMA* 1986;256:47–50.
213. Barzilai B, Gessler C, Perez JE, et al. Significance of Doppler-detected mitral regurgitation in acute myocardial infarction. *Am J Cardiol* 1988;61:220–223.
214. Lehmann KG, Francis CK, Dodge HT, et al. Mitral regurgitation in early myocardial infarction: incidence, clinical detection, and prognostic implications. TIMI Study Group. *Ann Intern Med* 1992;117:10–17.
215. Tcheng JE, Jackman JD, Nelson CL, et al. Outcome of patients sustaining acute ischemic mitral regurgitation during myocardial infarction. *Ann Intern Med* 1992;117:18–24.
216. Bursi F, Enriquez-Sarano M, Nkomo VT, et al. Heart failure and death after myocardial infarction in the community: the emerging role of mitral regurgitation. *Circulation* 2005;111:295–301.
217. Thompson CR, Christopher BE, Sleeper LA, et al. Cardiogenic shock due to acute severe mitral regurgitation complicating acute myocardial infarction: a report for the SHOCK Trial Registry. *J Am Coll Cardiol* 2000;36:1104–1109.
218. Nishimura RA, Shub C, Tajik AJ. Two-dimensional echocardiographic diagnosis of partial papillary muscle rupture. *Br Heart J* 1982;48:598–600.
219. Moursi MH, Bhatnagar SK, Vilacosta I, et al. Transesophageal echocardiographic assessment of papillary muscle rupture. *Circulation* 1996;94:1003–1009.
220. Fuchs RM, Heuser RR, Yin FCP, et al. Limitations of pulmonary wedge V waves in diagnosing mitral regurgitation. *Am J Cardiol* 1982;49:849–854.
221. Moore CA, Nygard TW, Kaser DI, et al. Postinfarction ventricular septal rupture: the importance of location of infarction and right ventricular function in determining survival. *Circulation* 1986;74:45–55.
222. Menon V, Webb JG, Hillis D, et al. Outcome and profile of ventricular septal rupture with cardiogenic shock after myocardial infarction: a report from the SHOCK Registry. *J Am Coll Cardiol* 2000;36:1110–1117.
223. Gershaw BS, Granger CB, Bunbaum Y, et al. Risk factors, angiographic patterns and outcomes in patients with ventricular septal defect complicating acute myocardial infarction. GUSTO I Investigators. *Circulation* 2000; 101:27–32.
224. Edwards BS, Edwards WD, Edwards JE. Ventricular septal rupture complicating acute myocardial infarction: identification of simple and complex types in 53 autopsied hearts. *Am J Cardiol* 1984;54:1201–1205.
225. Parry G, Goudevenos J, Adams PC, et al. Septal rupture after myocardial infarction: is very early surgery really worthwhile? *Eur Heart J* 1992;13:373–382.
226. Giuliani ER, Danielson GK, Pluth JR, et al. Postinfarction ventricular septal rupture: surgical considerations and results. *Circulation* 1974;49:455–459.
227. Cummings RG, Califf R, Jones RN, et al. Correlates of survival in patients with postinfarction ventricular septal defect. *Ann Thorac Surg* 1989;47: 824–830.
228. Davies RH, Dawkins KD, Skillington PD, et al. Late functional results after surgical closure of acquired ventricular septal defect. *J Thorac Cardiovasc Surg* 1993;106:592–598.
229. Muehrcke DD, Blank S, Daggett WM. Survival after repair of postinfarction ventricular septal defects in patients over the age of 70. *J Cardiac Surg* 1992; 7:290–300.
230. Held AC, Cole PL, Lipton B, et al. Rupture of the interventricular septum complicating acute myocardial infarction: a multicenter analysis of clinical findings and outcome. *Am Heart J* 1988;116:1330–1336.
231. Holzer R, Balzer D, Amin Z, et al. Transcatheter closure of postinfarction ventricular septal defects using the new Amplatzer muscular VSD occluder: Results of a U.S. Registry. *Catheter Cardiovasc Interv* 2004;61:196–201.
232. Barker TA, Ramnarine IR, Woo EB, et al. Repair of post-infarct ventricular septal defect with or without coronary artery bypass grafting in the northwest of England: a 5-year multi-institutional experience. *Eur J Cardiothorac Surg* 2003;24:940–946.
233. Krainin FM, Flessas AP, Spodick DH. Infarction-associated pericarditis: rarity of diagnostic electrocardiogram. *N Engl J Med* 1984;311:1211–1214.
234. Oliva PB, Hammill SC, Talano JV. Effect of definition on incidence of postinfarction pericarditis: is it time to redefine postinfarction pericarditis? *Circulation* 1994;90:1537–1541.
235. Widimsky P, Gregor P. Pericardial involvement during the course of myocardial infarction: a long-term clinical and echocardiographic study. *Chest* 1995;108:89–93.
236. Tofler GH, Muller JE, Stone PH, et al. Pericarditis in acute myocardial infarction: characterization and clinical significance. *Am Heart J* 1989; 117:86–92.
237. Van de Werf F, for the investigators of the European Cooperative Study Group for recombinant tissue-type plasminogen activation. Lessons from the European Cooperative Recombinant Tissue-Type Plasminogen Activator (rt-PA) versus Placebo Trial. *J Am Coll Cardiol* 1988;12:14A–19A.
238. Moscucci M, Eagle KA, Share D, et al. Public reporting and case selection for percutaneous coronary interventions: an analysis from two large multicenter percutaneous coronary intervention databases. *J Am Coll Cardiol* 2005;45:1759–1765.
239. Velazquez EJ, Francis GS, Armstrong PW, et al. VALIANT registry. An international perspective on heart failure and left ventricular systolic dysfunction complicating myocardial infarction: the VALIANT registry. *Eur Heart J* 2004;25:1911–1919.
240. Moller JE, Brendorp B, Ottesen M, et al. Bucindolol Evaluation in Acute Myocardial Infarction Trail Group. Congestive heart failure with preserved left ventricular systolic function after acute myocardial infarction: clinical and prognostic implications. *Eur J Heart Fail* 2003;5:811–819.
241. Rott D, Behar S, Leor J, et al. Working Group on Intensive Cardiac Care, Israel Heart Society. Effect on survival of acute myocardial infarction in Killip classes II or III patients undergoing invasive coronary procedures. *Am J Cardiol* 2001;88:618–623.

CHAPTER 21 ■ POST–MYOCARDIAL INFARCTION MANAGEMENT

DEEPAK L. BHATT AND L. KRISTIN NEWBY

OVERVIEW

The management of acute myocardial infarction (MI) has been revolutionized in the past decade. Advances in pharmacologic and mechanical reperfusion therapy have improved the survival of patients who experience ST-segment elevation MI, and as more patients survive the initial myocardial insult, subsequent medical care has increased in importance. An appreciation of pathologic left ventricular (LV) remodeling after MI has permitted the study of medications that preserve LV function. The role of plaque stabilization with lipid-lowering therapy has been established, and the use of antiplatelet therapy to prevent recurrent atherothrombotic events continues to grow. Appropriate control of risk factors such as obesity, metabolic syndrome, diabetes, and hypertension remains prominent. Additionally, inflammation has been identified as having a significant role in the pathogenesis of ischemic events. Controversy over noninvasive risk stratification versus the need for invasive assessment continues, although the pendulum seems to be swinging toward aggressive management. Despite impressive technological advances, lifestyle modification remains a key component of secondary prevention after MI.

GLOSSARY

Acute coronary syndrome: Plaque rupture leading to various degrees of coronary artery thrombosis and occlusion along with distal platelet microembolism. Most often refers to unstable angina and non– ST-segment elevation MI, although sometimes meant also to include ST-segment elevation MI.

Non–Q-wave myocardial infarction: Older nomenclature for MI believed to be caused by nonocclusive coronary arterial thrombus. Now referred to as *non–ST-segment elevation MI*.

Q-wave myocardial infarction: Older term for MI meant to imply transmural myocardial necrosis.

Remodeling: The process of LV cellular and geometric adaptation to compensate for damage sustained during MI.

ST-segment elevation myocardial infarction: MI resulting from coronary arterial occlusion by thrombus, manifested on the surface electrocardiogram as ST-segment elevation.

GENERAL PRINCIPLES

Historical Perspective

Because of the use of fibrinolytic therapy and, in communities where it is available, primary percutaneous coronary intervention (PCI), the past decade has seen dramatic decreases in deaths resulting from MI. However, in the Global Utilization of Streptokinase and t-PA for Occluded Coronary Arteries III (GUSTO III) trial of acute MI, in which two different fibrinolytic regimens were tested, the 1-year mortality rate was still 11% (1), and mortality rates in the Hirulog and Early Reperfusion or Occlusion (HERO) trial were even higher (10.8% at 30 days), reflecting global differences in outcomes after acute

MI (2). Further, the additional 4% mortality rate observed in GUSTO III between 30 days and 1 year illustrates the importance of initiating secondary prevention efforts during a patient's hospitalization for acute MI. Mortality rates in unselected populations included in MI registries are even higher: 9.4% in-hospital mortality in the National Registry of Myocardial Infarction (NRMI) (3). Furthermore, mortality rates in the United States Medicare database are more than twofold higher than mortality rates that have been observed in clinical trials. Therefore, despite improved therapies for acute MI, risk stratification, and secondary prevention are critically important in improving the outcomes of patients with acute MI by decreasing the likelihood of recurrent ischemic events, in both the short term and the long term.

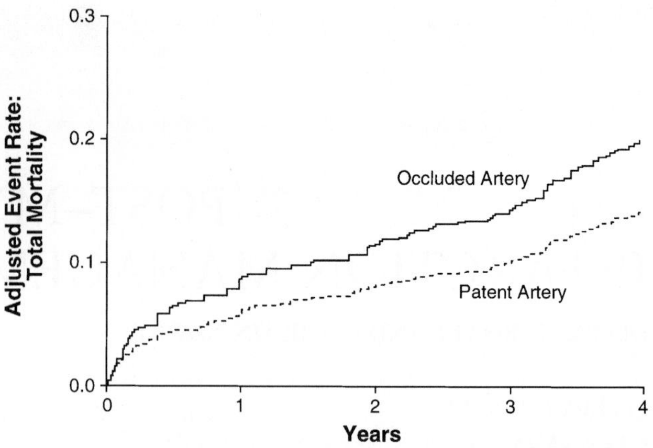

FIGURE 21.1. An occluded coronary artery is associated with a much lower survival rate, as illustrated by these data from the Survival and Ventricular Enlargement (SAVE) Trial, which provides indirect evidence supporting the "open-artery hypothesis." (*Source:* From Lamas GA, Flaker GC, Mitchell G, et al. Effect of infarct artery patency on prognosis after acute myocardial infarction. The Survival and Ventricular Enlargement Investigators. *Circulation* 1995;92:1101–1109, with permission.)

Pathophysiology

An appreciation of the pathophysiology of acute MI is necessary to understand how specific therapies may be used to target different components of the cascade of events that lead to acute MI. Plaque rupture, arterial thrombosis, myocardial necrosis, and adverse LV remodeling are parts of the continuum that leads to symptomatic manifestations and long-term sequelae of acute MI.

Plaque Rupture and Thrombosis

The inciting event of acute MI is plaque rupture. Numerous factors, which are only partially understood, determine the occurrence of plaque rupture in a susceptible individual. Production of matrix metalloproteinases leads to degradation of the shoulder of a coronary plaque, resulting in exposure of its lipid-rich core to flowing blood (4–6). This triggers formation of platelet-rich thrombus. When the degree of thrombus is flow occlusive or platelet microemboli occlude distal flow, ischemia occurs, and myocardial stunning and necrosis follow.

The 3-hydroxy-3-methylglutaryl coenzyme A reductase inhibitors (statins) may exert part of their benefit by decreasing the lipid content of plaques, rendering them less prone to rupture (7,8). Antithrombotic therapy decreases the tendency for occlusive thrombus formation; in particular, antiplatelet therapy decreases platelet aggregation at the site of ruptured plaque. Thus, in concert, statin therapy and antiplatelet therapy decrease the chance of MI occurring.

Left Ventricular Remodeling

When occlusive thrombus has developed and caused ischemia for as little as 45 to 60 minutes, myocardium is irreversibly damaged. When this necrosis is transmural, the left ventricle may undergo a process called *remodeling*. This adaptation occurs at both the cellular level (destruction of connective tissue with slippage of myofilaments) and the whole-organ level (changes in the size and shape of the left ventricle) and results from adaptive (or maladaptive) mechanisms, such as apoptosis and fibroblast and myocyte hypertrophy triggered by increased wall stress from the inciting cellular changes (9). Angiotensin-converting enzyme (ACE) inhibitors greatly decrease this process of adverse remodeling, and it appears that angiotensin receptor blockers (ARBs) share this property. This explains, at least in part, the marked benefits of ACE inhibition or angiotensin receptor blockade among patients who have ventricular dysfunction after MI.

Arrhythmogenic Substrate

The zone of myocardium surrounding the infarcted area is particularly prone to electrical instability. This often manifests as premature ventricular contractions (PVCs) and predisposes the patient to ventricular arrhythmia. β-Blockers are useful in reducing the electrical irritability of the damaged myocardium. Implantable cardioverter-defibrillators (ICDs) are the best line of defense in treating electrical excitability that causes potentially lethal arrhythmia, particularly in the setting of impaired LV function.

Open-Artery Hypothesis

Even if the LV muscle supplied by an occluded artery is dead, revascularization may still favorably effect ventricular remodeling and promote electrical stability. Depending on the duration of ischemia, among other factors, the myocardial cells either die or go into a state of hibernation. In this latter stage, revascularization can restore contractile functionality to what otherwise appears to be dead myocardium. Thus, there are a number of reasons, both established and theoretical, why vessel patency can improve prognosis (Fig. 21.1) (10).

CLINICAL MANAGEMENT

Exercise stress testing, noninvasive imaging, and coronary angiography are all used to risk stratify patients and determine their subsequent management. Risk stratification models may help to determine the most appropriate in-hospital and long-term management of patients with acute MI (11).

Noninvasive Assessment of Left Ventricular Function and Reperfusion

Transthoracic echocardiography is a standard technique used not only to determine the presence of mechanical complications of MI, but also to provide an estimate of LV systolic and diastolic function. Indeed, at least on a population level, LV ejection fraction has been shown to be a powerful predictor of outcome (Fig. 21.2) (12). Another alternative for post-MI assessment of LV systolic function that also allows an assessment of infarct size and remaining myocardial viability is cardiac magnetic resonance imaging (MRI). Cardiac MRI has been used successfully to predict recovery of systolic function at 6 months (13). A number of new modalities are being investigated as aids for

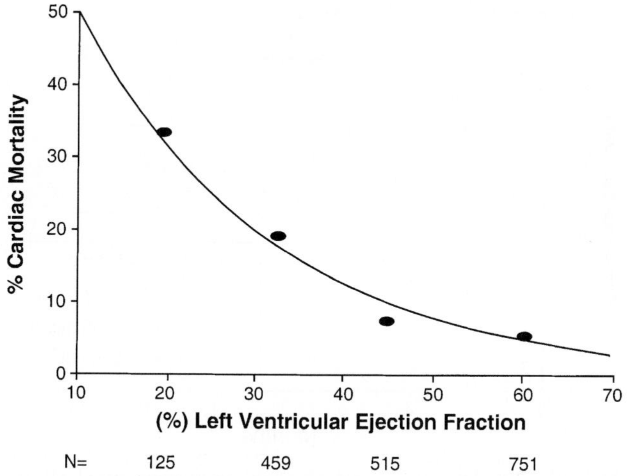

FIGURE 21.2. Diminished LV ejection fraction after MI is a powerful predictor of death after MI. (From Gottlieb S, Moss AJ, McDermott M, et al. Interrelation of left ventricular ejection fraction, pulmonary congestion and outcome in acute myocardial infarction. *Am J Cardiol* 1992;69:977–984, with permission.)

determination of tissue level reperfusion after MI, but none are widely available for routine use. Contrast echocardiography is one such modality (14,15), and in conjunction with ST-segment resolution may be useful in gauging reperfusion (16). MRI may be even more sensitive than contrast echocardiography in detection of microvascular obstruction (17), and such modalities may ultimately be important adjuncts to more conventional determinants of infarct size (18). These newer modalities may refine assessment of LV function so that an evaluation of microvascular integrity will become part of analyzing the state of the infarcted myocardium, at both a whole-organ and a cellular level.

Stress Testing

The role of stress testing in the management of patients after MI has been extensively studied. The value of exercise stress testing depends greatly on whether the patient has undergone revascularization (19). Guidelines have been developed to aid in the appropriate use of stress testing (20). Data from NRMI show that predischarge stress testing currently is performed in fewer than 10% of American patients, with the majority undergoing in-hospital revascularization or outpatient stress testing (3).

Certain features on a stress test identify patients at high risk of recurrent ischemic events. LV dilatation, pulmonary uptake of thallium-201, ejection fraction less than 40%, and reversible defects in the territory of the infarction are all markers of high risk on postexercise nuclear imaging scans. Additionally, large fixed defects and multivessel disease considerably raise the risk profile of the patient. Normal or low-risk results of a dipyridamole stress test predict an annual rate of death, MI, or urgent revascularization of less than 2%.

The Danish Trial in Acute Myocardial Infarction (DANAMI) randomly assigned 1,008 patients who had received fibrinolysis for MI and had inducible ischemia on stress testing to receive either invasive or conservative treatment (21). Those patients assigned to the invasive arm had a statistically significant reduction in the primary end points of death, MI, or readmission for unstable angina. The authors appropriately concluded that patients who have inducible ischemia detected before discharge should undergo coronary angiography.

Exercise stress testing can provide valuable information, primarily because the inability to exercise confers a poor prognosis (22,23). Although rare, myocardial rupture is possible during exercise stress testing or dobutamine stress testing in the post-MI period (24). As an alternative to submaximal exercise stress testing before hospital discharge, pharmacologic stress testing with dipyridamole 2 to 4 days after MI may be performed safely (25). In one study, dipyridamole stress testing outperformed submaximal exercise testing with nuclear imaging in its ability to predict postdischarge cardiac events (25).

Coronary Angiography

As noted, the DANAMI study showed that patients with inducible ischemia after acute MI had better outcomes if they were treated with an invasive strategy as opposed to a conservative one (21). Revascularization, either percutaneously or surgically, was found to be beneficial. An analysis of the patients from the DANAMI study who underwent coronary artery bypass grafting (CABG) was performed (26). The median time to CABG after acute MI was approximately 6 weeks. Patients who had inducible ischemia, including silent ischemia, after acute MI benefited from CABG.

Similarly, spontaneous ischemia in the form of postinfarction angina is a serious development that warrants invasive investigation. Armstrong et al. (27) reported on the incidence and consequences of recurrent ischemia across the spectrum of ST-segment elevation MI and non–ST-segment elevation acute coronary syndrome (ACS) in an analysis from the GUSTO-IIb trial database (27). In this cohort, 35% of patients with non–ST-segment elevation ACS had recurrent ischemia compared with 23% of patients with ST-segment elevation MI. Particularly when recurrent ischemia was classified as refractory, both 30-day and 1-year survivals were substantially lower than if no recurrent ischemia occurred. Similarly, the Gruppo Italiano per lo Studio della Sopravvivenza nell'Infarto Miocardico 3 (GISSI-3) trial analyzed the outcomes of patients with early angina after MI who were managed conservatively (28). Patients with post-MI angina had more in-hospital reinfarction, but despite successful medical management while in the hospital in many cases, these patients had a higher rate of death or reinfarction at 6 months. In fact, the presence of early post-MI angina was an independent predictor of the 6-month reinfarction or death. Among patients with early angina, the rate of reinfarction was 12%, versus 5% among patients without early angina ($P < .0001$). The rate of death was also higher among patients with early angina than in those without early angina (13% versus 7%, respectively; $P < .0001$). Based on these observations, angiography for ischemic symptoms after MI is given a class I indication in the American College of Cardiology/American Heart Association guidelines for coronary arteriography (29).

Indirect evidence from comparative studies favors an invasive approach to treatment of MI. Compared with Canadian patients, American patients are more likely to undergo catheterization and angioplasty. This difference in approach appears to lead to better outcomes in American patients (30). A study comparing outcomes after MI in areas in France and Spain with different rates of angiography reached a similar conclusion regarding the superiority of an invasive approach (31).

However, older, randomized studies such as the Treatment of Post-Thrombolytic Stenoses trial do not favor routine angiography after successful fibrinolysis, even when angiography demonstrates a "significant" stenosis (32). The Should We Intervene following Thrombolysis trial did not find a benefit for routine angiography after fibrinolysis either (33). Likewise, the Thrombolysis in Myocardial Infarction (TIMI) II-B and European Cooperative Study Group trials were unable to demonstrate an advantage to a routine invasive approach (34,35). The

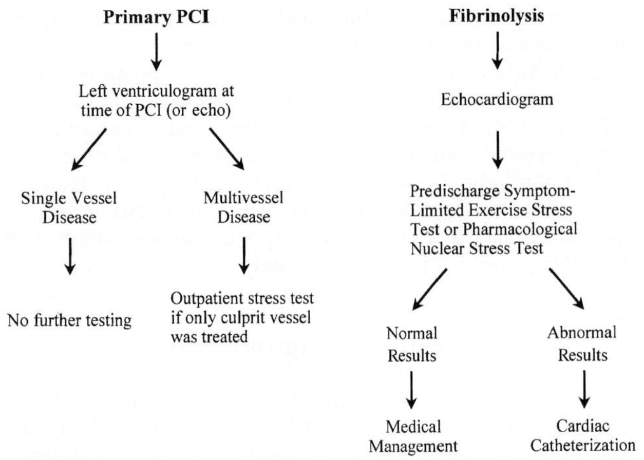

FIGURE 21.3. Risk assessment algorithm for the post–MI patient, depending on the primary mode of reperfusion. *Abbreviations:* echo, echocardiogram; PCI, percutaneous coronary intervention.

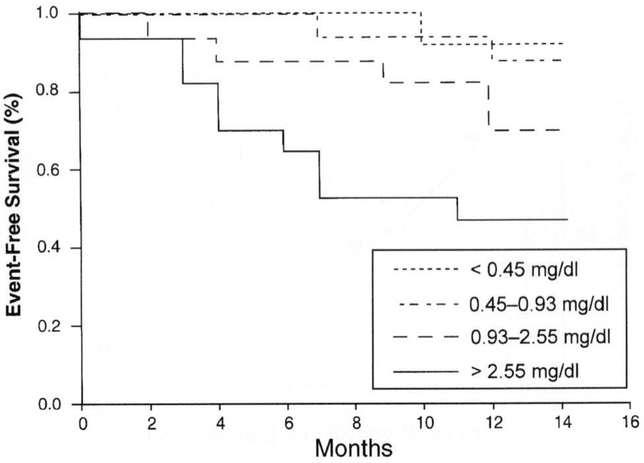

FIGURE 21.4. Even in patients who have an uncomplicated MI, the risk of subsequent cardiac events increases with each successive quartile elevation of the C-reactive protein level. (*Source:* From Tommasi S, Carluccio E, Bentivoglio M, et al. C-reactive protein as a marker for cardiac ischemic events in the year after a first, uncomplicated myocardial infarction. *Am J Cardiol* 1999;83:1595–1599, with permission.)

Thrombolysis and Angioplasty in Myocardial Infarction study found no advantage to immediate angioplasty after fibrinolysis in comparison with delayed angioplasty 5 to 10 days later (36). Perhaps the prothrombotic effects at the site of ruptured plaque that systemic fibrinolysis can create, coupled with further arterial trauma from balloon angioplasty, led to lack of favorable outcomes with invasive therapy (37). Therefore, the results of these trials may no longer apply in an era marked by greater use of stents and IV glycoprotein IIb/IIIa inhibition, but this issue needs to be examined prospectively (38). Recently, the ASSENT IV trial results were presented. This trial showed an increased risk of ischemic events and also major bleeding in patients who received a full dose of fibrinolysis followed by PCI versus primary PCI without antecedent lytic use (39). Therefore, in patients who appear to have successfully reperfused after fibrinolysis, or those who have received no reperfusion therapy acutely, it is still reasonable to use noninvasive risk stratification before invasive therapy, with its attendant risk.

One of the benefits of an invasive strategy is that it can provide diagnostic information and definitive therapy in the form of PCI. Whereas Fragmin and Fast Revascularisation during Instability in Coronary Artery Disease II (FRISC-II) and Treat Angina with Aggrastat and Determine Cost of Therapy with an Invasive or Conservative Strategy were studies demonstrating the superiority of an invasive approach over a conservative strategy in non–ST-segment elevation ACSs, it may prove to be legitimate to extrapolate these results to the management of patients after acute ST-segment elevation MI (40–45).

In the future, ST-segment resolution after fibrinolytic therapy may be used to guide the need for invasive therapy. Contrast echocardiography or perfusion MRI may also prove to have clinical usefulness in assessing lack of tissue-level perfusion and the need for invasive therapy. An algorithm for risk stratification is shown in Figure 21.3.

Assessment of Inflammatory Activity

Although an assessment of myocardial necrosis and microvascular obstruction is useful, measures of heightened inflammation, such as an elevated C-reactive protein (CRP) level, may provide additional ability to risk stratify patients (46,47). The value of CRP levels was examined in a study of 64 patients with an uncomplicated MI (48). All patients had normal LV function with no evidence of ischemia on a predischarge ergometer test. With each successive increase in quartile of CRP, the risk of cardiac death, recurrent MI, or new-onset angina in the ensuing year increased (Fig. 21.4). Even cruder indices of inflammation, such as the white blood cell (WBC) count, appear to help to risk stratify patients (49). A study of 975 patients with acute MI found that those who had angiographic thrombus were more likely to have an elevated WBC count, perhaps illustrating the interplay between inflammation and thrombosis (49). Furthermore, increasing elevation in levels of WBCs was associated with higher mortality.

Beyond their role in risk stratification, markers of inflammation may help to gauge the incremental benefit of invasive therapy, in a manner complementary to troponin elevation. This paradigm has been shown to be true for non–ST-segment elevation ACSs in two separate analyses, the results of which may apply to the acute MI setting. In an analysis of almost 12,000 patients with ACS, elevated WBC count correlated with 6-month mortality (50). However, in those patients undergoing in-hospital revascularization, the deleterious effect of an elevated WBC count were substantially lessened (50). Similarly, in FRISC-II, an invasive strategy (compared with a conservative approach) was seen to be of particular benefit in patients with elevated CRP, troponin T, or interleukin-6 levels (51).

Risk of Arrhythmia

The role of routine telemetry in patients after MI is well established. In fact, perhaps the major advance of the cardiac intensive care unit was the development of continuous monitoring for ventricular arrhythmia, allowing prompt defibrillation. High-grade heart block may develop after anterior wall MI, and permanent pacemaker implantation may be necessary. Atrial fibrillation may complicate MI, often as a result of concomitant ventricular dysfunction from a large infarction.

PVCs after MI are commonly observed on telemetry, and an increased frequency definitely increases the risk of subsequent arrhythmic death (52). Therefore, it was logical to think that decreasing or eliminating PVCs would be desirable. However, the Cardiac Arrhythmia Suppression Trial (CAST) I and CAST II showed that routine suppression of PVCs was not beneficial and that suppression with the agents studied was in fact associated with increased mortality (53–55). Therefore, routine suppression of asymptomatic ventricular arrhythmias was abandoned.

An ICD may be indicated to prevent life-threatening arrhythmia in certain high-risk patients after acute MI, particularly those with prior life-threatening ventricular arrhythmias or LV systolic dysfunction. The randomized clinical trials that have explored the use of ICD therapy were recently summarized by Al-Khatib et al. (56). In patients with prior ventricular fibrillation or symptomatic sustained ventricular tachycardia, the Antiarrhythmics versus Implantable Defibrillators Trial demonstrated the superiority of ICD over antiarrhythmic therapy, with a 3-year mortality rate of 24.6% versus 35.9%, respectively (57). Several trials have also randomized high-risk patients (defined clinically and/or guided by electrophysiologic testing) who were without prior life-threatening arrhythmias to prophylactic ICD therapy. All but two of these trials found a mortality benefit among patients receiving ICD therapy (57–64). In CABG-PATCH there was no mortality benefit from prophylactic ICD implantation at the time of CABG. The Defibrillator in Acute Myocardial Infarction Trial (DINAMIT), the other trial to show no benefit from ICD therapy, was the only trial to test prophylactic ICD implantation in the context of recent acute MI, and suggested that patients should not receive an ICD within one month of an MI (63). Interestingly, in a subanalysis of 14,609 patients from the VALIANT trial, which randomized acute MI patients with clinical evidence of heart failure or LV ejection fraction 40% or less to captopril, valsartan, or the combination, 7% died suddenly or had a resuscitated cardiac arrest within 6 months of their index MI, and 19% of all such events during the median 24.7 months of follow-up and 83% of all sudden deaths occurred within the first 30 days (65).

Thus, given that it is a very high-risk period for sudden death or resuscitated cardiac arrest, the reason for the failure to show a benefit of ICD implantation within 6 to 40 days of acute MI in the DINAMIT trial is unclear, but other competing factors may explain the overall mortality results observed in the trial. At present, recommendations are for prophylactic ICD implantation 1 month or more after MI in patients with an EF of less than 30% at that time, and many electrophysiologists wait at least 3 months and reassess LV function before deciding about prophylactic ICD implantation.

Concerns about the health economic implications of prophylactic ICD implantation in the hundreds of thousands of patients who would qualify for such therapy based on the results of these clinical trials were recently addressed in a study of the cost effectiveness of ICD therapy by Sanders et al. (66). Based on the results of six trials showing a mortality benefit from prophylactic ICD implantation in high-risk patients with reduced ejection fraction, it was estimated that prophylactic placement of an ICD would increase life expectancy by 2.12 to 6.21 years. Depending on the patient population, as defined by the individual trials' inclusion criteria, the cost effectiveness of prophylactic implantation was between $34,000 and $70,200 per quality-adjusted life-year and remained under $100,000 per quality-adjusted life-year across a broad range of sensitivity analyses. Thus, the use of ICD therapy in selected patient populations appears to have cost effectiveness in the range of other standard therapies for coronary artery disease. However, whereas ICD implantation definitely has a favorable impact on mortality rates in populations of patients and has been shown to be cost effective, the feasibility of such an approach, especially if it were applied broadly to all MI patients meeting trial criteria, remains to be determined. Methods to further define which patients are at highest risk and will receive most benefit from ICD therapy are needed. Home automatic external defibrillators are being evaluated in an ongoing randomized trial in patients with an anterior MI in the past month, a period of time that has been identified as being particularly high-risk for sudden cardiac death (65).

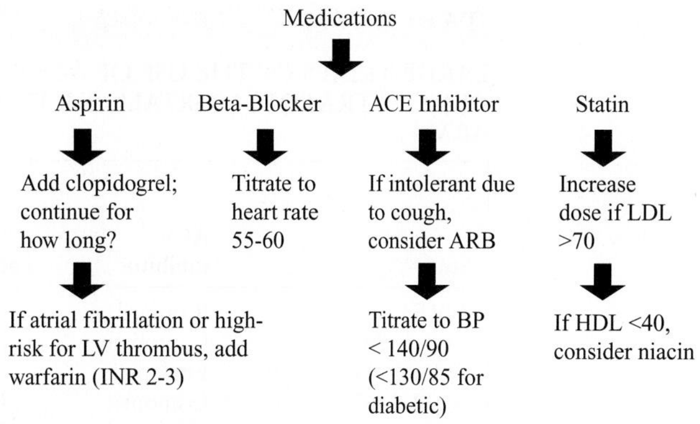

FIGURE 21.5. Flow chart for appropriate medications in patients after MI. If left ventricular (LV) dysfunction is not present, it is not clear whether both β-blockers and angiotensin-converting enzyme (ACE) inhibitors are necessary. *Abbreviations:* ARB, angiotensin-receptor blocker; BP, blood pressure; HDL, high-density lipoprotein; INR, international normalized ratio; LDL, low-density lipoprotein.

MEDICAL THERAPY

Several classes of medications designed to improve outcomes after acute MI have undergone rigorous evaluation in large, randomized, controlled trials. It is imperative that physicians screen post-MI patients for criteria that indicate that specific medications should be prescribed (Fig. 21.5).

Afterload Reduction

Angiotensin-Converting Enzyme Inhibitors

Use of ACE inhibitors after acute MI is supported by a vast amount of evidence (Table 21.1) (67–69). The Acute Infarction Ramipril Efficacy study found that ramipril decreased mortality after MI among patients with heart failure (70), and the Survival and Ventricular Enlargement trial demonstrated the significant mortality benefit from administration of captopril after MI among patients with asymptomatic LV dysfunction (71). The Trandolapril Cardiac Evaluation study showed that the benefit of ACE inhibition persisted through 2 years of therapy, suggesting that ACE inhibition should be continued indefinitely (72). In fact, the results of the Heart Outcomes Prevention Evaluation (HOPE) study suggest that ACE inhibitors may be indicated in all patients who have had an MI (73). Further, the EUROPA trial also found a reduction in cardiovascular events in patients with stable coronary artery disease without LV dysfunction who were randomized to the ACE inhibitor perindopril versus placebo (74). However, the PEACE trial did not find a significant benefit of ACE inhibition with trandolapril versus placebo in patients with stable heart disease; this may reflect that the patients enrolled in this trial were lower risk than in the prior two trials (75).

Early initiation of oral ACE inhibitors is recommended for these patients, unless hypotension is present (76–78). However, the data do not support the early administration of IV ACE inhibitors (79). The early benefit of ACE inhibition on minimizing LV dilatation is most marked when reperfusion has not occurred, but other beneficial effects of ACE inhibitors likely apply to all patients (80). Despite these favorable data, ACE inhibitors are underprescribed after acute MI (81). Unless systolic blood pressure is lower than 100 mm Hg, ACE inhibition should generally be initiated within 24 hours of acute MI (78).

TABLE 21.1

LARGE TRIALS OF THE USE OF ACE INHIBITORS AFTER ACUTE MI, DEMONSTRATING MORTALITY RATES FOR PLACEBO AND ACE INHIBITOR ARMS

Study	ACE inhibitor	Patients (*n*)	Length of follow-up	Mortality rates (%) Placebo	Mortality rates (%) ACE inhibitor
AIRE (70)	Ramipril	2,006	15 mo	22.4	16.8
CCS-1 (76)	Captopril	13,634	4 wk	9.6	9.1
CONSENSUS II (79)	Enalapril	6,090	6 mo	10.2	11.0
GISSI-3 (67)	Lisinopril	18,895	6 wk	7.1	6.3
ISIS-4 (68)	Captopril	58,050	5 wk	7.7	7.2
SAVE (71)	Captopril	2,231	42 mo	24.6	20.4
SMILE (300)	Zofenopril	1,556	1 yr	14.1	10.0
TRACE (301)	Trandolapril	1,749	24–50 mo	42.3	34.7

Abbreviations: AIRE, Acute Infarction Ramipril Efficacy Study; CCS-1, Chinese Cardiac Study; CONSENSUS II, Cooperative New Scandinavian Enalapril Survival Study II; GISSI-3, Gruppo Italiano per lo Studio della Sopravvivenza nell'Infarto Miocardico 3; ISIS-4, Fourth International Study of Infarct Survival; SAVE, Survival and Ventricular Enlargement Trial; SMILE, Survival of Myocardial Infarction Long-Term Evaluation Study; TRACE, Trandolapril Cardiac Evaluation Study.

Angiotensin-Receptor Blockers

At present, ARBs appear to be an acceptable alternative to ACE inhibitors, particularly for patients who are unable to tolerate ACE inhibitors because of side effects such as cough. Whether any incremental benefit occurs with the addition of an ARB to the treatment regimen for patients who are on an ACE inhibitor has been evaluated in the Valsartan in Acute Myocardial Infarction Trial, which compared the ARB valsartan, the ACE inhibitor captopril, or the combination in MI patients with heart failure (82). In this population, there was no difference in mortality between the captopril and valsartan groups, and the combination did not provide any greater benefit than either agent alone, but did increase the incidence of drug-related side effects. However, in a more broad population of patients with systolic dysfunction in the Candasartan in Heart failure Assessment of Reduction in Mortality (CHARM)-Added trial, the ARB, candasartan, added to ACE inhibitor was found to be superior to the use of ACE inhibitor alone (83). Importantly, in the CHARM-Alternative Trial, Granger et al. (84) showed that candasartan alone reduced mortality and morbidity by nearly 30% among patients with systolic dysfunction but intolerant of ACE inhibitors, supporting the use of ARBs as an alternative to ACE inhibitors in ACE inhibitor intolerant patients.

β-Blockers

The role of β-blockers in patients who have experienced MI is well established (Table 21.2) (85). Beneficial effects result from decreases in heart rate, blood pressure, myocardial oxygen demand, and arrhythmogenesis (86). Newer evidence suggests a favorable influence on LV remodeling as well (87). In aggregate, the data suggest that β-blockade reduces nonfatal MI by approximately 25%, which is paralleled by a 25% reduction in mortality (88,89). Although these data were gathered largely before the fibrinolytic era, TIMI II-B found that even in patients who had received fibrinolysis, compared with later administration of β-blockers, early β-blockade reduced recurrent chest pain and reinfarction (90). Furthermore, early β-blockade has been associated with a lower incidence of

TABLE 21.2

EVENT RATES FOR SELECTED LARGE TRIALS OF THE USE OF β-BLOCKERS VERSUS PLACEBO AFTER ACUTE MI

Study	β-Blocker	Patients (*n*)	Length of follow-up	Endpoint	Event rate (%) Placebo	Event rate (%) β-Blocker
BHAT (302)	Propranolol	3,837	24 mo	Death	9.8	7.2
COMMIT (93)	Metoprolol	45,849	16 d	Death	7.8	7.7
Goteborg Trial (303)	Metoprolol	1,395	3 mo	Death	8.9	5.7
ISIS-1 (304)	Atenolol	16,027	7 d	Vascular death	4.6	3.9
MIAMI (305)	Metoprolol	5,778	15 d	Death	4.9	4.3
Norwegian Multicenter Study (86,306)	Timolol	1,884	7 yr	Death	32.3	26.4
TIMI II-B (90)	Metoprolol	1,434	6 d	Reinfarction	5.1[a]	2.7

Abbreviations: BHAT, Beta-Blocker Heart Attack Trial; COMMIT, Clopidogrel and Metoprolol in Myocardial Infarction Trial; ISIS-1, First International Study of Infarct Survival; MIAMI, Metoprolol in Acute Myocardial Infarction Trial; TIMI II-B, Thrombolysis in Myocardial Infarction II-B Study.

[a]The placebo was delayed administration of metoprolol on day 6 after MI versus immediate IV administration followed by oral dosing on day 1.

intracranial hemorrhage after fibrinolysis (91). Conversely, in a secondary analysis from the GUSTO-1 trial database, Pfisterer et al. (92) raised concerns about the safety and efficacy of early IV β-blockade. In their analysis, they observed that patients treated with atenolol at any point were generally at lower risk, but that their adjusted 30-day mortality was significantly lower that those not receiving atenolol. However, patients treated with early intravenous then oral atenolol versus oral treatment alone had an increased odds of mortality (1.3; 95% confidence interval, 1.0–1.5; $P = .02$). Patients treated with IV atenolol had more heart failure, shock, recurrent ischemia, and pacemaker use than those treated with oral atenolol, but there were no significant differences in the rates of stroke, intracranial hemorrhage, and reinfarction. More recently, the COMMIT randomized trial also suggested that very early initiation of β-blockade was deleterious among patients who have a low blood pressure at admission and may be in impending cardiogenic shock (93). In COMMIT, early initiation of metoprolol increased the risk of cardiogenic shock, although it decreased recurrent infarction. Overall, though, there was no reduction in mortality. However, once patients were stabilized, β-blockers appeared to decrease the risk of sudden cardiac death. The lesson from these studies appears to be that in high-risk patients with hypotension or signs of heart failure, it is best not to initiate β-blockade, until the patient has stabilized.

β-Blockers remain underused after MI, sometimes because of unfounded concerns regarding relative contraindications such as diabetes or chronic obstructive pulmonary disease (94–96). β-Blockers have a similar relative benefit in the presence and absence of heart failure, although the absolute benefit is magnified in those with heart failure (97). Although numerous studies have confirmed the benefit and safety of β-blockade in the elderly, underuse remains a problem (98–100). The optimal dose of β-blockade in elderly patients, is not known, but doses lower than those that were used in several of the early randomized trials may be just as effective (101,102).

The limited available evidence suggests that β-blockade and ACE inhibition are complementary (103–108). In patients who experience congestive heart failure after MI, both classes of medication seem to be indicated. At the other end of the spectrum, in patients with normal LV function, perhaps only one of these classes of medication is needed. Without prospective data examining the incremental value of combination therapy, other patient factors, such as history of arrhythmia or diabetes, should also be considered in deciding which of these agents to use.

Aldosterone Antagonism

The Randomized Aldactone Evaluation Study found a 30% reduction in mortality among patients with severe heart failure randomized to spironolactone (109). Subsequently, the Eplerenone Post-AMI Heart Failure Efficacy and Survival Study demonstrated a 15% reduction in mortality among patients with acute MI complicated by heart failure (110). However, without close monitoring, hyperkalemia can be a potentially lethal complication of aldosterone antagonism (111).

Calcium Channel Blockers

Given the abundance of mortality data supporting the use of ACE inhibitors and β-blockers, calcium channel blockers should not be considered first-line therapy in post-MI patients (112). The short-acting calcium channel blockers, especially nifedipine, should not be used for acute or chronic therapy, because these agents do not decrease mortality rates and appear to raise the risk of cardiac events (113–117). Without further supportive evidence, the main role of calcium channel blockers is for control of persistent hypertension in post-MI patients, or as primary therapy in the very rare patient with coronary artery spasm (118). The calcium channel blocker amlodipine does have strong data supporting its role as an antihypertensive and it appears to have a role in decreasing plaque regression and preventing cardiovascular events in patients with coronary artery disease without hypertension (119). Because it does not affect heart rate, it can be safely combined with a β-blocker.

Nitrates

No study has provided compelling evidence that nitroglycerin reduces mortality rates after acute MI. GISSI-3 found no mortality advantage or decrease in the incidence of LV dysfunction from the use of transdermal nitroglycerin (67). The Fourth International Study of Infarct Survival found no mortality benefit from use of an oral mononitrate preparation in any subgroup examined (68). Nevertheless, because of the acute antiischemic effect of these agents, every patient who has experienced an MI should be instructed to carry a bottle of sublingual nitroglycerin at all times and should be instructed in its safe use.

3-Hydroxy-3-Methylglutaryl Coenzyme A Reductase Inhibitors

Statins are strongly indicated for use as secondary prevention after acute MI. The Cholesterol and Recurrent Events (CARE) trial demonstrated that pravastatin, compared with placebo, reduced the rate of death or MI in patients with previous MI (120). In addition to beneficial effects on reinfarction, the CARE study showed that statin use decreased the risk of stroke in survivors of acute MI (121,122). Several other trials have validated the role of statins in secondary and even primary prevention (123). Whether there are benefits specific to one statin over another remains to be elucidated. The Pravastatin or Atorvastatin Evaluation and Infection Therapy—Thrombolysis in Myocardial Infarction 22 trial randomized over 4,000 patients with ACS to receive atorvastatin 80 mg/d versus pravastatin 40 mg/d for a mean duration of 24 months and demonstrated a 16% reduction in ischemic events with a more aggressive LDL cholesterol reduction strategy with atorvastatin 80 mg (124). Whether this was due to greater degree of LDL reduction or differential CRP reduction or both remains a matter of debate (125).

Timing of Initiation of Therapy

Until recently, the appropriate time at which to measure lipid parameters was controversial (126). MI, as is true of most acute illnesses, can lower total cholesterol and LDL cholesterol levels temporarily. This led many doctors to avoid measurement of lipids during the hospitalization phase and defer decisions regarding lipid-lowering therapy to a subsequent outpatient evaluation. However, lipid-lowering therapy may not be started by the outpatient physician, who may assume that if it were necessary, it would have been started by the hospital specialist (127). The effect of MI on lipid values is minimized if blood tests are drawn within 48 hours of hospital admission for acute MI (126). Furthermore, in a study of 294 MI patients, in-hospital cholesterol levels were higher than the National Cholesterol Education Program target LDL for secondary prevention in 83.7% of patients anyway. Thus, there is no good reason to defer cholesterol measurements, although repeating them in the outpatient setting is not unreasonable. The argument can now be made that all patients should be treated with a statin, regardless of the initial in-hospital cholesterol measurement.

Data from a Swedish registry of post-MI patients indicated that the combination of statin therapy for hyperlipidemia initiated during the hospitalization and revascularization within 14 days dramatically reduced 1-year mortality after MI by two thirds (128). After adjustment for baseline differences, the investigators found a 25% reduction in mortality with early statin use and also reported a 36% reduction with early revascularization, both of which were highly statistically significant.

Additionally, the Myocardial Ischemia Reduction with Aggressive Cholesterol Lowering (MIRACL) trial suggested a benefit from initiation of statin therapy in the acute setting (129,130). MIRACL randomly assigned more than 3,000 patients who had ACSs to receive 80 mg of atorvastatin within 4 days. Patients who had recent or planned revascularization were excluded from the trial. A reduction in the composite endpoint of nonfatal MI, cardiac arrest with resuscitation, or angina requiring hospitalization was found ($P = .048$), driven almost entirely by a reduction in rehospitalization for angina. Although these results were not overwhelming, the trial adds to the evidence supporting a benefit from early initiation of statin therapy, with no downside.

Although the rate of statin use has been increasing, many patients still do not receive them. The National Registry of Myocardial Infarction 3 found that in 1999, only 36.2% of patients with acute MI were discharged while a statin was being administered (3). Statins are cost effective even in elderly patients who have had an MI, although they are particularly underused in this population (131). The Maximal Individual Therapy in Acute Myocardial Infarction (MITRA) project in Germany has demonstrated that statin use after an acute MI can be increased by dissemination of practice guidelines and physician-directed interventions. Early statin use after acute MI had increased in the MITRA registry from 15% to 76% between 1994 and 2000 (132).

Other Lipid-Directed Therapy

Decreased LDL levels may not be the only important result of lipid-directed therapy (133). The Bezafibrate Coronary Atherosclerosis Intervention Trial randomly assigned male patients younger than 45 years who had previously experienced an MI to receive bezafibrate or placebo and found a significant reduction in the number of coronary events (134). This beneficial effect was not accompanied by a reduction in LDL levels, but rather by reductions in triglyceride and fibrinogen levels and increases in high-density lipoprotein (HDL) cholesterol levels. Whether patients with elevated triglyceride levels derive particular benefit from fibrates still needs to be confirmed (135). The Veterans Affairs High-Density Lipoprotein Cholesterol Intervention Trial randomly assigned men with coronary artery disease and a low HDL level to receive gemfibrozil or placebo and found that gemfibrozil reduced the rate of cardiac death or MI (136,137). This study validated the importance of treating low HDL levels, although it is still not clear whether this relationship holds true if a patient is also receiving a statin to decrease LDL levels. Extended-release niacin may be even more effective at increasing HDL levels than gemfibrozil (137). Statins may also have a modest effect on increasing the HDL level (138).

Therefore, if a post-MI patient has an LDL level higher than 70 mg/dL, a statin should be prescribed, and its use should be initiated in the acute phase; even below this LDL level, likely statin initiation would be prudent. If the HDL level is lower than 40 mg/dL despite statin therapy, use of niacin or gemfibrozil should be considered. If triglyceride levels are elevated, gemfibrozil, rather than niacin, is preferred; otherwise niacin, because of its effects on decreasing fibrinogen and lipoprotein(a) levels, may be preferable (138).

Antithrombotic Therapy

Because of the important role that thrombosis plays in acute MI, much research has been done on the use of antithrombotic therapy for the secondary prevention of MI (139).

Antiplatelet Therapy

Aspirin. With its metaanalysis of 174 randomized trials of antiplatelet therapy for cardiovascular disease, the Antiplatelet Trialists' Collaboration conclusively demonstrated the value of aspirin use after MI (140). Approximately 20,000 patients with acute MI were included in this metaanalysis; aspirin reduced the rate of recurrent ischemic events from 14% to 10%. Because the majority of trials included in this metaanalysis lasted an average of 2 years and a significant benefit of aspirin therapy was found between years 1 and 3, aspirin should be continued for at least several years after MI, and, in the absence of bleeding complications, should be continued indefinitely. The Second International Study of Infarct Survival found that aspirin therapy given for 1 month after acute MI was beneficial (141). The benefit was on the same order of magnitude as the benefit of administration of fibrinolysis with streptokinase. The dose of aspirin should be no greater than 325 mg/day, although it is unclear whether more than 81 mg/day is actually necessary for chronic therapy (142). Thus, aspirin is a simple, highly cost-effective intervention in MI patients. Nevertheless, aspirin remains underused after MI (143).

Clopidogrel. Clopidogrel is an antiplatelet agent that works by blocking the adenosine diphosphate receptor. In the Clopidogrel versus Aspirin in Patients at Risk of Ischaemic Events (CAPRIE) study, 19,185 patients with established atherosclerosis of the coronary, cerebral, or peripheral circulation were randomly assigned to undergo secondary prevention with either aspirin or clopidogrel (144). After a mean follow-up period of 1.9 years, this trial found an overall 8.7% relative risk reduction in the primary end point of vascular death, MI, or ischemic stroke ($P = .043$). Interestingly, the CAPRIE study found a 19.2% relative risk reduction in fatal or nonfatal MI ($P = .008$) (145). Thus, compared with aspirin, clopidogrel's ability to reduce the incidence of MI in patients with previous ischemic events is particularly notable. In a subgroup analysis from CAPRIE, patients who were on statin therapy and randomly assigned to clopidogrel had a lower rate of recurrent ischemic events than patients who were randomly assigned to aspirin (146). Furthermore, the relative risk reduction for MI was slightly greater than 50% with this combination. Thus, the benefits of statin therapy and clopidogrel appear to be complementary. In patients who have had an MI while taking aspirin or who are intolerant to aspirin, it is reasonable to consider long-term therapy with clopidogrel, in addition to statin therapy (147).

COMMIT recently enrolled over 45,000 patients within 24 hours of acute ST-elevation MI in China and randomly assigned them to therapy with either clopidogrel or placebo, in addition to aspirin, for up to 4 weeks. Whereas CAPRIE showed that clopidogrel was more effective than aspirin in secondary prevention of MI, COMMIT demonstrated that clopidogrel decreased mortality and reinfarction in the acute setting in combination with aspirin (148). Similarly, the Clopidogrel as Adjunctive Reperfusion Therapy trial also found a reduction in ischemic events when clopidogrel was added to aspirin (149). Taken together, these two trials support use of clopidogrel in addition to aspirin for at least a month in patients with ST-elevation MI (150).

The results from the Clopidogrel in Unstable Angina to Prevent Recurrent Ischemic Events (CURE) trial demonstrate that clopidogrel plus aspirin was superior to aspirin alone in patients presenting with non–ST-elevation ACSs (151). After an average of 9 months, the rate of cardiovascular death, MI, or stroke was reduced from 11.5% in the aspirin-only group to 9.3% in the group assigned to receive both aspirin and clopidogrel ($P = .00005$). Furthermore, the rate of life-threatening bleeding was low: 2.1% in the dual antiplatelet therapy group versus 1.8% in the aspirin group. These findings from CURE regarding longer term clopidogrel are likely applicable to the ST-segment elevation MI population as well. The Clopidogrel for High Atherothrombotic Risk and Ischemic Stabilization, Management, and Avoidance trial seeks to determine whether the combination of clopidogrel plus aspirin should be used indefinitely in all patients with a history of MI (152,153).

Warfarin

When atrial fibrillation is present, the role of warfarin is established (154). Although less common in the reperfusion era, in the case of a large anterior wall MI with anterior akinesis or dyskinesis, warfarin may be considered. Whether warfarin should have a larger role in the routine secondary prevention of post-MI patients has been extensively studied, although with no clear conclusion.

The Sixty Plus Reinfarction Study Research Group found that anticoagulation was more effective after MI than placebo in reducing rates of recurrent MI and death (155). The Warfarin Re-Infarction Study (WARIS) also found that, compared with placebo, anticoagulation reduced mortality rates after MI, as well as rates of reinfarction (156). Additionally, the occurrence of stroke was reduced with warfarin therapy, perhaps because of the decreased occurrence of embolization of LV thrombus. The Anticoagulants in the Secondary Prevention of Events in Coronary Thrombosis (ASPECT) trial also found warfarin to be better than placebo in reducing recurrent MI and stroke, but again, an increase in bleeding complications was observed (157). The optimal international normalized ratio (INR) to minimize both thromboembolic and bleeding events in ASPECT was between 2 and 4 (158). However, in the postfibrinolytic patient with an initially patent artery, the Antithrombotics in the Prevention of Reocclusion in Coronary Thrombolysis (APRICOT) study demonstrated the superiority of aspirin over warfarin (159), and the Coumadin Aspirin Reinfarction Study found that aspirin plus a fixed dose of either 1 or 3 mg of warfarin was no better than aspirin alone (160). Similarly, the Combination Hemotherapy and Mortality Prevention study found no benefit with the use of warfarin adjusted to an INR of 1.5 to 2.0 in addition to aspirin after MI, although the addition of warfarin did cause more gastrointestinal bleeding (161).

Recent studies have revisited the role of warfarin in MI patients. The 308-patient APRICOT-2 study found that the combination of warfarin, with a dose calculated to achieve an INR of 2 to 3, and aspirin was superior to the use of aspirin alone in maintaining the angiographic patency of culprit infarct arteries (162). ASPECT-2 found that warfarin use either with or without aspirin was superior to aspirin alone in reducing ischemic events (163). WARIS-II examined warfarin anticoagulation with or without aspirin versus aspirin alone after MI and found that a regimen including warfarin was superior to aspirin alone in reducing ischemic events, although with far greater bleeding complications (164). The oral direct thrombin inhibitor ximelegatran was found to be effective in acute MI patients in the Efficacy and Safety of the Oral Direct Thrombin Inhibitor Ximelagatran in Patients with Recent Myocardial Damage trial, but this drug was not approved because of concerns over potential hepatotoxicity (165). However, other direct thrombin and factor Xa inhibitors are being evaluated in ACS patients (166).

Compared with placebo, adjusted-dose warfarin does appear to be beneficial in patients after MI if the patients are compliant and the dose of warfarin is carefully regulated, although bleeding remains a concern. Aspirin appears to be superior to warfarin as an antithrombotic strategy after MI, particularly if patients have undergone reperfusion therapy and are at lower risk for thrombus formation in a dyskinetic left ventricle. Potentially, a strategy of dual antiplatelet therapy with aspirin and clopidogrel would enhance the benefits seen with aspirin alone, without the large bleeding penalty incurred by warfarin. The value of a strategy including clopidogrel and aspirin over a strategy including warfarin and aspirin would be further enhanced in the setting of aggressive percutaneous revascularization with stent use, where dual antiplatelet therapy has been proven superior to warfarin plus aspirin (167,168). The management of atrial fibrillation in patients who have received a stent for management of their acute coronary event is challenging, especially in the era of drug-eluting stents. The STent Anti-thrombotic Regimen Study showed that thienopyridine plus aspirin therapy was superior to warfarin plus aspirin in preventing stent thrombosis (167), but recently, the aspirin plus clopidogrel versus warfarin arm of the ACTIVE trial of atrial fibrillation was stopped early owing to excess events in the clopidogrel arm. Thus, further prospective data are needed to define the treatment regimen that best balances benefits and risks in patients with atrial fibrillation in the setting of recent stenting, especially when they are at high risk for embolic stroke.

Hormone Replacement Therapy

Estrogen replacement in postmenopausal women can no longer be recommended for the secondary prevention of ischemic heart disease (169). Despite favorable effects on LDL and HDL cholesterol levels, estrogen replacement raises CRP and does not decrease progression of angiographic coronary artery disease, nor does it reduce clinical cardiovascular events (170–172). It appears that the use of conjugated equine estrogens actually increases the risk of thrombotic events; thus, it is particularly inappropriate for a woman with a recent MI (171).

The Heart and Estrogen/Progestin Replacement Study found no cardiovascular benefit to estrogen replacement versus placebo after 4.1 years of therapy (171). An increased risk of cardiovascular events was observed in the first year of estrogen therapy, possibly as a result of a prothrombotic effect or a proinflammatory effect, followed by fewer events after 2 years of estrogen replacement therapy in the treated group, possibly as a result of beneficial effects on lipid levels and endothelial function. The Women's Health Initiative provided further evidence against any cardiovascular benefit of estrogen replacement (173,174). Other doses and formulations of estrogen, phytoestrogens, or selective estrogen-receptor modulators may yet have a role in secondary prevention, but no randomized clinical data are currently available to evaluate them in this regard (175).

Antioxidants

The HOPE study did not find any benefit from use of vitamin E among patients with vascular disease (73). Although vitamins are relatively inexpensive and reasonably safe at normal doses, they do require patients to take even more pills, potentially instead of prescribed medication that has proven benefit. Therefore, at this time, routine vitamin supplementation in the healthy patient with an adequate diet cannot be recommended.

RISK FACTORS

Hypertension

Hypertension is a risk factor for death after MI (176–178). Additionally, hypertension places patients at greater risk for development of heart failure after MI (179). Treatment with ACE inhibitors seems particularly important in this subgroup of patients (180). In addition to benefits from long-term secondary prevention, immediate treatment of hypertension may decrease the risk of hemorrhagic stroke after fibrinolysis (181).

Diabetes

The use of effective medical therapies to treat hyperglycemia and concomitant risk factors is suboptimal in the post-MI patient with diabetes (182). Other risk factors that may be present in diabetic patients should be identified and aggressively treated (183). Subgroup analyses of major trials have confirmed that diabetic patients may benefit from the use of β-blockers, ACE inhibitors, statins, and aspirin (184,185). For example, a retrospective analysis of 2,790 diabetic patients from GISSI-3 demonstrated a reduction in mortality rates with ACE inhibition that was significantly larger than for patients without diabetes (186). Similarly, clopidogrel was shown to be superior to aspirin in a subgroup analysis of diabetic patients from CAPRIE, further illustrating that high-risk patients derive amplified benefit from aggressive pharmacotherapy (187). Tight glycemic control appears to have a beneficial effect in preventing both micro- and macrovascular events in patients with diabetes mellitus (188).

Inflammation

The role of inflammation in MI is being investigated, with identification of several markers that appear to correlate with adverse outcome after episodes of coronary instability (189,190). The possibility of using agents to treat inflammation to decrease the risk of recurrent ischemic events is appealing. Potential targets include tumor necrosis factor-α, CD40 ligand, and peroxisome proliferator–activated receptor-α and -γ (191). Additionally, agents already in use may have beneficial effects on inflammatory pathways. Statins may possess clinically relevant antiinflammatory properties (192). Antiplatelet agents such as clopidogrel and low-dose aspirin may have secondary antiinflammatory actions mediated through their ability to interfere with platelet activation and subsequent triggering of inflammatory processes. Ultimately, revascularization may prove to be the best "antiinflammatory" therapy (50,51).

Infection

Administration of influenza vaccine during the influenza season was shown in a case-controlled study of 218 patients to decrease independently the risk of recurrent MI (193). Therefore, vaccinating all eligible patients before hospital discharge seems prudent. Whether infection per se is a cause of MI is unclear. Perhaps, more likely, infection is one pathway that leads to inflammation, which may trigger MI. PROVE-IT did not find any benefit in post-ACS patients to support routine use of antibiotics, and other negative antibiotic trials in patients with coronary artery disease have also now been reported (194,195).

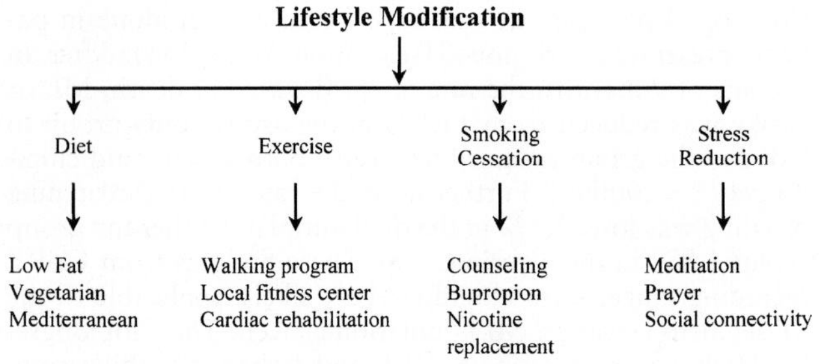

FIGURE 21.6. Lifestyle modification should consist of a multipronged effort to eliminate behaviors that are likely to contribute to adverse cardiac events. Although a comprehensive approach is mandatory, substantial latitude exists in specific recommendations, which allows therapy to be tailored to individual patients.

LIFESTYLE MODIFICATION

The post-MI patient must incorporate several elements of lifestyle modification into daily practice (Fig. 21.6). Physician involvement in this process is crucial. Although counseling a patient and family can be time consuming for the busy clinician, the likelihood of effecting change is highest during the first few days after MI, and this opportunity must not be lost.

Smoking Cessation

It is critical for patients who smoke to stop. The physician must always counsel the patient about the importance of this step, emphasizing the immediate cardiovascular and other health benefits associated with smoking cessation. The message should be repeated often during hospitalization and subsequent outpatient visits, and smoking status should be documented on follow-up (196). The patient is particularly receptive to such messages while in the cardiac care unit (197). The risk of recurrent MI is greatly increased if smoking is continued. However, if the post-MI patient ceases smoking, the risk of death is decreased by almost one half (198,199). In fact, the increased cardiovascular risk attributable to smoking decreases immediately after cessation, approaching the same level of risk as that of a nonsmoker by 4 years (200–205). Immediate economic benefits are also seen in terms of health care use (206).

Living in a household in which other members smoke decreases the chances of successful smoking cessation. The physician should counsel family members who smoke to stop as well. Patient concerns regarding possible weight gain after smoking cessation should also be addressed. Cigar smoking and the chewing of tobacco are also to be avoided. Additionally, illicit drug use, such as cocaine, should also be considered in the etiology of MI and, if present, should be discontinued; referral to formal drug rehabilitation is warranted. Passive smoking should also be avoided (207).

Rates of relapse after smoking cessation are high. Formal smoking cessation programs are useful in increasing long-term abstinence. A study of 100 post-MI patients with a history of smoking randomly assigned participants to receive either conventional care or inpatient counseling with telephone follow-up (208). At 1 year, 34% of the patients receiving conventional care were abstinent, versus 55% of those who were enrolled in the hospital-based counseling program ($P < .05$). Furthermore, smoking cessation programs are highly cost effective (209). Thus, smoking cessation programs do improve cessation rates, and methods to promote and fund such programs are needed.

The use of pharmacologic adjuncts such as nicotine replacement and bupropion can help increase the rates of smoking cessation, especially when combined with behavioral counseling (210). Transdermal nicotine appears to be safe in patients who have cardiac disease and decreases the rates of smoking cessation in the short term, although this benefit diminishes with time (211). Nicotine gum, nicotine nasal spray, and nicotine inhalers are other nicotine replacement options. The patient should be reminded not to smoke while receiving nicotine replacement, because there is some evidence that it might trigger MI (212). Bupropion is an antidepressant that has been shown to be more effective than placebo at maintaining abstinence at 1 year (213). It may even be more effective than transdermal nicotine (214). Persistent smoking after MI has been linked with depression and anxiety, and this may be one reason that bupropion is effective (215). The endocannabinoid receptor antagonist rimonabant has recently been demonstrated to increase significantly smoking cessation rates (216), but is not yet available.

Exercise

Ambulation in the hallways should begin as soon as the patient is hemodynamically stable and shows no evidence of ischemia. Prolonged bed rest is undesirable and leads to deconditioning and an increase in the risk of deep vein thrombosis. Simple measures, such as a daily walking program, may lead to weight loss (217). Exercise can trigger acute MI, which is something patients fear, but this occurs most often from sudden bursts of exercise, rather than from a gradual increase in the intensity of an exercise program. If a patient has been revascularized, the decision to proceed with an exercise program is simplified. Some have asserted that a pre-entrance exercise test may not be absolutely necessary in an appropriately monitored cardiac rehabilitation program (218). However, if no invasive investigation has occurred, standard practice consists of use of an exercise stress test to guide the decision about beginning an exercise program. Even a structured weight-training program appears safe when it is started 6 or more weeks after acute MI in low-risk patients, with a rate of complications lower than that for aerobic exercise (219). The importance of exercise training is most pronounced in post-MI patients who have LV dysfunction. Exercise training improves exercise capacity without causing LV dilatation or increasing LV wall thickness, which were concerns raised by older studies (220). β-Blockade does not attenuate the benefits of exercise training (221).

Exercise rehabilitation has been studied extensively, although the overall quality of the studies has been less than rigorous (222). Furthermore, many studies of cardiac rehabilitation consisted of exercise as well as other behavioral and risk factor modifications, thus making it impossible to determine the individual contribution of a specific intervention (223–225). Some analyses suggest that cardiac rehabilitation can decrease the risk of death in post-MI patients by up to 25% (226–228). Long-term follow-up showed a reduction in sudden death and cardiac mortality rates in another study (229). The benefits of exercise training extend to elderly patients, although high-risk patients appear to be referred to cardiac rehabilitation infrequently (230,231). A cost-effectiveness analysis found that cardiac rehabilitation costs as little as $4,950 per life-year saved, making it very economically attractive (232,233). One area in which there is a paucity of data is the effect of exercise training among patients with systolic dysfunction. The HF-ACTION trial will randomize approximately 3,000 patients to either an exercise program or encouragement to exercise but without a formal program. The primary outcome measure is death or hospitalization for any reason.

Resumption of Sexual Activity

An often unspoken fear of patients (and their spouses) is that sexual activity may trigger an acute MI (234,235). Both men and women describe decreased frequency of sexual activity and diminished satisfaction after MI (236). Sexual activity may be resumed 6 weeks after an infarction, or after 2 weeks if the risk of residual ischemia is low and no symptomatic heart failure or arrhythmia is present (237). If a patient has an exercise capacity of at least 6 metabolic equivalents, sexual activity should be well tolerated (238). The possibility of medication-induced sexual dysfunction, such as can be caused by β-blockers, should be investigated during outpatient follow-up. For men (or women) taking sildenafil (Viagra), tadalafil (Cialis), or vardenafil (Levitra), the patient should be educated about the possible interaction with nitrates (oral, topical, or sublingual) that can cause life-threatening hypotension and trigger MI. No convincing evidence exists that sildenafil or any related drug itself causes MI, although the subsequent sexual activity may rarely trigger MI (239,240). In fact, the actual risk of MI as a result of sexual activity, even in patients who have prior MI, is small, and regular exercise appears to decrease this risk further (241,242). Thus, in almost all patients who have had an MI, sexual activity can be resumed safely. Furthermore, some evidence suggests that regular sexual activity can even reduce cardiovascular risk, although the data are not compelling (243).

Return to Work

How soon a patient is able to return to work depends on the patient and the exact degree of physical exertion required by the patient's job, although occupation per se does not appear to influence the risk of MI (244). A major determinant of returning to work is the perception by the patient of the severity of the MI (245). Importantly, cardiac rehabilitation increases the likelihood of returning to work (246).

Driving is permissible, but air travel is not immediately recommended, although it is probably safe 2 to 3 weeks after an MI, if reversible ischemia has been excluded (247).

Alcohol and Coffee Consumption

Patients often ask whether resumption of alcohol consumption is permitted. Consumption of moderate quantities should not be problematic. Moderate consumption of any type of alcoholic beverage, not just red wine, appears to decrease the risk for cardiovascular death in patients with a history of MI, perhaps in part as a result of beneficial effects on the HDL cholesterol level (248,249). However, one study found that consumption of more than two drinks per day was associated with a 50% increase in mortality among men with prior MI (250). Thus, it appears that two or fewer drinks per day are safe for patients who have experienced an MI and may even be protective against future MI. An alternative hypothesis is that concomitant psychosocial factors, such as lower degrees of stress, account for the observed benefits of moderate alcohol consumption, or that alcohol abstainers have other medical comorbidities (251–253). No compelling data suggest that patients who do not drink should start consuming alcohol.

Although moderate, regular consumption of alcohol may have antiplatelet effects and may enhance endogenous fibrinolytic activity, ingestion of a large amount of alcohol may increase platelet activation transiently (254–256). Therefore, binge drinking is to be avoided (257,258). Regular heavy drinking leads to elevations in blood pressure and is associated with increases in MI, stroke, and mortality and should be avoided as well (259–261). Alcohol may also have untoward effects on systolic performance of recently infarcted myocardium (262).

Coffee consumption has been linked to an excess risk of MI, although this association is in part confounded by concomitant cigarette smoking (263,264). Increased cholesterol levels in coffee drinkers may also account for some of the association (265). Heavy coffee consumption—four or more cups per day—is probably best avoided (266,267).

Diet

Diet is an important part of realigning the patient's lifestyle after MI. Ideally, nutritional change should be implemented in the cardiac unit setting to emphasize the importance of this component of the patient's care. Consultation with a nutritionist can help the patient to make practical changes and can ensure that the person who is most involved with food preparation in the household also understands the changes that must take place.

The usual recommendation is for a low-fat, low-cholesterol diet in patients with coronary artery disease. A Mediterranean diet seems to confer cardioprotection and may even reduce mortality after MI (268). Fish consumption does not convincingly decrease the risk of MI, although it may have an effect on reducing sudden cardiac death owing to omega-3 fatty acid content (269). Vegetarianism does appear to decrease the risk of an MI, in part by favorable effects on glucose intolerance and the waist-to-hip ratio (270). Rimonabant is a medication that has been found to lead to significant weight loss (271). It is being evaluated to see what effect it may have on cardiovascular morbidity and mortality.

Psychosocial Aspects

Patients who have completed a high school education fare better after MI than those who have not graduated from high school (272). Higher rates of smoking only partially accounted for this difference in outcome between patients who graduated from high school and those who did not. Thus, a patient's socioeconomic background does influence the outcome after MI.

Whether mental stress has a role in MI has been debated, and data are available that support both sides of the argument. Psychological distress does appear to increase the risk of rehospitalization, MI, cardiac death, and sudden death in patients who have had acute coronary events (273,274). In fact, psychological distress may have more to do with the failure to return to previous levels of functioning than the extent of myocardial damage (275). Patients' self-perception of their level of functioning after MI contributes to actual levels of function (276).

Depression appears to increase the risk of MI. Similarly, MI can lead to depression. Therefore, the physician must be vigilant for signs of depression and not merely assume that it is "normal" for a patient to be depressed after a heart attack. The options for treating depression pharmacologically include the use of selective serotonin reuptake inhibitors (277). Although concerns exist over the cardiac side effects of tricyclic antidepressants, use of selective serotonin reuptake inhibitors after acute MI appears safe (278). Additionally, the social support provided by a spouse can have substantial effects on recovery after MI. Interestingly, the social support provided by a pet is associated with a positive influence on survival after MI as well (279).

Ideally, all these aspects of lifestyle modification can be incorporated into a comprehensive cardiac rehabilitation program. Whether this will be a formal or informal program depends largely on patient preference and local availability of resources, but in either case, the commitment to change on the part of the patient and physician is most critical.

CONTROVERSIES AND PERSONAL PERSPECTIVES

For the patient who appears to have experienced clinical reperfusion after fibrinolysis, the value of routine angiography remains controversial. Newer methods to assess microvascular reperfusion, such as electrocardiographic ST-segment resolution, contrast echocardiography, and MRI, may help to further clarify which patients will benefit from early angiography. Patients with recurrent spontaneous ischemia or abnormal results of a stress test should definitely undergo cardiac catheterization, with the goal of performing revascularization. After initial treatment, much of the distinction between therapy for ST-segment elevation MI and non–ST-segment elevation ACSs will continue to be blurred as an early invasive approach becomes the standard treatment for chest pain syndromes associated with electrocardiographic deviation or elevated markers of myocardial necrosis and inflammation.

Efforts to increase the use of β-blockers and ACE inhibitors or ARBs should continue, given the widespread availability of these proven medications. Whether both β-blockers and ACE inhibitors are necessary in every patient requires clarification from clinical trials. Because β-blockade has been shown to decrease adverse ventricular remodeling and ACE inhibition has been shown to decrease sudden death, the two classes of drugs may have overlapping protective effects, and both may not be necessary in the patient who has normal LV function after MI. The role of warfarin in acute MI should be limited to specific indications, such as atrial fibrillation or LV thrombus. Instead, oral antiplatelet therapy should be continued after acute MI. Aggressive identification and treatment of hypertension, hypercholesterolemia, obesity, metabolic syndrome, and diabetes should occur, with medical therapy begun in the hospital phase.

Quality improvement initiatives directed at the physician and the patient can increase the use of appropriate medications and lifestyle measures (280). Measures to improve quality do appear to be able to affect "hard" endpoints such as mortality rates (281). Communication between the hospital-based specialist and the outpatient physician is necessary to ensure a smooth transition of care for the patient. Effective methods to enhance such communication need to be developed and integrated into health care delivery systems (282). The availability of guidelines to aid the practitioner in management of MI should be welcomed (283,284). In fact, one of the few measurable differences between treatment of patients with MI in "top" hospitals and mediocre hospitals appears to be a difference in the use of medications such as aspirin and β-blockers, and this appears to translate into better outcomes, including reduced mortality rates (285). Although physician resistance to implementation of guidelines is often the result of a perceived intrusion into the "art" of medicine, in reality, much of the variation in physician practice stems from a failure to incorporate new data (286). For example, a large degree of geographic variation exists in the prescription of medications that have been proven to be effective in multiple, randomized clinical trials (287,288). Payer status also appears to influence management after acute MI (289). A comprehensive approach that integrates care at multiple levels in the health care system will help to standardize and optimize the care of patients after MI.

THE FUTURE

Early revascularization will become the favored strategy throughout Western health care systems. Optimal medical management begun early in the hospital course after MI will include statin therapy, β-blockade, ACE inhibition, or angiotensin receptor blockade, and dual antiplatelet therapy. The coupling of early revascularization with aggressive medical therapy will lead to dramatically improved outcomes after MI. The relative effectiveness, cost effectiveness, incremental benefit, and potential for interaction of all these different medications in combination remain to be determined (290,291). Inflammatory markers will help to stratify risk beyond current measures, and therapies directed specifically at inflammatory pathways will be developed. A more refined understanding of the role of inflammation will complement efforts directed at treating thrombosis. Clinical proteomics and metabolomics will open the door to new biomarkers or panels of biomarkers for identification of risk and targeted treatment to optimize the balance of benefits and risks of new and existing therapies. Potentially, pharmacogenomics will allow targeting of patients most likely to benefit from therapy. Initially, based on the knowledge of the human genome, efforts will be directed toward the development of pharmaceuticals tailored to specific genotypes. For example, factor VII, glycoprotein IIIa (PlA2 allele), and thrombospondin genes have all been demonstrated to have clinically relevant single-nucleotide polymorphisms that could guide the use of different antithrombotic cocktails (292–298). Eventually, therapies designed to modify or enhance an individual's genetic structure will be created. Lifestyle modification will remain an important part of secondary preventive efforts, although pharmaceutical adjuncts to aid in smoking cessation and weight loss will continue to be tested. The appreciation of psychosocial factors in the well-being of post-MI patients will grow. The aging of the population will continue to challenge the health care system. The mortality rate among aged patients with acute MI remains extremely high, and a shift toward more aggressive management in both the acute and chronic phases of therapy will be necessary (299). Use of practice guidelines and critical care pathways, aided by developments in medical informatics, will play an even larger role in reducing variability in physician management and improving the care of the post-MI patient.

As Western society focuses primarily on rational, guideline-based, cost-efficient delivery of the treatment options that advanced technology and drug development have made possible and will continue to deliver, there will be a growing burden of coronary disease in poor, developing nations. In these regions, such expensive treatments and technology will simply not be available because of costs. However, it is in these developing regions that the opportunity for primary prevention in the form of diet, exercise, and smoking cessation is perhaps greatest and should be a priority. Ensuring the best in treatment and secondary prevention will require a concerted effort by and collaboration among the medical communities in Western and developing countries, to define basic guidelines for therapy (e.g., aspirin and β-blockers) that are highly effective but not cost prohibitive, and the drug/device industry to ensure that their products are broadly applicable and available.

References

1. Topol EJ, Ohman EM, Armstrong PW, et al. Survival outcomes 1 year after reperfusion therapy with either alteplase or reteplase for acute myocardial infarction: results from the Global Utilization of Streptokinase and t-PA for Occluded Coronary Arteries (GUSTO) III Trial. *Circulation* 2000;102:1761–1765.
2. Hirulog and Early Reperfusion or Occlusion (HERO)-2 Trial Investigators. Thrombin-specific anticoagulation with bivalirudin versus heparin in patients receiving fibrinolytic therapy for acute myocardial infarction: the HERO-2 randomised trial. *Lancet* 2001;358:1855–1863.
3. Rogers WJ, Canto JG, Lambrew CT, et al. Temporal trends in the treatment of over 1. 5 million patients with myocardial infarction in the US from 1990 through 1999: the National Registry of Myocardial Infarction 1, 2 and 3. *J Am Coll Cardiol* 2000;36:2056–2063.
4. Nikkari ST, O'Brien KD, Ferguson M, et al. Interstitial collagenase (MMP-1) expression in human carotid atherosclerosis. *Circulation* 1995;92:1393–1398.
5. Ikeda U, Shimpo M, Ohki R, et al. Fluvastatin inhibits matrix metalloproteinase-1 expression in human vascular endothelial cells. *Hypertension* 2000;36:325–329.
6. Loftus IM, Naylor AR, Goodall S, et al. Increased matrix metalloproteinase-9 activity in unstable carotid plaques. A potential role in acute plaque disruption. *Stroke* 2000;31:40–47.
7. Huang Y, Mironova M, Lopes-Virella MF. Oxidized LDL stimulates matrix metalloproteinase-1 expression in human vascular endothelial cells. *Arterioscler Thromb Vasc Biol* 1999;19:2640–2647.
8. Rabbani R, Topol EJ. Strategies to achieve coronary arterial plaque stabilization. *Cardiovasc Res* 1999;41:402–417.
9. Dietz R, Osterziel KJ, Willenbrock R, et al. Ventricular remodeling after acute myocardial infarction. *Thromb Haemost* 1999;82[Suppl 1]:73–75.
10. Lamas GA, Flaker GC, Mitchell G, et al. Effect of infarct artery patency on prognosis after acute myocardial infarction. The Survival and Ventricular Enlargement Investigators. *Circulation* 1995;92:1101–1109.
11. Newby LK, Califf RM. Identifying patient risk: the basis for rational discharge planning after acute myocardial infarction. *J Thromb Thrombolysis* 1996;3:107–115.
12. Gottlieb S, Moss AJ, McDermott M, et al. Interrelation of left ventricular ejection fraction, pulmonary congestion and outcome in acute myocardial infarction. *Am J Cardiol* 1992;69:977–984.
13. Bodi V, Sanchis J, Lopez-Lereu MP, et al. Usefulness of a comprehensive cardiovascular magnetic resonance imaging assessment for predicting recovery of left ventricular wall motion in the setting of myocardial stunning. *J Am Coll Cardiol* 2005;46:1747–1752.
14. Brochet E, Czitrom D, Karila-Cohen D, et al. Early changes in myocardial perfusion patterns after myocardial infarction: relation with contractile reserve and functional recovery. *J Am Coll Cardiol* 1998;32:2011–2017.
15. Sakuma T, Hayashi Y, Sumii K, et al. Prediction of short- and intermediate-term prognoses of patients with acute myocardial infarction using myocardial contrast echocardiography one day after recanalization. *J Am Coll Cardiol* 1998;32:890–897.
16. Santoro GM, Valenti R, Buonamici P, et al. Relation between ST-segment changes and myocardial perfusion evaluated by myocardial contrast echocardiography in patients with acute myocardial infarction treated with direct angioplasty. *Am J Cardiol* 1998;82:932–937.
17. Wu KC, Kim RJ, Bluemke DA, et al. Quantification and time course of microvascular obstruction by contrast-enhanced echocardiography and magnetic resonance imaging following acute myocardial infarction and reperfusion. *J Am Coll Cardiol* 1998;32:1756–1764.
18. Wu KC, Zerhouni EA, Judd RM, et al. Prognostic significance of microvascular obstruction by magnetic resonance imaging in patients with acute myocardial infarction. *Circulation* 1998;97:765–772.
19. Abboud L, Hir J, Eisen I, et al. Long-term value of exercise testing after acute myocardial infarction: influence of thrombolytic therapy. *Chest* 2000;117:556–561.
20. Gibbons RJ, Balady GJ, Beasley JW, et al. ACC/AHA guidelines for exercise testing: a report of the American College of Cardiology/American Heart Association Task Force on Practice Guidelines (Committee on Exercise Testing). *J Am Coll Cardiol* 1997;30:260–311.
21. Madsen JK, Grande P, Saunamaki K, et al. Danish multicenter randomized study of invasive versus conservative treatment in patients with inducible ischemia after thrombolysis in acute myocardial infarction (DANAMI). Danish Trial in Acute Myocardial Infarction. *Circulation* 1997;96:748–755.
22. Chaitman BR, McMahon RP, Terrin M, et al. Impact of treatment strategy on predischarge exercise test in the Thrombolysis in Myocardial Infarction (TIMI) II Trial. *Am J Cardiol* 1993;71:131–138.
23. Zaret BL, Wackers FJ, Terrin ML, et al. Value of radionuclide rest and exercise left ventricular ejection fraction in assessing survival of patients after thrombolytic therapy for acute myocardial infarction: results of Thrombolysis in Myocardial Infarction (TIMI) phase II study. The TIMI Study Group. *J Am Coll Cardiol* 1995;26:73–79.
24. Joao I, Cotrim C, Duarte JA, et al. Cardiac rupture during exercise stress echocardiography: a case report. *J Am Soc Echocardiogr* 2000;13:785–787.
25. Brown KA, Heller GV, Landin RS, et al. Early dipyridamole (99m)Tc-sestamibi single photon emission computed tomographic imaging 2 to 4 days after acute myocardial infarction predicts in-hospital and postdischarge cardiac events: comparison with submaximal exercise imaging. *Circulation* 1999;100:2060–2066.
26. Hjelms E, Alstrup P, Paulsen PK, et al. CABG shortly after AMI treated with thrombolysis: an analysis of the surgical group and a comparison with PTCA in the DANAMI study. Danish Multicenter Randomized Study of

Invasive Versus Conservative Treatment in Patients with Inducible Ischemia after Thrombolysis in Acute Myocardial Infarction. *Eur J Cardiothorac Surg* 1998;13:555–558.
27. Armstrong PW, Fu Y, Chang WC, et al. Acute coronary syndromes in the GUSTO-IIb trial: prognostic insights and impact of recurrent ischemia. The GUSTO-IIb Investigators. *Circulation* 1998;98:1860–1868.
28. Early and six-month outcome in patients with angina pectoris early after acute myocardial infarction (the GISSI-3 APPI [angina precoce post-infarto] study). The GISSI-3 APPI Study Group. *Am J Cardiol* 1996;78:1191–1197.
29. Scanlon PJ, Faxon DP, Audet AM, et al. ACC/AHA guidelines for coronary angiography: a report of the American College of Cardiology/American Heart Association Task Force on practice guidelines (Committee on Coronary Angiography). Developed in collaboration with the Society for Cardiac Angiography and Interventions. *J Am Coll Cardiol* 1999;33:1756–1824.
30. Langer A, Fisher M, Califf RM, et al. Higher rates of coronary angiography and revascularization following myocardial infarction may be associated with greater survival in the United States than in Canada. The CARS Investigators (Coumadin/Aspirin Reinfarction Study). *Can J Cardiol* 1999;15:1095–1102.
31. Marrugat J, Ferrieres J, Masia R, et al. Differences in use of coronary angiography and outcome of myocardial infarction in Toulouse (France) and Gerona (Spain). The MONICA-Toulouse and REGICOR Investigators. *Eur Heart J* 2000;21:740–746.
32. Ellis SG, Mooney MR, George BS, et al. Randomized trial of late elective angioplasty versus conservative management for patients with residual stenoses after thrombolytic treatment of myocardial infarction. Treatment of Post-Thrombolytic Stenoses (TOPS) Study Group. *Circulation* 1992;86: 1400–1406.
33. SWIFT trial of delayed elective intervention v conservative treatment after thrombolysis with anistreplase in acute myocardial infarction. The Should We Intervene following Thrombolysis Group. *BMJ* 1991;302:555–560.
34. Terrin ML, Williams DO, Kleiman NS, et al. Two- and three-year results of the Thrombolysis in Myocardial Infarction (TIMI) Phase II clinical trial. *J Am Coll Cardiol* 1993;22:1763–1772.
35. de Bono DP. The European Cooperative Study Group trial of intravenous recombinant tissue-type plasminogen activator (rt-PA) and conservative therapy versus rt-PA and immediate coronary angioplasty. *J Am Coll Cardiol* 1988;12:20A–23A.
36. Topol EJ, Califf RM, George BS, et al. A randomized trial of immediate versus delayed elective angioplasty after intravenous tissue plasminogen activator in acute myocardial infarction. *N Engl J Med* 1987;317:581–588.
37. Duber C, Jungbluth A, Rumpelt HJ, et al. Morphology of the coronary arteries after combined thrombolysis and percutaneous transluminal coronary angioplasty for acute myocardial infarction. *Am J Cardiol* 1986;58: 698–703.
38. Miller JM, Smalling R, Ohman EM, et al. Effectiveness of early coronary angioplasty and abciximab for failed thrombolysis (reteplase or alteplase) during acute myocardial infarction (results from the GUSTO-III trial). Global Use of Strategies to Open Occluded Coronary Arteries. *Am J Cardiol* 1999;84:779–784.
39. Van de Werf, F. ASSENT IV Results. *European Society of Cardiology*. Stockholm, Sweden, September 2005.
40. Fragmin and Fast Revascularisation during Instability in Coronary Artery Disease Investigators. Invasive compared with non-invasive treatment in unstable coronary-artery disease: FRISC II prospective randomised multicentre study. *Lancet* 1999;354:708–715.
41. Cannon CP, Weintraub WS, Demopoulos LA, et al. Invasive versus conservative strategies in unstable angina and non-Q-wave myocardial infarction following treatment with tirofiban: rationale and study design of the international TACTICS-TIMI 18 Trial. Treat Angina with Aggrastat and Determine Cost of Therapy with an Invasive or Conservative Strategy. Thrombolysis in Myocardial Infarction. *Am J Cardiol* 1998;82:731–736.
42. Cannon CP, Weintraub WS, Demopoulos LA, et al. Comparison of early invasive and conservative strategies in patients with unstable coronary syndromes treated with the glycoprotein IIb/IIIa inhibitor tirofiban. *N Engl J Med* 2001;344:1879–1887.
43. Mehta SR, Cannon CP, Fox KA, et al. Routine vs selective invasive strategies in patients with acute coronary syndromes: a collaborative meta-analysis of randomized trials. *JAMA* 2005;293:2908–2917.
44. Bhatt DL. To cath or not to cath: that is no longer the question. *JAMA* 2005: 2935–2937.
45. Bhatt DL, Roe MT, Peterson ED, et al. Utilization of early invasive management strategies for high-risk patients with non-ST-segment elevation acute coronary syndromes: results from the CRUSADE Quality Improvement Initiative. *JAMA* 2004;292:2096–2104.
46. Bhatt DL, Topol EJ. Need to test the arterial inflammation hypothesis. *Circulation* 2002;106:136–140.
47. Mills R, Bhatt DL. The Yin and Yang of arterial inflammation. *J Am Coll Cardiol* 2004;44:50–52.
48. Tommasi S, Carluccio E, Bentivoglio M, et al. C-reactive protein as a marker for cardiac ischemic events in the year after a first, uncomplicated myocardial infarction. *Am J Cardiol* 1999;83:1595–1599.
49. Barron HV, Cannon CP, Murphy SA, et al. Association between white blood cell count, epicardial blood flow, myocardial perfusion, and clinical outcomes in the setting of acute myocardial infarction: a thrombolysis in myocardial infarction 10 substudy. *Circulation* 2000;102:2329–2334.
50. Bhatt DL, Chew DP, Lincoff AM, et al. Effect of revascularization on mortality associated with an elevated white blood cell count in acute coronary syndromes. *Am J Cardiol* 2003;92:136–140.
51. Jernberg T, Lindahl B, Siegbahn A, et al. N-terminal pro-brain natriuretic peptide in relation to inflammation, myocardial necrosis, and the effect of an invasive strategy in unstable coronary artery disease. *J Am Coll Cardiol* 2003;42:1909–1916.
52. Bigger JT, Fleiss JL, Kleiger R, et al. Effect of revascularization on mortality associated with an elevated white blood cell count in acute. The relationships among ventricular arrhythmias, left ventricular dysfunction, and mortality in the 2 years after myocardial infarction. *Circulation* 1984;69:250–258.
53. The Cardiac Arrhythmia Suppression Trial (CAST) Investigators. Preliminary report: effect of encainide and flecainide on mortality in a randomized trial of arrhythmia suppression after myocardial infarction. *N Engl J Med* 1989;321:406–412.
54. Echt DS, Liebson PR, Mitchell LB, et al. Mortality and morbidity in patients receiving encainide, flecainide, or placebo. The Cardiac Arrhythmia Suppression Trial. *N Engl J Med* 1991;324:781–788.
55. Effect of the antiarrhythmic agent moricizine on survival after myocardial infarction. The Cardiac Arrhythmia Suppression Trial II Investigators. *N Engl J Med* 1992;327:227–233.
56. Al-Khatib SM, Sanders GD, Mark DB, et al. Expert panel participating in a Duke Clinical Research Institute-sponsored conference. Implantable cardioverter defibrillators and cardiac resynchronization therapy in patients with left ventricular dysfunction: randomized trial evidence through 2004. *Am Heart J* 2005;49:1020–1034.
57. A comparison of antiarrhythmic-drug therapy with implantable defibrillators in patients resuscitated from near-fatal ventricular arrhythmias. The Antiarrhythmics Versus Implantable Defibrillators (AVID) Investigators. *N Engl J Med* 1997;337:1576–1583.
58. Moss AJ, Hall WJ, Cannom DS, et al. Improved survival with an implanted defibrillator in patients with coronary disease at high risk for ventricular arrhythmia. Multicenter Automatic Defibrillator Implantation Trial Investigators. *N Engl J Med* 1996;335:1933–1940.
59. Buxton AE, Lee KL, DiCarlo L, et al. Electrophysiologic testing to identify patients with coronary artery disease who are at risk for sudden death. Multicenter Unsustained Tachycardia Trial Investigators. *N Engl J Med* 2000;342:1937–1945.
60. Buxton AE, Lee KL, Fisher JD, et al. A randomized study of the prevention of sudden death in patients with coronary artery disease. Multicenter Unsustained Tachycardia Trial Investigators. *N Engl J Med* 1999;341:1882–1890.
61. Moss AJ, Zareba W, Hall WJ, et al. Prophylactic implantation of a defibrillator in patients with myocardial infarction and reduced ejection fraction. *N Engl J Med* 2002;346:877–883.
62. Bardy GH, Lee KL, Mark DB, et al. Amiodarone or an implantable cardioverter-defibrillator for congestive heart failure. *N Engl J Med* 2005; 352:225–237.
63. Hohnloser SH, Kuck KH, Dorian P, et al. Prophylactic use of an implantable cardioverter-defibrillator after acute myocardial infarction. *N Engl J Med* 2004;351:2481–2488.
64. Bigger JT Jr, for The Coronary Artery Bypass Graft (CABG) Patch Trial Investigators. Prophylactic use of implanted cardiac defibrillators in patients at high risk for ventricular arrhythmias after coronary-artery bypass graft surgery. Coronary Artery Bypass Graft (CABG) Patch Trial Investigators. *N Engl J Med* 1997;337:1569–1575.
65. Solomon SD, Zelenkofske S, McMurray JJ, et al, for the Valsartan in Acute Myocardial Infarction Trial (VALIANT) Investigators. Sudden death in patients with myocardial infarction and left ventricular dysfunction, heart failure, or both. *N Engl J Med* 2005;352:2581–2588. *Erratum in N Engl J Med* 2005;353:744.
66. Sanders GD, Hlatky MA, Owens DK. Cost-effectiveness of implantable cardioverter-defibrillators. *N Engl J Med* 2005;353:1471–1480.
67. GISSI-3: effects of lisinopril and transdermal glyceryl trinitrate singly and together on 6-week mortality and ventricular function after acute myocardial infarction. Gruppo Italiano per lo Studio della Sopravvivenza nell'Infarto Miocardico. *Lancet* 1994;343:1115–1122.
68. ISIS-4: a randomised factorial trial assessing early oral captopril, oral mononitrate, and intravenous magnesium sulphate in 58,050 patients with suspected acute myocardial infarction. ISIS-4 (Fourth International Study of Infarct Survival) Collaborative Group. *Lancet* 1995;345:669–685.
69. Young JB. Angiotensin-converting enzyme inhibitors post-myocardial infarction. *Cardiol Clin* 1995;13:379–390.
70. The Acute Infarction Ramipril Efficacy (AIRE) Study Investigators. Effect of ramipril on mortality and morbidity of survivors of acute myocardial infarction with clinical evidence of heart failure. *Lancet* 1993;342:821–828.
71. Pfeffer MA, Braunwald E, Moye LA, et al. Effect of captopril on mortality and morbidity in patients with left ventricular dysfunction after myocardial infarction: results of the survival and ventricular enlargement trial. The SAVE Investigators. *N Engl J Med* 1992;327:669–677.
72. Torp-Pedersen C, Kober L. Effect of ACE inhibitor trandolapril on life expectancy of patients with reduced left-ventricular function after acute myocardial infarction. TRACE Study Group. Trandolapril Cardiac Evaluation. *Lancet* 1999;354:9–12.

73. Yusuf S, Sleight P, Pogue J, et al. Effects of an angiotensin-converting-enzyme inhibitor, ramipril, on cardiovascular events in high-risk patients. The Heart Outcomes Prevention Evaluation Study Investigators. *N Engl J Med* 2000;342:145–153.
74. Fox KM. Efficacy of perindopril in reduction of cardiovascular events among patients with stable coronary artery disease: randomised, double-blind, placebo-controlled, multicentre trial (the EUROPA study). *Lancet* 2003;362:782–788.
75. Braunwald E, Domanski MJ, Fowler SE, et al. Angiotensin-converting-enzyme inhibition in stable coronary artery disease. *N Engl J Med* 2004;351:2058–2068.
76. Oral captopril versus placebo among 13,634 patients with suspected acute myocardial infarction: interim report from the Chinese Cardiac Study (CCS-1). *Lancet* 1995;345:686–687.
77. Flather MD, Lonn EM, Yusuf S. Effects of ACE inhibitors on mortality when started in the early phase of myocardial infarction: evidence from the larger randomized controlled trials. *J Cardiovasc Risk* 1995;2:423–428.
78. Indications for ACE inhibitors in the early treatment of acute myocardial infarction: systematic overview of individual data from 100,000 patients in randomized trials. ACE Inhibitor Myocardial Infarction Collaborative Group. *Circulation* 1998;97:2202–2212.
79. Swedberg K, Held P, Kjekshus J, et al. Effects of the early administration of enalapril on mortality in patients with acute myocardial infarction: results of the Cooperative New Scandinavian Enalapril Survival Study II (CONSENSUS II). *N Engl J Med* 1992;327:678–684.
80. de Kam PJ, Voors AA, van den Berg MP, et al. Effect of very early angiotensin-converting enzyme inhibition on left ventricular dilation after myocardial infarction in patients receiving thrombolysis: results of a meta-analysis of 845 patients. FAMIS, CAPTIN and CATS Investigators. *J Am Coll Cardiol* 2000;36:2047–2053.
81. Barron HV, Michaels AD, Maynard C, et al. Use of angiotensin-converting enzyme inhibitors at discharge in patients with acute myocardial infarction in the United States: data from the National Registry of Myocardial Infarction 2. *J Am Coll Cardiol* 1998;32:360–367.
82. Pfeffer MA, McMurray JJ, Velazquez EJ, et al. Valsartan, captopril, or both in myocardial infarction complicated by heart failure, left ventricular dysfunction, or both. *N Engl J Med.* 2003;349:1893–1906.
83. McMurray JJ, Ostergren J, Swedberg K, et al., CHARM Investigators and Committees. Effects of candesartan in patients with chronic heart failure and reduced left-ventricular systolic function taking angiotensin-converting-enzyme inhibitors: the CHARM-Added trial. *Lancet* 2003;362:767–771.
84. Granger CB, McMurray JJ, Yusuf S, et al, for the CHARM Investigators and Committees. Effects of candesartan in patients with chronic heart failure and reduced left-ventricular systolic function intolerant to angiotensin-converting-enzyme inhibitors: the CHARM-Alternative trial. *Lancet* 2003;362:772–776.
85. Yusuf S, Peto R, Lewis J, et al. Beta blockade during and after myocardial infarction: an overview of the randomized trials. *Prog Cardiovasc Dis* 1985;27:335–371.
86. Timolol-induced reduction in mortality and reinfarction in patients surviving acute myocardial infarction. *N Engl J Med* 1981;304:801–807.
87. Groenning BA, Nilsson JC, Sondergaard L, et al. Antiremodeling effects on the left ventricle during beta-blockade with metoprolol in the treatment of chronic heart failure. *J Am Coll Cardiol* 2000;36:2072–2080.
88. Goldstein S. Propranolol therapy in patients with acute myocardial infarction: the Beta-Blocker Heart Attack Trial. *Circulation* 1983;67:I53–I57.
89. Furberg CD, Bell RL. Effect of beta-blocker therapy on recurrent nonfatal myocardial infarction. *Circulation* 1983;67:I83–I85.
90. Roberts R, Rogers WJ, Mueller HS, et al. Immediate versus deferred beta-blockade following thrombolytic therapy in patients with acute myocardial infarction: results of the Thrombolysis in Myocardial Infarction (TIMI) II-B Study. *Circulation* 1991;83:422–437.
91. Barron HV, Rundle AC, Gore JM, et al. Intracranial hemorrhage rates and effect of immediate beta-blocker use in patients with acute myocardial infarction treated with tissue plasminogen activator. Participants in the National Registry of Myocardial Infarction-2. *Am J Cardiol* 2000;85:294–298.
92. Pfisterer M, Cox JL, Granger CB, et al. Atenolol use and clinical outcomes after thrombolysis for acute myocardial infarction: the GUSTO-I experience. Global Utilization of Streptokinase and TPA (alteplase) for Occluded Coronary Arteries. *J Am Coll Cardiol* 1998;32:634–640.
93. Collins R. The COMMIT trial. Presented at the American College of Cardiology, March 2005.
94. Woods KL, Ketley D, Lowy A, et al. Beta-blockers and antithrombotic treatment for secondary prevention after acute myocardial infarction: towards an understanding of factors influencing clinical practice. The European Secondary Prevention Study Group. *Eur Heart J* 1998;19:74–79.
95. Gottlieb SS, McCarter RJ, Vogel RA. Effect of beta-blockade on mortality among high-risk and low-risk patients after myocardial infarction. *N Engl J Med* 1998;339:489–497.
96. Phillips KA, Shlipak MG, Coxson P, et al. Health and economic benefits of increased beta-blocker use following myocardial infarction. *JAMA* 2000;284:2748–2754.
97. Houghton T, Freemantle N, Cleland JG. Are beta-blockers effective in patients who develop heart failure soon after myocardial infarction? A meta-regression analysis of randomised trials. *Eur J Heart Fail* 2000;2:333–340.
98. Gurwitz JH, Goldberg RJ, Chen Z, et al. Beta-blocker therapy in acute myocardial infarction: evidence for underutilization in the elderly. *Am J Med* 1992;93:605–610.
99. Krumholz HM, Radford MJ, Wang Y, et al. Early beta-blocker therapy for acute myocardial infarction in elderly patients. *Ann Intern Med* 1999;131:648–654.
100. Chen J, Marciniak TA, Radford MJ, et al. Beta-blocker therapy for secondary prevention of myocardial infarction in elderly diabetic patients: results from the National Cooperative Cardiovascular Project. *J Am Coll Cardiol* 1999;34:1388–1394.
101. Barron HV, Viskin S, Lundstrom RJ, et al. Beta-blocker dosages and mortality after myocardial infarction: data from a large health maintenance organization. *Arch Intern Med* 1998;158:449–453.
102. Rochon PA, Tu JV, Anderson GM, et al. Rate of heart failure and 1-year survival for older people receiving low-dose beta-blocker therapy after myocardial infarction. *Lancet* 2000;356:639–644.
103. Flather MD, Yusuf S, Kober L, et al. Long-term ACE-inhibitor therapy in patients with heart failure or left-ventricular dysfunction: a systematic overview of data from individual patients. ACE-Inhibitor Myocardial Infarction Collaborative Group. *Lancet* 2000;355:1575–1581.
104. Vaur L, Danchin N, Genes N, et al. Epidemiology of myocardial infarction in France: therapeutic and prognostic implications of heart failure during the acute phase. *Am Heart J* 1999;137:49–58.
105. McAlister FA. Trial is needed of ACE inhibitors plus beta blockers in survivors of myocardial infarction. *BMJ* 1998;317:751.
106. Anthonio RL, van Veldhuisen DJ, van Gilst WH. Left ventricular dilatation after myocardial infarction: ACE inhibitors, beta-blockers, or both? *J Cardiovasc Pharmacol* 1998;32:S1–S8.
107. Coletta C, Ricci R, Ceci V, et al. Effects of early treatment with captopril and metoprolol singly or together on six-month mortality and morbidity after acute myocardial infarction: results of the RIMA (Rimodellamento Infarto Miocardico Acuto) study. The RIMA researchers. *G Ital Cardiol* 1999;29:115-124; discussion 125–129.
108. Frishman WH, Cheng A. Secondary prevention of myocardial infarction: role of beta-adrenergic blockers and angiotensin-converting enzyme inhibitors. *Am Heart J* 1999;137:S25–S34.
109. Pitt B, Zannad F, Remme WJ, et al. The effect of spironolactone on morbidity and mortality in patients with severe heart failure. Randomized Aldactone Evaluation Study Investigators. *N Engl J Med* 1999;341:709–717.
110. Pitt B, Remme W, Zannad F, et al. Eplerenone, a selective aldosterone blocker, in patients with left ventricular dysfunction after myocardial infarction. *N Engl J Med* 2003;348:1309–1321.
111. Juurlink DN, Mamdani MM, Lee DS, et al. Rates of hyperkalemia after publication of the Randomized Aldactone Evaluation Study. *N Engl J Med* 2004;351:543–551.
112. Skolnick AE, Frishman WH. Calcium channel blockers in myocardial infarction. *Arch Intern Med* 1989;149:1669–1677.
113. Muller JE, Morrison J, Stone PH, et al. Nifedipine therapy for patients with threatened and acute myocardial infarction: a randomized, double-blind, placebo-controlled comparison. *Circulation* 1984;69:740–747.
114. The Danish studies on verapamil in acute myocardial infarction. The Danish Study Group on Verapamil in Myocardial Infarction. *Br J Clin Pharmacol* 1986;21:197S-204S.
115. Goldbourt U, Behar S, Reicher-Reiss H, et al. Early administration of nifedipine in suspected acute myocardial infarction. The Secondary Prevention Reinfarction Israel Nifedipine Trial 2 Study. *Arch Intern Med* 1993;153:345–353.
116. Ishikawa K, Nakai S, Takenaka T, et al. Short-acting nifedipine and diltiazem do not reduce the incidence of cardiac events in patients with healed myocardial infarction. Secondary Prevention Group. *Circulation* 1997; 95:2368–2373.
117. Reicher-Reiss H, Behar S, Boyko V, et al. Long-term mortality follow-up of hospital survivors of a myocardial infarction randomized to nifedipine in the SPRINT study. Secondary Prevention Reinfarction Israeli Nifedipine Trial. *Cardiovasc Drugs Ther* 1998;12:171–176.
118. Psaty BM, Heckbert SR, Koepsell TD, et al. The risk of myocardial infarction associated with antihypertensive drug therapies. *JAMA* 1995;274:620–625.
119. Nissen SE, Tuzcu EM, Libby P, et al. Effect of antihypertensive agents on cardiovascular events in patients with coronary disease and normal blood pressure: the CAMELOT study: a randomized controlled trial. *JAMA* 2004; 292:2217–2225.
120. Sacks FM, Pfeffer MA, Moye LA, et al. The effect of pravastatin on coronary events after myocardial infarction in patients with average cholesterol levels. Cholesterol and Recurrent Events Trial investigators. *N Engl J Med* 1996;335:1001–1009.
121. Plehn JF, Davis BR, Sacks FM, et al. Reduction of stroke incidence after myocardial infarction with pravastatin: the Cholesterol and Recurrent Events (CARE) study. The CARE Investigators. *Circulation* 1999;99:216–223.
122. White HD, Simes RJ, Anderson NE, et al. Pravastatin therapy and the risk of stroke. *N Engl J Med* 2000;343:317–326.
123. LaRosa JC, He J, Vupputuri S. Effect of statins on risk of coronary disease: a meta-analysis of randomized controlled trials. *JAMA* 1999;282:2340–2346.

124. Cannon CP, Braunwald E, McCabe CH, et al. Intensive versus moderate lipid lowering with statins after acute coronary syndromes. *N Engl J Med* 2004;350:1495–1504.
125. Karha J, Bhatt DL. Plaque regression-A new target for antiatherosclerotic therapy. *Am Heart J* 2005;149:384–387.
126. Gaziano JM, Hennekens CH, Satterfield S, et al. Clinical utility of lipid and lipoprotein levels during hospitalization for acute myocardial infarction. *Vasc Med* 1999;4:227–231.
127. Shepherd J. From best evidence to best practice: what are the obstacles? *Atherosclerosis* 1999;147[Suppl 1]:S45–S51.
128. Stenestrand U, Wallentin L. Early statin treatment following acute myocardial infarction and 1-year survival. *JAMA* 2001;285:430–435.
129. Schwartz GG, Oliver MF, Ezekowitz MD, et al. Rationale and design of the Myocardial Ischemia Reduction with Aggressive Cholesterol Lowering (MIRACL) study that evaluates atorvastatin in unstable angina pectoris and in non-Q-wave acute myocardial infarction. *Am J Cardiol* 1998;81:578–581.
130. Schwartz GG, Olsson AG. The myocardial ischemia reduction with aggressive cholesterol lowering (MIRACL) trial: effects of intensive atorvastatin treatment on early recurrent events after an acute coronary syndrome. American Heart Association Annual Meeting 2000.
131. Ganz DA, Kuntz KM, Jacobson GA, et al. Cost-effectiveness of 3-hydroxy-3-methylglutaryl coenzyme A reductase inhibitor therapy in older patients with myocardial infarction. *Ann Intern Med* 2000;132:780–787.
132. Schiele R, Gitt AK, Schneider S, et al. Early statin use in acute myocardial infarction is associated with a reduced hospital mortality: results of MITRA-2. *Eur Heart J* 2000;21:155.
133. Gylling H, Radhakrishnan R, Miettinen TA. Reduction of serum cholesterol in postmenopausal women with previous myocardial infarction and cholesterol malabsorption induced by dietary sitostanol ester margarine: women and dietary sitostanol. *Circulation* 1997;96:4226–4231.
134. de Faire U, Ericsson CG, Grip L, et al. Secondary preventive potential of lipid-lowering drugs. The Bezafibrate Coronary Atherosclerosis Intervention Trial (BECAIT). *Eur Heart J* 1996;17[Suppl F]:37–42.
135. Secondary prevention by raising HDL cholesterol and reducing triglycerides in patients with coronary artery disease: the Bezafibrate Infarction Prevention (BIP) study. *Circulation* 2000;102:21–27.
136. Rubins HB, Robins SJ, Collins D, et al. Gemfibrozil for the secondary prevention of coronary heart disease in men with low levels of high-density lipoprotein cholesterol. Veterans Affairs High-Density Lipoprotein Cholesterol Intervention Trial Study Group. *N Engl J Med* 1999;341:410–418.
137. Krakoff J, Vela BS, Brinton EA. The role of fibric acid derivatives in the secondary prevention of coronary heart disease. *Curr Cardiol Rep* 2000;2:452–458.
138. Guyton JR, Blazing MA, Hagar J, et al. Extended-release niacin vs gemfibrozil for the treatment of low levels of high-density lipoprotein cholesterol. Niaspan-Gemfibrozil Study Group. *Arch Intern Med* 2000;160:1177–1184.
139. Bhatt DL, Topol EJ. Antiplatelet and anticoagulant therapy in the secondary prevention of ischemic heart disease. *Med Clin North Am* 2000;84:163–179, ix.
140. Antiplatelet Trialists' Collaboration. Collaborative overview of randomised trials of antiplatelet therapy: I. Prevention of death, myocardial infarction, and stroke by prolonged antiplatelet therapy in various categories of patients. *BMJ* 1994;308:81–106.
141. Randomised trial of intravenous streptokinase, oral aspirin, both, or neither among 17,187 cases of suspected acute myocardial infarction: ISIS-2. ISIS-2 (Second International Study of Infarct Survival) Collaborative Group. *Lancet* 1988;2:349–360.
142. Bhatt DL. Aspirin resistance: more than just a laboratory curiosity. *J Am Coll Cardiol* 2004;43:1127–1129.
143. Aronow WS. Underutilization of aspirin in older patients with prior myocardial infarction at the time of admission to a nursing home. *J Am Geriatr Soc* 1998;46:615–616.
144. CAPRIE Steering Committee. A randomised, blinded, trial of clopidogrel versus aspirin in patients at risk of ischaemic events (CAPRIE). *Lancet* 1996;348:1329–1339.
145. Cannon CP. Effectiveness of clopidogrel versus aspirin in preventing acute myocardial infarction in patients with symptomatic atherothrombosis (CAPRIE trial). *Am J Cardiol* 2002;90:760–762.
146. Bhatt DL, Hirsch AT, Ringleb PA, et al. Reduction in the need for hospitalization for recurrent ischemic events and bleeding with clopidogrel instead of aspirin. CAPRIE investigators. *Am Heart J* 2000;140:67–73.
147. Bhatt DL, Foody JM, Hirsch AT, et al. Complementary, additive benefit of clopidogrel and lipid-lowering therapy in patients with atherosclerosis. *J Am Coll Cardiol* 2000;35[Suppl A]:326.
148. Chen ZM. The COMMIT trial. Presented at the American College of Cardiology, March 2005.
149. Sabatine MS, Cannon CP, Gibson CM, et al. Addition of clopidogrel to aspirin and fibrinolytic therapy for myocardial infarction with ST-segment elevation. *N Engl J Med* 2005;352:1179–1189.
150. Fathi RB, Bhatt DL. Enhancing reperfusion therapy for myocardial infarction with dual antiplatelet therapy: breaking the glass ceiling. *Am Heart J* 2005;149:947–949.
151. Yusuf S, Zhao F, Mehta SR, et al. Effects of clopidogrel in addition to aspirin in patients with acute coronary syndromes without ST-segment elevation. *N Engl J Med* 2001;345:494–502.
152. Bhatt DL, Topol EJ. Clopidogrel added to aspirin versus aspirin alone in secondary prevention and high-risk primary prevention: rationale and design of the Clopidogrel for High Atherothrombotic Risk and Ischemic Stabilization, Management, and Avoidance (CHARISMA) trial. *Am Heart J* 2004;148:263–268.
153. Bhatt DL, Topol EJ. Scientific and therapeutic advances in antiplatelet therapy. *Nat Rev Drug Discov* 2003;2:15–28.
154. Hart RG, Benavente O, McBride R, et al. Antithrombotic therapy to prevent stroke in patients with atrial fibrillation: a meta-analysis. *Ann Intern Med* 1999;131:492–501.
155. A double-blind trial to assess long-term oral anticoagulant therapy in elderly patients after myocardial infarction. Sixty Plus Reinfarction Study Research Group. *Lancet* 1980;2:989–994.
156. Smith P. Long-term anticoagulant treatment after acute myocardial infarction. The Warfarin Re-Infarction Study. *Ann Epidemiol* 1992;2:549–552.
157. Effect of long-term oral anticoagulant treatment on mortality and cardiovascular morbidity after myocardial infarction. Anticoagulants in the Secondary Prevention of Events in Coronary Thrombosis (ASPECT) Research Group. *Lancet* 1994;343:499–503.
158. Azar AJ, Cannegieter SC, Deckers JW, et al. Optimal intensity of oral anticoagulant therapy after myocardial infarction. *J Am Coll Cardiol* 1996;27:1349–1355.
159. Meijer A, Verheugt FW, Werter CJ, et al. Aspirin versus coumadin in the prevention of reocclusion and recurrent ischemia after successful thrombolysis: a prospective placebo-controlled angiographic study. Results of the APRICOT Study. *Circulation* 1993;87:1524–1530.
160. Randomised double-blind trial of fixed low-dose warfarin with aspirin after myocardial infarction. Coumadin Aspirin Reinfarction Study (CARS) Investigators. *Lancet* 1997;350:389–396.
161. Fiore LD, Ezekowitz MD, Brophy MT, et al. Department of Veterans Affairs Cooperative Studies Program Clinical Trial comparing combined warfarin and aspirin with aspirin alone in survivors of acute myocardial infarction: primary results of the CHAMP study. *Circulation* 2002;105:557–563.
162. Brouwer MA, van den Bergh PJ, Aengevaeren WR, et al. Aspirin plus coumarin versus aspirin alone in the prevention of reocclusion after fibrinolysis for acute myocardial infarction: results of the Antithrombotics in the Prevention of Reocclusion In Coronary Thrombolysis (APRICOT)-2 Trial. *Circulation* 2002;106:659–665.
163. van Es RF, Jonker JJ, Verheugt FW, et al. Aspirin and coumadin after acute coronary syndromes (the ASPECT-2 study): a randomised controlled trial. *Lancet* 2002;360:109–113.
164. Hurlen M, Abdelnoor M, Smith P, et al. Warfarin, aspirin, or both after myocardial infarction. *N Engl J Med* 2002;347:969–974.
165. Wallentin L, Wilcox RG, Weaver WD, et al. Oral ximelagatran for secondary prophylaxis after myocardial infarction: the ESTEEM randomised controlled trial. *Lancet* 2003;362:789–797.
166. Rajagopal V, Bhatt DL. Factor Xa inhibitors in acute coronary syndromes: moving from mythology to reality. *J Thromb Haemost* 2005;3:436–438.
167. Leon MB, Baim DS, Popma JJ, et al. A clinical trial comparing three antithrombotic-drug regimens after coronary-artery stenting. Stent Anticoagulation Restenosis Study Investigators. *N Engl J Med* 1998;339:1665–1671.
168. Bhatt DL, Bertrand ME, Berger PB, et al. Meta-analysis of randomized and registry comparisons of ticlopidine with clopidogrel after stenting. *J Am Coll Cardiol* 2002;39:9–14.
169. The Writing Group for the PEPI Trial. Effects of estrogen or estrogen/progestin regimens on heart disease risk factors in postmenopausal women. The Postmenopausal Estrogen/Progestin Interventions (PEPI) Trial. *JAMA* 1995;273:199–208.
170. Herrington DM, Reboussin DM, Brosnihan KB, et al. Effects of estrogen replacement on the progression of coronary-artery atherosclerosis. *N Engl J Med* 2000;343:522–529.
171. Hulley S, Grady D, Bush T, Furberg C, et al. Randomized trial of estrogen plus progestin for secondary prevention of coronary heart disease in postmenopausal women. Heart and Estrogen/progestin Replacement Study (HERS) Research Group. *JAMA*. 1998;280:605–613.
172. Cushman M, Legault C, Barrett-Connor E, et al. Effect of postmenopausal hormones on inflammation-sensitive proteins: the Postmenopausal Estrogen/Progestin Interventions (PEPI) Study. *Circulation* 1999;100:717–722.
173. Rossouw JE, Anderson GL, Prentice RL, et al. Risks and benefits of estrogen plus progestin in healthy postmenopausal women: principal results From the Women's Health Initiative randomized controlled trial. *JAMA* 2002;288:321–333
174. Anderson GL, Limacher M, Assaf AR, et al. Effects of conjugated equine estrogen in postmenopausal women with hysterectomy: the Women's Health Initiative randomized controlled trial. *JAMA* 2004;291:1701–1712.
175. Herrington D. Role of estrogens, selective estrogen receptor modulators and phytoestrogens in cardiovascular protection. *Can J Cardiol* 2000;16[Suppl E]:5E–9E.
176. Rakugi H, Yu H, Kamitani A, et al. Links between hypertension and myocardial infarction. *Am Heart J* 1996;132:213–221.
177. Gustafsson F, Kober L, Torp-Pedersen C, et al. Long-term prognosis after acute myocardial infarction in patients with a history of arterial hypertension. TRACE study group. *Eur Heart J* 1998;19:588–594.

178. Haider AW, Chen L, Larson MG, et al. Antecedent hypertension confers increased risk for adverse outcomes after initial myocardial infarction. *Hypertension* 1997;30:1020–1024.
179. Fresco C, Avanzini F, Bosi S, et al. Prognostic value of a history of hypertension in 11,483 patients with acute myocardial infarction treated with thrombolysis. GISSI-2 Investigators. Gruppo Italiano per lo Studio della, Sopravvivena nell'Infarto Miocardico. *J Hypertens* 1996;14:743–750.
180. Gustafsson F, Torp-Pedersen C, Kober L, et al. Effect of angiotensin converting enzyme inhibition after acute myocardial infarction in patients with arterial hypertension. TRACE Study Group, Trandolapril Cardiac Event. *J Hypertens* 1997;15:793–798.
181. Aylward PE, Wilcox RG, Horgan JH, et al. Relation of increased arterial blood pressure to mortality and stroke in the context of contemporary thrombolytic therapy for acute myocardial infarction: a randomized trial. GUSTO-I Investigators. *Ann Intern Med* 1996;125:891–900.
182. Chowdhury TA, Lasker SS, Dyer PH. Comparison of secondary prevention measures after myocardial infarction in subjects with and without diabetes mellitus. *J Intern Med* 1999;245:565–570.
183. Tenenbaum A, Fisman EZ, Boyko V, et al. Prevalence and prognostic significance of unrecognized systemic hypertension in patients with diabetes mellitus and healed myocardial infarction and/or stable angina pectoris. *Am J Cardiol* 1999;84:294–298.
184. Zuanetti G, Latini R, Maggioni AP, et al. Effect of the ACE inhibitor lisinopril on mortality in diabetic patients with acute myocardial infarction: data from the GISSI-3 study. *Circulation* 1997;96:4239–4245.
185. MacDonald TM, Butler R, Newton RW, et al. Which drugs benefit diabetic patients for secondary prevention of myocardial infarction? DARTS/MEMO Collaboration. *Diabet Med* 1998;15:282–289.
186. Zuanetti G, Latini R. Impact of pharmacological treatment on mortality after myocardial infarction in diabetic patients. *J Diabetes Complications* 1997;11:131–136.
187. Bhatt DL, Marso S, Hirsch A, et al. Amplified benefit of clopidogrel versus aspirin in patients with diabetes mellitus. *Am J Cardiol* 2002;90:625–628.
188. Klein L, Gheorghiade M. Management of the patient with diabetes mellitus and myocardial infarction: clinical trials update. *Am J Med* 2004;116[Suppl 5A]:47S-63S.
189. Ridker PM, Rifai N, Pfeffer M, et al. Elevation of tumor necrosis factor-alpha and increased risk of recurrent coronary events after myocardial infarction. *Circulation* 2000;101:2149–2153.
190. Phipps RP. Atherosclerosis: the emerging role of inflammation and the CD40-CD40 ligand system. *Proc Natl Acad Sci U S A* 2000;97:6930–6932.
191. Takano H, Nagai T, Asakawa M, et al. Peroxisome proliferator–activated receptor activators inhibit lipopolysaccharide-induced tumor necrosis factor-alpha expression in neonatal rat cardiac myocytes. *Circ Res* 2000; 87:596–602.
192. Ferro D, Parrotto S, Basili S, et al. Simvastatin inhibits the monocyte expression of proinflammatory cytokines in patients with hypercholesterolemia. *J Am Coll Cardiol* 2000;36:427–431.
193. Naghavi M, Barlas Z, Siadaty S, et al. Association of influenza vaccination and reduced risk of recurrent myocardial infarction. *Circulation* 2000;102:3039–3045.
194. Cannon CP, Braunwald E, McCabe CH, et al. Antibiotic treatment of *Chlamydia pneumoniae* after acute coronary syndrome. *N Engl J Med* 2005;352:1646–1654.
195. O'Connor CM, Dunne MW, Pfeffer MA, et al. Azithromycin for the secondary prevention of coronary heart disease events: the WIZARD study: a randomized controlled trial. *JAMA* 2003;290:1459–1466.
196. van Berkel TF, Boersma H, De Baquer D, et al. Registration and management of smoking behaviour in patients with coronary heart disease. The EUROASPIRE survey. *Eur Heart J* 1999;20:1630–1637.
197. Rigotti NA, Singer DE, Mulley AG Jr, et al. Smoking cessation following admission to a coronary care unit. *J Gen Intern Med* 1991;6:305–311.
198. Wilson K, Gibson N, Willan A, et al. Effect of smoking cessation on mortality after myocardial infarction: meta-analysis of cohort studies. *Arch Intern Med* 2000;160:939–944.
199. Greenwood DC, Muir KR, Packham CJ, et al. Stress, social support, and stopping smoking after myocardial infarction in England. *J Epidemiol Community Health* 1995;49:583–587.
200. Fisher SD, Zareba W, Moss AJ, et al. Effect of smoking on lipid and thrombogenic factors two months after acute myocardial infarction. *Am J Cardiol* 2000;86:813–818.
201. Dobson AJ, Alexander HM, Heller RF, et al. How soon after quitting smoking does risk of heart attack decline? *J Clin Epidemiol* 1991;44:1247–1253.
202. McElduff P, Dobson A, Beaglehole R, et al. Rapid reduction in coronary risk for those who quit cigarette smoking. *Aust N Z J Public Health* 1998;22:787–791.
203. Rosenberg L, Palmer JR, Shapiro S. Decline in the risk of myocardial infarction among women who stop smoking. *N Engl J Med* 1990;322:213–217.
204. Negri E, La Vecchia C, D'Avanzo B, et al. Acute myocardial infarction: association with time since stopping smoking in Italy. GISSI-EFRIM Investigators. Gruppo Italiano per lo Studio della Sopravvivenza nell'Infarto. Epidemiologia dei Fattori di Rischio dell'Infarto Miocardico. *J Epidemiol Community Health* 1994;48:129–133.
205. Kawachi I, Colditz GA, Stampfer MJ, et al. Smoking cessation and time course of decreased risks of coronary heart disease in middle-aged women. *Arch Intern Med* 1994;154:169–175.
206. Lightwood JM, Glantz SA. Short-term economic and health benefits of smoking cessation: myocardial infarction and stroke. *Circulation* 1997; 96:1089–1096.
207. Glantz SA, Parmley WW. Passive smoking and heart disease: epidemiology, physiology, and biochemistry. *Circulation* 1991;83:1–12.
208. Dornelas EA, Sampson RA, Gray JF, et al. A randomized controlled trial of smoking cessation counseling after myocardial infarction. *Prev Med* 2000;30:261–268.
209. Krumholz HM, Cohen BJ, Tsevat J, et al. Cost-effectiveness of a smoking cessation program after myocardial infarction. *J Am Coll Cardiol* 1993; 22:1697–1702.
210. Goldstein MG, Niaura R. Methods to enhance smoking cessation after myocardial infarction. *Med Clin North Am* 2000;84:63-80, viii.
211. Joseph AM, Norman SM, Ferry LH, et al. The safety of transdermal nicotine as an aid to smoking cessation in patients with cardiac disease. *N Engl J Med* 1996;335:1792–1798.
212. Dacosta A, Guy JM, Tardy B, et al. Myocardial infarction and nicotine patch: a contributing or causative factor? *Eur Heart J* 1993;14:1709–1711.
213. Hurt RD, Sachs DP, Glover ED, et al. A comparison of sustained-release bupropion and placebo for smoking cessation. *N Engl J Med* 1997;337: 1195–1202.
214. Jorenby DE, Leischow SJ, Nides MA, et al. A controlled trial of sustained-release bupropion, a nicotine patch, or both for smoking cessation. *N Engl J Med* 1999;340:685–691.
215. Huijbrechts IP, Duivenvoorden HJ, Deckers JW, et al. Modification of smoking habits five months after myocardial infarction: relationship with personality characteristics. *J Psychosom Res* 1996;40:369–378.
216. Cleland JG, Ghosh J, Freemantle N, et al. Clinical trials update and cumulative meta-analyses from the American College of Cardiology: WATCH, SCD-HeFT, DINAMIT, CASINO, INSPIRE, STRATUS-US, RIO-Lipids and cardiac resynchronisation therapy in heart failure. *Eur J Heart Fail* 2004;6:501–508.
217. Mertens DJ, Kavanagh T, Campbell RB, et al. Exercise without dietary restriction as a means to long-term fat loss in the obese cardiac patient. *J Sports Med Phys Fitness* 1998;38:310–316.
218. McConnell TR, Klinger TA, Gardner JK, et al. Cardiac rehabilitation without exercise tests for post-myocardial infarction and post-bypass surgery patients. *J Cardiopulm Rehabil* 1998;18:458–463.
219. Daub WD, Knapik GP, Black WR. Strength training early after myocardial infarction. *J Cardiopulm Rehabil* 1996;16:100–108.
220. Dubach P, Myers J, Dziekan G, et al. Effect of exercise training on myocardial remodeling in patients with reduced left ventricular function after myocardial infarction: application of magnetic resonance imaging. *Circulation* 1997;95:2060–2067.
221. Pavia L, Orlando G, Myers J, et al. The effect of beta-blockade therapy on the response to exercise training in postmyocardial infarction patients. *Clin Cardiol* 1995;18:716–720.
222. Jolliffe JA, Rees K, Taylor RS, et al. Exercise-based rehabilitation for coronary heart disease (Cochrane Review). *Cochrane Database Syst Rev* 2000; CD001800.
223. Oldridge NB, Guyatt GH, Fischer ME, et al. Cardiac rehabilitation after myocardial infarction: combined experience of randomized clinical trials. *JAMA* 1988;260:945–950.
224. O'Connor GT, Buring JE, Yusuf S, et al. An overview of randomized trials of rehabilitation with exercise after myocardial infarction. *Circulation* 1989;80:234–244.
225. van Dixhoorn J, Duivenvoorden HJ, Staal JA, et al. Cardiac events after myocardial infarction: possible effect of relaxation therapy. *Eur Heart J* 1987;8:1210–1214.
226. Miller TD, Balady GJ, Fletcher GF. Exercise and its role in the prevention and rehabilitation of cardiovascular disease. *Ann Behav Med* 1997;19:220–229.
227. Pashkow FJ. Rehabilitation in the patient after myocardial infarction with or without surgical management. *Semin Thorac Cardiovasc Surg* 1995; 7:240–247.
228. Hedback B, Perk J, Wodlin P. Long-term reduction of cardiac mortality after myocardial infarction: 10-year results of a comprehensive rehabilitation programme. *Eur Heart J* 1993;14:831–835.
229. Hamalainen H, Luurila OJ, Kallio V, et al. Reduction in sudden deaths and coronary mortality in myocardial infarction patients after rehabilitation: 15 year follow-up study. *Eur Heart J* 1995;16:1839–1844.
230. Stahle A, Mattsson E, Ryden L, et al. Improved physical fitness and quality of life following training of elderly patients after acute coronary events: a 1 year follow-up randomized controlled study. *Eur Heart J* 1999;20:1475–1484.
231. Melville MR, Packham C, Brown N, et al. Cardiac rehabilitation: socially deprived patients are less likely to attend but patients ineligible for thrombolysis are less likely to be invited. *Heart* 1999;82:373–377.
232. Ades PA, Pashkow FJ, Nestor JR. Cost-effectiveness of cardiac rehabilitation after myocardial infarction. *J Cardiopulm Rehabil* 1997;17:222–231.
233. Oldridge N, Furlong W, Feeny D, et al. Economic evaluation of cardiac rehabilitation soon after acute myocardial infarction. *Am J Cardiol* 1993;72: 154–161.
234. Muller JE. Sexual activity as a trigger for cardiovascular events: what is the risk? *Am J Cardiol* 1999;84:2N–5N.

235. Papadopoulos C, Larrimore P, Cardin S, et al. Sexual concerns and needs of the postcoronary patient's wife. *Arch Intern Med* 1980;140:38–41.
236. Papadopoulos C, Beaumont C, Shelley SI, et al. Myocardial infarction and sexual activity of the female patient. *Arch Intern Med* 1983;143:1528–1530.
237. DeBusk R, Drory Y, Goldstein I, et al. Management of sexual dysfunction in patients with cardiovascular disease: recommendations of The Princeton Consensus Panel. *Am J Cardiol* 2000;86:175–181.
238. DeBusk RF. Evaluating the cardiovascular tolerance for sex. *Am J Cardiol* 2000;86:51F–56F.
239. Porter A, Mager A, Birnbaum Y, et al. Acute myocardial infarction following sildenafil citrate (Viagra) intake in a nitrate-free patient. *Clin Cardiol* 1999;22:762–763.
240. Kloner RA. Cardiovascular risk and sildenafil. *Am J Cardiol* 2000;86:57F–61F.
241. Johnston BL, Cantwell JD, Watt EW, et al. Sexual activity in exercising patients after myocardial infarction and revascularization. *Heart Lung* 1978;7:1026–1031.
242. Muller JE, Mittleman A, Maclure M, et al. Triggering myocardial infarction by sexual activity: low absolute risk and prevention by regular physical exertion. Determinants of Myocardial Infarction Onset Study Investigators. *JAMA* 1996;275:1405–1409.
243. Kimmel SE. Sex and myocardial infarction: an epidemiologic perspective. *Am J Cardiol* 2000;86:10F–13F.
244. Hebert PR, Buring JE, O'Connor GT, et al. Occupation and risk of nonfatal myocardial infarction. *Arch Intern Med* 1992;152:2253–2257.
245. Petrie KJ, Weinman J, Sharpe N, et al. Role of patients' view of their illness in predicting return to work and functioning after myocardial infarction: longitudinal study. *BMJ* 1996;312:1191–1194.
246. Boudrez H, De Backer G, Comhaire B. Return to work after myocardial infarction: results of a longitudinal population based study. *Eur Heart J* 1994;15:32–36.
247. Zahger D, Leibowitz D, Tabb IK, et al. Long-distance air travel soon after an acute coronary syndrome: a prospective evaluation of a triage protocol. *Am Heart J* 2000;140:241–242.
248. Muntwyler J, Hennekens CH, Buring JE, et al. Mortality and light to moderate alcohol consumption after myocardial infarction. *Lancet* 1998;352: 1882–1885.
249. Gaziano JM, Hennekens CH, Godfried SL, et al. Type of alcoholic beverage and risk of myocardial infarction. *Am J Cardiol* 1999;83:52–57.
250. Shaper AG, Wannamethee SG. Alcohol intake and mortality in middle aged men with diagnosed coronary heart disease. *Heart* 2000;83:394–399.
251. Kaufman DW, Rosenberg L, Helmrich SP, et al. Alcoholic beverages and myocardial infarction in young men. *Am J Epidemiol* 1985;121:548–554.
252. Cleophas TJ, Tuinenberg E, van der Meulen J, et al. Wine consumption and other dietary variables in males under 60 before and after acute myocardial infarction. *Angiology* 1996;47:789–796.
253. La Vecchia C, Decarli A, Franceschi S, et al. Prevalence of chronic diseases in alcohol abstainers. *Epidemiology* 1995;6:436–438.
254. Ridker PM, Vaughan DE, Stampfer MJ, et al. Association of moderate alcohol consumption and plasma concentration of endogenous tissue-type plasminogen activator. *JAMA* 1994;272:929–933.
255. Serebruany VL, Lowry DR, Fuzailov SY, et al. Moderate alcohol consumption is associated with decreased platelet activity in patients presenting with acute myocardial infarction. *J Thromb Thrombolysis* 2000;9:229–234.
256. Numminen H, Syrjala M, Benthin G, et al. The effect of acute ingestion of a large dose of alcohol on the hemostatic system and its circadian variation. *Stroke* 2000;31:1269–1273.
257. Moreyra AE, Kostis JB, Passannante AJ, et al. Acute myocardial infarction in patients with normal coronary arteries after acute ethanol intoxication. *Clin Cardiol* 1982;5:425–430.
258. Fraser GE, Upsdell M. Alcohol and other discriminants between cases of sudden death and myocardial infarction. *Am J Epidemiol* 1981;114:462–476.
259. Bergstrand R, Vedin A, Wilhelmsson C, et al. Characteristics of males with myocardial infarction below age 40. *J Chronic Dis* 1983;36:289–296.
260. Wannamethee SG, Shaper AG. Patterns of alcohol intake and risk of stroke in middle-aged British men. *Stroke* 1996;27:1033–1039.
261. Bianchi C, Negri E, La Vecchia C, et al. Alcohol consumption and the risk of acute myocardial infarction in women. *J Epidemiol Community Health* 1993;47:308–311.
262. Gould L, Gopalaswamy C, Yang D, et al. Effect of oral alcohol on left ventricular ejection fraction, volumes, and segmental wall motion in normals and in patients with recent myocardial infarction. *Clin Cardiol* 1985;8:576–582.
263. Yano K, Rhoads GG, Kagan A. Coffee, alcohol and risk of coronary heart disease among Japanese men living in Hawaii. *N Engl J Med* 1977;297:405–409.
264. D'Avanzo B, La Vecchia C, Tognoni G, et al. Coffee consumption and risk of acute myocardial infarction in Italian males. GISSI-EFRIM. Gruppo Italiano per lo Studio della Sopravvivenza nell'Infarto, Epidemiologia dei Fattori di Rischio del'Infarto Miocardico. *Ann Epidemiol* 1993;3:595–604.
265. Kleemola P, Jousilahti P, Pietinen P, et al. Coffee consumption and the risk of coronary heart disease and death. *Arch Intern Med* 2000;160:3393–3400.
266. La Vecchia C, Gentile A, Negri E, et al. Coffee consumption and myocardial infarction in women. *Am J Epidemiol* 1989;130:481–485.
267. Klatsky AL, Friedman GD, Armstrong MA. Coffee use prior to myocardial infarction restudied: heavier intake may increase the risk. *Am J Epidemiol* 1990;132:479–488.
268. Barzi F, Woodward M, Marfisi RM, et al. Mediterranean diet and all-causes mortality after myocardial infarction: results from the GISSI-Prevenzione trial. *Eur J Clin Nutr* 2003;57:604–611.
269. Morris MC, Manson JE, Rosner B, et al. Fish consumption and cardiovascular disease in the physicians' health study: a prospective study. *Am J Epidemiol* 1995;142:166–175.
270. Pais P, Pogue J, Gerstein H, et al. Risk factors for acute myocardial infarction in Indians: a case-control study. *Lancet* 1996;348:358–363.
271. Van Gaal LF, Rissanen AM, Scheen AJ, et al. Effects of the cannabinoid-1 receptor blocker rimonabant on weight reduction and cardiovascular risk factors in overweight patients: 1-year experience from the RIO-Europe study. *Lancet* 2005;365:1389–1397.
272. Tofler GH, Muller JE, Stone PH, et al. Comparison of long-term outcome after acute myocardial infarction in patients never graduated from high school with that in more educated patients. Multicenter Investigation of the Limitation of Infarct Size (MILIS). *Am J Cardiol* 1993;71:1031–1035.
273. Allison TG, Williams DE, Miller TD, et al. Medical and economic costs of psychologic distress in patients with coronary artery disease. *Mayo Clin Proc* 1995;70:734–742.
274. Hoffmann A, Pfiffner D, Hornung R, et al. Psychosocial factors predict medical outcome following a first myocardial infarction. Working Group on Cardiac Rehabilitation of the Swiss Society of Cardiology. *Coron Artery Dis* 1995;6:147–152.
275. Friedman S. Cardiac disease, anxiety, and sexual functioning. *Am J Cardiol* 2000;86:46F–50F.
276. Bar-On D, Gilutz H, Maymon T, et al. Long-term prognosis of low-risk, post-MI patients: the importance of subjective perception of disease. *Eur Heart J* 1994;15:1611–1615.
277. Shores MM, Pascualy M, Veith RC. Major depression and heart disease: treatment trials. *Semin Clin Neuropsychiatry* 1998;3:87–101.
278. Roose SP, Spatz E. Treating depression in patients with ischaemic heart disease: which agents are best to use and to avoid? *Drug Saf* 1999;20:459–465.
279. Friedmann E, Thomas SA. Pet ownership, social support, and one-year survival after acute myocardial infarction in the Cardiac Arrhythmia Suppression Trial (CAST). *Am J Cardiol* 1995;76:1213–1217.
280. Mehta RH, Das S, Tsai TT, et al. Quality improvement initiative and its impact on the management of patients with acute myocardial infarction. *Arch Intern Med* 2000;160:3057–3062.
281. Marciniak TA, Ellerbeck EF, Radford MJ, et al. Improving the quality of care for Medicare patients with acute myocardial infarction: results from the Cooperative Cardiovascular Project. *JAMA* 1998;279:1351–1357.
282. Jolly K, Bradley F, Sharp S, et al. Randomised controlled trial of follow up care in general practice of patients with myocardial infarction and angina: final results of the Southampton heart integrated care project (SHIP). The SHIP Collaborative Group. *BMJ* 1999;318:706–711.
283. Ryan TJ, Anderson JL, Antman EM, et al. ACC/AHA guidelines for the management of patients with acute myocardial infarction: a report of the American College of Cardiology/American Heart Association Task Force on Practice Guidelines (Committee on Management of Acute Myocardial Infarction). *J Am Coll Cardiol* 1996;28:1328–1428.
284. Ryan TJ, Antman EM, Brooks NH, et al. 1999 update: ACC/AHA guidelines for the management of patients with acute myocardial infarction. A report of the American College of Cardiology/American Heart Association Task Force on Practice Guidelines (Committee on Management of Acute Myocardial Infarction). *J Am Coll Cardiol* 1999;34:890–911.
285. Chen J, Radford MJ, Wang Y, et al. Do "America's Best Hospitals" perform better for acute myocardial infarction? *N Engl J Med* 1999;340:286–292.
286. Ellerbeck EF, Jencks SF, Radford MJ, et al. Quality of care for Medicare patients with acute myocardial infarction: a four-state pilot study from the Cooperative Cardiovascular Project. *JAMA* 1995;273:1509–1514.
287. Pilote L, Califf RM, Sapp S, et al. Regional variation across the United States in the management of acute myocardial infarction. GUSTO-1 Investigators. Global Utilization of Streptokinase and Tissue Plasminogen Activator for Occluded Coronary Arteries. *N Engl J Med* 1995;333:565–572.
288. O'Connor GT, Quinton HB, Traven ND, et al. Geographic variation in the treatment of acute myocardial infarction: the Cooperative Cardiovascular Project. *JAMA* 1999;281:627–633.
289. Canto JG, Rogers WJ, French WJ, et al. Payer status and the utilization of hospital resources in acute myocardial infarction: a report from the National Registry of Myocardial Infarction 2. *Arch Intern Med* 2000;160:817–823.
290. Hall D, Zeitler H, Rudolph W. Counteraction of the vasodilator effects of enalapril by aspirin in severe heart failure. *J Am Coll Cardiol* 1992; 20:1549–1555.
291. Peterson JG, Topol EJ, Sapp SK, et al. Evaluation of the effects of aspirin combined with angiotensin-converting enzyme inhibitors in patients with coronary artery disease. *Am J Med* 2000;109:371–377.
292. Beer JH, Pederiva S, Pontiggia L. Genetics of platelet receptor single-nucleotide polymorphisms: clinical implications in thrombosis. *Ann Med* 2000;32[Suppl 1]:10–14.

293. Mrozikiewicz PM, Cascorbi I, Ziemer S, et al. Reduced procedural risk for coronary catheter interventions in carriers of the coagulation factor VII-Gln353 gene. *J Am Coll Cardiol* 2000;36:1520–1525.
294. Vijayan KV, Goldschmidt-Clermont PJ, Roos C, et al. The Pl(A2) polymorphism of integrin beta(3) enhances outside-in signaling and adhesive functions. *J Clin Invest* 2000;105:793–802.
295. Undas A, Sanak M, Musial J, et al. Platelet glycoprotein IIIa polymorphism, aspirin, and thrombin generation. *Lancet* 1999;353:982–983.
296. Walter DH, Schachinger V, Elsner M, et al. Platelet glycoprotein IIIa polymorphisms and risk of coronary stent thrombosis. *Lancet* 1997;350:1217–1219.
297. Nurden AT. Platelet glycoprotein IIIa polymorphism and coronary thrombosis. *Lancet* 1997;350:1189–1191.
298. Topol EJ, McCarthy J, Gabriel S, et al. Single nucleotide polymorphisms in multiple novel thrombospondin genes may be associated with familial premature myocardial infarction. *Circulation* 2001;104:2641–2644.
299. Haase KK, Schiele R, Wagner S, et al. In-hospital mortality of elderly patients with acute myocardial infarction: data from the MITRA (Maximal Individual Therapy in Acute Myocardial Infarction) registry. *Clin Cardiol* 2000;23:831–836.
300. Ambrosioni E, Borghi C, Magnani B. The effect of the angiotensin-converting-enzyme inhibitor zofenopril on mortality and morbidity after anterior myocardial infarction. The Survival of Myocardial Infarction Long-Term Evaluation (SMILE) Study Investigators. *N Engl J Med* 1995; 332:80–85.
301. Kober L, Torp-Pedersen C, Carlsen JE, et al. A clinical trial of the angiotensin-converting-enzyme inhibitor trandolapril in patients with left ventricular dysfunction after myocardial infarction. Trandolapril Cardiac Evaluation (TRACE) Study Group. *N Engl J Med* 1995;333:1670–1676.
302. A randomized trial of propranolol in patients with acute myocardial infarction: I. Mortality results. *JAMA* 1982;247:1707–1714.
303. Hjalmarson A, Elmfeldt D, Herlitz J, et al. Effect on mortality of metoprolol in acute myocardial infarction: a double-blind randomised trial. *Lancet* 1981;2:823–827.
304. Randomised trial of intravenous atenolol among 16,027 cases of suspected acute myocardial infarction: ISIS-1. First International Study of Infarct Survival Collaborative Group. *Lancet* 1986;2:57–66.
305. Metoprolol in acute myocardial infarction (MIAMI): a randomised placebo-controlled international trial. The MIAMI Trial Research Group. *Eur Heart J* 1985;6:199–226.
306. Pedersen TR. Six-year follow-up of the Norwegian Multicenter Study on Timolol after Acute Myocardial Infarction. *N Engl J Med* 1985;313:1055–1058.

CHAPTER 22 ■ MITRAL VALVE DISEASE

LEONARDO RODRIGUEZ AND A. MARC GILLINOV

With the widespread availability of echocardiography, there has been an increase in the number of patients diagnosed with mitral valve dysfunction. Although the prevalence of mitral stenosis caused by rheumatic disease has decreased in recent years in the United States and Europe, the prevalence of mitral regurgitation (MR) has increased. In adults, the most common causes of MR are degenerative, ischemic, endocarditic, and rheumatic processes (1). The etiology of mitral valve dysfunction influences the therapeutic approach, timing of intervention, results of treatment intervention, and long-term survival. Therefore, after a brief review of mitral valve anatomy, we discuss the management of mitral valve disease, focusing on the etiologies of mitral valve dysfunction.

MITRAL VALVE ANATOMY

The mitral apparatus includes the leaflets, annulus, chordae tendineae, papillary muscles, and left ventricle.

Leaflets

The mitral valve has two leaflets, the anterior (aortic) and posterior (mural). The leaflets are attached to the mitral annulus and the to the papillary muscles by primary and secondary chordae. The anterior mitral leaflet is in direct continuity with the fibrous skeleton of the heart.

The posterior leaflet is rectangular. The free margin of the posterior leaflet has two clefts that divide the posterior leaflet into three scallops: the largest or middle scallop, the posteromedial scallop, and the anterolateral scallop. Motion of the posterior leaflet is more restricted than that of the anterior leaflet; however, both mitral leaflets contribute to effective valve closure.

Annulus

The mitral annulus is the site of leaflet attachment to muscular fibers of the atrium and ventricle. The annulus is a nonplanar, saddle-shaped structure (2). It is flexible and decreases in diameter during systole by approximately 26% (3,4). Anteriorly, the annulus is attached to the fibrous skeleton of the heart (2). This limits flexibility and the capacity of the anterior annulus to dilate with MR, although dilatation of the anterior annulus has recently been documented in patients with MR (5,6). Important anatomic relations of the mitral annulus include the circumflex coronary artery, the coronary sinus, the aortic valve, and the bundle of His.

Chordae Tendineae

The chordae tendineae are chords of fibrous connective tissue that attach the mitral leaflets to either the papillary muscles or the left ventricular (LV) free wall. The chordae are divided into primary, secondary, and tertiary chordae. Primary chordae attach to the fibrous band running along the free edge of the leaflets, ensuring that the contact surfaces of the leaflets coapt without leaflet prolapse or flail. Secondary chordae attach to the ventricular surface of the leaflets and contribute to ventricular function (7,8). Tertiary chordae are unique to the posterior leaflet. They arise directly from the LV wall or from small trabeculae to insert into the ventricular surface of the leaflet near the annulus.

Papillary Muscles

The anterolateral and posteromedial papillary muscles each supply chordae tendineae to both leaflets. The anterolateral papillary muscle receives a dual blood supply from the anterior descending coronary artery and either a diagonal branch or a marginal branch of the left circumflex artery (9,10). The posteromedial papillary muscle receives its blood supply from either the left circumflex artery or a distal branch of the right coronary artery. Because of its single blood supply, the posteromedial papillary muscle is more commonly affected by myocardial infarction (MI).

ACUTE AND CHRONIC MITRAL REGURGITATION

Acute Mitral Regurgitation

Pathophysiology

The pathophysiologic consequences of acute, severe MR—such as that observed in patients following rupture of a papillary muscle—differ from those of chronic MR. With acute MR, a sudden volume overload is imposed on the nondilated, nonhypertrophied left ventricle and left atrium causing a sudden increase in left atrial pressure. Preload is increased, whereas afterload decreases as a result of the newly developed low-pressure runoff to the left atrium during systole (11). In the absence of coronary artery disease or MI, LV contractile function can be normal or even supranormal secondary to augmented sympathetic nervous stimulation of the myocardium (11,12).

Despite increased LV preload and contractility and decreased afterload, overall LV pump function declines in acute MR. Total LV stroke volume increases, but much of this flow is directed into the left atrium diminishing the effective, forward stroke volume through the aorta. The clinical impact of acute MR is largely determined by the compliance of the left atrium. In a normal, relatively noncompliant left atrium, acute MR results in high left atrial pressure, which can rapidly lead to pulmonary edema.

Diagnosis

Acute MR is usually associated with the sudden development of severe LV failure. Patients are often in pulmonary edema when initially seen, and cardiogenic shock is common. Severe acute MR secondary to acute inferoposterior MI is seen more often in women (13).

The physical examination is dominated by findings associated with LV failure; tachycardia and tachypnea are common. The murmur is usually loud if normal LV function is present. The murmur may be soft if LV function is markedly reduced.

Echocardiographic studies demonstrate the etiology of the acute regurgitant lesion: vegetations in patients with infectious endocarditis, ruptured chordae in individuals with mitral valve prolapse, or papillary muscle rupture in AMI. In many patients in critical condition, transthoracic echocardiography may show the presence of MR, but tachycardia or poor windows in a ventilated patient may obscure the precise structural mechanism. Transesophageal echocardiographic examination reveals the cause of the acute MR in almost all cases. Transesophageal echocardiography also allows evaluation of left and right ventricular function and other valvular lesions.

Bedside right heart catheterization is useful in these patients, allowing measurement of right-sided and capillary wedge pressures, as well as cardiac index. Patients with acute MR have marked elevation of filling pressures and low cardiac index. Large, regurgitant CV waves are observed in the pulmonary capillary wedge pressure tracing. Catheterization is also helpful in monitoring response to aggressive therapy.

Treatment

In patients with acute MR, IV vasodilator therapy with nitroprusside can produce dramatic benefit with reductions in ventricular cavity dilatation, diastolic filling pressures, and mitral regurgitant orifice (14,15). The nitroprusside infusion is continued until the patient is stabilized by either surgical intervention (14,16) or long-term oral medical therapy (e.g., angiotensin-converting enzyme inhibitors, digoxin, and diuretics). IV nitroglycerin is often effective in reducing pulmonary vascular congestion in these patients, particularly if the underlying etiology for MR is ischemic heart disease. Surgical therapy is almost always required in patients with acute severe MR. Intraaortic balloon counterpulsation can be helpful in stabilizing the patient before definitive therapy is instituted (13).

The surgical approach and results depend on the underlying pathology. Patients with MR secondary to AMI have a high surgical mortality (13). Patients with acute endocarditis may have elevated morbidity, particularly if there is multivalvular involvement, septic shock, or multiple septic emboli.

Chronic Mitral Regurgitation

The vast majority of patients present with chronic MR at the time of diagnosis with LV and left atrial adaptation to volume overload. The causes of MR are listed in Table 22.1.

Pathophysiology

MR causes LV and left atrial volume overload. The degree of volume overload depends on the regurgitant volume. The regurgitant volume is determined by the size of the regurgitant orifice area (ROA), the duration of systole and the systolic pressure gradient between the left ventricle and left atrium:

$$MRV = MROA \times C \times TS \times \sqrt{LVP - LAP}$$

where MRV is the regurgitant volume, MROA is the regurgitant orifice area, C is a constant, TS is the duration of systole, LVP is the mean LV pressure, and LAP is mean LA pressure (17).

Initially, as the severity of MR increases there is progressive enlargement of the left atrium and left ventricle to compensate for the regurgitant volume. LV dilatation occurs as a result of remodeling of the extracellular matrix with rearrangement of myocardial fibers, in association with the addition of new sarcomeres in series and the development of eccentric LV hypertrophy (17). In patients with severe, chronic MR, the left atrium is markedly dilated and atrial compliance is increased. Although there is fibrosis of the atrial wall, left atrial pressure can be normal or only slightly elevated.

The ejection fraction may be normal or even hyperdynamic as the ventricle empties into the lower pressure left atrium. The increase in end-diastolic volume and the small end systolic volume help to maintain a normal forward stroke volume.

TABLE 22.1

CAUSES OF MR

CHRONIC
Inflammatory
Rheumatic heart disease
Systemic lupus erythematosus
Progressive systemic sclerosis
Methysergide therapy
Degenerative
Myxomatous degeneration of the valve
Calcification of the mitral valve annulus
Marfan syndrome
Ehlers-Danlos syndrome
Pseudoxanthoma elasticum
Ankylosing spondylitis
Infiltrative amyloidosis
Infectious
Infectious endocarditis
Structural
Ruptured chordae tendineae (acute MR that can become chronic)
Dysfunction of a papillary muscle: ischemia (acute MR that can become chronic)
Dilatation of mitral valve annulus secondary to LV dilatation (cardiomyopathy)
Hypertrophic cardiomyopathy
Paravalvular prosthetic valve leak
Congenital
Cleft mitral valve (associated with other congenital heart diseases [e.g., primum atrial septal defect])
Parachute mitral valve (associated with other congenital heart diseases [e.g., endocardial cushion defect, endocardial fibroelastosis, transposition of the great arteries])
ACUTE
Structural
Trauma
Dysfunction or rupture of a papillary muscle (ischemic heart disease)
Prosthetic valve malfunction with paravalvular leak or leaflet malfunction or disruption
Infectious
Infectious endocarditis
Acute rheumatic fever
Degenerative
Myxomatous degeneration with chordal rupture

Abbreviation: LV, left ventricular; MR, mitral regurgitation.

In the absence of primary myocardial damage, diastolic function of the dilated ventricle is normal with decreased chamber stiffness but normal myocardial stiffness. In the compensated phase, total stroke volume is enhanced and ventricular afterload normalizes. Over time, and for poorly understood reasons, the ventricle progressively dilates, has increased diastolic pressure and afterload, and reduced ejection fraction (17). During this decompensated phase, there is also significant left atrial enlargement, increase in capillary wedge pressure, and development of pulmonary hypertension and right ventricular dysfunction.

The assessment of contractility in the presence of severe MR remains problematic; ejection phase indices overestimate contractile state (18). Ejection fraction is the most common parameter used to assess LV function but does not detect early changes in LV function. A recognized drop in LV ejection fraction is a late event. Several complex methods such as end systolic stress and elastance have been used to assess LV function but are impractical for routine evaluation and serial follow up of patients (19).

Diagnosis

Echocardiography is the main diagnostic tool in patients with MR because it displays in real time valvular anatomy and function and provides information about left and right ventricular function. The left ventricle can be normal in size or dilated depending on the severity and duration of MR. The left atrium is also enlarged, more severely in the presence of atrial fibrillation.

A systematic and comprehensive approach using transthoracic echo is of critical importance (20) (Fig. 22.1). The complete mitral valve apparatus must be interrogated by two-dimensional echo and Doppler. Assessment of global and regional LV function is important to understand the mechanism and prognosis of MR. New techniques such as tissue Doppler or strain have been applied in asymptomatic patients to assess subclinical LV dysfunction. The initial results are encouraging (21,22). In experienced echo laboratories transthoracic echocardiography may be adequate for diagnostic evaluation in the majority of patients with MR. Transesophageal echocardiography offers a better definition of the anatomy, and is indicated in cases with suboptimal transthoracic windows or unclear etiology, mechanism, or severity of the MR.

The severity of MR can be assessed by semiquantitative methods based on the size (length, width, or area) of the regurgitant jet or the width of the vena contracta or, alternatively, by quantitative techniques that attempt to quantify the regurgitant volume and fraction and the size of the ROA (23). The importance of quantification has been reinforced by recent data suggesting that large ROAs are associated with poor prognosis even in asymptomatic patients (24) (Fig. 22.2). Patients with ischemic MR have a risk ratio of cardiac death of 2.38 if the regurgitant orifice is larger than 20 mm^2 (25,26). Comparatively, patients with degenerative MR and ROA greater than 40 mm^2 carry an unfavorable prognosis. This difference can be partially explained by reduced ejection fraction in the ischemic group (24,27).

A consensus on quantification of native valvular regurgitation using echocardiography has been published (23) (Table 22.2). A regurgitant volume greater than or equal to 60 mL and an effective ROA greater than or equal to 40 mm^2 characterize severe MR. In most patients, a comprehensive evaluation using multiple techniques and parameters is necessary for accurate determination of the severity of MR. Very eccentric jets of MR are always a challenge for quantification and require considerable expertise.

Stress echocardiography can be used to determine the functional significance of MR, particularly in patients with minimal or no symptoms. It is also helpful to uncover latent LV dysfunction (28). Exercise ejection fraction predicts postoperative LV function better than does the resting ejection fraction (28). An increased end systolic volume with exercise is also a predictor of diminished post operative ejection fraction (28). In patients with tricuspid regurgitation, it is also possible to assess the development of pulmonary hypertension with exercise.

Treatment

All patients with MR should receive antibiotic prophylaxis before dental and other invasive procedures according to American Heart Association/American College of Cardiology guidelines (29). In addition, without antibiotic prophylaxis patients with mitral valve prolapse have a three- to eightfold (29) higher risk of developing infective endocarditis (30).

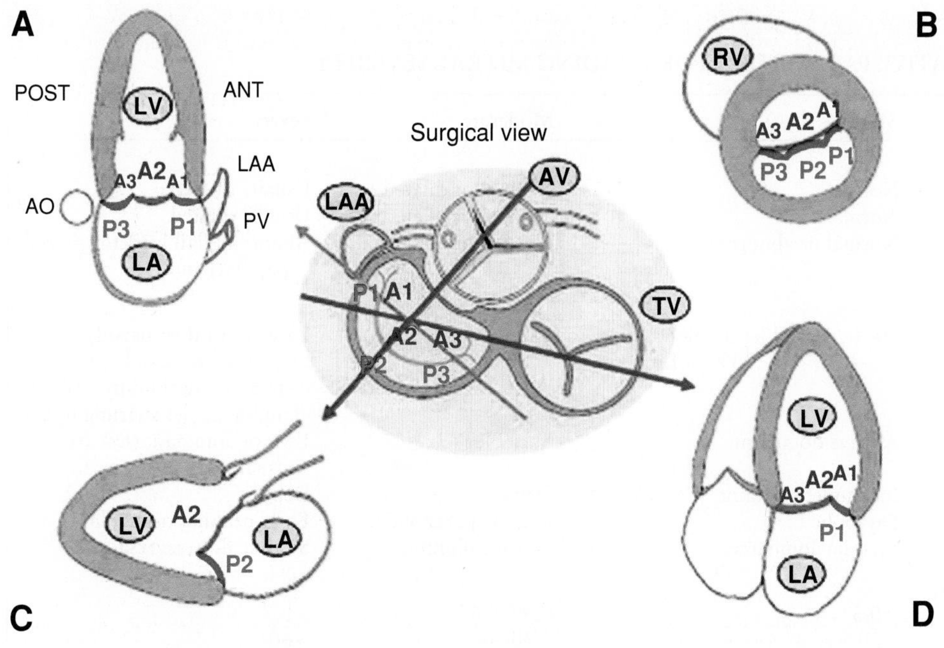

FIGURE 22.1. Four imaging planes to assess the location of prolapsed or flail segments. (A) Intercommissural plane. (B) Parasternal short-axis view showing the anterior leaflet and the three scallops of the posterior leaflet. (C) Parasternal long-axis view showing the middle segments of the anterior and posterior leaflets. (D) Apical four-chamber view. *Abbreviations:* ANT, anterior; AO, descending aorta; AV, aortic valve; LA, left atrium; LAA, left atrial appendage; LV, left ventricle; POST, posterior; PV, pulmonary vein; RV, right ventricle; TV, tricuspid valve. (*Source:* From Monin JL, Dehant P, Roiron C, et al. Functional assessment of mitral regurgitation by transthoracic echocardiography using standardized imaging planes diagnostic accuracy and outcome implications. *J Am Coll Cardiol* 2005; 46:302–309, by permission from the Journal of the American College of Cardiology.)

Optimal blood pressure control is important. Hypertension is a risk factor for development of severe MR in patients with mitral prolapse (31) and negatively affects LV performance in patients with ischemic heart disease or dilated cardiomyopathy.

Restriction of physical activity is recommended only in symptomatic patients and in those with LV dysfunction. Isometric exercise should be discouraged. The 2005 task force 3 issued recommendation for athletes with MR. Athletes with severe MR and definite LV enlargement ($\geq$60 mm), pulmonary hypertension, or any degree of LV systolic dysfunction at rest should not participate in competitive sports (32).

Management of underlying disease is fundamental in patients with ischemic heart disease or infective endocarditis. Other less frequent causes of secondary MR are affected by progression of the underlying process such as lupus or other inflammatory processes.

The most important goals of surgical intervention are improvement of symptoms, preservation of LV function, and increased longevity. Other considerations include preservation of the native mitral valve apparatus, avoidance of chronic anticoagulation, maintenance and/or restoration of sinus rhythm, and prevention/improvement of pulmonary hypertension and right ventricular dysfunction.

DEGENERATIVE MITRAL VALVE DISEASE

Degenerative mitral valve disease includes myxomatous mitral disease, mitral leaflet flail or prolapse, and Barlow syndrome. The Framingham Heart Study employed strict echocardiographic criteria to determine the prevalence of mitral valve prolapse. They noted a prevalence of 2.4% in their population; 60% of the patients with mitral valve prolapse were women (33).

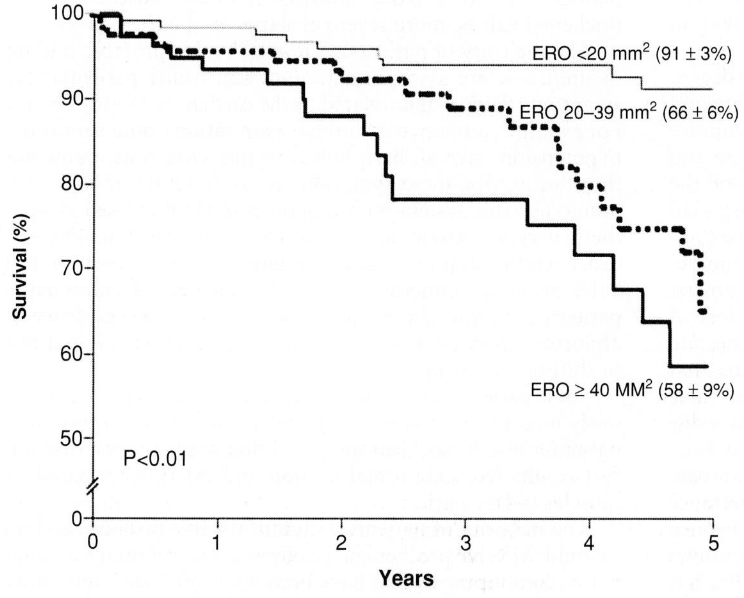

FIGURE 22.2. Kaplan-Meier estimates of the mean rates of overall survival among patients with asymptomatic MR under medical management, according to the effective orifice area (ERO). (*Source:* From Enriquez-Sarano M, Avierinos JF, Messika-Zeitoun D, et al. Quantitative determinants of the outcome of asymptomatic mitral regurgitation. *N Engl J Med* 2005;352:875–883, by permission of the New England Journal of Medicine.)

TABLE 22.2

QUALITATIVE AND QUANTITATIVE PARAMETERS FOR GRADING MITRAL SEVERITY

	Mild	Moderate	Severe
STRUCTURAL PARAMETERS			
LA size	Normal*	Normal or dilated	Usually dilated
LV size	Normal*	Normal or dilated	Usually dilated
Mitral leaflets or support apparatus	Normal or abnormal	Normal or abnormal	Abnormal/flail leaflet/ruptured papillary muscle
DOPPLER PARAMETERS			
Color flow jet area	Small, central jet usually <4 cm^2 or <20% of LA area	Variable	Large central jet usually <10cm^2 or <40% of LA area or variable size wall impinging jet swirling in LA
Mitral inflow—PW	A wave dominant	Variable	E wave dominant (E wave usually 1.2 m/s)
Jet density—CW	Incomplete or faint	Dense	Dense
Jet contour—CW	Parabolic	Usually parabolic	Early peaking triangular
Pulmonary vein flow	Systolic dominance	Systolic blunting	Systolic flow reversal
QUANTITATIVE PARAMETERS			
VC width (cm)	<0.3	0.30–0.69	>0.7
R Vol (mL/beat)	<30	30–44 45–59	>60
RF (%)	<30	30–39 40–49	>50
EROA (cm^2)	<0.20	0.20–0.29 0.30–0.39	>0.40

Abbreviations: CW: continuous wave Doppler; EROA: effective refractive orifice area; LA: left atrial; LV: left ventricular; PW: pulsed wave; RF: regurgitant fraction; VC: vena contractor.
Reproduced with permission from reference 23, Elsevier.

Etiology and Pathology

Pathologic changes associated with degenerative mitral valve disease may include annular dilatation, leaflet thickening, myxoid degeneration, chordal elongation, chordal rupture, and annular and leaflet calcification (34). In patients with degenerative disease, the mitral leaflets and chordae have 3% to 9% higher water contents and 30% to 150% higher concentrations of glycosaminoglycans than do normals (35). There are lower collagen concentrations in the leaflets compared with normals. The biochemical effects are more pronounced in chordae than in leaflets.

Disruption of the collagen bundles may explain why degenerative leaflets and chordae exhibit enhanced extensibility and decreased stiffness compared to normal valves. Chordal rupture is one of the causes of severe MR in degenerative disease and is secondary to mechanical weakening of the chordae and the abnormal stresses imparted by the redundant leaflet (36). Flail leaflet is more common in patients with unileaflet prolapse (37).

Mitral valve prolapse has been associated with a number of different conditions, including Marfan syndrome, Ehlers-Danlos syndrome, acute rheumatic carditis, and a variety of congenital cardiac anomalies. A number of these entities are the result of genetic defects in connective tissue structure that produce, among other anatomic abnormalities, mitral valve prolapse. Although most cases of degenerative mitral valve disease are sporadic, a familial basis for the condition has been recognized. This form of mitral valve prolapse has an autosomal dominant mode of inheritance with variable penetrance and is influenced by age and gender. There is marked heterogeneity of clinical presentation (36). A locus for autosomal dominant myxomatous mitral valve prolapse, *MMVP1,* has been mapped to chromosome 16p11.2-p12.1 (38) and a second locus, *MMVP2*, to chromosome 11p15.4 (39).

Natural History

The clinical spectrum of patients with degenerative valve disease is wide. Two distinct clinical groups appear to exist. One consists of young women with a midsystolic click and mild echocardiographic prolapse; they often have multiple complaints. The other group consists of middle-aged men with thickened valves, more severe prolapse, and MR.

The majority of patients with mitral valve prolapse and no or mild MR are asymptomatic (40–42). Many patients have symptoms that seem unrelated to the cardiac pathophysiology. For example, anxiety, easy fatigue, palpitations, and orthostatic hypotension have all been linked to this syndrome. Some authorities ascribe these symptoms to dysfunction of the autonomic nervous system with inappropriately increased sympathetic nervous activity at rest and with mild exertion (43). The exact relationship of these autonomic abnormalities to mitral valve prolapse is unclear. Studies that included asymptomatic patients with mitral valve prolapse have found no evidence of abnormal autonomic or neuroendocrine function either at rest or during tilt testing.

Some patients report chest discomfort that, at times, is obviously musculoskeletal in origin and at other times seems anginal in nature. It has been suggested that anginal chest discomfort results from abnormal tension and traction on papillary muscles (44).

The majority of patients with mitral valve prolapse and no or mild MR have a benign prognosis, but there are a number of complications that have been associated with this entity including arrhythmias, sudden death, cerebrovascular events, and MR.

Arrhythmias are common in patients with mitral valve prolapse. Both supraventricular and ventricular arrhythmias have been reported; however, it is unclear to what degree mitral valve prolapse is the actual cause of these rhythm disturbances.

Mitral valve prolapse carries a small but real risk of sudden death. The presence of severe MR with ruptured chordae and a flail segment increases the risk of sudden death. In Mayo Clinic data based on 348 patients with a follow-up of 48 months, the rate of sudden death was 1.8% per year (45). By multivariate analysis, independent predictors were functional class, ejection fraction, and atrial fibrillation. In patients with no or minimal symptoms, sinus rhythm and normal LV function, a linearized rate of 0.8% per year was observed; in patients in functional class III or IV, the incidence of sudden death was 7.8% (45).

Cerebral embolism occasionally occurs in patients with mitral valve prolapse. Formation of platelet–fibrin thrombi on severely myxomatous valves has been proposed as the embolic source. AMI can be another manifestation of arterial embolism in these patients. Zuppiroli et al. (40) followed 300 patients with mitral valve prolapse for more than 8 years and found a serious complication rate of only 1% per year in this population. The increased risk of cerebrovascular events in patients with mitral valve prolapse appears to be limited to older patients with thickened valves and MR (46,47–49).

Increasingly severe MR occurs in 10% to 15% of patients and can require mitral valve surgery if symptoms or LV dysfunction develop (40,42). Severe MR requiring surgery is three times more common in men than in women. Correlates with severe MR and the need for mitral valve surgery include male gender, older age, and the presence of obesity and hypertension (31).

Diagnosis

Physical Examination

Patients with mitral valve prolapse are often asthenic in habitus with low body weights. Arterial blood pressure is frequently low and orthostatic hypotension may be present. Straight-back syndrome, pectus excavatum, scoliosis, and a narrow thoracic anteroposterior diameter may be present. If severe MR is present, the carotid pulse may be brisk in upstroke with a hint of rapid fall off. Palpation of the precordium may reveal a brief inward movement of the apical impulse in midsystole coinciding with the occurrence of the midsystolic click.

Auscultation of these patients is best performed using the diaphragm of the stethoscope with the patient lying and standing. The usual finding is a sharp, systolic click heard 0.14 seconds or more after the S1. This click differs from the ejection click of aortic valve disease because it occurs well after the onset of the carotid arterial upstroke. At times, more than one click is heard. It is thought that clicks are generated by tensing of the chordae tendineae and billowing of the mitral valve leaflets. The click(s) is usually, but not always, followed by a mid- to late systolic crescendo murmur heard best at the apex. The duration of the murmur correlates directly with the severity of MR; the earlier and more prolonged the murmur, the more severe the regurgitation. The auscultatory findings are dynamic and change depending on loading conditions. Thus, maneuvers or conditions that modify LV size affect the timing and duration of the murmur. A decrease in cavity size moves the click and murmur earlier in systole because the valvular prolapse occurs earlier. Smaller ventricular size occurs with dehydration, standing, amyl nitrate administration, and the Valsalva maneuver. Although the murmur is longer in duration, its intensity may be less because the severity of MR diminishes in these conditions. Maneuvers that increase LV cavity size (increases in systemic blood volume, decreases in myocardial contractility, and increases in venous return) move the click and murmur later in systole.

Echocardiography

Echocardiography is the primary diagnostic modality in patients with degenerative mitral valve disease and confirms the diagnosis of mitral valve prolapse by demonstrating more than a 2-mm systolic posterior displacement of one or both leaflets into the left atrium in the parasternal long axis view (50,51). The echocardiogram determines the mechanism(s) and severity of MR and enables assessment of other valves and measurement of LV function and dimensions. In patients with classic prolapse, the leaflets are thick and redundant with variable degrees of billowing into the left atrium. Patients with mitral valve prolapse but without leaflet thickening have a more benign prognosis (52).

The ejection fraction is usually high and an ejection fraction below 60% should be considered abnormal in patients with severe MR. In cases of severe mitral valve prolapse, it is possible to observe a coaptation gap during systole. In many patients it is also possible to visualize ruptured chordae and flail segments using transthoracic echocardiography. A systematic approach using standard transthoracic echocardiography allows determination of the mechanism and severity of MR in most cases (20) (see Fig. 22.1). Transesophageal echocardiography is helpful in cases of suboptimal windows and, for better definition of the size and extent of the flail segment (Fig. 22.3). Intraoperative transesophageal echocardiography is an essential tool in patients undergoing mitral valve repair.

Color Doppler echocardiography allows visualization of the origin, direction, and severity of the regurgitant jet. In most cases the jet has a central origin with involvement of either the central scallop of the posterior leaflet (P2) or the central portion of the anterior leaflet (A2). The direction of the jet is typically opposite to the leaflet involved. In cases of predominant posterior leaflet involvement, the jet is anteriorly directed, and the jet is posteriorly directed when the prolapse is anterior. In cases of balanced bileaflet prolapse the jet is central. Involvement of commissural scallops may direct the jet in any direction.

When surgical therapy is planned, knowledge of the coronary artery anatomy is essential. In patients at low risk for coronary artery disease, this may be achieved with multislice CT scanning. In patients at high risk for coronary artery disease, coronary angiography is indicated (53,54).

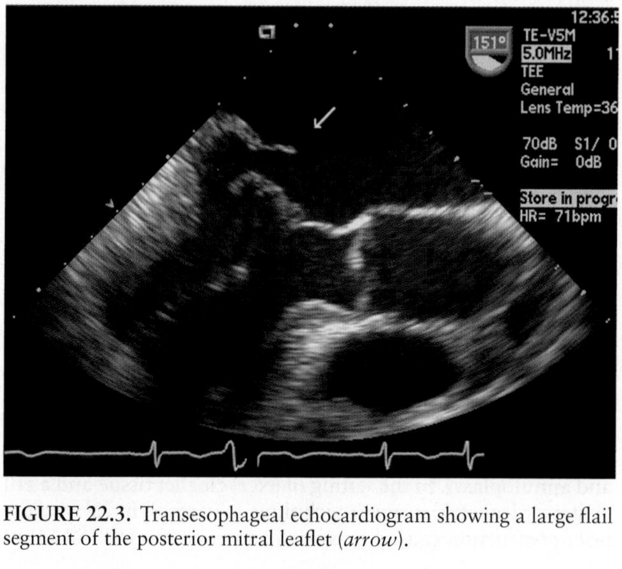

FIGURE 22.3. Transesophageal echocardiogram showing a large flail segment of the posterior mitral leaflet (*arrow*).

Medical Treatment

As mentioned, patients with MR or thickened leaflets should receive antibiotic prophylaxis. Patients with mitral valve prolapse but without regurgitation have an excellent prognosis. They usually do not progress to severe MR. Periodic echocardiographic follow-up in these patients is prudent.

The routine use of vasodilators in patients with MR remains controversial. Although there is agreement that this therapy is of value in patient with LV dysfunction (55–57), its indication in asymptomatic patients with normal ventricular function is less clear (57). In dogs with myxomatous disease, enalapril does not delay the onset of congestive heart failure (58). There is concern that vasodilators could mask the development of LV dysfunction and delay mitral valve surgery. Therefore, in the absence of adequate randomized clinical trials, the use of vasodilator therapy in asymptomatic patients with severe MR and normal LV function should be determined on a case by case basis taking into account LV size and systemic blood pressure. In patients with LV dysfunction at presentation therapy with vasodilators should be started and surgical correction performed without delay.

Surgical Treatment

Indications

Surgery should be considered in all patients with severe MR caused by degenerative mitral valve disease. More liberal indications for surgery are the result of increased understanding of the unfavorable natural history of patients with severe MR, extremely low operative risk in most patients with degenerative mitral valve disease, and excellent long-term results obtained with mitral valve repair (1,34,59). Definite indications for surgery in patients with severe MR are presence of symptoms or LV dysfunction (ejection fraction <0.60, end-systolic dimension >40–45 mm). Surgery should also be offered to patients with severe MR and new-onset atrial fibrillation.

There is some controversy concerning the role of surgery in asymptomatic patients with normal LV function. Recent data demonstrate high repair rates (>90%) and virtually no operative mortality in such patients (34,59,60). Furthermore, natural history studies demonstrate that asymptomatic patients with severe MR (effective ROA $\geq$ 40 mm^2) have reduced survival; surgical repair in such patients is associated with improved survival (24). In this group of patients, the 5-year probability of death or late cardiac surgery was 84% (24). Such patients frequently have a flail leaflet, which is a marker of severe MR (61). These data support the use of quantitative echocardiography to assess the severity of MR in asymptomatic patients and early surgery in those with severe MR.

In summary, the decision for surgical repair in patients with degenerative MR should be based on symptoms, LV function (at rest and exercise), severity of MR and local operative mortality and rate of successful repair.

Approach

Mitral valve repair is preferred to mitral valve replacement in patients with degenerative mitral valve disease (60,62,63). The probability of valve repair depends on the experience of the surgical team and the pathology encountered. Segmental posterior leaflet prolapse is the most common finding, affecting 60% to 80% of patients with severe MR caused by degenerative disease (1,59,64). This is usually repaired by quadrangular resection and annuloplasty. In the setting of excess leaflet tissue and a tall posterior leaflet, this repair technique may result in LV outflow tract obstruction caused by systolic anterior motion (SAM) of the mitral valve. SAM is avoided by reducing the height of the posterior leaflet with a sliding repair, which moves the point of leaflet coaptation posteriorly, away from the LV outflow tract (65,66). Anterior leaflet repair is more challenging. Anterior leaflet pathology may be corrected with a variety of repair techniques including creation of artificial chordae, chordal transfer, the edge-to-edge repair, chordal shortening, and anterior leaflet resection (67–72). All mitral valve repairs include annuloplasty. Functions of the annuloplasty include improved leaflet coaptation by reduction of the septal-lateral dimension of the valve, reduced tension on suture lines, and prevention of future annular dilatation (73–75). A variety of annuloplasty techniques are available (partial versus complete; flexible versus rigid), and all appear to function well in patients with degenerative disease (64). However, failure to incorporate an annuloplasty in the repair jeopardizes durability (34). In rare instances, mitral valve repair is not feasible. When this occurs, chordal-sparing mitral valve replacement is performed.

Results

The operative mortality for isolated mitral valve repair in degenerative disease is less than 1%; in contrast, most series report somewhat higher mortality for mitral valve replacement (1,62,63,76–79). In patients with degenerative mitral valve disease, preserved LV function, and minimal symptoms, long-term survival after repair is similar to that of age-matched patients in the general population (59). Long-term survival is influenced by patient age and ventricular dysfunction (34). Patients receiving mitral valve repair have better survival rates when compared to patients undergoing mitral valve replacement (62,63).

Durability of mitral valve repair for degenerative disease is excellent. In patients with posterior leaflet prolapse, 10- and 20-year freedoms from reoperation exceed 90% (34,59,60,64). In contrast, 10- and 20-year freedoms from reoperation after correction of anterior prolapse are 80% to 90% (34,59,60,64). Increased surgical experience and advances in surgical technique are responsible for recent improvements in repair durability (60). However, these reoperation rates likely overestimate repair durability; some patients develop recurrent MR but do not undergo cardiac reoperation (80). Therefore, annual echocardiographic surveillance is indicated in all patients after mitral valve repair for degenerative disease.

ISCHEMIC AND CARDIOMYOPATHIC MITRAL REGURGITATION

Etiology and Pathology

Ischemic and cardiomyopathic MR occurs in patients with normal mitral leaflets and chordae and no significant intrinsic mitral valve disease. Rather, changes in ventricular, annular, and/or papillary muscle geometry cause leaflet malcoaptation and resultant MR (4,80–83). Ischemic MR occurs as a consequence of coronary artery disease and should be distinguished from coexisting organic mitral valve disease and coronary artery disease (4,84,85). Ischemic MR may be caused by papillary muscle rupture or elongation, which cause leaflet flail or prolapse. More commonly, however, patients have restricted leaflet motion caused by changes in ventricular and annular geometry; this is termed *functional MR*. Patients with functional ischemic MR generally have completed MIs in the distribution of the right or circumflex coronary arteries (4,81–85). Regional changes in ventricular geometry and function, including apical and posterior displacement of the papillary muscles, cause leaflet restriction and tenting, which usually affects the posterior leaflet most severely and causes a central or posterior jet of MR (4,81–85). In contrast, patients with functional MR caused by idiopathic dilated cardiomyopathy have symmetrical changes in LV geometry resulting in more symmetrical mitral valve dysfunction (82). Functional MR, whether from ischemic disease or idiopathic dilated cardiomyopathy, is associated with annular dilatation (5,6).

Functional MR in patients with LV dysfunction is associated with poor prognosis. The impact of MR in such patients is graded; the more severe the MR, the lower the long-term survival (25,85–88). Patients with severe ischemic MR (regurgitant volume ≥30 mL/beat) have a 5-year survival rate of 35%; in contrast, similar patients with ischemic heart disease but without MR have a 5-year survival rate of 61% (25). The graded impact of MR on survival has been demonstrated in patients undergoing percutaneous coronary intervention, suggesting the possibility that treatment of both the coronary artery disease and the MR might improve outcomes (88).

In addition to impacting survival (25), functional MR influences quality of life and functional class (26). After MI, patients who develop ischemic MR are more likely to develop congestive heart failure than are similar patients without MR (26). These data suggest that quantification of MR in patients with coronary artery disease might be useful for risk stratification, with implications both for survival and for development of heart failure (25,26).

Diagnosis

Whereas the patient with a ruptured papillary muscle caused by MI usually presents in extremis with pulmonary edema and shock, most patients with ischemic and cardiomyopathic MR present with symptoms of congestive heart failure.

Physical Examination

The degree of congestive heart failure dominates physical exam findings. A prominent jugular venous pulse secondary to right ventricular dysfunction is common. The LV apical impulse is displaced laterally and a right ventricular heave may be appreciated. A holosystolic murmur is heard at the apex with radiation to the axilla and back. An S3 and S4 are common. In some cases of severe MR, a mid-diastolic rumble following an S3 is audible at the apex. This is the result of increase diastolic mitral flow and should not be confused with mitral stenosis.

Echocardiography

Diagnosis of ischemic and cardiomyopathic MR is established by echocardiography. Echo provides information about the mechanisms involved. Papillary muscle elongation occurs in some patients with completed MI. The involved papillary muscle shows increased echogenicity. The infarcted and elongated papillary muscle results in mitral leaflet prolapse, often involving the commissure (89). This mechanism is not always readily apparent and can be mistaken for degenerative disease, particularly when regional motion abnormalities are subtle. Regurgitant jets are eccentric and directed away from the involved prolapsing leaflet.

In patients with functional MR, regional remodeling with thinning and hypokinesis/akinesis of the inferior wall can be appreciated by two-dimensional echo and magnetic resonance imaging (MRI) (90) (Fig. 22.4). Regional dilatation displaces the papillary muscles inferiorly and laterally, tethering the leaflets and displacing the point of coaptation apically (83).

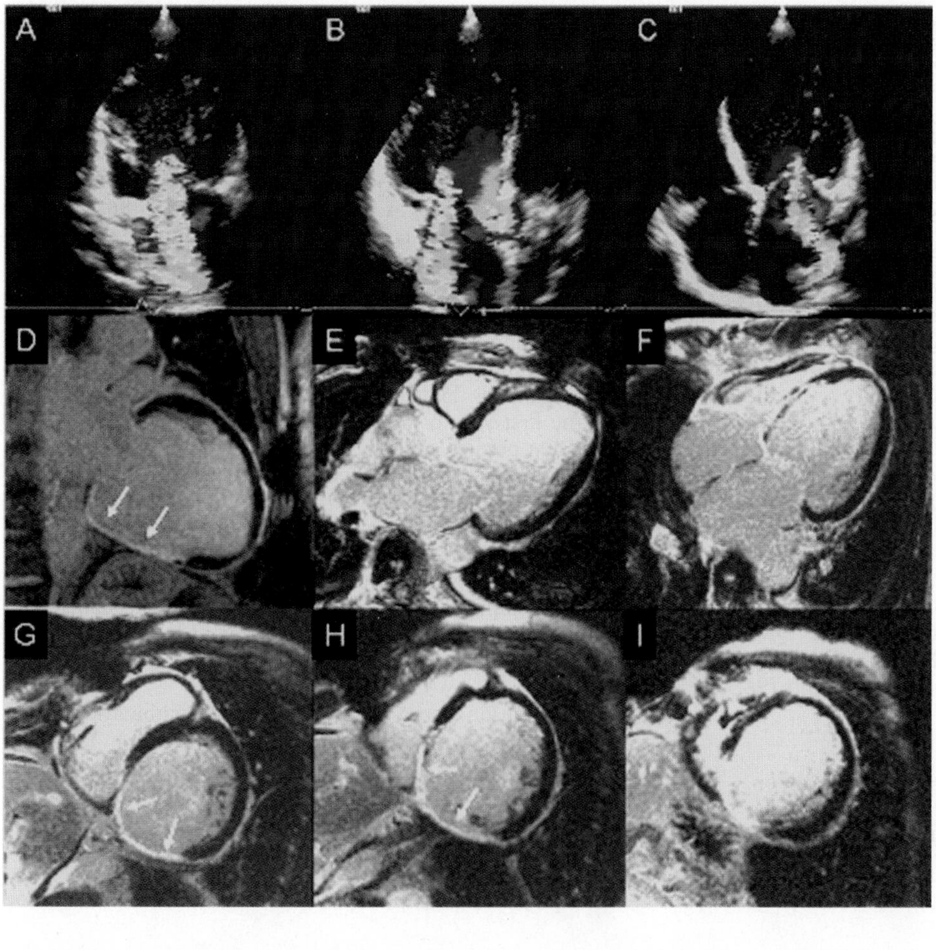

FIGURE 22.4. Transthoracic color Doppler echo images in the two-chamber (A), three-chamber (B), and four-chamber (C) views demonstrating severe MR. Delayed-enhancement magnetic resonance images in the two-chamber (D), three-chamber (E), and four-chamber (F) long-axis views as well as basal (G), middle (H), and apical (I) short-axis views demonstrating severe myocardial scarring localized to the inferior-posterior region as seen by the hyperenhanced areas (*arrows*). (*Source:* From Srichai MB, Grimm RA, Stillman AE, et al. Ischemic mitral regurgitation: impact of the left ventricle and mitral valve in patients with left ventricular systolic dysfunction. *Ann Thorac Surg* 2005; 80:170–178, by permission from Elsevier Inc.)

The degree of tenting of the leaflets caused by chordal tethering has been correlated with the severity of MR (90,91). Ischemic MR is related not only to inferior wall motion abnormalities, but also to the presence of scarred myocardium in the anterior wall, as recently demonstrated in a study using MRI (90).

In patients with global LV dysfunction, the left ventricle is dilated with increased sphericity. Annular dilatation, chordal tethering, and decreased mitral valve closing force are responsible for the MR (92). Mitral valve tethering gives a unique leaflet configuration in the parasternal long axis view (93). In this view, the leaflets appear concave toward the atrium, reflecting papillary muscle displacement with tethering exerted at the leaflet tips by marginal chordae and by intermediate chordae attached more basally, creating an angulated appearance (93). This particular leaflet morphology is associated with the presence of MR and is a rapid and reliable indication of functional MR (93).

Most patients with ischemic MR have two separate jets of MR—one from the medial side and the other from the lateral side of the valve—while in dilated cardiomyopathy a single, wide, central jet extending from the medial to the lateral is more common (81).

Cardiac Catheterization

Cardiac catheterization is essential to define the coronary anatomy and the need for revascularization. Usually, LV end-diastolic pressure is elevated. In cases where noninvasive determination of the severity of the MR is inconclusive or inconsistent with the history or clinical findings, ventriculography can be useful.

Medical Treatment

Medical treatment is the mainstay of therapy for patients with functional MR and LV dysfunction. Optimal blood pressure control and use of vasodilators and β-blockers at maximal tolerated dosages are important. MR is frequently dynamic and may be diminished by optimization of volume status and hemodynamic indices. These patients should undergo stress testing to rule out active ischemia. In patients with significant global LV dysfunction, additional testing to assess viable myocardium is also necessary. Patients with severe MR and more than five segments of viable myocardium have better 6-month survival rates after surgical repair than do those with more scarring (94). If significant ischemia or viability is present, revascularization should be considered. In some of these patients, severity of MR improves after ischemia has been relieved. However, most patients with severe MR who require coronary revascularization should be considered for surgery to address both issues (86).

In patients who are not candidates for coronary artery revascularization, mitral valve repair should be reserved for severe symptoms of congestive heart failure or significant limitations in daily activities after maximal medical therapy. It has been difficult to prove that mitral valve repair has a clear or demonstrable mortality benefit in patients with significant MR and severe LV dysfunction (95). Cardiac resynchronization therapy has an increasing role in patients with wide QRS and LV dysfunction. This pacing modality has been shown to improve LV function and to reduce MR in selected patients (96,97).

Surgical Treatment

Indications

In patients who require coronary artery bypass grafting, a mitral valve procedure is indicated if the MR is 3+ or greater on a preoperative study (84). The decision to perform mitral valve surgery should be based on a preoperative study; intraoperative echocardiography on a patient under general anesthesia is frequently associated with downgrading of the MR (86). There is considerable controversy concerning the management of mild to moderate ischemic MR in patients who require coronary artery bypass grafting (98–101). For such patients, revascularization alone does not reliably eliminate the MR, and 40% to 50% have residual MR that is 2+ or greater if the mitral valve is not addressed at the time of bypass surgery (98,99). However, there are few data demonstrating clinical benefit to mitral valve surgery in patients with mild to moderate MR (100). Currently, we favor mitral valve repair in patients with 2+ MR unless the patient is an extremely high-risk candidate or the operation is otherwise complex.

Procedure

In patients with ischemic MR caused by papillary muscle infarction leading to rupture or elongation, mitral valve replacement with a bioprosthetic valve is indicated. In patients with functional MR of ischemic or cardiomyopathic origin, mitral valve repair is usually the procedure of choice. In such patients, mitral valve repair generally consists of an undersized surgical annuloplasty (84,86,102). The annuloplasty reduces MR by decreasing the septal-lateral dimension of the mitral valve, thereby increasing leaflet coaptation (85). In most patients with functional ischemic MR, valve repair by undersized annuloplasty results in improved survival when compared to valve replacement (4,84). However, in the most critically ill patients, valve repair offers no survival advantage when compared to valve replacement (84). In addition, in patients with severe bileaflet restriction, an eccentric jet of MR, or pronounced annular dilatation, repair durability is limited, and a chordal sparing bioprosthetic mitral valve replacement should be performed (103).

Results

Ischemic Mitral Regurgitation. In the past, hospital mortality was 10% to 20% when combined coronary artery and mitral valve surgery was performed on patients with ischemic MR (85,103). More recently, hospital mortality in such patients has been 5% or less at experienced centers (85,86,103). Improved hospital results are attributable to better surgical techniques and patient selection. Patients with myocardial viability in regions subserved by diseased coronary arteries have particularly good early and late survival after coronary artery bypass grafting and mitral valve repair. However, repair durability is limited in some patients. After annuloplasty alone, approximately 25% of patients develop recurrent MR during the first year of follow-up (103). Preoperative characteristics that predict return of MR include severe bileaflet restriction, severe annular dilatation, more severe LV dysfunction, and higher degree of preoperative MR (103). Return of MR is influenced by continued LV remodeling, with increasing LV sphericity associated with greater degree of late MR (104). This observation highlights a limitation of annuloplasty; this approach fails to address directly ventricular mechanisms of MR. Adjunctive surgical techniques that address the geometry of the ventricle and papillary muscles may improve repair durability.

Observational studies suggest that the combination of annuloplasty and coronary revascularization results in favorable reverse ventricular remodeling (105). However, there is controversy concerning the survival impact of mitral valve surgery in patients with ischemic MR. Most studies fail to demonstrate improved survival as a result of correction of MR in these patients (95). LV dysfunction and comorbid conditions have a more pronounced impact on survival than does the addition of mitral valve surgery or the type of mitral valve procedure (106,107).

Dilated Cardiomyopathy. In patients with MR and dilated cardiomyopathy, mitral valve repair results in clinical benefits that include improved LV function and reduced heart failure symptoms (95,108,109). However, as with ischemic MR, data suggest that mitral valve repair in such patients does not confer a demonstrable mortality benefit (95). Large, randomized trials are necessary to discern the clinical impact of mitral valve repair in patients with functional MR caused by LV dysfunction.

ENDOCARDITIS

Etiology

Native mitral valve endocarditis (see Chapter 26) is usually caused by streptococcal or staphylococcal species (110,111). Although the inciting bacteremia can often be traced to a particular event (e.g., dental procedures), frequently the cause of bacteremia cannot be identified.

Diagnosis

The diagnosis of endocarditis depends on echocardiographic demonstration of vegetation and/or perforation, positive blood cultures, clinical history, physical examination, and laboratory studies (112–115). Patients frequently report fever and malaise. Physical examination may reveal elevated temperature, a murmur of MR, and peripheral stigmata of embolic events. With active infection, elevations of the white blood cell count and sedimentation rate are the norm. Echocardiography may reveal chordal rupture (70%), vegetation (62%), leaflet perforation (53%), and abscess (7%) (116). Transesophageal echocardiography is necessary in many patients for better definition of valvular morphology. Echocardiographic size (>10 mm) and mobility of the vegetation have been related to embolic complications (117,118).

Medical and Surgical Treatment

Treatment begins with antibiotic therapy. In many cases, a 6-week course of antibiotics is sufficient to cure the patient of infection, although there may be residual mitral valve dysfunction. Surgery is indicated in certain instances, including severe MR, uncontrolled sepsis, multiple embolic events, vegetations greater than 1 cm in diameter, and extension of the infectious process causing an abscess, heart block, or intracardiac fistula (116,119,120). In addition, patients with endocarditis caused by fungus, *Staphylococcus aureus,* or gram-negative bacilli should be considered for early surgery. If a surgical indication exists, patients should be taken to the operating room regardless of the duration of preoperative antimicrobial therapy. However, recent neurologic events may necessitate a delay in surgery. If a nonhemorrhagic stroke has occurred, surgery should be delayed for 2 weeks (121); if hemorrhagic, surgery should be delayed for at least 4 weeks (111).

The infected mitral valve can be repaired in up to 80% of patients (116,122). Potential advantages of mitral valve repair in the setting of infection include preservation of the native, living valve apparatus, which is resistant to infection, and corresponding avoidance of prosthetic material. At operation, all infected material is removed. If there is sufficient valvular tissue remaining after debridement, repair is performed.

Early and late results of surgical treatment of endocarditis are excellent. Hospital mortality is generally 2% to 5% and depends primarily on the patient's preoperative clinical condition (116). Repair is associated with lower hospital mortality than replacement (116). Recurrent endocarditis is rare, and 10-year survival is 80% (116). These excellent results, coupled with the high probability of valve repair, support consideration of early surgery in patients with native mitral valve endocarditis and surgical indications.

RHEUMATIC AND OTHER CAUSES OF MITRAL REGURGITATION

Etiologies

A variety of less common disease processes can cause MR. These include rheumatic involvement, use of anorexigenic drugs, connective tissue disease, and trauma. Patients with rapid atrial fibrillation and secondary LV dysfunction may develop significant MR; if the mitral valve is structurally normal in such patients, the severity of MR may improve significantly once sinus rhythm is reestablished particularly in those with tachycardia-related cardiomyopathy.

Diagnosis

Rheumatic Mitral Regurgitation

Pure rheumatic MR is uncommon in the United States, but remains a common cause of MR around the world. The valve has thickening of the leaflets and subvalvular apparatus. The posterior leaflet is typically restricted more than the anterior leaflet. There is mild diastolic doming and minimal commissural fusion. The MR jet is usually posteriorly directed. Chordal rupture can occur in rheumatic disease, particularly in patients with a history of endocarditis (123).

In most cases, the combination of severe MR and symptoms or changes in LV size or function should lead to surgical consideration. Durability of repair for pure rheumatic MR is limited (124,125). In such patients, repair may be offered as a palliative option, particularly if there are compelling reasons to provide a period of time during which the patient will not require anticoagulation (e.g., childbearing).

Anorexiant Valvular Disease

In 1997 it was reported that drugs that suppress appetite are related to a valve disorder similar to that caused by ergot derivatives and carcinoid syndrome (126). The pathophysiology of the valve disorder appears to be related to activation of serotonin receptors. All of these anorexiant agents affect central serotonergic receptors. A causal relationship of serotonin to this disorder is also suggested by its similarity to carcinoid heart disease. Because of the widespread use of these medications, it was feared that a large number of patients were affected by severe valvular disease, and the agents were withdrawn from the market in September 1997. More recently, the prevalence of clinically symptomatic valve disease in patients receiving these drugs has been reported to be 1 in 1,000 (127).

Anorexiant drug valvulopathy affects mainly the aortic and less commonly the mitral valve. Leaflet thickening, restricted leaflet motion, chordal thickening, and valve regurgitation without stenoses are the typical abnormalities (126). In most instances, the valve lesion is mild or moderate in severity. In the study by Jollis et al. (128), moderate or greater MR was present in 2.6% of the cases and in 1.5% of the controls. Factors thought to increase the likelihood of more severe disease are longer duration (>6 months) of treatment with anorexiant therapy and higher dose treatment. In most cases valvular lesions improve or remain stable after the drug is discontinued. Anorexiant drug valvulopathy is a rare indication for surgery. Patients with echocardiographic evidence of valvular involvement should receive prophylactic antibiotics for dental and other procedures associated with bacteremia.

Radiation Valvular Disease

Radiation valvular disease is a complicated problem that may involve the pericardium, aortic valve, mitral valve, and coronary arteries (129). The left ventricle can also be affected with interstitial fibrosis and restrictive physiology (129). The mitral valve shows signs of scarring and there is usually significant calcification of leaflet and annulus. Theses valve are not suitable for repair and require mitral valve replacement. Surgery in these cases carries a substantial morbidity.

Connective Tissue Disease

The mitral valve can be involved in connective tissue disease. In lupus erythematosus, the leaflets are scarred and Libman Sacks vegetations may be present (130,131). An association of lupus and mitral valve prolapse has been described (132). Indications for surgical intervention are individualized based on degree of valvular dysfunction and patient presentation.

MITRAL STENOSIS

Etiology and Pathophysiology

Rheumatic cardiac disease is an immunologic phenomenon that may affect any of the heart valves and the myocardium and is by far the most common cause of mitral stenosis. Pathologic features of rheumatic mitral valve disease include thickening of the leaflets with fusion of the edges at the commissures. The initial valvular pathologic lesion in acute rheumatic fever consists of inflammation manifesting as a series of translucent nodules along the line of closure of the mitral valve. Rarely, mitral stenosis is the result of entities other than rheumatic heart disease. Massive mitral annular calcification extending onto the leaflets is seen now more frequently with the aging of the population. Congenital mitral stenosis and a variety of rare inborn errors of metabolism can all lead to clinically important mitral stenosis (133). Other rare causes of mitral stenosis include malignant carcinoid syndrome, systemic lupus erythematosus, and rheumatoid arthritis, all of which can lead to mitral valvular fibrosis (134,135). Left atrial myxoma and ball-valve thrombus of the left atrium reproduce the pathophysiologic changes of mitral stenosis, although the valve itself is often normal (136).

Mitral valvulitis associated with an episode of acute rheumatic fever leads to abnormal flow patterns across the valve, placing increased tension on an already damaged valve. Valve inflammation leads to fibrin deposition on the valve surface, further increasing abnormal flow patterns across the valve. The eventual outcome from years of abnormal tension and stress placed on the mitral valve is fibrosis and thickening. Smoldering rheumatic immunologic activity may also continue to damage the valve, leading to progressive fibrosis (137).

The normal mitral valve area is 4 to 5 cm^2. As mitral stenosis progressively narrows the valve orifice, a gradient develops between the left atrium and the left ventricle. This gradient is usually small and clinically unimportant until the mitral valve area is less than 2.0 cm^2. The transmitral gradient is also affected by the diastolic mitral flow (square of transvalvular flow rate) and the duration of diastole. Therefore, increased cardiac output and faster heart rate (e.g., in exercise, pregnancy, fever, anemia) result in higher gradients at a give mitral valve area. Atrial fibrillation with fast ventricular response markedly shortens the diastolic filling time, thereby leading to a large increase in the mitral valve gradient.

When the mitral orifice is reduced to 1.0 cm^2 or less, severe mitral stenosis is present (Table 22.3). At this point, a gradient across the valve of approximately 20 mm Hg is necessary to maintain a normal cardiac output. Because normal LV mean diastolic pressure is usually 5 mm Hg, left atrial and pulmonary capillary wedge pressures in these patients are approximately 25 mm Hg (137). Pulmonary capillary wedge pressure in this range leads to interstitial pulmonary edema. The pulmonary lymphatic drainage increases in capacity in response to the increased volume of interstitial fluid. Despite this increase in lymphatic capacity, total lung water increases and pulmonary compliance declines. The increase in left atrial pressure results in a passive rise in pulmonary venous and arterial pressures. Later in the natural history there are reactive pulmonary vasoconstriction and morphologic changes in the pulmonary vasculature (138). Marked increase in pulmonary pressures cause right ventricular pressure overload and eventually lead to right ventricular dilatation and failure, often associated with tricuspid regurgitation.

TABLE 22.3

CLASSIFICATION OF THE SEVERITY OF MITRAL STENOSIS

Class	Mitral valve area (cm^2)	Resting pulmonary capillary pressure (mm Hg)	Cardiac output at rest	Symptoms
Class I: mild	>2.0	<10–12	Normal	Asymptomatic
Class II: moderate	1.6–2.0	~10–17	Normal	Mild dyspnea on exertion
Class III: Moderate to severe	1.1–1.5	>18	Decreased	Dyspnea with mild moderate exertion; may have pulmonary hypertension
Class IV: severe	≤1.0	>20–25	Markedly decreased	Dyspnea at rest; severe fatigue; pulmonary edema; pulmonary hypertension; right ventricular failure

Natural History

The progression of mitral stenosis is generally slow. Recent serial hemodynamic and Doppler echocardiographic studies have demonstrated annual mitral valve area loss ranging from 0.09 to 0.32 cm^2 (139–141). The rate of progression of mitral valve narrowing is variable among individuals, and difficult to predict based on initial valve area or gradients (140,141).

Complications of rheumatic mitral disease are attributable to the abnormal hemodynamic state produced by severe mitral stenosis. Pulmonary edema develops when the pulmonary capillary pressure exceeds 25 mm Hg, causing transudation of fluid from the capillary lumen into the pulmonary interstitium and alveoli. Atrial fibrillation is the result of left atrial dilatation and hypertrophy. Systemic embolism occurs as a result of left atrial thrombosis, which, in turn, is the result of slow flow in the dilated, fibrillating left atrium and appendage. Platelet activation has been reported and may contribute to thrombus formation (142). Hemoptysis results from rupture of small venules secondary to sudden increases in pulmonary venous pressure, such as might occur in a patient with moderate to severe mitral stenosis who performs strenuous exercise. An unusual complication of mitral stenosis is hoarseness (Ortner syndrome) that develops secondary to compression of the left recurrent laryngeal nerve by a dilated left pulmonary artery, leading to vocal cord paralysis. Rarely, patients report dysphagia, resulting from esophageal compression by a dilated left atrium.

Diagnosis

Fifty percent or more of patients with mitral stenosis do not recall an episode of rheumatic fever. In midlife, these patients report dyspnea on exertion. Younger female patients may report an unusual degree of dyspnea during pregnancy. The onset of atrial fibrillation with a rapid ventricular response may be the initial presentation with acute dyspnea and even pulmonary edema. This is the result of a marked decrease in the diastolic filling period, resulting in a concomitant increase in left atrial pressure. Cardiac output may also decrease, producing the sensation of fatigue.

Physical Examination

Patients with mitral stenosis have a number of characteristic physical findings. The malar flush may be observed in patients with fair complexions. Jugular venous distension is seen in advanced cases with right ventricular failure, and prominent cardiovascular waves are noted in patients with concomitant tricuspid regurgitation. The dilated hypertrophied right ventricle may be palpated during systole along the left sternal border. A systolic impulse from the dilated pulmonary artery can occasionally be felt in the second or third left intercostal space.

The classic auscultatory findings of mitral stenosis are a loud S1, an opening snap (OS) and a diastolic rumble. The low-pitched, diastolic rumble of mitral stenosis is best heard at the apex with the patient in the left lateral decubitus position. The intensity of the murmur does not correlate with the severity of mitral stenosis, but the duration of the murmur does (143). The rumbling diastolic murmur may be difficult to hear in patients with severe end-stage mitral stenosis accompanied by low cardiac output and right ventricular failure.

The OS is the most characteristic auscultatory feature of mitral stenosis. It occurs when the mitral valve reaches its maximum opening excursion into the LV cavity. The OS may occur between 0.03 and 0.13 seconds after the S2. The interval between the second heart sound and the OS (143) shortens with increasing severity of mitral stenosis. As the stenotic valve becomes progressively fibrotic, calcified, and less mobile, the intensity of the S1 diminishes and the OS may become inaudible. The OS can also be heard in patients with MR, heart block, ventricular septal defect, and other congenital anomalies (144,145). In patients with pulmonary hypertension, the pulmonic closure sound is prominent. When severe pulmonary hypertension is present, a short, early diastolic murmur of pulmonic regurgitation may be appreciated, the *Graham Steell murmur.* However, early diastolic murmurs are related more often to associated aortic regurgitation.

Electrocardiogram

Many patients with mitral stenosis are in atrial fibrillation. Those in sinus rhythm usually demonstrate left atrial enlargement on electrocardiography (ECG). Left atrial enlargement by ECG correlates more closely with atrial volume than with atrial pressure (146). LV hypertrophy is notably absent. When pulmonary hypertension leads to right ventricular hypertrophy and dilatation, the pattern of right ventricular hypertrophy may be seen in the ECG.

Chest X-Ray

Chest roentgenographic findings in mitral stenosis include left atrial enlargement, redistribution of pulmonary vascular flow to the upper lung fields, calcification of the mitral valve, an enlarged pulmonary artery, and an enlarged right ventricle (137). Other signs of elevated pulmonary venous pressure may be present, such as Kerley A and B lines and interstitial pulmonary edema. Right ventricular enlargement is best identified on the lateral view.

Echocardiography

Two-dimensional Doppler echocardiographic examination of the heart characterizes the severity and extent of the pathologic process in patients with mitral stenosis. In addition, it assesses right and LV function, left atrial size, and associated valvular abnormalities. The typical abnormalities of rheumatic mitral stenosis are diastolic doming of the leaflets, commissural fusion and chordal shortening. A comprehensive echo Doppler examination of the mitral valve includes anatomic aspects (thickening, calcification, restriction of leaflet motion, and subvalvular apparatus) and functional parameters (peak and mean gradients, presence and severity of MR), and calculation of mitral valve area. The mitral valve area can be measured by direct planimetry using the two-dimensional short axis. More recently, use of three-dimensional echo for visualization of the mitral valve orifice for planimetry has improved the accuracy of this method (147) (Fig. 22.5). Another common method for estimating valve area is the pressure half time obtained from the continuous Doppler spectrum. This method is less accurate in patients with associated severe aortic regurgitation. Transthoracic echocardiography is sufficient for diagnosis in most patients with mitral stenosis. Transesophageal echocardiography is very accurate in identifying thrombus in the left atrium and the left atrial appendage. Presence of spontaneous echoes in the left atrial cavity is a predictor of thrombus formation and embolic events (148). Echo Doppler allows determination of systolic pulmonary pressure from the velocity of the tricuspid regurgitant jet. Many patients do not require invasive study once a thorough Doppler echocardiographic examination is completed and its findings are consistent with the clinical presentation.

The morphologic information provided by echocardiography is important for evaluating potential candidates for percutaneous balloon valvuloplasty. Several scoring systems have been proposed that assign points to the degrees of leaflet

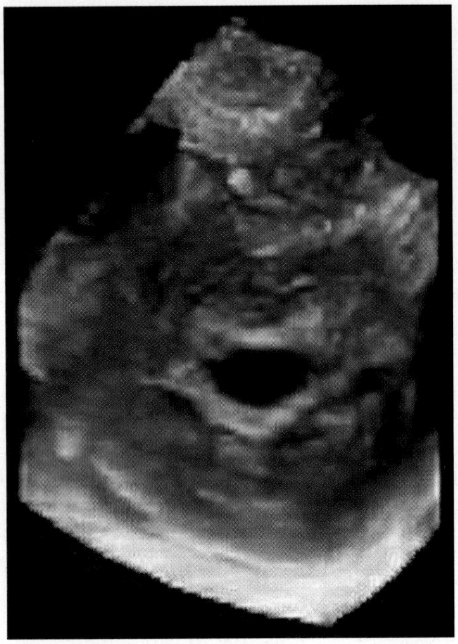

FIGURE 22.5. Real-time three-dimensional echocardiography showing the mitral valve orifice in short axis. Notice the fusion of the commissures and the precise delineation of the mitral valve orifice.

immobility, calcification, thickening, and involvement of the subvalvular apparatus (149–151). The Wilkins score from the Massachusetts General Hospital assigns up to 4 points to each component for a possible maximal score of 16 (150,152). The higher the score, the worse is the structural abnormality. Patients with low scores ($\leq$8) are ideal candidate for percutaneous valvuloplasty (153).

In patients with moderate to severe mitral stenosis with questionable symptoms, stress echocardiography using exercise can be very helpful. This test enables the clinician to objectively assess functional capacity and reproduce symptoms, to evaluate resting and exercise transmitral gradients, and often to assess the development of pulmonary hypertension with exercise. An exercise mean transmitral gradient 20 mm Hg or more and peak right ventricular systolic pressure 60 mm Hg or higher, particularly in the presence of symptoms, represents hemodynamically significant mitral stenosis and the patient should be evaluated for percutaneous mitral valvuloplasty (154). For patients unable to exercise, dobutamine echo is an alternative. Reis et al. (154a) studied 53 patients with mitral stenosis using dobutamine echo. They found that a mean transmitral gradient above 18 mm Hg at peak dobutamine infusion identified patients at risk of cardiovascular events during follow-up.

Cardiac Catheterization

The accuracy of Doppler echocardiographic techniques has resulted in selective use of cardiac catheterization in patients with mitral stenosis, primarily to identify concomitant coronary artery disease. However, in some patients cardiac catheterization provides useful information about the mitral valve, particularly in those whose symptoms are out proportion or inconsistent with the echocardiographic findings. A full hemodynamic and angiographic study for mitral stenosis consists of left and right heart catheterization with determination of the pressures in all four cardiac chambers. Special attention is paid to measurement of the diastolic gradient across the mitral valve. Heart rate and cardiac output are also determined, and the mitral valve area is calculated using the Gorlin formula (155). Coronary angiography is performed in older patients with risk factors for coronary artery disease.

Medical Treatment

Medical therapy for mitral stenosis seeks to prevent and treat complications associated with the disease. In general, relieving the mitral valvular obstruction with balloon valvuloplasty or surgical intervention is the best treatment for symptomatic mitral stenosis. However, prevention or treatment of a variety of complications associated with mitral stenosis is often necessary.

Prophylactic antibiotics are administered to patients with mitral stenosis before dental work and other interventions (see Chapter 26) to minimize the risk of developing infective endocarditis. Younger patients with a history of rheumatic fever are at risk of recurrence and continuous antibiotic therapy is recommended.

Mild dyspnea can be ameliorated with diuretics, as well as short- or long-acting nitrate preparations, but these agents are usually only of temporary benefit. Mitral valvuloplasty or replacement is indicated in symptomatic patients with mitral stenosis.

Cerebral embolism is a devastating complication of mitral stenosis, accounting for 60% to 70% of episodes of systemic embolism (156). Episodes of systemic embolism can occur in patients with severe, moderate, or even mild mitral stenosis; the risk of this complication increases markedly when atrial fibrillation develops. In the series of patients with mitral stenosis followed by Rowe et al. (157) 19% of the deaths were attributed to arterial embolism. Increasing age and left atrial size increase the risk of systemic embolism (158,159).

Atrial fibrillation is a common complication in patients with mitral stenosis. Initially, it develops as transient paroxysms; later in the course of the illness, atrial fibrillation is sustained. Often the ventricular response is rapid (>140 beats/min), resulting in a shortened diastolic filling period with concomitant pulmonary venous hypertension. Many of these patients complain of dyspnea at rest, and pulmonary edema may develop. The loss of atrial contraction has little effect on mitral valve flow in the patient with mitral stenosis in whom left atrial pressure is already elevated (160). Patients with mitral stenosis and atrial fibrillation (paroxysmal or permanent) should receive prophylactic anticoagulation with warfarin unless a strong contraindication exists. Patients in sinus rhythm with a very large left atrium or with spontaneous echo contrast on transesophageal echocardiography should also be considered for anticoagulation. Patients with a history of embolism should receive anticoagulation even if they are in sinus rhythm. An international normalized ratio between 2.0 and 3.0 should be maintained long term (161).

Attempts to maintain sinus rhythm with antiarrhythmic medication are often unrewarding and carry the risk of proarrhythmia. Rate control with digoxin, β-blockers, or calcium channel blockers constitutes a valid alternative. Patients who develop pulmonary edema secondary to rapid ventricular response are candidates for urgent electrical cardioversion. In selected cases, IV antiarrhythmic therapy with amiodarone may be effective. If the clinical decision is in favor of elective cardioversion, patients who have been in atrial fibrillation for 48 hours or more should be anticoagulated with warfarin for 3 to 4 weeks before and for 4 weeks after cardioversion. If heart rate is difficult to control and cardioversion is needed before completing 3 to 4 weeks of anticoagulation, transesophageal echocardiography must be performed before cardioversion to rule out left atrial thrombus.

Use of β-blockers in patients in sinus rhythm to prolong diastolic filling period has been employed empirically. However, this practice is controversial. Alan et al. (162) found that metoprolol improved symptoms and exercise time in some patients, but Monmeneu et al. (163) did not find improvement in exercise capacity. The studies are too small to draw definite conclusions. It is possible that patients with an elevated heart rate at rest and those with a rapid increase in heart rate with exercise benefit the most from β-blockers.

A recent task force has issued recommendations for athletic activity in patients with mitral stenosis (32). Athletes with severe mitral stenosis or those with peak pulmonary artery pressure greater than 50 mm Hg during exercise should not participate in competitive sports (32).

Catheter and Surgical Interventions

Indications

Symptomatic patients in functional class III or IV with severe mitral stenosis [mitral valve area (MVA) <1.0 cm^2] should be considered for percutaneous valvuloplasty or surgery. In younger patients with thin and pliable valves and no or minimal calcification, percutaneous valvuloplasty should be considered, even if the patient is in functional class II. The same applies to patient with severe symptoms but valve areas greater than 1.0 to 1.5 cm^2. In these patients, a complete workup, including stress echocardiography and right and left heart catheterization, is necessary to ensure that symptoms are related to the mitral stenosis.

Percutaneous Balloon Mitral Commissurotomy

Percutaneous transvenous valvotomy is performed with specially designed balloon catheters that are advanced across the stenotic mitral valve from the left atrium using a transseptal technique. The balloon is inflated, thereby separating the stenotic leaflets and splitting the commissures (164–166). A percutaneous technique employing a metallic valvulotome attached to a catheter has produced excellent short-term results, although the risk of hemopericardium appears to be higher (167). A small randomized trial showed similar results at 3 years when compared with the Inoue balloon technique (168).

Mitral valve area usually increases to 2.0 cm^2 or more following balloon valvuloplasty, left atrial pressure declines, and cardiac output increases (169). If the procedure is successful, patients experience marked symptomatic improvement. Relief of mitral stenosis is associated with improvement in both systolic and diastolic measures of LV performance (170, 171). The incidence of restenosis, as assessed by sequential echocardiography, is around 40% after 7 years (172). The success of the procedure is influenced by the experience of the operators performing the procedure and the degree of structural abnormalities (echo score). Age is also a predictor (173), and some inflammatory markers have also been related to procedural success (174).

Percutaneous balloon valvotomy is safe in experienced hands. Procedural mortality ranges from 0% to 3%. The incidence of pericardial effusion varies from 0.5% to 12.0%. Embolism occurs in 0.5% to 5.0% of cases. Severe MR occurs in 2% to 10% of patients and results from leaflet tearing, primarily in cases with unfavorable anatomy with heterogeneous distribution of thickening and calcifications. Urgent surgery for complications is necessary in less than 1% in experienced centers. Small interatrial shunts are present in 40% to 80% of cases by color Doppler; these tend to close in successful cases with the decrease in left atrial pressure.

Late results are quite good when compared with surgical valve repair (164–166). Palacios et al. (153) reported long-term follow-up in 879 patients. Patients with favorable anatomy did significantly better with improved survival (82% versus 57%) and event-free survival (38% versus 22%) at 12 years compared to the group with unfavorable echocardiographic features. Other independent factors affecting the long-term prognosis included presence of moderate or worse MR, age, prior surgical commissurotomy, New York Heart Association functional class IV, and higher postvalvotomy pulmonary artery pressure (153).

Technical contraindications for percutaneous valvuloplasty includes presence of 3 or 4+ MR, left atrial thrombus or a heavily calcified valve. Thrombus limited to the left atrial appendage is usually not a contraindication, provided that it is fixed and the procedure can be guided with transesophageal echocardiography.

Pregnancy and Mitral Stenosis

Pregnant women with severe mitral stenosis may develop significant symptoms owing to the increased physiologic demands of pregnancy. Cardiac output increases by 70% in the second trimester (175). Although this may be of no consequence in mild mitral stenosis, it may markedly increase gradients and left atrial pressure in moderately severe or severe mitral stenosis. Cardiac complications have been reported in 35% to 74% of pregnant patients with mitral stenosis (176). Percutaneous balloon valvuloplasty can be performed with abdominal and pelvic shielding in patients with severe mitral stenosis and progressive symptoms refractory to medical treatment (177). This should be discussed with all young women with mitral stenosis considering pregnancy. In already symptomatic patients, it may be advisable to perform valvuloplasty before pregnancy.

Surgery for Mitral Stenosis

In recent years, percutaneous balloon commissurotomy has largely replaced surgical repair of the stenotic mitral valve with pliable leaflets. Ben Farhat et al. (178) performed a randomized controlled trial comparing percutaneous balloon mitral commissurotomy with surgical closed and open commissurotomy in 90 patients with mitral stenosis and pliable valves. The best long-term results were obtained with balloon and open surgical commissurotomy, with only a 6.6% restenosis rate after 7 years as compared with a 37% restenosis rate for closed mitral commissurotomy. Moreover, larger initial mitral valve areas were obtained with the percutaneous and open surgical techniques as compared with the closed surgical procedure. The authors concluded that the procedure of first choice was the percutaneous balloon technique because of lower costs and elimination of the need for thoracotomy and cardiopulmonary bypass. Ommen et al. (179) observed no difference in long-term, event-free survival between patients with mitral stenosis treated by percutaneous balloon versus closed surgical mitral commissurotomy.

Although patients with mitral stenosis and low echocardiographic scores should have percutaneous balloon valvotomy, patients with higher echo scores ($\geq$10) should be offered surgery. For such patients, if the anterior leaflet and chordae are pliable, repair is considered (180). In contrast, if the valve is severely distorted, the leaflets heavily calcified, or the papillary muscles fused to the leaflet edges, the valve should be replaced.

Patients with mixed rheumatic stenosis and regurgitation present a particular technical challenge and are least amenable to repair (181). If valve distortion is not severe and the anterior leaflet and chordae are pliable, repair may be considered.

In North America, most patients who present for surgical treatment of rheumatic mitral valve disease have severely deformed valves that are best suited to replacement (180). Patients with combined mitral stenosis and regurgitation are also usually best served by replacement.

Mitral valve repair may confer a survival advantage when compared to mitral valve replacement in patients with rheumatic disease (180). Overall, 10-year freedom from reoperation in patients with repaired rheumatic valves is 72% (180). However, the feasibility and durability of repair are influenced strongly by valve pathology. In appropriately selected patients with pure mitral stenosis, open mitral commissurotomy provides excellent results, with 78% to 91% 10-year freedom from reoperation (182).

MINIMALLY INVASIVE MITRAL VALVE SURGERY

A variety of less invasive approaches have been developed to perform isolated mitral valve surgery or combined mitral and aortic valve surgery. Chest wall incisions include right parasternal (183), right thoracotomy (184,185), partial lower sternotomy (186), and partial upper sternotomy (186). Adjunctive techniques employed for mitral valve surgery include Port-Access instrumentation (187), video assistance (184,185), and robotic assistance (188). Excellent results have been reported with each of these approaches.

We favor partial upper sternotomy access for isolated valve surgery. This approach affords the surgeon a familiar orientation. Through a 6- to 8-cm skin incision, a partial upper sternotomy extends from the sternal notch to the left fourth intercostal space. The mitral valve is approached through a transseptal incision extended onto the dome of the left atrium. This exposure of the mitral valve facilitates both simple and complex repair procedures.

This approach has been used in more than 2,000 mitral valve procedures at The Cleveland Clinic Foundation; 90% of these patients had mitral valve repair. Conversion to full sternotomy was necessary in 1% of cases. Hospital mortality was 0.3%. This is now our approach of choice in patients with isolated heart valve disease.

MITRAL VALVE REPAIR VERSUS REPLACEMENT

With the exception of selected patients with mitral stenosis, definitive treatment of mitral valve dysfunction currently entails cardiac surgery. Indications for mitral valve surgery depend on the etiology and severity of valvular dysfunction and the patient's clinical condition. When mitral valve surgery is indicated, valve repair is generally preferable to replacement. Advantages to valve repair over replacement include improved early and late survivals, avoidance of long-term anticoagulation, and greater freedoms from endocarditis and thromboembolism (1). In experienced centers, the majority of regurgitant mitral valves are repaired. However, in certain situations, the valve may not be amenable to repair, and mitral valve replacement is indicated. When replacement is performed, preservation of the subvalvular apparatus is associated with better long-term preservation of LV function. There are two general categories of prostheses for mitral valve replacement—bioprosthetic valves and mechanical valves.

Bioprosthetic mitral valves are manufactured from bovine or porcine tissue. These stented valves do not require long-term anticoagulation if the patient is in sinus rhythm. The main issue with bioprosthetic valves is the possibility of reoperation for structural valve dysfunction. However, recent improvements in manufacturing and tissue fixation have resulted in improved durability of these valves. The risk of reoperation varies with patient age and is influenced strongly by the competing risk of death. The actual 16-year freedom from explant for structural valve dysfunction after mitral valve replacement with a bovine pericardial valve is 99% in a 70-year-old and 89% in a 60-year-old patient (189). With this valve, the annual risk of thromboembolism is 1%, similar to that observed with mechanical valves (189,190).

Mechanical valves are available in three different configurations: bileaflet valves, tilting single disc valves, and ball-and-cage valves. The bileaflet valves dominate clinical practice. These valves almost never suffer structural failure, but do require lifelong anticoagulation to reduce the risk of thromboembolism. As a result of this anticoagulation, the risk of major hemorrhage with mechanical valve is 0.5% to 1.5% per year (191).

Choice of replacement prosthesis depends on patient life expectancy, ability to take anticoagulants, and lifestyle. Postoperative survival is not influenced by type of mitral valve inserted (191). Recently, there has been a trend toward more use of tissue valves, likely attributable to improved durability of newer prostheses. Patient age has long been the key factor used to determine type of replacement valve; mechanical valves were generally inserted in patients over 70 years of age, and bioprosthetic valves in patients 70 years old or younger. However, patient life expectancy (rather than age) and lifestyle are of particular importance in deciding the type of replacement prosthesis when valve repair is not feasible.

MITRAL VALVE REPAIR AND ATRIAL FIBRILLATION

Thirty to fifty percent of patients presenting for mitral valve surgery have atrial fibrillation (192). In such patients, an important goal of the procedure is ablation of atrial fibrillation in addition to mitral valve repair. Failure to treat the atrial fibrillation leaves the patient with the requirement for lifelong anticoagulation and increased late risks of death and stroke (193).

There are a variety of surgical procedures available for ablation of atrial fibrillation, ranging from the Cox-Maze III procedure to pulmonary vein isolation using alternate energy sources (192–195). Alternate energy sources currently available to create lines of conduction block include microwave, radiofrequency, cryothermy, ultrasound, and laser. These are generally used to create left atrial lesion sets that include pulmonary vein isolation and connecting lesions to the left atrial appendage and to the mitral annulus. This is based on current concepts regarding the pulmonary veins and left atrium in the genesis of atrial fibrillation (196). In addition, the left atrial appendage is excluded or excised. Right atrial lesions are frequently omitted, because atrial fibrillation rarely arises from the right atrium.

The Cox-Maze III procedure cures atrial fibrillation in 70% to 95% of patients having concomitant mitral valve surgery (194,197). Increased left atrial size, longer duration of preoperative atrial fibrillation, and rheumatic disease may limit success. Early data suggest that use of alternate energy sources to create left atrial lesion sets ablates atrial fibrillation in 70% to 80% of patients (197). Given these data, patients with preoperative atrial fibrillation should have surgical ablation of atrial fibrillation at the time of mitral valve surgery.

PERCUTANEOUS MITRAL VALVE REPAIR

There is increasing interest in developing technologies for the percutaneous treatment of valvular lesions. The initial clinical experience in patients with MR is promising. The Everest 1 (198) was the first clinical trial using a percutaneous device for the treatment of MR. In this trial, 27 patients with MR underwent insertion of special clip designed to grasp and approximate the middle scallops of the anterior and posterior mitral leaflets, creating a double orifice. In this initial series, 93% of the patients had degenerative MR. There were no deaths or emergency surgery. Three patients had partial detachment of the clip, but none of them embolized. At 1 month 58% of the patients have 2+ or lower MR (198). A second randomized trial is underway to evaluate this new therapy against the surgical gold standard. Percutaneous annuloplasty (via the coronary sinus) is under active investigation and early preclinical and clinical experiences are promising.

CONTROVERSIES AND PERSONAL PERSPECTIVES

Quantification of Mitral Regurgitation

The available data strongly support the use of quantitative measurements to grade the severity of MR. The use of these techniques should diminish the interobserver variability and identify patients with severe MR. A few caveats do exist, however. Use of proximal convergence to measure ROA has limitations. Both technical factors and theoretical considerations make this technique prone to errors. Echocardiographic laboratories need to improve their expertise in all technical aspects of quantification of valvular dysfunction.

Timing of Mitral Valve Surgery

The timing of surgery in patients with degenerative mitral valve disease, no symptoms, and normal LV size and function remains controversial. In the absence of a randomized trial, a practical approach prevails. We favor early surgery in such patients when (a) degenerative MR is severe as assessed by quantitative methods and (b) repair is highly probable. The operative mortality for isolated mitral valve repair at The Cleveland Clinic Foundation has been 0 since 2003. Ninety-five percent of degenerative valves have been repaired, and long-term durability is excellent. Finally, 75% or more of these procedures were minimally invasive, reducing trauma, thereby hastening hospital discharge and return to normal function.

In patients with functional MR there is more uncertainty, and surgery is indicated for symptomatic patients after maximal medical therapy has been instituted. In patients with coronary artery disease, ischemia and viability need to be thoroughly investigated. If extensive viability/ischemia exist, aggressive revascularization and mitral repair are indicated.

The surgical techniques for treating functional regurgitation need to be improved to increase the success rate. Chordal cutting for the treatment of leaflet tethering and procedures that address the ventricle directly should be considered as adjuncts to annuloplasty.

THE FUTURE

Percutaneous Mitral Valve Repair and Replacement

A variety of ingenious, catheter-based approaches to mitral valve repair are in preclinical and clinical testing. These include percutaneous annuloplasty (via the coronary sinus or directly via the left atrium), techniques to reproduce the edge-to-edge repair (Alfieri stitch), and valve replacement. The primary controversies surrounding these efforts include patient selection, effectiveness necessary before clinical application, and clinical trial design.

It is likely that the next decade will see development of many new techniques for percutaneous mitral valve repair and replacement. Clinical trials using leaflet repairing devices or percutaneous annuloplasty are now beginning. Indications for each device and potential complications will be learned from these trials. Over time, many of these new procedures will be validated, and their availability will enable physicians to extend direct treatment of mitral valve dysfunction to large numbers of patients, beginning with those who are not currently candidates for surgical repair. As the initial experience suggests, extensive training will be necessary for the safe and effective applications of these new devices.

Other key advances are likely to involve cardiac imaging. Improvements in real-time three-dimensional echocardiography will enable earlier detection of valvular heart disease and more precise determination of the mechanism of valvular dysfunction. The latter will facilitate improvements in interventional and surgical techniques for valve repair. These advances may be of particular benefit in the development of new approaches to functional MR.

References

1. Carpentier A. Cardiac valve surgery—the "French correction". *J Thorac Cardiovasc Surg* 1983;86:323–337.
2. Levine RA, Triulzi MO, Harrigan P, et al. The relationship of mitral annular shape to the diagnosis of mitral valve prolapse. *Circulation* 1987;75: 756–767.
3. Ormiston JA, Shah PM, Tei C, et al. Size and motion of the mitral valve annulus in man. I. A two-dimensional echocardiographic method and findings in normal subjects. *Circulation* 1981;64:113–120.
4. Ahmad RM, Gillinov AM, McCarthy PM, et al. Annular geometry and motion in human ischemic mitral regurgitation: novel assessment with three-dimensional echocardiography and computer reconstruction. *Ann Thorac Surg* 2004;78:2063–2068.
5. Hueb AC, Jatene FB, Moreira LF, et al. Ventricular remodeling and mitral valve modifications in dilated cardiomyopathy: new insights from anatomic study. *J Thorac Cardiovasc Surg* 2002;124:1216–1224.
6. Gorman JH 3rd, Gorman RC, Jackson BM, et al. Annuloplasty ring selection for chronic ischemic mitral regurgitation: lessons from the ovine model. *Ann Thorac Surg* 2003;76:1556–1563.
7. David TE, Ho EC. The effect of preservation of chordae tendineae on mitral valve replacement for postinfarction mitral regurgitation. *Circulation* 1986;74:I116–120.
8. Rozich JD, Carabello BA, Usher BW, et al. Mitral valve replacement with and without chordal preservation in patients with chronic mitral regurgitation. Mechanisms for differences in postoperative ejection performance. *Circulation* 1992;86:1718–1726.
9. Estes EH Jr, Dalton FM, Entman ML, et al. The anatomy and blood supply of the papillary muscles of the left ventricle. *Am Heart J* 1966;71:356–362.
10. James TN. Anatomy of the coronary arteries in health and disease. *Circulation* 1965;32:1020–1033.
11. Ross J Jr. Afterload mismatch and preload reserve: a conceptual framework for the analysis of ventricular function. *Prog Cardiovasc Dis* 1976; 18:255–264.
12. Kass DA, Maughan WL, Guo ZM, et al. Comparative influence of load versus inotropic states on indexes of ventricular contractility: experimental and theoretical analysis based on pressure-volume relationships. *Circulation* 1987;76:1422–1436.
13. Thompson CR, Buller CE, Sleeper LA, et al. Cardiogenic shock due to acute severe mitral regurgitation complicating acute myocardial infarction: a report from the SHOCK Trial Registry. Should we use emergently revascularize occluded coronaries in cardiogenic shock? *J Am Coll Cardiol* 2000;36[3 Suppl A]:1104–1109.
14. Goodman DJ, Rossen RM, Holloway EL, et al. Effect of nitroprusside on left ventricular dynamics in mitral regurgitation. *Circulation* 1974;50: 1025–1032.
15. Chatterjee K, Parmley WW, Swan HJ, et al. Beneficial effects of vasodilator agents in severe mitral regurgitation due to dysfunction of subvalvar apparatus. *Circulation* 1973;48:684–690.
16. Horstkotte D, Schulte HD, Niehues R, et al. Diagnostic and therapeutic considerations in acute, severe mitral regurgitation: experience in 42

consecutive patients entering the intensive care unit with pulmonary edema. *J Heart Valve Dis* 1993;2:512–522.
17. Gaasch WH, Aurigemma GP. Inhibition of the renin-angiotensin system and the left ventricular adaptation to mitral regurgitation. *J Am Coll Cardiol* 2002;39:1380–1383.
18. Berko B, Gaasch WH, Tanigawa N, et al. Disparity between ejection and end-systolic indexes of left ventricular contractility in mitral regurgitation. *Circulation* 1987;75:1310–1319.
19. Starling MR, Kirsh MM, Montgomery DG, et al. Impaired left ventricular contractile function in patients with long-term mitral regurgitation and normal ejection fraction. *J Am Coll Cardiol* 1993;22:239–250.
20. Monin JL, Dehant P, Roiron C, et al. Functional assessment of mitral regurgitation by transthoracic echocardiography using standardized imaging planes diagnostic accuracy and outcome implications. *J Am Coll Cardiol* 2005;46:302–309.
21. Haluska BA, Short L, Marwick TH. Relationship of ventricular longitudinal function to contractile reserve in patients with mitral regurgitation. *Am Heart J* 2003;146:183–188.
22. Agricola E, Galderisi M, Oppizzi M, et al. Pulsed tissue Doppler imaging detects early myocardial dysfunction in asymptomatic patients with severe mitral regurgitation. *Heart* 2004;90:406–410.
23. Zoghbi WA, Enriquez-Sarano M, Foster E, et al. Recommendations for evaluation of the severity of native valvular regurgitation with two-dimensional and Doppler echocardiography. *J Am Soc Echocardiogr* 2003;16:777–802.
24. Enriquez-Sarano M, Avierinos JF, Messika-Zeitoun D, et al. Quantitative determinants of the outcome of asymptomatic mitral regurgitation. *N Engl J Med* 2005;352:875–883.
25. Grigioni F, Enriquez-Sarano M, Zehr KJ, et al. Ischemic mitral regurgitation: long-term outcome and prognostic implications with quantitative Doppler assessment. *Circulation* 2001;103:1759–1764.
26. Grigioni F, Detaint D, Avierinos JF, et al. Contribution of ischemic mitral regurgitation to congestive heart failure after myocardial infarction. *J Am Coll Cardiol* 2005;45:260–267.
27. Enriquez-Sarano M, Schaff HV, Orszulak TA, et al. Valve repair improves the outcome of surgery for mitral regurgitation. A multivariate analysis. *Circulation* 1995;91:1022–1028.
28. Leung DY, Griffin BP, Stewart WJ, et al. Left ventricular function after valve repair for chronic mitral regurgitation: predictive value of preoperative assessment of contractile reserve by exercise echocardiography. *J Am Coll Cardiol* 1996;28:1198–1205.
29. Dajani AS, Taubert KA, Wilson W, et al. Prevention of bacterial endocarditis. Recommendations by the American Heart Association. *Circulation* 1997;96:358–66.
30. Clemens JD, Horwitz RI, Jaffe CC, et al. A controlled evaluation of the risk of bacterial endocarditis in persons with mitral-valve prolapse. *N Engl J Med* 1982;307:776–781.
31. Singh RG, Cappucci R, Kramer-Fox R, et al. Severe mitral regurgitation due to mitral valve prolapse: risk factors for development, progression, and need for mitral valve surgery. *Am J Cardiol* 2000;85:193–198.
32. Bonow RO, Cheitlin MD, Crawford MH, et al. Task Force 3: valvular heart disease. *J Am Coll Cardiol* 2005;45:1334–1340.
33. Freed LA, Levy D, Levine RA, et al. Prevalence and clinical outcome of mitral-valve prolapse. *N Engl J Med* 1999;341:1–7.
34. Mohty D, Orszulak TA, Schaff HV, et al. Very long-term survival and durability of mitral valve repair for mitral valve prolapse. *Circulation* 2001;104[12 Suppl 1]:I1–I7.
35. Grande-Allen KJ, Griffin BP, Ratliff NB, et al. Glycosaminoglycan profiles of myxomatous mitral leaflets and chordae parallel the severity of mechanical alterations. *J Am Coll Cardiol* 2003;42:271–277.
36. Hayek E, Gring CN, Griffin BP. Mitral valve prolapse. *Lancet* 2005;365:507–518.
37. Mills WR, Barber JE, Skiles JA, et al. Clinical, echocardiographic, and biomechanical differences in mitral valve prolapse affecting one or both leaflets. *Am J Cardiol* 2002;89:1394–1399.
38. Disse S, Abergel E, Berrebi A, et al. Mapping of a first locus for autosomal dominant myxomatous mitral-valve prolapse to chromosome 16p11.2-p12.1. *Am J Hum Genet* 1999;65:1242–1251.
39. Freed LA, Acierno Jr JS, Dai D, et al. A locus for autosomal dominant mitral valve prolapse on chromosome 11p15.4. *Am J Hum Genet* 2003;72:1551–1559.
40. Zuppiroli A, Rinaldi M, Kramer-Fox R, et al. Natural history of mitral valve prolapse. *Am J Cardiol* 1995;75:1028–1032.
41. Levy D., Savage D. Prevalence and clinical features of mitral valve prolapse. *Am Heart J* 1987;113:1281–1290.
42. Wilcken DE, Hickey AJ. Lifetime risk for patients with mitral valve prolapse of developing severe valve regurgitation requiring surgery. *Circulation* 1988;78:10–14.
43. Gaffney FA, Karlsson ES, Campbell W, et al. Autonomic dysfunction in women with mitral valve prolapse syndrome. *Circulation* 1979;59:894–901.
44. Sanfilippo AJ, Harrigan P, Popovic AD, et al. Papillary muscle traction in mitral valve prolapse: quantitation by two-dimensional echocardiography. *J Am Coll Cardiol* 1992;19:564–571.
45. Grigioni F, Enriquez-Sarano M, Ling LH, et al. Sudden death in mitral regurgitation due to flail leaflet. *J Am Coll Cardiol* 1999;34:2078–2085.
46. Orencia AJ, Petty GW, Khandheria BK, et al. Risk of stroke with mitral valve prolapse in population-based cohort study. *Stroke* 1995;26:7–13.
47. Gilon D, Buonanno FS, Joffe MM, et al. Lack of evidence of an association between mitral-valve prolapse and stroke in young patients. *N Engl J Med* 1999;341:8–13.
48. Avierinos JF, Brown RD, Foley DA, et al. Cerebral ischemic events after diagnosis of mitral valve prolapse: a community-based study of incidence and predictive factors. *Stroke* 2003;34:1339–1344.
49. Petty GW, Orencia AJ, Khandheria BK, et al. A population-based study of stroke in the setting of mitral valve prolapse: risk factors and infarct subtype classification. *Mayo Clin Proc* 1994;69:632–634.
50. Levine RA, Handschumacher MD, Sanfilippo AJ, et al. Three-dimensional echocardiographic reconstruction of the mitral valve, with implications for the diagnosis of mitral valve prolapse. *Circulation* 1989;80:589–598.
51. Levine RA, Stathogiannis E, Newell JB, et al. Reconsideration of echocardiographic standards for mitral valve prolapse: lack of association between leaflet displacement isolated to the apical four chamber view and independent echocardiographic evidence of abnormality. *J Am Coll Cardiol* 1988;11:1010–1019.
52. Marks AR, Choong CY, Sanfilippo AJ, et al. Identification of high-risk and low-risk subgroups of patients with mitral-valve prolapse. *N Engl J Med* 1989;320:1031–1036.
53. Ohnesorge BM, Hofmann LK, Flohr TG, et al. CT for imaging coronary artery disease: defining the paradigm for its application. *Int J Cardiovasc Imaging* 2005;21:85–104.
54. Achenbach S, Ropers D, Pohle FK, et al. Detection of coronary artery stenoses using multi-detector CT with 16 × 0. 75 collimation and 375 ms rotation. *Eur Heart J* 2005;26:1978–1986.
55. Hamilton MA, Stevenson LW, Child JS, et al. Sustained reduction in valvular regurgitation and atrial volumes with tailored vasodilator therapy in advanced congestive heart failure secondary to dilated (ischemic or idiopathic) cardiomyopathy. *Am J Cardiol* 1991;67:259–263.
56. Weiland DS, Konstam MA, Salem DN, et al. Contribution of reduced mitral regurgitant volume to vasodilator effect in severe left ventricular failure secondary to coronary artery disease or idiopathic dilated cardiomyopathy. *Am J Cardiol* 1986;58:1046–1050.
57. Grayburn PA. Vasodilator therapy for chronic aortic and mitral regurgitation. *Am J Med Sci* 2000;320:202–208.
58. Kvart C, Haggstrom J, Pedersen HD, et al. Efficacy of enalapril for prevention of congestive heart failure in dogs with myxomatous valve disease and asymptomatic mitral regurgitation. *J Vet Intern Med* 2002;16:80–88.
59. Braunberger E, Deloche A, Berrebi A, et al. Very long-term results (more than 20 years) of valve repair with Carpentier's techniques in nonrheumatic mitral valve insufficiency. *Circulation* 2001;104[12 Suppl 1]:I8–11.
60. Mohty D, Enriquez-Sarano M. The long-term outcome of mitral valve repair for mitral valve prolapse. *Curr Cardiol Rep* 2002;4:104–110.
61. Ling LH, Enriquez-Sarano M, Seward JB, et al. Clinical outcome of mitral regurgitation due to flail leaflet. *N Engl J Med* 1996;335:1417–1423.
62. Akins CW, Hilgenberg AD, Buckley MJ, et al. Mitral valve reconstruction versus replacement for degenerative or ischemic mitral regurgitation. *Ann Thorac Surg* 1994;58:668–675; discussion 675–676.
63. Gillinov AM, Faber C, Houghtaling PL, et al. Repair versus replacement for degenerative mitral valve disease with coexisting ischemic heart disease. *J Thorac Cardiovasc Surg* 2003;125:1350–1362.
64. Gillinov AM, Cosgrove DM, Blackstone EH, et al. Durability of mitral valve repair for degenerative disease. *J Thorac Cardiovasc Surg* 1998;116:734–743.
65. Perier P, Clausnizer B, Mistarz K. Carpentier "sliding leaflet" technique for repair of the mitral valve: early results. *Ann Thorac Surg* 1994;57:383–386.
66. Gillinov AM, Cosgrove 3rd DM. Modified sliding leaflet technique for repair of the mitral valve. *Ann Thorac Surg* 1999;68:2356–2357.
67. Gillinov AM, Cosgrove 3rd DM. Current status of mitral valve repair. *Am Heart Hosp J* 2003;1:47–54.
68. Gillinov AM, Cosgrove 3rd DM, Wahi S, et al. Is anterior leaflet repair always necessary in repair of bileaflet mitral valve prolapse? *Ann Thorac Surg* 1999;68:820–823; discussion 824.
69. David TE. Replacement of chordae tendineae with expanded polytetrafluoroethylene sutures. *J Card Surg* 1989;4:286–290.
70. von Oppell UO, Mohr FW. Chordal replacement for both minimally invasive and conventional mitral valve surgery using premeasured Gore-Tex loops. *Ann Thorac Surg* 2000;70:2166–2168.
71. Spencer FC, Galloway AC, Grossi EA, et al. Recent developments and evolving techniques of mitral valve reconstruction. *Ann Thorac Surg* 1998;65:307–313.
72. Maisano F, Caldarola A, Blasio A, et al. Midterm results of edge-to-edge mitral valve repair without annuloplasty. *J Thorac Cardiovasc Surg* 2003;126:1987–1997.
73. Gillinov AM, Cosgrove 3rd DM, Shiota T, et al. Cosgrove-Edwards Annuloplasty System: midterm results. *Ann Thorac Surg* 2000;69:717–721.
74. Carpentier A, Deloche A, Dauptain J, et al. A new reconstructive operation for correction of mitral and tricuspid insufficiency. *J Thorac Cardiovasc Surg* 1971;61:1–13.

75. Duran CG, Ubago JL. Clinical and hemodynamic performance of a totally flexible prosthetic ring for atrioventricular valve reconstruction. *Ann Thorac Surg* 1976;22:458–463.
76. Hetzer R, Bougioukas G, Franz M, et al. Mitral valve replacement with preservation of papillary muscles and chordae tendineae—revival of a seemingly forgotten concept. I. Preliminary clinical report. *Thorac Cardiovasc Surg* 1983;31:291–296.
77. Grossi EA, Galloway AC, Miller JS, et al. Valve repair versus replacement for mitral insufficiency: when is a mechanical valve still indicated? *J Thorac Cardiovasc Surg* 1998;115:389–394; discussion 394–396.
78. Lee EM, Shapiro LM, Wells FC. Superiority of mitral valve repair in surgery for degenerative mitral regurgitation. *Eur Heart J* 1997;18:655–663.
79. Adams DH, Filsoufi F. Another chapter in an enlarging book: repair degenerative mitral valves. *J Thorac Cardiovasc Surg* 2003;125:1197–199.
80. Flameng W, Herijgers P, Bogaerts K. Recurrence of mitral valve regurgitation after mitral valve repair in degenerative valve disease. *Circulation* 2003;107:1609–1613.
81. Kwan J, Shiota T, Agler DA, et al. Geometric differences of the mitral apparatus between ischemic and dilated cardiomyopathy with significant mitral regurgitation: real-time three-dimensional echocardiography study. *Circulation* 2003;107:1135–1140.
82. Yiu SF, Enriquez-Sarano M, Tribouilloy C, et al. Determinants of the degree of functional mitral regurgitation in patients with systolic left ventricular dysfunction: a quantitative clinical study. *Circulation* 2000;102: 1400–1406.
83. Otsuji Y, Handschumacher MD, Schwammenthal E, et al. Insights from three-dimensional echocardiography into the mechanism of functional mitral regurgitation: direct in vivo demonstration of altered leaflet tethering geometry. *Circulation* 1997;96:1999–2008.
84. Gillinov AM, Wierup PN, Blackstone EH, et al. Is repair preferable to replacement for ischemic mitral regurgitation? *J Thorac Cardiovasc Surg* 2001;122:1125–141.
85. Miller DC. Ischemic mitral regurgitation redux—to repair or to replace? *J Thorac Cardiovasc Surg* 2001;122:1059–1062.
86. Adams DH, Filsoufi F, Aklog L. Surgical treatment of the ischemic mitral valve. *J Heart Valve Dis* 2002;11[Suppl 1]:S21–25.
87. Trichon BH, Felker GM, Shaw LK, et al. Relation of frequency and severity of mitral regurgitation to survival among patients with left ventricular systolic dysfunction and heart failure. *Am J Cardiol* 2003;91:538–543.
88. Ellis SG, Whitlow PL, Raymond RE, et al. Impact of mitral regurgitation on long-term survival after percutaneous coronary intervention. *Am J Cardiol* 2002;89:315–318.
89. Jouan J, Tapia M, C Cook R, et al. Ischemic mitral valve prolapse: mechanisms and implications for valve repair. *Eur J Cardiothorac Surg* 2004; 26:1112–1117.
90. Srichai MB, Grimm RA, Stillman AE, et al. Ischemic mitral regurgitation: impact of the left ventricle and mitral valve in patients with left ventricular systolic dysfunction. *Ann Thorac Surg* 2005;80:170–178.
91. Watanabe N, Ogasawara Y, Yamaura Y, et al. Quantitation of mitral valve tenting in ischemic mitral regurgitation by transthoracic real-time three-dimensional echocardiography. *J Am Coll Cardiol* 2005;45:763–769.
92. Levine RA, Hung J, Otsuji Y, et al. Mechanistic insights into functional mitral regurgitation. *Curr Cardiol Rep* 2002;4:125–129.
93. Nesta F, Otsuji Y, Handschumacher MD, et al. Leaflet concavity: a rapid visual clue to the presence and mechanism of functional mitral regurgitation. *J Am Soc Echocardiogr* 2003;16:1301–1308.
94. Pu M, Thomas JD, Gillinov MA, et al. Importance of ischemic and viable myocardium for patients with chronic ischemic mitral regurgitation and left ventricular dysfunction. *Am J Cardiol* 2003;92:862–864.
95. Wu AH, Aaronson KD, Bolling SF, et al. Impact of mitral valve annuloplasty on mortality risk in patients with mitral regurgitation and left ventricular systolic dysfunction. *J Am Coll Cardiol* 2005;45:381–387.
96. Breithardt OA, Sinha AM, Schwammenthal E, et al. Acute effects of cardiac resynchronization therapy on functional mitral regurgitation in advanced systolic heart failure. *J Am Coll Cardiol* 2003;41:765–770.
97. Kanzaki H, Bazaz R, Schwartzman D, et al. A mechanism for immediate reduction in mitral regurgitation after cardiac resynchronization therapy: insights from mechanical activation strain mapping. *J Am Coll Cardiol* 2004;44:1619–1625.
98. Lam BK, Gillinov AM, Blackstone EH, et al. Importance of moderate ischemic mitral regurgitation. *Ann Thorac Surg* 2005;79:462–470; discussion 462–470.
99. Aklog L, Filsoufi F, Flores KQ, et al. Does coronary artery bypass grafting alone correct moderate ischemic mitral regurgitation? *Circulation* 2001;104[12 Suppl 1]:I68–75.
100. Tolis GA Jr, Korkolis DP, Kopf GS, et al. Revascularization alone (without mitral valve repair) suffices in patients with advanced ischemic cardiomyopathy and mild-to-moderate mitral regurgitation. *Ann Thorac Surg* 2002;74:1476–80; discussion 1480–1481.
101. Duarte IG, Shen Y, MacDonald MJ, et al. Treatment of moderate mitral regurgitation and coronary disease by coronary bypass alone: late results. *Ann Thorac Surg* 1999;68:426–430.
102. Bolling SF, Pagani FD, Deeb GM, et al. Intermediate-term outcome of mitral reconstruction in cardiomyopathy. *J Thorac Cardiovasc Surg* 1998;115:381–386; discussion 387–388.
103. McGee EC, Gillinov AM, Blackstone EH, et al. Recurrent mitral regurgitation after annuloplasty for functional ischemic mitral regurgitation. *J Thorac Cardiovasc Surg* 2004;128:916–924.
104. Hung J, Papakostas L, Tahta SA, et al. Mechanism of recurrent ischemic mitral regurgitation after annuloplasty: continued LV remodeling as a moving target. *Circulation* 2004;110[11 Suppl 1]:II85–90.
105. Bax JJ, Braun J, Somer ST, et al. Restrictive annuloplasty and coronary revascularization in ischemic mitral regurgitation results in reverse left ventricular remodeling. *Circulation* 2004;110[11 Suppl 1]:II103–108.
106. Glower DD, Tuttle RH, Shaw LK, et al. Patient survival characteristics after routine mitral valve repair for ischemic mitral regurgitation. *J Thorac Cardiovasc Surg* 2005;129:860–868.
107. Trichon BH, Glower DD, Shaw LK, et al. Survival after coronary revascularization, with and without mitral valve surgery, in patients with ischemic mitral regurgitation. *Circulation* 2003;108[Suppl 1]:II103–110.
108. Calafiore AM, Gallina S, Di Mauro M, et al. Mitral valve procedure in dilated cardiomyopathy: repair or replacement? *Ann Thorac Surg* 2001; 71:1146–1152; discussion 1152–1153.
109. Bishay ES, McCarthy PM, Cosgrove DM, et al. Mitral valve surgery in patients with severe left ventricular dysfunction. *Eur J Cardiothorac Surg* 2000;17:213–221.
110. Middlemost S, Wisenbaugh T, Meyerowitz C, et al. A case for early surgery in native left-sided endocarditis complicated by heart failure: results in 203 patients. *J Am Coll Cardiol* 1991;18:663–667.
111. Suryapranata H, Roelandt J, Haalebos M, et al. Early cardiac valve replacement in infective endocarditis: a 10-year experience. *Eur Heart J* 1987; 8:464–470.
112. Durack DT, Lukes AS, Bright DK. New criteria for diagnosis of infective endocarditis: utilization of specific echocardiographic findings. Duke Endocarditis Service. *Am J Med* 1994;96:200–209.
113. Heinle S, Wilderman N, Harrison JK, et al. Value of transthoracic echocardiography in predicting embolic events in active infective endocarditis. Duke Endocarditis Service. *Am J Cardiol* 1994;74:799–801.
114. Dodds GA 3rd, Durack DT. Criteria for the diagnosis of endocarditis and the role of echocardiography. *Echocardiography* 1995;12:663–668.
115. Dodds GA, Sexton DJ, Durack DT, et al. Negative predictive value of the Duke criteria for infective endocarditis. *Am J Cardiol* 1996;77:403–407.
116. Muehrcke DD, Cosgrove DM 3rd, Lytle BW, et al. Is there an advantage to repairing infected mitral valves? *Ann Thorac Surg* 1997;63:1718–1724.
117. Sanfilippo AJ, Picard MH, Newell JB, et al. Echocardiographic assessment of patients with infectious endocarditis: prediction of risk for complications. *J Am Coll Cardiol* 1991;18:1191–1199.
118. Thuny F, Disalvo G, Belliard O, et al. Risk of embolism and death in infective endocarditis: prognostic value of echocardiography: a prospective multicenter study. *Circulation* 2005;112:69–75.
119. Enriquez-Sarano M. Timing of mitral valve surgery. *Heart* 2002;87:79–85.
120. Enriquez-Sarano M, Schaff HV, Frye RL. Early surgery for mitral regurgitation: the advantages of youth. *Circulation* 1997;96:4121–4123.
121. Gillinov AM, Shah RV, Curtis WE, et al. Valve replacement in patients with endocarditis and acute neurologic deficit. *Ann Thorac Surg* 1996;61:1125–1129; discussion 1130.
122. Zegdi R, Debieche M, Latremouille C, et al. Long-term results of mitral valve repair in active endocarditis. *Circulation* 2005;111:2532–2536.
123. Kaymaz C, Ozdemir N, Ozkan M. Differentiating clinical and echocardiographic characteristics of chordal rupture detected in patients with rheumatic mitral valve disease and floppy mitral valve: impact of the infective endocarditis on chordal rupture. *Eur J Echocardiogr* 2005;6:117–126.
124. Duran CM, Gometza B, Balasundaram S, et al. A feasibility study of valve repair in rheumatic mitral regurgitation. *Eur Heart J* 1991;12[Suppl B]:34–38.
125. Skoularigis J, Sinovich V, Joubert G, et al. Evaluation of the long-term results of mitral valve repair in 254 young patients with rheumatic mitral regurgitation. *Circulation* 1994;90:II167–74.
126. Connolly HM, Crary JL, McGoon MD, et al. Valvular heart disease associated with fenfluramine-phentermine. *N Engl J Med* 1997;337:581–588.
127. Jick H, Vasilakis C, Weinrauch LA, et al. A population-based study of appetite-suppressant drugs and the risk of cardiac-valve regurgitation. *N Engl J Med* 1998;339:719–724.
128. Jollis JG, Landolfo CK, Kisslo J, et al. Fenfluramine and phentermine and cardiovascular findings: effect of treatment duration on prevalence of valve abnormalities. *Circulation* 2000;101:2071–2077.
129. Lee PJ, Mallik R. Cardiovascular effects of radiation therapy: practical approach to radiation therapy-induced heart disease. *Cardiol Rev* 2005; 13:80–86.
130. Bulkey BH, Roberts WC. Systemic lupus erythematosus as a cause of severe mitral regurgitation. New problem in an old disease. *Am J Cardiol* 1975;35:305–308.
131. Galve E, Candell-Riera J, Pigrau C, et al. Prevalence, morphologic types, and evolution of cardiac valvular disease in systemic lupus erythematosus. *N Engl J Med* 1988;319s:817–823.
132. Evangelopoulos ME, Alevizaki M, Toumanidis S, et al. Mitral valve prolapse in systemic lupus erythematosus patients: clinical and immunological aspects. *Lupus* 2003;12:308–311.

133. Waller BF, Howard J, Fess S. Pathology of mitral valve stenosis and pure mitral regurgitation-part I. *Clin Cardiol* 1994;17:330–336.
134. Bortolotti U, Valente M, Agozzino L, et al. Rheumatoid mitral stenosis requiring valve replacement. *Am Heart J* 1984;107:1049–1051.
135. Misch KA. Development of heart valve lesions during methysergide therapy. *Br Med J* 1974;2:365–366.
136. Wrisley D, Giambartolomei A, Lee I, et al. Left atrial ball thrombus: review of clinical and echocardiographic manifestations with suggestions for management. *Am Heart J* 1991;121:1784–1790.
137. Dalen JE, Fenster PE. Mitral stenosis. In: Alpert JS, Dalen JE, Rahimtoola SH, eds. *Valvular heart disease*. Philadelphia: Lippincott Williams & Wilkins; 2000.
138. Otto CM. *Valvular heart disease*. Philadelphia: Saunders; 1999.
139. Dubin AA, March HW, Cohn K, et al. Longitudinal hemodynamic and clinical study of mitral stenosis. *Circulation* 1971;44:381–389.
140. Gordon SP, Douglas PS, Come PC, et al. Two-dimensional and Doppler echocardiographic determinants of the natural history of mitral valve narrowing in patients with rheumatic mitral stenosis: implications for follow-up. *J Am Coll Cardiol* 1992;19:968–973.
141. Sagie A, Freitas N, Padial LR, et al. Doppler echocardiographic assessment of long-term progression of mitral stenosis in 103 patients: valve area and right heart disease. *J Am Coll Cardiol* 1996;28:472–479.
142. Chen MC, Wu CJ, Yip HK, et al. Left atrial platelet activity with rheumatic mitral stenosis: correlation study of severity and platelet P-selectin expression by flow cytometry. *Chest* 2003;124:1663–1669.
143. Craige E. Phonocardiographic studies in mitral stenosis. *N Engl J Med* 1957;257:650–654.
144. Nixon PG, Wooler GH, Radigan LR. The opening snap in mitral incompetence. *Br Heart J* 1960;22:395–402.
145. Millward DK, McLaurin LP, Craige E. Echocardiographic studies to explain opening snaps in presence of nonstenotic mitral valves. *Am J Cardiol* 1973;31:64–70.
146. Cooksey JD, Dunn M, Massie E, eds. *Clinical vectorcardiography and electrocardiography,* 2nd ed. Chicago: Year Book Medical, 1977:272.
147. Zamorano J, Cordeiro P, Sugeng L, et al. Real-time three-dimensional echocardiography for rheumatic mitral valve stenosis evaluation: an accurate and novel approach. *J Am Coll Cardiol* 2004;43:2091–2096.
148. Daniel WG, Nellessen U, Schroder E, et al. Left atrial spontaneous echo contrast in mitral valve disease: an indicator for an increased thromboembolic risk. *J Am Coll Cardiol* 1988;11:1204–1211.
149. Reid CL, Chandraratna PA, Kawanishi DT, et al. Influence of mitral valve morphology on double-balloon catheter balloon valvuloplasty in patients with mitral stenosis. Analysis of factors predicting immediate and 3-month results. *Circulation* 1989;80:515–524.
150. Wilkins GT, Weyman AE, Abascal VM, et al. Percutaneous balloon dilatation of the mitral valve: an analysis of echocardiographic variables related to outcome and the mechanism of dilatation. *Br Heart J* 1988;60:299–308.
151. Iung B, Cormier B, Ducimetiere P, et al. Functional results 5 years after successful percutaneous mitral commissurotomy in a series of 528 patients and analysis of predictive factors. *J Am Coll Cardiol* 1996;27:407–414.
152. Abascal VM, Wilkins GT, Choong CY, et al. Echocardiographic evaluation of mitral valve structure and function in patients followed for at least 6 months after percutaneous balloon mitral valvuloplasty. *J Am Coll Cardiol* 1988;12:606–615.
153. Palacios IF, Sanchez PL, Harrell LC, et al. Which patients benefit from percutaneous mitral balloon valvuloplasty? Prevalvuloplasty and postvalvuloplasty variables that predict long-term outcome. *Circulation* 2002;105:1465–1471.
154. Lev EI, Sagie A, Vaturi M, et al. Value of exercise echocardiography in rheumatic mitral stenosis with and without significant mitral regurgitation. *Am J Cardiol* 2004;93:1060–1063.
154a. Reis G, Motta MS, Barbosa MM, et al. Dobutamine stress echocardiography for noninvasive assessment and risk stratification of patients with rheumatic mitral stenosis. *J Am Coll Cardiol* 2004;43:393–401.
155. Gorlin R, Gorlin SG. Hydraulic formula for calculation of the area of the stenotic mitral valve, other cardiac valves, and central circulatory shunts. I. *Am Heart J* 1951;41:1–29.
156. Selzer A, Cohn KE. Natural history of mitral stenosis: a review. *Circulation* 1972;45:878–890.
157. Rowe JC, Bland EF, Sprague HB, et al. The course of mitral stenosis without surgery: ten- and twenty-year perspectives. *Ann Intern Med* 1960; 52:741–749.
158. Sherrid MV, Clark RD, Cohn K. Echocardiographic analysis of left atrial size before and after operation in mitral valve disease. *Am J Cardiol* 1979; 43:171–178.
159. Coulshed N, Epstein EJ, McKendrick CS, et al. Systemic embolism in mitral valve disease. *Br Heart J* 1970;32:26–34.
160. Meisner JS, Keren G, Pajaro OE, et al. Atrial contribution to ventricular filling in mitral stenosis. *Circulation* 1991;84:1469–1480.
161. Hirsh J, Dalen J, Guyatt G. The sixth (2000) ACCP guidelines for antithrombotic therapy for prevention and treatment of thrombosis. American College of Chest Physicians. *Chest* 2001;119[1 Suppl]:1S–2S.
162. Alan S, Ulgen MS, Ozdemir K, et al. Reliability and efficacy of metoprolol and diltiazem in patients having mild to moderate mitral stenosis with sinus rhythm. *Angiology* 2002;53:575–581.
163. Monmeneu Menadas JV, Marin Ortuno F, Reyes Gomis F, et al. Beta-blockade and exercise capacity in patients with mitral stenosis in sinus rhythm. *J Heart Valve Dis* 2002;11:199–203.
164. Patel JJ, Shama D, Mitha AS, et al. Balloon valvuloplasty versus closed commissurotomy for pliable mitral stenosis: a prospective hemodynamic study. *J Am Coll Cardiol* 1991;18:1318–1322.
165. Turi ZG, Reyes VP, Raju BS, et al. Percutaneous balloon versus surgical closed commissurotomy for mitral stenosis. A prospective, randomized trial. *Circulation* 1991;83:1179–1185.
166. Reyes VP, Raju BS, Wynne J, et al. Percutaneous balloon valvuloplasty compared with open surgical commissurotomy for mitral stenosis. *N Engl J Med* 1994;331:961–967.
167. Cribier A, Eltchaninoff H, Koning R, et al. Percutaneous mechanical mitral commissurotomy with a newly designed metallic valvulotome: immediate results of the initial experience in 153 patients. *Circulation* 1999;99:793–799.
168. Guerios EE, Bueno RR, Nercolini DC, et al. Randomized comparison between Inoue balloon and metallic commissurotome in the treatment of rheumatic mitral stenosis: immediate results and 6-month and 3-year follow-up. *Catheter Cardiovasc Interv* 2005;64:301–311.
169. Chen CR, Cheng TO. Percutaneous balloon mitral valvuloplasty by the Inoue technique: a multicenter study of 4832 patients in China. *Am Heart J* 1995;129:1197–1203.
170. Goto S, Handa S, Akaishi M, et al. Left ventricular ejection performance in mitral stenosis, and effects of successful percutaneous transvenous mitral commissurotomy. *Am J Cardiol* 1992;69:233–237.
171. Stefanadis C, Dernellis J, Stratos C, et al. Effects of balloon mitral valvuloplasty on left atrial function in mitral stenosis as assessed by pressure-area relation. *J Am Coll Cardiol* 1998;32:159–168.
172. Hernandez R, Banuelos C, Alfonso F, et al. Long-term clinical and echocardiographic follow-up after percutaneous mitral valvuloplasty with the Inoue balloon. *Circulation* 1999;99:1580–1586.
173. Shaw TR, Sutaria N, Prendergast B. Clinical and haemodynamic profiles of young, middle aged, and elderly patients with mitral stenosis undergoing mitral balloon valvotomy. *Heart* 2003;89:1430–1436.
174. Krasuski RA, Bush A, Kay JE, et al. C-reactive protein elevation independently influences the procedural success of percutaneous balloon mitral valve commissurotomy. *Am Heart J* 2003;146:1099–1104.
175. Carabello BA.*Modern management of mitral stenosis Circulation* 2005; 112:432–437.
176. Elkayam U, Bitar F. Valvular heart disease and pregnancy part I: native valves. *J Am Coll Cardiol* 2005;46:223–230.
177. Nercolini DC, da Rocha Loures Bueno R, Eduardo Guerios E, et al. Percutaneous mitral balloon valvuloplasty in pregnant women with mitral stenosis. *Catheter Cardiovasc Interv* 2002;57:318–322.
178. Ben Farhat M, Ayari M, Maatouk F, et al. Percutaneous balloon versus surgical closed and open mitral commissurotomy: seven-year follow-up results of a randomized trial. *Circulation* 1998;97:245–250.
179. Ommen SR, Nishimura RA, Grill DE, et al. Comparison of long-term results of percutaneous mitral balloon valvotomy with closed transventricular mitral commissurotomy at a single North American Institution. *Am J Cardiol* 1999;84:575–577.
180. Yau TM, El-Ghoneimi YA, Armstrong S, et al. Mitral valve repair and replacement for rheumatic disease. *J Thorac Cardiovasc Surg* 2000;119:53–60.
181. Nakano S, Kawashima Y, Hirose H, et al. Reconsiderations of indications for open mitral commissurotomy based on pathologic features of the stenosed mitral valve. A fourteen-year follow-up study in 347 consecutive patients. *J Thorac Cardiovasc Surg* 1987;94:336–342.
182. Hickey MS, Blackstone EH, Kirklin JW, et al. Outcome probabilities and life history after surgical mitral commissurotomy: implications for balloon commissurotomy. *J Am Coll Cardiol* 1991;17:29–42.
183. Cosgrove DM 3rd, Sabik JF, Navia JL. Minimally invasive valve operations. *Ann Thorac Surg* 1998;65:1535–1538; discussion 1538–1539.
184. Chitwood WR Jr. Video-assisted and robotic mitral valve surgery: toward an endoscopic surgery. *Semin Thorac Cardiovasc Surg* 1999;11:194–205.
185. Chitwood WR Jr, Elbeery JR, Chapman WH, et al. Video-assisted minimally invasive mitral valve surgery: the "micro-mitral" operation. *J Thorac Cardiovasc Surg* 1997;113:413–414.
186. Gillinov AM, Banbury MK, Cosgrove DM. Is minimally invasive heart valve surgery a paradigm for the future? *Curr Cardiol Rep* 1999;1:318–322.
187. Mohr FW, Falk V, Diegeler A, et al. Minimally invasive port-access mitral valve surgery. *J Thorac Cardiovasc Surg* 1998;115:567–574; discussion 574–576.
188. Falk V, Walther T, Autschbach R, et al. Robot-assisted minimally invasive solo mitral valve operation. *J Thorac Cardiovasc Surg* 1998;115:470–471.
189. Marchand MA, Aupart MR, Norton R, et al. Fifteen-year experience with the mitral Carpentier-Edwards PERIMOUNT pericardial bioprosthesis. *Ann Thorac Surg* 2001;71[5 Suppl]:S236–239.
190. Grunkemeier GL, Starr A, Rahimtoola SH. Prosthetic heart valve performance: long-term follow-up. *Curr Probl Cardiol* 1992;17:329–406.
191. Hammer HF, Eber B, Schumacher M, et al. Evaluation of the role of coronary heart disease and left ventricular contractile function in systolic mitral valve displacement. *Wien Klin Wochenschr* 1993;105:488–491.

192. Cox JL. Intraoperative options for treating atrial fibrillation associated with mitral valve disease. *J Thorac Cardiovasc Surg* 2001;122:212–215.
193. Bando K, Kasegawa H, Okada Y, et al. Impact of preoperative and postoperative atrial fibrillation on outcome after mitral valvuloplasty for nonischemic mitral regurgitation. *J Thorac Cardiovasc Surg* 2005;129:1032–1040.
194. Cox JL, Ad N, Palazzo T, et al. Current status of the Maze procedure for the treatment of atrial fibrillation. *Semin Thorac Cardiovasc Surg* 2000;12:15–19.
195. McCarthy PM, Gillinov AM, Castle L, et al. The Cox-Maze procedure: the Cleveland Clinic experience. *Semin Thorac Cardiovasc Surg* 2000;12:25–29.
196. Haissaguerre M, Jais P, Shah DC, et al. Spontaneous initiation of atrial fibrillation by ectopic beats originating in the pulmonary veins. *N Engl J Med* 1998;339:659–666.
197. Gillinov AM, McCarthy PM. Advances in the surgical treatment of atrial fibrillation. *Cardiol Clin* 2004;22:147–157.
198. Feldman T, Wasserman HS, Herrmann HC, et al. Percutaneous mitral valve repair using the edge-to-edge technique: 6 month results of the EVEREST phase I clinical trial. *J Am Coll Cardiol* 2005;46:2141–2142.

CHAPTER 23 ■ AORTIC VALVE DISEASE

WILLIAM J. STEWART AND BLASE A. CARABELLO

AORTIC STENOSIS

Historical Perspective

Until about 1960, patients with aortic stenosis (AS) who developed classic symptoms of angina, syncope, or congestive heart failure (CHF) had only a few years to live, and survival was unaffected by medical therapy. Now the age-corrected survival after successful aortic valve replacement (AVR) mimics the normal population (1). Excellent outcome is predicated on proper timing of reliably safe surgery, and use of dependable "substitute" valves with excellent hemodynamic profiles. AS is primarily a disease of aging, and its incidence is increasing in our population, occurring in approximately 3,000,000 Americans.

Diagnosis of aortic valve disease has also undergone substantial refinement. The physician's bedside assessment of the severity of stenosis remains the first stage of diagnosis. Doppler echo provides accurate noninvasive measures of the transvalvular gradient (2,3), based on valvular velocity and the modified Bernoulli equation, and the aortic valve area (AVA) (4), based on the continuity equation. Left ventricular (LV) catheterization using the retrograde approach provides direct measurement of gradients and estimation of AVA.

After the development of cardiopulmonary bypass in 1953, Harken et al. (5) were first to perform successful AVR with a subcoronary mechanical prosthesis in 1960. Ross pioneered the aortic valve homograft in 1962 (6), and in 1967 transfer of the pulmonary valve to the aortic position (pulmonary autograft) (7), an approach that gained appreciable acceptance in the 1980s and 1990s before declining in popularity more recently.

Many aortic valve prostheses have been used and discarded over the years. The Starr-Edwards ball-and-cage prosthesis remained popular for most of the last 30 years, declining recently with the advent of lower profile mechanical valves. Carpentier et al. (8) developed a glutaraldehyde-preserved porcine heterograft in 1969. The bovine pericardial heterograft, after the first series developed early failure (9), was improved and is among the most widely used today (10). Tissue valves available today include stent-mounted pericardial valves, stent-mounted porcine valves (now declining in usage), stentless porcine valves, cryopreserved homografts (allografts), and pulmonary autografts.

Etiology

An Inflammatory Process Similar to Atherosclerosis

Several etiologies of valvular AS have been described, including senile calcific, bicuspid, rheumatic, and congenital varieties. In developed countries, the most common cause of adult-acquired AS at present is a chronic inflammatory and fibrotic process of the aortic valve very similar to arterial atherosclerosis. The progressive fibrosis and calcification (11) can occur on a bileaflet or a trileaflet valve, it just occurs earlier in life in the bicuspid valve.

About one percent of Americans are born with a bicuspid aortic valve. In most of these, the valve opens well at birth, but gradual and progressive fibrosis leads to stenosis in approximately one third (12,13), presumably because of flow characteristics of the bicuspid architecture increase chronic subclinical injury of the valve tissue and accelerate the atherogenic

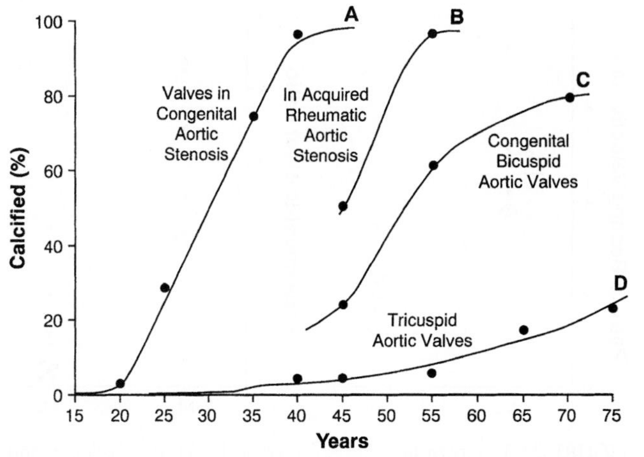

FIGURE 23.1. Timing of onset of symptoms and significantly calcified and stenotic valves versus the major etiologies of AS, including (**A**) congenital, (**B**) bicuspid, (**C**) rheumatic, and (**D**) senile. (*Source:* From Campbell M. Calcific aortic stenosis and congenital bicuspid aortic valves. *Br Heart J* 1968;30:606–616, with permission.)

process. Because bicuspid aortic valves occur more frequently in men, AS also has a male predominance. When it occurs, clinically significant stenosis of a bicuspid valve typically develops in the fifth or sixth decades of life, although it may occur earlier or later. In contrast, rheumatic AS, on average, becomes symptomatic in the fourth decade, and congenital AS becomes symptomatic in the first to third decades (Fig. 23.1) (14). Although the exact incidence of AS in patients born with tricuspid aortic valves is unknown, it is probably less than 1%, but is increasing with our aging population. In patients with a previously normal tricuspid aortic valve who eventually develop AS, the same atherosclerosis-like process, involving inflammation and calcification, leads to symptomatic stenosis, occurring typically in the seventh and eighth decades (14).

Otto et al. (15) have noted that the early lesion of AS is characterized by subendothelial thickening on the aortic side of the leaflet. Thickening occurs as the elastic lamina is displaced by the accumulation of cellular lipid infiltration and extracellular mineralization. There is proliferation of smooth muscle cells and lipid-laden foam cells resembling the plaque of coronary atherosclerosis (12).

Standard risk factors for coronary atherosclerosis are associated with acceleration of the thickening of the aortic valve. In fact, even mild degrees of fibrosis, termed *aortic sclerosis*, is a manifestation of an atherosclerotic process on the aortic valve that eventually leads to AS (16–19). Aortic sclerosis itself is associated with a significantly worse prognosis, possibly also owing to its link to atherosclerosis in all parts of the cardiovascular system (19).

Cholesterol, lipoprotein disorders, smoking, male gender, and age may accelerate the fibrotic effects (20) and development of AS. In patients with familial hypercholesterolemia, duration of exposure to high cholesterol concentrations correlates with development of AS (21). Acquired AS involves the same atherosclerosis-like histology and pathophysiology, and the same ultimate outcome, in bicuspid and tricuspid valves, only at an earlier age in the former.

Rheumatic Valvular Disease

In developed countries, rheumatic fever is the cause of AS in a minority of patients, accounting for less than 20% of the total (11). When rheumatic fever is the cause of AS, the mitral valve is also affected in most patients. Thus, the diagnosis of rheumatic AS should probably not be made in the presence of a completely normal-appearing mitral valve by echocardiography unless a diagnosis of previous rheumatic fever is ironclad (13).

Radiation-Induced Aortic Stenosis

There is an increased prevalence of AS following mediastinal radiation occurring two decades or more after therapy, sometimes associated also with radiation-induced disease of the coronary arteries, pericardium, myocardium, lungs, esophagus, or thyroid gland (22).

Congenital Aortic Stenosis

Congenital LV outflow tract obstruction occurs at valvular, subvalvular, and supravalvular levels. Williams syndrome is the association of supravalvular AS with elfin facies and hypercalcemia. It is sometimes associated with peripheral pulmonary arterial stenosis, which tends to improve with time, whereas the supravalvular AS tends to progress with time, probably owing to failure of growth of the sinotubular junction (23).

Subvalvular AS can be caused by a membranous ring or by a fibromuscular tunnel. In addition, some patients are born with small aortic roots, representing a mild form of aortic atresia (see Chapter 30). Congenital valvular AS is usually caused by cusp fusion of bicuspid, or unicuspid valves, and may present with severe heart failure in infancy. Congenital valvular AS differs greatly from adult-acquired AS, with more common incidence of normal or supernormal ejection performance (24,25), often with extensive hypertrophy, and more frequent sudden cardiac death (26). Thus, in pediatric patients, valve replacement should be recommended if the mean transvalvular gradient exceeds 50 mm Hg, even in the absence of symptoms. Because the commissural fusions are not densely calcified in congenital valvular AS, balloon aortic valvotomy is a reasonable option in asymptomatic patients with noncalcified congenital AS whose mean transvalvular gradient exceeds 50 mm Hg (27).

Clinical Presentation

Natural History. The natural history of acquired AS was depicted by Ross and Braunwald (Fig. 23.2) and confirmed by recent studies (28–31). The patient who eventually develops severe AS remains asymptomatic with a nearly normal survival for a long latency period. During this time, the valve slowly

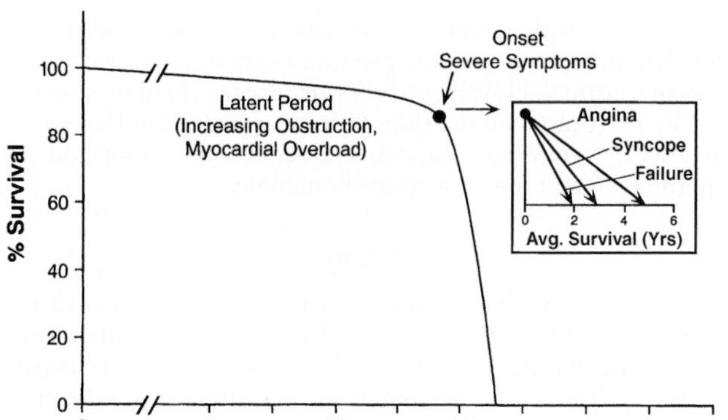

FIGURE 23.2. The natural history of AS. A long latent period with a nearly normal survival rate is present until the symptoms of angina, syncope, or CHF develop. At that time, a precipitous decline in survival occurs unless the problem is surgically corrected. *Inset*: The prognosis is worst with presenting symptoms of CHF, second worst with syncope. (*Source:* From Ross J Jr, Braunwald E. Aortic stenosis. *Circulation* 1968;38[Suppl 5]:V–61, with permission.)

develops fibrosis, inflammation, and calcification, but the patient remains well. However, once the symptoms of angina, syncope, or CHF develop, survival is dramatically shortened. Approximately 35% of patients who become symptomatic present with angina (32). In this group, 50% survive for only 5 years unless AVR is performed. In the 15% of patients who present with syncope, 50% survive for only 3 years; for the 50% with AS who present with symptoms of CHF, mean survival is less than 2 years unless the aortic valve is replaced. The risk of sudden cardiac death in asymptomatic or minimally symptomatic patients is rare, about 0.5% per year, whereas it increases to 2% per month after the development of symptoms (30,31). If the risk of death without surgery in a few years is less than that associated with AVR with available therapies, it seems reasonable to wait until the development of symptoms. However, declining surgical mortality rates have changed this, with earlier operation becoming more common (see section on AVR in asymptomatic AS).

The progression of AS is more rapid, and prognosis without AVR is worse, in patients who have moderate or severe valvular calcification and also in those who have a rapid increase in their Doppler-derived gradient (33–35). Similarly, smoking, hypercholesterolemia, and elevated serum creatinine and calcium levels have been associated with a more rapid rate of progression of AS (36).

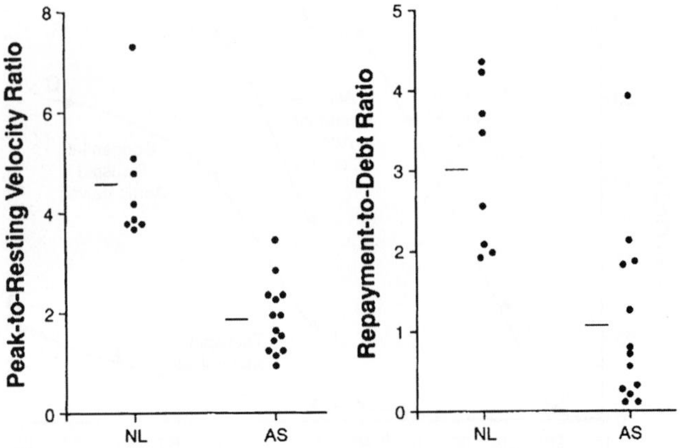

FIGURE 23.3. Shown here are ratios of peak-to-resting velocity and of repayment to debt, demonstrating the coronary reactive hyperemia responses (after a 20-second occlusion of the left anterior descending coronary artery in control patients [NL] and in patients with AS). (*Source:* From Marcus ML, Doty DB, Hiratzka LF, et al. Decreased coronary reserve: a mechanism for angina pectoris in patients with aortic stenosis and normal coronary arteries. *N Engl J Med* 1982;307:1362–1367, with permission.)

Pathophysiology of Aortic Stenosis and Its Relation to Symptoms

As AS worsens and the gradient increases, a progressive pressure overload is placed on the left ventricle. Increased systolic wall stress signals development of concentric LV hypertrophy (LVH) (37), accompanied by a dissociated and complex modulation of various genes responsible for contraction and relaxation. LVH also involves the renin–angiotensin system (38,39), and other pathways involving LV remodeling (40) associated with altered myocardial matrix metalloproteinase activity and expression. Increased muscle mass allows the ventricle to generate increased pressure while maintaining normal wall stress to compensate for the pressure load. The Laplace equation for wall stress is used to approximate afterload on a given area of myocardium.

$$\text{Stress} = \frac{\text{Pressure} \times \text{Radius}}{2 \times \text{thickness}}$$

As pressure in the numerator increases, increased thickness in the denominator offsets the pressure overload, and wall stress remains normal. However, as the pressure overload progresses, the hypertrophy that develops becomes involved in the pathogenesis of symptoms (e.g., subendocardial ischemia and arrhythmias), and thus a worsened outcome.

Angina

Angina, representing myocardial ischemia, occurs in AS because myocardial oxygen supply decreases and is outstripped by demand, which increases (41). With concentric hypertrophy, coronary flow reserve (during stress) becomes reduced from its normal five- to eightfold increase above baseline to a two- to threefold increase (Fig. 23.3) (42). Reduced flow reserve results from the endocardial compression by increased diastolic pressure, possibly with inadequate capillary ingrowth (43,44). In addition, outflow obstruction reduces diastolic perfusion time (45,46). Myocardial oxygen demand is increased in AS by increased systolic pressure and wall stress (47). Although LVH initially helps to normalize wall stress in AS, it becomes inadequate during exercise and later in the disease (48).

Syncope

Syncope in patients with AS, almost always precipitated by exertion, may be caused by an inability to increase in cardiac output during exercise, coupled with the normal decrease in total peripheral resistance. Alternatively increased intraventricular pressure during exercise may trigger a vasodepressor response (32,49,50). Supraventricular or ventricular arrhythmias may precipitate hypotension and syncope.

Congestive Heart Failure

Both systolic and diastolic myocardial dysfunction may occur in AS. This is detected by physical exam, chest radiography, and elevation of brain natriuretic peptide (BNP). The concentric hypertrophy requires a higher diastolic pressure for filling. Despite increased overall chamber stiffness because of LVH, the stiffness of each unit of myocardial volume remains normal (51) initially. However, as the disease progresses, increased collagen deposition reduces muscle compliance causing impaired LV filling with intrinsically stiffer myocardium (51,52).

Ventricular shortening depends on both afterload and contractility. Of patients with AS, 80% have excess afterload with increased peak systolic stress (Fig. 23.4) (53). The increase in pressure, the numerator of the Laplace equation, has not been normalized because of an inadequate increase in wall thickness in the denominator. Increased afterload reduces ejection performance and cardiac output and eventually decreases contractile function. Why the degree of hypertrophic compensation varies from patient to patient is only partially understood (54). Perhaps there is an inherent variability in the set point for pressure regulation of cardiac growth (55). The etiology of the decrease in contractility may include impaired calcium handling and subendocardial ischemia (56–58). Densification of microtubules comprising the myocardial cytoskeleton occurs in the context of inadequate hypertrophy and persistently increased systolic wall stress (59,60).

In addition to imaging studies that assess systolic dysfunction or ejection fraction (EF) in standard ways, diastolic dysfunction assessed using Doppler echocardiography, correlates with prognosis (61). The "Tei index," which calculates isovolumic contraction time plus isovolumic relaxation time divided by LV ejection time, helps to differentiate between symptomatic AS patients with depressed and less symptomatic AS patients with preserved systolic LV function (62).

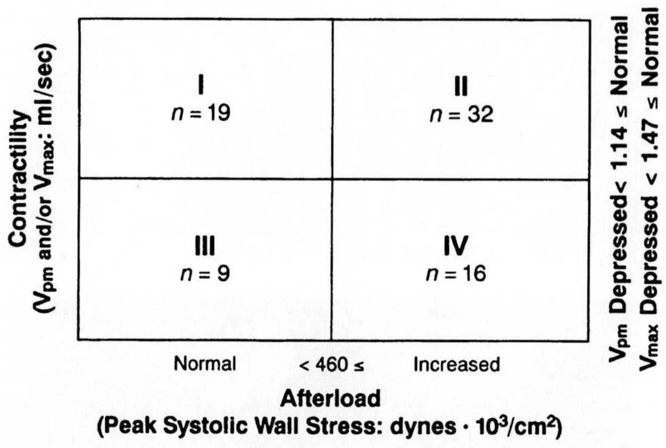

FIGURE 23.4. Here, contractility assessed as maximum dP/dT/P (V_{pm} and/or V_{max}) is plotted against afterload assessed as peak systolic wall stress in 76 patients with AS. Of the 57 patients with some abnormality, 48 (85%) had increased afterload. (*Source:* From Huber D, Grimm J, Koch R, Krayenbuehl HP. Determinants of ejection performance in aortic stenosis. *Circulation* 1981;64:126, with permission.)

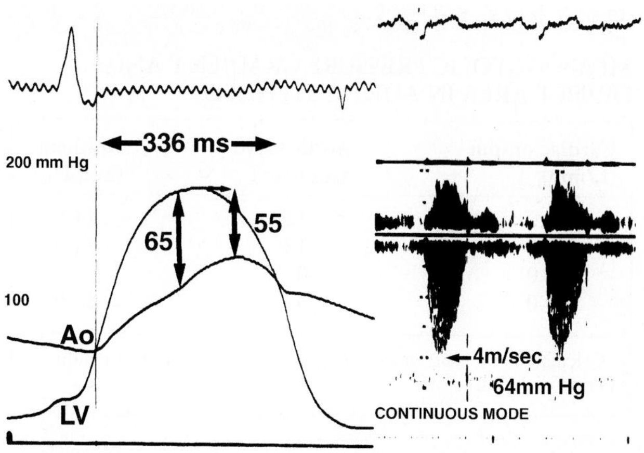

FIGURE 23.5. Micromanometer recordings of LV and ascending aortic pressure tracing (*left*) and continuous-wave Doppler velocity envelope (*right*) demonstrate correspondence of Doppler-derived peak instantaneous gradient (64 mm Hg) with peak instantaneous gradient determined by catheter measurements (65 mm Hg), which differs from the peak-to-peak gradient (55 mm Hg). The catheter- and Doppler-derived mean gradients matched perfectly (42 mm Hg). (*Source:* From Assey ME, Usher BW, Carabello BA, Spann JF Jr. The patient with valvular heart disease. In: Pepine CJ, Hill JA, Lambert CR, eds. *Diagnostic and therapeutic cardiac catheterization*, 2nd ed. Baltimore: Williams & Wilkins, 1994:692, with permission.)

Gastrointestinal Bleeding

Patients with AS have an increased risk of gastrointestinal bleeding (63,64), termed *Heyde syndrome*. Angiodysplasia, or arteriovenous malformations of the intestines, can occur, although they are difficult to find by standard methods (63). When unexplained anemia or occult blood in stool is present, an operative strategy that requires postoperative anticoagulation seems ill advised (64).

Hemodynamics

The best measurements for assessing the severity of AS are the mean systolic gradient and AVA, which are obtained accurately both by catheterization and Doppler methods, which are both derived from similar principles. The Gorlin formula uses direct pressure measurements from a catheter and pressure manometer. The continuity equation uses direct velocity measurements from Doppler echocardiographic instruments (4). Both methods derive AVA from Torricelli's equation:

$$F = A \times V \quad \text{or} \quad A = F/V$$

where F is flow, A is orifice area, and V is velocity. Using Doppler methods, velocity is measured directly by determining the amount of shift in the frequency of reflected ultrasound, both in the valve orifice (by continuous wave Doppler) and in the LV outflow tract (by pulsed Doppler). The area in the LV outflow tract is calculated by measuring its diameter directly from a two-dimensional echo image and assuming circular symmetry. Outflow tract area multiplied by outflow tract velocity are divided by valvular velocity to obtain the valve area using the continuity equation.

Using catheter methods, cardiac output is measured using the Fick or indicator dilution (thermodilution) technique. Pressure gradient is measured and converted to velocity:

$$V = \sqrt{g \times h}$$

where g is acceleration owing to gravity and h is mean gradient. These are combined in the Gorlin formula for calculating AVA (65), which is the following:

$$AVA = \frac{Q}{K\sqrt{h}}$$

where Q is cardiac output and h is the mean valve gradient. An alternative, third method for determining AVA is by careful planimetry of the systolic short-axis views of the aortic valve on a transesophageal echocardiography (TEE) (66), although this is not generally as accurate as the continuity equation. In some patients, TEE from deep transgastric views can record velocities representative of the transvalvular pressure gradients, although gradients derived in this way may miss the highest ones present.

To record pressure gradients invasively, a catheter is used to record pressure on both sides of the valve, ideally with a simultaneous recording, from which the average pressure difference during the systolic interval is measured. For Doppler methods, valvular velocity recorded by continuous wave Doppler is converted to gradient (G) using the simplified Bernoulli equation (Fig. 23.5) (2,3,67).

$$G = 4 \times V^2$$

Both Doppler and catheter methods can accurately derive the mean systolic gradient, averaged over the systolic interval. Peak instantaneous gradient measured by Doppler has no convenient direct-pressure measurement counterpart, and specifically is not the same as peak-to-peak gradient.

Progression of Aortic Stenosis

As shown in Table 23.1, reduction in aortic orifice area from its normal 3.0 to 4.0 cm^2 to approximately 1.5 cm^2 results in only a small gradient. However, after that degree of stenosis has developed, small additional reductions in the orifice area lead to progressively more dramatic increases in gradient. The average increase in gradient is 7 to 10 mm Hg per year (68) but with a large and unpredictable individual variation, as much as 25 mm Hg in 1 year in occasional patients (69).

A rapid rate of progression of stenosis, as reflected by an increase in aortic-jet maximum velocity of more than 0.3 m/second in the course of a year, occurs more often in patients who have clinical cardiac events (33).

TABLE 23.1

MEAN SYSTOLIC PRESSURE GRADIENT AND ORIFICE AREA IN AORTIC STENOSIS

Cardiac output (L/min)	Aortic valve area (cm^2)	Gradient[a] (mm Hg)
5.0	1.5	14.0
5.0	1.0	21.0
5.0	0.7	42.0
5.0	0.5	82.0

[a]Calculated at a heart rate of 76 beats/min and a systolic ejection period of 330 ms.

The unpredictable rate of progression of stenosis mandates careful follow-up. Patients should be educated about the cardinal symptoms of the disease and counseled to inform the physician of the onset of symptoms as soon as they occur. Most patients with critical AS who develop symptoms have an AVA of less than 0.7 cm^2 and a mean systolic gradient above 50 mm Hg. However, some patients may develop symptoms and therefore require surgery before or after reaching those thresholds. Some authorities would attribute symptoms to AS at valve areas below a threshold of 1.0 cm^2 or even higher (70). Some favor correction of this value for body surface area, especially in women with smaller body size; most patients who require surgery for critical AS have an AVA index below 0.4 cm^2/m^2.

A

B

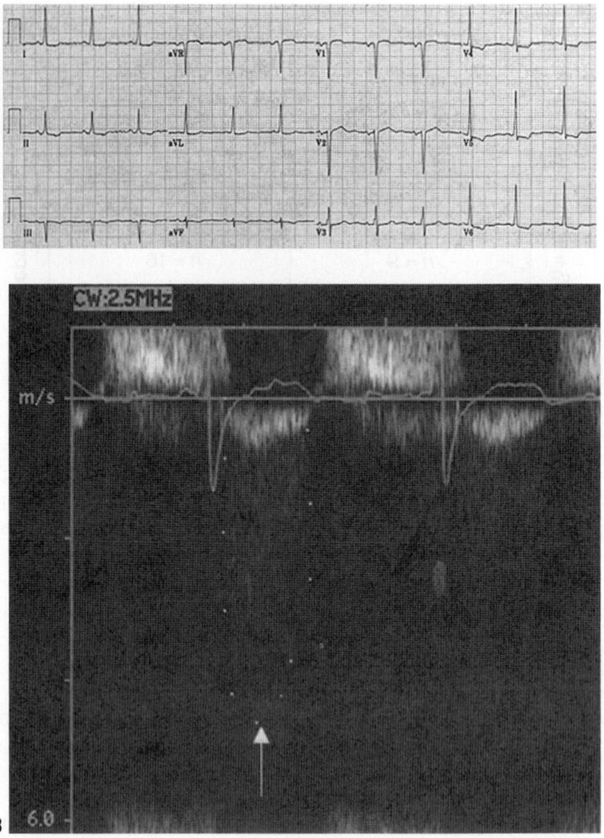

FIGURE 23.6. Typical ECG from a patient with severe symptomatic AS showing LV hypertrophy (**A**), and a continuous-wave Doppler spectrum from the same patient (**B**) showing a mean gradient of 47 mm Hg, derived from tracing the velocity envelope (*dots*), and a maximum instantaneous gradient of 70 mm Hg, calculated from the highest velocity (*arrow*) using the Bernoulli equation ($G = 4 \times V^2$).

Diagnosis

Physical Examination

Early in course of AS, the murmur typically peaks in early to midsystole and is associated with a systolic thrill. Harsh in quality and frequently lower in pitch than the blowing sound of mitral regurgitation, the murmur of AS is often loudest at the base of the heart and radiates to the neck. As AS becomes severe, the murmur peaks progressively later until it becomes loudest in the latter half of systole. The murmur may become softer as cardiac output decreases. The murmur is frequently well heard in the aortic area, disappears over the sternum, and becomes louder again over the apex, thus mimicking coexisting mitral regurgitation (Gallivardin phenomenon).

The severity of AS is best estimated at the bedside by palpation of the carotid arteries. In severe AS, the carotid upstroke becomes reduced in amplitude and delayed in timing (parvus et tardus) (see Fig. 23.5), because of work loss at the stenotic valve. Occasionally in elderly patients, inelasticity of the carotid arteries causes the carotid contour to maintain a more brisk upstroke, which can cause the examiner to underestimate the severity of the disease.

In moderate to severe AS, the aortic component of the second heart sound typically becomes diminished in intensity (because leaflet mobility is reduced), which may also be helpful in assessing the severity of AS. In severe congenital AS, the valve is still quite mobile, so both components of the S2 are preserved, and the murmur is usually preceded by an early ejection sound.

In severe AS, palpation of the cardiac apex reveals a powerful, enlarged, and sustained point of maximum impulse, which is usually not displaced much from normal position. A fourth heart sound is common. Evidence of pulmonary artery hypertension and right ventricular failure occurs only with far-advanced disease.

Electrocardiogram

The electrocardiogram (ECG) in AS usually demonstrates LVH and sometimes left atrial abnormality (Fig. 23.6). However, ECG signs of LVH may be absent in patients with AS even though severe LVH exists (Fig. 23.7).

Chest X-Ray

The cardiac silhouette is usually normal in size, but may demonstrate a boot-shaped silhouette consistent with concentric LVH. A prominent ascending aorta is common. Calcification in the aortic valve occasionally may be visualized in the lateral view. Significant cardiomegaly and pulmonary venous congestion occur later in the course of the disease.

Doppler Echocardiographic Studies

Ultrasonic examination of the heart in AS is the most important diagnostic modality for confirming the diagnosis and quantifying disease severity. Two-dimensional echocardiography demonstrates thickened and calcified aortic valve leaflets with reduced leaflet motion, sometimes with calcification of the aortic annulus. Distinction between bicuspid and tricuspid anatomy is often possible (Fig. 23.8) when the amount of calcification is small, but this distinction is difficult to make

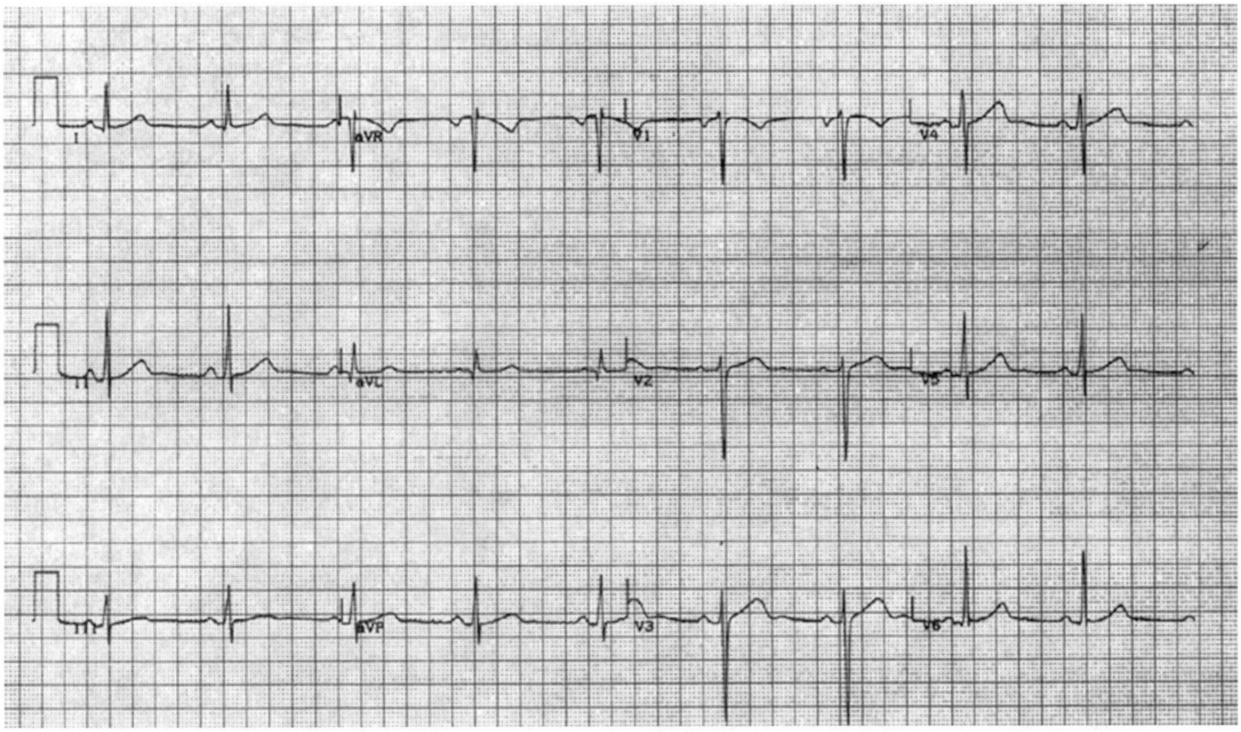

FIGURE 23.7. Atypical ECG from a patient with severe symptomatic AS whose Doppler study showed a mean systolic aortic valve gradient of 90 mm Hg. Except for slightly increased QRS voltage, the ECG is remarkably normal.

when there is significant fibrosis and calcification. In addition, the extent of concentric LVH can be quantitated by calculating LV mass from the echocardiographic images (71). LV ejection performance can be evaluated and the EF measured. Doppler studies (2,3,67,72,73) can accurately quantify the transvalvular pressure gradient (Fig. 23.9) and the valve area, using the given formulas. Doppler assessment of diastolic dysfunction is also useful, often defining the presence of abnormal LV relaxation (74).

When AS is first suspected, an initial Doppler echocardiographic study can confirm the diagnosis and assess hemodynamics. Clinical follow-up should be frequent enough to ascertain development of symptoms. Echocardiographic follow-up should be frequent enough to detect the development or worsening of problems such as LV dysfunction, LVH, or mitral regurgitation (68). A case can be made for periodic echocardiographic examination of asymptomatic patients, namely, yearly in patients with severe AS, every 2 years or so in patients with moderate AS, and every 5 years or so in patients with mild AS (75). Once symptoms develop, repeat Doppler echocardiography helps to confirm worsening of disease severity.

Stress Testing

In the past, stress testing was avoided in AS for fear of complications (76). Indeed, stress testing should be avoided in obviously symptomatic patients. However, stress testing can be performed safely in patients with AS. It is particularly useful when symptoms are uncertain by history alone, and to objectify the degree of exercise tolerance (77,78). Nuclear imaging has also been used to evaluate the presence of coronary disease, which may coexist with AS; one study of perfusion imaging (79) suggests a sensitivity and specificity of approximately 80% for concomitant coronary disease. Dobutamine echo is often a useful way to redefine valve area and gradient at a higher cardiac output, especially useful in patients with moderate to severe AS with a low gradient and depressed LV function (80,81).

Cardiac Catheterization

Because all of the information needed to quantify the extent and severity of AS can usually be obtained by physical examination combined with Doppler echocardiographic studies, the need to perform invasive hemodynamics in this population has declined to a small number of patients for whom the data conflict (82,83). Coronary disease may be present in as many as 25% of AS patients who do not complain of angina, and it is present in 40% to 80% of AS patients who complain of angina (84–86). Coronary revascularization of severe coronary stenoses is conventionally performed at the time of AVR and is probably beneficial (87–89). Thus, coronary arteriography is performed in most adult patients with AS to assess coronary anatomy. If the severity of AS is in doubt, the transvalvular gradient should be measured using a two-transducer technique, and right heart catheterization should be performed to measure cardiac output for the AVA calculation.

Differential Diagnosis of Aortic Stenosis Versus Hypertrophic Cardiomyopathy

Valvular AS may be confused clinically with hypertrophic obstructive cardiomyopathy (HOCM), which has very different management and outcomes. Fortunately, the issue is almost always settled by Doppler echocardiography. Compared to the fixed obstruction of valvular AS, HOCM is a myocardial

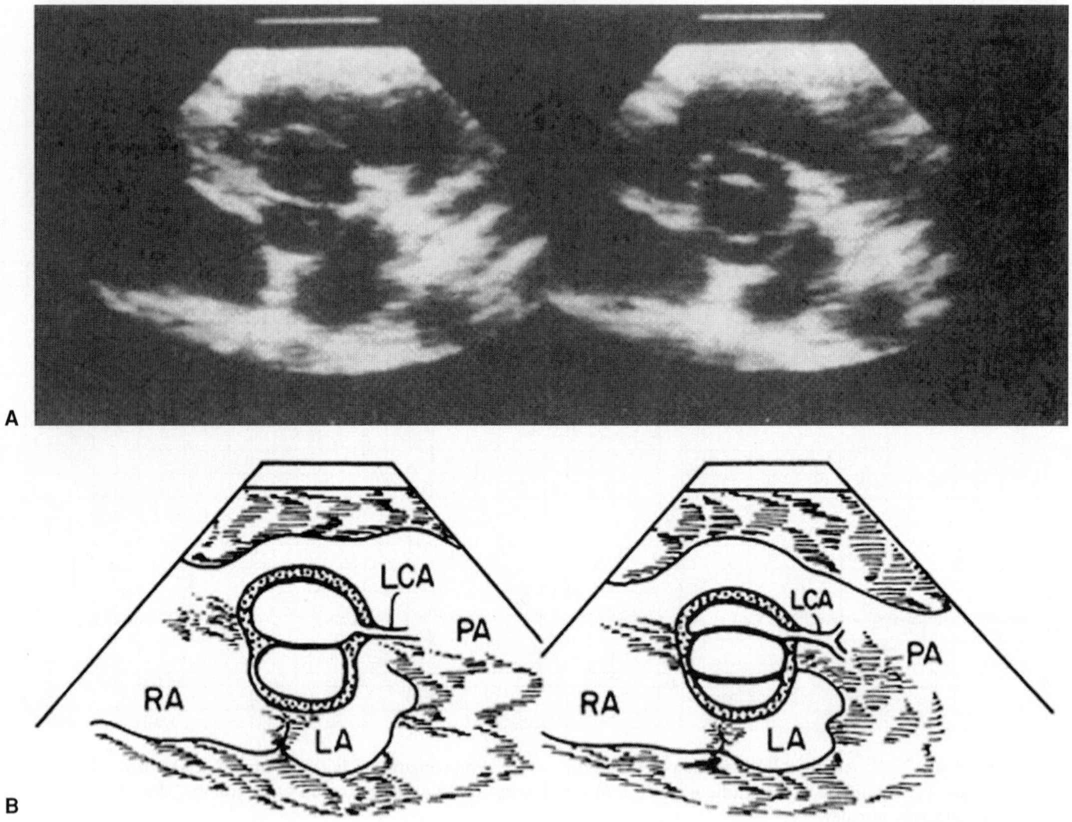

FIGURE 23.8. Echocardiographic images (A) and schematics (B) taken from the parasternal short-axis view from a patient with a bicuspid aortic valve in diastole (*left*) and in systole (*right*). *Abbreviations:*LA, left atrium; LCA, left coronary artery; PA, pulmonary artery; RA, right atrium. (*Source:* From Stewart WJ, King ME, Weyman AE. Prevalence of aortic valve prolapse with bicuspid aortic valve and its relation to aortic regurgitation: a cross-sectional echocardiographic study. *Am J Cardiol* 1984;54:1277–1282, with permission.)

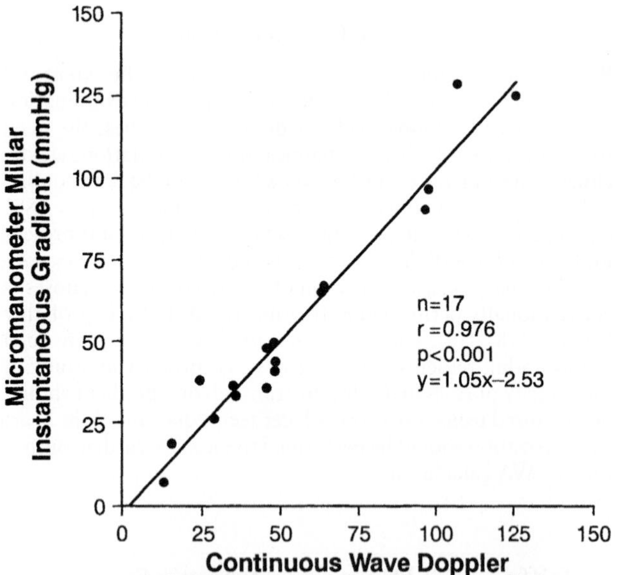

FIGURE 23.9. Correlation of peak instantaneous aortic valve gradient determined at cardiac catheterization using a micromanometer catheter technique with Doppler-derived estimated peak instantaneous gradient. (Data from the Medical University of South Carolina.) (*Source:* From Assey ME, Usher BW, Carabello BA, Spann JF Jr. The patient with valvular heart disease. In: Pepine CJ, Hill JA, Lambert CR, eds. *Diagnostic and therapeutic cardiac catheterization*, 2nd ed. Baltimore: Williams & Wilkins, 1994:693, with permission.)

disease with dynamic obstruction that varies indirectly with LV volume and directly with contractility. In HOCM, obstruction to outflow is from systolic anterior motion of the mitral valve, which contacts the hypertrophied intraventricular septum. Conditions that reduce ventricular volume or increase contractility worsen the obstruction in HOCM, in contrast to valvular AS (Table 23.2).

Management

Medical Therapy

There is no effective medical treatment for symptomatic AS. Most asymptomatic patients do not require therapy designed to alter hemodynamics. However, the presence of AS, or even sclerosis, is probably an indication for aggressive risk factor modification, including smoking cessation, cholesterol lowering, diabetes management, and hypertension control. As mentioned, the inflammatory nature of AS progression suggests that lipid-lowering goals appropriate for patients with known coronary disease are indicated. Statin use may reduce the rapidity of progression of AS (90,91), but this is controversial (92).

The onset of symptoms should lead to AVR promptly in most cases (93). In some patients who are deemed not to be surgical candidates, digitalis and diuretics may transiently improve CHF, and nitrates may be used cautiously to treat angina pectoris. However, these therapies provide no long-term benefit. Prophylactic antibiotics are indicated as pretreatment for dental or surgical procedures.

TABLE 23.2

VALVULAR AORTIC STENOSIS VERSUS HYPERTROPHIC CARDIOMYOPATHY: A COMPARISON

Characteristic	Aortic stenosis	Hypertrophic cardiomyopathy
Orifice area	Relatively fixed	Varies with ventricular volume
Carotid upstroke	Upstroke delayed	Sharp upstroke with spike and dome quality
Valsalva maneuver	Murmur decreases in intensity	Murmur increases in intensity
Post–extrasystolic beat	Obstruction unchanged	Obstruction worsens
	Stroke volume increases	Stroke volume decreases (increased contractility)
	Pulse pressure increases	Pulse pressure decreases
	Murmur increases	Murmur increases
Electrocardiogram	Sometimes normal	Almost always shows LVH
Hypertrophy	Concentric	Asymmetric septal hypertrophy, or concentric LVH
Angina	Typical	Often atypical
Syncope	With exertion	Postexertion
Congestive heart failure and preload reduction	Diuretics helpful	May worsen obstruction

Abbreviation: LVH, left ventricular hypertrophy.

Vasodilators, such as angiotensin-converting enzyme inhibitors, have been considered to be relatively contraindicated in AS. Dilation of systemic venous capacitance vessels may cause hypotension and a drop in cardiac output because the hypertrophied LV requires increased preload to maintain adequate forward flow. However, this traditional dogma has been challenged in AS patients presenting in cardiogenic shock, who have been treated successfully with nitroprusside and hemodynamic monitoring (197).

Balloon Valvotomy (Valvuloplasty)

After considerable initial interest, enthusiasm for aortic balloon valvotomy (valvuloplasty) in treating adult-acquired AS has waned. Although balloon valvotomy may be effective in relieving congenital AS as mentioned, results have proved disappointing in adults, most of whom have valve calcification. In most patients, balloon valvotomy reduces severe AS to moderately severe AS (94), producing an AVA of 0.8 to 1.0 cm^2 at best. The gradient typically is reduced by 50% and averages approximately 35 mm Hg after the procedure. Unfortunately, in 50% of patients, restenosis occurs within 6 months (95). Overall, balloon valvotomy has not reduced the high mortality seen in patients who do not undergo surgery for symptomatic AS (Fig. 23.10) (96). At present, balloon valvotomy should be reserved for patients with advanced CHF who are not candidates for surgery because of other comorbid conditions or because of unacceptably high perioperative risk. In these patients, balloon valvotomy may be performed, carrying a 2% to 5% risk of mortality; it may be effective in allowing bedridden patients to be discharged from the hospital. It may also be used palliatively in patients with treatable acute illnesses that are likely to resolve, thus eventually permitting elective aortic valve surgery.

Aortic Valve Replacement: Surgical Procedures

AVR is the definitive therapy for symptomatic AS and is mandatory unless there are compelling contraindications for operation. AVR is usually accomplished using a bioprosthetic or mechanical valve, performed through a median sternotomy incision, although recently less invasive techniques have been carried out through smaller hemisternotomy incisions or anterior

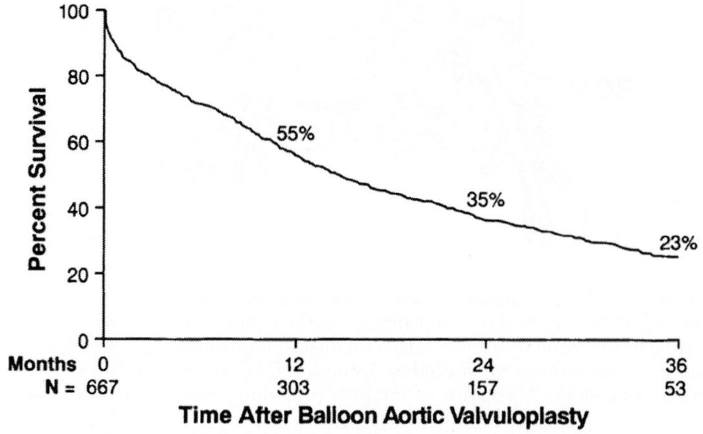

FIGURE 23.10. Plot of survival after balloon aortic valvuloplasty in 674 patients with AS, censored at the time of aortic valve surgery. Numbers below the x-axis indicate the number of patients surviving at each time point. (*Source:* From Otto CM, Mickel MC, Kennedy JW, et al. Three-year outcome after balloon aortic valvuloplasty: insights into prognosis of valvular aortic stenosis. *Circulation* 1994;89:642–650, with permission.)

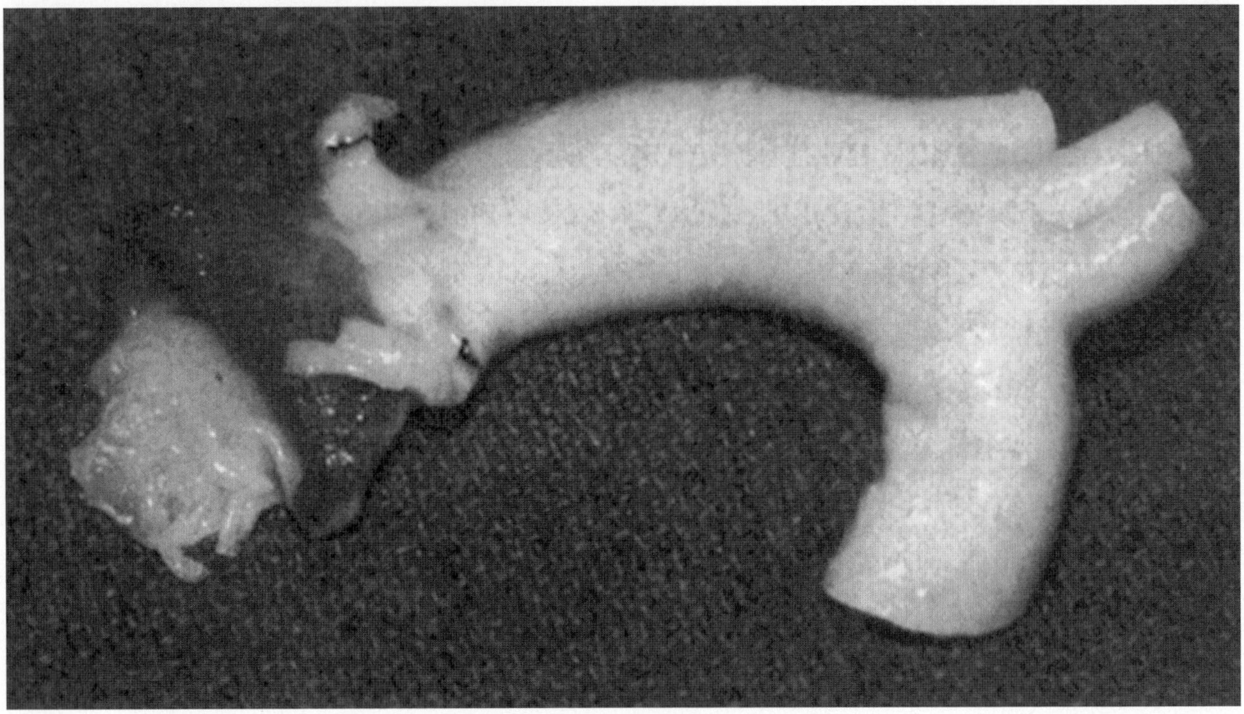

FIGURE 23.11. Homograft conduit before implantation. Most homografts are implanted as a miniroot that includes only a few centimeters of the tubular ascending aorta above the sinotubular junction, excluding the great vessels. In this example, the great vessels are still attached.

thoracotomies in the right second or third intercostal space (97) (see the section on Minimally Invasive Procedures).

Aortic Valve Replacement with Homograft (Allograft) Valve replacement with homograft (allograft) valves is more complex because the tissue implanted is entirely biologic (Fig. 23.11) without a stiff stent or sewing ring. Today, nearly all are inserted as a miniroot replacement, implanting the homograft and proximal aortic root as a unit, although this also requires that the patient's coronary arteries be reimplanted into the sinuses of Valsalva of the homograft aortic root.

Aortic Valve Replacement with Pulmonary Autograft (Ross Procedure). Use of the pulmonary autograft (Ross procedure) is even more complex (Fig. 23.12). The patient's own pulmonary valve and root are excised and reimplanted as an autograft into the aortic position, similar to that used with homografts. A pulmonary homograft is usually implanted as a miniroot to

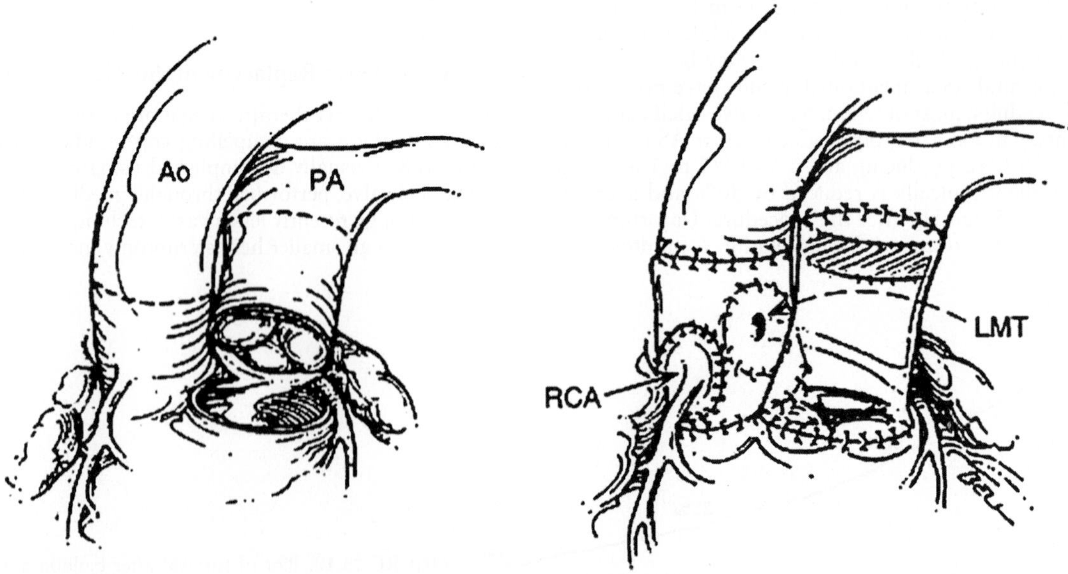

FIGURE 23.12. Methods of performing the Ross procedure. Schematic at left shows resection of the pulmonic valve and main pulmonary artery (*PA*). (*Right*) Schematic shows implantation of the pulmonary autograft in the aortic position (with reimplantation of the coronary arteries) and a homograft implanted as another miniroot to replace the pulmonic valve. *Abbreviations:* Ao, ascending aorta; LMT, left main trunk; RCA, right coronary artery. (*Source:* From DeLeon SY. Adaptation of the Ross procedure. *Ann Thorac Surg* 1995;59:1007, with permission.)

replace the pulmonic valve and the main pulmonary artery. Because significant coronary artery disease may be present in 25% to 30% of patients undergoing aortic valve surgery, especially in those with AS, it is frequently necessary to combine coronary artery bypass of the diseased vessels at the time of AVR.

Results

Mortality

Postoperative mortality should be 1% to 3%, depending on a variety of factors, including the individual surgeon's skill. The risk of operative mortality is higher in elderly or debilitated patients, in the presence of significantly impaired LV function, in patients with extensive coronary artery disease other valvular disease, and in patients with noncardiac comorbidities. After surgery there is an improvement in symptoms, a gradual decrease in LV mass, and an increase in EF, although not necessarily an increase in exercise capacity (98). Actuarial survival is approximately 80% to 85% at 5 years and 70% at 10 years postoperatively. As noted, coronary artery disease that is not treated at the time of AVR adversely affects long-term survival.

Postoperative Valve-Related Complications

Postoperative valve-related complications include (a) structural deterioration of the prosthetic valve; (b) hemodynamic prosthetic dysfunction; (c) prosthetic valve thrombosis; (d) thromboembolism; (e) anticoagulant-related bleeding; (f) infection; (g) prosthetic valve endocarditis; (h) hemolysis; and (i) heart block.

Structural Deterioration

Structural deterioration of currently available mechanical prostheses is extremely unusual (99–102). In contrast, virtually all tissue valves are prone to progressive, gradual deterioration, usually owing to leaflet calcification. Porcine valves in the aortic position may begin to fail at 7 to 8 years postoperatively (103), but freedom from hemodynamically significant structural deterioration is 54% to 58% at 15 years (104–106). Aortic bovine pericardial valve bioprostheses are somewhat better, with 91% to 96% free of significant structural deterioration at 10 years (10,107,108). Biologic valves deteriorate more rapidly in infants, children, and young adults than in older adults.

Homograft AVR also undergo fairly rapid structural deterioration, calcification, and development of aortic regurgitation, with some dependence on the technique of valve procurement, preservation, and implantation (109–111). Degeneration of even this human valve alternative is more accentuated in younger patients (112), in whom homografts are otherwise an attractive alternative. Ross (113) has estimated that the useful life of a homograft valve is approximately 15 years, but sometimes it is shorter.

The Ross procedure involves placing a pulmonary autograft and replacing the pulmonic valve with a homograft. However, both valves undergo progressive structural deterioration, and the patient is susceptible to postoperative problems with valve replacements in both the pulmonic and the aortic position (114,115).

Relative Stenosis and Patient–Prosthesis Mismatch

All standard prosthetic valves (mechanical valves as well as standard stented tissue valves) are inherently stenotic compared with the native aortic valve because part of the potential orifice area of prosthetic valves is occupied by struts, stents, hinge mechanisms, sewing rings, or valve leaflets. Accordingly, all of these valves have a measurable gradient, which is inversely proportional to prosthesis size. In contrast, because they are stentless, the aortic valve homograft, pulmonary autograft, and stentless porcine valves have better hemodynamic function because of the absence of sewing ring (116,117). There is less long-term experience with the stentless porcine valves.

Small-sized standard aortic prostheses (sizes 19 and 21) may be associated with gradients that are unacceptable in adult patients, particularly when the patient's body size is larger or their activity level and requisite cardiac output are greater. Patient–prosthesis mismatch involves the reality that a normally functioning valve implant may be too small for a patient whose body mass index is large in proportion to the aortic annulus. Patient–prosthesis mismatch is associated with an increased incidence of heart failure, pulmonary hypertension, prosthesis-related morbidity, and mortality (118–120). The prosthesis should be matched to the patient's needs. When the aortic annulus is found to be small, a stentless valve such as a homograft might be chosen, especially in younger patients with a large body surface area who are more physically active. Alternatively, insertion of a larger prosthesis may be feasible, combined with an annulus-enlarging procedure, such as the Nicks or the Konno procedures (121–123), the increased risks of which must be weighed against the increased risks of the mismatched smaller valve with relative stenosis.

Doppler echocardiography remains the best way to assess postoperative hemodynamics and to follow the function of an AVR noninvasively, but provides a numerically higher gradient compared with a catheter-derived gradient. Part of this difference is due to the pressure recovery phenomenon, analogous to the "airplane wing" effect (124,125). This discrepancy between catheter- and Doppler-derived gradients is most substantial in small aortic mechanical prosthetic valves such as bileaflet valves, where there is a localized area of low pressure at the downstream end of the smaller orifice between the two open prosthetic leaflets, creating higher velocity recordings.

Thromboembolism

Systemic thromboembolism after AVR with a modern mechanical prosthesis occurs at a rate of 1% to 2% per patient-year, even with adequate anticoagulation (99). The incidence is lower in patients with bioprostheses, homografts, and pulmonary autografts, who do not usually required anticoagulation (10,104,105,107,109,112,114,115).

Thrombosis of mechanical valves, often associated with inadequate anticoagulation, may occur suddenly and be fatal, or it may occur gradually. The thrombus material, or tissue ingrowth that ensues, may prevent normal movement of the valve leaflets, causing valve dysfunction and, subsequently, CHF (126). Early valve thrombosis has been treated successfully by administering thrombolytic agents, although there is a significant incidence of thromboembolism, bleeding, and stroke associated with this form of treatment (127). Reoperation for repeat valve replacement is often necessary, although there is increased operative risk compared to first-time operations.

Anticoagulation is required in all patients with mechanical prostheses, with a target range of the internationalized normalized ratio of 2.5 to 3.5, although this is associated with a rate of bleeding complications of 1% to 3% per patient-year. Anticoagulation is usually not necessary with porcine or pericardial bioprostheses, homografts, and pulmonary autografts, unless it is indicated for other reasons such as atrial fibrillation.

Heart Block

Because the conduction system is near the junction of the non- and right coronary leaflets, heart block occurs in about 1% of patients after AVR, and is higher among patients with perianular infection or abscesses.

Hemolysis

Clinically unimportant, mild hemolysis after uncomplicated mechanical AVR is common, associated with an lactate dehydrogenase level of 1.5 or 2.0 times normal. Clinical hemolysis and anemia after uncomplicated AVR is most frequently associated with a paravalvular leak and may be well tolerated.

Infection

Early postoperative prosthetic valve endocarditis occurs in about 2% of patients, and frequently requires reoperation. Late prosthetic valve endocarditis occurs in 0.5% to 1.0% per patient-year (128). Infection is uncommon in homograft and autograft valves.

Choice of Valve

There is no perfect aortic valve substitute. Each alternative has significant advantages and disadvantages. Multiple factors, including patient age, anatomy, ventricular function, lifestyle, fear of reoperation, and possible contraindications to anticoagulation, must be considered when choosing the most appropriate option for each individual patient. This decision should be made jointly, after careful discussion, before surgery and involve the patient, cardiologist, and surgeon.

Bovine Pericardial Bioprostheses

Pericardial bioprostheses do not require anticoagulation, and appear to be more durable than porcine bioprostheses, particularly in older patients. These valves also eventually deteriorate (10,107,108).

Mechanical Valves

Mechanical aortic prostheses in use today include the double-leaflet tilting disc valves named *St. Jude* (99,96,97) and *Carbomedics* (131), and the single-leaflet tilting disc valve named *Medtronic-Hall* (102,132,133). These prostheses are extremely durable (99), but have the aforementioned problems with valve thrombosis, thromboembolism, and need for anticoagulation with the associated increase in risks of bleeding.

Porcine Bioprostheses

Porcine bioprosthetic valves are associated with more rapid structural dysfunction, which increasingly appears after 8 to 10 years, especially in young patients and in those with renal dysfunction.

Stentless Porcine Prostheses

Stentless porcine prostheses are relatively new, and afford improved hemodynamic function (lower gradients) and a low incidence of thromboembolism. However, long-term durability remains undetermined (117).

Cryopreserved Homograft Valves

Cryopreserved homograft valves show excellent hemodynamic function. Thromboembolism and endocarditis are extremely uncommon (109,110,113). However, homografts are in short supply, not available in all sizes, and more difficult to implant. They also undergo structural deterioration at a higher rate than previously appreciated. Furthermore, reoperation is much more difficult than with standard valves because of the frequency of calcification of the walls of the implanted aortic root.

Pulmonary Autograft

Although technically difficult, the Ross procedure affords excellent hemodynamics and a very low incidence of thromboembolism and endocarditis. The aortic autograft (excised from the patient's own pulmonary position) has the potential for growth (114,115) in children. However, this operation trades one abnormal valve for two postoperative prosthetic valves. Aortic regurgitation and/or pulmonic stenosis have led to reoperation more commonly than previously expected.

Management of Aortic Stenosis in Patients With a Small Hyperdynamic Ventricle

As noted, the law of Laplace states that

$$\text{Stress} = \frac{\text{Pressure} \times \text{Radius}}{2 \times \text{thickness}}$$

If LVH were perfectly regulated, then just enough of it would develop to normalize wall stress. However, in some patients the hypertrophy that develops is inadequate, wall stress increases, and ejection performance decreases (134). In other patients with AS, particularly women, wall thickness increases markedly, wall stress actually becomes subnormal, LV systolic performance becomes supernormal, and the LV is small and hyperdynamic (135), with some associated increase in mortality (136). Their diastolic dysfunction may require high filling pressure to achieve adequate forward output postoperatively.

Management of Aortic Stenosis Patients With Low Cardiac Output, Low Ejection Fraction, and Low Transvalvular Gradient

In most patients with even far-advanced AS that has resulted in reduced LV EF and severe CHF, outcome after surgery is

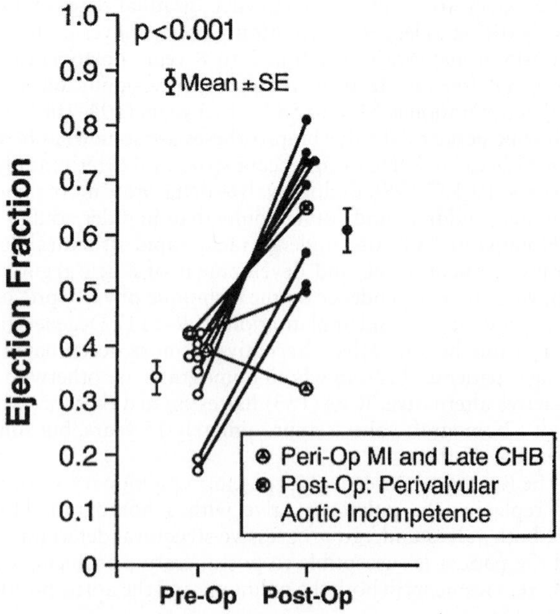

FIGURE 23.13. In patients with AS and poor LV function, reduced EF (preoperative) increased dramatically after AVR (postoperative), except for one patient ◬ who had a perioperative myocardial infarction (MI). *Abbreviation:* CHB, complete heart block. (*Source:* From Smith N, McAnulty JH, Rahimtoola SH. Severe aortic stenosis with impaired left ventricular function and clinical heart failure: results of valve replacement. *Circulation* 1978;58:255–264, with permission.)

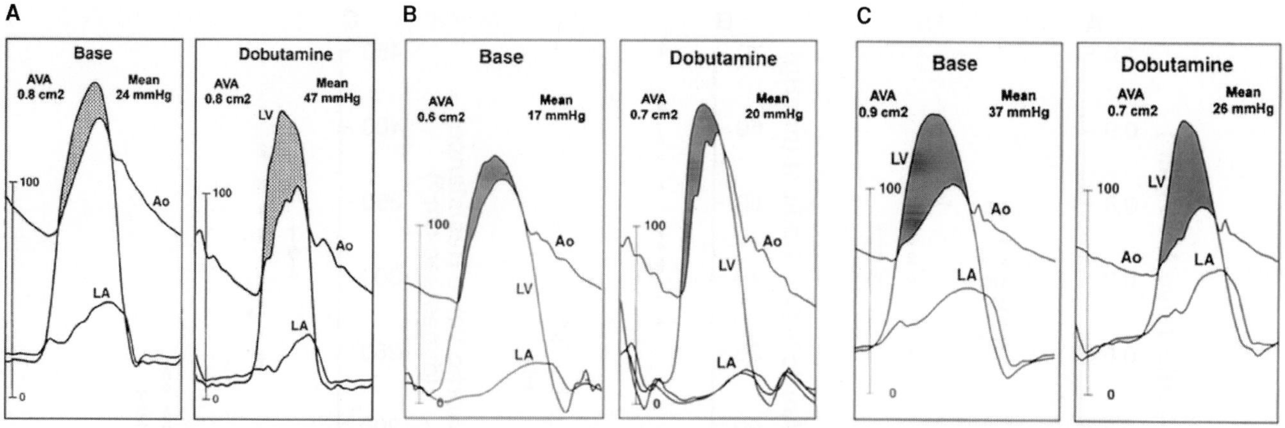

FIGURE 23.14. Representative hemodynamic tracings from three patients representing three different responses to dobutamine. (**A**) This patient responded to dobutamine infusion with an increase in cardiac output and an increase in aortic valvular mean gradient from 24 to 47 mm Hg. The AVA remained 0.8 cm^2. This patient had severe AS at the time of AVR and is alive in NYHA class I after operation. (**B**) The patient responded to dobutamine infusion with an increase in cardiac output and an increase in mean aortic valvular gradient from 17 to 20 mm Hg. The final AVA was 0.7 cm^2. This patient was found to have only mild AS at the time of operation. (**C**) This patient had no change in cardiac output, and the mean aortic valvular gradient decreased from 37 to 26 mm Hg in response to dobutamine infusion. The test was terminated because of hypotension. This patient had severe AS at the time of AVR but died 2 years postoperatively because of heart failure. *Abbreviations:* Ao, aortic; LA, left atrial; LV, left ventricular; base, baseline. (*Source:* From Nishimura RA, Grantham JA, Connolly HM, et al. Low-output, low-gradient aortic stenosis in patients with depressed left ventricular systolic function: the clinical utility of the dobutamine challenge in the catheterization laboratory. *Circulation* 2002;106:809–813.)

remarkably good (137). Surgical intervention relieves the afterload excess on the left ventricle, allowing an increase in LV performance (Fig. 23.13), which results in a stable postoperative course and rapid improvement in the symptoms of CHF. Unfortunately, this positive outlook is less universal in patients with severe AS and severe LV dysfunction. Various studies have shown 6% to 21% perioperative mortality with substantial postoperative death in the first few years, and a substantial number whose symptoms do not improve postoperatively (134,138–142). However, some patients with this condition do benifit from AVR.

The obvious challenge is to distinguish preoperatively those patients who have severe AS and may benefit from AVR while avoiding surgery in patients for whom the outcome will be poor. Some patients may have aortic "pseudostenosis" (143–145), where the severely impaired heart does not have the power to open the aortic valve, which is mild or moderately narrowed, and correcting the valve lesion may not improve the patient's condition. A useful diagnostic test is to cautiously give a dobutamine or nitroprusside infusion (80) to improve cardiac output, then recalculate AVA using either echocardiography (146) or cardiac catheterization (147). If the gradient stays the same and the AVA rises (>0.3 cm^2), the valve is not probably not severely stenotic (pseudostenosis), and the advisability of AVR is questionable. The ability to mount a contractile reserve itself has an important on survival (143,148). If cardiac output and gradient increase concomitantly, the calculated AVA remains small and severe AS probably exists (80) (Fig. 23.14).

Aortic valve resistance is another parameter that may help distinguish AS from aortic pseudostenosis (146,149–151) (Fig. 23.15). Aortic valve resistance (R) is proportional to mean transvalvular gradient and inversely proportional to systolic flow:

$$\text{Resistance} = \frac{\text{Mean gradient} \times \text{heart rate} \times \text{systolic ejection period} \times 1.33}{\text{Cardiac output}}$$

Valve resistance does not assume any discharge coefficients, and is less flow dependent than AVA. An R of less than 250 dynes/sec/cm^{-5} usually indicates milder stenosis.

Prophylactic Valve Replacement in Patients With Coronary Disease

In many cases, severe coronary disease requiring revascularization is present when the patient has only mild or moderate AS or regurgitation. Prophylactic valve replacement should be considered if their AS will progress to require reoperation for AVR in just a few years. These reoperations have a higher mortality rate (152) with some chance of damage to bypass grafts implanted during the first surgery. However, "prophylactic" surgery results in an unneeded valve prosthesis with all of its attendant risks and limited durability. Balaban et al. (153) suggested that aortic valve surgery should be done with the initial operation if the AS is at least moderate in severity. Smith et al. (154) suggested that patients under age 70 years should undergo "incidental AVR" even for mild AS, whereas those older than 70 should have AVR only if the AS is severe.

Aortic Valve Surgery: Minimally Invasive Procedures

The minimally invasive procedures are a group of cardiac procedures done through a smaller incision than the usual midsternal thoracotomy. The hemisternotomy, using an 8- to 10-cm vertical incision at the lower sternum (Fig. 23.16) (97), is feasible in most patients undergoing first-time isolated single valve repair or replacements. Minimally invasive procedures avoid splitting the entire sternum, reduce perioperative pain

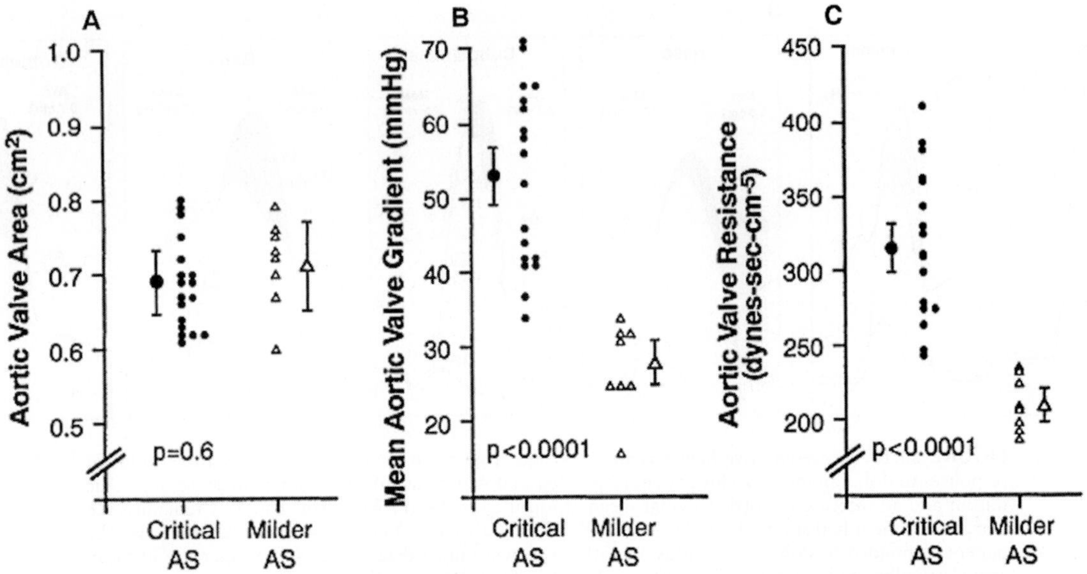

FIGURE 23.15. (**A**) AVA for patients with severe AS (*circles*) is compared with that of patients with milder AS (*triangles*) appearing to be aortic pseudostenosis. AVA calculated at catheterization was nearly identical in the two groups. (**B**) Aortic valve gradient for the same patient groups. The gradient was substantially higher in the group with severe AS. (**C**) Aortic valve resistance for the same two patient groups. Nearly complete separation is provided by this measure of severity of stenosis. (*Source:* From Cannon JD Jr, Zile MR, Crawford FA Jr, Carabello BA. Aortic valve resistance as an adjunct to the Gorlin formula in assessing the severity of aortic stenosis in symptomatic patients. *J Am Coll Cardiol* 1992;20:1517–1523, with permission.)

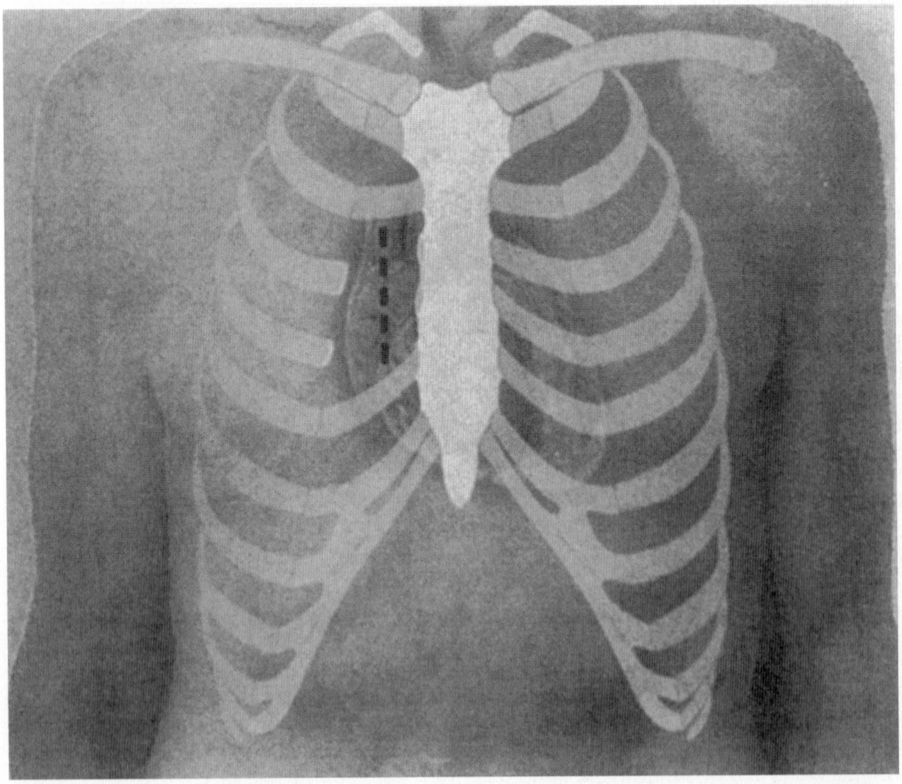

FIGURE 23.16. Location of incision for the minimally invasive procedure for aortic valve operations. A vertical incision approximately 3 to 4 inches long is made through the third and fourth ribs to the right of the sternum. (*Source:* From Cosgrove DM, Sabik JF. Minimally invasive approach for aortic valve operations. *Ann Thorac Surg* 1996;62: 596–597, with permission.)

and bleeding, and shorten length of hospital stay without increasing perioperative risk (97).

CHRONIC AORTIC REGURGITATION

Etiologies

Aortic regurgitation results from failure of leaflet coaptation, either because of diseased valve cusps or a diseased aortic root, which distorts cusp suspension (Fig. 23.17) (155). Common causes of cusp disease include congenital bicuspid aortic valve, rheumatic heart disease, infective endocarditis, all of which cause fibrosis and calcification of the leaflets, which often causes mixed AS and aortic regurgitation. Although a congenitally bicuspid aortic valve frequently leads to AS in adulthood, approximately 10% of bicuspid valve patients who require surgery present with pure aortic regurgitation without stenosis; these patients are usually younger, averaging approximately 40 years of age. Aortic regurgitation from a bicuspid aortic valve often results from leaflet prolapse, especially when one cusp is larger than the other (156). Although rheumatic heart disease primarily attacks the mitral valve, leading to mitral stenosis, many patients with rheumatic involvement also have some degree of aortic regurgitation, and in some patients aortic regurgitation is the predominant lesion. As mentioned, the presence of rheumatic mitral valve findings is the hallmark of diagnosing rheumatic aortic valve involvement. Infective endocarditis is the most common cause of acute aortic regurgitation.

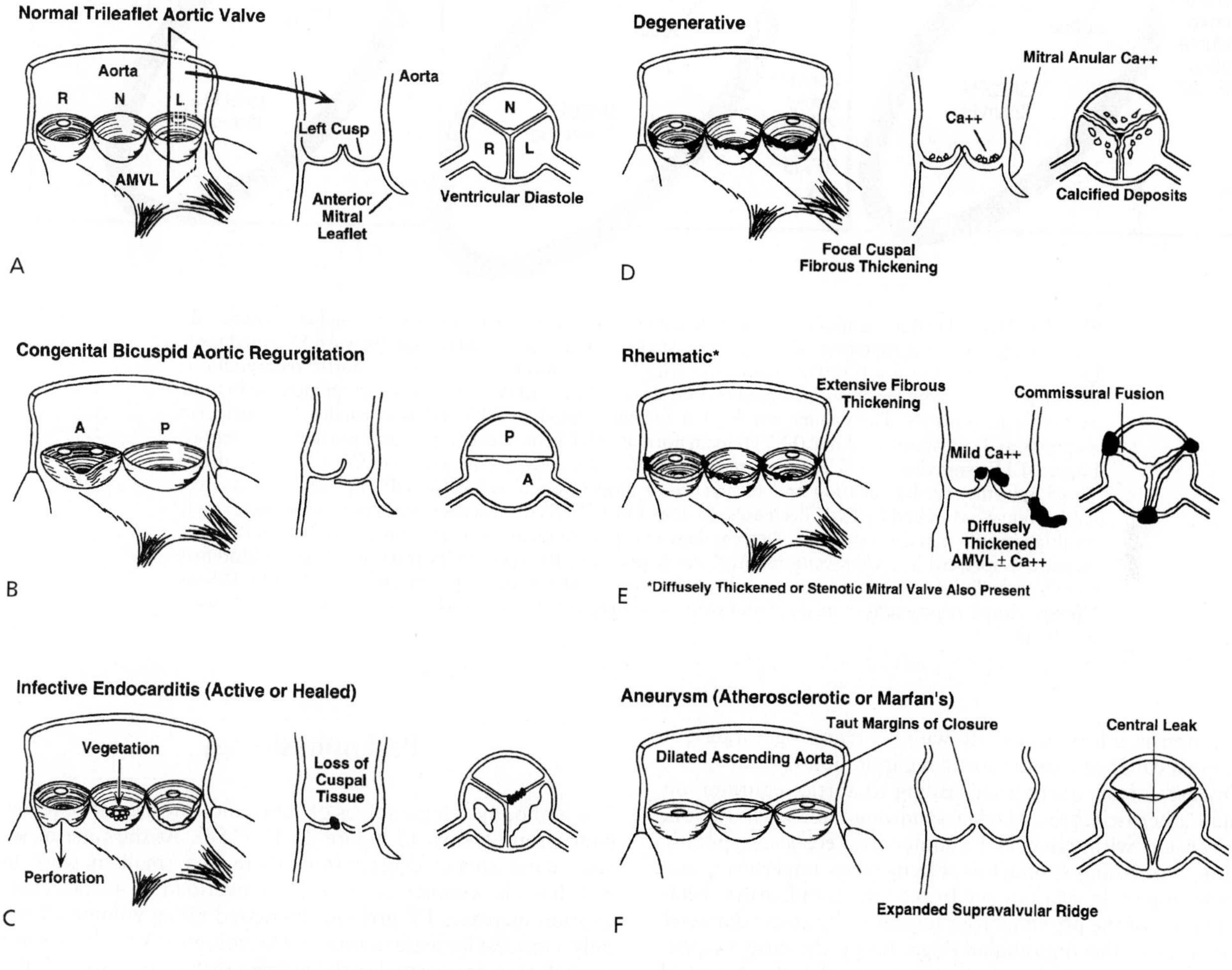

FIGURE 23.17. Various etiologies of aortic regurgitation. Each of the six panels shows a long axis of the aortic root opened up to show all the leaflets (*left*), a schematic of the long axis of the sinus of Valsalva (*middle*), and a schematic of the short axis of the aortic valve (*right*). (**A**) Normal trileaflet aortic valve. (**B**) Congenital bicuspid valve with a raphe between what would be the right and left coronary cusps in an anterior cusp that is larger than the posterior cusp, causing prolapse and aortic regurgitation. (**C**) Endocarditis causes aortic regurgitation through disruption of valve suspension or leaflet perforation. (**D**) Degenerative changes cause aortic regurgitation by restricting leaflet motion and coaptation. (**E**) Rheumatic valvulitis causes aortic regurgitation with postinflammatory leaflet fusion and fibrosis. (**F**) Aneurysms from atherosclerosis or cystic medial necrosis (Marfan type) cause aortic regurgitation by outward displacement of the leaflet suspension, with central noncoaptation, or by dissection causing failure of leaflet support. *Abbreviations:* A, anterior; AMVL, anterior mitral valve leaflet; Ca^{++}, calcification; L, left; N, noncoronary cusp; P, posterior; R, right coronary cusp. (*Source:* Modified from Frankl WS, Brest AN, eds. Valvular heart disease: comprehensive evaluation and management. *Cardiovasc Clin* 1986;30–31, with permission.)

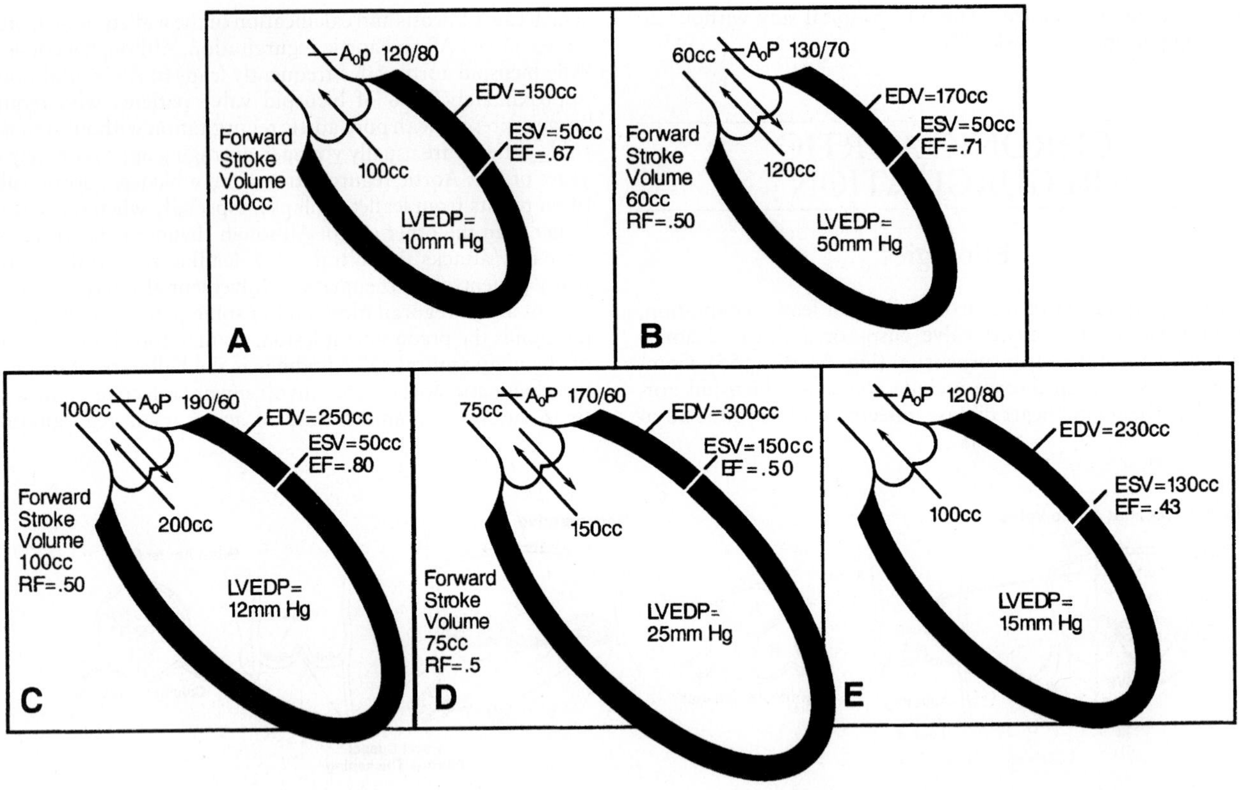

FIGURE 23.18. Hemodynamics of the clinical stages of aortic regurgitation. (**A**) Normal conditions. (**B**) Severe acute aortic regurgitation, although total stroke volume (SV) is increased, forward SV is reduced. LV end-diastolic pressure (LVEDP) rises dramatically. (**C**) Chronic, compensated aortic regurgitation. Eccentric hypertrophy produces increased end-diastolic volume (EDV), which permits an increase in total as well as forward SV. The volume overload is accommodated, and LVEDP is normalized. Ventricular emptying and end-systolic volume (ESV) remain normal. (**D**) Chronic, decompensated aortic regurgitation. Impaired LV emptying produces an increase in ESV and a decrease in EF, total SV, and forward SV. There is further cardiac dilation and recurrence of moderately elevated LVEDP. (**E**) Immediately after AVR, preload estimated by EDV decreases, as does LVEDP. ESV is also decreased, but to a lesser extent, resulting in an initial decrease in EF. Despite these changes, elimination of aortic regurgitation leads to an increase in forward SV. *Abbreviations:* AoP, aortic pressure; RF, regurgitant fraction. (*Source:* Modified from Carabello BA. Aortic regurgitation: hemodynamic determinants of prognosis. In: Cohn LH, DiSesa VJ, eds. *Aortic regurgitation: medical and surgical management.* New York: Marcel Dekker, 1986, with permission.)

If infection is tolerated acutely without requiring surgery, it becomes a cause of chronic aortic regurgitation.

Diseases of the aortic root leading to aortic regurgitation include atherosclerosis, Marfan syndrome, aortic dissection, hypertension with associated annuloaortic ectasia, syphilitic aortitis, ankylosing spondylitis, osteogenesis imperfecta, and systemic lupus. In Marfan syndrome and annuloaortic ectasia, dilation of the proximal root increases the aortic diameter at the level of the sinotubular ridge, lifting the cusp suspension superiorly, causing cusp separation and lack of central coaptation (157). Although annuloaortic ectasia is often associated with hypertension, its presence usually correlates better with age than elevated blood pressure. In Marfan syndrome, hypertension, and some patients with bicuspid aortic valves, cystic medial necrosis of the aorta occurs, and in some patients, it arises in isolation. Whether an aneurysm is caused by atherosclerosis or cystic medial necrosis, an intimal tear can occur, producing aortic dissection. Proximal dissection may undermine aortic valve cusp or commissural support. Ankylosing spondylitis, aortitis, and syphilis also cause ascending aortic dilation, but they also produce aortic wall thickening, which itself may distort the commissures and prevent leaflet coaptation.

Pathophysiology

The pathophysiologic stages of acute and chronic aortic regurgitation are shown in Figure 23.18 (158). At the time of severe acute aortic regurgitation, there is a small increase in end-diastolic volume as the volume overload of aortic regurgitation increases LV preload. Increased filling volume allows only a modest increase in total stroke volume (SV), which is not enough to compensate for the volume that is regurgitated. Because pulse pressure is proportional to SV, which is only slightly increased, there is usually no perceptible increase in pulse pressure at this stage of the disease. The large regurgitant volume entering the relatively small LV chamber greatly increases LV and left atrial diastolic pressure, leading to pulmonary congestion.

If the aortic regurgitation develops slowly, and the patient enters the chronic compensated phase, eccentric cardiac hypertrophy with the increased preload allows a large increase in LV end-diastolic volume. Because muscle function remains normal in this phase, normal performance of an enlarged ventricle permits ejection of a very large total SV. The large total SV allows forward SV to be normal despite a large regurgitant volume.

TABLE 23.3

HYPERTROPHY IN HUMAN LEFT-SIDED OVERLOAD VALVE LESSIONS

Valve lesions	Mass index: g/m^2 (patients analyzed, *n*)	Ratio of LV radius to thickness (patients analyzed, *n*)	Ratio of LV mass to volume (patients analyzed, *n*)
Normal subject	86 (259)	3.05 (88)	1.25 (225)
Mitral regurgitation	158 (146)	4.03 (64)	0.87 (117)
Aortic regurgitation	230 (148)	3.52 (31)	1.00 (141)
Aortic stenosis	178 (302)	2.35 (93)	1.55 (296)

Abbreviation: LV, left ventricular.
Source: From Carabello BA. The relationship of left ventricular geometry and hypertrophy to left ventricular function in valvular heart disease. *J Heart Valve Dis* 1995;4[Suppl II]:S132–S139, with permmission.

The enlarged compliant left ventricle accommodates filling at a lower pressure, more normal than in acute aortic regurgitation. In this stage, the patient may be entirely asymptomatic even during fairly strenuous activity. The large total SV interacts with the aorta to produce a wide pulse pressure, causing systolic hypertension. The wide pulse pressure produces most of the physical signs of aortic regurgitation.

The combined pressure and volume overload stimulates the development of both concentric and eccentric hypertrophy (Table 23.3). In this regard, aortic regurgitation differs markedly from mitral regurgitation, which usually has a pure volume overload (159) without pressure overload, and normal LV wall thickness. Aortic regurgitation also differs from AS, which is a pure pressure overload without volume overload. The hypertrophy that occurs in both appears to be related to changes in LV myocardial matrix metalloproteinase activity and inhibitory control, but with some differences—for example, in interstitial collagenase activity and stromelysin levels (40).

Sometimes after many years, LV dysfunction eventually develops, with further LV dilation, elevation of LV filling pressure, decreased EF, and reduced total and forward SV. Although most patients develop symptoms at this time, some still may enter this decompensated phase without complaints.

The final panel of Figure 23.18 depicts the patient after AVR has been performed. Shortly after AVR, there is a fall in both end-diastolic volume and end-systolic volume, with a greater decrease in the former. This results in a temporary reduction in ejection performance. However, if AVR is performed before LV dysfunction becomes permanent, additional remodeling occurs, resulting in an additional fall in end-systolic volume, with a return of ejection performance toward normal (160).

To summarize, in chronic aortic regurgitation, there is a large increase in total SV ejected into the aorta, which produces a widened pulse pressure and systolic hypertension accounting for the physical signs of the disorder; the widened pulse pressure and systolic hypertension are responsible for adding a pressure overload to this volume-overloaded state. Although initially compensated for by cardiac dilation to increase total SV, eventually afterload mismatch and contractile dysfunction lead to reduced ejection performance and cardiac decompensation (161). If aortic regurgitation is recognized and corrected surgically in a timely fashion, decompensation is reversed after AVR, afterload is reduced, and EF returns to normal (Fig. 23.19).

Clinical Profile: Symptoms

Congestive Heart Failure

Patients with aortic regurgitation in the chronic compensated phase are often entirely asymptomatic and can remain so for many years, even after myocardial dysfunction develops. As LV decompensation proceeds, in many patients symptoms occur, typically including dyspnea on exertion, orthopnea, and in advanced cases, paroxysmal nocturnal dyspnea and peripheral edema.

Angina and Aortic Regurgitation

Angina with normal epicardial coronary arteries is less frequent in aortic regurgitation than in AS (162). Aortic regurgitation results in a rapid fall in aortic diastolic pressure. Diastolic hypotension may be responsible for impaired coronary flow, leading to angina. In addition, the increased LV muscle mass increases the resistance to coronary flow. Other less common symptoms of aortic regurgitation include angina associated with vasoactive flushing (a pseudo-Nothnagel attack), an unpleasant awareness of the heartbeat, and carotid artery pain.

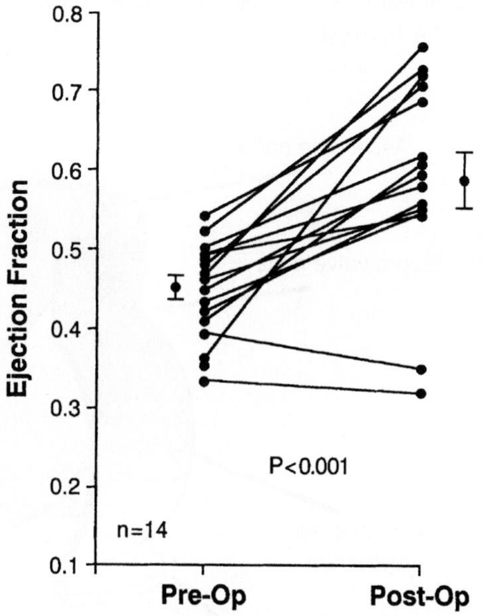

FIGURE 23.19. Preoperative and postoperative EF from 14 patients with aortic regurgitation. (*Source:* From Carabello BA, Usher BW, Hendrix GH, et al. Predictors of outcome for aortic valve replacement in patients with aortic regurgitation and left ventricular dysfunction: a change in the measuring stick. *J Am Coll Cardiol* 1987;10:991–997, with permission.)

TABLE 23.4

SIGNS OF AORTIC INSUFFICIENCY

Sign	Finding
Corrigan pulse	Rapid forceful carotid upstroke followed by rapid decline
Quincke pulse	Systolic plethora and diastolic blanching in nail bed when nail is slightly compressed
de Musset sign	Bobbing of head
Duroziez sign	Systolic and diastolic bruit heard over femoral artery when it is compressed
Hill sign	Augmentation of systolic blood pressure in leg by $\geq$30 mm Hg compared with that in arm

Physical Examination

Chronic severe aortic regurgitation results in cardiac dilation, large total SV, and a hyperdynamic circulation. The apical impulse is enlarged, sustained, and displaced laterally. The typical murmur of aortic regurgitation is a diastolic, blowing, decrescendo murmur heard best at the left sternal border with the patient sitting upright. The length of the murmur is somewhat related to the severity of the aortic regurgitation. In mild disease a short, early diastolic murmur is the rule. As the degree of valvular regurgitation worsens, the murmur may become pandiastolic. With the late onset of LV dysfunction and in acute, severe aortic regurgitation, high LV diastolic pressure causes earlier equilibration of the aortic and LV diastolic pressures in mid-diastole, reshortening the length of the diastolic murmur. Many patients with aortic regurgitation also have a systolic murmur even if they do not have AS because of the increase in antegrade flow. A second diastolic murmur, an apical mitral rumble (Austin-Flint murmur), may occur in severe aortic regurgitation, probably from the aortic regurgitation jet impinging on the mitral valve, causing diastolic turbulence without true LV inflow obstruction.

The large forward SV and wide pulse pressure cause numerous named signs (Table 23.4). Hill sign and Durozier sign are the most useful as a bedside gauge of aortic regurgitation severity. In blood pressure measurement with a sphygmomanometer, Korotkoff sounds may be heard down to a pressure of zero. When LV decompensation occurs, the pulse pressure may narrow again, and a third heart sound (S3) may occur.

Electrocardiogram

The ECG in chronic aortic regurgitation is nonspecific, but it almost always demonstrates LVH.

Echocardiography and Doppler Examination

Echocardiography with Doppler is the most important test to diagnose this disease. By two-dimensional echocardiography, normal leaflets are thin and mobile, opening to an orientation parallel to flow during systole, and suspended like a hammock in diastole, with the cusp belly hanging down to meet in the center, with an oval-shaped segment of overlap between each adjacent leaflet (Fig. 23.20).

With each etiology of aortic regurgitation—bicuspid aortic valve, rheumatic heart disease, infective endocarditis, calcific degeneration of leaflets, and aortic dilation—echocardiography-defined features have become well recognized. Echocardiography also gauges LV performance, chamber dimensions, and the extent of LVH, which are used with clinical data to time aortic valve surgery (see Aortic Valve Replacement and Repair).

Doppler interrogation is used to gauge the degree of aortic regurgitation in several ways. First, the spatial extent of the color Doppler aliasing in the outflow tract is used as a rough guide to the severity of aortic regurgitation (163). A semiquantitative scale of mild, moderate, moderately severe, and severe regurgitation is predicated primarily on the width (in long axis) and the area (in short axis) of the proximal portion of the jet of disturbed flow in the outflow tract. Continuous-wave Doppler interrogation of the aortic jet with measurement of the pressure half-time illustrates the decay of the diastolic velocity, and therefore gradient, across the aortic valve. In mild aortic regurgitation, the decay of the gradient is gradual, whereas in severe aortic regurgitation the decay occurs rapidly, reflecting equilibration of LV and aortic pressures in mid-diastole (164)

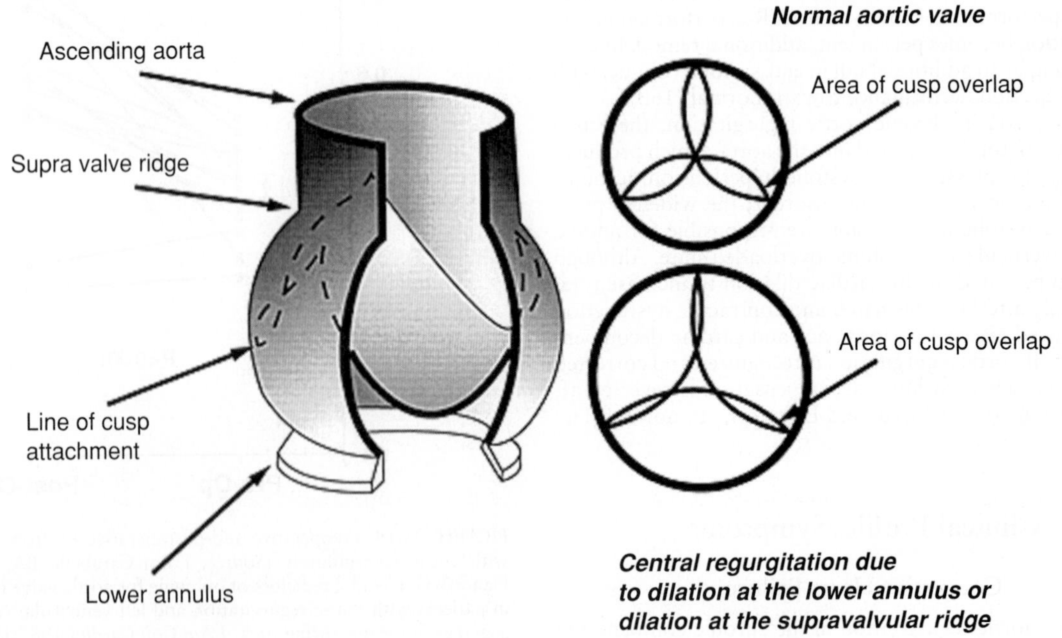

FIGURE 23.20. Aortic regurgitation in normal and thoracic aortic aneurysms.

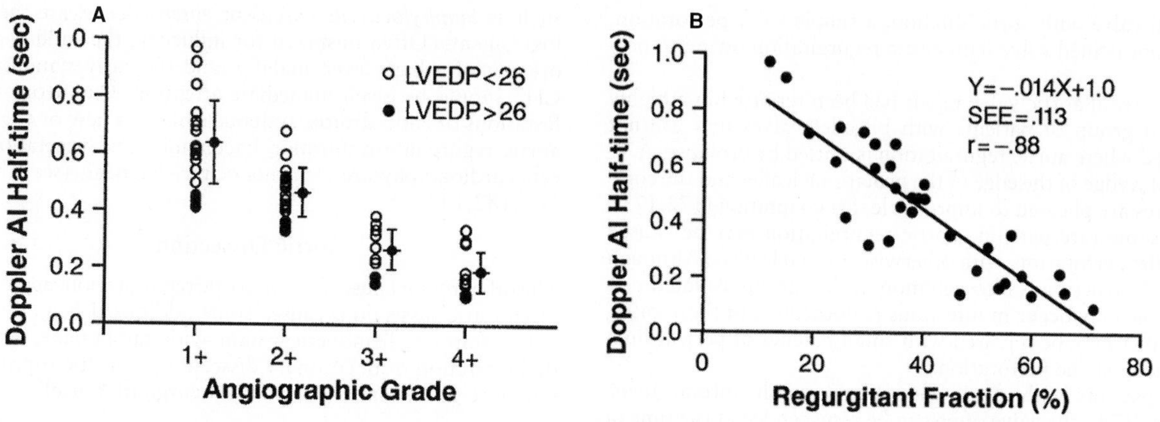

FIGURE 23.21. (A, B) Correlation of aortic insufficiency (AI) pressure half-time by continuous wave Doppler, in seconds, with the degree of regurgitation on angiography. Note inverse correlations. Patients with left ventricular end-diastolic pressure (LVEDP) of more than 26 mm Hg are indicated by the filled circles in (A). (*Source:* From Teague SM, Marty W, Sandatmanesh V, et al. The effects of mean pressure gradient, chamber compliance, and orifice size upon the Doppler half-time method. *J Am Coll Cardiol* 1988;11:204A, with permission.)

(Fig. 23.21). Descending aortic flow, measured by pulsed Doppler, shows pandiastolic reversal in diastole in severe aortic regurgitation.

Cardiac Catheterization

In patients with severe aortic regurgitation diagnosed by physical examination and ultrasound, cardiac catheterization need not be performed before AVR. Valve surgery without catheterization is more reasonable in men younger than 40 years or in women younger than 50 years, but atherosclerotic risk factors and symptoms should also be considered in this decision. In addition to the issue of defining concomitant coronary disease, when the severity of aortic regurgitation is in question, aortography can be useful. Unlike echocardiography, which visualizes the velocity of flow, aortography visualizes the opacification of the left ventricle with contrast injected into the aorta, which is more dense in more severe aortic regurgitation (165).

Management

Timing of Surgery

Recommendations for the timing of surgery in patients with relatively asymptomatic aortic regurgitation must be made individually based on the benefits and risks of the surgical and the medical approaches. AVR should be recommended if the patient either becomes symptomatic or if echocardiography demonstrates that LV dysfunction is developing, indicated by an end-systolic diameter approaching 50 to 55 mm or by an EF of less than 0.55.

Severe chronic aortic regurgitation may be tolerated for years in many patients; however, the combined LV pressure and volume overload eventually leads to muscle damage and LV dysfunction. Aortic valve surgery should be performed when symptoms develop, even NYHA class II symptoms of CHF. Surgery should also be performed in the asymptomatic patients with contractile dysfunction (166–169). However, individual differences among patients in loading conditions and the patient's hemodynamic response to aortic regurgitation confound standard clinical indices of contractile dysfunction, such as EF. Despite these problems, reliable guides to the timing of surgery have been developed.

Use of Echocardiography

Echocardiography interrogation of LV size and function, as a repeatable, noninvasive method, has become preeminent in predicting outcome and in timing surgery. Shortening fraction and systolic diameter, the minor axis one-dimensional equivalents of EF, and end-systolic volume, respectively, are the most useful indices for predicting outcome in patients with chronic minimally symptomatic aortic regurgitation (166–169). A shortening fraction less of than 27% or a resting EF of less than 55% should prompt consideration of AVR, even in the asymptomatic patient. End-systolic diameter or volume, indices that are more preload independent than EF, have also proved helpful in timing surgery (166–168). When the end-systolic diameter is 50 mm or greater, surgery should be strongly considered; postoperative survival is significantly decreased when it is 55 mm or larger. If surgery is performed within 18 months or so after these thresholds are crossed, systolic function is likely to return to normal (170). Regarding frequency of follow-up echocardiographic studies, when the end-systolic diameter is less than 40 mm, echocardiography should be performed biannually, when it is 40 to 50 mm, yearly follow-up is recommended (167).

Use of Exercise Ejection Fraction

Use of exercise EF (171) for the timing of surgery in asymptomatic or minimally symptomatic patients with aortic regurgitation is predicated on finding a fall in exercise EF, which may indicate an exhaustion of myocardial reserve, as opposed to the normal increase in EF with exercise. However, this parameter is controversial because a fall in EF may also result from changes in loading conditions that occur during exercise, especially when excessive afterload and hypertension develop during exercise owing to failure to vasodilate and decrease peripheral resistance.

Aortic Valve Replacement and Repair

Today, surgical treatment of most cases of aortic regurgitation entails valve replacement. Options for aortic valve surgery include (a) bioprosthetic valves of the standard stented variety; (b) mechanical prosthetic valves; (c) homograft valves; (d) pulmonary autografts; (e) stentless bioprosthetic valves; and (f) aortic valve repair. Transthoracic echocardiography may be used to determine anatomic information that may predict the likelihood of which surgical option can be used, particularly important in valve repair.

AVR is performed identically as discussed in the section on AS. However, unlike the situation in AS, valve repair may be possible in some patients with aortic regurgitation. The best candidates for successful aortic valve repair are a highly selected group with one of three types of anatomy: a structurally normal valve with aortic dilation, a simple valve perforation, or a noncalcified valve with aortic regurgitation owing to prolapse.

Successful aortic valve repair has been reported in a highly selected group of patients with bileaflet valves that are not calcified where aortic regurgitation is caused by prolapse. A V-shaped wedge of the edge of the prolapsing leaflet and the commissures are plicated to improves leaflet coaptation (172,173).

In some rare patients, aortic regurgitation may be caused by leaflet perforation, with otherwise normal leaflets. Although leaflet destruction is also common in that group, isolated perforations may occur in infectious endocarditis. In these cases, the leaflet may be repaired with small patches of pericardium sutured over the perforation.

In patients with aortic root dilation with normal aortic leaflets (174), the valve often can be resuspended at the time of aortic root replacement with a conduit (see Fig. 23.20) whether in the supracoronary position or with reconstruction of the sinuses of Valsalva (175).

In any technically more difficult aortic valve surgery, such as valve repair, the Ross procedure, or aortic homograft implantation, results should be assessed immediately in the operating room with transesophageal echocardiography to detect unsuccessful repair. This intraoperative echocardiography provides a safety net, allowing further surgery to be performed during the same thoracotomy to ensure a good clinical outcome.

Medical Therapy

Use of vasodilators, such as hydralazine, nifedipine, and angiotensin-converting enzyme inhibitors, in treating patients with asymptomatic chronic aortic regurgitation is controversial, especially the debate over whether that therapy forestalls the development of LV dysfunction. The premise is that arteriolar vasodilation reduces regurgitant flow and diminishes the aortic regurgitation severity. In a randomized 2-year study of hydralazine (176), asymptomatic patients given hydralazine had less ventricular dilation and better ejection performance than did a placebo group. Similar results have been reported with angiotensin-converting enzyme inhibitors (177). Nifedipine delayed the time when surgery was required (178) and improved 10-year survival and EF after surgery (179). However a more recent study found no efficacy of vasodilators in chronic aortic regurgitation (180). Thus, there is still controversy regarding long-term use of vasodilators in asymptomatic patients with severe, chronic aortic regurgitation who do not yet have LV dysfunction or other clear indications for surgery.

ACUTE AORTIC REGURGITATION

Background

Severe, acute aortic regurgitation frequently constitutes a surgical emergency. Mortality may be as high as 75% in medically treated patients, but is only 25% with surgery. Thus, recognition of acute aortic regurgitation and its proper management are crucial in ensuring good patient outcomes (181).

Etiology

Infective Endocarditis

The most common cause of acute aortic regurgitation, acute infective endocarditis, may develop on a previously bicuspid valve or a normal valve, especially if aggressive organisms, such as *Staphylococcus aureus* or *enterococcus*, are the etiologic agents. Often mistaken for influenza, the sudden development of a high fever, malaise, and the early symptoms of CHF should be given immediate attention. Cutaneous manifestations of endocarditis, systemic emboli, a new or changing aortic regurgitation murmur, bacteremia, and vegetations by echocardiography are elements of the diagnosis (see Chapter 26) (182,183).

Aortic Dissection

The other major cause of acute aortic regurgitation, acute proximal aortic dissection, causes some additional hemodynamic manifestations; hemopericardium with tamponade, myocardial infarction from coronary dissection, or aortic rupture, often more problematic than aortic regurgitation itself.

Pathophysiology

In contrast to chronic aortic regurgitation, with its large total SV and wide pulse pressure causing the bedside physical signs, in acute regurgitation, the eccentric LVH and compensatory LV dilation have not yet developed. Indeed, the only clue that this deadly disease is present may be the new murmur of aortic regurgitation (184), which may be quite short in early diastole because of rapid equilibration of LV and aortic pressures. In acute severe aortic regurgitation, the first heart sound (S1) may be soft because the high LV diastolic pressure closes the mitral valve before the onset of LV systole, an ominous sign that often indicates the need for urgent surgery.

Management

Echocardiography

Once acute aortic regurgitation is suspected, echocardiography should be performed immediately to help determine the etiology and severity of the valve dysfunction. Vegetations are key to the diagnosis in endocarditis. In aortic dissection, enlargement of the aorta, and the intimal flap separating flow (by color Doppler) in the true and false lumens, which may be better shown by transesophageal than transthoracic echocardiography (Chapter 52). M-mode echocardiography may demonstrate premature mitral closure as a sign of high LV diastolic pressure (185) and Doppler may show diastolic mitral regurgitation. Transesophageal echocardiography is particularly helpful in diagnosing endocarditis, perivalvular abscesses, and aortic dissection (182,183).

Medical Therapy

In suspected endocarditis, multiple blood cultures should be drawn before antibiotics are started. Thereafter, broad-spectrum antibiotics are begun empirically and are adjusted later when blood cultures identify the least toxic antibiotic regimen to which the organism is sensitive. In the absence of CHF, mitral preclosure, emboli, and progressive heart block, endocarditis patients with severe aortic regurgitation may be followed medically, with careful daily assessment for progression. Prolongation of the PR interval is an early sign of aortic ring abscess. Repeat echocardiography is useful to look for changes in vegetation size and worsening of aortic regurgitation. Vasodilator therapy may stabilize hemodynamics, but should not be used to delay surgery.

Surgical Therapy

Although there is always a concern that early implantation of a prosthesis in an infected patient may lead to prosthetic endocarditis, persistence of infection occurs in 10%, irrespective of timing of surgery (186). Therefore, once the need for surgery is established further delay is unwarranted and risks spread of the infection or embolization. In patients with extension of the infection into tissue around the aortic valve (annular ring abscess), an aortic homograft may be advantageous because it has reduced postoperative infection (187).

CONTROVERSIES AND PERSONAL PERSPECTIVES

Aortic Valve Replacement in Asymptomatic Aortic Stenosis Patients

Change has occurred recently in our understanding of the optimum time for surgery for AS (70,93) mostly because of improved surgical techniques and improved definition of the disease process. The question has arisen whether asymptomatic patients should have surgery. The 0.5% annual risk of sudden death without surgery (31) must be weighted against the mortality and morbidity of AVR. Although most patients have antecedent symptoms, many patients have insufficient symptoms to bring them to medical attention before death, an outcome just as bad as sudden mortal collapse.

Patients with LV dysfunction and AS who are asymptomatic pose the problem of whether the latter is the cause of the former. When AS is severe and no other cause of the myocardial process is evident, one should assume causality and proceed with surgery.

Factors associated with worse prognosis include severe valvular calcification and a rapid increase in aortic jet velocity over several echo studies (33). BNP and *N*-terminal BNP are elevated in proportion to severity of AS and symptomatic status (188,189). BNP decreases after successful surgery (190). BNP serum level above 66 pg/mL detected symptomatic patients and those at risk for cardiovascular death (188). Patients with elevated LDL or C-reactive protein have a higher risk of rapid AS progression.

Exercise stress testing in AS may reveal latent symptoms or hemodynamic instability, as a way of predicting future outcome. In patients who minimize their symptoms, exercise-limiting symptoms may be revealed by provocative testing (191).

In summary, as the risk for adverse outcomes within a few years with medical management becomes greater than the risk of surgery, early valve replacement in selected asymptomatic patients is appropriate. Elective surgery may be worth considering in asymptomatic patients whose stress tests show cardiac symptoms, hypotension, or ventricular tachycardia; and in those with elevated biomarkers, significant valve calcification, LV dysfunction, concomitant coronary disease, and rapid progression of aortic jet velocity. At a minimum, these patients require aggressive primary prevention and closer follow-up than other patients (192).

THE FUTURE

Future research regarding factors contributing to the "atherosclerosis-like" process of AS will fuel prevention strategies. Innovations in cardiac surgery and perioperative medical management will promote the ongoing trend for less perioperative mortality and morbidity. Surgery should not be put off until the patient's symptoms cannot be managed medically. New valvular replacement options will become more physiologic, with less prosthetic valve "penalty" in terms of persistent gradients, postoperative hypertrophy, and limited durability.

Percutaneous valve replacement has gone from the drawing board (193,194) to the pilot phase (195,196) and will become a reality for highly selected patients. It is uncertain whether percutaneous valve replacement will have any role for surgical candidates, like balloon valvotomy for mitral stenosis. At this point, percutaneous valve replacement is mostly a rescue procedure for desperately ill patients, similar to percutaneous balloon valvotomy for AS.

Reoperations for a second, third, or even sixth time will continue to become more common and with acceptable operative risk. Noninvasive monitoring of valve hemodynamics will allow further understanding of the disease processes affecting the aortic valve. All these factors will further improve the prognosis for patients with aortic valve disease. The progress continues.

ACKNOWLEDGMENT

We are indebted to Fred A. Crawford, Jr, MD, who contributed to the first edition of this chapter, published in the first edition of this book in 1998. His wisdom and experience are still an integral part of this manuscript.

References

1. Lindblom D, Lindblom U, Qvist J, Lundstrom H. Long-term relative survival rates after heart valve replacement. *J Am Coll Cardiol* 1990;15:566.
2. Hatle L. Noninvasive assessment and differentiation of left ventricular outflow obstruction with Doppler ultrasound. *Circulation* 1981;64:381–387.
3. Hegrenaes L, Hatle L. Aortic stenosis in adults: noninvasive estimation of pressure differences by continuous wave Doppler echocardiography. *Br Heart J* 1985;54:396–404.
4. Skjaerpe T, Hegrenaes L, Hatle L. Noninvasive estimation of valve area in patients with aortic stenosis by Doppler ultrasound and two-dimensional echocardiography. *Circulation* 1985;72:810–881.
5. Harken DE, Soroff HS, Taylor WJ, et al. Partial and complete prostheses in aortic insufficiency. *J Thorac Cardiovasc Surg* 1960;40:744.
6. Ross DN. Homograft replacement of the aortic valve. *Lancet* 1962;2:487.
7. Ross DN. Replacement of aortic and mitral valves with a pulmonary autograft. *Lancet* 1967;2:956.
8. Carpentier A, Lemaigre G, Robert L, et al. Biologic factors affecting long-term results of valvular heterografts. *J Thorac Cardiovasc Surg* 1969;58: 467.
9. Ionescu MI, Pakrashi BC, Holden MP, et al. Results of aortic valve replacement with frame-supported fascia lata and pericardial grafts. *J Thorac Cardiovasc Surg* 1972;64:340.
10. Cosgrove DM, Lytle BW, Taylor PC, et al. The Carpentier-Edwards pericardial aortic valve: ten-year results. *J Thorac Cardiovasc Surg* 1995;110: 653.
11. Passik CS, Ackermann DM, Pluth JR, et al. Temporal changes in the causes of aortic stenosis: a surgical pathologic study of 646 cases. *Mayo Clin Proc* 1987;62:119.
12. Fenoglio JJ Jr, McAllister HA Jr, DeCastro CM, et al. Congenital bicuspid aortic valve after age 20. *Am J Cardiol* 1977;39:164.
13. Roberts WC. The congenitally bicuspid aortic valve: a study of 85 autopsy cases. *Am J Cardiol* 1970;26:72.
14. Campbell M. Calcific aortic stenosis and congenital bicuspid aortic valves. *Br Heart J* 1968;30:606–616.
15. Otto CM, Kuusisto J, Reichenbach DD, et al. Characterization of the early lesion of "degenerative" valvular aortic stenosis: histological and immunohistochemical studies. *Circulation* 1994;90:844.
16. Juvonen J, Laurila A, Juvonen T, et al. Detection of *Chlamydia pneumoniae* in human nonrheumatic stenotic aortic valves. *J Am Coll Cardiol* 1997; 29:1054–1059.
17. Wierzbicki A, Shetty C. Aortic stenosis: an atherosclerotic disease? *J Heart Valve Dis* 1999;8:416–423.
18. Carabello BA. Aortic sclerosis—a window to the coronary arteries? *N Engl J Med* 1999;341:193–195.
19. Otto CM, Lind BK, Kitzman DW, et al. Association of aortic-valve sclerosis with cardiovascular mortality and morbidity in the elderly. *N Engl J Med* 1999;341:142–147.
20. Stewart BF, Siscovick D, Lind BK, et al. Clinical factors associated with calcific aortic valve disease. Cardiovascular Health Study. *J Am Coll Cardiol* 1997;29:630–634.
21. Rallidis L, Naoumova RP, Thompson GR, et al. Extent and severity of atherosclerotic involvement of the aortic valve and root in familial hypercholesterolaemia. *Heart* 1998;80:583–590.

22. Heidenreich PA, Hancock SL, Lee BK, et al. Asymptomatic cardiac disease following mediastinal irradiation. *J Am Coll Cardiol* 2003;42:743–749.
23. Kim YM, Yoo SJ, Choi JY, et al. Natural course of supravalvar aortic stenosis and peripheral pulmonary arterial stenosis in Williams' syndrome. *Cardiol Young* 1999;9:37–41.
24. Donner RM, Carabello BA, Black I, et al. Left ventricular wall stress in compensated aortic stenosis in children. *Am J Cardiol* 1983;51:946.
25. Assey ME, Wisenbaugh T, Spann JF Jr, et al. Unexpected persistence into adulthood of low wall-stress in patients with congenital aortic stenosis: is there a fundamental difference in the hypertrophic response to a pressure overload present from birth? *Circulation* 1987;75:973.
26. Keane JF, Driscoll DJ, Gersony WM, et al. Second natural history study of congenital heart defects: results of treatment of patients with aortic valvular stenosis. *Circulation* 1993;87[Suppl 2]:116.
27. Witsenburg M, Cromme-Dijkhuis AH, Frohn-Mulder IM, et al. Short- and midterm results of balloon valvuloplasty for valvular aortic stenosis in children. *Am J Cardiol* 1992;69:945.
28. Ross J Jr, Braunwald E. Aortic stenosis. *Circulation* 1968;38[Suppl 5]:61–67.
29. Kelly TA, Rothbart RM, Cooper CM, et al. Comparison of outcome of asymptomatic to symptomatic patients older than 20 years of age with valvular aortic stenosis. *Am J Cardiol* 1988;61:123.
30. Pellikka PA, Nishimura RA, Bailey KR, et al. The natural history of adults with asymptomatic, hemodynamically significant aortic stenosis. *J Am Coll Cardiol* 1990;15:1012.
31. Pellikka PA, Sarano ME, Nishimura RA, et al. Outcome of 622 adults with asymptomatic, hemodynamically significant aortic stenosis during prolonged follow-up. *Circulation* 2005;111:3290–3295.
32. Lombard JT, Selzer A. Valvular aortic stenosis: a clinical and hemodynamic profile of patients. *Ann Intern Med* 1987;106:292.
33. Rosenhek R, Binder T, Porenta G, et al. Predictors of outcome in severe, asymptomatic aortic stenosis. *N Engl J Med* 2000;343:611–617.
34. Bahler RC, Desser DR, Finkelhor RS, et al. Factors leading to progression of valvular aortic stenosis. *Am J Cardiol* 1999;84:1044–1048.
35. Otto CM, Burwash IG, Legget ME, et al. Prospective study of asymptomatic valvular aortic stenosis. *Circulation* 1997;95:2262–2270.
36. Palta S, Pai AM, Gill KS, et al. New insights into the progression of aortic stenosis: implications for secondary prevention. *Circulation* 2000;101:2497–2502.
37. Grossman W, Jones D, McLaurin LP. Wall stress and patterns of hypertrophy in the human left ventricle. *J Clin Invest* 1975;56:56.
38. Hamawaki M, Coffman TM, Lashus A, et al. Pressure-overload hypertrophy is unabated in mice devoid of AT1A receptors. *Am J Physiol* 1998;274[3 Pt 2]:H868–H873.
39. Koide M, Carabello BA, Conrad CC, et al. Hypertrophic response to hemodynamic overload: role of load vs. renin-angiotensin system activation. *Am J Physiol* 1999;276[2 Pt 2]:H350–H358.
40. Nagatomo Y, Carabello BA, Coker ML, et al. Differential effects of pressure or volume overload on myocardial MMP levels and inhibitory control. *Am J Physiol Heart Circ Physiol* 2000;278:H151–H161.
41. Gould KL, Carabello BA. Why angina in aortic stenosis with normal coronary arteriograms? *Circulation* 2003;107:3121–3123.
42. Marcus ML, Doty DB, Hiratzka LF, et al. Decreased coronary reserve: a mechanism for angina pectoris in patients with aortic stenosis and normal coronary arteries. *N Engl J Med* 1982;307:1362–1367.
43. Dunn RB, Griggs DM. Ventricular filling pressure as a determinant of coronary blood flow during ischemia. *Am J Physiol* 1983;244:H429.
44. Breisch EA, Houser SR, Carey RA, et al. Myocardial blood flow and capillary density in chronic pressure overload of the feline left ventricle. *Cardiovasc Res* 1980;14:469.
45. Rajappan K, Rimoldi OE, Camici PG, et al. Functional changes in coronary microcirculation after valve replacement in patients with aortic stenosis. *Circulation* 2003;107:3170–3175.
46. Gould LK, Carabello BA. Why angina in aortic stenosis with normal coronary arteriograms? *Circulation* 2003;107:3121–3123.
47. Julius BK, Spillman M, Vassali G, et al. Angina pectoris in patients with aortic stenosis and normal coronary arteries: mechanisms and pathophysiologic concepts. *Circulation* 1997;95:892–898.
48. Strauer BE. Ventricular function and coronary hemodynamics in hypertensive heart disease. *Am J Cardiol* 1979;44:999.
49. Schwartz LS, Goldfischer J, Sprague GJ, et al. Syncope and sudden death in aortic stenosis. *Am J Cardiol* 1969;23:647.
50. Richards AM, Nicholls MG, Ikram A, et al. Syncope in aortic valvular stenosis. *Lancet* 1984;2:1113.
51. Peterson KL, Tsuji J, Johnson A, et al. Diastolic left ventricular pressure-volume and stress-strain relations in patients with valvular aortic stenosis and left ventricular hypertrophy. *Circulation* 1978;58:77.
52. Hess OM, Ritter M, Schneider J, et al. Diastolic stiffness and myocardial structure in aortic valve disease before and after valve replacement. *Circulation* 1984;69:855.
53. Huber D, Grimm J, Koch R, et al. Determinants of ejection performance in aortic stenosis. *Circulation* 1981;64:126.
54. Lorell BH, Carabello BA. Left ventricular hypertrophy: pathogenesis, detection, and prognosis. *Circulation* 2000;102:470–479.
55. Koide M, Nagatsu M, Zile MR, et al. Premorbid determinants of left ventricular dysfunction in a novel model of gradually induced pressure overload in the adult canine. *Circulation* 1997;95:1601–1610.
56. Herzig JW, Ruegg JC, Solaro RJ. Myocardial excitation contraction coupling as influenced through modulation of the calcium sensitivity of the contractile proteins. *Heart Failure* 1991;6:244.
57. Nakano K, Corin WJ, Spann JF Jr, et al. Abnormal subendocardial blood flow in pressure overload hypertrophy is associated with pacing-induced subendocardial dysfunction. *Circ Res* 1989;65:1555.
58. Tsutsui H, Ishihara K, Cooper G IV. Cytoskeletal role in the contractile dysfunction of hypertrophied myocardium. *Science* 1993;260:682.
59. Tagawa H, Koide M, Sato H, et al. Cytoskeletal role in the transition from compensated to decompensated hypertrophy during adult canine left ventricular pressure overloading. *Circ Res* 1998;82:751–761.
60. Koide M, Hamawaki M, Narishige T, et al. Microtubule depolymerization normalizes in vivo myocardial contractile function in dogs with pressure-overload left ventricular hypertrophy. *Circulation* 2000;102:1045–1052.
61. Gjertsson P, Caidahl K, Farasati M, et al. Preoperative moderate to severe diastolic dysfunction: a novel Doppler echocardiographic long-term prognostic factor in patients with severe aortic stenosis. *J Thorac Cardiovasc Surg* 2005;129:890–896.
62. Bruch C, Schmermund A, Dagres N, et al. Severe aortic valve stenosis with preserved and reduced systolic left ventricular function: diagnostic usefulness of the Tei index. *J Am Soc Echocardiogr* 2002;15:869–876.
63. Pate GE, Chandavimol M, Naiman SC, et al. Heyde's syndrome: a review. *J Heart Valve Dis* 2004;13:701–712.
64. Batur P, Stewart WJ, Isaacson H. Increased prevalence of aortic stenosis in patients with arteriovenous malformations of the gastrointestinal tract in Heyde syndrome. *Arch Intern Med* 2003;163:1821–1824.
65. Gorlin R, Gorlin SG. Hydraulic formula for calculation of the area of the stenotic mitral valve, other cardiac valves, and central circulatory shunts. *Am Heart J* 1951;41:1.
66. Blumberg FC, Pfeifer M, Holmer SR, et al. Quantification of aortic stenosis in mechanically ventilated patients using multiplane transesophageal Doppler echocardiography. *Chest* 1998;114:94–97.
67. Assey ME, Usher BW, Carabello BA, et al. The patient with valvular heart disease. In: Pepine CJ, Hill JA, Lambert CR, eds. *Diagnostic and therapeutic cardiac catheterization,* 2nd ed. Baltimore: Williams & Wilkins, 1989:471–507.
68. Brener SJ, Duffy CI, Thomas JD, et al. Progression of aortic stenosis in 394 patients. Relation to changes in myocardial and mitral valve dysfunction. *J Am Coll Cardiol* 1995;25:305–310.
69. Otto CM, Pearlman AS, Gardner CL. Hemodynamic progression of aortic stenosis in adults assessed by Doppler echocardiography. *J Am Coll Cardiol* 1989;13:545.
70. Carabello B. Evaluation and management of patients with aortic stenosis. *Circulation* 2002;105:1746–1750.
71. Wyatt H, Heng MK, Meerbaum S, et al. Cross-sectional echocardiography: I. Analysis of mathematic models for quantifying mass of the left ventricle in dogs. *Circulation* 1977;60:1104–1110.
72. Warth DC, Stewart WJ, Bloch PC, et al. A new method to calculate aortic valve area without left heart catheterization. *Circulation* 1984;70:978–983.
73. Currie PJ, Seward JB, Reeder GS, et al. Continuous-wave Doppler echocardiographic assessment of severity of calcific aortic stenosis: a simultaneous Doppler-catheter correlative study in 100 adult patients. *Circulation* 1985;71:1162.
74. Vanoverschelde JL, Essamri B, Michel X, et al. Hemodynamic and volume correlates of left ventricular diastolic relaxation and filling in patients with aortic stenosis. *J Am Coll Cardiol* 1992;20:813–821.
75. ACC/AHA guidelines for the management of patients with valvular heart disease. A report of the American College of Cardiology/American Heart Association. Task Force on Practice Guidelines (Committee on Management of Patients with Valvular Heart Disease). *J Am Coll Cardiol* 1998;32:1486–1588.
76. Schlant RC, Friesinger GC II, Leonard JJ. Clinical competence in exercise testing: a statement for physicians from the ACP/ACC/AHA Task Force on Clinical Privileges in Cardiology. *J Am Coll Cardiol* 1990;16:1061.
77. Areskog NH. Exercise testing in the evaluation of patients with valvular aortic stenosis. *Clin Physiol* 1984;4:201.
78. Linderholm H, Osterman G, Teien D. Detection of coronary artery disease by means of exercise ECG in patients with aortic stenosis. *Acta Med Scand* 1985;218:181.
79. Samuels B, Kiat H, Friedman JD, et al. Adenosine pharmacological stress myocardial perfusion tomographic imaging in patients with significant aortic stenosis: diagnostic efficacy and comparison of clinical, hemodynamic, and electrocardiographic variables with 100 age-matched control subjects. *J Am Coll Cardiol* 1995;25:99.
80. deFilippi CR, Willett DL, Brickner E, et al. Usefulness of dobutamine echocardiography in distinguishing severe from nonsevere valvular aortic stenosis in patients with depressed left ventricular function and low transvalvular gradients. *Am J Cardiol* 1995;75:191.
81. Pop C, Metz D, Tassan-Mangina S, et al. Dobutamine Doppler echocardiography in severe aortic stenosis with left ventricular dysfunction. Comparison with postoperative examination. *Arch Mal Coeur Vaiss* 1999;92:1487–1493.

82. Popovic AD, Thomas JD, Neskovic AN, et al. Time-related trends in the preoperative evaluation of patients with valvular stenosis. *Am J Cardiol* 1997;80:1464–1468.
83. Roger V, Tajik AJ, Reeder GS, et al. Effect of Doppler echocardiography on utilization of hemodynamic cardiac catheterization in the preoperative evaluation of aortic stenosis. *Mayo Clin Proc* 1996;71:141–149.
84. Vandeplas A, Willems JL, Piessens J, et al. Frequency of angina pectoris and coronary artery disease in severe isolated valvular aortic stenosis. *Am J Cardiol* 1988;62:117.
85. Garcia-Rubira JC, Lopez V, Cubero J. Coronary arterial disease in patients with severe isolated aortic stenosis. *Int J Cardiol* 1992;35:121.
86. Alexopoulos D, Kolovou G, Kyriakidis M, et al. Angina and coronary artery disease in patients with aortic valve disease. *Angiology* 1993;44:707.
87. Lytle BW. Impact of coronary artery disease on valvular heart surgery. *Cardiol Clin* 1991;9:301.
88. Czer LS, Gray RJ, Stewart ME, et al. Reduction in sudden late death by concomitant revascularization with aortic valve replacement. *J Thorac Cardiovasc Surg* 1988;95:390.
89. Di Lello F, Flemma RJ, Anderson AJ, et al. Improved early results after aortic valve replacement analysis by surgical time frame. *Ann Thorac Surg* 1989;47:51.
90. Novaro GM, Tiong IY, Pearce GL, et al. Effect of hydroxymethylglutaryl coenzyme A reductase inhibitors on the progression of calcific aortic stenosis. *Circulation* 2001;104:2205–2209.
91. Rosenhek R, Rader F, Loho N, et al. Statins but not angiotensin-converting enzyme inhibitors delay progression of aortic stenosis. *Circulation* 2004;110:1291.
92. Cowell SJ, Newby DE, Prescott RJ, et al. A randomized trial of intensive lipid-lowering therapy in calcific aortic stenosis. *N Engl J Med* 2005;352:2389–2397.
93. Carabello BA. Timing of valve replacement in aortic stenosis. Moving closer to perfection. *Circulation* 1997;95:2241–2243.
94. Safian RD, Berman AD, Diver DJ, et al. Balloon aortic valvuloplasty in 170 consecutive patients. *N Engl J Med* 1988;319:125.
95. Litvack F, Jakubowski AT, Buchbinder NA, et al. Lack of sustained clinical improvement in an elderly population after percutaneous aortic valvuloplasty. *Am J Cardiol* 1988;62:270.
96. Otto CM, Mickel MC, Kennedy JW, et al. Three-year outcome after balloon aortic valvuloplasty: insights into prognosis of valvular aortic stenosis. *Circulation* 1994;89:642–650.
97. Cosgrove DM, Sabik JF. Minimally invasive approach for aortic valve operations. *Ann Thorac Surg* 1996;62:596–597.
98. Munt BI, Legget ME, Healy NL, et al. Effects of aortic valve replacement on exercise duration and functional status in adults with valvular aortic stenosis. *Can J Cardiol* 1997;13:346–350.
99. Akins CW. Results with mechanical cardiac valvular prostheses. *Ann Thorac Surg* 1995;60:1836.
100. Emery RW, Arom KV, Nicoloff DM. Utilization of the St. Jude medical prosthesis in the aortic position. *Semin Thorac Cardiovasc Surg* 1996;8:231.
101. Copeland JG. The Carbo-Medics prosthetic heart valve: a second generation bileaflet prosthesis. *Semin Thorac Cardiovasc Surg* 1996;8:237.
102. Akins CW. Medtronic-Hall prosthetic aortic valve. *Semin Thorac Cardiovasc Surg* 1996;8:242.
103. Hammermeister K, Sethi GK, Henderson WG, et al. Outcomes 15 years after valve replacement with a mechanical versus a bioprosthetic valve: final report of the veterans affairs randomized trial. *J Am Coll Cardiol* 2000;36:1152–1158.
104. Jamieson WR, Munro IA, Miyagishima RT, et al. Carpentier-Edwards standard porcine bioprosthesis: clinical performance to seventeen years. *Ann Thorac Surg* 1995;60:999.
105. Yun KL, Miller DC, Moore KA, et al. Durability of the Hancock MO bioprosthesis compared with standard aortic valve bioprostheses. *Ann Thorac Surg* 1995;60:S221.
106. Fann JI, Miller DC. Porcine valves: Hancock and Carpentier-Edwards aortic prostheses. *Semin Thorac Cardiovasc Surg* 1996;8:259.
107. Aupart MR, Sirinelli AL, Diemont FF, et al. The last generation of pericardial valves in the aortic position: ten-year follow-up in 589 patients. *Ann Thorac Surg* 1996;61:615.
108. Cosgrove DM. Carpentier pericardial valve. *Semin Thorac Cardiovasc Surg* 1996;8:269.
109. Jones EL, Shah VB, Shanewise JS, et al. Should the freehand allograft be abandoned as a reliable alternative for aortic valve replacement? *Ann Thorac Surg* 1995;59:1397.
110. Doty DB. Aortic valve replacement with homograft and autograft. *Semin Thorac Cardiovasc Surg* 1996;8:249.
111. Barratt-Boyes BG, Roche AHG, Subramanyan R, et al. Long-term follow-up of patients with antibiotic-sterilized aortic homograft inserted freehand in the aortic position. *Circulation* 1987;75:768–777.
112. Clarke DR, Campbell DN, Hayward AR, et al. Degeneration of aortic valve allografts in young recipients. *J Thorac Cardiovasc Surg* 1993;105:934.
113. Ross DN. Evolution of the homograft valve. *Ann Thorac Surg* 1995;59:565.
114. Gerosa G, Ross DN, Brucke PE, et al. Aortic valve replacement with pulmonary homografts: early experience. *J Thorac Cardiovasc Surg* 1994;107:424.
115. Elkins RC. Congenital aortic valve disease: evolving management. *Ann Thorac Surg* 1995;59:269.
116. David TE, Feindel CM, Bos J, et al. Aortic valve replacement with a stentless porcine aortic valve: a six-year experience. *J Thorac Cardiovasc Surg* 1994;108:1030.
117. Kon ND, Westaby S, Amarasena N, et al. Comparison of implantation techniques using freestyle stentless porcine aortic valve. *Ann Thorac Surg* 1995;59:857.
118. Kratz JM, Sade RM, Crawford FA Jr, et al. The risk of small St. Jude aortic valve prostheses. *Ann Thorac Surg* 1994;59:1114.
119. Li M, Dumesnil JG, Mathieu P, et al. Impact of valve prosthesis-patient mismatch on pulmonary arterial pressure after mitral valve replacement. *J Am Coll Cardiol* 2005;45:1034–1040.
120. Flais C, Dumesnil JG, Simard S, et al. Impact of valve prosthesis-patient mismatch on short-term mortality after aortic valve replacement. *Circulation* 2003: 108;983–988.
121. Nicks R, Cartmill T, Bernstein L. Hypoplasia of the aortic root: the problem of aortic valve replacement. *Thorax* 1970;25:339.
122. Manouguian S, Seybold-Epting W. Patch enlargement of the aortic valve ring by extending the aortic incision into the anterior mitral leaflet. *J Thorac Cardiovasc Surg* 1979;78:402.
123. Konno S, Imai Y, Iida Y, et al. A new method for prosthetic valve replacement in congenital aortic stenosis associated with hypoplasia of the aortic valve ring. *J Thorac Cardiovasc Surg* 1975;70:909.
124. Niederberger J, Schima H, Maurer G, et al. Importance of pressure recovery for the assessment of aortic stenosis by Doppler ultrasound: role of aortic size, aortic valve area, and direction of the stenotic jet in vitro. *Circulation* 1996;94:1934–1940.
125. Baumgartner H, Stefenelli T, Niederberger J, et al. "Overestimation" of catheter gradients by Doppler ultrasound in patients with aortic stenosis: a predictable manifestation of pressure recovery. *J Am Coll Cardiol* 1999;33:1655–1661.
126. Horstkotte D, Burckhardt D. Prosthetic valve thrombosis. *J Heart Valve Dis* 1995;4:141.
127. Birdi I, Angelini GD, Bryan AJ. Thrombolytic therapy for left-sided prosthetic heart valve thrombosis. *J Heart Valve Dis* 1995;4:154.
128. Agnihotri AK, McGriffin DC, Galbraith AJ, et al. The prevalence of infective endocarditis after aortic valve replacement. *J Thorac Cardiovasc Surg* 1995;110:1708.
129. Khan S, Chaux A, Matloff J, et al. The St. Jude medical valve: experience with 1000 cases. *J Thorac Cardiovasc Surg* 1994;108:1010.
130. Baudet EM, Puel V, McBride JT, et al. Long-term results of valve replacement with the St. Jude medical prosthesis. *J Thorac Cardiovasc Surg* 1995;109:858.
131. Fiane AE, Saatvedt K, Svennevig JL, et al. The CarboMedics valve: midterm follow-up with analysis of risk factors. *Ann Thorac Surg* 1995;60:1053.
132. Masters RG, Pipe AL, Walley VM, et al. Comparative results of the St. Jude medical and Medtronic-Hall mechanical valves. *J Thorac Cardiovasc Surg* 1995;110:663.
133. Akins CW. Long-term results with the Medtronic-Hall valvular prosthesis. *Ann Thorac Surg* 1996;61:806.
134. Carabello BA, Green LH, Grossman W, et al. Hemodynamic determinants of prognosis of aortic valve replacement in critical aortic stenosis and advanced congestive heart failure. *Circulation* 1980;62:42.
135. Carroll JD, Carroll EP, Feldman T, et al. Sex-associated differences in left ventricular function in aortic stenosis of the elderly. *Circulation* 1992;86:1099.
136. Aurigemma GP, Silver KH, McLaughlin M, et al. Impact of chamber geometry and gender on left ventricular systolic function in patients >60 years of age with aortic stenosis. *Am J Cardiol* 1994;74:794.
137. Smith N, McAnulty JH, Rahimtoola SH. Severe aortic stenosis with impaired left ventricular function and clinical heart failure: results of valve replacement. *Circulation* 1978;58:255.
137a. Tam JW, Masters RG, Burwash IG, et al. Management of patients with mild aortic stenosis undergoing coronary artery bypass grafting. *Ann Thorac Surg* 1998;65:1215–1219.
138. Lund O. Preoperative risk evaluation and stratification of long-term survival after valve replacement for aortic stenosis: reasons for earlier operative intervention. *Circulation* 1990;82:124.
139. Brogan WC III, Grayburn PA, Lange RA, et al. Prognosis after valve replacement in patients with severe aortic stenosis and a low transvalvular pressure gradient. *J Am Coll Cardiol* 1993;21:1657.
140. Connolly HM, Oh JK, Orszulak TA, et al. Aortic valve replacement for aortic stenosis with severe left ventricular dysfunction. *Circulation* 1999;795:2395–2400.
141. Connolly HM, Oh JK, Schaff HV, et al. Severe aortic stenosis with low transvalvular gradient and severe left ventricular dysfunction, result of aortic valve replacement in 52 patients. *Circulation* 2000;101:1940–1946.
142. Pereira J, Lauer MS, Bashir M, et al. Survival after aortic valve replacement for severe aortic stenosis with low transvalvular gradients and severe left ventricular dysfunction. *J Am Coll Cardiol* 2002;39:1356–1363.
143. Carabello BA, Ballard WL, Gazes PC. Patient #65. In: Sahn SA, Heffner JE, eds. *Cardiology pearls*. Philadelphia: Hanley & Belfus, 1994: 142.

144. Carabello BA, Crawford FA. Valvular heart disease. *N Engl J Med* 1997; 337:32–41.
145. Marcus R, Bednarz J, Abruzzo J, et al. Mechanism underlying flow-dependency of valve orifice area determined by the Gorlin formula in patients with aortic valve obstruction. *Circulation* 1993;88:I-103.
146. Schwammenthal E, Vered Z, Moshkowitz Y, et al. Dobutamine echocardiography in patients with aortic stenosis and left ventricular dysfunction: predicting outcome as a function of management strategy. *Chest* 2001; 119:1766–1777.
147. Nishimura RA, Grantham JA, Connolly HM, et al. Low-output, low-gradient aortic stenosis in patients with depressed left ventricular systolic function: the clinical utility of the dobutamine challenge in the catheterization laboratory. *Circulation* 2002;106:809–813.
148. Monin JL, Monchi M, Gest V, et al. Aortic stenosis with severe left ventricular dysfunction and low transvalvular pressure gradients. *J Am Coll Cardiol* 2001;37:2101–2107.
149. Ford LE, Feldman T, Chiu YC, Carroll JD. Hemodynamic resistance as a measure of functional impairment in aortic valvular stenosis. *Circ Res* 1990;66:1.
150. Cannon JD Jr, Zile MR, Crawford FA Jr, et al. Aortic valve resistance as an adjunct to the Gorlin formula in assessing the severity of aortic stenosis in symptomatic patients. *J Am Coll Cardiol* 1992;20:1517–1523.
151. Faggiano P, Gualeni A, Antonini-Canterin F, et al. Doppler echocardiographic assessment of hemodynamic progression of valvular aortic stenosis over time: comparison between aortic valve resistance and valve area. *G Ital Cardiol* 1999;29:1131–1136.
152. Odell JA, Mullany CJ, Schaff HV, et al. Aortic valve replacement after previous coronary artery bypass grafting. *Ann Thorac Surg* 1996;62:1424–1430.
153. Balaban KW, Pereira JJ, Bashir M, et al. Aortic valve replacement improves survival in patients undergoing coronary bypass surgery with mild to moderate aortic valve stenosis [abstract]. *Circulation* 2000;102:I-371.
154. Smith WT 4th, Ferguson TB Jr, Ryan T, et al. Should coronary artery bypass graft surgery patients with mild or moderate aortic stenosis undergo concomitant aortic valve replacement? A decision analysis approach to the surgical dilemma. *J Am Coll Cardiol* 2004;44:1241–1247.
155. Waller BF, Howard J, Fess S. Pathology of aortic valve stenosis and pure aortic regurgitation: II: a clinical morphologic assessment. *Clin Cardiol* 1994;17:150.
156. Stewart WJ, King ME, Weyman AE. Prevalence of aortic valve prolapse with bicuspid aortic valve and its relation to aortic regurgitation: a cross-sectional echocardiographic study. *Am J Cardiol* 1984;54:1277–1282.
157. Roberts WC, Dangel JC, Bulkley BH. Nonrheumatic valvular cardiac disease: a clinicopathological survey of 27 different conditions causing valvular dysfunction. *Cardiovasc Clin* 1973;5:334.
158. Carabello BA. Aortic regurgitation: hemodynamic determinants of prognosis. In: Cohn LH, DiSesa VJ, eds. *Aortic regurgitation: medical and surgical management*. New York: Marcel Dekker, 1986.
159. Wisenbaugh T, Spann JF, Carabello BA. Differences in myocardial performance and load between patients with similar amounts of chronic aortic versus chronic mitral regurgitation. *J Am Coll Cardiol* 1984;3:916.
160. Bonow RO, Dodd JT, Maron BJ, et al. Long-term serial changes in left ventricular function and reversal of ventricular dilatation after valve replacement for chronic aortic regurgitation. *Circulation* 1988;78:1108.
161. St. John-Sutton M, Plappert T, Spiegel A, et al. Early postoperative changes in left ventricular chamber size, architecture, and function in aortic stenosis and aortic regurgitation and their relation to intraoperative changes in afterload: a prospective two-dimensional echocardiographic study. *Circulation* 1987;76:77.
162. Timmermans P, Willems JL, Piessens J, et al. Angina pectoris and coronary artery disease in severe aortic regurgitation. *Am J Cardiol* 1988;61:826.
163. Perry GJ, Helmcke F, Nanda NC, et al. Evaluation of aortic insufficiency by Doppler color flow mapping. *J Am Coll Cardiol* 1987;9:952.
164. Teague SM, Heinsimer JA, Anderson JL, et al. Quantification of aortic regurgitation utilizing continuous wave Doppler ultrasound. *J Am Coll Cardiol* 1986;8:592.
165. Sellers RD, Levy MJ, Amplatz K. Left retrograde cardioangiography in acquired cardiac disease: technique, indications, and interpretations in 700 cases. *Am J Cardiol* 1964;14:437.
166. Henry WL, Bonow RO, Borer JS, et al. Observations on the optimum time for operative intervention for aortic regurgitation: I. Evaluation of the results of aortic valve replacement in symptomatic patients. *Circulation* 1980;61:471.
167. Bonow RO, Lakatos E, Maron BJ, et al. Serial long-term assessment of the natural history of asymptomatic patients with chronic aortic regurgitation and normal left ventricular systolic function. *Circulation* 1991;84:1625.
168. Carabello BA, Usher BW, Hendrix GH, et al. Predictors of outcome for aortic valve replacement in patients with aortic regurgitation and left ventricular dysfunction: a change in the measuring stick. *J Am Coll Cardiol* 1987;10:991.
169. Carabello BA, Crawford FA Jr. Valvular heart disease (review). *N Engl J Med* 1997;337:32–41.
170. Bonow RO, Rosing DR, Maron BJ, et al. Reversal of left ventricular dysfunction after aortic valve replacement for chronic regurgitation: influence of duration of preoperative left ventricular dysfunction. *Circulation* 1984;70:570.
171. Borer JS, Herrold EM, Hochreiter C, et al. Natural history of left ventricular performance at rest and during exercise after aortic valve replacement for aortic regurgitation. *Circulation* 1991;84[Suppl III]:III133–III139.
172. Cosgrove DM, Rosenkranz ER, Hendren WG, et al. Valvuloplasty for aortic insufficiency. *J Thorac Cardiovasc Surg* 1991;102:571–576.
173. Fraser CD Jr, Wang N, Mee RBB, et al. Repair of insufficient bicuspid aortic valves. *Ann Thorac Surg* 1994;58:386.
174. Movsowitz HD, Levine RA, Hilgenberg AD, et al. Transesophageal description of the mechanisms of aortic regurgitation in acute type A aortic dissection—implications for aortic valve repair. *J Am Coll Cardiol* 2000; 3:884–890.
175. David TE, Feindel CM, Bos J. Repair of the aortic valve in patients with aortic insufficiency and aortic root aneurysm. *J Thorac Cardiovasc Surg* 1995;109:345–351.
176. Greenberg BH, DeMots H, Murphy E, et al. Beneficial effects of hydralazine on rest and exercise hemodynamics in patients with chronic severe aortic insufficiency. *Circulation* 1980;62:49.
177. Schon HR. Hemodynamic and morphologic changes after long-term angiotensin-converting enzyme inhibition in patients with chronic valvular regurgitation. *J Hypertension* 1994;12[Suppl 4]:S95.
178. Scognamiglio R, Rahimtoola SH, Fasoli G, et al. Nifedipine in asymptomatic patients with severe aortic regurgitation and normal left ventricular function. *N Engl J Med* 1994;331:689.
179. Scognamiglio R, Negut C, Palisi M, et al. Long-term survival and functional results after aortic valve replacement in asymptomatic patients with chronic severe aortic regurgitation and left ventricular dysfunction. *J Am Coll Cardiol* 2005;45:1025–1030.
180. Evangelista A, Tornos P, Sambola A, et al. Long-term vasodilator therapy in patients with severe aortic regurgitation. *N Engl J Med* 2005;353:1342–1349.
181. Cohn LH, Birjiniuk V. Therapy of acute aortic regurgitation. *Cardiol Clin* 1991;9:339.
182. Roe MT, Abramson MA, Li J, et al. Clinical information determines the impact of transesophageal echocardiography on the diagnosis of infective endocarditis by the Duke criteria. *Am Heart J* 2000;139:945–951.
183. Habib G, Derumeaux G, Avierinos JF, et al. Value and limitations of the Duke criteria for the diagnosis of infective endocarditis. *J Am Coll Cardiol* 1999;33:2023–2029.
184. Mann T, McLaurin L, Grossman W, et al. Assessing the hemodynamic severity of acute aortic regurgitation due to infective endocarditis. *N Engl J Med* 1975;293:108.
185. Sareli P, Klein HO, Schamroth CL, et al. Contribution of echocardiography and immediate surgery to the management of severe aortic regurgitation from active infective endocarditis. *Am J Cardiol* 1986;57:413.
186. al Jubair K, al Fagih MR, Ashmeg A, et al. Cardiac operations during active endocarditis. *J Thorac Cardiovasc Surg* 1992;104:487.
187. Glazier JJ. Treatment of complicated prosthetic aortic valve endocarditis with annular abscess formation by homograft aortic root replacement. *J Am Coll Cardiol* 1991;17:1177–1182.
188. Lim P, Monin JL, Monchi M, et al. Predictors of outcome in patients with severe aortic stenosis and normal left ventricular function: role of B-type natriuretic peptide. *Eur Heart J* 2004;25:1972–1973.
189. Gerber IL, Stewart RA, Legget ME, et al. Increased plasma natriuretic peptide levels reflect symptom onset in aortic stenosis. *Circulation* 2003; 107:1884–1890.
190. Weber M, Arnold R, Rau M, et al. Relation of N-terminal pro B-type natriuretic peptide to progression of aortic valve disease. *Eur Heart J* 2005;26:1023–1030.
191. Das P, Rimington H, Chambers J. Exercise testing to stratify risk in aortic stenosis. *Eur Heart J* 2005;26:1309–1313.
192. Rosenhek R, Klaar U, Schemper M, et al. Mild and moderate aortic stenosis. Natural history and risk stratification by echocardiography. *Eur Heart J* 2004;25:199–205.
193. Lutter F, Ardehali R, Cremer J, et al. Percutaneous valve replacement: current state and future prospects. *Ann Thorac Surg* 2004;78:2199–2206.
194. Cribier A, Eltchaninoff H, Bash A, et al. Percutaneous transcatheter implantation of an aortic valve prosthesis for calcific aortic stenosis: first human case description. *Circulation* 2002;106:3006–3008.
195. Vassiliades TA Jr, Block PC, Cohn LH, et al. The clinical development of percutaneous heart valve technology: a position statement of the Society of Thoracic Surgeons (STS), the American Association for Thoracic Surgery (AATS), and the Society of Cardiovascular Angiography and Intervention (SCAI). *J Am Coll Cardiol* 2005;45:1554–1560.
196. Cribier A, Eltchaninoff H, Tron C, et al. Early experience with percutaneous transcatheter implantation of heart valve prosthesis for the treatment of end-stage inoperable patients with calcific aortic stenosis. *J Am Coll Cardiol* 2004;43:698–703.
197. Khot UN, Navarro GM, Poponic ZB, et al. Nitroprusside in critically ill patients with left ventricular dysfunction and aortic stenosis. *N Engl J Med* 2003;348:1756–1763.

CHAPTER 25 ■ PROSTHETIC VALVE DISEASE

MARIO J. GARCIA

HISTORICAL PERSPECTIVE

For many patients with valvular heart disease, prosthetic valve replacement is the only effective therapy. Hufnagel successfully implanted the first prosthetic valve in 1952 (1) in the descending aorta of a patient with aortic regurgitation. The first in situ aortic valve replacement was performed by Harken (2) in 1953 and the first mitral valve by Starr (3) in 1960. These bare-strut ball valves led to the development of the Starr-Edwards ball-and-cage valve. Tilting-disc valves were developed in the late 1960s and represented a significant advance by demonstrating a far superior hemodynamic performance over the ball-and-cage valves. Double-leaflet hingeless tilting valves were developed in the early 1970s, and since then have become the most commonly used mechanical valves. The first tissue valve was an aortic homograft inserted by Ross in 1962 (4). Stented porcine valve xenografts were first implanted in 1965 by Carpentier (5), which led to the development of the Hancock and the Carpentier-Edwards valves. Stentless porcine valves were later introduced, and these have gained increasing popularity over the last decade. Percutaneously deployed aortic prosthetic valves and mitral valve repair devices have been recently implanted with success and are poised to revolutionize the management of valvular heart disease.

NORMAL PROSTHETIC VALVE ANATOMY AND FUNCTION

Examples of common models of prosthetic valves are shown in Figure 25.1. Most mechanical and tissue valve prostheses have distinct components: a sewing ring, supporting struts, and an occluder device. Sewing rings are constructed from metallic alloys or plastics and are covered with a cloth through which sutures are passed to implant the valve. The size of the prosthesis is determined by the diameter of the suture ring. The supporting struts hold the occluders in place. The occluders may be composed of plastic, metal, or biologic tissue. Each type of prosthesis has specific features that may permit their recognition by means of auscultation, two-dimensional and Doppler echocardiography, and/or cinefluoroscopy. Occasionally, invasively obtained catheter gradients are needed to determine prosthetic valve dysfunction. Retrograde catheter crossing of tissue prostheses and ball-and-cage prosthesis may be performed safely to determine transvalvular gradients. Tilting-disc prostheses should not be crossed with these catheters because of the risk of catheter entrapment (6).

Stented tissue valves and mechanical prostheses have smaller effective orifices than normal native valves of the same size. This reduction in effective orifice is caused by the profile of the suture ring and the supporting struts. For this reason, most tissue and mechanical prostheses in a semilunar position will generate a systolic flow murmur. Diastolic murmurs in atrioventricular prosthetic valves are uncommonly heard unless there is prosthetic stenosis or high forward flow due to severe valvular regurgitation (7). The normal auscultatory findings of prosthetic valves may be altered by factors such as chest wall thickness, emphysema, stroke volume, and heart rate.

Some prosthetic valves may be identified from plain chest radiography (Fig. 25.2). Suture rings are often radiopaque, as are prosthetic cages and some tissue-valve-supporting stents. Tilting discs may or may not be seen in a plain film depending on the angle of the prosthesis, the construction material, and the x-ray penetration. Cinefluoroscopy may be useful for evaluating the mobility of the occluder of mechanical valves in patients with suspected obstruction. Prosthetic valve suture rings, cages, discs, and stents may produce echocardiographic shielding or lead to an inability to visualize structures or flow beyond the location of the ultrasound-reflecting surface. This limits the ability to detect transvalvular or paravalvular regurgitation, thrombi, or vegetations of infective endocarditis in mitral prostheses by transthoracic echocardiography (8). In those cases, transesophageal echocardiography offers superior visualization.

The effective orifice of the prosthesis and the cardiac output determine the magnitude of the transvalvular gradients. Transvalvular gradients are most commonly estimated

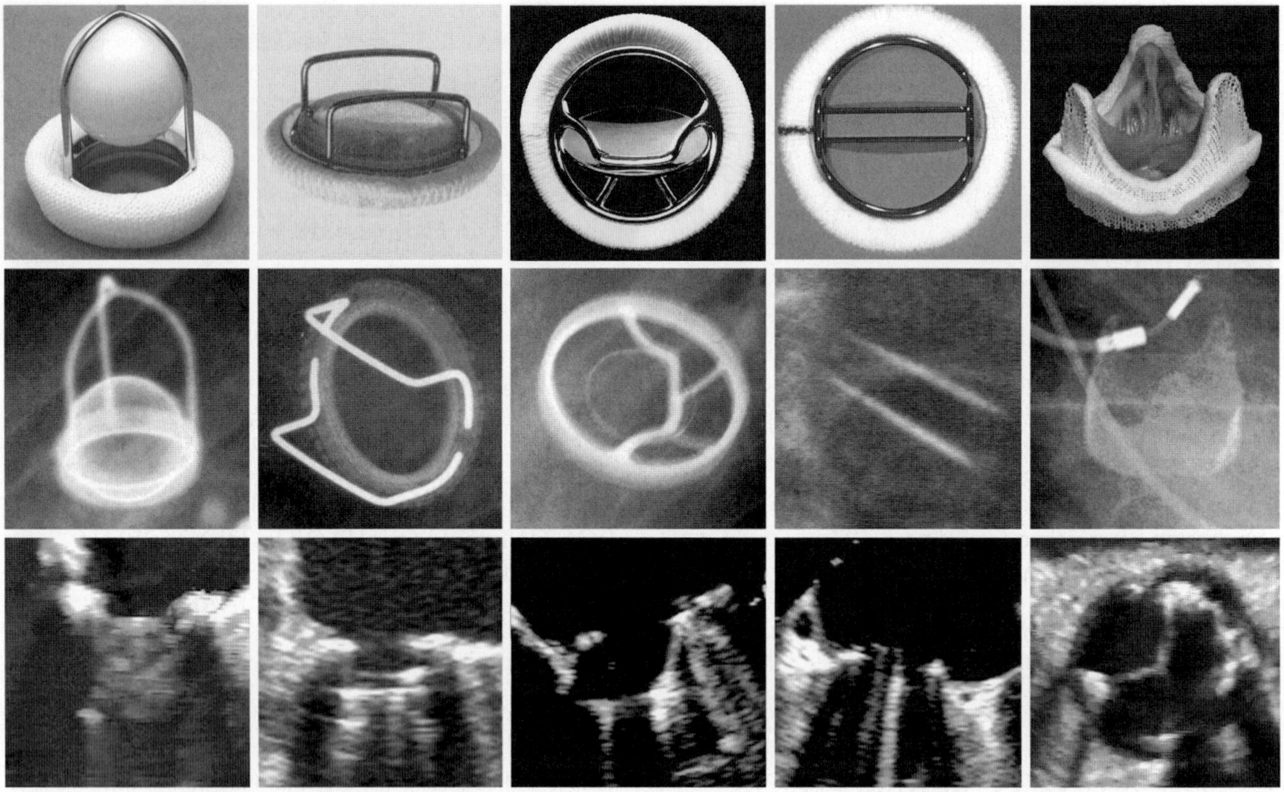

FIGURE 25.1. Photographic (**top row**), radiographic (**middle row**), and echocardiographic (**bottom row**) appearance of different mechanical and bioprosthetic valves. From left to right: Starr-Edwards ball-and-cage, Kay-Suzuki disc-and-cage, Björk-Shiley single-tilting-disc, and St. Jude's Medical bileaflet tilting-disc mechanical valves and Carpentier-Edwards xenograft. (Radiographs provided by courtesy of Dr. Carolyn van Dyke.)

from continuous-wave Doppler velocities by means of the modified Bernoulli equation ($\Delta P = 4V^2$). In most instances, Doppler-derived and catheter-derived gradients are comparable. However, Doppler measurement often overestimates the gradients of small mechanical valves in the aortic position (9). This discrepancy between catheter-derived and Doppler gradients is the result of pressure recovery upstream from the prosthesis. All mechanical and most biologic stented valves have a certain amount of intravalvular regurgitation.

Mechanical Valves

The first mechanical valves had a ball-and-cage design with a metallic alloy ring attached to a cage in which either a metallic or Silastic ball moves from a closed position occluding the ring to an open position in the outer end of the cage. Flow across the prosthesis is directed circumferentially around the ball, assuming a lateral angle. The Starr-Edwards ball-and-cage prosthesis has excellent durability, in many instances exceeding 30 years (10). A major disadvantage of ball-and-cage valves is their suboptimal hemodynamic profile. The mean transvalvular gradient for Starr-Edwards ball-and-cage prostheses in the mitral position is 4.6 + 2.4 mm Hg and the estimated effective orifice is 1.4 to 2.9 cm^2 (11,12,13,14,15). In the aortic position, mean gradient is 23 + 8 mm Hg and estimated effective orifice is 1.2 to 1.6 cm^2 (16,17). On auscultation, the ball-and-cage valves produce a loud opening click followed by multiple clicks of variable intensity produced by the ball bouncing in the cage and a flow murmur in the aortic position. A less intense click occurs with the closing of the valve. Radiographically, the support ring and cage can be detected in plain films. In certain models of ball-and-cage prostheses the ball is metallic or barium-impregnated, allowing its visualization. Two-dimensional echocardiography can demonstrate the highly reflective echoes produced by the metallic struts and the less intense reflective echoes produced by the proximal surface of the ball. In the disc-and-cage valves, such as the Kay-Suzuki valve, a flat disc replaces the ball occluder, providing a lower profile. These valves, however, have been discontinued due to the gradual erosion and often fatal embolization of the disc.

Tilting-disc valves consist of a metallic ring attached to a single or to two flat or concave discs that pivot from the occluded position to an open position at an angle of 60 to 85 degrees. The Björk-Shiley valve has been manufactured in six different models, four of which are available in the United States. The original models had a flat disc made of Delrin or pyrolytic carbon; this was later replaced with a convexoconcave disc. Fracture of the welded struts and embolization of the disc led to the withdrawal of these valves from the market. The Omniscience tilting-disc valve (18) has a free-floating concave-convex disc in titanium housing. This valve, no longer in use, has considerably higher risk of thrombosis, probably due to the smaller built-in volume of regurgitation (19). The Medtronic-Hall valve has a one-piece housing manufactured from titanium and a rotatable Teflon sewing ring and is still in use. A small orifice in the center permits regurgitant flow to "wash" potentially thrombogenic material from the disc. Currently available single tilting-disc valves have excellent hemodynamics and low risk of mechanical failure. The St. Jude Medical (20) and the Carbomedics (21) valves are bileaflet tilting-disc valves. The

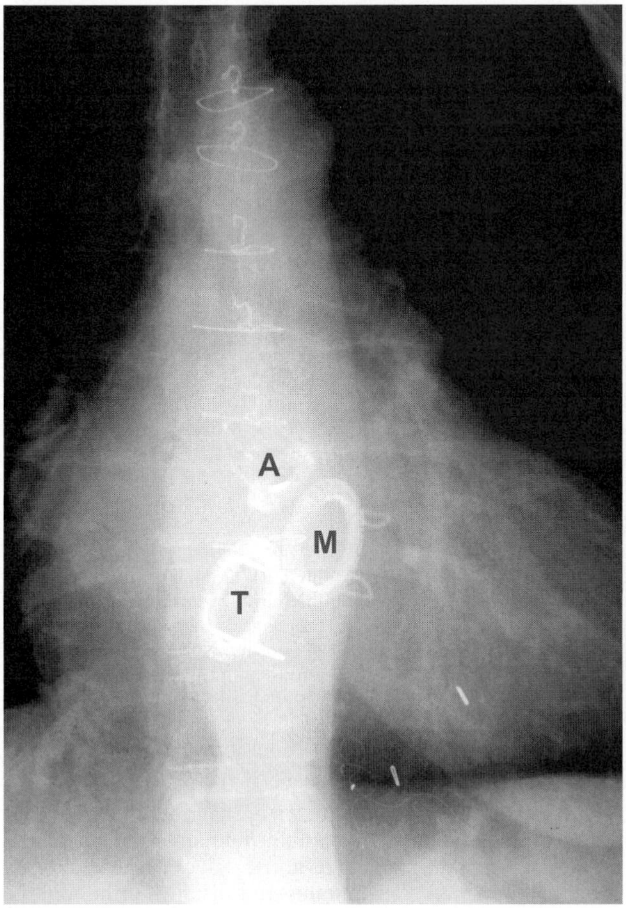

FIGURE 25.2. Radiographic appearance in the anteroposterior projection of mechanical valves in the aortic (A), mitral (M), and tricuspid (T) positions.

leaflets of the St. Jude Medical prosthesis are manufactured from pyrolytic carbon impregnated with tungsten for radiopacity. These semicircular leaflets open to an 85-degree angle, leaving two larger lateral orifices and a narrow rectangular slit between them. The flow across bileaflet tilting-disc valves is symmetric, providing excellent hemodynamic performance (22). The rates of mechanical failure and thromboembolism are very low. The Carbomedics bileaflet valve has similar characteristics and hemodynamic performance. Their mean transvalvular gradient is significantly lower than equally sized Starr-Edwards ball-and-cage valves, from 6 to 15 mm Hg in the aortic and from 2 to 7 mm Hg in the mitral position. Durability at 15 years has been shown to be excellent for this valve (23). The estimated effective orifices range from 2.1 to 3.9 cm^2 for mitral and 1.3 to 2.5 cm^2 for aortic prostheses. The auscultatory findings of tilting-disc prostheses include a loud single or double closing click and a soft midsystolic ejection murmur in the aortic or a low-frequency diastolic rumble in the mitral position. Tilting-disc prostheses also produce a softer opening click. These valves have different radiographic appearance based on the number and position of the struts and the tilting discs. In some valves, such as the Björk-Shiley and Wada-Cutter valves, the discs may be radiolucent. The two half-discs of bileaflet valves can be observed from a tangential plane (Fig. 25.3). The motion of the valve ring and the opening angle of the discs can be evaluated under fluoroscopic guidance. Color Doppler may help to identify the type of prosthesis. The Medtronic-Hall tilting-disc valve has a characteristic regurgitant flow jet through its central orifice. The St. Jude's Medical valve has two central divergent and multiple peripheral convergent regurgitant jets that may be visualized depending on the imaging angle (Fig. 25.4).

Tissue Valves

The biologic nonhuman tissue valves currently available are manufactured from either porcine valvular tissue or bovine pericardium mounted in supporting stents or preserved in situ in a segment of the porcine ascending aorta. The Carpentier-Edwards porcine valve (24) consists of a cloth-covered silicone-rubber sewing ring attached to three cloth-covered steel alloy flexible stents (25). The Hancock porcine valve has very similar characteristics, but the stents are manufactured of polypropylene. Bioprosthetic valves are structurally similar to human semilunar valves. Despite their human anatomic resemblance, these valves have suboptimal hemodynamic performance in

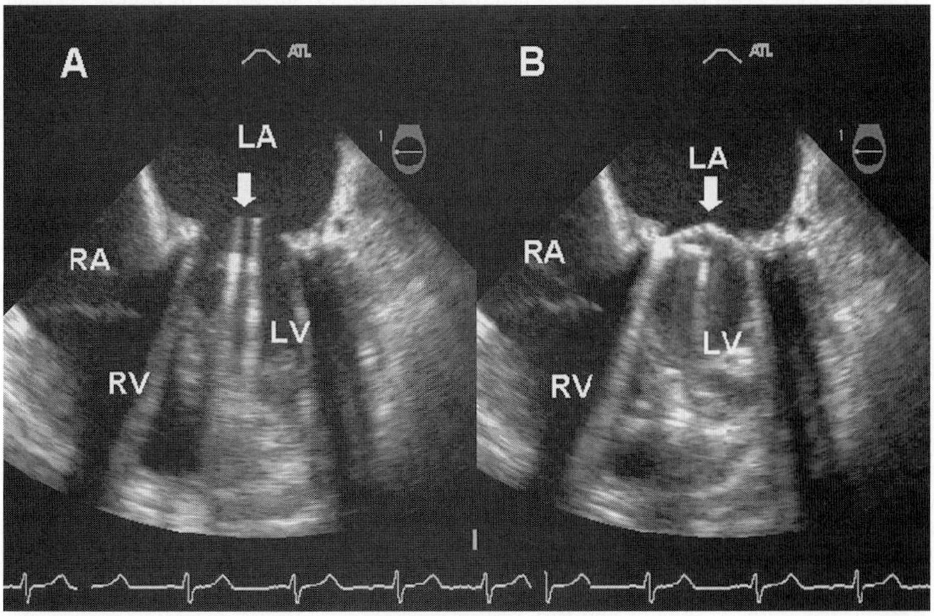

FIGURE 25.3. St. Jude's valve in the mitral position shown by transesophageal echocardiography during opening (A) and closing (B). LA, left atrium; LV, left ventricle; RA, right atrium; RV, right ventricle.

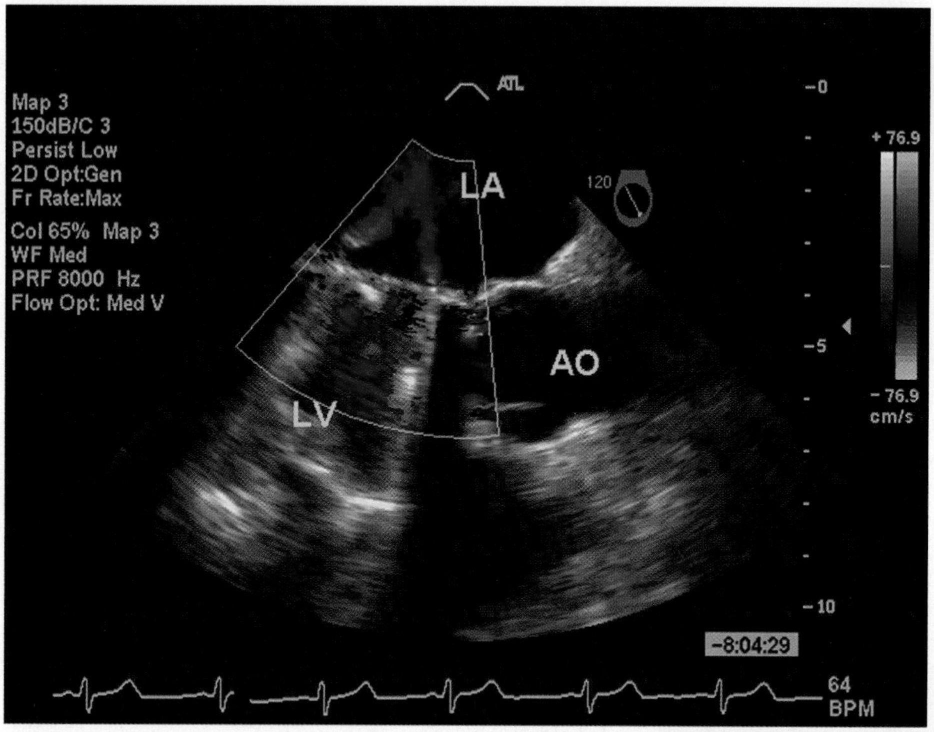

FIGURE 25.4. St. Jude's valve in the mitral position shown by transesophageal echocardiography during closure. Normal intravalvular regurgitant jets are seen in the left atrium (LA). AO, aorta; LV, left ventricle.

comparison to tilting-disc mechanical prostheses of the same diameter (26,27). This limitation results primarily from the reduction in their profile caused by the interposed stents and is more significant in valves smaller than 23 mm. The bioprosthetic leaflets are also stiffer than normal native human semilunar valves, exhibiting an incomplete opening at low flow rates. The durability of porcine bioprosthetic valves has improved significantly with newer changes in design and preservation techniques. Actuarial probability of freedom from structural valve degeneration at 5, 10, and 15 years has been reported at 99%, 79% and 57%, respectively (28). Durability is reduced in mitral prostheses because of the greater closing pressure in this position in younger patients and patients with increased calcium metabolism (29,30). Bovine, and more recently equine (31), pericardial bioprostheses were designed to improve the hemodynamic profile of the porcine valves. The Carpentier-Edwards bovine pericardial valve (32) resembles structurally the porcine tissue valves but appears to have superior hemodynamic performance, demonstrating lower transvalvular gradients during exercise (33). Intermediate follow-up of the Hancock II porcine bioprostheses suggests that their durability will be superior to that of their predecessors. Freedom from reoperation has been reported to be 100%, 97%, and 89% after aortic, mitral, and combined valve replacement, respectively, after 7 years of follow-up (34). Bioprosthetic valves are available in diameters of 19 to 31 mm. The effective orifice area for bioprostheses ranges from 1.4 to 2.5 cm^2 in the mitral and 0.9 to 1.8 cm^2 in the aortic position. The auscultatory findings of bioprosthetic valves include a systolic ejection murmur in the aortic position. Frequently, a systolic murmur is also heard in patients with mitral bioprostheses, caused by turbulent flow in the left ventricular outflow track. The bioprosthetic valve sewing ring is radiopaque in x-ray films. In some models wire-framed stents may also be seen. The three equidistant stents are the hallmark of bioprostheses by two-dimensional echocardiography. The three leaflets can also be imaged, although they are less echogenic than the native aortic valve. Normal bioprostheses may show mild intravalvular regurgitation by color Doppler (35).

Stentless heterograft and human homograft prostheses consist of a tubular segment of a porcine/human proximal ascending aorta containing its in situ aortic valve, which is sutured proximally to the aortic annulus and distally to the mid ascending aorta. Short-term and intermediate-term follow-up of stentless valves have demonstrated better hemodynamics with smaller resting and exercise gradients and greater regression of left ventricular (LV) hypertrophy when compared to stented tissue valves of similar size (36,37). Nevertheless this has not been shown to translate into improved clinical outcomes (38). Stentless aortic root bioprosthesis can be used safely to replace the aortic root for aortic valve and aortic root pathology (39). Freedom from structural valve degeneration has been reported to be about 85% at 9 years (40). Human aortic valves are harvested from cadaveric hearts and cryopreserved (41). Similar to stentless heterografts, these are supported by a short segment of the donor's aortic root, in which the recipient's coronary arteries are reimplanted. The homograft endothelial cells and fibroblasts are antigenic (42) and are gradually destroyed by immunologic reactions. Freedom from structural valve degeneration at 10, 15, and 20 years has been reported to be 81%, 62%, and 31%, respectively (43). The flow characteristics, auscultatory findings, and radiographic appearance of stentless valves are similar to those of native aortic valves. Homografts have a reduced rate of reinfection, as low as 95% after 20 years, when used to replace valves with endocarditis (44,45). Pulmonary allografts consist of healthy pulmonary valves transplanted to the aortic position to substitute a diseased aortic valve while a cadaveric homograft is then placed in the pulmonic position. Late follow-up has shown no evidence of primary tissue degeneration and normal cusp cellularity. This evidence suggests that the cusps not only survive permanently, but also can grow with the patient, making the operation ideal for children. Freedom from reoperation and actuarial patient survival has been reported at 85% and 80%, respectively, after 20 years. However, aortic insufficiency, degeneration of the implanted homograft in the pulmonary position, and stenosis of the pulmonary trunk anastomotic site are not infrequent causes of reoperation in these patients.

Selection of Prosthetic Valve Type

The selection of a prosthetic valve should always be individualized to each patient based on age, anatomic considerations, lifestyle, expected longevity, and relative risks of anticoagulation. The in-hospital mortality and complication rates after valve replacement are similar with mechanical and bioprostheses (46) and thus should not be considered determining factors in the selection of a valve. Several retrospective and prospective studies have shown that patient survival is comparable at long-term follow-up. Structural failure requiring reoperation is more common with prosthetic valves, whereas thromboembolic and bleeding complications are more common with mechanical valves. Children requiring valve replacement benefit most from mechanical prostheses (47). Tilting-disc mechanical valves provide better hemodynamic performance than bioprostheses particularly at smaller size, thus prolonging the need for reoperation. Structural valve deterioration of bioprosthetic valves also occurs more rapidly in children and young adults (46,48). Therefore, as a general rule, mechanical valves are preferred in younger patients, whereas bioprosthetic valves are recommended in older patients in whom the risk of anticoagulation is higher. Both mechanical and bioprosthetic valves have a disadvantage in women of childbearing age. Pregnant women with mechanical valves require rigorous control of their anticoagulation and are at higher risk for thromboembolism and for fetal hemorrhage and embryopathy (49,50). Bioprosthetic valves may obviate the need for anticoagulation (49,51), but they have the disadvantage of their limited durability. Obviously, bioprosthetic valves should be used in patients at higher risk for anticoagulation-related hemorrhage, including those with intestinal angiodysplasia, familial polyposis, inflammatory bowel disease, liver disease, and hereditary blood dyscrasias.

PATHOPHYSIOLOGY OF PROSTHETIC VALVES

Complications related to prosthetic heart valves can occur as early as in the immediate postoperative period. Their relative frequency and timing vary with each type of prosthesis and determine the manner in which patients with prosthetic valves should be clinically followed.

Thromboembolic Complications

Thromboembolism represents one of the most important causes of morbidity and mortality in patients with prosthetic valves. The incidence of thromboembolic events is significantly high in non-anticoagulated patients with mechanical prosthetic valves, ranging from 7% to 34% per year (52,53,54). Involved mechanisms include platelet activation by the synthetic surfaces, flow stagnation, increased shear stress, and activation of intrinsic clotting factors by the prosthetic material or the damaged endothelium (55). Thromboembolic complications are more common in older patients, patients in atrial fibrillation, and patients with left ventricular dysfunction (56). The risk of thromboembolism is higher for both mechanical and bioprostheses in the early postoperative period, declining after the first 3 months for bioprosthetic valves. Oral anticoagulation with warfarin significantly reduces the risk of thromboembolism in patients with mechanical heart valves. Improved prosthetic design and anticoagulation reduced the embolic rates to 2.5% to 4% per patient-year in anticoagulated patients with Starr-Edwards valves implanted after 1970 (57). The incidence of thromboembolic complications with Björk-Shiley tilting-disk valves is about 4% per year in the mitral and 2.5% per year in the aortic position, and the incidence is 1% to 3% average with Medtronic-Hall valves in anticoagulated patients (58). Bileaflet mechanical valves have a risk of about 2.5% per year in the mitral and 1% per year in the aortic position (59,60,61). Regardless of their type of mechanical prosthesis, the incidence of thromboembolism is less than 1% in those patients that maintain therapeutic anticoagulation (62). Unfortunately, chronic anticoagulation therapy increases the long-term hemorrhagic complications (Table 25.1). Pooled data from 46 studies including more than 13,000 patients with mechanical heart valves studied for more than 50,000 patient-years showed an incidence of major bleeding complications of about 1.4 per 100 patient-years (63). Hemorrhagic complications occur more frequently in patients with an International Normalized Ratio (INR) above therapeutic range (64) (Fig. 25.5). The intensity of anticoagulation should vary according to the type of the mechanical valve and the presence of other predisposing factors (Fig. 25.6). Antiplatelet therapy may be used in combination with warfarin in patients with mechanical heart valves. Low-dose aspirin (100 mg/day) in patients with a target INR of 3 to 4.5 has been shown to reduce the annualized risk of death and major systemic thromboembolic events from 11.7% to 4.2% (65). The additive benefit of aspirin is greater in patients with previous embolic events and those with coronary artery disease, but it is less clear in others in whom the increased risk of bleeding exceeds a low risk of thromboembolism.

Because pregnancy causes relative hypercoagulability (66), rigorous anticoagulation is required throughout gestation in patients with mechanical valve prostheses. Anticoagulant therapy is associated, however, with higher fetal morbidity and mortality, especially if the drugs are administered during the first trimester (67). Warfarin has teratogenic effects in the embryo and may result in fetal death when the embryo is exposed between the sixth and ninth weeks of gestation. Pregnant women with mechanical valves that receive warfarin during

TABLE 25.1

INCIDENCE OF ADVERSE EVENTS (THROMBOEMBOLISM, MAJOR BLEEDING, AND STROKE) IN PATIENTS WITH MECHANICAL VALVES RECEIVING CHRONIC ANTICOAGULATION

Event	Number	Incidence (per 100 patient-years)[a]
Thromboembolism		
Cerebral infarction	43	0.68
Peripheral embolism	2	0.03
Valve thrombosis	0	—
Any thromboembolism	45	0.71
Fatal thromboembolism	2	0.03
Bleeding episode		
Intracranial and spinal bleeding	36	0.57
Extracranial bleeding	128	2.11
Any bleeding	64	2.68
Fatal bleeding	20	0.30
Unclassified stroke	14	0.23
First events	210	3.50

[a]Because follow-up ended when the event of interest occurred, the denominators differ for the various endpoints.
Adapted from Cannegieter SC, Rosendaal FR, Wintzen AR, et al. Optimal oral anticoagulant therapy in patients with mechanical heart valves. *N Engl J Med* 1995;333:14. By permission of The Massachusetts Medical Society.

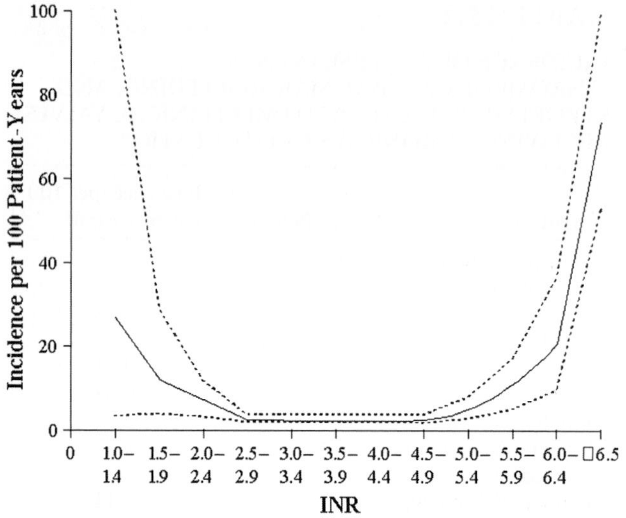

FIGURE 25.5. Incidence of adverse events (thromboembolism, major bleeding, and stroke) in patients with mechanical valves according to the International Normalized Ratio (INR). (From Cannegieter SC, Rosendaal FR, Wintzen AR, et al. Optimal oral anticoagulant therapy in patients with mechanical heart valves. *N Engl J Med* 1995;333:14. By permission of The Massachusetts Medical Society.)

this period carry a risk of embryopathy as high as 30% and a risk of spontaneous abortion of 25% to 30% (68). Therapeutic abortion should be considered if advanced gestation is discovered accidentally while receiving this drug. Anticoagulation should be maintained during pregnancy with either continuous intravenous or subcutaneous heparin administered twice daily starting at 17,500 to 20,000 units and adjusted to a target activated partial thromboplastin time (aPTT) greater than two times control 6 hours after administration (69). Subtherapeutic doses of heparin are associated with a significant risk of thromboembolism. The risk of major hemorrhagic complications in pregnant patients treated with heparin is about 2% (70). Substituting heparin from week 6 until week 12 of gestation eliminates the risk of embryopathy in pregnant women with mechanical valves (50). Warfarin should be substituted again by heparin from after week 38 until delivery because warfarin crosses the placenta and may cause fetal intracranial hemorrhage in the peripartum period (71). Heparin should be discontinued before elective induction of labor. Low-molecular-weight heparins have been shown to be safe and effective for the prevention and treatment of deep venous thrombosis in pregnant women (72), but they have been associated with a 12% risk of thromboembolic complications in pregnant women with mechanical valves (73).

Patients with mechanical valves undergoing minor surgical procedures in which blood loss is anticipated to be minimal and easily controlled do not require discontinuation of their anticoagulation. Otherwise, warfarin should be discontinued 3 days before major surgical procedures during which significant bleeding is expected. This is based on the half-life of warfarin, which varies from 18 to 36 hours. Although the overall risk of thromboembolism when anticoagulation is discontinued for less than 10 days is reported to be low (74), the risk may be significantly higher in cases of mitral prostheses, ball-and-cage valves, and atrial fibrillation. Therefore, in these cases and in patients with left ventricular dysfunction, with history of prior embolic events, or otherwise considered at high risk, warfarin should be substituted by intravenous heparin until 3 hours before the procedure and resumed postoperatively.

Prosthetic valve thrombosis is a serious complication of both mechanical and bioprosthetic valves (Fig. 25.7). Mechanical prostheses receiving adequate anticoagulation, regardless of their type, have a lower risk of 0.1% to 2% per 100 patient-years, similar to non-anticoagulated bioprosthetic valves. Valve thrombosis occurs more commonly with prostheses in the mitral than with those in the aortic position. The incidence of thrombosis appears to be much higher (4% per year) with prostheses in the tricuspid valve position (75). Most patients with prosthetic thrombosis also have redundant endocardial tissue growth (pannus) partially obstructing the prosthesis. Patients with prosthetic valve thrombosis manifest systemic or pulmonary embolization and symptoms of congestive heart failure and cardiovascular collapse. The onset of symptoms may be insidious, over a period of several weeks or, more commonly, abrupt, presenting as cardiovascular collapse (76). A murmur

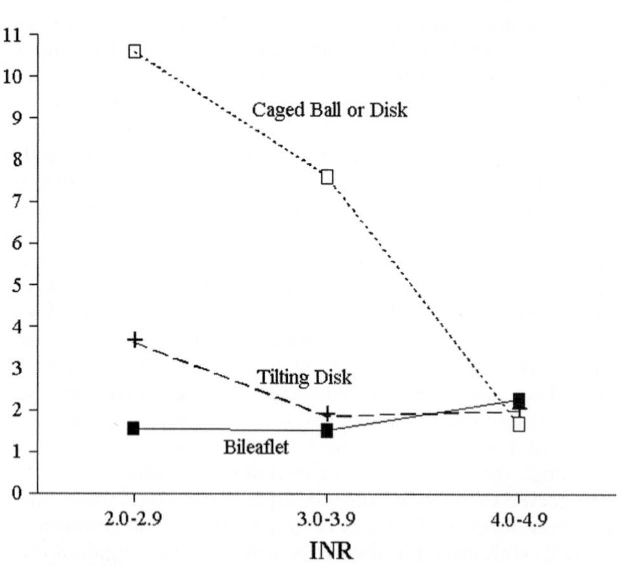

FIGURE 25.6. Incidence of adverse events (thromboembolism, major bleeding, and stroke) according to mechanical valve type. INR, International Normalized Ratio. (From Cannegieter SC, Rosendaal FR, Wintzen AR, et al. Optimal oral anticoagulant therapy in patients with mechanical heart valves. *N Engl J Med* 1995;333:15. By permission of The Massachusetts Medical Society.)

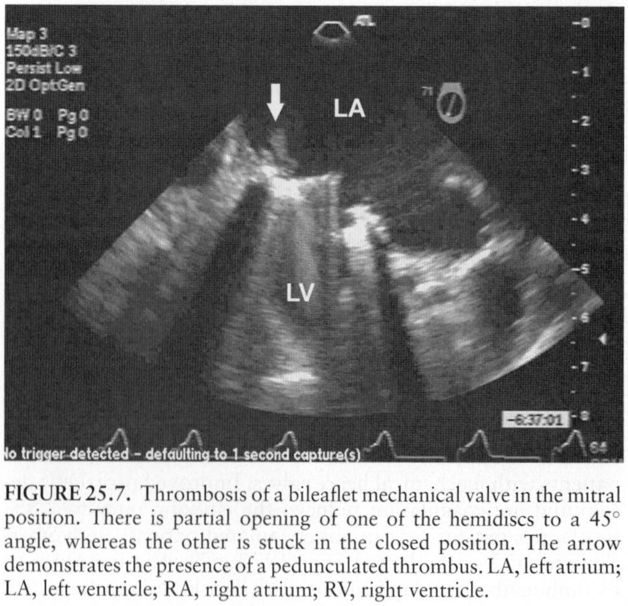

FIGURE 25.7. Thrombosis of a bileaflet mechanical valve in the mitral position. There is partial opening of one of the hemidiscs to a 45° angle, whereas the other is stuck in the closed position. The arrow demonstrates the presence of a pedunculated thrombus. LA, left atrium; LA, left ventricle; RA, right atrium; RV, right ventricle.

of prosthetic stenosis and/or regurgitation and decreased or absent opening and closing sound are found by auscultation. The diagnosis is easily established by two-dimensional and Doppler echocardiography, frequently requiring transesophageal imaging. Single- or multiple-echo densities representing thrombus are often visualized within the valve. Incomplete or intermittent opening and closing of the occluder mechanism may be detected by echocardiography or fluoroscopy. Prosthetic valve thrombosis carries a significant morbidity and mortality. Small thrombi of less than 5 mm in diameter often resolve with intravenous heparin if they are not obstructing the occluding mechanism of the valve (77). Thrombi of larger size, particularly if they interfere with the mechanical function of the prostheses, are associated with a high incidence of embolization and death by cardiovascular collapse and are rarely resolved with intravenous heparin alone. Thrombolytic therapy or surgery is required in these patients. Successful thrombolysis has been reported with intravenous streptokinase, urokinase, and tissue plasminogen activator (t-PA) (78,79,80,81,82). Thrombolysis is effective and has a low complication rate in the treatment of right-heart prosthetic thrombosis. Thrombolytic therapy is effective in the treatment of aortic and mitral valve thrombosis, with an initial success rate of 70% to 80%. However, it carries a significant morbidity and mortality. Pool data from several retrospective studies (78,79,80,81,82,83,84,85) have shown an incidence of embolism of 5% to 22% and a 5% to 12% risk of disabling stroke/death. Recent studies have shown a higher success rate and a lower complication rate for thrombolytic therapy guided by transesophageal echocardiographic monitoring when treating nonobstructive, small, and nonmobile thrombi (86,87,88). Pooled data from large surgical series (76,84,89) show a combined risk of death or stroke of 9%, although it is higher in class IV patients (14 of 86 [16%] vs. 3 of 63 [5%] in class I to III patients). Surgery carries a low morbidity and mortality in patients who are hemodynamically stable and have no other significant comorbidities and should be the treatment of choice in patients with large, mobile, and obstructive thrombi (78–90).

Patients with heterograft bioprostheses have an increased risk of thromboembolism during the first 3 months after implantation. This risk is attributed to the thrombogenic surface of the prosthetic sewing ring cloth, transient hypercoagulable state after surgery, platelet activation during cardiopulmonary bypass, flow stagnation due to chamber enlargement, and postoperative atrial fibrillation. The risk of thromboembolism appears to be higher for mitral (7%) than for aortic prostheses (3%) during this period (91). Anticoagulation with warfarin at a target INR of 2 to 3 has been shown to significantly reduce the thromboembolic risk in patients with mitral (91,92) but not in those with aortic bioprostheses (93,94).

Structural Degeneration

Structural failure occurs more commonly in bioprosthetic valves and eventually leads to prosthetic replacement (Table 25.2). Structural valve failure can occur as early as 4 years after implantation and increases linearly thereafter, approaching about 30% at 10 years and up to 60% at 15 years. Failure rate is higher in prosthesis in the mitral position (95,96) and in younger patients. About 50% of patients who are in their second decade of life at the time of surgery experience structural valve deterioration requiring valve replacement before 6 years. Thereafter, the incidence of structural failure of heterograft bioprostheses decreases linearly with increasing age. Bioprosthetic valve failure is usually insidious, presenting as progressive heart failure. Severe intravalvular prosthetic regurgitation tends to be clinically more significant than stenosis (97). Auscultation may reveal a stenotic and/or a regurgitant murmur and a soft or absent closing sound. Leaflet thickening, calcification, and restricted motion are seen with stenotic valves by two-dimensional echocardiography. Leaflet fracture will appear as excessive mobility and fluttering during opening and closing (98). Increased transvalvular gradients can be detected by continuous-wave Doppler or by catheterization. Color Doppler may demonstrate intravalvular regurgitation. Bending of the polypropylene stents may occur in certain models of the Hancock bioprosthesis and lead to functional stenosis (99). The incidence of this phenomenon, known as stent "creep," is unknown, but should be suspected when transvalvular gradients are elevated in the presence of apparently normal prosthetic leaflets.

TABLE 25.2

CAUSES OF REOPERATION IN PATIENTS WITH MECHANICAL AND BIOPROSTHETIC VALVES[a]

Cause	Mechanical prostheses	Bioprostheses
Operations	46	662
Prostheses	49	717
Structural valve degeneration	1 (2.0%)	518 (72.2%)
Nonstructural dysfunction	32 (65.3%)	82 (11.4%)
Prosthetic valve endocarditis	9 (18.4%)	74 (10.3%)
Thromboembolism	5 (10.2%)	10 (1.4%)
Incidental removal	1 (2.0%)	31 (4.3%)
Miscellaneous	1 (2.0%)	2 (0.3%)

[a]Percentages relate to operations, not number of prostheses replaced. Adapted from Tyers GF, Jamieson WR, Munro AI, et al. Reoperations in biological and mechanical valve populations: fate of the reoperative patient. *Ann Thorac Surg* 1995;60:S465. By permission of Elsevier Science Inc.

Malfunction of mechanical valve prostheses is relatively uncommon, but it is often abrupt and catastrophic. It may occur as a result of ball degeneration, strut fracture, or impaired mechanical function due to thrombus, pannus formation, or infection. The Starr-Edwards ball-and-cage prosthesis has a low incidence of mechanical failure (100). However, ball degeneration, also referred to as "ball variance," was common in Silastic valve models manufactured before 1965 (Fig. 25.8). Auscultatory findings that suggest malfunction of a ball-and-cage valve include decreased intensity or absence of the opening and/or closing clicks, new diastolic murmurs indicating incomplete closure, and regurgitation with valves in the aortic position, and new diastolic rumbling murmurs and/or systolic regurgitant murmurs with valves in the mitral position. Two-dimensional and M-mode echocardiography may reveal diminished mobility of the ball. It is of paramount importance to register extended Doppler and/or M-mode recordings of the prosthesis because obstruction may occur intermittently.

Tilting-disc valves may fail for a variety of reasons due to their complex structure. Immobilization of a disc can result from entrapment of the pivoting mechanism by free-floating sutures or chordae tendineae (101), resulting in valvular stenosis and/or regurgitation. Intermittent closure of the disc and/or a reduced opening angle are diagnostic features on echocardiographic and cinefluoroscopic examinations. Abnormal intravalvular regurgitation may be observed by color Doppler. Although dislodgment and embolization of a disc has been reported with the Harken (102), the Duromedics (103), and the Omnicarbon (104) tilting-disc valves, most instances of disc

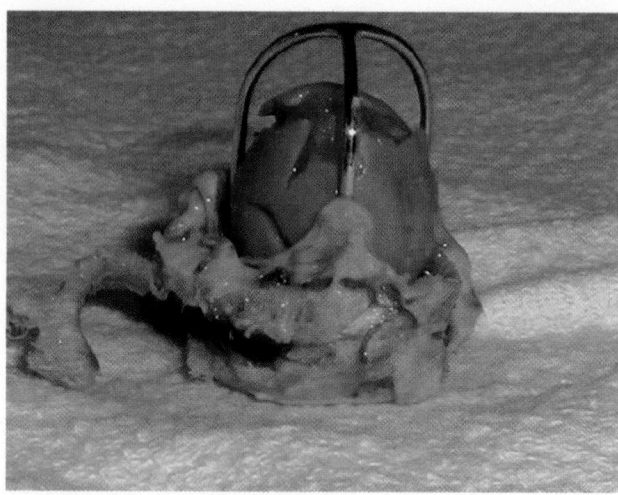

FIGURE 25.8. Structural degeneration of a Silastic ball in a Starr-Edwards valve.

escape due to strut fracture have been associated primarily with the Björk-Shiley convexoconcave tilting-disc valve. By 1987, there were 213 reports of fracture of the valve ring strut, which led to withdrawal of the Björk-Shiley tilting-disc valve from the market. By December 1994, 564 complete strut fractures were reported, two thirds of which were fatal (105). The risk of strut fracture is greater in larger-diameter Björk-Shiley prostheses, particularly in those manufactured in 1981 to 1982. Valves with a diameter between 21 and 27 mm and a 60-degree opening angle carry the lowest risk, about 0.02% per year. Larger valves (29 to 33 mm) with a 60-degree opening angle manufactured between February 1, 1981, and June 30, 1982, have an intermediate risk of fracture (0.32% per year). Large valves (>29 mm) with a 70-degree opening angle carry the highest risk, about 2% per year. This risk is also higher in patients younger than 50 years old at the time of implantation (105,106). Prophylactic valve replacement should be considered in those patients in whom the risk of embolization exceeds the risk of reoperation. In May 1994, the U.S. District Court in Cincinnati, Ohio, approved a settlement agreement between a worldwide class of Björk-Shiley heart valve patients and Shiley Incorporated. Under this agreement, a supervisory expert panel was appointed to establish guidelines for prophylactic valve replacement. Under these guidelines, recipients of Bjork-Shiley concave-convex valves qualify for monetary benefits to cover for prophylactic valve replacement if their estimated risk of outlet strut fracture exceeds their life-expectancy-adjusted risk of reoperation.

Prosthetic Valve Endocarditis

Approximately 3% to 6% of patients with prosthetic heart valves will experience prosthetic valve endocarditis during their lifetime (107,108). Prosthetic valve endocarditis represents about 15% of the cases of endocarditis in developed countries (109). The incidence of prosthetic valve endocarditis peaks at 5 weeks after surgery and levels off at 9 months after surgery. This probably occurs because of different factors related to the initial perioperative period including contamination of the surgical wound, exposure to nosocomial pathogens, and depressed immunologic system. The different frequencies and types of causative organisms support this concept and lead to the arbitrary classification of prosthetic valve endocarditis into early and late endocarditis. The overall risk of endocarditis is similar for mechanical and heterograft bioprostheses, although some studies suggest that the early endocarditis is more frequent in mechanical valves, whereas late endocarditis is more common in heterograft bioprostheses (109,110). The diagnosis of prosthetic valve endocarditis is based on the Duke criteria requiring the combination of two major criteria (evidence of endocarditis by echocardiography and positive blood cultures), one major plus three minor criteria (predisposition, fever, embolism, immunologic phenomena, suggestion of endocarditis by echocardiography, suggestive microbiology), or five minor criteria. Major echocardiographic criteria include the appearance of a new oscillating mass with independent motion attached to the prosthetic material, the detection of perivalvular tissue swelling indicative of an abscess, dehiscence of the prosthetic suture ring, or the appearance of new paravalvular or intravalvular regurgitation.

Early prosthetic valve endocarditis, by definition, occurs during the initial 60 days after valve implantation. It carries a higher mortality, ranging between 20% and 70% (109,110, 111). The classic signs of endocarditis may be masked by the signs of extracardiac sites of infection such as sternal osteomyelitis and in-dwelling catheter infections. Symptoms are usually less typical in early prosthetic valve endocarditis. Fever is the most common symptom, occurring in 97% of the patients. The clinical course tends to be more fulminant, with congestive heart failure observed in 60% and shock in 33% of the cases (109). *Staphylococcus epidermidis* is the most common causative organism of early prosthetic endocarditis, accounting for about 40% of the cases (112). The majority of infections caused by *S. epidermidis* during the first year (80%) are resistant to methicillin. Late prosthetic valve endocarditis resembles endocarditis of native valves. The incidence of late prosthetic valve endocarditis for mechanical valves is about 0.45% per patient-year in the mitral position, 0.54% in the aortic position, and 0.64% in double implants (110). The incidence for bioprosthetic valves is 0.49% in mitral, 0.91% in aortic, and 0.90% in double implants. A probable source of infection can be found in 25% to 80% of patients with late prosthetic valve endocarditis (110). Dental procedures, urinary tract infections, and urologic procedures are the commonest identifiable sources. Late prosthetic endocarditis is caused by similar organisms that cause endocarditis in native valves. Streptococci are the most common, followed by gram-negative bacteria, enterococci and *S. epidermidis*, organisms usually found in the dental, gastrointestinal, and skin flora. Culture-negative endocarditis, caused by fastidious gram-negative organisms, is also more frequent during the late period. In patients with mechanical valves, prosthetic valve endocarditis is associated with a high rate (50%–60%) of annular tissue invasion (109). Transthoracic and transesophageal echocardiography are very useful in establishing the diagnosis in patients with culture-negative endocarditis due to fastidious organisms or the use of antibiotics and in detecting the presence of complications (Fig. 25.9). The sensitivity of transthoracic echocardiography in detecting vegetations is significantly lower than in native valve endocarditis (113). For imaging infective vegetations, the sensitivity and specificity of transesophageal echocardiography are about 95% and 90%, respectively. Transesophageal imaging is also superior for detecting small vegetations, tissue invasion, and fistula formation (114,115,116). Transesophageal echocardiography may fail to detect vegetations in patients who present early after the onset of symptoms (117). In these patients one should consider performing a repeated study 48 to 72 hours later.

The treatment of prosthetic valve endocarditis often requires surgery, although medical cure can occur for uncomplicated infections with streptococci and less aggressive organisms. Surgical replacement should be promptly performed if (a) there is persistent bacteremia after 5 days of intravenous

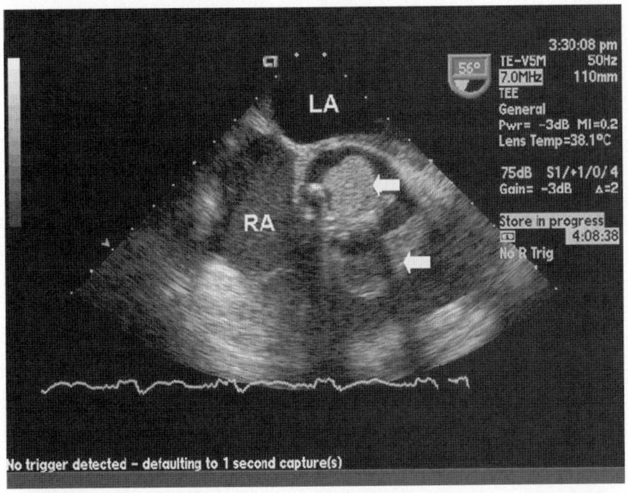

FIGURE 25.9. Endocarditis involving a Carpentier-Edwards bioprosthesis in the aortic position demonstrated by transesophageal echocardiography. The arrows indicate a large vegetation and a paravalvular abscess, respectively. LA, left atrium; RA, right atrium.

antibiotic therapy, (b) infection recurs after discontinuation of antibiotic therapy, (c) there is evidence of tissue invasion or fistulous tracks, (d) recurrent embolization occurs on antibiotic therapy, (e) infection is caused by a fungal organism, and (f) prosthetic obstruction, dehiscence, heart block, or congestive heart failure develop (118,119). The stentless aortic homograft is an excellent choice for replacement of infected aortic prostheses. The risk of recurrent endocarditis in aortic homografts is very low (120). Antibiotic treatment should be given for 6 weeks after surgery. In experienced centers, most patients with prosthetic valve endocarditis surgically treated have a favorable outcome. Of 146 patients reoperated for the treatment of prosthetic valve endocarditis by Lytle et al. (121) from 1975 through 1992, only 13% died in-hospital. In this study, surgical mortality decreased from 20% between 1975 and 1984 to 10% between 1984 and 1992. No adequate controlled studies testing the effectiveness of prophylactic antibiotics in patients with prosthetic valve endocarditis have been done. Antibiotics are recommended, however, based on observations determining that (a) transient bacteremia occurs after certain invasive procedures and (b) patients with prosthetic valve in whom bacteremia is documented have a 10% risk of developing late endocarditis (122). Antibiotic prophylaxis is recommended during invasive procedures that carry a high risk of bacteremia, including dental extractions and professional cleaning and gastrointestinal, genitourinary, and oral surgery. Prophylaxis is no longer recommended during flexible endoscopy or bronchoscopy or normal vaginal delivery (123).

Prosthetic Valve–Associated Hemolysis

Several mechanisms may contribute to the development of hemolysis in normal and malfunctioning prosthetic valves, including shear stress, turbulence, pressure fluctuations, interaction with foreign surfaces, and intrinsic abnormalities of the erythrocyte membrane (124). Subclinical hemolysis (increased reticulocyte count and lactate dehydrogenase, decreased haptoglobin) is found in most patients with mechanical valves, but it rarely results in significant anemia. Clinically significant hemolysis is commonly found in association with paravalvular regurgitant leaks. Flow acceleration, deceleration, and fragmentation may be important causes of increased shear stress with periprosthetic leaks (125). Abnormal flow through a partially thrombosed prosthetic valve may cause hemolytic anemia. Hemolytic anemia is also a common finding in prosthetic valve endocarditis (126) and in bioprosthetic valves with structural failure (127). Mild hemolytic anemia may be treated medically with erythropoietin, iron, and folic acid supplementation and blood transfusions. Control of hypertension with β-blockers may reduce the severity of hemolysis, probably by reducing the velocity of regurgitant flows and thus the shear stress (128). Closure of paravalvular regurgitant leaks or valve replacement is indicated in those patients with severe hemolysis requiring repeated blood transfusions or in those with congestive heart failure.

Prosthetic Valve Dehiscence

Separation of the sewing ring from the annular tissue may occur in the early postoperative period from loose sutures in patients with excessive calcification and fragility of the annular tissue. Late dehiscence occurs commonly as the result of infective endocarditis. A new regurgitant murmur may herald the presence of prosthetic valve dehiscence. Abnormal rocking of the sewing ring relative to the annular tissue is the characteristic finding observed by means of two-dimensional echocardiography or cinefluoroscopy (129,130). Color Doppler echocardiography demonstrates abnormal paravalvular flow seen as a regurgitant jet distal to the prosthesis or a region of proximal flow convergence.

Other Complications

Embolization of air through the right coronary artery is a relatively common cause of perioperative infarction of the inferior wall myocardium but rarely results in permanent systolic dysfunction. Myocardial infarction may rarely occur due to obstruction or dissection of the coronary ostia after reimplantation of the coronary trunks in stentless aortic homografts or prosthetic valve conduits. Intraoperative echocardiography is useful for demonstrating the presence of postoperative wall-motion abnormalities and the patency of flow in the coronaries of these patients (131). Myocardial infarction may also occur from coronary embolization of thrombotic material or infective and aseptic vegetations of endocarditis (132). Coexisting coronary artery disease represents, however, the most common cause of myocardial infarction in patients with prosthetic heart valves. Heart block may occur after replacement of severely calcified aortic valves as a result of trauma to the bundle of His by removal of calcium from the region of the right trigone, beneath the commissure between the noncoronary and the right coronary cusp. Fortunately, complete heart block is uncommon and is usually transient due to postoperative edema of the periannular tissue.

Perforation of the posterior mitral annular region may occur after mitral valve replacement, particularly when severe calcification of the mitral annulus is present (133). The posterior pericardium may initially contain the rupture, avoiding cardiac tamponade and death. The diagnosis of this infrequent complication is often incidentally done from a routine echocardiogram. Pseudoaneurysms detected early after mitral valve prosthetic implantation require prompt surgical repair.

Patient–Prosthesis Mismatch

All prosthetic valves with the exception of the stentless aortic homograft have effective orifices that are smaller than those

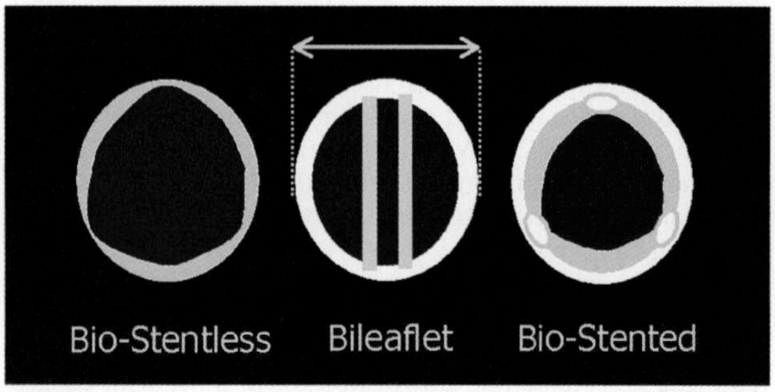

FIGURE 25.10. Illustration comparing bio-stentless, mechanical bileaflet, and bio-stented valves. For the same external diameter, the bio-stented valve has the smallest effective orifice.

of native valves of the same annular dimensions (Fig. 25.10). Thus, prosthetic valves are inherently stenotic and have a residual transvalvular pressure gradient. Occasionally this gradient is significant enough to cause symptoms, particularly when small prostheses are implanted in large patients. Pressure gradients that are of moderate magnitude at rest may increase significantly during exercise. Patient–prosthetic valve mismatch occurs most frequently after valve replacement for aortic stenosis. The aortic annulus is often small in these patients, and after replacement, the effective orifice may have an area between 1 and 1.5 cm^2. Dobutamine or exercise echocardiography may be useful for evaluating patients who have persisting symptoms after valve replacement by obtaining an estimate of the transvalvular gradients at high cardiac outputs and evaluating the effect of these gradients in left ventricular systolic function (134). In patients with small annular size, special consideration should be given to the hemodynamic profile when selecting the replacement valve. Stented bioprosthetic valves and ball-and-cage mechanical prostheses are intrinsically more stenotic. Patients with small tilting mechanical aortic prostheses often have increased resting and exercise gradients. However, recent studies have failed to demonstrate aerobic exercise impairment in these patients in comparison to age-matched healthy cohorts (135). Surgical techniques including supraannular implantation and supraannular and annular enlargement may be performed at several institutions to permit the implantation of larger prosthetic devices and avoid patient–prosthesis mismatch (136,137). Stentless valves are probably the best choice for active patients who want to avoid anticoagulation. Studies have shown better exercise hemodynamics and greater regression of LV hypertrophy in patients receiving stentless compared to those receiving stented valve prostheses (36,37). In general, stented aortic valve prostheses smaller than 21 mm in diameter are not recommended in larger patients who are physically active (138,139).

ROUTINE FOLLOW-UP OF PATIENTS WITH PROSTHETIC VALVES

After replacement, a transthoracic echocardiographic examination is recommended before discharge to exclude potential postoperative complications such as cardiac tamponade, ventricular pseudoaneurysm, prosthetic paravalvular regurgitation, or perioperative myocardial infarction. A follow-up clinical and echocardiographic evaluation is also recommended after 6 to 8 weeks. At this time careful determination of the transvalvular gradient, effective valvular orifice, and dimensionless transvalvular velocity index should be made for future comparisons. Further echocardiographic studies should not be required for several years unless there is failure of functional recovery after surgery or development of new symptoms that may indicate myocardial or valvular dysfunction. Additional information obtained from the echocardiogram such as the left and right ventricular systolic function, chamber sizes, and the estimation of the right ventricular systolic pressure can help to determine the etiology of symptoms. Echocardiographic studies should be repeated periodically in patients with evidence of prosthetic degeneration such as leaflet thickening and calcification, intravalvular regurgitation, or stenotic flow or in those with ventricular dysfunction or other valvular lesions. Otherwise, the routine performance of echocardiographic studies in asymptomatic patients with well-functioning prosthetic valves is controversial. Transesophageal echocardiography provides a more accurate assessment when regurgitation is suspected with mitral prostheses or when unexplained congestive heart failure or pulmonary hypertension occurs.

CONTROVERSIES AND PERSONAL PERSPECTIVES

The choice of mechanical versus bioprosthetic valve should be an early point of discussion among the cardiologist, the cardiac surgeon, and the patient. Multiple factors need to be considered in the decision-making process, including age of the patient, the probability of future pregnancy in young women, occupation, lifestyle, and life expectancy. The risk of a future reoperation should also be considered, possibly being greater after more extensive surgery such as stentless valve or allograft replacements. When feasible, valve repair is the preferred option. Otherwise, with the exception of very few circumstances, such as when a patient is already receiving chronic anticoagulation or has a short anticipated life expectancy, there are no absolute advantages of a specific valve type. Mechanical valve prostheses have a longer durability but require a lifelong commitment to chronic anticoagulation. They should be the choice in younger patients without contraindications who are expected to be medically compliant. The relative benefit-to-risk balance shifts earlier toward bioprosthetic valves in the aortic position. As a general guideline, we recommend bioprosthetic valves for aortic replacement in most patients older than 60 years and for mitral valve replacement after 70 years of age, but in general, this decision should be individualized for each specific patient taking into account existing comorbidities, lifestyle, and patient preferences. Middle-age or younger subjects who wish to avoid long-term anticoagulation requiring aortic valve replacement are good candidates for homograft or allograft replacement because the durability of theses valves appears to be greater than that of bioprosthesis. It remains to be determined whether the durability of stentless porcine valves is comparable.

THE FUTURE

Even though prosthetic valve replacement prolongs survival and improves quality of life for many patients with valvular disease, these valves have limited durability and potential risks. Many patients with prosthetic valve disease are poor surgical candidates due to coexisting lung, renal, or hepatic disease. Minimally invasive surgical procedures can reduce patient discomfort (140) but carry the same risks associated with cardiopulmonary bypass. Percutaneous valve repair (141,142) and replacement (143,144,145) procedures have been developed and are now being tested in clinical trials. These techniques could potentially improve the outcomes for high-risk patients by becoming an alternative to open-chest procedures.

New prosthetic valve designs, components, and preservation techniques are needed to improve durability and reduce the risks of thrombosis and infection associated with prosthetic devices. The limited durability of current bioprosthetic valves may be attributed in part to the absence of "life" tissue able to regenerate itself. Successful tissue engineering of functioning autologous heart valves based on human marrow stromal cells has been recently demonstrated in experimental models (146). Thus, it is conceivable than in the near future, life-tissue heart valves could be custom manufactured using autologous cells.

References

1. Hufnagel CA, Harvey WP. The surgical correction of aortic regurgitation: preliminary report. *Bull Georgetown Univ Med Center* 1953;6:60–61.
2. Harken DE, Soroff HS, Taylor WJ, et al. Partial and complete prostheses in aortic insufficiency. *J Thorac Cardiovasc Surg* 1960;40:744–762.
3. Starr A, Edwards ML. Mitral replacement: clinical experience with a ball valve prosthesis. *Ann Surg* 1961;154:726.
4. Ross DN. Homograft replacement of the aortic valve. *Lancet* 1967;2: 487.
5. Carpentier A, Chanard JC, Laurens P, et al. Use of aortic heterografts in treatment of mitral valvulopathy. Experimental basis and 1st clinical case. *Mem Acad Chir* 1967;93(19):617–622.
6. Grossman W. Profiles in valvular heart disease. In: Bain DS, Grossman W. *Cardiac catheterization, angiography and intervention,* 5th ed. Baltimore: Williams & Wilkins, 1996:735–756.
7. Morton MJ, Rahimtoola SH. How to follow patients with prosthetic heart valves. *J Cardiovasc Med* 1980;5:475–495.
8. van den Brink RB, Visser CA, Basart DC, et al. Comparison of transthoracic and transesophageal color Doppler flow imaging in patients with mechanical prostheses in the mitral valve position. *Am J Cardiol* 1989;63(20):1471–1474.
9. Baumgartner H, Khan S, DeRobertis M, et al. Effect of prosthetic aortic valve design on the Doppler-catheter gradient correlation: an in vitro study of normal St. Jude, Medtronic-Hall, Starr-Edwards and Hancock valves. *J Am Coll Cardiol* 1992;19(2):324–332.
10. Hammermeister KE, Sethi GK, Henderson WG, et al. A comparison of outcomes in men 11 years after heart-valve replacement with a mechanical valve or bioprosthesis. Veterans Affairs Cooperative Study on Valvular Heart Disease. *N Engl J Med* 1993;328(18):1289–1296.
11. Gabbay S, McQueen DM, Yellin EL, et al. In vitro hydrodynamic comparison of mitral valve prostheses at high flow rates. *J Thorac Cardiovasc Surg* 1978;76(6):771–787.
12. Horstkotte D, Haerten K, Herzer JA, et al. Five-year results after randomized mitral valve replacement with Björk-Shiley, Lillehei-Kaster, and Starr-Edwards prostheses. *Thorac Cardiovasc Surg* 1983;31(4):206–214.
13. Sala A, Schoevaerdts JC, Jaumin P, et al. Review of 387 isolated mitral valve replacements by the Model 6120 Starr-Edwards prosthesis. *J Thorac Cardiovasc Surg* 1982;84(5):744–750.
14. Walker DK, Scotten LN, Modi VJ, et al. In vitro assessment of mitral valve prostheses. *J Thorac Cardiovasc Surg* 1980;79(5):680–688.
15. Schaff HV, Chesebro JH. Experience with the Starr-Edwards silastic ball valve. *Cardiol Clin* 1985;3:405–416.
16. Pyle RB, Mayer JE Jr, Lindsay WG, et al. Hemodynamic evaluation of Lillehei-Kaiser and Starr-Edwards prosthesis. *Ann Thorac Surg* 1978; 26(4):336–343.
17. Winter TQ, Reis RL, Glancy DL, et al. Current status of the Starr-Edwards cloth-covered prosthetic cardiac valves. *Circulation* 1972;45(5/Suppl 1): 14–24.
18. Reif TH, Huffstutler MC JR. Design considerations for the omniscience pivoting disc cardiac valve prosthesis. *Int J Artif Organs* 1983;6(3):131–138.
19. Scotten LN, Racca RG, Nugent AH, et al. New tilting disc cardiac valve prostheses. In vitro comparison of their hydrodynamic performance in the mitral position. *J Thorac Cardiovasc Surg* 1981;82(1):136–146.
20. Emery RW, Mettler E, Nicoloff DM. A new cardiac prosthesis: the St. Jude Medical cardiac valve: in vivo results. *Circulation* 1979;60(2 Pt 2):48–54.
21. Subotic S, Petrovic P, Boskovic D, et al. Clinical and functional evaluation of the Carbomedics prosthetic heart valve in the mitral position. Preliminary results. *J Cardiovasc Surg* 1990;31(4):509–511.
22. Wang JH. The design simplicity and clinical elegance of the St. Jude Medical heart valve. *Ann Thorac Surg* 1989;48:S55–S56.
23. Aagaard J, Tingleff J. Fifteen years' clinical experience with the CarboMedics prosthetic heart valve. *J Heart Valve Dis* 2005;14(1):82–88.
24. Carpentier A, Lemaigre G, Robert L, et al. Biological factors affecting long-term results of valvular heterografts. *J Thorac Cardiovasc Surg* 1969;58(4):467–483.
25. Logeais Y, Langanay T, Leguerrier A, et al. Aortic Carpentier-Edwards supraannular porcine bioprosthesis: a 12-year experience. *Ann Thorac Surg* 1999;68(2):421–425.
26. Lurie AJ, Miller RR, Maxwell KS, et al. Hemodynamic assessment of the glutaraldehyde-preserved porcine heterograft in the aortic and mitral positions. *Circulation* 1977;56(3 Suppl):II104-II110.
27. Stinson EB, Griepp RB, Oyer PE, Shumway NE. Long-term experience with porcine aortic valve xenografts. *J Thorac Cardiovasc Surg* 1977;73(1):54–63.
28. Cohn LH, Collins Jr JJ, Rizzo RJ, et al. Twenty-year follow-up of the Hancock modified orifice porcine aortic valve. *Ann Thorac Surg* 1998;66(6 Suppl):S30–S34.
29. Jamieson WR, Tyers GF, Janusz MT, et al. Age as a determinant for selection of porcine bioprostheses for cardiac valve replacement: experience with Carpentier-Edwards standard bioprosthesis. *Can J Cardiol* 1991;7(4):181–188.
30. Jamieson WR, Rosado LJ, Munro AI, et al. Carpentier-Edwards standard porcine bioprosthesis: primary tissue failure (structural valve deterioration) by age groups. *Ann Thorac Surg* 1988;46(2):155–162.
31. Mueller XM, von Segesser LK. A new equine pericardial stentless valve. *J of Thorac Cardiovasc Surg* 2003;125(6):1405–1411.
32. Cosgrove DM, Lytle BW, Williams GW. Hemodynamic performance of the Carpentier-Edwards pericardial valve in the aortic position in vivo. *Circulation* 1985;72(3 Pt 2):II146–II152.
33. Eichinger WB, Botzenhardt F, Keithahn A, et al. Exercise hemodynamics of bovine versus porcine bioprostheses: a prospective randomized comparison of the mosaic and perimount aortic valves. *J Thorac Cardiovasc Surg* 2005;129(5):961–965.
34. Bortolotti U, Milano A, Mazzaro E, et al. Hancock II porcine bioprosthesis: excellent durability at intermediate-term follow-up. *J Am Coll Cardiol* 1994;24(3):676–682.
35. Goetze S, Brechtken J, Agler DA, et al. In vivo short-term Doppler hemodynamic profiles of 189 Carpentier-Edwards Perimount pericardial bioprosthetic valves in the mitral position. *J Am Soc Echocardiogr* 2004;17(9):981–987.
36. Williams RJ, Muir DF, Pathi V, et al. Randomized controlled trial of stented and stentless aortic bioprotheses: hemodynamic performance at 3 years. *Semin Thorac Cardiovasc Surg* 1999;11(4 Suppl 1):93–97.
37. Pibarot P, Dumesnil JG, Jobin J, et al. Hemodynamic and physical performance during maximal exercise in patients with an aortic bioprosthetic valve: comparison of stentless versus stented bioprostheses. *J Am Coll Cardiol* 1999;34(5):1609–1617.
38. Gaudino M, Alessandrini F, Glieca F, et al. Survival after aortic valve replacement for aortic stenosis: does left ventricular mass regression have a clinical correlate? *Eur Heart J* 2005;26(1):51–57.
39. Kon ND, Cordell AR, Adair SM, et al. Aortic root replacement with the freestyle stentless porcine aortic root bioprosthesis. *Ann Thorac Surg* 1999; 67(6):1609–1615.
40. David TE, Feindel CM, Scully HE, et al. Aortic valve replacement with stentless porcine aortic valves: a ten-year experience. *J Heart Valve Dis* 1998;7(3):250–254.
41. Doty DB, Michielon G, Wang ND, et al. Replacement of the aortic valve with cryopreserved aortic allograft. *Ann Thorac Surg* 1993;56(2):228–235.
42. Heslop BF, Wilson SE, Hardy BE. Antigenicity of aortic valve allografts. *Ann Surg* 1973;177(3):301–306.
43. Langley SM, McGuirk SP, Chaudhry MA, et al. Twenty-year follow-up of aortic valve replacement with antibiotic sterilized homografts in 200 patients. *Semin Thorac Cardiovasc Surg* 1999;11(4 Suppl 1):28–34.
44. Petrou M, Wong K, Albertucci M, et al. Evaluation of unstented aortic homografts for the treatment of prosthetic aortic valve endocarditis. *Circulation* 1994;90(5 Pt 2):II198–II204.
45. Grinda JM, Jouan J, Latremouille CH, et al. Human valvular substitutes for the treatment of complex progressive endocarditis. Application to aortic, mitral and tricuspid valve. *Arch Mal Coeur Vaiss* 2000;93(10):1195–1201.
46. Bloomfield P, Wheatley DJ, Prescott RJ, Miller HC. Twelve-year comparison of a Björk-Shiley mechanical heart valve with porcine bioprostheses. *N Engl J Med* 1991;324(9):573–579.
47. Ibrahim M, Cleland J, O'Kane H, et al. St. Jude Medical prosthesis in children. *J Thorac Cardiovasc Surg* 1994;108(1):52–56.
48. Bernal JM, Rabasa JM, Cagigas JC, et al. Valve-related complications with the Hancock I porcine bioprosthesis. A twelve- to fourteen-year follow-up study. *J Thorac Cardiovasc Surg* 1991;101(5):871–880.
49. Sareli P, England MJ, Berk MR, et al. Maternal and fetal sequelae of anticoagulation during pregnancy in patients with mechanical heart valve prostheses. *Am J Cardiol* 1989;63(20):1462–1465.
50. Iturbe-Alessio I, Fonseca MC, Mutchinik O, et al. Risks of anticoagulant therapy in pregnant women with artificial heart valves. *N Engl J Med* 1986; 315(22):1390–1393.
51. Hammond GL, Geha AS, Kopf GS, Hashim SW. Biological versus mechanical valves. Analysis of 1,116 valves inserted in 1,012 adult patients with a 4,818 patient-year and a 5,327 valve-year follow-up. *J Thorac Cardiovasc Surg* 1987;93(2):182–198.
52. Moggio RA, Hammond GL, Stansel Jr HC, Glenn WW. Incidence of emboli with cloth-covered Starr-Edwards valve without anticoagulation and with varying forms of anticoagulation. Analysis of 183 patients followed for 3 1/2 years. *J Thorac Cardiovasc Surg* 1978;75(2):296–299.
53. Akbarian M, Austen G, Yurchak PM, Scannell JG. Thromboembolic complications of prosthetic cardiac valves. *Circulation* 1968;37(5):826–831.

54. Chaux A, Gray RJ, Matloff JM, et al. An appreciation of the new St. Jude valvular prosthesis. *J Thorac Cardiovasc Surg* 1981;81(2):202–211.
55. Dewanjee MK, Trastek VF, Tago M, et al. Noninvasive radioisotopic technique for detection of platelet deposition on bovine pericardial mitral-valve prosthesis and in vitro quantification of visceral microembolism in dogs. *Trans Am Soc Artif Intern Organs* 1983;29:188–193.
56. Burchfiel CM, Hammermeister KE, Krause-Steinrauf H, et al. Left atrial dimension and risk of systemic embolism in patients with a prosthetic heart valve. Department of Veterans Affairs Cooperative Study on Valvular Heart Disease. *J Am Coll Cardiol* 1990;15(1):32–41.
57. Miller DC, Oyer PE, Stinson EB, et al. Ten to fifteen year reassessment of the performance characteristics of the Starr-Edwards Model 6120 mitral valve prosthesis. *J Thorac Cardiovasc Surg* 1983;85(1):1–20.
58. Antunes MJ, Wessels A, Sadowski RG, et al. Medtronic Hall valve replacement in a third-world population group. A review of the performance of 1000 prostheses. *J Thorac Cardiovasc Surg* 1988;95(6):980–993.
59. Arom KV, Nicoloff DM, Kersten TE, et al. St. Jude Medical prosthesis: valve-related deaths and complications. *Ann Thorac Surg* 1987;43(6):591–598.
60. Czer LS, Matloff JM, Chaux A, et al. The St. Jude valve: analysis of thromboembolism, warfarin-related hemorrhage, and survival. *Am Heart J* 1987;114(2):389–397.
61. Duncan JM, Cooley DA, Reul GJ, et al. Durability and low thrombogenicity of the St. Jude Medical valve at 5-year follow-up. *Ann Thorac Surg* 1986;42(5):500–505.
62. Murphy DA, Levine FH, Buckley MJ, et al. Mechanical valves: a comparative analysis of the Starr-Edwards and Björk-Shiley prostheses. *J Thorac Cardiovasc Surg* 1983;86(5):746–752.
63. Cannegieter SC, Rosendaal FR, Briet E. Thromboembolic and bleeding complications in patients with mechanical heart valve prostheses. *Circulation* 1994;89(2):635–641.
64. Saour JN, Sieck JO, Mamo LA, Gallus AS. Trial of different intensities of anticoagulation in patients with prosthetic heart valves. *N Engl J Med* 1990;322(7):428–432.
65. Turpie AG, Gent M, Laupacis A, et al. A comparison of aspirin with placebo in patients treated with warfarin after heart-valve replacement. *N Engl J Med* 1993;329(8):524–529.
66. Laros Jr RK, Alger LS. Thromboembolism and pregnancy. *Clin Obstet Gynecol* 1979;22(4):871–878.
67. Stevenson RE, Burton OM, Ferlauto GJ, Taylor HA. Hazards of oral anticoagulants during pregnancy. *JAMA* 1980;243(15):1549–1551.
68. Lutz DJ, Noller KL, Spittell Jr JA, et al. Pregnancy and its complications following cardiac valve prostheses. *Am J Obstet Gynecol* 1978;131(4):460–468.
69. Ginsberg JS, Hirsh J. Use of antithrombotic agents during pregnancy. *Chest* 1995;108(4 Suppl):305S–311S.
70. Ginsberg JS, Kowalchuk G, Hirsh J, et al. Heparin therapy during pregnancy. *Arch Intern Med* 1989;149(10):2233–2236.
71. Hirsh J, Cade JF, Gallus AS. Anticoagulants in pregnancy: a review of indications and complications. *Am Heart J* 1972;83(3):301–305.
72. Rasmussen C, Wadt J, Jacobsen B. Thromboembolic prophylaxis with low molecular weight heparin during pregnancy. *Int J Gynaecol Obstet* 1994; 47(2):121–125.
73. Oran B, Lee-Parritz A, Ansell J. Low molecular weight heparin for the prophylaxis of thromboembolism in women with prosthetic mechanical heart valves during pregnancy. *Thromb Haemost* 2004; 92(4):747–751.
74. Tinker JH, Tarhan S. Discontinuing anticoagulant therapy in surgical patients with cardiac valve prostheses. Observations in 180 operations. *JAMA* 1978;239(8):738–739.
75. Thorburn CW, Morgan JJ, Shanahan MX, Chang VP. Long-term results of tricuspid valve replacement and the problem of prosthetic valve thrombosis. *Am J Cardiol* 1983;51(7):1128–1132.
76. Kontos Jr GJ, Schaff HV, Orszulak TA, et al. Thrombotic obstruction of disc valves: clinical recognition and surgical management. *Ann Thorac Surg* 1989;48(1):60–65.
77. Gueret P, Vignon P, Fournier P, et al. Transesophageal echocardiography for the diagnosis and management of nonobstructive thrombosis of mechanical mitral valve prosthesis. *Circulation* 1995;91(1):103–110.
78. Vasan RS, Kaul U, Sanghvi S, et al. Thrombolytic therapy for prosthetic valve thrombosis: a study based on serial Doppler echocardiographic evaluation. *Am Heart J* 1992;123(6):1575–1580.
79. Kurzrok S, Singh AK, Most AS, Williams DO. Thrombolytic therapy for prosthetic cardiac valve thrombosis. *J Am Coll Cardiol* 1987;9(3):592–598.
80. Reddy NK, Padmanabhan TN, Singh S, et al. Thrombolysis in left-sided prosthetic valve occlusion: immediate and follow-up results. *Ann Thorac Surg* 1994;58(2):462–470.
81. Roudaut R, Labbe T, Lorient-Roudaut MF, et al. Mechanical cardiac valve thrombosis. Is fibrinolysis justified? *Circulation* 1992;86(5 Suppl):II8–II15.
82. Jost CM, Yancy Jr CW, Ring WS. Combined thrombolytic therapy for prosthetic mitral valve thrombosis. *Ann Thorac Surg* 1993;55(1):159–161.
83. Guerrero Lopez F, Vazquez Mata G, Reina Toral A, et al. Thrombolytic treatment for massive thrombosis of prosthetic cardiac valves. *Int Care Med* 1993;19(3):145–150.
84. Vitale N, Renzulli A, Cerasuolo F, et al. Prosthetic valve obstruction: thrombolysis versus operation. *Ann Thorac Surg* 1994;57(2):365–370.
85. Roudaut R, Lafitte S, Roudaut MF, et al. Fibrinolysis of mechanical prosthetic valve thrombosis: a single-center study of 127 cases. *J Am Coll Cardiol* 2003;41(4):653–658.
86. Ozkan M, Kaymaz C, Kirma C, et al. Intravenous thrombolytic treatment of mechanical prosthetic valve thrombosis: a study using serial transesophageal echocardiography. *J Am Coll Cardiol* 2000;35(7):1881–1889.
87. Shapira Y, Herz I, Vaturi M, et al. Thrombolysis is an effective and safe therapy in stuck bileaflet mitral valves in the absence of high-risk thrombi. *J Am Coll Cardiol* 2000;35(7):1874–1880.
88. Tong AT, Roudaut R, Ozkan M, et al. Transesophageal echocardiography improves risk assessment of thrombolysis of prosthetic valve thrombosis: results of the International PRO-TEE Registry. *J Am Coll Cardiol* 2004; 43(1):77–84.
89. Deviri E, Sareli P, Wisenbaugh T, Cronje SL. Obstruction of mechanical heart valve prostheses: clinical aspects and surgical management. *J Am Coll Cardiol* 1991;17(3):646–650.
90. Husebye DG, Pluth JR, Piehler JM, et al. Reoperation on prosthetic heart valves. An analysis of risk factors in 552 patients. *J Thorac Cardiovasc Surg* 1983;86(4):543–552.
91. Heras M, Chesebro JH, Fuster V, et al. High risk of thromboemboli early after bioprosthetic cardiac valve replacement. *J Am Coll Cardiol* 1995; 25(5):1111–1119.
92. Turpie AG, Gunstensen J, Hirsh J, et al. Randomised comparison of two intensities of oral anticoagulant therapy after tissue heart valve replacement. *Lancet* 1988;1(8597):1242–1245.
93. Gherli T, Colli A, Fragnito C, et al. Comparing warfarin with aspirin after biological aortic valve replacement: a prospective study. *Circulation* 2004;110(5):496–500.
94. Sundt TM, Zehr KJ, Dearani JA, et al. Is early anticoagulation with warfarin necessary after bioprosthetic aortic valve replacement? *J Thorac Cardiovasc Surg* 2005;129(5):1024–1031.
95. Oyer PE, Stinson EB, Reitz BA, et al. Long-term evaluation of the porcine xenograft bioprosthesis. *J Thorac Cardiovasc Surg* 1979;78(3):343–350.
96. Cohn LH, Mudge GH, Pratter F, Collins Jr JJ. Five to eight-year follow-up of patients undergoing porcine heart-valve replacement. *N Engl J Med* 1981;304(5):258–262.
97. Jones EL, Weintraub WS, Craver JM, et al. Ten-year experience with the porcine bioprosthetic valve: interrelationship of valve survival and patient survival in 1,050 valve replacements. *Ann Thorac Surg* 1990;49(3):370–383.
98. Bansal RC, Morrison DL, Jacobson JG. Echocardiography of porcine aortic prosthesis with flail leaflets due to degeneration and calcification. *Am Heart J* 1984;107(3):591–593.
99. Akiyama K, Sawatani O, Imamura E, et al. Stent creep of porcine bioprosthesis in the mitral position. *Ann Thorac Surg* 1988;46(1):73–78.
100. Grunkemeier GL, Starr A. Twenty-five year experience with Starr-Edwards heart valves: follow-up methods and results. *Can J Cardiol* 1988;4(7):381–385.
101. Williams DB, Pluth JR, Orszulak TA. Extrinsic obstruction of the Björk-Shiley valve in the mitral position. *Ann Thorac Surg* 1981;32(1):58–62.
102. Berger RL. Retrograde disc escape in a Harken mitral valve prosthesis. *Ann Thorac Surg* 1992;54(2):394–395.
103. Dimitri WR, Williams BT. Fracture of the Duromedics mitral valve housing with leaflet escape. *J Cardiovasc Surg* 1990;31(1):41–46.
104. Kornberg A, Wildhirt SM, Schulze C, Kreuzer E. Leaflet escape in Omnicarbon monoleaflet valve. *Eur J Cardiothorac Surg* 1999;15(6):867–869.
105. Birkmeyer JD, Marrin CA, O'Connor GT. Should patients with Björk-Shiley valves undergo prophylactic replacement? *Lancet* 1992;340(8818):520–523.
106. van der Meulen JH, Steyerberg EW, van der Graaf Y, et al. Age thresholds for prophylactic replacement of Björk-Shiley convexo-concave heart valves. A clinical and economic evaluation. *Circulation* 1993;88(1):156–164.
107. Calderwood SB, Swinski LA, Waternaux CM, et al. Risk factors for the development of prosthetic valve endocarditis. *Circulation* 1985;72(1):31–37.
108. Wilson WR, Danielson GK, Giuliani ER, Geraci JE. Prosthetic valve endocarditis. *Mayo Clinic Proc* 1982;57(3):155–161.
109. Ivert TS, Dismukes WE, Cobbs CG, et al. Prosthetic valve endocarditis. *Circulation* 1984;69(2):223–232.
110. Horstkotte D, Piper C, Niehues R, et al. Late prosthetic valve endocarditis. *Eur Heart J* 1995;16(Suppl B):39–47.
111. Chastre J, Trouillet JL. Early infective endocarditis on prosthetic valves. *Eur Heart J* 1995;16(Suppl B):32–38.
112. Conte Jr JE, Cohen SN, Roe BB, Elashoff RM. Antibiotic prophylaxis and cardiac surgery. A prospective double-blind comparison of single-dose versus multiple-dose regimens. *Ann Intern Med* 1972;76(6):943–949.
113. Effron MK, Popp RL. Two-dimensional echocardiographic assessment of bioprosthetic valve dysfunction and infective endocarditis. *J Am Coll Cardiol* 1983;2(4):597–606.
114. Erbel R, Rohmann S, Drexler M, et al. Improved diagnostic value of echocardiography in patients with infective endocarditis by transoesophageal approach. A prospective study. *Eur Heart J* 1988;9(1):43–53.
115. Daniel WG, Mugge A, Grote J, et al. Comparison of transthoracic and transesophageal echocardiography for detection of abnormalities of prosthetic and bioprosthetic valves in the mitral and aortic positions. *Am J Cardiol* 1993;71(2):210–215.

116. Daniel WG, Mugge A, Martin RP, et al. Improvement in the diagnosis of abscesses associated with endocarditis by transesophageal echocardiography. *N Engl J Med* 1991;324(12):795–800.
117. Sochowski RA, Chan KL. Implication of negative results on a monoplane transesophageal echocardiographic study in patients with suspected infective endocarditis. *J Am Coll Cardiol* 1993;21(1):216–221.
118. Threlkeld MG, Cobbs CG. Infectious disorders of prosthetic valves and intravascular devices. In: Mandell GL, Bennett JE, Dolin R, eds. *Mandell, Douglas and Bennett's principles and practice of infectious diseases,* Vol. 1, 4th ed. New York: Churchill Livingstone, 1995:783–793.
119. Baumgartner WA, Miller DC, Reitz BA, et al. Surgical treatment of prosthetic valve endocarditis. *Ann Thorac Surg* 1983;35(1):87–104.
120. Kirklin JK, Kirklin JW, Pacifico AD. Aortic valve endocarditis with aortic root abscess cavity: surgical treatment with aortic valve homograft. *Ann Thorac Surg* 1988;45(6):674–677.
121. Lytle BW, Priest BP, Taylor PC, et al. Surgical treatment of prosthetic valve endocarditis. *J Thorac Cardiovasc Surg* 1996;111(1):198–207.
122. Fang G, Keys TF, Gentry LO, et al. Prosthetic valve endocarditis resulting from nosocomial bacteremia. A prospective, multicenter study. *Ann Intern Med* 1993;119(7 Pt 1):560–567.
123. Dajani AS, Taubert KA, Wilson W, et al. Prevention of bacterial endocarditis. Recommendations by the American Heart Association. *JAMA* 1997;277(22):1794–1801.
124. Weed RI, Reed CF. Membrane alterations leading to red cell destruction. *Am J Med* 1966;41:681–698.
125. Garcia MJ, Vandervoort P, Stewart W, et al. Mechanisms of hemolysis with mitral prosthetic regurgitation: A study using transesophageal echo and fluid dynamic simulation. *J Am Coll Cardiol* 1996;27:399–406.
126. Gradon JD, Hirschbein M, Milligan J. Fragmentation hemolysis: an unusual indication for valve replacement in native valve infective endocarditis. *South Med J* 1996;89(8):818–820.
127. Enzenauer RJ, Berenberg JL, Cassell Jr PF. Microangiopathic hemolytic anemia as the initial manifestation of porcine valve failure. *South Med J* 1990;83(8):912–917.
128. Okita Y, Miki S, Kusuhara K, et al. Propranolol for intractable hemolysis after open heart operation. *Ann Thorac Surg* 1991;52(5):1158–1160.
129. Schapira JN, Martin RP, Fowles RE, et al. Two dimensional echocardiographic assessment of patients with bioprosthetic valves. *Am J Cardiol* 1979;43(3):510–519.
130. Kotler MN, Goldman A, Parry WR. Noninvasive evaluation of cardiac valve prostheses. *Cardiovasc Clin* 1986;17(1):201–241.
131. Redberg RF, Schiller NB. Use of transesophageal echocardiography in evaluating coronary arteries. *Cardiol Clin* 1993;11(3):521–528.
132. Herzog CA, Henry TD, Zimmer SD. Bacterial endocarditis presenting as acute myocardial infarction: a cautionary note for the era of reperfusion. *Am J Med* 1991;90(3):392–397.
133. Waller BF, Taliercio CP, Clark M, Pless J. Rupture of the left ventricular free wall following mitral valve replacement for mitral stenosis: a cause of complete (fatal) or contained (false aneurysm) cardiac rupture. *Clin Cardiol* 1991;14(4):341–345.
134. Zabalgoitia M, Kopec K, Abochamh DA, et al. Usefulness of dobutamine echocardiography in the hemodynamic assessment of mechanical prostheses in the aortic valve position. *Am J Cardiol* 1997;80(4):523–526.
135. Becassis P, Hayot M, Frapier JM, et al. Postoperative exercise tolerance after aortic valve replacement by small-size prosthesis: functional consequence of small-size aortic prosthesis. *J Am Coll Cardiol* 2000;36(3):871–877.
136. David TE, Uden DE. Aortic valve replacement in adult patients with small aortic annuli. *Ann Thorac Surg* 1983;36(5):577–583.
137. Piehler JM, Danielson GK, Pluth JR, et al. Enlargement of the aortic root or anulus with autogenous pericardial patch during aortic valve replacement. Long-term follow-up. *J Thorac Cardiovasc Surg* 1983;86(3):350–358.
138. Jaffe WM, Coverdale HA, Roche AH, et al. Rest and exercise hemodynamics of 20 to 23 mm allograft, Medtronic Intact (porcine), and St. Jude Medical valves in the aortic position. *J Thorac Cardiovasc Surg* 1990; 100(2):167–174.
139. Foster AH, Tracy CM, Greenberg GJ, et al. Valve replacement in narrow aortic roots: serial hemodynamics and long-term clinical outcome. *Ann Thorac Surg* 1986;42(5):506–516.
140. Grossi EA, Galloway AC, Ribakove GH, et al. Impact of minimally invasive valvular heart surgery: a case–control study. *Ann Thorac Surg* 2001;71: 807–810.
141. Liddicoat JR, Mac Neill BD, Gillinov AM, et al. Percutaneous mitral valve repair: a feasibility study in an ovine model of acute ischemic mitral regurgitation. *Catheter Cardiovasc Interv* 2003;60:410–416.
142. St. Goar FG, Fann JI, Komtebedde J, et al. Endovascular edge-to-edge mitral valve repair: short-term results in a porcine model. *Circulation* 2003; 108:1990–1993.
143. Andersen HR, Knudsen LL, Hasenkam JM. Transluminal implantation of artificial heart valves. Description of new expandable aortic valve and initial results with implantation by catheter technique in closed chest pigs. *Eur Heart J* 1992;13:704–708.
144. Bonhoeffer P, Boudjemline Y, Saliba Z, et al. Transcatheter implantation of a bovine valve in pulmonary position: A lamb study. *Circulation* 2000;102:813–816.
145. Cribier A, Eltchaninoff H, Bash A, et al. Percutaneous trans-catheter implantation of an aortic valve prosthesis for calcific aortic stenosis: first human case description. *Circulation* 2002;106:3006–3008.
146. Hoerstrup SP, Kadner A, Melnitchouk S, et al. Tissue engineering of functional trileaflet heart valves from human marrow stromal cells. *Circulation* 2002;106:I143–1150.

CHAPTER 26 ■ INFECTIVE ENDOCARDITIS

JENNIFER S. LI, G. RALPH COREY, AND VANCE G. FOWLER, JR.

Infectious endocarditis (IE) denotes infection of the endocardial surface of the heart and implies the physical presence of microorganisms in the lesion. Although the heart valves are most commonly affected, the disease may also occur within septal defects or on the mural endocardium. Infections of arteriovenous shunts and of arterioarterial shunts (patent ductus arteriosus) as well as infection related to coarctation of the aorta can also be included in this definition because of their similar clinical manifestations. Unfortunately, variability in the clinical presentation continues to make the diagnosis of IE challenging. Diagnostic criteria have been recently developed that utilize clinical findings, pertinent laboratory data, and echocardiography to diagnose IE with a high degree of sensitivity and specificity. Transesophageal echocardiography (TEE) has become a major advance in evaluating vegetations particularly in patients with prosthetic valve disease and in those with complications such as annular abscesses and intracardiac fistulae.

Yet, despite improvements in diagnosis and treatment, IE continues to be associated with high morbidity and mortality. Reasons for this are several. The patient with IE is often increasingly complex. For example, patients are often older with nosocomial bloodstream infections, infected prosthetic valves, or even congenital heart disease. In addition, *Staphylococcus aureus* has become a major pathogen in nosocomial IE. Targeted antibiotic treatment is the ideal approach to the pharmacologic management of IE. Prevention remains the standard of care. Successful management depends on the close cooperation of cardiologists, cardiothoracic surgeons, and infectious disease specialists.

GLOSSARY

Endarteritis: Inflammation of the intima of an artery.

Janeway lesion: Erythematous, nontender lesions on fingers, palm, or sole.

Mycotic aneurysms: Aneurysmal dilatation of a vessel caused by invasion of the vascular wall from infective endocarditis.

Osler nodes: Small, tender, purple erythematous subcutaneous nodules visibly found on the pulp of digits.

Roth spots: Retinal hemorrhages with a clear center.

Splinter hemorrhage: An embolic subungual hemorrhage located proximally in the nail bed.

Vegetations: Growth consisting of fused platelets, fibrin, and other bacteria adherent to a heart valve or other vascular structure.

HISTORICAL PERSPECTIVE

The first description of infection of the heart valves in humans appeared over 300 years ago (1). Riveriere described autopsy findings associated with IE in 1723 and Morgagni provided classical descriptions in 1761. In 1806, Jean Nicolause Corvisart first used the term *vegetations* to describe the characteristic macroscopic excrescences seen in IE (2). Laennec, Bouillaud, Charcot, and Vichow described many clinical and pathological features of IE over the next 75 years. However, it was not until 1937 that Gross concluded that heart valves were avascular structures involved in an inflammatory response (3).

Experiments by Rosenbach, Wyssokowitsch, and Weichselbaum subsequently demonstrated that most patients with IE had preexisting damage to their heart valves and that the initiating event was the entry of microbes into the bloodstream from a site of local infection or a mucosal surface (2).

In his series of famous Gulstonian lectures in 1885, William Osler became the first person to systematically describe the clinical features of IE by identifying four cardinal manifestations. These manifestations remain the hallmarks of clinical diagnosis in the present era: persistent bacteremia, active valvulitis, large-vessel emboli, and immunologic vascular phenomena (4). He coined the term *mycotic aneurysm* to describe the focal endarteritis that may complicate IE and described emboli to multiple organs such as the brain, spleen, kidney, and retina. He also described the Osler nodes, "small swollen areas, some the size of a pea, others a centimeter and a half in diameter, raised, red with a whitish spot in the center . . . the commonest situation is near the tip of the finger" (5).

A famous early case of IE was reported by Soma Weiss, who described a medical student who had chronic rheumatic heart disease and then developed *S. viridans* IE. In his diary, the student noted clubbing of his finger beds and peripheral embolic phenomenon. On discovering these cutaneous manifestations of his disease, he turned to his sister-in-law and prophetically proclaimed, "I shall be dead in 6 months" (6).

Although invariably fatal until the discovery of penicillin and other antimicrobial agents, steady advances in medical and surgical therapy have had a large impact on this disease. New methods in echocardiography and imaging as well as molecular tools have improved the ability to diagnose IE. However, the heterogeneous population of patients who develop IE and the growing development of resistant organisms continue to make IE a challenging disease for clinicians.

EPIDEMIOLOGY

The incidence of IE is difficult to determine because the criteria for diagnosis and the methods of reporting vary with different series (7,8). An analysis based on strict case definitions often reveals that only a small proportion (~20%) of clinically diagnosed cases are categorized as definite. Nevertheless, IE accounted for approximately 1 case per 1,000 hospital admissions, with a range of 0.16 to 5.40 cases per 1,000 admissions, in a review of 10 large surveys (7,9). This incidence has not changed appreciably over the past 30 years (10). Estimates from the American Heart Association (AHA) place the annual incidence of IE in the United States at 10,000 to 20,000 new cases.

Men are more commonly affected than women (mean male: female ratio 1.7:1 in 18 large series) (11). However, in patients under the age of 35 years, more cases occur in women. The disease remains uncommon in children and infants, in whom it is associated primarily with nosocomial bacteremia in the setting of underlying structural congenital heart disease (12,13).

There is general agreement that new trends in the epidemiology of IE have occurred during the past 30 years. These changes are mainly due to the types of susceptible hosts rather than to shifts in the virulence of the infecting microorganisms. Patients with IE are typically older. In 1926, the median age was less than 30 years; this had increased to 39 years by 1943, and currently over 50% of the patients are older than 50 years (14–16). A number of factors may relate to this shift in age distribution. First, there has been a change in the nature of the underlying heart disease owing to a decline in the incidence of acute rheumatic fever and rheumatic heart disease and a simultaneous rise in the frequency of degenerative heart disease. Second, the age of the population has been steadily increasing, and people with rheumatic or congenital heart disease are surviving longer.

In addition, such patients increasingly undergo prosthetic valve surgery, an important risk factor for IE. More than 150,000 heart valves are implanted annually worldwide (17). Prosthetic valve IE (PVE) develops in 1% to 4% of prosthetic valve recipients in the first year following valve replacement and in approximately 1% of recipients annually thereafter (18,19). The risk of IE in patients with mechanical or bioprosthetic valves is similar. In a multicenter follow-up study of over 1,000 patients who were randomized to receive mechanical or bioprosthetic valves, the overall rate of PVE was similar in both groups (0.8 cases per year of follow-up) (18). Mechanical prosthetic valves may be more susceptible to IE initially, whereas after 1 year, bioprosthetic valves are more likely to develop IE (20,21).

A new form of the disease—nosocomial IE—secondary to new therapeutic modalities (intravenous catheters, hyperalimentation lines, pacemakers, dialysis shunts, etc.) has emerged (22). Nosocomial IE is usually a complication of bacteremia induced by an invasive procedure or a vascular device. Of 125 cases of IE reviewed in Seattle, 35 were nosocomial in origin (28%) (23). Although nosocomial IE accounted for only 14.3% of cases in another recent study, 64% of patients were over 60 years of age, and mortality was high (24). The emerging importance of nosocomial IE in industrialized nations has influenced the microbiology of IE, with an increasing prevalence of *S. aureus* and decreasing prevalence of viridans streptococci among U.S. tertiary care centers (22). *S. aureus* is now a leading cause of bacteremia and IE. Over the past several years, the frequency of *S. aureus* bacteremia (SAB) has increased dramatically. This increasing frequency, coupled with increasing rates of antibiotic resistance, has renewed interest in this serious, common infection. *S. aureus* is a unique pathogen because of its virulent properties, protean manifestations, and ability to cause IE on architecturally normal cardiac valves (25).

The rise in the incidence of injection drug use has also had a major impact on the epidemiology of IE. The incidence of IE in intravenous drug users (IDU) may be 30 times higher than the general population and 4 times higher than the risk of IE in adults with rheumatic heart disease (26). In some areas of the United States, drug addiction is the most common predisposing cause for IE in patients less than 40 years old (27). *S. aureus* is the predominant organism. Tricuspid valve involvement is noted in 78%, mitral in 24%, and aortic in 8% of drug abusers with IE (28). More than one valve is involved in approximately 20% of cases and some of these infections are polymicrobial (29,30).

HEMODYNAMIC AND ANATOMIC CONSIDERATIONS

IE characteristically occurs on the atrial surface of the atrioventricular and the ventricular surface of the semilunar valve when associated with valvular insufficiency. Rodbard (31) showed that this localization is related to a decrease in lateral pressure (presumably with decreased perfusion of the intima) immediately "downstream" from the regurgitant flow. Lesions with high degrees of turbulence (small ventricular septal defect with a jet lesion, high-velocity jets across stenotic or regurgitant valves) readily create conditions that lead to bacterial colonization, whereas defects with a large surface area (large ventricular septal defect), low flow (ostium secundum atrial septal defect), or attenuation of turbulence (chronic congestive heart failure [CHF] with atrial fibrillation) are rarely implicated in IE. Cures of IE achieved with ligation alone of an arteriovenous fistula or patent ductus arteriosus also highlight the importance of hemodynamic factors.

The degree of mechanical stress exerted on the valve also affects the location of the IE (32). In 1,024 autopsy cases of IE reviewed through 1952, the incidence of valvular lesions was as follows: mitral, 86%; aortic, 55%; tricuspid, 19.6%; and pulmonic, 1.1%. This correlates with the pressure resting on the closed valve: 116, 72, 24, and 5 mm Hg, respectively.

Previous studies have shown that approximately three fourths of all patients with IE have a preexisting structural cardiac abnormality at the time that IE begins (33). However, the increasing incidence of *S. aureus* in nosocomial and IDU-associated IE has altered this pattern.

Aortic valve disease has been a predisposing cause for IE in 12% to 30% of cases (34). The peak gradient across the aortic valve is linked to the risk of IE; the higher the gradient, the higher the risk of developing IE (35). Patients with aortic regurgitation have an approximately 50% lower incidence of IE than those with aortic stenosis (36). Mitral valve disease has become relatively more important as a predisposing cause for IE. Preexisting mitral valve prolapse was the underlying cardiac lesion in 22% to 29% of IE in two cases series (37,38). The risk of IE is clearly higher in patients with mitral valve prolapse. In a careful retrospective epidemiologic matched case-control analysis, the calculated odds ratio (OR) 8.2 (95% confidence interval [CI], 2.4–28.4) indicates a substantially higher risk for the development of IE in these patients than in controls (39). Historically, rheumatic heart disease was the underlying lesion in 37% to 76% of the infections, and the mitral valve is involved in more than 85% of these cases (40). The tricuspid valve is rarely involved (0% to 6% of the cases), and the pulmonary valve even less often (<1%).

Congenital heart disease is now the underlying lesion in 10% to 20% of cases of IE (41). The most common congenital heart lesions predisposing to IE include bicuspid aortic valve, patent ductus arteriosus, ventricular septal defect, coarctation of the aorta, and tetralogy of Fallot. Unlike most other congenital defects, secundum atrial septal defects are not associated with an increased risk (42).

IE in patients with hypertrophic cardiomyopathy is virtually confined to those patients with outflow obstruction. In the subset of patients with hypertrophic cardiomyopathy who have outflow obstruction, the incidence of IE is 3.8 per 1,000 person-years with a probability of IE of 4.3% at 10 years. In patients with both outflow obstruction and left atrial dilatation (≥50 mm), the incidence of IE increases to 9.2 per 1,000 person-years (43).

The "degenerative" cardiac lesions (calcified mitral annulus, calcific nodular lesions secondary to arteriosclerotic cardiovascular disease) assume the greatest importance in patients without any demonstrable underlying valvular disease. The actual contribution made by these lesions is unknown, but they occur with an increased incidence in the elderly. In one series, degenerative lesions were present in 50% of patients over 60 years old with native valve IE (44).

PATHOPHYSIOLOGY

The endothelial lining of the heart and its valves is normally resistant to infection with bacteria and fungi. In vitro observations and studies in experimental animals have demonstrated that the development of IE requires the simultaneous occurrence of several independent events, each of which may be influenced by a host of separate factors (45–48). The valve surface must first be altered to produce a suitable site for bacterial attachment and colonization. Surface changes may be produced by various local and systemic stresses, including blood turbulence. These alterations result in the deposition of platelets and fibrin and in the formation of so-called sterile vegetation—the lesions of nonbacterial thrombotic endocarditis (NBTE).

Bacteria must then reach this site and adhere to the involved tissue to produce colonization. Transient bacteremia occurs whenever a mucosal surface heavily colonized with bacteria is traumatized, such as with certain dental, gastrointestinal, urologic, and gynecologic procedures. Certain strains of bacteria appear to have a selective advantage in adhering to platelets and/or fibrin and thus produce the disease with a lower inoculum. The ability of these organisms to adhere to NBTE lesions is a crucial early step in the development of IE. Gould et al. (49) showed that organisms frequently associated with IE (enterococci, viridans streptococci, *S. aureus, S. epidermidis, Pseudomonas aeruginosa*) adhered more avidly to normal canine aortic leaflets in vitro than did organisms uncommon in IE (*Klebsiella pneumoniae, Escherichia coli*) (49). In addition, *S. aureus* and the viridans streptococci produced IE more readily than did *E. coli* in the rabbit model of IE (50). This observation correlates with the relative frequency with which these organisms produce the disease in humans. Microbial adherence is mediated by several factors, including the amount of dextran in the cell wall of the microorganism, the ability of the organism to bind fibronectin, the presence of surface adhesions such as Fim A, and the presence of other compounds that may mediate bacterial adherence, including fibrinogen, laminin, and type 4 collagen (51–54).

After colonization, the surface is rapidly covered with a protective sheath of platelets and fibrin to produce an environment conducive to further bacterial multiplication and vegetation growth. Microbial growth results in the secondary accumulation of more platelets and fibrin until a macroscopic excrescence or vegetation is present (Fig. 26.1). The culmination of this process is mature vegetation consisting of an amorphous collection of fibrin, platelets, leukocytes, red blood cell debris, and dense clusters of bacteria. The surface of most vegetations consists of fibrin and scant numbers of leukocytes. Clumps of bacteria, histiocytes, and monocytes are usually found deep within the vegetation. Giant cells containing phagocytic bacteria may be found in some vegetations. Extremely high concentrations of bacteria (e.g., 10^9–10^{11} bacteria per gram of tissue) may accumulate deep within vegetations. Some of these bacteria exist in a state of reduced metabolic activity. Following

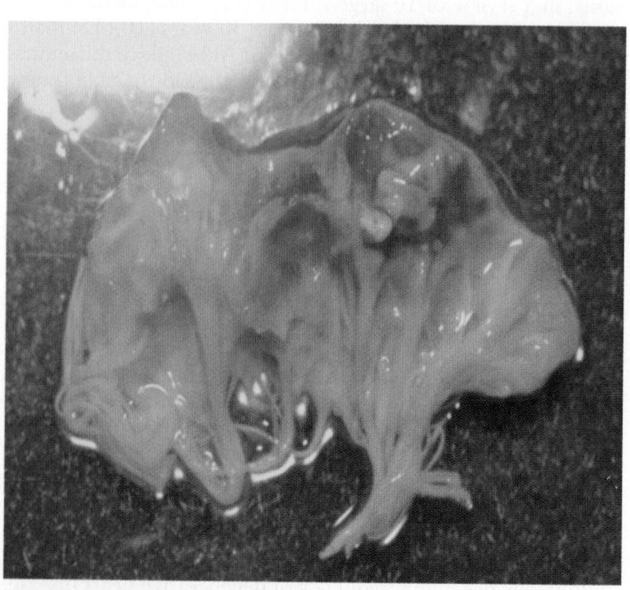

FIGURE 26.1. Pathologic specimen of a mitral valve and vegetation infected with *S. aureus*. Courtesy of Vance G. Fowler, Jr. MD.

therapy and during the process of healing, capillaries and fibroblasts appear within vegetations, but without treatment, vegetations are avascular structures (55).

Vegetations often prevent proper valvular leaflet or cusp coaptation, resulting in worsening valvular incompetence and CHF. Vegetation growth may result in leaflet perforation that can manifest as acute CHF (56). Patients with mitral or tricuspid valve vegetations may develop chordal rupture when infection progresses beyond the valve orifice. Extension of infection may also occur into surrounding structures such as the valve ring, the adjacent myocardium, the cardiac conduction system, or the mitral–aortic intravalvular fibrosa (57). Rarely, cavitation of periaortic abscesses may occur into the adjacent aortic wall, resulting in the formation of a diverticulum or aneurysm. Even more rarely, such aneurysms may perforate into surrounding structures resulting in aortic-atrial or aortic–pericardial fistulae (58).

IE causes the stimulation of both humoral and cellular immunity as manifested by hypergammaglobulinemia, splenomegaly, and the presence of macrophages in the peripheral blood. Rheumatoid factor (anti-immunoglobulin (Ig) G IgM antibody) develops in about 50% of patients with IE of longer than 6 weeks duration (59). Antinuclear antibodies also occur in IE and may contribute to the musculoskeletal manifestations, low-grade fever, or pleuritic pain (60). Opsonic (IgG), agglutinating (IgG, IgM), and complement-fixing (IgG, IgM) antibodies and cryoglobulins (IgG, IgM, IgA, C3, fibrinogen), various antibodies to bacterial heat shock proteins, and macroglobulins all have been described in IE (61,63). Circulating immune complexes have been found in high titers in virtually all patients with IE and may cause a diffuse glomerulonephritis (64). Some of the peripheral manifestations of IE, such as Osler nodes, may also result from a deposition of circulating immune complexes. Pathologically, these lesions resemble an acute Arthus reaction. However, the finding of positive culture aspirates in Osler nodes suggests that they may in fact be due to septic emboli rather than immune complex deposition (65).

CLINICAL MANIFESTATIONS AND COMPLICATIONS

The clinical presentation of IE ranges from subtle, chronic fatigue with low-grade fevers, weight loss, and malaise, to an abrupt onset of fulminant acute pulmonary edema brought on by massive acute aortic regurgitation. Although the virulence of the infecting organism can influence the acuity of the presentation, the interval from onset of infection to onset of symptoms is usually short. Most patients with IE develop symptoms within 2 weeks of the inciting bacteremia (66). Symptoms in staphylococcal IE may even begin within a few days of the onset of infection.

The symptoms and signs are protean, and essentially any organ system may be involved. Four processes contribute to the clinical picture: (a) the infectious process on the valve, including the local intracardiac complications; (b) septic or aseptic embolization to virtually any organ; (c) constant bacteremia, often with metastatic foci of infection; and (d) circulating immune complexes and other immunopathologic factors (67,68). As a result, the clinical presentation of patients with IE is highly variable and the differential diagnosis often broad. Because of the protean manifestations, the diagnosis of IE may be delayed or occasionally not clinically suspected and identified only on post-mortem examination (69,70).

In more recent years, because of a higher incidence of nosocomial IE and more rapid diagnostic modalities, the patient with low-grade fever, malaise, and peripheral stigmata from long-standing IE is not as common a presentation as it was previously. Fever is usually present in the current era, but may be absent (5% of the cases), especially in the setting of CHF or other comorbid condition, immunosuppressive therapy, advanced age, or previous antibiotic therapy (71,72). Nonspecific symptoms such as anorexia, weight loss, malaise, fatigue, chills, weakness, nausea, vomiting, and night sweats are not unusual. These nonspecific symptoms may result in an incorrect diagnosis of malignancy, collagen vascular disease, tuberculosis, or other chronic disease.

Audible heart murmurs occur in over 85% of the cases, but may be absent with right-sided or a mural infection. The classic "changing murmur" and the development of a new regurgitant murmur (usually aortic insufficiency) are uncommon and occur in 5% to 10% and in 3% to 5% of the cases, respectively. When present, these are diagnostically useful signs and usually complicate acute staphylococcal disease. Over 90% of patients who demonstrate a new regurgitant murmur develop CHF. The incidence of CHF appears to be increasing (approximately 25% in 1966 and 67% in 1972) and is now the leading cause of death in IE (23). Unless valve replacement or repair is undertaken, most patients with this complication die even if effective antimicrobial therapy is administered. Although valvular regurgitation is the most important hemodynamic complication of IE, hemodynamically significant valvular obstruction requiring surgery may occur rarely, even without a prior history of valvular stenosis (73).

The classic peripheral manifestations were previously found in up to one half of the cases with IE of prolonged duration; however, the prevalence has significantly decreased in recent years. Clubbing may be present if the disease is of long duration, and may recede with therapy. The complete syndrome of hypertrophic osteoarthropathy is rare. Splinter hemorrhages are linear red to brown streaks in the fingernails or toenails. They are a nonspecific finding and are often seen in the elderly or in people experiencing occupation-related trauma. Petechiae are found after a prolonged course, and usually appear in crops on the conjunctivae, buccal mucosa, palate, and extremities. These lesions are initially red and nonblanching, but become brown and barely visible in 2 to 3 days. Petechiae may result from either local vasculitis or emboli. Osler nodes are small, painful, nodular lesions usually found in the pads of fingers or toes and occasionally in the thenar eminence. They are 2 to 15 mm in size and are frequently multiple and evanescent, disappearing in hours to days. Osler nodes are rare in acute cases of IE. They are not specific for IE because they may be seen in systemic lupus erythematosus, marantic endocarditis, hemolytic anemia, and gonococcal infections and in extremities with cannulated radial arteries. Janeway lesions are hemorrhagic, macular, painless plaques with a predilection for the palms or soles. They persist for several days and are thought to be embolic in origin. They occur with greater frequency in staphylococcal IE. Roth spots are oval, pale, retinal lesions surrounded by hemorrhage and are usually located near the optic disk. They occur in less than 5% of the cases of IE and may also be found in anemia, leukemia, and connective tissue disorders such as systemic lupus erythematosus. Splenomegaly is more common in patients with IE of prolonged duration. Splenic septic emboli are common during IE, but localized signs and symptoms may be absent in approximately 90% of patients with this complication (74).

Abscess in or adjacent to the valve annulus is often heralded by the appearance of first- or second-degree heart block and/or fever that persists despite appropriate therapy. Annular abscesses are more common in patients with aortic valvular infection than in those with mitral valve involvement. Pericarditis is rare but, when present, is usually accompanied by myocardial abscess formation as a complication of staphylococcal infection. Myocarditis may occur as a result of coronary vasculitis, embolic coronary occlusion, or the effects of microbial toxins or immune complex deposition.

Musculoskeletal manifestations are common in IE; 44% of the patients in one series demonstrating musculoskeletal symptoms (75). These symptoms usually occurred early in the disease and were the only initial complaint in 15% of the cases. They included proximal oligo- or monoarticular arthralgias (38%), lower extremity mono- or oligoarticular arthritis (31%), low back pain (23%), and diffuse myalgias (19%). The back pain may be severe, limiting movement, and is the initial complaint in 5% to 10% of cases.

Major embolic episodes, as a group, are second only to CHF as a complication of IE and occur in at least one third of cases. Splenic artery emboli with infarction may result in left upper quadrant abdominal pain with radiation to the left shoulder, a splenic or pleural rub, or a left pleural effusion. Renal infarctions may be associated with microscopic or gross hematuria, but renal failure, hypertension, and edema are uncommon. Retinal artery emboli are rare (occurring in <2% of cases) and may be manifested by a sudden complete loss of vision. Pulmonary emboli can be a complication of right-sided IE. Coronary artery emboli usually arise from the aortic valve and may cause myocarditis with arrhythmias or myocardial infarction. Major vessel emboli (affecting the femoral, brachial, popliteal, or radial artery) are more frequent in fungal endocarditis.

Neurologic manifestations occur in 20% to 40% of the cases and may dominate the clinical picture, especially in staphylococcal IE. Stroke is the most common neurologic complication of IE, occurring in 9.6% of patients. Patients with mitral valve IE have a greater risk of stroke than patients with aortic valve IE (OR 2.0, 95% CI 1.1–3.9) (76). Of those patients with neurologic complications, up to 50% present with neurologic signs and symptoms as the heralding features of their illness (77,78). The development of clinical neurologic deterioration during IE is associated with a two- to fourfold increase in mortality. Mycotic aneurysms of the cerebral circulation occur in 2% to 10% of the cases. They are usually single, small, and peripheral, and may lead to devastating subarachnoid hemorrhage. Other features include seizures, severe headache, visual changes (particularly homonymous hemianopsias), choreoathetoid movements, mononeuropathy, and cranial nerve palsies. A toxic encephalopathy with symptoms ranging from a mild change in personality to frank psychosis may occur, especially in elderly patients.

Patients with IE may have symptoms of uremia. In the preantibiotic era, renal failure developed in 25% to 35% of the patients, but presently fewer than 10% are affected. When uremia does develop, diffuse glomerulonephritis with hypocomplementemia is usually found, but focal glomerulonephritis has also been implicated. Renal failure is more common with long-standing disease, but is usually reversible with appropriate antimicrobial treatment alone.

LABORATORY TESTING

Blood Cultures

The blood culture is the single most important laboratory test performed in a diagnostic workup for IE. The bacteremia is usually continuous and low-grade (80% of the cases have less than 100 CFU/mL of blood) (79). In approximately two thirds of the cases, all blood specimens drawn yield positive results on culture (23). When bacteremia is present, the first two blood cultures yield the etiologic agent more than 90% of the time. The sensitivity of blood cultures for the detection of streptococci is particularly susceptible to prior antibiotic therapy and is also affected by the media employed (80). Continuous monitoring blood culture systems (e.g., BACTEC, BacT/ALERT) are significantly more sensitive than conventional methods (81). In addition, blood culture media containing neutralizing resin particles have improved the detection of staphylococci from patients receiving antimicrobial therapy at the time of culture (82).

On the basis of these studies, the following procedures for culturing blood are recommended. At least three blood culture sets (no more than two bottles per venipuncture) should be obtained in the first 24 hours. More specimens may be necessary if the patient has received antibiotics in the preceding 2 weeks. Blood cultures drawn within 4 hours may yield equal results to those drawn 12 to 24 hours apart. In general, culture of arterial blood offers no advantage over use of venous blood. The constancy of bacteremia in patients with IE makes it unnecessary to await fever spikes or chills to obtain blood cultures. At least 10 mL of blood in adults or 0.5 to 5.0 mL from infants and children (when feasible) should be injected into both trypticase soy (and brain–heart infusion) and thioglycolate broth (83). Supplementation with 15% sucrose (in an attempt to isolate cell wall–deficient forms) or the use of pre-reduced anaerobic media is unrewarding. Inspection for macroscopic growth should be performed daily and routine subcultures done on days 1 and 3. The cultures should be held for at least 3 weeks. When gram-positive cocci grow on the initial isolation but fail to grow on subculture, nutritionally variant (thiol-dependent) streptococci should be suspected (84). In this event, subculture inoculation should be onto media supplemented with either 0.05 to 0.1% L-cysteine or 0.001% pyridoxal phosphate.

The interpretation of positive blood cultures requires consideration of their likelihood of causing IE. The following organisms are considered to be likely causes of IE when isolated from two or more blood cultures: *S. aureus*, viridans streptococci, enterococci (if acquired in the community and not nosocomially), *S. sanguis*, and group G streptococci. False-positive results are likely to be present when organisms such as *Propionibacterium* spp, *Corynebacterium* spp, *Bacillus* spp, and coagulase-negative staphylococci are recovered from a single blood culture or a minority of blood culture results. However, because these organisms are also capable of causing IE, it is important to determine if there is persistent bacteremia present as opposed to contamination with skin flora. Persistent bacteremia is likely if (a) positive cultures form organisms likely to cause IE are obtained from two samples collected more than 12 hours apart or (b) if for all other organisms, all of three or a majority of four or more separate blood cultures are positive and if the first and last samples are collected at least 1 hour apart (85).

Other Blood Laboratory Tests

The utility of other blood laboratory tests in the diagnosis of IE is limited. Hematologic parameters are often abnormal in IE, but none is diagnostic. Anemia is nearly always present (70%–90% of cases), especially in subacute cases, and has the characteristics of the anemia of chronic disease, with normochromic, normocytic indices. Thrombocytopenia occurs in 5% to 15% of the cases and leukocytosis is present in 20% to 30% of cases. The differential count is usually normal, but there may be a slight shift to the left. The erythrocyte sedimentation rate (ESR) is nearly always elevated (90% to 100% of cases), with a mean value of 57 mm/hour found in one large series (23). Hypergammaglobulinemia is detected in 20% to 30% of cases and may be accompanied by a plasmacytosis in the bone marrow aspirate. A positive result on assay for rheumatoid factor is found in 40% to 50% of cases, especially when the duration of the illness is longer than 6 weeks (58). Hypocomplementemia (seen in 5%–15% of cases) parallels the incidence of abnormal renal function test results (elevated creatinine level in 5%–15%). Urinalysis is frequently abnormal; proteinuria occurs in 50% to 65% of cases, and microscopic hematuria in 30% to 60%. Red cell casts may be seen in as many as 12% of cases; gross hematuria, pyuria, white cell casts, and bacteriuria may also be found (23).

Circulating immune complexes and mixed-type cryoglobulins are detectable in most patients with IE, but also constitute a nonspecific finding. The C-reactive protein concentration is virtually always elevated in IE and is a nonspecific finding. Recently, procalcitonin has been shown to be a better diagnostic marker than C-reactive protein in patients with suspected IE (86).

Culture-Negative Infective Endocarditis

Blood cultures fail to isolate an etiologic agent in 3% to 23% of cases (88). Culture-negative IE is most often associated with antibiotic use within the previous 2 weeks. Less frequently, intracellular pathogens not detected using standard culture approaches may be the cause (88). If blood cultures are negative in definite or possible IE, consideration should be made to analyze serum for *Bartonella*, *Coxiella*, and *Chlamydia* species antibodies (87). If the patient requires valve surgery, 16S rRNA polymerase chain reaction amplification of valve tissue often yields an etiologic agent (87,89).

Echocardiography

Since its first use in the diagnosis of IE in 1973, echocardiography has become paramount in the process of evaluating IE (90). It is crucial in detecting vegetations, echogenic distinct masses from the adjacent valve with independent motion from the valve itself. Vegetations have characteristic findings of a shaggy dense band of irregular echoes in a nonuniform distribution on one or more leaflets (see Fig. 26.2). Echocardiography may not only confirm the presence of vegetations in the setting of bacteremia, but also provides important hemodynamic information regarding ventricular function and an estimate of the degree of valvular regurgitation. Many reports have evaluated the role of transthoracic echocardiography (TTE) in the diagnosis and management of suspected IE (91). In summary, TTE should be performed in all patients in whom IE appears to be a reasonable diagnosis. TTE is not, however, an appropriate screening test in the evaluation of febrile patients in whom IE is unlikely on clinical grounds, or in bacteremic patients with organisms that rarely cause IE, particularly if there is another obvious focus to explain the clinical syndrome (92). In addition, (a) TTE has variable sensitivity for the detection of vegetations (<50% to >90% positive), indicating that a negative study does not exclude IE; (b) the sensitivity of TTE for detecting vegetations is highest in right-sided IE; (c) false-positive results are extremely rare; (d) only technically adequate studies are of value, a characteristic that heavily depends on the experience of the person performing the examination; and (e) patients with a "vegetation" identified by echocardiography are at an increased risk for subsequent systemic emboli, CHF, the need for emergency surgery, and death, especially with aortic valve involvement. Positive findings on the echocardiogram in a patient with IE should serve as adjunctive evidence, together with clinical parameters, in indicating surgical intervention. Although still controversial, larger vegetation size (>1 cm) has been associated with an increased risk of cerebral emboli (93). Some studies suggest that highly mobile vegetations constitute an independent increase in risk for complications in IE (94). However, in other studies, vegetation mobility on echocardi-

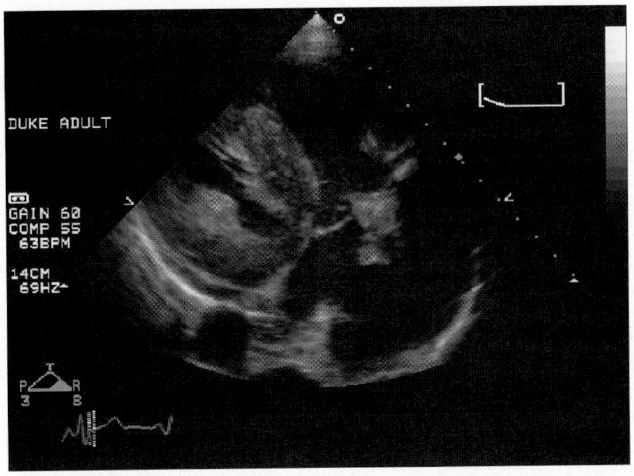

FIGURE 26.2. TTE of a large tricuspid valve vegetation.

ography has not been an important independent risk factor for embolic events in IE, because it is, in turn, strongly correlated with vegetation size (95). One problem in considering the significance of these echocardiographic characteristics is the high degree of interobserver variability in interpreting the echocardiography images (96).

TEE has significantly altered the diagnostic approach to patients with suspected IE (Fig. 26.3). TEE is more sensitive than conventional TTE in the detection of intracardiac vegetations (approximately 95% versus 60%–65%), particularly in the setting of prosthetic valves (97). TEE is particularly useful in visualizing masses on pacemaker leads or intravenous lines. The superiority of TEE over TTE is evident in the detection of small vegetations; therefore, TEE should be considered in patients with suspected IE and negative results on TTE. Potential sources of false-negative TEE studies include very small vegetations and previous embolization of vegetations. TEE is the procedure of choice for the detection of perivalvular abscesses with a diagnostic sensitivity and specificity of 87% and 95% for TEE versus 28% and 99% for TTE and, therefore, should be performed (unless contraindicated) in all IE patients when perivalvular abscess is suspected (98). Other recent investigations have demonstrated TEE to be superior in the diagnosis of valvular perforation and pacemaker IE (99,100). TEE has

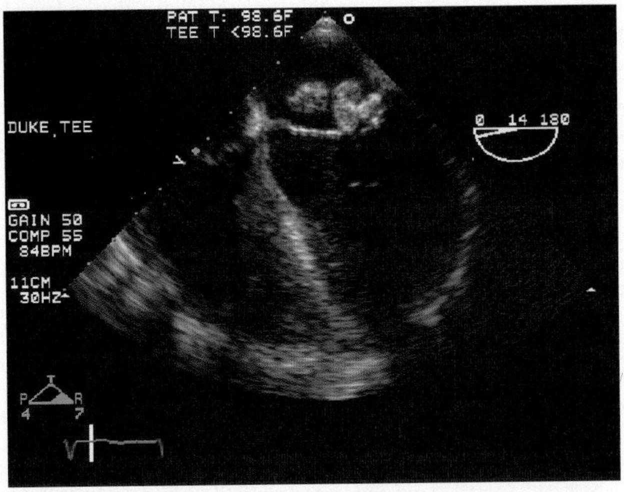

FIGURE 26.3. TEE revealing multiple mitral valve vegetations.

been shown to be a cost-effective method for defining the duration of antibiotic therapy (2 versus 4 weeks) compared to empiric courses of either 2 or 4 weeks in patients with intravascular catheter associated SAB (101). Similarly, a recent decision analysis found TEE to be more cost-effective than TTE among patients with a high pre-test probability of IE (102).

Electrocardiography

An electrocardiogram should be part of the evaluation of a patient with suspected IE, although it is usually unrevealing. The presence or new appearance of heart block is an important evidence of extension of infection to the valve annulus and conduction system (103). The presence of new prolongation of the PR interval in a patient with IE is virtually diagnostic of the presence of a ring abscess.

Other Imaging Modalities and Tests

Computed tomography and magnetic resonance imaging appear promising for the detection of perivalvular abscess, but clinical experience is limited (104,105). Other investigational techniques include the detection of vegetations by gallium 67, technetium 99m-labeled antibacterial antibody, or indium 111-labeled platelets, which have shown promise in experimental settings (106–108).

The role of cardiac catheterization in the evaluation of patients with IE remains controversial. It has been argued that intracardiac vegetations should not be crossed with intracardiac catheters. Cardiac catheterization may occasionally be useful to visualize abnormal flow if these features are uncertain after routine clinical assessment and TEE. Coronary angiography is recommended in patients prior to surgery for IE based on risk factors for coronary artery disease. In younger patients, the anatomic information provided by TEE usually is adequate to proceed to surgical repair or valve replacement without the need for invasive studies (55).

DIAGNOSTIC CRITERIA

IE is typically a syndrome diagnosis based on the presence of multiple findings rather than a single definitive test result. Practical and logical case definitions for IE are important for both clinicians and researchers who study this complex disease. Accurate identification and classification of patients of IE are important in defining the natural history, complications, epidemiology, and treatment outcomes.

The first diagnostic criteria for IE, developed by Pellitier and Petersdorf in 1977 (23), were specific, but lacked sensitivity. Subsequent diagnostic criteria for IE were published in 1982 by von Reyn et al. (109) (Beth Israel criteria), but did not incorporate echocardiographic findings into the case definitions. In addition, the isolation of a "typical" IE pathogen from blood cultures was not considered in the Beth Israel definitions. With improved methodology and recognition of the central role of echocardiography in the evaluation of suspected IE, new case definitions and diagnostic criteria (the Duke criteria) proposed in 1994, are now widely used and have been accepted by most clinicians (85). The definitions retain, in slightly modified form, the pathologic parameters of the Beth Israel. The Duke criteria build on the Beth Israel criteria by including echocardiographic evidence of IE (vegetations or paravalvular complications), as well as the isolation of typical IE pathogens from blood cultures, as "major criteria" for the clinically definite categorization of IE. In addition, the presence of recent IDU is included in the Duke criteria as a "minor criterion" for diagnosing IE, recognizing the increased risk of IE in this patient population. Direct comparisons of the Duke and Beth Israel criteria have now been carried out in 11 major studies, including nearly 1,400 patients. Patient populations from diverse geographic areas with presumed IE that have been studied include young,

TABLE 26.1

DEFINITION OF IE ACCORDING TO THE MODIFIED DUKE CRITERIA

DEFINITE INFECTIVE ENDOCARDITIS

Pathologic criteria

1. Microorganisms demonstrated by culture or histologic examination of a vegetation, a vegetation that has embolized, or an intracardiac abscess specimen; or
2. Pathologic lesions; vegetation or intracardiac abscess confirmed by histologic examination showing active endocarditis

Clinical criteria

1. Two major criteria; or
2. One major criterion and three minor criteria; or
3. Five minor criteria

POSSIBLE INFECTIVE ENDOCARDITIS

1. One major criterion and one minor criterion; or
2. Three minor criteria

REJECTED

1. Firm alternate diagnosis explaining evidence of infective endocarditis; or
2. Resolution of infective endocarditis syndrome with antibiotic therapy for $\leq$4 days; or
3. No pathologic evidence of infective endocarditis at surgery or autopsy, with antibiotic therapy for $\leq$4 days; or
4. Does not meet criteria for possible infective endocarditis, as above

Source: Adapted from Li JS, et al. Proposed modifications to the Duke criteria for the diagnosis of infective endocarditis. *Clin Infect Dis* 2000;30:633–638.

TABLE 26.2

DEFINITION OF TERMS USED IN THE MODIFIED DUKE CRITERIA FOR THE DIAGNOSIS OF IE

MAJOR CRITERIA
Blood culture positive for IE
Typical microorganisms consistent with IE from two separate blood cultures:
Viridans streptococci, *Streptococcus bovis,* Hacek group, *S. aureus;* or
Community-acquired enterococci, in the absence of a primary focus; or
Microorganisms consistent with IE from persistently positive blood cultures, defined as follows:
At least two positive cultures of blood samples drawn >12 h apart; or
All of three or a majority of ≤4 separate cultures of blood (with first and last sample drawn at least 1 h apart)
Single positive blood culture for *Coxiella burnetii* or antiphase I IgG antibody titer >1:800
EVIDENCE OF ENDOCARDIAL INVOLVEMENT
Echocardiogram positive for IE (TEE recommended in patients with prosthetic valves, rated at least "possible IE" by clinical criteria, or complicated IE [paravalvular abscess]; TTE as first test in other patients), defined as follows:
Oscillating intracardiac mass on valve or supporting structures, in the path of regurgitant jets, or on implanted material in the absence of an alternative anatomic explanation; or
Abscess; or
New partial dehiscence of prosthetic valve
New valvular regurgitation (worsening or changing of preexisting murmur not sufficient)
MINOR CRITERIA
Predisposition, predisposing heart condition or IDU
Fever >38°C
Vascular phenomena, major arterial emboli, septic pulmonary infarcts, mycotic aneurysm, intracranial hemorrhage, conjunctival hemorrhages, and Janeway lesions
Immunologic phenomena: glomerulonephritis, Osler nodes, Roth spots, and rheumatoid factor
Microbiological evidence: positive blood culture, but does not meet a major criterion as noted above or serologic evidence of active infection with organism consistent with IE

Source: Adapted from Li JS, et al. Proposed modifications to the Duke criteria for the diagnosis of infective endocarditis. *Clin Infect Dis* 2000;30:633–638.

middle-aged, and geriatric adults; pediatric patients; patients with native or prosthetic valve involvement; and both IDU and non-IDU patients. These studies confirmed the increased sensitivity of the Duke criteria in clinically diagnosing IE and the diagnostic utility of echocardiography in identifying clinically definite cases (110). Modifications of the Duke criteria have recently yielded more specificity to the schema (111). The modified Duke Criteria for the diagnosis of IE are provided in Tables 26.1 and 26.2.

TREATMENT

General Guidelines

Following the establishment of a diagnosis using clinical, microbiological, and echocardiographic methods, antibiotics should be administered in a dosage designed to give sustained bactericidal serum concentrations throughout much or the entire dosing interval. Certain general principles have been accepted that provide the framework for the current recommendations for treatment of IE. A prolonged course of therapy is necessary to eradicate microorganisms growing in valvular vegetations. Bactericidal, rather than bacteriostatic, antibiotics should be chosen to decrease the possibility of treatment failure or relapses. Parenteral antibiotics are recommended over oral drugs in most circumstances because of the importance of sustained antibacterial activity. Likewise, antibiotic combinations can produce a rapid bactericidal effect. This is seen with synergistic combinations such as penicillin plus an aminoglycoside effective against most viridans streptococci or enterococci. Recently, guidelines for outpatient parenteral antibiotic therapy for IE have been published. These guidelines outline a conservative approach (inpatient or daily outpatient follow-up) during the critical phase (weeks 0–2 of treatment) when complications are most likely, followed by outpatient parenteral therapy for the continuation phase of antibiotic therapy (112). Patients selected for outpatient therapy should respond clinically to inpatient therapy and be without evidence of metastatic or intracardiac complications. They also should be hemodynamically stable, compliant, and capable of managing the technical aspects of intravenous therapy. Such patients require careful, regular monitoring and should have prompt access to medical care should complications occur.

The AHA recently updated specific treatment guidelines based on the microbiologic etiologic agent (113). General therapeutic considerations are discussed below and summarized in Tables 26.3 through 26.5 (113–116).

MEDICAL THERAPY

Staphylococci

The great majority of staphylococci, regardless of their acquisition route (nosocomial or community), produce β-lactamase, and therefore are highly resistant to penicillin G. The drugs of choice for native valve methicillin-susceptible *S. aureus* (MSSA) are semisynthetic, penicillinase-resistant penicillins such as nafcillin or oxacillin sodium. The addition of gentamicin for the first 3 to 5 days of treatment is optional and may increase rates of nephrotoxicity and ototoxicity. In patients without a history

TABLE 26.3

ANTIMICROBIAL THERAPY FOR ENDOCARDITIS CAUSED BY STAPHYLOCOCCI

Pathogen	Antibiotic	Dosage and intervals	Duration
STAPHYLOCOCCUS-METHICILLIN SENSITIVE			
Native valve	Nafcillin or oxacillin	2 g IV q4h	4–6 weeks
	± gentamicin	1 mg/kg IM or IV q8h	First 3–5 days
Native valve-β-lactam allergic	Cefazolin	2 g IV q8h	4–6 weeks
	± gentamicin	1 mg/kg IM or IV q8h	First 3–5 days
	or		
	vancomycin	30 mg/kg/24 h IV in 2 equally divided doses not to exceed 2 g/24 h unless serum levels are monitored	4–6 weeks
Prosthetic valve	Nafcillin or oxacillin	2 g IV q4h	≥6 weeks
	or cefazolin	2 g IV q8h	≥6 weeks
	+ rifampin	300 mg PO q8h	≥6 weeks
	+ gentamicin	1 mg/kg IM or IV q8h	2 weeks
STAPHYLOCOCCUS-METHACILLIN RESISTANT			
Native valve	Vancomycin	30 mg/kg/24 h IV in 2 equally divided doses not to exceed 2 g/24 h unless serum levels are monitored	4–6 weeks
	± gentamicin	1 mg/kg IM or IV q8h	First 3–5 days
Prosthetic valve	Vancomycin	30 mg/kg/24 h IV in 2 or 4 equally divided doses not to exceed 2 g/24 h unless serum levels are monitored	≥6 weeks
	+ rifampin	300 mg PO q8h	≥6 weeks
	+ gentamicin	1 mg/kg IM or IV q8h	2 weeks

Source: Adapted from references 113–116.

of type 1 penicillin allergic reactions, a first-generation cephalosporin such as cefazolin is indicated. In patients with MSSA and allergies to β-lactams as well for patients infected with methicillin-resistant *S. aureus* (MRSA), vancomycin is the drug of choice. However, it must be noted that some evidence suggests than vancomycin is an inferior drug in the treatment of MSSA IE predominantly because of its slow bactericidal activity as well as its poor tissue penetration (117). Selected patients with uncomplicated, IDU-associated, native valve, right-sided MSSA IE can be successfully treated with a 2-week treatment regimen of a semisynthetic penicillin combined with an aminoglycoside (118).

Coagulase-negative staphylococci are usually methicillin resistant. Because of cross-resistance, cephalosporins should not be used in these patients. Vancomycin is usually given for at least 6 weeks. Gentamicin may be added during the first 3 to 5 days of treatment.

Staphylococcal PVE is associated with high mortality and requires aggressive management. The current recommendation for MSSA PVE favors the use of nafcillin or oxacillin, in combination with rifampin for 6 to 8 weeks, and low-dose gentamicin during the first 2 weeks. For PVE, vancomycin is used in combination with rifampin for 6 to 8 weeks, and gentamicin is again added during the first 2 weeks. Rifampin has been shown in animal models to have a unique ability to kill staphylococci adherent to prosthetic materials, but selection of resistant strains is common when a high burden of bacteria is exposed to the drug. To minimize resistance to rifampin, this medication should be added only after antibiotics active against staphylococci, such as β-lactam or vancomycin and aminoglycosides, have been started and the infection burden of bacteria significantly reduced. For strains resistant to gentamicin or other aminoglycosides, a fluoroquinolone may be used if the strain is susceptible. Surgical valve replacement is often required for the management of the infection because the mortality in patients with PVE treated with antibiotics alone ranges from 56% to 76%. Performing valve replacement surgery early in the course of antibiotic therapy may be associated with improved outcomes, although even with aggressive management the mortality rates are still almost 40%. Many medically managed patients with PVE are not surgical candidates because of complications with stroke. Strong consideration should be given to discontinuing anticoagulation in patients with *S. aureus* PVE because of the high incidence of intracerebral hemorrhage (116).

Viridans Group Streptococci, *Streptococcus bovis*, and Other Non-Enterococcal Streptococci

The taxonomic classification of *viridans* group streptococci includes a variety of streptococcal species including *S. sanguis, S. oralis (mitis), S. mutans,* and others. The treatment for streptococcal endocarditis is based on in vitro minimum inhibitory concentration (MIC) for penicillin.

1. Highly penicillin-susceptible *viridans* (MIC ≤0.12 μg/mL): Streptococci with an MIC of penicillin ≤0.12 μg/mL are considered highly susceptible and are usually treated with

TABLE 26.4

ANTIMICROBIAL THERAPY FOR ENDOCARDITIS CAUSED BY STREPTOCOCCI AND *STREPTOCOCCUS BOVIS*

Pathogen	Antibiotic	Dosage and intervals	Duration
STREPTOCOCCI-PENICILLIN SENSITIVE (MIC ≤0.12 μg/mL) (*S. viridans, S. bovis,* and other streptococci)			
Native valve	Penicillin G or	12–18 million U/24 h IV either continuously or in 6 equally divided doses	4 weeks
	ceftriaxone or	2 g IV or IM qd	4 weeks
	Penicillin G or	12–18 million U/24 h IV either continuously or in 6 equally divided doses	2 weeks
	ceftriaxone plus	2 g IV or IM qd	2 weeks
	gentamicin	1 mg/kg IM or IV q8h	2 weeks
Native valve-β lactam allergic	Vancomycin	30 mg/kg/24 h IV in 2 equally divided doses, not to exceed 2 g/24 h unless serum levels are monitored	4 weeks
Prosthetic valve	Penicillin G (vancomycin for patients allergic to β-lectams) plus	12–18 million U/24 h IV either continuously or in 6 equally divided doses	6 weeks
	gentamicin	1 mg/kg IM or IV q8h	2 weeks
STREPTOCOCCI-RELATIVELY PENICILLIN RESISTANT (MIC >0.1–0.5 μg/mL)			
Native valve	Penicillin G or	24 million U/24 h IV either continuously or in 6 equally divided doses	4 weeks
	ceftriaxone plus	2 g IV or IM qd	4 weeks
	gentamicin	1 mg/kg IM or IV q8h	2 weeks
Native valve β-lactam allergic	Vancomycin	30 mg/kg/24 h IV in 2 equally divided doses, not to exceed 2 g/24 h unless serum levels are monitored	4–6 weeks
Prosthetic valve	Penicillin G or	12–18 million U/24 h IV either continuously or in 6 equally divided doses	6 weeks
	ceftriaxone (vancomycin for patients allergic to β-lactams) plus	2 g IV or IM qd	6 weeks
	gentamicin	1 mg/kg IM or IV q8h	6 weeks
NON-ENTEROCOCCAL STREPTOCOCCI-RESISTANT TO PENICILLIN (MIC >0.5 μg/mL)			
Native and prosthetic valve	Penicillin G or	18–30 million U/24 h IV either continuously or in 6 equally divided doses	4–6 weeks for native; ≥6 for prosthetic
	ampicillin or	2–3 g IV q4h	
	vancomycin plus	30 mg/kg IV in 24 h in 2 equally divided doses	
	gentacicin	1 mg/kg IM or IV q8h	

Source: Adapted from references 113–116.

penicillin G or ceftriaxone for 4 weeks. Ceftriaxone, given in a single daily dose, is particularly useful for outpatient therapy. A very high cure rate (98%) is obtained with these regimens. Comparable cure rates can be achieved for uncomplicated cases with a combination of penicillin or ceftriaxone with low-dose aminoglycoside for 2 weeks. Cefazolin or other first-generation cephalosporins may be substituted for penicillin in patients whose penicillin hypersensitivity is not of the immediate type. Vancomycin is recommended for patients allergic to β-lactams. Doses should be adjusted

TABLE 26.5

ANTIMICROBIAL THERAPY FOR ENDOCARDITIS CAUSED BY ENTEROCOCCI

Pathogen	Antibiotic	Dosage and intervals
ENTEROCOCCI-PENICILLIN RESISTANT		
Native and prosthetic valves	Vancomycin	30 mg/kg/24 h in 2 equally divided doses
	or	
	ampicillin-sulbactam	3 mg IV q4h
	plus	
	gentamicin	1 mg/kg IM or IV q8h
ENTEROCOCCI-AMINOGLYCOSIDE RESISTANT		
Native and prosthetic valves	Penicillin G	20–40 million U IV/24 h either continuously or in 6 equally divided doses
	or	
	ampicillin	2–3 g IV q4h
	or	
	ampicillin	2 g IV q4h
	plus	
	ceftriaxone	2 g IV q12h
ENTEROCOCCI-VANCOMYCIN RESISTANT		
Native and prosthetic valves	Penicillin G	20–40 million U IV/24 h either continuously or in 6 equally divided doses
	or	
	ampicillin	2–3 g IV q4h
	plus	
	gentamicin	1 mg/kg IM or IV q8h
ENTEROCOCCI-PENICILLIN, AMINOGLYCOSIDE AND VANCOMYCIN RESISTANT		
Native and prosthetic valves	Ampicillin	2 g IV q4h
	plus	
	ceftriaxone	2 g IV q12h
	or	
	linezolid	600 mg PO or IV q12h
	or	
	quinupristin-dalfopristin	7.5 mg/kg IV q8h
	plus	
	imipenen/cilastatin	500 mg IV q6h

Source: Adapted from references 113–116.

to obtain peak vancomycin levels of 30 to 40 μg/mL and trough levels of 15 to 20 μg/mL.

2. Relatively penicillin-resistant *streptococci* (MIC >0.12 to 0.5 μg/mL): When IE is due to streptococcal strains with MIC for penicillin >0.12 μg/mL and <0.5 μg/mL, combination therapy with penicillin and gentamicin is indicated. Low-dose gentamicin is given for the first 2 weeks of the 4-week course of penicillin. In patients allergic to β-lactams, a 4-week course of vancomycin is recommended.
3. *Streptococcus* spp. with MIC of penicillin >0.5 μg/mL, or *Abiotrophia* spp: When IE is due to streptococcal strains with MIC for penicillin >0.5 μg/mL or nutritionally variant streptococci (now classified as *Abiotrophia* species), a regimen for penicillin-resistant enterococcal IE is appropriate. These regimens consist of 4 to 6 weeks of vancomycin combined with low-dose gentamicin. Renal function should be closely monitored when vancomycin is used in combination with aminoglycosides. To avoid nephrotoxicity, high-dose penicillin or ampicillin plus gentamicin can be used. For patients with symptoms lasting longer than 3 months, a 6-week course of treatment is preferred. The length of therapy for the aminoglycoside is debated. Vancomycin is substituted for β-lactams in patients allergic to those compounds.

Patients with viridans streptococci PVE can be treated with antibiotics alone if no other indications for surgery are present (e.g., unstable prosthesis, heart failure, new or progressive paravalvular leak, perivalvular extension of infection or persistent infection after 7 to 10 days of appropriate antibiotic therapy). For highly penicillin-susceptible streptococci PVE (MIC ≤0.12 μg/mL) penicillin G for 6 weeks and gentamicin for 2 weeks are usually indicated. When PVE is due to relatively penicillin-resistant streptococci (MIC >0.12–0.5 μg/mL) penicillin G is recommended for 6 weeks and gentamicin for 4 weeks. IE owing to nutritionally variant streptococci (now classified as *Abiotrophia* spp.) or viridans streptococci with MIC for penicillin above 0.5 μg/mL should be treated with 4 to 6 weeks of penicillin, ampicillin, or vancomycin combined with gentamicin. Vancomycin therapy is indicated for patients with confirmed immediate hypersensitivity to β-lactam antibiotics.

Enterococci

IE caused by enterococci is usually associated with *Enterococcus faecalis* and uncommonly with *E. faecium*. Enterococci are resistant to most classes of antibiotics, which make treatment difficult. Because of a defective bacterial autolytic enzyme system, cell wall-active agents are bacteriostatic against enterococci and should not be given alone to treat IE. In combination with gentamicin, penicillin G and ampicillin facilitate the intracellular uptake of the aminoglycoside, which subsequently results in a bactericidal effect against enterococci. There is a better outcome, measured by bacteriologic cure or survival, with a synergistic combination of a cell wall-active agent and aminoglycoside than with single-drug therapy. Although ampicillin is more active than penicillin G in vitro against enterococci, clinical data supporting the use of this antibiotic is not nearly as extensive as with penicillin. Before embarking on therapy susceptibility of the enterococcus should be determined for penicillin (or ampicillin), vancomycin, and aminoglycosides. For strains with intrinsic high-level resistance to penicillin (MIC >16 μg/mL), vancomycin is indicated. Vancomycin is also synergistic with aminoglycosides, particularly with gentamicin. MICs for gentamicin should be measured to guide treatment. When high level resistance to aminoglycosides is detected (500–2,000 μg/mL for gentamicin) combination with cell wall-active agents is no longer synergistic and therefore not recommended. Few data are available to guide therapy in these difficult cases; however, many experts attempt a long course of an active cell wall agent in the highest doses or combination therapy with 2 β-lactam antibiotics (e.g., ampicillin 20 g/d for 8–12 weeks combined with ceftriaxone).

IE caused by vancomycin-resistant enterococci (VRE) is difficult to treat. The optimal therapy of such infections is unknown. Most vancomycin-resistant strains of *E. faecalis* as well as a few of *E. faecium* are susceptible to achievable concentrations of ampicillin. In such cases, the recommended therapy is ampicillin or penicillin combined with gentamicin (unless high-level resistance is present). Even when enterococci are considered resistant to ampicillin (MIC ≥ 16 μg/mL), higher doses, in the range of 18 to 30 g/d, can be used to achieve sustained plasma levels of more than 100 to 150 μg/mL. To date, there has been little toxicity when employing high doses of ampicillin, but more experience is still needed with such doses. In 1999, the U.S. Food and Drug Administration approved quinupristin/dalfopristin as the first antibacterial drug to treat infections associated with vancomycin-resistant *E. faecium* bacteremia when no alternative treatment is available. However, quinupristin/dalfopristin alone is unlikely to be curative in VREF IE because the antibacterial is not usually bactericidal against *E. faecium*. Endocarditis models suggest that the association of quinupristin/dalfopristin with ampicillin may be beneficial. It is important to note that *E. faecalis* is not susceptible to quinupristin/dalfopristin. In 2000, the U.S. Food and Drug Administration approved linezolid to treat infections associated with vancomycin-resistant *E. faecium*, including cases with bloodstream infection. However, linezolid is bacteriostatic against VRE and therefore cannot be recommended for VRE IE. Newer agents such as daptomycin, telavancin, and dalbavancin show promise in clinical trials but are not yet approved in the US.

Gram-Negative Organisms

HACEK organisms, including *Haemophilus* spp. (*Haemophilus parainfluenzae, H. aphrophilus,* and *H. paraphrophilus*), *Actinobacillus actinomycetemcomitans, Cardiobacterium hominis, Eikenella corrodens,* and *Kingella kingae* account for 5% to 10% of native valve IE in nonintravenous drug abusers. A characteristic of the group is their fastidious growth characteristics. Thus, when standard microbiological techniques are used, incubation for 2 to 3 weeks is recommended for those cases in which IE is suspected and the initial blood cultures are negative. Third-generation cephalosporins such as ceftriaxone and cefotaxime are the drugs of choice for the treatment of HACEK IE. The recommended duration is 3 to 4 weeks for native valves and 6 weeks for PVE (115). Ampicillin monotherapy is no longer recommended because many strains produce β-lactamase. HACEK microorganisms are susceptible in vitro to fluoroquinolones. However, because clinical data are lacking, they should be used as alternative therapy in patients who cannot tolerate β-lactams. The same principles apply for the use of aztreonam and trimethoprim–sulfamethoxazole.

Pseudomonas aeruginosa causes IE primarily in IV drug abusers. The usual antibiotic treatment regimen consists of two antimicrobials such as antipseudomonal penicillin in large dose (e.g., piperacillin 18 g/d) along with a high dose-aminoglycoside (e.g., tobramycin 5–8 mg/kg/d to achieve levels of 8–10 μg/mL) for 6 weeks (116). Alternative regimens can be used as long as they are supported by in vitro susceptibility results. Examples of such alternative regimens are the combination of imipenem plus an aminoglycoside or a quinolone based-regimen with the addition of a second drug. However, the clinical experience is limited with both and they are not recommended as first-line therapy.

Coxiella burnetti

Q fever is caused by *C. burnetti*, a strict intracellular pathogen. Although rare in many parts of the world, in selected locations (e.g., southern France) infection with this organism is a relatively common cause of IE on native or prosthetic valves. The intracellular location of the microorganism is associated with frequent relapses and makes eradication extremely difficult. To achieve cure, valve replacement is commonly required along with an extended course of antibiotics. Some experts favor antibiotic treatment for a minimum of 3 years once IgG antibody titers drop below 1:400 and IgA phase I antibodies are undetectable. Several regimens are recommended including doxycycline with trimethoprim/sulfamethoxazole, rifampin, or fluoroquinolones. However, recent evidence suggests that combination of doxycycline and hydroxychloroquine allows therapy to be shortened and decreases relapses (116).

Fungal Infective Endocarditis

The incidence of fungal sepsis and fungal IE has undergone a striking increase in the past decade. Fungal IE occurs principally in a setting of narcotic addiction, after cardiac surgery, after the prolonged IV administration of drugs (especially broad-spectrum antibiotics), and in the compromised host (including preterm neonates). Although the survival rate in patients treated prior to 1974 was less than 20%, survival in the current era has increased to about 60%, coincident with improved diagnostic techniques (119). The preferred mode of therapy has not been determined. The use of antifungal agents alone has been often been unsuccessful in achieving a cure of this disease. The addition of surgical measures to antifungal therapy may result in an improvement in prognosis (120). Although previous recommendations strongly favor a combined medical–surgical approach, the introduction of new fungicidal agents has brought the need for universal surgery into question.

A mainstay of antifungal drug therapy is liposomal amphotericin B. This agent is much less toxic than routine amphotericin B, which produces multiple side effects, including fever, chills, phlebitis, headache, anorexia, anemia, hypokalemia, renal tubular acidosis, nephrotoxicity, nausea, and vomiting. After 1 to 2 weeks of liposomal amphotericin B therapy at full dosages, surgery is often required. Valve replacement is often necessary for left-sided fungal IE. The duration of antifungal therapy after surgery is empirical, but 6 to 8 weeks is usually recommended.

It is possible that combination antifungal therapy may improve the poor survival with fungal IE. Some strains of *Candida* spp. and *Cryptococcus neoformans* are inhibited in vitro by concentrations of 5-fluorocytosine achieved with the oral administration of 150 mg/kg per day in six divided doses. Synergism between 5-fluorocytosine and amphotericin B has been documented for these yeasts in vitro. Potentiation of amphotericin B activity by rifampin has been noted for virtually all strains of *Candida* spp. and for a few isolates of *Histoplasma capsulatum*. The therapeutic advantage of the addition of 5-fluorocytosine or rifampin to amphotericin for fungal IE requires further investigation. The use of fluconazole has apparently led to long-term cures of *Candida* IE in a limited number of patients when valve replacement was considered to be contraindicated (121). This agent should be tried after an initial course of amphotericin B in this setting and used for long-term suppressive therapy in patients who are not able to undergo surgery. The role of amphotericin–lipid–liposomal complexes, voriconazole, or caspofungin in the treatment of fungal IE is as yet unclear though at least two patients with left-sided fungal endocarditis have been cured using the liposomal amphotericin B along with caspofungin, both of which are fungicidal.

Culture-Negative Infective Endocarditis

The primary considerations for therapy are directed against staphylococci, streptococci, enterococci, and the HACEK organisms. This consists of a combination of penicillin, 20 million units IV daily in divided doses, or ampicillin, 2 g IV every 4 hours, plus gentamicin, 1 mg/kg IM or IV every 8 hours, plus ceftriaxone, 2 g IV once daily. When staphylococcal IE is likely (as in narcotic addicts), a penicillinase-resistant penicillin or a cephalosporin in full dosage should be substituted in the above regimen. If clinical improvement occurs, some authorities recommend discontinuation of treatment with the aminoglycoside after 2 weeks. The other agent(s) should be continued for the full 6 weeks of treatment. Continued surveillance for the causative agent and careful follow-up are mandatory, including evaluations for fastidious organisms such as bartonella, coxiella, legionella, and chlamydia (122).

SURGICAL THERAPY

Valve replacement has become an important adjunct to medical therapy in the management of IE and is now used in at least 25% of the cases. The generally accepted indications for surgical intervention during active IE are as follows: (1) refractory CHF; (2) more than one serious systemic embolic episode; (3) uncontrolled infection; (4) physiologically significant valve dysfunction as demonstrated by echocardiography; (5) ineffective antimicrobial therapy (e.g., as in fungal IE); (6) resection of mycotic aneurysms; (7) many cases of PVE caused by more antibiotic-resistant pathogens (e.g., staphylococci, enteric gram-negative bacilli); and (8) local suppurative complications including perivalvular or myocardial abscesses. The major indications in the past have been persistent infection and CHF in both adults and children. The AHA Committee on IE, working from data reported in the recent literature, has identified the following echocardiographic features in IE as associated with a potential increased need for surgical intervention: (1) persistent vegetations after a major systemic embolic episode, (2) large (>1 cm in diameter) anterior mitral valve vegetations, (3) 1 or more embolic events during first 2 weeks of antimicrobial therapy, (4) increase in vegetation size after 4 weeks of antibiotic therapy, (5) acute aortic or mitral insufficiency with signs of ventricular failure, (6) heart failure unresponsive to medical therapy, (7) valve perforation or rupture, (8) valvular dehiscence, rupture, or fistula, (9) new heart block, and (10) large abscess (113,123). The most frequent causes of death in IE, in approximate order, are neurologic and septic complications, CHF, embolic phenomena, rupture of a mycotic aneurysm, complications of cardiac surgery, lack of response to antimicrobial therapy, and PVE (122).

The hemodynamic status of the patient, not the activity of the infection, is the critical determining factor in the timing of cardiac valve replacement. Surgery should not be delayed because a full course of antibiotic therapy has not been completed or the patient is still bacteremic.

Indeed, the incidence of reinfection of a prosthetic valve after surgery is below 1%. Thus, when CHF is diagnosed in patients with aortic valve IE or persists despite therapy in mitral valve IE, surgery is indicated. Although not systematically studied, most authorities suggest that if there is evidence of active IE at the time of valve replacement surgery, antibiotic therapy should be continued postoperatively for 2 to 6 weeks (122).

In contrast to left-sided IE in which CHF is the usual indication for surgical intervention, persistent infection is the indication for surgery in over 70% of patients with right-sided IE. Most of the patients are narcotic addicts, with IE caused by organisms that are difficult to eradicate with antimicrobial therapy alone (e.g., fungi, gram-negative aerobic bacilli). Tricuspid valvulectomy or "vegetectomy" with valvuloplasty is now the procedure of choice for refractory right-sided IE. Combination antimicrobial therapy should be continued for 4 to 6 weeks postoperatively. These patients may develop mild to moderate right-sided heart failure, but this is easily tolerated, and the success rate with this approach is over 70%. Valve replacement as a second operation is advised only when medical management fails to control the hemodynamic manifestations and the patient has ceased using illicit drugs. However, eventual tricuspid valve replacement is usually required for progressive right heart failure (124,125).

Most patients with PVE (except those with late disease caused by penicillin-sensitive viridans streptococci) require valve replacement. Valve replacement is also necessary in a significant proportion of patients with IE on native valves after a medical cure; aortic involvement is a predictor of the need for surgery.

Medical therapy alone is inadequate and virtually all patients with periannular extension should undergo cardiac surgery. A small number of patients with significant comorbidities can be treated without surgical intervention, especially those without heart block, echocardiographic evidence of progression, or valvular dehiscence or insufficiency. Issues surrounding the surgical options can be complex, especially if there has been neurologic bleeding or significant comorbid disease.

PREVENTION

Antimicrobial prophylaxis before selected dental and invasive surgical and diagnostic procedures has become standard and routine in most countries, despite the fact that no prospective study has been performed that proves that such therapy is clearly beneficial. Only half of all patients who develop IE have a cardiac disorder that would have prompted IE prophylaxis in the first place. Furthermore, follow-up incidence of IE is low even if patients with predisposing valvular lesions do not receive prophylactic antibiotics: it has been estimated that only one in five untreated patients develops IE after having had an invasive procedure (55). Thus, perhaps only 1 in 10 IE episodes can be prevented by the appropriate use of antibiotic prophylaxis before an invasive procedure (55).

Maintenance of meticulous dental hygiene is of equal importance to antibiotic prophylaxis in the prevention of IE. Vigorous brushing of teeth or even chewing gum may result in transient bacteremia in patients with periodontal disease; it

TABLE 26.6

CARDIAC CONDITIONS AND THE NEED FOR ENDOCARDITIS PROPHYLAXIS[a]

ENDOCARDITIS PROPHYLAXIS RECOMMENDED
High risk
Prosthetic cardiac valves, including bioprosthetic and homograft valves
Previous bacterial endocarditis, even in the absence of heart disease
Complex cyanotic congenital heart disease (e.g., single ventricle states, transposition of the great arteries, tetralogy of Fallot)
Surgically constructed systemic–pulmonary shunts or conduits
Moderate risk
Rheumatic and other acquired valvular dysfunction, even after valvular surgery
Hypertrophic cardiomyopathy
Mitral valve prolapse with valvular regurgitation and/or thickened leaflets
Most other congenital cardiac malformations (other than the above and below)
ENDOCARDITIS PROPHYLAXIS NOT RECOMMENDED
Isolated secundum atrial septal defect
Surgical repair without residua beyond 6 mo of secundum atrial septal defect, ventricular septal defect, and patent ductus arteriosus
Previous coronary artery bypass graft surgery
Mitral valve prolapse without valvular regurgitation
Physiologic, functional, or innocent heart murmurs
Previous Kawasaki disease without valvular dysfunction
Previous rheumatic fever without valvular dysfunction
Cardiac pacemakers and implanted defibrillators

[a]This table lists selected conditions but is not meant to be all inclusive.
Source: Adapted from Dajani AS, et al: Prevention of bacterial endocarditis: recommendations by the American Heart Association. *JAMA* 1997;277:1794–1801.

is important to emphasize to the patient that maintenance of good dental hygiene is vital. In addition, it is advisable to instruct all patients to avoid gingival trauma with toothpicks and high-pressure water irrigation devices.

The guidelines for antimicrobial prophylaxis for IE formulated by an expert committee of the AHA are the regimens most widely used by clinicians in the United States (126). The guidelines are based on results of in vitro studies, clinical experience, data from experimental animal models, and clinical assumptions concerning the bacteria most likely to produce bacteremia and cause IE. These recommendations should not be assumed to be the standard of care in all clinical situations. Clinicians can reasonably deviate from these guidelines in individual cases.

Table 26.6 outlines the current clinical situations wherein antibiotic prophylaxis is recommended based on the risk involved. The precise risk of IE following invasive dental or surgical procedures in patients with any of the listed conditions cannot be precisely measured; in fact, differences in opinions continue to exist as to whether even patients with each of the listed predisposing conditions should receive antibiotic therapy before an invasive procedure. There is general agreement, however, that those patients with a prior history of IE and those with prosthetic heart valves are at higher risk than patients with congenital and valvular lesions.

In general, risk of IE is considered to be highest for oral or dental procedures in which the oral mucosa is penetrated and in which gingival or mucosal bleeding is likely to occur. Invasive dental procedures for which the risk of transient bacteremia is above 50% include tooth extractions, periodontal surgery, and cleaning of teeth with removal of tartar. The risk of bacteremia is substantially lower for invasive genitourinary procedures such as dilation of strictures, insertion of endoscopes and catheters, and prostatectomy. The risk of bacteremia following invasive gastrointestinal procedures such as colonoscopy with biopsy and endoscopic retrograde cholangiopancreatography is generally less than 5% to 10%. The AHA has listed those invasive procedures in which IE prophylaxis is and is not recommended (Table 26.6). Clinicians may choose to use antimicrobial prophylaxis in some patients with a high risk for IE who undergo a procedure with a low or intermediate risk of bacteremia, yet reasonably forego antimicrobial prophylaxis in patients with a very low risk of IE (e.g., those with a history of drug allergy) who undergo a procedure with an intermediate or high risk of bacteremia (Table 26.7).

The antimicrobial regimens suggested by the AHA for IE prophylaxis are listed in Table 26.8. Although the evidence supporting the routine use of antibiotic prophylaxis is spotty, failure to adhere to these guidelines in the current medicolegal climate may invite litigation.

CONTROVERSIES AND PERSONAL PERSPECTIVES

What Is the Appropriate Timing for Surgery in a Patient With Infective Endocarditis?

Early surgery, before deterioration in the clinical condition of the patient occurs, improves prognosis. However, this recommendation is based on retrospective data with results confounded by selection bias. There are currently no randomized trials comparing outcomes in patients treated with early versus delayed surgery. Timing of surgery is also affected by the causative agent of IE, with *S. aureus* infection requiring surgery earlier than infection with more indolent streptococcal species.

CHF secondary to valve dysfunction carries a worse prognosis for patients treated with medical therapy and also increases operative mortality following valve replacement. Heart failure

TABLE 26.7

DENTAL OR SURGICAL PROCEDURES AND ENDOCARDITIS PROPHYLAXIS

ENDOCARDITIS PROPHYLAXIS RECOMMENDED

Dental procedures known to induce gingival or mucosal bleeding, including professional cleaning
Tonsillectomy, adenoidectomy, or both
Surgical operations that involve intestinal or respiratory mucosa
Bronchoscopy with a rigid bronchoscope
Sclerotherapy for esophageal varices
Esophageal dilatation
Gallbladder surgery
Cystoscopy
Urethral dilatation
Urethral catheterization if urinary tract infection is present
Prostatic surgery
Incision and drainage of infected tissue
Vaginal delivery in the presence of infection

ENDOCARDITIS PROPHYLAXIS NOT RECOMMENDED

Dental procedures not likely to induce gingival bleeding, such as simple adjustment of orthodontic appliances or fillings above the gum line
Injection of local intraoral anesthetic (except intraligamentary injections)
Shedding of primary teeth
Tympanostomy tube insertion
Endotracheal intubation
Bronchoscopy with a flexible bronchoscope, with or without biopsy
Cardiac catheterization
TEE
Endoscopy with or without gastrointestinal biopsy
Cesarean section
In the absence of infection for urethral catheterization, dilatation and curettage, uncomplicated vaginal delivery, therapeutic abortion, sterilization procedures, or insertion or removal of intrauterine devices

Abbreviation: TEE, transesophageal echocardiography.
Source: Adapted from Dajani AS, et al: Prevention of bacterial endocarditis: recommendations by the American Heart Association. *JAMA* 1997;277:1794–1801.

TABLE 26.8

RECOMMENDED BACTERIAL ENDOCARDITIS PROPHYLAXIS REGIMENS

STANDARD REGIMEN FOR DENTAL/ORAL/UPPER RESPIRATORY TRACT PROCEDURES

Standard regimen in patients at risk (includes those with prosthetic heart valves and other high-risk patients): amoxicillin, 2.0 g, orally 1 h before procedure
For amoxicillin/penicillin-allergic patients: clindamycin (600 mg orally), cephalexin or cefadroxil (2 g orally), or azithromycin (500 mg orally) taken 1 h before procedure
Alternate standard regimens for dental/oral/upper respiratory tract procedures
For patients unable to take oral medications: ampicillin, 2.0 g IV (or IM) 30 min before procedure; then ampicillin, 1.0 g IV (or IM) 6 h after initial dose
For ampicillin/amoxicillin/penicillin-allergic patients unable to take oral medications: clindamycin, 600 mg IV, or cefazolin, 1 g IV, 30 min before procedure

STANDARD REGIMEN FOR GENITOURINARY/GASTROINTESTINAL PROCEDURES

Standard regimen in patients at high risk: ampicillin, 2.0 g IV (or IM), plus gentamicin, 1.5 mg/kg IV (or IM) (not to exceed 120 mg) 30 min before procedure; then amoxicillin, 1 g orally, IM or IV 6 h after initial dose
For amoxicillin/ampicillin/penicillin-allergic patients: vancomycin, 1.0 g IV administered over 1 h, plus gentamicin, 1.5 mg/kg IV (or IM) (not to exceed 120 mg) 1 h before procedure
Alternate oral regimen for genitourinary/gastrointestinal patients at moderate risk: amoxicillin, 3.0 g orally; ampicillin, 2 g IV; or vancomycin, 1 g IV to be completed 30 min before the procedure

secondary to acute aortic regurgitation is particularly poorly tolerated and requires emergent surgery.

Duration of antibiotic therapy before surgery does not affect operative mortality, and the incidence of recurrent IE is extremely low even after only a few doses of antibiotics. Therefore, delaying surgery to provide a longer course of antibiotic therapy is not indicated.

What Is the Appropriate Timing of Surgery Following Embolic Stroke in Patients With Infective Endocarditis?

Any patient with IE in whom neurologic symptoms develop should undergo contrasted computed tomography or magnetic resonance imaging of the head to identify the nature and extent of the lesion as well as the presence of hemorrhage. Patients with evidence of intracranial hemorrhage should undergo cerebral angiography to evaluate for possible neurosurgical intervention before cardiac surgery. Concerns about postoperative neurologic complications include the immediate risk of intracranial bleeding during cardiopulmonary bypass, as well as the risk associated with short- and long-term anticoagulation. In the absence of hemorrhagic infarction, valve replacement should be performed at least 72 hours after a stroke has occurred. In stable patients, a delay of 2 weeks is reasonable. Patients with evidence of hemorrhage on CT scan have an increased risk of intracranial bleeding during surgery and therefore should be operated on at least 2 to 4 weeks after the neurologic event has occurred.

What Is the Risk of Infective Endocarditis for Patients With *S. aureus* Bacteremia?

S. aureus is a leading cause of bacteremia and IE, with an increasing incidence because of the use of indwelling catheters. We recently performed a prospective observational study evaluating risk factors for complicated SAB demonstrating a 12% prevalence of IE in 724 consecutive patients admitted with one or more positive blood cultures (127). This is significantly lower than a previous study at our institution, in which the incidence of IE was almost 25% (128). This disparity is likely secondary to selection bias; only patients undergoing both TTE and TEE evaluation were included in the latter study.

We have followed patients with one or more positive blood cultures for *S. aureus* for a period of 12 weeks. Risk factors for development of complicated SAB were identified as positive follow-up blood cultures 48 to 96 hours following admission (OR, 5.58), persistent fevers 72 hours postadmission (OR, 2.23), community acquisition (OR, 3.10), and skin findings suggestive of acute systemic infection (OR, 2.04) (38). A risk scoring system based on these four criteria predicted a complication rate of 16% in the absence of all risk factors and 90% when all risk factors were present. Outcomes for patients with MRSA bacteremia were similar to those for patients with MSSA bacteremia in this study, although differing results have been observed in other studies (127).

We feel that it is therefore essential that patients with SAB undergo aggressive evaluation, including follow-up blood cultures 48 hours postadmission as well as TEE to exclude the presence of IE, even in the absence of physical examination findings or metastatic foci.

THE FUTURE

Because of the variability in clinical presentation and the heterogeneity in both microbiologic etiology and the patient population, IE remains a challenging disease for clinicians. In the current era, the morbidity and mortality of IE remains high. Close collaboration between the cardiologist, infectious disease specialist, and cardiothoracic surgeon is essential. Until recently, most series of patients with IE were from single centers. The International Collaboration on Endocarditis (ICE) (see http://endocarditis.org/ice) is a large group of collaborative investigators recently formed to perform collaborative studies to improve the outcome of patients with IE. Currently, the ICE studies include over 100 investigators at 50 centers in 20 countries. The multinational nature of the collaboration should also provide a global view of IE and opportunities for studies such as randomized trials of therapeutic treatment strategies.

References

1. Major RH. Notes on the history of endocarditis. *Bull Hist Med* 1945;17:351–359.
2. Contrepois A. Notes on the early history of infective endocarditis and the development of an experimental model. *Clin Infect Dis* 1995;20:461–466.
3. Gross L. Significance of blood vessels in human heart valves. *Am Heart J* 1937;13:275–280.
4. Gulstonian Lectures "On Malignant Endocarditis," Royal College of Physicians, London. *Br Med J*, 1885;1:467–70, 522–526, 577–579.
5. Osler W. Chronic infective endocarditis. *Q J Med* 1901;2:219.
6. Weiss S. Self-observations and psychologic reactions of medical student A. S. R. to the onset and symptoms of subacute bacterial endocarditis. *J Mount Sinai Hosp* 1941;42:79–94.
7. von Reyn CF, Levy BS, Arbeit RD, et al. Infective endocarditis: an analysis based on strict case definitions. *Ann Intern Med* 1982;94:505.
8. Steckelberg JM, Melton LJ III, Ilstrup DM, et al. Influence of referral bias on the apparent clinical spectrum of infective endocarditis. *Am J Med* 1990;88:582.
9. Harris SL. Definitions and demographic characteristics. In: Kaye D, ed. *Infective endocarditis*. New York: Raven Press; 1992:1.
10. Durack DT, Petersdorf RG. Changes in the epidemiology of endocarditis. In: Kaplan EL, Taranta AV, eds. *Infective endocarditis. An American Heart Association symposium*. Dallas, TX: American Heart Association, 1977:3.
11. Harris SL. Definitions and demographic characteristics. In: Kaye D, ed. *Infective endocarditis*. New York: Raven Press; 1992:1.
12. Baltimore RS. Infective endocarditis in children. *Pediatr Infect Dis J* 1992;11:907.
13. Valente AM, Jain R, Scheurer M, Fowler V, et al. Staphylococcus aureus bacteremia in childhood: who is at risk for endocarditis? *Pediatrics* 2005;115:e15–19.
14. Thayer WS. Studies on bacterial (infective) endocarditis. *Johns Hopkins Hosp Rep* 1926;22:1.
15. Garvey GJ, Neu HC. Infective endocarditis: an evolving disease. *Medicine (Baltimore)* 1978;57:105.
16. Lien EA, Solberg CO, Kalager T. Infective endocarditis 1973–1984 at the Bergen University Hospital: clinical features, treatment and prognosis. *Scand J Infect Dis* 1988;20:239–246.
17. Edwards MB, Taylor KM. A profile of valve replacement surgery in the UK (1986–1997): a study from the UK heart valve registry. *J Heart Valve Dis* 1999;8:697–701.
18. Grover FL, Cohen DJ, Oprian C, et al. Determinants of the occurrence of and survival from prosthetic valve endocarditis. Experience of the Veterans Affairs Cooperative Study on Valvular Heart Disease. *J Thorac Cardiovasc Surg* 1994;108:207–214.
19. Kassai B, Gueyffier F, Cucherat M, et al. Comparison of bioprosthesis and mechanical valves; meta-analysis of randomized clinical trials. *Cardiovasc Surg* 2000;8:477–483.
20. Calderwood SB, Swinski LA, Waternaux CM, et al. Risk factors for the development of prosthetic valve endocarditis. *Circulation* 1985;72:31–37.
21. Piper C, Korfer R, Horstkotte D. Prosthetic valve endocarditis. *Heart* 2001;85:590–593.
22. Cabell CH, Jollis JG, Peterson GE, et al. Changing patient characteristics and the effect on mortality in endocarditis. *Arch Intern Med* 2002;162:90–94.
23. Pelletier LL, Petersdorf RG. Infective endocarditis: a review of 125 cases from the University of Washington Hospitals, 1963–72. *Medicine (Baltimore)* 1977;56:287.
24. Terpenning MS, Buggy BP, Kaufmann CA. Hospital-acquired infective endocarditis. *Arch Intern Med* 1988;148:1601–1603.
25. Petti CA, Fowler VG Jr. Staphylococcus aureus bacteremia and endocarditis. *Cardiol Clin* 2003;21:219–233.
26. Cerubin CE, Baden M, Favaler F, et al. Infectious endocarditis in narcotic addicts. *Ann Intern Med* 1968;69:1091.

27. Terpenning MS, Buggy BP, Kauffman CA. Infective endocarditis: clinical features in young and elderly patients. *Am J Med* 1987;83:626–634.
28. Levine DP, Crane LR, Zervos MJ. Bacteremia in narcotic addicts at the Detroit Medical Center. II. Infectious endocarditis: a prospective comparative study. *Rev Infect Dis* 1986;8:374–396.
29. Mathew J, Addai T, Anand A, et al. Clinical features, site of involvement, bacteriologic findings, and outcome of infective endocarditis in intravenous drug users. *Arch Intern Med* 1995;155:1641–1648.
30. Saravolatz LP, Burch KH, Quinn EL. Polymicrobial infective endocarditis: an increasing clinical entity. *Am Heart J* 1978;95:163.
31. Rodbard S. Blood velocity and endocarditis. *Circulation* 1963;27:18.
32. Lepeschkin E. On the relation between the site of valvular involvement in endocarditis and the blood pressure resting on the valve. *Am J Med Sci* 1952;224:318.
33. McKinsey DS, Ratts TE, Bisno AL. Underlying cardiac lesions in adults with infective endocarditis. The changing spectrum. *Am J Med* 1987;82:681–688.
34. Michel PL, Acar J. Native cardiac disease predisposing to infective endocarditis. *Eur Heart J* 1995;16[Suppl B]:2–6.
35. Gersony WM, Hayes CJ, Driscoll DJ, et al. Bacterial endocarditis in patients with aortic stenosis, pulmonary stenosis, or ventricular septal defect. *Circulation* 1993;87:1121–1126.
36. Horstkotte D. Prosthetic valve endocarditis. In: Horstkotte D, Bodnar E, eds. *Infective endocarditis*. London: IRC Publishers, 1991:229–261.
37. McKinsey DS, Ratts TE, Bisno AL. Underlying cardiac lesions in adults with infective endocarditis. The changing spectrum. *Am J Med* 1987;82:681–688.
38. Weinberger I, Rotenberg Z, Zacharovitch D, et al. Native valve infective endocarditis in the 1970s versus the 1980s: underlying cardiac lesions and infecting organisms. *Clin Cardiol* 1990;13:94–98.
39. Clemens JD, Horwitz RI, Jaffe CC, et al. A controlled evaluation of the risk of bacterial endocarditis in persons with mitral-valve prolapse. *N Engl J Med* 1982;307:776.
40. Harris SL. Definitions and demographic characteristics. In: Kaye D, ed. *Infective endocarditis*. New York: Raven Press; 1992:1.
41. Bansal RC. Infective endocarditis. *Med Clin North Am* 1995;79:1205–1240.
42. Michel PL, Acar J. Native cardiac disease predisposing to infective endocarditis. *Eur Heart J* 1995;16[Suppl B]:2–6.
43. Spirito P, Rapezzi C, Bellone P, et al. Infective endocarditis in hypertrophic cardiomyopathy: prevalence, incidence, and indications for antibiotic prophylaxis. *Circulation* 1999;99:2132–2137.
44. McKinsey DS, Ratts TE, Bisno AL. Underlying cardiac lesions in adults with infective endocarditis. The changing spectrum. *Am J Med* 1987;82:681–688.
45. Scheld WM. Pathogenesis and pathophysiology of infective endocarditis. In: Sande MA, Kaye D, Root RK, eds. *Endocarditis*. Vol. 1: *Contemporary issues in infectious diseases*. London: Churchill Livingstone, 1984:1–32.
46. Freedman LR. The pathogenesis of infective endocarditis. *J Antimicrob Chemother* 1987;20[Suppl A]:1–6.
47. Livornese LL Jr, Korzeniowski OM. Pathogenesis of infective endocarditis. In: Kaye D, ed. *Infective endocarditis*. New York: Raven Press, 1992:19.
48. Tunkel AR, Scheld WM. Experimental models of endocarditis. In: Kaye D, ed. *Infective endocarditis*. New York: Raven Press; 1992;37.
49. Gould K, Ramirez-Ronda CH, Holmes RK, et al. Adherence of bacteria to heart valves in vitro. *J Clin Invest* 1975;56:1364.
50. Freedman LR, Valone J Jr. Experimental infective endocarditis. *Prog Cardiovasc Dis* 1979;22:169.
51. Ramirez-Ronda CH. Effects of molecular weight of dextran on the adherence of *Streptococcus sanguis* to damaged heart valves. *Infect Immun* 1980;29:1.
52. Lowrance JH, Baddour LM, Simpson WA. The role of fibronectin binding in the rat model of experimental endocarditis caused by *Streptococcus sanguis*. *J Clin Invest* 1990;86:7.
53. Becker RC, DiBello PM, Lucas FV. Bacterial tissue tropism: an in vitro model for infective endocarditis. *Cardiovasc Res* 1987;21:813–820.
54. Fenno JC, LeBlanc DJ, Fives-Taylor P. Nucleotide sequence analysis of a type 1 fimbrial gene of *Streptococcus sanguis* FW213. *Infect Immun* 1989; 57:3527–3533.
55. Sexton DJ, Bashore TM. Infective endocarditis. In: Topol EJ, ed. *Comprehensive cardiovascular medicine*. Philadelphia: Lippincott-Raven, 1998.
56. Weinstein L. Life-threatening complications of infective endocarditis and their management. *Arch Intern Med* 1986;146:953–957.
57. Karalis DG, Bansal RC, Hauck AJ, et al. Transesophageal echocardiographic recognition of subaortic complications in aortic valve endocarditis. Clinical and surgical implications. *Circulation* 1992;86:353–362.
58. Anguera I, Miro JM, Vilacosta I, et al. Aorto-cavitary Fistula in Endocarditis Working Group. Aorto-cavitary fistulous tract formation in infective endocarditis: clinical and echocardiographic features of 76 cases and risk factors for mortality. *Eur Heart J* 2005;26:288–97. Epub 2004 Nov 30.
59. Williams RC, Kunkel HG. Rheumatoid factors and their disappearance following therapy in patients with SBE. *Arthritis Rheum* 1962;5:126.
60. Bacon PA, Davidson C, Smith B. Antibodies to *Candida* and autoantibodies in subacute bacterial endocarditis. *Q J Med* 1974;43:537.
61. Qoronfleh MW, Weraarchakul W, Wilkinson BJ. Antibodies to a range of *Staphylococcus aureus* and *Escherichia coli* heat shock proteins in sera from patients with *S. aureus* endocarditis. *Infect Immun* 1993;61: 1567.
62. Laxdal T, Messner RP, Williams RC. Opsonic, agglutinating, and complement-fixing antibodies in patients with subacute bacterial endocarditis. *J Lab Clin Med*. 1968;71:638.
63. Horwitz D, Quismorio FP, Friou GJ. Cryoglobulinemia in patients with infectious endocarditis. *Clin Exp Immunol* 1975;19:131.
64. Bayer AS, Theofilopoulos AN, Eisenberg R, et al. Circulating immune complexes in infective endocarditis. *N Engl J Med* 1976;295:1500.
65. Alpert JS, Krous HF, Dalen JE, et al. Pathogenesis of Osler's nodes. *Ann Intern Med* 1976;85:471.
66. Tzukert AA, Leviner E, Sela M. Prevention of infective endocarditis: not by antibiotics alone. A 7-year follow-up of 90 dental patients. *Oral Surg Oral Med Oral Pathol* 1986;62:385–388.
67. Freedman LR. Infective endocarditis and other intravascular infections. In: Braude AI, David CE, Fierer J, eds. *Medical microbiology and infectious diseases*. Philadelphia: WB Saunders, 1981:1511.
68. Livornese LL Jr, Korzeniowski OM. Pathogenesis of infective endocarditis. In: Kaye D, ed. *Infective endocarditis*. New York: Raven Press, 1992:19.
69. Roder BL, Wandall DA, Frimodt-Moller N, et al. Clinical features of *Staphylococcus aureus* endocarditis: a 10-year experience in Denmark. *Arch Intern Med* 1999;159:462–469.
70. Figueiredo LT, Ruiz-Junior E, Schirmbeck T. Infective endocarditis (IE) first diagnosed at autopsy: analysis of 31 cases in Ribeirao Preto, Brazil. *Rev Inst Med Trop Sao Paulo* 2001;43:213–216.
71. Bradley, SF. *Staphylococcus aureus* infections and antibiotic resistance in older adults. *Clin Infect Dis* 2002;34:211–216.
72. Terpenning MS, Buggy BP, Kauffman CA. Infective endocarditis: clinical features in young and elderly patients. *Am J Med* 1987;83:626–634.
73. Charney R, Keltz TN, Attai L, et al. Acute valvular obstruction from streptococcal endocarditis. *Am Heart J* 1993;125:544.
74. Ting W, Silverman NA, Arzaman DA, et al. Splenic septic emboli in endocarditis. *Circulation* 1990;82[Suppl IV]:IV–105.
75. Churchill MA, Geraci JE, Hunder GG. Musculoskeletal manifestations of bacterial endocarditis. *Ann Intern Med* 1977;87:754.
76. Anderson DJ, Goldstein LB, Wilkinson WE, et al. Stroke location, characterization, severity, and outcome in mitral vs aortic valve endocarditis. *Neurology* 2003;61:1341–1346.
77. Selky AK, Roos KL. Neurologic complications of infective endocarditis. *Semin Neurol* 1995;12:225.
78. Heiro M, Nikoskelainen J, Engblom E, et al. Neurologic manifestations of infective endocarditis: a 17-year experience in a teaching hospital in Finland. *Arch Intern Med* 2000;160:2781–2787.
79. Beeson PB, Brannon ES, Warren JV. Observations on the sites of removal of bacteria from the blood of patients with bacterial endocarditis. *J Exp Med* 1945;81:9–23.
80. McKenzie R, Reimer LG. Effect of antimicrobials on blood cultures in endocarditis. *Diagn Microbiol Infect Dis* 1987;8:165–172.
81. Wilson ML, Harrell LJ, Mirrett S, et al. Controlled evaluation of BACTEC PLUS 27 and Roche Septi-Chek anaerobic blood culture bottles. *J Clin Microbiol* 1992;30:63–66.
82. Doern GV, Gantz NM. Detection of bacteremia in patients receiving antimicrobial therapy: an evaluation of the antimicrobial removal device and 16B medium. *J Clin Microbiol* 1983;18:43–48.
83. Aronson MD, Bos DH. Blood cultures. *Ann Intern Med* 1987;106:246–253.
84. Carey RB, Gross KC, Roberts RB. Vitamin-B_6–dependent *Streptococcus mitior (mitis)* isolated from patients with systemic infections. *J Infect Dis* 1975;131:722.
85. Durack DR, Lukes AS, Bright DK. New criteria for diagnosis of infective endocarditis: utilization of specific echocardiographic findings. Duke Endocarditis Service. *Am J Med* 1994;96:200–209.
86. Mueller C, Huber P, Laifer G, et al. Procalcitonin and the early diagnosis of infective endocarditis. *Circulation* 2004;109:1707–1710.
87. Greub G, Lepidi H, Rovery C, et al. Diagnosis of infectious endocarditis in patients undergoing valve surgery. *Am J Med* 2005;118:230–238.
88. Lamas CC, Eykyn SJ. Blood culture negative endocarditis; analysis of 63 cases presenting over 25 years. *Heart* 2003;89:258–262.
89. Gauduchon V, Chalabreysse L, Etienne J, et al. Molecular diagnosis of infective endocarditis by PCR amplification and direct sequencing of DNA from valve tissue. *J Clin Microbiol* 2003;41:763–766.
90. Dillan JC, Feigenbaum H, Konecke LL, et al. Echocardiographic manifestations of valvular vegetations. *Am Heart J* 1973;86:698.
91. Sachdev M, Peterson GE, Jollis JG. Imaging techniques for diagnosis of infective endocarditis. *Infect Dis Clin North Am* 2002;16:319–337.
92. Kuruppu JC, Corretti M, Mackowiak P, Roghmann MC. Overuse of transthoracic echocardiography in the diagnosis of native valve endocarditis. *Arch Intern Med* 2002;162:1715–1720.
93. Tischler MD, Vaitkus PT. The ability of vegetation size on echocardiography to predict clinical complications: a meta-analysis. *J Am Soc Echocardiogr* 1997;10:562–568.
94. SanFilippo AJ, Picard MH, Newell JB, et al. Echocardiographic assessment of patients with infective endocarditis. *J Am Coll Cardiol* 1991;18:1191–1199.
95. Davis RS, Strom JA, Frishman W, et al. The demonstration of vegetations by

echocardiography in bacterial endocarditis. An indication for early surgical intervention. *Am J Med* 1980;57:69.
96. Heinle S, Wilderman N, Harrison JK, et al. 1994 Value of transthoracic echocardiography in predicting embolic events in active infective endocarditis. Duke Endocarditis Service. *Am J Cardiol* 1994;74:799–801.
97. Erbel R, Rohmann S, Drexler M, et al. Improved diagnostic value of echocardiography in patients with infective endocarditis by transesophageal approach: a prospective study. *Eur Heart J* 1988;9:43.
98. Daniel WG, Mügge A, Martin RP, et al. Improvement in the diagnosis of abscesses associated with endocarditis by transesophageal echocardiography. *N Engl J Med* 1991;324:795.
99. De Castro S, Cartoni D, d'Amati G, et al. Diagnostic accuracy of transthoracic and multiplane transesophageal echocardiography for valvular perforation in acute infective endocarditis: correlation with anatomic findings. *Clin Infect Dis* 2000;30:825–826.
100. Rallidis LS, Komninos KA, Papasteriadis EG. Pacemaker-related endocarditis: the value of transesophageal echocardiography in diagnosis and treatment. *Acta Cardiologica* 2003;58:31–34.
101. Rosen AB, Fowler VGJ, Corey GR, et al. Cost-effectiveness of transesophageal echocardiography to determine the duration of therapy for intravascular catheter-associated *Staphylococcus aureus* bacteremia. *Ann Intern Med* 1999;130:810–820.
102. Heidenreich PA, Masoudi FA, Maini B, et al. Echocardiography in patients with suspected endocarditis: a cost-effectiveness analysis. *Am J Med* 1999;107:198–208.
103. Meine TJ, Nettles RE, Anderson DJ, et al. Cardiac conduction abnormalities in endocarditis defined by the Duke criteria. *Am Heart J* 2001;142:280–285.
104. Cowan JC, Patrick D, Reid DS. Aortic root abscess complicating bacterial endocarditis. Demonstration by computed tomography. *Br Heart J* 1984;52:591–593.
105. Akins EW, Slone RM, Wiechmann BN, et al. Perivalvular pseudoaneurysm complicating bacterial endocarditis: MR detection in five cases. *AJR Am J Roentgenol* 1991;1155–1158.
106. Wiseman J, Rouleau J, Rigo P, et al. Gallium-67 myocardial imaging for the detection of bacterial endocarditis. *Radiology* 1976;120:135.
107. Wong DW, Dhawan VK, Tanaka T, et al. Imaging endocarditis with technetium 99m-labeled antibody—an experimental study: concise communication. *J Nucl Med* 1982;23:229.
108. Riba AL, Thakur ML, Gottschalk A, et al. Imaging experimental infective endocarditis with indium-111—labeled blood cellular components. *Circulation* 1979;59:336.
109. von Reyn CF, Levy BS, Arbeit RD, et al. Infective endocarditis: an analysis based on strict case definitions. *Ann Intern Med* 1982;94:505.
110. Bayer AS, Bolger AF, Taubert KA, et al. Diagnosis and management of infective endocarditis and its complications. *Circulation* 1998;2936–2948.
111. Li JS, Sexton DJ, Mick N, et al. Proposed modifications to the Duke criteria for the diagnosis of infective endocarditis. *Clin Infect Dis* 2000;30:633–638.
112. Andrews MM, von Reyn CF. Patient selection criteria and management guidelines for outpatient parenteral antibiotic therapy for native valve infective endocarditis. *Clin Infect Dis* 2001;33:203–209.
113. Baddour LM, Wilson WR, Bayer AR, et al. Infective endocarditis, diagnosis, antimicrobial therapy, and management of complications. A statement for healthcare professionals from the Committee on rheumatic fever, endocarditis, and Kawasaki disease, Council on cardiovascular disease in the young, and the Councils on clinical cardiology, stroke, and cardiovascular surgery and anesthesia, American Heart Association—executive summary. *Circulation* 2005;111:3167–3184.
114. Wilson WR, Karchmer AW, Dajani AS, et al. Antibiotic treatment of adults with infective endocarditis due to streptococci, enterococci, staphylococci and HACEK microorganisms. *JAMA* 1995;274:1706–1713.
115. Le T, Bayer AS. Combination antibiotic therapy for infective endocarditis. *Clin Infect Dis* 2003;36:615–621.
116. Stryjewski ME, Corey GE. Treatment protocols for bacterial endocarditis and infection of electrophysiologic cardiac devices Biofilms, Infection, and antimicrobial therapy, eds, Pace, Rupp, and Finch. Boca Raton: CRC Press; 2005:428–449.
117. Levine DP, Fromm BS, Reddy BR. Slow response to vancomycin or vancomycin plus rifampin in methicillin-resistant *Staphylococcus aureus* endocarditis. *Ann Intern Med* 1991;115:674–680.
118. DiNubile MJ. Short-course antibiotic therapy for right sided *Staphylococcus aureus* endocarditis in injection drug users. *Ann Intern Med* 1994; 121:873–876.
119. Ellis ME, Al Abdely H, Sandridge A, et al. Fungal endocarditis: evidence in the world literature, 1965–1995. *Clin Infect Dis* 2001;32:50–62.
120. Benjamin DK Jr, Miro JM, Hoen B, et al. , and the ICE-MD Study Group. Candida endocarditis: contemporary cases from the International Collaboration of Infectious Endocarditis Merged Database (ICE-mD). *Scand J Infect Dis* 2004;36:453–455.
121. Steinbach WJ, Perfect JR, Cabell CH, et al. A meta-analysis of medical versus surgical therapy for *Candida* endocarditis. *J Infect* 2005;51:230–247.
122. Fowler VG Jr, Scheld WM, Bayer AS. Cardiovascular infections: endocarditis and intravascular infections. InMandell GL, Bennett JE, Rolin R, eds. *Principles and practice of infectious diseases*. 6th ed. London: Churchill Livingstone, 2004.
123. Bayer AS, Bolger AF, Taubert KA, et al. Diagnosis and management of infective endocarditis and its complications. *Circulation* 1998;2936–2948.
124. Straumann E, Stulz P, Jenzer HR. Tricuspid valve endocarditis in the drug addict: a reconstructive approach ("vegetectomy"). *Thorac Cardiovasc Surg* 1990;38:291.
125. DiNubile M. Surgery for addiction-related tricuspid valve endocarditis: caveat emptor. *Am J Med* 1987;82:811–813.
126. Dajani AS, Taubert KA, Wilson W, et al. Prevention of bacterial endocarditis: recommendations by the American Heart Association. *JAMA* 1997;227:1794–1801.
127. Fowler VG Jr, Olsen MK, Corey GR, et al. Clinical identifiers of complicated *Staphylococcus aureus* bacteremia. *Arch Intern Med* 2003;163:2066–2072.
128. Fowler V, Li J, Corey G, et al. Role of echocardiography in the evaluation of patients with *Staphylococcus aureus* bacteremia: experience in 103 patients. *J Am Coll Cardiol* 1997;30:1072–1078.

CHAPTER 27 ■ DISEASES OF THE PERICARDIUM, RESTRICTIVE CARDIOMYOPATHY, AND DIASTOLIC DYSFUNCTION

ALLAN L. KLEIN AND CRAIG R. ASHER

OVERVIEW

Diseases of the pericardium and restrictive cardiomyopathies cause impairment of the diastolic function of the heart. Myriad underlying etiologies, via several mechanisms, result in final common clinical presentations, making specific diagnosis difficult. Historically, these disorders have been within the realm of invasive cardiac investigation (1); however, they have recently become illuminated by several evolving noninvasive techniques, including echocardiography (2,3) and magnetic resonance imaging (MRI) (4). This chapter discusses the general principles of diastolic heart failure including its biology and physiology, clinical presentation, epidemiology, investigation, and treatment. It also reviews specific diseases of the myocardium and pericardium that may cause diastolic dysfunction.

GENERAL PRINCIPLES OF DIASTOLIC HEART DISEASE

Definition of Diastolic Dysfunction

Congestive heart failure is most often secondary to impairment of left ventricular systolic function. Diastolic heart failure is increasingly common and can be associated with significant morbidity and mortality (5). Clinically, it is important to distinguish these conditions, although in a given patient, combined systolic and diastolic dysfunction is frequently observed (6,7). Table 27.2 compares the structure and function of systolic and diastolic heart failure. The main differences are that in systolic heart failure, there is LV cavity enlargement, eccentric hypertrophy and abnormal systolic and diastolic function. While in diastolic heart failure, there is normal cavity sizes, concentric hypertrophy and abnormal diastolic function (7a). Several pathophysiologic definitions of diastolic heart failure have been proposed: (a) impaired capacity of the ventricles to fill without a compensatory increase in left atrial pressure (8); (b) abnormal ventricular filling that would produce inadequate cardiac output with a mean pulmonary venous pressure of less than 12 mm Hg (9), and (c) resistance to filling of one or both ventricles with an inappropriate upward shift of the pressure–volume loop, especially with exercise (10). These definitions have in common an abnormal resistance to filling, causing elevated left-sided filling pressures and congestion. Diastolic dysfunction impairs filling of the ventricle by impairing relaxation (early diastole), reducing compliance (early to late diastole), or leading to external constraint from the pericardium (10–12). Many pathologic processes and disease states can produce the clinical constellation of diastolic dysfunction (Table 27.1).

Diagnostic criteria for patients with diastolic heart failure have been proposed as a framework for designing and implementing treatment trials. To diagnose diastolic heart failure, the 1998 European Study Group on Diastolic Heart Failure required (a) clinical evidence of congestive heart failure, (b) normal or mild left ventricular dysfunction, and (c) the presence of impaired relaxation, filling, or compliance (13) (Table 27.2). All three components, as assessed by noninvasive testing or cardiac catheterization, were necessary for a diagnosis. Vasan

TABLE 27.1

CONDITIONS INVOLVING DIASTOLIC HEART FAILURE

Condition	Mechanism of diastolic dysfunction
Restrictive cardiomyopathy (idiopathic restrictive cardiomyopathy, cardiac amyloidosis)	Increased resistance to ventricular inflow
Constrictive pericarditis	Increased resistance to ventricular inflow, with decreased ventricular diastolic capacity
Ischemic heart disease	
Flash pulmonary edema, dyspnea during angina	Impaired myocardial relaxation Diastolic calcium overload
Postinfarction scarring and hypertrophy (remodeling)	Increased resistance to ventricular inflow
Hypertrophic heart disease (hypertrophic cardiomyopathy, chronic hypertension, aortic stenosis)	Impaired myocardial relaxation Diastolic calcium overload Increased resistance to ventricular inflow due to thick chamber walls, altered collagen matrix Activation of renin–angiotensin system
Volume overload (aortic or mitral regurgitation, arteriovenous fistula)	Increased diastolic volume relative to ventricular capacity Myocardial hypertrophy, fibrosis
Dilated cardiomyopathy	Impaired myocardial relaxation Diastolic calcium overload Myocardial fibrosis or scar
Mitral or tricuspid stenosis	Increased resistance to atrial emptying

Adapted from Grossman W. Diastolic dysfunction in congestive heart failure. *N Engl J Med* 1991;325:1557–1564.

and Levy subsequently proposed less rigid criteria using similar inclusions but defining diastolic heart failure as definite, probable, or possible depending on the number of elements present (14). There is a controversy whether measurements of LV relaxation or compliance by cardiac catheterization or Doppler echocardiography are actually needed in the presence of LV hypertrophy or concentric remodeling (14a).

Pathophysiology of Diastolic Function

Phases of Diastole

Diastole is the period from the closure of the aortic valve to the end of mitral inflow; it is divided into two periods, an isovolumic relaxation period and an auxotonic period, which includes rapid filling, diastasis (slow filling), and atrial systole (15). These phases are shown in Figure 27.1 relating left ventricular and left atrial pressure tracings and mitral, tricuspid, pulmonary, and hepatic venous Doppler echocardiography profiles. Each phase may be influenced by multiple factors including the effects of myocardial relaxation (16), the passive filling characteristics of the left ventricle (17), the dynamics of the left atrium (18–20), characteristics of the pulmonary veins (21) and the mitral valve (22), and the heart rate (23).

Isovolumic Relaxation. The isovolumic relaxation time period occurs from the time of aortic valve closure to mitral valve opening with no change in left ventricular volume (24). During this period, active, energy-dependent myocyte relaxation occurs until mid-diastole. Ventricular pressure (P_v) decay during the isovolumic period follows an approximately exponential curve that can be characterized by its starting pressure (P_0) and its time constant (tau, τ) (25). This curve can be fitted with the assumption of either a zero asymptote, $P_v = P_0 e^{-t/\tau}$ (25), or a nonzero asymptote, $P_v = P_0 e^{-t/\tau} + P_b$ (to account for subatmospheric pressure and the effects of pericardial pressure) (9,26), where P_b is the left ventricular pressure at the time of aortic closure or peak negative dp/dt, t is the time after the onset of relaxation, and τ is the time constant of relaxation.

A low value of τ is indicative of fast relaxation, whereas a high value represents slow relaxation. The duration of isovolumic duration can be obtained invasively and by several noninvasive modalities including phonocardiography and M-mode and Doppler echocardiography (27–29). Newer measures, including the color M-mode slope (Vp) (30) and the annular early velocity of tissue Doppler echocardiography, have been shown to relate closely to the time constant of relaxation (31). Isovolumic relaxation ends when the left ventricular pressure falls below the left atrial pressure, resulting in mitral valve opening and the start of the rapid-filling phase (9).

Rapid Filling. The auxotonic period occurs from mitral valve opening until mitral valve closing (15). The rapid-filling phase begins at mitral valve opening when the left ventricular pressure falls below the left atrial pressure. Left ventricular pressure continues to fall because of ongoing relaxation and elastic recoil, with blood accelerating due to the development of a left-atrial-to-left-ventricular pressure gradient (9). This gradient is influenced by the level of left atrial pressure at mitral valve opening and the rate of decline of left ventricular pressure (32). Blood rapidly enters the left ventricle from the left atrium during the early filling period, with approximately 70% of the stroke volume received by the left ventricle during the first one third of diastole (2). Active ventricular suction (pulling of blood) may play an important role in the rapid-filling phase (33,34). Ventricular suction may occur because of the recoil of the compressed elastic elements during contraction (35). Rapid filling ends as atrial and ventricular pressures equilibrate (9).

Diastasis (Slow Filling). Diastasis, or the slow-filling period, occurs between the rapid-filling phase and atrial contraction and accounts for less than 5% of filling. After rapid filling, left atrial and ventricular pressures are almost equal, yielding no immediate forward driving gradient (9).

Atrial Filling (Contraction). The atrial filling phase of diastole occurs when the left atrial pressure rises above the

TABLE 27.2

COMPARISON BETWEEN SHF AND DHF: LV STRUCTURAL AND FUNCTIONAL FEATURES

Characteristic	SHF	DHF
Remodeling		
LV end-diastolic volume	↑	N
LV end-systolic volume	↑	N
LV mass	↑ eccentric LVH	↑ concentric LVH
Relative wall thickness	↓	↑
Cardiomyocyte	↑ length	↑ diameter
Extracellular matrix collagen	↓	↑
Diastolic properties		
LV end-diastolic pressure	↑ ↑	↑ ↑
Relaxation time constant	↑	↑ ↑
Filling rate	↓	↓ ↓
Chamber stiffness	N-↓	↑
Myocardial stiffness	N-↑	↑
Systolic properties		
Performance		
Stroke volume	↓	N-↓
Stroke work	↓	N
Function		
Ejection fraction	↓	N
Ejection rate	↓	N
PRSW	↓	N
Contractility		
(+)*dP/dt*	↓	N
Ees	↓	N-↑
FS vs stress	↓	N
Preload reserve	Exhausted	Limited
Ea	↓	↑
Arterial-venticular coupling (Ea/Ees)	↓	N

Abbreviations: PRSW, preload-recruitable stroke work; Ees, end-systolic elastance; FS, fractional shortening; Ea, Effective arterial elastance.

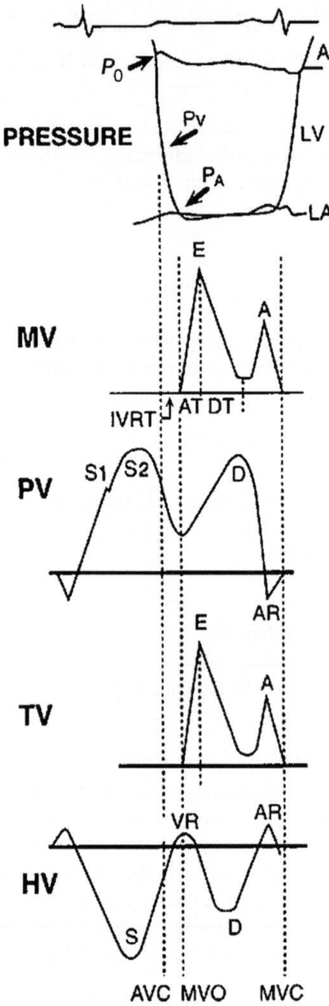

FIGURE 27.1. Diastole using Doppler echocardiography: combined schematic displaying left atrial (LA), left ventricular (LV), and aortic (Ao) pressures during diastole. Instantaneous LV pressure (P_v) falls exponentially through the isovolumic relaxation period (IVRT) from the P_0 (LV pressure at aortic valve closure (AVC) to P_A (LV pressure at mitral valve opening [MVO]) via the equation $P_v = P_0e^{-t/\tau}$. Transmitral (MV) Doppler demonstrates an early rapid-filling wave (E) broken into an acceleration time (AT) and a deceleration time (DT); a diastasis period with very little inflow; and an atrial contraction wave (A) associated with an elevation of LA pressure above LV pressure until mitral valve closure (MVC) is induced by the onset of ventricular systole. Pulmonary vein (PV) demonstrates a systolic wave (S1) related to atrial relaxation and mitral annular descent (S2), a diastolic wave (D) associated with atrial emptying through an open mitral valve, and an atrial reversal wave (AR) associated with atrial systole causing regurgitation of flow back up the pulmonary veins. Transtricuspid (TV) inflow has a similar pattern velocity to transmitral. Hepatic vein (HV) flow is similar to pulmonary vein flow, with a more prominent reversal of flow between the S and D waves associated with ventricular systole (VR).

ventricular pressure, forcing or pushing blood across the mitral valve and a small amount of regurgitation into the pulmonary veins. This late diastolic transmitral flow increases ventricular end-diastolic volume by 25% in normal individuals with only a small rise in mean pulmonary venous pressure. Diastole ends with onset of ventricular systole when the rapid increase in ventricular pressure closes the mitral valve (9).

Determinants of Diastolic Function

Diastolic function depends on four major factors: (a) active myocardial relaxation, (b) passive pressure–volume relationships (i.e., left ventricular compliance), (c) left atrium (including atrial function), pulmonary vein, and mitral valve characteristics, and (d) heart rate (9). Each variable can in turn be affected by different physiologic states and organic heart diseases. The physiology of ventricular diastolic function is exceedingly complex, involving interactions at the subcellular, myocyte, myocardial tissue, and whole-chamber levels (11,36). Pericardial contributions to diastolic physiology are discussed later in the chapter.

Myocardial relaxation is mediated by intracellular ATP and calcium (37,38). Contraction is initiated by calcium release in large quantities from the sarcoplasmic reticulum. This free ionized calcium ion binds to the troponin–tropomyosin complex, removing the inhibitory effect of that complex on the actin–myosin myofilaments (39). Active cross-bridges form between actin and myosin with consequent contraction of the myofilaments. This rapid increase of intracellular calcium is countered by calcium sequestration into the sarcoplasmic reticulum by the calcium-ATPase pump (40), which is tonically inhibited by the phospholamban. It has been demonstrated that relaxation is asynchronous, occurring earliest in apical segments and resulting in the intracavitary suction of blood from mid and basal regions toward the apex (41). Because relaxation is an energy-dependent process, it is influenced by many factors, including ischemia and left ventricular mass (42–44).

The passive filling characteristics of the ventricle describe the late diastolic volume–pressure relationship of the chamber. This is determined by the viscoelastic nature of the myocardium, the chamber size, the shape and thickness of the wall, the right and left ventricular pressure–volume interaction, the intrathoracic pressure and pericardial restraint, and any active myocardial relaxation that remains incomplete (17). *Compliance,* the ratio of change in volume per change in pressure, quantifies the net result of all of these factors. Intrinsic myocardial stiffness relates to the amount of collagen within the myocardium. Collagen plays an essential role in converting the contractile force of the myocytes into intraventricular pressure, as well as determining overall ventricular size and shape (45,46). Collagen fibrils coil around myofibrils. Little force is needed initially to stretch the coil, whereas large forces are required at full stretch, yielding an exponential stress–strain relationship (47). Pressure-induced hypertrophy is associated with increased collagen content and secondarily increased overall stiffness. Local collagen scarring after myocardial infarction is threefold stiffer than the surrounding myocardium (48).

Diastolic properties of the ventricle have been studied and quantified extensively using pressure–volume loops (Fig. 27.2) (49–51). Simultaneous recording of ventricular pressures and volumes (contrast angiography, radionuclide imaging, or echocardiography) yields the loops, which have traditionally been the benchmarks for quantifying the systolic and diastolic function of the heart.

There is a curvilinear relationship between the volume and pressure in the ventricle that is determined by the stress–strain

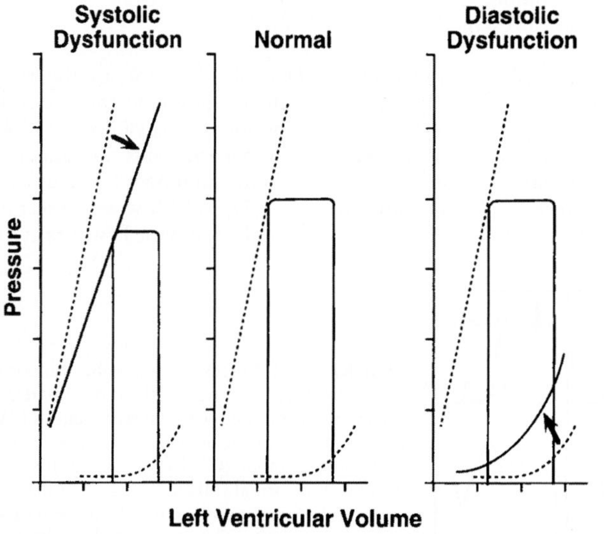

FIGURE 27.2. Schematic representation of ventricular pressure–volume loops. The center panel demonstrates the normal situation. Note the exponential nature of the curve through late diastole. In systolic dysfunction (**left**), the end-systolic pressure line is displayed downward and is manifested by a decreased ability of the LV to generate high pressures for a given volume. Diastolic dysfunction involves an upward and leftward shift of the exponential curve, a result of elevated filling pressures for a given volume. (From Katz AM. Influence of altered inotropy and lusitropy on ventricular pressure volume loops. *J Am Coll Cardiol* 1988;11:438.)

relationship. As the volume increases in the left ventricle during diastole, there is an increase in left ventricular (LV) pressure (47). The slope of the pressure–volume curve during diastole (dp/dV) is the chamber *stiffness*, and the inverse of this relation is the chamber *compliance* (52). The slope (dp/dV), or stiffness, of the left ventricle is not constant but rather follows an exponential curve upward as volume increases. Thus, when end-diastolic volume increases without intrinsic change in the mural stress–strain relationship, stiffness increases along this exponential curve. Conversely, an increase in stiffness constant E will move the loop to a steeper curve with no change in volume. Finally, it can be seen that increasing the loading pressure without changing the volume moves the loop directly upward with no change in dp/dV or stiffness.

Pulmonary vein/left atrium and mitral valve characteristics determine the volume of blood that enters the left ventricle (9). Early rapid filling is largely dependent on the pressure gradient between the pulmonary veins/left atrium and the left ventricle and the rate of myocardial relaxation and ventricular suction (33,34,53,54). Diseases of the mitral valve, such as mitral stenosis, delay left ventricular filling and prevent early rapid filling (9).

The left atrium acts as a reservoir of blood, as a passive conduit during early LV filling, and as an active pump at end-diastole (55). Atrial systolic function (active phase) may be essential to maintaining cardiac output in disease states (56,57). Atrial function relates to its compliance (58), preload, afterload, and intrinsic contractility. Atrial contractile performance varies considerably in health and disease (56,57). In young and healthy normal individuals, the atrial contribution is less than 20% of the total volume, whereas in older normal individuals, the atrial "kick" accounts for a greater proportion of the total LV filling (59). Atrial contractile function has delayed recovery after electrical cardioversion (20). Decreased atrial systolic function due to infiltration plays a role in the reduction in forward transmitral atrial contraction wave by Doppler echocardiography as seen in advanced amyloidosis (60).

Heart rate bears directly on cardiac output in cases of diastolic dysfunction (23,61). As heart rate increases, the diastolic filling period preferentially decreases with respect to the systolic ejection period. As ventricular filling is functionally delayed, adequacy of inflow deteriorates and cardiac output paradoxically falls.

Neurohormonal activation, conduction abnormalities, and pericardial constraint may also influence diastolic function. Catecholamines may enhance relaxation and increase heart rate, thus decreasing the diastolic period (62). Conduction abnormalities may also influence diastole (63). LV relaxation may be impaired by conduction abnormalities causing segmental asynchrony (64,65). This may contribute to decreased exercise tolerance in patients with left-bundle-branch block or right ventricular paced rhythms. The pericardium (see later discussion) considerably affects diastolic function, notably in constrictive pericarditis (66).

Diastolic Filling Patterns

Extensive literature exists regarding the empirically observed patterns of transmitral flow observed in normal individuals and patients with diastolic dysfunction. These patterns are the end result of the complex events only briefly described earlier and are nonspecific for any particular physiologic perturbation. Diastolic filling patterns may be influenced by technical factors (sample volume placement) and hemodynamic factors (heart rate, volume status, or conduction disorders) and are not always concordant with diastolic function (67).

Most simply, investigators have measured the peak velocity of the E wave and A wave by transmitral pulsed-wave Doppler and their relationship, the E/A ratio (68). These basic

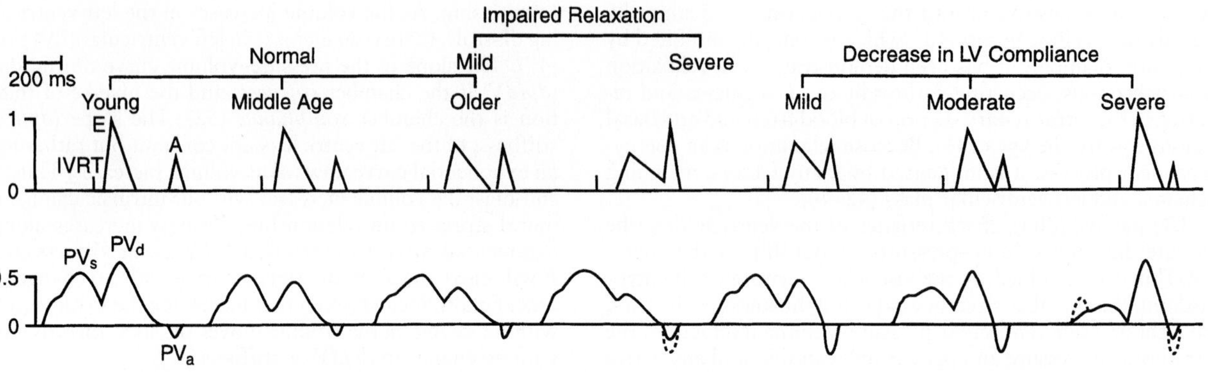

FIGURE 27.3. Schematic representation of transmitral and pulmonary venous Doppler profiles demonstrating the progression of the patterns with the normal aging process and with diseases of diastolic function, showing impaired relaxation and decrease in left ventricular (LV) compliance. Isovolumic relaxation time (IVRT), E-wave (E), A-wave (A) filling, pulmonary venous systolic (PV_s), diastolic (PV_d), and atrial reversal waves (PV_a) are shown. **Left:** In young normal individuals, the E/A is greater than 1, the deceleration time and IVRT are short, and there is mild blunting of pulmonary venous systolic flow. With age, ventricular relaxation becomes impaired and the E/A ratio reverses, the A wave increases, and the mitral deceleration time and IVRT lengthens and the pulmonary venous systolic flow increases. **Middle:** With diseases showing impaired relaxation, there may be similar findings with a further decrease in E/A ratio. **Right:** With more severe derangements of diastolic function, as chamber compliance decreases, left atrial pressure rises, deceleration time decreases, E/A ratio increases, and IVRT becomes shorter (restrictive physiology). Pulmonary venous systolic flow (PV_s) becomes progressively blunted as mean left atrial pressure and the atrial reversal (Pv_a) increase, helping to differentiate the "pseudonormal" pattern from normal. (From Appleton CP, Hatle LK. The natural history of left ventricular filling abnormalities: assessment by two dimensional and Doppler echocardiography. *Echocardiography* 1992;9:453.)

parameters vary with age and within the spectrum of diastolic filling (Fig. 27.3) (59,69). Taken alone, the normal situation (E/A ratio >1) passes through a reversed phase (E/A ratio <1), then through a "pseudonormal" pattern (E/A ratio >1) to the most abnormal "restrictive" pattern (E/A ratio >2). Thus, the E/A ratio demonstrates a U-shaped curve, making it impossible to tell from this single parameter where in the spectrum a given patient lies (31). The pulmonary venous pattern is an important source of added information (21) that may overcome the limitations of the E/A ratio for determining diastolic function in many patients. The finding of an increased pulmonary atrial reversal flow reversal velocity or width as well as a significant change in the E/A ratio with the Valsalva maneuver may aid to differentiate "pseudonormal" from normal diastolic function, corresponding to elevation of mean left atrial or left ventricular diastolic pressures, respectively (69–71).

Still, exceptions and limitations to the utility of pulmonary venous flow diminish the capability of distinguishing diastolic flow patterns in all individuals. Some patients may not have adequate pulmonary venous flow profiles; in particular, the atrial reversal wave may not be well delineated. Blunting of pulmonary venous systolic waves may be present in young individuals due to rapid diastolic "suction," and atrial reversal may be absent in advanced diastolic dysfunction due to the loss of atrial function with amyloid infiltration (69,72). Therefore, other modalities for assessment of diastolic function, including color M-mode Doppler and tissue Doppler echocardiography, have evolved that provide important adjunct information in determining diastolic function and left ventricular filling pressures (31) (Fig. 27.4 and Table 27.3).

Right-Sided Doppler Flows. Diastolic function of the right heart can be evaluated by the interrogation of the tricuspid inflow, hepatic vein flow, and superior vena cava flow (73,74). The Doppler flow patterns in the hepatic veins and superior vena cava are somewhat similar to the pulmonary venous flow patterns (3,75). In addition to the S, D, and AR waves, a second reversed flow is often seen between the S and the D waves at the

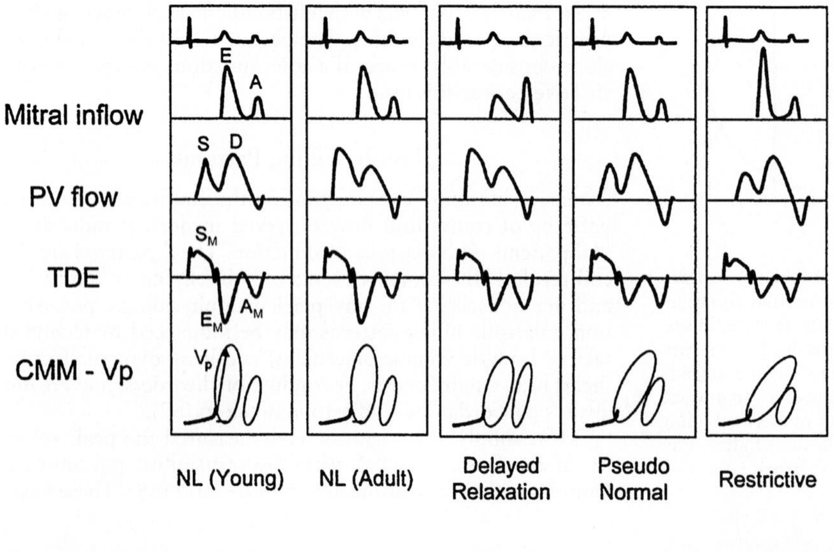

FIGURE 27.4. Stages of diastolic function. Schematic representation of the typical patterns seen with mitral inflow, pulmonary venous (PV) flow, tissue Doppler echocardiography (TDE), and color M-mode (CMM) propagation velocity (Vp) for normal (NL, young and adult), impaired relaxation, pseudonormal, and restrictive diastolic function. The stages of diastolic dysfunction can be determined using an integrated approach with these four different modalities for assessment of diastolic flow pattern: A, late mitral filling; A_M, diastolic filling during atrial contraction; D, diastolic filling; E, early mitral filling; E_M, early diastolic; S, systolic filling; S_M, systolic. (Adapted from Garcia MJ, Thomas JD, Klein AL. New Doppler echocardiographic applications for the study of diastolic function. *J Am Coll Cardiol* 1998;32:865–875.)

TABLE 27.3

DIASTOLIC FILLING VARIABLES

Left ventricular filling	Right ventricular filling
Left ventricular inflow	Right ventricular inflow
E-wave velocity (cm/s)	E-wave velocity (cm/s)
A-wave velocity (cm/s)	A-wave velocity (cm/s)
E/A ratio	E/A ratio
Deceleration time (ms)	Deceleration time (ms)
Isovolumic relaxation time (ms)	Superior vena cava and hepatic vein
Pulmonary vein flow	Forward flow
Forward flow	S-wave velocity (cm/s)
S-wave velocity (cm/s)	D-wave velocity (cm/s)
D-wave velocity (cm/s)	Reverse flow
Reverse flow	V-wave reversal (cm/s)
Atrial reversal wave velocity (cm/s)	Atrial reversal wave velocity (cm/s)
Atrial reversal wave duration (ms)	Tissue Doppler echocardiography (cm/s) of tricuspid annulus
Tissue Doppler echocardiography (cm/s) of mitral annulus	
Color M-mode flow propagation velocity (cm/s)	

end of ventricular contraction (VR) (74). Right-sided flow velocities normally increase during inspiration and decrease with the Valsalva maneuver (74,76).

As with the pulmonary venous flow, the S wave is related to right atrial (RA) relaxation and tricuspid annular descent and the D is related to early right ventricular (RV) filling velocity (E). The magnitudes of AR and VR vary according to RV stiffness, RA contractility, and central venous pressure (77). The effect of respiration of the right-sided flows is useful in differentiating constriction from restriction and estimating right-sided filling pressures (3,75).

Color M–Mode Doppler. A number of investigators have studied the use of the color Doppler M–mode (CMM) to characterize the spatiotemporal distribution of blood velocity throughout the ventricular inflow region in diastole (30,31,78–81).

A typical CMM echocardiogram has a temporal resolution of 5 msec, a spatial resolution of 300 μm, and a velocity resolution of approximately 4 cm/second. In normal sinus rhythm from the apical four-chamber view, the CMM demonstrates a characteristic pattern consisting of two filling waves propagating from the left atrium to the left ventricle, corresponding to the E and A waves. The velocities are highest above the mitral valve and lowest as they approach the apex, as shown by the change in color. The onset of flow occurs earlier at the mitral valve level than at the apex (31). The flow does not propagate instantaneously but rather propagates with a velocity (Vp) given by the slope of the leading edge of the blood wave.

Several qualitative and quantitative parameters have been proposed to characterize transmitral filling by the CMM echocardiogram. These studies have been used to characterize ventricular relaxation compared to cardiac catheterization (30,82). Brun et al. identified the leading edge of the E wave as representing the propagation velocity (30). This parameter is measured by identifying the boundary of the leading edge of color as it propagates into the ventricle, drawing a tangent to this line, and measuring its slope on the M-mode. A negative correlation was demonstrated between this propagation velocity and the time constant of relaxation τ in patients with coronary disease and cardiomyopathy. This propagation velocity parameter has been reported to be altered in conditions of delayed relaxation and ischemia, with a more rapid fall in ventricular pressure allowing a greater propagation of flow into the left ventricle (30,82). Another approach quantifying the propagation velocity (78) measured the delay required for the point of maximum velocity to traverse from the mitral valve to the apex.

In contrast to the standard mitral inflow velocities, the CMM propagation velocity has been determined to be relatively preload independent, as validated by hemodynamic measurements in humans and animals (80,83). When coupled with the ratio of the mitral inflow E wave to the CMM propagation velocity in intensive care unit patients, it provided a good estimate of pulmonary capillary wedge pressure (PCWP) (84). A study showed that an E/Vp ratio of 1.5 or greater was the best predictor of in-hospital clinical heart failure in patients with their first myocardial infarction (81). It appears that the propagation velocity may also be a discriminating feature between restrictive and constrictive diseases. Constrictive pericarditis is characterized by relatively normal early diastolic relaxation (and thus early diastolic filling) with an abrupt mid-diastolic cessation of inflow. Restrictive diseases have abnormal relaxation and impaired inflow from the opening of the mitral valve. These pathophysiologies seem to be reflected in the propagation velocity profile. Constrictive pericarditis is associated with extremely rapid flow propagation (a slope of $>$100 cm/sec), whereas restrictive cardiomyopathy shows markedly slowed propagation of the E wave (75,85).

Tissue Doppler imaging. Tissue Doppler imaging (TDI) quantifies the low velocity and high amplitude of tissue such as the ventricular myocardium or the motion of the mitral annulus (86–88). It provides a detailed spatial map of velocity in the myocardium, which can be further temporally enhanced with the CMM Doppler and pulsed-wave Doppler.

The TDI myocardial velocities are composed of several waves. After the electrocardiographic QRS, a short-amplitude multiphasic signal coincides with the closure of the mitral and tricuspid valve (89) and is caused by translational motion and geometric LV changes, assuming a more spherical shape during isovolumic contraction. After this signal, a larger, positive wave represents ventricular systole (S_M). A second, multiphasic signal during isovolumic relaxation coincides with aortic valve closing and tricuspid valve opening. In sinus rhythm, two waves corresponding to early filling (E_M) and atrial contraction (A_M) appear as a mirror image of the mitral inflow early (E) and atrial (A) filling velocities. In normal subjects, the peak of the E_M occurs earlier than the peak mitral inflow E wave (20 msec), suggesting that fast relaxation of the myocardium generates suction that pulls blood into the ventricle (E wave).

However, in patients with diastolic dysfunction, the mitral inflow E wave coincides with or precedes the E_M, suggesting more passive filling (31).

A major limitation of TDI is the effect of translation and rotation of the heart, in particular from the parasternal long-axis view. Thus, motion of the LV myocardium and annulus in the longitudinal plane can be measured from the apical four-chamber view. Because the apex is relatively fixed throughout the cardiac cycle and the axial plane of motion of the LV myocardium is parallel with the axis of the transducer, the velocities obtained from this acoustic window represent motion secondary to contraction and relaxation and do not require angle correction (31).

Color Doppler TDI provides a color map with high spatial resolution that is able to provide velocity data simultaneously from multiple segments of the myocardium. In contrast, pulsed-wave TDI is much simpler, providing high temporal and velocity resolution, with the data being stored using digital or video format. A limitation is that it measures only one point in time compared to the multiple information obtained from color Doppler TDI (90).

In normal individuals, the TDI velocities are mirror images of the mitral inflow velocities. With the aging process, there is an inverse effect on the E_M/A_M ratio similar to that reported for the mitral inflow (89). However, there are significant differences in patients with organic disease, distinct from transmitral flow velocities (91). In patients with impaired relaxation, the E_M velocity decreases when the E_M/A_M ratio is less than 1. In patients with advanced diastolic dysfunction (see later discussion) the E_M remains low even in the presence of elevated filling pressures (89).

Tissue Doppler E_M is less affected by preload than standard Doppler LV filling indices similar to CMM, and it has been shown to correlate with the time constant of relaxation in patients with normal or increased preload (92–94). In hemodynamic studies performed by Oki et al. the time constant of relaxation correlated well with E_M in all patients independent of filling pressures (83,92,93,95). In patients with various degrees of diastolic function, the tissue Doppler E_M was the best discriminator between normal individuals (16 cm/second) and patients with abnormal diastolic function (7.5 cm/second) compared to the standard mitral inflow or pulmonary vein flow (96). Other groups have confirmed that a TDI E_M of 8 cm/second is a useful cut-off between normal and abnormal filling pressures (97).

TDI myocardial velocities can be used to differentiate constrictive pericarditis from restriction. In patients with restriction, both relaxation and compliance is abnormal, whereas relaxation is normal in constriction. Patients with restriction have very slow early diastolic motion of the annulus, whereas patients with constriction have normal or very rapid early diastolic annular velocity (>8 cm/sec), suggesting preserved relaxation (85,86).

Strain imaging is another new modality that measures the deformation properties of a myocardial segment independent of translation or tethering. It is given by the equation $S = (L_0 - L_1)/L_0$, where L_0 is initial length and L_1 is compressed length (87,98). The strain rate measures the velocity in a certain direction over time dv/dx (sec^{-1}) of the longitudinal or circumferential fibers of the myocardium from parasternal or apical views. This technique has been used in patients with various diseases including hypertrophic cardiomyopathy (99) and patients with coronary artery disease (87,100,101,101a).

Interpretation of Diastolic Filling Patterns. Based on information from mitral inflow, pulmonary vein flow, CMM, and TDI, four patterns of diastolic function can be determined (Fig. 27.4). These patterns depend on age and hemodynamic conditions and represent stages of relaxation and compliance abnormalities and filling pressures. A recent classification proposed that diastolic dysfunction be graded in four stages that correlate with diastolic impairment and symptom class (102) (Fig. 27.5).

Normal. The normal filling pattern is seen in normal individuals with normal relaxation, compliance, and filling pressures. Normal individuals demonstrate a briskly accelerating E

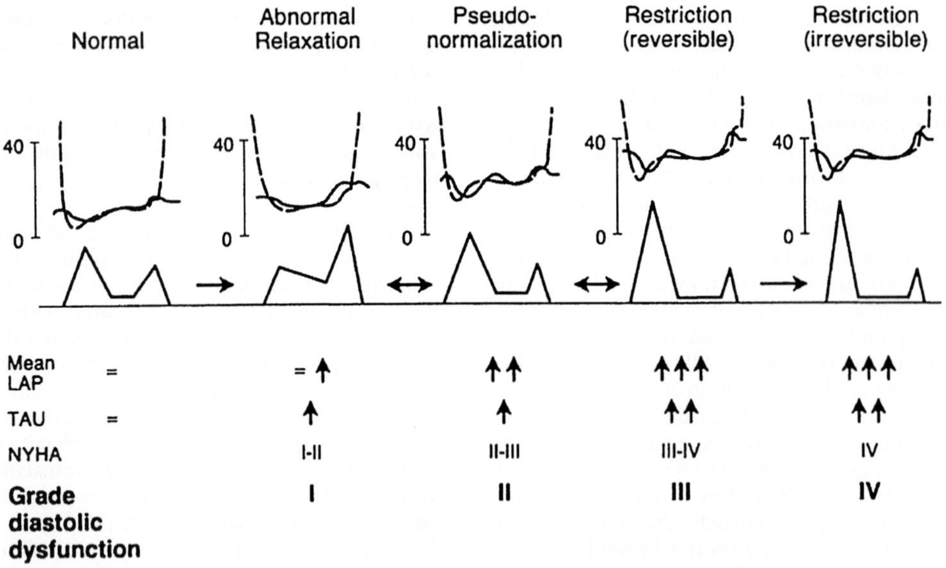

FIGURE 27.5. Proposed grading system for diastolic dysfunction based on progression of clinical disease patterns. Top row shows the high-fidelity left atrial and left ventricular pressure curves for the four grades of diastolic dysfunction, graded on a scale of I to IV, representing a progression from abnormal relaxation, to pseudonormalization, to restrictive (reversible), to restrictive (irreversible) disease. Below are the corresponding mitral flow velocity profiles; below these are the mean left atrial pressure (LAP), time constant of relaxation (TAU), and New York Heart Association (NYHA) class. Measurements are given in mm Hg. (From Nishimura RA, Tajik AJ. Evaluation of diastolic filling of the left ventricle in health and disease: Doppler echocardiography is the clinician's Rosetta Stone. *J Am Coll Cardiol* 1997;30:8–18).

wave, relatively rapid deceleration, and an A wave significantly smaller in magnitude than the E wave. The E/A ratio is greater than 1, the mitral deceleration time is typically between 150 and 220 msec, and the isovolumic relaxation time (IVRT) is greater than 100 msec. The S/D ratio is generally greater than 1, and the AR wave should be less than 35 cm/second. The CMM propagation is relatively fast (>45 cm/sec), and the tissue Doppler E_M is greater than 8 cm/sec, consistent with normal ventricular relaxation (31).

In young normal individuals, there is a greater predominance of early diastolic filling due to the rapid "suction" effect of the ventricle (more enhanced relaxation with Vp >55 cm/second and E_M >10 cm/second) and little additional filling during atrial contraction. This results in an even greater E/A ratio with further shortening of the deceleration time. Because atrial contribution is minimal, the mitral inflow A wave and pulmonary vein AR are very small. The S/D ratio may be less than 1, representing the large contribution of early filling.

Delayed relaxation pattern (stage I). This pattern is seen in patients with delayed LV relaxation but with relatively normal compliance and filling pressures. As a consequence of normal aging and various pathologic states with early stages of diastolic dysfunction, the time constant of relaxation is lengthened, and the E wave shows a slower acceleration, a lower peak velocity, and a prolonged deceleration time (>220 msec) and isovolumic relaxation time (>100 msec). To the extent that emptying may not be complete by the end of diastasis, an increased left atrial volume will be present at the time of atrial contraction, leading to a larger A wave, compensating in large part for the smaller E wave. Thus, the E/A ratio is less than 1, and concomitantly the S/D ratio is greater than 1 because if E is small, the corresponding D is small. Because relaxation is impaired, the color M-mode Vp is prolonged (<45 cm/second) and E_M is decreased (<8 cm/second).

Impaired relaxation may occur with normal or elevated filling pressures. If left ventricular end-diastolic pressure is normal, pulmonary vein AR is less than 35 cm/second, though if it is elevated, the AR is greater than 35 cm/second, or the duration of AR is greater than the duration of the mitral inflow A (103,104).

This pattern is seen in normal aging (3,59), ischemia (105), and hypertrophic cardiomyopathy (106,107) and secondary hypertrophy (108), and is usually seen in patients who typically have only mild symptoms or are asymptomatic (71). It can also be seen with hypovolemia due to a decreased left-atrial-to-left-ventricular pressure gradient with greater filling during atrial systole (75,109).

"Pseudonormal" pattern (stage II). This pattern is difficult to recognize because it is similar to the "normal" pattern. As left atrial pressure increases further to compensate for deteriorating diastolic function, the peak E-wave velocity increases. Therefore, abnormalities of relaxation and compliance and elevated filling pressures are present. This is associated with a normal appearance of the transmitral inflow with an E/A ratio between 1 and 2, a deceleration time between 150 and 220 msec, and an isovolumic relaxation time between 60 and 100 msec (69,71,75). One important feature to distinguish this pattern from the normal one is the pulmonary venous AR wave, which in pseudonormal filling displays a prolonged and increased AR of greater than 35 cm/second (59), whereas the pulmonary vein S/D ratio could be normal or less than 1. The AR wave prominence may not be present if atrial systolic failure occurs, although the duration of AR may still be greater than that of the mitral A wave. In addition, the Valsalva maneuver may be useful in differentiating normal from "pseudonormal" by reducing the preload, causing the normal-appearing E/A ratio to be less than 1, and thus exposing a delayed relaxation pattern (3,69,70,110). CMM propagation velocities and TDI are particularly helpful in detecting pseudonormal filling with a Vp of less than 45 cm/second and an E_M of less than 8 cm/second (96).

Usually in patients with pseudonormal patterns, the left atrial size is increased, the left ventricular function may be impaired or wall thickness increased, and the patient may have dyspnea (111). This pattern may represent an intermediate stage between impaired relaxation and restrictive filling as a result of disease progression, ischemia, or a change in loading conditions (71,75,112).

Restrictive filling pattern (stage III). This pattern is seen in the presence of severely reduced LV compliance and elevated filling pressures and ongoing delayed relaxation. It is characterized by a very elevated peak E-wave velocity with extremely rapid deceleration indicative of increased LV operating stiffness and diminutive (often absent) A wave. The E/A ratio is usually greater than 2 with a deceleration time of less than 150 msec and an isovolumic relaxation time of less than 60 msec (75). Pulmonary venous flow usually shows markedly blunted systolic flows with large and prolonged atrial reversals (except in conditions of atrial systolic failure) (3). A pulmonary venous systolic fraction that is 40% the sum of the systolic and diastolic fractions is consistent with significant elevation of PCWP (113). Similar to what is found in pseudonormal patterns, the CMM propagation velocity and E_M are reduced.

The restrictive filling pattern is equivalent to the "square root sign" or "dip-and-plateau" pattern seen in the ventricular pressure tracing at cardiac catheterization (69). The association between the restrictive filling pattern and the need for elevated filling pressures perhaps explains the poor prognosis connoted by the restrictive pattern (114). This pattern can be seen in patients with advanced stages of diastolic dysfunction due to restrictive, dilated, or ischemic cardiomyopathy, and usually the patients have dyspnea at rest and high New York Heart Association (NYHA) functional class (71). Severe enlargement and hypocontractility of the left atrium may be seen, and this pattern carries a poor prognosis in ischemic (115), dilated (116,117), and restrictive cardiomyopathies (114). In hypertrophic cardiomyopathy, there is a less clear prognostic potential of the filling patterns due to the complex interplay among systolic outflow tract obstruction, mitral regurgitation, and diastolic dysfunction (118).

Restrictive filling pattern (stage IV). As noted earlier, restrictive filling patterns are associated with a poor prognosis for patients with various types of cardiac disease. Additional prognostic information can be obtained in patients with restrictive filling patterns evaluated under different hemodynamic conditions. Failure to convert a restrictive mitral inflow filling pattern to a nonrestrictive pattern substantially increased the risk of death twofold in a study of patients with chronic heart failure (119,120).

Estimating Left Atrial and Left Ventricular Filling Pressures

Transmitral inflow and pulmonary venous flow by Doppler echocardiography has been used to noninvasively estimate left heart filling pressures, including mean pulmonary capillary wedge and left atrial pressure, and left ventricular end-diastolic pressure, primarily in patients with cardiac disease (104,111, 113,121–123). A notable exception is in patients with hypertrophic cardiomyopathy, where Doppler mitral flow patterns do not correlate well with left ventricular filling pressures due mainly to the exaggerated relaxation abnormalities and other variables affecting diastolic function in this disease (118).

An increased E/A ratio, a shortened deceleration and isovolumic relaxation time, a decreased atrial filling fraction, a decreased pulmonary venous systolic fraction, an elevated and prolonged atrial reversal flow velocity, and an increased left atrial volume may suggest an elevated mean left atrial pressure. Because these parameters are influenced by left atrial pressure and ventricular relaxation, these correlations work best for patients with abnormalities of left ventricular relaxation where left atrial pressure is the only variable. This includes mostly patients with structural heart disease. By combining the mitral E wave, a variable that correlates modestly with left atrial pressure, with one that is associated with ventricular relaxation (CMM propagation velocity or tissue Doppler echocardiography early-filling velocity), one can obtain closer approximations of left atrial pressure.

Using a regression equation, one can estimate PCWP from $PCWP = 5.27(E/Vp) + 4.6$, with $r = .80$, $p < .001$ (84). Similar studies have confirmed these findings and included patients with atrial fibrillation (124,125). In a study of 100 patients undergoing cardiac catheterization, ratios of E/E_M greater than 15 were associated with increased left ventricular filling pressure, whereas E/E_M less than 8 correlated with normal pressures. These associations were best for patients with left ventricular dysfunction (97). Algorithms for assessment of left atrial and left ventricular diastolic pressure have been proposed (Fig. 27.6).

Left ventricular filling pressures can be estimated even in patients with atrial fibrillation, with a correlation between PCWP and mitral deceleration time for patients with left ventricular dysfunction and atrial fibrillation (124). Even stronger correlations with the initial deceleration slope of the pulmonary venous diastolic wave have been reported (126).

End-diastolic left ventricular pressure has been estimated by echocardiography independent of left atrial pressure. Several studies have shown that the difference between the duration of the pulmonary venous atrial reversal and transmitral inflow A-wave duration can be used as an estimate of elevated left ventricular end-diastolic pressure (104,111,127). If the duration of the pulmonary venous reversal wave is prolonged with respect to that of the forward mitral A wave (>20 msec), left ventricular end-diastolic pressure is elevated (>15 mm Hg) (104). This variable has shown to be relatively age independent (128). Studies have demonstrated that a difference in duration of 30 msec or more between a pulmonary venous atrial reversal and the mitral inflow A wave is a predictor of severity of disease in cardiac amyloidosis (129) and cardiac mortality in patients with coronary artery disease (130).

Clinical Presentation and Significance

Patients with impaired diastolic function present with the typical syndromes of congestive heart failure including dependent edema, limited exercise tolerance, ascites and effusions,

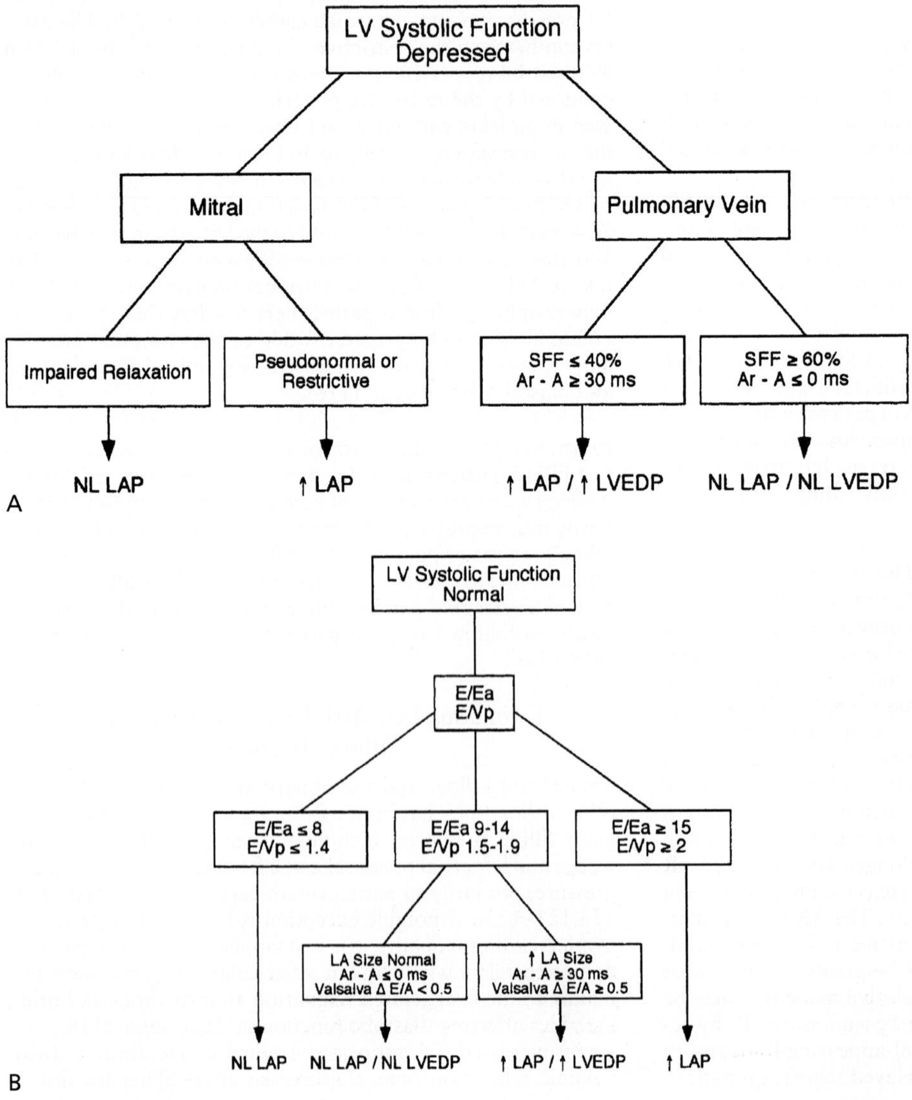

FIGURE 27.6. **A:** An algorithm for assessment of left atrial (LA) pressure and left ventricular (LV) end-diastolic pressure (LVEDP) in patients with depressed LV systolic function. Ar-A, difference in duration of the atrial reversal wave (pulmonary vein) and of the atrial wave of mitral inflow; NL LAP, normal left atrial pressure; SFF, systolic filling fraction; LAP, increased left atrial pressure. **B:** Algorithm for estimation of LAP and LVEDP in individuals with normal LV systolic function using the new indices of diastolic function, mitral inflow E velocity (E), pulmonary vein velocity, and left atrial size. Ea, early diastolic velocity at the mitral annulus; Vp, flow propagation velocity. (Adapted from Nagueh SF, Zoghbi WA. Clinical assessment of LV diastolic filling by Doppler echocardiography. *ACC Curr J Rev* 2001;10:45–49.)

orthopnea, and flash pulmonary edema. In general, the clinical exam is unreliable in differentiating systolic from diastolic dysfunction. The jugular veins will be distended, and dependent pitting edema may be very severe. Rales may be present on chest auscultation. Cardiac auscultation may demonstrate an S3 or S4 or a pericardial knock (8,75). Typical clinical patients with diastolic heart failure are the elderly, women, African Americans, and patients with hypertension, diabetes, and renal dysfunction (131). A study in Olmsted County, Minnesota, of patients with diastolic heart failure found that nearly 50% of patients were 80 years of age or older (132). The presentation of heart failure may be with flash pulmonary edema and hypertensive heart disease (133,134), advanced ischemic heart disease, or hypertensive hypertrophic cardiomyopathy (135). Patients who do not respond to treatment for heart failure include patients with diseases such as aortic stenosis or hypertrophic cardiomyopathy, infiltrative cardiomyopathy, and constrictive pericarditis (136). A recent study showed that older patients (≥45 years) may often have pre-clinical diastolic dysfunction as assessed by tissue Doppler imaging. They found that on average 28% of the patients had diastolic dysfunction with 20.7% having mild, 6.6% having moderate, and 0.7% having severe diastolic dysfunction with a normal ejection fraction. This was compared to 6% of patients with systolic dysfunction having had an EF of ≤0.50 and 2% of patients having had an EF of ≤0.40 (101a). More specific signs of individual disease states are discussed in subsequent sections.

Management of Diastolic Heart Failure

The general goal of treatment is twofold: to reduce the variables responsible for the underlying diastolic dysfunction and to reduce the clinical manifestations of the process. Treatment consists of reducing elevated filling pressures, maintaining atrial contraction, decreasing heart rate, preventing ischemia, improving relaxation, and causing the regression of ventricular hypertrophy (10,38,137,138). Therapy must be targeted to the specific pathologic process because some medications may be inappropriate for certain conditions. For instance, a β-blocker or calcium channel blocker would be preferable to an angiotensin-receptor blocker in patients with hypertrophic cardiomyopathy because the latter medication may contribute to left ventricular outflow obstruction (12,139,140).

Diuretics produce symptomatic relief but should be used judiciously because noncompliant ventricles, by definition, require higher pressures to achieve adequate filling. β-Blocking agents slow heart rate, decrease myocardial oxygen demand, control blood pressure, and produce regression of left ventricular hypertrophy. Calcium channel blockers have multiple benefits as negative chronotropic agents, controlling blood pressure, decreasing myocardial oxygen demand, dilating the coronary arteries, and leading to regression of hypertrophy (8). Angiotensin-converting-enzyme (ACE) inhibitors and angiotensin-receptor blockers have direct and indirect effects. These effects include blood pressure control and substantial ventricular mass regression. The degree of myocardial mass regression with these agents appears to be more significant than any other antihypertensive agent for similar blood pressure reduction (141). Improvement in diastolic function has been shown with both losartan and lisinopril by reduction in myocardial fibrosis (including decreased collagen volume) independent of left ventricular regression (142,143). Early data support further investigation of NO donors, which produce improved myocardial relaxation (138,144).

Doppler flow patterns may be useful in guiding therapy (75). Patients with abnormal relaxation with fusion of the E and A waves may need a calcium channel blocker or β-blocker to slow the heart rate, whereas patients with "pseudonormal" or restrictive filling may need diuretics or ACE inhibitors to lower the elevated filling pressures. If there is a prolonged PR interval in the setting of dilated cardiomyopathy, dual-chamber pacing may be beneficial (145). There may be some additional benefit in the use of Doppler flow patterns in the evaluation of biventricular pacing (146).

Prognosis

Patients with congestive heart failure secondary to diastolic dysfunction generally have a better prognosis than patients with systolic dysfunction (147); however, they may have recurrent congestive heart failure, hospitalizations, and recurrent chest pain despite coronary revascularization (5,134,148). The prognosis of diastolic heart failure varies depending on the population studied, with an annual mortality rate of approximately 10% per year, which is lower than the rate of 19% for patients with systolic dysfunction (149,150). The lower mortality for patients with diastolic function has been shown in a large number of population-based studies including the Veterans Administration Cooperative Study (V-HeFT) and the Coronary Artery Surgery Study (CASS) (149,151). The addition of coronary artery disease in patients with congestive heart failure adds considerable risk to diastolic dysfunction; however, it does not approach the risk of patients with low ejection fractions (147). A study by Senni et al. showed similar mortality in older patients with diastolic and systolic dysfunction (132). Left atrial volume indexed to body surface area has been shown to be a strong correlate of advanced diastolic impairment and a predictor of mortality (152). Other predictors of poor outcome determined from patients with preserved systolic function in the Digitalis Investigation Group Trial include impaired renal function, worse functional state, advanced age, and male gender (153).

Large prospective epidemiologic studies have provided significant insight into the clinical outcomes of patients with diastolic heart failure. A study group of 2,498 patients with functional class II to IV symptoms and left ventricular ejection fractions of greater than 40% was analyzed from the Duke [University] Databank for Cardiovascular Disease. A 5-year mortality rate of 28% was observed, with predictors of mortality in a multivariable model including advanced age, minority status, coronary artery disease, severe heart failure or lower ejection fraction, diabetes, and peripheral vascular disease (154).

The Candesartan in Heart Failure Assessment of Reduction in Mortality and Morbidity (CHARM)—Preserved Trial is the only prospective, randomized study of patients with heart failure class II to IV and preserved ejection fractions (>40%). In this study, 32 mg of candesartan, an angiotensin-receptor blocker, was compared versus placebo at a median follow-up of 36.6 months. Treatment with candesartan resulted in fewer hospital readmissions for congestive heart failure and a trend toward the reduction of the combined endpoint of cardiovascular death and readmissions for congestive heart failure (155) (Fig. 27.7).

RESTRICTIVE CARDIOMYOPATHY

Classification

Restrictive cardiomyopathy is defined as a disease of the myocardium that is characterized by "restrictive filling and reduced diastolic volume of either or both ventricles with normal or near-normal systolic function" (156). Systolic function may be normal in the early stage of disease, whereas wall thickness

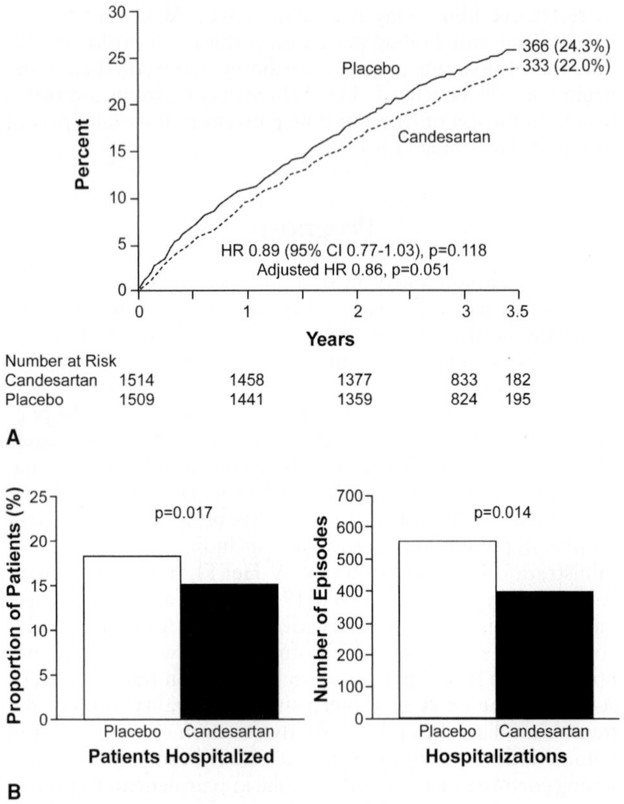

FIGURE 27.7. A. Time to cardiovascular (CV) death or hospital admission for congestive heart failure (CHF) according to the Candesartan in Heart Failure: Assessment of Reduction in Mortality and Morbidity (CHARM)-Preserved Trial. There was a trend toward a reduction of the primary outcome of CV death and CHF hospitalizations. B. There was a statistically significant reduction in the secondary endpoint of CHF hospitalizations. CI, confidence interval; HR, hazard rain.

may be normal or increased depending on the etiology of the disease (156–158). The disease may be idiopathic or associated with other diseases such as amyloidosis (156,157).

Restrictive cardiomyopathies are recognized as primary and secondary, with the secondary forms including the specific heart muscle diseases in which the heart is affected as part of a multisystem disorder, for example, infiltrative, storage, and noninfiltrative diseases (159). A working classification of restrictive cardiomyopathy is shown in (Fig. 27.8) (157,159). Restrictive cardiomyopathies can be further characterized into *interstitial* and *storage* disorders. In interstitial diseases, the infiltrates localize to the interstitium (between myocardial cells) as with cardiac amyloidosis and sarcoidosis, whereas in storage disorders, the deposits are within cells as with hemochromatosis and glycogen storage diseases (29). Secondary forms of restrictive cardiomyopathies are more common than the primary form (160) and display the classic restrictive hemodynamics only in their advanced form. The prototypical secondary restrictive cardiomyopathy is cardiac amyloidosis (29).

Anatomic Considerations

In idiopathic restrictive cardiomyopathy, pathologic studies have shown mild to moderate degrees of hypertrophy and fibrosis (161), with the hemodynamic findings unrelated to the histopathologic abnormalities detected (161). In cardiac amyloidosis (see later discussion), there is interstitial infiltration of amyloid fibrils in the ventricles and atria causing a firm, rubbery consistency of the heart (162,163), whereas in endomyocardial diseases, there is an endocardial fibrotic shell with extension into the myocardium (164).

Pathophysiology

The characteristic feature of restrictive cardiomyopathy is a marked increased stiffness of the myocardium or endocardium, which causes the ventricular pressure to rise dramatically with only small changes in volume, causing an upward shift of the left ventricular pressure–volume relationship and a dip-and-plateau or square root hemodynamic pattern (165,166). As mentioned, there is a controversy on whether this restrictive hemodynamic pattern is necessary (167,168) for this to be included as a restrictive cardiomyopathy; however, the 1995 World Health Organization/International Society and Federation of Cardiology (WHO/ISFC) classification does include restrictive hemodynamics as an absolute criterion for the diagnosis. Both ventricles are affected with the restrictive process, but usually the pressures are higher on the left than the right (169), which may reflect the relatively decreased compliance of the left ventricle compared to the right ventricle. An exception may be tropical endomyocardial fibrosis, in which the right ventricle may be predominantly involved (170).

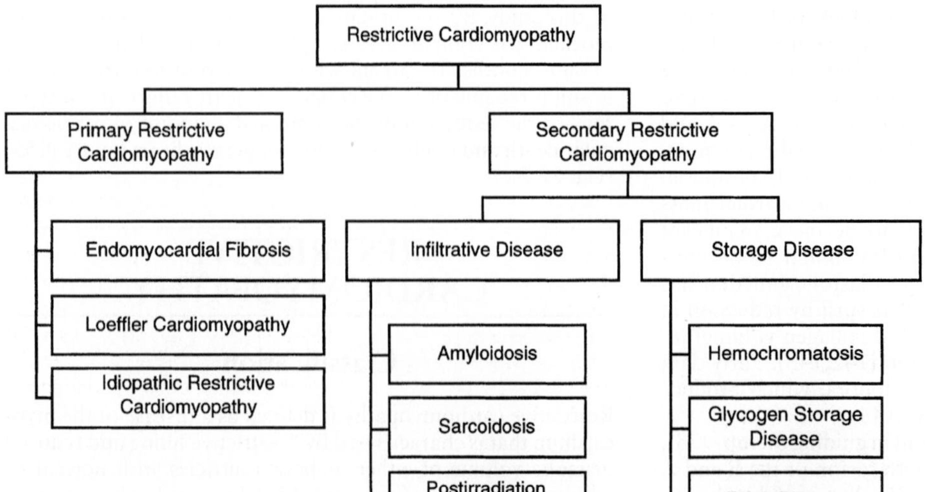

FIGURE 27.8. Working classification of restrictive cardiomyopathy. (From Leung DY, Klein AL. Restrictive cardiomyopathy; diagnosis and prognostic implications. In: Otto CM. *Practice of clinical echocardiography.* Philadelphia: WB Saunders 1997: 474.)

Clinical Profile

The clinical signs and symptoms of restrictive cardiac diseases relate closely to the degree of left atrial hypertension required to compensate for poor ventricular filling (171). This gives rise to the typical clinical features of exercise intolerance in early cases and dyspnea at rest and symptoms of low cardiac output, such as fatigue, in advanced cases (159). Left atrial dilation, pulmonary congestion, distention of central veins, hepatic distention, ascites, peripheral edema, and anasarca are seen in advanced cases. Exertional chest pain is usually absent. Atrial fibrillation is common due to the atrial enlargement. Ventricular arrhythmias or heart block are not uncommonly present in advanced cases and are often the cause of death in these patients. Symptoms of the underlying multisystem disorder, if present, may also be evident (159). Examination may reveal jugular venous distention, S4, or S3, depending on the filling characteristics (172). Kussmaul's sign (169) can be detected, whereas apical retraction (as in constrictive pericarditis) is not seen (173).

In our experience, the main laboratory test for diagnosing restrictive cardiomyopathy is echocardiography (3). Transthoracic or transesophageal echocardiography with respirometry has been used successfully to differentiate restriction from constriction (174,175). There will not be significant respiratory variation in patients with restriction as in those who have constriction (66,174). TDI and CMM Doppler (31,75,85,86) aid to further distinguish these disorders. Magnetic resonance imaging (MRI) and computed tomography (CT) scanning may also be useful for excluding increased pericardial thickness (176–179). Cine MRI may show an abnormal filling pattern in early and advanced stages of restrictive cardiomyopathy similar to echocardiography (180). MRI may also be capable of distinguishing tissue characteristics of infiltrative processes such as amyloid, differentiating it from other forms of cardiomyopathy (181).

Management

The prognosis of restrictive cardiomyopathy depends on whether there is evidence of an early or advanced stage of the disease as shown with cardiac amyloidosis (114). The prognosis is variable but usually progressive (182). Diuresis may help with symptomatic relief, whereas ACE inhibitors may be of benefit with LV dysfunction. Vasodilators should be used cautiously because they may cause hypotension. Reversible underlying conditions, such as hemochromatosis, should be addressed. Transplantation can be considered; however, often the restrictive cardiomyopathy is part of a systemic illness including skeletal myopathy (183). Signs or symptoms of ischemia in children with restrictive cardiomyopathy predict sudden death and should be managed aggressively with β-blockers, an implantable defibrillator, or consideration for transplantation (184).

PRIMARY RESTRICTIVE CARDIOMYOPATHY

Idiopathic Restrictive Cardiomyopathy

Idiopathic restrictive cardiomyopathy is a disease in patients with diastolic heart failure that is often characterized by familial transmission and the association with skeletal myopathies (161,185,186). It was first described by Benotti et al. (187), who described nine patients with heart failure, elevated right and left ventricular filling pressures, normal systolic function, and dip-and-plateau hemodynamic tracing.

Other investigators described similar findings using strict hemodynamic criteria (188–190). Some series excluded patients with hypertrophy and others did not show the dip-and-plateau pattern in all patients (168,186). Thus, there is a lack of consensus on the type of diastolic filling pattern and the degree of left ventricular hypertrophy in this disease (161).

Pathophysiology

The classic hemodynamic filling pattern is the dip-and-plateau pattern (187). The pathogenesis of the stiff ventricle may be secondary to myocyte abnormalities including abnormal calcium handling, accumulation of desmin, which is a cytoskeletal component, and myofiber disarray, as well as abnormalities of the extracellular matrix including proliferation of collagen fibers and elastic elements (170). As mentioned, it is believed that a restrictive filling pattern should not be an absolute requirement for the diagnosis. However, there must be abnormalities of diastolic filling, whether restrictive or abnormal relaxation, on Doppler echocardiography or abnormal filling pressures on cardiac catheterization (161,191).

Clinical Presentation

Idiopathic restrictive cardiomyopathy is usually a sporadic disease, but it can occur in families, with autosomal dominant transmission. The presence of a distal skeletal myopathy and heart block in this condition has been reported in five generations of an Italian family (157,185,186). Another restrictive cardiomyopathy with autosomal dominance with variable penetrance is associated with Noonan syndrome (192).

There may be differences in idiopathic restrictive cardiomyopathy in children compared to adults. In children, the disease may be more common in girls (193,194), and children may have a worse prognosis with the disease than adults (193,194).

Diagnosis

Cardiac catheterization and/or echocardiography and endomyocardial biopsy should be done to make the diagnosis. Atrial enlargement with nondilated ventricles with near-normal systolic function is uniformly present on echocardiography. In one series, the ejection fraction ranged from 40% to 55% in patients with advanced disease needing heart transplantation (195). Variable degrees of hypertrophy may be present (161,188,189,196). Cardiac catheterization and Doppler echocardiography may show restrictive hemodynamics; however, other patterns may be present as well (161). Biopsy is important in order to exclude other diseases and to assess myocyte hypertrophy and interstitial fibrosis (161,197).

Management

Most small series show a protracted clinical course in adults with a mean survival of 4 to 14 years (mean 9 years) (187,196). Patients have symptoms of congestive heart failure, elevated jugular veins, and mitral and tricuspid regurgitation (196). Progressive heart failure that responds poorly to medical management and complete heart block requiring a pacemaker may occur (185,196). In one series, the mean follow-up time to transplantation or death was 117 months compared to 44 months for cardiac amyloidosis (186). In a large series of 94 patients with echocardiographically defined idiopathic restrictive cardiomyopathy, predictors of poor prognosis included advanced age, male gender, left atrial enlargement, and advanced functional class (197). The 5-year survival rate for this group was 64%. Heart transplantation can be considered in patients with idiopathic restrictive cardiomyopathy; however, an associated skeletal myopathy may affect prognosis (186).

Endomyocardial Disease

There are two forms of the hypereosinophilic syndrome: endomyocardial fibrosis and Loffler endocarditis (198). Endomyocardial fibrosis (Davies disease) is a disease endemic to equatorial countries (e.g., Uganda, Nigeria, and Brazil) with rare appearance in nontropical countries (171,199). In contrast, Loffler endocarditis is a disease of temperate countries but occurs sporadically across the world (200). The common theme to these diseases is an abnormal eosinophilia in the blood and the endocardium causing a restrictive cardiomyopathy with endocardial fibrotic thickening at the apex and subvalvular regions causing impairment of ventricular inflow (198,201).

It has generally been thought that the two conditions are different forms of the same disease that result from tissue damage from the toxic effect of eosinophils and result in identical pathologic findings in advanced disease (198,202). However, despite the similarities of the two conditions, there are important differences. Loffler endocarditis is associated with cyanosis, advanced congestive heart failure, thromboembolic disease, and elevated right atrial pressures. Eosinophilia is present in this disease (203). In contrast, endomyocardial fibrosis affects younger patients without regard for gender and has no significant eosinophilia (198,203).

Loffler Endocarditis

This disease is considered to be part of the idiopathic hypereosinophilic syndrome, which is characterized by persistently elevated blood eosinophil counts without recognizable cause (171,204,205). Cardiac involvement occurs in more than 75% of the cases of the syndrome (198).

The etiology of the eosinophilia is unknown, but it may be related to parasitic and protozoal infections, malignancy (leukemia), or allergic or autoimmune reactions (206,207). For example, the eosinophilia-myalgia syndrome is associated with eosinophilia and restrictive cardiomyopathy, supporting the role of the eosinophil in the pathogenesis of this disorder (208).

Clinical Manifestation. The typical presenting patient is a male patient younger than 50 years of age who lives in a temperate climate and has the hypereosinophilic syndrome (171,200). Right- and left-sided congestive heart failure, mitral regurgitation, systemic embolism, cardiac enlargement on chest x-ray, and T-wave inversions on electrocardiogram are the main clinical manifestations of this disorder depending on the stage of the disease (160,209).

Echocardiography commonly demonstrates mural thrombosis. There may be obliteration of the apex and immobility of the posterior leaflet of the mitral valve with entrapment against the thickened posterobasal endocardium, resulting in mitral regurgitation (160,210). These findings were recently described in a review of 29 patients with classic echocardiographic features of the hypereosinophilic syndrome (211). Left ventricular systolic function is often preserved, and restrictive physiology may be demonstrated by Doppler echocardiography, usually in the fibrotic phase (212). Transesophageal echocardiography may be useful for assessing the diastolic dysfunction (213).

Cardiac catheterization typically shows the dip-and-plateau physiology with reduced left ventricular compliance due to the dense scarring of the ventricle. Mitral and tricuspid regurgitation may be present as well (198,205). Endomyocardial biopsy may be necessary to confirm the diagnosis; however, it may be difficult to obtain an adequate tissue sample (205).

Management. The treatment options depend on the stage of the disease. Early Loffler disease is treated medically with steroids, whereas surgery is reserved for the fibrotic stages. Corticosteroids and hydroxyurea may be used to treat the myocarditis when it is associated with the hypereosinophilia (206,214). Interferon has been used in a limited number of patients with promising results (207,215). Standard supportive medical therapy should include digoxin, diuretics, afterload reducers, and anticoagulants (198,205). Surgical treatment involves debriding the fibrous plaque from the endocardial surface, replacing the valves, and inserting a pacemaker (200,205, 206).

Endomyocardial Fibrosis

Endomyocardial fibrosis is endemic to tropical and subtropical Africa and occurs less frequently in South America and Asia (216–218). It is a common cause of congestive heart failure and death in equatorial Africa, accounting for 15% to 25% of the deaths secondary to heart disease (171,200). Endomyocardial fibrosis involves both ventricles in 50% of the cases, followed by involvement of the left ventricle in 40% and of the right ventricle in 10% of the cases (171,202).

Endomyocardial fibrosis occurs in three distinct areas: the left ventricular apex, the subvalvular apparatus, and the right ventricular apex (171,219). The fibrosis at the ventricular apex extends to the lower ventricular septum and to the posteromedial papillary muscle. The fibrosis also extends in the area behind the posterior mitral valve, causing tethering of the chordae tendinae and resulting in mitral regurgitation. The anterior leaflet of the mitral valve and the outflow tract is often spared. It also may involve the right ventricular apex, causing impairment of filling of the tricuspid inflow, and encasement of the papillary muscles of the tricuspid valve, resulting in tricuspid regurgitation (202,211).

A classification scheme according to the location of fibrosis was proposed by Shaper et al. (220). Usually, the right ventricle becomes more obliterated than the left ventricle (202). Microscopically, there is a thick layer of collagen tissue over a layer of connective tissue in the endocardium, with granulation tissue extending into the myocardium (221).

Clinical Profile. The clinical presentation in the endomyocardial fibrosis depends on whether the left, right, or both ventricles are involved. The disease affects both male and female individuals, usually children and young adults (203). Left-sided disease results in pulmonary congestion, whereas right-sided disease results in right heart failure simulating constrictive pericarditis. Often mitral and tricuspid regurgitation is present due to the involvement of the valves. Atrial fibrillation is not uncommon, occurring in one fourth of patients with endomyocardial fibrosis, especially when there is right ventricular involvement. Embolism is a frequent finding with endomyocardial fibrosis. A pericardial and pleural effusion may also be present (171,200,218).

Echocardiography shows the obliteration of the apices of the ventricles and dilated atria, and Doppler echocardiography shows evidence of mitral and tricuspid regurgitation. The posterior leaflet has decreased mobility in left-sided disease (171,200). The basal ventricle may be hypercontractile due to the obliterated apex "merlon sign" (222). Cardiac catheterization and Doppler echocardiography may show the restrictive hemodynamics of the disease.

Management. In endomyocardial fibrosis, the prognosis is poor, with progressive disease and death due to heart failure, or sudden death (171,200,220). The 2-year mortality is between 35% and 50% in patients with advanced disease (203,223). Surgery may improve symptoms in the fibrotic stage with excision of the fibrous endocardium and repair or replacement of the mitral and tricuspid valves (207,224,225), although operative mortality has been reported in the range of 15% to 25% (226,227). However, a study of 11 patients undergoing surgery with endocardial resection and valve replacement reported a 10-year survival of near 70% (228).

SECONDARY RESTRICTIVE MYOCARDIAL DISEASES

Infiltrative Conditions

Interstitial

Cardiac Amyloidosis

Cardiac amyloidosis is the prototype of restrictive myocardial diseases and the one most frequently encountered in clinical practice (29,229,230). There are several types of cardiac amyloidosis, each with its own clinical presentations and treatment strategies (231).

Etiology and Classification of Amyloidosis. Amyloidosis is a multisystem disease in which linear, nonbranching, aggregated fibrils with a cross-β pleated configuration are deposited in various organs of the body, including the heart (231,232). The fibrils deposit between cells (interstitial) with a replacement of the normal tissue structures. When stained with Congo red, this material shows apple-green birefringence when viewed under a polarizing microscope. Alcian blue can also be used to diagnose amyloid. Amyloidosis can be classified by the type of protein deposited (231) (Table 27.4). The primary type is the most common form, occurring in 85% of patients, with fibrils composed of κ or λ immunoglobulin light chains (AL type), often associated with multiple myeloma. There may be extracellular deposition of amyloid protein in the kidney, heart, liver, nerve, skin, and tongue resulting in tissue damage and organ malfunction (233). The most common manifestations include nephrotic syndrome or renal failure, congestive heart failure, sensorimotor peripheral neuropathy, and orthostatic hypotension. Most of the following discussion will focus on cardiac amyloidosis (AL type).

Familial amyloidosis results from the production of a mutant prealbumin protein (transthyretin [TTR]) (234), and there are different types that present with a cardiomyopathy, neuropathy, or nephropathy. TTR is made up of 125 pairs of amino acids, and more than 70 mutations have been recognized (231). This type of amyloid is important to recognize because liver transplantation may be lifesaving (231). Senile systemic amyloidosis occurs in elderly men from the production of a wild-type TTR and has been associated with congestive heart failure without noncardiac involvement (231). Secondary amyloidosis (AA type) is rare, with the fibrils consisting of protein A, a non-immunoglobulin (235,236). Isolated atrial amyloidosis is often found limited to the atria at autopsy in the elderly and derives from atrial natriuretic peptide (231). It is more common in female patients and seems to be associated with the presence of atrial fibrillation (237).

TABLE 27.4

SUMMARY OF THE MAIN FORM OF AMYLOIDOSIS THAT AFFECT THE HEART

Nomenclature	Precursor of amyloid fibril	Organ Involvement	Treatment	Comment
AL	Immunoglobulin light chain	Heart Kidney Liver Peripheral/Autonomic Nerves Soft Tissue Gastrointestinal System	Chemotherapy	Plasma cell dyscrasia related to (but usually not associated with) multiple myeloma Heart disease occurs in 1/3 to 1/2 of AL patients; heart failure tends to progress rapidly and has a very poor prognosis
ATTR (familial)	Mutant transthyretin	Peripheral/Autonomic Nerves Heart	Liver transplantation ? New pharmacological strategies to stabilize the TTR	Autosomal dominant; amyloid derived from a mixture of mutant and wild-type TTR; if present before, cardiac amyloid may progress despite liver transplantation
AapoA1	Mutant apolipoprotein	Kidney Heart	? Liver transplantation	Kidney disease is the commonest presentation; heart involvement is rare
Senile systemic amyloid	Wild-type transthyretin	Heart	Supportive ? New pharmacological strategies to stabilize the TTR	Almost exclusively found in elderly men; slowly progressive symptoms
AA	Serum amyloid A	Kidney Heart (rarely)	Treat underlying inflammatory process	Heart disease rare and, if present, rarely clinically significant
AANP	Atrial natriuretic peptide	Localized to the atrium	None required	Very common; may increase risk of atrial fibrillation and/or be deposited in greater amounts in the fibrillating atrium

AL, amyloid produced from clonal light chains; TTR, transthyretin; ATTR, amyloid produced from a mutant transthyretin; AapoA1, amyloid produced from mutant apolipoprotein; AA, amyloid produced from serum amyloid A protein; AANP, amyloid produced from atrial natriuretic peptide. Falk RH. Diagnosis and Management of the Cardiac Amyloidoses. *Circulation* 2005;112:2047–2060.

The heart is commonly involved in primary amyloidosis (AL type) and is associated with a plasma cell dyscrasia with the production of clonal light chains (231,232). Nearly half of patients have cardiac involvement including congestive heart failure; however, the heart is involved in almost all patients by pathologic examination (238). Death from cardiac involvement secondary to congestive heart failure or arrhythmia occurs in greater than 50% of patients with systemic amyloidosis (232). In familial amyloidosis, cardiac involvement occurs in 28% of patients at the time of diagnosis; however, it usually presents late in the course of the disease (234). Peripheral neuropathy and renal failure are the usual presenting features; however cardiac features may predominate (239). The disease was reported more than 30 years ago in a Danish family (240) but has also been described in a family from Appalachia (241) and in an Italian family (239). Cardiac failure or cardiac arrhythmia is responsible for the deaths in greater than 50% of patients (234). Familial amyloidosis has been reported in elderly blacks in the United States as a cause of heart failure secondary to a mutation in transthyretin isoleucine-122 (242,243).

Senile cardiac amyloidosis may involve extensive deposits in the heart producing congestive heart failure or may have minor deposits in the atria with no symptoms (232). It is important to differentiate senile cardiac amyloidosis from nonsecretory immunoglobulin-derived amyloidosis (AL type) and familial amyloidosis due to different treatment regimens (232,244). Cardiac involvement is unusual in secondary amyloidosis, with the renal manifestations being more predominant (235).

Clinical Presentation. Cardiac amyloidosis usually presents in men older than 30 years of age (236,238) and occurs in older patients in the familial form (234). Patients with cardiac amyloidosis present with diastolic heart failure and the "stiff heart syndrome" resulting from amyloid infiltration. Patients may present with various degrees of progressive biventricular heart failure depending on the stage of the disease as shown by two-dimensional and Doppler echocardiography (172). In early cardiac amyloidosis, patients may be asymptomatic, whereas patients with advanced disease have the typical evidence of restrictive cardiomyopathy with severe right heart failure, ascites, and peripheral edema (200). During cardiac catheterization, a square root sign will be present, and restrictive hemodynamics by Doppler echocardiography is detected only in the advanced stages of the disease (172). In addition, there may be an intermediate stage in which patients have more symptoms as left atrial pressure increases. Individual patients may actually evolve through the different stages of involvement (112). Often, it may be difficult to differentiate advanced cardiac amyloidosis from constrictive pericarditis (86,174). As the disease progresses, there will be both systolic and diastolic heart failure (245). Chest pain resembling angina pectoris may also be present despite normal epicardial coronary arteries during cardiac catheterization (246), or there may be partial obliteration of the distal coronary arteries by amyloid infiltration (163,239,247). Involvement of the intramyocardial vessels may be another explanation for this presentation (219,248). In 10% to 15% of cases, orthostatic hypotension is detected in patients with cardiac amyloidosis. This is secondary to amyloid infiltration of the autonomic nervous system, with symptoms of syncope, diarrhea, lack of sweating, and impotence (233). Kidney, adrenal, and cardiac involvement with amyloid deposition may aggravate the postural hypotension. Macroglossia, periorbital edema, peripheral neuropathy, and carpal tunnel syndrome are other characteristic findings (231,249). Refractory supraventricular and ventricular arrhythmias or conduction defects may be another mode of presentation (250). Sudden death secondary to arrhythmias may also be the cause of death, especially in familial amyloidosis (234).

Physical examination may reveal an S4 (early disease) or S3 (advanced disease) on auscultation depending on the stage of the illness (172). Mitral and tricuspid valvular regurgitation may also be present (29). There will be evidence of biventricular heart failure with often predominant right heart failure (200), with an elevated jugular venous pulse with a prominent y descent, hepatomegaly, ascites, and peripheral edema especially in the advanced disease. The blood pressure may be decreased, especially in patients with a history of hypertension (231). The cardiac silhouette on chest x-ray is usually enlarged in patients with advanced disease with evidence of pulmonary congestion (251). The electrocardiogram typically is of low voltage and shows a pseudoinfarction pattern with Q waves simulating a myocardial infarction in the precordial leads (219,252,253). Arrhythmias, especially atrial fibrillation, are common (30% of patients), and a sick-sinus syndrome may be present (219).

Atrioventricular conduction defects may be present especially in familial amyloidosis associated with polyneuropathy (234). Ventricular arrhythmias consisting of ventricular tachycardia may be present in advanced disease and may be a forewarner of death (239).

Investigations

Echocardiography. Use of two-dimensional and Doppler echocardiography is the procedure of choice in the noninvasive diagnosis, serial follow-up, and prognosis of patients with cardiac amyloidosis (29,73,112,114,172,245,254). Cardiac amyloidosis gives a distinctive appearance on two-dimensional echocardiography and is associated with abnormal left and right ventricular diastolic function. The classic presentation is the finding of a normal or small left ventricular cavity size with markedly thickened myocardium associated with a highly abnormal texture, which is often described as "granular sparkling" in appearance (29) (Fig. 27.9).

The sparkling granular appearance is thought to be due to the acoustic mismatch between the highly reflective amyloid deposits in the endocardium, myocardium, and pericardium and the normal tissue (255). Moreover, autopsy and clinical biopsy series have demonstrated the presence of amyloid fibrils in the myocardium at the site of the granular sparkling echoes. Ultrasonic tissue characterization has been used to identify patients with cardiac amyloidosis (256).

Global left ventricular systolic function is usually preserved in early disease, whereas systolic function is usually impaired in advanced disease. The interatrial septum and valve leaflets are also thickened. Both atria are enlarged, and small to moderate pericardial effusions are usually present (245,254).

Patients with cardiac amyloidosis have a low ratio of electrocardiographic voltage to left ventricular wall thickness that is thought to be specific to cardiac amyloidosis and suggested to be predictive of clinical symptoms and prognosis (257–259). However, the usefulness of this ratio is limited by the presence of other coexisting diseases that may result in decreased electrocardiographic voltage.

Left Ventricular Diastolic Dysfunction. Cardiac amyloidosis has traditionally been considered to be associated with a restrictive pattern of ventricular filling (260). However, a spectrum of left ventricular filling abnormalities using pulsed-wave Doppler echocardiography is detected in patients with cardiac amyloidosis (29,172,260). In a study of 53 patients with the classic echocardiographic features of cardiac amyloidosis (172), patients with advanced disease demonstrated a mean left ventricular wall thickness of greater than 15 mm and a "restrictive" physiology pattern of left ventricular filling. Furthermore, in serial studies of individual patients, those patients with the "impaired relaxation" pattern gradually evolved into a "restrictive" pattern through a "pseudonormal" or intermediate

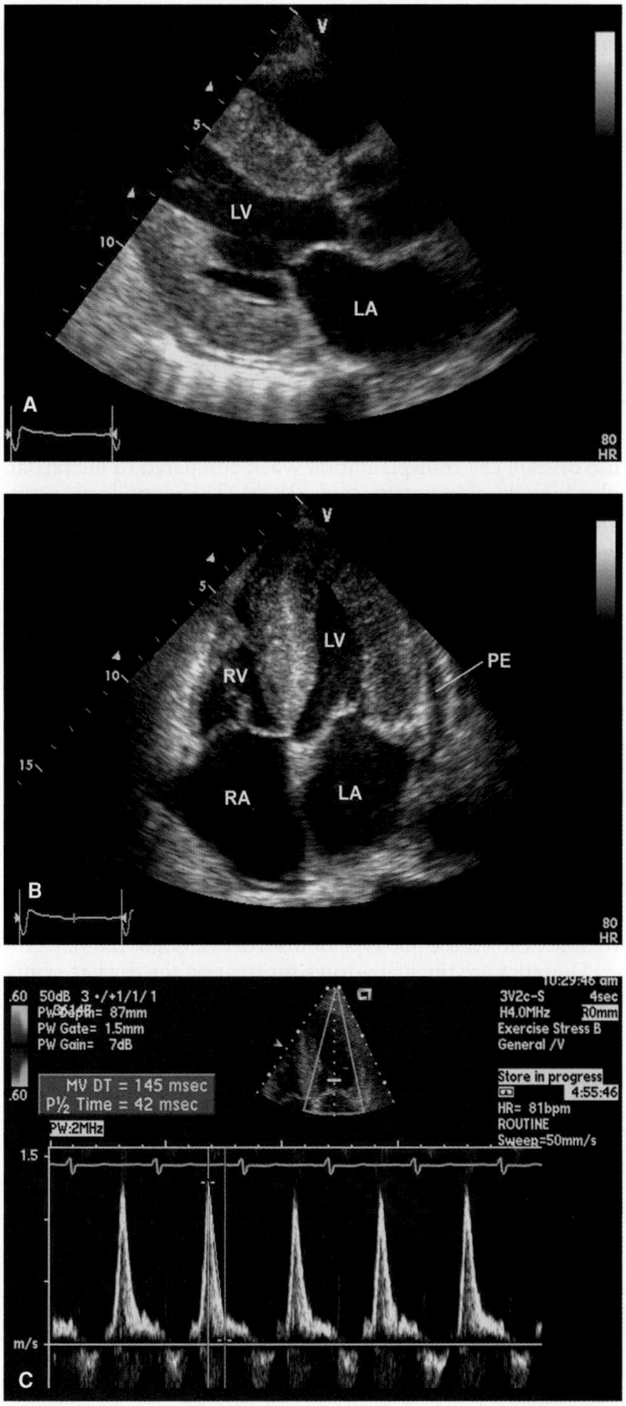

FIGURE 27.9. Parasternal long (A) and apical four-chamber (B) and mitral inflow (C) in advanced cardiac amyloidosis. Note that the left ventricular size is normal with markedly thickened ventricular walls and has its characteristic granular sparkling appearance. DT, deceleration time; LA, left atrium; LV, left ventricle; PE, pericardial effusion; PL EFF, pleural effusion; pm, papillary muscle; RA, right atrium; RV, right ventricle.

phase with the progression of the disease (112). The mechanism for this serial change in left ventricular filling pattern is thought to be due to the gradual decrease in the compliance of the left ventricle with progressive deposition of amyloid fibrils in the myocardium leading to subsequent loss of myocardial cells from pressure necrosis (261). When the duration of the pulmonary venous atrial reversal wave is longer than the mitral A-wave duration, filling pressures are elevated and the disease is advanced with restrictive physiology (129).

Patients with cardiac amyloidosis also have been shown to have abnormalities of right ventricular diastolic function (73). The right ventricular filling pattern is often similar to that of the left ventricle or may be less advanced. In early cases, that is, patients with right ventricular free wall thickness of less than 7 mm, there is abnormal relaxation. In advanced cases, when the right ventricular wall is 7 mm or greater in thickness, restrictive physiology is present. The systolic forward flows by Doppler echocardiography in the superior vena cava and hepatic vein also decreased and the diastolic flow increased compatible with restrictive physiology (73).

Newer diagnostic tools, including TDI and strain and strain rate imaging, have been used to characterize the longitudinal contraction in patients with cardiac amyloidosis before the onset of congestive symptoms with preserved left ventricular function. These tools showed that there was early impairment of longitudinal contraction before impairment in ejection fraction in these patients (262,263).

Prognostic Stratification. It has been suggested that the mean left ventricular wall thickness is a useful variable in assessing the degree of cardiac involvement and prognosis (264). In a study of 132 patients with biopsy-proven amyloidosis, patients with a mean wall thickness of 15 mm had a median survival of 0.4 years compared to a median survival of 2.4 years for those with a mean wall thickness of 12 mm. Doppler echocardiography has also been shown to be useful in prognostic stratification of patients with cardiac amyloidosis (114). Patients with a deceleration time of the mitral early-filling wave at baseline study of 150 msec or less had a significantly reduced survival compared to those whose deceleration time was greater than 150 msec (1-year probability of survival 49% vs. 92%; $p < .001$) (Fig. 27.10). Bivariate analysis showed that the combination of shortened deceleration time of 150 msec or less and an increased mitral E/A ratio was a stronger predictor of cardiac death than two-dimensional variables of mean left ventricular wall thickness and fractional shortening.

A new Doppler index (TEI index) combining systolic and diastolic performance has been determined to have significant

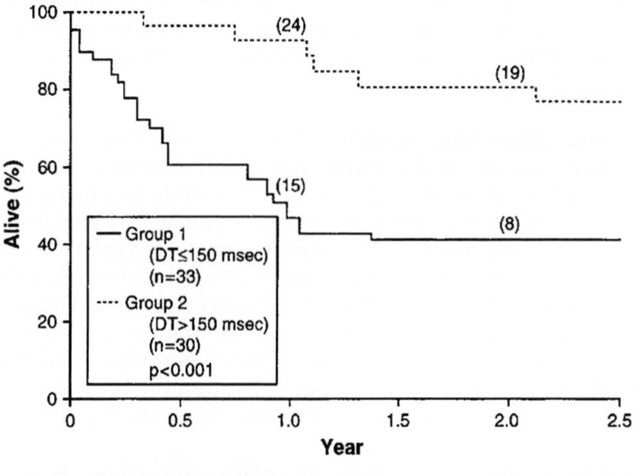

FIGURE 27.10. Survival in 63 patients with cardiac amyloidosis subdivided on the basis of the deceleration time (DT) of 150 msec. Patients with a shortened deceleration time of less than 150 msec (*bold line*) had a significantly reduced survival compared with patients with a deceleration time of greater than 150 msec. (From Klein AL, Hatle LK, Taliercio CP, et al. Prognostic significance of Doppler measures of diastolic function in cardiac amyloidosis. A Doppler echocardiographic study. *Circulation* 1991;83:808–816.)

prognostic importance in cardiac amyloidosis (265). Right ventricular enlargement has also been identified as an independent predictor of poor outcomes among patients with primary amyloidosis (266). Both elevated troponins and brain natriuretic peptide levels have been associated with a poorer prognosis (267).

Differentiation from Hypertrophic Cardiomyopathy. Left ventricular hypertrophy and hypertrophic cardiomyopathy are also associated with an increased myocardial wall thickness, and differentiation from cardiac amyloidosis may be important because treatment and prognosis of these conditions are very different (268). The presence of low voltage on the electrocardiogram favors a diagnosis of amyloidosis rather than hypertrophic cardiomyopathy; however, endomyocardial biopsy may be necessary in some cases to give a definitive diagnosis due to the grim prognostic implications of a diagnosis of cardiac amyloidosis (268).

Nuclear medicine techniques may also be useful in the diagnosis of cardiac amyloidosis, and these include radionuclide angiography and technetium-99m pyrophosphate scintigraphy and indium-labeled antimyosin antibodies (181,269–271).

Cardiac amyloidosis can be diagnosed noninvasively antemortem in most cases from the classic appearance on two-dimensional echocardiography, electrocardiogram, and an abdominal fat aspirate showing systemic amyloidosis (29,238). Other sites of biopsy can include the rectum, gingiva, bone marrow, kidney, and liver (238). Fat aspirate and bone marrow biopsy may detect amyloidosis in most patients (272). If the echocardiogram is not diagnostic or the fat pad aspirate is negative and cardiac amyloidosis is still suspected, an endomyocardial biopsy can be performed to make the diagnosis. This may be especially salient in the presence of poorly controlled hypertension in which the increased wall thickness on echocardiography may be due to amyloid deposition or hypertensive heart disease (231).

Serum and urine protein immunofixation and electrophoresis are recommended for assessing for the secretion of a monoclonal protein (231,232). In 10% of cases, there is no monoclonal protein secreted (nonsecretory primary amyloidosis). For accurate classification of the type of amyloid, antisera against TTR, the κ and λ light chains, and protein A in the biopsy should be performed (232). Recently, serum free-light-chain assay has been introduced to assess the ratio of κ to λ free light chains and has been more sensitive than immunofixation (273). The combination of a positive serum immunofixation and an abnormal κ-to-λ ratio could diagnose 99% of AL amyloidosis cases (274).

Magnetic Resonance Imaging. MRI can be used to identify the increased myocardial thickness and small LV cavity in cardiac amyloidosis. It can be used to demonstrate the lack of increased pericardial thickening with the ancillary findings of biatrial enlargement and inferior cava dilation, similar to echocardiography (275). Usually, the myocardial image has normal MRI properties (T2-weighted images) (276). Myocardial wall thickening due to hypertrophy or amyloid infiltration may be distinguishable (181). A pattern of global and subendocardial late gadolinium enhancement and specific features of T1 mapping are seen in patients with suspected amyloidosis (277).

Management. The prognosis of cardiac amyloidosis is uniformly poor, but it does depend on the type of disease, with AL amyloidosis having the worse prognosis (232,234–236,238). In a series of more than 800 patents with primary amyloidosis over a 10-year period, the median survival was 2.1 years (278). Management of cardiac amyloidosis involves two goals: treatment of the underlying disease and treatment of cardiac symptoms.

The definitive treatment for cardiac amyloidosis (AL type) involves antiplasma cell therapy that stops production of the light chains and includes alkylating agents such as melphalan and prednisone (231,278). Two randomized trials of chemotherapy have shown benefit in AL amyloid (279–281). A trial of 100 patients with primary amyloidosis using melphalan, prednisone, and colchicine showed improvement of systemic disease when the major features were not cardiac or renal (282). Colchicine has also been used to prevent amyloidosis associated with familial Mediterranean fever (278); however, there is no evidence that it halts the progression of amyloid deposition in primary amyloidosis. Dose-intensive melphalan with blood stem-cell support is being evaluated (283). Autologous stem cell transplantation has shown promise as a treatment option with an organ remission rate of 50% (283a). However, preliminary results from a randomized trial in France showed no difference in the overall survival rate in the use of stem cell transplantation when compared to melphalan plus high dose dexamethasone (283b). Thalidomide plus dexamethasone may be another approach for treatment of cardiac amyloidosis. Recently lenalidomide (analogue of thalidomide with less toxicity) is being studied as another treatment option (283c).

Cardiac transplantation is generally not performed for patients with AL type amyloid because this is a systemic illness with progressive amyloidosis in other organs (183). However, it has been considered in select patients without extracardiac disease (<5% of cases) because the transplanted heart is usually not clinically affected (284,285). Recently, liver transplantation has been suggested for the familial type (TTR variant) because the circulating transthyretin is produced in the liver. Thus, the new liver will replace the variant TTR with a normal TTR. Drugs such as nonsteroidal antiinflammatory drugs (e.g., diflunisal) that can stabilize TTR and prevent the formation of amyloid are being evaluated (286). There is no specific treatment for the senile type of disorder (231,287,288).

Diuretics are the main drugs for treating the cardiac symptoms (231). Avoidance of digoxin is recommended because digoxin-induced arrhythmias may occur due to binding of digoxin to the amyloid fibrils (200,289). However, with careful monitoring it has been used to control heart rate in patients with atrial fibrillation (236). In addition, patients with cardiac amyloidosis may be very sensitive to the negative inotropic effects of calcium channel blockers either because of their abnormal binding to amyloid fibrils or vasodilator effects (200,290). Vasodilator agents such as ACE inhibitors or angiotensin II inhibitors are poorly tolerated and have a risk of significant hypotension (231). Pacemakers may be useful in treating symptomatic high atrioventricular (AV) block (291), and anticoagulation should be considered because of the risk of thrombus formation with atrial amyloid involvement and atrial standstill (72,292).

Cardiac Sarcoidosis

Sarcoidosis is a noncaseating granulomatous disorder of unknown etiology that may involve the lung, lymph nodes, skin, liver, spleen, parotid glands, and heart (293,294). Pulmonary manifestations are the predominant finding, with pulmonary hypertension and pulmonary fibrosis, resulting in right heart failure (295). Sarcoid granulomata are found in the myocardium at autopsy in up to 25% of patients with sarcoidosis and are often clinically silent (296–299).

Clinical Manifestations. The clinical presentation of cardiac sarcoidosis is variable and may depend on the amount of myocardium replaced with granulomata as well as the amount and the location of scar tissue (160,300,301). Granulomatous involvement is typically found in the left ventricular free wall and the superior interventricular septum, although other areas, including the papillary muscles, atria, conduction system, and pericardium, can also be affected (300,302). Clinical evidence of heart disease is only seen in about 5% of patients with sarcoidosis, whereas 25% have microscopic evidence (296). Most patients are asymptomatic; however, rhythm abnormalities and conduction disorders may predominate (160,300). The most common arrhythmia is ventricular tachycardia (301,303,304), whereas complete heart block is the most common conduction disorder (299). Sudden death is the most feared complication (302,305) and occurs in 17% of patients when there is extensive myocardial involvement. Valvular dysfunction and pericardial effusions are less common manifestations in this disease (300,301).

Patients with congestive heart failure may show clinical features of restrictive cardiomyopathy and/or dilated cardiomyopathy (299). Patients with marked disease may develop aneurysm formation, papillary dysfunction, and mitral regurgitation (299,306). The electrocardiogram may show T-wave abnormalities, AV block, or Q waves mimicking myocardial infarction (299,307).

The echocardiographic findings consist of systolic and diastolic ventricular dysfunction, left ventricular aneurysm formation, small to moderate pericardial effusions, and abnormal ventricular wall thickness (29,308–311). Regional wall-motion abnormalities (suggestive of coronary artery disease) may be detected in the basal septum with sparing of the apex (312). There may be right ventricular dilation and increased wall thickness consistent with cor pulmonale (295). Left ventricular diastolic function abnormalities may be present in 14% of patients with pulmonary sarcoidosis without evidence of cardiac disease, suggesting subclinical sarcoid cardiomyopathy (313).

Thallium-201, gallium-67, or fluorine-18 fluorodeoxyglucose positron emission tomography scanning may show segmental defects suggestive of sarcoid infiltration (314–317). The gallium-67 uptake in the myocardium may be able to predict the efficacy of corticosteroids. MRI may also be useful for identifying areas of high intensity in the left ventricular septum and the free wall of the ventricle in the inflammatory phase while detecting thinning and aneurysm formation in the chronic phase (318). The basal and lateral left ventricular walls are the most common sites of enhancement (319). The findings on MRI may be useful in guiding endomyocardial biopsy (320). Endomyocardial biopsy may be useful, although the sensitivity is reported to be in the range of 20% to 30% and thus will not exclude the diagnosis if negative (299,307).

Management. The finding of pulmonary involvement with bilateral hilar adenopathy and evidence of myocardial disease may suggest sarcoidosis involving the heart in a young person (299). Echocardiography will show left ventricular dilation, regional wall-motion abnormalities, or aneurysm formation (160,311). Treatment of sarcoidosis may include the use of corticosteroids, especially when myocardial involvement, conduction abnormalities, and ventricular arrhythmias are present; however, this remains controversial (307,321–323). Permanent pacemakers may be needed to treat the conduction abnormalities (298,299). Implantable defibrillators may be needed to prevent sudden death (324,325), whereas heart transplantation is reserved for intractable heart failure (298,324).

Storage Diseases

Hemochromatosis

Hemochromatosis is an iron storage disease that affects the heart, pancreas, liver, gonads, and skin (326). Primary idiopathic hemochromatosis is an autosomal recessive disorder related to the human leukocyte antigen on chromosome 6, whereas secondary hemochromatosis results from hemoglobin synthesis abnormalities leading to ineffective erythropoiesis, chronic liver disease, excessive intake of iron, or multiple blood transfusions (326,327).

Clinical Presentation. Manifestations of cardiac involvement occur when there is a large amount of iron deposited over a long period of time. One third of patients manifest cardiac symptoms with evidence of congestive heart failure, supraventricular or ventricular arrhythmias, and conduction defects (326). One third of patients die from cardiac involvement. A dilated or restrictive cardiomyopathy may be present with evidence of systolic and diastolic dysfunction. Cardiomegaly may be seen on chest x-ray. Electrocardiographic findings have included arrhythmias, conduction disorders, and low voltages (29,326).

Echocardiography is a useful noninvasive technique in assessing cardiac involvement in primary hemochromatosis, detecting clinically occult heart involvement, following patients serially, and assessing left ventricular function after phlebotomy (328–330). Specific Doppler filling indexes and TDI are useful for differentiating hereditary hemochromatosis and normal individuals (331).

Olson et al. described 19 patients with primary hemochromatosis and demonstrated that 7 (37%) had chamber dilation and systolic dysfunction secondary to hemochromatosis, whereas 12 patients did not (332). Increased ventricular wall thickness and mass may also be observed, although Olson and coworkers suggested that increased ventricular wall thickness is not always present with cardiac hemochromatosis (332). Patterns consistent with dilated or restrictive cardiomyopathy have also been described in patients with primary hemochromatosis (333). Ventricular dysfunction and increased ventricular mass may normalize after successful phlebotomy (333). The presence of systolic dysfunction usually signifies poor prognosis (330). Secondary hemochromatosis manifestations in the heart include increased left ventricular wall thickness and mass, increased cavity dimension, and left atrial enlargement. Most patients have normal systolic function, and those with the depressed systolic function have the worse prognosis (334).

Other noninvasive tests, including CT scan and MRI, may be useful in demonstrating subclinical involvement of hemochromatosis (335). The MRI may show a low myocardial signal on the cine gradient echo consistent with myocardial iron deposition. Endomyocardial biopsy may be useful for excluding the diagnosis especially when the echocardiographic or clinical features are not evident (336,337). Laboratory tests will show an elevated serum ferritin and increased ratio of plasma iron level to total iron-binding capacity, urinary iron, liver iron, and saturation of transferrin (337).

Management. Treatment by repeat phlebotomies in primary hemochromatosis or the use of chelating agents (desferrioxamine) in secondary hemochromatosis may result in improvement of the cardiac involvement, thus making early diagnosis important (326,338,339). Heart transplantation may be considered when the heart involvement is life-threatening (339), or combined heart and liver transplantation may be useful in patients with heart and liver failure (340,341).

Fabry Disease

Fabry disease is a rare X-linked recessive disorder of glycolipid metabolism secondary to a deficiency of the lysosomal enzyme α-galactosidase A. This disease severely affects homozygous male individuals with milder symptoms occurring in female individuals (226,342). Abnormal deposition of glycolipid occurs in the heart, skin, and kidney (343). Histologic examination shows diffuse involvement of the myocardium, conduction system, vascular endothelium, and the mitral valve secondary to deposition in the lysosomes of the affected tissue.

Patients may develop angina and myocardial infarction with normal epicardial coronary vessels, mitral regurgitation, and congestive heart failure and increased wall thickness on echocardiography, mimicking hypertrophic cardiomyopathy and cardiac amyloidosis (343–345). Recent studies have shown that Fabry disease may be the cause of left ventricular hypertrophy in 6% of men with late-onset hypertrophic cardiomyopathy (346,347). Furthermore, 12% of female patients with late-onset hypertrophy were demonstrated to have Fabry disease by endomyocardial biopsy despite echocardiographic appearances of hypertrophic cardiomyopathy (348).

The electrocardiogram may show atrioventricular block and a short PR interval (349). Studies in adult patients have shown a correlation between age, the degree of α-galactosidase activity, and the degree of left ventricular hypertrophy (350). Similarities in the structure of the glycolipid ceramide trihexoside and the amyloid fibril may account for their similar appearance (344). MRI may show mildly increased signal intensity in the myocardium (351). Endomyocardial biopsy may show low α-galactosidase A levels (171,352,353). Treatment with enzyme replacement has been shown to decrease left ventricular hypertrophy (354).

Noninfiltrative Diseases

Carcinoid Heart Disease

Carcinoid heart disease is a rare cause of restrictive cardiomyopathy (355,356). Carcinoid syndrome results from metastatic carcinoid tumors that cause cutaneous flushing, diarrhea, bronchoconstriction and fibrous endocardial plaques in the heart (357,358). Cardiac disease is detected by echocardiography in greater than 50% of patients with carcinoid syndrome, whereas clinically apparent heart disease with right heart failure is detected in one fourth of patients (357,359).

The carcinoid tumors most commonly originate in the small bowel and appendix in greater than 60% of cases, but also may arise in the bronchus, biliary tract, pancreas, testis, and ovary (356,357). Carcinoid tumors from the ileum are the ones that metastasize to the liver and lymph nodes. These tumors contain cytoplasmic granules that take up and reduce silver salts (356). Carcinoid heart disease results from hepatic metastases that produce large amounts of humoral substances that can reach the right heart and are not inactivated by the liver but by the lungs (357). The humoral substances may include 5-hydroxytryptamine (5-HT), serotonin, bradykinin, and other substances. Rarely, left-sided disease may occur when the humoral substances can cross right to left through a patent foramen ovale, when produced by carcinoid tumor of the bronchus, or when there is extensive right-sided involvement (358,360,361).

Clinical Presentation

Carcinoid heart disease is difficult to diagnose until there is evidence of right heart failure with an elevated jugular venous pulse with a prominent v wave and tricuspid regurgitation (356). A systolic murmur along the left sternal border that shows inspiratory augmentation (tricuspid regurgitation) followed by an early diastolic sound and a diastolic rumble (tricuspid stenosis) may be detected. In addition, there may be murmurs of pulmonic stenosis and regurgitation (357). The chest x-ray may show cardiac enlargement, pleural effusions, and nodules. The pulmonary trunk is normal in size. The electrocardiogram is nonspecific, with evidence of right atrial enlargement, nonspecific ST and T-wave abnormalities, and sinus tachycardia (357). The hemodynamic findings are that of significant tricuspid regurgitation with a large right atrial v wave and diastolic gradient (357).

Echocardiography is a very sensitive technique for documenting the combined tricuspid and pulmonic abnormalities and right ventricular overload as well as for following the progression and detecting subclinical involvement (357,362).

In one series, echocardiography detected right-sided disease in 66% of patients with carcinoid syndrome, and the patients with more severe valvular disease were more associated with higher levels of bradykinins and serotonin (359,363). In another series of 132 patients with carcinoid syndrome, 56% of patients had cardiac involvement, which was associated with higher levels of 5-hydroxyindolacetic acid. The 3-year survival rate of patients with echocardiographic evidence of carcinoid heart disease was reduced compared to that of patients without cardiac involvement (357). Other studies have shown a correlation between posttreatment 5-hydroxyindolacetic acid levels and the progression of disease assessed by an echocardiographic score of valvular involvement (364).

The echocardiographic features of cardiac involvement are remarkable (365). The tricuspid valve leaflets were thickened, shortened, and retracted and showed incomplete coaptation and decreased excursion, resulting in stenosis and regurgitation. The pulmonic valve also showed thickening, retraction, and commissural fusion and stayed open in a partly fixed position, resulting in both stenosis and regurgitation. The predominant lesions seen are tricuspid regurgitation and pulmonary stenosis (366). Carcinoid plaques causing these lesions are usually seen on the ventricular surface of the tricuspid valve and the pulmonary artery surface of the pulmonic valve (366). The Doppler findings showed severe tricuspid regurgitation with a distinctive dagger-shaped Doppler spectral profile with an early peak pressure and rapid decline. In addition, the pressure half-time was prolonged, which was consistent with associated tricuspid stenosis (357). In addition, there was evidence of right ventricular volume overload from the associated tricuspid regurgitation (160). Transesophageal echocardiography may be useful in assessing the thickness of the valvular leaflets and the superficial wall layers on the cavity side of both atria (362,367).

Management

Carcinoid heart disease can be diagnosed in the presence of the right heart findings with the classic systemic features. There may also be urinary excretion of 5-hydroxyindoleacetic acid, the principal metabolite of serotonin (356,366).

The long-term prognosis is poor regardless of treatment modality (368). Chemotherapy may be partially effective in treating the hepatic metastasis, whereas removal of the primary tumor is rarely indicated. Occasionally, removal of the liver metastasis is performed, but more commonly hepatic arterial embolization is performed (356,369). Medical therapy often includes digitalis and diuretics for mild congestive heart failure. The effects of the carcinoid syndrome can be treated with the use of somatostatin analogues, serotonin antagonists, and α-adrenergic blockers (356,370–372). Levels of 5-hydroxyindoleacetic acid are directly linked to progression of carcinoid heart disease (373).

Interventional and surgical therapies have also been performed on patients with carcinoid valvular heart disease. Balloon valvuloplasty of the tricuspid stenosis and pulmonic stenosis can also be performed (374–377). Tricuspid valve replacement and pulmonary valvotomy is recommended with advanced disease (378,379). Implantation of a biologic valve or allograft is not recommended due to the development of carcinoid on the new valve (356,366,380). Surgical mortality for symptomatic patients with severe valve disease is high (381);

however there can be marked improvement in symptoms in survivors (368). A recent study from the Mayo Clinic on 200 patients with carcinoid heart disease showed that a better prognosis may be related to valve replacement surgery (382).

PERICARDIAL DISEASE

Anatomic Considerations

The pericardium is a closed, fibroserous membrane sac in the middle mediastinum posterior to the sternum and the second to sixth costal cartilages and anterior to the fifth to eighth vertebrae (383). During embryologic development, the heart invaginates the sac, based on a pedicle of the great vessels, cavae, and pulmonary veins. A layer of the serous sac becomes densely adherent to the myocardium, forming the visceral pericardium or epicardium. This layer envelops the entire heart apart from a bare area on the posterior aspect of the left atrium between the pulmonary veins—the oblique sinus. The visceral layer reflects back on itself and is continuous with the parietal pericardium. This reflection forms a second cleft between the great vessels and the left atrium—the transverse sinus (384).

The parietal pericardium consists of an outer fibrous layer composed of multiple layers of collagen, aligned in different directions, interspersed with elastin fibrils. This fibrous layer has ligamentous attachments with the central tendon of the diaphragm inferiorly, the sternum anteriorly by the superior and inferior sternopericardial ligaments, and the pleural membranes laterally. The inner layer of the parietal pericardium is a serous mesothelial membrane, with microvilli, to aid fluid secretion (385). The normal pericardium contains about 50 mL of pale serous fluid to minimize friction and restrict excessive cardiac motion. The fluid is low in protein and has a relatively high proportion of albumin, consistent with a transudate.

The pericardium is innervated by branches of C4–5 via the phrenic nerve. This may explain the perception of pericardial pain in the left shoulder tip. Arterial supply to the pericardium is via the internal (thoracic) mammary arteries and multiple branches of the bronchial, esophageal, and phrenic arteries. Venous drainage is via the azygous system.

Normal Physiology of Pericardium

For the pericardium as a whole, there is an exponential stress–strain relationship. At normal cardiac volumes, the pericardium is on the flat portion of the curve, and physiologic changes in volume are associated with minimal changes in intrapericardial pressure. However, with abrupt large increases in volume (such as in acute overhydration or valve rupture), the pericardium quickly reaches the exponential portion of the curve and significantly restricts further cardiac dilation. In this way, it can be argued that the pericardium has a very little role in limiting cardiac filling at normal physiologic volumes and only exerts a constraining effect on filling when abrupt changes in volume occur (Fig. 27.11). The pericardial pressure usually approximates pleural pressure and varies with the respiratory cycle, being approximately −6 mm Hg at end-inspiration and −3 mm Hg at end-expiration. The lowering of pericardial pressure more than atrial pressure and transmural pressures in inspiration allows increased filling of the right heart while there is increased aortic transmural pressures and pooling of the right ventricular output and consequently decreased left heart filling (386,387).

As the heart slowly enlarges in the face of a chronic process such as cardiomyopathy or chronic valvular insufficiency, so too the pericardium increases in volume and mass (388). Thus,

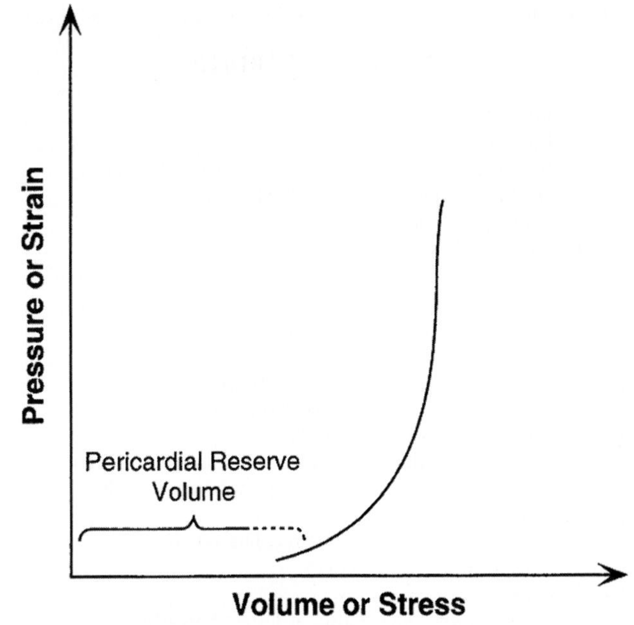

FIGURE 27.11. Schema of stress–strain and pressure–volume curves of the normal pericardium. After the relatively small pericardial reserve volume (the volume by which the unstressed pericardium exceeds the cardiac volume) is exhausted by filling of the pericardial sinuses and recesses, the curve at first rises gently; with continued filling at some point the curve rises more acutely. (From Spodick DH. *The pericardium: A comprehensive textbook*. New York: Marcel Dekker, 1997:19.)

even in cardiomegalic states, the pericardial stress–strain curve shifts to the right; during normal daily living, it exerts very little constraining effect to filling. Similarly, abrupt changes in cardiac volume superimposed on a chronically dilated heart will move the pericardium into the steep portion of the pressure–volume curve, and a constrictive effect on cardiac filling will be observed.

When the cardiac volume causes the pericardium to reach the steep portion of its pressure–volume curve, a phenomenon of ventricular interdependence is observed (389). Put simply, the ventricles, with their common interventricular septum, are forced to exist in a finite-volume cavity. Therefore, increased filling of one chamber (e.g., right ventricle during inspiration) will shift the septum into the left ventricle, impeding its filling and therefore output. A similar effect is seen in cardiac tamponade and constrictive pericarditis and is the pathophysiologic mechanism underlying pulsus paradoxus and "flow paradoxus" (66,390–392).

Clinical Presentations of Pericardial Disease

Acute Pericarditis

Inflammation of the layers of the pericardium from any of a myriad of causes yields a common clinical syndrome termed *acute pericarditis*. The causes of acute pericarditis are listed in Table 27.5. The classical symptom complex represents an important differential diagnosis in the assessment of chest pain presentations. However, the relatively common finding of pericardial inflammation at autopsy suggests that the majority of cases are subclinical.

Clinical Presentation. Acute pericarditis classically presents with progressive, often severe, chest pain over hours (393). This mechanical pain is typically postural, being worse on lying supine and relieved by sitting forward. It is often pleuritic and aggravated by coughing, motion, and swallowing. It

TABLE 27.5

AETIOLOGY OF ACUTE PERICARDITIS

I. **Idiopathic**
II. **Infectious**
Bacterial, Tuberculous, Viral: *Coxsackie, Influenza, HIV, etc.* Fungal, Rickettsial, Mycoplasma, Leptospira, Listeria, Parasitic, Other
III. **Vasculitis/Connective Tissue Disease:** Rheumatoid Arthritis, Rheumatic Fever, SLE, Scleroderma Sjögren's Syndrome, Reiter Syndrome, Ankylosing Spondylitis, Wegener's Granulomatosis, Giant Cell Arteritis, Polymyositis (Dermatomyositis), Behcet Syndrome, Familial Mediterraneun Fever, Dermatomyositis, Polyarteritis, Churg-Strause Syndrome, TTP, Leukoclastic Vasculitis, Other
IV. **Diseases in Adjacent Structures:** myocardial infarction, aortic dissection, pneumonia, pulmonary embolism, empyema
V. **Metabolic Disorders:** Uraemic, Dialysis-Related, Myxoedema, Gout, Scurvy
VI. **Neoplastic**
A. *Secondary* (Metastatic, or Direct Spread): Carcinoma, Lymphoma, Carcinoid, Other
B. *Primary* Mesothelioma, Sarcoma, Fibroma, Lipoma, Other
VII. **Trauma**
Direct: 1. Pericardial Perforation: Penetrating Injury, Esophageal or Gastric Perforation
2. Cardiac Injury: Cardiac Surgery, Percutaneous Procedures
Indirect: Radiation, Non-Penetrating Chest Injury
VIII. **Association with Other Syndromes**
Post-Myocardial and Pericardial Injury Syndromes, Inflammatory Bowel Disease, Loffler Syndrome, Stevens-Johnson Syndrome, Giant Cell Aortitis, Hypereosinophilic Syndromes, Acute Pancreatitis, etc.

Modified from Spodick DH. Pericardial Diseases. In: Braunwald E, Zipes DP, Libby P, eds. *Heart Disease: A Textbook of Cardiovascular Medicine*, 6th ed. Philadelphia, PA: W.B. Saunders, 2001.

is described as sharp, "stabbing," or "knifelike" in character. The pain may radiate to the neck or shoulder in the region of the trapezius ridge and less frequently to the arms and back and even left shoulder, making differentiation from coronary ischemic pain more difficult. There is often a low-grade fever associated with viral and idiopathic pericarditis, whereas purulent pericarditis is associated with very high fevers and systemic sepsis.

The presence of a pericardial rub is pathognomonic for pericarditis, although its absence does not exclude the syndrome. This "to-and-fro" rasping sound has a timing consistent with the cardiac cycle and is creaking in nature, like the sound of leather on leather. It is best appreciated with the diaphragm of the stethoscope applied to the lower left sternal edge and with the patient leaning forward in end-expiration. The sound classically has a triple cadence (394) with components related to (a) atrial systole, (b) ventricular systole, and (c) ventricular diastole. The rub is triphasic in nearly 50% of the cases, biphasic in 33% of the cases, and monophasic in 10% of the cases. The intensity of the sound can be attenuated by subcutaneous tissue thickness and hyperinflated lung volume. Furthermore, the development of a pericardial effusion as part of the inflammatory syndrome can lead to waxing and waning of the rub over days, although a loud pericardial rub can still be heard occasionally in the presence of a significant effusion. The sound should be differentiated from a pleural rub (which is similar in character and timed with the respiratory cycle), subcutaneous emphysema (which may be an associate in postsurgical or traumatic cases), and loud intracardiac murmurs (such as ventricular septal defects).

Investigations. The electrocardiogram represents the most useful diagnostic test in acute pericarditis. Inflammation of the subepicardial myocardium is thought to be the mechanism producing ST and T-wave changes, whereas inflammation of the atrium is thought to cause the PR-segment changes (395). The PR-segment deviations may precede the ST changes (396). In contrast to the regional ST changes of myocardial ischemia, pericarditis generally produces widespread electrocardiogram (ECG) changes in limb and precordial leads. Four phases of ECG abnormalities have been recognized (Table 27.6) (395,397): ST elevation and upright T waves (stage 1) is present in 90% of cases. Over time, the ST changes resolve and the ECG may look normal (stage II). There may be further evolution to T-wave inversion (stage III) and finally to normal (stage IV).

TABLE 27.6

FOUR-STAGE ("TYPICAL") ELECTROCARDIOGRAPHIC EVOLUTION OF ACUTE PERICARDITIS

Sequence stage	Leads of "epicardial" derivation: at least I, II, aV_L, aV_F, V_3–V_6			Leads reflecting "endocardial" potential: aV_R, often V_1, sometimes V_2		
	J-ST	T waves	PR segment	ST segment	T waves	PR segment
I	Elevated	Upright	Depressed or isoelectric	Depressed	Inverted	Elevated or isoelectric
II early	Isoelectric	Upright	Isoelectric or depressed	Isoelectric	Inverted	Isoelectric or elevated
II late	Isoelectric	Low to flat to inverted	Isoelectric or depressed	Isoelectric	Shallow to flat to upright	Isoelectric or elevated
III	Isoelectric	Inverted	Isoelectric	Isoelectric	Upright	Isoelectric
IV	Isoelectric	Upright	Isoelectric	Isoelectric	Inverted	Isoelectric

J-ST, junction of S (or T) wave with the end of the QRS complex.
Modified from Spodick DH. Electrocardiogram in acute pericarditis. Distributions of morphologic and axial changes by stages. *Am J Cardiol* 1974;33:470–474.

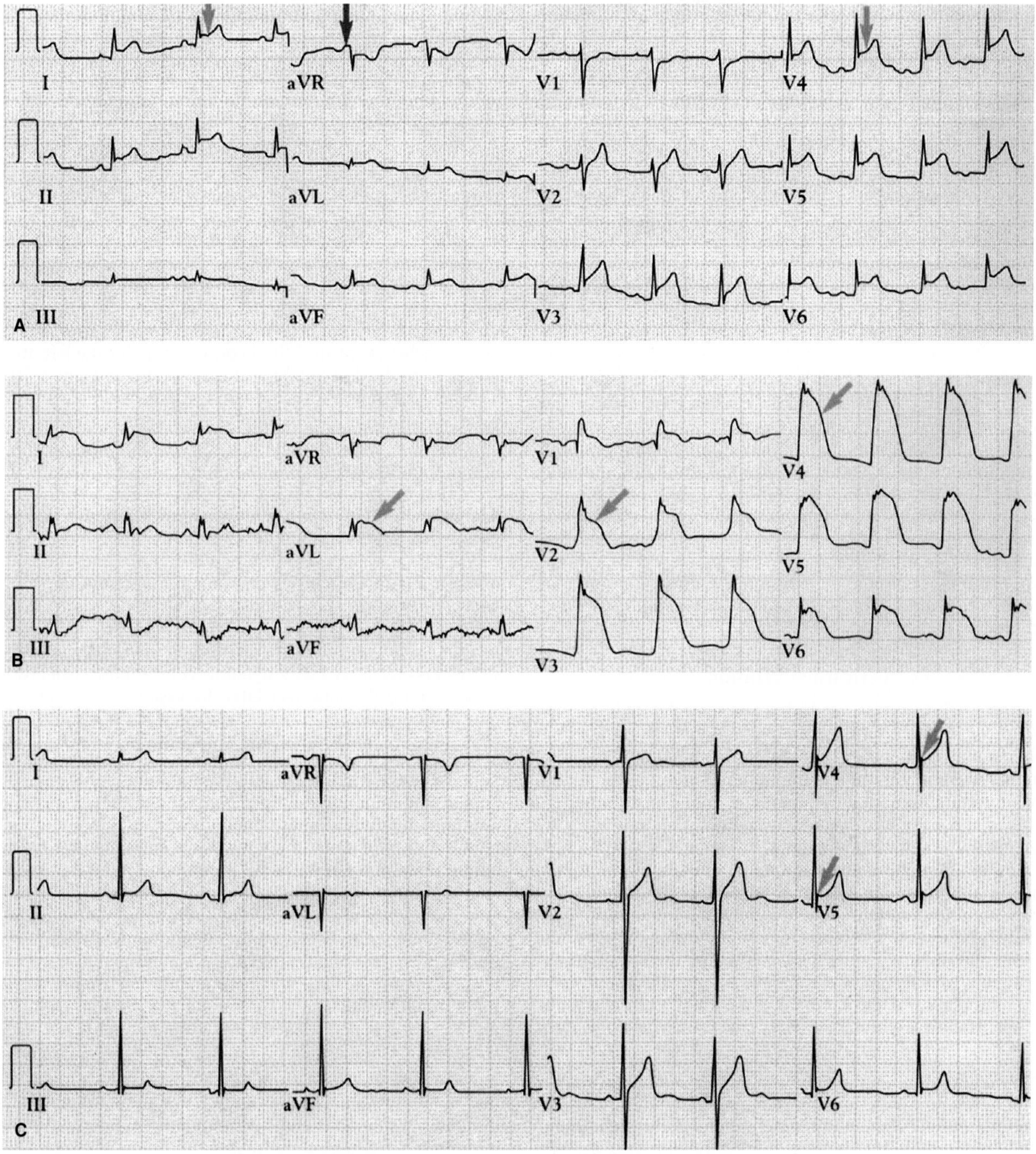

FIGURE 27.12. Differential diagnosis of acute pericarditis. **A:** Acute pericarditis. Note the upwardly concave ST elevations in limb leads I, II, aVF, and aVL and in precordial leads V3–V6 (*blue left and right arrows*) and the PR-segment elevation in aVR (*green middle arrow*). **B:** Acute myocardial infarction. Note the convex ST elevation in leads I, aVL, V1–V6 (*blue left, right, middle arrows*), indicating a large anterior myocardial infarction. **C:** Early repolarization. Note the elevation of the J point (*blue right arrows*) with pseudonormalization of the ST segment in V4–V6. (From Aikat S, Ghaffari S. A review of pericardial diseases: clinical, ECG and hemodynamic features and management. *Cleve Clin J Med* 2000;67:903–914.)

The ECG abnormalities should be differentiated most importantly from acute myocardial ischemia (Fig. 27.12). The ST changes are more widespread in pericarditis and have a typical "saddle-shaped" or upward concave appearance. Unlike myocardial infarction, there are no Q waves or loss of R-wave progression. The other important differential diagnosis of these ECG changes is the "early-repolarization" pattern. Although difficult without clinical correlation, differentiation can be made by the presence of PR-segment elevation (especially aVR) and ST elevation in V6, which is uncommon in the early-repolarization syndrome (398). Most patients with acute pericarditis remain in sinus rhythm (399).

Chest radiography contributes relatively little to the diagnosis of acute pericarditis. The presence of cardiomegaly may be seen in the minority of cases where a significant pericardial effusion has accumulated. Laboratory analysis of blood often shows a modest leukocytosis and raised C-reactive protein and sedimentation rate.

Radionuclide scanning with indium-111 (400) and gallium-67 (401,402) has been reported to be useful in identifying the pericardium as the source of an inflammatory syndrome of unknown diagnosis in some patients. MRI with gadolinium diethylenetriamine pentaacetic acid (Gd-DTPA) enhancement has identified specific regions of the pericardium involved in the inflammatory process (403).

Serum troponin I has been reported to be elevated in patients with ST elevation and acute pericarditis, reflecting a degree of epicardial myocardial injury (404). Elevations in troponin I among patients with viral or idiopathic pericarditis are most common in younger patients, men, and patients with ST elevations and pericardial effusions at presentation. However, for patients with acute pericarditis, elevated troponin I is not a negative prognostic marker (405).

Diagnostic algorithm. The following sequence has been proposed (406). All patients should have a complete history and physical examination, electrocardiography, and chest radiography. Diagnostic specific testing may include tuberculin skin testing, rheumatoid factor and antinuclear antibody, and viral studies. HIV testing should be considered. In more complex cases (i.e., symptoms and signs lasting >1 week, clinical evidence of tamponade, or purulent pericarditis), echocardiography and blood cultures *should be considered*. Pericardiocentesis (either percutaneous or surgical) is indicated for clinical tamponade, evidence for purulent pericarditis, high suspicion of tumor, or illness lasting longer than 1 week.

Pericardial Effusion

Pericardial effusion is diagnosed in routine echocardiography practice in almost 1 in 10 patients (407–409). Large pericardial effusions that develop slowly can be remarkably asymptomatic, whereas rapidly accumulating smaller effusions can present with tamponade.

Massive chronic pericardial effusion is a diagnosis ascribed to a syndrome consisting of a large pericardial effusion present for at least 3 months and not attributable to any systemic cause (410). These effusions can be present for many years and were well tolerated in one series, with tamponade a rarity (411). However, in two series, cardiac tamponade occurred in near one third of patients (410,412). In the larger study, 28 patients with large idiopathic chronic pericardial effusions were followed for a median of 7 years. Unexpected tamponade occurred in 8 patients (29%), and pericardiectomy was performed in 20 patients. Chronic nonspecific pericarditis was found in all patients evaluated by histology (412).

Clinical Presentation. Pericardial effusions that are not causing hemodynamic embarrassment to the heart are usually asymptomatic. Patients may describe dyspnea or dysphagia due to space-occupying effects in the chest. Physical compression may cause hoarseness (recurrent laryngeal nerve), hiccups (phrenic nerve), or nausea (diaphragm). Physical examination of patients with large effusions demonstrate muffled heart sounds. Ewart's sign, dullness on auscultation under the left scapula, is a result of compression of the base of the left lung. This may be associated with coarse crepitations due to local atelectasis. Chest x-ray findings include cardiomegaly, which may be massive, often with a characteristic globular shape to the heart silhouette. The cardiac margins are unusually sharp because the pericardium is free of the cardiac motion that usually blurs the silhouette radiographically. Electrocardiography demonstrates diminished QRS and T-wave voltages. Electrical alternans is a marker of massive pericardial effusion.

Echocardiography is the diagnostic tool of choice for pericardial effusion. Initially, M-mode was the standard, with a high sensitivity for posterior pericardial fluid (408). The advent of two-dimensional echocardiography has shown the various presentations of effusion, including circumferential, posterior, and loculated. The last are more common when scarring has supervened, for example, after surgery, trauma, or purulent pericarditis. The size of effusions can be graded as small (<10 mm of echo-free space in systole and diastole), moderate (≥10 mm at least posteriorly), large (≥20 mm), or very large (compression of the heart) (413). Furthermore, two-dimensional echocardiography can give information about the nature of the fluid, suggesting the presence of fibrin, clot, tumor, air, and calcium. Care must be taken to differentiate pericardial fluid from pleural fluid and ascites. Left pleural effusions can be difficult to differentiate from pericardial fluid. By transthoracic echocardiography in the parasternal long-axis view, pericardial fluid can be seen to reflect at the posterior atrioventricular groove, whereas pleural fluid continues under the left atrium, posterior to the descending aorta. Spin-echo and cine MRI can also be used to assess the size and extent of simple and complex pericardial effusions similar to echocardiography (414). The effusions seen by MRI may tend to be larger than those detected by echocardiography (415).

Management. The action taken after the finding of a significant pericardial fluid collection depends on the underlying etiology, the presence of hemodynamic compromise, and the volume of fluid. Pericardiocentesis may not be necessary in all cases, particularly when the diagnosis can be made based on other systemic features. Where doubt remains, particularly where malignancy or purulent pericarditis is suspected, pericardiocentesis is indicated. Hemodynamic compromise is an absolute indication for drainage (see later discussion).

Pericardial Tamponade

Fluid accumulation in the finite pericardial space will cause an increase in pressure with subsequent cardiac compression. Tamponade is not a binary phenomenon, and exhibits a spectrum from mild cardiac compression and embarrassment to cardiovascular collapse.

Pathophysiology. Systemic venous flow occurs in two phases: *systolic*, related to filling of the atrium with a closed tricuspid valve (x descent on central venous pressure trace, S wave on hepatic venous Doppler), and *diastolic*, related to filling of the right atrium as it empties through the open tricuspid valve (y descent on central venous pressure trace, D wave on hepatic venous Doppler). In tamponade, the heart is compressed and remains in a finite volume. Ventricular ejection decreases the relative proportion of the pericardial space occupied by the heart, allowing a fall in intrapericardial and atrial pressure and a rapid inflow of blood (large x descent and S wave). During diastole, the pericardium contains filled ventricles, which increases its pressure and thus decreases forward flow from the systemic veins (blunted y descent and D waves) (392,416). The systemic venous flow in cardiac tamponade should be distinguished from constrictive pericarditis with prominent x and y descent (S and D on hepatic venous Doppler) (3,75).

Pulsus paradoxus, defined as an inspiratory drop of systolic blood pressure of greater than 10 mm Hg, is a hallmark of cardiac tamponade. With inspiration, intrathoracic pressure becomes subatmospheric. Intrapericardial pressure, pathologically high in this syndrome, is reduced during inspiration (as it is physiologically reduced in the normal state), allowing increased right ventricular filling. Systemic venous diastolic flow (y descent, hepatic vein D wave) increases and right ventricular size and stroke volume increase. Again, due to the finite volume of the pericardium, the left ventricle is partially compressed by the enlarging right ventricle (due to leftward displacement of the intraventricular septum), causing an inspiratory decrease in systemic stroke volume (417). An alternative mechanism is that the pulmonary venous-to-left atrial pressure gradient is decreased because the changes in intrathoracic pressure are not transmitted to the left ventricle due to shielding by the pericardial fluid and the increased pulmonary vascular compliance. There is reciprocally increased flow on the right side of the heart due to interventricular interdependence (418,419). Pulsus paradoxus can also be detected in noncardiac conditions such as severe lung disease (in which intrathoracic pressure swings are supraphysiologic) as well as pulmonary embolus (in which right ventricular filling pressures are disproportionately higher than left pressures) (417,420).

Clinical Presentation. The spectrum of presentation of patients with cardiac tamponade ranges from dyspnea and edema to frank circulatory collapse. The classic triad of cardiac tamponade is (a) hypotension, (b) elevated jugular venous pressure, and (c) distant heart sounds (421). Early tamponade is manifested by tachycardia, tachypnea, dyspnea, edema, elevated venous pressure, and quiet cardiomegaly. Examination of the central venous waveform shows a prominent x descent and absence of the y descent.

Pulsus paradoxus is examined using the stethoscope over the brachial pulse and measuring the pressure gap between the appearance of the Korotkoff sounds during expiration only and their continuous presence. It is defined by an inspiratory fall in systolic blood pressure of 10 mm Hg with inspiration, an exaggeration of the normal situation. False-positive pulsus paradoxus without cardiac tamponade may occur with obstructive lung disease, right ventricular infarction, and pulmonary embolism; and a false-negative finding may occur with high left ventricular pressures as with left ventricular dysfunction or hypertrophy, severe hypotension, and severe aortic regurgitation or in the case of an atrial septal defect (422).

Profound circulatory collapse or shock is more common in patients with acute tamponade related to cardiac or pericardial trauma. In the most extreme cases, such as acute aortic dissection into the pericardium, patients may present with electromechanical dissociation. Patients who develop the syndrome subacutely tend to present in a less dire status and manifest signs of right heart failure with edema, hepatomegaly, ascites, and pleural effusion. Rarely, low-pressure cardiac tamponade without the typical signs can develop in the presence of dehydration and hypovolemia (423). Other variant forms of tamponade may include hypertensive cardiac tamponade (with high blood pressure), tamponade with ventricular dysfunction (right or left ventricular dysfunction), regional cardiac tamponade (localized effusions), or effusive constriction (413).

With an increase in invasive cardiac procedures in the electrophysiology and cardiac catheterization laboratories, the complication of cardiac tamponade is more frequent. A report of nearly 7,000 patients undergoing percutaneous coronary intervention found an incidence of 0.2%, with cardiac tamponade developing 2 to 36 hours after the procedure (424).

Investigations. The electrocardiogram and chest x-ray do not differentiate tamponade from noncompressive pericardial effusion. Large pericardial effusions allow "swinging" of the heart on its vascular pedicle, causing electrical alternans in some cases.

Echocardiography is a fast and noninvasive modality for accurately diagnosing tamponade (392) (Table 27.7). The presence of pericardial fluid should be documented and its location defined. The classic signs of cardiac tamponade are right atrial and right ventricular collapse (425–427). Postsurgical effusions may be loculated (e.g., behind the left atrium) and sometimes difficult to visualize from the transthoracic window. Indeed, if the diagnosis of tamponade is suspected in this scenario, transesophageal echocardiography is indicated (3). Two-dimensional echocardiography can also exclude pericardial masses and ventricular and valvular dysfunction as the cause of hemodynamic compromise. Doppler echocardiography allows direct quantitation of mitral and tricuspid inflows, pulmonary venous and systemic venous flows, and, with the use of a respirometer, their variation with respiration (428). Respiratory variation of transmitral E waves is minimal in normal individuals, and greater than 25% variation (increasing on the first beat of expiration and conversely on inspiration) is highly suggestive of significant tamponade. Tricuspid E waves often will exhibit some degree of respiratory variation in normal individuals, and greater than 40% variation is required (opposite pattern to the left side), and prominent hepatic venous flow reversals in expiration is required to suggest tamponade (392).

TABLE 27.7

ECHOCARDIOGRAPHIC FINDINGS IN PATIENTS WITH CARDIAC TAMPONADE

Abnormal inspiratory increase of right ventricular dimension with abnormal inspiratory decrease of left ventricular dimension
Inspiratory decrease of mitral valve DE excursion (M-mode) (anterior leaflet opening) and ejection fraction slope (initial anterior leaflet closing)
Right atrial collapse
Right ventricular early diastolic collapse
Left atrial collapse
"Flow paradoxus" with abnormal inspiratory increase of tricuspid valve flow and abnormal inspiratory decrease of mitral valve flow
Inferior vena cava plethora (failure to decrease proximal diameter by 50% or more on sniff or deep inspiration)
Loss of the hepatic vein D wave in expiration

Modified from Fowler NO. Pericardial disease. *Heart Dis Stroke* 1992;1:85–94.

Cardiac catheterization has historically been the diagnostic standard for tamponade and remains useful, particularly when noninvasive modalities are inconclusive. Right heart catheterization is often performed simultaneously with pericardiocentesis, allowing monitoring of improvement as the effusion is drained. Typically, patients demonstrate an elevated right atrial pressure, with a prominent x descent and diminished or absent y descent (416). The PCWP is also elevated and is often equal to intrapericardial and right atrial pressure. As pericardial fluid is drained, intrapericardial pressure falls below biatrial pressure. If this does not occur, the diagnosis of effusive constrictive disease should be considered (see later discussion).

Pericardiocentesis. While the equipment for pericardiocentesis is being prepared, the patient in tamponade may be supported with cautious fluid loading and inotropes. Percutaneous pericardiocentesis should be performed in an environment in which advanced cardiac life support equipment and personnel are immediately available. Historically, these procedures have been performed in the cardiac catheterization lab with arterial and right heart catheters in situ. More recently, the procedure has tended to be performed in the procedure room of the cardiac or intensive care unit, or even at the bedside, using echocardiographic guidance (429–431). Surgical drainage of the pericardium (either by a subxiphoid approach or utilizing a complete pericardiectomy) is indicated for loculated effusions, patients at risk of excessive bleeding, and in situations in which fluid has recurred after previous drainage procedures (432).

Echocardiography can demonstrate the most accessible window for passage of the needle (429,430,433). Historically, the subxiphoid approach has been used most commonly with a long needle passed under the xiphoid and directed toward the left shoulder at a 30° angle to the skin. Echocardiography performed at the cardiac apex can often identify a window through which the pericardium can be entered (usually in the sixth or seventh rib space in the anterior axillary line) without risk of cardiac puncture. A short needle is passed through the rib space under constant negative pressure until fluid is aspirated. It is important to confirm that the fluid aspirated is intrapericardial, that is, the blood should not clot.

Once the pericardial space is reached by either approach, a soft-tipped guide wire is passed and the needle removed. A multiholed catheter is then introduced and the pericardial fluid suctioned out. It is prudent to drain the fluid in steps of less than 1 liter at a time to allow cardiovascular equilibrium to be restored at each stage and to avoid the rare complication of acute right ventricular dilation (434,435). Clinical improvement usually occurs after the aspiration of only 100 to 200 mL of fluid. The fluid should be drained completely and specimens sent for chemistry, cytology, culture, cell counts, and acid-fast bacilli (AFB) staining. It is common practice to leave the catheter in for some hours, connected to a free drainage bag, to allow further drainage as the patient assumes different postures. It is important to avoid the allowance of air into the pericardium because this is most uncomfortable for the patient.

Percutaneous pericardiocentesis is a rapid and safe procedure when performed by trained personnel (433). In a recent study of patients undergoing urgent pericardiocentesis after cardiac perforation, tamponade was relieved in 99% of patients. A major complication rate of 3% occurred and included pneumothorax and right ventricular laceration. No deaths resulted directly from pericardiocentesis (436). A similar review of 245 pericardiocenteses performed in patients with postoperative effusions showed that anticoagulant therapy was the most common contributing factor to early pericardial effusions (<7 days), and postpericardiotomy syndrome contributed most often to late effusions (437). The rate of major complications from pericardiocentesis was 2% in this study.

Surgical Procedures. A median sternotomy or anterolateral thoracotomy approach provides good visualization for pericardial surgery including pericardiectomy for constrictive and effusive disease (438). However, less invasive procedures are available for drainage of pericardial effusions when pericardiocentesis is not feasible or recurrent fluid accumulates.

Subxiphoid pericardiectomy is a safe and efficacious method of draining large pericardial effusions. A small incision is made in the upper epigastrium and the pericardium is approached by posterior retraction of the diaphragm from the sternum. A pleuropericardial window is often created to allow ongoing drainage (439). This approach, although still safe, has the advantage over pericardiocentesis due to a higher diagnostic yield, allowing for fluid analysis and pericardial biopsy (440).

Alternative nonthoracotomy techniques for formation of a pericardial window include percutaneous pericardiotomy using an inflatable balloon from a subxiphoid approach (441–448) and a video-assisted thoracic surgical (VATS) pericardiectomy. These procedures are effective for the management of malignant and other large pericardial effusions. In addition, pericardial biopsy can be performed via a pericardioscopy technique, establishing a diagnosis or etiology in near 50% of patients (449).

Constrictive Pericarditis

Dense fibrosis and adhesion of the parietal and visceral layers of the pericardium creates a rigid "case" around the heart, limiting its filling and causing profound disturbances of cardiac function. This final common pathway may be the end result of one (or more) of many etiologic agents, including infection, post cardiac surgery, and radiation. The constrictive process can follow the etiology acutely, subacutely (months), or chronically (years) (413). The clinical presentation is well recognizable, with debilitating right heart failure and a poor prognosis. A voluminous literature exists about the many methods of differentiating this constellation from that of restrictive cardiomyopathy, which presents with similar clinical signs and symptoms (Table 27.8).

Pathophysiology. The fundamental abnormality in constrictive pericarditis is the limited filling and enhanced interventricular dependence of the heart due to the rigid encasement of the heart by a thickened pericardium, which effectively isolates it from the normal respiratory swings in pressure and allows a finite filling volume for the ventricles (66). Within the pericardium, the myocardium is intrinsically normal (unless there is a combined abnormality such as in radiation myocarditis), with no specific abnormality of systolic or diastolic function. In constriction, the ventricle fills abruptly on valve opening (often more abruptly than normal due to elevated atrial filling pressures). However, in mid-diastole, the chambers reach the maximum volume that the constraining pericardium will allow and filling abruptly ceases. This can be appreciated visually on two-dimensional echocardiography as wall motion ceases with a shudder in mid-diastole. In contrast, restrictive myocardial diseases involve abnormal ventricular filling from the very onset of diastole as the chamber relaxes slowly and stiffness increases with a compensatory increase in left atrial pressure (169).

However, it is the effect of respiration on cardiac flows that is the major hallmark for differentiating constrictive from restrictive cardiac diseases. Because the heart is effectively isolated from the thorax by its rigid encasement, it does not experience marked respiratory swings in pressure. Thus, on inspiration, intrathoracic (and therefore pulmonary vein) pressure decreases but left atrial pressure does not. Thus, the pulmonary vein-to-left atrial pressure gradient that drives left atrial inflow diminishes, as does mitral inflow. The resultant decreased left ventricular filling during diastole allows more room for right ventricular filling due to a septal shift and enhanced ventricular interdependence, and thus right-sided inflows increase. The exact opposite sequence occurs in expiration (3,66,174,450,451).

Filling pressures rise to compensate for the decrease in cardiac output via renal retention of salt and water. The finite space of the pericardium causes the filling pressure of the four chambers (and the pulmonary wedge pressure) to equalize. Intraventricular pressure recordings demonstrate the classic dip-and-plateau or square-root sign morphologies (Fig. 27.13). The "dip" represents the abrupt early filling at the atrioventricular valve opening related to high filling pressures and corresponds to a deep y descent on the central venous tracing. The "plateau" phase represents a period of unchanging pressure and volume related to the finite volume of the pericardial encasement. The x descent on the venous trace may also be prominent as systolic emptying of the ventricles allows filing of the atria. The x and y descents are sometimes referred to as the "W" pattern (452).

Differentiating Restriction from Constrictive Pericarditis

Hemodynamics. Cardiac catheterization has been traditionally the gold standard in distinguishing between these two

TABLE 27.8

DIFFERENTIAL DIAGNOSIS OF RESTRICTIVE CARDIOMYOPATHY AND CONSTRICTIVE PERICARDITIS

Type of evaluation	Restrictive cardiomyopathy	Constrictive pericarditis
Physical examination	Kussmaul's sign may be present Apical impulse may be prominent S_3 (advanced disease), S_4 (early disease) Regurgitant murmurs common Pulsus paradoxus absent	Kussmaul's sign usually present Apical impulse usually not palpable Pericardial knock may be present Regurgitant murmurs uncommon Pulsus paradoxus rare[a]
Electrocardiography	Low voltage (especially in amyloidosis), pseudoinfarction, left-axis deviation, atrial fibrillation, conduction disturbances common	Low voltage (<50%)
Chest radiography	Absent calcification	Calcification sometimes
Echocardiography	Small LV cavity with large atria Increased wall thickness sometimes present (especially thickened interatrial septum in amyloidosis) Thickened cardiac valves (amyloidosis) Granular sparkling texture (amyloidosis)	Normal wall thickness Pericardial thickening seen; prominent early diastolic filling with abrupt displacement of interventricular septum
Doppler studies		
Mitral inflow	No respiration variation of mitral inflow E wave, IVRT E/A ratio ≥2 Short DT Diastolic regurgitation	*With inspiration* Decreased mitral inflow E wave, prolonged IVRT *With expiration*, opposite changes Short DT Diastolic regurgitation
Pulmonary vein	Blunted S/D ratio (0.5), prominent and prolonged AR No respiration variation D wave	S/D ratio = 1 *With inspiration* Decreased PV S and D waves *With expiration*, opposite changes
Tricuspid inflow	Mild respiration variation of tricuspid inflow E wave E/A ratio ≥2 TR peak velocity, no significant respiration change Short DT with inspiration Diastolic regurgitation	*With inspiration* Increased tricuspid inflow E wave, increased TR peak velocity *With expiration*, opposite changes Short DT Diastolic regurgitation
Hepatic vein	Blunted S/D ratio, increased inspiratory reversals	*With inspiration* Minimally increased HV S and D *With expiration*, decreased diastolic flow and increased reversals
Inferior vena cava	Plethoric	Plethoric
Color M-mode	Slow flow propagation	Rapid flow propagation (≥100 cm/s)
Mitral annular motion	Low-velocity early filling (<8 cm/s)	High-velocity early filling (≥8 cm/s)
Cardiac catheterization	Dip and plateau LVEDP often >5 mm Hg greater than RVEDP, but may be identical RV systolic pressure >50 mm Hg RVEDP less than one-third of RV systolic pressure	Dip and plateau RVEDP and LVEDP usually equal *With inspiration* Increase in RV systolic pressure Decrease in LV systolic pressure *With expiration*, opposite changes
Endomyocardial biopsy	May reveal specific cause of restrictive cardiomyopathy	May be normal or show nonspecific myocyte hypertrophy or myocardial fibrosis
Computed tomography/magnetic resonance imaging	Pericardium usually normal	Pericardium may be thickened

AR, atrial reversal flow velocity; DT, deceleration time; IVRT, isovolumic relaxation time; LV, left ventricular; LVEDP, left ventricular end-diastolic pressure; RV, right ventricular; RVEDP, right ventricular end-diastolic pressure; TR, tricuspid regurgitation.
[a] Unless effusive or subacute constrictive pericarditis is present.
Modified from Kushwaha SS, Fallon JT, Fuster V. Restrictive cardiomyopathy. *N Engl J Med* 1997;336:267–276.

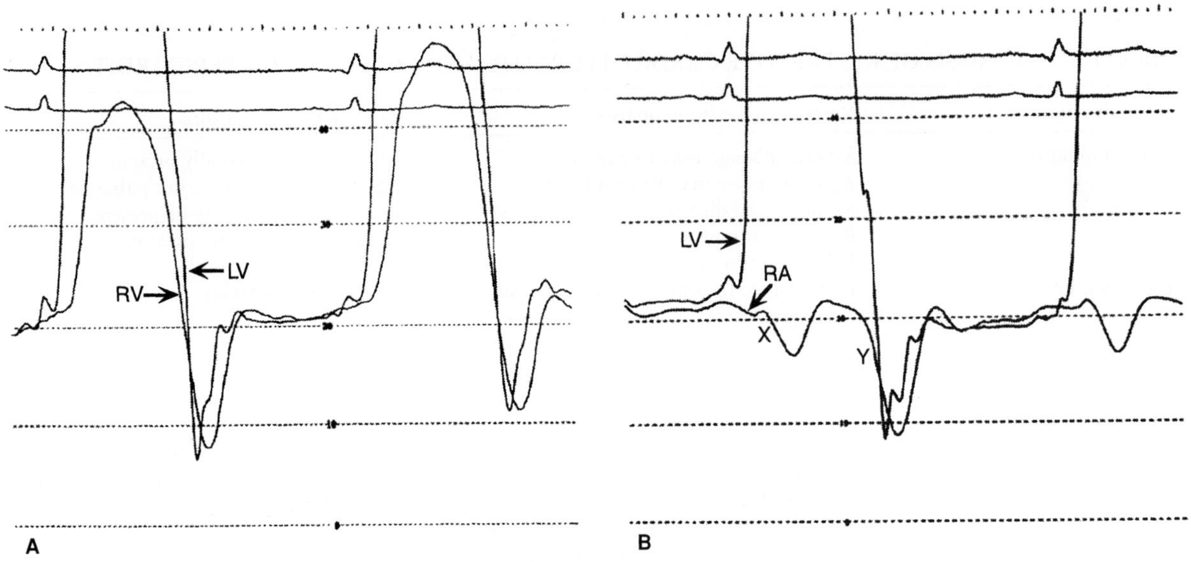

FIGURE 27.13. **A:** Simultaneous right ventricular (RV) and left ventricular (LV) pressure recordings demonstrating equalization of diastolic pressures and dip-and-plateau physiology. **B:** Simultaneous right atrial (RA) and LV pressure recordings demonstrating equalization during diastole and prominent X and Y descents in the RA tracing. (From Vaitkus PV, Cooper KA, Shuman WP, et al. Constrictive pericarditis. *Circulation* 1996;93:834–835.)

similar diseases; however, there can be overlap of the hemodynamics (66). Simultaneous recordings of the right and left heart pressures have revealed elevation and equalization (within 5 mm Hg) of the right atrial pressure, right ventricle diastolic pressure, PCWP, and pre-a-wave left ventricular diastolic pressure. The right atrial pressure contour typically shows an M or W configuration with a preserved systolic x descent and a prominent y descent and with small a and v waves. The right ventricular and left ventricular pressure tracings show a dip-and-plateau contour. The right ventricular and pulmonary artery systolic pressure is mildly elevated at less than 50 mm Hg compared to greater than 50 mm Hg in restriction. Administration of saline over 6 to 8 minutes can enhance the classic findings of constriction in a patient with occult constriction (416).

One small study of 11 patients with hemodynamic correlation demonstrated that brain natriuretic peptide (BNP) levels in isolated constrictive pericarditis are near normal compared to significantly elevated levels in patients with restriction (453).

Echocardiography. There have been many M-mode and two-dimensional signs that have been used to differentiate these two conditions; however, these signs have proven to be nonspecific and insensitive (454–457). The important two-dimensional echocardiographic features of constriction that may provide clues to the diagnosis include pericardial thickening, myocardial tethering, a septal bounce with respiration, and inferior vena cava plethora (169,458).

Doppler echocardiography. As described earlier, Doppler echocardiography with respirometry has emerged as a useful tool in these conditions (66,174,459). Limited ventricular filling and enhanced ventricular interaction account for the Doppler findings in constrictive pericarditis, whereas decreased distensibility of the ventricles accounts for the Doppler findings in restriction (66).

The classic Doppler echocardiographic findings are shown in Figures 27.14 and 27.15. The similarities with restriction examined by Doppler echocardiography include a short deceleration time indicative of the dip-and-plateau hemodynamic pattern and limited filling. The main differences include enhanced respiratory variation in mitral inflow and pulmonary venous flow ($\geq 25\%$) (at the onset of inspiration and expiration) in constriction but not restriction (unless a concomitant pericardial effusion accounting for respiratory variation is present). In restriction, there is a markedly blunted pulmonary venous systolic flow, with greater diastolic forward flow indicative of a prominent y descent and elevated left atrial pressures; in constriction, usually both systolic and diastolic flows are present (3). Due to enhanced ventricular interdependence, there is a decreased transtricuspid flow in expiration and enhanced expiratory flow reversals in the hepatic vein with constriction; there is increased inspiratory flow reversal in restriction. Respiratory variation in the tricuspid regurgitation peak velocity and velocity duration has been noted in constriction but not in restriction (460). Superior vena cava Doppler can help to distinguish respiratory variation of mitral inflow in patients with chronic obstructive lung disease and constrictive pericarditis (461). The systolic forward component of superior vena cava flow varies significantly with chronic obstructive lung disease, whereas there is little change with constrictive pericarditis. Color M-mode Doppler and tissue Doppler echocardiography have provided complimentary information in the evaluation of patients with constrictive pericarditis (85,86,462,463) (Fig. 27.16). The velocity of propagation from color M-mode and the tissue Doppler E annular velocity are normal or supranormal ($Vp \geq 100$ cm/s, $E_{annular} \geq 8$ cm/s) in constriction, representing normal compliance but abnormal relaxation. Exceptions to the finding of a normal tissue Doppler E annular velocity include patients with extensive annular calcification, LV dysfunction, or segmental differences in velocities (464).

There are several pitfalls in using Doppler echocardiography with respiratory monitoring for distinguishing constriction from restriction. Factors including depth of respiration, position of the sample volume, level of left atrial pressure, presence of concomitant myocardial disease or tricuspid regurgitation, and atrial fibrillation may influence the accuracy of the diagnosis. Transesophageal echocardiography may be used to delineate the anatomy (pericardial thickening) as well describe the physiology better than transthoracic echocardiography (174).

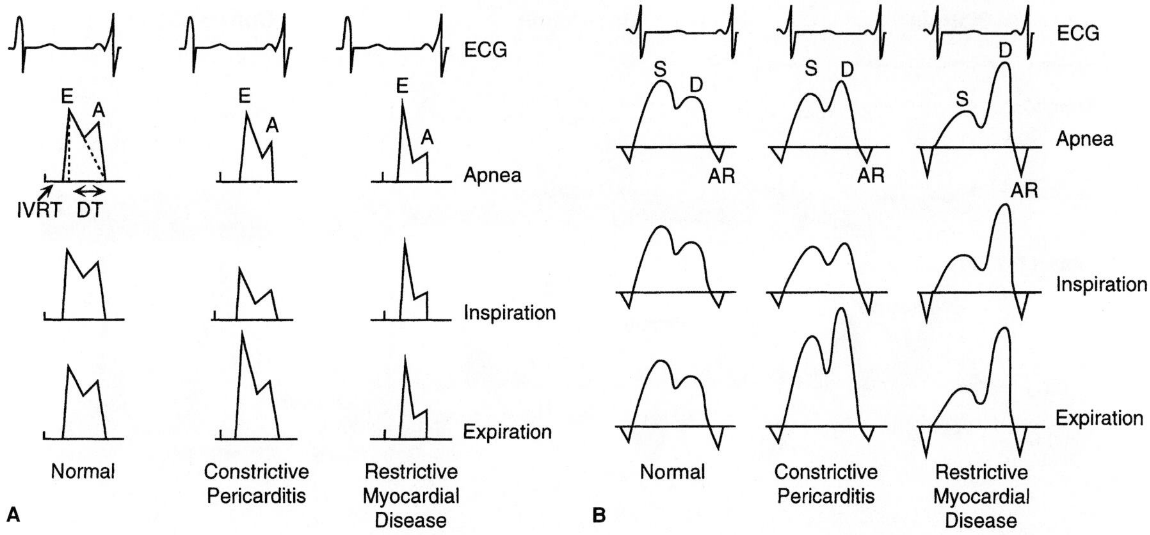

FIGURE 27.14. Left ventricular inflow velocities and pulmonary venous flow during different phases of respiration. AA, A wave velocity; AR, atrial reversal velocity; D, diastolic wave velocity; DT, deceleration time; E, E wave velocity; ECG, electrocardiogram; IVRT, isovolumic relaxation time; S, systolic wave velocity. (From Klein AL, Cohen GI. Doppler echocardiographic assessment of constrictive pericarditis, cardiac amyloidosis, and cardiac tamponade. *Cleve Clin J Med* 1992;59:278–290.)

Preload reduction maneuvers may be useful in lowering the left atrial pressure to enhance the respiratory variation, and volume loading may be used if the filling pressures are decreased (465,466). Mixed restriction/constriction may occur postirradiation and may have features of localized pericardial thickening with restrictive physiology (175,175a). In addition, atrial fibrillation may make it difficult to perform a Doppler evaluation of constriction and restriction. However, a series of 31 patients with constrictive pericarditis showed a similar respiratory variation of pulmonary venous flow and mitral inflow in patients with atrial fibrillation compared to normal sinus rhythm (467). Occasionally, ventricular pacing can be used to regularize the RR intervals in patients with atrial fibrillation. Constrictive pericarditis can also be evaluated in the operating room during mechanical ventilation. In a study with 15 patients, it was noted that positive-pressure ventilation reversed the pattern of respiratory variation of the mitral inflow and pulmonary venous flow velocities (468).

Magnetic Resonance Imaging for Pericardial Disease. Direct visualization of the pericardium is possible with MRI in healthy (469,470) and diseased states (471,472). This imaging modality is evolving as part of the routine work-up of suspected pericardial disease (4,451,473). In constrictive pericarditis, the pericardium is seen as a thickened, low-intensity signal band related to its fibrocalcific nature (474) (Fig. 27.17).

The increased pericardial thickening can be measured easily by MRI but does not necessarily indicate pericardial constriction (414). Ancillary findings by MRI include the conical or tubular narrowing of the ventricular cavities by the thickened

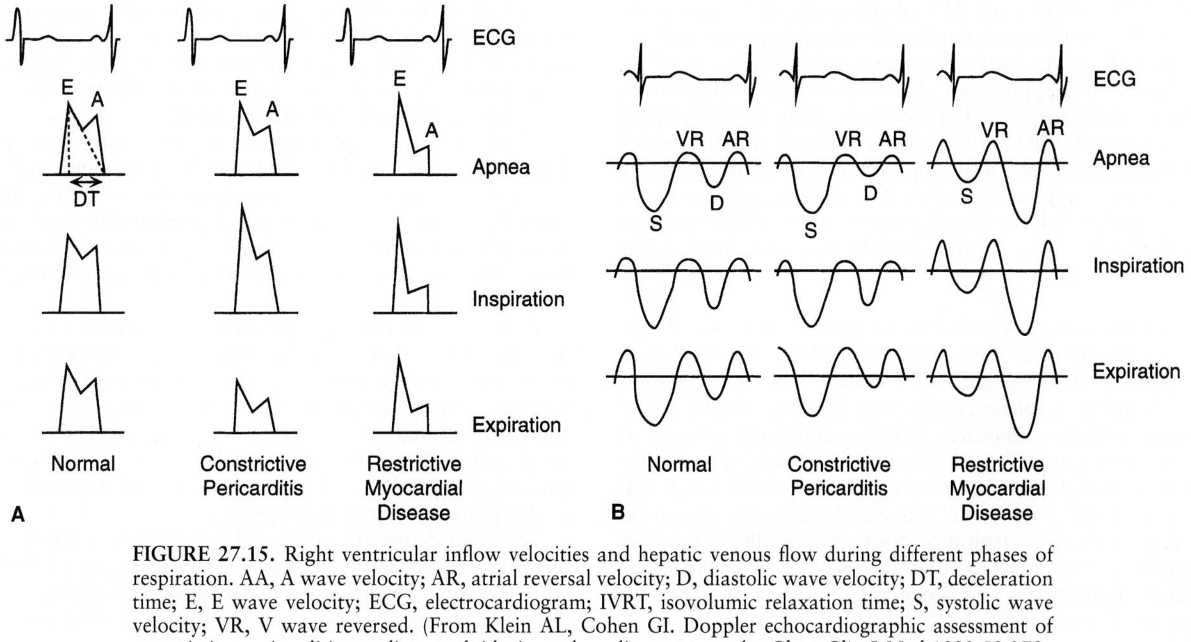

FIGURE 27.15. Right ventricular inflow velocities and hepatic venous flow during different phases of respiration. AA, A wave velocity; AR, atrial reversal velocity; D, diastolic wave velocity; DT, deceleration time; E, E wave velocity; ECG, electrocardiogram; IVRT, isovolumic relaxation time; S, systolic wave velocity; VR, V wave reversed. (From Klein AL, Cohen GI. Doppler echocardiographic assessment of constrictive pericarditis, cardiac amyloidosis, and cardiac tamponade. *Cleve Clin J Med* 1992;59:278–290.)

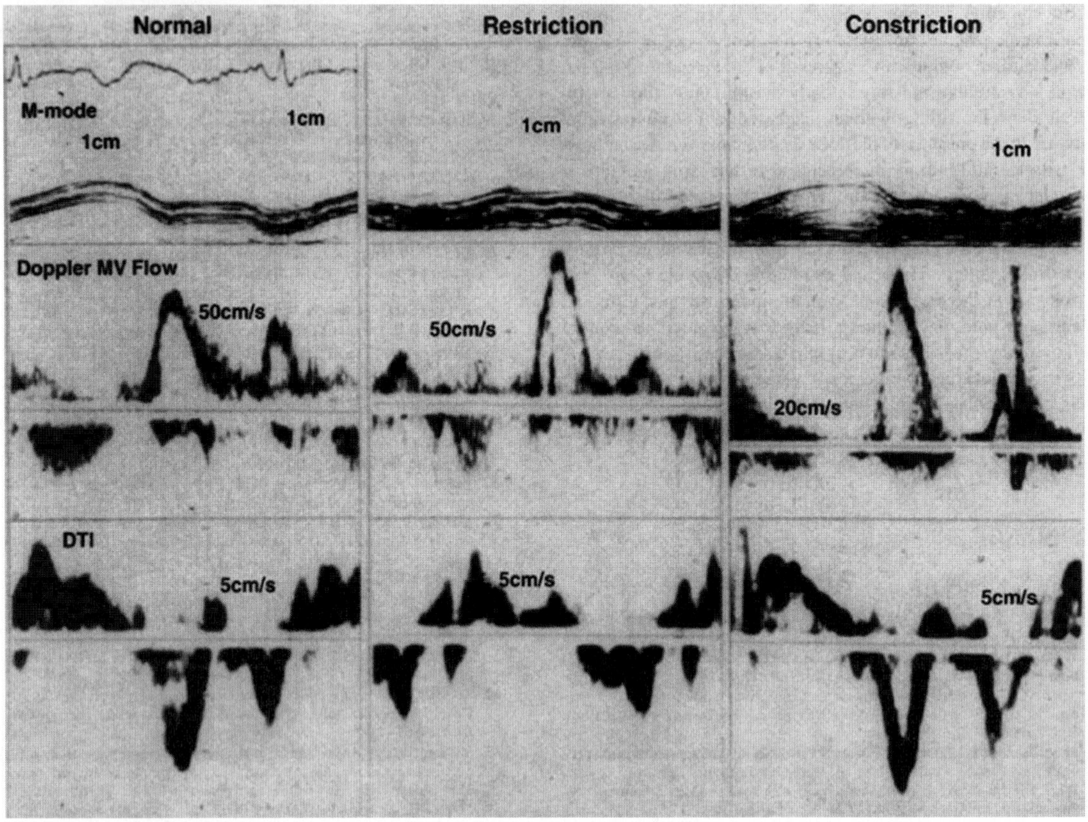

FIGURE 27.16. Samples of mitral annular M-mode tracings, Doppler tissue imaging (DTI) velocities in the longitudinal axis, and transmitral Doppler flow velocities in a normal volunteer, a patient with restrictive cardiomyopathy, and a patient with constrictive pericarditis. A marked difference is seen in early diastolic longitudinal axis velocities, despite similar early transmitral flow velocities. MV, mitral valve. (From Garcia MJ, Rodriguez L, Ares M, et al. Differentiation of constrictive pericarditis from restrictive cardiomyopathy; assessment of left ventricular diastolic velocities in longitudinal axis by Doppler tissue imaging. *J Am Coll Cardiol* 1996;27:108–114.)

pericardium, atrial dilation, inferior vena cava enlargement, hepatomegaly, and ascites. The sensitivity, specificity, and accuracy of MRI imaging in the diagnosis of constrictive pericarditis were 88%, 100%, and 93%, respectively, in one study (4). Cine MRI is useful in assessing the functional impairment of the abnormal filling in constriction compared to restriction (475), and phase flow mapping may show abnormal flow patterns in the superior vena cava that improve after pericardial stripping (476). However, MRI may have difficulty in distinguishing between calcification and fibrous tissue; thus, CT scanning may be better for assessing pericardial thickening when calcification is present (450,477,478). Gadolinium-enhanced MRI has been used in the diagnosis of tuberculous constrictive pericarditis (479).

Clinical Presentation. Patients with significant pericardial constriction present with congestive heart failure. Gross dependent edema, effusions, and ascites (480), hepatic congestion with dysfunction, splenomegaly, poor exercise tolerance, and cachexia constitute anasarca, of which constriction is one of the few remaining causes in developed nations. Jugular venous distention is common, with a prominent y descent (Friedreich's sign) (481); the classic Kussmaul sign (a rise in central venous pressure with inspiration due to the inability of the right atrium to receive additional volume) is seen in some cases. The syndrome is relentless and progressive, responding poorly to conservative medical therapy.

Pulsus paradoxus is seen when effusive constriction is present. Auscultation of the chest reveals quiet heart sounds, often with a pericardial knock, which correlates with the abrupt cessation of early diastolic filling (E wave) when the ventricles reach their finite-volume limit.

The ECG demonstrates low voltages with nonspecific T-wave changes. Atrial fibrillation is seen in a minority of patients. Chest roentgenography may demonstrate "egg shell" calcification of the pericardium, particularly in tuberculous pericarditis, and pleural effusions (482).

There may be variation in the presentation of constriction. These variants include localized constriction (localized scarring) (483), effusive constriction (after the pericardial fluid is drained), elastic constriction (thick pericardial fluid), latent or occult constriction (volume depleted), transient constriction (484), and constriction with normal pericardial thickness (485).

Effusive-constrictive pericarditis is a variation of constrictive pericarditis that is infrequently recognized. Confirmation of this diagnosis requires pericardiocentesis and cardiac catheterization. Patients present with predominant cardiac tamponade with elevated intrapericardial and intracardiac pressures. After pericardiocentesis with a fall to baseline intrapericardial pressure, the hemodynamics of constriction remains. Pericardiectomy is often required (486).

Transient constrictive pericarditis occurs in a subset of patients presenting with constrictive physiology due to almost all etiologies with the possible exception of radiation. Complete resolution of hemodynamic abnormalities and symptoms occurs after medical therapy for approximately 3 months. Pericardiectomy is not required (487,488).

A

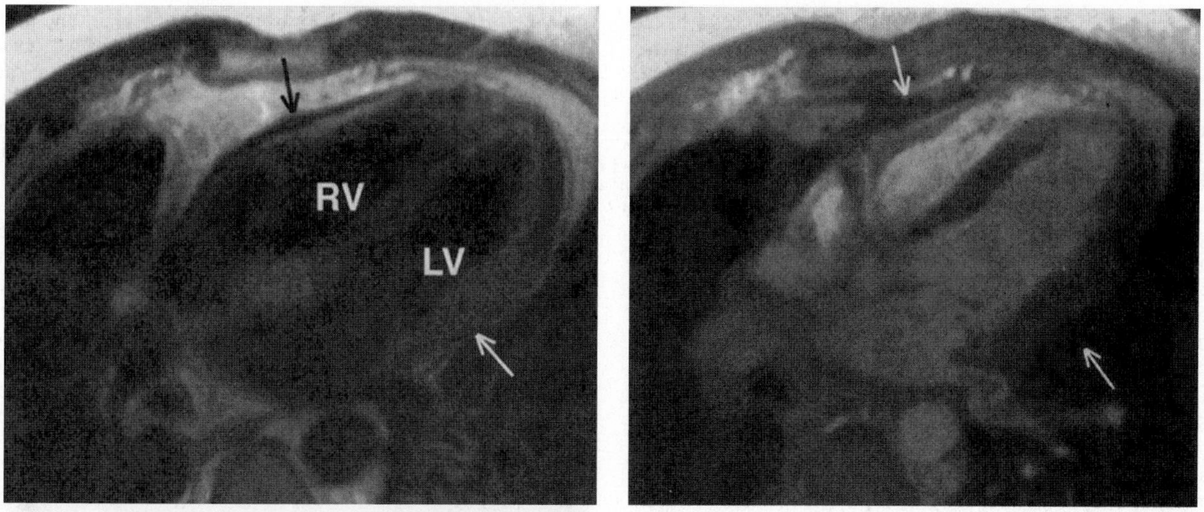

B

C

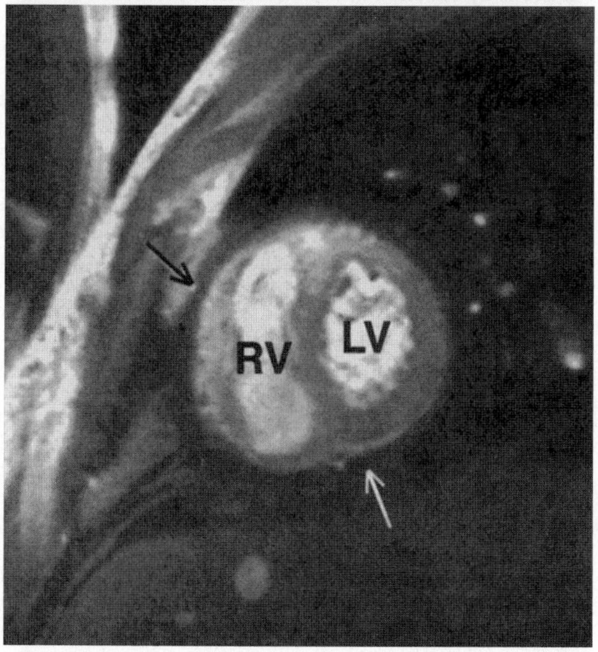

FIGURE 27.17. Constrictive pericarditis. Spin-echo and cine magnetic resonance imaging; horizontal long-axis and short-axis views. On the "dark blood" image (**A**), thickened pericardium is represented by a curvilinear signal void (*arrows*) separated by the bright signal of the epicardial and pericardial fat. There is an associated conical/tubular compression deformity of the basal and middle portions of the right ventricle (RV) and left ventricle (LV). On the "bright blood" images (**B, C**), the fibrous/calcified nature of the pericardium is confirmed by the dark appearance of the pericardium (*arrows*). The abnormal pericardium caused abrupt limitation of diastolic filling of the ventricles on the cine image loops. (Courtesy of R. D. White, MD, Cleveland Clinic Foundation.)

Treatment. Conservative medical management of constrictive pericarditis is at best palliative, with no substantial effect on the natural history of the disease. Diuretics decrease the intensity of fluid overload symptoms, and atrioventricular blocking agents and antiarrhythmics are useful for the management of atrial fibrillation. Surgical pericardiectomy remains the only definitive management of this problem and should be performed before calcification and myocardial involvement progress (450,489–491). In one series, a worse prognosis following pericardiectomy was associated with inadequate resection, higher NYHA functional class, radiation, myocardial involvement, residual coronary artery disease, older age, chronic disease, and arrhythmias (484). A second contemporary series of 135 patients with constrictive pericarditis found a 6% 30-day perioperative mortality for pericardiectomy and 78% and 57% 5- and 10-year survival, respectively, with improvement in functional class in most patients. Similar to prior studies, predictors of poor prognosis included advanced age, NYHA class, and postradiation etiology. Symptomatic benefit postpericardiectomy has been correlated with improvement in diastolic filling pattern and shorter duration of symptoms (492). Furthermore, the prognosis of patients after pericardiectomy largely depends on etiology, with a 30-day perioperative mortality of 2.7% for idiopathic constriction, 8.3% for postsurgical constriction, and 21.4% for postradiation constriction (overall 6%) (493).

Idiopathic and Viral Pericarditis

The majority of cases of acute pericarditis have no specific cause detected and are designated idiopathic. Many of these cases represent acute viral pericarditis. Attacks of this syndrome follow the seasonal epidemics of enterovirus infection (Coxsackie B and echovirus) (494). Proven viral cases are more likely to occur in immunocompromised hosts. Cytomegalovirus pericarditis has increased in frequency in association with immunocompromised hosts and early HIV infection (495–497). Most recently, myopericarditis has been reported associated with smallpox vaccination (498).

Clinical Presentation. Idiopathic or viral pericarditis in the immunocompetent host is typically self-limited beginning with a nonspecific flulike illness. There is often a history of a prodromal upper respiratory tract infection. There may be associated arthralgias and myalgias. Patients present with a syndrome of chest pain as described earlier. The pain is often severe, distressing, and associated with sympathetic activation—clamminess, pallor, and tremor. There is often an associated low-grade fever. Significant dyspnea is uncommon in simple cases unless there is hemodynamic compromise by a large pericardial effusion or associated viral pneumonitis (499).

The specific diagnosis of viral pericarditis should be entertained in all cases after other etiologic agents have been considered. However, the identification of the viral agent from serologic markers or from pericardial fluid occurs infrequently in clinical practice. A fourfold rise in serum antibody levels is highly suggestive of an underlying viral cause. Associated myocarditis is often associated with modest elevation of cardiac isozymes (404,494,500).

Uncomplicated acute pericarditis is a self-limited benign illness with few sequelae and a course ranging from days to a few weeks. Complications are infrequent and include (a) relapsing attacks of acute pericarditis (see later discussion), (b) acute tamponade, (c) acute myocarditis with ventricular dysfunction and late cardiomyopathy, and (d) chronic constrictive pericarditis (499).

Management. Specific antiviral therapy is not indicated for viral/idiopathic pericarditis in the immunocompetent host. Treatment is directed toward symptomatic relief. The mainstay of therapy centers on the oral antiinflammatory drugs, particularly aspirin (650 mg twice daily or three times daily) or most often on the nonsteroidal antiinflammatory agents (501) indomethacin (25 to 50 mg four times daily) and ibuprofen (800 mg three times daily). Most regimens are given for 7 to 10 days followed by a gradual tapering over 2 to 4 weeks to reduce recurrence and include gastric protection for patients at high risk of bleeding. Indomethacin should be reserved in adults due to deleterious effects on coronary blood flow and myocardial infarcts. Thus, other nonsteroidal agents are commonly used. No specific studies have used the COX-2 inhibitor agents. Colchicine (0.6 mg every 12 hours), with or without a load of 2 to 3 mg, may be used when added to the antiinflammatory agent or by itself in treating the initial attack or preventing recurrences (502–504). The COPE (Colchicine for Acute Pericarditis) trial randomized 120 patients with a first episode of acute pericarditis to aspirin versus aspirin plus colchicine (maintenance dose 0.5 to 1.0 mg daily) for 3 months. Patients receiving the colchicine regimen had a reduction in recurrence rate from 32.5% to 10.5%. Colchicine was discontinued in 8% of patients due to diarrhea (505).

There is no role for antibiotics unless purulent pericarditis has been documented. Systemic steroid therapy with prednisone has been used in severe and intractable cases but generally should be avoided during a first episode due to concern for recurrence after tapering (499,506). Some patients may have recurrent or incessant pericarditis that may be related to an immunopathic etiology (507). Not infrequently, these patients may be steroid dependent. Colchicine may be an effective drug to use when attempting to wean patients off steroids (508,509). Outpatient management of acute pericarditis is safe in patients without poor prognostic predictors, which include fever greater than 38°C, subacute onset, immunodepression, trauma, oral anticoagulants, myopericarditis, severe effusion, and cardiac tamponade (510).

CONTROVERSIES AND PERSONAL PERSPECTIVES

Decades ago the study of diastology, restrictive cardiomyopathy, and pericardial disease was largely limited to tertiary centers, required invasive diagnostic procedures, and was associated with poor outcomes and few treatment options. Now it is recognized that disorders of diastology are highly prevalent and that diastolic heart failure occurs often as a manifestation of common clinical problems. Over the last several years, many pivotal basic and clinical studies have furthered our understanding of the pathophysiology of diastolic dysfunction, aided in the characterization of specific disorders, and advanced the management of patients with diastolic heart failure.

Although some investigators have supported a broader classification of "heart failure with a normal ejection fraction (HFNEF)," recent work using invasively determined pressure–volume loops has confirmed that abnormalities in active relaxation and passive stiffness are operative in patients with heart failure and a normal ejection fraction. Therefore, diastolic heart failure should be accepted as a well-defined entity with heart failure symptoms, abnormalities of diastolic impairment, and normal or near-normal ejection fraction.

Echocardiography remains the cornerstone of the study of diastology. Additional lessons regarding the fundamentals of diastolic dysfunction have been learned with the use of newer, ultrasound-based technologies including strain, strain rate, tissue-tracking, and torsion imaging (511). These technologies have allowed for earlier recognition of diastolic dysfunction as well as aided in distinguishing primary forms of pathologic hypertrophy and restrictive cardiomyopathies and predicting preclinical deterioration to heart failure in select patient groups.

Concomitant with advances in cardiac ultrasound technology is the emergence of computed tomography and most notably cardiac magnetic resonance imaging for the evaluation and diagnosis of pericardial disease and restrictive cardiomyopathy. MRI with gadolinium enhancement has become an important test for the diagnosis of cardiac sarcoidosis, hemochromatosis, and amyloidosis and may predict cardiac events among patients with hypertrophic cardiomyopathy. Although these technological advances are not available to all clinicians, simple laboratory tests, such as BNP, have helped in the diagnosis of diastolic abnormalities including diastolic heart failure and correlated with filling pressures and stages of diastolic dysfunction.

Still dwarfed by the multitude of studies performed on patients with systolic heart failure, the CHARM-Preserved Trial represents a landmark first large-scale prospective study of patients with diastolic heart failure. Rather than treatment based solely on fluid regulation, optimization of hemodynamics, and correction of inciting factors, the use of angiotensin-receptor blockers in the CHARM study targeted the underlying pathophysiologic derangement of diastolic dysfunction. Overall, heart failure readmissions were decreased and there was a trend toward reduction in the combined endpoint of cardiac death and hospitalizations.

THE FUTURE

Although it is expected that echocardiographic techniques, cardiac MRI, CT, and the measurement of BNP levels will continue to elucidate the pathophysiology of diastology and related diseases and improve diagnosis and management strategies, we anticipate that the next frontier in diastology will occur in the development of better treatment options.

An evolution from a hemodynamic to a neurohormonal treatment paradigm for diastolic heart failure is expected. Aldosterone, angiotensin-converting-enzyme, and angiotensin-receptor antagonists require further investigation spurred by the findings of the CHARM Trial. Although currently limited to patients with systolic dysfunction, cardiac resynchronization therapy may have a role in the treatment of some patients with predominant diastolic heart failure. Stem cell and enzyme replacement therapies hold promise for specific primary diseases of diastology and require further study.

Genetic characterization of disorders of diastolic function remains limited and may have important clinical ramifications in the future. For example, there are few distinguishing features between late-onset hypertrophic cardiomyopathy and Fabry disease, two disorders with very different treatments. Genetic testing will help to diagnose patients with diseases of diastolic dysfunction and further select patients and relatives at high risk for cardiac events and help in tailoring treatment. A reclassification of cardiomyopathies based on genetic and cellular etiologies has been proposed by an AHA task force and will help to refocus emphasis on pre-clinical identification and targeted therapy (512).

References

1. Yellin EL, Nikolic S, Frater RW. Left ventricular filling dynamics and diastolic function. *Prog Cardiovasc Dis* 1990;32(4):247–271.
2. Thomas JD, Weyman AE. Echocardiographic Doppler evaluation of left ventricular diastolic function. Physics and physiology. *Circulation* 1991;84(3):977–990.
3. Klein AL, Cohen GI. Doppler echocardiographic assessment of constrictive pericarditis, cardiac amyloidosis, and cardiac tamponade. *Cleve Clin J Med* 1992;59(3):278–290.
4. Masui T, Finck S, Higgins CB. Constrictive pericarditis and restrictive cardiomyopathy: evaluation with MR imaging. *Radiology* 1992;182(2):369–373.
5. Brogan 3rd WC, Hillis LD, Flores Ed, et al. The natural history of isolated left ventricular diastolic dysfunction. *Am J Med* 1992;92(6):627–630.
6. Gaasch WH. Diagnosis and treatment of heart failure based on left ventricular systolic or diastolic dysfunction. *JAMA* 1994;271(16):1276–1280.
7. Little WC, Applegate RJ. Congestive heart failure: systolic and diastolic function. *J Cardiothorac Vasc Anesth* 1993;7(4 Suppl 2):2–5.

7a. Zile MR, Balcu CF, Bonnema DD. Diastolic heart failure: definitions and terminology. *Prog Cardiovasc Dis* 2005;47:307–313.

8. Gaasch WH. Diastolic dysfunction of the left ventricle: importance to the clinician. *Adv Intern Med* 1990;35:311–340.
9. Little WC, Downes TR. Clinical evaluation of left ventricular diastolic performance. *Prog Cardiovasc Dis* 1990;32(4):273–290.
10. Brutsaert DL, Sys SU, Gillebert TC. Diastolic failure: pathophysiology and therapeutic implications. *J Am Coll Cardiol* 1993;22(1):318–325.
11. Thomas JD, Klein AL. Doppler-echocardiographic evaluation of diastolic function. In: Skorton DJ, Schelbert HR, Wolf GL, Brundage BH, eds. *Marcus' cardiac imaging: a companion to Braunwald's heart disease*, 2nd ed. Philadelphia: WB Saunders, 1996;336–364.
12. Zile MR, Baicu CF, Gaasch WH. Diastolic heart failure—abnormalities in active relaxation and passive stiffness of the left ventricle. *N Engl J Med* 2004;350(19):1953–1959.
13. European Study Group on Diastolic Heart Failure. How to diagnose diastolic heart failure. *Eur Heart J* 1998;19(7):990–1003.
14. Vasan RS and Levy D. Defining diastolic heart failure: a call for standardized diagnostic criteria. *Circulation* 2000;101(17):2118–2121.

14a. Zile MR, Gaasch WH, Carroll JD, et al. Heart failure with a normal ejection fraction: Is measurement of diastolic function necessary to make the diagnosis of diastolic heart failure? *Circulation* 2001;104:779–782.

15. Zile MR. Diastolic dysfunction: detection, consequences and treatment. Part 1: Definition and determinants of diastolic function. *Mod Concepts Cardiovasc Dis* 1989;58(12):67–72.
16. Lorell BH, Apstein CS, Weinberg EO, et al. Diastolic function in left ventricular hypertrophy: clinical and experimental relationships. *Eur Heart J* 1990;11(Suppl G):54–64.
17. Gaasch WH, Quinones MA, Waisser E, et al. Diastolic compliance of the left ventricle in man. *Am J Cardiol* 1975;36(2):193–201.
18. Flachskampf FA, Weyman AE, Guerrero JL, et al. Calculation of atrioventricular compliance from the mitral flow profile: analytic and in vitro study. *J Am Coll Cardiol* 1992;19(5):998–1004.
19. Keren G, Bier A, Sherez J, et al. Atrial contraction is an important determinant of pulmonary venous flow. *J Am Coll Cardiol* 1986;7(3):693–695.
20. Grimm RA, Leung DY, Black IW, et al. Left atrial appendage "stunning" after spontaneous conversion of atrial fibrillation demonstrated by transesophageal Doppler echocardiography. *Am Heart J* 1995;130(1):174–176.
21. Klein AL, Tajik AJ. Doppler assessment of pulmonary venous flow in healthy subjects and in patients with heart disease. *J Am Soc Echocardiogr* 1991;4(4):379–392.
22. Keren G, Meisner JS, Sherez J, et al. Interrelationship of mid-diastolic mitral valve motion, pulmonary venous flow, and transmitral flow. *Circulation* 1986;74(1):36–44.
23. Appleton CP. Influence of incremental changes in heart rate on mitral flow velocity: Assessment in lightly sedated, conscious dogs. *J Am Coll Cardiol* 1991;17(1):227–236.
24. Thomas JD, Flachskampf FA, Chen C, et al. Isovolumic relaxation time varies predictably with its time constant and aortic and left atrial pressures: implications for the noninvasive evaluation of ventricular relaxation. *Am Heart J* 1992;124(5):1305–1313.
25. Weiss JL, Frederikson JW, Weisfeldt JL. Hemodynamic determinants of the time-course of fall in canine left ventricular pressure. *J Clin Invest* 1976;58(3):751–760.
26. Raaf G, Glantz S. Volume loading slows left ventricular isovolumic relaxation rate. Evidence of load-dependent relaxation in the intact dog heart. *Circ Res* 1981;48(6 Pt 1):813–824.
27. Lee CH, Vancheri F, Josen MS, et al. Discrepancies in the measurement of isovolumic relaxation time: a study comparing M mode and Doppler echocardiography. *Br Heart J* 1990;64(3):214–218.
28. Lewis BS, Lewis N, Sapoznikov D, et al. Isovolumic relaxation period in man. *Am Heart J* 1980;100(4):490–499.
29. Klein AL, Oh JK, Miller FA, et al. Two-dimensional and Doppler echocardiographic assessment of infiltrative cardiomyopathy. *J Am Soc Echocardiogr* 1988;1(1):48–59.
30. Brun P, Tribouilloy C, Duval AM, et al. Left ventricular flow propagation during early filling is related to wall relaxation: a color M-mode Doppler analysis. *J Am Coll Cardiol* 1992;20(2):420–432.
31. Garcia MJ, Thomas JD, Klein AL. New Doppler echocardiographic applications for the study of diastolic function. *J Am Coll Cardiol* 1998;32(4):865–875.
32. Choong CY, Abascal VM, Thomas JD, et al. Combined influence of ventricular loading and relaxation in the transmitral flow velocity profile in dogs measured by Doppler echocardiography. *Circulation* 1988;78(3):672–683.
33. Robinson TF, Factor SM, Sonnenblick EH. The heart as a suction pump. *Sci Am* 1986;254(6):84–91.
34. Suga H, Goto Y, Igarashi Y, et al. Ventricular suction under zero source pressure for filling. *Am J Physiol* 1986;251(1 Pt 2):H47–H55.
35. Nikolic S, Yellin EL, Tamura K, et al. Passive properties of the canine left ventricle: diastolic stiffness and restoring forces. *Circ Res* 1988;62(6):1210–1222.
36. Thomas JD, Newell JB, Choong CY, et al. Influence of ventricular loading, compliance, and relaxation on transmitral velocity: hydrodynamic and numerical analysis. *Am J Physiol* 1991;260(5 Pt 2):H1718–H1731.
37. Pouleur H. Diastolic dysfunction and myocardial energetics. *Eur Heart J* 1990;11(Suppl C):30–34.
38. Bonow RO, Udelson JE. Left ventricular diastolic dysfunction as a cause of congestive heart failure. Mechanisms and management. *Ann Intern Med* 1992;117(6):502–510.
39. Morgan JP, Erny RE, Allen PD, et al. Abnormal intracellular calcium handling, a major cause of systolic and diastolic dysfunction in ventricular myocardium from patients with heart failure. *Circulation* 1990;81(2 Suppl): III21–III32.
40. Cunningham MJ, Apstein CS, Weinberg EO, et al. Deleterious effect of ouabain on myocardial function during hypoxia. *Am J Physiol* 1989;256 (3 Pt 2):H681–H687.
41. Courtois M, Kovacs Jr SJ, Ludbrook PA. Transmitral pressure–flow velocity relation: importance of regional pressure gradients in the left ventricle during diastole. *Circulation* 1988;78(3):661–671.
42. Lorell BH, Grossman W. Cardiac hypertrophy: the consequences for diastole. *J Am Coll Cardiol* 1987;9(5):1189–1193.
43. Ling D, Rankin JS, Edwards 2nd CH, et al. Regional diastolic mechanics of the left ventricle in the conscious dog. *Am J Physiol* 1979;236(2):H323–H330.
44. Courtois M, Kovacs SJ, Ludbrook PA. Physiological early diastolic intraventricular pressure gradient is lost during acute myocardial ischemia. *Circulation* 1990;81(5):1688–1696.
45. Janicki J, Matsubara B. Myocardial collagen and left ventricular diastolic function. In: Gaasch W, LeWinter M, eds. *Left ventricular diastolic dysfunction and heart failure*. Philadelphia: Lea & Febiger, 1994:125–140.
46. Matsubara B, Hennigar J, Janicki J. Structural and functional role of myocardial collagen. *Circulation* 1991;84(4):II212.
47. Factor SM, Flomenbaum M, Zhao MJ, et al. The effect of acutely increased ventricular cavity pressure on intrinsic myocardial connective tissue. *J Am Coll Cardiol* 1988;12(6):1582–1589.
48. Lerman RH, Apstein CS, Kagan HM, et al. Myocardial healing and repair after experimental infarction in the rabbit. *Circ Res* 1983;53(3):378–388.
49. Gilbert JC, Glantz SA. Determinants of left ventricular filling and the diastolic pressure–volume relation. *Circ Res* 1989;64(5):827–852.
50. Cheng CP, Igarashi Y, Little WC. Mechanism of augmented rate of left ventricular filling during exercise. *Circ Res* 1992;70(1):9–19.
51. Tyberg JV, Misbach GA, Glantz SA, et al. A mechanism for shifts in the diastolic, left ventricular, pressure–volume curve: the role of the pericardium. *Eur J Cardiol* 1978;7(Suppl):163–175.
52. Shah PM, Pai RG. Diastolic heart failure. *Curr Probl Cardiol* 1992; 17(12):781–868.
53. Cheng CP, Freeman GL, Santamore WP, et al. Effect of loading conditions, contractile state, and heart rate on early diastolic left ventricular filling in conscious dogs. *Circ Res* 1990;66(3):814–823.

54. Ishida Y, Meisner JS, Tsujioka K, et al. Left ventricular filling dynamics: influence of left ventricular relaxation and left atrial pressure. *Circulation* 1986;74(1):187–196.
55. Toutouzas P, Stefanadis C, Boudoulas H. 1st international symposium on left atrial function: introduction. *Eur Heart J* 2000;2(Suppl):K1–K3.
56. Ito T, Suwa M, Hirota Y, et al. Influence of left atrial function on Doppler transmitral and pulmonary venous flow patterns in dilated and hypertrophic cardiomyopathy: evaluation of left atrial appendage function by transesophageal echocardiography. *Am Heart J* 1996;131(1):122–130.
57. Pollick C, Taylor D. Assessment of left atrial appendage function by transesophageal echocardiography. Implications for the development of thrombus. *Circulation* 1991;84(1):223–231.
58. Lau VK, Sagawa K, Suga H. Instantaneous pressure volume relationship of right atrium during isovolumic contraction in the canine heart. *Am J Physiol* 1979;236(5):H672–H679.
59. Klein AL, Burstow DJ, Tajik AJ, et al. Effects of age on left ventricular dimensions and filling dynamics in 117 normal persons. *Mayo Clin Proc* 1994;69(3):212–224.
60. Plehn JF, Friedman BJ. Diastolic dysfunction in amyloid heart disease: restrictive cardiomyopathy or not? *J Am Coll Cardiol* 1989;13(1):54–56.
61. Harrison MR, Clifton GD, Pennell AT, et al. Effect of heart rate on left ventricular diastolic transmitral flow velocity patterns assessed by Doppler echocardiography in normal subjects. *Am J Cardiol* 1991;67(7):622–627.
62. Walsh RA. Sympathetic control of diastolic function in congestive heart failure. *Circulation* 1990;82(2 Suppl):I52–I58.
63. Panidis IP, Ross J, Munley B, et al. Diastolic mitral regurgitation in patients with atrioventricular conduction abnormalities: a common finding by Doppler echocardiography. *J Am Coll Cardiol* 1986;7(4):768–774.
64. Tanabe A, Mohri T, Ohga M, et al. The effects of pacing-induced left bundle branch block on left ventricular systolic and diastolic performances. *Jpn Heart J* 1990;31(3):309–317.
65. Xiao HB, Lee CH, Gibson DG. Effect of left bundle branch block on diastolic function in dilated cardiomyopathy. *Br Heart J* 1991;66(6):443–447.
66. Hatle LK, Appleton CP, Popp RL. Differentiation of constrictive pericarditis and restrictive cardiomyopathy by Doppler echocardiography. *Circulation* 1989;79(2):357–370.
67. Appleton CP, Jensen JL, Hatle LK, et al. Doppler evaluation of left and right ventricular diastolic function: a technical guide for obtaining optimal flow velocity recordings. *J Am Soc Echocardiogr* 1997;10(3):271–292.
68. Mantero A, Gentile F, Gualtierotti C, et al. Left ventricular diastolic parameters in 288 normal subjects from 20 to 80 years old. *Eur Heart J* 1995;16(1):94–105.
69. Appleton CP, Hatle LK, Popp RL. Relation of transmitral flow velocity patterns to left ventricular diastolic function: new insights from a combined hemodynamic and Doppler echocardiographic study. *J Am Coll Cardiol* 1988;12(2):426–440.
70. Dumesnil JG, Gaudreault G, Honos GN, et al. Use of Valsalva maneuver to unmask left ventricular diastolic function abnormalities by Doppler echocardiography in patients with coronary artery disease or systemic hypertension. *Am J Cardiol* 1991;68(5):515–519.
71. Appleton CP, Hatle LK. The natural history of left ventricular filling abnormalities: assessment by two-dimensional and Doppler echocardiography. *Echocardiography* 1992;9(4):437–457.
72. Plehn JF, Southworth J, Cornwell 3rd GG. Brief report: atrial systolic failure in primary amyloidosis. *N Engl J Med* 1992;327(22):1570–1573.
73. Klein AL, Hatle LK, Burstow DJ, et al. Comprehensive Doppler assessment of right ventricular diastolic function in cardiac amyloidosis. *J Am Coll Cardiol* 1990;15(1):99–108.
74. Klein AL, Leung DY, Murray RD, et al. Effects of age and physiologic variables on right ventricular filling dynamics in normal subjects. *Am J Cardiol* 1999;84(4):440–448.
75. Cohen GI, Pietrolungo JF, Thomas JD, et al. A practical guide to assessment of ventricular diastolic function using Doppler echocardiography. *J Am Coll Cardiol* 1996;27(7):1753–1760.
76. Appleton CP, Hatle LK, Popp RL. Superior vena cava and hepatic vein Doppler echocardiography in healthy adults. *J Am Coll Cardiol* 1987; 10(5):1032–1039.
77. Zoghbi WA, Habib GB, Quinones MA. Doppler assessment of right ventricular filling in a normal population. Comparison with left ventricular filling dynamics. *Circulation* 1990;82(4):1316–1324.
78. Stugaard M, Smiseth OA, Risoe C, et al. Intraventricular early diastolic filling during acute myocardial ischemia, assessment by multigated color m-mode Doppler echocardiography. *Circulation* 1993;88(6):2705–2713.
79. Stugaard M, Steen T, Lundervold A, et al. Visual assessment of intra ventricular flow from colour M-mode Doppler images. *Int J Card Imaging* 1994; 10(4):279–287.
80. Takatsuji H, Mikami T, Urasawa K, et al. A new approach for evaluation of left ventricular diastolic function: spatial and temporal analysis of left ventricular filling flow propagation by color M-mode Doppler echocardiography. *J Am Coll Cardiol* 1996;27(2):365–371.
81. Moller JE, Sondergaard E, Seward JB, et al. Ratio of left ventricular peak E-wave velocity to flow propagation velocity assessed by color M-mode Doppler echocardiography in first myocardial infarction: prognostic and clinical implications. *J Am Coll Cardiol* 2000;35(2):363–370.
82. Duval-Moulin AM, Dupouy P, Brun P, et al. Alteration of left ventricular diastolic function during coronary angioplasty–induced ischemia: a color M-mode Doppler study. *J Am Coll Cardiol* 1997;29(6):1246–1255.
83. Garcia MJ, Smedira NG, Greenberg NL, et al. Color M-mode Doppler flow propagation velocity is a preload insensitive index of left ventricular relaxation: animal and human validation. *J Am Coll Cardiol* 2000;35(1): 201–208.
84. Garcia MJ, Ares MA, Asher C, et al. An index of early left ventricular filling that combined with pulsed Doppler peak E velocity may estimate capillary wedge pressure. *J Am Coll Cardiol* 1997;29(2):448–454.
85. Rajagopalan N, Garcia MJ, Rodriguez L, et al. Comparison of new Doppler echocardiographic methods to differentiate constrictive pericardial heart disease and restrictive cardiomyopathy. *Am J Cardiol* 2001; 87(1):86–94.
86. Garcia MJ, Rodriguez L, Ares M, et al. Differentiation of constrictive pericarditis from restrictive cardiomyopathy: assessment of left ventricular diastolic velocities in longitudinal axis by Doppler tissue imaging. *J Am Coll Cardiol* 1996;27(1):108–114.
87. Hatle L, Sutherland GR. Regional myocardial function—a new approach. *Eur Heart J* 2000;21(16):1337–1357.
88. Trambaiolo P, Tonti G, Salustri A, et al. New insights into regional systolic and diastolic left ventricular function with tissue Doppler echocardiography: from quantitative analysis to a quantitative approach. *J Am Soc Echocardiogr* 2001;14(2):85–96.
89. Garcia MJ, Rodriguez L, Ares M, et al. Myocardial wall velocity assessment by pulsed Doppler tissue imaging: characteristic findings in normal subjects. *Am Heart J* 1996;132:648–656.
90. Garcia MJ, Thomas JD. Tissue Doppler to assess diastolic left ventricular function. *Echocardiography* 1999;16(5):501–508.
91. Rodriguez L, Garcia M, Ares M, et al. Assessment of mitral annular dynamics during diastole by Doppler tissue imaging: comparison with mitral Doppler inflow in subjects without heart disease and in patients with left ventricular hypertrophy. *Am Heart J* 1996;131(5):982–987.
92. Oki T, Tabata T, Yamada H, et al. Clinical application of pulsed Doppler tissue imaging for assessing abnormal left ventricular relaxation. *Am J Cardiol* 1997;79(7):921–928.
93. Sohn DW, Chai IH, Lee DJ, et al. Assessment of mitral annulus velocity by Doppler tissue imaging in the evaluation of left ventricular diastolic function. *J Am Coll Cardiol* 1997;30(2):474–480.
94. Nagueh SF, Sun H, Kopelen HA, et al. Hemodynamic determinants of the mitral annulus diastolic velocities by tissue Doppler. *J Am Coll Cardiol* 2001;37:278–285.
95. Firstenberg MS, Greenberg NL, Main ML, et al. Determinants of diastolic myocardial tissue Doppler velocities: influences of relaxation and preload. *J Appl Physiol* 2001;90(1):299–307.
96. Farias CA, Rodriguez L, Garcia MJ, et al. Assessment of diastolic function by tissue Doppler echocardiography: comparison with standard transmitral and pulmonary venous flow. *J Am Soc Echocardiogr* 1999;12(8):609–617.
97. Ommen SR, Nishimura RA, Appleton CP, et al. Clinical utility of Doppler echocardiography and tissue Doppler imaging in the estimation of left ventricular filling pressures: a comparative simultaneous Doppler-catheterization study. *Circulation* 2000;102(15):1788–1794.
98. Urheim S, Edvardsen T, Torp H, et al. Myocardial strain by Doppler echocardiography. Validation of a new method to quantify regional myocardial function. *Circulation* 2000;102(10):1158–1164.
99. Greenberg NL, Lever H, Castro P, et al. Evaluation of segmental myocardial strain rate by tissue Doppler echocardiography in a feline model of hypertrophic cardiomyopathy. *J Am Coll Cardiol* 1999;33:458A.
100. Sutherland GR, Kukulski T, Voight JU, et al. Tissue Doppler echocardiography: future developments. *Echocardiography* 1999;16(5):509–520.
101. Stoylen A, Heimdal A, Bjornstad K, et al. Strain rate imaging by ultrasonography in the diagnosis of coronary artery disease. *J Am Soc Echocardiogr* 2000;13(12):1053–1064.
101a. Marwick TH. Measurement of strain and strain rate by echocardiography: Ready for prime time? *J Am Coll Cardiol* 2006;47:1313–1327.
102. Nishimura RA, Tajik AJ. Evaluation of diastolic filling of left ventricle in health and disease: Doppler echocardiography is the clinician's Rosetta Stone. *J Am Coll Cardiol* 1997;30(1):8–18.
103. Rakowski H, Appleton C, Chan KL, et al. Canadian consensus recommendations for the measurement and reporting of diastolic dysfunction by echocardiography: from the Investigators of Consensus on Diastolic Dysfunction by Echocardiography. *J Am Soc Echocardiogr* 1996;9(5):736–760.
104. Rossvoll O, Hatle LK. Pulmonary venous flow velocities recorded by transthoracic Doppler ultrasound: relation to left ventricular diastolic pressures. *J Am Coll Cardiol* 1993;21(7):1687–1696.
105. Iliceto S, Amico A, Marangelli V, et al. Doppler echocardiographic evaluation of the effect of atrial pacing–induced ischemia on left ventricular filling in patients with coronary artery disease. *J Am Coll Cardiol* 1988; 11(5):953–961.
106. Takenaka K, Dabestani A, Gardin JM, et al. Left ventricular filling in hypertrophic cardiomyopathy: a pulsed Doppler echocardiographic study. *J Am Coll Cardiol* 1986;7(6):1263–1271.
107. Bryg RJ, Pearson AC, Williams GA, et al. Left ventricular systolic and diastolic flow abnormalities determined by Doppler echocardiography in

obstructive hypertrophic cardiomyopathy. *Am J Cardiol* 1987;59(9):925–931.
108. Otto CM, Pearlman AS, Amsler LC. Doppler echocardiographic evaluation of left ventricular diastolic filling in isolated valvular aortic stenosis. *Am J Cardiol* 1989;63(5):313–316.
109. Choong CY, Herrmann HC, Weyman AE, et al. Preload dependence of Doppler-derived indexes of left ventricular diastolic function in humans. *J Am Coll Cardiol* 1987;10(4):800–808.
110. Hurrell DG, Nishimura RA, Ilstrup DM, et al. Utility of preload alteration in assessment of left ventricular filling pressure by Doppler echocardiography: a simultaneous catheterization and Doppler echocardiographic study. *J Am Coll Cardiol* 1997;30(2):459–467.
111. Appleton CP, Galloway JM, Gonzalez MS, et al. Estimation of left ventricular filling pressures using two-dimensional and Doppler echocardiography in adult patients with cardiac disease. Additional value of analyzing left atrial size, left atrial ejection fraction and the difference in duration of pulmonary venous and mitral flow velocity at atrial contraction. *J Am Coll Cardiol* 1993;22(7):1972–1982.
112. Klein AL, Hatle LK, Taliercio CP, et al. Serial Doppler echocardiographic follow-up of left ventricular diastolic function in cardiac amyloidosis. *J Am Coll Cardiol* 1990;16(5):1135–1141.
113. Kuecherer HF, Muhiudeen IA, Kusumoto FM, et al. Estimation of mean left atrial pressure from transesophageal pulsed Doppler echocardiography of pulmonary venous flow. *Circulation* 1990;82(4):1127–1139.
114. Klein AL, Hatle LK, Taliercio CP, et al. Prognostic significance of Doppler measures of diastolic function in cardiac amyloidosis. A Doppler echocardiography study. *Circulation* 1991;83(3):808–816.
115. Oh JK, Ding ZP, Gersh BJ, et al. Restrictive left ventricular diastolic filling identifies patients with heart failure after acute myocardial infarction. *J Am Soc Echocardiogr* 1992;5(5):497–503.
116. Pinamonti B, Di Lenarda A, Sinagra G, et al. Restrictive left ventricular filling pattern in dilated cardiomyopathy assessed by Doppler echocardiography: clinical, echocardiographic and hemodynamic correlations and prognostic implications. Heart Muscle Disease Study Group. *J Am Coll Cardiol* 1993;22(3):808–815.
117. Rihal CS, Nishimura RA, Hatle LK, et al. Systolic and diastolic dysfunction in patients with clinical diagnosis of dilated cardiomyopathy. Relation to symptoms and prognosis. *Circulation* 1994;90(6):2772–2779.
118. Nishimura RA, Appleton CP, Redfield MM, et al. Noninvasive Doppler echocardiographic evaluation of left ventricular filling pressures in patients with cardiomyopathies: a simultaneous Doppler echocardiographic and cardiac catherization. *J Am Coll Cardiol* 1996;28(5):1226–1233.
119. Pozzoli M, Traversi E, Cioffi G, et al. Loading conditions improve the prognostic value of Doppler evaluation of mitral flow in patients with chronic heart failure. *Circulation* 1997;95(5):1222–1230.
120. Pinamonti B, Zecchin M, Di Lenarda A, et al. Persistence of restrictive left ventricular filling pattern in dilated cardiomyopathy: an ominous prognostic sign. *J Am Coll Cardiol* 1997;29(3):604–612.
121. Stork TV, Muller RM, Piske GJ, et al. Noninvasive measurement of left ventricular filling pressures by means of transmitral pulsed Doppler ultrasound. *Am J Cardiol* 1989;64(10):655–660.
122. Vanoverschelde JL, Robert AR, Gerbaux A, et al. Noninvasive estimation of pulmonary arterial wedge pressure with Doppler transmitral flow velocity pattern in patients with known heart disease. *Am J Cardiol* 1995; 75(5):383–389.
123. Nagueh SF, Middleton KJ, Kopelen HA, et al. Doppler tissue imaging: a noninvasive technique for evaluation of left ventricular relaxation and estimation of filling pressures. *J Am Coll Cardiol* 1997;30(6):1527–1533.
124. Nagueh SF, Kopelen HA, Quinones MA. Assessment of left ventricular filling pressures by Doppler in the presence of atrial fibrillation. *Circulation* 1996;94(9):2138–2154.
125. Gonzalez-Vilchez F, Ares M, Ayuela J, et al. Combined use of pulsed and color M-mode Doppler echocardiography for the estimation of pulmonary capillary wedge pressure: an empirical approach based on an analytical relation. *J Am Coll Cardiol* 1999;34(2):515–523.
126. Chirillo F, Brunazzi MC, Barbiero M, et al. Estimating mean pulmonary wedge pressure in patients with chronic atrial fibrillation from transthoracic Doppler indexes of mitral and pulmonary venous flow velocity. *J Am Coll Cardiol* 1997;30(1):19–26.
127. Brunazzi MC, Chirillo F, Pasqualini M, et al. Estimation of left ventricular diastolic pressures from precordial pulsed-Doppler analysis of pulmonary venous and mitral flow. *Am Heart J* 1994;128(2)293–300.
128. Klein AL, Abdalla I, Murray RD, et al. Age independence of the difference in duration of pulmonary venous atrial reversal flow and transmitral A-wave flow in normal subjects. *J Am Soc Echocardiogr* 1998;11(5):458–465.
129. Abdalla I, Murray RD, Lee JC, et al. Duration of pulmonary venous atrial reversal flow velocity and mitral inflow a wave: new measure of severity of cardiac amyloidosis. *J Am Soc Echocardiogr* 1998;11(12):1125–1133.
130. Dini FL, Dell'Anna R, Micheli A, et al. Impact of blunted pulmonary venous flow on the outcome of patients with left ventricular systolic dysfunction secondary to either ischemic or idiopathic dilated cardiomyopathy. *Am J Cardiol* 2000;85(12):1455–1460.
131. Devereux RB, Roman MJ, Liu JE, et al. Congestive heart failure despite normal left ventricular systolic function in a population-based sample: the Strong Heart Study. *Am J Cardiol* 2000;86(10):1090–1096.
132. Senni M, Tribouilloy CM, Rodeheffer RJ, et al. Congestive heart failure in the community: a study of all incident cases in Olmsted County, Minnesota, in 1991. *Circulation* 1998;98(21):2282–2289.
133. Gandhi SK, Powers JC, Nomeir AM, et al. The pathogenesis of acute pulmonary edema associated with hypertension. *N Engl J Med* 2001;344(1): 17–22.
134. Kramer K, Kirkman P, Kitzman D, et al. Flash pulmonary edema: association with hypertension and reoccurrence despite coronary revascularization. *Am Heart J* 2000;140(3):451–455.
135. Grossman W. Diastolic dysfunction in congestive heart failure. *N Engl J Med* 1991;325(22):1557–1564.
136. Grossman W. Diastolic dysfunction and congestive heart failure. *Circulation* 1990;81(2 Suppl):III1–III7.
136a. Redfield MM, Jacobsen SJ, Burnett JC Jr, et al. Burden of systolic and diastolic ventricular dysfunction in the community: Appreciating the scope of the heart failure epidemic. *JAMA* 2003;289:194–202.
137. Litwin SE, Grossman W. Diastolic dysfunction as a cause of heart failure. *J Am Coll Cardiol* 1993;22(4 Suppl A):49A–55A.
138. Mandinov L, Eberli FR, Seiler C, et al. Diastolic heart failure. *Cardiovasc Res* 2000;45(4):813–825.
139. Zile MR, Brutsaert DL. New concepts in diastolic dysfunction and diastolic heart failure: Part I: diagnosis, prognosis, and measurements of diastolic function. *Circulation* 2002;105(11):1387–1393.
140. Zile MR, Brutsaert DL. New concepts in diastolic dysfunction and diastolic heart failure: Part II: Causal mechanisms and treatment. *Circulation* 2002;105(12):1503–1508.
141. Kahan T. The importance of left ventricular hypertrophy in human hypertension. *J Hypertens Suppl* 1998;16(7):S23–S29.
142. Brilla CG, Funck RC, Rupp H. Lisinopril-mediated regression of myocardial fibrosis in patients with hypertensive heart disease. *Circulation* 2000;102(12):1388–1393.
143. Diez J, Querejeta R, Lopez B, et al. Losartan-dependent regression of myocardial fibrosis is associated with reduction of left ventricular chamber stiffness in hypertensive patients. *Circulation* 2002;105(21):2512–2517.
144. Matter CM, Mandinov L, Kaufmann PA, et al. Effect of NO donors on LV diastolic function in patients with severe pressure-overload hypertrophy. *Circulation* 1999;99(18):2396–2401.
145. Nishimura RA, Hayes DL, Holmes DR, et al. Mechanism of hemodynamic improvement by dual-chamber pacing for severe left ventricular dysfunction: an acute Doppler and catheterization hemodynamic study. *J Am Coll Cardiol* 1995;25(2):281–288.
146. Breithardt OA, Stellbrink C, Franke A, et al. Echocardiographic evidence of hemodynamic and clinical improvement in patients paced for heart failure. *Am J Cardiol* 2000;86(9A):133K–137K.
147. Vasan RS, Benjamin EJ, Levy D. Prevalence, clinical features and prognosis of diastolic heart failure: an epidemiologic perspective. *J Am Coll Cardiol* 1995;26(7):1565–1574.
148. Smith GL, Masoudi FA, Vaccarino V, et al. Outcomes in heart failure patients with preserved ejection fraction: mortality, readmission, and functional decline. *J Am Coll Cardiol* 2003;41(9):1510–1518.
149. Cohn JN, Johnson G. Heart failure with normal ejection fraction. The V-HeFT Study. Veterans Administration Cooperative Study Group. *Circulation* 1990;81(2 Suppl):III48–III53.
150. Hogg K, Swedberg K, McMurray J. Heart failure with preserved left ventricular systolic function; epidemiology, clinical characteristics, and prognosis. *J Am Coll Cardiol* 2004;43(3):317–327.
151. Judge KW, Pawitan Y, Caldwell J, et al. Congestive heart failure symptoms in patients with preserved left ventricular systolic function: analysis of the CASS registry. *J Am Coll Cardiol* 1991;18(2):377–382.
152. Pritchett AM, Mahoney DW, Jacobsen SJ, et al. Diastolic dysfunction and left atrial volume: a population-based study. *J Am Coll Cardiol* 2005;45(1):87–92.
153. Jones RC, Francis GS, Lauer MS. Predictors of mortality in patients with heart failure and preserved systolic function in the Digitalis Investigation Group trial. *J Am Coll Cardiol* 2004;44(5):1025–1029.
154. O'Connor CM, Gattis WA, Shaw L, et al. Clinical characteristics and long-term outcomes of patients with heart failure and preserved systolic function. *Am J Cardiol* 2000;86(8):863–867.
155. Yusuf S, Pfeffer MA, Swedberg K, et al. Effects of candesartan in patients with chronic heart failure and preserved left-ventricular ejection fraction: the CHARM-Preserved Trial. *Lancet* 2003;362(9386):777–781.
156. Richardson P, McKenna W, Bristow M, et al. Report of the 1995 World Health Organization/International Society and Federation of Cardiology Task Force on the Definition and Classification of Cardiomyopathies. *Circulation* 1996;93:841–842.
157. Kushawa SS, Fallon JT, Fuster V. Restrictive cardiomyopathy. *N Engl J Med* 1997;336:267–276.
158. Angelini A, Calzolari V, Thiene G, et al. Morphologic spectrum of primary restrictive cardiomyopathy. *Am J Cardiol* 1997;80(8):1046–1050.
159. Leung DY, Klein AL. Restrictive cardiomyopathy: diagnosis and prognostic implications. In: Otto CM, ed. *The practice of clinical echocardiography.* Philadelphia: WB Saunders, 1997;473–493.
160. Click RL, Olson LJ, Edwards WD, et al. Echocardiography and systemic diseases. *J Am Soc Echocardiogr* 1994;7(2):201–216.
161. Keren A, Popp RL. Assignment of patients into the classification of cardiomyopathies. *Circulation* 1992;86(5):1622–1633.

162. Roberts WC, Waller BF. Cardiac amyloidosis causing cardiac dysfunction: analysis of 54 necropsy patients. *Am J Cardiol* 1983;52(1):137–146.
163. Buja LM, Khoi NB, Roberts WC. Clinically significant cardiac amyloidosis. Clinicopathologic findings in 15 patients. *Am J Cardiol* 1970;26(4):394–405.
164. Spry CJ, Take M, Tai PC. Eosinophilic disorders affecting the myocardium and endocardium: a review. *Heart Vessels Suppl* 1985;1:240–242.
165. Abelmann WH, Lorell BH. The challenge of cardiomyopathy. *J Am Coll Cardiol* 1989;13(6):1219–1239.
166. Shabetai R. Controversial issues in restrictive cardiomyopathy. *Postgrad Med J* 1992;68(Suppl 1):S47–S51.
167. Hirota Y, Kohriyama T, Hayashi T, et al. Idiopathic restrictive cardiomyopathy: differences of left ventricular relaxation and diastolic wave forms from constrictive pericarditis. *Am J Cardiol* 1983;52(3):421–423.
168. Hirota Y, Shimizu G, Kita Y, et al. Spectrum of restrictive cardiomyopathy: report of the national survey in Japan. *Am Heart J* 1990;120(1):188–194.
169. Appleton CP, Popp RL, Hatle LK. Differentiation of constrictive pericarditis and restrictive cardiomyopathy: general overview and new insights from two-dimensional and Doppler echocardiographic studies. In: Soler-Soler J, Permanyer-Miralda G, Sagrista-Sauleda J, eds. *Pericardial disease: new insights and old dilemmas*. Dordrecht, Netherlands: Kluwer, 1990: 59–93.
170. Hirota Y. Restrictive cardiomyopathy, cardiac amyloidosis and hypereosinophilic heart disease. In: Abelmann WH, Braunwald E, eds. *Cardiomyopathies, myocarditis, and pericardial disease. Atlas of heart diseases*. Philadelphia: Current Medicine, 1995:5.1–5.15.
171. Child JS, Perloff JK. The restrictive cardiomyopathies. *Cardiol Clin* 1988; 6(2):289–316.
172. Klein AL, Hatle LK, Burstow DJ, et al. Doppler characterization of left ventricular diastolic function in cardiac amyloidosis. *J Am Coll Cardiol* 1989;13(5):1017–1026.
173. Wynne J, Braunwald E. The cardiomyopathies and myocarditides. In: Braunwald E, ed. *Heart disease. A textbook of cardiovascular medicine*, 5th ed. Philadelphia: WB Saunders, 1997:1426–1434.
174. Klein AL, Cohen GI, Pietrolungo JF, et al. Differentiation of constrictive pericarditis from restrictive cardiomyopathy by Doppler transesophageal echocardiographic measurements of respiratory variations in pulmonary venous flow. *J Am Coll Cardiol* 1993;22(7):1935–1943.
175. Klein AL, Canale MP, Rajagopalan N, et al. Role of transesophageal echocardiography in assessing diastolic dysfunction in a large clinical practice: a 9-year experience. *Am Heart J* 1999;138(5 Pt 1):880–889.
175a. Yamada H, Tabata T, Drinko JK, et al. Clinical features of mixed physiology of constriction and restriction: Echocardiographic characteristics and clinical outcome. *Eur J Echocardiogr* 2006 (in press).
176. Oren RM, Grover-McKay M, Stanford W, et al. Accurate preoperative diagnosis of pericardial constriction using cine computed tomography. *J Am Coll Cardiol* 1993;22(3):832–838.
177. White CS. MR evaluation of the pericardium. *Top Magn Reson Imaging* 1995;7(4):258–266.
178. Ling LH, Oh JK, Tei C, et al. Pericardial thickness measured with transesophageal echocardiography: feasibility and potential clinical usefulness. *J Am Coll Cardiol* 1997;29(6):1317–1323.
179. Soler R, Rodriguez E, Remuinan C, et al. Magnetic resonance imaging of primary cardiomyopathies. *J Comput Assist Tomogr* 2003;27(5):724–734.
180. Soldo SJ, Norris SL, Gober JR, et al. MRI-derived ventricular volume curves for the assessment of left ventricular function. *Magn Reson Imaging* 1994;12(5):711–717.
181. Celletti F, Fattori R, Napoli G, et al. Assessment of restrictive cardiomyopathy of amyloid or idiopathic etiology by magnetic resonance imaging. *Am J Cardiol* 1999;83(5):798–801, A10.
182. Wilmshurst PT, Katritsis D. Restrictive cardiomyopathy. *Br Heart J* 1990;63(6):323–324.
183. Hosenpud JD, DeMarco T, Frazier OH, et al. Progression of systemic disease and reduced long-term survival in patients with cardiac amyloidosis undergoing heart transplantation. Follow-up results of a multicenter survey. *Circulation* 1991;84(5 Suppl):III338–III343.
184. Rivenes SM, Kearney DL, Smith EO, et al. Sudden death and cardiovascular collapse in children with restrictive cardiomyopathy. *Circulation* 2000;102(8):876–882.
185. Fitzpatrick AP, Shapiro LM, Rickards AF, et al. Familial restrictive cardiomyopathy with atrioventricular block and skeletal myopathy. *Br Heart J* 1990;63(2):114–118.
186. Katritsis D, Wilmshurst PT, Wendon JA, et al. Primary restrictive cardiomyopathy: clinical and pathologic characteristics. *J Am Coll Cardiol* 1991;18(5):1230–1235.
187. Benotti JR, Grossman W, Cohn PF. Clinical profile of restrictive cardiomyopathy. *Circulation* 1980;61(6):1206–1212.
188. McManus BM, Bren GB, Robertson EA, et al. Hemodynamic cardiac constriction without anatomic myocardial restriction or pericardial constriction. *Am Heart J* 1981;102(1):134–136.
189. Keren A, Billingham ME, Weintraub D, et al. Mildly dilated congestive cardiomyopathy. *Circulation* 1985;72(2):302–309.
190. Artz G, Wynne J. Restrictive cardiomyopathy. *Curr Treat Options Cardiovasc Med* 2000;2(5):431–438.
191. Gewillig M, Mertens L, Moerman P, et al. Idiopathic restrictive cardiomyopathy in childhood. A diastolic disorder characterized by delayed relaxation. *Eur Heart J* 1996;17(9):1413–1420.
192. Cooke RA, Chambers JB, Curry PV. Noonan's cardiomyopathy: a non-hypertrophic variant. *Br Heart J* 1994;71(6):561–565.
193. Lewis AB. Clinical profile and outcome of restrictive cardiomyopathy in children. *Am Heart J* 1992;123(6):1589–1593.
194. Cetta F, O'Leary PW, Seward JB, et al. Idiopathic restrictive cardiomyopathy in childhood: diagnostic features and clinical course. *Mayo Clin Proc* 1995;70(7):634–640.
195. Keren A, Billingham ME, Popp RL. Features of mildly dilated congestive cardiomyopathy compared with idiopathic restrictive cardiomyopathy and typical dilated cardiomyopathy. *J Am Soc Echocardiogr* 1988; 1(1):78–87.
196. Siegel RJ, Shah PK, Fishbein MC. Idiopathic restrictive cardiomyopathy. *Circulation* 1984;70(2):165–169.
197. Ammash NM, Seward JB, Bailey KR, et al. Clinical profile and outcome of idiopathic restrictive cardiomyopathy. *Circulation* 2000;101(21):2490–2496.
198. Parrillo JE. Heart disease and the eosinophil. *N Engl J Med* 1990;323 (22):1560–1561.
199. Valiathan SM, Kartha CC. Endomyocardial fibrosis—the possible connexion with myocardial levels of magnesium and cerium. *Int J Cardiol* 1990;28(1):1–5.
200. Spyrou N, Foale R. Restrictive cardiomyopathies. *Curr Opin Cardiol* 1994;9(3):344–348.
201. Davies J, Spry CJ, Sapsford R, et al. Cardiovascular features of 11 patients with eosinophilic endomyocardial disease. *Q J Med* 1983;52(205):23–39.
202. Ribeiro PA, Muthusamy R, Duran CM. Right-sided endomyocardial fibrosis with recurrent pulmonary emboli leading to irreversible pulmonary hypertension. *Br Heart J* 1992;68(3):326–329.
203. Gupta PN, Valiathan MS, Balakrishnan KG, et al. Clinical course of endomyocardial fibrosis. *Br Heart J* 1989;62(6):450–454.
204. Fausi AS, Harley JB, Roberts WC, et al. NIH conference. The idiopathic hypereosinophilic syndrome. Clinical, pathophysiologic, and therapeutic considerations. *Ann Intern Med* 1982;97(1):78–92.
205. Weller PF, Bubley GJ. The idiopathic hypereosinophilic syndrome. *Blood* 1994;83(10):2759–2779.
206. Arnold M, McGuire L, Lee JC. Loeffler's fibroplastic endocarditis. *Pathology* 1988;20(1):79–82.
207. Felice PV, Sawicki J, Anto J. Endomyocardial disease and eosinophilia. *Angiology* 1993;44(11):869–874.
208. Berger PB, Duffy J, Reeder GS, et al. Restrictive cardiomyopathy associated with the eosinophilia-myalgia syndrome. *Mayo Clin Proc* 1994;69(2):162–165.
209. Parrillo JE, Borer JS, Henry WL, et al. The cardiovascular manifestations of the hypereosinophilic syndrome; prospective study of 26 patients with review of the literature. *Am J Med* 1979;67(4):572–582.
210. Acquatella H, Schiller NB. Echocardiographic recognition of Chagas' disease and endomyocardial fibrosis. *J Am Soc Echocardiogr* 1988;1(1):60–68.
211. Ommen SR, Seward JB, Tajik AJ. Clinical and echocardiographic features of hypereosinophilic syndromes. *Am J Cardiol* 2000;86(1):110–113.
212. Acquatella H, Rodriguez-Salas LA, Gomez-Mancebo JR. Doppler echocardiography in dilated and restrictive cardiomyopathies. *Cardiol Clin* 1990;8(2):349–367.
213. Garcia-Pascual J, Gonzalez-Gallarza RD, Jimenez MP, et al. Loffler's syndrome: pulmonary vein and transmitral Doppler flow analysis by transesophageal echocardiography—report of a case. *J Am Soc Echocardiogr* 2000;13(7):690–692.
214. Uetsuka Y, Kasahara S, Tanaka N, et al. Hemodynamic and scintigraphic improvement after steroid therapy in a case with eosinophilic heart disease. *Heart Vessels Suppl* 1990;5:8–12.
215. Butterfield JH, Gleich GJ. Interferon-alpha treatment of six patients with the idiopathic hypereosinophilic syndrome. *Ann Intern Med* 1994;121(9):648–653.
216. Conner DH, et al. Endomyocardial fibrosis in Uganda (Davies' disease). 1. An epidemiologic, clinical, and pathologic study. *Am Heart J* 1967; 74(5):687–709.
217. Seward JB. Restrictive cardiomyopathy: reassessment of definitions and diagnosis. *Curr Opin Cardiol* 1988;3:391–395.
218. Valiathan MS. Endomyocardial fibrosis. *Natl Med J India* 1993;6(5):212–216.
219. Johnson RA, Palacios I. Nondilated cardiomyopathies. *Adv Intern Med* 1984;30:243–274.
220. Shaper AG, Hutt MS, Coles RM. Necropsy study of endomyocardial fibrosis and rheumatic heart disease in Uganda 1950–1965. *Br Heart J* 1968; 30(3):391–401.
221. Chopra P, Narula J, Talwar KK, et al. Histomorphologic characteristics of endomyocardial fibrosis: An endomyocardial biopsy study. *Hum Pathol* 1990;21(6):613–616.
222. Berensztein CS, Pineiro D, Marcotegui M, et al. Usefulness of echocardiography and Doppler echocardiography in endomyocardial fibrosis. *J Am Soc Echocardiogr* 2000;13(5):385–392.
223. Barretto AC, da Luz PL, de Oliveira SA, et al. Determinants of survival in endomyocardial fibrosis. *Circulation* 1989;80(3 Pt 1):I177–I182.

224. Mady C, Pereira Barretto AC, de Oliveira SA, et al. Effectiveness of operative and nonoperative therapy in endomyocardial fibrosis. *Am J Cardiol* 1989;63(17):1281–1282.
225. deOliveira SA, Pereira Barretto AC, Mady C, et al. Surgical treatment of endomyocardial fibrosis: a new approach. *J Am Coll Cardiol* 1990;16(5): 1246–1251.
226. Uva MS, Jebara VA, Acar C, et al. Mitral valve repair in patients with endomyocardial fibrosis. *Ann Thorac Surg* 1992;54(1):89–92.
227. Martinez EE, Venturi M, Buffolo E, et al. Operative results in endomyocardial fibrosis. *Am J Cardiol* 1989;63(9):627–629.
228. Schneider U, Jenni R, Turina J, et al. Long-term follow up of patients with endomyocardial fibrosis: effects of surgery. *Heart* 1998;79(4):362–367.
229. Gertz MA, Rajkumar SV. Primary systemic amyloidosis. *Curr Treat Options Oncol* 2002;3(3):261–271.
230. Kholova I, Niessen HW. Amyloid in the cardiovascular system: a review. *J Clin Pathol* 2005;58(2):125–133.
231. Falk RH. Diagnosis and management of the cardiac amyloidoses. *Circulation* 2005;112(13):2047–2060.
232. Kyle RA. Amyloidosis. *Circulation* 1995;91(4):1269–1271.
233. Kyle RA, Greipp PR. Amyloidosis (AL). Clinical and laboratory features in 229 cases. *Mayo Clin Proc* 1983;58(10):665–683.
234. Gertz MA, Kyle RA, Thibodeau SN. Familial amyloidosis: a study of 52 North American–born patients examined during a 30-year period. *Mayo Clin Proc* 1992;67(5):428–440.
235. Gertz MA, Kyle RA. Secondary systemic amyloidosis: response and survival in 64 patients. *Medicine* (Baltimore) 1991;70(4):246–256.
236. Gertz MA, Lacy MQ, Dispenzieri A. Amyloidosis. *Hematol Oncol Clin North Am* 1999;13(6):1211–1233, ix.
237. Goette A, Rocken C. Atrial amyloidosis and atrial fibrillation: a gender-dependent "arrhythmogenic substrate"? *Eur Heart J* 2004;25(14):1185–1186.
238. Gertz MA, Kyle RA. Primary systemic amyloidosis—a diagnostic primer. *Mayo Clin Proc* 1989;64(12):1505–1519.
239. Booth DR, Tan SY, Hawkins PN, et al. A novel variant of transthyretin, 59Thr→Lys, associated with autosomal dominant cardiac amyloidosis in an Italian family. *Circulation* 1995;91(4):962–967.
240. Frederiksen T, Gotzsche H, Harboe N, et al. Familial primary amyloidosis with severe amyloid heart disease. *Am J Med* 1962;33:328–348.
241. Benson MD, Wallace MR, Tejada E, et al. Hereditary amyloidosis: description of a new American kindred with late onset cardiomyopathy. Appalachian amyloid. *Arthritis Rheum* 1987;30(2):195–200.
242. Jacobson DR, Pastore RD, Yaghoubian R, et al. Variant-sequence transthyretin (isoleucine 122) in late-onset cardiac amyloidosis in black Americans. *N Engl J Med* 1997;336(7):466–473.
243. Benson MD. Aging, amyloid, and cardiomyopathy. *N Engl J Med* 1997; 336(7):502–504.
244. Olson LJ, Gertz MA, Edwards WD, et al. Senile cardiac amyloidosis with myocardial dysfunction. Diagnosis by endomyocardial biopsy and immunohistochemistry. *N Engl J Med* 1987;317(12):738–742.
245. Cueto-Garcia L, Tajik AJ, Kyle RA, et al. Serial echocardiographic observations in patients with primary systemic amyloidosis: an introduction to the concept of early (asymptomatic) amyloid infiltration of the heart. *Mayo Clin Proc* 1984;59(9):589–597.
246. Benson MD. Hereditary amyloidosis and cardiomyopathy. *Am J Med* 1992;93(1):1–2.
247. Barth RF, Willerson JT, Buja LM, et al. Amyloid coronary artery disease, primary systemic amyloidosis and paraproteinemia. *Arch Intern Med* 1970;126(4):627–630.
248. Mueller PS, Edwards WD, Gertz MA. Symptomatic ischemic heart disease resulting from obstructive intramural coronary amyloidosis. *Am J Med* 2000;109(3):181–188.
249. Rubinow A, Cohen AS. Skin involvement in generalized amyloidosis. A study of clinically involved and uninvolved skin in 50 patients with primary and secondary amyloidosis. *Ann Intern Med* 1978;88(6):781–785.
250. Hesse A, Altland K, Linke RP, et al. Cardiac amyloidosis: a review and report of a new transthyretin (prealbumin) variant. *Br Heart J* 1993;70(2): 111–115.
251. Shabetai R. Pathophysiology and differential diagnosis of restrictive cardiomyopathy. *Cardiovasc Clin* 1988;19(1):123–132.
252. Dubrey SW, et al. Familial and primary (AL) cardiac amyloidosis: echocardiographically similar diseases with distinctly different clinical outcomes. *Heart* 1997;78(1):74–82.
253. Murtagh B, Hammill SC, Gertz MA, et al. Electrocardiographic findings in primary systemic amyloidosis and biopsy-proven cardiac involvement. *Am J Cardiol* 2005;95(4):535–537.
254. Siqueira-Filho AG, Cunha CL, Tajik AJ, et al. M-mode and two-dimensional echocardiographic features in cardiac amyloidosis. *Circulation* 1981;63(1):188–196.
255. Chiaramida SA, Goldman MA, Zema MJ, et al. Real-time cross-sectional echocardiographic diagnosis of infiltrative cardiomyopathy due to amyloid. *J Clin Ultrasound* 1980;8(1):58–62.
256. Chandrasekaran K, Aylward PE, Fleagle SR, et al. Feasibility of identifying amyloid and hypertrophic cardiomyopathy with the use of computerized quantitative texture analysis of clinical echocardiographic data. *J Am Coll Cardiol* 1989;13(4):832–840.
257. Carroll JD, Gaasch WH, McAdam KP. Amyloid cardiomyopathy: characterization by a distinctive voltage/mass relation. *Am J Cardiol* 1982; 49(1):9–13.
258. Falk RH, Plehn JF, Deering T, et al. Sensitivity and specificity of the echocardiographic features of cardiac amyloidosis. *Am J Cardiol* 1987; 59(5):418–422.
259. Rahman JE, Helou EF, Gelzer-Bell R, et al. Noninvasive diagnosis of biopsy-proven cardiac amyloidosis. *J Am Coll Cardiol* 2004;43(3):410–415.
260. Chew C, Ziady GM, Raphael MJ, et al. The functional defect in amyloid heart disease. The "stiff heart" syndrome. *Am J Cardiol* 1975;36(4):438–444.
261. St. John Sutton MG, Reichek N, Kastor JA, et al. Computerized M-mode echocardiographic analysis of left ventricular dysfunction in cardiac amyloid. *Circulation* 1982;66(4):790–799.
262. Koyama J, Ray-Sequin PA, Davidoff R, et al. Usefulness of pulsed tissue Doppler imaging for evaluating systolic and diastolic left ventricular function in patients with AL (primary) amyloidosis. *Am J Cardiol* 2002; 89(9):1067–1071.
263. Koyama J, Ray-Sequin PA, Falk RH. Longitudinal myocardial function assessed by tissue velocity, strain, and strain rate tissue Doppler echocardiography in patients with AL (primary) cardiac amyloidosis. *Circulation* 2003;107(19):2446–2452.
264. Cueto-Garcia L, Reeder GS, Kyle RA, et al. Echocardiographic findings in systemic amyloidosis: spectrum of cardiac involvement and relation to survival. *J Am Coll Cardiol,* 1985;6(4):737–743.
265. Tei C, Dujardin KS, Hodge DO, et al. Doppler index combining systolic and diastolic myocardial performance: clinical value in cardiac amyloidosis. *J Am Coll Cardiol* 1996;28(3):658–664.
266. Patel AR, Dubrey SW, Mendes LA, et al. Right ventricular dilation in primary amyloidosis: an independent predictor of survival. *Am J Cardiol* 1997;80(4):486–492.
267. Dispenzieri A, Kyle RA, Gertz MA, et al. Survival in patients with primary systemic amyloidosis and raised serum cardiac troponins. *Lancet* 2003;361(9371):1787–1789.
268. Oh JK, Tajik AJ, Edwards WD, et al. Dynamic left ventricular outflow tract obstruction in cardiac amyloidosis detected by continuous-wave Doppler echocardiography. *Am J Cardiol* 1987;59(9):1008–1010.
269. Hongo M, Fujii T, Hirayama J, et al. Radionuclide angiographic assessment of left ventricular diastolic filling in amyloid heart disease: a study of patients with familial amyloid polyneuropathy. *J Am Coll Cardiol* 1989; 13(1):48–53.
270. Hongo M, Hirayama J, Fujii T, et al. Early identification of amyloid heart disease by technetium-99m-pyrophosphate scintigraphy: a study with familial amyloid polyneuropathy. *Am Heart J* 1987;113(3):654–662.
271. Lekakis J, Nanas J, Moustafellou C, et al. Cardiac amyloidosis detected by indium-111 antimyosin imaging. *Am Heart J* 1992;124(6):1630–1631.
272. Gertz MA, Lacy MQ, Dispenzieri A. Amyloidosis: recognition, confirmation, prognosis, and therapy. *Mayo Clin Proc* 1999;74(5):490–494.
273. Abraham RS, Katzmann JA, Clark RJ, et al. Quantitative analysis of serum free light chains. A new marker for the diagnostic evaluation of primary systemic amyloidosis. *Am J Clin Pathol* 2003;119(2):274–278.
274. Katzmann JA, Abraham RS, Dispenzieri A, et al. Diagnostic performance of quantitative kappa and lambda free light chain assays in clinical practice. *Clin Chem* 2005;51(5):878–881.
275. von Kemp K, Beckers R, Vandenweghe, et al. Echocardiography and magnetic resonance imaging in cardiac amyloidosis. *Acta Cardiol* 1989;44(1): 29–36.
276. Sechtem U, Higgins CB, Sommerhoff BA, et al. Magnetic resonance imaging of restrictive cardiomyopathy. *Am J Cardiol* 1987;59(5):480–482.
277. Maceira AM, Joshi J, Prasad SK, et al. Cardiovascular magnetic resonance in cardiac amyloidosis. *Circulation* 2005;111(2):186–193.
278. Gertz MA, Kyle RA. Amyloidosis: prognosis and treatment. *Semin Arthritis Rheum* 1994;24(2):124–138.
279. Skinner M, Anderson J, Wang M, et al. Treatment of patients with primary amyloidosis. In: Kisilevsky R, Benson MD, Frangione B, et al., eds. *Amyloid and amyloidosis 1993.* New York: Parthenon, 1994: 232–234.
280. Kyle RA, Gertz MA, Garton JP, et al. Primary systemic amyloidosis (AL): randomized trial of colchicine vs melphalan and prednisone vs melphelan, prednisone, and colchicine. In: Kisilevsky R, Benson MD, Frangione B, et al., Eds. *Amyloid and amyloidosis 1993.* New York: Parthenon, 1994: 648–650.
281. Kronzon I, Fedor M, Schwartz D, et al. A 58-year-old man with shortness of breath, ascites and leg edema. *Circulation.* 1996;94(6):1483–1488.
282. Skinner M, Anderson J, Simms R, et al. Treatment of 100 patients with primary amyloidosis; a randomized trial of melphalan, prednisone, and colchicine versus colchicine alone. *Am J Med* 1996;100(3):290–298.
283. Comenzo RL, Vosburgh E, Falk RH, et al. Dose-intensive melphalan with blood stem-cell support for the treatment of AL (amyloid light-chain) amyloidosis: survival and responses in 25 patients. *Blood* 1998;91(10):3662–3670.
283a. Gertz MA, Blood E, Vesole DH, et al. A multicenter phase 2 trial of stem cell transplantation for immunoglobulin light-chain amyloidosis (E4A97): An Eastern Cooperative Oncology Group Study. *Bone Marrow Transplant* 2004;34:149–154.

283b. Jaccard A, Moreau P, Leblond V, et al. Autologous stem cell transplantation (ASCT) versus oral melphalan and high-dose dexamethasone in patients with AL (primary) amyloidosis: Results of the French Multicentric Randomized Trial (MAG and IFM Intergroup) [abstract]. *Blood* 2005; 106:421a.
283c. Rajkumar SV, Dispenzieri A, Kyle RA. Monoclonal gammopathy of undetermined significance, Waldenstrom macroglobulinemia, AL amyloidosis, and related plasma cell disorders: Diagnosis and treatment. *Mayo Clin Proc* 2006;81:693–703.
284. Dubrey S, Simms RW, Skinner M, et al. Recurrence of primary (AL) amyloidosis in a transplanted heart with four-year survival. *Am J Cardiol* 1995;76(10):739–741.
285. Pelosi Jr F, Capehart J, Roberts WC. Effectiveness of cardiac transplantation for primary (AL) cardiac amyloidosis. *Am J Cardiol* 1997;79(4):532–535.
286. Miller SR, Sekijima Y, Kelly JW. Native state stabilization by NSAIDs inhibits transthyretin amyloidogenesis from the most common familial disease variants. *Lab Invest* 2004;84(5):545–552.
287. Holmgren G, Ericzon BG, Groth CG, et al. Clinical improvement and amyloid regression after liver transplantation in hereditary transthyretin amyloidosis. *Lancet* 1993;341(8853):1113–1116.
288. Skinner M, Lewis WD, Jones LA, et al. Liver transplantation as treatment for familial amyloidotic polyneuropathy. *Ann Intern Med* 1994;120:133–134.
289. Rubinow A, Skinner M, Cohen AS. Digoxin sensitivity in amyloid cardiomyopathy. *Circulation* 1981;63(6):1285–1288.
290. Pollak A, Falk RH. Left ventricular systolic dysfunction precipitated by verapamil in cardiac amyloidosis. *Chest* 1993;104(2):618–620.
291. Wright JR, Calkins E. Clinical-pathologic differentiation of common amyloid syndromes. *Medicine* (Baltimore) 1981;60(6):429–448.
292. Willens HJ, Levy R, Kessler KM. Thromboembolic complications in cardiac amyloidosis detected by transesophageal echocardiography. *Am Heart J* 1995;129(2):405–406.
293. Zelitch SR, Israel HL. Sarcoidosis. *Am Fam Physician* 1988;38(2):127–139.
294. Alton M, Juhlin-Dannfelt A, Pehrsson SK, et al. Sarcoid heart disease. *Sarcoidosis* 1992;9(2):147–149.
295. Rizzato G, et al. Right heart impairment in sarcoidosis: haemodynamic and echocardiographic study. *Eur J Respir Dis* 1983;64(2):121–128.
296. Silverman KJ, Hutchins GM, Bulkley BH. Cardiac sarcoid: a clinicopathologic study of 84 unselected patients with systemic sarcoidosis. *Circulation* 1978;58(6):1204–1211.
297. Gibbons WJ, Levy RD, Nava S, et al. Subclinical cardiac dysfunction in sarcoidosis. *Chest* 1991;100(1):44–50.
298. Sharma OP. Myocardial sarcoidosis. A wolf in sheep's clothing. *Chest* 1994;106(4):988–990.
299. Sharma OP, Maheshwari A, Thaker K. Myocardial sarcoidosis. *Chest* 1993;103(1):253–258.
300. Roberts WC, McAllister Jr HA, Ferrans VJ. Sarcoidosis of the heart. A clinicopathologic study of 35 necropsy patients (group 1) and review of 78 previously described necropsy patients (group 11). *Am J Med* 1977;63(1):86–108.
301. Jain A, Starek PJ, Delany DL. Ventricular tachycardia and ventricular aneurysm due to unrecognized sarcoidosis. *Clin Cardiol* 1990;13(10): 738–740.
302. Bohle W, Schaefer HE. Predominant myocardial sarcoidosis. *Pathol Res Pract* 1994;190(2):212–217; discussion, 217–219.
303. Huang PL, Brooks R, Carpenter C, et al. Antiarrhythmic therapy guided by programmed electrical stimulation in cardiac sarcoidosis with ventricular tachycardia. *Am Heart J* 1991;121(2 Pt 1):599–601.
304. Winters SL, Cohen M, Greenberg S, et al. Sustained ventricular tachycardia associated with sarcoidosis: assessment of the underlying cardiac anatomy and the prospective utility of programmed ventricular stimulation, drug therapy and an implantable antitachycardia device. *J Am Coll Cardiol* 1991;18(4):937–943.
305. Kavanagh T, Huang S. Cardiac sarcoidosis: an unforeseen cause of sudden death. *Can J Cardiol* 1995;11(2):136–138.
306. Shammas RL, Movahed A. Sarcoidosis of the heart. *Clin Cardiol* 1993; 16(6):462–472.
307. Sekiguchi M, Yazaki Y, Isobe M, et al. Cardiac sarcoidosis: diagnostic, prognostic, and therapeutic considerations. *Cardiovasc Drugs Ther* 1996; 10(5):495–510.
308. Gregor P, Widimsky P, Sladkova T, et al. Echocardiography in sarcoidosis. *Jpn Heart J* 1984;25(4):499–508.
309. Kinney EL, Jackson GL, Reeves WC, et al. Thallium-scan myocardial defects and echocardiographic abnormalities in patients with sarcoidosis without clinical cardiac dysfunction. An analysis of 44 patients. *Am J Med* 1980;68(4):497–503.
310. Lewin RF, Mor R, Spitzer S, et al. Echocardiographic evaluation of patients with systemic sarcoidosis. *Am Heart J* 1985;110(1 Pt 1):116–122.
311. Burstow DJ, Tajik, AJ, Bailey KR, et al. Two-dimensional echocardiographic findings in systemic sarcoidosis. *Am J Cardiol* 1989;63(7):478–482.
312. Valantine H, McKenna WJ, Nihoyannopoulos P, et al. Sarcoidosis: a pattern of clinical and morphological presentation. *Br Heart J* 1987;57(3): 256–263.
313. Fahy GJ, Marwick T, McCreery CJ, et al. Doppler echocardiographic detection of left ventricular diastolic dysfunction in patients with pulmonary sarcoidosis. *Chest* 1996;109(1):62–66.
314. Tawarahara K, Kurata C, Okayama K, et al. Thallium-201 and gallium 67 single photon emission computed tomographic imaging in cardiac sarcoidosis. *Am Heart J* 1992;124(5):1383–1384.
315. Yamamoto N, Gotoh K, Yagi Y, et al. Thallium-201 myocardial SPECT findings at rest in sarcoidosis. *Ann Nucl Med* 1993;7(2):97–103.
316. Taki J, Nakajima K, Bunko H, et al. Cardiac sarcoidosis demonstrated by Tl-201 and Ga-67 SPECT imaging. *Clin Nucl Med* 1990;15(9):636–639.
317. Fields CL, Ossorio MA, Roy TM, et al. Thallium-201 scintigraphy in the diagnosis and management of myocardial sarcoidosis. *South Med J* 1990;83(3):339–342.
318. Riedy K, Fisher MR, Belic N, et al. MR imaging of myocardial sarcoidosis. *AJR Am J Roentgenol* 1988;151(5):915–916.
319. Smedema JP, Snoep G, van Kroonenburgh MP, et al. Evaluation of the accuracy of gadolinium-enhanced cardiovascular magnetic resonance in the diagnosis of cardiac sarcoidosis. *J Am Coll Cardiol* 2005;45(10):1683–1690.
320. Matsuki M, Matsuo M. MR findings of myocardial sarcoidosis. *Clin Radiol* 2000;55(4):323–325.
321. Schaedel H, Kirsten D, Schmidt A, et al. Sarcoid heart disease—results of follow-up investigations. *Eur Heart J* 1991;12(Suppl D):26–27.
322. Shammas RL, Movahed A. Successful treatment of myocardial sarcoidosis with steroids. *Sarcoidosis* 1994;11(1):37–39.
323. Chiu CZ, Nakatani S, Zhang G, et al. Prevention of left ventricular remodeling by long-term corticosteroid therapy in patients with cardiac sarcoidosis. *Am J Cardiol* 2005;95(1):143–146.
324. Bajaj AK, Kopelman HA, Echt DS. Cardiac sarcoidosis with sudden death: treatment with the automatic implantable cardioverter defibrillator. *Am Heart J* 1988;116(2 Pt 1):557–560.
325. Paz HL, McCormick DJ, Kutalek SP, et al. The automated implantable cardiac defibrillator. Prophylaxis in cardiac sarcoidosis. *Chest* 1994;106(5):1603–1607.
326. Hauser SC. Hemochromatosis and the heart. *Heart Dis Stroke* 1993; 2(6):487–491.
327. Buja LM, Roberts WC. Iron in the heart, etiology, and clinical significance. *Am J Med* 1971;51(2):209–221.
328. Candell-Riera J, Lu L, Seres L, et al. Cardiac hemochromatosis: beneficial effects of iron removal therapy. An echocardiographic study. *Am J Cardiol* 1983;52(7):824–829.
329. Short EM, Winkle RA, Billingham ME. Myocardial involvement in idiopathic hemochromatosis. Morphologic and clinical improvement following venesection. *Am J Med* 1981;70(6):1275–1279.
330. Olson LJ, Baldus WP, Tajik AJ. Echocardiographic features in idiopathic hemochromatosis. *Am J Cardiol* 1987;60(10):885–889.
331. Palka P, Macdonald G, Lange A, et al. The role of Doppler left ventricular filling indexes and Doppler tissue echocardiography in the assessment of cardiac involvement in hereditary hemochromatosis. *J Am Soc Echocardiogr* 2002;15(9):884–890.
332. Olson LJ, Edwards WD, Holmes Jr DR, et al. Endomyocardial biopsy in hemochromatosis: clinicopathologic correlates in six cases. *J Am Coll Cardiol* 1989;13(1):116–120.
333. Dabestani A, Child JS, Henze E, et al. Primary hemochromatosis: anatomic and physiologic characteristics of the cardiac ventricles and their response to phlebotomy. *Am J Cardiol* 1984;54(1):153–159.
334. Henry WL, Nienhuis AW, Wiener M, et al. Echocardiographic abnormalities in patients with transfusion-dependent anemia and secondary myocardial iron deposition. *Am J Med* 1978;64(4):547–555.
335. Blankenberg F, Eisenberg S, Scheinman MN, et al. Use of cine gradient echo (GRE) MR in the imaging of cardiac hemochromatosis. *J Comput Assist Tomogr* 1994;18(1):136–138.
336. Przybojewski JZ. Endomyocardial biopsy: a review of the literature. *Cathet Cardiovasc Diagn* 1985;11(3):287–330.
337. Porter J, Cary N, Schofield P. Haemochromatosis presenting as congestive cardiac failure. *Br Heart J* 1995;73(1):73–75.
338. Rivers J, Garrahy P, Robinson W, et al. Reversible cardiac dysfunction in hemochromatosis. *Am Heart J* 1987;113(1):216–217.
339. Westra WH, Hruban RH, Baughman KL, et al. Progressive hemochromatotic cardiomyopathy despite reversal of iron deposition after liver transplantation. *Am J Clin Pathol* 1993;99(1):39–44.
340. Case records of the Massachusetts General Hospital. Weekly clinicopathological exercises. Case 31-1994. A 25-year-old man with the recent onset of diabetes mellitus and congestive heart failure. *N Engl J Med* 1994;331:460–466.
341. Caines AE, Kpodonu J, Massad MG, et al. Cardiac transplantation in patients with iron overload cardiomyopathy. *J Heart Lung Transplant* 2005;24(4):486–488.
342. Sakuraba H, Yanagawa Y, Igarashi T, et al. Cardiovascular manifestations in Fabry's disease. A high incidence of mitral valve prolapse in hemizygotes and heterozygotes. *Clin Genet* 1986;29(4):276–283.
343. Bass JL, Shrivastava S, Grabowski GA, et al. The M-mode echocardiogram in Fabry's disease. *Am Heart J* 1980;100(6 Pt 1):807–812.
344. Cohen IS, Fluri-Lundeen J, Wharton TP. Two dimensional echocardiographic similarity of Fabry's disease to cardiac amyloidosis: a function of ultrastructural analogy? *J Clin Ultrasound* 1983;11(8):437–441.

345. Tanaka H, Adachi K, Yamashita Y, et al. Four cases of Fabry's disease mimicking hypertrophic cardiomyopathy. *J Cardiol* 1988;18(3):705–718.
346. Nakao S, Takenaka T, Maeda M, et al. An atypical variant of Fabry's disease in men with left ventricular hypertrophy. *N Engl J Med* 1995;333(5):288–293.
347. Sachdev B, Takenaka T, Teraguchi H, et al. Prevalence of Anderson-Fabry disease in male patients with late onset hypertrophic cardiomyopathy. *Circulation* 2002;105(12):1407–1411.
348. Chimenti C, Pieroni M, Morgante E, et al. Prevalence of Fabry disease in female patients with late-onset hypertrophic cardiomyopathy. *Circulation* 2004;110(9):1047–1053.
349. Pochis WT, Litzow JT, King BG, et al. Electrophysiologic findings in Fabry's disease with a short PR interval. *Am J Cardiol* 1994;74(2):203–204.
350. Linhart A, Palecek T, Bultas J, et al. New insights in cardiac structural changes in patients with Fabry's disease. *Am Heart J* 2000;139(6):1101–1108.
351. Matsui S, Murakami E, Takekoshi N, et al. Myocardial tissue characterization by magnetic resonance imaging in Fabry's disease. *Am Heart J* 1989;117(2):472–474.
352. von Scheidt W, Eng CM, Fitzmaurice TF, et al. An atypical variant of Fabry's disease with manifestations confined to the myocardium. *N Engl J Med* 1991;324(6):395–399.
353. Maben P, Evans R, Lin J, et al. Endomyocardial biopsy. Diagnosis of Fabry's disease in congestive cardiomyopathy. *J Kans Med Soc* 1983;84(11):556–557.
354. Weidemann F, Breunig F, Beer M, et al. Improvement of cardiac function during enzyme replacement therapy in patients with Fabry disease: a prospective strain rate imaging study. *Circulation* 2003;108(11):1299–1301.
355. McGuire MR, Pugh DM, Dunn MI. Carcinoid heart disease. Restrictive cardiomyopathy as a late complication. *J Kans Med Soc* 1978;79(12):661–665.
356. Strickman NE, Hall RJ. Carcinoid heart disease. In: Kapoor AS, Reynolds RD, eds. *Cancer and the heart.* New York: Springer-Verlag, 1986: 135–156.
357. Pellikka PA, Tajik AJ, Khandheria BK, et al. Carcinoid heart disease. Clinical and echocardiographic spectrum in 74 patients. *Circulation* 1993; 87(4):1188–1196.
358. Robiolio PA, Rigolin VH, Wilson JS, et al. Carcinoid heart disease. Correlation of high serotonin levels with valvular abnormalities detected by cardiac catheterization and echocardiography. *Circulation* 1995;92(4):790–795.
359. Lundin L. Carcinoid heart disease. A cardiologist's viewpoint. *Acta Oncol* 1991;30(4):499–502.
360. Millward MJ, Blake MP, Byrne MJ, et al. Left heart involvement with cardiac shunt complicating carcinoid heart disease. *Aust N Z J Med* 1989; 19(6):716–717.
361. Blick DR, Zoghbi WA, Lawrie GM, et al. Carcinoid heart disease presenting as right-to-left shunt and congestive heart failure: successful surgical treatment. *Am Heart J* 1988;115(1 Pt 1):201–203.
362. Lundin L, Landelius J, Andren B, et al. Transesophageal echocardiography improves the diagnostic value of cardiac ultrasound in patients with carcinoid heart disease. *Br Heart J* 1990;64(3):190–194.
363. Lundin L, Norheim I, Landelius J, et al. Carcinoid heart disease: relationship of circulating vasoactive substances to ultrasound-detectable cardiac abnormalities. *Circulation* 1988;77(2):264–269.
364. Denney WD, Kemp Jr WE, Anthony LB, et al. Echocardiographic and biochemical evaluation of the development and progression of carcinoid heart disease. *J Am Coll Cardiol* 1998;32(4):1017–1022.
365. Callahan JA, Wroblewski EM, Reeder GS, et al. Echocardiographic features of carcinoid heart disease. *Am J Cardiol* 1982;50(4):762–768.
366. Roberts WC. A unique heart disease associated with a unique cancer: carcinoid heart disease. *Am J Cardiol* 1997;80(2):251–256.
367. Le Metayer P, Constans J, Bernard N, et al. Carcinoid heart disease: two cases of left heart involvement diagnosed by transthoracic and transoesophageal echocardiography. *Eur Heart J* 1993;14(12):1721–1723.
368. Connolly HM, Nishimura RA, Smith HC, et al. Outcome of cardiac surgery for carcinoid heart disease. *J Am Coll Cardiol* 1995;25(2):410–416.
369. Ruszniewski P, Malka D. Hepatic arterial chemoembolization in the management of advanced digestive endocrine tumors. *Digestion* 2000;62(Suppl 1):79–83.
370. Kvols LK. Metastatic carcinoid tumors and the malignant carcinoid syndrome. *Ann N Y Acad Sci* 1994;733:464–470.
371. Oates JA. The carcinoid syndrome. *N Engl J Med* 1986;315:702–704.
372. O'Toole D, Ducreux M, Bommelaer G, et al. Treatment of carcinoid syndrome: a prospective crossover evaluation of lanreotide versus octreotide in terms of efficacy, patient acceptability, and tolerance. *Cancer* 2000;88(4):770–776.
373. Moller JE, Connolly HM, Rubin J, et al. Factors associated with progression of carcinoid heart disease. *N Engl J Med* 2003;348(11):1005–1015.
374. Mullins PA, Hall JA, Shapiro LM. Balloon dilatation of tricuspid stenosis caused by carcinoid heart disease. *Br Heart J* 1990;63(4):249–250.
375. Grant SC, Scarffe JH, Levy RD, et al. Failure of balloon dilatation of the pulmonary valve in carcinoid pulmonary stenosis. *Br Heart J* 1992;67(6): 450–453.
376. Onate A, Alcibar J, Inguanzo R, et al. Balloon dilation of tricuspid and pulmonary valves in carcinoid heart disease. *Tex Heart Inst J* 1993;20(2):115–119.
377. Hargreaves AD, Pringle SD, Boon NA. Successful balloon dilatation of the pulmonary valve in carcinoid heart disease. *Int J Cardiol* 1994;45(2):150–151.
378. Lundin L, Hansson HE, Landelius J, et al. Surgical treatment of carcinoid heart disease. *J Thorac Cardiovasc Surg* 1990;100(4):552–561.
379. Knott-Craig CJ, Schaff HV, Mullany CJ, et al. Carcinoid disease of the heart. Surgical management of ten patients. *J Thorac Cardiovasc Surg* 1992; 104(2):475–481.
380. Ohri SK, Schofield JB, Hodgson H, et al. Carcinoid heart disease: early failure of an allograft valve replacement. *Ann Thorac Surg* 1994;58(4):1161–1163.
381. Robiolio PA, Rigolin VH, Harrison JK, et al. Predictors of outcome of tricuspid valve replacement in carcinoid heart disease. *Am J Cardiol* 1995; 75(7):485–488.
382. Moller JE, Pellikka PA, Bernheim AM, et al. Prognosis of carcinoid heart disease: analysis of 200 cases over two decades. *Circulation* 2005;112(21): 3320–3327.
383. Moore KL. *Clinically oriented anatomy.* Baltimore: Williams & Wilkins, 1980:1257.
384. Holt JP. The normal pericardium. *Am J Cardiol* 1970;26(5):455–465.
385. Ishihara T, Ferrans VJ, Jones M, et al. Histologic and ultrastructural features of normal human parietal pericardium. *Am J Cardiol* 1980;46(5):744–753.
386. Shabetai R. Pericardial and cardiac pressure. *Circulation* 1988;77(1):1–5.
387. Spodick DH. Macrophysiology, microphysiology, and anatomy of the pericardium: a synopsis. *Am Heart J* 1992;124(4):1046–1051.
388. Freeman GL, LeWinter MM. Pericardial adaptations during chronic cardiac dilation in dogs. *Circ Res* 1984;54(3):294–300.
389. Janicki JS. Influence of the pericardium and ventricular interdependence on left ventricular diastolic and systolic function in patients with heart failure. *Circulation* 1990;81(2 Suppl):III15–III20.
390. Elzinga G, van Grondelle R, Westerhof N, et al. Ventricular interference. *Am J Physiol* 1974;226:941–947.
391. Appleton CP, Hatle LK, Popp RL. Cardiac tamponade and pericardial effusion: respiratory variation in transvalvular flow velocities studied by Doppler echocardiography. *J Am Coll Cardiol* 1988;11(5):1020–1030.
392. Burstow DJ, Oh JK, Bailey KR, et al. Cardiac tamponade: characteristic Doppler observations. *Mayo Clin Proc* 1989;64(3):312–324.
393. Troughton RW, Asher CR, Klein AL. Pericarditis. *Lancet* 2004;363 (9410):717–727.
394. Spodick DH. Acoustic phenomena in pericardial disease. *Am Heart J* 1971;81(1):114–124.
395. Spodick DH. Electrocardiogram in acute pericarditis. Distributions of morphologic and axial changes by stages. *Am J Cardiol* 1974;33(4):470–474.
396. Baljepally R, Spodick DH. PR-segment deviation as the initial electrocardiographic response in acute pericarditis. *Am J Cardiol* 1998;81(12): 1505–1506.
397. Spodick DH. Diagnostic electrocardiographic sequences in acute pericarditis. Significance of PR segment and PR vector changes. *Circulation* 1973;48(3):575–580.
398. Spodick DH. Differential characteristics of the electrocardiogram in early repolarization and acute pericarditis. *N Engl J Med* 1976;295(10):523–526.
399. Spodick D. Arrhythmias during acute pericarditis: A prospective study of 100 cases. *JAMA* 1976;235(1):39–41.
400. Coupland DB, Terriff B, Fung AY, et al. The 'hot halo' sign. Pyogenic pericarditis on In-111 leukocyte scintigraphy. *Clin Nucl Med* 1992;17(7):579–580.
401. Parry R, Akhtar N, Hartnell GG. Case report: unsuspected pericarditis diagnosed with gallium67 scan. *Clin Radiol* 1993;48(5):332–333.
402. Kodama K, Igase M, Funada J, et al. Gallium-67 citrate scintigraphy in idiopathic pericarditis—report of a case. *Jpn Circ J* 1994;58(4):298–302.
403. Matsuoka H, Hamada M, Honda T, et al. Precise assessment of myocardial damage associated with secondary cardiomyopathies by use of Gd-DTPA-enhanced magnetic resonance imaging. *Angiology* 1993;44(12): 945–950.
404. Bonnefoy E, Godon P, Kirkorian G, et al. Serum cardiac troponin I and ST-segment elevation in patients with acute pericarditis. *Eur Heart J* 2000;21(10):832–836.
405. Imazio M, Demichelis B, Cecchi E, et al. Cardiac troponin I in acute pericarditis. *J Am Coll Cardiol* 2003;42(12):2144–2148.
406. Permanyer-Miralda G, Sagrista-Sauleda J, Soler-Soler J. Primary acute pericardial disease: a prospective series of 231 consecutive patients. *Am J Cardiol* 1985;56(10):623–630.
407. Berger M, Bobak L, Jelveh M, et al. Pericardial effusion diagnosed by echocardiography. Clinical and electrocardiographic findings in 171 patients. *Chest* 1978;74(2):174–179.
408. Horowitz MS, Schultz CS, Stinson EB, et al. Sensitivity and specificity of echocardiographic diagnosis of pericardial effusion. *Circulation* 1974; 50(2):239–247.
409. Riba AL, Morganroth J. Unsuspected substantial pericardial effusions detected by echocardiography. *JAMA* 1976;236(23):2623–2625.

410. Soler-Soler J. Massive chronic pericardial effusion. In: Soler-Soler J, Permanyer-Miralda G, Sagrista-Sauleda J, eds. Pericardial diseases—old dilemmas and new insights. Dordrecht, Netherlands: Kluwer, 1990:153–165.
411. Fowler N. Chronic pericarditis. In: No F, ed. *The pericardium in health and disease.* Mount Kisco, NY: Futura, 1985:217–334.
412. Sagrista-Sauleda J, et al. Long-term follow-up of idiopathic chronic pericardial effusion. *N Engl J Med* 1999;341(27):2054–2059.
413. Spodick DH. Pericarditis, pericardial effusion, cardiac tamponade, and constriction. *Crit Care Clin* 1989;5(3):455–476.
414. Sechtem U, Tscholakoff D, Higgins CB. MRI of the abnormal pericardium. *AJR. Am J Roentgenol* 1986;147(2):245–252.
415. Mulvagh SL, Rokey R, Vick 3rd GW, et al. Usefulness of nuclear magnetic resonance imaging for evaluation of pericardial effusions, and comparison with two-dimensional echocardiography. *Am J Cardiol,* 1989; 64(16):1002–1009.
416. Lorell BH, Grossman W. Profiles in constrictive pericarditis, restrictive cardiomyopathy and cardiac tamponade. In: Baim DS, Grossman W, eds. *Cardiac catherization, angiography and intervention.* Baltimore: Williams & Wilkins, 1996:801–857.
417. Shabetai R. The pathophysiology of cardiac tamponade. *Cardiovasc Clin* 1976;7(3):67–89.
418. Gauchat HW, Katz LN. Observations of pulsus paradoxus (with special reference to pericardial effusions) I. Clinical. *Arch Intern Med* 1924; 33:350–370.
419. Katz LN, Gauchat HW. Observations of pulsus paradoxus (with special reference to pericardial effusions) II. Experimental. *Arch Intern Med* 1924;33:371–393.
420. Fowler NO. Pulsus paradoxus. *Heart Dis Stroke* 1994;3(2):68–69.
421. Beck CS. Two cardiac compression triads. *JAMA* 1935;104:714–716.
422. Spodick DH. *The pericardium: A comprehensive textbook.* New York: Marcel Dekker, 1997:153–179.
423. Antman EM, Cargill V, Grossman W. Low-pressure cardiac tamponade. *Ann Intern Med* 1979;91(3):403–406.
424. Von Sohsten R, Kopistansky C, Cohen M, et al. Cardiac tamponade in the "new device" era: evaluation of 6999 consecutive percutaneous coronary interventions. *Am Heart J* 2000;140(2):279–283.
425. Armstrong WF, Schilt BF, Helper DJ, et al. Diastolic collapse of the right ventricle with cardiac tamponade: an echocardiographic study. *Circulation* 1982;65(7):1491–1496.
426. Kronzon I, Cohen ML, Winer HE. Diastolic atrial compression: a sensitive echocardiographic sign of cardiac tamponade. *J Am Coll Cardiol* 1983; 2(4):770–775.
427. Singh S, Wann LS, Schuchard GH, et al. Right ventricular and right atrial collapse in patients with cardiac tamponade—a combined echocardiographic and hemodynamic study. *Circulation* 1984;70(6):966–971.
428. Schutzman JJ, Obarski TP, Pearce GL, et al. Comparison of Doppler and two-dimensional echocardiography for assessment of pericardial effusion. *Am J Cardiol* 1992;70(15):1353–1357.
429. Callahan JA, Seward JB, Nishimura RA, et al. Two-dimensional echocardiographically guided pericardiocentesis: experience in 117 consecutive patients. *Am J Cardiol* 1985;55(4):476–479.
430. Callahan JA, Seward JB, Tajik AJ. Cardiac tamponade: pericardiocentesis directed by two-dimensional echocardiography. *Mayo Clin Proc* 1985; 60(5):344–347.
431. Salem K, Mulji A, Lonn E. Echocardiographically guided pericardiocentesis—the gold standard for the management of pericardial effusion and cardiac tamponade. *Can J Cardiol* 1999;15(11):1251–1255.
432. Schiavone WA, Rice TW. Pericardial disease: current diagnosis and management methods. *Cleve Clin J Med* 1989;56(6):639–645.
433. Tsang TS, Freeman WK, Sinak LJ, et al. Echocardiographically guided pericardiocentesis: evolution and state-of-the-art technique. *Mayo Clin Proc* 1998;73(7):647–652.
434. Van Dyke Jr WH, Cure J, Chakko CS, et al. Pulmonary edema after pericardiocentesis for cardiac tamponade. *N Engl J Med* 1983;309:595–596.
435. Armstrong WF, Feigenbaum H, Dillon JC. Acute right ventricular dilation and echocardiographic volume overload following pericardiocentesis for relief of cardiac tamponade. *Am Heart J* 1984;107(6):1266–1270.
436. Tsang TS, El-Najdawi EK, Seward JB, et al. Percutaneous echocardiographically guided pericardiocentesis in pediatric patients: evaluation of safety and efficacy. *J Am Soc Echocardiogr* 1998;11(11):1072–1077.
437. Tsang TS, Barnes ME, Hayes SN, et al. Clinical and echocardiographic characteristics of significant pericardial effusions following cardiothoracic surgery and outcomes of echo-guided pericardiocentesis for management: Mayo Clinic experience, 1979–1998. *Chest* 1999;116(2):322–331.
438. Flores RM, Jaklitsch MT, DeCamp Jr MM, et al. Video-assisted thoracic surgery pericardial resection for effusive disease. *Chest Surg Clin North Am* 1998;8(4):835–851.
439. Sugimoto JT, Little AG, Ferguson MK, et al. Pericardial window: mechanisms of efficacy. *Ann Thorac Surg* 1990;50(3):442–445.
440. Van Trigt P, Douglas J, Smith PK, et al. A prospective trial of subxiphoid pericardiotomy in the diagnosis and treatment of large pericardial effusion. A follow-up report. *Ann Surg* 1993;218(6):777–782.
441. Kouvaras G, Polydorou A, Hatziantoniou G. Percutaneous balloon pericardiotomy for management of cardiac tamponade in a patient with lung cancer and large pericardial effusion. *Acta Cardiol* 1994;49(6):549–553.
442. Fakiolas CN, Beldekos DI, Foussas SG, et al. Percutaneous balloon pericardiotomy as a therapeutic alternative for cardiac tamponade and recurrent pericardial effusion. *Acta Cardiol* 1995;50(1):65–70.
443. Vora AM, Lokhandwala YY, Kale PA. Echocardiography guided creation of balloon pericardial window. *Cathet Cardiovasc Diagn* 1992;25(2):164–165.
444. Galli M, Politi A, Pedretti F, et al. Percutaneous balloon pericardiotomy for malignant pericardial tamponade. *Chest* 1995;108(6):1499–1501.
445. Di Segni E, Lavee J, Kaplinsky E, et al. Percutaneous balloon pericardiostomy for treatment of cardiac tamponade. *Eur Heart J* 1995;16(2):184–187.
446. Bahl VK, Bhargava B, Chandra S. Percutaneous pericardiotomy using Inoue balloon catheter. *Cathet Cardiovasc Diagn* 1995;36(1):98–99.
447. Bahl VK, Juneja R, Wasir HS. Percutaneous balloon pericardiotomy for cardiac tamponade. *Indian Heart J* 1994;46(2):115–116.
448. Ziskind AA, Pearce AC, Lemmon CC, et al. Percutaneous balloon pericardiotomy for the treatment of cardiac tamponade and large pericardial effusions: description of technique and report of the first 50 cases. *J Am Coll Cardiol* 1993;21(1):1–5.
449. Seferovic PM, Ristic AD, Maksimovic R, et al. Diagnostic value of pericardial biopsy: improvement with extensive sampling enabled by pericardioscopy. *Circulation* 2003;107(7):978–983.
450. Oh JK, Hatle LK, Seward JB, et al. Diagnostic role of Doppler echocardiography in constrictive pericarditis. *J Am Coll Cardiol* 1994;23(1):154–162.
451. Myers RB, Spodick DH. Constrictive pericarditis: clinical and pathophysiologic characteristics. *Am Heart J* 1999;138(2 Pt 1):219–232.
452. Grossman W, Baim D. *Cardiac catheterization, angiography and intervention.* Philadelphia: Lea & Febiger, 1991:644–698.
453. Leya FS, Arab D, Joyal D, et al. The efficacy of brain natriuretic peptide levels in differentiating constrictive pericarditis from restrictive cardiomyopathy. *J Am Coll Cardiol* 2005;45(11):1900–1902.
454. Candell-Riera J, Gutierrez-Palau L, et al. "Atrial systolic notch" and "early diastolic notch" on the interventricular septal echogram in constrictive pericarditis. *J Am Coll Cardiol* 1985;5(4):1020–1021.
455. Chandraratna PA, Aronow WS, Imaizumi T. Role of echocardiography in detecting the anatomic and physiologic abnormalities of constrictive pericarditis. *Am J Med Sci* 1982;283(3):141–146.
456. D'Cruz IA, Dick A, Gross CM, et al. Abnormal left ventricular–left atrial posterior wall contour: a new two-dimensional echocardiographic sign in constrictive pericarditis. *Am Heart J* 1989;118(1):128–132.
457. Engel PJ, Fowler NO, Tei CW, et al. M-mode echocardiography in constrictive pericarditis. *J Am Coll Cardiol* 1985;6(2):471–474.
458. Ling LH, Oh JK, Boonyaratavej S, et al. Diagnostic cases in 135 cases of constrictive pericarditis. *Circulation* 1996;94(Suppl I):I667.
459. Mertens LL, Denef B, DeGeest H. The differentiation between restrictive cardiomyopathy and constrictive pericarditis. *Echocardiography* 1993;10(5):497–508.
460. Klodas E, Nishimura RA, Appleton CP, et al. Doppler evaluation of patients with constrictive pericarditis: use of tricuspid regurgitation velocity curves to determine enhanced ventricular interaction. *J Am Coll Cardiol* 1996;28(3):652–657.
461. Boonyaratavej S, Oh JK, Tajik AJ, et al. Comparison of mitral inflow and superior vena cava Doppler velocities in chronic obstructive pulmonary disease and constrictive pericarditis. *J Am Coll Cardiol* 1998;32(7):2043–2048.
462. Oki T, Tabata T, Yamada H, et al. Right and left ventricular wall motion velocities as diagnostic indicators of constrictive pericarditis. *Am J Cardiol* 1998;81(4):465–470.
463. Palka P, Lange A, Donnelly JE, et al. Differentiation between restrictive cardiomyopathy and constrictive pericarditis by early diastolic Doppler myocardial velocity gradient at the posterior wall. *Circulation* 2000;102(6):655–662.
464. Sengupta PP, Mohan JC, Mehta V, et al. Accuracy and pitfalls of early diastolic motion of the mitral annulus for diagnosing constrictive pericarditis by tissue Doppler imaging. *Am J Cardiol* 2004;93(7):886–890.
465. Oh JK, Tajik AJ, Appleton CP, et al. Preload reduction to unmask the characteristic Doppler features of constrictive pericarditis: a new observation. *Circulation* 1997;95:796–799.
466. Klein AL, Al-Assaad AN, Pietrolungo JF, et al. Does rapid volume loading during transesophageal echocardiography differentiate constrictive pericarditis from restrictive cardiomyopathy? *J Am Soc Echocardiogr* 1994; S38:7C.
467. Tabata T, Kabbani SS, Murray RD, et al. Difference in the respiratory variation between mitral inflow and pulmonary venous flow Doppler velocities in patients with constrictive pericarditis. *J Am Soc Echocardiogr* 2000;13:435.
468. Abdalla IA, Murray RD, Awad HE, et al. Reversal of the pattern of respiratory variation of Doppler inflow velocities in constrictive pericarditis during mechanical ventilation. *J Am Soc Echocardiogr* 2000;13(9):827–831.
469. Pennell DJ, Underwood R. Magnetic resonance imaging of the heart. *Br J Hosp Med* 1993;49(2):90–95, 98–102.
470. Duvernoy O, Larsson SG, Thuren J, et al. Epicardial fat causing pitfalls in CT and MR imaging of the pericardium. *Acta Radiol* 1992;33(1):1–5.

471. Harasawa H, Li KS, Nakamoto T, et al. Ventricular coupling via the pericardium: normal versus tamponade. *Cardiovasc Res* 1993;27(8):1470–1476.
472. Glockner JF. Imaging of pericardial disease. *Magn Reson Imaging Clin North Am* 2003;11(1):149–162, vii.
473. Frank H, Globits S. Magnetic resonance imaging evaluation of myocardial and pericardial disease. *J Magn Reson Imaging* 1999;10(5):617–626.
474. Furber A, Pezard P, Jeune JJ, et al. Radionuclide angiography and magnetic resonance imaging: complementary non-invasive methods in the diagnosis of constrictive pericarditis. *Eur J Nucl Med* 1995;22(11):1292–1298.
475. White RD, Zisch RJ. Magnetic resonance imaging of pericardial disease and paracardiac and intracardiac masses. In: Elliot LP, ed. *The fundamentals of cardiac imaging in children and adults*. Philadelphia: Lippincott, 1991:420–430.
476. White RD, Hardy PA, Van Dyke CW, et al. Diastolic dysfunction: dynamic MRI velocity-mapping of related flow patterns in the superior vena cava. *J Magn Reson Imag* 1993;3(Suppl.):65.
477. O'Keeffe D, McCarthy P, O'Regan P. Computed tomography in constrictive pericarditis. *Ir Med J* 1984;77(6):172–174.
478. Olson MC, Posniak HV, McDonald V, et al. Computed tomography and magnetic resonance imaging of the pericardium. *Radiographics* 1989; 9(4):633–649.
479. Hayashi H, Kawamata H, Machida M, et al. Tuberculous pericarditis: MRI features with contrast enhancement. *Br J Radiol* 1998;71(846):680–682.
480. Van der Merwe S, Dens J, Daenen W, et al. Pericardial disease is often not recognised as a cause of chronic severe ascites. *J Hepatol* 2000;32(1):164–169.
481. Abrams J. The jugular venous pulse. In: Abrams J, ed. *Essentials of cardiac physical diagnosis*. Philadelphia: Lea & Febiger, 1987:41–54.
482. Ling LH, Oh JK, Breen JF, et al. Calcific constrictive pericarditis: is it still with us? *Ann Intern Med* 2000;132(6):444–450.
483. Hasuda T, Satoh T, Yamada N, et al. A case of constrictive pericarditis with local thickening of the pericardium without manifest ventricular interdependence. *Cardiology* 1999;92(3):214–216.
484. Spodick DH. *The pericardium: A comprehensive textbook*. New York: Marcel Dekker, 1997:214–259.
485. Talreja DR, Edwards WD, Danilson GK, et al. Constrictive pericarditis in 26 patients with histologically normal pericardial thickness. *Circulation* 2003;108(15):1852–1857.
486. Sagrista-Sauleda J, Angel J, Sanchez A, et al. Effusive-constrictive pericarditis. *N Engl J Med* 2004;350(5):469–475.
487. Haley JH, Tajik AJ, Danielson GK, et al. Transient constrictive pericarditis: causes and natural history. *J Am Coll Cardiol* 2004;43(2):271–275.
488. Sagrista-Sauleda J, Permanyer-Miralda G, Candell-Riera J, et al. Transient cardiac constriction: an unrecognized pattern of evolution in effusive acute idiopathic pericarditis. *Am J Cardiol* 1987;59(9):961–966.
489. Aagaard MT, Haraldsted VY. Chronic constrictive pericarditis treated with total pericardiectomy. *Thorac Cardiovasc Surg* 1984;32(5):311–314.
490. Astudillo R, Ivert T. Late results after pericardectomy for constrictive pericarditis via left thoracotomy. *Scand J Thorac Cardiovasc Surg* 1989;23(2): 115–119.
491. Tona IC, Danielson GK. Surgical management of pericardial diseases. *Cardiol Clin* 1990;8:683–696.
492. Senni M, Redfield MM, Ling LH, et al. Left ventricular systolic and diastolic function after pericardiectomy in patients with constrictive pericarditis: Doppler echocardiographic findings and correlation with clinical status. *J Am Coll Cardiol,* 1999;33(5):1182–1188.
493. Bertog SC, Thambidorai SK, Parakh K, et al. Constrictive pericarditis: etiology and cause-specific survival after pericardiectomy. *J Am Coll Cardiol* 2004;43(8):1445–1452.
494. Shabetai R. Acute pericarditis. *Cardiol Clin* 1990;8(4):639–644.
495. Saatci U, Ozen S, Ceyhan M, et al. Cytomegalovirus disease in a renal transplant recipient manifesting with pericarditis. *Int Urol Nephrol* 1993; 25(6):617–619.
496. Campbell PT, Li JS, Wall TC, et al. Cytomegalovirus pericarditis: a case series and review of the literature. *Am J Med Sci* 1995;309(4):229–234.
497. Acierno LJ. Cardiac complications in acquired immunodeficiency syndrome (AIDS): a review. *J Am Coll Cardiol* 1989;13(5):1144–1154.
498. Halsell JS, Riddle JR, Atwood JE, et al. Myopericarditis following smallpox vaccination among vaccinia-naive US military personnel. *JAMA* 2003;289(24):3283–3289.
499. Spodick DH. *The pericardium: a comprehensive textbook*. New York: Marcel Dekker, 1997:260–290.
500. Newby LK, Ohman EM. Troponins in pericarditis: implications for diagnosis and management of chest pains patients. *Eur Heart J* 2000;21(10): 798–800.
501. Sternbach GL. Pericarditis. *Ann Emerg Med* 1988;17(3):214–220.
502. Adler Y, Zandman-Goddard G, Ravid M, et al. Usefulness of colchicine in preventing recurrences of pericarditis. *Am J Cardiol* 1994;73(12):916–917.
503. Spodick DH. Diagnosis and management of acute noneffusive pericarditis. *Cardiol Board Rev* 1994;11(3):13–16.
504. Adler Y, Finkelstein Y, Guindo J, et al. Colchicine treatment for recurrent pericarditis. A decade of experience. *Circulation* 1998;97(21):2183–2185.
505. Imazio M, Bobbio M, Cecchi E, et al. Colchicine in addition to conventional therapy for acute pericarditis: results of the COlchicine for acute PEricarditis (COPE) trial. *Circulation* 2005;112(13):2012–2016.
506. Melchior TM, Ringsdal V, Hildebrandt P, et al. Recurrent acute idiopathic pericarditis treated with intravenous methylprednisolone given as pulse therapy. *Am Heart J* 1992;123(4 Pt 1):1086–1088.
507. Fowler NO, Harbin 3rd AD. Recurrent acute pericarditis: follow-up study of 31 patients. *J Am Coll Cardiol* 1986;7(2):300–305.
508. Brucato A, Cimaz R, Balla E. Prevention of recurrences of corticosteroid-dependent idiopathic pericarditis by colchicine in an adolescent patient. *Pediatr Cardiol* 2000;21(4):395–396.
509. Imazio M, Bobbio M, Cecchi E, et al. Colchicine as first-choice therapy for recurrent pericarditis: results of the CORE (COlchicine for REcurrent pericarditis) trial. *Arch Intern Med* 2005;165(17):1987–1991.
510. Imazio M, Demichelis B, Cecchi E, et al. Cardiac troponin I in acute pericarditis. *J Am Coll Cardiol* 2003;42(12):2144–2148.
511. Notomi Y, Setser RM, Shiota T, et al. Assessment of left ventricular torsional deformation by Doppler tissue imaging: validation study with tagged magnetic resonance imaging. *Circulation* 2005;111(9):1141–1147.
512. Maron BJ, Towbin JA, Thiene G, et al. Contemporary definitions and classification of the cardiomyopathies: An American Heart Association Scientific Statement from the Council on Clinical Cardiology, Heart Failure and Transplantation Committee; Quality of Care and Outcomes Research and Functional Genomics and Translational Biology Interdisciplinary Working Groups; and Council on Epidemiology and Prevention. *Circulation* 2006; 113:1807–1816.

CHAPTER 28 ■ PULMONARY HYPERTENSION

SRINIVAS MURALI

INTRODUCTION

Pulmonary hypertension (PH) is associated with a group of heterogeneous but distinct disorders and is characterized by complex proliferation of the pulmonary vascular endothelium and progressive pulmonary vascular remodeling (1,2). Clinically, PH is defined as a mean pulmonary arterial pressure that is greater than 25 mm Hg at rest or greater than 30 mm Hg during exercise along with a pulmonary capillary wedge pressure or left atrial pressure less than 15 mm Hg, measured at cardiac catheterization. Morphologic evidence for right ventricular remodeling must accompany the hemodynamic derangement (3). This definition was first used in the National Institutes of Health Registry on primary pulmonary hypertension and is now widely accepted by most specialists in the field. Noninvasively, based on echocardiography, PH is defined as a measured Doppler tricuspid regurgitation velocity of greater than 2.8 m/second, which estimates a right ventricular and pulmonary artery systolic pressure of at least 40 mm Hg from the Bernoulli equation (4–7).

The right ventricle is a low-pressure pump that accommodates well to changes in volume but not pressure (8). The increased afterload to the right ventricle in PH initially results in the normal adaptive response of hypertrophy and dilation. Eventually, the right ventricular contractile function declines when it is unable to further respond and tolerate this hemodynamic burden. Cor pulmonale is defined as right ventricular dysfunction and failure that directly results from PH associated with chronic parenchymal lung disease (9,10).

CLASSIFICATION OF PULMONARY HYPERTENSION

Even though PH was first described more than 100 years ago, a comprehensive classification for improving clinical understanding was not developed until 1998 (Evian classification). The earlier description of "primary" and "secondary" PH was abandoned and replaced by a classification in an effort to group disorders that share similarities in pathophysiology, clinical presentation, and treatment options (11). It separated conditions that directly affected the pulmonary arterial bed (PAH) from disorders that either involved the pulmonary venous circulation or affected the pulmonary circulation indirectly with involvement of respiratory structure or function. This classification was confusing, however, and had many shortcomings, and did not gain wide acceptance in clinical practice. With improved understanding of the pathogenesis of PAH, a revision to the nomenclature in the classification was proposed in 2003 (Venice classification) not only to reflect current understanding and perspective, but also to permit the widespread use and acceptance of the classification in clinical practice (Table 28.1). The term "primary" pulmonary hypertension (PPH) was replaced by "idiopathic" pulmonary hypertension (IPAH), and, when there was a genetic basis, "familial" pulmonary hypertension. PAH that occurred along with other conditions was referred to as "associated" pulmonary hypertension. This revised classification is accepted by the American College of Chest Physicians (12).

The classification emphasized the role of functional assessment in patients with PH, and a functional classification (WHO Classification), modified from the New York Heart Association functional classification, was adopted to aid clinical definition of the functional limitation (Table 28.2).

TABLE 28.1

REVISED VENICE NOMENCLATURE AND CLASSIFICATION OF PULMONARY HYPERTENSION—2003

1. Pulmonary arterial hypertension (PAH)
   - Sporadic (idiopathic) (IPAH)
   - Familial (FPAH)
   - Associated with:
     - Collagen vascular disease
     - Congential systemic-to-pulmonary shunts
     - Portal hypertension
     - HIV infection
     - Drugs and toxins
     - Other
   - Associated with significant venous or capillary involvement
     - Pulmonary venoocclusive disease
     - Pulmonary capillary hemangiomatosis
   - Persistent pulmonary hypertension of the newborn
2. Pulmonary venous hypertension
   - Left-sided artial or ventricular heart disease
   - Left-sided valvular heart disease
3. Pulmonary hypertension associated with hypoxemia
   - Chronic obstructive pulmonary disease
   - Interstitial lung disease
   - Sleep-disordered breathing
   - Alveolar hypoventilation disorders
   - Chronic exposure to high altitude
4. Pulmonary hypertension due to chronic thrombotic and/or embolic disease
   - Thromboembolic obstruction of proximal pulmonary arteries
   - Thromboembolic obstruction of distal pulmonary arteries
5. Miscellaneous
   - Sarcoidosis
   - Histiocytosis X
   - Lymphangiomatosis
   - Compression of pulmonary vessels

TABLE 28.2

WORLD HEALTH ORGANIZATION (WHO) CLASSIFICATION OF FUNCTIONAL STATUS IN PULMONARY ARTERIAL HYPERTENSION

Class	Description
I	No limitation of usual physical activity; ordinary physical activity does not cause increased dyspnea, fatigue, chest pain, or presyncope
II	No symptoms at rest; mild limitation of physical activity; normal physical activity causes increased dyspnea, fatigue, chest pain, or presyncope
III	No symptoms at rest; marked limitation of physical activity; less-than-ordinary physical activity causes increased dyspnea, fatigue, chest pain, or presyncope
IV	Unable to perform any physical activity at rest; signs of right ventricular failure; dyspnea, fatigue, chest pain, or presyncope present at rest and symptoms are increased by any physical activity

EPIDEMIOLOGY OF PULMONARY ARTERIAL HYPERTENSION

Idiopathic Pulmonary Arterial Hypertension

The prevalence of idiopathic pulmonary arterial hypertension (IPAH) is not known, and data are somewhat elusive (13–15). The prevalence is approximately 1 to 4 new cases per 1 million population. According to World Health Organization (WHO) estimates, there are 5,000 patients with IPAH in the United States and Europe. However, the prevalence may be increasing because of heightened awareness and early recognition in minimally symptomatic patients. According to the National Institutes of Health Registry of 187 patients with primary pulmonary hypertension (PPH) who were followed for 7 years, the mean age at diagnosis was 36 years and the female-to-male preponderance was 2:1 (3). The mean duration of symptoms before diagnosis was 2 years. One-year survival was 68%, 3-year survival was 48%, and 5-year survival was 34%; the median survival was 2.8 years from diagnosis (16). This registry was discontinued, however, before current treatments for PAH

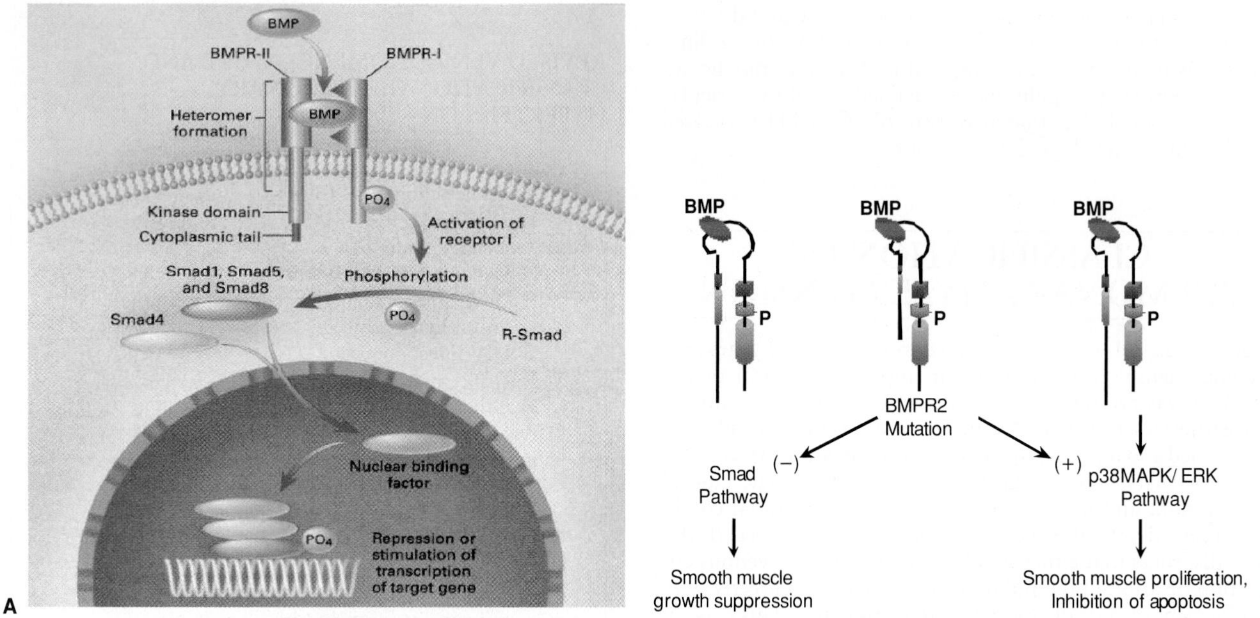

FIGURE 28.1. **A:** Bone morphogenetic protein (BMP) receptor type 2 (BMPR-2) function. BMPR-1 and BMPR-2 are adjacent on cell membranes. BMP binds to the extracellular domain (ligand binding) of BMPR-2, resulting in the formation of a heteromeric complex with BMPR-1. BMPR-2 then phosphorylates the transmembrane region of BMPR-1, activating the kinase domain. The activated BMPR-1 phosphorylates receptor Smad (R-Smad), thus activating a family of signalling molecules (Smad1, Smad5, and Smad8), which bind with Smad4 and migrate to the nucleus. The phosphorylated Smad complex attaches to a binding factor in the nucleus, and the resulting assembly either stimulates or represses gene transcription by ineracting with DNA. **B:** Effect of BMPR-2 mutations on intracellular signaling. Normal and abnormal signalling of BMPR-2. Normal pathway: BMPR-2 combines with BMPR-1 and signals through Smad pathway which is not affected by BMPR-2 mutations. This leads to smooth muscle growth suppression. An alternative pathway, through p38 MAP kinase/ERK pathway is the predominant way that mutated BMPR-2 signals leading to smooth muscle proliferation and inhibition of apoptosis. (Adapted from Newman JH, Wheeler L, Lane KB. Mutation in the gene for bone morphogenetic protein receptor II as a cause of primary pulmonary hypertension in a large kindred. *N Engl J Med* 2001;345:319–324.)

became available. Plans are underway to begin two new registries (funded by industry) that will help to ascertain the prevalence of IPAH in the United States.

Familial Pulmonary Arterial Hypertension

This condition accounts for 6% to 10% of IPAH patients. Mutations in two receptors of the TGF-β superfamily of growth factors have been identified in patients with familial PAH (17–19). Greater than 50% of familial cases and nearly 20% of sporadic cases have exonic mutations of the bone morphogenetic protein receptor type 2 (BMPR-2). Bone morphogenetic protein (BMP) is an osteoinductive cytokine that regulates smooth muscle cell growth and apoptosis (Fig. 28.1). It binds to a heteromeric complex of two receptors, BMPR-1 and BMPR-2, phosphorylating a family of signaling molecules (Smad proteins) that translocate to the nucleus and interact with specific proteins messaging suppression of smooth muscle cell growth. In the presence of BMPR-2 mutations, there is disruption of this normal Smad pathway, leading to signaling via an alternate p38 mitogen-activated protein kinase/extracellular signal-regulated kinase (MAPK/ERK) pathway that results in smooth muscle proliferation and inhibition of apoptosis (20–22). The entire interaction linking BMPR-2 mutations to the developmentof PAH is incompletely understood. Because the presence of the BMPR-2 mutation confers only a 15% to 20% lifetime risk of developing PAH, a second hit may be required to complete the interaction between this mutation and the development of PAH. Further studies are needed to delineate all the interactions among genes that may regulate the development of PAH and the environment in persons carrying this mutation (23).

Germline mutations of other genes in the TGF-β receptor family, such as the activin-like kinase type-1 (ALK-1) gene and endoglin (ENG) in patients with hereditary hemorrhagic telangiectasia (Osler-Weber-Rendu disease), also confer susceptibility to PAH (24). Autoantibodies to BMPR-2 or ALK-1 may also play a role in the development of PAH associated with connective tissue disease (25). Genetic polymorphisms of the serotonin transporter (5-HTT) have been implicated in the pathogenesis of PH (26–28). The long (L) allele is associated with increased 5-HTT transcription, and homozygosityfor the L-allele (LL) leads not only to an increased risk of developing PAH, but also to early onset of the disease in affected individuals. Whether this functional polymorphism confers susceptibility to PAH associated with other disorders is not known. Genetic testing and counseling have been recommended for relatives of patients with familial PAH.

Besides genetic risk factors there are other risk factors associated with the development of PAH (29) (Table 28.3).

Collagen Vascular Diseases

These are associated with both pulmonary involvement and the development of PAH. About 40% of patients with collagen vascular disease have no interstitial lung disease or pulmonary vascular disease. In the remaining 60%, about 19% have isolated PAH, 22% have interstitial lung disease, and

TABLE 28.3

RISK FACTORS FOR PULMONARY ARTERIAL HYPERTENSION

Genetic risk factors	Other risk factors
Major	Connective tissue disease
Mutations in BMPR-2	High-flow states
ALK-1	Female gender
Minor	Drugs/toxins
Serotonin transporter polymorphisms	Viral infections
	Environmental?
Other vascular genes?	

BMPR-2, bone morphogenetic protein receptor-2; ALK-1, activin-like kinase type-1.

the rest have both. PAH associated with systemic sclerosis or mixed connective tissue disease is present in 37% of patients, equally divided between diffuse and limited (CREST syndrome) disease; in 14% of patients with systemic lupus erythematosus; and in 5% of patients with rheumatoid arthritis (30–35). In a community rheumatology practice setting, approximately 13% of patients with collagen vascular disease were found to have undiagnosed PAH. In another series from Canada, 21% of patients with limited systemic sclerosis and 26% with diffuse sclerosis had associated PAH on a screening echocardiogram. The mean duration of systemic sclerosis was 9 years at the time of diagnosis of PAH. It is not known why only some patients with connective tissue disease develop PAH, and there are no biologic or inflammatory markers that can identify susceptible individuals reliably. Complex interactions among genes, environment, and the immune system are perhaps involved in the initial insult to the pulmonary vasculature in these patients. When PAH develops in patients with systemic sclerosis, it portends a very poor prognosis, far worse than in those with and without interstitial lung disease. The 1-year survival in patients with PAH is 50% and the 3-year survival 30%, compared to greater than 90% and greater than 80%, respectively, in patients without pulmonary hypertension (36).

Patients with systemic sclerosis who are most likely to acquire isolated PAH generally have limited disease (CREST syndrome), anticentromere antibodies, antinucleolar antibodies including U3RNP, B23, Th/To, and U1RNP, disease onset after menopause, and marked decreases in diffusing capacity to carbon monoxide.

Congenital Systemic-Pulmonary Shunts

The prevalence of PAH in patients with congenital systemic-to-pulmonary shunts is not known. Congenital heart anomalies are present in 0.8% of live births, and there are approximately 1 million adult patients with congenital heart disease in the United States. This number is likely to increase further as operative techniques are refined and definitive surgical repairs are performed in childhood. The high pressure and flow through the pulmonary circulation from a left-to-right shunt leads to the development of PAH. The size and duration of the shunt, genetic factors, and vasoactive mediators all predict the development of PAH in congenital heart disease. BMPR-2 mutations are present in 6% of patients, and high circulating levels of endothelin-1 and norepinephrine are associated with the development of PAH. Actuarial survival in PAH associated with congenital heart disease is better than that seen in other conditions. The 1-year survival is 92%, 2-year survival is 89%, 3-year survival is 77%, and 5-year survival is 77% (37,38).

Pulmonary Arterial Hypertension Associated with Liver Disease

Pulmonary-hepatic vascular disorders in advanced liver disease include hepatopulmonary syndrome and portopulmonary hypertension. Hepatopulmonary syndrome is present in 20% of liver disease patients and is characterized by progressive hypoxemia due to an oxygenation defect from intrapulmonary vascular dilations. It does not cause pulmonary hypertension and resolves after liver transplantation. Portopulmonary hypertension is characterized by pulmonary hypertension but not hypoxemia, and is also present in about 20% of advanced liver disease patients. Three hemodynamic subsets are noted: (a) a hyperdynamic circulatory state is common and is associated with moderate increases in pulmonary pressures, a severe increase in cardiac output, a normal pulmonary capillary wedge pressure, and a reduced pulmonary vascular resistance; (b) excess volume subset is also common and is associated with moderate increases in pulmonary pressure and cardiac output, severe increases in pulmonary capillary wedge pressure, and a normal pulmonary vascular resistance; (c) a vasoproliferative state is rare and is associated with severe increases in pulmonary pressures and vascular resistance, a mild decrease in pulmonary capillary wedge pressure, and a moderate increase followed by a decrease in cardiac output. Liver transplantation generally results in resolution of PH, although it can be risky. The vasoproliferative hemodynamic subset in particular is a contraindication to liver transplantation (39–43).

HIV-Associated Pulmonary Arterial Hypertension

There are more than 1 million people with human immunodeficiency virus (HIV) infection in the United States. HIV-associated PAH is seen in 0.5% of patients. Infection with human herpesvirus-8 (HHV-8), which causes Kaposi sarcoma, has been implicated in the pathogenesis of PH associated with HIV infection. The use of highly active antiretroviral therapy may improve PH associated with HIV infection. The actuarial survival is 58% at 1 year, 39% at 2 years, and 21% at 3 years (44–50).

Pulmonary Arterial Hypertension Associated with Drugs

Drugs and toxins associated with the development of PAH include fenfluramine anorexinogens, aminorex, amphetamines, and cocaine. The use of these drugs for more than 3 months confers a 30-fold higher risk of PAH than in the general population. The development of PAH is thought to be mediated through interactions with the serotonin transporter located in the pulmonary vascular smooth muscle cell. Individuals with higher baseline serotonin expression related to the L allele of the serotonin gene (LL variant) are thought to be susceptible to anorexinogen-induced PAH. Insufficiency of the K_V 1.5 channel activity may also predispose to the development of PAH by augmenting the vasoconstrictor response (51–54).

Pulmonary Arterial Hypertension Associated with Hemoglobinopathies

It is estimated that 20% to 40% of patients with β-thalassemia and sickle cell anemia are prone to developing pulmonary hypertension. Mortality in sickle cell anemia with pulmonary hypertension is markedly worse than in sickle cell anemia with normal pulmonary pressures (55,56).

OTHER CAUSES OF PULMONARY HYPERTENSION

Chronic Obstructive Lung Disease

Severe chronic obstructive lung disease is frequently associated with PH. It is the most common cause of pulmonary parenchymal disease in the Unites States. According to the Global Initiative for Chronic Obstructive Lung Disease, it is a disease state characterized by progressive, irreversible airflow obstruction and abnormal inflammatory response and fibrosis in the lungs to noxious particles and gases. The progressive airflow limitation is both from bronchiolitis and from loss of elastic recoil from parenchymal destruction, elastolysis, and loss of alveolar attachments. Morphologically, it is characterized by chronic bronchitis, bronchiolitis, and emphysema. There is permanent air space enlargement in emphysema involving the terminal bronchioles and alveoli. It can either be centrilobular, as seen in smokers, or panacinar, as occurs in α1-antitrypsin deficiency. The parenchymal destruction is driven by an imbalance between proteases and antiproteases along with inflammation that predominantly involves CD 8+ T lymphocytes but also neutrophils and macrophages. The proteases that are upregulated include leukocyte elastase, cathepsin G, matrix metalloproteinases, and cysteine proteinases. The counterbalancing antiproteases, including α1antitrypsin, secretory leukocyte protease inhibitor, and tissue inhibitors of metalloproteinases, are decreased. The inflammatory cells also secrete reactive oxygen species, which provokes release of several proinflammatory cytokines, through the activation of intracellular inflammatory pathways. Endothelin-1 (ET-1) expression is also increased in the pulmonary vasculature in chronic obstructive lung disease, particularly during exacerbations (57–59).

Pulmonary Hypertension Associated with Interstitial Lung Disease

Interstitial lung disease may be from connective tissue disease, as previously described, or from idiopathic pulmonary fibrosis. Rarely, pulmonary sarcoidosis can cause interstitial lung disease. Depending on the etiology, the prevalence of PH varies in interstitial lung disease. It has been reported in 31% of patients with idiopathic pulmonary fibrosis. When it is present, patients with idiopathic pulmonary fibrosis have lower diffusing capacity for carbon monoxide and are more likely to require supplemental oxygen. Presence of PH results in greater functional limitation, with lower 6-minute walk distance and higher mortality. There is a linear inverse correlation between pulmonary pressures and clinical outcome, with patients with PH having a threefold higher mortality. In idiopathic pulmonary fibrosis, there is repeated lung injury with progressive fibrotic reaction. The levels of the antioxidant glutathione are markedly depleted, and the resulting imbalance between oxidants and antioxidants promotes fibrosis. There is increased endothelin expression, and progression is not related to inflammation (60,61).

Pulmonary Hypertension and Sleep-Disordered Breathing

Obstructive sleep apnea (OSA) is the most common type of sleep-disordered breathing and affects 5% to 15% of the adult population. Its physiologic consequences include systemic hypertension, stroke, coronary disease, heart failure, atrial arrhythmias, and pulmonary hypertension, especially when there is preexisting pulmonary disease. The precise link between OSA and the aforementioned conditions is unknown. Autonomic dysfunction, increased daytime and nocturnal sympathetic activity, endothelial dysfunction, enhanced leukocyte adhesion, increased platelet aggregation, and activation of proinflammatory and prothrombotic factors such as interleukin-6, fibrinogen, and plasminogen activator inhibitor are present in patients with OSA. Patients with OSA and PH are older and heavier and have worse lung function. Apnea-hypopnea index is a poor predictor of PH. Patients with OSA and PH have decreased nitric oxide activity. The apneic spells associated with OSA are associated with hypoxemia and elevations in pulmonary artery pressures, which resolve with restoration of ventilation. The reasons for persistent PH in OSA are not very clear. However, PH in OSA is generally mild and moderately responds to continuous positive-airway-pressure therapy (62–65).

Chronic Thromboembolic Pulmonary Hypertension

This form of PH develops in only 0.1% to 4% of patients who survive an acute pulmonary embolism. However, its prevalence may be underappreciated. A history of thromboembolic events is present in 60% of patients, and coagulation disorders, most notably a positive lupus anticoagulant titer, is present in 30% of patients. Serotonin transporter gene polymorphism is seen in 30% of patients with chronic thromboembolic PH. The presence of this genetic polymorphism may unfavorably modulate the clinical course of the disease. Appropriate diagnosis of this form of PH is critical because some patients can be cured with surgical thromboendarterectomy (66–71).

Pulmonary Hypertension Associated with Left Heart Disease

Chronic left ventricular failure is a common and important cause of PH. In the United States, there are more than 5 million people affected by left ventricular failure, and approximately 550,000 new cases are diagnosed annually. Heart failure affects 10% of the population older than 65 years of age and is the leading cause of hospitalization among adults. Approximately two thirds of heart failures are secondary to diminished left ventricular contractility or systolic dysfunction, and the remainder are due to impaired left ventricular filling or diastolic dysfunction. Coronary artery disease and primary cardiomyopathy are the most common causes of systolic left ventricular failure, whereas hypertension is the leading cause of diastolic failure.

Advanced heart failure accounts for at least 10% of all heart failure (approximately 500,000 patients) and its prevalence is increasing particularly because of emphasis and monitoring of evidence-based medical therapies and reduction in sudden cardiac death due to prophylactic defibrillator implantation. PH may be either mild or moderate, although it can be

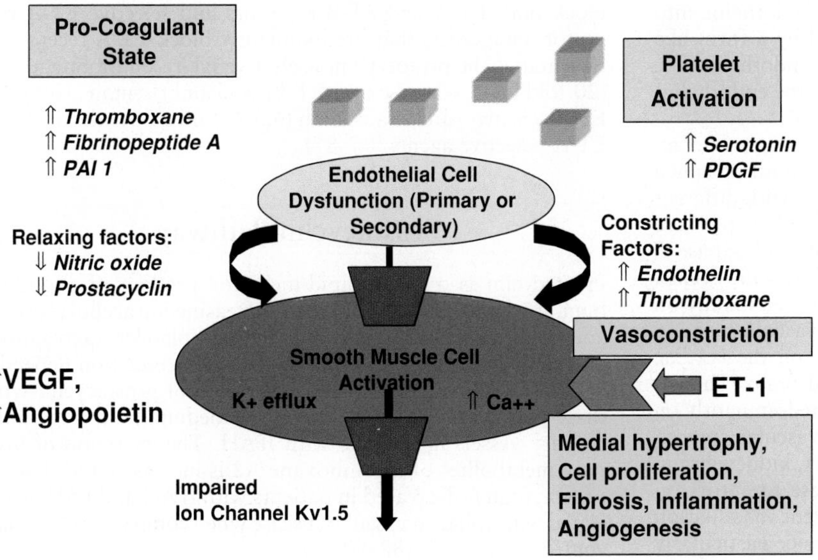

FIGURE 28.2. Pathogenetic mechanisms in pulmonary arterial hypertension. ET-1, endothelin-1; PAI 1, plasminogen activator inhibitor-1; PDGF, platelet-derived growth factor; VEGF, vascular endothelial growth factor. (Adapted and modified from Gaine SP, Rubin LJ. Primary pulmonary hypertension. *Lancet* 1998;352:719–725.)

severe in up to one third of the patients. It is critical that every heart failure patient with advanced symptoms undergo a thorough evaluation to ascertain the presence and severity of PH (72–75).

PATHOPHYSIOLOGY OF PULMONARY ARTERIAL HYPERTENSION

The pathogenesis of PAH involves several key biologic events (Fig. 28.2). Endothelial cell dysfunction, whether inherited or from other risk factors, results in increased intracellular transcription of constricting factors such as endothelin-1 and thromboxane A2 and decreased activity of relaxing factors like nitric oxide and prostacyclin. This imbalance favors vasoconstriction and signals smooth muscle cell activation and dysfunction, hyperplasia and hypertrophy, inhibition of apoptosis, fibroblast proliferation, collagen deposition, activation of proinflammatory cytokines, and angiogenesis. A number of growth factors including vascular endothelial growth factor and angiopoietin are upregulated, which also promotes cell proliferation and angiogenesis. Impaired function or insufficiency of the voltage-gated potassium-ion channels (K_V 1.5) on the pulmonary vascular smooth muscle cell results in efflux of potassium and increased intracellular calcium, which induces further pulmonary vasoconstriction. Platelet activation releases platelet-derived growth factor and serotonin into the circulation. Increased availability of thromboxane A2, fibrinopeptide A, and plasminogen activator inhibitor-1 creates a procoagulant milieu within the pulmonary circulation predisposing to in situ thrombosis. Vasoconstriction, cell proliferation, fibrosis, angiogenesis, and thrombosis combine to produce progressive and deleterious pulmonary vascular remodeling. The list of mediators that are dysregulated in PAH are shown in Table 28.4. Of these, endothelin (ET-1), prostacyclin, and nitric oxide have been studied extensively (76,77).

The Endothelin System

ET-1 is synthesized and released not only by the endothelial cell, but also by other cell types such as leukocytes, macrophages, cardiomyocytes, vascular and airway smooth muscle cells, and mesangial cells. Physicochemical factors such as hypoxemia, pulsatile stretch, low shear stress, and other factors including proinflammatory cytokines, transforming growth factor-β, endotoxin, and a number of circulating neurohormones promote endothelin synthesis and release. Both nitric oxide and prostacyclin inhibit endothelin synthesis. The message for endothelin synthesis from the nucleus results in

TABLE 28.4

CURRENT PHARMACOLOGIC TREATMENTS FOR PULMONARY ARTERIAL HYPERTENSION

Adjuvant therapy	Other therapy	FDA-approved therapy	Investigational therapy
Digoxin (oral) Diuretics (oral or IV) Oxygen Anticoagulation (oral)	Calcium channel blockers (oral)	Bosentan (oral) Sildenafil (oral) Iloprost (inhaled) Treprostinil (SC or IV) Epoprostenol (IV)	Sitaxsentan (oral) Ambrisentan (oral) Treprostinil (inhaled, oral) Vardenafil, tadalafil (oral) Vasoactive intestinal polypeptide (inhaled) Adrenomedullin (IV or inhaled) Simvastatin (oral)

FDA, Food and Drug Administration; IV, intravenous; SC, subcutaneous.

Pulmonary Hypertension

the release of an inactive precursor prepro-endothelin into the cytoplasm. This precursor is then cleaved by a furin-like enzyme into an inactive intermediate called big-endothelin. The big-endothelin (big ET-1) is further cleaved by the endothelin-converting enzyme (ECE) to active ET-1 (78–84).

After release, ET-1 mediates its effects through interaction with two classes of cell surface receptors, both of which are G protein–coupled transmembrane proteins, with different molecular and physiologic functions. ET-1 binding to these receptors activates the phosphatidyl inositol phospholipase C pathway, which in turn signals several key cell-specific events. The endothelin type A (ET-A) receptors are located mainly on the vascular smooth muscle cells and mediate vasoconstriction and cell proliferation. They are also present on the cardiac myocyte, cardiac fibroblast, lung, kidney, and brain. The endothelin type B (ET-B) receptors are present predominantly on endothelial cells but are also located on the vascular smooth muscle cells and other organs such as the heart, kidney, brain, intestine, and melanocytes. Activation of these receptors on endothelial cells mediates nitric oxide–dependent vasodilation and prostacyclin release as well as ET-1 clearance particularly in the pulmonary and renal vascular beds, whereas those on the smooth muscle cells mediate vasoconstriction. The net biologic effect of ET-1 depends on the density of ET-A receptors on the vascular smooth muscle cell and the ET-B receptors on the endothelial cell. ET-B receptors are also important for sodium and water absorption in the distal renal tubules.

Under physiologic conditions, ET-1 causes vasoconstriction, cell proliferation, and differentiation determined by a complex interplay between its effects on ET-A and ET-B receptors. ET-1 is important for maintenance of basal tone in many vascular beds. Other effects of ET-1 include a reduction in heart rate, a decrease in coronary blood flow and coronary sinus oxygen saturation, and an increase in cardiac contractility. In pathologic states, the ET receptors are regulated differently, which results in different acute and chronic biologic effects. The acute effects involve vasoconstriction and inflammation, whereas the chronic effects include fibroblast proliferation, synthesis of extracellular matrix components, hypertrophy of cardiac myocytes, neurohormonal secretion, and cell proliferation. ET-1 increases plasma renin activity, enhances conversion of angiotensin I to angiotensin II, and augments the synthesis and release of aldosterone from the adrenal glands. In patients with chronic heart failure, plasma ET-1 levels are increased and correlate directly with functional impairment and inversely with left ventricular ejection fraction. There is a direct correlation between plasma ET-1 levels and left ventricular filling pressures and an indirect correlation with survival and need for transplantation in chronic heart failure patients. Unlike other neurohormones, however, plasma ET-1 also correlates with the severity of pulmonary hypertension in chronic heart failure patients. ET-1 expression in the pulmonary vasculature is increased in patients with PAH. Plasma ET-1 levels are elevated not only in patients with IPAH, but also in patients with pulmonary hypertension associated with connective tissue diseases and congenital heart disease. The high plasma levels of ET-1 in chronic heart failure and pulmonary hypertension may be not only from increased synthesis, but also from reduced clearance in the lung.

Antagonism of the ET system can be achieved either by ECE inhibition or by blocking ET-A and ET-B receptors. Most ECE inhibitors also inhibit neutral endopeptidase (NEP), and so they not only inhibit ET-1 production, but also prevent the metabolism of vasodilating mediators such as atrial natriuretic peptide and bradykinin. The effectiveness of ECE inhibitors may be limited by non-ECE–mediated conversion of big ET-1 to ET-1 (ECE escape). ET-receptor antagonists either selectively block ET-A or ET-B receptor or block both. There are "mixed" or "dual," nonselective ET receptor antagonists that block both ET-A and ET-B receptors and selective ET-A receptor antagonists that predominantly block ET-A receptors. Bosentan is the prototype nonselective ET-receptor antagonist (20-fold ET-A selective over ET-B), and ambrisentan (100-fold ET-A selective) and sitaxsentan (6,500-fold ET-A selective) are ET-A–selective agents (85–87).

Prostacyclin Pathway

Prostacyclin is a major lipid-mediator product of endothelium. It relaxes smooth muscle by increasing intracellular cyclic adenosine monophosphate and inhibits platelet aggregation and smooth muscle cell proliferation. Its production depends on prostacyclin synthase. The expression of prostacyclin synthase is downregulated in the small, medium, and large pulmonary vessels in patients with IPAH. The excretion of urinary metabolites of thromboxane A2 is increased and that of prostacyclin is decreased in patients with IPAH and PAH associated with collagen vascular disease when compared to normal control individuals (88–90).

Nitric Oxide Pathway

The expression of endothelial NO synthase (eNOS)is reduced in lungs of patients with pulmonary hypertension, suggesting that reduced bioavailability of NO is important in the pathogenesis. In response to L-arginine, PAH patients have impaired NO production. Exhaled NO and urinary NO metabolites are also reduced in PAH patients. Treatment with endothelin antagonists partially reverses these abnormalities, which suggests that ET-1 may be partly responsible for the decreased eNOS activity in PAH (91–95). Other potential causes for reduced bioavailability of NO in PAH include oxidant stress, increased levels of asymmetric dimethyl arginine (ADMA), which inhibits NOS activity, and decreased L-arginine levels due to increased activity of arginase released from erythrocytes and endothelial cells (96–99).

NO mediates its biologic effects through an intracellular second messenger called cyclic guanosine monophosphate (cGMP), which is broken down and inactivated by phosphodiesterases (PDEs), especially the isozymes PDE1 and PDE5. Because PDE5 is abundant in the pulmonary vasculature, its inhibition is an attractive therapeutic target in PAH. Impaired activity of soluble guanylate cyclase (sGC) because of oxidation may cause hyporesponsiveness to NO in PAH (100,101).

Pathways Mediating Pulmonary Hypertension in Left Heart Disease

Left ventricular injury leading to structural remodeling and dysfunction is the seminal event in the progression of heart failure. The translation of injury to remodeling depends on the upregulation and downregulation of several neurohormone and cytokine pathways that results in neurohormonal imbalance (102–105). The renin–angiotensin–aldosterone system, the sympathetic nervous system, and endothelin are the vasoconstrictor systems that are activated, whereas endogenous vasodilator systems, such as nitric oxide and kinins, are deactivated. All of these systems extensively interact with each other, resulting in pulmonary vascular endothelial cell dysfunction. This triggers pulmonary vasoconstriction and vascular remodeling through multiple mechanisms, leading to the development of pulmonary hypertension. The translation from endothelial cell dysfunction to intimal thickening and medial hypertrophy is not well understood, but it involves endothelin-1 and nitric oxide, both of which play a critical role in the maintenance of vascular tone in health. Plasma endothelin-1 levels vary directly with pulmonary artery pressures and pulmonary vascular resistance and inversely with stroke volume in heart failure patients with PH. Plasma endothelin-1 level is a direct correlate of mortality in heart failure patients. Left ventricular remodeling also results in mitral regurgitation, which causes left atrial hypertension and further triggers pulmonary vascular endothelial dysfunction.

Other Pathways

Vasoactive intestinal polypeptide (VIP) is an important neurohormone that is involved in the water and electrolyte secretion in the gut. It inhibits platelet activation and vascular smooth muscle cell proliferation. It is a pulmonary vasodilator, bronchodilator and decreases pulmonary artery pressures and pulmonary vascular resistance in experimental models of PAH. Its biologic action is mediated through activation of two specific VIP receptors (VPAC-1 and VPAC-2), which in turn, promotes cAMP and cGMP signalling. Serum VIP levels are reduced in PAH patients compared to normal subjects and patients with parenchymal lung disease. VIP expression in the tunica media is also reduced in PAH.

Platelet derived growth factor (PDGF) is a mitogen that is up regulated in PAH. PDGF signalling promotes pulmonary vascular smooth muscle cell proliferation in experimental models of pulmonary hypertension. PDGF receptor inhibition has been shown to reverse pulmonary vascular remodeling. Angiopoietin expression has also been shown to be increased in the lung of patients with chronic thrombo–embolic PH. Additionally, matrix metallo-proteinases (MMP) 1 and 9 are also upregulated in the lung tissue. As in chronic heart failure, sympathetic nervous system, renin-angiotensin aldosterone, and B-type natriuretic peptide activity are all increased in patients with PAH.

CLINICAL DIAGNOSIS OF PULMONARY HYPERTENSION

Screening and Early Detection

Patients who have conditions that are associated with PAH should be screened for early recognition (106–108). Family members of affected patients or patients who have a history of use of fenfluramine appetite suppressants, current or prior use of amphetamines, or cocaine should also be screened. Accordingly, PAH should be suspected particularly if patients develop unexplained dyspnea. However, many of these patients are either asymptomatic or minimally symptomatic. Although exertional dyspnea is the most frequently encountered symptom, it is sometimes accompanied by exertional fatigue and exercise intolerance. Patients with a history of acute pulmonary embolism should be carefully evaluated for chronic thromboembolic pulmonary hypertension. Similarly, patients with chronic obstructive lung disease, interstitial lung disease, and sleep-disordered breathing should be screened for development of PH if they develop worsening symptoms. Patients with left heart disease who deteriorate on medical therapy or who become refractory to medical therapy should be suspected to have developed associated PH. Transthoracic echocardiogram is the most commonly used screening test for PH. If the resting study is normal, an exercise echocardiogram should be considered to look for exercise-induced PH. The key is to have a high index of suspicion in all patients with the aforementioned conditions (37).

Signs and Symptoms

Although exertional dyspnea and reduced exercise capacity are frequent symptoms, some patients have very nonspecific complaints, such as persistent fatigue, weight gain, and abdominal bloating. Angina and syncope are less common symptoms and frequently portend a poor prognosis. In the later stages, orthopnea, paroxysmal nocturnal dyspnea, and peripheral edema develop indicating the presence of right ventricular failure. Of course, symptoms related to the associated conditions may be present (37).

Physical findings of PH can be elusive unless the patient has advanced disease. The intensity of the pulmonic component of the second heart sound is accentuated and the second sound is widely split. Murmurs of tricuspid regurgitation and pulmonic regurgitation may be present. Parasternal heave or a third or fourth heart sound along the left sternal border indicates right ventricular hypertrophy or dilation. When right ventricular failure develops, other signs such as jugular venous distension, peripheral edema, ascites, hepatomegaly, and hepatojugular reflux are present. Physical findings related to the associated conditions may be present.

Diagnostic Evaluation

Each patient with suspected PAH must undergo a careful, comprehensive diagnostic work-up to clarify the diagnosis, ascertain the severity, and identify the etiology (Fig. 28.3).

Electrocardiogram

This may show right ventricular hypertrophy, right atrial enlargement, right-axis deviation, and incomplete or complete right-bundle-branch block. Secondary repolarization changes may also be present (109).

Chest X-Ray

Findings on a chest radiograph include enlargement of the main and hilar pulmonary arteries, pruning or attenuation of peripheral vascular markings, and displacement of the right ventricle anteriorly into the retrosternal space that can be seen in the lateral view. Findings associated with coexistent conditions such as chronic obstructive lung disease, interstitial lung disease, and left heart disease may be present (110).

Echocardiogram

The echocardiogram is the most important diagnostic test in PAH patients (111). Pulmonary artery systolic pressure is estimated by measuring the Doppler systolic tricuspid regurgitant flow velocity and applying the Bernoulli equation. In experienced laboratories, quantifiable tricuspid regurgitant flow signals are recorded in 74% of cases; the sensitivity of this method in estimating the pulmonary artery systolic pressure ranges between 0.79 and 1.00, and the specificity ranges from 0.60 to 0.98. The echocardiographic estimate is inaccurate, however, in the presence of severe right ventricular failure and pulmonary regurgitation. Perhaps more important than the estimated pulmonary artery systolic pressure, the echocardiogram provides important information regarding the right atrial and right ventricular morphology, right and left ventricular function, the mitral and tricuspid valve structure, and the integrity of the interatrial and interventricular septum. A transesophageal study or a contrast study may be needed to define the anatomy

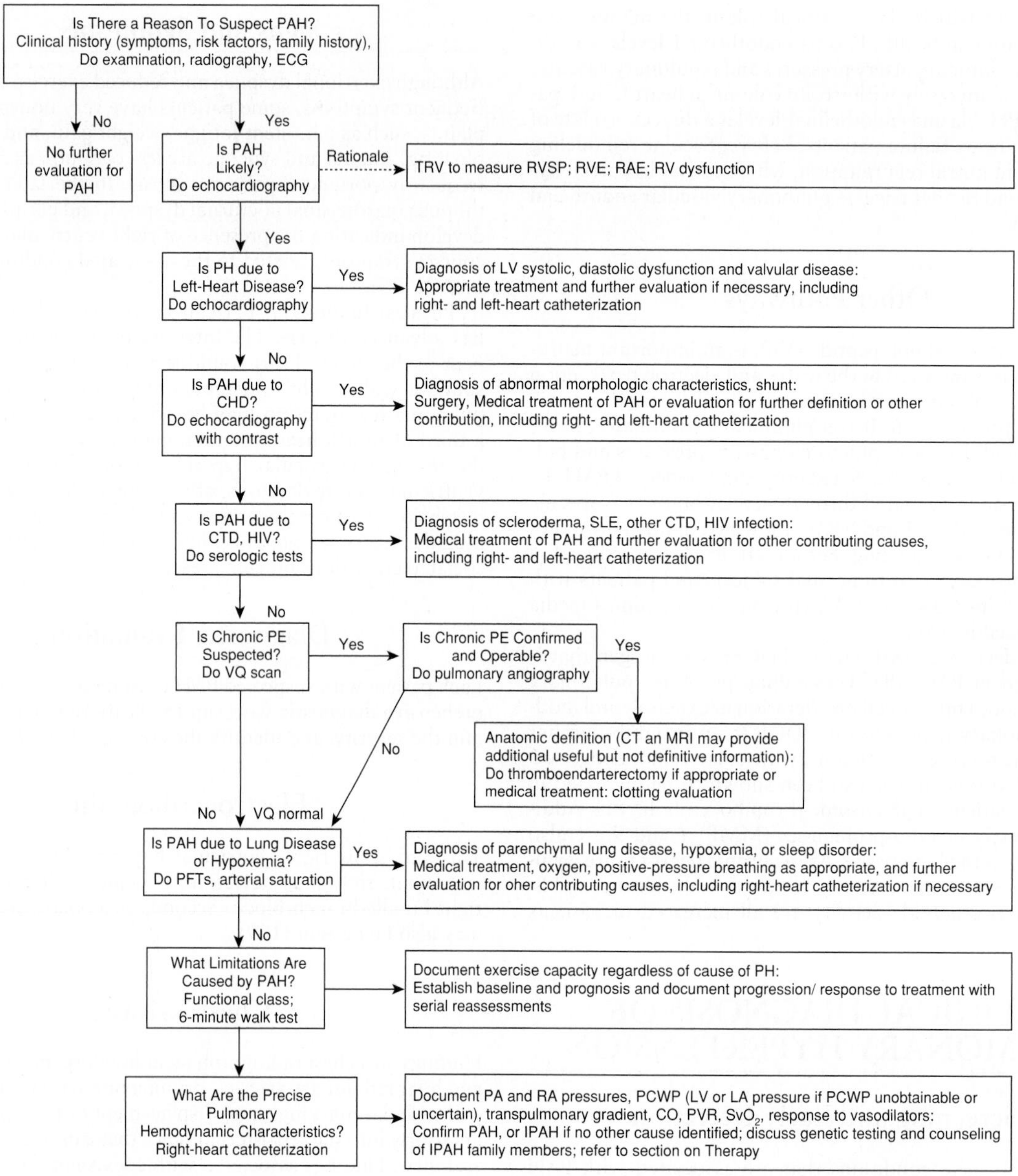

FIGURE 28.3. Algorithm for a diagnostic approach in pulmonary hypertension. CHD, Congenital heart disease; CO, cardiac output; CT, Computed tomography; CTD, Connective tissure disease; ECG, Electrocardiogram; IPAH, idiopathic pulmonary arterial hypertension; LA, left atrium; LV, Left ventricle; MRI, Magnetic resonance imaging; PA, Pulmonary artery; PAH, Pulmonary arterial hypertension; PCWP, Pulmonary capillary wedge pressure; PE, Pulmonary embolism; PFT, Pulmonary function tests; PH, Pulmonary hypertension; PVR, Pulmonary vascular resistance; RAE, Right atrial enlargement; RVE, Right ventricular enlargement; RVSP, Right ventricular systolic pressure; SLE, Systemic lupus erythematosus; SvO2, Mixed venous oxygen saturation; TRV, Tricuspid regurgitation velocity; VQ, Ventilation perfusion. (Adapted from Rubin LJ, Badesch DB. Evaluation and management of the patient with pulmonary arterial hypertension. *Ann Internal Med* 2005;143:288–292.)

in patients who have congenital systemic-pulmonary shunts (4–7).

Pulmonary Function Test

This helps to exclude and characterize airway and pulmonary parenchymal disease. Patients with chronic obstructive lung disease and those with interstitial pulmonary fibrosis have mild to moderate PH and marked obstructive and restrictive ventilatory defects. Mild restrictive defects are present in up to 20% of patients with IPAH. Mild to moderate restrictive defects can also be seen in patients with chronic thromboembolic pulmonary hypertension. In patients with systemic sclerosis, isolated reductions in diffusing capacity for carbon dioxide is present in 25% of patients. The greater the reduction in diffusing capacity, the worse is the prognosis. When the diffusing capacity in a patient with systemic sclerosis is less than 50% of predicted, there is a high likelihood that PAH is present (37).

Arterial Blood Gases

It is important to ascertain the presence of hypoxemia at rest. This may indicate the presence of a right-to-left intracardiac or intrapulmonary shunt. Overnight oximetry and exercise oxygen desaturation study may be needed to determine whether supplemental oxygen therapy is required. Nocturnal hypoxemia may be seen in up to 75% of IPAH patients (37).

Ventilation–Perfusion Lung Scan

This is the preferred test for assessing for chronic thromboembolic pulmonary hypertension. The diagnostic criteria require the presence of a segmental or larger perfusion defect with mismatched ventilation. Some patients may have subsegmental or patchy perfusion defects, which are less specific findings. A normal ventilation–perfusion scan essentially rules out surgically correctible chronic thromboembolic PH, whereas an abnormal scan can sometimes be present in vasculitis, extrinsic compression, and pulmonary venoocclusive disease. A positive scan generally underestimates the degree and extent of vascular obstruction (112,113).

Computed Tomographic Scan

This noninvasive test can give valuable information regarding the lung parenchyma, pulmonary arteries, right ventricle, bronchial collateral flow, and pulmonary vascular obstruction. Patients with pulmonary venoocclusive disease may have a ground glass pattern in the lower lobes. Pulmonary infarctions and pulmonary fibrosis can be evaluated reliably with this test (114,115).

Pulmonary Angiography

This is the definitive test for the diagnosis of chronic thromboembolic PH. Because it is invasive and carries a risk, it should only be performed in experienced centers. It is necessary to accurately define the pulmonary vascular anatomy when surgical treatment is contemplated for chronic thromboembolic PH (113).

Cardiac Catheterization

This is the most important diagnostic test for PAH patients. It gives an accurate measurement of pulmonary artery pressures and cardiac output from which the pulmonary vascular resistance and transpulmonary gradient can be calculated. It can help to detect and define intracardiac shunts, rule out the presence of left heart disease, and help to guide therapy (37,116).

Vasoreactivity testing can be combined with right heart catheterization to ascertain whether the PAH is "vasoreactive" or "fixed." This finding is critical to both making treatment decisions and determining prognosis. Inhaled nitric oxide, intravenous adenosine, or prostacyclin is frequently used to determine vasoreactivity. The reported incidence of vasoreactivity is between 8.6% and 26.5%. When the mean pulmonary artery pressure decreases by at least 10 mm Hg to 40 mm Hg or less with an increase or unchanged cardiac output with acute vasodilator challenge, the patient is labeled "vasoreactive" or a "responder." Vasoreactivity testing is recommended in IPAH patients only because patients with PAH associated with other conditions are rarely responders. A positive vasoreactivity test suggests a good prognosis.

In a patient with PH associated with left heart failure, acute vasoreactivity testing should be done particularly if the patient is to be considered for cardiac transplantation. Intravenous sodium nitroprusside, milrinone, prostacyclin, or inhaled nitric oxide is generally used for this purpose. Although there is no standard definition by which to identify a "responder," the goal is to see whether the transpulmonary gradient and pulmonary vascular resistance can be decreased appreciably without raising pulmonary capillary wedge pressure or lowering cardiac output or causing systemic hypotension. Patients who are acutely vasoreactive and are listed for transplantation will require serial testing every 6 to 8 weeks to ensure that they remain vasoresponsive (37).

Other Tests

This includes routine blood work, testing for HIV titer, and serologic testing for antinuclear antibodies and other antibodies that may indicate the presence of an underlying autoimmune–collagen vascular disorder. Elevated titers of antinuclear antibody in a nonspecific pattern are seen in up to 40% of IPAH patients. Sleep study is necessary for patients in whom sleep apnea is suspected. Cardiac magnetic resonance imaging (MRI) is a very useful ancillary test in selected patients. It may be particularly useful in the assessment of right ventricular mass and function, especially because the echocardiogram is limited in this regard. Thoracoscopic or open-lung biopsy may be indicated for patients with vasculitis, pulmonary venoocclusive disease, granulomatous, and interstitial lung disease. Lung biopsy is a risky procedure that can cause pulmonary hemorrhage, hypoxemia, and death and should be done only in experienced centers (117–119).

PROGRESSION AND PROGNOSIS

Hemodynamic Progression in Pulmonary Arterial Hypertension

The human pulmonary circulation, unlike the systemic circulation, is a low-resistance vascular bed (120). According to the hydrodynamic equation, which draws an analogy from Ohm's law, the resistance to flow (R) varies directly with the pressure drop (ΔP) and inversely with the rate of flow (Q) across the pulmonary vascular bed such that $R = \Delta P/Q$. The pressure drop in the pulmonary vascular bed is also known as the transpulmonary pressure gradient (TPG), which is the difference between the measured mean pulmonary artery pressure and pulmonary capillary wedge pressure (PCWP). Pulmonary vascular resistance (PVR) is calculated by dividing TPG by flow or cardiac output. It is important to remember that TPG is a measured variable, whereas PVR is calculated.

The rate of disease progression can vary among patients (38). From the histopathologic standpoint, progression in the pulmonary arterioles involves continued intimal proliferation, medial hypertrophy, intimal and adventitial fibrosis, thrombosis in situ, angiogenesis, and development of plexiform lesions. Hemodynamic progression is a useful clinical surrogate of disease progression and consists of a progressive rise in pulmonary vascular resistance (Fig. 28.4). There is associated increase in mean pulmonary artery pressure, until right ventricular failure sets in. Because the failing right ventricle can no longer generate the pulmonary artery pressure that it previously did while pumping blood into a high-resistance pulmonary circulation, the flow or cardiac output that was preserved until this point starts to fall along with some drop in pulmonary artery

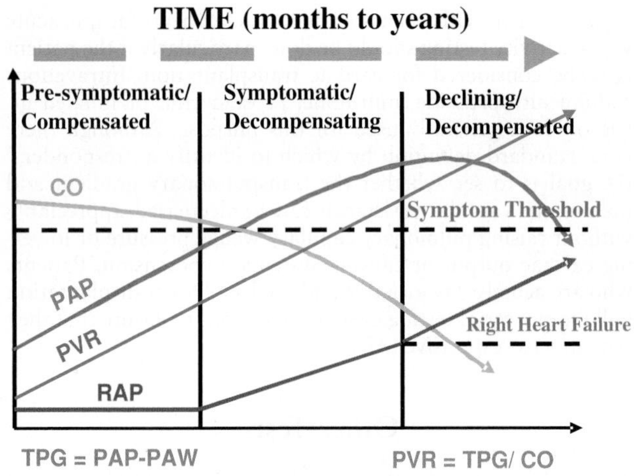

FIGURE 28.4. Hemodynamic progression of pulmonary arterial hypertension over time. CO, cardiac output; PAP, mean pulmonary artery pressure; PAW, pulmonary artery wedge pressure; PVR, pulmonary vascular resistance; RAP, right atrial pressure; TPG, transpulmonary pressure gradient.

pressure. Overt right ventricular failure with marked symptom limitation develops, characterized by decreasing pulmonary artery pressure, declining cardiac output, rising right atrial pressure, and progressively increasing pulmonary vascular resistance. Recognizing clinical and hemodynamic progression is critical to the selection of treatment for PAH (121).

Progression of Pulmonary Hypertension Associated with Left Heart Failure

PH in heart failure patients is "postcapillary" characterized by an elevated PCWP (>15 mm Hg) and PVR. Initially, the TPG is normal, although over time it increases (>10 mm Hg). Initially, PH in heart failure is "vasoreactive" and is readily reversed acutely with vasodilator challenge. Over time, PH becomes "nonvasoreactive" or "fixed" with reduced responsiveness or unresponsiveness to pharmacologic treatments. Hemodynamic progression from "vasoreactive" to "fixed" disease is accompanied by progressive structural pulmonary vascular remodeling. Plexiform lesions, which are the histologic signature of IPAH, are not typically seen in left heart failure patients with associated PH (122).

In heart failure patients the presence of significant PH is a contraindication to orthotopic cardiac transplantation (123,124). The donor right ventricle will fail acutely, resulting in allograft failure and death, if it is required to pump into a high-resistance pulmonary circulation. A normal right ventricle cannot acutely generate a pressure in excess of 50 mm Hg. The risk posed by PH in transplant candidates is a continuous risk that is directly proportional to both PVR and TPG. Nonetheless, for clinical reasons, thresholds have been defined for PVR and TPG beyond which the risk is considered excessive, and orthotopic transplantation is contraindicated. These thresholds vary among transplant programs and are higher in experienced, high-volume transplant centers. Heart failure patients with a TPG of 12 mm Hg or a PVR of 3 Wood units are considered suitable with an acceptable risk in most transplant centers, whereas patients with a TPG of 15 mm Hg or greater or a PVR of 5 Wood units or greater despite acute vasoreactive testing are clearly not appropriate candidates. The posttransplant mortality is threefold higher in the latter high-risk group, and even higher if the gender is female. In these patients, heterotopic transplantation or heart-lung transplantation may be considered. Because long-term outcomes with heterotopic heart transplantation are inferior to those with orthotopic transplantation, this procedure is not performed in most transplant centers. Heart-lung transplantation is limited by the lack of adequate donors. Data from the International Society for Heart and Lung Transplantation (ISHLT) registry demonstrate that pretransplantation PH is an independent risk factor of outcome after transplantation (125–127). This risk exists even with oversizing of the donor allograft.

Heart failure patients with PH who undergo transplantation will have gradual, complete resolution of their PH during the first 6 to 12 months. The greater the severity of PH before surgery, the longer is the time to resolution. In some patients with severe PH, there is incomplete resolution, with residual elevations in pulmonary pressures and PVR. Even those patients who undergo heterotopic heart transplantation have some resolution of PH over time. Remodeling of the allograft right ventricle and development of tricuspid insufficiency accompany the resolution of PH after transplantation.

Prognosis

The presence of pulmonary hypertension carries with it a poor prognosis, irrespective of the cause (38). Patients with connective tissue disease and PH have a worse clinical outcome than do those who do not have pulmonary hypertension. The same is true for sickle cell disease, interstitial lung disease, and left heart disease. When PH complicates left heart failure, both morbidity and mortality are increased. Patients complain of worsening fatigue and dyspnea and declining exercise tolerance. The peak exercise oxygen consumption (peak VO_2) correlates inversely with mean pulmonary pressure and pulmonary vascular resistance and correlates directly with resting right ventricular ejection fraction. Atrial arrhythmias are more frequent, which further compromises cardiac output. As right ventricular failure sets in, cardiorenal syndrome with progressive renal insufficiency, hyponatremia, and diuretic resistance develops. In the advanced stages, patients have anasarca, severe tricuspid regurgitation secondary to annular dilation, and chronic hepatic congestion that can lead to cardiac cirrhosis. Rarely, patients develop hypoxemia either at rest or with activity because of a right-to-left shunt through a patent foramen ovale. Left heart failure patients with PH have increased frequency of hospitalizations, increased risk of cardiovascular events, and a higher mortality compared to patients without PH. The risk of death is directly proportional to the pulmonary vascular resistance.

EVIDENCE-BASED THERAPY FOR PULMONARY ARTERIAL HYPERTENSION

The goals of treatment of PAH include improvement of symptoms, quality of life, and survival and the prevention of disease progression. Once the diagnosis is established, medical therapy should commence as outlined in the treatment guidelines established by the American College of Chest Physicians (Fig. 28.5). This treatment algorithm was developed based on the functional class of the patient, the cause of PAH, and the weight of evidence for benefit with each therapy. Treatments for PAH are listed in Table 28.4 (128).

General Measures

PAH patients must avoid heavy exertion, bending over and rising quickly, cigarette smoking, high sodium intake, and use of appetite suppressants or diet pills. Estrogen-containing

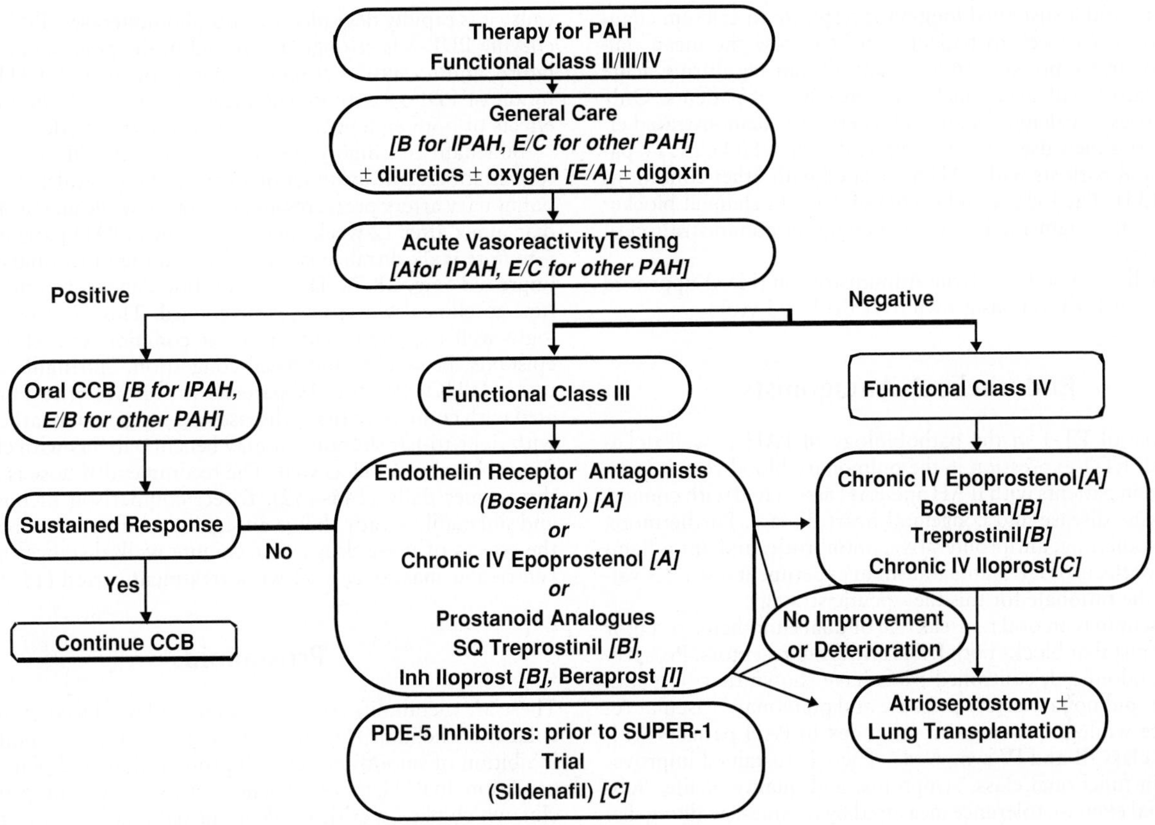

FIGURE 28.5. American College of Chest Physicians (ACCP) evidence-based clinical practice guidelines. There are no recommendations for class II patients. Sildenafil was not approved by the Food and Drug Administration at the time these guidelines were published. CCB, calcium channel blockers; IPAH, idiopathic pulmonary arterial hypertension; Inh, inhaled; IV, intravenous; PAH, pulmonary arterial hypertension; PDE-5, phosphodiesterase-5; SQ, subcutaneous. The grading of recommendations is given in the square brackets: A, strong; B, moderate; C, weak; D, negative; E, based on expert opinion; I, inconclusive. (From Badesch DB, Abman SH, Ahearn GS. Medical therapy for pulmonary arterial hypertension. ACCP evidence-based clinical practice guidelines. *Chest* 2004;126:35S–62S.)

contraceptives should not be prescribed because they increase the risk for venous thromboembolism. Pregnancy must be avoided because the maternal mortality risk exceeds 50%. Patients should not take over-the-counter medications or herbal preparations that contain vasoconstrictive substances such as pseudoephedrine or ephedrine. When migraine headaches are present, serotonergic medications should not be used. Prophylactic influenza vaccine should be recommended for all patients. Patients with PAH are particularly prone to vasovagal syncope, and appropriate precautions must be taken to prevent vasovagal events during invasive procedures and surgery. General anesthesia and intubation can be risky because not only can they cause hypoxemia and hypercarbia and precipitate vasovagal events, but they also cause shifts in both intrathoracic and intracardiac filling pressures (129–131).

Chronic adjuvant therapies include digoxin, diuretics, supplemental oxygen, and anticoagulation. There are no prospective, randomized clinical trials evaluating the chronic use of digoxin in PAH patients. Short-term use of digoxin in one small, uncontrolled study was beneficial and reduced circulating catecholamines. Digoxin may also be useful for rate control in patients who have atrial arrhythmias (132).

Diuretics are recommended for alleviating systemic congestion. The response to diuretic therapy is variable, and doses should be individualized. Renal function and electrolyte balance should be monitored because overdiuresis can cause serious hypotension and renal failure by impairing right ventricular function. The aldosterone antagonist spironolactone may be particularly useful in patients with right heart failure.

Supplemental oxygen should be used to correct hypoxemia, which can aggravate pulmonary vasoconstriction. Some patients may only have hypoxemia with activity or sleep or at high altitudes. The goal is to maintain oxygen saturation greater than 90%. Patients with congenital heart disease and right-to-left shunting may not benefit from supplemental oxygen, although this may reduce the frequency of phlebotomies. Patients should avoid exposure to high altitudes (>1,800 m above sea level) and should recognize the potential need for supplemental oxygen during airplane flights (129).

Chronic anticoagulation with warfarin is controversial in PAH patients. There are no prospective data supporting its routine use, although there is retrospective evidence demonstrating improved outcomes in IPAH patients who receive chronic anticoagulation. The current consensus is that warfarin therapy should only be prescribed to IPAH patients and not to patients with PAH associated with other conditions. Routine anticoagulation in patients with collagen vascular disease and congenital heart disease carries the risk of gastrointestinal bleeding and hemoptysis, respectively. The target International Normalized Ratio (INR) is 1.5 to 2.5 (134).

Calcium Channel Blockers

These drugs benefit only IPAH patients who demonstrate acute reduction (>20%) in mean pulmonary artery pressure and pulmonary vascular resistance during acute vasoreactivity testing. Acute vas-reactivity to this degree is observed in only 12% of patients, and a sustained long-term response to calcium channel blockers is seen in patients who decrease the mean pulmonary artery pressure to less than 40 mm Hg during acute vasodilator challenge, which is about 6.8% of patients. Only high doses of calcium channel blockers have demonstrated efficacy, and their use is not recommended in WHO class IV patients and patients with PAH associated with other conditions (134,135). The long-term benefits of calcium channel blocker therapy are augmented by the concomitant administration of warfarin.

The list of Food and Drug Administration (FDA)-approved treatments for PAH has grown over the last 5 years.

Endothelin-1 Antagonists

The role of ET-1 in the pathobiology of PAH is well documented. ET-1 expression in the pulmonary blood vessels is increased in patients with IPAH and PAH associated with connective tissue disease and congenital heart disease. Furthermore, the vasodilating, antiproliferative, antifibrotic, and antiinflammatory effects of ET-1 antagonism in experimental studies validates the rationale for this therapeutic strategy.

Bosentan is an oral nonselective or dual endothelin-receptor antagonist that blocks both ET-A and ET-B receptors. Prospective, randomized, controlled trials have shown that bosentan reduces pulmonary artery pressure and pulmonary vascular resistance while improving cardiac index in PAH patients with WHO class III and IV symptoms. There is sustained improvement in functional class, symptoms, and quality of life. Submaximal exercise tolerance measured by 6-minute walking distance increases significantly by 44 m (placebo corrected) on bosentan therapy. Time to clinical worsening is prolonged, and progressive right ventricular remodeling is prevented during long-term therapy. The observed 1-year and 2-year survival (96% and 89%, respectively) in bosentan-treated IPAH patients is significantly better than the predicted survival (69% and 57%, respectively) from the National Institutes of Health (NIH) survival equation (Fig. 28.6). Bosentan is effective in WHO class III and IV patients with IPAH or PAH associated with connective tissue disease, congenital systemic-to-pulmonary shunting, drugs and toxins, and HIV infection. Its use in WHO class II patients is under investigation (136–144).

Dosing starts at 62.5 mg twice daily with uptitration to 125 mg twice daily after 4 weeks. Both doses are clinically effective, and there is no true dose–response effect. Reversible hepatic aminotransferase enzyme elevation to greater than three times normal occurs in approximately 12.8% of bosentan-treated patients. These elevations are typically seen during the first 16 weeks of treatment in greater than 90% of the patients. These are dose dependent and are usually reversible with dose reduction, although discontinuation of therapy is needed in 1% to 2% of patients. Monthly assessments of liver function are therefore recommended. This effect is due to inhibition of the bile acid transport pump in the hepatocyte. Bosentan is metabolized in the liver through the P450 enzymes CYP2C9 and CYP3A4. Other side effects, such as lower-extremity edema, anemia, and nasal congestion, are less frequent. Because bosentan may decrease the efficacy of hormonal contraception, dual mechanical barrier contraceptive techniques are recommended in women of childbearing age who are prescribed this medication.

Phosphodiesterase-5 Inhibitors

The biologic effects of nitric oxide are mediated through augmentation of cyclic guanosine monophosphate (cGMP) in the vascular smooth muscle cell. The activity of cGMP is short because it is rapidly degraded by phosphodiesterases (PDEs). The enzyme PDE-5 is strongly expressed in the pulmonary vasculature, and its activity is increased in patients with PAH. Inhibition of PDE -5 activity enhances and prolongs the biologic effects of both endogenous and inhaled nitric oxide.

Sildenafil is a highly specific inhibitor of PDE-5; it is prescribed for erectile dysfunction in men. This drug also decreases pulmonary artery pressures and resistance while increasing cardiac index after 12 weeks of oral therapy in PAH patients. The 6-minute walk distance is increased and the functional class is improved (Fig. 28.7). There is no dose-dependent effect, and time to clinical worsening is prolonged. This drug is surprisingly well tolerated, and the most common side effects are epistaxis, headache, and nasal congestion. Sildenafil is effective in WHO class II to IV patients with IPAH or PAH associated with connective tissue disease and congenital heart disease with right-to-left shunting. It may benefit patients with chronic thromboembolic PH as well. The recommended dose is 20 mg three times daily (145–152). Direct comparison of bosentan and sildenafil therapy shows no significant differences between the effects of these drugs on 6-minute walk distance or right ventricular mass over a 12-week treatment period (153).

Prostanoids

These are metabolites of arachidonic acid produced in the vascular endothelium. Their main biologic effects are vasodilation, inhibition of smooth muscle cell proliferation, and platelet aggregation. In PAH, there is a deficiency of endogenous prostacyclin, which plays a critical role in the pathogenesis. Exogenous prostacyclin given orally, parenterally, or as an inhalation can therefore provide therapeutic benefit in PAH patients.

Intravenous epoprostenol therapy for 12 weeks improves hemodynamics, symptoms, quality of life, and 6-minute walk distance. Progressive right ventricular remodeling is attenuated, and these benefits are sustained during long-term therapy. Observed survival in IPAH patients receiving chronic intravenous epoprostenol infusions is significantly better than the expected survival from the NIH survival equation (Fig. 28.8). Adverse effects of this therapy include flushing, nausea, vomiting, diarrhea, jaw pain, musculoskeletal pain, erythematous rash, and central line–related complications. Intravenous epoprostenol therapy is effective in patients with IPAH, PAH associated with connective tissue disease, congenital heart disease with right-to-left shunting, or drugs and WHO class III to IV symptoms. The starting dose is 2 ng/kg/minute with uptitration as tolerated and based on symptoms to 30 ng/kg/minute. Higher doses can be used, but this can be limited by the development of adverse effects. Because of the complexities of this therapy, it should only be prescribed at experienced centers (154–159).

Treprostinil is a tricyclic benzidine analogue of prostacyclin that can be administered either subcutaneously or intravenously. Continuous subcutaneous delivery over 12 weeks increases 6-minute walk distance in a dose-dependent manner (Fig. 28.9). Additional benefits include improvement in symptoms, hemodynamics, and quality of life. Subcutaneous treprostinil is effective in IPAH, PAH associated with connective tissue disease, and congenital heart disease with right-to-left shunting and WHO class II to IV symptoms. Adverse effects of this therapy include pain at the site of injection, diarrhea, jaw pain, and edema. The starting dose is 1.25 ng/kg/minute with gradual uptitration to 22.5 ng/kg/minute using a positive-pressure, microinfusion pump. Higher doses can be used, if tolerated (160). Intravenous treprostinil administration for 12 weeks improves hemodynamics similar to subcutaneous therapy in IPAH patients with WHO class III or IV symptoms. The adverse effect profile of intravenous treprostinil therapy is

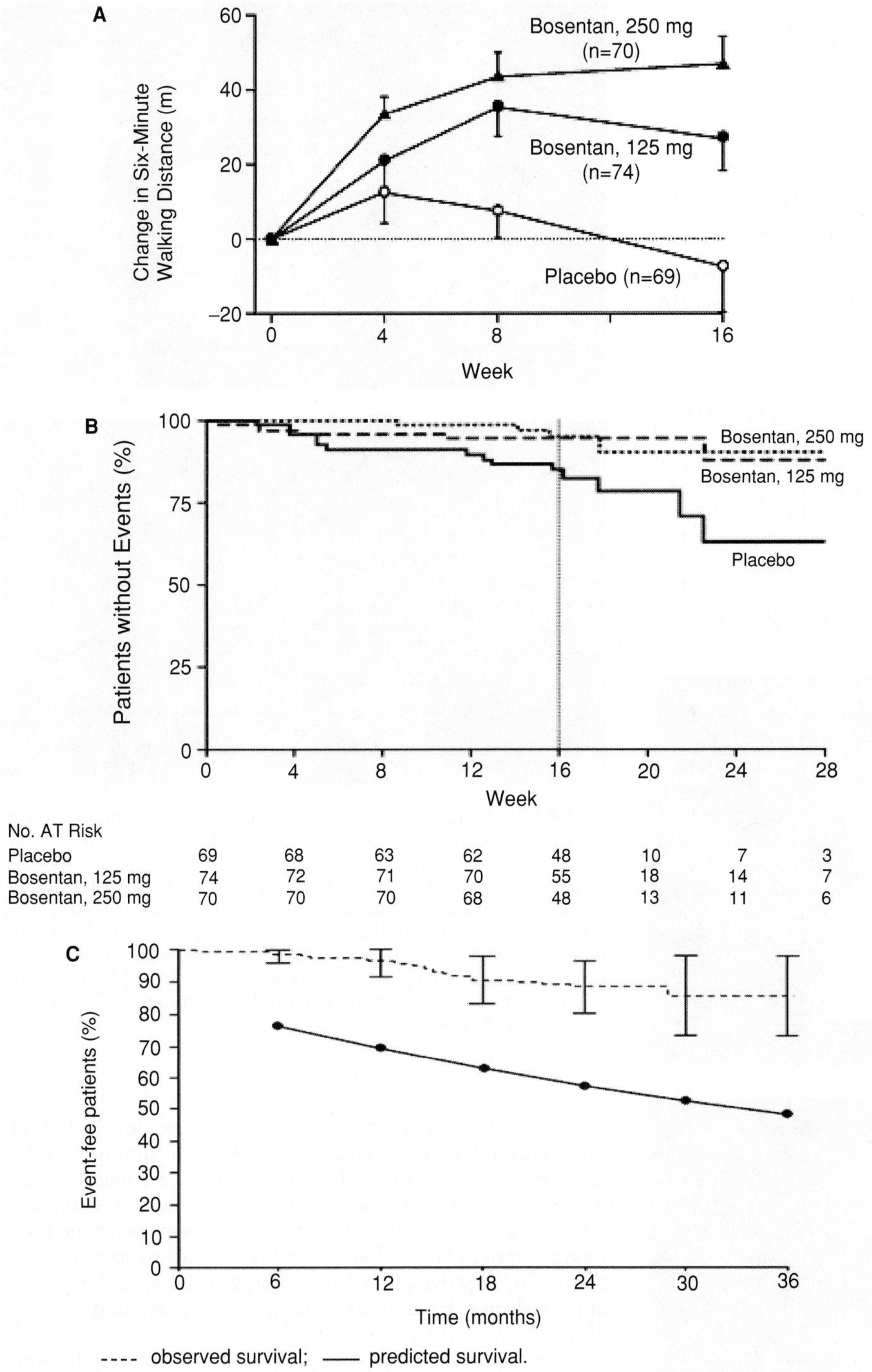

FIGURE 28.6. Bosentan therapy for pulmonary arterial hypertension. **A:** Mean ($\pm$SE) change in 6-minute walk distance from baseline to week 16. $p < .01$ for a 125-mg dose of bosentan versus placebo and $p < .001$ for a 250-mg bosentan dose versus placebo by the Mann–Whitney U test. There was no significant difference between the two bosentan groups ($p = 0.18$ by the Mann–Whitney U test). **B:** Kaplan–Meier estimates of the proportion of patients with clinical worsening. $p < .05$ for bosentan groups versus placebo group at weeks 16 and 28 by the log-rank test. There was no significant difference between the two bosentan groups at weeks 16 and 28 ($p = .87$). **C:** Observed survival on bosentan therapy versus predicted survival in idiopathic pulmonary arterial hypertension patients only. Observed survival (*dashed line*) and predicted survival (*solid line*). Kaplan–Meier estimates are given with 99.9% confidence intervals and predicted survival is calculated using the D'Alonzo (National Institutes of Health) equation. There was a significant difference between the two curves at each 6-month interval.

similar, and the starting dose is 5 ng/kg/minute with gradual uptitration as tolerated to 60 ng/kg/minute. This drug should also be prescribed only by experienced centers (161).

Inhaled iloprost (prostanoid) therapy also improves 6-minute walk distance, functional class, hemodynamics, dyspnea, and quality of life after 12 weeks (Fig. 28.9). Side effects include increased cough, flushing, headache, jaw pain, nausea, and hypotension. This therapy is effective in patients with IPAH, PAH associated with connective tissue disease, drugs, or chronic thromboembolic disease and WHO class III and IV symptoms. The recommended dosage is six to nine inhalations of 2.5 μg of iloprost daily using a portable nebulizer with uptitration to 5 μg, if tolerated (162–165). Oral prostanoid has short-term benefit, but this is not sustained during long-term therapy (166,167).

The therapeutic effects of all FDA approved pharmacologic agents used in PAH and calcium channel blockers are compared in Table 28.5.

FUTURE PHARMACOLOGIC TREATMENTS

The investigational therapies in clinical trials include the selective oral ET-A antagonists sitaxsentan and ambrisentan, the long-acting oral PDE-5 inhibitors vardenafil and tadalafil, inhaled and oral treprostinil, inhaled vasoactive intestinal peptide (VIP), and intravenous or inhaled adrenomedullin (168,169).

Sitaxsentan therapy has been shown to improve hemodynamics, symptoms, WHO class, 6-minute walk distance,

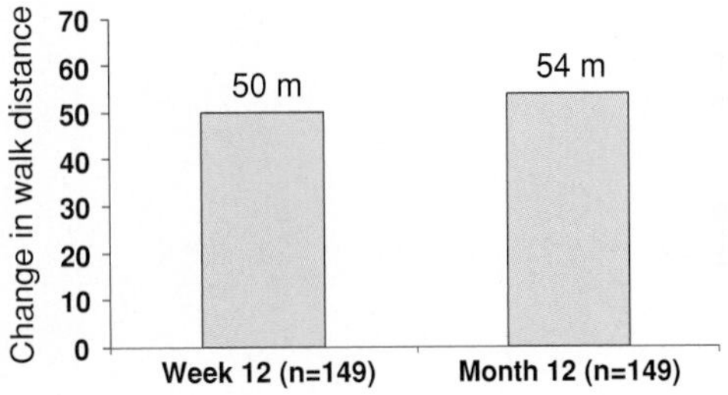

FIGURE 28.7. Effect of sildenafil on exercise tolerance in PAH. Change in walk distance from baseline (From Galie N, Ghofrani HA, Trobicki A, et al. Sildenafil citrate therapy for pulmonary arterial hypertension. *N Engl J Med* 2005;353:2148–2153).

and peak exercise oxygen consumption in IPAH and PAH associated with connective tissue disease and congenital heart disease. The benefits of sitaxsentan were comparable to that seen with bosentan in a prospective, randomized trial. Hepatic aminotransferase elevations are seen in only 3% of sitaxsentan-treated patients, but because sitaxsentan inhibits the cytochrome P450 (CYP) oxidase CYP2C19, it inhibits the metabolism of warfarin. The INR needs close monitoring when this drug is used concomitantly with warfarin (170,171).

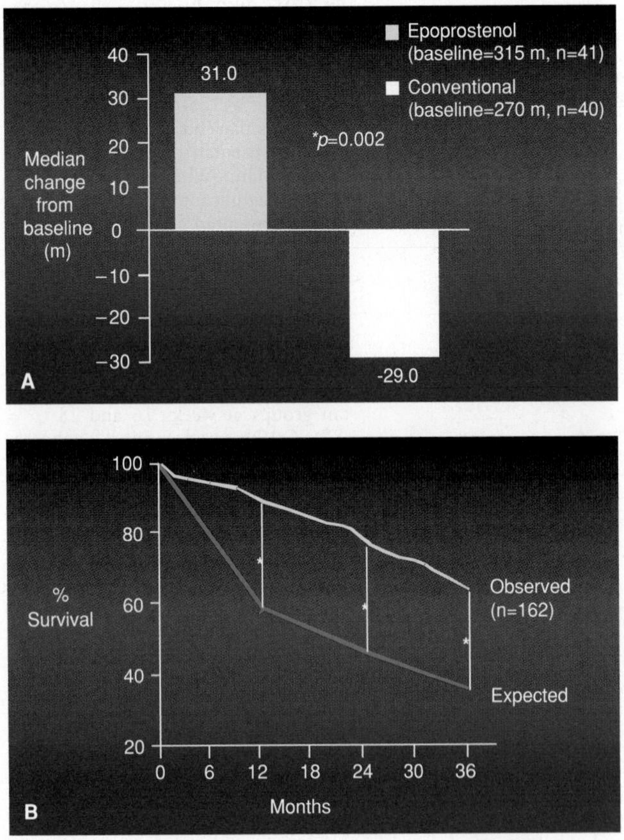

FIGURE 28.8. Epoprostenol therapy in pulmonary arterial hypertension. **Top:** Median change in 6-minute walk exercise test, baseline and week 12. The *p* value is between treatment groups. (From Barst RJ, Rubin LJ, McGoon MD, et al. A comparison of continuous intravenous epoprostenol (prostacyclin) with conventional therapy for primary pulmonary hypertension. The Primary Pulmonary Hypertension Study Group. *N Engl J Med* 1996;334:296–302.) **Bottom:** Survival in primary pulmonary hypertension: effect of epoprostenol. Asterisks indicate $p < .001$. The expected survival is based on the D'Alanzo NIH survival equation. (From McLaughlin VV, Shillington A, Rich S. Survival in primary pulmonary hypertension: the impact of epoprostenol therapy. *Circulation* 2002;106:1477–1482.)

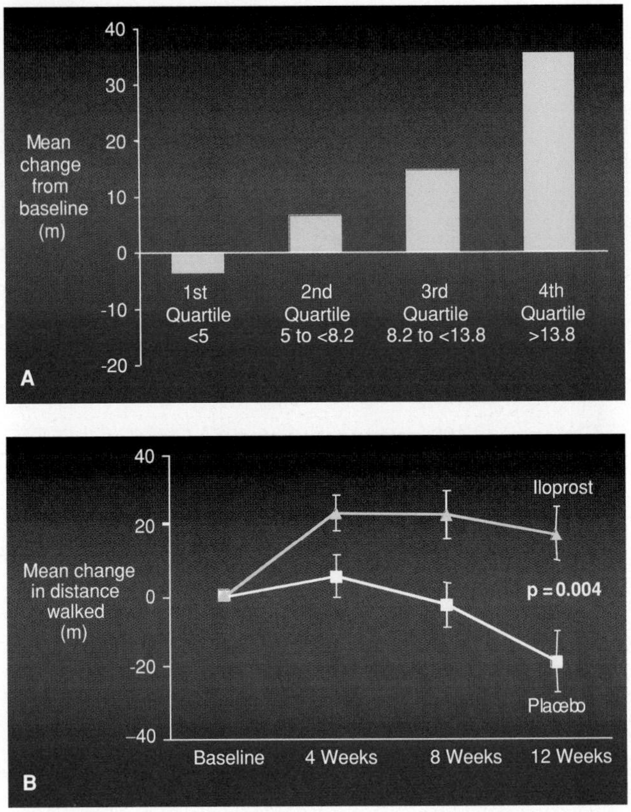

FIGURE 28.9. **A:** Exercise response as a function of subcutaneous treprostinil dose. (From Simonneau G, Barst RJ, Galie N, et al. Continuous subcutaneous infusion of treprostinil, a prostacyclin analogue, in patients with pulmonary arterial hypertension: a double blind, randomized, placebo controlled trial. *Am J Respir Crit Care Med* 2002;165:800–804.) **B:** Effect of inhaled iloprost and placebo on mean change in 6-minute walk. (From Olschewski H, Simonneau G, Galiè N, et al., for the Aerosolized Iloprost Randomized Study Group. Inhaled iloprost for severe pulmonary hypertension. *N Engl J Med* 2002;347:322–329.)

Ambrisentan is another selective ET-A antagonist that improves hemodynamics, functional class, and 6-minute walk distance in IPAH and in PAH associated with collagen vascular disease, anorexinogen use, and HIV infection. This drug does not have any significant interaction with the cytochrome P450 oxidase system (172). The clinical trials with these two investigational, selective ET-A antagonists and those with the FDA approved dual ET agonist, Bostentan are compared in Table 28.6.

A recent case series showed promising results with simvastatin therapy in PAH patients. Besides reducing serum cholesterol, statins have antiproliferative and antiinflammatory effects and induce nitric oxide synthase expression in the pulmonary vasculature. Statins have also been shown to increase expression of BMPR-2 receptors on the vascular smooth muscle cell. Prospective, clinical trials are needed to clarify the role of statins in the treatment of PAH (173,174).

An open label 12 week trial of aerosolized VIP inhaled four times daily has been shown to decrease pulmonary pressures and vascular resistance and increase cardiac output and six minute walk distance in IPAH patients who are "non–vasoreactive" to inhaled nitric oxide. A double-blind, prospective, controlled trial assess the clinical benefits of inhaled VIP in PAH is in progress.

Imatinib, which is an oral PDGF receptor inhibitor and approved for treatment in patients with chronic myeloid

TABLE 28.5

BENEFICIAL EFFECTS OF DRUGS USED IN PULMONARY ARTERIAL HYPERTENSION

	Improvement on therapy					
	Hemodynamics	Six-minute walk	WHO class	One-year survival	Three-year survival	Right ventricle remodeling[a]
Calcium channel blockers[b]	Yes			Yes	Yes	
Epoprostenol	Yes	Yes	Yes	Yes	Yes	Yes
Treprostinil	Yes	Yes	Yes	Yes		
lloprost	Yes	Yes	Yes			
Sildenafil	Yes	Yes	Yes			
Bosentan	Yes	Yes	Yes	Yes	Yes	Yes

[a]Right ventricle remodeling effects are based on two-dimensional echocardiograms.
[b]In vasoreactive patients with idiopathic pulmonary arterial hypertension only.

leukemia, has been shown to improve hemodynamics, clinical staus and six minute walk test in patients with PAH, in an uncontrolled trial. A prospective, double-blind clinical trial is currently underway.

Combination Drug Therapy

Few clinical trials have evaluated prospectively the use of combination therapy in PAH patients. The common clinical practice is to add a second therapy when there is subjective and/or objective evidence for clinical deterioration or disease progression on the initial therapy. However, targeting more than one biologic pathway that is critical to the pathogenesis of PAH makes intuitive sense for all patients, not just for those who are deteriorating.

Several small pilot trials have shown both safety and efficacy of various combination strategies. Hemodynamics, exercise capacity, and functional class improved in both the epoprostenol and combination of epoprostenol and bosentan treatment groups in one study with no statistically significant difference. There were more study withdrawals in the combination therapy group because of adverse effects. In another trial, the addition of inhaled iloprost therapy to patients on chronic bosentan therapy demonstrated a significant improvement in 6-minute walk distance and WHO functional class. There were no major safety issues, and the drugs were well tolerated. There appears to be no clinically significant pharmacologic interaction between prostanoid and endothelin-receptor-antagonist therapy in PAH patients (175).

Several small studies have also evaluated the clinical benefits of combining a PDE-5 inhibitor and a prostanoid. The acute hemodynamic effects of oral sildenafil in combination with inhaled iloprost are significantly greater than those with sildenafil or iloprost alone. In yet another study, long-term (9 to 12 months) adjunctive therapy with oral sildenafil improved hemodynamics and 6-minute walk distance in PAH patients demonstrating clinical deterioration on chronic (>3 months) inhaled iloprost therapy. A double-blind, prospective, placebo-controlled trial of oral sildenafil in combination with intravenous epoprostenol is underway. Another prospective, randomized trial evaluating the combination of inhaled iloprost

TABLE 28.6

PLACEBO-CONTROLLED CLINICAL TRIALS WITH ENDOTHELIN ANTAGONISTS IN PULMONARY ARTERIAL HYPERTENSION

Trial	Condition	Drug studied	*N*	Effect on primary endpoint
Bosentan pilot	IPAH, PAH associated with CTD	Bosentan 125 mg BID for 12 weeks	32	Significant increase in 6-minute walk distance
BREATHE-1	IPAH, PAH associated with CTD	Bosentan 125 or 250 mg BID for 16 weeks	213	Significant increase in 6-minute walk distance
STRIDE-1	IPAH, PAH associated with CTD or CHD	Sitaxsentan 100 or 300 mg daily for 12 weeks	178	Significant increase in percentage, predicted peak excercise VO_2 (300-mg dose only) and 6-minute walk distance
STRIDE-2	IPAH, PAH associated with CTD or CHD	Sitaxsentan 50 or 100 mg daily or bosentan 125 mg BID for 18 weeks	246	Significant increase in 6-minute walk distance with 100-mg daily of sitaxsentan and bosentan
Ambrisentan pilot	IPAH, PAH associated with CTD or HIV or anorexinogen use	Ambrisentan 1, 2.5, 5, or 10 mg daily for 12 weeks	64	Significant increase in 6-minute walk distance

BID, twice daily; IPAH, idiopathic pulmonary arterial hypertension; CTD, connective tissue disease; CHD, congenital right to left intracardiac shunt; HIV, human inmmunodeficiency virus.

and oral sildenafil is being planned. There are no known pharmacologic or clinical interactions during coadministration of a prostanoid and PDE-5 inhibitor in PAH patients (176–178).

The combination of bosentan and sildenafil therapy increased 6-minute walk distance, and this improvement was sustained for 6 to 12 months. The changes in peak exercise oxygen consumption (peak VO_2) were concordant with the 6-minute walk distance data. A prospective, randomized, clinical trial evaluating the combination of bosentan and sildenafil therapy in PAH patients is being planned. Bosentan significantly decreases plasma concentrations of sildenafil in a dose-dependent fashion when the two drugs are used concomitantly. The clinical relevance of this pharmacologic interaction is unknown (179,180).

There are several unanswered questions with combination therapy in PAH patients. Besides the issue of long-term efficacy and safety, it is not known whether a combination strategy of coadministration of two or more drugs at the same time is different than the sequential combination therapy in which a second drug is added after several weeks of therapy with the initial agent. Carefully designed clinical trials are needed to answer these questions. Combination therapy with oral and inhaled agents may permit partial or complete withdrawal of parenteral therapy in some PAH patients. One of the important limitations of polypharmacy in PAH is the cost of treatment. All FDA-approved therapies for PAH are expensive, and the cost of care can be exorbitant when two or more drugs are used in the same patient. It is therefore critically important that the benefit of combination therapy is not only conclusive and significant, but also that it is robust when compared to monotherapy, so that the incremental cost can be justified.

Interventional and Surgical Therapies

Pulmonary endarterectomy is a potentially curative treatment option for severely symptomatic patients with chronic thromboembolic PH. Careful patient selection is a key to successful outcome because it is vital to correlate the thrombus burden with the degree of PH. Eligible patients must have thromboembolic PH on pulmonary angiography and pulmonary vascular resistance greater than 300 dynes·sec·cm^{-5} without significant noncardiac comorbid disease. The magnitudes of preoperative pulmonary pressures or resistance are not contraindications for surgery because some of the greatest benefits are noted in patients with extreme PH. Operative mortality rates in experienced centers range between 5% and 11%. Although there are no randomized, prospective, controlled studies evaluating the benefits of pulmonary thromboendarterectomy, significant and persistent decreases in pulmonary pressures and resistance can be seen along with markedly improved functional status, quality of life, and right ventricular function in 80% to 95% of patients. Five-year survival rates of 75% have been reported in experienced centers (181,182).

For patients with persistent WHO class IV symptoms on medical therapy, balloon atrial septostomy can provide palliation. In this interventional procedure, a right-to-left interatrial shunt is created to help decompress a severely dysfunctional right ventricle and increase cardiac output and systemic oxygen delivery despite a fall in the systemic arterial oxygen saturation. This procedure carries a mortality risk of 5.6% and should only be done at experienced centers. The long-term benefits of balloon atrial septostomy are unknown (183–185).

Lung and heart-lung transplantation are options for carefully selected PAH patients who are failing other therapies. Appropriate timing of transplant listing is critical because the waiting period for donor organs is unpredictable and often long. The lung allocation score used by the United Network for Organ Sharing (UNOS) does not prioritize patients with PAH. Double-lung transplantations are recommended, but heart-lung transplantation may be necessary when severe right ventricular failure is present. However, there is no consensus on when heart-lung transplantation should be considered in PAH patients. Right ventricular remodeling and dysfunction will reverse gradually after double-lung transplantation. In general, patients with severe right ventricular failure requiring intravenous inotropic therapy are considered candidates for heart-lung rather than double-lung transplantation. One-, 3-, and 5-year survival rates after double-lung transplantation are 64%, 54%, and 44%, respectively, for IPAH patients. Results are inferior in patients with PAH associated with congenital systemic-to-pulmonary shunts (186–188).

Cell and Gene Therapy

Use of bone marrow derived endothelial progenitor cells (EPC) in combination with endothelial nitric oxide synthase (eNOS) gene therapy has shown to decrease pulmonary pressures and pulmonary vascular resistance and reverse pulmonary vascular remodeling in a rat model of PAH. Pre-treatment with these cells can also prevent the development of PAH. Thus, these cells can not only help repair endothelial injury but can also induce microvascular angiogenesis, which may be the mechanism by which they prevent the development of PAH. Similar cell based gene transfer strategies in animal models with other vasodilator (adrenomedullin gene) and angiogenic genes (vascular endothelial growth factor and angiopoietin-1 genes) have also yielded promising results. We look forward to future hybrid cell-gene therapy studies in the human PAH phenotype.

Monitoring Disease Activity

After patients have begun evidence-based therapy, it is important to monitor the clinical course of their PH and the long-term effects of therapy (38). Assessment of WHO class and 6-minute walk tests are useful in defining disease stability or progression. The distance walked in 6 minutes is an independent predictor of outcome (190). Echocardiograms should be repeated to monitor for progressive right ventricular remodeling. Right ventricular size, eccentricity index, right atrial size, and pericardial effusion are some of the echocardiographic variables that are predictors of survival (191,192). Some centers have advocated the use of metabolic exercise testing with measurement of peak exercise oxygen consumption. If these noninvasive measures suggest clinical deterioration, then right heart catheterization should be done to assess hemodynamics and guide changes in therapy. Pulmonary pressures, pulmonary vascular resistance, right atrial pressure, and cardiac output are hemodynamic predictors of clinical outcome. The role of serum biologic markers such as brain natriuretic peptide, cardiac troponin, serum uric acid, and serum neurohormone levels in monitoring disease activity is not very clear (193). Serial pulmonary function testing may be useful in monitoring PAH associated with collagen vascular disease.

Most centers do clinical assessment and 6-minute walk tests every 3 months with a echocardiogram every 6 months. Cardiac catheterization is done if there is symptomatic progression or a decline in the noninvasive studies.

Treatment for Other Forms of Pulmonary Hypertension

None of the therapies for PAH have shown benefit in other forms of PH. In patients with chronic obstructive pulmonary disease (COPD), the goal is to maximize lung function and dilate obstructed airways. The bronchodilators that are used include theophylline derivatives, β-adrenergic receptor agonists, ipratropium bromide, and steroids. Diastolic right ventricular dysfunction may precede the development of impaired systolic function. Atrial fibrillation must be avoided because this is generally poorly tolerated. Digoxin may be used for rate control. Statins may have a role in PH associated with COPD because these drugs appear to limit pulmonary parenchymal destruction and progression of PH in an experimental model of emphysema (194).

Patients with idiopathic pulmonary fibrosis may benefit from treatment with a combination of steroids and azathioprine. In patients who have progressive disease on combination therapy, treatment with interferon-γ1b should be considered (195). All patients who have left heart failure from systolic dysfunction, whether they have associated PH or not, should be on evidence-based drug treatments, which include digoxin, diuretics, angiotensin-converting inhibitors, β-adrenergic blockers, and aldosterone antagonists (196,197). If PH is acutely "vasoreactive," the patient may be considered for transplantation, provided there are no other contraindications. Every effort must be made to prevent progression of PH until transplantation, and frequent monitoring (every 6 to 8 weeks) with right heart catheterization may be necessary. If PH is not acutely "vasoreactive," then one might consider chronic infusions of neseritide (48 to 72 hours) or milrinone given intravenously as a continuous infusion (up to 2 weeks) or as an aerosolized inhalation to decrease pulmonary pressures, TPG, and PVR. Chronic left ventricular unloading with a left ventricular assist device (either continuous flow or pulsatile) may also be considered in selected patients to reverse PH. If there is significant improvement in pulmonary hemodynamics with any of these strategies, cardiac transplantation may be feasible (198–200).

None of the therapies that are approved for the treatment of PAH have shown benefit in chronic left heart failure patients. Although acute administration of endothelin antagonists induces pulmonary vasodilation in left heart failure patients, chronic therapy has no proven survival benefit in randomized, controlled trials (201,202). Likewise, intravenous epoprostenol infusions failed to show survival benefit in patients with chronic severe left heart failure. Incidentally, several patients in this study experienced reductions in pulmonary pressures, PCWP, and PVR on therapy (203). Unfortunately, none of these clinical trials selectively evaluated the long-term clinical benefits in patients with PH associated with chronic left heart failure. Sildenafil has been shown to decrease pulmonary pressures and pulmonary vascular resistance in PH associated with left heart failure (204). This hemodynamic effect is augmented when the drug is coadministered with inhaled nitric oxide (205). Whether chronic treatment with sildenafil can cause sustained benefits in PH associated with left heart failure is unknown.

SUMMARY

Pulmonary hypertension, irrespective of the associated condition, causes substantial morbidity and mortality. The revised nomenclature in the clinical classification has helped clinicians to group disorders that share a common pathophysiology. We now recognize the risk factors for the development of PH and have the ability to screen high-risk patient groups. New diagnostic tools have improved our ability to diagnose and risk stratify PH patients. Significant advances in our understanding of the biology of PAH in the last two decades has led to the development of several therapeutic targets in this disease. These include prostanoids, endothelin-receptor antagonists, and phosphodiesterase-5 inhibitors. Prospective, randomized clinical trials have demonstrated both the efficacy and safety of each of these treatments in PAH patients. Patients with PAH are living longer with better quality of life than in the past. Because hemodynamic and clinical progression continues in many patients on therapy, it has been advocated that multiple treatment targets have to be addressed to achieve optimal benefit. Preliminary pilot trials have supported this hypothesis by showing synergistic benefit and safety of combination therapy. Larger, long-term clinical trials are in progress to validate these preliminary observations. Surgical therapy has yielded excellent results for patients with chronic thromboembolic PH. However, treatment of PH associated with other relatively common conditions, such as COPD and left heart failure, remains a challenge. Recognizing newer treatments that add to the current menu of medical therapy for PAH patients and bring hope to other forms of associated PH patients will be an important challenge for the future.

CONTROVERSIES AND PERSONAL PERSPECTIVES

Pulmonary hypertension is rapidly evolving as a distinct specialty in medicine. Unlike many other illnesses, PH crosses the traditional borders that exist among medical specialties. A number of disparate, distinct conditions are associated with PH, and therefore it is critical that all clinicians be familiar with this illness. It is important that this disease be suspected and appropriate steps taken to ensure proper treatment. Delay in treatment can have disastrous consequences. Once diagnosis is established, medical treatment guided by the American College of Chest Physicians (ACCP) practice guidelines should be immediately initiated. Recognition of PH in its earliest stages is the key to an optimal outcome. A number of strategies for promoting education in the physician community are underway, and these have yielded favorable results. The Pulmonary Hypertension Association (PHA) has played a pivotal role in this regard. Once the condition is recognized, it is important to refer the patient to the closest pulmonary hypertension program in a timely fashion. The names of the programs and the physicians involved are listed on the PHA website. All of the programs have dedicated teams of physicians, nurses, and physician extenders who can provide specialized care and work in collaboration with the community physicians. The number of pulmonary hypertension programs has doubled in the last few years, which attests to the increasing numbers of PH patients. Some programs are led by cardiologists and others by pulmonary medicine specialists. Through the PHA, the different programs and their members have the opportunity to network, and this has led to collaborative research and fostered the evolution of new therapeutic ideas.

Despite the tremendous progress in this field, PH remains a challenging disease to treat. The most common causes of PH, which are COPD and left heart failure, do not yet have specific treatments. All the drugs that are effective in PAH do not offer any sustained benefit to these groups of patients. Furthermore, disease progression occurs on therapy in many PAH patients. Perhaps other biologic pathways are critical to COPD and left heart failure patients that may be different than the ones that are involved in PAH. Clearly, much work needs to be done to help discern the mechanisms involved so that newer strategies for treatment can be developed to benefit all patients who have PH. We also need better treatments for right ventricular failure. Much of the research in heart failure has focused on the left ventricle, which has led to the development of a number of drugs for left heart failure. There is no approved therapy for right ventricular failure.

PH is a very expensive illness to treat. The detailed diagnostic work-up necessary and the FDA-approved treatments are very expensive. As we move toward combining drugs to maximize treatment benefit, the cost burden will escalate further. As new drugs are developed, newer combinations will be considered. All PAH therapies are needed lifelong, and because many of them prolong survival, the cost of care per patient is exorbitant. Furthermore, all the efforts to promote early recognition and early treatment of the disease will add to this already high cost. Clearly, the prices of drugs used in treating PAH have to come down drastically, if we are to continue with our mission to find treatments that benefit all patients who suffer from this disease.

THE FUTURE

The future for patients with PH looks bright. The field as a whole is advancing rapidly, and our understanding of the pathogenesis continues to evolve. Several new agents that have shown the potential for preventing or reversing vascular injury in experimental animal models may soon be ready for human clinical testing. With the evolution of new therapies, it is the hope that we may be able to individualize treatment algorithms rather than treat everyone the same way. Genetic factors play a major role in the variation of treatment responses and the incidence of adverse effects to medications in cardiovascular diseases. Pharmacogenetics helps to elucidate this genetic heterogeneity, which is determined by genetic polymorphisms. The polymorphisms may involve drug-metabolizing enzymes, transporters, or pharmacologic targets of drugs that influence not only the treatment effect, but also the dose–response relationship in individuals. The study of genetic polymorphisms and their modulating effects on treatment response and clinical outcomes in PAH is just beginning. The hope for the future is that pharmacogenetics will provide physicians with both the knowledge and the tools needed to allow for an individualized, cost-effective treatment approach so that the best drug therapy can be prescribed for each PAH patient.

References

1. Gaine SP, Rubin LJ. Primary pulmonary hypertension. *Lancet* 1998;352:719–725.
2. Rubin LJ. Primary pulmonary hypertension. *N Engl J Med* 1997;336:111–117.
3. Rich S, Dantzer DR, Ayers SM, et al. Primary pulmonary hypertension: a national prospective study. *Ann Intern Med* 1987;107:216–228.
4. Cheitlin MD, Armstrong WF, Aurigemma GP, et al. ACC/AHA/ASE 2003 guideline update for the clinical application of echocardiography: summary article; a report of the American College of Cardiology/American Heart Association Task Force on Practice Guidelines (ACC/AHA/ASE Committee to Update the 1997 Guidelines for the Clinical Application of Echocardiography). *Circulation* 2003;108:1146–1162.
5. Bossone E, Rubenfire M, Bach DS, et al. Range of tricuspid regurgitation velocity at rest and during exercise in normal adult men: implications for the diagnosis of pulmonary hypertension. *J Am Coll Cardiol* 1999;33:1662–1666.
6. Brecker SJ, Gibbs JS, Fox KM, et al. Comparison of Doppler derived haemodynamic variables and simultaneous high fidelity pressure measurements in severe pulmonary hypertension. *Br Heart J* 1994;72:384–389.
7. Denton CP, Cailes JB, Phillips GD, et al. Comparison of Doppler echocardiography and right heart catheterization to assess pulmonary hypertension in systemic sclerosis. *Br J Rheumatol* 1997;36:239–243.
8. Gaynor SL, Maniar HS, Bloch JB, et al. Right atrial and ventricular adaptation to chronic right ventricular pressure overload. *Circulation* 2005; 112:I212–I218.
9. Chaouat A, Bugnet AS, Kadaoui N, et al. Severe pulmonary hypertension and chronic obstructive pulmonary disease. *Am J Respir Crit Care Med* 2005;172:189–194.
10. Yilmaz R, Gencer M, Ceylan E, Demirbag R. Impact of chronic obstructive pulmonary disease with pulmonary hypertension on both left ventricular systolic and diastolic performance. *J Am Soc Echocardiogr* 2005;18:873–881.
11. Simonneau G, Galie N, Rubin LJ, et al. Clinical classification of pulmonary hypertension. *J Am Coll Cardiol* 2004;43(Suppl S):5S–12S.
12. Rubin LJ. Diagnosis and management of pulmonary arterial hypertension: ACCP evidence-based clinical practice guidelines. *Chest* 2004;126:7S–10S.
13. Pietra GG, Capron F, Stewart S, et al. Pathologic assessment of vasculopathies in pulmonary hypertension. *J Am Coll Cardiol* 2004;43(Suppl S): 25S–32S.
14. Wagenvoort CA, Wagenvoort H. Primary pulmonary hypertension: a pathologic study of the lung vessels in 156 classically diagnosed cases. *Circulation* 1970;42:1163–1184.
15. Newman JH. Pulmonary hypertension. *Am J Respir Crit Care Med* 2005; 172:1072–1077.
16. D'Alonzo GE, Barst RJ, Ayers SM, et al. Survival in patients with primary pulmonary hypertension: results from a national prospective registry. *Ann Intern Med* 1991;115:343–349.
17. Lane KB, Machado RD, Pauciulo MW, et al. Heterozygous germ line mutations in a TGF-β receptor, BMPR2, are the cause of familial primary pulmonary hypertension. *Nat Genet* 2000;26:81–84.
18. Richter A, Yeager ME, Zaiman A, et al. Impaired transforming growth factor-β signaling in idiopathic pulmonary arterial hypertension. *Am J Respir Crit Care Med* 2004;170:1340–1348.
19. Harrison RE, Berger R, Haworth SG, et al. Transforming growth factor-beta receptor mutations and pulmonary arterial hypertension in childhood. *Circulation* 2005;111:435–441.
20. Du L, Sullivan CC, Chu D, et al. Signalling molecules in nonfamilial pulmonary hypertension. *N Engl J Med* 2003;348:500–509.
21. Yu PB, Beppu H, Kawai N, et al. Bone morphogenetic protein (BMP) type II receptor deletion reveals BMP ligand-specific gain of signaling in pulmonary artery smooth muscle cells. *J Biol Chem* 2005;280:24443–24450.
22. Yang X, Long L, Southwood M, et al. Dysfunctional Smad signaling contributes to abnormal smooth muscle cell proliferation in familial pulmonary arterial hypertension. *Circ Res* 2005;96:1053–1063.
23. Song Y, Jones JE, Beppu H, et al. Increased susceptibility to pulmonary hypertension in heterozygous BMPR2-mutant mice. *Circulation* 2005;112: 553–562.
24. Trembath JRC, Thompson JR, Machado RD, et al. Clinical and molecular genetic features of pulmonary hypertension in patients with hereditary hemorrhagic telangiectasia. *N Engl J Med* 2001;345:325–334.
25. Satoh T, Kimura K, Okano Y, et al. Lack of circulating autoantibodies to bone morphogenetic protein receptor-II or activin receptor-like kinase 1 in mixed connective tissue disease patients with pulmonary arterial hypertension. *Rheumatology (Oxford)* 2005;44:192–196.
26. Eddahibi S, Humbert M, Fadel E, et al. Serotonin transporter overexpression is responsible for pulmonary artery smooth muscle hyperplasia in primary pulmonary hypertension. *J Clin Invest* 2001;108:1141–1150.
27. Eddahibi S, Chaouat A, Morrell N, et al. Polymorphism of the serotonin transporter gene and pulmonary hypertension in chronic obstructive pulmonary disease. *Circulation* 2003;108:1839–1844.
28. Vachharajani A, Saunders S. Allelic variation in the serotonin transporter (5HTT) gene contributes to idiopathic pulmonary hypertension in children. *Biochem Biophys Res Commun* 2005;334:376–379.
29. Humbert M, Nunes H, Sitbon O, et al. Risk factors for pulmonary arterial hypertension. *Clin Chest Med* 2001;22:459–475.
30. Battle RW, Davitt MA, Cooper SM, et al. Prevalence of pulmonary hypertension in limited and diffuse scleroderma. *Chest* 1996;110:1515–1519.
31. Ungerer RG, Tashkin DP, Furst D, et al. Prevalence and clinical correlates of pulmonary arterial hypertension in progressive systemic sclerosis. *Am J Med* 1983;75:65–74.
32. Tanaka E, Harigai M, Tanaka M, et al. Pulmonary hypertension in systemic lupus erythematosus: evaluation of clinical characteristics and response to immunosuppressive treatment. *J Rheumatol* 2002;29:282–287.
33. Fagan KA, Badesch DB. Pulmonary hypertension associated with connective tissue disease. In: Peacock AJ, Rubin LJ, eds. *Pulmonary circulation.* London: Arnold, 2004:181–190.
34. Macgregor AJ, Canavan R, Knight C, et al. Pulmonary hypertension in systemic sclerosis: risk factors for progression and consequences for survival. *Rheumatology (Oxford)* 2001;40:453–459.
35. Love PE, Santoro SA. Antiphospholipid antibodies: anticardiolipin and the lupus anticoagulant in systemic lupus erythematosus (SLE) and in non-SLE disorders. Relevance and clinical significance. *Ann Intern Med* 1990;112:682–698.
36. Stupi AM, Steen VD, Owens GR, et al. Pulmonary hypertension in the CREST variant of systemic sclerosis. *Arthritis Rheum* 1986;29:515–524.
37. McGoon M, Gutterman D, Steen V, et al. Screening, early detection, and diagnosis of pulmonary arterial hypertension. ACCP evidence-based clinical practice guidelines. *Chest* 2004;126:14S–34S.
38. McLaughlin VV, Presberg KW, Doyle RL, et al. Prognosis of pulmonary arterial hypertension. ACCP evidence-based clinical practice guidelines. *Chest* 2004;126;78S–92S.
39. Edwards BS, Weir EK, Edwards WD, et al. Co-existent pulmonary and portal hypertension: morphologic and clinical features. *J Am Coll Cardiol* 1987;10:1233–1238.
40. Krowka MJ. Hepatopulmonary syndrome and portopulmonary hypertension: implications for liver transplantation. *Clin Chest Med* 2005;26:587–597.

41. Krowka MJ. Portopulmonary hypertension and the issue of survival. *Liver Transpl* 2005;11:1026–1027.
42. Rodriguez-Roisin R, Krowka MJ, Herve P, et al. Highlights of the ERS Task Force on Pulmonary-Hepatic Vascular Disorders (PHD). *J Hepatol* 2005;42:924–927.
43. Chun PK, San Antonio RP, Davia JE. Laennec's cirrhosis and primary pulmonary hypertension. *Am Heart J* 1980;99:779–782.
44. Cool CD, Rai PR, Yeager MF, et al. Expression of human herpesvirus 8 in primary pulmonary hypertension. *N Engl J Med* 2003;349:1113–1122.
45. Henke-Gendo C, Mengel M, Hoeper MM, et al. Absence of Kaposi's sarcoma–associated herpesvirus in patients with pulmonary arterial hypertension. *Am J Respir Crit Care Med* 2005;172:1581–1585.
46. Katano H, Hogaboam CM. Herpesvirus-associated pulmonary hypertension? *Am J Respir Crit Care Med* 2005;172:1485–1486.
47. Montani D, Marcelin AG, Sitbon O, et al. Human herpes virus 8 in HIV and non-HIV infected patients with pulmonary arterial hypertension in France. *AIDS* 2005;19:1239–1240.
48. Nicastri E. Human herpesvirus 8 and pulmonary hypertension. *Emerg Infect Dis* 2005;11:1480–1482.
49. Laney AS, De Marco T, Peters JS, et al. Kaposi sarcoma–associated herpesvirus and primary and secondary pulmonary hypertension. *Chest* 2005;127:762–767.
50. Hsue PY, Waters DD. What a cardiologist needs to know about patients with human immunodeficiency virus Infection. *Circulation* 2005: 112:3947–3957.
51. Abenheim L, Moride Y, Brenot F, et al. Appetite suppressant drugs and the risk of primary pulmonary hypertension: International Primary Pulmonary Hypertension Study Group. *N Engl J Med* 1996;335:609–616.
52. Rich S, Rubin LJ, Walker AM, et al. Anorexinogens and pulmonary hypertension in the United States: results from the surveillance of North American Pulmonary Hypertension. *Chest* 2000;117;870–874.
53. Gomez-Sanchez MA, Saenz DLC, Gomez-Pajuelo C, et al. Clinical and pathologic manifestations of pulmonary vascular disease in toxic oil syndrome. *J Am Coll Cardiol* 1991;18:1539–1545.
54. Belohlavkova S, Simak J, Kokesova A, et al. Fenfluramine-induced pulmonary vasoconstriction: role of serotonin receptors and potassium channels. *J Appl Physiol* 2001: 91:755–761.
55. Gladwin MT, Sachdev V, Jison ML, et al. Pulmonary hypertension as a risk factor for death in patients with sickle cell disease. *N Engl J Med* 2004;350:886–895.
56. Castro O, Hoque M. Pulmonary hypertension in sickle cell disease: cardiac catheterization results and survival. *Blood* 2003;101:1257–1261.
57. Cromie JB. Correlation of anatomic pulmonary emphysema and right ventricular hypertrophy. *Am Rev Respir Dis* 1961;84:657–667.
58. Dinh-Xuan AT, Higgenbotham TW, Cleland JA, et al. Impairment of endothelium dependent pulmonary artery relaxation in chronic obstructive lung disease. *N Engl J Med* 1991;324:1539–1547.
59. Szilasi M, Dolinay T, Nemes Z, et al. Pathology of chronic obstructive pulmonary disease. *Pathol Oncol Res* 2006;12:52–60.
60. Nadrous HF, Pellikka PA, Krowka MJ, et al. Pulmonary hypertension in patients with idiopathic pulmonary fibrosis. *Chest* 2005;128:2393–2399.
61. Nadrous HF, Pellikka PA, Krowka MJ, et al. The impact of pulmonary hypertension on survival in patients with idiopathic pulmonary fibrosis. *Chest* 2005;128:616S–617S.
62. Strollo Jr PJ, Rogers R. Obstructive sleep apnea. *N Engl J Med* 1996; 334:99–104.
63. Bady E, Achkar A, Pascal S, et al. Pulmonary arterial hypertension in patients with sleep apnea syndrome. *Thorax* 2000;55:934–939.
64. Ip MSM, Lam B, Chan LY, et al. Circulating nitric oxide is suppressed in obstructive sleep apnea and is reversed by nasal continuous positive airway pressure. *Am J Respir Crit Care Med* 2000;162:2166–2171.
65. Sajkov D, Wang T, Saunders NA, et al. Continuous positive airway pressure treatment improves pulmonary hemodynamics in patients with obstructive sleep apnea. *Am J Respir Crit Care Med* 2002;165:152–158.
66. Atwood Jr CW, McCrory D, Garcia JG, et al. Pulmonary artery hypertension and sleep-disordered breathing: ACCP evidence-based clinical practice guidelines. *Chest* 2004;126:72S–77S.
67. Fedullo PF, Auger WR, Kerr KM, et al. Chronic thromboembolic pulmonary hypertension. *N Engl J Med* 2001;345:1465–1472.
68. Morris TA, Auger WR, Ysrael MZ, et al. Parenchymal scarring is associated with restrictive spirometric defects in patients with chronic thromboembolic pulmonary hypertension. *Chest* 1996;110:399–403.
69. Azarian R, Wartski M, Collignon MA, et al. Lung perfusion scans and hemodynamics in acute and chronic pulmonary embolism. *J Nucl Med* 1997;38:980–983.
70. Ryan KL, Fedullo PF, Davis GB, et al. Perfusion scan findings understate the severity of angiographic and hemodynamic compromise in chronic thromboembolic pulmonary hypertension. *Chest* 1988;93:1180–1185.
71. Chapman PJ, Bateman ED, Benatar SR. Primary pulmonary hypertension and thrombo-embolic pulmonary hypertension: similarities and differences. *Respir Med* 1990;84:485–488.
72. Barker WH, Mulloly JP, Getchell W. Changing incidence and survival for heart failure in a well-defined older population, 1970–1974 and 1990–1994. *Circulation* 2006;113:799–805.
73. Abramson SV, Burke JF, Kelly Jr JJ, et al. Pulmonary hypertension predicts mortality and morbidity in patients with dilated cardiomyopathy. *Ann Intern Med* 1992;116:888–895.
74. Rabinovitch M. Pulmonary hypertension: pathophysiology as a basis for clinical decision making. *J Heart Lung Transplant* 1999;18:1041–1053.
75. Moraes DL, Colucci WS, Givertz MM. Secondary pulmonary hypertension in chronic heart failure: the role of the endothelium in pathophysiology and management. *Circulation* 2000;102:1718–1723.
76. Humbert M, Morrell NW, Archer SL, et al. Cellular and molecular pathobiology of pulmonary arterial hypertension. *J Am Coll Cardiol* 2004;43(Suppl S):13S–24S.
77. Eddahibi S, Humbert M, Fadel E, et al. Serotonin transporter overexpression is responsible for pulmonary artery smooth muscle hyperplasia in primary pulmonary hypertension. *J Clin Invest* 2001;108:1141–1150.
78. Wedgwood S, Black SM. Endothelin-1 decreases endothelial NOS expression and activity through ETA receptor-mediated generation of hydrogen peroxide. *Am J Physiol Lung Cell Mol Physiol* 2005;288:L480–L487.
79. Migneault A, Sauvageau S, Villeneuve L, et al. Chronically elevated endothelin levels reduce pulmonary vascular reactivity to nitric oxide. *Am J Respir Crit Care Med* 2005;171:506–513.
80. Giaid A, Saleh D. Reduced expression of endothelial nitric oxide synthase in the lungs of patients with pulmonary hypertension. *N Engl J Med* 1995;333:214–221.
81. Kim H, Yung GL, Marsh JJ, et al. Endothelin mediates pulmonary vascular remodelling in a canine model of chronic embolic pulmonary hypertension. *Eur Respir J* 2000;15:640–648.
82. Rubens C, Ewert R, Halank M, et al. Big endothelin-1 and endothelin-1 plasma levels are correlated with the severity of primary pulmonary hypertension. *Chest* 2001;120:1562–1569.
83. Giaid A, Yanagisawa M, Langleben D, et al. Expression of endothelin-1 in the lungs of patients with pulmonary hypertension. *N Engl J Med* 1993;328:1732.
84. Galie N, Grigioni F, Bacchi-Reggiani L, et al. Relation of endothelin-1 to survival in patients with primary pulmonary hypertension. *Eur J Clin Invest* 1996;26:273.
85. Farber HW, Loscalzo J. Pulmonary arterial hypertension. *N Engl J Med* 2004: 351:1655–1665.
86. Miyauchi T, Masaki T. Pathophysiology of endothelin in the cardiovascular system. *Annu Rev Physiol* 1999: 61:391–415.
87. Levin ER. Endothelins. *N Engl J Med* 1995;333:356–363.
88. Tuder RM, Cool CD, Geraci MW, et al. Prostacyclin synthase expression is decreased in lungs from patients with severe pulmonary hypertension. *Am J Respir Crit Care Med* 1999;159:1925–1932.
89. Christman BW, McPherson CD, Newman JH, et al. An imbalance between the excretion of thromboxane and prostacyclin metabolites in pulmonary hypertension. *N Engl J Med* 1992;327:70–75.
90. Tuder RM, Cool CD, Geraci MW, et al. Prostacyclin synthase expression is decreased in lungs from patients with severe pulmonary hypertension. *Am J Respir Crit Care Med* 1999;159:1925–1932.
91. Xu W, Kaneko FT, Zheng S, et al. Increased arginase II and decreased NO synthesis in endothelial cells of patients with pulmonary arterial hypertension. *FASEB J* 2004;18:1746–1748.
92. Demoncheaux EA, Higenbottam TW, Kiely DG, et al. Decreased whole body endogenous nitric oxide production in patients with primary pulmonary hypertension. *J Vasc Res* 2005;42:133–136.
93. Mason NA, Springall DR, Burke M, et al. High expression of endothelial nitric oxide synthase in plexiform lesions of pulmonary hypertension. *J Pathol* 1998;185:313–318.
94. Girgis RE, Champion HC, Diette GB, et al. Decreased exhaled nitric oxide in pulmonary arterial hypertension: response to bosentan therapy. *Am J Respir Crit Care Med* 2005;172:352–357.
95. Lara AR, Erzurum SC. A urinary test for pulmonary arterial hypertension? *Am J Respir Crit Care Med* 2005;172:262–263.
96. Pullamsetti S, Kiss L, Ghofrani HA, et al. Increased levels and reduced catabolism of asymmetric and symmetric dimethylarginines in pulmonary hypertension. *FASEB J* 2005;19:1175–1177.
97. Sydow K, Munzel T. ADMA and oxidative stress. *Atheroscler Suppl* 2003; 4:41–51.
98. Kielstein JT, Bode-Boger SM, Hesse G, et al. Asymmetrical dimethylarginine in idiopathic pulmonary arterial hypertension. *Arterioscler Thromb Vasc Biol* 2005;25:1414–1418.
99. Morris CR, Kato GJ, Poljakovic M, et al. Dysregulated arginine metabolism, hemolysis-associated pulmonary hypertension, and mortality in sickle cell disease. *JAMA* 2005;294:81–90.
100. Braner DA, Fineman JR, Chang R, Soifer SJ. M&B 22948, a cGMP phosphodiesterase inhibitor, is a pulmonary vasodilator in lambs. *Am J Physiol* 1993;264:H252–H258.
101. Corbin JD, Beasley A, Blount MA, et al. High lung PDE5: a strong basis for treating pulmonary hypertension with PDE5 inhibitors. *Biochem Biophys Commun* 2005;334:930–938.
102. Cody RJ, Haas GJ, Binkley PF, et al. Plasma endothelin correlates with the extent of pulmonary hypertension in patients with chronic congestive heart failure. *Circulation* 1992;85:504–509.
103. Hiroe M, Hirata Y, Fujita N, et al. Plasma endothelin-1 levels in idiopathic dilated cardiomyopathy. *Am J Cardiol* 1991;68:114–115.

104. McMurray JJ, Ray SG, Abdullah I, et al. Plasma endothelin in chronic heart failure. *Circulation* 1992;85:1374–1379.
105. Wei CM, Lerman A, Rodeheffer RJ, et al. Endothelin in human congestive heart failure. *Circulation* 1994;89:1580–1586.
106. Barst RJ, McGoon M, Torbicki A, et al. Diagnosis and differential assessment of pulmonary arterial hypertension. *J Am Coll Cardiol* 2004;43(Suppl S);40S–47S.
107. Galie N, Torbicki A, Barst R, et al. Guidelines on diagnosis and treatment of pulmonary arterial hypertension. The Task Force on Diagnosis and Treatment of Pulmonary Arterial Hypertension of the European Society of Cardiology. *Eur Heart J* 2004;25:2243–2278.
108. Grunig E, Janssen B, Mereles D, et al. Abnormal pulmonary artery pressure response in asymptomatic carriers of primary pulmonary hypertension gene. *Circulation* 2000;102:1145–1150.
109. Bossone E, Paciocco G, Iarussi D, et al. The prognostic role of the ECG in primary pulmonary hypertension. *Chest* 2002;121:513–518.
110. Lupi E, Dumont C, Tejada VM, et al. A radiologic index of pulmonary arterial hypertension. *Chest* 1975;68:28–31.
111. Bossone E, Duong-Wagner TH, Paciocco G, et al. Echocardiographic features of primary pulmonary hypertension. *J Am Soc Echocardiogr* 1999;12:655–662.
112. Bailey CL, Channick RN, Auger WR, et al. "High probability" perfusion lung scans in pulmonary veno-occlusive disease. *Am J Respir Crit Care Med* 2000;162:1974–1978.
113. Fishman AJ, Moser KM, Fedullo PF. Perfusion lung scans versus pulmonary angiography in evaluation of suspected primary pulmonary hypertension. *Chest* 1983;84:679–683.
114. King MA, Ysrael M, Bergin CJ. Chronic thromboembolic pulmonary hypertension: CT findings. *AJR Am J Roentgenol* 1998;170:955–960.
115. Swensen SJ, Tashjian JH, Myers JL, et al. Pulmonary veno-occlusive disease: CT findings in eight patients. *AJR Am J Roentgenol* 1996;167:937–940.
116. Rich S, D'Alonzo GE, Dantzker DR, et al. Magnitude and implications of spontaneous hemodynamic variability in primary pulmonary hypertension. *Am J Cardiol* 1985;55:159–163.
117. Boxt LM. MR imaging of pulmonary hypertension and right ventricular dysfunction. *Magn Reson Imaging Clin North Am* 1996;4:307–325.
118. Sun XG, Hansen JE, Oudiz RJ, et al. Pulmonary function in primary pulmonary hypertension. *J Am Coll Cardiol* 2003;41:1028–1055.
119. Nicod P, Moser KM. Primary pulmonary hypertension: the risk and benefit of lung biopsy. *Circulation* 1989;80:1486–1488.
120. Murali S. Pulmonary hypertension, cardiac transplantation, and the cardiomyopathies. In: Uretsky BF, ed. *Cardiac catheterization; concepts, techniques, and applications*. Malden, MA: Blackwell Science, 1997:461–495.
121. Hoeper MM, Rubin LJ. Update in pulmonary hypertension 2005. *Am J Respir Crit Care Med* 2006;173:499–505.
122. Enriquez-Sarano M, Rossi A, Seward JB, et al: Determinants of pulmonary hypertension in left ventricular dysfunction. *J Am Coll Cardiol* 1997;29:153–159.
123. Costard-Jackle A, Fowler MB. Influence of preoperative pulmonary artery pressure on mortality after heart transplantation: testing of potential reversibility of pulmonary hypertension with nitroprusside is useful in defining a high risk group. *J Am Coll Cardiol* 1992;19:48–54.
124. Abramson SV, Burke JF, Kelly Jr JJ, et al. Pulmonary hypertension predicts mortality and morbidity in patients with dilated cardiomyopathy. *Ann Intern Med* 1992;116:888–895.
125. Murali S, Kormos RL, Uretsky BF, et al. Preoperative pulmonary hemodynamics and early mortality after orthotopic cardiac transplantation: the Pittsburgh experience. *Am Heart J* 1993;126:896–904.
126. Kirklin JK, Naftel DC, Kirklin JW, et al. Pulmonary vascular resistance and the risk of heart transplantation, *J Heart Transplant* 1988;7:331–336.
127. Hosenpud JD, Bennett LE, Keck BM. The registry of the International Society for Heart and Lung Transplantation: eighteenth official report—2001. *J Heart Lung Transplant* 2001;20:805–815.
128. Badesch DB, Abman SH, Ahearn GS. Medical therapy for pulmonary arterial hypertension. ACCP evidence-based clinical practice guidelines. *Chest* 2004;126:35S–62S.
129. Rubin LJ, Badesch DB. Evaluation and management of the patient with pulmonary arterial hypertension. *Ann Int Med* 2005;143:288–292.
130. Humbert M, Sitbon O, Simonneau G. Treatment of pulmonary arterial hypertension. *N Engl J Med* 2004;351:1425–1436.
131. Galie N, Seeger W, Naeije R, et al. Comparative analysis of clinical trials and evidence-based treatment algorithm in pulmonary arterial hypertension. *J Am Coll Cardiol* 2004;43(Suppl S):81S–88S.
132. Rich S, Seidlitz M, Dodin E, et al. The short-term effects of digoxin in patients with right ventricular dysfunction from pulmonary hypertension. *Chest* 1998;114:787–792.
133. Fuster V, Steele PM, Edwards WD, et al. Primary pulmonary hypertension: natural history and the importance of thrombosis. *Circulation* 1984;70:580–587.
134. Rich S, Kaufmann E, Levy PS. The effect of high doses of calcium-channel blockers on survival in primary pulmonary hypertension. *N Engl J Med* 1992;327:76–81.
135. Sitbon O, Humbert M, Jas X, et al. Long-term response to calcium channel blockers in idiopathic pulmonary arterial hypertension. *Circulation* 2005;111:3105–3111.
136. Channick RN, Sitbon O, Barst RJ, et al. Endothelin receptor antagonists in pulmonary arterial hypertension. *J Am Coll Cardiol* 2004;43(Suppl S):62S–67S.
137. Channick RN, Simonneau G, Sitbon O, et al. Effects of the dual endothelin receptor antagonist bosentan in patients with pulmonary hypertension: a randomized, placebo-controlled study. *Lancet* 2001;358:1119–1123.
138. Rubin LJ, Badesch DB, Barst RJ, et al. Bosentan therapy for pulmonary arterial hypertension. *N Engl J Med* 2002;346:896–903.
139. McLaughlin VV, Sitbon O, Badesch DB, et al. Survival with first-line bosentan in patients with primary pulmonary hypertension. *Eur Respir J* 2005;25:244–249.
140. Sitbon O, McLaughlin VV, Badesch DB, et al. Survival in patients with class III idiopathic pulmonary arterial hypertension treated with first line oral bosentan compared with an historical cohort of patients started on intravenous epoprostenol. *Thorax* 2005;60:1025–1030.
141. Schulze-Neick I, Gilbert N, Ewert R, et al. Adult patients with congenital heart disease and pulmonary arterial hypertension: first open prospective multicenter study of bosentan therapy. *Am Heart J* 2005;150:716.
142. Hoeper MM, Halank M, Marx C, et al. Bosentan therapy for portopulmonary hypertension. *Eur Respir J* 2005;25:502–508.
143. Hoeper MM, Kramm T, Wilkens H, et al. Bosentan therapy for inoperable chronic thromboembolic pulmonary hypertension. *Chest* 2005;128:2363–2367.
144. Bonderman D, Nowotny R, Skoro-Sajer N, et al. Bosentan therapy for inoperable chronic thromboembolic pulmonary hypertension. *Chest* 2005;128:2599–2603.
145. Hoeper MM. Drug treatment of pulmonary arterial hypertension: current and future agents. *Drugs* 2005;65:1337–1354.
146. Richalet JP, Gratadour P, Robach P, et al. Sildenafil inhibits altitude-induced hypoxemia and pulmonary hypertension. *Am J Respir Crit Care Med* 2005;171:275–281.
147. Machado RF, Martyr S, Kato GJ, et al. Sildenafil therapy in patients with sickle cell disease and pulmonary hypertension. *Br J Haematol* 2005;130:445–453.
148. Wharton J, Strange JW, Moller GM, et al. Antiproliferative effects of phosphodiesterase type 5 inhibition in human pulmonary artery cells. *Am J Respir Crit Care Med* 2005;172:105–113.
149. Galiè N, Ghofrani HA, Torbicki A, et al. Sildenafil citrate therapy for pulmonary arterial hypertension. *N Engl J Med* 2005;353:2148–2153.
150. Michelakis E, Tymchak W, Lien D, et al. Oral sildenafil is an effective and specific pulmonary vasodilator in patients with pulmonary arterial hypertension: comparison with inhaled nitric oxide. *Circulation* 2002;105:2398–2403.
151. Lepore JJ, Maroo A, Pereira NL, et al. Effect of sildenafil on the acute pulmonary vasodilator response to inhaled nitric oxide in adults with primary pulmonary hypertension. *Am J Cardiol* 2002;90:677–680.
152. Ghofrani HA, Schermuly RT, Rose F, et al. Sildenafil for long-term treatment of nonoperable chronic thromboembolic pulmonary hypertension. *Am J Respir Crit Care Med* 2003;167:1139–1141.
153. Wilkins MR, Paul GA, Strange JW, et al. Sildenafil versus Endothelin Receptor Antagonist for Pulmonary Hypertension (SERAPH) study. *Am J Respir Crit Care Med* 2005;171:1292–1297.
154. Barst RJ, Rubin LJ, McGoon MD, et al. A comparison of continuous intravenous epoprostenol (prostacyclin) with conventional therapy for primary pulmonary hypertension. The Primary Pulmonary Hypertension Study Group. *N Engl J Med* 1996;334:296–302.
155. McLaughlin VV, Genthner DE, Panella MM, et al. Reduction in pulmonary vascular resistance with long-term epoprostenol (prostacyclin) therapy in primary pulmonary hypertension. *N Engl J Med* 1998;338:273–277.
156. McLaughlin VV, Shillington A, Rich S. Survival in primary pulmonary hypertension: the impact of epoprostenol therapy. *Circulation* 2002;106:1477–1482.
157. Sitbon O, Humbert M, Nunes H, et al. Long-term intravenous epoprostenol infusion in primary pulmonary hypertension: prognostic factors and survival. *J Am Coll Cardiol* 2002;40:780–788.
158. Badesch DB, Tapson VF, McGoon MD, et al. Continuous intravenous epoprostenol for pulmonary hypertension due to the scleroderma spectrum of disease. A randomized, controlled trial. *Ann Intern Med* 2000;132:425–434.
159. Barst RJ, Rubin LJ, McGoon MD, et al. Survival in primary pulmonary hypertension with long-term continuous intravenous prostacyclin. *Ann Intern Med* 1994;121:409–415.
160. Simonneau G, Barst RJ, Galie N, et al. Continuous subcutaneous infusion of treprostinil, a prostacyclin analogue, in patients with pulmonary arterial hypertension: a double blind, randomized, placebo controlled trial. *Am J Respir Crit Care Med* 2002;165:800–804.
161. Gomberg-Maitland M, Tapson VF, Benza RL, et al. Transition from Intravenous to intravenous treprostinil in pulmonary hypertension. *Am J Respir Crit Care Med* 2005;172:1586–1589.
162. Hoeper MM, Olschewski H, Ghotrani HA, et al. A comparison of acute hemodynamic effects of inhaled nitric oxide and aerosolized iloprost in primary pulmonary hypertension. German PPH Study Group. *J Am Coll Cardiol* 2000;35:176–182.
163. Olschewski H, Simonneau G, Galiè N, et al., for the Aerosolized Iloprost Randomized Study Group. Inhaled iloprost for severe pulmonary hypertension. *N Engl J Med* 2002;347:322–329.

164. Olschewski H, Ghofrani HA, Schmehl T, et al. Inhaled iloprost to treat severe pulmonary hypertension. An uncontrolled trial. German PPH Study Group. *Ann Intern Med* 2000;132:435–443.
165. Hoeper MM, Schwarze M, Ehlerding S, et al. Long-term treatment of primary pulmonary hypertension with aerosolized iloprost, a prostacyclin analogue. *N Engl J Med* 2000;342:1866–1870.
166. Barst RJ, McGoon M, McLaughlin V, et al. Beraprost therapy for pulmonary arterial hypertension. *J Am Coll Cardiol* 2003;41:2119–2125.
167. Galie N, Humbert M, Vachiery JL, et al. Effects of beraprost sodium, an oral prostacyclin analogue, in patients with pulmonary arterial hypertension: a randomized, double-blind, placebo-controlled trial. *J Am Coll Cardiol* 2002;39:1496–1502.
168. Petkov V, Mosgoeller W, Ziesche R, et al. Vasoactive intestinal peptide as a new drug for treatment of primary pulmonary hypertension. *J Clin Invest* 2003;111:1339–1346.
169. Ghofrani HA, Voswinckel R, Reichenberger F, et al. Differences in hemodynamic and oxygenation responses to three different phosphodiesterase-5 inhibitors in patients with pulmonary arterial hypertension: a randomized prospective study. *J Am Coll Cardiol* 2004;44:1488–1496.
170. Wilkins MR. Selective or nonselective endothelin receptor blockade inpulmonary arterial hypertension. *Am J Respir Crit Care Med* 2004;169:433–434.
171. Barst RJ, Langleben D, Frost A, et al. Sitaxsentan therapy for pulmonary arterial hypertension. *Am J Respir Crit Care Med* 2004;169:441–447.
172. Galié N, Badesch D, Oudiz R, et al. Ambrisentan therapy for pulmonary arterial hypertension. *J Am Coll Cardiol* 2005;46:529–535.
173. Nishimura T, Vaszar LT, Faul JL, et al. Simvastatin rescues rats from fatal pulmonary hypertension by inducing apoptosis of neointimal smooth muscle cells. *Circulation* 2003;108:1640–1645.
174. Kao PN. Simvastatin treatment for pulmonary hypertension: an observational case series. *Chest* 2005;127:1446–1452.
175. Humbert M, Barst RJ, Robbins IM, et al. Combination of bosentan with epoprostenol in pulmonary arterial hypertension: BREATHE-2. *Eur Respir J* 2004;24:353–359.
176. Ghofrani HA, Wiedemann R, Rose F, et al. Combination therapy with oral sildenafil and inhaled iloprost for severe pulmonary hypertension. *Ann Intern Med* 2002;136:515–522.
177. Wilkens H, Guth A, Konig J, et al. Effect of inhaled iloprost plus oral sildenafil in patients with primary pulmonary hypertension. *Circulation* 2001;104:1218–1222.
178. Ghofrani HA, Rose F, Schermuly RT, et al. Oral sildenafil as long-term adjunct therapy to inhaled iloprost in severe pulmonary arterial hypertension. *J Am Coll Cardiol* 2003;42:158–164.
179. Hoeper MM, Faulenbach C, Golpon H, et al. Combination therapy with bosentan and sildenafil in idiopathic pulmonary arterial hypertension. *Eur Respir J* 2004;24:1007–1010.
180. Paul GA, Gibbs JS, Boobis AR, et al. Bosentan decreases the plasma concentration of sildenafil when coprescribed in pulmonary hypertension. *Br J Clin Pharmacol* 2005;60:107–112.
181. Archibald CJ, Auger WR, Fedullo PF et al. Long-term outcome after pulmonary thromboendarterectomy. *Am J Respir Crit Care Med* 1999;160: 523–528.
182. Thistlethwaite PA, Kemp A, Du L, et al. Outcomes of pulmonary endarterectomy for treatment of extreme thromboembolic pulmonary hypertension. *J Thorac Cardiovasc Surg* 2006;131:307–313.
183. Sandoval J, Gaspar J, Pulido T, et al. Graded balloon dilation atrial septostomy in severe primary pulmonary hypertension. A therapeutic alternative for patients non-responsive to vasodilator treatment. *J Am Coll Cardiol* 1998;32:297–304.
184. Sandoval J, Rothman A, Pulido T. Atrial septostomy for pulmonary hypertension. *Clin Chest Med* 2001;22:547–560.
185. Rothman A, Sklansky MS, Lucas VW, et al. Atrial septostomy as a bridge to lung transplantation in patients with severe pulmonary hypertension. *Am J Cardiol* 1999;84:682–686.
186. Bando K, Armitage JM, Paradis IL, et al. Indications for and results of single, bilateral and heart-lung transplantation for pulmonary hypertension. *J Thorac Cardiovasc Surg* 1994;108:1056–1065.
187. Christie JD, Kotloff RM, Pochettino A, et al. Clinical risk factors for primary graft failure following lung transplantation. *Chest* 2003;124:1232–1241.
188. Mendeloff EN, Meyers BF, Sundt TM, et al. Lung transplantation for pulmonary vascular disease. *Ann Thorac Surg* 2002;73:209–299.
189. Pielsticker EJ, Martinez FJ, Rubenfire M. Lung and heart-lung transplant practice patterns in pulmonary hypertension centers. *J Heart Lung Transplant* 2001;20:1297–1304.
190. Miyamoto S, Nagaya N, Satoh T, et al. Clinical correlates and prognostic significance of six minute walk test in patients with primary pulmonary hypertension: comparison with cardio-pulmonary exercise testing. *Am J Respir Crit Care Med* 2000;161:487–492.
191. Bossone E, Rubenfire M, Bach DS, et al. Range of tricuspid regurgitation velocity at rest and during exercise in normal adult men: implications for the diagnosis of pulmonary hypertension. *J Am Coll Cardiol* 1999;33:1662–1666.
192. Hinderliter AL, Willis 4th PW, Barst RJ, et al. Effects of long-term infusion of prostacyclin (epoprostenol) on echocardiographic measures of right ventricular structure and function in primary pulmonary hypertension. Primary Pulmonary Hypertension Study Group. *Circulation* 1997;95:1479–1486.
193. Nagaya N, Nishikimi T, Uematsu M, et al. Plasma brain natriuretic peptide as a prognostic indicator in patients with primary pulmonary hypertension. *Circulation* 2000;102:865–870.
194. Lee JH, Lee DS, Kim EK, et al. Simvastatin inhibits cigarette smoking–induced emphysema and pulmonary hypertension in rat lungs. *Am J Respir Crit Care Med* 2005;172:987–993.
195. Demedts M, Behr J, Buhl R, et al. High-dose acetylcysteine in idiopathic pulmonary fibrosis. *N Engl J Med* 2005: 353:2229–2242.
196. Heart Failure Society of America. Executive summary: HFSA 2006 comprehensive heart failure practice guideline. *J Card Fail* 2006;12:10–38.
197. Nohria A, Lewis E, Stevenson LW. Medical management of advanced heart failure. *JAMA* 2002;287:628–640.
198. Hill JA, Hsu K, Aranda Jr JM, et al. Sustained use of nesiritide to aid in bridging to heart transplant. *Clin Cardiol* 2003;26:211–214.
199. Sablotzki A, Strazmann W, Scheubel R, et al. Selective pulmonary vasodilation with inhaled aerosolized milrinone in heart transplant candidates. *Can J Anaesth* 2005;52(10):1076–1082.
200. Salzberg SP, Lachat ML, von Harbou K, et al. Normalization of high pulmonary vascular resistance with LVAD support in heart transplantation candidates. *Eur J Cardiothorac Surg* 2005;27:222–225.
201. Givertz MM, Colucci WS, LeJemtel TH, et al. Acute endothelin A receptor blockade causes selective pulmonary vasodilation in patients with chronic heart failure. *Circulation* 2000;101:2922–2927.
202. Teerlink JR. Recent heart failure trials of neurohormonal modulation (OVERTURE and ENABLE): approaching the asymptote of efficacy? *J Card Fail* 2002;8:124–127.
203. Califf RM, Adams KF, McKenna WJ, et al. A randomized, controlled trial of epoprostenol therapy for severe congestive heart failure: the Flolan International Randomized Survival Trial (FIRST). *Am Heart J* 1997;134:44–54.
204. Alaeddini J, Uber P, Park MH, et al. Efficacy and safety of sildenafil in the evaluation of pulmonary hypertension in severe heart failure. *Am J Cardiol* 2004;94:1475–1477.
205. Lepore, JJ, Maroo, A, Bigatello, LM, et al. Hemodynamic effects of sildenafil in patients with congestive heart failure and pulmonary hypertension: combined administration with inhaled nitric oxide. *Chest* 2005;127:1647–1653.

CHAPTER 29 ■ HYPERTROPHIC CARDIOMYOPATHY

WILLIAM J. McKENNA AND PERRY M. ELLIOTT

INTRODUCTION

Hypertrophic cardiomyopathy (HCM) is a phenotypically heterogeneous condition that affects individuals of all ages. The disease is typically inherited in an autosomal dominant fashion with variable clinical penetrance. In adults, the majority of cases are caused by mutations in one of 12 cardiac sarcomeric protein genes; in infants and children, left ventricular hypertrophy is often associated with congenital malformations and syndromes, inherited disorders of metabolism, and neuromuscular diseases.

The disease is characterized by myocardial hypertrophy, most commonly affecting the interventricular septum, disorganization ("disarray") of cardiac myocytes and myofibrils, myocardial fibrosis, and small-vessel disease. Twenty-five percent of patients have resting left ventricular outflow tract obstruction.

Patients present throughout life with chest pain, dyspnea, palpitations, and syncope; the most important complication of the disease is sudden death, which occurs with an annual incidence of approximately 1%. Other complications include atrial arrhythmia, thromboembolism, infective endocarditis, and congestive cardiac failure. Symptoms can be improved with pharmacologic therapy or relief of left ventricular outflow tract obstruction using alcohol ablation or surgery; cardiac transplantation is required in a small minority of cases. Sudden death prevention is based on the identification of clinical risk markers; patients with multiple risk factors are treated with implantable cardioverter defibrillators.

HISTORICAL PERSPECTIVE

Asymmetric hypertrophy of the interventricular septum was first described in 1869 by Liouville (1) and Hallopeau (2), but it was only in the 1950s that hypertrophic cardiomyopathy was established as a discrete clinical entity with the description of "functional obstruction of the left ventricle" by Sir Russell Brock (3) and asymmetric septal hypertrophy by Donald Teare (4). There followed a period of intense clinical investigation in which the characteristic morphologic and hemodynamic features of the disease were defined. In the 1960s (5–9), reliance on stethoscope and cardiac catheterization meant that left ventricular outflow tract obstruction was considered to be the diagnostic hallmark of HCM, a fact reflected in the many pseudonyms for the disease used during this period (e.g., idiopathic hypertrophic subaortic stenosis [IHSS]); in the 1970s, M-mode echocardiography (10–12) reemphasized asymmetric septal hypertrophy (ASH) as the diagnostic hallmark of the disease, but the advent of two-dimensional echocardiographic imaging demonstrated that virtually any pattern of unexplained myocardial hypertrophy is consistent with the diagnosis (13,14).

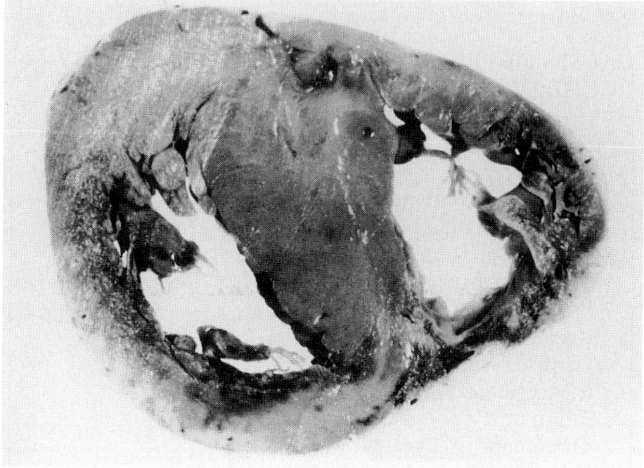

FIGURE 29.1. Myocardial section demonstrating the classic appearance of severe asymmetric septal hypertrophy in a patient with hypertrophic cardiomyopathy. (From Teare D. Asymmetrical hypertrophy of the heart in young adults. *Br Heart J* 1958;20:1–8.)

In the 1980s, work on the clinical pathophysiology of the disease continued, but the growing recognition that the majority of cases were familial led to the identification of the first genetic mutation in the gene encoding the β-myosin heavy chain (15). Since then, numerous mutations in this and other sarcomeric proteins have been reported, leading to the modern concept of the disease as a disorder of the myocyte contractile apparatus. This remains the current view, but genetic characterization has illustrated the diversity of clinical expression and is beginning to show that similar mutations can cause dilated and restrictive cardiomyopathy in the absence of hypertrophy (16,17).

PATHOLOGY

Macroscopic

Hypertrophic cardiomyopathy (HCM) is defined by the presence of unexplained myocardial hypertrophy (18,19), typically involving the interventricular septum more than the posterior or free wall of the left ventricle (4–14,19–21) (Fig. 29.1). Hypertrophy is less commonly concentric and can be confined to the left ventricular apex (19–23); right ventricular hypertrophy is also common but has not been reported in isolation (24). The cut surface of involved myocardium has a characteristic appearance with abnormally short and broad muscle fibers running in different directions. A patch of subendocardial thickening on the septum caused by repeated contact with the anterior leaflet of the mitral valve may be seen in patients who have had outflow tract obstruction (20,21).

Microscopic

Microscopically HCM is characterized by myocyte disarray (18–21,25–27) (Fig. 29.2), in which there is loss of the normal parallel arrangement of cardiomyocytes, cells instead forming circles or whorls around foci of connective tissue. The myofibrillar architecture within cells is also disrupted (myofibrillar disarray). Individual myocytes vary in shape and have pleomorphic nuclei and abnormal intercellular connections (28). Myocyte disarray is not specific to HCM, and it occurs in other syndromic causes of left ventricular hypertrophy such as Noonan syndrome and Friedreich ataxia as well as congenital heart disease, hypertension, and aortic stenosis (20,21,25–27,29–30). In HCM, it is typically more extensive, occupying 20% or more of at least one ventricular tissue block and more than 5% of total myocardium at postmortem. Disarray is often associated with myocardial fibrosis in the form of extensive scarring or a more diffuse interstitial pattern (20,21,25–27,29–33). Abnormal small intramural arteries are common, particularly in patients with ventricular dilation and reduced systolic function (20,21,27,34–36) (Fig. 29.3).

MOLECULAR GENETICS

Many cases of left ventricular hypertrophy in infants and young children are associated with congenital malformations and syndromes, inherited metabolic disorders, and neuromuscular diseases (Table 29.1) (18,19,26,29,30,37–43). The majority of adolescents and adults with HCM have familial disease with an autosomal dominant pattern of inheritance; approximately 50% to 60% of patients have mutations in one of eight genes that encode different components of the cardiac sarcomere (Fig. 29.4): β-myosin heavy chain (chromosome 14); cardiac troponin T (chromosome 1); cardiac troponin I (chromosome 19);

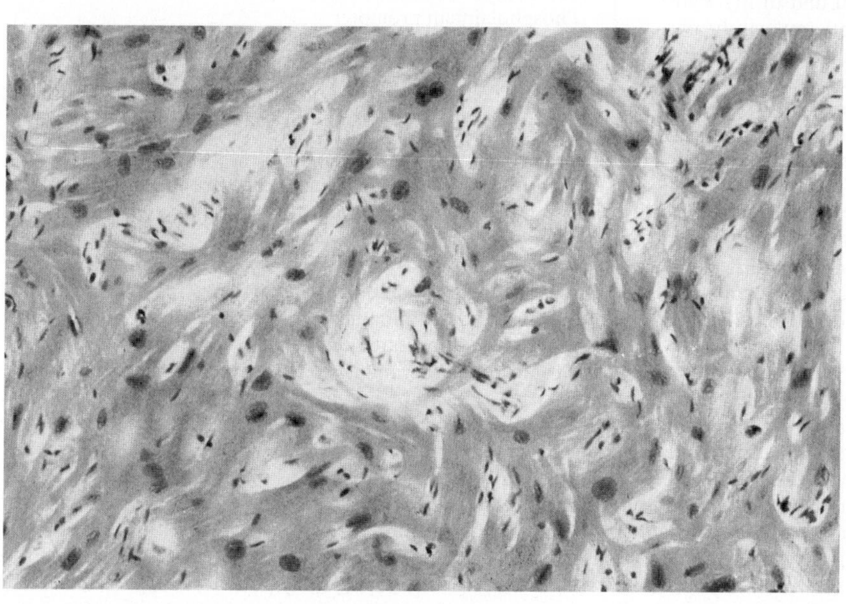

FIGURE 29.2. Myocyte disarray. Myocytes cross at right angles and display abnormal intercellular connections. Myocyte nuclei are large and of different sizes. There are foci of fibrosis containing spindle-shaped connective tissue cells. There is also evidence of marked disorganization of the intracellular myobrillar structure. Hematoxylin and eosin stain. (Courtesy of Prof. M. Davies, St. George's Hospital Medical School, London.)

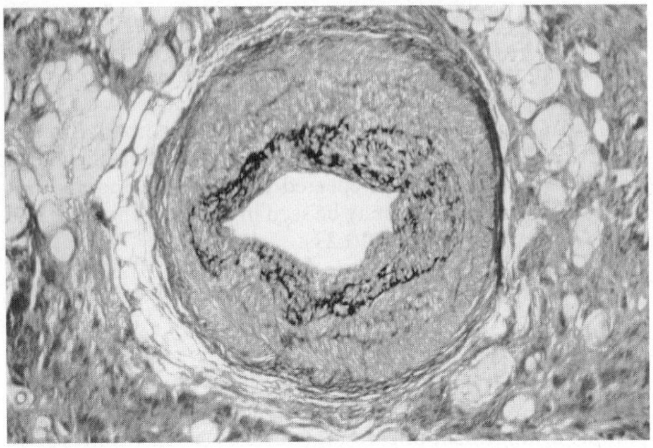

FIGURE 29.3. Section through a small artery demonstrating smooth muscle disorganization in the intima and media, resulting in an abnormally high ratio of medial width to lumen. In the adjacent myocardium there is extensive replacement of myocytes (*yellow*) by fibrous tissue (*red*). Elastica van Gieson stain. (Courtesy of Prof. M. Davies, St. George's Hospital Medical School, London.)

α-tropomyosin (chromosome 15); cardiac myosin-binding protein C (chromosome 11); the essential and regulatory myosin light chains (chromosomes 3 and 12, respectively); and cardiac actin (chromosome 15). Mutations in three other sarcomeric protein genes have been reported: titin (62), troponin C (63), and α-cardiac myosin heavy chain (19,44–62). Some adult patients with apparently unexplained ventricular hypertrophy have diseases such as Anderson-Fabry disease (63), mitochondrial disease (64), and a rare phenotype comprising HCM, Wolff-Parkinson-White syndrome, and premature conduction disease caused by mutations in the gene encoding the γ-subunit of AMP kinase, an important regulator of cellular energy homeostasis (65–67). Other examples of nonsarcomeric gene mutations that can result in HCM phenocopies include LAMP-2 (Danon disease) (67,68), human muscle LIM protein (69), and phospholamban promoter (70).

Pathophysiology of Sarcomeric Protein Gene Mutations

The proteins of the sarcomere, the functional unit of myocyte contraction, are organized into thick filaments (myosin heavy chain, myosin-binding protein C, and myosin essential and regulatory light chains) and thin filaments (actin, troponins T, I, and C, and tropomyosin) (44–46,71–73) (Fig. 29.4). Myocyte contraction occurs as the myofilaments slide over each other in a repetitive cycle of myosin and actin attachment, energy-dependent conformational changes in myosin, and actin–myosin release. The globular head of myosin heavy chain, connected through a flexible hinge region to the rod, contains enzymatic activity for ATP hydrolysis and actin-binding sites. Contraction is initiated following a rise in cytosolic calcium, which then binds the troponin complex and α-tropomyosin; this releases the inhibitory effect of troponin I on actin–myosin interaction, allowing actin to bind tightly to the myosin head; ATP then binds myosin, altering the conformation of the actin-binding sites and displacing the myosin head along the thin filament. ATP hydrolysis and release of ADP and Pi results in force generation (the power stroke) and restoration of the unbound conformation of myosin (44–46,72). Force transmission to the myocyte cytoskeleton is mediated via a complex of molecules including cardiac myosin-binding protein C, titin, dystrophin, and the sarcoglycan complex (44–46,73).

TABLE 29.1

CAUSES OF LEFT VENTRICULAR HYPERTROPHY IN CHILDREN AND ADULTS

Sarcomeric protein gene mutations
β-Myosin heavy chain
Cardiac myosin-binding protein C
Cardiac troponin I
Troponin T
α-Tropomyosin
Essential myosin light chain
Regulatory myosin light chain
Cardiac α-actin
α-Myosin heavy chain
Titin
Troponin C
Syndromes
Noonan syndrome
LEOPARD syndrome
Costello syndrome
Friedreich ataxia
Beckwith-Wiedemann syndrome
Swyer syndrome (pure gonadal dysgenesis)
Metabolic disorders
Glycogen storage disease II (Pompe disease)
Glycogen storage disease III (Forbes disease)
Danon disease
Anderson-Fabry disease
Carnitine deficiency
Phosphorylase B kinase deficiency
Infants of diabetic mother
AMP kinase (Wolff-Parkinson-White syndrome, hypertrophic cardiomyopathy, conduction disease)
Debrancher enzyme deficiency
Hurler syndrome
Hurler-Scheie disease
Hunter syndrome
Mannosidosis
Fucosidosis
Total lipodystrophy
Mitochondrial cytopathy
Other
Obesity
Athletic training
Muscle LIM protein
Phospholamban promoter
Amyloidosis
Pheochromocytoma

Mutations in genes encoding sarcomere proteins might interfere with sarcomeric function in a number of ways (44–46;71–95). Inactivation of an allele can result in a reduced amount of functional protein (haploinsufficiency), whereas others produce a mutant protein that interferes with normal protein function (dominant negative) or has a novel function. Animal models of mutated myosin heavy chain (75,83,87,94), myosin-binding protein C (76,84), and troponin T (78,82) mimic some aspects of human disease, including cardiac hypertrophy, myocyte disarray, and interstitial fibrosis (74). Most transgenic models suggest that HCM results from the dominant negative effects of mutant proteins on sarcomere function and not haploinsufficiency or altered stoichiometry of sarcomere components. In addition, there seems to be a dose response, the levels of mutant sarcomere protein expressed within the heart correlating with myocyte dysfunction (76). Some effects

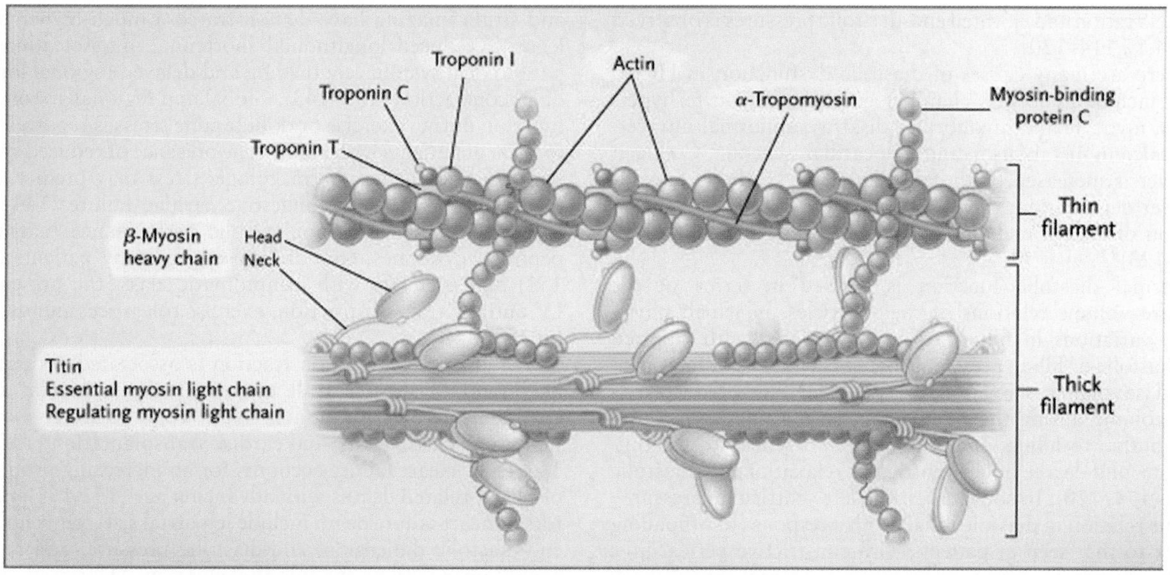

FIGURE 29.4. Structure of the human sarcomere. Cardiac contraction occurs as a consequence of actin–myosin interaction. This is initiated by the binding of calcium to the troponin complex (C, I, and T) and α-tropomyosin. Actin then stimulates ATPase activity in the globular myosin head, resulting in the generation of contractile force. Cardiac myosin-binding protein C binds to myosin and modulates contraction. (From Nabel EG. Cardiovascular disease. *N Engl J Med* 2003;349:60–72, Fig. 3.)

of human hypertrophic mutations relate to their proximity to critical binding sites; for example, in the myosin head domain, where affected residues interfere with the actin-binding site or the nucleotide (ATP)-binding pocket (71–94).

The time course of functional abnormalities has been studied in animal models (74–78,82–84,87). Altered calcium sensitivity, myocyte disarray, and abnormal myocardial contraction and relaxation velocities appear to be early manifestations, with hypertrophy and fibrosis developing predominantly during puberty in conjunction with activation of stress-related signaling kinases. In most models, global cardiac function declines with aging.

Although it is clear that sarcomere mutations are associated with activation of myocyte growth pathways, the underlying mechanisms remain poorly understood. Disturbed calcium homeostasis, activation of the renin–aldosterone–angiotensin system, and abnormal myocardial energetics have been implicated (44–46,65–67,80,94–99). Some isolated fiber experiments have suggested that reduced contractile function is the stimulus to hypertrophy; however, most studies show that the force and velocity of myocyte contraction are in fact increased rather than decreased, declining with age after the development of the hypertrophic phenotype. Adverse effects of this gain in function include uncoordination between myosin heads and higher levels of energy consumption (44–46).

Whatever the mechanisms underlying expression of sarcomere protein gene mutations, individual mutations show marked heterogeneity in expression among individuals and even among myocardial fibers. Potential genetic modifiers of disease expression include renin–angiotensin–aldosterone system gene polymorphism (96–99); rare examples of homozygotes and compound heterozygotes also have been described (86,100–102).

Clinical Genotype–Phenotype Correlations

Reports suggest that mutations in some genes tend to be associated with a common phenotype; for example, some families with cardiac troponin T mutations have mild hypertrophy and a high risk of sudden death, whereas myosin-binding protein C mutations are associated with late-onset disease (44–46,57,58,61,81,82,91,103–105). However, detailed family studies have shown that the expression of these mutations is heterogeneous, with examples of severe hypertrophy and benign clinical outcomes in the case of troponin T mutations and childhood disease in myosin-binding protein C (44–46,57,58,61,81,82,91,103–107). The fact that disease expression for all of the described sarcomeric genes varies not only among unrelated individuals, but also within the same family means that HCM should be seen as a complex inherited trait influenced by other genetic and environmental factors.

Gender Effects

Most large clinical series show a predominance of male patients, and some animal models of sarcomeric protein gene mutations have reported earlier disease expression, greater left ventricular dilation, more severe systolic impairment, and a higher propensity to ventricular arrhythmia in response to adrenergic stress in male animals (82,83,108). In humans, postmortem analyses suggest that male patients have more fibrosis (36). In vivo data are less consistent, demonstrating lesser wall thicknesses in older women (109) and larger cavity dimensions and reduced systolic function in men (110). Regional differences in LV systolic function in men and women may be explained by differences in regional wall thickness and wall stress (111).

PATHOPHYSIOLOGY

Diastolic Dysfunction

Symptoms in nonobstructive HCM are often caused by abnormal diastolic function. In a minority of patients, a "restrictive" hemodynamic picture may predominate, with elevation of filling pressures, biatrial dilation, and signs of right heart failure, often in the absence of substantial myocardial hypertrophy (112,113). In the majority of cases, a mixed picture with slow relaxation and elevated end-diastolic pressures is observed (10–14,17,114–120).

There are many causes of diastolic dysfunction in HCM. These include abnormal chamber geometry, myocyte hypertrophy, myocyte and myofibrillar disarray, abnormal intracellular calcium metabolism, and myocardial ischemia. Collagen turnover is increased, with collagen type I synthesis prevailing over degradation; there is also evidence for abnormal inhibition of matrix metalloproteinases (MMP-1 and MMP-2) (121–123).

Normal diastolic function is defined in terms of the pressure–volume relations of the ventricles, in which physiologic variations in filling are not associated with elevated end-diastolic or filling pressures. Patients with HCM have prolonged isovolumic relaxation, delayed peak filling, reduced relative volume during the rapid filling period, increased atrial contribution to filling, and regional heterogeneity in the timing, rate, and degree of left ventricular relaxation and diastolic filling (114–120). In some cases, the left ventricular pressure–volume relation in diastole is flat, with a response to offloading similar to that seen in patients with constrictive pericarditis, which suggests the presence of increased external constraint to left ventricular filling (119).

Left Ventricular Outflow Tract Obstruction

Approximately 25% of patients with HCM have a resting pressure gradient in the outflow tract of the left ventricle (5–14,19) caused by systolic anterior motion (SAM) of the mitral valve leaflets. Some patients without evidence of outflow obstruction at rest develop gradients during physiologic and pharmacologic interventions that diminish left ventricular end-diastolic volume or augment left ventricular contractility. In general, clinically significant obstruction should only be considered when the outflow gradient is at least 30 mm Hg and probably more than 50 mm Hg (14).

The accepted explanation for SAM is that septal hypertrophy and consequent outflow tract narrowing produce a high-velocity stream anterior to the mitral valve that causes the tip of the anterior mitral valve leaflet to be sucked against the septum by the Venturi effect (5–14,19,124–133). Experimental and observational data suggest that anterior papillary muscle displacement and primary mitral valve abnormalities are also necessary to create sufficient leaflet slack to allow SAM (127–133). Occasionally outflow tract obstruction may be caused by contact between the interventricular septum and an anomalously inserted papillary muscle (134). Pressure gradients may also occur in the mid-cavity in association with cavity obliteration, sometimes associated with paradoxical diastolic flow in the sequestered apical segment (135).

Mitral regurgitation occurs in almost all patients with obstructive HCM as a consequence of SAM and abnormal mitral leaflet coaptation (5–14,124–133,136). The regurgitant jet is usually posteriorly directed; when the jet is centrally or anteriorly directed, intrinsic mitral valve disease (including calcification of the mitral valve annulus, leaflet fibroelastosis caused by repeated traumatic septal contact, mitral valve prolapse, and rheumatic valve disease) should be suspected.

Systolic Dysfunction

Symptoms of congestive cardiac failure are common in patients with HCM, but conventional measurements of ejection fraction are normal in the majority of patients. M-mode assessments of short-axis left ventricular dimensions have shown a low prevalence of systolic impairment (<3%) with an annual incidence of less than 1% (10–14,137–143). Tissue Doppler and strain imaging have demonstrated a much higher prevalence of reduced longitudinal shortening in association with paradoxical systolic lengthening and delayed regional longitudinal contraction (139–143). Global and regional systolic dysfunction during exercise or dobutamine stress is reported in up to 50% of patients with HCM. The presence of reduced systolic performance during pharmacologic stress may predict subsequent development of congestive cardiac failure (144–146). Systemic markers of poor systolic performance (natriuretic peptides, cytokines, etc.) are present in many patients (147–151) and correlate with symptomatic class, the presence of LV outflow tract obstruction, exercise tolerance, and diastolic function.

A reduction in ejection fraction is associated with greater likelihood of greater wall thinning, left ventricular cavity enlargement, deterioration in New York Heart Association functional class, death, and cardiac transplantation (137,138, 152,153). Heart failure accounts for an increasing proportion of HCM-related deaths with advancing age (152,153); predictors of heart failure death include left atrial size, left ventricular end-diastolic dimension, end-diastolic pressure, and reduced exercise capacity at the initial evaluation. Depressed cardiac function may contribute to the high prevalence of atrial fibrillation in patients who die from heart failure (152).

Myocardial Ischemia

Patients with HCM have reduced coronary flow reserve and metabolic evidence for myocardial ischemia during pacing and pharmacologic stress (154–164). A number of pathophysiologic mechanisms have been suggested as causes of myocardial ischemia, including small-vessel disease, reduced capillary density, epicardial coronary compression, and increased oxygen demand caused by myocardial hypertrophy and myocyte disarray. It is likely that myocardial ischemia contributes to chest pain and dyspnea in many individuals, and there are limited data to suggest that myocardial ischemia may be a trigger for fatal ventricular arrhythmia and may contribute to long-term morbidity and mortality (159,162,164).

CLINICAL PROFILE

Epidemiology

The prevalence of HCM has been reported in many countries and racial groups in the United States and Canada, Europe, Israel, South America, and the Far East. The majority of studies suggest that HCM has a population prevalence of approximately 1 in 500 (165–174). The prevalence of unexplained left ventricular hypertrophy in children is unknown, but an incidence of left ventricular hypertrophy between 0.3 and 0.5 per 100,000 is reported from medical centers in the United States and Australia (37–39). The frequency is highest in the first year of life and shows a male predominance.

Age at Presentation

In the majority of cases, ventricular hypertrophy develops during periods of rapid somatic growth, sometimes during the first year of life, but more typically during adolescence (175). De novo myocardial hypertrophy can occur throughout life (176–179), but the pattern of disease in some middle-aged and elderly patients differs from that observed in younger patients with HCM in that they have mild hypertension and a number of morphologic differences including restricted anterior excursion of the mitral valve, mitral annular calcification, and a crescent-shaped left ventricular cavity (176–179). It is uncertain whether the majority of patients with this so-called elderly phenotype have a separate disease entity.

Symptoms

Because most patients with HCM have few if any symptoms, the diagnosis is often made incidentally or during family screening. Exertional chest pain and dyspnea are the most common symptoms, with characteristic day-to-day variation (5–9,14,19,137,138,142,148,152–162,172,177–184). Prolonged chest pain may occur at rest and is often precipitated by large meals (184). Patients less commonly present with paroxysmal nocturnal dyspnea and orthopnea, sometimes in the presence of apparently mild disease. A minority of patients complain of syncope or presyncope that can be exertional or occur at rest; the causes of syncope include left ventricular outflow tract obstruction, paroxysmal arrhythmia, conduction system disease, and abnormal vascular responses during exercise. Alcohol can precipitate exertional symptoms or syncope by exacerbating outflow tract obstruction (185).

Examination

In the majority of patients physical examination is normal. There may be a rapid upstroke to the arterial pulse, sometimes followed by a secondary peak, reflecting hyperdynamic left ventricular contraction (5–9,14). The left ventricular impulse may be forceful, and a palpable left atrial beat may be present. In approximately one third of patients there is a prominent a wave in the jugular venous pressure wave caused by reduced right ventricular compliance. On auscultation, the first and second heart sounds are usually normal, but a fourth heart sound, reflecting atrial systole into a poorly compliant left ventricle, may be heard in patients who are in sinus rhythm. Occasionally there may be reverse splitting of the second heart sound in patients with severe left ventricular outflow tract obstruction. In one fourth of patients, a systolic murmur caused by left ventricular outflow obstruction can be heard at the left sternal edge, radiating to the aortic and mitral areas but not into the neck or axilla. Physiologic and pharmacologic maneuvers that decrease afterload or venous return (standing, Valsalva, amyl nitrate) increase the intensity of the murmur, whereas interventions that increase afterload and venous return (squatting and phenylephrine) reduce it. The majority of patients with significant left ventricular outflow gradients also have mitral regurgitation. This can be difficult to distinguish clinically from the outflow gradient (5–9,14,124–126,136), but its presence is suggested by the length of the murmur (starting 30 to 40 msec before the onset of the outflow gradient), radiation to the axilla, and, in patients with severe regurgitation, a middiastolic rumble. Rarely, a systolic murmur may be heard in the pulmonary area as a consequence of right ventricular outflow obstruction.

Electrocardiogram

More than 95% of patients with HCM have an abnormal echocardiogram (ECG) (186–194); an abnormal ECG in the young is a sensitive marker of early disease expression (193,194). The most frequent ECG changes are left atrial enlargement, repolarization abnormalities, and pathologic Q waves, most commonly in the inferolateral leads. Voltage criteria for left ventricular hypertrophy alone are nonspecific and are often seen in normal young adults. Giant negative T waves in the mid-precordial leads are characteristic of hypertrophy confined to the left ventricular apex (22–23,186–

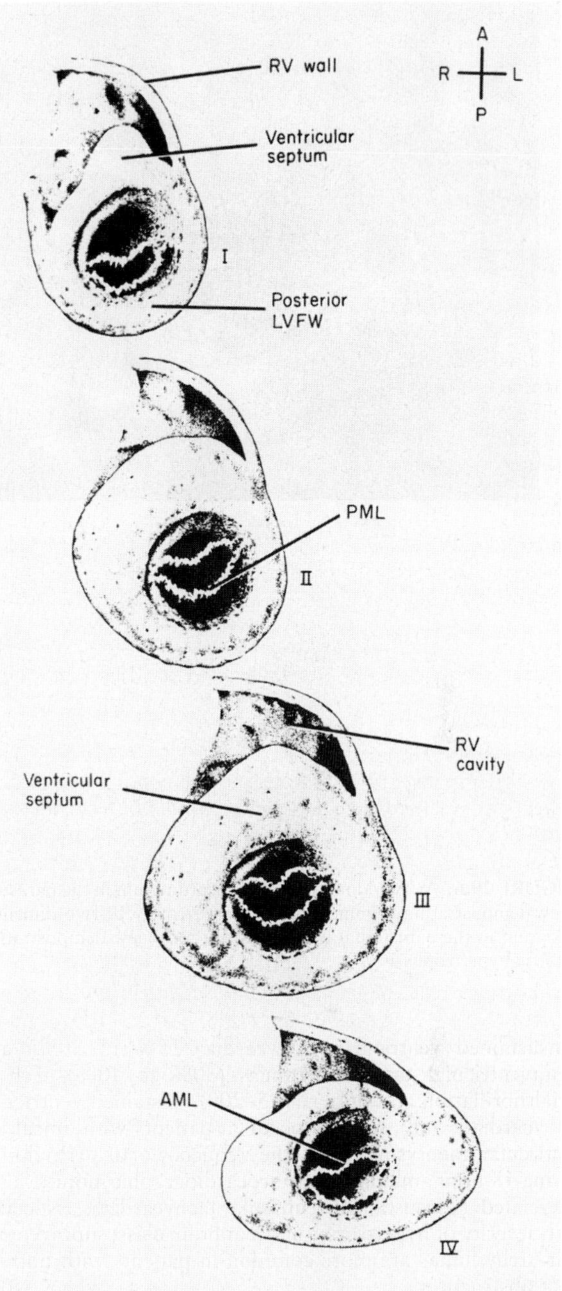

FIGURE 29.5. Maron classification. Artist's impression of four patterns of hypertrophy identified in 153 patients using two-dimensional echocardiography shown in the short-axis plane at mitral valve level. (A, anterior; AML, anterior mitral leaflet; L, patient's left; LVFW, left ventricular free wall; P, posterior; PML, posterior mitral leaflet; R, patient's right; RV, right ventricular). Type I (10% of patients) hypertrophy confined to the anterior portion of the ventricular septum. Type II (20% of patients) hypertrophy involving the anterior and posterior septum. Type III (52% of patients) hypertrophy involving the anterior and posterior septum as well as the lateral free wall. Type IV (18% of patients) hypertrophy involving left ventricular regions other than the anterior septum and the posterior free wall. (From Maron BJ Wolfson JK, Ciro E, Spirito P. Relation of electrocardiographic abnormalities and patterns of left ventricular hypertrophy identified by 2-dimensional echocardiography in patients with hypertrophic cardiomyopathy. *Am J Cardiol* 1983;51:189–194.)

192). Some patients have a short PR interval with a slurred QRS upstroke, not usually associated with Wolff-Parkinson-White syndrome. Ambulatory electrocardiographic monitoring frequently reveals premature ventricular complexes (88%),

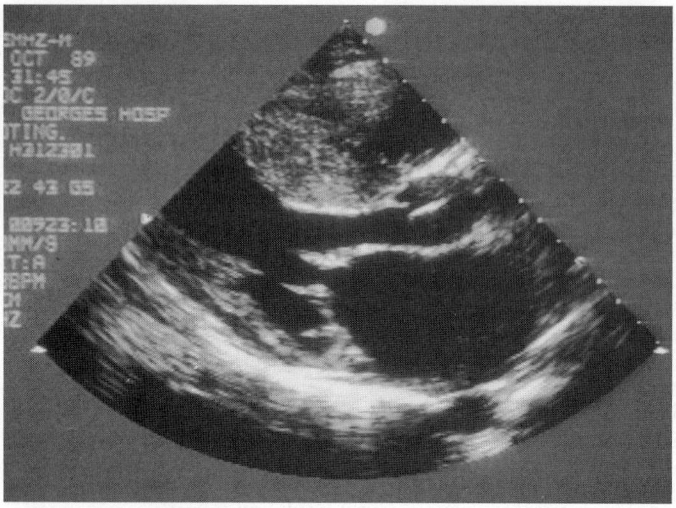

A

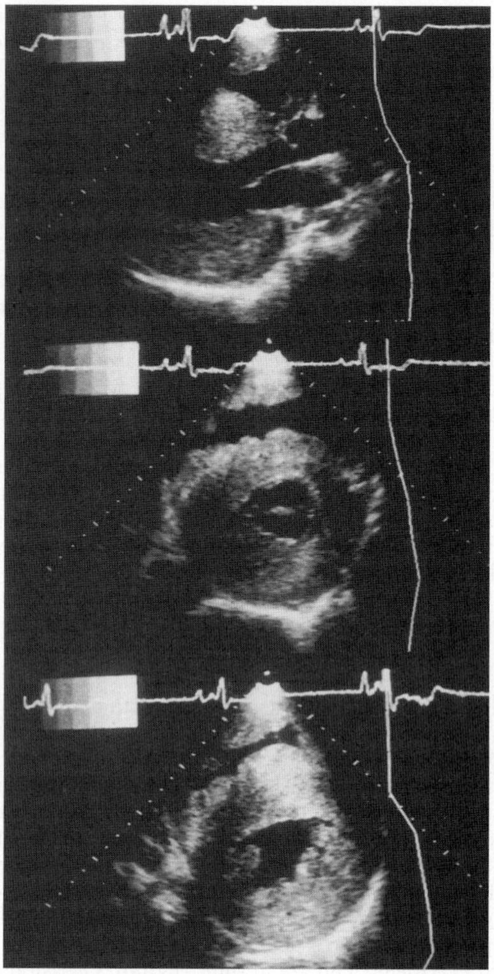

B

FIGURE 29.6. **A:** Two-dimensional echocardiogram in the parasternal long-axis view demonstrating asymmetric septal hypertrophy. **B:** Two-dimensional echocardiogram in the parasternal long and short-axis view demonstrating severe concentric hypertrophy.

nonsustained ventricular tachycardia (25% to 30%) and supraventricular tachyarrhythmias (30% to 40%) such as atrial fibrillation and flutter (195–200). Sustained ventricular tachycardia is rare, but can occur in patients with apical left ventricular aneurysms (198). The frequency of all arrhythmias during 48-hour ambulatory electrocardiographic monitoring is age related. Nonsustained ventricular tachycardia is associated with severity of hypertrophy and symptom class; supraventricular arrhythmias are more common in patients with outflow tract obstruction.

Echocardiography

Diagnostic criteria in adults are based on the demonstration of unexplained left ventricular hypertrophy on echocardiography (18,19). Some relatives of patients with unequivocal disease do not fulfill conventional echocardiographic criteria, but in the context of familial disease, nondiagnostic ECG and echo abnormalities may be sufficient to diagnose HCM (19,193–194,201). A diastolic wall thickness greater than two standard deviations from the mean corrected for age, sex, and height (typically $\geq$1.5 cm in an adult) is generally accepted as diagnostic for HCM (19). Right ventricular hypertrophy is diagnosed when at least two right ventricular wall measurements exceed two standard deviations from the mean recorded in normal individuals. The most common abnormalities seen on M-mode echocardiography (10–14,124–132,202,203) include asymmetric septal hypertrophy (ASH), systolic anterior motion (SAM) of the mitral valve, a small left ventricular cavity, septal immobility, and premature closure of the aortic valve. Various patterns of hypertrophy can be observed on two-dimensional imaging (Figs. 29.5 and 29.6). When a ratio of septal to free wall thickness of 1.3:1 is used to define asymmetry (13), concentric hypertrophy is present in only 1% to 2% of patients; this rises to approximately 30% when a ratio of septal to free wall thickness of 1.5:1 is used (203). The severity of HCM can be scored in several ways; the most frequent method (14) uses the apical four-chamber view to determine the extent of septal involvement and the parasternal short-axis view at the level of the mitral valve leaflet tips to assess anterolateral wall involvement. A simpler method defines the extent of hypertrophy as mild if only one left ventricular segment is involved, moderate if two segments are involved, and severe if three or more segments are involved. Right ventricular hypertrophy occurs in greater than one third of patients with HCM (204).

Approximately 25% of patients with HCM have a resting pressure gradient between the cavity and outflow tract of the left ventricle (10–14,19,124–133,202) (Fig. 29.7). This is nearly always accompanied by SAM characterized by an abrupt anterior movement of the mitral valve that reaches its maximum when approximately two thirds of systole is completed and before maximum anterior movement of the posterior left ventricular wall (Fig. 29.7). "Pseudo-SAM" is an exaggeration of the normal anterior movement of the mitral valve in systole, reaching its peak at the end of systole when the posterior left ventricular wall has fully contracted (205). Left ventricular outflow tract obstruction is typically dynamic, varying in response to activity, alcohol use, and heavy meals. For this reason, many laboratories routinely perform provocation maneuvers and,

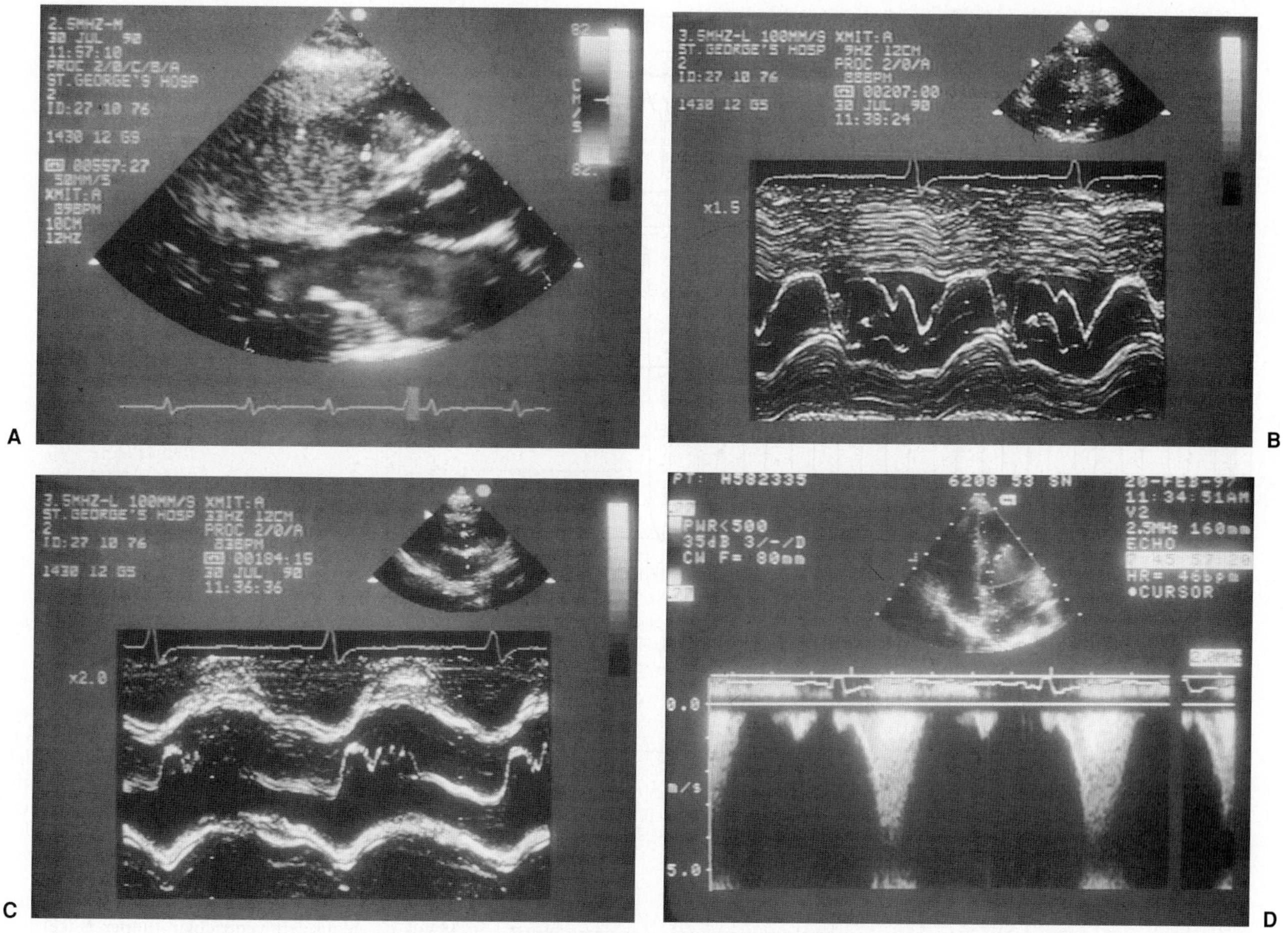

FIGURE 29.7. **A:** Two-dimensional echo in the parasternal long-axis view demonstrating complete systolic anterior motion of the mitral valve and contact between the anterior mitral valve leaflet and the interventricular septum. **B:** M-mode echocardiogram demonstrating asymmetric septal hypertrophy, systolic anterior motion of the mitral valve, and contact between the anterior mitral valve leaflet and the interventricular septum. **C:** M-mode echocardiogram demonstrating midsystolic closure of the aortic valve in a patient with left ventricular outflow obstruction. **D:** Continuous-wave Doppler demonstrating characteristic "dynamic" left ventricular outflow tract obstruction.

increasingly, upright exercise testing in symptomatic patients to detect inducible gradients. Gradients provoked by dobutamine stress may not be reproducible during physiologic conditions and can be poorly tolerated.

The use of conventional pulsed-wave Doppler to assess diastolic function in HCM has a number of limitations, most notably the fact that mitral flow velocity curves cannot be used reliably to determine filling pressures (206). There is also a poor correlation between exercise capacity and conventional Doppler indices of diastolic function (142,143,207–210). Tissue Doppler imaging (TDI) of mitral annular motion measured from the apical window has been proposed as a load-independent parameter of diastolic function. TDI can detect subclinical systolic and diastolic dysfunction in transgenic animal models and patients with disease-causing sarcomeric protein genes (211–214). There is a reasonable correlation between the transmitral E/septal Ea ratio, left ventricular filling pressures, and exercise capacity (142,214,215); it also predicts children with HCM who are at risk of adverse clinical outcomes including death, cardiac arrest, ventricular tachycardia, and the development of severe cardiac symptoms (214). Peak negative myocardial velocity gradients can differentiate pathologic hypertrophy from physiologic adaptation (216–218). Peak negative myocardial velocity gradient may reflect regional variations in myocardial fatty acid metabolism (219).

Cardiac Catheterization

Echocardiography has replaced cardiac catheterization in the diagnosis of HCM. Catheterization is indicated when planning therapy (e.g., in severe mitral regurgitation) and in excluding coronary atherosclerosis in older patients with chest pain. The characteristic left ventricular outflow gradient may be demonstrated during pullback across the aortic valve (Fig. 29.8) or by measuring simultaneous aortic and left ventricular inflow pressures. An outflow gradient can be associated with an initial early spike in the aortic pressure wave, followed by a secondary, dome-shaped tidal wave prior to the dicrotic notch (Fig. 29.8). In addition, the aortic pressure wave often fails to show post-extrasystolic potentiation, and may reduce in amplitude following an extrasystole. Right atrial and right ventricular pressures are usually normal except in patients with right ventricular outflow gradients or severe restrictive physiology. Pulmonary capillary wedge pressure may be elevated, particularly when mitral regurgitation is severe. An increased V wave can also be seen in the pulmonary capillary wedge tracing in the absence of significant mitral regurgitation, when there is reduced left atrial compliance.

Left ventriculography may show a septal bulge encroaching on the left ventricular outflow tract during systole together with

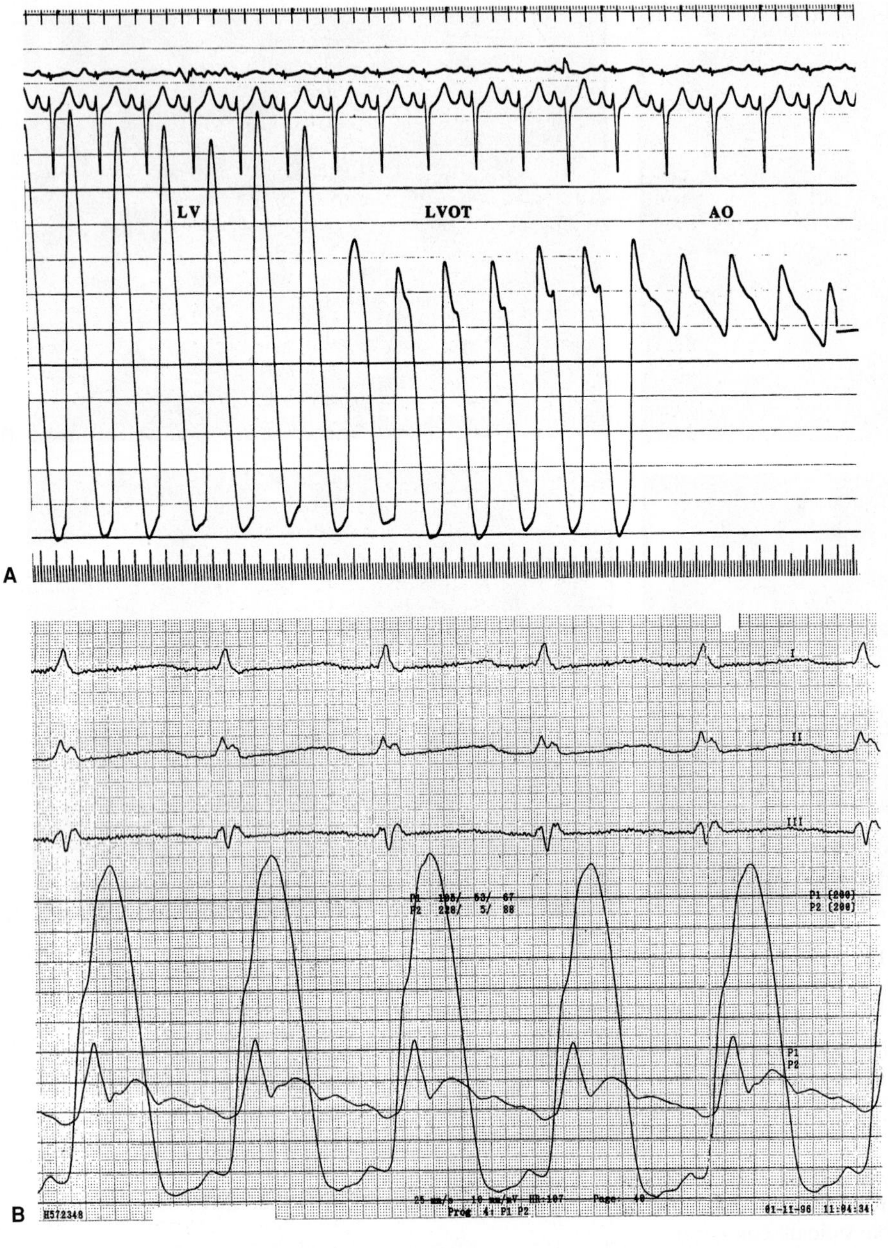

FIGURE 29.8. **A:** Pullback pressure tracing showing sequential pressure pulses in the body of the left ventricle (LV), the left ventricular outflow tract (LVOT), and the aorta (AO). There is a pressure gradient between the body and outflow of the left ventricle, and pulsus alternans is observed in the left ventricular pressure trace before the level of obstruction. **B:** Simultaneous left ventricular (**upper trace**) and aortic (**lower trace**) pressure tracings in a patient with severe left ventricular outflow obstruction. In the LV tracing there is a prominent atrial contraction wave contributing to elevated LV end-diastolic pressure. The aortic trace demonstrates a rapid upstroke with a second peak in late systole ("spike and dome") before the incisura. The notch on the upstroke of the LV pressure tracing corresponds approximately with the time of systolic anterior motion-septal contact.

systolic anterior motion of the anterior mitral valve leaflet and mitral regurgitation. In patients with hypertrophy confined to the left ventricular apex, the ventricular angiogram may show a characteristic "spade-shaped" appearance in the right anterior oblique projection.

Radionuclide Scanning

Fixed and reversible perfusion defects are seen during stress thallium imaging in greater than 25% of patients (154,155,157,158,160,220–222). Fixed thallium-201 defects, believed to represent myocardial scars, are associated with increased left ventricular cavity dimensions, reduced shortening fraction, and impaired exercise capacity. Reversible regional thallium-201 defects correlate poorly with symptomatic status. "Apparent cavity dilation" possibly representing subendocardial hypoperfusion is described in some patients (154,220).

Positron emission tomography (PET) has shown that myocardial blood flow in the interventricular septum and in the left ventricular free wall is similar to that in normal controls at baseline, but is significantly less during dipyridamole-induced coronary vasodilation (156). Data on the relation of flow abnormalities to myocardial metabolism are conflicting, with some showing blood flow/fluorodeoxyglucose (FDG) mismatch (believed to indicate the presence of ischemic myocardium) and others only matched reductions in myocardial blood flow and FDG uptake in the septum (223,224). Heterogeneous FDG uptake may relate to regional systolic function and age (225,226).

Magnetic Resonance Imaging

Cardiac magnetic resonance imaging (CMR) can be used to determine the severity and distribution of left ventricular hypertrophy and provides information on systolic and diastolic ventricular function. Up to 80% of patients with HCM have patchy areas of late hyperenhancement on gadolinium-enhanced magnetic resonance (Fig. 29.9) (227–233); correlation with histologic data indicates that late enhancement is caused by myocardial fibrosis (227). The extent of hyperenhancement correlates with wall thickness, regional systolic

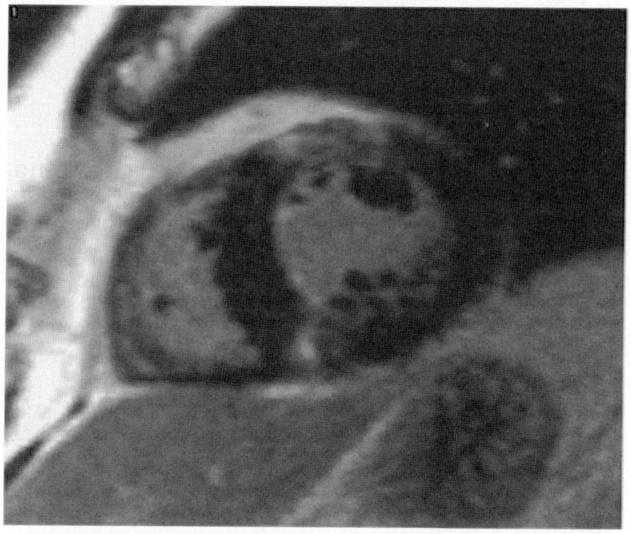

FIGURE 29.9. Gadolinium-enhanced cardiac magnetic resonance image showing a short-axis view of the left ventricle. Late gadolinium enhancement is seen at the junction of the interventricular septum extending into the anterior septum. (Courtesy of Dr. S. Prasad, Cardiac Magnetic Resonance Imaging Unit, Royal Brompton Hospital, London.)

function, and the presence of risk markers for sudden cardiac death (232). Extensive hyperenhancement is associated with progressive remodeling of the left ventricle (227,228,231).

PRINCIPLES OF CLINICAL MANAGEMENT

Symptomatic Treatment in Obstructive Hypertrophic Cardiomyopathy

Patients with moderate to severe left ventricular outflow tract obstruction may experience exertional chest pain, dyspnea, or syncope. β-Blockers improve symptoms in up to 70% of patients by decreasing heart rate, thereby improving passive ventricular filling, and reducing myocardial oxygen demand (234–239). β-Blockers are limited by side effects of fatigue, impotence, and sleep disturbance; they may also paradoxically reduce exercise capacity by inducing chronotropic incompetence. It has been suggested that very high dose therapy (propranolol 1,000 mg/day) is associated with improved survival in children (239), but this finding must be weighed against the effects of very high dose β-blockade on growth and psychosocial performance.

Verapamil in doses up to 480 mg/day (sustained release) is widely used in patients with nonobstructive and obstructive HCM and may be particularly useful in the treatment of chest pain (240–246). Its principal actions are to improve ventricular relaxation and filling, reduce myocardial ischemia, and decrease left ventricular contractility. The most frequent side effect is constipation, but verapamil can occasionally cause hemodynamic deterioration and even death in patients with severe disabling symptoms, elevated pulmonary arterial pressure, and severe outflow tract obstruction (235). Current practice is to use β-blockers before verapamil, but there are no data suggesting the superiority of one drug over the other.

The type I-A antiarrhythmic agent disopyramide can also be effective in symptomatic patients with obstruction. Doses of 300 to 600 mg/day can decrease outflow obstruction and mitral regurgitant volume (247–252). Its major limitations are anticholinergic side effects such as dry mouth and eyes, constipation, difficulty in micturition, and accelerated atrioventricular (AV) nodal conduction that increases ventricular rate during atrial fibrillation (AF). The last problem can be minimized by coadministration of β-blockers. There is no evidence for an adverse effect on prognosis in HCM patients caused by its proarrhythmic effects (252); however, QT interval should be monitored, and coadministration of other QT-prolonging drugs avoided. An alternative class I antiarrhythmic, cibenzoline, which has fewer anticholinergic side effects, may be equally effective (253).

Surgical Treatment of Outflow Tract Obstruction

Surgery should be considered in all patients with outflow tract gradients greater than 50 mm Hg (resting or with provocation) and symptoms refractory to medical therapy (254–276). The aim of surgical intervention is to eliminate systolic anterior motion of the mitral valve and septal-mitral contact by widening the left ventricular outflow tract. The most commonly performed procedure is a ventricular septal myotomy-myectomy (Morrow procedure), in which a trough of septal muscle (typically 5 to 10 g in weight), extending from just below the base of the aortic valve to a point approximately 1 cm beyond the distal margins of mitral leaflets, is removed via an aortotomy. This procedure results in a significant reduction in outflow gradient in 95% of cases, reduced mitral regurgitation, and long-term symptomatic improvement in up to 70% of patients. Operative mortality figures are less than 1% to 2% in experienced centers. Complications such as atrioventricular block and ventricular septal defects can occur, but they have become less frequent with modification of surgical technique and the use of peri-operative transesophageal echocardiography (265). Aortic regurgitation may occur in patients postoperatively but is not usually of hemodynamic significance (266).

The conventional myectomy can be extended distally into the left ventricle together with mobilization of the anterolateral papillary muscle. This reduces anterior tethering of the mitral apparatus (276) and may relieve midcavity obstruction. Mitral valve replacement (277) can also abolish outflow tract obstruction but should only be considered in patients with other intrinsic mitral valve abnormalities because of the long-term risks of anticoagulation and prosthetic valve dysfunction. Mitral valve plication in conjunction with myotomy-myectomy has been advocated as an alternative to mitral valve replacement in patients with elongation of the anterior mitral leaflet (278). More recently elongation of the horizontal diameter of the mitral valve using a glutaraldehyde-preserved autologous pericardial patch has been proposed (279).

Some young patients (often in association with Noonan syndrome) have obstruction to the right ventricular outflow due to hypertrophy of trabeculae or crista supraventricularis muscle (280). This can be treated by resection of the right ventricular outflow tract muscle and insertion of an outflow tract patch.

Dual-Chamber Pacing

Several studies have suggested that dual-chamber (DDD) pacing using a short programmed atrioventricular delay to ensure constant activation of the right ventricle from its apex improves symptoms in patients with left ventricular outflow tract gradients (281–298). Success depends on achieving an AV delay that gives maximum preexcitation while maintaining effective atrial transport. Although preliminary data indicated that pacing is capable of reducing gradients by approximately 50%, several multicenter trials have shown that pacemaker insertion is associated with a substantial placebo effect and little objective improvement in exercise capacity. There are few comparative data for DDD pacing and myectomy, but one small nonrandomized study suggested that gradient reduction and exercise duration are greater after surgery (291). Nevertheless a minority (10% to 20%) of patients do respond to pacing, and thus pacemaker insertion remains an option in patients with an unacceptable operative risk. Pacemaker insertion may also facilitate the use of higher doses of β-blockers in some patients (287). Long-term reductions in outflow gradient and wall thinning are described, but it is unclear whether this reflects true reverse remodeling or the natural history of the disease (298).

Septal Alcohol Ablation

Septal alcohol ablation (also termed percutaneous transcoronary septal myocardial ablation [PTSMA] and transcoronary alcohol septal ablation [TASH]) involves selective injection of alcohol into one or more septal perforator branches of the left anterior descending coronary artery to create a localized septal scar (299–326). Published data suggest that procedure-related mortality is approximately 1% in experienced centers, but deaths due to conduction system damage, inadvertent injection of alcohol into other myocardial segments, myocardial trauma, and coronary dissection are recognized. Excessive myocardial damage is prevented by intracoronary injection of echo contrast agent before injection of alcohol to ensure that only the septal bulge at the point of SAM-septal contact is opacified. Alcohol injection is contraindicated if there is opacification of other regions of the myocardium such as the distal septum, right ventricle, or papillary muscles. The amount of ethanol injected is determined subjectively from the septal anatomy and the rate of contrast washout; typically 1 to 3 mL of desiccated ethanol is injected, resulting in creatinine phosphokinase levels between 400 and 2,500 units.

Alcohol septal ablation can be associated with a substantial reduction in resting outflow gradient at the time of injection, but a biphasic response in which the acute response resolves before discharge is common. Irrespective of the initial response, successful alcohol ablation is associated with a progressive decrease in the gradient over a period of 6 to 12 months.

Septal ablation results in a transmural infarction of the basal midseptum and adjacent right bundle tissue, whereas surgical myectomy affects the endocardial portion of the basal anterior septum and adjacent left bundle tissue. Consequently, most patients develop right- and not left-bundle-branch block after alcohol ablation. Higher degrees of AV block can occur transiently but persist in only 10% to 15% of patients. Prolonged or recurrent AV block after the procedure should prompt consideration of permanent dual-chamber pacing.

Results from the largest series show that gradients can be abolished or substantially reduced in 80% of patients. This reduction is paralleled by an improvement in symptom class and exercise tolerance, diastolic function, and left ventricular synchrony. Interim results suggest that left ventricular cavity dimensions increase slightly after alcohol ablation, but progressive ventricular dilation and late arrhythmic complications have not been described. Late freedom from pacing may be higher after surgery than after alcohol ablation (319).

Treatment of Symptoms in Nonobstructive Hypertrophic Cardiomyopathy

β-blockade may improve chest pain and dyspnea, but the response is usually suboptimal. Verapamil, often in high doses (240 to 480 mg/day) is a useful alternative, particularly in patients with exertional chest pain (240–246). Diltiazem (327) also has beneficial effects on symptoms and left ventricular function and provides a useful alternative to verapamil when side effects are problematic. Nifedipine (328) has been advocated, but the potential hazards of vasodilation, particularly in patients with latent outflow gradients, preclude its general use. Although diuretics, sometimes in combination with β-blockers or calcium antagonists, may alleviate symptoms caused by pulmonary congestion, they can be dangerous in patients with severe diastolic impairment.

Management of Supraventricular Arrhythmia

Atrial fibrillation is the most common sustained arrhythmia in HCM (182,195–200,329–333). Paroxysmal or persistent AF occurs in up to 25% of HCM patients; predisposing factors include left atrial size, age, and left ventricular outflow tract obstruction. Atrial fibrillation can trigger life-threatening ventricular arrhythmias (334,335) and cause syncope or heart failure. Atrial fibrillation is independently associated with heart failure–related death, fatal and nonfatal stroke, and progressive heart failure symptoms. The risk of associated complications is increased when the arrhythmia presents before 50 years of age and in the presence of left ventricular outflow tract obstruction. Atrial fibrillation should be electrically or pharmacologically cardioverted in accordance with current guidelines. Amiodarone can be effective in maintaining sinus rhythm; β-blockers, with or without class III action, may also be effective; class 1 agents are not recommended (except for disopyramide in the context of outflow tract obstruction). Where restoration of sinus rhythm is not possible, control of the ventricular rate with β-blockers or calcium antagonists will improve symptoms in most patients (199). Atrial fibrillation in HCM is associated with a significant risk of thromboembolism and oral anticoagulation should be considered in all patients with paroxysmal or persistent atrial fibrillation (199,330).

Atrial flutter should be treated in a similar manner to AF. Treatment is not usually indicated for other asymptomatic and self-limiting supraventricular arrhythmias, but if they are sustained or associated with symptoms, then specific medical therapy (or electrophysiologic testing) should be considered.

SUDDEN CARDIAC DEATH

The reported annual incidence of sudden cardiac death in patients with hypertrophic cardiomyopathy has declined from 2% to 4% per annum in early series to 1% or less as a consequence of evolving diagnostic criteria, family screening, and modern treatment protocols (5–9,19,152,159,180–183,336–355). Sudden cardiac death occurs throughout life, with a peak in adolescence and young adulthood, and may be the initial disease presentation (152,159,180–183,336–355), occurring without warning signs or symptoms. Sudden cardiac death occurs most commonly during mild exertion or sedentary activities.

The mechanism underlying sudden cardiac death is believed to be sudden ventricular arrhythmia, but other causes including AV block and thromboembolism probably account for some cases. Clinical observations suggest that a number of trigger factors can initiate cardiac arrest, specifically, atrial fibrillation, ventricular tachycardia, and myocardial ischemia.

Clinical Risk Markers

Numerous clinical features have been proposed as markers of increased sudden death risk; the most readily determined in clinical practice include unexplained syncope, a family history of premature sudden deaths (19,181,336;347;351), nonsustained ventricular tachycardia during 48-hour ambulatory ECG monitoring (19,181,195–197,336,345–347), an abnormal blood pressure response during upright exercise (failure of blood pressure to rise appropriately by more than 20 to 30 mm Hg from baseline) (19,336,341,348–350,356,357), and severe left ventricular hypertrophy (maximum wall thickness of

≥30 mm) (19,340,351,352). The risk associated with all these risk factors is greatest in younger patients. Two studies have suggested that left ventricular outflow tract obstruction may be associated with an increased risk of death (353,354); in one study, outflow obstruction was associated with a twofold increase in the risk of cardiovascular death (particularly from stroke) that related to symptoms at initial evaluation but not the severity of obstruction (354). In patients developing severe symptoms, functional class III/IV was more predictive of outcome than obstruction alone.

The largest published series of invasive electrophysiologic testing in HCM suggests that patients with inducible ventricular arrhythmias have an increased risk of sudden death, with a positive predictive accuracy of less than 20% (355). However, most patients studied have been those already thought to be at high risk, and there are few data in low-risk patients. Moreover, polymorphic ventricular tachycardia and ventricular fibrillation (the most commonly provoked arrhythmias) are nonspecific electrophysiologic testing responses to multiple ventricular extrastimuli (358).

Prevention of Sudden Cardiac Death

Approximately one third of patients with a history of syncopal ventricular tachycardia or ventricular fibrillation have a further event during follow-up and should be referred for implantable cardioverter defibrillator (ICD) therapy (359,360). The recommended risk assessment for patients without such a history consists of clinical history (syncope), family pedigree analysis (premature sudden death), echocardiogram (hypertrophy, outflow gradient), 48-hour ambulatory ECG (nonsustained ventricular tachycardia), and a symptom-limited exercise test with careful measurement of blood pressure (abnormal blood pressure response) (19). Pedigree analysis may require involvement of a clinical geneticist or specialists with expertise in the assessment of inherited cardiovascular disease.

Although most individual clinical risk markers in patients have a relatively low positive predictive accuracy, the presence of multiple clinical risk factors substantially increases the risk of sudden death. It is recommended that patients with multiple risk factors for sudden cardiac death should be considered for ICD therapy (19,361–364). Patients with only one risk factor represent a difficult group; judgment on whether such individuals require an ICD depends on the clinical context, including other markers of disease severity (19).

The absence of risk factors and potential "triggers" for sudden death accurately identifies a cohort of patients with a low risk of sudden cardiac death (the majority of patients with HCM). In young patients, the rapid changes in cardiac structure and apparent risk of sudden death that accompany somatic growth mean that periodic reassessment should be performed, at least until early adulthood. In spite of the lack of prospective data, regular evaluation of low-risk adults with Holter monitoring and exercise testing is recommended. Changes in symptoms, particularly sustained palpitation or syncope, warrant urgent reevaluation at any age.

EXERCISE AND HYPERTROPHIC CARDIOMYOPATHY

The Athlete's Heart

Although HCM is the most common cause of death in young athletes in the United States (365–369), its diagnosis in individuals who regularly participate in competitive sports can be problematic (366,368–377) because the physiologic adaptation to athletic training can mimic HCM. Pure strength training is associated with an increase in left ventricular mass and wall thickness relative to the left ventricular cavity size but is rarely associated with an increase in absolute wall thickness (375).

Fewer than 2% of all elite athletes develop a wall thickness greater than 13 mm, and none have wall thicknesses greater than 16 mm (366,368–377). In female athletes, maximum wall thickness is usually no more than 14 mm. A diagnosis of HCM in an elite athlete is more likely when an individual has a maximum left ventricular wall thickness exceeding these values and/or when he or she is symptomatic and has a family history of HCM and premature sudden death. The athlete's ECG is characterized by voltage criteria for left ventricular hypertrophy, sinus bradycardia, and sinus arrhythmia. Although marked repolarization abnormalities are described in some elite athletes (366,369,376,377), they are uncommon and should always raise suspicion of myocardial disease. Echocardiographic features favoring HCM include small left ventricular cavity dimensions (athletes tending to have increased left ventricular end-diastolic dimensions), left atrial enlargement, left ventricular outflow gradients, and Doppler evidence of diastolic impairment. Metabolic exercise testing may be useful in differentiating physiologic hypertrophy from HCM; a peak oxygen consumption greater than 50 mL/min/kg or more than 20% above the predicted maximum oxygen consumption favors athletic adaptation (378).

Exercise in Patients with Hypertrophic Cardiomyopathy

Although many HCM sudden deaths occur after moderate to severe exertion, the increase in the relative risk of sudden death incurred by regular participation in vigorous exercise is unknown. There are no systematic data to prove that abstention from vigorous physical activity prevents death, but consensus guidelines recommend that athletes with unequivocal HCM should be advised not to take part in most competitive events, irrespective of symptoms or the presence of left ventricular outflow obstruction (379,380). There is no evidence to suggest that genetically affected but phenotypically normal family members should be subjected to the same restrictions as patients with unequivocal disease.

SPECIAL PROBLEMS IN HYPERTROPHIC CARDIOMYOPATHY

Hypertrophic Cardiomyopathy and Pregnancy

For most women with HCM, pregnancy (with normal vaginal delivery) is associated with a very low risk of serious complications (381,382). Caution is advised when administering cardioactive drugs during pregnancy because of their potential effects on the fetus, and the peripheral vasodilation associated with conventional epidural anesthesia poses a theoretical risk in the presence of left ventricular outflow tract obstruction. All women with HCM should be offered specialized obstetric care during pregnancy.

Infective Endocarditis

Patients with left ventricular outflow tract obstruction or with intrinsic mitral valve disease are at risk of infective endocarditis (383,384). Vegetations usually develop on the anterior mitral valve leaflet but can also occur in the outflow tract endocardial at the point of mitral-septal contact or on the aortic valve. American Heart Association recommendations for antibiotic prophylaxis should be followed before dental or high-risk surgical procedures.

CONTROVERSIES AND PERSONAL PERSPECTIVES

The modern era of HCM began with Donald Teare's landmark pathologic report in 1958 and the subsequent clinical papers of Braunwald, Goodwin and others in the early 1960s. In these early days, HCM was entirely a clinical diagnosis, relying on the detection of asymmetric hypertrophy of the interventricular septum and a left ventricular outflow tract gradient in the absence of other hemodynamic or systemic causes of myocardial hypertrophy. Over subsequent decades, the familial nature of the disease was recognized and following the identification of mutations in contractile proteins in the 1980s and 90s, HCM was redefined as a disease of the cardiac sarcomere. Adoption of this paradigm focused investigators on disease pathways and potential therapeutic targets and resulted in important changes in the management of patients and families affected by HCM. This narrow view of the disease does, however, have many limitations, the most notable of which is the recognition that between 30% and 50% of patients who fulfill current diagnostic criteria do not have a mutation in any of the sarcomeric protein genes. The nosologic confusion that this generates is exacerbated by the recognition that sarcomeric protein gene mutations can also cause dilated and restrictive cardiomyopathy.

One response to these difficulties is to redefine all the cardiomyopathies according to their underlying genetic etiology (if known) or by the presence of other characteristic pathologic features. An alternative strategy might be to move away from attempts to confine the term hypertrophic cardiomyopathy to a distinct disease entity, and to recognize instead that HCM is more appropriately viewed as a syndrome with many possible causes and manifestations. While this lacks the preciseness and clarity of a more detailed classification system, it provides a more realistic starting point for diagnostic and management algorithms, much in the same way a diagnosis of 'heart failure' is the beginning of a clinical process rather than its end. We may also learn other lessons from the experience of patients with congestive heart failure; in particular, the adoption of prospective randomized controlled studies of therapeutic interventions in areas of therapeutic uncertainty such as asymptomatic outflow tract obstruction.

THE FUTURE

Over the last half century, the concept of hypertrophic cardiomyopathy has evolved from a rare esoteric heart muscle disease of the young associated with a poor prognosis to a relatively common genetic syndrome with protean clinical manifestations. The genetic, pathologic, and clinical heterogeneity that is the hallmark of HCM continues to present clinicians with diagnostic and treatment challenges, most notably the diagnosis of disease in relatives and children, and the prevention of disease related complications such as sudden death, stroke, and heart failure. The ability to diagnose the disease is improving with advances in imaging technology and genomics. The identification of patients who are at risk of disease-related complications has been improved by the adoption of systematic clinical risk assessment and the discovery of new risk markers. The prevention of sudden death in patients with HCM has been facilitated by the development of effective defibrillator technology. In the future, drugs that prevent ventricular remodeling should reduce other disease related complications.

References

1. Liouville H. Retrecissement cardiaque sous aortique. *Gaz Med Paris* 1869; 24:161.
2. Hallopeau L. Retrecissement ventriculo-aortique. *Gaz Med Paris* 1869; 24:683.
3. Brock R. Functional obstruction of the left ventricle. *Guy's Hospital Rep* 1957;106:221.
4. Teare D. Asymmetrical hypertrophy of the heart in young adults. *Br Heart J* 1958;20:1–8.
5. Frank S, Braunwald E. Idiopathic hypertrophic subaortic stenosis: Clinical analysis of 126 patients with emphasis on the natural history. *Circulation* 1968;37:759–788.
6. Goodwin JF, Hollman A, Cleland WP, Teare D. Obstructive cardiomyopathy simulating aortic stenosis. *Br Heart J* 1960;22:403–414.
7. Braunwald E, Morrow AG, Cornell WP, et al. Idiopathic hypertrophic subaortic stenosis. Clinical, hemodynamic and angiographic manifestations. *Am J Med* 1960;29:924–945.
8. Wigle ED, Heimbecker RO, Gunton RW. Idiopathic ventricular septal hypertrophy causing muscular subaortic stenosis. *Circulation* 1962;26:325–340.
9. Bevegard S, Jonsson B, Karloff I. Low subvalvular aortic and pulmonic stenosis caused by asymmetrical hypertrophic and derangement of muscle bundles of the ventricular wall. *Acta Med Scand* 1962;172:269–283.
10. Henry WL, Clarke CE, Epstein SE. Asymmetrical septal hypertrophy (ASH): Echocardiographic identification of the pathognomonic anatomic abnormality of IHSS. *Circulation* 1973;43:225–233.
11. Shah PM, Gramiak R, Kramer DH. Ultrasound localization of left ventricular outflow obstruction in hypertrophic obstructive cardiomyopathy. *Circulation* 1969;40:3–11.
12. Popp RL, Harrison DC. Ultrasound in the diagnosis and evaluation of therapy of idiopathic hypertrophic subaortic stenosis. *Circulation* 1969; 40:905–914.
13. Maron BJ, Gottdiener JS, Epstein SE. Patterns and significance of the distribution of left ventricular hypertrophy in hypertrophic cardiomyopathy: A wide angle, two-dimensional echocardiographic study of 125 patients. *Am J Cardiol* 1981;48:418–428.
14. Wigle ED, Sasson Z, Henderson MA, et al. Hypertrophic cardiomyopathy: The importance of the site and extent of hypertrophy: A review. *Prog Cardiovasc Dis* 1985;28:1–83.
15. Geisterfer-Lowrance AAT, Kass S, Tanigawa G, et al. A molecular basis for familial hypertrophic cardiomyopathy: A β-cardiac myosin heavy chain gene missense mutation. *Cell* 1990;62:999–1006.
16. Kamisago M, Sharma SD, DePalma SR, et al. Mutations in sarcomere protein genes as a cause of dilated cardiomyopathy. *N Engl J Med.* 2000; 34:1688–1696.
17. Mogensen J, Kubo T, Duque M, et al. Idiopathic restrictive cardiomyopathy is part of the clinical expression of cardiac Troponin I mutations. *J Clin Invest* 2003;111:209–216.
18. Report of the 1995 World Health Organization/International Society and Federation of Cardiology Task Force on the Definition and Classification of Cardiomyopathies. *Circulation* 1996;93:841–842.
19. Maron BJ, McKenna WJ, Danielson GK, et al. American College of Cardiology/European Society of Cardiology Clinical Expert Consensus Document on Hypertrophic Cardiomyopathy. A report of the American College of Cardiology Foundation Task Force on Clinical Expert Consensus Documents and the European Society of Cardiology Committee for Practice Guidelines. *J Am Coll Cardiol* 2003;42:1687–1713.
20. Hughes SE. The pathology of hypertrophic cardiomyopathy. *Histopathology* 2004;44:412–427.
21. Davies MJ, McKenna WJ. Hypertrophic cardiomyopathy: Pathology and pathogenesis. *Histopathology* 1995;26:493–500.
22. Yamaguchi H, Ishimura T, Nishiyama S, et al. Hypertrophic nonobstructive cardiomyopathy with giant negative T-waves (apical hypertrophy): Ventriculographic and echocardiographic features in 30 patients. *Am J Cardiol* 1979;44:401–412.
23. Kitaoka H, Doi Y, Casey SA, et al. Comparison of prevalence of apical hypertrophic cardiomyopathy in Japan and the United States. *Am J Cardiol* 2003;92:1183–1186.
24. Mozaffarian D, Caldwell JH. Right ventricular involvement in hypertrophic cardiomyopathy: A case report and literature review. *Clin Cardiol* 2001;24:2–8.
25. Maron BJ, Roberts WC. Quantitative analysis of cardiac muscle cell disorganisation in the ventricular septum of patients with hypertrophic cardiomyopathy. *Circulation* 1979;59:689–706.
26. Maron BJ, Sato N, Roberts WC, et al. Quantitative analysis of cardiac muscle cell disorganisation in the ventricular septum: Comparison of fetuses and infants with and without congenital heart disease and patients with hypertrophic cardiomyopathy. *Circulation* 1979;60:685–696.

27. Varnava AM, Elliott PM, Mahon N, et al. Relation between myocyte disarray and outcome in hypertrophic cardiomyopathy. *Am J Cardiol* 2001; 88:275–279.
28. Sepp R, Severs NJ, Gourdie RG. Altered patterns of cardiac intercellular junction distribution in hypertrophic cardiomyopathy. *Heart* 1996;76:412–417.
29. Burch M, Mann JM, Sharland M, et al. Myocardial disarray in Noonan syndrome. *Br Heart J* 1992;68:586–588.
30. Brumback RA, Panner BJ, Kingston WJ. The heart in Friedreich's ataxia. Report of a case. *Arch Neurol* 1986;43:189–192.
31. Maron BJ, Epstein SE, Roberts WC. Hypertrophic cardiomyopathy and transmural infarction without significant atherosclerosis of the extramural coronary arteries. *Am J Cardiol* 1979;43:1086–1102.
32. Factor SM, Butany J, Sole MJ, et al. Pathological fibrosis and matrix connective tissue in the subaortic myocardium of patients with hypertrophic cardiomyopathy. *J Am Coll Cardiol* 1991;17:1343–1351.
33. Shirani J, Pick R, Roberts WC, Maron BJ. Morphology and significance of the left ventricular collagen network in young patients with hypertrophic cardiomyopathy and sudden cardiac death. *J Am Coll Cardiol* 2000;35:36–44.
34. Maron BJ, Wolfson JK, Epstein SE, Roberts WC. Intramural ("small vessel") coronary artery disease in hypertrophic cardiomyopathy. *J Am Coll Cardiol* 1986;8:545.
35. Tanaka M, Fujiwara H, Onodera T, et al. Quantitative analysis of narrowings of intramyocardial small arteries in normal hearts, hypertensive hearts, and hearts with hypertrophic cardiomyopathy. *Circulation* 1987;75:1130–1139.
36. Varnava AM, Elliott PM, Sharma S, et al. Hypertrophic cardiomyopathy: The interrelation of disarray, fibrosis, and small vessel disease. *Heart* 2000;84:476–482.
37. Lipshultz SE, Sleeper LA, Towbin JA, et al. The incidence of pediatric cardiomyopathy in two regions of the United States. *N Engl J Med* 2003; 348:1647–1655.
38. Nugent AW, Daubeney PEF, Chondros P, et al. The epidemiology of childhood cardiomyopathy in Australia. *N Engl J Med* 2003;348:1639–1646.
39. Maron BJ. Hypertrophic cardiomyopathy in childhood. *Pediatr Clin North Am* 2004;51:1305–1346.
40. Barker D, Wright E, Nguyen K, et al. Gene for von Recklinghausen neurofibromatosis is in the pericentric region of chromosome 17. *Science* 1987; 236:1100.
41. Kimberling WJ, Taylor RA, Chapman RG, Lubs HA. Linkage and gene localisation of hereditary spherocytosis (HS). *Blood* 1978;52:859.
42. Gilgenkrantz S, Vigneron C, Gregoire MJ, et al. Association of del(11) (p15.1 p12), aniridia, catalase deficiency and cardiomyopathy. *Am J Med Genet* 1982;13:39.
43. Burch M, Sharland M, Shinebourne E, et al. Cardiologic abnormalities in Noonan syndrome: Phenotypic diagnosis and echocardiographic assessment of 118 patients. *J Am Coll Cardiol* 1993;22:1189–1192.
44. Seidman JG, Seidman C. The genetic basis for cardiomyopathy: From mutation identification to mechanistic paradigms. *Cell* 2001;104:557–567.
45. Marian AJ, Roberts R. The molecular genetic basis for hypertrophic cardiomyopathy. *J Mol Cell Cardiol* 2001;33:655–670.
46. Schwartz K, Carrier L, Guicheney P, Komajda M. Molecular basis of familial cardiomyopathies. *Circulation* 1995;91:532–540.
47. Jarcho JA, McKenna WJ, Pare JA, et al. Mapping a gene for familial hypertrophic cardiomyopathy to chromosome 14q1. *N Engl J Med* 1989; 321:1372–1378.
48. Watkins H, Conner D, Thierfelder L, et al. Mutations in the cardiac myosin binding protein-C gene on chromosome 11 cause familial hypertrophic cardiomyopathy. *Nat Genet* 1995;11:434–437.
49. Thierfelder L, MacRae C, Watkins H, et al. A familial hypertrophic cardiomyopathy locus maps to chromosome 15q2. *Proc Natl Acad Sci USA* 1993;90:6270–6274.
50. Carrier L, Hengstenberg C, Beckmann JS, et al. Mapping of a novel gene for familial hypertrophic cardiomyopathy to chromosome 11. *Nat Genet* 1993;4:311–313.
51. Mogensen J, Klausen IC, Pedersen AK, et al. Alpha-cardiac actin is a novel disease gene in familial hypertrophic cardiomyopathy. *J Clin Invest* 1999;103:R39–R43.
52. Kimura A, Harada H, Park JE, et al. Mutations in the cardiac troponin I gene associated with hypertrophic cardiomyopathy. *Nat Genet* 1997; 16:379–382.
53. Poetter K, Jiang H, Hassanzadeh S, et al. Mutations in either the essential or regulatory light chains of myosin are associated with a rare myopathy in human heart and skeletal muscle. *Nat Genet* 1996;13:63–69.
54. Satoh M, Takahashi M, Sakamoto T, et al. Structural analysis of the titin gene in hypertrophic cardiomyopathy: Identification of a novel disease gene. *Biochem Biophys Res Commun* 1999;262:411–447.
55. Hoffmann B, Schmidt-Traub H, Perrot A, et al. First mutation in cardiac troponin C, L29Q, in a patient with hypertrophic cardiomyopathy. *Hum Mutat* 2001;17:524.
56. Niimura H, Patton KK, McKenna WJ, et al. Sarcomere protein gene mutations in hypertrophic cardiomyopathy of the elderly. *Circulation* 2002; 105:446–451.
57. Richard P, Charron P, Carrier L, et al. Hypertrophic cardiomyopathy: Distribution of disease genes, spectrum of mutations and implications for a molecular diagnosis strategy. *Circulation* 2003;107:2227–2232.
58. Watkins H, McKenna WJ, Thierfelder L, et al. Mutations in the genes for cardiac troponin T and alpha-tropomyosin in hypertrophic cardiomyopathy. *N Engl J Med* 1995;332:1058–1064.
59. Thierfelder L, Watkins H, MacRae C, et al. Alpha-tropomyosin and cardiac troponin T mutations cause familial hypertrophic cardiomyopathy: A disease of the sarcomere. *Cell* 1994;77:701–712.
60. Bonne G, Carrier L, Bercovici J, et al. Cardiac myosin binding protein C gene splice acceptor site mutation is associated with familial hypertrophic cardiomyopathy. *Nat Genet* 1995;11:438–440.
61. Niimura H, Bachinski LL, Sangwatanaroj S, et al. Mutations in the gene for cardiac myosin-binding protein C and late-onset familial hypertrophic cardiomyopathy. *N Engl J Med* 1998;338:1248–1257.
62. Sanbe A, Nelson D, Gulick J, et al. In vivo analysis of an essential myosin light chain mutation linked to familial hypertrophic cardiomyopathy. *Circ Res* 2000;87:296–302.
63. Sachdev B, Takenaka T, Teraguchi H, et al. Prevalence of Anderson-Fabry disease in male patients with late onset hypertrophic cardiomyopathy. *Circulation* 2002;105:1407–1411.
64. DiMauro S, Schon EA. Mitochondrial respiratory-chain diseases. *N Engl J Med* 2003;348:2656–2668.
65. Blair E, Redwood C, Ashrafian H, et al. Mutations in the gamma(2) subunit of AMP-activated protein kinase cause familial hypertrophic cardiomyopathy: Evidence for the central role of energy compromise in disease pathogenesis. *Hum Mol Genet* 2001;10:1215–1220.
66. Murphy RT, Mogensen J, McGarry K, et al. Adenosine monophosphate-activated protein kinase disease mimicks hypertrophic cardiomyopathy and Wolff-Parkinson-White syndrome: Natural history. *J Am Coll Cardiol* 2005;45:922–930.
67. Arad M, Maron BJ, Gorham JM, et al. Glycogen storage diseases presenting as hypertrophic cardiomyopathy. *N Engl J Med* 2005;352:362–372.
68. Charron P, Villard E, Sebillon P, et al. Danon's disease as a cause of hypertrophic cardiomyopathy: A systematic survey. *Heart* 2004;90:842–846.
69. Geier C, Perrot A, Özcerlik C, et al. Mutations in the human muscle LIM protein gene in families with hypertrophic cardiomyopathy. *Circulation* 2003;107:1390–1395.
70. Minamisawa S, Sato Y, Tatsuguchi Y, et al. Mutation of the phospholamban promoter associated with hypertrophic cardiomyopathy. *Biochem Biophys Res Commun* 2003;304:1–4.
71. Rayment I, Holden HM, Sellers JR, et al. Structural interpretation of the mutations in the beta-cardiac myosin that have been implicated in familial hypertrophic cardiomyopathy. *Proc Natl Acad Sci USA* 1995;92:3864–3868.
72. Rayment I, Holden HM, Whittaker M, et al. Structure of the actin–myosin complex and its implications for muscle contraction. *Science* 1993;261:58–65.
73. Schiaffino S, Reggiani C. Molecular diversity of myofibrillar proteins: Gene regulation and functional significance. *Physiol Rev* 1996;76:371–396.
74. Marian AJ, Wu Y, Lim DS, et al. A transgenic rabbit model for human hypertrophic cardiomyopathy. *J Clin Invest* 1999;104:1683–1692.
75. Geisterfer-Lowrance AA, Christe M, Conner DA, et al. A mouse model of familial hypertrophic cardiomyopathy. *Science* 1996;272:731–734.
76. Yang Q, Sanbe A, Osinka H, et al. A mouse model of myosin binding protein C human familial hypertrophic cardiomyopathy. *J Clin Invest* 1998; 102:1292–1300.
77. Oberst L, Zhao G, Park JT, et al. Dominant-negative effect of a mutant cardiac troponin T on cardiac structure and function in transgenic mice. *J Clin Invest* 1998;102:1498–1505.
78. Tardiff JC, Factor SM, Tompkins BD, et al. A truncated cardiac troponin T molecule in transgenic mice suggests multiple cellular mechanisms for familial hypertrophic cardiomyopathy. *J Clin Invest* 1998;101:2800–2811.
79. Redwood CS, Moolman-Smook JC, Watkins H. Properties of mutant contractile proteins that cause hypertrophic cardiomyopathy. *Cardiovasc Res* 1999;44:20–36.
80. Watkins H. Genetic clues to disease pathways in hypertrophic and dilated cardiomyopathies. *Circulation* 2003;107:1344–1346.
81. Gomes AV, Potter JD. Molecular and cellular aspects of troponin cardiomyopathies. *Ann N Y Acad Sci* 2004;1015:214–224.
82. Knollmann BC, Kirchhof P, Sirenko SG, et al. Familial hypertrophic cardiomyopathy–linked mutant troponin T causes stress-induced ventricular tachycardia and Ca2+-dependent action potential remodelling. *Circ Res* 2003;92:428–436.
83. Olsson MC, Palmer BM, Stauffer BL, et al. Morphological and functional alterations in ventricular myocytes from male transgenic mice with hypertrophic cardiomyopathy. *Circ Res* 2004;94:201–207.
84. Harris SP, Bartley CR, Hacker TA, et al. Hypertrophic cardiomyopathy in cardiac myosin binding protein-C knockout mice. *Circ Res* 2002;90:594–601.
85. Kirschner SE, Becker E, Antognozzi M, et al. Hypertrophic cardiomyopathy–related beta-myosin mutations cause highly variable calcium sensitivity with functional imbalances among individual muscle cells. *Am J Physiol Heart Circ Physiol* 2005;288:H1242–H1251.
86. Alpert NR, Mohiddin SA, Tripodi D, et al. Molecular and phenotypic effects of heterozygous, homozygous, and compound heterozygote myosin heavy-chain mutations. *Am J Physiol Heart Circ Physiol* 2005;288:H1097–H1102.

87. Nagueh SF, Chen S, Patel R, et al. Evolution of expression of cardiac phenotypes over a 4-year period in the beta-myosin heavy chain–Q403 transgenic rabbit model of human hypertrophic cardiomyopathy. *J Mol Cell Cardiol* 2004;36:663–673.
88. Doolan A, Tebo M, Ingles J, et al. Cardiac troponin I mutations in Australian families with hypertrophic cardiomyopathy: Clinical, genetic and functional consequences. *J Mol Cell Cardiol* 2005;38:387–393.
89. Gomes AV, Harada K, Potter JD. A mutation in the N-terminus of troponin I that is associated with hypertrophic cardiomyopathy affects the Ca(2+)-sensitivity, phosphorylation kinetics and proteolytic susceptibility of troponin. *J Mol Cell Cardiol* 2005;39:754–765.
90. Gomes AV, Liang J, Potter JD. Mutations in human cardiac troponin I that are associated with restrictive cardiomyopathy affect basal ATPase activity and the calcium sensitivity of force development. *J Biol Chem* 2005; 280:30909–30915.
91. Gomes AV, Barnes JA, Harada K, Potter JD. Role of troponin T in disease. *Mol Cell Biochem* 2004;263:115–129.
92. Gomes AV, Potter JD. Cellular and molecular aspects of familial hypertrophic cardiomyopathy caused by mutations in the cardiac troponin I gene. *Mol Cell Biochem* 2004;263:99–114.
93. Redwood C, Lohmann K, Bing W, et al. Investigation of a truncated cardiac troponin T that causes familial hypertrophic cardiomyopathy: Ca(2+) regulatory properties of reconstituted thin filaments depend on the ratio of mutant to wild-type protein. *Circ Res* 2000;86:1146–1152.
94. Spindler M, Saupe KW, Christe ME, et al. Diastolic dysfunction and altered energetics in the a-MHC403/+ mouse model of familial hypertrophic cardiomyopathy. *J Clin Invest* 1998;101:1775–1783.
95. Crilley JG, Boehm EA, Blair E, et al. Hypertrophic cardiomyopathy due to sarcomeric gene mutations is characterized by impaired energy metabolism irrespective of the degree of hypertrophy. *J Am Coll Cardiol* 2003;41:1776–1782.
96. Pfeufer A, Osterziel KJ, Urata H, et al. Angiotensin converting enzyme and heart chymase gene polymorphisms in hypertrophic cardiomyopathy. *Am J Cardiol* 1996;78:362–364.
97. Yoneya K, Okamoto H, Machida M, et al. Angiotensin converting enzyme gene polymorphism in Japanese patients with hypertrophic cardiomyopathy. *Am Heart J* 1995;130:1089–1093.
98. Lechin M, Quinones MA, Omran A, et al. Angiotensin converting enzyme genotypes and left ventricular hypertrophy in patients with hypertrophic cardiomyopathy. *Circulation* 1995;92:1808–1812.
99. Tesson F, Dufour C, Moolman JC, et al. The influence of the angiotensin I converting enzyme genotype in familial hypertrophic cardiomyopathy varies with the disease gene mutation. *J Mol Cell Cardiol* 1997;29:831–838.
100. Richard P, Charron P, Leclercq C, et al. Homozygotes for a R869G mutation in the beta-myosin heavy chain gene have a severe form of familial hypertrophic cardiomyopathy. *J Mol Cell Cardiol* 2000;32:1575–1583.
101. Richard P, Isnard R, Carrier L, et al. Double heterozygosity for mutations in the beta-myosin heavy chain and in the cardiac myosin binding protein C genes in a family with hypertrophic cardiomyopathy. *J Med Genet* 1999;36:542–545.
102. Ho CY, Lever HM, DeSanctis R, et al. Homozygous mutation in cardiac troponin T: Implications for hypertrophic cardiomyopathy. *Circulation* 2000;102:1950–1955.
103. Watkins H, Rosenzweig A, Hwang DS, et al. Characteristics and prognostic implications of myosin missense mutations in familial hypertrophic cardiomyopathy. *N Engl J Med* 1992;326:1108–1114.
104. Moolman JC, Corfield VA, Posen B, et al. Sudden death due to troponin T mutations. *J Am Coll Cardiol* 1997;29:549–555.
105. Charron P, Dubourg O, Desnos M, et al. Clinical features and prognostic implications of familial hypertrophic cardiomyopathy related to the cardiac myosin-binding protein C gene. *Circulation* 1998;97:2230–2236.
106. Elliott PM, D'Cruz L, McKenna WJ. Late-onset hypertrophic cardiomyopathy caused by a mutation in the cardiac troponin T gene. *N Engl J Med.* 1999;341:1855–1856.
107. Anan R, Shono H, Kisanuki A, et al. Patients with familial hypertrophic cardiomyopathy caused by a Phe110Ile missense mutation in the cardiac troponin T gene have variable cardiac morphologies and a favorable prognosis. *Circulation* 1998;98:391–397.
108. Maass AH, Ikeda K, Oberdorf-Maass S, et al. Hypertrophy, fibrosis, and sudden cardiac death in response to pathological stimuli in mice with mutations in cardiac troponin T. *Circulation* 2004;110:2102–2109.
109. Maron BJ, Casey SA, Hurrell DG, Aeppli DM. Relation of left ventricular thickness to age and gender in hypertrophic cardiomyopathy. *Am J Cardiol* 2003;91:1195–1198.
110. Dimitrow PP, Czarnecka D, Kawecka-Jaszcz K, Dubiel JS. The influence of age on gender-specific differences in the left ventricular cavity size and contractility in patients with hypertrophic cardiomyopathy. *Int J Cardiol* 2003;88:11–16.
111. Frielingsdorf J, Franke A, Hess OM, Flachskampf FA. Are there sex differences in regional systolic function and wall stress in hypertrophic obstructive cardiomyopathy? A three-dimensional echocardiography study. *J Am Soc Echocardiogr* 2004;17:638–643.
112. Waller BF, Maron BJ, Morrow AG, Roberts WC. Hypertrophic cardiomyopathy mimicking pericardial constriction or myocardial restriction. *Am Heart J* 1981;102:790–792.
113. McKenna WJ, Stewart JT, Nihoyannopoulos P, et al. Hypertrophic cardiomyopathy without hypertrophy: Two families with myocardial disarray in the absence of increased myocardial mass. *Br Heart J* 1990;63:287–290.
114. Maron BJ, Spirito P, Green KJ, et al. Noninvasive assessment of left ventricular diastolic function by pulsed Doppler echocardiography in patients with hypertrophic cardiomyopathy. *J Am Coll Cardiol* 1987;10:733–742.
115. Betocchi S, Bonow RO, Bacharach SL, et al. Isovolumic relaxation period in hypertrophic cardiomyopathy: Assessment by radionuclide angiography. *J Am Coll Cardiol* 1986;7:74–81.
116. Bonow RO, Frederick TM, Bacharach SL, et al. Atrial systole and left ventricular filling in hypertrophic cardiomyopathy: Effect of verapamil. *Am J Cardiol* 1983;51:1386–1391.
117. Newman H, Sugrue DD, Oakley CM, et al. Relation of left ventricular function and prognosis in hypertrophic cardiomyopathy. An angiographic study. *J Am Coll Cardiol* 1985;5:1064–1074.
118. Betocchi S, Hess OM. LV hypertrophy and diastolic heart failure. *Heart Fail Rev* 2000;5:333–336.
119. Pak PH, Maughan L, Baughman KL, Kass DA. Marked discordance between dynamic and passive diastolic pressure–volume relations in idiopathic hypertrophic cardiomyopathy. *Circulation* 1996;94:52–60.
120. Ito T, Suwa M, Imai M, et al. Assessment of regional left ventricular filling dynamics using color kinesis in patients with hypertrophic cardiomyopathy. *J Am Soc Echocardiogr* 2004;17:146–151.
121. Fassbach M, Schwartzkopff B. Elevated serum markers for collagen synthesis in patients with hypertrophic cardiomyopathy and diastolic dysfunction. *Z Kardiol* 2005;94:328–335.
122. Lombardi R, Betocchi S, Losi MA, et al. Myocardial collagen turnover in hypertrophic cardiomyopathy. *Circulation* 2003;108:1455–1460.
123. Mundhenke M, Schwartzkopff B, Stark P, et al. Myocardial collagen type I and impaired left ventricular function under exercise in hypertrophic cardiomyopathy. *Thorac Cardiovasc Surg* 2002;50:216–222.
124. Maron BJ, Harding AM, Spirito P, et al. Systolic anterior motion of the posterior mitral valve leaflet: A previous unrecognized cause of dynamic subaortic obstruction in patients with hypertrophic cardiomyopathy. *Circulation* 1983;68:282–293.
125. Spirito P, Maron BJ. Patterns of systolic anterior motion of the mitral valve in hypertrophic cardiomyopathy: Assessment by two-dimensional echocardiography. *Am J Cardiol* 1984;54:1039–1046.
126. Spirito P, Maron BJ. Significance of left ventricular outflow tract cross-sectional area in hypertrophic cardiomyopathy; a two-dimensional echocardiographic assessment. *Circulation* 1983;67:1100–1108.
127. Reis RL, Bolton MR, King JF, et al. Anterior-superior displacement of papillary muscles producing obstruction and mitral regurgitation in idiopathic hypertrophic subaortic stenosis. *Circulation* 1974;49/50(Suppl II): 181–188.
128. Klues HG, Maron BJ, Dollar AL, Roberts WC. Diversity of structural mitral valve alterations in hypertrophic cardiomyopathy. *Circulation* 1992;85:1651–1660.
129. Klues HG, Roberts WC, Maron BJ. Morphological determinants of echocardiographic patterns of mitral valve systolic anterior motion in obstructive hypertrophic cardiomyopathy. *Circulation* 1993;87:1570–1579.
130. Klues HG, Proschan MA, Dollar AL, et al. Echocardiographic assessment of mitral valve size in obstructive hypertrophic cardiomyopathy. Anatomic validation from mitral valve specimen. *Circulation* 1993;88:548–555.
131. Yock PG, Hatle L, Popp RL. Patterns and timing of Doppler-detected intracavitary and aortic flow in hypertrophic cardiomyopathy. *J Am Coll Cardiol* 1986;8:1047–1058.
132. Wigle ED, Henderson M, Rakowski H, Wilansky S. Muscular (hypertrophic) subaortic stenosis (hypertrophic obstructive cardiomyopathy): The evidence for true obstruction to left ventricular outflow. *Postgrad Med J* 1986;62:531–536.
133. Levine RA, Vlahakes GJ, Lefebvre, et al. Papillary muscle displacement causes systolic anterior motion of the mitral valve. Experimental validation and insights into the mechanism of subaortic obstruction. *Circulation* 1995;91:1189–1195.
134. Maron BJ, Nishimura RA, Danielson GK. Pitfalls in clinical recognition and a novel operative approach for hypertrophic cardiomyopathy with severe outflow obstruction due to anomalous papillary muscle. *Circulation* 1998;98:2505–2508.
135. Nakamura T, Matsubara K, Furukawa K, et al. Diastolic paradoxic jet flow in patients with hypertrophic cardiomyopathy: Evidence of concealed apical asynergy with cavity obliteration. *J Am Coll Cardiol* 1992;19:516–524.
136. Wigle ED, Adleman AG, Auger P, et al. Mitral regurgitation in muscular subaortic stenosis. *Am J Cardiol* 1969;24:698.
137. Thaman R, Gimeno JR, Murphy RT, et al. Prevalence and clinical significance of systolic impairment in hypertrophic cardiomyopathy. *Heart* 2005;91:920–925.
138. Thaman R, Gimeno JR, Reith S, et al. Progressive left ventricular remodeling in patients with hypertrophic cardiomyopathy and severe left ventricular hypertrophy. *J Am Coll Cardiol* 2004;44:398–405.
139. Sengupta PP, Mehta V, Arora R, et al. Quantification of regional nonuniformity and paradoxical intramural mechanics in hypertrophic cardiomyopathy by high frame rate ultrasound myocardial strain mapping. *J Am Soc Echocardiogr* 2005;18:737–742.

140. Tabata T, Oki T, Yamada H, et al. Subendocardial motion in hypertrophic cardiomyopathy: Assessment from long- and short-axis views by pulsed tissue Doppler imaging. *J Am Soc Echocardiogr* 2000;13:108–115.
141. Yamada H, Oki T, Tabata T, et al. Assessment of left ventricular systolic wall motion velocity with pulsed tissue Doppler imaging: Comparison with peak dP/dt of the left ventricular pressure curve. *J Am Soc Echocardiogr* 1998;11:442–449.
142. Matsumura Y, Elliott PM, Virdee MS, et al. Left ventricular diastolic function assessed using Doppler tissue imaging in patients with hypertrophic cardiomyopathy: Relation to symptoms and exercise capacity. *Heart* 2002;87:247–251.
143. Nagueh SF, Bachinski LL, Meyer D, et al. Tissue Doppler imaging consistently detects myocardial abnormalities in patients with hypertrophic cardiomyopathy and provides a novel means for an early diagnosis before and independently of hypertrophy. *Circulation* 2001;104:128–130.
144. Losi MA, Betocchi S, Aversa M, et al. Dobutamine stress echocardiography in hypertrophic cardiomyopathy. *Cardiology* 2003;100:93–100.
145. Okeie K, Shimizu M, Yoshio H, et al. Left ventricular systolic dysfunction during exercise and dobutamine stress in patients with hypertrophic cardiomyopathy. *J Am Coll Cardiol* 2000;36:856–863.
146. Kawano S, Iida K, Fujieda K, et al. Response to isoproterenol as a prognostic indicator of evolution from hypertrophic cardiomyopathy to a phase resembling dilated cardiomyopathy. *J Am Coll Cardiol* 1995;25:687–692.
147. Briguori C, Betocchi S, Manganelli F, et al. Determinants and clinical significance of natriuretic peptides and hypertrophic cardiomyopathy. *Eur Heart J* 2001;22:1328–1336.
148. Maron BJ, Tholakanahalli VN, Zenovich AG, et al. Usefulness of B-type natriuretic peptide assay in the assessment of symptomatic state in hypertrophic cardiomyopathy. *Circulation* 2004;109:984–989.
149. Noji Y, Shimizu M, Ino H, et al. Increased circulating matrix metalloproteinase-2 in patients with hypertrophic cardiomyopathy with systolic dysfunction. *Circ J* 2004;68:355–360.
150. Zen K, Irie H, Doue T, et al. Analysis of circulating apoptosis mediators and proinflammatory cytokines in patients with idiopathic hypertrophic cardiomyopathy. *Int Heart J* 2005;46:231–244.
151. Hogye M, Mandi Y, Csanady M, et al. Comparison of circulating levels of interleukin-6 and tumor necrosis factor-alpha in hypertrophic cardiomyopathy and in idiopathic dilated cardiomyopathy. *Am J Cardiol* 2004;94:249–251.
152. Maron BJ, Olivotto I, Spirito P, et al. Epidemiology of hypertrophic cardiomyopathy–related death: Revisited in a large non–referral-based patient population. *Circulation* 2000;102:858–864.
153. Ikeda H, Maki S, Yoshida N, et al. Predictors of death from congestive heart failure in hypertrophic cardiomyopathy. *Am J Cardiol* 1999;83:1280–1283, A9.
154. Cannon RO, Dilsizian V, O'Gara P, et al. Myocardial metabolic, hemodynamic, and electrocardiographic significance of reversible thallium-201 abnormalities in hypertrophic cardiomyopathy. *Circulation* 1991;83:1660–1667.
155. Pasternac A, Noble J, Streulens Y, et al. Pathophysiology of chest pain in patients with cardiomyopathies and normal coronary arteriograms. *Circulation* 1982;65:778
156. Camici P, Chiriatti G, Lorenzoni R, et al. Coronary vasodilatation is impaired in both hypertrophied and non hypertrophied myocardium of patients with hypertrophic cardiomyopathy: A study with nitrogen-13 ammonia and positron emission tomography. *J Am Coll Cardiol* 1991;17:879–886.
157. Elliott PM, Rosano GMC, Gill JS, et al. Changes in coronary sinus pH during dipyridamole stress in patients with hypertrophic cardiomyopathy. *Heart* 1996;75:179–183.
158. Cannon RO, Rosing DR, Maron BJ, et al. Myocardial ischemia in patients with hypertrophic cardiomyopathy: Contribution of inadequate vasodilator reserve and elevated left ventricular filling pressures. *Circulation* 1985;71:234–437.
159. Nicod P, Polikar R, Peterson KL. Hypertrophic cardiomyopathy and sudden death. *N Engl J Med* 1988;318:1255–1257.
160. Morioka N, Shigematsu Y, Hamada M, Higaki J. Circulating levels of heart-type fatty acid–binding protein and its relation to thallium-201 perfusion defects in patients with hypertrophic cardiomyopathy. *Am J Cardiol* 2005;95:1334–1337.
161. Elliott PM, Kaski JC, Prasad K, et al. Chest pain during daily life in patients with hypertrophic cardiomyopathy: An ambulatory electrocardiographic study. *Eur Heart J* 1996;17:1056–1064.
162. Cecchi F, Olivotto I, Gistri R, et al. Coronary microvascular dysfunction and prognosis in hypertrophic cardiomyopathy. *N Engl J Med* 2003; 349:1027–1235.
163. Shimizu M, Ino H, Okeie K, et al. Exercise-induced ST-segment depression and systolic dysfunction in patients with nonobstructive hypertrophic cardiomyopathy. *Am Heart J* 2000;140:52–60.
164. Dilsizian V, Bonow RO, Epstein SE, Fananapazir L. Myocardial ischemia detected by thallium scintigraphy is frequently related to cardiac arrest and syncope in young patients with hypertrophic cardiomyopathy. *J Am Coll Cardiol* 1993;22:796–804.
165. Hada Y, Sakamoto T, Amano K, et al. Prevalence of hypertrophic cardiomyopathy in a population of adult Japanese workers as detected by echocardiographic screening. *Am J Cardiol* 1987;59:183–184.
166. Savage DD, Castelli WP, Abbott RD, et al. Hypertrophic cardiomyopathy and its markers in the general population: The great masquerader revisited: The Framingham Study. *J Cardiovasc Ultrasonogr* 1983;2:41–47.
167. Maron BJ, Gardin JM, Flack JM, et al. Prevalence of hypertrophic cardiomyopathy in a population of young adults. Echocardiographic analysis of 4111 subjects in the CARDIA study. Coronary Artery Risk Development in (Young) Adults. *Circulation* 1995;92:785–789.
168. Codd MB, Sugrue DD, Gersh BJ, Melton LJ. Epidemiology of idiopathic dilated and hypertrophic cardiomyopathy: A population based study in Olmsted County, Minnesota, 1975–1984. *Circulation* 1989;80:564–572.
169. Maron BJ, Peterson EE, Maron MS, Peterson JE. Prevalence of hypertrophic cardiomyopathy in an outpatient population referred for echocardiographic study. *Am J Cardiol* 1994;73:577–580.
170. Maron BJ, Spirito P, Roman MJ, et al. Prevalence of hypertrophic cardiomyopathy in a population-based sample of American Indians aged 51 to 77 years (the Strong Heart Study). *Am J Cardiol* 2004;93:1510–1514.
171. Nistri S, Thiene G, Basso C, et al. Screening for hypertrophic cardiomyopathy in a young male military population. *Am J Cardiol* 2003;91:1021–1023.
172. Maron BJ, Schiffers A, Klues HG. Comparison of phenotypic expression of hypertrophic cardiomyopathy in patients from the United States and Germany. *Am J Cardiol* 1999;83:626–627.
173. Maron BJ, Mathenge R, Casey SA, et al. Clinical profile of hypertrophic cardiomyopathy identified de novo in rural communities. *J Am Coll Cardiol* 1999;33:1590–1595.
174. Zou Y, Song L, Wang Z, et al. Prevalence of idiopathic hypertrophic cardiomyopathy in China: A population-based echocardiographic analysis of 8080 adults. *Am J Med* 2004;116:14–18.
175. Maron BJ, Spirito P, Wesley Y, Arce J. Development or progression of left ventricular hypertrophy in children with hypertrophic cardiomyopathy: Identification by two-dimensional echocardiography. *N Engl J Med* 1986;315:610–614.
176. Topol EJ, Traill TA, Fortuin NJ. Hypertensive hypertrophic cardiomyopathy of the elderly. *N Engl J Med* 1985;312:277–283.
177. Faye WP, Taliercio CP, Ilstrup DM, et al. Natural history of hypertrophic cardiomyopathy in the elderly. *J Am Coll Cardiol* 1990;16:821–826.
178. Lewis JF, Maron BJ. Clinical and morphology expression of hypertrophic cardiomyopathy in patients ≥65 years of age. *Am J Cardiol* 1994;73:1105–1111.
179. Chikamori T, Doi YL, Yonezawa Y, et al. Comparison of clinical features in patients greater than or equal to 60 years of age to those less than or equal 40 years of age with hypertrophic cardiomyopathy. *Am J Cardiol* 1990;66:875–878.
180. McKenna WJ, Deanfield J, Faruqui A, et al. Prognosis in hypertrophic cardiomyopathy. Role of age and clinical, electrocardiographic and haemodynamic features. *Am J Cardiol* 1981;47:532–538.
181. McKenna WJ, Franklin RCG, Nihoyannopoulos P, et al. Arrhythmia and prognosis in infants, children and adolescents with hypertrophic cardiomyopathy. *J Am Coll Cardiol* 1988;11:147–153.
182. Maron BJ, Casey SA, Poliac LC, et al. Clinical course of hypertrophic cardiomyopathy in a regional United States cohort. *JAMA* 1999;281:650–655.
183. Spirito P, Chiarella F, Carratino L, et al. Clinical course and prognosis of hypertrophic cardiomyopathy in an outpatient population. *N Engl J Med* 1989;320:749–755.
184. Gilligan DM, Chan WL, Ang EL, Oakley CM. Effects of a meal on hemodynamic function at rest and during exercise in patients with hypertrophic cardiomyopathy. *J Am Coll Cardiol* 1991;18:429–436.
185. Paz R, Jortner R, Tunick PA, et al. The effect of the ingestion of ethanol on obstruction of the left ventricular outflow tract in hypertrophic cardiomyopathy. *N Engl J Med* 1996;335:938–941.
186. Savage DD, Seides SF, Clark CE, et al. Electrocardiographic findings in patients with obstructive and non-obstructive hypertrophic cardiomyopathy. *Circulation* 1978;58:402–409.
187. Montgomery JV, Harris KM, Casey SA, et al. Relation of electrocardiographic patterns to phenotypic expression and clinical outcome in hypertrophic cardiomyopathy. *Am J Cardiol* 2005;96:270–275.
188. Maron BJ, Wolfson JK, Ciro E, Spirito P. Relation of electrocardiographic abnormalities and patterns of left ventricular hypertrophy identified by 2-dimensional echocardiography in patients with hypertrophic cardiomyopathy. *Am J Cardiol* 1983;51:189–194.
189. Lemery R, Kleinebenne A, Nihoyannopoulos P, et al. Q-waves in hypertrophic cardiomyopathy in relation to the distribution and severity of right and left ventricular hypertrophy. *J Am Coll Cardiol* 1990;16:368–374.
190. Cosio FG, Moro C, Alonso M, et al. The Q-waves of hypertrophic cardiomyopathy. *N Engl J Med* 1980;302:96–99.
191. Panza JA, Maron BJ. Relation of electrocardiographic abnormalities to evolving left ventricular hypertrophy in hypertrophic cardiomyopathy during childhood. *Am J Cardiol* 1989;63:1258–1265.
192. Alfonso F, Nihoyannopoulos P, Stewart J, et al. Clinical significance of giant negative T waves in hypertrophic cardiomyopathy. *J Am Coll Cardiol* 1990;15:965–971.
193. Rosenweig A, Watkins H, Hwang DS, et al. Preclinical diagnosis of familial hypertrophic cardiomyopathy by genetic analysis of blood lymphocytes. *N Engl J Med* 1991;325:1753–1760.
194. Al-Mahdawi S, Chamberlain S, Chojnowska L, et al. The electrocardiogram is a more sensitive indicator than echocardiography of hypertrophic

cardiomyopathy in families with a mutation in the MYHA7 gene. *Br Heart J* 1994;72:105–111.
195. Adabag AS, Casey SA, Kuskowski MA, et al. Spectrum and prognostic significance of arrhythmias on ambulatory Holter electrocardiogram in hypertrophic cardiomyopathy. *J Am Coll Cardiol* 2005;45:697–704.
196. McKenna WJ, England D, Doi Y, et al. Arrhythmia in hypertrophic cardiomyopathy. 1. Influence on prognosis. *Br Heart J* 1981;46:168–172.
197. Maron BJ, Savage DD, Wolfson JK, Epstein SE. Prognostic significance of 24 hour ambulatory electrocardiographic monitoring in patients with hypertrophic cardiomyopathy: A prospective study. *Am J Cardiol* 1981; 48:252–257.
198. Alfonso F, Frenneaux MP, McKenna WJ. Clinical sustained uniform ventricular tachycardia in hypertrophic cardiomyopathy: Association with left ventricular apical aneurysm. *Br Heart J* 1989;61:178–181.
199. Robinson K, Frenneaux MP, Stockins B, et al. Atrial fibrillation in hypertrophic cardiomyopathy: A longitudinal study. *J Am Coll Cardiol* 1990; 15:1279–1285.
200. Losi MA, Betocchi S, Aversa M, et al. Determinants of atrial fibrillation development in patients with hypertrophic cardiomyopathy. *Am J Cardiol* 2004;94:895–900.
201. McKenna WJ, Spirito P, Desnos M, et al. Experience from clinical genetics in hypertrophic cardiomyopathy: Proposal for new diagnostic criteria in adult members of affected families. *Heart* 1997;77:130–132.
202. Doi YL, McKenna WJ, Gehrke J, et al. M-mode echocardiography in hypertrophic cardiomyopathy: Diagnostic criteria and prediction of obstruction. *Am J Cardiol* 1980;45:6–14.
203. Shapiro LM, McKenna WJ. Distribution of left ventricular hypertrophy in hypertrophic cardiomyopathy: A two-dimensional echocardiographic study. *J Am Coll Cardiol* 1983;2:437–444.
204. McKenna WJ, Kleinebenne A, Nihoyannopoulos O, Foale R. Echocardiographic measurement of right ventricular wall thickness in hypertrophic cardiomyopathy: Relation to clinical and prognostic features. *J Am Coll Cardiol* 1988;11:351–358.
205. Doi YL, McKenna WJ, Oakley CM, et al. "Pseudo SAM" in patients with hypertensive heart disease. *Eur Heart J* 1983;4:838–845.
206. Nishimura RA, Appleton CP, Redfield MM, et al. Noninvasive Doppler echocardiographic evaluation of left ventricular filling pressures in patients with cardiomyopathies: A simultaneous Doppler echocardiographic and cardiac catheterization study. *J Am Coll Cardiol* 1996;28:1226–1233.
207. Lele SS, Thomson HL, Seo H, et al. Exercise capacity in hypertrophic cardiomyopathy: Role of stroke volume limitation, heart rate, and diastolic filling characteristics. *Circulation* 1995;92:2886–2894.
208. Briguori C, Betocchi S, Romano M, et al. Exercise capacity in hypertrophic cardiomyopathy depends on left ventricular diastolic function. *Am J Cardiol* 1999;84:309–315.
209. Nihoyannopoulos P, Karatasakis G, Frenneaux M, et al. Diastolic function in hypertrophic cardiomyopathy: Relation to exercise capacity. *J Am Coll Cardiol* 1992;19:536–540.
210. Losi MA, Betocchi S, Grimaldi M, et al. Heterogeneity of left ventricular filling dynamics in hypertrophic cardiomyopathy. *Am J Cardiol* 1994;73:987–990.
211. Nagueh SF, McFalls J, Meyer D, et al. Tissue Doppler imaging predicts the development of hypertrophic cardiomyopathy in subjects with subclinical disease. *Circulation* 2003;108:395–398.
212. Cardim N, Perrot A, Ferreira T, et al. Usefulness of Doppler myocardial imaging for identification of mutation carriers of familial hypertrophic cardiomyopathy. *Am J Cardiol* 2002;90:128–132.
213. Ho CY, Sweitzer NK, McDonough B, et al. Assessment of diastolic function with Doppler tissue imaging to predict genotype in preclinical hypertrophic cardiomyopathy. *Circulation* 2002;105:2992–2997.
214. McMahon CJ, Nagueh SF, Pignatelli RH, et al. Characterization of left ventricular diastolic function by tissue Doppler imaging and clinical status in children with hypertrophic cardiomyopathy. *Circulation* 2004;109:1756–1762.
215. Nagueh SF, Lakkis NM, Middleton KJ, et al. Doppler estimation of left ventricular filling pressures in patients with hypertrophic cardiomyopathy. *Circulation* 1999;99:254–261.
216. Kato T, Noda A, Izawa H, et al. Myocardial velocity gradient as a noninvasively determined index of left ventricular diastolic dysfunction in patients with hypertrophic cardiomyopathy. *J Am Coll Cardiol* 2003;42:278–285.
217. Palka P, Lange A, Fleming AD, et al. Differences in myocardial velocity gradient measured throughout the cardiac cycle in patients with hypertrophic cardiomyopathy, athletes and patients with left ventricular hypertrophy due to hypertension. *J Am Coll Cardiol* 1997;30:760–768.
218. Vinereanu D, Florescu N, Sculthorpe N, et al. Differentiation between pathologic and physiologic left ventricular hypertrophy by tissue Doppler assessment of long-axis function in patients with hypertrophic cardiomyopathy or systemic hypertension and in athletes. *Am J Cardiol* 2001;88:53–58.
219. Yamada H, Oki T, Yamamoto T, et al. Potential application of tissue Doppler imaging to assess regional left ventricular diastolic function in patients with hypertrophic cardiomyopathy: Comparison with 123I-beta-methyl iodophenyl pentadecanoic acid myocardial scintigraphy. *Clin Cardiol* 2004;27:33–39.
220. O'Gara PT, Bonow RO, Maron BJ, et al. Myocardial perfusion abnormalities in patients with hypertrophic cardiomyopathy: Assessment with thallium-201 emission computed tomography. *Circulation* 1987;76:1214–1223.
221. Yamada M, Elliott PM, Kaski JC, et al. Dipyridamole stress thallium-201 perfusion abnormalities in patients with hypertrophic cardiomyopathy. Relationship to clinical presentation and outcome. *Eur Heart J* 1998;19:500–507.
222. Von Dohlen TW, Prisant LM, Frank MJ. Significance of positive or negative thallium-201 scintigraphy in hypertrophic cardiomyopathy. *Am J Cardiol* 1989;64:498–503.
223. Nienaber CA, Gambhir SS, Mody FV, et al. Regional myocardial blood flow and glucose utilisation in symptomatic patients with hypertrophic cardiomyopathy. *Circulation* 1993;87:1580–1590.
224. Grover-McKay M, Schwaiger M, Krivokapich J, et al. Regional myocardial blood flow and metabolism at rest in mildly symptomatic patients with hypertrophic cardiomyopathy. *J Am Coll Cardiol* 1989;13:317–324.
225. Perrone-Filardi P, Bacharach SL, Dilsizian V, et al. Regional systolic function, myocardial blood flow and glucose uptake at rest in hypertrophic cardiomyopathy. *Am J Cardiol* 1993;72:199–204.
226. Kagaya Y, Ishide N, Takeyama D, et al. Differences in myocardial fluro-18 2-deoxyglucose uptake in young versus old patients with hypertrophic cardiomyopathy. *Am J Cardiol* 1992;69:242–246.
227. Moon JC, Reed E, Sheppard MN, et al. The histologic basis of late gadolinium enhancement cardiovascular magnetic resonance in hypertrophic cardiomyopathy. *J Am Coll Cardiol* 2004;43:2260–2264.
228. Amano Y, Takayama M, Takahama K, Kumazaki T. Delayed hyperenhancement of myocardium in hypertrophic cardiomyopathy with asymmetrical septal hypertrophy: Comparison with global and regional cardiac MR imaging appearances. *J Magn Reson Imaging* 2004;20:595–600.
229. Moon JC, Mogensen J, Elliott PM, et al. Myocardial late gadolinium enhancement cardiovascular magnetic resonance in hypertrophic cardiomyopathy caused by mutations in troponin I. *Heart* 2005;91:1036–1040.
230. Teraoka K, Hirano M, Ookubo H, et al. Delayed contrast enhancement of MRI in hypertrophic cardiomyopathy. *Magn Reson Imaging* 2004;22:155–161.
231. Sipola P, Lauerma K, Jaaskelainen P, et al. Cine MR imaging of myocardial contractile impairment in patients with hypertrophic cardiomyopathy attributable to Asp175Asn mutation in the α–tropomyosin gene. *Radiology* 2005.
232. Moon JC, McKenna WJ, McCrohon JA, et al. Toward clinical risk assessment in hypertrophic cardiomyopathy with gadolinium cardiovascular magnetic resonance. *J Am Coll Cardiol* 2003;41:1561–1567.
233. Choudhury L, Mahrholdt H, Wagner A, et al. Myocardial scarring in asymptomatic or mildly symptomatic patients with hypertrophic cardiomyopathy. *J Am Coll Cardiol* 2002;40:2156–2164.
234. Cohen LS, Braunwald E. Amelioration of angina pectoris in idiopathic hypertrophic subaortic stenosis with beta-adrenergic blockade. *Circulation* 1967;35:847–851.
235. Wigle ED, Rakowski H, Kimball BP, Williams WG. Hypertrophic cardiomyopathy. Clinical spectrum and treatment. *Circulation* 1995;92:1680–1692.
236. Spirito P, Seidman CE, McKenna WJ, Maron BJ. The management of hypertrophic cardiomyopathy. *N Engl J Med* 1997;336:775–778.
237. Gilligan DM, Chan WL, Joshi J, et al. A double-blind, placebo-controlled crossover trial of nadolol and verapamil in mild and moderately symptomatic hypertrophic cardiomyopathy. *J Am Coll Cardiol* 1993;21:1672–1679.
238. Sherrid MV, Pearle G, Gunsburg DZ. Mechanism of benefit of negative inotropes in obstructive hypertrophic cardiomyopathy. *Circulation* 1998; 97:41–47.
239. Ostman-Smith I, Wettrell G, Riesenfeld T. A cohort study of childhood hypertrophic cardiomyopathy: Improved survival following high-dose beta-adrenoceptor antagonist treatment. *J Am Coll Cardiol* 1999;34:1813–1822.
240. Kaltenbach M, Hopf R, Kober G, et al. Treatment of hypertrophic obstructive cardiomyopathy with verapamil. *Br Heart J* 1979;42:35–42.
241. Rosing DR, Kent KM, Maron BJ, Epstein SE. Verapamil therapy: A new approach to the pharmacological treatment of hypertrophic cardiomyopathy. II. Effects on exercise capacity and symptomatic status. *Circulation* 1979;60:1208–1213.
242. Bonow RO, Dilsizian V, Rosing DR, et al. Verapamil induced improvement in left ventricular filling and increased exercise tolerance in patients with hypertrophic cardiomyopathy. Short and long-term effects. *Circulation* 1985; 72:853–864.
243. Bonow RO, Rosing DR, Bacharach SL, et al. Effects of verapamil on left ventricular systolic function and diastolic filling in patients with hypertrophic cardiomyopathy. *Circulation* 1981;64:787–796.
244. Spicer RL, Rocchini AP, Crowley DC, Rosenthal A. Chronic verapamil therapy in pediatric and young adult patients with hypertrophic cardiomyopathy. *Am J Cardiol* 1984;53:1614–1619.
245. Udelson JE, Bonow RO, O'Gara PT, et al. Verapamil prevents silent myocardial perfusion abnormalities during exercise in asymptomatic patients with hypertrophic cardiomyopathy. *Circulation* 1989;79:1052–1060.
246. Gistri R, Cecchi F, Choudhury L, et al. Effect of verapamil on absolute myocardial blood flow in hypertrophic cardiomyopathy. *Am J Cardiol* 1994;74:363–368.
247. Pollick C. Muscular subaortic stenosis: Hemodynamic and clinical improvement after disopyramide. *N Engl J Med* 1982;307:997–999.

248. Pollick C, Kimball B, Henderson M, Wigle ED. Disopyramide in hypertrophic cardiomyopathy. I. Hemodynamic assessment after intravenous administration. *Am J Cardiol* 1988;62:1248–1251.
249. Pollick C. Disopyramide in hypertrophic cardiomyopathy II. Non-invasive assessment after oral administration. *Am J Cardiol* 1988;62:1252–1255.
250. Sherrid MV, Pearle G, Gunsburg DZ. Mechanism of benefit of negative inotropes in obstructive hypertrophic cardiomyopathy. *Circulation* 1998;97:41–47.
251. Matsubara H, Nakatani S, Nagata S, et al. Salutary effect of disopyramide on left ventricular diastolic function in hypertrophic obstructive cardiomyopathy. *J Am Coll Cardiol* 1995;26:768–775.
252. Sherrid MV, Barac I, McKenna WJ, et al. Multicenter study of the efficacy and safety of disopyramide in obstructive hypertrophic cardiomyopathy. *J Am Coll Cardiol* 2005;45:1251–1258.
253. Hamada M, Shigematsu Y, Ikeda S, et al. Class Ia antiarrhythmic drug cibenzoline: A new approach to the medical treatment of hypertrophic obstructive cardiomyopathy. *Circulation* 1997;96:1520–1524.
254. Morrow AG, Reitz BA, Epstein SE, et al. Operative treatment in hypertrophic subaortic stenosis: Techniques and the results of pre and postoperative assessments in 83 patients. *Circulation* 1975;52:88–102.
255. Maron BJ, Epstein SE, Morrow AG. Symptomatic status and prognosis of patients after operation for hypertrophic cardiomyopathy: Efficacy of ventricular septal myotomy/myectomy. *Eur Heart J* 1983;4(Suppl F):175–180.
256. Schulte D, Borisov K, Gams E, et al. Management of symptomatic hypertrophic obstructive cardiomyopathy—long-term results after surgical therapy. *Thorac Cardiovasc Surg* 1999;47:213–218.
257. ten Berg JM, Suttorp MJ, Knaepen PJ, et al. Hypertrophic obstructive cardiomyopathy. Initial results and long-term follow-up after Morrow septal myectomy. *Circulation* 1994;90:1781–1785.
258. Theodoro DA, Danielson GK, Feldt RH, Anderson BJ. Hypertrophic obstructive cardiomyopathy in pediatric patients: Results of surgical treatment. *J Thorac Cardiovasc Surg* 1996;112:1589–1597.
259. Yu EH, Omran AS, Wigle ED, et al. Mitral regurgitation in hypertrophic obstructive cardiomyopathy: Relationship to obstruction and relief with myectomy. *J Am Coll Cardiol* 2000;36:2219–2225.
260. Williams WG, Wigle ED, Rakowski H, et al. Results of surgery for hypertrophic obstructive cardiomyopathy. *Circulation* 1987;76:V104–V108.
261. Rothlin ME, Gobet D, Habere T, et al. Surgical treatment versus medical treatment in hypertrophic obstructive cardiomyopathy. *Eur Heart J* 1983;4(Suppl F):215–223.
262. McCully RB, Nishimura RA, Baily KR, et al. Hypertrophic obstructive cardiomyopathy: Preoperative echocardiographic predictors of outcome after septal myectomy. *J Am Coll Cardiol* 1996;27:1491–1496.
263. Redwood DR, Goldstein RE, Hirshfeld J, et al. Exercise performance after septal myotomy and myectomy in patients with obstructive hypertrophic cardiomyopathy. *Am J Cardiol* 1979;44:215–220.
264. Schoendube FA, Klues HG, Reith S, et al. Long-term clinical and echocardiographic follow-up after surgical correction of hypertrophic obstructive cardiomyopathy with extended myectomy and reconstruction of the subvalvular mitral apparatus. *Circulation* 1995;92:II122–II127.
265. Grigg LE, Wigle ED, Williams WG, et al. Transesophageal Doppler echocardiography in obstructive hypertrophic cardiomyopathy: Clarification of pathophysiology and importance in intraoperative decision making. *J Am Coll Cardiol* 1992;20:42–52.
266. Sasson Z, Prieur T, Skrobik Y, et al. Aortic regurgitation: A common complication after surgery for hypertrophic obstructive cardiomyopathy. *J Am Coll Cardiol* 1989;13:63–67.
267. Bigelow WG, Trimble AS, Wigle DE, et al. The treatment of muscular subaortic stenosis. *J Thorac Cardiovasc Surg* 1974;68:384–390.
268. Heric B, Lytle BW, Miller DP, et al. Surgical management of hypertrophic obstructive cardiomyopathy. Early and late results. *J Thorac Cardiovasc Surg* 1995;110:195–206.
269. Cohn LH, Trehan H, Collins JJ. Long-term follow-up of patients undergoing myotomy/myectomy for obstructive hypertrophic cardiomyopathy. *Am J Cardiol* 1992;70:657–660.
270. Krajcer Z, Leachman RD, Cooley DA, Coronado R. Septal myotomy-myomectomy versus mitral valve replacement in hypertrophic cardiomyopathy. Ten-year follow-up in 185 patients. *Circulation* 1989;80:I57–I64.
271. Maron BJ, Merrill WH, Freier PA, et al. Long-term clinical course and symptomatic status of patients after operation for hypertrophic subaortic stenosis. *Circulation* 1978;57:1205–1213.
272. McCully RB, Nishimura RA, Tajik AJ, et al. Extent of clinical improvement after surgical treatment of hypertrophic obstructive cardiomyopathy. *Circulation* 1996;94:467–471.
273. Merrill WH, Friesinger GC, Graham Jr TP, et al. Long–lasting improvement after septal myectomy for hypertrophic obstructive cardiomyopathy. *Ann Thorac Surg* 2000;69:1732–1735.
274. Mohr R, Schaff HV, Danielson GK, et al. The outcome of surgical treatment of hypertrophic obstructive cardiomyopathy. Experience over 15 years. *J Thorac Cardiovasc Surg* 1989;97:666–674.
275. Robbins RC, Stinson EB. Long-term results of left ventricular myotomy and myectomy for obstructive hypertrophic cardiomyopathy. *J Thorac Cardiovasc Surg* 1996;111:586–594.
276. Minakata K, Dearani JA, Nishimura RA, et al. Extended septal myectomy for hypertrophic obstructive cardiomyopathy with anomalous mitral papillary muscles or chordae. *J Thorac Cardiovasc Surg* 2004;127:481–489.
277. McIntosh CL, Greenberg GJ, Maron BJ, et al. Clinical and hemodynamic results after mitral valve replacement in patients with hypertrophic cardiomyopathy. *Ann Thorac Surg* 1989;47:236–246.
278. McIntosh CL, Maron BJ, Cannon RO 3rd, Klues HG. Initial results of combined anterior mitral leaflet plication and ventricular septal myotomy-myectomy for relief of left ventricular outflow tract obstruction in patients with hypertrophic cardiomyopathy. *Circulation* 1992;86(5 Suppl):II60–II67.
279. Kofflard MJ, van Herwerden LA, Waldstein DJ, et al. Initial results of combined anterior mitral leaflet extension and myectomy in patients with obstructive hypertrophic cardiomyopathy. *J Am Coll Cardiol* 1996;28:197–202.
280. Maron BJ, McIntosh CL, Klues HG, et al. Morphologic basis for obstruction to right ventricular outflow in hypertrophic cardiomyopathy. *Am J Cardiol* 1993;71:1089–1094.
281. Hassenstein P, Storch HH, Schmitz W. Results of electrical pacing in patients with hypertrophic obstructive cardiomyopathy [in German]. *Thoraxchir Vask Chir* 1975;23:496–498.
282. Duck HJ, Hutschenreiter W, Pankau H, Trenckmann H. Atrial synchronous ventricular stimulation with reduced AV delay time as a therapeutic principle in hypertrophic obstructive cardiomyopathy [in German]. *Z Gesamte Inn Med* 1984;39:437–447.
283. McDonald K, McWilliams E, O'Keefe B, Maurer B. Functional assessment of patients treated with permanent dual chamber pacing as a primary treatment for hypertrophic cardiomyopathy. *Eur Heart J* 1988;9:893–898.
284. Slade AKB, Sadoul N, Shapiro L, et al. DDD pacing in hypertrophic cardiomyopathy: A multicentre clinical experience. *Heart* 1996;75:44–49.
285. Jeanrenaud X, Goy JJ, Kappenberger L. Effects of dual-chamber pacing in hypertrophic obstructive cardiomyopathy. *Lancet* 1992;339:1318–1323.
286. Fananapazir L, Epstein ND, Curiel RV, et al. Long-term results of dual chamber (DDD) pacing in obstructive hypertrophic cardiomyopathy. Evidence for progressive symptomatic and hemodynamic improvement and reduction of left ventricular hypertrophy. *Circulation* 1994;90:2731–2742.
287. Nishimura RA, Trusty JM, Hayes DL, et al. Dual chamber pacing for hypertrophic cardiomyopathy: A randomised double-blind crossover trial. *J Am Coll Cardiol* 1997;29:435–441.
288. Kappenberger L, Linde C, Daubert C, et al. Pacing in hypertrophic obstructive cardiomyopathy. A randomized crossover study. PIC Study Group. *Eur Heart J* 1997;18:1249–1256.
289. Gadler F, Linde C, Daubert C, et al. Significant improvement of quality of life following atrioventricular synchronous pacing in patients with hypertrophic obstructive cardiomyopathy. Data from 1 year of follow-up. PIC Study Group. Pacing In Cardiomyopathy. *Eur Heart J* 1999;20:1044–1050.
290. Maron BJ, Nishimura RA, McKenna WJ, et al. Assessment of permanent dual-chamber pacing as a treatment for drug-refractory symptomatic patients with obstructive hypertrophic cardiomyopathy. A randomized, double-blind, crossover study (M-PATHY). *Circulation* 1999;99:2927–2933.
291. Ommen SR, Nishimura RA, Squires RW, et al. Comparison of dual-chamber pacing versus septal myectomy for the treatment of patients with hypertropic obstructive cardiomyopathy: A comparison of objective hemodynamic and exercise end points. *J Am Coll Cardiol* 1999;34:191–196.
292. Nishimura RA, Hayes DL, Ilstrup DM, et al. Effect of dual-chamber pacing on systolic and diastolic function in patients with hypertrophic cardiomyopathy. Acute Doppler echocardiographic and catheterization hemodynamic study. *J Am Coll Cardiol* 1996;27:421–430.
293. Posma JL, Blanksma PK, Van Der Wall EE, et al. Effects of permanent dual chamber pacing on myocardial perfusion in symptomatic hypertrophic cardiomyopathy. *Heart* 1996;76:358–362.
294. Cannon RO, Tripodi D, Dilsizian V, et al. Results of permanent dual-chamber pacing in symptomatic nonobstructive hypertrophic cardiomyopathy. *Am J Cardiol* 1994;73:571–576.
295. Rishi F, Hulse JE, Auld DO, et al. Effects of dual–chamber pacing for pediatric patients with hypertrophic obstructive cardiomyopathy. *J Am Coll Cardiol* 1997;29:734–740.
296. Betocchi S, Elliott PM, Briguori C, et al. Dual chamber pacing in hypertrophic cardiomyopathy: Long-term effects on diastolic function. *Pacing Clin Electrophysiol* 2002;25:1433–1440.
297. Betocchi S, Losi MA, Piscione F, et al. Effects of dual-chamber pacing in hypertrophic cardiomyopathy on left ventricular outflow tract obstruction and on diastolic function. *Am J Cardiol* 1996;77:498–502.
298. Megevand A, Ingles J, Richmond DR, Semsarian C. Long-term follow-up pf patients with obstructive hypertrophic cardiomyopathy treated with dual chamber pacing. *Am J Cardiol* 2005;95:991–993.
299. Sigwart U. Non-surgical myocardial reduction for hypertrophic obstructive cardiomyopathy. *Lancet* 1995;346:211–214.
300. Lakkis NM, Nagueh SF, Dunn JK, et al. Nonsurgical septal reduction therapy for hypertrophic obstructive cardiomyopathy: One-year follow-up. *J Am Coll Cardiol* 2000;36:852–855.
301. Ruzyllo W, Chojnowska L, Demkow M, et al. Left ventricular outflow tract gradient decrease with non-surgical myocardial reduction improves exercise capacity in patients with hypertrophic obstructive cardiomyopathy. *Eur Heart J* 2000;21:770–777.
302. Faber L, Seggewiss H, Gleichmann U. Percutaneous transluminal septal myocardial ablation in hypertrophic obstructive cardiomyopathy: Results

with respect to intraprocedural myocardial contrast echocardiography. *Circulation* 1998;98:2415–2421.
303. Gietzen FH, Leuner CJ, Raute-Kreinsen U, et al. Acute and long-term results after transcoronary ablation of septal hypertrophy (TASH). Catheter interventional treatment for hypertrophic obstructive cardiomyopathy. *Eur Heart J* 1999;20:1342–1354.
304. Nagueh SF, Lakkis NM, He ZX, et al. Role of myocardial contrast echocardiography during nonsurgical septal reduction therapy for hypertrophic obstructive cardiomyopathy. *J Am Coll Cardiol* 1998;32:225–229.
305. Knight C, Kurbaan AS, Seggewiss H, et al. Nonsurgical septal reduction for hypertrophic obstructive cardiomyopathy: Outcome in the first series of patients. *Circulation* 1997;95:2075–2081.
306. Seggewiss H, Gleichmann U, Faber L, et al. Percutaneous transluminal septal myocardial ablation in hypertrophic obstructive cardiomyopathy: Acute results and 3-month follow-up in 25 patients. *J Am Coll Cardiol* 1998; 31:252–258.
307. Maron BJ. Role of alcohol septal ablation in treatment of obstructive hypertrophic cardiomyopathy. *Lancet* 2000;355:425–426.
308. Faber L, Meissner A, Ziemssen P, Seggewiss H. Percutaneous transluminal septal myocardial ablation for hypertrophic obstructive cardiomyopathy: Long-term follow up of the first series of 25 patients. *Heart* 2000;83:326–331.
309. Flores-Ramirez R, Lakkis NM, Middleton KJ, et al. Echocardiographic insights into the mechanisms of relief of left ventricular outflow tract obstruction after nonsurgical septal reduction therapy in patients with hypertrophic obstructive cardiomyopathy. *J Am Coll Cardiol* 2001;37:208–214.
310. Gietzen FH, Leuner CJ, Obergassel L, et al. Transcoronary ablation of septal hypertrophy for hypertrophic obstructive cardiomyopathy: Feasibility, clinical benefit, and short-term results in elderly patients. *Heart* 2004;90:638–644.
311. Kim JJ, Lee CW, Park SW, et al. Improvement in exercise capacity and exercise blood pressure response after transcoronary alcohol ablation therapy of septal hypertrophy in hypertrophic cardiomyopathy. *Am J Cardiol* 1999;83:1220–1122.
312. Kuhn H, Gietzen FH, Schafers M, et al. Changes in the left ventricular outflow tract after transcoronary ablation of septal hypertrophy (TASH) for hypertrophic obstructive cardiomyopathy as assessed by transoesophageal echocardiography and by measuring myocardial glucose utilization and perfusion. *Eur Heart J* 1999;20:1808–1817.
313. Qin JX, Shiota T, Lever HM, et al. Outcome of patients with hypertrophic obstructive cardiomyopathy after percutaneous transluminal septal myocardial ablation and septal myectomy surgery. *J Am Coll Cardiol* 2001; 38:1994–2000.
314. Kuhn H, Gietzen FH, Leuner C, et al. Transcoronary ablation of septal hypertrophy (TASH): A new treatment option for hypertrophic obstructive cardiomyopathy. *Z Kardiol* 2000;89:IV41–IV54.
315. Mazur W, Nagueh SF, Lakkis NM, et al. Regression of left ventricular hypertrophy after nonsurgical septal reduction therapy for hypertrophic obstructive cardiomyopathy. *Circulation* 2001;103:1492–1496.
316. Fernandes VL, Nagueh SF, Wang W, et al. A prospective follow-up of alcohol septal ablation for symptomatic hypertrophic obstructive cardiomyopathy—the Baylor experience (1996–2002). *Clin Cardiol* 2005; 28:124–130.
317. Park TH, Lakkis NM, Middleton KJ, et al. Acute effect of nonsurgical septal reduction therapy on regional left ventricular asynchrony in patients with hypertrophic obstructive cardiomyopathy. *Circulation* 2002;106:412–415.
318. Chang SM, Lakkis NM, Franklin J, et al. Predictors of outcome after alcohol septal ablation therapy in patients with hypertrophic obstructive cardiomyopathy. *Circulation* 2004;109:824–827.
319. Ralph-Edwards A, Woo A, McCrindle BW, et al. Hypertrophic obstructive cardiomyopathy: Comparison of outcomes after myectomy or alcohol ablation adjusted by propensity score. *J Thorac Cardiovasc Surg* 2005;129:351–358.
320. Talreja DR, Nishimura RA, Edwards WD, et al. Alcohol septal ablation versus surgical septal myectomy: Comparison of effects on atrioventricular conduction tissue. *J Am Coll Cardiol* 2004;44:2329–2332.
321. Chojnowska L, Ruzyllo W, Witkowski A, et al. Early and long-term results of non-surgical septal reduction in patients with hypertrophic cardiomyopathy. *Kardiol Pol* 2003;59:269–282.
322. Nagueh SF, Lakkis NM, Middleton KJ, et al. Changes in left ventricular filling and left atrial function six months after nonsurgical septal reduction therapy for hypertrophic obstructive cardiomyopathy. *J Am Coll Cardiol* 1999;34:1123–1128.
323. Firoozi S, Elliott PM, Sharma S, et al. Septal myotomy-myectomy and transcoronary septal alcohol ablation in hypertrophic obstructive cardiomyopathy: A comparison of clinical, hemodynamic and exercise outcomes. *Eur Heart J* 2002;20:1617–1624.
324. Boekstegers P, Steinbigler P, Molnar A, et al. Pressure-guided nonsurgical myocardial reduction induced by small septal infarctions in hypertrophic obstructive cardiomyopathy. *J Am Coll Cardiol* 2001;38:846–853.
325. Gietzen FH, Leuner CJ, Obergassel L, et al. Role of transcoronary ablation of septal hypertrophy in patients with hypertrophic cardiomyopathy, NYHA functional class III or IV and outflow obstruction only under provocable conditions. *Circulation* 2002;106:454–459.
326. Sitges M, Shiota T, Lever HM, et al. Comparison of left ventricular diastolic function in obstructive hypertrophic cardiomyopathy in patients undergoing percutaneous septal alcohol ablation versus surgical myotomy/myectomy. *Am J Cardiol* 2003;91:817–821.
327. Iwase M, Sobotata I, Takagi S, et al. Effects of diltiazem on left ventricular diastolic behaviour in patients with hypertrophic cardiomyopathy: Evaluation with pulsed Doppler echocardiography. *J Am Coll Cardiol* 1987;9:1099.
328. Betocchi S, Cannon RO, Watson RM, et al. Effects of sublingual nifedipine on hemodynamics and systolic and diastolic function in patients with hypertrophic cardiomyopathy. *Circulation* 1985;72:1001–1007.
329. Bauer F, Shiota T, White RD, et al. Determinants of left atrial dilation in patients with hypertrophic cardiomyopathy: A real-time 3-dimensional echocardiographic study. *J Am Soc Echocardiogr* 2004;17:968–975.
330. Maron BJ, Olivotto I, Bellone P, et al. Clinical profile of stroke in 900 patients with hypertrophic cardiomyopathy. *J Am Coll Cardiol* 2002;39:301–330.
331. Spirito P, Lakatos E, Maron BJ. Degree of left ventricular hypertrophy in patients with hypertrophic cardiomyopathy and chronic atrial fibrillation. *Am J Cardiol* 1992;69:1217–1222.
332. Olivotto I, Cecchi F, Casey SA, et al. Impact of atrial fibrillation on the clinical course of hypertrophic cardiomyopathy. *Circulation* 2001;104:2517–2524.
333. Cecchi F, Olivotto I, Montereggi A, et al. Hypertrophic cardiomyopathy in Tuscany: Clinical course and outcome in an unselected regional population. *J Am Coll Cardiol* 1995;26:1529–1536.
334. Boriani G, Rapezzi C, Biffi M, et al. Atrial fibrillation precipitating sustained ventricular tachycardia in hypertrophic cardiomyopathy. *J Cardiovasc Electrophysiol* 2002;13:954.
335. Stafford WJ, Trohman RG, Bilsker M, et al. Cardiac arrest in an adolescent with atrial fibrillation and hypertrophic cardiomyopathy. *J Am Coll Cardiol* 1986;7:701–704.
336. Elliott PM, Poloniecki J, Dickie S, et al. Sudden death in hypertrophic cardiomyopathy: Identification of high risk patients. *J Am Coll Cardiol* 2000;36:2212–2218.
337. Kofflard MJ, Ten Cate FJ, van der Lee C, van Domburg RT. Hypertrophic cardiomyopathy in a large community-based population: Clinical outcome and identification of risk factors for sudden cardiac death and clinical deterioration. *J Am Coll Cardiol* 2003;41:987–989.
338. Maron BJ, Roberts WC, Epstein SE. Sudden death in hypertrophic cardiomyopathy: A profile of 78 patients. *Circulation* 1982;65:1388–1394.
339. Maron BJ, Kogan J, Proschan MA, et al. Circadian variability in the occurrence of sudden cardiac death in patients with hypertrophic cardiomyopathy. *J Am Coll Cardiol* 1994;23:1405–1409.
340. Spirito P, Bellone P, Harris KM, et al. Magnitude of left ventricular hypertrophy and risk of sudden death in hypertrophic cardiomyopathy. *N Engl J Med* 2000;342:1778–1785.
341. Maki S, Ikeda H, Muro A, et al. Predictors of sudden cardiac death in hypertrophic cardiomyopathy. *Am J Cardiol* 1998;82:774–778.
342. McKenna WJ, Deanfield JE. Hypertrophic cardiomyopathy: An important cause of sudden death. *Arch Dis Child* 1984;59:971–975.
343. Cannan CR, Reeder GS, Bailey KR, et al. Natural history of hypertrophic cardiomyopathy. A population based study, 1976 through 1990. *Circulation* 1995;92:2488–2495.
344. Maron BJ, Tajik AJ, Ruttenberg HD, et al. Hypertrophic cardiomyopathy in infants: Clinical features and natural history. *Circulation* 1982;65:7–17.
345. Yetman AT, McCrindle BW, MacDonald C, et al. Myocardial bridging in children with hypertrophic cardiomyopathy—a risk factor for sudden death. *N Engl J Med* 1998;339:1201–1209.
346. Monserrat L, Elliott PM, Gimeno JR, et al. Non-sustained ventricular tachycardia in hypertrophic cardiomyopathy: An independent marker of sudden death risk in young patients. *J Am Coll Cardiol* 2000;42:873–879.
347. Spirito P, Rapezzi C, Autore C, et al. Prognosis of asymptomatic patients with hypertrophic cardiomyopathy and nonsustained ventricular tachycardia. *Circulation* 1994;90:2743–2747.
348. Sadoul N, Prasad K, Elliott PM, et al. Prospective prognostic assessment of blood pressure response during exercise in patients with hypertrophic cardiomyopathy. *Circulation* 1997;96:2987–2991.
349. Isobe N, Toyama T, Taniguchi K, et al. Failure to raise blood pressure during exercise is a poor prognostic sign in patients with hypertrophic nonobstructive cardiomyopathy. *Circ J* 2003;67:191–194.
350. Olivotto I, Maron BJ, Montereggi A, et al. Prognostic value of systemic blood pressure response during exercise in a community based population with hypertrophic cardiomyopathy. *J Am Coll Cardiol* 1999;33:2044–2051.
351. Elliott PM, Gimeno Blanes JR, Mahon NG, McKenna WJ. Relation between the severity of left ventricular hypertrophy and prognosis in patients with hypertrophic cardiomyopathy. *Lancet* 2001;357:420–424.
352. Olivotto I, Gistri R, Petrone P, et al. Maximum left ventricular thickness and risk of sudden death in patients with hypertrophic cardiomyopathy. *J Am Coll Cardiol* 2003;41:315–321.
353. Maron MS, Olivotto I, Betocchi S, et al. Effect of left ventricular outflow tract obstruction on clinical outcome in hypertrophic cardiomyopathy. *N Engl J Med* 2003;348:295–303.
354. Autore C, Bernabo P, Barilla CS, et al. The prognostic importance of left ventricular outflow obstruction in hypertrophic cardiomyopathy varies in relation to the severity of symptoms. *J Am Coll Cardiol* 2005;45:1076–1080.

355. Fananapazir L, Chang AC, Epstein SE, McAreavey D. Prognostic determinants in hypertrophic cardiomyopathy: Prognostic evaluation of a therapeutic strategy based on clinical, Holter, hemodynamic and electrophysiological findings. *Circulation* 1992;86:730–740.
356. Frenneaux MP, Counihan PJ, Caforio A, et al. Abnormal blood pressure response during exercise in hypertrophic cardiomyopathy. *Circulation* 1990;82:1995–2002.
357. Counihan PJ, Frenneaux MP, Webb DJ, McKenna WJ. Abnormal vascular responses to supine exercise in hypertrophic cardiomyopathy. *Circulation* 1991;84:686–696. Fananapazir L, Chang AC, Epstein SE, McAreavey D. Prognostic determinants in hypertrophic cardiomyopathy: Prognostic evaluation of a therapeutic strategy based on clinical, Holter, hemodynamic and electrophysiological findings. *Circulation* 1992;86:730–740.
358. Wellens HJJ, Brugada P, Stevenson WG. Programmed electrical stimulation of the heart in patients with life threatening ventricular arrhythmias. What is the significance of induced arrhythmias and what is the correct stimulation protocol? *Circulation* 1985;72:1–7.
359. Elliott PM, Sharma S, Varnava A, et al. Survival after cardiac arrest or sustained ventricular tachycardia in patients with hypertrophic cardiomyopathy. *J Am Coll Cardiol* 1999;33:1596–1601.
360. Cecchi F, Maron BJ, Epstein SE. Long-term outcome of patients with hypertrophic cardiomyopathy successfully resuscitated after cardiac arrest. *J Am Coll Cardiol* 1989;13:1283–1288.
361. Silka MJ, Kron J, Dunnigan A, Dick M. Sudden cardiac death and the use of implantable cardioverter-defibrillators in pediatric patients. *Circulation* 1993;87:800–807.
362. Kron J, Oliver RP, Norsted S, Silka MJ. The automatic implantable cardioverter defibrillator in young patients. *J Am Coll Cardiol* 1990;16:896–902.
363. Maron BJ, Shen WK, Link MS, et al. Efficacy of implantable cardioverter-defibrillators for the prevention of sudden death in patients with hypertrophic cardiomyopathy. *N Engl J Med* 2000;342:365–373.
364. Primo J, Geelen P, Brugada J, et al. Hypertrophic cardiomyopathy: Role of the implantable cardioverter defibrillator. *J Am Coll Cardiol* 1998;31:1081–1085.
365. Maron BJ, Roberts WC, McAllister HA, et al. Sudden death in young athletes. *Circulation* 1980;62:218–229.
366. Firoozi S, Sharma S, McKenna WJ. Risk of competitive sport in young athletes with heart disease. *Heart* 2003;89:710–714.
367. Burke AP, Farb A, Virmani R, et al. Sports-related and non–sports-related sudden cardiac death in young adults. *Am Heart J* 1991;121:568–575.
368. Maron BJ, Carney KP, Lever HM, et al. Relationship of race to sudden cardiac death in competitive athletes with hypertrophic cardiomyopathy. *J Am Coll Cardiol* 2003;41:974–980.
369. Maron BJ. Sudden death in young athletes. *N Engl J Med* 2003;349:1064–1075.
370. Pellicia A, Maron BJ, Spataro A, et al. The upper limit of physiologic cardiac hypertrophy in highly trained elite athletes. *N Engl J Med* 1991;324:295.
371. Shapiro LM, Kleinebenne A, McKenna WJ. The distribution of left ventricular hypertrophy in hypertrophic cardiomyopathy: Comparison to athletes and hypertensives. *Eur Heart J* 1985;6:967–974.
372. Maron BJ, Pellicia A, Spirito P. Cardiac disease in young trained athletes. Insights into methods for distinguishing athlete's heart from structural heart disease, with particular emphasis on hypertrophic cardiomyopathy. *Circulation* 1995;91:1569–1601.
373. Lewis JF, Spirito P, Pellicia A, Maron BJ. Usefulness of Doppler echocardiographic assessment of diastolic filling in distinguishing "athlete's heart" from hypertrophic cardiomyopathy. *Br Heart J* 1992;68:296–300.
374. Spirito P, Pellicia A, Proschan MA, et al. Morphology of the "athletes heart" assessed by echocardiography in 947 elite athletes representing 27 sports. *Am J Cardiol* 1994;74:802–806.
375. Pelliccia A, Spataro A, Caselli G, Maron BJ. Absence of left ventricular wall thickening in athletes engaged in intense power training. *Am J Cardiol* 1993;72:1048–1054.
376. Serra-Grima R, Estorch M, Carrio I, et al. Marked ventricular repolarization abnormalities in highly trained athletes' electrocardiograms: Clinical and prognostic implications. *J Am Coll Cardiol* 2000;36:1310–1316.
377. Pelliccia A, Maron BJ, Culasso F, et al. Clinical significance of abnormal electrocardiographic patterns in trained athletes. *Circulation* 2000;102:278–284.
378. Sharma S, Elliott PM, Whyte G, et al. Utility of metabolic exercise testing in distinguishing hypertrophic cardiomyopathy from physiologic left ventricular hypertrophy in athletes. *J Am Coll Cardiol* 2000;36:864–870.
379. Maron BJ, Douglas PS, Graham TP, et al. Task Force 1: Preparticipation screening and diagnosis of cardiovascular disease in athletes. *J Am Coll Cardiol* 2005;45:1322–1326.
380. Maron BJ, Zipes DP. Introduction: Eligibility recommendations for competitive athletes with cardiovascular abnormalities–general considerations. *J Am Coll Cardiol* 2005;45:1318–1321.
381. Thaman R, Varnava A, Hamid MS, et al. Pregnancy related complications in women with hypertrophic cardiomyopathy. *Heart* 2003;89:752–756.
382. Autore C, Conte MR, Piccininno M, et al. Risk associated with pregnancy in hypertrophic cardiomyopathy. *J Am Coll Cardiol* 2002;40:1864–1869.
383. Spirito P, Rapezzi C, Bellone P, et al. Infective endocarditis in hypertrophic cardiomyopathy: Prevalence, incidence, and indications for antibiotic prophylaxis. *Circulation* 1999;99:2132–2137.
384. Roberts WC, Kishel JC, McIntosh CL, et al. Severe mitral or aortic valve regurgitation, or both, requiring valve replacement for infective endocarditis complicating hypertrophic cardiomyopathy. *J Am Coll Cardiol* 1992;19:365–371.

CHAPTER 30 ■ CONGENITAL HEART DISEASE

M. ELIZABETH BRICKNER

INTRODUCTION

Congenital heart disease (CHD) is defined as a gross structural abnormality of the heart, great arteries, or great veins that is present at birth (1). Congenital cardiac malformations are relatively uncommon. Multiple studies have demonstrated an incidence of 0.6% of live births for moderate to severe defects (2). The prevalence is higher in stillbirths and spontaneous abortions (3). There are approximately 32,000 new cases per year in the United States and greater than 1,000,000 new cases per year worldwide (4). Although the prevalence is low, the population of patients with CHD continues to expand. Because of the dramatic advances made in medical, surgical, and interventional device therapy, survival into adulthood is now the rule for the vast majority of patients with congenital cardiac defects.

ETIOLOGY

The etiology of CHD is multifactorial. Recurrence risks vary with the gender of the proband and the specific cardiac defect (5), with an overall recurrence risk of 3% to 5% in the offspring of patients with congenital heart disease (6–8). The exact proportion of patients with a specific genetic etiology is unknown. There are reports of familial defects following Mendelian patterns of inheritance (9). Certain chromosomal abnormalities are associated with congenital heart defects. The most common of these is trisomy 21 (Down syndrome). At least 50% of patients with Down syndrome have CHD (most commonly atrioventricular septal defects or ventricular septal defects), often associated with early pulmonary vascular obstructive disease (1,11). Despite the identification of many candidate genes on chromosome 21, the key genes contributing to the cardiac phenotype in Down syndrome have yet to be defined (12). Other syndromes associated with CHD include Turner syndrome, Noonan syndrome, Williams syndrome, Marfan syndrome, and trisomy 13, 14, 15, and 18.

Deletions of 22q11 are seen in DiGeorge syndrome (thymic aplasia, hypoparathyroidism, congenital heart defects involving the outflow tracts, and a dysmorphic appearance) (13,14). From transgenic studies with a mouse model, *TBX1* has been identified as the likely gene responsible for the cardiac and hypoparathyroid phenotype (15). 22q11 deletions are now recognized as the cause of a broader group of defects and are seen in 50% of patients with conotruncal abnormalities (14). CATCH-22, a syndrome due to microdeletion at chromosome 22q11, consists of cardiac conotruncal abnormalities, abnormal facies, thymic abnormalities, cleft palate, and hypocalcemia. Some patients may have the gene deletion without accompanying syndromic features (13).

Mutations in a few specific genes have been identified in some cases of congenital heart defects. Mutations in *TBX5* are seen in the majority of patients with Holt-Oram syndrome, an autosomal disorder with cardiac septal defects and upper limb defects (16). Mutations in the elastin gene (*ELN*) have been identified as a cause of supravalvular aortic stenosis (17). Mutations in *NKX2.5* have been associated with the autosomal dominant phenotype of atrial septal defect or tetralogy of Fallot (18).

FETAL AND NEONATAL CIRCULATION

In fetal life, the placenta is a low-resistance structure that acts as a respiratory organ and receives the largest amount of fetal blood flow. Blood from the placenta returns to the fetus through the ductus venosus, entering the inferior vena cava (IVC) to the right atrium (RA). A portion of the IVC blood flow is directed across the patent foramen ovale (PFO) to the left atrium (LA), bypassing the right heart. Blood from the superior vena cava (SVC) is directed into the right ventricle (RV) along with the remaining blood return from the IVC and is then pumped out into the pulmonary artery. Because of high pulmonary vascular resistance in the fetus, most pulmonary blood flow crosses the ductus arteriosus and enters the descending thoracic aorta. At birth, the relatively low resistance placental circulation is removed, and systemic vascular resistance increases within minutes. With respiration, the pulmonary vascular bed dilates in response to inspired oxygen, and pulmonary vascular resistance decreases while pulmonary blood flow increases. Pulmonary venous blood return increases, which increases systemic ventricular output and helps to close the foramen ovale. The ductus arteriosus is patent at birth, but begins to constrict shortly after birth and usually closes within hours to several days (1). Defects in which pulmonary blood flow depends on flow through the ductus are characterized as ductal dependent. With closure of the ductus in these patients, progressive hypoxemia, acidosis, and death invariably occur. Prostaglandin E_1 infusion to maintain patency of the ductus is used as a temporizing measure until more definitive therapy can be undertaken (19).

DIAGNOSTIC TOOLS

The physical exam is critical in the evaluation of patients with known or suspected CHD and includes elements that may not be routinely performed in patients with acquired forms of heart disease. In addition to precordial palpation, assessment of venous waveforms, and careful cardiac auscultation, it is also important to assess for cyanosis (including differential cyanosis), palpate pulses and measure blood pressure in both upper and lower extremities, and check oxygen saturation. Evidence of phenotypes associated with CHD (e.g., Down syndrome, William syndrome) should be sought. Although the electrocardiogram (ECG) and chest x-ray (CXR) are a routine part of the evaluation of patients with CHD, they are not specific enough for diagnostic purposes. Imaging studies by qualified personnel play a critical role in the evaluation of these patients. A careful review of prior data, including catheterization data, imaging, and operative reports, is essential as well.

Transthoracic echocardiography (TTE) is the most widely used diagnostic tool for establishing the initial diagnosis and following patients serially (20,21). Studies in these patients are complex and time-consuming and should be performed by sonographers and physicians with expertise in CHD. Transesophageal echocardiography (TEE) is particularly useful in adults with poor acoustic windows, providing excellent visualization of the atrial septum, pulmonary veins, interatrial baffles, and Fontan connections (22,23). Intraoperative TEE plays a critical role for patients undergoing surgical repair (24). TEE is also used to guide catheter interventions and device deployment. Increasingly, intracardiac echocardiography is being used for these procedures. Three-dimensional echocardiography is an evolving technology that may be helpful in evaluating patients with congenital heart disease (25,26).

Cardiac magnetic resonance imaging (MRI) is an extremely useful tool for the assessment of patients with congenital heart disease, providing high-quality images with a wide field of view in nearly all patients. MRI is particularly useful for assessment of extracardiac anatomy, including delineation of the great vessels, branch pulmonary arteries, and surgical shunts, as well as systemic and pulmonary venous connections (27–29). MRI allows quantitation of ventricular mass, volumes, and ejection fraction and can be used to calculate shunt flow and regurgitant flow. Contrast is not required for routine imaging but may be particularly useful in assessing vascular structures. The role of cardiac computed tomography (CT) imaging is evolving. Cardiac CT provides excellent visualization of anatomy (particularly extracardiac anatomy) but does use ionizing radiation (30).

Cardiac catheterization plays a critical role in the management of patients with congenital heart disease, as both a diagnostic and a therapeutic tool (31,32). Due to the complex hemodynamic data and difficult anatomy in many of these patients, catheterization is best performed by experienced personnel. There is an expanding role for interventional catheterization procedures, including closure of shunts, pulmonary and aortic valvotomy, pulmonary artery stenting, stenting of conduits, and balloon aortoplasty for aortic coarctation. (See Chapter 83.)

SPECIFIC DEFECTS

Left-to-Right Shunts

Atrial Septal Defect

An atrial septal defect (ASD) is a direct communication between the atrial chambers. ASDs are common, accounting for 5% to 10% of all congenital heart defects and one third of all congenital defects diagnosed in adulthood (33,34). They are usually sporadic, but familial cases have been reported. They are more common in female than male individuals (2:1) (35). An associated congenital defect may be seen in up to 30% of cases. ASDs are seen in association with skeletal deformities of the upper extremities, including Holt-Oram syndrome (36). Ostium secundum and primum defects are also associated with Down syndrome.

There are several morphologic types of ASDs. The most common is the ostium secundum defect (seen in 75% of cases). Secundum defect occurs in the region of the fossa ovalis, may extend in any direction, and may be multiple. Partial anomalous pulmonary venous connections are seen in 2% of patients with secundum defects. Ostium primum defects account for 15% of ASDs. Primum defects are part of the spectrum of atrioventricular (AV) septal defects and are associated with a common AV junction. A common AV valve is usually present with fusion of the inferior and superior bridging leaflets, leading to separate mitral and tricuspid orifices. This results in a trileaflet appearance of the "anterior" mitral leaflet, sometimes referred to as "cleft" in the anterior leaflet. Mitral regurgitation may be associated with this abnormal valve. Sinus venosus defects account for 10% of ASDs. Sinus venosus defects occur in the superior portion of the septum near the insertion of the SVC and are frequently associated with anomalous pulmonary venous drainage of the right pulmonary veins, most commonly the right upper pulmonary vein. Inferior sinus venosus defects are rare. They occur at the mouth of the IVC and may have right-to-left shunting and cyanosis due to preferential shunting of IVC blood to the LA. The rarest form of ASD is the coronary sinus defect, which may occur at the mouth of the coronary sinus or in the body of the coronary sinus itself (known as "unroofing" of the coronary sinus). Coronary sinus ASDs are often associated with a persistent left superior vena cava connecting to the LA (37). Some patients may have absence of most of the interatrial septum, resulting in a "common atrium."

With unrestricted defects, there is no pressure gradient between the atria. Left-to-right shunting across the ASD occurs in late systole and diastole. The magnitude of the shunt depends on the size of the defect and the relative of compliance of the right and left ventricles as well as the pulmonary and systemic vascular resistance. Diseases that affect left ventricular (LV) compliance (e.g., hypertension, coronary artery disease) can increase the magnitude of the left-to-right shunt. The left-to-right shunt results in right ventricular volume overload with increased pulmonary blood flow (Fig. 30.1). Large shunts may result in pulmonary hypertension. Spontaneous closure of ASDs may occur (38–40). Small ASDs (<3 mm) usually close by 18 months, and as many as 80% of defects in the range

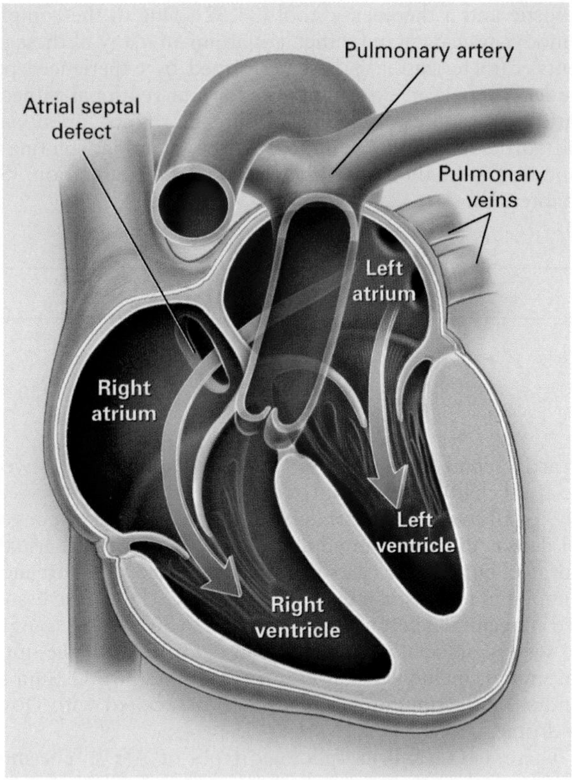

FIGURE 30.1. Left-to-right shunting across an ostium secundum atrial septal defect, causing right ventricular volume overload. (From Brickner ME, Hillis LD, Lange RA. Congenital heart disease in adults. *N Engl J Med* 2000;342:340.)

of 5 to 8 mm close by 18 months. Larger defects rarely close spontaneously.

The cardiac exam demonstrates a right ventricular lift with significant volume overload. S1 is normal. S2 is widely split and does not vary with respiration, although this pathognomonic finding is not universally present. A systolic flow murmur is common due to increased flow across the right ventricular outflow tract. A diastolic rumble across the tricuspid valve may be heard with large shunts. With the development of pulmonary hypertension, splitting of S2 narrows and the intensity of P2 increases. With shunt reversal (the Eisenmenger syndrome), cyanosis and clubbing develop. Cyanosis may also be seen in the absence of pulmonary hypertension in patients with very large defects, a prominent Eustachian valve, a coronary sinus defect, or in association with pulmonic stenosis, RV dysfunction, or Ebstein's anomaly. Typical ECG findings include right-axis deviation (except in ostium primum defects) and an rSR″ or rsR′ pattern in lead V1. There may be evidence of right ventricular hypertrophy (RVH). Some patients have prolongation of the PR interval. Inverted P waves in the inferior leads suggest a sinus venosus type of defect. A superior QRS axis (extreme right- or left-axis deviation) suggests a primum atrial septal defect. The CXR shows right-sided chamber enlargement, a dilated pulmonary artery, and increased pulmonary vascular markings in patients with significant shunts.

The diagnosis is made by echocardiography, which demonstrates the location and size of the defect as well as the direction of shunting. The presence of a dilated RA and RV consistent with right-sided volume overload should suggest the presence of an ASD, prompting thorough interrogation of the atrial septum and a bubble study. Ostium secundum and primum defects are well visualized by transthoracic imaging, particularly on subcostal views. Sinus venosus defects may be more difficult to demonstrate and require additional views (41,42). TEE is frequently used in the adult populations to fully interrogate the interatrial septum (43).

Cardiac catheterization is not usually required in patients with an ASD unless there is associated pulmonary hypertension or the noninvasive assessment is inconclusive (44). The presence of an ASD is confirmed by catheter passage across the atrial septum and a "step up" in oxygen saturation at the level of the atrium. Systemic and pulmonary blood flow, ratio of pulmonary to systemic blood flow (Qp/Qs), pulmonary pressure, and pulmonary vascular resistance should be assessed. If anomalous pulmonary venous drainage is suspected, levophase pulmonary artery injections should be obtained. Coronary angiography is usually performed for patients over the age of 40 years if surgical correction is planned. ASDs can also be diagnosed by cardiac MRI, which is also excellent for assessing pulmonary venous connections.

ASDs are often diagnosed in childhood, but they can also present in adulthood. Patients with an ASD are usually asymptomatic in childhood, but patients may have decreased exercise tolerance and increased respiratory infections. Symptoms usually occur in adulthood by the third or fourth decade. Seventy percent of patients will have symptoms by the fifth decade, and annual mortality increases to 10% by the sixth decade for patients with untreated ASDs (45). The most common symptoms are dyspnea and decreased exercise tolerance. Patients may present with atrial arrhythmias, congestive heart failure, or symptoms associated with pulmonary vascular disease. There is some increased risk of stroke due to paradoxical embolism, but this is usually seen only in patients with atrial arrhythmias and/or right ventricular dysfunction. Pulmonary vascular obstructive disease (the Eisenmenger syndrome) is uncommon with ASDs, occurring in 5% to 10% of cases, more commonly in female patients (45,46). Patients with the Eisenmenger syndrome secondary to an ASD typically present in their twenties or thirties.

Closure of the defect is recommended for ASDs with a Qp/Qs greater than 1.5:1 and a pulmonary to systemic vascular resistance ratio less than 0.7 (47–50). In children, closure is usually recommended between the ages of 2 and 4 years to allow for spontaneous closure. In adolescents and adults, closure is usually undertaken when the diagnosis is made. The surgical approach has low morbidity and mortality (<1%) and is done by patching the defect or with direct suture closure.

Surgical closure of an ASD in childhood or early adulthood (before the age of 25 years) results in a long-term mortality similar to that of an age- and sex-matched control population (47). These patients can be considered cured. Patients undergoing surgery after the age of 25 years have reduced survival compared to control subjects, most strikingly in those older than the age of 40 years. Surgical closure between the ages of 25 and 40 years in asymptomatic patients is controversial but is generally presumed to prevent symptomatic deterioration (49,51,52). For symptomatic patients older than the age of 40 years, surgical closure improves exercise capacity, improves survival compared to medically managed patients, and prevents further deterioration in functional capacity (47,53). However, it does not reduce the risk of supraventricular arrhythmias, heart failure, or cerebrovascular accidents (48,53–57). Surgical closure in symptomatic patients with a significant shunt who are over the age of 60 years results in symptomatic improvement in 80% (54). Patients with older age at repair require surveillance for atrial arrhythmias, heart failure, stroke, and progressive pulmonary vascular disease. Seventy percent of patients with preoperative arrhythmias have persistent arrhythmias postoperatively, and 10% to 25% of patients without arrhythmias will develop them postoperatively. An increased risk of systemic arterial hypertension of unclear etiology has been demonstrated after ASD closure in older patients (54).

Preoperative pulmonary vascular resistance (PVR) is predictive of outcome. Patients with a PVR of less than 7 Wood units have improvement in symptoms and New York Heart Association (NYHA) functional class, whereas a PVR of greater than 15 Wood units is associated with a high surgical mortality (50). If PVR is greater than two thirds of systemic vascular resistance, patients must have a large shunt or evidence of pulmonary vascular reactivity before surgery is considered.

The role of device closure is increasing (56). First attempted in 1976, device systems (57) have undergone continuous evolution in terms of material, design, shape, and delivery method. Devices available or in clinical trials include the Amplatzer septal occluder, the Atrial Septal Defect Occlusion System (ASDOS), the Buttoned Device, the Guardian Angel, the Helex Septal occluder, and the Cardioseal. Success rates vary but generally are in the range of 90% to 97% for initial successful deployment. Residual leaks are common on initial assessment but usually decrease or disappear with longer-term follow-up. Choice of the device type depends on the location of the defect and the degree of aortic rim tissue (must have 4- to 5-mm rim). There are no comparative studies between device and surgical closure. (See Chapter 83.)

There is no consensus for long-term follow-up after device closure, and long-term outcomes are largely unknown (including the risk for atrial arrhythmias, heart failure, and stroke). Because there is ongoing morbidity and mortality in adults undergoing surgical closure of ASDs, it is reasonable to postulate that a similar outcome may be seen in adults undergoing device closure. Potential complications specific to device closure include the potential for obstruction of pulmonary or systemic venous drainage, interference with the mitral valve, and erosion of the atrial wall or the aortic wall.

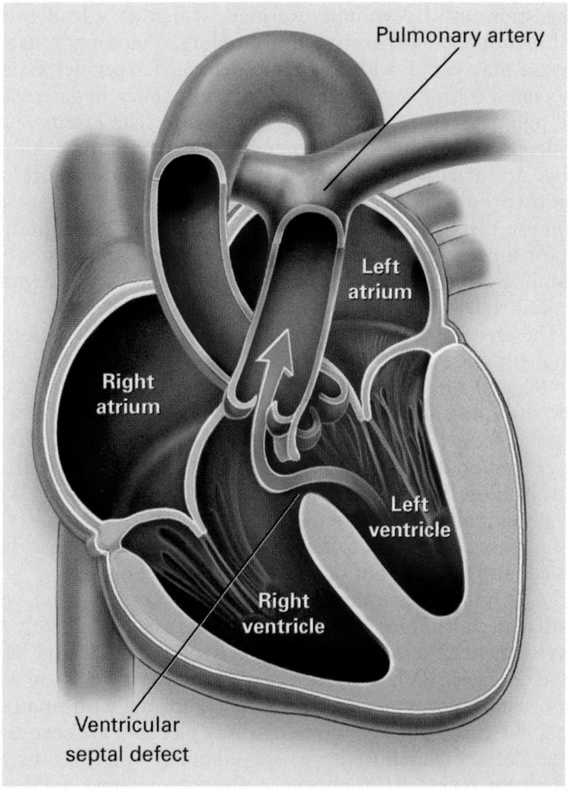

FIGURE 30.2. Left-to-right shunting across a perimembranous ventricular septal defect. (From Brickner ME, Hillis LD, Lange RA. Congenital heart disease in adults. *N Engl J Med* 2000;342:340.)

Ventricular Septal Defect

Ventricular septal defects (VSDs) are the most common form of congenital heart defect, accounting for 25% to 30% of all patients with congenital heart disease (33). The male:female ratio is 1. VSDs are the most common defect seen in the pediatric population. VSDs are usually a single defect, but they can occur in the setting of more complex congenital heart defects. Defects can be divided into restrictive defects (flow restricted between the LV and the RV with right ventricular pressure less than half of systemic levels) or nonrestrictive defects (with equal left and right ventricular pressures) (58,59). From 70% to 80% of VSDs can be characterized as restrictive, with the potential to close or become smaller (60,61). Nearly half of all VSDs are small, and up to 75% may close spontaneously. Even large defects can decrease in size (62–65). VSDs usually close by the age of 10 years. Spontaneous closure in adults is rare but has been reported (65).

The ventricular septum consists of the trabecular muscular septum, the inlet septum (formed from the endocardial cushion), the outlet or infundibular septum, and the membranous septum. Failure of growth, alignment, or fusion of these components results in a VSD. Perimembranous VSDs are the most common type, accounting for 75% to 80% of cases (Fig. 30.2). A perimembranous defect occurs at the junction of the inlet, outlet, and trabecular septum and may extend variably into these regions. The perimembranous VSD underlies the septal leaflet of the tricuspid valve and may decrease in size or close spontaneously due to adherence of septal leaflet tissue to the defect, resulting in a ventricular septal aneurysm. Inlet septal defects account for 5% to 10% of VSDs. They occur in the muscular septum, under the mitral and tricuspid leaflets, due to deficiency of tissue from the endocardial cushion. Inlet VSDs rarely close spontaneously. Muscular defects or defects of the trabecular septum account for 20% of all VSDs. They may be located in various positions within the trabecular septum and may be multiple. Muscular VSDs tend to decrease in size with muscle growth and may close spontaneously. Outlet defects (also known as doubly committed subarterial defects or supracristal VSDs) account for 5% of all VSDs. They occur in the right ventricular outlet or conal portion of the septum, underlying both the pulmonary and aortic valves. Outlet defects do not close spontaneously, but their size can decrease due to prolapse of aortic cusp tissue through the defect (also resulting in aortic regurgitation).

The degree of left-to-right shunting depends on the size of the defect and the relative resistance of the systemic and pulmonary vascular beds. VSDs are characterized as small when the defect size is less than one-third of the aortic root size, and these are always restrictive. Pulmonary vascular resistance remains normal. With moderate restrictive defects, the defect is approximately half the size of the aortic valve, and there is moderate to severe left-to-right shunting. Patients with moderate defects may develop symptoms associated with LV volume overload and are at risk for developing pulmonary vascular disease. Large VSDs are nonrestrictive, with equal pressures in the left and right ventricles. There is a large left-to-right shunt initially, and the pulmonary circulation is exposed to systemic pressures early in the course of the disease. Patients with nonrestrictive VSDs usually develop irreversible pulmonary vascular disease within the first decade of life, eventually resulting in shunt reversal and Eisenmenger physiology.

The natural history of VSDs depends on the size and location of the defect. Small, restrictive defects with a Qp/Qs less than 1.5 to 1 do not place a hemodynamically significant load on the LV. Moderate or large defects cause pulmonary congestion and LV volume overload, which may lead to LV dysfunction and congestive heart failure. Pulmonary hypertension may occur with moderate defects. Larger defects are associated with a significant risk of pulmonary hypertension and pulmonary vascular obstructive disease. The Eisenmenger syndrome occurs in 10% of patients with VSDs (65). All patients are at risk for bacterial endocarditis and require antibiotic prophylaxis. Other complications include aortic cusp prolapse through the defect, resulting in aortic regurgitation and/or subaortic obstruction, and the development of a double-chambered RV due to hypertrophy of muscle bundles within the mid-right ventricular cavity.

The physical exam findings vary with the size of the defect. A patient with a small defect has a normal PMI, a normal S1 and S2, and a harsh pansystolic murmur associated with a systolic thrill. In addition to the murmur and thrill, patients with larger defects have evidence of LV enlargement with prominence and/or displacement of the apical impulse, a diastolic mitral inflow rumble, and frequently a gallop rhythm. With the development of pulmonary hypertension, the intensity of P2 increases, splitting of the second heart sound becomes narrowed, and the murmur decreases or disappears.

ECG findings are nonspecific. The ECG is normal with small defects. Larger defects are usually associated with the development of left ventricular hypertrophy (LVH) and ST-T wave changes. RVH may be seen with large defects or with the Eisenmenger syndrome. The CXR is normal with small defects, but cardiomegaly and pulmonary plethora are seen with larger defects. Patients with severe pulmonary vascular disease and shunt reversal (Eisenmenger physiology) have mild cardiomegaly or normal heart size with large central pulmonary arteries, peripheral pruning of the pulmonary vessels, and oligemic lung fields.

The diagnosis can be made by echocardiography with Doppler color flow mapping. With careful interrogation of the septum, the site and size of defects can be demonstrated (66–68). The pressure gradient between the LV and the RV can be assessed by continuous-wave Doppler interrogation of the VSD jet, and right ventricular systolic pressure can be indirectly estimated from continuous-wave Doppler interrogation of the tricuspid regurgitation (TR) jet (69,70). Care must be taken with the latter approach because the TR jet may be contaminated by the VSD jet (particularly with perimembranous defects), resulting in inaccurate right ventricular pressure estimation. The interventricular pressure gradient may be inaccurate in the setting of tortuous or serpiginous defects where the modified Bernoulli equation is not applicable. Echocardiography may also reveal other associated defects, including aortic regurgitation.

Cardiac catheterization is generally reserved for patients in whom there is uncertainty regarding the size of the shunt and the pulmonary vascular resistance. The reversibility of pulmonary hypertension can be assessed with the administration of oxygen, nitric oxide, prostaglandins, or adenosine. Selective coronary angiography is usually performed for patients older than the age of 40 years if surgical repair is planned.

The clinical presentation depends on the size of the shunt. Patients with small defects are asymptomatic and have normal growth and development. The diagnosis in usually made on the basis of finding a loud holosystolic murmur. Larger shunts may result in symptoms of congestive heart failure in infancy as well as an increased susceptibility to pulmonary infections. The diagnosis of a VSD in adulthood is usually based on the incidental finding of a murmur or the development of a complication related to the VSD (e.g., endocarditis, aortic valve prolapse and regurgitation, or the Eisenmenger syndrome) (71). Overall, the 25-year survival for all patients is 87% (65). Mortality increases with the size of the VSD.

Patients with symptomatic heart failure initially are treated with medical therapy, including diuretics and afterload reduction. Digoxin is often used in the pediatric setting. There are no randomized trials of medical therapy, but its use is indicated to stabilize the patient until surgical repair can be performed. Indications for surgery include severe intractable heart failure within the first 3 months of life, the presence of symptoms in older infants and children, and the presence of a moderate or large defect with a Qp/Qs greater than 2:1. Repair is also recommended for subarterial defects regardless of the shunt size due to the risk of aortic valve prolapse. Pulmonary vascular resistance should be below 8 Wood units (less than two-thirds systemic vascular resistance) for surgery to have long-term success. Repair is usually performed from the RA but occasionally through the RV, with placement of a patch or direct suture closure. Pulmonary artery banding is rarely performed. It is used to decrease pulmonary blood flow in patients with multiple defects or complex malformations that are not otherwise amenable to repair. Transcatheter device closure of VSDs appears to be feasible in some cases but is not widely available (72–75).

The prognosis is normal for patients with spontaneous closure of their VSD. Unoperated patients with an isolated small VSD and normal PVR have an excellent long-term prognosis, although they remain at risk for endocarditis (65,76). Unoperated patients with moderate to large shunts are at risk for multiple complications, including endocarditis, aortic regurgitation, LV dysfunction from chronic volume overload, arrhythmias, development of the Eisenmenger syndrome, and sudden death. Patients with subarterial VSDs (and occasionally perimembranous defects) may develop prolapse of the aortic cusp through the defect with the development of progressive aortic regurgitation (65,71,77).

Overall, late outcome after early surgical closure of a VSD is excellent. Residual shunts are common, seen in up to 20% of cases after surgery, but are usually small (78). Late complications after surgical repair include endocarditis (if a residual shunt persists after surgery), surgically induced aortic or pulmonary regurgitation, and tricuspid regurgitation (if the septal leaflet was manipulated during the VSD repair). Arrhythmias and conduction disturbances may be seen (79,80). Right-bundle-branch block occurs in 30% to 60% of patients after surgical closure, first-degree AV block is seen in 10%, and complete heart block in 1% to 3% over long-term follow-up (71,78). Patients may have LV dysfunction with late repair of the defect or with significant aortic regurgitation. Patients may have persistent pulmonary hypertension after surgery or may develop progressive pulmonary hypertension despite successful closure of their shunt (65). There is an increased risk of sudden cardiac death after VSD closure, seen in 2% of patients (65,71). The etiology for sudden death has not been defined.

In general, patients undergoing early repair without a residual shunt, evidence of pulmonary hypertension, arrhythmias, or conduction block do not require long-term follow-up. Later repair of VSDs is associated with a risk of pulmonary hypertension and LV dysfunction, making long-term follow-up of these patients mandatory.

Patent Ductus Arteriosus

Patent ductus arteriosus (PDA) refers to continued patency of a normal structure in fetal circulation (Fig. 30.3). The ductus arteriosus is derived from the left sixth aortic arch and is usually a left-sided structure, but may be right sided or bilateral. PDA occurs in 5% to 10% of congenital defects and is often present in premature infants (3,81,82). An increased incidence is also seen in cases of maternal rubella.

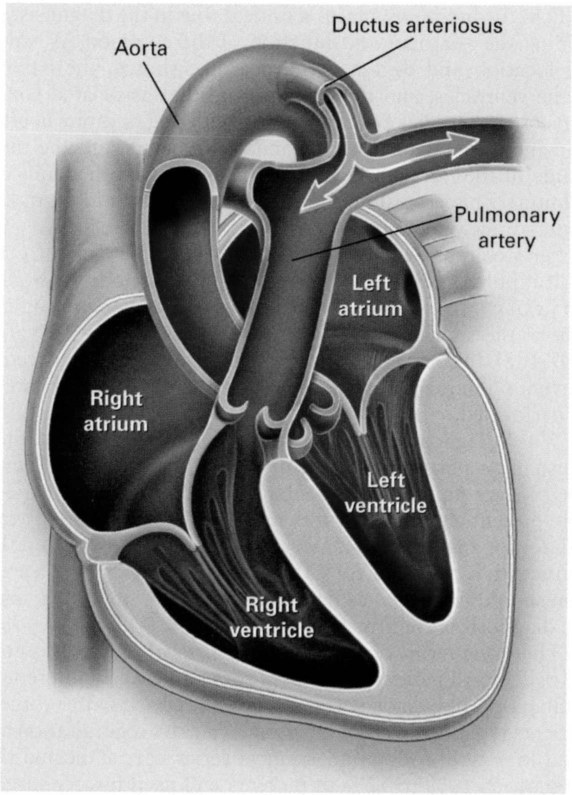

FIGURE 30.3. Patent ductus arteriosus with left-to-right shunting. (From Brickner ME, Hillis LD, Lange RA. Congenital heart disease in adults. *N Engl J Med* 2000;342:340.)

A PDA is associated with a left-to-right shunt that is predominantly systolic in early infancy but becomes continuous as PVR decreases. Thus, in the newborn with a significant shunt, there is an active precordium and only a systolic murmur. In older children and adults, a continuous "machinery" murmur is present at the left upper sternal border. A PDA may close spontaneously before the age of 6 months.

The clinic presentation of a PDA is similar to that of a VSD. With small shunts, there is a loud murmur but the ECG and CXR are normal. In patients with a moderate to large shunt, the clinical exam is remarkable for an enlarged apical impulse and bounding pulses in addition to the continuous murmur from the shunt. With a moderate to large shunt, the ECG may show LVH and the CXR will demonstrate cardiac enlargement and pulmonary plethora. Patients with moderate to large shunts may develop atrial arrhythmias, left heart failure, and pulmonary hypertension, including the development of the Eisenmenger syndrome. In patients with the Eisenmenger syndrome, the continuous murmur disappears as the aortic-to-pulmonary pressure gradient decreases. Patients with Eisenmenger syndrome secondary to a PDA have preferential shunting of deoxygenated blood to the descending thoracic aorta through the ductus while oxygenated blood is ejected into the ascending aorta. This leads to the differential cyanosis, with cyanosis and clubbing in the feet but not in the upper extremities. Because of the proximity of the left subclavian artery to the ductus, there may be some clubbing and cyanosis in the left hand. All patients are at risk for endarteritis, regardless of the size of the shunt. An exception to this rule is the "silent ductus," which refers to a trivial shunt seen by color flow Doppler without an associated murmur. A "silent ductus" has no hemodynamic significance, and the risk of endocarditis is extremely low (83).

Echocardiography demonstrates continuous flow from the aorta to the pulmonary artery by color Doppler. Direct visualization of the ductus by echocardiography is usually possible in children but difficult in adults. The aortic-to-pulmonary artery pressure gradient can be measured from the continuous-wave Doppler tracings. The presence of other associated congenital defects should be a routine part of the exam. The diagnosis can also be made and/or confirmed at cardiac catheterization by the presence of an oxygen saturation step-up at the level of the pulmonary artery and demonstration of the ductus by aortography.

In premature infants, closure of the ductus arteriosus can be promoted with the use of indomethacin (once coarctation and ductal-dependent congenital defects are excluded) (84). Closure of the ductus is generally recommended for all shunt sizes (except silent PDA) to reduce the risk of endarteritis as well as that of LV volume overload in moderate to large shunts (85). Closure of a PDA is contraindicated in the setting of Eisenmenger physiology.

Closure of a PDA can usually be accomplished with percutaneous closure devices. The Rashkind double umbrella device was introduced in 1979 and had an occlusion rate of 82.5% at 1 year and 94.8% at 20 months but a fairly high rate of complications. The device is not currently approved by the Food and Drug Administration (FDA) (86). Coils may be used to close a PDA. Coils have been available since 1976 (never applied for FDA approval) and can be deployed using small delivery systems. Closure rates of 93% to 97% have been reported with coil embolization after 6-month follow-up (87,88). Embolization into the pulmonary circulation was reported in 3% to 8% of initial studies (87–89), but the incidence is lower after modifications in technique (90–93). The Amplatzer duct occluder has shown excellent early outcomes, with a 98% closure rate at 6 months (94). The U.S. experience with the Amplatzer device reported in 2004 demonstrated a 99% success rate for device implant, with 76% occlusion on initial angiogram, 89% occlusion by postprocedure day 1, and 99.7% occlusion at 1 year. Serious adverse events were seen in 2.3% of cases (95). Patients after device closure still require bacterial endocarditis prophylaxis for at least 6 months, lifelong if there is a residual shunt. There are rare reported cases of hemolysis after device implant (96,97).

Surgical ligation and division of the ductus can be done with low morbidity and mortality but is rarely needed (98–100). Surgical closure is required for a PDA that is too large for device closure and for those patients with distorted ductal anatomy (e.g. aneurysm or calcification).

A patient with a PDA repaired in childhood can be considered "cured." Patients repaired in adolescence or adulthood remain at risk for complications such as pulmonary hypertension, LV dysfunction, and arrhythmias and should have routine follow-up. Although rare, an aneurysm of the PDA may occur with risk of rupture. The natural history of device closure is unknown. Intermittent follow-up is advisable.

Atrioventricular Septal Defects

Partial and complete atrioventricular septal defects (AVSDs) are seen in 2% to 3% of patients with congenital heart disease. Also known as AV canal defects or endocardial cushion defects, they are characterized by a common atrioventricular junction guarded by a common atrioventricular valve. There is absence of the atrioventricular septum that separates the RA from the LV. The aorta is "unwedged" from its usual position between the atrioventricular orifices, which results in a narrowing of the subaortic region and a longer outflow dimension of the interventricular septum. There is considerable variation in the features of AVSDs, including variations in the common atrioventricular valve, differences in the degree and direction of shunting, and the relative "balance" of the atrioventricular valves and the ventricles (101). With a partial atrioventricular septal defect (partial AVSD), the common AV valve is divided into separate right and left orifices, which are separated by fusion between the superior and inferior bridging leaflets. This gives a three-leaflet appearance to the mitral valve, often mistaken as a cleft in the anterior leaflet. On echocardiography, the mitral and tricuspid valves appear at the same level at the AV junction. Partial AVSDs may have attachment of the bridging leaflets of the common AV valve to the ventricular septum, resulting in only interatrial shunting (the so-called ostium primum defect). Alternatively, the bridging leaflets may be attached to the atrial septum, resulting in only an interventricular shunt (inlet-type VSD).

With a complete atrioventricular septal defect (complete AVSD), the common AV valve "floats" between the atrial and ventricular septum, allowing shunting at both atrial and ventricular levels. Patients with a complete AVSD may have a common valve with a single orifice or may have separate left and right orifices. When the common AV valve is equally committed to both ventricles, this is referred to as a balanced defect. In unbalanced forms, there is commitment of the common AV valve to one ventricle with resultant hypoplasia of the other ventricle. Many other associated malformations may coexist, including left ventricular outflow obstruction, other congenital deformities of the AV valve, and association with other forms of congenital heart disease (e.g., tetralogy of Fallot, double-outlet right ventricle, etc.). There is a distorted arrangement of atrioventricular node (located in the posterior atrial wall) and the bundle of His (located under the inferior bridging leaflet), which makes these patients prone to conduction block.

AVSDs are particularly common in patients with Down syndrome (seen in 30% to 40% of Down patients with CHD), usually as the complete form of AVSD. Conversely, Down syndrome is present in 70% to 80% of patients with a complete AVSD (10,11). The risk of developing associated pulmonary vascular disease appears to be greater and more rapidly progressive in patients with Down syndrome (102). This is due, at least in part, to a tendency toward airway obstruction (due to macroglossia, a small hypopharynx, and poor pharyngeal muscle tone), abnormal capillary bed morphology in the lungs, and possible pulmonary hypoplasia (103,104).

The clinical presentation depends on the specific malformation (105). Partial AVSDs of the ostium primum type present similar to other ASDs, except for the unusual QRS axis (leftward and superior counterclockwise axis). Patients may have first-degree AV block as well. Partial AVSDs of the inlet VSD type present similar to other VSDs. Patients with complete AVSDs typically present with breathlessness and heart failure in infancy due to excessive pulmonary blood flow. Symptoms usually becomes manifest after PVR falls, usually within a few weeks of birth. These patients are also at significant risk for pulmonary hypertension if not repaired. The magnitude of left-to-right shunting and the degree of regurgitation through the common AV valve determine the clinical presentation. Patients with large shunts and/or significant AV valve regurgitation present earlier with symptoms of heart failure and/or evidence of pulmonary hypertension. Varying degrees of cyanosis may be present if there is significant right-to-left shunting.

The ECG in patients with a complete AVSD shows left-axis deviation due to an abnormal activation sequence of the ventricles (due to deficiency of intermediation radiation of left bundle branch). First-degree AV block is common, and right-bundle-branch block and right ventricular hypertrophy (RVH) are invariably present. Left ventricular hypertrophy (LVH) may be present as well. The CXR shows cardiomegaly and pulmonary plethora.

Echocardiography places a critical role in the diagnosis, including the anatomy and function of the common AV valve, the location and degree of intracardiac shunts, the balance of the ventricles, and the presence of other associated conditions (106). Cardiac catheterization with angiography is often warranted to assess hemodynamic parameters and the magnitude of the intracardiac shunts. In patients with significant pulmonary hypertension, a lung biopsy is occasionally required to determine operability.

Surgical repair should be undertaken at the time of diagnosis if pulmonary vascular disease is not prohibitive. Surgical repair of complete AV septal defects is complex, requiring closure of the shunts and creation of two competent AV valves (107,108). In some cases, a pulmonary artery band is placed to prevent pulmonary hypertension if repair of the defect cannot be performed.

When diagnosis of made in adolescence or adulthood, there is usually a partial AV septal defect or the patient has developed severe pulmonary vascular obstructive disease. Patients who present in adulthood with a partial AVSD are usually candidates for surgery (109). Device closure is not an option. Patients with a complete AVSD and severe pulmonary hypertension should be treated as having Eisenmenger physiology once the diagnosis is confirmed.

The long-term outcome after surgical repair is good (110,111). All patients are at risk for endocarditis and require antibiotic prophylaxis. Despite a good prognosis after surgery, patients remain at risk for left-sided AV valve regurgitation and need long-term follow-up. Surgical series have indicated that as many as 10% to 12% of patients will need further surgery for left-sided AV valve regurgitation. Patients may also have a residual VSD, may develop subaortic or subpulmonary obstruction, or may develop progressive pulmonary vascular disease (especially with "late" closure of VSD). Patients are also at risk for development of complete heart block, sinus node dysfunction, and atrial arrhythmias. Sudden death has been reported, although the risk is largely unknown.

Aortopulmonary Window

The aortopulmonary window is a rare form of congenital heart disease, manifested by a communication between the ascending aorta and the pulmonary trunk above the level of the coronary arteries (112,113). An aortopulmonary window can occur as an isolated defect but is often associated with other anomalies. The defect is usually very large, resulting in a large left-to-right shunt and a high likelihood of developing pulmonary hypertension. Thus, patients usually present in infancy with symptoms of heart failure or with cyanosis due to pulmonary hypertension with right-to-left shunting. The diagnosis is made by echocardiography demonstrating the defect and the associated shunting. Occasionally, defects may be small enough to be closed with catheter intervention (114), but surgical closure is required for the majority (115–117). Presentation in adulthood is nearly always associated with the Eisenmenger syndrome.

Partial Anomalous Pulmonary Venous Connection

Partial anomalous pulmonary venous connection is defined as one or more (but not all) pulmonary veins connecting to a systemic vein, the RA, or the coronary sinus. Examples include connection of the right upper lobe and right middle lobe veins to the SVC, right upper lobe and right middle lobe veins to the RA, right pulmonary veins to the IVC, right lower lobe vein to the IVC (scimitar syndrome), left upper or lower pulmonary veins to the coronary sinus, and left lower pulmonary veins to the RA or IVC (118–120).

Partial anomalous pulmonary venous connection is relatively uncommon, accounting for less than 1% of all congenital defects. An ASD is usually present, and the clinical presentation is similar to that of an uncomplicated ASD. Partial anomalous pulmonary venous connection can be seen with any type of ASD but is most commonly associated with the sinus venosus type of ASD. Other associated defects may occur. The exam findings, ECG, and CXR findings in patients with partial anomalous pulmonary venous connection are similar to those of a secundum ASD. The CXR findings in the scimitar syndrome are addressed later.

Patients are usually asymptomatic in childhood. They may remain undiagnosed in adulthood if the anomalous pulmonary venous connection is an isolated defect. If more than 50% of the total pulmonary blood flow drains to the right heart, symptoms are common. Thus, symptomatic patients usually have more than one anomalous connection or an associated lesion. Symptoms are similar to those of ASD, with dyspnea, arrhythmias, and (rarely) pulmonary hypertension. The diagnosis can be made by echocardiography if care is taken to identify the pulmonary vein connections. TEE is usually required in adult patients to adequately define the pulmonary vein anatomy (121). Cardiac MRI is an excellent tool for the diagnosis of partial anomalous pulmonary venous connections (122).

Treatment depends on the magnitude of shunting. Isolated anomalous pulmonary venous connection with a small shunt does not require surgery. For larger shunts, surgical closure of the ASD and rerouting of pulmonary venous return to the left atrium is performed to prevent long-term complications such as atrial arrhythmias, right heart failure, and pulmonary hypertension (123,124). Pulmonary venous drainage should be assessed in any patient with an ASD who is being considered for either device or surgical closure. The presence of an anomalous pulmonary venous connection is a contraindication to device closure. Inspection of the pulmonary venous connections should be a routine part of surgical closure of an ASD, and anomalous pulmonary venous connections should be repaired when present.

The long-term outcome after surgical repair of partial anomalous pulmonary venous connection is excellent. Bacterial endocarditis prophylaxis is not required after surgical repair. Obstruction of the reimplanted pulmonary veins or obstruction of the vena cava at the site of pulmonary vein explantation is uncommon but may require surgical or catheter intervention (127).

Scimitar Syndrome

The scimitar syndrome refers to the presence of anomalous drainage of the right pulmonary veins to the IVC with a characteristic appearance on CXR resembling a scimitar or Turkish sword. There is usually some degree of hypoplasia of the right lung and the right pulmonary artery, usually with an aberrant systemic artery from thoracic aorta supplying part of the right lung. Surgical correction removes the left-to-right shunt and may improve blood flow to the right lung. There is a risk of postoperative pulmonary venous obstruction (126).

Obstructive Lesions

Pulmonary Stenosis

Pulmonary stenosis (PS) is a common defect, occurring in 7% to 10% of patients with congenital heart disease. Obstruction may be subvalvular, valvar, or supravalvular. Valvar stenosis is the most common (90%). The pulmonary valve morphology varies. The valve may be unicommissural with an eccentric orifice (extremely rare), bicuspid or trileaflet with commissural fusion, or dysplastic. Dysplastic valves have markedly thickened leaflets with disorganized myxomatous tissue but minimal commissural fusion. Bicuspid or trileaflet valves with commissural fusion are usually amenable to balloon dilation or surgical valvotomy, whereas dysplastic valves are less amenable to these procedures. Dysplastic valves are commonly associated with Noonan syndrome (127). PS is usually an isolated lesion. Associated cardiac and noncardiac malformations are more common when the valve is dysplastic (128). Chronic obstruction of the right ventricular outflow tract leads to RVH, which may be particularly prominent in the infundibular region, further contributing to RV outflow tract obstruction. Severe PS presenting in infancy is associated with severe RVH and a small right ventricular cavity size. Lesser degrees of PS are associated with RVH, but the RV cavity is usually well formed. The degree of stenosis is classified by peak systolic gradient, with trivial stenosis defined as a peak gradient less than 25 mm Hg, mild stenosis with a gradient of 25 to 49 mm Hg, moderate stenosis with a gradient of 50 to 79 mm Hg, and severe stenosis with a peak gradient above 80 mm Hg.

Infants with critical PS present in neonatal period, usually with cyanosis due to right-to-left shunting across a PFO or ASD. Mortality is high in neonates with critical PS unless intervention is prompt (129). Lesser degrees of stenosis usually present later in childhood or in adulthood. Patients with trivial or mild stenosis with a peak gradient of less than 25 mm Hg have a good outcome. There is usually no significant progression of disease, and therefore no treatment is warranted. Patients with more significant stenosis may present with exertional dyspnea, chest pain, fatigue, or syncope, occasionally with cyanosis (130).

The physical exam findings in valvar PS include an RV lift, a thrill along the left sternal border, and a harsh crescendo-decrescendo systolic ejection murmur in the pulmonary area, which is louder in expiration. A systolic ejection click is often present. The intensity of P2 is reduced in patients with severe stenosis. The ECG reflects the degree of RVH (except in the neonatal period). The ECG is normal with mild degrees of obstruction and shows right-axis deviation and RVH with moderate to severe obstruction. Poststenotic dilation of the main pulmonary artery and the left pulmonary artery (due to a more parallel take-off of the left pulmonary artery) may be seen on CXR with all degrees of PS (131,132). Heart size is normal with mild to moderate obstruction, but right-sided enlargement is seen with severe stenosis. Echocardiography is the diagnostic method of choice and can demonstrate valvular and infundibular anatomy. Continuous-wave Doppler is used to quantitate the transvalvular gradient. A complete study includes an assessment of the integrity of atrial septum as well as assessment of RV size and function.

In the Second Natural History Study of Congenital Heart Defects, patients with mild PS (peak gradient 25 to 49 mm Hg) had a 20% chance of requiring intervention at some point. Patients with moderate stenosis treated medically were at risk for progressive obstruction with symptoms warranting intervention. Most patients with a peak gradient greater than 50 mm Hg required intervention, with better outcomes demonstrated in those patients undergoing intervention than in those treated medically (132).

The earliest surgical interventions on the pulmonary valve were performed using a closed technique with blunt dilation of the right ventricular outflow tract (Brock procedure). Currently, pulmonary valvotomy is performed using cardiopulmonary bypass (133). Transcatheter intervention with balloon valvuloplasty has now largely replaced operative intervention and has become the therapy of choice (134–137). Balloon valvuloplasty can be performed with a low rate of complications and outcomes similar to surgery with a similar reduction in gradient (138). An infundibular gradient may be present after successful pulmonary valvotomy but often regresses over 3 to 12 months.

Long-term outcomes for both surgical and balloon valvotomy are excellent. Long-term complications of both procedures include pulmonary regurgitation and residual or recurrent RV outflow tract obstruction. Reintervention is required in some cases for recurrent RV outflow obstruction with symptoms or significant arrhythmias. The presence of severe pulmonary regurgitation with decreasing exercise capacity, deteriorating RV function, or the development of significant arrhythmias is an indication for pulmonary valve replacement (133).

Subpulmonary stenosis is usually seen in complex defects, such as tetralogy of Fallot. Isolated subpulmonary stenosis is rare.

Supravalvular obstruction with pulmonary arterial stenosis may be seen in rubella syndrome and Williams syndrome and in association with other complex congenital cardiac defects (e.g., tetralogy of Fallot). Pulmonary arterial stenosis may also occur as an isolated defect (139,140). Stenosis may occur in the main pulmonary artery, at the bifurcation of the pulmonary artery branches, and at the secondary or more distal branches. The obstruction may be focal or diffuse (often a manifestation of more widespread vasculopathy such as rubella, cutis laxa, or Ehlers-Danlos syndrome) (141).

The clinical presentation is similar to that of valvar PS. Patients have a systolic ejection murmur, but there is no ejection click, and P2 is normal. The ECG and CXR findings are usually nonspecific. Echocardiography may demonstrate the presence of RV pressure overload and may demonstrate the site of stenosis, but the branch pulmonary arteries may be difficult to visualize by TTE. Doppler study of the main and branch pulmonary arteries is used to quantitate the severity of stenosis. CT or MRI scans offer excellent visualization of the main pulmonary artery trunk and the pulmonary artery branches (142). Angiography can also be used to demonstrate the obstruction, and the localized pressure gradient can be demonstrated at catheterization. Perfusion imaging helps in assessing perfusion imbalance. Although pulmonary artery stenosis may be managed surgically with pericardial or prosthetic patch repair to enhance stenotic vessels, stenting of pulmonary vessels is playing an increasing role (143–146).

Obstruction of the Left Ventricular Outflow Tract

Left ventricular outflow tract obstruction may occur at the level of the valve, below the valve, or in the ascending aorta. Valvar aortic stenosis (AS) is the most common cause of congenital LV outflow obstruction, and bicuspid valves are by far the most common type. The bicuspid aortic valve is usually not included in epidemiologic studies of congenital heart disease but is the most common type of congenital cardiac defect, seen in 1% to 2% of the general population (147–149). A bicuspid aortic valve results from fusion of two commissures, resulting in two rather than three valve leaflets. There is a high incidence of bicuspid valves in a mouse model of nitric oxide synthase deficiency, suggesting a role of nitric oxide in the development of the normal trileaflet aortic valve (150). Bicuspid aortic valves may be familial, but most appear to be spontaneous mutations. Bicuspid valves and coarctation of the aorta are the most common defects found in patients with Turner syndrome (XO) (151).

Considered a normal variant by some, a bicuspid aortic valve may function normally throughout life or may develop either stenosis or regurgitation. There are autopsy reports of normally functioning bicuspid valves in octogenarians (147,148). The abnormal opening of the valve leaflets is presumed to cause an abnormal flow profile across the valve, resulting in valve thickening, fibrosis, and calcification. This, in turn, may result in either progressive stenosis or regurgitation. Although it is usually an isolated abnormality, associated cardiac defects are seen in up to 20% of patients (including coarctation of the aorta, PDA, and VSD). Left-dominant coronary circulation is seen in 30% to 60% of cases. Patients with bicuspid aortic valves may have associated abnormalities within the media of the aorta, placing them at risk for aortic root dilation and dissection (149,152). The degree of aortic root abnormality may be out of proportion to the severity of the valvular dysfunction (153).

Congenital AS presenting in infancy is unusual (occurs in 10% to 15% of patients with congenital AS) and may be associated with other lesions. The valve morphology in isolated valvar AS in the neonate may be bicuspid, unicuspid, or severely dysplastic. Neonates with severe AS typically present with severe decompensation, and prompt intervention is required (154,155).

Children with less severe degrees of AS are usually asymptomatic, and the diagnosis is usually made based on the presence of a murmur. Bicuspid aortic valves are often seen in adults as an incidental finding.

Children and adults with congenital AS usually have a systolic ejection click and a systolic ejection murmur. The aortic closure sound (A2) may be normal or decreased due to decreased leaflet mobility. The second heart sound may be normal or narrowly split. Paradoxical splitting of the second heart sound may be present with severe obstruction. The ECG may be normal or may demonstrate LVH. There is poor correlation between the degree of stenosis and the ECG findings. The CXR may demonstrate a normal heart size or cardiomegaly. Poststenotic dilation of the ascending aorta may be seen.

The clinical manifestations of AS are similar for congenital and acquired forms. Chest pain, congestive heart failure symptoms, and syncope (often exertional or postexertional) are the presenting symptoms. Unlike acquired forms of AS, symptomatic congenital AS tends to present earlier in life (in the forties or fifties). In the adult population, bicuspid aortic valves account for half of all surgical cases of isolated AS. Patients with associated abnormalities of the aortic media may present with aortic root dilation, dissection, and rupture. All patients are at risk for endocarditis, particularly those with bicuspid aortic valves.

Echocardiography is the diagnostic tool of choice for the diagnosis of AS (156). Patients with a bicuspid aortic valve typically have two unequal-size aortic cusps with an eccentric closure line. Valve anatomy can be determined, and the presence of associated regurgitation or stenosis can also be demonstrated and quantitated, with assessment of the transvalvular gradient, and calculation of valve area. LVH and LV function (both systolic and diastolic) should be assessed.

Cardiac catheterization is usually reserved for patients in whom either surgical or catheter intervention is contemplated or for additional quantitation of the severity of valvular disease. Coronary angiography is usually performed in patients older than the age of 40 years. Visualization of the aortic root by echo, angiography, or MRI is an important part of the diagnostic evaluation. All patients with congenital AS need bacterial endocarditis prophylaxis. The indications for catheter or surgical intervention differ between the pediatric and adult populations. In children, there is a risk of sudden death in the absence of definable symptoms related to the aortic valve disease. For this reason, catheter or surgical intervention is recommended for those patients with severe stenosis as defined by a valve area of less than 0.5 cm^2/m^2 or a mean gradient of greater than 50 mm Hg (157). Exercise testing is also used, with the development of ST-segment depression or significant ventricular ectopy considered to be a reasonable indication for intervention. For mild stenosis (gradient $<$40 mm Hg), observation is recommended because the risk of sudden death is low.

In the adult population, the indications for surgical intervention are the same as for those patients with acquired forms of AS, namely chest pain, congestive heart failure, and syncope.

Unlike the pediatric population, sudden death occurs rarely in asymptomatic adult patients with AS (158). In symptomatic adults, survival is poor without surgical intervention, with 5-year survival rates ranging from 15% to 50%. Because of the associated aortic root abnormalities, the initial presentation of a patient with a bicuspid aortic valve may be in the setting of aortic dissection or rupture (149,153).

In the pediatric and adolescent populations, balloon valvotomy is a reasonable option for many patients. Successful balloon valvotomy requires a pliable, noncalcified valve. Surgical options in the pediatric age group include valvotomy and valve replacement. The Ross procedure is usually preferred in the pediatric population because of the potential for growth of the "neoaortic" valve in proportion to patient's somatic growth. In adolescents and young adults, balloon valvotomy may be an option if the valve appears pliable and has little or no calcification. In most adult patients, there is usually significant calcification and leaflet thickening, making balloon and surgical valvotomy unattractive. Thus, aortic valve replacement is usually required. Late complications of both balloon valvotomy and surgical valvotomy are well recognized. Series of surgical valvotomy have similar outcomes to catheter-based procedures, with a 40% to 50% incidence of reoperation for recurrent stenosis or regurgitation (159–168). Aortic regurgitation is common postvalvuloplasty (either surgical or balloon). The degree of aortic regurgitation (AR) is usually mild, but it is moderate in 20% to 30% of cases, with a potential to progress over time. LV dysfunction may occur, usually in patients with a later age at repair and/or a history of prolonged, severe obstruction. The reported risk of sudden death in the postsurgical valvotomy population is 0.4% per year, usually associated with residual or progressive aortic valve disease (169). All patients remain at risk for endocarditis.

Subaortic stenosis may take many forms, ranging from a discrete fibrous or muscular ridge to a more diffuse (tunnel) form of muscular hypertrophy (170–174). Subaortic obstruction may be isolated or may occur in association with other defects (in 60%). The most common associated defects are VSD, coarctation, Shone syndrome, PDA, and valvar AS. Subaortic obstruction occurs due to an accumulation of fibroelastic tissue and may be an acquired lesion. Subtle abnormalities of the LV outflow tract may result in altered shear stress, triggering cell proliferation (175). Progression of stenosis is common, although the rate of progression is variable and often difficult to predict (176–180). Downstream turbulent flow may result in damage to the aortic leaflets, resulting in aortic regurgitation in as many as 50% of patients (181).

The clinical presentation varies. Patients with mild obstruction are usually asymptomatic. Dyspnea, chest pain, or syncope is seen with moderate to severe obstruction. The diagnosis is made by echocardiography demonstrating narrowing of the LV outflow tract. A discrete membrane may be visualized, or there may be more diffuse narrowing and obstruction. Measurement of the severity of subaortic stenosis by Doppler is accurate, with discrete forms of obstruction, but it may be inaccurate in long, tunnel-like stenosis. Cardiac catheterization is used to measure the subaortic gradient and to visualize the subvalvular anatomy by angiography. Management is controversial for asymptomatic patients. Patients are at risk for progressive obstruction and progressive aortic valve damage. Some experts suggest waiting for symptoms, whereas others propose early intervention to prevent aortic valve damage (182–185). In general, a resting gradient greater than 50 mm Hg and/or progressive AR are indications for surgery. Surgery is more complicated for tunnel-type stenosis, which has a higher operative mortality (186). In addition to resection of subaortic tissue, some patients may need augmentation of the LV outflow tract (aortoventriculoplasty or Konno procedure). These patients are at risk for complete AV block as a complication of surgery. All patients are at risk for progressive AR, even after successful relief of subaortic obstruction, which occurs in as many as 25% to 40% of cases. Recurrence of LV outflow tract obstruction after successful surgical excision occurs frequently, and is reported to be as high as 27% (182–187).

Supravalvular AS is the rarest form of LV outflow tract obstruction, and is caused by a variety of different pathologic lesions. All forms of supravalvular obstruction tend to progress over time. Supravalvular AS is frequently seen in Williams syndrome (supravalvar AS, intellectual impairment, and distinct facial features) (188,189). Supravalvular stenosis may also occur as an isolated sporadic case and occasionally in familial form. The most common manifestation is narrowing of aorta at the level of the sinotubular junction. There is potential for involvement of the coronary artery ostia, including dilation of coronary arteries and obstruction (190,191), aneurysms of the ascending aorta (192), pulmonary artery stenosis (193), and involvement of other major arterial branches, including the cerebral circulation (194,195). The aortic valve is abnormal in 35% to 50% of cases, with bicuspid valves and aortic regurgitation or stenosis. The diagnosis of supravalvar obstruction may be made by echocardiography, MRI, or catheterization.

Surgery is performed for all symptomatic patients. Other indications for intervention include a gradient of greater than 50 mm Hg or progressive aortic valve dysfunction in asymptomatic patients. Surgery involves relieving obstruction while preserving aortic root geometry and aortic valve function. The Ross procedure is often recommended for those patients requiring aortic valve replacement. Recurrence of supravalvular stenosis is uncommon after repair. Reoperation is required in 17% to 40% of patients undergoing surgery at an early age, usually aortic valve replacement for progressive AR (196–199).

Coarctation of the Aorta

Coarctation of the aorta is defined as a narrowing or obstruction of the aortic arch. Coarctation is a common defect and occurs in 8% to 10% of all congenital defects; it is more common in male than in female individuals (2:1) (33,200). Aortic coarctation may occur in isolation but is often associated with other congenital defects (bicuspid aortic valve in up to 85% of cases; also VSD and mitral valve abnormalities). Aortic coarctation is common in Turner syndrome, occurring in 30% of cases.

Aortic obstruction usually occurs at the level of the ligamentum arteriosus and is due to thickened intima and increased tissue in the media consisting of collagen, smooth muscle cells, and varying degrees of elastin. A more diffuse arteriopathic process appears to be involved because some patients have a propensity to aortic aneurysm formation and dissection or may have associated aneurysms in the circle of Willis (seen in 10% of cases) (201).

The clinical presentation depends on the location and severity of the obstruction. More than half of patients present with symptoms in the first year of life. In the infantile type, systemic blood flow depends on flow through the ductus to the descending thoracic aorta. In these infants, ductal closure can result in circulatory collapse. The use of prostaglandin E_1 to maintain ductal flow is a temporizing measure, and immediate intervention is required due to the absence of adequate collateral circulation. After repair in infancy, these patients remain at risk for premature atherosclerosis, late hypertension, and premature death (202–204).

Presentation in older children and adults is different. In these patients, blood flow to the descending thoracic aorta is supplied by the LV through the ascending aorta. Collateral circulation gradually develops between the proximal and distal aorta (Fig. 30.4). These patients are usually asymptomatic and present with upper limb hypertension.

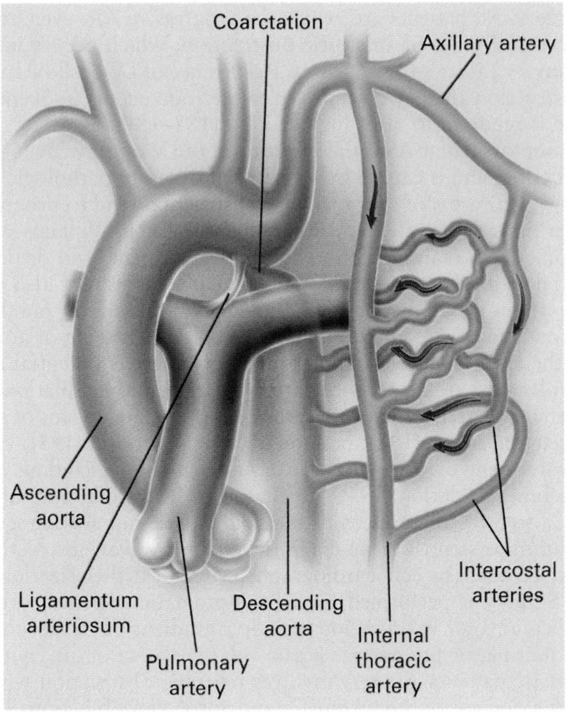

FIGURE 30.4. Coarctation of the aorta with development of extensive collaterals (internal mammary and intercostal arteries). (From Brickner ME, Hillis LD, Lange RA. Congenital heart disease in adults. *N Engl J Med* 2000;342:340.)

The physical exam findings depend on the age of presentation. In the infantile form, the infant is usually in circulatory shock and may have differential cyanosis. In adolescents and adults, the exam is remarkable for a blood pressure difference between the upper and lower extremities and diminished or absent femoral pulses. A short systolic murmur from the coarctation is common and may be heard in the left interscapular area. Faint, continuous murmurs from collateral vessels may also be audible. The ECG is often normal but may show LVH. On CXR, the heart size may be normal or mildly enlarged. Rib notching from the fourth to eighth ribs may be seen in older children and adults due to hypertrophied intercostal arteries as part of the collateral circulation (205). A "3" sign representing a pre- and poststenotic dilation of the aorta at the level of the coarctation may be seen.

Echocardiography is a good technique for the diagnosis of coarctation, demonstrating the area of obstruction in the aorta and demonstrating disturbed flow by Doppler techniques. Continuous-wave Doppler with the expanded Bernoulli equation is needed to accurately assess the degree of obstruction. For patients with severe stenosis and extensive collaterals, the Doppler gradient may underestimate the degree of obstruction due to decreased blood flow through the coarctation segment (206). MRI is excellent for demonstrating aortic anatomy and is particularly useful in the adult population in whom echocardiographic imaging of the aortic arch and descending thoracic aorta may be difficult (207,208).

The long-term outcome for patients with coarctation of the aorta is poor without intervention. Sixty percent of patients with symptomatic coarctation and 90% with complicated coarctation (associated with other lesions) will die within the first year of life without intervention (209). The average life expectancy for simple coarctation without surgery is 35 years. Presentation in adulthood suggests mild to moderate postductal coarctation.

Indications for intervention beyond the neonatal period include congestive heart failure, the presence of upper extremity hypertension, and/or a gradient greater than 20 mm Hg across the obstruction. Exercise testing may be used to provoke a gradient across the area of obstruction.

Surgery for "native" coarctation in children can be done with an end-to-end anastomosis, a subclavian flap (to augment the aortic arch), or an interposition graft (210–212). In adults, resection of the obstructed segment with end-to-end anastomosis is the procedure of choice (213–215). An interposition tube graft may be needed if there is a long segment of coarctation. A bypass jump graft is occasionally required in older patients with fragile aortic tissue or a long segment of obstruction. Postoperative complications include hypertension, abdominal pain, chylothorax, late aneurysm formation, and, rarely, spinal cord ischemia.

Percutaneous transcatheter angioplasty of native or recurrent coarctation has an increasing role. In native coarctation, balloon procedure with or without stent placement is a treatment alternative. Acute and long-term results for native aortic coarctation are similar to those of surgery (216–221), but aortoplasty is associated with higher rates of aneurysm formation and restenosis than surgery. Balloon aortoplasty appears to be a better option than surgery for recurrent coarctation (222–224). Complications of catheter procedures include femoral artery injury and thrombosis, aneurysm formation, embolic events, and, rarely, aortic rupture. Hypertension is common, even after successful relief of obstruction (202,225–227). Hypertension is seen in as many as 75% of patients after repair and is more common in those patients with older age at repair. The incidence of hypertension appears to increase with longer follow-up. Patients with normal resting blood pressure often demonstrate an abnormal blood pressure response to exercise as well as increased left ventricular mass. Although the pathophysiology is not well understood, the hypertension is likely to be related to structural changes in the central and peripheral vessel walls, abnormalities of endothelial reactivity, and alterations in the renin–angiotensin system. In some patients, there is persistent hypoplasia of the aortic arch, which contributes to persistent hypertension. Chronic hypertension places patients at risk for premature coronary artery disease (CAD), LV dysfunction, rupture of aortic or cerebral aneurysms, and sudden death. Meticulous blood pressure control is mandatory. β-Blockers are usually recommended as first-line therapy, although there are no randomized trials.

Lifelong follow-up with imaging of the aorta is mandatory but not often employed. Even after successful "repair," there is evidence of ongoing morbidity and mortality in these patients (203,228). In one long-term follow-up of postoperative coarctation repair, the overall 30-year survival was only 72%. Thirteen percent of patients required reoperation for either aortic valve replacement or recurrent coarctation (228). Residual or recoarctation may be seen in 3% to 41% of patients and can occur with any surgical technique or after angioplasty (seen in 8% to 11% of patients undergoing angioplasty for native coarctation). Residual or recurrent obstruction is associated with hypertension, increased LV mass, and the development of CAD and congestive heart failure (229). Angioplasty is usually recommended for recoarctation after previous surgery, with a good success rate (65% to 100%) and an acceptable (13%) complication rate (222–224). Stents are increasingly being used for recurrent coarctation, although only short-term data are available (230,232).

Patients may have aneurysm formation at site of repair (seen in 5% to 9% of surgical patients and 4% to 12% of patients after balloon procedures) and are also at risk for dissection and rupture. Both repaired and unrepaired patients may have evidence of a diffuse arteriopathy of the aorta of unclear etiology and may develop aneurysm formation and dissection at a site remote from the original site of coarctation (201). All patients (repaired and unrepaired) are at risk for endarteritis or endocarditis on an associated bicuspid valve. As many as 10% of patients with coarctation of the aorta will have aneurysms of circle of Willis. Their growth appears to be promoted by uncontrolled hypertension. Screening for intracranial aneurysms is not routinely recommended.

Interruption of the Aortic Arch

Interruption of the aortic arch is defined as the absence of continuity between the transverse arch and the descending thoracic aorta. This uncommon defect produces symptoms in the neonatal period as the ductus arteriosus closes (233). There are rare cases of survival to adulthood. Interrupted aortic arch may be associated with DiGeorge syndrome (234,235) and is nearly always associated with other defects (e.g.,VSD, PDA, and complex defects). The diagnosis is made by echocardiography. Prostaglandin E_1 is administered to maintain ductal patency and to temporize until surgery can be performed (236–238). After repair, patients may develop LV outflow obstruction and obstruction at the site of the surgical repair (239).

Other Obstructive Lesions

Shone Syndrome. Left ventricular inflow and outflow obstructive lesions frequently occur together. Shone syndrome was originally described as supravalvular mitral membrane, parachute mitral valve, subaortic stenosis, and coarctation of the aorta. Currently, the term Shone syndrome is applied to patients with some or all of these features (240).

Congenital Mitral Stenosis. Congenital mitral stenosis is rare. When present, it often coexists with other left-sided stenotic lesions (i.e., LV outflow tract obstruction and coarctation of the aorta) (241). The obstruction may be supravalvular, at the annulus, at the leaflet margins, or at the level of the chordae and papillary muscle. Typically, congenital mitral stenosis has rolled leaflet edges, short, thick chordae, and hypoplastic papillary muscles. If the papillary muscles fuse to form a single papillary muscle, the term "parachute" mitral valve is applied (242). The age at presentation depends on the severity of obstruction and the presence of other associated lesions. Congenital mitral stenosis is usually diagnosed in childhood, rarely in adulthood. Patients typically present with symptoms of heart failure and signs of pulmonary hypertension. Echocardiography is diagnostic (243). Treatment consists of medical management, with surgery for symptoms refractory to medical management (244,245). Balloon valvotomy may be considered, but results are less satisfactory than for rheumatic mitral stenosis (246–248). There are limited data on long-term surgical outcomes (249).

Cor Triatriatum. Cor triatriatum is a rare congenital defect in which a membrane divides the LA into a superior pulmonary venous chamber and an inferior chamber including the LA appendage and inflow portion of the LA. This occurs due to embryologic failure of the common pulmonary vein to become incorporated into the LA. An associated ASD is common, either above or below the membrane, but the atrial septum may be intact (250–252). From 70% to 80% of patients have other associated defects. The clinical presentation depends on the severity of obstruction (size of the orifice) and the presence of associated defects (253).

Patients may present in infancy or adulthood. Patients presenting in infancy have dyspnea, cyanosis, exercise intolerance, and failure to thrive. Patients who present in adulthood may have atrial arrhythmias, dyspnea, syncope, chest pain, or symptoms caused by pulmonary hypertension. The diagnosis may be also be made incidentally during echocardiography. TTE or TEE demonstrates a nonmobile membrane in the left atrium. Echocardiography is also used to define the location, size, and number of membrane openings, the transmembrane gradient, and the presence of associated defects including anomalies of pulmonary venous connection. In some cases, it may be necessary to volume load the patient in order to assess the significance of the transmembrane gradient. Surgical excision is therapy of choice (254). There is a high mortality in symptomatic patients who do not undergo intervention. Reoperation is rarely necessary.

Pulmonary Vein Stenosis. Congenital pulmonary vein stenosis and atresia is uncommon, usually consisting of diffuse hypoplasia of the pulmonary veins. Surgical results are disappointing, with recurrence of stenosis and progressive pulmonary hypertension commonly seen after surgery (255–259). Transcatheter approaches with balloon dilation have also been disappointing. There is some preliminary data suggesting that cutting balloon technology may be helpful.

Vascular Rings. Vessels encircling the trachea and the esophagus cause vascular rings. In contrast, vascular slings partially encircle these structures. Compression of the trachea and esophagus may cause dysphagia, wheezing, and respiratory distress, or these vascular abnormalities may be incidental findings. Imaging by echocardiography or magnetic resonance imaging is usually diagnostic (260,261).

Complex Lesions

Transposition Complexes

In transposition complexes, the great arteries arise from the wrong ventricles (ventriculoarterial discordance), with the aorta arising from the RV and the pulmonary artery from the LV. The aorta is usually anterior to the pulmonary artery, and there are many variations in the spatial relationship of the two great vessels. The terms D and L refer to the cardiac loop or position of the ventricles.

Complete Transposition

In complete transposition of the great arteries (also known as D-transposition), there is atrioventricular concordance (the RA connected to the RV and the LA to the LV) but ventriculoarterial discordance (the RV connected to the aorta and the LV to the pulmonary artery). This results in two parallel circulations. Complete transposition is the second-most-common cyanotic lesion overall and the most common cyanotic lesion presenting in neonates (33,200). Two thirds of patients are male.

Most cases are not associated with a specific gene defect. There is an increased incidence in infants of diabetic mothers, leading to speculation that complete transposition may be related to a maternal intrauterine hormone imbalance (262). Associated defects are common. From 60% to 70% of patients with complete transposition have an intact ventricular septum, whereas 30% to 40% have a moderate to large VSD (263). Other abnormalities may be present, including LV outflow tract obstruction (subpulmonary obstruction), which is seen in 25% of cases, and coarctation of the aorta, which is seen in 5%.

With complete transposition and intact ventricular septum, there is complete separation of the pulmonary and systemic circulations, and the only intracardiac mixing occurs through the foramen ovale and the ductus arteriosus (Fig. 30.5). Because the foramen ovale allows only limited interatrial shunting, the infant is dependent on shunting through the ductus arteriosus.

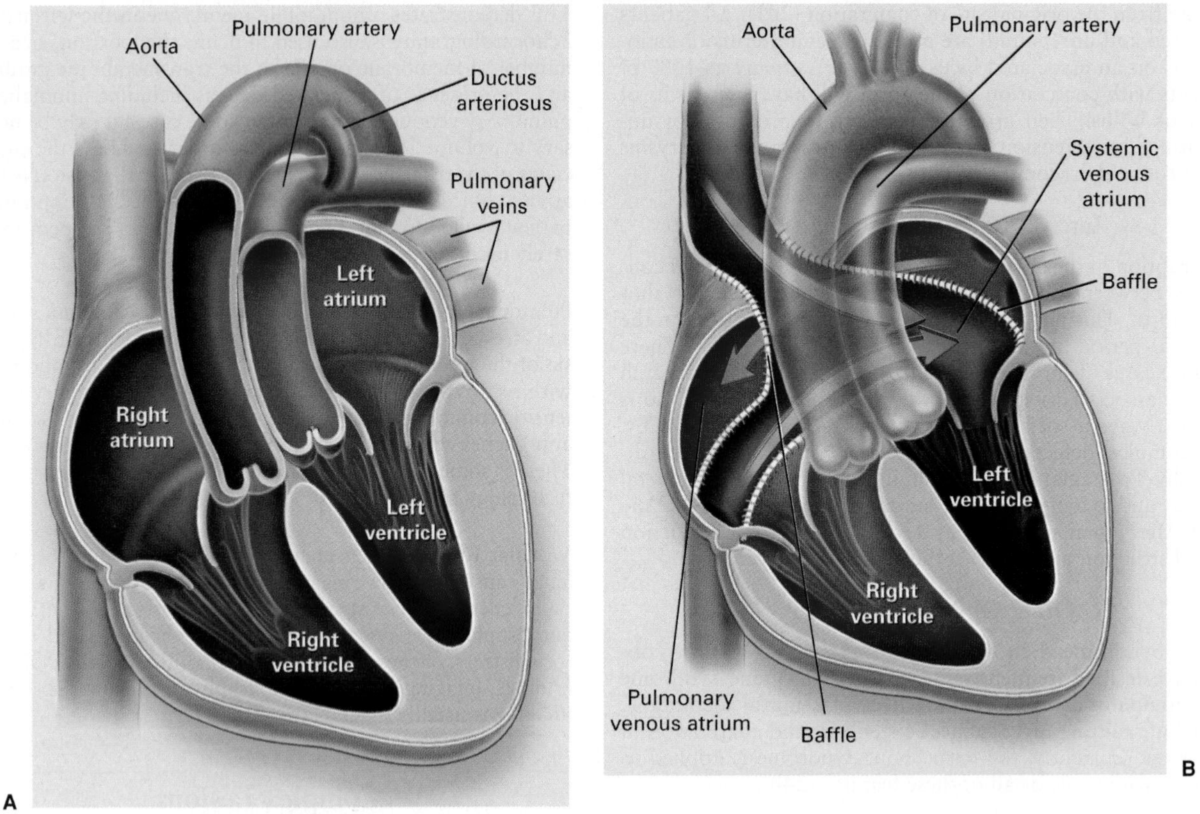

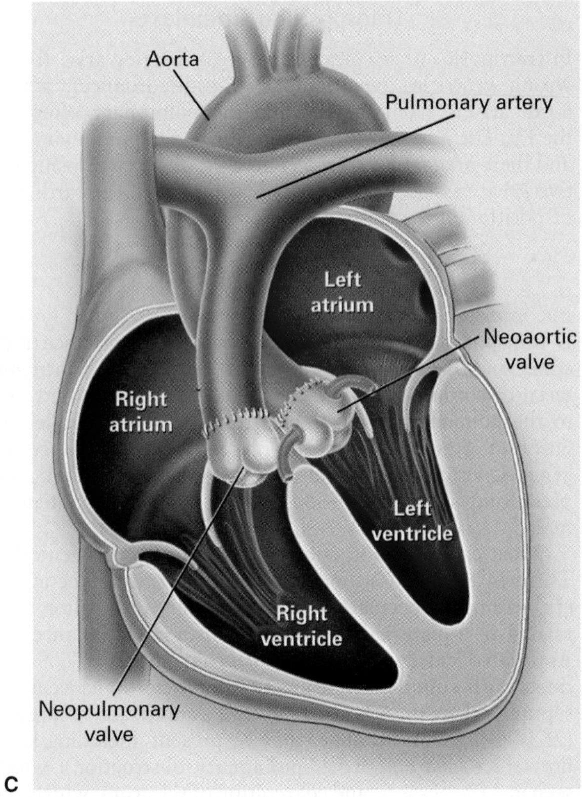

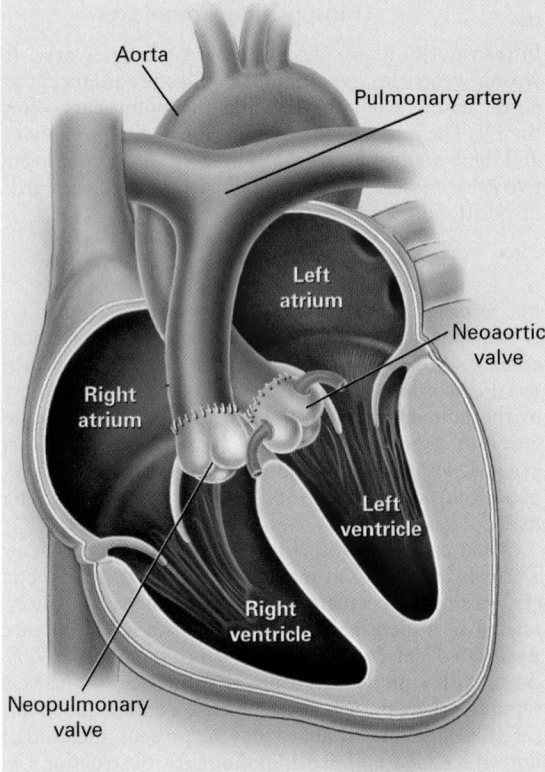

FIGURE 30.5. Complete transposition and operative repair. **A:** Basic anatomy of complete transposition with intact ventricular septum. Systemic venous blood returns to the right ventricle and to the aorta while pulmonary venous blood returns to the left ventricle and the pulmonary artery. There is complete separation of systemic and pulmonary circulations. **B:** The atrial switch procedure redirects systemic venous blood to the pulmonary artery (through the left ventricle) and pulmonary venous blood to the aorta (through the right ventricle). **C:** The arterial switch operation results in complete physiologic repair with creation of neoaortic and neopulmonary vessels. Coronary arteries are relocated to the neoaorta. (From Brickner ME, Hillis LD, Lange RA. Congenital heart disease in adults. *N Engl J Med* 2000;342:340.)

These infants are severely cyanotic within hours to days after birth. Without intervention, mortality is 90% in the first year of life (264). Treatment involves prostaglandin E_1 to maintain patency of ductus and balloon atrial septostomy to improve oxygenation by increasing intracardiac mixing (265–267). Patients with complete transposition and a VSD tend to have less cyanosis and be less critically ill in the neonatal period.

The cardiac exam in neonates with complete transposition is remarkable for severe cyanosis, no murmur, and a single S2. The ECG typically shows RVH and right-axis deviation, and the CXR shows cardiomegaly with increased pulmonary vascular markings. Although the ECG and CXR findings are suggestive, the diagnosis is made by echocardiography (268–270). Cardiac catheterization may be performed to define anatomy but is usually not required.

Surgery during the late 1950s and early 1960s was performed using the atrial switch procedure (the Senning or Mustard procedure) (271,272) (Fig. 30.5B). These procedures rerouted venous return to allow systemic venous flow to be returned to the LV and then ejected into the pulmonary artery and pulmonary venous blood to be returned to the RV and ejected into the aorta. The Senning procedure used right atrial wall and atrial septal tissue to create the baffle, whereas the Mustard procedure used pericardium or synthetic material to create the baffle. Although they were lifesaving, many long-term complications of these procedures have been described.

Sinus node dysfunction is common after the atrial switch procedure. Late loss of sinus rhythm has been estimated to occur at a rate of 2.4% per year (273). In one series, 72% of patients remained in sinus rhythm at 1 year after surgery, 56% at 5 years, 50% at 10 years, and 43% at 13 years (274). The heart rate response to exercise is variable. Exercise capacity in post–atrial switch patients is usually reduced relative to normal, with chronotropic incompetence the most common limitation (275). In the absence of symptoms, a resting heart rate less than 40 beats per minute while awake or less than 30 beats per minute while asleep has been proposed as an indication for permanent pacing (276). Pacemaker implantation is usually done by a transvenous approach. In post–atrial switch patients, it is critical to evaluate for baffle leaks (transvenous leads relatively contraindicated) or SVC baffle stenosis before attempting transvenous lead placement (277). When present, baffle obstruction can frequently be managed with balloon dilation and stenting (278). Transvenous lead placement may be challenging due to the postoperative anatomy and is best performed by an operator experienced in congenital heart disease.

Supraventricular tachycardia, often an intraatrial reentrant tachycardia or atrial fibrillation, occurs in up to 50% of patients after the atrial switch procedure (273,274,279–281). Although catheter ablation may be successful in these patients, it is technically very challenging due to the postoperative anatomy (276).

Right ventricular dysfunction is major concern in post–atrial switch patients. In most series, 10% to 20% of patients are reported to develop severe RV dysfunction (280–287). Abnormal coronary perfusion in the setting of RVH has been suggested as a possible etiology for the development of RV dysfunction (288). Tricuspid regurgitation is common after the atrial switch operation, usually seen in the setting of systemic ventricular dysfunction. Although medical therapy (angiotensin-converting-enzyme inhibitors and β-blockers) for RV dysfunction is commonly used, there are no systematic studies of their efficacy (289,290). Attempts to convert these patients to a late arterial switch (removal of atrial baffle, recreation of atrial septum, and "switching" the great arteries) has been proposed by some but appears to be associated with high mortality (291–293). Transplantation remains the other surgical option for patients with symptomatic systemic ventricular dysfunction.

Reoperation is needed in as many as 20% of cases for baffle complications (usually obstruction), progressive subpulmonary outflow obstruction, or tricuspid (systemic AV valve) insufficiency (277,294). Late development of pulmonary vascular disease occurs in 7% of cases and is more common in patients undergoing late repair or in patients with a ventricular septal defect (295).

Late-term studies have demonstrated an increased mortality after the atrial switch operation. The 20-year survival rate was 76% in one series and 80% in another series (281,285). The most common mechanism of death was sudden death, followed by systemic RV failure. The incidence of late death is 2.7 times higher for patients with complete transposition and a VSD as compared to patients with an intact ventricular septum. The incidence of sudden death has been reported to range from 2% to 3% (273) to as high as 16% (296). Risk factors for sudden death include systemic (right) ventricular dysfunction, tricuspid regurgitation (systemic AV valve), and atrial arrhythmias.

Patients who have undergone an atrial switch procedure are challenging to manage. Routine arrhythmia surveillance with Holter and exercise treadmill testing every 1 to 2 years is recommended. Pacemakers are indicated for symptomatic bradycardia, and electrophysiologic study is recommended for patients with syncope. New arrhythmias should also prompt a search for hemodynamic derangement, often a change in right ventricular function. Serial imaging studies to follow RV function are recommended, and serial cardiopulmonary stress tests are useful for following functional capacity (297).

In 1975, the arterial switch operation with coronary relocation began to replace the atrial switch procedure (Fig. 30.5C). With this procedure, the great arteries are transected above the aortic and pulmonary valves and "switched," then the coronaries are removed from the aorta and implanted into the neoaorta. Since the 1980s, the arterial switch has been performed in infancy (often in the neonatal period) with very low mortality (298–301). Although it is technically challenging, there are far fewer long-term complications than with the atrial switch procedure. Potential long-term complications of the arterial switch operation include pulmonary artery stenoses, supraaortic obstruction (rare), and abnormalities of the neoaortic valve and aortic root. Neoaortic valve regurgitation and mild degrees of aortic root dilation are possible but are usually mild (302). Patients have a potential risk of coronary abnormalities (including ostial narrowing if ostial growth is impaired). In one prospective angiographic study, coronary artery abnormalities were seen in 18% of patients, including coronary occlusions and major stenoses. Coronary abnormalities may be related to specific surgical techniques and may be treated with surgical revascularization or catheter techniques (303,304). After the arterial switch operation, the LV is left in the systemic circulation, and normal LV function is seen in greater than 95% of patients postoperatively.

There is limited long-term survival data. One review of more than 1,000 survivors showed an 88% survival at 10 and 15 years with isolated complete transposition and 80% for transposition with associated lesions (302). Sinus node dysfunction and heart block are uncommon. Supraventricular arrhythmias are uncommon (seen in 5% or cases in one series), and ventricular tachycardia is rare (0.5%) (305). Sudden death is unusual. Most cases of sudden death are related to coronary obstruction and myocardial infarction.

The Rastelli operation is used for patients with complete transposition complicated by pulmonary outflow obstruction and a VSD (306). This procedure involves baffling blood flow from the LV through the VSD to the aorta and inserting a conduit between the RV and the pulmonary artery while the pulmonary valve/subpulmonary region is oversewn. Although the LV is left in the systemic circulation, the development of conduit stenosis is inevitable, necessitating further surgeries for conduit replacement. Long-term survival rate after the Rastelli operation is 82% at 5 years, 80% at 10 years, 68% at 15 years, and 52% at 20 years (307). Patients undergoing the Rastelli operation are at risk for supraventricular and ventricular arrhythmias, heart block, and sudden death. Left ventricular dysfunction occurs in up to 25% of patients at late follow-up. Right ventricular dysfunction is also common, often related to conduit dysfunction (307).

Congenitally Corrected Transposition

Congenitally corrected transposition is characterized by atrioventricular and ventriculoarterial discordance, resulting in systemic venous return to the RA, LV, and pulmonary artery, and pulmonary venous return to the LA, RV, and aorta (308–311). Thus, the tricuspid valve and the RV are in the systemic circulation. The aorta is positioned anterior and leftward of the pulmonary artery. Also known as L-transposition or ventricular inversion, congenitally corrected transposition is uncommon, occurring in less than 1% of patients. Associated defects are common, with VSD, pulmonary outflow tract obstruction, and morphologic abnormalities of the tricuspid valve seen most commonly. An Ebstein-type malformation of the tricuspid valve may be seen, and tricuspid regurgitation (systemic AV valve regurgitation) is likely to progress with time (312–317). Other defects may occur, including ASD, PDA, double-outlet right ventricle, and subaortic stenosis. The AV node and bundle of His are abnormally located in patients with congenitally corrected transposition, placing patients at risk for conduction system abnormalities. Patients are particularly prone to develop spontaneous heart block (occurs in 2% to 4% of patients per year) (318) or complete heart block with surgery (318–320). Left-sided accessory bypass tracts with preexcitation and AV reentrant tachycardia are seen in 2% to 4% of cases. Dextrocardia is present in 20%. The diagnosis may be made by echocardiography, angiography, and cardiac MRI.

Infants and children with congenitally corrected transposition may present with congestive heart failure, usually in the setting of a large VSD or severe tricuspid regurgitation. Treatment includes initial medical management, followed by surgical repair. VSD closure is performed with sutures placed on the RV side to avoid heart block. Tricuspid valve repair is rarely successful in these patients, and tricuspid valve replacement is usually required. Children with a VSD and severe pulmonary outflow obstruction usually present with cyanosis. Initial management often includes a shunt in infancy, followed by surgical repair done at a later stage (321). These patients often require placement of a conduit to relieve pulmonary outflow obstruction and thus will require further surgery for conduit replacement at some point. The "double-switch" operation may be undertaken, which includes an atrial switch combined with a baffle to direct blood from the LV to the aorta (intraventricular Rastelli) and a RV-to-pulmonary artery conduit (322–324). The double-switch operation is complicated, and the long-term outcome is largely unknown. Complications include conduit obstruction, baffle obstruction, and rhythm problems.

Patients with isolated congenitally corrected transposition (no associated defects) may remain symptom-free until well into adulthood. There are some cases of survival into the seventh and eight decades. Symptoms occur in more than 50% of patients in adulthood, with heart block, tricuspid regurgitation, congestive heart failure, and supraventricular arrhythmias commonly seen (314,325,326). Complete heart block is seen in 24% to 39% of cases, tricuspid regurgitation in 40% to 44%, and congestive heart failure in 17% to 34%. From 30% to 50% of adults with congenitally corrected transposition will require surgery over long-term follow-up (315–329). All patients are at risk for progressive dysfunction of the systemic ventricle (morphologic RV), regardless of the presence of associated anomalies (326,329).

Permanent pacing is required for complete heart block, with DDD mode preferred due to the presence of the RV as the systemic ventricle. Transvenous pacing should be avoided in the presence of an uncorrected shunt. Surgery is indicated for closure of a VSD, relief of subpulmonary obstruction, and repair or replacement of tricuspid valve for severe regurgitation. (330). The timing of tricuspid valve surgery is difficult due in part to the difficulty in assessing RV function. The presence of moderate or greater tricuspid regurgitation in the face of diminishing RV function is an indication for tricuspid valve surgery. The preoperative ejection fraction is predictive of postoperative survivorship, with a poor outcome associated with an RV ejection fraction less than 40% to 45%, thus emphasizing the importance of timely surgical referral (327). Some surgeons have proposed the "double-switch" operation to restore the LV to the systemic circulation. This complicated procedure involves rerouting the systemic and pulmonary venous return to the right and left atria, respectively (atrial switch), and connecting the LV to the aorta and the RV to the pulmonary artery (arterial switch). In many cases, a pulmonary artery band must be placed first to promote hypertrophy of the LV and "prepare" it to tolerate systemic pressure. Surgical procedures may be quite complex, and experience is limited (331–334).

Tetralogy of Fallot

Tetralogy of Fallot is the most common cyanotic malformation, accounting for 10% of all congenital heart disease (33,200). There is a slight male preponderance. Fifteen percent of patients with tetralogy of Fallot have a deletion on chromosome 22q11 (335). Tetralogy of Fallot is characterized by malalignment of the infundibular outlet septum, which results in a VSD, obstruction of the right ventricular outflow tract, and an aorta that overrides the VSD. Right ventricular hypertrophy, the fourth component, occurs as a consequence of both RV outflow obstruction and the large nonrestrictive VSD (336–338) (Fig. 30.6). Multiple variations of RV outflow obstruction can be seen, including infundibular stenosis, hypoplastic pulmonary valve annulus, bicuspid pulmonary valve, and varying

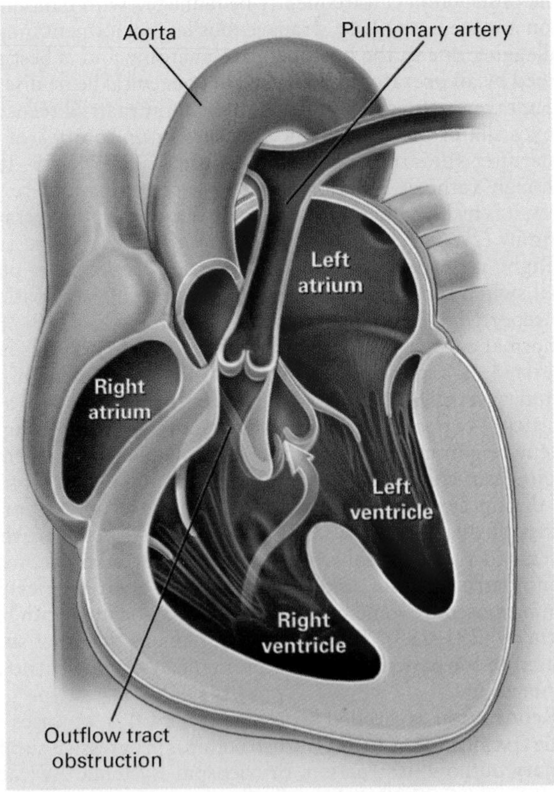

FIGURE 30.6. Tetralogy of Fallot with a large ventricular septal defect (VSD), overriding aorta, obstruction of the right ventricular outflow tract, and right ventricular hypertrophy. Right-to-left shunting is present across the VSD. (From Brickner ME, Hillis LD, Lange RA. Congenital heart disease in adults. *N Engl J Med* 2000;342:340.)

degrees of hypoplasia of the main pulmonary trunk and its branches. The branch pulmonary arteries may be confluent or nonconfluent, with origin of one vessel from the ductus or from the aorta. Alternatively, one branch pulmonary artery may be absent. Extreme variants of tetralogy of Fallot may be seen with an absent pulmonary valve (seen in DiGeorge syndrome and velocardiofacial syndrome) or with pulmonary atresia (339,340). Coronary anomalies are present in 3% of cases. The most significant of these is origin of the left coronary artery from the right coronary artery, with the left coronary artery crossing the right ventricular outflow tract (important surgical implications). From 25% to 30% of cases have a right-sided aortic arch. Multiple VSDs are seen in 5% to 7% of cases. An ASD or PFO may be present as well (pentalogy of Fallot).

Most patients present with cyanosis in infancy. Cyanosis occurs due to the right-to-left shunt across the nonrestrictive VSD and the obstruction to pulmonary blood flow. The severity of the RV outflow tract obstruction determines the severity of cyanosis. With mild degrees of RV outflow tract obstruction, patients usually have minimal cyanosis ("pink tetralogy") and may present in adulthood. In most cases, survival to adolescence and adulthood is uncommon without treatment. Only 10% of patients with unoperated tetralogy of Fallot survive to 10 years of age (341,342).

Prior to the era of surgical repair, shunts were commonly used to increase pulmonary blood flow and decrease cyanosis. Shunts used included the Pott shunt (descending thoracic aorta to left pulmonary artery), the Waterston shunt (ascending aorta to right pulmonary artery), and the Blalock-Taussig shunt (subclavian artery to pulmonary artery). These shunts were designed to decrease cyanosis but did not result in physiologic cure. Long-term complications of these shunts include pulmonary hypertension (especially with the Potts shunt), distortion of pulmonary artery branches, and LV dysfunction from chronic volume overload. Cardiologists may encounter adults with tetralogy of Fallot who have had only a palliative shunt procedure. These patients remain cyanotic and are at risk for pulmonary hypertension, biventricular dysfunction, and premature death due to heart failure or sudden cardiac death. Currently, shunts may be performed as a bridge to total repair or in patients not amenable to complete repair. Currently, most patients undergo complete repair at the time of diagnosis (343–347). Surgery involves closure of the VSD and relief of RV outflow obstruction. Corrective surgery was first performed in 1955 (348), and surgical techniques have evolved over time. Earlier approaches involved large incisions across the RV outflow tract with a transannular patch. This approach often leads to progressive pulmonary regurgitation and also places patients at risk for reentrant ventricular tachycardia originating around the patch. Current surgical techniques are designed to avoid annular incisions (349–351). Preoperative assessment for coronary anomalies is important to avoid coronary injury during surgery.

Long-term follow-up after tetralogy of Fallot repair has been reported in more than 1,000 patients, with 90% to 95% survival at an average of 10 years (352–354). The best long-term results are seen with repair before the age of 5 years. Thus, early repair is advocated without prior palliative shunts (354,355). There are smaller series of adult patients undergoing repair of tetralogy with low mortality and favorable long-term outcomes (356).

Despite fairly good long-term outcomes, patients are at risk for multiple complications, including pulmonary regurgitation, residual RV outflow obstruction, residual shunts, atrial and ventricular arrhythmias, AR with or without aortic root dilation, left and right ventricular dysfunction, and late sudden death (352,353,356). RV dysfunction is usually related to residual lesions in the RV outflow tract (obstruction or regurgitation). LV dysfunction may be secondary to chronic volume overload from prior shunts or a residual VSD or from inadequate myocardial preservation at the time of surgical repair. Reintervention is needed in approximately 10% of patients over a 20-year follow-up (357).

Pulmonary regurgitation is a particular problem in patients with repaired tetralogy of Fallot, particularly in patients with large transannular incisions or placement of a transannular patch. Pulmonary regurgitation is usually well tolerated but results in chronic volume overload of the RV, ultimately resulting in deterioration of RV function. Patients are often asymptomatic until significant RV dysfunction is present. They may present with arrhythmias (atrial or ventricular), symptoms of right heart failure, or sudden death. The timing of pulmonary valve replacement is controversial. The presence of progressive RV enlargement, worsening tricuspid regurgitation, arrhythmias, and evidence of deteriorating exercise tolerance are all indications for pulmonary valve replacement (358–363). Although pulmonary valve replacement in symptomatic patients usually results in subjective improvement, there may not be a significant change in RV volumes or systolic function. Some authors advocate early pulmonary valve replacement to reduce the risk of late morbidity and mortality (362,363).

Right-bundle-branch block is present in 80% to 90% of patients after repair, related to the right ventriculotomy. Bifasicular block is seen in 15%. The presence of bifasicular block with PR prolongation suggests a risk of high-grade block, and a permanent pacemaker is warranted. The overall risk of sudden death is small, with a reported incidence of 2% to 6%. A recent study reported a risk of sudden death of 1.2% after 10 years, 2.2% at 20 years, 4% at 25 years, and 6% at 35 years (364). A QRS width greater than 180 msec has been shown to be predictive of increased risk for sustained ventricular tachycardia and sudden death (365). The QRS width corresponds to the degree of RV enlargement and the severity of pulmonary insufficiency. The rate of QRS change with time or the QT dispersion (a difference of >60 msec between the longest and shortest QT intervals on 12-lead ECG) may be a better predictor of patients at risk for sustained ventricular arrhythmia and sudden death than QRS duration alone (365,366).

Premature ventricular contractions (PVCs) are common after repair of tetralogy of Fallot, and are seen in 40% and 60% of cases on Holter monitoring (365,367,368). Sustained ventricular tachycardia is seen in 4% to 7% of cases and may originate as a reentrant tachyarrhythmia from the right ventricular outflow tract scar (369). The prognostic significance of PVCs and nonsustained ventricular tachycardia is unclear. Currently, treatment is only recommended for symptomatic patients (368,370). The role of electrophysiologic studies is unclear. Such studies are largely used for evaluation of syncope. Failure to induce ventricular arrhythmias with programmed stimulation does not accurately predict the subsequent development of clinical ventricular arrhythmias (371). Reentrant ventricular tachycardia originating around the RV outflow tract scar may be successfully treated with ablation. However, it is not clear whether ablation will protect patients from sudden death. Current indications for implantable cardioverter defibrillator (ICD) implantation include secondary prevention of sudden death in survivors of sudden cardiac death, patients with syncope and inducible ventricular tachycardia, and those patients with sustained monomorphic ventricular tachycardia. The role of ICDs for primary prevention of sudden death has not been explored.

Atrial arrhythmias are an important cause of morbidity in patients after tetralogy repair, and are often correlated with congestive heart failure and tricuspid regurgitation (372,373). Patients may have reentrant atrial tachycardia (incision tachycardia) or atrial fibrillation or flutter. Atrial arrhythmias are seen in up to one third of adult patients and are associated with long-standing shunts, older age at surgical repair, reoperation, and the presence of moderate to severe tricuspid regurgitation. There are no good data on the choice of antiarrhythmic therapy. Reentrant atrial tachycardia and atrial flutter have been successfully ablated. The new onset of an arrhythmia should always prompt investigation of the patient's hemodynamic status, with correction of lesions as indicated (pulmonary valve replacement or tricuspid valve replacement/repair) with concomitant intraoperative cryoablation (286,373).

Recommendations vary for follow-up. Serial ECGs, Holter monitoring, and exercise testing may be useful. The patient's hemodynamic status may be a better predictor of arrhythmias and other adverse outcomes. The presence of residual/recurrent pulmonary obstruction or severe pulmonary regurgitation with RV volume overload predicts worse outcome, and these complications should be evaluated with serial imaging (374).

Ventricular Septal Defect with Pulmonary Atresia

Ventricular septal defect with pulmonary atresia is a rare lesion. It is characterized by a biventricular heart with a VSD and no continuity between the ventricular chambers and the pulmonary arterial tree. Patients must have some source of pulmonary blood supply (usually via the ductus or from collateral vessels from the aorta or its branches) (375–377). The native pulmonary arteries are often hypoplastic and may or may not communicate with one another. Some of these sources of pulmonary blood flow will be underperfused due to small size or stenosis within the vessel, whereas other sources may be "unprotected," with excessive pulmonary blood flow resulting in pulmonary vascular obstructive disease (378). Most unoperated patients die in infancy or childhood, although some survive to adulthood (379). Surgical repair is complicated due to the fragile pulmonary circulation. Multiple surgeries may be required (379–386). Long-term prognosis for these patients is more guarded than that for patients with repaired tetralogy of Fallot. Long-term surgical after repair has been reported to be 92% at 5 years, 86% at 10 years, 83% at 15 years, and 75% at 20 years in one series (387).

Pulmonary Atresia with Intact Ventricular Septum

Pulmonary atresia with intact ventricular septum is another rare congenital defect. There is either an imperforate pulmonary valve (80%) or muscular obliteration of the RV infundibulum with no pulmonary valve. There are varying degrees of hypoplasia of the tricuspid valve and the RV cavity. Pulmonary blood flow is provided through the ductus (or, less commonly, through aortopulmonary collaterals) with an obligatory right-to-left shunt at the atrial level (388). The severity of the defect ranges. Some patients have a nearly normal RV cavity with mild infundibular narrowing that is amendable to pulmonary valvotomy or catheter perforation of valve. Other patients have more significant RV hypoplasia with tricuspid stenosis. In other patients, the tricuspid valve is dysplastic or absent, with severe tricuspid regurgitation and a thinned, underdeveloped RV. In patients with severe RV hypoplasia, the high-pressure RV is decompressed through a dilated coronary circulation, the coronary sinusoids. Echocardiography is critical in the initial diagnosis (389–391), but cardiac catheterization is usually required to define the coronary circulation (392). Surgical options are complicated, and long-term survival is poor, with only 30% to 35% survival at 15 to 20 years of age (393–395). There are preliminary reports of intervention in the fetus (perforation of pulmonary valve) to permit normal growth of RV and improve long-term outcome (396).

Double-Chambered Right Ventricle

Double-chambered RV is an uncommon defect. The RV is divided or septated by muscular or fibrous structures into a high-pressure proximal chamber and a lower-pressure distal chamber (397). The RV outflow obstruction appears to be an acquired lesion, but probably results from a congenitally abnormal substrate. A double-chambered RV is often associated with a perimembranous VSD (seen in >75% of cases) (397,398). A double-chambered RV may also be seen with other abnormalities of the RV outflow tract, including valvar PS, tetralogy of Fallot, and double-outlet right ventricle. The degree of RV outflow obstruction ranges from trivial to severe. The clinical presentation depends on the size of the VSD and the degree of RV outflow obstruction, with a clinical appearance similar to that of tetralogy of Fallot. In some cases, the VSD may close spontaneously, and these patients present similarly to patients with isolated PS. Symptoms associated with double-chambered RV include exertional dyspnea, cyanosis, angina, dizziness, and syncope. The clinical exam includes an RV heave and a harsh systolic ejection murmur with a thrill. Unlike patients with tetralogy, the second heart sound is normal, with physiologic splitting. Patients may be cyanotic due to right-to-left shunting across an ASD, or PFO or may shunt right to left across the VSD proximal to the RV obstruction.

The diagnosis is made by echocardiography or MRI. The severity of obstruction can be assessed by Doppler or at catheterization. Operative intervention is recommended for those patients with "significant" obstruction. Surgery consists of resection of the obstructing muscle bundles in the RV and RV outflow tract, closure of the VSD, and repair of other associated defects (399,400).

Tricuspid Atresia

Tricuspid atresia is defined as the absence of a right-sided atrioventricular connection, usually associated with underdevelopment of the RV (absence of inlet portion). An ASD is invariably present for the obligatory right-to-left shunt. If the interatrial communication is restrictive, patients have severe cyanosis in infancy. A nonrestrictive ASD may become restrictive over time. The great arteries may be normally related (70%) or transposed (30%). With normally related great arteries, the pulmonary artery arises from the RV and there is usually valvular or subvalvular PS. With transposed great arteries, the aorta arises from the RV and there may be associated PS, pulmonary atresia, and subaortic obstruction (due to a small VSD restricting blood flow into the RV) (401).

Tricuspid atresia is an uncommon lesion (seen in 1% to 3% of all congenital defects) (33) and is usually sporadic, although some familial cases have been described. The diagnosis is suspected in a cyanotic infant with decreased pulmonary blood flow on CXR. Echocardiography is diagnostic. Catheterization may be required to define hemodynamics before surgical intervention.

Tricuspid atresia has a very high mortality in infancy, with few patients surviving beyond 6 months of age without some type of palliation (402). Rare survival into adulthood without surgery has been reported. In critically ill infants, medical therapy with prostaglandin E_1 is used to maintain patency of the ductus, and a balloon atrial septostomy may be used for patients with restrictive ASDs to improve right atrial-to-left atrial shunting. Patients with tricuspid atresia are now routinely treated with staged palliative surgical procedures. A palliative shunt may be required initially to improve pulmonary blood flow in patients with severe PS. A systemic-to-pulmonary artery shunt (Blalock-Taussig or modified Blalock-Taussig shunt) or a cavopulmonary shunt (bidirectional Glenn shunt) is used.

The Fontan procedure is now considered the definitive procedure for patients with tricuspid atresia. First done in 1971 (403), the Fontan procedure separates the pulmonary and systemic circulation by creating a direct connection of the systemic venous blood to the lungs without an intervening ventricle. Multiple modifications of the surgical technique have been made. Overall, the Fontan procedure is excellent for long-term palliation (404–410). The procedure is most commonly performed with direct anastomosis of the systemic venous return to the pulmonary arterial circulation, bypassing the systemic venous ventricle (modified Fontan) or completely bypassing both the systemic venous atrium and ventricle with a total cavopulmonary anastomosis using an intracardiac or extracardiac conduit (411–413). The Fontan operation is typically performed at the age of 2 to 3 years. Risk factors for poor outcome from the Fontan operation include high pulmonary vascular resistance (>2 Wood units/m^2), high mean pulmonary artery pressure (>18 mm Hg), distorted pulmonary artery anatomy, systolic or diastolic dysfunction with an LV end-diastolic pressure greater than 12 mm Hg, and atrioventricular regurgitation. A patient with two or more risk factors is considered to be at high risk (406,410,413,414).

Multiple long-term complications of the Fontan procedure may occur, including RA enlargement, atrial arrhythmias, thrombus formation within the Fontan circuit, conduit obstruction due to deterioration of prosthetic materials, hepatic congestion potentially leading to cirrhosis, progressive ventricular dysfunction, atrioventricular valve regurgitation, development of systemic venous collaterals and/or pulmonary arteriovenous fistula, right-to-left shunts at the atrial level, and protein-losing enteropathy (415). Older versions of the Fontan procedure with a direct RA-to-pulmonary artery anastomosis often result in progressive dilation of the RA, contributing to arrhythmogenesis. Atrioventricular valve regurgitation and ventricular dysfunction also contribute to arrhythmias. Sinus node dysfunction is common after the Fontan operation and is seen in 10% to 15% of cases. For patients requiring permanent pacing, epicardial lead placement is required for ventricular pacing and may be required for atrial pacing because the placement of transvenous atrial leads may be complicated. Sinus node dysfunction and bradycardia increase the risk for atrial tachycardias.

Reentrant atrial tachycardia, atrial fibrillation, and atrial flutter are reported in nearly half of Fontan patients in long-term outcome studies (276,416,417). Sustained atrial arrhythmias tend to be poorly tolerated and may result in the development of atrial thrombus (occasionally causing Fontan pathway obstruction) as well as congestive heart failure. Anticoagulation is critical in these patients. TEE is particularly useful for visualizing thrombus within the Fontan circuit. Catheter ablation of arrhythmias in patients after the Fontan operation is technically very challenging. Multiple circuits are usually present, and ablation may have limited effectiveness due to extensive fibrosis and scarring. Although acute success rates are good in small series, arrhythmia recurrence is common in long-term follow-up. Drug therapy is likewise complicated for these patients. They often require a combination of drug therapy and pacing. Amiodarone may have an increased incidence of thyroid and hepatic toxicity in the Fontan population (418,419). On occasion, patients with refractory arrhythmias may require surgical revision to a total cavopulmonary connection with intraoperative electrophysiologic mapping to guide surgical cryoablation.

Protein-losing enteropathy is an uncommon complication that is presumed to result from increased systemic venous pressure causing intestinal lymphangiectasia. Patients develop a debilitating gastrointestinal protein loss resulting in malnutrition, edema, effusions, ascites, and hypogammaglobulinemia. Protein-losing enteropathy is very difficult to treat. Multiple treatments have been tried with varying success (417). The 5-year survival rate is less than 50% (420).

The 5- to 10-year survival is reported to be 60% to 70% after a Fontan operation (406,408,411,414,421). Patients usually report good functional status but have abnormal exercise capacity with a lower maximal workload, lower maximal oxygen consumption, and a blunted heart rate response (422). Patients are at risk of developing cyanosis due to pulmonary arteriovenous fistulas in the setting of a classic Glenn shunt or may have anomalous systemic venous connections. Patients have an ongoing mortality after the Fontan procedure despite a successful operation, with the precise mechanism of death not clearly identified. A small number of successful pregnancies have been reported after the Fontan operation (423).

Total Anomalous Pulmonary Venous Connection

Total anomalous pulmonary venous connection is defined as connection of all of the pulmonary veins to one or more of the systemic veins, draining to the RA or coronary sinus (424,425). There is no direct communication of the pulmonary veins to the LA. Pulmonary venous drainage may return to the heart above the level of the diaphragm (supracardiac type) or below the diaphragm (infracardiac type), or it may occur in a mixed pattern. An ASD or PFO is necessary for survival, allowing blood to enter the LA and LV. There may be associated obstruction of the common pulmonary venous channel, which is more commonly seen with the infracardiac types. Patients with obstructed forms of total anomalous pulmonary venous connection present in the neonatal period with progressive hypoxemia, marked pulmonary edema, and a small heart on chest x-ray. Patients with unobstructed total anomalous pulmonary venous connection usually present in infancy with congestive heart failure and mild hypoxemia. Less commonly, they may present later in childhood or adolescence, rarely in adulthood (426).

The diagnosis is made by echocardiography. Cardiac catheterization with angiography is usually not required unless pulmonary venous drainage patterns are complex. MRI is an excellent tool for defining the pulmonary venous connections. Corrective surgery to redirect the pulmonary venous return to the LA and close the associated ASD is necessary for all patients with this condition (427). For severely ill infants with the obstructed form, medical therapy with digoxin, diuretics, and mechanical ventilation may help to stabilize the patient until corrective surgical repair can be accomplished. The development of postoperative pulmonary venous obstruction is uncommon but carries a poor prognosis.

Ebstein's Anomaly

Ebstein's anomaly is an uncommon defect (<1.0% of all congenital defects), and is characterized by varying degrees of dysplasia and apical displacement of the septal and mural (posterior) leaflets of the tricuspid valve. The anterior leaflet is often malformed and excessively large and may be adherent to the RV free wall. Tricuspid leaflet displacement results in "atrialization" of the inlet portion of the RV. The "true" RV or functional RV (apical and outflow segments) may be quite small (Fig. 30.7). The degree of leaflet displacement varies, resulting in wide differences in the clinical presentation. Patients have varying degrees of tricuspid regurgitation, whereas tricuspid stenosis is unusual (428). There is an increased incidence in Ebstein's malformation in the offspring of mothers treated with lithium carbonate in the first trimester of pregnancy.

Ebstein's malformation may occur as an isolated defect or in association with other complex congenital heart defects (e.g., tetralogy of Fallot, AV septal defect, etc.). Ebstein's anomaly is commonly seen with congenitally corrected transposition (429,430). The most common associated congenital defect is an ostium secundum ASD or a PFO, which is present in greater than 50% of patients (431). Poor RV compliance and elevated RA pressure cause right-to-left shunting across the ASD. In addition, patients may have some degree of RV outflow obstruction. Wolff-Parkinson-White (WPW) syndrome is frequently seen in Ebstein's anomaly and is often associated with multiple pathways (usually right-sided) due to discontinuity of the central fibrous body associated with the septal leaflet displacement (432).

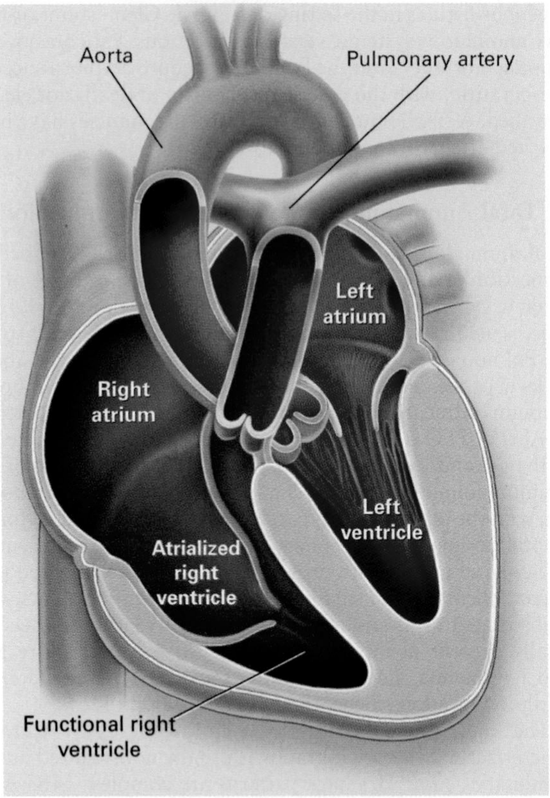

FIGURE 30.7. Ebstein's anomaly. Apical displacement of the tricuspid leaflets results in atrialization of a portion of the right ventricle. The functional right ventricle is small. An interatrial communication is usually present. (From Brickner ME, Hillis LD, Lange RA. Congenital heart disease in adults. *N Engl J Med* 2000;342:340.)

The clinical spectrum of patients with Ebstein's anomaly varies from severe disease presenting in utero or in infancy to an incidental diagnosis made in the seventh to eighth decades of life (433). The clinical exam demonstrates variable degrees of cyanosis. A soft systolic murmur of tricuspid regurgitation is usually present, and a middiastolic murmur may be present. The characteristic triple or quadruple gallop rhythm is caused by splitting of S1, wide splitting of S2, and the presence of an S3 and S4. Multiple clicks may be heart. The ECG is usually abnormal, with tall P waves and right-bundle-branch block seen frequently. First-degree AV block is seen in 40% to 50% of cases, and 25% have WPW. On CXR, heart size varies from normal to massively enlarged. Echocardiography is diagnostic. Specific criteria have been defined for the diagnosis of Ebstein's anomaly, requiring septal leaflet displacement greater than 8 mm/m^2 from the annulus (431). The size of the functional RV, the degree of tricuspid valve regurgitation or stenosis, and the presence of an interatrial shunt can be demonstrated.

The long-term prognosis depends on the age at presentation. Presentation in infancy with cyanosis and congestive heart failure is usually associated with a poor prognosis (432–434). Adolescents and adults are more likely to present with arrhythmias, usually SVT (reentrant supraventricular tachycardia, atrial fibrillation, and atrial flutter) (433). There is an increased risk of sudden death in patients with Ebstein's anomaly, occurring in 3% to 4% of patients (433). Predictors of poor outcome include a diagnosis in infancy, NYHA class III or IV, systemic arterial saturation less than 90%, and a cardiothoracic ratio greater than 0.65 (435).

WPW syndrome is present in 20% to 25% of patients with Ebstein's anomaly (432). The bypass tracts are usually right-sided or posterior septal, along the atrialized portion of the RV, and multiple bypass tracts are seen in 30% to 50% of cases. Ablation of these accessory pathways in Ebstein's anomaly is often complicated, with the success rate for ablation lower than that for ablation of WPW in the general population (75% vs. 95%). The recurrence rate is also higher (436). For patients with WPW syndrome who require tricuspid valve surgery (repair/replacement) and/or closure of their ASD, intracardiac mapping and surgical elimination of pathway has a high success rate with low risk of recurrence (276).

Morbidity and mortality for neonates with severe Ebstein's anomaly is quite high. Indications for surgery include critically ill neonates who fail intensive medical therapy, advanced functional class (III or IV) with significant cardiomegaly, the presence of significant cyanosis, and paradoxical emboli. The initial surgical approach may be creation of a palliative systemic-to-pulmonary artery shunt to relieve cyanosis, with later conversion to a Fontan-type operation. The mortality for surgical repair remains significant, particularly in the neonatal population (6% to 14%) (437,438). Less than 20% of patients require surgery within first decade of life, and surgical outcomes are much better in older patients (who tend to be less ill, with more suitable valve anatomy). For older children, adolescents, and adults, the surgical options include tricuspid valve repair or tricuspid valve replacement (bioprosthesis preferred) along with closure of the atrial septal defect. For some patients, cardiac transplantation may be appropriate. It is unclear whether surgery affects the risk of sudden death.

For patients with significant cyanosis, closure of the ASD or PFO is usually done at the time of surgical repair of the tricuspid valve. ASD device closure has been rarely reported and may result in hemodynamic deterioration.

Double-Outlet Right Ventricle

Double-outlet right ventricle (DORV) is an uncommon defect in which more than half of each great artery is connected to the morphologic RV (439,440). DORV is nearly always associated with a large, nonrestrictive VSD, which provides the only outlet from the LV. There is a wide variety of spatial orientations of the great arteries, as well as variation in the location of the VSD. The VSD may be subaortic, subpulmonary, doubly committed (beneath both great arteries), or noncommitted. Patients may have pulmonary or aortic outflow obstruction, abnormalities of the atrioventricular junction, and ventricular hypoplasia. The clinical presentation depends on the specific morphology of the VSD and the presence or absence of PS. Patients may present with a large left-to-right shunt and congestive heart failure or may have cyanosis. There are only rare survivors to adulthood without prior surgical repair.

The diagnosis requires echocardiography and cardiac catheterization with angiography. Surgical treatment is a primary repair for most patients.

There are four major types of DORV, each of which requires a different type of surgical repair (441–445). The most common form is the subaortic VSD without associated PS. In this case, oxygenated blood from the LV is directed through the VSD into the aorta. These patients present with mild or no cyanosis. Their clinical presentation resembles that of a large VSD, with patients at risk for congestive heart failure and pulmonary hypertension. Surgical treatment involves a primary repair, tunneling left ventricular blood through the VSD to the aorta. Surgery is performed early in infancy to prevent the development of pulmonary hypertension. Patients with a subaortic VSD may have valvar or subvalvar PS (so-called Fallot type), causing desaturated blood to enter the aorta. The clinical presentation with this type is similar to that of tetralogy of Fallot. Surgical treatment includes an intraventricular tunnel from the LV to the aorta, along with relief of pulmonary obstruction by a patch graft or extracardiac conduit. This surgery is done in older infants and children. With a subpulmonary VSD (the Taussig-Bing malformation), oxygenated blood from the LV is directed into the pulmonary artery while desaturated blood is directed to the aorta. The clinical picture resembles that of complete transposition of the great arteries. Patients are at risk for severe pulmonary vascular obstructive disease early in life. Surgical treatment is performed early in infancy, usually by tunneling left ventricular blood through the VSD to the pulmonary artery combined with an arterial switch operation. Patients with DORV with a remote VSD (located away from the aorta and pulmonary artery) usually present with mild cyanosis and increased pulmonary blood flow. There may be associated abnormalities of the atrioventricular valves, including AV valve straddling, making surgical repair complex. Patients with ventricular hypoplasia or severe AV valve straddling may not be candidates for biventricular repair and may require a Fontan-type operation.

Single Ventricle

Single ventricle is an uncommon defect in which both atria are connected to one ventricle (446–448). There are usually two atrioventricular valves (double inlet), although rarely there may be a common atrioventricular valve (common inlet). The morphology of the single ventricle is usually that of an LV with a rudimentary RV (outlet chamber). On occasion, the single ventricle may have the morphology of an RV, often associated with a double outlet (both aorta and pulmonary artery arising from the RV). In some cases, the ventricular morphology is indeterminate. The great arteries are transposed in the majority of cases, with the aorta arising anteriorly from the rudimentary outlet chamber. The connection between the single ventricle and the outlet chamber (the bulboventricular foramen) may become obstructed, causing decreased systemic blood flow and increased pulmonary blood flow.

There is complete mixing of blood in the common ventricle, and the degree of cyanosis is determined by the amount of pulmonary blood flow. Infants without PS have markedly increased pulmonary blood flow with symptoms of heart failure. These patients are at risk for the development of pulmonary vascular obstructive disease and have a high mortality in infancy. Infants may have valvar or subvalvar PS, which "protects" the pulmonary circulation by limiting pulmonary blood flow but results in more severe cyanosis.

Surgical management for patients with a single ventricle is complex. Patients with severe cyanosis often require a palliative shunt to increase pulmonary blood flow. Patients without PS may have a pulmonary artery band to decrease pulmonary blood flow, but this procedure may worsen obstruction of the bulboventricular foramen. Patients with a single ventricle are usually treated with a Fontan-type repair (449). On occasion, a patient may have biventricular repair with creation of a ventricular septum, although this operation carries a high operative risk.

Long-term outcomes for unoperated and palliated patients with a single ventricle have been reported (450,451). For unoperated patients, survival is only 30% to 50% at 14 to 16 years. Survival depends on the morphology of the ventricle, with better survival seen in patients with an LV morphology. Two thirds of palliated patients were alive at 15 years.

Common Arterial Trunk

Common arterial trunk or persistent truncus arteriosus is an uncommon defect (33,200), and is characterized by a single great vessel arising from the ventricular mass that gives rise to the coronary arteries, at least one pulmonary artery, and the brachiocephalic arteries (452). A VSD is invariably present, directly below the truncus. The pulmonary arteries may arise from a common pulmonary trunk off the ascending portion of the arterial trunk or may have separate origins of the branch pulmonary arteries from either the ascending portion of the truncus, the descending aorta, the ductus arteriosus, or an aortopulmonary collateral. The truncal valve may be bicuspid, tricuspid, or quadricuspid and may be stenotic, regurgitant, or both (453). The coronary artery origins have a variety of abnormalities (454,455). Some forms are associated with other severe anomalies of the aorta, including coarctation, aortic arch atresia, and aortic interruption.

In most patients, there is excessive pulmonary blood flow that ultimately leads to congestive heart failure and severe pulmonary vascular obstructive disease. Mortality is high in childhood without surgical intervention, and only rare patients survive to adulthood (456). Surgery is the only definitive therapy and is usually undertaken shortly after diagnosis. Surgery includes separation of the pulmonary arteries from the arterial trunk, creation of continuity between the RV and the pulmonary arteries with a valved conduit, and closure of the VSD (457,458). Long-term survival after initial successful repair is good (85% at 20 years in one series), but reoperation rates are high (90% at 10 years) (459,460). Reoperation is most commonly performed for conduit replacement or for truncal valve insufficiency. Reoperation is the most important predictor of late death, with 50% of late deaths occurring at time of reoperation (458,460).

Hypoplastic Left Heart Syndrome

Hypoplastic left heart syndrome (HLHS) occurs in 1% of all congenital defects and is the most common cardiac cause of death in the first month of life (33,200). HLHS is characterized by aortic atresia or severe stenosis, mitral atresia or severe stenosis, and left ventricular hypoplasia with varying amounts of endocardial fibroelastosis. An ASD is seen in 15% to 20% of cases, a VSD in 10%, and coarctation of the aorta in 70% to 80%. In most cases, the entire circulation depends on flow through the ductus arteriosus from the RV. With closure of the ductus in the first few hours to days, the neonate develops a relentless low-output state with metabolic acidosis and death. An immediate diagnosis can be made by echocardiography, and prostaglandin E_1 therapy is initiated to maintain ductal flow (461). A balloon atrial septostomy may provide some temporary relief to improve oxygenation, but surgery is required for survival. Two major surgical options are the Norwood procedure (462–465) and cardiac transplantation (466,467). The Norwood operation is a complex staged surgical therapy, culminating in a Fontan operation. In stage 1, an atrial septectomy is performed to allow intracardiac mixing, the main pulmonary artery is divided with the distal stump closed, and a neo-ascending aorta is created from the proximal main pulmonary trunk and the native ascending aorta. Augmentation of the aortic isthmus may be performed to relieve coarctation. A modified Blalock-Taussig shunt (Gore-Tex graft) is used to provide pulmonary blood flow to the distal confluent pulmonary arteries. In stage 2, a bidirectional Glenn shunt is created (SVC to the right pulmonary artery). Stage 3 is the creation of a modified Fontan. The long-term outcome and complications from these complicated repairs are only beginning to be studied. There are preliminary data on fetal intervention for HLHS, with intrauterine perforation of the fetal aortic valve to permit normal growth of the LV and improve long-term outcome (468).

Heterotaxy Syndromes

Heterotaxy refers to an abnormal arrangement of the viscera, with incompletely or nonlateralized abdominal viscera (469–472). The liver is symmetric and midline, and the thoracic contents are more symmetric (either bilateral trilobed lungs with bilateral eparterial bronchi or bilateral bilobed lungs with bilateral hyparterial bronchi). Visceral heterotaxy is frequently associated with severe cardiac malformations. Atrial isomerism (bilateral right- or left-sidedness) is usually present. In patients with right atrial isomerism (bilateral morphologic right atria), the spleen is often absent (asplenia). The most commonly associated cardiac lesions in right atrial isomerism are total anomalous pulmonary venous connection, a common atrioventricular valve, and abnormalities of ventriculoarterial connections. In patients with left atrial isomerism (bilateral morphologic left atria), there are usually multiple spleens (polysplenia). The most common associated cardiac lesions with left atrial isomerism are anomalous systemic venous connections (absence of the IVC, bilateral SVC, absence of the coronary sinus, and partial anomalous pulmonary venous connections), AVSD, VSD, and DORV (473).

Eisenmenger Syndrome

Eisenmenger syndrome is a term applied to any large communication between the systemic and pulmonary circulation that results in irreversible changes in the pulmonary vascular bed, with reversal of the shunt direction (474) (Fig. 30.8). The Eisenmenger syndrome may occur with any congenital defect that results in a large left-to-right shunt, with aortopulmonary collaterals, and with surgically created aortopulmonary anatomizes.

The pulmonary vascular changes begin in childhood (often within the first 2 years of life) and are progressive. Any nonrestrictive communication at any level will result in increased pulmonary blood flow and transmission of near-systemic pressures to the pulmonary circulation, resulting in the development of pulmonary vascular disease. Increased activity of endogenous vascular elastase in the pulmonary vascular bed has been shown to induce other mediators, resulting in smooth muscle migration and hypertrophy and stimulation of elastin and collagen synthesis. These steps are critical in the formation of irreversible pulmonary vascular disease (475).

The pathologic changes in the pulmonary vascular bed correlate with the hemodynamic status and can be graded in terms of severity. Grade A is characterized by increased pulmonary blood flow but normal mean pulmonary artery pressure. Pathologically, extension of muscle into nonmuscular peripheral arteries is seen. Grade B is characterized by increased mean pulmonary artery pressure. Pathologically, medial hypertrophy is seen in more proximal vessels as a result of smooth muscle hypertrophy and proliferation as well as increased connective tissue elements. With grade C, there is increased pulmonary vascular resistance, which correlates pathologically with a reduced concentration of distal pulmonary vessels (476). The Heath-Edwards classification has been used to grade the severity of pulmonary vascular obstructive disease on a histopathologic basis (grades I to VI) (477). The presence of grade II changes or greater predicts persistence of pulmonary vascular resistance in the postoperative state.

The Eisenmenger syndrome is most commonly seen in association with large communications such as large VSDs, large PDA, and aortopulmonary windows. The Eisenmenger syndrome was seen in only 9% of patients with ASD in Wood's initial description (474). Early and progressive pulmonary vascular disease leading to the Eisenmenger syndrome is frequently seen in patients with Down syndrome (102). The prevalence of the Eisenmenger syndrome is declining with improved diagnosis and therapy for congenital defects. In large adult congenital heart disease clinics, approximately 4% of patients have the Eisenmenger syndrome (478). The prevalence is higher in clinics with a concentration in cyanotic lesions, and is seen in 19% of one such clinic (479).

Although the pathologic changes of pulmonary vascular obstructive disease are present in childhood, the age at diagnosis varies. Patients with large shunts at the ventricular or aortopulmonary level are usually diagnosed in childhood, whereas

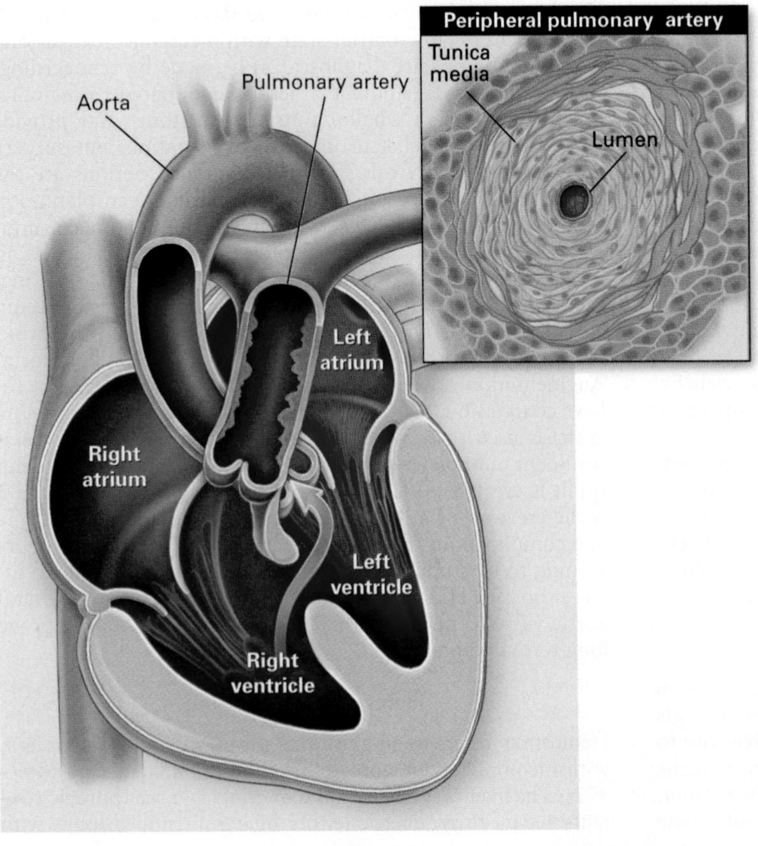

FIGURE 30.8. Eisenmenger syndrome with a nonrestrictive ventricular septal defect and severe pulmonary vascular obstructive disease, leading to shunt reversal. (From Brickner ME, Hillis LD, Lange RA. Congenital heart disease in adults. *N Engl J Med* 2000;342:340.)

those with shunts at the atrial level are more likely to be diagnosed in adulthood. A history of congestive heart failure in childhood suggests a large left-to-right shunt. Symptoms disappear as pulmonary vascular resistance increases and the magnitude of the shunt decreases. Shunt reversal and cyanosis appear later. Patients may have minimal symptoms in childhood and present with severe pulmonary vascular disease in adulthood. Pulmonary vascular disease may also occur as a late complication of palliative shunts performed for cyanotic lesions in childhood.

Because the development of pulmonary vascular disease is gradual, symptoms related to the Eisenmenger syndrome usually occur gradually. While most patients are symptomatic, they usually report fairly good functional capacity (480). The most common symptoms are dyspnea, fatigue, palpitations, edema, and syncope. The physical findings in the Eisenmenger syndrome include cyanosis and clubbing, an RV heave (and often a palpable pulmonary artery impulse), a pulmonary ejection sound, and a loud P2. The pulmonary component of the second heart sound moves earlier as pulmonary pressures increase, and the second heart sound may be single (fusion of A2 and P2). Murmurs of pulmonary and tricuspid regurgitation may be present secondary to pulmonary hypertension. The murmurs associated with the original shunt are absent. Differential cyanosis is present in patients with the Eisenmenger syndrome secondary to a PDA.

The natural history of patients with the Eisenmenger syndrome is significantly different from that of patients with primary pulmonary hypertension. Despite high pulmonary pressures, patients with the Eisenmenger syndrome have more favorable hemodynamics and a better prognosis than those with primary pulmonary hypertension. In one study comparing the two patient populations, the actuarial survival was 77% at 3 years for Eisenmenger syndrome as compared to 35% for patients with primary pulmonary hypertension (481). In one case series, the actuarial survival rate for 201 Eisenmenger patients was 80% at 10 years and 77% at 15 years after the initial diagnosis (482). In another series with a combined pediatric and adult population, the actuarial survival was 75% at 30 years of age, 70% survival at 40 years, and 55% survival at 50 years. Simple defects had better survival than complex defects (481). There are no prospective studies of long-term outcome in patients with the Eisenmenger syndrome.

Risk factors that have been identified from retrospective studies include syncope, age at presentation, poor functional class, complex underlying disease, supraventricular arrhythmias, oxygen saturation less than 85%, increased serum creatinine, RV dysfunction, and increased serum uric acid concentration (480–485).

Many of the complications seen in the Eisenmenger syndrome are related to the presence of chronic cyanosis and are discussed in a subsequent section. Supraventricular arrhythmias are common, and are seen in 36% of Eisenmenger patients on Holter monitoring (479,480). The development of supraventricular arrhythmias predicts clinical deterioration and death in some series (480,483). In general, sinus rhythm should be restored promptly when possible. Ventricular arrhythmias are less common. There is no published experience with implantable cardiodefibrillators in the Eisenmenger population.

The management of patients with the Eisenmenger syndrome is deceptively simple. Physicians should "avoid therapies not proven to be beneficial, alleviate symptoms, [and] intervene only when needed" to avoid destabilizing the "balanced physiology" (486). Afterload reduction should be avoided because it may worsen right-to-left shunting. Arterial hypertension should be treated, however, because untreated hypertension may increase the risk of intrapulmonary bleeding and hemoptysis. β-Blockers are usually well tolerated. Pregnancy is associated with a high maternal mortality and a high risk of fetal complications and should be avoided, preferably with permanent sterilization (487–489).

Hemoptysis may occur in patients with the Eisenmenger syndrome and may be life-threatening. The amount of hemoptysis does not necessarily reflect the extent of intrapulmonary hemorrhage. Therefore, CXR and CT scans of the chest are required to define the extent of pulmonary hemorrhage. Treatment is conservative in most cases, consisting of bed rest, cough suppressants, avoidance of antiplatelet and anticoagulant agents, and treatment of hypovolemia. For severe or incessant bleeding, aortography with selective embolization of bleeding source may be successful in some cases.

Routine phlebotomy should be avoided (see management of chronic cyanosis). Potentially nephrotoxic agents (including nonsteroidal antiinflammatory drugs) should be avoided.

Patients with the Eisenmenger syndrome have increased morbidity and mortality during noncardiac surgery (490). Careful anesthetic management is required for these patients (491). Medical therapy for patients with the Eisenmenger syndrome differs from that for patients with primary pulmonary hypertension. Anticoagulation has a proven role in primary pulmonary hypertension, but there are no data to support its use in the Eisenmenger syndrome. Anticoagulation is generally avoided in these patients due to their increased risk of bleeding. However, anticoagulation is indicated for atrial fibrillation, atrial flutter, recurrent thromboembolic events, mechanical heart valves, or other high-risk anatomy. Obviously, anticoagulation in this patient population requires meticulous management. Although it is often used, oxygen therapy does not have proven efficacy in patients with the Eisenmenger syndrome. In a single small study of nocturnal oxygen therapy in Eisenmenger patients, there were no benefits in terms of exercise capacity, quality of life, or degree of erythrocytosis (492). The drying effects on the nasal mucosa may predispose patients to epistaxis.

Pulmonary vasoactive therapy has been extensively studied in patients with primary pulmonary hypertension but there is only limited experience in the Eisenmenger population. Rosenzweig et al. studied continuous intravenous prostacyclin therapy in 20 patients with Eisenmenger syndrome over a 1-year period. Exercise capacity improved, pulmonary pressures decreased slightly, and 8 of 12 patients listed for transplant were removed from the transplant list (493). In three small, nonrandomized reports of patients with Eisenmenger syndrome treated with bosentan, an endothelin antagonist, improvement in functional class and improved exercise capacity were seen without obvious adverse effects (494–496). Preliminary results from the BREATHE-5 trial have been released in the news media. In this randomized, double-blind, placebo-controlled trial of bosentan in 54 patients with the Eisenmenger syndrome, treatment with bosentan improved exercise capacity and decreased pulmonary vascular resistance without worsening oxygen saturation.

The role of transplantation for patients with the Eisenmenger syndrome is controversial. Patients are invariably symptomatic with decreased exercise tolerance, but the long-term outcomes for patients with the Eisenmenger syndrome are better than often appreciated and referral may be premature. One report suggests that patients with the Eisenmenger syndrome awaiting transplant have a very low mortality, raising the issue of the appropriateness of transplant for some of these patients (497). Patients require either lung transplantation with repair of the cardiac defect or heart-lung transplantation. With 3- to 5-year survival rates in the range of 50% to 60% for combined heart-lung transplant, transplant should be considered only in those patients whose predicted life expectancy without transplant is less than 2 years.

Miscellaneous Defects

Congenital Anomalies of the Coronary Arteries

Congenital anomalies of the coronary arteries may occur in isolation or in association with other congenital anomalies. Multiple variations exist. A rare but potentially lethal condition is the anomalous origin of the left coronary artery from the pulmonary artery. As pulmonary pressures fall in newborns with this condition, myocardial perfusion becomes dependent on collaterals from the right coronary circulation. These infants may present with ischemic symptoms or symptoms of heart failure from an ischemic cardiomyopathy. They may present in the neonatal period or later in infancy or childhood (498). This coronary anomaly is rarely seen in adults. In children, the diagnosis of coronary anomalies may often be made by echocardiography with color flow Doppler (499–501). Other patients may require catheterization with aortography and angiography. The treatment is surgical, with reimplantation of the anomalous coronary or aortocoronary bypass (502–504). Postoperatively, patients may have persistent problems with abnormal myocardial perfusion (505,506).

Congenital Pericardial Defects

Congenital pericardial defects may be partial or complete. Partial absence of the left side of the pericardium may cause chest pain. An unusual cardiac silhouette may be seen on CXR due to herniation of the left atrial appendage or the ventricles through the defect. Herniation of the right lung through a partial right-sided defect may result in obstruction of the SVC. Alternatively, right heart structures may herniate through right-sided defects (507–511).

Sinus of Valsalva Aneurysms

Sinus of Valsalva aneurysms are defined as enlargement of one of the aortic sinuses between the valve annulus and sinotubular ridge (512). Absence of the elastic lamellae results in focal weakening of the aortic wall. This leads to aneurysmal dilation of the weakened portion and may ultimately lead to rupture. Sinus of Valsalva aneurysms are rare, and are seen in 0.09% of the general population at autopsy (513). They are four times more common in male individuals. Aneurysms occur in the right coronary sinus in 65% to 85% of cases, in the noncoronary sinus in 10% to 30%, and in the left coronary sinus in less than 5% (512–514). Sinus of Valsalva aneurysms may be associated with VSD, AR, bicuspid aortic valve, or connective tissue disorders such as Marfan syndrome or Ehlers-Danlos syndrome. The diagnosis can be made by echocardiography demonstrating the aneurysm and color flow mapping to demonstrate flow in ruptured aneurysms. Patients are usually asymptomatic until the aneurysm ruptures, which usually occurs in the third and fourth decades. A sinus of Valsalva aneurysm may cause local obstructive symptoms (compression of the right ventricular outflow tract or the coronary ostium).

Classically, rupture of a sinus of Valsalva aneurysm occurs with exertion or after trauma (514). The usual site of rupture is into the RV (in 90% of cases). Patients typically present with chest pain, cough, and breathlessness. Over time, they may develop LV volume overload and symptoms of congestive heart failure and may present late. Patients often have a continuous/machinery murmur, but this is not invariably present. Without surgical intervention, there is usually progressive deterioration with LV failure. Surgical repair is recommended for ruptured aneurysms or symptomatic aneurysms with compression, arrhythmias, or evidence of infection. Unruptured aneurysms without symptoms do not warrant surgical intervention.

Absent Pulmonary Valve

The absent pulmonary valve syndrome is an uncommon defect usually associated with tetralogy of Fallot or a ventricular septal defect. When the defect occurs in isolation, it may result in fetal heart failure and death or may be associated with survival to the seventh or eight decade (515). Pulmonary valve replacement is indicated for right heart failure.

SPECIAL MANAGEMENT ISSUES IN CONGENITAL HEART DISEASE

Postoperative Patients

Truly corrective surgery for congenital heart disease is uncommon. Most patients have had reparative or palliative surgery and require lifelong surveillance for long-term complications. Table 30.1 lists common surgical procedures in CHD patients, including the anatomy and associated complications. Palliative procedures include pulmonary artery banding (to decrease pulmonary blood flow) and the creation of shunts to increase pulmonary blood flow. Both systemic venous-to-pulmonary artery or arterial-to-pulmonary artery shunts may be used. Older systemic arterial-to-pulmonary artery shunts were fraught with complications. Currently, the modified Blalock-Taussig shunt or a systemic venous-to-pulmonary artery shunt is used to provide a controlled source of pulmonary blood flow (516,517). The modified Blalock-Taussig shunts use a prosthetic tube graft between the subclavian artery and the pulmonary artery to provide a controlled source of blood flow. The Glenn shunt diverts part of the systemic venous return to the lungs (SVC to the pulmonary artery with an end-to-side anastomosis). Actuarial survival with the Glenn shunt in patients with a single ventricle is 84% at 10 years and 66% at 20 years (517). Patients may develop pulmonary arteriovenous malformations (AVMs) in the lung with the shunt due to the exclusion of inferior vena cava blood from that lung (518). Pulmonary AVMs may result in cyanosis due to intrapulmonary shunting. The bidirectional Glenn shunt consists of an end-to-side anastomosis of the SVC to the pulmonary artery, leaving the right and left pulmonary arteries in continuity. The bidirectional Glenn shunt is often used en route to the Fontan procedure (415). Venous-to-pulmonary shunts are favored and have fewer complications and more balanced pulmonary blood flow than the systemic arterial-to-pulmonary artery shunts (519).

Physiologic repair of congenital defects results in separation of the pulmonary and systemic circulations. Examples of physiologic repairs include the atrial switch operations for complete transposition and the Fontan procedure for tricuspid atresia. Prosthetic materials are usually used, resulting in a risk for long-term complications associated with these prosthetic materials. Physicians caring for these postoperative patients must understand the specific details of the operative repair in order to monitor for long-term complications.

Management of Patients with Chronic Cyanosis

Chronic cyanosis associated with the Eisenmenger syndrome or other cyanotic congenital heart defect is a multisystem disorder (520,521). Erythrocytosis (an isolated increase in the red cell line) occurs in chronic cyanosis as a physiologic response to hypoxia, resulting in increased oxygen-carrying capacity. The increase in red cell mass also increases whole-blood viscosity and may result in symptoms of hyperviscosity such as headaches, fatigue, myalgias, paresthesias, and transient visual disturbances.

TABLE 30.1

GLOSSARY OF SURGICAL TERMS

Name	Anatomy	Complications
PALLIATIVE SHUNTS FOR INCREASING PULMONARY BLOOD FLOW		
Classic Glenn shunt	SVC to RPA, disconnect RPA	Pulmonary AVMs in the right lung
Bidirectional Glenn shunt	SVC to RPA, pulmonary arteries left in continuity	
Bilateral Glenn shunt	Right SVC to RPA, left SVC to LPA	
Classic Blalock-Taussig shunt	Subclavian artery to ipsilateral PA	Pulmonary hypertension (uncommon), kinking of pulmonary artery
Modified Blalock-Taussig shunt	Prosthetic tube graft from subclavian artery to PA	May obstruct
Potts shunt	Descending aorta to LPA	Pulmonary hypertension, LV volume overload, distortion of LPA
Waterson shunt	Ascending aorta to RPA	Pulmonary hypertension, LV volume overload, distortion of RPA
Central shunt	Prosthetic graft from ascending aorta to PA	May obstruct
PALLIATIVE PROCEDURE FOR DECREASING PULMONARY BLOOD FLOW AND PREVENTING PULMONARY VASCULAR DISEASE		
Pulmonary artery band	—	Inadequate banding, migration of band, obstruction of branch PA
PALLIATIVE PROCEDURES FOR INCREASING INTRACARDIAC MIXING AT THE ATRIAL LEVEL		
Blalock-Hanlon atrial septectomy	Surgical excision of atrial septum	—
Rashkind procedure	Balloon atrial septostomy	—
PHYSIOLOGIC REPAIR–SEPARATION OF PULMONARY AND SYSTEMIC CIRCULATION		
Mustard and Senning procedures	Atrial switch, baffling of systemic venous return to LV, pulmonary venous return to RV	RV dysfunction, baffle leaks, obstruction, arrhythmias, sinus node dysfunction
Arterial switch	Relocation of aorta and pulmonary artery trunks, reimplantation of coronaries in neoaorta for CTGA	Minimal, coronary abnormalities, aortic root dilation, AR
Double-switch procedure	Atrial switch and arterial switch	—
Lecompte maneuver	PA brought anterior to aorta during arterial switch	—
Rastelli	LV outflow baffled through VSD to aorta, RV to PA conduit	Conduit obstruction, baffle obstruction, arrhythmias
Fontan	Diversion of systemic venous return to pulmonary artery, usually without subpulmonary ventricle	Multiple; see text
Classic Fontan	Valved conduit from RA to PA or direct anastomosis of RA to PA	—
Extracardiac Fontan	IVC connected to PA via extracardiac conduit, SVC to PA via bidirectional Glenn	—
Lateral tunnel Fontan	IVC flow to PA, most of RA excluded, bidirectional Glenn	—
Damus-Kaye-Stansel	Transect main PA, anastomose proximal PA to ascending aorta to provide systemic blood flow, oversew aorta, close VSD, conduit from RV to PA	—
Norwood procedure	Multistage operation for HLHS, systemic to PA shunt, followed by staged Fontan operation, results in RV as dominant ventricle	—
1.5 Ventricle repair	Bidirectional cavopulmonary connection, IVC flow via small pulmonary ventricle to PA	—
MISCELLANEOUS PROCEDURES		
Brock procedure	Resection of RV infundibulum with blunt instrument, without cardiopulmonary bypass	Pulmonary regurgitation
Unifocalization	Surgical technique to create a common trunk for multiple direct aortopulmonary collaterals	—
Ross procedure	Autograft transplant of PV, annulus, and pulmonary trunk to aorta, reimplantation of coronaries, RVOT reconstruction with homograft	—
Konno procedure	Aortoventriculoplasty, enlargement of LVOT with patch in ventricular system, enlargement of aortic annulus and ascending aorta, AVR	—

AR, aortic regurgitation; AVM, arteriovenous malformation; AVR, aortic valve replacement; CTGA, corrected transposition of the great arteries; HLHS, hypoplastic left heart syndrome; IVC, inferior vena cava; LPA, pulmonary artery; LV, left ventricle; LVOT, left ventricular outflow tract; PA, pulmonary artery; RPA, right pulmonary artery; RVOT, right ventricular outflow tract; SVC, superior vena cava; VSD, ventricular septal defect.

Most patients with chronic cyanosis are in a compensated state, with a stable hemoglobin and hematocrit and minimal symptoms of hyperviscosity. Phlebotomy is not appropriate for these patients. Patients may develop decompensated erythrocytosis with an unstable, rising hematocrit associated with severe hyperviscosity symptoms. Phlebotomy is indicated only for severe symptoms with a hematocrit greater than 65 in a well-hydrated patient in an iron-replete state. Patients with chronic cyanosis may have anemia with a hemoglobin level above 15 g/dL, often due to iron deficiency from phlebotomy or heavy menses. Because iron-deficient red cells are less deformable than normal biconcave red cells, patients with iron deficiency may have hyperviscosity symptoms with lower hematocrit levels. Careful iron repletion may be indicated in iron-deficient patients (522). Certain laboratory precautions are necessary for patients with erythrocytosis. The relatively low plasma volume in patients with a high hemoglobin and hematocrit may give spurious results for hematocrit unless appropriate adjustments are made. Measurements of blood glucose may also be spuriously low due to increased glycolysis from the increased number of red blood cells (521,523).

Patients with cyanotic congenital heart disease are at increased risk for both bleeding and thrombosis. Thrombocytopenia is commonly seen due to shortened platelet survival (increased peripheral consumption or destruction). Chronic cyanosis is associated with qualitative platelet disorders and also affects coagulation factors (decreased levels of factors V, VII, IX, and X), leading to an increased risk of bleeding (524,525). Increased blood viscosity stimulates the release of endothelium-derived nitric oxide and prostaglandins, leading to increased tissue vascularity, which further contributes to an increased risk of bleeding (521). The measured prothrombin time and partial thromboplastin time are usually normal. The bleeding time is often normal as well, despite abnormal platelet function. Fortunately, bleeding is usually mild and self-limited in patients with chronic cyanosis. The exception is hemoptysis, which may be life-threatening.

Patients with chronic cyanosis are also at increased risk of thrombosis, which may be promoted by sluggish flow through cardiac chambers and the presence of prosthetic material such as valves and conduits. Although there is some increased risk of cerebral venous thrombosis in cyanotic children with elevated hematocrits, there is no increased risk of arterial thrombosis in either children or adults (526–528). Prophylactic phlebotomy is contraindicated and actually increases the risk of stroke (528).

Hyperuricemia is common in patients with chronic cyanosis and occurs as a consequence of increase urate production and decreased renal clearance. Arthralgias are common, and gout may occur. However, urate nephropathy and uric acid stones are uncommon (529). The degree of hyperuricemia is useful as a marker of impaired renal function in these patients (479,523,530). Functional and structural abnormalities of the kidneys are common in patients with chronic cyanosis. Serum creatinine is usually a poor indicator of renal function, and significant renal dysfunction may be seen in patients with a normal serum creatinine.

Patients with right-to-left shunts are at risk for paradoxical embolization, and meticulous care must be taken when intravenous access is used. Filters should be used on all intravenous lines. These patients are also at increased risk of cerebral abscess due to the potential for paradoxical embolization of infected material. Patients commonly present with a headache.

Endocarditis

All patients are at increased risk for endocarditis. This is particularly true for those patients with bicuspid aortic valves, prosthetic shunts and conduits, and restrictive ventricular septal defects. Low-pressure lesions (e.g., ASDs) tend to have low risk. In a series of CHD patients with endocarditis, LV outflow tract obstruction was most common underlying cardiac defect, followed by unoperated small VSDs, then cyanotic congenital heart disease (531). Antibiotic prophylaxis is required for most patients with CHD (532).

Contraception and Pregnancy

Most patients with CHD will reach child-bearing age and will need to address the risks of pregnancy (533,534). Patients can be stratified into high, moderate, and low risk for complications during pregnancy (535,536). The highest-risk group includes patients with the Eisenmenger syndrome (487–489), severe pulmonary hypertension, severe LV outflow tract obstruction (including unrepaired coarctation of the aorta), Marfan syndrome with a dilated aortic root, and class III or IV congestive heart failure (523,534). Low-risk lesions include uncomplicated left-to-right shunts, mild left-sided obstructive lesions, isolated pulmonic or tricuspid valve disease, and repaired tetralogy of Fallot. Nearly all other types of congenital heart defects fall in the moderate-risk category. There are only limited data regarding pregnancy outcomes for specific cardiac defects.

Maternal functional class is also a risk factor for fetal outcome, with fetal mortality rates of 30% for mothers in New York Heart Association class IV. Cyanosis is a significant risk factor for fetal and maternal complications. In one series of pregnancy in mothers with chronic cyanosis, live births occurred in only 43% of pregnancies, and maternal complications occurred in 32% (536). Fetal risks are strongly related to the degree of maternal cyanosis.

A risk stratification scheme has been proposed to predict cardiac events in pregnancy that can be applied to mothers with CHD (537). Preconceptual counseling is important so that a potential mother can understand the risks to herself and her fetus. Offspring of patients with CHD have a higher risk of congenital heart defects, generally in the range of 5% to 6% (533,534). The defect in the offspring is usually not the same as in the mother except for autosomal dominant and familial syndromes. Prenatal cardiac ultrasound is recommended to screen for fetal cardiac malformations (262).

Contraception is complicated in patients with CHD, and the risks of different forms of contraception must be understood (538). Barrier methods have a high failure rate (10% to 20%). Intrauterine devices have a lower failure rate (4%) but are associated with an increased risk of infection and are generally contraindicated in patients with CHD. Oral contraceptives have a low failure rate (1% to 3%) but are associated with increased risk for thromboembolism and are contraindicated in patients with cyanosis or pulmonary hypertension. Progesterone-only contraceptives are associated with a risk of fluid retention and irregular bleeding. Sterilization is the most effective means of contraception and is recommended for high-risk patients.

Management of pregnancy, labor, and delivery is discussed further in Chapter 31.

Functional Capacity and Exercise Limitations

Despite reported good functional class, many patients with CHD have significant exercise limitations. Even patients with "simple lesions" and "repaired" lesions usually have decreased exercise capacity when formally tested (539–541). In general, patients with "simple shunts" who are status post repair with no evidence of pulmonary hypertension can participate in all sports. In the presence of pulmonary hypertension, intense activity should be prohibited, and competitive sports are not permitted. For patients with obstructive lesions, exercise limitations depend on the severity of stenosis. The presence of pulmonary hypertension, ventricular dysfunction, and rhythm abnormalities must be considered. Specific exercise recommendations were recently updated (542).

Noncardiac Surgery

Patients with CHD may be at increased risk for noncardiac surgery due to abnormal cardiac anatomy, the presence of shunts (both systemic-to-pulmonary and pulmonary-to-systemic shunts), cyanosis, and the presence of poor ventricular function, clinical heart failure, or pulmonary hypertension (543,544). There may be a poor correlation between clinical status and functional reserve. Cardiac anatomy must be clearly defined before surgery, and anesthesia must be carefully planned, based on the cardiac anatomy and hemodynamic state (489). Antibiotic prophylaxis against bacterial endocarditis is usually recommended. Preoperative phlebotomy to a hematocrit less than 65 may be considered to improve hemostatic function. Dehydration should be avoided in patients with cyanosis or severe pulmonary hypertension.

In patients with severe pulmonary hypertension, any decrease in systemic vascular resistance will cause systemic output to fall or will increase the magnitude of the right-to-left shunt in patients with a pulmonary to systemic shunt. Patients with a Fontan circulation pose a particular challenge. Because pulmonary blood flow depends on systemic preload, pulmonary blood flow and oxygenation may be adversely affected by changes in pulmonary vascular resistance, hemorrhage, vasodilator drugs, inadequate volume replacement, and positive-pressure ventilation causing increased intrathoracic pressure. Intravenous access must be meticulously managed in all patients with shunts to avoid paradoxical embolization.

Transplantation in Congenital Heart Disease

Patients with complex CHD may require heart transplant, lung transplant with cardiac repair, or a combined heart-lung transplant, depending on their particular anatomy and hemodynamics. Complex anatomy may make transplant surgery technically more challenging. Cyanotic patients and other patients with complex anatomy are at increased risk of bleeding from collaterals. Significant comorbidities may be present, including pulmonary vascular disease, renal dysfunction, and liver disease. The optimal timing of transplant is difficult. Maximum oxygen uptake is usually abnormal in patients with CHD, even in the absence of symptoms. A specific cutoff predicting poor outcome in CHD patients has not been defined. Because many patients are not candidates for ventricular assist devices, late referral may pose a significant problem because there is only limited therapy to "bridge" the patient to transplant (545).

There are limited data for outcome of transplantation in these patients. In the 2001 Registry of the International Society for Heart Lung Transplantation (ISHLT), only 1.6% of adult heart transplants were performed for CHD (546). Similar data was reported for lung transplant, whereas CHD accounted for one third of all heart-lung transplants. The most common diagnoses were the Eisenmenger syndrome and postoperative complex CHD (including the Fontan operation and postoperative atrial baffle for transposition of the great arteries). In the pediatric population, survival for patients with transplanted for CHD is not different from those with cardiomyopathy (547). However, in adults, survival is worse for patients with CHD than for patients with acquired heart disease (548,549).

CONTROVERSIES AND PERSONAL PERSPECTIVES

The majority of patients with CHD will survive to adulthood, with a population of nearly one million in the United States. The population of adult patients with CHD is estimated to be larger than the pediatric population (550). Although many patients who underwent intervention in childhood may consider themselves "cured," few can be truly considered cured. Most patients are at risk for long-term complications and will require long-term follow-up. At least half of these patients will have "significant defects," and more than 25% will have "complex defects" requiring long-term expert care (551). Traditionally, pediatric cardiologists have provided the care for most of these patients.

Adult patients with CHD often have little knowledge about their disease or its complications and may mistakenly consider themselves cured (552). When these patients develop complications related to their CHD, they frequently present to adult cardiologists who traditionally have had little training or exposure to patients with more complicated forms of CHD, and thus these patients may receive suboptimal care.

The Thirty-Second Bethesda Conference recommended the close collaboration of adult and pediatric cardiologists and the establishment of regional referral centers to provide expert care for this patient population (553). Such regional referral centers are designed to optimize the care of adult patients with congenital heart disease, as well as facilitate research and training in this area. Although there is an increasing number of adult CHD centers, access to expert care for most patients is limited.

Many questions remain regarding the optimal treatment of these patients. There are no large randomized, controlled trials in this patient population, and most of the literature involves case series or retrospective case–control series. The role of angiotensin-converting-enzyme inhibitors and β-blockers for patients with ventricular dysfunction in the setting of a single ventricle or a systemic RV is unknown. Optimal treatment of arrhythmias is largely undefined, and the role of ICDs in primary prevention of sudden death is completely unknown. Because of the relatively small numbers of patients, collaborative efforts are needed to create large databases, potentially even a national CHD database to effectively address clinical questions.

THE FUTURE

Many challenges remain. The genetic control of cardiac development is being intensely studied with efforts aimed at identifying specific gene defects and altered signals that result in cardiac malformations. Although gene therapy ultimately holds tremendous potential for altering cardiac development in the future, current possibilities of using interventional techniques on the fetal heart provide a unique opportunity for altering the morphology of the developing heart. Although there have been dramatic advances in the care of infants and children with CHD, there is still significant mortality for some patients and inadequate surgical options for some complex defects. Further advances in both surgical and catheter techniques will widen the spectrum of defects that can be treated and potentially minimize the long-term risk of complications.

Survivors of palliative or reparative procedures remain at risk for complications and sequelae of their original operation(s). Advances in our diagnostic tools (including echocardiography, cardiac MRI, and CT scanning) have improved our ability to define cardiac anatomy and may ultimately allow us to identify patients at risk for complications so that treatment interventions may be made in a timelier manner. Dramatic advances have been made in transcatheter techniques, and the role of the catheterization lab as a therapeutic location continues to evolve. Because arrhythmias are one of the most common complications seen in adult patients with CHD, advances in catheter ablation techniques, pacemaker technology, and defibrillators will likely contribute to significant improvements in the long-term outcomes of this patient population.

References

1. Perloff JK. *Clinical recognition of congenital heart disease,* 5th ed. Philadelphia: WB Saunders, 2003:1–5.
2. Hoffman JIE, Kaplan S. The incidence of congenital heart disease. *J Am Coll Cardiol* 2002;39:1890–1900.
3. Mitchell SC, Korones SB, Berendes HW. Congenital heart disease in 56,109 births. *Circulation* 1971;43:323–332.
4. Perloff JK, Warnes CA. Challenges posed by adults with repaired congenital heart disease. *Circulation* 2001;103:2637–2643.
5. Nora JJ. From generational studies to a multilevel genetic–environmental interaction. *J Am Coll Cardiol* 1994;23:1468–1471.
6. Pyeritz RE, Murphy EA. Genetics and congenital heart disease: perspectives and prospects. *J Am Coll Cardiol* 1989;13:1458–1468.
7. Payne RM, Johnson MC, Grant JW, et al. Toward a molecular understanding of congenital heart disease. *Circulation* 1995;91:494–504.
8. Johnson MC, Payne RM, Grant JW, et al. The genetic basis of pediatric heart disease. *Ann Intern Med* 1995;27:289–300.
9. Burn J, Brennan P, Holloway S, et al. Recurrence risks in offspring of adults with major heart defects: results from first cohort of British collaborative study. *Lancet* 1998;351:311–315.
10. Spicer RL. Cardiovascular disease in Down syndrome. *Pediatr Clin North Am* 1984;31:1331–1343.
11. Park SC, Mathews RA, Zuberbuhler JR, et al. Down's syndrome with congenital heart disease. *Am J Dis Child* 1977;131:29–33.
12. Barlow GM, Chen XN, Shi ZY, et al. Down syndrome congenital heart disease: a narrowed region and a candidate gene. *Genet Med* 2001;3(2):91–101.
13. Wilson DI, Goodship JA, Burn J, et al. Deletions within chromosome 22q11 in familial congenital heart disease. *Lancet* 1992;340:573–575.
14. Wilson DI, Cross IE, Goodship JA, et al. A prospective cytogenetic study of 36 cases of DiGeorge syndrome. *Am J Hum Genet* 1992;51(5):957–963.
15. Lindsay EA, Vitelli F, Su H, et al. *Tbx1* haploinsufficiency in the DiGeorge syndrome region causes aortic arch defects in mice. *Nature* 2001;4:97–101.
16. Li QY, Newbury-Ecob RA, Terrett JA, et al. Holt-Oram syndrome is caused by mutations in *TBX5*, a member of the Brachyury (T) gene family. *Nat Genet* 1997;15(1):21–29.
17. Metcalfe K, Rucka AK, Smoot L, et al. Elastin: mutational spectrum in supravalvular aortic stenosis. *Eur J Hum Genet* 2000;8(12):955–963.
18. Schott JJ, Benson DW, Basson CT, et al. Congenital heart disease caused by mutations in the transcription factor NKX2-5. *Science* 1998;281(5373):32–34.
19. Freed MD, Heymann MA, Lewis AB, et al. Prostaglandin E_1 in infants with ductus arteriosus–dependent congenital heart disease. *Circulation* 1981;64:899–905.
20. Tworetzky W, McElhinney DB, Brook MM, et al. Echocardiographic diagnosis alone for the complete repair of major congenital heart defects. *J Am Coll Cardiol* 1999;33:228–233.
21. Ho SY, McCarthy KP, Josen M, et al. Anatomic–echocardiographic correlates: an introduction to normal and congenitally malformed hearts. *Heart* 2001;86(Suppl II):II3–II11.
22. Marelli AJ, Child JS, Perloff JK. Transesophageal echocardiography in congenital heart disease in the adult. *Cardiol Clin* 1993;3:505–520.
23. Stumpfer O, Sutherland GR, eds. *Transesophageal echocardiography in congenital heart disease.* London, Edward Arnold; 1994:31–277.
24. Ungerleider R, Kisslo J, Greeley W, et al. Intraoperative echocardiography during congenital heart operations: experience from 1000 cases. *Ann Thorac Surg* 1995;60:S539–S542.
25. Salustri A, Spitaels S, McGhie J, et al. Transthoracic three-dimensional echocardiography in the adult patient with congenital heart disease. *J Am Coll Cardiol* 1995;26:759–767.
26. Vogel M, Ho S, Lincoln C, et al. Three-dimensional echocardiography can simulate intraoperative visualization of congenitally malformed hearts. *Ann Thorac Surg* 1995;60:1282–1288.
27. Geva T, Sahn DJ, Powell AJ. Magnetic resonance imaging of congenital heart disease in adults. *Prog Pediatr Cardiol* 2003;17:21–39.
28. Nienaber CA, Rehders TC, Fratz S. Detection and assessment of congenital heart disease by magnetic resonance techniques. *J Cardiovasc Magn Reson* 1999;1(2):169–184.
29. de Roos A, Roest AA. Evaluation of congenital heart disease by magnetic resonance imaging. *Eur Radiol* 2000;10:2–6.
30. Goon HW, Park IS, Ko JK, et al. Computed tomography for the diagnosis of congenital heart disease in pediatric and adult patients. *Int J Cardiovasc Imaging* 2005;21:347–365.
31. Moore JD, Doyle TP. Interventional catheter therapy in adults with congenital heart disease. *Prog Pediatr Cardiol* 2003;(17):61–71.
32. Holzer R, Cao QL, Hijazi ZM. State of the art catheter interventions in adults with congenital heart disease. *Expert Rev Cardiovasc Ther* 2004;2: 699–711.
33. Ferencz C, Rubin JD, Loffredo CA, et al. Epidemiology of congenital heart disease: the Baltimore–Washington Infant Study 1981–1989. In: Anderson RH, ed. *Perspectives in pediatric cardiology,* Vol. 4. Mount Kisco, NY: Futura, 1993:353.
34. Grabitz RG, Joffres MR, Collins-Nikai RI. Congenital heart disease: incidence in the first year of life. The Alberta Heritage pediatric cardiology program. *Am J Epidemiol* 1988;128:381–388.
35. Feldt R, Avasthey P, Yoshimasu F, et al. Incidence of congenital heart disease in children born to residents of Olmstead County, Minnesota, 1950–1969. *Mayo Clinic Proc* 1971;46:794–799.
36. Holt AR, Oram S. Familial heart disease with skeletal malformations. *Br Heart J* 1960;22:236–242.
37. Bourdillon PD, Foale RA, Somerville J. Persistent left superior vena cava with coronary sinus and left atrial connections. *Eur J Cardiol* 1980;11: 227–234.
38. Cockerham JT, Martin TC, Giutierrez FR, et al. Spontaneous closure of secundum atrial septal defect in infants and children. *Am J Cardiol* 1983;52:1267–1271.
39. Cayler GC. Spontaneous closure of symptomatic atrial septal defects. *N Engl J Med* 1967;276:65–73.
40. Cumming GR. Functional closure of atrial septal defects. *Am J Cardiol* 1968;22:888–892.
41. Muhler EG, Engelhardt W, von Bernuth G. Detection of sinus venosus atrial septal defect by two-dimensional echocardiography. *Eur Heart J* 1992;13: 453–456.
42. Mehta RH, Helmcke F, Nanda NC, et al. Uses and limitations of transthoracic echocardiography in the assessment of atrial septal defect in the adult. *Am J Cardiol* 1991;67:288–294.
43. Morimoto K, Matsuzki M, Tohma Y, et al. Diagnosis and quantitative evaluation of secundum-type atrial septal defect by transesophageal echocardiography. *Am J Cardiol* 1990;66:85–91.
44. Lipshultz SE, Sanders SP, Mayer JE, et al. Are routine perioperative cardiac catheterization and angiography necessary before repair of ostium primum atrial septal defect? *J Am Coll Cardiol* 1988;11:373–378.
45. Campbell M. Natural history of atrial septal defect. *Br Heart J* 1970; 1970:820–826.
46. Haworth SG. Pulmonary vascular disease in secundum atrial septal defect in childhood. *Am J Cardiol* 1983;51:265–272.
47. Murphy JG, Gersh BJ, McGoon MD, et al. Long-term outcome after surgical repair of isolated atrial septal defect. Follow-up at 27 to 32 years. *N Engl J Med* 1990;323:1645–1650.
48. Konstantinides S, Geibel A, Olschewski M, et al. A comparison of medical and surgical therapy for atrial septal defect in adults. *N Engl J Med* 1995;333:469–473.
49. Gatzoulis M, Redington A, Somerville J, et al. Should atrial septal defects in adults be closed? *Ann Thorac Surg* 1996;61:657–659.
50. Steele PM, Fuster V, Cohen M, et al. Isolated atrial septal defect with pulmonary vascular obstructive disease: long term follow-up and prediction of outcome after surgical correction. *Circulation* 1987;76:1037–1042.
51. Shah D, Azhar M, Oakley CM, et al. Natural history of secundum atrial septal defect in adults after medical or surgical treatment: a historical perspective study. *Br Heart J* 1994;71:224–228.
52. Horvath KA, Burke RP, Collins Jr JJ, et al. Surgical treatment of adult atrial septal defect: early and long-term results. *J Am Coll Cardiol* 1992;20: 1156–1159.
53. Marelli AJ, Alejos JC. Exercise response in atrial septal defect. *Prog Pediatr Cardiol* 1993;2:20–23.
54. St John Sutton MG, Tajik AJ, McGoon DC. Atrial septal defect in patients ages 60 years or older: Operative results and long-term postoperative follow-up. *Circulation* 1981;64:402–409.
55. Gatzoulis MA, Freeman MA, Siu SC, et al. Atrial arrhythmia after surgical closure of atrial septal defects in adults. *N Engl J Med* 1999;340:839–846.
56. Rigby M. The era of transcatheter closure of atrial septal defects. *Heart* 1999;81:227–228.
57. King TD, Mills NL. Secundum atrial septal defect: non-operative closure during cardiac catheterization. *JAMA* 1976;235:2506–2509.
58. Soto B, Ceballos R, Kirklin J. Ventricular septal defects: a surgical viewpoint. *J Am Coll Cardiol* 1989;14:1291–1297.
59. Van Praagh R, Geva T, Kreutzer J. Ventricular septal defects: how shall we describe, name and classify them? *J Am Coll Cardiol* 1989;14:1298–1299.
60. Nadas AS, ed. Report from the Joint Study on the Natural History of Congenital Heart Defects. *Circulation* 1977;56:1–87.
61. O'Fallon WM, Wediman WH. Report from the Second Joint Study on the Natural History of Congenital Heart Defects. *Circulation* 1993;87:1–126.
62. Ramaciotti C, Vetter JM, Bornemeier RA, et al. Prevalence, relation to spontaneous closure and association of muscular ventricular septal defects with other cardiac defects. *Am J Cardiol* 18995;75:61–65.
63. Moe DG, Guntheroth WG. Spontaneous closure of uncomplicated ventricular septal defect. *Am J Cardiol* 1987;60:674–678.
64. Frontera IP, Cabezuelo HG. Natural and modified history of isolated ventricular septal defect: a 17-year study. *Pediatr Cardiol* 1992;13:193–197.

65. Kidd L, Driscoll DJ, Gersony WM, et al. Second natural history study of congenital heart defects. Results of treatment of patients with ventricular septal defects. *Circulation* 1993;87:I38–I59.
66. Sutherland G, Godman M, Smallhorn J, et al. Ventricular septal defects. Two-dimensional echocardiographic and morphological correlations. *Br Heart J* 1982;47:315–328.
67. Gnanapragasam JP, Houston AB, Doig WB, et al. Influence of colour Doppler echocardiography on the ultrasonic assessment of congenital heart disease: a prospective study. *Br Heart J* 1991;66:238–243.
68. Krabill KA, Ring WS, Foker JE, et al. Echocardiographic versus cardiac catheterization diagnosis of infants with congenital heart disease requiring cardiac surgery. *Am J Cardiol* 1987;69:351–354.
69. Ge Z, Zhang Y, Kang W, et al. Noninvasive evaluation of right ventricular and pulmonary artery systolic pressures in patients with ventricular septal defects: simultaneous study of Doppler and catheterization data. *Am Heart J* 1993;125:1073–1081.
70. Murphy DJ, Ludomirsky A, Huhta JC. Continuous-wave Doppler in children with ventricular septal defect: noninvasive estimation of interventricular pressure gradient. *Am J Cardiol* 1986;57:428–432.
71. Kaplan S. Natural and postoperative history across age groups. *Cardiol Clin* 1993;11:543–556.
72. Bridges ND, Perry SB, Keane JF, et al. Preoperative transcatheter closure of congenital muscular ventricular septal defects. *N Engl J Med* 1991;324:1312–1317.
73. Lock JE, Block PC, McKay RG, et al. Transcatheter closure of ventricular septal defects. *Circulation* 1988;78:361–368.
74. O'Laughlin MP, Mullins CE. Transcatheter occlusion of ventricular septal defect. *Cathet Cardiovasc Diagn* 1989;17:175–179.
75. Rigby ML, Redington AN. Primary transcatheter umbrella closure of perimembranous ventricular septal defect. *Br Heart J* 1994;72:368–371.
76. Weidman WH, DuShane JW, Ellison RC. Clinical course in adults with ventricular septal defects. *Circulation* 1977;56:178–179.
77. Rhodes LA, Keane JF, Keane JP, et al. Long term follow-up (to 43 years) of ventricular septal defect with audible aortic regurgitation. *Am J Cardiol* 1990;66:340–345.
78. Moller JH, Patton C, Varco RL, et al. Late results (30 to 35 years) after operative closure of isolated ventricular septal defect from 1954 to 1960. *Am J Cardiol* 1991;68:1491–1497.
79. Blackstone EH, Kirklin JW, Bradley EL, et al. Optimal age and results in repair of large ventricular septal defects. *J Thorac Cardiovasc Surg* 1976;72:661–679.
80. Rizzoli G, Blackstone EH, Kirklin JW, et al. Incremental risk factors in hospital mortality after repair of ventricular septal defects. *J Thorac Cardiovasc Surg* 1980;80:494–505.
81. Hoffman JIE. Incidence of congenital heart disease: I. Postnatal incidence. *Pediatr Cardiol* 1995;16:103–113.
82. Hoffman JIE. Incidence of congenital heart disease: II. Prenatal incidence. *Pediatr Cardiol* 1995;16:155–165.
83. Mullins CE, Pagotto L. Patent ductus arteriosus. In: Garson Jr A, Bricker JT, Fisher DJ, Neish SR, eds. *The science and practice of pediatric cardiology*, Vol. 1. Baltimore: Williams & Wilkins, 1998:1181–1196.
84. Fyler DC. Patent ductus arteriosus. In: Fyler DC, ed. *Nadas' pediatric cardiology*. St. Louis: Mosby-Year Book, 1992:525–534.
85. Therrien J, Dore A, Gersony W, et al. CCS Consensus Conference 2001 update: recommendations for the management of adults with congenital heart disease. Part I. *Can J Cardiol* 2001;17:940–959.
86. Tynam M. Transcatheter occlusion of persistent arterial duct: European registry. *Lancet* 1992;340:1062–1066.
87. Bulbul ZR, Fahey JT, Doyle TP, et al. Transcatheter closure of the patent ductus arteriosus: a comparative study between occluding coils and the Rashkind umbrella device. *Cathet Cardiovasc Diagn* 1996;39:355–363.
88. Lloyd TR. Patent ductus arteriosus closure: devices and techniques. In: Imai Y, Kazuo M, eds. *Proceedings of the Second World Congress of Pediatric Cardiology and Cardiac Surgery*. New York: Futura, 1998;315–317.
89. Uzun O, Hancock S, Parsons JM, et al. Transcatheter occlusion of the arterial duct with Cook detachable coils: early experience. *Heart* 1996;76:269–273.
90. Dalvi B, Goyal V, Narula D, et al. New technique using temporary balloon occlusion for transcatheter closure of patent ductus arteriosus with Gianturco coils. *Cathet Cardiovasc Diagn* 1997;41:62–70.
91. Sommer RJ, Gutierrez A, Lai WW, et al. Use of preformed nitinol snare to improve transcatheter coil delivery in occlusion of patent ductus arteriosus. *Am J Cardiol*. 1994;74:836–839.
92. Hays MD, Hoyer MH, Glasow PF. New forceps delivery technique for coil occlusion of patent ductus arteriosus. *Am J Cardiol* 1996;77:209–211.
93. Berdjis F, Moore JW. Balloon occlusion delivery technique for closure of patent ductus arteriosus. *Am Heart J* 1997;133:601–604.
94. Masura J, Walsh KP, Tahnoupoulous B, et al. Catheter closure of moderate to large-sized patent ductus arteriosus using the new Amplatzer duct occluder; immediate and short-term results. *J Am Coll Cardiol* 1998;31:878–882.
95. Pass RH, Hijazi ZM, Hsy D, et al. Multicenter USA Amplatzer Patent Ductus Arteriosus Occlusion Device Trial: initial and one-year results. *J Am Coll Cardiol* 2004;44:513–519.
96. Ladusans EJ, Murduch I, Franciosis J. Severe hemolysis after percutaneous closure of a ductus arteriosus (arterial duct). *Br Heart J* 1989;61:548–560.
97. Hayes AM, Redington AN, Rigby ML. Severe haemolysis after transcatheter duct occlusion: a non-surgical remedy. *Br Heart J* 1992;67:321–322.
98. Panagopoulus PH, Tatooles CJ, Abedeen E, et al. Patent ductus arteriosus in infants: a review of 936 operations (1946–1969). Thorax 1971;26:137–144.
99. Trippestad A., Efskind L. Patent ductus arteriosus surgical treatment in 686 patients. *Scand J Thorac Cardiovasc Surg* 1972;6:38–42.
100. Mavroudis C, Backer CL, Gevitz M. Forty-six years of patent ductus arteriosus division at Children's Memorial Hospital of Chicago: standards for comparison. *Ann Surg* 1994;1220:402–409.
101. Siew YH, Baker EJ, Rigby ML, et al. Atrioventricular septal defect. In: *Color atlas of congenital heart disease; morphologic and clinical correlations*. London: Mosby-Wolfe, 1995:65–75.
102. Clapp S, Perry BL, Farooki ZQ, et al. Down's syndrome, complete atrioventricular canal, and pulmonary vascular obstructive disease. *J Thorac Cardiovasc Surg* 1900;100:115–121.
103. Cooney TP, Thurlbeck WM. Pulmonary hypoplasia in Down's syndrome. *N Engl J Med* 1982;307:1170–1173.
104. Chi TPL, Krovetz LJ. The pulmonary vascular bed in children with Down syndrome. *J Pediatr* 1975;86:533–538.
105. Shinebourne EA, Ho SY. Atrioventricular septal defect: complete and partial (ostium primum atrial septal defect). In: Gatzoulis MA, Webb GD, Daubeney PEF, eds. *Diagnosis and management of adult congenital heart disease*. Edinburgh: Churchill Livingstone: 2003:179–187.
106. Smallhorn JF, Tommasini G, Anderson RH, et al. Assessment of atrioventricular septal defects by two-dimensional echocardiography. *Br Heart J* 1982;47:109–121.
107. Carpentier A. Surgical anatomy and management of the mitral component of atrioventricular canal defects. In: Anderson RH, Shinebourne RA, eds. *Paediatric cardiology*. Edinburgh: Churchill Livingstone 1977:477–486.
108. Capouya ER, Laks H, Drinkwater DC, et al. Management of the left atrioventricular valve in the repair of complete atrioventricular septal defects. *J Thorac Cardiovasc Surg* 1992;104:196–201.
109. Gatzoulis MA, Hechters S, Webb GD, et al. Surgery for partial atrioventricular septal defect in the adult. *Ann Thorac Surg* 1999;67:504–510.
110. Gunther T, Mazzitelli D, Hachnel CJ, et al. Long term results after repair of complete atrioventricular septal defects: analysis of risk factors. *Ann Thorac Surg* 1988;65:754–759.
111. Bergin ML, Warnes CA, Tajik AJ, et al. Partial atrioventricular canal defect: long term follow up after initial repair in patients ≥40 years old. *J Am Coll Cardiol* 1995;25:1189–1194.
112. Yen Ho S, Gerlis LM, Anderson C, et al. The morphology of aortopulmonary windows with regard to their classification and morphogenesis. *Cardiol Young* 1994;4:146–155.
113. Gerlis LM, MacGregor CC d'A, Yen Ho S. An anatomical study of 110 cases with deficiency of the aorticopulmonary septum with emphasis on the role of the arterial duct. *Cardiol Young* 1992;2:342–352.
114. Stamato T, Benson LN, Smallhorn JF, et al. Transcatheter closure of an aortopulmonary window with a modified double umbrella occluder system. *Cathet Cardiovasc Diagn* 1995;35:165–167.
115. van Som JAM, Puga FJ, Danielson GK, et al. Aortopulmonary window: factors associated with early and late success after surgical treatment. *Mayo Clinic Proc* 1993;68:128–133.
116. Bertonlini A, Dalmonte P, Bava GL, et al. Aortopulmonary septal defects. A review of the literature and report of ten cases. *J Cardiovasc Surg* 1994;35(3):207–213.
117. Kirklin JW, Barratt-Boyes BG. Aortopulmonary window. *Cardiac Surg* 1993;1:1153–1157.
118. Cohen AJ, Sell JE, Zurcher RP, et al. Anomalous pulmonary venous drainage of the right lung. *Ann Thorac Surg* 1993;56:1397–1399.
119. Jennings JG, Serwer GA. Partial anomalous pulmonary venous connection to the azygos vein with intact atrial septum. *Pediatr Cardiol* 1986;7:116–117.
120. Mullen JC, Razzouk AJ, Williams WG, et al. Partial anomalous pulmonary venous connection to the azygos vein with atrial septal defect. *J Thorac Surg* 1991;52:1164–1165.
121. Wong ML, McCrindle BW, Mota C, et al. Echocardiographic evaluation of partial anomalous pulmonary venous drainage. *J Am Coll Cardiol* 1995;50:503–507.
122. Masui T, Seelos K, Kersting-Sommerhoff BA, et al. Abnormalities of the pulmonary veins: evaluation with MR imaging and comparison with cardiac angiography and echocardiography. *Radiology* 1991;181:645–649.
123. Gaynor JW, Burch M, Dollery C, et al. Repair of anomalous pulmonary venous connection to the superior vena cava. *Ann Thorac Surg* 1995;59:1471–1475.
124. Van Meter Jr C, LeBlanc JG, Culpepper WS, et al. Partial anomalous pulmonary venous return. *Circulation* 1990;82(Suppl IV):195–198.
125. Saalouke MG, Shapiro SR, Perry LW. Isolated partial anomalous pulmonary venous drainage associated with pulmonary vascular obstructive disease. *Am J Cardiol* 1977;39:398–407.
126. Vogel M. Partial anomalous pulmonary venous connection and the scimitar syndrome. In: Gatzoulis MA, Webb GD, Daubeney PEF, eds. *Diagnosis and management of adult congenital heart disease*. Edinburgh: Churchill Livingstone, 2003:205–210.

127. Mendez HMM, Opitz JM. Noonan syndrome: a review. *Am J Med Genet* 1985;21:493–506.
128. Schieken RM, Freedman S, Pierce WS. Severe congenital pulmonary stenosis with pulmonary valvular dysplasia syndrome. *Ann Thorac Surg* 1973;15:570–577.
129. Hanley FL, Sade RM, Freedom RM, et al. Outcomes in critically ill neonates with pulmonary stenosis and intact ventricular septum: a multiinstitutional study. Congenital Heart Surgeons Society. *J Am Coll Cardiol* 1993;22:183–192.
130. Hayes CJ, Gersony WM, Driscoll DJ, et al. Second Natural History Study of Congenital Heart Defects: results of treatment of patients with pulmonary valvar stenosis. *Circulation* 1993;87(Suppl I):I28–I37.
131. Shindo T, Kuroda T, Watanabe S, et al. Aneurysmal dilatation of the pulmonary trunk with mild pulmonic stenosis. *Intern Med* 1995;34:199–202.
132. Tami LF, McElderry MW. Pulmonary artery aneurysm due to severe congenital pulmonic stenosis: case report and literature review. *Angiology* 1994;45:383–390.
133. Kopecky SL, Gersh BJ, McGoon MD, et al. Long-term outcome of patients undergoing surgical repair of isolated pulmonary valve stenosis. Follow-up at 20–30 years. *Circulation* 1988;78:1150–1156.
134. McCrindle BW. Independent predictors of longterm results after balloon pulmonary valvuloplasty. Valvuloplasty and Angioplasty of Congenital Anomalies (VACA) Registry Investigators. *Circulation* 1994;89:1751–1759.
135. Lau KW, Hung JS. Controversies in percutaneous balloon pulmonary valvuloplasty: timing, patient selection and technique. *J Heart Valve Dis* 1993;2:321–325.
136. Rao PS. Balloon pulmonary valvuloplasty for isolated pulmonic stenosis. In: Rao PS, ed. *Transcatheter therapy in pediatric cardiology*. New York: Wiley-Liss, 1993:59–104.
137. David SW, Goussous YM, Harbi N, et al. Management of typical and dysplastic pulmonic stenosis, uncomplicated or associated with complex intracardiac defects, in juveniles and adults: use of percutaneous balloon pulmonary valvuloplasty with eight-month hemodynamic follow-up. *Cathet Cardiovasc Diagn* 1993;29:105–112.
138. Stanger P, Cassidy SC, Girod DA, et al. Balloon pulmonary valvuloplasty: results of the Valvuloplasty and Angioplasty of Congenital Anomalies Registry. *Am J Cardiol* 1990;65:775–783.
139. Tang JS, Kauffman SL, Lynfield J. Hypoplasia of the pulmonary arteries in infants with congenital rubella. *Am J Cardiol* 1971;27:491–496.
140. Kreutzer J, Landzberg MJ, Preminger TJ, et al. Isolated peripheral pulmonary artery stenoses in the adult. *Circulation* 1996;93:1417–1423.
141. Tanoue LT. Pulmonary involvement in collagen vascular disease: a review of the pulmonary manifestations of the Marfan syndrome, ankylosing spondylitis, Sjögren's syndrome, and relapsing polychondritis. *J Thorac Imaging* 1992;7:62–77.
142. Jeang MK, Adyanthaya A, Kuo L, et al. Multiple pulmonary artery aneurysms: new use for magnetic resonance imaging. *Am J Med* 1986;81:1001–1004.
143. O'Laughlin MP, Perry SB, Lock JE, Mullins CE. Use of endovascular stents in congenital heart disease. *Circulation* 1991;83:1923–1939.
144. Hijazi ZM, al-Fadley F, Geggel RL, et al. Stent implantation for relief of pulmonary artery stenosis: immediate and short-term results. *Cathet Cardiovasc Diagn* 1996;38:16–23.
145. Shaffer KM, Mullins CE, Grifka RG, et al. Intravascular stents in congenital heart disease: short- and long-term results from a large single-center experience. *J Am Coll Cardiol* 1998;31:661–667.
146. Fogelman R, Nykanen D, Smallhorn JF, et al. Endovascular stents in the pulmonary circulation. Clinical impact on management and medium-term follow-up. *Circulation* 1995;92:881–885.
147. Roberts WC. The congenitally bicuspid aortic valve. *Am J Cardiol* 1970;26:72–83.
148. Fenoglio JJ, McAllister HA, deCastro CM, et al. Congenital bicuspid aortic valve after age 20. *Am J Cardiol* 1977;39:164–169.
149. Ward C. Clinical significance of the bicuspid aortic valve. *Heart* 2000;83:81–85.
150. Lee TC, Zhao YD, Coutman DW, et al. Abnormal aortic valve development in mice lacking endothelial nitrate oxide synthase. *Circulation* 2000;101:2345–2348.
151. Ogata T, Matsuo N. Turner syndrome and female sex chromosome aberrations: deduction of the principle factors involved in the development of clinical features. *Hum Genet* 1995;95:607–629.
152. Niwa K, Perloff JK, Bhuta SM, et al. Structural abnormalities of great arterial walls in congenital heart disease: light and electron microscopic analysis. *Circulation* 2001;103:393–400.
153. Keane MG, Wiegers WE, Plapper T, et al. Bicuspid aortic valves are associated with aortic dilatation out of proportion to coexistent valvular lesions. *Circulation* 2000;102(Suppl III):III35–III39.
154. Rhodes LA, Colan SD, Perry SB, et al. Predictors of survival in neonates with critical aortic stenosis. *Circulation* 1991;84:2325–2335.
155. Mosca RS, Iannettoni MD, Schwartz SM, et al. Critical aortic stenosis in the neonate: a comparison of balloon valvuloplasty and transventricular dilatation. *J Thorac Cardiovasc Surg* 1995;109:147–154.
156. Hagler DJ, Tajik AJ, Seward JB, et al. Noninvasive assessment of pulmonary valve stenosis, aortic valve stenosis and coarctation of the aorta in critically ill neonates. *Am J Cardiol* 1986;57:369–372.
157. Bonow RO, Carabello B, de Leon AC, et al. ACC/AHA guidelines for the management of patients with valvular heart disease: a report of the American College of Cardiology/American Heart Association Task Force on Practical Guidelines (Committee on Management of Patients with Valvular Heart Disease). *J Am Coll Cardiol* 1998;12:1486–1488.
158. Kelly TA, Rothbart RM, Cooper CM, et al. Comparison of outcome of asymptomatic to symptomatic patients older than 20 years of age with valvular aortic stenosis. *Am J Cardiol* 1988;61:123–130.
159. Bauer EP, Schmidli J, Vogt PR, et al. Valvotomy for isolated congenital aortic stenosis in children: prognostic factors for outcome. *Thorac Cardiovasc Surg* 1992;40:334–339.
160. Justo RN, McCrindle BW, Benson LH, et al. Aortic valve regurgitation after surgical versus percutaneous balloon valvotomy for congenital aortic valve stenosis. *Am J Cardiol* 1996;77:1332–1338.
161. Hawkins JA, Minich LL, Shaddy RE, et al. Aortic valve repair and replacement after balloon valvuloplasty in children. *Ann Thorac Surg* 1996;61:1355–1358.
162. Moore P, Egito E, Mowrey H, et al. Midterm results of balloon dilatation of congenital aortic stenosis: predictors of success. *J Am Coll Cardiol* 1996;27:1257–1263.
163. Rocchini AP, Beekman RH, Ben SG, et al. Balloon aortic valvuloplasty in the young adult with congenital aortic stenosis. *Am J Cardiol* 1994;7:1112–1117.
164. Sandhu SK, Lloyd TR, Crowley DC, et al. Effectiveness of balloon valvuloplasty in the young adult with congenital aortic stenosis. *Cathet Cardiovasc Diagn* 1995;36:122–127.
165. Shaddy RE, Boucek MM, Sturtevant JE, et al. Gradient reduction, aortic valve regurgitation and prolapse after balloon aortic valvuloplasty in 32 consecutive patients with congenital aortic stenosis. *J Am Coll Cardiol* 1990;16:451–456.
166. Sholler GF, Keane JF, Perry SB, et al. Balloon dilatation of congenital aortic valve stenosis: results and influence of technical and morphological features on outcome. *Circulation* 1988;78:351–360.
167. Rocchini AP, Beekman RH, Schachar GB, et al. Balloon aortic valvuloplasty: results of the Valvuloplasty and Angioplasty of Congenital Anomalies Registry. *Am J Cardiol* 1990;65:784–789.
168. Keane JF, Driscoll DJ, Gersony WM, et al. Second Natural History Study of Congenital Heart Defects: results of treatment of patients with aortic valve stenosis. *Circulation* 1993;87(Suppl I):I16–I27.
169. Pihkala J, Nykanen D, Freedom RM, et al. Interventional cardiac catheterization. *Pediatr Clin North Am* 1999;45:441–464.
170. Choi JY, Sullivan ID. Fixed subaortic stenosis: anatomical spectrum and nature of progression. *Br Heart J* 1991;65:280–286.
171. Freedom RM, Pelech A, Brand A, et al. The progressive nature of subaortic stenosis in congenital heart disease. *Int J Cardiol* 1985;8:137–143.
172. Leichter DA, Sullivan I, Gersony WM. "Acquired" discrete subvalvular aortic stenosis: natural history and hemodynamics. *J Am Coll Cardiol* 1989;14:1539–1544.
173. Maginot KR, Williams RG. Fixed subaortic stenosis. *Prog Pediatr Cardiol* 1994;3:141–149.
174. Sommerville J. Fixed subaortic stenosis: a frequently misunderstood lesion. *Int J Cardiol* 1985;8:145–148.
175. Cape EG, Vanauker MD, Sigfusson G, et al. Potential role of mechanical stress in the etiology of pediatric heart disease: septal shear stress in subaortic stenosis. *J Am Coll Cardiol* 1997;30:247–254.
176. Shem-Tov A, Schneeweiss A, Motro M, et al. Clinical presentation and natural history of mild discrete subaortic stenosis: follow-up of 1–17 years. *Circulation* 1982;66:509–512.
177. van Son JA, Schaff HV, Danielson GK, et al. Surgical treatment of discrete and tunnel subaortic stenosis: late survival and risk of reoperation. *Circulation* 1993;88:159–169.
178. Wright GB, Kean JF, Nadas AS, et al. Fixed subaortic stenosis in the young: medical and surgical course in 83 patients. *Am J Cardiol* 1983;52:830–835.
179. Coleman DM, Smallhorn JF, McCrindle BW, et al. Postoperative follow-up of fibromuscular subaortic stenosis. *J Am Coll Cardiol* 1994;24:1558–1564.
180. Ashraf H, Cotroneo J, Dhar N, et al. Long-term results after excision of fixed subaortic stenosis. *J Thorac Cardiovasc Surg* 1985;90:864–871.
181. Feigl A, Lucas Jr RV, Edwards JE. Involvement of the aortic valve cusps in discrete subaortic stenosis. *Pediatr Cardiol* 1984;5:185–190.
182. Keane JF, Fellows KE, LaFarge CG, et al. The surgical management of discrete and diffuse supravalvular aortic stenosis. *Circulation* 1976;54:112–117.
183. Brauner R, Laks H, Drinkwater DCJ, et al. Benefits of early surgical repair in fixed subaortic stenosis. *J Am Coll Cardiol* 1991;18:1499–1505.
184. Lupinetti FM, Pridjian AK, Callow LB, et al. Optimum treatment of discrete subaortic stenosis. *Ann Thorac Surg* 1992;54:467–470.
185. Rayburn ST, Netherland DE, Heath BJ. Discrete membranous subaortic stenosis: improved results after resection and myectomy. *Ann Thorac Surg* 1997;64:105–109.
186. van Son JA, Schaff HV, Danielson GK, et al. Surgical treatment of discrete and tunnel subaortic stenosis. Later survival and risk of reoperation. *Circulation* 1993;88:III59–III69.
187. Serraf A, Zoghby J, Lacour-Gayet F, et al. Surgical treatment of subaortic stenosis: a seventeen-year experience. *J Thorac Cardiovasc Surg* 1999;117:669–678.

188. Zalzstein E, Moes CA, Musewe NN, et al. Spectrum of cardiovascular anomalies in Williams-Beuren syndrome. *Pediatr Cardiol* 1991;12:219–223.
189. Giddens NG, Finley JP, Nanton MA, et al. The natural course of supravalvular aortic stenosis and peripheral pulmonary artery stenosis in Williams syndrome. *Br Heart J* 1989;62:315–319.
190. Terhune PE, Buchino JJ, Rees AH. Myocardial infarction associated with supravalvular aortic stenosis. *J Pediatr* 1985;106:251–254.
191. van Son JA, Edwards WD, Danielson GK. Pathology of coronary arteries, myocardium, and great arteries in supravalvular aortic stenosis: report of five cases with implications for surgical treatment. *J Thorac Cardiovasc Surg* 1994;108:21–28.
192. Beitzke A, Becker H, Rigler B, et al. Development of aortic aneurysms in familial supravalvular aortic stenosis. *Pediatr Cardiol* 1986;6:227–229.
193. Bleiden LC, Lucas Jr RV, Carter JB, et al. A developmental complex including supravalvular stenosis of the aorta and pulmonary trunk. *Circulation* 1974;49:585–590.
194. Rein AJJT, Preminger TJ, Perry SB, et al. Generalized arteriopathy in Williams syndrome: an intravascular ultrasound study. *J Am Coll Cardiol* 1993;21:1727–1730.
195. Kaplan P, Levinson M, Kaplan BS. Cerebral artery stenoses in Williams syndrome causes strokes in childhood. *J Pediatr* 1995;126:943.
196. McElhinney DB, Petrossian E, Tworetzky W, et al. Issues and outcomes in the management of supravalvular aortic stenosis. *Ann Thorac Surg* 1998;66:1337–1342.
197. Delius RS, Samyn MM, Behrednt DM. Should a bicuspid aortic valve be replaced in the presence of subvalvar or supravalvar aortic stenosis? *Ann Thorac Surg* 1998;66:1137–1142.
198. Stamm C, Kreutzer C, Zurakowski D, et al. Forty-one years of surgical experience with congenital supravalvular aortic stenosis. *J Thorac Cardiovasc Surg* 1999;118:874–885.
199. Sharma BK, Fujiwara H, Halman GL, et al. Supravalvar aortic stenosis: a 20-year review of surgical experience. *Ann Thorac Surg* 1991;51;1031–1039.
200. Fyler DC, Buckly LP, Hellenbrand WE, et al. Report of the New England Regional Infant Cardiac Program. *Pediatrics* 1980;65(Suppl):375–461.
201. Warnes CA. Bicuspid aortic valve and coarctation: two villains part of a diffuse problem. *Heart* 2003;89:965–966.
202. Gardiner HM, Celermajer DS, Sorensen KE, et al. Arterial reactivity is significantly impaired in normotensive young adults after successful repair of aortic coarctation in childhood. *Circulation* 1994;89:1745–1750.
203. Cohen M, Fuster V, Steele PM, et al. Coarctation of the aorta: Long–term follow–up and prediction of outcome after surgical correction. *Circulation* 1989;80:840–845.
204. Brouwer RM Erasmus ME, Ebels T, et al. Influence of age on survival, late hypertension, and recoarctation in elective aortic coarctation repair: Including long-term results after elective aortic coarctation repair with a follow-up from 25 to 44 years. *J Thorac Cardiovasc Surg* 1994;108:525–531.
205. Martin EC, Strattford MA, Gersony WM. Initial detection of coarctation of the aorta: an opportunity for the radiologist. *AJR Am J Roentgenol* 1981;137:1015–1017.
206. Shaddy RE, Snider AR, Silverman NH, et al. Pulsed Doppler findings in patients with coarctation of the aorta. *Circulation* 1986;73:82–88.
207. Stern HC, Locher D, Wallnofer K, et al. Noninvasive assessment of coarctation of the aorta: comparative measurements by two-dimensional echocardiography, magnetic resonance, and angiography. *Pediatr Cardiol* 1991;12:1–5.
208. Simpson IA, Chung KJ, Glass RF, et al. Cine magnetic resonance imaging for evaluation of anatomy and flow relations in infants and children with coarctation of the aorta. *Circulation* 1988;78:142–148.
209. Kaplan S. Long term survival patterns. *J Am Coll Cardiol* 1991;18:319–320.
210. Quaegebeur JM, Jonas RA, Weinberg AD, et al. Outcomes in seriously ill neonates with coarctation of the aorta: a multiinstitutional study. *J Thorac Cardiovasc Surg* 1994;108:841–851.
211. Zehr KJ, Gillinov AM, Redmond JM, et al. Repair of coarctation of the aorta in neonates and infants: a thirty-year experience. *Ann Thorac Surg* 1995;59:33–41.
212. Rubay JE, Sluysmans T, Alexandrescu V, et al. Surgical repair of coarctation of the aorta in infants under one year of age: long-term results in 146 patients comparing subclavian flap angioplasty and modified end-to-end anastamosis. *J Cardiovasc Surg* 1992;33:216–222.
213. Bouchart F, Dubar A, Tabley A, et al. Coarctation of the aorta in adults: surgical results and long-term follow-up. *Ann Thorac Surg* 2000;70:1483–1488.
214. Bauer M, Alexi-Meskishvili VV, Bauer U, et al. Benefits of surgical repair of coarctation of the aorta in patients older than 50 years. *Ann Thorac Surg* 2001;72:2060–2064.
215. Carr JA, Amaato JJ, Higgins RS. Long-term results of surgical coarctectomy in the adolescent and adult with 18-year follow-up. *Ann Thorac Surg* 2005;79:1950–1955.
216. Fletcher SE, Nihill MR, Grifka RG, et al. Balloon angioplasty of native coarctation of the aorta: midterm follow-up and prognostic factors. *J Am Coll Cardiol* 1995;25:730–734.
217. Mendelsohn AM, Lloyd TR, Crowley DC, et al. Late follow-up of balloon angioplasty in children with a native coarctation of the aorta. *Am J Cardiol* 1994;74:696–700.
218. Shaddy RE, Boucek MM, Sturtevant JE, et al. Comparison of angioplasty and surgery for unoperated coarctation of the aorta. *Circulation* 1993;87:793–797.
219. Johnson MC, Canter CE, Strauss AW, et al. Repair of coarctation of the aorta in infancy: comparison of surgical and balloon angioplasty. *Am Heart J* 1993;125:464–468.
220. Fawzy ME, Dunn B, Galal O, et al. Balloon coarctation angioplasty in adolescents and adults: early and intermediate results. *Am Heart J* 1992;124:167–171.
221. Rao PS, Galal O, Smith PA, et al. Five- to nine-year follow-up results of balloon angioplasty of native aortic coarctation in infants and children. *J Am Coll Cardiol* 1996;27:462–470.
222. Hellenbrand WE, Allen HD, Golinko RJ, et al. Balloon angioplasty for aortic recoarctation: results of valvuloplasty and angioplasty of Congenital Anomalies Registry. *Am J Cardiol* 1990;65:790–792.
223. Hijazi ZM, Fahey JT, Kleinman CS, et al. Balloon angioplasty for recurrent coarctation of the aorta. Immediate and long-term results. *Circulation* 1991;84:1150–1156.
224. Rao PS, Wilson AD, Chopra PS. Immediate and follow-up results of balloon angioplasty of postoperative recoarctation in infants and children. *Am Heart J* 1990;120:1315–1320.
225. Leandro J, Smallhorn JF, Benson L, et al. Ambulatory blood pressure monitoring and left ventricular mass and function after successful repair of coarctation of the aorta. *J Am Coll Cardiol* 1992;20:197–204.
226. Presbitero P, Demarie D, Villani M, et al. Long term results (15 to 30 years) of surgical repair of aortic coarctation. *Br Heart J* 1987;7:462–467.
227. de Divitis M, Pilla C, Kattenhorn M, et al. Ambulatory blood pressure, left ventricular mass, and conduit artery function late after successful repair of coarctation of the aorta. *J Am Coll Cardiol* 2003;41:2259–2265.
228. Celermajer DS, Greaves K. Survivors of coarctation repair: fixed but not cured. *Heart* 2002;88:113–114.
229. Kaemmerer H, Oelert F, Bahlmann J, et al. Arterial hypertension in adults after surgical treatment of aortic coarctation. *Thorac Cardiovasc Surg* 1998;46:121–125.
230. Suarez DLJ, Pan M, Romero M, et al. Balloon-expandable stent repair of severe coarctation of aorta. *Am Heart J* 1995;129:1002–1008.
231. Redington AN, Hayes AM, Ho SY. Transcatheter stent implantation to treat aortic coarctation in infancy. *Br Heart J* 1993;69:80–82.
232. Rosenthal E, Quershi SA, Tynan M. Stent implantation for aortic recoarctation. *Am Heart J* 1995;129:1220–1221.
233. Immagoulou A, Anderson RC, Moller JH. Interruption of the aortic arch: clinical features in 20 patients. *Chest* 1972;51:549–553.
234. Finley JP, Collins GF, De Chadarevian JP, et al. DiGeorge syndrome presenting as severe congenital heart disease in the newborn. *Can Med Assoc J* 1977;116:635–640.
235. Van Microp LHS, Kutsche LM. Cardiovascular anomalies in DiGeorge syndrome and importance of neural crest as a possible pathogenic factor. *Am J Cardiol* 1986;58:133–137.
236. Sell JE, Jonas RA, Mayer JE, et al. The results of a surgical program for interrupted aortic arch. *J Thorac Cardiovasc Surg* 1988;96:864–877.
237. Serraf A, Lacour-Gayet F, Robotin M, et al. Repair of interrupted aortic arch: a ten-year experience. *J Thorac Cardiovasc Surg* 1996;112;1150–1160.
238. Jonas RA, Quaegebeur JM, Kirklin JW, et al. Outcomes in patients with interrupted aortic arch and ventricular septal defect: a multiinstitutional study. *J Thorac Cardiovasc Surg* 1994;107:1099–1113.
239. Geva T, Hornberger LK, Sanders SP, et al. Echocardiographic predictors of left ventricular outflow tract obstruction after repair of interrupted aortic arch. *J Am Coll Cardiol* 1993;22:1953–1960.
240. Shone JD, Sellers RD, Anderson RC, et al. The developmental complex of "parachute mitral valve," supravalvular ring of left atrium, subaortic stenosis, and coarctation of the aorta. *Am J Cardiol* 1963;11:714–725.
241. Shone JD, Sellers RD, Anderson RC, et al. The developmental complex of "parachute mitral valve," supravalvar ring of the left atrium, subaortic stenosis, and coarctation of the aorta. *Am J Cardiol* 1963;11:14.
242. Ruckman RN, Van Praagh R. Anatomic types of congenital mitral stenosis: report of 49 autopsy cases with consideration of the diagnosis and surgical implications. *Am J Cardiol* 1978;42:592–601.
243. Banerfee A, Kohl T, Silverman NH. Echocardiographic evaluation of congenital mitral valve anomalies in children. *Am J Cardiol* 1995;76:1284–1291.
244. Aharon AS, Laks H, Drinkwater DC, et al. Early and late results of mitral valve repair in children. *J Thorac Cardiovasc Surg* 1994;107:1262–1270.
245. Coles JG, Williams WG, Watanabe T, et al. Surgical experience with reparative techniques in patients with congenital mitral valvular anomalies. *Circulation* 1987;76:117–122.
246. Alday LE, Juaneda E. Percutaneous balloon dilatation in congenital mitral stenosis. *Br Heart J* 1987;57:479–482.
247. Grifka RG, O'Laughlin MP, Nihill MR, et al. Double-transseptal, double-balloon valvuloplasty for congenital mitral stenosis. *Circulation* 1992;85:123–129.
248. Kveselis DA, Rocchini AP, Beekman R, et al. Balloon angioplasty for congenital and rheumatic mitral stenosis. *Am J Cardiol* 1986;57:348–350.

249. Collins-Nakai RI, Rosenthal A, Castaneda AR, et al. Congenital mitral stenosis. A review of 20 years' experience. *Circulation* 1977;56:1039–1047.
250. Van Praagh R, Corsini I. Cor triatriatum: pathologic anatomy and a consideration of morphogenesis based on 13 postmortem cases and a study of normal development of the pulmonary vein and atrial septum in 83 human embryos. *Am Heart J* 1968;78:379–405.
251. Anderson RH. Understanding the nature of congenital division of the atrial chambers. *Br Heart J* 1992;68:1–3.
252. Feld H, Shani J, Rudyat HW, et al. Initial presentation of cor triatriatum in a 55-year old woman. *Am Heart J* 1992;124:788–791.
253. Murphy D. Cor triatriatum and mitral stenosis. In: Gatzoulis MA, Webb GD, Daubeney PEF, eds. *Diagnosis and management of adult congenital heart disease*. Edinburgh: Churchill Livingstone: 2003:191–197.
254. Rorie M, Xie GY, Miles H, et al. Diagnosis and surgical correction of cor triatriatum in an adult: combined used of transesophageal echocardiography and catheterization. *Cathet Cardiovasc Interv* 2000;51:83–86.
255. Bini RM, Cleveland DC, Ceballos R, et al. Congenital pulmonary vein stenosis. *Am J Cardiol* 1984;54:369–375.
256. Sun CC, Doyle T, Ringel PE. Pulmonary vein stenosis. *Hum Pathol* 1995; 26:880–886.
257. Driscoll DJ, Hesslein PS, Mullins CE. Congenital stenosis of individual pulmonary veins: clinical spectrum and unsuccessful treatment by transvenous balloon dilatation. *Am J Cardiol* 1982;49:1767–1772.
258. van Son JAM, Danielson GK, Puga FJ, et al. Repair of congenital and acquired pulmonary vein stenosis. *Ann Thorac Surg* 1995;60:144–150.
259. Park SC, Neches WH, Lenox CC, et al. Diagnosis and surgical treatment of bilateral pulmonary vein stenosis. *J Thorac Cardiovasc Surg* 1974;67:755–761.
260. Moes CAF, Freedom RM. Rings, slings and other things contributing to a neonatal noose. In: Freedom RM, Benson LN, Smallhorn JF, eds. *Neonatal heart disease*. London: Springer-Verlag, 1992:731–749.
261. Abrams D, Gerlis L, Daubeney P. Tracheoesophageal compression in congenital heart disease: vascular rings, pulmonary slings, and other vascular abnormalities. In: Gatzoulis MA, Webb GD, Daubeney PEF, eds. *Diagnosis and management of adult congenital heart disease*. Edinburgh: Churchill Livingstone: 2003:273–280.
262. Bromley B, Estroff JA, Sanders SP, et al. Fetal echocardiography: accuracy and limitations in a population at high and low risk for heart defects. *Am J Obstet Gynecol* 1992;166:1473–1481.
263. Freedom RM, Smallhorn JF, Trusler GA. Transposition of the great arteries. In: Freedom RM, Benson LN, Smallhorn JF, eds. *Neonatal heart disease*. London: Springer-Verlag, 1992:179–212.
264. Liebman J, Cullum L, Belloc N. Natural history of transposition of the great arteries: anatomy and birth and death characteristics. *Circulation* 1969;40:237–362.
265. Lang P, Freed MD, Bierman FZ, et al. Use of prostaglandin E_1 in infants with d-transposition of the great arteries and intact ventricular septum. *Am J Cardiol* 1977;44:76–81.
266. Benson LN, Olley PM, Patel RG, et al. Role of prostaglandin E_1 in the management of transposition of the great arteries. *Am J Cardiol* 1979;44:691–696.
267. Baylen BG, Grzeszczak M, Gleason ME, et al. Role of balloon atrial septostomy before early arterial switch repair of transposition of the great arteries. *J Am Coll Cardiol* 1992;19:1025–1031.
268. Pasquini L, Sanders SP, Parness IA, et al. Coronary echocardiography in 406 patients with d-loop transposition of the great arteries. *J Am Coll Cardiol* 1994;24:763–768.
269. Chin AJ, Yeager SB, Sanders SP, et al. Accuracy of prospective two-dimensional echocardiographic evaluation of left ventricular outflow tract in complete transposition of the great arteries. *Am J Cardiol* 1985;55;759–764.
270. Snider AR, Serwer GB, Ritter SB. *Echocardiography in pediatric heart disease*. St. Louis, MO: Mosby, 1997:297–342.
271. Senning A. Surgical correction of transposition of the great vessels. *Surgery* 1959;45:966–975.
272. Mustard WT. Successful two-stage correction of transposition of the great vessels. *Surgery* 1964;55:469–473.
273. Flinn CJ, Wolff GS, Dick MI, et al. Cardiac rhythm after the mustard operation for complete transposition of the great arteries. *N Engl J Med* 1984;310:1635–1638.
274. Puley G, Siu S, Connelly M, et al. Arrhythmia and survival in patients >18 years of age after the Mustard procedure for complete transposition of the great arteries. *Am J Cardiol* 1999;83:1080–1084.
275. Paul MH, Wessel HU. Exercise studies in patients with transposition of the great arteries after atrial repair operations (Mustard/Senning): a review. *Pediatr Cardiol* 1999;20:49–55.
276. Harris L, Balaji S. Arrhythmias in the adult with congenital heart disease. In: Gatzoulis MA, Webb GD, Daubeney PEF, eds. *Diagnosis and management of adult congenital heart disease*. Edinburgh: Churchill Livingstone: 2003:105–113.
277. Cobanoglu A, Abbruzzese PA, Freimanis I, et al. Pericardial baffle complications following the mustard operation. *J Thorac Cardiovasc Surg* 1984; 87:371–378.
278. Bu'Lock FA, Tometzki AJ, Kitchiner DJ, et al. Balloon expandable stents for systemic venous pathway stenosis late after Mustard's operation. *Heart* 1998;79:225–229.
279. Deanfield J, Camm J, Macartney FJ, et al. Arrhythmia and late mortality after Mustard and Senning operation for transposition of the great arteries. An eight-year prospective study. *J Thorac Cardiovasc Surg* 1988;96:569–576.
280. Garson AJ, Bink-Boelkens M, Hesslein PS. Atrial flutter in the young. A collaborative study of 380 cases. *J Am Coll Cardiol* 1985;6:871–878.
281. Gelatt M, Hamilton RM, McCrindle BW, et al. Arrhythmia and mortality after the Mustard procedure: a 30-year single center experience. *J Am Coll Cardiol* 1997;29:194–201.
282. Hagler DJ, Ritter DG, Mair DD, et al. Right and left ventricular function after the mustard procedure in transposition of the great arteries. *Am J Cardiol* 1979;44:276–283.
283. Murphy JH, Barlai-Kovach MM, Mathews RA, et al. Rest and exercise right and left ventricular function late after the mustard operation: assessment by radionuclide ventriculography. *Am J Cardiol* 1983;51:1520–1526.
284. Hurwitz RA, Caldwell RL, Girod DA, et al. Right ventricular systolic function in adolescents and young adults after Mustard operation for transposition of the great arteries. *Am J Cardiol* 1996;77:294–297.
285. Wilson NJ, Clarkson PM, Barratt-Boyes BG, et al. Long-term outcome after the Mustard repair for simple transposition of the great arteries. 28 year follow-up. *J Am Coll Cardiol* 1998;32:758–765.
286. Oeschlin EN, Jenni R. Forty years after the first atrial switch procedure in patients with transposition of the great arteries: long-term results in Toronto and Zurich. *Thorac Cardiovasc Surg* 2000;48:233–237.
287. Turina MI, Siebenmann R, von Segesser I, et al. Late functional deterioration after atrial correction for transposition. *Circulation* 1989;80:II62–II67.
288. Millane T, Bernard EJ, Jaeggi E, et al. Role of ischemia and infarction in late right ventricular dysfunction after atrial repair of transposition of the great arteries. *J Am Coll Cardiol* 2000;35:1661–1668.
289. Lester SJ, McElhinney DB, Viloria E, et al. Effects of losartan in patients with a systemically functioning morphologic right ventricle after atrial repair of transposition of the great arteries. *Am J Cardiol* 2001;88:1314–1316.
290. Muhill IV, Liu P, Webb G. Applying new standard therapies to new targets. The use of ACE inhibitors and B-blockers for heart failure in adults with congenital heart disease. *Int J Cardiol* 2004;97:25–33.
291. Mee RBB. Severe right ventricular failure after Mustard or Senning operation. *J Thorac Cardiovasc Surg* 1986;92:385–390.
292. Poirier NC, Yu JH, Brizard CP, et al. Long-term results of left ventricular reconditioning and anatomic correction for systemic right ventricular dysfunction after atrial switch procedures. *J Thorac Cardiovasc Surg* 2004;127:975–981.
293. Chang AC, Wernovsky G, Wessel DL, et al. Surgical management of late right ventricular failure after Mustard or Senning repair. *Circulation* 1992;86:II140–II149.
294. Webb GD, McLaughlin PR, Gow RM, et al. Transposition complexes. *Cardiol Clin* 1993;11:651–664.
295. Park SC, Neches WH, Matthews RA, et al. Haemodynamic function after the Mustard operation for transposition of the great arteries. *Am J Cardiol* 1985;55:1238–1239.
296. Gewillig M, Cullen S, Mertens B, et al. Risk factors for arrhythmia and death after mustard operation for simple transposition of the great arteries. *Circulation* 1991;84:III187–III192.
297. Therrien J, Warnes C, Daliento L, et al. CCS Consensus Conference 2001 Update: Recommendations for the management of adults with congenital heart disease Part III. *Can J Cardiol* 2001;17:1138–1158.
298. Kirklin JW, Blackstone EH, Tcherenkov CI, et al. Clinical outcomes after the arterial switch operation for transposition: patient, support, procedural, and institutional risk factors. Congenital Heart Surgeons Society. *Circulation* 1992;86:1501–1515.
299. Norwood WI, Dobell AR, Freed MD, et al. Intermediate results of the arterial switch repair. A 20-institution study. *J Thorac Cardiovasc Surg* 1988;96:854–863.
300. Wernovsky G, Mayer JE, Jonas RA, et al. Factors influencing early and late outcome of the arterial switch operation for transposition of the great arteries. *J Thorac Cardiovasc Surg* 1995;109:289–302.
301. Di Donato RM, Wernovsky G, Walsh EP, et al. Results of the arterial switch operation for transposition of the great arteries with ventricular septal defect: surgical considerations and midterm follow-up data. *Circulation* 1989;80:1689–1705.
302. Losay J, Touchot A, Serraf A, et al. Late outcome after arterial switch operation for transposition of the great arteries. *Circulation* 1001;104(Suppl I):I21–I26.
303. Bonhoeffer P, Bonnet D, Piechaud JT, et al. Coronary artery obstruction after the arterial switch operation for transposition of the great arteries in newborns. *J Am Coll Cardiol* 1997;29:202–206.
304. Legendre A, Losay J, Touchot-Kone A, et al. Coronary events after arterial switch operation for transposition of the great arteries. *Circulation* 2003;108:II186–II190.
305. Rhodes LA, Wernovsky G, Keane JF, et al. Arrhythmias and intracardiac conduction after the arterial switch operation. *J Thorac Cardiovasc Surg* 1995;109:303–310.
306. Rastelli GC, McGoon DC, Wallace RB. Anatomic correction of transposition of the great arteries with ventricular septal defect and sub-pulmonary stenosis. *J Thorac Cardiovasc Surg* 1969;58:545–552.

307. Kreutzer C, De Vive J, Oppido G, et al. Twenty-five year experience with Rastelli repair for transposition of the great arteries. *J Thorac Cardiovasc Surg* 2000;120:211–223.
308. Scheibler GL, Edwards JE, Burchell HB, et al. Congenital corrected transposition of the great vessels: a study of 35 cases. *Pediatrics* 1961;27:851–888.
309. Anderson RC, Lillehei CW, Lester RG. Corrected transposition of the great vessels of the heart. *Pediatrics* 1957;20:626–646.
310. Friedberg DZ, Nadas AS. Clinical profile of patients with congenital corrected transposition of the great arteries: a study of 60 cases. *N Engl J Med* 1970;282:1053–1059.
311. Cohen DM, Freedom RM, Williams WL. Congenitally corrected transposition of the great arteries. In: Caugill LD, ed. *Cardiac surgery: cyanotic congenital heart disease.* Philadelphia: Hanley & Belfus, 1989:225–240.
312. Anderson KR, Danielson GK, McGoon DW, et al. Ebstein's anomaly of the left-sided tricuspid valve: pathological anatomy of the valvular malformation. *Circulation* 1978;58:87–91.
313. Horvath P, Szufladowicz M, de Leval MR, et al. Tricuspid valve abnormalities in patients with atrioventricular discordance: surgical implications. *Ann Thorac Surg* 1994;57:941–945.
314. Presbitero P, Somerville J, Rabajoli F, et al. Corrected transposition of the great arteries without associated defects in adult patients: clinical profile and follow-up. *Br Heart J* 1995;74:57–59.
315. Connelly MS, Liu PP, Williams WG, et al. Congenitally corrected transposition of the great arteries in the adult: functional status and complications. *J Am Coll Cardiol* 1996;27:1238–1243.
316. Webb CL. Congenitally corrected transposition of the great arteries: clinical features, diagnosis, and prognosis. *Prog Pediatr Cardiol* 1999;10:17–30.
317. Lundstrom U, Bull C, Wyse RKH, et al. The natural and 'unnatural' history of congenitally corrected transposition. *Am J Cardiol* 1990;65:1222–1229.
318. Kurosawa H, Becker AE. *Atrioventricular conduction in congenital heart disease.* London: Springer-Verlag, 1987:225–252.
319. Anderson RH, Arnold R, Wilkinson JL. The conducting system in congenitally corrected transposition. *Lancet* 1973;1:1286–1288.
320. Anderson RH, Becker AE, Arnold R, et al. The conducting tissues in congenitally corrected transposition. *Circulation* 1974;50:911–924.
321. Bove E. Congenitally corrected transposition of the great arteries: surgical options for biventricular repair. *Prog Pediatr Cardiol* 1999;10:45–49.
322. Yagihara T, Kishimoto H, Isobe F, et al. Double switch operation in cardiac anomalies with atrioventricular and ventriculoarterial discordance. *J Thorac Cardiovasc Surg* 1994;107:351–358.
323. Imai Y, Sawatari K, Hoshino S, et al. Ventricular function after anatomic repair in patients with atrioventricular discordance. *J Thorac Cardiovasc Surg* 1994;107:1272–1283.
324. Ibarwi MN, Deleon SY, Backer CL, et al. An alternative approach to the surgical management of physiologically corrected transposition with ventricular septal defect and pulmonary stenosis or atresia. *J Thorac Cardiovasc Surg* 1990;100:410–415.
325. Graham TP Jr, Bernard YD, Mellen BG, et al. Long-term outcome in congenitally corrected transposition of the great arteries: a multi-institutional study. *J Am Coll Cardiol* 2000;36:255–261.
326. Lundstrom U, Bull C, Wyse RK, et al. The natural and "unnatural" history of congenitally corrected transposition. *Am J Cardiol* 1990;65:1222–1229.
327. Esper W, Moodie D, Gill C, et al. Congenitally corrected transposition of the great arteries in adults. *J Am Coll Cardiol* 1983;1:663–670.
328. Masden RR, Franch RH. Isolated congenitally corrected transposition of the great arteries. In: Hurst JW, ed. *The heart, update III.* New York: McGraw-Hill: 1980:59–83.
329. Warnes CA. Congenitally corrected transposition: the uncorrected misnomer. *J Am Coll Cardiol* 1996;27:1244–1245.
330. Kirklin JW, Barratt-Boyes BG. *Cardiac surgery,* 2nd ed. New York: Churchill Livingstone, 1993:1263–1300.
331. Di Donato R, Troconis CJ, Marino B, et al. Combined Mustard and Rastelli operations. An alternative approach for repair of associated anomalies in congenitally corrected transposition in situs inversus (I,D,D). *J Thorac Cardiovasc Surg* 1992;104:1246–1248.
332. Stumper O, Wright JG, De Giovanni JV, et al. Combined atrial and arterial switch procedure for congenital corrected transposition with ventricular septal defect. *Br Heart J* 1995;73:479–482.
333. Yamagishi Y, Imai Y, Hoshino S, et al. Anatomic correction of atrioventricular discordance. *J Thorac Cardiovasc Surg* 1993;105:1067–1076.
334. Yagihara T, Kishimoto H, Isobe F, et al. Double switch operation in cardiac anomalies with atrioventricular and ventriculoarterial discordance. *J Thorac Cardiovasc Surg* 1994;107:351–358.
335. Goldmuntz E, Clark BJ, Mitchell LE, et al. Frequency of 22q11 deletions in patients with conotruncal defects. *J Am Coll Cardiol* 1998;32:492–498.
336. Anderson RH, Tynan M. Tetralogy of Fallot: a centennial review. *Int J Cardiol* 1988;21:219–232.
337. Becker AE, Connor M, Anderson RH. Tetralogy of Fallot: a morphometric and geometric study. *Am J Cardiol* 1975;35:402–412.
338. Geva T, Ayres NA, Pac FA, et al. Quantitative morphometric analysis of progressive infundibular obstruction in tetralogy of Fallot: a prospective longitudinal echocardiographic study. *Circulation* 1995;92:886–892.
339. Rose JS, Levin DC, Goldstein S, et al. Congenital absence of the pulmonary valve associated with congenital aplasia of the thymus (DiGeorge's syndrome). *AJR Am J Roentgenol* 1974;122:97–102.
340. Scambler PJ, Kelly D, Lindsay E, et al. Velo-cardio-facial syndrome associated with chromosome 22 deletions encompassing the DiGeorge locus. *Lancet* 1992;339:1138–1139.
341. Mitchell SC, Korones SB, Berendes HW. Congenital heart disease in 56,109 births: incidence and natural history. *Circulation* 1971;43:323–332.
342. Bertranou EG, Blackstone EH, Hazelrig JB, et al. Life expectancy without surgery in tetralogy of Fallot. *Am J Cardiol* 1978;42:458–466.
343. Castaneda AR. Tetralogy of Fallot: advantages of early repair. *Saudi Heart Bull* 1989;1:24–26.
344. Kirklin JW, Barratt-Boyes BG. *Cardiac surgery,* 2nd ed. New York: Churchill Livingstone, 1993:861–1012.
345. Di Donato RM, Jonas RA, Lang P, et al. Neonatal repair of tetralogy of Fallot with and without pulmonary atresia. *J Thorac Cardiovasc Surg* 1991;101:126–131.
346. Kirklin JW, Blackstone E, Kirklin JK, et al. Surgical results and protocols in the spectrum of tetralogy of Fallot. *Ann Surg* 1983;198:251–261.
347. Kirklin JW, Blackstone EH, Pacifico AD, et al. Risk factors of early and late failure after repair of tetralogy of Fallot, and their neutralization. *Thorac Cardiovasc Surg* 1984;32:208–214.
348. Lillehei CW, Cohen M, Warden HE. Direct vision intracardiac surgical correction of the tetralogy of Fallot, pentalogy of Fallot, and pulmonary atresia defects: Report of the first 10 cases. *Ann Surg* 1995;142:418–423.
349. Kawashima Y, Kitamura S, Nakano S, et al. Corrective surgery for tetralogy of Fallot without or with minimal right ventriculotomy and with repair of the pulmonary valve. *Circulation* 1981;64:147–153.
350. Karl TR, Porniviliwan S, Mee RBB. Tetralogy of Fallot: favourable outcome on nonneonatal transatrial, transpulmonary repair. *Ann Thorac Surg* 1992;54:903–907.
351. Reddy VM, Liddicoat JR, McElhinney DB, et al. Routine repair of tetralogy of Fallot in neonates and infants less than three months of age. *Ann Thorac Surg* 1995;60:S592–S596.
352. Murphy JG, Gersh BJ, Mair DD, et al. Long-term outcome in patients undergoing surgical repair of tetralogy of Fallot. *N Engl J Med* 1993;329:593–599.
353. Katz NM, Blackstone EH, Kirklin JW, et al. Late survival and symptoms after repair of tetralogy of Fallot. *Circulation* 1982;65:403–410.
354. Fuster V, McGoon DC, Kennedy MA, et al. Long-term evaluation (12 to 22 years) of open heart surgery for tetralogy of Fallot. *Am J Cardiol* 1980; 46:635–642.
355. Castaneda AR, Jonas R, Mayer JE, et al. *Tetralogy of Fallot: Cardiac surgery of the neonate and infant.* Philadelphia: WB Saunders, 1994:215–235.
356. Presbitero P, Demarie D, Aruta E, et al. Results of total correction of tetralogy of Fallot performed in adults. *Ann Thorac Surg* 1988;46:297–301.
357. Oechslin EN, Harrison DA, Harris L, et al. Reoperation in adults with repair of tetralogy of Fallot: indications and outcomes. *J Thorac Cardiovasc Surg* 1999;118:245–251.
358. Vliegen HW, van Straten A, de Roos A, et al. Magnetic resonance imaging to assess the hemodynamic effects of pulmonary valve replacement in adults late after repair of tetralogy of Fallot. *Circulation* 2002;106:1703–1707.
359. Yemets IM, Williams, WG, Webb GD, et al. Pulmonary valve replacement late after repair of tetralogy of Fallot. *Ann Thorac Surg* 1977;64:526–530.
360. Bove El, Byrum CJ, Thomas FD, et al. The influence of pulmonary insufficiency on ventricular function following repair of tetralogy of Fallot. *J Thorac Cardiovasc Surg* 1983;85:691–696.
361. Warner KG, Anderson JE, Fulton DR, et al. Restoration of the pulmonary valve reduces right ventricular volume overload after previous repair of tetralogy of Fallot. *Circulation* 1993;88:II189–II197.
362. Therrien J, Siu S, McGlaughlin PR, et al. Pulmonary valve replacement in adults late after repair of tetralogy of Fallot: are we operating too late? *J Am Coll Cardiol* 2000;36:1670–1675.
363. Davlouros PA, Karatza AA, Gatzoulis MA, et al. Timing and type of surgery for severe pulmonary regurgitation after repair of tetralogy of Fallot. *Int J Cardiol* 2004;47:91–101.
364. Nollert G, Fischlein T, Bouterwek S, et al. Long-term survival in patients with repair of tetralogy of Fallot: 36-year follow-up of 490 survivors of the first year after surgical repair. *J Am Coll Cardiol* 1997;30:1374–1383.
365. Gatzoulis M, Balaji S, Webber S, et al. Risk factors for arrhythmia and sudden death in repaired tetralogy of Fallot: a multi-centre study. *Lancet* 2000;356:975–981.
366. Gatzoulis M, Till JA, Redington AN. Depolarisation–repolarisation inhomogeneity after repair of tetralogy of Fallot. *Circulation* 1997;95:401–404.
367. Deanfield JE, McKenna WJ, Hallidie-Smith KA. Detection of late arrhythmias and conduction disturbances after correction of tetralogy of Fallot. *Br Heart J* 1980;44:248–253.
368. Cullen S, Celermajer DS, Franklin RCG, et al. Prognostic significance of ventricular arrhythmia after repair of tetralogy of Fallot: a 12-year prospective study. *J Am Coll Cardiol* 1994;23:1151–1155.
369. Harrison D, Harris L, Siu S, et al. Sustained VT in adult patients later after repair of tetralogy of Fallot. *J Am Coll Cardiol* 1997;30:1368–1373.
370. Garson AJ, Randall DC, Gillette PC, et al. Prevention of sudden death after repair of tetralogy of Fallot: treatment of ventricular arrhythmias. *J Am Coll Cardiol* 1985;6:221–227.
371. Khairy P, Landzberg MJ, Gatzoulis MA, et al. Value of programmed ventricular stimulation after tetralogy of Fallot repair: a multicenter study. *Circulation* 2004;109:1994–2000.

372. Roos-Heeslink J, Perlroth M, McGhie J, et al. Atrial arrhythmias in adults after repair of tetralogy of Fallot. Correlations with clinical, exercise, and echocardiographic findings. *Circulation* 1995;91:2214–2219.
373. Theodoro D, Danielson G, Porter C, et al. Right-sided Maze procedure for right atrial arrhythmias in congenital heart disease. *Ann Thorac Surg* 1998;65:149–154.
374. Therrien J, Gatzoulis M, Graham T, et al. CCS Consensus Conference 2001 update: recommendations for the management of adults with congenital heart disease Part II. *Can J Cardiol* 2001;17:1032–1050.
375. Anderson RH, Seo JW, Ho SY. The pulmonary arterial supply in tetralogy of Fallot with pulmonary atresia. In: Yacoub MH, Pepper JR, eds. *Annual of cardiac surgery 1990–1991*. London: Current Science, 1991:77–83.
376. Thiene G, Anderson RH. Pulmonary atresia with VSD: anatomy. In: Anderson RH, Macartney FJ, Shinebourne EA, et al., eds. *Paediatric cardiology,* Vol. 5. Edinburgh: Churchill Livingstone, 1983:81–101.
377. Marino B, Calabro R, Gagliardi MG, et al. Patterns of pulmonary arterial anatomy and blood supply in complex congenital heart disease with pulmonary atresia. *J Thorac Cardiovasc Surg* 1987;94:518–520.
378. Burrows PE, Freedom RM, Rabinovitch M, et al. The investigation of abnormal pulmonary arteries in congenital heart disease. *Radiol Clin North Am* 1985;23:689–717.
379. Marelli AJ, Perloff JK, Child JS, et al. Pulmonary atresia with ventricular septal defect in adults. *Circulation* 1994;89:243–251.
380. Puga FJ. Surgical treatment of pulmonary atresia and ventricular septal defect. *Prog Pediatr Cardiol* 1992;1:37–49.
381. Rome JJ, Mayer JE, Castaneda AR, et al. Tetralogy of Fallot with pulmonary atresia: rehabilitation of diminutive pulmonary arteries. *Circulation* 1993;88:1691–1698.
382. Shanley CJ, Lupinetti FM, Shah NL, et al. Primary unifocalization for the absence of intrapericardial pulmonary arteries in the neonate. *J Thorac Cardiovasc Surg* 1993;106:237–247.
383. Reddy VN, Liddicoat JR, Hanley FM. Midline one-stage complete unifocalization and repair of pulmonary atresia with ventricular septal defect and major aortopulmonary collaterals. *J Thorac Cardiovasc Surg* 1995;109:832–845.
384. Puga FJ, McGoon DC, Julsrud PR, et al. Complete repair of pulmonary atresia with nonconfluent pulmonary arteries. *Ann Thorac Surg* 1983;35:36–44.
385. Barbero-Marcial M, Jatene AD. Surgical management of the anomalies of the pulmonary arteries in the tetralogy of Fallot with pulmonary atresia. *Semin Thorac Cardiovasc Surg* 1990;2:93–107.
386. Iyer KS, Mee RBB. Staged repair of pulmonary atresia with ventricular septal defect and major systemic to pulmonary artery collaterals. *Ann Thorac Surg* 1991;51:65–72.
387. Cho JM, Puga FJ, Danielson GK, et al. Early and long-term results of the surgical treatment of tetralogy of Fallot with pulmonary atresia, with or without major aortopulmonary collaterals. *J Thorac Cardiovasc Surg* 2002;124:70–81.
388. Freedom RM. *Pulmonary atresia and intact ventricular septum.* Mount Kisco, NY: Futura, 1989;262.
389. Hanseus K, Bjorkhem G, Lundstron NR, et al. Cross-sectional echocardiographic measurements of right ventricular size and growth in patients with pulmonary atresia and intact ventricular septum. *Pediatr Cardiol* 1991;12:135–142.
390. Musewe N, Smallhorn JF. Echocardiographic evaluation of pulmonary atresia with intact ventricular septum. In: Freedom RM, ed. *Pulmonary atresia and intact ventricular septum.* Mount Kisco, NY: Futura, 1989:33–155.
391. Leung MP, Mok CK, Hui PW. Echocardiographic assessment of neonates with pulmonary atresia and intact ventricular septum. *J Am Coll Cardiol* 1988;12:719–725.
392. Burrows PE, Freedom RM, Benson LN, et al. Coronary angiography of pulmonary atresia, hypoplastic right ventricle, and ventriculocoronary communications. *AJR Am J Roentgenol* 1990;154:789–795.
393. Coles JG, Freedom RM, Lightfoot NE, et al. Long-term results in neonates with pulmonary atresia and intact ventricular septum. *Ann Thorac Surg* 1989;47:213–237.
394. Lightfoot NE, Coles JG, Dasmahapatra HK, et al. Analysis of survival in patients with pulmonary atresia and intact ventricular septum treated surgically. *Int J Cardiol* 1989;24:159–164.
395. Hanley FL, Sade RM, Blackstone EH, et al. Outcomes in neonatal pulmonary atresia with intact ventricular septum. *J Thorac Cardiovasc Surg* 1993;105:406–427.
396. Arzt W, Franklin RC, Loughna P, et al. Fetal pulmonary valvuloplasty for critical pulmonary stenosis or atresia with intact septum. *Lancet* 2002; 360:1567–1568.
397. Restivo A, Cameron AH, Anderson RH, et al. Divided right ventricle: a review of its anatomical varieties. *Pediatr Cardiol* 1984;5:197–204.
398. Ward CJB, Culham JAC, Patterson MWH, et al. The trilogy of double-chambered right ventricle, perimembranous ventricular septal defect and subaortic narrowing: a more common association than previously recognized. *Cardiol Young* 1995;5:140–146.
399. Galal O, al-Halees Z, Solymar L, et al. Double-chambered right ventricle in 73 patients: spectrum of the disease and surgical results of transatrial repair. *Can J Cardiol* 2000;16:167–174.
400. McElhinney DB, Chatterjee KM, Reddy VM. Double-chambered right ventricle presenting in adulthood. *Ann Thorac Surg* 2000;70:124–127.
401. Sade RM, Fyfe DA. Tricuspid atresia: current concepts in diagnosis and treatment. *Pediatr Clin North Am* 1990;37:151–169.
402. Dick M, Fyler DC, Nadas AS. Tricuspid atresia: clinical course in 101 patients. *Am J Cardiol* 1975;36:327–337.
403. Fontan F, Baudet E. Surgical repair of tricuspid atresia. *Thorax* 1971; 26:240–248.
404. De Brux JL, Zannini L, Binet JP, et al. Tricuspid atresia: results of treatment of 115 children. *J Thorac Cardiovasc Surg* 1983;85:440–446.
405. Fontan F, Deville C, Quaegebeur J, et al. Repair of tricuspid atresia in 100 patients. *J Thorac Cardiovasc Surg* 1983;85;647–659.
406. Mair DD, Hagler DJ, Puga FJ, et al. Fontan operation in 176 patients with tricuspid atresia: results and a proposed new index for patient selection. *Circulation* 1990;82(Suppl IV):164–169.
407. Patel MM, Overy DC, Kozonis MC, et al. Long-term survival in tricuspid atresia. *J Am Coll Cardiol* 1987;9:38–40.
408. Tam CKH, Lightfoot NE, Finlay CD, et al. Course of tricuspid atresia in the Fontan era. *Am J Cardiol* 1989;63:589–593.
409. Franklin RCG, Spiegalhalter DJ, Sullivan ID, et al. Tricuspid atresia presenting in infancy: survival and suitability for the Fontan operation. *Circulation* 1993;87:427–439.
410. Kirklin JK, Blackstone EH, Kirklin JW, et al. The Fontan operation: ventricular hypertrophy, age and date of operation as risk factors. *J Thorac Cardiovasc Surg* 1986;92:1049–1064.
411. Humes RA, Mair DD, Porter CJ, et al. Results of the modified Fontan operation in adults. *Am J Cardiol* 1988;612:602–604.
412. DeLaval M, Killner P, Gewillig M, et al. Total cavopulmonary connection. A logical alternative to atriopulmonary connection for complex Fontan operation. *J Thorac Cardiovasc Surg* 1988;96:682–695.
413. Castaneda AR. From Glenn to Fontan: a continuing evolution. *Circulation* 1992;86(Suppl II):II80–II84.
414. Laks H, Milliken JC, Perloff JK, et al. Experience with the Fontan procedure. *J Thorac Cardiovasc Surg* 1984;88:939–951.
415. Constantine M, Backer CL, Deal BJ. Venous shunts and the Fontan circulation in adult congenital heart disease. In: Gatzoulis MA, Webb GD, Daubeney PEF, eds. *Diagnosis and management of adult congenital heart disease.* Edinburgh: Churchill Livingstone: 2003:79–83.
416. Porter CJ, Garson A. Incidence and management of dysrhythmia after Fontan procedure. *Herz* 1993;18:318–327.
417. Balaji S, Johnson T, Sade R, et al. Management of atrial flutter after the Fontan procedure. *J Am Coll Cardiol* 1994;23:1209–1215.
418. Thorne S. Atrioventricular valve atresia. In: Gatzoulis MA, Webb GD, Daubeney PEF, eds. *Diagnosis and management of adult congenital heart disease.* Edinburgh: Churchill Livingstone: 2003:405–411.
419. Thorne SA, Barnes J, Cullinan P. et al. Amiodarone-associated thyroid dysfunction in adults with congenital heart disease. *Circulation* 1999;100: 149–154.
420. Feldt RH, Dricoll DJ, Offord KP, et al. Protein-losing enteropathy after the Fontan operation. *J Thorac Cardiovasc Surg* 1996;112:672–680.
421. Mair DD, Danielson GK, Schaff HU, et al. The Fontan procedure in adults: Operative and late results with 121 patients. *J Am Coll Cardiol* 1994;1A-48A:119A.
422. Grand GP, Mansell AL, Garafano RP, et al. Cardiorespiratory response to exercise after the Fontan procedure for tricuspid atresia. *J Am Cardiol* 1995;26:1016–1021.
423. Canobbio MM, Mair DD, van der Valde, et al. Pregnancy outcomes after the Fontan repair. *J Am Coll Cardiol* 1996;28:763–767.
424. Auer J. Development of human pulmonary veins and its major variations. *Anat Rec* 1948;101:581–594.
425. Brody H. Drainage of the pulmonary veins into the right side of the heart. *Arch Pathol* 1942;33:221–240.
426. Gathman GE, Nadas AS. Total anomalous pulmonary venous connection: clinical and physiologic observations in 75 pediatric patients. *Circulation* 1970;42:143–154.
427. Lupinetti FM, Kulik TJ, Beekman RH, et al. Correction of total anomalous pulmonary venous connection in infancy. *J Thorac Cardiovasc Surg* 1993;106:880–885.
428. Rusconi PG, Zuberbuhler JR, Anderson RH, et al. Morphologic-echocardiographic correlates of Ebstein's malformation. *Eur Heart J* 1991;12:784–790.
429. Freedom RM, Benson LN. Neonatal expression of Ebstein's anomaly. *Prog Pedatr Cardiol* 1993;2:22–27.
430. Watson H. The natural history of Ebstein's anomaly in childhood and adolescence: a preliminary report on the first 100 cases. *Proc Assoc Eur Cardiol* 1970;6:35–39.
431. Shina A, Seward J, Edwards W, et al. Two-dimensional echocardiographic spectrum of Ebstein's anomaly: detailed anatomic assessment. *J Am Coll Cardiol* 1984;3:356–370.
432. Perloff JK. *The clinical recognition of congenital heart disease.* Philadelphia: WB Saunders, 1994:247–272.
433. Celemajer D, Bull C, Till J, et al. Ebstein's anomaly: presentation and outcome from fetus to adult. *J Am Coll Cardiol* 1994;23:170–176.
434. Watson H. Natural history of Ebstein's anomaly of tricuspid valve in childhood and adolescence: an international co-operative study of 505 cases. *Br Heart J* 1974;36:417–427.
435. Gentles T, Calder A, Clarkson P, et al. Predictors of long-term survival with Ebstein's anomaly of the tricuspid valve. *Am J Cardiol* 1992;69:377–381.

436. Cappato R, Schluter M, Weiss C, et al. Radiofrequency current catheter ablation of accessory atrioventricular pathways in Ebstein's anomaly. *Circulation* 1996;94:376–383.
437. Carpentier A. A new reconstructive operation for Ebstein's anomaly of the tricuspid valve. *J Thorac Cardiovasc Surg* 1988;96:92–101.
438. Nair D, Seward J, Driscoll D, et al. Surgical repair of Ebstein's anomaly; selection of patients and early and late operative results. *Circulation* 1985;72:72–76.
439. Siew YH, Baker EJ, Rigby ML, Anderson RH. Double outlet right ventricle. In: *Color atlas of congenital heart disease; morphologic and clinical correlations*. London: Mosby-Wolfe, 1995:157–164.
440. Van Praagh S, Davidoff MD, Chin A, et al. Double outlet right ventricle: anatomic types and development implications based on a study of 101 autopsied cases. *Coeur* 1982;8:389–440.
441. Lecompte Y, Batisse A, Di Carlo D. Double-outlet right ventricle: a surgical synthesis. *Adv Cardiac Surg* 1993;4:109–136.
442. Capuani A, Uemura H, Yen Ho S, et al. Anatomic spectrum of abnormal ventriculoarterial connections: surgical implications. *Ann Thorac Surg* 1885;59:352–360.
443. Rubay J, Lecompte Y, Batisse A, et al. Anatomic repair of anomalies of ventriculo-arterial connection: results of a new technique in cases associated with pulmonary outflow obstruction. *Eur J Cardiothorac Surg* 1988; 2:305–311.
444. Sakata R, Lecompte Y, Batisse A, et al. Anatomic repair of anomalies of ventriculoarterial connection associated with ventricular septal defect. I. Criteria of surgical decision. *J Thorac Cardiovasc Surg* 1988;95:90–95.
445. Williams WG, Freedom RM. Double-outlet right ventricle and double-outlet left ventricle. In: Baue AE, Geha AS, Hammond GI, et al., eds. *Glenn's thoracic and cardiovascular surgery*, 5th ed. Norwalk, CT: Appleton & Lange, 1991:1243–1258.
446. Van Praagh R, Plett JA, Van Praagh S. Single ventricle: pathology, embryology, terminology and classification. *Herz* 1979;4:113–150.
447. Van Praagh R, Ongley PA, Swan HJC. Anatomic types of single or common ventricle in man: morphologic and geometric aspects of 60 necropsied cases. *Am J Cardiol* 1964;13:367–386.
448. Van Praagh R, Van Praagh S, Vlad P, et al. Diagnosis of the anatomic types of single or common ventricle. *Am J Cardiol* 1965;15:345–359.
449. Franklin RC, Speigelhalter DJ, Rossi Filho RI, et al. Double inlet-ventricle presenting in infancy. III. Outcome and potential for definitive repair. *J Thorac Cardiovasc Surg* 1991;101:924–934.
450. Moodie DS, Ritter DG, Tajik AJ, et al. Long-term follow-up in the unoperated univentricular heart. *Am J Cardiol* 1994;635–658.
451. Moodie DS, Ritter DG, Tajik AJ, et al. Long-term follow-up after palliative operation for univentricular heart. *Am J Cardiol* 1984;53:1648–1651.
452. Van Praagh R. Truncus arteriosus: what is it and how should it be classified? *Eur J Cardiothorac Surg* 1987;1:65–70.
453. Gelband H, Van Meter S, Gersony WM. Truncal valve abnormalities in infants with persistent truncus arteriosus. *Circulation* 1972;45:397–403.
454. de la Cruz MV, Cayre R, Angelini P, et al. Coronary arteries in truncus arteriosus. *Am J Cardiol* 1990;66:1482–1486.
455. Suzuki A, Ho SY, Anderson RH, et al. Coronary arterial and sinusal anatomy in hearts with a common arterial trunk. *Ann Thorac Surg* 1989; 48:792–797.
456. Stanger P. Truncus arteriosus. In: Moller JH, Neal WA, eds. *Fetal, neonatal, and infant cardiac disease*. Norwalk, CT: Appleton & Lange, 1989:587–602.
457. Hanley FL, Heinemann MK, Jonas RA, et al. Repair of truncus arteriosus in the neonate. *J Thorac Cardiovasc Surg* 1993;105:1047–1056.
458. Bove EL, Lupinetti FM, Pridjian AK, et al. Results of a policy of primary repair of truncus arteriosus in the neonate. *J Thorac Cardiovasc Surg* 1993;105:1057–1066.
459. Rajasinghe HA, McElhinney DB, Reddy VM, et al. Long term follow up of truncus arteriosus repaired in infancy: a 20 year experience. *J Thorac Cardiovasc Surg* 1997;113:869–879.
460. Williams JM, De Leeuw M, Black MD, et al. Factors associated with outcomes of persistent truncus arteriosus. *J Am Coll Cardiol* 1999;34:545–553.
461. Hastreiter AR, Van Der Horst RL, Sepehri B, et al. Prostaglandin E_1 infusion in newborns with a hypoplastic left ventricle and aortic atresia. *Pediatr Cardiol* 1982;2:95–98.
462. Norwood Jr WI, Jacobs MJ, Murphy JD. Fontan procedure for hypoplastic left heart syndrome. *Ann Thorac Surg* 1992;54:1025–1030.
463. Norwood WI Jr. Hypoplastic left heart syndrome. *Ann Thorac Surg* 1991;52:688–695.
464. Puga FJ. Modified Fontan procedure for hypoplastic left heart syndrome after palliation with the Norwood operation. *J Am Coll Cardiol* 1991; 17:1150–1151.
465. Forbess JM, Cook N, Serraf A, et al. An institutional experience with second- and third-stage palliative procedures for hypoplastic left heart syndrome: the impact of the bi-directional cavopulmonary shunt. *J Am Coll Cardiol* 1997;29:665–670.
466. Bailey LL, Nehlsen-Cannarella SL, Doroshow RW, et al. Cardiac allotransplantation in newborns as therapy for hypoplastic left heart syndrome. *N Engl J Med* 1986;315:949–963.
467. Razzouk AJ, Chinnock RE, Gundry SR, et al. Transplantation as a primary treatment for hypoplastic left heart syndrome: intermediate term results. *Ann Thorac Surg* 1996;62:1–8.
468. Tworetzky W, Wilkins-Haug L, Jennings RW, et al. Balloon dilatation of severe aortic stenosis in the fetus: potential for prevention of hypoplastic left heart syndrome: candidate selection, technique, and results of successful intervention. *Circulation* 2004;110:125–131.
469. Van Praagh S, Kakou-Guikahue M, Kim HS, et al. Atrial situs in patients with visceral heterotaxy and congenital heart disease: conclusions based on findings in 104 postmortem cases. *Coeur* 1988;19:484–502.
470. Van Praagh S, Kreutzer J, Alday L, et al. Systemic and pulmonary venous connections in visceral heterotaxy, with emphasis on the diagnosis of the atrial situs: a study of 109 postmortem cases. In: Clark EB, Takao A, eds. *Developmental cardiology. Morphogenesis and function*. Mount Kisco, NY: Futura, 1990:671–727.
471. Freedom RM, Smallhorn JF. Syndromes of right or left atrial isomerism. In: Freedom RM, Benson LN, Smallhorn JF, eds. *Neonatal heart disease*. London: Springer-Verlag, 1992;543–560.
472. Anderson C, Devine WA, Anderson RH, et al. Abnormalities of the spleen in relation to congenital malformations of the heart: a survey of necropsy findings in children. *Br Heart J* 1990;63:122–128.
473. Norgard G, Berg A. Isomerism (heterotaxia). In: Gatzoulis MA, Webb GD, Daubeney PEF, eds. *Diagnosis and management of adult congenital heart disease*. Edinburgh: Churchill Livingstone: 2003:413–421.
474. Wood P. The Eisenmenger syndrome or pulmonary hypertension with reversed central shunt. *BMJ* 1958;ii:701–709,755–762.
475. Rabinovitch M. Elastase and the pathobiology of unexplained pulmonary hypertension. *Chest* 1998;114:213S–224S.
476. Rabinovitch M, Haworth SG, Castaneda AR, et al. Lung biopsy in congenital heart disease: a morphometric approach to pulmonary vascular disease. *Circulation* 1978;58:1107–1122.
477. Heath D, Edwards JE. The pathology of hypertensive pulmonary vascular disease: a description of six grades of structural changes in the pulmonary arteries with special reference to congenital cardiac septal defects. *Circulation* 1958;18:533–547.
478. Oechslin EN, Harrison DA, Connelly MS, et al. Mode of death in adults with congenital heart disease. *Am J Cardiol* 2000;86:1111–1116.
479. Niwa K, Perfloff JK, Kaplan S, et al. Eisenmenger syndrome in adults: ventricular septal defect, truncus arteriosus, univentricular heart. *J Am Coll Cardiol* 1999;34:223–232.
480. Daliento L, Somerville J, Presbitero P, et al. Eisenmenger syndrome. Factors relating to deterioration and death. *Eur Heart J* 1998;19:1845–1855.
481. Hopkins WE, Ochoa LL, Richardson GW. Comparison of the hemodynamics and survival of adults with severe primary pulmonary hypertension or Eisenmenger syndrome. *J Heart Lung Transplant* 1996;15:100–105.
482. Saha A, Balakrishnan KG, Jaiswal PK, et al. Prognosis for patients with Eisenmenger syndrome of various aetiology. *Int J Cardiol* 1994;45:199–207.
483. Cantor WJ, Harrison DA, Moussadji JS, et al. Determinants of survival and length of survival in adults with Eisenmenger syndrome. *Am J Cardiol* 1999;84:677–681.
484. Young D, Mark H. Fate of the patient with the Eisenmenger syndrome. *Am J Cardiol* 1971;28:658–669.
485. Oya H, Nagaya N, Satoh T, et al. Haemodynamic correlates and prognostic significance of serum uric acid in adult patients with Eisenmenger syndrome. *Heart* 2000;84:53–58.
486. Somerville J. How to manage the Eisenmenger syndrome. *Int J Cardiol* 1998;63:1–8.
487. Jones AM, Howitt G. Eisenmenger's syndrome in pregnancy. *Br Med J* 1965;1:1627–1633.
488. Avila W, Brinberg M, Snitcowsky R, et al. Maternal and fetal outcome in pregnant women with Eisenmenger's syndrome. *Eur Heart J* 1995;16:460–464.
489. Gleicher N, Midwall J, Hochberger D, et al. Eisenmenger's syndrome and pregnancy. *Obstet Gynecol Surv* 1979;43:721–741.
490. Ammash NM, Connolly HM, Abel MD, et al. Noncardiac surgery in Eisenmenger syndrome. *J Am Coll Cardiol* 1999;33:222–227.
491. Baum VC, Perloff JK. Anesthetic implications of adults with congenital heart disease. Review article. *Anesth Analg* 1993;76:1342–1358.
492. Sandoval J, Aguirre JS, Pulido T, et al. Nocturnal oxygen therapy in patients with the Eisenmenger syndrome. *Am J Respir Crit Care Med* 2001; 164:1682–1687.
493. Rosenzweig EB, Kerstein D, Barst RJ. Long-term prostacyclin for pulmonary hypertension with associated congenital heart defects. *Circulation* 1999;99:1856–1865.
494. Gatzoulis MA, Rogers P, Li W, et al. Safety and tolerability of bosentan in adults with Eisenmenger physiology. *Int J Cardiol* 2005;98(1):147–151.
495. Apostolopoulou SC, Magninas A, Cokkinos DV, et al. Effect of the oral endothelin antagonist bosentan on the clinical, exercise, and haemodynamic status of patients with pulmonary arterial hypertension related to congenital heart disease. *Heart* 2005;91:1447–1452.
496. Christensen DD, McConnell ME, Book WM, et al. Initial experience with bosentan therapy in patients with the Eisenmenger syndrome. *Am J Cardiol* 2005;95:435–436.
497. Meester JD, Smits JA, Persijn GG, et al. Lung transplant waiting list: differential outcome of type of end-stage lung-disease, one year after registration. *J Heart Lung Transplant* 1999;18:563–571.

498. Johnsrude CL, Perry JC, Cecchin F, et al. Differentiating anomalous left main coronary artery originating from the pulmonary artery in infants from myocarditis and dilated cardiomyopathy by electrocardiogram. *Am J Cardiol* 1995;75:71–74.
499. Holley DG, Sell JE, Hougen TJ, et al. Pulsed Doppler echocardiographic and color flow imaging detection of retrograde filling of anomalous left coronary artery from the pulmonary artery. *J Am Soc Echocardiogr* 1992;5:85–88.
500. Houston AB, Pollock JC, Doig WB, et al. Anomalous origin of the left coronary artery from the pulmonary trunk: elucidation with colour Doppler flow mapping. *Br Heart J* 1990;63:50–54.
501. Jureidini SB, Nouri S, Crawford CJ, et al. Reliability of echocardiography in the diagnosis of anomalous origin of the left coronary artery from the pulmonary trunk. *Am Heart J* 1991;122:61–68.
502. Raanani E, Abramov D, Abramov Y, et al. Individual anatomy demands various techniques in correction of an anomalous origin of the left coronary artery in the pulmonary artery. *Thorac Cardiovasc Surg* 1995;3:99–103.
503. Cherian KM, Bharati S, Rao SG. Surgical correction of anomalous origin of the left coronary artery from the pulmonary artery. *J Card Surg* 1994;9:386–391.
504. Kirklin JW, Barratt-Boyes BG. *Cardiac surgery*. New York: Wiley, 1993:1635–1654.
505. Seguchi M, Nakanishi T, Nakazawa M, et al. Myocardial perfusion after aortic implantation for anomalous origin of the left coronary artery from the pulmonary artery. *Eur Heart J* 1990;11:213–218.
506. Paridon SM, Farooki ZQ, Kuhns LR, et al. Exercise performance after repair of anomalous origin of the left coronary artery from the pulmonary artery. *Circulation* 1990;81:1287–1292.
507. Gehlmann HR, van Ingen GJ. Symptomatic congenital complete absence of the left pericardium: case report and review of the literature. *Eur Heart J* 1989;10:670–675.
508. Van Son JA, Danielson GK, Schaff HV, et al. Congenital partial and complete absence of the pericardium. *Mayo Clinic Proc* 1993;68:743–747.
509. Connolly HM, Click RL, Schattenberg TT, et al. Congenital absence of the pericardium: echocardiography as a diagnostic tool. *J Am Soc Echocardiogr* 1995;8:87–92.
510. Jacob JL, Souza Jr AS, Parro JA. Absence of the left pericardium diagnosed by computed tomography. *Int J Cardiol* 1995;47:293–296.
511. Gassner I, Judmaier W, Fink C, et al. Diagnosis of congenital pericardial defects, including a pathognomonic sign for dangerous apical ventricular herniation, on magnetic resonance imaging. *Br Heart J* 1995;74:60–66.
512. Sakakibara S, Konno S. Congenital aneurysm of sinus of Valsalva: anatomy and classification. *Am Heart J* 1962;63:405–424.
513. Takach TJ, Reul GJ, Duncan JM, et al. Sinus of Valsalva aneurysm or fistula: management and outcome. *Ann Thorac Surg* 1999;68:1573–1577.
514. Swan L. Sinus of Valsalva aneurysms. In: Gatzoulis MA, Webb GD, Daubeney PEF, eds. *Diagnosis and management of adult congenital heart disease*. Edinburgh: Churchill Livingstone: 2003:239–243.
515. Mori K, Hayabuchi Y, Kuroda Y. Diagnosis and natural history of isolated congenital pulmonary regurgitation in fetal life. *Cardiol Young* 2000;10:162–165.
516. Stewart S, Alexson C, Manning J. Long-term palliation with the classic Blalock-Taussig shunt. *J Thorac Cardiovasc Surg* 1988;96:117–121.
517. Kopf GS, Laks H, Stansel HC, et al. Thirty-year follow-up of superior vena-pulmonary artery (Glenn) shunts. *J Thorac Cardiovasc Surg* 1990;106: 662–671.
518. Ashrafian H, Swan L. The mechanism of formation of pulmonary arteriovenous malformations associated with the class Glenn shunt (superior cavopulmonary anatomists). *Heart* 2002;88:369.
519. Lee C, Hartzell V, Danielson G, et al. Comparison of atriopulmonary versus atriaventricular connections for modified Fontan/Kretuzer repair of tricuspid valve atresia. *J Thorac Cardiovasc Surg* 1986;92:1032–1048.
520. Perloff JK. Systemic complications of cyanosis in adults with congenital heart disease. Hematologic derangements, renal function, and urate metabolism. *Cardiol Clin* 1993;11:689–699.
521. Perloff JK, Rosove MH, Child JS, et al. Adults with cyanotic congenital heart disease: hematologic management. *Ann Int Med* 1988;109:406–413.
522. Oeschslin E. Hematologic management of the cyanotic adult with congenital heart disease. *Int J Cardiol* 2004;97:109–115.
523. Perloff JK, Rosove MH, Siestema KE, et al. Cyanotic congenital heart disease: a multisystem disorder. In: Perloff JK, Child JS, eds. *Congenital heart disease in adults,* 2nd ed. Philadelphia: WB Saunders: 1998: 199–226.
524. Gill J, Wilson A, Brooks J, et al. Loss of the largest von Willebrand factor multimers from the plasma of patients with congenital cardiac defects. *Blood* 1986;67:758–761.
525. Rabinovitch M, Andrew M, Thoma H, et al. Abnormal endothelial factor VIII associated with pulmonary hypertension and congenital heart defects. *Circulation* 1987;76:1043–1052.
526. Perloff JK, Marelli AJ, Miner PD. Risk of stroke in adults with cyanotic congenital heart disease. *Circulation* 1993;87:1954–1959.
527. Phornphutkul C, Rosenthal A, Nadas AS, et al. Cerebrovascular accidents in infants and children with cyanotic congenital heart disease. *Am J Cardiol* 1973;32:329–334.
528. Ammash N, Warnes CA. Cerebrovascular events in adult patients with cyanotic congenital heart disease. *J Am Coll Cardiol* 1996;28:768–772.
529. Yung D. Hyperuricemia and congenital heart disease. *Am J Dis Child* 1980;134:902–903.
530. Perloff JK, Latta H, Barsotti P. Pathogenesis of the glomerular abnormalities in cyanotic congenital heart disease. *Am J Cardiol* 2000;86:1198.
531. Li W, Somerville J. Infective endocarditis in the grown-up congenital heart (GUCH) population. *Eur Heart J* 1998;19:166–173.
532. Child JS, Perloff JK. Infective endocarditis: risks and prophylaxis. In: Perloff JK, Childs JS, eds. *Congenital heart disease in adults*. Philadelphia: WB Saunders; 1991: 129–143.
533. Connolly HM, Warnes CA. Pregnancy and contraception. In: Gatzoulis MA, Webb GD, Daubeney PEF, eds. *Diagnosis and management of adult congenital heart disease*. Edinburgh: Churchill Livingstone: 2003: 135–144.
534. Pitkin R, Perloff J, Kood B, et al. Pregnancy and congenital heart disease. *Ann Intern Med* 1990;112:445–454.
535. Whittemore R, Hobbins JC, Engle MA. Pregnancy and its outcome in women with and without surgical treatment of congenital heart disease. *Am J Cardiol* 1982;50;641.
536. Presbitero P, Somerville J, Stone S, et al. Pregnancy in cyanotic congenital heart disease. Outcome of mother and fetus. *Circulation* 1994;89:2673–2676.
537. Siu S, Sermer M, Harrison D, et al. Risk and predictors for pregnancy-related complications in women with heart disease. *Circulation* 1997;96: 2789–2794.
538. Sciscione AC, Callan NA. Pregnancy and contraception. *Cardiol Clin* 1993;4:701–709.
539. Fredriksen PM, Veldtman G, Hechter S, et al. Aerobic capacity in adults with various congenital heart diseases. *Am J Cardiol* 2991;87:310–314.
540. Fredriksen PM, Chen A, Veldtman G, et al. Exercise capacity in adult patients with congenitally corrected transposition of the great arteries. *Heart* 2001;85:191–195.
541. Fredriksen PM, Therrien J, Veldtman G, et al. Lung function and aerobic capacity in adult patients following modified Fontan procedure. *Heart* 2000;85:295–299.
542. Graham TP, Driscoll DJ, Gersony WM, et al. 36th Bethesda conference. Eligibility recommendations for competitive athletes with cardiovascular abnormalities. Task Force 2: Congenital heart disease. *J Am Coll Cardiol* 2005;45:1326–1333.
543. Perloff JK, Sangwan S. Noncardiac surgery. In: Perloff JK, Child JS, eds. *Congenital heart disease in adults*. Philadelphia: WB Saunders, 1988: 291–299.
544. Colman JM. Noncardiac surgery in adult congenital heart disease. In: Gatzoulis MA, Webb GD, Daubeney PEF, eds. *Diagnosis and management of adult congenital heart disease*. Edinburgh: Churchill Livingstone: 2003: 99–104.
545. Webber SA, Pigular FA. Heart and lung transplantation in adult congenital heart disease. In: Gatzoulis MA, Webb GD, Daubeney PEF, eds. *Diagnosis and management of adult congenital heart disease*. Edinburgh: Churchill Livingstone: 2003: 93–98.
546. Hosenpud JD, Bennett LE, Berkeley M, et al. The Registry of the International Society for Heart and Lung Transplantation: 18th Official Report—2001. *J Heart Lung Transplant* 2001;20:805–851.
547. Webber SA, Fricker FJ, Michael M, et al. Orthotopic heart transplantation in children with congenital heart disease. *Ann Thorac Surg* 1994;58:1664–1669.
548. Saeed I, Rogers CA, Murday AJ. The UK Cardiothoracic Transplant Audit: intrathoracic organ transplantation in adults with congenital heart disease. *J Heart Lung Transplant* 2001;20:261.
549. Stoica SC, Perreas K, Sharples LD, et al. Heart-lung transplantation for Eisenmenger's syndrome: operative risks and late outcomes of 51 consecutive cases from a single institution [Abstract]. *J Heart Lung Transplant* 2001;20:173–174.
550. Warnes CA, Liberthson R, Danielson GK, et al. 32nd Bethesda conference: Care of the adult with congenital heart disease. Task force I: The changing profile of congenital heart disease in adult life. *J Am Coll Cardiol* 2001;37:1170–1175.
551. Wren C, O'Sullivan JJ. Survival with congenital heart disease and need for follow up in adult life. *Heart* 2001;85:438–443.
552. Warnes CA. The adult with congenital heart disease: born to be bad? *J Am Coll Cardiol* 2005;46:1–8.
553. Webb GD, Williams RG. 32nd Bethesda conference: Care of the adult with congenital heart disease. Summary of recommendations—care of the adult with congenital heart disease. *J Am Coll Cardiol* 1002;37:1167–1169.

CHAPTER 31 ■ THE HEART AND PREGNANCY

KENNETH L. BAUGHMAN

OVERVIEW

Pregnancy normally induces significant physiologic adaptation in the cardiovascular system, including increases in heart rate, left ventricular size, stroke volume, and left ventricular mass. Systemic vascular resistance decreases during pregnancy. The maximal increase in hemodynamic burden for the pregnant woman is achieved at the end of the second trimester. Uterine contractions and the sympathetic discharge associated with delivery further increase cardiovascular demands, with the greatest increase in cardiac output achieved in the final stages of delivery. These alterations are resolved approximately 6 weeks after delivery. Moderate aerobic exercise during pregnancy is safe, increasing maximal aerobic power and the capacity for sustained submaximal exercise, as well as preserving aerobic capacity in late gestation have been demonstrated.

Hypertension complicates 10% of pregnancies, is rarely due to secondary causes, and is classified as chronic hypertension, gestational hypertension, or preeclampsia. Preeclampsia, the most worrisome of these disorders, involves hypertension, proteinuria, edema, and possibly coagulopathy and liver dysfunction. If preeclampsia is severe, the condition may lead to eclampsia, a seizure disorder associated with high morbidity and mortality. The HELLP syndrome (*h*emolysis, *e*levated *l*iver function tests, and *l*ow *p*latelet levels) is a preeclampsia variant that has the same potential for malignant degeneration to eclampsia.

Peripartum cardiomyopathy is the presence of a new cardiomyopathy, without any other cause of congestive heart failure or preexisting heart muscle disorder, that appears in the final month of the pregnancy or in the first 5 months postpartum. Older patients, patients experiencing multibirth pregnancies, patients with toxemia, and patients carrying a first child are somewhat more likely to experience this condition. Most patients with this condition present within 1 to 2 months of delivery. Myocarditis is frequently found in patients who undergo endomyocardial biopsy early after presentation.

All forms of chronic anticoagulation may result in bleeding between the uterus and placenta and subsequent pregnancy loss. Heparin may cause osteoporosis if it is administered at a high dose for long periods, and warfarin (Coumadin) may be associated with an embryopathy or central nervous system abnormalities. Patients who require anticoagulants should receive heparin or low-molecular-weight heparin in the first trimester and in the terminal stages of pregnancy. Coumadin can usually be safely administered through the remainder of pregnancy until just before delivery.

Bioprosthetic heart valves may degenerate during or after pregnancy and require replacement. Pregnant patients who have mechanical prostheses have a lower live birth rate and higher incidence of thromboembolic complications.

Myocardial infarctions associated with pregnancy are unusual; however, pregnancy is associated with an increased incidence of vasospasm and coronary dissection. Pregnant patients are also predisposed to aortic dissection, particularly if they have aortic disease, including Marfan syndrome or Takayasu aortitis.

Patients who have congenital heart disease, even if it is corrected, must be screened carefully before they become pregnant to ensure that their pulmonary vascular resistance, ventricular function, valvular insufficiency, prosthetic devices, and aortopathy will be able to tolerate the cardiovascular strains of pregnancy.

Tocolytic therapy consists primarily of the use of β-sympathomimetic agents to decrease uterine contraction and allow fetal lung maturation. Approximately 5% of exposed mothers develop pulmonary edema, which appears to be a capillary leak syndrome.

Because antiarrhythmic agents pose a significant risk to the patient and fetus, they must be chosen carefully.

GLOSSARY

Bioprosthesis: An artificial valve made of biologic material, including either homograft (human) or heterograft (pig) tissue.
Embryopathy: Damage to the embryo, usually as a result of maternal exposure, typically in the first trimester of pregnancy.
HELLP syndrome: Hemolysis, elevated liver function tests, and low platelet levels in pregnant patients. Considered to be a variant of preeclampsia.
Myocarditis: Inflammation of the myocardium, characterized by a significant inflammatory infiltrate associated with myocyte necrosis.
Peripartum cardiomyopathy: Cardiomyopathy appearing in the final month of pregnancy or the first 5 months postpartum, with no preexisting heart muscle disorder and absence of any other cause of congestive heart failure.
Preeclampsia: The appearance of hypertension, proteinuria, and edema in a patient of more than 20 weeks' gestation.
Teratogenic risk: Risk of an induced fetal abnormality, usually caused by maternal exposure in the first trimester of pregnancy.
Tocolytic therapy: Sympathomimetic therapy used to decrease uterine contractions; usually initiated to prolong gestation and increase fetal lung maturation.

INTRODUCTION

Cardiologists and internists are increasingly being consulted in the management of cardiovascular complications associated with pregnancy. A greater number of women with known or potential cardiovascular disease are becoming pregnant, and cardiovascular complications in pregnant women are increasingly recognized.

This chapter discusses the normal morphologic and physiologic changes that occur during pregnancy, as well as the pathophysiology and management of hypertension associated with pregnancy and peripartum cardiomyopathy. Treatment of pregnant patients who have congenital heart disease or artificial heart valves and of those who require anticoagulation during pregnancy is outlined. Detection and management of coronary artery disease and coronary dissection, as well as the use of a cardiopulmonary bypass during pregnancy, are reviewed. Avoidance of fetal risk factors during pregnancy, including toxic drinking water, is addressed, as are the potential cardiac dangers of the use of tocolytic therapy to retard uterine contraction. Finally, management of both supraventricular and ventricular tachycardia in pregnancy is reviewed.

NORMAL PHYSIOLOGIC AND MORPHOLOGIC CHANGES IN PREGNANCY

Striking adaptations occur in the maternal cardiovascular system in response to pregnancy. An appreciation of these changes is mandatory to allow appropriate treatment of pregnant patients who have cardiovascular disease. Hunter and Robson (1) summarized hemodynamic and structural changes in maternal subjects based on echocardiographic studies. Longitudinal studies of cardiac output began before conception and continued into the postnatal period. Cardiac output increases as early as 5 weeks after the last menstrual period and rises to 45% above baseline at 24 weeks' gestation. Increased cardiac output is achieved by an increase in heart rate, which rises progressively until 32 weeks' gestation, and in stroke volume, which begins to increase by 8 weeks and peaks as early as 20 weeks (Fig. 31.1). Twin pregnancies result in an additional 15% rise in cardiac output in mothers. The cardiovascular system is taxed further by stage 1 of labor, which is associated with an additional 12% increase in demand for cardiac output. This demand increases to a mean of 34% above the already increased baseline value as labor progresses to its final stages. After delivery stroke volume decreases by 2 weeks postpartum. Heart rate remains elevated for 2 days postpartum and returns to baseline by 10 days after delivery. Cardiac output similarly decreases from pregnancy levels to normal levels between 24 hours and 10 days postpartum. The magnitude of these echocardiographic changes was confirmed by Mabie et al. (2) and Vered et al. (3), who in addition documented an increase in left ventricular mass during pregnancy.

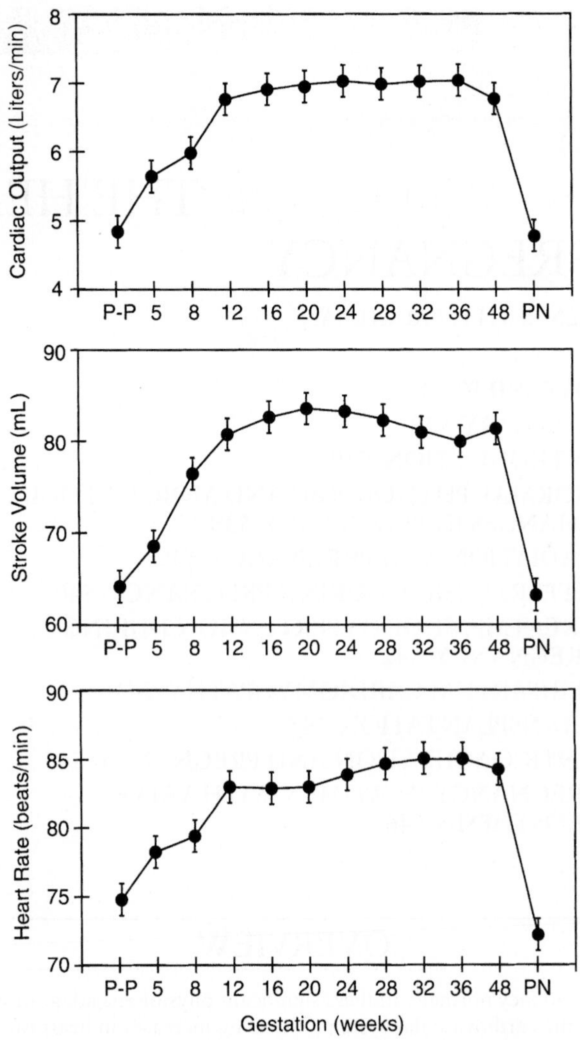

FIGURE 31.1. Serial echocardiographically determined changes in heart rate, stroke volume, and cardiac output during pregnancy and the early postpartum period. P-P, peripartum; PN, postnatal. (From Hunter S, Robson SC. Adaptation of the maternal heart in pregnancy. *Br Heart J* 1992;68:540–543.)

The structural changes noted by echocardiography are secondary to the alterations in intravascular volume and neurohumoral stimulation that are associated with pregnancy. Plasma volume increases approximately 40% and red blood

TABLE 31.1

PHYSICAL FINDINGS DURING NORMAL PREGNANCY

Mild jugular venous distention
Class 1–2+ lower-extremity edema
Decreased breath sounds at bases
Upward and leftward deviation of point of maximal impulse
Volume-loaded ventricle (active precordium)
Increased valve closure sounds
"Flow" murmurs (pulmonic and aortic)
Mammary soufflé (left sternal border)
Wide pulse pressure
Increased heart rate

cell volume 30% above baseline prepregnancy levels, resulting in mild relative anemia (4). Estrogen-mediated stimulation of the renin–angiotensin axis results in increased renal tubular absorption of sodium and an increase in total body salt and water, contributing to the increased plasma volume. Systemic vascular resistance and diastolic blood pressure decrease as a result of changes in aortic compliance and arterial venous shunting in the uterus.

The normal physiologic changes associated with pregnancy result in alterations in the physical examination of the pregnant patient (Table 31.1). Because of the increase in total body salt and water, as well as plasma volume, the central venous pressure may be slightly increased and the pregnant patient may have 1 to 2+ lower-extremity edema. As pregnancy progresses, increased uterus size forces both diaphragms upward, which may decrease pulmonary vital capacity and total lung volume. The previously documented changes in left ventricular size and mass result in a mildly displaced and diffuse point of maximal impulse of the left ventricle and increased valve closure sounds. Because of the insulation of the atrioventricular sounds by the abdomen, only the aortic and pulmonic closure sounds are characteristically louder on examination. Increased flow through the pulmonic valve causes a "functional" early systolic murmur and slight widening of the physiologic variation of closure of the pulmonic component of the second heart sound. Ventricular gallop rhythms and diastolic murmurs are unexpected. Occasionally, a normal physiologic diastolic murmur can be heard at the left sternal border in pregnant patients. This physiologic murmur is usually generated by increased diastolic flow through the internal mammary artery. This "mammary soufflé" may persist in lactating mothers, even after delivery. The expected decrease in aortic diastolic pressure during pregnancy that is associated with the decreased systemic vascular resistance results in a widened pulse pressure and pulsatile fingertips, warm hands, and occasional Quincke sign in the extremity nail beds. These findings are also suggestive of aortic regurgitation that may be confused by the diastolic murmur of the mammary soufflé at the sternal border. Echocardiography may be required to distinguish the presence or absence of aortic valve disease.

The physiologic changes associated with pregnancy may also alter the results of noninvasive evaluations of the heart (Table 31.2). The increase in size and left ventricular mass seen by echocardiography has already been described. The electrocardiogram may also be altered. Upward movement of the diaphragm results in a leftward shift of the electrical axis of ventricular depolarization, and increased ventricular mass may result in increased ventricular voltage. Heart rate may be increased, particularly late in pregnancy, and atrial as well as ventricular arrhythmias may increase in frequency in patients predisposed to such events. Chest radiographic studies reveal

TABLE 31.2

CHANGES IN NONINVASIVE TEST RESULTS THAT OCCUR DURING PREGNANCY

Test	Change
Electrocardiography	Leftward axis deviation Increased ventricular voltage Increased rate Repolarization changes
Chest x-ray film	Upward diaphragm displacement Horizontal heart placement Enlarged pulmonary silhouette
Echocardiography	Increased left ventricular diastolic dimension Increased left ventricular wall thickness Mild increase in contractility

a mild increase in cardiac size, a horizontal shift of the heart that increases with the duration of pregnancy, and fullness of the left cardiac border and pulmonary vascular supply (5).

Exercise can usually be maintained throughout pregnancy. Potential risks of exercise include hyperthermia-induced neural tube defects and decreased placental/fetal oxygen and substrate, which theoretically could alter fetal growth. Aerobic exercise to 69% maximal heart rate in pregnant patients does not alter core temperature, and oxygen saturation does not fall below 95% (6,7). Maternal exercise does increase fetal heart rate and fetal heart rate variability in the 20-minute postexercise interval (8,9). Potential exercise benefits include maintenance of aerobic capacity, enhanced cardiopulmonary reserve, and improved psychologic well-being and may help to prevent low back pain and gestational glucose intolerance (10,11). The increase in maternal resting heart rate and decreased maximal heart rate in pregnancy narrow the window of exercise heart rate response. Although there are no controlled trials, exercise is considered safe in pregnancy if there are no contraindications, nonballistic aerobic exercise is chosen, and excess ambient temperature and extremes of exertion are avoided (12–14).

RADIATION AND PREGNANCY

X-rays produce direct and indirect damage to cells. Direct damage results from the effect of the high-energy radiation beam on cellular and molecular structure. Indirect damage is the result of ionized water and free radical generation. The strength and potential damage of x-rays are measured by the amount of ionic charge created per unit mass of air. One R (roentgen) creates more than 2 billion ion pairs per cubic centimeter of exposures to air. The absorbed dose of radiation is measured in rad, calculated by the energy imparted per unit mass of tissue. One rad is equivalent to the deposition of .01 J of energy per kilogram of tissue. One R of radiation usually produces 1 rad in tissue. Roentgen-equivalent-man (REM) is a measure of absorbed radiation modified by local tissue characteristics, which better delineates the risk of radiation damage to a given organ (15).

Radiation is harmful to all living tissue and particularly to the conceptus. Increasing radiation exposure is associated with a range of tissue defects, beginning with isolated cellular damage and progressing to growth impairment, structural deformity, neoplasia, and gonadal damage. Environmental radiation results in 50 to 100 mREM of exposure during the 9 months of childbearing. The amount of radiation considered

TABLE 31.3

PERCENTAGE LIKELIHOOD THAT CHILDHOOD CANCER WILL NOT DEVELOP AFTER PRENATAL IRRADIATION

Gestational age	None	1 rad	5 rad	10 rad
First trimester	99.93	99.75	99.12	98.25
Second and third trimesters	99.93	99.88	99.70	99.48

to be "safe" is unclear; however, virtually no data have demonstrated significant fetal damage after exposure to less than 1 rad (16).

Several features alter the amount of radiation exposure that occurs during radiologic procedures, including the nature of the radiation source, the equipment used, the size of the patient, the depth of the uterus and conceptus, and the distance from the area being investigated, as well as the extent of the radiologic study. The dose of radiation received by the uterus may vary 50-fold depending on these features and whether appropriate uterus shielding is performed.

The increased risk of development of a subsequent malignancy by children receiving radiation in utero was reported by the Childhood Cancer Research Group in 1956 and confirmed in 1975 (15). Bithell and Stewart (16) demonstrated a relative risk of 1.47 for the development of subsequent malignancy in children whose mothers underwent radiographs during pregnancy. Furthermore, the relative risk increased progressively from 1.26 for one film exposure to 2.32 for five or more x-rays, indicating a dose response. A first-trimester exposure resulted in a relative risk of malignancy of 8.95, falling to 1.25 and 1.41 in the second and third trimesters, respectively. The risk of childhood cancer from radiation exposure is displayed in Table 31.3 (16).

The risk of radiation must be evaluated relative to the benefit to the mother. It is imperative that the clinician define (a) the dose of radiation to the conceptus (Tables 31.4 and 31.5), (b) the age and development of the conceptus, (c) the radiation risk from the radiation source, (d) the risk associated with delaying or not performing the test, and (e) the potential for alternative means of answering the question with nonradiation studies (17,18).

TABLE 31.4

AVERAGE DOSE (MRAD) TO UTERUS BASED ON 1,000-mREM Exposure

	Beam quality, half-value layer (mm aluminum)	
Exposed area, position	1.5	4.0
Chest		
PA	0.3	4.5
Lateral	0.1	1.8
Pelvis		
AP	142.0	486.0
Lateral	13.0	97.0
Thoracic spine		
AP	0.2	3.0
Lateral	0.04	0.8
Intravenous pyelogram or barium enema, AP	133.0	451.0
Renal angiogram, lateral	13.0	91.0

AP, anteroposterior; PA, posteroanterior.
From Rosenstein M. *Organ doses in diagnostic radiology.* Washington, D.C.: U.S. Department of Health, Education, and Welfare, 1976.

HYPERTENSION DURING PREGNANCY

High blood pressure may complicate as many as 10% of all pregnancies and remains a major cause of maternal and fetal morbidity and mortality (19,20). In normal pregnancy, diastolic blood pressure falls, often by as much as 10 mm Hg in the first and second trimesters as a result of decreased systemic vascular resistance. Blood pressure then increases gradually at or near term and may transiently rise higher than nonpregnant values in the immediate puerperium. Rarely is high blood pressure in pregnancy the result of secondary causes. The categories for high blood pressure in pregnancy are (a) chronic hypertension, (b) gestational hypertension, and (c) preeclampsia, with or without preexisting high blood pressure.

Chronic high blood pressure is categorized as preexistent hypertension or a blood pressure of at least 140/90 mm Hg before 20 weeks' gestation. If the diastolic blood pressure is 110 mm Hg or greater, severe hypertension is diagnosed. Pregnant women with a diastolic blood pressure higher than 75 mm Hg in the second trimester and 95 mm Hg in the third trimester should be observed carefully (21). The maternal and fetal outcomes are good unless preeclampsia or abruptio placentae complicates the final stages of gestation. Clear evidence exists (22) that treatment of diastolic blood pressure of greater than 110 mm Hg during pregnancy lowers the risk of stroke and cardiovascular complications, although the benefit of lowering blood pressure in mild chronic hypertension during pregnancy is less clearly defined.

Gestational hypertension is defined as asymptomatic blood pressure elevation after 20 weeks' gestation. Unless this elevation of pressure reflects early preeclampsia or unrecognized chronic hypertension, the maternal and fetal outcomes are usually very good, even without treatment.

Preeclampsia is the most feared hypertensive disorder of pregnancy and may lead to life-threatening eclampsia, a convulsive disorder. Preeclampsia is characterized by hypertension, proteinuria (levels >300 mg in 24 hours), and edema but may include coagulopathy and altered liver function in pregnant patients after 20 weeks' gestation (Table 31.6). Preeclampsia may be mild or severe, depending on the degree of blood pressure elevation and proteinuria. In preeclampsia, plasma volume and cardiac output fail to rise, and systemic resistance does not fall. There is an initial alteration in placental perfusion and angiogenic growth factors that leads to generalized damage to the endothelium (23) and release of placental debris in the circulation (24). This appears to be related to failure of the uterine spiral arteries to develop, preventing the anticipated arteriovenous shunting. Some researchers believe that the primary abnormality causing preeclampsia is the result of prostaglandin

TABLE 31.5

CONCEPTUS DOSE ESTIMATES FROM RADIONUCLIDE EXPOSURE

Radionuclide	Conceptus age (wk)	Organ	Dose per unit maternally administered activity (rad/mCi)
^{99m}Tc-sodium pertechnetate	1.5–6.0	Whole	0.0027–0.048
^{99m}Tc-polyphosphate	1.5–6.0	Whole	0.025
^{67}Ga-citrate	1.5–6.0	Whole	0.25
^{131}I	1.5–6.0	Whole	0.1–3.0

^{67}Ga, gallium 67; ^{131}I, iodine 131; ^{99m}Tc, technetium 99m.
From Wegnerckileser RG, Saldana LR. *Exposure of the pregnant patient to diagnostic radiation: a guide to medical management.* Philadelphia: JB Lippincott, 1985.

deficiency; endothelial cell dysfunction; immune, genetic, or sodium/calcium membrane disorders; increase in sympathetic nervous system activity (25); and increased levels of platelet-activating factor (26), plasma levels of prostaglandin isoforms (27), and angiotensin-1 receptor autoantibodies (28). These observations may have ramifications for treatment. There may be a genetic susceptibility for preeclampsia/eclampsia, and preliminary data indicate chromosome 2 as the likely location (29). The maternal risks of preeclampsia include cerebral hemorrhage, pulmonary edema, disseminated intravascular coagulopathy, liver failure, renal failure, convulsions, and death. These risks are correlated with the severity of the complications and level of gestation at the onset of the condition. The fetus may suffer hypoxemia, acidosis, growth retardation, and death.

Mild preeclampsia may be managed at home; however, development of progressive symptoms such as headache, visual disturbances, and abdominal pain requires hospitalization (Table 31.7). The use of antihypertensive or anticonvulsant therapy to treat mild preeclampsia remains questionable. Treatment of severe preeclampsia, on the other hand, may require termination of the pregnancy, regardless of fetal viability, if the mother's life is in jeopardy. Two recent large prospective, randomized trails have demonstrated the superiority of magnesium sulfate over phenytoin (anticonvulsant) and namodipine (calcium channel blocker with cerebral vasodilating properties) in prevention of eclampsia in women with severe preeclampsia (30–32). Antihypertensive therapy should be initiated with hydralazine, labetalol, or nifedipine to lower mean blood pressure and diastolic blood pressure to 126 and 90 mm Hg, respectively. Because these patients are already volume depleted, use of diuretics should be avoided. Intravenous magnesium should be given during labor and delivery and for 24 hours postpartum for patients who have severe preeclampsia to avoid convulsions.

There is no known mechanism for avoidance of preeclampsia, although sodium chloride restriction, diuretics, low-dose aspirin, and increased dietary calcium have been attempted.

A variant of preeclampsia, the HELLP syndrome, is characterized by minimal or no elevation of blood pressure, mild decreases in platelet levels, hemolysis, mild liver function abnormalities, and absence of renal impairment at the onset (20,22). This syndrome may progress rapidly, resulting in hemolysis, thrombocytopenia, and liver failure. Recognition of this syndrome prepartum should prompt immediate delivery. O'Brien and coworkers (33) suggested that corticosteroids may be of some benefit in this unusual disorder; however, a subsequent randomized, placebo-controlled trial comparing dexamethazone to saline control did not reduce disease severity or duration (34). Both the HELLP syndrome and preeclampsia may occur up to 10 days postpartum.

TABLE 31.6

TYPICAL FINDINGS IN PATIENTS WITH PREECLAMPSIA

- Definition
  - Hypertension
  - Proteinuria
  - Edema
  - Coagulopathy
  - Liver dysfunction
- After 20 wk of gestation
- Categories
  - Mild
  - Severe

TABLE 31.7

OMINOUS SIGNS AND SYMPTOMS IN WOMEN WITH PREECLAMPSIA

- Blood pressure $\geq$160 mm Hg systolic or $\geq$110 mm Hg diastolic
- Proteinuria of new onset at a rate of $\geq$2 g per 24 h or $\geq$100 mg/dL in a randomly collected specimen
- Increasing serum creatinine levels [especially >177 mmol/L (2 mg/dL) unless the level was known to be elevated previously]
- Platelet count <100,000 cells/liter or evidence of microangiopathic hemolytic anemia (e.g., schistocytes or increase in lactic acid dehydrogenase and direct bilirubin levels)
- Upper abdominal pain, especially epigastric and right-upper-quadrant pain
- Headache, vision disturbances, or other cerebral signs
- Cardiac decompensation (e.g., pulmonary edema, usually associated with underlying heart disease or chronic hypertension)
- Retinal hemorrhage, exudates, or papilledema (these signs are extremely rare in the absence of other indicators of severity and, when present, almost always indicate underlying chronic hypertension)
- Fetal growth retardation

From Cunningham FG, Lindheimer MD. Hypertension in pregnancy. *N Engl J Med* 1992;326:927–932.

Long-term follow-up (24 to 36 years postpartum) of patients with preeclampsia demonstrated an increased risk for death (2.1, 95% confidence interval [CI] 1.8 to 2.5) with deaths from cardiovascular events contributing most strongly to this increase (35).

TREATMENT OF HYPERTENSION DURING PREGNANCY

Medications commonly used to treat chronic, gestational, and preeclamptic hypertension are listed in Tables 31.8 and 31.9. Appropriate medical management of pregnancy-related hypertension depends on an understanding of the pathophysiology outlined in the previous sections. Some changes are unique to alterations in kidney handling of sodium and water.

The mean increase in total body water and sodium during pregnancy is 6 to 8 liters and 500 to 900 mEq, respectively, approximately one-half of which is extracellular (36). Many factors alter sodium excretion in pregnancy; despite a 50% increase in the glomerular filtration rate, elevated levels of progesterone and aldosterone result in a 40% increase in plasma volume. The result is that more than 80% of all healthy pregnant women develop physiologic-dependent or generalized edema. Edema may be a normal physiologic response; hypertension and preeclampsia are not. Despite the increase in interstitial volume that occurs with preeclampsia, the intraventricular volume is reduced, and oliguria and hemoconcentration are typically present. There is no evidence that the use of sodium restriction or diuretics prevents preeclampsia or other hypertensive complications of pregnancy, and use of such agents may cause additional volume contraction, alkalosis, electrolyte abnormalities, pancreatitis, and bleeding or hyponatremia in the neonate (21,36). Use of diuretics in women with preeclampsia should be avoided, and these agents are of limited benefit for treatment of pregnancy-related hypertension. Patients who have taken diuretics chronically before pregnancy or who are extremely sensitive to salt may derive some benefit from them (36).

Among agents used to treat chronic hypertension in pregnancy, Aldomet (methyldopa) is safe and preferable to other drugs. Randomized trials have demonstrated that Aldomet improves fetal survival, and it is the only drug with long-term

TABLE 31.8

GUIDELINES FOR TREATING SEVERE HYPERTENSION NEAR TERM OR DURING LABOR

Regulation of blood pressure
- The degree to which blood pressure should be decreased is disputed; we recommend maintaining diastolic levels between 90 and 110 mm Hg.

Drug therapy
- Hydralazine administered intravenously is the drug of choice. Start with low doses (5 mg as an intravenous bolus), then administer 5 to 10 mg every 20 to 30 min to avoid precipitous decreases in pressure. Side effects include tachycardia and headache.
- Diazoxide is recommended for women whose hypertension is refractory to hydralazine. Use 30-mg miniboluses because precipitous hypotension may result if higher doses are used. Side effects include arrest of labor and neonatal hypoglycemia.
- The experience with labetalol is growing, and some physicians use this agent instead of diazoxide as a second-line drug.
- Favorable results have been reported with calcium channel blockers. If magnesium sulfate is being infused, magnesium may potentiate the effects of calcium channel blockers, resulting in precipitous and severe hypotension.
- Refrain from using sodium nitroprusside because fetal cyanide poisoning has been reported in animals. However, maternal well-being should dictate the choice of therapy.

Prevention of convulsions
- Parenteral magnesium sulfate is the drug of choice for preventing eclamptic convulsions. Therapy should be continued for 12 to 24 h postpartum because one third of women with eclampsia have convulsions during this period.

From Cunningham FG, Lindheimer MD. Hypertension in pregnancy. *N Engl J Med* 1992;326:927–932.

TABLE 31.9

ANTIHYPERTENSIVE DRUGS USED TO TREAT CHRONIC HYPERTENSION IN PREGNANT WOMEN

α_2-Adrenergic receptor agonists
- Methyldopa is the most extensively used drug in this group. Its safety and efficacy are supported by evidence from randomized trials, and a 7.5-yr follow-up study has been made of children born to mothers treated with methyldopa.

β-Adrenergic receptor antagonists
- These drugs, especially atenolol and metoprolol, appear to be safe and efficacious when used in late pregnancy, but fetal growth retardation has been reported when treatment was started in early or mid-gestation. Fetal bradycardia can occur, and animal studies suggest that the fetus's ability to tolerate hypoxic stress may be compromised.

α-Adrenergic receptor and β-adrenergic receptor antagonists
- Labetalol appears to be as effective as methyldopa, but no follow-up studies have been conducted in children born to mothers given labetalol, and concern about maternal hepatotoxicity exists.

Arteriolar vasodilators
- Hydralazine is frequently used as adjunctive therapy with methyldopa and β-adrenergic receptor antagonists. Rarely, neonatal thrombocytopenia has been reported. Trials with calcium channel blockers look promising. The experience with minoxidil is limited, and this drug is not recommended.

Angiotensin-converting-enzyme inhibitors
- Captopril causes fetal death in diverse animal species, and several converting enzyme inhibitors have been associated with oligohydramnios and neonatal renal failure when administered to humans. *Do not use in pregnant women.*

Diuretics
- Many authorities discourage the use of diuretics, but others continue these medications if they were prescribed before conception or if a woman with chronic hypertension appears to be quite sensitive to salt.

From Cunningham FG, Lindheimer MD. Hypertension in pregnancy. *N Engl J Med* 1992;326:927–932.

follow-up (7.5 years), in which no difference in health, physical, or intellectual outcomes was seen (37,38). The use of β-receptor–blocking agents during pregnancy has been studied. Growth retardation, acute fetal distress, high perinatal mortality, and hypoglycemia have been found to be nearly nonexistent in controlled trials, and use of these agents are now considered nearly as safe as administration of Aldomet (38,39). Type II calcium channel blockers are potent vasodilators and have been used to treat hypertension during pregnancy. Uterine blood flow is minimally affected by nitrindipine and nifedipine, and the drug may decrease uterine contractions as a result of its smooth muscle relaxant properties; therefore, it may serve as a successful tocolytic agent (40).

Angiotensin-converting-enzyme (ACE) inhibitors are the agents of choice for use in nonpregnant patients who have cardiomyopathy or congestive heart failure and after myocardial infarction, but this class of antihypertensive drugs should *never* be used during pregnancy (41). Fetal complications include growth retardation, renal tubular dysplasia, renal failure, bone malformations (hypocalvaria, limb contractures), oligohydramnios, patent ductus arteriosis, pulmonary hypoplasia, respiratory distress, and neonatal death (42–45). The U.S. Food and Drug Administration (FDA) issued a warning against the use of ACE inhibitors during pregnancy after the first trimester (46). Most authorities favor avoiding these agents even in patients who are contemplating pregnancy.

Preeclampsia requires prompt control of accelerated hypertension. Because of its long history of use for preeclampsia, hydralazine remains the drug of choice for most physicians. The drug can be given intravenously, intramuscularly, or orally and titrated to achieve maximal effect (21). Labetalol combines α- and β-blocking properties, can be given intravenously, and incurs a prompt response. Nifedipine has been used sublingually and, when compared with hydralazine in a small, controlled trial, resulted in improved blood pressure control (40). Type II calcium channel blockers are tocolytic, which may be advantageous for treatment of patients who have premature contractions but deleterious for patients in whom delivery should be hastened. Nitroprusside probably should be avoided because of the potential for thiocyanate accumulation. Magnesium sulfate has been demonstrated to be beneficial during preeclampsia and for up to 24 hours after delivery.

PERIPARTUM CARDIOMYOPATHY

Peripartum cardiomyopathy, a relatively infrequent dilated cardiomyopathy that occurs in women of reproductive age, is defined as "a disorder of heart muscle, which presents clinically with the onset of heart failure in the last month of pregnancy or the first 5 postpartum months" (47,48). Established diagnostic criteria include (a) absence of a determinable cause for cardiac failure, (b) absence of preexisting heart muscle disease, and (c) time limitations of onset of illness. Other causes of congestive heart failure in pregnancy should be ruled out, as well as preeclampsia and pulmonary emboli, which may complicate late pregnancy and delivery. Some recent literature on this topic is tainted by the inclusion of patients who were in the last trimester of gestation rather than the final month. This expansion of the definition encompasses the response of patients with preexistent heart disease to the volume load imposed by pregnancy, which clouds the clinical observations about this unique disorder. Such patients should be excluded.

Peripartum cardiomyopathy complicates 1 in 1,300 to 1 in 4,000 deliveries in the United States (49–51). This condition may affect women of any race or age or with any number of prior deliveries; however, pregnancies in older age, multigravida pregnancies, African American race, and twin pregnancies are thought to represent predisposing features (Fig. 31.2).

The etiology of peripartum cardiomyopathy is unknown. Melvin et al. (52) in 1982 demonstrated myocarditis by endomyocardial biopsy in three of three patients presenting with peripartum cardiomyopathy. Sanderson et al. (53) performed biopsies on 11 women with peripartum cardiomyopathy in Nairobi and found healing myocarditis in 5, and O'Connell et al. (54) found myocarditis in 4 of 14 consecutive patients in the United States. Midei et al. (55) reported that 14 (78%) of 18 consecutive patients with peripartum cardiomyopathy had myocarditis found on endomyocardial biopsy. Felker et al. (56) expanded their study to include 42 women with peripartum cardiomyopathy who underwent biopsy. Despite a delay in biopsy of 1 to 2 weeks after presentation, the incidence of myocarditis remained high (62%). In addition, this group demonstrated that the prognosis for mothers with peripartum cardiomyopathy is good relative to patients with idiopathic

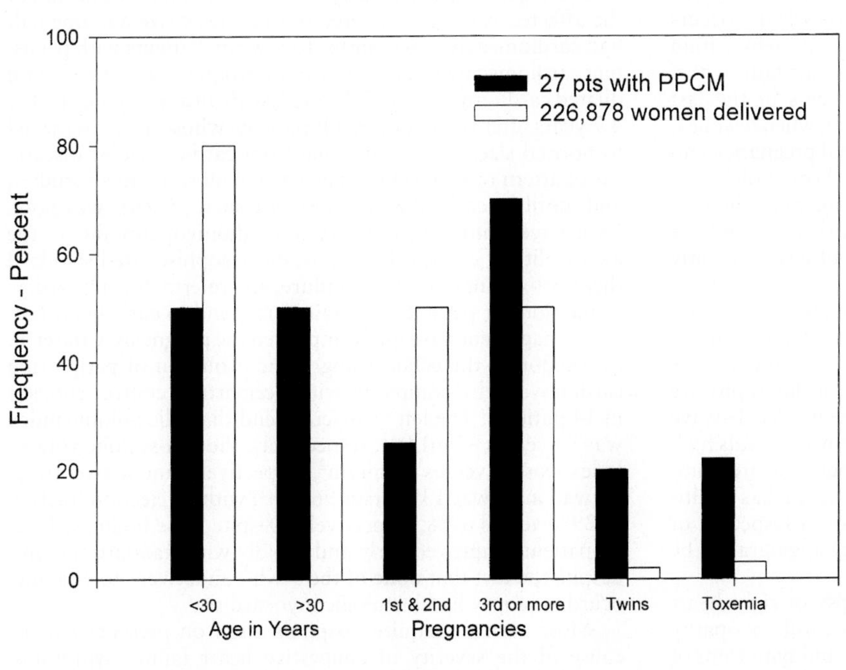

FIGURE 31.2. Risk factors for the development of peripartum cardiomyopathy (PPCM). pts, patients. (From Demakis JG, Rahimtoola SH. Peripartum cardiomyopathy. *Circulation* 1971;44:964–968.)

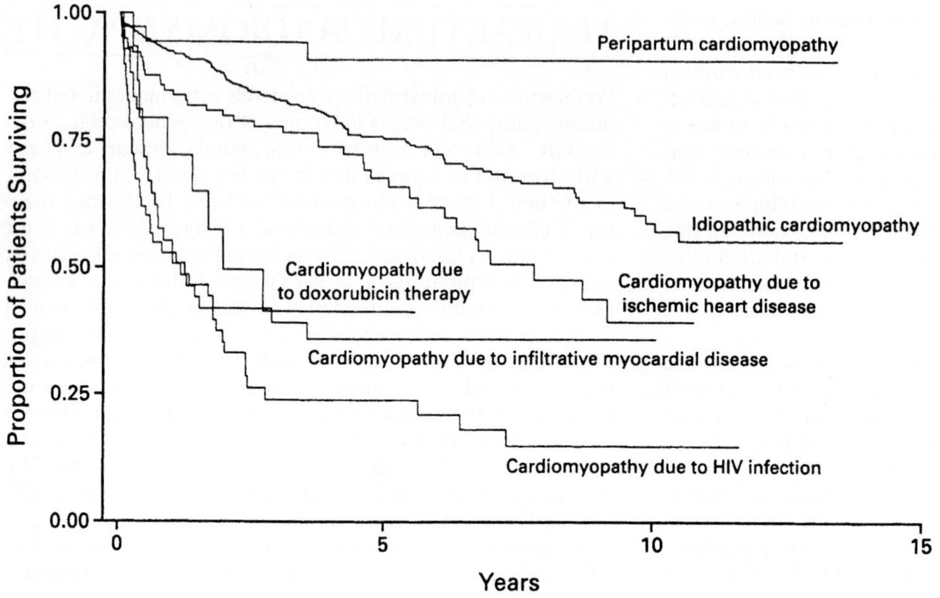

FIGURE 31.3. Adjusted Kaplan-Meier estimates of survival according to the underlying cause of cardiomyopathy. Only idiopathic cardiomyopathy and cardiomyopathy resulting from causes for which survival was significantly different from that among patients with idiopathic cardiomyopathy are shown. HIV, human immunodeficiency virus. (From Felker GM, Thompson RE, Hare JM, et al. Underlying causes and long-term survival in patients with initially unexplained cardiomyopathy. *N Engl J Med* 2000; 342:1077–1084.)

dilated cardiomyopathy (57) (Fig. 31.3). Of 42 patients included in that study, only 3 died (7%), and 3 underwent orthotopic heart transplantation (7%) (56). Ventricular function improved in most patients. In our experience, patients presenting early after delivery had more profound congestive heart failure and dramatic myocarditis found by endomyocardial biopsy, but they also had a greater chance of spontaneous resolution. These studies suggest that peripartum cardiomyopathy is immunologic in origin. Whether the inciting agent is an inapparent viral infection or an aberrant immunologic response to a placental or fetal antigen is unknown. As is true of the other cardiomyopathies that present with heart failure, patients with peripartum cardiomyopathy display elevated levels of tumor necrosis factor-α, interleukins, and apoptosis-signaling receptors (58). Data from the Centers for Disease Control and prevention evaluating 245 recently pregnant patients who died with cardiomyopathy (70% peripartum cardiomyopathy) showed that 48% died within 42 days of delivery and 50% between 43 days and 1 year (59).

Patients who have peripartum cardiomyopathy typically present with heart failure, which is more profound near the time of delivery and more subtle in presentation when it occurs months later. Approximately 80% of patients present within the first 3 months postpartum. Symptoms of heart failure may be particularly difficult to diagnose for patients in the last month of pregnancy and very early postpartum, when dyspnea, edema, and fatigue may be the result of normal pregnancy and delivery. The physical findings of congestive heart failure are manifest, including jugular venous distention, rales, hepatic congestion, and edema. Patients presenting early may not have cardiomegaly, and the point of maximal impulse is frequently superiorly placed.

The chest x-ray confirms the presence of pulmonary congestion and usually cardiomegaly. Echocardiography demonstrates markedly decreased contractility with variable degrees of cardiac enlargement. The results of electrocardiography are almost always abnormal and show nonspecific ST-T–wave changes. Right heart catheterization (if performed) reveals high filling pressures and decreased cardiac output that are compatible with cardiomyopathy. Only if the patient has multiple risk factors for coronary artery disease or is suspected of having a coronary dissection should coronary angiography be performed.

We do not perform endomyocardial biopsy or right heart catheterization on patients with peripartum cardiomyopathy unless they fail to show improvement in signs and symptoms of congestive heart failure and in echocardiographic ventricular function after 2 weeks of standard management therapy for congestive heart failure. If patients with peripartum cardiomyopathy who have failed to respond to standard heart failure treatement have myocarditis by endomyocardial biopsy, consideration should be given to treatment with immunosuppressive agents. Although endomyocardial biopsy can define the presence and severity of myocarditis in patients who have peripartum cardiomyopathy, it is unclear that this offers any therapeutic advantage because immunosuppressive therapy is likely ineffective in influencing long-term left ventricular function (60).

Standard management of heart failure should be applied to these patients postpartum, with careful attention to the potential influence of drugs on the uterus and, for patients in the last month of pregnancy, the fetus. Standard treatment includes afterload reduction therapy, diuresis, administration of digoxin (if signs or symptoms of congestive heart failure persist despite preload and afterload reduction therapy), and anticoagulation therapy (if ventricular compromise persists).

In Demakus' initial series (47,48) approximately one half of the affected patients recovered normal heart size and one half had cardiomegaly at 6 months' follow-up. Patients with persistent cardiomegaly had the same poor prognosis as patients with dilated cardiomyopathy; 80% died, with an average survival of 4.7 years after presentation. Of patients whose hearts returned to normal size, 14% died, none from cardiovascular disease. This pattern of survival has persisted in all subsequent studies, and, until recently, the prognosis for such patients was poor. Earlier recognition of peripartum cardiomyopathy due to the availability of echocardiography, more sophisticated standard therapy for congestive heart failure, and referral for full cardiac evaluation for patients who fail to respond to early heart failure management have likely improved the prognosis. Cole et al. (61) reported the echocardiographic evolution of peripartum cardiomyopathy compared with peripartum control subjects in 14 patients. The left ventricular end-diastolic volume index was 95 versus 67 mL/m^2, respectively; the end-systolic volume index was 66 versus 27 mL/m^2, respectively; and left ventricular wall mass was 139 versus 96 g/m^2, with an ejection fraction of 29% versus 67%, respectively. Despite these findings, 13 of 14 patients improved early and rapidly with standard therapy, despite the fact that none of the 5 who underwent to endomyocardial biopsy had histologic myocarditis.

Most patients require hospitalization on presentation because of the severity of congestive heart failure symptoms.

Appropriate therapy is administered until the patient's condition is stabilized. This can usually be accomplished with standard medical therapy, but occasionally extraordinary therapy is needed, including intraaortic balloon counterpulsation or use of a left ventricular assist device. Because the degree of reversibility of left ventricular dysfunction associated with peripartum cardiomyopathy is high and because the patients are young, all means necessary should be applied to ensure the mother's survival. Once discharged from the hospital, patients are followed every 2 weeks with clinical evaluation and an echocardiogram until left ventricular function is stabilized and no longer improving. Echocardiograms are repeated at 3 months and 6 months postpartum. The ventricular function at 6 months will likely be the ventricular performance that the patient maintains. Vigorous activity and nursing are discouraged during this interval to avoid left ventricular stress, which might alter ventricular remodeling during recovery. No other noninvasive tests are helpful in follow-up.

Recurrent pregnancies in patients who have experienced peripartum cardiomyopathy remain problematic. Demakis et al. (48) reported that of 14 patients whose hearts returned to normal, 8 attempted 21 subsequent pregnancies. Of these 8 patients, 3 experienced transient cardiac decompensation responsive to heart failure management. Of the 13 patients whose hearts failed to recover, 6 attempted repeat pregnancy, with 3 experiencing deterioration and death. Through a survey mechanism, Elkayam et al. (62) identified 44 patients who attempted 60 subsequent pregnancies after documented peripartum cardiomyopathy. Patients presenting in the last trimester—as opposed to the last month of pregnancy—were included. Of the 28 patients who normalized ventricular function at rest, there was a significant decrease in ejection fraction (from 56% to 49%), and 21% experienced congestive heart failure with subsequent pregnancies. Of the 16 patients with abnormal resting ventricular function, ejection fraction decreased (from 36% to 32%), and 44% developed symptomatic congestive heart failure with repeat pregnancy. Mortality was not noted in those with normalized ventricular function but was 19% in those with persistent dysfunction. Lampert et al. (63) studied ventricular reserve in patients with peripartum cardiomyopathy who normalized ventricular function. These authors used an echocardiographic load and heart rate–independent mechanism to assess ventricular contractility and reserve in response to methoxamine and dobutamine infusion. Contractile reserve, even in patients with ventricular recovery, was impaired.

There are, therefore, three categories of patients after peripartum cardiomyopathy: those with persistent abnormal cardiac function, those with normal resting but abnormal cardiac reserve with stress, and those with normal resting and stress ventricular performance. For patients who do not recover left ventricular function, pregnancy is contraindicated and standard long-term management for congestive heart failure should be undertaken. For those whose congestive heart failure is unresponsive to treatment, cardiac transplantation can be done (64,65) with a favorable long-term survival and morbidity comparable to that in age-matched control subjects. For patients with normal resting but abnormal stress ventricular response, pregnancy can be undertaken; however, cardiac decompensation may occur. Fortunately, this decompensation is usually responsive to medical management, and maternal mortality is not expected. In patients with normal resting and stress ventricular response after peripartum cardiomyopathy, repeat pregnancy can be undertaken with less risk of decompensation.

TRANSPLANTATION

The transplanted heart is denervated and may have limitations in ventricular dilation, making the hemodynamic burden of pregnancy more difficult to manage (66). Cardiac transplant patients are usually hypertensive and hypercholesterolemic, and they face the potential that accelerated atherosclerosis will develop in the transplanted heart's coronary arteries, increasing the risk of cardiovascular compromise. Pregnancy may interrupt routine surveillance endomyocardial biopsy procedures because of the risk of fetal radiation exposure, thereby limiting the transplant cardiologist's ability to diagnose and treat rejection successfully before hemodynamic compromise develops. Immunosuppressive agents pose a potential risk to the fetus of genetic alterations and to the mother's renal function (cyclosporine) and bone, skin, and adrenal integrity (prednisone). Scott et al. (67) reviewed the experience of 30 posttransplant patients who became pregnant. Overall, 48% had chronic hypertension, 24% had preeclampsia, and 28% had preterm labor. Six episodes of rejection required increased immunosuppressive therapy, and 9 required increased cyclosporine dose to maintain therapeutic levels. Of 27 live births, 10 infants were preterm (<36 weeks), 5 infants were small for gestational age, and 4 infants had neonatal complications. No congenital abnormalities were reported. Data from the National Transplantation Pregnancy Registry (68) confirmed a high incidence of premature and low-birth-weight infants born to 35 transplant recipients with 47 pregnancies. The risks appear to be similar in heart-lung transplant recipients (69). Pregnancy in cardiac transplant recipients must be considered high risk for mother and fetus and is discouraged.

ANTICOAGULATION AND PREGNANCY

Occasionally, pregnant patients require systemic anticoagulation for prophylaxis and treatment of venous or arterial thromboembolic disease or because of the presence of an artificial heart valve. Systemic anticoagulation exposes the mother and fetus to significant risks. Both heparin and warfarin may cause in utero placental bleeding, resulting in spontaneous abortion. Long-term systemic heparinization may cause osteoporosis. Heparin and low-molecular-weight heparin do not cross the placental barrier and have no effect on the fetus. Warfarin does cross the placental membrane and causes fetal anticoagulation. Administration of warfarin during the first trimester may cause an embryopathy, and exposure at any time in gestation may cause central nervous system abnormalities in the fetus. Weeks 6 to 12 of gestation appear to be the critical time interval for embryopathy caused by warfarin exposure, resulting in nasal hypoplasia or stippled epiphysis. Central nervous system abnormalities caused by warfarin exposure include hemorrhage and dorsal or ventral midline dysplasia. Data concerning low-molecular-weight heparin are limited. Ellison et al. (70) found a low incidence of complications with use of 40 mg of low-molecular-weight heparin once per day for prophylasis. Satisfactory anti–factor Xa levels and prevention of thromboembolism were achieved (70).

Systemic heparinization during pregnancy traditionally has been thought to result in high risk to the fetus and mother. Ginsberg and Hirsh (71) reviewed the published literature in 1989 and reported a summary of 106 studies that evaluated 1,325 pregnancies in women who were receiving anticoagulation therapy. After excluding comorbid conditions, the risk of maternal death was 2.5% (7 of 278 patients) for women receiving heparin and 16.8% (95 of 567 patients) for patients treated with oral anticoagulants. These authors also carried out a prospective study of 77 women with 100 pregnancies, among whom heparin was given for prevention or treatment of venous thromboembolism in 98 pregnancies and because of a prosthetic valve replacement in 2 (72). The rates of prematurity, abortion, stillbirths, neonatal deaths, and congenital abnormalities were similar to those in normal populations. In addition, no symptomatic thromboembolisms and only two episodes of bleeding were seen after a mean of 18 weeks of treatment per pregnancy. Osteoporosis is a potential complication of heparin therapy. In a prospective study of heparin use in pregnant patients (73), using bone densitometry to evaluate osteoporosis in 14 patients, 36% experienced a greater than 10% decrease in femur bone density measurements from baseline to immediately postpartum, compared with 14 pregnant control subjects. These data confirm that one third of pregnant patients treated with prolonged heparin are likely to develop osteoporosis, even at doses as low as 15,000 units/day. In addition, patients rarely may develop heparin-associated antibodies during pregnancy, resulting in thrombosis and thrombocytopenia (74,75).

In their literature review, Ginsberg and Hirsh (71) reported warfarin embryopathy in 45 of 970 exposed fetuses and central nervous system abnormalities in 26 of 970 patients. Of 22 cases of heparin osteoporosis that have been reported, 7 have occurred in pregnant patients. Development of osteoporosis may be related to total exposure and has been reported in patients receiving 15,000 to 20,000 units daily for more than 6 months.

Low-molecular-weight heparin is increasingly being used in pregnant patients. Low-molecular-weight heparin is more convenient, is associated with a lower incidence of osteoporosis and heparin-induced thrombocytopenia (HIT), and appears to be at least equally efficacious compared with unfractionated heparin (UFH) (76). Because the volume of distribution and body weight change during pregnancy, at least monthly assessment of anti–factor Xa should be done (77).

Based on these data, most authors recommend systemic heparinization or low-molecular-weight heparinization during the critical weeks 6 to 12 of gestation and in the last 2 weeks of pregnancy to allow rapid reversal for delivery. A dose of 10,000 units twice per day subcutaneously is the recommended treatment. Activated partial thromboplastin time should be measured 6 hours after administration of heparin and should be 1.5 to 2.0 times control. Warfarin can be administered during the remainder of gestation with little risk of embryopathy.

PREGNANCY IN WOMEN WITH VALVE PROSTHESES

Cardiologists are often asked to evaluate and manage the condition of patients with prosthetic heart valves during pregnancy or to advise young women on the selection of an appropriate artificial valve designed to maximize the potential for a future successful and uncomplicated pregnancy (78,79). However, limited data are available for assisting in these tasks (Table 31.10) (80–87).

Recently, Vongpatanasin et al. (88) recommended that administration of warfarin be discontinued in patients attempting pregnancy and that administration of subcutaneous heparin be substituted, twice per day at a dose that prolongs the activated partial thromboplastin time by more than two times control 6 hours after administration. After week 12 of gestation, warfarin can be safely substituted until "the middle of the third trimester, after which warfarin should be discontinued and heparin resumed until delivery."

Based on limited experience, the FDA initially issued a warning that enoxaparin should not be used in patients with prosthetic heart valves due to apparent risk of valve thrombosis. Ginsberg et al. (89) and Topol (90) issued strong rebuttals and recommend (a) aggressive UFH throughout, (b) adjusted low-molecular-weight heparin (LMWH) throughout, and (c) UFH or LMWH until week 13 and again before delivery. Both authors cautioned that UFH and LWMH must be maintained at therapeutic doses, failure of which likely resulted in the early valve thrombosis experience.

In summary, (a) pregnancy in a woman with an artificial valve prosthesis poses significant risks to the mother and fetus; (b) pregnancy is a hypercoagulable state, and valve thrombosis or thromboembolic complications are not rare, particularly in women with mechanical prostheses and especially in women with mitral valve replacement; (c) bioprostheses may degenerate in an accelerated fashion during or shortly after delivery; (d) maternal and fetal risks are increased by the presence of advanced congestive heart failure, and pregnancy is inadvisable for women with artificial heart valves and symptoms of significant heart failure; and (e) heparin cannot be recommended for use as the sole anticoagulating agent during pregnancy and should be combined with warfarin after week 12 of gestation for women with mechanical heart prostheses who require anticoagulation therapy.

CARDIOPULMONARY BYPASS DURING PREGNANCY

Severe native or prosthetic valvular heart disease and, rarely, symptomatic coronary atherosclerosis may require cardiac surgical intervention in pregnant women. A mortality rate as high as 20% may be seen among pregnant patients with native valvular heart disease and class III to IV congestive heart failure (91). Although balloon commissurotomy of mitral stenosis or percutaneous transluminal coronary angioplasty of coronary atherosclerosis may be beneficial for pregnant women who have appropriate mitral or coronary anatomy, most other valve and coronary disease patients require more than medical treatment and should undergo cardiopulmonary bypass.

TABLE 31.10

STUDIES OF THE USE OF VALVE PROSTHESES IN PREGNANT WOMEN

Reference	Type of prosthesis	Number of pregnancies	Live births (%)	Thromboembolic complications (%): Valve thrombi	Emboli	Valve degeneration (%)
Hanania et al. (80)	Mechanical	95	53	11	9	0
Sbarouni et al. (81)	Mechanical	151	73	9	5	0
Born et al. (82)	Mechanical	35	63	8	3	0
Hanania et al. (80)	Bioprosthesis	60	80	0	0	18
Sbarouni et al. (81)	Bioprosthesis	63	83	0	0	35
Born et al. (82)	Bioprosthesis	25	100	0	5	16

Valve-related risk factors during pregnancy. Both thromboembolic and valve degeneration problems may appear.

Pomini et al. (92) examined 59 reports of cardiac surgery performed with the aid of cardiopulmonary bypass from 1958 through 1992. Cardiopulmonary bypass may compromise the placenta and fetus as a result of hypothermia, decreased arterial perfusion, and alterations in coagulation as well as acid–base balance. The reported fetal and maternal mortality rates were 2.9% and 20.2% overall, respectively, but 0% and 12%, respectively, for the 40 most recently reported subjects (1975 through 1991). Hypothermia alters placental oxygen exchange and has been demonstrated to initiate uterine contractions. Embryo fetal mortality associated with hypothermic cardiopulmonary bypass was 24%, and mortality associated with normothermic perfusion was 0%. Increased rates of pump flow diminished evidence of fetal cardiac distress, and higher-volume cardiopulmonary bypass flow is recommended, with the appropriate fetal monitoring to ensure adequacy. Therefore, normothermic bypass at high-flow volumes is recommended.

In addition, it is recommended that patients whose pregnancies are past 20 weeks' gestation be positioned in the left lateral decubitus position during surgery to ensure that the uterus does not obstruct venous return as a result of direct inferior vena cava compression. Hyperkalemic arrest solutions may reach the fetal circulation and should be avoided, if possible. Finally, the duration of cardiopulmonary bypass should be minimized, and the operating room must be prepared for emergency cesarean section (78).

MYOCARDIAL INFARCTION ASSOCIATED WITH PREGNANCY

Symptomatic coronary artery disease and myocardial infarction occur infrequently during pregnancy (approximately 1 in 36,000 deliveries) (93). Nevertheless (94–99) because pregnant patients may display spontaneous coronary artery dissection (100–102) and because the population of women attempting pregnancy is progressively older (103), cardiologists must be familiar with this potential problem. Other risk factors for myocardial infraction in pregnancy are chronic hypertension, diabetes, eclampsia, and severe preeclampsia (93).

PREGNANCY IN WOMEN WITH CONGENITAL OR ACQUIRED CARDIAC DISEASE

Women who have congenital or acquired cardiac disease with or without surgical correction require cardiology assistance in management of their pregnancy. Siu et al. (104) examined prospectively the maternal and neonatal risks associated with pregnancy in women with known heart disease. Investigators enrolled 562 consecutive patients and determined outcome in 599 pregnancies. Maternal cardiac complications (pulmonary edema, arrhythmia, stroke, or cardiac death) complicated 13% of pregnancies and were predicted by prior cardiac events or arrhythmia, poor functional class or cyanosis, left heart obstruction, and left ventricular systolic function. Patients experienced a 4%, 31%, and 68% risk of primary or secondary cardiac events with no, one, and more than one predictor, respectively. Neonatal complications occurred in 20% of pregnancies and were associated with poor maternal functional class or cyanosis, left heart obstruction, anticoagulation, smoking, and multiple gestations. Long-term databases confirm the increased proportion of high-risk pregnancies associated with congenital as opposed to rheumatic heart disease (105). Wooley and Sparks (106) summarized five clinical studies of 490 patients who had congenital heart disease and were undergoing pregnancy, and reported a maternal mortality of 0.53% and a fetal mortality of 18.90%. Congenital defects considered to place patients at a higher risk included Eisenmenger complex, pulmonary hypertension, cyanotic cardiac defects, and aortopathy associated with Marfan syndrome (107) and coarctation. Perloff (108) identified potential residual changes after congenital surgical correction that increased concern about maternal and fetal outcomes, including (a) residual elevation of pulmonary vascular resistance, (b) residual aortic stenosis or regurgitation, (c) persistent right or left ventricular dysfunction, (d) aortopathy after aorta or aortic valve repair or replacement, (e) uncertain capability of prosthetic material, and (f) cleft mitral valve residual defects after endocardial cushion repair (109–112) (Table 31.11). Selected acquired heart disease may also increase risk during pregnancy (113–117).

TABLE 31.11

AREAS OF POTENTIAL CONCERN FOR PATIENTS WITH "CORRECTED" CONGENITAL HEART DISEASE WHO ARE CONTEMPLATING PREGNANCY

Residual elevation of pulmonary vascular resistance
Persistent ventricular dysfunction
Residual valvular insufficiency
Prosthetic devices or material
Aortopathy

CARDIOVASCULAR COMPLICATIONS OF TOCOLYTIC THERAPY

Tocolytic agents decrease uterine contractility and are used to prolong gestation, usually beyond week 34, to allow fetal lung maturation (118). These agents are used in up to 5% of all pregnancies (118). Few data exist to support long-term use of these agents (118). Drugs used include magnesium, β-sympathetic medications, and recently calcium channel blocking agents. (118,119). In one study, as many as 4.4% of the female patients exposed to tocolytic drugs developed pulmonary edema (120). The peculiar nature of this life-threatening complication must be understood by cardiologists so they can assist obstetricians in intelligent management.

Pisani and Rosenow (120) reviewed 22 years of medical literature and reported 58 cases. The most commonly used agents were β-sympathomimetics; corticosteroids were used in two thirds of the patients to accelerate fetal lung maturation. The average duration of treatment was 54 hours, but the syndrome can appear after less than 24 hours of exposure, and, in a few cases, symptoms appear up to 12 hours after drug discontinuation. Patients complained of dyspnea (76%), chest pain (24%), and cough (17%). Affected women sometimes had fever (temperature higher than 38°C; 14%), were rarely hypotensive, and uniformly had pulmonary rales. Chest x-rays showed bilateral pulmonary infiltrates (81%) and rarely showed effusion. Echocardiography, in only 7 patients, revealed normal left ventricular function. Right heart catheterization demonstrated elevated filling pressures in only 2 of 9 cases, and the cardiac index was greater than 6 L/minutes/m^2.

Treatment includes discontinuation of tocolytic therapy and administration of supplemental oxygen and intravenous diuretics; response is usually rapid. Maternal and fetal mortality is rare, unless the woman's condition is complicated by sepsis or full-blown acute respiratory distress syndrome. The etiology of tocolytic pulmonary edema is unknown but does not appear to be related to myocardial failure.

Other entities that may present similarly include peripartum cardiomyopathy, pulmonary embolism, aspiration with acute respiratory distress syndrome, pneumomediastinum, and amniotic fluid embolization. Amniotic fluid embolization, although rare (incidence of 1 in 8,000 to 1in 80,000 deliveries), is associated with cardiovascular collapse, respiratory distress, disseminated intravascular coagulopathy, and coma and is rapidly fatal in more than 80% of patients (121). A recent population based study of more than 1 million deliveries revealed a frequency of amniotic fluid embolization of 1 in 20,646 with a maternal mortality of 26.4%. Of those with a diagnosis of amniotic fluid embolization, 66% displayed disseminated intravascular coagulation (DIC), 72% hemorrhaged, and 47% showed obstetric shock (122). A similar registry recorded a maternal mortality of 61% with neurologically intact survival of only 15% (123). In this series, 70% of amniotic fluid embolization occurred during labor, 19% during cesarean section after delivery, and 11% after routine vaginal delivery (123). Therefore, amniotic fluid embolization presents as a spectrum and accounts for up to one third of maternal deaths (124). Management is directed to oxygenation, circulatory support, and coagulative treatment (125).

The risks for development of tocolytic therapy pulmonary edema appear to be related in part to the dose, the number of agents used, and the form of delivery (intravenous vs. subcutaneous). Perry and colleagues (126) studied 8,709 women who were given continuous subcutaneous infusions of terbutaline to arrest preterm labor. Patients were followed daily in the hospital or at home. Pulmonary edema developed in only 0.32% of cases (28 of 8,709 patients). Of the 28 patients affected, 17 were receiving one to three tocolytic agents and aggressive intravenous hydration. It appears that tocolytic therapy can be administered relatively safely; however, patients receiving certain dosages, multiple drug infusions, and supplemental intravenous hydration must be watched carefully.

ARRHYTHMIAS IN PREGNANT WOMEN

Page (127), Cox and Gardner (39), Joglar and Richard (128), and Rutherford (129) recently reviewed the treatment of arrhythmia during pregnancy. The hemodynamic stress of pregnancy may exacerbate arrhythmias, and treatment of rhythm disorders poses a risk to the mother as well as to the fetus (130–132).

Pregnancy significantly alters drug absorption and metabolism as a result of (a) altered gastrointestinal motility, (b) expanded plasma volume, (c) decreased plasma protein, (d) progesterone-induced alterations of hepatic metabolism, and (e) increased renal blood flow. Therefore, frequent measurement of drug levels may be necessary (127–130). The teratogenic risk of drug exposure is greatest in the first trimester of pregnancy; use of drugs should be avoided during this time if possible (Table 31.12).

ANTIPHOSPHOLIPID SYNDROME

The antiphospholipid syndrome should be suspected in mothers with arterial or venous thrombosis, thrombocytopenia, neurologic disease, or recurrent abortion. Fetal loss is associated with thrombosis of the uteroplacental vasculature. Antiphospholipid antibodies recognize a plasma cofactor on the trophoblast and/or endothelial cell surface that produces a procoagulant state (133). Women with systemic lupus erythematosus who have the lupus anticoagulant or antiphospholipid antibodies have a greater than 60% chance of pregnancy loss, compared with a 15% loss among women with systemic lupus erythematosus who do not have these antibodies. It is believed that the antiphospholipid antibody results in placental infarction or thromboses, with subsequent pregnancy loss.

Silveria et al. (134) treated 11 consecutive patients who had positive anticardiolipin (antiphospholipid) assays and had experienced at least one pregnancy loss with prednisone and aspirin. This resulted in an improved live birth rate, from 15.6% before treatment to 100% after treatment, without significant adverse effects to the mother or fetus. Heparin, low-dose aspirin, and intravenous immunoglobulin have been proposed as treatment options for the antiphospholipid syndrome. In a prospective, double-blind, placebo-controlled trial involving only 50 patients who had antiphospholipid antibodies and three or more fetal losses, 75 mg/day of aspirin had no influence on the live birth rate compared with placebo (80% vs. 85%, respectively) (135). Similarly, Branch et al. (136) found no difference in maternal or fetal outcomes when intravenous immunoglobulin was added to a regimen including aspirin and heparin for patients who had antiphospholipid antibodies. Interruption of the anticardiolipin cycle of thrombosis may be important because patients with this syndrome may develop ventricular diastolic dysfunction over the course of time (137).

CONTROVERSIES AND PERSONAL PERSPECTIVES

Peripartum cardiomyopathy remains a controversial area in the management of the pregnant or peripartum patient. The etiology of the syndrome is unknown. On the assumption that the condition is associated with myocardial inflammation, the antigen to which the immune response is directed is unknown. It is also evident that in a high proportion of patients, peripartum cardiomyopathy, with or without myocarditis, resolves spontaneously. We have, therefore, taken the stance that once peripartum cardiomyopathy is recognized, patients should be treated with standard heart failure therapy for 2 weeks. If clear echocardiographic evidence of improvement in the myopathic state is seen, patients need not undergo endomyocardial biopsy. If the myopathic state does not improve or deteriorates, the patients undergo endomyocardial biopsy, and those with myocarditis are treated with immunosuppressive agents in the hope of improving left ventricular function. Patients with ejection fractions in the exceedingly low range (<15%) and those who are more than 4 months from delivery are unlikely to respond, even if myocarditis is demonstrated. Patients in whom ventricular function does not return to normal at rest and with stress exercise after peripartum cardiomyopathy should be should be discouraged from additional pregnancies.

A second controversial area is the use of anticoagulants in pregnant patients. Some authors recommend heparin or LMWH throughout the pregnancy to avoid any warfarin-related embryopathy or central nervous system abnormality. Other authors have observed such a low rate of embryopathy and central nervous system disorders with use of warfarin that they use the agent throughout the pregnancy, until delivery. Unless the patient declares her desire for a pregnancy and switches from warfarin to heparin before conceiving, most patients receiving chronic anticoagulants present to their physician already pregnant. These patients have already sustained most of the potential risk for embryopathy by the time the physician is aware of the pregnancy. On balance, the risk to the patient and fetus seems least if warfarin is discontinued before pregnancy is initiated and if heparin or LMWH is used throughout at least the first 12 weeks of gestation. Thereafter, warfarin can be used

TABLE 31.12

PHARMACODYNAMICS AND ADVERSE EFFECTS OF CARDIOVASCULAR DRUGS IN PREGNANCY

Drug	Classification (Vaughan-Williams)	Therapeutic concentration	Protein binding (%)	Fetal to maternal ratio	Breast milk to plasma ratio	FDA pregnancy category	Adverse effects
Digoxin		0.5–2.0 ng/mL	20–25	~1	0.6–0.9	C	Low birth weight
Adenosine		NA	NA	ND	ND	C	None
Quinidine	1A	3–6 μg/mL	70–80	0.24–1.40	0.71	C	Low platelet levels
Procainamide	1A	4–8 μg/mL	15–20	0.28–132	~1	C	None
Disopyramide	1A	2–4 μg/mL	35–90	0.39	0.9	C	Uterine contraction
Lidocaine	1B	1.5–5.0 μg/mL	60–80	0.5–0.6	~1	B	Cardiovascular system side effects
Mexiletine	1B	0.5–2.0 μg/mL	60–75	1.0	0.78–1.89	C	Decreased heart rate, low birth weight, low APGAR score
Tocainide	1B	4–10 μg/mL	10–15	ND	ND	C	ND
Phenytoin	1B	10–20 μg/mL	90	0.65–1.00	0.12–0.45	C	Mental and growth retardation
Flecainide	1C	<0.2–1.0 μg/mL	40	0.70–0.83	1.57–2.18	C	None
Encainide	1C	0.5–1.0 μg/mL	75–85	ND	ND	B	None
Propafenone	1C	0.2–3.0 μg/mL	~95	0.14–0.20	0.14–0.20	C	None
β-Blockers	2	Variable	Variable	Variable	Variable	C	Possible low heart rate, hypoglycemia
Amiodarone	3	1.0–2.5 μg/mL	96	0.09–0.14	2.25–9.00	C	Low thyroid, growth retardation, premature birth
Sotalol	3	ND	ND	ND	ND	B	β-Blocker effect
Bretylium	3	0.5–1.0 μg/mL	0–8	ND	ND	—	ND
Verapamil	4	15–30 ng/mL	90	0.17–0.40	0.23–0.94	C	Heart block, hypotension
Diltiazem	4	50–300 ng/mL	80–90	ND	ND	C	Teratogenic?
Furosemide		NA	NA	Placental transfer		C	Low Na^+, K^+, glucose levels
Heparin		NA	NA	No placental transfer		C	Abortion
Coumadin		NA	NA	Placental transfer		D	Abortion, hemorrhage

APGAR, activity, pulse, grimace, appearance, respiration; FDA, U.S. Food and Drug Administration; NA, not applicable; ND, not determined.
From Rutherford JD. Management of cardiovascular disease during pregnancy. In: Smith TW, ed. *Cardiovascular therapeutics*. Philadelphia: WB Saunders, 1996:695–701; and Cox JL, Gardner MJ. Treatment of cardiac arrhythmias during pregnancy. *Prog Cardiovasc Dis* 1993;36:137–178.

until just before delivery, when heparin must be substituted to allow delivery without substantial bleeding.

The choice of artificial heart valves is a third controversial area of management in pregnant patients. Patients with bioprostheses have a much higher live birth rate and usually do not require chronic anticoagulation. However, the natural degeneration of bioprostheses in patients in this age group may complicate pregnancy and delivery. Mechanical prostheses do not degenerate but are associated with a higher rate of thromboembolic complications, including valve thrombosis and embolic phenomena in the central nervous system and periphery. Most of these thromboembolic complications have occurred in patients receiving an inadequate anticoagulation therapy. I favor the implantation of a mechanical prosthesis, even for the patient who desires a subsequent pregnancy. On the patient declares an intent for pregnancy, conversion from warfarin to adequate heparin or LMWH anticoagulation until after the first trimester, and then careful management of warfarin therapy, should diminish the potential for thromboembolic complications.

Not all clinicians are willing to follow patients who have undergone corrected congenital or acquired heart disease through pregnancy. These patients have often sustained life-threatening complications before surgery, and the surgery itself is usually high risk. Once patients have survived these risks, many clinicians are wary of the patient's decision to incur what some would consider an unnecessary additional risk. There is also the potential that the mother's genetic disorder may be passed on to any children. Other clinicians empathize with the patient's desire to bear and raise children despite the risk to the patient. We ensure that the patient is informed of the potential risk that her cardiac disorder could be transmitted to her offspring. If a patient is willing to accept this risk, a full cardiovascular evaluation is undertaken to evaluate the patient's cardiopulmonary capability to sustain the cardiovascular stress of normal pregnancy and delivery. Occasionally, the risk is determined to be too great, based on elevated pulmonary vascular resistance, high filling pressures, left or right ventricular dysfunction, aortopathy, or inadequate correction of congenital abnormalities (16,17). Most patients are willing to accept the decision to avoid pregnancy after a thorough evaluation.

THE FUTURE

An increased understanding of the pathophysiology of disorders such as preeclampsia and peripartum cardiomyopathy will lead to more effective therapies. With advances in vascular biology, more-effective anticoagulation regimens can be used in patients who have thrombogenic abnormalities. More-thorough prepregnancy cardiovascular evaluations, including stress or dobutamine echocardiography and magnetic resonance imaging, will better identify patients with acquired or corrected congenital heart disease who are able to proceed safely with pregnancy and delivery.

Little controversy exists about the risks of use of antiarrhythmic agents, regardless of the state of pregnancy. Drugs are infrequently used, and when used are carefully chosen to avoid teratogenic and maternal problems.

It is likely that an increasing proportion of high-risk pregnancies will be undertaken by older women or women with preexisting heart disease. These factors will result in continued growth and development of the already strong relationships between physicians in cardiology and those in high-risk obstetrics.

It is also likely that the etiology of preeclampsia will be discovered in the near future. An increased understanding of vascular biology and alterations of vascular biology that occur in pregnant women will allow an appropriate recognition of the underlying abnormality associated with this potentially fatal complication of pregnancy. Once the pathophysiology is understood, it is almost certain that an effective therapy can be introduced, significantly reducing maternal and fetal morbidity and mortality.

We are only beginning to understand the pathophysiology of peripartum cardiomyopathy. If the condition is associated with myocarditis, it seems logical that the etiology is immunologic. It is unlikely that the causative agent is viral and more likely that it is related to an altered placental antigen. Understanding the pathophysiology of the condition will allow better recognition and treatment of patients with this disorder. Once the pathophysiology is understood, it is anticipated that almost all patients who have peripartum cardiomyopathy will recover, as opposed to the approximately 50% recovery rate that is currently achieved.

Although new forms of anticoagulants are available, including low-molecular-weight heparin, antiplatelet agents, direct thrombin inhibitors, and platelet IIb/IIIa glycoprotein inhibitors, it is unlikely that any significant improvement will be made in the risk to patients who are pregnant and require anticoagulant therapy. Progress in this regard again depends on advances in vascular biology. Estrogen, progesterone, and other pregnancy-related hormone alterations that affect vascular and platelet reactivity may serve as a nidus for thrombus formation. Effective anticoagulant therapy depends on the physician understanding these alterations and providing appropriate interruption of pregnancy-related changes. Once these thrombogenic abnormalities are recognized and understood, it is expected that pregnancy can be more safely undertaken by women with mechanical valve prostheses.

Although earlier correction of congenital and acquired heart disease is possible, it is unlikely that the early repair of these disorders will significantly alter the risk to the patient associated with pregnancy and delivery. More thorough prepregnancy cardiovascular evaluations, including stress or dobutamine echocardiography and magnetic resonance imaging with or without exercise, will likely better identify patients who are capable of proceeding safely with pregnancy and delivery.

Safer doses and durations of tocolytic therapy are already being used. The lack of understanding of pulmonary edema related to tocolytic therapy is the result primarily of inadequate investigation into the condition of these relatively rare patients. Despite the small number of patients who experience this disorder, the nature of the disorder can be ascertained, and appropriate treatment regimens can be designed.

The increased risk associated with use of antiarrhythmic agents has been recognized in nonpregnant patients. This risk is increased further with the pregnant state because drug absorption and metabolism both change in association with pregnancy. Therefore, drug therapy should be avoided if possible during pregnancy, and, if it is used, agents should be used that carry no teratogenic risk. Our knowledge of medication treatment in pregnancy is rudimentary and based primarily on animal data with limited human trials. Obstetricians, cardiologists, pharmacologists, and pharmacoepidemiologists must provide data concerning the risk/benefit ratio, the maternal, breast, and fetal levels of medications used, and how they are altered during pregnancy if we are to improve our understanding of the treatment of these cardiac patients.

References

1. Hunter S, Robson SC. Adaptation of the maternal heart in pregnancy. *Br Heart J* 1992;68:540–543.
2. Mabie WC, DiSessa TG, Crocker LG, et al. A longitudinal study of cardiac output in normal human pregnancy. *Am J Obstet Gynecol* 1994;170:849–856.
3. Vered Z, Poler SM, Gibson P, et al. Noninvasive detection of the morphologic and hemodynamic changes during normal pregnancy. *Clin Cardiol* 1991;14:327–334.
4. Hess DB, Hess LW. Management of cardiovascular disease in pregnancy. *Obstet Gynecol Clin North Am* 1992;19:679–695.
5. Elkayam U, Gleicher N. Changes in cardiac findings during normal pregnancy. In: Elkayam U, Gleiden N, eds. *Cardiac problems in pregnancy: diagnosis and management of maternal and fetal disease,* 2nd ed. New York: Alan R. Liss, 1990:31.
6. Clapp JF. Influence of endurance exercise and diet on human placental development and fetal growth. *Placenta* 2006;27:527–534.
7. Larsson L, Lindqvist PG. Low-impact exercise during pregnancy—a study of safety. *Acta Obstet Gynecol Scand* 2005;84(1):34–38.
8. MacPhail A, Davies GA, Victory R, et al. Maximal exercise testing in late gestation: fetal responses. *Obstet Gynecol* 2000;96(4):565–570.
9. Wolfe LA, Weissgerber TL. Clinical physiology of exercise in pregnancy: a literature review. *J Obstet Gynaecol Can* 2003;25(6):473–483.
10. Wolfe LA, Hall P, Webb KA, et al. Prescription of aerobic exercise during pregnancy. *Sports Med* 1989;8(5):273–301.
11. Wang TW, Apgar BS. Exercise during pregnancy. *Am Fam Physician* 1998; 57(8):1857.
12. Sady MA, Haydon BB, Sady SP, et al. Cardiovascular response to maximal cycle exercise during pregnancy and at two and seven months post partum. *Am J Obstet Gynecol* 1990;162:1181–1185.
13. Lotgering FK, Struijk PC, Van Doorn MB, et al. Errors in predicting maximal oxygen consumption in pregnant women. *J Appl Physiol* 1992;72: 562–567.
14. Lotgering FK, Struijk PC, Van Doorn MB, et al. Anaerobic threshold and respiratory compensation in pregnant women. *J Appl Physiol* 1995;78: 1772–1777.
15. Wegnerckileser RG, Saldana LR. *Exposure of the pregnant patient to*

diagnostic radiation: a guide to medical management. Philadelphia: Lippincott, 1985.
16. Bithell JF, Stewart AM. Pre-natal irradiation and childhood malignancy: a review of British data from the Oxford survey. *Br J Cancer* 1975;31:271–287.
17. Rosenstein M. *Organ doses in diagnostic radiology*. Washington, DC: U.S. Department of Health, Education, and Welfare, 1976.
18. Elkayam U, Kawanishi D, Reid CL, et al. Contrast echocardiography to reduce ionizing radiation associated with cardiac catheterization during pregnancy. *Am J Cardiol* 1983;52:213–214.
19. Lindheimer MD. Hypertension in pregnancy. *Hypertension* 1993;22:127–137.
20. Sibai BM. Treatment of hypertension in pregnant women. *N Engl J Med* 1996;335:257–265.
21. Cunningham FG, Lindheimer MD. Hypertension in pregnancy. *N Engl J Med* 1992;326:927–932.
22. Collins R, Peto R, MacMahon S, et al. Blood pressure, stroke and coronary heart disease. 2. Short term reductions in blood pressure: overview of randomized drug trials in their epidemiologic context. *Lancet* 1990;335:827–838.
23. Bar J, Ben-Haroush A, Feldberg D, et al. The pharmacologic approach to the prevention of preeclampsia: from antiplatelet, antithrombosis and antioxidant therapy to anticonvulsants. *Curr Med Chem Cardiovasc Hematol Agents* 2005;3(3):181–185.
24. Sibai B, Dekker G, Kupferminc M. Pre-eclampsia. *Lancet* 2005;26; 365(9461):785–799.
25. Schobel HP, Fischer T, Heuszer K, et al. Preeclampsia: a state of sympathetic overactivity. *N Engl J Med* 1996;335:1480–1485.
26. Rowland BL, Vermillion ST, Roudebush WE. Elevated circulating concentrations of platelet activating factor in preeclampsia. *Am J Obstet Gynecol* 2000;183:930–932.
27. McKinney ET, Shouri R, Hunt RS, et al. Plasma, urinary and salivary 8-epi-prostaglandin f2alpha levels in normotensive and preeclamptic pregnancies. *Am J Obstet Gynecol* 2000;183:874–877.
28. Dechend R, Homuth V, Wallukat G, et al. AT(1) receptor agonistic antibodies from preeclamptic patients cause vascular cells to express tissue factor. *Circulation* 2000;101:2382–2387.
29. Fitzpatrick E, Goring HH, Liu H, et al. Fine mapping and SNP analysis of positional candidates at the preeclampsia susceptibility locus (PREG1) on chromosome 2. *Hum Biol* 2004;76(6):849–862.
30. Lucas MJ, Leveno KJ, Cunningham FG. A comparison of magnesium sulfate with phenytoin for the prevention of eclampsia. *N Engl J Med* 199; 333(4):201–205.
31. Belfort MA, Anthony J, Saade GR, et al. A comparison of magnesium sulfate and nimodipine for the prevention of eclampsia. *N Engl J Med* 2003; 348(4):304–311.
32. Greene MF. Magnesium sulfate for preeclampsia. *N Engl J Med* 2003; 348(4):275–276.
33. O'Brien JM, Milligan DA, Barton JR. Impact of high-dose corticosteroid therapy for patients with HELLP (hemolysis, elevated liver enzymes, and low platelet count) syndrome. *Am J Obstet Gynecol* 2000;183: 921–924.
34. Barrilleaux PS, Martin Jr JN, Klauser CK, et al. Postpartum intravenous dexamethasone for severely preeclamptic patients without hemolysis, elevated liver enzymes, low platelets (HELLP) syndrome: a randomized trial. *Obstet Gynecol* 2005;105(4):843–848.
35. Funai EF, Friedlander Y, Paltiel O, et al. Long-term mortality after preeclampsia. *Epidemiology* 2005;16(2):206–215.
36. Lindheimer MD, Katz AI. Sodium and diuretics in pregnancy. *N Engl J Med* 1976;288:891–894.
37. Cockburn J, Ounsted M, Moar VA, et al. Final report of study on hypertension during pregnancy: the effects of specific treatment on the growth and development of the children. *Lancet* 1982;647–649.
38. Sweit M. Antihypertensive drugs in pregnancy. *BMJ* 1985;291:3565–3566.
39. Cox JL, Gardner MJ. Treatment of cardiac arrhythmias during pregnancy. *Prog Cardiovasc Dis* 1993;36:137–178.
40. Childress CH, Katz VL. Nifedipine and its indications in obstetrics and gynecology. *Obstet Gynecol* 1994;83:616–624.
41. Shotan A, Widerhorn J, Hurst A, et al. Risks of angiotensin-converting enzyme inhibition during pregnancy: experimental and clinical evidence, potential mechanisms, and recommendations for use. *Am J Med* 1994;96:451–456.
42. Sedman AB, Kershaw DB, Bunchman TE. Recognition and management of angiotensin converting enzyme inhibitor fetopathy. *Pediatr Nephrol* 1995; 9(3):382–385.
43. Shotan A, Widerhorn J, Hurst A, et al. Risks of angiotensin-converting enzyme inhibition during pregnancy: experimental and clinical evidence, potential mechanisms, and recommendations for use. *Am J Med* 1994; 96(5):451–456.
44. Buttar HS. An overview of the influence of ACE inhibitors on fetal-placental circulation and perinatal development. *Mol Cell Biochem* 1997;176(1–2): 61–71.
45. Centers for Disease Control and Prevention. Postmarketing surveillance for angiotensin-converting enzyme inhibitor use during first trimester pregnancy—United States, Canada and Israel, 1987-1995. *MMWR Morb Mortal Wkly Rep* 1997;46(11):240–242.
46. Nightingale SL. From the Food and Drug Administration. *JAMA* 1992; 267:2445.
47. Demakis JG, Rahimtoola SH. Peripartum cardiomyopathy. *Circulation* 1971;44:964–968.
48. Demakis JG, Rahimtoola SH, Sutton GC, et al. Natural course of peripartum cardiomyopathy. *Circulation* 1971;44:1053–1061.
49. Lampert MB, Lang RM. Peripartum cardiomyopathy. *Am Heart J* 1995; 130:860–870.
50. Homans DC. Current concepts: peripartum cardiomyopathy. *N Engl J Med* 1985;312:1432–1437.
51. Reimold SC, Rutherford JD. Peripartum cardiomyopathy. *N Engl J Med* 2001;24:1629–1630.
52. Melvin KR, Richardson PJ, Olsen EGJ, et al. Peripartum cardiomyopathy due to myocarditis. *N Engl J Med* 1982;307:731–734.
53. Sanderson JE, Olsen EGJ, Gate D. Peripartum heart disease: an endomyocardial biopsy study. *Br Heart J* 1986;56:285–291.
54. O'Connell JB, Costanzo-Nordin MR, Subramanian R, et al. Peripartum cardiomyopathy: clinical, hemodynamic, histologic and prognostic characteristics. *J Am Coll Cardiol* 1986;8:52–55.
55. Midei MG, DeMent SH, Feldman AM, et al. Peripartum myocarditis and cardiomyopathy. *Circulation* 1990;81:922–928.
56. Felker GM, Jaeger CJ, Klodas E, et al. Myocarditis and long-term survival in peripartum cardiomyopathy. *Am Heart J* 2000;140:785–791.
57. Felker GM, Thompson RE, Hare JM, et al. Underlying causes and long-term survival in patients with initially unexplained cardiomyopathy. *N Engl J Med* 2000;342:1077–1084.
58. Sliwa K, Skudicky D, Bergemann A, et al. Peripartum cardiomyopathy: analysis of clinical outcome, ventricular function, plasma levels of cytokines and Fas/APO-1. *J Am Coll Cardiol* 2000;35:701–705.
59. Whitehead SJ, Berg CJ, Chang J. Pregnancy-related mortality due to cardiomyopathy. *Obstet Gynocol* 2003;102(6):1326–1331.
60. Felker GM, Jaeger CJ, Klodas E, et al. Myocarditis and long-term survival in peripartum cardiomyopathy. *Am Heart J* 2000;140(5):785–791.
61. Cole P, Cook F, Plappert T, et al. Longitudinal changes in left ventricular architecture and function in peripartum cardiomyopathy. *Am J Cardiol* 1987;60:871–876.
62. Elkayam U, Tummala P, Rao K, et al. Maternal and fetal outcomes with subsequent pregnancies in women with peripartum cardiomyopathy. *N Engl J Med* 2001;344:1567–1571.
63. Lampert MD, Winert L, Hibbard J, et al. Contractile reserve in patients with peripartum cardiomyopathy and recovered left ventricular function. *Am J Obstet Gynecol* 1997;176:189–195.
64. Rickenbacher PR, Rizeq MN, Hunt SA, et al. Long-term outcome after heart transplantation for peripartum cardiomyopathy. *Am Heart J* 1994; 127:1318–1323.
65. Liljestrand J, Lindstrom B. Childbirth after post partum cardiac insufficiency treated with cardiac transplant. *Acta Obstet Gynecol Scand* 1993; 72:406–408.
66. Laifer SA, Yeagley CJ, Armitage JM. Pregnancy after cardiac transplantation. *Am J Perinatol* 1994;11:217–219.
67. Scott JR, Wagoner LE, Olsen SL, et al. Pregnancy in heart transplant recipients: management and outcome. *Obstet Gynecol* 1993;82:324–327.
68. Branch KR, Wagoner LE, McGrory CH, et al. Risks of subsequent pregnancies on mother and newborn in female heart transplant recipients. *J Heart Lung Transplant* 1998;17:698–702.
69. Troche V, Ville Y, Fernandez H. Pregnancy after heart or heart-lung transplantation: a series of 10 pregnancies. *Br J Obstet Gynaecol* 1998;105:454–458.
70. Ellison J, Walker ID, Greer IA. Antenatal use of enoxaparin for prevention and treatment of thromboembolism in pregnancy. *BJOG* 2000;107:1116–1121.
71. Ginsberg JS, Hirsh J. Anticoagulants during pregnancy. *Annu Rev Med* 1989;40:79–86.
72. Ginsberg JS, Kowalchuk G, Hirsh J, et al. Heparin therapy during pregnancy: risks to the fetus and mother. *Arch Intern Med* 1989;149:2233–2236.
73. Barbour LA, Kick SD, Steiner JF, et al. A prospective study of heparin-induced osteoporosis in pregnancy using bone densitometry. *Am J Obstet Gynecol* 1994;170:862–869.
74. Calhoun BC, Hesser JW. Heparin-associated antibody with pregnancy: discussion of two cases. *Am J Obstet Gynecol* 1987;156:964–966.
75. Greinacher A, Eckhardt T, Mussmann J, et al. Pregnancy complicated by heparin associated thrombocytopenia: management by a prospectively in vitro selected heparinoid (Org 10172). *Thromb Res* 1993;71(2): 123–126.
76. McRae SJ, Ginsberg JS. Initial treatment of venous thromboembolism. *Circulation* 2004;110(9):I3–I9.
77. Barbour LA, Oja JL, Schultz LK. A prospective trial that demonstrates that dalteparin requirements increase in pregnancy to maintain therapeutic levels of anticoagulation. *Am J Obstet Gynecol* 2004;191(3): 1024–1029.
78. Reimold SC, Rutherford JD. Valvular heart disease in pregnancy. *N Engl J Med* 2003;349(1):52–59.
79. Hung L, Rahimtoola S. Prosthetic heart valves and pregnancy. *Circulation* 2003;107:1240–1246.
80. Hanania G, Thomas D, Michel PL, et al. Pregnancy and prosthetic heart

valves: a French cooperative retrospective study of 155 cases. *Eur Heart J* 1994;15:1651–1658.
81. Sbarouni E, Oakley CM. Outcome of pregnancy in women with valve prostheses. *Br Heart J* 1994;71:196–201.
82. Born D, Martinez EE, Almeida PAM, et al. Pregnancy in patients with prosthetic heart valves: the effects of anticoagulation on mother, fetus, and neonate. *Am Heart J* 1992;124:413–417.
83. Chan WS, Anand S, Ginsberg JS. Anticoagulation of pregnant women with mechanical heart valves: a systematic review of the literature. *Arch Intern Med* 2000;160(2):191–196.
84. Lev-Ran O, Kramer A, Gurevitch J, et al. Low-molecular-weight heparin for prosthetic heart valves: treatment failure. *Ann Thorac Surg* 2000; 69(1):264–265.
85. Sadler L, McCowan L, White H, et al. Pregnancy outcomes and cardiac complications in women with mechanical, bioprosthetic and homograft valves. *BJOG* 2000;107(2):245–253.
86. Salazar E, Espinola N, Roman L, et al. Effect of pregnancy on the duration of bovine pericardial bioprostheses. *Am Heart J* 1999;137:714–720.
87. Mangione JA, Lourenco RM, dos Santos ES, et al. Long-term follow-up of pregnant women after percutaneous mitral valvuloplasty. *Catheter Cardiovasc Interv* 2000;50:413–417.
88. Vongpatanasin W, Hillis LD, Lange RA. Prosthetic heart valves. *N Engl J Med* 1996;335:407–416.
89. Ginsberg JS, Chan WS, Bates SM, et al. Anticoagulation of pregnant women with mechanical heart valves. *Intern Med* 2003;163(6):694–698.
90. Topol EJ. Anticoagulation with prosthetic cardiac valves. *Intern Med* 2003;163(18):2251–2252.
91. Sullivan HJ. Valvular heart surgery during pregnancy. *Surg Clin North Am* 1995;75:59–75.
92. Pomini F, Mercogliano D, Cavalletti C, et al. Cardiopulmonary bypass in pregnancy. *Ann Thorac Surg* 1996;61:259–268.
93. Ladner HE, Danielson B, Gilbert WM. Acute myocardial infraction in pregnancy and the puerperium: a population-based study. *Obstet Gynecol* 105(3):480–484.
94. Sheikh AU, Harper MA. Myocardial infarction during pregnancy: management and outcome of two pregnancies. *Am J Obstet Gynecol* 1993;169: 279–284.
95. Donnelly S, McKenna P, McGing P, et al. Myocardial infarction during pregnancy. *Br J Obstet Gynaecol* 1993;100:781–782.
96. Roth A, Elkayam U. Acute myocardial infarction associated with pregnancy. *Ann Intern Med* 1996;125:751–762.
97. Hennekens CH, Albert CM, Godfried SL, et al. Adjunctive drug therapy of acute myocardial infarction: evidence from clinical trials. *N Engl J Med* 1996;335:1660–1667.
98. Cowan NC, de Belder MA, Rothman MT. Coronary angioplasty in pregnancy. *Br Heart J* 1988;59:588–592.
99. Mather PJ, Hansen CL, Goldman B, et al. Postpartum multivessel coronary dissection. *J Heart Lung Transplant* 1994;13:533–537.
100. Coulson CC, Kuller JA, Bowes Jr WA. Myocardial infarction and coronary artery dissection in pregnancy. *Am J Perinatol* 1995;12:328–330.
101. Kearney P, Singh H, Huttr J, et al. Spontaneous coronary artery dissection: a report of three cases and review of the literature. *Postgrad Med J* 1993;69:940–945.
102. Rensing BJ, Kofflard M, van den Brand MJ, et al. Spontaneous dissections of all three coronary arteries in a 33-week-pregnant woman. *Catheter Cardiovasc Interv* 1999;48(2):207–210.
103. Pombar X, Strassner HT, Fenner PC. Pregnancy in a woman with class H diabetes mellitus and previous coronary artery bypass graft: a case report and review of the literature. *Obstet Gynecol* 1995;85:825–829.
104. Siu S, Sermer M, Colman JM, et al. Prospective multicenter study of pregnancy outcomes in women with heart disease. *Circulation* 2001;104:515–521.
105. Allan LD, Sharland GK, Milburn A, et al. Prospective diagnosis of 1,006 consecutive cases of congenital heart disease in the fetus. *J Am Coll Cardiol* 1994;23:1452–1458.
106. Wooley CF, Sparks EH. Congenital heart disease, heritable cardiovascular disease, and pregnancy. *Prog Cardiovasc Dis* 1992;35:41–60.
107. Pyeritz RE. Maternal and fetal complications of pregnancy in the Marfan syndrome. *Am J Med* 1981;71:784–790.
108. Perloff JK. Pediatric congenital cardiac becomes a postoperative adult: the changing population of congenital heart disease. *Circulation* 1973;47:606–619.
109. Presbitero P, Somerville J, Stone S, et al. Pregnancy in cyanotic congenital heart disease: outcome of mother and fetus. *Circulation* 1994;89:2673–2676.
110. Connolly HM, Warnes CA. Ebstein's anomaly: outcome of pregnancy. *J Am Coll Cardiol* 1994;23:1194–1198.
111. Clarkson PM, Wilson NJ, Neutze JM, et al. Outcome of pregnancy after the Mustard operation for transposition of the great arteries with intact ventricular septum. *J Am Coll Cardiol* 1994;24:190–193.
112. Connolly HM, Grogan M, Warnes CA. Pregnancy among women with congenitally corrected transposition of great arteries. *J Am Coll Cardiol* 1999;33:1692–1695.
113. Pelliccia F, Cianfrocca C, Gaudio C, et al. Sudden death during pregnancy in hypertrophic cardiomyopathy. *Eur Heart J* 1992;13:421–423.
114. Oakley GDG, McGarry K, Limb DG, et al. Management of pregnancy in patients with hypertrophic cardiomyopathy. *BMJ* 1979;1:1749–1750.
115. Tang LCH, Chan SYW, Wong VCW, et al. Pregnancy in patients with mitral valve prolapse. *Int J Gynaecol Obstet* 1985;23:217–221.
116. Lao TT, Sermer M, MaGee L, et al. Congenital aortic stenosis and pregnancy—a reappraisal. *Am J Obstet Gynecol* 1993;169:540–545.
117. Al Kasab SM, Sabag T, Al Zaibag M, et al. Beta-adrenergic receptor blockade in the management of pregnant women with mitral stenosis. *Am J Obstet Gynecol* 1990;163:37–40.
118. Berkman N, Thorp J, Lohr K, et al. Tocolytic treatment for the management of preterm labor: a review of the evidence. 2003;188(6):1648–1659.
119. Carr DB, Clark AL, Kernek K, et al. Maintenance oral nifedipine for preterm labor: a randomized clinical trial. *Am J Obstet Gynecol* 1999;181: 822–827.
120. Pisani RJ, Rosenow 3rd EC. Pulmonary edema associated with tocolytic therapy. *Ann Intern Med* 1989;110:714–718.
121. Morgan M. Amniotic fluid embolism. *Anaesthesia* 1979;34:20–32.
122. Gilbert WM, Danielsen B. Amniotic fluid embolism: decreased mortality in a population-based study. *Obstet Gynecol* 1999;93(6):973–977.
123. Clark SL, Hankins GD, Dudley DA, et al. Amniotic fluid embolism: analysis of the national registry. *Am J Obstet Gynecol* 1995;172(4 Pt 1):1158–1167.
124. Davies S. Amniotic fluid embolus: a review of the literature. *Can J Anaesth* 2001;48(1):88–98.
125. Tuffnell DJ. Amniotic fluid embolism. *Curr Opin Obstet Gynecol* 2003; 15(2):119–122.
126. Perry KG, Morrison JC, Rust OA, et al. Incidence of adverse cardiopulmonary effects with low-dose continuous terbutaline infusion. *Am J Obstet Gynecol* 1995;173:1273–1277.
127. Page RL. Treatment of arrhythmias during pregnancy. *Am Heart J* 1995; 130:871–876.
128. Joglar JA, Page RL. Antiarrhythmic drugs in pregnancy. *Cardiology* 2001; 16(1):40–45.
129. Rutherford JD. Management of cardiovascular disease during pregnancy. In: Smith TW, ed. *Cardiovascular therapeutics*. Philadelphia: WB Saunders, 1996:695–701.
130. American Academy of Pediatrics Committee on Drugs. The transfer of drugs and other chemicals into human milk. *Pediatrics* 1994;93:137–150.
131. Afridi I, Moise Jr KJ, Rokey R. Termination of supraventricular tachycardia with intravenous adenosine in a pregnant woman with Wolff-Parkinson-White syndrome. *Obstet Gynecol* 1992;80:481–483.
132. Brodsky M, Doria R, Allen B, et al. New-onset ventricular tachycardia during pregnancy. *Am Heart J* 1992;123:933–941.
133. Caruso A, De Carolis S, Di Simone N. Antiphospholipid antibodies in obstetrics: new complexities and sites of action. *Hum Reprod Update* 1999; 5(3):267–276.
134. Silveria LH, Huggle CL, Jara LJ, et al. Prevention of anticardiolipin antibody–related pregnancy losses with prednisone and aspirin. *Am J Med* 1992;93:403–411.
135. Pattison NS, Chamley LW, Birdsall M, et al. Does aspirin have a role in improving pregnancy outcome for women with the antiphospholipid syndrome? A randomized controlled trial. *Am J Obstet Gynecol* 2000;183: 1008–1012.
136. Branch DW, Peaceman AM, Druzin M, et al. A multicenter, placebo-controlled pilot study of intravenous immune globulin treatment of antiphospholipid syndrome during pregnancy. The Pregnancy Loss Study Group. *Am J Obstet Gynecol* 2000;182(1 Pt 1):122–127.
137. Hasnie AMA, Stoddard MF, Gleason CB, et al. Diastolic dysfunction is a feature of the antiphospholipid syndrome. *Am Heart J* 1995;129:1009–1013.

CHAPTER 32 ■ WOMEN AND HEART DISEASE

JUDITH HSIA AND JOANN E. MANSON

OVERVIEW

Heart disease remains the leading cause of death for women in the United States (Table 32.1); coronary heart disease (CHD) alone accounts for 241,622 deaths annually (1). Despite public education efforts, only 46% of women identified heart disease as the leading cause of death in 2003, although this was improved from 30% in 1997 (2). CHD risk factors are similar in men and women, although the magnitude of risk associated with some risk factors differs between genders. For example, diabetes mellitus confers greater risk (3) and high-density lipoprotein-cholesterol greater protection in women (4). Once women develop CHD, they are less prompt in seeking medical attention for acute coronary symptoms than men (5) and have poorer outcomes following myocardial infarction (6).

CORONARY HEART DISEASE RISK FACTORS IN WOMEN

The prevalence of modifiable risk factors generally increases with age (Table 32.2). Cigarette smoking is an exception. In 2002, 25%, 22%, 24%, 21%, and 9%, respectively, of women aged 18 to 24, 25 to 34, 35 to 44, 45 to 64, and 65 years or older smoked, slightly lower than rates for men (7).

Mean age at menopause in the United States is 51 years. Consequently, the postmenopausal years constitute a significant proportion of a woman's lifespan. A relatively hypoestrogenic state is attained at menopause, unfavorably affecting several CHD risk factors. Thus, although interventions directed at CHD prevention should be undertaken at all ages, the need for effective prevention measures is particularly acute during and after menopause.

In a longitudinal study of premenopausal women undergoing natural menopause, total plasma cholesterol rose by 6%, triglycerides by 11%, and low-density lipoprotein cholesterol (LDL-C) by 10%, all significantly higher than premenopausal levels (9). High-density lipoprotein cholesterol (HDL-C) began to fall 2 years prior to the last menses and declined gradually, but significantly, with menopause. Other unfavorable lipid changes with menopause include smaller LDL-C particle size (10) and an increase in plasma lipoprotein (a) levels (11).

Weight gain is common during midlife among women, but appears to be independent of menopausal status (12). Menopause is associated with a steeper increase in diastolic blood pressure, independent of age (13). Studies of glucose and insulin levels during menopause have provided mixed results.

PRIMORDIAL PREVENTION

Primordial, primary, and secondary prevention measures can reduce CHD risk across a woman's lifespan. The goal of primordial prevention is to deter development of coronary risk factors, usually through healthy lifestyle practices. Women are unlikely to receive lifestyle counseling; fewer than 5% of physicians advise women to engage in physical activity at least 6 days per week as recommended by national guidelines (14).

In 2004, the American Heart Association and American College of Cardiology (AHA/ACC) jointly endorsed cardiovascular prevention guidelines for women (15). Lifestyle interventions, generally appropriate for primordial, primary, and secondary prevention purposes, and which were categorized as class I recommendations, that is, useful and effective for cardiovascular disease prevention in women, included (a) not smoking, (b) obtaining at least 30 minutes of moderate-intensity physical activity on most days, (c) maintaining a healthy body

TABLE 32.1

CAUSES OF DEATH IN WOMEN, UNITED STATES 2001

Age (y)	25–34	35–44	45–54	55–64	65–74	75–84	≥85	All[a]
Number of deaths from all causes	12,926	33,510	63,217	99,181	189,379	361,187	447,998	1,233,004
PERCENT OF TOTAL DEATHS								
Heart disease	8.4	11.9	16.0	20.1	34.5	30.0	38.2	29.3
Cancer	16.5	27.7	38.7	41.3	24.1	22.0	9.8	21.6
Cerebrovascular disease	2.2	3.7	4.3	4.4	5.8	9.0	10.7	8.1
Chronic respiratory disease	1.1	1.5	2.6	5.5	7.9	6.7	3.7	5.1
Diabetes mellitus	2.0	2.3	3.5	4.4	4.4	3.6	2.2	3.1
Alzheimer disease					1.0	3.3	5.4	3.1
Accidents	21.3	12.9	5.7	2.5	1.6	1.7	1.7	2.9
Homicide/suicide	14.8	7.7	3.3	0.8	<0.4	<0.7	<0.7	<0.6

[a]Includes children, adolescents, and young adults <25 years.
Source: Data from CDC/NCHS, National Vital Statistics System. Available: www.cdc.gov/nchs/data/dvs/LCWK2_2001.pdf.

weight, and (d) consumption of a heart-healthy diet, which includes a variety of fruits, vegetables, grains, low-fat or nonfat dairy products, fish, legumes, and sources of protein low in saturated fat.

Adherence to a prudent lifestyle reduces coronary risk. During 14-year follow-up of the Nurses' Health Study cohort (16), the incidence of CHD was 80% lower among women who did not smoke cigarettes, were not overweight, maintained a prudent diet, engaged in moderate to vigorous physical activity for 30 minutes daily, and consumed alcohol in moderation, compared to women not adhering to these lifestyle practices.

The hypothesis that reducing saturated fat and cholesterol consumption, preventing weight gain, and increasing physical activity would prevent a rise in LDL-C during menopause was tested in a randomized trial of 535 women (12). LDL-C was 10 mg/dL lower at 6 months among women randomized to cognitive–behavioral intervention, and 5.4 mg/dL lower at 54 months ($p = .009$). The intervention group lost 1 pound, whereas the comparison group gained 5.2 pounds ($p < .001$).

PHYSICAL ACTIVITY AND DIET FOR RISK FACTOR PREVENTION

Among the 2,191 women with prediabetes randomized in the Diabetes Prevention Program, physical activity of moderate intensity for 150 minutes/week in conjunction with 7% weight loss reduced progression to diabetes by 54% (95% confidence interval [CI] 40%–64%) (17).

Exercise alone has not been shown to prevent hypertension, although a multicomponent lifestyle intervention which included exercise (180 minutes/week) reduced systolic blood pressure 1.2 mm Hg in African-American women and 4.5 mm Hg in non–African-American women with above-optimal blood pressure or stage I hypertension (18).

Weight loss prevented hypertension in the Trials of Hypertension Prevention, Phase II. Among 381 women randomized to a weight loss intervention of dietary change, physical activity, and social support, or no intervention, those with the greatest weight loss had the largest reductions in diastolic blood pressure. For the entire cohort of men and women, the risk of

TABLE 32.2

PREVALENCE OF RISK FACTORS AND HEALTHY WEIGHT, OVERWEIGHT, AND OBESITY AMONG WOMEN IN THE UNITED STATES BY AGE (%)

Age (y)	Hypertension	Physician-diagnosed diabetes	High cholesterol	Healthy weight	Overweight	Obese	Physically active	Sedentary
20–34	3	1	30	43	53	28	49	12
35–44	15	4	43	37	61	32	47	13
45–54	32	7	68	33	65	37		
55–64	54	13	79	28	72	42	42	16
65–74	73		85	26	71	39		
≥75	83	16	74	37	60	24	32	32

Hypertension and weight data from NHANES 1999–2002 (7); Healthy weight, body mass index (BMI) 18.5 to <25 kg/m^2; overweight, BMI 25–29.9; obese, BMI ≥30.
Cholesterol data from NHANES 1999–2000 (8). Hypercholesterolemia defined as total cholesterol ≥5.2 mmol/L (200 mg/dL) or using cholesterol-lowering medication.
Diabetes data from 2002 Behavior Risk Factor Surveillance System (Available: www.cdc.gov/mmwr/preview).
Physical activity data from 2003 Behavior Risk Factor Surveillance Systemy (Available: www.cdc.gov/nccdphp/dnpa/physical/stats/index.htm). Physically active indicates moderate-intensity activity for at least 30 minutes on ≥5 days per week or vigorous-intensity activity for at least 20 minutes ≥3 days per week. Sedentary indicates <10 minutes total per week of moderate- or vigorous-intensity activity. Youngest age group for physical activity data is age 25–34.

TABLE 32.3

PHYSICAL ACTIVITY IN OLDER WOMEN ACROSS ETHNIC GROUPS

	White (*n* = 74,240)	African American (*n* = 6,465)	Hispanic (*n* = 3,231)	Asian (*n* = 2,445)	American Indian[a] (*n* = 327)
ENERGY EXPENDITURE FROM WALKING (%)					
		*	*		
0 MET hr/wk (referent)	28.2	39.0	31.7	30.3	31.8
0.5–2.5	18.0	17.8	18.9	18.2	19.3
2.6–5.0	18.0	13.9	15.9	15.9	13.5
5.1–10.0	118.3	14.7	14.8	17.3	16.8
10.1–40.8	16.5	13.7	15.0	17.7	17.1
Missing data	1.0	0.9	3.7	0.7	1.5
MINUTES/WEEK OF MODERATE-TO-STRENUOUS PHYSICAL ACTIVITY (%)					
		*	*	*	
0 (referent)	33.3	45.2	45.3	41.5	40.1
10–69	16.4	19.4	16.8	14.2	18.7
70–149	15.6	12.9	12.1	14.7	10.4
150–249	16.6	10.2	9.8	13.7	12.5
250–1330	17.2	11.4	12.3	15.2	16.8
Missing	1.0	0.9	3.7	0.7	1.5

[a]Comparison with white women not performed.
*$P < .05$ for comparison between white women and particular ethnic group.
Source: Adapted from Hsia J, Wu L, Allen C, et al. Physical activity and diabetes risk in postmenopausal women. *Am J Prev Med* 2005;28:19–25.

developing hypertension was lower in the intervention group (risk ratio 0.79, 95% CI 0.65–0.96) (19).

The current popularity of low-carbohydrate diets has increasing interest in their impact on plasma lipids. Isocaloric low-fat and very-low-carbohydrate diets were compared in normal weight, normolipemic women (20). The low-fat diet contained less than 10% of calories from saturated fat and less than 300 mg of daily cholesterol. The very-low-carbohydrate diet contained 30% of calories from protein, 60% from fat, and 10% from carbohydrates. LDL-C, HDL-C, and triglycerides were not changed after 4 weeks on the low-fat diet. In contrast, LDL-C increased 15% after 4 weeks on the very-low-carbohydrate diet; HDL-C increased 33% and triglycerides fell 33% (all $p < .05$). LDL-C subclasses and C-reactive protein levels were not affected by either diet.

DRUG TREATMENT FOR PRIMORDIAL PREVENTION

Although less effective than lifestyle modification, metformin reduced progression to diabetes by 28% (95% CI 10%–43%) among women with prediabetes (17). In a post hoc analysis from the Heart Outcomes Prevention Evaluation trial, 27 of 1,201 women assigned to placebo developed diabetes compared with 16 of 1,279 women in the ramipril group (relative risk 0.57, 95% CI 0.31–1.07) (21). Incidence of diabetes was also reduced by conjugated estrogens with medroxyprogesterone acetate in post hoc analysis from the Women's Health Initiative randomized trial (hazard ratio 0.79, 95% CI 0.67–0.93) (22). Neither ramipril nor postmenopausal hormone therapy (HT) is currently recommended, however, for the primary prevention of type 2 diabetes.

PRIMARY PREVENTION

Primary prevention interventions delay or prevent onset of disease.

Exercise

Physically active women generally demonstrate lower CHD rates than sedentary women (23–26), although the association is not as well established as for men. Nonetheless, only 27% of women exercise regularly, and 41% engage in no leisure-time physical activity at all (27). Patterns of physical activity differ among ethnic groups (Table 32.3). Asian women, for example, walk as much as white women, but are less likely to engage in moderate-to-strenuous physical activity (28). Several studies indicate that moderate-intensity exercise (such as brisk walking) and vigorous exercise are associated with similar CHD risk reduction in women (23,24,28).

Aspirin

In a randomized trial of 39,876 women without known cardiovascular disease, aspirin 100 mg every other day did not prevent the primary outcome of myocardial infarction/stroke/cardiovascular death during 10.1-year follow up (relative risk 0.91, 95% CI 0.80–1.03) (29). Stroke, a prespecified secondary outcome, was reduced by aspirin (relative risk 0.83, 95% CI 0.69–0.99), but gastrointestinal bleeding, peptic ulcer, hematuria, and epistaxis were all significantly increased. Women aged 65 and older had a reduced risk of myocardial infarction, stroke, and major cardiovascular events with aspirin, but women younger than age 65 did not have clear cardiovascular benefits (Table 32.4). The AHA/ACC Prevention Guidelines for Women, developed before the Women's Health Study aspirin trial results were published, categorized routine use of aspirin in low-risk women as a class III intervention, that is, not useful/effective and may be harmful (15).

Hypertension

About 60% of heart failure cases and first strokes, and about half of first myocardial infarctions in women are attributable

TABLE 32.4

LOW-DOSE ASPIRIN AND THE PRIMARY PREVENTION OF CARDIOVASCULAR EVENTS IN WOMEN ACCORDING TO AGE GROUP: THE WOMEN'S HEALTH STUDY

Age (y)	Total (*N*)	Major CVD events[a] RR (95% CI)	Stroke RR (95% CI)	Myocardial infarction RR (95% CI)
45–54	24,025	1.01 (0.81–1.26)	0.85 (0.63–1.16)	1.23 (0.87–1.75)
55–64	11,754	0.98 (0.80–1.20)	0.84 (0.62–1.14)	1.17 (0.86–1.59)
≥65	4,097	0.74 (0.59–0.92)	0.78 (0.57–1.08)	0.66 (0.44–0.97)

[a]Major cardiovascular (CVD) event was defined as nonfatal myocardial infarction, nonfatal stroke, or death from cardiovascular causes.
Source: Adapted from Ridker PM, Cook NR, Lee I-M, et al. A randomized trial of low-dose aspirin in the primary prevention of cardiovascular disease in women. *New Engl J Med* 2005;352:1293–1304.

to hypertension (30). A diet high in fruits, vegetables, and low-fat dairy products with reduced total and saturated fat lowered systolic blood pressure by 6.2 mm Hg (97.5% CI 3.3–9.2 mm Hg) and diastolic blood pressure by 2.7 mm Hg (97.5% CI 0.7–4.8 mm Hg) in the 225 hypertensive women enrolled in the Dietary Approaches to Stop Hypertension trial (31).

With regard to choosing among antihypertensive drugs, the relative risk of myocardial infarction/CHD death was similar among the 15,638 women randomized to lisinopril, chlorthalidone, or amlodipine-based therapy in the Antihypertensive and Lipid-Lowering treatment to prevent Heart Attack Trial (32). Stroke risk was higher with lisinopril (relative risk 1.22, 95% CI 1.01–1.46) than chlorthalidone (referent), and heart failure risk was higher with amlodipine (relative risk 1.33, 95% CI 1.14–1.55) and with lisinopril (relative risk 1.23, 95% CI 1.05–1.43) than with chlorthalidone.

Dyslipidemia

The importance of physical activity combined with prudent diet for lipid management was supported by a year-long trial that included 180 postmenopausal women with moderately elevated LDL-C and euglycemia (33). Participants were randomized into four groups: no intervention, AHA step II diet, exercise alone, or step II diet plus exercise. The goal of the exercise program was to achieve at least 10 miles of brisk walking or jogging each week. After 1 year, body weight for women in the exercise alone group was no different from the control group. The step II diet group had lost 2.7 ± 3.5 kg ($p < .001$ versus control, $p < .05$ versus exercise alone) and the step II diet plus exercise group had lost 3.1 ± 3.7 kg ($p < .001$ versus control, $p < .01$ versus exercise alone). LDL-C, which was 161 mg/dL at baseline, was no different in the control, exercise alone, and step II diet groups at 1 year. In the step II diet plus exercise group, LDL fell 14.5 ± 22.2 mg/dL ($p < .05$ versus control). HDL-C and triglycerides were unchanged in all groups at 1 year.

Although primary prevention trials of hydroxymethylglutaryl coenzyme A reductase inhibitors (statins) have included women, the number enrolled and their lower clinical event rate have limited the utility of gender-specific subgroup analyses (Table 32.5) (34,35). It would not be appropriate to conclude from the limitations of available data that women do not benefit from statin therapy.

Fibrate and/or niacin therapy are recommended for high-risk women on statin therapy with low HDL-C or elevated non–HDL-C (Table 32.6). For primary prevention specifically

TABLE 32.5

WOMEN IN TRIALS OF HYDROXYMETHYL GLUTARYL COENZYME A REDUCTASE INHIBITORS

	Event rate in placebo group (%/y)		No. women with events/ No. women in treatment group		RR (95% CI) in women
	Women	Men	Active	Placebo	
PRIMARY PREVENTION					
AFCAPs/TexCAPS (lovastatin)	0.49	1.20	7/499	13/498	0.54 (0.22–1.35)
ASCOT – LLA (atorvastatin)	0.53	1.03	19/979	17/963	1.10 (0.57–2.12)
SECONDARY PREVENTION					
4S (simvastatin)	2.04	2.72	60/407	91/420	0.66 (0.48–0.91)
CARE (pravastatin)	2.69	2.62	23/286	39/290	0.57 (0.34–0.96)
LIPID (pravastatin)	1.10	1.43	39/756	50/760	0.82 (0.54–1.24)
HPS (simvastatin)	3.54	5.52	367/2542	450/2540	0.81 (not stated)

Abbreviations: AFCAPs/TexCAPS, Air Force/Texas Coronary Atherosclerosis Prevention Study; ASCOT – LLA, Anglo-Scandinavian Cardiac Outcomes Trial – Lipid Lower Arm; 4S, Scandinavian Simvastatin Survival Study; CARE, Cholesterol and Recurrent Events trial; LIPID, Long-Term Intervention with Pravastatin in Ischemic Disease study; HPS, Heart Protection Study.
Primary outcome for each study: AFCAPS/TexCAPS (34) – myocardial infarction/unstable angina/sudden death; ASCOT-LLA (35), CARE (50) – myocardial infarction/coronary death; 4S (49) – myocardial infarction/coronary death/resuscitated sudden death; LIPID (51) – coronary death; HPS (52) (prespecified primary outcome for subgroup analyses) – myocardial infarction/coronary death/fatal or nonfatal stroke/revascularization
Estimates of event rates assume equal duration of follow up for men and women.

TABLE 32.6

AHA/ACC CV PREVENTION GUIDELINES FOR WOMEN

High-risk women[a]: initiate statin therapy unless contraindicated. Niacin or fibrate therapy should be initiated for low HDL-C or elevated non–HDL-C.
Intermediate-risk women[b]: LDL-lowering therapy, preferably with a statin, should be initiated for LDL-C $\geq$ 130 mg/dL and niacin or fibrate therapy initiated when HDL-C is low or non–HDL-C elevated after LDL-C goal is achieved.
Low-risk women[c]: LDL-lowering therapy should be considered when LDL-C $\geq$ 190 mg/dL or if multiple risk factors are present, when LDL-C $\geq$ 160 mg/dL. Niacin or fibrate therapy should be considered when HDL-C is low or non–HDL-C elevated after LDL-C goal is achieved.

[a]CHD, cerebrovascular or peripheral arterial disease, diabetes, chronic kidney disease, 10-year Framingham risk of myocardial infarction/CHD death >20%, some women with subclinical cardiovascular disease (e.g., coronary calcification).
[b]Ten-year Framingham risk 10–20%, metabolic syndrome, some women with multiple risk factors or subclinical cardiovascular disease.
[c]Ten-year Framingham risk <10%.
Source: Adapted from Mosca L, Appel LJ, Benjamin EJ, et al. Evidence-based guidelines for cardiovascular disease prevention in women. *Circulation* 109;2004:672–692.

in women, no randomized clinical outcomes trials of fibrates or niacin have been conducted. A metaanalysis of lipid effects of extended release niacin found slightly better LDL-C lowering efficacy in women than men, 6.8% versus 0.2% ($p = .006$) at 1 g daily, 11.3% versus 5.6% at 1.5 g ($p = .013$), and 14.8% versus 6.9% at 2 g ($p = .01$). Changes in other lipid parameters were similar in women and men (36).

Diabetes

CHD risk increases with duration of diabetes, and is higher for women than for men (Figure 32.1). Intensive multiple risk factor management reduces cardiovascular events in patients with type 2 diabetes, but gender-specific data are limited (38–40). Intensive blood glucose control did not significantly reduce myocardial infarction in patients with type 1 or 2 diabetes (41,42).

Postmenopausal Hormone Therapy

Although observational studies suggested that HT confers cardioprotection, randomized clinical trials have demonstrated no CHD risk reduction (and a possible short-term increase in risk) with HT (43,44). Although recent analyses support that younger women may have more favorable CHD outcomes

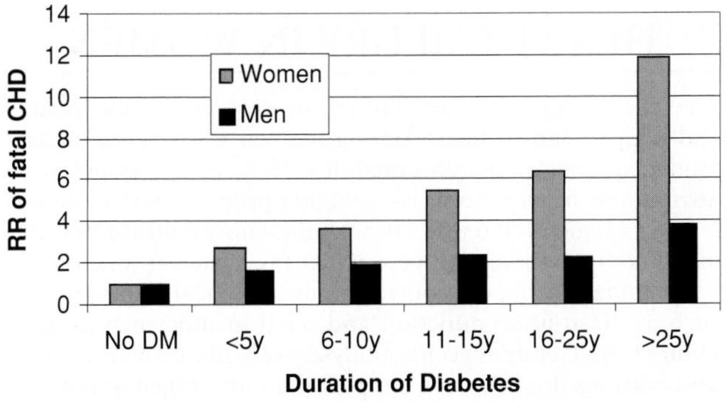

FIGURE 32.1. Multivariate-adjusted relative risk of fatal CHD according to duration of diabetes in the Nurses' Health Study and Health Professionals' Follow-up Study by gender. (*Source:* Adapted from Bassuk SS, Manson JE. Gender and its impact on risk factors for cardiovascular disease. In: Legato MJ, ed. *Principles of gender-specific medicine.* Boston: Elsevier, 2004:193–214.)

with unopposed estrogen than older women, current national guidelines do not recommend HT for the prevention of CHD in women (15).

SECONDARY PREVENTION IN WOMEN

Aspirin

The AHA/ACC Guidelines for Cardiovascular Prevention in Women (15) recommend aspirin, 75 to 162 mg/d, and clopidogrel in high-risk women intolerant to aspirin, as class I recommendations in high-risk women, including those with atherosclerotic vascular disease, diabetes, chronic kidney disease, or a 10-year risk of myocardial infarction/CHD death more than 20% as estimated by the Framingham algorithm (45). In a meta-analysis of 287 trials of antiplatelet therapy, aspirin reduced the composite outcome of myocardial infarction/stroke/vascular death by 23% ($p < .0001$). Among patients with prior myocardial infarction, subsequent nonfatal myocardial infarction was reduced by 18% ($p < .0001$), although gender-specific data were not provided (46). No data are available on clopidogrel in women.

β-Blockers

β-Blockade is of demonstrated benefit in women with CHD and those with congestive heart failure (47). The AHA/ACC Guidelines for Cardiovascular Prevention in Women include a class I recommendation that β-blockers be continued indefinitely in women with prior myocardial infarction or who have chronic ischemic syndromes (15).

Angiotensin-Converting Enzyme Inhibition and Angiotensin-Receptor Blockade

Three trials have evaluated angiotensin-converting enzyme inhibition for secondary coronary prevention. In the first, 2480 women (and 6,817 men) with vascular disease or diabetes, and at least one other risk factor, were randomized to ramipril or placebo for 4.5 years. Eighty percent qualified for randomization with antecedent CHD. In women, ramipril reduced the primary end point of myocardial infarction/stroke/cardiovascular death from 14.9% to 11.3% (relative risk 0.77, 95% CI 0.62–0.96) (21).

In the second trial, perindopril reduced cardiovascular death/non-fatal myocardial infarction/resuscitated cardiac arrest by 22% in 1,779 women at least 60 years of age with stable coronary artery disease (48). In the third trial, trandolapril did not reduce the primary outcome of cardiovascular death/myocardial infarction/coronary revascularization in 8,290 CHD patients (18% women) with documented normal left ventricular function during 4.8-year follow-up (hazard ratio 0.96, 95% CI 0.88–1.06) (49). Gender-specific analyses were not provided. The lack of treatment benefit was attributed to the low-risk profile of the cohort, which was predominantly optimally treated with aspirin, statins, β-blockers, and coronary revascularization. Taken together, these three trials suggest that angiotensin-converting enzyme inhibition reduces coronary events in higher risk women with CHD, but may not further reduce risk in those already receiving optimal management.

Secondary prevention trials with angiotensin-receptor blockers have not been performed. The AHA/ACC Guidelines for Cardiovascular Disease Prevention in Women include a class I recommendation for angiotensin-converting enzyme inhibitor use among high-risk women. Angiotensin-receptor blockers are recommended in high-risk women with heart failure or reduced ejection fraction who are intolerant to angiotensin-converting enzyme inhibitors (15).

Lipid-Lowering Therapy

The benefits of statin therapy for secondary coronary prevention in women are well established and similar to those in men (Table 32.5) (50–53). Too few women were enrolled in niacin or fibrate trials to permit subgroup analysis by gender (54–57).

Postmenopausal Hormone Therapy

Secondary prevention trials of HT, like the primary prevention trials, have not demonstrated cardioprotection (15,58). HT is not recommended for secondary prevention of CHD (15).

DIAGNOSIS OF CORONARY HEART DISEASE IN WOMEN

Presenting symptoms of women and men with acute coronary syndromes are similar (59); about 70% report chest pain (60). On the other hand, atypical symptoms are more common in women and many women with symptoms have neither obstructive coronary disease nor demonstrable ischemia. Among 406 women undergoing coronary angiography for suspected coronary ischemia in the Women's Ischemia Syndrome Evaluation study, 68 had obstructive CHD and ischemia demonstrated by noninvasive testing, 52 had CHD without ischemia, 105 had ischemia without CHD, and 181 had neither CHD nor ischemia (61). Overall, greater number, intensity, and duration of anginal symptoms were associated with lower quality of life.

Identifying women who should undergo noninvasive screening for coronary disease depends on the presence of symptoms and some form of global risk assessment, using either the Framingham risk score, coronary calcium score or other means such as C-reactive protein (62,63). In general, stress testing is not recommended for low-risk, asymptomatic women. High-risk, asymptomatic women such as those with diabetes, known atherosclerotic cardiovascular disease, or chronic kidney disease should be screened. For intermediate risk, asymptomatic women, growing evidence supports the utility of noninvasive testing (64,65). For symptomatic women, noninvasive testing is recommended for those at intermediate and high risk. Low-risk women with symptoms incur a considerable risk of false-positive results.

Treadmill stress electrocardiography in women with normal resting electrocardiograms and who are able to exercise adequately has lower sensitivity (61%) and specificity (77%) than for men (66). Use of imaging, either with echocardiography or scintigraphy, improves the diagnostic accuracy of stress testing. Accuracy of stress echocardiography appeared gender neutral, whereas perfusion imaging, particularly with thallium, may be slightly less accurate in women because of the breast attenuation artifact and small left ventricular size (67).

Women with CHD are more likely to present with angina than with myocardial infarction (68). Female gender is, however, an independent predictor of delay in seeking medical attention (5). Reasons for women's delay in seeking treatment included symptoms' severity, perceived seriousness, atypical character, confusion due to presence of other chronic illnesses, low self-perceived vulnerability to CHD, and engagement in various other coping mechanisms (69).

TREATMENT OF CORONARY HEART DISEASE IN WOMEN

Women with myocardial infarction have higher in-hospital mortality than men at all ages up to 80 years (70), even after multivariate adjustment. In the United States, revascularization for either angina or myocardial infarction is widespread (49). Age and medical history-adjusted rates of referral for coronary angiography and percutaneous coronary intervention appear similar in women and men in a Washington state registry (71). In-hospital mortality following percutaneous coronary intervention appears higher for women, both for elective procedures and in the setting of acute myocardial infarction. Following adjustment for age, size, comorbidity, and treatment delay, the gender difference is attenuated, but persists. Vascular complication rates in women remain 1.5 to 4 times higher than in men (72).

Referral patterns for coronary artery bypass surgery were similar for women and men in a New York state registry (73). Women undergoing surgery had higher perioperative mortality, greater transfusion requirement, were more likely to need prolonged mechanical ventilation and had longer average intensive care unit and overall hospital stays than men (74). The higher surgical risk in women has been attributed to their age, size, and concurrent medical conditions.

HEART FAILURE IN WOMEN

The prevalence of heart failure in women is age related and higher than in men. Among women in the Framingham Study, hypertension accounted for 59% of the population-attributable heart failure risk, a higher proportion than in men (75). In a registry of 65,275 heart failure hospitalizations (52% in women), preserved left ventricular function was identified in 46%, underscoring the contributions of clinical characteristics such as diastolic dysfunction and renal insufficiency to heart failure (76). Gender-specific analyses were not provided. These observations do, however, support the importance of risk factor management for heart failure prevention.

Metaanalyses of β-blocker trials for left ventricular systolic dysfunction showed similar benefits in women and men (47,77). Long-acting metoprolol reduced death or all-cause hospitalization by 21% among 898 women with class II to

IV heart failure and left ventricular ejection fraction of 40% or lower ($p = .044$) (78).

Peripartum cardiomyopathy is a form of heart failure peculiar to women. Although the etiology remains uncertain (79), it appears that left ventricular function returns to normal in about half (80). Maternal mortality in one recent series was 9%. Subsequent pregnancy should be strongly discouraged, however; the risk of recurrence is high.

CONTROVERSIES AND PERSONAL PERSPECTIVES

Gender disparities in referral for evaluation and treatment of CHD have largely been resolved. On the other hand, implementation of proven CHD prevention strategies could be improved for both men and women. In a recent survey, obstetrician-gynecologists reported that they provided primary care to 67% of their patients (14). This may represent a particular obstacle to CHD prevention in women, because awareness and use of national prevention guidelines was lower among obstetrician-gynecologists compared with other primary care physicians or cardiologists.

When seeing a woman referred for a specific symptom such as palpitations, cardiologists might seize that opportunity for global risk assessment, as the patient's primary care provider may be an obstetrician-gynecologists, a specialty that self-reports greater barriers to CHD risk assessment and management (14).

THE FUTURE

Two areas of focus to improve cardiovascular care for women might be (a) reducing women's delay in seeking medical attention for acute coronary syndromes and (b) increasing the ease and accuracy of global risk assessment in women. Suitable cohorts should be characterized, particularly among ethnic minorities, in which to develop and validate risk models.

References

1. American Heart Association. Heart disease and stroke statistics—2005 update. Available: www.americanheart.org. Accessed May 31, 2005.
2. Mosca L, Ferris A, Fabunmi R, et al. Tracking women's awareness of heart disease. An American Heart Association National Study. *Circulation* 2004;109:573–579.
3. Barrett-Connor E, Giardina E-GV, Gitt AK, et al. Women and heart disease. The role of diabetes and hyperglycemia. *Arch Intern Med* 2004;164:934–942.
4. Gordon DJ, Probstfield JL, Garrison RJ, et al. High-density lipoprotein cholesterol and cardiovascular disease. Four prospective American studies. *Circulation* 1989;79:8–15.
5. Schmidt SB, Borsch MA. The prehospital phase of acute myocardial infarction in the era of thrombolysis. *Am J Cardiol* 1990;65:1411–1415.
6. Andrikopoulos GK, Tzeis SE, Pipilis AG, et al. Younger age potentiates post myocardial infarction survival disadvantage of women. *Int J Cardiol* 2006;108:320–325.
7. National Center for Health Statistics. *Health, United States, 2004 (with chartbook on trends in the health of Americans)*. Hyattsville, MD: National Center for Health Statistics, 2004.
8. Ford ES, Mokdad AH, Giles WH, et al. Serum total cholesterol concentrations and awareness, treatment, and control of hypercholesterolemia among US adults. Findings from the National Health and Nutrition Examination Survey, 1999–2000. *Circulation* 2003;107:2185–2189.
9. Jensen J, Nilas L, Christiansen C. Influence of menopause on serum lipids and lipoproteins. *Maturitas* 12:1990;321–331.
10. Campos H, McNamara JR, Wilson PW, et al. Differences in low density lipoprotein subfractions and apolipoproteins in premenopausal and postmenopausal women. *J Clin Endocrinol Metab* 1988;67:30–35.
11. Abbey M, Owen A, Suzakawa M, et al. Effects of menopause and hormone replacement therapy on plasma lipids, lipoproteins and LDL-receptor activity. *Maturitas* 1999;33:259–269.
12. Kuller LH, Simkin-Silverman LR, Wing R, et al. Women's Healthy Lifestyle Project: A randomized clinical trial: results at 54 months. *Circulation* 2001; 103:32–37.
13. Staessen J, Bulpitt CJ, Fagard R, et al. The influence of menopause on blood pressure. *J Hum Hypertens* 1989;3:427–433.
14. Mosca L, Linfante AH, Benjamin EJ, et al. National study of physician awareness and adherence to cardiovascular disease prevention guidelines. *Circulation* 2005;111:499–510.
15. Mosca L, Appel LJ, Benjamin EJ, et al. Evidence-based guidelines for cardiovascular disease prevention in women. *Circulation* 109:2004;672–692.
16. Stampfer MJ, Hu FB, Manson JE, et al. Primary prevention of coronary heart disease in women through diet and lifestyle. *N Engl J Med* 2000;343:16–22.
17. Diabetes Prevention Program Research Group. Reduction in the incidence of type 2 diabetes with lifestyle intervention or metformin. *N Engl J Med* 2002; 346:393–403.
18. Svetkey LP, Erlinger TP, Vollmer WM, et al. Effect of lifestyle modifications on blood pressure by race, sex, hypertension status, and age. *J Hum Hypertens* 2005;19:21–31.
19. Stevens VJ, Obarzanek E, Cook NR, et al. Long-term weight loss and changes in blood pressure: results of the Trials of Hypertension Prevention, Phase II. *Ann Intern Med* 2001;134:1–11.
20. Bolek JS, Sharman MJ, Gómez AL, et al. An isoenergetic very low carbohydrate diet improves serum HDL cholesterol and triacylglycerol concentrations, the total cholesterol to HDL cholesterol ratio and postprandial lipemic responses compared with a low fat diet in normal weight, normolipidemic women. *J Nutr* 2003;133:2756–2761.
21. Lonn E, Roccaforte R, Yi Q, et al. Effect of long-term therapy with ramipril in high-risk women. *J Am Coll Cardiol* 2002;40:693–702.
22. Margolis KL, Bonds DE, Rodabough RJ, et al. Effect of oestrogen plus progestin on the incidence of diabetes in postmenopausal women: results from the Women's Health Initiative Hormone Trial. *Diabetologia* 2004;47:1175–1187.
23. Manson JE, Hu FB, Rich-Edwards JW, et al. A prospective study of walking as compared with vigorous exercise in the prevention of coronary heart disease in women. *N Engl J Med* 1999;341:650–658.
24. Manson JE, Greenland P, LaCroix AZ, et al. Walking compared with vigorous exercise for the prevention of cardiovascular events in women. *N Engl J Med* 2002;347:716–725.
25. Lee IM, Rexrode KM, Cook NR, et al. Physical activity and coronary heart disease in women: Is 'no pain, no gain' passé? *JAMA* 2001;285:1447–1454.
26. Sesso HD, Paffenbarger RS, Ha T, et al. Physical activity and cardiovascular disease risk in middle-aged and older women. *Am J Epidemiol* 1999;150: 408–416.
27. Schoenborn CA, Barnes PM. *Leisure-time physical activity among adults: United States, 1997–8* [Advance Data from Vital and Health Statistics; No. 325]. Hyattsville, MD: National Center for Health Statistics, 2002.
28. Hsia J, Wu L, Allen C, et al. Physical activity and diabetes risk in postmenopausal women. *Am J Prev Med* 2005;28:19–25.
29. Ridker PM, Cook NR, Lee I-M, et al. A randomized trial of low-dose aspirin in the primary prevention of cardiovascular disease in women. *N Engl J Med* 2005;352:1293–1304.
30. Thom TJ, Kannel WB, Silbershatz H, et al. Cardiovascular disease in the United States and prevention approaches. In: Fuster V, Alexander RW, O'Rourke RA, eds. *Hurst's the heart*. New York: McGraw-Hill, 2001:3–17.
31. Sacks FM, Svetkey LP, Vollmer WM, et al. Effects on blood pressure of reduced dietary sodium and the Dietary Approaches to Stop Hypertension (DASH) diet. *N Engl J Med* 2001;344:3–10.
32. The ALLHAT Officers and Coordinators for the ALLHAT Collaborative Research Group. Major outcomes in high-risk hypertensive patients randomized to angiotensin-converting enzyme inhibitor or calcium channel blocker vs diueretic. *JAMA* 2002;288:2981–2997.
33. Stefanick ML, Mackey S, Sheehan M, et al. Effects of diet and exercise in men and postmenopausal women with low levels of HDL cholesterol and high levels of LDL cholesterol. *N Engl J Med* 1998;339:12–20.
34. Clearfield M, Downs JR, Weis S, et al. Air Force/Texas Coronary Atherosclerosis Prevention Study (AFCAPS/TexCAPS): efficacy and tolerability of long-term treatment with lovastatin in women. *J Womens Health Gend Based Med* 2001;10:971–981.
35. Sever PS, Dahlof B, Poulter NR, et al. Prevention of coronary and stroke events with atorvastatin in hypertensive patients who have average or lower-than-average cholesterol concentrations, in the Anglo-Scandinavian Cardiac Outcomes Trial—Lipid Lowering Arm (ASCOT-LLA): a multicentre randomised controlled trial. *Lancet* 2003;361:1149–1158.
36. Goldberg AC. A meta-analysis of randomized controlled studies on the effects of extended-release niacin in women. *Am J Cardiol* 2004;94:121–124.
37. Bassuk SS, Manson JE. Gender and its impact on risk factors for cardiovascular disease. In: Legato MJ, ed. *Principles of gender-specific medicine*. Boston: Elsevier, 2004:193–214.
38. Gaede P, Vedel P, Larsen N, et al. Multifactorial intervention and cardiovascular disease in patients with type 2 diabetes. *N Engl J Med* 2003;348:383–393.
39. Armitage J, Bowman L. Cardiovascular outcomes among participants with diabetes in the recent large statin trials. *Curr Opin Lipidol* 2004;15:439–446.

40. Tuomilehto J, Rastenyte D, Birkenhager WH, et al. Effects of calcium-channel blockade in older patients with diabetes and systolic hypertension. *N Engl J Med* 1999;340:677–684.
41. The DCCT Research Group. Effect of intensive diabetes management on macrovascular events and risk factors in the Diabetes Control and Complications Trial. *Am J Cardiol* 1995;75:894–903.
42. UKPDS Group. Intensive blood-glucose control with sulphonylureas or insulin compared with conventional treatment and risk of complications in patients with type 2 diabetes (UKPDS 33). *Lancet* 1998;352:837–853.
43. Manson JE, Hsia J, Johnson KC, et al., for the Women's Health Initiative Investigators. Estrogen plus progestin and the risk of coronary heart disease. *N Engl J Med* 2003;349:523–534.
44. Hsia J, Langer RD, Manson JE, et al. Conjugated esquire estrogens and the risk of coronary heart disease. *Arch Intern Med* 2006;166:357–365.
45. US Department of Health and Human Services, Public Health Service, National Institutes of Health, National Heart, Lung, and Blood Institute. *ATP III guidelines at-a-glance quick desk reference* [NIH Publication No. 01-3305]. Washington, DC: USDHHS, 2001.
46. Antithrombotic Trialists' Collaboration. Collaborative meta-analysis of randomised trials of antiplatelet therapy for prevention of death, myocardial infarction and stroke in high risk patients. *BMJ* 2002;324:71–86.
47. Hjalmarson A. International beta-blocker review in acute and postmyocardial infarction. *Am J Cardiol* 1988;61:26B–29B.
48. EUROPA Investigators. Efficacy of perindopril in reduction of cardiovascular events among patients with stable coronary artery disease: randomised, double-blind, placebo-controlled, multicentre trial (the EUROPA study). *Lancet* 2003;362:782–788.
49. Braunwald E, Domanski MJ, Fowler SE, et al. Angiotensin-converting-enzyme inhibition in stable coronary artery disease. *N Engl J Med* 2004; 351:2058–2068.
50. Miettinen TA, Pyorala K, Olsson AG, et al. Cholesterol-lowering therapy in women and elderly patients with myocardial infarction or angina pectoris: findings from the Scandinavian Simvastatin Survival Study (4S). *Circulation* 1997;96:4211–4218.
51. Lewis SJ, Sacks FM, Mitchell JS, et al. Effect of pravastatin on cardiovascular events in women after myocardial infarction: the cholesterol and recurrent events (CARE) trial. *J Am Coll Cardiol* 1998;32:140–146.
52. Hague W, Forder P, Simes J, et al. Effect of pravastatin on cardiovascular events and mortality in 1516 women with coronary heart disease: results from the Long-Term Intervention with Pravastatin in Ischemic Disease (LIPID) study. *Am Heart J* 2003;145:643–651.
53. HPS Collaborative Group. MRC/BHF Heart Protection Study of cholesterol lowering with simvastatin in 20,536 high-risk individuals: a randomized placebo-controlled trial. *Lancet* 2002;360:7–22.
54. Brown BG, Zhao XQ, Chait A, et al. Simvastatin and niacin, antioxidant vitamins, or the combination for the prevention of coronary disease. *N Engl J Med* 2001;345:1583–1592.
55. BIP Study Group. Secondary prevention by raising hdl cholesterol and reducing triglycerides in patients with coronary artery disease. *Circulation* 2000;102:21–27.
56. Canner PL, Berge KG, Wenger NK, et al. Fifteen year mortality in Coronary Drug Project patients: long-term benefit with niacin. *J Am Coll Cardiol* 1986;8:1245–1255.
57. Rubins HB, Robins SJ, Collins D, et al. Gemfibrozil for the secondary prevention of coronary heart disease in men with low levels of high-density lipoprotein cholesterol. *N Engl J Med* 1999;341:410–418.
58. Hulley S, Grady D, Bush T, et al., for the Heart and Estrogen/progestin Replacement Study (HERS) Research Group. Randomized trial of estrogen plus progestin for secondary prevention of CHD in postmenopausal women. *JAMA* 1998;280:605–613.
59. Kudenchuk PJ, Maynard C, Martin JS, et al. Comparison of presentation, treatment, and outcome of acute myocardial infarction in men versus women (the Myocardial Infarction Triage and Intervention Registry). *Am J Cardiol* 1996;78:9–14.
60. Milner KA, Funk M, Richards S, et al. Gender differences in symptom presentation associated with coronary heart disease. *Am J Cardiol* 1999;84:396–399.
61. Olson MB, Kelsey SF, Matthews K, et al. Symptoms, myocardial ischaemia and quality of life in women: Results from the NHLBI-sponsored WISE Study. *Eur Heart J* 2003;24:1506–1514.
62. Wenger NK. Coronary heart disease: the female heart is vulnerable. *Prog Cardiovasc Dis* 2003;46:199–229.
63. Cushman M, Arnold AM, Psaty BM, et al. C-reactive protein and the 10-year incidence of coronary heart disease in older men and women. The Cardiovascular Health Study. *Circulation* 2005;112:25–31.
64. Conroy RFM, Pyorala K, Fitzgerald AP, et al. Estimation of ten-year risk of fatal cardiovascular disease in Europe: the SCORE project. *Eur Heart J* 2003;24:987–1003.
65. Pasternak RC, Abrams J, Greenland P, et al. Identification of coronary heart disease risk: is there a detection gap? *J Am Coll Cardiol* 2003;41:1863–1874.
66. Kwok Y, Kim C, Grady D, et al. Meta-analysis of exercise testing to detect coronary artery disease in women. *Am J Cardiol* 1999;83:660–666.
67. Mieres JH, Shaw LJ, Hendel RCD, et al. Writing Group on Perfusion Imaging in Women. American Society of Nuclear Cardiology consensus statement: Task Force on Women and Coronary Artery Disease—the role of myocardial perfusion imaging in the clinical evaluation of coronary artery disease in women. *J Nucl Cardiol* 2003;10:95–101.
68. Hochman JS, Tamis JE, Thompson TD, et al. Sex, clinical presentation, and outcome in patients with acute coronary syndromes. *N Engl J Med* 1999; 341:226–232.
69. Lefler LL, Bondy KN. Women's delay in seeking treatment with myocardial infarction: a meta-synthesis. *J Cardiovasc Nurs* 2004;19:251–268.
70. Vaccarino V, Parsons L, Every NR, et al. Sex-based differences in early mortality after myocardial infarction. *N Engl J Med* 1999;341:217–225.
71. Kim C, Shaaf CH, Maynard C, et al. Unstable angina in the myocardial infarction triage and intervention registry (MITI): short- and long-term outcomes in men and women. *Am Heart J* 2001;141:73–77.
72. Lansky AJ, Hochman JS, Ward PA, et al. Percutaneous coronary intervention and adjunctive pharmacotherapy in women. A statement for healthcare professionals from the American Heart Association. *Circulation* 2005;111:940–953.
73. Hannan EL, van Ryan M, Burke J, et al. Access to coronary artery bypass surgery by race/ethnicity and gender among patients who are appropriate for surgery. *Med Care* 1999;37:3–4.
74. Fox AA, Nussmeier NA. Does gender influence the likelihood or types of complications following cardiac surgery? *Semin Cardiothorac Vasc Anesth* 2004;8:283–295.
75. Levy D, Larson MG, Vasan RS, et al. The progression from hypertension to congestive heart failure. *JAMA* 1996;275:1557–1562
76. Fonarow GC, Adams KF, Abraham WT, et al. Risk stratification for in-hospital mortality in acutely decompensated heart failure. Classification and regression tree analysis. *JAMA* 2005;293:572–580.
77. Shekelle PG, Rich MW, Morton SC, et al. Efficacy of angiotensin-converting enzyme inhibitors and beta-blockers in the management of left ventricular systolic dysfunction according to race, gender, and diabetic status: a meta-analysis of major clinical trials. *J Am Coll Cardiol* 2003;41:1529–1538.
78. Ghali JK, Pina IL, Gottlieb SS, et al. Metoprolol CR/XL in female patients with heart failure: analysis of the experience in the Metoprolol Controlled Release Randomized Intervention Trial in Heart Failure (MERIT-HF). *Circulation* 2002;105:1585–1591.
79. Pearson GD, Veille J-C, Rahimtoola S, et al. Peripartum cardiomyopathy. Proceedings of a Workshop Sponsored by the National Heart, Lung, and Blood Institute and the Office of Rare Diseases, NIH. *JAMA* 2000;283:1183–1188.
80. Elkayam U, Akhter MW, Singh H, et al. Pregnancy-associated cardiomyopathy. Clinical characteristics and a comparison between early and late presentation. *Circulation* 2005;111:2050–2055.

CHAPTER 33 ■ THE ELDERLY AND AGING

KAREN P. ALEXANDER AND CHRISTOPHER M. O'CONNOR

OVERVIEW

The extraordinary increase in older persons, coupled with their high prevalence of cardiovascular disease, makes understanding the age-related changes in the cardiovascular system and disease manifestations in the elderly an important endeavor. According to the American College of Cardiology, the percentage of elderly patients treated per cardiologist will continue to increase through the year 2020 (1). Demand for services coupled with the high cost of cardiovascular care necessitates the careful consideration of treatment benefits across patient age, and the heterogeneity of aging requires careful consideration of treatment risks.

Although randomized controlled trials provide treatment-specific information, they do not clarify the value of treatments applied to populations differing from those studied, like the elderly. Age-related changes in the cardiovascular system modify presentation and outcome of cardiovascular disease, and age-related changes in other systems alter the pharmacokinetics and pharmacodynamics of cardiovascular drugs. In addition, treatments known to be effective, safe, and inexpensive are often underused (e.g., aspirin and β-blockers), while others with less evidence to clarify their risk and expense are used frequently (e.g., catheter-based interventions). Because patient-centered evidence-based medicine in the elderly is of enormous importance, more information on drug efficacy and safety as well as functional and health status outcomes across age is needed. This broader perspective along with consideration of patient preferences should guide treatment selection from among evidence-supported options. In so doing, cardiologists can provide the best cardiovascular care within the global health context of the elderly patient.

Historical Perspective

Never has a society had as many elderly, nor committed so large a share of community resources to their well-being. The absolute and proportional number of older Americans in the population is increasing at a remarkable rate (Fig. 33.1). Since the beginning of the twentieth century, longevity has increased by about 30 years (2). In 1900, life expectancy in the United States at birth was 47 years. In 2002, life expectancy at birth in the United States reached a high of 77.3 years (3). Despite

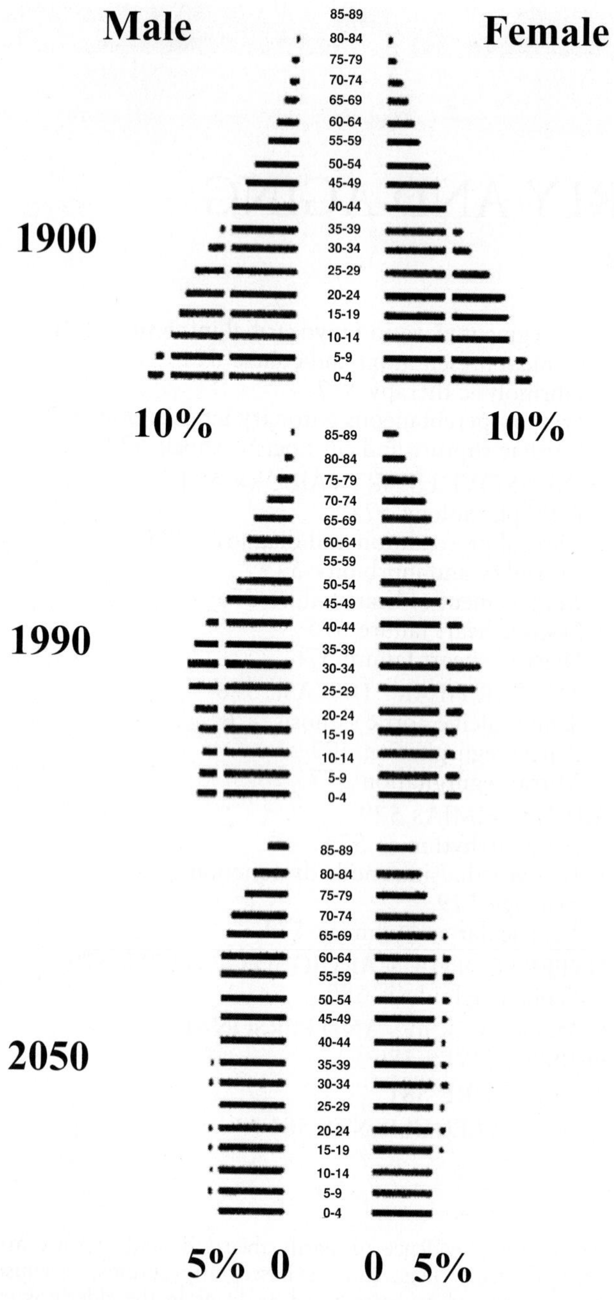

FIGURE 33.1. Distribution of the U.S. population by 5-year age categories for 1900 and 1990, and projections for 2050 (6). The distribution becomes rectangular as the proportion of the population achieving old age increases and (projected) birth rates stabilize. (*Source:* From U.S. Census Bureau. *J NIH Res* 1995;7:29.)

longer life expectancies, maximum life span remains limited at 85 to 90 years (4,5). The proportion of people aged 65 years or older is projected to increase from 12.4% to 19.6% in the United States between 2000 and 2030 (6). During this same time interval the absolute number of the oldest old in the United States—age 85 years or older—will increase most dramatically, doubling from 9.3 million to 19.5 million. Thus, it is the larger number of individuals living into later life that accounts for the current demographic shift. The key outcome for treatment of cardiovascular disease in the elderly has shifted to a focus on compression of morbidity.

More than 40% of the annual U.S. budget is spent on Medicare and Medicaid (7). Congestive heart failure (CHF) is the most common diagnosis-related group in the Medicare population (8). In addition, 60% of hospital admissions for myocardial infarction (MI) are among Medicare eligible patients (age ≥65) (9). Atrial fibrillation occurs at a median age of 75 years, and is present in 9% of the population between ages 80 and 89 years (10,11). Not surprisingly, 25.8% of elderly nursing home residents age 65 or older had a primary cardiovascular diagnosis at the time of admission to long-term care (8).

Despite the greater burden of disease in the elderly, cardiovascular therapies have primarily been studied in younger populations. Until recently, older patients were explicitly excluded from therapeutic trials (12). Accordingly, the average age in heart failure trials ranges from 59 to 64 years (13–15). In addition, fewer than 20% of elderly dwelling in the community with heart failure would meet other inclusion criteria for trials, resulting in limited information on CHF in this population (16). The average age in acute coronary syndrome (ACS) trials ranges from 57 to 62 years, also representing a younger and healthier population than their community treated counterparts (17–21). The data emphasize that the medical system spends the least money studying cardiovascular patients who account for the greatest health care expenditures.

In this chapter, the diagnosis and management of cardiovascular disease in the elderly is addressed considering three key concepts. First, age-related *cardiovascular changes*, including degenerative changes in the conduction system, alterations in the myocardium and left ventricular (LV) function, and senile calcification of the aortic valve, are discussed. These and other changes are the consequences of the aging process, but substantially alter the clinical presentation and course of cardiovascular disease. Second, consideration of altered *pharmacokinetics* and *pharmacodynamics* related to patient age are discussed. The third issue is the *heterogeneity* of the aging process, which dictates the need for highly individualized decisions in the elderly, particularly in those beyond age 75 years. For many older persons, quality of life and functional independence, rather than longevity, become primary therapeutic targets. To integrate these subjective aspects of care into the patient's entire health context requires substantial time and attention. The charge of cardiovascular health care providers with regard to the aging population must be to develop best approaches to cardiovascular care that exists, which optimizes quality of life within the entire health context of the elderly individual.

THE OLDER CARDIAC PATIENT

Cardiovascular Changes Related to Aging

Age-related changes in the cardiovascular system parallel age-related changes elsewhere in the body. However, age-related changes in a single organ or group of organs, such as the brain, lungs, or kidneys, may predominate, while, other organs remain unaffected. Age-related changes in the cardiovascular system are specific and enumerable (Tables 33.1 and 33.2). First, elderly hearts experience myocyte hypertrophy along with an increase in the connective tissue matrix (22). On the cellular level, total number of myocytes decreases and remaining myocytes hypertrophy (23). The weight of the heart increases 1.5 g/year between 30 and 90 years of age because of this hypertrophy and connective tissue deposition (24,25). With aging, ventricular chamber dimensions decrease with septal hypertrophy because of increased ventricular septal thickness and decreased base-to-apex dimensions. The "sigmoid septum" of aging is another morphologic manifestation of the senescent heart resulting from the reduction in the ventricular cavity

TABLE 33.1

AGE-RELATED CHANGES IN CARDIAC ANATOMY

MYOCARDIUM
Increased heart weight, LV mass, LV wall thickness
Increased myocyte size, decreased myocyte number
Fibrosis with deposition of less distensible form of collagen
CHAMBERS
Decreased LV cavity size, shortened long axis
Rightward shift and dilatation of the aorta
Dilatation of left atrium, senile septum
VALVES
Calcific and fatty degeneration of valve leaflets and annuli
CORONARY ARTERIES
Atherosclerosis
Dilation, tortuosity, and Monckeberg calcific arteriosclerosis
CONDUCTION SYSTEM
Fibrosis of atrioventricular node and left anterior fascicle
Loss of specialized cells and fibers

Abbreviation: LV, left ventricular.

size and rightward shift of the ascending aorta (26). Although not hemodynamically significant, this curved septum simulates asymmetric hypertrophic cardiomyopathy. Despite structural changes, systolic function of the heart at rest remains essentially normal. However, alterations that impair peak systolic function do occur at the subcellular level of myocardial function. These include availability of energy stores, intracellular calcium handling, and transmembrane action potential (27). Changes in receptor density, receptor coupling, and postreceptor mechanisms reduce the response of myocardial cells to β-adrenergic stimulation with age (28). Intriguing studies in isolated cardiac muscles from older animals show a reduction in inotropic response to catecholamines and digitalis (which require a receptor) but an unchanged response of myofibrils to direct exposure to calcium (after chemical removal of the cell membrane). The altered pattern of Ca^{2+} regulation allows the myocardium of older hearts to generate force for a longer period of time following excitation (29). This enables the continued ejection of blood during late systole, a beneficial adaptation with respect to enhanced vascular stiffness and early reflected pulse waves. Older persons have higher levels of catecholamines and greater release of catecholamines with stress, but reduced chronotropic and inotropic responses.

In contrast to systolic function, which is preserved at rest, diastolic function is impaired. Connective tissue matrix becomes replaced with a less distensible form of collagen. This causes greater stiffness of the senescent heart, requiring greater filling pressures to adapt via the Frank–Starling mechanism (30). Progressive cellular disarray, myocyte asynchrony, and abnormal calcium handling further affect the compliance and filling parameters during diastole. From a study of senescent animal models, the most predictable change in cardiac muscle function is longer duration of relaxation. This impaired relaxation with senescence is attributable to slower intracellular handling of calcium and longer action potentials, in addition to the stiffness from altered collagen. Echocardiographic Doppler studies in humans confirm prolonged relaxation and slower early diastolic filling with aging (31). However, end-systolic volumes are usually maintained by augmentation of late diastolic filling evidenced by exaggerated A wave and altered E:A ratio through the mitral valve (32). Diastolic function of the aging heart may be worsened by coexisting structural changes, such as mitral or aortic valvular disease, hypertension, atrial arrhythmias, or senile amyloidosis, which further alter hemodynamic conditions.

Age-related changes in the arterial system begin in the 30s and accelerate through midlife. Increased collagen deposition and weakened vascular elastin result in altered elasticity, distensibility, and dilatation. These changes, particularly in the intima, appear to resemble those that occur during atherosclerosis (33,34). Within the vascular media, there is progressive growth of smooth muscle, as well as deposition of lipids and calcium in the elastic lamella. Stiffening of the central arteries results in higher pulse wave velocities and augmentation in systolic arterial pressure, and whereas the lower elasticity results in a diminished contribution of arterial recoil to forward arterial perfusion. As arterial distensibility decreases, the speed of travel of the pulse along an arterial segment, referred to as the *pulse wave velocity*, increases. The forward cardiac ejection wave travels through central compliance arteries until it meets forward resistance. The pulse wave is then reflected (reflection wave), where it sums with continuing forward cardiac ejection increasing systolic pressures. Less compliant vasculature returns the reflection wave sooner, making a greater contribution to systolic pressure. Cyclic fatiguing and elastase activity also result in a reduction and fragmentation of vascular elastin (35). Vascular remodeling therefore takes place and results in dilatation and elongation of the aorta and major arteries. These changes are accompanied by impaired endothelial function owing to reduced prostacyclin production by cells which remain. With age, the endothelium undergoes apoptosis, progressive irregularity in cell size and shape, and increased multinucleated giant cells. Endothelial-dependent responses to agonists such as acetylcholine are therefore impaired (36,37). The impaired endothelial function of aging is difficult to separate

TABLE 33.2

AGE-RELATED CHANGES IN CARDIOVASCULAR PHYSIOLOGY

VASCULAR IMPEDENCE INCREASES IN LARGE AND MEDIUM-SIZE ARTERIES
Pulse wave velocity and pulse pressure increases
Systolic blood pressure increases
Impaired endothelial function
MYOCARDIAL RELAXATION DECREASES
Diastolic dysfunction develops
Peak EF maintained by a larger diastolic volume
Cardiac output and stroke volume are preserved at rest
ELECTRICAL CONDUCTION AND HEART RATE RESPONSE TO STIMULI IS IMPAIRED
PR, QRS, and QT are prolonged
Peak exercise HR declines
Sensitivity to β-agonists is decreased
Reactivity to chemoreceptors and baroreceptors is diminished
INTEGRATED PERFORMANCE DURING CARDIOVASCULAR EXERCISE IS IMPAIRED
Decrease peripheral muscle mass; increased adipose tissue
Diminished respiratory capacity
Diminished Vo_2 max reserves

Abbreviations: EF, ejection fraction; HR, heart rate.

from that which results from coexisting hypertension, hypercholesterolemia, and atherosclerosis.

Age-related changes in the conduction system result from apoptosis and the deposition of collagenous and fatty tissue. Fat accumulates around the sinoatrial node, sometimes producing partial or complete separation of the node from the atrial musculature. There is also a pronounced decrease in the number of pacemaker cells in the sinoatrial node beginning at age 60. At age 75, less than 10% of the cell number found in the young adult remains. Calcification of the atrioventricular node and left and right bundle branches also occur. Thus, older patients often have modest increases in electrocardiographic PR and QT intervals, increased QRS duration and bundle branch blocks, and decreased T-wave amplitude (38). The maximum predicted heart rate (HR) in an octogenarian is 30 beats per minute lower than it was at age 50, and HR in older individuals is also less responsive to β-adrenergic stimulation. In the Framingham cohort, variability in RR intervals declines by 38% between age 40 and 70, reflecting the lesser contribution of autonomic tone to cardiac function with aging (39). Altered autonomic regulation is also demonstrated by reduced heart rate variability (HRV) to head-up tilt testing and impaired baroreflex (40). The Framingham study demonstrated the gradual increase in the prevalence of atrial fibrillation in the population between age 50 and 80 (<0.5%–8.8%) (41). In addition, there is an increase in ambient rate of premature atrial and ventricular contractions as evidenced by holter monitors in healthy adults. Short runs of supraventricular tachycardia occur in up to 33% of healthy individuals over age 60 (42).

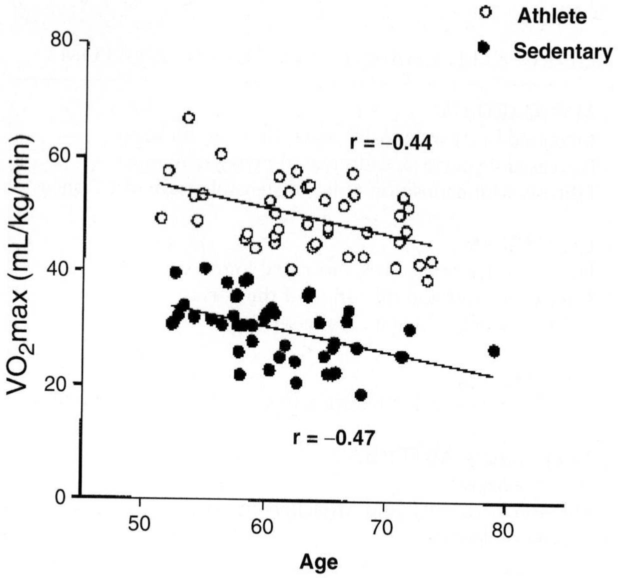

FIGURE 33.2. Aerobic capacity as a function of exercise and aging. Vo_2 max for athletes (*open circles*) and sedentary individuals (*closed circles*) across age. Lines reflect the slope of decline of peak aerobic capacity with age. Athletes demonstrate similar slope of decline but maintain significantly higher aerobic capacity at all ages. (*Source:* From Katzel LI, Sorkin JD, Fleg JL. A comparison of longitudinal changes in aerobic fitness in older endurance athletes and sedentary men. *J Am Geriatr Soc* 2001;49:1657–1664, with permission.)

Integrated Cardiovascular Performance

Aerobic capacity (Vo_2 max) declines with normal aging due to diminished cardiac reserve. Age-related changes in heart function must be differentiated from those resulting from a sedentary lifestyle or other disease processes. Many older patients become inactive, both physically and mentally, which accelerates deterioration and loss of function (43). Early studies found a steady decline in overall cardiovascular performance with aging as judged from exercise training (44). Cardiovascular performance and multiple gated acquisition (MUGA) cardiac volumes were assessed during upright cycle exercise in 40 healthy volunteers (45). Although total exercise duration was similar in young and old, there were age-associated deficits in chronotropic and LV systolic reserve performance. At 10 minutes of exercise in the steady state, older subjects had lower HR and Vo_2, but higher end-diastolic and end-systolic volume indices than younger subjects. Therefore, maximum cardiac output was preserved because of increased cardiac volumes (preload), despite lower HR, contractility, and greater impedance (afterload) in older subjects. Interestingly, β-blockade in younger individuals also blunts HR response and increases end-diastolic volume with exercise in a similar fashion. This suggests that age-related differences in cardiac performance may be related to a reduction in β-adrenergic responsiveness in the elderly (46). In addition, changes in the periphery, such as decreased muscle mass and increased body fat impair O_2 extraction from circulating blood volume in older patients. When Vo_2 max is normalized for markers of peripheral muscle mass, the proportion of the decline in aerobic capacity attributed to age itself decreased by about 50% (47). More recent work comparing maximum aerobic capacity (Vo_2 max) in older athletes and sedentary individuals demonstrated that athletes started at higher levels of aerobic capacity, but both groups had similar declines over time (48) (Fig. 33.2). Therefore, there is an inevitable decline in peak performance with age. However, older individuals can derive benefit from successful physical training in the same ways as younger persons in terms of increased exercise tolerance, muscle mass, and improved ventricular performance (49). In fact, motivated fit older persons can also achieve the same peak cardiac output as younger cohorts, albeit by different mechanisms (50).

In summary, the changes in cardiac structure and function with aging certainly have important implications for physiologic responses to exertion as well as clinical responses to disease. Diastolic dysfunction, left ventricular hypertrophy (LVH), and conduction disease may remain below the clinical threshold until coexisting cardiovascular conditions like ischemia, valvular disease, arrhythmia, or hypertension unmask this diminished capacity and trigger symptomatic presentation.

Clinical Pharmacology in the Elderly

Pharmacotherapy is one of the most important interventions in the treatment of elderly patients, but age-related alterations in pharmacokinetics (what the drug does in the patient) and pharmacodynamics (what the drug does to the patient) are important to consider (Table 33.3). Three key components of pharmacokinetics—distribution, metabolism, and excretion—are affected by the aging process. Drug absorption from the gastrointestinal tract does not appear to be affected unless altered by frequently used drugs such as antacids or anticholinergic agents. Once absorbed, however, age-related changes begin to impact drug handling.

First, the liver, which is a major site of oxidative and synthetic drug metabolism, undergoes changes with aging. Autopsy and ultrasound studies have shown a progressive decrease in liver mass after the age of 50. Regional blood flow to the liver at age 65 is reduced by 45% relative to that in a 25-year-old individual. Important changes are also attributed specific hepatic enzyme systems (particularly the cytochrome

TABLE 33.3

AGE-RELATED PHARMACOLOGIC CHANGES IN THE ELDERLY

GENERAL CONSIDERATIONS
Multiple drugs usual (drug interactions common)
Memory problems and confusion (lack of consistent use)
PHARMACOKINETICS (BIOAVAILABILITY)
Decreased drug absorption (usually not important)
Decreased mucosal absorptive surface (small bowel)
Reduced splanchnic blood flow
Reduced gastric emptying time and gastrointestinal motility
Altered volume of distribution (based on lipid solubility of drug)
Less muscle mass and increased body fat
Decreased total body water
Reduced drug metabolism (biotransformation)
Less liver mass, reduced blood flow
Reduced cellular enzyme activity (primarily affects oxidation)
Reduced drug elimination (major factor)
Reduced glomerular filtration rate and tubular secretion
Altered protein binding
Increased α-acid glycoprotein (owing to inflammation, illness)
Reduced hepatic albumin synthesis and serum protein levels
PHARMACODYNAMICS (ALTERED SENSITIVITY TO DRUGS)
Receptor change(s)
Reduced β_1-adrenergic responsiveness
Blunted reflex responses
Reduced baroreceptor reflex activity
Altered fluid and electrolyte balance

P-450 system) (52). These changes are likely responsible for the reduction in hepatic metabolism of drugs that can be as great as 25% over the human lifespan.

Glomerular filtration rate declines by 40% between age 20 and age 70 owing to diminished renal blood flow and renal mass. One common mistake is overestimating renal function by evaluating the blood urea nitrogen and creatinine in older patients. Because blood urea nitrogen reflects protein ingestion and serum creatinine is produced by the muscle, it is not uncommon for malnourished elderly patients with diminished muscle mass to have normal blood urea nitrogen and creatinine levels even in the presence of significant renal impairment. Even estimated creatinine clearance may not account for reduction in muscle mass component of total body mass, but this remains the best estimate for clinical practice (53). Many standard cardiovascular drugs (low-molecular-weight heparin, GP IIB/IIIA inhibitors, digoxin, diuretics, angiotensin-converting enzyme [ACE] inhibitors, atenolol, nadolol, and clonidine) are affected by renal clearance and adjustments for reduced renal function are recommended. The Cockroft–Gault formula should be applied routinely to estimate renal function in older patients receiving drugs excreted by the kidneys. Changes in creatinine clearance or volume of distribution may prolong half-life and increase drug side effects in the elderly.

Age-related alterations in drug distribution from changes in body composition and plasma proteins have more minor implications. The increase in adipose tissue results in a more extensive distribution and longer half-life of lipid-soluble drugs. The decrease in total body water and reduced volume of distribution leads to higher serum concentrations of water-soluble drugs (54,55). Decreases in serum albumin with age minimally impact drug distribution. However, many drug assays measure the total amount of drug. Because it is the unbound concentration that is pharmacologically active, patients who are hypoalbuminic may actually have unacceptably high drug levels. For example, levels of phenytoin, which is highly bound to albumin, may be misleading interpreting serum levels in the setting of malnourishment or chronic illness.

Drug Use in the Elderly

Drugs can improve function and quality of life in elderly patients, but constant vigilance remains necessary for adverse reactions and interactions. Reduced metabolism and slower elimination increase the propensity for drug complications. Age-related changes in pharmacodynamics further expose the elderly to therapeutic effects and toxicity. Drug use in the elderly cardiovascular patient is also complicated by drug interactions, with many elderly taking as many as 8 to 15 drugs on a daily basis (51). With altered distribution and elimination, diminished reflex and end-organ responses, and exposure to interactions, lower dosages of drugs are intuitive and advisable. Although the ability to distinguish adverse drug effects (e.g., drowsiness, altered cognition, constipation, and falls) from manifestations of disease can be problematic, a basic understanding of pharmacologic principles and simplification of regimens can minimize risks of medication errors and improve compliance.

Heterogeneity of Aging

Data obtained from clinical trial populations may not be generalizable to a heterogeneous elderly population (56). Among older populations with heart disease, large subgroups of individuals also have multiple comorbidities, frailty, or are disabled. One in five (20%) of Medicare beneficiaries have five or more chronic conditions, and 50% take more than five daily medications (57). Similarly, one in five (19.6%) community dwelling elders age 65 years or older depend on others for assistance with activities of daily living (58). In the Women's Health Initiative, 16.3% of women over 65 years were frail (59). *Frailty* is a decline in physiologic reserves associated with an increased vulnerability to adverse outcomes and diminished resistance to stress. Frailty often overlaps with cardiovascular disease, comorbid conditions, depression, and inflammatory dysregulation, all of which may contribute to cardiovascular risk and outcomes (60). In addition to physiologic impairments, the Heart Protection Study (HPS) found that 34% of community-dwelling elderly over age 70 had mild cognitive impairment (61). The Cardiovascular Health Study confirmed a prevalence of mild cognitive impairment in those age 75 years or older of 29% by detailed neuropsychological testing (62). For these vulnerable elderly, face value extension of all practice guidelines may divert attention from the key aspects of care in this population or even result in unintended harm (63). Yet treatment gaps in vulnerable elderly remain a significant problem (64). Patient-specific customization of care is needed to minimize the problem of overtreatment, drug–drug interactions, and medical errors in the vulnerable elderly.

CARDIOVASCULAR RISK FACTORS

The role of conventional cardiovascular risk factors in determining risk in the elderly has been debated. Conventional wisdom held that conventional risk factors such as smoking, hypertension, and dyslipidemia were less important in the aged because of their diminished relative impact on risk. Yet, although relative risk (RR) associated with a given factor may decline, the higher prevalence of these risk factors, and of cardiovascular disease at older ages, yields greater absolute and attributable risk in the elderly. Therefore, because coronary heart disease (CHD) is the leading cause of death in older individuals, even small reductions in RR may result in a substantial number of lives saved. Chronologic age also stands as a surrogate for unmeasured comorbidity and marks duration of exposure to conventional risk factors. Guidelines still emphasize modification of conventional risk factors regardless of patient age (65).

In the elderly, overall risk is best determined by the severity and combination of risk factors. Traditional risk factors (e.g., hypertension, smoking, dyslipidemia, diabetes mellitus) often act as risk multipliers in the setting of end-organ impairment (e.g., LVH, chronic kidney disease). Grids developed from epidemiologic data are available to help estimate long-term risks in specific patients (10-year risk), but are quite limited past age 75 (66). In elderly populations, the overall risk must include consideration of subclinical cardiovascular disease as well as existing end-organ impairments. Indicators of subclinical disease include peripheral arterial bruits, electrocardiographic (ECG) abnormalities, low ankle–brachial indices, or atherosclerosis on carotid ultrasound. Newer risk factors are also emerging which reflect declining reserves in organ function (e.g., creatinine clearance, pulse pressure, LVH, and anemia).

Hypertension

Morphologic changes in the aorta and the peripheral vessels make systolic hypertension an inevitable consequence of aging (67,68). Population trends demonstrate increased systolic blood pressure and decreased diastolic blood pressure with aging (Fig. 33.3). Hypertension, defined as systolic pressure above 140 mm Hg, alone or in association with diastolic pressure above 90 mm Hg, occurs in more than 50% of the elderly population (69). Isolated systolic hypertension affects 30% of adults age 80 years or older (70). Thus, hypertension is a hallmark of aging, but is also a modifiable cardiovascular risk factor in the elderly.

Multiple studies have assessed the risks of elevated systolic blood pressure in the elderly (71–73). In the Framingham study, participants aged 65 to 94 years with a systolic pressure higher than 180 mm Hg had a three- to fourfold increased risk of CHD compared to patients with a systolic pressure lower than 120 mm Hg (67). Wide pulse pressure has been identified as a marker for arterial stiffness and important risk indicator for cardiovascular complications in the elderly (74–76). The prognostic importance of wide pulse pressure is greater than either systolic blood pressure or diastolic blood pressure. The Framingham Heart Study found that the risk of cardiovascular events increased by 16% per 10–mm Hg rise in systolic blood pressure, but by 23% per 10–mm Hg rise in pulse pressure (77). After adjusting for demographics, morbidity, and risk factors, each 10–mm Hg increase in pulse pressure was associated with a 12% increase in CHD death and a 14% increase in CHF. The National Health and Nutrition Examination Survey (NHANES) and pooled European and Chinese Trials confirmed the positive associations between pulse pressure and MI, stroke, cardiovascular mortality, and all-cause mortality (78–80). Treatment of hypertension reduces the rate of stroke, CHF, chronic renal failure, and CHD as well as all-cause mortality (81,82).

Nonpharmacologic treatment should be pursued in all hypertensive patients with salt restriction, exercise, abstinence from alcohol, and weight reduction when appropriate. The Trial of Nonpharmacologic Interventions in the Elderly (TONE) enrolled 975 hypertensive patients between the ages of 60 and 80. Patients were randomly assigned to undergo a reduction in dietary sodium, weight reduction, both, or neither. Each intervention significantly reduced blood pressure, but the combination was most successful (83).

Antihypertensive medication is justified if systolic pressures are 160 mm Hg or higher, and between 140 and 159 mm Hg based on individual risk assessments (84,85). A greater benefit from the treatment of systolic hypertension is also seen among those with wide pulse pressure. The number of hypertensives needed to treat to prevent one cardiovascular death was 119 when pretreatment pulse pressure were between 65 and 89 mm Hg, and just 63 when pretreatment pulse pressure were greater than 90 mm Hg (86). The Systolic Hypertension in the Elderly Program (SHEP) was the first randomized, controlled trial of the treatment of isolated systolic hypertension (87). Nearly 450,000 patients older than age 60 were screened, and 4,736 were randomly assigned to treatment (stepwise chlorthalidone or atenolol) or placebo and followed for approximately 5 years.

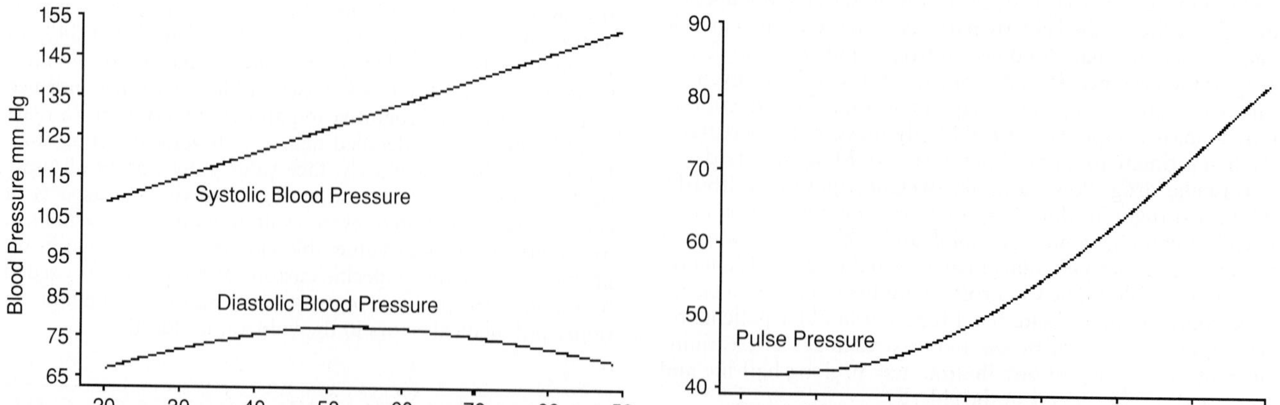

FIGURE 33.3. Association between age and systolic and diastolic blood pressure and pulse pressure in NHANES III. (*Source:* From Hajjar IM, Grim CE, George V, et al. Impact of diet on blood pressure and age-related changes in blood pressure in the US population: analysis of NHANES III. *Arch Intern Med* 2001;161:589–593.)

Baseline systolic blood pressure ranged from 160 to 219 mm Hg and diastolic blood pressure were less than 90 mm Hg. Active treatment lowered the risk of stroke (36% risk reduction) and MI (28% risk reduction) and improved survival. A recent metaanalysis combining eight trials of systolic hypertension in the elderly further confirms the enduring benefit from treatment (88). In this metaanalysis, treatment lowered systolic blood pressure by an average of 10 mm Hg and diastolic blood pressure by 4 mm Hg. In so doing, the treatment group had a lower risk of stroke (30% risk reduction), cardiovascular events (23% risk reduction), and mortality (13% risk reduction) (Fig. 33.4). Greatest treatment benefit was again seen in subgroups including men, those aged 70 years or older, with wider pulse pressure, or prior cardiovascular complications. In a subgroup analysis of 1,670 subjects over 80 years of age, antihypertensive therapy reduced stroke by 34% and heart failure by 39%, although there was a nonsignificant 6% increase in mortality (89). The Hypertension in the Very Elderly Trial (HYVET) will enroll 2,100 patients older than 80 years of age and will compare two groups randomized to indapamide with or without perindopril for a primary end point of stroke at 5 years. This study should answer lingering questions about whether active antihypertensive therapy is associated with significant reductions in cardiovascular morbidity and mortality in the very elderly age group as it clearly is in young elderly (90).

Pharmacologic treatment in older persons follows the same principles outlined for the general care of hypertension in JNC VII (91). The choice of agents in elderly hypertensives is as broad as in younger patients, although the best studied drugs are diuretics and β-blockers. The large National Institutes of Health–funded Antihypertensive and Lipid-lowering Treatment to Prevent Heart Attack Trial (ALLHAT) compared treatment with a diuretic, calcium channel blocker, and ACE inhibitor across 33,357 participants over 5 years of follow up. There were no differences in mortality between groups, but

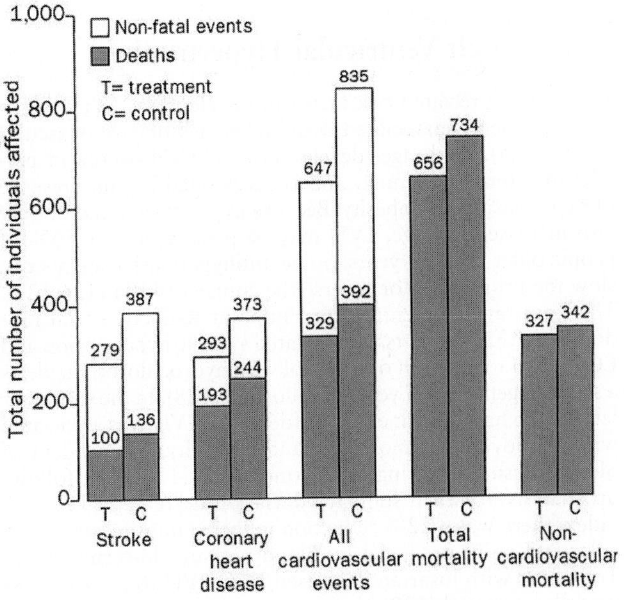

FIGURE 33.4. Metaanalysis-isolated systolic hypertension. Total number of individuals affected in this metaanalysis of more than 16,000 patients with mean age of 70.3 years. Treatment (*T*) with antihypertensive therapy lowers number of individuals affected compared with control (*C*). Improvement shown for nonfatal (*open bar*) and fatal (*solid bar*) events. (*Source:* From Staessen JA, Gasowski J, Wang JG, et al. Risks of untreated and treated isolated systolic hypertension in the elderly: meta-analysis of outcome trials. *Lancet* 2000;355:865–872, with permission.)

patients treated with thiazide diuretics achieved a lower systolic blood pressure, and demonstrated advantages in rates of CHF, stroke, and combined cardiovascular events (92). Interestingly, a subanalysis of losartan versus atenolol in the elderly found that angiotensin receptor blockers resulted in better end point reduction in the subgroup with high pulse pressures (93). Certain agents may also be selected for elderly with coexisting conditions. For example, ACE inhibitors may be preferred for elderly diabetics, or those with renal disease or heart failure because of their favorable effects on neurohumoral state. In addition, drug intolerances often dictate selection of agents among available choices. In summary, the evidence that systolic hypertension and pulse pressure are risk factors for cardiovascular and cerebrovascular complications in the elderly is clear, and evidence that treatment lowers risk is robust.

Dyslipidemia

The importance of dyslipidemia as a risk factor in the elderly has been debated. This relates, in part, to epidemiologic studies looking at hypercholesterolemia as a risk factor in the elderly that were confounded by older people with coexisting noncardiac illness and frailty who had low cholesterol levels (94,95). Perhaps the best evidence linking cholesterol and risk in the elderly comes from the Rotterdam study, a population-based study of 6,006 individuals older than 55 years (96). Men and women age 70 years or older with total cholesterol in the top quartile had a greater risk of MI compared with those in the lowest quartile, RR 3.2 (95% confidence interval [CI], 1.3–7.7) and RR 2.9 (95% CI, 1.3–6.6), respectively. Likewise, men and women age 70 years or older with high-density lipoprotein in the top quartile had a lower risk of MI compared with those in the lowest quartile, RR 0.5 (95% CI, 0.3–0.9) and RR 0.4 (95% CI, 0.2–0.9), respectively. The findings in this study have been confirmed by other studies and evidence now supports that dyslipidemia continues to be a risk factor in the elderly, although data past age 75 are sparse.

Evidence for the treatment for dyslipidemia in the elderly is stronger for secondary prevention. The large secondary prevention trials, Cholesterol and Recurrent Events Trial (CARE) and Long-term Intervention with Pravastatin in Ischemic Disease (LIPID), excluded patients older than 75 years, and the Scandinavian Simvastatin Survival Study Group trial (45) set an upper age limit of 69 years (97–99). Trials confirmed the benefit of statins for secondary prevention in young elderly (100,101). However, two recent studies have added to the evidence base in the elderly. The Heart Protection Study (HPS), which compared simavastatin to placebo in high-risk secondary prevention, enrolled patients up to age 80, and specifically targeted an older population (52% age $\geq$65 years) (102). In this study, the 5,806 patients aged 70 years or more had the same absolute risk reduction with simvastatin as was demonstrated in patients younger than age 65 years (5.1% versus 5.2%). This resulted in a number needed to treat in the oldest subgroup of 20 patients to prevent one cardiovascular death or MI. The Pravastatin in Elderly Individuals at Risk of Vascular Disease (PROSPER) trial was performed exclusively in the elderly. In this trial, 5,804 high-risk individuals age 70 years or older (range, 70–82; mean, 75) were randomized to pravastatin or placebo (103). Pravastatin treatment was associated with a 15% relative and a 2.1% absolute risk reduction compared with placebo at 3.2 years of follow up. The magnitude of risk reduction was less than anticipated, but could not be compared to a younger subgroup. Observational studies also show that those elderly with heart disease treated with statins do better than those without statin therapy. The Intermountain Heart Collaborative Study followed a cohort of 7,220 individuals with coronary artery disease by statin treatment over a mean follow-up duration of 3.3 years (104). Elderly patients were less likely to receive statins, but mortality was similarly decreased with statin use across all age groups. For those age 80 years or more, mortality was 29.5% among statin nonusers and 8.5% among statin users (hazard ratio 0.5, $P < .036$). In addition, these studies have shown the tolerability of lipid lowering medications in the elderly to be similar to younger patients.

Many primary prevention trials do not permit meaningful elderly subgroup analyses. The oldest patient in West of Scotland Coronary Prevention Study (WOSCOPS) was age 65, and the oldest patient in AFCAPS/TexCAPS was 73 (105,106). The Anglo-Scandinavian Cardiac Outcomes Trial (ASCOT), which enrolled patients up to age 79 years, found that primary prevention treatment with atorvastatin significantly reduced the risk of cardiovascular death and nonfatal MI in patients older than 60 years (hazard ratio 0.64, 0.47–0.86), but only trended to reduction in those age 60 years or younger (hazard ratio 0.66, 0.41–1.06) (107). With these data, the easiest group in which to pursue primary prevention is the young old, namely, those between 65 and 75 years of age. High-risk elderly patients with substantial remaining life-years are likely to benefit from primary prevention, but definitive data are yet to be obtained.

Diabetes Mellitus

Diabetes and metabolic syndrome are powerful predictors of primary and secondary cardiovascular events in patients of all ages. Total body fat and visceral adiposity increase until age 65, and are often accompanied by insulin resistance and diabetes (108). The elderly are also susceptible to glucose intolerance owing to diminished reserves in the mechanisms to lower glucose, and susceptible to hypoglycemia because of lower levels of regulatory hormones that raise glucose, like glucagon and growth hormone (109). NHANES III determined that metabolic syndrome is prevalent in approximately 44% of the general U.S. population older than 50 years (110). Metabolic syndrome is associated with an increase in incidence of cardiovascular disease and future cardiovascular events over four years after accounting for other factors (odds ratio [OR] 1.38; 95% CI 1.07–1.79). The metabolic syndrome has also been shown to be an independent predictor of arterial stiffness in the Baltimore Longitudinal Study of Aging (111).

Type 2 diabetes is less common in older persons, occurring in approximately 15% of the general population older than age 70, with a peak incidence at age 75 to 84 in men (16.5%) and women (12.8%) (112). However, in a population with ACS, the prevalence of diabetes is higher, and peaks 10 years earlier (29.6% age <65; 38.8% ages 65–74; 35.5% ages 75–84; and 24.7% age ≥85) (113). Insulin resistance rather than insulin deficiency is the hallmark of diabetes in older age (114,115). Risk stratification is of particular importance in older diabetics because of the variability in their outcomes related to other risk factors, as well as the common occurrence of unrecognized MI (108). Although randomized trials for diabetic treatment were conducted in younger cohorts, abundant epidemiologic evidence suggests glucose control is equally beneficial in the elderly (116,117).

Smoking

The prevalence of smoking dramatically decreases with age. For example, almost half of patients with ACS under age 65 are smokers (46.6%), compared with just 4% of patients age 85 or older (113). Similarly, smoking is a stronger relative risk factor for cardiovascular events in the young (118). Smoking cessation post-MI is shown to reduce mortality by 25% to 50%, most of which occurs in the first year (119). Thus, the few smokers who continue to smoke in their later years will still benefit from smoking cessation.

Life Style

Diet, exercise, and psychological well-being determine the pace of aging as well as the quality of life in later years. Dietary intake in the elderly should mirror that recommended for health, yet total caloric needs decline over time. In fact, the only lifestyle intervention proven to lengthen life (albeit in animals) is caloric restriction by 30% (120). This level of dietary restriction would be poorly tolerated in humans, but emphasizes the role of dietary intake on metabolic activity (insulin secretion, body temperature) and other process central to aging and disease. However, the epidemiologic data between diet and cardiovascular outcomes are not strong. The Cardiovascular Health Study was able to document a weak relationship between healthier dietary patterns (low fat, low cholesterol) and longer 10-year survival (121).

Exercise has tremendous value in reducing the risk of CHD mortality and morbidity and slowing the decline in physical function. The Honolulu Heart Program, which studied 2,678 physically capable elderly men aged 71 to 93, demonstrated a relationship between lower risk of CHD and longer distance walked (122). Men who walked more than 1.5 miles per day had half the risk of CHD as those who walked less than 0.25 miles a day (2.5% versus 5.1%). Combined with the evidence that an active life style reduces the risk of CHD in younger individuals, these data suggests that walking has disease prevention value for the elderly.

Social isolation and depression are also common in elderly patients, and are independently associated with recurrent events after MI and death from cardiovascular disease (123,124). Emerging evidence indicates that treatment of these factors also improves outcomes; however, clinical trials are difficult to control in the psychosocial area.

Left Ventricular Hypertrophy

A poorly appreciated risk factor in the elderly is LVH, which is independently associated with higher risk of cardiovascular events (125). With age, development of LVH occurs in parallel to arterial stiffening, and is accelerated by the presence of hypertension and obesity. Because hypertension and obesity also increase with age, LVH may be present in over 50% of people older than 65 years. Some antihypertensive agents can slow the progression or reverse the course of LVH (126,127). The Losartan Intervention for Endpoint Reduction trial randomized 1,326 patients with isolated systolic hypertension and ECG–LVH to losartan or atenolol with hydrochlorothiazide as a second agent for 4.5 years of follow up (128). In the subpopulation who had LVH at entry, the degree of LVH was associated with cardiovascular morbidity and mortality, independent of blood pressure lowering or treatment arm (129). In a follow-up analysis, for each standard deviation decrease in LV mass index, there was a 22% reduction in the composite cardiovascular end point predicted by blood pressure–lowering effect. Treatment with losartan decreased ECG-LVH to a greater extent than atenolol (130).

Chronic Kidney Disease

Abnormal renal function is a significant predictor of all-cause and cardiovascular mortality, cardiovascular disease, claudication, and CHF in elderly individuals. The National Kidney Foundation KDOQI Guidelines have named five stages of chronic kidney disease (CKD) (131). Risk for adverse outcomes increases notably in stage III and beyond (creatinine clearance <60 cc/min). In the Cardiovascular Health study, 11.2% of participants had an elevated serum creatinine level (≥1.3 mg/dL for women or ≥1.5 mg/dL for men) (132). In a large epidemiologic study, CKD stage III or greater was present in 7.4% of the population. Individuals with CKD were more likely to reach a composite outcome of MI, stroke, or death over 10 years of follow up than were those without CKD (30.1% versus 13.2%, respectively) (133). CKD also predicts a higher risk of mortality and bleeding following acute MI (134,135). Patients with CKD have a greater degree of subclinical cardiovascular disease, metabolic derangements, and longer exposure to risk factors (136). Patients with CKD have also been shown to have small LDL particles, hyperfibrinoginemia, homocysteinemia, increased inflammatory markers, and are often anemic (137–139).

CORONARY HEART DISEASE

The incidence of cardiovascular disease, peripheral arterial disease, stroke, and CHF all increase with age. Although not inevitable, atherosclerosis is often present and increasingly severe in the elderly. At autopsy, more than 50% of people older than the age of 50 were found to have significant stenosis of at least one coronary artery. The severity and number of stenoses increase with each age decile (140). The relationship between gender and risk for cardiovascular disease reverses past age 65. Although cardiovascular disease has a greater prevalence in men prior to this age, its prevalence in women exceeds that in men past this age (Fig. 33.5).

The classic description of symptomatic coronary artery disease is from the perspective of young white men, yet more than half of acute MIs occur past age 65 years and in women. In these groups, chest pain diminishes in favor of other ischemic symptoms, particularly dyspnea, dizziness, and fatigue. Coexisting inactivity or comorbid illness further delay recognition of ischemic symptoms or modify its character. The ECG of an elderly patient may show nonspecific changes or intraventricular conduction delays at baseline, making interpretation in the acute setting more challenging. With unclear symptoms and nondiagnostic ECGs, diagnostic testing is often the next step. When the diagnosis of CHD remains questionable, angiography should be considered. However, because atherosclerosis is apt to be present in the absence of symptomatic CHD, the coronary arteriogram may provide a false-positive result in reference to symptoms, even though it may establish a cardiac diagnosis.

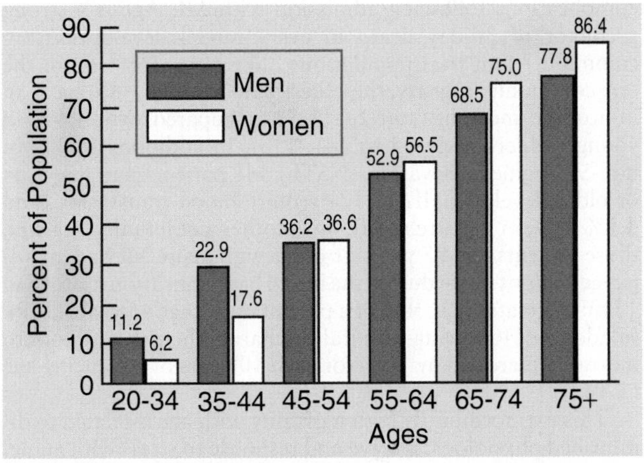

FIGURE 33.5. Prevalence of cardiovascular diseases in Americans age 20 or older by age and gender. From NHANES: 1999–2002. (*Source:* From *AHA statistical update 2004*. Available: www.amheart.org. Accessed August 18, 2005.)

Stable Angina

Stable angina is reported in 10% of people older than age 65. The diagnosis of ischemic heart disease becomes increasingly difficult as symptoms are atypical, vague, or silent. Of the 5,888 participants in the Cardiovascular Health Study, 15.3% evidenced a prior MI, and 201 (22.3%) of these were clinically unrecognized. Predictors of unrecognized or "silent" MIs include female gender, older age, absence of preceding angina, and self-assessed health as good or excellent (141). Prognosis of patients with unrecognized MIs is the same if not higher than those with recognized MIs. Therefore, detailed information on functional capacity and recent changes in activities of daily living are of importance in identifying symptoms and directing evaluation.

Noninvasive Testing

In the elderly, symptoms are the key factor in the decision to pursue testing. Exercise ECG testing is the simplest and least expensive approach (142,143). However, exercise protocols may need to be modified with regard to speed and incline. Although HR may not reach 85% predicted, increases in systolic blood pressure frequently occur, and therefore adequate HR–blood pressure product may still be achieved. The high incidence of resting ECG abnormalities in this age group lowers the sensitivity and specificity of the ECG portion of the study; however, duration of exercise is more important than ST-segment depression (144,145). Nuclear and echocardiographic imaging are often added to increase diagnostic yield. Older patients may have musculoskeletal or balance problems that limit their ability to engage in full treadmill exercise, in which case pharmacologic stress tests (dipyridamole, adenosine, and dobutamine hydrochloride) are performed.

Coronary Arteriography

Coronary arteriography is the standard for establishing the presence and extent of coronary atherosclerosis. The decision to use coronary arteriography is complicated by the high prevalence of significant coronary atherosclerosis, which makes attribution of functional or symptomatic significance challenging. In light of its limited diagnostic clarity in the elderly, angiography should primarily be undertaken to assess the suitability of coronary anatomy for revascularization. The complication rate for arteriography is not much increased in the elderly, provided that the patient is stable and has no major comorbidity that would alter their risk (146).

Revascularization

Because of the extent of disease, symptoms in the elderly may be refractory to medical therapy. Furthermore, the elderly patient may be intolerant of the dose increases in medication necessary for symptom relief. Therefore, mechanical revascularization is an attractive option when symptoms persist and limit function or quality of life. Randomized clinical trials comparing revascularization strategies have included few elderly patients, but analyses of retrospective studies provide descriptive information (147–151). Morbidity and mortality from procedures in the elderly depends greatly on case selection. In a large registry of nearly 110,000 patients, the 7,472 octogenarians undergoing coronary artery bypass grafting (CABG) had an in-hospital mortality of 3.8% compared to 1.1% in the younger patients. They also had a slightly higher rate of Q-wave MI, stroke, renal failure, and vascular complications (152). In this study, however, the mortality for octogenarians varied 10-fold depending on the presence of comorbidities (0.8%–7.2%). In a study of the Medicare database, 24,461 octogenarians who underwent isolated CAGB had a 30-day mortality of 10.5% compared to 4.3% in the cohort 65 to 80 years old (153). Another registry of 22 centers and 64,467 patients (4,306 of whom were older than 80 years), found that mortality following isolated CABG was 8.1% among octogenarians and 3% in younger patients (154). In addition to having advanced atherosclerosis, the octogenarians also had more comorbid conditions, including peripheral vascular disease, pulmonary disease, and renal disease, yet among those octogenarians without associated comorbidity, mortality following CABG was just 4.2%. However, aortic valve replacement (10.1%) and mitral valve replacement (19.6%) performed with CABG markedly increased in-hospital mortality for octogenarians. A recent analysis pooled the observational outcomes of patients aged 75 years or older who underwent revascularization with either percutaneous coronary intervention (PCI; n = 48,439) or CABG (n = 180,709) between 1990 and 1999. During this interval, the proportion of patients aged 75 years or older undergoing revascularization rose by 10%. Composite estimates for in-hospital mortality following PCI was 3.0% (range 1.5%–5.2%), and following CABG was 5.9% (range 4.9%–8.4%). Age remained a major determinant of procedural risk, along with procedural urgency, LV dysfunction, and prior CABG (155).

The heterogeneity of the aging process and competing risks makes assessment of the total patient, as well as the extent of disease, key to successful decision making and outcomes (156). Although better case selection and technical advances will undoubtedly improve mortality and morbidity, substantially higher risks will certainly persist in the elderly. It is also fair to say that the key determinant of short- and long-term outcomes is preexisting functional status, more than the extent of coronary artery disease (157,158).

ACUTE CORONARY SYNDROMES

Unstable Angina and Non–ST-Segment Elevation Myocardial Infarction

Non–ST-segment elevation MI is the most common form of myocardial infarction in the elderly, accounting for 55% of MIs in patients above age 85 but less than 40% of MIs in patients below age 65 (159). The higher proportion non–ST-segment elevation MIs in the elderly has been attributed to the higher prevalence of prior MIs, multivessel disease, hypertension, and ventricular hypertrophy, all of which contribute to increased subendocardial ischemia. With progressively older age, patients with ACS are more likely to be female; from 30% below age 65 to 62% over age 85 years (113). In addition, traditional risk factors (e.g., hypertension, diabetes, smoking, hyperlipidemia) diminish in the oldest groups compared to younger counterparts, whereas comorbidities (e.g., CHF, stroke, renal dysfunction) become increasingly common (113).

Clinical Presentation and Course

Presenting symptoms of acute MI differ in the elderly from those in younger patients. Complaints other than pain, particularly dyspnea, syncope, acute confusion, or vague constitutional symptoms, are common in the group over age 75 (160). In the Worcester Heart Attack Study, chest pain was reported in 63% of the overall population, but was reported in less than half of the women over age 75 years (45.5%). In fact, respiratory complaints (22%; dyspnea or cough) and other symptoms were more common (32%; dizziness, arm numbness, headache, syncope, sweating, palpitations, nausea, weakness, or other) (161). Dyspnea in the elderly MI patient may be due to age-related diastolic dysfunction, lung changes, or associated pulmonary disease. Neurologic symptoms, syncope, stroke, and acute confusion are likely the result of acute reduction in cardiac output in the setting of an aging central nervous system (CNS) or associated cerebrovascular disease. Dizziness may also relate to diminished autonomic responsiveness. Of course, delirium may accompany any acute illness in the elderly and may predominate as the presenting complaint. When pain is the presenting complaint, it may be atypical in character or location, and sometimes appears as an upper abdomen pain rather than a crushing or squeezing substernal sensation. Elderly patients have changes in pain perception and altered ischemic thresholds, but the exact explanation for atypical pain syndromes is not known. In addition, the ECG of older patients may demonstrate a variety of abnormalities, and enzyme elevations may be no more than minimal. ACS is also more likely to develop in elderly patients who present with another acute illness or worsening of a comorbid condition (e.g., pneumonia, chronic obstructive pulmonary disease, or hip fracture). These "secondary" coronary events occur in the setting of increased myocardial oxygen demand or hemodynamic stress in patients with underlying atherosclerotic disease.

Delay in hospital presentation is common in elderly patients with ACSs, possibly related to diminished chest pain sensation, cognitive impairment, comorbid illness, or social constraints. In the Global Registry of Acute Coronary Events (GRACE) registry, the median time from symptom onset to presentation was 2.3 hours in those under 45 years, but 3.0 hours over age 85 (159). Those with ST-segment elevation MI were more likely to present promptly than those with non–ST-segment elevation MI (median 2.3 hours versus 3.0 hours). Older and male patients, diabetics, and those with prior angina were more likely to delay, whereas patients with diaphoresis, acute heart failure, severe chest pain, or traveling by ambulance were less likely to delay (162,163). In addition, in-hospital delays in treatment persist in patients of older age and female gender (164). Atypical presentations have been shown to portend a worse prognosis with a threefold higher risk of in-hospital mortality due in part to delays in diagnosis and treatment as well as less use of evidence-based medication (13% versus 4%, $P < .001$) (165).

The elderly have a higher rate of mortality, CHF, and other complications following admission with MI. Age is a strong predictor of 30-day death in every model developed from community and trial populations alike (166–169). From the one community registry, the oldest patients (age ≥85) have an in-hospital mortality rate of 11.5% compared with 4.6% in younger elderly (age 65 to 74) (113). In addition, 16.7% of non-ST segment elevation (NSTE) MI patients age 85 years or older develop CHF, 15.7% require blood transfusion, and 4.1% have a recurrent MI. In another community registry, those patients age 85 years or older with acute MI had an adjusted odds of death during the initial hospitalization more than 15 times greater than that of a patient under age 45 years (159). In addition, following hospital discharge, the risk of 6-month mortality increases by 70% for each 10 years of advancing age (170).

This extraordinarily high mortality with age is related to diminished physiologic reserve and response to stress with aging. Diastolic dysfunction and altered baroreceptor and β-receptor responses diminish HR and increase blood pressure during the acute event; reduced lung and renal function make these organs prone to complications.

Antiplatelet and Antithrombotic Therapy

Community practice patterns continue to demonstrate a decline in the use of early and discharge cardiac medications among eligible ACS patients with advancing age (113,159). Limited randomized data coupled with lingering uncertainty regarding benefits and risks are likely modulators of this practice. The American Heart Association/American College of Cardiology (AHA/ACC) Guidelines for Unstable Angina and Non–ST-segment MI recommend antiplatelet and antithrombin therapy as evidenced by clinical trials. Recommendations are not altered by patient age, but the guidelines do state that management decisions should consider general health, comorbidities, cognitive status, and life expectancy in the elderly. In addition, altered pharmacokinetics and sensitivity to hypotensive drugs should trigger caution and observation for adverse effects (171). Aspirin's relative benefit is not affected by age; in fact its absolute benefit is greatest in populations at highest risk, such as the elderly (172). In the Clopidogrel in Unstable angina to prevent Recurrent Events (CURE) trial, the addition of clopidogrel to aspirin therapy was significantly better than placebo across all subgroups (173). Compared with younger patients, the subgroup age 65 years or more had a similar absolute (2.0% versus 2.2%) benefit with clopidogrel. From a safety perspective in the elderly, the combination of aspirin and clopidogrel increased bleeding, but is lowest when aspirin doses are under 100 mg/d (174). Relative cardiovascular benefits of the GP IIb/IIIa inhibitors have been more varied across older populations studied. Although worse outcomes are seen in some older age subgroups, similar benefits are observed in others. An age–subgroup analysis from the Platelet Glycoprotein in Unstable Angina: Receptor Suppression using Integration Therapy (PURSUIT) trial explored these issues in depth and found a reversal of the treatment effect in 500 patients aged 80 years or more, accompanied by an increase in bleeding above age 70 years (175). Although younger patients experienced benefit, eptifibatide was associated with a 5.6% absolute and 23.6% relative increase in death or MI in patients age 80 years or more, along with a 7.2% absolute and 71.3% relative increase in moderate or severe bleeding (175). Clarification of the benefit of GP IIb/IIIa inhibitors with and without revascularization and attention to dose adjustments is of great importance to the elderly.

The efficacy of antithrombin therapy may be altered by age-related changes in thrombosis and fibrinolysis (176). Observational studies have also linked advanced age with higher heparin levels and greater risk of bleeding (177). Unfractionated heparin dose is weight adjusted; however, alterations in body composition may result in overestimates of the required dose in the elderly (178). Anticoagulant activity (anti-Xa levels) of renally cleared low-molecular-weight heparins, have also been shown to be higher in the elderly (179). Subgroup data from randomized trials of antithrombin therapy regarding efficacy in patients of advanced age is lacking. Correct weight (unfractionated heparin) and renal adjustment (low-molecular-weight heparin) of antithrombin dose is also of great importance for safe use in the elderly.

Early Invasive Versus Ischemia-Guided Therapy

Despite their higher risk, community practice patterns also demonstrate a decrease in the use of cardiac catheterization among eligible elderly (113,159). Many of the randomized comparisons demonstrate a more favorable treatment effect of early invasive care among the elderly (180,181). The TACTICS-TIMI 18 trial assigned patients to early invasive or conservative treatment (182). The age subgroup analysis found that a substantial treatment effect for the reduction of death and MI persisted with the invasive strategy (183). In fact, compared with younger patients, the invasive strategy yielded a greater absolute (4.1% versus 1.0%) and relative (42.0% versus 20.4%) risk reduction in death or MI at 30 days in the subgroup aged 65 years or more, and a 10.8% absolute and 56% relative reduction in death and nonfatal MI among patients aged 75 years or older. An age–treatment interaction was significant in favor of better outcomes with invasive care over the age of 75 years ($P = .044$) (Fig. 33.6). This benefit coexisted with a threefold higher risk of major bleeding with the early invasive strategy in patients aged 75 years or older (16.6% versus 6.5%; $P = .009$). From a clinical perspective, the number needed to treat to prevent one death or MI with invasive care was 250 among those aged less than 65 years, but just 9 for those aged 75 years or more. This emphasizes that selection of patients continues to be crucial to their observed benefits. Rather than focusing on patient age or procedural risks alone, careful selection of elderly for invasive care should focus on the overall opportunity for benefit, with features indicating high cardiovascular risk (e.g., positive cardiac markers, ECG changes, CHF) all being important.

ST-Segment Elevation Myocardial Infarction

The pivotal decision and determinant of survival in the elderly with ST-segment elevation MI is reperfusion therapy early following symptom onset (thrombolytic therapy or percutaneous catheter-based intervention). Older age, however, is one of the main predictors of no reperfusion therapy. The proportion of elderly with ST-elevation MI receiving reperfusion is 65% between age 65 and 69 years, but just 20% for those age 85 years or older (184). Delay in presentation is a common problem in the elderly with acute MI (185). Because therapeutic interventions carry risks, the potential benefits of interventions in the elderly must be carefully considered and judged to be present. In addition, treatment outcomes consistent with the patients' values and wishes—although challenging to assess in an urgent situation—must also be considered. In one community registry, of the 70.5% of ST-elevation MI patients eligible for reperfusion; 8% presented more than 12 hours after symptom onset, and 12.8% had contraindications (186). However, reperfusion therapy was given to 61% (43% thrombolytic therapy, 13% direct PCI, and 6% both). Predictors of no reperfusion included age 75 years or older (OR 2.63; 95% CI 2.04–3.38), female gender, no chest pain, diabetes, CHF, prior MI, prior CABG, and treatment in teaching hospitals or those with catheterization laboratories (186). In a large Medicare analysis, only 23.2% of eligible elderly patients with ST-elevation acute MI received thrombolysis within 6 hours of arrival, and only 2.5% underwent primary angioplasty (187). Elderly patients often do not meet standard eligibility criteria for reperfusion therapy for ST-segment elevation MI (e.g., ST-segment elevation, arrival within 6 hours of the event, and no contraindications). In one study, 10% of patients older than age 75 met eligibility criteria because the rest lacked ST-segment elevation or had late arrival (188). An analysis of very elderly patients with ST-elevation MI (age $\geq$89 years), found that 60% presented more than 9 hours after symptom onset, 22% refused or had a clinical exclusion to thrombolysis, and 8% had no chest pain (189).

Clinical Presentation and Course

The elderly are less likely to present with chest pain and more likely to have ECGs demonstrating preexisting conduction disease. Right or left bundle branch block occurs in 5% to 10%

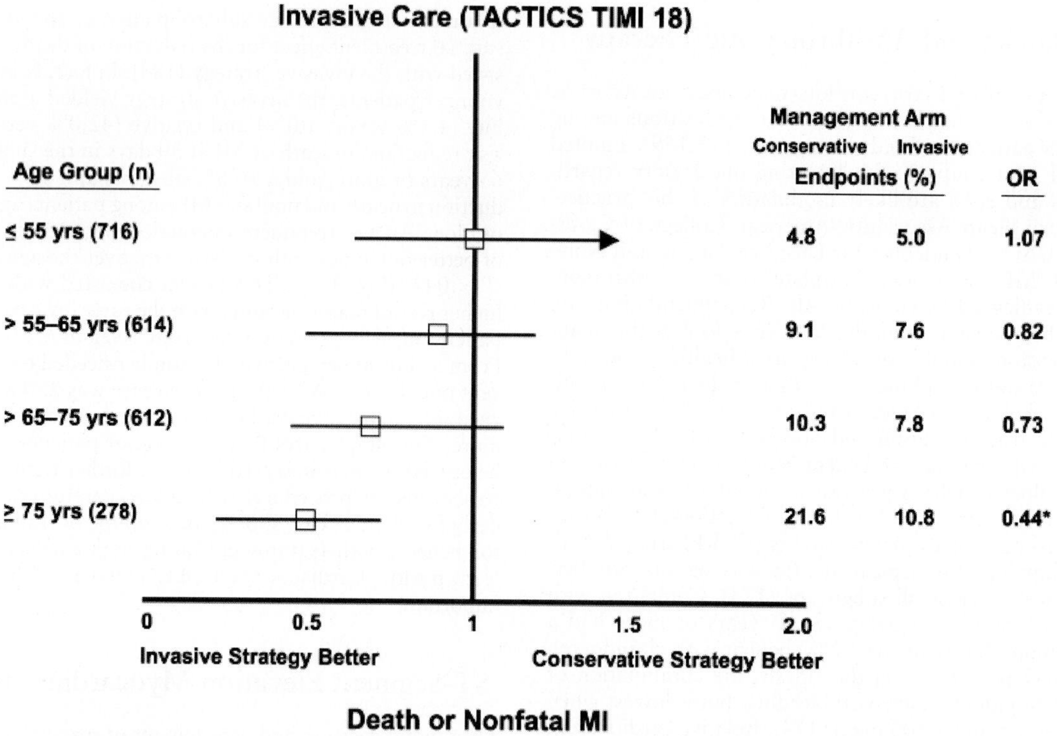

FIGURE 33.6. Benefit of Early Invasive Strategy by Age in the TACTICS-TIMI 18 Trial. Event rates and adjusted OR of death or MI shown for an early invasive vs. conservative strategy. (*Source:* Adapted from Bach RG, Cannon CP, Weintraub WS, et al. The effect of routine, early invasive management on outcome for elderly patients with non–ST-segment elevation acute coronary syndromes. *Ann Intern Med* 2004;141:186–195.)

of AMI cases overall and is more common in the elderly. In 29,585 acute MI patients with left bundle branch block in the Second National Registry of Myocardial Infarction, mean age was 76.4 years (190). As expected, only 8.4% of this high-risk group of acute MI patients were given reperfusion therapy, in part because only 50% had chest pain, and their mortality was high (22%). Elderly hospital survivors of ST-segment elevation MI have an extremely high 1-year mortality, in the range of 30% to 40%, with most deaths occurring in the first 30 days. By far, the most common adverse outcome is death at 30 days, which increases 10-fold between age under 65 and age 85 years or more (Fig. 33.7). Mortality is increased in the setting of cardiogenic shock, LV dysfunction, right ventricular infarction, residual myocardial ischemia, or ventricular arrhythmias (191–193).

Fibrinolytic Therapy

Elderly patients are underrepresented in fibrinolytic trials because of explicit age exclusions, in addition to absence of inclusion criteria (194–198). The greatest concern with fibrinolytic therapy in the elderly is the increased risk of intracranial hemorrhage, thought due to weakened cerebrovascular integrity, prior ischemic events, or amyloid angiopathy. Large, randomized, controlled trials and case-control studies all demonstrate a higher risk of cerebral hemorrhage in the elderly with tissue-type plasminogen activator (t-PA) than with streptokinase treatment (199–201). Although risks from fibrinolytic therapy are increased in the elderly, risks from untreated MI remain higher. For this reason, most studies document equal, if not greater, benefits from fibrinolytic therapy in the elderly compared with younger patients (187,202). The rate of hemorrhagic stroke with fibrinolytic therapy, even in those age 85 years or older, is diminutive (1.7%) compared to risk of 30-day mortality (30.3%) (166). The small rate of hemorrhagic events must be weighed against the mortality reduction possible with fibrinolytic therapy. However, although reperfusion therapy is favorable regardless of age, small sample size results in less certainty of benefit for those aged over 85 years.

In the Fibrinolytic Therapy Trialists' overview of randomized fibrinolytic trials, the greatest absolute benefit of fibrinolytic therapy was seen in patients older than age 75 (194). Particularly, a 26% RR in mortality in patients under 55 years of age yielded 11 lives saved per thousand treated, whereas a 15% RR in mortality in patients 75 years or older yielded 34 lives saved (194). Observational studies from the Cooperative Cardiovascular Project by two different groups of investigators had different patient selection and methodologies but raise concerns about safety of thrombolysis in the elderly. The first study evaluated 15,940 patients age 65 or older who received fibrinolytic therapy or primary PCI (187). Patients who underwent reperfusion had lower 1-year mortality than those who did not undergo reperfusion. The second study evaluated 7,864 patients who received thrombolytic therapy (203). A survival benefit with thrombolytic therapy was seen in younger patients, but a disadvantage was seen in patients aged 76 to 86 years. Two other observational studies also found that the benefit from thrombolytic therapy in younger patient groups did not extend to the extremes of age (>80 years and ≥85 years, respectively) (204,205). In a group of very elderly patients with ST-elevation MI (age ≥89 years), those receiving thrombolytic therapy had a 44% mortality rate, largely owing to myocardial rupture. In this population, those who were admitted to a cardiac care unit but given no reperfusion, and those undergoing primary angioplasty, did equally well (189). Hence, concerns persist in observational data that very elderly patients may experience short-term adverse effects from thrombolytic

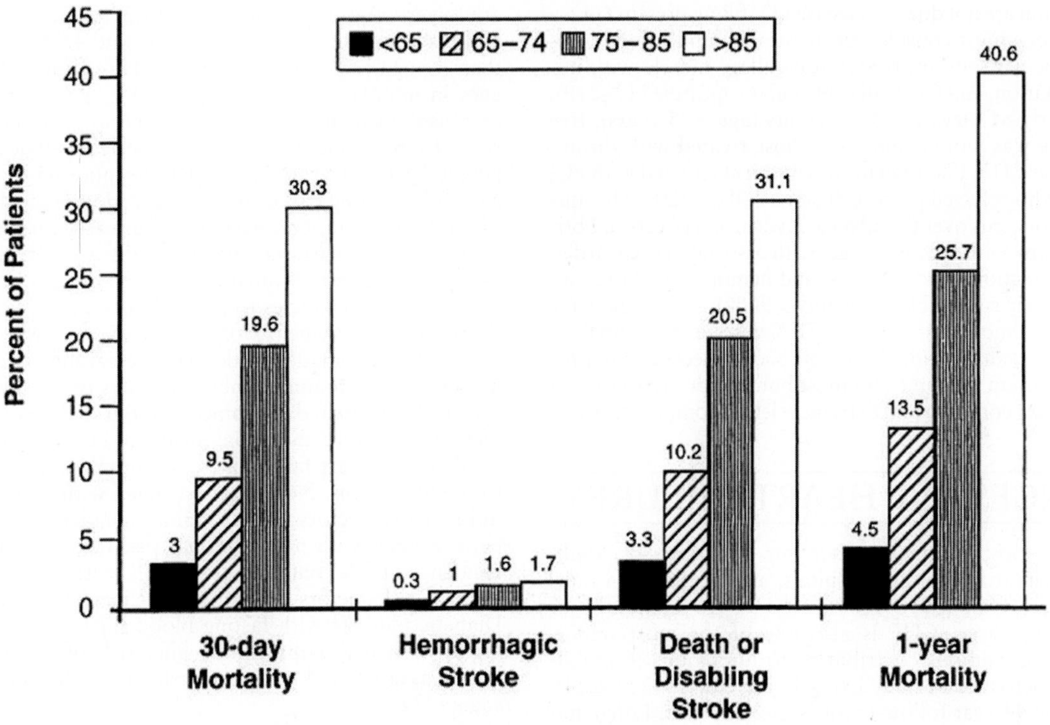

FIGURE 33.7. Profound effects of age on mortality and stroke in a very large sample of 41,021 patients from the GUSTO-I trial (95). Of the total, 24,708 were under age 65; 11,201 were 65 to 74; 4,625 were 75 to 85; and 412 were older than 85 years. All patients had ST-segment elevation and were treated with thrombolytic agents. Postdischarge 1-year mortality remained high in the oldest group (6.1% and 10.3%) and continued to be low (1.5%) in the under-65 group. (*Source:* From White HD, Barbash GI, Califf RM, et al. Age and outcome with contemporary thrombolytic therapy: results from the GUSTO-I trial. *Circulation* 1996;94:1826–1833, with permission.)

therapy sufficient to counterbalance benefits. Nevertheless, in a long-term observational cohort of 6,891 ST-elevation MI patients aged 75 years or older, those who received thrombolytic therapy ($n = 3{,}897$) still had a 13% relative advantage in death and cerebral bleeding complications at 1 year compared with those who received no therapy (206). In fact, the updated AHA/ACC guidelines no longer classify thrombolytic therapy recommendations for ST elevation or left bundle branch block within 12 hours of onset differently on the basis of patient age (previously class Ia indication age <75, class IIa indication age ≥75) (207).

Primary Percutaneous Coronary Interventions

Primary angioplasty is particularly appealing for the elderly because it can be applied without ST-segment elevation or chest pain, and is preferable in the setting of hypotension or shock. Pooled analyses of randomized controlled trials of PCI versus fibrinolytic therapy find a general mortality advantage in patients assigned to angioplasty, with a lower cerebral complication rate (208). In the Primary Angioplasty in Myocardial Infarction (PAMI) study, there was a lower rate of recurrent MI and death in elderly patients (age ≥65 years) who underwent angioplasty compared with those who received fibrinolytic therapy (209). The Global Use of Strategies to Open Occluded Coronary Arteries in Acute Coronary Syndromes–IIb (GUSTO IIb) trial also showed trends to lower 30-day mortality with primary PCI among patients age 70 years or older (210). The Primary Coronary Angioplasty Trialist's investigators studied 2,635 patients enrolled in 10 randomized trials of primary angioplasty versus fibrinolysis (211). They found that among patients 70 years of age or older, primary angioplasty was more effective than fibrinolysis in reducing 30-day mortality. Relative Risk (RR) reductions were similar across age, but 23 patients needed to be treated with angioplasty over fibrinolytic therapy below age 60 compared with only 8 patients over age 70 (212).

Observational data from National Registry of Myocardial Infarction also suggests that primary PCI yields more favorable outcomes than fibrinolytic therapy (213). Among patients older than 75 years, mortality was 16.5% in the t-PA group and 14.4% in those undergoing PCI. Combined rates of mortality or disabling stroke were 18.4% in the t-PA group and 14.6% in those undergoing PCI. Among 20,683 patients who received reperfusion therapy in the Cooperative Cardiovascular Project database, primary PCI was also associated with modest short- and long-term mortality benefits compared to fibrinolytic therapy (187). Therefore, PCI remains a preferable alternative to fibrinolytic therapy in elderly patients with acute MI if performed in a timely fashion. The decision to use PCI, fibrinolytic therapy, or neither—particularly in patients older than the age of 75—remains a highly individualized decision.

Cardiac Rupture and Cardiogenic Shock

The catastrophic complications of ST-elevation MI are more frequent in the elderly, specifically free wall rupture and cardiogenic shock. These risks mirror age-related fundamental changes in cardiac anatomy (214). The outcome for patients age 75 or older with shock is poor, and revascularization has an adverse effect compared with medical therapy in this population (215,216). In addition to confirming that hypotension and hypoperfusion are not due to decreased LV filling pressure or arrhythmias, one must consider mechanical complications (ruptured ventricular septum, ruptured papillary muscle with mitral regurgitation, and free wall ventricular rupture) (217–219). In 706 elderly ST-elevation MI patients (age ≥75 years), free wall rupture was more common in those treated with thrombolytic therapy (17.1%) than in either patients treated with PCI (4.9%) or who received no reperfusion (7.9%) (220). This further raises concerns over the adverse myocardial effects of fibrinolytic therapy with advanced age, with associated myocardial edema, contraction band necrosis, and hemorrhage. Free wall rupture is rarely survivable (mortality >90%), and cardiogenic shock carries a mortality of at least 50% despite optimum therapy. Therefore, an individualized approach is necessary to provide the optimum outcome and most humanistic alternative in these relatively common and extremely lethal complications.

CONGESTIVE HEART FAILURE

CHF is the most common reason for admission of Medicare recipients to acute care hospitals, and readmission rates are extremely high (30%–50%) within 3 to 6 months of the initial discharge. CHF is also one of the most important chronic conditions contributing to limitations in mobility and the activities of daily living in the elderly (221–224). Based on the 44-year follow-up of National Heart, Lung, and Blood Institute's Framingham Health Study, CHF incidence approaches 10/1,000 after the age of 65. In a study conducted in Minnesota, 5.6% had moderate to severe diastolic dysfunction and normal ejection fraction (EF). Prevalence of systolic dysfunction was 6%, and moderate or severe systolic dysfunction was present in 2%. Clinical CHF was more common among those with systolic or diastolic dysfunction as compared to those with normal ventricular function, but even in those with moderate to severe systolic or diastolic function, less than half had been diagnosed with CHF. Heart failure with preserved systolic function occurs in at least 30% to 40% of elderly patients, and at even higher rates in the oldest of old (225,226) (Fig. 33.8).

Age is a powerful risk factor for the development of CHF. The annual rates per thousand of new and recurrent CHF events in the population increase with advancing age (65–74 years, 75–84 years, and ≥85 years) (see Fig. 33.8). These rates are lower in nonblack women at 11.2%, 26.3%, and 64.9%, and black women at 18.9%, 33.5%, and 48.4%, respectively, than in men (227). There is more CHF diagnosed at younger ages in nonblack men, namely, 21.5%, 43.3%, and 73.1%, and black men, at 21.1%, 52%, and 66.7%, respectively. The risk of developing heart failure was nearly twice as high in people 75 to 85 years of age than in those 65 to 74 years of age. Other strong risk factors associated with the development of CHF are LVH, coronary artery disease, cardiomegaly, reduced vital capacity, valvular heart disease, elevated baseline body mass index, elevated pulse pressure, MI, and diabetes mellitus (223). Diabetes is a particularly strong risk factor for heart failure in women. Women with diabetes who had an elevated body mass index or depressed creatinine clearance were highest risk with annual incidence rates of 7% and 13%, respectively, compared to women without diabetes or other risk factors, who have an annual incidence rate of just 0.4%. The incidence of heart failure increases in proportion to risk factor combinations. Nondiabetic women with at least three additional risk factors had an annual incidence of 3.4%, diabetic women with no additional risk factors had an annual incidence of 3%, but diabetic women with three or more additional risk factors had an annual incidence rate of 8.2%. Diabetic patients with fasting blood sugars greater than 300 mg/dL also had a threefold higher risk of developing heart failure as compared to diabetic patients with controlled blood sugars (228).

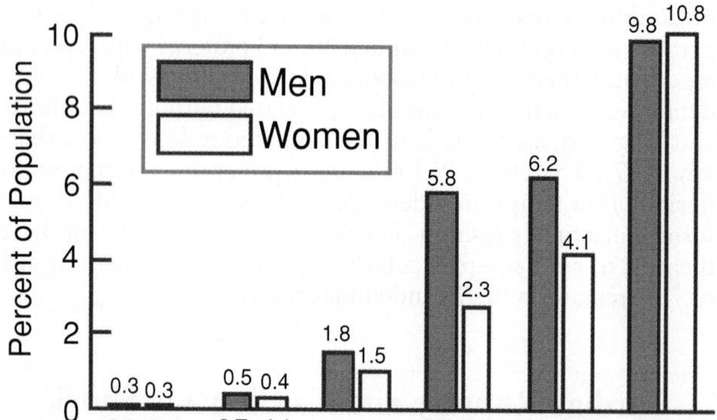

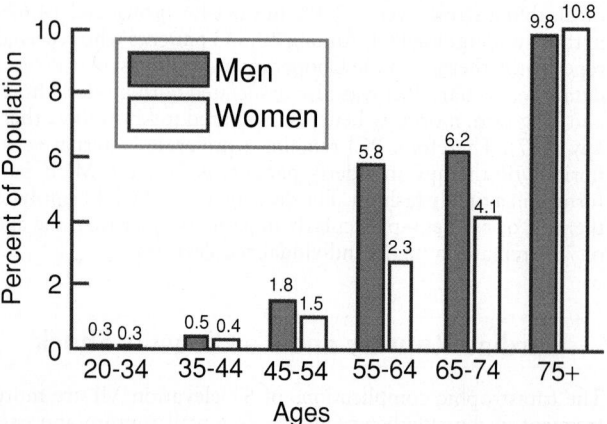

FIGURE 33.8. Prevalence of congestive heart failure by age and gender. Data from NHANES 1999–2002. The prevalence of CHF rises significantly with patient age, and is common in both men and women over the age of 75 years. (From *AHA heart statistics 2005*. Available: www.americanheart.org.)

Pathophysiology

CHF is a syndrome with diverse causes despite its well-known signs and symptoms. The unifying pathophysiology is best described as an inability of the heart to adequately supply the oxygenation and metabolic needs of the body at normal intracardiac filling pressures, sometimes at rest, but especially with exercise (229–231). The syndrome may result from systolic or diastolic myocardial dysfunction, abnormal loading conditions, valvular disease, arrhythmias, or hypertension (all common conditions in the elderly). Rarely, a restrictive process, such as pericarditis, is responsible. In fact, the etiology of CHF in the elderly is often multifactorial and pulmonary edema has been noted in patients with EFs across the spectrum from less than 10% to more than 55% (Fig. 33.9). Furthermore, in any individual patient, congestion may or may not be present, so the term *heart failure* is more encompassing and accurate than *congestive heart failure*.

Regardless of the precipitating cause, age-related changes in the cardiovascular system contribute to CHF and complicate its diagnosis and treatment (232). This is particularly true for older patients with CHF and preserved systolic function (225,227,233–236). First, amyloid deposits may worsen diastolic dysfunction. Diastolic dysfunction coupled with CHD is particularly devastating because myocardial ischemia worsens diastolic function and can produce sudden, dramatic increases in LV filling pressure and pulmonary venous pressure. Atrial fibrillation also produces a substantial increase in LV filling pressure, which may result in pulmonary congestion and heart failure (237). The contribution of atrial contraction in maintaining a low LV filling pressure is especially important when diastolic dysfunction is present (229,234,236). Current concepts regarding the decompensation of chronic heart failure include the importance of transient elevation in blood pressure. Recent studies have suggested that blood pressure can reach systolic levels as high as 200 mm Hg in the prehospital period, resulting in acute diastolic dysfunction even in the setting of low EF and pulmonary edema (238). Additionally, as many as 20% to 30% of patients with CHF decompensation have elevations in markers of myocardial injury suggesting ischemia may

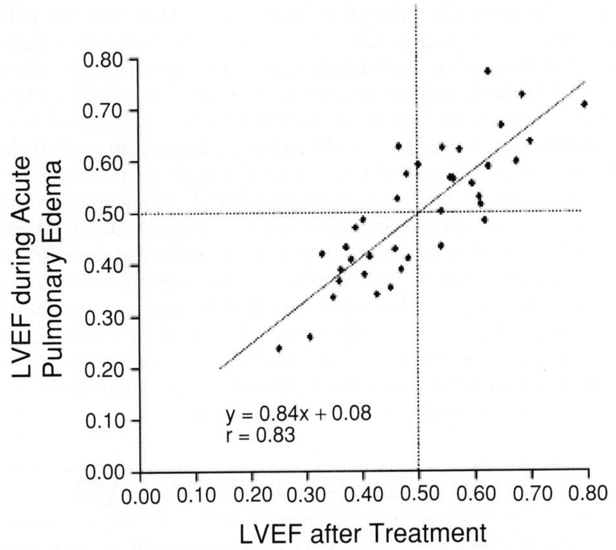

FIGURE 33.9. Changes in EF during recovery from pulmonary edema. The LVEF during acute pulmonary edema and following treatment are correlated and span the spectrum of EF. *Abbreviation:* LVEF, left ventricular ejection fraction. (*Source:* Adapted from Gandhi SK, Powers JC, Nomeir AM, et al. The pathogenesis of acute pulmonary edema associated with hypertension. *N Engl JMed* 2001;344:17–22.)

contribute to the pathophysiology of acute decompensation (239).

Clinical Presentation and Diagnosis

As is true for all cardiovascular syndromes in the elderly, the diagnosis of heart failure can be challenging. The usual symptoms of dyspnea, cough, paroxysmal nocturnal dyspnea, and orthopnea may be present, but other symptoms often predominate (230). Nonspecific complaints such as weakness, fatigue, anorexia, or subtle deterioration in CNS function presenting as somnolence, confusion, or disorientation may confuse the diagnosis. Objective data are therefore valuable because the pathophysiology of heart failure in the elderly is complex. ECG and chest radiography are always useful, but echocardiography is the most valuable imaging technique because it determines both LV systolic and diastolic function. In addition, the echocardiogram can precisely define valvular abnormalities, and give clues to rare abnormalities that occur in the elderly, such as amyloid infiltration. Additional imaging modalities such as cardiac magnetic resonance imaging and multislice computed tomography scan provide a less invasive approach for determining the presence or absence of coronary artery disease. Cardiac magnetic resonance imaging, with its ability to perform tissue characterization, can help to distinguish among the several different etiologies of heart failure, such as iron overload, amyloid, or ischemic etiologies (240).

The difficulties in diagnosing heart failure in elderly patients have led to an interest in the use of neurohormonal markers as well as for diagnosis and to assess prognosis. One of the more widely studied markers is brain (B-type) natrietic peptide (BNP) (241–244). The routine use of BNP is now part of the ACC/AHA guidelines in the diagnosis of patients with unexplained dyspnea. However, the determination and understanding of BNP in the elderly is challenging. The available assays are altered by age and compromised renal function. Whereas a level of 500 ng/dL would clearly be abnormal in a population less than 55 years of age, it may be normal in an elderly population.

Mortality and Morbidity

The prognosis for elderly patients with CHF varies greatly (1-year mortality rates from <10% to >50%), depending on the cause of their CHF, their age, presence of atrial fibrillation, and presence of comorbidities (225,233,245–247). The 2001 overall death rate for heart failure was 18.7%; 19.6% for white men, 21.7% for black men, 18.1% for white women, and 18.8% for black women. Fortunately, a community-based study conducted in Olmstead County, Minnesota, showed that although the incidence of heart failure has not declined, survival has improved over the past two decades. Yet, the absolute number of deaths from CHF has also increased by 35.3% between 1999 and 2002 owing to improvements in AMI care and the aging population. In addition, these improvements in survival have been more limited among women and the elderly (248). Patients with primarily diastolic dysfunction tend to fare better than those with principally systolic dysfunction or a combination of the two. Female gender and diabetes worsen prognosis (249). In randomized trials, the oldest patients tend to benefit most from therapy because their mortality rate is much higher (247), but mortality and morbidity remain at high levels despite this therapy benefit. The OPTIMIZE Registry of acute decompensated heart failure demonstrates two important points. First, elderly patients receive evidence-based therapies, such as β-blockers, ACE inhibitors, and spironolactone, less often than younger cohorts. Second, their short-term mortality is markedly increased independently from treatment factors based on age. The associated comorbidities that the elderly carry also increase their risk for short-term mortality.

Not only is heart failure a condition associated with high mortality, but also with high morbidity. Hospital discharges for heart failure increased by 150% between 1979 and 2002. Heart failure carries an in-hospital mortality rate of 3% to 4%, a 3-month mortality of 10%, and a 20% to 30% risk of rehospitalization at 3 months (250–252). The cost of heart failure is staggering, with a $27.9 billion dollar price tag for direct and indirect costs of heart failure in the United States in 2005 (AAA Factbook).

Management of Heart Failure

As mentioned, randomized controlled trials of CHF that define treatment provide limited insight with regard to older patients (253–259). In addition, older patients included in trials do not reflect the typical older patient. The Acute Decompensated Heart Failure National Registry enrolled more than 150,000 patients, and the OPTIMIZE Registry more than 35,000 patients (260). Although randomized, controlled clinical trials of therapies in heart failure enrolled patients in their 60s, these registries had a median age of over 70 years. Careful assessment of pathophysiology is the key to appropriate management. Calcific aortic stenosis, CHD, hypertension, or diastolic dysfunction—or some combination of these disorders—may be simultaneously present, emphasizing the importance of individualized evaluation and the complexity of treatment.

Systolic Heart Failure

In elderly patients, systolic dysfunction is treated the same as in younger cohorts, with allowances made for the comorbidities and altered pharmacology of aging. ACE inhibitor and β-blocker therapy remain the cornerstone of treatment for heart failure in the elderly. Although intolerance to ACE inhibitors is higher than initially thought, particularly among the elderly, angiotensin receptor blockers are an acceptable alternative to

ACE-inhibitor therapy. β-Blocker therapy has also shown consistent evidence of benefit in the elderly (261,262). The Study of the Effects of Nebivolol Intervention on Outcomes and Rehospitalization in Seniors with Heart Failure (SENIORS) trial suggested that heart failure patients should be given β-blockade regardless of age. In this study, 2,128 elderly CHF patients ($\geq$70 years) were randomized to nebivolol or placebo and followed for a primary endpoint of all-cause mortality and hospital admission. Nebivolol significantly reduced the endpoint by 14% ($P = .039$). All-cause mortality was reduced by 12% but did not reach statistical significance. The results did not vary by LVEF (<35 or $\geq$35), age (<75 years or $\geq$75 years), or gender subgroups who all received similar end point reductions with nebivolol. Thus, the results suggest that β-blockers are effective in the elderly and those with preserved systolic function (263). In addition, a metaanalysis of 12,729 patients in five trials of CHF, the elderly showed a similar reduction in mortality on β-blockers as nonelderly patient (RR = 0.76 [0.64–0.90] for the elderly versus RR = 0.66 [0.52–0.85] for the nonelderly) (264). Recent data from Cardiac Insufficiency Bisoprolol Study-III (CIBIS-III) trial suggest that there is a slight advantage with respect to clinical outcomes if β-blocker therapy is initiated prior to ACE inhibition. The risks and benefits of additional comorbidities in these patients should be assessed to determine which agents should be added next. Diuretics are the cornerstone for controlling congestive symptoms. Digitalis preparations are of limited value in systolic and diastolic heart failure (265), but are still used for refractory symptoms with careful dosing in the elderly (15). Digitalis preparations have been useful in controlling the ventricular rate in atrial fibrillation, but age-related atrioventricular nodal dysfunction often limits ventricular response anyway in the elderly. Recent data from the Digitalis Investigation Group (DIG) study suggest that digitalis levels below 1.0 may improve survival and reduce heart failure hospitalization, particularly in the New York Heart Association class III population (266).

Device therapy with biventricular pacemakers and implantable cardioverter defibrillators are now a class Ia recommendation in appropriate patients. However, given the cost of the device, therapy in the elderly should be reserved for those who are expected to have some reasonable residual life expectancy and no overwhelming life– or quality-of-life–limiting comorbidities.

Diastolic Heart Failure

When diastolic heart failure is the primary problem, pulmonary congestion can be relieved by diuresis. The steep diastolic pressure–volume relationship indicates that even a modest decrease in circulating blood volume can markedly reduce LV filling pressure, resulting in hypotension, fatigue, and reduced renal perfusion. Hence, the use of diuretics requires individualized decisions with regard to dosage and duration of treatment. Diastolic heart failure remains one of the important areas of investigation in the elderly. Four randomized control clinical trials have been conducted in elderly patients with diastolic heart failure. In the CHARM-Preserve Study in which the angiotensin receptor blocker candesartan was used in patients with preserved systolic function with an LVEF less than 40%, showed a strong trend toward improvement in CHF hospitalization or cardiovascular death. This trend, when adjusted for baseline differences proved to be important, although did not reach statistical significance, perhaps because of the high rate of death from noncardiac causes in this population. The ongoing Irbesartan in Heart Failure with Preserved Systolic Function study has completed enrollment of over 4,500 patients with a mean age of 71 years, and will provide additional information regarding the value of irbesartan in elderly patients with diastolic heart failure (267). As stated, the SENIORS study demonstrated that the β-blocker nebevilol afforded a trend toward clinical benefit in patients with preserved or mild LV systolic dysfunction. Finally, an National Heart, Lung, and Blood Institute–sponsored trial of aldosterone antagonism in diastolic heart failure is expected to have results in the next 5 years.

Diastolic dysfunction with impaired LV filling may be improved by the use of β-blockers and calcium channel blockers, which may enhance compliance and also reduce atrioventricular node conduction. ACE inhibitors are probably valuable for most patients with diastolic dysfunction because the nonhemodynamic effects of these drugs may be useful in reducing the collagen deposition of diastolic heart disease and because most elderly patients have an element of systolic, as well as diastolic, dysfunction related to systolic hypertension.

VALVULAR HEART DISEASE

Systolic murmurs are extremely common in elderly patients, with a prevalence of 60% or greater. Most murmurs do not carry important clinical implications and are the result of age-related aortic valve thickening and sclerosis or minor mitral regurgitation secondary to papillary muscle dysfunction caused by CHD, hypertensive or idiopathic cardiomyopathy, or age-related mitral valve changes (268). The primary valvular heart disease among patients ages 26 to 84 is aortic valve disease, which accounts for the majority of morbidity and mortality. In 2002, an estimated 93,000 valve procedures were performed in the United States (269).

Senile Calcific Aortic Stenosis

Aortic valve disease is the most common valvular heart disease in the elderly. The murmur of aortic stenosis is present in about 50% of patients over the age of 75. A Finnish epidemiologic study in patients aged more than 55 years demonstrated a progressive increase in the degree of aortic valve calcification and stenosis with age (270). In the group aged 55 to 71 years, only 7% had severe calcification, whereas 19% had severe calcification in the group older than 85 years. In addition, 13.7% of this over-85 age group had an aortic valve area less than 1 cm^2, and 4% had a valve area less than 0.6 cm^2 (Table 33.4).

TABLE 33.4

HELSINKI AGING STUDY: AORTIC VALVE AREA AND AGE

	Age group (y)		
Aortic valve area (cm 2)	75–76 (n = 197)	80–81 (n = 155)	85–86 (n = 124)
≤1.2	2.5%	3.9%	8.1%
<1.0	2.6%	2.6%	8.1%
<0.8	0.5%	2.6%	5.6%
<0.6	None	1.9%	3.2%
<0.4	None	None	0.8%

Note: Critical as +2.9; moderate as +4.8.
Source: From Lindroos M, Kupari M, Heikkila J, et al. Prevalence of aortic valve abnormalities in the elderly: an echocardiographic study of a random population sample. *J Am Coll Cardiol* 1993;21: 1220–1225.

Age-related changes in the aortic ring may result in a systolic murmur that must be differentiated from aortic valve stenosis. Although congenital bicuspid aortic valve is the most frequent cause of calcific aortic stenosis into the sixth decade (271), by age 70 age-related changes are responsible for stenosis. Early fibrotic changes in the valve apparatus are followed by calcium deposition resulting in cuspal stiffness (272). Calcium deposits do not involve or compromise the commissures, which distinguishes senile stenosis from rheumatic and congenital lesions. Calcific deposits reduce cuspal mobility and heavy deposits immobilize cusps with resultant stenosis. The loss of collagen fibrils, development of fatty changes, and calcification may also result in annuloaortic ectasia and sometimes mild or moderate aortic regurgitation.

The clinical diagnosis of senile calcific aortic stenosis can be difficult. The murmur of significant senile calcific aortic stenosis may not be prominent. However a diminished aortic second sound is virtually always present because of the restricted movement and heavy calcification. A high level of suspicion and a careful search for physical findings is needed. It should be considered in all elderly patients with angina, dyspnea, or subtle CNS symptoms, and echocardiography should be performed if doubt exists. Doppler echocardiography is the ideal approach to assess systolic murmurs and follow the course of senile aortic stenosis. Because of age-dependent lessening of compensatory hypertrophy, LVH may not be as great in elderly patients (273).

Management of senile calcific aortic stenosis is similar to the management of calcific aortic stenosis in younger patients, but is more complicated because of the frequent presence of associated atherosclerotic disease and comorbidities. Patients with a significant gradient and symptoms of angina, syncope, or CHF should be considered for surgery. In addition, those who are undergoing CABG with moderate or greater aortic stenosis, or with significant LV dysfunction should be considered for valve surgery; however, operative mortality and morbidity are considerably higher in older patients. The operative risk increases from 5% in the young old (age 65–75) to greater than 13% in those older than 85. CABG or mitral valve surgery doubles the risk. The decision to operate is therefore determined by cardiac factors as well as the physical and cognitive function, nutritional status, and other individual comorbidities. Valve selection is also important in the elderly. Those patients who are good candidates for warfarin and are expected to live 10 years should be considered for a mechanical valve. The guidelines make a strong case that once the patient reaches the age of 65 the risks associated with mechanical valves and the exposure to anticoagulation exceed the risk of tissue valves wearing out.

As in younger patients, postponing valve replacement until the appearance of major symptoms of aortic stenosis—CHF, angina, and syncope (or equivalent symptoms)—is usually appropriate, but interpreting these symptoms in elderly patients can be very difficult. Angina may be more related to CHD; CHF to hypertensive disease or diastolic dysfunction; and syncope to conduction-system disease, arrhythmias, or cerebral vascular disease. When symptoms are clear and mean gradient is more than moderate (>50 mm Hg), the decision to proceed with valve replacement is more straightforward. Even if associated CHD and important comorbidities are present, the decision is justified if the patient wishes to proceed, with the understanding that mortality is high (up to 50% in the oldest patients) during the following 3 or 4 years (274).

Aortic Regurgitation

Aortic regurgitation is much less common than aortic stenosis in the elderly and is usually the result of hypertension, valvular deformity, or changes in the aortic root. Occasionally, it results from a variety of other causes like infectious endocarditis, Marfan syndrome, ankylosing spondylitis, or collagen vascular diseases (275). For aortic regurgitation in the elderly to be severe enough to justify surgery is unusual; aortic regurgitation secondary to dissection and endocarditis are the exceptions. As with all valvular disease, echocardiography allows a precise determination of cause and severity, as well as an estimate of LV function. Classic clinical findings of severe aortic regurgitation include widened pulse pressure, peripheral findings, and a diastolic murmur, but these may be altered in the elderly because of associated conditions. In addition, the regurgitant murmur may be difficult to hear because of associated pulmonary disease or high LV end-diastolic pressure.

Because LV dysfunction can occur in the absence of symptoms, operation to correct severe aortic regurgitation is often recommended before the development of symptoms. A variety of clinical predictions have been developed to aid this decision to perform surgery and use LVEF and end-systolic dimension criteria (276). When the EF is under 55% or the LV end-systolic dimension is greater than 55 mm Hg, or both, aortic valve surgery should be performed, because waiting may result in increased mortality and poorer outcomes. In elderly patients, particularly those older than the age of 75, postponing surgery in this situation also seems reasonable, because the risk of surgery and long-term outcomes are not well characterized. Medical therapy with afterload reduction is a reasonable alternative in older patients. In younger patients, nifedipine therapy has been shown to postpone and reduce the need for surgery in a randomized, controlled trial (277), and afterload reduction using ACE inhibition is strongly suspected to be the treatment of choice in the elderly (278).

Mitral Regurgitation

Mitral regurgitation is common in the elderly but usually is mild, representing an incidental finding unlikely to ever require medical or surgical therapy. However, in a substantial minority of the elderly with mitral regurgitation, the degree of regurgitation poses a dilemma in regard to its importance in the patient's syndrome. Age-related changes in the mitral valve and degenerative changes in the fibrous ring are characterized by fragmentation and disorganization of elastic and collagen fibers, and deposition of lipids and calcium. Severe calcification of the mitral ring may immobilize the posterior mitral leaflet, and results in moderate mitral regurgitation. Extensive calcific deposits in the mitral ring may affect the conduction system and produce heart block, ulcerate and embolize, or become the site of infectious endocarditis (Fig. 33.10). Mitral annular calcification occurs almost exclusively among the elderly (279). Mitral regurgitation that occurs with mitral valve prolapse (MVP) is rare in older persons. A minority of patients with MVP have progressive regurgitation, and in older age a few experience spontaneous chordal rupture with marked mitral regurgitation (280,281). MVP with myxomatous degeneration of the mitral valve is an increasingly common indication for mitral valve replacement in older patients (282). In a report of 266 patients undergoing mitral valve surgery for severe mitral regurgitation (mean age, 64 years), slightly over 60% had MVP. The underlying morphologic changes (expansion of the leaflets, stretching and thinning of the chordae tendineae, and increased mucopolysaccharides in the spongiosa layer of the leaflets) are similar to those observed in younger patients but are more extensive, which makes mitral valve repair less likely (282).

The threshold for the use of afterload-reducing agents, particularly ACE inhibitors, should be low in elderly patients with

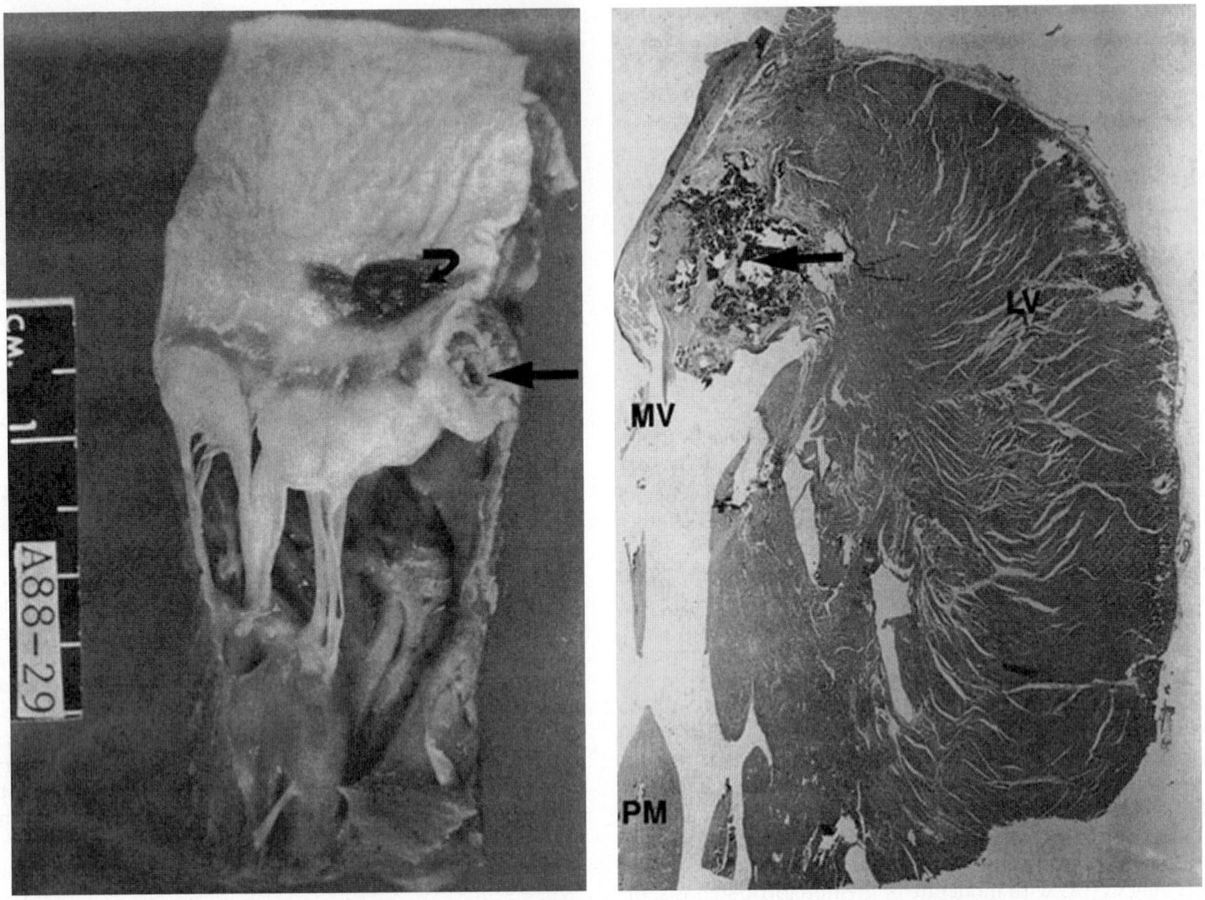

A B

FIGURE 33.10. Age-related changes in the mitral valve (MV) apparatus. (**A**) Longitudinal section of the posterior wall of the left atrium, posterior mitral leaflet, and posterior LV wall. Note massive calcification of the mitral annulus (*straight arrow*) and the ulceration through the atrial endocardium. The latter is covered by a thrombus (*curved arrow*). (**B**) Microscopic longitudinal section of posterior LV wall, posterior mitral leaflet, and posteromedial papillary muscle (PM). Massive calcification of the mitral annulus (*arrow*) is apparent, extending also into the adjacent myocardium. (*Source:* From Kitzman DW, Scholz DG, Hagen PT, et al. Age-related changes in normal human hearts during the first 10 decades of life. Part II (maturity): a quantitative anatomic study of 765 specimens from subjects 20 to 99 years old. *Mayo Clin Proc* 1988;63:137–146, with permission.)

regurgitant lesions, particularly because of associated hypertension and CHD. In well-compensated moderate-to-severe mitral regurgitation, the LVEF should be normal and should not affect the use of afterload-reducing agents. Watchful waiting, use of afterload-reducing agents, and serial echocardiography are key to monitoring patients prior to surgical intervention. The indications for mitral valve surgery in the elderly are similar to those in the young, with greater emphasis on symptom relief. In mitral regurgitation, pump function can be maintained in the normal range while contractility is deteriorating. The LV end-systolic pressure–volume relationship provides a conceptual framework to allow differentiation of muscle dysfunction and pump function. A variety of indices have been developed relating preoperative LV echocardiographic dimension to allow prediction of postoperative EF, which is the most important determinant of long-term outcome. One popular algorithm calls for operating when the LV end-systolic dimension is greater than 45 mm (282,283). The elderly have shortened life expectancy, increased mortality, and increased complication rate after valve surgery, so decisions must be highly individualized. Biologic valves, subject to degeneration and calcification in younger patients, are frequently the valves of choice in older individuals, in whom prosthesis longevity is increased (284). Mitral valve repair instead of replacement is effective and popular, and is always desirable when feasible. Preserving the valve, and particularly the valvular apparatus including the papillary muscles, lessens postoperative complications and greatly improves long-term outcome, and should always be encouraged; however, it is not always possible in the elderly (284).

As with aortic stenosis, a large proportion of elderly patients with mitral regurgitation have accompanying CHD. Most of these elderly patients are in a situation in which the conventional measures predict a poor outcome with EF substantially reduced (often ≤35%), and end-systolic dimension over the desirable limit (285–289). In patients in whom CABG is clearly indicated because of ischemia, the preferred approach usually is to perform the bypass and not to include mitral valve repair if the regurgitation is only mild or moderate and not associated with pulmonary hypertension. The thinking is that in these patients mitral regurgitation may improve postoperatively owing to the improved myocardial blood flow. In those patients in whom the clinical problem is primarily severe mitral regurgitation related to CHD, anecdotal experience and reports of small series indicate that patients can undergo surgery with a relatively low surgical mortality (range, 10%–15%) and that in some instances the EF, surprisingly, is improved with mitral valve repair. Long-term follow-up information is limited, however, and postoperative mortality remains high.

ARRHYTHMIAS

Cardiac arrhythmias are common in the elderly population and present in a number of different clinical conditions, but are discussed only briefly here. Cardiac arrhythmias include acute disturbances such as palpitations, syncope, or sudden cardiac death. Alternatively, cardiac arrhythmias may be chronic and persistent, causing intermittent symptoms and impacting quality of life. The entire spectrum of arrhythmias, both tachyarrhythmias and bradyarrhythmias, can be seen in the elderly population. Age-related changes in the heart and autonomic nervous system discussed in earlier sections of this chapter, especially those involving the conduction system, are important in arrhythmias. Drugs commonly used in older patients, including β-blockers, calcium channel blockers, digitalis, and antihypertensives (such as α-methyldopa), can produce some of the same ECG changes as degenerative conduction system disease. This further illustrates the need to carefully differentiate abnormalities and findings caused by adverse drug reactions from those related to disease in the elderly.

Atrial Arrhythmias

Atrial fibrillation is most commonly sustained arrhythmia in elderly patients. It is predominantly a disease of the elderly, and 75% of individuals with atrial fibrillation are between 65 and 85 years old. The main objectives when treating patients with atrial fibrillation are to control symptoms, restore sinus rhythm, prevent embolic events (particularly stroke), and reduce the risk of developing heart failure. The Atrial Fibrillation Follow-up Investigation of Rhythm management (AFFIRM) trial, a large multicenter randomized trial, compared rate control to rhythm control using antiarrhythmic drugs in patients with recent onset atrial fibrillation with background anticoagulation therapy and found no difference in mortality or stroke between the two approaches. Thus, it is reasonable to offer either strategy as first-line treatment for new onset atrial fibrillation. In most elderly patients, rate control with anticoagulation is the preferred method to prevent stroke. Anticoagulation with warfarin is the mainstay of atrial fibrillation treatment. Careful attention to levels of anticoagulation, avoiding bleeding complication, and maintaining an international normalized ratio of 2.0 to 3.0, preferably on the lower side, is preferred in the elderly population. Elderly patients who are prone to fall because of seizure disorders, gait disorders, syncope, and other conditions may not be candidates for warfarin therapy. New approaches to the treatment of atrial fibrillation are exciting and may be even more advantageous in the elderly. These include device therapies such as pacemakers or atrial defibrillators and catheter ablation techniques. Linear atrial ablation and pulmonary vein ablation appears to be safe and appropriate in selected elderly patients. Device strategies are currently reserved for patients who have drug-refractory atrial fibrillation and difficult-to-achieve rhythm control, which is felt to be necessary.

Atrial flutter is also a common arrhythmia in the elderly and may coexist with atrial fibrillation in up to 15% of patients. The risk of stroke with this arrhythmia was once considered low, but recent data suggest that it is an intermediate risk compared to atrial fibrillation. Anticoagulation should be considered in appropriate patients. Ablation is now widely used as a common first-line approach. Because of the safety of the procedure and the ability to come off of medications, ablative therapy should be considered in the elderly population. Randomized controlled clinical trials are needed to confirm this strategy as a first-line approach.

Bradycardia/Sinus Node Dysfunction

Sinus node dysfunction is a major indication for pacemaker implantation in the elderly. The spectrum of difficulties includes sinus bradycardia, sinus node exit block, to sinus arrest. Symptom relief is usually obtained with permanent pace making, yet 10% of patients may have recurrent syncope, which is then probably due to vasodepressor mechanisms. In the previously reported Mode Selection Trial, 2010 elderly patients with sinus node dysfunction but normal sinus rhythm were randomized to receive rate-adaptive pacemakers programmed to either the dual-chamber rate modulated (DDDR) or single-chamber ventricular rate modulated mode. Those paced to DDDR mode showed significantly reduced rates of atrial fibrillation and heart failure hospitalizations over 4 years as well as improvements in subjective heart failure and quality of life indices. Over the 4-year follow-up, period the DDDR strategy was cost effective by standard criteria (290). Recent evidence shows that more physiologic pacing and reducing the total amount of time paced can help patients to improve their functional status and prevent heart failure down the road (Dual Chamber and VVI Implantable Defibrillator Trial) (291). Current trials investigating this question are underway.

Syncope

Orthostasis is common in the elderly patients and is aggravated by medical therapy for hypertension or heart failure. When persistent and progressive despite optimization of medical therapy, treatment becomes quite difficult. Hydration and support stockings to increase venous return are first line. Drugs including β-blockers, α-antagonists (midodrine), volume expanders (fludrocortisone or erythropoietin) or serotonin reuptake inhibitors have all been tried with variable success. In refractory patients, dual-chamber pacing combined with drug therapy has been attempted.

Ventricular Arrhythmias

Although ventricular ectopic beats and nonsustained ventricular tachycardia confer an increased risk, they do not mandate direct treatment. However, ventricular tachyarrhythmias with syncope or cardiac arrest warrant aggressive intervention. Data amassed from a number of clinical trials suggest that elderly patients will benefit to the same or greater extent as younger patients from defibrillator therapy as well as correction of significant ischemia. The recent AHA/ACC guidelines for CHF suggest that implantable cardioverter defibrillator therapy is a class Ia recommendation for patients with an EF less than 35% with previous MI or patients with nonischemic cardiomyopathy with an EF less than 35% and CHF symptoms. Results from the Sudden Cardiac Death in Heart Failure Trial (SCDHeft) suggest that long-term amiodarone therapy is not effective in reducing the risk of death in patients with reduced EF as a prophylactic strategy (292).

HYPERTROPHIC CARDIOMYOPATHIES

Hypertrophic cardiomyopathy has a different genetic basis, morphology, and prognosis in elderly patients than in younger patients. Studies have found that more than 50% of patients with hypertrophic cardiomyopathy are older than 50 and as many as 40% are older than 60 (293). Echocardiographic studies have shown similar asymmetric hypertrophy of the septum, systolic anterior motion of the mitral valve, and severity of an outflow tract gradient in young and elderly patients, although younger patients have more severe hypertrophy (294,295). Ventricular cavity contours differ; the septum in the young is more hypertrophied, has reversed curvature, and thus creates a crescent-shaped LV cavity, whereas elderly patients have normally shaped left and right ventricles and less hypertrophy overall.

In a majority of elderly patients with obstructive hypertrophic cardiomyopathy who are women, the dynamic subaortic obstruction is the result of atypical systolic contact between the mitral valve and the intraventricular septum (295). Sizable calcium deposits in the mitral valve annulus in these patients contributed to the outflow tract narrowing. Another subset of patients, who were African American, and many of whom had longstanding hypertension, had severe concentric hypertrophy with a small LV cavity, increased EF (80%), and diastolic dysfunction (296). Although hypertension may aggravate the underlying cardiomyopathy, hypertension is not the primary cause of hypertrophic cardiomyopathy. These observations reflect the spectrum of hypertrophic cardiomyopathic disease in the elderly.

The long-term survival rate of elderly patients with hypertrophic cardiomyopathy is very similar to that of an age- and gender-matched control group (293–297). Although adequate studies on the genetic transmission of hypertrophic cardiomyopathy in elderly patients are lacking, the genotypes are different from those that occur in the more malignant syndrome seen in younger patients (298,299), especially patients with a family history of disease and, most important, when the family history involves sudden cardiac death (298–302).

Senile Amyloidosis

Autopsy studies indicate that amyloid is commonly present in patients older than the age of 75, and up to two thirds of patients older than age 85 may show evidence of amyloidosis (303). Among these patients, approximately one third may show extensive ventricular involvement; CHF is present in approximately half the patients and may be attributable primarily to the amyloidosis (304). Amyloidosis was judged to be an important contributor to death (perhaps the primary cause) in one group of patients (305). The biochemical properties of amyloid in old hearts and its relationship to the amyloid of familial amyloidosis or multiple myeloma need further clarification (293). Immunohistochemical studies recognize three distinct types of senile cardiovascular amyloidosis: isolated atrial amyloidosis, senile aortic amyloidosis, and senile systemic amyloidosis, in which organs such as lungs, liver, and kidneys are involved, in addition to the heart (306). The latter, although rare, may cause significant cardiovascular morbidity. Distinguishing between nonsecretory, immunoglobulin-derived primary amyloidosis with cardiac involvement and senile systemic amyloidosis is possible only with immunohistochemical techniques. Although it is rarely diagnosed clinically, definitive diagnosis has been made by biopsy or autopsy (307).

Diastolic dysfunction increases as amyloid deposits progress. Patients often present with pulmonary congestion and right heart failure with edema. Conduction defects and atrial fibrillation, although common in older patients with amyloid deposits, are not due to amyloid infiltration of the conducting system. Patients with senile amyloidosis may be more sensitive to the effects of digitalis and have more episodes of digitalis toxicity (308,309). The outcome of patients with senile amyloidosis is grave, and such patients have a mortality rate of 50% by 6 months from the time of endomyocardial biopsy diagnosis. Not surprisingly, their CHF responds poorly to all interventions. Much remains to be learned about the characteristics, occurrence, and pathophysiologic effects of senile amyloidosis.

CONTROVERSIES AND PERSPECTIVES

The amount and cost of cardiovascular care provided to elderly patients will continue to increase because of the growing number of elderly patients, the larger number of services and procedures provided per patient, and the increased cost of the sophisticated care given. The pressure to control costs will continue (310). Physicians will feel obligated to use the considerable fiscal resources available for elderly care appropriately. In order to do this, they will require better outcome data for all major cardiovascular syndromes, which will lead to an understanding of the widely disparate practice patterns, especially in the use of procedures. Data on such outcomes must extend to long-term follow up and include information on quality of life and function. These studies will highlight the need for a philosophical approach emphasizing quality of life and the patient's individual health care priorities. In addition, randomized, controlled trials are less likely to resolve management dilemmas in the elderly because of the extraordinary heterogeneity in this population. However, every effort must be made to include elderly patients in clinical trials evaluating cardiovascular therapies. In fact, the National Institutes of Health and other sponsors of clinical trials should require representation of elderly patients to better understand risk benefit; however, registries with prospectively collected key variables will likely be the best approach. The Centers for Medicare and Medicaid Services will continue to be a big stakeholder in these studies. Critical characterization of complications of procedures and adverse drug reactions, and collection of follow-up data on functional status are key areas for registry studies.

The heterogeneity of aging will serve as a stimulus for physicians to characterize elderly patients more objectively in relation to their ability to withstand the stress of procedures and complications of disease, with emphasis on physiologic reserve and biologic age rather than chronologic age. Biologic age is multifactorial, involving cognitive, emotional, physical, and nutritional attributes as well as the function of specific organs including the lungs, kidneys, and liver. With better characterization of biologic age, more precise estimates of outcomes can be made, patients can be given better information, and they will have more realistic expectations. Genetic profiling of risk in the elderly may be particularly helpful in determining specific treatment strategies. No single feature can characterize the total elderly patient. The concept of competing risks will evolve, because even the most successful therapy will have limited effect on longevity in the very old.

Although research at the cellular and molecular level will characterize and provide better understanding of the aging process, this basic information is not likely to be immediately useful in the management of the large number of elderly patients with major cardiovascular disease. Preventive measures, physical exercise, mental stimulation, avoidance of depression, good nutrition, and abstinence from tobacco use, are helpful approaches to postpone or ameliorate the consequences of aging and allow patients to better tolerate cardiovascular diseases when these become manifest.

THE FUTURE

Advances in medicine will result in a progressively larger elderly population. These patients require a more philosophical approach with emphasis on quality of life and choice. Data from "long-term" outcome studies and randomized, controlled clinical trials will guide the physician in making appropriate choices and providing realistic expectations for the elderly patient. Prevention and postponement of cardiovascular disease will be emphasized as the most effective approaches.

ACKNOWLEDGMENTS

The authors thank Ethel Hardy and Crystal Crawford for excellent editorial assistance.

References

1. Fuster V. Where am I going? The future of academic cardiovascular medicine. *J Am Coll Cardiol* 2005;46[Suppl 7]:A1–A4.
2. US Bureau of the Census. *Demographics and socioeconomic aspects of aging in the United States.* Washington, D.C.: US Bureau of the Census; 1984.
3. National Center for Health Statistics. *With chartbook on trends in the health of Americans.* Hyattsville, MD: National Center for Health Statistics; 2004.
4. Fries JF. Aging, natural death, and the compression of morbidity. *N Engl J Med* 1980;303:130–135.
5. Olshansky SJ, Carnes BA, Cassel C. In search of Methuselah: estimating the upper limits to human longevity. *Science* 1990;250:634–640.
6. Centers for Disease Control and Prevention. Public Health and aging: trends in aging—United States and worldwide. *MMWR* 2003;52:101–106.
7. The Quality of Health Care Received by Older Adults. *Rand Health* 2004.
8. United States Department of Health and Human Services. *National nursing home survey.* Washington, D.C.: USDHHS; 1997.
9. Graves EJ. 1992 Summary: National hospital discharge survey. Advance data from vital and health statistics [report no. 249]. Hyattsville, MD: National Center for Health Statistics; 1994.
10. Kannel WB, Wolf PA, Benjamin EJ, Levy D. Prevalence, incidence, prognosis, and predisposing conditions for atrial fibrillation: population-based estimates. *Am J Cardiol* 1998;82:2N–9N.
11. Feinberg WM, Blackshear JL, Laupacis A, et al. Prevalence, age distribution, and gender of patients with atrial fibrillation. Analysis and implications. *Arch Intern Med* 1995 Mar;155:469–473.
12. Lee P, Alexander K, Hammill B, et al. Representation of elderly person and women in published randomized trials of acute coronary syndromes. *JAMA* 2001;286:708–713.
13. Packer M, Bristow MR, Cohn JN, et al. The effect of carvedilol on morbidity and mortality in patients with chronic heart failure. U.S. Carvedilol Heart Failure Study Group. *N Engl J Med* 1996;334: 1349–1355.
14. Packer M, O'Connor CM, Ghali JK, et al. Effect of amlodipine on morbidity and mortality in severe chronic heart failure. Prospective Randomized Amlodipine Survival Evaluation Study Group. *N Engl J Med* 1996;335: 1107–1114.
15. Pitt B, Zannad F, Remme WJ, et al. The effect of spironolactone on morbidity and mortality in patients with severe heart failure. Randomized Aldactone Evaluation Study Investigators. *N Engl J Med* 1999;341:709–717.
16. Masoudi FA, Havranek EP, Wolfe P, et al. Most hospitalized older persons do not meet the enrollment criteria for clinical trials in heart failure. *Am Heart J* 2003;146:250–257.
17. Prashat J, Deboer D, Sykora K, et al. Characteristics and mortality outcomes of thrombolysis trial participants and non-participants: a population comparison. *J Am Coll Cardiol* 1996;27:1335.
18. Gusto IIb Investigators. A comparison of recombinant hirudin with heparin for the treatment of acute coronary syndromes. The Global Use of Strategies to Open Occluded Coronary Arteries (GUSTO) IIb investigators. *N Engl J Med* 1996;335:775–782.
19. GUSTO III Investigators. A comparison of reteplase with alteplase for acute myocardial infarction. The Global Use of Strategies to Open Occluded Coronary Arteries (GUSTO III) Investigators. *N Engl J Med* 1997;337:1118–1123.
20. PURSUIT Trial Investigators. Inhibition of platelet glycoprotein IIb/IIIa with eptifibatide in patients with acute coronary syndromes. The PURSUIT Trial Investigators. Platelet Glycoprotein IIb/IIIa in Unstable Angina: Receptor Suppression Using Integrilin Therapy. *N Engl J Med* 1998;339:436–443.
21. Kandzari DE, Roe MT, Chen AY, et al. Influence of clinical trial enrollment on the quality of care and outcomes for patients with non-ST-segment elevation acute coronary syndromes. *Am Heart J* 2005;149:474–481.
22. Burns TR, Klima M, Teasdale TA, Kasper K. Morphometry of the aging heart. *Mod Pathol* 1990;3:336–342.
23. Olivetti G, Melissari M, Capasso JM, Anversa P. Cardiomyopathy of the aging human heart. Myocyte loss and reactive cellular hypertrophy. *Circ Res* 1991;68:1560–1568.
24. Kitzman DW, Scholz DG, Hagen PT, et al. Age-related changes in normal human hearts during the first 10 decades of life. Part II (Maturity): A quantitative anatomic study of 765 specimens from subjects 20 to 99 years old. *Mayo Clin Proc* 1988;63:137–146.
25. Lie JT, Hammond PI. Pathology of the senescent heart: anatomic observations on 237 autopsy studies of patients 90 to 105 years old. *Mayo Clin Proc* 1988;63:552–564.
26. Goor D, Lillehei CW, Edwards JE. The "sigmoid septum". Variation in the contour of the left ventricular outt. *Am J Roentgenol Radium Ther Nucl Med* 1969;107:366–376.
27. Laketta EG, Gerstemblith G, Weisfeldt ML. The aging heart: structure, function, and disease. In: Braunwald E, ed., *Heart disease.* 5th ed. Philadelphia: Saunders; 1997:1687–1700.
28. Lakatta EG, Sollott SJ. Perspectives on mammalian cardiovascular aging: humans to molecules. *Comp Biochem Physiol* 2002;132:699–721.
29. Wei JY, Spurgeon HA, Lakatta EG. Excitation-contraction in rat myocardium: alterations with adult aging. *Am J Physiol* 1984;246:H784–H791.
30. Nixon JV, Hallmark H, Page K, et al. Ventricular performance in human hearts aged 61 to 73 years. *Am J Cardiol* 1985;56:932–937.
31. Spirito P, Maron BJ. Influence of aging on Doppler echocardiographic indices of left ventricular diastolic function. *Br Heart J* 1988;59:672–679.
32. Benjamin EJ, Levy D, Anderson KM, et al. Determinants of Doppler indexes of left ventricular diastolic function in normal subjects (the Framingham Heart Study). *Am J Cardiol* 1992;70:508–515.
33. Lakatta EG. Cardiovascular aging research: the next horizons. *J Am Geriatr Soc* 1999;47:613–625.
34. Taddei S, Virdis A, Mattei P, et al. Aging and endothelial function in normotensive subjects and patients with essential hypertension. *Circulation* 1995;91:1981–1987.
35. Robert L. Aging of the vascular wall and atherogenesis: role of the elastin-laminin receptor. *Atherosclerosis* 1996;123:169–179.
36. Vanhoutte PM, Boulanger CM, Mombouli JV. Endothelium-derived relaxing factors and converting enzyme inhibition. *Am J Cardiol* 1995;76:3E–12E.
37. Celermajer DS, Sorensen KE, Spiegelhalter DJ, et al. Aging is associated with endothelial dysfunction in healthy men years before the age-related decline in women. *J Am Coll Cardiol* 1994;24:471–476.
38. Furberg CD, Manolio TA, Psaty BM, et al. Major electrocardiographic abnormalities in persons aged 65 years and older (the Cardiovascular Health Study). Cardiovascular Health Study Collaborative Research Group. *Am J Cardiol* 1992;69:1329–1335.
39. Tsuji H, Venditti FJJ, Manders ES, et al. Reduced heart rate variability and mortality risk in an elderly cohort. The Framingham Heart Study. *Circulation* 1994;90:878–883.
40. Laitinen T, Niskanen L, Geelen G, et al. Age dependency of cardiovascular autonomic responses to head-up tilt in healthy subjects. *J Appl Physiol* 2004;96:2333–2340.
41. Kannel WB, Wolf PA, Benjamin EJ, et al. Prevalence, incidence, prognosis, and predisposing conditions for atrial fibrillation: population-based estimates. *Am J Cardiol* 1998;82:2N–9N.
42. Fleg JL, Kennedy HL. Long-term prognostic significance of ambulatory electrocardiographic findings in apparently healthy subjects. *Am J Cardiol* 1992;70:748–751.
43. Friesinger GC, Gravanis ME. Aging and the cardiovascular system. In: Gravanis ME, ed., *Health and disease in cardiovascular disorders.* St. Louis: Mosby; 1995.
44. Brandfonbrener M, Landowne M, Shock NW. Changes in cardiac output with age. *Circulation* 1955;12:557–566.
45. Correia LC, Lakatta EG, O'Connor FC, et al. Attenuated cardiovascular reserve during prolonged submaximal cycle exercise in healthy older subjects. *J Am Coll Cardiol* 2002;40:1290–1297.
46. Fleg JL, Schulman S, O'Connor F, et al. Effects of acute beta-adrenergic receptor blockade on age-associated changes in cardiovascular performance during dynamic exercise. *Circulation* 1994;90:2333–2341.
47. Fleg JL, Lakatta EG. Role of muscle loss in the age-associated reduction in VO_2 max. *J Appl Physiol* 1988;65:1147–1151.
48. Katzel LI, Sorkin JD, Fleg JL. A comparison of longitudinal changes in aerobic fitness in older endurance athletes and sedentary men. *J Am Geriatr Soc* 2001;49:1657–1664.
49. Ades PA, Ballor DL, Ashikaga T, et al. Weight training improves walking endurance in healthy elderly persons. *Ann Intern Med* 1996;124: 568–572.
50. Vaitkevicius PV, Ebersold C, Shah MS, et al. Effects of aerobic exercise training in community-based subjects aged 80 and older: a pilot study. *J Am Geriatr Soc* 2002;Soc:2009–2013.
51. Woodhouse K. Drugs and the liver. Part III: ageing of the liver and the metabolism of drugs. *Biopharm Drug Dispos* 1992;13:311–320.

52. Fliser D, Bischoff I, Hanses A, et al. Renal handling of drugs in the healthy elderly. Creatinine clearance underestimates renal function and pharmacokinetics remain virtually unchanged. *Eur J Clin Pharmacol* 1999;55:205–211.
53. Chutka DS, Evans JM, Fleming KC, et al. Symposium on geriatrics—part I: drug prescribing for elderly patients. *Mayo Clin Proc* 1995;70:685–693.
54. Podrazik PM, Schwartz JB. Cardiovascular pharmacology of aging. *Cardiol Clin* 1999;17:17–34.
55. Chutka DS, Evans JM, Fleming KC, et al. Symposium on geriatrics—part I: drug prescribing for elderly patients. *Mayo Clin Proc* 1995;70:685–693.
56. Tinetti ME, Bogardus STJ, Agostini JV. Potential pitfalls of disease-specific guidelines for patients with multiple conditions. *N Engl J Med* 2005;351:2870–2874.
57. Kaufman DW, Kelly JP, Rosenberg L, et al. Recent patterns of medication use in the ambulatory adult population of the United States: the Slone survey. *JAMA* 1916;287:337–344.
58. Fried TR, Bradley EH, Williams CS, et al. Functional disability and health care expenditures for older persons. *Arch Intern Med* 2001;161:2602–2607.
59. Fugate W, Lacroix AZ, Gray SL, et al. Frailty: emergence and consequences in women aged 65 and older in the Women's Health Initiative Observational Study. *J Am Geriatr Soc* 2005;53:1321–1330.
60. Walston J, McBurnie MA, Newman A, et al. Frailty and activation of the inflammation and coagulation systems without clinical comorbidities. *Arch Intern Med* 2002;16:2333–2341.
61. Collins R, Armitage J, Parish S, et al., for the Heart Protection Collaborative Group. MRC/BHF Heart Protection Study of cholesterol-lowering with simvastatin in 5963 people with diabetes: a randomised placebo-controlled trial. *Lancet* 2005;361:2005–2016.
62. Lopez OL, Jaqust WJ, DeKosky ST, et al. Prevalence and classification of mild cognitive impairment in the Cardiovascular Health Study Cognition Study. *Arch Neurol* 2003;60:1385–1389.
63. Boyd CM, Darer J, Boult C, et al. Clinical practice guidelines and quality of care for older patients with multiple comorbid diseases: implications for pay for performance. *JAMA* 1910;294:716–724.
64. Wenger NS, Solomon DH, Roth CP, et al. The quality of medical care provided to vulnerable community-dwelling older patients. *Ann Intern Med* 2004;139:740–747.
65. Williams MA, Fleg JL, Ades PA, et al. Secondary prevention of coronary heart disease in the elderly (with emphasis on patients > or =75 years of age): an American Heart Association scientific statement from the Council on Clinical Cardiology Subcommittee on Exercise, Cardiac Rehabilitation, and Prevention. *Circulation* 1909;105:1735–1743.
66. Grundy SM, Pasternak R, Greenland P, et al. Assessment of cardiovascular risk by use of multiple-risk-factor assessment equations: a statement for healthcare professionals from the American Heart Association and the American College of Cardiology. *Circulation* 1999;100:1481–1492.
67. Hedner T. The problem of hypertension in the elderly. *Blood Press Suppl* 2000;2:4–6.
68. Rehman HU. Age and the cardiovascular system. *Hosp Med* 1999;60:645–652.
69. Kannel WB. Fifty years of Framingham Study contributions to understanding hypertension. *J Hum Hypertens* 2000;14:83–90.
70. Staessen JA, Gasowski J, Wang JG, et al. Risks of untreated and treated isolated systolic hypertension in the elderly: meta-analysis of outcome trials. *Lancet* 2000;355:865–872.
71. Staessen JA, Fagard R, Thijs L, et al. Randomised double-blind comparison of placebo and active treatment for older patients with isolated systolic hypertension. The Systolic Hypertension in Europe (Syst-Eur) Trial Investigators. *Lancet* 1997;350:757–764.
72. Liu L, Wang JG, Gong L, et al. Comparison of active treatment and placebo in older Chinese patients with isolated systolic hypertension. Systolic Hypertension in China (Syst-China) Collaborative Group. *J Hypertens* 1998;16:1823–1829.
73. Staessen JA, Gasowski J, Wang JG, et al. Risks of untreated and treated isolated systolic hypertension in the elderly: meta-analysis of outcome trials. *Lancet* 2000;355:865–872.
74. Blacher J, Staessen JA, Girerd X, et al. Pulse pressure not mean pressure determines cardiovascular risk in older hypertensive patients. *Arch Intern Med* 2000;160:1085–1089.
75. Chae CU, Pfeffer MA, Glynn RJ, et al. Increased pulse pressure and risk of heart failure in the elderly. *JAMA* 1999;281:634–639.
76. Vaccarino V, Berger AK, Abramson J, et al. Pulse pressure and risk of cardiovascular events in the systolic hypertension in the elderly program. *Am J Cardiol* 2001;88:980–986.
77. Franklin SS, Khan SA, Wong ND, et al. Is pulse pressure useful in predicting risk for coronary heart Disease? The Framingham heart study. *Circulation* 1999;100:354–360.
78. Domanski M, Norman J, Wolz M, et al. Cardiovascular risk assessment using pulse pressure in the first national health and nutrition examination survey (NHANES I). *Hypertension* 2001;38:793–797.
79. Staessen JA, Fagard R, Thijs L, et al. Randomised double-blind comparison of placebo and active treatment for older patients with isolated systolic hypertension. The Systolic Hypertension in Europe (Syst-Eur) Trial Investigators. *Lancet* 1997;350:757–764.
80. Liu L, Wang JG, Gong L, et al. Comparison of active treatment and placebo in older Chinese patients with isolated systolic hypertension. Systolic Hypertension in China (Syst-China) Collaborative Group. *J Hypertens* 1998;16:1823–1829.
81. Guidelines Subcommittee. 1999 World Health Organization-International Society of Hypertension guidelines for the management of hypertension. Guidelines Subcommittee. *J Hypertens* 1999;17:151–183.
82. Staessen JA, Gasowski J, Wang JG, et al. Risks of untreated and treated isolated systolic hypertension in the elderly: meta-analysis of outcome trials. *Lancet* 2000;355:865–872.
83. Whelton PK, Appel LJ, Espeland MA, et al. Sodium reduction and weight loss in the treatment of hypertension in older persons: a randomized controlled trial of nonpharmacologic interventions in the elderly (TONE). TONE Collaborative Research Group. *JAMA* 1998;279:839–846.
84. Chaudhry SI, Krumholz HM, Foody JM. Systolic hypertension in older persons. *JAMA* 2004;292:1074–1080.
85. Vaccarino V, Berger AK, Abramson J, et al. Pulse pressure and risk of cardiovascular events in the systolic hypertension in the elderly program. *Am J Cardiol* 2001;88:980–986.
86. Staessen JA, Gasowski J, Wang JG, et al. Risks of untreated and treated isolated systolic hypertension in the elderly: meta-analysis of outcome trials. *Lancet* 2000;355:865–872.
87. Systolic Hypertension in the Elderly Program Cooperative Research Group. Prevention of stroke by antihypertensive drug treatment in older persons with isolated systolic hypertension. Final results of the Systolic Hypertension in the Elderly Program (SHEP). SHEP Cooperative Research Group. *JAMA* 1991;265:3255–3264.
88. Staessen JA, Gasowski J, Wang JG, et al. Risks of untreated and treated isolated systolic hypertension in the elderly: meta-analysis of outcome trials. *Lancet* 2000;355:865–872.
89. Staessen JA, Gasowski J, Wang JG, et al. Risks of untreated and treated isolated systolic hypertension in the elderly: meta-analysis of outcome trials. *Lancet* 2000;355:865–872.
90. Beckett NS, Connor M, Sadler JD, et al. Orthostatic fall in blood pressure in the very elderly hypertensive: results from the hypertension in the very elderly trial (HYVET)—pilot. *J Hum Hypertens* 1999;13:839–840.
91. Chobanian AV, Bakris GL, Black HR, et al. The Seventh Report of the Joint National Committee on Prevention, Detection, Evaluation, and Treatment of High Blood Pressure. The JNC 7 report. *JAMA* 2003;289:2560–2572.
92. Major outcomes in high-risk hypertensive patients randomized to angiotensin-converting enzyme inhibitor or calcium channel blocker vs diuretic: The Antihypertensive and Lipid-Lowering Treatment to Prevent Heart Attack Trial (ALLHAT). *JAMA* 2002;288:2981–2997.
93. Fyhrquist F, Dahlof B, Devereux RB, et al. Pulse pressure and effects of losartan or atenolol in patients with hypertension and left ventricular hypertrophy. *Hypertension* 2005;45:580–585.
94. Hall KM, Luepker RV. Is hypercholesterolemia a risk factor and should it be treated in the elderly? *Am J Health Promot* 2000;14:347–356.
95. Schatz IJ, Masaki K, Yano K, et al. Cholesterol and all-cause mortality in elderly people from the Honolulu Heart Program: a cohort study. *Lancet* 2001;358:351–355.
96. Houterman S, Verschuren WM, Hofman A, et al. Serum cholesterol is a risk factor for myocardial infarction in elderly men and women: the Rotterdam Study. *J Intern Med* 1999;246:25–33.
97. Scandinavian Simvastatin Survival Study Group. Randomised trial of cholesterol lowering in 4444 patients with coronary heart disease: the Scandinavian Simvastatin Survival Study (4S). *Lancet* 1994;344:1383–1389.
98. Sacks FM, Pfeffer MA, Moye LA, et al. The effect of pravastatin on coronary events after myocardial infarction in patients with average cholesterol levels. *N Engl J Med* 1996;335:1001–1009.
99. The Long-term Intervention with Pravastatin in Ischemic Disease (LIPID) Study Group. Prevention of cardiovascular events and death with pravastatin in patients with coronary heart disease and a broad range of initial cholesterol levels. *N Engl J Med* 1998;339:1349–1357.
100. Miettinen TA, Pyorala K, Olsson AG, et al. Cholesterol-lowering therapy in women and elderly patients with myocardial infarction or angina pectoris. Findings from the Scandinavian Simvastatin Survival Study (4S). *Circulation* 1997;96:4211–4218.
101. Hunt D, Young P, Simes J, et al. Benefits of pravastatin on cardiovascular events and mortality in older patients with coronary heart disease are equal to or exceed those seen in younger patients: results from the LIPID trial. *Ann Intern Med* 2001;134:931–940.
102. Heart Protection Study Collaborative Group. Heart Protection Study of cholesterol lowering with simvastatin in 20 536 high-risk individuals: a randomised placebo-controlled trial. *Lancet* 2002;360:7–22.
103. Shepherd J, Blauw GJ, Murphy MG, et al. Pravastatin in elderly individuals at risk of vascular disease (PROSPER): a randomised controlled trial. *Lancet* 2002;360:1623–1630.
104. Maycock CAA, Muhlestein JB, Horne BD, et al. Statin therapy is associated with reduced mortality across all age groups of individuals with significant coronary disease, including very elderly patients. *J Am Coll Cardiol* 2002;40:1777–1785.

105. Shepherd J, Cobbe SM, Ford I, et al. Prevention of coronary heart disease with pravastatin in men with hypercholesterolemia. West of Scotland Coronary Prevention Study Group. *N Engl J Med* 1995;333: 1301–1307.
106. Downs JR, Clearfield M, Weis S, et al. Primary prevention of acute coronary events with lovasatin in men and women with average cholesterol levels: results of AFCAPS/TexCAPS. Air Force/Texas Coronary Atherosclerosis Prevention Study. *JAMA* 1998;279:1615–1622.
107. Sever PS, Dahlor B, Poulter NR, et al. Prevention of coronary and stroke events with atorvastatin in hypertensive patients who have average or lower-than-average cholesterol concentrations, in the Anglo-Scandinavian Cardiac Outcomes Trial—Lipid Lowering Arm (ASCOT-LLA): a multicentre randomised controlled trial. *Lancet* 2003;361:1149–1158.
108. Wilson PWF, Kannel WB. Obesity, diabetes, and risk of cardiovascular disease in the elderly. *Am J Geriatr Cardiol* 2002;11:119–123, 125.
109. Meneilly GS. Pathophysiology of type 2 diabetes in the elderly. *Clin Geriatr Med* 1999;15:239–253.
110. Ford ES, Giles WH, Dietz WH. Prevalence of the metabolic syndrome among US adults: findings from the third National Health and Nutrition Examination Survey. *JAMA* 2002;287:356–359.
111. Scuteri A, Najjar SS, Muller DC, et al. Metabolic syndrome amplifies the age-associated increases in vascular thickness and stiffness. *J Am Coll Cardiol* 2004;43:1388–1395.
112. Morley JE. An overview of diabetes mellitus in older persons. *Clin Geriatr Med* 1999;15:211–224.
113. Alexander K, Roe MT, Kulkarni SP, et al. Evolution of cardiovascular care for elderly patients with non-ST-segment elevation acute coronary syndromes: results from CRUSADE. *J Am Coll Cardiol* 2005;46:I490–I495.
114. Meneilly GS. Pathophysiology of type 2 diabetes in the elderly. *Clin Geriatr Med* 1999;15:239–253.
115. Mooradian AD, Thurman JE. Glucotoxicity: potential mechanisms. *Clin Geriatr Med* 1999;15:255.
116. Diabetes Control and Complications Trial Research Group. The effect of intensive treatment of diabetes on the development and progression of long-term complications in insulin-dependent diabetes mellitus. *N Engl J Med* 1993;329:977–986.
117. United Kingdom Prospective Diabetes Study (UKPDS) Group. Intensive blood-glucose control with sulphonylureas or insulin compared with conventional treatment and risk of complications in patients with type 2 diabetes (UKPDS 33). *Lancet* 1998;352:837–853.
118. Burns DM. Cigarette smoking among the elderly: disease consequences and the benefits of cessation. *Am J Health Promot* 2000;14:357–361.
119. Sparrow D, Dawber TR. The influence of cigarette smoking on prognosis after a first myocardial infarction. A report from the Framingham study. *J Chronic Dis* 1978;31:425–432.
120. Roth GS. Caloric restriction and caloric restriction mimetics: current status and promise for the future. *J Am Geriatr Soc* 2005;53[9 Suppl]:S280–S283.
121. Diehr P, Beresford SA. The relation of dietary patterns to future survival, health, and cardiovascular events in older adults. *J Clin Epidemiol* 2003;56:1224–1235.
122. Hakim AA, Curb JD, Petrovitch H, et al. Effects of walking on coronary heart disease in elderly men: the Honolulu Heart Program. *Circulation* 1999;100:9–13.
123. Frasure-Smith N, Lesperance F, Talajic M. Depression and 18-month prognosis after myocardial infarction. *Circulation* 1995;91:999–1005.
124. Ariyo AA, Haan M, Tangen CM, et al. Depressive symptoms and risks of coronary heart disease and mortality in elderly Americans. Cardiovascular Health Study Collaborative Research Group. *Circulation* 2000;102:1773–1779.
125. Levy D, Garrison RJ, Savage DD, et al. Prognostic implications of echocardiographically determined left ventricular mass in the Framingham Heart Study. *N Engl J Med* 1990;322:1561–1566.
126. Devereux RB, Dahlof B, Levy D, et al. Comparison of enalapril versus nifedipine to decrease left ventricular hypertrophy in systemic hypertension (the PRESERVE trial). *Am J Cardiol* 1996;78:61–65.
127. Strauer BE, Schwartzkopff B. Objectives of high blood pressure treatment: left ventricular hypertrophy, diastolic function, and coronary reserve. *Am J Hypertens* 1998;11:879–881.
128. Kjeldsen SE, Dahlof B, Devereaux RB, et al. Effects of losartan on cardiovascular morbidity and mortality in patients with isolated systolic hypertension and left ventricular hypertrophy: a Losartan Intervention for Endpoint Reduction (LIFE) substudy. *JAMA* 2002;288:1491–1498.
129. Okin PM, Devereaux RB, Jern S, et al. Regression of electrocardiographic left ventricular hypertrophy during antihypertensive treatment and the prediction of major cardiovascular events. *JAMA* 2004;292:2343–2349.
130. Devereaux RB, Wachtell K, Gerdts E, et al. Prognostic significance of left ventricular mass change during treatment of hypertension. *JAMA* 2004; 292:2350–2356.
131. Levey AS, Coresh J, Balk E, et al. National Kidney Foundation practice guidelines for chronic kidney disease: evaluation, classification, and stratification. *Ann Intern Med* 2003;139:137–147.
132. Fried LF, Shlipak MG, Crump C, et al. Renal insufficiency as a predictor of cardiovascular outcomes and mortality in elderly individuals. *J Am Coll Cardiol* 2003;41:1364–1372.
133. Weiner DE, Tighiouart H, Amin MG, et al. Chronic kidney disease as a risk factor for cardiovascular disease and all-cause mortality: a pooled analysis of community-based studies. *J Am Soc Nephrol* 2004;15: 1307–1315.
134. Santopinto JJ, Fox KAA, Goldberg RJ, et al. Creatinine clearance and adverse hospital outcomes in patients with acute coronary syndromes: findings from the global registry of acute coronary events (GRACE). *Heart* 2003;89:1003–1008.
135. Gibson CM, Dumaine RL, Gelfand EV, et al. Association of glomerular filtration rate on presentation with subsequent mortality in non-ST-segment elevation acute coronary syndrome; observations in 13,307 patients in five TIMI trials. *Eur Heart J* 2004;25:1998–2005.
136. Shlipak MG, Fried LF, Stehman-Breen C, et al. Chronic renal insufficiency and cardiovascular events in the elderly: findings from the Cardiovascular Health Study. *Am J Geriatr Cardiol* 2004;13:81–90.
137. Catena C, Zingaro L, Casaccio D, et al. Abnormalities of coagulation in hypertensive patients with reduced creatinine clearance. *Am J Med* 2000; 109:556–561.
138. Wanner C, Krane V, Metzger T, et al. Lipid changes and statins in chronic renal insufficiency and dialysis. *J Nephrol* 2001;14[Suppl 4]:S76–S80.
139. Shlipak MG, Fried LF, Crump C, et al. Elevations of inflammatory and procoagulant biomarkers in elderly persons with renal insufficiency. *Circulation* 2003;107:87–92.
140. Sugiura M, Hiraoka K, Ohkawa S. Severity of coronary sclerosis in the aged: a pathological study in 968 consecutive autopsy cases. *Jpn Heart J* 1976;17:471–478.
141. Sheifer SE, Gersh BJ, Yanez ND, et al. Prevalence, predisposing factors, and prognosis of clinically unrecognized myocardial infarction in the elderly. *J Am Coll Cardiol* 2000;35:119–126.
142. Goraya TY, Jacobsen SJ, Pellikka PA, et al. Prognostic value of treadmill exercise testing in elderly persons. *Ann Intern Med* 2000;132:862–870.
143. Schulman SP, Fleg JL. Stress testing for coronary artery disease in the elderly. *Clin Geriatr Med* 1996;12:101–119.
144. Gaul G. Stress testing in persons above the age of 65 years: applicability and diagnostic value of a standardized maximal symptom-limited testing protocol. *Eur Heart J* 1984;5[Suppl E]:51–53.
145. Schulman SP, Fleg JL. Stress testing for coronary artery disease in the elderly. *Clin Geriatr Med* 1996;12:101–119.
146. Guadagnoli E, Landrum MB, Peterson EA, et al. Appropriateness of coronary angiography after myocardial infarction among Medicare beneficiaries. Managed care versus fee for service. *N Engl J Med* 2000;343:1460–1466.
147. Peterson ED, Cowper PA, Jollis JG, et al. Outcomes of coronary artery bypass graft surgery in 24,461 patients aged 80 years or older. *Circulation* 1995;92[9 Suppl]:II85–II91.
148. Tu JV, Pashos CL, Naylor CD, et al. Use of cardiac procedures and outcomes in elderly patients with myocardial infarction in the United States and Canada. *N Engl J Med* 1997;336:1500–1505.
149. Batchelor WB, Anstrom KJ, Muhlbaier LH, et al. Contemporary outcome trends in the elderly undergoing percutaneous coronary interventions: results in 7,472 octogenarians. National Cardiovascular Network Collaboration. *J Am Coll Cardiol* 2000;36:723–730.
150. Alexander KP, Anstrom KJ, Muhlbaier LH, et al. Outcomes of cardiac surgery in patients > or = 80 years: results from the National Cardiovascular Network. *J Am Coll Cardiol* 2000;35:731–738.
151. Chauhan MS, Kuntz RE, Ho KL, et al. Coronary artery stenting in the aged. *J Am Coll Cardiol* 2001;37:856–862.
152. Batchelor WB, Anstrom KJ, Muhlbaier LH, et al. Contemporary outcome trends in the elderly undergoing percutaneous coronary interventions: results in 7,472 octogenarians. National Cardiovascular Network Collaboration. *J Am Coll Cardiol* 2000;36:723–730.
153. Peterson ED, Cowper PA, Jollis JG, et al. Outcomes of coronary artery bypass graft surgery in 24,461 patients aged 80 years or older. *Circulation* 1995;92[9 Suppl]:II85–II91.
154. Alexander KP, Anstrom KJ, Muhlbaier LH, et al. Outcomes of cardiac surgery in patients > or = 80 years: results from the National Cardiovascular Network. *J Am Coll Cardiol* 2000;35:731–738.
155. Peterson ED, Alexander K, Malenka DJ, et al. Multicenter experience in revascularization of very elderly patients. *Am Heart J* 2004;148:486–492.
156. Welch HG, Albertsen PC, Nease RF, et al. Estimating treatment benefits for the elderly: the effect of competing risks. *Ann Intern Med* 1996;124:577–584.
157. Pressley JC, Patrick CH. Frailty bias in comorbidity risk adjustments of community-dwelling elderly populations. *J Clin Epidemiol* 1999;52:753–760.
158. Rumsfeld JS, MaWhinney S, McCarthy M Jr, et al. Health-related quality of life as a predictor of mortality following coronary artery bypass graft surgery. Participants of the Department of Veterans Affairs Cooperative Study Group on Processes, Structures, and Outcomes of Care in Cardiac Surgery. *JAMA* 1999;281:1298–1303.
159. Avezum A, Makdisse M, Spencer F, et al. Impact of age on management and outcome of acute coronary syndrome: observations from the Global Registry of Acute Coronary Events (GRACE). *Am Heart J* 2005;149:67–73.

160. Aronow WS. Prevalence of presenting symptoms of recognized acute myocardial infarction and of unrecognized healed myocardial infarction in elderly patients. *Am J Cardiol* 1987;60:1182.
161. Milner KA, Vaccarino V, Arnold AL, et al. Gender and age differences in chief complaints of acute myocardial infarction (Worcester Heart Attack Study). *Am J Cardiol* 2004;93:606–608.
162. Goldberg RJ, Steg PG, Sadiq I, et al. Extent of, and factors associated with, delay to hospital presentation in patients with acute coronary disease (The GRACE Registry). *Am J Cardiol* 2002;89:791–796.
163. Ottesen MM, Kober L, Jorgensen S, et al. Determinants of delay between symptoms and hospital admission in 5978 patients with acute myocardial infarction. The TRACE Study Group. Trandolapril Cardiac Evaluation. *Eur Heart J* 1996;17:429–437.
164. Berglin, Blohm M, Hartford M, et al. Factors associated with pre-hospital and in-hospital delay time in acute myocardial infarction: a 6-year experience. *J Intern Med* 1998;243:243–250.
165. Brieger D, Eagle K, Goodman S, et al. Acute coronary syndromes without chest pain, an underdiagnosed and undertreated high-risk group. *Chest* 2004;126:461–469.
166. White HD, Barbush GI, Califf RM, et al. Age and outcome with contemporary thrombolytic therapy. Results from the GUSTO-I Trial. *Circulation* 1996;94:1826–1833.
167. Goldberg RJ, Gore JM, Gurwitz JH, et al. The impact of age on the incidence and prognosis of initial acute myocardial infarction: the Worcester Heart Attack Study. *Am Heart J* 1989;117:543–549.
168. Lee KL, Woodlief LH, Topol EJ, et al. Predictors of 30-day mortality in the era of reperfusion for acute myocardial infarction. Results from an international trial of 41,021 patients. GUSTO-I Investigators. *Circulation* 1995;91:1659–1668.
169. Boersma E, Pieper KS, Steyerberg EW, et al. Predictors of outcome in patients with acute coronary syndromes without persistent ST-segment elevation. Results from an international trial of 9461 patients. *Circulation* 2000;101:2557–2567.
170. Eagle KA, Lim MJ, Dabbons OH, et al. A validated prediction model for all forms of acute coronary syndrome. Estimating the risk of 6-month postdischarge death in an international registry. *JAMA* 2004;291:2727–2733.
171. Braunwald E, Antman EM, Beasley JW, et al. ACC/AHA guidelines for the management of patients with unstable angina and non-ST-segment elevation myocardial infarction: executive summary and recommendations: a report of the American College of Cardiology/American Heart Association Task Force on Practice Guidelines (Committee on Management of Patients with Unstable Angina)-summary article. *J Am Coll Cardiol* 2002;40:1366–1374.
172. Antiplatelet Trialists' Collaboration. Collaborative overview of randomized trials of antiplatelet therapy—I: prevention of death, myocardial infarction, and stroke by prolonged antiplatelet therapy in various categories of patients. *BMJ* 1994;308:81–106.
173. The Clopidogrel in Unstable Angina to Prevent Recurrent Events Trial Investigators. Effects of clopidogrel in addition to aspirin in patients with acute coronary syndromes without ST-segment elevation. *N Engl J Med* 2001;345:494–502.
174. Peters RJ, Mehta SR, Fox KA, et al. Effects of aspirin dose when used alone or in combination with clopidogrel in patients with acute coronary syndromes: observations from the Clopidogrel in Unstable angina to prevent Recurrent Events (CURE) study. *Circulation* 2003;108:1682–1687.
175. Hasdai D, Holmes DR Jr, Criger DA, et al. Cigarette smoking status and outcome among patients with acute coronary syndromes without persistent ST-segment-elevation: effect of inhibition of platelet glycoprotein IIb/IIIa with eptifibatide. The PURSUIT Trial Investigators. *Am Heart J* 2000;139:454–460.
176. Mari D, Mannucci P, Coppola R, et al. Hypercoagulability in centenarians: the paradox of successful aging. *Blood* 1995;85:3144–3149.
177. Campbell NR, Hull RD, Brant R, et al. Aging and heparin-related bleeding. *Arch Intern Med* 1996;156:857–860.
178. Spinler S, Evans CM. Update in unfractionated heparin, low-molecular-weight heparins, and heparinoids in the elderly (age >64 years). *J Thromb Thrombolysis* 2000;9:117.
179. Toss H, Wallentin L, Siegbahn A. Influences of sex and smoking habits on anticoagulant activity in low-molecular-weight heparin treatment of unstable coronary artery disease. *Am Heart J* 1999;137:72–78.
180. Wallentin L, Lagergvst B, Husted S, et al. Outcome at 1 year after an invasive compared with a non-invasive strategy in unstable coronary-artery disease: the FRISC II invasive randomised trial. *Lancet* 2000;356: 9–16.
181. Fox K, Poole-Wilson PA, Henderson RA, et al. Interventional versus conservative treatment for patients with unstable angina or non-ST-elevation myocardial infarction: the British Heart Foundation RITA 3 randomised trial. *Lancet* 2002;360:743–751.
182. Cannon CP, Weintraub WS, Demopoulos LA, et al. Comparison of early invasive and conservative strategies in patients with unstable coronary syndromes treated with the glycoprotein IIb/IIIa inhibitor tirofiban. *N Engl J Med* 2001;344:1879–1887.
183. Bach RG, Cannon CP, Weintraub WS, et al. The effect of routine, early invasive management on outcome for elderly patients with non-ST-segment elevation acute coronary syndromes. *Ann Intern Med* 2004;141:186–195.
184. Rathore SS, Mehta RH, Wang Y, et al. Age and quality of care provided to elderly patients with acute myocardial infarction. *Am J Med* 2003;114:307–315.
185. Sheifer SE, Rathore SS, Gersh BJ, et al. Time to presentation with acute myocardial infarction in the elderly. Associations with race, sex, and socioeconomic characteristics. *Circulation* 2000;102:1651–1656.
186. Eagle K, Goodman S, Avezum A, et al. Practice variation and missed opportunities for reperfusion in ST-segment-elevation myocardial infarction: findings from the Global Registry of acute Coronary Events (GRACE). *Lancet* 2002;369:373–377.
187. Berger AK, Schulman KA, Gersh BJ, et al. Primary coronary angioplasty vs thrombolytics for the management of acute myocardial infarction in elderly patients. *JAMA* 1999;282:341–348.
188. Berger AK, Radford MJ, Krumholz HM. Factors associated with delay in reperfusion therapy in elderly patients with acute myocardial infarction: analysis of the cooperative cardiovascular project. *Am Heart J* 2000;139:985–992.
189. Martinez-Selles M, Datino T, Bueno H. Influence of reperfusion therapy on prognosis in patients aged >89 years with acute myocardial infarction. *Am J Cardiol* 2005;95:1232–1234.
190. Shlipak MG, Go AS, Frederick PD, et al. Treatment and outcomes of left bundle-branch block patients with myocardial infarction who present without chest pain. National Registry of Myocardial Infarction 2 Investigators. *J Am Coll Cardiol* 2000;36:706–712.
191. Califf RM, White HD, Van de Werf F, et al. One-year results from the Global Utilization of Streptokinase and TPA for Occluded Coronary Arteries (GUSTO-I) trial. GUSTO-I Investigators. *Circulation* 1996;94:1233–1238.
192. Volpi A, De Vita C, Franzosi MG, et al. Determinants of 6-month mortality in survivors of myocardial infarction after thrombolysis. Results of the GISSI-2 data base. The Ad hoc Working Group of the Gruppo Italiano per lo Studio della Sopravvivenza nell'Infarto Miocardico (GISSI)-2 Data Base. *Circulation* 1993;88:416–429.
193. Bueno H, Lopez-Palop R, Bermejo J, et al. In-hospital outcome of elderly patients with acute inferior myocardial infarction and right ventricular involvement. *Circulation* 1997;96:436–441.
194. Fibrinolytic Therapy Trialists' (FTT) Collaborative Group. Indications for fibrinolytic therapy in suspected acute myocardial infarction: collaborative overview of early mortality and major morbidity results from all randomized trials of more than 1,000 patients. *Lancet* 1994;343:311–322.
195. ISIS-2 (Second International Study of Infarct Survival) Collaborative Group. Randomised trial of intravenous streptokinase, oral aspirin, both, or neither among 17,187 cases of suspected acute myocardial infarction: ISIS-2. *Lancet* 1988;2:349–360.
196. Italiano per lo Studio della Sopravvivenza nell'Infarto Miocardico. GISSI-2: a factorial randomised trial of alteplase versus streptokinase and heparin versus no heparin among 12,490 patients with acute myocardial infarction. *Lancet* 1990;336:65–71.
197. Third International Study of Infarct Survival) Collaborative Group. ISIS-3: a randomised comparison of streptokinase vs tissue plasminogen activator vs anistreplase and of aspirin plus heparin vs aspirin alone among 41,299 cases of suspected acute myocardial infarction. *Lancet* 1992;339:753–770.
198. The GUSTO investigators. An international randomized trial comparing four thrombolytic strategies for acute myocardial infarction. *N Engl J Med* 1993;329:673–682.
199. O'Connor CM, Califf RM, Massey EW, et al. Stroke and acute myocardial infarction in the thrombolytic era: clinical correlates and long-term prognosis. *J Am Coll Cardiol* 1990;16:533–540.
200. Gore JM, Granger CB, Simoons ML, et al. Stroke after thrombolysis.Mortality and functional outcomes in the GUSTO-I trial. Global Use of Strategies to Open Occluded Coronary Arteries. *Circulation* 1995;92: 2811–2818.
201. Simoons ML, Maggioni AP, Knatterud G, et al. Individual risk assessment for intracranial haemorrhage during thrombolytic therapy. *Lancet* 1993;342:1523–1528.
202. White H. Thrombolytic therapy in the elderly: weighing up the risks and benefits. *Lancet* 2000;356:2028.
203. Thiemann DR, Coresh J, Schulman SP, et al. Lack of benefit for intravenous thrombolysis in patients with myocardial infarction who are older than 75 years. *Circulation* 2000;101:2239–2246.
204. Soumeral SB, McLaughlin TJ, Ross-Degnan D, et al. Effectiveness of thrombolytic therapy for acute myocardial infarction in the elderly: cause for concern in the old-old. *Arch Intern Med* 2002;161:561–568.
205. Angeja BG, Rundle AC, Gurwitz JH, et al. Death or nonfatal stroke in patients with acute myocardial infarction treated with tissue plasminogen activator. Participants in the National Registry of Myocardial Infarction-2. *Am J Cardiol* 2001;87:627–630.
206. Stenestrand U, Wallentin L, for the Register of Information and Knowledge About Swedish Heart Intensive Care Admissions (RIKS-HIA). Fibrinolytic therapy in patients 75 years and older with ST-segment-elevation myocardial infarction.One year follow-up of a large prospective cohort. *Arch Intern Med* 2003;163:965–971.
207. Antman EM, Anbe DT, Armstrong PW, et al. ACC/AHA guidelines for the management of patients with ST-elevation myocardial infarction: executive summary: a report of the ACC/AHA Task Force on Practice Guidelines

(Writing Committee to Revise the 1999 Guidelines for the Management of Patients With Acute Myocardial Infarction). *Circulation* 2004;10:588–636.
208. Keeley EC, Boura JA, Grines CL. Primary angioplasty versus intravenous thrombolytic therapy for acute myocardial infarction: a quantitative review of 23 randomized trials. *Lancet* 2003;361:13–20.
209. Grines CL, Browne KF, Marco J, et al., for the Primary Angioplasty in Myocardial Infarction Study Group. A comparison of immediate angioplasty with thrombolytic therapy for acute myocardial infarction. *N Engl J Med* 1993;328:673–679.
210. A clinical trial comparing primary coronary angioplasty with tissue plasminogen activator for acute myocardial infarction. The Global Use of Strategies to Open Occluded Coronary Arteries in Acute Coronary Syndromes (GUSTO IIb) Angioplasty Substudy Investigators. *N Engl J Med* 1997;336:1621–1628.
211. Zijlstra F, Patel A, Jones M, et al. Clinical characteristics and outcome of patients with early (<2 h), intermediate (2–4 h) and late (>4 h) presentation treated by primary coronary angioplasty or thrombolytic therapy for acute myocardial infarction. *Eur Heart J* 2002;23:550–557.
212. PCAT Collaborators'. Primary coronary angioplasty compared with intravenous thrombolytic therapy for acute myocardial infarction: six-month follow up and analysis of individual patient data from randomized trials. *Am Heart J* 2003;145:47–57.
213. Tiefenbrunn AJ, Chandra NC, French WJ, et al. Clinical experience with primary percutaneous transluminal coronary angioplasty compared with alteplase (recombinant tissue-type plasminogen activator) in patients with acute myocardial infarction: a report from the Second National Registry of Myocardial Infarction (NRMI-2). *J Am Coll Cardiol* 1998;31:1240–1245.
214. Goldberg RJ, Gore JM, Gurwitz JH, et al. The impact of age on the incidence and prognosis of initial acute myocardial infarction: the Worcester Heart Attack Study. *Am Heart J* 1989;117:543–549.
215. Hochman JS, Buller CE, Sleeper LA, et al. Cardiogenic shock complicating acute myocardial infarction—etiologies, management and outcome: a report from the SHOCK Trial Registry. SHould we emergently revascularize Occluded Coronaries for cardiogenic shocK? *J Am Coll Cardiol* 2000;36[3 Suppl A]:1063–1070.
216. Hochman JS, Sleeper LA, Webb JG, et al. Early revascularization in acute myocardial infarction complicated by cardiogenic shock. SHOCK Investigators. Should We Emergently Revascularize Occluded Coronaries for Cardiogenic Shock. *N Engl J Med* 1999;341:625–634.
217. Thompson CR, Buller CE, Sleeper LA, et al. Cardiogenic shock due to acute severe mitral regurgitation complicating acute myocardial infarction: a report from the SHOCK Trial Registry. SHould we use emergently revascularize Occluded Coronaries in cardiogenic shocK? *J Am Coll Cardiol* 2000;36[3 Suppl A]:1104–1109.
218. Menon V, Webb JG, Hillis LD, et al. Outcome and profile of ventricular septal rupture with cardiogenic shock after myocardial infarction: a report from the SHOCK Trial Registry. SHould we emergently revascularize Occluded Coronaries in cardiogenic shocK? *J Am Coll Cardiol* 2000;36[3 Suppl A]:1110–1116.
219. Slater J, Brown RJ, Antonelli TA, et al. Cardiogenic shock due to cardiac free-wall rupture or tamponade after acute myocardial infarction: a report from the SHOCK Trial Registry.Should we emergently revascularize occluded coronaries for cardiogenic shock? *J Am Coll Cardiol* 2000;36[3 Suppl A]:1117–1122.
220. Bueno H, Martinez-Selles M, Perez-David E, et al. Effect of thrombolytic therapy on the risk of cardiac rupture and mortality in older patients with first acute myocardial infarction. *Eur Heart J* 2005;26:1705–1711.
221. Schocken DD, Sharma K, Schwartz S, et al. Population-based prevalence and mortality of heart failure in the United States: data from NHANES II with 12–16 year follow-up. *Circulation* 1999;100[Suppl I]:I-396.
222. Senni M, Tribouilloy CM, Rodeheffer RJ, et al. Congestive heart failure in the community: trends in incidence and survival in a 10-year period. *Arch Intern Med* 1999;159:29–34.
223. Chen YT, Vaccarino V, Williams CS, et al. Risk factors for heart failure in the elderly: a prospective community-based study. *Am J Med* 1999;106: 605–612.
224. Rich MW, Beckham V, Wittenberg C, et al. A multidisciplinary intervention to prevent the readmission of elderly patients with congestive heart failure. *N Engl J Med* 1995;333:1190–1195.
225. Vasan RS, Larson MG, Benjamin EJ, et al. Congestive heart failure in subjects with normal versus reduced left ventricular ejection fraction: prevalence and mortality in a population-based cohort. *J Am Coll Cardiol* 1999;33:1948–1955.
226. Adams KF Jr, Fonarow GC, Emerman CL, et al. Characteristics and outcomes of patients hospitalized for heart failure in the United States: rationale, design, and preliminary observations from the first 100,000 cases in the Acute Decompensated Heart Failure National Registry (ADHERE). *Am Heart J* 2005;149:209–216.
227. Gottdiener JS, Arnold AM, Aurigemma GP, et al. Predictors of congestive heart failure in the elderly: the Cardiovascular Health Study. *J Am Coll Cardiol* 2000;35:1628–1637.
228. Bibbins-Domingo K, Lin F, Vittinghoff E, et al. Predictors of heart failure among women with coronary disease. *Circulation* 2004;110:1424–1430.
229. Gaasch WH. Diagnosis and treatment of heart failure based on left ventricular systolic or diastolic dysfunction. *JAMA* 1994;271:1276–1280.
230. Guidelines for the diagnosis of heart failure. The Task Force on Heart Failure of the European Society of Cardiology. *Eur Heart J* 1995;16:741–751.
231. Cowie MR, Wood DA, Coats AJ, et al. Incidence and aetiology of heart failure; a population-based study. *Eur Heart J* 1999;20:421–428.
232. Cody RJ, Torre S, Clark M, et al. Age-related hemodynamic, renal, and hormonal differences among patients with congestive heart failure. *Arch Intern Med* 1989;149:1023–1028.
233. Ghali JK, Kadakia S, Bhatt A, et al. Survival of heart failure patients with preserved versus impaired systolic function: the prognostic implication of blood pressure. *Am Heart J* 1992;123:993–997.
234. Gandhi SK, Powers JC, Nomeir AM, et al. The pathogenesis of acute pulmonary edema associated with hypertension. *N Engl J Med* 2001;344:17–22.
235. Fleg JL, Kitzman DW, Aronow WS, et al. Physician management of patients with heart failure and normal versus decreased left ventricular systolic function. Council on Geriatric Cardiology. *Am J Cardiol* 1998;81:506–509.
236. Gardin JM, Arnold AM, Bild DE, et al. Left ventricular diastolic filling in the elderly: the cardiovascular health study. *Am J Cardiol* 1998;82:345–351.
237. Rutherford JD, Pfeffer MA, Moye LA, et al. Effects of captopril on ischemic events after myocardial infarction.Results of the Survival and Ventricular Enlargement trial. SAVE Investigators. *Circulation* 1994;90:1731–1738.
238. Cotter G, Moshkovitz Y, Kaluski E, et al. The role of cardiac power and systemic vascular resistance in the pathophysiology and diagnosis of patients with acute congestive heart failure. *Eur J Heart Fail* 2003;5:443–451.
239. Gattis WA, O'Connor CM, Hasselblad V, et al. Usefulness of an elevated troponin-I in predicting clinical events in patients admitted with acute heart failure and acute coronary syndrome (from the RITZ-4 trial). *Am J Cardiol* 2004;93:1436–1437.
240. Patel MR, Baeza RG, Goyal A, et al. Highlights from the American College of Cardiology Annual Scientific Session 2005: March 6 to 9, 2005, Orlando, Florida. *Am Heart J* 2005;149:1009–1019.
241. Dao Q, Krishnaswamy P, Kazanegra R, et al. Utility of B-type natriuretic peptide in the diagnosis of congestive heart failure in an urgent-care setting. *J Am Coll Cardiol* 2001;37:379–385.
242. Cheng V, Kazanagra R, Garcia A, et al. A rapid bedside test for B-type peptide predicts treatment outcomes in patients admitted for decompensated heart failure: a pilot study. *J Am Coll Cardiol* 2001;37:386–391.
243. Maisel A. B-type natriuretic peptide measurements in diagnosing congestive heart failure in the dyspneic emergency department patient. *Rev Cardiovasc Med* 2002;3[Suppl 4]:S10–S17.
244. McCullough PA, Nowak RM, McCord J, et al. B-type natriuretic peptide and clinical judgment in emergency diagnosis of heart failure: analysis from Breathing Not Properly (BNP) Multinational Study. *Circulation* 2002;106:416–422.
245. Furberg CD, Psaty BM, Manolio TA, et al. Prevalence of atrial fibrillation in elderly subjects (the Cardiovascular Health Study). *Am J Cardiol* 1994;74:236–241.
246. O'Connor CM, Gattis WA, Shaw L, et al. Clinical characteristics and long-term outcomes of patients with heart failure and preserved systolic function. *Am J Cardiol* 2000;86:863–867.
247. Swedberg K, Held P, Kjekshus J, et al. Effects of the early administration of enalapril on mortality in patients with acute myocardial infarction.Results of the Cooperative New Scandinavian Enalapril Survival Study II (CONSENSUS II). *N Engl J Med* 1992;327:678–684.
248. Roger VL, Weston SA, Redfield MM, et al. Trends in heart failure incidence and survival in a community-based population. *JAMA* 2004;292:344–350.
249. Aronow WS, Ahn C. Incidence of heart failure in 2,737 older persons with and without diabetes mellitus. *Chest* 1999;115:867–868.
250. Cuffe MS, Califf RM, Adams KF Jr, et al. Short-term intravenous milrinone for acute exacerbation of chronic heart failure: a randomized controlled trial. *JAMA* 2002;287:1541–1547.
251. Fonarow GC. The Acute Decompensated Heart Failure National Registry (ADHERE): opportunities to improve care of patients hospitalized with acute decompensated heart failure. *Rev Cardiovasc Med* 2003;4[Suppl 7]:S21–S30.
252. Fonarow GC. Strategies to improve the use of evidence-based heart failure therapies: OPTIMIZE-HF. *Rev Cardiovasc Med* 2004;5[Suppl 1]:S45–S54.
253. Packer M, Bristow MR, Cohn JN, et al. The effect of carvedilol on morbidity and mortality in patients with chronic heart failure. U.S. Carvedilol Heart Failure Study Group. *N Engl J Med* 1996;334:1349–1355.
254. The Digitalis Investigation Group. The effect of digoxin on mortality and morbidity in patients with heart failure. *N Engl J Med* 1997;336:525–533.
255. Pitt B, Segal R, Martinez FA, et al. Randomised trial of losartan versus captopril in patients over 65 with heart failure (Evaluation of Losartan in the Elderly Study, ELITE). *Lancet* 1997;349:747–752.
256. Packer M, O'Connor CM, Ghali JK, et al. Effect of amlodipine on morbidity and mortality in severe chronic heart failure. Prospective Randomized Amlodipine Survival Evaluation Study Group. *N Engl J Med* 1996;335:1107–1114.
257. MERIT-HF Study Group. Effect of metoprolol CR/XL in chronic heart failure: Metoprolol CR/XL Randomised Intervention Trial in Congestive Heart Failure (MERIT-HF). *Lancet* 1999;353:2001–2007.

258. Pitt B, Zannad F, Remme WJ, et al. The effect of spironolactone on morbidity and mortality in patients with severe heart failure. Randomized Aldactone Evaluation Study Investigators. *N Engl J Med* 1999;341:709–717.
259. Pitt B, Poole-Wilson PA, Segal R, et al. Effect of losartan compared with captopril on mortality in patients with symptomatic heart failure: randomised trial—the Losartan Heart Failure Survival Study ELITE II. *Lancet* 2000;355:1582–1587.
260. Fonarow GC, Corday E. Overview of acutely decompensated congestive heart failure (ADHF): a report from the ADHERE registry. *Heart Fail Rev* 2004;9:179–185.
261. Cohn JN, Anand IS, Latini R, et al. Sustained reduction of aldosterone in response to the angiotensin receptor blocker valsartan in patients with chronic heart failure: results from the Valsartan Heart Failure Trial. *Circulation* 2003;108:1306–1309.
262. Pfeffer MA, Swedberg K, Granger CB, et al. Effects of candesartan on mortality and morbidity in patients with chronic heart failure: the CHARM-Overall programme. *Lancet* 2003;362:759–766.
263. Flather MD, Shibata MC, Coats AJ, et al. Randomized trial to determine the effect of nebivolol on mortality and cardiovascular hospital admission in elderly patients with heart failure (SENIORS). *Eur Heart J* 2005;26:215–225.
264. Dulin BR, Haas SJ, Abraham WT, Krum H. Do elderly systolic heart failure patients benefit from beta blockers to the same extent as the non-elderly? Meta-analysis of >12,000 patients in large-scale clinical trials. *Am J Cardiol* 2005;95:896–898.
265. The effect of digoxin on mortality and morbidity in patients with heart failure. The Digitalis Investigation Group. *N Engl J Med* 1997;336:525–533.
266. Adams KF Jr, Patterson JH, Gattis WA, et al. Relationship of serum digoxin concentration to mortality and morbidity in women in the digitalis investigation group trial: a retrospective analysis. *J Am Coll Cardiol* 2005;46:497–504.
267. Carson P, Massie BM, McKelvie R, et al. The Irbesartan in Heart Failure With Preserved Systolic Function (I-PRESERVE) Trial: rationale and design. *J Card Fail* 2005;11:576–585.
268. Sahasakul Y, Edwards WD, Naessens JM, et al. Age-related changes in aortic and mitral valve thickness: implications for two-dimensional echocardiography based on an autopsy study of 200 normal human hearts. *Am J Cardiol* 1988;62:424–430.
269. American Heart Association. *Heart disease and stroke statistics—2005 update*. Dallas, TX: American Heart Association; 2005.
270. Lindroos M, Kupari M, Heikkila J, et al. Prevalence of aortic valve abnormalities in the elderly: an echocardiographic study of a random population sample. *J Am Coll Cardiol* 1993;21:1220–1225.
271. Passik CS, Ackermann DM, Pluth JR, et al. Temporal changes in the causes of aortic stenosis: a surgical pathologic study of 646 cases. *Mayo Clin Proc* 1987;62:119–123.
272. Otto CM, Kuusisto J, Reichenbach DD, et al. Characterization of the early lesion of 'degenerative' valvular aortic stenosis. Histological and immunohistochemical studies. *Circulation* 1994;90:844–853.
273. Isoyama S, Wei JY, Izumo S, et al. Effect of age on the development of cardiac hypertrophy produced by aortic constriction in the rat. *Circ Res* 1987;61:337–345.
274. Sprigings DC, Forfar JC. How should we manage symptomatic aortic stenosis in the patient who is 80 or older? *Br Heart J* 1995;74:481–484.
275. Akasaka T, Yoshikawa J, Yoshida K, et al. Age-related valvular regurgitation: a study by pulsed Doppler echocardiography. *Circulation* 1987;76:262–265.
276. Bonow RO. Asymptomatic aortic regurgitation: indications for operation. *J Card Surg* 1994;9[Suppl]170–173.
277. Scognamiglio R, Rahimtoola SH, Fasoli G, et al. Nifedipine in asymptomatic patients with severe aortic regurgitation and normal left ventricular function. *N Engl J Med* 1994;331:689–694.
278. Evangelista A, Tornos P, Sambola A, et al. Long-term vasodilator therapy in patients with severe aortic regurgitation. *N Engl J Med* 2005;353:1342–1349.
279. Korn D, Desanctis RW, Sell S. Massive calcification of the mitral annulus. A clinicopathological study of fourteen cases. *N Engl J Med* 1962;267:900–909.
280. Devereux RB. Recent developments in the diagnosis and management of mitral valve prolapse. *Curr Opin Cardiol* 1995;10:107–116.
281. Leibovitch ER. Cardiac valve disorders: growing significance in the elderly. *Geriatrics* 1989;44:91–99.
282. Enriquez-Sarano M, Tajik AJ, Schaff HV, et al. Echocardiographic prediction of left ventricular function after correction of mitral regurgitation: results and clinical implications. *J Am Coll Cardiol* 1994;24:1536–1543.
283. Ross J Jr. Left ventricular function and the timing of surgical treatment in valvular heart disease. *Ann Intern Med* 1981;94:498–504.
284. Jamieson WR, Munro AI, Miyagishima RT, et al. Carpentier-Edwards standard porcine bioprosthesis: clinical performance to seventeen years. *Ann Thorac Surg* 1995;60:999–1006.
285. Enriquez-Sarano M, Schaff HV, Orszulak TA, et al. Valve repair improves the outcome of surgery for mitral regurgitation. A multivariate analysis. *Circulation* 1995;91:1022–1028.
286. Azar H, Szentpetery S. Mitral valve repair in patients over the age of 70 years. *Eur J Cardiothorac Surg* 1994;8:298–300.
287. Jebara VA, Dervanian P, Acar C, et al. Mitral valve repair using Carpentier techniques in patients more than 70 years old. Early and late results. *Circulation* 1992;86[Suppl]II53–II59.
288. Chen FY, Adams DH, Aranki SF, et al. Mitral valve repair in cardiomyopathy. *Circulation* 1998;98[9 Suppl]II124–II127.
289. Christenson JT, Simonet F, Maurice J, et al. Mitral regurgitation in patients with coronary artery disease and low left ventricular ejection fractions. How should it be treated? *Tex Heart Inst J* 1995;22:243–249.
290. Link MS, Hellkamp AS, Estes NA III, et al. High incidence of pacemaker syndrome in patients with sinus node dysfunction treated with ventricular-based pacing in the Mode Selection Trial (MOST). *J Am Coll Cardiol* 2004;43:2066–2071.
291. Wilkoff BL, Cook JR, Epstein AE, et al. Dual-chamber pacing or ventricular backup pacing in patients with an implantable defibrillator: the Dual Chamber and VVI Implantable Defibrillator (DAVID) Trial. *JAMA* 2002;288:3115–3123.
292. Bardy GH, Lee KL, Mark DB, et al. Amiodarone or an implantable cardioverter-defibrillator for congestive heart failure. *N Engl J Med* 2005;352:225–237.
293. Zieman SJ, Fortuin NJ. Hypertrophic and restrictive cardiomyopathies in the elderly. *Cardiol Clin* 1999;17:159–172.
294. Backes RJ, Gersh BJ. Cardiomyopathies in the elderly. *Cardiovasc Clin* 1992;22:105–125.
295. Lewis JF, Maron BJ. Elderly patients with hypertrophic cardiomyopathy: a subset with distinctive left ventricular morphology and progressive clinical course late in life. *J Am Coll Cardiol* 1989;13:36–45.
296. Topol EJ, Traill TA, Fortuin NJ. Hypertensive hypertrophic cardiomyopathy of the elderly. *N Engl J Med* 1985;312:277–283.
297. Fay WP, Taliercio CP, Ilstrup DM, et al. Natural history of hypertrophic cardiomyopathy in the elderly. *J Am Coll Cardiol* 1990;16:821–826.
298. Watkins H. Multiple disease genes cause hypertrophic cardiomyopathy. *Br Heart J* 1994;72[Suppl]S4–S9.
299. Schwartz K, Carrier L, Guicheney P, et al. Molecular basis of familial cardiomyopathies. *Circulation* 1995;91:532–540.
300. Haugland H, Ohm OJ, Boman H, et al. Hypertrophic cardiomyopathy in three generations of a large Norwegian family. A clinical, echocardiographic, and genetic study. *Br Heart J* 1986;55:168–175.
301. Davies MJ, McKenna WJ. Hypertrophic cardiomyopathy: an introduction to pathology and pathogenesis. *Br Heart J* 1994;72[Suppl]S2–S3.
302. Niimura H, Bachinski LL, Sangwatanaroj S, et al. Mutations in the gene for cardiac myosin-binding protein C and late-onset familial hypertrophic cardiomyopathy. *N Engl J Med* 1998;338:1248–1257.
303. Pomerance A. Senile cardiac amyloidosis. *Br Heart J* 1965;27:711–718.
304. Lie JT, Hammond PI. Pathology of the senescent heart: anatomic observations on 237 autopsy studies of patients 90 to 105 years old. *Mayo Clin Proc* 198863:552–564.
305. Johansson B, Westermark P. Senile systemic amyloidosis: a clinicopathological study of twelve patients with massive amyloid infiltration. *Int J Cardiol* 1991;32:83–92.
306. Pitkanen P, Westermark P, Cornwell GG III. Senile systemic amyloidosis. *Am J Pathol* 1984;117:391–399.
307. Olson LJ, Gertz MA, Edwards WD, et al. Senile cardiac amyloidosis with myocardial dysfunction. Diagnosis by endomyocardial biopsy and immunohistochemistry. *N Engl J Med* 1987;317:738–742.
308. Kyle RA, Gertz MA. Cardiac amyloidosis. *Int J Cardiol* 1990;28:139–141.
309. Rubinow A, Skinner M, Cohen AS. Digoxin sensitivity in amyloid cardiomyopathy. *Circulation* 1981;63:1285–1288.
310. Centers for Medicare & Medicaid Services OoIS. Data from the Medicare decision support access facility. Available: www.cms hhs gov/review/supp/2003/table19.pdf. Accessed November 16, 2005.

CHAPTER 34 ■ END-OF-LIFE CARE

GARY S. FRANCIS AND JULIE LAVEGLIA

OVERVIEW

Life in the coronary care unit (CCU) is changing. Once a comfortable "laboratory" for conducting studies of physiology and pharmacology, as well as a bastion of medical education, the modern CCU has become a vastly different place over the course of the last 15 to 20 years. This is particularly true in large, tertiary teaching hospitals. The patients are older and sicker, and they have more multiorgan dysfunction than before. They frequently require multiple-team, interdisciplinary management. Patients who have routine, uncomplicated myocardial infarction continue to be admitted, but many such patients are now well cared for in large suburban hospitals by highly qualified cardiologists. Tertiary teaching hospitals more often receive elderly patients with highly complex conditions who are transferred on day 2 or 3 of acute myocardial infarction complicated by acute pulmonary edema, stroke, refractory ventricular tachycardia, cardiogenic shock, severe mitral regurgitation, ruptured interventricular septum, critical aortic stenosis, acute renal failure, sepsis, or some combination. Such patients can usually be stabilized and their conditions managed, but they not uncommonly languish for days in the CCU, obtunded, unable to be easily weaned from the ventilator. Anxious families understandably become frustrated, and uncertainty about prognosis only serves to further fracture the bond between the medical team and family members.

The dilemma is made worse by the inability of many patients to participate in the decision-making process. Families may be absent. Occasionally, competing interests and desires may emerge among family members. Decisions about the end of life are seemingly more complex in today's world. Resources are often constrained, and economic pressures exist to reduce the length of stay in the CCU. The overall daily charges for the CCU range from \$2,000 to \$10,000 per day. To put the economic burden into perspective, it is estimated that critical care costs in the United States are more than \$80 billion per year, or approximately 1% of the gross domestic product (1). Of course, the high cost of care is a global problem, certainly not unique to the United States.

The aging CCU patient population, complexity of disease, high prevalence of multiorgan dysfunction, unrealistic expectations of patients and families, and persistence of taboos regarding discussions of the end of life in most cultures mean that physicians who work in the CCU must be familiar with certain guiding principles regarding the withholding and withdrawal of life support systems. The decision to withhold or withdraw life-sustaining support from a critically ill patient is an increasingly difficult but necessary part of providing care in the CCU. The preciousness of human life is embedded in nearly every religion and culture. The natural tendency of every physician is to nurture the patient back to health, and therefore to preserve life without regard to age, cost, or other culturally imposed boundaries. It is clear that in a small number of cases, death is inescapable. In such cases, the wise physician turns attention to the family, while ensuring that the patient is made comfortable. But mostly there are gray zones, in which outcomes are uncertain and decisions about continued aggressive treatments are extremely difficult. Uncertainty becomes champion.

How are these decisions made? Who makes these decisions? What are the ethical principles that underlie these decisions? How does a physician actually withdraw life support? The goal of this chapter is to provide CCU physicians with practical advice that will help to guide them through this difficult process.

HISTORICAL PERSPECTIVE

For many years, the ethical and legal consensus in the United States has been that patients and their surrogates have the right to refuse life-prolonging therapy. This stems from the common law right of self-determination (the principles of autonomy), which was upheld by the U.S. Supreme Court in 1891 (2). Despite agreement on this general principle, dying patients in the United States frequently receive unwanted interventions (3,4). The patient's right to autonomy, although sacred and carefully guarded, sometimes competes with the staff member's skill in providing aggressive life-extending treatment. Physicians and nurses are often poorly trained in withholding or withdrawing intensive life support. It is sometimes easier for them to continue aggressive care than to struggle with the difficult decision to withdraw life support. This issue came to a head in the landmark case of Karen Ann Quinlan (1976), and the courts ultimately forged a legal consensus based on the principle of patient autonomy. This principle establishes the right of patients (or their surrogates) to determine which medical interventions to accept or refuse, even when the absence of treatment results in death. It was affirmed by the U.S. Supreme Court in the case of Nancy Cruzan in 1990. The court acknowledged that patients who die after life support is withheld or withdrawn die of the underlying disease process. Such deaths are not assisted suicides or euthanasia. The courts have also reasoned that the spouse and children are the most appropriate surrogates because they are best positioned to know the patient's feelings and desires about treatment.

In fact, next of kin are no better than physicians in estimating what the patient would want with regard to end-of-life care (5). Therefore, the physician, acting on behalf of the patient, must assess the validity of the surrogates' preferences and the commonality of belief structure. Friends or family members may hold power of attorney to make decisions for the patient, as directed by a living will or advanced directive. However, living wills have not had a major impact on decision making or costs associated with end-of-life care because they are so nonspecific. Patients frequently express different beliefs when they are healthy than when they face decisions about withdrawal of life support measures (6). The U.S. Supreme Court has unanimously ruled that there is no constitutional right to physician-assisted suicide, but has also effectively required all states to ensure that their laws do not obstruct the provision of palliative care—including the administration of drugs as needed to avoid pain at the end of life (7). The provision of morphine or other medications at the end of life to control pain and suffering has the full force of the judiciary behind it.

From a historical context, these rulings have come at a time when modern technology can sustain organ function for prolonged periods, and thus they are of great importance to physicians working in the CCU. Lay people, through the print media and television, have come to expect full recovery after illness. Families and patients often seem mystified when informed of the details of an illness and become alarmed when they realize that meaningful recovery may not be possible. The gap between family expectations and medical reality can only be closed by frequent empathetic and effective communication between the medical team, the family, and, when appropriate, the patient.

The widely publicized case of Terri Schiavo has reinforced the concept that people should carefully consider and discuss with spouses and family members how they want to be managed in case there is a life-threatening injury or illness. Most important, a power of attorney should be identified who can speak for the critically ill patient in the event of incapacitation.

ETHICAL PRINCIPLES

Some fundamental principles of medical ethics have evolved over centuries and are generally accepted (Table 34.1).

TABLE 34.1

FUNDAMENTAL PRINCIPLES OF MEDICAL ETHICS

Autonomy
Preservation of life
Alleviation of suffering
First do no harm
Justice: ensure that medical resources are allocated fairly
Telling the truth
The rule of double effect

Autonomy

The term *autonomy* is derived from the Greek words *auto* (self) and *nomos* (rule or law). The principle is the source of the common law right of self-determination and lies behind the constitutional right of privacy. No right is held more sacred, and the U.S. Supreme Court has used this principle in asserting the right of patients to refuse life-saving treatment. If an adult patient is heavily sedated or unconscious, a surrogate decision maker (usually a spouse or family member) should authorize decisions about care. Health care providers need to realize that decisions about care are in the hands of the patient, not the medical team. The attending physician and other members of the medical team determine treatment strategy on the basis of scientific principles and then decide on the best course of action based on discussion with the patient or the families. The patient (or the surrogate decision maker) almost always accepts the team's advice, but the relationship is one of partnership, not paternalism. The ethical principle of autonomy states that the patient has a right to self-determination that supersedes the desires of the medical team—even if it means that death of the patient will result. In the United States, minors do not have autonomy under the law, and parents become the decision makers.

The CCU environment does not always allow for the luxury of time, and lengthy discussions with multiple family members are sometimes not possible. Management of cardiogenic shock, recurrent ventricular fibrillation, acute pulmonary edema, or acute aortic dissection requires quick, reasoned actions. In such emergencies, the principle of preservation of life guides the team of caregivers, provided there are no antecedent instructions from the patient or family to withhold life support.

Although end-of-life issues are best discussed in the privacy of the outpatient clinic when the patient is medically stable, many patients misunderstand the process of advanced life support or are apprehensive about discussing death. Moreover, people's views change when they become acutely ill (6), so the outpatient view may not be synonymous with the view when faced with the actual end of life. There is a nearly universal taboo against discussing death, which is particularly common among the older generation. A significant number of people prefer a less dominant autonomous role in end-of-life decisions and put their trust in their doctors and the health care system (8). To approach a critically ill patient in the CCU with heartless questions about cardiopulmonary resuscitation and intubation is a grotesque distortion of what should be a very private, reasoned dialogue. Trying to berate a sick patient into being autonomous near end of life is a tragic mistake. Our practice is always to discuss end of life in the outpatient setting when appropriate, but recognizing that views may change. When this is not possible, which is often the case, it is helpful to talk to the patient with a nurse or alone at the bedside and attempt to have them understand and make distinctions between short-term aggressive care and prolonged life support.

In the end, the informed patient can usually make an autonomous decision. Physicians must guard against imposing their own values and should not slant the discussion in such a way as to mirror their own feelings about the end of life. It must be recognized that some cultures object to informing patients of a terminal diagnosis. It may be believed that the family, not the patient, should make life support decisions. Violating a patient's cultural values should be avoided. This is a serious problem that defies a simple solution. It is often useful to have serious dialogue with the family and then the patient as soon as possible—usually within 48 hours of admission to the CCU.

Preservation of Life

All physicians and nurses are aware of this ethical principle, and it requires no explanation. Problems may arise when preservation of life competes with beneficence or alleviation of suffering. For a dying patient, alleviation of suffering may be more important than prolonging the end of life. However, the sanctity of life is of great importance and has its roots in most religions. Many believe that every second of life is sacred and must be preserved at all cost.

Alleviation of Suffering (Beneficence)

To restore health and relieve suffering is one of the most time-honored goals of physicians. It is the fundamental duty of all doctors. Beneficence supersedes the perceived beliefs of society or the personal values of the physician. Relief of suffering may supersede preservation of life (see the section Rule of Double Effect), particularly when death is inescapable.

First Do No Harm (Nonmaleficence)

Primum non nocere is an ancient principle of medicine and is embedded in the Hippocratic oath: "I will use treatment to help the sick according to my ability and judgment, but I will never use it to injure or wrong them." This principle underlies the physician's decision to recognize that death is inescapable and to proceed with comfort care. However, the Hippocratic oath's injunction to "do no harm" seldom applies in today's environment. It is unethical to continue aggressive care for patients who have no hope for recovery; the physician's goal is to provide comfort, not to prolong dying. Likewise, inappropriate drug use and the ordering of diagnostic tests that are potentially risky but not likely to help the patient are unethical under certain circumstances. On the other hand, there may be pressure from families to "keep going." Such a dilemma requires frequent and careful dialogue with the family. It may take days for some family members to realize that death is imminent. In the CCU, it is not always possible to know when death is inescapable, and it is important for the physician to convey a sense of hope, when appropriate. Families and patients sometimes have unrealistic expectations and will request that "everything be done," even though the patient has little or no hope for meaningful recovery. Some families will put a highly spiritual spin on the problem and insist that the medical team should hold out for a "miracle." Sometimes, the patient wants more aggressive care than the family thinks is appropriate (9). Physicians may be inaccurately overly pessimistic, whereas patients tend to be inaccurately overly optimistic (8). Frequent, careful assessment of the patient and the prognosis coupled with frequent communication with family becomes even more important.

An experienced CCU team can often sense when multiorgan failure is beginning to emerge and is keenly aware of this when each day brings a new struggle to keep the patient alive. Such patients are often intubated, sedated, and unable to carry on meaningful dialogue. It is the caregivers who have specialized knowledge of the natural history of disease, not the family. It is the medical team who must use this powerful knowledge to help guide families when making decisions about withdrawal of life support. Families often want certainty, but there is no certainty in most instances, only judgments. Medical teams should clearly describe what will likely happen if aggressive treatments are continued and contrast this information with what will likely happen if comfort-only care is begun. A combination of objective quantitative information and the team's judgment about outcome is better than either alone (8).

Justice: Ensure That Medical Resources Are Allocated Fairly

It is clear that some economically deprived populations are underserved and as a consequence may have higher morbidity and mortality rates. Decisions regarding care should be blind to economic circumstances, ethnicity, perceived societal views, political persuasion, gender, and age. As care becomes more rationed in our society, the principle of justice takes on more practical importance. Heart transplantation, for example, is a highly rationed form of treatment with generally accepted medical indications and contraindications. If a heart is transplanted into a patient who does not comply with treatment and who dies quickly of rejection, two people die: the noncompliant patient and the anonymous patient on the transplant list who dies awaiting a heart transplant. In our society, end-stage heart failure and the need for heart transplants occurs in cocaine dealers, prisoners, pedophiles, and wealthy elderly people who are beyond the usual age limit for heart transplantation. The principle of justice would assume that only medical need determines care. However, outcomes for heart transplantation are affected by social issues, medical compliance, age, family support, and underlying general health. If there were a surplus of donor hearts, decisions about who should receive a heart transplant would be less difficult. As all therapy becomes more rationed in an era of harsh cost containment, the principle of justice becomes more applicable in the CCU. The principle of justice will become more difficult to apply as competition for scarce resources intensifies. Some evidence exists that justice has been ignored and that racial bias has entered the decision-making process (9).

Telling the Truth

Honest communication between physician and patient is very important and is a major principle of ethics in Western society (10). In some societies, it is considered inappropriate to tell a patient that he or she has cancer; the stigma and fear associated with knowing one has cancer outweigh the active withholding of information about diagnosis and prognosis. In the United States, it is assumed that patients and families want to understand the diagnosis, prognosis, and risks and benefits of various diagnostic and therapeutic procedures, but the level of understanding desired by patients and families is highly variable (5). This principle is particularly important to uphold in the CCU, where the presence of many different teams and fellows can greatly fragment the care of the patient. It is important to try to personally explain to the patient the risks and benefits of cardiac catheterization, percutaneous coronary interventions, and cardiac surgery, fully understanding that someone else will obtain direct informed consent and will further expound on the risks and benefits of these procedures. Patients tend to view the CCU team and the attending physician as "their" doctors. This is who they see on rounds daily and know and trust most explicitly, and this is who should explain to the patient and family what diagnostic and therapeutic plans are evolving—what the strategy will be for the next 24 to 72 hours. Consultants may be asked to discuss the case with families on occasion. For example, when complex noncardiac complications occur, such as intracerebral hemorrhage or severe hypoxic encephalopathy, it is reasonable for the neurology team to have a discussion with the family. If an internist or family doctor has a long-standing relationship with the patient, that person should be consulted and engaged with the decision when possible.

Rule of Double Effect

The rule of double effect may be the ethical principle least understood by medical personnel and lay people. Many are not even aware of the principle. According to the rule of double effect, outcomes that would be morally wrong if intentionally provoked are permissible if foreseen but unintended (11–13). Specifically, administering opioids to treat a terminally ill patient's dyspnea or pain may be acceptable even if the medication contributes to or causes the patient's death. A harmful effect of treatment, even death, is permissible if death is not intended but occurs only as a side effect of a beneficial action. It is not uncommon for dying or terminally ill patients in the CCU to receive morphine as part of comfort care. It is usually given in small doses (an initial drip of 1–2 mg/h or repeated boluses ranging from 10–30 mg/h) to alleviate air hunger or dyspnea, supplemented by benzodiazepines to treat anxiety or agitation. Patients with renal dysfunction may be best treated with fentanyl; morphine may accumulate and lead to undesired respiratory depression. Appropriate use of opioids for symptom control does not usually shorten life, and there is generally little or no need to invoke the rule of double effect (14).

The rule of double effect was developed by moral theologians of the Roman Catholic Church in the Middle Ages (15,16). The underlying logic is that it is impossible for a person to avoid all harmful actions. Failure to intervene to comfort a dying patient harms the patient by allowing treatable discomfort to continue. If the intent of treatment is to relieve suffering, the foreseen but unintended risk of earlier death is permissible. The U.S. Supreme Court has demonstrated support for this principle by requiring all states to ensure that their laws do not obstruct the provision of adequate palliative care, especially for alleviation of the physical discomfort of patients who are facing death (17,18). The physician's goal under these circumstances is to relieve the patient's discomfort (in this case, air hunger or dyspnea). Neither the physician nor the patient intends for the patient to die. If death occurs from the opioids (rare), it is foreseen but unintended. The rule of double effect and subsequent legal rulings supporting the principle have served to reassure physicians that prescribing morphine drips and other opioids for terminally ill patients is morally and legally permissible and is the proper thing to do (19).

FAMILY CONFLICTS

The decision to withdraw advanced life-support measures is one of the most difficult decisions that clinicians and families must make. Often the prognosis is not absolutely certain. The patient's judgment should be involved when possible, although most patients who are on advanced life support are not mentally competent. Only a small minority are able to participate in the initial decision to limit treatment (4% in a surgical intensive care unit [ICU] versus 27% in an oncology service) (20). It is important to provide hope to families, but hope is a double-edged sword. Hard questions need to be asked of families: What has been the family's experience with other dying patients? What do they consider "suffering"? What is their concept of "meaningful recovery"? The medical team should avoid offering guarantees and certainties regarding death or recovery. The worst thing a medical team can do is give mixed messages or abdicate responsibility. Families need time to deal with the devastating thought of withdrawal of life support systems and death. A useful tactic is to get the family together in a quiet, private room and discuss the issue at length. Give them room to vent. Allow the family to verbalize their grief. Make sure their spiritual needs are attended to by a hospital chaplain. Warring siblings with polarized desires for aggressive care versus comfort care are a particularly difficult problem, and an ethics consultation is usually in order. When our CCU team is first contemplating withdrawal of advanced life support, we take the following steps:

1. Determine the prognosis as carefully as possible. Unfortunately, Acute Physiologic Assessment and Chronic Health Evaluation scores do not apply to CCU patients. One must be able to deal with the uncertainty of dying.
2. Assess the patient's competence; engage them when possible. Patients receiving advanced life support are generally not mentally competent.
3. Discuss the case with the whole team and reach consensus about a decision. The bedside nurse often has a more expansive knowledge of the family and the patient's needs and wants.
4. Do not rush the families! A useful strategy is to tell them that if things do not improve over the next 48 to 72 hours, withdrawal of life support may be appropriate. It should be stressed that repeated procedures and diagnostic tests can be uncomfortable and can be a form of suffering. Emphasize that comfort care may allow the patient to have a more peaceful and dignified death. The time-limited goal often allows the family time to contemplate a most difficult decision.
5. Families need assurances that comfort care will be maintained and that the CCU team will not abandon them. However, in some cases, transferring the patient out of the CCU after withdrawal of life support is appropriate, and this should be explained to the family in anticipation of such a move.

When family members or legal surrogates want "everything done," the medical team should comply with this request. A direct challenge by the medical team usually fails to convince the family of the futility of further treatment, but repeated, compassionate discussions can result in ethical decisions that will benefit the patient.

FUTILITY

The concept of medical futility has been controversial and remains vague. It attempts to establish the principle that physicians may use their judgment and skills to determine when treatment is futile. Once such a determination has been made, the physician can unilaterally withhold or withdraw treatment, even if the patient or family objects. The principle of autonomy is thus essentially expunged. Futility is not an objective entity, but embraces many judgment-based values (21). There is no clear definition of medical futility (22). Such decisions, other than about physiologic futility (e.g., treating hypertension with an antibiotic) or an absolute inability to prevent death, always involve judging value. Whose value counts?

In reality, physicians can only frame choices for the patient; they cannot make unilateral decisions. Moreover, the courts have not recognized the right of physicians to act unilaterally in cases in which they believe further care would be futile (23). This is not to say that physicians do not recognize clinical situations in which care is futile. It simply means they cannot act unilaterally. Their obligation is to speak with the patient or the family, frame the issue, and have the patient or the family participate fully in the decision regarding further care. Judgments about anything other than physiologic futility are vague; imposed value judgments, imprecise definitions, a lack of concrete data, and great uncertainty about the definition of "futility" allow for an ambiguous concept. Communication of information to the family such as the success rate of resuscitation, long-term meaningful recovery, and likelihood of discharge from the hospital must be clear and consistent.

WITHHOLDING OR WITHDRAWAL OF LIFE-SUSTAINING THERAPY

Once the medical team and the patient or family have decided that the patient is dying and that further aggressive care is unwarranted, there is precious little guidance about how the process should be implemented. Physicians seem poorly trained in managing the transition from aggressive care to comfort care. The following steps should be considered:

- A final decision should be made after careful discussion with the patient (if appropriate), the family, and the nursing staff. It is vital that the team and family include discussion of comfort measures to be put into place and any resuscitative efforts, if any, to be carried out. Generally, no resuscitation effort is carried out.
- Such patients are frequently intubated, and therefore a do-not-resuscitate order should also be written. If the patient is not intubated, a do-not-intubate order should be written. A Do Not Resuscitate/Do Not Intubate (DNR/DNI) order should always be placed in the medical record to support the patient's and family's final decision.
- A morphine drip should be started. Patients in the CCU often suffer dyspnea as the primary discomfort, and morphine, 1 mg/h, usually alleviates this symptom. Presumed respiratory distress can be treated with a 5- to 10-mg bolus of morphine, followed by an increase in the infusion to 2 to 5 mg/h. Patients with renal insufficiency should probably not receive morphine. Fentanyl, which is hepatically metabolized, may be more appropriate.
- Conscious patients who manifest anxiety should be treated with intravenous lorazepam (1–4 mg every 30 minutes), and patients with delirium should be treated with intravenous haloperidol if necessary. If tolerance to these medications has developed, the hypnotic drug propofol may be used, provided profound left ventricular function is not present.
- Ventilation: In most cases, we prefer to leave the endotracheal tube in place while gradually decreasing the ventilator rate, positive end-expiratory pressure, oxygen therapy, and tidal volume until the patient is spontaneously breathing room air through the endotracheal tube. This way, secretions can be suctioned to prevent rattling, which may be perceived as suffering by the family. The gradual turning off of the ventilator (30 minutes to 3 hours) allows the family to spend time at the bedside if desired, but there is no merit in prolonging the dying process by very slow weaning over the course of many hours. Many intensivists prefer to give the patient a drying agent and then remove the endotracheal tube. Patients who are receiving neuromuscular blocking drugs should cease receiving such treatment before the ventilator is withdrawn. Such agents should not be introduced when the ventilator is being withdrawn, and neuromuscular function should be restored before life support is withdrawn (24). It is believed that withdrawal of life support can ethically occur in the presence of pharmacologic neuromuscular blockade when death is expected to be rapid, but it is usually safest to stop neuromuscular blockade before withdrawing the ventilator, because assessment of comfort is impossible. When discontinuation of neuromuscular blockade is not possible because the burden on the family of waiting for neuromuscular blockade to wane exceeds the benefits of allowing better assessment of the patient's comfort level, sedatives and analgesics can be skillfully administered.
- Some patients or families will specifically request that the endotracheal tube be removed. This can be done after appropriate suctioning. Humidified air can be given to prevent drying of the airway.
- Pressors should be stopped.
- Intraaortic balloon pumps should be turned off.
- Antibiotic therapy should be stopped.
- Artificial nutrition should be stopped.
- Blood draws should be stopped.
- Intravenous fluids should be reduced and used to facilitate analgesics and sedation.
- Restraints should be removed, monitors discontinued, and alarms silenced.
- Excess secretions should be suctioned.

Sometimes families do want to suddenly stop "everything." There is often confusion regarding the process of dying. They may ask to leave the monitors on, or inquire about vital signs, to know how close the patient is to dying. It is best to try to accommodate them. Comfort measures, DNR status, continuation of lab tests, tube feedings, and antibiotics are issues that should be discussed with families. Escalation of intravenous medications (i.e., pressors) should be discussed. Eventually, most families come to realize that there is little rationale for only partial removal of life support, except to give the principals time to grieve and accept that death may be imminent.

In specific cases where an implantable cardioverter defibrillator (ICD) has been in place, clinicians should discuss with patients, legal surrogates and next of kin the deactivation of the ICD. Recurrent shocks can be uncomfortable and may complicate and prolong the dying process. By discussing the option of deactivating the ICD, shared decision making is facilitated and patient control over health care choices is further ensured.

The median time between withdrawal of life support and death was 3.5 hours in one study, but varied from 5 minutes to 5.5 days (25). Families should be told that death may not be instantaneous, and that patients are sometimes transferred to a palliative care unit where they will be kept comfortable. Rarely, patients may even spontaneously recover.

Withdrawal of artificial nutrition and hydration is often very difficult for health care workers and families to accept (26). However, both ethical guidelines and court decisions support the practice (27,28). Recent information supports the conclusion that tube feeding seldom achieves the intended medical aims and that it may cause, rather than prevent, suffering (29). Continued nutrition and hydration may lead to considerable volume overload and pulmonary edema in a patient who is not otherwise being monitored carefully (30). Emerging consensus now suggests that dying patients experience little or no discomfort on withdrawal of tube feedings, parenteral nutrition, and intravenous hydration (31).

There is a growing recognition that nephrologists should maintain a low threshold for initiating dialysis on a trial basis, and a similarly low threshold for discontinuing dialysis that fails to appreciably improve the quality of life. Death occurs, on average, 9.6 days after discontinuation of chronic dialysis treatment (32).

Last, it must be emphasized that forgoing life-sustaining treatment is usually not a single-point decision, but one that evolves over the course of several days (20). In two large academic surgical ICUs (Moffitt-Long Hospital, San Francisco, and San Francisco General Hospital), the median time from ICU admission to death in patients undergoing withholding or withdrawal of life support varied from 4 to 8 days (median time period at Moffitt-Long Hospital and San Francisco General Hospital, respectively) (33). This suggests that it takes time for the decision to evolve and for the patient to die after the

TABLE 34.2

LIMITATIONS OF PROGNOSTIC MODELS FOR END-OF-LIFE DECISION-MAKING IN THE CORONARY CARE UNIT

Prognostic models give probabilities of survival or death rather than a "yes" or "no" answer; because of 95% confidence intervals, no model can statistically exclude survival even in the most severely ill patients.

Individual accuracy of these predictions depends on whether a specific patients's medical condition was reasonably well represented in the population from which the model was derived.

Most models derive their predictions from factors present at or shortly after admission to the intensive care unit and do not provide updated mortality estimates as the patient's condition changes.

Some patients have inherently unpredictable courses.

Conventional models of patients in the intensive care unit predict only hospital survival, not long-term survival, functional status, or quality of life after hospital discharge.

Modified from Faber-Lagendoer K, Lanken PN. Dying patients in the intensive care unit: foregoing treatment, maintaining care. *Ann Intern Med* 2000;133:886–893, with permission.

TABLE 34.3

WAYS IN WHICH INTENSIVE CARE UNITS CAN SIMULATE A HOME ENVIRONMENT FOR DYING PATIENTS

Transportable aspects of a patient's home	Ways to provide these aspects in the intensive care unit
Privacy	Provide a private room
	Close doors and curtains
Ready access to family	Suspend restrictive visiting hours
	Provide comfortable chairs, recliners, and cots for family members in the patient's room
Access to patient's own possessions and amenities	Allow family to bring in favorite music, clothes, religious icons, food, and pets
Family serving as personal caregivers	When appropriate, allow family to assist with patient care
Access to religious rituals and spiritual support	Provide religious and spiritual resources
	Encourage religious and other family rituals at the bedside before and after death

Modified from Faber-Lagendoer K, Lanken PN. Dying patients in the intensive care unit: foregoing treatment, maintaining care. *Ann Intern Med* 2000;133:886–893, with permission.

decision is made. However, surgical ICUs are quite different from CCUs. No such data are yet available from CCUs. At the Cleveland Clinic Foundation, the CCU mortality rate is 7.5%. Approximately one half of the deaths result from withholding or withdrawing of life support and one half result from "natural" causes. Current prognostic models have limitations (Table 34.2), but should be used as an adjunct to the process of shared decision making.

The withholding or withdrawal of life support is a difficult, often agonizing process. It requires careful scrutiny and rests on important ethical and legal principles that are continually evolving (34). There are no absolute guidelines for deciding when to withdraw advanced life support. Each patient and clinical situation must be considered in their own contexts. Frequent communication with patients, families, or legal surrogates; open sharing of data; and careful assessment of the changing prognosis are critical to the process.

EUTHANASIA

Euthanasia is the act of putting to death without pain a person suffering from an incurable and painful condition. It is a vague and emotionally provocative term and best describes an act such as giving a lethal injection. It is not to be confused with withholding or withdrawing life support in a dying patient. The U.S. Supreme Court has unanimously ruled that there is no constitutional right to physician-assisted suicide (euthanasia) (17,18). There is no constitutional right to suicide, and there is no legal or historical support for such a right. The right to abortion or the right to refuse treatment is different from the right to assisted suicide. Limiting physician-assisted suicide to terminally ill patients also has no basis in constitutional principles. Only 6% of medical students, house staff, or faculty physicians surveyed in one study were willing to terminate the life of a patient deliberately by administering medication to cause respiratory arrest, and only 1.1% of those surveyed were willing to do so if it causes a cardiac arrest (35). Of course, it is possible that these numbers might increase if legal restraints were removed. However, there is a long and impressive list, starting with Hippocrates and including leading physicians, philosophers, and biomedical ethicists, of professionals who are opposed to euthanasia. One humane alternative is to simulate a home environment for dying patients in the ICU (Table 34.3).

Strong popular support for euthanasia exists in Holland, which legalized euthanasia in 2000 (36). It is estimated that 5,000 to 10,000 Dutch citizens die each year after administration of a barbiturate followed by a lethal injection of a paralytic agent. In 1994, Oregon voters passed the Death with Dignity Act. This act does not permit euthanasia, but it allows state residents to receive prescriptions for self-administered lethal medications from their physicians. A 1-year follow-up indicated that only 23 patients received such prescriptions, 15 patients died after taking them, 6 died from underlying illness, and 2 patients who received such prescriptions were still alive (37). Some good has come out of the euthanasia movement—it has forced physicians to deal with death and dying.

SUMMARY

People in the United States are uncomfortable discussing death. They do not know how to start the conversation and in some cases do not want to discuss it at all. People remain confused about what constitutes a "good death" (Table 34.4). A good death includes management of pain and symptoms, clear decision making, preparation for death, and completion. The language is not always precise—a feeding tube is not the same as food and water. Only frequent, clear, and open dialogue will overcome this hurdle. Eventually, society needs to understand end-of-life issues in a more realistic light and to realize that what they see on the television series *ER* does not mimic the real world. Patients will die despite our best efforts. Our job as physicians is to help patients and their families through the dying process, just as we help them achieve meaningful recovery.

TABLE 34.4

PRINCIPLES OF A GOOD DEATH

To know when death is coming, and to understand what can be expected
To be able to retain control of what happens
To be afforded dignity and privacy
To have control over pain relief and other symptom control
To have a choice and control over where death occurs (at home or elsewhere)
To have access to information and expertise as necessary
To have access to any spiritual or emotional support required
To have access to hospice care in any location, not only in the hospital
To have control over who is present and who shares the end
To be able to issue advance directives that ensure wishes are respected
To have time to say goodbye and control over other aspects of timing
To be able to leave when it is time to go, and not to have life prolonged pointlessly
Modified from Brown M. A good death. Principles of palliative care are yet to be applied in acute hospitals. *BMJ* 2000;320:1206, with permission.

CONTROVERSIES AND PERSONAL PERSPECTIVES

The concept of futility is controversial (21). It is supported by neither scientific principle nor the justice system. When continued aggressive life support seems futile, it is best to discuss the likely outcome of continued support versus comfort care with the family. The final outcome—death—may be the same, but how the patient dies may be quite different. It is best that the family not perceive that the team is giving up, but rather that passive comfort care may be preferable to the potential suffering associated with continued life support. It must be stressed that such a decision is based on experience and judgment, not on the certainty of death. The family needs to understand and agree that the patient's best interests are served by such a strategy. Medical futility cannot be easily defined and is value laden.

It has also been our personal experience that partial withdrawal of life support or "slow codes" confuse the issue and can prolong suffering. Decisions to withdraw or withhold life support should generally be complete. Only those measures that offer comfort should be continued. Occasionally families ask that care not be escalated, which may provide the needed time for them to grieve until a decision to withdraw life support can be made.

THE FUTURE

We have room for improvement in training our residents and fellows in end-of-life issues. Dying is part of living, and to ignore the management of dying is as grievous an error as ignoring methods of managing a major illness. We need to improve and develop the education of our trainees and ourselves about these uncomfortable issues.

Times are changing. In the past, left ventricular assist devices (LVADs) meant transplant. Now, some patients are receiving permanent or so-called "destination therapy" LVADs. Who should have these devices? The ethics and selection criteria are still emerging. The CardioWest Total Artificial Heart is now being implanted at multiple centers. Selection criteria are still emerging. These devices are being used by some as a bridge to transplant in patients with rapid biventricular decompensation. Devices are only a small component of cardiology, but the decisions to implant them are often difficult and sometimes occur in the dark of night when there is little time for reflection and extensive consultation. As more experience is gained, selection criteria may become more standardized. At our institution, we have end-of-life, small group seminars as part of our didactic curriculum in the CCU. Bioethicists, nurses, pharmacists, and cardiologists assigned to the CCU participate in these lectures, which are often centered around a specific case history. We need to educate the public about death and dying. Expectations for individual patients must be framed carefully and repeatedly. Above all, families must be drawn into these important dialogues. Hope for meaningful recovery must in some cases be replaced with hope for comfort and caring.

References

1. Snider G. Allocation of intensive care: the physician's role. *Am J Respir Crit Care Med* 1994;150:575–580.
2. Raffin TA. Ethics and withdrawal of support. In: Murray JF, Nadel JA, eds. *Textbook of respiratory medicine,* 2nd ed. Philadelphia: Saunders, 1994: 2487–2503.
3. Solomon M, O'Donnell L, Jennings B, et al. Decisions near the end of life: professional views on life-sustaining treatments. *Am J Public Health* 1993; 83:14–23.
4. A controlled trial to improve care for seriously ill hospitalized patients. The Study to Understand Prognoses and Preferences for Outcomes and Risks of Treatments (SUPPORT). The SUPPORT Principal Investigators. *JAMA* 1995;274:1591–1598. [Published erratum appears in *JAMA* 1996;275: 1232].
5. Puchalski CM, Zhong Z, Jacobs MM, et al. Patients who want their family and physician to make resuscitation decisions for them: observations from SUPPORT and HELP. Study to Understand Prognoses and Preferences for Outcomes and Risks of Treatments. Hospitalized Elderly Longitudinal Project. *J Am Geriatr Soc* 2000;48[Suppl]:S84–S90.
6. Rosenfeld KE, Wenger NS, Phillips RS, et al. Factors associated with change in resuscitation preference of seriously ill patients. The SUPPORT Investigators. Study to Understand Prognoses and Preferences for Outcomes and Risks of Treatments. *Arch Intern Med* 1996;156:1558–1564.
7. Burt RA. The Supreme Court speaks: not assisted suicide but a constitutional right to palliative care. *N Engl J Med* 1997;337:1234–1236.
8. Knaus WA, Harrell FE Jr, et al. The SUPPORT prognostic model: objective estimates of survival for seriously ill hospitalized adults. Study to Understand Prognoses and Preferences for Outcomes and Risks of Treatments. *Ann Intern Med* 1995;122:191–203.
9. Phillips RS, Hamel MB, Teno JM, et al. Race, resource use, and survival in seriously ill hospitalized adults. The SUPPORT Investigators. *J Gen Intern Med* 1996;11:387–396.
10. Bok S. *Lying: moral choice in public and private life.* New York: Pantheon Books, 1978:xxii,326.
11. Decisions near the end of life. Council on Ethical and Judicial Affairs, American Medical Association. *JAMA* 1992;276:2229–2233.
12. Good care of the dying patient. Council on Scientific Affairs, American Medical Association. *JAMA* 1996;275:474–478.
13. Quill TE, Dresser R, Brock DW. The rule of double effect: a critique of its role in end-of-life decision making. *N Engl J Med* 1997;337:1768–1771.
14. Thorns A, Sykes N. Opioid use in last week of life and implications for end-of-life decision-making [letter]. *Lancet* 2000;356:398–399.
15. Kenny AJP. *The anatomy of the soul: historical essays in the philosophy of mind.* Oxford: Basil Blackwell, 1973:ix,146[1].
16. Mangan J. A historical analysis of the principle of double effect. *Theol Studies* 1949;10:41–61.
17. Coleson RE. *Washington v. Glucksberg. Issues Law Med* 1997;13:315–321.
18. Coleson RE. *Vacco v. Quill. Issues Law Med* 1997;13:323–328.
19. Foley KM. Competent care for the dying instead of physician-assisted suicide [editorial]. *N Engl J Med* 1997;336:54–58.
20. Faber-Langendoen K, Bartels DM. Process of foregoing life-sustaining treatment in a university hospital: an empirical study. *Crit Care Med* 1992; 20:570–577.
21. Helft PR, Siegler M, Lantos J. The rise and fall of the futility movement. *N Engl J Med* 2000;343:293–296.
22. Youngner SJ. Who defines futility?. *JAMA* 1988;260:2094–2095.
23. Daar JF. Medical futility and implications for physician autonomy. *Am J Law Med* 1995;21:221–240.

24. Truog RD, Burns JP, Mitchell C, et al. Pharmacologic paralysis and withdrawal of mechanical ventilation at the end of life. *N Engl J Med* 2000;342: 508–511.
25. Wilson WC, Smedira NG, Fink C, et al. Ordering and administration of sedatives and analgesics during the withholding and withdrawal of life support from critically ill patients. *JAMA* 1992;267:949–953.
26. Slomka J. What do apple pie and motherhood have to do with feeding tubes and caring for the patient? *Arch Intern Med* 1995;155:1258–1263.
27. Center H. *Guidelines on the termination of life-sustaining treatment and the care of the dying: a report*. Briarcliff Manor, NY: The Center, 1987:xii, 159.
28. Weir RF, Gostin L. Decisions to abate life-sustaining treatment for nonautonomous patients: ethical standards and legal liability for physicians after Cruzan. *JAMA* 1990;264:1846–1853.
29. Gillick MR. Rethinking the role of tube feeding in patients with advanced dementia. *N Engl J Med* 2000;342:206–210.
30. Rousseau P. Why give IV fluids to the dying? *Patient Care* 1992;26:71–74.
31. Brody H, Campbell ML, Faber-Langendoen K, Ogle KS. Withdrawing intensive life-sustaining treatment: recommendations for compassionate clinical management. *N Engl J Med* 1997;336:652–657.
32. Cohn LM, McCue JD, Germain M, et al. Dialysis discontinuation: a "good" death? *Arch Intern Med* 1995;155:42–47.
33. Smedira NG, Evans BH, Grais LS, et al. Withholding and withdrawal of life support from the critically ill. *N Engl J Med* 1990;322:309–315.
34. Ruark JE, Raffin TA. Initiating and withdrawing life support: principles and practice in adult medicine. *N Engl J Med* 1988;318:25–30.
35. Caralis PV, Hammond JS. Attitudes of medical students, housestaff, and faculty physicians toward euthanasia and termination of life-sustaining treatment. *Crit Care Med* 1992;20:683–690.
36. de Wachter MA. Active euthanasia in the Netherlands. *JAMA* 1989; 262:3316–3319.
37. Chin AE, Hedberg K, Higginson GK, Fleming DW. Legalized physician-assisted suicide in Oregon: the first year's experience. *N Engl J Med* 1999; 340:577–583.

CHAPTER 35 ■ THE HEART AND OTHER ORGAN SYSTEMS

ROBERT M. CALIFF

INTRODUCTION

Cardiovascular specialists are often consulted to evaluate patients with diseases that emanate from organ systems remote from the heart but with substantial cardiac manifestations. At some point the cardiovascular system becomes a factor in most major systemic diseases. In this section, commonly encountered problems involving an interaction of the heart and other organ systems are reviewed. The goal is to focus on the cardiovascular manifestations of these problems without providing a comprehensive review of the illnesses per se.

Increasing attention is being focused on the interaction between the cardiovascular system and the central nervous system. Ranging from genetic diseases associated with neuromuscular degeneration to atherosclerotic disease of the cerebrovascular circulation, considerable knowledge about cardiovascular manifestations is required to understand the manifestations of neurologic disorders.

Myocarditis, endocarditis, and pericarditis are covered in detail in other portions of the book, but the enormous number of infectious causes of these problems, each with specific implications for treatment, requires discussion here. In addition, the rapidly growing knowledge base concerning the effects of the human immunodeficiency virus on the cardiovascular system will increasingly require the attention of cardiovascular specialists.

Although cardiovascular manifestations of rheumatic diseases are not common compared with atherosclerosis, some of the most striking cardiovascular problems arise from rheumatic diseases. The management of vasculitis, pericarditis, or aortic valve difficulties associated with rheumatic diseases requires a thorough understanding of both areas.

As with cerebrovascular disease, the basic approaches to atherosclerosis (medical management, percutaneous intervention, and surgical intervention) create a close tie between the most common type of renal disease and the cardiovascular system. In addition, the rapid growth of angiography with its associated problem of contrast nephropathy creates an iatrogenic condition requiring careful evaluation and treatment by the angiographer.

Finally, in many respects, cardiovascular disease is an endocrine disease in the sense that a major contributor to disease progression and outcome in cardiovascular diseases is the neuroendocrine status. In particular, diabetes has become the focus of activity in understanding factors associated with increased risk.

We hope that these sections in combination with specific disease-oriented chapters throughout the book will provide the reader with a comprehensive view of the interaction of the cardiovascular system with other organ systems in the development and progression of human disease.

CHAPTER 35A ■ ENDOCRINE SYSTEMS AND THE HEART

MARCO ROFFI AND FABIO CATTANEO

THE THYROID

The major secretory product of the thyroid gland is thyroxine (T_4), a relatively inactive hormone. Subsequently, T_4 is converted by the enzyme 5′-monodeiodinase to the biologically active compound triiodothyronine (T_3). Both thyroid hormone excess and depletion may affect the cardiovascular system. Cardiovascular involvement in thyroid dysfunction may be the result of direct hormone effects at the cellular level, interactions with the sympathetic nervous system, or alterations of peripheral circulation and metabolism (1). At the cellular level, thyroid hormones act mainly through binding to specific nuclear receptors and activation of gene transcription. Additionally, they activate extranuclear sites as mitochondrial- and membrane-bound enzymes (1). Women are more likely to develop thyroid dysfunction, with an estimated 2.7% prevalence of hyperthyroidism and 1.9% prevalence of hypothyroidism in an unselected population (2).

Thyrotoxicosis

The terms *hyperthyroidism* and *thyrotoxicosis* can be differentiated, but are frequently used interchangeably. *Hyperthyroidism* is increased formation and release of thyroid hormones from the thyroid gland, whereas *thyrotoxicosis* is the clinical syndrome that results from thyroid hormone excess. The most frequent cause of thyrotoxicosis is Graves disease, which accounts for 60% to 90% of cases and occurs in women 10 times more frequently than in men. This disorder is characterized by autoantibodies activating the thyroid-stimulating hormone (TSH) receptor. Other causes of thyrotoxicosis include toxic adenoma, toxic multinodular goiter, thyroiditis, and thyroid autonomy.

Cardiovascular symptoms of thyroid hormone excess are nonspecific. Palpitations are usually caused by sinus tachycardia and, occasionally, by atrial fibrillation. Exercise intolerance and dyspnea on exertion may be a result of the combination of inability to raise cardiac output and skeletal and/or respiratory muscle weakness. The hemodynamic changes occurring in thyrotoxicosis are summarized in Table 35A.1 and include tachycardia, increased cardiac output and stroke volume, and decreased systemic vascular resistance (3,4). In the elderly, cardiovascular involvement may be limited to arrhythmias such as sinus tachycardia or atrial fibrillation, which occasionally trigger angina or heart failure. In contrast to hypothyroidism, which is characterized by diastolic hypertension, hyperthyroidism is associated with systolic hypertension in the presence of normal or low diastolic blood pressure. It is speculated that isolated systolic hypertension is secondary to the inability of the vasculature to accommodate increased cardiac output and stroke volume. Several studies have demonstrated that hyperthyroidism is associated with increased cardiovascular morbidity and mortality. In an English cohort of 7,203 patients treated for hyperthyroidism the standardized mortality ratio was 1.1 in comparison with the general population and an excess of cardiovascular deaths was identified (5). Similarly, a standardized mortality rate of 1.3 over 14 years was identified among 1,762 women treated for hyperthyroidism at a U.S. center (6). Moreover, a Swedish study following 10,522 patients for 15 years after radioiodine treatment detected a standardized mortality rate of 1.5 for women and 1.3 for men (7). Even in the absence of symptoms, low TSH has been identified as an independent predictor of mortality (2.1 standardized mortality ratio) among 1,191 individuals followed for 10 years (8). The observed increase was largely accounted for by cardiovascular mortality.

Sympathetic Nervous System and Ventricular Function

Many of the cardiovascular signs and symptoms of thyrotoxicosis mimic a high-adrenergic state and respond to β-blockade, suggesting an underlying dysfunction of the catecholamine metabolism or, alternatively, an increased sensitivity to catecholamines. However, patients with thyrotoxicosis have low or normal plasma catecholamine levels, normal urinary catecholamine excretion, and normal response to catecholamine infusion (9). In addition, there is no conclusive evidence of increased β-adrenergic receptor density in the myocardium, increased catecholamine turnover at neural synapses, or increased affinity of adrenergic receptor for catecholamines. Finally, recent animal studies support the notion that the cardiovascular effects of hyperthyroidism are largely independent from adrenergic activation (10).

Short-term hyperthyroidism is associated with increased cardiac contractility and improved diastolic function, which

TABLE 35A.1

CARDIOVASCULAR HEMODYNAMICS IN THYROID DYSFUNCTION

	Thyrotoxicosis	Hypothyroidism
Systemic vascular resistance	↓	↑
Cardiac output	↑	↓
Systolic blood pressure	↑	↓ or →
Diastolic blood pressure	↓	↑ or →
Heart rate	↑	↓
Systolic function	↑	↓
Diastolic function	↑	↓
Blood volume	↑	↓

↑, increased; ↓, decreased; →, unchanged.

may be the result of augmented activity of the sarcoplasmic reticulum calcium ATPase pump (11). In both humans and animals, chronic thyrotoxicosis causes variable degrees of left ventricular hypertrophy (LVH). It has been demonstrated that thyroid hormones induce cardiac protein synthesis, leading to the hypothesis that this anabolic pathway may be the trigger of LVH (12). However, β-adrenergics effectively block or reverse hypertrophy, suggesting that increased cardiac workload is the mediator of LVH (13). In addition to the effects on the myocardium, T_3 shows vasodilator properties by acting directly on vascular smooth muscle cells, potentially explaining the decreased systemic vascular resistance observed in hyperthyroidism (14).

It remains a source of debate whether thyrotoxicosis per se may lead to heart failure. In the majority of cases, heart failure can be explained by the combination of underlying heart disease, arrhythmias, and chronically increased cardiac output. However, myocardial dysfunction has been described in absence of underlying cardiac disease (15) and improvement in myocardial contractility after restoration of euthyroidism has been reported (16). Therefore, thyroid hormone excess should be excluded in patients with unexplained heart failure. Several factors may contribute to heart failure in thyrotoxicosis (3,4). Diastolic function deteriorates in the course of the disease owing to LVH and progressive left ventricular (LV) stiffness, leading to LV filling impairment, in particular in the setting of tachycardia or atrial fibrillation (Fig. 35A.1). In addition, thyrotoxic patients may present with intravascular volume expansion, possibly secondary to a decrease in renal perfusion with subsequent renin-angiotensin system-mediated increase in sodium reabsorption (17). Occasionally, the decreased systemic resistance may overwhelm the cardiac capacity and cause high output failure. More frequently however, the high-output state may unmask coronary artery disease, and heart failure is precipitated by ischemia.

Arrhythmias

Sinus tachycardia at rest, during sleep, and during exercise is the most common arrhythmia in thyrotoxicosis. Other common rhythm disturbances include atrial premature contractions and atrial fibrillation. Less frequently, patients present with paroxysmal atrial tachycardia and atrial flutter. Ventricular arrhythmias are rare. It is speculated that thyroid hormones have direct effects on the conduction system, possibly via cellular changes in cation transport, this may trigger a decrease of atrial excitation threshold, an increase of sinoatrial node firing, and the shortening of conduction tissue refractory with subsequent rapid ventricular rate response in the presence of supraventricular arrhythmias (18). Although thyrotoxicosis is the underlying etiology in less than 5% of atrial fibrillation cases, this rhythm disturbance may occur in 5% to 15% of hyperthyroid patients. In one recent population-based study that included 40,628 patients with clinical hyperthyroidism, atrial fibrillation or flutter were found in 8.3% of cases (19). Atrial fibrillation related to thyrotoxicosis is more frequently detected in the elderly and in males, probably reflecting the increased prevalence of intrinsic heart disease. Because atrial fibrillation, particularly in the elderly, may be the only manifestation of thyrotoxicosis, thyroid hormone excess should be excluded in this setting. Accordingly, one report showed subtle hyperthyroidism in 12.5% of elderly patients with atrial fibrillation previously considered idiopathic (20). Major complications of atrial fibrillation include heart failure and embolic events. In the absence of chronic atrial fibrillation or underlying heart disease, most patients convert spontaneously to sinus rhythm within 8 to 12 weeks of antithyroid treatment (21). Conversely, reversion into atrial fibrillation is likely in persistently thyrotoxic patients. Patients in atrial fibrillation should be anticoagulated and cardioversion should be deferred until euthyroidism is restored.

Subclinical Hyperthyroidism

Cardiovascular manifestations of subclinical hyperthyroidism include sinus tachycardia, LVH, diastolic dysfunction, reduced

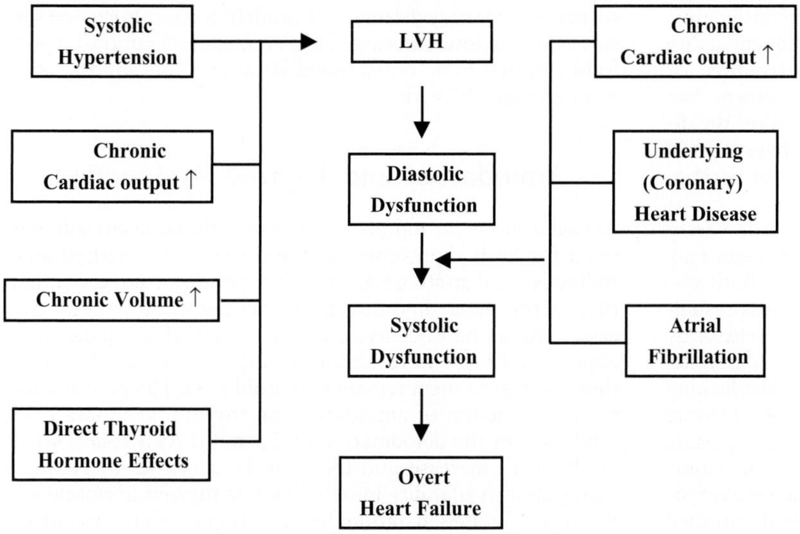

FIGURE 35A.1. Pathophysiology of heart failure in thyrotoxicosis. (*Source:* From Roffi M, Cattaneo F, Topol EJ. Thyrotoxicosis and the cardiovascular system: subtle but serious effects. *Cleve Clin J Med* 2003;70:57–63, with permission.)

Endocrine Systems and the Heart

exercise performance, and atrial fibrillation (22). A study including 2,002 patients older than 60 years of age with serum TSH levels of 0.1 mU/L or lower reported a threefold increased risk of atrial fibrillation over 10 years (23). Similarly, in a cross-sectional study involving 23,638 patients, low serum TSH was associated with a fivefold higher prevalence of atrial fibrillation compared with individuals with normal levels (13.3% and 2.3%, respectively), with no difference between subclinical or overt thyroid hormone excess (24). Recently proposed guidelines for the diagnosis and management of subclinical thyroid disease have summarized the impact of subclinical hyperthyroidism on cardiovascular outcomes and the benefit of treatment (22). The investigators, underscoring the paucity of data, advised against routine treatment for patients whose TSH is mildly decreased (serum TSH 0.1–0.45 mU/L), even in the presence of atrial fibrillation. Accordingly, there is only limited evidence that antithyroid therapy may facilitate spontaneous conversion to sinus rhythm or be helpful in maintaining sinus rhythm following cardioversion in this setting.

Diagnosis and Therapy

Measurement of serum TSH is the most sensitive screening test for hyperthyroidism. An undetectable value is the hallmark of the disease, whereas normal TSH virtually excludes it. Elevated serum levels of free T_4, free T_3, or total T_3 confirm the diagnosis. β-Adrenergic blockers provide relief of symptoms such as tachycardia, tremor, anxiety, and heat intolerance. Alternatively, calcium channel blockers such as verapamil or diltiazem have been administered. However, caution is warranted, because these agents may cause hemodynamic instability by further reducing systemic vascular resistance and contractility. The discussion of therapy strategies to reduce thyroid hormone synthesis is beyond the scope of the chapter. It remains to be determined whether an early and aggressive control of hyperthyroidism may positively influence the increased morbidity and mortality associated with this condition. Encouraging are the findings of a large-scale study documenting that the cardiovascular mortality excess noted among hyperthyroid patients undergoing radioiodine treatment was highest in the first year following treatment and then declined (5).

Hypothyroidism

Hypothyroidism is the clinical syndrome associated with decreased secretion of thyroid hormones. This condition reflects in over 90% of cases a disease of the gland itself (primary hypothyroidism). Rarely, hypothyroidism can be caused by pituitary disease (secondary hypothyroidism) or hypothalamic disease (tertiary hypothyroidism). The most frequent cause of hypothyroidism in adults is autoimmune thyroiditis, or Hashimoto disease, which affects mainly older women. The slow and progressive nature of hypothyroidism makes the diagnosis difficult, particularly in the elderly. Most hypothyroid patients present with nonspecific symptoms caused by psychological or skeletal muscle dysfunction.

Longstanding hypothyroidism may affect the cardiovascular system. Bradycardia is common. Pericardial effusion may occur, but rarely causes hemodynamic compromise. Both systolic and diastolic LV performance may be decreased, presumably because of alterations in calcium uptake and release by cardiac myocytes (4). An increase in systemic vascular resistance has been described, possibly as the result of the lacking direct vasodilatory effect of thyroid hormones (14). Despite symptoms suggesting a decreased sympathetic tone, plasma catecholamines are increased (25). The resulting hemodynamic changes are opposite but less marked than in thyrotoxicosis (see Table 35A.1). Characteristic features include diminished cardiac output, decreased stroke volume, impaired ventricular function, decreased intravascular volume, increased systemic vascular resistance, and decreased peripheral oxygen consumption (26). Heart failure may occur when the metabolic demand cannot be matched by adequate cardiac output. As in patients with thyrotoxicosis, overt heart failure in hypothyroidism generally represents exacerbation of intrinsic cardiac disease. Rarely, thyroid hormone depletion may cause cardiomyopathy. Therefore, unexplained heart failure should prompt determination of thyroid hormones. In the absence of underlying heart disease, the decreased myocardial contractility observed in hypothyroidism may be reversible after hormone replacement.

Coronary Artery Disease

Patients with hypothyroidism are burdened by an increased prevalence of hyperlipidemia, hypertension, and atherosclerosis. Total cholesterol, low-density lipoprotein cholesterol, very-low-density lipoprotein cholesterol, lipoprotein (a), and apolipoprotein B concentrations are often elevated in hypothyroidism, and some patients have high serum triglycerides. It has been demonstrated that patients with hypothyroidism have an intrinsic low-density lipoprotein cholesterol catabolism dysfunction, which is reversible after hormone replacement (27). In a review of 12 studies, the prevalence of hypertension in this patient population was 21% (28). In large series of hypertensive patients, hypothyroidism accounted for 3% to 5% of the cases (29,30). Although the pathophysiology remains unknown, a causal link between thyroid hormone deficiency and hypertension is confirmed by the observation that hormone replacement may lower blood pressure in these patients (30). Additional interactions between hypothyroidism and atherosclerosis include the thyroid hormone's regulatory function on homocysteine metabolism, the effects on vascular reactivity, and possibly the interaction with newer cardiovascular risk factors such as C-reactive protein (31). A population-based cross-sectional has confirmed previous case-control studies by showing that even subclinical hypothyroidism predisposes to coronary artery disease in women (32). However, the findings could not be replicated in another large-scale trial among subclinical hypothyroid men and women (33).

Diagnosis and Therapy

An elevated TSH combined with a low free T_4 is diagnostic of primary hypothyroidism. Antimicrosomal and antithyroglobulin antibodies are characteristic of Hashimoto disease. Hypothyroidism is preferentially treated with T_4 because of its long half-life. In the elderly, as well as in patients with known or suspected coronary disease, it is prudent to start hormone substitution at a lower dosage. However, exacerbation of angina following hormone replacement is rare and responds well to β-adrenergic blockade.

Amiodarone and Thyroid Dysfunction

Amiodarone is an iodine-rich antiarrhythmic agent administered for both supraventricular and ventricular arrhythmias. Iodine is a substrate necessary for thyroid hormone synthesis that at the same time directly influences intrathyroidal processes. As a consequence, more than half of the patients on amiodarone may have abnormal thyroid function tests, although most of them remain euthyroid (34). The predominant peripheral action of amiodarone on thyroid hormones is the inhibition of the deiodination of T_4 to T_3. As a result, serum levels of T_4 increase and levels of T_3 decrease. In addition, high iodide availability initially inhibits thyroid hormone synthesis (the Wolff–Chaikoff effect). During the first 3 months of

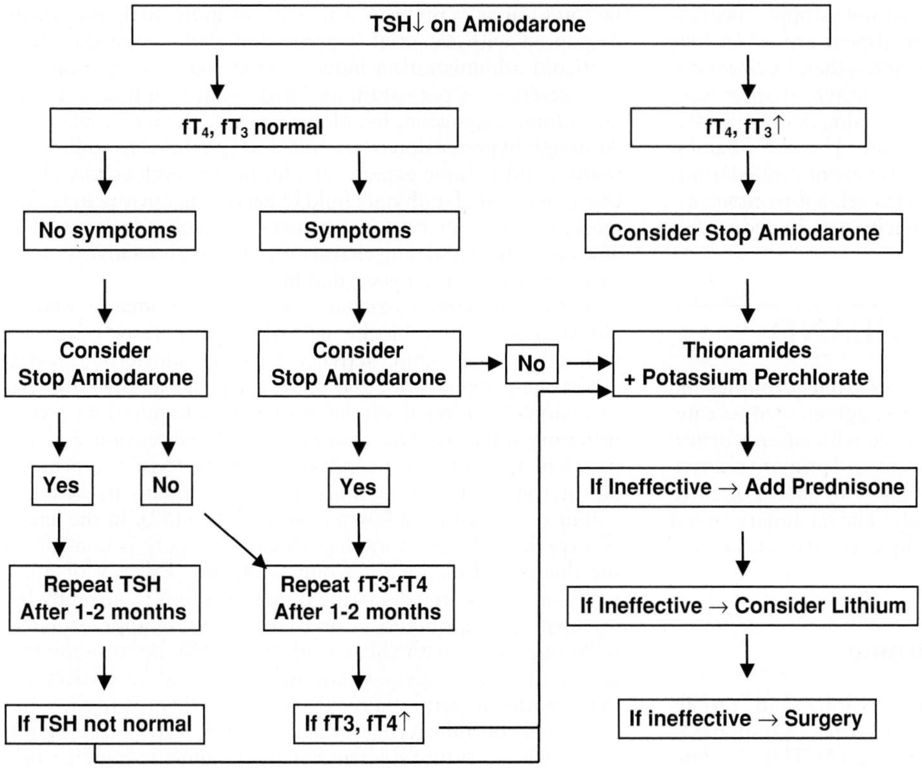

FIGURE 35A.2. Management algorithm for amiodarone-induced thyrotoxicosis. *Abbreviations:* fT_3, free triiodothyronine; fT_4, free thyroxine; TSH, thyroid-stimulating hormone.

therapy, TSH levels are commonly slightly elevated but tend to normalize during long-term administration. Amiodarone-induced thyroid hormone excess prevails in areas with low iodine intake, whereas hypothyroidism is more frequent in countries with high iodine intake.

Amiodarone-Induced Thyrotoxicosis

The incidence of amiodarone-induced thyrotoxicosis (AIT) is directly related to the iodine intake of the population, ranging from 2% in countries with high iodine intake to 10% in the presence of iodine deficiency (35). Because antiadrenergic effects of amiodarone may partially conceal thyrotoxic symptoms, clinical manifestations of AIT may be subtle and a high degree of suspicion is required for the diagnosis. AIT should be considered in the presence of new or recurrent atrial arrhythmias and unexplained weight loss or fatigue. Thyrotoxicosis may occur throughout the treatment period with amiodarone and, because of its long terminal half-life, up to several months after drug discontinuation. The pathogenesis of AIT is complex and not completely understood. Three mechanisms have been postulated (36). First, iodine may affect thyroid autoregulatory mechanisms and may lead, particularly in patients with underlying thyroid autonomy, to excessive hormone synthesis. Second, destructive inflammatory histologic changes and increased cytokines and thyroglobulin levels have been identified, suggesting a direct cytotoxic effect of amiodarone. The third and more controversial mechanism involves amiodarone as a trigger of an autoimmune response to the thyroid gland. Diagnosis of AIT relies on low TSH in the presence of normal or elevated free T_4 and free T_3, and negative thyrotropin-receptor antibodies. In the presence of AIT, amiodarone should be discontinued whenever possible. Nonetheless, successful treatment of this condition despite continuation of amiodarone therapy has been described (37). Because of the long terminal half-life of amiodarone, symptomatic treatment with β-adrenergic antagonists in patients with AIT should be cautious even after discontinuation of the drug to prevent bradycardia or atrioventricular conduction abnormalities. The management of AIT is summarized in Figure 35A.2 and discussed in detail elsewhere (38,39).

Amiodarone-Induced Hypothyroidism

Hypothyroidism is a frequent sequela of amiodarone therapy, with a reported incidence ranging from 13% in iodine-replete countries to 6% in countries with low or intermediate iodine intake (40). The risk of developing hypothyroidism is increased in the elderly and women, particularly in the presence of autoimmune thyroiditis. Accordingly, women on amiodarone with microsomal and/or thyroglobulin autoantibodies have a greater than 10-fold risk of developing hypothyroidism (41). Possible mechanisms include failure to escape the Wolff–Chaikoff effect and iodine-mediated exacerbation of preexisting autoimmune thyroid disease. TSH levels above 10 to 15 mU/L in patients on amiodarone are usually diagnostic for hypothyroidism. The diagnosis is confirmed by low T_4 or free T_4. The assessment of T_3 or free T_3 adds little information, because these parameters may be diminished even in euthyroid patients on amiodarone. Once the diagnosis of hypothyroidism is established, amiodarone can be safely continued and T_4 replacement added in increasing doses at 4- to 6-week intervals until TSH returns to within normal limits and symptoms resolve. Drug discontinuation leads to frequent recovery of thyroid function among patients with no thyroid antibodies, whereas patients with antibodies usually do not recover (40).

Noniodinated Amiodarone Analogs

Dronedarone is a noniodinated amiodarone analog that has been developed to obviate the thyroid dysfunction associated with amiodarone therapy. The electrophysiologic and antiarrhythmic properties of the two compounds are similar. A small, randomized, dose-ranging study to assess safety and efficacy of dronedarone in maintaining sinus rhythm following cardioversion for atrial fibrillation showed a modest efficacy in the absence of thyroid function abnormalities (42). Of concern, a placebo-controlled randomized clinical trial testing the drug in patients with heart failure was prematurely stopped because of a death rate excess in the active treatment arm (43). Like amiodarone, dronedarone is lipophilic and is therefore prone to tissue accumulation and, potentially, to nonthyroid organ toxicity. Another noniodinated amiodarone analog (SSR149744C) is currently in phase III clinical trial testing. This compound is believed to be less lipophilic than amiodarone or dronedarone. As a consequence, long-term side effects related to tissue accumulation such as the pulmonary toxicity may be reduced or suppressed.

THE ADRENAL GLAND

The cortex of the adrenal gland produces steroid hormones and the medulla, functionally a sympathetic ganglion, secretes catecholamines. Clinical syndromes associated with adrenocortical hypersecretion include Cushing syndrome and primary aldosteronism (Conn syndrome), and result from an excess of cortisol and mineralocorticoids, respectively. The medullary tumor pheochromocytoma is characterized by excessive synthesis of catecholamines.

Cushing Syndrome

Cortisol, a central element of carbohydrate and protein metabolism, is synthesized in the adrenal cortex in response to the pituitary adrenocorticotropic hormone (ACTH). *Cushing syndrome* denotes glucocorticoid excess, which can be either endogenous or exogenous. ACTH-secreting pituitary tumor—Cushing disease—accounts for about 80% of the cases of endogenous hypercorticism. In 10% of cases, an ectopic ACTH-producing tumor is identified. In the remaining cases, glucocorticoid excess is caused by adrenal pathologies such as adenoma, carcinoma, or bilateral hyperplasia. The association of Cushing disease, premature atherosclerosis, and increased cardiovascular morbidity and mortality has long been recognized (44). In a recent study, the prevalence of hypertension, diabetes, and hyperlipidemia in this patient populations was 85%, 47%, and 37%, respectively (45). Hypertension has been related to volume expansion, increased production of vasoactive substances, and increased reactivity of vascular smooth muscle cells. LVH may be more frequent and severe in Cushing disease than in essential hypertension (46). In addition, an hypercoagulable state underlies the fourfold increase in thromboembolic complications observed in this patient population (47). In individuals with clinical features suggestive of hypercorticism screening can be performed with a 24-hour urine collection for free cortisol, among others. Other useful tests in the initial evaluation of this condition include the dexamethasone suppression test and the measurement of midnight salivary cortisol levels (48). Specific treatment, which may include surgical removal and pharmacologic or radiation therapy, is chosen depending on the underlying process. Cardiovascular morbidity and mortality remain higher than in the general population even following surgery.

Primary Aldosteronism

A benign cortical tumor of the adrenal gland is found in about two thirds of the cases of primary aldosteronism (Conn syndrome); the remaining are due to bilateral adrenal hyperplasia (idiopathic hyperaldosteronism). Primary aldosteronism has traditionally been considered a rare cause of hypertension, with an estimated prevalence ranging between 0.05% and 2.20% among unselected hypertensive individuals (49). However, recent prospective data suggest that primary aldosteronism may be found in as many as 6% to 10% of individuals previously diagnosed with essential hypertension (50). Acute mineralocorticoid administration induces renal sodium retention and the excretion of potassium and hydrogen, resulting in vascular volume expansion, hypokalemia, and metabolic alkalosis. Although hypertension is presumed to be related to sodium retention and volume expansion, chronic mineralocorticoid excess is associated with only mild hypervolemia owing to escape mechanisms. Primary aldosteronism is associated with cardiac and vascular remodeling characterized by perivascular fibrosis, excessive LVH, and myocardial fibrosis (51).

Because mineralocorticoid excess is asymptomatic, primary aldosteronism is a biochemical diagnosis. Tests of choice include plasma renin activity, plasma aldosterone levels, aldosterone–renin ratio, and fludrocortisone suppression test. Occasionally, adrenal venous sampling is required as a confirmatory analysis. The association of hypertension and hypokalemia, if not diuretic induced, is characteristic of primary aldosteronism. However, more than 50% of patients with this condition do not have low potassium levels (52). In the hands of experienced operators, laparoscopic surgery is considered the therapy of choice for Conn syndrome. Efficacy of minimally invasive adrenal-sparing tumor excisions is currently being investigated. Surgery cures hypertension in approximately 60% of patients with solitary adenoma (53). Because the rate of hypertension regression following bilateral adrenalectomy in idiopathic hyperplasia is extremely low, therapy in these patients relies on aldosterone antagonists (i.e., spironolactone and possibly in the future eplerenone), potassium-sparing diuretics, angiotensin-converting enzyme inhibitors, and angiotensin II receptor blockers.

Pheochromocytoma

Pheochromocytoma is located in about 90% in the adrenal glands, whereas extraadrenal tumors, originating from chromaffin tissue of any sympathetic paraganglion (paragangliomas), account for the remaining 10% of cases. The classic presentation of pheochromocytoma, encountered in only a minority of patients, is expression of episodic catecholamine releases and is characterized by a paroxysm of palpitations, diaphoresis, and headache. The spells begin abruptly, may last for minutes to hours, and subside gradually. Hypertension, another hallmark of pheochromocytoma, is paroxysmal in only about half of the cases (54). Prolonged exposure to high levels of catecholamines results in arterial and venous vasoconstriction and in plasma volume contraction, leading to orthostatic hypotension. Electrocardiographic findings are nonspecific. Ischemic changes may be detected, particularly during hypertensive episodes. It has been postulated that pheochromocytoma affects the myocardium in the form of catecholamine-induced cardiomyopathy (55). Tumor removal has been associated with regression of both LV dilatation and LVH. Because pheochromocytoma is the cause of hypertension in less than 1% of unselected patients, routine screening is not warranted.

With respect to diagnosis, assessment of 24-hour urinary metanephrines and plasma metanephrines show comparable sensitivity and specificity. The biochemical diagnosis is usually clear cut, with values exceeding 5 to 20 times the upper limit of normal. The preferred imaging tools are computer tomography or magnetic resonance imaging. Metaiodobenzylguanidine or octreotide scintigraphy may be useful for localization of metastatic, recurrent, or extraadrenal tumors. Laparoscopic adrenalectomy is the therapy of choice. Adrenergic blockade for a few weeks is indicated prior to tumor resection, although on rare occasions urgent surgery may be necessary. The α-blocker phenoxybenzamine, an irreversible noncompetitive antagonist predominantly of the α_1-receptor, has been the mainstay of pre- and perioperative control of blood pressure. In patients intolerant to phenoxybenzamine, the α_1-selective antagonists prazosin, terazosin, or doxazosin have been administered (56). To achieve optimal control of hypertension and tachyarrhythmias β-blockers can be added. However, β-blockade should not be started in patients not pretreated with α-blockers to prevent unopposed α_1-mediated vasoconstriction with subsequent exacerbation of hypertension. Hypertensive crisis may be managed with intravenous nitroprusside or the α_1/α_2-blocker phentolamine. Over 90% of pheochromocytomas are benign and cured with surgery at a low operative mortality (56). Following tumor removal, up to 25% of patients may remain hypertensive. Life-long follow up is mandatory because the disease may show late recurrence.

ACROMEGALY

Acromegaly is a rare disorder caused by a growth hormone (GH)-secreting pituitary tumor. Main signs and symptoms associated with this condition are either due to mass effect (headaches, visual field defects, cranial nerve palsy, and hypopituitarism) or to GH excess (acral and soft tissue overgrowth). Patients with acromegaly have a two- to threefold increase in mortality compared to the general population, mainly from cardiovascular causes (57,58). An insight into cardiovascular morbidity and risk factors of acromegalic patients is provided by the Spanish Acromegaly Registry (58). Among 1,219 patients, the prevalence of hypertension, diabetes, and dyslipidemia were 39%, 38%, and 26%, respectively. Overt cardiovascular disease was present in 14% of patients. The pathophysiology of hypertension remains incompletely understood. Increased plasma volume is a common finding in the absence of disturbances of the renin–angiotensin–aldosterone system or the catecholamine metabolism (59). The salt-sensitive nature of hypertension suggests that, at least in part, it may be due to a direct GH effect on the renal sodium pump, leading to sodium retention. Despite optimal acromegaly control, most of the patients remain hypertensive. Conversely, diabetes is cured in approximately two thirds of the patients undergoing successful tumor removal (60).

Myocardial trophic properties of GH have been documented in both in vitro and in vivo animal models showing LV hypertrophic response and enhanced cardiac function associated with GH excess (61). Controversy surrounds the notion of acromegalic cardiomyopathy, partly because of frequent associated confounding conditions such as hypertension and coronary artery disease. Nonetheless, echocardiographic studies in patients with acromegaly of recent onset and no associated cardiovascular abnormalities have demonstrated LVH (62). Additional arguments in favor of an acromegalic cardiomyopathy include the observation that LVH and LV dysfunction may improve with therapy (63). Finally, one autopsy series of acromegalic patients demonstrated myocardial interstitial fibrosis and inflammatory infiltrates (64). It is speculated that elevated GH and/or insulin-like growth factor (IGF)-1 levels may lead to LVH, followed by fibrosis, diastolic dysfunction, and later in the process, systolic dysfunction and overt heart failure (65). Overall, current evidence suggests that, although most cardiac disease in acromegaly is explained by coexisting hypertension and coronary artery disease, a small proportion of patients may have a cardiomyopathy.

With respect to diagnosis, measurements of IGF-1 levels represent the screening test of choice. The presumptive diagnosis is confirmed by a glucose tolerance test showing no decrease of serum GH level following oral glucose load. The goals of therapy in acromegaly are to reverse or prevent tumor mass effects and to reduce the long-term morbidity and mortality, possibly without inducing hypopituitarism. Current treatment strategies include transsphenoidal surgery, radiation therapy, and drug therapy. In the Spanish registry, the cure rates after surgery and radiation therapy were 40% and 28%, respectively (58). The low cure rate among patients undergoing surgery is due to incomplete tumor resection. Preliminary data on stereotactic radiotherapy and radiosurgery appear promising. Dopamine agonists adequately lower GH levels in only a minority of patients, and adverse effects limit tolerability and compliance (66). The somatostatin analogs octreotide and lanreotide, which effectively inhibit GH secretion and reduce tumor size, are regarded by many investigators as first-line treatment of acromegaly. However, normal GH and IGF-1 levels are achieved in only about half of the patients (67). The genetically engineered GH receptor antagonist pegvisomant has been recently shown to be effective and well tolerated (68). Should these promising results be confirmed, GH receptor antagonism may become a cornerstone of the medical management of acromegaly, perhaps in combination with somatostatin analogs (69).

HYPERPARATHYROIDISM

In primary hyperparathyroidism (PHPT) inappropriate secretion of parathormone (PTH) causes excessive renal calcium reabsorption, phosphaturia, 1,25 $(OH)_2D$ synthesis, and increased bone reabsorption. Hypercalcemia, hypercalciuria, hypophosphatemia, and loss of cortical bone are typical associated findings. Females are affected about twice as frequently as males, and after the age of 40 years the incidence of the disease sharply increases. A single parathyroid adenoma, hyperplasia of all parathyroid glands, and parathyroid carcinoma are the underlying pathologies in over 80%, 10% to 20%, and less than 2% of patients, respectively (70). PHPT is often diagnosed following incidental plasma calcium measurements. At the time of diagnosis most patients are either asymptomatic or have nonspecific symptoms, such as fatigue, weakness, or mental disturbances. Epidemiologic studies linking PHPT with an increased cardiovascular mortality have given conflicting results. With respect to cardiovascular morbidity, patients with PHPT have a higher incidence of LVH, cardiac calcific deposits in the myocardium, and calcification of the aortic and mitral valve compared to the general population (71). Approximately 30% to 40% of PHPT patients are hypertensive, which represents an about twofold increased incidence compared to the general population of the same age and gender (72). In an unselected population of hypertensive patients, approximately 1% may have PHPT (49). Because no direct correlation between hypertension and elevated PTH or calcium levels has been found, the pathophysiology of hypertension in this setting remains unclear. A regression of LVH after parathyroidectomy has been described (73).

The finding of hypercalcemia in the presence of an elevated PTH is the key to diagnosis, although in the initial phase of the disease normocalcemic PHPT may be present. Parathyroidectomy remains the therapy of choice for younger patients and in the presence of severe hypercalcemia. High-volume centers report virtually no perioperative mortality and a cure rate ranging between 90% and 98% (74). Older patients and individuals with mild PHPT may not require surgery. Although prospective randomized trials are lacking, the conservative approach is supported by long-term studies showing a remarkable stability of the disease and has been reinforced in the guidelines (75). Cinacalcet, the prototype of a novel class of drugs, the calcimimetics, has recently undergone clinical testing. These agents bind to the calcium-sensing receptor located on the cells of the parathyroid gland and induce conformational changes of the receptor that increase its sensitivity to extracellular calcium. As a consequence, PTH secretion is reduced. Long-term reduction in serum calcium and PTH concentrations in patients with PHPT receiving cinacalcet has been documented in a small randomized trial (76).

CONTROVERSIES AND PERSONAL PERSPECTIVES

Cardiovascular involvement is frequent in endocrine disease. However, it is often controversial whether hormonal imbalances have direct deleterious effects on the cardiovascular system or whether cardiovascular disease results from the frequently observed increased prevalence of associated cardiovascular risk factors. Little is known about the mechanisms of interaction between hormones and the cardiovascular tissue or the pathways leading to associated conditions such as hypertension or hyperlipidemia. In addition, it remains often unproven that effective endocrine control reduces cardiovascular morbidity and mortality. The limited data available are explained by the low prevalence of many endocrine disorders. From a clinical standpoint, one of the most challenging steps in treating endocrine disease remains the diagnosis. Clinical suspicion is essential; endocrine pathologies, and in particular the associated cardiovascular manifestations, may present subtly and nonspecifically.

THE FUTURE

The use of amiodarone as antiarrhythmic agent is limited by side effects and in particular by thyroid dysfunction. Iodine-free amiodarone analogs such as dronedarone are currently being tested with promising results and may become a valuable alternative. Novel drug classes may in the future be able to control inappropriate hormone secretion and may be administered to patients who do not qualify for surgery or have a recurrence of the disease. In acromegaly, the administration of genetically engineered GH receptor antagonists may turn into a cornerstone of therapy, perhaps in combination with somatostatin analogs. In PHPT, calcimimetics may be used to achieve long-term control of serum calcium and PTH levels. On a broader perspective, newer innovative therapeutic modalities including applications of pharmacogenomics may modulate endocrinologic diseases prior to cardiovascular involvement. In addition, delineation of the responsible genes will allow a better understanding of pathophysiology and potentially lead to newer therapeutic strategies.

References

1. Polikar R, Burger AG, Scherrer U, et al. The thyroid and the heart. *Circulation* 1993;87:1435–1441.
2. Tunbridge WM, Evered DC, Hall R, et al. The spectrum of thyroid disease in a community: the Whickham survey. *Clin Endocrinol* 1977;7:481–493.
3. Woeber KA. Thyrotoxicosis and the heart. *N Engl J Med* 1992;327:94–98.
4. Klein I, Ojamaa K. Thyroid hormone and the cardiovascular system. *N Engl J Med* 2001;344:501–509.
5. Franklyn JA, Maisonneuve P, Sheppard MC, et al. Mortality after the treatment of hyperthyroidism with radioactive iodine. *N Engl J Med* 1998;338:712–718.
6. Goldman MB, Maloof F, Monson RR, et al. Radioactive iodine therapy and breast cancer. A follow-up study of hyperthyroid women. *Am J Epidemiol* 1988;127:969–980.
7. Hall P, Lundell G, Holm LE. Mortality in patients treated for hyperthyroidism with iodine-131. *Acta Endocrinol* 1993;128:230–234.
8. Parle JV, Maisonneuve P, Sheppard MC, et al. Prediction of all-cause and cardiovascular mortality in elderly people from one low serum thyrotropin result: a 10-year cohort study. *Lancet* 2001;358:861–865.
9. Levey GS, Klein I. Catecholamine-thyroid hormone interactions and the cardiovascular manifestations of hyperthyroidism. *Am J Med* 1990;88:642–646.
10. Bachman ES, Hampton TG, Dhillon H, et al. The metabolic and cardiovascular effects of hyperthyroidism are largely independent of beta-adrenergic stimulation. *Endocrinology* 2004;145:2767–2774.
11. Mintz G, Pizzarello R, Klein I. Enhanced left ventricular diastolic function in hyperthyroidism: noninvasive assessment and response to treatment. *J Clin Endocrinol Metab* 1991;73:146–150.
12. Sanford CF, Griffin EE, Wildenthal K. Synthesis and degradation of myocardial protein during the development and regression of thyroxine-induced cardiac hypertrophy in rats. *Circ Res* 1978;43:688–694.
13. Klein I, Hong C. Effects of thyroid hormone on cardiac size and myosin content of the heterotopically transplanted rat heart. *J Clin Invest* 1986;77:1694–1698.
14. Park KW, Dai HB, Ojamaa K, et al. The direct vasomotor effect of thyroid hormones on rat skeletal muscle resistance arteries. *Anesth Analg* 1997;85:734–738.
15. Ebisawa K, Ikeda U, Murata M, et al. Irreversible cardiomyopathy due to thyrotoxicosis. *Cardiology* 1994;84:274–277.
16. Bauerlein EJ, Chakko CS, Kessler KM. Reversible dilated cardiomyopathy due to thyrotoxicosis. *Am J Cardiol* 1992;70:132.
17. Das KC, Mukherjee M, Sarkar TK, et al. Erythropoiesis and erythropoietin in hypo- and hyperthyroidism. *J Clin Endocrinol Metab* 1975;40:211–220.
18. Freedberg AS, Papp JG, Williams EM. The effect of altered thyroid state on atrial intracellular potentials. *J Physiol* 1970;207:357–369.
19. Frost L, Vestergaard P, Mosekilde L. Hyperthyroidism and risk of atrial fibrillation or flutter: a population-based study. *Arch Intern Med* 2004;164:1675–1678.
20. Forfar JC, Miller HC, Toft AD. Occult thyrotoxicosis: a correctable cause of "idiopathic" atrial fibrillation. *Am J Cardiol* 1979;44:9–12.
21. Nakazawa HK, Sakurai K, Hamada N, et al. Management of atrial fibrillation in the post-thyrotoxic state. *Am J Med* 1982;72:903–906.
22. Surks MI, Ortiz E, Daniels GH, et al. Subclinical thyroid disease: scientific review and guidelines for diagnosis and management. *JAMA* 2004;291:228–238.
23. Sawin CT, Geller A, Wolf PA, et al. Low serum thyrotropin concentrations as a risk factor for atrial fibrillation in older persons. *N Engl J Med* 1994;331:1249–1252.
24. Auer J, Scheibner P, Mische T, et al. Subclinical hyperthyroidism as a risk factor for atrial fibrillation. *Am Heart J* 2001;142:838–842.
25. Polikar R, Kennedy B, Ziegler M, et al. Plasma norepinephrine kinetics, dopamine-beta-hydroxylase, and chromogranin-A, in hypothyroid patients before and following replacement therapy. *J Clin Endocrinol Metab* 1990;70:277–281.
26. Wieshammer S, Keck FS, Waitzinger J, et al. Left ventricular function at rest and during exercise in acute hypothyroidism. *Br Heart J* 1988;60:204–211.
27. Thompson GR, Soutar AK, Spengel FA, et al. Defects of receptor-mediated low density lipoprotein catabolism in homozygous familial hypercholesterolemia and hypothyroidism in vivo. *Proc Natl Acad Sci USA* 1981;78:2591–2595.
28. Gomberg-Maitland M, Frishman WH. Thyroid hormone and cardiovascular disease. *Am Heart J* 1998;135:187–196.
29. Anderson GH, Jr., Blakeman N, Streeten DH. The effect of age on prevalence of secondary forms of hypertension in 4429 consecutively referred patients. *J Hypertens* 1994;12:609–615.
30. Streeten DH, Anderson GH, Howland T, et al. Effects of thyroid function on blood pressure. Recognition of hypothyroid hypertension. *Hypertension* 1988;11:78–83.
31. Cappola AR, Ladenson PW. Hypothyroidism and atherosclerosis. *J Clin Endocrinol Metab* 2003;88:2438–2444.
32. Hak AE, Pols HA, Visser TJ, et al. Subclinical hypothyroidism is an independent risk factor for atherosclerosis and myocardial infarction in elderly women: the Rotterdam Study. *Ann Intern Med* 2000;132:270–278.
33. Heinonen OP, Gordin A, Aho K, et al. Symptomless autoimmune thyroiditis in coronary heart-disease. *Lancet* 1972;1:785–786.
34. Albert SG, Alves LE, Rose EP. Thyroid dysfunction during chronic amiodarone therapy. *J Am Coll Cardiol* 1987;9:175–183.
35. Martino E, Safran M, Aghini-Lombardi F, et al. Environmental iodine intake and thyroid dysfunction during chronic amiodarone therapy. *Ann Intern Med* 1984;101:28–34.
36. Harjai KJ, Licata AA. Effects of amiodarone on thyroid function. *Ann Intern Med* 1997;126:63–73.
37. Osman F, Franklyn JA, Sheppard MC, et al. Successful treatment of amiodarone-induced thyrotoxicosis. *Circulation* 2002;105:1275–1277.
38. Bartalena L, Brogioni S, Grasso L, et al. Treatment of amiodarone-induced thyrotoxicosis, a difficult challenge: results of a prospective study. *J Clin Endocrinol Metab* 1996;81:2930–2933.
39. Roffi M, Cattaneo F, Brandle M. Thyrotoxicosis and the cardiovascular system. *Minerva Endocrinol* 2005;30:47–58.
40. Newman CM, Price A, Davies DW, et al. Amiodarone and the thyroid: a practical guide to the management of thyroid dysfunction induced by amiodarone therapy. *Heart* 1998;79:121–127.
41. Trip MD, Wiersinga W, Plomp TA. Incidence, predictability, and pathogenesis of amiodarone-induced thyrotoxicosis and hypothyroidism. *Am J Med* 1991;91:507–511.
42. Touboul P, Brugada J, Capucci A, et al. Dronedarone for prevention of atrial fibrillation: a dose-ranging study. *Eur Heart J* 2003;24:1481–1487.

43. Doggrell SA, Hancox JC. Dronedarone: an amiodarone analogue. *Expert Opin Investig Drugs* 2004;13:415–426.
44. Plotz CM, Knowlton AI, Ragan C. The natural history of Cushing's syndrome. *Am J Med* 1952;13:597–614.
45. Mancini T, Kola B, Mantero F, et al. High cardiovascular risk in patients with Cushing's syndrome according to 1999 WHO/ISH guidelines. *Clin Endocrinol* 2004;61:768–777.
46. Sugihara N, Shimizu M, Kita Y, et al. Cardiac characteristics and postoperative courses in Cushing's syndrome. *Am J Cardiol* 1992;69:1475–1480.
47. Jacoby RC, Owings JT, Ortega T, et al. Biochemical basis for the hypercoagulable state seen in Cushing syndrome. *Arch Surg* 2001;136:1003–1006.
48. Yaneva M, Mosnier-Pudar H, Dugue MA, et al. Midnight salivary cortisol for the initial diagnosis of Cushing's syndrome of various causes. *J Clin Endocrinol Metab* 2004;89:3345–3351.
49. Dluhy RG, Williams GH. Endocrine hypertension. In: Wilson JD, Foster DW, Kronenberg HM, Larsen PR, eds. *Williams textbook of endocrinology.* 9th ed. Philadelphia: Saunders; 1998:729–749.
50. Khan U, Gomez-Sanchez CE, Celso E. Primary aldosteronism: evolving concepts in diagnosis and treatment. *Curr Opin Endocrinol Diabetes* 2004;11: 153–157.
51. Campbell SE, Diaz-Arias AA, Weber KT. Fibrosis of the human heart and systemic organs in adrenal adenoma. *Blood Press* 1992;1:149–156.
52. Mulatero P, Stowasser M, Loh KC, et al. Increased diagnosis of primary aldosteronism, including surgically correctable forms, in centers from five continents. *J Clin Endocrinol Metab* 2004;89:1045–1050.
53. Harris DA, Au-Yong I, Basnyat PS, et al. Review of surgical management of aldosterone secreting tumours of the adrenal cortex. *Eur J Surg Oncol* 2003; 29:467–474.
54. Bravo EL. Evolving concepts in the pathophysiology, diagnosis, and treatment of pheochromocytoma. *Endocr Rev* 1994;15:356–368.
55. Sardesai SH, Mourant AJ, Sivathandon Y, et al. Phaeochromocytoma and catecholamine induced cardiomyopathy presenting as heart failure. *Br Heart J* 1990;63:234–237.
56. Prys-Roberts C. Phaeochromocytoma—recent progress in its management. *Br J Anaesth* 2000;85:44–57.
57. Molitch ME. Clinical manifestations of acromegaly. *Endocrinol Metab Clin North Am* 1992;21:597–614.
58. Mestron A, Webb SM, Astorga R, et al. Epidemiology, clinical characteristics, outcome, morbidity and mortality in acromegaly based on the Spanish Acromegaly Registry. *Eur J Endocrinol* 2004;151:439–446.
59. Davies DL, Beastall GH, Connell JM, et al. Body composition, blood pressure and the renin-angiotensin system in acromegaly before and after treatment. *J Hypertens Suppl* 1985;3:S413–S415.
60. Nabarro JD. Acromegaly. *Clin Endocrinol* 1987;26:481–512.
61. Cittadini A, Stromer H, Katz SE, et al. Differential cardiac effects of growth hormone and insulin-like growth factor-1 in the rat. A combined in vivo and in vitro evaluation. *Circulation* 1996;93:800–809.
62. Fazio S, Cittadini A, Biondi B, et al. Cardiovascular effects of short-term growth hormone hypersecretion. *J Clin Endocrinol Metab* 2000;85:179–182.
63. Colao A, Marzullo P, Cuocolo A, et al. Reversal of acromegalic cardiomyopathy in young but not in middle-aged patients after 12 months of treatment with the depot long-acting somatostatin analogue octreotide. *Clin Endocrinol* 2003;58:169–176.
64. Lie JT. Pathology of the heart in acromegaly: anatomic findings in 27 autopsied patients. *Am Heart J* 1980;100:41–52.
65. Bihan H, Espinosa C, Valdes-Socin H, et al. Long-term outcome of patients with acromegaly and congestive heart failure. *J Clin Endocrinol Metab* 2004;89:5308–5313.
66. Barkan AL. Acromegaly. Diagnosis and therapy. *Endocrinol Metab Clin North Am* 1989;18:277–310.
67. Flogstad AK, Halse J, Bakke S, et al. Sandostatin LAR in acromegalic patients: long-term treatment. *J Clin Endocrinol Metab* 1997;82:23–28.
68. van der Lely AJ, Hutson RK, Trainer PJ, et al. Long-term treatment of acromegaly with pegvisomant, a growth hormone receptor antagonist. *Lancet* 2001;358:1754–1759.
69. Feenstra J, de Herder WW, ten Have SM, et al. Combined therapy with somatostatin analogues and weekly pegvisomant in active acromegaly. *Lancet* 2005;365:1644–1646.
70. Shane E. Parathyroid carcinoma. *Curr Ther Endocrinol Metab* 1994;5:522–525.
71. Stefenelli T, Abela C, Frank H, et al. Cardiac abnormalities in patients with primary hyperparathyroidism: implications for follow-up. *J Clin Endocrinol Metab* 1997;82:106–112.
72. Sivula A, Pelkonen R. Long-term health risk of primary hyperparathyroidism: the effect of surgery. *Ann Med* 1996;28:95–100.
73. Stefenelli T, Mayr H, Bergler-Klein J, et al. Primary hyperparathyroidism: incidence of cardiac abnormalities and partial reversibility after successful parathyroidectomy. *Am J Med* 1993;95:197–202.
74. Walgenbach S, Hommel G, Junginger T. Outcome after surgery for primary hyperparathyroidism: ten-year prospective follow-up study. *World J Surg* 2000;24:564–569.
75. Bilezikian JP, Potts JT Jr, Fuleihan Gel H, et al. Summary statement from a workshop on asymptomatic primary hyperparathyroidism: a perspective for the 21st century. *J Clin Endocrinol Metab* 2002;87:5353–5361.
76. Peacock M, Bilezikian JP, Klassen PS, et al. Cinacalcet hydrochloride maintains long-term normocalcemia in patients with primary hyperparathyroidism. *J Clin Endocrinol Metab* 2005;90:135–141.

CHAPTER 35B ■ HEMATOLOGIC DISORDERS AND THE HEART

AYALEW TEFFERI AND ANGELA DISPENZIERI

INTRODUCTION

The hematopoietic and cardiovascular systems are intimately connected from the standpoint of embryogenesis, anatomy, and pathophysiology. The hematopoietic stem cell (HSC) and endothelium share a common embryonic precursor cell from the mesoderm-derived aorta-gonad-mesonephros (AGM) region: the hemangioblast (1). It is therefore not completely surprising that HSCs were recently shown to have the potential to participate in the neovascularization of ischemic myocardium and improve heart function (2). Blood, a suspension of cells in plasma, resides in the intravascular compartment and is in close contact with vascular endothelium, which facilitates the physiologic as well as pathologic (e.g., thrombosis) interaction between the two. Furthermore, the heart is either directly or indirectly affected during most instances of both neoplastic and nonneoplastic diseases of the blood.

Hematology is broadly defined as the study of blood cells and coagulation proteins. The hematopoietic system is comprised of the bone marrow, peripheral blood, lymph nodes, spleen, liver, and thymus. Under normal conditions, the bone marrow is the exclusive site of postnatal hematopoiesis. All blood cells are derived from HSCs that normally reside in the bone marrow and depend on growth factors and supporting stroma for their development. HSCs are capable of self-renewal as well as differentiation into either myeloid or lymphoid cells. The former include granulocytes, erythrocytes, platelets, and monocytes. The latter include lymphocytes and plasma cells. All stages of myelopoiesis occur in the bone marrow, whereas B- and T-cell lymphopoiesis, although it starts in the bone marrow, is completed in lymph nodes/spleen and thymus, respectively.

An operational classification of hematologic disorders considers both neoplastic (hematologic malignancies) and nonneoplastic conditions. Table 35B.1 outlines the current classification of hematologic malignancies. Nonneoplastic diseases of the blood include quantitative and qualitative blood cell abnormalities, coagulation disorders, and certain complications of blood component transfusion. Examples of the former include anemia and other cytopenias, polycythemia and other cytosis, and sickle cell disease. Coagulation disorders include both thromboembolic and hemorrhagic diseases. Transfusion medicine deals with the indications, process, and complications of blood component transfusion. This chapter focuses on selected topics in hematology that are either frequently encountered in cardiology practice or associated with direct myocardial injury (Table 35B.2).

ANEMIA

Evaluation of anemia should start with examination of the red blood cell (RBC) indices, that is, mean corpuscular volume (MCV), red cell distribution width (RDW), and the peripheral blood smear (PBS) (Fig. 35B.1). Accordingly, anemia is first classified according to the MCV as microcytic (MCV <80 fL), normocytic (MCV 80 to 100 fL), and macrocytic (MCV >100 fL) (3).

Microcytic Anemia

The three major diagnostic possibilities for microcytic anemia are iron-deficiency anemia (IDA), thalassemia, and anemia of chronic disease (ACD). Because the most common of these is IDA, we recommend the determination of serum ferritin as the initial step for all cases of microcytic anemia (Table 35B.3). A low serum ferritin is diagnostic of IDA. In contrast, the diagnosis of IDA is unlikely in the presence of persistently normal or elevated serum ferritin (4). If the serum ferritin level is not decreased, the next step involves either a hemoglobin electrophoresis if the microcytosis is of long standing or consideration of ACD otherwise. Hematologic consultation is required to accurately interpret the results from hemoglobin electrophoresis.

Normocytic Anemia

The first step in approaching normocytic anemia is to exclude relatively easily treatable causes: nutrient-deficient

TABLE 35B.1

CLASSIFICATION OF HEMATOLOGIC DISORDERS

1. Myeloid disorders
   a. Acute myeloid leukemia
   b. Chronic myeloid disorders
      i. Myelodysplastic syndrome
      ii. Myeloproliferative disorders
         A. Classic myeloproliferative disorders
            (1) Chronic myeloid leukemia
            (2) Essential thrombocythemia
            (3) Polycythemia vera
            (4) Myelofibrosis with myeloid metaplasia
         B. Atypical myeloproliferative disorders
            (1) Primary eosinophilic disorders
            (2) Systemic mastocytosis
            (3) Chronic neutrophilic leukemia
            (4) Chronic basophilic leukemia
            (5) Chronic myelomonocytic leukemia
            (6) Juvenile myelomonocytic leukemia
            (7) Unclassified myeloproliferative disorder
2. Lymphoid disorders
   a. Acute lymphocytic leukemia
   b. Chronic lymphoid disorders
      ii. Hodgkin and non-Hodgkin lymphoma
      iii. Myeloma, amyloidosis, and other plasma cell proliferative disorders
      iv. Chronic lymphocytic leukemia and other chronic lymphoid leukemias

anemia, anemia of renal insufficiency, and hemolysis (Table 35B.4). In this regard, it is underscored that both iron and vitamin B12/folate deficiencies are possible causes of "normocytic" anemia despite their usual association with microcytic and macrocytic anemia, respectively (5,6). Initial laboratory tests that should be ordered when hemolysis is suspected include reticulocyte count and serum levels of haptoglobin, lactate dehydrogenase (LDH), and indirect bilirubin. In addition, a urinary hemosiderin test should be ordered if valvular hemolysis is suspected. The differential diagnosis of a normocytic anemia that is not linked to any one of the foregoing possibilities includes ACD and a primary bone marrow disorder. Patient history and information from the PBS provide the most helpful information in distinguishing the two.

Macrocytic Anemia

Drugs, including hydroxyurea and zidovudine, and excess alcohol consumption must first be ruled out as the cause of macro-

TABLE 35B.2

HEMATOLOGY IN CARDIOLOGY PRACTICE

1. Hematologic problems that are frequently encountered in cardiology practice
   a. Anemia
   b. Thrombocytopenia
   c. Neutropenia
   d. Polycythemia
   e. Thrombocytosis
2. Hematologic conditions that directly affect the myocardium
   a. Eosinophilia
   b. Amyloidosis
   c. Hemochromatosis

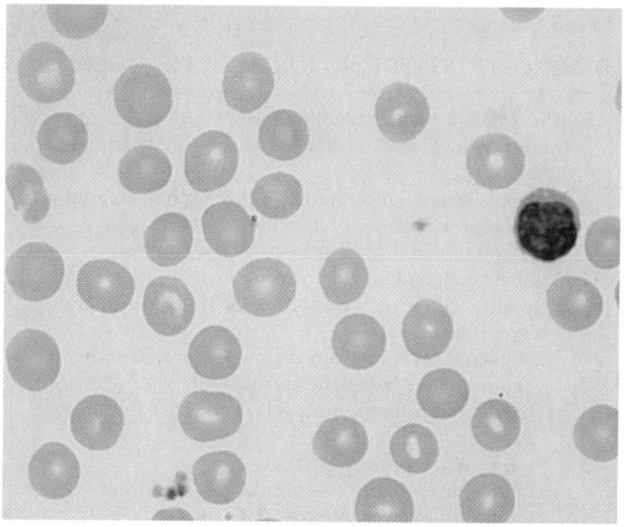

FIGURE 35B.1. A peripheral blood smear showing morphologically normal red blood cells, platelets, and a small lymphocyte.

cytic anemia (Table 35B.5). The next step is to rule out nutritional causes (B12 or folate deficiency), and we prefer to use both serum homocysteine and B12 levels for initial screening for optimal sensitivity (5,7). If one of the two tests is abnormal, a serum methylmalonic acid level should be checked; an increased level suggests B12 deficiency. Further investigation of macrocytic anemia that is neither drug-induced nor nutritional is simplified by subcategorizing the process into either a marked (MCV >110 fL) or mild (MCV 100 to 110 fL) subtype (Table 35B.5). Markedly macrocytic anemia is almost always associated with a primary bone marrow disease, whereas mildly macrocytic anemia can also be associated with more benign conditions (Table 35B.5).

THROMBOCYTOPENIA

The differential diagnosis of thrombocytopenia should always include heparin-induced thrombocytopenia (HIT) and thrombotic thrombocytopenic purpura/hemolytic-uremic syndrome

TABLE 35B.3

DIAGNOSTIC STEPS FOR MICROCYTIC ANEMIA

Step 1. Check serum ferritin level
   1. Decreased—iron-deficiency anemia
   2. Persistently normal or elevated—go to step 2
Step 2. Determine duration of microcytosis
   1. Chronic—consider thalassemia, and order hemoglobin electrophoresis
   2. Acquired—consider anemia of chronic disease
      a. Usual causes
         i. Temporal arteritis
         ii. Rheumatoid arthritis
         iii. Chronic inflammation
         iv. Chronic infection
      b. Unusual causes
         i. Renal cell carcinoma
         ii. Hodgkin lymphoma
         iii. Castleman disease
         iv. Myelofibrosis

TABLE 35B.4

DIAGNOSTIC STEPS FOR NORMOCYTIC ANEMIA

Step 1. Rule out easily treatable causes
  1. Nutrient-deficiency anemia—check serum ferritin and homocysteine
  2. Anemia of renal insufficiency—check serum creatinine
Step 2. Look for evidence of hemolysis by checking haptoglobin, lactate dehydrogenase, indirect bilirubin, and reticulocyte count
  1. Results suggestive of hemolysis—look for peripheral blood smear clues
    a. Spherocytes on the blood smear—consider either autoimmune hemolytic anemia (AIHA) or hereditary spherocytosis (HS) and order Coombs test
      i. Coombs-positive—AIHA
      ii. Coombs-negative—consider SA, and order osmotic fragility test
    b. Schistocytes on the blood smear—consider the following;
      i. Thrombotic thrombocytopenic purpura/hemolytic-uremic syndrome (TTP/HUS)—hematology consultation
      ii. Disseminated intravascular coagulation (DIC)—hematology consultation
      iii. Valvular hemolysis—order urine hemosiderin test
    c. Other findings—hematologic consultation
  2. Not suggestive of hemolysis—consider either anemia of chronic disease (ACD) or primary bone marrow disorder—evaluate peripheral blood smear
    a. Suggestive of primary marrow disorder—hematology consultation
    b. Not suggestive of marrow disease—consider other clinical and laboratory findings to determine need for hematology consultation

(TTP/HUS) because of the urgency for specific therapy for the particular diagnoses (Table 35B.6).

Any patient exposed to heparin in any form or dose, including heparin flushes, is at risk of HIT. Both unfractionated heparin and low-molecular-weight heparin (LMWH) can cause HIT (8). There are two types of HIT; a non–immune-mediated type I (benign) and an immune-mediated type II (potentially catastrophic). Although type I HIT occurs in the first few days and type II after usually 5 days of exposure to heparin, we favor considering all HIT as being type II until proven otherwise, especially in patients with previous exposure history to heparin (9). When HIT is suspected (platelet count $<150 \times 109$/liter or a decrease of $\geq 50\%$ from baseline), discontinuation of all forms of heparin is highly recommended, and such an action should be accompanied by both laboratory testing for HIT (10) and an immediate consultation with a hematologist for institution of alternative anticoagulation (11). A negative enzyme-linked immunosorbent assay (ELISA) test for HIT makes the diagnosis unlikely (10). However, a positive test is not always diagnostic of HIT unless corroborated by a functional assay.

Both TTP/HUS and disseminated intravascular coagulation (DIC) are characterized by microangiopathic hemolytic anemia (MAHA): presence of schistocytes in the PBS associated with anemia, increased LDH, and decreased haptoglobin. However, the absence of "schistocytes" does not rule out the possibility of MAHA, and the results should always be interpreted within the context of the clinical scenario. In general, thrombocytopenia accompanies MAHA that is associated with both TTP/HUS

TABLE 35B.5

DIAGNOSTIC STEPS FOR MACROCYTIC ANEMIA

Step 1. Rule out drug-induced macrocytosis
  1. Hydroxyurea
  2. Zidovudine
  3. Other drugs
Step 2. Rule out B12/folate deficiency—check homocysteine and B12 levels
  1. Both normal—B12/folate deficiency unlikely—use mean corpuscular volume (MCV) to guide further investigation
    a. MCV >110—consider primary bone marrow disease
      i. Myelodysplastic syndrome
      ii. Aplastic anemia
      iii. Large granular lymphocytic disorder
    b. MCV <110—consider both marrow disease and other causes
      i. Myelodysplastic syndrome
      ii. Aplastic anemia
      iii. Large granular lymphocyte disorder
      iv. Excess alcohol consumption
      v. Liver disease
      vi. Reticulocytosis from hemolysis
  2. At least one abnormal—check serum methylmalonic acid (MMA)
    a. MMA increased—consider B12 deficiency
    b. MMA normal—consider folate deficiency and check serum folate

TABLE 35B.6

DIAGNOSTIC STEPS FOR THROMBOCYTOPENIA

Step 1. Rule out heparin-induced thrombocytopenia (HIT)
Step 2. Rule out microangiopathic hemolytic anemia (MAHA); schistocytes in blood smear, increased lactate dehydrogenase, and decreased haptoglobin; differential diagnosis of MAHA includes
  1. Thrombotic thrombocytopenic purpura/hemolytic-uremic syndrome (TTP/HUS)
  2. Disseminated intravascular coagulation (DIC)
  3. Valvular hemolysis—usually not associated with thrombocytopenia
Step 3. Rule out the possibility of both drug- and virus-associated thrombocytopenias
  1. Drug-associated thrombocytopenia—glycoprotein IIa/IIIb inhibitors, quinine, and others
  2. Virus-associated thrombocytopenia—HIV and others
Step 4. Consider other immune- and non–immune-mediated thrombocytopenias
  1. Immune mediated
    a. Idiopathic thrombocytopenic purpura—should be diagnosis of exclusion
    b. Lymphoproliferative disease-associated thrombocytopenia
    c. Autoimmune disease-associated thrombocytopenia
  2. Non-immune mediated
    a. Hypersplenism—should be suspected in all patients with cirrhosis
    b. Bone marrow disease
      i. Myelodysplastic syndrome—only occasionally presents with isolated thrombocytopenia
      ii. Amegakaryocytic thrombocytopenia—very rare
    c. Hereditary thrombocytopenia
    d. Posttransfusion purpura

and DIC but not valvular hemolysis-associated MAHA. On the other hand, clotting times (prothrombin time [PT] and partial thromboplastin time [PTT]) are often prolonged in DIC but not in TTP/HUS.

In addition to HIT, TTP/HUS, and DIC, the differential diagnosis of thrombocytopenia should include both immune-mediated and non–immune-mediated causes. In both instances, both drugs and viruses must be considered as potential causes. Included in the former are platelet glycoprotein (GP) IIb/IIIa inhibitors, in cases of which acute thrombocytopenia can occur within hours of drug exposure (12). Other causes of drug-associated thrombocytopenia include quinidine, quinine, procainamide, sulfa drugs, anticonvulsants, antirheumatic drugs, diuretics, and nonsteroidal antiinflammatory drugs (NSAID) (13). Human immunodeficiency virus and other virus infections should always be part of the differential diagnosis of thrombocytopenia (14). In contrast, idiopathic thrombocytopenic purpura (ITP) should be a diagnosis of exclusion. Other immune-mediated causes include lymphoproliferative and autoimmune disorders. Non–immune-mediated causes of thrombocytopenia include hypersplenism, the hereditary thrombocytopenias that might be associated with giant platelets, and posttransfusion purpura (15).

NEUTROPENIA

Neutropenia is clinically most relevant when it is severe (absolute neutrophil count [ANC] $<500 \times 106$/liter) because of the associated risk of infection (16). The most frequent cause of acquired neutropenia is drug therapy. In this regard, the most commonly recommended agents are listed in Table 35B.7, including those that are used in cardiology practice (17). Other frequent causes of neutropenia include both viral and bacterial infections. Less frequent causes include immune neutropenia and large granular lymphocyte (LGL) leukemia (18). Diagnostic evaluation in the latter cases includes PBS examination, lymphocyte immunophenotyping by flow cytometry, T-cell receptor (TCR) gene rearrangement studies, and antineutrophil antibody testing. Immune neutropenia might or might not be associated with an autoimmune disease (e.g., Felty syndrome), and the detection of an antineutrophil antibody supports the diagnosis.

TABLE 35B.7

DRUGS THAT ARE FREQUENTLY IMPLICATED IN NEUTROPENIA

Drug category	Individual drugs
Anticonvulsants	Carbamazepine, valproic acid, diphenylhydantoin
Thyroid inhibitors	Carbimazole, methimazole, propylthiouracil
Antibiotics	Penicillins, cephalosporins, sulfonamides, chloramphenicol, vancomycin, trimethoprim-sulfamethoxazole
Antipsychotics	Clozapine
Antiarrhythmics	Procainamide
Antirheumatics	Gold Salts, hydroxychloroquine, penicillamine
Aminosalicylates	
Nonsteroidal antiinflammatory drugs	

TABLE 35B.8

A STEPWISE DIAGNOSTIC APPROACH TO POLYCYTHEMIA VERA (PV)

Step 1. Check serum erythropoietin (Epo) level
1. Elevated serum Epo—PV diagnosis unlikely
2. Decreased serum Epo—proceed with bone marrow biopsy and JAK2 mutation screening[a]
3. Normal serum Epo—proceed with bone marrow biopsy only in the presence of either clinical (e.g., splenomegaly, thrombosis, pruritus) or laboratory (e.g., thrombocytosis, leukocytosis, increased leukocyte alkaline phosphatase score) features of PV; otherwise repeat blood count in 3 mo

Step 2. Consider the following after bone marrow biopsy and JAK2 mutation screening:
1. Either JAK2 mutation screening positive or consistent histology—PV diagnosis likely
2. Both JAK2 mutation screening and histology negative—PV diagnosis unlikely

Step 3. Note that a positive JAK2 mutation cannot distinguish between PV and other myeloproliferative disorders

[a] JAK2 mutation screening refers to the JAK2 V617F mutation that is found in approximately 90% of PV patients but not in normal volunteers.

POLYCYTHEMIA

In routine clinical practice, the term polycythemia is used to indicate the perception of an increased red cell mass (RCM). This perception might be real (true polycythemia) or spurious (apparent polycythemia [AP]). True polycythemia is caused by either polycythemia vera (PV) or a nonclonal increase in RCM that is often, but not always, driven by erythropoietin (secondary polycythemia [SP]). The management approaches to PV (at least phlebotomy and aspirin) versus SP (phlebotomy often not required) versus AP (no phlebotomy) are different enough to warrant accurate distinction among them (19). Table 35B.8 outlines a way of accomplishing this without the need for measuring the red cell mass (20).

THROMBOCYTOSIS

Similar to the aforementioned situation with polycythemia, one needs to approach thrombocytosis in a stepwise fashion and first distinguish between reactive thrombocytosis (RT) and clonal thrombocytosis (CT). RT is known to accompany a variety of conditions including IDA, surgical asplenia, infection, chronic inflammation, hemolysis, tissue damage, and nonmyeloid malignancy (21). The initial laboratory tests that help to distinguish RT from CT include PBS, serum ferritin, and C-reactive protein (CRP) (22). For example, PBS might reveal the presence of Howell-Jolly bodies in case of asplenia, anisocytosis and poikilocytosis in case of IDA, and polychromasia in case of hemolysis. A normal serum ferritin level excludes the possibility of IDA-associated RT. The measurement of CRP is helpful in attending to the possibility of an occult inflammatory or malignant process as a cause for RT (22). If the clinical scenario is not consistent with RT, a bone marrow biopsy with chromosome studies and JAK2 mutation screening is advised (Table 35B.9) (23). The results would be consistent with chronic myeloid leukemia in the presence of the Philadelphia

TABLE 35B.9

A STEPWISE DIAGNOSTIC APPROACH TO ESSENTIAL THROMBOCYTHEMIA (ET)

Step 1. Rule out reactive thrombocytosis with history, physical examination, and laboratory studies as elaborated in the text

Step 2. If reactive thrombocytosis appears to be unlikely, proceed with bone marrow biopsy and JAK2 mutation screening[a]

1. Either JAK2 mutation screening positive or consistent histology—ET diagnosis likely
2. Both JAK2 mutation screening and histology negative—ET diagnosis unlikely

Step 3. Note that a positive JAK2 mutation cannot distinguish between ET and other myeloproliferative disorders

[a]JAK2 mutation screening refers to the JAK2 V617F mutation that is found in approximately 90% of PV patients but not in normal volunteers.

(Ph) chromosome and a Ph-negative myeloproliferative disorder (MPD), including essential thrombocythemia (ET), in the presence of the JAK2 V617F mutation. However, ET is still a possibility in the absence of molecular markers as long as the bone marrow histology is consistent with MPD.

EOSINOPHILIA

Eosinophilia is generally classified into a primary and a secondary process. Secondary eosinophilia accompanies either certain infections (tissue-invasive parasitosis) or noninfectious conditions (drugs, toxins, allergic or inflammatory conditions, lymphoma, metastatic cancer). Primary eosinophilia is operationally classified into two categories, clonal and idiopathic. Clonal eosinophilia occurs in the context of an otherwise classified hematologic malignancy including acute leukemia and chronic myeloid disorders (Table 35B.1). Idiopathic eosinophilia represents a third category that is neither reactive nor clonal. Hypereosinophilic syndrome (HES) is a subcategory of idiopathic eosinophilia and is characterized by the triad of prominent eosinophilia (absolute eosinophil count $\geq$1,500/liter), chronic course ($\geq$6 months), and eosinophil-mediated tissue injury (e.g., cardiomyopathy, pneumonitis, dermatitis, sinusitis, gastrointestinal inflammation, stroke) (24). We now outline a stepwise approach to the patient with eosinophilia.

1. Rule out reactive eosinophilia. The first step in approaching the patient with blood eosinophilia is to exclude the possibility of secondary eosinophilia. In this regard, the PBS is not helpful (Fig. 35B.2), and work-up beyond stool examination for ova and parasites is recommended only if the history dictates it.
2. Distinguish between clonal eosinophilia and hypereosinophilic syndrome. If reactive eosinophilia is considered unlikely, a bone marrow examination with appropriate cytogenetic and molecular studies is advised. Furthermore, bone marrow examination in patients with suspected HES should be accompanied by immunohistochemical stains for tryptase and mast cell immunophenotyping so as not to miss occult systemic mastocytosis. Standard cytogenetic methods are not always capable of revealing treatment-relevant molecular lesions, and therefore should be accompanied by fluorescent in situ hybridization or reverse transcriptase-polymerase chain reaction (RT-PCR)–based laboratory testing to detect the imatinib-sensitive *FIP1L1-PDGFRA* mutation (Fig. 35B.3) (25).

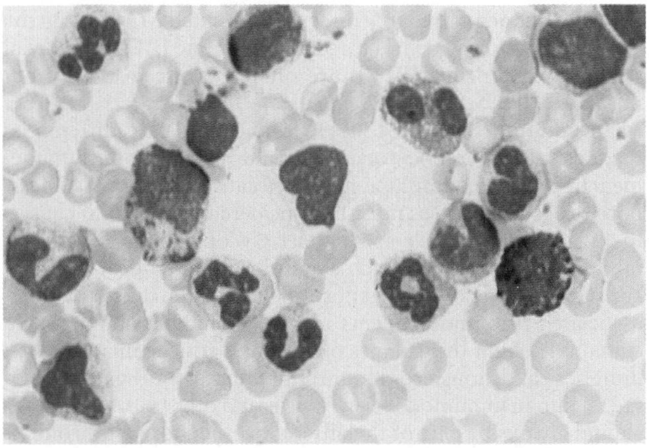

FIGURE 35B.2. A peripheral blood smear showing a typical eosinophil in the right upper corner and a basophil two cells below it.

3. Assess eosinophilia-associated tissue damage including cardiac disease. In addition to looking for the cause of eosinophilia, initial evaluation of the patient with eosinophilia should include laboratory tests to assess for eosinophilic-mediated tissue damage. In this regard, lung involvement is suggested by chest radiography that typically shows transient and migrating opacities that are prominent in the lung periphery. The corresponding computed tomography (CT) findings are characterized by small peripheral nodules. Cardiac involvement is suggested by either elevated serum troponin level or echocardiogram. Increased level of serum cardiac troponin has been shown to correlate with the presence of cardiomyopathy in HES, and recent studies have suggested a predictive role for drug-induced cardiogenic shock during treatment with imatinib (26). In a systematic study of echocardiographic findings in 51 HES patients seen at the Mayo Clinic, abnormalities were noted in 49% of the patients and included left (24%) and right (20%) ventricular apical thrombus, posterior mitral leaflet involvement (20%), tricuspid involvement (10%), endocardial thickening (12%), dilated left ventricle (14%), and pericardial effusion (18%) (27). Tissue biopsy typically reveals eosinophilic infiltrates, deposition of eosinophil granule proteins, as well as cell necrosis and apoptosis.
4. Provide management of primary eosinophilia. Tissue injury in HES is mediated by material released from eosinophilic granules including major basic protein (MBP), eosinophil cationic protein (ECP), and eosinophil-derived neurotoxin (EDN) (28). It is also conceivable that such eosinophil-derived molecules, either directly or indirectly, contribute to thromboembolic complications associated with HES (29). Therefore, the major goal of therapy in HES is to debulk the blood and tissue eosinophil burden.

The most appealing drug for the treatment of primary eosinophilia is imatinib (Gleevec) (30). However, the drug is effective only in the presence of a mutation that involves either *PDGFRA* or *PDGFRB*. Most such patients will respond completely and durably to low dose levels (100 mg/day). Treatment with imatinib is recommended even in the absence of symptoms because of the potential for preventing cardiovascular complications (31). Imatinib therapy has occasionally been associated with drug-induced cardiogenic shock that is reversible with systemic corticosteroid therapy (32). Therefore, concomitant corticosteroid use (1 mg/kg/day) for 1 to 2 weeks is advised in the presence of either an abnormal echocardiogram or elevated serum troponin levels (26,32).

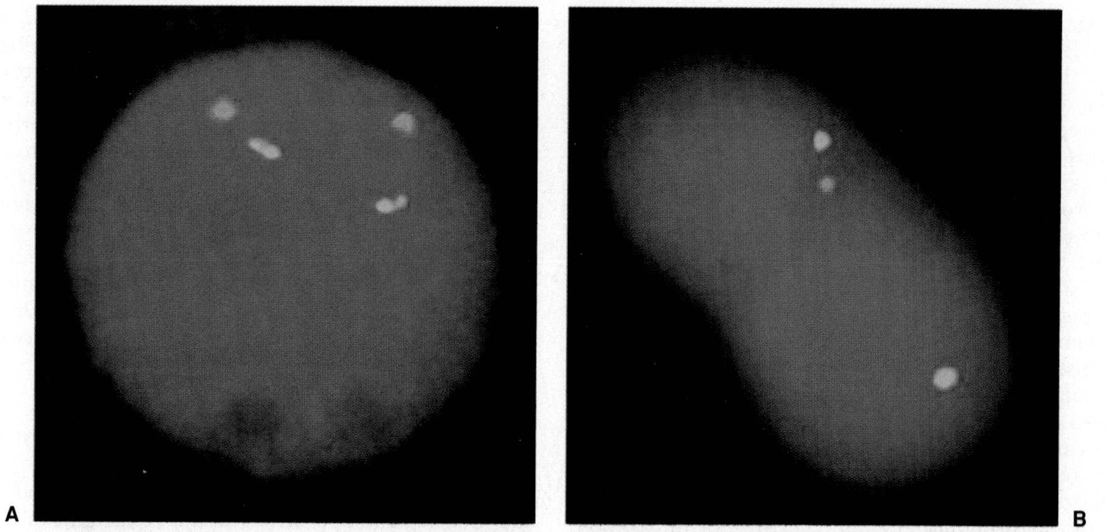

FIGURE 35B.3. Fluorescent in situ hybridization slides showing (A) two orange signals (normal) and (B) only one orange signal (abnormal) indicating the loss of a DNA region in the latter instance that is consistent with the occurrence of a *FIP1L1-PDGFRA* fusion on chromosome 4q12 that is associated with an imatinib-sensitive primary eosinophilic disorder (see text for further elaboration).

Initial therapy for molecularly undefined HES, in case of symptomatic disease, consists of prednisone alone (1 mg/kg/day) or in combination with hydroxyurea (starting dose 500 mg twice daily) (33). However, most patients relapse during the steroid taper and often require additional drug therapy. In this regard, interferon-α is considered the second-line treatment of choice based on numerous reports of well-documented long-lasting remissions in the majority of treated patients (34). For cases that are refractory to usual drug therapy, higher-dose imatinib (400 mg/day), cladribine, and monoclonal antibodies to either interleukin-5 (mepolizumab) or CD52 (alemtuzumab) can be considered (34). In truly drug-refractory cases, nonmyeloablative allogeneic stem cell transplantation is a viable treatment option (34).

AMYLOIDOSIS

Amyloidosisis an infiltrative disease that is either hereditary or acquired and is characterized by tissue deposition of insoluble amyloid fibrils made up of monoclonal immunoglobulin light chain fragments (systemic AL amyloidosis), serum amyloid A protein (secondary AA amyloidosis), β2-microglobulin (dialysis-associated amyloidosis), wild-type transthyretin (senile systemic amyloidosis), and a spectrum of mutant proteins found in hereditary amyloidoses including mutant transthyretin (TTR)-associated familial amyloid polyneuropathy, cystatin C–associated cerebral amyloid angiopathy, and others (35). At diagnosis, amyloidosis is generally widespread with diffuse involvement of blood vessels even in tissues without clinical evidence of involvement (36). The most common amyloid syndromes are nephrotic syndrome, restrictive cardiomyopathy, hepatomegaly, and peripheral neuropathy.

Cardiac Amyloidosis

Symptoms and signs of cardiac amyloidosis include arrhythmias, conduction blocks, and congestive heart failure (CHF) (Fig. 35B.4). The typical electrocardiogram findings include

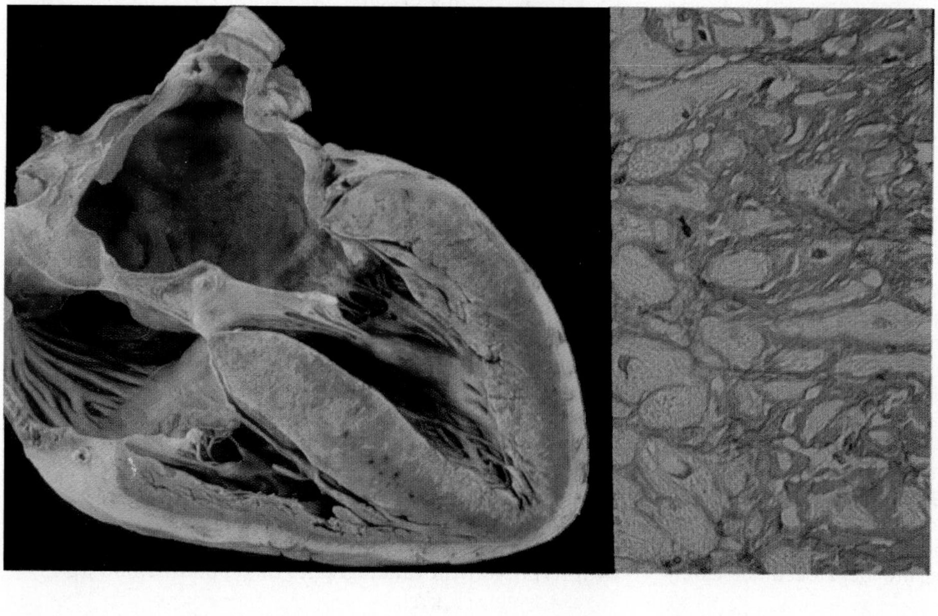

FIGURE 35B.4. Amyloid involving the heart. **Left:** Gross specimen (four-chamber view). The lighter tan material is amyloid and the darker tan material is normal myocardium. **B:** Photomicrograph (sulfated Alcian blue stain). Amyloid is green, and myocytes are yellow. (Courtesy of Dr. William Edwards, Professor of Pathology, Mayo Clinic College of Medicine, Rochester, Minnesota.)

low voltage in standard limb leads and QS pattern in right precordial leads. The typical echocardiogram findings include symmetric thickening of ventricular walls and septum and left ventricular diastolic dysfunction. Cardiac involvement in amyloidosis is seen mostly with either systemic AL or senile systemic amyloidosis (37). Senile systemic amyloidosis is a disease of elderly men, usually limited to the heart, and is characterized by a slowly progressive CHF (38). In contrast, death in most patients with systemic AL amyloidosis is of a cardiac cause, either progressive CHF or sudden cardiac death.

The most common complaints in patients with cardiac amyloidosis are fatigue and dyspnea on exertion. Cardiac AL amyloidosis mimics both ischemic and cardiomyopathic heart disease because amyloid fibrils are deposited in both coronary microvasculature and extracellular matrix. The outcome in systemic AL amyloidosis patients is usually determined by the extent of cardiac involvement. Increased left ventricular wall thickness, reduced systolic function, and diastolic dysfunction are all adverse prognostic factors (36,39,40). Syncope is a powerful predictor of imminent sudden death (41). In addition, both symptomatic CHF and elevations of cardiac troponins (cTnT, cTnI) and N-terminal brain natriuretic peptide have been shown to be powerful predictors of survival in systemic AL amyloidosis (42–45).

Diagnosis of Amyloidosis

Amyloidosis should be in the differential diagnosis of cardiomyopathy, intractable arrhythmias, nephrotic syndrome with or without renal insufficiency, autonomic or peripheral neuropathy, bowel dysfunction associated with malabsorption, severe fatigue associated with weight loss, unexplained hepatomegaly, periorbital purpura or abnormal bruising, macroglossia, and monoclonal gammopathy (43). Initial laboratory testing should include serum and urinary protein electrophoresis with immunofixation; serum immunoglobulin free light chain estimation; subcutaneous fat aspirate or affected tissue biopsy with Congo red or sulfated Alcian blue staining; immunohistochemical typing of the amyloid fibrils; and DNA analysis when hereditary amyloidosis is suspected (46). If the immunohistochemical typing is not fruitful, the specific type of the amyloid fibrils can be characterized by amino acid sequencing.

Treatment of Amyloidosis

There is no known cure for systemic AL amyloidosis, although both chemotherapy and autologous stem cell transplantation can produce organ responses in approximately 50% of patients (47). Liver transplantation is an established treatment modality for treatment of certain types of hereditary TTR amyloidosis (48).

HEMOCHROMATOSIS

Hemochromatosis is broadly defined as the state of excess tissue iron deposition that is associated with demonstrable organ dysfunction (49). Causes of hemochromatosis include hereditary hemochromatosis (HH), chronic red blood cell transfusion therapy, and excessive oral iron intake over a long period of time (50,51).

Clinical Features

The clinical features of symptomatic hemochromatosis include liver cirrhosis that might progress into hepatocellular carcinoma, diabetes mellitus from pancreatic islet cell iron deposition, skin pigmentation, hypogonadotropic hypogonadism, arthritis from chondrocalcinosis and synovial hemosiderosis, cardiomyopathy, and arrhythmias (52).Treatment with phlebotomy ameliorates all manifestations except arthropathy and insulin-dependent diabetes (52). Cardiac manifestations of hemochromatosis include congestive and restrictive cardiomyopathy and arrhythmias (53). Echocardiogram findings include increases in left ventricular (LV) end-diastolic and end-systolic diameters and decrease in ejection fraction without increased wall thickness (54,55). Treatment with phlebotomy has been shown to reverse some of these changes (54). On the other hand, hemochromatosis does not appear to increase the risk of ischemic heart disease (56).

Genetics of Hereditary Hemochromatosis

Causes of HH include mutations of genes that encode for different iron-regulating proteins. In this regard, the most frequent mutant alleles involve the *HFE* gene, which is located on the short arm of chromosome 6 (e.g., C282Y and H63D mutations) (57). For example, in previously diagnosed American patients with phenotypically overt HH, homozygous C282Y was seen in approximately 80% of the cases, whereas an additional 8% to 10% were compound heterozygotes for C282Y/H63D (58). The genetic basis for the remainder of cases is slowly being unfolded and includes several non–*HFE*-associated HH subtypes including juvenile HH involving the hemojuvelin and hepcidin proteins, transferrin receptor 2–related HH, and ferroportin-related iron overload (49).

Although most non-Hispanic white patients with previously established diagnosis of hemochromatosis carry the homozygous C282Y mutant allele, less than 10% of the control population-derived C282Y homozygotes develop the disease over their lifetime (57). This is an important point in view of the relatively high incidence of homozygous C282Y in the general non-Hispanic white population (0.44%) (50). Similarly, although approximately 0.4% of the general population might display serum ferritin levels of greater than 1000 μg/L, only 13% of such cases have been shown to carry the homozygous C282Y mutation (50). These two scenarios as well as information from other studies indicate that homozygous *HFE* gene mutations have very low penetrance and may not account for the majority asymptomatic iron overload states. Of particular importance to cardiology, the incidence of *HFE* mutations among patients with idiopathic dilated cardiomyopathy was not found to be different than in the control population (59).

Diagnosis and Treatment of Hemochromatosis

The diagnosis of hemochromatosis depends on what is considered as the disease phenotype: presence of symptoms with evidence for organ involvement, presence of evidence for organ involvement regardless of symptoms, or presence of abnormal iron studies even in the absence of organ involvement. The issue is further confounded by the information from molecular tests. In any event, it is reasonable to suspect hemochromatosis on the grounds of either clinical suspicion or a transferrin saturation of greater than 45%. At that point, we recommend both serum ferritin determination and *HFE* mutation screening. A liver biopsy is not necessary unless the serum ferritin is greater than 1,000 μg/L because values lower than 1,000 μg/L are usually not associated with cirrhosis (58). Phlebotomy is the cornerstone of therapy in hemochromatosis and is indicated in the presence of symptoms as well as in asymptomatic cases with serum ferritin values greater than 500 to 1,000 μg/L.

CONTROVERSIES AND PERSONAL PERSPECTIVES

The advent of electronic cell counters has made complete blood count (CBC) one of the most frequently ordered laboratory tests in most disciplines of medicine. For example, at our institution, approximately 1,800 CBCs are ordered every day, and 10% to 20% of the results are reported as being abnormal. The cardiologist often encounters abnormalities on the CBC that he or she should be able to address without resorting to a hematology consultation. This chapter was written to provide guidance in this regard. As a general rule, it is prudent to perform a peripheral blood smear in most instances of abnormal CBC. In addition, we consider the serum ferritin to be the most reliable test for evaluating body iron stores in the context of both iron-deficiency anemia and hemochromatosis. Accordingly, we do not recommend other iron studies, including serum iron concentration and transferrin saturation, during the diagnostic work-up of iron-deficiency anemia. Similarly, we do not endorse the long-standing textbook dogma that iron deficiency could be masked by an elevated serum ferritin from an acute-phase reaction.

THE FUTURE

The molecular pathogenesis of primary eosinophilia is being unraveled, and it is becoming evident that most instances of HES represent a myeloproliferative disorder. At the same time, pathogenesis-targeted therapy is being developed and should result in effective therapy with subsequent prevention of eosinophilia-associated heart disease. Similarly, the genetic characterization of hemochromatosis has already resulted in both early diagnosis and institution of phlebotomy, which should prevent target organ damage from iron overload. However, there has not been as much progress in either the pathogenesis or therapy of systemic AL amyloidosis, and the management of affected patients remains a major challenge.

References

1. Hamaguchi I, Huang XL, Takakura N, et al. In vitro hematopoietic and endothelial cell development from cells expressing TEK receptor in murine aorta-gonad-mesonephros region. *Blood* 1999;93:1549–1556.
2. Wollert KC, Meyer GP, Lotz J, et al. Intracoronary autologous bone-marrow cell transfer after myocardial infarction: the BOOST randomised controlled clinical trial. *Lancet* 2004;364:141–148.
3. Tefferi A, Hanson CA, Inwards DJ. How to interpret and pursue an abnormal complete blood cell count in adults. *Mayo Clin Proc* 2005;80:923–936.
4. Barron BA, Hoyer JD, Tefferi A. A bone marrow report of absent stainable iron is not diagnostic of iron deficiency. *Ann Hematol* 2001;80:166–169.
5. Pruthi RK, Tefferi A. Pernicious anemia revisited. *Mayo Clin Proc* 1994;69:144–150.
6. Ho CH. The differential diagnostic values of serum transferrin receptor, serum ferritin and related parameters in the patients with various causes of anemia. *Haematologica* 2001;86:206–207.
7. Tefferi A, Pruthi RK. The biochemical basis of cobalamin deficiency. *Mayo Clin Proc* 1994;69:181–186.
8. Prandoni P, Siragusa S, Girolami B, et al. for the BELZONI Investigators Group. The incidence of heparin-induced thrombocytopenia in medical patients treated with low-molecular-weight heparin: a prospective cohort study. *Blood* 2005;106:3049–3054.
9. Warkentin TE, Kelton JG. Temporal aspects of heparin-induced thrombocytopenia. *N Engl J Med* 2001;344:1286–1292.
10. Warkentin TE. New approaches to the diagnosis of heparin-induced thrombocytopenia. *Chest* 2005;127:35S–45S.
11. Warkentin TE, Greinacher A. Heparin-induced thrombocytopenia: recognition, treatment, and prevention: the Seventh ACCP Conference on Antithrombotic and Thrombolytic Therapy. *Chest* 2004;126:311S–337S.
12. Aster RH. Immune thrombocytopenia caused by glycoprotein IIb/IIIa inhibitors. *Chest* 2005;127:53S–59S.
13. van den Bemt PM, Meyboom RH, Egberts AC. Drug-induced immune thrombocytopenia. *Drug Saf* 2004;27:1243–1252.
14. Evatt BL. HIV Infection and thrombocytopenia. *Curr Hematol Rep* 2005;4:149–153.
15. Cines DB, Bussel JB, McMillan RB, Zehnder JL. Congenital and acquired thrombocytopenia. *Hematology* (Am Soc Hematol Educ Program) 2004;390–406.
16. Bodey GP, Buckley M, Sathe YS, Freireich EJ. Quantitative relationships between circulating leukocytes and infection in patients with acute leukemia. *Ann Intern Med* 1966;64:328–340.
17. van Staa TP, Boulton F, Cooper C, et al. Neutropenia and agranulocytosis in England and Wales: incidence and risk factors. *Am J Hematol* 2003;72:248–254.
18. Dhodapkar MV, Li CY, Lust JA, et al. Clinical spectrum of clonal proliferations of T-large granular lymphocytes: a T-cell clonopathy of undetermined significance?. *Blood* 1994;84:1620–1627.
19. Tefferi A. Polycythemia vera: a comprehensive review and clinical recommendations. *Mayo Clin Proc* 2003;78:174–194.
20. Sirhan S, Fairbanks VF, Tefferi A. Red cell mass and plasma volume measurements in polycythemia. *Cancer* 2005;104:213–215.
21. Tefferi A. Thrombocytosis and essential thrombocythemia. In Michelson AD, ed., *Platelets*. Orlando, FL: Academic Press, 2002:667–679.
22. Tefferi A, Ho TC, Ahmann GJ, et al. Plasma interleukin-6 and C-reactive protein levels in reactive versus clonal thrombocytosis. *Am J Med* 1994;97:374–378.
23. Tefferi A, Gilliland DG. The JAK2V617F tyrosine kinase mutation in myeloproliferative disorders: status report and immediate implications for disease classification and diagnosis. *Mayo Clin Proc* 2005;80:947–958.
24. Chusid MJ, Dale DC, West BC, Wolff SM. The hypereosinophilic syndrome: analysis of fourteen cases with review of the literature. *Medicine* (Baltimore) 1975;54:1–27.
25. Cools J, DeAngelo DJ, Gotlib J, et al. A tyrosine kinase created by fusion of the PDGFRA and FIP1L1 genes as a therapeutic target of imatinib in idiopathic hypereosinophilic syndrome. *N Engl J Med* 2003;348:1201–1214.
26. Pitini V, Arrigo C, Azzarello D, et al. Serum concentration of cardiac troponin T in patients with hypereosinophilic syndrome treated with imatinib is predictive of adverse outcomes. *Blood* 2003;102:3456–3457; author reply, 3457.
27. Ommen SR, Seward JB, Tajik AJ. Clinical and echocardiographic features of hypereosinophilic syndromes. *Am J Cardiol* 2000;86:110–113.
28. Gleich GJ, Adolphson CR, Leiferman KM. The biology of the eosinophilic leukocyte. *Annu Rev Med* 1993;44:85–101.
29. Vargas CA, Maldonado O, Botero RC, et al. Budd-Chiari syndrome associated with the hypereosinophilic syndrome. *Am J Gastroenterol* 1993;88:1802–1803.
30. Pardanani A, Tefferi A. Imatinib targets other than bcr/abl and their clinical relevance in myeloid disorders. *Blood* 2004;104:1931–1939.
31. Klion AD, Robyn J, Akin C, et al. Molecular remission and reversal of myelofibrosis in response to imatinib mesylate treatment in patients with the myeloproliferative variant of hypereosinophilic syndrome. *Blood* 2004;103:473–478.
32. Pardanani A, Reeder T, Porrata LF, et al. Imatinib therapy for hypereosinophilic syndrome and other eosinophilic disorders. *Blood* 2003;101:3391–3397.
33. Parrillo JE, Fauci AS, Wolff SM. Therapy of the hypereosinophilic syndrome. *Ann Intern Med* 1978;89:167–172.
34. Tefferi A. Modern diagnosis and treatment of primary eosinophilia. *Acta Haematol* 2005;114:52–60.
35. Hirschfield GM. Amyloidosis: a clinico-pathophysiological synopsis. *Semin Cell Dev Biol* 2004;15:39–44.
36. Cueto-Garcia L, Tajik AJ, Kyle RA, et al. Serial echocardiographic observations in patients with primary systemic amyloidosis: an introduction to the concept of early (asymptomatic) amyloid infiltration of the heart. *Mayo Clinic Proc* 1984;59:589–597.
37. Ikeda S. Cardiac amyloidosis: heterogenous pathogenic backgrounds. *Intern Med* 2004;43:1107–1114.
38. Ng B, Connors LH, Davidoff R, et al. Senile systemic amyloidosis presenting with heart failure: a comparison with light chain-associated amyloidosis. *Arch Intern Med* 2005;165:1425–1429.
39. Klein AL, Hatle LK, Taliercio CP, et al. Prognostic significance of Doppler measures of diastolic function in cardiac amyloidosis. A Doppler echocardiography study. *Circulation* 1991;83:808–816.
40. Hongo M, Yamamoto H, Kohda T, et al. Comparison of electrocardiographic findings in patients with AL (primary) amyloidosis and in familial amyloid polyneuropathy and anginal pain and their relation to histopathologic findings. *Am J Cardiol* 2000;85:849–853.
41. Chamarthi B, Dubrey SW, Cha K, et al. Features and prognosis of exertional syncope in light-chain associated AL cardiac amyloidosis. *Am J Cardiol* 1997;80:1242–1245.
42. Dispenzieri A, Kyle RA, Gertz MA, et al. Survival in patients with primary systemic amyloidosis and raised serum cardiac troponins. *Lancet* 2003;361:1787–1789.
43. Kyle RA, Gertz MA. Primary systemic amyloidosis: clinical and laboratory features in 474 cases. *Semin Hematol* 1995;32:45–59.
44. Dispenzieri A, Gertz MA, Kyle RA, et al. Serum cardiac troponins and N-terminal pro–brain natriuretic peptide: a staging system for primary systemic amyloidosis. *J Clin Oncol* 2004;22:3751–3757.

45. Dispenzieri A, Gertz MA, Kyle RA, et al. Prognostication of survival using cardiac troponins and N-terminal pro–brain natriuretic peptide in patients with primary systemic amyloidosis undergoing peripheral blood stem cell transplantation. *Blood* 2004;104:1881–1887.
46. Guidelines on the diagnosis and management of AL amyloidosis. *Br J Haematol* 2004;125:681–700.
47. Gertz MA, Lacy MQ, Dispenzieri A, Hayman SR. Amyloidosis. *Best Pract Res Clin Haematol* 2005;18:709–727.
48. Suhr OB, Herlenius G, Friman S, Ericzon BG. Liver transplantation for hereditary transthyretin amyloidosis. *Liver Transpl* 2000;6:263–276.
49. Pietrangelo A. Hereditary hemochromatosis—a new look at an old disease. *N Engl J Med* 2004;350:2383–2397.
50. Adams PC, Reboussin DM, Barton JC, et al. Hemochromatosis and iron-overload screening in a racially diverse population. *N Engl J Med* 2005;352:1769–1778.
51. Bell H, Berg JP, Undlien DE, et al. The clinical expression of hemochromatosis in Oslo, Norway. Excessive oral iron intake may lead to secondary hemochromatosis even in HFE C282Y mutation negative subjects. *Scand J Gastroenterol* 2000;35:1301–1307.
52. Niederau C, Strohmeyer G, Stremmel W. Epidemiology, clinical spectrum and prognosis of hemochromatosis. *Adv Exp Med Biol* 1994;356:293–302.
53. Cutler DJ, Isner JM, Bracey AW, et al. Hemochromatosis heart disease: an unemphasized cause of potentially reversible restrictive cardiomyopathy. *Am J Med* 1980;69:923–928.
54. Candell-Riera J, Lu L, Seres L, et al. Cardiac hemochromatosis: beneficial effects of iron removal therapy. An echocardiographic study. *Am J Cardiol* 1983;52:824–829.
55. Olson LJ, Baldus WP, Tajik AJ. Echocardiographic features of idiopathic hemochromatosis. *Am J Cardiol* 1987;60:885–889.
56. Ellervik C, Tybjaerg-Hansen A, Grande P, et al. Hereditary hemochromatosis and risk of ischemic heart disease: a prospective study and a case–control study. *Circulation* 2005;112:185–193.
57. Waalen J, Nordestgaard BG, Beutler E. The penetrance of hereditary hemochromatosis. *Best Pract Res Clin Haematol* 2005;18:203–220.
58. Morrison ED, Brandhagen DJ, Phatak PD, et al. Serum ferritin level predicts advanced hepatic fibrosis among U.S. patients with phenotypic hemochromatosis. *Ann Intern Med* 2003;138:627–633.
59. Hannuksela J, Leppilampi M, Peuhkurinen K, et al. Hereditary hemochromatosis gene (HFE) mutations C282Y, H63D and S65C in patients with idiopathic dilated cardiomyopathy. *Eur J Heart Fail* 2005;7:103–108.

CHAPTER 35C ■ THE HEART AND THE RENAL SYSTEM

DEREK P. CHEW AND LYNDA A. SZCZECH

INTRODUCTION

Patients with renal impairment experience a disproportionately large burden of cardiovascular morbidity and mortality, largely the result of accelerated atherogenesis, a hallmark characteristic of significant renal dysfunction (1,2). This elevated risk extends across the entire spectrum of renal insufficiency, with the magnitude of risk correlating with the degree of renal impairment (3). Among patients with end-stage renal failure, cardiac mortality accounts for approximately half of all deaths, and of these, over 50% occur as a result of acute myocardial infarction, with an incidence three to five times higher than in the general population (4). Also contributing to symptomatic myocardial ischemia is small vessel disease, reduced capillary density, volume overload, and altered myocyte bioenergetics. Several factors underlie this increased risk, including a greater prevalence and consequence of traditional coronary risk factors such as diabetes, lipid abnormalities, and hypertension (5,6).

Cardiac failure is observed in approximately 35% to 40% of the renal dialysis population (6). Among dialysis patients, concentric left ventricular (LV) hypertrophy is evident in 42%, eccentric LV hypertrophy in 23%, and systolic dysfunction in 16% of patients (7,8). In addition, high-output states associated with atrioventricular (AV) fistulas, salt and water overload, and anemia lead to ventricular overload and LV hypertrophy. Chronic ischemia and increased myocardial oxygen demand, hyperparathyroidism, uremia, and malnutrition all contribute to cardiomyocyte loss, fibrosis, and systolic dysfunction (9–12).

This chapter focuses on the effect of the numerous metabolic derangements associated with chronic kidney disease (CKD) and end-stage renal disease (ESRD), including secondary hyperparathyroidism, vitamin D deficiency, phosphorus, calcium, and lipid abnormalities. These disturbances may be causal in changes of cardiac structure and function responsible for the high cardiovascular morbidity and mortality within this population. Diagnosis and treatment of cardiac disease in this unique population is also discussed, along with a description of the cardiovascular effects of renal replacement therapies modalities.

RENAL IMPAIRMENT AS A RISK FACTOR IN CARDIAC DISEASE

Even a modest decline in renal function are now recognized as a potent and common risk factor for adverse short- and long-term outcome among patients with coronary artery disease (3). Not surprisingly, given the prevalence of advanced age, diabetes, and hypertension, moderate renal impairment (creatinine clearance <60 mL/min) is evident in up to one quarter of patients enrolled in acute coronary syndrome (ACS), cardiac failure, and coronary revascularization clinical trials and an even greater proportion of registry patients. As a risk factor for ischemic and bleeding events among cardiac patients, this degree of renal dysfunction has been associated with a two- to fourfold increased in adverse outcome, including late mortality (13–16). Other emerging measures of renal function associated with increased cardiovascular risk include microalbuminuria, the urinary albumin:creatinine ratio, and the serum blood urea nitrogen (BUN) level, although the incremental clinical value of these clinical markers requires further clarification (17–19). Recently, a relationship between cystatin C, a renal marker independent of age and gender, and late mortality has also been demonstrated (20).

Long-term morbidity and mortality from cardiac disease among patients with significant renal impairment remains high. Mortality is observed at a rate of approximately 1% per year among patients with renal insufficiency not treated with dialysis. Following renal transplantation, annual mortality of 0.54% or about twofold greater than the general population is documented. Among patients receiving renal replacement therapy, cardiac mortality accounts for over 40% of all deaths with an annual cardiovascular mortality 10- to 30-fold higher than the general population. The annual incidence of myocardial infarction among hemodialysis patients is 8%, with a similar annual incidence of developing pulmonary edema or requirement for extra hemofiltration. Salient data from the 34,189-patient U.S. registry of long-term dialysis demonstrates that myocardial infarction was associated with a 59% 1-year, 73% 2-year, and 90% 5-year mortality (21). LV function remains an important determinant of survival. Among patients starting dialysis therapy, systolic dysfunction portends a median survival of approximately 3 years; outcomes for those with LV dilation or concentric LV hypertrophy are slightly better. The development of new-onset cardiac failure when on hemodialysis therapy is associated with a median survival of 18 months (8).

METABOLIC CHANGES ASSOCIATED WITH CHRONIC RENAL FAILURE

Overview

Secondary hyperparathyroidism is a multifaceted process and is highly prevalent among both CKD and ESRD patients. The reduced production of 1,25-$(OH)_2$ D_3 and phosphorus excretion by the kidney increases serum phosphorus–calcium complexes, leading to hypocalcemia. This downregulates the 1α-hydroxylase that is responsible for the renal conversion of 25-(OH) D_3 to 1,25-$(OH)_2$ D_3. Coronary artery calcification is greater among CKD and ESRD, but the mechanism of this increased burden is not entirely clear (22).

Cardiovascular Changes

In experimental and animal models, parathyroid hormone (PTH) has been shown to be associated with several changes in cardiovascular structure and function. These include increased force and frequency of contraction of cardiomyocytes, increased blood pressure by increases in intravascular smooth muscle cell calcium, increased intracellular cardiomyocyte calcium concentration, increased LV mass via cardiomyocyte hypertrophy and interstitial fibrosis, increased atherosclerosis via increases in insulin resistance, calcium and phosphorus deposition in vessel walls, disturbed lipoprotein metabolism, hypertension, and increased intravascular smooth muscle cell calcium concentration (23,24).

In humans with CKD, secondary hyperparathyroidism, or its markers, has been associated with increased myocardial calcium content, impaired ventricular systolic and diastolic function (25). Plasma PTH concentration and LV dysfunction are not universally reversed with parathyroidectomy, suggesting long-standing severe hyperparathyroidism is irreversible, or that other factors are more important than PTH excess (23).

Treatment

Hyperphosphatemia is associated with increased mortality risk in observational studies (26). Current clinical practice guidelines suggest that phosphorus levels be maintained between 3.5 and 5.5 mg/dL through dietary restriction and phosphate binders (both calcium containing and non–calcium containing). Longer dialysis sessions and daily nocturnal dialysis can also improve clearance (27).

In addition, hypocalcemia, hypercalcemia, and an elevated calcium–phosphorus product have both associated with an increased mortality risk (25,26). Although hypercalcemia may be associated with vitamin D analogs or calcium-containing phosphate binders and hypocalcemia may be associated with the use of calcimimetics, clinical decisions on how to treat these derangements should be made based on the clinical scenario of each patient. Hypocalcemia may be treated using supplemental calcium or vitamin D analogs; hypercalcemia may be treated through the addition of calcimimetics, lowering or discontinuing the dose of vitamin D analogs, or the conversion from calcium- to non–calcium-containing phosphate binders. Although the management of these derangements is complex, few studies provide evidence on the association between agents on outcomes of morbidity and mortality.

Among phosphate binders, the Treat to Goal study demonstrated similar control of hyperphosphatemia among ESRD patients treated with sevelamer HCL as compared to phosphorus-containing phosphate binders (28). However, patients randomized to sevelamer HCL experienced statistically significant reductions in coronary artery calcification scores, but an effect on lipid profiles with this agent may also be a significant contributor. Also, correlation with morbidity and mortality has not been examined.

In one study, 26% of patients with New York Heart Association congestive heart failure class III or IV had low serum concentrations of 1,25-$(OH)_2$ D_3 (29). The administration of vitamin D to patients with CKD has improved cardiac function (30). The effects of vitamin D on cardiovascular structure and function include regression of LV hypertrophy and decreased coronary artery calcification (31,32). Although a number of different vitamin D analogs are available, recent observational cohort studies suggest that the use of paricalcitol may be associated with an improved survival and decreased morbidity (33–35). These findings need to be confirmed in a prospective randomized trial.

LIPID ABNORMALITIES

Abnormal lipid metabolism is common in patients with CKD and ESRD (36). Abnormalities include those that are demonstrated among patients with nephrotic syndrome as well as the seemingly paradoxical relationship between lipid and outcomes among patients with ESRD.

The two most common lipid abnormalities in the nephrotic syndrome are hypercholesterolemia and hypertriglyceridemia potentially through a reduction in plasma oncotic pressure (36,37). For reasons that are not clear, hepatic synthesis of lipoproteins containing apolipoprotein B and cholesterol increases. Raising the plasma oncotic pressure with albumin or dextran produces a rapid reduction in lipid levels in nephrotic patients. New techniques suggest that diminished catabolism, rather than increased hepatic protein synthesis, is primarily responsible for hypercholesterolemia in patients with the nephrotic syndrome (38). Impaired metabolism is primarily responsible for the elevated triglyceride levels. The delipidation cascade, in which very-low-density lipoproteins are converted to intermediate-density lipoproteins and then to LDL by lipoprotein lipases is slowed in the nephrotic syndrome (39).

Interventional trials in patients with nephrotic syndrome have not been performed; however, patients with persistent, long-standing hyperlipidemia are at increased risk for atherosclerotic disease (40). Among nephrotic patients without diabetes mellitus, the relative risk of death from coronary artery disease may be as high as 5.5-fold (41). Although optimal treatment for patients with long-standing, persistent nephrotic syndrome is uncertain, angiotensin-converting enzyme (ACE) inhibitors or angiotensin receptor blockers may be a potential adjunctive therapy (42). The reduction in proteinuria seen with these agents may be associated with a 10% to 20% decline in the plasma levels of total and LDL cholesterol and lipoprotein (a) (43,44).

Among patients with CKD not specifically related to nephrotic syndrome and ESRD, lipid abnormalities are common. Although the primary finding is hypertriglyceridemia, malnutrition must be considered in the evaluation of patients with normal or low total cholesterol concentrations (45). Triglyceride levels can be elevated because of diminished clearance related to both an alteration in the composition of circulating triglycerides (which become enriched with apolipoprotein C-III) and reduction in the activity of lipoprotein lipase and hepatic triglyceride lipase (46,47). Lipoprotein lipase activity may be reduced owing to PTH secretion or retention of a circulating lipase inhibitor (48). Other alterations in lipids include a decline in high-density lipoprotein cholesterol and an elevation in lipoprotein(a) (49–51). This may be accentuated among patients on peritoneal dialysis related presumably to absorption of glucose from the dialysate solution. Therapeutic interventions for the hypertriglyceridemia include fibric acids; however, no long-term benefit of drug therapy with these agents has been demonstrated. The increased risk of rhabdomyolysis among patients with renal disease must be noted.

With regard to cholesterol-lowering and statin therapy, three trials address the long-term effects among patients with either CKD or ESRD. The Prevention of Renal and Vascular Endstage Disease Intervention Trial (PREVEND IT) randomized patients with microalbuminuria and creatinine clearance of less than 60% of the normal age-adjusted value to receive fosinopril versus placebo and pravastatin versus placebo evaluating the effect of both medications on a primary outcome of cardiovascular mortality and hospitalization for cardiovascular morbidity (52). Subjects treated with fosinopril showed a 40% lower incidence of the primary end point (hazard ratio [HR] = 0.60, $P = .01$), subjects treated with pravastatin did not show similar significant reduction (HR = 0.87, $P = .65$). Among patients with type 2 diabetes mellitus and ESRD, the Die Deutsche Diabetes Dialyse (4D) trial randomized subjects to receive 20 mg/d of atorvastatin or placebo and followed patients for the primary end point of cardiovascular death, nonfatal myocardial infarction, or stroke (53). Although there was no significant difference in outcomes among treatment groups with respect to the primary composite endpoint (relative risk [RR], 0.92; 95% confidence interval [CI], 0.77 to 1.10; $P = .37$), differences between treatment groups existed when each event was analyzed separately. Fatal stroke was more likely among those receiving atorvastatin (RR = 2.03, $P = .04$), and all cardiac events were less likely among patients receiving the drug (RR = 0.82, $P = .03$). Last, among patients with CKD, the ongoing trial Study of Heart and Renal Protection (SHARP) will assess the effects of cholesterol-lowering therapy with a combination of simvastatin and the cholesterol absorption inhibitor ezetimide on nonfatal myocardial infarction or cardiac death, nonfatal or fatal stroke, or revascularization.

Current Kidney Disease Outcomes Quality Initiative guidelines that do not yet incorporate the results of these two negative trials recommend a goal LDL cholesterol of less than 100 mg/dL (<2.6 mmol/L) in patients with CKD using dietary modification, exercise, weight loss, and drug therapy to include statins. As the results of the SHARP study become available and additional interpretation of the results from both PREVEND IT and the 4D trial take place, a reevaluation of current lipid lowering guidelines may be required.

Hyperhomocysteinemia

Moderate hyperhomocysteinemia is a recognized independent risk factor for coronary artery disease in patients with normal renal function (53,54). Homocysteine levels have been shown to be elevated two- to fourfold among patients with chronic renal failure and hyperhomocysteinemia has also been associated with coronary artery disease among patients with renal failure (increase in mortality risk of 1% per μmol/L increase in total homocysteine concentration) (55–57).

Homocysteine metabolism depends on vitamin B_6, vitamin B_{12}, and folic acid. In renal failure, poor nutrition coupled with removal of water-soluble vitamins by dialysis may partially explain a tendency to deficiencies of these vitamins and the high prevalence of hyperhomocysteinemia. In non-ESRD populations, treatment with folic acid alone or in combination with vitamins B_{12} and B_6 has been shown to lower homocysteine levels. However, the effects have not been as pronounced in ESRD patients and outcome data are limited (58). One trial randomized 510 ESRD patients to 1, 5, or 15 mg of folic acid to evaluate the effect of supplementation in preventing mortality and cardiovascular events at 24 months (59). Rates of mortality and cardiovascular events among the folic acid groups did not differ (at 24 months: 43.7% in the 1-mg group, 38.6% in the 5-mg group, and 47.1% in the 15-mg group; log-rank $P = .47$). Furthermore, although not specifically within a renal disease population, a recent large-scale trial of folate and vitamin B_6 has failed to demonstrate any attenuation of cardiovascular risk, and the routine use of these agents cannot be currently recommended.

UREMIC AND DIALYSIS-ASSOCIATED PERICARDITIS

Pericarditis associated with chronic renal failure accounts for 3% to 4% of all deaths in ESRD patients due to tamponade, cardiac arrhythmias, or heart failure. Pericarditis may be divided into two types, namely, uremic pericarditis seen among patients not yet receiving dialysis and dialysis-associated pericarditis among patients receiving adequate doses of maintenance dialysis.

Uremic pericarditis is observed in 6% to 10% of patients with advanced renal failure (acute or chronic) before or shortly after dialysis is initiated (60). The pathogenesis is poorly understood but may include fluid overload, bleeding diatheses related to uremia, serositis, decreased fibrinolytic activity, and hyperparathyroidism.

Dialysis-associated pericarditis occurs in approximately 13% of patients on maintenance hemodialysis and may occasionally be seen with chronic peritoneal dialysis (61). The pathogenesis may be related to inadequate dialysis, volume overload, accumulation of middle molecules, malnutrition, hyperparathyroidism, heparin therapy, viral infection, and possibly, immune mechanisms.

Clinically, these two entities are very similar. In uremic pericarditis, typical diffuse ST- and T-wave elevation is typically not seen, presumably because epicardial injury is uncommon (61). The majority of these patients respond quickly to dialysis, and this should be initiated in the absence of circulatory compromise or impending tamponade. Because of the risk of hemorrhage into the pericardial space, heparin should be avoided. Intensified dialysis therapy usually leads to resolution of the pericarditis within 1 to 2 weeks (62). Antiinflammatory medications and systemic corticosteroids have been tried with limited success. Surgical drainage may be necessary prior to the initiation of dialysis if the effusion is significantly large (estimated to exceed 250 mL by echocardiography) or mandatory when overt tamponade appears, and is the treatment of choice if it enlarges or fails to resolve after a trial of intensified dialysis.

DIAGNOSIS AND MANAGEMENT OF ISCHEMIC HEART DISEASE AND CONGESTIVE HEART FAILURE

Diagnosis

Clinical history remains the cornerstone of diagnosis in coronary artery disease among patients with ESRD. However, reduced physical capacity and significant comorbidities often obscure the clinical manifestations. Similarly, specific interpretation of the resting or stress/exercise electrocardiogram (ECG) is often limited by changes related to presence of long-standing hypertension, LV hypertrophy, and electrolyte abnormalities, compromising their diagnostic utility in excluding significant myocardial ischemia in renal failure patients.

Cardiac Markers

Among patients with significant renal insufficiency, cardiac marker elevations are common in the absence of clinical ischemia. These marker elevations appear unrelated to the type of dialysis (peritoneal dialysis versus hemodialysis) or the level of uremia, but may be due to reduced renal clearance of degradation fragments (63). Among dialysis-dependent patients, troponin is detectable in between 30% to 50% of patients depending on the assay used, and less commonly, among patients with chronic renal impairment not requiring renal replacement (10%–20%). Elevations in troponin T and I have been correlated with increased LV muscle mass as well as with increased coronary calcium scores on CT scanning (64–66). Among dialysis patients, elevations in creatine kinase (CK)-MB are detectable with lower prevalence in prospective studies (<10%). Serum myoglobin levels have limited diagnostic utility because of their presence in skeletal muscle and its reduced renal clearance.

In the context of substantial reductions in renal function, asymptomatic elevations in troponin T or I and CK-MB portend in increased risk of mortality and cardiovascular events. Among chronic renal disease patients without symptoms of ACS, a pooled analysis of 39 studies suggests that troponin I (>0.15 ng/mL) has a high sensitivity for ACS (>95%), and an elevated troponin T (>0.1 ng/mL) was associated with an increased likelihood ratio for mortality over 12 to 24 months of 4.5, (95% CI, 2.9–7.1) (67). Among patients presenting with ACS, elevations in serum troponin T are associated with increased mortality and recurrent myocardial infarction at all degrees of renal impairment (Fig. 35C.1) (68). Furthermore, among renal patients with troponin elevation, concurrent elevations in C-reactive protein portend an even greater risk of all-cause mortality (69). Whether the degree of troponin elevation is associated with a gradation of mortality risk has yet to be clearly defined with either troponin I or T. The utility of troponin in assessing outcome post-coronary intervention has not been established (70).

Thallium Scintigraphy

Initial reports demonstrating reduced sensitivity, specificity and clinical utility of thallium scintigraphy in the diagnosis of coronary artery disease and risk stratification prior to renal transplantation may be attributable to a high prevalence of inadequate tests resulting from reduced exercise tolerance, inadequate heart rate response, concurrent β-blockade and LV hypertrophy (71). More recently, improved diagnostic utility has been associated with dipyridamole or combined

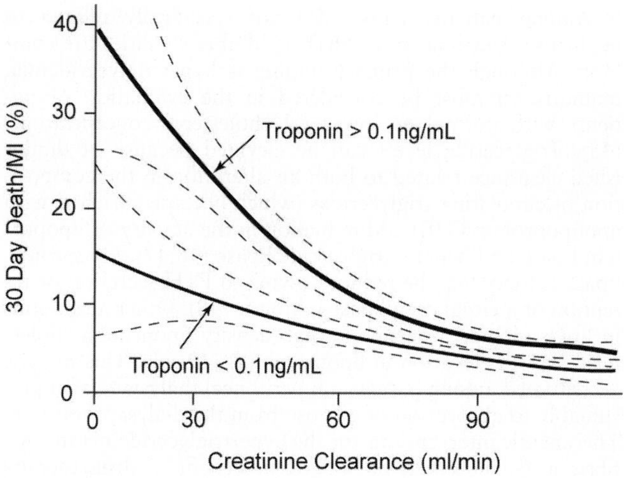

FIGURE 35C.1. Relationship between 30-day death or myocardial infarction with declining creatinine clearance: Observations from the Global Utilization of Strategies to open Occluded arteries (GUSTO) IV. (*Source:* Adapted with permission from Aviles RJ, Askari AT, Lindahl B, et al. Troponin T levels in patients with acute coronary syndromes, with or without renal dysfunction. *N Engl J Med* 2002;346:2047–2052.)

dipyridamole-exercise testing in some studies. Of note, Dahan et al. (72) demonstrated 92% sensitivity, 89% specificity, and 71% positive predictive value with dipyridamole–exercise thallium scanning in patients undergoing hemodialysis. Within this study, the negative predictive value of a normal scan was 91% during 2.8 years of follow up (72).

Stress Echocardiography

Stress echocardiography (with or without dobutamine) has emerged as useful for the diagnosis of coronary artery disease among patients with end-stage renal failure and risk stratifying candidates for renal transplantation. Initial studies documented 95% sensitivity and 89% specificity for the detection of coronary artery disease among candidates for renal transplantation, with a normal scan predicting a 97% 12-month event-free survival (73,74). This investigation also appears to be cost effective for risk stratifying patients undergoing renal transplantation (75). Utility has also been documented in the dialysis population. Compared with an 84% event-free survival observed among patients without ischemia, a 66% event-free survival over a mean of 38 months of follow up was documented among end-stage renal failure patients with ischemia on dobutamine echocardiography. Importantly, this study observed a prominent increase in events after 2 years in those without initial ischemia, potentially highlighting the duration of prognostic information provided by diagnostic testing in these patients with aggressive coronary artery disease (76).

Angiography and Contrast-Induced Nephropathy

The indications for coronary angiography within this population are similar to those in the general population. However, in the patient with significant renal impairment not managed with renal replacement therapy, the additional risk of contrast-induced nephropathy (CIN) requires careful consideration and preparation. Coronary angiography should be undertaken only when the information provided is vital to the planning of ongoing management.

CIN is a leading cause of in-hospital acute renal failure, and is clearly associated with increased incidence of permanent dialysis and late mortality. Depending on the associated comorbidities, this complication is reported in about 5% to 10% of patients with substantial renal impairment undergoing coronary angiography (77,78). Total volume of contrast, elevated baseline creatinine, functioning renal allografts, concomitant nephrotoxins such as nonsteroidal antiinflammatory drugs, and cardiac failure are associated with an increased risk of this complication (79). Diabetes mellitus is a potent risk factor for the development of CIN, although most of this risk relates to the presence of associated diabetic nephropathy. In diabetic patients with concurrent renal dysfunction, the risk is approximately fourfold that of diabetics without documented renal dysfunction (80).

The precise mechanism of CIN has not been clearly defined. Direct toxic effects on proximal renal tubular epithelium and mitochondrial function have been observed (81). Glomerular hyperfiltration with mismatch between perfusion and filtration, leading to a hypoxic insult to the renal medulla, has been observed in diabetes and may help to explain the susceptibility of these patients to CIN (82). Heightened endothelial release of endothelin-1 may have a role in this response, with endothelin release increased with ionic compared with nonionic contrast media (83). Other potential contributing mechanisms include increased red cell rigidity and white cell margination affecting blood viscosity and rheology within the renal vasculature.

Clinically, CIN manifests as a rise in serum creatinine, occurring 24 to 48 hours after angiography, peaking over 3 to 5 days, with slow resolution over 7 to 10 days. Oliguria is common among patients with reduced baseline renal function. In addition, urinary sodium excretion is low, as is the fractional excretion of sodium (<1). A persistent nephrogram on abdominal x-ray and renal cortical attenuation on CT scanning are also frequently observed for more than 24 hours. Up to 50% of patients require permanent dialysis.

Hydration with half-normal saline remains the key proven strategy for reducing the incidence of CIN. Enhanced diuresis with either furosemide or mannitol is of no greater benefit compared to saline hydration alone, but forced diuresis with intravenous crystalloid infusion, furosemide, or mannitol with or without dopamine may also reduce the risk of CIN if a high level of urinary volume can be achieved (84,85). However, caution must be exercised in those with reduced cardiac function. Routine use of dopamine is not associated with a lower risk of CIN in high-risk populations (86). Evidence with theophylline, as an antagonist of adenosine, is supportive but inconclusive (87). *N*-acetylcysteine has been extensively investigated as a therapy to prevent CIN. This agent probably acts as a free radical scavenger and induces intrarenal nitric oxide–mediated vasodilation. Doses studied include 600 mg twice daily for 48 hours beginning the day prior to angiography and intravenous regimens have also been described (88). Metaanalyses of these studies with *N*-acetylcysteine suggests an overall benefit, but these analyses are hampered by substantial heterogeneity in study design (89,90). Other possible strategies of potential benefit include prehydration with sodium bicarbonate and pretreatment with high-dose ascorbic acid (3 g/d) (91,92). Although the results from these studies are encouraging, confirmation with corroborative studies is required.

In patients with reduced renal function, low osmolar contrast agents appear to be associated with a reduced incidence of CIN when the data are considered collectively (93). No differences were observed when patients with normal renal function were studied. Likewise, ionicity appears to impact on the development of CIN, again predominantly among patients with renal insufficiency (80). Thus, the use of low osmolar nonionic agents is advocated among those with renal impairment at substantial risk of CIN. Some studies suggest that the low osmolar nonionic dimer, iodixanol, is associated with lower rates of CIN than the low osmolar nonionic monomer, iohexol (79). However, small comparisons with other monomeric contrast agents have demonstrated little difference. Regardless of the contrast agent used, limiting the dose of contrast in these patients remains an important clinical practice.

Treatment

Medical Therapy

The medical management of ischemic heart disease and cardiac failure among patients with substantial renal impairments parallels the guidelines developed for the general population, although several aspects warrant special consideration. Anemia contributes to myocardial ischemia, altering the balance between oxygen supply and demand. While decreasing oxygen delivery, anemia also contributes to increased cardiac work by volume overload, reduced coronary filling times, and reduced vasodilator reserve. Correction of uremic anemia with erythropoietin improves cardiac performance and reduces angina in the short term, although no reduction in fatal or nonfatal cardiac events has been shown and an excess risk may exist (94,95). Hyperparathyroidism also results in increased cardiomyocyte calcium content, impacting myocardial oxidative metabolism and increasing the susceptibility of myocytes to injury (96). The value of rigorous control of calcium metabolism on cardiac endpoints requires prospective study.

Observational evidence also documents an underutilization of proven therapies within this population. Among patients presenting with non–ST-elevation ACS, patients with renal insufficiency are less likely to receive invasive management, although an increased risk of bleeding events among those invasively management is recognized (97–99). In the setting of acute myocardial infarction, thrombolytic therapy, aspirin, β-blockers, and ACE inhibition remain underutilized (100–102). Similar observations have been made among patients with cardiac failure despite comparable efficacy of these agents (103). Nevertheless, specific evidence supporting the efficacy of many therapies used in the management of cardiac disease among patients with renal dysfunction is currently lacking, particularly therapies such as antiarrhythmics and inotropes. Evidence supporting the use of the commonly prescribed therapies is presented in Table 35C.1.

In addition to the underutilization of therapies is the problem of inappropriate dosing of pharmaceuticals among these patients where impairment of renal function is often underappreciated. A literature review of prescription-related adverse events indicates that cardiovascular drugs are the most commonly implicated medications associated with adverse events and that inappropriate dosing is the most common form of error (104). Hence, the importance of accurate measures of renal function, using calculated creatinine clearance, and appropriate adjustment of dosing of cardiovascular medications in the face of reduced renal function cannot be understated.

Indications for Revascularization

The principles of revascularization among patients with renal impairment are similar to nonrenal patients, although the impact of renal disease on both short- and long-term outcomes bears careful consideration (14,105). Although the choice between revascularization strategies remains at times contentious within the general population, the poor long-term results associated with percutaneous coronary intervention (PCI) has lead many to recommend coronary artery bypass grafting as the preferred strategy for patients with significant renal impairment (106–108). Recent analysis from the United States Renal System database reported an increased risk of in-hospital

TABLE 35C.1

RENAL CONSIDERATIONS FOR COMMON THERAPIES USED IN ACUTE CORONARY SYNDROMES, STABLE ANGINA AND CARDIAC FAILURE

	Elimination and dose modification	Evidence in patients with renal impairment
THERAPIES USED IN ACS		
Aspirin	No dose reduction recommended	Observational data supporting comparable efficacy with some studies showing increased bleeding (102).
Thienopyridines Clopidogrel Ticlopidine	No dose reduction recommended; extensively metabolized in the liver	Currently no specific data.
Unfractionated heparin	No dose reduction recommended: Renal elimination at higher doses	Currently no specific data.
Low-molecular-weight heparin	Dose reduction and monitoring of factor Xa levels recommended; clearance by renal mechanisms	Comparable suppression of ischemic events observed among conservatively managed patients with increased bleeding events reported (184).
Glycoprotein IIb/IIIa inhibition Abciximab Tirofiban Eptifibatide	Abciximab—no dose reduction required; tirofiban and epitifibatide—renal clearance, dose reduction recommended	Greater absolute suppression of ischemic events with moderate increase in bleeding events associated with tirofiban use in among ACS patients undergoing invasive management (185). Suppression of ischemic events with modest increases in bleeding have been observed among patients undergoing PCI in clinical trials and registries (186–188). Similar rates of bleeding events observed among patients receiving abciximab and tirofiban in the setting of PCI (189).
Direct thrombin inhibitors	Degree of renal elimination varies among the agents	Greater suppression of ischemic events and reduction in bleeding event when compared to heparin among patients undergoing PCI (190). Comparable suppression of ischemic events and fewer bleeding events compared with heparin and glycoprotein IIb/IIIa inhibition in PCI (191). Trials of bivalirudin in ACS currently ongoing.
Fibrinolysis	Dose reduction not recommended	Retrospective studies suggest improved outcome associated with reperfusion therapy among patients with renal failure (192). Adequate controlled data currently lacking
THERAPIES USED IN STABLE ISCHEMIC HEART DISEASE AND CARDIAC FAILURE		
Angiotensin converting enzyme inhibitor	Renal elimination varies among agents	Reduction in mortality and progression of renal disease among patients with diabetic nephropathy (193,194). Retard progression of renal dysfunction in hypertensive renal disease (195). Caution should be exercised during initiation among the elderly, those with acute renal dysfunction, diabetics, hypertensive nephrosclerosis, cardiac failure with renal insufficiency, and volume depletion, where GFR is maintained by efferent arteriolar vasoconstriction.
Angiotensin receptor antagonists	Renal elimination varies among agents	Comparable retardation of renal disease progression as observed with ACE inhibition (196,197). Attenuation of mincroalbuminuria has been demonstrated independent of an effect on blood pressure (198). Mortality benefit yet to be defined in the renal impairment population. Similar caution as with ACE inhibition.
β-Blockers	Renal elimination varies among agents	Observational data supports reduction in hospitalization and cardiac and all-cause mortality among dialysis patients (199).
Calcium antagonists	Hepatic metabolism—no specific dosing recommendations	Renoprotective effects suggested but data from small studies demonstrate conflicting results (200,201). Evidence indicating effects on mortality or progression to dialysis currently lacking.

(continued)

TABLE 35C.1

RENAL CONSIDERATIONS FOR COMMON THERAPIES USED IN ACUTE CORONARY SYNDROMES, STABLE ANGINA AND CARDIAC FAILURE (CONTINUED)

	Elimination and dose modification	Evidence in patients with renal impairment
Digoxin	Renal elimination 70%—dose reduction recommended	Reductions in loading and maintenance doses owing to a lower volume of distribution and prolonged half-life. Caution in hemodialysis there digoxin-induced arrhythmias may resulting from rapid reductions in plasma potassium, magnesium, and hydrogen ions leading to elevated ionized calcium concentrations. Digoxin–Fab fragments are useful in the treatment of digoxin-induced arrhythmias, renal elimination of the digoxin–Fab fragment is prolonged. Both digoxin and the Fab immune fragment are removed by CAVH.
Nitrates	Vascular and hepatic metabolism—no dose reduction recommended	Currently no specific data are available.
HMG CoA-reductase inhibition	Hepatic metabolism—no dose reduction recommended	Among patients with mild to moderate renal impairment appears to be comparable to the general population and has been associated with a reduction in mortality (202,203). Randomized comparisons in renal patients suggest modest benefit if any (52,53).

Abbreviations: ACE, angiotensin-converting enzyme; ACS, acute coronary syndromes; CAVH, continuous arterio-venous haemofiltration; GFR, glomerular infiltration rate; PCI, percutaneous coronary intervention.

mortality among patients receiving coronary artery bypass grafting with internal mammary artery grafting compared with patients receiving coronary stents (5.0% versus 2.3%). However, when assessing long-term cardiac death or myocardial infarction, coronary artery bypass grafting with the internal mammary artery was associated with a substantially lower risk of late events (HR, 0.52; 95% CI, 0.37–0.73) when compared with percutaneous transluminal coronary angioplasty, and a less prominent benefit when compared with coronary stenting (HR, 0.90; 95% CI, 0.69–1.17) (108). The relative merits among patients with less advanced renal impairment requires further evaluation. Furthermore, whether the continued evolution in mechanical revascularization strategies, specifically drug-eluting coronary stenting, is able to bridge the gap between percutaneous and surgical revascularization awaits adequately designed prospective trials.

Percutaneous Coronary Intervention

Despite improvements in procedural results with more modern technology, PCI outcomes among patients with moderate and severe renal disease are still inferior to the general population, and an increased rate of in-hospital major adverse ischemic and bleeding events persists (109,110). Long-term recurrent angina, myocardial infarction, target vessel revascularization, and mortality remain a substantial problem among these patients (15,111,112). Factors contributing to these adverse events include a higher degree of residual stenosis, less procedural success, smaller vessel size, extensive calcification reflecting the diffuse atheromatous disease process and a prothrombotic tendency (113–116). Furthermore, patients experiencing a decline in renal function following PCI experience an increased risk of late mortality even when the baseline creatinine is normal (117,118).

In observational data from patients with baseline creatinine of more than 1.5 mg/dL undergoing PCI, coronary stenting appears to be associated with an improved procedural success rate and reduced long-term death, myocardial infarction, or revascularization (119). However, coronary stenting has also been associated with an increased rate of in-hospital cardiac events compared with balloon angioplasty (stents 11% versus 5% percutaneous transluminal coronary angioplasty) among dialysis patients. Within this study, target vessel revascularization was required in 22% of dialysis-dependent patients receiving stents, a rate that was comparable a contemporaneous non–renal failure population, but late mortality and disease progression resulted in a poor late event-free survival (116). Observational data comparing 1,080 patients receiving sirolimus-eluting stents compared with bare metal stents demonstrate a reduction in target vessel revascularization (HR, 0.59; 95% CI, 0.39–0.90; P = .01), but no reduction in 1-year mortality (120). Whether contemporary catheter-based revascularization (drug-eluting stents and GP IIb/IIIa inhibition offers results comparable to coronary artery bypass grafting remains to be clarified.

Coronary Artery Bypass Grafting

The adverse prognostic impact of renal insufficiency on the outcomes following coronary artery bypass grafting is well established and extends to include those with moderate renal dysfunction (creatinine >2.0 mg/dL) (121). Among patients with more advanced renal insufficiency, a threefold increased risk of mortality has been observed (122). In addition to an increased prevalence of risk factors such as extensive coronary artery disease, LV dysfunction, diabetes, and prior myocardial infarction, elevated BUN appears to impart increased risk of perioperative mortality and a low cardiac output postoperative state. The mortality risk associated with BUN may be partly attributable to the presence of associated comorbid conditions, such as uremia-induced platelet dysfunction and fluid, electrolyte and acid–base disturbances contributing to perioperative cardiac failure and arrhythmias. Depressed immune function also increases the rate of infection. These patients experience an increased incidence of prolonged ventilation, mediastinitis, and stroke, contributing to increased intensive care and in-hospital stays as well as an in-hospital mortality rate ranging from 4% to 14% or approximately three times the rate observed in the general population. Cardiopulmonary bypass has been associated with a deterioration in renal function leading to the 26% rate of permanent dialysis observed in one series of patients with mild to moderate renal impairment following coronary artery bypass grafting (123). Importantly, however, in a large series of patients, the requirement for postoperative dialysis was associated with a 64% mortality rate (124). Among renal transplant patients, a relatively small deterioration in renal function is also observed (125). Furthermore, combined coronary artery bypass grafting and valvular surgery appears to be associated with an even greater risk of in-hospital mortality and the presence of cardiac failure prior to coronary artery bypass grafting is associated with a three- to fourfold risk of increased late mortality (126,127).

The use of peritoneal dialysis or hemodialysis on the day prior to surgery and following the operation is practiced in some centers. Minimizing fluid shifts and electrolyte disturbance during the procedure with intraoperative dialysis has also been suggested. Similarly, developments in operative techniques and increased use of arterial conduits may benefit these high-risk patients. Several studies now report less deterioration in renal function and lower rates of in-hospital morbidity among patients receiving "off-pump" versus "on-pump" surgery (128–130).

RENAL REPLACEMENT THERAPY

Among patients undergoing renal transplantation, the incidence of coronary artery disease is increased and associated with a greater mortality, especially in high-risk groups (131). Risk stratification and subsequent revascularization appears to reduce long-term cardiac events (132). Therefore, a diagnostic strategy among these patients is warranted. Coronary angiography is advocated for the screening of coronary artery disease given its prevalence within this population. However, strategies among asymptomatic patients identifying intermediate and low-risk groups may allow some patient to proceed to transplantation without invasive testing (133). Patients considered at intermediate risk include those older than 50 years or with diabetes in the absence clinical cardiac disease and may warrant initial noninvasive investigations. In a metaanalysis of 12 studies (8 thallium scintigraphy and 4 dobutamine stress echocardiography) a significantly increased risk of myocardial infarction (RR, 2.73; 95% CI, 1.25–5.97; $P = .01$) and cardiac death (RR, 2.92; 95% CI, 1.66–5.12; $P < .001$) was observed among patients awaiting renal or pancreatorenal transplantation with an ischemic test result (134). Intermediate and high-risk patients with equivocal noninvasive tests may warrant coronary angiography (135). Patients less than 45 years old with no history of smoking, without diabetes for more than 25 years, and no ST-T–wave changes on ECG, again without clinical cardiac disease, appear to be at low risk of coronary artery disease, and transplantation without prior cardiac investigation may be safe (133).

Management of Coronary Artery Disease Prior to Renal Transplantation

Hemodialysis

The acute hemodynamic consequences of hemodialysis and the long-term effects of renal replacement therapy both have an impact on cardiovascular disease. This discussion focuses primarily on the intradialytic element of the interaction between renal replacement therapy and cardiovascular disease, highlighting the special considerations of necessary to provide renal replacement therapy to patients with cardiovascular disease.

Hemodynamic Concerns

Hemodialysis alters both intracellular and extracellular composition and volume. These alterations may have the hemodynamic effects of hypotension, dysrhythmias, and ischemia. Hypotension is the most common complication of hemodialytic therapy. Ultrafiltration of intravascular fluid during hemodialysis reduces plasma volume, resulting in a decline in cardiac output and blood pressure. Hypotension, however, is not merely a reflection of ultrafiltration and its rate of removal. There are a number of other factors and processes relevant to dialysis-associated hypotension including plasma refill rate, dialysate-related factors, dialysis membrane factors, and autonomic and cardiac function.

Plasma refill rate is the rate at which plasma volume removed by ultrafiltration is restored from intracellular and interstitial fluid compartments. Although there is wide interpatient variation, the size of the interstitial component has a direct relationship with refill rates (136). One mechanism driving plasma refill rate is the increase in intravascular oncotic pressure secondary to hypotonic fluid removal by ultrafiltration (137). Therefore, patients with low plasma protein levels are predisposed to intradialytic hypotension (138). Greater ultrafiltration rates (required to manage greater weight gains between dialysis) and removal of a greater solute load contribute to hypotension.

Dialysate may also play a role in dialysis hypotension. The inclusion of acetate as a buffer in dialysate lowers the plasma refill rate and may have a negative inotropic effect (139,140). The widespread replacement of acetate with bicarbonate, however, has largely obviated this concern. Low sodium concentration in dialysate is associated with hypotension, and elevated dialysate sodium is used therapeutically for intradialytic hypotension (141,142). Modeling of sodium concentration in the dialysate over the course of a dialysis treatment may be of value. The long-term benefits of such interventions are not clear; most studies report positive sodium balance, temporary decreases in intradialytic hypotension, less blood volume reduction, and a subsequent increase in thirst and body weight (141,143). Increased calcium concentration in the dialysate generally results in an increased serum ionized calcium concentration and improved LV contractility (144,145). Intradialytic hypotension is less common with low dialysate magnesium.

Other factors that influence blood pressure include anemia, membrane interactions, and dialysate temperature. Intradialytic hypotensive episodes are significantly reduced in anemic patients after transfusion (146). Although the issue of biocompatibility and hypotension is controversial, it arose from the observation that hemofiltration is association with a greater hemodynamic stability than hemodialysis (147). Although data suggest that the use of dialysis membranes that are considered biocompatible may be associated with less hypotension, this finding is not consistent across all studies (148,149). Maintenance of core temperature during isolated ultrafiltration and hemodialysis optimizes hemodynamic stability during dialysis (150).

The autonomic nervous system should provide an increase in systemic vascular resistance during ultrafiltration (151). Patients with cardiovascular disease may be more prone to hypotension if their sympathetic compensatory mechanisms are already maximized or if the use of certain medications, such as β-blockers or ACE inhibitors, further compromise compensatory mechanisms.

Hypotension among patients with ESRD may also be an early sign of pericarditis or pericardial effusions. Treatment for pericarditis usually involves increasing dialysis dose, but large effusions may benefit from drainage; aggressive ultrafiltration may further predispose these patients to hypotension and cardiovascular collapse (152). In addition, 70% of incident hemodialysis patients have LV hypertrophy (7). LV hypertrophy is associated with reduced LV compliance and rapid lowering of preload impairs LV filling. Among patients who have narrow volume ranges because of these factors, modalities using longer durations such as continuous renal replacement therapy or peritoneal dialysis have been suggested (153).

Dysrhythmias

Dysrhythmias are seen frequently among patients during hemodialysis (154). The etiology of intradialytic dysrhythmias may be related to fluid, acid–base, or electrolyte shifts. Patients with ESRD and LV hypertrophy or following coronary artery revascularization have significant increased risk of sudden death, with up to 75% of such deaths attributable to ventricular fibrillation (155). Bicarbonate dialysate is associated with less frequent dysrhythmia than acetate dialysate (156). Hypokalemia precipitates dysrhythmias and patients taking digoxin are more susceptible (157). Prevention of hypomagnesemia may also reduce intradialytic ventricular ectopy.

Ischemia

Fluctuations in blood pressure and heart rate during dialysis may lead to alterations in coronary perfusion. Hypoxemia and a decreased systemic vascular resistance are common intradialytic problems compounding ischemia (158). The presence of LV hypertrophy and coronary artery disease among patients undergoing hemodialysis may further undermine coronary reserve. Intradialytic ischemia can be complicated by the sudden release of adenosine, which further compounds hypotension.

Chest pain on dialysis may be related to ischemic disease, but other etiologies include reactions to dialyzers (membranes) or chemicals required for sterilization or processing such as ethylene oxide. Intradialytic ST depression on ECG is predictive of future cardiac morbidity (159). Patients with recurrent ischemia should be prescribed a tight fluid restriction to minimize ultrafiltration requirements. Although continuous blood volume monitoring has theoretical benefits in minimizing ischemia, a randomized trial did not demonstrate a benefit to either morbidity or mortality among hemodialysis patients not selected for the presence of cardiac disease (160). Its use in hemodialysis patients with ischemic disease should be considered in light of these findings.

Arteriovenous fistulae are associated with cardiac enlargement and hypertrophy among patients with ESRD (161). The extent to which they contribute to high-output failure is unclear as the occurrence of failure is unusual.

Peritoneal Dialysis

Among patients with advanced LV systolic failure, peritoneal dialysis has been advocated as the therapy of choice. Because fluid shifts occur gradually, a more constant volume status is maintained. In addition, the need for an AV fistula with its consequent high-output state is obviated (161). Although the intermittent nature of hemodialysis may contribute to an increased rate of sudden and cardiac death early in the treatment cycle, sudden cardiac deaths are more evenly distributed among patients on peritoneal dialysis (162).

Peritoneal dialysis is associated with a large absorption of glucose across the peritoneal membrane, which may contribute to abnormal glucose and insulin metabolism, glucose intolerance, hyperinsulinemia, reduced peripheral sensitivity to insulin, and hyperlipidemia (163,164). These factors may contribute to the development and progression of atherogenesis. Hyperinsulinemia and hyperlipidemia are important factors to consider among patients with preexisting atherosclerotic disease and should play at least some role in modality selection (165). Nonenzymatic glycation of proteins in the peritoneal cavity with the resultant formation of advanced glycation end products may also play a role in genesis and progression of cardiovascular disease (166). Such concerns have contributed to the advent of alternative peritoneal dialysis solutions such as amino acid–containing solutions.

Transplantation

Although transplantation is considered the treatment of choice for management of ESRD and has been associated with regression of cardiovascular disease and particularly LV hypertrophy, atherosclerotic disease is still a major cause of morbidity and mortality in transplant recipients (62,167). Two-year mortality following myocardial infarction for transplant recipients has recently been reported at 33.6% (168). The increasing prevalence of atherosclerotic disease in the transplant population may be related to the increase in age and increasing proportion of diabetics currently undergoing transplantation. There are, however, a number of factors specifically related to immunosuppressive therapies that predispose to development and progression of atherosclerotic heart disease.

Calcineurin inhibitors, reduced renal blood flow, and increased systemic vascular resistance are associated with hypertension (169,170). This has been linked to accelerated atherosclerotic disease through mechanisms including the induction of heat shock proteins, enhancing endothelial sensitivity, and alteration of cardiac vascular remodeling (171–173). These drugs have been shown to potentiate the atherosclerotic effects of hyperlipidemia in mice and to increase LDL oxidation in humans (174,175).

Sirolimus (Rapamune, rapamycin), a macrocyclic triene antibiotic, is associated with hyperlipidemia and hypercholesterolemia in a dose-related manner, as a result of lipoprotein lipase inhibition (176). Hypertriglyceridemia exceeding 454 mg/dL was seen in 75% of patients in one study where sirolimus was added to cyclosporine-based regimens (177). A reduction in trough levels led to a return to pretreatment status after 6 months. Electrolyte abnormalities have also been reported with this agent (178–180).

The development of diabetes mellitus posttransplantation is associated with the use of corticosteroids, cyclosporine, and tacrolimus and may contribute significantly to increased cardiovascular risk (181). Tacrolimus suppresses insulin production in the pancreatic β-cells and the introduction of tacrolimus has been associated with a significantly higher incidence of this problem (182,183).

THE FUTURE

The interactions between cardiac disease and impaired renal function are complex. The large contribution that cardiac disorders add to the morbidity and mortality of patients with advanced degrees of renal impairment is well recognized. However, the association between modest degrees of renal dysfunction and poor outcomes across the spectrum of common cardiac presentations including ACS, PCI, coronary artery bypass grafting, and cardiac failure can no longer be ignored by clinical cardiologists. As a marker of risk, reduced renal dysfunction arbitrarily defined as a creatinine clearance of less than 60 mL/min is more prevalent and more potent than many of the novel risk factors currently under investigation. Given the ease and lack of expense with which this risk factor can be assessed, incorporating an assessment of renal function in to the routine management of patients with cardiovascular disease should provide a more accurate representation of clinical risk.

The central unanswered question pertaining to renal impairment patients is whether the underlying pathophysiology of cardiac disease is different to that seen among patients with normal creatinine clearance, or whether the development of renal dysfunction simply promotes a more aggressive clinical manifestation of the same basic pathology. Answering such questions would aid in the development of novel approaches to the treatment of patients with both cardiac and renal disease. Despite the prevalence of renal impairment and the broad array of pharmacologic and device therapies available for the care of cardiac patients, adequate well-controlled studies evaluating the magnitude of efficacy and the relative safety of many of these therapies are currently lacking. Specific randomized controlled trials focused on patients with various degrees of renal impairment are urgently needed to inform the optimal management of these high-risk patients.

Nevertheless, beyond the treatment of established cardiovascular and renal disease, is the need for greater awareness and prevention. With the increasing prevalence of diabetes and the metabolic syndrome, coupled with the extended life expectancy now enjoyed by many industrialized societies, strategies to slow the development of renal dysfunction remain of paramount importance.

References

1. Baigent C, Burbury K, Wheeler D. Premature cardiovascular disease in chronic renal failure. *Lancet* 2000;356:147–152.
2. Foley RN, Parfrey PS, Sarnak MJ. Clinical epidemiology of cardiovascular disease in chronic renal disease. *Am J Kidney Dis* 1998;32[5 Suppl 3]:S112–119.
3. Gupta R, Birnbaum Y, Uretsky BF. The renal patient with coronary artery disease: current concepts and dilemmas. *J Am Coll Cardiol* 2004;44:1343–1353.
4. Held PJ, Port FK, Webb RL, et al. Excerpts from United States Renal Data System 1995 Annual Data Report. *Am J Kidney Dis* 1995;26(4 Suppl 2):S1–186.
5. Marso SP, Ellis SG, Gurm HS, et al. Proteinuria is a key determinant of death in patients with diabetes after isolated coronary artery bypass grafting. *Am Heart J* 2000;139:939–944.
6. Parfrey PS, Foley RN. The clinical epidemiology of cardiac disease in chronic renal failure. *J Am Soc Nephrol* 1999;10:1606–1615.
7. Foley RN, Parfrey PS, Harnett JD, et al. Clinical and echocardiographic disease in patients starting end-stage renal disease therapy. *Kidney Int* 1995; 47:186–192.
8. Parfrey PS, Foley RN, Harnett JD, et al. Outcome and risk factors of ischemic heart disease in chronic uremia. *Kidney Int* 1996;49:1428–1434.
9. Foley RN, Parfrey PS, Harnett JD, et al. The prognostic importance of left ventricular geometry in uremic cardiomyopathy. *J Am Soc Nephrol* 1995;5:2024–2031.
10. Foley RN, Parfrey PS, Harnett JD, et al. Hypoalbuminemia, cardiac morbidity, and mortality in end-stage renal disease. *J Am Soc Nephrol* 1996;7: 728–736.
11. Foley RN, Parfrey PS, Harnett JD, et al. The impact of anemia on cardiomyopathy, morbidity, and mortality in end-stage renal disease. *Am J Kidney Dis* 1996;28:53–61.
12. Foley RN, Parfrey PS, Morgan J, et al. Effect of hemoglobin levels in hemodialysis patients with asymptomatic cardiomyopathy. *Kidney Int* 2000;58:1325–1335.
13. Al Suwaidi J, Reddan DN, Williams K, et al. Prognostic implications of abnormalities in renal function in patients with acute coronary syndromes. *Circulation* 2002;106:974–980.
14. Szczech LA, Best PJ, Crowley E, et al. Outcomes of patients with chronic renal insufficiency in the bypass angioplasty revascularization investigation. *Circulation* 2002;105:2253–2258.
15. Azar RR, Prpic R, Ho KK, et al. Impact of end-stage renal disease on clinical and angiographic outcomes after coronary stenting. *Am J Cardiol* 2000; 86:485–489.
16. McCullough PA, Soman SS, Shah SS, et al. Risks associated with renal dysfunction in patients in the coronary care unit. *J Am Coll Cardiol* 2000;36: 679–684.
17. Anavekar NS, Gans DJ, Berl T, et al. Predictors of cardiovascular events in patients with type 2 diabetic nephropathy and hypertension: a case for albuminuria. *Kidney Int Suppl* 2004;S50–55.
18. Kirtane AJ, Leder DM, Waikar SS, et al. Serum blood urea nitrogen as an independent marker of subsequent mortality among patients with acute coronary syndromes and normal to mildly reduced glomerular filtration rates. *J Am Coll Cardiol* 2005;45:1781–1786.
19. Marso SP, Ellis SG, Tuzcu M, et al. The importance of proteinuria as a determinant of mortality following percutaneous coronary revascularization in diabetics. *J Am Coll Cardiol* 1999;33:1269–1277.
20. Shlipak MG, Sarnak MJ, Katz R, et al. Cystatin C and the risk of death and cardiovascular events among elderly persons. *N Engl J Med* 2005; 352:2049–2060.
21. Herzog CA, Ma JZ, Collins AJ. Poor long-term survival after acute myocardial infarction among patients on long-term dialysis. *N Engl J Med* 1998;339:799–805.
22. Goodman WG, Goldin J, Kuizon BD, et al. Coronary-artery calcification in young adults with end-stage renal disease who are undergoing dialysis. *N Engl J Med* 2000;342:1478–1483.
23. Rostand SG, Drueke TB. Parathyroid hormone, vitamin D, and cardiovascular disease in chronic renal failure. *Kidney Int* 1999;56:383–392.
24. Wang R, Wu L, Karpinski E, Pang PK. The changes in contractile status of single vascular smooth muscle cells and ventricular cells induced by bPTH-(1-34). *Life Sci* 1993;52:793–801.
25. Lowrie EG, Lew NL. Death risk in hemodialysis patients: the predictive value of commonly measured variables and an evaluation of death rate differences between facilities. *Am J Kidney Dis* 1990;15:458–482.
26. Block GA, Hulbert-Shearon TE, Levin NW, Port FK. Association of serum phosphorus and calcium x phosphate product with mortality risk in chronic hemodialysis patients: a national study. *Am J Kidney Dis* 1998;31:607–617.
27. Mucsi I, Hercz G, Uldall R, et al. Control of serum phosphate without any phosphate binders in patients treated with nocturnal hemodialysis. *Kidney Int* 1998;53:1399–1404.
28. Chertow GM, Burke SK, Raggi P. Sevelamer attenuates the progression of coronary and aortic calcification in hemodialysis patients. *Kidney Int* 2002;62:245–252.
29. Shane E, Mancini D, Aaronson K, et al. Bone mass, vitamin D deficiency, and hyperparathyroidism in congestive heart failure. *Am J Med* 1997; 103:197–207.
30. Coratelli P, Petrarulo F, Buongiorno E, et al. Improvement in left ventricular function during treatment of hemodialysis patients with 25-OHD3. *Contrib Nephrol* 1984;41:433–437.
31. Park CW, Oh YS, Shin YS, et al. Intravenous calcitriol regresses myocardial hypertrophy in hemodialysis patients with secondary hyperparathyroidism. *Am J Kidney Dis* 1999;33:73–81.
32. Watson KE, Abrolat ML, Malone LL, et al. Active serum vitamin D levels are inversely correlated with coronary calcification. *Circulation* 1997;96: 1755–1760.
33. Teng M, Wolf M, Lowrie E, et al. Survival of patients undergoing hemodialysis with paricalcitol or calcitriol therapy. *N Engl J Med* 2003;349:446–456.
34. Teng M, Wolf M, Ofsthun MN, et al. Activated injectable vitamin D and hemodialysis survival: a historical cohort study. *J Am Soc Nephrol* 2005;16:1115–1125.
35. Dobrez DG, Mathes A, Amdahl M, et al. Paricalcitol-treated patients experience improved hospitalization outcomes compared with calcitriol-treated patients in real-world clinical settings. *Nephrol Dial Transplant* 2004;19:1174–1181.
36. Appel G. Lipid abnormalities in renal disease. *Kidney Int* 1991;39:169–183.
37. Joven J, Villabona C, Vilella E, et al. Abnormalities of lipoprotein metabolism in patients with the nephrotic syndrome. *N Engl J Med* 1990;323: 579–584.
38. Demant T, Mathes C, Gutlich K, et al. A simultaneous study of the metabolism of apolipoprotein B and albumin in nephrotic patients. *Kidney Int* 1998;54:2064–2080.
39. Vega GL, Toto RD, Grundy SM. Metabolism of low density lipoproteins in nephrotic dyslipidemia: comparison of hypercholesterolemia alone and combined hyperlipidemia. *Kidney Int* 1995;47:579–586.
40. Radhakrishnan J, Appel AS, Valeri A, Appel GB. The nephrotic syndrome, lipids, and risk factors for cardiovascular disease. *Am J Kidney Dis* 1993;22:135–142.
41. Ordonez JD, Hiatt RA, Killebrew EJ, Fireman BH. The increased risk of coronary heart disease associated with nephrotic syndrome. *Kidney Int* 1993;44:638–642.
42. Hollenberg NK, Raij L. Angiotensin-converting enzyme inhibition and renal protection. An assessment of implications for therapy. *Arch Intern Med* 1993;153:2426–2435.
43. Keilani T, Schlueter WA, Levin ML, Batlle DC. Improvement of lipid abnormalities associated with proteinuria using fosinopril, an angiotensin-converting enzyme inhibitor. *Ann Intern Med* 1993;118:246–254.
44. de Zeeuw D, Gansevoort RT, de Jong PE. Losartan in patients with renal insufficiency. *Can J Cardiol* 1995;11[Suppl F]:41F–44F.
45. Weiner DE, Sarnak MJ. Managing dyslipidemia in chronic kidney disease. *J Gen Intern Med* 2004;19:1045–1052.

46. Attman PO, Samuelsson O, Alaupovic P. Lipoprotein metabolism and renal failure. *Am J Kidney Dis* 1993;21:573–592.
47. Senti M, Romero R, Pedro-Botet J, et al. Lipoprotein abnormalities in hyperlipidemic and normolipidemic men on hemodialysis with chronic renal failure. *Kidney Int* 1992;41:1394–1399.
48. Cheung AK, Parker CJ, Ren K, Iverius PH. Increased lipase inhibition in uremia: identification of pre-beta-HDL as a major inhibitor in normal and uremic plasma. *Kidney Int* 1996;49:1360–1371.
49. Kronenberg F, Konig P, Neyer U, et al. Multicenter study of lipoprotein(a) and apolipoprotein(a) phenotypes in patients with end-stage renal disease treated by hemodialysis or continuous ambulatory peritoneal dialysis. *J Am Soc Nephrol* 1995;6:110–120.
50. Levine DM, Gordon BR. Lipoprotein(a) levels in patients receiving renal replacement therapy: methodologic issues and clinical implications. *Am J Kidney Dis* 1995;26:162–169.
51. Seres DS, Strain GW, Hashim SA, et al. Improvement of plasma lipoprotein profiles during high-flux dialysis. *J Am Soc Nephrol* 1993;3:1409–1415.
52. Asselbergs FW, Diercks GF, Hillege HL, et al. Effects of fosinopril and pravastatin on cardiovascular events in subjects with microalbuminuria. *Circulation* 2004;110:2809–2816.
53. Wanner C, Krane V, Marz W, et al. Atorvastatin in patients with type 2 diabetes mellitus undergoing hemodialysis. *N Engl J Med* 2005;353:238–248.
54. Clarke R, Daly L, Robinson K, et al. Hyperhomocysteinemia: an independent risk factor for vascular disease. *N Engl J Med* 1991;324:1149–1155.
55. Bachmann J, Tepel M, Raidt H, et al. Hyperhomocysteinemia and the risk for vascular disease in hemodialysis patients. *J Am Soc Nephrol* 1995;6: 121–125.
56. Chauveau P, Chadefaux B, Coude M, et al. Hyperhomocysteinemia, a risk factor for atherosclerosis in chronic uremic patients. *Kidney Int Suppl* 1993;41:S72–77.
57. Moustapha A, Naso A, Nahlawi M, et al. Prospective study of hyperhomocysteinemia as an adverse cardiovascular risk factor in end-stage renal disease. *Circulation* 1998;97:138–141.
58. Bostom AG, Shemin D, Lapane KL, et al. High dose-B-vitamin treatment of hyperhomocysteinemia in dialysis patients. *Kidney Int* 1996;49:147–152.
59. Wrone EM, Hornberger JM, Zehnder JL, et al. Randomized trial of folic acid for prevention of cardiovascular events in end-stage renal disease. *J Am Soc Nephrol* 2004;15:420–426.
60. Rostand SG, Rutsky EA. Pericarditis in end-stage renal disease. *Cardiol Clin* 1990;8:701–707.
61. Rutsky EA, Rostand SG. Treatment of uremic pericarditis and pericardial effusion. *Am J Kidney Dis* 1987;10:2–8.
62. Braun WE. Long-term complications of renal transplantation. *Kidney Int* 1990;37:1363–1378.
63. Diris JH, Hackeng CM, Kooman JP, et al. Impaired renal clearance explains elevated troponin T fragments in hemodialysis patients. *Circulation* 2004;109:23–25.
64. Abaci A, Ekici E, Oguzhan A, et al. Cardiac troponins T and I in patients with end-stage renal disease: the relation with left ventricular mass and their prognostic value. *Clin Cardiol* 2004;27:704–709.
65. Duman D, Tokay S, Toprak A, et al. Elevated cardiac troponin T is associated with increased left ventricular mass index and predicts mortality in continuous ambulatory peritoneal dialysis patients. *Nephrol Dial Transplant* 2005;20:962–967.
66. Jung HH, Ma KR, Han H. Elevated concentrations of cardiac troponins are associated with severe coronary artery calcification in asymptomatic haemodialysis patients. *Nephrol Dial Transplant* 2004;19:3117–123.
67. Needham DM, Shufelt KA, Tomlinson G, et al. Troponin I and T levels in renal failure patients without acute coronary syndrome: a systematic review of the literature. *Can J Cardiol* 2004;20:1212–1218.
68. Aviles RJ, Askari AT, Lindahl B, et al. Troponin T levels in patients with acute coronary syndromes, with or without renal dysfunction. *N Engl J Med* 2002;346:2047–2052.
69. Boulier A, Jaussent I, Terrier N, et al. Measurement of circulating troponin Ic enhances the prognostic value of C-reactive protein in haemodialysis patients. *Nephrol Dial Transplant* 2004;19:2313–2318.
70. Kini AS, Lee P, Marmur JD, et al. Correlation of postpercutaneous coronary intervention creatine kinase-MB and troponin I elevation in predicting midterm mortality. *Am J Cardiol* 2004;93:18–23.
71. Marwick TH, Steinmuller DR, Underwood DA, et al. Ineffectiveness of dipyridamole SPECT thallium imaging as a screening technique for coronary artery disease in patients with end-stage renal failure. *Transplantation* 1990;49:100–103.
72. Dahan M, Viron BM, Poiseau E, et al. Combined dipyridamole-exercise stress echocardiography for detection of myocardial ischemia in hemodialysis patients: an alternative to stress nuclear imaging. *Am J Kidney Dis* 2002;40:737–744.
73. Reis G, Marcovitz PA, Leichtman AB, et al. Usefulness of dobutamine stress echocardiography in detecting coronary artery disease in end-stage renal disease. *Am J Cardiol* 1995;75:707–710.
74. Herzog CA, Marwick TH, Pheley AM, et al. Dobutamine stress echocardiography for the detection of significant coronary artery disease in renal transplant candidates. *Am J Kidney Dis* 1999;33:1080–1090.
75. Brennan DC, Vedala G, Miller SB, et al. Pretransplant dobutamine stress echocardiography is useful and cost-effective in renal transplant candidates. *Transplant Proc* 1997;29:233–234.
76. Marwick TH, Lauer MS, Lobo A, et al. Use of dobutamine echocardiography for cardiac risk stratification of patients with chronic renal failure. *J Intern Med* 1998;244:155–161.
77. Sterner G, Nyman U, Valdes T. Low risk of contrast-medium-induced nephropathy with modern angiographic technique. *J Intern Med* 2001;250: 429–434.
78. Parfrey PS, Griffiths SM, Barrett BJ, et al. Contrast material-induced renal failure in patients with diabetes mellitus, renal insufficiency, or both. A prospective controlled study. *N Engl J Med* 1989;320:143–149.
79. Bettmann MA. Contrast medium-induced nephropathy: critical review of the existing clinical evidence. *Nephrol Dial Transplant* 2005;20[Suppl 1]: i12–17.
80. Rudnick MR, Goldfarb S, Wexler L, et al. Nephrotoxicity of ionic and nonionic contrast media in 1196 patients: a randomized trial. The Iohexol Cooperative Study. *Kidney Int* 1995;47:254–261.
81. Spinler SA, Goldfarb S. Nephrotoxicity of contrast media following cardiac angiography: pathogenesis, clinical course, and preventive measures, including the role of low-osmolality contrast media. *Ann Pharmacother* 1992;26:56–64.
82. Heyman SN, Rosenberger C, Rosen S. Regional alterations in renal haemodynamics and oxygenation: a role in contrast medium-induced nephropathy. *Nephrol Dial Transplant* 2005;20[Suppl 1]:i6–11.
83. Wang A, Holcslaw T, Bashore TM, et al. Exacerbation of radiocontrast nephrotoxicity by endothelin receptor antagonism. *Kidney Int* 2000;57: 1675–1680.
84. Solomon R, Werner C, Mann D, et al. Effects of saline, mannitol, and furosemide to prevent acute decreases in renal function induced by radiocontrast agents. *N Engl J Med* 1994;331:1416–1420.
85. Stevens MA, McCullough PA, Tobin KJ, et al. A prospective randomized trial of prevention measures in patients at high risk for contrast nephropathy: results of the P.R.I.N.C.E. Study. Prevention of Radiocontrast Induced Nephropathy Clinical Evaluation. *J Am Coll Cardiol* 1999;33: 403–411.
86. Gare M, Haviv YS, Ben-Yehuda A, et al. The renal effect of low-dose dopamine in high-risk patients undergoing coronary angiography. *J Am Coll Cardiol* 1999;34:1682–1688.
87. Ix JH, McCulloch CE, Chertow GM. Theophylline for the prevention of radiocontrast nephropathy: a meta-analysis. *Nephrol Dial Transplant* 2004;19:2747–2753.
88. Tepel M, van der Giet M, Schwarzfeld C, et al. Prevention of radiographic-contrast-agent-induced reductions in renal function by acetylcysteine. *N Engl J Med* 2000;343:180–184.
89. Kshirsagar AV, Poole C, Mottl A, et al. *N*-Acetylcysteine for the prevention of radiocontrast induced nephropathy: a meta-analysis of prospective controlled trials. *J Am Soc Nephrol* 2004;15:761–769.
90. Misra D, Leibowitz K, Gowda RM, et al. Role of *N*-acetylcysteine in prevention of contrast-induced nephropathy after cardiovascular procedures: a meta-analysis. *Clin Cardiol* 2004;27:607–610.
91. Merten GJ, Burgess WP, Gray LV, et al. Prevention of contrast-induced nephropathy with sodium bicarbonate: a randomized controlled trial. *JAMA* 2004;291:2328–2334.
92. Spargias K, Alexopoulos E, Kyrzopoulos S, et al. Ascorbic acid prevents contrast-mediated nephropathy in patients with renal dysfunction undergoing coronary angiography or intervention. *Circulation* 2004;110:2837–2842.
93. Barrett BJ, Carlisle EJ. Metaanalysis of the relative nephrotoxicity of high- and low-osmolality iodinated contrast media. *Radiology* 1993;188:171–178.
94. Fellner SK, Lang RM, Neumann A, et al. Cardiovascular consequences of correction of the anemia of renal failure with erythropoietin. *Kidney Int* 1993;44:1309–1315.
95. Rostand SG. Coronary heart disease in chronic renal insufficiency: some management considerations. *J Am Soc Nephrol* 2000;11:1948–1956.
96. Massry SG, Smogorzewski M. Mechanisms through which parathyroid hormone mediates its deleterious effects on organ function in uremia. *Semin Nephrol* 1994;14:219–231.
97. Bhatt DL, Roe MT, Peterson ED, et al. Utilization of early invasive management strategies for high-risk patients with non-ST-segment elevation acute coronary syndromes: results from the CRUSADE Quality Improvement Initiative. *JAMA* 2004;292:2096–2104.
98. Chertow GM, Normand SL, McNeil BJ. "Renalism": inappropriately low rates of coronary angiography in elderly individuals with renal insufficiency. *J Am Soc Nephrol* 2004;15:2462–2468.
99. Januzzi JL, Cannon CP, DiBattiste PM, et al. Effects of renal insufficiency on early invasive management in patients with acute coronary syndromes (The TACTICS-TIMI 18 Trial). *Am J Cardiol* 2002;90:1246–1249.
100. Shlipak MG, Heidenreich PA, Noguchi H, et al. Association of renal insufficiency with treatment and outcomes after myocardial infarction in elderly patients. *Ann Intern Med* 2002;137:555–562.
101. Herzog CA. Acute myocardial infarction in patients with end-stage renal disease. *Kidney Int Suppl* 1999;71:S130–133.
102. Berger AK, Duval S, Krumholz HM. Aspirin, beta-blocker, and angiotensin-converting enzyme inhibitor therapy in patients with end-stage renal disease and an acute myocardial infarction. *J Am Coll Cardiol* 2003;42:201–208.

103. McAlister FA, Ezekowitz J, Tonelli M, Armstrong PW. Renal insufficiency and heart failure: prognostic and therapeutic implications from a prospective cohort study. *Circulation* 2004;109:1004–1009.
104. Kanjanarat P, Winterstein AG, Johns TE, et al. Nature of preventable adverse drug events in hospitals: a literature review. *Am J Health Syst Pharm* 2003;60:1750–1759.
105. Hemmelgarn BR, Southern D, Culleton BF, et al. Survival after coronary revascularization among patients with kidney disease. *Circulation* 2004;110:1890–1895.
106. Szczech LA, Reddan DN, Owen WF, et al. Differential survival after coronary revascularization procedures among patients with renal insufficiency. *Kidney Int* 2001;60:292–299.
107. Herzog CA, Ma JZ, Collins AJ. Comparative survival of dialysis patients in the United States after coronary angioplasty, coronary artery stenting, and coronary artery bypass surgery and impact of diabetes. *Circulation* 2002;106:2207–2211.
108. Herzog CA, Ma JZ, Collins AJ. Long-term outcome of renal transplant recipients in the United States after coronary revascularization procedures. *Circulation* 2004;109:2866–2871.
109. Best PJ, Lennon R, Ting HH, et al. The impact of renal insufficiency on clinical outcomes in patients undergoing percutaneous coronary interventions. *J Am Coll Cardiol* 2002;39:1113–1119.
110. Reinecke H, Trey T, Matzkies F, et al. Grade of chronic renal failure, and acute and long-term outcome after percutaneous coronary interventions. *Kidney Int* 2003;63:696–701.
111. Mueller C, Neumann FJ, Perruchoud AP, Buettner HJ. Renal function and long term mortality after unstable angina/non-ST segment elevation myocardial infarction treated very early and predominantly with percutaneous coronary intervention. *Heart* 2004;90:902–907.
112. Naidu SS, Selzer F, Jacobs A, et al. Renal insufficiency is an independent predictor of mortality after percutaneous coronary intervention. *Am J Cardiol* 2003;92:1160–1164.
113. Schoebel FC, Gradaus F, Ivens K, et al. Restenosis after elective coronary balloon angioplasty in patients with end stage renal disease: a case-control study using quantitative coronary angiography. *Heart* 1997;78: 337–342.
114. Schwarz U, Buzello M, Ritz E, et al. Morphology of coronary atherosclerotic lesions in patients with end-stage renal failure. *Nephrol Dial Transplant* 2000;15:218–223.
115. Le Feuvre C. Angioplasty and stenting in patients with renal disease. *Heart* 2000;83:7–8.
116. Le Feuvre C, Dambrin G, Helft G, et al. Comparison of clinical outcome following coronary stenting or balloon angioplasty in dialysis versus non-dialysis patients. *Am J Cardiol* 2000;85:1365–1368.
117. Gruberg L, Mintz GS, Mehran R, et al. The prognostic implications of further renal function deterioration within 48 h of interventional coronary procedures in patients with pre-existent chronic renal insufficiency. *J Am Coll Cardiol* 2000;36:1542–1548.
118. Lindsay J, Apple S, Pinnow EE, et al. Percutaneous coronary intervention-associated nephropathy foreshadows increased risk of late adverse events in patients with normal baseline serum creatinine. *Catheter Cardiovasc Interv* 2003;59:338–343.
119. Rubenstein MH, Harrell LC, Sheynberg BV, et al. Are patients with renal failure good candidates for percutaneous coronary revascularization in the new device era? *Circulation* 2000;102:2966–2972.
120. Lemos PA, Arampatzis CA, Hoye A, et al. Impact of baseline renal function on mortality after percutaneous coronary intervention with sirolimus-eluting stents or bare metal stents. *Am J Cardiol* 2005;95:167–172.
121. Hirose H, Amano A, Takahashi A, Nagano N. Coronary artery bypass grafting for patients with non-dialysis-dependent renal dysfunction (serum creatinine > or =2.0 mg/dl). *Eur J Cardiothorac Surg* 2001;20: 565–572.
122. Liu JY, Birkmeyer NJ, Sanders JH, et al. Risks of morbidity and mortality in dialysis patients undergoing coronary artery bypass surgery. Northern New England Cardiovascular Disease Study Group. *Circulation* 2000;102:2973–2977.
123. Samuels LE, Sharma S, Morris RJ, et al. Coronary artery bypass grafting in patients with chronic renal failure: a reappraisal. *J Card Surg* 1996;11:128–133; discussion 34–35.
124. Chertow GM, Levy EM, Hammermeister KE, et al. Independent association between acute renal failure and mortality following cardiac surgery. *Am J Med* 1998;104:343–348.
125. Ferguson ER, Hudson SL, Diethelm AG, et al. Outcome after myocardial revascularization and renal transplantation: a 25-year single-institution experience. *Ann Surg* 1999;230:232–241.
126. Frenken M, Krian A. Cardiovascular operations in patients with dialysis-dependent renal failure. *Ann Thorac Surg* 1999;68:887–893.
127. Khaitan L, Sutter FP, Goldman SM. Coronary artery bypass grafting in patients who require long-term dialysis. *Ann Thorac Surg* 2000;69:1135–1139.
128. Ascione R, Nason G, Al-Ruzzeh S, et al. Coronary revascularization with or without cardiopulmonary bypass in patients with preoperative nondialysis-dependent renal insufficiency. *Ann Thorac Surg* 2001;72:2020–2025.
129. Beauford RB, Saunders CR, Niemeier LA, et al. Is off-pump revascularization better for patients with non-dialysis-dependent renal insufficiency? *Heart Surg Forum* 2004;7:E141–146.
130. Bucerius J, Gummert JF, Walther T, et al. On-pump versus off-pump coronary artery bypass grafting: impact on postoperative renal failure requiring renal replacement therapy. *Ann Thorac Surg* 2004;77:1250–1256.
131. Le A, Wilson R, Douek K, et al. Prospective risk stratification in renal transplant candidates for cardiac death. *Am J Kidney Dis* 1994;24:65–71.
132. Manske CL, Wang Y, Rector T, et al. Coronary revascularisation in insulin-dependent diabetic patients with chronic renal failure. *Lancet* 1992;340 (8826):998–1002.
133. Manske CL, Thomas W, Wang Y, Wilson RF. Screening diabetic transplant candidates for coronary artery disease: identification of a low risk subgroup. *Kidney Int* 1993;44:617–621.
134. Rabbat CG, Treleaven DJ, Russell JD, et al. Prognostic value of myocardial perfusion studies in patients with end-stage renal disease assessed for kidney or kidney-pancreas transplantation: a meta-analysis. *J Am Soc Nephrol* 2003;14:431–439.
135. De Lima JJ, Sabbaga E, Vieira ML, et al. Coronary angiography is the best predictor of events in renal transplant candidates compared with noninvasive testing. *Hypertension* 2003;42:263–268.
136. Koomans HA, Geers AB, vd Meiracker AH, et al. Effects of plasma volume expansion on renal salt handling in patients with the nephrotic syndrome. *Am J Nephrol* 1984;4:227–234.
137. Mellander S, Oberg B. Transcapillary fluid absorption and other vascular reactions in the human forearm during reduction of the circulating blood volume. *Acta Physiol Scand* 1967;71:37–46.
138. Degoulet P, Reach I, Di Giulio S, et al. Epidemiology of dialysis induced hypotension. *Proc Eur Dial Transplant Assoc* 1981;18:133–138.
139. Iseki K, Onoyama K, Maeda T, et al. Comparison of hemodynamics induced by conventional acetate hemodialysis, bicarbonate hemodialysis and ultrafiltration. *Clin Nephrol* 1980;14:294–298.
140. Jaraba M, Rodriguez-Benot A, Guerrero R, et al. Cardiovascular response to hemodialysis: the effects of uremia and dialysate buffer. *Kidney Int Suppl* 1998;68:S86–91.
141. Henrich WL, Woodard TD, McPhaul JJ Jr. The chronic efficacy and safety of high sodium dialysate: double-blind, crossover study. *Am J Kidney Dis* 1982;2:349–353.
142. Levine J, Falk B, Henriquez M, Raja RM, et al. Effects of varying dialysate sodium using large surface area dialyzers. *Trans Am Soc Artif Intern Organs* 1978;24:139–141.
143. Churchill DN. Sodium and water profiling in chronic uraemia. *Nephrol Dial Transplant* 1996;11[Suppl 8]:38–41.
144. Henrich WL, Hunt JM, Nixon JV. Increased ionized calcium and left ventricular contractility during hemodialysis. *N Engl J Med* 1984;310:19–23.
145. Leunissen KM, van den Berg BW, van Hooff JP. Ionized calcium plays a pivotal role in controlling blood pressure during haemodialysis. *Blood Purif* 1989;7:233–239.
146. Sherman RA, Torres F, Cody RP. The effect of red cell transfusion on hemodialysis-related hypotension. *Am J Kidney Dis* 1988;11:33–35.
147. Ritz E, Bosch J, Henderson LW, et al. Hemofiltration and vascular stability. *Contrib Nephrol* 1982;32:200–217.
148. Chanard J, Brunois JP, Melin JP, et al. Long-term results of dialysis therapy with a highly permeable membrane. *Artif Organs* 1982;6:261–266.
149. Locatelli F, Mastrangelo F, Redaelli B, et al. Effects of different membranes and dialysis technologies on patient treatment tolerance and nutritional parameters. The Italian Cooperative Dialysis Study Group. *Kidney Int* 1996;50:1293–1302.
150. van der Sande FM, Gladziwa U, Kooman JP, et al. Energy transfer is the single most important factor for the difference in vascular response between isolated ultrafiltration and hemodialysis. *J Am Soc Nephrol* 2000;11:1512–1517.
151. Hampl H, Paeprer H, Unger V, Kessel MW. Hemodynamics during hemodialysis, sequential ultrafiltration and hemofiltration. *J Dial* 1979; 3:51–71.
152. Renfrew R, Buselmeier TJ, Kjellstrand CM. Pericarditis and renal failure. *Annu Rev Med* 1980;31:345–360.
153. Wizemann V, Kramer W. Choice of ESRD treatment strategy according to cardiac status. *Kidney Int Suppl* 1988;24:S191–195.
154. Shapira OM, Bar-Khayim Y. ECG changes and cardiac arrhythmias in chronic renal failure patients on hemodialysis. *J Electrocardiol* 1992; 25:273–279.
155. D'Elia JA, Weinrauch LA, Gleason RE, et al. Application of the ambulatory 24-hour electrocardiogram in the prediction of cardiac death in dialysis patients. *Arch Intern Med* 1988;148:2381–2385.
156. Fantuzzi S, Caico S, Amatruda O, et al. Hemodialysis-associated cardiac arrhythmias: a lower risk with bicarbonate? *Nephron* 1991;58:196–200.
157. Morrison G, Michelson EL, Brown S, Morganroth J. Mechanism and prevention of cardiac arrhythmias in chronic hemodialysis patients. *Kidney Int* 1980;17:811–819.
158. Burns CB, Scheinhorn DJ. Hypoxemia during hemodialysis. *Arch Intern Med* 1982;142:1350–1353.
159. Nakamura S, Uzu T, Inenaga T, Kimura G. Prediction of coronary artery disease and cardiac events using electrocardiographic changes during hemodialysis. *Am J Kidney Dis* 2000;36:592–599.
160. Steuer RR, Leypoldt JK, Cheung AK, et al. Reducing symptoms during hemodialysis by continuously monitoring the hematocrit. *Am J Kidney Dis* 1996;27:525–532.

161. London GM, Parfrey PS. Cardiac disease in chronic uremia: pathogenesis. *Adv Ren Replace Ther* 1997;4:194–211.
162. Bleyer AJ, Russell GB, Satko SG. Sudden and cardiac death rates in hemodialysis patients. *Kidney Int* 1999;55:1553–1559.
163. Mak RH, DeFronzo RA. Glucose and insulin metabolism in uremia. *Nephron* 1992;61:377–382.
164. Ramos JM, Heaton A, McGurk JG, Ward MK, Kerr DN. Sequential changes in serum lipids and their subfractions in patients receiving continuous ambulatory peritoneal dialysis. *Nephron* 1983;35:20–23.
165. Prichard S. Major and minor risk factors for cardiovascular disease in peritoneal dialysis. *Perit Dial Int* 2000;20[Suppl 2]:S154–159.
166. Dawnay A, Millar DJ. The pathogenesis and consequences of AGE formation in uraemia and its treatment. *Cell Mol Biol* (Noisy-le-grand) 1998;44:1081–1094.
167. Burt RK, Gupta-Burt S, Suki WN, et al. Reversal of left ventricular dysfunction after renal transplantation. *Ann Intern Med* 1989;111:635–640.
168. Herzog CA, Ma JZ, Collins AJ. Long-term survival of renal transplant recipients in the United States after acute myocardial infarction. *Am J Kidney Dis* 2000;36:145–152.
169. Charnick SB, Nedelman JR, Chang CT, et al. Description of blood pressure changes in patients beginning cyclosporin A therapy. *Ther Drug Monit* 1997;19:17–24.
170. Murray BM, Paller MS, Ferris TF. Effect of cyclosporine administration on renal hemodynamics in conscious rats. *Kidney Int* 1985;28:767–774.
171. Amberger A, Hala M, Saurwein-Teissl M, et al. Suppressive effects of anti-inflammatory agents on human endothelial cell activation and induction of heat shock proteins. *Mol Med* 1999;5:117–128.
172. Bouchard D, Despatis MA, Buluran J, Cartier R. Vascular effects of cyclosporin A and acute rejection in canine heart transplantation. *Ann Thorac Surg* 1997;64:1325–1330.
173. Jenkins JT, Boyle JJ, McKay IC, et al. Vascular remodelling in intramyocardial resistance vessels in hypertensive human cardiac transplant recipients. *Heart* 1997;77:353–356.
174. Emeson EE, Shen ML. Accelerated atherosclerosis in hyperlipidemic C57BL/6 mice treated with cyclosporin A. *Am J Pathol* 1993;142:1906–1915.
175. Varghese Z, Fernando RL, Turakhia G, et al. Calcineurin inhibitors enhance low-density lipoprotein oxidation in transplant patients. *Kidney Int Suppl* 1999;71:S137–140.
176. Kraemer FB, Takeda D, Natu V, Sztalryd C. Insulin regulates lipoprotein lipase activity in rat adipose cells via wortmannin- and rapamycin-sensitive pathways. *Metabolism* 1998;47:555–559.
177. Brattstrom C, Wilczek HE, Tyden G, et al. Hypertriglyceridemia in renal transplant recipients treated with sirolimus. *Transplant Proc* 1998;30:3950–3951.
178. Adu D, Turney J, Michael J, McMaster P. Hyperkalaemia in cyclosporin-treated renal allograft recipients. *Lancet* 1983;2(8346):370–372.
179. Scoble JE, Freestone A, Varghese Z, et al. Cyclosporin-induced renal magnesium leak in renal transplant patients. *Nephrol Dial Transplant* 1990;5:812–815.
180. Zazgornik J, Shaheen FA, Kopsa H, et al. Severe hyperkalaemia, hyperchloraemia, hyporeninaemia and hyperaldosteronism in a cyclosporin-treated renal-transplant patient. *Nephrol Dial Transplant* 1988;3:826–829.
181. Jindal RM, Sidner RA, Milgrom ML. Post-transplant diabetes mellitus. The role of immunosuppression. *Drug Saf* 1997;16:242–257.
182. A comparison of tacrolimus (FK 506) and cyclosporine for immunosuppression in liver transplantation. The U.S. Multicenter FK506 Liver Study Group. *N Engl J Med* 1994;331:1110–1115.
183. Tamura K, Fujimura T, Tsutsumi T, et al. Transcriptional inhibition of insulin by FK506 and possible involvement of FK506 binding protein-12 in pancreatic beta-cell. *Transplantation* 1995;59:1606–1913.
184. Spinler SA, Inverso SM, Cohen M, et al. Safety and efficacy of unfractionated heparin versus enoxaparin in patients who are obese and patients with severe renal impairment: analysis from the ESSENCE and TIMI 11B studies. *Am Heart J* 2003;146:33–41.
185. Januzzi JL Jr, Snapinn SM, DiBattiste PM, et al. Benefits and safety of tirofiban among acute coronary syndrome patients with mild to moderate renal insufficiency: results from the Platelet Receptor Inhibition in Ischemic Syndrome Management in Patients Limited by Unstable Signs and Symptoms (PRISM-PLUS) trial. *Circulation* 2002;105:2361–2366.
186. Best PJ, Lennon R, Gersh BJ, et al. Safety of abciximab in patients with chronic renal insufficiency who are undergoing percutaneous coronary interventions. *Am Heart J* 2003;146:345–350.
187. Best P, Lennon R, Ting H, et al. The Safety of Abciximab Before Percutaneous Coronary Revascularization in Patients With Chronic Renal Insufficiency. *J Am Coll Cardiol* 2001;37(2 Suppl A).
188. Reddan DN, O'Shea JC, Sarembock IJ, et al. Treatment effects of eptifibatide in planned coronary stent implantation in patients with chronic kidney disease (ESPRIT Trial). *Am J Cardiol* 2003;91:17–21.
189. Berger PB, Best PJ, Topol EJ, et al. The relation of renal function to ischemic and bleeding outcomes with 2 different glycoprotein IIb/IIIa inhibitors: the do Tirofiban and ReoPro Give Similar Efficacy Outcome (TARGET) trial. *Am Heart J* 2005;149:869–875.
190. Chew DP, Bhatt DL, Kimball W, et al. Bivalirudin provides increasing benefit with decreasing renal function: a meta-analysis of randomized trials. *Am J Cardiol* 2003;92:919–923.
191. Chew DP, Lincoff AM, Gurm H, et al. Bivalirudin versus heparin and glycoprotein IIb/IIIa inhibition among patients with renal impairment undergoing percutaneous coronary intervention (a subanalysis of the REPLACE-2 trial). *Am J Cardiol* 2005;95:581–585.
192. Wright RS, Reeder GS, Herzog CA, et al. Acute myocardial infarction and renal dysfunction: a high-risk combination. *Ann Intern Med* 2002;137:563–570.
193. Strippoli GF, Craig M, Deeks JJ, et al. Effects of angiotensin converting enzyme inhibitors and angiotensin II receptor antagonists on mortality and renal outcomes in diabetic nephropathy: systematic review. *BMJ* 2004;329:828.
194. Lewis EJ, Hunsicker LG, Clarke WR, et al. Renoprotective effect of the angiotensin-receptor antagonist irbesartan in patients with nephropathy due to type 2 diabetes. *N Engl J Med* 2001;345:851–860.
195. Agodoa LY, Appel L, Bakris GL, et al. Effect of ramipril vs amlodipine on renal outcomes in hypertensive nephrosclerosis: a randomized controlled trial. *JAMA* 2001;285:2719–2728.
196. Barnett AH, Bain SC, Bouter P, et al. Angiotensin-receptor blockade versus converting-enzyme inhibition in type 2 diabetes and nephropathy. *N Engl J Med* 2004;351:1952–1961.
197. Brenner BM, Cooper ME, de Zeeuw D, et al. Effects of losartan on renal and cardiovascular outcomes in patients with type 2 diabetes and nephropathy. *N Engl J Med* 2001;345:861–869.
198. Zandbergen AA, Baggen MG, Lamberts SW, et al. Effect of losartan on microalbuminuria in normotensive patients with type 2 diabetes mellitus. A randomized clinical trial. *Ann Intern Med* 2003;139:90–96.
199. Abbott KC, Trespalacios FC, Agodoa LY, et al. Beta-blocker use in long-term dialysis patients: association with hospitalized heart failure and mortality. *Arch Intern Med* 2004;164:2465–2471.
200. Herlitz H, Harris K, Risler T, et al. The effects of an ACE inhibitor and a calcium antagonist on the progression of renal disease: the Nephros Study. *Nephrol Dial Transplant* 2001;16:2158–2165.
201. Kumagai H, Hayashi K, Kumamaru H, Saruta T. Amlodipine is comparable to angiotensin-converting enzyme inhibitor for long-term renoprotection in hypertensive patients with renal dysfunction: a one-year, prospective, randomized study. *Am J Hypertens* 2000;13:980–985.
202. Tonelli M, Moye L, Sacks FM, et al. Pravastatin for secondary prevention of cardiovascular events in persons with mild chronic renal insufficiency. *Ann Intern Med* 2003;138:98–104.
203. Tonelli M, Isles C, Curhan GC, et al. Effect of pravastatin on cardiovascular events in people with chronic kidney disease. *Circulation* 2004;110:1557–1563.

CHAPTER 35D ■ CARDIAC MANIFESTATIONS OF SELECTED NEUROLOGIC DISORDERS

KENNETH W. MAHAFFEY AND DANIEL LASKOWITZ

INTRODUCTION

Cardiac manifestations of neurologic disorders are common and diverse. Understanding the pathophysiology of cardiac and neurologic disorders is critical for physicians caring for patients with cardiovascular and neurologic disease states and investigators attempting to develop therapies and management strategies for disorders that have both central nervous system and cardiovascular components. The importance of interactions between cardiology and neurology are exemplified by ongoing collaborative efforts between cardiologists and neurologists in several key clinical areas, including stroke prevention in atrial fibrillation, percutaneous intervention in cerebrovascular occlusive disease, and the use of thrombolytic and antiplatelet therapies in nonhemorrhagic stroke. Many of these specific issues are discussed in other chapters. In this chapter, the focus is on cardiac manifestations of specific central nervous system events and the cardiac anomalies associated with hereditary and acquired neuromuscular disorders.

CARDIAC MANIFESTATIONS OF NEUROLOGIC EVENTS

It was over 70 years ago that Beattie et al. (1) recognized that the central nervous system had neurogenic input in cardiac arrhythmias. Soon after, Aschenbrenner and Bodechtel (2) reported electrocardiographic (ECG) abnormalities in young patients with brain lesions and presumed normal cardiac structure. It is now commonly known that ECG abnormalities can occur in the setting of central nervous system abnormalities such as ischemic stroke, intracranial hemorrhage, seizure, headache, meningitis, encephalitis, and cranial trauma. Generally, these ECG features can be interpreted correctly in the setting of known or suspected neurologic disease. However, the erroneous diagnosis of primary cardiac disease can occur and more importantly result in inappropriate therapy or delay in proper treatment. Substantial work has been done to attempt to understand the pathophysiology of these cardiac manifestations.

Acute Ischemic Stroke

Cardiovascular complications are extremely common following stroke and represent a major form of morbidity. These complications may be caused by focal cerebral injury or may be a manifestation of preexisting cardiac disease, which is common.

Several studies have documented a high prevalence of ECG changes and arrhythmias in patients with acute ischemic stroke. Common ECG changes include QT prolongation, T-wave abnormalities, prominent U waves, and ST-segment abnormalities (Table 35D.1) (3–7). The prevalence of asymptomatic coronary artery disease in patients with symptomatic cerebrovascular disease has been reported to be as high as 28% to 65% (8,9). Thus, cerebrovascular disease may be a marker for coronary artery disease that becomes clinically apparent during the physiologic stress of acute ischemic stroke. Few studies have systematically examined old tracings to establish if the ECG changes were new (10).

Arrhythmias are also common after acute ischemic stroke (see Table 35D.1). Atrial fibrillation has been most frequently described, although it is often unclear whether the atrial fibrillation was the cause of a cardioembolic event or secondary to cerebral infarction (3,10,11). Ventricular ectopy has also been frequently reported, although episodes of sustained ventricular tachycardia are distinctly uncommon. Atrioventricular (AV) block has been reported and has been attributed to excessive vagal stimulation (12). Intensive monitoring of patients presenting with acute stroke has increased the recognition of these arrhythmias, but has not been shown to reduce morbidity or mortality. Because life-threatening arrhythmias in these patients are uncommon, it may be difficult to show a clear benefit. Prolonged cardiac monitoring, however, may be a useful diagnostic tool and routine ECG evaluation may identify the approximately 15% of patients with acute ischemic stroke who may suffer a myocardial infarction (13,14).

TABLE 35D.1

REPORTED ELECTROCARDIOGRAPHIC CHANGES AND ARRHYTHMIAS IN PATIENTS WITH INTRACRANIAL HEMORRHAGE OR ISCHEMIC STROKE

Electrocardiographic changes
QT prolongation
T-wave inversion
Increased T-wave amplitude
Prominent U waves
ST-segment elevation
ST-segment depression
Premature atrial complexes
Premature ventricular complexes
Atrioventricular block (first-, second-, and third-degree)
Fascicular block
Bundle branch blocks
Arrhythmias
Sinus tachycardia
Sinus bradycardia
Sinus arrest
Asystole
Supraventricular tachycardia
Wandering atrial pacemaker
Atrial fibrillation
Atrial flutter
Ventricular tachycardia
Ventricular flutter
Ventricular fibrillation
Idioventricular rhythm
Torsades de pointes

Intracranial Hemorrhage

Byer in 1947 (15) first reported large T waves and QT prolongation in a patient with subarachnoid hemorrhage. The first systematic review of ECGs in patients with intracerebral or subarachnoid hemorrhage was done in 1954 and reported that QT prolongation, increased T-wave amplitude, and abnormal U waves were the most common abnormalities (16). Others have reported similar changes (see Table 35D.1) (17,18).

The precise incidence of specific ECG abnormalities is not known because reports have included patients with diverse baseline clinical characteristics and lesion types but rates vary from 50% to 98% (3,10,17,19). Although there is no definitive correlation between hemorrhage location and specific ECG changes, several studies have noted an association between frontal lobe hemorrhage and QT prolongation (5,20).

The largest comparative series evaluating ECG abnormalities in stroke patients included 150 stroke patients and 150 age- and gender-matched controls: 92% of stroke patients and 65% of controls had abnormal ECGs. Abnormal ECGs were found in 43 (98%) patients with intracranial hemorrhage. Few ECG findings characterized a particular stroke type. Atrial fibrillation was significantly more common in patients with cerebral embolus (47% versus 9% for other stroke type), and QT prolongation was most common in patients with subarachnoid hemorrhage (71% versus 39% for other stroke types). U waves were more common in patients with intracranial hemorrhage than in patients with other stroke types (25% versus 8%).

Supraventricular and ventricular arrhythmias as well as conduction abnormalities have been well documented in patients with intracranial hemorrhage (see Table 35D.1). Several observational series have reported arrhythmias in 47% to 90% of patients (10,11,21,22) and serious or life-threatening arrhythmias in 20% to 50% of patients with intracranial hemorrhage (21,23–25).

A comprehensive evaluation of arrhythmias in stroke patients was reported by Di Pasquale et al. (21). Twenty-four-hour Holter monitor recordings were performed on 120 patients with subarachnoid hemorrhage: 96 of 107 patients (90%) with adequate recordings had arrhythmias (Table 35D.2). In general, arrhythmias are more frequent and severe in patients with recordings in the first 48 hours after onset of bleeding. The QT_c interval more often prolonged with malignant ventricular arrhythmias. Hypokalemia is common and potassium levels were significantly lower in patients with ventricular arrhythmias. The presence of malignant ventricular arrhythmias or asystole has been reported as a univariable predictor of mortality after intracranial hemorrhage (10,26–31).

Management of Arrhythmias in Patients With Intracranial Hemorrhage or Ischemic Stroke

Management of patients with arrhythmias in the setting of intracranial hemorrhage has not been studied rigorously. Because of the high incidence of arrhythmias, continuous ECG monitoring is recommended, but there is no consensus about its required duration. Patients with QT prolongation should be monitored closely and possible causative factors such as medications or electrolyte abnormalities should be identified and corrected. Patients with Torsade de Pointes have been treated with atrial or ventricular overdrive pacing or isoproterenol. Left stellate ganglion block has also been proposed in patients with recurrent arrhythmias (32).

Intracranial Hemorrhage and Electrocardiographic Changes Consistent With Acute Myocardial Infarction

Multiple cases of patients with intracranial hemorrhage and ECG changes consistent with acute myocardial infarction and normal coronary anatomy by cardiac catheterization or at autopsy have been reported (33–38). Although a rare clinical entity, physicians need to be aware that ECG changes and symptoms consistent with myocardial ischemia or acute infarction may coexist with intracranial hemorrhage and a thorough history and physical examination are essential to avoid the catastrophic consequences of administering thrombolytic or anticoagulant therapy.

Mechanisms of Electrocardiographic Changes and Arrhythmias in Patients With Intracranial Hemorrhage or Ischemic Stroke

Substantial work in experimental models and humans has been done to try to understand the pathogenesis of the ECG changes seen in patients with cerebrovascular events. The first comprehensive report of central nervous system control of cardiovascular function was proposed over a century ago by Jackson (39). The most widely accepted mechanism by which lesions in the central nervous system result in changes in the ECG is a direct result of alterations in the autonomic nervous system control on cardiac electrophysiology. Several other processes are considered contributory, including a direct effect on the myocardium, consequences of the associated hemodynamic derangements, electrolyte abnormalities, alterations in circulating catecholamine levels, or concurrent coronary artery disease.

Experimental animal studies have strongly supported the belief that ECG changes associated with neurologic lesions are due, at least in part, to altered sympathetic tone. Stimulation of various brain structures has resulted in specific ECG changes similar to those seen in patients with ischemic stroke and intracranial hemorrhage (40–51).

TABLE 35D.2

CARDIAC ARRHYTHMIAS AND TRANSIENT ST-SEGMENT CHANGES IN 107 PATIENTS WITH SUBARACHNOID HEMORRHAGE AND TECHNICALLY ADEQUATE HOLTER RECORDING

Holter findings	Early stage (n = 62)	Late stage (n = 45)	*p* value
Ventricular premature complex	34	15	<.05
Nonsustained ventricular tachycardia	5	0	NS
Supraventricular premature complex	14	15	NS
Paroxysmal atrial fibrillation	2	0	NS
Paroxysmal supraventricular tachycardia	4	3	NS
Sinus bradycardia <50/min	19	23	NS
Sinus tachycardia >120/min	29	3	<.05
Sinus arrhythmia	18	14	NS
Wandering pacemaker	5	2	NS
Sinoatrial block	14	9	NS
Sinoatrial arrest >3 sec	4	2	NS
Atrioventricular dissociation	4	0	NS
Second-degree atrioventricular block	1[a]	0	NS
Idioventricular rhythm	2	0	NS
Torsades de pointes	4	0	NS
Ventricular flutter	1	0	NS
Ventricular fibrillation	1	0	NS
Asystole	5	0	NS
ST-segment depression[a]	4	3	NS
ST-segment elevation[b]	1	0	NS
Negative recording	3	8	NS

NS, not significant.
[a]Decreased ST ≥1.5 mm.
[b]Increased ST, 1.5 mm.
From Di Pasquale G, Pinelli G, Andreoli A, et al. Holter detection of cardiac arrhythmias in intracranial subarachnoid hemorrhage. *Am J Cardiol* 1987;59:596–600, with permission.

A few studies performed during neurosurgery have investigated the cardiac effects of cortical stimulation. The cingulate gyrus, insula, areas of the temporal lobes, and the frontal cortex have all been shown to have cardiovascular effects when stimulated (52–57). ECG changes similar to those seen in acute central nervous system events have been reported after right radical neck dissection (58). Sympathetic trunk ablation or stimulation of vagal centers supports the hypothesis that centrally mediated alterations in sympathetic or vagal tone result in the ECG changes.

The ECG abnormalities in cats caused by cortical stimulation were reversed with transection of the spinal cord above the level of the sympathetic outflow tracts, suggesting that alterations in autonomic outflow may cause the cardiac findings (59). Others have proposed that changes in sympathetic and vagal tone, noradrenaline, or catecholamine levels are contributing factors for the ECG changes (60,61). ECG abnormalities in dogs after brain stimulation have been reversed by propranolol administration (46). Others believe that ECG abnormalities are independent of elevated plasma norepinephrine levels (62), and measurements of urinary catecholamines in humans after cerebrovascular events have been inconclusive (63).

Patients with cerebrovascular disease are also at risk for cardiovascular disease from atherosclerotic processes. Hertzer et al. (64) performed cardiac catheterization on 1,000 patients undergoing vascular surgery. In the subgroup of 295 patients with a primary diagnosis of cerebrovascular disease, 59% of the patients had significant coronary artery disease, and almost half (44%) of the patients without symptoms of coronary disease had significant stenosis, severe operable coronary atherosclerotic disease, or severe inoperable coronary atherosclerotic disease.

The pathogenic mechanism for arrhythmias has also not been well characterized. Experimental studies have demonstrated that injection of blood into the subarachnoid space is associated with the rapid onset of arrhythmias. Chronic elevations of intracranial pressure, however, typically cause bradyarrhythmias (65–67). Based on animal models and clinical observations, several mechanisms for the arrhythmias have been proposed. Sudden increases in intracranial pressure cause compression on the brainstem and diencephalic structures, which results in increased sympathetic or vagal stimulation of the heart. Alterations in cerebral vascular tone may cause changes in systemic hemodynamics. Underlying coronary artery disease and hypertensive heart disease, which is common in patients with cerebrovascular disease, may be a contributing factor in some patients (11). Hypoxia owing to respiratory compromise, elevated catecholamines, and electrolyte imbalances, particularly hypokalemia, may also contribute to the arrhythmias (21).

Myocardial Damage in Patients With Intracranial Hemorrhage and Ischemic Stroke

Some controversy remains about whether the ECG abnormalities observed in patients with acute ischemic stroke or intracranial hemorrhage may represent primary myocardial changes. Experimental studies have shown pathologic myocardial changes following intracranial blood injection in mice (68,69). Focal myocardial lesions consisting of infiltrates of lymphocytes or histiocytes were seen in 45% of rats with experimentally induced intracranial hemorrhage (70). Subendocardial hemorrhages have been reported following subarachnoid hemorrhage and stellate ganglion stimulation in animals, which have been reduced in rats treated with propanolol (71–74). Several investigators have shown focal necrosis, myofibrillar degeneration, and inflammatory cell infiltration in animals following catecholamine infusions or hypothalamic stimulation (73,75–81).

Despite numerous reports of patients with normal myocardium after stroke even in the presence of ECG changes (18,20,35,82), data from human autopsy series suggest that patients with acute ischemic stroke or intracranial hemorrhage have an increased incidence of abnormal myocardial pathology. In two autopsy series, 8% to 12% of patients with intracranial hemorrhage, tumor, infection, or head injury had foci of myocytolysis predominantly in the left ventricle, without evidence of infarction (63,83). Focal myocytolysis is often seen with myocardial infarction, but is a distinctive lesion characterized by loss of sarcoplasm from focal areas of myocardium with retention of the cellular nuclei and sarcolemma (84). Others have also reported myocytolysis or foci of necrosis (85–87). The cause of these findings is unknown, but may be due to sympathetic cardiac stimulation or excessive catecholamine levels or increased corticosteroid levels that may potentiate catecholamine effects on the myocardium (88,89).

Epilepsy

Cardiac arrhythmias are common during partial and generalized seizure activity, and may be associated with significant morbidity and mortality. In several series, sinus tachycardia was the most common arrhythmia, and was present during 97% of ictal episodes. By contrast, severe or life-threatening arrhythmias were present in only 5% of patients (90–93). There have been numerous reports of cardiac arrest and asystole associated with seizure activity; undiagnosed seizure disorders have presented as unexplained syncope (94–104).

Even when accidental deaths from seizures are discounted, epileptic patients are at significantly higher risk of sudden death (99,100). Several epidemiologic studies have suggested that sudden unexplained death may account for more than 10% of deaths in an epileptic population (99,100). A correlation between type of arrhythmia and seizure focus has never been established, although some studies have suggested that temporal lobe seizures may be more arrhythmogenic (105,106).

Migraine Headache

The precise etiology of migraine headaches is unknown. Migraine headaches are generally thought to be associated with arterial vasomotor and autonomic nervous system abnormalities. There are reports of typical anginalike chest pain and myocardial infarction in patients during the acute phase of a migraine headache. A generalized vasospastic disorder has been suggested to explain these findings (107,108). Sympathetic dysfunction, vasospasm and altered autonomic innervation of the heart are reported in patients with migraine headaches (107–112).

Common medications used to treat migraine headaches can also have cardiac effects. Ergot compounds and sumatriptan are the two most common therapies used in aborting migraine headache. Dihydroergotamine has a high affinity for 5-HT_1, 5-HT_2, dopamine, and other catecholamine receptors (113). Ergotamine has been shown to precipitate coronary spasm and chest pain in patients with migraine (114). Sumatriptan has a more specific agonist of the pre- and postsynaptic 5-$HT_{1B/D}$ receptor, and works by constricting large intracranial vessels and blocking neurogenic inflammation (115). Sumatriptan has produced chest pain syndromes (116), and although it may affect blood pressure, the symptoms are generally not associated with ECG changes (117,118). Both agents have the potential for coronary vasoconstriction, and are contraindicated in patients with ischemic heart disease or variant angina. Patients with multiple risk factors for ischemic heart disease should undergo cardiac evaluation prior to therapy. Although experience with newer agents in the same drug class is limited, all of these drugs maintain the same precautions and contraindications regarding administration to patients with coronary artery disease.

Meningitis and Encephalitis

Cardiac abnormalities may occur in patients with meningitis and encephalitis. Alterations in central nervous system function due to increased intracranial pressure or involvement of specific neurologic centers known to be key in autonomic control of the heart can result in ST, T-wave, and QT abnormalities as well as atrial and ventricular arrhythmias (82,119–124).

Cranial Trauma

Patients with cranial trauma can have ECG changes and arrhythmias similar to patients with intracranial hemorrhage. In an extensive review, ECG tracings from 164 patients under the age of 40 and without history of cardiovascular disorder were compared with those from 100 patients with limb injury, and 164 healthy age- and gender-matched controls. Patients with head injury had an increased frequency of QT_c prolongation (15% versus 0%–1% in other groups), increased P-wave amplitude (24% versus 2%–14% in the other groups), and T-wave inversion (10% versus 0%–6% in other groups). The incidence of ECG abnormalities increased with worsening level of consciousness (125). Others have reported ECG changes in a patient with severe cranial trauma suggestive of acute myocardial infarction, but no autopsy evidence of heart disease (126).

Experimental models of head trauma in mice replicate the clinical findings and suggest the role of vagal stimulation in the genesis of arrhythmias in the setting of head trauma because arrhythmias appear to be attenuated by atropine pretreatment (127).

NEUROMUSCULAR DISORDERS WITH CARDIAC MANIFESTATIONS

Cardiac disease may be associated with the major types of diseases of the peripheral nerves, the neuromuscular junction, and the muscles with varying characteristics and severity. The cardiac manifestations and the clinical features of the neuromuscular disorders are heterogeneous. In some disorders, the most distinguishing feature is a cardiomyopathy, whereas in other disorders conduction abnormalities are prominent (Table 35D.3). The cardiac involvement can be minimal or life threatening. Several of the more common and clinically important diseases are reviewed below.

Disorders of Peripheral Nerves

Guillain–Barré Syndrome

Guillain–Barré syndrome is an acute autoimmune polyneuropathy that involves inflammation and demyelination of

TABLE 35D.3

CARDIAC MANIFESTATIONS OF NEUROMUSCULAR DISORDERS

Neuromuscular disorders commonly associated with electrocardiographic abnormalities
Guillain-Barré syndrome
Duchenne's muscular dystrophy
Becker's muscular dystrophy
Kearns-Sayre syndrome
Myotonic muscular dystrophy
Scapuloperoneal syndrome
Periodic paralysis
Myasthenia gravis
Peroneal muscular atrophy
Neuromuscular disorders commonly associated with cardiomyopathy
Duchenne's muscular dystrophy
Becker's muscular dystrophy
Centronuclear myopathy
Myasthenia gravis

nerves, and is classically characterized by ascending motor weakness and areflexia. The diagnosis is supported by a compatible clinical presentation, cerebral spinal fluid findings of albuminocytologic dissociation, and electrodiagnostic evidence of acute demyelination. Autonomic and cardiac complications in patients with Guillain–Barré syndrome are more common than generally recognized, and may significantly complicate medical management.

Cardiac involvement in Guillain–Barré syndrome was initially described by Sir William Osler in 1892, who made the observation that some patients with "acute febrile neuritis" succumbed to "paralysis of the heart" (128). Cardiac arrhythmias are also common. Sinus tachycardia has been reported in 45% to 79% of patients (129), but atrial fibrillation, atrial flutter, paroxysmal atrial tachycardia, and ventricular tachycardia are also noted (130–132). Bradyarrhythmias, sinus pauses, and asystole are also common and may portend cardiac arrest (130). Some authors recommend prophylactic pacemaker insertion for patients with clinically significant bradycardias or sinus pauses (131,133,134). Although bradyarrhythmias may occur spontaneously, patients often exhibit vagal hypersensitivity to suctioning, and care should be taken to preoxygenate adequately, suction gently, and administer atropine when appropriate. Cardiac involvement usually parallels severity of disease, and patients at highest risk for malignant arrhythmias often have more fulminant disease progression.

Autonomic neuropathy is commonly associated with Guillain–Barré syndrome and may be associated with cardiac dysfunction. Early evidence of autonomic dysfunction may become clinically manifest as abnormalities of bladder function, gastroparesis, abnormal pseudomotor activity, or blood pressure lability. Formal autonomic testing has revealed subclinical evidence of neuropathy in two thirds of patients with Guillain–Barré syndrome. It is difficult to obtain a true measure of the clinically relevant autonomic neuropathy in Guillain–Barré syndrome because most of the published observations are case reports or small series. Hypertension is common, with a reported incidence of 5% to 79%. Clinically significant hypotension may also occur, and is often exacerbated by impaired venous return to the heart caused by positive pressure ventilation and paralysis of the calf and abdominal musculature. The occurrence of dysautonomia in Guillain–Barré syndrome is most likely due to a failure of baroreflex buffering mechanisms due to deafferentiation of baroreceptor impulses.

Recognition of the features of early dysautonomia in the setting of Guillain–Barré syndrome is important. Patients with these symptoms are at increased risk for developing cardiac arrhythmias, especially AV block. Identification of this population with autonomic screening tests has met with limited success (135,136). It is probable that fulminant autonomic neuropathy, with inflammation of the small intramyocardial nerves, is responsible for the focal myocarditis described in Guillain–Barré syndrome (137). A dysautonomia-induced hypersympathetic state may also be responsible for acute reversible left ventricular dysfunction in these patients (138).

Friedreich Ataxia

Friedreich ataxia is an autosomal recessive neurodegenerative disease characterized by progressive ataxia, areflexia, proprioceptive loss, and upper motor neuron findings. When strict neurologic and genetic criteria for this disorder were met, cardiac involvement was reported in greater than 90% of the patients (139,140). No correlation between severity of neurologic and cardiac disease has been confirmed.

The most common cardiac abnormality in patients with Friedreich ataxia is concentric left ventricular hypertrophy (141,142). The cardiac pathology in this disorder is differentiated from genetic hypertrophic cardiomyopathy by the lack of cellular disorganization in the ventricular septum. Echocardiographic assessment of systolic and diastolic function is usually normal. The concentric hypertrophy associated with Friedreich ataxia also tends to have a more benign course than hypertrophic cardiomyopathy, and malignant arrhythmias are distinctly uncommon (143).

Although much less common than concentric left ventricular hypertrophy, a minority of patients with Friedreich ataxia may develop a dilated cardiomyopathy associated with global hypokinesis. This carries a worse prognosis, and patients usually experience progressive deterioration of cardiac function (144).

Peroneal Muscular Atrophy

Peroneal muscular atrophy includes two autosomal dominant genetic disorders collectively called Charcot–Marie–Tooth neuropathy. The clinical features include progressive distal lower extremity muscle weakness that begins in the second or third decade of life. Peroneal muscular atrophy does not normally involve the heart. Atrial flutter has been reported (145), but more common findings are conduction disturbances with complete heart block and right bundle branch block, which have been reported in several members of a family (146–148).

Disorders of the Neuromuscular Junction

Myasthenia Gravis

Myasthenia gravis is caused by an autoimmune process that results in a decrease in the number of acetylcholine receptors at the neuromuscular junction. It affects women more frequently than men, and can appear at any age with increased frequency in the third and fourth decades in women, and the sixth and seventh decades in men. Weakness and fatigue are the classic symptoms, with weakness worsening after repeated use and improving following periods of rest.

Substantial data support the association with myocardial disease, particularly with malignant thymoma, although the nature and pathology of this process is unresolved. The cardiac abnormalities may represent a progressive autoimmune process or coincidental findings from other disease processes. Typical cardiac manifestations include nonspecific ECG changes, arrhythmias, and heart failure. The ECG changes have been reversed with neostigmine treatment. Drugs used to treat arrhythmias and cardiac disease, such as quinidine, procainamide, lidocaine, and calcium channel blockers, should be used with caution because they can exacerbate symptoms of myasthenia gravis (149,150).

Disorders of Muscle

Cardiac dysfunction is relatively common with primary disorders of muscle. In some circumstances, these cardiac abnormalities are potentially life threatening, and cardiac evaluation is an important aspect of the clinical management of these patients. In Duchenne muscular dystrophy, a dilated cardiomyopathy is present in virtually all patients by the age of 18, and management of associated heart failure is an important component of care. In other conditions, such as myotonic dystrophy and polymyositis, the conduction system is preferentially affected, and may lead to clinically important arrhythmias or sudden cardiac death. Table 35D.4 summarizes the key neurologic features and cardiac manifestations of these primary muscle disorders.

Duchenne and Becker Muscular Dystrophy

Duchenne muscular dystrophy is an X-linked recessive disorder with an incidence of 1:3,300 male births (151). This disorder, which is caused by a mutation in the dystrophin gene, usually presents in early childhood with severe and progressive muscle wasting. Death usually occurs by the third decade of life and is caused by respiratory and cardiac compromise.

Cardiac abnormalities are common in Duchenne muscular dystrophy and include ECG changes, dilated cardiomyopathy, and arrhythmias. Up to 90% of patients with Duchenne muscular dystrophy have characteristic electrographic abnormalities, which include the presence of tall precordial R waves, an increase in R/S ratio in V_1, and deep, narrow Q waves in the left precordial leads (152,153). Rhythm disturbances are also common. The majority of patients have sinus tachycardia, which may be either sustained or labile (14). AV block is less common, but has been reported. Accelerated AV conduction may lead to a decrement in the PR interval (154). Dilated cardiomyopathy is also common in Duchenne muscular dystrophy, and heart failure may be the terminal event in 10% of patients (155). Pathologically, patients with Duchenne muscular dystrophy demonstrate extensive myocardial fibrosis, most prominently in the posterobasal left ventricular wall (154,156,157). There is usually selective sparing of the septum, right ventricle, and atrium. Degenerative changes of the conduction system have also been described (152). Given the absence of dystrophin in all cells, it is unclear why this pattern of selective myocardial involvement occurs.

Clinical management of cardiac complications in patients with Duchenne muscular dystrophy is an important aspect of their care. In a large, longitudinal study of over 300 patients, preclinical evidence of cardiac involvement was present in approximately one quarter of patients under the age of 6. Clinically apparent cardiomyopathy typically appeared by the age of 10, and was present in virtually all patients by 18 years of age (158). Surprisingly, given the prevalence and severity of these cardiac abnormalities, most patients usually remain relatively asymptomatic until late in the course of their disease. This may be due to the disproportionate involvement of the muscles of respiration, and that these cardiac abnormalities develop slowly enough to allow some degree of compensation (159). In approximately 10% of patients, the proximal cause of death is directly referable to a cardiac cause (155). Female carriers are not usually symptomatic, although ECG abnormalities have been reported (160).

Becker muscular dystrophy is a milder variant of Duchenne muscular dystrophy and is also caused by a mutation of the dystrophin gene. Becker dystrophy is characterized by a much later onset of weakness, and less fulminant progression. Only 10% of patients are wheelchair bound by the fifth decade of life (161). Cardiac abnormalities are similar to those seen in Duchenne muscular dystrophy, although usually not as severe. Up to 75% of patients with Becker muscular dystrophy develop cardiac abnormalities, although the majority of these are subclinical. A subset of patients may develop severe cardiomyopathy, often disproportionate to the degree of skeletal muscle weakness (162,163). It is usual for congestive heart failure to be a presenting symptom (164). Thus, longitudinal noninvasive assessment of cardiac function is warranted in patients with Becker muscular dystrophy. When cardiac failure occurs, symptoms may develop precipitously. Initial management should include diuretics and afterload reduction. Because Becker muscular dystrophy is associated with a near-normal life expectancy, cardiac transplantation has been performed in these circumstances (165).

Myotonic Dystrophy

Myotonic dystrophy is characterized by myotonia, muscle weakness, frontal balding, cataracts, and gonadal dysfunction. It is an autosomal dominant disease caused by an unstable triple repeat expansion in chromosome 19. A variety of cardiac disturbances have been associated with myotonic dystrophy, including conduction abnormalities, mitral valve prolapse, and cardiomyopathy. These usually become clinically symptomatic several years after the onset of other symptoms associated with myotonic dystrophy.

Conduction disturbances account for the most common abnormality in this condition. Approximately 90% of patients with myotonic dystrophy eventually have ECG abnormalities (166). The most frequent abnormalities are first-degree AV block and intraventricular conduction delay (167,168). In one series, first-degree AV block was seen in approximately two thirds of patients, and one third had right bundle branch block or left anterior hemiblock. Left bundle branch block was less common (169). These conduction disturbances are probably progressive, but only a few small longitudinal studies have evaluated the natural history.

Approximately one quarter of patients have evidence of mitral valve prolapse, although the significance of this is unclear given the high prevalence of this condition in the general population (170,171). In one of the few series examining the cardiac pathology of patients with myotonic dystrophy, fibrosis, and fatty infiltrate of the sinoatrial and AV nodes, conduction system, and ventricular walls were noted (172). Recognition of the high incidence of cardiac pathology plays an important role in the management of patients with myotonic dystrophy. In general, the cardiac abnormalities associated with myotonic dystrophy are relatively well tolerated, although 7% of patients will have clinical evidence of heart failure, and sudden cardiac death has been reported (173,174).

Periodic Paralysis

There are several forms of familial, or primary, periodic paralysis (175). Hypokalemic periodic paralysis is associated with low potassium at the onset of the paralytic attack. Hyperkalemic periodic paralysis is characterized by increased potassium concentrations at the initiation of the episodes, but normal serum potassium concentrations are common (176). These primary periodic paralyses have some common features. They are generally inherited as autosomal dominant traits with symptoms first recognized early in life and uncommonly after the third decade. Attacks of paralysis are characterized by weakness of the limbs, proximal more than distal, with respiratory

TABLE 35D.4

DISORDERS OF MUSCLE ASSOCIATED WITH CARDIAC MANIFESTATIONS

Disease	Genetic association	Neurologic and medical presentation	Cardiac manifestations
Duchenne muscular dystrophy	X-linked recessive	Presents in early childhood with severe and disabling muscle wasting; pseudohypertrophy	ECG abnormalities: tall precordial R-waves, deep narrow Q-waves in left precordial leads *Rhythm abnormalities:* sinus tachycardia, AVB, decreased PR interval *Anatomic abnormalities:* myocardial fibrosis, dilated cardiomyopathy
Becker muscular dystrophy	X-linked recessive	Less fulminant course than Duchenne MD; only 10% wheelchair bound by fifth decade of life	Similar to Duchenne MD, except less severe and often subclinical; Dilated cardiomyopathy may be severe in a subset
Myotonic dystrophy	Autosomal dominant caused by unstable triple repeat expansion in chromosome 19	Myotonia, muscle weakness, frontal balding, cataracts, and gonadal dysfunction	*Conduction abnormalities:* first-degree AVB, intraventricular conduction delay, LAHB, RBBB <LBBB *Anatomic abnormalities:* mitral valve prolapse, fibrosis and fatty infiltrate of SA and AV nodes, dilated cardiomyopathy
Periodic paralysis	Autosomal dominant; usually present in the first decade of life; hyperkalemic form mapped to chromosome 17	Episodes of proximal < distal muscle weakness may be associated with hypokalemia or hyperkalemia; muscles of respiration rarely involved	ECG abnormalities and arrhythmias associated with alterations in serum potassium; ventricular tachycardia; prolonged QT
Limb-girdle dystrophy	Variable; autosomal recessive and autosomal dominant variants have been reported	Muscle weakness begins in first to fourth decades, often first becoming symptomatic in the proximal lower extremities	Cardiac involvement uncommon but ECG abnormalities, conduction disturbances, and cardiomyopathy with CHF have been reported
Facioscapuloperoneal dystrophy	Autosomal dominant; mapped to long arm of chromosome 4	Facial weakness in first or second decade progressing to upper and lower extremities	Cardiac involvement uncommon; atrial standstill has been reported
Scapuloperoneal	X-linked	Myopathy of shoulder girdle and distal lower extremities	*Conduction abnormalities:* complete heart block and SCD reported in third and fourth decade
Centronuclear myopathy	No definitive inheritance pattern	Ptosis, hyporeflexia, slowly progressive myopathy	Dilated cardiomyopathy, myocardial fibrosis, congestive heart failure, SCD reported
Polymyositis	No definitive inheritance pattern; triggered by viral infections, autoimmune	Proximal muscle weakness	Rhythm abnormalities common and include atrial fibrillation, atrial flutter, frequent APCs, VPCs Conduction abnormalities common. Anatomic abnormalities include fibrosis, diffuse interstitial and perivascular mononuclear infiltrates, muscle fiber degeneration, mitral valve prolapse, and cardiomyopathy.
Kearns-Sayre Syndrome	Mitochondrial cytopathy	Progressive external ophthalmoplegia, retinal pigmentary degeneration, myopathy	Conduction abnormalities include RBBB, LAHB, AVB. SCD reported. Often selective infra-nodal involvement with normal PR interval

Abbreviations: AV, atrioventricular; AVB, atrioventricular block; APC, atrial premature contraction; CHF, congestive heart failure; ECG, electrocardiogram; LAHB, left anterior hemiblock; LBBB, left bundle branch block; MD, muscular dystrophy; RBBB, right bundle branch block; SA, sinoatrial; SCD, sudden cardiac death; VPC, ventricular premature contraction.

muscles rarely involved. Other common features include susceptibility after strenuous exercise, termination of attacks with mild exercise, normal function between attacks (although persistent weakness may develop after years of repeated episodes), and precipitation of attacks with cold.

Cardiac manifestations include the classic ECG abnormalities associated with alterations in serum potassium concentrations. Ventricular electrical instability can occur with premature ventricular complexes, fusion beats, multiple ventricular complexes, and ventricular tachycardias including bidirectional ventricular tachycardia, which can be treated with potassium supplementation in the hypokalemic variety and epinephrine or glucose and insulin for the hyperkalemic or normokalemic types (177–180).

Limb-Girdle Dystrophies

The limb-girdle dystrophies include several disorders. Autosomal recessive and autosomal dominant inheritance has been reported in different families. Muscle weakness begins in the first to fourth decades, generally in the proximal lower extremity first and the upper extremities later with variable progression (181). Cardiac involvement is uncommon, but can include nonspecific ECG changes, arrhythmias, and conduction system disturbances. Rarely, a cardiomyopathy can occur with heart failure (182,183).

Facioscapulohumeral Dystrophy

Facioscapulohumeral dystrophy is an autosomal dominant disorder characterized by onset of weakness in the first or second decade. Facial muscle weakness is generally the initial manifestation. Subsequent involvement of the upper extremities is followed by proximal lower extremity weakness. Cardiac involvement is extremely uncommon. There are sporadic cases of cardiomyopathy and conduction abnormalities. The rare entity of atrial paralysis or standstill has been reported with a familial occurrence associated with facioscapulohumeral dystrophy (184–187).

X-Linked Humeroperoneal Dystrophy

Typical clinical presentation is proximal upper extremity and distal lower extremity weakness beginning in the first decade of life. Progression is slow and often stabilizes by the second decade, but contractures may develop. Cardiac involvement is common and appears to exclusively affect the atrium (188). Atrial fibrosis and myocyte degeneration may occur. ECG abnormalities include small P waves, atrial fibrillation, atrial flutter, atrial paralysis, and varying degrees of AV block. Permanent ventricular pacing is recommended.

Scapuloperoneal Syndrome

Scapuloperoneal syndrome is an X-linked myopathy characterized by weakness of the shoulder girdle and distal lower extremities. Cardiac abnormalities appear to be isolated to the conduction system, and complete heart block and sudden cardiac death have been reported, generally in the third or fourth decade (189,190).

Centronuclear Myopathy

Centronuclear myopathy is a slowly progressive disease characterized by skeletal muscle wasting and characteristic central nuclei on histologic examination (191). There are several forms of the disease with onsets at birth, early childhood, or later in early adulthood. Familial occurrence is reported, but there is no definitive inheritance pattern established. Ptosis of the eyelids is almost universal, as well as hyporeflexia or areflexia. A cardiomyopathy has been described with extensive fibrosis, dilatation, and focal compensatory hypertrophy (192–194). Progressive heart failure and death can occur at an early age (192).

Polymyositis

Polymyositis is a nonsuppurative inflammatory process of skeletal muscle and thought to be caused by genetic factors, viral infections, and autoimmune mechanisms. The heart is infrequently involved. The myocardium can have diffuse interstitial and perivascular mononuclear infiltrates, muscle fiber degeneration, and fibrosis (195,196). The conduction system, including the sinoatrial node, His bundle, and left and right bundle branches, can be involved with similar histologic changes (197,198). Several series have found ECG changes and arrhythmias in more than half of the patients (199,200).

ECG abnormalities include atrial fibrillation, atrial flutter, atrial and ventricular premature complexes, AV conduction delay, and bundle branch blocks. Echocardiographic or cardiac catheterization findings include mitral valve prolapse and enhanced cardiac function (200,201). Contrary to these data, a cardiomyopathy with congestive heart failure also has been reported (196,202). The cardiac abnormalities observed in polymyositis may be due to the same process involving the skeletal muscle, a coincidental finding, or associated with therapy such as corticosteroids.

Kearns-Sayre Syndrome

The mitochondrial myopathies are a heterogeneous collection of diseases characterized by abnormal muscle fibers. Cardiac involvement is rare. The Kearns-Sayre syndrome, however, is characterized by the triad of progressive external ophthalmoplegia, retinal pigmentary degeneration, and heart block (203). The syndrome is generally thought to be acquired, afflicting both sexes equally, with onset before the age of 20. Common features include ataxia, hearing loss, dementia, short stature, delayed secondary sexual characteristics, peripheral neuropathy, and endocrine abnormalities.

Cardiac abnormalities almost exclusively involve the conduction system. Characteristic conduction abnormalities are right bundle branch block, left anterior fascicular block, and AV block (204–206). A normal P-R is common due to the selective infranodal involvement. Sudden death has been recognized and pacemaker insertion is recommended (207).

CARDIOVASCULAR ABNORMALITIES IN NEURODEGENERATIVE DISEASES

Parkinson Disease

Cardiovascular abnormalities are common in Parkinson disease (PD) and may be challenging to manage. In particular, autonomic dysfunction is prevalent and orthostatic hypotension often exacerbates postural instability, one of the hallmarks of this neurodegenerative disorder. Lewy bodies, the eosinophilic cytoplasmic inclusions characteristic of PD pathology, have been identified throughout the autonomic nervous system, including the hypothalamus, sympathetic system (thoracic intermediolateral nucleus and sympathetic ganglia), and parasympathetic system (dorsal vagal nucleus and parasympathetic nuclei). Of note, there is also evidence of cardiac sympathetic denervation, and Lewy bodies have been identified in the cardiac plexus (208). Myocardial imaging with ^{123}I-metaiodobenzylguanidine (MIBG) has demonstrated functional loss of cardiac sympathetic tone associated with these anatomic abnormalities (209). Interestingly, the marked decrease in myocardial MIBG uptake appears to be specific for PD and may have some diagnostic value in differentiating atypical PD from other neurodegenerative disorders associated with extrapyramidal features (209). These abnormalities in cardiac autonomic tone seen in PD may also have contributed to several sporadic cases of sudden cardiac death associated with a prolonged QTc interval (210).

Alzheimer Disease

Although less systematically studied, dysautonomia has also been described in Alzheimer disease (AD) (211). Vascular disease is also associated with dementia and is often difficult to clinically distinguish from AD. A large, population-based study in Rotterdam explored the relationship between atherosclerosis and dementia. Evaluation of 284 demented patients and 1,698 normal controls revealed that the odds ratio for AD in those with severe disseminated atherosclerosis compared to those with normal vasculature was 3.0 (212). Although the biology for the association between atherosclerosis and AD remains undefined, presence of the apolipoprotein-E4 allele appears to be a risk factor. Patients with atherosclerotic cerebrovascular disease and AD have a higher prevalence of the apolipoprotein-E4 genotype.

PERSONAL PERSPECTIVES

Over the past several years, tremendous advances have occurred because of the collaborative efforts between cardiology and neurology specialists. A growing appreciation of the similar pathophysiology and treatments for acute coronary disease and acute cerebrovascular events has strengthened the relationships of clinicians and clinical investigators. As cardiac and neurologic intensivists, we continue to focus on providing continued support for alignment of our subspecialties because with this approach we will advance our treatments and improve patient care.

THE FUTURE

The current focus on unraveling the genetic predisposition to disease will eventually provide tremendous advances in our understanding of disease mechanisms and help to identify potential new therapeutic interventions. In addition, studies evaluating the ability of the brain to withstand ischemic insults and the possible role for cerebral and myocardial protectants are under evaluation. Combinations of antiplatelet and antithrombin therapies that have been proven effective in acute and chronic cardiac diseases are being investigated in cerebrovascular disease populations. Finally, the investigation of diagnostic strategies with various biomarkers and imaging studies to diagnose stroke and myocardial infarction are being conducted. Work in the basic sciences on genetics, pharmaceuticals, and biomarkers as well as work being done in clinical trials will result in key translations of scientific discoveries to the bedside. There are ample opportunities in the coming years for continued collaboration of cardiologists and neurologists.

References

1. Beattie J, Brow GR, Long CNH. Physiological and anatomical evidence for the existence of nerve tracts connecting hypothalamus with spinal sympathetic centers. *Proc R Soc Lond Biol* 1930;106:253–275.
2. Aschenbrenner R, Bodechtel G. Uber EKG veranderungen bei hirntumorkranken. *Klin Wschr* 1938;17:298–302.
3. Dimant J, Grob D. Electrocardiographic changes and myocardial damage in patients with acute cerebrovascular accidents. *Stroke* 1977;8:448–455.
4. Ramani A, Shetty U, Kindaje GN. Electrocardiographic abnormalities in cerebrovascular accidents. *Angiology* 1990;41:681–686.
5. Yamour BJ, Sridharan MR, Rice JF, et al. Electrocardiographic changes in cerebrovascular hemorrhage. *Am Heart J* 1980;99:294–300.
6. Sainani GS, Andarkar SW. Electrocardiographic changes in cerebrovascular accidents. *Indian J Med Sci* 1976;30:331–333.
7. Miura T, Tsuchihashi K, Yoshida E, et al. Electrocardiographic abnormalities in cerebrovascular accidents. *Jpn J Med* 1984;23:22–26.
8. Rokey R, Rolak LA, Harati Y, et al. Coronary artery disease in patients with cerebrovascular disease: a prospective study. *Ann Neurol* 1984;16:50–53.
9. Hertzer NR, Young JR, Beven EG, et al. Coronary angiography in 506 patients with extracranial cerebrovascular disease. *Arch Intern Med* 1985;145:849–852.
10. Goldstein DS. The electrocardiogram in stroke: relationship to pathophysiological type and comparison with prior tracings. *Stroke* 1979;10:253–259.
11. Norris JW, Froggatt GM, Hachinski VC. Cardiac arrhythmias in acute stroke. *Stroke* 1978;9:392–396.
12. Chhetri MK, De B. Electrocardiographic changes in cerebrovascular accident. Role of vagal hyperactivity and intracranial hypertension. *Indian Heart J* 1965;17:347–355.
13. Chin PL, Kaminski J, Rout M. Myocardial infarction coincident with cerebrovascular accidents in the elderly. *Age Ageing* 1977;6:29–37.
14. Rogers FB. Unsuspected cardiac infarction with cerebrovascular accidents. *J Am Geriatr Soc* 1955;3:714–719.
15. Byer E, Ashman R, Toth LA. Electrocardiograms with large upright T-waves and long Q-T intervals. *Am Heart J* 1947;33:796–806.
16. Burch GE, Meyers R, Abildskov JA. A new electrocardiographic pattern observed in cerebrovascular accidents. *Circulation* 1954;9:719–723.
17. Fentz V, Gormsen J. Electrocardiographic patterns in patients with cerebrovascular accidents. *Circulation* 1962;25:22–28.
18. Wasserman F, Choquette G, Cassinelli R, et al. Electrocardiographic observations in patients with cerebrovascular accidents. *Am J Med Sci* 1956;231:502–510.
19. Stern S, Lavy S, Carmon A, et al. Electrocardiographic patterns in haemorrhagic stroke. *J Neurol Sci* 1969;8:61–67.
20. Cropp GJ, Manning GW. Electrocardiographic changes simulating myocardial ischemia and infarction associated with spontaneous intracranial hemorrhage. *Circulation* 1960;22:25–38.
21. Di Pasquale G, Pinelli G, Andreoli A, et al. Holter detection of cardiac arrhythmias in intracranial subarachnoid hemorrhage. *Am J Cardiol* 1987;59:596–600.
22. Lavy S, Yaar I, Melamed E, et al. The effect of acute stroke on cardiac functions as observed in an intensive stroke care unit. *Stroke* 1974;5:775–780.
23. Estanol Vidal B, Badui Dergal E, Cesarman E, et al. Cardiac arrhythmias associated with subarachnoid hemorrhage: prospective study. *Neurosurgery* 1979;5:675–680.
24. Sen S, Stober T, Burger L, et al. Long-term recording electrocardiogram in intracranial hemorrhage. *Jpn Heart J* 1982;23:659–661.
25. Mikolich JR, Jacobs WC, Fletcher GF. Cardiac arrhythmias in patients with acute cerebrovascular accidents. *JAMA* 1981;246:1314–1317.
26. Parizel G. Life-threatening arrhythmias in subarachnoid hemorrhage. *Angiology* 1973;24:17–21.
27. Estanol BV, Marin OS. Cardiac arrhythmias and sudden death in subarachnoid hemorrhage. *Stroke* 1975;6:382–386.
28. Carruth JE, Silverman ME. Torsade de Pointes atypical ventricular tachycardia complicating subarachnoid hemorrhage. *Chest* 1980;78:886–888.
29. Sen S, Strober T, Burger L, et al. Recurrent Torsade de Pointes type ventricular tachycardia in intracranial hemorrhage. *Intens Care Med* 1984;10:263–264.
30. Hust MH, Nitsche K, Hohnloser S, et al. Q-T prolongation and Torsades de Pointes in a patient with subarachnoid hemorrhage. *Clin Cardiol* 1984;7:44–48.
31. Chao CL, Chen WJ, Wu CC, et al. Torsade de Pointes and T-wave alternans in a patient with brainstem hemorrhage. *Int J Cardiol* 1995;51:199–201.
32. Grossman MA. Cardiac arrhythmias in acute central nervous system disease. Successful management with stellate ganglion block. *Arch Intern Med* 1976;136:203–207.
33. Levine H. Non-specificity of the electrocardiogram associated with coronary artery disease. *Am J Med* 1953;15:344–354.
34. Katta SR, Berk WA. Hypertensive intracerebral hemorrhage simulating acute myocardial infarction. *Ann Emerg Med* 1992;21:1002–1005.
35. Menon S. Electrocardiographic changes simulating myocardial infarction in cerebrovascular accident. *Lancet* 1964;11:433–434.
36. Beard EF, Robertson JW, Robertson RCL. Spontaneous subarachnoid hemorrhage simulating acute myocardial infarction. *Am Heart J* 1959;58:755–759.
37. Kitching AD, Bernstein M, O'Kelly BF. Primary intracranial hemorrhage presenting as acute myocardial infarction: a contraindication to thrombolytic therapy. *Can Med Assoc J* 1994;150:519–522.

38. Ashby DW, Chadha JS. Electrocardiographic abnormalities simulating myocardial infarction in intracerebral hemorrhage and cerebral thrombosis. *Br Heart J* 1968;30:732–734.
39. Jackson HJ. On the anatomical and physiological localization of movements in the brain. In: Taylor J, ed. *Selected Writings of John Hughlings Jackson*. London: Staples Press; 1958: 37–76.
40. Fulton JF. *Functional Localization in the Frontal Lobes and Cerebellum*. London: Oxford University Press; 1949: 66.
41. Kortiweg GCJ, Boeles JTF, TenCate J. Influence of stimulation of some subcortical areas on the electrocardiogram. *J Neurophysiol* 1957;20:100–107.
42. Manning JW, Cotten MD. Mechanism of cardiac arrhythmias induced by diencephalic stimulation. *Am J Physiol* 1962;203:1120–1124.
43. Fuster JM, Weinberg SJ. Bioelectrical changes of the heart cycle induced by stimulation of diencephalic regions. *Exp Neurol* 1960;2:26–39.
44. Weinberg SJ, Fuster JM. Electrocardiographic changes produced by localized hypothalamic stimulations. *Ann Intern Med* 1960;53:332–341.
45. Hoff EC, Kell JF, Carroll MN. Effects of cortical stimulation and lesions on cardiovascular function. *Physiol Rev* 1963;43:68–114.
46. Hockman CH, Mauck HP Jr, Hoff EC. ECG changes resulting from cerebral stimulation. II. A spectrum of ventricular arrhythmias of sympathetic origin. *Am Heart J* 1966;71:695–700.
47. Ruggiero DA, Mraovitch S, Granata AR, et al. A role of insular cortex in cardiovascular function. *J Comp Neurol* 1987;257:189–207.
48. Mesulam MM, Mufson EJ. Insula of the old world monkey. III: Efferent cortical output and comments on function. *J Comp Neurol* 1982;212:38–52.
49. Oppenheimer SM, Cechetto DF. Cardiac chronotropic organization of the rat insular cortex. *Brain Res* 1990;533:66–72.
50. Yanowitz F, Preston JB, Abildskov JA. Functional distribution of right and left stellate innervation to the ventricles. Production of neurogenic electrocardiographic changes by unilateral alteration of sympathetic tone. *Circ Res* 1966;18:416–428.
51. Ueda H, Yanai Y, Murao S, et al. Electrocardiographic and vectorcardiographic changes produced by electrical stimulation of the cardiac nerves. *Jpn Heart J* 1964;5:359–372.
52. Chapman WP, Livingston RB, Livingston KE. Frontal lobotomy and electrical stimulation of orbital surface of frontal lobes. *Arch Neurol Psych* 1949;62:701–716.
53. Chapman WP, Livingston KE, Poppen JL. Effect upon blood pressure of electrical stimulation of tips of temporal lobes in man. *J Neurophysiol* 1950;13:65–71.
54. Delgado JMR. Circulatory effects of cortical stimulation. *Physiol Rev* 1960;40:146–170.
55. Pool JL, Ransohoff J. Autonomic effects on stimulating rostral portion of cingulate gyri in man. *J Neurophysiol* 1949;12:385–392.
56. Oppenheimer SM, Gelb A, Girvin JP, et al. Cardiovascular effects of human insular cortex stimulation. *Neurology* 1992;42:1727–1732.
57. Svigelj V, Grad A, Tekavcic I, et al. Cardiac arrhythmia associated with reversible damage to insula in a patient with subarachnoid hemorrhage. *Stroke* 1994;25:1053–1055.
58. Hugenholz PG. Electrocardiographic changes typical for central nervous system disease after right radical neck dissection. *Am Heart J* 1967;74:438–441.
59. Porter RW, Kamikawa K, Greenhoot JH. Persistent electrocardiographic abnormalities experimentally induced by stimulation of the brain. *Am Heart J* 1962;64:815–820.
60. Melville KI, Blum B, Shister HE, et al. Cardiac ischemic changes and arrhythmias induced by hypothalamic stimulation. *Am J Cardiol* 1963;12:781–791.
61. Meyer JS, Stoica E, Pascu I, et al. Catecholamine concentrations in CSF and plasma of patients with cerebral infarction and haemorrhage. *Brain* 1973; 96:277–288.
62. Grad A, Kiauta T, Osredkar J. Effect of elevated plasma norepinephrine on electrocardiographic changes in subarachnoid hemorrhage. *Stroke* 1991;22:746–749.
63. Connor RC. Heart damage associated with intracranial lesions. *Br Med J* 1968;3:29–31.
64. Hertzer NR, Beven EG, Young JR, et al. Coronary artery disease in peripheral vascular patients. A classification of 1000 coronary angiograms and results of surgical management. *Ann Surg* 1984;199:223–233.
65. Smith M, Ray CT. Cardiac arrhythmias, increased intracranial pressure, and the autonomic nervous system. *Chest* 1972;61:125–133.
66. Estanol BV, Loyo MV, Mateos JH, et al. Cardiac arrhythmias in experimental subarachnoid hemorrhage. *Stroke* 1977;8:440–449.
67. Lacy PS, Earle AM. A small animal model for electrocardiographic abnormalities observed after an experimental subarachnoid hemorrhage. *Stroke* 1983;14:371–377.
68. Burch GE, Sun SC, Colcolough HL, et al. Acute myocardial lesions; following experimentally-induced intracranial hemorrhage in mice: a histological and histochemical study. *Arch Pathol* 1967;84:517–521.
69. Burch GE, Sohal RS, Sun SC, et al. Effects of experimental intracranial hemorrhage on the ultrastructure of the myocardium of mice. *Am Heart J* 1969;77:427–429.
70. Hunt D, Gore I. Myocardial lesions following experimental intracranial hemorrhage: Prevention with propanolol. *Am Heart J* 1972;83:232–236.
71. Koskelo P, Punsar S, Sipila W. Subendocardial haemorrhage and ECG changes in intracranial bleeding. *Br Med J* 1964;1:1479–1480.
72. Kay MP, McDonald RH, Randall WC. Systolic hypertension and subendocardial hemorrhages produced by electrical stimulation of the stellate ganglion. *Circ Res* 1961;9:1164–1170.
73. Mehes G, Papp G, Rajkovits K. Effect of adrenergic alpha- and beta-receptor blocking drugs on the myocardial lesions induced by sympathomimetic amines. *Acta Physiol Hung* 1967;32:175–184.
74. Lehr D, Krukowski M, Colon R. Electrolyte changes in Isoproterenol-induced myocardial necrosis and the preventive effect of B-adrenergic blockade. *Fed Proc* 1965;24:561. Abstract.
75. Raab W. Key position of catecholamines in functional and degenerative cardiovascular pathology. *Am J Cardiol* 1960;5:571–578.
76. Chappel CI, Rona G, Balazs T, et al. Comparison of cardiotoxic action of certain sympathetic amines. *Can J Biochem* 1969;37:35.
77. Szakacs JE, Mehlman B. Pathologic changes induced by I-norepinephrine. *Am J Cardiol* 1960;5:619–627.
78. Ferrans VJ, Hibbs RG, Black WC, et al. Isoproterenol-induced myocardial necrosis. A histochemical and electron microscopic study. *Am Heart J* 1964;68:71–90.
79. Bajusz E, Jasmin G. Influence of variations in electrolyte intake upon the development of cardiac necrosis produced by vasopressor amines. *Lab Invest* 1964;13:757–766.
80. Bloom S, Cancilla PA. Myocytolysis and mitochondrial calcification in rat myocardium after low doses of isoproterenol. *Am J Pathol* 1969;54:373–391.
81. Schenk EA, Moss AJ. Cardiovascular effects of sustained norepinephrine infusions. II. Morphology. *Circ Res* 1966;18:605–615.
82. Hersch C. Electrocardiographic changes in subarachnoid haemorrhage, meningitis, and intracranial space-occupying lesions. *Br Heart J* 1964;26: 785–793.
83. Connor RC. Fuchsinophilic degeneration of myocardium in patients with intracranial lesions. *Br Heart J* 1970;32:81–84.
84. Schlesinger MJ, Reiner L. Focal myocytolysis of the heart. *Am J Pathol* 1955;31:443–459.
85. Greenhoot JH, Reichenbach DD. Cardiac injury and subarachnoid hemorrhage. A clinical, pathological, and physiological correlation. *J Neurosurg* 1969;30:521–531.
86. Hammermeister KE, Reichenbach DD. QRS changes, pulmonary edema, and myocardial necrosis associated with subarachnoid hemorrhage. *Am Heart J* 1969;78:94–100.
87. Castleman B. Case records of the Massachusetts General Hospital: Case 1—970. *N Engl J Med* 1970;282:38–44.
88. Van Vliet PD, Burchell HB, Titus JL. Focal myocarditis associated with pheochromocytoma. *N Engl J Med* 1966;274:1102–1108.
89. Jenkins JS, Buckell M, Carter AB, et al. Hypothalamic-pituitary-adrenal function after subarachnoid hemorrhage. *Br Med J* 1969;4:707–709.
90. Howell SJ, Blumhardt LD. ECG abnormalities in epileptics. *Neurology* 1988;38:1168.
91. Keilson MJ, Hauser WA, Magrill JP. Electrocardiographic changes during electrographic seizures. *Arch Neurol* 1989;46:1169–1170.
92. Keilson MJ, Hauser WA, Magrill JP, et al. ECG abnormalities in patients with epilepsy. *Neurology* 1987;37:1624–1626.
93. Keilson MJ, Magrill JP. Simultaneous ambulatory cassette EEG/ECG monitoring. In: Ebersole JS, ed. *Ambulatory EEG Monitoring*. New York: Raven Press; 1989: 171–193.
94. Wilder-Smith E. Complete atrio-ventricular conduction block during complex partial seizure. *J Neurol Neurosurg Psychiatry* 1992;55:734–736.
95. Liedholm LJ, Gudjonsson O. Cardiac arrest due to partial epileptic seizures. *Neurology* 1992;42:824–829.
96. Howell SJ, Blumhardt LD. Cardiac asystole associated with epileptic seizures: a case report with simultaneous EEG and ECG. *J Neurol Neurosurg Psychiatry* 1989;52:795–798.
97. Dasheiff RM, Dickinson LJ. Sudden unexpected death of epileptic patient due to cardiac arrhythmia after seizure. *Arch Neurol* 1986;43:194–196.
98. Reeves AL, Nollet KE, Klass DW, et al. The ictal bradycardia syndrome. *Epilepsia* 1996;37:983–987.
99. Earnest MP, Thomas GE, Eden RA, et al. The sudden unexplained death syndrome in epilepsy: demographic, clinical, and postmortem features. *Epilepsia* 1992;33:310–316.
100. Terrence CF Jr, Wisotzkey HM, Perper JA. Unexpected, unexplained death in epileptic patients. *Neurology* 1975;25:594–598.
101. Terrence CF, Rao GR, Perper JA. Neurogenic pulmonary edema in unexpected, unexplained death of epileptic patients. *Ann Neurol* 1981;9:458–464.
102. Falconer B, Rajs J. Post-mortem findings of cardiac lesions in epileptics: a preliminary report. *Forensic Sci Int* 1976;8:63–71.
103. Panidis IP, Morganroth J. Initiating events of sudden cardiac death. *Cardiovasc Clin* 1985;15:81–92.
104. Hirsch CS, Martin DL. Unexpected death in young epileptics. *Neurology* 1971;21:682–690.
105. Epstein MA, Sperling MR, O'Connor MJ. Cardiac rhythm during temporal lobe seizures. *Neurology* 1992;42:50–53.
106. Galimberti CA, Marchioni E, Barzizza F, et al. Partial epileptic seizures of different origin variably affect cardiac rhythm. *Epilepsia* 1996;37:742–747.

107. Wayne VS. A possible relationship between migraine and coronary artery spasm. *Aust N Z J Med* 1986;16:708–710.
108. Lafitte C, Even C, Henry-Lebras F, et al. Migraine and angina pectoris by coronary artery spasm. *Headache* 1996;36:332–334.
109. Pogacnik T, Sega S, Pecnik B, et al. Autonomic function testing in patients with migraine. *Headache* 1993;33:545–550.
110. Appel S, Kuritzky A, Zahavi I, et al. Evidence for instability of the autonomic nervous system in patients with migraine headache. *Headache* 1992; 32:10–17.
111. Rozentryt P, Durko A, Kozubski W, et al. Automatic regulation of sinus rhythm in patients with migraine. *Neurol Neurochir Pol* 1995;29:889–900.
112. Prusinski A, Trzos S, Rozentryt P, et al. Studies of heart rhythm variability in migraine. Preliminary communication. *Neurol Neurochir Pol* 1994; 28(Suppl 1):23–27.
113. Touchon J, Bertin L, Pilgrim AJ, et al. A comparison of subcutaneous sumatriptan and dihydroergotamine nasal spray in the acute treatment of migraine. *Neurology* 1996;47:361–365.
114. Snell NJ, Russell-Smith C, Coysh HL. Myocardial ischemia in migraine sufferers taking ergotamine. *Postgrad Med J* 1978;54:37–39.
115. Dechant KL, Clissold SP. Sumatriptan: a review of its pharmacodynamic and pharmacokinetic properties, and therapeutic efficacy in the treatment of migraine and cluster headache. *Drugs* 1992;43(Suppl):776–798.
116. Walton-Shirley M, Flowers K, Whiteside JH. Unstable angina pectoris associated with Imitrex therapy. *Cathet Cardiovasc Diagn* 1995;34:188.
117. Paterna S, Parrinello G, Pinto A, et al. Effect of sumatriptan on facial temperature variations, blood pressure and electrocardiogram in healthy subjects and patients with migraine without aura. *Clin Ter* 1995;146:469–476.
118. Brown EG, Endersby CA, Smith RN, et al. The safety and tolerability of sumatriptan: an overview. *Eur Neurol* 1991;31:339–344.
119. Chandra R, Tandon RN, Singhal A. Reversible sick sinus syndrome with junctional and ventricular escape and fusion beats in a case of tuberculous meningitis. *Indian Heart J* 1981;33:37–39.
120. Brubakk O. Non-invasive assessment of cardiac function in meningitis. *Acta Med Scand* 1979;205:67–72.
121. Detsky AS, Salit IE. Complete heart block in meningococcemia. *Ann Emerg Med* 1983;12:391–393.
122. Bisht DB. Cardiac manifestations of encephalitis with special reference to ECG changes. *Indian Heart J* 1967;19:340–345.
123. De Keyser J, De Boel S, Ceulemans L, et al. Torsade de pointes as a complication of brainstem encephalitis. *Intens Care Med* 1987;13:76–77.
124. Uemura A, Morimoto S, Hiramitsu S, et al. A case of brain stem encephalitis complicated with bifascicular block caused by rubella virus. *Kokyu To Junkan* 1992;40:499–503.
125. Hersch C. Electrocardiographic changes in head injuries. *Circulation* 1961;23:853–860.
126. Brunninkhuis LG. Electrocardiographic abnormalities suggesting myocardial infarction in a patient with severe cranial trauma. *Pacing Clin Electrophysiol* 1983;6:1336–1340.
127. Jacobson SA, Danufsky P. Marked EKG changes produced by experimental head trauma. *J Neuropath Exp Neurol* 1954;13:462–466.
128. Osler W. *The Principles and Practice of Medicine.* New York: Appleton-Century-Crofts; 1892: 777.
129. Krone A, Reuther P, Fuhrmeister U. Autonomic dysfunction in polyneuropathies: a report on 106 cases. *J Neurol* 1983;230:111–121.
130. Greenland P, Griggs RC. Arrhythmic complications in the Guillain–Barré syndrome. *Arch Intern Med* 1980;140:1053–1055.
131. Emmons PR, Blume WT, DuShane JW. Cardiac monitoring and demand pacemaker in Guillain–Barré syndrome. *Arch Neurol* 1975;32:59–61.
132. Stewart IM. Arrhythmias in Guillain–Barré syndrome. *Br Med J* 1973;2: 665–666.
133. Narayan D, Huang MT, Mathew PK. Bradycardia and asystole requiring permanent pacemaker in Guillain–Barré syndrome. *Am Heart J* 1984;108: 426–428.
134. Favre H, Foex P, Guggisberg M. Use of demand pacemaker in a case of Guillain–Barré syndrome. *Lancet* 1970;1:1062–1063.
135. Winer JB, Hughes RA. Identification of patients at risk of arrhythmia in the Guillain–Barré syndrome. *Q J Med* 1988;68:735–739.
136. Flachenecker P, Mullges W, Wermuth P, et al. Eyeball pressure testing in the evaluation of serious bradyarrhythmias in Guillain–Barré syndrome. *Neurology* 1996;47:102–108.
137. Feiden W, Gerhard L, Borchard F. Neuritis cordis due to the acute polyneuritis of the Guillain–Barré syndrome. *Virchows Arch A Pathol Anat Histopathol* 1988;413:573–580.
138. Iga K, Himura Y, Izumi C, et al. Reversible left ventricular dysfunction associated with the Guillain–Barré syndrome: an expression of catecholamine cardiotoxicity? *Jpn Circ J* 1995;59:236–240.
139. Brumback RA, Panner BJ, Kingston WJ. The heart in Friedreich's ataxia. Report of a case. *Arch Neurol* 1986;43:189–192.
140. Child JS, Perloff JK, Bach PM, et al. Cardiac involvement in Friedreich's ataxia: a clinical study of 75 patients. *J Am Coll Cardiol* 1986;7:1370–1378.
141. Gottdiener JS, Hawley RJ, Maron BJ, et al. Characteristics of the cardiac hypertrophy in Friedreich's ataxia. *Am Heart J* 1982;103:525–531.
142. Smith ER, Sangalang VE, Heffernan LP, et al. Hypertrophic cardiomyopathy: the heart disease of Friedreich's ataxia. *Am Heart J* 1977;94:428–434.
143. Palagi B, Picozzi R, Casazza F, et al. Biventricular function in Friedreich's ataxia: a radionuclide angiographic study. *Br Heart J* 1988;59:692–695.
144. Alboliras ET, Shub C, Gomez MR, et al. Spectrum of cardiac involvement in Friedreich's ataxia: clinical, electrocardiographic and echocardiographic observations. *Am J Cardiol* 1986;58:518–524.
145. Leak D. Paroxysmal atrial flutter in peroneal muscular atrophy. *Br Heart J* 1961;23:326–328.
146. Littler WA. Heart block and peroneal muscular atrophy. *Q J Med* 1970;39:431–440.
147. Kay JM, Littler WA, Meade JB. Ultrastructure of the myocardium in familial heart block and peroneal muscular atrophy. *Br Heart J* 1972;34:1081–1084.
148. Lowry PJ, Littler WA. Peroneal muscular atrophy associated with cardiac conducting tissue disease: further observations. *Postgrad Med J* 1983;59: 530–532.
149. Luomanmaki K, Hokkanen E, Heikkila J. Electrocardiogram in myasthenia gravis. Analysis of a series of 97 patients. *Ann Clin Res* 1969;1:236–245.
150. Gibson TC. The heart in myasthenia gravis. *Am Heart J* 1975;90:389–396.
151. Engel AG. Duchenne dystrophy. In: Engel AG, Banker BQ, eds. *Myology Basic and Clinical.* New York: McGraw Hill; 1986: 1185–1240.
152. Sanyal SK, Johnson WW. Cardiac conduction abnormalities in children with Duchenne's progressive muscular dystrophy: electrocardiographic features and morphologic correlates. *Circulation* 1982;66:853–863.
153. Perloff JK. Cardiac rhythm and conduction in Duchenne's muscular dystrophy: a prospective study of 20 patients. *J Am Coll Cardiol* 1984;3:1263–1268.
154. Perloff JK, Roberts WC, de Leon AC Jr, et al. The distinctive electrocardiogram of Duchenne's progressive muscular dystrophy: an electrocardiographic-pathologic correlative study. *Am J Med* 1967;42:179–188.
155. Quinlivan RM, Dubowitz V. Cardiac transplantation in Becker muscular dystrophy. *Neuromuscul Disord* 1992;2:165–167.
156. Frankel KA, Rosser RJ. The pathology of the heart in progressive muscular dystrophy: epimyocardial fibrosis. *Hum Pathol* 1976;7:375–386.
157. Nomura H, Hizawa K. Histopathological study of the conduction system of the heart in Duchenne progressive muscular dystrophy. *Acta Pathol Jpn* 1982;32:1027–1033.
158. Nigro G, Comi LI, Politano L, et al. The incidence and evolution of cardiomyopathy in Duchenne muscular dystrophy. *Int J Cardiol* 1990;26:271–277.
159. Farah MG, Evans EB, Vignos PJ Jr. Echocardiographic evaluation of left ventricular function in Duchenne's muscular dystrophy. *Am J Med* 1980; 69:248–254.
160. Perloff JK, Henze E, Schelbert HR. Alterations in regional myocardial metabolism, perfusion, and wall motion in Duchenne muscular dystrophy studied by radionuclide imaging. *Circulation* 1984;69:33–42.
161. Walton JN, Gardner-Medwin D. Progressive muscular dystrophy and the myotonic disorders. In: Walton J, ed. *Disorders of Voluntary Muscle.* 4th ed. Edinburgh: Churchill Livingstone; 1981: 481–524.
162. Kinoshita H, Goto Y, Ishikawa M, et al. A carrier of Duchenne muscular dystrophy with dilated cardiomyopathy but no skeletal muscle symptoms. *Brain Dev* 1995;17:202–205.
163. Katiyar BC, Misra S, Somani PN, et al. Congestive cardiomyopathy in a family of Becker's X-linked muscular dystrophy. *Postgrad Med J* 1977;53:12–15.
164. Sakata C, Sunohara N, Nonaka I, et al. A case of Becker muscular dystrophy presenting cardiac failure as an initial symptom. *Rinsho Shinkeigaku* 1990;30:210–213.
165. Casazza F, Brambilla G, Salvato A, et al. Cardiac transplantation in Becker muscular dystrophy. *J Neurol* 1988;235:496–498.
166. Motta J, Guilleminault C, Billingham M, et al. Cardiac abnormalities in myotonic dystrophy. Electrophysiologic and histopathologic studies. *Am J Med* 1979;67:467–473.
167. Church SC. The heart in myotonia atrophica. *Arch Intern Med* 1967;119: 176–181.
168. Fisch C. The heart in dystrophia myotonica. *Am Heart J* 1951;41:525–538.
169. Griggs RC, Davis RJ, Anderson DC, et al. Cardiac conduction in myotonic dystrophy. *Am J Med* 1975;59:37–42.
170. Gottdiener JS, Hawley RJ, Gay JA, et al. Left ventricular relaxation, mitral valve prolapse, and intracardiac conduction in myotonia atrophica: assessment by digitized echocardiography and noninvasive His bundle recording. *Am Heart J* 1982;104:77–85.
171. Hawley RJ, Gottdiener JS, Gay JA, et al. Families with myotonic dystrophy with and without cardiac involvement. *Arch Intern Med* 1983;143: 2134–2136.
172. Nguyen HH, Wolfe JT III, Holmes DR Jr, et al. Pathology of the cardiac conduction system in myotonic dystrophy: a study of 12 cases. *J Am Coll Cardiol* 1988;11:662–671.
173. Harper PS. *Myotonic Dystrophy.* Philadelphia: WB Saunders; 1979.
174. Orndahl G, Thulesius O, Enestrom S, et al. The heart in myotonic disease. *Acta Med Scand* 1964;176:479.
175. Egan TJ, Klein R. Hyperkalemic familial periodic paralysis. *Pediatrics* 1959; 24:761–773.
176. Conn JW, Streeten DHP. Periodic paralysis. In: Stanbury JB, Fredrickson DS, Wyngaarden JB, ed. *The Metabolic Basis of Inherited Disease.* New York: McGraw-Hill; 1960:867–918.

177. Klein R, Ganelin R, Marks JF, et al. Periodic paralysis with cardiac arrhythmia. *J Pediatr* 1963;62:371–385.
178. Kastor JA, Goldreyer BN. Ventricular origin of bidirectional tachycardia. Case report of a patient not toxic from digitalis. *Circulation* 1973;48:897–903.
179. Lisak RP, Lebeau J, Tucker SH, et al. Hyperkalemic periodic paralysis and cardiac arrhythmias. *Neurology* 1972;22:810–815.
180. Fukuda K, Ogawa S, Yokozuka H, et al. Long-standing bidirectional tachycardia in a patient with hypokalemic periodic paralysis. *J Electrocardiol* 1988;21:71–75.
181. Jackson CE, Strehler DA. Limb-girdle muscular dystrophy: Clinical manifestations and detection of preclinical disease. *Pediatrics* 1968;41:495–502.
182. Perloff JK, de Leon AC Jr, O'Doherty D. The cardiomyopathy of progressive muscular dystrophy. *Circulation* 1966;33:625–648.
183. Fairfax AJ, Lambert CD. Neurological aspects of sinoatrial heart blocks. *J Neurol Neurosurg Psychiatry* 1976;39:576–580.
184. James TN. Observations on the cardiovascular involvement, including the cardiac conduction system, in progressive muscular dystrophy. *Am Heart J* 1962;63:48–56.
185. Baldwin BJ, Talley RC, Johnson C, et al. Permanent paralysis of the atrium in a patient with facioscapulohumeral muscular dystrophy. *Am J Cardiol* 1973;31:649–653.
186. Caponnetto S, Pastorini C, Tirelli G. Persistent atrial standstill in a patient affected with facioscapulohumeral dystrophy. *Cardiologia* 1968;53:341–350.
187. Allensworth DC, Rice GJ, Lowe GW. Persistent atrial standstill in a family with myocardial disease. *Am J Med* 1969;47:775–784.
188. Waters D, Nutter DO, Hopkins LC, et al. Cardiac features of an unusual X-linked humeroperoneal neuromuscular disease. *N Engl J Med* 1975;293:1017–1022.
189. Thomas PK, Calne DB, Elliott CF. X-linked scapuloperoneal syndrome. *J Neurol Neurosurg Psychiatry* 1972;35:208–215.
190. Thomas PK, Schott GD, Morgan-Hughes JA. Adult onset scapuloperoneal myopathy. *J Neurol Neurosurg Psychiatry* 1975;38:1008–1015.
191. Sher JH, Rimalovski AB, Athanassiades TJ, et al. Familial centronuclear myopathy: A clinical and pathological study. *Neurology* 1967; 17:727–742.
192. Verhiest W, Brucher JM, Goddeeris P, et al. Familial centronuclear myopathy associated with "cardiomyopathy." *Br Heart J* 1976;38:504–509.
193. Bethlem J, van Wijngaarden GK, Meijer AE, et al. Neuromuscular disease with type I fiber atrophy, central nuclei, and myotube-like structures. *Neurology* 1969;19:705–710.
194. Shafiq SA, Sande MA, Carruthers RR, et al. Skeletal muscle in idiopathic cardiomyopathy. *J Neurol Sci* 1972;15:303–320.
195. Kinney TD, Maher MM. Dermatomyositis: a study of five cases. *Am J Pathol* 1940;16:561–594.
196. Hill DL, Barrows HS. Identical skeletal and cardiac muscle involvement in a case of fatal polymyositis. *Arch Neurol* 1968;19:545–551.
197. Schaumburg HH, Nielsen SL, Yurchak PM. Heart block in polymyositis. *N Engl J Med* 1971;284:480–481.
198. Lynch PG. Cardiac involvement in chronic polymyositis. *Br Heart J* 1971;33:416–419.
199. Diessner GR, Howard FM Jr, Winkelmann RK, et al. Laboratory tests in polymyositis. *Arch Intern Med* 1966;117:757–763.
200. Gottdiener JS, Sherber HS, Hawley RJ, et al. Cardiac manifestations in polymyositis. *Am J Cardiol* 1978;41:1141–1149.
201. Babka JC, Pepine CJ. Hyperkinetic cardiovascular state in polymyositis. *Chest* 1973;64:243–246.
202. Winkelmann RK, Mulder DW, Lambert EH, et al. Course of dermatomyositis-polymyositis: Comparison of untreated and cortisone-treated patients. *Mayo Clin Proc* 1968;43:545–556.
203. Kearns TP, Sayer GP. Retinitis pigmentosa, external ophthalmoplegia, and complete heart block. *Arch Ophthalmol* 1958;60:280–289.
204. Clark DS, Myerburg RJ, Morales RR, et al. Heart block in Kearns-Sayre syndrome, electrophysiologic-pathologic correlation. *Chest* 1975;68:727–730.
205. Roberts NK, Perloff JK, Kark RA. Cardiac conduction in the Kearns-Sayre syndrome (a neuromuscular disorder associated with progressive external ophthalmoplegia and pigmentary retinopathy). *Am J Cardiol* 1979;44: 1396–1400.
206. Charles R, Holt S, Kay JM, et al. Myocardial ultrastructure and the development of atrioventricular block in Kearns-Sayre syndrome. *Circulation* 1981;63:214–219.
207. McComish M, Compston A, Jewitt D. Cardiac abnormalities in chronic progressive external ophthalmoplegia. *Br Heart J* 1976;38:526–529.
208. Wakabayashi K, Takahashi H. Neuropathology of autonomic nervous system in Parkinson's disease. *European Neurology* 1997;38(Suppl 2):2–7.
209. Sato H, Serita T, Seto M, et al. Loss of 123I-MIBG uptake in Parkinson's disease: Assessment of cardiac sympathetic denervation and diagnostic value. *J Nuclear Med* 1999;40:371–375.
210. Ishizaki F, Harada T, Yoshinaga H, et al. Prolonged QTc intervals in Parkinson's disease–relation to sudden death and autonomic dysfunction. *Shinkei Brain Nerve* 1996;48:443–448.
211. Francheschi M, Ferini-Strambi L, Minicucci F, et al. Signs of cardiac dysfunction during sleep in patients with Alzheimer's disease. *Gerontology* 1986;32:327–334.
212. Hofman A, Ott A, Breteler MM, et al. Atherosclerosis, apolipoprotein E, and prevalence of dementia and Alzheimer's disease in the Rotterdam Study. *Lancet* 1997;349:151–154.

CHAPTER 35E ■ CARDIOVASCULAR MANIFESTATIONS OF RHEUMATIC DISEASES

NICOLA J. GOODSON AND DANIEL H. SOLOMON

INTRODUCTION

The rheumatic diseases encompass a broad spectrum of conditions, all of which primarily cause joint and musculoskeletal pathology. It has long been recognized that cardiac pathology occurs in association with many rheumatic conditions. Until recently, most accepted that cardiac involvement took the form of structural abnormalities such as pericardial disease or valvulopathies. However, many chronic inflammatory rheumatic conditions appear to be associated with premature atherosclerotic disease and a reduced life expectancy. There is emerging evidence that chronic inflammation is associated with the occurrence of cardiac events in people both with and without chronic inflammatory joint disease. However, both atherosclerosis and many rheumatic diseases have a complicated etiology and it is likely that inflammation contributes to other environmental and host risk factors in these patients.

Cardiovascular disease (CVD) is common in many inflammatory arthritides and, as much of this remains clinically silent, it is difficult to measure the true incidence and prevalence of cardiovascular involvement in each rheumatic condition (Table 35E.1). This chapter discusses the cardiovascular involvement in many of the more common rheumatologic conditions. Many treatments used in rheumatic conditions also have potential cardiovascular effects, and these are discussed later.

CARDIAC INVOLVEMENT IN OSTEOARTHRITIS

It is unclear whether there is a direct link between osteoarthritis and CVD. Obesity is a common risk factor for both conditions. The sedentary lifestyle that often accompanies osteoarthritis of the lower extremities may predispose toward CVD. There are some data to suggest that the cardiovascular risk profile in patients with osteoarthritis is more severe than the non-osteoarthritis population (1). However, one large population-based study did not find an increase in the risk of cardiovascular outcomes in patients with osteoarthritis compared with non-arthritis subjects (2).

CARDIAC INVOLVEMENT IN RHEUMATOID ARTHRITIS

Rheumatoid arthritis (RA) is one of the more common rheumatic conditions, affecting approximately 0.5% to 1.0% of the adult population. The incidence of RA rises with

TABLE 35E.1

PREVALENCE OF RHEUMATIC DISORDERS AND SUMMARY OF CARDIOVASCULAR INVOLVEMENT

Disorder	Prevalence of rheumatic condition/100,000	Pericardium	Valvular	Myocardium	Coronary artery	Conducting system
Osteoarthritis	8,000	Not described	Not affected	Not affected	? Increased prevalence of IHD	Not affected
Rheumatoid arthritis	1,000	Pericardial effusion and thickening 1%–20%	Mitral and aortic insufficiency 5%–30%	LV dysfunction and CCF 5%	Coronary arteritis is rare ATS and CAD is common	CHB rare. Autonomic disturbance uncommon
Ankylosing spondylitis	1,000	Pericardial thickening 5%	Aortic regurgitation in 10%; mitral regurgitation rare	Diastolic dysfunction 55%	40% increased rate of MI	First-degree AV block 15%; CHB 1%
Gout	275–800	Not described	Rare reports of valve tophi	Not described	Associated with CAD	Not described
Systemic lupus erythematosis	20–80	Clinical pericarditis 25%, subclinical 60%	Valve thickening 50%; Libman Sacks endocarditis 30%	Myocarditis in 1%–10%	Coronary arteritis is rare, ATS common, CAD prevalence is 1–8 times higher in SLE	Rare
Systemic sclerosis	8	Rare clinical presentation, effusion seen in 30%–80% at autopsy	Rare	Myocarditis, myofibrosis and diastolic dysfunction 10%–30%	Coronary artery spasm, and small vessel occlusions. 60% have cold-induced ischemia	AV block 10%
Giant cell arteritis	200 (aged >50 y)	Rare	Rare	Rare	ATS CAD common	Rare
Takayasu	0.2–0.6	Rare	Extension of aortic dilatation may involve aortic valve	Dilated cardiomyopathy; occurs rarely	Coronary artery stenoses and aneurismal dilatation occur rarely	Not described
Polyarteritis nodosa	6.3/100,000	Subclinical pericarditis 33%		Congestive cardiac failure 10%	Myocardial infarction 5%–10%	Uncommon
Kawasaki disease	Incidence in U.S.: 10/100,000; incidence in Japan: 100/100,000	Pericardial effusion common in acute febrile phase	Mitral and tricuspid regurgitation in 30%–50%	Myocarditis common in acute febrile phase	Coronary artery aneurysms in subacute phase 20%; sudden death due to MI	Contribute to sudden death
Wegeners granulomatosis	3–5	Pericarditis common 10%–50%	Aortic and mitral regurgitation	Granulomatous invasion of myocardium common 25%. CCF and dilated cardiomyopathy are rare.	Coronary arteritis is commonly seen in 50%, but rarely causes MI; accelerated ATS	Atrial Arrhythmias and CHB
Churg–Strauss	1.3	Common 20%–30%	Valvular insufficiency is rare	Myocarditis, Myofibrosis, and ischemic cardiomyopathy are common	Coronary arteritis and MI is a common cause of death	Supraventricular and ventricular arrhythmias occur

Abbreviations: ATS, atherosclerosis; CAD, coronary artery disease; CCF, congestive cardiac failure; CHB, complete heart block; LV, left ventricular; MI, myocardial infarction.

increasing age, and females are affected two to three times more frequently than males. The underlying etiology is not known. However, genetic, host, and environmental risk factors for RA have been identified that influence susceptibility and progression of the disease (3).

RA is characterized by widespread chronic inflammation of synovial tissues, in a symmetrical distribution, that leads to joint damage and disability. Although RA is primarily an inflammatory disease of joint tissues, it has systemic effects and can involve many organ systems including the cardiovascular system.

Patients with RA have a reduced life expectancy when compared to the general population. This equates to an average loss of 4 to 8 years of life. Although it is known that RA patients have increased mortality from infections, renal disease, gastrointestinal disorders, and lymphoproliferative disease, these causes of death represent only a small proportion of all RA deaths (4). CVD is responsible for 35% to 50% of all RA deaths and most of the excess mortality observed in RA cohorts is due to increased rates of CVD mortality (5–8).

Excess mortality is not just limited to clinic based cohorts of established RA patients as study of community based RA cohorts and early inflammatory polyarthritis cohorts have also demonstrated excess CVD mortality (9,10). This suggests that mechanisms which promote CVD mortality are not restricted to patients with severe RA and are also present early in the RA disease process (11).

Structural cardiac lesions including pericarditis and nonspecific mitral and aortic valve abnormalities are commonly described in autopsy series and echocardiographic studies of RA patients. However, these lesions usually remain clinically silent and rarely lead to significant hemodynamic disturbances. Therefore, it is difficult to record the prevalence of this "rheumatoid heart disease" and assess how it contributes to the excess CVD mortality observed in RA patients.

More recently, there has been much interest in coronary heart disease (CHD) in RA. This condition has been shown to be highly prevalent in RA cohorts. It is also often asymptomatic and frequently diagnosed at autopsy. However, CHD in RA is not a benign disease and appears to be responsible for much of the observed excess mortality. Indeed, CHD appears be the single largest cause of CVD deaths in RA populations (8,12,13).

Pericardial Disease

Rheumatoid pericarditis was first described by Charcot in 1881 (14) and is thought to be a common CVD manifestation of RA (Fig. 35E.1). Autopsy studies have reported pericardial disease in up to 50% of RA patients (15) and more recently echocardiographic studies have reported that pericardial disease occurs in up to 30% of RA cases (16). However, clinically significant pericarditis is observed infrequently in RA, affecting fewer than 2% of patients (17,18). It is possible that the prevalence of pericarditis in RA is declining because of more effective disease-modifying antirheumatic drugs (DMARD) or because RA is becoming a less severe disease (19). Pericarditis is associated with increased disease severity and is more common in male RA patients. Patients are usually rheumatoid factor positive and they frequently have rheumatoid nodules and erosive joint disease. Systemic symptoms are common and include fatigue, weight loss, and other extraarticular system involvement (18).

The pericardial fluid is classically exudative containing leukocytes, elevated levels of lactate dehydrogenase, and a low concentration of glucose, but these findings are not universal (18). Chronic inflammation can cause thickening of the pericardium that can lead to constrictive pericarditis, which is a rare sequela of severe or recurrent pericarditis in RA (20). Calcification of the pericardium is rarely seen in RA pericarditis (21). Pericardial effusions that develop owing to infection are rarely seen in RA. However, if there is any suspicion that the pericarditis may be infectious, cultures for tuberculosis and fungi as well as standard culture of pericardial fluid should be obtained; many RA patients are immunosuppressed by their DMARDs.

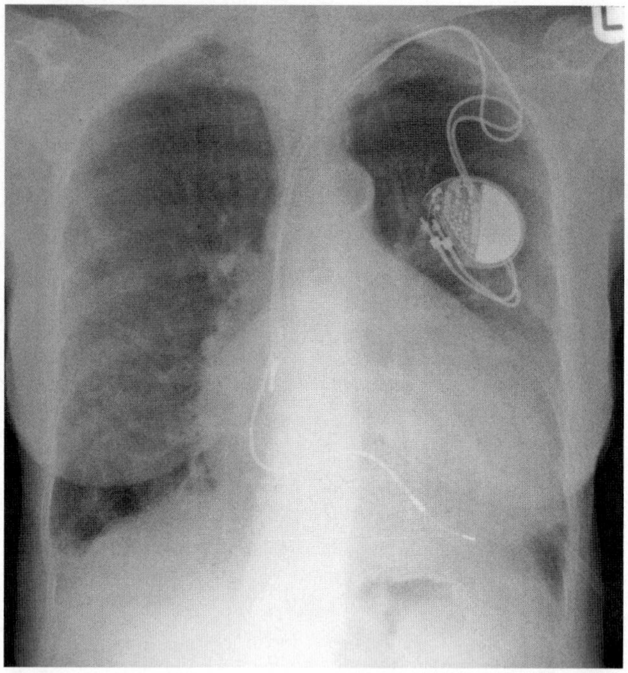

FIGURE 35E.1. Pericardial effusion in RA. The globular cardiomegaly represents a modest pericardial effusion that was due to pericarditis in this seropositive RA patient. The dual chamber pacemaker was inserted for CHB. (*Source:* Reproduced with kind permission from Dr John Curtis, Consultant Radiologist, University Hospital Aintree.)

The vast majority of patients respond to treatment with non-steroidal anti-inflammatory drugs (NSAIDs). After infection has been ruled out, short courses of oral steroids may be used, and DMARD therapy should be increased to control active rheumatoid disease. Colchicine has been used to treat recurrent non-RA pericarditis; however, it is not clear whether this is beneficial in RA pericarditis (22).

Endocardial and Valve Involvement

There are rare case reports of rheumatoid nodules affecting the endocardium or heart valves causing valve dysfunction. In particular, there have been several reports of aortic valve nodulosis causing regurgitation requiring aortic valve replacement (23,24) and mitral valve nodules causing embolic disease (25). There has also been one report in the literature of an endocardial nodule mimicking an atrial myxoma (26).

Based on autopsy studies, diffuse endocardial involvement in RA appears to be a relatively common manifestation of RA (27). Valvular abnormalities are frequently seen on echocardiographic studies and it has been hypothesized that heart valve involvement may be an additional extraarticular manifestation of RA (28). Hospital-based studies report a prevalence of nonspecific aortic and/or minimal mitral regurgitation in 5% to 30% of RA patients (29–31). Mitral valve insufficiency seems to be associated with nodular RA, which suggests that heart valve involvement reflects more severe RA disease (32). It appears that the valve lesion is due to infiltration of inflammatory cells that leads to thickening and calcification at the base of the valve and valve ring (27,33). However, symptomatic valve disease is a very rare manifestation of RA.

Myocardial and Conduction System Involvement

Myocarditis occurs in RA either as the result of focal granulomatous disease affecting the myocardium or more diffuse fibrosing lesions, and is a common finding at autopsy (33). It is commonly asymptomatic, but may lead to the development of cardiac failure or disruption of the conducting system of the heart.

It seems that ECG evidence of conduction abnormalities and arrhythmias are common in patients with RA. One study reported that 50% of RA patients had evidence of cardiac arrhythmias on 24-hour ECG monitoring, although this arrhythmia prevalence was similar to that seen in a hospital-based non-RA control group (34). Another study reported a higher prevalence of abnormal ventricular repolarization in RA patients compared to control patients (35). Complete heart block (CHB) has been described in association with RA, possibly due to disruption of the atrioventricular (AV) node by rheumatoid granulomata (36,37). Autonomic nervous system disturbance has been observed in RA cohorts (38,39), which may be a risk factor for silent CVD events (40,41).

Coronary Artery Disease

There is increasing evidence that RA patients have an increased prevalence of CHD due to atherosclerosis. This appears to be responsible for much of the excess CVD mortality observed in RA. Several studies have shown that RA patients have a two- to threefold increase in rates of myocardial infarction (MI) when compared to the general population (42,43). In addition, Maradit-Kremers et al. (41) have highlighted that RA patients are more likely to experience silent ischemia and sudden cardiac death. In one UK RA cohort cardiovascular admissions were not increased despite increased cardiovascular mortality (8). Therefore, it is possible that the true prevalence of CHD events in RA is underestimated by these hospital-based studies. Also patients who fail to present with typical CHD symptoms are unlikely to benefit from interventions to improve CHD outcomes. There is a need to educate both physicians and patients to be more aware that CHD events may not present typically in association with RA.

Several CVD risk factors, including cigarette smoking and obesity, have also been identified as risk factors for the development of RA (44). Some of these, including age, smoking, hypertension, and lipid levels have been associated with subclinical atherosclerosis in RA (45). Cigarette smoking is associated with more severe RA and it may be this disease severity and inflammation that promotes atherosclerosis in RA. However, studies of RA populations have not found that traditional CVD risk factors explain the increased CVD events seen in these patients (42,43). One study revealed that a low body mass index (BMI) was associated with increased CVD mortality and it has been hypothesized that a low BMI reflects increased inflammatory disease burden in RA (46). This demonstrates how difficult it is to separate the effects of the RA disease activity from the effects of CVD risk factors when investigating CVD in RA.

CVD epidemiology in the general population has revealed the importance of several novel CHD risk factors including homocysteine, thrombotic markers, insulin resistance, and markers of inflammation (47). There is a high prevalence of these "novel" risk factors in patients with inflammatory joint disease. Patients with RA have been found to have abnormal homocysteine metabolism (48), which may be exacerbated further by the use of methotrexate or sulphasalazine (49). However, it is not known whether elevated homocysteine levels predict future CHD events in RA patients. Thrombotic markers may be increased in RA due to systemic inflammation and have been associated with CHD events in RA (50). Insulin resistance has been recognized to complicate RA. It is also associated with inflammation, obesity, steroid use, and CVD (51). Of particular interest in RA is the association between inflammation and CVD. Atherosclerosis is now thought to be an inflammatory condition (52) and prospective study has recognized markers of inflammation, including C-reactive protein (CRP), are predictors of future CHD events in both the general (53) and in inflammatory polyarthritis populations (54). Other studies have found that erythrocyte sedimentation rate (ESR) measurements predict CHD events in RA (55). It seems that in RA an elevated CRP is associated with endothelial dysfunction (56), which may promote atherosclerosis in RA patients.

Understanding the pathogenesis of CHD in RA is complicated; several factors, including inflammation, RA disease severity, and cardiovascular risk factors, all interact with each other. It may be that with a combined approach, allowing for modification of CHD risk factors and reduction of inflammation using immunosuppressive agents, the cardiovascular mortality in RA can be reduced. Although coronary arteritis is observed at autopsy in 10% of RA cases (27), this rarely leads to MI or damage.

CARDIAC INVOLVEMENT IN ANKYLOSING SPONDYLITIS

Ankylosing spondylitis (AS) is a common chronic inflammatory disease that involves the sacroiliac joints and the axial skeleton and may cause enthesitis and peripheral joint inflammation. Extraarticular organ and peripheral joint involvement are markers of more severe AS. Although acute anterior uveitis is the most common extraarticular manifestation, occurring in 20% to 30% of cases, clinically significant cardiovascular involvement occurs in approximately 10% of patients with AS. The prevalence of AS is higher in males than females and the condition is more common in populations with a higher prevalence of HLA B27; that is, higher among Caucasians and Native Americans than African Americans and Asians.

A number of clinic-based studies have demonstrated increased mortality rates and excess CVD mortality in AS patients compared to the general population (57,58). Much of this excess CVD mortality was due to AS-specific cardiovascular complications (57).

Several characteristic cardiovascular lesions are described as being complications of AS. These include valvular heart disease, which occurs in approximately 10% of patients. However, the cardiovascular system may also be affected by the systemic inflammation associated with AS. Pericarditis is rarely seen in association with AS, although echocardiographic studies have revealed pericardial thickening and effusion in 5% of asymptomatic patients (59).

Valvular Involvement

Clinically significant aortic regurgitation occurs in approximately 2% to 10% of patients with AS. The prevalence of valve disease increases with longer disease duration and AS severity. Stenotic aortic valve lesions have not been described in association with AS. Inflammation of the ascending aorta at the level of the sinuses of Valsalva causes distortion and dilatation of the aortic ring. Fibrotic thickening and downward retraction of the valve cusp bases with inward rolling of the edges of the valve cusps occur, and these factors contribute to the development of aortic incompetence (60). These "characteristic" pathologic findings have also been described in association with other seronegative spondarthropathies. Fibrosis may extend down from the nonseptal portion of the aorta to involve the mitral leaflet. This can occasionally give rise to mitral valve insufficiency. Mitral insufficiency may also develop secondary to left ventricular dilatation caused by aortic regurgitation. Asymptomatic mitral prolapse is observed in approximately 10% of patients with AS.

Arrhythmias

AV conduction blocks have been reported in association with AS and other spondarthropathies and are thought to represent the most common cardiac complication of AS. However, the prevalence of these conduction defects varies markedly between studies. One early study of 190 patients described first-degree AV block in 15% of AS patients whereas another study found ECG evidence of AV block in only 6% (61). It seems that HLA B27 related disease processes are more prevalent in cardiology patients requiring permanent pacemakers (62) and there is some evidence that AV block may occur intermittently in AS patients. This suggests that the conduction disturbance may be initially due to a reversible inflammatory process rather than disruption owing to fibrosis (60). Other arrhythmias include increased frequencies of both atrial and ventricular arrhythmias with evidence of prolonged QT dispersion being noted in nearly 60% of AS patients in one study (61). This suggests that the whole conducting system may be affected in AS and damage is not limited to AV nodal tissue.

Disturbance of the autonomic nervous system has been described in AS, with evidence of decreased parasympathetic activity (63). These findings were more marked in AS patients with active inflammatory disease and as similar findings have been observed in other systemic inflammatory conditions this disturbance of the autonomic nervous system may be related to systemic inflammation rather than specifically due to AS.

Myocardium

Although patients with known aortic valve insufficiency may develop ventricular failure as a secondary phenomenon, myocardial involvement in AS may also occur in the absence of aortic valve disease. Left ventricular dilatation and impaired diastolic function of the left ventricle have been described in association with AS (64) and diastolic ventricular dysfunction is observed even in patients with less severe AS disease.

Coronary Artery Disease

AS is not typically associated with accelerated atherosclerosis. One small study revealed ECG evidence of ischemic heart disease in 18% of AS patients (65). However, a study utilizing data from the UK General Practice Research Database did reveal that men with AS had a 40% increase in rates of first MI compared to men without AS (66). Rates of traditional CVD risk factors appear to be similar in AS patients (64), so it is possible that chronic inflammation associated with AS may promote accelerated atherosclerosis in this condition. NSAIDs are the main treatment for AS symptom control and many patients will have long-term exposure to these drugs. Therefore, these patients may be at increased risk of NSAID-associated cardiovascular side effects, including hypertension (67), and congestive cardiac failure given the association between AS and left ventricular dysfunction (68).

CARDIAC INVOLVEMENT IN GOUT

Gout is a common rheumatic disease with a prevalence of 2.8 to 8 per 1,000 population. It is more common in men and premenopausal women are usually spared. Its classical clinical presentation is with acute, exquisitely painful swelling affecting the first metatarsophalangeal joint, although other joints can be affected. Gout is a crystal arthropathy and demonstration of monosodium urate crystals in the joint fluid or soft tissues is required for a firm diagnosis.

Apart from rare case reports of valvular pathology owing to gouty tophi (69), there is little evidence of any other structural cardiac involvement that develops in association with gout. Hyperuricemia is the common metabolic abnormality that leads to the development of gout in some people and there is a substantial body of research that has linked hyperuricemia and gout with CVD. It is widely accepted that diuretic use and hypertension are both risk factors for developing gout (70). However, there are also data linking gout and hyperuricemia to an elevated risk of CVD (71,72). It is not clear in which direction the causal arrow should be drawn. Other factors including obesity, the metabolic syndrome, and renal impairment may also contribute to the development of both gout and coronary artery disease.

There has been growing interest in the link between uric acid levels, xanthine oxidoreductase, and CVD. Xanthine oxidoreductase exists in two forms, xanthine oxidase and xanthine dehydrogenase. Both of these enzymes are responsible for metabolizing uric acid from hypoxanthine and xanthine. Allopurinol, a drug commonly used to treat gout, lowers serum uric acid by inhibiting xanthine oxidoreductase.

Xanthine oxidoreductase is also an important source of reactive oxygen species in the cardiovascular system (73). Through this role, it has been linked with hypertension, endothelial dysfunction, and congestive heart failure (74). Trials of new inhibitors of this enzyme are currently underway to test whether they may be beneficial in congestive heart failure.

Finally, the link between gout and heart disease is nowhere more apparent than in the organ transplant patient. One large study found that 19% of post-transplant patients experienced a gout attack (75). Common anti-rejection immunosuppressives are partly to blame for this association. Cyclosporine and azathioprine both reduce the excretion of uric acid from the distal tubules and are associated with hyperuricemia and gout attacks (76,77). Preventing attacks is difficult. Allopurinol can be used to help prevent further attacks of gout. However, there is concern over the use of allopurinol in patients concomitantly taking azathioprine. Xanthine oxidase is not only an important enzyme in uric acid production, but also in metabolism of azathioprine. Thus, inhibition of xanthine oxidase by allopurinol generally increases the levels of 6-mercaptopurine, the active form of azathioprine, by two- to threefold. Therefore, azathioprine doses should be cut in half and 6-mercaptopurine levels should be measured after initiating allopurinol. Some clinicians avoid this potential interaction by using mycophenolate mofetil, rather than azathioprine, as an immunosuppressive drug in transplant patients.

Colchicine myoneuropathic toxicity is not uncommon in patients with borderline renal function concomitantly taking azathioprine or tacrolimus (78). In addition, cyclosporine inhibits the enterohepatic circulation of colchicine and thus toxicity is

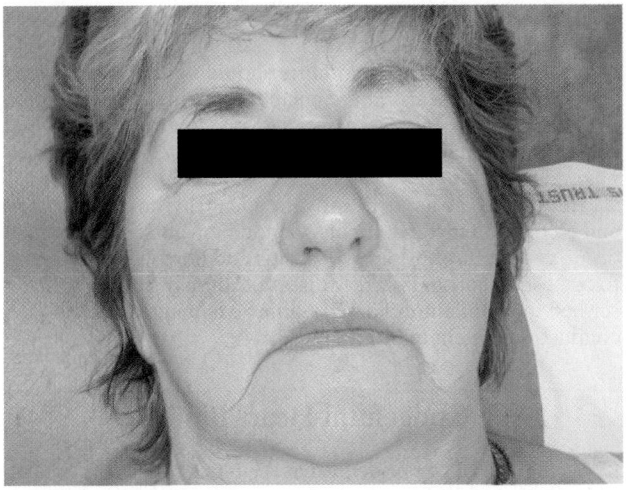

FIGURE 35E.2. Lupus facial rash. This patient with SLE developed a typical erythematous rash in a butterfly distribution over the cheeks. (*Source:* Reproduced with kind permission from Dr Jeffrey S. Marks, Consultant Rheumatologist, Stepping Hill Hospital.)

more common in patients using both medications concurrently. Thus, despite their own set of toxicities, short-term administration of NSAIDs and/or higher dose glucocorticoids may be considered in acute gout attacks in the posttransplant patient.

CARDIAC INVOLVEMENT IN SYSTEMIC LUPUS ERYTHEMATOSIS

Systemic lupus erythematosis (SLE) is a chronic inflammatory autoimmune condition of unknown origin. It can affect nearly every organ system in the body but commonly involves the skin (Fig. 35E.2); musculoskeletal, cardiorespiratory, and neurologic systems; kidneys; and serous membranes. Like many inflammatory rheumatic diseases the clinical course can be extremely variable with episodes of both acute and chronic relapse interspersed by periods of remission.

Clinical cardiac involvement is relatively common in SLE, developing in 50% of patients during the course of their illness, although cardiac symptoms are rarely a feature at disease presentation. Autopsy studies have revealed that many SLE patients have evidence of subclinical CVD and nearly all the structures of the heart can be affected by lupus. Clinical symptoms due to pericarditis, myocarditis, and valve involvement are seen, but much of the excess mortality observed in lupus patients is due to the effects of accelerated atherosclerosis. Although the overall prognosis has improved for lupus patients over recent years (79), these patients still experience a reduced life expectancy. Urowitz et al. (80) described a bimodal mortality pattern in SLE. Early mortality occurs due to the direct effects of the lupus disease process or secondary infection; a later peak of increased mortality occurs due to the effects of accelerated atherosclerosis causing premature myocardial infarct or stroke. Because premenopausal women have a very low incidence of CHD and a low incidence of stroke, the relative risk of these events in SLE women is strikingly high.

Pericardial Disease

Approximately one quarter of patients with SLE experience symptomatic pericarditis at some point in their disease course. Most cases of pericarditis occur as part of a generalized serositis with associated pleural effusion or ascites.

Although pericardial disease in lupus is frequently asymptomatic, it is one of the most common echocardiographic lesions observed in patients with SLE. Scarring and pericardial thickening in the absence of effusion may be seen in healed disease. The pericardial fluid may be a fibrinous exudate or less commonly a transudate and contains a normal glucose concentration. The white cell count is usually increased with predominantly polymorphonuclear cells. Autoantibodies including antinuclear antibodies, and anti–double-stranded DNA as well as immune complexes and lupus erythematosis cells may also be seen. Occasionally, a hemorrhagic effusion is seen (81).

Pericarditis in SLE is usually benign and responds to NSAIDs, although courses of corticosteroids (0.5–1 mg/kg prednisolone) are sometimes required. Tamponade and constrictive pericarditis are rare. However, purulent pericarditis in the immunosuppressed SLE patient can give rise to large effusions and occasionally tamponade. Drainage is recommended where infection is suspected (82).

Valvular Disease

Anatomic and functional valve abnormalities are frequently described in association with SLE. A longitudinal study utilized transesophageal echocardiography to examine 69 lupus patients (83). The most frequent abnormality described was thickening of the valve cusps, which was seen in 51% of patients. This valve thickening had a similar predilection for the mitral and aortic valves, but was rarely seen in the tricuspid valve. Valve thickening was diffuse and frequently associated with decreased mobility. Calcification of the valve was rarely seen.

Libman–Sacks endocarditis is the most characteristic valve lesion associated with SLE. This was originally described as "atypical verrucous endocarditis" by Libman and Sacks in the 1920s (84). These valvular vegetations were seen in 43% of SLE patients on the initial echocardiograph (83). The vegetations are characterized by ovoid verrucae, which are rather flattened and smaller than the lesions seen in infective endocarditis or rheumatic fever (Fig. 35E.3) They usually have a diameter

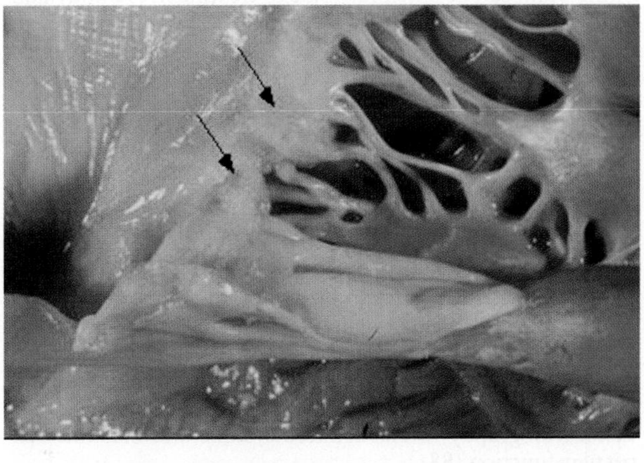

FIGURE 35E.3. Libman–Sacks endocarditis. This patient was observed to have a cardiac murmur. However, the valvular vegetations found at autopsy were not observed on prior echocardiography. (*Source:* Schur PH. Cardiac manifestations of systemic erythematosis in adults. In: Rose BD, ed. *UpToDate.* Waltham, MA: UpToDate; 2005. Copyright 2005 UpToDate, Inc. For more information visit www.uptodate.com.)

of 1 to 4 mm and tend to gather in clumps on the atrial side of the mitral valve closing edges and on the vessel side of the aortic valve, although they do occur in other sites in smaller numbers (83). Histology reveals that the lesions may be active with focal necrosis and infiltrates of mononuclear cells or healed with vascularized fibrous tissue, which occasionally become calcified (85). These valvular pathologies were observed to change over time and were not related temporally to the clinical features of SLE (83). Some studies have suggested an association between valvular heart disease and antiphospholipid antibodies (86).

The clinical features of valve involvement are varied. Both verrucous endocarditis and valve thickening can be associated with a systolic murmur and valvular regurgitation has been reported in up to 74% of SLE patients. Although most patients remain asymptomatic, a significant number go on to develop moderate to severe regurgitation; valve stenosis is rarely seen (87). Mitral valve prolapse is observed more commonly in SLE patients. Systolic murmurs occur as a result of increased cardiac output in association with fever, tachycardia or anemia as part of active systemic disease.

Complications of valve disease include mitral valve cord rupture, infective endocarditis, ischemic cerebrovascular stroke, and heart failure. It is thought that valve pathology in SLE significantly contributes to the excess CVD mortality observed in these patients. The prevalence of infective endocarditis in SLE patients is thought to be similar to that in patients with prosthetic valves. The signs and symptoms of infective endocarditis including fever, cardiac murmurs, and splinter hemorrhages may also observed in a lupus flare in patients with Libman–Sacks endocarditis. Therefore, repeated blood cultures are essential. Patients with a lupus flare tend to have a reduced white cell count, serologic markers of lupus activity, elevated ESR, but relatively low levels of CRP and repeatedly negative blood cultures. Management of the lupus patient with valve pathology includes antibiotic prophylaxis prior to high-risk procedures, and some recommend this for all lupus patients (87). Because the incidence of ischemic cerebrovascular accidents is increased among SLE patients with valvulopathy, these patients should be considered for antiaggregant therapy, particularly in the presence of antiphospholipid antibodies. Another difficult differential diagnosis, in the sick lupus patient with new onset of neurologic symptoms, is the distinction between cerebral vasculitis caused by active lupus and cerebral thromboembolic disease. In this situation transesophageal echocardiography and magnetic resonance imaging of the brain can be a helpful guide to treatment. Hemodynamically significant valve disease requires valve replacement. There is an increased preoperative mortality and recurrent valve inflammation can occur on bioprosthetic valves.

Myocardium and Conduction Abnormalities

The myocarditis associated with SLE occurs in less than one quarter of patients and is often asymptomatic. However, it can present acutely with tachycardia disproportionate to body temperature, chest discomfort, and symptoms of cardiac failure. Acute myocarditis is commonly accompanied by pericarditis. Cardiomegaly may occur and ST- and T-wave electrocardiographic abnormalities and evidence of conduction disturbance may be seen in association with elevated cardiac enzymes. Echocardiography reveals reduced systolic and diastolic ventricular function (88).

Histologic examination in the acute stage of the illness reveals myocardial infiltration by mononuclear cells. This inflammatory damage can lead to significant myocardial fibrosis and the development of a dilated cardiomyopathy after treatment. Treatment of acute myocarditis in lupus should be instituted early and includes use of high-dose parenteral methylprednisolone 1,000 mg/d for 3 days followed by high doses of oral corticosteroids. In addition, standard supportive treatment of congestive cardiac failure should be used and factors that may worsen heart failure, including anemia, hypertension, and infections, should be corrected (88). Other treatments that have been used in acute lupus myocarditis include cyclophosphamide, azathioprine, and intravenous immunoglobulins.

Sinus tachycardia is the most frequent rhythm abnormality and is common in SLE patients. Conduction abnormalities may occur as a result of prior myocarditis and fibrosis or secondary to coexisting coronary artery disease. Autopsy studies have described focal inflammation and fibrotic damage disrupting the conduction system in SLE (81).

Congenital Heart Block

Congenital CHB can be defined as AV block that exists at birth or is diagnosed in utero or within the neonatal period (89). It is a rare disorder that is strongly associated with the presence of maternal antibodies anti-Ro/SSA and anti-La/SSB that cross the placenta. Nearly 85% of mothers of children with congenital CHB have these antibodies. However, only 1 in 50 pregnant women with the candidate serology goes on to have an affected child. The recurrence rate in subsequent pregnancies is about 18% (90). Prenatal diagnosis has allowed interventions in utero to try and prevent progression of AV block. Current guidelines recommend use of serial fetal echocardiography every 2 weeks from the 16th week of gestation in high-risk patients. If any incomplete AV block or recent onset third-degree AV block is detected, therapy with dexamethasone (4 mg/d) or betamethasone is instituted. Other glucocorticoids should be avoided because they are metabolized by the placenta. This treatment has been shown to reverse the severity of AV block in some cases, although persistent third-degree AV block is unlikely to resolve. Other treatments that have been used with some success in utero include plasmapheresis and immunoglobulins.

Currently, there is no supporting evidence to suggest use of prophylactic treatment, even in high-risk mothers (91). Studies have revealed that use of prednisolone early in pregnancy does not influence antibody titers or prevent the development of CHD. The intrauterine and perinatal mortality rate is high for this condition. However, use of fetal echocardiography, measurement of maternal serology, and the use of pacemakers have lead to marked improvements in life expectancy for a number of affected children.

Coronary Heart Disease

Over recent years, CHD has been increasingly recognized as a major cause of mortality and morbidity in patients with SLE. Most of this CHD is due to atherosclerosis rather than to local vasculitis affecting the coronary arteries. This accelerated atherosclerosis in SLE was first recognized in the 1970s by Urowitz et al. (80,92). They described a marked increase in deaths from atherosclerosis in patients with SLE. Much of this excess CVD mortality is due to MI and sudden cardiac death. However, coronary artery disease in lupus may remain clinically silent or present with atypical symptoms (93). Younger women with SLE have been reported to have a 52-fold increase in rates of MI compared to women of the same age in the general population (94).

CHD seems to develop in younger patients with longstanding disease (95). Studies have revealed that SLE patients have more traditional cardiovascular risk factors, including hypertension, smoking, dyslipidemia, diabetes mellitus, and obesity than healthy controls (96). However, one study revealed a 10-fold increase in risk of nonfatal MI after adjusting for the Framingham risk factors (97). SLE patients appear to have a distinct pattern of dyslipidemia, with elevated triglycerides, low high-density lipoprotein cholesterol, and normal low-density lipoprotein cholesterol. There is also evidence of increased low-density lipoprotein oxidation and elevated levels of lipoprotein(a) (98). In addition, the presence of inflammation and cytokines seems to be associated with the development of atherosclerotic lesions in SLE. Other potential CHD risk factors that have been identified include elevated homocysteine and endothelial cell antibodies (98). It is thought that a combination of traditional and novel risk factors contribute to the high CVD risk in SLE patients. The role of treatment in promoting CHD in SLE is interesting. Studies have shown that hydroxychloroquine use was associated with a reduction in total cholesterol concentration whereas high-dose prednisolone use was associated with adverse effects on serum cholesterol, hypertension, and body weight (99). However, steroid use was not associated with the development of atherosclerotic plaque in SLE patients (100). In this study, women with lupus were four times more likely to have evidence of subclinical atherosclerosis than controls, and SLE was identified as an independent predictor of atherosclerosis. Therefore, it seems reasonable to recommend regular assessment and modification of CHD risk factors in SLE patients (101).

CARDIAC INVOLVEMENT IN SYSTEMIC SCLEROSIS

Systemic sclerosis (SSc) has a reported UK prevalence of 8 in 100,000, a female to male ratio of 5.2:1 and an onset in the 5th to 6th decades of life (102). The prevalence has been reported to be higher in the U.S. population (103). However, this remains a rare condition. It can manifest as several subtypes with the major divisions being between limited (Fig. 35E.4) or diffuse disease. Diffuse SSc often has a younger age at onset and is characterized by Raynaud's phenomenon, cutaneous involvement proximal to the forearms, and a positive anti–Scl-70 antibody. Gastrointestinal, respiratory, renal, and cardiac fibrosis often occur. Limited SSc occurs more commonly than diffuse disease, is often preceded by Raynaud's phenomenon, and is associated with a positive anticentromere antibody. This condition also affects the gastrointestinal tract and cardiorespiratory systems. Both diffuse and limited disease are associated with a substantial reduction in life expectancy.

Cardiac Involvement

Cardiac involvement in SSc includes ischemic damage, myocarditis, myocardial fibrosis, pericarditis, systemic hypertension, and pulmonary hypertension. Studies have revealed that myocardial fibrosis and pericardial effusions have been seen in 30% to 80% of patients at autopsy. This is patchy and is thought to represent connective tissue infiltration into damaged myocardium. This low-grade myocardial inflammation may lead to diastolic dysfunction and disturbance of the conduction system. Arrhythmias and heart block are relatively common and contribute to the decreased life expectancy of these patients (104).

There are several mechanisms by which ischemic damage may occur in SSc, including coronary artery vasospasm, small vessel disease, and occlusive coronary artery disease. Endothelial dysfunction and fibroproliferation have been proposed as pathobiological models of scleroderma and it has been suggested that macrovascular coronary artery disease occurs as a result of these processes (105).

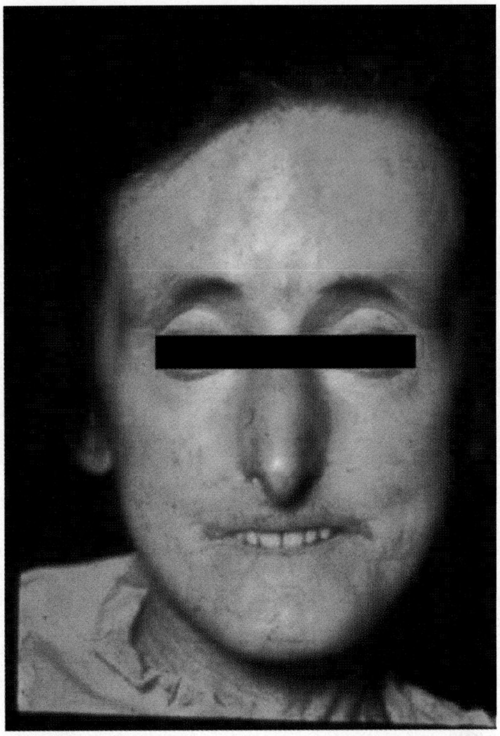

FIGURE 35E.4. Woman with limited SSc of the CREST variant. She had skin tightening around her mouth and nose and telangectasia on her face. Other features of this condition, not shown in this image, include sclerodactyly, calcinosis, Raynaud's and esophageal involvement. (*Source:* Reproduced with kind permission from Dr Jeffrey S. Marks, Consultant Rheumatologist, Stepping Hill Hospital.)

Renal involvement is a major cause of mortality in SSc. Scleroderma renal crisis with accelerated hypertension with oliguric renal failure and high levels of renin occurs in 12% of diffuse SSc and 2% of limited SSc patients (106). Use of angiotensin-converting enzyme inhibitors at maximal dose, aiming for a decrease of systolic blood pressure of 20 mm Hg/24 hours has transformed the survival of these patients. Concurrent prostacyclin administration helps to control blood pressure and potentially improves renal blood flow and endothelial function. Some centers advocate the use of angiotensin-converting enzyme inhibitors early in the course of diffuse SSc to try to prevent renal crisis. However, currently there is little evidence to support this approach (106).

Pulmonary Hypertension

Pulmonary artery hypertension (PAH) is a common manifestation of SSc. Although PAH in SSc may occur secondary to lung fibrosis (Fig. 35E.5), it is more commonly associated with limited SSc. PAH occurs in 10% of SSc patients. Symptoms of PAH include dyspnea on exertion and ankle swelling. Initial investigations include ECG and a plain chest radiograph that may show pruning of the pulmonary arteries. Use of doppler echocardiography with estimation of the pulmonary artery pressure along with pulmonary function testing are recommended regular screening tests in patients with SSc (106). However, because of a relative lack of specificity, right heart catheterization is required to confirm the diagnosis of PAH. Treatment of PAH has progressed over recent years and now includes parenteral continuous infusion of prostacyclin and the orally active endothelin receptor blocker Bosantin (106). This

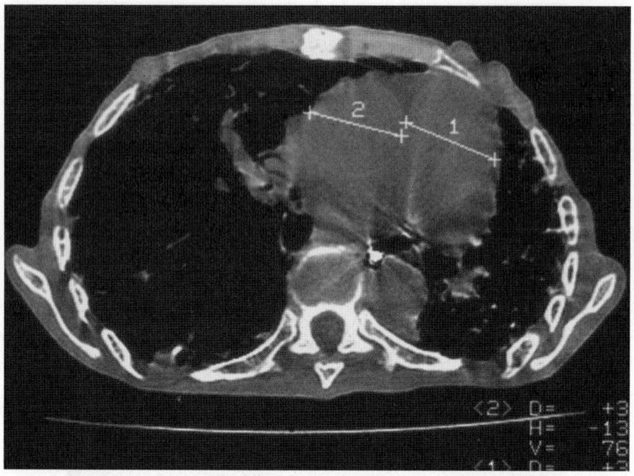

FIGURE 35E.5. PAH in systemic sclerosis. This CT image demonstrates gross dilatation of the right pulmonary artery. This patient with SSc had severe pulmonary fibrosis and had developed pulmonary hypertension secondary to this. (*Source:* Reproduced with kind permission from Dr John Curtis, Consultant Radiologist, University Hospital Aintree.)

latter drug has been shown to be very effective at treating PAH and its symptoms in SSc.

CARDIAC INVOLVEMENT IN VASCULITIS

Inflammation of the blood vessels is termed *vasculitis* and can affect all parts of the vascular tree. Different forms of vasculitis affect different types and sizes of blood vessels. Vasculitis may also occur secondary to other conditions like SLE and RA. However, this section concentrates on the cardiovascular manifestations of some of the primary systemic vasculitides.

Giant Cell Arteritis

Giant cell arteritis (GCA) is a common granulomatous arteritis that has a predilection for the extracranial branches of the carotid artery and the aorta. This disease occurs in the elderly and is very rarely seen in patients under the age of 50 years. The cause of this condition is unknown. However, it appears to be a systemic inflammatory disease that leads to macrophage-induced oxidative damage. Diagnosis is based on new onset of headaches in a patient aged 50 or above, elevated ESR, abnormal thickening of the temporal artery, and diagnostic temporal artery histology. High-dose oral prednisolone is used to treat this condition. The dose of steroids is gradually reduced, although most patients require several years of treatment. The age- and gender-adjusted incidence in people aged over 50 was 19 in 100,000 with a higher incidence in women (24/100,000) than in men (10/100,000) (107). There was no increased mortality in these patients. However, other studies have reported that death from CVD is increased in these patients compared to the general population (Standardized Mortality Ratio [SMR] 1.5 in females and 1.6 in males) (108).

Occasionally, the coronary arteries are involved in the vasculitic process. One study observed a twofold increase in CVD events in GCA patients and these included increased rates of CHD events, peripheral vascular disease, and aortic dissection (109). There are several potential mechanisms that could explain this increased rate of CVD in GCA. Focal vasculitis can lead to vessel occlusion and damage to the vessel wall can lead to dissection or aneurysm formation. Heavy cigarette smoking appears to be a risk factor for the development of GCA (110) and may promote CAD. Although one might expect that corticosteroids would increase the risk of CVD events by their influence on CHD risk factors, it is interesting to note that corticosteroid use in GCA was actually associated with a lower rate of CVD in the study reported by Ray et al. (109). This suggests that treatment of inflammation may be beneficial in preventing CVD in these patients. With regard to prevention of CVD in these patients, it seems reasonable to recommend assessment and treatment of modifiable CVD risk factors, both at the time of diagnosis and, consider use of low dose aspirin during their disease treatment.

Takayasu's Arteritis

Takayasu arteritis (TA) is a large vessel vasculitis of unknown etiology that involves the aorta and its primary braches. TA is extremely rare, although it is more common in the Far East. In Japan, an autopsy study identified TA in 1 out of every 3,000 postmortems. TA affects women 10 times more frequently than men. Infiltration of the vessel wall by inflammatory cells via the vasa vasorum leads to local inflammation and vessel damage. Migration and proliferation of smooth muscle cells cause increased intimal thickness and luminal stenosis. However, if smooth muscle destruction occurs, aneurysms may develop. Collateral vessel formation occurs around stenoses. The clinical manifestations of TA vary; many patients present with an indolent onset of disease. The most common presentation is upper extremity claudication, which is often associated with blood pressure asymmetry between limbs, absent pulses, and bruits detected over the carotid, subclavian, and aortic vessels. Nonspecific systemic features include fever malaise and generalized myalgia and arthralgia. Hypertension commonly occurs due to renal artery stenosis.

The cardiac manifestations of this condition include aortic valve regurgitation resulting from dilatation of the ascending aorta and a dilated cardiomyopathy (111). Most patients respond to oral corticosteroids, which tend to be used at a high dose initially. Unfortunately, a proportion of patients relapse as the steroid dose is reduced and often other immunosuppressive drugs need to be added (112).

Polyarteritis Nodosa

Polyarteritis nodosa (PAN) is a necrotizing nongranulomatous vasculitis of medium-sized and small arteries. The lesions are segmental and, in the acute stage, inflammation affects the whole of the vessel wall. This is then followed by fibrinoid necrosis. Aneurysms of the blood vessels are a characteristic finding in PAN. This rare condition is associated with prior hepatitis B infection in some patients. Historical data show that this condition had a 1-year survival rate of less than 20%. However, introduction of immunosuppressive agents including corticosteroids and cyclophosphamide have improved the 5-year survival rate to 80%. The major causes of mortality in PAN are renal failure and infection, although CVD morbidity contributes to the excess mortality. Diagnosis is based on the presence of arterial aneurysms on angiography. Multiple organ involvement is seen. However, favored sites include the gut, the kidneys, peripheral nerves, and the heart. Hypertension often occurs secondary to renal cortical infarction. Treatments include high-dose glucocorticoids that can be combined with cyclophosphamide in severe cases. In patients with underlying hepatitis B infection, use of antiviral treatment is required in combination with glucocorticoids and plasma exchange (113).

Pericarditis is noted at autopsy in nearly one third of PAN patients, but rarely presents clinically. More frequent clinical cardiac presentations are with congestive cardiac failure and MI (114). Coronary arteritis with necrotizing inflammation and aneurysms has been described in PAN and it is thought that vessel occlusion at these sites of inflammation may lead to MI (115,116). MI, although often clinically silent in PAN, occurs in approximately 5% of cases (114). Atherosclerosis is promoted by hypertension, renal impairment, and high-dose corticosteroids. Cardiac failure occurs in 10% and may be due to local inflammatory myocarditis. However, more commonly, cardiac failure develops secondary to coronary artery disease, hypertension, and renal failure.

Kawasaki Disease

Kawasaki disease (KD) is an arteritis of unknown etiology that occurs in young children and represents the commonest form of acquired heart disease in the United States. KD is more prevalent in Japan and in children of Japanese origin (117). It affects large, medium, and small arteries; the coronary arteries are usually affected. The disease presents with fever, conjunctival injection, and erythema of the oral and pharyngeal mucosa. A macular polymorphous rash on the trunk and erythema and indurative edema of the palms and soles may be seen. Swollen cervical lymph nodes are typical features of this condition. Desquamation of the fingertips occurs after the acute febrile stage of the illness has settled. During the acute febrile stage of the illness, which usually lasts 1 to 2 weeks, myocarditis and pericardial effusion are common. Mitral and tricuspid regurgitation may occur secondary to the myocarditis or due to local valvular inflammation (118). In the subacute phase, which occurs after the fever settles, coronary artery aneurysms may develop. During this subacute phase of KD, patients are at risk of sudden death. Death is usually due to MI (119). KD patients often have a high platelet count and are prone to thrombosis in areas of coronary artery aneurysm formation. Patients surviving the subacute phase enter a convalescent phase of the illness where all clinical signs resolve and inflammation levels return to normal. About 20% of patients develop coronary artery abnormalities and these structural lesions may increase the risk of future MI.

Treatment of KD in the acute stage includes high-dose intravenous immunoglobulin, which, if administered in the early stages of the illness, reduces the prevalence of coronary artery abnormalities (117). High-dose aspirin may be used in the acute febrile stage of the illness. This is then switched to low-dose aspirin when the patient becomes afebrile and enters the subacute phase of the illness. Patients with coronary artery abnormalities are often instructed to remain on low-dose aspirin indefinitely (117). Corticosteroids have been used to treat KD patients who have not responded to intravenous immunoglobulin.

Churg–Strauss Syndrome

This is a rare systemic allergic granulomatous vasculitis affecting predominantly small vessels. To classify a disease as Churg-Strauss syndrome (CSS), four out of six of the following American College of Rheumatology classification criteria need to be met: (i) asthma; (ii) eosinophilia; (iii) mono- or polyneuropathy; (iv) transient pulmonary infiltrates; (v) paranasal sinus abnormality; and (vi) extravascular eosinophils. Rashes with purpura, urticaria, and subcutaneous nodules may be seen. Approximately 25% of patients do not have any antineutrophil cytoplasmic antibodies (ANCA), 25% are positive for cANCA, and 50% are positive for pANCA. Cardiovascular involvement is commonly seen in CSS. One case series reported that 22 out of 28 patients with CSS had evidence of CVD involvement (120). Cardiovascular complications of CSS contribute to the excess mortality observed in this condition with older reports commonly recording cardiac failure as a frequent cause of death (121). However, the recent study by Lane et al. (120) did not report any increased deaths due to CVD (120) and it is not clear whether this difference in mortality causality represents changes in the way deaths are coded or an effect of immunosuppressive treatment modifying the disease course. Many patients respond to corticosteroids alone, although occasionally cyclophosphamide is added. Asthma requires conventional treatment (113). There is some concern about the use of leukotriene receptor antagonist drugs; they have been associated with the development of CSS. However, recent studies have failed to support this (122).

Cardiac involvement in CSS seems to predominantly affect the pericardium and myocardium. Autopsy series have frequently described myocarditis, coronary arteritis, and pericarditis (121). Valve involvement is rarely seen. The cardiac failure described in CSS seems to be the result of cardiac damage induced by myocarditis, with necrotizing granulomata and eosinophilic infiltration being observed during the acute stages of the illness (121). Myocardial fibrosis tends to develop later in the disease process. Interestingly, marked improvements in left ventricular function have been described when immunosuppressive therapy is introduced during the acute inflammatory stage of this illness (123). Pericarditis is present clinically in 20% to 30% of patients with CSS (124). Again, necrotizing granulomata, eosinophils, and fibrosis may occur. Constrictive pericarditis is a rare complication. Coronary arteritis occurs in the larger epicardial coronary arteries and in smaller intramural arteries. It may occasionally lead to MI and coronary vasculitis is a common finding at autopsy (121).

Wegener Granulomatosis

Wegener granulomatosis (WG) is characterized by chronic granulomatous inflammation and small vessel vasculitis. Upper respiratory tract disease is seen in 90% of cases and lung involvement is also common. The kidneys are affected in 80% of cases and urine should be examined for blood, protein, and casts. Other disease features include purpuric rashes, nail fold infarcts, gastrointestinal tract hemorrhage, sensory neuropathy, or mononeuritis multiplex and cardiac involvement (113). Medical therapy with corticosteroids and cytotoxic agents has improved survival rates. However, recent studies have highlighted that WG is now being diagnosed in older patients (125) and increasing age at diagnosis is a poor prognostic marker (126). Mortality rates remain high compared to the general population.

Pericarditis is the most commonly reported cardiovascular manifestation of WG, affecting 50% of patients at autopsy. It commonly presents as an acute pericarditis and this may occur with a systemic flare of WG with other organ involvement (127). Treatment of the pericarditis in this situation should involve increasing the dose of corticosteroids and cytotoxic drug therapy. Occasionally large effusions and tamponade occur, but more frequently the effusions are small and often subclinical (128). Constrictive pericarditis is rare.

Myocardial disease can occur due to granulomatous invasion of the myocardium. This has been reported to occur in 25% of cases. However, congestive heart failure and dilated cardiomyopathy are rare complications (127). Several arrhythmias have been described in association with WG and these include CHB due to granulomatous invasion of the conduction system, and atrial arrhythmias that may occur because of disturbance of the sinoatrial node by pericardial inflammation (127).

Valvular involvement is increasingly recognized as a complication of WG. It seems that the aortic and mitral valves are more frequently affected (129). It is thought that endocardial inflammation damages the heart valves and causes myxomatous degeneration and valve regurgitation (127).

Coronary vasculitis is seen in 50% of cases at autopsy, but rarely presents as an acute MI. However, death from MI is relatively common in WG (130). A recent study, examining carotid intima media thickness in WG patients, revealed that WG patients had increased intima media thickness when compared to age-matched controls and this difference was not explained by an increased prevalence of traditional CVD risk factors. The authors suggest that WG patients have accelerated atherosclerosis that is promoted by inflammation and vascular remodeling associated with this disease (131).

CARDIOVASCULAR EFFECTS OF RHEUMATIC DISEASE TREATMENTS

There is increasing evidence that inflammation plays an important role in the pathogenesis of many cardiovascular conditions. Several medications commonly used for treatment of rheumatic diseases also impact on the cardiovascular system (Table 35E.2). Moreover, the major role of eicosanoids and Tumor Necrosis Factor (TNF)-alpha in arthritis and CVD assure that treatments for one condition may also influence the other. Some of these effects appear to be beneficial and may be related to the immunosuppressive effects of anti-rheumatic drugs whilst other effects appear deleterious. In this section, we will review the effects of specific anti-rheumatic medications on the cardiovascular system.

Nonsteroidal Antiinflammatory Drugs

The nonaspirin NSAIDs have come under close scrutiny because of several large randomized controlled trials of the selective cyclooxygenase-2 inhibitors (coxibs) (Table 35E.3) (132–139).

All of the coxibs appear to be associated with an increase in thrombotic cardiovascular events. However, interpretation of these studies is made more difficult by changing comparator groups. For example, when coxibs are compared with naproxen, they have uniformly been found to increase the risk of events. However, several observational studies suggest that naproxen is cardioprotective (140). Rofecoxib and celecoxib have also been found to increase the risk of events compared with placebo.

The data regarding NSAIDs are much less clear. As mentioned, naproxen has been found in several observational studies and randomized controlled trials to be associated with a reduced risk of thrombotic cardiovascular events. However, some observational data and the randomized controlled trials that show equal risk in coxibs and NSAIDs could be interpreted to mean that all NSAIDs, selective and nonselective, are associated with thrombotic cardiovascular risk.

The mechanisms for the risk associated with selective cyclooxygenase-2 inhibitors, and possibly nonselective NSAIDs,

TABLE 35E.2

CARDIOVASCULAR EFFECTS OF RHEUMATIC DISEASE MEDICATIONS

	Reported effects in cardiovascular system	
Medication	Potential benefit	Potential toxicity
Glucocorticoids	Reduction in endovascular inflammation.	Increase blood pressure and atherosclerosis. Worsen lipid profile.
NSAIDs		
a) Nonselective NSAIDs	Naproxen associated with a reduction in thrombotic cardiovascular outcomes. Naproxen twice daily has an effect on platelets similar to aspirin.	All agents raise blood pressure. Some agents may increase the risk of CHF. Some agents may increase the risk of thrombotic cardiovascular events.
b) Selective COX-2 inhibitors		Hypertension occurs with all agents. All agents are associated with thrombotic cardiovascular events.
Cyclosporine		Hypertension and hyperlipidemia occur in a small percentage of patients.
Hydroxychloroquine (Plaquenil)	Several reports of improved lipid profiles.	Hypertension occurs in a small percentage of patients. Cardiomyopathy is a very rare complication.
Leflunomide (Arava)		Hypertension and hyperlipidemia occur in a small percentage of patients.
Methotrexate (Rheumatrex)	Several epidemiologic studies suggest that cardiovascular mortality is reduced.	Hyperhomocysteinemia is a known complication of treatment.
TNF-α antagonists		
Etanercept (Enbrel)	Improved flow mediated dilatation in several small studies in patients with long-standing RA.	
Infliximab (Remicade)		Increased mortality in class III and class IV CHF.
Xanthine oxidase inhibitors (allopurinol)	May reduce free radical generation.	

Abbreviations: RA, rheumatoid arthritis.

TABLE 35E.3

CARDIOVASCULAR EVENTS OBSERVED IN LONG-TERM TRIALS OF COXIBS AND NSAIDS

Trial (reference)	Patient population	Follow-up (mo)[a]	Aspirin (%)	Coxib arm				Comparator arm				Relative risk (95% CI)
				n	Dosage	Events	Rate[b]	*n*	Dosage	Events	Rate[b]	
ROFECOXIB TRIALS												
VIGOR (133)	RA	9	0	4,047	Rofecoxib 50 mg qd	45	1.67	4,029	Naproxen 500 mg bid	19	0.70	2.38 (1.39–4.00)
APPROVe (134)	Adenomatous polyp	30	16	1,287	Rofecoxib 25 mg qd	46	1.50	1,299	Placebo	26	0.78	1.92 (1.19–3.11)
CELECOXIB TRIALS												
CLASS (135)	OA and RA	9	22	3,987	Celecoxib 400 mg bid	34	1.5	1,985	Ibuprofen 800 mg tid	20	1.8	0.83[c]
								1,996	Diclofenac 75 mg bid	15	1.4	1.07[c]
APC (136)	Adenomatous polyp	≥33	30	685	Celecoxib 200 mg bid	16	0.78	679	Placebo	7	0.34	2.3 (0.9–5.5)
				671	Celecoxib 400 mg bid	23	1.14	...	...	...	...	3.4 (1.4–2.8)
PreSAP (137)	Adenomatous polyp	≥33	16	933	Celecoxib 400 mg qd	20	0.72	628	Placebo	12	0.64	1.1 (0.6–2.3)
AD 97-02-001 (137)	Mild-to-moderate AD	12	NA	285	Celecoxib 200 mg bid	11	NA	140	Placebo	3	NA	1.80[c]
VALDECOXIB TRIALS												
CABG I (138)	Post-CABG	44 days	100	311	Parecoxib/valdecoxib 20 mg bid[d]	24	NA	151	Placebo/placebo	4	NA	2.91[c]
CABG II (139)	Post-CABG	40 days	100	555	Parecoxib/valdecoxib 20 mg bid[d]	11	NA	560	Placebo/ Placebo	3	NA	2.0 (0.5–8.1)
				556	Placebo/valdecoxib 20 mg bid[d]	6	NA	...	...	...	...	3.7 (1.0–13.5)
LUMIRACOXIB TRIAL												
TARGET (140)	OA	12	22	4,376	Lumiracoxib 40 mg	19	0.59	4,397	Ibuprofen 800 mg tid	23	0.74	0.76 (0.41–1.40)
			25	4,741	Lumiracoxib 40 mg	40	1.10	4,730	Naproxen 500 mg bid	27	0.76	1.46 (0.89–2.37)

Abbreviations: AD, Alzheimer's disease; CABG, coronary artery bypass graft; NA, not available; OA, osteoarthritis; RA, rheumatoid arthritis.
The ellipse (...) signifies that the data are the same as the row above. Some of the cardiovascular events were not adjudicated in the references noted. When post-publication adjudication changed numbers, the revised numbers from the FDA reviewer's reports were used (http://www.fda.gov/ohrms/dockets).
[a]Median duration of follow-up, unless noted.
[b]Rate refers to cardiovascular events per 100 person-years. The definition of event differed by study (see text for definitions).
[c]When not available, the relative risks were calculated as the crude event rate in coxib users divided by the crude event rate in the comparator group.
[d]In CABG I and CABG II, medications were administered by intravenous route (parecoxib) for the first 3 days and then by mouth for 11 more days in CABG I and for 7 more days in CABG II.
Source: Solomon DH. Selective cyclooxygenase 2 inhibitors and cardiovascular events. In: Lockshin MD, ed., *Arthritis & Rheumatism.* Copyright 2005 Wiley-Liss Inc. Reprinted with permission of Wiley-Liss Inc., a subsidiary of John Wiley & Sons, Inc

have not been well established. Several mechanisms have been proposed. Animal models suggest that selective cyclooxygenase-2 inhibition may be associated with thrombosis and vasoconstriction because of an imbalance between thromboxane and prostacyclin (141). Hypertension associated with coxibs and NSAIDs is common and partly due to inhibition of prostaglandin-dependent counterregulatory mechanisms (67). Acute and chronic elevations in blood pressure may explain some of the increased cardiovascular risk associated with these agents. Preexisting heart failure may be exacerbated by NSAIDs because they cause sodium and water retention by their action on the kidney (68). As well, some data point to cyclooxygenase-independent oxidative stress as a mechanism associated with several of the selective cyclooxygenase-2 inhibitors. These mechanisms could explain both short- and long-term risks, similar to what has been suggested by the clinical trial and observational data.

Clinical pharmacology studies have also raised the possibility that some NSAIDs may block the benefits of aspirin (142). In one study, ibuprofen was shown to block aspirin's ability to inhibit platelet function. This may occur because of competitive inhibition by ibuprofen at the acetylation site in the platelet cyclooxygenase-1 enzyme. Without access to this site, aspirin is unable to irreversibly inhibit thromboxane A_2 production in the platelet. Some clinical studies of this issue have found an increased risk of cardiovascular events in patients taking aspirin and concomitant ibuprofen, but not all (Table 35E.4) (143–149).

Glucocorticoids

Exogenous glucocorticoids are commonly used in many rheumatic diseases. The diabetogenic, hypertensive, and volume-overloading effects of these agents at high dosages are widely recognized (150). However, the long-term effects of low-dose glucocorticoids in the context of systemic inflammation are not well understood.

Autopsy studies conducted in the 1970s in young women with SLE alerted the medical community to the atherogenic potential of these agents (151). These women had been treated with chronic moderate to high doses of glucocorticoids (e.g., 20 mg/d of prednisone). Another study of RA patients revealed that cumulative glucocorticoid dosage was associated with carotid plaque and arterial incompressibility (152). However, one study demonstrated that SLE patients with atherosclerotic carotid plaque were less likely to have received cyclophosphamide and steroids, suggesting that effective immunosuppression may actually provide some cardioprotective mechanism (153). Therefore, it is difficult to know whether in the context of treatment of systemic inflammatory conditions the cardiovascular effects of corticosteroids are all detrimental.

Methotrexate

Methotrexate is the most common drug used worldwide for RA. Because methotrexate is a folic acid antagonist, it influences several metabolic pathways, including the homocysteine–methionine pathway. Its use is associated with hyperhomocysteinemia, a known risk factor for CVD. In the United States, many patients are treated concomitantly with daily folic acid to reduce the adverse effects of methotrexate. The effect of methotrexate on CVD is difficult to study because use of this agent may be associated with more severe RA, and the severity of arthritis may worsen CVD. Landewe et al. (154) reported results from an observational study that suggested methotrexate use by RA patients with CVD was associated with a marked increase in mortality. However, this study may not have adequately controlled for RA severity. Another observational study has attempted to control for disease severity in a time-varying manner (155). These investigators found that patients with RA who took methotrexate were at a reduced risk of cardiovascular mortality compared with patients who never took this agent. It has been suggested that methotrexate may reduce CVD mortality by effectively reducing the inflammatory disease burden in these patients. Although other studies have found results in line with a potential cardioprotective effect of methotrexate, this finding is still somewhat controversial. Because of the risk of hyperhomocysteinemia and gastrointestinal side effects, folic acid should be given concomitantly with methotrexate.

TNF-α Antagonists

Although the pathophysiology of rheumatic diseases is far from well understood, TNF-α appears to play a central role in the ongoing inflammatory reaction associated with RA, AS, and psoriatic arthritis. Not surprisingly, blocking TNF-α with several different pharmacologic antagonists (adalimumab, etanercept, infliximab) has proven a very effective strategy for controlling these conditions (156). These agents have also been investigated for congestive heart failure because of the recognized role of TNF-α in this condition (157). However, subjects with class III or IV congestive heart failure who were randomized to receive etanercept or infliximab had higher rates of mortality than patients taking placebo (158,159). Thus, these agents are contraindicated in patients with severe congestive heart failure.

On the other hand, there are some data to suggest that these agents may improve vascular endothelial function in patients with RA. Several studies have found that infliximab treatment was associated with improvements, albeit transient, in flow-mediated dilatation (160,161). All of these studies were small and were not conducted in subjects with early disease. Thus, although there is some promise that TNF-α blockade may reverse some of the endothelial dysfunction of RA, it is not clear that this will impact clinical outcomes. Nor is it clear that this strategy has a role in nonrheumatic disease patients.

Hydroxychloroquine

The antimalarial agent hydroxychloroquine is commonly used in SLE and RA. This agent has some weak antiplatelet effects and has been shown to have some benefit on the lipid profile (162,163). However, there are no data that associate this drug with improved cardiovascular outcomes.

CONTROVERSIES AND PERSONAL PERSPECTIVES

One area of drug treatment that may facilitate improvements in cardiovascular survival in patients with inflammatory joint disease is the use of HMG-CoA reductase inhibitors (statins). Statins have long been used in the treatment of hyperlipidemia and in the prevention of CVD. In addition to their lipid-lowering effects, statins have also been found to have pleiotropic effects that may contribute to their mortality reduction. These include atherosclerosis plaque stabilization, modification of endothelial function, and reduction of cytokine synthesis and CRP concentrations (164). It is this reduction in inflammation that has stimulated much interest in the use of statins as an adjunctive treatment for inflammatory rheumatic diseases. Two studies have demonstrated that statins have an antiinflammatory effect and reduce disease activity in patients

TABLE 35E.4

EPIDEMIOLOGIC STUDIES OF A POTENTIAL INTERACTION BETWEEN IBUPROFEN AND ASPIRIN

Author (reference)	Study population	Study design	Source of drug information	Outcome of interest	Exposure of interest	n	Events (n)	Results adjusted[a]
STUDIES DEMONSTRATING A POSSIBLE INCREASED RISK OF CVD EVENTS WITH IBUPROFEN[b] AND ASPIRIN COMBINATIONS								
MacDonald (144)	Tayside general practice	Cohort	Medicines monitoring unit-prescription dispensing	CVD mortality	ASA (Reference)	6,285	1,350	HR (95% CI)
					ASA and ibuprofen	187	39	1.73 (1.05, 2.84)
					ASA and diclofenac	206	44	0.80 (0.49, 1.31)
Kimmel (145)	Hospital discharge after MI and community controls	Case control	Retrospective survey including OTC medications	First hospitalized nonfatal MI	ASA (reference)	1,059	288	OR (95% CI)
					ASA and NSAID users	366	74	0.83 (0.58, 1.17)
					ASA and frequent ibuprofen[c]	NA	NA	2.03 (0.60, 6.84)
Kurth (146)	Male primary prevention (Physicians Health Study)	Randomized controlled trial	Prospective survey via mailed questionnaire every 6-12 mo	First MI	ASA (reference)	10,780	107	HR (95% CI)
					ASA and NSAID[d] (1–59 d)	195	26	1.19 (0.77, 1.85)
					ASA and NSAID[d] (≥60 d)	25	6	2.84(1.24, 6.52)
STUDIES DEMONSTRATING NO INCREASED RISK OF CVD EVENTS WITH IBUPROFEN[a] AND ASPIRIN COMBINATIONS								
Curtis (147)	Medicare patients post-MI (Cooperative Cardiovascular Project)	Cohort	Hospital discharge medications	1-year mortality	ASA (reference)	66,739	11,546	HR (95% CI)
					ASA and NSAIDs	2,733	432	0.96 (0.86, 1.06)
					ASA and ibuprofen	844	118	0.84 (0.70,1.01)
Patel (148)	Veterans Affairs patients	Cohort	Pharmacy records	MI	ASA (reference)	10,239	684	RR (95% CI)
					ASA and ibuprofen	3,859	138	0.61 (0.50, 0.73)
Garcia-Rodriguez (149)	Primary care (GPRD)	Nested case control	Primary care prescriptions	MI and CVD mortality	ASA (reference)	3,515	1,119	OR (95% CI)
					ASA and NSAID	466	163	1.10 (0.89, 1.37)
					ASA and ibuprofen	132	46	1.08 (0.74, 1.58)
Fischer (150)	Primary care (GPRD)	Nested case control	Primary care prescriptions	MI	No use of NSAIDS or ASA	7,450	6,706	OR (95% CI)
					ASA and NSAID	251	69	0.76 (0.56, 1.04)
					ASA and ibuprofen	95	27	0.69 (0.42, 1.15)

Abbreviations: ASA, aspirin; CI, confidence interval; GPRD, general practice research database; HR, hazard ratio; MI, myocardial infarction; NA, not available; OR, odds ratio;; RR, relative risk.

[a]Adjusted for demographics and measures of CVD risk in all but the Patel study.

[b]Some studies did not examine ibuprofen separately.

[c]Frequent ibuprofen use was defined as use ≥4 times/week.

[d]Type of NSAID not known. Duration of NSAID use was estimated for each year of the study from the frequency of use in the preceeding month.

Source: Solomon DH. The cardiovascular system in rheumatic disease: the newest "extraarticular" manifestation? In: *Journal of Rheumatology*. Duncan A Gordon (Ed), (c) 2000-2005. The Journal of Rheumatology Publishing Company Limited. Reprinted with permission of The Journal of Rheumatology Publishing Company Limited.

with RA (165,166). This raises questions about whether statins should be used in all RA patients to reduce inflammation and CHD events. Because the disease activity reduction noted with statin use is only modest, it is probably hard to justify use of these drugs as inflammatory disease modifiers. Further study is required to examine to what extent statins reduce CVD events in inflammatory rheumatic diseases. As with all drugs, the potential benefits should outweigh the risks of using medications. There are concerns about identifying statin hepatotoxicity in patients treated with methotrexate and leflunomide, and the risk of muscular toxicity is elevated by concomitant cyclosporine use in females and elderly patients. Therefore, it is difficult to know which inflammatory joint disease patients would derive the most benefit from statin therapy.

It will be interesting to see whether more effective suppression of chronic inflammation will lead to a reduction in CVD morbidity, as well as improved musculoskeletal function. It may be that combining modification of traditional risk factors with active suppression of inflammation will lead to greater improvements. It is also important to educate both the physician and the patient about the cardiovascular complications associated with rheumatic diseases to enable more timely diagnosis and treatment of CVD events.

THE FUTURE

The debate over the cardiovascular safety of selective coxibs and nonselective NSAIDs continues. These drugs have been the mainstay of symptom control in many rheumatic diseases for many years. Although simple analgesics like paracetamol and codeine provide excellent pain relief, they are not as effective at controlling the morning stiffness experienced by many inflammatory arthritis sufferers. Therefore a promising development for the future is the nitric oxide–releasing NSAIDs and cyclooxygenase-inhibiting nitric oxide donors. These drugs are currently in development and appear to have a safe gastrointestinal and cardiovascular profile (167), although they still cause some renal side effects (168). They appear to be as efficacious as traditional nonselective NSAIDs (167). However, some of the lessons learnt from the initial launch of the coxibs may result in a more cautious introduction of these new drugs.

ACKNOWLEDGMENT

James Rossi provided excellent assistance in compiling figures and tables.

References

1. Singh G, Miller JD, Lee FH, et al. Prevalence of cardiovascular disease risk factors among US adults with self-reported osteoarthritis: data from the Third National Health and Nutrition Examination Survey. *Am J Manag Care* 2002;8:383–391.
2. Watson DJ, Rhodes T, Guess HA. All-cause mortality and vascular events among patients with rheumatoid arthritis, osteoarthritis, or no arthritis in the UK General Practice Research Database. *J Rheumatol* 2003;30:1196–1202.
3. Symmons DPM. Epidemiology of rheumatoid arthritis: determinants of onset, persistence and outcome. *Best Pract Res Clin Rheumatol* 2002;16:707–722.
4. Pincus T, Callahan LF. What is the natural history of rheumatoid arthritis. *Rheum Dis Clin North Am* 1993;19:123–146.
5. Wolfe F, Mitchell DM, Sibley JT, et al. The mortality of rheumatoid arthritis. *Arthritis Rheum* 1994;37:481–494.
6. Symmons DPM, Jones MA, Scott DL, et al. Longterm mortality outcomes in patients with rheumatoid arthritis: Early presenters continue to do well. *J Rheumatol* 1998;25:1072–1077.
7. Bjornadal L, Baecklund E, Yin L, et al. Decreasing mortality in patients with rheumatoid arthritis: results from a large population based cohort in Sweden, 1964–95. *J Rheumatol* 2002;29:906–912.
8. Goodson N, Marks J, Lunt M, et al. Cardiovascular admissions and mortality in an inception cohort of patients with rheumatoid arthritis with an onset in the 1980s and 1990s. *Ann Rheum Dis* 2005;64:1595–1601.
9. Gabriel SE, Crowson CS, Kremers HM, et al. Survival in rheumatoid arthritis: a population-based analysis of trends over 40 years. *Arthritis Rheum* 2003;48:54–58.
10. Goodson NJ, Wiles NJ, Lunt M, et al. Mortality in early inflammatory polyarthritis: cardiovascular mortality is increased. *Arthritis Rheum* 2002;46: 2010–2019.
11. Kaplan MJ, Clune WJ. New evidence for vascular disease in patients with early rheumatoid disease. *Lancet* 2003;316:1068–1069.
12. Myllykangas-Luosujärvi R, Aho K, Kautianen H, et al. Cardiovascular mortality in women with rheumatoid arthritis. *J Rheumatol* 1995;22:1065–1067.
13. Wallberg-Jonsson S, Ohman ML, Dahlqvist SR. Cardiovascular morbidity and mortality in patients with seropositive rheumatoid arthritis in Northern Sweden. *J Rheumatol* 1997;24:445–451.
14. Charcot JM. *Clinical lectures on senile and chronic disease*. London: New Syddenham Society; 1881:95:164–179.
15. Bonfiglio T, Atwater EC. Heart disease in patients with seropositive rheumatoid arthritis; a controlled autopsy study and review. *Arch Intern Med* 1969;124:714–719.
16. Goodson NJ. Cardiac involvement in rheumatoid arthritis. In: Doria A, Pauletto P, eds. *The heart in systemic autoimmune diseases*. Amsterdam: Elsevier; 2004:121–144.
17. Gordon DA, Stein JL, Broder I. The extra-articular features of rheumatoid arthritis: a systematic analysis of 127 cases. *Am J Med* 1973;54:445–452.
18. Hara KS, Ballard DJ, Ilstrup DM, et al. Rheumatoid pericarditis: clinical features and survival. *Medicine* 1990;69:81–91.
19. Silman AJ. Trends in the incidence and severity of rheumatoid arthritis. *J Rheumatol Suppl* 1992;32:71–73.
20. Thould AK. Constrictive pericarditis in rheumatoid arthritis. *Ann Rheum Dis* 1986;45:89–94.
21. Manji H, Raven P. Calcific constrictive pericarditis due to rheumatoid arthritis. *Postgrad Med J* 1990;66:57–58.
22. Fernandez-Muixi J, Vidal F, Bardaji A, et al. Recurrent pericarditis and cardiac tamponade in rheumatoid arthritis: effectiveness of colchicine. *Br J Rheumatol* 1994;33:596–597.
23. Levine AJ, Dimitri WR, Bonser RS. Aortic regurgitation in rheumatoid arthritis necessitating aortic valve replacement. *Eur J Cardiothorac Surg* 1999;15:213–214.
24. Chand EM, Freant LJ, Rubin JW. Aortic valve rheumatoid nodules producing clinical aortic regurgitation and a review of the literature. *Cardiovasc Pathol* 1999;8:333–338.
25. Mounet F, Soula P, Concina P, et al. Specific valvular heart disease of rheumatoid arthritis: two case reports. *Arch Mal Coeur Vaiss* 1997;90: 987–989.
26. Webber MD, Selsky EJ, Roper PA. Identification of a mobile intracardiac rheumatoid nodule mimicking an atrial myxoma. *J Am Soc Echocardiogr* 1995;8:961–964.
27. Bely M, Apathy A, Beke-Martos E. Cardiac changes in rheumatoid arthritis. *Acta Morphologica Hungarica* 1992;40:149–186.
28. Bacon PA, Gibson DG. Cardiac involvement in rheumatoid arthritis. An echocardiographic study. *Ann Rheum Dis* 1974;33:20–24.
29. Nomeir AM, Turner RA, Watts LE. Cardiac involvement in rheumatoid arthritis. Followup study. *Arthritis Rheum* 1979;22:561–564.
30. Mody GM, Stevens JE, Meyers OL. The heart in rheumatoid arthritis—a clinical and echocardiographic study. *Q J Med* 1987;65:921–928.
31. Toumanidis ST, Papamichael CM, Antoniades LG, et al. Cardiac involvement in collagen diseases. *Eur Heart J* 1995;16:257–262.
32. Wislowska M, Sypula S, Kowalik I. Echocardiographic findings and 24-h electrocardiographic Holter monitoring in patients with nodular and nonnodular rheumatoid arthritis. *Rheumatol Int* 1999;18(s-6):163–169.
33. Liebowitz WB. The heart in rheumatoid arthritis: a clinical and pathological study of 62 cases. *Ann Intern Med* 1963;58:102–110.
34. Tlustochowicz W, Piotrowicz R, Cwetsch A, et al. 24-h ECG monitoring in patients with rheumatoid arthritis. *Eur Heart J* 1995;16:848–851.
35. Goldeli O, Dursun E, Komsuoglu B. Dispersion of ventricular repolarization: a new marker of ventricular arrhythmias in patients with rheumatoid arthritis. *J Rheumatol* 1998;25:447–450.
36. Ahern M, Lever JV, Cosh J. Complete heart block in rheumatoid arthritis. *Ann Rheum Dis* 1983;42:389–397.
37. Okada Y, Nakanishi I, Kajikawa K, et al. An autopsy case of rheumatoid arthritis with an involvement of the cardiac conduction system. *Jpn Circ J* 1983;47:671–676.
38. Leden I, Eriksson A, Lilja B, et al. Autonomic nerve function in rheumatoid arthritis of varying severity. *Scand J Rheumatol* 1983;12:166–170.
39. Toussirot E, Serratrice G, Valentin P. Autonomic nervous-system involvement in rheumatoid-arthritis-50 cases. *J Rheumatol* 1993;20:1508–1514.
40. Curtis BM, O'Keefe JH Jr. Autonomic tone as a cardiovascular risk factor: the dangers of chronic fight or flight. *Mayo Clin Proc* 2002;77:45–54.

41. Maradit-Kremers H, Crowson CS, Nicola PJ, et al. Increased unrecognized coronary heart disease and sudden deaths in rheumatoid arthritis: a population-based cohort study. *Arthritis Rheum* 2005;52:402–411.
42. Solomon DHM, Karlson EWM, Rimm EBS, et al. Cardiovascular morbidity and mortality in women diagnosed with rheumatoid arthritis. *Circulation* 2003;107:1303–1307.
43. del Rincon ID, Williams K, Stern MP, et al. High incidence of cardiovascular events in a rheumatoid arthritis cohort not explained by traditional cardiac risk factors. *Arthritis Rheum* 2001;44:2737–2745.
44. Symmons DPM, Bankhead CR, Harrison BJ, et al. Blood transfusion, smoking and obesity as risk factors for development of rheumatoid arthritis: results from a primary care based incident case-control study in Norfolk, England. *Arthritis Rheum* 1997;40:1955–1961.
45. Dessein PH, Joffe BI, Veller MG, et al. Traditional and nontraditional cardiovascular risk factors are associated with atherosclerosis in rheumatoid arthritis. *J Rheumatol* 2005;32:435–442.
46. Maradit-Kremers H, Nicola PJ, Crowson CS, et al. Prognostic importance of low body mass index in relation to cardiovascular mortality in rheumatoid arthritis. *Arthritis Rheum* 2004;50:3450–3457.
47. Ridker P, Stampher M. Novel risk factors for systemic atherosclerosis: a comparison of C-reactive protein, fibrinogen, homocysteine, lipoprotein(a) and standard cholesterol screening as predictors of peripheral arterial disease. *JAMA* 2001;285:2481–2485.
48. Roubenoff R, Dellaripa P, Nadeau M, et al. Abnormal homocysteine metabolism in rheumatoid arthritis. *Arthritis Rheum* 1997;40:718–722.
49. Haagsma CJ, Blom HJ, van Riel PLCM, et al. Influence of sulphasalazine, methotrexate, and the combination of both on plasma homocysteine concentrations in patients with rheumatoid arthritis. *Ann Rheum Dis* 1999;58:79–84.
50. Wållberg-Jonsson S, Cederfelt M, Rantapaa DS. Hemostatic factors and cardiovascular disease in active rheumatoid arthritis: an 8 year followup study. *J Rheumatol* 2000;27:71–75.
51. Dessein PH, Joffe BI, Stanwix AE. Inflammation, insulin resistance, and aberrant lipid metabolism as cardiovascular risk factors in rheumatoid arthritis. *J Rheumatol* 2003;30:1403–1405.
52. Tracy RP. Inflammation markers and coronary heart disease. *Curr Opin Lipidol* 1999;10:435–441.
53. Ridker PM. Connecting the role of C-reactive protein and statins in cardiovascular disease. *Clin Cardiol* 2003;26(4 Suppl 3):III39–44.
54. Goodson NJ, Symmons DPM, Scott DGI, et al. Baseline C-reactive protein and prediction of death from cardiovascular disease in patients with inflammatory polyarthritis. *Arthritis Rheum* 2005;52:2293–2299.
55. Maradit-Kremers H, Nicola PJ, Crowson CS, et al. Cardiovascular death in rheumatoid arthritis: a population-based study. *Arthritis Rheum* 2005;52:722–732.
56. Vaudo G, Marchesi S, Gerli R, et al. Endothelial dysfunction in young patients with rheumatoid arthritis and low disease activity. *Ann Rheum Dis* 2004;63:31–35.
57. Lehtinen K. Mortality and causes of death in 398 patients admitted to hospital with ankylosing spondylitis. *Ann Rheum Dis* 1993;52:174–176.
58. Radford EP, Doll R, Smith PG. Mortality among patients with ankylosing spondylitis not given x-ray therapy. *N Engl J Med* 1977;297:572–576.
59. O'Neil TW, King G, Molony J, et al. Echocardiographic abnormalities in ankylosing spondylitis. *Ann Rheum Dis* 1992;51:652–654.
60. Bergfeldt L. HLA-B27-associated cardiac disease. *Ann Intern Med* 1997;127:621–629.
61. Yildirir A, Aksoyek S, Calguneri M, et al. QT dispersion as a predictor of arrhythmic events in patients with ankylosing spondylitis. *Rheumatology (Oxford)* 2000;39:875–879.
62. Bergfeldt L. HLA B27-associated rheumatic diseases with severe cardiac bradyarrhythmias. Clinical features and prevalence in 223 men with permanent pacemakers. *Am J Med* 1983;75:210–215.
63. Toussirot E, Bahjaoui-Bouhaddi M, Poncet JC, et al. Abnormal autonomic cardiovascular control in ankylosing spondylitis. *Ann Rheum Dis* 1999;58:481–487.
64. Peters MJ, van der Horst-Bruinsma I, Dijkmans BA, et al. Cardiovascular risk profile of patients with spondylarthropathies, particularly ankylosing spondylitis and psoriatic arthritis. *Semin Arthritis Rheum* 2004;34:585–592.
65. Sukenic S, Pras A, Buskila D, et al. Cardiovascular manifestations of ankylosing spondylitis. *Clin Rheumatol* 1987;6:588–592.
66. Symmons DPM, Goodson NJ, Cook MN, et al. Men with ankylosing spondylitis have an increased risk of myocardial infarction. *Arthritis Rheum* 2004;50(9 Suppl):1216.
67. Armstrong EP, Malone DC. The impact of nonsteroidal anti-inflammatory drugs on blood pressure, with an emphasis on newer agents. *Clin Ther* 2003;25:1–18.
68. Bleumink GS, Feenstra J, Sturkenboom MC, et al. Nonsteroidal anti-inflammatory drugs and heart failure. *Drugs* 2003;63:525–534.
69. Iacobellis G, Iacobellis G. A rare and asymptomatic case of mitral valve tophus associated with severe gouty tophaceous arthritis. *J Endocrinol Invest* 2004;27:965–966.
70. Choi HK, Atkinson K, Karlson EW, et al. Obesity, weight change, hypertension, diuretic use, and risk of gout in men: the health professionals follow-up study. *Arch Intern Med* 2005;165:742–748.
71. Mikuls TR, Farrar JT, Bilker WB, et al. Gout epidemiology: results from the UK General Practice Research Database, 1990-1999. *Ann Rheum Dis* 2005;64:267–272.
72. Niskanen LK, Laaksonen DE, Nyyssonen K, et al. Uric acid level as a risk factor for cardiovascular and all-cause mortality in middle-aged men: a prospective cohort study. *Arch Intern Med* 2004;164:1546–1551.
73. Maxwell AJ, Bruinsma KA. Uric acid is closely linked to vascular nitric oxide activity. Evidence for mechanism of association with cardiovascular disease. *J Am Coll Cardiol* 2001;38:1850–1858.
74. Berry CE, Hare JM. Xanthine oxidoreductase and cardiovascular disease: molecular mechanisms and pathophysiological implications. *J Physiol (Lond)* 2004;555:589–606.
75. Wluka AE, Ryan PF, Miller AM, et al. Post-cardiac transplantation gout: incidence of therapeutic complications. *J Heart Lung Transplant* 2000;19:951–956.
76. Burack DA, Griffith BP, Thompson ME, et al. Hyperuricemia and gout among heart transplant recipients receiving cyclosporine. *Am J Med* 1992;92:141–146.
77. Pascual E. Gout update: from lab to the clinic and back. *Curr Opin Rheumatol* 2000;12:213–218.
78. Rana SS, Giuliani MJ, Oddis CV, et al. Acute onset of colchicine myoneuropathy in cardiac transplant recipients: case studies of three patients. *Clin Neurol Neurosurg* 1997;99:266–270.
79. Urowitz MB, Gladman DD, Abu-Shakra M, et al. Mortality studies in systemic lupus erythematosus. Results from a single center. III. Improved survival over 24 years. *J Rheumatol* 1997;24:1061–1065.
80. Urowitz MB, Bookman AA, Koehler BE, et al. The bimodal mortality pattern of systemic lupus erythematosus. *Am J Med* 1976;60:221–225.
81. Moder KGM, Miller TDM, Tazelaar HDM. Cardiac involvement in systemic lupus erythematosus. *Mayo Clin Proc* 1999;74:275–284.
82. Cauduro SA, Moder KG, Tsang TS, et al. Clinical and echocardiographic characteristics of hemodynamically significant pericardial effusions in patients with systemic lupus erythematosis. *Am J Cardiol* 2003;92:1370–1375.
83. Roldan CA, Shively BK, Crawford MH. An echocardiographic study of valvular heart disease associated with systemic lupus erythematosus. *N Engl J Med* 1996;335:1424–1430.
84. Libman E, Sacks B. A hitherto undescribed form of valvular and mural endocarditis. *Arch Intern Med* 1924;33:701.
85. Bulkley BH, Roberts WC. The heart in systemic lupus erythematosus and the changes induced in it by corticosteroid therapy. A study of 36 necropsy patients. *Am J Med* 1975;58:243–264.
86. Nesher G, Ilany J, Rosenmann D, et al. Valvular dysfunction in antiphospholipid syndrome: prevalence, clinical features, and treatment. *Semin Arthritis Rheum* 1997;27:27–35.
87. Fluture A, Chaudhari S, Frishman WH. Valvular heart disease and systemic lupus erythematosus: therapeutic implications. *Heart Disease* 2003;5:349–353.
88. Wijetunga M, Rockson S. Myocarditis in systemic lupus erythematosus. *Am J Med* 2002;113:419–423.
89. Brucato A, Jonzon A, Friedman D, et al. Proposal for a new definition of congenital complete atrioventricular block. *Lupus* 2003;12:427–435.
90. Buyon JP, Clancy RM. Neonatal lupus syndromes. *Curr Opin Rheumatol* 2003;15:535–541.
91. Bracato A, Buyon J. Neonatal lupus syndromes: clinical features. In: Doria A, Pauletto P, eds. *The heart in systemic autoimmune diseases*. Amsterdam: Elsevier; 2004:163–188.
92. Rubin LA, Urowitz MB, Gladman DD. Mortality in systemic lupus erythematosus: the bimodal pattern revisited. *Q J Med* 1985;55:87–98.
93. Sun SS, Shiau YC, Tsai SC, et al. The role of technetium-99m sestamibi myocardial perfusion single-photon emission computed tomography (SPECT) in the detection of cardiovascular involvement in systemic lupus erythematosus patients with non-specific chest complaints. *Rheumatology* 2001;40:1106–1111.
94. Manzi S, Meilahn EN, Rairie JE, et al. Age-specific incidence rates of myocardial infarction and angina in women with systemic lupus erythematosus: comparison with the Framingham Study. *Am J Epidemiol* 1997;145:408–415.
95. Bjornadal L, Yin L, Granath F, et al. Cardiovascular disease a hazard despite improved prognosis in patients with systemic lupus erythematosus: results from a Swedish population based study 1964–95. *J Rheumatol* 2004;31:713–719.
96. Bruce IN, Urowitz MB, Gladman DD, et al. Risk factors for coronary heart disease in women with systemic lupus erythematosus: the Toronto Risk Factor Study. *Arthritis Rheum* 2003;48:3159–3167.
97. Esdaile JM, Abrahamowicz M, Grodzicky T , et al. Traditional Framingham risk factors fail to fully account for accelerated atherosclerosis in systemic lupus erythematosus [see comment]. *Arthritis Rheum* 2001;44:2331–2337.
98. Svenungsson E, Jensen-Urstad K, Heimburger M, et al. Risk factors for cardiovascular disease in systemic lupus erythematosus. *Circulation* 2001;104:1887–1893.
99. Petri M, Lakatta C, Magder L, et al. Effect of prednisone and hydroxychloroquine on coronary artery disease risk factors in systemic lupus erythematosus: a longitudinal data analysis. *Am J Med* 1994;96:254–259.

100. Roman MJ, Shanker BA, Davis A, et al. Prevalence and correlates of accelerated atherosclerosis in systemic lupus erythematosus. *N Engl J Med* 2003;349:2399–2406.
101. Wajed J, Ahmad Y, Durrington PN, et al. Prevention of cardiovascular disease in systemic lupus erythematosus–proposed guidelines for risk factor management. *Rheumatology (Oxford)* 2004;43:7–12.
102. Allcock RJ, Forrest I, Corris PA, et al. A study of the prevalence of systemic sclerosis in northeast England. *Rheumatology* 2004;43:589–602.
103. Mayes MD. Scleroderma epidemiology. *Rheum Dis Clin North Am* 2003; 29:239–254.
104. Candell-Riera J, Armadans-Gil L, Simeon CP, et al. Comprehensive noninvasive assessment of cardiac involvement in limited systemic sclerosis. *Arthritis Rheum* 1996;39:1138–1145.
105. Coghlan JG, Denton CP. Cardiac involvement in scleroderma. In: Doria A, Pauletto P, eds. *The heart in systemic autoimmune diseases*. Amsterdam: Elsevier; 2004:189–195.
106. Denton CP, Black M. Scleroderma—clinical and pathological advances. *Best Pract Res Clin Rheumatol* 2004;18:271–290.
107. Salvarani C, Crowson CS, O'Fallon W, et al. Reappraisal of the epidemiology of giant cell arteritis in Olmsted County, Minnesota, over a fifty-year period. *Arthritis Rheum* 2004;51:264–268.
108. Uddhammar A, Eriksson AL, Nystrom L, et al. Increased mortality due to cardiovascular disease in patients with giant cell arteritis in northern Sweden. *J Rheumatol* 2002;29:737–742.
109. Ray JG, Mamdani MM, Geerts WH. Giant cell arteritis and cardiovascular disease in older adults. *Heart* 2005;91:324–328.
110. Duhaut P, Pinede L, Demolombe-Rague S, et al. Giant cell arteritis and cardiovascular risk factors: a multicenter, prospective case-control study. Groupe de Recherche sur l'Arterite a Cellules Geantes. *Arthritis Rheum* 1998;41:1960–1965.
111. Johnston SL, Lock RJ, Gompels MM. Takayasu arteritis: a review. *J Clin Pathol* 2002;55:481–486.
112. Liang P, Hoffman GS. Advances in the medical and surgical treatment of Takayasu arteritis. *Curr Opin Rheumatol* 2005;17:16–24.
113. Savage CO, Harper L, Cockwell P, et al. ABC of arterial and vascular disease: vasculitis. *Br Med J* 2000;320:1325–1328.
114. Lhote F, Cohen P, Guillevin L. Polyarteritis nodosa, microscopic polyangiitis and Churg-Strauss syndrome. *Lupus* 1998;7:238–258.
115. Chu KH, Menapace FJ, Blankenship JC, et al. Polyarteritis nodosa presenting as acute myocardial infarction with coronary dissection. *Cathet Cardiovasc Diagn* 1998;44:320–324.
116. Kastner D, Gaffney M, Tak T. Polyarteritis nodosa and myocardial infarction. *Can J Cardiol* 2000;16:515–518.
117. Newburger JW, Takahashi M, Gerber MA, et al. Diagnosis, treatment, and long-term management of Kawasaki disease: a statement for health professionals from the Committee on Rheumatic Fever, Endocarditis and Kawasaki Disease, Council on Cardiovascular Disease in the Young, American Heart Association. *Circulation* 2004;110:2747–2771.
118. Suzuki A, Kamiya T, Tsuchiya K, et al. Tricuspid and mitral regurgitation detected by color flow Doppler in the acute phase of Kawasaki disease. *Am J Cardiol* 1988;61:386–90.
119. Rowley AH, Shulman ST. Kawasaki syndrome. *Clin Microbiol Rev* 1998;11:405–414.
120. Lane SE, Watts RA, Shepstone L, et al. Primary systemic vasculitis: clinical features and mortality. *Q J Med* 2005;98:97–111.
121. Kozak M, Gill EA, Green LS. The Churg-Strauss syndrome. A case report with angiographically documented coronary involvement and a review of the literature. *Chest* 1995;107:578–580.
122. Keogh KA, Specks U. Churg-Strauss syndrome: clinical presentation, antineutrophil cytoplasmic antibodies, and leukotriene receptor antagonists. *Am J Med* 2003;115:284–290.
123. Frustaci A, Gentiloni N, Chimenti C, et al. Necrotizing myocardial vasculitis in Churg-Strauss syndrome: clinicohistologic evaluation of steroids and immunosuppressive therapy. *Chest* 1998;114:1484–1489.
124. Guillevin L, Cohen P, Gayraud M, et al. Churg-Strauss syndrome. Clinical study and long-term follow-up of 96 patients. *Medicine* 1999;78:26–37.
125. Harper L, Savage CO. ANCA-associated renal vasculitis at the end of the twentieth century–a disease of older patients. *Rheumatology (Oxford)* 2005;44:495–501.
126. Bligny D, Mahr A, Toumelin PL, et al. Predicting mortality in systemic Wegener's granulomatosis: a survival analysis based on 93 patients. *Arthritis Rheum* 2004;51:83–91.
127. Korantzopoulos P, Papaioannides D, Siogas K. The heart in Wegener's granulomatosis. *Cardiology* 2004;102:7–10.
128. Morelli S, Gurgo Di Castelmenardo AM, Conti F, et al. Cardiac involvement in patients with Wegener's granulomatosis. *Rheumatol Intl* 2000; 19:209–212.
129. Davenport A, Goodfellow J, Goel S, et al. Aortic valve disease in patients with Wegener's granulomatosis. *Am J Kidney Dis* 1994;24:205–208.
130. Matteson EL, Gold KN, Bloch DA, et al. Long-term survival of patients with Wegener's granulomatosis from the American College of Rheumatology Wegener's Granulomatosis Classification Criteria Cohort. *Am J Med* 1996;101:129–134.
131. de Leeuw K, Sanders JS, Stegeman C, et al. Accelerated atherosclerosis in patients with Wegener's granulomatosis. *Ann Rheum Dis* 2005;64:753–759.
132. Bombardier C, Laine L, Reicin A, et al. Comparison of upper gastrointestinal toxicity of rofecoxib and naproxen in patients with rheumatoid arthritis. VIGOR Study Group. *N Engl J Med* 2000;343:1520–1528.
133. Bresalier RS, Sandler RS, Quan H, et al. Cardiovascular events associated with rofecoxib in a colorectal adenoma chemoprevention trial. *N Engl J Med* 2005;352:1092–1102.
134. Silverstein FE, Faich G, Goldstein JL, et al. Gastrointestinal toxicity with celecoxib vs nonsteroidal anti-inflammatory drugs for osteoarthritis and rheumatoid arthritis: the CLASS study: A randomized controlled trial. Celecoxib Long-term Arthritis Safety Study. *JAMA* 2000;284:1247–1255.
135. Solomon SD, McMurray JJ, Pfeffer MA, et al. Cardiovascular risk associated with celecoxib in a clinical trial for colorectal adenoma prevention. *N Engl J Med* 2005;352:1071–1080.
136. Arthritis advisory committee, Drug safety and risk management advisory committee. Advisory committee briefing document. Celecoxib and valdecoxib safety. Available: www.fda.gov. Accessed January 22,2005.
137. Ott E, Nussmeier NA, Duke PC, et al. Efficacy and safety of the cyclooxygenase 2 inhibitors parecoxib and valdecoxib in patients undergoing coronary artery bypass surgery. *J Thorac Cardiovasc Surg* 2003;125:1481–1482.
138. Nussmeier NA, Whelton AA, Brown MT, et al. Complications of the COX-2 inhibitors parecoxib and valdecoxib after cardiac surgery. *N Engl J Med* 2005;352:1081–1091.
139. Farkouh ME, Kirshner H, Harrington RA, et al. Comparison of lumiracoxib with naproxen and ibuprofen in the Therapeutic Arthritis Research and Gastrointestinal Event Trial (TARGET), cardiovascular outcomes: randomised controlled trial. *Lancet* 2004;364:675–685.
140. Juni P, Nartey L, Reichenbach S, et al. Risk of cardiovascular events and rofecoxib: cumulative meta- analysis. *Lancet* 2004;364:2021–2029.
141. Cheng Y, Austin SC, Rocca B, et al. Role of prostacyclin in the cardiovascular response to thromboxane A2. *Science* 2002;296:539–541.
142. Catella-Lawson F, Reilly MP, Kapoor SC, et al. Cyclooxygenase inhibitors and the antiplatelet effects of aspirin. *N Engl J Med* 2001;345:1809–1817.
143. MacDonald TM, Wei L. Effect of ibuprofen on cardioprotective effect of aspirin. *Lancet* 2003;361:573–574.
144. Kimmel SE, Berlin JA, Reilly M, et al. The effects of nonselective non-aspirin non-steroidal anti-inflammatory medications on the risk of nonfatal myocardial infarction and their interaction with aspirin. *J Am Coll Cardiol* 2004;43:985–990.
145. Kurth T, Glynn RJ, Walker AM, et al. Inhibition of clinical benefits of aspirin on first myocardial infarction by non-steroidal antiinflammatory drugs. *Circulation* 2003;108:1191–1195.
146. Curtis JP, Wang YF, Portnay EL, et al. Aspirin, ibuprofen, and mortality after myocardial infarction: retrospective cohort study. *Br Med J* 2003;327: 1322–1323.
147. Patel TN, Goldberg KC. Use of aspirin and ibuprofen compared with aspirin alone and the risk of myocardial infarction. *Arch Intern Med* 2004;164: 852–856.
148. Garcia Rodriguez LA, Varas-Lorenzo C, Maguire A, et al. Nonsteroidal antiinflammatory drugs and the risk of myocardial infarction in the general population. *Circulation* 2004;109:3000–3006.
149. Fischer LM, Schlienger RG, Matter CM, et al. Current use of nonsteroidal antiinflammatory drugs and the risk of acute myocardial infarction. *Pharmacotherapy* 2005;25:503–510.
150. Maxwell SR, Moots RJ, Kendall MJ. Corticosteroids: do they damage the cardiovascular system?. *Postgrad Med J* 1994;70:863–870.
151. Haider YS, Roberts WC. Coronary arterial disease in systemic lupus erythematosus; quantification of degrees of narrowing in 22 necropsy patients (21 women) aged 16 to 37 years. *Am J Med* 1981;70:775–781.
152. del Rincon, I, O'Leary DH, Haas RW, et al. Effect of glucocorticoids on the arteries in rheumatoid arthritis. *Arthritis Rheum* 2004;50:3813–3822.
153. Roman MJ, Shanker B, Davis A, et al. Prevalence and correlates of accelerated atherosclerosis in systemic lupus erythematosus. *N Engl J Med* 2003;349:2399–2406.
154. Landewe RB, van den Borne BE, Breedveld FC, et al. Methotrexate effects in patients with rheumatoid arthritis with cardiovascular comorbidity. *Lancet* 2000;355:1616–1617.
155. Choi HK, Hernan MA, Seeger JD, et al. Methotrexate and mortality in patients with rheumatoid arthritis: a prospective study. *Lancet* 2002;359: 1173–1177.
156. Olsen NJ, Stein CM. New drugs for rheumatoid arthritis. *N Engl J Med* 2004;350:2167–2179.
157. Agnoletti L, Curello S, Bachetti T, et al. Serum from patients with severe heart failure downregulates eNOS and is proapoptotic: role of tumor necrosis factor-alpha. *Circulation* 1999;100:1983–1991.
158. Chung ES, Packer M, Lo KH, et al. Anti-TNF Therapy Against Congestive Heart Failure Investigators. Randomized, double-blind, placebo-controlled, pilot trial of infliximab, a chimeric monoclonal antibody to tumor necrosis factor-alpha, in patients with moderate-to-severe heart failure: results of the anti-TNF Therapy Against Congestive Heart Failure (ATTACH) trial. *Circulation* 2003;107:3133–3144.
159. Mann DL, McMurray JJ, Packer M, et al. Targeted anticytokine therapy in patients with chronic heart failure: results of the Randomized Etanercept Worldwide Evaluation (RENEWAL). *Circulation* 2004;109:1594–1602.
160. Hurlimann D, Forster A, Noll G, et al. Anti-tumor necrosis factor-alpha treatment improves endothelial function in patients with rheumatoid arthritis. *Circulation* 2002;106:2184–2187.

161. Gonzalez-Juanatey C, Testa A, Garcia-Castelo A, et al. Active but transient improvement of endothelial function in rheumatoid arthritis patients undergoing long-term treatment with anti-tumor necrosis factor alpha antibody. *Arthritis Rheum* 2004;51:447–450.
162. Turpie AG. Antithrombotic effects of drugs which suppress platelet function: their potential in prevention growth of tumour cells. *Prog Clin Biol Res* 1982;89:31–62.
163. Kavanaugh A. Lipid profiles in patients with rheumatoid arthritis. *Ann Rheum Dis* 1998;57:175.
164. Costenbader KH, Kim DJ, Peerzada J, et al. Cigarette smoking and the risk of systemic lupus erythematosus: a meta-analysis. *Arthritis Rheum* 2004;50:849–857.
165. Kanda H, Hamasaki K, Kubo K, et al. Antiinflammatory effect of simvastatin in patients with rheumatoid arthritis. *J Rheumatol* 2002;29:2024–2026.
166. McCarey DW, McInnes IB, Madhok R, et al. Trial of Atorvastatin in Rheumatoid Arthritis (TARA): double-blind, randomised placebo-controlled trial. *Lancet* 2004;363:2015–2021.
167. Perini R, Fiorucci S, Wallace JL. Mechanisms of nonsteroidal anti-inflammatory drug-induced gastrointestinal injury and repair: a window of opportunity for cyclooxygenase-inhibiting nitric oxide donors. *Can J Gastroenterol* 2004;18:229–236.
168. Huledal G, Jonzon B, Malmenas M, et al. Renal effects of the cyclooxygenase-inhibiting nitric oxide donator AZD3582 compared with rofecoxib and naproxen during normal and low sodium intake. *Clin Pharmacol Ther* 2005;77:437–450.

CHAPTER 35F ■ THE HEART AND INFECTIOUS DISEASES

ANDREW BOYLE

OVERVIEW

Infectious myocarditis is an important etiology of both fulminant and chronic heart failure. Systemic infections such as the human immunodeficiency virus (HIV) and Chagas disease are common causes of profound heart failure, particularly in developing countries. A method for accurately diagnosing infectious myocarditis premortem is elusive, and diagnosis largely relies on circumstantial evidence such as rising serum antibody titers. Newer techniques such as gene amplification by reverse transcription polymerase chain reaction (rt-PCR) and nucleic acid hybridization of right ventricular endomyocardial biopsy (EMB) tissue suffer from a lack of sensitivity. Furthermore, once a diagnosis is made, treatment is mainly focused on hemodynamic support and symptom relief as opposed to counteracting the pathologic organism. Nevertheless, full recovery of cardiac function is common, although not uniform.

CLINICAL PRESENTATION IN INFECTIOUS MYOCARDITIS

There is a wide spectrum of clinical presentations of infectious myocarditis, ranging from a clinically silent syndrome with complete recovery to acutely or chronically decompensated irreversible heart failure leading to either death or cardiac transplantation. The symptoms of mild to moderate infectious myocarditis are relatively nonspecific, consisting of fevers, sweats, or chills associated with mild dyspnea and palpitations. In severe cases of infectious myocarditis, symptoms relate to hypoperfusion and cardiac congestion. Chest pain is relatively infrequent and usually results from accompanying pericarditis. The signs of infectious myocarditis are also nonspecific and include frequent atrial and ventricular ectopy, sinus tachycardia, and, in severe cases, ventricular arrhythmias and volume overload. Varying degrees of atrioventricular heart block may develop transiently and usually resolve spontaneously and completely (1). In the majority of cases, the initial infection remains completely unrecognized and full recovery of cardiac function ensues. However, for unclear reasons, in a minority of patients, the infectious insult leads to progressive myocardial dysfunction either acutely or, more commonly, many years later. This is believed to be one of the more common etiologies for dilated cardiomyopathy (DCM), accounting for 12.8% of all cases (2). Most commonly (in 51.2% of all cases), no etiology is discovered, and the cardiomyopathy is thus termed idiopathic.

DIAGNOSIS OF INFECTIOUS MYOCARDITIS

In light of the lack of specific signs and symptoms for infectious myocarditis, an accurate and early diagnosis of this condition relies on a high clinical suspicion by the practitioner. Often the earliest evidence of active myocarditis is nonspecific changes on the resting electrocardiogram. These changes usually involve the ST segment and the T wave, but in severe cases, significant intraventricular conduction delays can develop either transiently or permanently. A pseudoinfarction electrocardiographic pattern with Q waves and ST-segment elevation offers a particularly poor prognosis, often with a rapidly fatal course (3). Abnormal QRS morphology and left-bundle-branch block are also indicative of a worse prognosis, although usually from progressive congestive heart failure over a more protracted time course (1). There electrocardiographic changes are obviously more helpful when a baseline electrocardiogram is available for comparison.

Serum troponin levels (4) can be elevated as a reflection of ongoing myocardial necrosis from the inflammatory process. The degree of their elevation, indeed whether they are elevated at all, is a function of both the severity of the inflammatory insult as well as its acuity. Both the sensitivity and specificity of these markers of myonecrosis are particularly poor.

A documented fourfold rise in serum viral antibody titers from the acute to the convalescent stage of the infection is indirect evidence of viral infection, which does not assist in the management of the patient in the acute phase of the illness

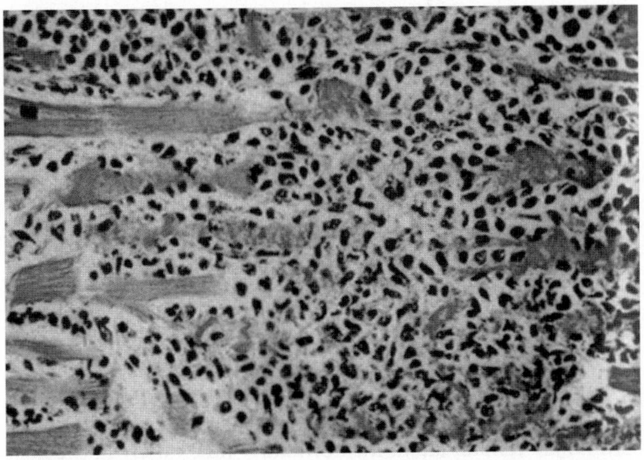

FIGURE 35F.1. Example of severe diffuse lymphocytic myocarditis in a human right ventricular endomyocardial biopsy sample. An extensive interstitial lymphocytic infiltrate and myocyte necrosis are readily seen. (From Hauck AJ, Kearney DL, Edwards WD. Evaluation of postmortem endomyocardial biopsy specimens from 38 patients with lymphocytic myocarditis: implications for role of sampling error. *Mayo Clin Proc* 1989;64:1235–1245.

(5). A significant rise in viral-specific immunoglobulin M (IgM) antibody titers is an earlier serologic finding, although it is still not rapid enough to have therapeutic implications.

Echocardiography is of limited use in the diagnosis of acute infectious myocarditis and serves mainly to confirm left ventricular systolic dysfunction as well as to eliminate other potential etiologies, particularly valvular cardiomyopathies and anatomic abnormalities such as atrial and ventricular septal defects. Gadolinium-enhanced magnetic resonance imaging (MRI) has proven to be relatively sensitive in the detection of acute myocarditis (6). However, it lacks specificity in that abnormal myocardial enhancement reflects only active inflammation regardless of its etiology, including after a myocardial infarction (MI) and various other cardiomyopathic processes.

The gold standard for diagnosis of acute viral myocarditis remains the EMB, despite its many imperfections. The Dallas criteria were created by a panel of cardiac pathologists in 1986 to standardize the pathologic requirements for a diagnosis of IM (7). In brief, a diagnosis of IM in this classification system requires the simultaneous finding of lymphocyte infiltration and myocyte necrosis (Fig. 35F.1). EMB samples in which one criterion is met but not the other are deemed borderline myocarditis. Despite this attempt to create uniformity in histologic diagnosis, there remains significant interobserver variability (8). Furthermore, lymphocytic myocarditis is a patchy disease and is unevenly distributed throughout the myocardium (9). In some patients, the pathologic myocardium is not easily accessible by the bioptome, which, by definition, is limited to sampling subendocardial tissue. Even when the inflammatory process involves the subendocardium, there is a tremendous sampling error when only three to five biopsies are obtained (10). The rate of false-negative EMB is as high as 83% for individual biopsies and 55% when five biopsy samples are obtained in a single patient with autopsy-proven IM (9). In addition, there is a high rate of false-positive EMB because of the presence of small numbers of lymphocytes normally present in the interstitium and because of the difficulty in distinguishing among lymphocytes, interstitial macrophages, fibroblasts, endothelial cells, and pericytes by light microscopy (11). Newer techniques that have been developed to detect myocardial viral genome products in EMB samples using cloned DNA fragments complementary to the viral genome (in situ DNA hybridization) and rt-PCR have generally been successful (12,13). However, these techniques rely on having adequate biopsy samples and thus suffer from significant sampling errors as previously discussed. Furthermore, they have yet to be implemented in the clinical setting because there are few virus-specific therapies that could be initiated should a specific etiology be identified.

Because of the relatively low sensitivity and specificity of all the aforementioned diagnostic studies, the diagnosis of IM at this time and for the foreseeable future remains mainly a clinical one.

ETIOLOGIC AGENTS OF INFECTIOUS MYOCARDITIS

Viruses

Enteroviruses

The enteroviruses are a group of viruses pathogenic to the gastrointestinal and upper respiratory tracts (Table 35F.1). Coxsackie B virus (CBV) appears to be the most common pathogen. Serologic studies have revealed that 36% of all adults with acute myocarditis have demonstrable rises in either their serum anti-CBV antibody titers or IgM (14,15). The full epidemiologic impact of CBV-induced myocarditis is difficult to assess in light of the ubiquitous nature of this organism as evidenced by the high rate of similar findings in control populations (15).

TABLE 35F.1

THE PATHOGENS IN ACUTE INFECTIOUS MYOCARDITIS

Viruses	**Bacteria**
Enteroviruses	*Chlamydia pneumoniae*
Coxsackie A virus	*Chlamydia psittaci*
Coxsackie B virus	*Corynebacterium diphtheriae*
Echovirus	Whipple disease
Polio virus	*Neisseria meningitidis*
Herpes viruses	*Mycoplasma pneumoniae*
Cytomegalovirus	*Legionella pneumophila*
Epstein-Barr virus	*Brucella melitensis*
Herpes simplex	*Salmonella typhi*
Varicella zoster	*Vibrio cholerae*
Human immunodeficiency virus	**Spirochetes**
Other viruses	Lyme borreliosis
Hepatitis B virus	Syphilis
Hepatitis C virus	*Leptospira interrogans*
Adenovirus	**Rickettsiae**
Influenza A virus	Rocky Mountain spotted fever
Influenza B virus	Q fever
Rabies virus	Ehrlichiosis
Parvovirus B19	**Fungi**
Mumps	*Aspergillus*
Measles	*Candida albicans*
Rubella	*Histoplasma capsulatum*
	Cryptococcus neoformans
	Coccidioides immitis
	Mucormycosis
	Parasites
	Chagas disease
	Toxoplasma gondii
	Trichinella spiralis

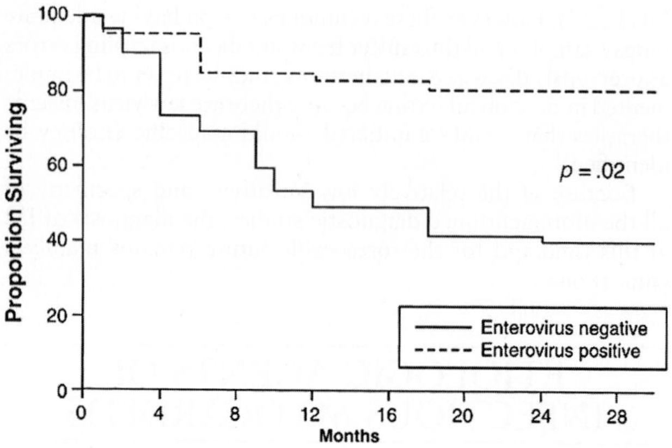

FIGURE 35F.2. Survival curves for patients for whom results of right ventricular endomyocardial biopsies, using in situ DNA hybridization, were enterovirus positive or enterovirus negative. (From Why HJ, Meany BT, Richardson PJ, et al. Clinical and prognostic significance of detection of enteroviral RNA in the myocardium of patients with myocarditis or dilated cardiomyopathy. *Circulation* 1994;89:2582–2589.)

Elements of the CBV genome have also been detected using rt-PCR in EMB of patients who met the Dallas criteria for diagnosis of acute myocarditis (16). The specificity of this finding is questionable, however, due to the unexpectedly high finding of enteroviral RNA in autopsy cases without cardiac disease (16). Furthermore, delineation of the exact viral species using this method is difficult due to significant nucleic acid sequence homology at the 5′-untranslated region of the RNA of all enteroviruses (17). However, probes do exist to species-specific regions of the RNA, which are thus able to differentiate among various species using in situ hybridization.

In the vast majority of patients infected with CBV, cardiac manifestations are not appreciated, although cardiac involvement has been estimated to be as high as 5.3% (18). In most cases, the signs and symptoms of infection are benign and resolve spontaneously. Some investigators have nevertheless proposed that some cases of nonischemic DCM may represent the end stage of either a previously detected (19) or undetected (20) enteroviral infection. Much of this speculation has arisen as a result of the frequent, although not uniform, detection of enteroviral RNA in EMB from patients with nonischemic DCM without clinical evidence of IM (16). In addition, patients with DCM in whom persistent enteroviral RNA can be detected in their EMB have a much worse clinical prognosis (Fig. 35F.2). However, due to the high prevalence of enteroviral infections in the community, these studies provide only circumstantial evidence of a possible link between enteroviral myocarditis and DCM without offering definitive proof. In fact, in one study, enteroviral RNA was detected more frequently in control patients undergoing either heart or lung transplantation for ischemic heart disease or primary lung disease than in patients with DCM (20). However, compelling evidence of a protease encoded by CBV mediating degradation of cardiac dystrophin in mice, thereby reducing myocardial structural integrity, suggests a potential pathogenic role for enteroviruses in DCM in humans (21,22).

Adenovirus

The adenovirus genome has recently been demonstrated in EMB and autopsy samples of myocardium from children and adults with acute myocarditis (23). It was found in a much greater proportion of patients than previously expected, although it may be less pathogenic than enteroviruses (24). The discovery of a common myocardial receptor, the so-called common CBV-adenovirus receptor, suggests a common portal of entry for these viruses and may explain their prominence as causative agents in acute myocarditis and DCM (25). The fact that this receptor appears to be upregulated in patients with DCM compared to controls is also supportive of this theory, albeit not conclusive (26).

Herpes Viruses

Cytomegalovirus (CMV) is readily identified in infected cells due to its characteristic microscopic nuclear and paranuclear inclusion bodies. CMV is a ubiquitous organism that, in the immunocompetent host, commonly produces an asymptomatic primary infection, as evidenced by the presence of circulating anti-CMV antibodies in the majority of the population (27). CMV may remain latent intracellularly indefinitely in the host waiting to become reactivated and lead to a systemic infection if the patient becomes immunocompromised, usually as a result of HIV infection, neoplasia, immunosuppression for rheumatologic or pulmonary disease, or posttransplantation. One component of this generalized infection may include CMV myocarditis, which can be adequately treated with ganciclovir (28). After cardiac transplantation, CMV has also been associated with accelerated cardiac allograft vasculopathy, which is generally believed to be reflective of chronic allograft rejection (29). This hypothesis also remains controversial because others have been unable to confirm this finding (30). Even more intriguingly, however, treatment of cardiac transplant recipients immediately postoperatively with ganciclovir appears to lower the incidence of allograft vasculopathy, regardless of whether or not they developed a systemic CMV illness (31).

Other Herpes Viruses. Epstein-Barr virus (EBV) can rarely cause symptomatic myocarditis (32). EBV has also been implicated in the development of posttransplantation lymphoproliferative disease (PTLD) after cardiac transplantation (33), which is a life-threatening complication often treated by lowering the patient's immunosuppression and possibly systemic chemotherapy.

Herpes simplex virus (24) and varicella zoster virus (34) have been implicated as rare etiologic agents of acute myocarditis.

Human Immunodeficiency Virus

Acquired immunodeficiency syndrome (AIDS) is the end-stage of HIV infection. As the number of worldwide HIV infections has reached epidemic proportions and because advances in medical therapies have enabled prolonged patient survival from both AIDS and various opportunistic infections, the cardiac manifestations of this disease have become more apparent. These cardiac manifestations include direct effects of HIV itself and effects resulting from opportunistic infections that arise as a consequence of an immunosuppressed state.

EMB-proven acute or chronic lymphocytic myocarditis is a frequent finding in patients with AIDS (35). Most frequently, this is a consequence of a superimposed opportunistic infection. HIV RNA and DNA has been detected in such biopsies but is usually very sparse, most often in areas of myocardium without an inflammatory infiltrate or ongoing myonecrosis, and is frequently associated with other opportunistic pathogens (36). A causal relationship has therefore not been firmly established between HIV and myocarditis. It must be noted, however, that no pathogen is identified in a large percentage of cases of AIDS-associated cardiomyopathy, a finding not dissimilar from that of patients whose cardiomyopathy is unrelated to AIDS. Some investigators have proposed that AIDS-associated cardiomyopathy may result from antiretroviral therapy (37). Regardless

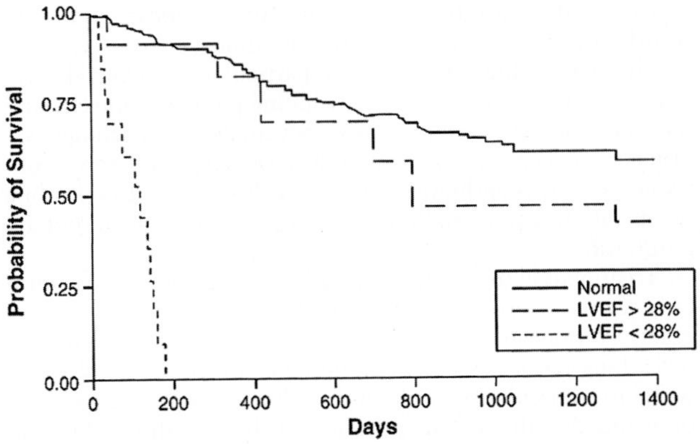

FIGURE 35F.3. Survival curves for 296 human immunodeficiency virus–positive patients who had structurally normal hearts or cardiac dysfunction. LVEF, left ventricular ejection fraction. (From Currie PF, Jacob AJ, Foreman AR, et al. A review of endocarditis in acquired immunodeficiency syndrome and human immunodeficiency virus infection. *Eur Heart J* 1994;309:1606.)

of the etiology of the cardiomyopathic process associated with AIDS, the diagnosis is a harbinger of a poor clinical prognosis, irrespective of the adequacy of the anti-HIV therapy itself (Fig. 35F.3).

Cardiac neoplasms also develop in patients with HIV. Cardiac Kaposi sarcomas are not usually isolated to the heart, but rather are part of a widely metastatic process (38). They are usually asymptomatic, and most cases are discovered unexpectedly at autopsy (Fig. 35F.4). Cardiac non-Hodgkin B-cell lymphoma is also usually associated with a widely disseminated malignant process in HIV patients, but can be a primary lesion as well (39).

Accelerated coronary atherosclerosis has also been observed at autopsy in relatively young HIV patients, although a causal relationship has yet to be established (40). Protease inhibitors, antiretroviral agents used to treat patients with HIV, have been implicated in the development of coronary atherosclerosis (41), likely as result of profound deleterious effects on lipid profiles and insulin metabolism. A recent short-term follow-up of Veteran's Administration patients with HIV failed to demonstrate an increase in cardiovascular (CV) events in patients treated with protease inhibitors (42). Given the potentially significant lag time between the development of hyperlipidemia and insulin resistance and the development of clinically significant cardiovascular disease, it would seem prudent to carefully manage all CV risk factors in all patients exposed to protease inhibitors. Nevertheless, protease inhibitors should not be withheld from HIV patients due to their potential cardiovascular complications given the dramatic improvement in survival and reduced HIV viremia with these agents. Statin therapy is appropriate for hyperlipidemic HIV patients, although lovastatin

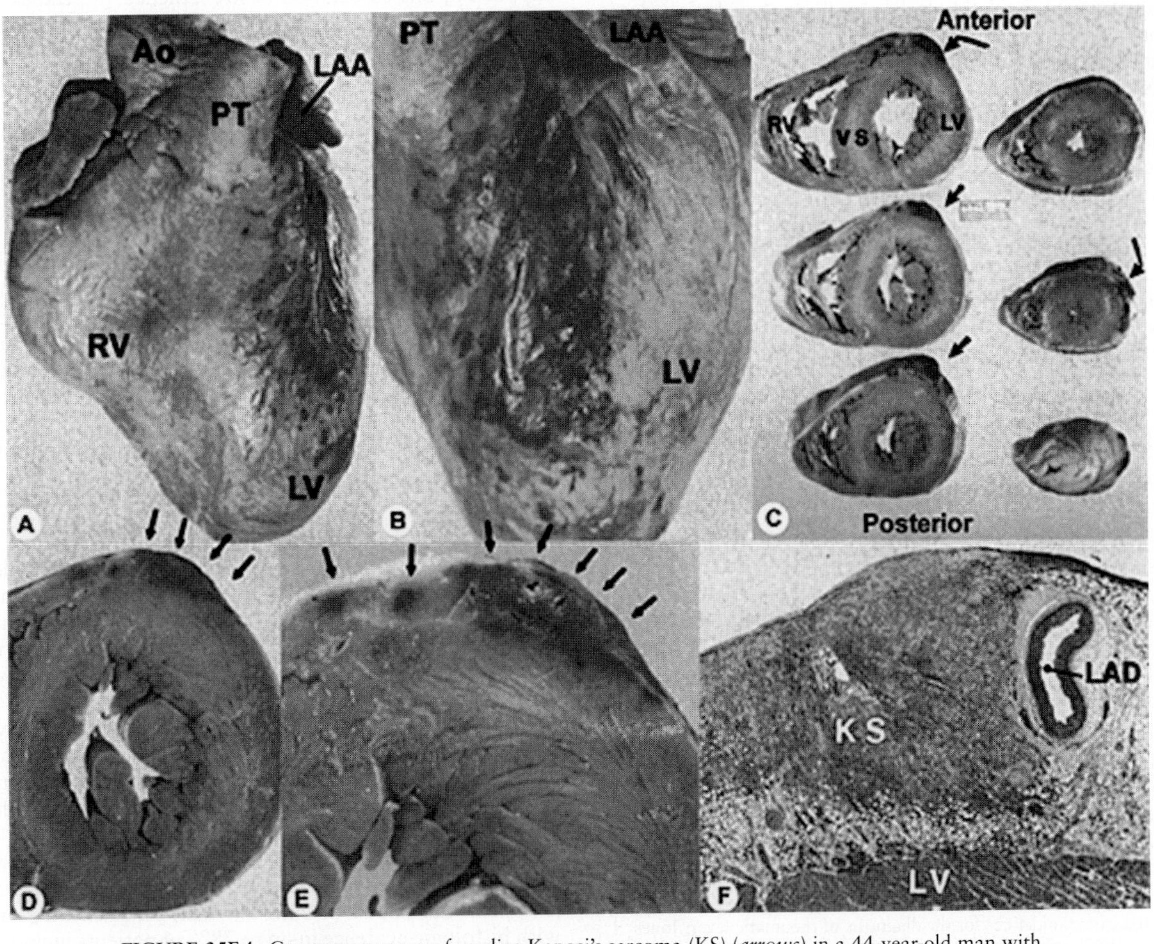

FIGURE 35F.4. Gross appearance of cardiac Kaposi's sarcoma (KS) (*arrows*) in a 44-year-old man with acquired immunodeficiency syndrome. LAA, left atrial appendage; LAD, left anterior descending coronary artery; LV, left ventricle; PT, pulmonary trunk; RV, right ventricle. [From Silver MA, Macher AM, Reichert CM, et al. Cardiac involvement by Kaposi's sarcoma in acquired immune deficiency syndrome (AIDS). *Am J Cardiol* 1984;53:983–985.]

and simvastatin are not recommended due to their interactions with protease inhibitors at the cytochrome P450 enzyme system (43). Care must also be taken when an HIV patient is receiving antifungals or macrolide antibiotics for either prophylaxis or treatment against a variety of opportunistic infections because these may also interact with the cytochrome P450 system.

Other Viruses

Several other viruses have also been proven to rarely cause acute myocarditis including hepatitis B virus (44), hepatitis C virus (45), influenza A (46) and B (47) viruses, rabies virus (48), and parvovirus B19 (49). Cases of mumps (50), measles (51), and rubella (52) myocarditis have all been reported, and fetal rubella infection, as a result of early gestational maternal transmission, can lead to multiple congenital heart defects. However, mumps, measles, and rubella have largely been eradicated as a result of widespread childhood immunization programs.

Bacteria

Rheumatic Fever

Acute rheumatic fever is characterized by a systemic inflammatory response approximately 3 weeks after an untreated group A streptococcal pharyngeal infection but never after a cutaneous infection. The incidence of acute rheumatic fever in the developed world is on the decline in light of widespread antistreptococcal antibiotic therapy for upper respiratory tract infections and general improvements in living conditions. The same is not true in the developing world. Appropriate antibiotic therapy during the preceding pharyngeal infection essentially eliminates the future risk of developing rheumatic fever (53).

The diagnosis of acute rheumatic fever is mainly a clinical one using the revised Jones criteria of 1992 (Table 35F.2). Evidence of two major criteria or one major criterion and at least two minor criteria are required for a presumptive diagnosis of rheumatic fever, which is enhanced by a history of a recent upper respiratory tract infection, a positive throat culture, or a positive antistreptococcal antibody test.

TABLE 35F.2

REVISED JONES CRITERIA FOR THE DIAGNOSIS OF ACUTE RHEUMATIC FEVER, 1992

Major criteria
Carditis
Polyarthritis
Chorea
Erythema marginatum
Subcutaneous nodules
Minor criteria
Arthralgia
Fever
Elevated erythrocyte sedimentation rate
Elevated C-reactive protein levels
First-degree atrioventricular block

Adapted from Guidelines for the diagnosis of rheumatic fever: Jones criteria, 1992 update. Special Writing Group of the Committee on Rheumatic Fever, Endocarditis, and Kawasaki Disease of the Council on Cardiovascular Disease in the Young of the American Heart Association. *JAMA* 1992;268:2069–2073, with permission.

Rheumatic carditis can involve the endocardium, myocardium, or pericardium. Most commonly, there is variable involvement of the cardiac valves, particularly the mitral valve and its subvalvular apparatus, including papillary muscles and their attached chordae tendineae. Severe clinical decompensation is the exception rather than the rule. The most feared consequence of this pathologic process is chronic scarring leading to mitral, and potentially aortic, valvular stenosis and/or regurgitation.

Treatment in mild cases is usually with high doses of aspirin (54). Corticosteroids can be added to this regimen in severe cases. To prevent recurrences of carditis and acute rheumatic fever, long-term, perhaps even life-long, antibiotic prophylaxis with intramuscular benzathine penicillin G every 3 weeks is recommended, although the duration of therapy should be individualized depending on the patient's risk of recurrence (55).

Chlamydia pneumoniae

Chlamydia pneumoniae (CP) has generated tremendous interest recently as a result of its purported association with the development of coronary atherosclerosis. Seroepidemiologic studies initially demonstrated increased anti-CP titers in patients with an acute MI (68%) or chronic angina (50%) compared to controls (17%) (56). This concept, however, remains controversial in light of the fact that several studies have since confirmed this finding (57,58) whereas others have refuted it (59,60), mainly because of high seropositivity prevalence in their control groups. Nevertheless, the potential evidence supporting this association is strengthened by studies readily demonstrating the presence of CP organisms in atherosclerotic plaques (61,62) but rarely in normal coronary arteries. This evidence is weakened, however, by the demonstration that CP DNA could be detected in the presence of coronary atherosclerosis but did not reflect either the extent or severity of the disease (63). CP DNA could be detected only at one site in one patient with severe diffuse atherosclerosis, whereas another patient with only mild coronary atherosclerosis had detectable DNA in every arterial segment examined.

A large meta-analysis of all randomized, controlled trials using antibiotic therapy against CP to treat patients with preexisting coronary atherosclerosis failed to show any clinical benefit with reductions in the incidence of acute coronary syndromes, MI, or mortality (64). At this time, the treatment of coronary atherosclerosis by antibiotics has been abandoned.

Chlamydia pneumoniae (65) and *Chlamydia psittaci* (66) have also both been implicated in cases of acute myocarditis, albeit rarely.

Other Bacteria

Corynebacterium diphtheriae infection can commonly lead to myocarditis by virtue of its exotoxin, which has a high affinity for the cardiac conduction system. Once myocardial involvement occurs, the patient has a much worse prognosis, with a mortality upward of 50% (67). This disease has largely been eradicated in the developed world due to widespread childhood immunization programs but persists in the developing world, where such programs have not been implemented. Treatment of this life-threatening condition must consist of both antitoxin toward the exotoxin as well as antibiotics against the infecting organism.

Whipple disease, or intestinal lipodystrophy, is a rare chronic systemic bacterial infection caused by *Tropheryma whippelii*. Cardiac involvement in Whipple disease is common, with histologic evidence in up to 78% of patients including the myocardium (68), although patients are rarely symptomatic.

Many other bacteria have also rarely been associated with myocarditis including *Neisseria meningitidis* (meningococcus) (69), *Mycoplasma pneumoniae* (70), *Legionella pneumophila*

(71), *Brucella melitensis* (72), *Salmonella typhi* (73), and *Vibrio cholerae* by way of its cholera toxin (74).

Spirochetes

Lyme Disease

Lyme disease is a systemic illness caused by the spirochete *Borrelia burgdorferi*, whose primary vector is the ixodid tick. Carditis is a common manifestation thought to occur in approximately 10% of all patients in the disseminated phase of the illness, often weeks to months after the initial infection (75). Because it can take up to 8 weeks for serologic conversion, signs and symptoms of Lyme borreliosis frequently precede positive serologic tests, yielding many false-negative results. The most common cardiac finding in patients with Lyme disease is varying degrees of atrioventricular block, which can fluctuate from normal to first-degree atrioventricular block to complete heart block in the same patient within minutes. Although patients are often asymptomatic, some may become syncopal during periods of high-degree atrioventricular block and may benefit from temporary transvenous pacing. Permanent pacing is rarely indicated, and complete resolution is the rule, usually within 1 to 2 weeks (76).

Lyme borreliosis can also less commonly cause acute myopericarditis (75), and *B. burgdorferi* has been isolated from EMB in patients with both acute (77) and chronic (78) cardiomyopathies. Furthermore, patients with DCM are more likely to have positive Lyme serologies than are controls (79), although this seems to be a weak association and has not been confirmed by others (80). This hypothesis is enhanced by the finding that ceftriaxone could reverse the cardiomyopathic process in 9 of 42 patients seropositive for *B. burgdorferi* (81), although others have been unable to demonstrate any such reversal (78). In summary, the evidence supporting an epidemiologic role for *B. burgdorferi* in DCM is very circumstantial, fails to prove causation, and is not currently the subject of major investigative efforts.

Current recommendations for the treatment of Lyme disease are listed in Table 35F.3. Antibiotic therapy during the early phase of the disease seems to eliminate the potential for development of future disseminated disease, including carditis (82). No evidence exists, however, demonstrating that antibiotic therapy once carditis has developed leads to more rapid resolution of the carditis because it is usually self-limited, with complete recovery in most cases. Nevertheless, antibiotic therapy is now common clinical practice mainly to prevent further dissemination of the disease including neurologic sequelae. Others have also advocated the use of corticosteroids and salicylates in severe cases (75), although this approach has not been proven prospectively to confer any therapeutic advantage.

TABLE 35F.3

RECOMMENDATIONS FOR THE TREATMENT OF LYME CARDITIS

Early Lyme disease
Doxycycline, 100 mg twice daily for 10–21 d; amoxicillin, 500 mg three times daily for 10–21 d
Lyme carditis
Ceftriaxone, 2 g i.v. daily for 14 d
Penicillin G, 20 million U i.v. daily for 14 d
Alternatives, for mild cases of Lyme carditis only
Doxycycline, 100 mg orally twice daily for 14–21 d
Amoxicillin, 500 mg three times daily for 14–21 d

Adapted from Rahn DW, Malawista SE. Lyme disease: recommendations for diagnosis and treatment. *Ann Intern Med* 1991;114:472–481, with permission.

Other Spirochetes

In the early part of the twentieth century, syphilitic aortitis, caused for the spirochete *Treponema pallidum*, was relatively common, resulting in aortic aneurysms, aortic valvular insufficiency, and coronary ostial stenoses (83). However, this condition has largely been eradicated with widespread public health measures aimed at stopping the spread of sexually transmitted diseases and the development of effect antibiotic therapy.

Patients with severe leptospirosis, caused by the spirochete *Leptospira interrogans*, often have transient electrocardiographic changes (84) and can develop acute myocarditis (85). Acute coronary arteritis and aortitis are also common postmortem findings in patients with severe leptospirosis (85).

Rickettsiae

Rocky Mountain spotted fever is a tick-transmitted systemic illness caused by *Rickettsia rickettsii* and is characterized by a generalized vasculitis. Acute myopericarditis and atrioventricular conduction disturbances are relatively common and can be fatal (86) but are usually not clinically significant (87).

Q fever is a systemic rickettsial illness caused by *Coxiella burnetii*, usually inhaled by humans after aerosolization from the placenta of farm animals. Valvular endocarditis is by far the most common clinical presentation of chronic Q fever infection (88). Conversely, acute myopericarditis is a rare phenomenon, although it portends a much worse prognosis (88).

Ehrlichiosis is a tick-borne rickettsial organism that infects circulating monocytes and granulocytes. It can also rarely cause acute myocarditis (89).

Fungi

Fungal infections of the heart are uncommon and generally occur only in patients who are immunosuppressed (90). Fungal endocarditis can also occur after cardiac surgery, intravenous (IV) drug abuse, or prolonged central venous access (91,92). Although disseminated *Aspergillus* and candidal infections are common after cardiac transplantation (93), involvement of the myocardium is exceedingly rare. Fungal myocarditis has been reported with *Aspergillus* (94), *Candida albicans* (95), *Histoplasma capsulatum* (90), *Cryptococcus neoformans* (90), *Coccidioides immitis* (96), and mucormycosis (97). In postmortem studies, myocardial fungal involvement is characterized by diffuse myocardial abscesses as well as coronary artery occlusion by fungal mycelia and thrombus (95,97). However, direct invasion via the mediastinum has also been observed (98).

Parasites

Chagas Disease (Trypanosomiasis)

Chagas disease is a protozoal infestation caused by *Trypanosoma cruzi* and is transmitted to humans in the feces of the reduviid bug as it bites. Chagas disease is endemic to Central and South America, where more than 20 million people are estimated to be infected (99). More rarely, it may be transmitted by blood transfusions from an infected donor (100). The

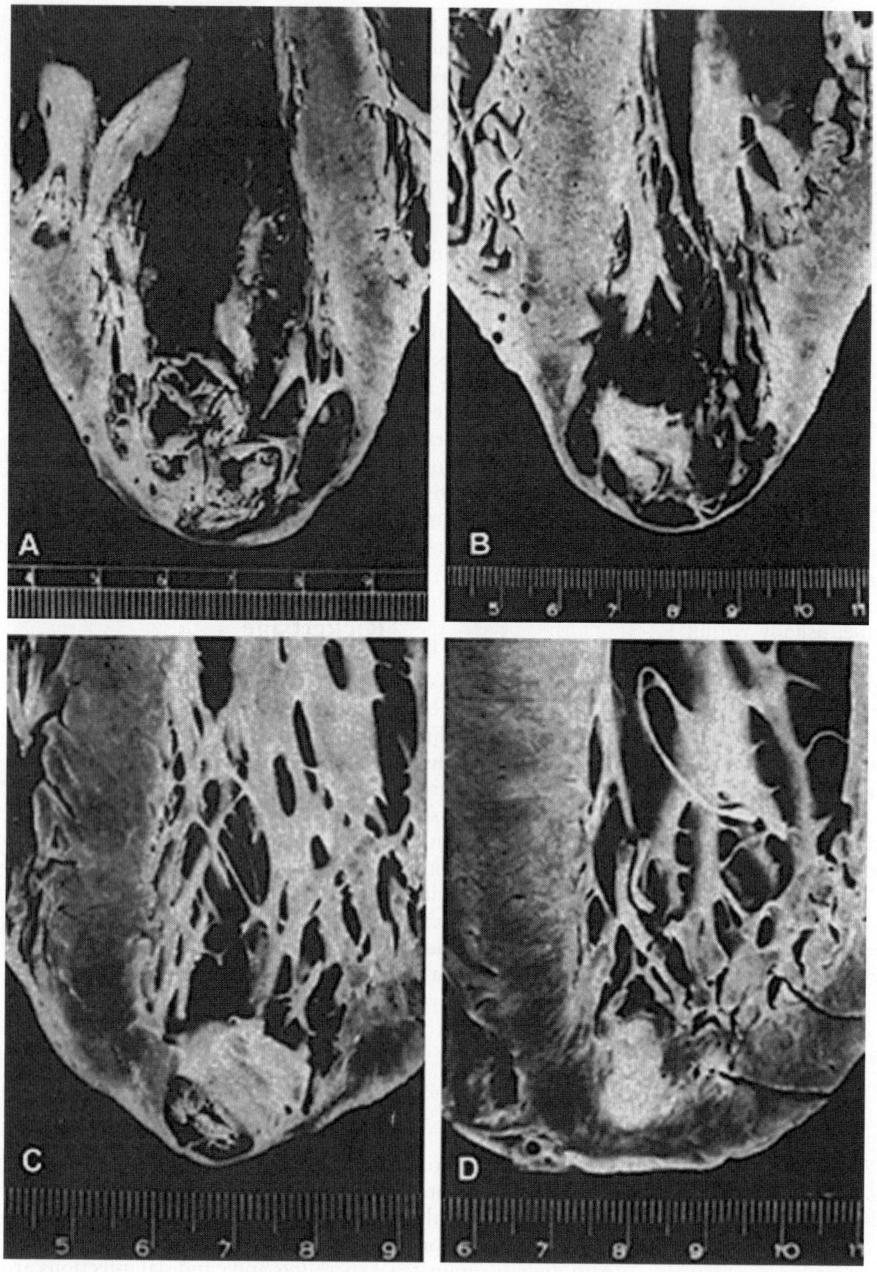

FIGURE 35F.5. Examples of left ventricular apical aneurysms in patients with Chagas disease. [From Samuel J, Oliveira M, Correa De Araujo RR, et al. Cardiac thrombosis and thromboembolism in chronic Chagas heart disease. *Am J Cardiol* 1983;52(1):147–151.]

acute phase of the human disease is usually benign and clinically asymptomatic other than a mild fever, although acute myocarditis can be demonstrated in EMB of most patients and can be fatal (101). More commonly, a slowly progressive cardiomyopathic process ensues that may remain clinically unrecognized for more than 20 years (99). During this indeterminate phase, 30% to 40% of infected patients (and >80% of those who go on to develop a cardiomyopathy) develop conduction abnormalities due to extensive myocardial fibrosis. A right-bundle-branch block and/or a left anterior hemiblock are the most frequent abnormalities and can progress to higher degrees of atrioventricular heart block (102).

Chronic Chagasic cardiomyopathy develops in approximately 10% to 30% of all infected patients. The pathogenesis of this disease is controversial, but it is likely multifactorial, including a continued direct parasitic effect on the myocardium (103), autoimmune-mediated myocyte injury (104), and parasite-mediated microvascular endothelial injury resulting in compromised myocardial perfusion (104). Anatomically, Chagas disease can be distinguished from other cardiomyopathies by the classic finding of apical thinning and aneurysm formation (Fig. 35F.5). Functionally, multiple segmental wall-motion abnormalities are common as well as global systolic dysfunction (102), highlighting the need to rule out a coronary etiology for the cardiomyopathy. These apical aneurysms and/or their accompanying left ventricular systolic dysfunction place patients at risk for thromboembolism and potentially lethal ventricular arrhythmias (105). Alternatively, the cardiomyopathic process may progress unrelentingly until the patient develops overt congestive heart failure, a harbinger of a very poor prognosis (Fig. 35F.6).

Antiparasitic therapy at this stage is generally thought to be ineffective, although studies have suggested that treatment may prevent disease progression in a minority of patients (106). Given the relatively poor prognosis of these patients, it would seem appropriate to attempt one course of antiparasitic therapy

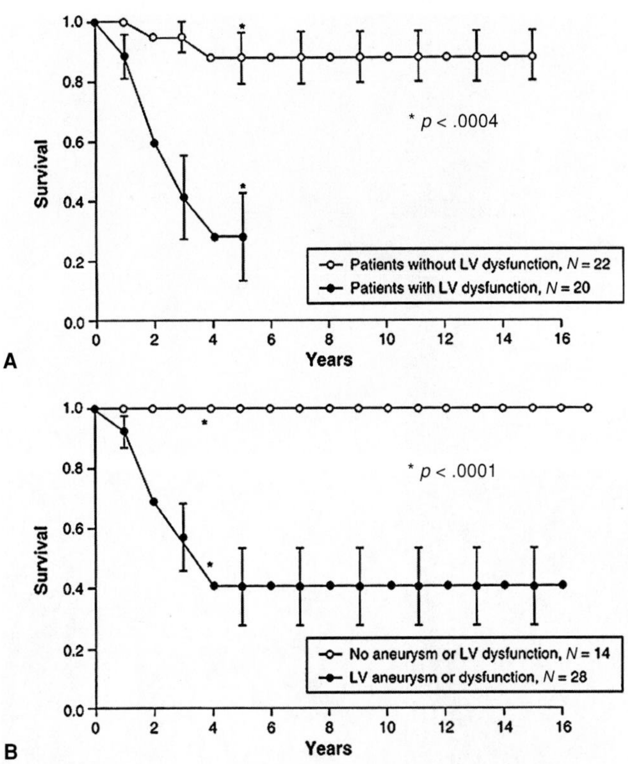

FIGURE 35F.6. **A:** Survival curves for patients who have Chagas disease with and without left ventricular (LV) dysfunction. (From Hagar JM, Rahimtoola SH. Chagas heart disease. *Curr Probl Cardiol* 1995;20:825–924.) **B:** Survival curves for patients who have Chagas disease with LV dysfunction or aneurysm or with neither. (From Hagar JM, Rahimtoola SH. Chagas heart disease in the United States. *N Engl J Med* 1991;325:763–768.)

in virtually all patients, although this is controversial. Despite the inflammatory nature of this disorder, immunosuppression is not advised due to potential reactivation of otherwise latent organisms (107). Because iatrogenic immunosuppression is used routinely to prevent rejection after cardiac transplantation, concerns have arisen with regard to the candidacy of end-stage Chagasic cardiomyopathy patients for transplantation. However, successful cardiac transplantation can be performed with careful serologic follow-up to detect and treat any reactivation of the disease, which occurs at some point in nearly all patients (108). However, the higher incidence of malignant neoplasms observed in these patients compared to controls is of concern and may be related to parasite reactivation or the antiparasitic therapy they received (109).

Other Parasites

Acute myocarditis as a result of parasitic infestation is a rare phenomenon, although multiple parasites have been implicated. *Toxoplasma gondii* may cause acute myocarditis in an immunocompromised patient (110). *Toxoplasma gondii* can be transmitted to a heart transplant recipient through the donor allograft (111), which shows the need for careful pre-operative serologic screening of both the donor and recipient.

Trichinella spiralis may also cause acute myocarditis (112). Acute cardiac decompensation can also rarely occur with *Plasmodium falciparum* (malaria) as a result of parasitic coronary occlusion (113). Patients with hepatosplenic schistosomiasis can develop portal hypertension, and consequently, via collateral circulation, *Schistosoma mansoni* eggs can embolize and occlude the pulmonary arteries, leading to pulmonary hypertension and cor pulmonale (114). Hydatid cysts can form within the myocardium, can compress or obstruct the adjacent chamber (115), and can be safely treated with surgical excision.

MECHANISM OF INJURY IN VIRAL MYOCARDITIS

The state of knowledge with regard to the pathogenesis of viral myocarditis is derived almost exclusively from animal studies and is controversial and incomplete (Fig. 35F.7). There are at least three phases of injury: (a) a direct effect of the viral pathogen on the myocyte, (b) an acute inflammatory response resulting in viral clearance and myocytolysis of infected cells, and (c) a chronic phase in animals unable to eradicate the virus. Although the time sequence in the murine viral myocarditis model is more rapid, it is felt to generally accurately reflect the sequence of events in humans.

The initial phase in this murine model is characterized by a direct cytotoxic effect of the virus on the myocyte during the first four days postinoculation. At this time, no inflammatory infiltrate is visualized histologically (116), yet myocyte necrosis is seen (Fig. 35F.8). This hypothesis is strongly supported by the finding that mice with severe combined immunodeficiency syndrome (SCID), and thus no B- or T-cell immunologic response, have widespread myonecrosis without accompanying inflammatory cells (117).

The second phase, usually from days 4 to 14, is characterized by a large increase in cytokine production leading to severe inflammatory cell infiltration and myocyte necrosis (Figure 35F.8). Similar cytokine elevations have been observed in humans with acute myocarditis (118). Natural killer cells appear

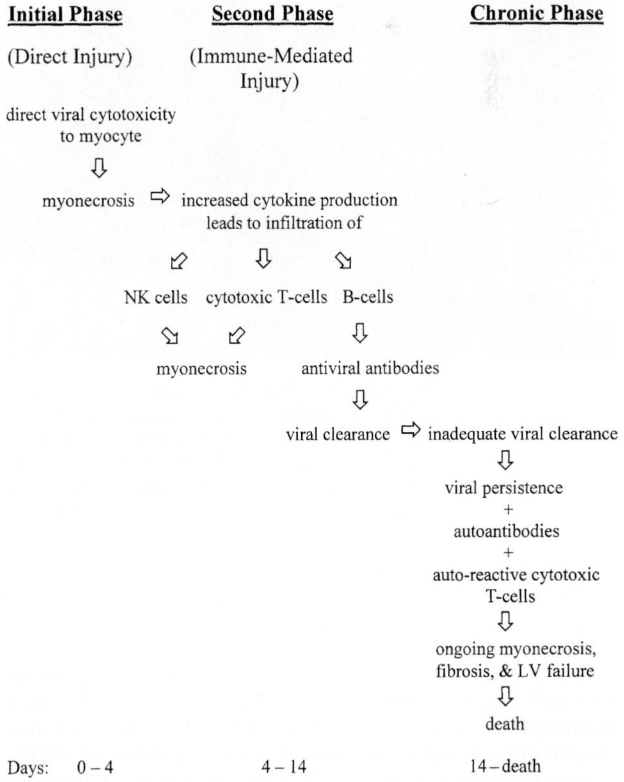

FIGURE 35F.7. Pathogenesis of acute infectious myocarditis. LV, left ventricular; NK, natural killer.

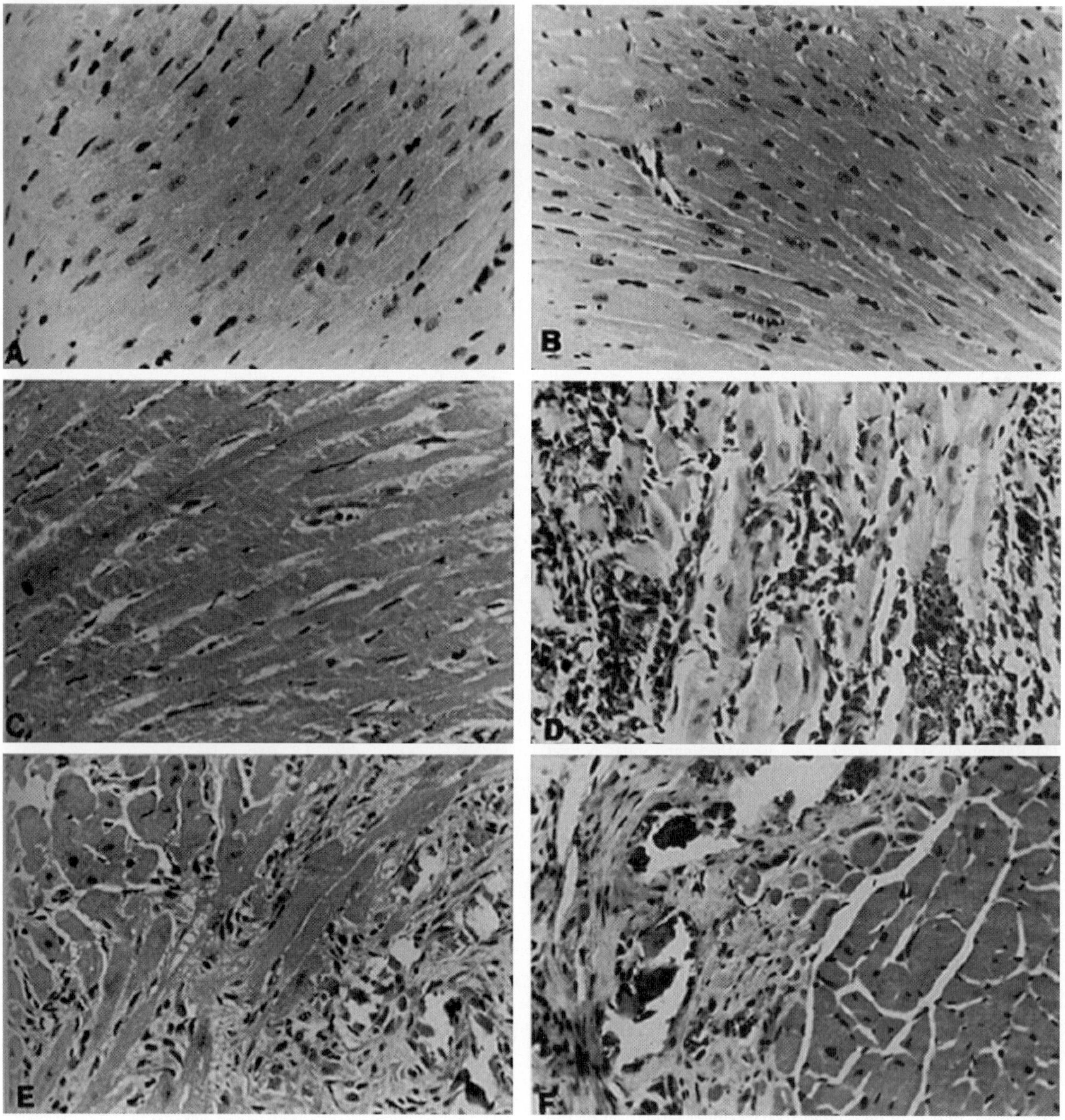

FIGURE 35F.8. Typical histopathologic findings in the murine experimental myocarditis model. **A:** Control subject. **B:** One day after inoculation, no histologic changes are seen. **C:** Three days after inoculation, small foci of degenerated myocytes can be seen. **D:** Seven days after inoculation, extensive cellular infiltration and myonecrosis are visible. **E:** Fourteen days after inoculation, reduced mononuclear cell infiltration and fibrosis around necrotic zones are present. **F:** Eighty days after inoculation, dense fibrosis surrounding calcification is visible. (From Shioi T, Matsumori A, Sasayama S. Persistent expression of cytokine in the chronic stage of viral myocarditis in mice. *Circulation* 1996;94:2930–2937.)

in this inflammatory milieu on approximately day 4 and inhibit viral replication, which also peaks at this time (119), resulting in cytolysis of infected cardiac myocytes (120). Viruses are also cleared via B lymphocyte–derived antiviral antibodies, which appear after day 4 with a rapidly rising titer (121). T lymphocytes are also crucial in this phase, with their concentration peaking on days 7 to 14, resulting in widespread myonecrosis of infected cells (122). The importance of lymphocytes to the process of viral load clearance is confirmed in mice with SCID, in which viremia persisted throughout the duration of the study (117). T lymphocytes recognize viral proteins expressed on the surface of infected myocytes, resulting in further myocytolysis (122). However, T lymphocytes are not critical for viral load clearance and seem to play a more harmful than helpful role by increasing the severity of the resulting myonecrosis, perhaps by also killing uninfected myocytes by autoimmune mechanisms (122), an effect that may be counterbalanced by increased production of interferon-β (123). Therefore, in this model, humoral immunity is responsible for viral clearance, whereas cellular immunity inflicts much of the pathologic damage to the myocardium.

The chronic phase is characterized by progressive left ventricular dysfunction and dilation. Several different mechanisms have been proposed to explain this deterioration, but in all likelihood, the process is multifactorial. With more sensitive diagnostic tools such as rt-PCR and in situ DNA hybridization, persistence of viral RNA has been demonstrated in chronic cardiomyopathic hearts, raising the possibility of ongoing virus-specific immune-mediated damage (124). Alternatively, ongoing myonecrosis may be caused by either autoantibodies that cross-react between viral antigens and cardiac myocyte antigens (125,126) or autoreactive cytotoxic T lymphocytes, which cross-react in a similar manner (122). In this scenario, noninfected cells are also irreversibly injured.

Recent evidence has suggested that cytokine-induced [perhaps through tumor necrosis factor-α (127)] increased de novo gene transcription of macrophage calcium-independent inducible nitric oxide synthase (iNOS) may have a dual role in the development of viral myocarditis (128). High concentrations of NO may help mediate the host's defense against the invading organism, but it may also be toxic to the surrounding tissues (129). However, intermediate levels of NO may have a protective role by inhibiting proteolytic activity against dystrophin and thereby maintaining structural integrity of the myocardium (130). The degree of a host's upregulation of iNOS activity may help to explain some of the individual variability in the severity of illness in response to a common viral pathogen.

TREATMENT OF INFECTIOUS MYOCARDITIS

Treatment, in general, for both acute and chronic infectious myocarditis is aimed at reducing congestion, improving cardiac hemodynamics, and prolonging survival, irrespective of its etiology. Guidelines exist and are updated regularly to assist in this endeavor (131). However, in contrast to other etiologies of congestive heart failure, it is important to note that, in murine models of acute myocarditis, high doses of digoxin increased mortality, presumably by increasing the production of various cytokines (132).

Immunosuppression with corticosteroids, cyclosporine, and/or azathioprine was once advocated for the treatment of new-onset myocarditis. However, the Myocarditis Treatment Trial showed no survival benefit or improved myocardial recovery in the treatment arm (Fig. 35F.9). Immunosuppression has also been shown to be clinically ineffective for patients with DCM (133). FTY720, a new experimental systemic immunosuppressant, affects lymphocyte trafficking by accelerating the sequestration of mature lymphocytes into lymph nodes and thereby reducing circulating lymphocytes without affecting their function. In a murine experimental model of acute viral myocarditis, FTY720 improved survival and attenuated histologic abnormalities without increasing viral replication (134). Human trials are needed, however, before this promising strategy can be implemented clinically.

IV immunoglobulin (IVIg) therapy had also been advocated for patients with acute myocarditis. However, the Intervention in Myocarditis and Acute Cardiomyopathy trial failed to demonstrate any therapeutic effect for IVIg therapy as compared to placebo, with most patients having a spontaneous recovery of left ventricular function (135).

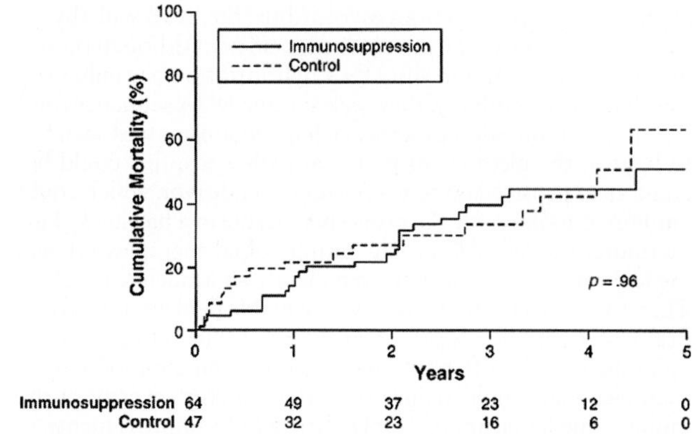

FIGURE 35F.9. Actuarial mortality in the Myocarditis Treatment Trial. The numbers of patients at risk are listed at the bottom. (From Mason JW, O'Connell JB, Herskowitz A, et al. A clinical trial of immunosuppressive therapy for myocarditis. The Myocarditis Treatment Trial Investigators. *N Engl J Med* 1995;333:269–275.)

Specific antimicrobial therapy should always be tried when available. This is particularly true in patients infected with CMV, bacteria, spirochetes, rickettsiae, or parasites. Unfortunately, the most common viral species have no specific antiviral therapy. Ribavirin, a nucleoside analogue with potent nonspecific antiviral activity, has been shown to prevent the development of viral myocarditis in a murine model (136). Ribavirin was only effective, however, if given before or simultaneously with the inoculation with the viral pathogen. Any delay in the administration of the ribavirin rendered it useless, which may explain its apparent ineffectiveness in humans (137).

Infrequently, acute myocarditis may become fulminant and lead to circulatory collapse and cardiogenic shock. Such patients can be hemodynamically supported with ventricular assist devices (VAD) (138). Most patients can be successfully weaned from these devices within a few days to weeks as ventricular function improves. If ventricular function does not improve, VADs can serve as a bridge to transplantation or as destination therapy. Initial concerns with regard to decreased survival after cardiac transplantation in the setting of active myocarditis (139) have been contradicted by a large retrospective analysis (140). However, a greater frequency of episodes of acute rejection is observed in patients with preoperative myocarditis, particularly in the first 4 months (99), which may predispose them to an increased risk of transplant vasculopathy (141). At this juncture, it seems prudent to try to stabilize a patient medically for as long as possible to allow him or her a chance to recover ventricular function or, at the very least, to transplant the patient in a less inflammatory or infectious milieu.

CONTROVERSIES AND PERSONAL PERSPECTIVES

It is unfortunate that a clinician's ability to accurately diagnose and specifically treat patients with acute infectious myocarditis has not progressed at the same rate as with various other cardiac ailments. This stems from four fundamental problems with this disease process: (a) patients fail to present to their physician before most of the damage is already completed, (b) clinicians have a low index of suspicion, (c) it is difficult to identify the exact pathogen in a time-efficient manner, and (d) there is a lack of availability of specific therapies once a pathogen is identified. Although it remains the current gold standard for the diagnosis of acute infectious myocarditis, the EMB will always suffer from a lack of sensitivity and specificity. Although the addition of rt-PCR and in situ DNA hybridization has enhanced this diagnostic modality, they seek specific DNA sequences and thus presume one already knows which organisms to search for. In light of the plethora of potential pathogens, this could become an expensive and time-consuming endeavor, which could amount to looking for the proverbial needle in a haystack. Furthermore, the lack of specific antimicrobial therapies renders the identification of the pathogen mainly an academic exercise. Therefore, it seems that any advance in this field would have to begin with the development of either specific effective therapies against the offending pathogen or immunomodulatory therapies that would reduce the extent and/or severity of the immune-mediated injury. Only then would improvements in diagnostics become clinically meaningful.

THE FUTURE

The greatest worldwide epidemiologic impact could be achieved via improved living and health standards in the developing world, including sexually transmitted disease prevention. Clearly, the incidence and prevalence of HIV and Chagasic cardiomyopathies could be significantly reduced with such measures.

The most exciting recent development in the treatment of acute infectious myocarditis is the demonstration that FTY720 could reduce circulating lymphocytes, improve survival, and attenuate histologic abnormalities without increasing viral replication (134). For the first time, there is a compound that offers promise for the treatment of acute myocarditis and appears to be pathogen independent. If the results obtained in animal models can be replicated in humans, this therapeutic approach holds a tremendous amount of promise, provided patients can be identified early enough to benefit from this therapy.

References

1. Morgera T, Di Lenarda A, Dreas L, et al. Electrocardiography of myocarditis revisited: clinical and prognostic significance of electrocardiographic changes. *Am Heart J* 1992;124(2):455–467.
2. Felker GM, Hu W, Hare JM, et al. The spectrum of dilated cardiomyopathy. The Johns Hopkins experience with 1,278 patients. *Medicine* 1999; 78(4):270–283.
3. Take M, Sekiguchi M, Hiroe M, et al. Long-term follow-up of electrocardiographic findings in patients with acute myocarditis proven by endomyocardial biopsy. *Jpn Circ J* 1982;46(11):1227–1234.
4. Lauer B, Niederau C, Kuhl U, et al. Cardiac troponin T in patients with clinically suspected myocarditis. *J Am Coll Cardiol* 1997;30(5):1354–1359.
5. See DM, Tilles JG. Viral myocarditis. *Rev Infect Dis* 1991;13(5):951–956.
6. Friedrich MG, Strohm O, Schulz-Menger J, et al. Contrast media–enhanced magnetic resonance imaging visualizes myocardial changes in the course of viral myocarditis. *Circulation* 1998;97(18):1802–1809.
7. Aretz HT, Billingham ME, Edwards WD, et al. Myocarditis. A histopathologic definition and classification. *Am J Cardiovasc Pathol* 1987;1(1): 3–14.
8. Shanes JG, Ghali J, Billingham ME, et al. Interobserver variability in the pathologic interpretation of endomyocardial biopsy results. *Circulation* 1987;75(2):401–405.
9. Hauck AJ, Kearney DL, Edwards WD. Evaluation of postmortem endomyocardial biopsy specimens from 38 patients with lymphocytic myocarditis: implications for role of sampling error. *Mayo Clin Proc* 1989.64(10):1235–1245.
10. Chow LH, Radio SJ, Sears TD, et al. Insensitivity of right ventricular endomyocardial biopsy in the diagnosis of myocarditis. *J Am Coll Cardiol* 1989;14(4):915–920.
11. Linder J, Cassling RS, Rogler WC, et al. Immunohistochemical characterization of lymphocytes in uninflamed ventricular myocardium. Implications for myocarditis. *Arch Pathol Lab Med* 1985;109(10):917–920.
12. Nicholson F, Ajetunmobi JF, Li M, et al. Molecular detection and serotypic analysis of enterovirus RNA in archival specimens from patients with acute myocarditis. *Br Heart J* 1995;74(5):522–527.
13. Jin O, Sole MJ, Butany JW, et al. Detection of enterovirus RNA in myocardial biopsies from patients with myocarditis and cardiomyopathy using gene amplification by polymerase chain reaction. *Circulation* 1990;82(1):8–16.
14. El-Hagrassy MM, Banatvala JE, Coltart DJ. Coxsackie B virus–specific IgM responses in patients with cardiac and other diseases. *Lancet* 1980; 2(8205):1160–1162.
15. Bell EJ, McCartney RA. A study of Coxsackie B virus infections, 1972–1983. *J Hygiene* 1984;93(2):197–203.
16. Ueno H, Yokota Y, Shiotani H, et al. Significance of detection of enterovirus RNA in myocardial tissues by reverse transcription polymerase chain reaction. *Int J Cardiol* 1995;51(2):157–164.
17. Hyypia T. Etiological diagnosis of viral heart disease. *Scand J Infect Dis Suppl* 1993;88:25–31.
18. Coxsackie B5 virus infections during 1965. A report to the Director of the Public Health Laboratory Service from various laboratories in the United Kingdom. *Br Med J* 1967;4(579):575–577.
19. Levi G, Scalvini S, Volterrani M, et al. Coxsackie virus heart disease: 15 years after. *Eur Heart J* 1988;9(12):1303–1307.
20. Muir P, Nicholson F, Illavia SJ, et al. Serological and molecular evidence of enterovirus infection in patients with end-stage dilated cardiomyopathy. *Heart* 1996;76(3):243–249.
21. Badorff C, Lee GH, Lamphear BJ, et al. Enteroviral protease 2A cleaves dystrophin: evidence of a cytoskeletal disruption in an acquired cardiomyopathy. *Nat Med* 1999;5(3):320–326.
22. Badorff C, Knowlton KU. Dystrophin disruption in enterovirus-induced myocarditis and dilated cardiomyopathy: from bench to bedside. *Med Microbiol Immunol* 2004;193:121–126.
23. Bowles NE, Ni J, Kearney DL, et al. Detection of viruses in myocardial tissues by polymerase chain reaction: evidence of adenovirus as a common cause of myocarditis in children and adults. *J Am Coll Cardiol* 2003;42(3): 466–472.
24. Martin AB, Webber S, Fricker FJ, et al. Acute myocarditis. Rapid diagnosis by PCR in children. *Circulation* 1994;90(1):330–339.
25. Roelvink PW, Lizonova A, Lee JG, et al. The coxsackievirus-adenovirus receptor protein can function as a cellular attachment protein for adenovirus serotypes from subgroups A, C, D, E, and F. *J Virol* 1998;72(10):7909–7915.
26. Noutsias M, Fechner H, de Jonge H, et al. Human coxsackievirus-adenovirus receptor is colocalized with integrins $\alpha_v\beta_3$ and $\alpha_v\beta_5$ on the cardiomyocyte sarcolemma and upregulated in dilated cardiomyopathy: implications for cardiotropic viral infections. *Circulation* 2001;104:275–280.
27. Lowry RW, Adam E, Hu C, et al. What are the implications of cardiac infection with cytomegalovirus before heart transplantation? *J Heart Lung Transpl* 1994;13(1 Pt 1):122–128.
28. Shabtai M, Luft B, Waltzer WC, et al. Massive cytomegalovirus pneumonia and myocarditis in a renal transplant recipient: successful treatment with DHPG. *Transplant Proc* 1988;20(3):562–563.
29. Grattan MT, Moreno-Cabral CE, Starnes VA, et al. Cytomegalovirus infection is associated with cardiac allograft rejection and atherosclerosis. *J Am Med Assoc* 1989;261(24):3561–3566.
30. Gulizia JM, Kandolf R, Kendall TJ, et al. Infrequency of cytomegalovirus genome in coronary arteriopathy of human heart allografts. *Am J Pathol* 1995;147(2):461–475.
31. Valantine HA, Gao SZ, Menon SG, et al. Impact of prophylactic immediate posttransplant ganciclovir on development of transplant atherosclerosis: a post hoc analysis of a randomized, placebo-controlled study. *Circulation* 1999;100(1):61–66.
32. Tyson Jr AA, Hackshaw BT, Kutcher MA. Acute Epstein-Barr virus myocarditis simulating myocardial infarction with cardiogenic shock. *Southern Med J* 1989;82(9):1184–1187.
33. Gray J, Wreghitt TG, Pavel P, et al. Ebstein-Barr virus infection in heart and heart-lung transplant recipients: incidence and clinical impact. *J Heart Lung Transpl* 1995;14(4):640–646.
34. Tsintof A, Delprado WJ, Keogh AM. Varicella zoster myocarditis progressing to cardiomyopathy and cardiac transplantation. *Br Heart J* 1993; 70(1):93–95.
35. Anderson DW, Virmani R, Reilly JM, et al. Prevalent myocarditis at necropsy in the acquired immunodeficiency syndrome. *J Am Coll Cardiol* 1988;11(4):792–799.
36. Herskowitz A, Wu TC, Willoughby SB, et al. Myocarditis and cardiotropic viral infection associated with severe LV dysfunction in late-stage infection with HIV. *J Am Coll Cardiol* 1994;24(4):1025–1032.
37. Herskowitz A, Willoughby SB, Baughman KL, et al. Cardiomyopathy associated with antiretroviral therapy in patients with HIV infection: a report of six cases. *Ann Intern Med* 1992;116(4):311–313.
38. Silver MA, Macher AM, Reichert CM, et al. Cardiac involvement by Kaposi's sarcoma in acquired immunodeficiency syndrome. *Am J Cardiol* 1984;53(7):983–985.
39. Duong M, Dubois C, Buisson M, et al. Non-Hodgkin's lymphoma of the heart in patients infected with human immunodeficiency virus. *Clinical Cardiol* 1997;20(5):497–502.
40. Joshi VV, Pawel B, Connor E, et al. Arteriopathy in children with acquired immunodeficiency syndrome. *Pediatr Pathol* 1987;7(3):261–275.
41. Henry K, Melroe H, Huebsch J, et al. Severe premature CAD with PI. *Lancet* 1998;351(9112):1328.

42. Bozette SA, Ake CF, Tam HK et al. Cardiovascular and cerebrovascular events in patients treated for human immunodeficiency virus infection. *N Engl J Med* 2003;348:702–710.
43. Corsini A. The safety of HMG-CoA reductase inhibitors in special populations at high cardiovascular risk. *Cardiovasc Drugs Ther* 2003;17:265–285.
44. Mahapatra RK, Ellis GH. Myocarditis and hepatitis B virus. *Angiology* 1985;36(2):116–119.
45. Matsumori A, Yutani C, Ikeda Y, et al. Hepatitis C virus from the hearts of patients with myocarditis and cardiomyopathy. *Lab Invest* 2000;80(7): 1137–1142.
46. Engblom E, Ekfors TO, Meurman OH, et al. Fatal influenza A myocarditis with isolation of virus from the myocardium. *Acta Med Scand* 1983; 213(1):75–78.
47. Craver RD, Sorrells K, Gohd R. Myocarditis with influenza B infection. *Pediatr Infect Dis J* 1997;16(6):629–630.
48. Cheetham HD, Hart J, Coghill NF, et al. Rabies with myocarditis. Two cases in England. *Lancet* 1970;1(7653):921–922.
49. Enders G, Dotsch J, Bauer J, et al. Life-threatening parvovirus B19–associated myocarditis and cardiac transplantation as possible therapy: two case reports. *Clin Infect Dis* 1998;26(2):355–358.
50. Ni J, Bowles NE, Kim YH, et al. Viral infection of the myocardium in endocardial fibroelastosis. Molecular evidence for the role of mumps virus as an etiologic agent. *Circulation* 1997;95(1):133–139.
51. Frustaci A, Abdulla AK, Caldarulo M, et al. Fatal measles myocarditis. *Cardiologia* 1990;35(4):347–349.
52. Kriseman T. Rubella myocarditis in a 9-year-old patient. *Clin Pediatr* 1984;23(4):240–241.
53. Davis J, Schmidt W. Benzathine penicillin G: its effectiveness in prevention of streptococcal infections in a heavily exposed population. *N Engl J Med* 1957;256(8):339–342.
54. Thatai D, Turi ZG. Current guidelines for the treatment of patients with rheumatic fever. *Drugs* 1999;57(4):545–555.
55. Lue HC, Wu MH, Wang JK, et al. Three- versus four-week administration of benzathine penicillin G: effects on incidence of streptococcal infections and recurrences of rheumatic fever. *Pediatrics* 1996;97(6 Pt 2):984–988.
56. Saikku P, Leinonen M, Mattila K, et al. Serological evidence of an association of a novel *Chlamydia*, TWAR, with chronic coronary heart disease and acute myocardial infarction. *Lancet* 1988;2(8618):983–986.
57. Thom DH, Grayston JT, Siscovick DS, et al. Association of prior infection with *Chlamydia pneumoniae* and angiographically demonstrated coronary artery disease. *J Am Med Assoc* 1992;268(1):68–72.
58. Linnanmaki E, Leinonen M, Mattila K, et al. *Chlamydia pneumoniae*-specific circulating immune complexes in patients with chronic coronary heart disease. *Circulation* 1993;87(4):1130–1134.
59. Ridker PM, Kundsin RB, Stampfer MJ, et al. Prospective study of *Chlamydia pneumoniae* IgG seropositivity and risks of future myocardial infarction. *Circulation* 1999;99(9):1161–1164.
60. Nieto FJ, Folsom AR, Sorlie PD, et al. *Chlamydia pneumoniae* infection and incident coronary heart disease: the Atherosclerosis Risk in Communities Study. *Am J Epidemiol* 1999;150(2):149–156.
61. Kuo CC, Shor A, Campbell LA, et al. Demonstration of *Chlamydia pneumoniae* in atherosclerotic lesions of coronary arteries. *J Infect Dis* 1993; 167(4):841–849.
62. Muhlestein JB, Hammond EH, Carlquist JF, et al. Increased incidence of *Chlamydia* species within the coronary arteries of patients with symptomatic atherosclerotic versus other forms of cardiovascular disease. *J Am Coll Cardiol* 1996;27(7):1555–1561.
63. Thomas M, Wong Y, Thomas D, et al. Relation between direct detection of *Chlamydia pneumoniae* DNA in human coronary arteries at postmortem examination and histological severity (Stary grading) of associated atherosclerotic plaque. *Circulation* 1999;99(21):2733–2736.
64. Andraws R, Berger JS, Brown DL. Effects of antibiotic therapy on outcomes in patients with coronary heart disease: a meta-analysis of randomized controlled trials. *J Am Med Assoc* 2005;293:2641–2647.
65. Bruu AL, Haukenes G, Aasen S, et al. *Chlamydia pneumoniae* infections in Norway 1981–87 earlier diagnosed as ornithosis. *Scand J Infect Dis* 1991; 23(3):299–304.
66. Schinkel AF, Bax JJ, van der Wall EE, et al. Echocardiographic follow-up of *Chlamydia psittaci* myocarditis. *Chest* 2000;117(4):1203–1205.
67. Stockins BA, Lanas FT, Saavedra JG, et al. Prognosis in patients with diphtheric myocarditis and bradyarrhythmias: assessment of results of ventricular pacing. *Br Heart J* 1994;72(2):190–191.
68. Silvestry FE, Kim B, Pollack BJ, et al. Cardiac Whipple disease: identification of Whipple bacillus by electron microscopy of a patient before death. *Ann Intern Med* 1997;126(3):214–216.
69. Hardman JM, Earle KM. Myocarditis in 200 fatal meningococcal infections. *Arch Pathol* 1969;87(3):318–325.
70. Chen SC, Tsai CC, Nouri S. Carditis associated with *Mycoplasma pneumoniae* infection. *Am J Dis Child* 1986;140(5):471–472.
71. Armengol S, Domingo C, Mesalles E. Myocarditis: a rare complication during *Legionella* infection. *Int J Cardiol* 1992;37(3):418–420.
72. Lubani M, Sharda D, Helin I. Cardiac manifestations in brucellosis. *Arch Dis Child* 1986;61(6):569–572.
73. Akdeniz H, Tuncer I, Irmak H, et al. *Salmonella* myocarditis in a patient with Wolf-Parkinson-White syndrome that was confused with an inferior myocardial infarction. *Clin Infect Dis* 1997;25(3):736–737.
74. Leon F, Badui E, Campos A, et al. Cholera and myocarditis—a case report. *Angiology* 1997;48(6):545–549.
75. Steere AC, Batsford WP, Weinberg M, et al. Lyme carditis: cardiac abnormalities of Lyme disease. *Ann Intern Med* 1980;93(1):8–16.
76. McAlister HF, Klementowicz PT, Andrews C, et al. Lyme carditis: an important cause of reversible heart block. *Ann Intern Med* 1989;110(5):339–345.
77. de Koning J, Hoogkamp-Korstanje JA, van der Linde MR, et al. Demonstration of spirochetes in cardiac biopsies of patients with Lyme disease. *J Infec Dis* 1989;160(1):150–153.
78. Stanek G, Klein J, Bittner R, et al. Isolation of *Borrelia burgdorferi* from the myocardium of a patient with longstanding cardiomyopathy. *N Engl J Med* 1990;322(4):249–252.
79. Klein J, Stanek G, Bittner R, et al. Lyme borreliosis as a cause of myocarditis and heart muscle disease. *Eur Heart J* 1991;12(Suppl D):73–75.
80. Rees DH, Keeling PJ, McKenna WJ, et al. No evidence to implicate *Borrelia burgdorferi* in the pathogenesis of dilated cardiomyopathy in the United Kingdom. *Br Heart J* 1994;71(5):459–461.
81. Gasser R, Dusleag J, Reisinger E, et al. Reversal by ceftriaxone of dilated cardiomyopathy *Borrelia burgdorferi* infection. *Lancet* 1992;339(8802): 1174–1175.
82. Steere AC, Hutchinson GJ, Rahn DW, et al. Treatment of the early manifestations of Lyme disease. *Ann Intern Med* 1983;99(1):22–26.
83. Jackman Jr JD, Radolf JD. Cardiovascular syphilis. *Am J Med* 1989; 87(4):425–433.
84. Watt G, Padre LP, Tuazon M, et al. Skeletal and cardiac muscle involvement in severe, late leptospirosis. *J Infect Dis* 1990;162(1):266–269.
85. de Brito T, Morais CF, Yasuda PH, et al. Cardiovascular involvement in human and experimental leptospirosis: pathologic findings and immunohistochemical detection of leptospiral antigen. *Ann Trop Med Parasitol* 1987;81(3):207–214.
86. Bradford WD, Hackel DB. Myocardial involvement in Rocky Mountain spotted fever. *Arch Pathol Lab Med* 1978;102(7):357–359.
87. Walker DH, Paletta CE, Cain BG. Pathogenesis of myocarditis in Rocky Mountain spotted fever. *Arch Pathol Lab Med* 1980;104(4):171–174.
88. Raoult D, Tissot-Dupont H, Foucault C, et al. Q fever 1985–1998. Clinical and epidemiologic features of 1,383 infections. *Medicine* 2000;79(2):109–123.
89. Jahangir A, Kolbert C, Edwards W, et al. Fatal pancarditis associated with human granulocytic Ehrlichiosis in a 44-year-old man. *Clin Infect Dis* 1998;27(6):1424–1427.
90. Altieri PI, Climent C, Lazala G, et al. Opportunistic invasion of the heart in Hispanic patients with acquired immunodeficiency syndrome. *Am J Trop Med Hyg* 1994;51(1):56–59.
91. Atkinson JB, Connor DH, Robinowitz M, et al. Cardiac fungal infections: review of autopsy findings in 60 patients. *Hum Pathol* 1984;15(10):935–942.
92. Walsh TJ, Hutchins GM, Bulkley BH, et al. Fungal infections of the heart: analysis of 51 autopsy cases. *Am J Cardiol* 1980;45(2):357–366.
93. Grossi P, Farina C, Fiocchi R, et al. Prevalence and outcome of invasive fungal infections in 1,963 thoracic organ transplant recipients: a multicenter retrospective study. Italian Study Group of Fungal Infections in Thoracic Organ Transplant Recipients. *Transplantation* 2000;70(1):112–116.
94. Williams AH. *Aspergillus* myocarditis. *Am J Clin Pathol* 1974;61(2):247–256.
95. Franklin WG, Simon AB, Sodeman TM. *Candida* myocarditis without valvulitis. *Am J Cardiol* 1976;38(7):924–928.
96. Schwartz EL, Waldmann EB, Payne RM, et al. Coccidioidal pericarditis. *Chest* 1976;70(5):670–672.
97. Benbow EW, McMahon RF. Myocardial infarction caused by cardiac disease in disseminated zygomycosis. *J Clin Pathol* 1987;40(1):70–74.
98. Berarducci L, Ford K, Olenick S, et al. Invasive intracardiac aspergillosis with widespread embolization. *J Am Soc Echocardiogr* 1993;6(5):539–542.
99. Hagar JM, Rahimtoola SH. Chagas' heart disease. *Curr Probl Cardiol* 1995;20(12):825–924.
100. Grant IH, Gold JW, Wittner M, et al. Transfusion-associated acute Chagas disease acquired in the United States. *Ann Intern Med* 1989;111(10):849–851.
101. Parada H, Carrasco HA, Anez N, et al. Cardiac involvement is a constant finding in acute Chagas' disease: a clinical, parasitological and histopathological study. *Int J Cardiol* 1997;60(1):49–54.
102. Hagar JM, Rahimtoola SH. Chagas' heart disease in the United States. *N Engl J Med* 1991;325(11):763–768.
103. Higuchi ML, de Brito T, Reis M, et al. Correlation between *Trypanosoma cruzi* parasitism and myocardial inflammatory infiltrate in human chronic Chagasic myocarditis: light microscopy and immunohistochemical findings. *Cardiovasc Pathol* 1993;2(2):101–106.
104. Rossi MA, Bestetti RB. The challenge of Chagasic cardiomyopathy. The pathologic roles of autonomic abnormalities, autoimmune mechanisms and microvascular changes, and therapeutic implications. *Cardiology* 1995; 86(1):1–7.
105. Bestetti RB, Freitas OC, Muccillo G, et al. Clinical and morphological characteristics associated with sudden cardiac death in patients with Chagas' disease. *Eur Heart J* 1993;14(12):1610–1614.
106. de Andrade AL, Zicker F, de Oliveira RM, et al. Randomised trial of efficacy of benznidazole in treatment of early *Trypanosoma cruzi* infection. *Lancet* 1996;348(9039):1407–1413.

107. Sinagra A, Riarte A, Lauricella M, et al. Reactivation of experimental chronic *T cruzi* infection after immunosuppressive treatment by cyclosporine A and betametasone. *Transplant* 1993;55(6):1431–1434.
108. Bocchi EA, Bellotti G, Mocelin AO, et al. Heart transplantation for chronic Chagas' heart disease. *Ann Thorac Surg* 1996;61(6):1727–1733.
109. Bocchi EA, Higuchi ML, Vieira ML, et al. Higher incidence of malignant neoplasms after heart transplantation for treatment of Chagas' heart disease. *J Heart Lung Transpl* 1998;17(4):399–405.
110. Hofman P, Drici MD, Gibelin P, et al. Prevalence of *Toxoplasma* myocarditis in patients with the acquired immunodeficiency syndrome. *Br Heart J* 1993;70(4):376–381.
111. Ryning FW, McLeod R, Maddox JC, et al. Probable transmission of *Toxoplasma gondii* by organ transplantation. *Ann Intern Med* 1979;90(1):47–49.
112. Compton SJ, Celum CL, Lee C, et al. Trichinosis with ventilatory failure and persistent myocarditis. *Clin Infect Dis* 1993;16(4):500–504.
113. Merkel W. *Plasmodium falciparum* malaria: the coronary and myocardial lesions observed at autopsy in two cases of acute fulminating *P. falciparum* infection. *Arch Pathol* 1946;41:290–298.
114. Sadigursky M, Andrade ZA. Pulmonary changes in schistosomal cor pulmonale. *Am J Trop Med Hyg* 1982;31(4):779–784.
115. Miralles A, Bracamonte L, Pavie A, et al. Cardiac echinococcosis. Surgical treatment and results. *J Thorac Cardiovasc Surg* 1994;107(1):184–190.
116. Henke A, Huber S, Stelzner A, et al. The role of CD8+ T lymphocytes in Coxsackie B3–induced myocarditis. *J Virol* 1995;69(11):6720–6728.
117. Chow LH, Beisel KW, McManus BM. Enteroviral infection of mice with severe combined immunodeficiency. Evidence for direct viral pathogenesis of myocardial injury. *Lab Invest* 1992;66(1):24–31.
118. Matsumori A, Yamada T, Suzuki H, et al. Increased circulating cytokines in patients with myocarditis and cardiomyopathy. *Br Heart J* 1994;72(6):561–566.
119. Godeny EK, Gauntt CJ. Involvement of natural killer cells in coxsackievirus B3–induced murine myocarditis. *J Immunol* 1986;137(5):1695–1702.
120. Seko Y, Shinkai Y, Kawasaki A, et al. Evidence of perforin-mediated cardiac myocyte injury in acute murine myocarditis caused by Coxsackievirus B3. *J Pathol* 1993;170(1):53–58.
121. Lodge PA, Herzum M, Olszewski J, et al. Coxsackievirus B3 myocarditis. Acute and chronic forms of the disease caused by different immunopathogenic mechanisms. *Am J Pathol* 1987;128(3):455–463.
122. Huber SA, Lodge PA. Coxsackievirus B3 myocarditis in Balb/c mice. Evidence for autoimmunity to myocyte antigens. *Am J Pathol* 1984;116(1):21–29.
123. Deonarain R, Cerullo D, Fuse K, et al. Protective role for interferon-(beta) in Coxsackievirus B3 infection. *Circulation* 2004;110(23):3540–3543.
124. Klingel K, Hohenadl C, Canu A, et al. Ongoing enterovirus-induced myocarditis is associated with persistent heart muscle infection: quantitative analysis of virus replication, tissue damage, and inflammation. *Proc Nat Acad Sci USA* 1992;89(1):314–318.
125. Maisch B, Bauer E, Cirsi M, et al. Cytolytic cross-reactive antibodies directed against the cardiac membrane and viral proteins in Coxsackievirus B3 and B4 myocarditis. Characterization and pathogenetic relevance. *Circulation* 1993;87(5 Suppl):IV49–IV65.
126. Lawson CM, O'Donoghue HL, Reed WD. Mouse cytomegalovirus infection induces antibodies which cross-react with virus and cardiac myosin: a model for the study of molecular mimicry in the pathogenesis of viral myocarditis. *Immunology* 1992;75(3):513–519.
127. Huber SA, Sartini D. Roles of tumor necrosis factor alpha and the p55 receptor in CD1d induction and Coxsackievirus B3–induced myocarditis. *J Virol* 2005;79(5):2659–2665.
128. Robinson NM, Zhang HY, Bevan AJ, et al. Induction of myocardial nitric oxide synthase by Coxsackievirus B3 in mice. *Eur J Clin Invest* 1999;29:700–707.
129. Heineke J, Kempf T, Kraft T, et al. Downregulation of cytoskeletal muscle LIM protein by nitric oxide: impact on cardiac myocyte hypertrophy. *Circulation* 2003;107(10):1424–1432.
130. Badorff C, Fichtlscherer B, Rhoads RE, et al. Nitric oxide inhibits dystrophin proteolysis by coxsackieviral protease 2A through s-nitrosylation: a protective mechanism against enteroviral cardiomyopathy. *Circulation* 2000;102(18):2276–2281.
131. Consensus recommendations for the management of chronic heart failure. On behalf of the membership of the Advisory Council to Improve Outcomes Nationwide in Heart Failure. *Am J Cardiol* 1999;83(2A):1A–38A.
132. Matsumori A, Igata H, Ono K, et al. High doses of digitalis increase the myocardial production of proinflammatory cytokines and worsen myocardial injury in viral myocarditis: a possible mechanism of digitalis toxicity. *Jpn Circ J* 1999;63(12):934–940.
133. Parrillo JE, Cunnion RE, Epstein SE, et al. A prospective, randomized, controlled trial of prednisone for dilated cardiomyopathy. *NEJM* 1989; 321(16):1061–1068.
134. Miyamoto T, Matsumori A, Hwang MW et al. Therapeutic effects of FTY720, a new immunosuppressive agent, in a murine model of acute viral myocarditis. *J Am Coll Cardiol* 2001;37(6):1713–1718.
135. McNamara DM, Holubkov R, Starling RC et al. Controlled trial of intravenous immune globulin in recent-onset dilated cardiomyopathy. *Circulation* 2001;103:2254–2259.
136. Kishimoto C, Crumpacker CS, Abelmann WH. Ribavirin treatment of murine Coxsackievirus B3 myocarditis with analyses of lymphocyte subsets. *J Am Coll Cardiol* 1988;12(5):1334–1341.
137. Ray CG, Icenogle TB, Minnich LL, et al. The use of intravenous ribavirin to treat influenza virus–associated acute myocarditis. *J Infect Dis* 1989; 159(5):829–836.
138. Reiss N, el-Banayosy A, Posival H, et al. Management of acute fulminant myocarditis using circulatory support systems. *Artif Organs* 1996;20(8): 964–970.
139. O'Connell JB, Dec GW, Goldenberg IF, et al. Results of heart transplantation for active lymphocytic myocarditis. *J Heart Transpl* 1990;9(4):351–356.
140. O'Connell JB, Breen TJ, Hosenpud JD. Heart transplantation in dilated heart muscle disease and myocarditis. *Eur Heart J* 1995;16(Suppl O):137–139.
141. Kobashigawa JA, Miller L, Yeung A, et al. Does acute rejection correlate with the development of transplant coronary artery disease? A multicenter study using intravascular ultrasound. *J Heart Lung Transpl* 1995;14(6): S221–S226.

CHAPTER 36 ■ SUBSTANCE ABUSE AND THE HEART

ROBERT A. KLONER AND SHEREIF H. REZKALLA

OVERVIEW

Cocaine may be associated with myocardial ischemia and myocardial infarction (MI). A physician who sees a young person with an unexplained MI should consider cocaine use to be a possible cause. Cocaine may also cause hypertension, cardiomyopathy, arrhythmias, and sudden death. Whether coffee is associated with cardiovascular disease remains highly controversial. However, tea, particularly green tea, may be beneficial. Anabolic steroids and amphetamines have been associated with cases of MI. Excessive alcohol consumption causes dilated cardiomyopathy and hypertension, but moderate consumption of alcohol may reduce coronary artery disease. Tobacco use is unquestionably a strong risk factor for coronary artery disease.

COCAINE CARDIOTOXICITY

Of the various substances of abuse that may affect the heart, cocaine has received the most attention over the last 10 years (1–9). This is largely a result of its widespread use, especially in large urban areas of the United States; the relative ease with which the substance can be obtained; and the occurrence of sudden death among athletes who have used cocaine. In this section, we review the history of cocaine use, describe the basic science of the effect of cocaine use on the heart, detail the results of clinical and autopsy reports of cocaine use in humans, and describe the clinical approach to and therapy for patients who have cocaine cardiotoxicity.

History

Cocaine is an alkaloid from the *Erythroxylon coca* plant, which grows primarily in South America (10). The Indians of South America have chewed coca leaves for thousands of years. During the time of the Inca empire, coca leaves were used as part of religious ceremonies and given as gifts for special services. In the eleventh century, coca leaves lost their religious significance, and chewing of the leaves spread across all social classes; the leaves were often used as payment for labor in the fields. Writings tell of the restorative powers of coca leaves, including their ability to satisfy hunger and provide a sense of strength and power to the weary. Albert Nieman identified cocaine as the active substance in coca leaves in the late 1850s, and as early as 1880, experimental studies in dogs showed that cocaine had a cardiac-accelerating effect. Sigmund Freud advocated the use of cocaine for a host of ailments, and Carl Koller and William Halstead demonstrated that cocaine had local anesthetic properties.

In the 1860s, a wine known as Vin Mariani, which contained cocaine as a stimulant, was introduced to the market, and in 1886, the drink Coca-Cola was introduced, with cocaine as the active ingredient in the original preparation. Cocaine has since been removed from Coca-Cola, but in the late 1800s, a number of wines and tonics contained cocaine. The first death associated with cocaine use was reported in the 1890s, and numerous reports of addiction and death—including death from use of cocaine as a local anesthetic—appeared in the early 1900s.

That cocaine could affect the human heart was suggested in an article by Lewin in 1931, who stated, "Experiments carried out years ago in Europe proved that drinking of an infusion of 12 g of coca leaves, occasioned—besides a greater frequency of pulse, palpitations of the heart, faintness, seeing of sparks and tinnitus aurium—a feeling of augmented power and a greater desire for activity" (11,12).

By the early 1900s, cocaine was regarded as a dangerous and addictive substance. President William Howard Taft, in an address to Congress in 1910, said that "cocaine posed the most dangerous drug problem that the United States ever faced." The Pure Food and Drug Act of 1906 required that cocaine be listed as an ingredient whenever it was included in a product, and the Harrison Narcotic Act of 1914 permitted sale of cocaine by prescription only and banned the use of cocaine in patented remedies. Public sentiment was in favor of these regulations, and medical problems caused by cocaine use were relatively infrequent until the 1970s, when cocaine gained prominence as a recreational drug. In the mid-1980s, several highly publicized cases of deaths in athletes who used cocaine and various reports (13) that linked the recreational use of cocaine to cardiac events stimulated renewed interest in the medical consequences of cocaine abuse. (The chewing of coca leaves is still common in South America, where, in general, serious medical consequences have not been reported; this may be because a lower dose of the substance is extracted when the plant leaves are chewed, because cocaine is degraded by gastric acid, and because only a small amount of gastrointestinal absorption occurs when cocaine is taken in this fashion.)

It is estimated that approximately 5 to 6 million people in the United States use cocaine on a regular basis, that approximately 1 million are addicted, and that 25 to 30 million Americans have tried cocaine at least once (2,3).

Forms of Cocaine

Cocaine hydrochloride is a water-soluble form of cocaine in which the alkaloid extract of the *E. coca* plant is dissolved in hydrochloric acid to form a white crystalline powder (14,15). Because the white powder can be absorbed by the mucous membranes, intranasal insufflation (snorting) of this white powder is the most common route of administration. The powder also can be injected intravenously. Cocaine is not readily absorbed gastrointestinally, and the low pH of the gastric mucosa may inactivate the alkaloid (14,15).

Crack cocaine is produced by mixing cocaine powder with baking soda and water and then heating the results. The alkaloid base precipitates into a soft mass that hardens and is then smoked. The term "crack" derives from the cracking or popping sound heard when the cocaine crystals are prepared in this fashion.

Freebase cocaine is made by mixing the cocaine powder with a base (such as ammonia) and a solvent (such as ether). The alkaloid base or "free base" is extracted from the ether by evaporation. Like crack, freebase cocaine is smoked. The flammability of ether poses yet another danger in the preparation of this form of cocaine. Freebase use has declined as crack has become more available and because crack does not pose the problem of flammability.

An estimated 90% of cocaine use in the United States is carried out through nasal snorting. In addition, approximately one third of cocaine users have smoked crack. Less than 10% have injected the drug intravenously. Because cocaine is rapidly absorbed through the respiratory tract, smoking of either crack or freebase cocaine rapidly delivers cocaine to the circulation. Cocaine enters the brain within 6 to 8 seconds by the respiratory route (smoking) and within 10 to 15 seconds by an intravenous route. Snorting cocaine results in peak cocaine concentrations in 30 to 60 minutes (15). The amount of cocaine that can be absorbed through the nasal route may be self-limited to some extent because of vasoconstriction of the nasal mucosa induced by cocaine itself.

Cocaine is often combined with other substances, most commonly ethanol. An estimated 9 to 12 million individuals use this combination on a recreational basis (16,17). Cocaethylene is the cocaine metabolite formed in the presence of ethyl alcohol and may be more potent than cocaine itself (see section on cocaethylene).

Pharmacology

The pharmacology of cocaine is complex and has been the subject of a vast amount of basic science research during the last 10 years. First, cocaine is a local anesthetic. It blocks sodium and potassium channels (6) and thus blocks initiation and conduction of electrical impulses. This effect accounts for prolongation of electrocardiographic (ECG) intervals and decreases in cardiac contractility and may lead to a proarrhythmic effect (18). Second, cocaine blocks the reuptake of neurotransmitters at the presynaptic endings of nerves. As a result, neurotransmitters such as dopamine and norepinephrine accumulate in the synaptic cleft, which results in an intense sympathomimetic effect (6). This second major action of cocaine accounts for increases in heart rate, blood pressure, and contractility, and, by stimulation of α-receptors in the vasculature, contributes to vasoconstriction. A third pharmacologic action of cocaine that affects the cardiovascular system is a decrease in vagal tone, which also contributes to an increase in heart rate (19). Thus, on one hand, cocaine may have a cardiodepressive effect resulting from its effect on sodium and potassium channels. On the other hand, it has a stimulatory effect because of its sympathomimetic properties. These opposing forces may result in very complex outcomes (20).

Effects of Cocaine Administration in Experimental Studies

Cocaine directly depresses the myocardium in experimental studies, resulting in both regional and global abnormalities (21–35). When administered intravenously to animals, it results in various degrees of conduction abnormalities and lethal ventricular arrhythmias (36–49). It results in significant myocardial ischemia because of its deleterious effects on platelet function (46–48) and the coronary arteries (49–54). Details of the various laboratory studies are summarized elsewhere (2).

Controlled Studies of Administration of Cocaine in Humans

Cocaine is known to increase both heart rate and blood pressure in awake individuals. Fischman and coworkers (55) demonstrated a dose-related increase in these parameters when patients received intravenous cocaine. Although small doses did not have a significant effect, an intravenous injection of cocaine, 16 and 32 mg, resulted in a significant rise in both heart rate and blood pressure in human volunteers. The changes peaked at 10 minutes after administration and returned to baseline in approximately 1 hour.

To examine the acute effects of cocaine in humans, investigators administered low doses (2 mg/kg) of intranasal cocaine to patients in the cardiac catheterization laboratory (3,56–58). They observed increases in heart rate and blood pressure but mild, diffuse reductions in coronary caliber (8% to 12% of normal), a 33% increase in coronary vascular resistance, and a 17% reduction in coronary sinus blood flow. Thus, even though myocardial oxygen demand increased—with an increase in double product—these patients exhibited a decrease in coronary blood flow. It is likely that in cocaine abusers, who often use much higher doses than those administered in this controlled study, the imbalance in oxygen supply and demand is even worse. It was shown that the cocaine-induced coronary vasoconstriction could be reversed with the α-adrenergic blocking agent phentolamine, suggesting that α-receptor stimulation by cocaine is a crucial aspect of the vasoconstriction. The vasoconstriction was worse at sites of atherosclerosis and could be relieved by nitroglycerin (59). The β-blocker propranolol potentiated the cocaine-induced vasoconstriction, presumably because the β-receptors were blocked, leaving the α-receptors unopposed. Investigators showed (60) that accumulation of cocaine metabolites may also contribute to coronary vasospasm. Addition of ethanol to intranasal cocaine did not worsen coronary vasospasm (16). Isolated human coronary arteries from patients undergoing cardiac transplantation have also been shown to undergo vasospasm when exposed to cocaine.

Administration of cocaine as a local anesthetic agent for use in laryngoscopy increased the frequency of ventricular premature beats (61). There have been occasional case reports of acute MI when intranasal cocaine was used as a topical anesthetic for nasal operative procedures. The effects of cocaine on human fetal left ventricles were studied (62). Cocaine reduced action potential amplitude, depressed the force of ventricular contraction, and, then, at 90 minutes of exposure, resulted in electrical and mechanical arrest, which also suggests that cocaine has a direct cardiodepressant effect on cardiac muscle. Finally, we observed that when human blood is exposed to cocaine, in approximately one half of the samples, platelet aggregation to adenosine diphosphate but not collagen or epinephrine is increased (Fig. 36.1) (47). Further studies showed that volunteers receiving cocaine at a dose of 2 mg/kg intranasally had platelet activation, α-granule release, and formation of platelet microaggregates (48).

In summary, controlled studies in humans receiving low doses of intranasal cocaine showed that cocaine increases heart rate and blood pressure but causes coronary vasoconstriction at the same time. Thus, the potential for ischemia through an imbalance between oxygen supply and demand may occur, especially when even higher doses of cocaine are used.

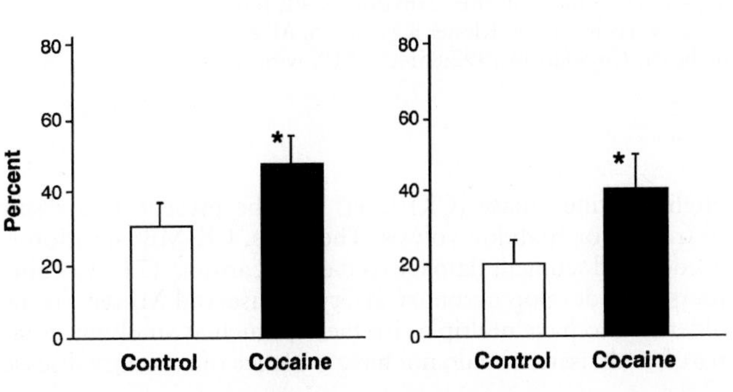

FIGURE 36.1. Platelet aggregation from humans (1 mg, adenosine diphosphate) after incubation with saline or cocaine. Peak aggregation (**left**) and aggregation at 15 minutes (**right**). Data are expressed as mean ± standard error of the mean; $^*p < .02$. (From Rezkalla SH, Mazza JJ, Kloner RA, et al. Effects of cocaine on human platelets in healthy subjects. *Am J Cardiol* 1993;72:243–246.)

TABLE 36.1

CARDIOVASCULAR COMPLICATIONS OF COCAINE USE

Myocardial infarction and myocardial ischemia
Myocarditis
Cardiomyopathy: dilated and hypertrophic
Arrhythmias: tachyarrhythmias and bradyarrhythmias
Hypertension
Aortic dissection
Endocarditis
Acceleration of atherosclerosis?

Cardiovascular Disease Associated with Cocaine Use

Most of our knowledge regarding the clinical complications of cocaine use in patients comes from clinical reports and autopsy studies. A number of cardiovascular diseases associated with cocaine use have been reported in the literature (63,64). These are summarized in Table 36.1, and mechanisms of cocaine action are illustrated in Figure 36.2.

Acute Myocardial Infarction

Four possible causes of MI are related to cocaine use. (a) Coronary artery spasm is caused by the intense α-sympathetic stimulation associated with use of cocaine. (b) Thrombus formation was observed in 24% of patients in whom coronary artery disease was absent (65). Thrombus may have occurred on top of an area of vasospasm that was then relieved, and increased platelet aggregability may contribute (47). Thrombus formation may also occur on top of atherosclerotic narrowing. Plaque fracture or rupture, which is common in most Q-wave MIs, is usually not observed in cocaine-related infarcts (53,66). (c) Increased myocardial oxygen demand may occur in the presence of a fixed lesion. Chronic use of cocaine may cause an acceleration of atherosclerosis, resulting in atherosclerotic narrowing in young patients (53). The sympathomimetic responses of increased heart rate and blood pressure, in addition to the stenosis, may contribute to infarction. (d) Some combination of the foregoing three factors may cause MI.

More than 100 cases of cocaine-related MI have been reported in the literature (67). Many more probably occur but are never reported. Clinical, angiographic, and autopsy features reveal some unique properties of cocaine-related infarction. MI after cocaine use typically occurs within 3 hours of use, but this period ranges from minutes to a few days. The median time of onset of chest pain in the infarct patient depends on the route of administration (65). Onset of chest pain occurred at a median time of 30 minutes with intravenous use, 90 minutes with use of crack cocaine, and 135 minutes with nasal insufflation. In a study of 3,946 patients with acute MI (68), 38 patients reported cocaine use before the clinical presentation. The risk appears to be higher in the 60 minutes after cocaine administration, and it rapidly decreases after the first hour. In one study, the description of chest pain was typical: "pressure, crushing, squeezing, tightness, discomfort, heaviness, and in one case, sharp." Forty-four percent of patients had a history of chest pain (65). There may be a vasospastic component to some of these cases, as suggested by Holter monitoring studies of cocaine use (69). In 1988, at Montefiore Medical Center in Bronx, New York, 35 patients were admitted for chest pain associated with cocaine use. Of these, 11 developed infarction (70). Chest pain after the use of cocaine is not always caused by

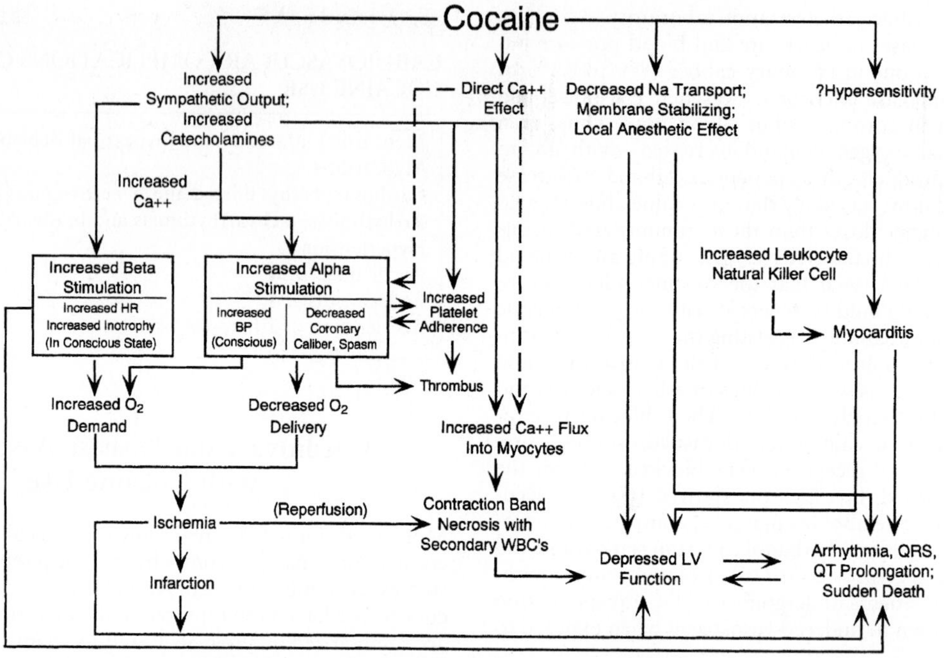

FIGURE 36.2. Schematic diagram showing potential mechanisms of the cardiotoxic effects of cocaine. Two primary mechanisms are suggested. First, cocaine inhibits presynaptic reuptake of catecholamines, resulting in a potentiation of the sympathetic nervous system and an increase in catecholamine levels. Second, cocaine inhibits sodium transport across the sarcolemmal membrane, leading to a membrane-stabilizing or local anesthetic effect that has been likened to a type I antiarrhythmic effect. In conscious preparations, increased sympathetic output and catecholamine levels result in an increase in heart rate and, in some studies, inotropy, which can increase oxygen demand. α-Stimulation of blood vessels causes a vasoconstrictor response with increase in blood pressure in conscious preparations, also resulting in increased oxygen demand. α-Sympathetic stimulation decreases coronary artery caliber, increases coronary vascular resistance, and may lead to coronary spasm in both conscious and anesthetized preparations, thus reducing oxygen supply. Repetitive bouts of coronary spasm might alter or damage the endothelium, contributing to accelerated atherosclerosis, which has been reported with use of cocaine. Increased platelet aggregability has been reported with use of cocaine (and may be related to increased catecholamine levels), which can contribute to thrombus formation. All of these factors contribute to an imbalance between oxygen supply and demand and may thus lead to myocardial ischemia with subsequent infarction and associated left ventricular dysfunction and arrhythmias. Increased sympathetic output may also contribute to tachyarrhythmias. Catecholamine excess is known to lead to contraction-band formation, and this is thought to be related to calcium overload. Isner and Chokshi (Isner JM, Chokshi SK. Cardiac complications of cocaine abuse. *Annu Rev Med* 1991;42:33–38) postulated that cocaine may have a direct effect on calcium flux into blood vessels (and perhaps myocytes), leading to vasoconstriction that may be independent of the sympathetic nervous system (*dashed lines*). The local anesthetic effect of cocaine may cause direct depression of inotropy (which in some studies surpasses any indirect positive inotropic response caused by sympathetic simulation) and can lead to a transient cardiomyopathic presentation. This local anesthetic effect can also lead to prolongation of electrocardiographic intervals, including QRS and QT duration, perhaps resulting in arrhythmias and sudden death, much like the proarrhythmic effects of agents such as quinidine. Hypersensitivity to cocaine has been postulated but not absolutely proved to be a cause of myocarditis. In addition, an increase in natural killer cell activity (which may be related to increased catecholamines) has been reported with cocaine and could lead to myocarditis. Scattered foci of myocarditis could lead to a cardiomyopathic presentation and form the nidus for arrhythmias. BP, blood pressure; HR, heart rate; LV, left ventricular; WBC's, white blood cells. (From Kloner RA, Hale S, Alker K, et al. The effects of acute and chronic cocaine use on the heart. *Circulation* 1992;85:407–419, with permission of the American Heart Association.)

MI and may indicate the presence of angina or be noncardiac in nature.

In one report, the mean age of patients with acute MI associated with cocaine was 33 years, and 92% of patients were male (70). The most common associated risk factor was cigarette smoking. There does not appear to be any clear-cut dose relationship between the use of cocaine and development of MI. Chronic, occasional, and first-time users may develop infarction. The ECG was abnormal in 90% or more of patients in the emergency department. ECG abnormalities included ST-segment elevation, T-wave inversion, and Q waves. Both Q- and non–Q-wave infarcts have been reported after cocaine use. High creatine kinase (CK) levels may be present as a result of trauma or rhabdomyolysis. Therefore, CK-MB elevation is needed to document damage to the myocardium (71). Cocaine users who develop coronary artery disease and MI tend to be older and to have multiple risk factors, such as smoking, compared with users who do not have evidence of coronary disease (72).

Coronary vasospasm has been well documented in only a few cocaine-related infarct patients. Coronary stenosis is present in 29% of cases. Thrombosis is present in approximately one fourth of cases. In an analysis of 92 cases in which either coronary angiographic or coronary anatomic data were collected at autopsy (67), 38% of patients had normal coronary arteries. Of those, 77% had infarcts of the anterior wall.

In a review of the literature (65), 22 of 91 cases of cocaine-induced infarction had some complication: 6 had congestive heart failure, 3 had cardiogenic shock, 11 had potentially life-threatening arrhythmias, 3 had ventricular fibrillation, 6 had ventricular tachycardia, and 2 had cardiac arrests. Three deaths occurred. In the series from Montefiore Hospital (70), among 22 patients with cocaine-related acute MI, no in-hospital deaths occurred, and only one episode of heart failure and ventricular tachycardia was seen. A case report of a patient who developed an intraventricular thrombus after cocaine-induced MI was described (73).

Management of Cocaine-Induced Myocardial Ischemia and Myocardial Infarction

No controlled, randomized, prospective trials clarify the best way to manage cocaine-induced ischemia or infarction. As stated earlier, not all episodes of chest pain associated with cocaine are necessarily MIs. The incidence of MIs associated with cocaine-induced chest pain was 0% to 31% in retrospective analysis and approximately 6% in prospective analyses (74). In addition, not all cocaine-related chest pain is necessarily ischemic; pleuritic pain has been reported. Chest radiographs should be obtained to rule out pneumothorax and pneumomediastinum, which have both been reported with cocaine use. Initiation of thrombolytic therapy should not be delayed while chest radiographs are awaited, however, unless physical examination strongly suggests conditions other than MI.

Patients who enter the emergency department with pain that suggests ischemia (but do not have evidence of infarction) after cocaine use should be observed (74–76). One report (74) favored a 12-hour observation period during which ECG and serial CK-MB measurements are obtained to rule out MI. Recent studies have further validated this concept (77,78). Total creatine phosphokinase level elevation appears to occur in a significant number of cocaine users. This is an unreliable screening test for the detection of myocardial injury (79). Myoglobin level is not reliable in detecting MI secondary to cocaine use, but troponin-1 and CK-MB appear to have a good specificity (80). If possible, previous ECGs should be obtained because cocaine users not infrequently also have early repolarization variants on their ECG or left ventricular (LV) hypertrophy. In a prospective study, dobutamine stress echocardiography was both beneficial and safe in the evaluation of chest pain in this group of patients (81).

Medical therapies for cocaine-related chest pain that is ischemic (anginal) but is not infarction include nitroglycerin, oxygen, aspirin, and benzodiazepines (74–76). Verapamil or other calcium channel blockers may be considered if pain continues (74). If the ECG suggests MI, administration of thrombolytic agents (intravenous or intracoronary) (82) and aspirin should be considered. Some investigators (76) suggest the use of two-dimensional echocardiography to assist in establishing the diagnosis. Thrombolytic therapy has, in fact, been used successfully, but no contraindications, such as severe hypertension, intracerebral hemorrhage, or seizures, all of which may occur with cocaine, should be present. A few case reports have raised some safety issues regarding thrombolytic agents in the setting of cocaine. One death occurred from intracerebral hemorrhage. Thus primary intervention, percutaneous coronary angioplasty, and stenting (83) may be the preferred approach in hospitals with such expertise. A recent case report described the efficacy of platelet glycoprotein IIb/IIIa inhibitor, given intravenously, with complete resolution of a thrombus in the coronary artery that was temporally related to use of crack cocaine (84).

Because β-blockers may exacerbate coronary vasospasm in cocaine-induced coronary ischemia secondary to unopposed α-receptor stimulation, they should be used with extreme caution, if at all, in the acute setting. The available data are from scattered case reports, and no final conclusion has been drawn (85). At the time of the patient's discharge, however, β-blockers should be considered part of routine postinfarction therapy (85). The benefits of β-blockers may outweigh the potential risk of increasing the vasomotor tone, particularly because the cocaine effect should be gone by the time of discharge. If, however, the patient begins to use cocaine again after discharge, β-blockers could worsen vasospasm. Labetalol might be a safer choice, but its primary effect is β-blockade, not α-blockade, and therefore even this agent is controversial.

The best therapy for cocaine-induced ventricular arrhythmias remains to be determined. In experimental studies, sodium bicarbonate reverses QRS prolongation caused by cocaine (86). The use of lidocaine is debated because it, a sodium channel blocker and local anesthetic, could theoretically worsen the proarrhythmic effect of cocaine. Some studies, however, suggest that lidocaine is safe when it is administered several hours after the use of cocaine.

It is crucial that patients stop using cocaine and that they be educated about the dangers of this substance. Concern that cocaine may accelerate atherosclerosis is an additional reason to recommend drug rehabilitation programs.

Our experience in an inner-city hospital was that acute MI occurring in an otherwise healthy young person may be related to cocaine, and a history of cocaine use and urine testing for cocaine should be considered. Urine testing may detect cocaine or its metabolites as long as 3 weeks after use. Various methods are used, including enzyme-multiplied immunoassay, gas chromatography, and mass spectrometry. A skin patch has recently been tested as an easy-to-use screening tool. When a young person has an MI, the physician should remember to ask whether the patient has been using cocaine (87).

Cocaine-Induced Cardiomyopathy and Myocarditis

Cases of transient congestive heart failure have occurred after use of cocaine (88). In some cases, this has involved global hypokinesis, typical of a cardiomyopathy, that may be accompanied by normal coronary angiograms (89,90). Clinically unrecognized reduction in LV function was reported in 7% of chronic cocaine users in one study (91). A case of recurrent dilated cardiomyopathy in a patient who quit and then began reusing cocaine was also reported (92).

In a controlled, randomized study, intracoronary cocaine or saline was administered to 20 patients during cardiac catheterization. Cocaine, but not saline infusion, led to an increase in LV end-diastolic pressure and a decrease in LV ejection fraction (93). These findings suggest that cocaine can induce a global toxic effect on myocytes. Autopsy reports have described a mononuclear cell–type myocarditis in chronic cocaine users (94). Lymphocytes and macrophages were observed in the region of myocyte necrosis. A second common morphologic finding among chronic cocaine users is the presence of contraction bands. Myocardial contraction-band necrosis occurs with catecholamine excess and calcium overload, as well as after reperfusion of ischemic tissue. In an experimental study involving rabbits, we observed that an acute infusion of cocaine caused foci of contraction-band necrosis in some of the animals (26).

As is true for MI, no controlled studies are available that clarify the best therapy for cocaine-induced cardiomyopathy. Limited data suggest that this condition may be reversible after cessation of cocaine use for 2 to 7 months. Administration of diuretics and angiotensin-converting-enzyme inhibitors (or angiotensin-receptor blockers) certainly should be utilized.

In addition to dilated cardiomyopathy, LV hypertrophy has been reported with chronic cocaine use. It is presumably caused at least in part by the elevations in blood pressure that occur with cocaine use (94).

Cocaine-Induced Hypertension

The hypertension induced by cocaine use is most likely secondary to the drug's sympathomimetic effect (95). Labetalol has been suggested as therapy because it blocks both α- and β-receptors. This agent is primarily a β-receptor blocker, however, and therefore unopposed α-receptor stimulation could increase both peripheral vascular and coronary vascular resistance. Calcium channel blockers and α-blocking agents such as prazosin and phentolamine might be a better choice.

Cocaine-Induced Arrhythmias

Case reports have described a variety of arrhythmias associated with cocaine use, including ventricular tachycardia, ventricular fibrillation, and sudden death (2,96) and supraventricular arrhythmias (42). Ventricular arrhythmias may be associated with MI. One case report described a patient who developed ventricular tachycardia and fibrillation after using cocaine but who had no infarct and had normal coronary arteries at catheterization. After defibrillation, the ECG showed ST-segment elevation in leads V_1 and V_2, suggesting that the arrhythmia may have been related to transmural ischemia (possibly caused by transient vasospasm). A case report of torsades de pointes in a patient with cocaine-related prolongation of the QT interval was described. On the basis of these and other case reports, six potential types of cocaine-induced arrhythmias in humans are thought to be likely: (a) those associated with structural damage (i.e., cocaine-induced MI or cardiomyopathy), (b) those caused by QT prolongation, the direct effect of cocaine on the myocardium, (c) those resulting from cocaine's sympathomimetic and vagolytic effects, (d) those resulting from cocaine-induced ischemia, (e) those caused by reperfusion after resolution of coronary artery vasospasm, and (f) those resulting from the systemic effects of cocaine, such as hyperthermia, seizures, and acidosis.

On rare occasions, bradyarrhythmias and sinus arrest have been described in cocaine users (97). This could be related to cocaine-induced myocardial ischemia. No controlled studies in humans have determined the best approach to cocaine-induced arrhythmia. In animal studies, sodium bicarbonate has been shown to reverse cocaine's prolongation of the QRS interval. Concerns about the use of β-blockers have been described. Antiarrhythmic agents, such as lidocaine, procainamide, and quinidine, have the potential to compound cocaine's depressant effects on the conduction system and prolongation of the QT interval. Calcium channel blockers, such as nitrendipine and verapamil, have shown promise in experimental animal studies. If the arrhythmia is thought to be caused by ischemia or infarction, then the antiischemic and antiinfarction agents described earlier should be used to relieve ischemia.

Acceleration of Atherosclerosis Associated with Cocaine Use

Severe atherosclerosis of the coronary arteries has been described in young patients who died from cocaine (53). In one study (52), the average age of patients who developed cocaine-induced thrombus was only 29 years. A more recent study showed that coronary calcifications are more prevalent among cocaine users, again suggesting an increased prevalence of atherosclerosis (98). When interpreting these studies, it is important to remember that cocaine users tend also to be cigarette smokers, which might contribute to acceleration of atherosclerosis. An increase in adventitial mast cells within the atherosclerotic coronary arteries of cocaine users has been described (52). It was suggested that release of vasoactive substances by the mast cells could explain the acceleration of atherosclerosis in cocaine users (99). Elevation of catecholamine levels can increase low-density-lipoprotein (LDL) uptake by the arterial wall. Hence, increases in catecholamine levels in cocaine users might also help explain this acceleration of atherosclerosis. Jones and colleagues observed that cocaine had a direct toxic effect on coronary endothelium, resulting in endothelial denudation (100). Repetitive episodes of coronary vasospasm might also eventually lead to endothelial damage.

In addition to an acceleration of atherosclerosis, a few cases of intimal hyperplasia have been described as a cause for coronary narrowing (101,102). Another study (103) described thickening of intramural coronary arteries in young men who had ischemic chest pain related to cocaine use and had epicardial coronary arteries of normal appearance. More recently, coronary artery aneurysms were shown to be more prevalent among cocaine users (104).

Aortic Dissection

Aortic dissection is an uncommon presentation in cocaine addicts, and is usually reported in an occasional case report. Although cocaine use is responsible for fewer than 1% of cases of aortic dissection (105), the percentage is as high as 37% in cities with high cocaine use (106). It is crucial to rule out aortic dissection with careful clinical assessment and chest x-ray before initiating therapies for other diseases, such as thrombolytic therapy for acute MI.

Miscellaneous Cardiac Conditions Reported with Cocaine Use

Intravenous cocaine use has been associated with bacterial endocarditis. It has been suggested that left-sided endocarditis is more common than right-sided endocarditis in this setting (4). Cocaine users are also prone to developing paravalvular abscesses.

The best way of avoiding cocaine-induced cardiovascular diseases is total abstinence. Various methods for treatment of cocaine addiction exist, including aversion therapy and narcotherapy. No long-term comparative studies on the usefulness of various programs are available, and the most optimistic success rate at 1 year is approximately 60%. It seems that greater efforts should be directed at preventing substance abuse before it starts, particularly in adolescents and in young adults.

Cocaine has also been shown to have a deleterious effect on other blood vessels, including peripheral (107,108), intestinal (109), and cerebral vessels (110,111). A summary of the effects of cocaine on the heart is shown in Figure 36.2.

COCAETHYLENE

Cocaethylene is a pharmacologically active cocaine metabolite that has been detected in patients who simultaneously abuse cocaine and ethanol. It has been estimated that 9 to 12 million people in the United States use a combination of cocaine and ethanol (16,17), which accounts for more than 1,000 yearly deaths. The combination may be more toxic than either agent alone. Studies suggested that their simultaneous use markedly increases the rate of sudden death (112) and that patients dying from the combination had cocaine blood concentrations lower (900 mg/mL) than patients dying of cocaine abuse alone (2,800 mg/mL), which suggests a synergistic effect (113). Other studies, however, suggested that blood cocaine concentrations become elevated when oral ethanol is given to people snorting cocaine (114). Cocaethylene was more potent in killing mice than as cocaine alone (115).

The mechanism(s) whereby cocaethylene has such deleterious effects have been studied. Combinations of cocaine and alcohol result in greater increases in heart rate, cardiac output, diastolic blood pressure, and myocardial depression than either agent alone (116–118). Although both cocaine and cocaethylene produced direct negative inotropic effects on isolated cardiac myocytes by decreasing the availability of calcium, the negative inotropic effect was more potent with cocaethylene, and this was related to an additional action, reduction of myofilament responsiveness to calcium (30).

Cocaethylene is more potent than cocaine in depressing contraction of myocardial cells in culture (17). In a study comparing cocaine, ethanol, and a combination of both, cocaine alone increased heart rate and blood pressure and, as previously observed, decreased coronary artery diameter (16). In patients who used both substances, rate–pressure product increased, but coronary diameter increased as well. Therefore, ethanol did not potentiate the vasoconstrictor effect of cocaine; in fact, it appeared to counteract it. This study suggested that the combination of cocaine and alcohol probably does not exacerbate ischemia. However, the doses of cocaine used were low.

Although the exact mechanism whereby the combination of cocaine and ethanol causes increased rates of sudden death in humans remains to be elucidated, it is a deadly combination with which physicians should be familiar.

CAFFEINE, COFFEE, AND TEA

Few areas in the medical literature are as confusing as the question of whether coffee and caffeine have deleterious effects on the cardiovascular system. Numerous studies describe data that conflict with others, and, in the end, it is difficult to draw conclusions. Recent reviews have described some of the difficulties in the papers published on this issue (119,120). Often, animal studies used doses of caffeine that are "hundreds to thousands of times those achieved by normal human consumption." In addition, tolerance to caffeine is common in humans who regularly drink coffee, and most animal studies do not include conditioning protocols. Coffee and caffeine consumption is often associated with other variables and risk factors for coronary artery disease that are not always taken into account. For example, coffee consumption is more common among people with higher education levels and incomes, more common among white people, and more common among Catholics. It is less common among Mormons and Seventh-Day Adventists, for religious reasons. Coffee is more commonly consumed among patients who are depressed and are experiencing anxiety and is commonly used by people who also smoke cigarettes. Most physiologic studies in humans and animals test the effects of caffeine and relate this to coffee use. However, coffee may have compounds other than caffeine that can affect the cardiovascular system. Nevertheless, caffeine is an important compound in coffee that has been implicated in cardiovascular events.

Physiology of Caffeine Use

Caffeine is a methylxanthine found in a variety of products, including coffee, tea, chocolate, soft drinks, and many over-the-counter medications. Coffee is the predominant source of caffeine in the Western hemisphere, and tea is the most common source in the rest of the world. Ninety-nine percent of caffeine from beverages is absorbed by the gastrointestinal tract and peaks in the serum within 30 to 60 minutes of ingestion. Caffeine is metabolized by the liver, and a very small percentage is excreted unchanged by the kidneys.

Caffeine's major mechanism of action is to antagonize adenosine receptors. A second action at the usual levels of consumption is phosphodiesterase inhibition. By antagonizing adenosine, caffeine blocks the vasodilatory effect of adenosine and adenosine's inhibitory effects on platelet aggregation, catecholamine levels, and renin release, as well as lipolysis. Thus, acute caffeine administration may increase blood pressure and increase levels of plasma catecholamine, renin (121), and free fatty acid. Tolerance develops within hours to days of caffeine use, and the effect of caffeine on any individual is highly dependent on the individual and the pattern of consumption.

In general, the effects of caffeine on heart rate and blood pressure in humans are quite variable, and contradictory statements about those effects can be found in the literature. In people who do not regularly drink caffeinated beverages, caffeine may initially increase blood pressure, but the effect is lessened or absent in those who regularly consume caffeine. In one study, a 10-mm Hg increase in blood pressure was seen after consumption of 3 to 5 mg/kg of caffeine. There was an initial *decrease* in heart rate during the first hour after consumption, followed by an *increase* from 2 to 3 hours after consumption (121). Prolonged exposure to caffeine results in tolerance, but chronic drinkers of caffeinated coffee may still exhibit small long-term increases in blood pressure, which seems to be worse among drinkers of boiled rather than filtered coffee (122,123). The increase in both systolic and diastolic blood pressure is more consistent in hypertensive patients, particularly in older men and women (124,125). Coffee drinking should be modified in hypertensive patients who, despite medication, still fall outside their goals (126). In one study of 499 hypertensive men, the risk of thromboembolic stroke increased significantly in coffee drinkers (127). However, this finding requires confirmation in larger-scale epidemiologic studies.

Coffee and Coronary Heart Disease

Debate about whether coffee consumption and coronary heart disease are associated continues. Some epidemiologic studies suggest that they are, and that the prevalence of coronary disease increases among coffee drinkers, especially those with intake of five or more cups of coffee per day. In a study of 1,130 male medical students older than 25 years, daily consumption of one to two cups of coffee resulted in a relative risk of coronary heart disease of 1.3; more than five cups of coffee daily increased the risk to 2.5 (128). The investigation did not fully control for all risk factors, but it did control for smoking. Other studies also suggested a relationship between increased coffee consumption and coronary events (129). Many studies (usually with a shorter period of follow-up), however, have been entirely negative. In a study of 45,589 men, daily consumption of four or more cups of coffee increased the risk of a cardiovascular event to only 1.04 (130). The study concluded that consumption of caffeinated coffee is in most cases unlikely to be a risk factor for cardiovascular disease.

Until the controversy regarding the effect of caffeinated coffee on coronary heart disease events is resolved, it might be prudent to limit patients with ischemic heart disease to fewer than four cups of coffee per day (131).

Tea and Cardiovascular Disease

Tea consumption, particularly green tea, was shown to decrease the risk of myocardial infarctions and is associated with less atherosclerosis (132,133). Most, but not all, studies show a benefit in decreasing cardiac events (134–136). Tea flavonoids and other polyphenols are the likely culprits for the benefit in tea drinking (137,138), and it appears that tea is better than other known sources, such as wine (139). These substances increase plasma antioxidant potential in humans (140), and may reverse endothelial dysfunction in patients with coronary artery disease (141). Tea consumption does not have any tangible effect on platelet aggregation (142).

Coffee and Lipid Alterations

There is also ongoing debate about whether coffee increases serum cholesterol levels. Many of the studies that have shown a correlation between coffee consumption and increases in serum cholesterol levels have been performed outside the United States, whereas some of the studies that showed no association were performed in the United States.

It has been suggested that the method of brewing the coffee may be important. In some of the European studies, coffee was prepared by boiling, whereas in the United States, coffee is brewed mainly by filtering. Boiled coffee appears to have a greater adverse effect than filtered coffee on total serum cholesterol, LDL-cholesterol, and apoprotein B levels. It has been postulated that caffeine plays a minimal role in altering lipid levels and that a surfactant in coffee (which is removed by filtration) is responsible for the elevation in lipid levels observed in some of the European studies (120,143). Other factors associated with boiled coffee that have been implicated in increasing serum lipids include cafestol and kahweal, two subfractions that can be found within the lipid fraction of coffee.

Studies in the United States did not report any increase in total or LDL-cholesterol levels in patients who consumed filtered coffee (144,145). Thus, at least in the United States, the use of filtered coffee does not seem to cause an increase in cholesterol levels, and in European studies in which boiled coffee did seem to have some effect, a component other than caffeine appeared to be the culprit.

Coffee and Homocysteine Levels

Several studies have demonstrated a positive correlation between heavy coffee consumption and elevated homocysteine levels. These studies included drinking of filtered and unfiltered coffee (146–148). In a controlled crossover study, 64 healthy volunteers were randomly assigned to receive 1 liter of unfiltered coffee daily for 2 weeks or to ingest a coffee-free diet (149). In the heavy-coffee-drinking group, plasma fasting homocysteine levels were elevated by 10%. These were short-term studies and did not investigate whether a concomitant increase in cardiovascular events occurred. The results may, however, explain the reported increase in cardiovascular events among people who consume large amounts of coffee, particularly unfiltered coffee, in some studies.

Coffee and Arrhythmias

Although a common belief exists that caffeine can exacerbate arrhythmias, the evidence supporting this in humans is limited. Animal studies have examined this question, but studies demonstrating an association between caffeine and arrhythmia have usually involved doses that were several times higher than those ingested by humans.

One study demonstrated that caffeine had little or no effect on cardiac conduction in humans but might exacerbate underlying susceptibilities to arrhythmias (150). Although earlier studies found an increase in ventricular premature beats on the ECGs of patients who drank nine or more cups of coffee or the equivalent amount of tea (151), more recent studies have been negative.

In a study that examined the effect of caffeine on 50 patients with histories of symptomatic ventricular arrhythmias, continuous ECG recordings at rest and during exercise revealed no increase in ventricular arrhythmias after caffeine consumption, despite an increase in plasma norepinephrine and epinephrine levels (152). During programmed ventricular stimulation, the effect of caffeine varied among the patients. Some patients required an increase, others a decrease, and others no change in the extra stimuli needed to induce arrhythmias during exposure to caffeine (153). Although moderate caffeine ingestion produces a slight prolongation of QRS complexes seen on signal-averaged ECG (154), many studies suggest that moderate ingestion of caffeine does not exacerbate arrhythmias (155–157).

ANABOLIC STEROIDS AND CARDIOVASCULAR DISEASE

It is estimated that approximately 1 million Americans use anabolic steroids (158). Recent case reports suggest that anabolic steroids used primarily among bodybuilders may be associated with MI. Kennedy (159) described a 24-year-old bodybuilder who presented with 3 days of dull chest pain. He had been taking anabolic steroids, including oral stanozolol, intramuscular nandrolone, and intramuscular sustanon. He also had a history of smoking. The patient developed a lateral-wall MI, demonstrated by ECG and enzyme criteria. He was found to be hypertensive, his total serum cholesterol level was observed to be high, and his high-density-lipoprotein (HDL) levels were low.

Acute MI was also reported in a young power lifter who was taking androgenic steroids (160). This patient had hypercholesterolemia, hyperaggregable platelets, and normal appearance of coronary arteries on angiography. Other cases have been documented in which MI, thrombotic occlusion of the coronary artery, and strokes were associated with use of anabolic steroids (160). In a literature review on the link between anabolic steroids and atherogenic changes, anabolic steroids were found to have caused a 52% decrease in HDL levels, a 78% decrease in HDL b levels, and a 36% increase in LDL levels (161). Some studies reported depression of apolipoprotein A-1 and increases in apolipoprotein B. Commonly used anabolic steroids were stanozolol, oxandrolone, testosterone, methandrostenolone, nandrolone decanoate, and oxymetholone—usually in various combinations.

Changes in serum lipid levels after administration of anabolic steroids are rapid, occurring within days to a week. Lipid levels return to baseline approximately 3 to 5 weeks after cessation of anabolic steroid use according to some reports, whereas other reports suggest that a prolonged residual effect may be seen, with lipid levels abnormal even at 6 months after steroid use ended.

It has been estimated that the deleterious effects of anabolic steroid use on serum lipid levels might increase the risk of coronary heart disease to three to six times normal (161). The actual incidence of cardiovascular events among anabolic steroid users is probably underreported, however, and is limited to occasional case reports. Moreover, many young patients likely conceal their use of anabolic steroids when questioned. It is important to point out that physiologic doses of testosterone do not seem to adversely affect lipid levels. No effect on HDL levels was seen after administration of such doses in older men, and epidemiologic studies actually suggest a positive correlation between endogenous testosterone and HDL levels (162).

Exogenous steroids can also increase blood pressure (163) and hence cause LV hypertrophy and possibly increase thrombosis. A link between androgen use and thrombus formation is largely derived from experimental animal studies. In experimental thrombosis models, administration of exogenous androgens resulted in development of a larger experimental thrombus and reduced time to blood vessel occlusion (164–167). Use of exogenous androgens has also been reported to enhance platelet aggregation (168).

QT dispersion is increased in athletes who take anabolic steroids (169). QT dispersion reflects the heterogeneity of ventricular repolarization and is known to be associated with increased risk of ventricular arrhythmias. Atrial fibrillation was also reported in young athletes who abuse anabolic steroids (170).

AMPHETAMINES

Amphetamines are stimulants that are sympathomimetic agents. Use of amphetamine and its derivatives may increase blood pressure and has been associated with lethal arrhythmias and MI (171–176). A 27-year-old man who developed an acute MI and ventricular fibrillation after intravenous amphetamine and was successfully cardioverted was shown to have normal coronary arteries during angiography (172). It was suggested that amphetamines might cause coronary artery vasospasm followed by thrombus formation (177). Cases of cardiomyopathy have also been reported with use of amphetamines (178,179), including smoking of crystal amphetamine, or "ice" (179).

DESIGNER DRUGS

A "designer" drug is a drug manufactured in a laboratory to produce a potent addictive psychedelic effect. The most popular designer drug is "Ecstasy," 3,4-methylenedioxymethamphetamine (MDMA), which is popular among young adults. The drug has potent sympathomimetic properties and has been linked to a variety of vascular emergencies. Intracerebral hemorrhage, stroke, hypertension, ventricular arrhythmias, and even death were reported with the use of this drug (180–183). *In vitro* studies suggest that MDMA may have a proliferative action on human cardiac valvular cells, similar to that of phentermine-fenfluramine (184). More recently a variety of other designer drugs have invaded the market, such as paramethoxyamphetamine ("death"), phenethylamine designer drugs, γ-hydroxybutyrate, and many others (185–187). They all have significant toxicities. Selling of designer drugs now has moved from street corners to the Internet, which presents new challenges for law enforcement (188). Young patients presenting with acute cardiac events should be asked about the use of designer drugs in addition to questions about cocaine use.

PHENTERMINE-FENFLURAMINE (PHEN-FEN)

Phentermine is a nonsympathomimetic stimulant that inhibits the clearance of serotonin in the lungs. Fenfluramine is a sympathomimetic amine that promotes the release of serotonin (189). Both drugs in combination were widely used as anorexigenic agents for management of obesity. Shortly after their release, a variety of side effects were reported, including valvular regurgitation, primary pulmonary hypertension, endomyocardial fibrosis, and retroperitoneal hemorrhages.

In 1997, the cases of a group of 24 women who developed valvular heart disease after phentermine-fenfluramine therapy were reported (190). Twenty patients presented with various cardiovascular symptoms, and a new murmur was discovered in 4 patients during physical examination. The most common valvular abnormalities were mitral regurgitation and aortic regurgitation. The valves showed a glistening appearance on inspection. On histopathologic examination, proliferation of fibroblasts and an increase in extracellular matrix were found. These patients were young and had no previous histories of heart disease. Surgical intervention was performed in five patients.

Further epidemiologic studies confirmed a relationship between phentermine and fenfluramine and valvular regurgitant lesions but to a much lesser extent (191–194). The incidence of valvular abnormalities ranges between 6% and 30% among patients who are taking phentermine-fenfluramine, with the most common lesion being aortic regurgitation. The incidence appears to be higher among patients who have undergone longer treatment with the drugs (195) and may stabilize or even regress after the cessation of therapy (196,197). The U.S. Department of Health and Human Services recommends that patients exposed to these medications undergo cardiovascular and echocardiographic examination and that antibiotic prophylaxis be administered when appropriate (198).

A less common but more serious complication of phentermine-fenfluramine therapy is primary pulmonary hypertension (199). This occurs after exposure of at least a few months and has a 3-year survival rate of 50% (200). In one study, histologic examination at autopsy revealed intimal hyperplasia, medial hypertrophy, intimal fibroelastosis, and plexogenic arteriopathy of the pulmonary arteries (201).

Another rare complication of phentermine-fenfluramine therapy is restrictive cardiomyopathy secondary to endomyocardial fibrosis (202). A case report of ruptured retroperitoneal aneurysm was described (203) and was felt to be secondary to enhanced sympathetic activity.

ALCOHOL

It is estimated that alcohol is consumed by two thirds of the adult population in the United States, which makes it one of the most widely used addictive drugs. It is also a unique substance in that a small amount may have some benefit on cardiovascular morbidity and mortality rates but consumption of larger amounts can have devastating effects. The toxic effect of alcohol extends to the brain, liver, skeletal muscle, and many other organs. In this section, we focus on its cardiovascular effects.

Epidemiology

Approximately two thirds of the adult population in the United States report alcohol consumption, and 10% of these are heavy drinkers. Men drink more than women, but women are more sensitive to the cardiac effects of alcohol (204). Alcohol consumption is also prevalent among adolescents, with rates ranging from 10% to 35% (205). It is more prevalent among young men than young women and among white students than black students; white male adolescents have the highest rate of consumption. Alcohol abuse is present in approximately 15% of the geriatric population (206).

Metabolism

Alcohol is absorbed from the stomach and small intestine. It is then distributed to tissues rich in water content and blood flow. Thus, the heart, liver, and brain are prime targets for alcohol's effects (207). In the liver, ethylalcohol is metabolized first to acetaldehyde and then to acetate. Acetate leaves the liver and is metabolized in extrahepatic tissues.

Cardiovascular Effects of Alcohol

Alcoholic Cardiomyopathy

Chronic ingestion of alcohol produces a decrease in both systolic and diastolic function of the myocardium. The condition is clinically indistinguishable from idiopathic dilated cardiomyopathy (208,209). Ethanol and its metabolites, acetaldehyde and acetate, exert direct cardiac toxic effects. Although the nutritional deficiencies associated with alcoholism may play some role in alcoholic cardiomyopathy, they probably are not the only source; dietary supplementation fails to prevent the condition.

Initially, loss of the integrity of the sarcolemmal membrane occurs, resulting in loss of its function. This leads to an increase in the concentration of intracellular calcium. Animal studies showed that alcohol administration for 12 weeks led to a threefold increase in intracellular calcium (210). Furthermore, investigators found that administration of verapamil prevents alcohol-induced LV dysfunction (211). Ethanol also affects the sarcoplasmic reticulum, the mitochondria, and contractile protein synthesis and may produce oxygen free radicals (212,213). All these adversely affect the structure and function of the myocardium.

The symptoms of alcoholic heart disease include dyspnea on exertion, orthopnea, fatigue, and peripheral edema. On examination, signs of right-sided and left-sided heart failure may be present. In addition, signs of chronic alcoholism, such as telangiectasia, spider angioma, and hepatic enlargement are a clue to the diagnosis. One clue to the diagnosis of alcoholic myopathy is the presence of skeletal myopathy presenting as muscle weakness (214). Chest radiography shows cardiomegaly and pulmonary congestion. A 12-lead ECG may show LV hypertrophy, nonspecific ST- and T-wave abnormality, and various cardiac arrhythmias.

Individuals who drink alcohol may have various nutritional deficiencies, among them thiamine deficiency. Thiamine deficiency may lead to beriberi, which may also present with dilated cardiomyopathy. It is, however, distinct from pure alcoholic myopathy in that it is a form of high cardiac output failure (215). The two conditions may coexist.

The most sensitive and clinically useful tool in management and diagnosis of alcoholic cardiomyopathy is echocardiography. This technique usually reveals dilation of all chambers of the heart, and Doppler echocardiography shows valvular regurgitation, particularly of the mitral and tricuspid valves. Alcohol affects both systolic and diastolic function. Studies have shown a decrease in ejection fraction and stroke index (216). Doppler echocardiography is quite sensitive in evaluating diastolic dysfunction, even before the development of clinically evident dysfunction (217,218).

The hearts of alcoholic cardiomyopathy patients may have an increased uptake of antimyosin antibody, which may decrease after alcohol withdrawal (219). The natural history of alcoholic cardiomyopathy depends largely on the patient's drinking habits. If treatment is started early and the patient stops drinking, it may be partially reversible (220). Well-developed disease, however, is usually fatal if the patient continues to consume alcohol.

Treatment of alcoholic cardiomyopathy includes correction of electrolyte abnormalities (221) and cessation of alcohol abuse (222,223) in addition to the usual treatment of congestive heart failure. The prognosis of alcoholic myopathy is similar to that of idiopathic dilated myopathy (224).

The prevalence of alcoholic cardiomyopathy in the community and how much a person can drink before developing the disease are not known. In the Framingham Heart Study no increase in the incidence of congestive heart failure was found in patients who had up to 15 alcoholic drinks per week (225). In patients with left ventricular dysfunction secondary to coronary artery disease, there was no increased risk for developing heart failure among alcohol drinkers (226). The same is true in older patients (227). Furthermore, patients with known alcoholic cardiomyopathy may improve their ventricular function when they limit drinking to a maximum of four drinks per day (228). Despite these data, one should be careful when discussing this issue with patients because not every person can control his or her drinking habits.

Hypertension

A link between alcohol use and high blood pressure has long been suspected (229). Social drinking is associated with a mild rise in systolic pressure, whereas those who drink heavily may have a substantial rise (230,231). Several mechanisms have been proposed. However, the exact mechanism is not clear. This may, at least in part, explain the increase in LV mass. However, even alcoholic individuals who are normotensive may have an increase in LV mass (232). Blood pressure may normalize after a short period of abstinence.

Cardiac Arrhythmias

Alcohol use is associated with a variety of atrial and ventricular arrhythmias, regardless of whether the patient has overt alcoholic heart disease. Possible mechanisms include electrolyte imbalance, the hypercatecholamine states often seen during alcohol withdrawal, and a patchy delay in conduction that results in increased reentry (233). The QT-interval prolongation seen in alcoholic patients may be implicated in the genesis of ventricular arrhythmias (234). The most common arrhythmia, however, appears to be atrial fibrillation (235–238).

In the Framingham study, long-term follow-up showed that the increased risk of developing atrial fibrillation is limited to subjects who consumed more than three drinks per day (239). The treatment is cessation of alcohol consumption; most rhythm disturbances disappear with little or no intervention.

Sudden Death

Heavy alcohol drinking is associated with an increase in sudden death (240,241). Lighter drinkers, however, were at a lower risk for death from cardiovascular diseases, particularly coronary artery disease. In a prospective 13-year follow-up of 12,321 male British doctors, the consumption of one or two drinks each day was associated with a significantly lower mortality rate than that seen among heavy drinkers or nondrinkers (242).

Coronary Artery Disease

Alcohol's effect on the incidence of coronary artery disease is biphasic. Heavy alcohol drinking increases the incidence, whereas mild to moderate drinking decreases the risk of myocardial infarction and cardiovascular death (243–246). This is related to a beneficial effect on HDL cholesterol, endogenous tissue plasminogen activator, and blood platelets (247,248).

What advice should physicians give their patients with regard to alcohol consumption? Alcohol is an addictive drug, and it may be difficult for some people to control their drinking. Heavy drinking increases overall mortality rates (249). Other risk factor modifications should be the priority in patients who have coronary artery disease. Mild alcohol drinking may, however, have a role in the subgroup of patients who have low HDL levels as the sole risk factor for coronary artery disease and in whom other measures to improve HDL levels have failed. Although mild to moderate alcohol drinking appears to decrease cardiac events in patients with known coronary artery disease, red wine appears to be superior to other types of drinks, likely secondary to the flavonoids and other components found in red wine (250–253).

Prevention of Alcohol Addiction

Attempts to cure alcohol addiction are not always successful and often begin after many years of drinking, when significant health problems have already developed. Thus, efforts toward prevention of drinking should be the goal. Various programs are already in place that have had some success (254).

TOBACCO

A cigarette is a controlled device that delivers nicotine and many other substances to the human body. With each puff, approximately 100 μg of nicotine is absorbed through the lungs, with an average drug delivery of 1 to 2 mg of nicotine per cigarette. With the widespread prevalence of smoking and its significant effects on the cardiovascular system, cigarette smoking has a major impact on public health (255).

Tobacco Addiction

Drug addiction or dependency is described as "a behavioral pattern in which the use of a given psychoactive drug is given a sharply higher priority over other behaviors which once had a significantly higher value" (256). In other words, addiction is defined as loss of control over use of the drug and an inability to quit despite obvious risks associated with its use. In the case of cigarette smoking, the drug is nicotine. Smokers report pleasure, relaxation, reduction of anxiety and stress, and improved attention after cigarette smoking (257). Within seconds of smoking a cigarette, nicotine is absorbed through the lung alveoli and taken up by the bloodstream to the brain and other tissues. In the brain, it acts at the nicotinic receptors, which are known to be increased in the brain tissues of smokers. As a result, dopamine, norepinephrine, acetylcholine, and endorphins are released. This results in the reported feelings of decreased anxiety and tension, pleasure and relaxation, and increased performance. Cigarette smoking may also be associated with a decrease in the enzyme monoamine oxidase, which is responsible for the breakdown of dopamine, in the brain (258). Thus, cigarette smoking not only increases the secretion of dopamine, but it also slows its metabolism.

With each cigarette smoked, tolerance to the effects of nicotine develops. With abstinence at night, however, the effects are renewed, so that the first cigarette of the day produces the maximal psychological effect. When smoking ceases, symptoms of restlessness, irritability, impatience, and increased anxiety occur. Most symptoms gradually disappear in 1 to 2 weeks, but the desire to smoke may persist for a very long time.

Despite a recent controversy regarding whether cigarettes should be considered addictive, the balance of the arguments strongly suggests that they are (259). It has also been suggested that an individual's genetic composition may influence smoking behavior (260).

Cardiovascular Effects

The main components of cigarettes that exert cardiovascular effects are nicotine and carbon monoxide. The former may lead to the release of norepinephrine, which increases pulse rate, blood pressure, and platelet aggregability. It may also cause endothelial injury and adversely affect events that occur during atherosclerotic plaque rupture (261). Carbon monoxide displaces the oxygen from hemoglobin, interfering with oxygen delivery to cardiac tissue. Cigarette smoking has also been associated with hyperfibrinogenemia and low levels of HDL (262). These mechanisms lead to the devastating effects of smoking, regardless of the method used.

In a major epidemiologic study, 10,914 subjects were followed to assess the progression of atherosclerotic disease (263). Carotid ultrasounds were performed on the subjects, and the intimal medial thickness was measured at baseline and at 3 years of follow-up. Current smokers had a 50% increase in the rate of progression of atherosclerosis compared to nonsmokers. Past smokers had a 25% increase in atherosclerosis. The increase in the rate of atherosclerosis progression associated with smoking was more marked in diabetic and hypertensive patients.

Smoking results in an increase in heart rate and blood pressure (264). In addition to an increased cardiovascular risk profile, this increase in myocardial oxygen demand may increase, at least theoretically, anginal episodes in patients who already have coronary artery disease.

Active Smoking

Although cigarette smoking had long been suspected to increase the risk of cardiovascular diseases, the two were formally linked in 1958 (265). Subsequently, pathologic studies showed more-advanced coronary artery disease among heavy smokers than among light smokers (266). Smoking is associated with a two- to fourfold increase in coronary artery disease and an increased risk of MI and sudden death (267). Furthermore, if patients with MI continue to smoke, the rate of reinfarction and death also increases. The risk appears to be related to the duration of smoking and the number of cigarettes smoked per day. However, this is not universally accepted (268). Smoking also has a synergistic effect with other coronary risk factors, particularly hypercholesterolemia.

Passive Smoking

Passive smoking is the involuntary inhalation of air contaminated by cigarette smoke. It affects both smokers and nonsmokers. Smokers have an increased risk of developing various cardiovascular effects, whereas nonsmokers may have an increased incidence of MI with chronic exposure and impaired cardiac performance with acute exposure. Investigators exposed patients who survived a first heart attack to passive smoking during an exercise stress test. During passive-smoking exposure, exercise tolerance decreased, time to recovery to baseline heart rate was prolonged, and the occurrence of cardiac arrhythmias increased (269).

Passive environmental smoking results in a 25% increase in the risk of coronary artery disease (270) and death (271) and is now estimated to be the third-leading preventable cause of death after active smoking and alcohol abuse (272). Controlled studies showed that passive smoking impairs endothelial-dependent coronary vasodilation (273), and this is only partially reversible after exposure has ended (274). Passive smoking also leads to accelerated lipid peroxidation and accumulation of LDL cholesterol in human macrophages (275). People exposed to passive smoking have higher levels of C-reactive protein, homocysteine, and fibrinogen (276). These effects contribute to accelerated atherosclerosis (263) and subsequently to increased mortality rates (272). Educating smokers about the risk of passive smoking appears to be more important than ever in the face of these data. Special attention should be given to children and adolescents of parents who smoke (277–279).

Cigar and Pipe Smoking

Although cigarette smoking overall is on the decline in the United States, cigar smoking is rising. Regular cigar smokers who inhale smoke or are heavy smokers have an increased risk of coronary artery disease (280). One prospective study, however, suggested that the cardiovascular risk associated with cigars is less than that associated with cigarettes (281).

Smokeless Tobacco

Smokeless tobacco refers to tobacco snuff, chewing tobacco, and the recently introduced smokeless cigarette. Smokeless tobacco delivers an average amount of nicotine similar to smoking and may produce similar cardiovascular effects. In addition, chewing tobacco leads to a variety of cancerous and precancerous conditions, commonly oral leukoplakia (282,283). An epidemiologic study from Sweden, however, failed to show an increased risk of MI in people who use tobacco snuff (284).

Smoking Cessation

Smoking cessation (285–290) and prevention (291–295) should be a priority for all health caregivers. This topic is discussed in detail in Chapter 8.

CANNABIS

Various forms of the plant are abused, including the plant leaves, the resin extracted from the buds, and the hash oil prepared from the resin. Cannabis is the most widely used illicit drug across the world. It may have some therapeutic potential, and it is considered a cornerstone in some religious ceremonies (296). The drug leads to a significant increase in pulse rate and a modest rise in blood pressure (297). Rarely has the drug been linked to acute myocardial infarction (298) and cerebrovascular events (299). We described a case of ventricular tachycardia and slow coronary flow temporarily related to marijuana smoking (300).

SUMMARY

Substance abuse remains an ongoing public health problem in the United States. Several common agents of abuse contribute to heart disease. The types and frequency of heart disease related to substance abuse probably vary depending on the prevalence and frequency of the type of drug being used. An acute dose of cocaine can have several adverse effects on the heart, including cardiodepressor effects, reductions in contractility and coronary artery blood flow, and conduction abnormalities, which are probably related to its local anesthetic properties. At the same time, cocaine has cardiostimulatory effects, increasing heart rate, blood pressure, contractility, ventricular excitability, and coronary vasoconstriction, related to its sympathomimetic and vagolytic effects. Cocaine has the potential for exacerbating ischemia in patients by increasing heart rate and blood pressure at the same time that it causes coronary vasoconstriction and, in some patients, increased platelet aggregation. The following common cardiovascular diseases have been associated with cocaine abuse in patients: acute MI and myocardial ischemia, dilated and hypertrophic cardiomyopathy, myocarditis, hypertension, arrhythmias, and possibly acceleration of atherosclerosis. Aortic dissection has been reported (301).

Controversy regarding the safety of caffeine and coffee use among coronary artery disease patients is ongoing. The consumption of filtered coffee does not cause an increase in cholesterol levels, whereas boiled coffee may negatively affect lipid levels. Moderate consumption of coffee probably is safe for most patients who have coronary artery disease. Anabolic steroid abuse has been associated with acute MI and lipid abnormalities. There are case reports of MI and cardiomyopathy after use of amphetamines. Small amounts of alcohol may have some benefit on cardiovascular morbidity and mortality rates, but excess use is associated with alcoholic cardiomyopathy, hypertension, arrhythmias, and sudden death.

Tobacco use is a risk factor for coronary artery disease. Both active smoking and exposure to passive smoke increase the risk of coronary artery disease events. Marijuana has been described as a trigger for MI. Substance abuse associated with injection of intravenous material results in a risk of infective endocarditis (covered elsewhere in the text).

The best approach to long-term therapy for heart disease related to substance abuse is to avoid the deleterious substances. Rehabilitation programs play an important role in this regard. Specific therapies for cardiotoxicity in general are lacking. Anecdotal reports regarding therapy for acute ischemic cocaine cardiotoxicity favor nitrates, oxygen, aspirin, benzodiazepines, α-blockers, and possibly calcium channel blockers. If acute MI is present in the setting of cocaine, use of thrombolytic agents and aspirin may be considered, unless a contraindication such as severe hypertension, intracerebral hemorrhage, or seizures is present. Percutaneous coronary intervention is probably the best approach. Future studies are necessary to help clarify the best therapy for cocaine cardiotoxicity.

Primary prevention of substance abuse is clearly the most important goal for our society—although a formidable one, it is worth striving for. The cardiotoxicity of substance abuse is generally serious and potentially life threatening, and treatment is far less optimal than preventing the behavior that causes disease in the first place.

CONTROVERSIES AND PERSONAL PERSPECTIVES

A few controversies persist regarding substance abuse and the heart. Some of the controversy regarding how an acute dose of cocaine affects the heart depends on the model being studied. When cocaine is administered to awake, conscious animals and humans, the sympathomimetic effects predominate, with increases in heart rate and blood pressure. When the drug is administered to pentobarbital-anesthetized animals, the sympathomimetic effects appear to be masked and the cardiodepressive effects predominate. This has caused some confusion in the literature regarding the acute effects of cocaine on the heart. Some debate exists as to whether cocaine actually accelerates atherosclerosis because many of the clinical reports suggesting such an effect involved patients who also have other risk factors, especially tobacco smoking. No general agreement exists regarding the best way to treat acute cocaine cardiotoxicity, and virtually no controlled studies have addressed this issue. The use of β-blockers remains controversial. Although they decrease the heart rate and blood pressure, they block the β-receptors, leaving the α-receptors unopposed, with the potential to worsen coronary artery vasospasm.

Based on the personal observation of one of us (R.A.K.) in a large inner-city county hospital, cocaine cardiotoxicity is probably more common than we realize, especially in that type of environment. When a younger person presents with an acute MI, especially if other risk factors are not present, it is very important to remember to ask about a history of substance abuse, especially cocaine. Initially, patients may be reluctant to divulge this information. However, eventually, with compassionate persistence, the story often emerges. Patients then need to be educated about the hazards of substance abuse. Most will not be aware that cocaine can affect the heart. Patients presenting with chest pain following cocaine use but without evidence of acute MI can be observed and undergo stress testing once stable. Not all chest pain following cocaine use is cardiac.

It is likely that the controversy regarding whether coffee and caffeine are deleterious to the cardiovascular system will continue for some time. Until the controversy is resolved, coffee should be consumed in moderation, especially by individuals with a history of coronary artery disease.

THE FUTURE

The association between substance abuse and heart disease has received increased attention, largely as a result of publicity surrounding the deaths of athletes and entertainment stars who used drugs such as cocaine. Given the prevalence of drug abuse in this country, it is a topic that likely will remain important over the next decade. Its importance may vary, depending on which drugs are most used at a given point in time.

ACKNOWLEDGMENT

We thank Alice Stargardt for a superb job and outstanding editorial assistance in preparing this chapter.

References

1. Isner JM, Chokshi SK. Cardiac complications of cocaine abuse. *Annu Rev Med* 1991;42:33–38.
2. Kloner RA, Hale S, Alker K, et al. The effects of acute and chronic cocaine use on the heart. *Circulation* 1992;85:407–419.
3. Lange RA, Willard JE. The cardiovascular effects of cocaine. *Heart Dis Stroke* 1993;2:136–141.
4. Om A. Cardiovascular complications of cocaine. *Am J Med Sci* 1992;303: 333–339.
5. Bunn WH, Giannini AJ. Cardiovascular complications of cocaine abuse. *Am Fam Physician* 1992;46:769–773.
6. Das G. Cardiovascular effects of cocaine abuse. *Int J Clin Pharmacol Ther Toxicol* 1993;31:521–528.
7. Perper JA, Van Thiel DH. Cardiovascular complications of cocaine abuse. *Recent Dev Alcohol* 1992;10:343–359.
8. Chakko S, Myerburg RJ. Cardiac complications of cocaine abuse. *Clin Cardiol* 1995;18:67–72.
9. Cregler LL. Cocaine: the newest risk factor for cardiovascular disease. *Clin Cardiol* 1991;14:449–456.
10. Billman GE. Cocaine: a review of its toxic actions on cardiac function. *Crit Rev Toxicol* 1995;25:113–132.
11. Rezkalla SH, Hale S, Kloner RA. Cocaine-induced heart disease. *Am Heart J* 1990;120:1403–1408.
12. Lewin L. *Phantastica, narcotics and stimulating drugs: their use and abuse.* New York: EP Dutton, 1931:79.
13. Isner JM, Estes 3rd NA, Thompson PD, et al. Acute cardiac events temporary related to cocaine abuse. *N Engl J Med* 1986;315:1438–1443.
14. Warner EA. Cocaine abuse. *Ann Intern Med* 1993;119:226–235.
15. Warner EA. Is your patient using cocaine? Clinical signs that should raise suspicion. *Postgrad Med* 1995;98:173–180.
16. Pirwitz MJ, Willard JE, Landau C, et al. Influence of cocaine, ethanol, or their combination on epicardial coronary arterial dimensions in humans. *Arch Intern Med* 1995;155:1186–1191.
17. Welder AA, Grammas P, Melchert RB. Cellular mechanisms of cocaine cardiotoxicity. *Toxicol Lett* 1993;69:227–238.
18. Bauman JL, Grawe JJ, Winecoff AP, et al. Cocaine-related sudden cardiac death: a hypothesis correlating basic science and clinical observations. *J Clin Pharmacol* 1994;34:902–911.
19. Newlin DB. Effect of cocaine on vagal tone: a common factors approach. *Drug Alcohol Depend* 1995;37:211–216.
20. Kloner RA, Hale S. Unraveling the complex effects of cocaine on the heart. *Circulation* 1993;87:1046–1047.
21. Hale SL, Alker KJ, Rezkalla S, et al. Adverse effects of cocaine on cardiovascular dynamics, myocardial blood flow, and coronary artery diameter in an experimental model. *Am Heart J* 1989;118:927–933.
22. Stambler BS, Komamura K, Ihara T, et al. Acute intravenous cocaine causes transient depression followed by enhanced left ventricular function in conscious dogs. *Circulation* 1993;87:1687–1697.
23. Garfinkel A, Raetz SL, Harper RM. Heart rate dynamics after cocaine administration. *J Cardiovasc Pharmacol* 1992;19:453–459.
24. Hale SL, Alker KJ, Rezkalla SH, et al. Nifedipine protects the heart from the acute deleterious effects of cocaine if administered before but not after cocaine. *Circulation* 1991;83:1437–1443.
25. Abel FL, Wilson SP, Zhao RR, et al. Cocaine depresses the canine myocardium. *Circ Shock* 1989;28:309–319.
26. Gardin JM, Wong N, Alker K, et al. Acute cocaine administration induces ventricular regional wall motion and ultrastructural abnormalities in an anesthetized rabbit model. *Am Heart J* 1994;128:1117–1129.
27. Pagel PS, Power MW, Kenny D, et al. Cocaine depresses myocardial contractility and prolongs isovolumetric relaxation in conscious dogs with partial autonomic nervous system blockade. *J Cardiovasc Pharmacol* 1992;20: 25–34.
28. Morcos NC, Fairhurst A, Henry WL. Direct myocardial effects of cocaine. *Cardiovasc Res* 1993;27:269–273.
29. Simkhovich BZ, Kloner RA, Alker KJ, et al. Time course of direct cardiotoxic effects of high cocaine concentration in isolated rabbit heart. *J Cardiovasc Pharmacol* 1994;23:509–516.
30. Qiu Z, Morgan JP. Differential effects of cocaine and cocaethylene on intracellular Ca^{2+} and myocardial contraction in cardiac myocytes. *Br J Pharmacol* 1993;109:293–298.
31. Fraker Jr TD, Temesy-Armos PN, Brewster PS, et al. Mechanism of cocaine-induced myocardial depression in dogs. *Circulation* 1990;81: 1012–1016.
32. Vitullo JC, Karam R, Mekhail N, et al. Cocaine-induced small vessel spasm in isolated rat hearts. *Am J Pathol* 1989;135:85–91.
33. Perreault CL, Hague NL, Ransil BJ, et al. The effects of cocaine on intracellular CA^{2+} handling and myofilament Ca^{2+} responsiveness of ferret ventricular myocardium. *Br J Pharmacol* 1990;101:679–685.
34. Tomita F, Bassett AL, Myerburg RJ, et al. Effects of cocaine on sarcoplasmic reticulum in skinned rat heart muscle. *Am J Physiol* 1993;264:H845–H850.
35. Stambler BS, Morgan JP, Mietus J, et al. Cocaine alters heart rate dynamics in conscious ferrets. *Yale J Biol Med* 1991;64:143–153.
36. Hale SL, Lehmann MH, Kloner RA. Electrocardiographic abnormalities after acute administration of cocaine in the rat. *Am J Cardiol* 1989;63: 1529–1530.
37. Przywara DA, Dambach GE. The direct actions of cocaine on cardiac cellular activity [Abstract]. *Circulation* 1988;78(Suppl II):II-47.
38. Billman GE, Lappi MD. The effects of cocaine on cardiac vagal tone before and during coronary artery occlusion: cocaine exacerbates the autonomic response to myocardial ischemia. *J Cardiovasc Pharmacol* 1993;22:869–876.
39. Kabas JS, Blanchard SM, Matsuyama Y, et al. Cocaine-mediated impairment of cardiac conduction in the dog: a potential mechanism for sudden death after cocaine. *J Pharmacol Exp Ther* 1990;252:185–191.
40. Schwartz AB, Janzen D, Jones RT, et al. Electrocardiographic and hemodynamic effects of intravenous cocaine in awake and anesthetized dogs. *J Electrocardiol* 1989;22:159–166.
41. Temesy-Armos PN, Fraker Jr TD, Brewster PS, et al. The effects of cocaine on cardiac electrophysiology in conscious, unsedated dogs. *J Cardiovasc Pharmacol* 1992;19:883–891.
42. Nanji AA, Filipenko JD. Asystole and ventricular fibrillation associated with cocaine intoxication. *Chest* 1984;85:132–133.
43. Watt TB, Pruitt RD. Cocaine-induced incomplete bundle branch block in dogs. *Circ Res* 1964;15:234–239.
44. Weidmann S. Effect of calcium ions and local anaesthetics on electrical properties of Purkinje fibres. *J Physiol (Lond)* 1955;129:568–582.
45. Grossie J. Ca-dependent action of cocaine on K current in freshly dissociated dorsal root ganglia from rats. *Am J Physiol* 1993;265(3 Pt 1):C674–C679.
46. Togna G, Tempesta E, Togna AR, et al. Platelet responsiveness and biosynthesis of thromboxane and prostacyclin in response to *in vitro* cocaine treatment. *Haemostasis* 1985;15:100–107.
47. Rezkalla SH, Mazza JJ, Kloner RA, et al. Effects of cocaine on human platelets in healthy subjects. *Am J Cardiol* 1993;72:243–246.
48. Heesch CM, Wilhelm CR, Ristich J, et al. Cocaine activates platelets and increases the formation of circulating platelet containing microaggregates in humans. *Heart* 2000;83:688–695.
49. Trulson ME, Epps LR, Joe JC. Cocaine: long-term administration depletes cardiac cellular enzymes in the rat. *Acta Anat* 1987;129:165–168.
50. Maillet M, Chiarasini D, Nahas G. Myocardial damage induced by cocaine administration of a week's duration in the rat. *Adv Biosci* 1991;80:187–197.
51. Kolodgie FD, Virmani R, Rice HE, et al. Intravenous cocaine accelerates atherosclerosis in cholesterol-fed New Zealand white rabbits [Abstract]. *J Am Coll Cardiol* 1990;15:217A.
52. Kolodgie FD, Virmani R, Cornhill JF, et al. Increase in atherosclerosis and adventitial mast cells in cocaine abusers: an alternative mechanism of cocaine-associated coronary vasospasm and thrombosis. *J Am Coll Cardiol* 1991;17:1553–1560.
53. Dressler FA, Malekzadeh S, Roberts WC. Quantitative analysis of amounts of coronary arterial narrowing in cocaine addicts. *Am J Cardiol* 1990;65: 303–308.
54. Chen Y, Ke Q, Xiao YF, et al. Cocaine and catecholamines enhance inflammatory cell retention in the coronary circulation of mice by upregulation of adhesion molecules. *Am J Physiol Heart Circ Physiol* 2005;288:H2323–H2331.

55. Fischman MW, Schuster CR, Resnekov L, et al. Cardiovascular and subjective effects of intravenous cocaine administration in humans. *Arch Gen Psychiatry* 1976;33:983–989.
56. Lange RA, Cigarroa RG, Yancy CW, et al. Cocaine-induced coronary-artery vasoconstriction. *N Engl J Med* 1989;321:1557–1562.
57. Lange RA, Cigarroa RG, Flores ED, et al. Potentiation of cocaine-induced coronary vasoconstriction by beta adrenergic blockade. *Ann Intern Med* 1990;112:897–903.
58. Flores ED, Lange RA, Cigarro RG, et al. Effect of cocaine on coronary artery dimensions in atherosclerotic coronary artery disease: enhanced vasoconstriction at sites of significant stenoses. *J Am Coll Cardiol* 1990; 16:74–79.
59. Brogan WC 3d, Lange RA, Kim AS, et al. Alleviation of cocaine-induced coronary vasoconstriction by nitroglycerin. *J Am Coll Cardiol* 1991;18: 581–586.
60. Brogan 3rd WC, Lange RA, Glamann DB, et al. Recurrent coronary vasoconstriction caused by intranasal cocaine: possible role for metabolites. *Ann Intern Med* 1992;116:556–561.
61. Orr D, Jones I. Anaesthesia for laryngoscopy. *Anaesthesia* 1968;23:194–202.
62. Richards IS, Kulkarni AP, Bremner WF. Cocaine-induced arrhythmia in human foetal myocardium *in vitro:* possible mechanism for foetal death *in utero*. *Pharmacol Toxicol* 1990;66:150–154.
63. Lange RA, Hillis LD. Cardiovascular complications of cocaine use. *N Engl J Med* 2001;345:351–358.
64. Kloner RA, Rezkalla SH. Cocaine and the heart. *N Engl J Med* 2003;348: 487–488.
65. Hollander JE, Hoffman RS. Cocaine-induced myocardial infarction: an analysis and review of the literature. *J Emerg Med* 1992;10:169–177.
66. Virmani R, Robinowitz M, Smialek JE, et al. Cardiovascular effects of cocaine: an autopsy study of 40 patients. *Am Heart J* 1988;115:1068–1075.
67. Minor RL, Brook BD, Brown DD, et al. Cocaine-induced myocardial infarction in patients with normal coronary arteries. *Ann Intern Med* 1991;115:797–806.
68. Mittleman MA, Mintzer D, Maclure M, et al. Triggering of myocardial infarction by cocaine. *Circulation* 1999;99:2737–2741.
69. Nademanee K, Gorelick DA, Josephson MA, et al. Myocardial ischemia during cocaine withdrawal. *Ann Intern Med* 1989;111:876–880.
70. Amin M, Gabelman G, Buttrick P. Cocaine-induced myocardial infarction: a growing threat to men in their 30s. *Postgrad Med* 1991;90:50–55.
71. Rubin RB, Neugarten J. Cocaine-induced rhabdomyolysis masquerading as myocardial ischemia. *Am J Med* 1989;86:551–553.
72. Hollander JE, Shih RD, Hoffman RS, et al. Predictors of coronary artery disease in patients with cocaine-associated myocardial infarction. *Am J Med* 1997;102:158–163.
73. Lee H, Eisenberg M, Drew D, et al. Intraventricular thrombus after cocaine-induced myocardial infarction. *Am Heart J* 1995;129:403–405.
74. Hollander JE. The management of cocaine-associated myocardial ischemia. *N Engl J Med* 1995;333:1267–1272.
75. Om A, Ellahham S, DiSciascio G. Management of cocaine-induced cardiovascular complications. *Am Heart J* 1993;125:469–475.
76. Olshaker JS. Cocaine chest pain. *Emerg Clin North Am* 1994;12:391–396.
77. Weber JE, Shofer FS, Larkin GL, et al. Validation of a brief observation period for patients with cocaine-associated chest pain. *N Engl J Med* 2003;348:510–517.
78. Hoey J. Cocaine-associated chest pain in the emergency department. *CMAJ* 2003;168:1017.
79. Counselman FL, McLaughlin EW, Kardon EM, et al. Creatine phosphokinase elevation in patients presenting to the emergency department with cocaine-related complaints. *Am J Emerg Med* 1997;15:221–223.
80. Hollander JE, Levitt MA, Young GP, et al. Effect of recent cocaine use on the specificity of cardiac markers for diagnosis of acute myocardial infarction. *Am Heart J* 1998;135:245–252.
81. Dribben WH, Kirk MA, Trippi JA, et al. A pilot study to assess the safety of dobutamine stress echocardiography in the emergency department evaluation of cocaine-associated chest pain. *Ann Emerg Med* 2001;38:42–48.
82. Yao SS, Spindola-Franco H, Menegus M, et al. Successful intracoronary thrombolysis in cocaine-associated acute myocardial infarction. *Cathet Cardiovasc Diagn* 1997;42:294–297.
83. Shah DM, Dy TC, Szto GY, et al. Percutaneous transluminal coronary angioplasty and stenting for cocaine-induced acute myocardial infarction: a case report and review. *Cathet Cardiovasc Interv* 2000;49:447–451.
84. Frangogiannis NG, Farmer JA, Lakkis NM. Tirofiban for cocaine-induced coronary artery thrombosis: a novel therapeutic approach. *Circulation* 1999;100:1939.
85. Leikin JB. Cocaine and b-adrenergic blockers: a remarriage after a decade-long divorce? *Crit Care Med* 1999;27:688–689.
86. Wang RY. pH-dependent cocaine-induced cardiotoxicity. *Am J Emerg Med* 1999;17:364–369.
87. Hollander JE, Brooks DE, Valentine SM. Assessment of cocaine use in patients with chest pain syndromes. *Arch Intern Med* 1998;158:62–66.
88. Chokshi SK, Moore R, Pandian NG, et al. Reversible cardiomyopathy associated with cocaine intoxication. *Ann Intern Med* 1989;111:1039–1040.
89. Weiner RS, Lockhart JT, Schwartz RG. Dilated cardiomyopathy and cocaine abuse: report of two cases. *Am J Med* 1986;81:699–701.
90. Hogya PT, Wolfson AB. Chronic cocaine abuse associated with dilated cardiomyopathy. *Am J Emerg Med* 1990;8:203–204.
91. Bertolet BD, Freund G, Martin CA, et al. Unrecognized left ventricular dysfunction in an apparently healthy cocaine abuse population. *Clin Cardiol* 1990;13:323–328.
92. Willens HJ, Chakko SC, Kessler KM. Cardiovascular manifestations of cocaine abuse: a case of recurrent dilated cardiomyopathy. *Chest* 1994;106:594–600.
93. Pitts WR, Vongpatanasin W, Cigarroa JE, et al. Effects of the intracoronary infusion of cocaine on left ventricular systolic and diastolic function in humans. *Circulation* 1998;97:1270–1273.
94. Brickner ME, Willard JE, Eichhorn EJ, et al. Left ventricular hypertrophy associated with chronic cocaine abuse. *Circulation* 1991;84:1130–1135.
95. Clyburn EB, DiPette DJ. Hypertension induced by drugs and other substances. *Semin Nephrol* 1995;15:72–86.
96. Benchimol A, Bantell H, Dressen KB. Accelerated ventricular rhythm and cocaine abuse. *Ann Intern Med* 1978;88:519–520.
97. Castro VJ, Nacht R. Cocaine-induced bradyarrhythmia: an unsuspected cause of syncope. *Chest* 2000;117:275–277.
98. Lai S, Lima JA, Lai H, et al. Human immunodeficiency virus 1 infection, cocaine, and coronary calcification. *Arch Intern Med* 2005;165:690–695.
99. Karch SB, Billingham ME. Coronary artery and peripheral vascular disease in cocaine users. *Coron Artery Dis* 1995;6:220–225.
100. Jones LF, Tackett RL. Chronic cocaine treatment enhances the responsiveness of the left anterior descending coronary artery and the femoral artery to vasoactive substances. *J Pharmacol Exp Ther* 1990;255:1366–1370.
101. Simpson R, Edwards W. Pathogenesis of cocaine induced ischemic heart disease: autopsy findings in a 21-year-old man. *Arch Pathol Lab Med* 1986;110:479–484.
102. Roh LS, Hamele-Bena D. Cocaine-induced ischemic myocardial disease. *Am J Forensic Med Pathol* 1990;11:130–135.
103. Majid PA, Patel B, Kim HS, et al. An angiographic and histologic study of cocaine-induced chest pain. *Am J Cardiol* 1990;65:812–814.
104. Satran A, Bart BA, Henry CR, et al. Increased prevalence of coronary artery aneurysms among cocaine users. *Circulation* 2005;111:2424–2429.
105. Eagle KA, Isselbacher EM, DeSanctis RW. Cocaine-related aortic dissection in perspective. *Circulation* 2002;105:1529–1530.
106. Hsue PY, Salinas CL, Bolger AF, et al. Acute aortic dissection related to crack cocaine. *Circulation* 2002;105:1592–1595.
107. Marder VJ, Mellinghoff IK. Cocaine and Buerger disease: is there a pathogenetic association? *Arch Intern Med* 2000;160:2057–2060.
108. Gutierrez A, England JD, Krupski WC. Cocaine-induced peripheral vascular occlusive disease: a case report. *Angiology* 1998;49:221–224.
109. Wattoo MA, Osundeko O. Cocaine-induced intestinal ischemia. *West J Med* 1999;170:47–49.
110. Kaufman MJ, Levin JM, Ross MH, et al. Cocaine-induced cerebral vasoconstriction detected in humans with magnetic resonance angiography. *JAMA* 1998;279:376–380.
111. Khellaf M, Fénelon G. Intracranial hemorrhage associated with cocaine abuse [Letter]. *Neurology* 1998;50:1519–1520.
112. Rose S, Hearn WL, Hime GW, et al. Cocaine and cocaethylene concentrations in human postmortem cerebral cortex [Abstract]. *Neuroscience* 1990;16:14.
113. Escobedo LG, Ruttenber AJ, Agocs MM, et al. Emerging patterns of cocaine use and the epidemic of cocaine overdose deaths in Dade County, Florida. *Arch Pathol Lab Med* 1991;115:900–905.
114. Perez-Reyes M, Jeffcoat R. Ethanol/cocaine interaction: cocaine and cocaethylene plasma concentrations and their relationship to subjective cardiovascular effects. *Life Sci* 1992;51:553–563.
115. Hearn WL, Rose S, Wagner J, et al. Cocaethylene is more potent than cocaine in mediating lethality. *Pharmacol Biochem Behav* 1991;39:531–533.
116. Uszenski RT, Gillis RA, Schaer GL, et al. Additive myocardial depressant effects of cocaine and ethanol. *Am Heart J* 1992;124:1276–1283.
117. Foltin RW, Fischman MW. Ethanol and cocaine interactions in humans: cardiovascular consequences. *Pharmacol Biochem Behav* 1988;31:877–883.
118. Farre M, de la Torre R, Llorente M, et al. Alcohol and cocaine interactions in humans. *J Pharmacol Exp Ther* 1993;266:1364–1373.
119. Chou T. Wake up and smell the coffee: caffeine, coffee, and the medical consequences. *West J Med* 1992;157:544–553.
120. Chou T, Benowitz NL. Caffeine and coffee: effects on health and cardiovascular disease. *Comp Biochem Physiol C Pharmacol Toxicol Endocrinol* 1994;109:173–189.
121. Robertson D, Frolich JC, Carr RK, et al. Effects of caffeine on plasma renin activity, catecholamines and blood pressure. *N Engl J Med* 1978;298:181–186.
122. van Dusseldorp M, Smits P, Thien T, et al. Effect of decaffeinated versus regular coffee on blood pressure: a 12-week, double-blind trial. *Hypertension* 1989;14:563–569.
123. van Dusseldorp M, Smits P, Lenders JW, et al. Boiled coffee and blood pressure: a 14-week controlled trial. *Hypertension* 1991;18:607–613.
124. Rachima-Maoz C, Peleg E, Rosenthal T. The effect of caffeine on ambulatory blood pressure in hypertensive patients. *Am J Hypertens* 1998; 11:1426–1432.

125. Rakic V, Burke V, Beilin LJ. Effects of coffee on ambulatory blood pressure in older men and women: a randomized controlled trial. *Hypertension* 1999;33:869–873.
126. James JE. Critical review of dietary caffeine and blood pressure: a relationship that should be taken more seriously. *Psychosom Med* 2004;66:63–71.
127. Hakim AA, Ross GW, Curb JD, et al. Coffee consumption in hypertensive men in older middle-age and the risk of stroke: the Honolulu Heart Program. *J Clin Epidemiol* 1998;51:487–494.
128. LaCroix AZ, Mead LA, Liang KY, et al. Coffee consumption and the incidence of coronary artery disease. *N Engl J Med* 1986;315:977–982.
129. Rosenberg L, Palmer Jr, Kelly JP, et al. Coffee drinking and nonfatal myocardial infarction in men under 55 years of age. *Am J Epidemiol* 1988;128:570–578.
130. Grobbee DE, Rimm EB, Giovannucci E, et al. Coffee, caffeine, and cardiovascular disease in men. *N Engl J Med* 1990;323:1026–1032.
131. Lynn LA, Kissinger JF. Coronary precautions: should caffeine be restricted in patients after myocardial infarction? *Heart Lung* 1992;21:365–371.
132. Sesso HD, Gaziano JM, Buring JE, et al. Coffee and tea intake and the risk of myocardial infarction. *Am J Epidemiol* 1999;149:162–167.
133. Geleijnse JM, Launer LJ, Hofman A, et al. Tea flavonoids may protect against atherosclerosis. The Rotterdam Study. *Arch Intern Med* 1999;159:2170–2174.
134. McKay DL, Blumberg JB. The role of tea in human health: an update. *J Am Coll Nutr* 2002;21:1–13.
135. Mennen LI, Sapinho D, de Bree A, et al. Consumption of foods rich in flavonoids is related to a decreased cardiovascular risk in apparently healthy French women. *J Nutr* 2004;134:923–926.
136. Peters U, Poole C, Arab L. Does tea affect cardiovascular disease? A meta-analysis. *Am J Epidemiol* 2001;154:495–503.
137. Huxley RR, Neil HA. The relation between dietary flavonol intake and coronary heart disease mortality: a meta-analysis of prospective cohort studies. *Eur J Clin Nutr* 2003;57:904–908.
138. Riemersma RA, Rice-Evans CA, Tyrrell RM, et al. Tea flavonoids and cardiovascular health. *Q J Med* 2001;94:277–282.
139. de Vries JH, Hollman PC, van Amersfoort I, et al. Red wine is a poor source of bioavailable flavonols in men. *J Nutr* 2001;131:745–748.
140. Langley-Evans S. Consumption of black tea elicits an increase in plasma antioxidant potential in humans. *Int J Food Sci Nutr* 2000;51:309–315.
141. Duffy SJ, Keaney Jr JF, Holbrook M, et al. Short- and long-term black tea consumption reverses endothelial dysfunction in patients with coronary artery disease. *Circulation* 2001;104:151–156.
142. Duffy SJ, Vita JA, Holbrook M, et al. Effect of acute and chronic tea consumption on platelet aggregation in patients with coronary artery disease. *Arterioscler Thromb Vasc Biol* 2001;21:1084–1089.
143. Stavric B. An update on research with coffee/caffeine (1989–1990). *Food Chem Toxicol* 1992;30:533–555.
144. Rosmarin PC. Coffee and coronary heart disease: a review. *Prog Cardiovasc Dis* 1989;32:239–245.
145. Rosmarin PC, Applegate WB, Somes GW. Coffee consumption and serum lipids: a randomized, crossover clinical trial. *Am J Med* 1990;88:349–356.
146. Nygård O, Refsum H, Ueland PM, et al. Coffee consumption and plasma total homocysteine: the Hordaland Homocysteine Study. *Am J Clin Nutr* 1997;65:136–143.
147. El-Khairy L, Ueland PM, Nygård O, et al. Lifestyle and cardiovascular disease risk factors as determinants of total cysteine in plasma: the Hordaland Homocysteine Study. *Am J Clin Nutr* 1999;70:1016–1024.
148. Stolzenberg-Solomon RZ, Miller 3rd ER, Maguire MG, et al. Association of dietary protein intake and coffee consumption with serum homocysteine concentrations in an older population. *Am J Clin Nutr* 1999;69:467–475.
149. Grubben MJ, Boers GH, Blom HJ, et al. Unfiltered coffee increases plasma homocysteine concentrations in healthy volunteers: a randomized trial. *Am J Clin Nutr* 2000;71:480–484.
150. Dobmeyer DJ, Stine RA, Leier CV, et al. The arrhythmogenic effects of caffeine in human beings. *N Engl J Med* 1983;308:814–816.
151. Prineas RJ, Jacobs Jr DR, Crow RS, et al. Coffee, tea and VPB. *J Chronic Dis* 1980;33:67–72.
152. Graboys TB, Blatt CM, Lown B. The effect of caffeine on ventricular ectopic activity in patients with malignant ventricular arrhythmia. *Arch Intern Med* 1989;149:637–639.
153. Chelsky LB, Cutler JE, Griffith K, et al. Caffeine and ventricular arrhythmias: an electrophysiological approach. *JAMA* 1990;264:2236–2240.
154. Donnerstein RL, Zhu D, Samson R, et al. Acute effects of caffeine ingestion on signal-averaged electrocardiograms. *Am Heart J* 1998;136:643–646.
155. Stamler JS, Goldman ME, Gomes J, et al. The effect of stress and fatigue on cardiac rhythm in medical interns. *J Electrocardiol* 1992;25:333–338.
156. Myers MG, Harris L. High dose caffeine and ventricular arrhythmias. *Can J Cardiol* 1990;6:95–98.
157. Myers MG. Caffeine and cardiac arrhythmias. *Ann Intern Med* 1991; 114:147–150.
158. Welder AA, Melchert RB. Cardiotoxic effects of cocaine and anabolic-androgenic steroids in the athlete. *J Pharmacol Toxicol Methods* 1993; 29:61–68.
159. Kennedy C. Myocardial infarction in association with misuse of anabolic steroids. *Ulster Med J* 1993;62:174–176.
160. Ferenchick GS. Anabolic/androgenic steroid abuse and thrombosis: is there a connection? *Med Hypotheses* 1991;35:27–31.
161. Glazer G. Atherogenic effects of anabolic steroids on serum lipid levels: a literature review. *Arch Intern Med* 1991;151:1925–1933.
162. Barrett-Connor EL. Testosterone and risk factors for cardiovascular disease in men. *Diabetes Metab* 1995;21:156–161.
163. Rockhold RW. Cardiovascular toxicity of anabolic steroids. *Annu Rev Pharmacol Toxicol* 1993;33:497–520.
164. Uzunova AD, Ramey ER, Ramwell PW. Arachidonate-induced thrombosis in mice: effects of gender or testosterone and estradiol administration. *Prostaglandins* 1977;13:995–1002.
165. Penhos JC, Rabbani F, Myers A, et al. The role of gonadal steroids in arachidonate-induced mortality in mice. *Proc Soc Exp Biol Med* 1981; 167:98–100.
166. Emms H, Lewis GP. Sex and hormonal influences on platelet sensitivity and coagulation in the rat. *Br J Pharmacol* 1985;86:557–563.
167. Myers A, Papadopoulos A, O'Day D, et al. Sexual differentiation of arachidonate toxicity in mice. *J Pharmacol Exp Ther* 1982;222:315–318.
168. Johnson M, Ramwell PW. Androgen mediated sex differences in platelet aggregation [Abstract]. *Physiologist* 1974;17:256.
169. Stolt A, Karila T, Viitasalo M, et al. QT interval and QT dispersion in endurance athletes and in power athletes using large doses of anabolic steroids. *Am J Cardiol* 1999;84:364–366.
170. Sullivan ML, Martinez CM, Gallagher EJ. Atrial fibrillation and anabolic steroids. *J Emerg Med* 1999;17:851–857.
171. Carson P, Oldroyd K, Phadke K. Myocardial infarction due to amphetamine. *BMJ (Clin Res Ed)* 1987;294:1525–1526.
172. Dowling GP, McDonough 3rd ET, Bost RO. "Eve" and "Ecstasy": a report of five deaths associated with the use of MDEA and MDMA. *JAMA* 1987;257:1615–1617.
173. Suarez RV, Riemersma R. "Ecstasy" and sudden cardiac death. *Am J Forensic Med Pathol* 1988;9:339–341.
174. Packe GE, Garton MJ, Jennings K. Acute myocardial infarction caused by intravenous amphetamine abuse. *Br Heart J* 1990;64:23–24.
175. Ragland AS, Ismail Y, Arsura EL. Myocardial infarction after amphetamine use. *Am Heart J* 1993;125:247–249.
176. Furst SR, Fallon SP, Reznik GN. Myocardial infarction after inhalation of methamphetamine [Letter]. *N Engl J Med* 1990;323:1147–1148.
177. Bashour TT. Acute myocardial infarction resulting from amphetamine abuse: a spasm-thrombus interplay? *Am Heart J* 1994;128:1237–1239.
178. Jacobs LJ. Reversible dilated cardiomyopathy induced by methamphetamine. *Clin Cardiol* 1989;12:725–727.
179. Hong R, Matsuyama E, Nur K. Cardiomyopathy associated with the smoking of crystal methamphetamine. *JAMA* 1991;265:1152–1154.
180. McEvoy AW, Kitchen ND, Thomas DGT. Intracerebral haemorrhage in young adults: the emerging importance of drug misuse. *BMJ* 2000;320: 1322–1324.
181. Perez Jr JA, Arsura EL, Strategos S. Methamphetamine-related stroke: four cases. *J Emerg Med* 1999;17:469–471.
182. Zahn KA, Li RL, Purssell RA. Cardiovascular toxicity after ingestion of "herbal ecstasy." *J Emerg Med* 1999;17:289–291.
183. Reneman L, Habraken JB, Majoie CB, et al. MDMA ("Ecstasy") and its association with cerebrovascular accidents: preliminary findings. *AJNR Am J Neuroradiol* 2000;21:1001–1007.
184. Setola V, Hufeisen SJ, Grande-Allen KJ, et al. 3,4-Methylene-dioxymethamphetamine (MDMA, "Ecstasy") induces fenfluramine-like proliferative actions on human cardiac valvular interstitial cells *in vitro*. *Mol Pharmacol* 2003;63:1223–1229.
185. de Boer D, Bosman I. A new trend in drugs-of-abuse; the 2C-series of phenethylamine designer drugs. *Pharm World Sci* 2004;26:110–113.
186. Staack RF, Maurer HH. New designer drug 1-(3,4-methylenedioxybenzyl) piperazine (MDBP): studies on its metabolism and toxicological detection in rat urine using gas chromatography/mass spectrometry. *J Mass Spectrom* 2004;39:255–261.
187. Ling LH, Marchant C, Buckley NA, et al. Poisoning with the recreational drug paramethoxyamphetamine ("death"). *Med J Aust* 2001;174:453–455.
188. DEA News Release July 22, 2004. DEA announces arrests of website operators selling illegal designer drugs. Available at http://www.usdoj.gov/dea/pubs/pressrel/pr072204p.html (accessed January 28, 2005).
189. Silvestry FE, St. John Sutton M. Anorectic therapy and valvular heart disease: a reappraisal. *Eur Heart J* 1999;20:917–920.
190. Connolly HM, Crary JL, McGoon MD, et al. Valvular heart disease associated with fenfluramine-phentermine. *N Engl J Med* 1997;337:581–588.
191. Jick H, Vasilakis C, Weinrauch LA, et al. A population-based study of appetite-suppressant drugs and the risk of cardiac-valve regurgitation. *N Engl J Med* 1998;339:719–724.
192. Khan MA, Herzog CA, St. Peter JV, et al. The prevalence of cardiac valvular insufficiency assessed by transthoracic echocardiography in obese patients treated with appetite-suppressant drugs. *N Engl J Med* 1998;339:713–718.
193. Burger AJ, Sherman HB, Charlamb MJ, et al. Low prevalence of valvular heart disease in 226 phentermine-fenfluramine protocol subjects prospectively followed for up to 30 months. *J Am Coll Cardiol* 1999;34:1153–1158.
194. Jick H. Heart valve disorders and appetite-suppressant drugs. *JAMA* 2000;283:1738–1740.
195. Jollis JG, Landolfo CK, Kisslo J, et al. Fenfluramine and phentermine and cardiovascular findings: effect of treatment duration on prevalence of valve abnormalities. *Circulation* 2000;101:2071–2077.

196. Cannistra LB, Cannistra AJ. Regression of multivalvular regurgitation after the cessation of fenfluramine and phentermine treatment. *N Engl J Med* 1998;339:771.
197. Mast ST, Jollis JG, Ryan T, et al. The progression of fenfluramine-associated valvular heart disease assessed by echocardiography. *Ann Intern Med* 2001;134:261–266.
198. Centers for Disease Control and Prevention. Cardiac valvulopathy associated with exposure to fenfluramine or dexfenfluramine: US Department of Health and Human Services interim public health recommendations, November 1997. *JAMA* 1997;278:1729–1731.
199. Rich S, Rubin L, Walker AM, et al. Anorexigens and pulmonary hypertension in the United States: results from the Surveillance of North American Pulmonary Hypertension. *Chest* 2000;117:870–874.
200. Simonneau G, Fartoukh M, Sitbon O, et al. Primary pulmonary hypertension associated with the use of fenfluramine derivatives. *Chest* 1998;114:195S–199S.
201. Mark EJ, Patalas ED, Chang HT, et al. Fatal pulmonary hypertension associated with short-term use of fenfluramine and phentermine. *N Engl J Med* 1997;337:602–606.
202. Fowles RE, Cloward TV, Yowell RL. Endocardial fibrosis associated with fenfluramine-phentermine. *N Engl J Med* 1998;338:1316.
203. Sobel RM. Ruptured retroperitoneal aneurysm in a patient taking phentermine hydrochloride. *Am J Emerg Med* 1999;17:102–103.
204. Urbano-Marquez A, Estruch R, Fernandez-Sola J, et al. The greater risk of alcoholic cardiomyopathy and myopathy in women compared with men. *JAMA* 1995;274:149–154.
205. Johnson CC, Myers L, Webber LS, et al. Alcohol consumption among adolescents and young adults: the Bogalusa Heart Study, 1981 to 1991. *Am J Public Health* 1995;85:979–982.
206. Gambert SR. Alcohol abuse: medical effects of heavy drinking in late life. *Geriatrics* 1997;52:30–37.
207. Goldstein D. *The pharmacology of alcohol*. New York: Oxford University Press,1983.
208. Piano MR, Schwertz DW. Alcoholic heart disease: a review. *Heart Lung* 1994;23:3–17.
209. Teragaki M, Takeuchi K, Takeda T. Clinical and histologic features of alcohol drinkers with congestive heart failure. *Am Heart J* 1993;125:808–817.
210. Polimeni PI, Otten MD, Hoeschen LE. *In vivo* effects of ethanol on the rat myocardium: evidence for a reversible, nonspecific increase of sarcolemmal permeability. *J Mol Cell Cardiol* 1983;15:113–122.
211. Wu S, White R, Wikman-Coffelt J, et al. The preventive effect of verapamil on ethanol-induced cardiac depression: phosphorus-31 nuclear magnetic resonance and high-pressure liquid chromatographic studies of hamsters. *Circulation* 1987;75:1058–1064.
212. Preedy VR, Atkinson LM, Richardson PJ, et al. Mechanisms of ethanol-induced cardiac damage. *Br Heart J* 1993;69:197–200.
213. Preedy VR, Siddiq T, Why H, et al. The deleterious effects of alcohol on the heart: involvement of protein turnover. *Alcohol* 1994;29:141–147.
214. Fernandez-Sola J, Estruch R, Grau JM, et al. The relation of alcoholic myopathy to cardiomyopathy. *Ann Intern Med* 1994;120:529–536.
215. Moushmoush B, Abi-Mansour P. Alcohol and the heart: the long-term effects of alcohol on the cardiovascular system. *Arch Intern Med* 1991;151:36–42.
216. Thomas AP, Rozanski DJ, Renard DC, et al. Effects of ethanol on the contractile function of the heart: a review. *Alcohol Clin Exp Res* 1994;18:121–131.
217. Kupari M, Koskinen P, Suokas A, et al. Left ventricular filling impairment in asymptomatic chronic alcoholics. *Am J Cardiol* 1990;66:1473–1477.
218. Lazarevic AM, Nakatani S, Neskovic AN, et al. Early changes in left ventricular function in chronic asymptomatic alcoholics: relation to the duration of heavy drinking. *J Am Coll Cardiol* 2000;35:1599–1606.
219. Ballester M, Martí V, Carrió I, et al. Spectrum of alcohol-induced myocardial damage detected by indium-111-labeled monoclonal antimyosin antibodies. *J Am Coll Cardiol* 1997;29:160–167.
220. Stöllberger C, Finsterer J. Reversal of dilated to hypertrophic cardiomyopathy after alcohol abstinence. *Clin Cardiol* 1998;21:365–367.
221. Machiels JP, Dive A, Donckier J, et al. Reversible myocardial dysfunction in a patient with alcoholic ketoacidosis: a role for hypophosphatemia. *Am J Emerg Med* 1998;16:371–373.
222. Jacob AJ, McLaren KM, Boon NA. Effects of abstinence on alcoholic heart muscle disease. *Am J Cardiol* 1991;68:805–807.
223. Gavazzi A, DeMaria R, Parolini M, et al. Alcohol abuse and dilated cardiomyopathy in men. The Italian Multicenter Cardiomyopathy Study Group. *Am J Cardiol* 2000;85:1114–1118.
224. Fauchier L, Babuty D, Poret P, et al. Comparison of long-term outcome of alcoholic and idiopathic dilated cardiomyopathy. *Eur Heart J* 2000;21:306–314.
225. Walsh CR, Larson MG, Evans JC, et al. Alcohol consumption and risk for congestive heart failure in the Framingham Heart Study. *Ann Intern Med* 2002;136:181–191.
226. Aguilar D, Skali H, Moyé LA, et al. Alcohol consumption and prognosis in patients with left ventricular systolic dysfunction after a myocardial infarction. *J Am Coll Cardiol* 2004;43:2015–2021.
227. Abramson JL, Williams SA, Krumholz HM, et al. Moderate alcohol consumption and risk of heart failure among older persons. *JAMA* 2001;285: 1971–1977.
228. Nicolás JM, Fernández Solà J, Estruch R, et al. The effect of controlled drinking in alcoholic cardiomyopathy. *Ann Intern Med* 2002;136:192–200.
229. Lian C. L'alcoholism cause d'hypertension arterielle. *Bull Acad Natl Med* 1915;74:525–528.
230. Regan TJ. Alcohol and the cardiovascular system. *JAMA* 1990;264:377–381.
231. Moreira LB, Fuchs FD, Moraes RS, et al. Alcohol intake and blood pressure: the importance of time elapsed since last drink. *J Hypertens* 1998;16:175–180.
232. Manolio TA, Levy D, Garrison RJ, et al. Relation of alcohol intake to left ventricular mass: the Framingham Study. *J Am Coll Cardiol* 1991;17:717–721.
233. Koskinen P, Kupari M. Alcohol and cardiac arrhythmias. *BMJ* 1992;304: 1394–1395.
234. Hendrickse MT. QT interval, autonomic neuropathy, and alcoholic liver disease. *Lancet* 1993;342:61.
235. Ettinger PO, Wu CF, DeLa Cruz Jr C, et al. Arrhythmias and the "holiday heart": alcohol-associated cardiac rhythm disorders. *Am Heart J* 1978;95:555–562.
236. Lowenstein SR, Gabow PA, Cramer J, et al. The role of alcohol in new-onset atrial fibrillation. *Arch Intern Med* 1983;143:1882–1885.
237. Koskinen P, Kupari M, Leinonen H. Role of alcohol in recurrences of atrial fibrillation in persons less than 65 years of age. *Am J Cardiol* 1990;66:954–958.
238. Engel TR, Luck JC. Effect of whiskey on atrial vulnerability and "holiday heart." *J Am Coll Cardiol* 1983;1:816–818.
239. Djoussé L, Levy D, Benjamin EJ, et al. Long-term alcohol consumption and the risk of atrial fibrillation in the Framingham Study. *Am J Cardiol* 2004;93:710–713.
240. Wannamethee G, Shaper AG. Alcohol and sudden cardiac death. *Br Heart J* 1992;68:443–448.
241. Klatsky AL, Armstrong MA, Friedman GD. Alcohol and mortality. *Ann Intern Med* 1992;117:646–654.
242. Doll R, Peto R, Hall E, et al. Mortality in relation to consumption of alcohol: 13 years' observations on male British doctors. *BMJ* 1994;309:911–918.
243. Gaziano JM, Buring JE, Breslow JL, et al. Moderate alcohol intake, increased levels of high-density lipoprotein and its subfractions, and decreased risk of myocardial infarction. *N Engl J Med* 1993;329:1829–1834.
244. Rimm EB, Klatsky A, Grobbee D, et al. Review of moderate alcohol consumption and reduced risk of coronary heart disease: is the effect due to beer, wine, or spirits. *BMJ* 1996;312:731–736.
245. Maclure M. Demonstration of deductive meta-analysis: ethanol intake and risk of myocardial infarction. *Epidemiol Rev* 1993;15:328–351.
246. Maclure M. Alcohol intake and risk of myocardial infarction. *N Engl J Med* 1994;330:1241–1242.
247. Ridker PM, Vaughan DE, Stampfer MJ, et al. Association of moderate alcohol consumption and plasma concentration of endogenous tissue-type plasminogen activator. *JAMA* 1994;272:929–933.
248. Rubin R, Rand ML. Alcohol and platelet function. *Alcohol Clin Exp Res* 1994;18:105–110.
249. Steinberg D, Pearson TA, Kuller LH. Alcohol and atherosclerosis. *Ann Intern Med* 1991;114:967–976.
250. Di Castelnuovo A, Rotondo S, Iacoviello L, et al. Meta-analysis of wine and beer consumption in relation to vascular risk. *Circulation* 2002;105:2836–2844.
251. Rimm EB, Stampfer MJ. Wine, beer, and spirits: are they really horses of a different color? *Circulation* 2002;105:2806–2807.
252. Cheng TO. Effect of red versus white wine on the heart. *Am J Cardiol* 2002;89:490.
253. Grønbæk M, Becker U, Johansen D, et al. Type of alcohol consumed and mortality from all causes, coronary heart disease, and cancer. *Ann Intern Med* 2000;133:411–419.
254. Pentz MA, Dwyer JH, MacKinnon DP, et al. A multicommunity trial for primary prevention of adolescent drug abuse: effects on drug use prevalence. *JAMA* 1989;261:3259–3266.
255. Vander Martin R, Cummings SR, Coates TJ. Ethnicity and smoking: differences in white, black, Hispanic, and Asian medical patients who smoke. *Am J Prev Med* 1990;6:194–199.
256. Edwards G, Arif A, Hadgson R. Nomenclature and classification of drug- and alcohol-related problems: a WHO memorandum. *Bull World Health Org* 1981;59:225–242.
257. Benowitz NL. Cigarette smoking and nicotine addiction. *Med Clin North Am* 1992;76:415–437.
258. Stephenson J. Clues found to tobacco addiction. *JAMA* 1996;275:1217–1218.
259. Schelling TC. Addictive drugs: the cigarette experience. *Science* 1992;255: 430–433.
260. Carmelli D, Swan GE, Robinette D, et al. Genetic influence on smoking: a study of male twins. *N Engl J Med* 1992;327:829–833.
261. Falk E. Why do plaques rupture? *Circulation* 1992;86(Suppl 6):III30–III42.
262. McCall MR, van den Berg JJ, Kuypers FA, et al. Modification of LCAT activity and HDL structure: new links between cigarette smoke and coronary heart disease risk. *Arterioscler Thromb* 1994;14:248–253.
263. Howard G, Wagenknecht LE, Burke GL, et al. Cigarette smoking and progression of atherosclerosis. The Atherosclerosis Risk in Communities (ARIC) Study. *JAMA* 1998;279:119–124.

264. Bolinder G, deFaire U. Ambulatory 24-h blood pressure monitoring in healthy, middle-aged smokeless tobacco users, smokers, and nontobacco users. *Am J Hypertens* 1998;11:1153–1163.
265. Hammond EC, Horn D. Smoking and death rates: report on forty-four months of follow-up of 187,783 men: II. Death rates by cause. *JAMA* 1958;166:1294–1308.
266. Auerbach O, Carter HW, Garfinkel L, et al. Cigarette smoking and coronary artery disease: a macroscopic and microscopic study. *Chest* 1976;70:697–705.
267. Lakier JB. Smoking and cardiovascular disease. *Am J Med* 1992;93(Suppl 1A):8S–12S.
268. Ambrose JA, Barua RS. The pathophysiology of cigarette smoking and cardiovascular disease. An update. *J Am Coll Cardiol* 2004;43:1731–1737.
269. Leone A. Cardiovascular damage from smoking: a fact or belief? *Int J Cardiol* 1993;38:113–117.
270. He J, Whelton PK. Passive cigarette smoking increases risk of coronary heart disease. *Eur Heart J* 1999;20:1764–1765.
271. Steenland K. Risk assessment for heart disease and workplace ETS exposure among nonsmokers. *Environ Health Perspect* 1999;107(Suppl 6):859–863.
272. Werner RM, Pearson TA. What's so passive about passive smoking? Secondhand smoke as a cause of atherosclerotic disease. *JAMA* 1998;279:157–158.
273. Sumida H, Watanabe H, Kugiyama K, et al. Does passive smoking impair endothelium-dependent coronary artery dilation in women? *J Am Coll Cardiol* 1998;31:811–815.
274. Raitakari OT, Adams MR, McCredie RJ, et al. Arterial endothelial dysfunction related to passive smoking is potentially reversible in healthy young adults. *Ann Intern Med* 1999;130:578–581.
275. Valkonen M, Kuusi T. Passive smoking induces atherogenic changes in low-density lipoprotein. *Circulation* 1998;97:2012–2016.
276. Panagiotakos DB, Pitsavos C, Chrysohoou C, et al. Effect of exposure to secondhand smoke on markers of inflammation: the ATTICA Study. *Am J Med* 2004;116:145–150.
277. Whincup PH, Gilg JA, Emberson Jr, et al. Passive smoking and risk of coronary heart disease and stroke: prospective study with cotinine measurement. *BMJ* 2004;329:200–205.
278. Burke V, Gracey MP, Milligan RA, et al. Parental smoking and risk factors for cardiovascular disease in 10- to 12-year-old children. *J Pediatr* 1998; 133:206–213.
279. Moskowitz WB, Schwartz PF, Schieken RM. Childhood passive smoking, race, and coronary artery disease risk: the MCV Twin Study. Medical College of Virginia. *Arch Pediatr Adolesc Med* 1999;153:446–453.
280. Satcher D. Cigars and public health. *N Engl J Med* 1999;340:1829–1831.
281. Wald NJ, Watt HC. Prospective study of effect of switching from cigarettes to pipes or cigars on mortality from three smoking related diseases. *BMJ* 1997;314:1860–1863.
282. Christen AG, McDaniel RK, McDonald Jr JL. The smokeless tobacco "time bomb." *Postgrad Med* 1990;87:69–74.
283. Asplund K. Smokeless tobacco and cardiovascular disease. *Prog Cardiovasc Dis* 2003;45:383–394.
284. Huhtasaari F, Lundberg V, Eliasson M, et al. Smokeless tobacco as a possible risk factor for myocardial infarction: a population-based study in middle-aged men. *J Am Coll Cardiol* 1999;34:1784–1790.
285. Schwartz JL. Methods of smoking cessation. *Med Clin North Am* 1992;76:451–476.
286. Kimmel SE, Berlin JA, Miles C, et al. Risk of acute first myocardial infarction and use of nicotine patches in a general population. *J Am Coll Cardiol* 2001;37:1297–1302.
287. Benowitz NL, Fitzgerald GA, Wilson M, et al. Nicotine effects on eicosanoid formation and hemostatic function: comparison of transdermal nicotine and cigarette smoking. *J Am Coll Cardiol* 1993;22:1159–1167.
288. Warner Jr JG, Little WC. Myocardial infarction in a patient who smoked while wearing a nicotine patch. *Ann Intern Med* 1994;120:695.
289. Arnaot MR. Treating heart disease: nicotine patches may not be safe. *BMJ* 1995;310:663–664.
290. Campbell IA. Smoking cessation. *Thorax* 2000;55(Suppl 1):S28–S31.
291. Kessler DA. Nicotine addiction in young people. *N Engl J Med* 1995;333: 186–189.
292. Lynch BS, Bonnie RJ, eds. *Growing up tobacco free: preventing nicotine addiction in children and youth*. Washington, DC: National Academy Press, 1994:8.
293. Department of Health and Human Services. *Preventing tobacco use among young people: a report of the Surgeon General*. Washington, DC: Government Printing Office, 1994:5–58.
294. Glynn TJ. Essential elements of school-based smoking prevention programs. *J Sch Health* 1989;59:181–188.
295. Whooley MA, Boyd AL, Gardin JM, et al. Religious involvement and cigarette smoking in young adults. The CARDIA Study. *Arch Intern Med* 2002;162:1604–1610.
296. Gupta BD, Jani CB, Shah PH. Fatal "Bhang" poisoning. *Med Sci Law* 2001; 41:349–352.
297. Sidney S. Cardiovascular consequences of marijuana use. *J Clin Pharmacol* 2002;42:64S–70S.
298. Mittleman MA, Lewis RA, Maclure M, et al, Triggering myocardial infarction by marijuana. *Circulation* 2001;103:2805–2809.
299. Moussouttas M. Cannabis use and cerebrovascular disease. *Neurologist* 2004;10:47–53.
300. Rezkalla SH, Sharma P, Kloner RA. Coronary no-flow and ventricular tachycardia associated with habitual marijuana use. *Ann Emerg Med* 2003; 42:365–369.
301. Rashid J, Eisenberg MJ, Topol EJ. Cocaine-induced aortic dissection. *Am Heart J* 1996;132:1301–1304.

CHAPTER 37 ■ THE ATHLETE'S HEART

PAUL D. THOMPSON AND N. A. MARK ESTES

OVERVIEW

The *athlete's heart* or the *athletic heart syndrome* is a constellation of clinical findings including sinus bradycardia, systolic flow murmurs, and cardiac chamber enlargement with normal or augmented function. All four cardiac chambers may be enlarged. Chamber enlargement may rarely exceed the upper limits of normal, but marked enlargement of the right ventricle or either atrium suggests a pathologic process. Clinical findings of the athletic heart syndrome are limited to athletes whose sports and training require a large aerobic or endurance exercise component. The left ventricular wall can be slightly thickened, but this thickening is generally restricted to athletes with left ventricular chamber enlargement and rarely reaches the thickness of pathologic, states such as hypertrophic cardiomyopathy (HCM). Physicians are often required to evaluate asymptomatic athletes prior to participation and to evaluate symptomatic athletes before permitting their return to vigorous exercise training. In these situations, the athletic heart syndrome must be differentiated from pathologic conditions associated with cardiac complications during exercise. These include HCM, coronary artery anomalies, aortic stenosis, and right or left ventricular cardiomyopathy in young athletes and coronary artery disease in adults.

GLOSSARY OF TERMS

Athlete's heart or athletic heart syndrome: A constellation of clinical, electrocardiographic, and echocardiographic variants of normal found in well-trained athletes who participate in sports requiring prolonged primarily aerobic exercise training.

Endurance or isotonic exercise: Generally rhythmic physical exertion such as running, swimming, or bicycling, which require significant sustained increases in oxygen uptake.

Strength exercise: Physical exertion requiring lifting or moving objects against resistance. Strength exercises can result in motion against resistance such as weight lifting or require exertion against a fixed object referred to as *isometric exercise*.

Maximal oxygen uptake: Physiologic and highly reproducible upper limit of an individual's ability to extract and utilize oxygen during progressive isotonic exercise.

Onset of blood lactate accumulation (OBLA): The point during exercise where the accumulation of lactate can be detected in blood samples. This point corresponds to an abrupt increase in the respiratory rate often referred to as the *anaerobic threshold*.

HISTORICAL PERSPECTIVE

The athlete's heart presently refers to normal cardiac adaptations that occur with prolonged, primarily endurance, exercise training, but the history of the athlete's heart reflects the historical debate about the risks and benefits of vigorous exercise training and competition (1). Vigorous sports competition in the pre-Victorian era was largely an activity of the laboring class who competed in rowing, bicycling, and running events to test the skills required in their employment. There was little interest in such intense competition among the aristocracy and therefore little concern about its health risks. This changed during the Victorian era, when interest in competitive athletics increased, in part because sports were believed to develop what has been called the "most prized of Victorian virtues, character" (2). The athlete's heart in this period was primarily a moral concept referring to the character developed from athletic competition (2). Concern about the possible health risk of extreme exertion increased with growing sports participation among the aristocracy, and the appearance of such events as the Oxford–Cambridge boat race, first held in 1829 (2). In 1867, the "mechanic clause" was added to the rules of the British Amateur Athletic Club to exclude competitors whose work required physical labor. This made amateur athletic competition an activity for the elite (3). Articles on the dangers of the rower's, runner's and bicyclist's heart soon followed (1). These concerns are understandable given the cardiac diagnostic techniques of the day, primarily by palpation of the pulse, percussion of the precordium for heart size, and auscultation for murmurs. The clinical characteristics of the athlete's heart including sinus bradycardia, cardiac enlargement, and pulmonic and aortic flow murmurs were interpreted as heart block, cardiomyopathy, and valvular obstruction, respectively, conditions with poor prognoses until the later half of the twentieth century. Indeed, it was not until 1942 that the famed Boston cardiologist, Paul Dudley White, reported four cases of marked bradycardia in endurance athletes and concluded that this could be normal in endurance athletes (4).

The term *athlete's heart* appears to have been coined by a Swedish physician, S. Henschen in 1899 (5). He percussed cardiac size in cross-country skiers before and after a ski race and concluded that skiing produce a physiologic cardiac enlargement, which enabled the heart to perform more work than the heart of an untrained individual. He also noted that both the right and left sides of the heart were enlarged. Subsequent studies using roentgenographic, echocardiographic, computed tomographic, and magnetic resonance imaging techniques have only confirmed Henschen's conclusion that exercise training produces a generalized cardiac enlargement.

How could Henschen, using only the "educated finger" for chest percussion, have reached such accurate conclusions? In sum, he picked the right athletes, and this fact highlights several clinical characteristics of the athletic heart syndrome. First, Henschen studied endurance trained athletes. Strength trained athletes, such as weight lifters, have increased cardiac dimensions, but their enlargement is related to body size and muscle mass (6). Only endurance trained athletes, or athletes training with both endurance and strength modalities, develop the athletic heart syndrome. Second, Henschen selected cross-country skiers, endurance athletes whose exercise uses both arm and leg muscles. Cardiac dimensions and stroke volume are greatest in those athletes whose training requires the use of the most muscle mass. This chapter summarizes the clinical principles of the athlete's heart developed since Henschen's report 100 years ago.

BASIC PRINCIPLES OF CARDIOVASCULAR EXERCISE PHYSIOLOGY

Successful endurance athletes, compared to the general population, have a higher ability to perform maximal dynamic exercise, which can be measured as maximal oxygen uptake (Vo_2 max) (7). Vo_2 max is physiologically limited by the ability of the cardiopulmonary system to deliver, and the ability of the exercising muscles to use, oxygen. Rearranging the Fick equation for cardiac output (cardiac output = $Vo_2/A - Vo_2$ difference) demonstrates that Vo_2 max is the product of maximal cardiac output and the maximal arteriovenous O_2 difference (7). Maximal cardiac output is the product of maximal heart rate and stroke volume. Because maximal heart rate among healthy individuals varies primarily by age and because the ability to increase the $A - Vo_2$ difference is limited, the major factor responsible for the higher Vo_2 max among endurance athletes is an increased stroke volume (7). The clinical findings typical of the athlete's heart are generally manifestations of this increased stroke volume.

Although higher Vo_2 max values distinguish endurance athletes from sedentary individuals, among endurance athletes, Vo_2 max is not a good discriminator of superior athletic performance because Vo_2 max does not measure an individual's ability to maintain exertion over a long period of time (7). Other factors including the athlete's mechanical efficiency and the athlete's anaerobic threshold or onset of blood lactate accumulation (OBLA) contribute to submaximal work capacity and are better discriminators of competitive exercise performance among athletes (7). Enhanced mechanical efficiency means that an athlete can perform a physical task while consuming less oxygen than a less efficient athlete. A higher OBLA means that the athlete can perform more mechanical work without producing lactate. OBLA is associated with a higher respiratory rate stimulated by the production of carbon dioxide from buffering lactic acid (HLactate + $HCO_3^- \rightarrow H_2CO_3$ + lactate$^- \rightarrow H_2O + CO_2$). In addition, the lactate production indicates a level of exertion requiring glycogen catabolism and glycogen depletion is one potential limiting factor in endurance performance. Finally, lactic acid itself contributes to fatigue.

The increase in heart rate early during exercise is due primarily to withdrawal of resting vagal tone. At approximately 50% of maximal heart rate, additional acceleration of heart rate is associated with increased sympathetic activity (8). Peak heart rate is estimated as 220—age with a standard deviation of the estimate of $\pm$11 to 22 beats per minute (BPM) (9) and 95% confidence limits of $\pm$22 to 44 BPM. This emphasizes the problem of estimating heart rate by age. The increase in $A - Vo_2$ diff in produced by redistribution of blood from nonexercising tissue to the exercising musculature, increased extraction of O_2 over the exercising muscle bed, and hemoconcentration (8). A change in any component of this system can affect exercise capacity. Cardiologists focus on changes in maximum heart rate and stroke volume, but changes in hemoglobin concentration, the ability to fully oxygenate the red cells, the capacity to shunt blood to exercising muscle, and the ability of the muscles to extract oxygen can affect exercise performance. All should be considered in evaluating athletes for problems with exercise performance.

CLINICAL COMPONENTS OF THE ATHLETE'S HEART SYNDROME

Variants Attributed to Enhanced Parasympathetic Tone

Several of the findings of the athletic heart syndrome including resting bradycardia, sinus arrhythmia, and atrioventricular (AV) conduction delay are attributed to changes in the sympathetic nervous system with enhanced parasympathetic and reduced sympathetic tone. Enhanced parasympathetic tone is most important (10). Athletes also may demonstrate ST-T wave changes of early repolarization and T inversions, which are also attributed to sympathetic nervous system alterations. Some of the T-wave changes can be quite bizarre and may be similar to those seen with conditions known to affect the parasympathetic nervous system such as subarachnoid hemorrhage (Figs. 37.1–37.3).

Many of the changes typical of the athletic heart syndrome, such as sinus arrhythmia and the ST changes of early repolarization, are also characteristic of young, healthy individuals,

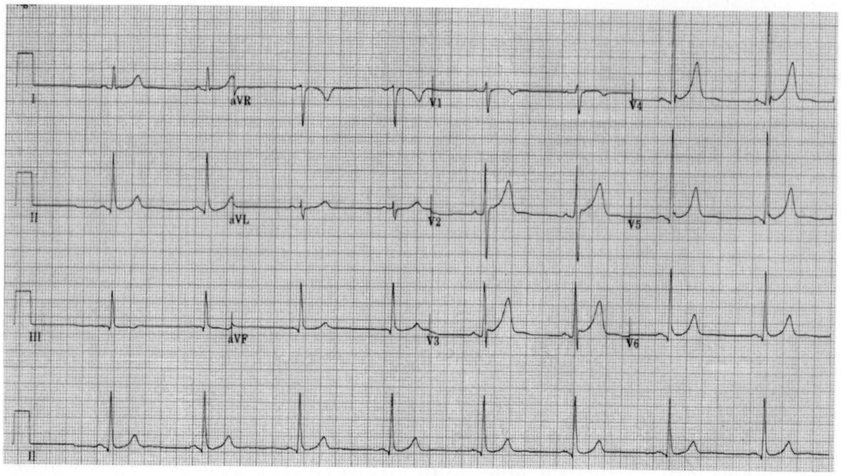

FIGURE 37.1. ECG from a 53-year-old physician who has run a minimum of 60 km weekly for 40 years. The axis is 70 degrees, somewhat unusual in a healthy individual in this age group, and there is ST elevation of early repolarization in leads V3–V6.

but are more marked or more frequent in athletes and may persist into middle age among physically active subjects. All of these abnormalities in sinus rate, A-V conduction, and the ST changes of early repolarization should resolve with exercise with its attendant withdrawal of vagal tone and increased sympathetic activity. This is not always true for marked T-wave inversions (11), however; thus, their failure to resolve does not necessarily imply a pathologic process.

Sinus Bradycardia

Maximal VO_2 and maximal cardiac output are increased in endurance athletes, but there is little change in resting oxygen consumption or cardiac output. Consequently, the larger resting stroke volume characteristic of endurance athletes permits a reduction in resting heart rate. Sinus bradycardia, generally defined as a heart rate less than 60 BPM, is typical of the athletic heart syndrome and reported in up to 91% of endurance athletes (12). The bradycardia in athletes can be profound, and a rate of 25 BPM has been reported in one distance runner (13). In addition to sinus bradycardia, sinus pauses or "sinus arrest" of more than 2 seconds have been documented during sleep in endurance athletes (12).

Sinus Arrhythmia

Sinus arrhythmia refers to variation in sinus rate with respiration. Specifically, the sinus rate decreases slightly at the start of the expiratory phase of the respiratory cycle. Sinus arrhythmia is common in young healthy subjects, but is more marked in endurance athletes.

Atrioventricular Conduction Delay

First-degree AV block, defined as a PR interval longer than 0.20 seconds is reported in 10% to 33% of endurance athletes (14). Second-degree AV block of the Mobitz I or Wenchebach pattern, characterized by progressive prolongation of the PR interval before a nonconducted P wave, is also seen more commonly in the athletic heart syndrome (14). Second-degree AV block with Mobitz II appearance, characterized by a nonconducted P wave without preceding PR prolongation, is not typical of the athletic heart syndrome. Mobitz type II block typically occurs at the level of the His–Purkinje system, whereas Mobitz type I block is due to progressive slowing of conduction in the AV node. AV block with Mobitz II appearance may occur in well-trained athletes owing to enhanced vagal tone, but this is rare (12). Its presence should prompt a search for other causes and should be attributed to the athletic training only if the athlete is asymptomatic and no other abnormalities are detected (Fig. 37.4).

The prolongation of the AV interval and decrease in AV conduction velocity described above may also unmask the ventricular preexcitation pattern, part of the Wolff–Parkinson–White (WPW) syndrome when accompanied by symptomatic arrhythmia. Indeed, a WPW conduction pattern is more common in endurance athletes (15). Cardiologists should be cognizant of this fact when evaluating athletes for an asymptomatic WPW conduction pattern because the risk of sudden death in asymptomatic subjects with this abnormality is low.

Vasovagal Syncope

Vasovagal syncope appears to occur more frequently in endurance-trained individuals related in part to their enhanced

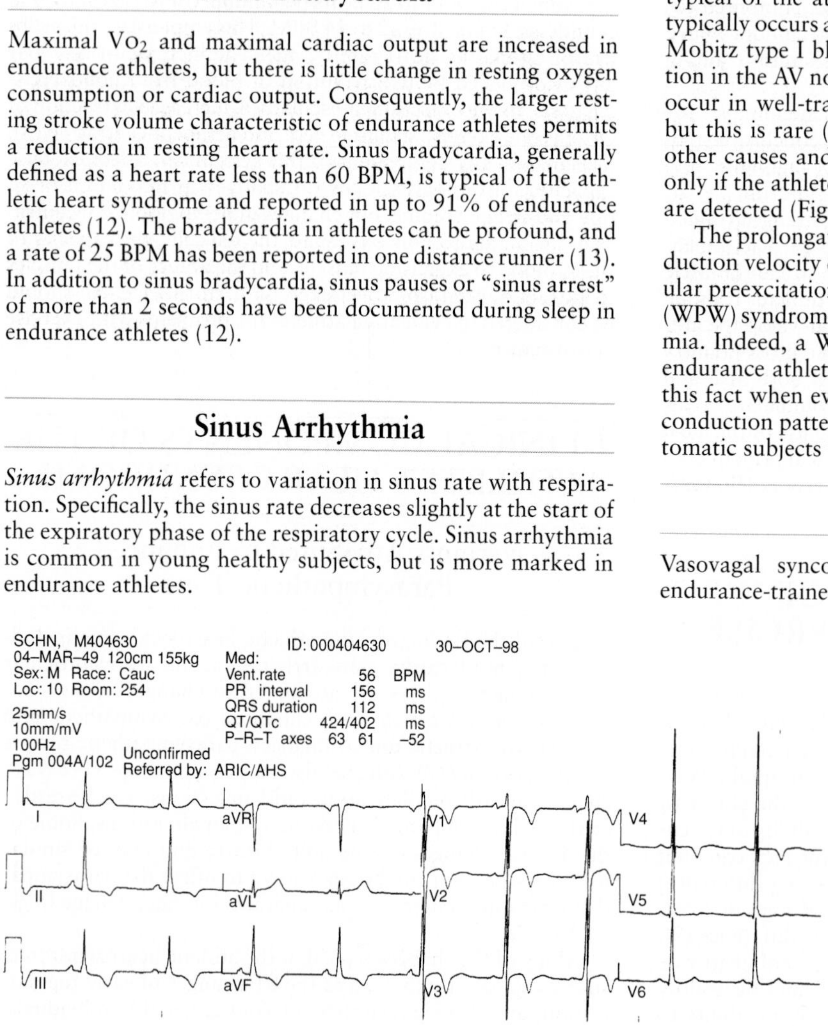

FIGURE 37.2. ECG from a 49-year-old Caucasian physician showing diffuse T-wave inversions. He had run 58 to 108 km weekly and ridden a bicycle 32 km weekly for 20 years. The ECG was obtained when he volunteered for a study of healthy subjects. An echocardiogram showed left ventricular internal dimensions at end diastole and systole of 50 and 20 mm, respectively, and left ventricular posterior and septal wall thickness of 12 mm each. He was not restricted from athletic competition.

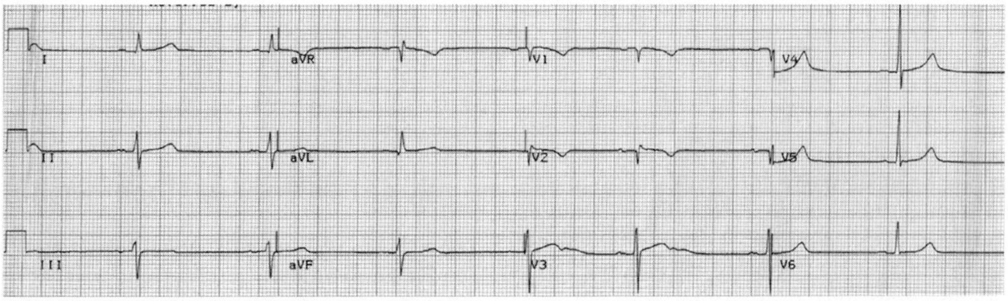

FIGURE 37.3. ECG from a 36-year-old physician showing marked bradycardia of 46 BPM, voltage criteria for left ventricular hypertrophy (note the $^1/_2$ standard calibration), and a prolonged QT interval in lead V3. He was 180 cm tall (5′10″) and weighed 67 kg (147 lbs). He had played college lightweight American football and rowed in lightweight crew. Over the past 5 years he had run 100 to 130 km weekly and competed in 42-km footraces. He was asymptomatic and had no family history of cardiac complications. His echocardiogram showed left ventricular internal dimensions at end diastole and systole to be 54 and 37 mm, respectively. The left ventricular posterior wall thickness was 10 mm and the septal thickness was 11 mm. He was not restricted from athletic participation despite the QT interval because he was totally asymptomatic.

vagal tone. Lower body negative pressure is a research technique used to examine blood pressure control and an individual's response to orthostatic stress. Compared to nonathletes and strength-trained athletes, endurance-trained individuals have a reduced ability to maintain blood pressure during lower body negative pressure (16). The clinical implications of this are that endurance trained individuals are more vulnerable to vasovagal syncope or simple fainting and that positive tilt table responses are almost the norm in well-trained endurance athletes. These athletes have a large venous capacity from exercise training, enhanced vagal tone, and reduced sympathetic tone, all of which make them vulnerable to postural hypotension and a positive tilt table response. Tilt table results should not be interpreted as an adequate explanation for syncope in athletes, therefore, unless the clinical situation also strongly supports this explanation.

Electrocardiographic ST-T Wave Changes

ST elevation of the "early repolarization pattern" is so common in endurance trained athletes that it should be considered the norm rather than the exception. Persistent training into advanced age can preserve this pattern in older athletes. ST depression, in contrast, is rare and should prompt a search for other causes. Peaked, biphasic, and inverted T waves in the precordial leads are also frequently seen in endurance athletes. The biphasic T waves typically occur in the precordial "transition" leads where the QRS complex is changing from a primarily negative deflection in the right precordial leads to primarily positive in the left-sided leads. Deeply inverted T waves can also be normal in athletes, but are rare and require the exclusion of significant disease (11). Among 952 healthy Italian national caliber athletes, only 27 athletes had marked T-wave inversions, 375 had abnormal or mildly abnormal electrocardiograms (ECGs), suggesting HCM in 11 and arrhythmogenic right ventricular cardiomyopathy in 16. Only one of these athletes actually had HCM, however (17).

CARDIAC ARRHYTHMIAS IN ATHLETES

Athletes frequently present for cardiac consultation because of palpitations. This is often sinus tachycardia, among the more

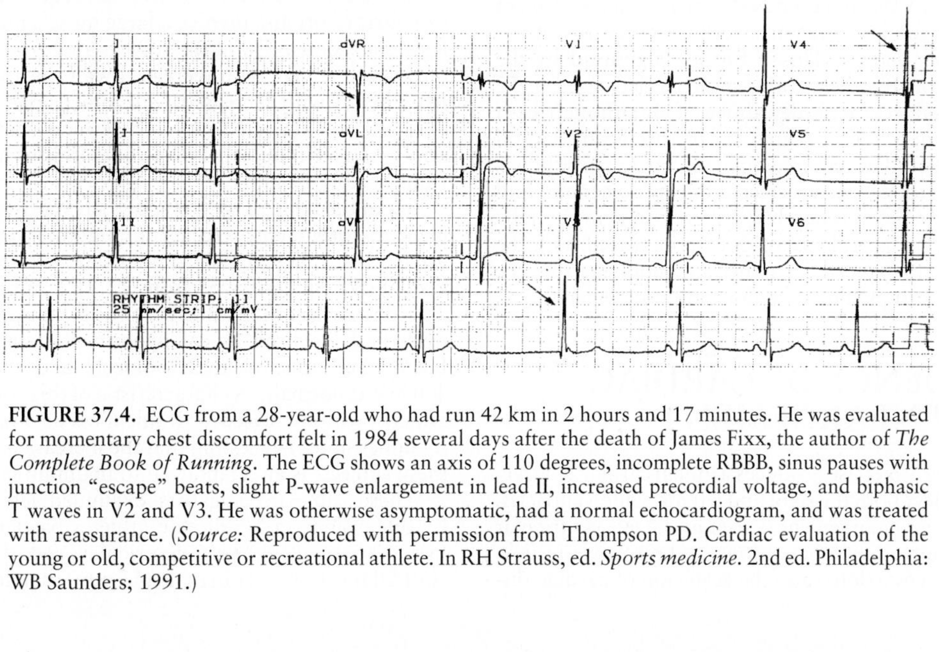

FIGURE 37.4. ECG from a 28-year-old who had run 42 km in 2 hours and 17 minutes. He was evaluated for momentary chest discomfort felt in 1984 several days after the death of James Fixx, the author of *The Complete Book of Running*. The ECG shows an axis of 110 degrees, incomplete RBBB, sinus pauses with junction "escape" beats, slight P-wave enlargement in lead II, increased precordial voltage, and biphasic T waves in V2 and V3. He was otherwise asymptomatic, had a normal echocardiogram, and was treated with reassurance. (*Source:* Reproduced with permission from Thompson PD. Cardiac evaluation of the young or old, competitive or recreational athlete. In RH Strauss, ed. *Sports medicine*. 2nd ed. Philadelphia: WB Saunders; 1991.)

nervous subjects, or premature atrial or ventricular depolarizations (PVDs) detected by heart rate monitoring or palpation during athletic training. Occasional PVDs may be more frequent in athletes because the prolonged diastole provides extra time for such beats to occur. Premature beats are best treated with reassurance alone, but some athletes may require β-adrenergic blocking or other agents for symptomatic relief. Physicians should avoid β-blockers in elite athletes because they may affect athletic performance and are prohibited in sports such as archery and shooting because they prolong diastole and thereby reduce body movement produced by cardiac contraction.

Atrial Fibrillation

Atrial fibrillation (AF) is unusual in young subjects, but may be more frequent in athletes (18). Among 1,160 individuals with AF, 70 (6%) had no evidence of heart disease, so-called lone AF, and 32 of these were endurance athletes (19). The onset of AF in athletes is often during sleep or postprandially, consistent with the concept that increased vagal tone from sleep and eating plus the exercise training contribute to its onset (19). AF in young, healthy endurance athletes is often transient and requires no treatment (18) once cardiac pathology is excluded usually by an ECG and echocardiography alone.

Ventricular Arrhythmias

It is not clear whether frequent or complex ventricular arrhythmias are a component of the athlete's heart syndrome. Biffi et al. (20) divided 355 athletes with three or more PVDs on 12-lead resting ECG ($n = 337$) or palpitations ($n = 18$) into three groups based on ventricular arrhythmias (20). Arrhythmia in 230 athletes were detected by routine screening, whereas 125 other athletes were referred for suspected disease. Group A had 2,000 or more PVDs in 24 hours and one or more burst of nonsustained ventricular tachycardia (NSVT) ($n = 71$). Group B had 100 to 2,000 PVDs and no NSVT ($n = 153$). Group C had fewer than 100 PVDs and no NSVT ($n = 131$). The presence of cardiac disease increased with the arrhythmia frequency and was 30%, 3%, and 0% in groups A, B, and C, respectively. Group A athletes were disqualified from competition. The only death during a mean 8 years of follow-up occurred in an athlete who ignored her disqualification. The authors suggest that frequent PVDs, and even NSVT, may be a component of the athlete's heart and have an excellent prognosis in the absence of cardiac disease. This is further supported by the observation that the frequency of arrhythmia decreased in 50 of the group A subjects with detraining (19), although such changes could simply reflect regression to the mean. Several points from these studies require emphasis. First, arrhythmias in most of these athletes were detected during screening, and the prognosis may be considerably different in symptomatic subjects. Second, the prevalence of disease increased with the frequency and complexity of the arrhythmia implying that the most extensive workups should be done in these athletes.

EVIDENCE OF CARDIAC ENLARGEMENT

Habitual endurance exercise produces a global cardiac enlargement that may affect both the right and left atria and ventricles. The most consistent enlargement is seen in the left ventricular chambers where intracavity dimensions, and rarely wall thickness, can be large enough to raise the suspicion of cardiac disease. Mild enlargement of both atria and the right ventricle can occur, but marked enlargement of these structures suggests a disease process and is not observed in the athletic heart syndrome.

ECG Evidence of Chamber Enlargement

The ECG in well-trained athletes may show mildly increased P-wave amplitude suggesting right atrial enlargement, P-wave notching suggesting left atrial enlargement, incomplete right bundle branch block (RBBB), and voltage criteria for right and left ventricular hypertrophy (12). Among endurance athletes, voltage criteria for right ventricular hypertrophy are noted in 18% to 69% of subjects (12). This ECG evidence for atrial and right ventricular enlargement does not usually suggest extreme enlargement so that marked evidence of atrial or right ventricular enlargement should prompt a search for pathologic causes. Similarly, although incomplete RBBB is common, complete heart block is not generally accepted as part of the athletic heart syndrome (12). In contrast to ECG evidence of atrial and right ventricular enlargement, the voltage criteria for left ventricular hypertrophy can be extreme in endurance athletes (Fig. 37.5).

Echocardiographic Evidence of Cardiac Enlargement

Thomas and Douglas (21) summarized the topic of echocardiographic dimensions in athletes. At least 59 studies have used echocardiography to examine cardiac dimensions in athletes (21). These studies consistently documented increased left ventricular dimensions. Thirteen studies demonstrated that the right ventricular transverse dimension was increased an average of 24% in the athletes compared to controls (22 versus 17 mm) (21). Fourteen studies comparing the left atria of athletes and controls demonstrated that the transverse dimension was 16% larger in the athletes. Only one study to our knowledge has documented a larger right atrial size in the athletes (21).

Pelliccia et al. (22) examined left ventricular wall thickness in 947 elite Italian athletes including 209 women. Only 16 athletes (1.7%) had a left ventricular wall thickness greater than 12 mm, the upper limit of normal. Fifteen of these athletes were rowers or canoeists, sports that require both isotonic and isometric effort and involve a large muscle mass. These 15 athletes represented 7% of the rowers and canoeists studied. The only other athlete with increased wall thickness was a cyclist. All athletes with increased wall dimensions had won medals in international competition. The largest wall thickness in any athlete was 16 mm. All of the female athletes had wall thickness values below 11 mm.

Six of the athletes with marked left ventricular wall enlargement discontinued exercise training and were restudied after 40 to 240 (average 90) days of reduced activity. Average wall thickness decreased from 12.8 ± 0.9 to 10.5 ± 0.4 mm, $P < .05$. Three of the athletes, none with increased wall thickness, had localized apical hypertrophy suggestive of apical HCM, but none of these subjects had the marked apical T-wave abnormalities characteristic of this condition. All of the athletes with increased wall thickness also had increased cavity dimensions, suggesting that the increase in wall thickness in these subjects is an adaptation to maintain normal wall stress.

These same investigators examined left ventricular cavity dimensions in 1,300 elite athletes participating in 38 different sports (23). Left ventricular end diastolic diameter (LVEDD) was greater in male (55 mm) than in female (48 mm)

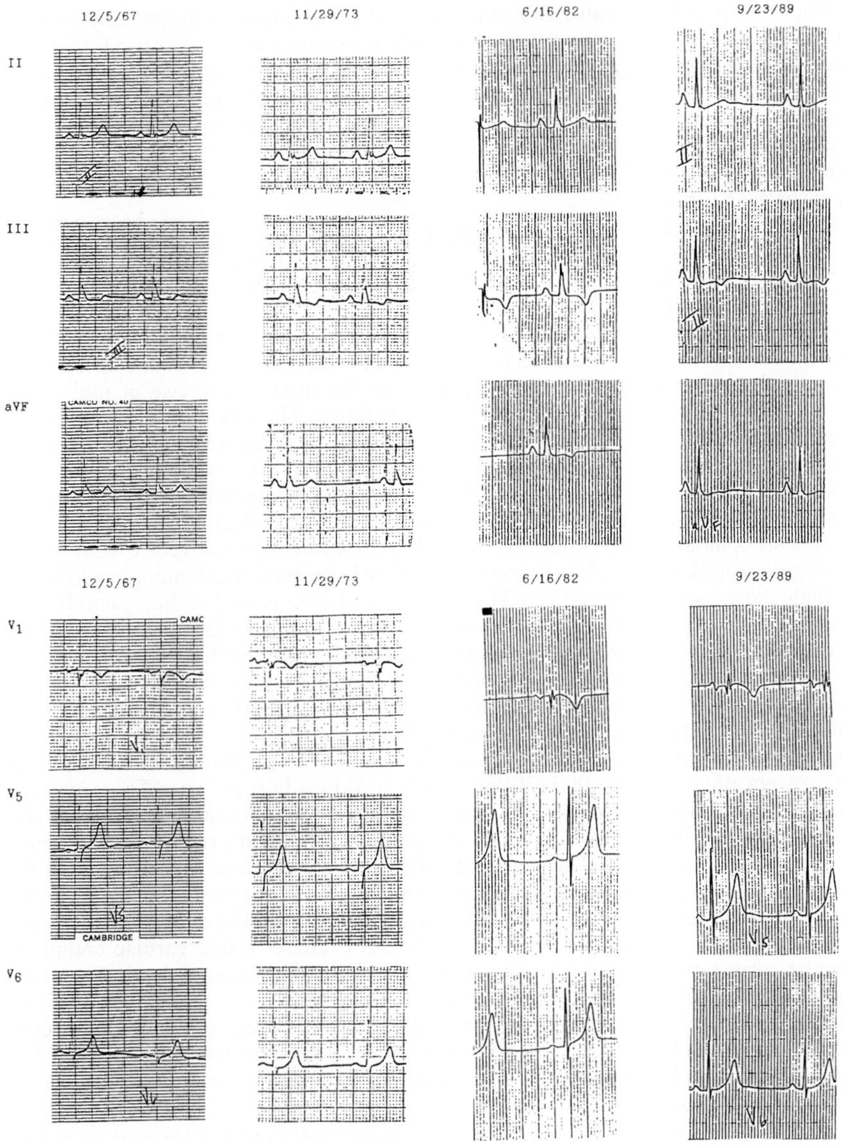

FIGURE 37.5. Selected leads from the serial ECGs of a 42-year-old physician who began running in the late 1960s and progressed to running multiple 42-km footraces. The tracings show the development of the classic ECG of the athletic heart syndrome including increased P-wave height (lead II), increased P-wave negativity (lead V1), increased right-sided R wave (lead V1), and increased precordial voltage (leads V5 and V6). These suggest right and left atrial and ventricular enlargement respectively. There are also progressive T-wave changes with increased precordial T waves (V5 and V6) and increasing negative T waves in the inferior leads (III and AVF). The presence of all of these findings in a single ECG is unusual even among well-trained elite athletes. This individual remains healthy in his mid-50s.

athletes. LVEDD was greater than 55 mm, the upper limits of normal, in 45% of the athletes and exceeded 60 mm in 14%. The largest cardiac dimensions observed were 66 mm for a female and 70 mm for a male athlete. Regression analysis demonstrated that body surface area ($r = 0.76$), heart rate ($r = -0.37$), and age ($r = 0.29$) correlated with LVEDD and together accounted for 60% of the variability in LVEDD. Adding gender and the type of sport to these factors accounted for 72% of the variability. Age may function in this group as a surrogate for the duration of training. The sports that were most associated with an LVEDD equal or greater than 60 mm were cycling (49% of cycling athletes), ice hockey (42%), basketball (40%), rugby (39%), canoeing (39%), and rowing (34%). All are sports that require a large endurance component or a combination of moderate endurance training and increased body size. Systolic and diastolic function was normal in the athletes. Once again, few athletes had evidence of left ventricular wall hypertrophy. Only 14 of the athletes (1.1%) had a septal thickness of more than 12 mm and only 4 athletes (0.3%) exceed this posterior wall thickness. Wall thickness among the athletes correlated with cavity dimensions. Athletes with increased cavity dimensions also tended to have larger left atrial and aortic root dimensions.

The results of these studies in the Italian athletes provide several useful principles in differentiating the athletic heart syndrome from pathologic conditions. Although many athletes had increased intracavitary dimensions, no athlete had a LVEDD greater than 70 mm. Left ventricular wall thickness greater than 12 mm was unusual even in elite athletes, and its presence should prompt a search for pathologic causes. No athlete had a left ventricular wall thickness greater than 16 mm and values above this range should raise the possibility of HCM. Wall hypertrophy above the normal range was not observed in female athletes. All athletes with wall hypertrophy also demonstrated increased cavity dimensions, which is not seen in diseases with pathologic wall thickening. Wall thickening in high-caliber athletes regressed with detraining.

The results of these Italian studies, however, should not be assumed to apply to the most extreme endurance athletes. The Italian studies included athletes from multiple disciplines, many of which had little endurance component. Results from studies of extreme endurance athletes demonstrate that athletic training can be associated with cardiac changes mimicking cardiac disease. Among 291 Japanese participants in a 100-km footrace, the mean and range (mm), respectively, of LVEDD (62 ± 7, 42–75), left ventricular end-systolic diameter (LVESD) (40 ± 6; 23–55), IVS (10 ± 2, 5–19), and posterior wall thickness (PWT) (10 ± 1, 5–15) suggest marked enlargement of these structure despite the men having a body surface area of only 1.66 ± 0.1 m^2 (24). A total of 33 (11%) had LVEDD values greater than 70 mm. Such LVEDD and LVESD values could create confusion in evaluating athletes with aortic or mitral regurgitation for valve repair or placement. Similarly, both the mean and range of their aortic and left atrial diameters were increased at 58 ± 4 (27-50) and 40 ± 5 (26–49) mm, respectively. Some endurance athletes may also demonstrate reduced left ventricular function. Among 147 cyclists participating in the Tour de France, 17 (11%) had a left ventricular ejection fraction of 52% or less calculated with the Teichholz formula (25). Such results suggest that extreme endurance athletes may occasionally demonstrate borderline left ventricular function.

We have emphasized that the largest changes in cardiac dimensions occur with endurance exercise training or the combination of endurance and strength training in large individuals. Many clinicians believe that endurance and strength exercise training produce different cardiac adaptations. Habitual dynamic exercise training is presumed to increase primarily left ventricular volume, whereas exercise with a high static component is presumed to increase left ventricular wall thickness. In the most comprehensive examination of this issue, Pluim et al. (26) performed a systematic review of 59 echocardiographic studies of athletes published from 1975 through 1998. They divided the 1,451 subjects into endurance trained (e.g., long distance runners), strength trained (e.g., weight lifters), and combined static and dynamic trained (e.g., rowers and cyclists) athletes. These reports included 31 studies of endurance athletes, 24 studies of strength athletes, and 23 studies of athletes trained by a combination of endurance and strength exercise. Septal thickness in endurance athletes (10.5 mm) was significantly greater than controls (8.8 mm), but less than strength-trained subjects (11.8 mm) and combination athletes (11.3 mm). Posterior wall thickness, in contrast, was actually greater in endurance athletes (10.3 mm) than controls (8.8 mm), but not different from combination (11 mm) or strength-trained (11 mm) subjects. These authors concluded that the differences in the cardiac dimensions of endurance and strength trained athletes are relatively minor and that there is no clear dichotomy in the cardiac adaptations to endurance or strength training. None of the cardiac dimensions are adjusted for body size nor are any of the included studies prospective, so it is possible that some of the septal thickness in strength-trained and combination-trained athletes results from body size and not the training modality.

The clinical significance of these findings is that clinicians should avoid ascribing cardiac wall hypertrophy to the effects of exercise training even among strength-trained athletes because the effects of such activity alone on cardiac wall thickness is relatively minor.

FUNCTIONAL CARDIAC MURMURS IN ATHLETES

Both young and old endurance athletes often have functional cardiac murmurs created by the cardiac adaptations to exercise training. Training does not change resting cardiac output, but this is delivered via a slower heart rate and a larger stroke volume. Much of the larger stroke volume is delivered more vigorously in early systole by a more dynamic ventricle. This increases blood velocity. The pulmonic and aortic valve orifices do not increase with exercise training so the increased blood velocity produces early systolic flow murmurs. Such flow murmurs in young athletes are caused by flow across the pulmonic valve and often vary with respiration. Athletes aged 50 years or more may have mild sclerosis of the aortic valve leaflets and their flow murmurs are often due to both aortic valve sclerosis and the turbulence mentioned above. These murmurs are less "innocent" because they may progress to important aortic stenosis (AS).

EXERCISE-RELATED CARDIAC EVENTS

Clinicians are often required to differentiate the athletic heart syndrome from life-threatening cardiac disease and to make recommendations about the risks of exercise in individuals with diagnosed abnormalities. There is little doubt that vigorous physical exertion increases the risk of cardiac events in children and adults with cardiovascular abnormalities. Van Camp et al. (27) estimated an absolute rate of exercise related death among U.S. high school and college athletes of only 1 per 133,000 men and 769,000 women, respectively. Corrado et al. (28) prospectively collected reports of SCDs among individuals ages 12 to 35 years over a 21-year period in the Veneto Region of Italy. There was approximately 1 sudden death per 33,000 young athletes per year, and this rate was 2.5-fold higher among athletes compared to nonathletes (28). Among adults vigorous exertion increases the risk of both sudden death (29,30) and acute myocardial infarction (31–33). The rate of exercise-related sudden death is estimated at 1 death per 15,000 (29) to 18,000 (30) previously healthy adults per year. These are relatively rare events, but in both children (28) and adults (29,30) vigorous exertion appears to increase the risk of cardiac events.

The causes of exertion-related cardiac events varies by the age of the subject. Among adults, variously defined as above 29 or above 39 years of age, atherosclerotic vascular disease is the cause of almost all exercise-related cardiac complications. Among younger subjects, the causes of death are usually congenital cardiac abnormalities or acquired myocarditis or cardiomyopathy. The prevalence of various causes of exercise-related events may vary by geographic distribution. HCM has repeatedly been shown to be the dominant cause of exercise related deaths in young American athletes (27,34), whereas right ventricular dysplasia is the primary cause of such events in Italian athletes especially in the Veneto region of Italy (28,35). The reasons for this discrepancy are unclear. It has been attributed to a required national screening program for Italian athletes, which has identified and excluded athletes with HCM (36), although other factors including a regional interest in the disease, an increased prevalence of the condition in the Mediterranean area (37) or recent international recognition of this entity may also contribute. Cardiac conditions commonly associated with exercise-related events in U.S. young athletes include HCM, coronary artery anomalies, myocarditis, AS, and dilated cardiomyopathy (Table 37.1). The coronary artery anomalies included anomalous origin, intramyocardial course, and an ostial ridge at the coronary origin. Some coronary anomalies such as an acute take-off of the artery from the aorta (38) may be overlooked or unappreciated during autopsy.

These reports do not include all of the cardiac conditions for which exercise increases the risk of sudden death and should not be used to decide to permit an individual with a diagnosed cardiac condition to participate in vigorous exercise and competitive sports. Cardiac arrhythmia and sudden death in the long QT syndromes, for example, are often associated with physical activity (39) especially swimming (40), but are not detectable by autopsy alone.

There are several clinically important lessons from these pathologic studies of exercise related events. Several of the conditions identified at autopsy could have been detected before

TABLE 37.1

CARDIOVASCULAR CAUSES (%) OF EXERCISE-RELATED SUDDEN DEATH IN YOUNG ATHLETES*

	Van Camp (27) ($n = 100$)[a]	Maron et al. (34) ($n = 134$)	Corrado (28) ($n = 55$)[b]
HCM	51	36	1
Probable HCM	5	10	—
Coronary anomaly[c]	18	23	9
Valvular and subvalvular aortic stenosis	8	4	—
Possible myocarditis	7	3	5
Dilated and nonspecific CM	7	3	1
Atherosclerotic CAD	3	2	10
Aortic rupture	2	5	1
Arrhythmogenic right ventricular CM	1	3	11
Myocardial scarring	—	3	—
Mitral valve prolapse	1	2	6
Other congenital abnormalities	—	1.5	—
Long QT syndrome	—	0.5	1
WPW syndrome	1	—	1
Cardiac conduction disease	—	—	3
Cardiac sarcoidosis	—	0.5	—
Coronary artery aneurysm	1	—	—
Normal heart at necropsy	7	2	1
Pulmonary thromboembolism	—	—	1

*Ages ranged from 13–24 (27), 12–40 (34), and 12–35 (28) years. All (27), 90% (34), and 89% (28) had symptom onset during or within an hour of training or competition.
[a]Total exceeds 100% because several athletes had multiple abnormalities.
[b]Includes some athletes whose deaths were not associated with recent exertion.
[c]Includes aberrant artery origin and course, tunneled arteries, and other abnormalities.
Abbreviations: CAD, coronary artery disease; CM, cardiomyopathy; HCM, hypertrophic cardiomyopathy; WPW, Wolf–Parkinson–White.

death. These include valvular and subvalvular aortic stenosis, Marfan syndrome as a cause of aortic rupture, and possibly HCM, although a murmur in the later condition is detected in only 25% of cases. Few of the victims were women, consistent with other observations that women are protected to some extent from sudden death (41).

PREPARTICIPATION SCREENING OF COMPETITIVE ATHLETES

There is ongoing debate about the value of screening competitive athletes and the components of such screening. Cardiologists are frequently asked to evaluate athletes with possible abnormalities detected during screening. These abnormalities are often normal variants of no significance, including bradycardia and functional murmurs, but on rare occasions a completely asymptomatic athlete with a major cardiac abnormality is identified.

The American Heart Association recommends cardiovascular screening for high school and college athletes prior to athletic participation and repeated at 2- to 4-year intervals (42,43). The examination should include a personal and family history and a physical examination focused on detecting conditions associated with exercise-related events (42). The American Heart Association does not recommend routine, additional noninvasive testing such as a routine ECG. This is controversial; a subsection of the study group on Sports Cardiology of the European Society of Cardiology has recommended that routine ECGs be obtained on all athletes as part of a preparticipation evaluation (44). We have not advocated routine ECG screening of all competitive athletes because of the rarity of exercise-related events, the high likelihood of false-positive results in a low-risk population, the requirement for further testing once an abnormality is detected, and the addition financial burden this would impose on athletic participation. Also, screening programs often generate a high rate of false-positive results. Fuller et al. (45) obtained a medical history, had a cardiologist perform cardiac auscultation, and recorded a resting ECG on 5,615 athletes (45). Possible cardiovascular abnormalities were detected in 10.4% of the athletes. These included an abnormal cardiac history in 2%, abnormal auscultatory findings in 3%, hypertension in 0.3%, and an abnormal ECG in 2.6% of the athletes, but only 22 athletes were ultimately denied participation for severe aortic insufficiency (AI) ($n = 1$), severe hypertension ($n = 5$), WPW ECG pattern ($n = 6$), premature ventricular contractions ($n = 5$), RBBB ($n = 4$), and supraventricular tachycardia ($n = 1$). The reasons for excluding the athletes with WPW, premature ventricular contractions, and RBBB were not provided. Among the 22 excluded athletes, the patient with severe AI underwent valve replacement, the hypertensive patients were treated, and the patient with supraventricular tachycardia underwent therapeutic ablation. Fifteen of the excluded subjects were lost to follow-up, greatly reducing the value of the study. Over the 3 years of the study, there was one cardiac arrest in an athlete, but this occurred in an athlete with an anomalous right coronary artery who had passed screening. The authors reason that including ECGs in the evaluation of high school athletes increases the detection of cardiac abnormalities. An alternative interpretation is that sphyngomanometry and auscultation alone could have detected most important abnormalities and that the ECG only increases the detection of asymptomatic abnormalities unlikely to be of major significance. Additional studies of screening and its utility are clearly needed before firm conclusions are possible.

Others suggest that echocardiography should be routinely included in the preparticipation screening of athletes because HCM is the predominant cause of exercise-related sudden death in young Americans. Italian investigators are among the more enthusiastic supporters of this approach (36). Italy has had a national law since 1971 requiring athletes to undergo an examination including a medical history, physical examination, ECG, and step test. Those athletes with abnormal findings are referred for other testing including a 24-hour ECG recording, an echocardiogram, and a formal exercise test. This program has screened 33,735 athletes and referred 3,016 for echocardiography (36), an abnormality rate similar to that reported by Fuller et al. (45). Of the referred athletes, 621 were disqualified from competition, 58.7% because of cardiac issues including 22 athletes with HCM. Four disqualified athletes died over 8.2 ± 5 years (mean $\pm$ SD) of follow-up. None of the 22 athletes with HCM died. A total of 49 nondisqualified athletes died, yielding an annual death rate of 1 per 62,500 athletes. The authors compared the frequency of HCM as a cause of exercise deaths in the United States and in Italy and concluded that the low prevalence of HCM among their athletes who died was most likely a result of the screening program.

Several problems limit the widespread application of these results. The prevalence of HCM in this population is low. Only 0.06% of the athletes had this diagnosis, whereas the expected prevalence in a sample of healthy young Americans is 0.2% (46). Only 4 of 365 athletes who were excluded form participation died of a cardiac condition. We do not know how these excluded athletes were medically managed, but the death rate is low, raising the possibility that screening prohibited individuals who were not at great risk. The annual death rate of 1 per 62,500 athletes is similar to, if not higher than, the death rate of 1 per 133,000 male athletes reported for American athletes who presumably underwent far less screening (27). Consequently, these results actually raise questions about the effectiveness of routine, extensive screening.

CARDIAC EXAMINATION OF COMPETITIVE ATHLETES

The components of the cardiovascular examination are detailed elsewhere in this text and a consensus statement on the components of the preparticipation cardiac examination has been published (42,43). The following emphasizes clinical principles useful in examining athletes as part of a preparticipation examination or when evaluating athletes for suspected cardiac abnormalities.

Preparticipation Screening of Athletes

The preparticipation screening of athletes should include (42) an inquiry about (a) exertional symptoms including chest discomfort, syncope, dyspnea, and fatigue; (b) past cardiac murmurs, hypertension, or cardiac diagnoses; and (c) a family history of sudden death or of any of the conditions known to be associated with sudden death. The physical examination should include (a) brachial artery blood pressure measurement; (b) precordial auscultation with the athlete supine and standing; (c) simultaneous palpation of the radial and femoral pulses to exclude coarctation; and (d) an assessment for stigmata of Marfan syndrome.

Examining Athletes for Suspected Disease

The examination of athletes for suspected cardiac disease should be considerably more detailed than the preparticipation examination. The cardiac evaluation remains an important part of evaluating athletes even with modern diagnostic techniques. A careful physical examination can eliminate the need for additional testing. The severity of valvular lesions can be both over- and underestimates by echocardiography, cardiac catheterization, and physical examination. The best decisions are made when the results of several examination techniques are compared for agreement or discrepancies and the cardiologist does not rely on clinical, echocardiographic, or catheterization data alone. We have seen multiple athletes with clinical symptoms and physical examination findings of severe aortic stenosis who were not repaired because the catheterization data did not indicate a "critical" valve area. Mild, moderate, and severe aortic stenosis are classified as a calculated aortic valve area less than 1.5, 1 to 1.5, and less than 1.0 cm^2, respectively, but these values are not normalized for body surface area (47) and may severely underestimate the severity of the stenosis in large individuals such as athletes in some sports.

A complete review of the physical examination is beyond the scope of this chapter, but there are several points important in examining athletes. A systolic pressure more than 15 mm higher in the right arm if associated with a systolic ejection murmur suggests supravalvular aortic stenosis. A widened pulse pressure more than 40 mm Hg suggests a regurgitant murmur and should prompt auscultation for aortic insufficiency (AI). Elevated blood pressure in a young athlete requires simultaneous palpation of the radial and femoral pulses to exclude a radial–femoral pulse delay suggestive of aortic coarctation. It is often incorrectly assumed that the mere presence of a femoral pulse excludes coarctation, but some patients can reconstitute a palpable, but delayed, femoral pulse via collaterals.

Palpating the carotid pulse is an important maneuver in athletes because aortic stenosis remains a frequent, easily identified cause of sudden cardiac death. A carotid pulse that is low volume, has a slow upstroke, or is difficult to locate should increase suspicion of important AS.

S_2 is produced by closure of the aortic followed by the pulmonic valves. During inspiration filling of the right ventricle is augmented. The larger volume of blood in the right ventricle shifts the intraventricular septum leftward, compromises (left ventricular) filling, and reduces left ventricular stroke volume. This hastens aortic closure so that the aortic valve closes earlier in the cardiac cycle during inspiration. On the right side, the larger right ventricular volume delays pulmonic valve closure. Both the earlier aortic closure and the delayed pulmonic closure increase the splitting of S_2 during inspiration. This is best appreciated in the seated position. In the supine position venous return from the legs can nearly maximize right ventricular filling so that any additional increase in the splitting of S_2 is difficult to detect. This is especially true in endurance athletes whose plasma volume can average 800 mL larger than comparison subjects (48). Some of this increased plasma volume shifts to the central circulation in the supine position. During the expiratory phase of the cardiac cycle, aortic and pulmonic closure occurs almost simultaneously and S_2 should be single or nearly so. If there is an intracardiac connection between the right and left sides of the heart such as an atrial septal defect (ASD), a common problem in young subjects, there is no or little differential in right and left cardiac filling during respiration. Right ventricular filling is also increased from left to right intracardiac shunting, which increases the right ventricular stroke volume. S_2, therefore, is often widely split, does not move during respiration, and fails to close during expiration. Several clinical characteristics of ASDs are also found in the athletic heart syndrome, including a systolic murmur similar to the benign pulmonic flow murmur common in athletes and right ventricular conduction delay on the ECG. The behavior of S_2 is useful in athletes for distinguishing an ASD from the athletic heart syndrome. S_3 and S_4 gallops are common in athletes and are of no importance unless the gallops are loud or associated with other abnormalities.

The initial auscultatory examination of the athlete is performed with the athlete seated. This reduces the chance of producing a flow murmur, facilitates hearing AI, and maximizes splitting of the second sound. The upright position also reduces ventricular volume and increases the chance of detecting a murmur in obstructive HCM. Auscultation should be repeated with the athlete in the supine and left lateral positions. The athletes should also be examined standing and squatting if there is any suspicion of HCM. Squatting increases ventricular afterload, which decrease the murmur of obstructive HCM, whereas standing often increases the murmur if obstruction is present.

Recommendations for Athletes With Diagnosed Disease

Guidelines for determining athletic eligibility among children and adults with diagnosed cardiovascular disease have been expertly presented in the 36th Bethesda Conference on this topic (49) and need not be repeated here. These guidelines are necessarily conservative because they serve as a standard of practice. Physicians can use these guidelines to be more or less restrictive of athletic participation given the individual's disease severity, patient preference, the physician's appreciation of risk, and the patient and family's willingness to tolerate that risk.

PERFORMANCE-ENHANCING SUBSTANCES IN ATHLETES

Anabolic steroids, stimulants, peptide hormones, and other substances are used by athletes to improve athletic performance (50). Anabolic–androgenic steroids include more than 30 natural and synthetic testosterone derivatives. Anabolic steroids have atherogenic, thrombotic, vasospastic, and potential direct myocardial effects (50). Several studies and case reports suggest that anabolic steroids can cause thromboembolism and cardiomyopathy (50). The oral anabolic steroid, stanozolol, but not intramuscular testosterone, produces remarkable reductions in high-density lipoprotein cholesterol and increases in low-density lipoprotein cholesterol probably via a first-pass hepatic effect (51). Case reports have implicated anabolic steroids as the primary cause of myocardial infarction and sudden death from coronary artery thrombosis even in the absence of atherosclerotic plaque (50). Stimulants used by athletes include amphetamines, cocaine, ephedra, dexedrine, ritalin, adderall, β_2-agonists, and others (52). Cocaine use has been associated with "catecholamine" cardiomyopathy, myocardial infarction, premature atherosclerosis, ventricular arrhythmias, and aortic dissection (53). Ephedra, derived from the ephedra plant family, contains several ephedrine alkaloids. These substances increase heart rate, cardiac output, and peripheral vascular resistance; promote short-term weight loss; and are ergogenic for anaerobic exercise (54). Ephedra has been associated with ischemic and hemorrhagic stroke, cardiac arrhythmias including ventricular tachycardia, coronary vasospasm, acute myocardial infarction, tachycardia-induced cardiomyopathy, and sudden death (54). The U.S. Food and Drug Administration banned all ephedra sales in 2004 (50), but "ephedra-free" and "ephedra-like" products containing "bitter orange" have been marketed as ephedra's replacement. Bitter orange is derived from *Citrus aurantium* contains synephrine, an α-adrenergic sympathomimetic agent, and likely has safety issues similar to ephedra (50). Autologous and homologous blood transfusion or "blood doping" has been used by endurance athletes to increase oxygen-carrying capacity and endurance exercise performance. Potential adverse effects include polycythemia, hypertension, congestive heart failure, and hyperviscosity, which increases the risk of stroke (50). Recombinant erythropoietin has been used as a pharmacologic alternative to blood doping (50), and has probably replaced transfusion procedures among athletes. Recombinant erythropoietin can produce extremely high hematocrits thereby increasing the risk of thrombotic vascular events (50). Human growth hormone, chorionic gonadotropin (hGH), is reportedly used by athletes to improve athletic performance by increasing fat-free mass, muscular strength, and recovery from exercise (50). Athletes may also attempt to induce endogenous GH production by using such medications as clonidine, levodopa, amino acid supplements, or propranolol (50). Adverse cardiac effects from excessive hGH use include hypertension, cardiomegaly, ventricular hypertrophy, and dyslipidemia (50). The use of ergogenic aids is reportedly widespread among athletes, and cardiovascular effects from such drugs and techniques should be considered when evaluating young athletes with cardiovascular problems.

CONTROVERSIES AND PERSONAL PERSPECTIVE

The major controversy involving the athlete's heart is not whether athletes should be screened prior to competition; nearly all experts recommend such screening, but how extensive this screening should be. Deaths during athletic participation are rare, but each is a tragedy and prompts a call for more widespread and complex cardiovascular screening. What is not clear is the cost effectiveness of such screening once the evaluation of false-positive results is considered. This debate is highlighted by the recent recommendation from the Sports Cardiology Study Group of the European Society of Cardiology that an ECG should be routinely obtained on all athletes prior to sports participation. At present, we recommend that all athletes be evaluated prior to participation by a knowledgeable examiner preferably someone who knows the athlete and his family well, and can examine the athlete in a setting conducive to a careful evaluation. Testing beyond the history and physical examination should be prompted by findings on this initial examination.

Our perspective on the athlete heart is indeed personal. One of us (PDT) started training for competitive distance running events at age 12 and ultimately qualified for the 1972 U.S. Olympic Marathon Trials as a medical student. However, during the first year of medical school, he had a murmur detected during a demonstration of cardiac auscultation. His subsequent ECG showed left ventricular hypertrophy and early repolarization changes, prompting an interest in cardiology and the medical problems of endurance athletes. The other author (NAME III) developed his interest in the athletic heart syndrome in part from his experiences as a secondary school and collegiate athlete. We have had the privilege of providing advice and medical care to hundreds of competitive athletes including two medalists in the Olympic marathon. The opportunity to combine our personal interest in athletics with our professions as cardiologists has enriched our academic careers.

In evaluating athletes for cardiac abnormalities, we make a strong distinction between abnormalities discovered during screening examinations and those discovered during the evaluation of symptoms. Most screening examinations do not detect real disease, but do detect a high frequency of normal variants common in young healthy subjects and part of the athletic heart syndrome. In our personal experience, physicians frequently overreact to mild abnormalities detected on screening because of legal concerns and the lack of appreciation for the magnitude of changes that can be produced by extreme endurance exercise.

On the other hand, symptomatic athletes require a very thorough examination. We are repeatedly impressed with the number of well-known athletes who die during exercise after having presented with exercise symptoms that were ignored or inadequately evaluated. Excluding important cardiac disease in symptomatic athletes may be the most efficient way to prevent exercise-related complications.

In evaluating symptoms, it is extremely important to evaluate any possible cardiovascular disease in the context of the athlete's total physical and psychological situation. Many young competitive athletes face enormous pressure from coaches, parents, and peers. Failure to achieve the desired level of success is extremely stressful on competitors at any age. Young athletes who present with fainting, for example, may be simply seeking a medical way out of a difficult, stressful situation. It is easier to claim a medical reason for failure than to simply not be good enough. We refer to this condition as *the athletic swoon syndrome*. Typically this is a young athlete in an individual sport who competes well when winning but collapses dramatically when losing often within sight of the finish line. We do not mean to minimize the importance of this problem. The athlete often needs reassurance both medically and personally to place winning and losing in a more healthy perspective. Also, this athletic swoon syndrome must be differentiated from true exercise-induced syncope and from the prolonged QT syndrome. True exercise-induced syncope is a threatening symptom associated with important cardiac disease, and patients with long QT are occasionally misdiagnosed as having hysterical syncope (55).

We also strongly recommend that individuals who serve as trainers and coaches or who officiate at sporting events should learn and update yearly their cardiopulmonary resuscitation skills and that automatic defibrillators be available in areas where athletes train and compete. Coaches and officials are often present when athletes collapse. If properly trained in resuscitation and the use of automatic defibrillators, coaches and trainers may be able to resuscitate potential victims of exercise-related sudden death. We believe that competency in these skills should be a prerequisite for physical educators, coaches, and sports officials.

THE FUTURE

The future of research and treatment of the athletic heart syndrome will likely be a combination of a basic science and a practical approach to the problem. The basic science will be driven by new molecular biology techniques to rapidly screen DNA samples from individuals. This will permit an increased understanding of the genetic variants producing cardiovascular disease and may ultimately permit the identification of the most dangerous genotypes. This information should permit more specific recommendations for athletes with phenotypically diagnosed disease. For example, rather than excluding all athletes with HCM from athletic participation, only those with genotypes known to be associated with the exercise-induced events would be restricted. Genetics will also be used to screen family members of index cases to facilitate the decision as to whether other members of a family with cardiac disease can participate in competitive athletics.

The practical approach will require a more careful cost–benefit analysis of potential screening strategies. Present recommendations vary among expert groups and some consensus must be established. Present discussions on the cost versus benefit of this subject often deal solely with the costs of the tests and the number of athletes to be screened, but do little to evaluate the cost for evaluating false-positive results, which are possibly the most costly aspect of any screening procedure. A more complete assessment of the costs and benefits will permit a more rationale approach to the problem.

References

1. Thompson PD. D. Bruce Dill Historical lecture. Historical concepts of the athlete's heart. *Med Sci Sports Exerc* 2004;36:363–370.
2. Wharton J. "Athlete's Heart": the medical debate over athleticism, 1870–1920 Sport and exercise science, essays in the history of sports medicine. In: Berryman JW, Park RJ, eds. *Sport and exercise science, essays in the history of sports medicine.* Urbana and Chicago: University of Illinois Press; 1992.
3. Park RJ. High-protein diets, "damaged hearts," and rowing men: antecedents of modern sports medicine and exercise science, 1867–1928. *Exerc Sport Sci Rev* 1997;25:137–169.
4. White P. The pulse after a marathon race. *JAMA* 1918;71:1047–1048.
5. Rost R. The athlete's heart. Historical perspectives—solved and unsolved problems. *Cardiol Clin* 1997;15:493–512.
6. Longhurst JC, Kelly AR, Gonyea WJ, et al. Chronic training with static and dynamic exercise: cardiovascular adaptation, and response to exercise. 1. *Circ Res* 1981;48:I171–I178.
7. Levine BD. Exercise physiology for the clinician. In: Thompson PD, ed. *Exercise and sports cardiology.* New York: McGraw-Hill; 2001.
8. Rowell LB. *Human circulation: regulation during physical stress.* New York: Oxford University Press; 1986.
9. Ferguson CM, Meyers J, Froelicher VF. Overview of exercise testing. In: Thompson P, ed. *Exercise and sports cardiology.* New York: McGraw-Hill; 2000.
10. Kenney WL. Parasympathetic control of resting heart rate: relationship to aerobic power 1. *Med Sci Sports Exerc* 1985;17:451–455.
11. Serra-Grima R, Estorch M, Carrio I, et al. Marked ventricular repolarization abnormalities in highly trained athletes' electrocardiograms: clinical and prognostic implications. *J Am Coll Cardiol* 2000;36:1310–1316.
12. Estes III NAM, Link MS, Hamoud M, et al. Electrocardiographic variants and cardiac rhythm and conduction disturbances in the athlete. In: Thompson P, ed. *Exercise and sports cardiology.* New York: McGraw-Hill; 2000.
13. Chapman J. Profound sinus bradycardia in the athletic heart syndrome. *J Sports Med Physical Fitness* 1981;22:294–298.
14. Ingelfinger FJ. Editorial: Paul Dudley White, 1886–1973. *N Engl J Med* 1973;289:1251.
15. Huston TP, Puffer JC, Rodney WM. The athletic heart syndrome. *N Engl J Med* 1985;313:24–32.
16. Smith ML, Graitzer HM, Hudson DL, et al. Baroreflex function in endurance- and static exercise-trained men. 1. *J Appl Physiol* 1988;64:585–591.
17. Pelliccia A, Maron BJ, Culasso F, et al. Clinical significance of abnormal electrocardiographic patterns in trained athletes. *Circulation* 2000;102: 278–284.
18. Furlanello F, Bertoldi A, Dallago M, et al. Atrial fibrillation in elite athletes. *J Cardiovasc Electrophysiol* 1998;9:S63–S68.
19. Biffi A, Maron BJ, Verdile L, et al. Impact of physical deconditioning on ventricular tachyarrhythmias in trained athletes. *J Am Coll Cardiol* 2004; 44:1053–1058.
20. Biffi A, Pelliccia A, Verdile L, et al. Long-term clinical significance of frequent and complex ventricular tachyarrhythmias in trained athletes. *J Am Coll Cardiol* 2002;40:446–452.
21. Thomas LR, Douglas PS. Echocardiographic findings in athletes. In: Thompson PD, ed. *Exercise and sports cardiology.* New York: McGraw-Hill; 2000.
22. Pelliccia A, Maron BJ, Spataro A, et al. The upper limit of physiologic cardiac hypertrophy in highly trained elite athletes. *N Engl J Med* 1991;324: 295–301.
23. Pelliccia A, Culasso F, Di Paolo FM, et al. Physiologic left ventricular cavity dilatation in elite athletes. *Ann Intern Med* 1999;130:23–31.
24. Nagashima J, Musha H, Takada H, et al. New upper limit of physiologic cardiac hypertrophy in Japanese participants in the 100-km ultramarathon. *J Am Coll Cardiol* 2003;42:1617–1623.

25. Abergel E, Chatellier G, Hagege AA, et al. Serial left ventricular adaptations in world-class professional cyclists: implications for disease screening and follow-up. *J Am Coll Cardiol* 2004;44:144–149.
26. Pluim BM, Zwinderman AH, van der Laarse A, et al. The athlete's heart. A meta-analysis of cardiac structure and function. *Circulation* 2000; 101:336–344.
27. Van Camp SP, Bloor CM, Mueller FO, et al. Nontraumatic sports death in high school and college athletes. *Med Sci Sports Exerc* 1995;27:641–647.
28. Corrado D, Basso C, Rizzoli G, et al. Does sports activity enhance the risk of sudden death in adolescents and young adults? *J Am Coll Cardiol* 2003; 42:1959–1963.
29. Thompson PD, Funk EJ, Carleton RA, et al. Incidence of death during jogging in Rhode Island from 1975 through 1980. *JAMA* 1982;247: 2535–2538.
30. Siscovick DS, Weiss NS, Fletcher RH, et al. The incidence of primary cardiac arrest during vigorous exercise. *N Engl J Med* 1984;311:874–877.
31. Mittleman MA, Maclure M, Tofler GH, et al. Triggering of acute myocardial infarction by heavy physical exertion. Protection against triggering by regular exertion. Determinants of Myocardial Infarction Onset Study Investigators. *N Engl J Med* 1993;329:1677–1683.
32. Willich SN, Lewis M, Lowel H, et al. Physical exertion as a trigger of acute myocardial infarction. Triggers and Mechanisms of Myocardial Infarction Study Group. *N Engl J Med* 1993;329:1684–1690.
33. Giri S, Thompson PD, Kiernan FJ, et al. Clinical and angiographic characteristics of exertion-related acute myocardial infarction. *JAMA* 1999;282: 1731–1736.
34. Maron BJ, Shirani J, Poliac LC, et al. Sudden death in young competitive athletes. Clinical, demographic, and pathological profiles. *JAMA* 1996; 276:199–204.
35. Thiene G, Nava A, Corrado D, et al. Right ventricular cardiomyopathy and sudden death in young people. *N Engl J Med* 1988;318:129–133.
36. Corrado D, Basso C, Schiavon M, et al. Screening for hypertrophic cardiomyopathy in young athletes. *N Engl J Med* 1998;339:364–369.
37. McKoy G, Protonotarios N, Crosby A, et al. Identification of a deletion in plakoglobin in arrhythmogenic right ventricular cardiomyopathy with palmoplantar keratoderma and woolly hair (Naxos disease). *Lancet* 2000; 355:2119–2124.
38. Virmani R, Chun PK, Goldstein RE, et al. Acute takeoffs of the coronary arteries along the aortic wall and congenital coronary ostial valve-like ridges: association with sudden death. *J Am Coll Cardiol* 1984;3:766–771.
39. Chiang CE, Roden DM. The long QT syndromes: genetic basis and clinical implications. *J Am Coll Cardiol* 2000;36:1–12.
40. Ackerman MJ, Tester DJ, Porter CJ, et al. Molecular diagnosis of the inherited long-QT syndrome in a woman who died after near-drowning. *N Engl J Med* 1999;341:1121–1125.
41. Kannel WB, Thomas HE Jr. Sudden coronary death: the Framingham Study. *Ann N Y Acad Sci* 1982;382:3–21.
42. Maron BJ, Thompson PD, Puffer JC, et al. Cardiovascular preparticipation screening of competitive athletes. A statement for health professionals from the Sudden Death Committee (clinical cardiology) and Congenital Cardiac Defects Committee (cardiovascular disease in the young), American Heart Association. *Circulation* 1996;94:850–856.
43. Maron BJ, Thompson PD, Puffer JC, et al. Cardiovascular preparticipation screening of competitive athletes: addendum: an addendum to a statement for health professionals from the Sudden Death Committee (Council on Clinical Cardiology) and the Congenital Cardiac Defects Committee (Council on Cardiovascular Disease in the Young), American Heart Association. *Circulation* 1998;97:2294.
44. Corrado D, Pelliccia A, Bjornstad HH, et al. Cardiovascular preparticipation screening of young competitive athletes for prevention of sudden death: proposal for a common European protocol. Consensus Statement of the Study Group of Sport Cardiology of the Working Group of Cardiac Rehabilitation and Exercise Physiology and the Working Group of Myocardial and Pericardial Diseases of the European Society of Cardiology. *Eur Heart J* 2005;26:516–524.
45. Fuller CM, McNulty CM, Spring DA, et al. Prospective screening of 5,615 high school athletes for risk of sudden cardiac death. *Med Sci Sports Exerc* 1997;29:1131–1138.
46. Maron BJ, Gardin JM, Flack JM, et al. Prevalence of hypertrophic cardiomyopathy in a general population of young adults. Echocardiographic analysis of 4111 subjects in the CARDIA Study. Coronary Artery Risk Development in (Young) Adults. *Circulation* 1995;92:785–789.
47. Bonow RO, Carabello B, de Leon AC Jr, et al. Guidelines for the management of patients with valvular heart disease: executive summary. A report of the American College of Cardiology/American Heart Association Task Force on Practice Guidelines (Committee on Management of Patients with Valvular Heart Disease). *Circulation* 1998;98:1949–1984.
48. Herbert PN, Bernier DN, Cullinane EM, et al. High-density lipoprotein metabolism in runners and sedentary men. *JAMA* 1984;252:1034–1037.
49. Maron BJ, Zipes DP. 36th Bethesda Conference: eligibility recommendations for competitive athletes with cardiovascular abnormalities. *J Am Coll Cardiol* 2005;45:2–64.
50. Dhar R, Stout CW, Link MS, et al. Cardiovascular toxicities of performance-enhancing substances in sports. *Mayo Clin Proc* 2005;80: 1307–1315.
51. Thompson PD, Cullinane EM, Sady SP, et al. Contrasting effects of testosterone and stanozolol on serum lipoprotein levels. *JAMA* 1989;261:1165–1168.
52. Samenuk D, Link MS, Homoud MK, et al. Adverse cardiovascular events temporally associated with ma huang, an herbal source of ephedrine. *Mayo Clin Proc* 2002;77:12–16.
53. Gordon NM, Thompson PD. Cardiac complications of recreational cocaine use. *Cardiovasc Rev Rep* 1987;8:29–32.
54. Estes NA III, Kloner R, Olshansky B, et al. Task Force 9: drugs and performance-enhancing substances. *J Am Coll Cardiol* 2005;45:1368–1369.
55. Viskin S, Fish R, Roth A, et al. Clinical problem-solving. QT or not QT? *N Engl J Med* 2000;343:352–356.

CHAPTER 38 ■ CARDIAC TRAUMA

SAMIR R. KAPADIA AND ERIC J. TOPOL

OVERVIEW

Among young people, trauma is the most common cause of death, with cardiovascular mortality being the major contributor. Patients with injury to the thorax, blunt or penetrating, should be transferred rapidly to a trauma center for fast and expert surgical evaluation. In unstable patients, echocardiography helps to identify critical injury and facilitates early surgical exploration, which can be lifesaving. In more stable patients, the goal of evaluation is to rule out significant occult cardiac and thoracic great vessel injury. Echocardiography, computed tomography (CT), thoracoscopy, and magnetic resonance imaging (MRI) can enable the clinician to make an accurate diagnosis of these injuries. Although a normal electrocardiogram (ECG) helps to identify low-risk patients with blunt cardiac injuries, the significance of an abnormal ECG and cardiac enzyme elevation in this setting remains unclear.

Trauma is a leading cause of death for young adults in the United States (1), with thoracic trauma accounting for 30% to 50% of 150,000 total deaths from trauma occurring annually (2–5). The heart and thoracic great vessels are commonly involved in blunt and penetrating trauma. Most serious injuries to these vital organs are rapidly fatal. Therefore, fast transport of these patients to trauma centers, rapid recognition of injury, and expeditious expert treatment are essential for better survival.

INJURY TO THE HEART

Classification of Cardiac Injury

Physical trauma to the heart can be penetrating or blunt. A penetrating injury results when a foreign object enters the body and pierces the heart. Blunt injury, conversely, results from physical forces acting externally on the body. Iatrogenic injuries to the heart and great vessels from invasive procedures are not uncommon. Electrical and radiation injuries are other uncommon mechanisms of cardiovascular trauma.

Penetrating Cardiac Injury

Historical Perspective

Penetrating cardiac injury has been well recognized for centuries, with earliest descriptions by Homer in *The Iliad* (6). In 1761, Morgagni (7) noted that blood in the pericardial sac could lead to compression of the heart. Fischer (8), in 1868, reported pericardial drainage after injury in 452 cases, with 10% survival. Even in this era, however, there was serious skepticism about the therapy. One of the prominent surgeons of this time, Billroth, stated the following: "The surgeon who should attempt to suture a wound of heart would lose respect of his colleagues" and "Let no man dare to operate on the heart" (9,10). In 1896, Cappelen performed the first repair of a human left ventricle and left anterior descending artery, but the patient did not survive. Rehn (11), at about the same time, is credited with the first right ventricular repair in which the patient survived. In 1902, Hill (12) became the first American surgeon to suture a myocardial injury, in a 13-year-old boy, by the flickering lights of kerosene lamps on a kitchen table.

Anatomic Considerations

The classic precordium is defined as an area of chest bounded by the sternal notch superiorly, the xiphoid process inferiorly, and the nipples laterally. Most stab wounds injuring the heart enter through the classic precordium. Most gunshot wounds strike the heart without entering this zone. The relative frequency of cardiac chamber involvement depends on the anatomic location of the chamber as well as the type of penetration. The right ventricle, with its maximum anterior exposure, is at the greatest risk for injury. In a series of penetrating wounds to the heart, the right ventricle was involved in 42%, the left ventricle in 33%, the left atrium in 6%, and the right atrium in 15% (13). Pericardial reflections are important to recognize because they are positioned on portions of the ascending aorta, the main pulmonary artery, portions of the right and left pulmonary arteries, portions of the pulmonary veins, and portions of the superior and inferior vena cava. This is important because even trivial injuries to the intrapericardial portions of these vessels can result in cardiac tamponade.

Etiology

Penetrating wounds to the heart commonly result from puncture wounds, knife wounds, and gunshot wounds (14). Puncture wounds are caused by ice picks, needles, or pellets from an air gun or a distant shotgun, typically involving a single chamber. Knife injuries also frequently involve a single chamber, producing a slitlike defect. Small-caliber gunshot wounds can cause multiple-chamber perforations along with injuries to the great vessels. In contrast, large-caliber gunshot wounds result in fatal gaping cardiac defects.

Pathophysiology

The size of pericardial defect and the severity of cardiac injury determine the clinical presentation and subsequent outcome. If the defect in the pericardium is small, a blood clot may seal this defect. If the bleeding from the heart or proximal vessels continues in the closed pericardial sac, intrapericardial pressure rapidly increases. Rapid accumulation of blood, even when small (about 100 mL), leads to a sufficient rise in intrapericardial pressure to cause tamponade. Conversely, if the defect in the pericardium is large, rapid exsanguination and death will occur. The number of cardiac structures involved determines the severity of cardiac injury. Multiple-chamber injury is usually fatal. Involvement of one or more cardiac valves with damage to the leaflets, annulus, chordae, or papillary muscle can lead to hemodynamic compromise (15). Conduction system damage (16) and coronary artery injury, although less common than in blunt trauma, have been reported with penetrating injury (17).

Clinical Profile

Patients presenting to the emergency room (ER) with penetrating cardiac injury may be dead on arrival, alive but hemodynamically compromised, or hemodynamically stable. A few patients who are dead on arrival can be revived with resuscitative thoracotomy in the ER. Identifying this small subgroup of patients is important to conserve resources because the yield of indiscriminate resuscitative thoracotomy is very low (<5%). Patients who show some signs of life on transport have up to a 30% chance of successful resuscitation (18). Patients with stab wounds compared with gunshot wounds and patients presenting with cardiac tamponade have a better chance of survival. In the second group of patients with hemodynamic compromise, it is important to recognize cardiac tamponade. Dyspnea, diaphoresis, agitation, confusion, apathy, or a feeling of strangling oppression should alert the physician to look for cardiac tamponade (19). Only 10% to 40% of trauma victims with tamponade present with the Beck triad of hypotension, jugular distention, and muffled heart sounds (20–22). Neck vein distention may be absent because of accompanying hypovolemia. Pulsus paradoxus is neither sensitive nor specific for tamponade in this situation.

The third, more stable group should be examined in detail after primary assessment of airway, breathing, and circulation. The entry site is especially important with stab wounds. An entrance wound high on the right side is likely to involve the aorta and right atrium. Lower right and left parasternal wounds involve the right ventricle, whereas inferolateral left parasternal wounds typically signify left ventricle involvement (23). In a gunshot wound, the entry site may be deceptive. If the entry site involves the "danger zone" of Suer and Mordax, which includes the precordium, epigastrium, and superior mediastinum, cardiac injury is typically present (13). The trajectory of the gunshot should also be determined. If the trajectory suggests juxtacardiac passage, the physician should keep a high index of suspicion for cardiac injury.

Management

Rapid transport of the patient to the trauma center is essential for better outcome. The so-called scoop and run policy, without an attempt to stabilize the patient in the field, is the best approach (24). Even roadside thoracotomy done by medical teams flown to the scene is without benefit (25). Intubation is beneficial for patients with cardiac arrest or hemodynamic instability (26,27). Closed chest cardiopulmonary resuscitation (CPR) is not only ineffective but also contraindicated if an impaling weapon is present. An intravenous line can be started en route to the hospital, although the role of intravenous fluids is controversial (28,29).

For patients who are dead on arrival, diagnostic and therapeutic endeavor consists of an ER thoracotomy with a goal to relieve tamponade, control hemorrhage, and restore cardiac function (27,30,31). After resuscitation, the patient should be rapidly transferred to the operating room for definitive surgery.

In patients with hemodynamic compromise, rapid operating room thoracotomy by a cardiothoracic trauma surgeon appears to be the most effective procedure. The role of ER thoracotomy has been a constant source of debate, but it should be restricted to patients who arrive in a moribund state or who rapidly deteriorate after arrival (32–35). ER thoracotomy with the use of staples to control cardiac bleeding and to minimize the risk of personal contamination from a needle stick remains controversial (36). Staples to the heart can enlarge the wound and at times are difficult to remove during definitive surgery. Definitive surgical treatment is detailed elsewhere, but the general principles are as follows (4,37,38). Myocardial rupture is repaired in all cases. In patients with distal coronary artery injury, ligation is sufficient. Definitive valve or shunt surgery is usually deferred until later. Approach to a foreign body is variable, but most commonly only those objects projecting into cavities or involving the left ventricle are removed.

In hemodynamically stable patients or those stabilized with volume, transthoracic echocardiography (TTE) should be performed rapidly to diagnose pericardial effusion (PE). PE, however small, serves as a marker for cardiac penetration (39). When compared prospectively with a surgical gold standard (subxiphoid window), echocardiography has high specificity and sensitivity in diagnosing PE (40). It has rapidly become a modality of choice to assess patients with thoracic trauma (41). However, in the presence of hemothorax, its sensitivity is significantly decreased (42). Transesophageal echocardiography (TEE) can overcome this limitation of TTE, but in many patients it either is not feasible because of other injuries or is not expeditiously available and hence is of limited usefulness (43–46). Subxiphoid pericardial window was the traditional way to rule out PE in patients with suspected penetrating wound to the heart. It is best performed in the operating room with the patient under light general anesthesia. Although it is a safe procedure and provides a definitive diagnosis of hemopericardium (47–50), it typically results in a negative exploration rate of 75% to 80% (49). The availability of TTE in the ER has significantly reduced the frequency of this operation, which is now used only in few difficult situations to complement echocardiography (51–53). Thoracoscopic pericardial window is another alternative that has been shown to be safe and effective in diagnosing cardiac injury (54). However, echocardiography has other advantages in that it is a reliable tool to localize foreign bodies (55–58) (Fig. 38.1) and helps in diagnosing and monitoring structural abnormalities such as valvular regurgitations and shunts (59,60) (Figs. 38.2 and 38.3). Therefore, the availability of TTE in the ER is shown to decrease time to definitive therapy, thus leading to a better outcome (61,62).

Importantly, the ECG is not helpful in evaluating penetrating injury. It inconsistently shows the injury pattern and, if negative, does not rule out significant injury (49). The chest radiograph may help by identifying patients with hemothorax who are difficult to image with ultrasound. However, other findings, such as an enlarged cardiac shadow or pneumopericardium, are infrequently present (20). Pericardiocentesis is not indicated for diagnosis in stable patients and can actually be harmful (63).

Prognosis

Various indices to categorize patients with penetrating cardiac trauma are available. Trauma indices describing anatomic

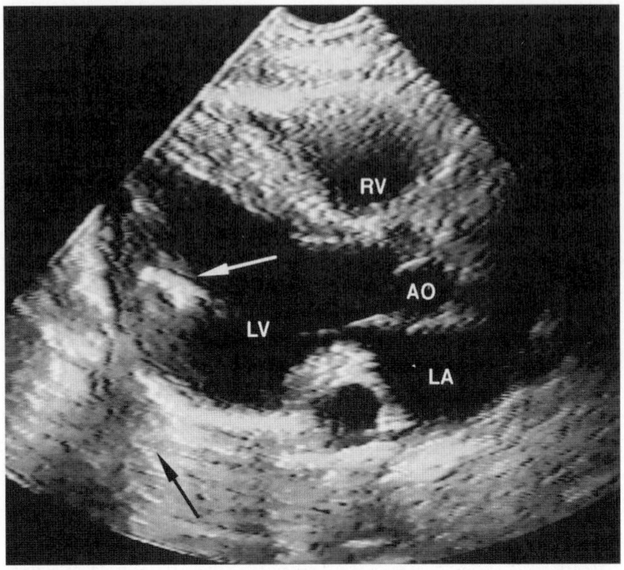

FIGURE 38.1. A transthoracic echocardiogram, a parasternal long-axis view, demonstrating a shotgun pellet (*white arrow*) in the distal posterior wall of the left ventricle. The pellet was identified years after the injury, and the patient was asymptomatic. Note how the pellet casts an acoustic shadow (*black arrow*). AO, aorta, LA, left atrium; LV, left ventricle; RV, right ventricle. (From Dr. Carlos Antonio Da Mota Silveira and Dr. Roberto Pereira, Pernambuco University, Brazil.)

severity, such as American Association for the Surgery of Trauma (AAST) Organ Injury Scaling (OIS), Heart Injury Scale, Penetrating Cardiac Trauma Index (PCTI), Penetrating Thoracic Trauma Index (PTTI), Penetrating Trauma Index (PTI), Cardiovascular-Respiratory Score (CVRS) component of Trauma Score, and Injury Severity Score (ISS), are good predictors of outcome. However, the general condition of the patient plays a significant role in determining the prognosis of cardiac trauma. For this reason, a general condition index such as the Physiologic Index (PI) can be combined with anatomic indices to categorize a patient more accurately.

Patients who reach the operating room without requiring ER thoracotomy have a favorable outcome (64,65). Overall, patients with stab wounds have a better prognosis than those with gunshot wounds (35,66,67). Single-chamber injury to the heart with hemodynamic stability, shorter duration of CPR before arriving at the hospital, successful intubation, and younger age are all factors associated with better outcome (27,68,69). The presence of pericardial tamponade is thought to be a favorable predictor because it possibly prevents exsanguination (70). Late sequelae such as pseudoaneurysm, ventricular septal defect, valvular regurgitation, and constrictive pericarditis have been reported (66,71–74). Surveillance for these anatomic sequelae with echocardiography is recommended (16,60,75,76) (Fig. 38.4).

Blunt Cardiac Injury

In civilian life, the most common cause of blunt cardiac injury is a motor vehicular accident (MVA). Falls from heights, falling objects, direct trauma from assault, and blast injury are other less common causes. Injury patterns in MVAs are governed by the location of the victim in the vehicle and the direction of impact. In a front impact, abrupt deceleration against the steering wheel is the most common cause of cardiovascular trauma. Side impact generates a high shearing force, more commonly causing an aortic injury. Seat belts and airbags also play a major role in determining the injury patterns. For unrestrained drivers, each cardiac and aortic injury occurs in approximately 20% of cases (77). Even in restrained drivers, significant thoracic injuries can still occur from contact with the steering wheel

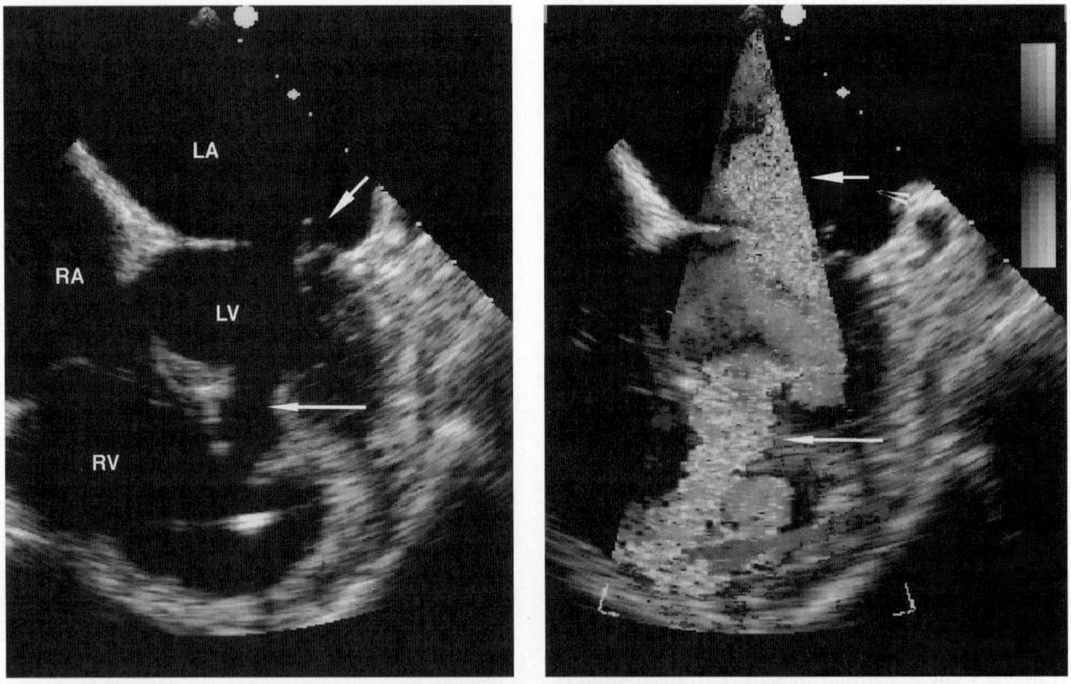

FIGURE 38.2. A transesophageal echocardiogram demonstrating a traumatic ventricular septal defect (*long arrow*) and mitral regurgitation (*short arrow*) from a gunshot wound. A Swan-Ganz catheter is seen in the right ventricle (RV). LA, left atrium; LV, left ventricle; RA, right atrium. (From the Digital Imaging and Communications in Medicine (DICOM) demonstration DISC 96.)

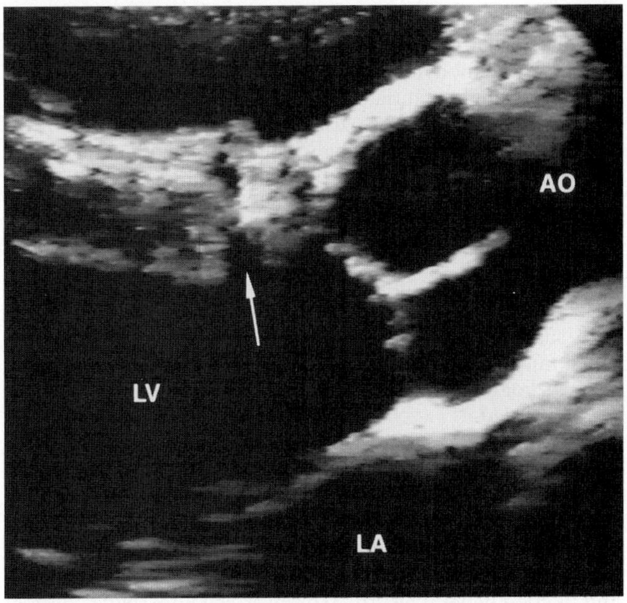

FIGURE 38.3. A transthoracic echocardiogram, a parasternal long-axis view, showing an interventricular septal defect from a stab wound. This was successfully repaired. AO, aorta; LA, left atrium; LV, left ventricle. (From Dr. Carlos Antonio Da Mota Silveira and Dr. Roberto Pereira, Pernambuco University, Brazil.)

and from deceleration, but the number of deaths from thoracic injuries is significantly lower (78–80). The air bag has been associated with rupture of the right atrium (81).

Myocardial Contusion

Historical Perspective. Myocardial contusion was first noted by Burch in 1676 in an 8-year-old boy. In 1859, Schnabel noted a hematoma with a right atrial tear in a 49-year-old man who died several hours after the blunt injury. In 1954, Burchell aptly observed "and always with heart contusion, arise both doubt and much confusion" (82). The confusion is still prevalent in literature because myocardial contusion is a pathologic diagnosis without an accurate clinical counterpart (83,84). It implies a bruise to a segment of myocardium that reveals subepicardial and intramyocardial hemorrhage, disruption of myocardial fibers, cellular infiltration, and interstitial edema on histologic examination. The definition by some includes the presence of myocardial necrosis with or without bleeding into the myocardium (85). In strict pathologic terms, contusion should not include necrosis as its integral part. Therefore, myocardial contusion is considered a less favorable term to describe this injury pattern (86). Commotio cordis is a term used to describe fatal cardiac arrest without detectable structural damage to the heart as a result of blunt impact to chest (87).

Anatomic Considerations. The anterior right ventricular wall is most commonly involved. The anterior interventricular septum and anterior-apical left ventricle are next in frequency. Blunt injury can also damage the conduction system of the heart, manifesting as a right bundle branch block (88).

Pathophysiology. Autopsy studies of patients who died of blunt cardiac injury show subendocardial and interstitial hemorrhage, large surrounding areas of focal myocardial edema, myofibrillar degeneration, myocytolysis, and infiltration with polymorphonuclear cells. In essence, the pathologic features resemble those of myocardial infarction (MI). The few distinguishing features of blunt injury are the more abrupt demarcation between normal and abnormal, more hemorrhage, and more frequent cellular laceration (89,90). Functionally, these changes present with a decrease in myocardial contractility and cardiac output (91,92). Right ventricular ejection fraction is more commonly decreased, probably owing to its anterior location and the acutely altered loading condition of the ventricle (93). At times, patients with mild injury present with regional wall motion abnormalities but negative chemical markers of myocardial necrosis. The term cardiac concussion has been used to describe this condition. The mechanism is not known, but local factors that impair cardiac contractility, such as hematoma and focal inflammation, are considered responsible. These patients have excellent short- and long-term prognoses.

A swine model that replicates commotio cordis has provided important insights into the mechanisms for this phenomenon. Determinants of ventricular fibrillation (VF) following a chest blow include impact delivered at a wide range of velocities directly over the heart and timing within a narrow 15- to-30-millisecond window just before the T-wave peak during the vulnerable phase of repolarization (94–97).

Clinical Profile. Cardiac contusion presents with a wide spectrum of severity. Patients with contusion can be hemodynamically unstable or stable. Pericardial tamponade and valvular regurgitation are important cardiac reasons for decompensation. Coronary artery injury, most typically right coronary

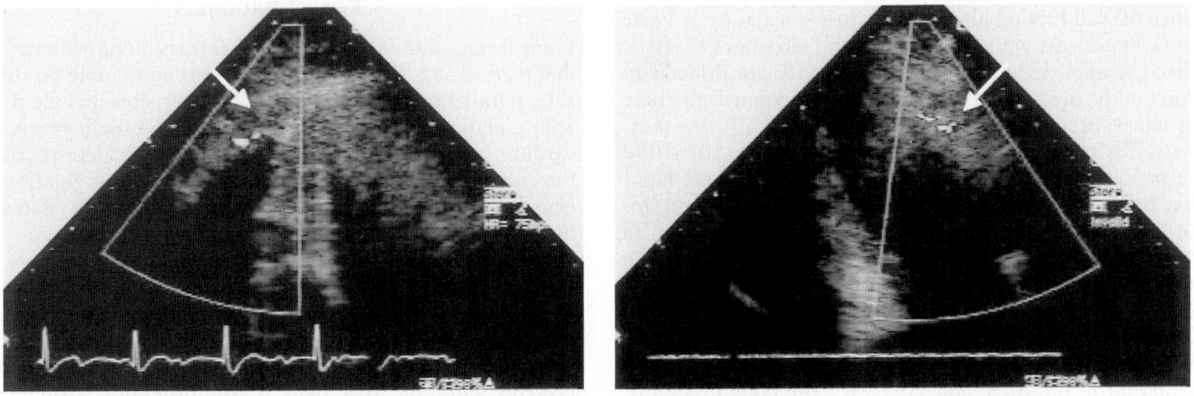

FIGURE 38.4. Patient with stab wound to the chest and right ventricle perforation. Perforation was repaired but on follow-up echocardiogram there was a very small pseudoaneurysm with some flow (*arrows*). Patient was conservatively managed without any complications.

artery, can present with acute MI. Arrhythmias are not infrequent, but their significance remains unclear. Atrial fibrillation, but not premature ventricular contractions and nonsustained ventricular tachycardia, has been associated with a worse outcome (91).

Hemodynamically unstable patients should be evaluated for the cardiac and noncardiac causes of hypotension. Noncardiac causes include hypovolemia and associated vascular injuries. Fluid challenge helps to identify significant hypovolemia. For patients with vascular injuries, blood pressure and pulses in both upper and lower extremities should be carefully checked for discrepancies. The cardiac cause of hypotension in this group is pericardial tamponade. Clinical signs of pericardial tamponade should be evaluated carefully. Muffled heart sounds and pulsus paradoxus are not specific for tamponade and are absent in a significant number of patients. Neck veins may not be distended as a result of associated bleeding and hypovolemia. Other mechanical causes of cardiac decompensation are valvular regurgitation and shunts. Any murmur, especially pansystolic or continuous, should point to one of these complications. Left or right ventricular failure can lead to hypotension and would manifest with an S_3 heart sound, rales, and increased jugular venous pressure. Coronary artery injury presents with chest pain similar to that caused by MI, but in the presence of trauma it may be difficult to ascertain the quality of chest pain. In hemodynamically stable patients, special attention should be given to complaints of chest pain, new murmur, early signs of pericardial tamponade, and heart failure.

Management. For hemodynamically unstable patients arriving after blunt chest trauma, echocardiography should be performed quickly. If echocardiography suggests a mechanical cause for hypotension, rapid appropriate surgical correction is mandatory. Fluid resuscitation in hypotensive patient is controversial; the role of colloid, crystalloid, hypertonic saline, and blood substitutes has been debated (97a). If the patient has severe ventricular dysfunction without myocardial rupture or pericardial effusion, right heart catheterization may be useful to manage fluids and inotropes. Intraaortic balloon pump counterpulsation, after ruling out aortic injury, has been effectively used in this situation (98). For the more stable group, various diagnostic tests including ECG, cardiac enzymes, and other imaging modalities are available to quantify cardiac damage. The goal of these investigations is to identify patients at risk of immediate and future cardiac complications, but no test is considered a gold standard. A normal ECG helps to identify a very low-risk population, but ECG changes are neither specific nor sensitive to identify presence of wall motion abnormalities. Although echocardiography can identify these wall motion abnormalities, its role in the management of stable patients after chest trauma has been questioned because the presence of wall motion abnormality does not signify a worse outcome in patients with normal ECG and enzymes (99–101). Cardiac enzymes, especially CK and CK-MB, are difficult to interpret in the presence of other injuries. Troponin T and I are much more specific, but the incremental value of these measures over ECG has not been extensively evaluated (102–105). In one prospective study of 333 consecutive patients with blunt cardiac trauma, the clinical significance of serial ECG and troponin I was evaluated. Significant clinical events were defined as the presence of cardiogenic shock, arrhythmias requiring treatment, or posttraumatic structural deficits. Of patients with abnormal ECG only or troponin I only, 22% and 7%, respectively, experienced clinical events. The positive and negative predictive values were 29% and 98% for ECG, 21% and 94% for troponin I, and 34% and 100% for the combination of ECG and troponin I. This study therefore suggested some incremental value of measuring troponin in patients with blunt trauma (105).

The approach to patients with blunt trauma has to be individualized according to hemodynamic stability and other injuries. In a hemodynamically stable patient, if no abnormalities are detected on initial detailed physical examination, ECG, and chest radiograph, the patient can be observed in the ER for 12 hours and then discharged. If the ECG shows nonspecific changes, 24 hours of observation with serial enzyme assay are advisable. If enzymes are negative after the period of observation, the patient can be discharged without further investigations. If on initial ECG there are specific abnormalities or if the chest radiograph is abnormal, echocardiography should be performed to further assess cardiac injury. If the patient with suspected cardiac contusion has to be operated on for other injuries and be under general anesthesia, preoperative echocardiography and intraoperative invasive monitoring are recommended.

Prognosis. Late complications such as arrhythmia, aneurysm, pseudoaneurysm, heart failure, valvular regurgitation, and shunts have been reported but are rare. Although similarities are drawn between MI and cardiac contusion, significant differences affect the outcome. Typically, trauma victims are younger and in good general health. Moreover, the underlying cause of myocardial damage (trauma) is episodic and is not an ongoing process (atherosclerosis). Therefore, the prognosis in these patients is much better than in those with MI (126).

Myocardial Rupture

Rupture of the cardiac chamber, the most severe form of blunt cardiac injury, is a common finding in the patients with fatal nonpenetrating cardiac trauma (90,107,108). The right-sided chambers rupture more frequently than the left-sided chambers. The atria are more commonly involved than the ventricles (90,109). Interventricular septal rupture, an uncommon event, involves the apical part of the muscular septum more than the membranous interventricular septum (110,111). Interatrial septal rupture occurs rarely (112). In another rare situation, patients with an isolated interventricular septal defect can present late with heart failure and a holosystolic murmur (113). A small muscular interventricular septal defect can be treated expectantly and repaired after 6 to 8 weeks, depending on the size of the shunt and intracardiac pressures. Percutaneous closure has been attempted in some patients (114). Myocardial rupture results in sudden cardiovascular collapse in most patients (115,116). On physical examination of rare survivors of free wall rupture, a sound resembling a splashing mill wheel (*bruit de moulin*) has been described. Rapid recognition of cardiac rupture with immediate thoracotomy can be lifesaving (117).

Pericardial Injury

Blunt trauma can lead to pericardial tears along with myocardial tears (118). These tears occur most commonly on the left side, parallel to the phrenic nerve. Other sites include the diaphragmatic surface of the pericardium, the right pleuropericardium, and the anterior pericardium (113). Irrespective of the site of the tear, cardiac herniation and strangulation can occur (119). With a diaphragmatic tear, abdominal viscera can herniate into the pericardial space (120).

With a pericardial tear, patients are unstable because of concomitant myocardial tear or cardiac herniation. Early diagnosis is important for survival and can be achieved only when the index of suspicion is high. The diagnosis is typically made at the time of thoracotomy. Intrapericardial diaphragmatic hernia presents with epigastric pain, gastric distention, palpitations, and shortness of breath. Gurgling sounds in the chest with muffled heart sounds and air bubbles in the pericardium on chest radiograph help in the diagnosis. Blunt trauma can lead to pericarditis without a tear. Depending on the size of the effusion, cardiac tamponade can develop. Some patients can develop late pericardial effusion owing to the postpericardiotomy syndrome.

Patients with hemodynamic instability should undergo thoracotomy. Myocardial tears are repaired, leaving the pericardium open. In the presence of significant hemopericardium, surgical drainage is recommended. With a small effusion, conservative management with echocardiographic follow-up is recommended. Rarely, constrictive pericarditis may develop within 6 months to a year.

Valve Injury

Valves are involved less commonly with blunt injury. Frequently involved valves are the aortic, mitral, and tricuspid, in that order. The pulmonary valve is rarely involved. Many patients have an underlying valvular disorder that predisposes the valves to rupture. The aortic valve is most vulnerable in the isovolumetric relaxation phase and the mitral valve in the isovolumetric contraction phase. Injury to the tricuspid valve results from a sudden increase in hydrostatic pressure on the right side of the heart from venous compression (121,122). With blunt trauma, the aortic valve tears at the leading edge of the cusp, more commonly near the commissures (Fig. 38.5). Bioprosthetic valves are particularly at risk (123). Mitral valve injury includes rupture or avulsion of a papillary muscle (most common), rupture of chordae, or, rarely, a tear of the valve leaflets. Tricuspid injury leads to regurgitation from rupture of the anterior papillary muscle, a tear in the anterior leaflet, or, rarely, a tear of the septal leaflet (124–129).

Valvular injuries present with acute regurgitation. Acute aortic regurgitation can present with left ventricular failure without signs of wide pulse pressure. In mitral regurgitation, harsh pansystolic murmur radiating to the base rather than the axilla with an apical systolic thrill can be present (130). Tricuspid regurgitation presents with hypotension and signs of right heart failure. TEE helps to delineate the mechanism and severity of valvular regurgitation (131). Acute severe valvular regurgitation requires surgical reconstruction (124,132). For mild to moderate regurgitation, follow-up with rest or stress echocardiography is recommended (133). Endocarditis prophylaxis is recommended in all cases.

Coronary Artery Injury

Coronary artery injury is rare in patients who die of blunt injury (90,134). If a patient presents with clinical signs of acute MI, cardiac catheterization should be considered (135,136). If coronary artery thrombosis is identified, percutaneous intervention or surgery should be considered, depending on the clinical situation (137). Posttraumatic arteriovenous and arteriocameral fistulae have been reported.

Electrical Injury

Historical Perspective

In 1750, Franklin showed, by flying a wired kite during a thunderstorm, that electric charge could be passed from the cloud to the primitive accumulator, the Leyden jar. This led to the discovery of the Franklin rod, a device designed to conduct atmospheric electricity safely to earth. Every day, 50,000 lightning bolts are estimated to hit the earth. The flash lasts 0.2 to 1 second, with an amplitude of 25,000 to 500,000 amp and voltage of more than 1,000 kV. Most of these lightning bolts enter the earth without destruction, and only unprotected people or structures are sometimes involved. In the United States, lightning injuries are more common on the eastern seaboard than in the west. Wyoming, owing to heavy outdoor activity, has the highest incidence of fatal lightning strikes in the United States. More men than women are more involved with lightning strikes (4:1). Interestingly, however, when a bolt comes through the telephone system, women are more likely to be the victims (138,139). In the United States, 100 to 300 persons die annually of lightning injury. Accidental exposure to household AC current leads to about 1,000 deaths annually in the United States (140).

Pathophysiology

There are major differences between injuries from AC and DC current. AC current changes the polarity of cells and depolarizes them. This results in acetylcholine release at the neuromuscular junction and subsequently tetanic spasm of the muscles. It leads to prolonged contact with the source, because the flexors

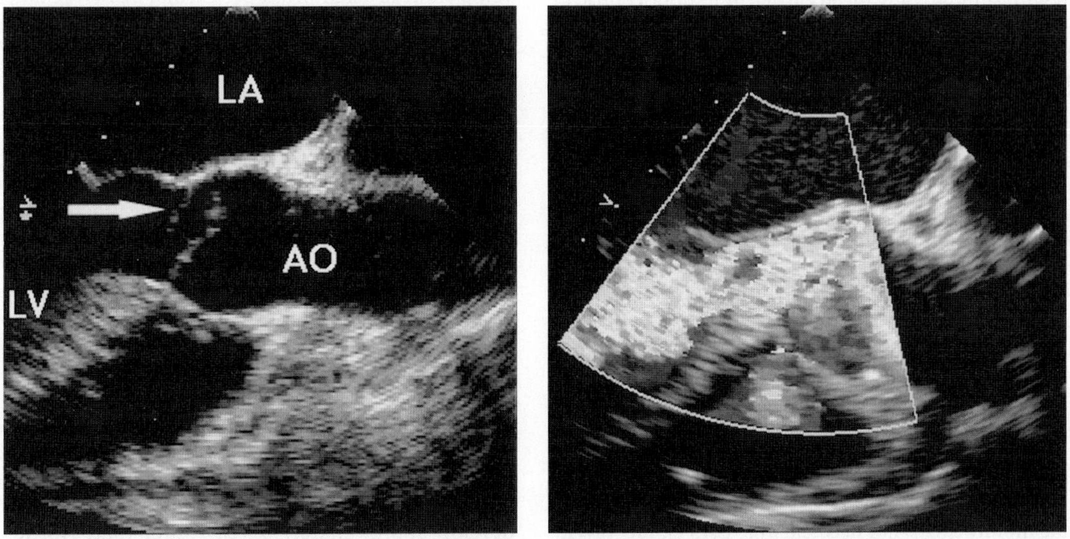

FIGURE 38.5. Aortic valve rupture from a blunt injury resulting from a motor vehicle accident. The intraoperative transthoracic echocardiogram in the long-axis view shows the flail left coronary cusp (**left,** *white arrow*) resulting in severe acute aortic regurgitation. AO, aorta; LA, left atrium; LV, left ventricle. (From Dr. Ellen Mayer and Dr. Joseph Sabik, Cleveland Clinic Foundation, Cleveland, Ohio.)

of the hand are more powerful than the extensors. The current also causes tetanic spasms of the blood vessels, leading to ischemia in the distal bed. In the heart, it causes direct tissue damage with contraction band necrosis. Conduction abnormalities are common because conduction tissue is sensitive to the AC current. The lower domestic frequency (50 Hz in Europe and 60 Hz in the United States) of AC current induces VF. Higher-frequency AC current, as used in diathermy, is thought to be relatively safe and causes only local tissue damage. DC current causes less direct tissue damage compared with similar-energy AC current. DC current, as in lightning stroke, can lead to VF or uniform depolarization of the left ventricle, causing asystole. Sometimes cardiac automaticity can be restored spontaneously after asystole. However, concomitant respiratory arrest may continue, and hypoxic cardiac arrest may occur. The path of AC or DC current through the body is also important in determining the severity of injury. Transthoracic current flow (e.g., hand-to-hand pathway) is more likely to be fatal from respiratory and cardiac arrest than vertical or straddle current path flow (141). However, vertical path flow can also cause significant myocardial injury because of the direct effect of the current on the heart and because of coronary vasospasm (142–144).

Clinical Profile

Electrical injuries present with VF, ventricular asystole, conduction system disturbances, transient myocardial ischemia, and myocardial damage. Cardiac arrest can result from primary VF or can be secondary to prolonged respiratory center arrest or muscle paralysis. Electrical injury has a predilection for the conduction system for unclear reasons. It presents with sinoatrial or atrioventricular node dysfunction. MI can result from coronary artery spasm because angiography is frequently normal in these patients (140). It presents with increased enzymes and wall motion abnormalities. The ECG may show typical ST-segment elevations, and Q waves can develop with evolution. QT prolongation has been noted in patients with electrical injury. The reason may be the direct effect of the current on myocardium or the indirect effect from injury to the central nervous system. Valve injury from electrical current has been reported (145).

Management

If the patient is in cardiopulmonary arrest, he or she should be resuscitated with standard advanced cardiac life support protocol. Because of the low metabolic rate, survival after prolonged arrest is better in patients with electrical injury, especially from lightning, than from other causes (146). Lightning victims who do not suffer cardiac arrest have an excellent chance of recovery because subsequent arrest is uncommon. Therefore, when multiple victims are struck simultaneously with lightning, usual triage priorities should be reversed. Rescuers should give highest priority to patients in respiratory or cardiac arrest. Patients who regain their vital signs after resuscitation have high survival rates (147,148).

After resuscitation, patients should be monitored for arrhythmia. They may develop significant tachycardia and hypertension owing to catecholamine surge that may require β-blocker therapy. Serial enzymes and echocardiography may help to estimate the extent of myocardial injury. Patients with significant myocardial damage should be monitored closely for complications. Treatment of post-MI complications is similar to that from other causes (149).

After AC shock, if the patients are stable and have a normal ECG, cardiac monitoring is not necessary (150,151). However, for patients struck with lightning, overnight monitoring is recommended even if they are stable and have a normal ECG. If the admission ECG is not normal (one-third of victims of electrical injury), irrespective of the cause of injury, echocardiographic assessment of left ventricular function and serial CK estimation are indicated (152).

Prognosis

The mortality with lightning is 20% to 30% (147). The mortality with domestic AC electrocution is difficult to estimate owing to variability in severity of the shock. For every three significant injuries, there is approximately one death (153). This amounts to 1,000 annual deaths in the United States (140). ECG abnormalities usually resolve in a few weeks (154). Ventricular dysfunction also improves in most patients (155,156). Patients tend to have a good long-term prognosis, but they should be monitored periodically for at least 1 year (150).

Radiation Injury

Until the middle of the twentieth century, the heart was thought to be resistant to radiation injury (157,158). High-dose radiation was delivered without proper cardiac shielding. Many reports of radiation-induced cardiac abnormalities changed the perception of safety of radiation to the heart. Radiation, when used in the treatment of mediastinal tumors, primarily Hodgkin and non-Hodgkin lymphoma, and spinal irradiation, can cause cardiac abnormality in as many as 40% of patients (159–161). This awareness and the availability of better radiation techniques in the 1990s led to careful use of high-dose radiation to the chest with proper cardiac shielding (162). A dose of more than 3,000 rad to the chest is usually not used. Therefore, the long-term effects of modern radiation may be less severe than before (163), although we are likely to continue to encounter these problems because of better long-term survival of patients who received radiation in the past and delayed manifestation of cardiac effects (164,165). Radiation-induced injuries involve various cardiac structures and can have acute or delayed manifestations.

Pericardium

Acute pericarditis resulting from radiation is rare (< 2%). Over the years, about half of the patients develop echocardiographically demonstrable abnormalities, and approximately 5% develop clinically significant pericardial disease. Clinical manifestations and management of radiation pericarditis are discussed in detail in Chapter 27.

Myocardium

Radiation causes progressive fibrin deposition and capillary destruction, leading to fibrosis in the myocardium (166,167). The result is mild left ventricular dysfunction not requiring specific treatment (166,168). Coronary artery disease should be ruled out when significant systolic dysfunction of the left ventricle is identified. Restrictive cardiomyopathy has also been described after radiation treatment (169,170).

Valves

Valvular thickening is present in many patients after radiation treatment, but significant valvular disease is an infrequent sequela (166). The mean time from radiation to clinically recognizable valvular disease is about 10 years, and the symptoms develop approximately 5 years after that. Aortic and mitral replacements from radiation-induced sclerosis with significant aortic stenosis or mitral regurgitation have been reported (171). Pulmonary and tricuspid valve disease is even less common (172–174).

Conduction System

Nodal and infranodal conduction abnormalities occur in patients with radiation injury. Although right bundle branch block is most common, complete heart block has been reported (169,173,175). Management of these abnormalities is similar to that from other causes.

Coronary Arteries

External radiation injury involves the proximal portion of coronary arteries (176–179). The left and right coronary ostia and the proximal left anterior descending and left circumflex arteries are involved in most cases. The lesions have an increased number of plasma cells with a paucity of lipids (180). Large bizarre fibroblasts are also present (181). Coronary artery disease commonly presents about 5 years after radiation, but it can present as late as 29 years later (179). Predisposing factors other than the total dose of radiation are not clearly identified. Patients can present with any ischemic complication, such as angina, MI, arrhythmia, or heart failure. Sudden death has been reported from left main stenosis or diffuse atherosclerosis (181a). Children treated with chest radiation have a higher risk of MI (182). For significant left main stenosis, coronary artery bypass grafting with a left internal mammary artery conduit is recommended, although surgery can be technically difficult because of excessive scarring. For other focal lesions, percutaneous transluminal coronary angioplasty can be useful. The long-term effects of intracoronary radiation commonly used to treat recurring in-stent restenosis remain unknown (183,184).

Iatrogenic Cardiac Injury

With the rapid increase in percutaneous interventions and devices, many procedural complications that lead to cardiac injury have been recognized. These are described in detail in discussions of individual procedures. In the catheterization laboratory, with myocardial biopsy or diagnostic catheterizations, significant vascular injuries, valve injuries, and myocardial injuries have been reported (185,186). With percutaneous coronary interventions, coronary artery perforation and accompanied complications have been well recognized (187,188). Cardiac perforation is a known complication of transseptal valvuloplasty (189). Central line–related cardiac injuries have been frequently reported (190,191). Pericardiocentesis can be complicated by ventricular perforation (192). In the electrophysiology laboratory, with transvenous pacemakers, defibrillators, lead extraction, and radiofrequency ablation catheters, ventricular perforation is encountered (193). Timely recognition of these complications is the key to appropriate management and better outcome.

INJURY TO THE GREAT VESSELS

Penetrating Injury

Thoracic great vessel injuries cause immediate death in a significant number of patients with penetrating injury. Gunshot wounds and knife wounds are the common causes of injury (194). Iatrogenic causes such as percutaneous placement of jugular venous lines, overinflation of a Swan-Ganz catheter balloon, and complications of intraaortic balloon pump use can also lead to injury to the intrathoracic vessels (195–197). Recently, cardiac and aortic perforations have been associated with devices to close atrial septal defects (198). These injuries can manifest with simple lacerations, pseudoaneurysm, or an arteriovenous fistula. A high suspicion for injury is warranted while evaluating all penetrating thoracic wounds, because clinical signs of pulse deficit or murmur may be absent despite significant vascular injury (199). The chest radiograph may show hemothorax, widened mediastinum, and cervical or supraclavicular widening. In stable patients, a multidetector CT scan helps to define the problem and has largely replaced conventional aortography (200). In unstable patients, surgical exploration with thoracotomy is indicated. Follow-up of these patients is recommended because some of them may develop late complications such as distal ischemia, edema, fistula, and pseudoaneurysms. Endovascular options are becoming more of a reality with the availability of various occluder devices and stent grafts (201).

Blunt Injury

Anatomic Considerations

MVAs are responsible for the majority of cases of aortic rupture (202–204). Because the blood vessels are fixed by their branches to the chest wall, the direction of the pull determines the site of the tear. The aorta is fixed superiorly to the thoracic outlet and posteriorly to the chest wall. Vertical deceleration pulls the heart down and to the left, which causes shear on the right side, leading to a tear at the origin of the innominate artery. Horizontal deceleration causes shear at the aortic isthmus, the junction between the relatively mobile arch and the fixed descending aorta (205–207). Aortic injury can result in rupture, medial tear, and intramural hematoma or only intimal disruption. Rupture of the thoracic aorta causes immediate death in 75% to 90% of patients. Patients with contained ruptures have an unpredictable course, with up to 30% mortality in the first 24 hours (90,208,209). Patients with intimal flap or mural hematomas have a benign course.

Clinical Profile

Aortic rupture alone does not cause shock because it quickly leads to exsanguination and death (210). Patients who arrive at the ER have sealed their defect with a clot. These patients may have reverse coarctation as a result of injury to the origin of subclavian artery, acute pseudocoarctation with upper extremity hypertension, and increased pulse amplitude (199,211). Injury to the branches of the aortic arch can cause cerebral ischemia, but limb ischemia is rare, owing to a rich collateral supply (212–215) (see Chapter 105).

Management

In unstable patients with suspected aortic injury, the cause of bleeding should be ascertained and treated before aortic surgery is performed (208,209). In stable patients with aortic rupture, the chest radiograph can show mediastinal widening ($\geq$8 cm), a blurred aortic knob, shift of the trachea or nasogastric tube when present, a left main bronchus depressed more than 40 degrees, the presence of an apical cap sign, obliteration of the aortopulmonary window, and multiple rib or sternal fractures (216,217). These signs are present in 70% to 95% of cases (218). If the chest radiograph is abnormal, TEE or multislice CT (MSCT) is performed to confirm the diagnosis. TEE is sensitive and specific for the diagnosis of aortic intimal disruption, medial tear, and perivascular hematoma. The advantages over aortography are its bedside availability, the noninvasive nature of the study, and the ability to evaluate the heart simultaneously. However, its limitations are an occasional inability to pass the probe in patients with cervical injury, a "blind spot" (this is the 3- to 5-cm portion of upper ascending aorta that is blinded by trachea) of ascending aorta, and operator variability (219–221). MSCT scan has a high sensitivity for screening purposes and is a very useful imaging tool that is at times complementary to TEE (222–228). If TEE/MSCT shows no abnormality, the patient should be observed, and chest radiography should be repeated in 6 hours. If TEE/MSCT shows rupture of the aorta, surgery is indicated. In patients with a small intramural hematoma or a small intimal flap, conservative medical management with close follow-up is justified. Biplane aortography is no longer considered to be the gold standard because, depending on the plane of projection, tears and perivascular hematomas can be missed. It is an invasive procedure with occasional serious complications. MRI is useful in this situation because it gives an excellent definition of anatomy, including the arch vessels. If the initial chest radiograph does not show any signs of aortic injury, further management should be guided by clinical judgment (229).

In stable patients, nonoperative management of an intimal tear of the thoracic aorta or delayed operative management of a full-thickness tear in patients with multiple injuries is favored. The use of β-blockers to control shear stress medically by controlling heart rate and blood pressure appears to be effective in these patients.

Prognosis

Patients treated for thoracic aortic rupture with surgery have a risk of paraplegia (4% to 10%) (230–232). This risk is lower with distal perfusion techniques at the time of repair compared with clamp-and-sew technique (233). Brain ischemia, MI, and other end-organ damage have been reported. The overall mortality is 10% to 25% when patients reach the hospital alive.

CONTROVERSIES AND PERSONAL PERSPECTIVE

Echocardiography has established its role in ER management of stable patients with penetrating cardiac injuries. TEE has proven to be useful in management of suspected great vessel injuries and is also helpful in difficult situations to complement TTE. MSCT angiography is increasingly used in the ER and may minimize the need for diagnostic invasive angiography. The role of echocardiography remains less clear in the management of blunt trauma in patients with stable hemodynamics. Percutaneous interventions with stent grafts may find their role in the management of a subgroup of patients with thoracic great vessel injuries. The role of thoracoscopy is increasing in the management of stable patients. Comparisons of various treatment strategies from different centers can be improved if data are reported using similar injury indices.

THE FUTURE

Emergency services with a special effort for rapid patient transport to a well-equipped trauma center can save patients with serious cardiovascular trauma. The concept of fluid resuscitation in the field and in the intensive care unit keeps evolving with better understanding of pathophysiology and availability of different crystalloids, colloids, and blood substitutes. Widespread use of MSCT angiography in the ER may improve early detection and management of great vessel injuries. Endovascular stent grafts use may increase in the management of injuries to thoracic great vessels including the ascending aorta and the arch.

References

1. National Center of Health Statistics, US Department of Health and Human Services, Service PH. *Monthly vital statistics report, advance report of final mortality statistics.* 1992;43:1–76.
2. Mattox KL, Feliciano DV, Burch J, et al. Five thousand seven hundred sixty cardiovascular injuries in 4459 patients: epidemiologic evolution 1958 to 1987. *Ann Surg* 1989;209:698–705.
3. Mattox KL. Thoracic vascular trauma. *J Vasc Surg* 1988;7:725–729.
4. Symbas PN. *Cardiothoracic trauma.* Philadelphia: WB Saunders, 1989: 160–231.
5. Redelmeier DA, Tibshirani RJ. Association between cellular-telephone calls and motor vehicular collisions. *N Engl J Med* 1997;336:453–458.
6. Homer. *The Iliad,* vol 16. New York: Macmillan, 1922:line 442, 299.
7. Morgagni JB. *De sedibus et causes morborum: lipsiae sumptibus Leopoldi Vossii,* 1829.
8. Fischer G. Die Wunden des Herzens und des Hertzbeutels. *Arch Klin Chir* 1868;9:571.
9. Richardson RG. *The scalpel and the heart.* New York: Scribner, 1970:27.
10. Billroth T. Offenes Schreiben an Herr der Wittelshofer uver die erste mil gustingen susgange ausgefuhrte pylorectomie. *Wein Med Wochenschr* 1881;31:161.
11. Rehn L. Ueber Penetrerende Herzwunden und Herznaht. *Arch Klin Chir* 1897;55:315.
12. Hill LL. A report of a case of successful suturing of the heart, and table of other cases of suturing by different operators with various terminations and conclusions drawn. *Med Rec* 1902;62:846.
13. Karrel R, Shaffer MA, Franaszek JB. Emergency diagnosis, resuscitation, and treatment of acute penetrating cardiac trauma. *Ann Emerg Med* 1982; 11:504–517.
14. Symbas PN, Symbas PJ. Missiles in the cardiovascular system. *Chest Surg Clin N Am* 1997;7:343–356.
15. Pate JW, Richardson RL Jr. Penetrating wounds of cardiac valves. *JAMA* 1969;207:309–311.
16. Cha EK, Mittal V, Allaben RD. Delayed sequelae of penetrating cardiac injury. *Arch Surg* 1993;128:836–839.
17. Espada R, Whisennand HH, Mattox KL, et al. Surgical management of penetrating injuries to the coronary arteries. *Surgery* 1975;78:755–760.
18. Ivatury RR, Shah PM, Ito K, et al. Emergency room thoracotomy for the resuscitation of patients with "fatal" penetrating injuries of the heart. *Ann Thorac Surg* 1981;32:377–385.
19. Porter JM, Page R, Wood AE, et al. Ventricular perforation associated with central venous introducer-dilator systems. *Can J Anaesth* 1997;44: 317–320.
20. Demetriades D, van der Veen BW. Penetrating injuries of the heart: experience over two years in South Africa. *J Trauma* 1983;23:1034–1041.
21. Symbas PN. Traumatic heart disease. *Curr Probl Cardiol* 1982;7:3–35.
22. Rogers FB, Leavitt BJ. Upper torso cyanosis: a marker for blunt cardiac rupture. *Am J Emerg Med* 1997;15:275–276.
23. Wilson RF, Bassett JS. Penetrating wounds of the pericardium or its contents. *JAMA* 1966;195:513–518.
24. Ivatury RR, Nallathambi MN, Roberge RJ, et al. Penetrating thoracic injuries: in-field stabilization vs. prompt transport. *J Trauma* 1987;27:1066–1073.
25. Purkiss SF, Williams M, Cross FW, et al. Efficacy of urgent thoracotomy for trauma in patients attended by a helicopter emergency medical service. *J R Coll Surg Edinb* 1994;39:289–291.
26. Hopson LR, Hirsh E, Delgado J, et al. Guidelines for withholding or termination of resuscitation in prehospital traumatic cardiopulmonary arrest. *J Am Coll Surg* 2003;196:475–481.
27. Durham LA 3rd, Richardson RJ, Wall MJ Jr, et al. Emergency center thoracotomy: impact of prehospital resuscitation. *J Trauma* 1992;32:775–779.
28. Bickell WH, Wall MJ Jr, Pepe PE, et al. Immediate versus delayed fluid resuscitation for hypotensive patients with penetrating torso injuries. *N Engl J Med* 1994;331:1105–1109.
29. Fowler R, Pepe PE. Prehospital care of the patient with major trauma. *Emerg Med Clin North Am* 2002;20:953–974.
30. Henderson VJ, Smith RS, Fry WR, et al. Cardiac injuries: analysis of an unselected series of 251 cases. *J Trauma* 1994;36:341–348.
31. Kavolius J, Golocovsky M, Champion HR. Predictors of outcome in patients who have sustained trauma and who undergo emergency thoracotomy. *Arch Surg* 1993;128:1158–1162.
32. Mattox KL, Beall AC Jr, Jordan GL Jr, et al. Cardiorrhaphy in the emergency center. *J Thorac Cardiovasc Surg* 1974;68:886–895.
33. Blake DP, Gisbert VL, Ney AL, et al. Survival after emergency department versus operating room thoracotomy for penetrating cardiac injuries. *Am Surg* 1992;58:329–332.
34. Attar S, Suter CM, Hankins JR, et al. Penetrating cardiac injuries. *Ann Thorac Surg* 1991;51:711–715; discussion 715–716.
35. Ivatury RR, Rohman M, Steichen FM, et al. Penetrating cardiac injuries: twenty-year experience. Am Surg 1987;53:310–317.
36. Macho JR, Markison RE, Schecter WP. Cardiac stapling in the management of penetrating injuries of the heart: rapid control of hemorrhage and decreased risk of personal contamination. *J Trauma* 1993;34:711–715.

37. Gao JM, Gao YH, Wei GB, et al. Penetrating cardiac wounds: principles for surgical management. *World J Surg* 2004;28:1025–1029.
38. Feliciano DV, Moore EE, Mattox KL, eds. *Trauma*. Stamford, CT: Appleton & Lange, 1996.
39. Bolton JW, Bynoe RP, Lazar HL, et al. Two-dimensional echocardiography in the evaluation of penetrating intrapericardial injuries. *Ann Thorac Surg* 1993;56:506–509.
40. Jimenez E, Martin M, Krukenkamp I, et al. Subxiphoid pericardiotomy versus echocardiography: a prospective evaluation of the diagnosis of occult penetrating cardiac injury. *Surgery* 1990;108:676–679.
41. Rozycki GS, Feliciano DV, Ochsner MG, et al. The role of ultrasound in patients with possible penetrating cardiac wounds: a prospective multicenter study. *J Trauma* 1999;46:543–551.
42. Meyer DM, Jessen ME, Grayburn PA. Use of echocardiography to detect occult cardiac injury after penetrating thoracic trauma: a prospective study. *J Trauma* 1995;39:902–907.
43. Mollod M, Felner JM. Transesophageal echocardiography in the evaluation of cardiothoracic trauma. *Am Heart J* 1996;132:841–849.
44. Catoire P, Orliaguet G, Liu N, et al. Systematic transesophageal echocardiography for detection of mediastinal lesions in patients with multiple injuries. *J Trauma* 1995;38:96–102.
45. Chirillo F, Totis O, Cavarzerani A, et al. Usefulness of transthoracic and transoesophageal echocardiography in recognition and management of cardiovascular injuries after blunt chest trauma. *Heart* 1996;75:301–306.
46. Pearson GD, Karr SS, Trachiotis GD, et al. A retrospective review of the role of transesophageal echocardiography in aortic and cardiac trauma in a level I pediatric trauma center. *J Am Soc Echocardiogr* 1997;10:946–955.
47. Andrade-Alegre R, Mon L. Subxiphoid pericardial window in the diagnosis of penetrating cardiac trauma. *Ann Thorac Surg* 1994;58:1139–1141.
48. Miller FB, Bond SJ, Shumate CR, et al. Diagnostic pericardial window: a safe alternative to exploratory thoracotomy for suspected heart injuries. *Arch Surg* 1987;122:605–609.
49. Brewster SA, Thirlby RC, Snyder WH. Subxiphoid pericardial window and penetrating cardiac trauma. *Arch Surg* 1988;123:937–941.
50. Duncan AO, Scalea TM, Sclafani SJ, et al. Evaluation of occult cardiac injuries using subxiphoid pericardial window. *J Trauma* 1989;29:955–959.
51. Symbas NP, Bongiorno PF, Symbas PN. Blunt cardiac rupture: the utility of emergency department ultrasound. *Ann Thorac Surg* 1999;67:1274–1276.
52. Nagy KK, Lohmann C, Kim DO, et al. Role of echocardiography in the diagnosis of occult penetrating cardiac injury. *J Trauma* 1995;38:859–862.
53. Mandavia DP, Hoffner RJ, Mahaney K, et al. Bedside echocardiography by emergency physicians. *Ann Emerg Med* 2001;38:377–382.
54. Morales CH, Salinas CM, Henao CA, et al. Thoracoscopic pericardial window and penetrating cardiac trauma. *J Trauma* 1997;42:273–275.
55. Hassett A, Moran J, Sabiston DC, et al. Utility of echocardiography in the management of patients with penetrating missile wounds of the heart. *J Am Coll Cardiol* 1986;7:1151–1156.
56. Font VE, Gill CC, Lammermeier DE. Echocardiographically guided removal of an intracardiac foreign body. *Cleve Clin J Med* 1994;61:228–231.
57. Mazzei WJ, Burzynski M. Transesophageal echocardiographic monitoring of an intraventricular foreign body. *J Cardiothorac Anesth* 1989;3:84–86.
58. Fry SJ, Picard MH, Tseng JF, et al. The echocardiographic diagnosis, characterization, and extraction guidance of cardiac foreign bodies. *J Am Soc Echocardiogr* 2000;13:232–239.
59. Porembka DT, Johnson DJ 2nd, Hoit BD, et al. Penetrating cardiac trauma: a perioperative role for transesophageal echocardiography. *Anesth Analg* 1993;77:1275–1277.
60. Mattox KL, Limacher MC, Feliciano DV, et al. Cardiac evaluation following heart injury. *J Trauma* 1985;25:758–765.
61. Plummer D, Brunette D, Asinger R, et al. Emergency department echocardiography improves outcome in penetrating cardiac injury. *Ann Emerg Med* 1992;21:709–712.
62. Rozycki GS, Feliciano DV, Schmidt JA, et al. The role of surgeon-performed ultrasound in patients with possible cardiac wounds. *Ann Surg* 1996;223:737–744.
63. Demetriades D, Rabinowitz B, Sofianos C. Emergency room thoracotomy for stab wounds to the chest and neck. *J Trauma* 1987;27:483–485.
64. Tyburski JG, Astra L, Wilson RF, et al. Factors affecting prognosis with penetrating wounds of the heart. *J Trauma* 2000;48:587–590.
65. Wall MJ Jr, Mattox KL, Chen CD, et al. Acute management of complex cardiac injuries. *J Trauma* 1997;42:905–912.
66. Wait MA, Mueller M, Barth MJ, et al. Traumatic coronary sinocameral fistula from a penetrating cardiac injury: case report and review of the literature. *J Trauma* 1994;36:894–897.
67. Harris DG, Papagiannopoulos KA, Pretorius J, et al. Current evaluation of cardiac stab wounds. *Ann Thorac Surg* 1999;68:2119–2122.
68. Asensio JA, Murray J, Demetriades D, et al. Penetrating cardiac injuries: a prospective study of variables predicting outcomes. *J Am Coll Surg* 1998;186:24–34.
69. Kaplan AJ, Norcross ED, Crawford FA. Predictors of mortality in penetrating cardiac injury. *Am Surg* 1993;59:338–341.
70. Moreno C, Moore EE, Majure JA, et al. Pericardial tamponade: a critical determinant for survival following penetrating cardiac wounds. *J Trauma* 1986;26:821–825.
71. Schwengel RH, Bennett SK, Sequeira AJ, et al. Late presentation of left ventricular pseudoaneurysm and ventricular septal defect after surgery for penetrating cardiac injury. *Am Heart J* 1994;127:930–932.
72. Symbas PN, DiOrio DA, Tyras DH, et al. Penetrating cardiac wounds: significant residual and delayed sequelae. *J Thorac Cardiovasc Surg* 1973;66:526–532.
73. Wilson WR, Coyne JT, Greer GE. Mitral regurgitation as a late sequela of penetrating cardiac trauma. *J Heart Valve Dis* 1997;6:171–173.
74. Scott CH, Ferrari VA, Mittal S, et al. Diagnosis of a persistent coronary fistula after ventricular septal defect patch closure. *J Am Soc Echocardiogr* 1997;10:573–575.
75. Duque HA, Florez LE, Moreno A, et al. Penetrating cardiac trauma: follow-up study including electrocardiography, echocardiography, and functional test. *World J Surg* 1999;23:1254–1257.
76. Demetriades D, Charalambides C, Sareli P, et al. Late sequelae of penetrating cardiac injuries. *Br J Surg* 1990;77:813–814.
77. Swierzewski MJ, Feliciano DV, Lillis RP, et al. Deaths from motor vehicle crashes: patterns of injury in restrained and unrestrained victims. *J Trauma* 1994;37:404–407.
78. Arajarvi E. A retrospective analysis of chest injuries in 280 seat belt wearers. *Accident Anal Prev* 1988;20:251–259.
79. Arajarvi E, Santavirta S, Tolonen J. Aortic ruptures in seat belt wearers. *J Thorac Cardiovasc Surg* 1989;98:355–361.
80. Arajarvi E, Santavirta S. Chest injuries sustained in severe traffic accidents by seatbelt wearers. *J Trauma* 1989;29:37–41.
81. Lancaster GI, DeFrance JH, Borruso JJ. Air-bag-associated rupture of the right atrium [letter]. *N Engl J Med* 1993;328.
82. Symbas PN. Contusion of the heart. In: Symbas PN, ed. *Cardiothoracic trauma*. Philadelphia: WB Saunders, 1989:55–76.
83. Sybrandy KC, Cramer MJ, Burgersdijk C. Diagnosing cardiac contusion: old wisdom and new insights. *Heart* 2003;89:485–489.
84. RuDusky BM. More on myocardial contusion: with additional insight on myocardial concussion. *Chest* 1997;112:570–572.
85. Tenzer ML. The spectrum of myocardial contusion: a review. *J Trauma* 1985;25:620–627.
86. Mattox KL, Flint LM, Carrico CJ, et al. Blunt cardiac injury [editorial]. *J Trauma* 1992;33:649–650.
87. Maron BJ, Poliac LC, Kaplan JA, et al. Blunt impact to the chest leading to sudden death from cardiac arrest during sports activities. *N Engl J Med* 1995;333:337–342.
88. Pontillo D, Capezzuto A, Achilli A, et al. Bifascicular block complicating blunt cardiac injury: a case report and review of the literature. *Angiology* 1994;45:883–890.
89. Saunders CR, Doty DB. Myocardial contusion. *Surg Gynecol Obstet* 1977;144:595–603.
90. Parmley LF, Manion WC, Mattingly TW. Nonpenetrating traumatic injury to the heart. *Circulation* 1958;18:371–396.
91. McLean RF, Devitt JH, Dubbin J, et al. Incidence of abnormal RNA studies and dysrhythmias in patients with blunt chest trauma. *J Trauma* 1991;31:968–970.
92. Doty DB, Anderson AE, Rose EF, et al. Cardiac trauma: clinical and experimental correlations of myocardial contusion. *Ann Surg* 1974;180:452–460.
93. Sutherland GR, Cheung HW, Holliday RL, et al. Hemodynamic adaptation to acute myocardial contusion complicating blunt chest injury. *Am J Cardiol* 1986;57:291–297.
94. Link MS, Maron BJ, Wang PJ, et al. Reduced risk of sudden death from chest wall blows (commotio cordis) with safety baseballs. *Pediatrics* 2002;109:873–877.
95. Link MS, Maron BJ, Wang PJ, et al. Upper and lower limits of vulnerability to sudden arrhythmic death with chest-wall impact (commotio cordis). *J Am Coll Cardiol* 2003;41:99–104.
96. Maron BJ, Gohman TE, Kyle SB, et al. Clinical profile and spectrum of commotio cordis. *JAMA* 2002;287:1142–1146.
97. Maron BJ, Estes NA 3rd, Link MS. Task Force 11: commotio cordis. *J Am Coll Cardiol* 2005;45:1371–1373.
97a. Moore FA, McKinley BA, Moore EE. The next generation in shock resuscitation. *Lancet* 2004;363:1988–1996.
98. Saunders CR, Doty DB. Myocardial contusion: effect of intra-aortic balloon counterpulsation on cardiac output. *J Trauma* 1978;18:706–708.
99. Mori F, Zuppiroli A, Ognibene A, et al. Cardiac contusion in blunt chest trauma: a combined study of transesophageal echocardiography and cardiac troponin I determination. *Ital Heart J* 2001;2:222–227.
100. Dubrow TJ, Mihalka J, Eisenhauer DM, et al. Myocardial contusion in the stable patient: what level of care is appropriate?. *Surgery* 1989;106:267–273; discussion 273–274.
101. Baxter BT, Moore EE, Moore FA, et al. A plea for sensible management of myocardial contusion. *Am J Surg* 1989;158:557–561; discussion 561–562.
102. Salim A, Velmahos GC, Jindal A, et al. Clinically significant blunt cardiac trauma: role of serum troponin levels combined with electrocardiographic findings. *J Trauma* 2001;50:237–243.

103. Collins JN, Cole FJ, Weireter LJ, et al. The usefulness of serum troponin levels in evaluating cardiac injury. *Am Surg* 2001;67:821–825; discussion 825–826.
104. Edouard AR, Felten ML, Hebert JL, et al. Incidence and significance of cardiac troponin I release in severe trauma patients. *Anesthesiology* 2004; 101:1262–1268.
105. Velmahos GC, Karaiskakis M, Salim A, et al. Normal electrocardiography and serum troponin I levels preclude the presence of clinically significant blunt cardiac injury. *J Trauma* 2003;54:45–50; discussion 50–51.
106. Sturaitis M, McCallum D, Sutherland G, et al. Lack of significant long-term sequelae following traumatic myocardial contusion. *Arch Intern Med* 1986;146:1765–1769.
107. Santavirta S, Arajarvi E. Ruptures of the heart in seatbelt wearers. *J Trauma* 1992;32:275–279.
108. Rodriguez A, Ong A. Delayed rupture of a left ventricular aneurysm after blunt trauma. *Am Surg* 2005;71:250–251.
109. Kato K, Kushimoto S, Mashiko K, et al. Blunt traumatic rupture of the heart: an experience in Tokyo. *J Trauma* 1994;36:859–863.
110. Moront M, Lefrak EA, Akl BF. Traumatic rupture of the interventricular septum and tricuspid valve: case report. *J Trauma* 1991;31:134–136.
111. Rollins MD, Koehler RP, Stevens MH, et al. Traumatic ventricular septal defect: case report and review of the English literature since 1970. *J Trauma* 2005;58:175–180.
112. Rao G, Garvey J, Gupta M, et al. Atrial septal defect due to blunt thoracic trauma. *J Trauma* 1977;17:405–406.
113. Fulda G, Brathwaite CE, Rodriguez A, et al. Blunt traumatic rupture of the heart and pericardium: a ten-year experience (1979–1989). *J Trauma* 1991;31:167–172.
114. Bauriedel G, Redel DA, Schmitz C, et al. Transcatheter closure of a post-traumatic ventricular septal defect with an Amplatzer occluder device. *Cathet Cardiovasc Interv* 2001;53:508–512.
115. Shalaby RI, Rajendran U, Regunathan R. Blunt traumatic rupture of the heart: case report and selected review. *Ann Thorac Cardiovasc Surg* 1999;5:123–129.
116. Fulton JO, Nel L, de Groot KM, et al. Blunt cardiac rupture. *S Afr J Surg* 1998;36:132–135.
117. Calhoon JH, Hoffmann TH, Trinkle JK, et al. Management of blunt rupture of the heart. *J Trauma* 1986;26:495–502.
118. Janson JT, Harris DG, Pretorius J, et al. Pericardial rupture and cardiac herniation after blunt chest trauma. *Ann Thorac Surg* 2003;75:581–582.
119. Carrillo EH, Heniford BT, Dykes JR, et al. Cardiac herniation producing tamponade: the critical role of early diagnosis. *J Trauma* 1997;43:19–23.
120. Meng RL, Straus A, Milloy F, et al. Intrapericardial diaphragmatic hernia in adults. *Ann Surg* 1979;189:359–366.
121. Jiang CL, Gu TX, Zhang ZW, et al. Diagnosis and treatment of traumatic tricuspid valve insufficiency. *Chin J Traumatol* 2003;6:379–381.
122. Bailey PL, Peragallo R, Karwande SV, et al. Mitral and tricuspid valve rupture after moderate blunt chest trauma. *Ann Thorac Surg* 2000;69:616–618.
123. Rumisek JD, Robinowitz M, Virmani R, et al. Bioprosthetic heart valve rupture associated with trauma. *J Trauma* 1986;26:276–279.
124. van Son JA, Danielson GK, Schaff HV, et al. Traumatic tricuspid valve insufficiency: experience in thirteen patients. *J Thorac Cardiovasc Surg* 1994;108:893–898.
125. Bayezid O, Mete A, Turkay C, et al. Traumatic tricuspid insufficiency following blunt chest trauma. *J Cardiovasc Surg* 1993;34:69–71.
126. Chiu WC, Shindler DM, Scholz PM, et al. Traumatic tricuspid regurgitation with cyanosis: diagnosis by transesophageal echocardiography. *Ann Thorac Surg* 1996;61:992–993.
127. Holper K, Hahnel C, Augustin N, et al. Operative correction of traumatic tricuspid insufficiency. *Herz* 1996;21:172–178.
128. Kleikamp G, Schnepper U, Kortke H, et al. Tricuspid valve regurgitation following blunt thoracic trauma. *Chest* 1992;102:1294–1296.
129. Linka A, Ritter M, Turina M, et al. Acute tricuspid papillary muscle rupture following blunt chest trauma. *Am Heart J* 1992;124:799–802.
130. Ronan JA Jr, Steelman RB, DeLeon AC Jr, et al. The clinical diagnosis of acute severe mitral insufficiency. *Am J Cardiol* 1971;27:284–290.
131. Petkov MP, Napolitano CA, Tobler HG, et al. A rupture of both atrioventricular valves after blunt chest trauma: the usefulness of transesophageal echocardiography for a life-saving diagnosis. *Anesth Analg* 2005;100: 1256–1258.
132. Dontigny L, Baillot R, Panneton J, et al. Surgical repair of traumatic tricuspid insufficiency: report of three cases. *J Trauma* 1992;33:266–269.
133. Leung DY, Griffin BP, Stewart WJ, et al. Left ventricular function after valve repair for chronic mitral regurgitation: predictive value of preoperative assessment of contractile reserve by exercise echocardiography. *J Am Coll Cardiol* 1996;28:1198–1205.
134. Banzo I, Montero A, Uriarte I, et al. Coronary artery occlusion and myocardial infarction: a seldom encountered complication of blunt chest trauma. *Clin Nucl Med* 1999;24:94–96.
135. Patel R, Samaha FF. Right coronary artery occlusion caused by blunt trauma. *J Invas Cardiol* 2000;12:376–378.
136. Liedtke AJ, Allen RP, Nellis SH. Effects of blunt cardiac trauma on coronary vasomotion, perfusion, myocardial mechanics, and metabolism. *J Trauma* 1980;20:777–785.
137. Ginzburg E, Dygert J, Parra-Davila E, et al. Coronary artery stenting for occlusive dissection after blunt chest trauma. *J Trauma* 1998;45:157–161.
138. Andrews CJ, Darveniza M. Telephone-mediated lightning injury: an Australian survey. *J Trauma* 1989;29:665–671.
139. Eriksson A, Ornehult L. Death by lightning. *Am J Forensic Med Pathol* 1988;9:295–300.
140. James TN, Riddick L, Embry JH. Cardiac abnormalities demonstrated postmortem in four cases of accidental electrocution and their potential significance relative to nonfatal electrical injuries of the heart. *Am Heart J* 1990;120:143–157.
141. Thompson JC, Ashwal S. Electrical injuries in children. *Am J Dis Child* 1983;137:231–235.
142. Chandra NC, Siu CO, Munster AM. Clinical predictors of myocardial damage after high voltage electrical injury. *Crit Care Med* 1990;18:293–297.
143. Ku CS, Lin SL, Hsu TL, et al. Myocardial damage associated with electrical injury. *Am Heart J* 1989;118:621–624.
144. Xenopoulos N, Movahed A, Hudson P, et al. Myocardial injury in electrocution. *Am Heart J* 1991;122:1481–1484.
145. Guler N, Ozkara C, Tuncer M, et al. Aortic valve rupture due to high-voltage electrical injury: case report. *J Heart Valve Dis* 2004;13:857–859.
146. Taussig HB. "Death" from lightning and the possibility of living again. *Am Sci* 1969;57:306–316.
147. Cooper MA. Lightning injuries: prognostic signs for death. *Ann Emerg Med* 1980;9:134–138.
148. Cooper MA. Lightning injuries. *Emerg Med Clin North Am* 1983;1:639–641.
149. Kirchmer JT Jr, Larson DL, Tyson KR. Cardiac rupture following electrical injury. *J Trauma* 1977;17:389–391.
150. Carleton SC. Cardiac problems associated with electrical injury. *Cardiol Clin* 1995;13:263–266.
151. Purdue GF, Hunt JL. Electrocardiographic monitoring after electrical injury: necessity or luxury. *J Trauma* 1986;26:166–167.
152. Solem L, Fischer RP, Strate RG. The natural history of electrical injury. *J Trauma* 1977;17:487–492.
153. Bernstein T. Electrical injury: electrical engineer's perspective and an historical review. *Ann N Y Acad Sci* 1994;720:1–10.
154. Kleiner JP, Wilkin JH. Cardiac effects of lightning stroke. *JAMA* 1978; 240:2757–2759.
155. McGill MP, Kamp TJ, Rahko PS. High-voltage injury resulting in permanent right heart dysfunction. *Chest* 1999;115:586–587.
156. Homma S, Gillam LD, Weyman AE. Echocardiographic observations in survivors of acute electrical injury. *Chest* 1990;97:103–105.
157. Warren S. Effects of radiation on the cardiovascular system. *Arch Pathol* 1942;34:1070–1079.
158. Leach JE. Effect of roentgen therapy on the heart: a clinical study. *Arch Intern Med* 1943;72:715–745.
159. Vallebona A. Cardiac damage following therapeutic chest irradiation: importance, evaluation and treatment. *Minerva Cardioangiol* 2000;48:79–87.
160. Lipshultz SE, Sallan SE. Cardiovascular abnormalities in long-term survivors of childhood malignancy [editorial]. *J Clin Oncol* 1993;11:1199–1203.
161. Jakacki RI, Goldwein JW, Larsen RL, et al. Cardiac dysfunction following spinal irradiation during childhood. *J Clin Oncol* 1993;11:1033–1038.
162. Gaya AM, Ashford RF. Cardiac complications of radiation therapy. *Clin Oncol (R Coll Radiol)* 2005;17:153–159.
163. Glanzmann C, Huguenin P, Lutolf UM, et al. Cardiac lesions after mediastinal irradiation for Hodgkin's disease. *Radiother Oncol* 1994;30:43–54.
164. Zinzani PL, Gherlinzoni F, Piovaccari G, et al. Cardiac injury as late toxicity of mediastinal radiation therapy for Hodgkin's disease patients. *Haematologica* 1996;81:132–137.
165. Prosnitz RG, Chen YH, Marks LB. Cardiac toxicity following thoracic radiation. *Semin Oncol* 2005;32:S71–80.
166. Kreuser ED, Voller H, Behles C, et al. Evaluation of late cardiotoxicity with pulsed Doppler echocardiography in patients treated for Hodgkin's disease. *Br J Haematol* 1993;84:615–622.
167. Corn BW, Trock BJ, Goodman RL. Irradiation-related ischemic heart disease. *J Clin Oncol* 1990;8:741–750.
168. Applefeld MM, Wiernik PH. Cardiac disease after radiation therapy for Hodgkin's disease: analysis of 48 patients. *Am J Cardiol* 1983;51:1679–1681.
169. Arsenian MA. Cardiovascular sequelae of therapeutic thoracic radiation. *Prog Cardiovasc Dis* 1991;33:299–311.
170. Gottdiener JS, Katin MJ, Borer JS, et al. Late cardiac effects of therapeutic mediastinal irradiation: assessment by echocardiography and radionuclide angiography. *N Engl J Med* 1983;308:569–572.
171. Mittal S, Berko B, Bavaria J, et al. Radiation-induced cardiovascular dysfunction. *Am J Cardiol* 1996;78:114–115.
172. Gustavsson A, Eskilsson J, Landberg T, et al. Late cardiac effects after mantle radiotherapy in patients with Hodgkin's disease. *Ann Oncol* 1990;1:355–363.
173. Pohjola-Sintonen S, Totterman KJ, Salmo M, et al. Late cardiac effects of mediastinal radiotherapy in patients with Hodgkin's disease. *Cancer* 1987;60:31–37.

174. Knight CJ, Sutton GC. Complete heart block and severe tricuspid regurgitation after radiotherapy: case report and review of the literature. *Chest* 1995;108:1748–1751.
175. Cohen SI, Bharati S, Glass J, et al. Radiotherapy as a cause of complete atrioventricular block in Hodgkin's disease: an electrophysiological-pathological correlation. *Arch Intern Med* 1981;141:676–679.
176. Om A, Ellahham S, Vetrovec GW. Radiation-induced coronary artery disease. *Am Heart J* 1992;124:1598–1602.
177. Brosius FC, Waller BF, Roberts WC. Radiation heart disease: analysis of 16 young (aged 15 to 33 years) necropsy patients who received over 3,500 rads to the heart. *Am J Med* 1981;70:519–530.
178. Boivin JF, Hutchison GB, Lubin JH, et al. Coronary artery disease mortality in patients treated for Hodgkin's disease. *Cancer* 1992;69:1241–1247.
179. McEniery PT, Dorosti K, Schiavone WA, et al. Clinical and angiographic features of coronary artery disease after chest irradiation. *Am J Cardiol* 1987;60:1020–1024.
180. McReynolds RA, Gold GL, Roberts WC. Coronary heart disease after mediastinal irradiation for Hodgkin's disease. *Am J Med* 1976;60:39–45.
181. Fajardo LF, Stewart JR, Cohn KE. Morphology of radiation-induced heart disease. *Arch Pathol* 1968;86:512–519.
181a. Yeh ET, Tong AT, Lenihan DJ, et al. Cardiovascular complications of cancer therapy: diagnosis, pathogenesis, and management. *Circulation* 2004;109:3122–3131.
182. Hancock SL, Tucker MA, Hoppe RT. Factors affecting late mortality from heart disease after treatment of Hodgkin's disease. *JAMA* 1993;270:1949–1955.
183. Williams DO, Sharaf BL. Intracoronary radiation: it keeps on glowing. *Circulation* 2000;101:350–351.
184. Taylor AJ, Gorman PD, Farb A, et al. Long-term coronary vascular response to (32)P beta-particle-emitting stents in a canine model. *Circulation* 1999;100:2366–2372.
185. Davis GK, Au J, Roberts D. Myocardial perforation associated with the use of the Gensini ventriculography catheter. *Int J Cardiol* 1996;53:103–106.
186. Katta S, Akosah K, Stambler B, et al. Atrioventricular fistula: an unusual complication of endomyocardial biopsy in a heart transplant recipient. *J Am Soc Echocardiogr* 1994;7:405–409.
187. Flynn MS, Aguirre FV, Donohue TJ, et al. Conservative management of guidewire coronary artery perforation with pericardial effusion during angioplasty for acute inferior myocardial infarction. *Cathet Cardiovasc Diagn* 1993;29:285–288.
188. Von Sohsten R, Kopistansky C, Cohen M, et al. Cardiac tamponade in the "new device" era: evaluation of 6999 consecutive percutaneous coronary interventions. *Am Heart J* 2000;140:279–283.
189. Manga P, Singh S, Brandis S. Left ventricular perforation during percutaneous balloon mitral valvuloplasty. *Cathet Cardiovasc Diagn* 1992;25:317–319.
190. Ingle RJ. Rare complications of vascular access devices. *Semin Oncol Nurs* 1995;11:184–193.
191. Reese JC. Cardiac tamponade caused by central venous catheter perforation of the heart: a preventable complication [letter]. *J Am Coll Surg* 1996;182:558.
192. Morgan CD, Marshall SA, Ross JR. Catheter drainage of the pericardium: its safety and efficacy. *Can J Surg* 1989;32:331–334.
193. Thakur RK, Klein GJ, Yee R, et al. Complications of radiofrequency catheter ablation: a review. *Can J Cardiol* 1994;10:835–839.
194. Gavant ML, Flick P, Menke P, et al. CT aortography of thoracic aortic rupture. *AJR Am J Roentgenol* 1996;166:955–961.
195. Childs D, Wilkes RG. Puncture of the ascending aorta: a complication of subclavian venous cannulation [letter]. *Anaesthesia* 1986;41:331–332.
196. Feliciano DV, Mattox KL, Graham JM, et al. Major complications of percutaneous subclavian vein catheters. *Am J Surg* 1979;138:869–874.
197. Pape LA, Haffajee CI, Markis JE, et al. Fatal pulmonary hemorrhage after use of the flow-directed balloon-tipped catheter. *Ann Intern Med* 1979;90:344–347.
198. Divekar A, Gaamangwe T, Shaikh N, et al. Cardiac perforation after device closure of atrial septal defects with the Amplatzer septal occluder. *J Am Coll Cardiol* 2005;45:1213–1218.
199. Calhoon JH, Grover FL, Trinkle JK. Chest trauma: approach and management. *Clin Chest Med* 1992;13:55–67.
200. Alkadhi H, Wildermuth S, Desbiolles L, et al. Vascular emergencies of the thorax after blunt and iatrogenic trauma: multi-detector row CT and three-dimensional imaging. *Radiographics* 2004;24:1239–1255.
201. Arora R, Trehan V, Rangasetty UM, et al. Transcatheter closure of ruptured sinus of Valsalva aneurysm. *J Interv Cardiol* 2004;17:53–58.
202. Strassman G. Traumatic rupture of aorta. *Am Heart J* 1947;33:508.
203. Parmley LF, Mattingly TW, Manion WC. Nonpenetrating traumatic injury of the aorta. *Circulation* 1958;17:1086.
204. Baker PB, Keyhani-Rofagha S, Graham RL, et al. Dissecting hematoma (aneurysm) of coronary arteries. *Am J Med* 1986;80:317–319.
205. Feczko JD, Lynch L, Pless JE, et al. An autopsy case review of 142 nonpenetrating (blunt) injuries of the aorta. *J Trauma* 1992;33:846–849.
206. Hunt JP, Baker CC, Lentz CW, et al. Thoracic aorta injuries: management and outcome of 144 patients. *J Trauma* 1996;40:547–555.
207. Ben-Menachem Y. Rupture of the thoracic aorta by broadside impacts in road traffic and other collisions: further angiographic observations and preliminary autopsy findings. *J Trauma* 1993;35:363–367.
208. Kipfer B, Leupi F, Schuepbach P, et al. Acute traumatic rupture of the thoracic aorta: immediate or delayed surgical repair? *Eur J Cardiothorac Surg* 1994;8:30–33.
209. Pate JW, Fabian TC, Walker W. Traumatic rupture of the aortic isthmus: an emergency?. *World J Surg* 1995;19:119–125.
210. Martin SK, Shatney CH, Sherck JP, et al. Blunt trauma patients with prehospital pulseless electrical activity (PEA): poor ending assured. *J Trauma* 2002;53:876–880; discussion 880–881.
211. Symbas PN, Tyras DH, Ware RE, et al. Rupture of the aorta: a diagnostic triad. *Ann Thorac Surg* 1973;15:405–410.
212. George SJ. Transoesophageal echocardiography in chest trauma [letter]. *Br J Anaesth* 1996;76:336–337.
213. Cogbill TH, Moore EE, Meissner M, et al. The spectrum of blunt injury to the carotid artery: a multicenter perspective. *J Trauma* 1994;37:473–479.
214. Rosenberg JM, Bredenberg CE, Marvasti MA, et al. Blunt injuries to the aortic arch vessels. *Ann Thorac Surg* 1989;48:508–513.
215. Johnson SF, Johnson SB, Strodel WE, et al. Brachial plexus injury: association with subclavian and axillary vascular trauma. *J Trauma* 1991;31:1546–1550.
216. Gundry SR, Williams S, Burney RE, et al. Indications for aortography in blunt thoracic trauma: a reassessment. *J Trauma* 1982;22:664–671.
217. Burney RE, Gundry SR, Mackenzie JR, et al. Chest roentgenograms in diagnosis of traumatic rupture of the aorta: observer variation in interpretation. *Chest* 1984;85:605–609.
218. Smith MD, Cassidy JM, Souther S, et al. Transesophageal echocardiography in the diagnosis of traumatic rupture of the aorta. *N Engl J Med* 1995;332:356–362.
219. Sparks MB, Burchard KW, Marrin CA, et al. Transesophageal echocardiography: preliminary results in patients with traumatic aortic rupture. *Arch Surg* 1991;126:711–713; discussion 713–714.
220. Saletta S, Lederman E, Fein S, et al. Transesophageal echocardiography for the initial evaluation of the widened mediastinum in trauma patients. *J Trauma* 1995;39:137–141.
221. Vlahakes GJ, Warren RL. Traumatic rupture of the aorta [editorial]. *N Engl J Med* 1995;332:389–390.
222. Feliciano DV, Rozycki GS. Advances in the diagnosis and treatment of thoracic trauma. *Surg Clin North Am* 1999;79:1417–1429.
223. Madayag MA, Kirshenbaum KJ, Nadimpalli SR, et al. Thoracic aortic trauma: role of dynamic CT. *Radiology* 1991;179:853–855.
224. Raptopoulos V. Chest CT for aortic injury: maybe not for everyone. *AJR Am J Roentgenol* 1994;162:1053–1055.
225. Agee CK, Metzler MH, Churchill RJ, et al. Computed tomographic evaluation to exclude traumatic aortic disruption. *J Trauma* 1992;33:876–881.
226. Durham RM, Zuckerman D, Wolverson M, et al. Computed tomography as a screening exam in patients with suspected blunt aortic injury. *Ann Surg* 1994;220:699–704.
227. Tomiak MM, Rosenblum JD, Messersmith RN, et al. Use of CT for diagnosis of traumatic rupture of the thoracic aorta. *Ann Vasc Surg* 1993;7:130–139.
228. LeBlang SD, Dolich MO. Imaging of penetrating thoracic trauma. *J Thorac Imaging* 2000;15:128–135.
229. Pretre R, Chilcott M. Blunt trauma to the heart and great vessels. *N Engl J Med* 1997;336:626–632.
230. Mauney MC, Tribble CG, Cope JT, et al. Is clamp and sew still viable for thoracic aortic resection?. *Ann Surg* 1996;223:534–540.
231. von Oppell UO, Dunne TT, De Groot KM, et al. Spinal cord protection in the absence of collateral circulation: meta-analysis of mortality and paraplegia. *J Card Surg* 1994;9:685–691.
232. Von Oppell UO, Brink J, Hewitson J, et al. Acute traumatic rupture of the thoracic aorta: a comparison of techniques. *S Afr J Surg* 1996;34:19–24.
233. Jahromi AS, Kazemi K, Safar HA, et al. Traumatic rupture of the thoracic aorta: cohort study and systematic review. *J Vasc Surg* 2001;34:1029–1034.
234. Pickens JJ, Copass MK, Bulger EM. Trauma patients receiving CPR: predictors of survival. *J Trauma* 2005;58:951–958.

CHAPTER 39 ■ CARDIAC TUMORS

ALLEN BURKE, JEAN JEUDY JR, AND RENU VIRMANI

OVERVIEW

Cardiac masses can be considered in three groups: nonneoplastic masses, such as mural thrombi, which can mimic neoplasms; primary neoplasms, either benign or malignant; and metastatic tumors, which may be endocardially based, simulating primary lesions. In surgical series, primary lesions are by far the most common. In autopsy series that include incidental cardiac or pericardial deposits, metastatic tumors are much more common. Pediatric cardiac tumors comprise a group of hamartomatous lesions that are best considered separately, because many of these tumors do not occur in adults and have no extracardiac counterparts; they are not discussed in this chapter.

The type of tumor expected in the heart varies greatly by patient age (Table 39.1) and site in the heart (Table 39.2). Overall, myxoma is by far the most common primary cardiac tumor.

The estimated frequency of primary cardiac neoplasms, based on population estimates, ranges from 0.0017% to 0.33% (1). Primary tumors may arise in adults most frequently from the endocardium, followed by the cardiac muscle, and, most infrequently, the pericardium. Interestingly, the rate of metastatic lesions is the reverse: the pericardium is by the most common site especially for epithelial malignancies, with endocardial lesions common only for those tumors growing into the great veins.

Echocardiography has the best spatial and temporal resolution of the cardiac imaging modalities, and it provides excellent anatomic and functional information (2,3). It is the optimal imaging modality for imaging small masses (<1 cm) or masses arising from valves. Echocardiography can image velocities with Doppler, which allows for assessment of presence, degree, and location of obstructions to blood flow or valve regurgitation. Magnetic resonance imaging (MRI) has the highest soft tissue contrast of the imaging modalities, and this property makes it the most sensitive modality for detection of tumor infiltration; it is also more manipulable than other imaging modalities (4). For example, a T2-weighted standard or fast spin echo sequence distinguishes tumors with high water content, such as hemangioma, from tumors with low water content, such as fibroma. MRI can characterize tumor vascularity with intravenous contrast and permits assessment of wall motion allowing for characterization of ventricular function, inflow or outflow obstruction, and valve regurgitation. Electrocardiographic (ECG)-gated CT scans with multidetector scanners or electron beam scanners are also very useful for cardiac imaging. The advantages and disadvantages of CT are intermediate between those of echocardiography and MRI (5). CT scanners have spatial resolution, better than that of MRI, but not as high echocardiography. CT has better soft tissue contrast than echocardiography and can be used to characterize fatty content and calcifications (Fig. 39.1) definitively; however, the overall soft tissue contrast and the ability to characterize tumor infiltration and tumor type are less than those of MRI. Catheterization provides indirect and nonspecific imaging based on filling defects within the cardiac chambers (6), allows endomyocardial biopsy for biopsy, and provides selective coronary angiography before surgical resection of an intramyocardial tumor.

BENIGN TUMORS AND TUMOR-LIKE LESIONS

Mural Thrombi

Most mural thrombi occur in association with underlying heart disease (7) or after cardiac surgery, including mitral valve replacement or the Maze procedure. Left atrial thrombi are frequently associated with mitral valvular disease, especially mitral stenosis, and thrombi occur in either atrium in patients with atrial fibrillation (7). Mural thrombi are occasionally removed surgically and may be clinically and pathologically misdiagnosed as myxomas (8).

Mural thrombi in the absence of heart disease occur in any chamber but are most common in the right atrium (7). In the majority of patients, a coagulation defect is either suspected or documented. One of the more common coagulopathies diagnosed in patients with mural thrombi is the antiphospholipid syndrome, but a wide variety of conditions may be a predisposing factor, including essential thrombocytosis and Behçet disease. If venous emboli become dislodged into the right ventricle, a mistaken preoperative diagnosis of right ventricular tumor may be made.

TABLE 39.1

PRIMARY CARDIAC TUMORS: FREQUENCY AND MEAN AGE AT PRESENTATION

Tumor type	Percentage (%)[a]	Mean age at presentation
Teratoma	<1	16 weeks
Rhabdomyoma	2	33 weeks
Fibroma	3	13 years
Rhabdomyosarcoma	2	15 years
Hemangioma	2	31 years
Atrioventricular nodal tumor	<1[b]	33 years
Sarcoma (all)	10	41 years
Myxoma	77	50 years
Papillary fibroelastoma	1	59 years
Lipomatous hypertrophy	3	64 years

[a]Percentage of primary cardiac tumors removed surgically.
[b]Atrioventricular nodal tumor has been anecdotally reported as a surgical specimen; most are autopsy findings.

Echocardiography, cineangiography,and MRI have been used to make a diagnosis of mural cardiac thrombus both in patients with organic heart disease and in patients with presumed coagulopathies and normal cardiac function. In some cases, the imaging findings are indistinguishable from primary cardiac tumors, such as myxoma, when the location is intra-atrial (Fig. 39.2).

On occasion, there can be a thin stalk at the attachment site, mimicking myxoma, or no attachment site at all (ball thrombus). Histologically, organized thrombi are characterized by layers of degenerated blood cells with a margin of granulation tissue and eventually fibrosis.

Ectopias

Cystic Tumor of the Atrioventricular Node

These curious endodermal inclusions may represent a form of ultimobranchial heterotopia (9). Most patients have congenital heart block, and almost three of four are female. Most tumors occur sporadically, but there is an association with cysts of endocrine organs and other midline defects, such as ventricular septal defect, nasal septal defect, encephalocele, thyroglossal duct cysts, and absent septum pellucidum (10).

TABLE 39.2

CARDIAC TUMORS, BY SITE AND GENERAL IMAGING CHARACTERISTICS

Site	Relation to chamber wall	Most likely	Others
Left atrium (cavitary mass)	Pedunculated or broad-based attachment	Myxoma	Thrombus Sarcoma Metastasis (extension of lung primary) Hemangioma
Left atrium, involving wall/pericardium	Infiltrating	Sarcoma (fibrous or myogenous differentiation)	Lymphoma Metastasis Hemangioma Paraganglioma
Right atrium (cavitary mass)	Pedunculated or broad-based attachment	Myxoma Thrombus Lipomatous hypertrophy	Metastasis (especially renal cell, hepatocellular carcinoma) Hemangioma
Right atrium, involving wall/pericardium	Infiltrating	Angiosarcoma Metastasis	Lymphoma Hemangioma Paraganglioma
Ventricle (cavitary mass)	Pedunculated or broad-based attachment	Thrombus Metastasis (right ventricle) Inflammatory myofibroblastic tumor	Sarcoma Lipoma Hemangioma Myxoma
Ventricle, involving wall	Infiltrating	Sarcoma, including rhabdomyosarcoma	Hemangioma Lipoma Lymphoma
Valve		Papillary fibroelastoma	Sarcoma Lipoma Hemangioma
Pericardium	Infiltrating	Metastasis Mesothelioma Lymphoma	Sarcoma (especially angiosarcoma, synovial sarcoma) Hemangioma
Pericardium	Localized	Metastasis Solitary fibrous tumor	Hemangioma Paraganglioma Lipoma Calcifying fibrous tumor

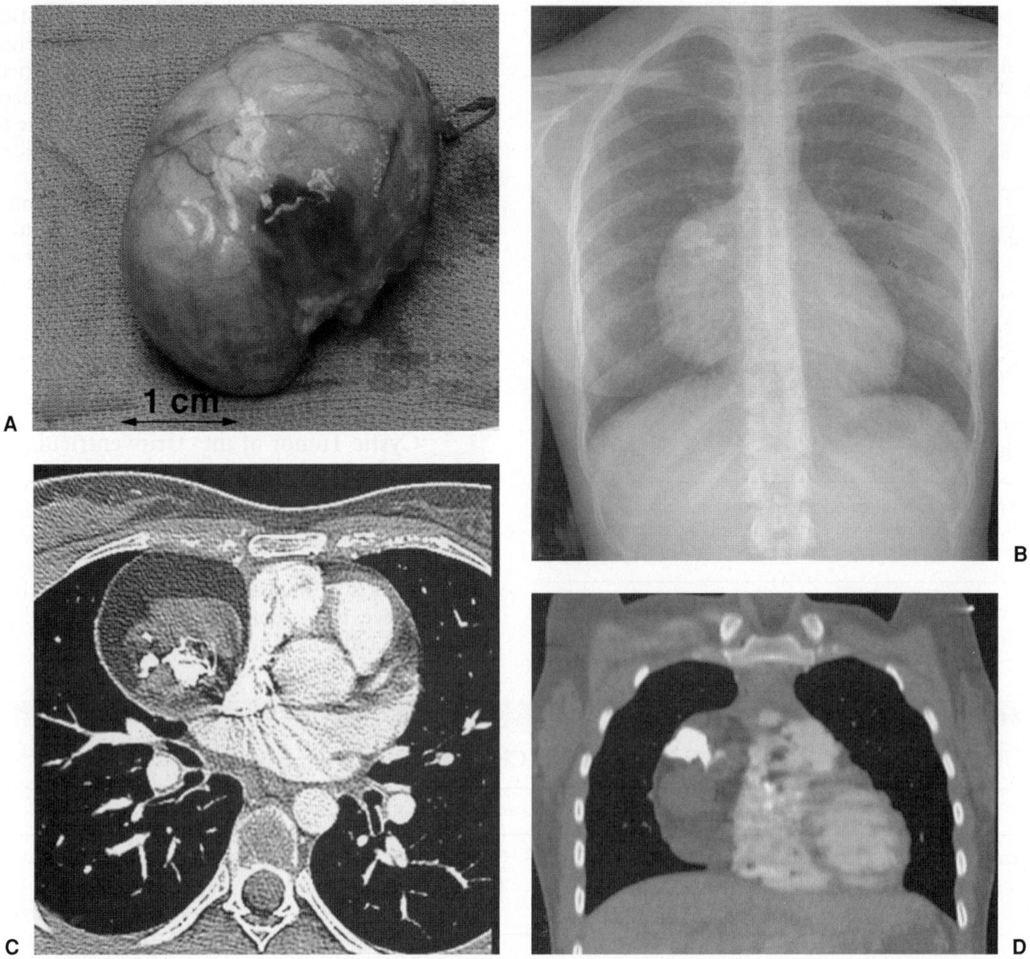

FIGURE 39.1. Pericardial teratoma. A. Gross photograph of an excised specimen, which at surgery was intrapericardial, demonstrates a smooth-surfaced tumor externally. B. Posteroanterior chest radiograph demonstrates a mediastinal mass projecting to the right of the heart with obvious calcification. C. Axial chest computed tomography (CT) demonstrates an anterior mediastinal mass with combination of soft tissue, fat, and calcification consistent with teratoma. D. Coronal reconstruction of CT data demonstrates a right pericardial mass with combined calcification soft tissue and fat densities.

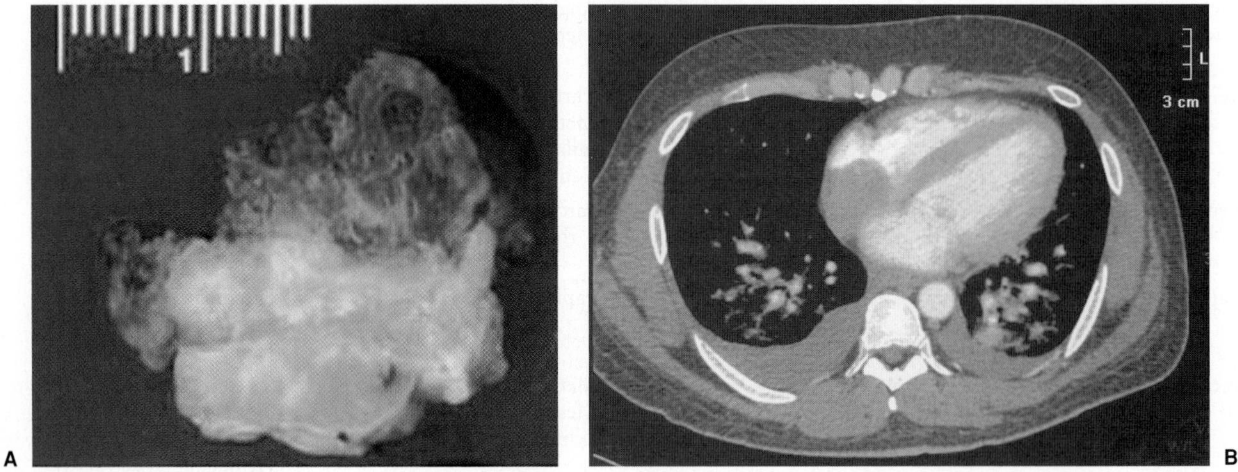

FIGURE 39.2. Right mural thrombus. A. Gross photograph of a resected specimen demonstrates surface thrombus (brown in fixed state), organized white thrombus underneath, and a portion of the excised atrial septum at the bottom. B. Axial chest computed tomography demonstrates a soft tissue mass contiguous with the posterior wall of the right atrium and the interatrial septum. The imaging impression was atrial myxoma; histology (not shown) was organized thrombus.

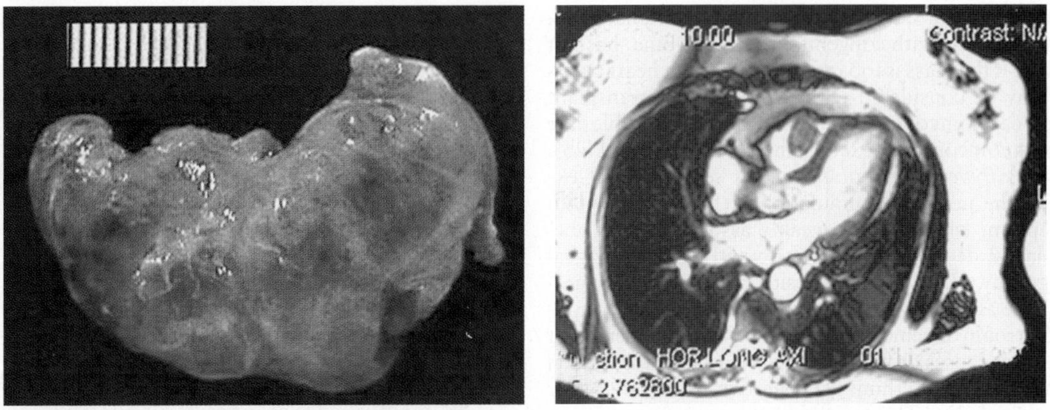

A B

FIGURE 39.3. Ectopic thyroid, intracavity, right ventricle. A. Gross specimen demonstrates an irregularly lobulated tumor with the gross appearance of thyroid. B. Axial magnetic resonance imaging with bright blood technique demonstrates a mass within the right ventricle.

Thyroid Heterotopia

When ectopic thyroid occurs in the myocardium, it is called *struma cordis*. The right ventricular outflow is generally involved (11) (Fig. 39.3), although left ventricular obstruction has been reported. The condition is believed to occur early in embryogenesis, when part or all of the functioning thyroid tissue becomes lodged in the ventricular outflow region. Radioiodide imaging is diagnostic (12). Although pulmonary stenosis with right ventricular hypertrophy may occur, most patients are asymptomatic (11). Histologically, one sees follicular structures containing colloid; if there is any difficulty in diagnosis, immunohistochemical stains for thyroglobulin may be performed.

Papillary Fibroelastomas

Also known as fibroelastic papilloma, this unusual lesion occurs exclusively on endocardial surfaces, most commonly on valve leaflets, like Lambl excrescences (13). No gender predominance is noted, and there is a wide range of age at presentation, with a mean age of approximately 60 years (13). Papillary fibroelastomas occasionally occur in areas of previous endocardial damage or in patients with preexisting heart disease (14). Most symptoms arise from left-sided lesions that shower fibrin clots into the cerebral circulation or prolapse into the coronary orifice. The most common symptoms are transient neurologic defects, myocardial ischemia (15), and, rarely, sudden death. Papillary fibroelastomas of the cardiac valves demonstrate typical echocardiographic features (16). Transesophageal echocardiography is helpful in cases of rare sites, such as the venae cavae or atria (17). Three-dimensional echocardiography may provide enhanced imaging (18). Unlike Lambl excrescences, papillary fibroelastomas can become quite large and occur on any valve surface or area of the endocardium (19). Thrombi may occur on the surface of the proliferation, and dislodged clots are responsible for embolic symptoms. Histologically, they are avascular papillary structures lined by endothelial cells. They are often mistaken for cardiac myxomas, which are vascular and of heterogeneous cell types. Papillary fibroelastoma is treated curatively by surgery, whether there are preexisting embolic symptoms or a lesion is incidentally discovered. Asymptomatic patients can be treated surgically if the tumor is mobile, because the tumor mobility is the independent predictor of death or nonfatal embolization. Asymptomatic patients with nonmobile lesions can be followed-up closely with periodic clinical evaluation and echocardiography, and they can receive surgical intervention when symptoms develop or the tumor becomes mobile (13). Recurrences are rare, and valve-sparing surgery should be considered whenever possible, because partially resected lesions do not always regrow (20).

Cardiac Hamartomas

The term *hamartoma* has no specific meaning, but it embraces a group of tumors that are not neoplasms, may be associated with syndromes involving extracardiac sites, and are composed of recognizable histologic issue types often in a haphazard or disorganized growth pattern. Recurrences are rare after excision, and the lesions have no metastatic potential. In the heart, the most common hamartomas include rhabdomyomas and Purkinje cell hamartomas/histiocytoid cardiomyopathy; because these lesions occur exclusively in children, they are not discussed further here. Hamartomas of mature cardiac myocytes and adult forms of rhabdomyomas are extraordinarily rare and are not addressed.

Cardiac fibroma is a nonneoplastic mass of fibrous tissue that occurs within the heart walls, usually ventricular free wall or interventricular septum. Most cardiac fibromas are discovered in children and often before 1 year of age (21). However, cases are also reported in adults and even as incidental finding in the elderly (21). Symptoms relate to the site of tumor, which is most commonly the ventricular septum, followed by the free walls of the left and right ventricle. Approximately 3% of patients with Gorlin syndrome have cardiac fibromas (22). At echocardiography, fibromas typically appear as a large, well-circumscribed, solitary mass in the septum or ventricular free wall (5), and in some cases they may be confused with hypertrophic cardiomyopathy (23). The tumors are frequently very large and may cause obstruction, which can be assessed by color Doppler. MRI likewise shows a large, solitary, homogeneous myocardial mass centered in the ventricles (5). Because of the fibrous nature of the tumor, the signal intensity is often less than that of adjacent uninvolved myocardium, and contrast-enhanced imaging usually demonstrates a hypoperfused tumor core. CT also shows a large, solitary, ventricular mass, which usually has low attenuation on CT, which may also detect calcification, a helpful feature in making a confident diagnosis (5). Cardiac fibroma is benign, but its nature of slow but continuous growth may cause conduction defects and arrhythmias. Extension into the ventricular free walls may result in atrioventricular valve inflow or arterial outflow obstruction. Spontaneous regression, as can occur with congenital rhabdomyoma, has not been observed. If the mass is too large for resection, heart transplantation may be considered with or without pretransplant palliation or cardiomyoplasty (24). However, favorable late results even after incomplete excision have been reported (25).

Lipomatous hypertrophy of the atrial septum is an exaggeration of the normal accumulation of brown fat within the atrial septum, which is only weakly associated with obesity. In the last 2 decades, transthoracic and transesophageal echocardiography, CT, MRI, and positron emission tomography (PET) have allowed antemortem diagnosis (26,27). Lipomatous hypertrophy is removed incidentally during open heart surgery for other causes or for relief of cardiac symptoms, such as supraventricular arrhythmias, congestive heart failure, or vena caval obstruction. The indications for surgery are somewhat controversial, because the detection of incidental masses may lead to unnecessary surgery for a benign lesion that may simply be an exaggeration of normal features. Histologically, there is a mixture of mature and brown fat, which ultrastructurally contains abundant mitochondria (28). Entrapped, enlarged myocytes are common and may lead to the false diagnosis of sarcoma, or the brown fat clusters may be mistaken for lipoblasts.

Cardiac Myxomas

In surgical series, cardiac myxomas account for almost 80% of heart tumors (29–31). Patient age ranges from 2 to 97 years. The mean age at presentation is 50 years (32). Ninety percent of individuals are between the ages of 30 and 60 years. A recent analysis of multiple surgical series including 1,195 individuals with myxomas revealed that 67% were female and 33% were male (33). Patients with the myxoma (Carney) complex are generally younger and more often male in comparison with patients with sporadic myxomas (34,35).

The clinical presentation is diverse and includes obstructive cardiac symptoms, embolic phenomena, and constitutional symptoms. Most patients have an abnormal physical examination, characteristically with a diastolic or systolic murmur. A "tumor plop" may be occasionally heard in early diastole.

In more than 50% of patients, left atrial myxomas cause symptoms of mitral valve stenosis or obstruction (dyspnea and orthopnea from pulmonary edema or heart failure). Right atrial myxomas may obstruct the tricuspid valve and cause symptoms of right-sided heart failure (32). Embolic phenomena occur in 30% to 40% of patients. Frequent sites of embolization include the central nervous system, kidney, spleen, and extremities. Coronary embolism is rare. Smooth-surfaced tumors are more likely to produce valvular obstruction, whereas polypoid and myxoid tumors are more likely to embolize (34). Anemia, leukocytosis, and elevated erythrocyte sedimentation rate are the most common laboratory findings. Constitutional symptoms (possibly related to interleukin-6 production by tumor cells), which are seen in approximately 20% of patients, include myalgia, muscle weakness, arthralgia, fever, fatigue, and weight loss (36). Although infection of a myxoma is rare, when present the initial manifestations mimic those of infective endocarditis. About 20% of cardiac myxomas are asymptomatic; incidental myxomas are usually smaller than 40 mm (37). Abnormal but nonspecific ECG changes may be identified in 20% to 40% of patients and include atrial fibrillation or flutter and left and right bundle branch block (32).

At echocardiography, cardiac myxomas typically appear as a mobile mass attached to the endocardial surface by a stalk, usually arising from the fossa ovalis (5). Myxomas with this appearance can be confidently diagnosed by echocardiography, and further imaging is not necessary. Because myxomas

A

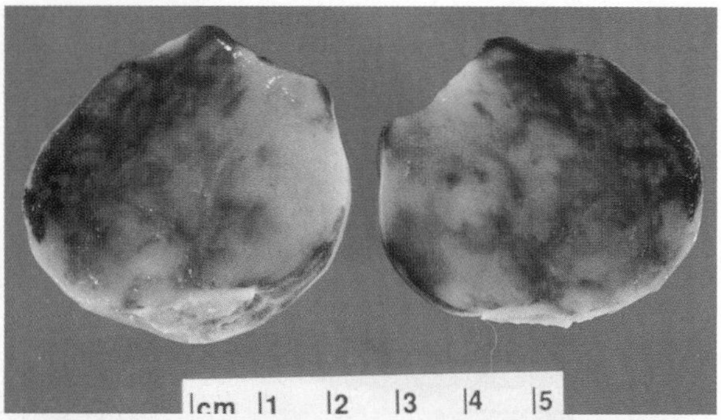

B

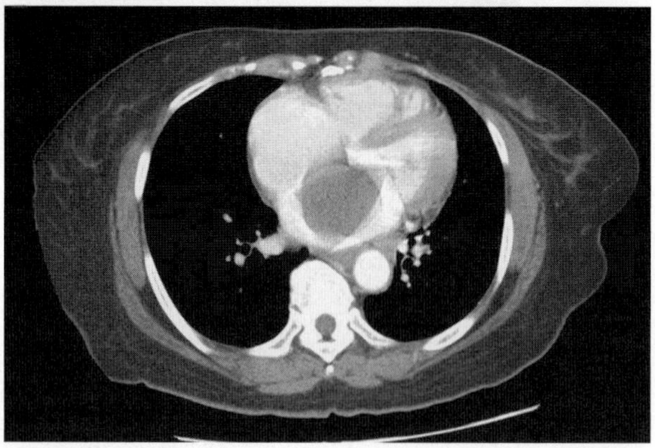

FIGURE 39.4. Cardiac myxoma. **A.** Gross photograph of a smooth-surfaced myxoma that has been sectioned down the middle. **B.** Axial chest computed tomography demonstrates a mass within the left atrium apparently attached to the interatrial septum.

are usually small and mobile, they are typically better defined by echocardiography than by either MRI or CT, given that echocardiography has the best spatial and temporal resolution. If the narrow stalk is not visible, the diagnosis cannot be made by echocardiography, and further imaging, usually MRI, will be necessary show the tumor's margins and to exclude tumor infiltration. By MRI and CT, myxoma appears as an intracavitary heterogeneous, lobular mass (38) (Fig. 39.4). As with echocardiography, if the narrow stalk is visible, myxoma can be diagnosed by MRI or CT.

Myxoma cells may arise from subendothelial vasoformative reserve cells or primitive cells that reside in the fossa ovalis and surrounding endocardium (32). They arise from the endocardium of the left atrial septum near the fossa ovalis in 85% to 90% of cases. Most of the remainder are located in the right atrium. Multiple tumors occurring at sites other than the fossa ovalis and the ventricles are generally found in the "familial" or "syndromic" form of cardiac myxoma. Myxomas are either sessile or pedunculated, but the site of attachment is always discrete and usually is in the region of the fossa ovalis. In approximately 2% of cardiac myxomas, heterologous elements, in the form of glandular structures, are identified (34).

Although most myxomas are sporadic, fewer than 5% of them form a component of the myxoma complex (32). This autosomal dominant syndrome, known as Carney syndrome, includes cardiac myxomas and extracardiac manifestations: abnormal skin pigmentation (lentigines and blue nevi), calcifying Sertoli-Leydig testicular tumors, cutaneous myxomas, myxoid breast fibroadenomas, pigmented adrenal cortical hyperplasia, pituitary hyperactivity, psammomatous melanotic schwannomas, and thyroid tumors.

Patients with sporadic tumors have a good prognosis, with a 1% recurrence rate. However, about 10% of patients with

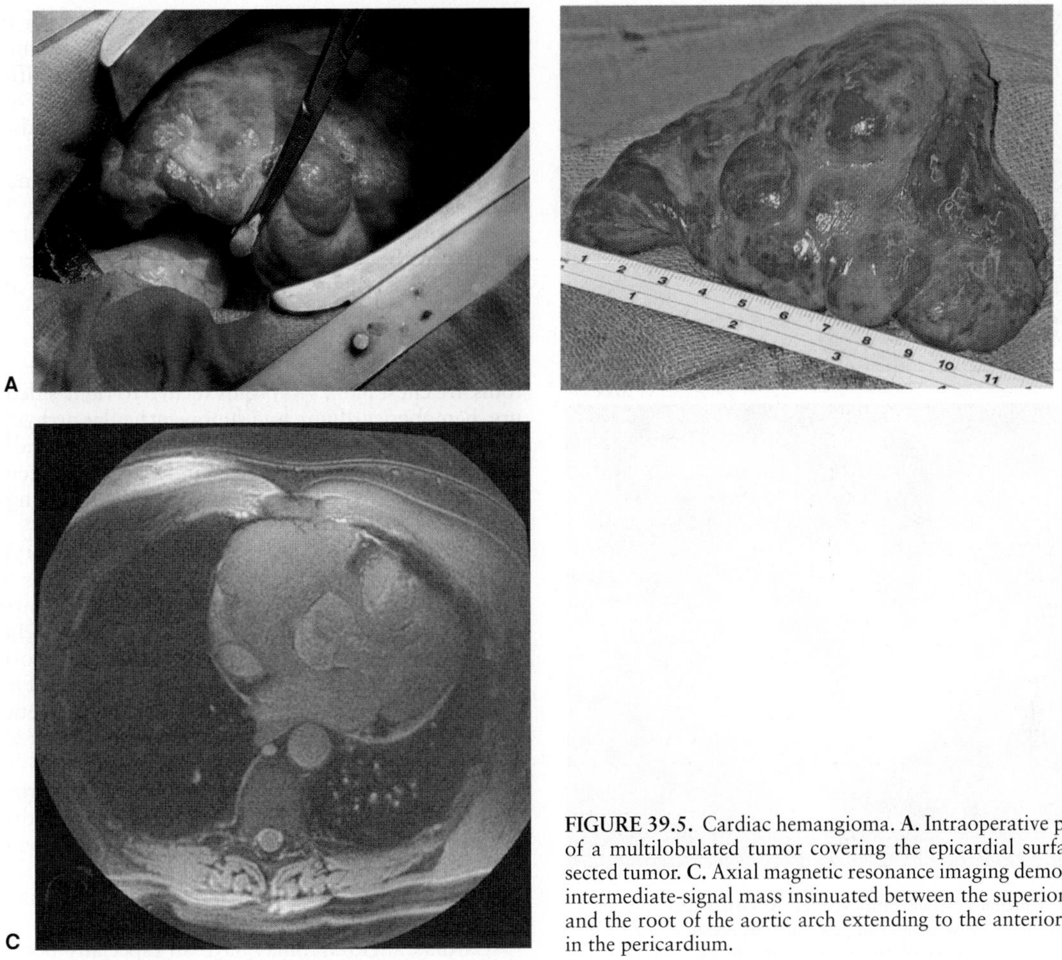

FIGURE 39.5. Cardiac hemangioma. A. Intraoperative photograph of a multilobulated tumor covering the epicardial surface. B. Resected tumor. C. Axial magnetic resonance imaging demonstrates an intermediate-signal mass insinuated between the superior vena cava and the root of the aortic arch extending to the anterior chest wall in the pericardium.

familial myxomas either have recurrent tumors or develop another tumor in a different location (34,35,39). Because embolization is the major complication of myxomas, especially of myxoid, friable, familial tumors, identification of first-degree relatives of patients with documented myxoma syndrome is important. Intracranial aneurysm resulting from embolization is also a rare, but potentially serious, complication. The origin of these aneurysms is unclear, but histologic verification of myxoma cells in arterial walls has been reported (40).

Because most left atrial myxomas arise from the interatrial septum, the tumors can be removed en bloc with a 5-mm margin of normal tissue. The fossa ovalis, where the pretumor cells of myxomas are thought likely to exist, should also be excised if possible. Although resection of the attachment and of 5 mm of normal tissue, including endocardium and underlying myocardium, has been recommended (41), no data support that documentation of negative margins at the time of surgery decreases the recurrence rate.

Hemangiomas

Hemangiomas are incidental lesions discovered during chest radiography or surgery for other purposes, or they may cause arrhythmias, pericardial effusions, congestive heart failure, or outflow tract obstruction, and rarely sudden death (42). Cardiac hemangiomas are of two basic pathologic types (43). Circumscribed lesions are histologically uniform and are composed of cavernous vascular spaces, often with a myxoid background. They may be easily shelled out at surgery and are often endocardially based masses that project into the lumen, but they may occur in the pericardium (Fig. 39.5). Infiltrating cardiac hemangiomas, in contrast to their circumscribed counterparts, are more likely to cause symptoms than circumscribed hemangiomas, and they often result in cardiac arrhythmias because of their intramural location (43). Cardiac hemangiomas are generally cured by surgical resection, occasionally requiring synthetic graft placement (43).

Paragangliomas/Pheochromocytomas

Paragangliomas of the heart, or pheochromocytomas, develop within the atria, are usually benign, and may be functional, resulting in systemic hypertension (44). Most patients are young or middle-aged adults. Functional tumors have been successfully removed with remission of symptoms. Complete surgical excision is recommended for all cardiac paragangliomas, often with an atrial graft repairing the portion of atrium or atrial septum removed. Echocardiography (45), computed tomography (CT) and MRI (Fig. 39.6) have been successfully used to delineate cardiac paragangliomas preoperatively. Somatostatin-receptor nuclear imaging may provide specific imaging (46). Malignant behavior of paragangliomas in the heart is rare. Pathologically, paragangliomas are poorly circumscribed masses measuring up to 15 cm. Paragangliomas of the heart are similar histologically and immunohistochemically to extracardiac paragangliomas. Treatment is surgical. In case of functional paragangliomas (pheochromocytomas), special anesthetic procedures to control cathecholamine release has been recommended (47).

A
B
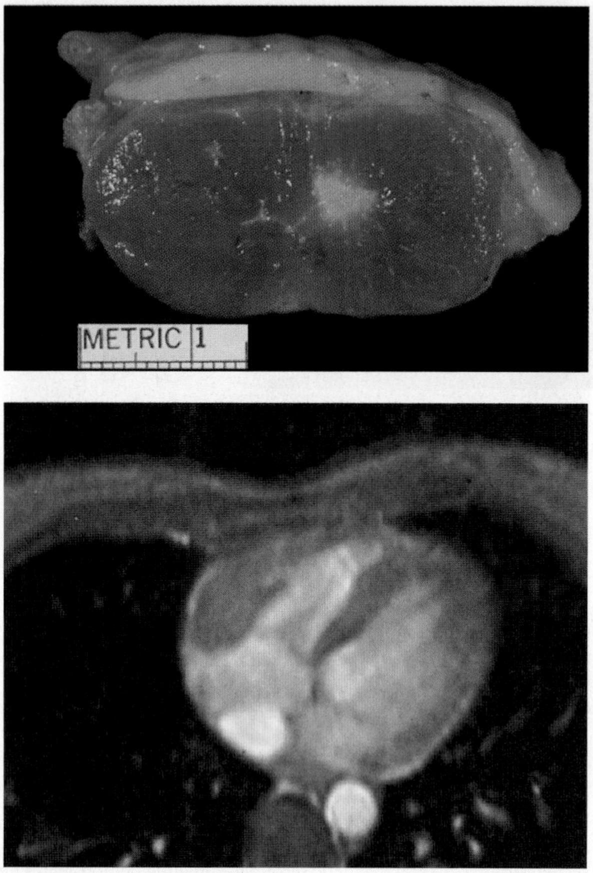

FIGURE 39.6. Cardiac pheochromocytoma. **A.** Gross specimen demonstrates the typical yellow-bronze appearance. **B.** Axial magnetic resonance imaging at the level of the right ventricle demonstrates an oblong mass bounded by the pericardium with compression of the right atrium and ventricle.

Lipomas

In series of heart tumors, lipomas generally account for 0.5% to 3% of surgically removed lesions. There is a predilection for the pericardium and epicardial surfaces. When these tumors involve the valves, the designation "fibrolipoma" has been used. Many cardiac lipomas are incidental findings, or they cause a variety of arrhythmias, syncope, and ECG abnormalities.

Lipomas in the pericardial space have variable echogenicity but are often hypoechoic, whereas intracavitary lipomas are typically echogenic (5). CT and MRI may establish the fatty nature of the tumor. As seen by echocardiography, intracavitary lipomas are usually circumscribed but cannot be differentiated from other circumscribed cardiac masses. However, MRI and CT both allow for very specific identification of fat and therefore can be used to diagnose lipomas definitively. Surgical excision is generally curative (48). Recurrences are rare (49). Large size may preclude complete excision; in such instances, incomplete resection or follow-up may be indicated (50).

MALIGNANT CARDIAC TUMORS

Primary Cardiac Sarcomas

Cardiac sarcomas are pathologically classified by histologic type (51): angiosarcomas, endomyocardially based tumors, which usually have features of smooth muscle or fibroblastic differentiation, and rhabdomyosarcoma (striated muscle differentiation). The sarcomas with myofibroblastic differentiation are the most pathologic diverse and may occur occasionally within the heart muscle and pericardium in addition to the more common endocardial or intimal origin.

Angiosarcomas are the most common malignant cardiac neoplasms with specific cell type differentiation. They occur over a wide age range (36 months to 80 years),with a peak incidence in the fourth decade (52), and with equal frequency in men and women. These tumors most often arise in the right atrium near the atrioventricular groove (80%), but they have been reported in the other three chambers as well as in the pericardium (52). The most common presenting symptoms are chest pain, symptoms related to right-sided heart failure, hemopericardium, and supraventricular arrhythmias (53). Sometimes, early pericardial involvement may lead to pericardial biopsy during emergency surgical cardiac decompression for tamponade or cardiac rupture (54). Familial angiosarcoma has been reported (55).

During echocardiography, an angiosarcoma typically appears as an echogenic, nodular, or lobulated mass in the right atrium with pericardial effusion or direct pericardial extension (5). MRI imaging sequences sensitive for hemorrhage (T1-weighted images) may show areas of hemorrhage that may be diffuse or nodular. After administration of intravenous contrast (gadolinium-diethylenetriamine pentaacetic acid), enhancement along vascular lakes may be seen, described as a "sun ray" appearance (56).

Pathologically, angiosarcomas are usually form lobulated variegated masses in the right atrial wall, protruding into the chamber. They range in size from 2.0 cm to several centimeters. The pericardium is frequently involved, occasionally as the dominant site, and hence a hemorrhagic pericardial effusion is a frequent accompaniment.

Cardiac angiosarcomas have an especially poor prognosis because patients typically present with metastasis, with survival typically measured in months. Metastases occur most frequently to the lung, then liver. Angiosarcoma is generally treated by a combination of surgery (sometimes with modifications including explantation and ex situ resection) and radiation with or without sarcoma-type chemotherapy; heart transplantation is a consideration if metastatic disease is not identified (57–60).

Sarcomas with myoblastic or fibroblastic differentiation form endoluminal masses that are most frequently found in the left atrium (51) (Fig. 39.7). No evidence indicates that they are related to cardiac myxomas (51). This type of sarcoma has been subclassified as malignant fibrous histiocytoma (recently designated undifferentiated pleomorphic sarcoma) (51), osteosarcoma, leiomyosarcoma (52) (Fig. 39.8), and fibrosarcoma or myxofibrosarcoma (52). Any of the histologic subtypes may be associated with myxoid change. Synovial sarcoma is characterized by the X;18 chromosomal translocations that account for approximately 5% of cardiac sarcomas (52) with a predilection for the atria and pericardium. Rhabdomyosarcomas, which have skeletal muscle differentiation, account for less than 5% of cardiac sarcomas (52,61) and occur most frequently in children and young adults. Extracardiac embryonal rhabdomyosarcoma imparts a relatively good prognosis in comparison with the alveolar subtype.

Cardiac sarcomas may be graded based on cell type, presence of necrosis, and mitotic activity (62). Complete resection of malignant primary cardiac tumors can rarely be achieved, but palliative surgery is usually undertaken because many patients present with mechanical obstruction. Adjunctive chemotherapy, radiation therapy, or both can sometimes be used, although the optimal protocol and efficacy are unclear.

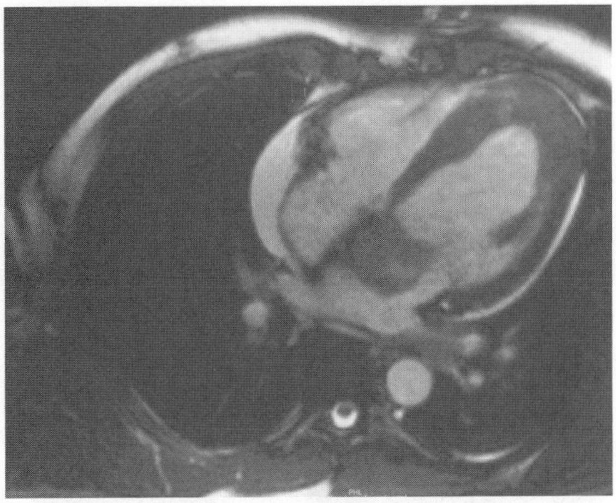
A

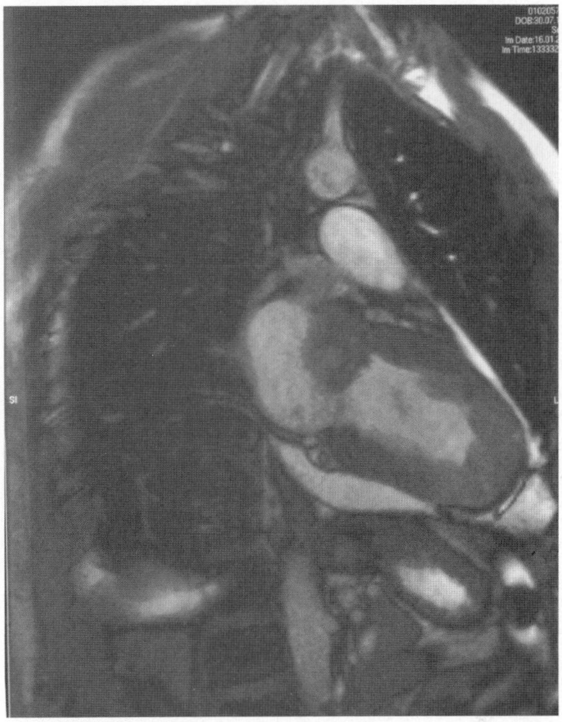
B

FIGURE 39.7. Cardiac sarcoma. **A.** Axial magnetic resonance imaging (MRI) of the heart demonstrates a mass with an intermediate signal attached to the interatrial septum just above the mitral valve. **B.** Two-chamber long-axis MRI demonstrating the lesion.

Cardiac Lymphomas

Cardiac lymphomas are usually part of disseminated disease; up to 20% of patients with disseminated non-Hodgkin lymphoma have evidence of cardiac involvement at autopsy (63). Because of the rise in immunocompromised patients, because of both human immunodeficiency virus infection or acquired immunodeficiency syndrome (AIDS) and allograft recipients, increasing proportions, although still comprising a small minority, of patients with cardiac lymphoma are in this category.

Primary cardiac lymphoma in immunocompetent patients is an uncommon malignancy, accounting for 1.3% of primary cardiac tumors and 0.5% of extranodal lymphomas (63). Symptoms include cardiac tamponade (64), heart failure (65), atrial fibrillation or flutter (66), heart block (67), right heart obstruction (65), and embolic phenomena. In a literature review of 40 patients, presenting symptoms included dyspnea, edema, arrhythmia, and pericardial effusion. There was a mild male predominance (male-to-female ratio of 23:17) with a mean age of 67 years. Lesions were found in the following locations, listed in order of frequency: right atrium, pericardium, right ventricle, left atrium, left ventricle, and other sites. Antemortem diagnosis was obtained in only 37 of the 40 patients (68).

Cardiac lymphomas comprise less than 5% of all lymphomas arising in patients with AIDS and organ transplants,

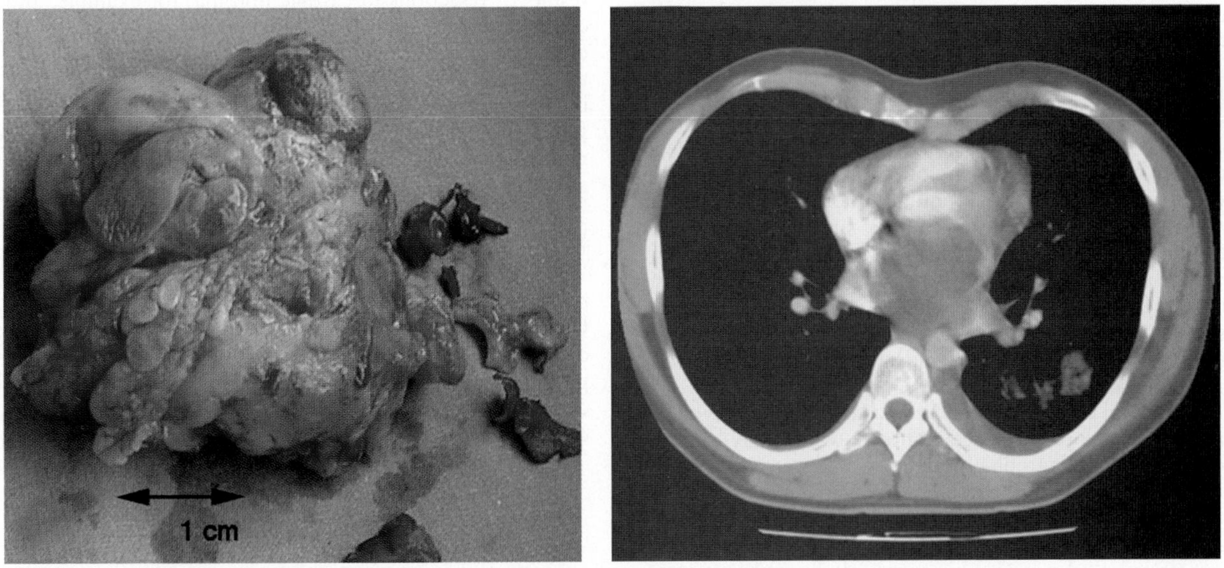

A B

FIGURE 39.8. Cardiac leiomyosarcoma. **A.** Gross specimen demonstrates a multilobulated irregular mass. **B.** Axial chest computed tomography demonstrates a large soft tissue mass, which fills the left atrium.

and location of the tumor in the donor heart is the exception rather than the rule in heart transplant recipients. In an autopsy series of 440 patients with AIDS, only one demonstrated myocardial involvement with lymphoma (69).

Lymphoma manifests as an ill-defined, infiltrative mass, in which case it is typically best depicted with MRI because of the technique's superior soft tissue contrast (5). Atrial location is typical, with infiltration of atrial or ventricular walls. Lymphomas may have high or low signal on MRI, they may have attenuation similar to that of muscle or lower attenuation than muscle on CT, and they may show increased or decreased contrast enhancement. In addition to echocardiography, MRI, and CT, nuclear medicine techniques may be useful procedures for the noninvasive assessment of cardiac lymphomas. Cardiac gadolinium-enhanced MRI (CMR) and fluorine-18 fluorodeoxyglucose PET may be useful to evaluate the response to chemotherapy (70).

Histologically, cardiac lymphomas span the spectrum of B-cell proliferations and include follicle center cell lymphomas, immunoblastic lymphomas, diffuse large cell lymphomas, and Burkitt lymphoma. Primary cardiac T-cell lymphomas are rare and occur only in immunocompetent patients.

Treatment is similar to that of B-cell lymphomas in extracardiac sites, specifically anthracycline-based chemotherapy, and it may include anti-CD20 (rituximab) (70). Chemotherapy has been used alone or combined with radiotherapy. Similarly, palliative cardiac surgery has been performed, mainly for tumor debulking. Irrespective of the treatment applied, 60% of the patients died of their tumor 1.8 months after diagnosis. The survival is generally less than a month without treatment but has been prolonged up to 5 years with palliative treatments in selected cases (63). Multimodality treatment may include autologous stem cell transplantation (71).

Metastatic Cardiac Tumors

Malignancies spread to the heart as follows: by direct extension, usually from mediastinal tumor; hematogenously; via lymphatics; and rarely by intracavitary extension from the inferior vena cava or pulmonary veins. Epithelial malignancies typically spread to the heart by the lymphatics. Melanoma, sarcomas, leukemia, and renal cell carcinoma metastasize to the heart by a hematogenous route. Melanomas, renal tumors, including Wilms tumor and renal cell carcinoma, adrenal tumors, liver tumors, and uterine tumors are the most frequent intracavitary tumors.

In a series of 133 surgically resected cardiac tumors, 14% were metastases (72). Surgically resected lesions are usually right sided and represent either cavoatrial extensions from abdominal tumors, such as renal cell carcinomas or hepatocellular carcinomas, or hematogenous metastases that may present months or years after initial tumor excision. Intracardiac masses are often unusual tumors, such as sarcomas and melanomas or germ cell tumors (Fig. 39.9). Carcinomas emanating from the lung may form cavitary left atrial masses mimicking a primary cardiac tumor. More frequently, epithelial malignancies involve the heart as pericardial studding; these tumors are infrequently resected and cause symptoms related to pericardial tamponade.

The clinical presentation of cardiac metastasis involving the pericardium includes shortness of breath, which may be out of proportion to radiographic findings in patients with pericardial effusion or may be the result of associated pleural effusion, cough, anterior thoracic pain, pleuritic chest pain, or peripheral edema. The differential diagnosis of pericardial effusion in a patient with known malignancy includes malignant pericardial effusion, radiation-induced pericarditis, drug-induced pericarditis, and idiopathic pericarditis (73). Tumors metastatic to the right side of the heart may cause a variety of symptoms (74). Right ventricular outlet obstruction is a complication of bulky right-sided metastases (75). Involvement of the right side of the heart and tricuspid valves may give rise to right-sided heart failure. Left-sided metastases may cause obstruction of the mitral or aortic valve and syncope.

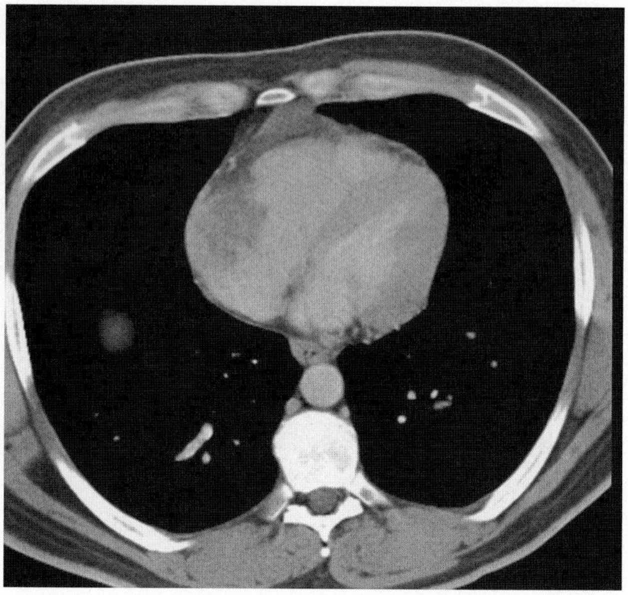

FIGURE 39.9. Metastatic seminoma. Axial chest computed tomography demonstrates an irregular soft tissue mass centered within the right atrium with apparent extension into the right ventricle.

CONTROVERSIES AND PERSONAL PERSPECTIVES

Treatment of cardiac tumors must often be tailored to the individual patient, because data from series of specific lesions are often not available. Until more experience is published on results of resections of cardiac fibroma, for example, and on combination chemotherapy with surgical resection of primary cardiac sarcomas, there will be no standardized treatment for these lesions. The role of extensive preoperative evaluations in patients with incidentally discovered cardiac masses is also somewhat controversial, and multimodality imaging, angiography, and even preoperative biopsy to establish a diagnosis are not uniformly necessary.

THE FUTURE

Optimal treatment of cardiac tumors awaits more sophisticated surgical techniques and chemotherapeutic regimens for primary malignancies. Cardiac transplantation will likely become a more established therapy for inoperable primary cardiac neoplasms, both benign and malignant.

References

1. Reynen K. Frequency of primary tumors of the heart. *Am J Cardiol* 1996; 77:107.

2. Lepper W, Shivalkar B, Rinkevich D, et al. Assessment of the vascularity of a left ventricular mass using myocardial contrast echocardiography. *J Am Soc Echocardiogr* 2002;15:1419–1422.
3. Schvartzman PR, White RD. Imaging of cardiac and paracardiac masses. *J Thorac Imaging* 2000;15:265–273.
4. Siripornpitak S, Higgins CB. MRI of primary malignant cardiovascular tumors. *J Comput Assist Tomogr* 1997;21:462–466.
5. Araoz PA, Eklund HE, Welch TJ, et al. CT and MR imaging of primary cardiac malignancies. *Radiographics* 1999;19:1421–1434.
6. Cheng TO. Role of selective coronary arteriography in patients with cardiac myxoma. *Cardiology* 2000;94:263.
7. Waller B, Grider L, Rohr T, et al. Intracardiac thrombi: frequency, location, etiology, and complications: a morphologic review. Part I. *Clin Cardiol* 1995;18:477–479.
8. Kmetzo J, Peters R, Plotnick G, et al. Left atrial mass: thrombus mimicking myxoma. *Chest* 1985;88:906–907.
9. Cameselle-Teijeiro J, Abdulkader I, Soares P, et al. Cystic tumor of the atrioventricular node of the heart appears to be the heart equivalent of the solid cell nests (ultimobranchial rests) of the thyroid. *Am J Clin Pathol* 2005;123:369–375.
10. Burke AP, Anderson PG, Virmani R, et al. Tumor of the atrioventricular nodal region: a clinical and immunohistochemical study. *Arch Pathol Lab Med* 1990;114:1057–1062.
11. Chosia M, Waligorski S, Listewnik MH, et al. Ectopic thyroid tissue as a tumour of the heart: case report and review of the literature. *Pol J Pathol* 2002;53:173–175.
12. Rieser GD, Ober KP, Cowan RJ, et al. Radioiodide imaging of struma cordis. *Clin Nucl Med* 1988;13:421–422.
13. Gowda RM, Khan IA, Nair CK, et al. Cardiac papillary fibroelastoma: a comprehensive analysis of 725 cases. *Am Heart J* 2003;146:404–410.
14. Kurup AN, Tazelaar HD, Edwards WD, et al. Iatrogenic cardiac papillary fibroelastoma: a study of 12 cases (1990 to 2000). *Hum Pathol* 2002;33:1165–1169.
15. Boulmier D, Ecke JE, Verhoye JP. Recurrent myocardial infarction due to obstruction of the RCA ostium by an aortic papillary fibroelastoma. *J Invasive Cardiol* 2002;14:686–688.
16. Bottio T, Pittarello D, Bonato R, et al. Echocardiographic diagnosis of aortic valve papillary fibroelastoma. *Tex Heart Inst J* 2004;31:322–323.
17. Vora TR. Unusual presentation of papillary fibroelastoma: utility of serial transesophageal echocardiograms. *Echocardiography* 2004;21:69–71.
18. Dichtl W, Muller LC, Pachinger O, et al. Images in cardiovascular medicine. Improved preoperative assessment of papillary fibroelastoma by dynamic three-dimensional echocardiography. *Circulation* 2002;106:1300.
19. Butany J, Nair V, Ahluwalia MS, et al. Papillary fibroelastoma of the interatrial septum: a case report. *J Card Surg* 2004;19:349–353.
20. Sumino S, Paterson HS. No regrowth after incomplete papillary fibroelastoma excision. *Ann Thorac Surg* 2005;79:e3–4.
21. Burke AP, Rosado-de-Christenson M, Templeton PA, et al. Cardiac fibroma: clinicopathologic correlates and surgical treatment. *J Thorac Cardiovasc Surg* 1994;108:862–870.
22. Vaughan CJ, Veugelers M, Basson CT. Tumors and the heart: molecular genetic advances. *Curr Opin Cardiol* 2001;16:195–200.
23. Veinot JP, O'Murchu B, Tazelaar HD, et al. Cardiac fibroma mimicking apical hypertrophic cardiomyopathy: a case report and differential diagnosis. *J Am Soc Echocardiogr* 1996;9:94–99.
24. Waller BR, Bradley SM, Crumbley AJ 3rd, et al. Cardiac fibroma in an infant: single ventricle palliation as a bridge to heart transplantation. *Ann Thorac Surg* 2003;75:1306–1308.
25. Agarwala BN, Starr JP, Walker E, et al. Surgical issues in giant right ventricular fibroma. *Ann Thorac Surg* 2004;78:328–330.
26. Fan CM, Fischman AJ, Kwek BH, et al. Lipomatous hypertrophy of the interatrial septum: increased uptake on FDG PET. *AJR Am J Roentgenol* 2005;184:339–342.
27. Tatli S, O'Gara PT, Lambert J, et al. MRI of atypical lipomatous hypertrophy of the interatrial septum. *AJR Am J Roentgenol* 2004;182:598–600.
28. Burke AP, Litovsky S, Virmani R. Lipomatous hypertrophy of the atrial septum presenting as a right atrial mass. *Am J Surg Pathol* 1996;20:678–685.
29. Burke AP, Virmani R. *Tumors of the heart and great vessels,* 3rd ed. Washington, DC: Armed Forces Institute of Pathology, 1996.
30. Perchinsky MJ, Lichtenstein SV, Tyers GF. Primary cardiac tumors: forty years' experience with 71 patients. *Cancer* 1997;79:1809–1815.
31. Veinot JP, Burns BF, Commons AS, et al. Cardiac neoplasms at the Canadian Reference Centre for Cancer Pathology. *Can J Cardiol* 1999;15:311–319.
32. Burke AP, Tazelaar H, Gomez Roman JJ, et al. Benign tumors of pluripotent mesenchyme. In: Travis W, ed. *Tumours of the lung, thymus, pleura and heart*. Lyon: Springer-Verlag; 2004:260–265.
33. Yoon DH, Roberts W. Sex distribution in cardiac myxomas. *Am J Cardiol* 2002;90:563–565.
34. Burke AP, Virmani R. Cardiac myxoma: a clinicopathologic study. *Am J Clin Pathol* 1993;100:671–680.
35. Carney JA. Differences between nonfamilial and familial cardiac myxoma. *Am J Surg Pathol* 1985;9:53–55.
36. Mochizuki Y, Okamura Y, Iida H, et al. Interleukin-6 and "complex" cardiac myxoma. *Ann Thorac Surg* 1998;66:931–933.
37. Yuda S, Nakatani S, Yutani C, et al. Trends in the clinical and morphological characteristics of cardiac myxoma: 20-year experience of a single tertiary referral center in Japan. *Circ J* 2002;66:1008–1013.
38. Grebenc ML, Rosado-de-Christenson ML, Green CE, et al. Cardiac myxoma: imaging features in 83 patients. *Radiographics* 2002;22:673–689.
39. McCarthy PM, Piehler JM, Schaff HV, et al. The significance of multiple, recurrent, and "complex" cardiac myxomas. *J Thorac Cardiovasc Surg* 1986; 91:389–396.
40. Watson JC, Stratakis CA, Bryant-Greenwood PK, et al. Neurosurgical implications of Carney complex. *J Neurosurg* 2000;92:413–418.
41. Ipek G, Erentug V, Bozbuga N, et al. Surgical management of cardiac myxoma. *J Card Surg* 2005;20:300–304.
42. Tazelaar H, Burke AP, Watanabe G, et al. Hemangioma. In: Travis W, ed. *Tumours of the lung, thymus, pleura and heart.* Lyon: Springer-Verlag, 2004:266–267.
43. Burke A, Johns JP, Virmani R. Hemangiomas of the heart: a clinicopathologic study of ten cases. *Am J Cardiovasc Pathol* 1990;3:283–290.
44. Lupinski RW, Shankar S, Agasthian T, et al. Primary cardiac paraganglioma. *Ann Thorac Surg* 2004;78:e43–44.
45. Osranek M, Bursi F, Gura GM, et al. Echocardiographic features of pheochromocytoma of the heart. *Am J Cardiol* 2003;91:640–643.
46. Cottin Y, Berriolo A, Guy F, et al. Somatostatin-receptor scintigraphy identifies a cardiac pheochromocytoma. *Circulation* 1999;100:2387–2388.
47. Ng JM. Desflurane and remifentanil use during resection of a cardiac pheochromocytoma. *J Cardiothorac Vasc Anesth* 2004;18:630–631.
48. Reynen K, Rein J, Wittekind C, et al. Surgical removal of a lipoma of the heart. *Int J Cardiol* 1993;40:67–68.
49. Wiese TH, Enzweiler CN, Borges AC, et al. Electron beam CT in the diagnosis of recurrent cardiac lipoma. *AJR Am J Roentgenol* 2001;176:1066–1068.
50. Hananouchi GI, Goff WB 2nd. Cardiac lipoma: six-year follow-up with MRI characteristics, and a review of the literature. *Magn Reson Imaging* 1990;8:825–828.
51. Burke AP, Tazelaar H, Butany JW, et al. Cardiac sarcomas. In: Travis W, ed. *Tumours of the lung, thymus, pleura and heart.* Lyon: Springer-Verlag, 2004: 273–281.
52. Burke AP, Cowan D, Virmani R. Primary sarcomas of the heart. *Cancer* 1992;69:387–395.
53. Butany J, Yu W. Cardiac angiosarcoma: two cases and a review of the literature. *Can J Cardiol* 2000;16:197–205.
54. Corso RB, Kraychete N, Nardeli S, et al. Spontaneous rupture of a right atrial angiosarcoma and cardiac tamponade. *Arq Bras Cardiol* 2003;81:611–613, 608–610. Epub 2004 Jan 2028.
55. Casha AR, Davidson LA, Roberts P, et al. Familial angiosarcoma of the heart. *J Thorac Cardiovasc Surg* 2002;124:392–394.
56. Economides EG, Singh A. Case of tumor neovascularization demonstrated by cardiac catheterization. *Cathet Cardiovasc Diagn* 1998;43:451–453.
57. Aoka Y, Kamada T, Kawana M, et al. Primary cardiac angiosarcoma treated with carbon-ion radiotherapy. *Lancet Oncol* 2004;5:636–638.
58. Hoffmeier A, Scheld HH, Tjan TD, et al. Ex situ resection of primary cardiac tumors. *Thorac Cardiovasc Surg* 2003;51:99–101.
59. Sinatra R, Brancaccio G, di Gioia CR, et al. Integrated approach for cardiac angiosarcoma. *Int J Cardiol* 2003;88:301–304.
60. Uberfuhr P, Meiser B, Fuchs A, et al. Heart transplantation: an approach to treating primary cardiac sarcoma? *J Heart Lung Transplant* 2002;21:1135–1139.
61. Tazelaar HD, Locke TJ, McGregor CG. Pathology of surgically excised primary cardiac tumors. *Mayo Clin Proc* 1992;67:957–965.
62. Burke AP, Veinot J, Loire R, et al. Tumors of the heart: introduction. In: Travis W, ed. *Tumours of the lung, thymus, pleura and heart*. Lyon: Springer-Verlag, 2004:251–253.
63. Gowda RM, Khan IA. Clinical perspectives of primary cardiac lymphoma. *Angiology* 2003;54:599–604.
64. Wilhite DB, Quigley RL. Occult cardiac lymphoma presenting with cardiac tamponade. *Tex Heart Inst J* 2003;30:62–64.
65. Chalabreysse L, Berger F, Loire R, et al. Primary cardiac lymphoma in immunocompetent patients: a report of three cases and review of the literature. *Virchows Arch* 2002;441:456–461. Epub 2002 Sep 2027.
66. Hayes D Jr, Liles DK, Sorrell VL. An unusual cause of new-onset atrial flutter: primary cardiac lymphoma. *South Med J* 2003;96:799–802.
67. Clifford SM, Guerra SM, Mangion JR. Massive metastatic intracardiac lymphoma presenting with complete heart block with resolution following chemotherapy. *Echocardiography* 2003;20:201–202.
68. Ikeda H, Nakamura S, Nishimaki H, et al. Primary lymphoma of the heart: case report and literature review. *Pathol Int* 2004;54:187–195.
69. Barbaro G, Di Lorenzo G, Grisorio B, et al. Cardiac involvement in the acquired immunodeficiency syndrome: a multicenter clinical-pathological study. Gruppo Italiano per lo Studio Cardiologico dei pazienti affetti da AIDS Investigators. *AIDS Res Hum Retroviruses* 1998;14:1071–1077.
70. Bley TA, Zeiser R, Ghanem NA, et al. High grade cardiac lymphoma vitality monitoring by gadolinium-enhanced magnetic resonance imaging (MRI). *In Vivo* 2005;19:689–693.
71. Lo SS, Yeager AM, Peel RL, et al. Multimodality treatment in a case of primary cardiac lymphoma. *Clin Lymphoma* 2003;4:112–114.

72. Murphy MC, Sweeney MS, Putnam JB Jr, et al. Surgical treatment of cardiac tumors: a 25-year experience. *Ann Thorac Surg* 1990;49:612–617; discussion 617–618.
73. Chiles C, Woodard PK, Gutierrez FR, et al. Metastatic involvement of the heart and pericardium: CT and MR imaging. *Radiographics* 2001;21: 439–449.
74. Bowman AR, Siegel RJ, Blanche C, et al. Metastatic pancreatic adenocarcinoma to the heart diagnosed antemortem. *J Am Soc Echocardiogr* 2000;13: 415–416.
75. Petropoulakis PN, Steriotis JD, Melanidis JG, et al. Metastatic malignant melanoma as an intracavitary obstructive mass in the right heart. *Eur J Cardiothorac Surg* 1998;14:538–540.

CHAPTER 41 ■ PERIOPERATIVE ANESTHETIC CONSIDERATIONS IN NONCARDIAC SURGERY FOR THOSE AT HIGH RISK OF CARDIOVASCULAR DISEASE

MICHAEL F. ROIZEN, JOHN ELLIS, SRINIVAS MANTHA, AND JOE FOSS

GOALS OF PERIOPERATIVE MANAGEMENT

The goals of anesthesia for those at risk of or with overt cardiovascular disease are similar for any procedure: to minimize patient morbidity and maximize surgical benefit. These goals should be achieved in the most cost-effective manner. The increasing age of the population in Western societies and the desire to restore functional status will likely increase the number of operative procedures performed in the elderly and consequently those with likely significant cardiovascular disease.

The changes in outcome after vascular procedures illustrate the magnitude of improvements in perioperative care in the last 40 years. Perioperative morbidity from such procedures has decreased dramatically, from a 6-day mortality of greater than 25% for major aortic reconstruction in the mid-1960s to less than 2.5% 6-day mortality today. We believe that advances in preoperative preparation and anesthetic management are responsible for a substantial portion of these beneficial changes (1–3). The anesthesiologist may have a greater influence in reducing the morbidity and costs of vascular surgery than in any other complex surgical procedure through the ability to affect outcome and resource utilization.

Nowhere in medicine is the team performance and function likely to be more important to patient outcome in complex surgery than with the combination of primary care physician; cardiologist; surgeon; anesthesiologist; critical care, pain therapy, and rehabilitation subspecialists; and nurse. Why do we specify complex surgery? Because the data are clear: advances in perioperative care have made anesthesia for minimally invasive procedures as safe as the other events in daily living encountered by such patients (4,5). This chapter intends to inform all team members of the perspectives and concerns of the anesthesiologist that bear on perioperative medical and surgical management in care of patients about to undergo complex surgery (we use anesthesia considerations for vascular procedures as the model because these are the best characterized).

The heart is the major focus of the anesthesiologist's attention in such patients because myocardial dysfunction is the most important cause of morbidity after vascular and other complex surgery in the elderly (1,2). Recent studies have identified and emphasized that improvements in outcome were due initially to improvements in fluid management and now to the refinement of preoperative risk-stratification and risk-reducing strategies and the management of the consequences of the stressful nature of the postoperative period to patients. These strategies protect the cardiovascular system and also help to preserve other organ systems (particularly renal and central nervous systems). Thus this chapter reviews current controversies in the selection of anesthetic techniques, monitoring modalities, guidelines (6), chronic medical therapy initiation and continuation, and organ protection strategies.

ASPECTS OF ATHEROSCLEROSIS IMPORTANT TO PERIOPERATIVE CONSIDERATIONS

Advances in the understanding of factors in the pathogenesis of atherosclerosis enhance the ability to assess and minimize risk in the individual patient. The realization that atherosclerosis is a generalized inflammatory disorder of the arterial tree with associated endothelial dysfunction (7) leads to very important risk reduction assessments and strategies.

The predisposing risk factors for atherosclerosis have been classified as "old," "old/new,"and "new" (Table 41.1) (8). The metabolic syndrome (9) and the six situations that contribute to the proinflammatory, prothrombotic state (10) each can be modified preoperatively. The components of the metabolic syndrome constitute a particular combination of what the Expert Panel on Detection, Evaluation, and Treatment of High Blood Cholesterol in Adults (ATP III) terms underlying, major, and emerging risk factors. According to ATP III, *underlying* risk factors for cardiovascular disease are obesity (especially abdominal obesity), physical inactivity, and atherogenic diet; the *major* risk factors are cigarette smoking, hypertension, elevated low-density-lipoprotein cholesterol (LDL-C), low high-density lipoprotein (HDL), family history of premature coronary heart disease, and aging; and the *emerging* risk factors include elevated triglycerides, small LDL particles, insulin resistance, and glucose intolerance. These might seem to require long-term treatment, but each can be modified even in as short a period as 2 weeks before surgery. Furthermore, even the hypertension- and stress-reducing therapies proposed by the Joint Commission on Prevention, Detection, Evaluation, and Treatment of High Blood Pressure (JNC 7) such as aiming at a blood pressure of 115/75 mm Hg lead to different perioperative strategies and tactics (11).

These understandings of various risk factors in the pathogenesis of atherosclerosis have enhanced our ability to assess long-term and perioperative risk in the individual patient. For example, a simple scoring system for calculating a 10-year risk of acute coronary events (12) influences assessment of perioperative management. The model incorporates the following eight independent risk variables ranked in order of importance: age, LDL cholesterol, smoking, HDL cholesterol, systolic blood pressure, family history of premature myocardial infarction (MI), diabetes mellitus, and triglycerides.

The natural history of cardiovascular disease causes further changes in therapies. Persons with cerebral atherosclerosis are at increased risk for ischemic stroke. Stroke is the third-leading cause of death and principal cause of long-term disability in the United States, with 600,000 new or recurrent strokes occurring annually. Presence of even asymptomatic carotid artery disease identifies patients at risk for fatal and nonfatal MI especially in the perioperative period. The prevalence of greater than 25% carotid stenosis in patients older than 65 years was 43% in men and 34% in women in one of the Framingham studies. Those with renal artery atherosclerosis are at risk for perioperative renal failure. Moreover, once disease is apparent in one vascular territory, there is increased risk for adverse events in other territories. For example, patients with peripheral arterial disease (PAD) have a fourfold greater risk of myocardial infarction and a two- to threefold greater risk of stroke than patients without PAD. Regardless of whether symptoms are evident, patients with PAD are six times more likely to die within 10 years than patients without PAD. Patients with symptomatic PAD have a 15-year accrued survival rate of approximately 22% compared with a survival rate of 78% in patients without PAD symptoms. Current U.S. disease-based data sets have been used to compare 5-year mortality rates from common malignancies with the rate of PAD, providing a "commonsense" yardstick of relative risk. This analysis demonstrated that the patient survival rate for PAD is worse than the outcome for breast cancer and Hodgkin disease.

Given the high morbidity and mortality related to PAD and its perioperative prognostic significance, several methods have been proposed for the detection of PAD. Among the several methods, use of the ankle–brachial index (ABI) is a very popular, simple, noninvasive, and inexpensive measurement for assessing the patency of the lower-extremity arterial system. The ABI is measured by having the patient lie in the supine position and then taking the ankle and brachial blood pressure measurements using a 5- to 7-MHz handheld Doppler device. In the lower extremity, posterior tibial and dorsalis pedis artery systolic pressures are measured and compared with the arm pressure. The ABI is calculated by dividing the higher of the ankle systolic pressures by the higher of two systolic brachial

TABLE 41.1

RISK FACTORS FOR ATHEROSCLEROSIS

Old	Old/new	New
Gender (men > women) Age Family history of premature cardiovascular disease Total cholesterol, LDL cholesterol, HDL cholesterol (negative risk factor) Hypertension Smoking Overweight/obesity	High-normal blood pressure Metabolic syndrome Diabetes mellitus, impaired glucose tolerance, impaired fasting glucose	Apolipoprotein B, apolipoprotein A-1, triglycerides, triglyceride-rich lipoprotein remnants, small, dense LDL, oxidized LDL, antibodies against oxidized LDL Lipoprotein(a) Homocysteine High-sensitivity C-reactive protein

HDL, high-density lipoprotein; LDL, low-density lipoprotein.

pressures. Measuring the ABI is the most effective, accurate, and practical method of PAD detection. An ABI value of 1.0 or greater is considered normal, whereas a value less than 0.9 indicates the presence of PAD and approaches 95% sensitivity in detecting angiogram-positive disease. It is almost 100% specific in excluding healthy individuals. The ABI also helps to evaluate the severity of the disease. For example, ABI values of 0.81 to 0.9 are consistent with mild disease and values of 0.5 to 0.81 with moderate disease, and values less than 0.5 are considered to indicate severe obstructive disease. Furthermore, a value less than 0.9 is highly predictive of morbidity and mortality from cardiovascular events linked with PAD. The major disadvantage of the ABI is that some elderly and diabetic patients have calcified arteries that prevent occlusion of blood flow by the blood pressure cuff, which may result in an unusually high ABI reading (>1.50). More recently, large observational studies and atherosclerosis regression trials of lipid-modifying pharmacotherapy have established that intima–media thickness of the carotid and femoral arteries, as measured noninvasively by B-mode ultrasound, is a valid surrogate marker for the progression of atherosclerotic disease (7).

CONSIDERATIONS FOR VASCULAR AND OTHER COMPLEX SURGERY PATIENTS

The goals of vascular surgery are to provide an enduring restoration of normal perfusion so as to prevent stroke, improve functional status, and prevent death from aneurysm rupture. Perioperative management is important because approximately 700,000 patients in the United States underwent vascular surgical procedures in 2002. Increasingly, randomized clinical trials are demonstrating the benefits to patient quality and length of life from revascularization procedures of the aorta, the carotids, the renal arteries, and the lower-extremity arteries (7,13). An explosive growth of less invasive procedures is changing surgery in the elderly, including vascular surgery. New treatment options include lasers, angioplasty, stenting, atherectomy (rotary and directional devices), gene therapy to help prevent restenosis and to promote angiogenesis, and thrombolysis, at times with concomitant or secondary surgery. Although outcome studies for many of these procedures just now are being completed, they appear to be associated with less short-term risk than traditional surgery. Less invasive approaches will invariably lead to procedures being performed in patients with such severe comorbidities that they would previously have been denied surgery. A recent randomized clinical trial involving 60 patients who underwent percutaneous transluminal coronary angioplasty (PTCA) for acute MI showed that intracoronary transfer of autologous bone marrow cells resulted in improvement of the left ventricular systolic function at 6 months' follow-up. As with this potential application, other developments are both promising and challenging, such as creation of a long-lasting arterial substitute for small-caliber vessels and performance of revascularization less invasively and with less morbidity.

Abdominal aortic aneurysms (AAAs) occur in up to 5% of men older than 65 years of age. Most AAAs are small and require only infrequent follow-up. There are two therapeutic options for AAA patients with lesions large enough to cause worry about rupture: open surgery and endovascular aortic aneurysm repair (EVAR) (3). The main impetus behind EVAR has been its potential for significantly reducing procedural mortality and morbidity, and it was expected to speed recovery and reduce cost through decreased use of hospital resources. The new technology has evoked a mixed response, with enthusiasts and detractors debating its value; unfortunately, bias and conflict of interest may be involved. EVAR seems to be an appropriate elective treatment in patients with AAAs with significant comorbid conditions and suitable anatomy and in patients with relatively limited life expectancy and larger or enlarging AAAs. A recent decision-analysis model suggests that EVAR is preferable in older patients at higher operative risk and open surgery is preferred in younger patients at low operative risk. For atherosclerotic disease of carotid arteries, studies have clearly shown an advantage for surgical endarterectomy compared to medical therapy. Carotid endarterectomy (CEA) is appropriate for symptomatic patients (transient ischemic attacks or nondisabling stroke) with 70% to 99% carotid stenosis and in selected asymptomatic patients with 60% or greater stenosis after careful consideration of additional risk factors. In experienced hands CEA and carotid stenting may have equivalent success and complication rates. Combined perioperative mortality and major morbidity rates should be less than 6% for symptomatic patients and less than 3% for asymptomatic patients for percutaneous procedures, as for CEA. Patients with restenosis after CEA and those with radiation-induced stenosis are at increased risk from surgery and thus good candidates for stenting.

Perioperative management has taken lessons from medical therapy for atherosclerotic vascular disease (AVD) in improving functional status, preventing stroke, preventing limb loss, and reducing potential atherosclerotic progression and cardiovascular morbidity. In general, medical measures typically include smoking cessation, lifestyle changes, antilipidemic therapy, control of blood pressure, control of diabetes mellitus, and antiplatelet therapy. Cessation of smoking is by far the most effective "medical" therapy. Although acute smoking cessation before surgery may not reduce perioperative respiratory complications, patients should be encouraged to stop smoking. Cessation rates are approximately 25% after major surgery. Despite the low success rates, the benefits of smoking cessation are so great that such perioperative programs are probably very cost-effective.

Lifestyle changes such as weight loss and exercise reduce perioperative complications in small randomized and nonrandomized studies. Nonlipid properties can be observed earlier (as early as 2 weeks of therapy) than lipid effects. Patients who were already taking statins when they presented to the hospital with acute coronary events and continued to receive them were less likely to experience more adverse complications or die than patients who never received statins (14). Statin use is also associated with improved graft patency and limb salvage and decreased amputation rate in patients undergoing infrainguinal bypass for AVD (15). Recently, angiotensin-converting-enzyme (ACE inhibitors) were shown to upregulate type III collagen synthesis, which could improve atherosclerotic plaque stabilization (16). Such action may explain the beneficial effects of ACE inhibitors with regard to acute vascular events (e.g., stroke) that are independent of their antihypertensive effect. For example, ACE inhibitor use was also associated with decreased long-term mortality in patients undergoing infrainguinal bypass for AVD (15).

CONSIDERATIONS IN MANAGEMENT OF CHRONIC AND PERIOPERATIVE RISK-REDUCING MEDICAL THERAPIES

Antiplatelet therapy is a mainstay of medical therapy for peripheral vascular disease. Chronic therapy with aspirin or other antiinflammatory drugs may retard the progression of atherosclerosis and prevent morbid cardiovascular events.

TABLE 41.2

CONCOMITANT MEDICAL THERAPY, SIDE EFFECTS OF POTENTIAL CONCERN PERIOPERATIVELY, AND OUR RECOMMENDATIONS

Medication or drug class	Side effect of potential concern in the perioperative period	Recommendation for perioperative use
Aspirin	Platelet inhibition may increase bleeding; decreased glomerular filtration rate	Continue through day of surgery; monitor fluid and urine status
HMG-CoA reductase inhibitors	Liver function test abnormalities	Assess liver function tests and continue through morning of surgery
β-Blockers	Bronchospasm	Continue through perioperative period
ACE inhibitors	Induction hypotension, cough	Continue through perioperative period; consider 1/2 dose on day of surgery
Diuretics	Hypovolemia, electrolyte abnormalities	Continue through morning of surgery; monitor fluid and urine status
Calcium channel blockers	Perioperative hypotension especially with amlodipine	Continue through perioperative period; consider withholding amlodipine on the morning of surgery
Oral hypoglycemics	Hypoglycemia pre- and intraoperatively	When feasible, switch to insulin preoperatively; monitor glucose status perioperatively

ACE, angiotensin-converting enzyme; HMG-CoA, 3-hydroxy-3-methylglutaryl–coenzyme A reductase.

Therefore, many patients presenting for vascular surgery will be taking aspirin, nonsteroidal antiinflammatory drugs (NSAIDs), and even COX-2 inhibitors, ticlopidine, or clopidogrel. Clopidogrel irreversibly inhibits adenosine diphosphate (ADP)-induced platelet aggregation and reduces formation of both arterial and venous thrombi. Oral platelet glycoprotein IIb/IIIa inhibitors may also be used acutely during percutaneous coronary intervention and as adjunctive treatment of acute coronary syndromes. Considerations of the adverse effects of aspirin, including increased bleeding tendency, gastritis, and renal vasoconstriction, as well as thrombotic thrombocytopenic purpura and neutropenia from ticlopidine must be weighed against potential benefits. In general, we recommend that patients continue to take aspirin through the day of surgery for all non–closed space, non–plastic surgical procedures. Other acute anticoagulant issues are addressed later (17,18).

There is substantial evidence that antihypertensive, plaque stress–reducing, lipid-lowering, and antiplatelet therapies decrease the stroke risk in the perioperative period as well as chronically. Our recommendations for management of concomitant medical therapy in the perioperative period are listed in Table 41.2.

RISK ASSESSMENT ALGORITHMS

Although the foregoing disorders associated with vascular disease and complex surgery (diabetes, smoking and its sequelae, chronic pulmonary disease, hypertension, renal insufficiency, and ischemic heart disease) are the most common, it is their consequences that are most important to perioperative outcome. Understanding the end-organ effects of these diseases can guide appropriate perioperative therapy. It would be suboptimal to administer anesthesia to patients with uncontrolled medical conditions such as severe hypertension, a recent myocardial infarction, uncontrolled diabetes and hyperglycemia, or untreated pulmonary infections. However, an expanding aneurysm, crescendo transient ischemic attacks, or threatened limb loss can force one's hand. In such situations, attempts to rapidly control chronically deranged blood pressure (which could precipitate cerebral ischemia) or electrolytes (which could, e.g., result in accidental administration of a bolus of potassium) may be more hazardous than leaving the condition untreated or trying to control the abnormality slowly. The National Veterans Affairs Surgical Risk Study found that low serum albumin values and high American Society of Anesthesiologists (ASA) physical classification were among the best predictors of morbidity and mortality after vascular surgery (19,20) (Table 41.3).

Whereas chronic medical conditions increase the likelihood of postoperative morbidity and mortality, postoperative complications have even greater predictive value for adverse outcomes (Table 41.4) (21). Other causes of morbidity after vascular and other complex surgery include bleeding, pulmonary infections, graft infections, renal insufficiency and failure, hepatic failure, cerebrovascular accidents, and spinal cord

TABLE 41.3

THE 10 MOST IMPORTANT PREOPERATIVE PREDICTORS OF POSTOPERATIVE 30-DAY MORTALITY AFTER VASCULAR SURGERY IN VETERAN'S AFFAIRS MEDICAL CENTERS

Predictor	Odds ratio
Ventilator dependent	2.71
American Society of Anesthesiologists class	1.89
Emergency operation	2.40
Do Not Resuscitate status	2.96
Blood urea nitrogen >40 mg/dL	1.47
Albumin	0.61
Age	1.03
Creatinine >1.2 mg/dL	1.48
Esophageal varices	4.30
Operative complexity score	1.32

All variables are statistically significant ($p < 0.05$) and were selected after stepwise multivariable analysis.
Modified from Khuri SF, Daley J, Henderson W, et al. Risk adjustment of the postoperative mortality rate for the comparative assessment of the quality of surgical care: results of the National Veterans Affairs Surgical Risk Study. *J Am Coll Surg* 1997;185(4):315.

TABLE 41.4

DEMOGRAPHICS, HOSPITAL CHARACTERISTICS, PREOPERATIVE CHRONIC MEDICAL CONDITIONS, AND POSTOPERATIVE COMPLICATIONS AND THEIR CONTRIBUTIONS TO MORTALITY PREDICTION

Variable	Prevalence (%)	Odds ratio (mortality)	*p* value
Demographic			
Higher income		0.93/octile	.0001
Older age		1.03/year	.0001
African American	5.0	0.62	.0012
Hispanic	1.9	0.62	.0012
Other insurance	1.5	1.35	.0005
Through emergency room	10.8	1.94	.0001
Transfer from another hospital	1.6	1.80	.0001
Emergency admit	13.9	2.44	.0001
Urgent admission	21.4	1.78	.0001
Hospital			
Urban	90.6	0.82	.0339
Investor	12.5	0.75	.0009
Midwest	21.3	1.34	.0063
South	40.0	1.27	.0038
Chronic medical condition			
Dysrhythmias	13.6	2.84	.0001
Chronic renal failure	1.3	2.60	.0001
Congestive heart failure	7.9	1.89	.0001
Cerebrovascular disease	12.6	1.38	.0001
Conduction defects	2.8	1.30	.0404
Coronary obstructive pulmonary disease	3.1	1.20	NS
Diabetes	21.1	1.01	NS
Coronary disease	30.2	0.82	.0006
Hypertension	44.5	0.65	.0001
Postoperative complications			
Respiratory failure	7.9	6.19	.0001
Acute renal failure	3.5	5.60	.0001
Myocardial infarction	1.4	5.22	.0001
Stroke	1.0	3.03	.0001
Peripheral vascular complications	0.8	3.03	.0001
Postoperative cardiac failure	5.1	2.50	.0001

NS, not significant.
From Ellis JE. Health sciences research and large database analysis in vascular surgery and anesthesia: confirming common sense? *Prob Anesth* 1999;11:238.

ischemia resulting in paraplegia. The incidence of these other causes of morbidity has declined substantially in the last 20 years. Although multisystem organ failure may account for an increasing proportion of deaths after vascular surgery and complex vascular surgery, we believe that maintaining adequate cardiac function and perfusion of vital organs remains a vital aspect of reducing perioperative mortality. The factors that affect patient prognosis after vascular and complex surgery remain primarily related to the heart (1). We will therefore examine more closely the effects of known or suspected coronary artery disease on patient management before, during, and after vascular and other complex surgery.

Coronary Artery Disease in Patients with Peripheral Vascular Disease

Hertzer et al. (22) performed coronary angiography in 1,001 consecutive patients presenting for vascular surgery and identified severe correctable coronary artery disease in 25% of the entire series. The incidence of significant coronary artery disease (stenosis >70%) detected by angiography was 78% in those with clinical indications of coronary artery disease and 37% in patients without any clinical indications. However, subsequent analysis demonstrated that clinical risk factors still predicted the severity of coronary artery disease (Fig. 41.1) (23). The absence of severe coronary stenoses can be predicted with a positive predictive value of 96% for patients who had none of the following risk factors: history of diabetes, prior angina, previous myocardial infarction, and congestive heart failure.

Short-term postoperative morbidity and mortality after vascular surgery is higher than after other types of complex noncardiac surgery (24). Long-term morbidity and mortality after vascular surgery are greatly influenced by the presence of coronary artery disease. The presence of uncorrected coronary artery disease appears to double 5-year mortality after vascular surgery. Coronary artery bypass graft (CABG) is associated with improved survival in peripheral vascular disease patients who have triple-vessel, but not single- or double-vessel, coronary artery disease (25). Previous percutaneous transluminal coronary angioplasty (PTCA) may protect against

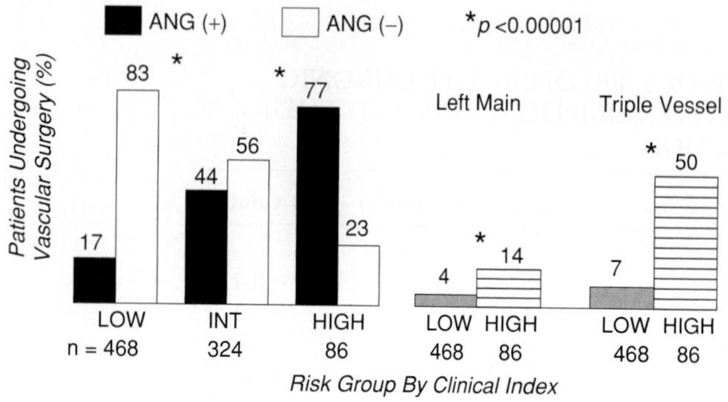

FIGURE 41.1. Clinical risk factors predicting severe (left main or triple vessel) coronary artery disease. A preoperative clinical index (diabetes mellitus, prior myocardial infarction, angina, age >70 years, congestive heart failure) was used to stratify patients. ANG(+), angiogram positive for coronary artery disease; ANG(–), angiogram negative for coronary artery disease; INT, intermediate. (Based on data from Paul SD, Eagle KA, Kuntz KM, et al. Concordance of preoperative clinical risk with angiographic severity of coronary artery disease in patients undergoing vascular surgery. *Circulation* 1966;94(7):1561. Secondary analysis of data from Hertzer NR, Beven EG, Young JR, et al. Coronary artery disease in peripheral vascular patients: a classification of 1000 coronary angiograms and results of surgical management. *Ann Surg* 1984;199:223.)

perioperative cardiac events after vascular surgery. The prevalence of asymptomatic coronary artery disease and the substantial short-term and long-term cardiac morbidity and mortality in patients undergoing vascular surgery have led investigators and clinicians to propose and undertake extensive preoperative evaluation to detect underlying coronary artery disease.

Before discussing preoperative workup for detecting underlying coronary artery disease (CAD) it is important to review the pathophysiology that leads to perioperative MI or postoperative cardiovascular dysfunction. In addition to CAD, other important etiologic factors for perioperative cardiovascular events are perioperative hypothermia; significant valvular heart disease, especially aortic stenosis; history of congestive heart failure (CHF); anemia; increased intraoperative bleeding as assessed by the amount of cell-salvaged blood; increased circulating catecholamines; exogenous vasoconstrictors; and hypercoagulability (easily activated platelets with a higher fibrinogen rate and decreased fibrinolysis) (26–30). A recent systematic review and meta-analysis of 30 observational studies ("level B evidence") failed to demonstrate an association between preoperative hypertension/hypertensive heart disease and perioperative adverse cardiac events (31).

The timing and character of perioperative MI reported in the literature seems to have shifted from a predominance of Q-wave MI peaking between postoperative days 2 and 3 with high mortality to earlier-occurring (operative day/day 1 postsurgery) non–Q-wave MI with lower mortality. MI occurring in the perioperative period is associated with sustained elevation of heart rate (greater by twofold if heart rate is more than 90 beats per minute, and especially greater if sustained at more than 110 beats per minute), an absence of chest pain, and prolonged premonitory episodes of ST-segment depression before overt MI (32). The pathophysiology of perioperative MI differs somewhat from that of MI occurring in the usual nonoperative setting. In contrast to the usual case, plaque rupture occurs only in about half of perioperative infarctions. The remainder is due to a prolonged imbalance between myocardial oxygen demand and supply in the setting of CAD. Myocardial oxygen supply may be diminished by anemia or hypotension, whereas oxygen demand may be increased by tachycardia and hypertension resulting from postoperative pain, withdrawal of anesthesia, or shifts in intravascular volume (33). That and validating studies lead to usual perioperative risk reduction with β-adrenergic blockade.

Previously abnormal endothelial function due to acute inflammatory responses was a well-recognized factor in the medical setting but not in the perioperative setting. Recent studies, however, have shown that endothelial dysfunction as evaluated preoperatively by noninvasive ultrasound assessment of dilation mediated by brachial artery flow is useful in predicting short-term as well as long-term adverse cardiovascular outcomes after vascular surgery (34). Decreased endothelium-dependent flow-mediated dilation reflects endothelial dysfunction in patients with AVD.

Controversy persists as to whether preoperative identification of patients most likely to have perioperative cardiovascular events related to myocardial ischemia benefits patients. Invasive interventions may benefit patients with vascular disease but are generally more risky than in other groups of patients. Many believe that preparatory coronary revascularization may be a "survival test" that is accompanied by increased short-term morbidity; others believe that these procedures lead to better long-term survival. Patients who have survived coronary revascularization have fewer cardiac complications after vascular surgery (24,27,35).

Three essential purposes are served by preoperative cardiac risk stratification. The first is to forgo surgery or perform a more conservative surgical procedure in those at high risk. The second is to determine which patients should undergo myocardial revascularization. This goal requires that we identify patients with left main coronary artery disease and those with triple-vessel coronary artery disease and poor left ventricular function because these patients are most likely to benefit from coronary revascularization in the long run (25). Finally, because most perioperative myocardial ischemia and infarction occur early in the postoperative period, a third rationale for preoperative segregation of high-risk patients is to target those who might benefit from preoperative drug therapy as well as aggressive therapy in the first 24 to 72 hours after surgery. The patient's history and bedside examination including electrocardiogram (ECG) before complex surgery serve to predict coronary anatomy and to provide important prognostic information. Based on these clinical criteria for risk stratification, patients who have three risk factors or more are considered to be at "high risk" (36). The need for emergency or urgent surgery identifies a group of patients at greatly increased risk for cardiac complications.

Studies have suggested that risk of reinfarction in the perioperative period depends primarily on the amount of time that has passed since infarction. Traditional recommendations suggested that at least 6 months must elapse after an MI before a patient is eligible for elective noncardiac surgery. However, advances in therapeutic modalities in patients with acute and prior ST-elevation MI (thrombolytic and other drug therapies—β-blockers, aspirin, statins, immunizations, and ACE inhibitors, listed in order of strength of data and importance of effect in the perioperative period—and primary angioplasty) are helping to limit the ventricular remodeling and its adverse consequences and thereby to promote early recovery. In addition, noninvasive testing (as described later) helps to identify patients at relatively low risk despite a recent infarction. Thus, the long waiting period of 6 months before surgery may no longer apply to most patients.

Exercise tolerance may also be a useful prognostic indicator, although claudication, orthopedic problems, and frailty may limit a patient's capabilities. Patients with limited exercise capacity (<4 metabolic equivalents [METS]) have greatly increased perioperative risk (24). The oxygen consumption of a 70-kg, 40-year-old man in a resting state is 3.5 mL/kg/minute or 1 MET. Taking care of oneself, eating, dressing, walking indoors, walking a block or two on level ground at 2 to 3 miles/hour (3.2 to 4.8 km/hour), and doing light household work such as dusting and washing clothes (and engaging in sexual activity) represent a functional capacity ranging from 1 to 4, respectively (surgery and sex are about equal in stress). Climbing a flight of stairs or walking up a hill, walking on level ground at 4 miles/hour, moving heavy furniture, participating in moderate recreational activities such as bowling, dancing, and so on, and participating in strenuous sports like swimming or football represent a functional capacity ranging from 4 to 10 in that order.

Because claudication in vascular surgery patients limits the evaluation of functional capacity and CAD evaluation by conventional exercise testing, other, noninvasive tests have become popular for cardiac risk stratification in these patients (37,38). The noninvasive tests include ambulatory ECG, radionuclide ventriculogram (RNV), dipyridamole scintigraphy (DTS), dobutamine stress echocardiography (DSE), and dipyridamole stress echocardiography. Our meta-analysis published in1994 attempted to evaluate the value of the first four of these tests in predicting adverse cardiac outcomes (MI or cardiac-related deaths) within 30 days after vascular surgery (37). The usefulness of the tests was as follows (highest to lowest): DSE, DTS, RNV, and ambulatory ECG. These results were confirmed in a recent meta-analysis (38). The high percentage of patients (at least 25% in our practice) with baseline ECG abnormalities further limits the usefulness of ambulatory ECG. The baseline ECG abnormalities typically include ventricular hypertrophy with "strain," bundle branch block, pacemakers, and the effects of digoxin. Congestive heart failure is a strong predictor of morbid postoperative events. Determination of systolic left ventricular function may therefore provide prognostic information.

Radionuclide ventriculography can be used to define systolic and diastolic function. Our meta-analysis showed that patients who have an ejection fraction less than 35% by radionuclide ventriculography are 3.7 times more likely to have a postoperative cardiac event. However, RNV has generally been supplanted by echocardiography, with definition of myocardial structure and pharmacologic stress. A recent meta-analysis demonstrated the limited value of routine preoperative left ventricular ejection fraction (LVEF) by multigated acquisition scanning (MUGA) as a general screening test before vascular surgery (39). RNV and MUGA differ in the way that radioactivity of blood-pool tracer (typically ^{99m}Tc-labeled red cells) is measured and imaging is performed. With both methods, assessment can be made of LVEF, right ventricular ejection fraction, LV regional wall motion, and LV volumes. Because preoperative LVEF plays a key role in defining the long-term cardiac outcome after vascular surgery (39,40), the recommendation for RNV and MUGA as a routine screening test appears to be for class III patients and for class IIa patients with current or history of CHF.

DTS is based on the principle of coronary steal. A new technique for imaging in DTS is single-photon emission computed tomography (SPECT). DTS is not suitable for patients with bronchospasm, critical carotid stenosis, or a condition that prevents their being withdrawn from theophylline preparations.

In a DSE test, oxygen consumption of the heart is increased by slow and graded infusion of dobutamine to see whether new regional wall-motion abnormalities develop. The infusion is continued until 85% of the maximum predicted heart rate for the patient's age is achieved. The maximum heart rate in men is 220 beats per minute minus age in years, and in women, some centers use 200 beats per minute minus age in years. Evaluation is based on the severity and number of myocardial segments manifesting new wall-motion abnormalities. Hypotension developing during the DSE is also considered a high-risk result and is useful in predicting adverse cardiac outcome after vascular or complex surgery in the elderly.

Dipyridamole stress echocardiography is another form of pharmacologic stress testing that can be useful in cardiac risk stratification in vascular and complex surgery in older patients. Both DTS and DSE have been used and studied extensively for this purpose (1,2,24,37,38). Because coronary angiography is impractical to use routinely before vascular surgery due to the costs and risks involved, the use of screening tests is controversial. Some studies show them to have great prognostic value, whereas others show that these tests do not perform better than the basic clinical evaluation. The essential reason could be lack of studies of ideal design. The ideal clinical trial to help to resolve these controversies would be prospective, collect data over a relatively short period of time, select patients consecutively, and blind clinicians caring for the patients to the test results. Ethical concerns about not making test results available to clinicians have precluded large-scale randomized trials.

CARDIAC RISK STRATIFICATION

The algorithm proposed by American College of Cardiology/American Heart Association (ACC/AHA) incorporates clinical history, exercise tolerance, and surgical procedure into the decision to perform further evaluation (24). The guidelines classify the clinical predictors of increased perioperative cardiovascular risk (MI, CHF, and death) as major, intermediate, and minor. The major risk factors include acute MI (<7 days), recent MI (7 to 30 days), unstable angina, decompensated CHF, and significant arrhythmias. The guidelines mandate intensive management for major risk factors, which may result in delay or cancellation of surgery unless it is emergent. The guidelines place vascular surgery (aortic and peripheral vascular surgery) in the high-risk surgery category, with an estimated cardiac risk (MI or cardiac-related death) exceeding 5%. Carotid endarterectomy and many complex operations done in the elderly are regarded as being of intermediate risk, with an estimated cardiac risk and mortality risk in the 30 days after surgery ranging from 1% to 5%. The following discussion deals with cardiac risk stratification for vascular and other complex surgery in the elderly.

As the prior probability of a disease in a population increases, the predictive value of a positive test increases and the predictive value of a negative test decreases (1). This allows us to eliminate testing in situations that do not provide additional information. Typically in a scenario of cardiac risk stratification in vascular and complex surgery in the elderly, studies have consistently identified current or prior angina pectoris, prior myocardial infarction, congestive heart failure, advanced age (70 years or older), severely limited exercise tolerance, chronic renal insufficiency (serum creatinine >2.0 mg%), cerebrovascular accident, and need for insulin therapy as risk factors for the development of perioperative cardiac morbidity (24,35,36). Generally patients presenting for surgery can be categorized by these clinical criteria as follows: at least one risk factor, low risk; two risk factors, intermediate risk; three or more risk factors, high risk. By applying the principles of Bayes' theorem, traditional recommendations made more than a decade ago proposed the use of noninvasive cardiac testing in patients with intermediate clinical risk, no testing in those at low clinical risk, and coronary angiography in those at high clinical risk and those tested positive by noninvasive testing. Such a strategy of risk stratification was also supported by decision analysis for cost-effectiveness that attempted to look at 5-year survival as an outcome measure (41). However, the current recommendations seem to have shifted the paradigm toward perioperative drug therapy aimed at reducing cardiac risk either with no noninvasive cardiac testing (33) or with highly selective noninvasive testing (36). Essential reasons for the change in cardiac risk stratification patterns derive from recent views on the usefulness of noninvasive tests (typically DTS/DSE) in predicting cardiac outcome; perioperative risk reducing strategies; semiquantitative interpretation of DTS or DSE; and coronary revascularization. The following discussion explains in detail each of these issues in relationship to the perioperative care of the vascular or complex surgery patient.

Usefulness of Noninvasive Tests (Typically Dipyridamole Scintigraphy/Dobutamine Stress Echocardiography) in Predicting Cardiac Outcome

To understand this issue, one needs to understand the application of Bayes' theorem (1). Recent recommendations suggest the use of likelihood ratios (LRs) for evaluating the usefulness of diagnostic tests (42). In risk stratification by noninvasive testing, computation of LRs reveals that no method reaches the ideal values for LRs (1,2,33). These findings support the argument for almost avoiding noninvasive testing while making the best use of risk-reducing drug therapy (33). Studies have also shown that the strategy of subjecting patients with positive noninvasive tests (DTS/DSE) to coronary angiography followed by coronary revascularization where indicated does not improve short- or intermediate-term outcome. Thus it has become apparent that further stratification before surgery by grading the positive noninvasive test results is needed.

Semiquantitative Interpretation of Dipyridamole Scintigraphy/Dobutamine Stress Echocardiography

Fortunately, the results of DTS/DSE are amenable to semiquantitative interpretation. Abnormality in five or more segments during DSE is considered a "strongly positive" test result for risk stratification with an LR of 13.09 (36). Similarly, for DTS, a recent meta-analysis demonstrated that greater extent of reversibility increased the risk, whereas defects in fewer than 20% of myocardial segments did not significantly alter the risk of perioperative cardiac complications (43). For practical purposes, to make it comparable to DSE on a three-grade scale, the results of DTS can be defined as follows: "normal" implies no distribution defects or involvement of fewer than 20% of the segments, "weakly positive" refers to involvement of 21% to 50% of the segments, and "strongly positive" holds when the involvement exceeds 50% of the segments.

Perioperative Cardiac Risk-Reducing Strategies

Of the various risk-reducing strategies, growing evidence suggests that perioperative β-blockade provides benefit in preventing cardiac morbidity and mortality (44). Benefits of the therapy are best observed when oral preoperative therapy is extended to intraoperative and postoperative periods by intravenous therapy to titrate the heart rate of 65 beats per minute or less. Typically, oral therapy can be initiated at least the day before surgery with either 50 to 100 mg of atenolol daily or 5 to 10 mg of bisoprolol, whereas intraoperative and postoperative periods are best managed by intravenous administration of 5 to 10 mg of atenolol twice daily. Alternatively, esmolol 500 μg/kg may be given intravenously over 1 minute followed by infusion of 50 to 200 μg/kg per minute to achieve the target heart rate. Patients already taking β-blockers continue to the day of surgery followed by intravenous therapy to achieve the target heart rate as described previously. A recent decision-analytic model that evaluated five different regimens of perioperative β-blockade found the therapy to be both cost-effective and efficacious from a short-term perspective (45). Although older literature warns against use with any degree of reactive airway disease, insulin-dependent diabetes, and even peripheral vascular disease, newer data suggest that careful titration of β1-selective agents is well tolerated in most such patients. However, severe asthma or a strong component with chronic obstructive airway disease remains a major relative contraindication, as do cardiac conduction disease in the absence of a pacemaker and previous documented drug sensitivities. Reviews show that hypovolemia can be poorly tolerated in the presence of β-blockade, and racial difference to β-blockade might exist (29).

α-2-Adrenergic blockers (clonidine or mivazerol) have been used to reduce perioperative cardiac morbidity and mortality for more than a decade. Our randomized, double-blind control study ($n = 61$; 82% vascular surgery patients) demonstrated beneficial effects of perioperative use of clonidine for this purpose. We used a regimen of a transdermal clonidine system (0.2 mg/day) the night before surgery, which was left in place for 72 hours, and 0.3 mg of oral clonidine administered 60 to 90 minutes before surgery. Clonidine reduced intraoperative myocardial ischemia (46). A recent meta-analysis demonstrated beneficial effects of perioperative α-blockers with regard to cardiac morbidity and death in patients undergoing vascular surgery (evidence level B) (47). Other studies used oral clonidine 4 to 6 μg/kg administered at 90 to 120 minutes before surgery with intravenous 3 μg/kg administered in the postoperative period to maintain the levels for 72 hours. The regimen for mivazerol includes intravenous administration of 4 μg/kg 20 minutes before surgery and 1.5 μg/kg/hr for 72 hours.

Statins have been proven to be useful for controlling adverse cardiac events perioperatively as well as during long-term follow-up for vascular surgery patients. A case-control study demonstrated decreased perioperative mortality after vascular surgery (48). A recent randomized trial demonstrated beneficial effects of statin use (atorvastatin 20 mg daily started 45 days before surgery) with regard to primary endpoints (cardiac-related death, nonfatal MI, unstable angina, stroke) at 6-month follow-up (49). Another observational study demonstrated that long-term statin use after successful abdominal aortic aneurysm repair was associated with reduced all-cause and cardiovascular mortality irrespective of clinical factors and β-blocker use (50).

ACE inhibitors have several beneficial actions with regard to acute vascular events independent of their antihypertensive action in patients with atherosclerotic vascular disease (7,15). No studies provide evidence for their independent ability to reduce perioperative cardiac problems in therapy aimed at risk reduction.

A recent meta-analysis demonstrated beneficial effects of calcium channel blockers in reducing perioperative adverse cardiac events (cardiac-related death, MI, ischemia, or supraventricular tachycardia) in patients undergoing different types of noncardiac surgery (51). The majority of these effects were attributable to diltiazem. Another extended meta analysis confirmed a reduction in the risk of restenosis and clinical events when calcium channel blockers were added to standard therapy after percutaneous coronary intervention (52). We do not recommend their use for perioperative cardiac risk reduction. Drug interventions are summarized in Table 41.5.

In addition to drug therapies, other interventions may also be beneficial in reducing adverse perioperative cardiovascular events. Perioperative maintenance of normothermia with a forced-air rewarming device is associated with a reduced incidence of morbid cardiac events and ventricular tachycardia

TABLE 41.5

DRUGS WITH PROVEN OR POTENTIAL BENEFITS WITH REGARD TO ACUTE VASCULAR EVENTS IN PATIENTS UNDERGOING VASCULAR OR COMPLEX SURGERY

Intervention	Regimen and remarks	Recommendation
Perioperative β-blockade (44)	Preoperative oral bisoprolol or atenolol initiated at least 30 d before surgery and intravenous therapy during intraoperative and postoperative period (atenolol or esmolol)	Class I
α-Blockers (46,47)	Pretreatment with oral clonidine 0.3 mg at least 90 min before surgery and therapy continued for 72 h (oral or transdermal, 0.2 mg/d) Intravenous clonidine clonideni 0.3 mg daily can also be administered for 72 h Alternatively, intravenous mivazerol 4 μg/kg bolus given 20 min before surgery followed by 1.5 μg/kg/h continued for 72 h	Class IIa
Statin therapy (49,50)	Typical dose of atorvastatin is 20 mg once daily initiated at least 45 d before surgery Continued use after surgery is associated with reduced cardiovascular events in the long-term follow-up Also improves graft survival, facilitates limb salvage, and decreases amputation rates Atherosclerotic plaque stabilization, resistance of low-density lipoprotein to oxidation antiinflammatory action, and reversal of endothelial dysfunction may explain some of these benefits Some of the beneficial effects are independent of their lipid-lowering properties and may be observed as early as 2 weeks after initiation of therapy	Class I
ACE inhibitors (15,16)	Potential benefits include decreased stroke rate (e.g., ramipril), limitation of ventricular remodeling that follows acute ST-elevation myocardial infarction, decreased long-term mortality following infrainguinal bypass surgery, and so on Ability to stabilize the atherosclerotic plaque by upregulating type III collagen of the fibrous cap of the unstable plaque may explain some of these benefits	Class IIb
Calcium channel blockers (51,52)	Reduced perioperative adverse cardiac events including supraventricular tachycardia in patients undergoing various types of noncardiac surgery Evidence is limited in patients undergoing vascular surgery Reduction in the incidence of restenosis and clinical events when added to standard therapy after percutaneous coronary intervention	Class IIb

See text for details. Refer to Figure 41.2 for the algorithm. Calcium channel blockers and angiotensin-converting-enzyme (ACE) inhibitors, although not recommended as independent agents for the purpose, should be continued should a patient be receiving them.
Refer to Table 41.2 for suggestions for precautions on their perioperative use. Statin use is also associated with improved graft patency limb salvage and decreased amputation rate in patients undergoing infrainguinal bypass for atherosclerotic vascular disease.

(26). Although invasive hemodynamic monitoring may be beneficial, the exact role of the pulmonary artery catheter (PAC) is controversial. A recent randomized control study failed to demonstrate benefits of perioperative hemodynamic optimization using PAC initiated the day before surgery in patients undergoing infrarenal abdominal aortic aneurysm repair. The endpoints measured were in-hospital mortality, cardiovascular morbidity, postoperative renal failure, and duration of hospital stay (53).

ANTICOAGULANT DRUGS IN THE PERIOPERATIVE PERIOD

When patients develop acute ischemia, systemic anticoagulation may be instituted. The agents used may range from dextran (to enhance microcirculatory blood flow) to heparin, Coumadin, and thrombolytics. Therefore, when patients present for urgent surgery to reverse acute ischemia, we specifically ask them and their surgeons about recent or planned anticoagulation. If the answer is "yes," forgoing regional anesthesia is usual. The implications of new antiplatelet agents for the use of regional anesthesia are unclear. However, the use of low-molecular-weight heparin (LMWH) is clearly dangerous when combined with regional anesthesia.

A primary concern with the use of anticoagulation and antiplatelet therapy is the risk of spinal hematoma after spinal-epidural anesthesia (neuraxial block) (17). Emergency decompressive laminectomy to evacuate the hematoma may become necessary. Cases of permanent paraplegia have also been reported. The diagnosis and treatment of spinal-epidural hematoma are often delayed. Neuraxial anesthetic techniques are attractive in vascular and complex surgery patients because they are believed to reduce morbidity and provide improved postoperative analgesia. Both needle puncture and neuraxial catheter removal pose a potential risk for development of spinal-epidural hematoma in such anticoagulated patients. Guidelines proposed to improve safety in such situations are based on the Second Consensus Conference on Neuraxial Anesthesia and Anticoagulation convened by the American Society of Regional Anesthesia and Pain Medicine (17,18). Ethical issues, the rarity of spinal hematoma, and the existence of multiple factors contributing to its occurrence preclude designing a prospective, randomized study to get level A evidence. In addition, there is no laboratory model for appropriate guidance.

The guidelines are therefore based on expert opinion (level C evidence) and on a review of several observational studies, case series, and case reports (level B evidence), and are presented in what follows.

Management of the Patient Receiving Unfractionated Heparin

1. During subcutaneous (minidose) prophylaxis there is no contraindication to the use of neuraxial techniques. The risk of neuraxial bleeding may be reduced by delay of the heparin injection until after the needle insertion and may be increased in debilitated patients after prolonged therapy. Because heparin-induced thrombocytopenia may occur during heparin administration, patients receiving heparin for greater than 4 days should have a platelet count assessed before neuraxial block and catheter removal.
2. Therapeutic anticoagulation with intravenous heparin is routine during vascular surgery and may be continued into the postoperative period as well. Three risk factors associated with increased risk were identified: a time interval less than 60 minutes between the administration of heparin and lumbar puncture, traumatic needle placement, and concomitant use of other anticoagulants (antiplatelet medications, LMWH, and oral anticoagulants). Combining neuraxial techniques with intraoperative anticoagulation with heparin during vascular surgery seems acceptable with the following cautions:
   - Avoid the technique when other coagulopathies are present.
   - Heparin administration is usually delayed for 1 hour after needle placement.
   - Indwelling neuraxial catheters can be removed 2 to 4 hours after the last heparin dose and the patient's coagulation status is evaluated; reheparinization can occur 1 hour after catheter removal.
   - It must be possible to monitor the patient postoperatively to provide early detection of motor blockade and consider the use of minimal concentration of local anesthetics to enhance the early detection of a spinal hematoma.
   - Although the occurrence of a bloody or difficult neuraxial needle placement may increase risk, there are no data to support mandatory cancellation of a case. Direct communication with the surgeon and a specific risk–benefit decision about proceeding in each case are warranted.

Management of the Patient Receiving Low-Molecular-Weight Heparin

The biochemical and pharmacologic properties of LMWH differ from those of unfractionated heparin. Most relevant are the lack of monitoring of anticoagulant response (anti-Xa level), prolonged half-life, and irreversibility with protamine. Prolonged LMWH therapy may be associated with an accumulation of anti-Xa activity and fibrinolysis. In addition, the plasma half-life of LMWH increases in patients with renal failure. Different types of LMWH vary both biochemically and pharmacologically in molecular weight, anti-IIa and anti-Xa activities, and plasma half-life. However, lack of adequate trials makes it impossible to recommend one specific LMWH. Experience in Europe suggests that the rate of spinal hematoma is similar among LMWH preparations. As with unfractionated heparin, the risk of spinal hematoma increases with concomitant use of other anticoagulants, including dextran. The following guidelines are applicable for a patient receiving LMWH.

1. Monitoring of the anti-Xa level is not recommended because it is not predictive of the risk of bleeding.
2. The presence of blood during needle and catheter placement does not necessitate postponement of surgery. However, initiation of LMWH therapy in this setting should be delayed for 24 hours postoperatively.
3. Preoperative LMWH:
   - Preoperative LMWH thromboprophylaxis can be assumed to have altered coagulation. In such patients, needle placement should occur at least 10 to 12 hours after the LMWH dose.
   - In patients receiving higher (treatment) doses of LMWH, such as enoxaparin 1 mg/kg every 12 hours, enoxaparin 1.5 mg/kg daily, dalteparin 120 U/kg every 12 hours, dalteparin 200 U/kg daily, or tinzaparin 175 U/kg daily, delay at least 24 hours to assure normal hemostasis at the time of needle insertion.
   - Neuraxial techniques should be avoided in patients administered a dose of LMWH within 2 hours preoperatively (general surgery patients) because needle placement would occur during peak anticoagulant activity.
4. Postoperative LMWH: Patients with postoperative initiation of LMWH thromboprophylaxis may safely undergo single-injection and continuous catheter techniques. Management is based on total daily dose, timing of the first postoperative dose, and dosing schedule.
   - *Twice-daily dosing.* This dosage regimen may be associated with an increased risk of spinal hematoma. The first dose of LMWH should be administered no earlier than 24 hours postoperatively, regardless of anesthetic technique, and only in the presence of adequate (surgical) hemostasis. Indwelling catheters should be removed before initiation of LMWH thromboprophylaxis. If a continuous technique is selected, the epidural catheter may be left indwelling overnight and removed the following day, with the first dose of LMWH administered at least 2 hours after catheter removal.
   - *Single-daily dosing.* This dosing regimen approximates the European application. The first postoperative LMWH dose should be administered 6 to 8 hours postoperatively. The second postoperative dose should occur no sooner than 24 hours after the first dose. Indwelling neuraxial catheters may be safely maintained. However, the catheter should be removed a minimum of 10 to 12 hours after the last dose of LMWH. Subsequent LMWH dosing should occur a minimum of 2 hours after catheter removal.

Management of the Patient Receiving Antiplatelet Medications

Antiplatelet medications, including NSAIDs, thienopyridine derivatives (ticlopidine and clopidogrel), and platelet glycoprotein (GP) IIb/IIIa antagonists (abciximab, eptifibatide, tirofiban) exert diverse effects on platelet function. The pharmacologic differences make it impossible to extrapolate among the groups of drugs in the practice of neuraxial techniques.

1. There is no wholly accepted test, including bleeding time, for guiding antiplatelet therapy. Careful preoperative assessment of conditions that might increase bleeding include a history of easy bruisability/excessive bleeding and female gender; increased age may be important, but we have no data on such.
2. NSAIDs appear to represent no added significant risk for the development of spinal hematoma in patients having epidural

or spinal anesthesia. The use of NSAIDs alone does not create a level of risk that will interfere with the performance of neuraxial blocks.

3. There seem to be no specific concerns as to the timing of single-shot or catheter techniques in the dosing of NSAIDs, postoperative monitoring, or the timing of neuraxial catheter removal.
4. The actual risk of spinal hematoma with ticlopidine and clopidogrel and the GP IIb/IIIa antagonists is unknown.
   - Based on labeling and surgical reviews, the suggested time interval between discontinuation of thienopyridine therapy and neuraxial blockade is 14 days for ticlopidine and 7 days for clopidogrel.
   - Platelet GP IIb/IIIa inhibitors have a profound effect on platelet aggregation. After administration, the time to normal platelet aggregation is 24 to 48 hours for abciximab and 4 to 8 hours for eptifibatide and tirofiban. Neuraxial techniques should be avoided until platelet function has recovered. GP IIb/IIIa antagonists are contraindicated within 4 weeks of surgery. Should one be administered in the postoperative period (after a neuraxial technique), the patient should be carefully monitored neurologically.

Management of the Patient Receiving Thrombolytic Therapy

Patients receiving fibrinolytic/thrombolytic medications are at risk of serious hemorrhagic events, particularly those who have undergone an invasive procedure. Consensus statements are based on the profound effect on hemostasis, the use of concomitant heparin and/or antiplatelet agent, and the potential for *spontaneous* neuraxial bleeding with these medications.

1. Ideally, before the use of thrombolytic therapy the patient should be queried for a recent history of lumbar puncture, spinal or epidural anesthesia, or epidural steroid injection to allow appropriate monitoring. Guidelines detailing original contraindications for thrombolytic drugs suggest avoidance of these drugs for 10 days after puncture of noncompressible vessels.
2. Patients receiving fibrinolytic and thrombolytic drugs should be cautioned against receiving spinal or epidural anesthetics except in highly unusual circumstances. Data are not available to allow a clear outline of the length of time neuraxial puncture should be avoided after discontinuation of these drugs.
3. In patients who have received neuraxial blocks at or near the time of fibrinolytic and thrombolytic therapy, neurologic monitoring should occur at least every 2 hours. Furthermore, if neuraxial blocks have been combined with fibrinolytic and thrombolytic therapy and ongoing epidural catheter infusion, the infusion should be limited to drugs minimizing sensory and motor block to facilitate assessment of neurologic function.
4. There is no definitive recommendation for removal of neuraxial catheters in patients who unexpectedly receive fibrinolytic and thrombolytic therapy during a neuraxial catheter infusion. The measurement of fibrinogen level (one of the last clotting factors to recover) may be helpful in making a decision about catheter removal or maintenance.

Management of the Patient Receiving Oral Anticoagulants

The management of patients receiving warfarin perioperatively remains controversial.

1. Caution should be used when performing neuraxial techniques in patients recently discontinued from chronic warfarin therapy. The anticoagulant therapy must be stopped (ideally 4 to 5 days before the planned procedure), and the prothrombin time/International Normalized Ratio (PT/INR) measured before initiation of neuraxial block.
2. Neurologic testing of sensory and motor function should be routine during epidural analgesia for patients on warfarin therapy. The type of analgesic solution should be tailored to minimize the degree of sensory and motor blockade. These assessments need be continued for 24 hours after catheter removal, and longer if the INR was greater than 1.5 at the time of catheter removal.
3. An INR greater than 3 should prompt the physician to withhold or reduce the warfarin dose in patients with indwelling neuraxial catheters.

Spinal and epidural anesthesia may be safely performed in a patient undergoing subsequent therapeutic heparinization provided heparinization occurs a minimum of 60 minutes after the needle placement. In addition, the heparin effect is monitored and maintained within acceptable levels (activated clotting time or activated partial thromboplastin time 1.5 to 2 times baseline), and indwelling catheters are removed at a time when heparin activity is low or completely reversed.

In patients who have previously undergone procedures during which heparin was administered, heparin antibodies may be present. When suspected, platelet aggregation tests may be performed with heparin in vitro before surgery. When undiagnosed patients with heparin antibodies receive heparin, platelet counts may drop after surgery. In the most severe cases, thrombosis may occur due to platelet activation. Heparin-induced thrombocytopenia (HIT) is a common immune-mediated adverse drug reaction. The central role of thrombin generation in this syndrome provides a rationale for the use of anticoagulants that reduce thrombin generation (danaparoid) or inhibit thrombin (lepirudin). Fondaparinux produces its antithrombotic effect through factor Xa inhibition. These drugs may be given to provide anticoagulation during surgery instead of heparin; however, their half-lives are longer than those of heparin, their metabolism depends on renal function, and their interactions with regional anesthesia are unclear. Until further clinical experience is available, performance of neuraxial techniques involves only single needle pass and avoidance of indwelling neuraxial catheters.

In summary, for any given scenario, concomitant use of other anticoagulants including antiplatelet medications and dextran increases the risk of spinal hematoma. It must be remembered that identification of risk factors and establishment of guidelines will not completely eliminate the complication of spinal hematoma. The type of analgesic solution should be tailored to minimize the degree of sensory and motor blockade. Vigilance in monitoring is critical to allow early evaluation of neurologic dysfunction and prompt intervention. The guidelines focus on prevention of spinal hematoma and optimization of neurologic outcome.

PREOPERATIVE CORONARY REVASCULARIZATION AS A RISK REDUCTION STRATEGY

This issue is highly controversial. The combined risk of coronary angiography and revascularization should not exceed the risk of proposed surgery, an issue in which institutional factors play a vital role. The range of options for preparatory coronary revascularization continues to expand rapidly. These include traditional surgical revascularization (CABG), transmyocardial laser therapy, percutaneous transluminal coronary angioplasty (PTCA), coronary stent placement, excimer laser, rotoblader, beating heart coronary bypass surgery, and endoscopic CABG. However, mortality rates associated with CABG are 2.4-fold higher in patients with peripheral vascular disease (7.7% vs. 3.2%) than in those without it and vary by center (currently more than sixfold variation in mortality for the same operation is reported by various centers). Higher complication rates can be anticipated for the newer revascularization techniques when performed in patients with peripheral vascular disease or diseases requiring complex surgery in the elderly.

Earlier observational studies noted the effect of preoperative coronary revascularization in reducing perioperative cardiac events. Recent data, however, from prospective studies show less benefit. In a prospective study, Back et al. (54) used the algorithm proposed by the ACC/AHA guidelines (24) in 425 patients scheduled for major vascular reconstructions and concluded that previous coronary revascularization provides only modest protection against perioperative adverse cardiac events and mortality. Another prospective study that evaluated cardiac troponin found larger beneficial effects of preoperative coronary revascularization (55). Even if one considers coronary revascularization to be protective, an obligate delay in performing the planned vascular or other complex surgical procedure must be considered. Once the patient has recovered from successful coronary revascularization (1 week after angioplasty, 6 weeks after coronary stent placement, and 6 to 8 weeks after CABG, typically), peripheral vascular or other complex surgery is usually then performed. The time delay after coronary stent placement is theoretical based on time for stent endothelialization and antiplatelet therapy to prevent stent thrombosis, especially in the prothrombotic period after complex surgery. High rates of mortality, MI, and stent thrombosis may be expected if noncardiac surgery is performed earlier than 6 weeks (56).

Proposed Algorithm

Given such abundant data and controversies, how can one summarize recommendations for preoperative cardiac risk stratification in a patient presenting for vascular or other complex surgery? We propose an algorithm keeping in mind the following important issues: perioperative MI is usually of non–Q-wave type (i.e., non–ST-elevation type), resulting in imbalance between oxygen supply and demand, as opposed to MI of Q-wave type (i.e., ST-elevation type), which results from plaque rupture followed by a cascade of events leading to thrombosis. Furthermore, a time delay between coronary revascularization (6 weeks for CABG or PTCA with coronary stenting) and noncardiac surgery may not be desirable in patients presenting for vascular or complex surgery because of resulting surgical problems such as ischemia and gangrene of extremities in case of AVD of aorta and iliofemoral vessels or rupture of aortic aneurysm or complications of other diseases such as cancer. In addition, anticoagulation that needs to be continued after coronary stenting may preclude the use of stress-reducing regional anesthesia. Advances in the medical management of atherosclerosis include the use of β-blocking agents, other antihypertensives, aspirin, and statin drugs, which diminish stress on endothelium and restore endothelial function, reduce ambulatory myocardial ischemia, may cause plaque regression, and may be equivalent or superior to coronary revascularization in patients with stable angina. Perioperative β-blockade or α-2 adrenergic blockers are best combined with statins and aspirin and perhaps preoperative walk or other exercise regimens and immunizations to achieve the best outcome. The rationale is to prevent any type of perioperative MI: non–ST-elevation MI, in which stress-reducing agents such as β-blockers or α-2 blockers are beneficial; and ST-elevation MI, in which statins and aspirin are more appropriate agents. We recommend additional thermal care for patients undergoing all complex surgery and use of pulmonary artery catheter for patients with poor left ventricular function or those with prior history of CHF. This algorithm is summarized in Figure 41.2 and Table 41.6.

COMBINED CORONARY ARTERY DISEASE AND CAROTID ARTERY OR OTHER COMPLEX SURGICAL DISEASE

The risks of cardiac and other complications after carotid endarterectomy (CEA) or other complex surgical disease states are less than after abdominal aortic or infrainguinal bypass procedures. ACC/AHA guidelines place the CEA in the intermediate-risk category (cardiac risk 1% to 5%) (24), as are most procedures including radical tumor removal and most bariatric procedures. The risk of stroke after CABG increases progressively with extent of objectively measured carotid stenosis and the extent of symptoms. Therefore the controversy over whether to perform combined CABG and CEA or to perform staged operation remains. "Staged" implies performing CEA followed by CABG; "reverse staged," CABG followed by CEA. A recent systematic review attempted to answer this question by evaluating the combined cardiovascular risk (death $\pm$ MI $\pm$ stroke) for the three types of surgical scenarios (57). From 10% to 12% of patients who underwent staged or synchronous procedures suffered death or major cardiovascular morbidity (stroke, MI) within 30 days of surgery. Overall, outcomes for staged and synchronous procedures were similarly poor. Carotid disease accounts for less than 50% of post-CABG strokes, with aortic arch atheroscleroembolism the most important cause.

SUMMARY

Surgery is one of, if not the most, complex team endeavors in health care; primary care physician; cardiologist; anesthesiologist; surgeon; critical care, pain management, and rehabilitation specialists; and nurses must work with the patient as an orchestrated group to gain the best outcome. Outcome studies have tested the ability of anesthesiologists to define those perioperative factors that foster best outcomes with least resources utilization. The variability in outcome across institutions for the same procedure in similar patients indicates that nothing has replaced the quality of the team and combined excellence in determining outcome. Some outcome studies for these patients, such as those receiving anticoagulant therapies, are largely unresolved, and only guidelines based on expert opinion can be offered. On the other hand, studies have resulted in fewer tests for preoperative risk assessments and indicate that simpler risk reduction strategies using aspirin, β-blockers, antihypertensives, statins, immunizations, and maybe diet and physical activity regimens may become routine.

CONTROVERSIES AND PERSONAL PERSPECTIVES

In the 35 years the senior author has practiced anesthesia, almost everything has radically changed; for example, only 2 of the 25 drugs routinely used in perioperative care in 1971 are still used with any frequency in such care now. Who back then would have thought of percutaneous mitral valve repairs or

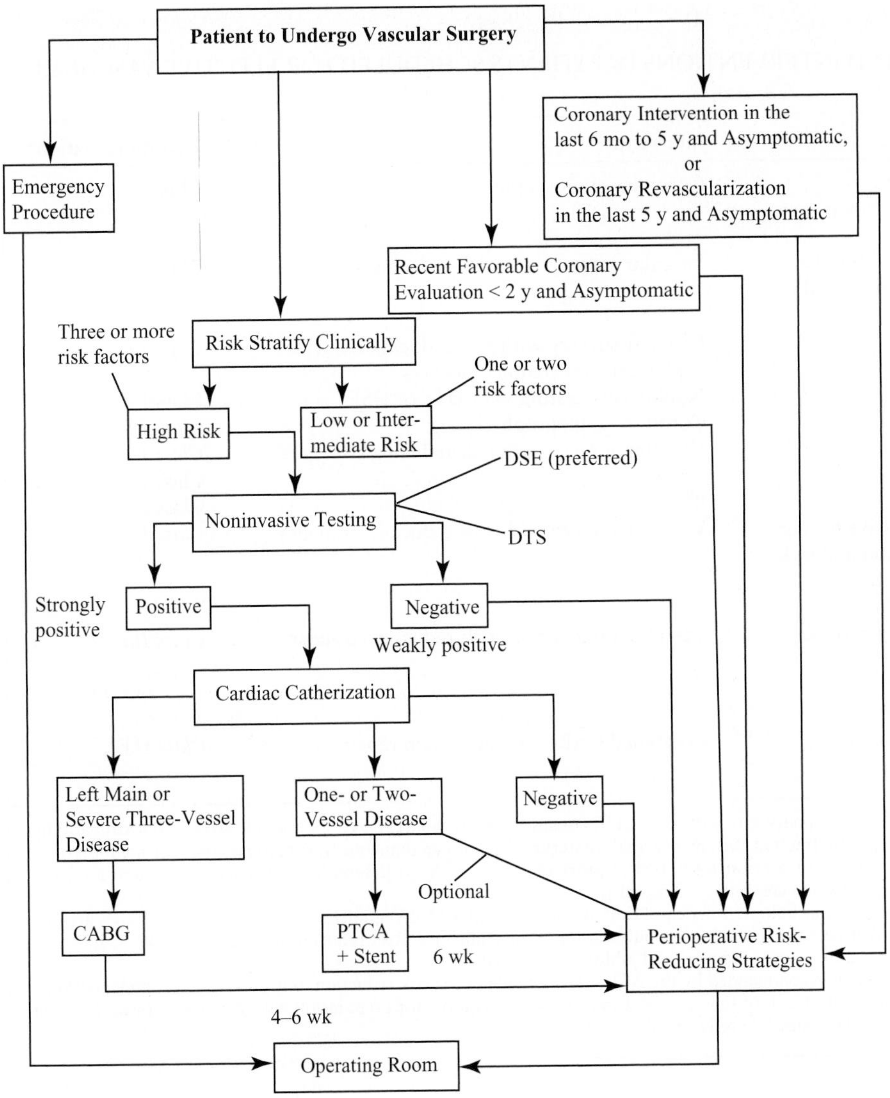

FIGURE 41.2. Our proposal for cardiac risk stratification. We recommend coronary revascularization only for highly selected cases. The patient is initially evaluated clinically for the following risk factors: age greater than 70 years, angina (current or previous), prior myocardial infarction, history of congestive heart failure, history of cerebrovascular accident, diabetes on insulin therapy, and renal insufficiency (serum creatinine >2 mg/dL). After clinical risk stratification, the patient is managed as proposed depending on the scenario. Risk-reducing strategies include statin therapy (at least 2 weeks of preparation is necessary) and perioperative β-blockade (if time permits, for 30 days of preparation; if time does not permit, for one night) or α-2-adrenergic blockade. Aspirin and antihypertensives are continued, and immunizations are rendered current. Additional thermal care (forced-air rewarming) is provided. If the patient has a history of prior coronary artery bypass graft within the last 5 years or coronary intervention in the last 6 months to 5 years and remains asymptomatic, then the patient can undergo vascular surgery. See text for details. CABG, coronary artery bypass graft; DSE, dobutamine stress echocardiography; DTS, dipyridamole thallium scintigraphy; PTCA, percutaneous transluminal coronary angioplasty.

thoracic aorta arterial stents? Patient age, comorbidity, and outcomes have radically changed too, patient age in a way that is more challenging, and morbidity and mortality for the better. We have gone from the 70-year-old with an ejection fraction of 30 being too sick to the 85-year-old with an ejection fraction of 20 being routine. Instead of measuring 30-day mortality rate decreases from the mid teens or higher, we now measure such changes from a logarithmically smaller number.

Such transformations have required great clinicians making superb efforts to treat the very sick and achieve "sub–single digit" mortality and morbidity. And the target—what surgery is being done for what person and for what disease—seems to be moving as technology promotes rapid change and the move from invasive to noninvasive procedures for vascular restorations and other complex disease states.

Perioperative therapies are becoming evidence based, and the focus is on excellent teams rather than excellent individual effort; routinely we are seeing surgery of the sickest vasculopaths and patients with ejection fractions in the 10% to 15% range undergoing complex surgery with 30-day mortality and morbidity rates less than 1%. We are witnessing not just a return to preoperative functional status, but also a restoration of functional status. This progress has occurred through the combination of better pharmaceuticals, better teamwork, better physiologic understanding, and the advent of evidence-based medicine. Progress has so far only occurred, however, in centers that have enough volume to develop excellent teams and despite the lack of care patients have given themselves.

THE FUTURE

When our team brought transesophageal echocardiography over from Germany in 1981, it was predicted that after the first case it would be routine, cost $5,000 or less per operating room, and be built into every monitor by 1986. One can take more confidence in predicting the changes that will help to shape the future. Will aspirin, statins, β-blockers, ACE inhibitors, immunization, and exercise and diet therapy become routine in the preoperative period, and will outcome studies allow us to choose those processes that promote return to functional status quicker and decrease resource utilization the most? The answer is yes, but how fast we get there will depend on how much administrative and motivational support is given by Medicare and the National Institutes of Health versus how much the pennywise, pound-foolish approach and sometimes limited focus of government bureaucracies interfere with the entrepreneurial spirit of physician scientists who want to radically improve outcomes and decrease resource use. The personalized medicine and genomic understanding of the next decade has the potential to radically change preoperative therapies and radically alter outcomes by the logarithm and a half that has

TABLE 41.6

CARDIAC RISK STRATIFICATION AND INTERVENTIONS IN PATIENTS SCHEDULED FOR ELECTIVE VASCULAR OR COMPLEX SURGERY

Presentation	Intervention	Recommendation[a]
Unstable angina, recent MI (7 d to 1 mo), decompensated CHF, significant arrhythmias (any one)	Coronary angiography	**Class 1**
Prior CABG in the last 5 y/prior PTCA within the last 6 mo to 5 y and asymptomatic with regard to cardiac problems	Vascular surgery with risk-reducing strategies	**Class I**
Prior PTCA within the last 6 mo	Vascular surgery with risk-reducing strategies plus calcium channel blockers	*Class I*
High clinical risk (3 or more risk factors)	Noninvasive testing with DTS or DSE	**Class I**
High-risk results of DTS/DSE	Coronary angiography	*Class I*
Intermediate-/low-risk results of DTS/DSE	Vascular surgery with risk-reducing strategies	*Class I*
"Critical" CAD or left main disease, EF <35%	CABG	**Class I**
One- or two-vessel CAD	PTCA	**Class I**
Documented CAD by clinical or noninvasive testing without prior coronary revascularization and lack of waiting time obligated by coronary revascularization	Vascular surgery with risk-reducing strategies	*Class I*
One or two-vessel disease documented by coronary angiography without prior coronary revascularization and lack of waiting time obligated by coronary revascularization	Vascular surgery with risk-reducing strategies	*Class IIa*
Severe CAD with impending rupture of aortic aneurysm	Combined CABG and aneurysm repair	*Class IIa*

CABG, coronary artery bypass graft surgery; CAD, coronary artery disease; CHF, congestive heart failure; DSE, dobutamine stress echocardiography; DTS, dipyridamole thallium scintigraphy; EF; ejection fraction; MI, myocardial infarction; PTCA, percutaneous transluminal coronary angioplasty.
Clinical risk factors include age >70 y, angina (current or previous), prior MI, history of congestive heart failure, history of cerebrovascular accident, diabetes on insulin therapy, and renal insufficiency (serum creatinine >2 mg/dL).
[a]Recommendations in bold are American College of Cardiology/American Heart Association (ACC/AHA) guidelines, whereas those in italics are our proposed recommendations based on evidence that became available after publication of the guidelines. Risk-reducing strategies typically include drug therapy (perioperative β-blockade + statins or α-2-blockers + statins) and additional thermal care.
Note that in addition to the perioperative β-blockade recommended by the ACC/AHA guidelines for risk reduction, our proposed recommendation also includes statin therapy. Furthermore, in the event of lack of time for the 1 month ideally required for preparation with β-blockers or in the event of absolute contraindication for their use, α-2-blockers may be used instead.

occurred in complex patients with high degrees of comorbidity undergoing complex surgery. We can hope that teams of physicians and nurses will be able to foster innovation and overcome government and insurance company obstacles to foster major improvements. Will we be able to motivate the individual to keep healthier arteries longer? That will be a major challenge, but if major food sellers insist on NO transfat in goods on their shelves, fast-food outlets earn more money from offering healthy food, and exercise shoes wear out before new styles are introduced, the transformation is possible and will change preoperative patient status and perioperative risk reduction strategies.

References

1. Mantha S. Rationale for cardiac risk stratification before peripheral vascular surgery: application of evidence-based medicine and Bayesian analysis. *Semin Cardiothorac Vasc Anesth* 2000;41:98.
2. Mantha S, Fleisher LA, Roizen MF, et al. Cost-effectiveness and benefit of preoperative work-up and preparation for vascular surgery. In: Youngberg JA. *Cardiac, vascular, and thoracic anesthesia.* New York: Churchill Livingston, 2000:20.
3. Rutherford RB, Krupski WC. Current status of open versus endovascular stent-graft repair of abdominal aortic aneurysm. *J Vasc Surg* 2004;39:1129.
4. Warner MA, Shields SE, Chute CG. Major morbidity and mortality within 1 month of ambulatory surgery and anesthesia. *JAMA* 1993;270:1437–1441.
5. Schein OD, Katz JU, Bass EB, et al. The value of routine preoperative medical testing before cataract surgery. *N Engl J Med* 2000;342:168–175.
6. Gibbons RJ, Smith S, Antman E. American College of Cardiology/American Heart Association clinical practice guidelines: Part I: Where do they come from? *Circulation* 2003;107:2979.
7. Faxon DP, Creager MA, Smith Jr SC, et al. Atherosclerotic Vascular Disease Conference: Executive summary: Atherosclerotic Vascular Disease Conference Proceeding for Healthcare Professionals from a Special Writing Group of the American Heart Association. *Circulation* 2004;109:2595.
8. Fruchart JC, Nierman MC, Stroes ES, et al. New risk factors for atherosclerosis and patient risk assessment. *Circulation* 2004;109:III15.
9. Grundy SM, Brewer Jr HB, Cleeman JI, et al. Definition of metabolic syndrome: Report of the National Heart, Lung, and Blood Institute/American Heart Association Conference on Scientific Issues Related to Definition. *Circulation* 2004;109:433.
10. Third report of the National Cholesterol Education Program (NCEP) Expert Panel on Detection, Evaluation, and Treatment of High Blood Cholesterol in Adults (Adult Treatment Panel III). Final report. *Circulation* 2002; 106:3143.
11. Chobanian AV, Bakris GL, Black HR, et al. Seventh report of the Joint National Committee on Prevention, Detection, Evaluation, and Treatment of High Blood Pressure. *Hypertension* 2003;42:1206.
12. Assmann G, Cullen P, Schulte H. Simple scoring scheme for calculating the risk of acute coronary events based on the 10-year follow-up of the Prospective Cardiovascular Munster (PROCAM) study. *Circulation* 2002;105:310.
13. Bettmann MA, Dake MD, Hopkins LN, et al. Atherosclerotic Vascular Disease Conference: Writing Group VI: revascularization. *Circulation* 2004; 109:2643.
14. Spencer FA, Allegrone J, Goldberg RJ, et al. Association of statin therapy with outcomes of acute coronary syndromes: the GRACE study. *Ann Intern Med* 2004;140:857.

15. Henke PK, Blackburn S, Proctor MC, et al. Patients undergoing infrainguinal bypass to treat atherosclerotic vascular disease are underprescribed cardioprotective medications: effect on graft patency, limb salvage, and mortality. *J Vasc Surg* 2004;39:357.
16. Claridge MW, Hobbs SD, Quick CR, et al. ACE inhibitors increase type III collagen synthesis: a potential explanation for reduction in acute vascular events by ACE inhibitors. *Eur J Vasc Endovasc Surg* 2004;28:67.
17. Horlocker TT, Wedel DJ, Benzon H, et al. Regional anesthesia in the anticoagulated patient: defining the risks (the Second ASRA Consensus Conference on Neuraxial Anesthesia and Anticoagulation). *Reg Anesth Pain Med* 2003;28:172.
18. Horlocker TT, Wedel DJ, Benzon H, et al. Regional anesthesia in the anticoagulated patient: defining the risks. *Reg Anesth Pain Med* 2004;29:1.
19. Khuri SF, Daley J, Henderson W, et al. Risk adjustment of the postoperative mortality rate for the comparative assessment of the quality of surgical care: results of the National Veterans Affairs Surgical Risk Study. *J Am Coll Surg* 1997;185:315.
20. Daley J, Khuri SF, Henderson W, et al. Risk adjustment of the postoperative morbidity rate for the comparative assessment of the quality of surgical care: results of the National Veterans Affairs Surgical Risk Study. *J Am Coll Surg* 1997;185:328.
21. Ellis JE. Health sciences research and large database analysis in vascular surgery and anesthesia. Confirming common sense? *Prob Anesth* 1999;11: 238.
22. Hertzer NR, Beven EG, Young JR, et al. Coronary artery disease in peripheral vascular patients. A classification of 1000 coronary angiograms and results of surgical management. *Ann Surg* 1984;199:223.
23. Paul SD, Eagle KA, Kuntz KM, et al. Concordance of preoperative clinical risk with angiographic severity of coronary artery disease in patients undergoing vascular surgery. *Circulation* 1996;94:1561; erratum, *Circulation* 1996;94(10):2668.
24. Eagle KA, Berger PB, Calkins H, et al. ACC/AHA guideline update for perioperative cardiovascular evaluation for noncardiac surgery—executive summary. A report of the American College of Cardiology/American Heart Association Task Force on Practice Guidelines (Committee to Update the 1996 Guidelines on Perioperative Cardiovascular Evaluation for Noncardiac Surgery). *J Am Coll Cardiol* 2002;39:542.
25. Rihal CS, Eagle KA, Mickel MC, et al. Surgical therapy for coronary artery disease among patients with combined coronary artery and peripheral vascular disease. *Circulation* 1995;91:46.
26. Frank SM, Fleisher LA, Breslow MJ, et al. Perioperative maintenance of normothermia reduces the incidence of morbid cardiac events. A randomized clinical trial. *JAMA* 1997;277:1127.
27. Sprung J, Abdelmalak B, Gottlieb A, et al. Analysis of risk factors for myocardial infarction and cardiac mortality after major vascular surgery. *Anesthesiology* 2000;93:129.
28. Kertai MD, Bountioukos M, Boersma E, et al. Aortic stenosis: an underestimated risk factor for perioperative complications in patients undergoing noncardiac surgery. *Am J Med* 2004;116:8.
29. London MJ, Zaugg M, Schaub MC, et al. Perioperative beta-adrenergic receptor blockade: physiologic foundations and clinical controversies. *Anesthesiology* 2004;100:170.
30. Samama CM, Thiry D, Elalamy I, et al. Perioperative activation of hemostasis in vascular surgery patients. *Anesthesiology* 2001;94:74.
31. Howell SJ, Sear JW, Foex P. Hypertension, hypertensive heart disease and perioperative cardiac risk. *Br J Anaesth* 2004;92:570.
32. Badner NH, Knill RL, Brown JE, et al. Myocardial infarction after noncardiac surgery. *Anesthesiology* 1998;88:572.
33. Grayburn PA, Hillis LD. Cardiac events in patients undergoing noncardiac surgery: shifting the paradigm from noninvasive risk stratification to therapy. *Ann Intern Med* 2003;138:506.
34. Gokce N, Keaney Jr JF, Hunter LM, et al. Predictive value of noninvasively determined endothelial dysfunction for long-term cardiovascular events in patients with peripheral vascular disease. *J Am Coll Cardiol* 2003;41: 1769.
35. L'Italien GJ, Paul SD, Hendel RC, et al. Development and validation of a Bayesian model for perioperative cardiac risk assessment in a cohort of 1,081 vascular surgical candidates. *J Am Coll Cardiol* 1996;27:779.
36. Boersma E, Poldermans D, Bax JJ, et al. Predictors of cardiac events after major vascular surgery: role of clinical characteristics, dobutamine echocardiography, and beta-blocker therapy. *JAMA* 2001;285:1865.
37. Mantha S, Roizen MF, Barnard J, et al. Relative effectiveness of four preoperative tests for predicting adverse cardiac outcomes after vascular surgery: a meta-analysis. *Anesth Analg* 1994;79:422.
38. Kertai MD, Boersma E, Bax JJ, et al. A meta-analysis comparing the prognostic accuracy of six diagnostic tests for predicting perioperative cardiac risk in patients undergoing major vascular surgery. *Heart* 2003;89:1327.
39. Karkos CD, Baguneid MS, Triposkiadis F, et al. Routine measurement of radioisotope left ventricular ejection fraction prior to vascular surgery: is it worthwhile? *Eur J Vasc Endovasc Surg* 2004;27:227.
40. Kazmers A, Kohler TR. Very late survival after vascular surgery. *J Surg Res* 2002;105:109.
41. Glance LG. Selective preoperative cardiac screening improves five-year survival in patients undergoing major vascular surgery: a cost-effectiveness analysis. *J Cardiothorac Vasc Anesth* 1999;13:265.
42. Stengel D, Bauwens K, Sehouli J, et al. A likelihood ratio approach to meta-analysis of diagnostic studies. *J Med Screen* 2003;10:47.
43. Etchells E, Meade M, Tomlinson G, et al. Semiquantitative dipyridamole myocardial stress perfusion imaging for cardiac risk assessment before noncardiac vascular surgery: a meta-analysis. *J Vasc Surg* 2002;36:534.
44. Auerbach AD, Goldman L. Beta-blockers and reduction of cardiac events in noncardiac surgery: scientific review. *JAMA* 2002;287:1435.
45. Fleisher LA, Corbett W, Berry C, et al. Cost-effectiveness of differing perioperative beta-blockade strategies in vascular surgery patients. *J Cardiothorac Vasc Anesth* 2004;18:7.
46. Ellis JE, Drijvers G, Pedlow S, et al. Premedication with oral and transdermal clonidine provides safe and efficacious postoperative sympatholysis. *Anesth Analg* 1994;79:1133.
47. Wijeysundera DN, Naik JS, Beattie WS. Alpha-2 adrenergic agonists to prevent perioperative cardiovascular complications: a meta-analysis. *Am J Med* 2003;114:742.
48. Poldermans D, Bax JJ, Kertai MD, et al. Statins are associated with a reduced incidence of perioperative mortality in patients undergoing major noncardiac vascular surgery. *Circulation* 2003;107:1848.
49. Durazzo AE, Machado FS, Ikeoka DT, et al. Reduction in cardiovascular events after vascular surgery with atorvastatin: a randomized trial. *J Vasc Surg* 2004;39:967.
50. Kertai MD, Boersma E, Westerhout CM, et al. Association between long-term statin use and mortality after successful abdominal aortic aneurysm surgery. *Am J Med* 2004;116:96.
51. Wijeysundera DN, Beattie WS. Calcium channel blockers for reducing cardiac morbidity after noncardiac surgery: a meta-analysis. *Anesth Analg* 2003; 97:634.
52. Dens J, Desmet W, Piessens J. An updated meta-analysis of calcium-channel blockers in the prevention of restenosis after coronary angioplasty. *Am Heart J* 2003;145:404.
53. Bonazzi M, Gentile F, Biasi GM, et al. Impact of perioperative haemodynamic monitoring on cardiac morbidity after major vascular surgery in low risk patients. A randomised pilot trial. *Eur J Vasc Endovasc Surg* 2002;23: 445.
54. Back MR, Stordahl N, Cuthbertson D, et al. Limitations in the cardiac risk reduction provided by coronary revascularization prior to elective vascular surgery. *J Vasc Surg* 2002;36:526.
55. Landesberg G, Mosseri M, Shatz V, et al. Cardiac troponin after major vascular surgery. The role of perioperative ischemia, preoperative thallium scanning, and coronary revascularization. *J Am Coll Cardiol* 2004;44:569.
56. Wilson SH, Fasseas P, Orford JL, et al. Clinical outcome of patients undergoing non-cardiac surgery in the two months following coronary stenting. *J Am Coll Cardiol* 2003;42:234.
57. Naylor AR, Cuffe RL, Rothwell PM, et al. A systematic review of outcomes following staged and synchronous carotid endarterectomy and coronary artery bypass. *Eur J Vasc Endovasc Surg* 2003;25:380.

CHAPTER 42 ■ MEDICAL ECONOMICS IN CARDIOVASCULAR MEDICINE

DANIEL B. MARK

OVERVIEW

During the late 1960s and 1970s (euphemistically termed the "open checkbook era" in health care), hospitals and physicians in the United States were paid essentially what they charged. Competition on price was nonexistent, but competition among hospitals to have the most modern, technologically up-to-date facilities was fierce. The resulting double-digit annual escalation in health care costs alarmed both policy makers and private businesses and led to the first concerted efforts to control the growth of medical spending (1).

The failure of modest efforts at medical cost control in the United States during the 1970s and 1980s convinced many payers that the medical establishment would not voluntarily become fiscally accountable. In the late 1980s, the business and insurance communities began an aggressive bid for control of health care costs and increased accountability in medicine that led to the "managed care era." The medical profession was caught largely by surprise (2). Many physicians had assumed that the value of the U.S. health care system was self-evident, and hence their dominant role in it was assured. Others believed that pathophysiologic reasoning or personal experience and judgment were sufficient to justify a course of action, regardless of the cost. Still others regarded any discussion of costs as demeaning to the profession. These attitudes largely became untenable when multiple outcome studies in the 1980s demonstrated that physicians practicing in different areas of the country made remarkably different management decisions for similar patients (3,4). Other studies from this period reported that physicians across the country performed significant numbers of unnecessary surgical procedures, particularly coronary artery bypass graft (CABG) surgery. Together, variability of practice and appropriateness of care studies suggested the presence of substantial waste in the medical care system and demonstrated that physicians and hospitals by themselves had no incentives to develop more standardized and efficient modes of practice.

For a brief period in the 1990s, managed care became the de facto national health care reform policy in the United States. However, by 2000, it was evident that managed care would not be an effective long-term solution to control medical spending. Further, because it was driven by market interests rather than carefully crafted policy, it did not address many key issues (e.g., access to care and funding of medical research and education).

Spending on health care has grown almost without any respite over the last 50 years in the United States, and by 2014, it is expected to reach \$3.6 trillion, or 18.7% of the gross domestic product (5). Although no absolute correct level of health care spending by a country can be identified, more money to health care means less for other societal priorities. Further, the major sources for the funds are taxpayers and employers, and neither group has an incentive to spend more subsidizing health care. Consequently, the pressure from payers to resist increases will continue to intensify, and more of the expense will be shifted back to the patient/employee. In order for clinicians to be responsible stewards of medical resources and effective advocates for the true value of medical care, they must understand both the outcomes of medical care and its costs (6). The purpose of this chapter is to provide a general introduction to the key concepts of medical cost analysis and an overview of the economic consequences of selected cardiovascular diagnostic and therapeutic technologies.

COST TERMINOLOGY GLOSSARY

Direct costs: Costs that can be unambiguously linked to the production of a given product or service. These costs are usually under the control of the health care provider.

Fixed costs: Costs that remain unchanged as production of health care services (e.g., tests, therapies) is increased or decreased. Note that costs are fixed relative to a defined time period. In the long run, virtually all costs become variable.

Incremental costs: The extra costs of shifting a group of patients from one diagnostic or therapeutic strategy to an alternative. Incremental costs are a fundamental component of cost-effectiveness analysis.

Indirect costs: Costs that cannot be traced to the production of specific goods and services. These costs are arbitrarily allocated among all goods and services using one of several standard accounting methods. These costs are usually not under the direct control of health care providers.

Indirect costs (economics): Economists sometimes use this term to refer to the societal costs associated with loss of productivity as a result of morbidity.

Induced costs and induced savings: The costs of tests or therapies added or averted, respectively, as a consequence of some initial management decision.

Productivity costs: A recently proposed substitute for the economic meaning of indirect costs.

Variable costs: Costs that change with each unit charge in service volume (e.g., tests, therapies).

CONCEPTS AND METHODOLOGY

Medical Economics: Major Concepts

To the average person, "cost" means money. The accountant has a more detailed notion of the resources required to produce the good or service underlying any given monetary payment (7,8). The economist, however, operates from a more theoretic position (9,10). A major economic axiom is that any societal decision to use resources in the production of goods or services is accompanied by forgone opportunities to do something else with those resources (11,12). Because each health service or program uses up some societal resources that could have been employed for some other purpose, it thereby involves a cost. Economists refer to this as "opportunity cost." When economists talk about cost, they usually have opportunity cost rather than dollars in mind.

Economics also holds as axiomatic that society's resources are finite. Hence, choices must be made among the competing goals that society has for its resources, and not all goals can be fulfilled (11,12). Economics provides a set of tools to help define alternatives and make choices. In this context, the health economist is concerned with answering three basic questions:

1. How much should be spent on health care, and what health care goods and services should be produced?
2. How shall these goods and services be produced?
3. For whom shall they be produced? (9,10)

Resources are typically divided into large generic categories, such as labor, land, and capital (e.g., machines, factories, stores of materials). The application of technology allows society to convert these raw resource inputs into desired goods and services, such as medical care. To compare societal choices for potential alternative uses of resources, it is necessary to assess the opportunity cost of health care, national defense, public education, and other societal priorities using some common metric. Some societies use barter, the transformation of one good into another of equivalent value through physical exchange, to match goods and services to individual needs. In industrialized societies, however, markets are used to match buyers and sellers, and money is employed as the exchange intermediary. The market price in these societies then represents the amount of money equivalent in value to the total resource inputs used in the production of each good or service. (Market prices also include a profit component that ideally is equivalent to a fair rate of return on investment.) The key concept to the economist is consumption of resources. The dollar cost is merely a convenient way of valuing all the disparate resources involved on a common scale.

The major concepts in a field are usually reflected in the use of specialized terminology. The earlier glossary is provided to define some of the more important terms used in medical cost analysis.

TABLE 42.1

METHODOLOGIC ISSUES IN MEDICAL COST STUDIES

STRUCTURAL FRAMEWORK OF THE STUDY
Observational study
Randomized controlled trial
Decision model
PERSPECTIVE(S) OF THE STUDY
Societal
Medicare, managed care organization, other third-party payers
State or local government
Integrated health care system
Hospitals, clinics, other providers
Patients
APPROACH TO COST MEASUREMENT
Bottom-up
Top-down
TIME EFFECTS
Discounting
Inflation
GENERALIZABILITY
Practice setting(s)
Geographic relevance

Methodology of Medical Cost Studies

The performance of a medical cost study requires that consideration be given to five issues (Table 42.1): (a) the structural framework for the cost analysis, (b) the perspective(s) of the analysis, (c) the approach to cost measurement, (d) the importance of time and the need for discounting costs in the analysis, and (e) issues related to generalizability of the findings.

Structural Framework

Cost studies generally fall into three major domains, based on the source of the data used in the analysis: observational studies, randomized controlled trials, and decision model-based studies. *Observational cost studies* include both descriptive series (which are sometimes referred to as cost finding or cost identification studies) and more complex analyses using regression models in nonrandomized comparisons. Descriptive cost series are primarily useful in areas where there are still few published data on costs. More complex observational studies are used to identify the major determinants of a particular treatment cost (cost drivers) or to make comparisons among providers or strategies for a particular condition. To identify the independent cost drivers in a data set, statistical multivariable models are used. In scorecarding or benchmarking applications, appropriate use of statistical adjustment techniques is critical to "level the playing field." Understanding the major cost drivers allows the analyst to account for the factors most important to creating a level playing field.

Since the early 1990s, increasing numbers of randomized trials have incorporated cost measurement into their design (13,14). Cost data are collected in a randomized trial primarily to answer the following question: "If the intervention under study is found to be effective, as hypothesized, is it also an efficient method of improving health benefits?" Because effectiveness is almost always the primary issue for the trial, cost is typically evaluated as a secondary end point or in an ancillary study. Whenever possible, the economic portion of the trial should be planned and conducted prospectively along with the clinical portion of the trial (15). This ensures that early consideration is given to inclusion of the most important economic variables on the case report form and that additional economic data required can be collected efficiently. Because follow-up on most trials is shorter than desired from an economic impact perspective, modeling is necessary to extrapolate within trial results to the necessary long-term perspective.

Not all randomized trials are suitable for economic analysis. The sample size requirements to obtain a precise estimate of the difference in costs between two treatment strategies may be surprisingly large. Even in a large clinical trial, economic analysis may be problematic if the clinical protocol specifies important additional testing or treatment that distorts standard patterns of care. Generally, the best trials for economic analysis are the large, simple randomized trials that attempt to mimic as closely as possible good clinical practice as it occurs in the medical community at large (16).

An intention-to-treat analysis in a randomized trial protects from unaccounted for treatment selection biases but not other types of potential biases. Some economic analysts have been critical of the use of economic analysis in randomized trials because these analyses do not provide a picture of the economic effects of the new therapy as it will be employed in the community at large. The providers and institutions in a trial are rarely representative of the medical communities in which they practice. Trial investigators may systematically steer certain eligible patients away from enrollment in the trial because these investigators feel certain that they already know what is best for these patients. Demographic and educational factors have been shown to affect patient willingness to be randomized in a trial. Whereas these biases may affect the generalizability of the economic substudy of a randomized trial, they also affect the generalizability of clinical results of that trial (17). These issues are discussed further in the section on generalizability later in the chapter.

The third major structural option for economic analysis is a decision model in which the analyst specifies the structure of the problem and then derives the data needed to populate the model from relevant and available sources. In the empiric options discussed earlier, the level of detail of the analysis is determined through the decisions about what to measure. In the model-based approach, the analyst determines the structure of the model and therefore the level of detail considered. This, in turn, is determined by the level of understanding of the problem being studied and the detail level of the data available for the model. Patient-level data are infrequently used in such models, but meta-analyses are being used with increasing frequency to characterize clinical outcomes.

Perspectives of Cost Analysis

A cost analysis always entails a perspective that is defined by identifying the buyers and sellers (or consumers or producers) of the medical care in question (11). Table 42.1 lists the most common perspectives used for cost studies. The importance of perspective (also referred to by some as the viewpoint for the analysis) is pragmatic: a particular medical care, good, or service may be a cost from one perspective but not from another. Most health economists and health policy analysts recommend the primary use of the societal perspective, supplemented by other perspectives of interest (11).

Resource Use and Cost Measurement

After the structure and objectives of the study have been defined and the perspectives have been agreed on, decisions must be made about what resources to include in the analysis and the method to be used for assigning costs to those resources. As mentioned at the outset of this chapter, "cost" means different things to different analysts and consumers of cost data. To measure cost, one must have a clear operational definition of what is to be measured. The economist's concept of opportunity cost represents the purest definition of "true cost." However, opportunity cost is a theoretic construct that does not have a practical measurement analog.

Accountants are more concerned with measurement than economists and consequently make some important simplifications. To measure true accounting costs requires us to determine all the individual resources consumed in the production of a particular medical good or service and assign market prices to each. Although measurement of true accounting costs is possible in some restricted situations, most cost analyses incorporate certain approximations to increase ease of measurement. Because collecting cost information itself has a cost, the analyst must decide how much detail is necessary to satisfy a particular cost accounting goal.

Two general approaches can be used to assess the cost of medical care services and products: "bottom-up" and "top-down" (Table 42.2) (1). They differ in the level of detail used to describe resource consumption and in the quality of the cost weights collected. The bottom-up methods all involve enumeration of individual resources consumed in an episode of medical care and the corresponding cost weights. The gold standard bottom-up approach (also known as microcosting) involves a detailed assessment of all the resources consumed by the medical care in question, detailed cost accounting estimates of individual resource cost weights, and assignment of appropriate cost weights to each resource (7). The sum of the resources multiplied by their unit cost yields the total cost. Unfortunately, this method can be quite laborious and expensive to employ and is therefore infrequently used.

A simplified version of the bottom-up approach involves enumeration and costing of "big ticket items." This method requires the identification of the subset of resources consumed that are considered the most important cost components ("the big tickets"). Use of this approach allows the analyst to concentrate on costing out only a subset of the entire resources consumed. The principal advantage of this approach is that it is less expensive. However, this approach also has several important potential limitations (Table 42.2).

The other major approach to cost estimation, particularly for hospital-based costs, is the top-down approach. At least two variants of this approach can be employed, one based on detailed hospital billing data and the other on summary episode-of-care descriptors. The method employing hospital billing records is suitable for use only in U.S. institutions that generate hospital bills (and, of course, analyses that involve hospitalizations). The medical charges that appear on U.S. hospital bills represent a tremendously inflated statement of the underlying true costs for the care in question (18). In the earlier (preprospective payment) era of Medicare, hospitals were reimbursed on the basis of their "reasonable and necessary" costs of providing care to patients. To define what proportion of hospital charges these reasonable costs were, Medicare developed an elaborate reporting system that required each hospital to file a cost report each year with the Centers for Medicare and Medicaid Services (CMS). This report provides a set of correction factors, known as the Medicare ratios of cost to charges (RCCs). The RCCs are used with a CMS-defined summary billing form, the Uniform Billing Form of 1992 (UB-92), to generate an estimate of hospital costs from hospital charge data for any hospital admission at an institution participating in the Medicare program. The major U.S. hospitals that do not generate the data necessary for these calculations include the Veterans Administration System, some other military hospitals, and some fully capitated HMOs. The strengths of this

TABLE 42.2

STRENGTHS AND LIMITATIONS OF COST MEASUREMENT METHODS

Method	Strengths	Limitations
BOTTOM-UP		
Full microcosting analysis	Most accurate	Most expensive and time-consuming
Hospital cost accounting system	Accuracy approaches microcosting	Variable levels of detail used Many key assumptions invisible to end user
Big ticket cost analysis	Efficient Less expensive	Estimates average (not marginal) cost May oversimplify, miss important cost differences Presumes uniform cost weights
TOP-DOWN		
Hospital bill charge to cost conversion	Efficient Based on detailed resource use data Can be used for most U.S. hospitals	Estimates average cost (not marginal cost) Variable methodologies used by different hospitals
DRG reimbursement rates	Efficient Least expensive	Not sensitive to resource use variations within a DRG category HCFA reimbursement rates may be lower than true costs

DRG, diagnosis-related group; HCFA, Health Care Financing Administration.

approach are severalfold (Table 42.2) (19). Most importantly, the approach is based on a detailed enumeration of resource consumption and thus tends to provide a sensitive measure of variations in resource use. In addition, this method is suitable for use in large-scale multicenter studies involving U.S. hospitals. The top-down charge-to-cost conversion also has several limitations that should be kept in mind (Table 42.2) (20).

Medicare diagnosis-related group (DRG) reimbursement rates provide an alternative top-down cost estimation method that does not depend on conversion of hospital charge data (1). Once the patient's DRG is defined, it becomes a straightforward matter to assign the "hospital costs." This method is not sensitive to variations in resource use intensity within a given type of hospitalization. Furthermore, the reimbursement rates that are set by CMS or that are provided by private insurers are only very loosely related to the resource costs of providing care. For these reasons, DRG reimbursement rates are primarily used for economic analyses done from the CMS or other payer's perspective. They are used for other cost analyses only when more accurate and appropriate cost weights cannot be obtained or the accuracy of such estimates is not particularly important to the overall analysis. Analogous DRG-based methods are available for use in some European countries.

Assignment of costs to physician services is typically done in one of three ways (1). In the past, physician fees (charges) were used. These numbers are determined by what the physician was historically able to bill for his or her services in the fee-for-service sector, rather than the true cost of the resource inputs. Thus, physician fees are a distorted and inflated measure of physician service costs analogous to hospital charges. However, unlike the situation with hospital charges, no Medicare conversion factors have been established to translate these numbers into true physician costs. Alternatively, physician services can be included in a bottom-up microcosting analysis (discussed earlier), although assigning costs remains problematic with this approach.

For this reason, most analysts now use the Medicare Fee Schedule, which is based in part on a resource-based relative value scale (RBRVS) developed by Hsiao and colleagues at Harvard University in Cambridge, Massachusetts (21). The underlying concept of the RBRVS is that the price of a physician service should reflect the long-term cost of providing that service. Thus, the resulting physician fees include both the variable costs of the service in question and a component of fixed costs reflecting practice overhead expenses (e.g., office staff and malpractice insurance). Medicare fees under this system are tied to the physician's Current Procedural Terminology (CPT) classification system. Thus, use of the system in a cost analysis starts with assignment of appropriate CPT codes to the relevant physician procedures and services. The detail with which a physician's work is recorded in a particular study determines whether this approach is more a microcosting estimation or a big ticket estimation method.

For cost analyses outside the United States, a variety of estimates of physician service cost may be available. In Canada, for example, the Provincial Health Authorities each generate their own Physician Fee Schedule that is similar in general outlines to the Medicare Fee Schedule.

Time Effects on Cost

Time has an important influence on medical costs that must be considered in economic studies. When medical care or its consequences take place over a period of years, there is broad agreement in the economic community that all future costs (as well as future health outcomes) should be expressed in terms of their "present value" to the decision maker (11). The mathematic procedure for calculating present value costs from a stream of costs that occur over a period of years is called discounting. The rationale for discounting costs can be easily illustrated. Given the choice between having $100 now and $100 5 years from now, the decision maker will always choose the former option. This reflects the decision maker's time preference for present value relative to future value. The time preference is logical because if the decision maker has the $100 now, he or she can invest it and have significantly more than $100 5 years from now. Conversely, receiving $100 5 years from now would be equivalent to receiving a sum less than $100 today.

Inflation is a separate issue from discounting (11). Inflation causes the value of money to diminish over time. As a simplifying step, most medical economists tend to ignore the effects of inflation. The implicit assumption is that inflation affects all components of the costs being studied or compared equivalently. However, inflation must be taken into account when comparing the results of (historical) cost studies from different years. For example, a study done in 1985 on the cost of CABG surgery would need to be adjusted for inflation to provide properly calibrated cost estimates relevant to 2006. The most common method for achieving this kind of inflation correction is through the use of the medical care component of the Consumer Price Index (CPI) or a relevant subcomponent.

Generalizability

The methodology we have reviewed so far relates to the assessment of the costs of medical care for a defined cohort of patients in the context of an observational study or a randomized trial. In either case, it is possible to collect empiric resource use and cost data on the patients in question and to draw conclusions about the economic effects of the given medical care from the empiric data available. Sometimes, however, the economic analyst is interested in a broader question: What is the economic impact of the therapy in question on an entire health system? The system in question may be a country, a state or province, a managed health care organization, or a chain of hospitals. There are clear trade-offs in moving from the empiric arena to the health system or policy arena. In particular, policy or systemwide projections typically involve far greater uncertainty and consequent imprecision. Typically, one of a number of surrogate sources is employed to estimate the relevant information, such as claims data or even expert opinion. When several such estimates of uncertain accuracy are employed together, the result may be little more than an elegant "back of the envelope" projection.

Medical Cost Drivers

Cost drivers can be considered conceptually to fall into four major categories (Table 42.3): patient-related factors, treatment-related factors, provider-related factors, geographic-economic factors (1). *Patient-related factors* affect cost primarily by influencing the likelihood of complications of various types and severity resulting from variations in the severity in the underlying disease process and the extent of comorbidity. *Treatment-related cost determinants* fall into two major categories. The first involves costs incident to management decisions made by the medical providers. Thus, an aggressive interventional management strategy for a patient with an acute coronary syndrome (ACS) will be associated with higher medical costs (over the short run at least) than a conservative strategy. Second, there is a more complex interaction between the management strategy selected and the patient characteristics, which may result in an increase or decrease in treatment-related complications and consequent cost. For example, timely aggressive intervention may prevent a serious complication that would have otherwise resulted from disease progression. Alternatively, use of an aggressive strategy may cause a previously unsuspected comorbidity to become clinically manifest and thus induce extra medical care costs.

TABLE 42.3

MAJOR CATEGORIES OF MEDICAL COST DRIVERS

PATIENT-RELATED FACTORS
Age
Sex
Cardiac disease severity (e.g., ejection fraction, extent of coronary artery disease)
Cardiac comorbidity (cardiac disease other than the principal condition under study)
Noncardiac comorbidity
TREATMENT-RELATED FACTORS
Aggressive versus conservative management
Complications
PROVIDER-RELATED FACTORS
Quality of care
Efficiency of care
Preferred management styles
GEOGRAPHIC/ECONOMIC FACTORS
Labor Costs
Supply Costs

Provider-related factors refer to quality and efficiency of care issues as well as overall preferred management styles for a particular clinical problem. Complications associated with medical care cannot be eliminated, but care that is of a very high technical quality can minimize those complications relative to care of lesser quality. Efficiency of care as it relates to a provider refers to the provision of the required care with a minimum set of necessary medical resources and thus the minimum amount of waste achievable. Multiple studies have now shown that some practitioners have a more resource-intensive style of practice than others; how these different styles related to quality and efficiency of care remains controversial (22–27).

Even after all the foregoing characteristics are accounted for, costs will still vary from one provider to the next because of *geographic-economic factors* that create true variations in the costs of the component resources required to provide the care in question. Variations in the cost of medical care labor in different geographic markets and variations in the purchase price of supplies can both affect cost in important ways. For example, low unemployment rates and a shortage of skilled registered nurses may drive up the salary rate for nurses in a particular region. Very large hospital chains or payers can negotiate discounts with medical suppliers and pharmaceutical companies that are not available to small independent providers.

Cost-Effectiveness Analysis

Cost-effectiveness analysis is a form of economic efficiency analysis (1,11,28,29). As described earlier in this chapter, economists are concerned with making decisions about the most efficient use of scarce societal resources. The principal agenda of the analysis is to define for the policy maker how to allocate finite health care dollars among the possible alternative programs. In its most general form, economic efficiency analysis attempts to help solve problems of allocation of resources across major sectors of the economy, such as education,

TABLE 42.4

COST-EFFECTIVENESS, COST-UTILITY, AND COST-BENEFIT RATIOS: SAMPLE CALCULATIONS

Strategy	Treatment costs	Effectiveness (life expectancy)	Utility (QOL)	QOL-adjusted life expectancy	Benefits[a]
Rx A	$20,000	4.5 y	0.80	3.60 QALYs	$4,000
Rx B	$10,000	3.5 y	0.90	3.15 QALYs	$2,000

$$\text{Incremental cost-effectiveness ratio} = \frac{\$20{,}000 - \$10{,}000}{4.5\ years - 3.5\ years} = \$10{,}000 \text{ per life-year saved}$$

$$\text{Incremental cost-utility ratio} = \frac{\$20{,}000 - \$10{,}000}{3.6\ QALYs - 3.15\ QALYs} = \$22{,}222 \text{ per QALY saved}$$

$$\text{Incremental cost-benefit ratio} = \frac{\$20{,}000 - \$10{,}000}{\$4{,}000 - \$2{,}000} = 5$$

QALY, quality-adjusted life-years; QOL, quality of life; Rx, prescription.
[a]Shows health benefits valued in dollars.
From Detsky AS, Naglie IG. A clinician's guide to cost-effectiveness analysis. *Ann Intern Med* 1990;113:147–154.

defense, public works, and health care. It is assumed in such analyses that the decision maker desires to maximize the benefits produced for society for a given investment of resources. Consequently, these techniques are insensitive to considerations about who gains and who loses as such trade-offs are made.

Types of Analyses

Economic efficiency analysis actually includes three related analytic techniques: cost-effectiveness analysis, cost-utility analysis, and cost-benefit analysis (Table 42.4) (30). These methods have several important features in common. First, all three explicitly evaluate the following decision maker's dilemma: "In moving from a reference therapy (strategy) to a new therapy (strategy), how much will be gained in additional benefits, how much additional cost will be incurred, and will the resource (monetary) investment required to produce an extra unit of benefit with this new therapy fall into an acceptable or worthwhile range judged according to past experience or other precedents?" The general formula for all three techniques is as follow:

$$\frac{C_{new} - C_{usual\ care}}{E_{new} - E_{usual\ care}}$$

Where C = costs and E = effectiveness.

Second, they all use the same calculation for the incremental costs of the new strategy or therapy (Table 42.4).

The three modes of economic efficiency analysis differ in the way they evaluate incremental health benefits (Table 42.4) (30). *Cost-effectiveness analysis* expresses incremental benefits in terms of natural units. Most commonly, incremental life-years are used. It is this form of the cost-effectiveness ratio for which most of the available benchmarks exist (Table 42.5). However, it is legitimate to calculate cost-effectiveness ratios using other medical end points. For example, a cost-effectiveness ratio of incremental dollars required to save an additional life or to produce an additional 30-day survivor or to discover one additional patient with left main coronary artery disease (CAD) could be calculated if such outcomes were deemed relevant to decision making. The difficulty is not in calculating such ratios, but rather in interpreting them. There is a general consensus that cost-effectiveness ratios less than $50,000 per added life-year are "economically attractive," whereas ratios above $100,000 per added life-year are "economically unattractive" (1,11). The middle zone represents an uncertain area. No such benchmarks exist for cost-effectiveness ratios constructed with other effectiveness measures such as those cited earlier. Thus,

TABLE 42.5

COST-EFFECTIVENESS AND USE OF SELECTED INTERVENTIONS IN THE MEDICARE POPULATION[a]

Intervention	Cost-effectiveness (cost/QALY)[b]
Influenza vaccine	Cost saving
Pneumococcal vaccine	Cost saving
β-Blockers after myocardial infarction	<$10,000
Mammographic screening	$10,000–$25,000
Colon-cancer screening	$10,000–$25,000
Osteoporosis screening	$10,000–$25,000
Management of antidepressant medications	Cost saving up to $30,000
Hypertension medication (DBP >105 mm Hg)	$10,000–$60,000
Cholesterol management, as secondary prevention	$10,000–$50,000
Implantable cardioverter-defibrillator	$30,000–$85,000
Dialysis in end-stage renal disease	$50,000–$100,000
Lung volume reduction surgery	$100,000–$300,000
Left ventricular assist devices	$500,000–$1.4 million
Positron emission tomography in Alzheimer disease	Dominated[c]

DBP, diastolic blood pressure; QALY, quality-adjusted life-year.
[a]Ranges are provided, rather than point estimates, because the actual cost effectiveness will vary according to the target populations and the strategies used.
[b]Calculation based on 2002 U.S. dollars.
[c]Benefits are lower and costs are higher than with the use of the standard workup.
Modified from Sanders GD, Hlatky MA, Owens DK. Cost-effectiveness of implantable cardioverter-defibrillators. *N Engl J Med* 2005;353:1471–1480.

these alternative cost-effectiveness ratios cannot be used for making broad-based trade-offs among alternatives for societal investment, and they can be problematic to interpret as isolated measures of value within a given health care system.

Cost-effectiveness ratios are not the precise figures they appear to be (31). Rather, they are estimates with varying (often large) degrees of uncertainty incorporated in their calculation. Furthermore, no single cost-effectiveness threshold separates the "worthwhile" from the "worthless" interventions. The figures discussed in the previous paragraph for dollars per added life-year are general guidelines, not absolute benchmarks. A cost-effectiveness analysis addresses a particular decision scenario for a particular time. Its results are not absolute for all scenarios at all times. A particular intervention may be judged economically attractive in the United States but not in the United Kingdom. Similar disparities may arise in the fee-for-service versus managed care segments of the U.S. health care system. These differences relate in part to variations in the costs of care in these different systems as well as to the different levels of willingness to spend additional dollars to buy more health care benefits.

Cost-utility analysis is a special case of cost-effectiveness analysis in which the benefit is expressed most often as a quality-adjusted life-year (QALY) (Table 42.4) (30). Calculation of such a quantity assumes that patients would be willing to give up extra survival to improve quality of life. The process of equating various quality of life states to equivalent survival durations is known as utility assessment. Utilities or utility weights are quantitative measures of the relative desirability of different health states. By convention, they are scored from 0 (death) to 1 (excellent health), although values less than 0 can be used to represent health states judged worse than death. Although this system is conceptually attractive, it has some important pragmatic problems in assessing utilities and incorporating them into an economic analysis. The two major methods of deriving utilities for use in economic analysis are direct assessment and use of a health utility index. Direct assessment typically involves interview- or questionnaire-based measurements using patients in a given health state of interest or, less commonly, other subjects who are asked to imagine (with the help of certain descriptive aids) being in the health state in question. The most commonly used direct assessment methods are the standard gamble and the time trade-off (11,32). The major alternatives to these direct utility assessment techniques are the health utility indexes. Each index consists of a set of discrete health states, typically defined in relatively simple generic terms, for which utility weights have been derived. Most often, utility weights are obtained from the general (nondiseased) population. The most widely used health utility index at present is the EuroQoL 5D (11,33).

Cost-benefit analysis requires that health benefits be converted to their monetary equivalent (Table 42.4) (30). Because physicians and patients are often uncomfortable with these conversions, and because the methodology for making such equations is vulnerable to important technical and ethical criticisms, this method of analysis is infrequently used in medicine. Its principal advantage over the other forms of economic analysis is that it can be used across the entire spectrum of societal decision making, whereas cost-effectiveness and cost-utility analyses are useful only for health policy decisions in which the goal is to maximize the added life-years (or added QALYs) produced. Cost-benefit analysis directly calculates the gain or loss for society of a particular program expressed in terms of dollars invested versus the monetary value of the return on investment. The results can be expressed as a ratio (as shown in Table 42.4) or (more preferably) as the net benefits of the program (the incremental benefits minus the incremental costs). If the cost-benefit ratio is greater than 1, or the net benefits are positive, the program is judged "worthwhile" from a societal perspective.

Several groups have proposed standards for cost-effectiveness analysis (11,34–36). The Panel on Cost Effectiveness in Health and Medicine convened by the U.S. Public Health Service published the most widely cited expert consensus standards for U.S. cost-effectiveness analysis (11,37–39). The special challenges of performing economic analyses alongside multicountry randomized clinical trials has received increased attention recently because of the rising proportions of all large trials that are now international (40).

ECONOMIC STUDIES OF CARDIOVASCULAR DISEASE

Acute Coronary Syndromes

General Considerations

ACSs (acute myocardial infarction (MI), unstable angina) share a common pathophysiology, similar clinical manifestations, a need for hospital-based management in most cases, and a self-limited course that extends typically 30 to 60 days from presentation (41,42). After this period, most (surviving) patients cycle back to a more stable phase of CAD. The economic analysis of ACSs and their treatments therefore is primarily focused on the events during the critical initial phase of presentation and care, particularly those occurring during the initial hospitalization.

Conceptually, hospitalization for an ACS can be divided into four major resource/cost components (Fig. 42.1). In patients eligible for reperfusion therapy, the reperfusion strategy selected (i.e., either thrombolytic therapy or primary coronary angioplasty) is a major cost component. Although streptokinase (SK) is relatively inexpensive (at around $300 per dose), tissue-type plasminogen activator (t-PA), recombinant t-PA (rt-PA), and tenecteplase (TNK) all cost more than $2,000 per dose, and the

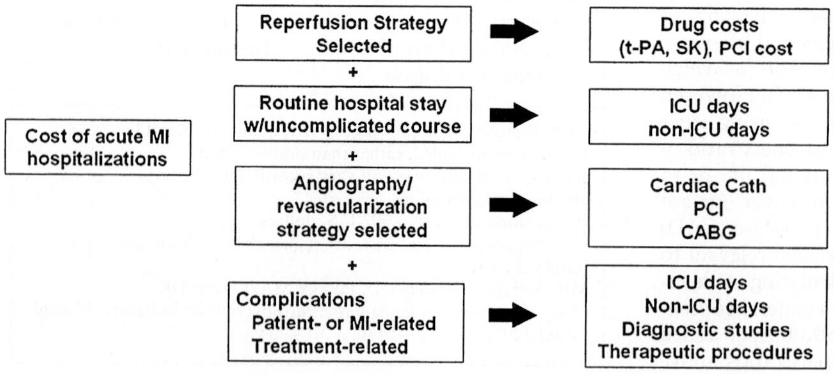

FIGURE 42.1. Cost components for an acute coronary syndrome hospitalization. CABG, coronary artery bypass grafting; Cath, catheterization; ICU, intensive care unit; MI, myocardial infarction; PCI, percutaneous coronary intervention.

procedural costs of primary percutaneous transluminal coronary angioplasty (PTCA) are even higher. A second component is the routine hospital stay required for the patient with an uncomplicated course. For patients with acute MI in the United States, this typically includes 1 or 2 days in the intensive care unit and 3 or 4 days more in a step-down or regular hospital floor setting. For patients with unstable angina, the course is typically shorter. The primary cost components for this type of care are the hospital room costs and the associated ancillary care costs (e.g., laboratory testing, medications administered, consultations obtained, radiology testing performed). A third major component is the risk stratification strategy selected. For many patients in the United States who have ACSs, diagnostic coronary angiography is the principal mode of risk stratification. Use of coronary revascularization techniques has been shown to track the use of coronary angiography with a fair degree of predictability (43). Need for revascularization is a major predictor of higher hospital costs (44). For some patients, one of several noninvasive testing strategies may be employed. These may eventually lead to coronary angiography and revascularization or may permit the patient to be discharged without undergoing such testing.

The last category of cost components for patients with ACSs is complications. These are of several different types and have varying cost implications. The reperfusion strategy selected, for example, can induce a variety of complications including minor bleeding (which may have no discernible cost effects) and major bleeding (which may induce a significant extra cost). Coronary angiography in the anticoagulated patient may lead to a major groin hematoma or other vascular complications, which, in turn, require additional days of care, testing, and consultation. Thrombolytic and anticoagulant drugs may induce gastrointestinal bleeding, sometimes because of previously undiagnosed gastrointestinal comorbidity. The ACS itself may produce complications (e.g., heart failure, arrhythmias, recurrent ischemia). Costs related to complications can be substantial and are difficult to predict.

Reperfusion Therapies

Following the demonstration by the Gruppo Italiano per lo Studio della Sopravvivenza nell'Infarto-1 (GISSI-1) and ISIS-2 trials of the survival enhancing benefit of thrombolysis with intravenous SK, intensive research focused on ways to improve reperfusion therapy over this "base case" strategy. That process is still ongoing. Early work focused on finding a better fibrinolytic drug regimen, one that offered more complete early reperfusion with a lowered risk of major bleeding, particularly intracranial hemorrhage. More recent work has explored mechanical reperfusion methods combined with various adjunctive drug regimens. As of 2006, primary percutaneous coronary intervention (PCI) continues to be favored at many centers in the United States and in parts of Europe, whereas thrombolysis is still used in centers and in situations where emergency PCI is not an option.

From an economics point of view, the main comparisons of interest have been with lytic therapy versus no reperfusion therapy and PCI versus lytic therapy. All the adjunctive strategies that have been tested can be viewed as attempting to improve the effectiveness, safety, or both of the two major reperfusion strategies.

Thrombolytic Therapy

The benefits of thrombolytic therapy for enhancing survival in acute ST-segment elevation MI are firmly established (45). As of 2005, U.S. market share for SK is only about 4%, that for t-PA is around 44%, and those for rt-PA and TNK are equivalent at around 25% each. Outside the United States, SK remains the most widely used thrombolytic agent, primarily because of affordability (46).

Unfortunately, none of the large-scale randomized trials of SK versus conservative (i.e., no reperfusion) therapy collected the empiric data on resource use or cost necessary to estimate the direct costs of these two strategies. Naylor and colleagues (47) used a model-based analysis and available clinical trial data to estimate that substitution of intravenous SK for no reperfusion therapy had a cost-effectiveness ratio of approximately $2,000 to $4,000 per added life-year, assuming that each additional survivor who received SK therapy had a life expectancy of approximately 10 years. These figures make SK therapy an extremely economically attractive intervention, probably falling into the category of "best buy."

The Global Utilization of Streptokinase and t-PA for Occluded Coronary Arteries I (GUSTO I) trial clearly established that t-PA was superior to intravenous SK in establishing Thrombolysis in Myocardial Ischemia-3 (TIMI-3) coronary flow and in saving lives (48). Because the cost of t-PA is substantially higher than that of SK, the question that directly emerged from the clinical results of GUSTO I was whether the added benefits of accelerated t-PA were sufficient to justify the added costs of this regimen. From a patient perspective (assuming that the patient does not bear the added cost of t-PA), the choice of thrombolytic regimen virtually always favors t-PA on medical grounds alone (i.e., additional survivors minus additional disabling strokes). Conversely, from the fee-for-service hospital perspective, t-PA is usually a losing financial proposition because the added costs of the therapy are often not reflected in the reimbursement received. The one added survivor per 100 generated by t-PA is a statistical survivor, and the individual patient who is actually "lost" when SK is used in lieu of t-PA cannot be identified clinically and is therefore invisible to the hospital. Furthermore, most of the added life-years generated by t-PA, as discussed later, occur after patients are discharged from the hospital.

In a detailed prospective economic, the GUSTO I trial estimated that cumulative medical costs (hospital costs plus physician fees) at 1 year averaged $24,575 for SK-treated patients and $24,990 for t-PA–treated patients exclusive of the costs of the thrombolytic agent (49). When the average wholesale drug costs for the two agents were added in, the incremental lifetime (undiscounted) costs for each patient who received t-PA was $2,845. Using the empiric 1-year GUSTO survival data, additional data from the Duke Cardiovascular Database, and statistical modeling, we projected a life expectancy for t-PA–treated patients of 15.41 years versus 15.27 for the SK-treated patients, an undiscounted increase in life expectancy for t-PA of 0.14 years per patient. This result can be more intuitively restated as follows: the one extra patient per 100 saved with accelerated t-PA lives an average of 14 additional years.

With an increased life expectancy of 0.14 years of life per patient for t-PA–treated patients, a cost of $270 for the SK and $2,216 for the t-PA, the cost-effectiveness ratio for t-PA was $27,115 per year of life saved (discounted at 5%) (49).

Both the cost-effectiveness analyses of SK versus no reperfusion and of t-PA versus SK make the critical assumption that the early survival benefits demonstrated in clinical trials are preserved indefinitely over the lifetime of the cohort. Strong evidence for this exists for SK, with follow-up of the GISSI trial out to 10 years and the Dutch Intracoronary Streptokinase Trial out to 20 years (50,51). The survival benefit of t-PA over SK has been documented out to 1 year (52).

The GUSTO III trial compared rt-PA with t-PA and found no difference in major cardiovascular events (including death, stroke, and bleeding) out to 1 year (53). The costs of these two agents are the same and although the nursing time and ancillary costs associated with a double-bolus regimen are likely smaller than with a bolus and 90-minute infusion, inefficiencies in the care process would likely eliminate these small theoretic savings.

TNK-tPA was compared with rt-PA in 16,999 patients in the Assessment of the Safety and Efficacy of a New Thrombolytic-2 (ASSENT-2) study (54). Mortality was identical in the two arms of the study, as was intracranial hemorrhage. Bleeding complications and the need for blood transfusion were modestly reduced by TNK. The cost of TNK is the same as that of t-PA, and the single-bolus administration regimen is attractive to a busy emergency department, if not cost saving. A formal economic analysis of ASSENT-2 has not been performed.

The ASSENT-3 trial compared full-dose TNK plus enoxaparin, full-dose TNK plus unfractionated heparin, and half-dose TNK plus abciximab plus unfractionated heparin (55). Both experimental regimens produced a decrease in the 30-day primary composite and point of death, reinfarction, or refractory ischemia. Unexpectedly, however, the early reduction in nonfatal MI did not translate into improved survival at 1 year. An economic analysis of ASSENT-3 found that the TNK enoxaparin arm was less expensive than the TNK unfractionated heparin arm in 80% of 1,000 bootstrap replications (56). The abciximab regimen was cost saving in 75% of bootstrap samples only with the assumption of efficient packaging of TNK in a 25-mg vial at half price.

Primary Percutaneous Coronary Reperfusion

A quantitative overview of 10 randomized trials conducted between 1989 and 1996, the Primary Coronary Angioplasty Trialists (PCAT) meta-analysis, showed a strong possibility direct angioplasty was actually superior to thrombolytic therapy in saving lives (57). At 30 days, primary balloon angioplasty reduced mortality from 6.5% to 4.4%, a 34% relative reduction ($p = .02$). Death and nonfatal reinfarction were reduced by 40% ($p < .001$). Furthermore, comparison of hospital charges in the Primary Angioplasty in Myocardial Infarction I (PAMI I) study and estimated hospital costs in the Mayo Clinic Randomized Trial both suggested that primary angioplasty may also be a less expensive reperfusion strategy (58–60). However, of the 10 trials included in the overview, 9 were quite small.

Six-month follow-up data on the PCAT trials showed preservation of the initial therapeutic advantage of PTCA (61). Further, 5-year follow-up data from the Dutch trial of 395 patients showed continued benefit for PTCA for both mortality and reinfarction (62).

Since the PCAT meta-analysis, 12 additional trials have compared a primary PCI strategy with a thrombolytic regimen. Most of these more recent trials included the use of stents, and some included glycoprotein IIb/IIIa inhibitors as well. Pooled analysis of the four trials that compared on-site thrombolysis with transport to a tertiary hospital for PCI showed a reduction in 30-day mortality from 9.6% with lytic therapy to 6.8% with PCI ($p = .01$) (63).

The economics of primary PCI versus thrombolysis has not been adequately examined for contemporary practice. One of the challenges has been that the PCI strategy costs have gone through several cycles. For example, bare metal stents were substantially more expensive in the early years of stenting than at present. Addition of the costs of a glycoprotein IIb/IIIa inhibitor, particularly abciximab, or the need for emergency transport to a tertiary hospital, or substitution of a drug-eluting stent as is the practice at present all increase costs. Although the cost of thrombolytic therapy itself has remained stable over the past decade, factors that can alter the cost of the thrombolysis strategy include the risk stratification strategy used (routine diagnostic catheterization versus noninvasive stress testing and selective catheterization) and the decision about when to discharge the patient.

An economic analysis of the largest single modern trial, DANish trial in Acute Myocardial Infarction-2 (DANAMI-2), is planned but has not yet been reported (64). Cost data are available for the Canadian Stenting versus Thrombolysis in Acute myocardial infarction Trial (STAT) study of 123 patients (65). Initial hospitalization costs (in 1999 U.S. dollars) were $6,354 for primary stenting versus $7,893 for t-PA ($p = .001$). The cost of the t-PA (in Canada) was $1,809, whereas the hospital costs of the PCI procedure were $2,129. However, the PCI strategy was associated with a 2-day reduction in the length of stay, which is problematic to interpret in an unblinded study because it may result either from improved disease course or from physician bias. In addition, 64% of the t-PA–treated group had an unscheduled coronary angiogram during the index hospitalization. In follow-up, PCI-treated patients had fewer readmissions, and by 6 months, PCI had $2,500 lower cumulative costs than t-PA.

The benefits of adding abciximab to primary stenting in acute MI were tested in the Controlled Abciximab and Device Investigation to Lower Late Angioplasty Complications (CADILLAC) trial. This trial enrolled 2,665 patients with acute MI who were within 12 hours of symptom onset and who were deemed eligible for stenting. Randomization used a factorial design: balloon PTCA versus stent and open-label abciximab versus no abciximab. Addition of abciximab reduced 30-day ischemia and ischemia-driven target revascularization for both stent-treated and PTCA-treated patients (66). On the cost side, abciximab increased initial procedural costs by $1,122 but reduced subsequent length of stay by 0.6 days, thus providing a partial cost offset (67). At 1 year, however, cumulative abciximab arm costs were $1,244 higher. Because there was no clear benefit of abciximab on survival or composite events at 12 months in this trial, the economic attractiveness of adjunctive abciximab in a primary PCI strategy remains uncertain.

Guidelines on the use of primary PCI in acute ST-segment elevation MI emphasize the importance of the "door-to-balloon" time, the level of experience of the operator and laboratory, and the patient's symptom duration in selecting the preferred reperfusion strategy. A recent analysis of the National Registry of Myocardial Infarction (NRMI) data showed that patients who presented in off hours (evenings, nights, weekends) had a 21-minute longer door-to-balloon time (68). Another recent analysis from NRMI showed only 4% of U.S. patients with acute ST-segment elevation MI who were transferred from one hospital to another for PCI had a door-to-balloon time of 90 minutes or less, as recommended by American College of Cardiology/American Heart Association (ACC/AHA) Guidelines (69). None of these nuances have been examined in economic models.

One of the main limitations of the primary angioplasty reperfusion strategy is that only about 20% of U.S. hospitals have catheterization facilities, and many of these are not staffed 24 hours a day (70). Building new interventional catheterization laboratories, training new personnel to staff them, and providing 24-hour coverage would substantially increase the long-term per case cost of the procedure (71).

Coronary Angiography and Predischarge Risk Stratification

Six large randomized trials have now compared different forms of invasive and conservative management strategies for patients with ACSs. TIMI IIIB compared these two strategies in 1,473 patients (72). Early invasive management involved routine angiography at 18 to 48 hours after presentation. Early conservative management employed angiography only if certain high-risk indicators were present. At 6 weeks, the two strategies had identical rates of death and MI. Hospital stay was shorted for the invasive arm of the study, and rehospitalization for recurrent unstable angina was also reduced in this arm. The Veterans Affairs Non–Q-Wave Infarction Strategies in Hospital (VANQWISH) study, in contrast, found that early conservative management in 920 patients with non–Q-wave MI was associated with lower mortality at hospital discharge and at 12 months (73). In the conservative arm of both TIMI IIIB and VANQWISH, catheterization was employed in about half of the assigned patients. In contrast, in the Fast Revascularisation during InStability in Coronary artery disease II (FRISC II) study, only 10% of conservatively treated patients received catheterization (74). This trial showed a significant 1.7% absolute reduction in mortality and an additional 2.0% absolute reduction in nonfatal MI with the early invasive strategy. In this Swedish study, the early invasive group had their average length of stay prolonged by 3.9 days (75), and cumulative costs at 1 year were approximately $3,100 higher. Costs per life-year added were not calculated but likely would fall into an economically attractive range. If such an extreme conservative strategy is the comparator, invasive therapy has clearly demonstrable benefits in patients with ACS. What is less clear is whether a policy that uses angiography about half the time is inferior to one that uses it almost all the time. In the Randomized Intervention Treatment of Angina-3 (RITA-3) trial, 1,810 patients with ACS were randomized to early invasive versus early conservative therapy (76). Similarly to FRISC II, the early conservative group had a low rate of coronary angiography during the index hospitalization (16%). With a median of 2 years of follow-up, no difference was observed in death or nonfatal MI. Refractory angina at 4 months and at 1 year was significantly lower in the early invasive arm of the study. At 5 years, the early invasive arm had a 22% lower rate of death or MI, with the treatment benefit largely concentrated in the highest-risk patients (77).

In the Treat Angina with Aggrastat and Determine Cost of Therapy with an Invasive or Conservative Strategy—Thrombolysis in Myocardial Infarction (TACTICS-TIMI) 18 trial, all patients received tirofiban, and bare metal coronary stents were used in more than 80% of PCI procedures (78). Fifty-one percent of the patients in the early conservative-treatment arm of the trial were referred for coronary angiography during the index hospitalization. At 6 months, death was equivalent in the two arms of the trial, and there was about a 2 per 100 reduction in the rate of MI. A cost analysis of this trial found that the invasive arm was modestly more expensive during the index hospitalization ($15,714 versus $14,047) but less expensive during the first 6 months of follow-up ($6,098 versus $7,180) (79). Thus, cumulative costs at 6 months were $12,813 for the invasive arm versus $21,227 for the conservative arm of this trial. Cost per life-year added for the invasive strategy was approximately $13,000, an economically attractive result.

The Invasive versus Conservative Treatment in Unstable Coronary Syndromes (ICTUS) trial randomized 1,200 patients with ACS who had an elevated troponin T level to early invasive versus selective invasive strategies (80). During the index hospitalization, 98% of the early invasive patients and 53% of the selective invasive strategy patients had a cardiac catheterization. At the end of 1 year, there was no difference in the mortality rate, whereas the selective invasive arm had fewer nonfatal MIs (10% versus 15%, $p = .005$), primarily attributable to revascularization procedures. Complementing these recent results, an observational study using data from 158,831 Medicare patients with acute MI (1994 to 1995) suggested that in regions of the United States with high rates of appropriate medical therapy, routine use of cardiac catheterization did not enhance survival (81).

If one takes the position that early invasive approach improves the outcome in at least a subset of patients with ACS, new data suggest an important disconnect between who receives the strategy and who should. The Can Rapid Risk Stratification of Unstable Angina Patients Suppress Adverse Outcomes with Early Implementation in the ACC/AHA guidelines (CRUSADE) registry recently examined the use of the early invasive strategy in 17,926 high-risk non–ST-segment elevation ACS patients who met ACC/AHA Guidelines for this management (82). Only 45% of the high-risk patients received an early invasive strategy. In general, early invasive management was reserved for younger patients with fewer comorbidities.

Antithrombin Therapy in Non–ST-Segment Elevation Acute Coronary Syndrome

Small randomized trials of heparin versus no heparin in patients with unstable angina or non–Q-wave MI have shown a reduction in short-term rates of death and nonfatal MI. Consequently, heparin has been adopted as a standard of care for these patients in the early phase of their presentation (41).

Several studies have now been conducted using low-molecular-weight heparins in patients with ACSs. In a systematic overview of six trials comparing enoxaparin with unfractionated heparin in 21,946 patients with ACS, death or nonfatal MI was reduced 9% at 30 days (83). No difference was seen in mortality alone or in major bleeding.

The economic analysis of one of these trials, Efficacy and Safety of Subcutaneous Enoxaparin as Non-Q-Wave Coronary Events (ESSENCE) (3,171 patients), showed that the low-molecular-weight heparin strategy was associated with a drug cost of $155 per patient (2.5 days of therapy) in the United States. After taking this cost into account, the enoxaparin strategy was associated with a cost savings of $760 to $1,170 per patient shifted from standard unfractionated heparin therapy owing to a reduction in use of invasive procedures and length of stay (84). However, given the more conservative incremental efficacy outcomes of the most recent enoxaparin trials, particularly Superior Yield of the New Strategy of Enoxaparin, Revascularization, and Glycoprotein IIb/IIIa inhibitors (SYNERGY) (2001 to 2003), it is unclear whether the cost savings seen in ESSENCE pertain to contemporary practice (85).

Intravenous Antiplatelet Therapy

Three compounds that block the platelet glycoprotein IIb/IIIa receptor have been approved for clinical use in the United States: abciximab (in patients undergoing or planned for percutaneous revascularization), eptifibatide, and tirofiban. The GUSTO IV trial surprisingly failed to show a benefit of abciximab therapy in patients with non–ST-segment elevation ACS (86). Tirofiban has been tested in two trials, PRISM and Platelet Receptor Inhibition in Ischemic Syndrome Management (PRISM)-PLUS.

The Platelet glycoprotein IIb/IIIa in Unstable angina: Receptor Suppression Using Intergrilin Therapy (PURSUIT) trial, with 10,948 patients, was the largest trial of an intravenous glycoprotein IIb/IIIa inhibitor in patients with non–ST-segment elevation ACS. At 30 days, the eptifibatide arm had a 1.5% absolute reduction in death or MI compared with placebo ($p = .04$) (87). A detailed prospective economic substudy in the 3,522 U.S. patients enrolled in PURSUIT showed two major findings (88). First, with a diagnostic catheterization rate of 85% as background, addition of eptifibatide did not alter the use of invasive cardiac procedures or hospital length of stay. Second, with a cost for the eptifibatide regimen ranging from $1,217 (average wholesale price) to $1,014 (hospital discounted price) and an incremental increase in life expectancy of 0.11 years attributable to eptifibatide therapy in U.S. patients, the cost per year of life added was between $13,700 and $16,500. This fulfills criteria cited earlier for an economically attractive therapy.

Coronary Revascularization

In the United States, approximately 1.5 million inpatient diagnostic cardiac catheterizations, 515,000 CABG operations (on 306,000 patients), and 657,000 percutaneous interventional procedures (on 640,000 patients) are performed annually (based on 2002 figures) (89). Thus, defining the clinical effectiveness, costs, and appropriate roles for these technologies has been a paramount research problem in clinical medicine over the last decade. Early outcomes research studies in cardiology found a surprising and substantial degree of variability in the use of these procedures in different geographic areas in the United States (90). More recent investigations have at least partially explained the sources of these variations. Two of the paramount determinants are the availability of cardiovascular specialists in the geographic area and the availability of angiographic and revascularization facilities (26,43). There are also strong correlations between the use of noninvasive diagnostic testing and the subsequent use of coronary angiography on the one hand and between the use of coronary angiography and subsequent revascularization procedures on the other (91). Early responses from health policy analysts to the observations about geographic variability in cardiac procedure use centered on the presumption that the high-use areas had a higher rate of inappropriate care (92). However, numerous studies using rigorous expert panel consensus guidelines for appropriate and necessary care have failed to confirm this supposition. In fact, the rate of unnecessary procedures in New York State is virtually equivalent to that in Ontario, Canada, a geographic area with approximately half the overall procedure rate of New York (93). Work by Hux and Naylor and their colleagues in Canada suggested that in areas of Ontario where the use of angiography and revascularization is higher, greater proportions of patients who receive the procedures have small predicted marginal health benefits in terms of survival or angina relief (94). Thus, the debate about the appropriate use of invasive cardiac procedures is shifting from a focus on wasteful and unnecessary care to the balance between incremental benefits and incremental costs. Unfortunately, although some recent studies have described the costs of different interventional strategies for CAD, very few studies have attempted to address their cost effectiveness. A comprehensive cost-effectiveness analysis in this area would, in fact, be quite difficult because of the complexity of the underlying clinical decisions, the difficulty in obtaining adequate outcome data, and the rapidly evolving technologies that comprise the set of currently used invasive cardiac procedures. Wong and colleagues made an attempt in 1990, but their model does not include more recent data or changes in current evidence or practice patterns (95).

Comparisons of Revascularization Strategies

Six trials have compared medical therapy with percutaneous revascularization (96). The Angioplasty Compared to Medical Therapy (ACME) trial found a very modest improvement among 212 patients with single-vessel disease in exercise treadmill time and physical functioning in the PTCA arm of the study (97). A preliminary economic analysis of ACME was conducted but was not published. The RITA-2 trial found that PTCA improved angina and exercise test performance but had a slight excess of procedure-related MIs. Quality of life was significantly better for the PTCA arm at 1 year, but these benefits were attenuated by 3 years (98). At least part of this attenuation appears to result from late revascularization procedures in the medical arm. An economic analysis of RITA-2 from the U.K. health system perspective has been published (99). Using the resource use data from the trial and unit costs derived from five U.K. centers, the investigators estimated that at 3 years, PTCA cost £2,685 more. A cost-effectiveness analysis was not performed. The Asymptomatic Cardiac Ischemia Pilot (ACIP) randomized 558 patients with clinically stable CAD and documented ischemia to one of three treatment strategies: angina-guided medical care, ischemia-guided medical care, and revascularization. The ischemia-guided therapy was adjusted on the basis of repeated ambulatory monitoring studies. The principal medical regimens used in this pilot study were either atenolol-nifedipine or diltiazem-isosorbide. Patients randomized to revascularization received either PTCA or CABG at the discretion of the principal investigator. Although an economic analysis was not initially planned for this study, the investigators performed a post hoc analysis using the available resource use data along with cost estimates taken from the GUSTO I analysis (100). At the end of 3 months, the average costs for the revascularization patients were $13,400 compared with $1,500 for the angina-guided patients and $900 for the ischemia-guided patients. However, between 3 months and 2 years, the costs for the medical arms of the trial significantly exceeded those for the revascularization arm, primarily owing to an increased need for revascularization procedures and rehospitalizations. At the end of 2 years, the cumulative costs for the angina-guided strategy were $7,735, those for the ischemia-guided strategy were $8,575 and those for the revascularization strategy were $16,782. No empiric data were collected past 2 years in ACIP. However, taking the second year costs as the best estimate of annual costs for each treatment arm, a simple linear extrapolation (discounting future costs at a 3% rate) suggested that at 10 years, patients in the medical arms of the trial would have cumulative costs of about $23,500, whereas those in the revascularization arm would average $25,300. Unfortunately, good empiric data on resource use patterns after 5 years in a modern cohort of CAD patients do not exist.

The on-going Clinical Outcomes Utilizing Percutaneous Coronary Revascularization and Aggressive Guideline-Driven Drug Evaluation (COURAGE) trial is comparing optimal medical therapy with a strategy of PCI, and an economic analysis of this trial is planned (101).

Two randomized trials have compared the costs of coronary angioplasty and CABG surgery in patients with multivessel coronary artery disease (CAD) in the United States. The Emory Angioplasty Surgery Trial (EAST) enrolled 392 patients between 1987 and 1990 (102). Patients were followed every 6 months for 3 years. Hospital costs were estimated from hospital bills with charges converted to costs using department-level cost-to-charge ratios (103). Physician fees were obtained from physician bills (i.e., charges). Hospital cost data were not collected for outside (i.e., non-EAST) hospitalization. Instead, EAST costs were applied to the follow-up hospitalizations reported on follow-up contacts. Costs were all deflated to 1987 dollars. For the initial hospitalization, hospital costs were $11,684 (median, $10,290) for PTCA and $14,579 (median, $13,991) for CABG ($p < 0.0001$) (103). With physician fees added in, total initial costs were $16,223 for PTCA and $24,005 for CABG ($p < 0.0001$) (Fig. 42.2). At the end of 3 years, cumulative costs for the PTCA arm of the study were $23,734 versus $25,310 for CABG ($p < 0.0001$) (Fig. 42.3). Thus, PTCA costs initially constituted 68% of CABG costs but after 3 years had risen to 94% of CABG costs (103). In multiple regression analysis, the major correlates of initial medical costs were randomization to CABG, heart failure, and male gender. Regression analysis of 3-year costs identified ejection fraction, hypertension, and male gender as the major cost correlates. Assignment to CABG was no longer an independent predictor. Between 3 and 8 years, the CABG-treated patients had $2,700 of extra medical costs versus $4,700 for those in the PTCA arm of the trial. With 8 years of follow-up, total costs were $46,348 for the CABG arm and $44,491 for the PTCA arm ($p = .37$) (104).

The Bypass Angioplasty Revascularization Investigation (BARI) enrolled 1,829 patients with multivessel CAD between 1988 and 1991 in 18 centers (105). The BARI Substudy of

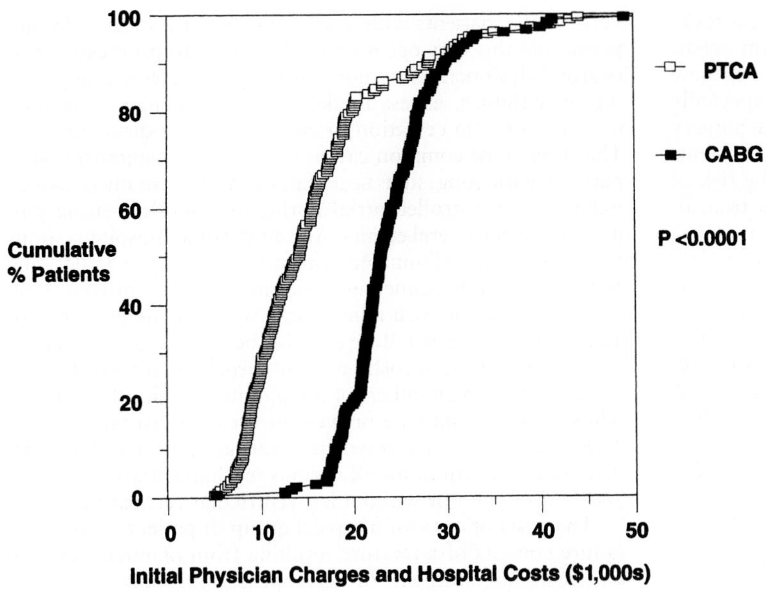

FIGURE 42.2. Cumulative distribution plot of total initial costs (hospital and physician) by treatment group in the Emory Angioplasty Versus Surgery Trial (EAST). CABG, coronary artery bypass grafting; PTCA, percutaneous transluminal coronary angioplasty. (From Weintraub WS, Mauldin PD, Becker E, et al. A comparison of the costs of and quality of life after coronary angioplasty or coronary surgery for multivessel coronary disease: results from the Emory Angioplasty Versus Surgery Trial (EAST). *Circulation* 1995;92:2831–2840.)

Economics and Quality of Life (SEQOL) was conducted in 7 of the 18 enrolling sites and collected cost data on 934 of the 1,829 total patients randomized in the trial (106). Detailed cost data were collected on all hospitalizations (regardless of diagnosis), as well as outpatient visits to 10 different types of health care providers and outpatient cardiac tests and procedures. Medication use was also collected in this trial. Initial length of stay was 9 days for the PTCA arm of the trial and 13.3 days for the CABG arm. Hospital costs were $14,415 versus $21,534, whereas physician fees were $6,698 versus $10,813 (106). In follow-up, PTCA-treated patients averaged 3.1 readmissions versus 2.7 for CABG-treated patients. Total inpatient follow-up costs (hospital plus physician) were $27,439 for PTCA and $19,529 for CABG. The number of outpatient visits was equivalent for the two therapies, as were outpatient costs ($1,656 versus $1,617). The PTCA-treated patients took an average of 4.1 cardiac medications at a cumulative 5-year cost of $4,948. The CABG-treated patients averaged 4.0 cardiac medications at a cost of $3,670. Outpatient diagnostic testing was equivalent in the two treatments, but CABG-treated patients had a slightly higher rate of nursing home admission (3.2% versus 2.6%) with higher associated costs ($1,027 versus $265). After 5 years of follow-up, total discounted costs in the CABG arm were 5% greater than those for PTCA ($58,889 versus $56,225). In subgroup analyses, patients with two-vessel disease had significantly lower costs with angioplasty ($52,390 versus $58,498 for CABG), whereas angioplasty costs were actually higher than CABG surgery in patients with three-vessel disease ($60,918 versus $59,430).

Cost analysis of the British RITA-1 trial of 1,011 patients confirmed the findings of EAST and BARI (107). The initial costs (estimated in British pounds) of treating with PTCA were about 52% that of CABG, but at the end of 5 years, PTCA and CABG costs differed by only about £400 (108).

Several trials have compared a percutaneous revascularization strategy including routine stenting with CABG. The Arterial Revascularization Therapies Study (ARTS) randomized 1,205 patients with multivessel CAD to stent versus CABG (109). At 1 year, there was no significant difference in mortality, stroke, or MI. Repeat revascularization occurred in 16.8% of stent-treated patients versus 3.5% of CABG-treated patients. Initial procedural costs (based on European practices and prices and converted to U.S. dollars) were lower in the stent arm of the trial ($6,400 versus $10,700). At 1 year, these differences had

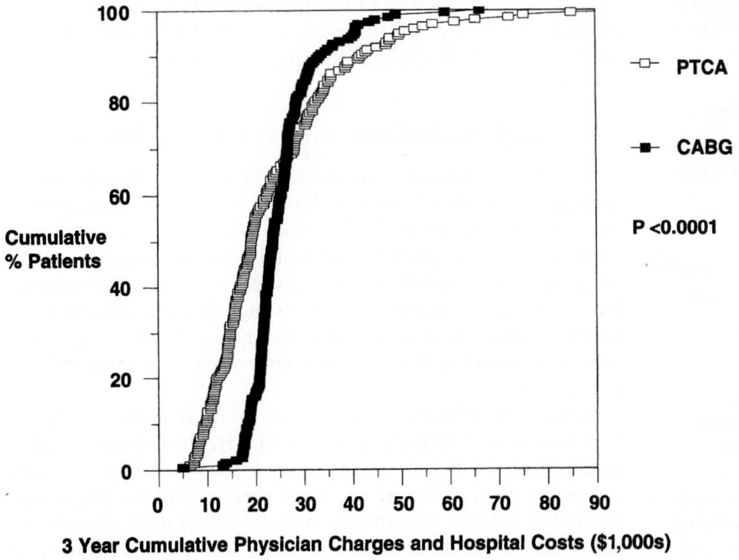

FIGURE 42.3. Cumulative distribution plot of 3 years costs by treatment group in the Emory Angioplasty Versus Surgery Trial (EAST). CABG, coronary artery bypass grafting; PTCA, percutaneous transluminal coronary angioplasty. (From Weintraub WS, Mauldin PD, Becker E, et al. A comparison of the costs of and quality of life after coronary angioplasty or coronary surgery for multivessel coronary disease: results from the Emory Angioplasty Versus Surgery Trial (EAST). *Circulation* 1995;92:2831–2840.)

narrowed somewhat because of the extra repeat procedures in the stent arm of the trial: $10,700 for the stent arm versus $13,600 for the CABG arm (p <.001). The relevance of these cost data for U.S. practice is uncertain, given the unexpectedly low cost estimates for CABG. The Canadian/European Surgery or Stent (SoS) study randomized 988 patients to CABG or stent-assisted PCI (110). At a median 2-year follow-up, the risk of death or nonfatal MI was similar in the two arms of the trial, although the CABG arm had fewer deaths than the PCI arm (2% versus 5%, p = .01). The need for additional revascularization procedures (the trial's primary end point) was 21% in the PCI arm versus 6% in the CABG arm (p <.001). Over the first year, quality of life improved significantly in both arms but to a greater extent in the CABG arm (111). Initial costs for CABG were £3,437 higher, and at 1 year the differential narrowed to £2,609 (112). Taking account of survival and quality of life, there were no differences in QALYs between the two arms of the trial in the first year (0.694 for PCI versus 0.695 for CABG).

Heart Failure

Approximately 4.7 million Americans carry a diagnosis of heart failure, and more than 550,000 new cases are identified each year (89). About 70% of cases are the result of CAD, with hypertension the next most common underlying disorder (113). The annual hospitalization volume for heart failure now approaches 1 million (1998 figure) with an associated annual cost in excess of $3.7 billion. The prevalence of heart failure rises with increasing age, and this disease is the single most frequent cause of hospitalization in the Medicare population (age ≥65) (89). After a first admission for heart failure, Medicare patients have a 44% chance of being readmitted at least once within 6 months (114).

Costs of Medical Care

To analyze the costs of heart failure and their determinants, it is useful to look at four cost components (Fig. 42.4): maintenance care, primary prevention of sudden cardiac death, care for episodes of decompensation, and procedures to reverse the heart failure state. Maintenance care includes the use of medications and routine medical follow-up for the patient with a stable, well-compensated course. The goals of maintenance therapy are to reduce symptoms and improve functional status to the extent possible, to improve survival, and to decrease the need for repeat hospitalizations. Primary prevention of sudden death in eligible patients with systolic dysfunction involves implantation of implantable cardioverter-defibrillators (ICDs).

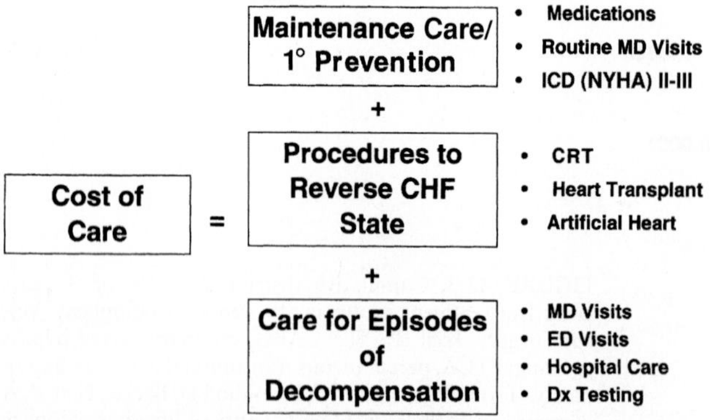

FIGURE 42.4. Cost components for heart failure care. CRT, cardiac resynchronization therapy; Dx, diagnosis; ED, emergency department; NYHA, New York Heart Association.

Periodically, patients with heart failure enter a state of decompensation; this may occur gradually owing to progressive myocardial dysfunction or more abruptly (e.g., from complicating arrhythmias, excess intake of dietary sodium, infection, or inappropriate cessation or reduction of medical therapy). The three most common causes of need for hospitalization in patients with congestive heart failure (CHF) are uncontrolled ischemia, uncontrolled atrial fibrillation, and increasing pulmonary or peripheral edema. Although not all hospitalizations for CHF can be eliminated without reversing the underlying heart failure state, some interventions have been proven to reduce the need for such admissions. Whether the efficiency of admissions for heart failure can also be improved (with a consequent reduction in costs) remains largely undefined. Finally, there are growing numbers of nonpharmacologic interventions whose goal is to stabilize or even reverse the heart failure state. These include cardiac resynchronization therapy (CRT), cardiac transplantation, use of various mechanical assist devices, and CABG (with or without left ventricular reconstruction).

The costs of care for a typical group of patients with heart failure consists of a mixture resulting from maintenance care and costs for treatment of decompensation. Only very small numbers of patients (2,016 in 2004) undergo cardiac transplantation (89). There are no "natural history" cost studies of heart failure, so it is difficult to define the cost of the disorder independently of the interventions used to treat it. In the National Heart, Lung and Blood Institute (NHLBI) Cardiovascular Health Study, involving 5,888 subjects aged 65 and older selected from four geographic communities, the presence of heart failure was associated with annual costs of about $8,500 (115).

Digoxin

Digoxin is one of the oldest pharmacologic interventions in cardiovascular medicine, but its clinical effectiveness remains controversial. The National Institutes of Health (NIH) Digitalis Investigation Group (DIG) trial found no survival benefit for digoxin but a significant 6% reduction in the need for hospitalization (116). Using DRG-based Medicare reimbursement rates, Eisenstein and colleagues performed a cost analysis of the DIG trial (116). Digoxin-treated patients averaged fewer all-cause (1.9 versus 2.0, p = .01) and heart failure (0.6 versus 0.8, p = .001) hospitalizations. Digoxin-treated patients had higher total medical costs ($12,648 versus $12,362, p = .001). Heart failure costs were lower ($3,122 versus $4,130, p = .001), but non–heart failure costs were higher. Interestingly, PTCAs were more frequent in the digoxin arm of the trial, a finding suggesting that these patients improved enough clinically to be treated more aggressively for their CAD. The average cost of the digoxin therapy over a mean of 37 months was $163.

Angiotensin-Converting Enzyme Inhibitors

Angiotensin-converting enzyme (ACE) inhibitor therapy is now recognized as one of the foundations of modern medical therapy for heart failure (117). Numerous large-scale clinical trials have clearly demonstrated that ACE inhibitors prolong survival in patients with heart failure caused by systolic dysfunction. Unfortunately, none of these trials included prospective measurement of costs. Two U.S. studies have used decision analysis models to estimate the cost effectiveness of this form of therapy (118,119).

Glick and colleagues used primary data from the Studies of Left Ventricular Dysfunction (SOLVD) treatment trial (mild to moderate heart failure and ejection fraction <35%) to model the cost effectiveness of enalapril therapy (118). The model evaluated both 48-month outcomes (from the available empiric data) and projected lifetime outcomes. Analysis was done from a societal perspective, and costs were expressed in 1992 U.S. dollars. On the health benefit side, this study estimated that patients randomized to enalapril gained 0.14 discounted years of life and 0.11 discounted QALYs during the 4-year follow-up of the trial. The life expectancy of these patients was estimated at 6.5 to 7.0 years, and over this period enalapril was projected to add 0.30 discounted years and 0.21 discounted QALYs.

On the cost side, the enalapril-treated patients averaged $11,840 in discounted costs of hospitalization, enalapril therapy, and outpatient visits during the 4 years of the study. The corresponding cost for the placebo-treated patients were $12,560. Thus, during the trial period, enalapril saved $720 per patient (118). Importantly, these savings occurred during the first 18 months of the trial, and costs after this point were similar. Over the projected life expectancy of the study cohort, enalapril-treated patients had discounted costs of $22,000, whereas placebo-treated patients had costs of $21,975. The lifetime incremental cost of enalapril therapy was therefore projected to be $25 per patient.

During the 4 years of the trial, enalapril improved survival and reduced medical costs. Projecting these data out to a lifetime cost-effectiveness perspective, enalapril saved an added life-year for $80 and an added QALY for $115 (118). These data demonstrate that, at a minimum, ACE inhibitor therapy with enalapril in mild to moderate CHF is in the "best buy" category of cost effectiveness. There are several reasons that it is likely that, in this population, ACE inhibitor therapy is actually cost saving over the patient's lifetime. First, sensitivity analysis on the long-term effects of enalapril show that if the drug continues to reduce hospitalizations after 18 months it would be cost saving (118). Second, the average wholesale price for a year's supply of enalapril 20 mg/day is $475. The advent of generic captopril makes an ACE inhibitor available for a substantially lower cost and would therefore make the therapy cost saving over a lifetime time horizon. Finally, the cost assigned to follow-up hospitalizations was based on Health Care Financing Administration DRG reimbursement rates and may have therefore underestimated the fair cost of such an event (and hence the value of preventing it).

β-Blocking Agents

Two important randomized trials have recently reported that β-blocker therapy in heart failure produces a clinically important and statistically significant reduction in both mortality and hospitalization. The Metoprolol CR/XL Randomized Intervention Trial in Congestive Heart Failure (MERIT-HF) randomized 3,991 patients with New York Heart Association (NYHA) class or higher II heart failure and an ejection fraction of up to 0.40 to metoprolol CR/XL or placebo (120). With an average follow-up of 1 year, metoprolol reduced death or heart transplantation by 32%. All-cause hospitalization was reduced from 33% to 29% ($p = .004$), and days in hospital were reduced from 6.1 to 5.1 per patient ($p = .004$). The discounted retail cost of metoprolol XL/CR therapy ranges from $26/month for the 50-mg dose ($312/year) to $59/month for the 200-mg dose ($708/year). Although a formal cost analysis of MERIT-HF has not yet been reported, the cost of metoprolol therapy should be largely offset by the approximate 1-day average reduction in hospital stay.

The Cardiac Insufficiency Bisoprolol Study II (CIBIS II) enrolled 2,647 patients with heart failure in class III or IV with an ejection fraction of up to 35% (121). All-cause mortality was reduced 34% by bisoprolol ($p < .001$). All-cause hospitalization was reduced 20% from 34% to 33% ($p < .001$). An economic analysis of CIBIS II from the perspective of a European third-party payer found that after accounting for the cost of the drug and the extra clinic visits for dose titration, bisoprolol was cost saving compared with no bisoprolol (122).

In contrast, the Beta-Blocker Evaluation of Survival Trial (BEST) randomized 2,708 patients with class III or IV heart failure to bucindolol or placebo (123). At an average of 2 years, no significant effect was noted on mortality overall, although there was a survival advantage in nonblack patients. Hospitalization was reduced by 8% in the bucindolol-treated group ($p = .08$).

Economic analysis of the smaller U.S. Carvedilol Heart Failure Trials Program was performed using a Markov decision model, clinical data from the trials, and published cost data (124). Trial data were projected out to a lifetime perspective. Projected lifetime costs of conventional CHF care in this model were $28,750. Costs for the carvedilol strategy were $36,420, or $7,600 more than conventional therapy. Carvedilol was projected to extend life expectancy by 0.31 to 0.95 years per patient over the life expectancy without such therapy (6.7 years). This range reflects different assumptions about the persistence of therapeutic benefit. The corresponding cost effectiveness of carvedilol therapy ranged from $30,000 per life-year added to $13,000 per life-year added. Current (2005) discounted retail price for carvedilol is approximately $45 to $50 per month, or $575 per year.

Defibrillator and Cardiac Resynchronization Therapy

Although ICDs are now well-established tools in the secondary prevention of sudden cardiac death (i.e., in patients with a cardiac arrest or symptomatic malignant arrhythmia), the data to support their use as primary prevention in the heart failure population are relatively recent (125,126). CRT, conversely, was developed to improve left ventricular function and thereby to ameliorate heart failure symptoms. Recent clinical trial data have persuasively demonstrated that CRT therapy without ICD can effectively prolong survival (127). One of the major residual uncertainties is whether (and under what circumstances) the two therapies have complementary survival benefits. The issue is of both clinical and economic importance because the cost differential for a CRT-P (pacemaker) device and a CRT-D (defibrillator) device is about $20,000 (device and leads only).

The economics of primary prevention with ICD therapy alone have been examined in the Sudden Cardiac Death in Heart Failure Trial (SCD-HeFT) and MADIT II trial populations and using a decision model (128,129). SCD-HeFT used a single-lead VVI ICD programmed for shock-only therapy, and by protocol, ICDs were to be implanted in an outpatient setting. These two factors served to minimize the upfront cost of the ICD arm of the trial. Although there is a modest incremental cost involved in following patients with an ICD, most of the incremental long-term costs of the ICD arm of the trial were due to the need for generator replacements and to complications requiring hospitalization. Survival modeling in the SCD-HeFT trial yielded a life expectancy for the placebo arm of 8.4 years and for the ICD arm of 10.9 years (both undiscounted) (128). Using the empiric data from SCD-HeFT as a basis for lifetime cost-effectiveness estimation yielded ratios less than $50,000 per life-year added under a wide variety of assumptions about the long-term benefits and costs. A cost-effectiveness model based on ICD effectiveness reflected in MADIT II and empiric data regarding long-term outcomes of MADIT II–eligible patients in the Duke Databank yielded a cost-effectiveness ratio of $50,000 per life-year gained (126). A model-based analysis using a metaanalysis of eight primary prevention trials calculated cost-effectiveness ratios of between $34,000 and $70,000 per QALY gained (129).

The economics of CRT devices has been less well studied. An economic analysis of the COMPANION trial using the Medicare perspective found that both CRT-P and CRT-D had cost-effectiveness ratios lower than $50,000 per QALY. The COMPANION trial, however, does not provide a clear bridge between the clinical benefits of CRT-P as reflected in the Cholesterol And Recurrent Events-Heart Failure (CARE-HF) trial and the benefits of ICD therapy as reflected in SCD-HeFT and MADIT II (130). Specifically, the incremental survival benefit of CRT-D over CRT-P in Comparison of medical therapy, pacing, and defibrillation in chronic heart failure (COMPANION) appears quite modest, thus making it unlikely that an incremental cost-effectiveness ratio of CRT-D relative to CRT-P would fall into an economically attractive range.

Surgical Approaches

Invasive approaches that have been used to reduce or reverse the heart failure state include CABG (with or without ventricular reconstruction), heart transplantation, and left ventricular assist devices (LVADs).

For patients with ischemic cardiomyopathy, CABG has offered a theoretically attractive but controversial approach. Although registry data suggest more favorable survival with CABG than with medical therapy, no randomized trial has validated these observations (131). Randomized trial and registry data from the 1970s comparing CABG and medication demonstrated a magnification in absolute terms of the survival benefits of surgery in patients with impaired left ventricular function (132). Whether these observations extend to patients with advanced heart failure (NYHA class ≥ III) and a severely impaired left ventricle (ejection fraction <35%) remains uncertain. In recent years, clinicians at some centers have begun using "viability" radiologic studies such as positron emission tomography or perfusion imaging to identify the subset with substantial ischemic viable myocardium who are presumed most likely to benefit from high-risk CABG. The ongoing STICH trial will be the first large-scale randomized trial of modern surgical versus optimal modern medical therapy in these difficult patients and will include an economic evaluation as well as substudies to define whether preoperative viability screening is of benefit (131).

Heart transplantation offers a radical but effective therapy for a small subset of patients with advanced heart failure. Although it has been estimated that more than 40,000 patients a year with advanced heart failure could benefit from cardiac replacement therapy, only about 2,300 donor hearts are available each year for transplantation. This shortage of organs available relative to organs needed creates some major inefficiencies in the care of patients on the heart transplant list. The availability of a suitable heart for a given patient is, of course, unpredictable, and because available organs are allocated on an illness severity–based priority scale, physicians face an incentive to keep their candidate patients hospitalized in the intensive care unit with intravenous inotropes and a balloon pump to preserve their position at the top of the list. As a consequence, patients may wait for months in the hospital.

No high-quality modern cost data on transplantation have been published, but claims (charge) data are available (133). In 1999, charges per transplant patient averaged $303,000 through the end of the first year (corresponding costs are likely to be about half that amount). Hospital charges were $181,000, physician charges were $23,000, and organ procurement expenses were $24,000. Follow-up care averaged $40,000, and immunosuppressive therapy charges were $11,400. The average medical charges for care after the first year (including angiography, biopsies, and drug therapy) are approximately $24,000. Thus, cumulative 5-year charges for heart transplantation are currently about $400,000 (representing probably about $200,000 in medical costs). Although no modern cost-effectiveness analysis of heart transplantation has been done, heart transplantation currently has a 1-year survival rate of more than 90% and a posttransplant life expectancy of approximately 9 to 11 years. This represents a huge increment in life-years over medical treatment of advanced heart failure, and the cost per added life-year is therefore likely to fall securely in the economically attractive zone.

Several LVADs have been approved by the U.S. Food and Drug Administration (FDA) as a bridge to transplantation. The acquisition cost of these devices is high, currently $50,000 to $75,000 (not counting costs of implantation or follow-up care). One small observational study suggested that, when used as a bridge to transplant, these devices pay for themselves (134). Of 90 consecutive patients on the heart transplant list who received LVADs, 44 were discharged to home to await their transplant. The cost for pretransplant care at home was $13,200 versus $165,200 for inpatient care. In addition, 30% of the outpatients resumed working, and all were independent in activities of daily living.

LVADs have recently also been approved by the FDA as "destination therapy" in patients who are not eligible for a heart transplant. The Randomized Evaluation of Mechanical Assistance Therapy for Congestive Heart Failure (REMATCH) trial randomized 129 class IV patients ineligible for transplantation to the HeartMate VE LVAD or optimal medical therapy (135). The LVAD arm of the trial reduced mortality by 48% ($p = .001$), and quality of life at 1 year was significantly improved. However, by 2 years, almost all patients in both arms of the trial had died. The hospital costs of the initial LVAD implant (including device costs) were $210,187 (136). Although REMATCH was small, there was evidence that survival with an LVAD in the second half of the trial's enrollment was improved compared with the first half ($p = .03$), a finding suggesting an important learning curve in the use of the LVAD (137).

Disease Management Approaches

Disease management is a composite strategy that seeks to reconfigure the medical care process to provide equal or better outcomes relative to conventional care at a lower net cost. It is based on the use of national peer-reviewed practice guidelines and locally created critical pathways to define standard care goals and the most efficient means of reaching them. Nonphysician medical staff is used to follow patients carefully (in clinic or over the telephone), to encourage compliance with prescribed therapies, and to solve problems before they reach a crisis stage. Often, problem solving requires formulating a fresh view of how the medical care system should operate (sometimes referred to as "re-engineering"). Outcome measurement and continuous quality improvement are other integral aspects of disease management.

There have now been at least 19 randomized trials, involving 5,752 patients with heart failure, of disease management strategies (138). Overall, these trials demonstrated a significant decrease in hospitalization with disease management, although the most effective components of such a program remain to be defined. Rich and colleagues at Jewish Hospital in St. Louis, Missouri, enrolled 182 hospitalized elderly patients with heart failure (mean age, 79; mean NYHA class, 2.4) at high-risk for readmission into a disease management trial (139). Enrollment occurred over a 4-year period. The intervention arm of the trial consisted of patient and family education by a registered nurse, dietary consultation by a registered dietitian, review and simplification of the medical regimen by a geriatric cardiologist, and intensive follow-up by telephone and home visits. The control arm consisted of standard care. Over the 90-day follow-up period, patients in the intervention group had a 44% reduction in all-cause rehospitalization ($p = .035$) and a significant improvement in quality of life. Economic assessment showed that the intervention arm was associated with a net $460 cost saving per patient. The cost of the program itself was $216 per patient. More than $1,000 per patient was saved by the reduced need for follow-up hospitalization (139). Compliance with prescribed medical therapy (as assessed by pill counts) was 88% in the intervention arm and 81% in the control arm ($p = .003$) (140).

A more recent trial compared usual care with a nurse-administered, telephone-based disease management program in a randomized trial of 151 patients (141). Specially trained nurses used guideline-based therapy and encouraged self-management, as well as screening for heart failure exacerbations. Patients in the intervention group had longer time to hospital readmission, significantly fewer admissions, and significantly lower costs at 6 months. Differences were not preserved at 1 year. Functional status was not affected.

Prevention of Coronary Heart Disease and Its Complications

Clinically overt coronary heart disease (CHD) has a prevalence of about 13 million persons in the United States and is the most common cause of death in this and other industrialized countries (89). It is also a major cause of morbidity and resulting disability. Approximately 2 to 2.3 million individuals with CHD in the United States have limitations in their daily activities because of the disease. CHD accounts for more than 2.2 million hospital admissions per year and for more than 10 million outpatient medical visits. The direct medical costs of caring for patients with CAD in the United States has been estimated at $70 billion, whereas the cost to society of the loss in productivity from morbidity and premature mortality has been assessed at $62 billion (89). For many years, it has been hypothesized that prevention may be a more cost-effective way of reducing the clinical and economic sequelae of CHD than treatment of symptomatic or decompensated disease. As discussed elsewhere in this text, epidemiologic studies have identified a set of major modifiable risk factors for CHD, and clinical trials have been conducted to define the relationship between modification of these risk factors and subsequent outcome. *Primary prevention* is usually defined as prevention in individuals at risk for the disease but without any clinical evidence that the disease has actually developed. *Secondary prevention* is prevention in patients with clinically manifest disease. In primary prevention, the risk factors that have been most often targeted are hypercholesterolemia, smoking, hypertension, diabetes, and physical inactivity. In secondary prevention programs, in addition to these risk factors, major emphasis is given to the use of aspirin, clopidogrel, β-blockers, and ACE inhibitors in appropriate patients.

In general, effective prevention programs for CHD improve outcomes at a net increased cost (142). Secondary prevention programs usually have more favorable cost-effectiveness ratios than primary programs. Some clinicians find this counterintuitive because, they argue, prevention programs are usually less expensive on a per patient basis than waiting until symptoms or complications develop that necessitate expensive high-technology therapies. Although this may be true, the total economics picture is very substantially influenced by the number of individuals who must be treated to prevent a single death or major complication. Because risk factors for CHD only define a propensity for future disease, many individuals who are enrolled in primary prevention programs will never develop the disease and consequently cannot benefit from the interventions applied. In contrast, secondary prevention programs target individuals with an established propensity to develop disease-related complications. Consequently, the number needed to treat to prevent one adverse event is small. For example, using data from the West of Scotland Coronary Prevention Study (WOSCOPS), which largely consisted of a primary prevention population, prevention of one additional death by cholesterol reduction with a statin agent would require treating 166 patients for 5 years (143). Using data from the CARE study of patients with established CHD and modestly elevated cholesterol, prevention of one death would require treating 91 patients for 5 years (144). Using the Scandinavian Simvastatin Survival Study (4S) results in patients with CHD and very elevated cholesterol levels, only 29 patients would have required 5 years of statin therapy to prevent one death (145). Because the direct costs of statin therapy would be similar in the foregoing three examples, it is clear that the largest "bang for the buck" (and the most favorable cost-effectiveness ratio) would be obtained in treating the highest-risk patients.

Hypercholesterolemia

Numerous observational studies have established a strong dose-response relationship between total cholesterol levels and CHD risk. The National Cholesterol Education Program has established a target desirable level of less than 220 mg/dL for adults without evidence of clinical CHD. The corresponding low-density lipoprotein (LDL) cholesterol level is less than 130 mg/dL. Earlier primary prevention trials tested diet and pharmacologic regimens that were able to achieve reductions in total cholesterol of around 10%. Associated reductions in all-cause mortality were small and largely nonsignificant. Consequently, early cost-effectiveness analysis based on these clinical data generally concluded that cholesterol reduction as a primary prevention strategy was not economically attractive (146).

WOSCOPS found that primary prevention with pravastatin at 40 mg/day reduced total cholesterol by 20% relative to placebo in 4,159 male patients who were more than 45 years old and who had LDL cholesterol levels of at least 155 mg/dL. Pravastatin-treated patients experienced a 22% reduction in all-cause mortality ($p = .051$) (143). Over 4.9 years of follow-up, for every 1,000 patients shifted to the pravastatin arm of the trial, there were 5 fewer deaths, 19 fewer MIs, 14 fewer diagnostic catheterizations, and 8 fewer revascularization procedures. An economic analysis using British costs and the WOSCOPS data was published (147). This analysis estimated that treating 10,000 men like those in the trial would prevent approximately 300 from developing CHD. The pravastatin therapy cost $3,700 per patient for 5 years and saved approximately $100 per patient as a result of reduced numbers of procedures and complications. Life expectancy was increased by pravastatin by 0.10 years, and the cost per year of life added was $32,600.

A cost-effectiveness model of cholesterol-lowering strategies in the United States reported that primary prevention with a statin compared with diet therapy has a cost-effectiveness ratio ranging from $54,000 per QALY to $1.4 million per QALY, depending on patient risk level (148). Importantly, the WOSCOPS economic model did not assume a preexisting secondary prevention program (i.e., wait to treat patients once they manifest clinical CAD), which may explain part of the difference with this U.S. model.

The Air Force/Texas Coronary Atherosclerosis Prevention Study (AFCAPS/TexCAPS) randomized 6,605 subjects without clinical CAD and with average cholesterol levels to lovastatin or placebo (149). Over 5 years of therapy, lovastatin reduced acute coronary events by 37% ($p < .001$). In absolute terms, for every 1,000 patients shifted to lovastatin therapy, there were 4 fewer cardiovascular deaths, 26 fewer MIs, 16 fewer unstable angina admissions, and 31 fewer revascularization procedures. The cumulative 5-year cost of lovastatin therapy was $4,654 per patient, and there was a $524 cost offset owing to reduced cardiac events and procedures (net cost of drug therapy, $4,130). A cost-effectiveness analysis of this trial has not yet been reported.

The National Cholesterol Education Program has identified an LDL cholesterol level of less than 100 mg/dL as optimal in patients with evidence of CHD. Although numerous important secondary prevention trials have been published, two of the most useful for assessing economic impact are 4S and CARE. The 4S trial randomized 4,444 patients of both sexes ages 35 to 60 years with a history of angina or prior MI and total cholesterol levels of 210 to 310 mg/dL to adjusted-dose simvastatin or placebo (145). The majority of patients received 20 mg of simvastatin, whereas 37% required 40 mg/day. Over a median of 5.4 years, simvastatin decreased total cholesterol 25%, decreased LDL cholesterol 35%, and decreased total mortality 30% ($p = .0003$) (145). The study also observed a 37% reduction in the need for revascularization in the simvastatin arm of the trial ($p < .0001$). In a subsequent analysis, the 4S investigators reported that simvastatin therapy reduced hospitalizations for acute cardiovascular disease, including revascularization (81% of which were CABG procedures), by 26% ($p < .0001$). Over the course of the study, total hospital days resulting from cardiovascular disease were reduced by 5,138 days in the simvastatin arm ($p < .0001$). The beneficial effect of simvastatin on hospitalization first became evident after 10 months of therapy and became statistically significant after 22 months. No effect was seen on the use of antianginal or other cardiovascular drugs.

Using U.S.-derived reimbursement rates as cost weights, the 4S investigators estimated that the observed reduction in hospitalizations would equal a $3,872 reduction in average cost per patient treated with simvastatin (150). With a wholesale price for simvastatin over the trial averaging $4,400 per patient ($4,879 undiscounted), the net cost of simvastatin therapy was estimated to be $528 per patient over the trial or $0.28 per day (an offset of 88% of the drug's cost). The cost of repeat laboratory measurement of lipids and transaminases (three to four in the first year, annually after year 1) added a discounted cost of $250 per patient or an additional $0.13 per day. Thus, the total net cost of the simvastatin strategy was estimated at $778 per patient over a mean of 1,915 days of follow-up (approximately $148 per year). As noted earlier, the benefits of simvastatin on follow-up medical care take 10 months to become clinically detectable and appear to increase progressively as treatment is continued.

Interestingly, three separate cost-effectiveness analyses have been conducted using the data from the 4S trial. One was conducted from a Swedish perspective (151). Two others were done from a U.S. perspective. Schwartz estimated a cost per year of life saved of $18,100 with a cost per QALY saved of $15,100 assuming costs and benefits only occurred for the duration of the trial (152). Extrapolating to a lifetime perspective yielded a cost per year of life saved of $5,800 with a cost per QALY saved of $6,100. The most recently published analysis used the empiric data from 4S in a Markov model to evaluate cost effectiveness of therapy for different subgroups (153). In this analysis, costs were derived from four hospitals in Sweden that had patient-based cost accounting systems. Swedish costs were converted to U.S. dollars. The patient's work status measured every 6 months was used to estimate productivity costs saved by simvastatin. This analysis estimated that for 59-year-old men, the cost effectiveness of 5 years of simvastatin therapy was $5,400 per year of life saved, whereas the corresponding figure for 59-year-old women was $10,500. Adding in the productivity costs related to time lost from work saved by simvastatin improved the cost-effectiveness ratios to $1,600 for men and $5,100 for women (153). Extensive sensitivity analyses showed that statin therapy was very economically attractive under a wide range of assumptions.

The CARE study evaluated pravastatin versus placebo in 4,159 patients who had experienced MI 3 to 20 months earlier and who had a total cholesterol level of less than 240 mg/dL and an LDL cholesterol level of 115 to 174 mg/dL (144). Similar to other statin trials, pravastatin reduced total cholesterol 20% and LDL cholesterol 28%. Death and nonfatal MI were reduced by 24%. The mean cost for 6 years of pravastatin therapy in CARE was $5,500, which was partially offset by a $1,660 savings from reduced cardiac events and procedures (154). A cost-effectiveness model using the CARE data estimated that to add a life-year with pravastatin therapy would cost between $16,000 and $31,000.

The Heart Protection Study (HPS) randomized 20,536 patients with vascular disease or diabetes to 40 mg of simvastatin or placebo for 5 years (155). Simvastatin therapy reduced all-cause mortality from 14.7% to 12.9% ($p < .001$), an 18% relative reduction. Death or nonfatal MI was reduced by one fourth. Simvastatin also reduced revascularization by 24% and hospitalization for vascular events by 22% ($p < .001$). Using 2001 prices, the cost of 5 years of simvastatin therapy was about £1,500. Initial cost-effectiveness estimates were calculated as cost per major vascular event avoided, which was £11,600 for the study overall and fell to £4,500 for the highest-risk quintile. Using a generic price for simvastatin (15% of the 2001 U.K. proprietary price) made statin therapy cost saving, and therefore economically dominant, in most risk groups. Lifetime cost-effectiveness ratios and a U.S. perspective analysis are under preparation.

Secondary Preventions with Antiplatelet Therapy

Long-term aspirin therapy is the mainstay of secondary prevention efforts in patients with manifest CAD (156). The clinical effectiveness is substantial, and the cost is minimal. Gaspoz and colleagues, using the Coronary Heart Disease Policy Model, estimated that routine use of lifetime aspirin therapy for secondary prevention would yield a cost-effectiveness ratio of about $11,000 per QALY gained (157).

The clopidrogrel in unstable angina to prevent recurrent ischemic events (CURE) trial randomly assigned 12,562 patients with non–ST-segment elevation ACS to either clopidogrel (300-mg load, 75 mg/day) or placebo (158). Over a mean follow-up of 9 months, the primary composite end point of cardiovascular death, MI, or stroke was reduced by clopidogrel from 11.4% to 9.3% ($p < .01$). Cardiovascular death was reduced from 5.5% to 5.1% ($p < .05$), and MI was reduced from 6.7% to 5.2% ($p < .05$). Several economic analyses of clopidogrel therapy for secondary prevention have been reported. Weintraub and colleagues used the empiric patient-level data from the trial along with Medicare DRG reimbursement rates to calculate incremental costs and cost effectiveness (159). The clopidogrel arm of the trial saved $325 on hospital costs over the average 9-month follow-up and spent $766 on the clopidogrel therapy, leaving a net incremental cost for the clopidogrel arm of $442. Using the Framingham Heart Study data to estimate the effect of events prevented with clopidogrel, the investigators estimated 0.069 life-years gained. The resulting incremental cost-effectiveness ratio was $6,318 per life-year gained. A second model-based analysis using the published CURE results examined 1 year of clopidogrel therapy found similar, economically attractive results (160). However, as therapy was projected beyond 2 years, particularly in lower-risk patients, economic attractiveness diminished substantially. A third model-based analysis of routine lifetime clopidogrel therapy added to aspirin therapy for secondary prevention found a cost per QALY of more than $130,000 (157). Importantly, these results were sensitive to the price of clopidogrel therapy.

Other Secondary Prevention Therapies

Long-term use of β-blockers following MI was modeled by Goldman and colleagues (161). Based on the earlier (prethrombolytic) β-blocker trials, these investigators estimated cost-effectiveness ratios of less than $15,000 per life-year added, with ratios less than $5,000 for moderate- or high-risk patients. Their model projected a 6-year course of therapy with 25% mortality reductions by β-blockers in years 1 to 3, 7% reduction in years 4 to 6, and gradual attenuation of treatment benefit over a subsequent 9-year period. Based on the data from the survival and ventricular enlargement (SAVE) trial, Tsevat and colleagues developed a decision model to assess the cost effectiveness of captopril therapy in 50- to 80-year-old survivors of acute MI with an ejection fraction of 40% or less (162). Under the assumption that survival benefits of captopril persisted more than 4 years, these investigators estimated cost-effectiveness ratios of $10,400 per QALY or less (1991 dollars), depending on age. Analysis of the cost effectiveness of early lisinopril use in acute MI based on GISSI-3 data yielded a cost-effectiveness ratio of $2,300 (U.S.) per 6-week death avoided (163). Assuming the clinical benefits observed in GISSI-3 were sustained over a 10- to 15-year life expectancy, these data suggest that 6 weeks of ACE inhibitor therapy for all post-MI patients may fall into a "best buy" category of economic attractiveness.

CONTROVERSIES AND PERSONAL PERSPECTIVES

Not too long ago, medical economics was viewed as a scholarly academic discipline that was largely irrelevant to the practice of medicine. Cost is now one of the dominant issues in almost all medical decisions, although it is the controlling issue in only a minority. Demands by payers that medicine demonstrate its value (benefits produced for dollars spent) have thrust economists into the mainstream of the revolution that is currently reshaping medical practice. However, just as clinicians found themselves woefully unprepared to prove the medical benefits of many of their decisions, economists were unprepared to provide the pragmatic sorts of data now required of them. As discussed earlier, medical economics is principally concerned with matters related to the efficient societal allocation of scarce resources. Economists have paid little attention to measuring the cost of health care and instead have preferred to discuss the abstract notion of "opportunity cost" while leaving the more pragmatic measurement issues to accountants. Payers and policy makers, however, are not interested in theories or abstract problems of resource allocation. Instead, they wish to understand the costs of care and how these costs can be reduced or at least controlled. Clinicians are also not interested in theoretic economic exercises. They want to be able to prove that the care they provide their patients is worth the money it costs. Cost-effectiveness ratios are the economists' measure of value and have some important strengths. However, the need to frame all cost-effectiveness ratios in terms of the long-term costs required to add an extra QALY (11) often stretches the available clinical and cost data beyond credibility.

New approaches are needed in this area to meet the demands for information and for relevant measures of medical value. Three major methodologic areas need intensive work over the next few years. First, we need to improve methods for costing out medical care accurately but efficiently (i.e., with a relatively low cost of data collection). Because many large clinical trials now involve a consortium of different countries, we particularly need to understand the strengths and limitations of such data for economic analysis (40). Second, we need to develop new measures of value that do not require extrapolation out to a lifetime perspective. These measures would not preclude traditional cost-effectiveness analysis but could be used to supplement it. Third, we need to understand the process of decision making better. Economics presumes rational decision makers seeking to maximize societal utility, but is this conceptual model too different from the messy real world to be useful? Finally, on the pragmatic side, we need more high-quality empiric cost and outcome data to enhance our insights and allow us to ask progressively better questions.

In the final analysis, no economic model can dictate how much resources society should expend on health care and what types of health care should be given priority. These are political and ethical questions that transcend medicine. However, the medical profession must constantly strive to achieve better outcomes at an acceptable cost and to continue the dramatic pace of technologic advances set over the last century.

References

1. Mark DB. Medical economics in interventional cardiology. In: Topol EJ, ed. *Textbook of interventional cardiology*. Philadelphia: Harcourt Health Sciences, 2002.
2. Anders G. *Health against wealth: HMOs and the breakdown of medical trust*. New York: Houghton Mifflin, 1996.
3. Wennberg JE, Freeman JL, Culp WJ. Are hospital services rationed in New Haven or over-utilised in Boston? *Lancet* 1987;1:1185–1189.
4. Wennberg JE. Outcomes research, cost containment, and the fear of health care rationing. *N Engl J Med* 1990;323:1202–1204.
5. Heffler S, Smith S, Keehan S, et al. Trends: U.S. health spending projections for 2004–2014. *Health Aff (Millwood)* 2005;W5-74–W5-85.
6. Neumann PJ, Rosen AB, Weinstein MC. Medicare and cost-effectiveness analysis. *N Engl J Med* 2005;353:1516–1522.
7. Finkler SA. *Essentials of cost accounting for health care organizations*. Gaithersburg, MD: Aspen, 1994.
8. Stewart RD. *Cost estimating*, 2 ed. New York: John Wiley & Sons, 1991.
9. Feldstein PJ. *Health care economics*, 4th ed. Albany, NY: Delmar, 1993.
10. Fuchs VR. *The health economy*. Cambridge, MA: Harvard University Press, 1986.
11. Gold MR, Siegel JE, Russell LB, et al. *Cost-effectiveness in health and medicine*. New York: Oxford University Press, 1996.
12. Drummond MF, O'Brien B, Stoddart GL, et al. *Methods for the economic evaluation of health care programmes*, 2nd ed. Oxford: Oxford Medical Publications, 1997.
13. Adams ME, McCall NT, Gray DT, et al. Economic analysis in randomized control trials. *Med Care* 1992;30:231–243.
14. Drummond MF, Davies L. Economic analysis alongside clinical trials: revisiting the methodological issues. *Int J Tech Assess Health Care* 1991; 7:561–573.
15. Rigby K, Silagy C, Crockett A. Can resource use be extracted from randomized controlled trials to calculate costs? *Int J Tech Assess Health Care* 1996;12:714–720.
16. Freemantle N, Drummond M. Should clinical trials with concurrent economic analyses be blinded? *JAMA* 1997;277:63–64.
17. Ellwein LB, Drummond MF. Economic analysis alongside clinical trials. *Int J Tech Assess Health Care* 1996;12:691–697.
18. Finkler SA. The distinction between costs and charges. *Ann Intern Med* 1982;96:102–109.
19. Shwartz M, Young DW, Siegrist RB. The ratio of costs to charges: how good a basis for estimating costs? *Inquiry* 1995;32:476–481.
20. Ashby JL. The accuracy of cost measures derived from Medicare cost report data. *Hospital* 1992;3:1–8.
21. Hsiao WC, Braun P, Yntema D, et al. Estimating physicians' work for a resource-based relative-value scale. *N Engl J Med* 1988;319:835–841.
22. Feit F, Mueller HS, Braunwald E, et al., the TIMI Research Group. Thrombolysis in myocardial infarction (TIMI) Phase II trial: outcome comparison of a "conservative strategy" in community versus tertiary hospitals. *J Am Coll Cardiol* 1990;16:1529–1534.
23. Every NR, Larson EB, Litwin PE, et al., for the Myocardial Infarction Triage and Intervention Project Investigators. The association between onsite cardiac catheterization facilities and the use of coronary angiography after acute myocardial infarction. *N Engl J Med* 1993;329:546–551.
24. Blustein J. High-technology cardiac procedures: the impact of service availability on service use in New York State. *JAMA* 1993;270:344–349.
25. Pilote L, Miller DP, Califf RM, et al. Determinants of the use of coronary angiography and revascularization after thrombolysis for acute myocardial infarction. *N Engl J Med* 1996;335:1198–1205.
26. Jollis JG, Delong ER, Peterson ED, et al. Outcome of acute myocardial infarction according to the specialty of the admitting physician. *N Engl J Med* 1996;335:1880–1887.
27. Mark DB, Naylor CD, Hlatky MA, et al. Use of medical resources and quality of life after acute myocardial infarction in Canada versus the United States. *N Engl J Med* 1994;331:1130–1135.
28. Drummond MF, Stoddart GL, Torrance GW. *Methods for the economic evaluation of health care programmes*. Oxford: Oxford University Press, 1987.

29. Eisenberg JM. Clinical economics: a guide to the economic analysis of clinical practices. *JAMA* 1989;262:2879–2886.
30. Detsky AS, Naglie IG. A clinician's guide to cost-effectiveness analysis. *Ann Intern Med* 1990;113:147–154.
31. Mason J, Drummond M, Torrance G. Some guidelines on the use of cost effectiveness league tables. *BMJ* 1993;306:570–572.
32. Sox HC Jr, Blatt MA, Higgins MC, et al. *Medical decision making*. Boston: Butterworths, 1988.
33. Patrick DL, Erickson P. *Health status and health policy: quality of life in health care evaluation and resource allocation*. New York: Oxford University Press, 1993.
34. Task Force on Principles for Economic Analysis of Health Care Technology. Economic analysis of health care technology: a report on principles. *Ann Intern Med* 1995;123:61–70.
35. Torrance GW, Blaker D, Detsky AS, et al. Canadian guidelines for economic evaluation of pharmaceuticals. *Pharmacoeconomics* 1996;9:535–559.
36. Langley PC. The November 1995 revised Australian guidelines for the economic evaluation of pharmaceuticals. *Pharmacoeconomics* 1996;9:341–352.
37. Weinstein MC, Siegel JE, Gold MR, et al., for the Panel on Cost-Effectiveness in Health and Medicine. Recommendations of the panel on cost-effectiveness in health and medicine. *JAMA* 1996;276:1253–1258.
38. Russell LB, Gold MR, Siegel JE, et al., for the Panel of Cost-Effectiveness in Health and Medicine. The role of cost-effectiveness analysis in health and medicine. *JAMA* 1996;276:1172–1177.
39. Siegel JE, Weinstein MC, Russell LB, et al. for the Panel on Cost-Effectiveness in Health and Medicine. Recommendations for reporting cost-effectiveness analyses. *JAMA* 1996;276:1339–1341.
40. Reed SD, Anstrom KJ, Bakhai A, et al. Conducting economic evaluations alongside multinational clinical trials: toward a research consensus. *Am Heart J* 2005;149:434–443.
41. Braunwald E, Antman EM, Beasley JW, et al. ACC/AHA 2002 guideline update for the management of patients with unstable angina and non-ST-segment elevation myocardial infarction: a report of the American College of Cardiology/American Heart Association Task Force on Practice Guidelines (Committee on the Management of Patients With Unstable Angina). www.acc.org/clinical/guidelines/unstable/incorporated/index htm 2002.
42. Mark DB. Assessment of prognosis in patients with coronary artery disease. In: Stack RS, ed. *Interventional cardiovascular medicine*. New York: Churchill Livingstone, 1999:161–182.
43. Pilote L, Califf RM, Sapp S, et al., for the GUSTO-1 Investigators. Regional variation across the United States in the management of acute myocardial infarction. *N Engl J Med* 1995;333:565–578.
44. Weintraub WS, Mauldin PD, Talley JD, et al. Determinants of hospital charges and costs in acute myocardial infarction: a report from the Myocardial Infarction Cost Study (MICS) Group. *Am J Manage Care* 1996;2:977–986.
45. Collins R, Peto R, Baigent C, et al. Aspirin, heparin, and fibrinolytic therapy in suspected acute myocardial infarction. *N Engl J Med* 1997;336: 847–860.
46. Armstrong PW, Collen D. Fibrinolysis for acute myocardial infarction: current status and new horizons for pharmacological reperfusion, part 1. *Circulation* 2001;103:2862–2866.
47. Naylor CD, Bronskill S, Goel V. Cost-effectiveness of intravenous thrombolytic drugs for acute myocardial infarction. *Can J Cardiol* 1993;9:553–558.
48. GUSTO Investigators. An international randomized trial comparing four thrombolytic strategies for acute myocardial infarction. *N Engl J Med* 1993; 329:673–682.
49. Mark DB, Hlatky MA, Califf RM, et al. Cost effectiveness of thrombolytic therapy with tissue plasminogen activator as compared with streptokinase for acute myocardial infarction. *N Engl J Med* 1995;332:1418–1424.
50. Franzosi MG, Santoro E, De Vita C, et al. Ten-year follow-up of the first megatrial testing thrombolytic therapy in patients with acute myocardial infarction: results of the Gruppo Italiano per lo Studio della Sopravvivenza nell'Infarto-1 study. The GISSI Investigators. *Circulation* 1998;98:2659–2665.
51. van Domburg RT, Sonnenschein K, Nieuwlaat R, et al. Sustained benefit 20 years after reperfusion therapy in acute myocardial infarction. *J Am Coll Cardiol* 2005;46:15–20.
52. Califf RM, White HD, Van de Werf F, et al., for the GUSTO-1 Investigators. One year results from the Global Utilization of Streptokinase and t-PA for Occluded Coronary Arteries (GUSTO-1) trial. *Circulation* 1996;94:1233–1238.
53. Topol EJ, Ohman EM, Armstrong PW, et al. Survival outcomes 1 year after reperfusion therapy with either alteplase or reteplase for acute myocardial infarction: results from the Global Utilization of Streptokinase and t-PA for Occluded Coronary Arteries (GUSTO) III trial. *Circulation* 2000;102:1761–1765.
54. Assessment of the Safety and Efficacy of a New Thrombolytic Investigators. Single-bolus tenecteplase compared with front-loaded alteplase in acute myocardial infarction: the ASSENT-2 double-blind randomised trial. *Lancet* 1999;354:716–722.
55. Assessment of the Safety and Efficacy of a New Thrombolytic investigators. Efficacy and safety of tenecteplase in combination with enoxaparin, abciximab, or unfractionated heparin: the ASSENT-3 randomised trial in acute myocardial infarction. *Lancet* 2001;358:605–613.
56. Kaul P, Armstrong PW, Cowper PA, et al. Economic analysis of the Assessment of the Safety and Efficacy of a New Thrombolytic regimen (ASSENT-3) study: costs of reperfusion strategies in acute myocardial infarction. *Am Heart J* 2005;149:637–644.
57. Weaver WD, Simes RJ, Betriu A, et al. Comparison of primary coronary angioplasty and intravenous thrombolytic therapy for acute myocardial infarction: a quantitative review. *JAMA* 1997;278:2093–2098.
58. Grines CL, Browne KF, Marco J, et al. A comparison of immediate angioplasty with thrombolytic therapy for acute myocardial infarction. *N Engl J Med* 1993;328:673–679.
59. Gibbons RJ, Holmes DR, Reeder GS, et al. Immediate angioplasty compared with the administration of a thrombolytic agent followed by conservative treatment for myocardial infarction. *N Engl J Med* 1993;328:685–691.
60. Reeder GS, Bailey KR, Gersh BJ, et al., for the Mayo Coronary Care Unit and Catheterization Laboratory Groups. Cost comparison of immediate angioplasty versus thrombolysis followed by conservative therapy for acute myocardial infarction: a randomized prospective trial. *Mayo Clin Proc* 1994;69:5–12.
61. Grines C, Patel A, Zijlstra F, et al. Primary coronary angioplasty compared with intravenous thrombolytic therapy for acute myocardial infarction: six-month follow up and analysis of individual patient data from randomized trials. *Am Heart J* 2003;145:47–57.
62. Zijlstra F, Hoorntje JC, de Boer MJ, et al. Long-term benefit of primary angioplasty as compared with thrombolytic therapy for acute myocardial infarction. *N Engl J Med* 1999;341:1413–1419.
63. Zijlstra F. Angioplasty vs thrombolysis for acute myocardial infarction: a quantitative overview of the effects of interhospital transportation. *Eur Heart J* 2003;24:21–23.
64. Andersen HR, Nielsen TT, Vesterlund T, et al. Danish multicenter randomized study on fibrinolytic therapy versus acute coronary angioplasty in acute myocardial infarction: rationale and design of the DANish trial in Acute Myocardial Infarction-2 (DANAMI-2). *Am Heart J* 2003;146:234–241.
65. Le May MR, Davies RF, Labinaz M, et al. Hospitalization costs of primary stenting versus thrombolysis in acute myocardial infarction: cost analysis of the Canadian STAT Study. *Circulation* 2003;108:2624–2630.
66. Tcheng JE, Kandzari DE, Grines CL, et al. Benefits and risks of abciximab use in primary angioplasty for acute myocardial infarction: the Controlled Abciximab and Device Investigation to Lower Late Angioplasty Complications (CADILLAC) trial. *Circulation* 2003;108:1316–1323.
67. Bakhai A, Stone GW, Grines CL, et al. Cost-effectiveness of coronary stenting and abciximab for patients with acute myocardial infarction: results from the CADILLAC (Controlled Abciximab and Device Investigation to Lower Late Angioplasty Complications) trial. *Circulation* 2003;108:2857–2863.
68. Magid DJ, Wang Y, Herrin J, et al. Relationship between time of day, day of week, timeliness of reperfusion, and in-hospital mortality for patients with acute ST-segment elevation myocardial infarction. *JAMA* 2005;294:803–812.
69. Nallamothu BK, Bates ER, Herrin J, et al. Times to treatment in transfer patients undergoing primary percutaneous coronary intervention in the United States: National Registry of Myocardial Infarction (NRMI)-3/4 analysis. *Circulation* 2005;111:761–767.
70. Faxon DP, Heger JW. Primary angioplasty: enduring the test of time. *N Engl J Med* 1999;341:1464–1465.
71. Lieu TA, Lundstrom RJ, Ray GT, et al. Initial cost of primary angioplasty for acute myocardial infarction. *J Am Coll Cardiol* 1996;28:882–889.
72. TIMI IIIB Investigators. Effects of tissue plasminogen activator and a comparison of early invasive and conservative strategies in unstable angina and non–Q-wave myocardial infarction: results of the TIMI IIIB Trial. Thrombolysis in Myocardial Ischemia. *Circulation* 1994;89:1545–1556.
73. Boden WE, O'Rourke RA, Crawford MH, et al. Outcomes in patients with acute non–Q-wave myocardial infarction randomly assigned to an invasive as compared with a conservative management strategy. Veterans Affairs Non–Q-Wave Infarction Strategies in Hospital (VANQWISH). *N Engl J Med* 1998;338:1785–1792.
74. FRagmin and Fast Revascularisation during InStability in Coronary artery disease Investigators. Invasive compared with non-invasive treatment in unstable coronary artery disease: FRISC II prospective randomised multicentre study. *Lancet* 1999;354:708–715.
75. Janzon M, Levin LA, Swahn E. Cost-effectiveness of an invasive strategy in unstable coronary artery disease; results from the FRISC II invasive trial: the Fast Revascularisation during InStability in Coronary artery disease. *Eur Heart J* 2002;23:31–40.
76. Fox KA, Poole-Wilson PA, Henderson RA, et al. Interventional versus conservative treatment for patients with unstable angina or non–ST-elevation myocardial infarction: the British Heart Foundation RITA 3 randomised trial. Randomized Intervention Trial of unstable Angina. *Lancet* 2002;360: 743–751.
77. Fox KA, Poole-Wilson P, Clayton TC, et al. 5-year outcome of an interventional strategy in non–ST-elevation acute coronary syndrome: the British Heart Foundation RITA 3 randomised trial. *Lancet* 2005;366:914–920.
78. Cannon CP, Weintraub WS, Demopoulos LA, et al. Comparison of early invasive and conservative strategies in patients with unstable coronary

syndromes treated with the glycoprotein IIb/IIIa inhibitor tirofiban. *N Engl J Med* 2001;344:1879–1887.
79. Mahoney EM, Jurkovitz CT, Chu H, et al. Cost and cost-effectiveness of an early invasive vs conservative strategy for the treatment of unstable angina and non–ST-segment elevation myocardial infarction. *JAMA* 2002; 288:1851–1858.
80. de Winter RJ, Windhausen F, Cornel JH, et al. Early invasive versus selectively invasive management for acute coronary syndromes. *N Engl J Med* 2005;353:1095–1104.
81. Stukel TA, Lucas FL, Wennberg DE. Long-term outcomes of regional variations in intensity of invasive vs medical management of Medicare patients with acute myocardial infarction. *JAMA* 2005;293:1329–1337.
82. Bhatt DL, Roe MT, Peterson ED, et al. Utilization of early invasive management strategies for high-risk patients with non–ST-segment elevation acute coronary syndromes: results from the CRUSADE Quality Improvement Initiative. *JAMA* 2004;292:2096–2104.
83. Petersen JL, Mahaffey KW, Hasselblad V, et al. Efficacy and bleeding complications among patients randomized to enoxaparin or unfractionated heparin for antithrombin therapy in non–ST-segment elevation acute coronary syndromes: a systematic overview. *JAMA* 2004;292:89–96.
84. Mark DB, Cowper PA, Berkowitz S, et al. Economic assessment of low molecular weight heparin (enoxaparin) versus unfractionated heparin in acute coronary syndrome patients: results from the ESSENCE randomized trial. *Circulation* 1998;97:1702–1707.
85. Ferguson JJ, Califf RM, Antman EM, et al. Enoxaparin vs unfractionated heparin in high-risk patients with non–ST-segment elevation acute coronary syndromes managed with an intended early invasive strategy: primary results of the SYNERGY randomized trial. *JAMA* 2004;292:45–54.
86. GUSTO IV-ACS Investigators. Effect of glycoprotein IIb/IIIa receptor blocker abciximab on outcome in patients with acute coronary syndromes without early coronary revascularisation: the GUSTO IV-ACS randomised trial. *Lancet* 2001;357:1915–1924.
87. PURSUIT Investigators. Inhibition of platelet glycoprotein IIb/IIIa with eptifibatide in patients with acute coronary syndromes without persistent ST-segment elevation. *N Engl J Med* 1998;339:436–443.
88. Mark DB, Harrington RA, Lincoff AM, et al. Cost effectiveness of platelet glycoprotein IIb/IIIa inhibition with eptifibatide in patients with non–ST elevation acute coronary syndromes. *Circulation* 2000;101:366–371.
89. American Heart Association. *2005 heart and stroke statistical update*. Dallas, TX: American Heart Association, 2005.
90. Wennberg JE, Freeman JL, Shelton RM, et al. Hospital use and mortality among Medicare beneficiaries in Boston and New Haven. *N Engl J Med* 1989;321:1168–1173.
91. Verrilli DK, Welch G. The impact of diagnostic testing on therapeutic interventions. *JAMA* 1996;275:1189–1191.
92. Chassin MR, Kosecoff J, Park RE, et al. Does inappropriate use explain geographic variations in the use of health care services? A study of three procedures. *JAMA* 1987;258:2533–2537.
93. McGlynn EA, Naylor CD, Anderson GM, et al. Comparison of the appropriateness of coronary angiography and coronary artery bypass graft surgery between Canada and New York State. *JAMA* 1994;272:934–940.
94. Hux JE, Naylor CD, the Steering Committee of the Provincial Adult Cardiac Care Network of Ontario. Are the marginal returns of coronary artery surgery smaller in high-rate areas? *Lancet* 1996;348:1202–1207.
95. Wong JB, Sonnenberg FA, Salem DN, et al. Myocardial revascularization for chronic stable angina: an analysis of the role of percutaneous transluminal coronary angioplasty based on data available in 1989. *Ann Intern Med* 1990;113:852–871.
96. Bucher HC, Hengstler P, Schindler C, et al. Percutaneous transluminal coronary angioplasty versus medical treatment for non–acute coronary heart disease: metaanalysis of randomised controlled trials. *BMJ* 2000; 321:73–77.
97. Parisi AF, Folland ED, Hartigan P. A comparison of angioplasty with medical therapy in the treatment of single-vessel coronary artery disease. *N Engl J Med* 1992;326:10–16.
98. Pocock SJ, Henderson RA, Clayton T, et al. Quality of life after coronary angioplasty or continued medical treatment for angina: three-year follow-up in the RITA-2 trial: Randomized Intervention Treatment of Angina. *J Am Coll Cardiol* 2000;35:907–914.
99. Sculpher M, Smith D, Clayton T, et al. Coronary angioplasty versus medical therapy for angina: health service costs based on the second Randomized Intervention Treatment of Angina (RITA-2) trial. *Eur Heart J* 2002;23:1291–1300.
100. Pepine CJ, Mark DB, Bourassa MG, et al. Cost estimates for treatment of cardiac ischemia (from the Asymptomatic Cardiac Ischemia Pilot [ACIP] study). *Am J Cardiol* 1999;84:1311–1316.
101. Weintraub WS, Barnett PCS, Hartigan P, et al. Economic methods in the Clinical Outcomes Utilizing Percutaneous Coronary Revascularization and Aggressive Guideline-Driven Drug Evaluation (COURAGE) trial. *Am Heart J* 2006;151:1180–1185.
102. King SB III, Lembo NJ, Weintraub WS, et al., for the Emory Angioplasty versus Surgery Trial. A randomized trial comparing coronary angioplasty with coronary bypass surgery. *N Engl J Med* 1994;331:1044–1050.
103. Weintraub WS, Mauldin PD, Becker E, et al. A comparison of the costs of and quality of life after coronary angioplasty or coronary surgery for multivessel coronary disease: results from the Emory Angioplasty Versus Surgery Trial (EAST). *Circulation* 1995;92:2831–2840.
104. Weintraub WS, Becker ER, Mauldin PD, et al. Costs of revascularization over eight years in the randomized and eligible patients in the Emory Angioplasty versus Surgery Trial (EAST). *Am J Cardiol* 2000;86:747–752.
105. BARI Investigators. Comparison of coronary bypass surgery with angioplasty in patients with multivessel disease. *N Engl J Med* 1996;335:217–225.
106. Hlatky MA, Rogers WJ, Johnstone I, et al., for the BARI Investigators. Medical care costs and quality of life after randomization to coronary angioplasty or coronary bypass surgery. *N Engl J Med* 1997;336:92–99.
107. Sculpher MJ, Seed P, Henderson RA, et al., for the RITA trial participants. Health service costs of coronary angioplasty and coronary artery bypass surgery: the Randomised Intervention Treatment of Angina (RITA) trial. *Lancet* 1994;344:927–930.
108. Henderson RA, Pocock SJ, Sharp SJ, et al. Long-term results of RITA-1 trial: clinical and cost comparisons of coronary angioplasty and coronary-artery bypass grafting. Randomised Intervention Treatment of Angina. *Lancet* 1998;352:1419–1425.
109. Serruys PW, Unger F, Sousa JE, et al., for the Arterial Revascularization Therapies Study Group. Comparison of coronary-artery bypass surgery and stenting for the treatment of multivessel disease. *N Engl J Med* 2001;344: 1117–1124.
110. SOS Investigators. Coronary artery bypass surgery versus percutaneous coronary intervention with stent implantation in patients with multivessel coronary artery disease (the Stent or Surgery trial): a randomised controlled trial. *Lancet* 2002;360:965–970.
111. Zhang Z, Mahoney EM, Stables RH, et al. Disease-specific health status after stent-assisted percutaneous coronary intervention and coronary artery bypass surgery: one-year results from the Stent or Surgery trial. *Circulation* 2003;108:1694–1700.
112. Weintraub WS, Mahoney EM, Zhang Z, et al. One year comparison of costs of coronary surgery versus percutaneous coronary intervention in the Stent or Surgery trial. *Heart* 2004;90:782–788.
113. Smith WM. Epidemiology of congestive heart failure. *Am J Cardiol* 1985; 55:3A–8A.
114. Krumholz HM, Parent EM, Tu N, et al. Readmission after hospitalization for congestive heart failure among Medicare beneficiaries. *Arch Intern Med* 1997;157:99–104.
115. Psaty BM, Furberg CD, Kuller LH, et al. Association between blood pressure level and the risk of myocardial infarction, stroke, and total mortality: the cardiovascular health study. *Arch Intern Med* 2001;161:1183–92.
116. Eisenstein EL, Yusuf S, Bourassa M, et al. What is the economic value of digoxin therapy in congestive heart failure patients? Results from the DIG trial. *J Card Fail* 2006;12:336–342.
117. Hunt SA, Baker DW, Chin MH, et al. ACC/AHA guidelines for the evaluation and management of chronic heart failure in the adult: executive summary a report of the American College of Cardiology/American Heart Association Task Force on Practice Guidelines (Committee to Revise the 1995 Guidelines for the Evaluation and Management of Heart Failure). *Circulation* 2001;104:2996–3007.
118. Glick H, Cook J, Kinosian B, et al. Costs and effects of enalapril therapy in patients with symptomatic heart failure: an economic analysis of the Studies of Left Ventricular Dysfunction (SOLVD) treatment trial. *J Card Fail* 1995;1:371–380.
119. Paul SD, Kuntz KM, Eagle KA, et al. Costs and effectiveness of angiotensin converting enzyme inhibition in patients with congestive heart failure. *Arch Intern Med* 1994;154:1143–1149.
120. Hjalmarson A, Goldstein S, Fagerberg B, et al. Effects of controlled-release metoprolol on total mortality, hospitalizations, and well-being in patients with heart failure: the Metoprolol CR/XL Randomized Intervention Trial in congestive heart failure (MERIT-HF). MERIT-HF Study Group. *JAMA* 2000;283:1295–1302.
121. CIBIS II Investigators. The Cardiac Insufficiency Bisoprolol Study II (CIBIS-II): a randomised trial. *Lancet* 1999;353:9–13.
122. CIBIS-II Investigators and Health Economics Group. Reduced costs with bisoprolol treatment for heart failure: an economic analysis of the second Cardiac Insufficiency Bisoprolol Study (CIBIS-II). *Eur Heart J* 2001; 22:1021–1031.
123. Beta-Blocker Evaluation of Survival Trial Investigators. A trial of the beta-blocker bucindolol in patients with advanced chronic heart failure. *N Engl J Med* 2001;344:1659–1667.
124. Delea TE, Vera-Llonch M, Richner RE, et al. Cost effectiveness of carvedilol for heart failure. *Am J Cardiol* 1999;83:890–896.
125. Bardy GH, Lee KL, Mark DB, et al. Amiodarone or an implantable cardioverter-defibrillator for congestive heart failure. *N Engl J Med* 2005; 352:225–237.
126. Al Khatib SM, Anstrom KJ, Eisenstein EL, et al. Clinical and economic implications of the multicenter automatic defibrillator implantation trial-II. *Ann Intern Med* 2005;142:593–600.
127. Cleland JG, Daubert JC, Erdmann E, et al. The effect of cardiac resynchronization on morbidity and mortality in heart failure. *N Engl J Med* 2005; 352:1539–1549.
128. Mark DB, Nelson CL, Anstrom KJ, et al. Cost effectiveness of defibrillator therapy or amiodarone in chronic stable heart failure: results from the sudden cardiac death in heart failure trial (SCD-Heft). *Circulation* 2006; in press.

129. Sanders GD, Hlatky MA, Owens DK. Cost-effectiveness of implantable cardioverter-defibrillators. *N Engl J Med* 2005;353:1471–1480.
130. Bristow MR, Saxon LA, Boehmer J, et al. Cardiac-resynchronization therapy with or without an implantable defibrillator in advanced chronic heart failure. *N Engl J Med* 2004;350:2140–2150.
131. Jones RH. Is it time for a randomized trial of surgical treatment of ischemic heart failure? *J Am Coll Cardiol* 2001;37:1210–1213.
132. Bounous EP Jr, Mark DB, Pollock BG, et al. Surgical survival benefits for coronary disease patients with left ventricular dysfunction. *Circulation* 1988;78(suppl I):151–157.
133. Evans RW. Economic impact of mechanical cardiac assistance. *Prog Cardiovasc Dis* 2000;43:81–94.
134. Morales DL, Catanese KA, Helman DN, et al. Six-year experience of caring for forty-four patients with a left ventricular assist device at home: safe, economical, necessary. *J Thorac Cardiovasc Surg* 2000;119:251–259.
135. Rose EA, Gelijns AC, Moskowitz AJ, et al. Long-term mechanical left ventricular assistance for end-stage heart failure. *N Engl J Med* 2001;345: 1435–1443.
136. Oz MC, Gelijns AC, Miller L, et al. Left ventricular assist devices as permanent heart failure therapy: the price of progress. *Ann Surg* 2003;238:577–583.
137. Park SJ, Tector A, Piccioni W, et al. Left ventricular assist devices as destination therapy: a new look at survival. *J Thorac Cardiovasc Surg* 2005;129:9–17.
138. Whellan DJ, Hasselblad V, Peterson E, et al. Metaanalysis and review of heart failure disease management randomized controlled clinical trials. *Am Heart J* 2005;149:722–729.
139. Rich MW, Beckham V, Wittenberg C, et al. A multidisciplinary intervention to prevent the readmission of elderly patients with congestive heart failure. *N Engl J Med* 1995;333:1190–1195.
140. Rich MW, Gray DB, Beckham V, et al. Effect of a multidisciplinary intervention of medication compliance in elderly patients with congestive heart failure. *Am J Med* 1996;101:270–276.
141. Dunagan WC, Littenberg B, Ewald GA, et al. Randomized trial of a nurse-administered, telephone-based disease management program for patients with heart failure. *J Card Fail* 2005;11:358–365.
142. Weinstein MC. Economics of prevention: the costs of prevention. *J Gen Intern Med* 1990;5(suppl):S89–S92.
143. Shepherd J, Cobbe SM, Ford I, et al., for the West of Scotland Coronary Prevention Study Group. Prevention of coronary heart disease with pravastatin in men with hypercholesterolemia. *N Engl J Med* 1995;333:1301–1307.
144. Sacks FM, Pfeffer MA, Moye LA, et al., for the CARE Investigators. Cholesterol And Recurrent Events (CARE). *N Engl J Med* 1996;335:1001–1009.
145. Scandinavian Simvastatin Survival Study Group. Randomised trial of cholesterol lowering in 4444 patients with coronary heart disease: the Scandinavian Simvastatin Survival Study (4S). *Lancet* 1994;344:1383–1389.
146. Morris S, McGuire A, Caro J, et al. Strategies for the management of hypercholesterolaemia: a systematic review of the cost-effectiveness literature. *J Health Serv Res Policy* 1997;2:231–250.
147. Caro J, Klittich W, McGuire A, et al. International economic analysis of primary prevention of cardiovascular disease with pravastatin in WOSCOPS. West of Scotland Coronary Prevention Study. *Eur Heart J* 1999;20:263–268.
148. Prosser LA, Stinnett AA, Goldman PA, et al. Cost-effectiveness of cholesterol-lowering therapies according to selected patient characteristics. *Ann Intern Med* 2000;132:769–779.
149. Downs JR, Clearfield M, Weis S, et al. Primary prevention of acute coronary events with lovastatin in men and women with average cholesterol levels: results of AFCAPS/TexCAPS. Air Force/Texas Coronary Atherosclerosis Prevention Study. *JAMA* 1998;279:1615–1622.
150. Pedersen TR, Kjekshus J, Berg K, et al., for the Scandinavian Simvastatin Survival Group. Cholesterol lowering and the use of healthcare resources: results of the Scandinavian Simvastatin Survival Group. *Circulation* 1996;93:1796–1802.
151. Jonsson B, Johannesson M, Kjekshus J, et al., for the Scandinavian Simvastatin Survival Group. Cost-effectiveness of cholesterol lowering: results from the Scandinavian Simvastatin Survival Study (4S). *Eur Heart J* 1996;17:1001–1007.
152. Schwartz JS. Economics and cost-effectiveness in evaluating the value of cardiovascular therapies: comparative economic data regarding lipid-lowering drugs. *Am Heart J* 1999;137:S97-S104.
153. Johannesson M, Jonsson B, Kjekshus J, et al., for the Scandinavian Simvastatin Survival Group. Cost effectiveness of simvastatin treatment to lower cholesterol levels in patients with coronary heart disease. *N Engl J Med* 1997;336:332–336.
154. Tsevat J, Kuntz KM, Orav EJ, et al. Cost-effectiveness of pravastatin therapy for survivors of myocardial infarction with average cholesterol levels. *Am Heart J* 2001;141:727–734.
155. Heart Protection Study Collaborative Group. MRC/BHF Heart Protection Study of cholesterol lowering with simvastatin in 20,536 high-risk individuals: a randomised placebo-controlled trial. *Lancet* 2002;360:7–22.
156. Antiplatelet Trialist's Collaboration. Collaborative overview of randomized trials of antiplatelet therapy. I. Prevention of death, myocardial infarction, and stroke by prolonged antiplatelet therapy in various categories of patients. *BMJ* 1994;308:81–106.
157. Gaspoz JM, Coxson PG, Goldman PA, et al. Cost effectiveness of aspirin, clopidogrel, or both for secondary prevention of coronary heart disease. *N Engl J Med* 2002;346:1800–1806.
158. Budaj A, Yusuf S, Mehta SR, et al. Benefit of clopidogrel in patients with acute coronary syndromes without ST-segment elevation in various risk groups. *Circulation* 2002;106:1622–1626.
159. Weintraub WS, Mahoney EM, Lamy A, et al. Long-term cost-effectiveness of clopidogrel given for up to one year in patients with acute coronary syndromes without ST-segment elevation. *J Am Coll Cardiol* 2005;45:838–845.
160. Schleinitz MD, Heidenreich PA. A cost-effectiveness analysis of combination antiplatelet therapy for high-risk acute coronary syndromes: clopidogrel plus aspirin versus aspirin alone. *Ann Intern Med* 2005;142:251–259.
161. Goldman L, Sia STB, Cook EF, et al. Costs and effectiveness of routine therapy with long-term beta-adrenergic antagonists after acute myocardial infarction. *N Engl J Med* 1988;319:152–157.
162. Tsevat J, Duke D, Goldman L, et al. Cost-effectiveness of captopril therapy after myocardial infarction. *J Am Coll Cardiol* 1995;26:914–919.
163. Franzosi MG, Maggioni AP, Santoro E, et al. Cost-effectiveness analysis of early lisinopril use in patients with acute myocardial infarction: results from GISSI-3 trial. *Pharmacoeconomics* 1998;13:337–346.

CHAPTER 45 ■ QUALITY OF CARE AND MEDICAL ERRORS IN CARDIOVASCULAR DISEASE

ERIC D. PETERSON AND ROBERT M. CALIFF

OVERVIEW

Definitions of Quality of Care and Patient Safety

Quality of care has been defined as "the degree to which health service for individuals and populations increase the likelihood of desired health outcomes and are consistent with current professional knowledge" (1). As characterized by the Institute of Medicine (IOM), quality of care has several dimensions, including safety, effectiveness, timeliness, efficiency, equitability, and patient-centeredness (2). Table 45.1 applies these principles to the care of cardiovascular patients. A medical error is defined as either having the wrong plan for an element of medical care or failure to execute the correct plan. These errors can be further subdivided into errors of omission, defined as a failure to apply therapies that are proven beneficial, and errors of commission, the inappropriate delivery of a medical treatment or intervention (3). Thus, quality of care and medical error avoidance are linked concepts, requiring caregivers both to do the right things and to do things right.

If asked a decade ago, most clinicians would have assumed cardiac care provided was nearly always appropriate and delivered in a safe, efficient manner. Careful scrutiny, however, has failed to confirm this rosy assumption. Patients often fail to receive lifesaving therapies (4–8), and still others are subjected to diagnostic and therapeutic procedures in situations where there is little proven benefit (9,10). Care delivery itself is often imperfect, burdened by unnecessary delays and technical mistakes (11–14). These and other studies prompted the IOM to conclude in 2002 that "there is not a gap between what healthcare is now and what could be, but rather a chasm" (2).

Such troubling findings have prompted government, payers, and the public to challenge physicians' autonomy (15). These external parties are now demanding our health care provider professions both to monitor and to improve the consistency and quality of health care. Quality assessment and medical error reports are now being posted for the public (16–19). Even more challenging, payers are now differentially reimbursing hospitals and physicians based on the quality of care they deliver, initiating the new era of "pay for performance" (P4P) (20–22). Although these new policies have the potential to revolutionize health care quality and safety, they also may lead to unintentional adverse consequences for patients and providers alike (23). The balance between these alternative futures will depend on the how these new policies are implemented and the response of health care providers to them.

Given the importance of improving patient outcomes and the likely impact on the practice and income of cardiovascular specialists, clinicians need to gain an understanding of the methodology used for quality assessment as well as the means of improving quality of care. This chapter provides a historical perspective on the field and defines the major concepts of quality and medical errors. We review the current quality indicators for cardiovascular care and procedures as well as identify many of the methodologic challenges that belie their measurement. We summarize available information on the state of cardiovascular quality of care and then review means by which this care may be improved in the future.

TABLE 45.1

DEFINING QUALITY IN CARDIOVASCULAR CARE

Timely: Rapid identification and treatment initiation
Effective: Implement evidence-based care
Safe: Ensure that care is delivered in a technically correct manner
Equitable: Treat all eligible patients, regardless of age, gender, race, insurance, or socioeconomic status
Cost-effective: Avoid overuse of tests or treatments where benefits are limited
Patient-centered: Always consider the risks and benefits of the above for the individual patient

Based on the dimensions of quality care developed by the Institute of Medicine (Committee on Quality of Health Care in America, Institute of Medicine. *Crossing the quality chasm: a new health system for the 21st century*. Washington, DC: National Academies Press, 2001).

Historical Perspective

Although the quality of care has been a part of the medical profession since its beginning, Florence Nightingale is generally credited with codifying many of its fundamental concepts in her book *Notes on Hospitals* (24). Published in 1863, this review of hospitals in London and the United Kingdom found a 91% death rate in the 24 hospitals in London, versus 40% in 55 county and regional facilities. She used these data to recommend sweeping changes in the operations, care processes, and location of the London hospitals (24,25). Her vision also extended to an understanding of the challenges involved with measuring quality of care when she wrote the following:

> Accurate hospital statistics are much more rare than is generally imagined, and at best they only give the mortality which has taken place in the hospitals, and take no cognizance of those cases which are discharged in a hopeless condition, to die immediately afterwards, a practice which is followed to a much greater extent by some hospitals than others. We have known incurable cases discharged from one hospital, to which the deaths ought to have been accounted and received into another hospital, to die there in a day or two after admission, thereby lowering the mortality rate of the first at the expense of the second (24).

Nearly 145 years later, we are still coping with many of the same issues—suboptimal data collection, lack of adequate follow-up, interhospital transfer of high-risk patients who are "lost" in current report card measurement systems, and less-than-expected accountability.

In 1914, Ernest Amory Codman, a surgeon in Boston, started his own center known as the End-Result Hospital, based on the philosophy that caregivers should both study their outcomes and be rewarded with higher reimbursement when their outcomes are documented to be superior to those of their peers (26,27). In 1917, he outlined these principles:

> So I am called eccentric for saying in public: that hospitals, if they wish to be sure of improvement, 1) must find out what their results are; 2) must analyze their results to find their strong and weak points; 3) must compare their results with those of other hospitals; 4) must welcome publicity not only for their successes but for their errors. Such opinions will not be eccentric in a few years hence (28).

Although Codman was a visionary in his outlook on quality, he slightly miscalculated the time course; it would take to the end of the century for these policy changes to take hold.

In 1986, the U.S. Health Care Financing Administration (HCFA) put quality concerns back in the spotlight when it analyzed and publicly released individual hospitals' mortality rates (29,30). Like Nightingale's analysis a century earlier, these data demonstrated substantial variability among centers. Yet similar concerns existed over the ability of these data to "adjust" for patients' disease severity (27,31). For example, the hospitals reported with the highest mortality rates were, not surprisingly, cancer hospice facilities. Risk adjustment was an imperfect and underdeveloped science. Because of these methodologic limitations, the HCFA ultimately stopped the release of hospital mortality reports (29), yet public reporting of provider results had been released from Pandora's box.

That clinicians can cause harm as well as cure has been understood since medicine's beginnings. In ancient Greek, the same word, *pharmakon,* meant both "drug" and "poison" (32). In the sixteenth century, Paracelsus, the father of clinical pharmacology, updated this concept when he said: "All drugs are poisons; the benefit depends on the dosage" (33). Thus, as we will see, many therapies can result in avoidable iatrogenic harm if they are delivered in an improper setting, dose, or manner.

The review of treatment "failures" has also been a means of understanding how to avoid potential mistakes in the future. Morbidity and mortality conferences were therefore designed to determine whether clinician care was the cause of an individual patient's poor outcomes. Similarly, systematic review of medical error also can lead to care improvements. As an example, in 1847, Dr. Semmelweis working in Vienna noticed that peripartum wound infection rates were killing 13% of women giving birth at his hospital, a rate four times that seen at a nearby hospital run by midwives. By following students in their daily care, Dr. Semmelweis noted that many went directly from the dissection room to deliveries without washing their hands. By establishing a new policy of strict disinfection between cases, he was able to drop infection rates to less than 2%, thus saving countless lives (34).

More recently, the impact of medical errors on public health was graphically summarized by the IOM report *To Err Is Human.* This study estimated that between 40,000 and 100,000 patients each year died in U.S. hospitals as a result of medical errors, and the financial cost of such events was estimated at 17 to 29 billion dollars (3). Although this estimate was hotly disputed by many health care providers, it is likely an underestimate, because it did not consider the full extent of errors of omission, especially for chronic cardiovascular disease. Multiple recent studies have estimated that at least 100,000 lives per year could be saved by optimizing the use of long-term cardiovascular medications.

THE QUALITY CYCLE

Cardiology has led the way in medicine in terms of amassing an evidence base for clinical decision making as well as for monitoring and improving care quality. The cycle of clinical therapeutics (Fig. 45.1) provides a model for the adoption of new findings into routine clinical practice (35). Large randomized clinical trials have become the standard in cardiology to define the safety and effectiveness of new therapies (36,37). The findings from these published trials are then reviewed by expert committees from the major cardiovascular professional societies and are summarized into evidence-based clinical practice recommendations. These recommendations define therapies for which the balance of safety and effectiveness is positive for a defined population (class I therapies) and those that are ineffective and perhaps harmful (class III). Most current therapies, unfortunately, are in an uncertain category (class II). These guidelines can be used to distill quality indicators that define specific situations when giving a therapy is uncontroversial; if not given, a quality concern exists. Based on these quantifiable quality indicators, the performance of the individual provider, provider group, hospital, or health system can be objectively measured (38). Such performance data can then be

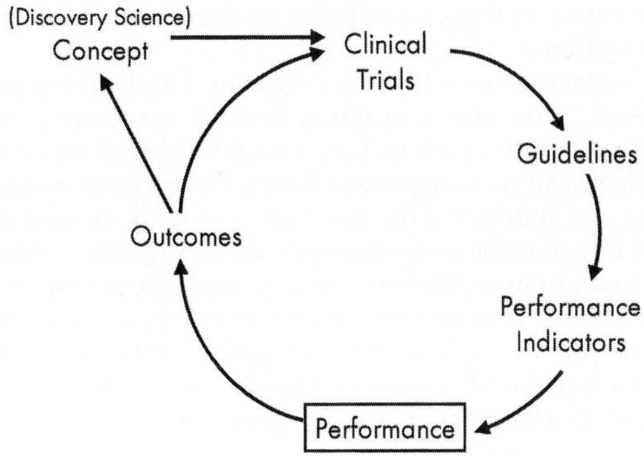

FIGURE 45.1. The cycle of clinical therapeutics. (Adapted from Califf RM, Peterson ED, Gibbons RJ, et al. Integrating quality into the cycle of therapeutic development. *J Am Coll Cardiol* 2002;40:1895–1901.)

benchmarked against peers and feedback given to providers as a means of driving care adoption (39). The ultimate goal of this cycle is to promote the consistent use of best practices to improve the outcomes of patients (see Fig. 45.1).

This idealized cycle of evidence-based care, however, can become derailed at multiple junctures. Unfortunately, many decisions in medicine have not or cannot be systematically studied (40). The studies on which the quality cycle is based often lack an appropriate design or control population, or they may be conducted in highly selected patient populations and clinical settings for inadequate time periods with end points that cannot be used to have assurance about the balance of benefit and risk for the therapy. These methodologic limitations thereby hinder the development of evidence-based care guidelines (37).

The guidelines process itself introduces further challenges. Not all medical decisions (or patients) fall into simple care algorithms, and reductionist strategies often result in oversimplification. Guideline developers often use subgroup analyses despite their known limitations (41). Conflict-of-interest issues may cloud the objectivity of the guidelines developers (42), and the process itself is slow. After multiple rounds of review and consensus building, the guidelines are often out of date soon after publication (43).

Performance measurement and feedback can create further distortions. Similar to the guidelines process, long delays occur before new study findings are incorporated into existing performance indicators. An accurate picture of provider quality emerges only after examining multiple performance metrics, yet current measurement sets are severely constrained by the shortage of adequate supporting clinical trials and the expense of data collection in practice (6). Substantial delays often occur between care delivery and performance feedback, and this feedback often fails to reach front-line caregivers (44). Finally, providers have traditionally lacked adequate incentives for reviewing these data and/or changing practice.

Data Sources for Quality Assessment

Data availability is in many ways the linchpin for quality assessment. Peter Drucker summarized it thus: "If you can't measure it, you can't manage it." This holds for medicine as well as for business. Yet the validity of quality of care measures cannot be understood without understanding where such data come from and their potential limitations. Specifically, there are major concerns that many of the data available to the public have previously relied on inaccurate sources and extrapolation beyond the limits of the data: *bad data in, bad data out.* Data sources for quality assessment include administrative databases (also known as claims or billing data), the patient's paper medical record, and more recently, electronic health records and multicenter clinical data registries.

Administrative Databases

The primary purpose for administrative databases is to allow for patient billing and tracking. The U.S. Medicare claims system provides an example of administrative data sources. Medicare Part A fields cover inpatient hospital claims, whereas Part B fields cover outpatient and physician claims. Claims databases, such as Medicare, generally capture patient demographic information (age, gender, race), a limited number of diagnostic codes (e.g., primary diagnosis and secondary diagnoses), major procedure codes, and a few outcomes (length of hospital stay, mortality). Claims databases, however, usually do not capture details regarding treatment (e.g., medications used), patient counseling information, or many contraindications for treatments. As such, these databases are often unable to examine many process-based quality of care indicators.

The accuracy of claims databases also limits their role in comparing provider outcomes. For example, in one study the rate of agreement between claims-coded databases and those found on chart review ranged from a low of 9% for unstable angina to a high of 83% for diabetes (45). Claims data also do not differentiate complications of care received from preexisting comorbid conditions (46–48). For example, if a patient undergoing bypass surgery had congestive heart failure (CHF) coded as a secondary diagnosis, one could not easily tell whether this was a preoperative risk factor or a postoperative complication. Although the provider's results should certainly be adjusted for the former, the latter should not, because the poor result represents an adverse outcome of the treatment. As such, administrative data sources cannot fully adjust for patient risk in provider outcome performance comparisons. Claims databases also generally do not capture detailed pharmacologic or laboratory information, although this is changing rapidly, and pharmaceutical quality is becoming a cornerstone of outpatient quality measurement. Until electronic health records are available, however, accurate information about patient counseling will not be available from claims data. As such, the use of this form of data has significant limitations for examining most process-based quality indicators.

Medical Record Review

Historically, the patient's paper chart has been a primary data source for clinical data abstraction. However, the chart review process also has many deficiencies as a tool for quality assessment. The nomenclature used to describe similar phenomena varies from practitioner to practitioner. Pertinent negatives are frequently not mentioned, so the reviewer must assume that if a finding or procedure is not mentioned in the medical record, it was not evaluated or done. In an adverse event reporting study, a chart audit missed more than half of adverse events related to medications (49). Beyond these limitations, chart review can be exorbitantly costly, thereby precluding it as a means of longitudinal large-scale quality assessment.

Clinical Databases and the Electronic Clinical Record

As an alternative to the paper chart, health care policy experts have attempted to drive the adoption of the integrated, interoperable electronic health record in hospital and physician offices (50,51). Such systems incorporate standard nomenclature and database architecture and thus have the capacity to export their information among databases. In the near future, such systems also may have unique patient identifiers that will enable one to track quality of care in a longitudinal fashion.

In parallel to the growth in the electronic collection of clinical information, cardiovascular registries have been growing in both North America and Europe. In general, these clinical registries collect standardized clinical elements regarding a specific procedure or disease state, as well as the patient's in-hospital care processes and outcomes. These data are then often provided back to individual sites as a means of benchmarking care and stimulating quality improvement (QI). The earliest examples of such registries were procedure-specific for coronary bypass graft (CABG) surgery and percutaneous coronary intervention (PCI) (52–57). More recently, disease-specific clinical data registries have been formed for those suffering myocardial infarction (MI), acute coronary syndromes, CHF, and stroke.

Although these multicenter clinical databases have considerable promise as a means of quality assessment and improvement, they also have certain limitations. Sites that elect to participate in these registries may not always be representative of community care providers. Indeed, providers with the worst quality and outcomes may be the least likely to participate voluntarily in a registry measuring quality. Additionally, not all clinical data registries have active auditing systems to ensure that all eligible patients are entered and that entered information is accurate and complete. Finally, patient privacy concerns often limit the ability of these registries to track patients after discharge or if they transfer between facilities.

Selecting Quality Indicators

The selection of indicators to be used to assess quality of care is also challenging. All measures have inherent strengths and limitations. The following are general proposed principles that can guide in this selection process (58).

1. The measure should be meaningful. Any potential quality indicator must either be directly or closely linked to an important patient or society outcome. The measure should be valid and reliable. To serve as a useful marker of quality, a measure must be able to be consistently measured among multiple providers, in a standard and reproducible fashion.
2. The measure needs to be able to account or adjust for differences in the type of patients treated by various providers. Specifically, if the metric looks at a given treatment, one needs to be able to define who is and is not eligible for therapy. If the metric examines outcomes, it must be able to risk-adjust these results to reflect any differences in patients' severity of illness or comorbidity.
3. The measure should be amenable to improvement. This requires that there be provider variablity in performance at baseline and room to improve. Second, ideally, there should be a known pathway or process for improving on the metric.
4. It should be economically feasible to measure provider performance over time and among systems. Specifically, although certain metrics such as longitudinal health status are certainly important quality measures, the economic burden of requiring all providers to collect these would be great for routine quality assessment. Advances in technologic and system delivery may alter a metric's feasibility status.

With these principles in mind, Donabedian, considered by many as the father of quality assessment, classified three principal forms of quality measures—structure, process, and outcome (59).

Structure

The structure of health care delivery refers to characteristics inherent to the treating physicians, nurses, and other health care providers, as well as the facilities and health care system in which care is delivered. Examples of provider structural features include their training and specialty status, as well as level of experience (e.g., years in practice or annual procedural volume). Hospital structural features include center size, academic affiliation, specialty equipment and services provided, nurse-to-patient ratios, and types of disease management or transitional services offered.

Three factors limit the use of structural measures as quality indicators. First, the association between structure and care quality is often incomplete. For example, although studies have often demonstrated a general relationship between procedural volume and outcomes, the association is weak enough that it breaks down at the individual provider level, where there are many exceptions to this rule (44). Second, the reasons for the link between a structural measure and quality are often poorly understood, so remedies for quality problems that are identified are not clear. Third, structural characteristics are usually less amenable to change than are care processes.

Process

Process refers to actions performed in the delivery of care to a patient, including the use of diagnostic and therapeutic modalities, and patient counseling. Process also refers to the timing and technical competency of their delivery. The study of process of care has gained much traction in quality assessment for several reasons. When it is known that one diagnostic or therapeutic strategy is superior to an alternative, it is usually straightforward to measure whether an individual provider or group of providers is using this strategy (60). Thus, measurements of the proportion of patients who are treated with aspirin or β-blocker drugs after MI and the timing of delivery of reperfusion therapy to patients with acute MI have become a standard means of assessing quality. This approach of using explicit process-based performance criteria derived from results of randomized trials has increasingly supplanted traditional nonquantitative chart-based peer review by an independent expert. In particular, the consistency of standardized performance indicators provides for a means of nationally or internationally benchmarking provider quality in an objective fashion.

Although measurement of care processes is growing, there are definite limitations. These include questions of accurately defining the right "denominator"—including those patients who are eligible for a therapy while excluding all those who have contraindications. Measurement of care processes credits "doing something," but it rarely attempts to gauge when no therapy is indicated. This can lead to overtreatment or rushed initiation of treatment. Additionally, process measures usually are binary (yes/no), with credit given if some treatment or procedure is given, without concern as to whether it was delivered in a technically competent and safe manner. However, this approach is amenable to rewarding giving the correct dose of a medication or behavioral intervention.

Outcomes

Outcomes refers to tangible measures of the consequences of care and can be considered in the categories of length of life, nonfatal adverse events (e.g., recurrent MI, stroke), and patient health status measures (symptoms, functional status, quality of life) (Fig. 45.2). On the positive side, patient outcome represents the summation of all structure and care processes, including the behavior of the patient/consumer. Improving this end product of what happens to the patient is ultimately the driving goal of medical care. On the negative side, however, the assessment of patient outcomes as quality metrics has its challenges. Adverse outcome events are often uncommon and therefore must be studied among large patient samples to detect stable provider differences. This limits what providers can compare or forces assessment over an extended period. Additionally, multiple factors beyond provider quality affect patient outcomes and must be accounted for before outcome comparisons are meaningful. Many important patient outcomes take years to manifest. This has led to increased use of intermediate outcome measures, surrogates closely associated with the

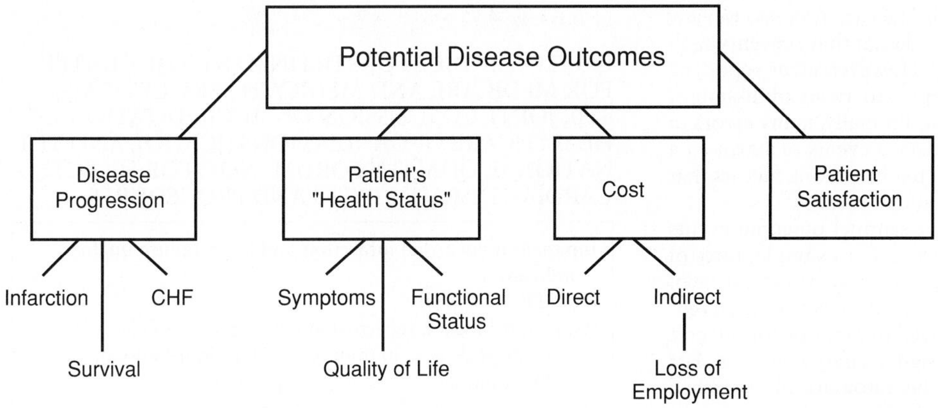

FIGURE 45.2. The spectrum of outcomes in acute myocardial infarction. CHF, congestive heart failure. (From Spertus JA, Radford MJ, Every NR, et al. Challenges and opportunities in quantifying the quality of care for acute myocardial infarction. *Circulation* 2003;107:1681–1691.)

care process and long-term outcomes. Examples of such intermediate measures include the percentage of patients reaching target goals for blood pressure control, cholesterol levels, or hemoglobin A1c values.

Beyond clinical events, there is increasing interest in assessing the impact of provider care on patients' symptoms, health status, and overall quality of life. Several validated mechanisms have been developed for quantifying health status for cardiac patients (61,62). These scales not only measure symptoms but also assess the degree to which these influence patients' perceptions of their well-being and activities of daily life. Although clearly meaningful to patients and society, collection of health status data is resource intensive, and methods for risk-adjusting these results are still under development (58). Furthermore, to the extent these types of measures are used for internal QI, they can be extremely variable, but in outpatients many factors other than the provider can influence the intermediate outcome, thereby leading to concern that "adverse selection" of patients (i.e., taking the most difficult patients into your clinic) can lead to inferior measures.

Patient Satisfaction

Patient perception of care (satisfaction) is a form of outcome of care delivery. Successful care should strive to leave the patient in the best condition possible, but also to have him or her satisfied with how the care was delivered. Such satisfaction data are gained through systematic survey of patients using standardized questionnaires (63). Patient satisfaction with providers has been linked to the likelihood of that patient returning to his or her provider and/or following medical advice. However, although it is important, patient satisfaction is a multidimensional feature that can be strongly influenced by factors not directly associated with the "hard" elements of care quality (safety and effectiveness). Instead, patient satisfaction often depends on elements such as staff friendliness, waiting delays, food services, and physical environment. Additionally, average responses to standardized patient satisfaction survey tools tend to vary by gender, race, and socioeconomic status; accordingly, just as with intermediate biologic measures, these measures may reflect the cultural composition of the patients served rather than the quality of the service delivered. For these reasons, satisfaction information should be complementary to other quality and safety data but not a substitute, because patients with a high satisfaction level can also have care that is poor in terms of safety and effectiveness.

Cost and Efficiency

Health care resource use or costs represent an outcome of great interest to payers, policy makers, and increasingly the patients who are being asked to shoulder more of the personal costs of health care. The term efficiency has been used to describe the provision of value for the resources used. Unfortunately, operational definitions of efficiency are difficult to establish, because a truly objective measure would require simultaneous definition of the safety, effectiveness, timeliness, and cost of the activity.

Because medical charges (bills) are not necessarily reflective of true costs in the United States, hospital charge information must first be adjusted using hospital-specific cost-to-charge ratios, conversion factors that allow for rough estimates of actual resources used (64). In many other countries, hospital bills do not exist (65). Alternative means of estimating costs are available for centers with more detailed microcost accounting systems (64). These systems collect and tally individual unit costs of health care inputs (e.g., labor, consumable materials, pharmacy, laboratories). Like patient satisfaction, measurement of the resources used in delivery of care should be a secondary or complementary metric relative to quality assessment. Yet as health care costs continue to escalate, there is increasing need for providers to improve both their effectiveness and their efficiency.

Medical Errors

Multiple types of medical errors exist (Table 45.2). Assessment of these errors can be captured as either process metrics (error reporting systems) or patient outcomes (adverse events). Each of these systems for identifying medical errors has promise and potential challenges. Voluntary provider reporting allows for

TABLE 45.2

TYPES OF MEDICAL ERRORS

DIAGNOSTIC
Failure to use, or delayed use of, indicated test
Use of inappropriate or outmoded technology
Failure to act on results in timely manner
TREATMENT
Failure to use, or delayed use of, indicated treatment
Error in dosing or delivery
Equipment or system failure
Interaction with other medications or treatments
Failure to personalize care (e.g., missed allergy)
Inadequate monitoring of treatment
Failure to communicate treatment directions to patient
Inappropriate (not indicated) care

Adapted from Kohn LT, Corrigan JM, Donaldson MS, eds. Committee on Quality of Health Care in America, Institute of Medicine. *To err is human: building a safer health system.* Washington, DC: National Academies Press, 1999.

staff to acknowledge breakdowns in the care process. Review of these data can promote process redesign that prevents such errors from occurring in the future. However, error reporting is subjective, and staff may underreport to avoid admission of guilt or out of fear of retribution. Additionally, many errors in processes of care do not lead to adverse events or harm to a patient. A great deal of work can be put into fixing factors that may or may not influence the outcome of care.

Adverse event systems search for sentinel outcome events as signals that a medical error occurred. For example, rates of pressure ulcer or in-hospital patient falls may be indicative of less than ideal nursing care. More recently, electronic surveillance systems have also been employed to monitor for adverse outcomes automatically that may signal safety concerns. For example, pharmacy databases can be automatically searched for the use of naloxone (Narcan) or digitalis antibodies, potentially indicative of opiate or digoxin overdosing, respectively. Like other forms of outcome reporting, the interpretation of the summary of adverse event reporting varies depending on the diligence of the institution and its personnel in reporting events and collecting relevant data. Thus, those most committed to case finding may falsely appear worse than those who intentionally or inadvertently miss such events. The mere identification of an adverse sentinel event does not lead to insight into the event's underlying cause or means of averting such events in the future.

An important construct in error analysis is that errors are far more common than adverse events; therefore, many adverse events are a subset of errors. Conversely, adverse events occur in the absence of errors when expected side effects or toxicities of therapy occur, so all adverse events are not a subset of errors. Newly funded active surveillance systems are now showing that fewer than 15% of adverse events are reported in voluntary reporting systems; therefore, many more errors occur.

Quality Indicators for Specific Cardiac Conditions

Table 45.3 summarizes current quality indicators defined by the Center for Medicare and Medicaid Services (CMS), the Joint Commission on Accreditation of Healthcare Organizations (JCAHO), and those set for by the National Quality Forum for selected cardiac disease states and procedures. As evident in these tables, in-hospital care processes tend to be the dominant metrics used to assess quality of care for disease states such as acute MI, CHF, or chronic cardiac disease. For revascularization procedures, less is known about what care process leads to better outcomes. Thus, for these conditions, quality tends to be assessed with structural measures (procedural volume) and/or outcomes (procedural mortality or morbidity).

Statistical Issues in Quality Assessment and Provider Profiling

Risk Adjustment

Patients' outcomes are influenced by a host of patient-specific factors, including patient demographics (e.g., age, gender), disease severity (e.g., underlying coronary anatomy, ventricular function), comorbid illness (e.g., diabetes, chronic obstructive pulmonary disease), treatment factors, and chance. The goal in quality assessment is to identify the modifiable, provider-related component from these other confounding clinical factors. The statistical methodology needed for appropriately risk-adjusting provider outcome comparisons has been the subject of several recent reviews and requires building multivariable statistical models to weight the most important patient-specific

TABLE 45.3

QUALITY INDICATORS DEFINED BY THE CENTER FOR MEDICARE AND MEDICAID SERVICES (CMS), THE JOINT COMMISSION ON ACCREDITATION OF HEALTHCARE ORGANIZATIONS (JCAHO), AND THE NATIONAL QUALITY FORUM (NQF) FOR SELECTED CARDIAC DISEASE STATES AND PROCEDURES

Inpatient myocardial infarction and heart failure quality indicators
ACUTE MI CARE
Aspirin, β-blocker, reperfusion prescription (STEMI): If lytic, door-drug <30 minutes; if PCI, door-balloon <90 minutes
DISCHARGE CARE
Aspirin, β-blocker, ACE inhibitor, lipid therapy (high LDL), smoking cessation
CORE HF MEASURES
Discharge instructions, assess LVEF, ACE inhibitor, ARB at discharge, smoking cessation
Coronary artery disease and heart failure outpatient quality indicators
RISK FACTOR MEASURES FOR CORONARY ARTERY DISEASE
Measure BP, document lipid profile, assess activity level, smoking cessation, screen for diabetes
RISK FACTOR MEASURES FOR HEART FAILURE
Measure BP, assess activity level, assess LVEF, weight measures, symptoms of volume excess, laboratory tests (chemistry, thyroid function test, etc)
THERAPIES FOR CORONARY ARTERY DISEASE
Antiplatelet therapy, β-blocker (MI), ACE inhibitor, drug therapy for lipids
THERAPIES FOR HEART FAILURE
β-Blocker, ACE inhibitor, warfarin for atrial fibrillation
NQF measures for cardiac surgery
STRUCTURE
Participation in database, surgical volume
PROCESS OF CARE
Perioperative antibiotics (timing/selection), β-blocker (preoperative, discharge), internal mammary artery use, antiplatelet therapy, lipid therapy
OUTCOMES
Prolonged ventilation, sternal wound infection, stroke, renal insufficiency, reoperation, in-hospital mortality, operative mortality

ACE, angiotensin-converting enzyme; BP, blood pressure; LDL, low-density lipoprotein; LVEF, left ventricular ejection fraction; MI, myocardial infarction; PCI, percutaneous coronary intervention; STEMI, ST-segment myocardial infarction.
Data selected from: Centers for Medicare and Medicaid Services (CMS) and the Joint Commission on Accreditation of Healthcare Organizations (JCAHO). *Specifications Manual* for *National Hospital Quality Measures, version 1:05:*2005; and: National Quality Fourm. *National Voluntary Consensus Standards for Hospital Care: An Initial Performance Measure Set.* Washington DC: 2003.

factors so deviations in outcome can be attributed to the care provided rather than to the patients receiving care (66–73).

Any statistical risk model must be scrutinized to determine whether it functions reliably (74). Model discrimination characterizes a risk model's ability to identify those having an event accurately from those not. This is summarized by a C-index or area under the receiver operator calibration (ROC) curve, which calculates for every pair of patients whether a patient with an event was predicted to be more likely to have an event than a patient without an event. Thus, by chance alone, a C-index would be 0.5 (no predictive value), whereas perfect discrimination would yield a C-index of 1.0 (perfect prediction) (75). Models published to date that predict outcome following acute cardiac events (e.g., MI) have had somewhat low discriminatory ability, particularly when applied in populations other than those in which they were developed (76). In contrast, models that predict outcomes of cardiac procedures have higher C-indexes. However, such a high C-index indicates that preprocedure severity of disease (i.e., how sick the patient was before the procedure) has much more impact on outcome than does provider quality (which is unmeasured by the model). A second model metric is measured by the degree to which the absolute probabilities of the outcomes predicted by the model are calibrated or match those actually observed in a given population. Model calibration is particularly important to assess when one is applying a previously developed model in a new population (71,72,77,78).

Impact of Chance and Sample Size on Patient Outcomes

The randomness in biologic systems makes accurate measurement of health care quality using outcomes challenging at best. Even if risk adjustment models were perfect, chance events could still obscure differences in provider outcome comparisons (79). When one has a low number of observations to compare, estimates of provider outcomes are unstable and prone to error (80). For example, if a provider performs one procedure and the patient lives, it is unlikely that his or her future success will be fully 100%. Confidence intervals are one means of expressing the uncertainty of a provider's outcomes when limited sample size exists (81). Hierarchic modeling has been recently proposed as a more accurate means of estimating provider performance (82). This statistical technique shrinks provider results toward the overall group average, in proportion to their sample size, thereby partially adjusting for variability in limited patient samples.

Although such statistical techniques provide a range of estimates, they do not avoid the challenges of assessing quality among low-volume providers. Specifically, providers with a low number of observations may avoid being classified as statistical outliers as a result of wide confidence intervals surrounding their outcome estimates. One means of addressing this problem is to increase provider sample size by following serial trends in performance over time. Alternatively, one can examine performance based on a broader series of provider quality metrics, thereby increasing the number of observations per patient treated.

Regression to the Mean

Because of the inherent variability in measurement of performance, providers with outlier results will often be found to have a value more similar to the group norm on future measurement. Although this concept of regression to the mean is well known, many who track care quality over time fail to account for it. When care is noted to be worse than average (e.g., a higher than normal complication rate), providers often respond with some change in care process. When subsequent care is found to be improved, providers often attribute this to the change in care versus a predictable return to a population average. Following trends over longer periods can help to distinguish these two possibilities in study designs that simply compare event frequencies with historical measures in the same institutions.

Impact of Patient Transfers

The current inability to track patients across health care settings can also distort assessments of provider quality of care. For example, patients evaluated for acute MI at small community hospitals are often later transferred to tertiary care centers. Preliminary studies have found that transferred patients tend to younger and healthier, leaving a high proportion of sick and elderly at the community hospital for outcome comparison (83). Although risk adjustment can partially compensate for these differences, unmeasured differences may persist. Additionally, the quality of care processes themselves may vary considerably among those transferred versus those not. For example, the time to treatment for patients with MI who receive primary PCI tends to vary widely depending on whether the patient presents de novo to a hospital or requires transfer (Fig. 45.3). Despite this, current quality metrics measure only those patients who initially present to a given hospital. As such, quality issues raised by inefficient systems of care are missed (84).

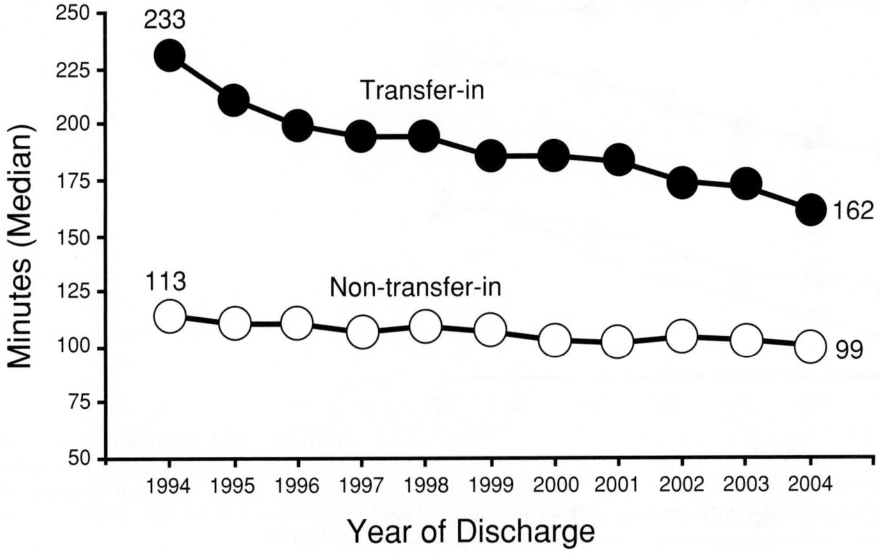

FIGURE 45.3. Median door-to-balloon times for primary percutaneous coronary intervention by transfer status. (Adapted from Gibson CM. NRMI and current treatment patterns for ST-elevation myocardial infarction. *Am Heart J* 2004;148 [suppl]:S29–S33.)

CURRENT CARDIOVASCULAR QUALITY OF CARE

In the following sections, we review aspects of care of patients with acute MI, CHF, and CABG to exemplify the current state of cardiovascular quality and care. This review is not meant to be complete, but rather to emphasize areas where there is evidence for the potential for improvement in care process and outcomes.

Myocardial Infarction Care

Multiple studies have documented a wide gap between American College of Cardiology (ACC)/American Heart Association (AHA) guideline recommendations and the care patients actually receive in community practice. Early studies from the Cooperative Cardiovascular Project (CCP), a survey of MI care among U.S. Medicare beneficiaries in 1993, reported that only 84% of "ideal patients" (without contraindications) received aspirin on admission, 70% received thrombolytics, and 47% were discharged on a β-blocker, despite their proven efficacy (85). Evidence-based MI care has improved since then (Figs. 45.4 and 45.5); however, between 10% and 30% of patients eligible for any given evidence-based treatment still fail to receive it, in both the United States (see Fig. 45.4) and Western Europe (see Fig. 45.5).

Consistency is another indicator of provider quality. Ideally, cardiovascular care should be standardized among providers and demonstrate consistent evidence-based practice for all patients. However, variability among providers predominates. Medicare studies have found that use of discharge β-blockers ranged from 51% to 93% among U.S. states (86). On a hospital level, Chen found that "best hospitals" (defined by *US News and World Report* rankings) more closely adhered to ACC/AHA guidelines than did average hospitals, a difference correlating with lower in-hospital mortality rates (87). Figure 45.6 shows wide variability in hospital performance between leading centers (top 25%) and those that are lagging behind (bottom 25%).

Even more variability in care can be found at the individual provider level. Studies have consistently found that patients with MI who were treated by a cardiologist were much more likely to receive appropriate therapies (88–90). Although evidence indicates that ongoing efforts to disseminate care guidelines and provide care feedback have narrowed this gap somewhat, studies still indicate that specialists treat cardiology patients in a more evidence-based manner, and their patients have better outcomes (91). Evidence-based cardiovascular care should also be provided to patients regardless of their age (92,93), race (94), gender (95,96), and socioeconomic or insurance status (97). Yet study after study has found disparities in each of these categories for cardiac patients. These gaps tend to be widest for resource-intensive cardiac procedures (e.g., catheterization, PCI, or CABG), but they also exist for routine use of secondary prevention medications and lifestyle modification patient education (Tables 45.4 to 45.6) (94).

Beyond frequent errors of omission, studies have also begun to document errors of commission, or safety concerns, in the care of patients with MI. Ten percent of patients admitted with acute coronary syndrome in the United States receive at least one transfusion during their hospital stay, a rate that doubles if the patient is more than 75 years old or has renal insufficiency (98). Although some of these events are unavoidable complications of therapies and laboratory-based interventions used in the treatment of patients with MI, drug dosing represents a potentially modifiable process. Specifically, studies have found that patients treated with fibrinolytic therapy, heparin, and glycoprotein IIb/IIIa inhibitors frequently receive these drugs at doses greater than that recommended. When patients' medicines are overdosed, risks of bleeding increase markedly (99), leaving an open window for improvement.

Heart Failure Care

Fewer studies have been published to date regarding the quality of care of patients with CHF as opposed to those receiving care for MI (100). Despite this, there is ample evidence of quality concerns in CHF care. In 1998 and 1999, a U.S. survey of patients with CHF (n = 37,000+) found that only 64%

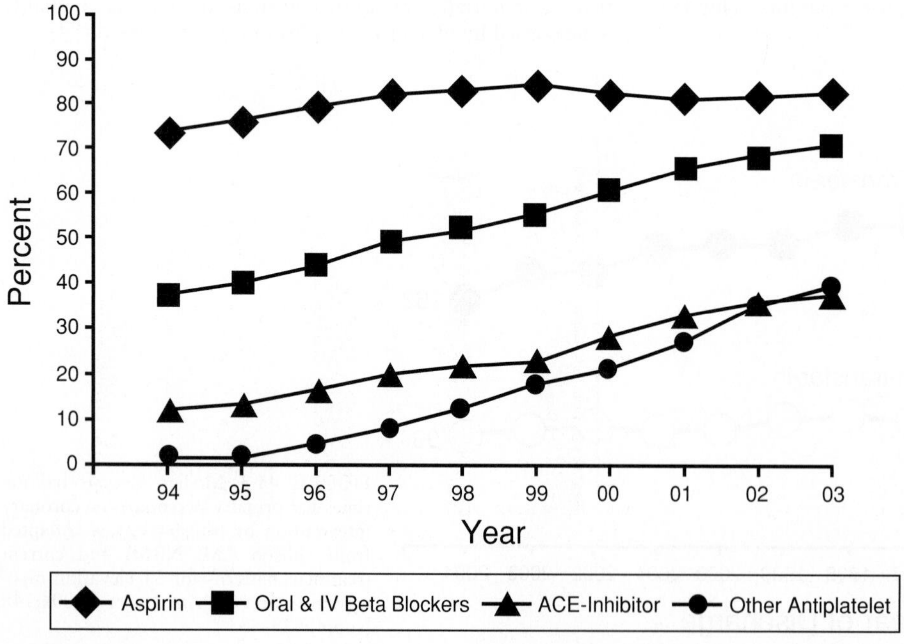

FIGURE 45.4. Medications received within first 24 hours among all eligible patients in the National Registry of Myocardial Infarction (NRMI) 1 to NRMI 4.

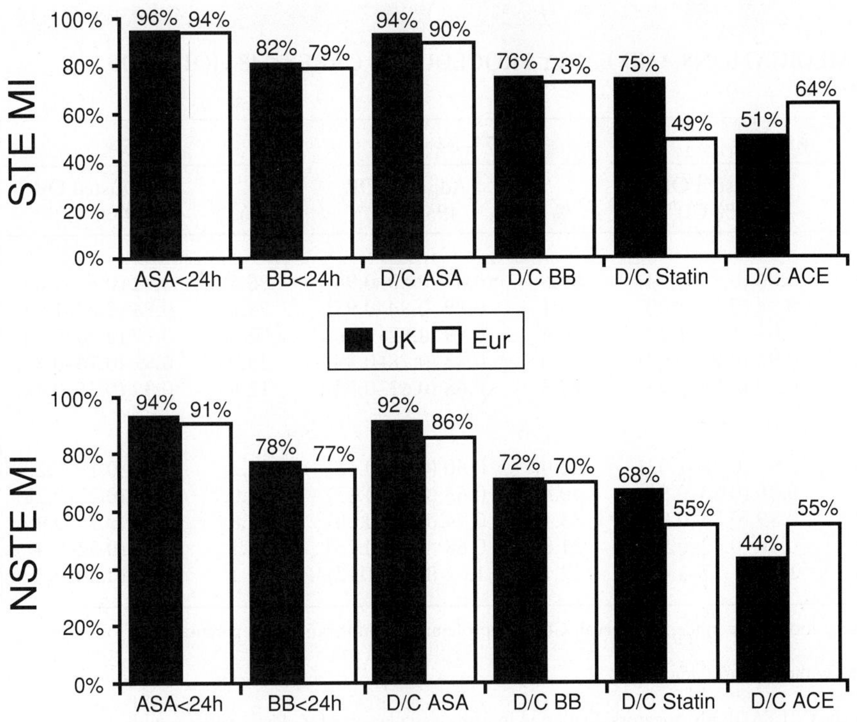

FIGURE 45.5. Care patterns for ST-elevation myocardial infarction (STE MI) (**upper panel**) and non–ST-elevation (NSTE) MI (**lower panel**) in the United Kingdom and the rest of Europe. ACE, angiotensin-converting enzyme inhibitor; ASA, aspirin; BB, β-blocker; D/C, discharge. (From Carruthers KF, Dabbous OH, Flather MD, et al., Contemporary management of acute coronary syndromes: does the practice match the evidence? The global registry of acute coronary events [GRACE]. *Heart* 2005;91:290–298.)

of patients with CHF had their left ventricular ejection fraction documented, whereas only 68% of those eligible received an angiotensin-converting enzyme (ACE) inhibitor (101). In a follow-up survey in 2000 and 2001, these rates were virtually unchanged at 69% and 64%, respectively. More recent data from voluntary registries have documented some improvement, but these rates remain lower than 80%, even among patients considered ideal for treatment (102). As with MI, care of patients with CHF varies significantly at the regional, hospital, and provider levels.

Safety concerns can also mar the quality of care of patients with HF. Recently, studies have found that the adoption of aldosterone blocking agents into clinical practice was associated with an increase in iatrogenic complications from the agent. If used in the wrong patients and/or not carefully monitored after drug initiation, aldosterone blockers can result in hyperkalemia or renal failure. Juurlink and colleagues found that after promotion of this therapy in Canada, there was a more than fourfold rise in admissions for hyperkalemia (103). In a U.S. study, Masoudi and colleagues found that many patients started on aldosterone blockers had frank contraindications for treatment (104).

Coronary Artery Bypass Graft Care

CABG remains the prototype for comparison of procedural mortality. Studies have consistently demonstrated significant

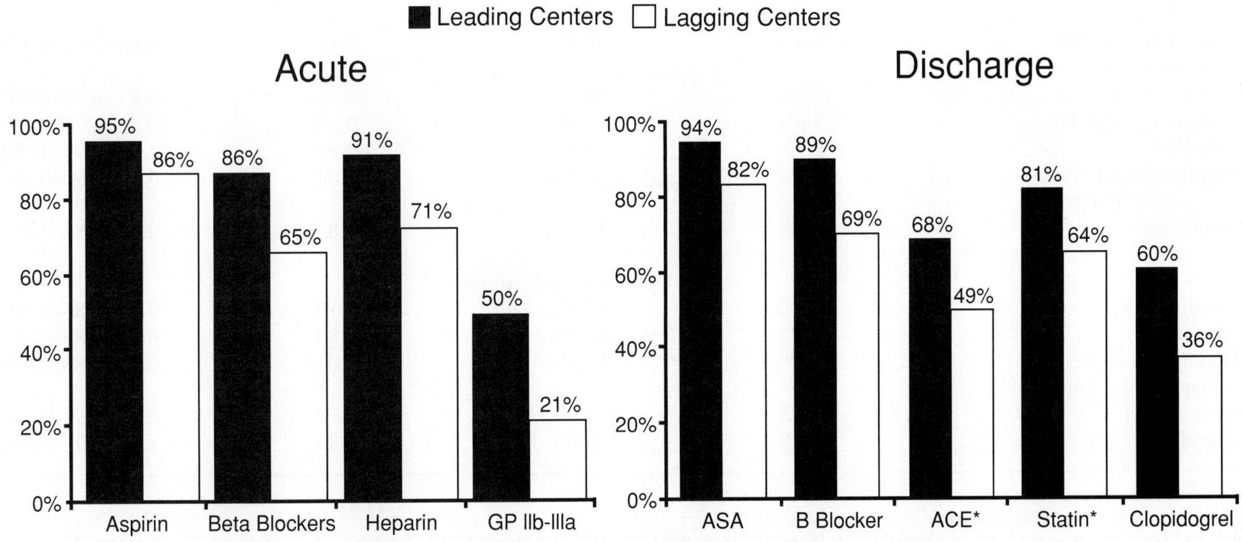

FIGURE 45.6. Variability in care quality between leading and lagging centers among 430 CRUSADE hospitals. ACE, angiotensin-converting enzyme inhibitor; ASA, aspirin; GP, glycoprotein. (Data from 89,500 patients with non–ST-segment acute coronary syndrome.)

TABLE 45.4

ACUTE (≤24 HOURS OF ADMISSION) MEDICATIONS AND EARLY PROCEDURAL CARE (≤48 HOURS OF ADMISSION) BY AGE GROUP IN CRUSADE[a]

	<65 y	65–74 y		75–84 y		≥85 y	
	%	%	Adjusted OR (95% CI)[b]	%	Adjusted OR (95% CI)[b]	%	Adjusted OR (95% CI)[b]
MEDICATIONS							
Aspirin	93.1	90.6	0.86 (0.80–0.94)	89.6	0.87 (0.80–0.96)	88.5	0.92 (0.81–1.04)
β-Blockers	79.7	78.1	0.94 (0.89–1.00)	76.1	0.89 (0.84–0.95)	75.8	0.96 (0.88–1.04)
Heparin, any	84.8	83.7	1.07 (1.00–1.14)	80.4	0.99 (0.92–1.06)	72.8	0.77 (0.70–0.85)
Clopidogrel	45.2	40.8	0.93 (0.88–0.98)	35.0	0.83 (0.78–0.88)	29.9	0.82 (0.76–0.87)
GP IIb/IIIa inhibitors	44.6	35.9	0.90 (0.84–0.95)	25.8	0.68 (0.63–0.73)	12.8	0.39 (0.35–0.44)
PROCEDURES							
Cath	83.1	77.8	0.95 (0.88–1.02)	64.0	0.60 (0.55–0.65)	32.2	0.20 (0.17–0.23)
Cath <48 hours	62.8	53.5	0.88 (0.83–0.94)	40.4	0.63 (0.59–0.67)	18.0	0.25 (0.22–0.28)
PCI	50.4	42.2	0.89 (0.84–0.95)	33.4	0.74 (0.68–0.80)	18.8	0.43 (0.39–0.49)
PCI <48 hours	38.7	29.6	0.88 (0.82–0.94)	21.0	0.68 (0.63–0.73)	10.1	0.37 (0.32–0.42)
CABG	14.5	16.8	1.37 (1.27–1.48)	12.1	1.02 (0.93–1.12)	3.1	0.25 (0.20–0.30)

CABG, coronary artery bypass graft; Cath, catheterization; CI, confidence interval; GP, glycoprotein; OR, odds ratio; PCI, percutaneous coronary intervention.
[a]All p values <.0001; all medication use in patients without contraindications.
[b]In comparison with patients <65 years of age.
From Alexander KP, Roe MT, Chen AY, et al., for the CRUSADE Investigators. Evolution in cardiovascular care for elderly patients with non–ST-segment elevation acute coronary syndromes: results from the CRUSADE National Quality Improvement Initiative. *J Am Coll Cardiol* 2005; 46:1479–1487.

TABLE 45.5

USE OF MEDICAL TREATMENT BY SEX WITH ODDS RATIOS FOR USE IN WOMEN RELATIVE TO MEN IN CRUSADE

Variable	Male (n = 21,323)	Female (n = 14,552)	Unadjusted OR	Adjusted[a] OR (95% CI)
		Treatment within 24 hours		
Aspirin	91.6%	89.6%	0.83	0.93 (0.86–1.01)
Heparin, any	84.0%	80.0%	0.80	0.91 (0.86–0.97)
Unfractionated heparin	54.8%	48.5%	0.81	0.91 (0.87–0.95)
Low-molecular-weight heparin	35.9%	37.7%	1.07	1.03 (0.98–1.08)
Glycoprotein IIb/IIIa inhibitor, any	38.6%	28.7%	0.68	0.86 (0.81–0.92)
Troponin-positive	39.9%	30.5%	0.69	0.87 (0.81–0.92)
Troponin-negative	29.0%	19.4%	0.68	0.81 (0.71–0.93)
β-Blocker	77.7%	75.8%	0.94	1.01 (0.95–1.06)
Angiotensin-converting enzyme inhibitor	42.2%	42.4%	1.03	0.95 (0.90–0.99)
Clopidogrel	41.0%	35.6%	0.82	0.97 (0.92–1.01)
		Discharge medications		
Aspirin	90.4%	87.5%	0.79	0.91 (0.85–0.98)
β-Blocker	82.7%	80.5%	0.89	0.94 (0.88–1.00)
Angiotensin-converting enzyme inhibitor	55.5%	55.3%	1.01	0.93 (0.88–0.98)
Statin	63.4%	55.9%	0.77	0.92 (0.88–0.98)
Clopidogrel	53.2%	48.0%	0.84	1.01 (0.96–1.06)

CI, confidence interval; OR, odds ratio.
[a]Reference is male; variables in model listed in methods.
Adapted from Blomkalns AL, Chen AY, Hochman JS, et al., for the CRUSADE Investigators. Sex disparities in the diagnosis and treatment of non–ST-segment elevation acute coronary syndromes: large scale observations from the CRUSADE Quality Improvement Initiative. *J Am Coll Cardiol* 2005;45:832–837.

TABLE 45.6

RATES AND ADJUSTED ODDS OF MEDICATION AND PROCEDURE USE BY RACE IN CRUSADE

	White	African American	Adjusted OR (95% CI)[a]
Aspirin	90%	88%	1.0 (0.89, 1.11)
β-Blocker	83%	81%	1.05 (0.95, 1.16)
Clopidogrel	41%	32%	0.83 (0.76, 0.90)
Glycoprotein IIb/IIIa	36%	29%	0.80 (0.73, 0.87)
Cath <48 hours	47%	36%	0.73 (0.67, 0.79)
CABG	12%	8%	0.74 (0.65, 0.83)
Lipid drug	79%	74%	0.83 (0.75, 0.90)

CABG, coronary artery bypass graft; Cath, catheterization; CI, confidence interval; OR, odds ratio.
[a]Comparison adjusted for gender, race, comorbidity, cardiac markers, insurance status, hospital features, and clustering effects.
Adapted from Sonel AF, Good CB, Mulgund J, et al., for the CRUSADE Investigators. Racial variations in treatment and outcomes of black and white patients with high risk non–ST-elevation acute coronary syndromes: insights from CRUSADE. *Circulation* 2005;111:1225–1232.

variability at the hospital and surgeon level in post-CABG mortality rates, even after stringent controlling for patient risk factors (105). Over time, however, serial efforts at feeding this information back to providers have reduced interprovider variability and have most likely contributed to marked declines in overall CABG risks (106).

Although overall outcomes are improving, studies also document that care process could be improved. Ferguson and colleagues found that as late as 2000, up to 15% of patients undergoing CABG surgery did not receive an internal mammary artery graft, despite the proven value of this technique (107). Similarly, preoperative β-blockers were not used in up to 40% of patients undergoing CABG (108). A study by Foody and colleagues noted that secondary prevention practices at discharge were less than ideal: Up to 45% did not receive long-term ACE inhibitors despite depressed left ventricular function, whereas 65% did not receive statin therapy (109).

Percutaneous Coronary Intervention Care

Measurement of PCI quality is even more challenging than for CABG surgery. Relatively few process measures differentiate high- and low-quality providers. Similarly, death is rare with PCI, and it is more often indicative of the stability of the patient entering the laboratory than of the quality of the care provided there. Nonfatal events (e.g., periprocedural MI) occur more commonly. Yet patient disease severity affects these outcome metrics as well, and they may be biased depending on the variability with which providers measure and interpret post-procedural cardiac enzymes as well as the local threshold for defining MI. With that said, the ACC currently measures PCI process and outcomes from more than 400 U.S. centers. This database has demonstrated that provider risk-adjusted mortality differs slightly based on procedural volume as well as highlighting the potential to improve the consistency of secondary prevention interventions (110). Appropriate dosing of antithrombotic drugs and consistent use of clopidogrel among patients discharged with a coronary stent represent areas for improving the safety of PCI in current clinical practice.

Procedural appropriateness, however, is perhaps more important for PCI than its technical quality. Specifically, concerns have been raised that PCI is often undertaken in situations when the anticipated benefits from the procedure are slim or when CABG would be a preferable alternative (111). This most prominently includes performing single-vessel PCI in asymptomatic patients or doing incomplete revascularization in patients with multivessel coronary artery disease. Under such conditions, PCI certainly either raises health care costs and thereby places patients at low but real risk with limited anticipated gain or offers inferior treatment.

Longitudinal Cardiac Care

Although the process gaps seen in acute cardiac care are wide, these are dwarfed by those seen in the outpatient setting. In 2002, only 79% of cardiac patients treated who were covered by managed care plans had cholesterol screened after hospital discharge, and 61% of these patients had a low-density lipoprotein value treated to a goal of less than 130 mg/dL (112). Similarly, 58% of managed care patients with hypertension had their blood pressure controlled to a goal of 140/90 mm Hg (112).

In a study from Duke University, even when evidence-based treatments were initiated at discharge, few patients reported taking these medications by 1 year (Fig. 45.7) (113). Similarly, other investigators have found that up to 50% of patients with MI who are prescribed statin therapy will not be taking these medications by 1 year (114). The issue here is not purely patients' ability to pay. In a study of 15,070 managed care patients, Kramer found that β-blocker adherence rates were only 50% at 1 year, even though all patients in the study had prescription drug coverage (115).

REASONS FOR THE QUALITY GAP

Although developing national guidelines for care is an important first step for promoting evidence-based care, as demonstrated in the previous section, the release of such guidelines does not guarantee full incorporation of these recommendations into clinical practice. Reasons for this "voltage gap" between evidence and practice are multiple (116). Busy clinicians may never review guideline recommendations. If the guidelines are read, they may be perceived as threatening to physician autonomy or viewed as "cookbook medicine" if the provider was not part of their creation (117). Systems are needed to encourage providers to be aware of the guidelines, agree with the guidelines, work through appropriate research methods to improve deficiencies in the guidelines, adopt the guidelines, and consistently adhere to the guidelines (118). At each of

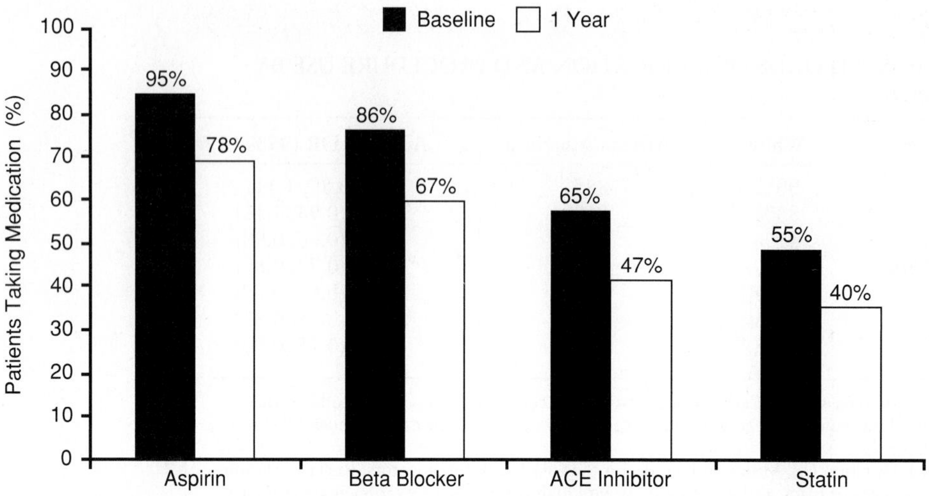

FIGURE 45.7. Long-term medical adherence: the Duke experience. Percentage of patients taking medication at baseline (*black bars*) and at 1 year (*white bars*). (Adapted from Newby LK, LaPointe NM, Chen AY, et al. Long-term adherence to evidence-based secondary prevention therapies in coronary artery disease. *Circulation* 2006;113:203–212.)

these stages, potential barriers exist, thus stressing the need for multimodal interventions, rather than a single "magic bullet" (119).

Understanding the specific barriers impeding implementation of specific guidelines in a specific practice setting is an important first step (Fig. 45.8). Cabana and colleagues grouped potential barriers into four general categories: knowledge (awareness, familiarity), attitudes (agreement with, empowerment, and motivation), behavior (inertia) and external forces (adequate time and resources, patient preferences) (120). To this list of barriers one needs to add challenges brought by the speed of medical progress itself. Clinicians can be overwhelmed with new studies and guideline recommendations (121). This is especially true for cardiac care, in which new findings are constantly released, demanding frequent review and revision of the guidelines. Rapidly incorporating these changes into routine care can be a challenge to clinicians (122).

MARKERS OF SUCCESS IN QUALITY IMPROVEMENT

Bradley and colleagues also attempted to identify factors present in hospitals that had successfully adopted care guidelines (namely, use of β-blockers in acute MI) (123). Specifically, she used open-ended interviews to identify four major themes that were associated with the greatest improvement in β-blockers use. Those common themes were (a) a high degree of goal sharing among clinicians and support staff regarding the use of evidence-based therapies, (b) substantial administrative support for QI, (c) strong physician leadership or a physician champion, and (d) high-quality data feedback. Additional factors that have been shown to improve adherence to practice guidelines include reminder systems such as critical care pathways or computerized support programs, patient-oriented interventions, and the use of local opinion leaders in the education of physicians.

QUALITY IMPROVEMENT STRATEGIES

Strategies for Overcoming Barriers

Many approaches to improving adherence with evidence-based care have been tried, with variable success (124–130). Before discussing these, however, it should be noted that the QI literature itself is far from high quality and suffers from substantial methodologic concerns. Most QI interventions were designed as observational studies, as opposed to more rigorous randomized trials. Further, many of these observational case series lacked a contemporary control group. Thus, it is often difficult or impossible to discern the degree to which changes in care process or outcome should be attributed to the intervention versus unrelated temporal trends. Studies also have tended to be limited in terms of sample size, evaluated under highly favorable settings, and studied within selected patient populations. Moreover, most work has assessed single rather than multimodal interventions. Finally, nearly all have limited time horizons, leaving the durability of these approaches unknown. Acknowledging these limitations, the most relevant strategies are summarized.

Educational Interventions

Didactic lecture format has been the traditional approach to clinician education. Although lectures often increase clinician knowledge, their effect on actual practice patterns and behavior changes has been difficult to demonstrate (131). For example, a systematic review of 160 studies found that a third of education

Practice environment: Organizational context	**Prevailing opinion:** Social context	**Knowledge and attitudes:** Professional context
■ Financial disincentives	■ Routines of practice	■ Clinical uncertainty
■ Organizational constraints • Lack of time	■ Opinion leaders	■ Sense of competence
■ Perception of liability	■ Medical training • Obsolete knowledge	■ Compulsion to act
■ Patient expectation	■ Advocacy • Sales reps	■ Information overload • Inability to recall evidence

FIGURE 45.8. Barriers to implementation of evidence-based medical care. (From Grol R, Grimshaw J. From best evidence to best practice: effective implementation of change in patients' care. *Lancet* 2003;362:1225–1230.)

programs failed to affect physician performance, and half failed to influence patient outcomes (132,133). Although educational initiatives overall have had inconsistent results, certain educational interventions have had success. For instance, Soumerai found that (a) targeting physicians with the greatest need of improvement, (b) assessing barriers to change, and (c) providing "person-to-person contact with credible experts" were three important predictors of the success of an educational intervention (134). Additionally, involvement of local opinion leaders and using teaching strategies that elicit target clinician input have had more consistent results (135).

Provider Feedback

Physicians are generally competitive and success-driven. Interventions that supply feedback on performance relative to peers can effectively motivate change (124,136–142). However, feedback interventions have also had variable impact on care patterns, depending on the form of feedback (119,127,129). Predictors of success with feedback include its accuracy and appropriateness of its measures, its source (credibility of measurer), and its timeliness (with the shortest delay from care to feedback) (123,143,144).

Root Cause Analysis

When medical errors occur, it is helpful to review the underlying causes for this breakdown in depth. Rather than finding personal culpability, root cause analysis stresses identifying system flaws that permitted the error to occur. As such, these reviews are undertaken to determine whether process or system redesign is an option to prevent future errors (145).

Using Tools to Promote Standardization of Care

The use of standardized order sets as a means of promoting consistent care has also met with variable success, depending on the setting. Studies have demonstrated that these simple tools can improve the consistency and quality of care (146). However, often obtaining initial agreement among physician groups to use a common algorithm of care is challenging. Even after such orders are drafted, implementing their consistent use can be undermined by other factors (e.g., hospital review committees, easy access to form).

Use of Electronic Health Records and Computer Physician Order Entry

Moving forward, computer- and Web-based support as well as patient order entry systems (with standardized order sets) could provide an answer for many of the operational issues noted earlier. Computer-based reminder systems have revealed short-term success (147). On-line, Web-based data collection can itself act as a reminder mechanism. Additionally, many have proposed Web-based educational programs as an excellent means of rapidly disseminating medical advances and promoting guideline adoption across broad clinician audiences (148,149). Finally, computer physician order entry (CPOE) has been proposed as an effective means of addressing reducing the frequency of serious medication errors (150), and although most of the literature supports the use of CPOE, new types of errors can be introduced by CPOE systems (151).

Continuous Quality Improvement

Investigators have suggested that health care needs to borrow from the industrial concept of continuous QI (CQI) (152,153). CQI begins, as with many programs, with quality measurement and benchmarking. However, once baseline measurements have occurred, the entire health care team is gathered and challenged to come up with new mechanisms to improve this performance. CQI also emphasizes that approaches for care will often need to be tailored specifically to an individual working environment. In other words, it is difficult to impose a specific plan for care (or process of care) from the outside without obtaining input from local caregivers and without modifying the approach to meet local needs. Finally, although repeat measurement of care practices is an integral part of CQI, its most important role is to motivate subsequent improvement efforts. This whole process is performed in successive waves of rapid-cycle improvement (152).

Although conceptually appealing, successful implementation of CQI principles into physician care of individual patients in health and disease has been difficult (154). Numerous reasons have been offered. Shortell and associates (155) classified these into *strategic* (Is the process important enough to improve quality?), *cultural* (Does the organization buy into the CQI concepts at all levels?), *technical* (Does an appropriately sophisticated information system exist?), and *structural* reasons (Do mechanisms to facilitate learning/education to disseminate process improvements exist?). All four are necessary for sustained CQI results, whether the effort is local, regional, or national. Assessed in this manner, QI requires a comprehensive approach to learning and knowledge building, in which technical skills, clinical expertise, a grasp of CQI principles and practices, and familiarity with organization theory and behavior are all necessary (156).

Voluntary Quality Improvement Initiatives in Cardiovascular Disease

Over the last decade, multiple voluntary efforts have been undertaken to improve cardiovascular care practice and outcomes. These have ranged in scope from single-center QI projects (157) to regional QI projects (158) and national programs (159–163).

Single-Center Quality Improvement

The University of California Los Angeles Cardiovascular Hospitalization Atherosclerosis Program (CHAMP) was an early prototype for a highly successful single-center QI effort (157). By instituting education and standardized order sets, CHAMP was able to markedly improve in-hospital care as well as reduce mortality rates for patients with acute MI (Table 45.7). This success has importantly been maintained and improved on over time (164).

Regional Quality Improvement

The Guidelines Applied in Practice (GAP) initiative was a series of ACC-run projects, each focused on a different guideline and designed to develop and test QI tools and strategies (158). The first GAP project, launched in 2000, focused on in-hospital MI care in 10 Michigan hospitals. GAP used a multifocal initiative, local opinion leaders, and cross-functional hospital QI teams to implement a set of "low-tech" QI tools, including pocket reminder cards and routine, standardized admission order sets and discharge checklists. The GAP pilot demonstrated a significant improvement in guidelines adherence on a range of MI quality indicators. In the first 6 months following implementation, GAP found significant increases in use of admission aspirin (81% to 87%, $p < .05$), β-blockers (65% to 74%, $p < .05$), discharge aspirin (84% to 92%, $p < .01$), and smoking cessation counseling (53% to 65%, $p < .05$). Other indicators (e.g., ACE inhibitors at discharge) noted nonsignificant but favorable trends toward improvement. Of note, elderly patients and women showed a more significant benefit when compared with younger and male patients (158).

TABLE 45.7

RESULTS OF THE UNIVERSITY OF CALIFORNIA LOS ANGELES CARDIOVASCULAR HOSPITALIZATION ATHEROSCLEROSIS PROGRAM (CHAMP) IN IMPROVING IN-HOSPITAL CARE AND REDUCING MORTALITY RATES FOR PATIENTS WITH ACUTE MYOCARDIAL INFARCTION

Discharge therapy	Pre-CHAMP (1992–1993) (n = 256)	Post-CHAMP (1994–1995) (n = 302)	*p*-value
Aspirin	78%	92%	<.001
β-Blockers	12%	61%	<.001
Nitrates	62%	34%	<.01
Calcium antagonists	68%	12%	<.001
Angiotensin-converting enzyme inhibitors	4%	56%	<.001
Statins	6%	86%	<.0001
1-year mortality	7.0%	3.3%	

Adapted from Fonarow GC, Gawlinski A. Rationale and design of the Cardiac Hospitalization Atherosclerosis Management Program at the University of California Los Angeles. *Am J Cardiol* 2000;85:10A–17A.

National Acute Coronary Syndrome Quality Improvement

The National Registry of Myocardial Infarction (NRMI) was initiated in July of 1990 to provide participating hospitals a means of tracking the characteristics, treatment, and outcome of patients with acute MI (159). In terms of QI, the NRMI provides hospitals with quarterly feedback on MI care processes and outcomes. In particular, the NRMI demonstrated that a high percentage of U.S. patients with MI failed to receive primary reperfusion therapy within guideline-recommended time limits (see Fig. 45.4). Over time, these metrics have improved considerably, in part because of the process of ongoing provider feedback. In the last few years, the NRMI has been joined by a series of other national acute coronary syndrome registries including the Can Rapid risk stratification of Unstable angina patients Suppress ADverse outcomes with Early implementation of the ACC/AHA guidelines (CRUSADE) initiative and the AHA's Get with the Guidelines (GWTG). CRUSADE was established to promote awareness and widespread use of the ACC/AHA clinical treatment guidelines in patients with acute coronary syndrome (161,165). CRUSADE also provides member sites with educational seminars, quarterly performance feedback, patient care materials, and a forum for sharing QI techniques. As of mid-2005, CRUSADE has documented consistent improvement in the use of evidence-based care among its 450 participating medical centers (Fig. 45.9).

The AHA's GWTG program is a similar hospital-based QI initiative targeting a broader cardiovascular patient population including those with MI, CHF, and stroke (160). GWTG uses a Web-based management tool for prospective data collection and feedback, and it provides real-time, guideline-based, online reminders specifically addressing discharge management. The GWTG program also has noted significant improvement in most quality metrics overtime for both MI and stroke, with its CHF program just getting under way (166).

Revascularization Quality Improvement

As noted previously, the infrastructure of regional and national revascularization registries has been used to support CQI. For example, the ACC National Cardiovascular Data Registry (ACC-NCDR) provides feedback to more than 400 interventional centers as a means of supporting QI. Most recently, this group has expanded their QI support with the release of CATHKIT, a tool to support catheterization laboratory accreditation and adoption of QI tools in interventional laboratories (167).

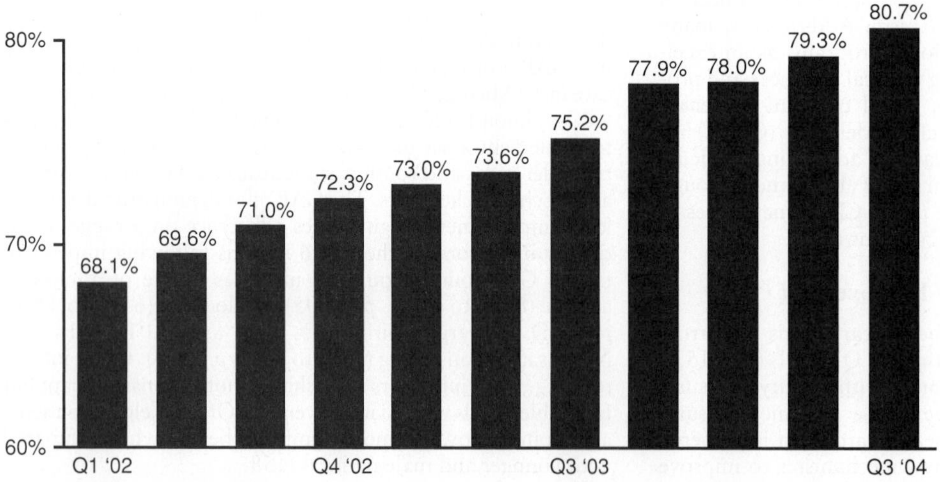

FIGURE 45.9. Trends in composite guidelines adherence by quarters among centers participating in CRUSADE, 2002 to 2004.

In a similar manner, the Society of Thoracic Surgery has used their bypass and valve registry as a means of supporting provider feedback and other QI activities. Between 2001 and 2003, this group conducted a national randomized clinical trial of CQI in CABG surgery (162). More than 400 hospitals were randomized to interventions designed to increase use of preoperative β-blockers or internal mammary artery grafts. In this rigorous, controlled study, Ferguson and colleagues found that simple interventions, including a "call to action," education documents, and systematic feedback, could improve the adoption of these process measures into clinical practice.

External Forces

Public Reporting of Provider Performance

To date, involvement in QI efforts has generally been a voluntary professional activity. Moving forward, however, external forces are rapidly changing the incentives for QI. Specifically, multiple entities, most notably government agencies (e.g., the Centers for Medicare and Medicaid Services in the United States and the British Health Service in the United Kingdom) and voluntary health agencies, many with accrediting power, such as the JCAHO, are now actively requiring providers to submit results on specific quality indicators (Table 45.8).

Profiling efforts have initially focused on hospital-based metrics (e.g., MI, CHF, CABG) but will soon expand to broader disease metrics (primary and secondary prevention) and outpatient treatment. Furthermore, many are committed to a policy of public disclosure of such data once collected. These data are analyzed relative to peer institutions and are placed on a public Web site (www.HospitalCompare.hhs.gov). In theory, public reporting of provider performance would facilitate patients' selection of best providers based on full disclosure. However, in many medical settings, provider choice is not an option either because care is required under urgent conditions (e.g., acute MI) or because alternative health care providers are not available (owing to distance or insurance constrains). It is also often difficult to summarize provider performance statistics in a manner that is both accurate and simple enough for public consumption. Even when outcomes have been prominently displayed and discussed in the newspapers, both patients and physicians have demonstrated limited interest in using such data in the selection of providers for given procedures (168–170).

Pay for Quality

Beyond increasing provider accountability via public profiling, payers have now begun to use provider performance information to alter payment. Initially, commercial insurers used performance data to influence referral patterns, by encouraging patients to go to providers whose care was either less expensive, higher quality, or both. More recently, payers have begun to use such data to alter the actual payment they give providers. The ongoing CMS P4P program is one example. The program, which began in March of 2003, includes approximately 300 hospitals that volunteered to participate in a pilot study that would benchmark care for five conditions (MI, CHF, CABG, pneumonia, and hip fractures). Participating centers are ranked by their performance. The top 20% of performers will receive a small financial reward, whereas the bottom performers will receive slightly less money. Over the next few years, this program is expected to expand to include nearly all U.S. hospitals and more conditions. In fact, current CMS director Mark McClellan has been quoted as saying that P4P-based compensation will account for up to 20% to 30% of physicians' total pay within the next 5 years (171).

These proposed decisions to pay providers differentially based on quality of care have already been implemented in the United Kingdom. As of 2005, U.K. primary care practitioners will receive bonus payments totaling more than 1.8 billion U.S. dollars as a reward for providing high-quality primary care—equaling more than 20% of their total prior salaries (172).

TABLE 45.8

ORGANIZATIONS INVOLVED IN THE MEASUREMENT OF QUALITY IN ACUTE MYOCARDIAL INFARCTION

Organization	Web site	Perspective	Most relevant activity
Centers for Medicare and Medicaid Services (CMS)	www.cms.gov	Payer	National Heart Care Project
Joint Commission on the Accreditation of Healthcare Organizations (JCAHO)	www.jcaho.org	Hospital	ORYX initiatives
American Medical Association (AMA)	www.ama-assn.org	Physician	Physician Consortium for Quality Improvement
National Quality Forum (NQF)	www.qualityforum.org	Payer	Hospital Performance Measures Project
American Heart Association (AHA)	www.americanheart.org	Hospital	Get With The Guidelines; ACC/AHA Task Force on Performance Measures
American College of Cardiology (ACC)	www.acc.org	Physician	Guidelines Applied in Practice (GAP); ACC/AHA Task Force on Performance Measures
Veterans Affairs (VA) Health System	www.va.gov	Hospital	Ischemic Heart Disease Quality Enhancement Research Initiative (IHD QUERI)
National Committee for Quality Assurance (NCQA)	www.ncqa.org	Health plan	Healthplan Employers Data and Information Set (HEDIS)

Adapted from Spertus JA, Radford MJ, Every NR, et al. Challenges and opportunities in quantifying the quality of care for acute myocardial infarction. *Circulation* 2003;107:1681–1691.

Over a short 18-month period, clinicians, academics, and the government developed consensus rules for defining quality as well as the scoring system used to define bonus pay. This system, based on both guidelines-based process measures and intermediate patient outcomes (e.g., reaching goal blood pressure control) provides a potential model for future systems.

Although it is intuitive that those providing higher quality of care should be paid more, physician response to these programs has been mixed. Concerns have been raised: What are the indicators of quality? Who defines these? How will they be adjusted for patient case mix? In addition to these difficult questions, it remains uncertain how best to structure these reward systems. Specifically, P4P could be a bonus for high-quality care in which all exceeding a certain threshold are rewarded. Alternatively, this could be a competition among peers in which only providers with the top performance receive additional pay. P4P may also be burdened with adverse unintended consequences (43). Providers may attempt to slant their results, by avoiding the tough cases while spending more time documenting reasons that certain care was not done (in short, doctoring the charts and not the patients). Providers may also adopt a test-taking mentality, concerning themselves with only what is measured and ignoring other areas of medicine that may need improvement. Similarly, care may become rushed or inappropriately begun in certain patients as providers attempt to implement all graded treatments in ever-shorter inpatient hospital stays. The resources required for implementing P4P are also considerable. The provider must invest in information technology and personnel time required to capture the data, whereas the profiler must also support data harvesting, analysis, and reporting functions. These are dollars that are not going directly into patient care or QI. Finally, P4P will take resources away from those providers whose care initially lags behind their peers. In doing so, P4P could accentuate existing care disparities.

CONTROVERSIES AND PERSONAL PERSPECTIVES

The issue of quality will provide much ammunition for controversy over the next 5 years. As noted earlier, differential reimbursement is a powerful tool to change the behavior of health care providers and their organizations and delivery systems. The rules for appropriate use of this powerful tool will need to developed as experiments are done in real time involving hundreds to millions of people at a time. The ethics of quality initiatives have not been addressed formally, although efforts are now under way (173).

Control of quality systems will also be hotly debated. Growing numbers of consumer organizations are pushing for public control, whereas most health care providers prefer to have internally driven quality efforts.

THE FUTURE

As was expressed by Nightingale more than a century ago, there is a need for better accountability in medicine. The study of quality parameters and methods of QI have built a compelling case that individual practitioners, groups of practitioners, hospitals, and health systems can improve their performance to the benefit of their patients. Internally, medical centers should consider developing risk-adjusted models for procedures such as CABG and PCI to monitor groups of physicians over an extended period, such that the number of operations or procedures is suitable for analysis. Until now, the outpatient arena has been spared from the scrutiny that has been placed on hospitals. This will change dramatically as more attention is paid to the importance of avoiding medication errors of omission and commission and to the critical centrality of disease management in improving the quality of life of patients with chronic cardiovascular disease.

The importance of quality assessment and its increasing effect on reimbursement will continue to generate tremendous controversy (174–180). The cost of information about quality care (181) and the cost of not delivering quality care (182) will remain contentious. The risks of risk adjustment (183–185) and release to the public of such data (186–190) will continue to be limitations. Fundamental issues such as defining the optimal way to measure quality (191–196), appropriateness of procedures (197,198), and physician competence (199,200) lie at the heart of debate and will continue to evolve over time. Without question, the effect of simply studying quality can have a salutary outcome (201), and as clinical trials continue to address major issues in medical therapy and information systems can measure the adoption of knowledge into practice, the amount of interest and controversy will only increase for the foreseeable future.

References

1. Lohr KN, Schroeder SA. A strategy for quality assurance in Medicare. *N Engl J Med* 1990;323:278–279.
2. Committee on Quality of Health Care in America, Institute of Medicine. *Crossing the quality chasm: a new health system for the 21st century*. Washington, DC: National Academies Press, 2001.
3. Kohn LT, Corrigan JM, Donaldson MS, eds. Committee on Quality of Health Care in America, Institute of Medicine. *To err is human: building a safer health system*. Washington, DC: National Academies Press, 1999.
4. McGlynn EA, Asch SM, Adams J, et al. The quality of health care delivered to adults in the United States. *N Engl J Med* 2003;348:2635–2645.
5. Williams SC, Schmaltz SP, Morton DJ, et al. Quality of care in U.S. hospitals as reflected by standardized measures, 2002–2004. *N Engl J Med* 2005; 353:255–264.
6. Jha AK, Li Z, Orav EJ, et al. Care in U.S. hospitals: the Hospital Quality Alliance program. *N Engl J Med* 2005;353:265–274.
7. Marciniak TA, Ellerbeck EF, Radford MJ, et al. Improving the quality of care for Medicare patients with acute myocardial infarction: results from the Cooperative Cardiovascular Project. *JAMA* 1998;279:1351–1357.
8. Ohman EM, Roe MT, Smith SC Jr, et al. , for the CRUSADE Investigators. Care of non–ST-segment elevation patients: insights from the CRUSADE national quality improvement initiative. *Am Heart J* 2004;148(suppl 5):S34–S39.
9. O'Connor GT, Quinton HB, Traven ND, et al. Geographic variation in the treatment of acute myocardial infarction: the Cooperative Cardiovascular Project. *JAMA* 1999;281:627–633.
10. Center for the Evaluative Clinical Sciences at Dartmouth Medical School. *The Dartmouth atlas of health care*. Chicago: Health Forum, 1999.
11. Lambrew CT, Bowlby LJ, Rogers WJ, et al. Factors influencing the time to thrombolysis in acute myocardial infarction: Time to Thrombolysis Substudy of the National Registry of Myocardial Infarction-1. *Arch Intern Med* 1997;157:2577–2582.
12. Brennan TA, Leape LL, Laird NM, et al. Incidence of adverse events and negligence in hospitalized patients: results of the Harvard Medical Practice Study I. *N Engl J Med* 1991;324:370–376.
13. Thomas EJ, Studdert DM, Burstin HR, et al. Incidence and types of adverse events and negligent care in Utah and Colorado. *Med Care* 2000;38:261–271.
14. Alexander KP, Chen AY, Roe MT, et al. Antiplatelet and antithrombin dose variation in patients with non–ST-segment elevation acute coronary syndromes. *Circulation* 2005;111:e310–e359(abst).
15. Relman A. Assessment and accountability: the third revolution in medical care. *N Engl J Med* 1988;319:1220–1222.
16. Topol E, Califf RM. Scorecard cardiovascular medicine. Its impact and future directions. *Ann Intern Med* 1994;120:65–70.
17. HealthGrades Web site. Available at: www.healthgrades.com. Accessed September 7, 2005.
18. *U.S. News & World Report* Web site. Available at: www.usnews.com/usnews/home.htm. Accessed September 7, 2005.
19. Solucient top 100 hospitals. Solucient Web site. Available at: http://www.100tophospitals.com. Accessed September 7, 2005.
20. Peterson ED. Should we link payment to quality? *Am Heart J* 2004;148 (suppl 5):S56–S58.
21. Roland M. Linking physicians' pay to the quality of care: a major experiment in the United Kingdom. *N Engl J Med* 2004;351:1448–1454.
22. Marshall M, Smith P. Rewarding results: using financial incentives to improve quality. *Qual Saf Health Care* 2003;12:397–398.

23. McElduff P, Lyratzopoulos G, Edwards R, et al. Will changes in primary care improve health outcomes? Modelling the impact of financial incentives introduced to improve quality of care in the UK. *Qual Saf Health Care* 2004; 13:191–197.
24. Nightingale F. *Notes on hospitals*, 3rd ed. London: Longman, Green, Longman, Roberts and Green, 1863.
25. Iezzoni LI. 100 Apples divided by 15 red herrings: a cautionary tale from the mid-19th century on comparing hospital mortality rates. *Ann Intern Med* 1996;124:1079–1085.
26. Codman EA. The product of a hospital. *Surg Gynecol Obstet* 1914;18:491–496.
27. Hammermeister KE. Risk, predicting outcomes, and improving care. *Circulation* 1995;91:899–900.
28. Codman EA. In: O'Leary DS, ed. *A study in hospital efficiency: as demonstrated by the case report of the first five years of a private hospital.* Oakbrook Terrace, IL: Joint Commission on Accreditation of Healthcare Organizations, 1996.
29. Brinkley J. US releasing lists of hospitals with abnormal mortality rates. *New York Times,* March 12, 1986:1.
30. Health Care Financing Administration. *Medicare hospital mortality information,* vol. 1, 1986. HCFA Publication No. 01-002. Washington, DC: US Government Printing Office, 1987.
31. Blumberg MS. Comments on HCFA hospital death rate statistical outliers. *Health Serv Res* 1987;21:715–740.
32. Derrida J. *Plato's pharmacy.* Barbara Johnson tr. Dissemination 1981; London: Athlone Press, 1981.
33. Pagel W. *Paracelsus: an introduction to philosophical medicine in the era of the Renaissance.* 2nd rev. ed. New York: Karger, 1982.
34. Semmelweis I. *The etiology, concept, and prophylaxis of childbed fever.* Carter KC, trans-ed.Madison, WI: University of Wisconsin Press, 1983.
35. Califf RM, Peterson ED, Gibbons RJ, et al. Integrating quality into the cycle of therapeutic development. *J Am Coll Cardiol* 2002;40:1895–1901.
36. Yusuf S, Collins R, Peto R. Why do we need some large, simple randomized trials? *Stat Med* 1984;3:409–422.
37. Califf RM, DeMets DL. Principles from clinical trials relevant to clinical practice: parts I and II. *Circulation* 2002;106:1015–1021, 1172–1175.
38. Spertus JA, Eagle KA, Krumholz HM, et al. American College of Cardiology and American Heart Association methodology for the selection and creation of performance measures for quantifying the quality of cardiovascular care. *Circulation* 2005;111:1703–1712.
39. Kiefe CI, Allison JJ, Williams OD, et al. Improving quality improvement using achievable benchmarks for physician feedback: a randomized controlled trial. *JAMA* 2001;285:2871–2879.
40. Hlatky MA, Califf RM, Harrell FE Jr, et al. Clinical judgment and therapeutic decision making. *J Am Coll Cardiol* 1990;15:1–14.
41. Lichtman JH, Roumanis SA, Radford MJ, et al. Can practice guidelines be transported effectively to different settings? Results from a multicenter interventional study. *Jt Comm J Qual Improv* 2001;27:42–53.
42. Choudhry NK, Stelfox HT, Detsky AS. Relationships between authors of clinical practice guidelines and the pharmaceutical industry. *JAMA* 2002; 287:612–617.
43. Shekelle P, Eccles MP, Grimshaw JM, et al. When should clinical guidelines be updated? *BMJ* 2001;323:155–157.
44. Peterson ED, Coombs LP, DeLong ER, et al., for the STS National Cardiac Database Investigators: procedural volume as a marker of quality for CABG surgery. *JAMA* 2004;291:195–201.
45. Jollis JG, Ancukiewicz M, DeLong ER, et al. Discordance of databases designed for claims payment versus clinical information systems. *Ann Intern Med* 1993;119:844–850.
46. Jencks SF, Huff ED, Cuerdon T. Change in the quality of care delivered to Medicare beneficiaries, 1998–1999 to 2000–2001. *JAMA* 2002;289:305–312.
47. McCarthy EP, Iezzoni LI, Davis RB, et al. Does clinical evidence support ICD-9-CM diagnosis coding of complications? *Med Care* 2000;38:868–876.
48. Lawthers AG, McCarthy EP, Davis RB, et al. Identification of in-hospital complications from claims data: is it valid?. *Med Care* 2000;38:785–795.
49. O'Neil AC, Petersen LA, Cook EF, et al. Physician reporting compared with medical-record review to identify adverse medical events. *Ann Intern Med* 1993;119:370–376.
50. Baron RJ, Fabens EL, Schiffman M, et al. Electronic health records: just around the corner? Or over the cliff? *Ann Intern Med* 2005;143:222–226.
51. Kaushal R, Blumenthal D, Poon EG, et al., for the Cost of National Health Information Network Working Group. The costs of a national health information network. *Ann Intern Med* 2005;143:165–173.
52. Grover FL, Shroyer AL, Edwards FH, et al. Data quality review program: the Society of Thoracic Surgeons Adult Cardiac National Database. *Ann Thorac Surg* 1996;62:1229–1231.
53. Hannan EL, Kilburn H Jr, O'Donnell JF, et al. Adult open heart surgery in New York State. An analysis of risk factors and hospital mortality rates. *JAMA* 1990;264:2768–2774.
54. O'Connor GT, Plume SK, Olmstead EM, et al. Multivariate prediction of in-hospital mortality associated with coronary artery bypass graft surgery: Northern New England Cardiovascular Disease Study Group. *Circulation* 1992;85:2110–2118.
55. O'Connor GT, Malenka DJ, Quinton H, et al. Multivariate prediction of in-hospital mortality after percutaneous coronary interventions in 1994–1996. *J Am Coll Cardiol* 1999;34:681–691.
56. Edwards FH, Grover FL, Shroyer AL, et al. The Society of Thoracic Surgeons National Cardiac Surgery Database: current risk assessment. *Ann Thorac Surg* 1997;63:903–908.
57. Brindis RG, Fitzgerald S, Anderson HV, et al. The American College of Cardiology–National Cardiovascular Data Registry (ACC-NCDR): building a national clinical data repository. *J Am Coll Cardiol* 2001;37:2240–2245.
58. Spertus JA, Radford MJ, Every NR, et al. Challenges and opportunities in quantifying the quality of care for acute myocardial infarction. *Circulation* 2003;107:1681–1691.
59. Donabedian A. Evaluating the quality of medical care. *Milbank Mem Fund Q* 1966;44(suppl):166–206.
60. Brook RH, McGlynn EA, Cleary PD. Part 2: measuring quality of care. *N Engl J Med* 1996;335:966–970.
61. Spertus JA, Winder JA, Dewhurst TA, et al. Development and evaluation of the Seattle Angina Questionnaire: a new functional status measure for coronary artery disease. *J Am Coll Cardiol* 1995;25:333–341.
62. Green CP, Porter CB, Bresnahan DR, Spertus JA. Development and evaluation of the Kansas City Cardiomyopathy Questionnaire: a new health status measure for heart failure. *J Am Coll Cardiol* 2000;35:1245–1255.
63. Consumer Assessment of Health Plans. Agency for Healthcare Research and Quality Web site. Available at: www.ahrq.gov/qual/cahpsix.htm. Accessed September 7, 2005.
64. Luce BR, Manning WG, Siegel JE, Lipscomb J. Estimating costs in cost-effectiveness analysis. In: Gold MR, Siegel JE, Russell LB, Weinstein MC, eds: *Cost-effectiveness in health and medicine.* New York: Oxford University Press, 1996:176–213.
65. Reed SD, Radeva JI, Weinfurt KP, et al., for the VALIANT Investigators. Resource use, costs, and quality of life among patients in the multinational Valsartan in Acute Myocardial Infarction Trial (VALIANT). *Am Heart J* 2005;150:323–329.
66. Buell HE, DeLong ER, Peterson ED, et al. When is a CABG mortality model complete, stable, and reliable? *J Am Coll Cardiol* 1999;33:548A.
67. DeLong ER, Muhlbaier LH, Cowper PA, et al. Highly accurate risk prediction models may not predict outcomes. *Circulation* 1999;100:13–18.
68. Iezzoni LI. The risks of risk adjustment. *JAMA* 1997;278:1600–1607.
69. Jencks SF, Daley J, Draper D, et al. Interpreting hospital mortality data: the role of clinical risk adjustment. *JAMA* 1988;260:3611–3616.
70. Halm EA, Chassin MR. Why do hospital death rates vary? *N Engl J Med* 2001;345:692–694.
71. Shahian DM, Normand SL, Torchiana DF, et al. Cardiac surgery report cards: comprehensive review and statistical critique. *Ann Thorac Surg* 2001; 72:2155–2168.
72. Shahian DM, Blackstone EH, Edwards FH, et al., for the STS workforce on evidence-based surgery. Cardiac surgery risk models: a position article. *Ann Thorac Surg* 2004;78:1868–1877.
73. Peterson ED, DeLong ER, Muhlbaier LH, et al. Challenges in comparing risk-adjusted bypass surgery mortality results: results from the Cooperative Cardiovascular Project. *J Am Coll Cardiol* 2000; 36:2174–2184.
74. Daley J. Criteria by which to evaluate risk-adjusted outcomes programs in cardiac surgery. *Ann Thorac Surg* 1994;58:1827–1835.
75. Grunkemeier GL, Jin R. Receiver operating characteristic curve analysis of clinical risk models. *Ann Thorac Surg* 2001;72:323–326.
76. Ohman EM, Granger CB, Harrington RA, et al. Risk stratification and therapeutic decision making in acute coronary syndromes. *JAMA* 2000; 284:876–878.
77. DeLong ER, Peterson ED, DeLong DM, et al. Comparing risk-adjustment methods for provider profiling. *Stat Med* 1997;16:2645–2664.
78. Justice AC, Covinsky KE, Berlin JA. Assessing the generalizability of prognostic information. *Ann Intern Med* 1999;130:515–524.
79. Thomas JW, Hofer TP. Accuracy of risk-adjusted mortality rate as a measure of hospital quality of care. *Med Care* 1999;37:83–92.
80. Dimick JB, Welch HG, Birkmeyer JD. Surgical mortality as an indicator of hospital quality: the problem with small sample size. *JAMA* 2004;292:847–851.
81. Localio AR, Berlin JA, Ten Have TR, et al. Adjustments for center in multicenter studies: an overview. *Ann Intern Med* 2001;135:112–123.
82. Shahian DM, Normand SL, Torchiana DF, et al. Cardiac surgery report cards: comprehensive review and statistical critique. *Ann Thorac Surg* 2001; 72:2155–2168.
83. Roe MT, Boden WE, Chen A, et al. Is the "hub-and-spoke" model working? Patterns of transfer for high-risk acute coronary syndromes patients from community hospitals without revascularization capacity. *J Am Coll Cardiol* 2004;43:1A (abst).
84. Califf RM, Faxon DP. Need for centers to care for patients with acute coronary syndromes. *Circulation* 2003;107:1467–1470.
85. Ellerbeck EF, Jencks SF, Radford MJ, et al. Quality of care for Medicare patients with acute myocardial infarction: a four-state pilot study from the Cooperative Cardiovascular Project. *JAMA* 1995;273:1509–1514.
86. Jencks SF, Cuerdon T, Burwen DR, et al. Quality of medical care delivered to Medicare beneficiaries: a profile at state and national levels. *JAMA* 2000;284:1670–1676.
87. Chen J, Radford MJ, Wang Y, et al. Do "America's Best Hospitals" perform better for acute myocardial infarction? *N Engl J Med* 1999;340:286–292.

88. Jollis JG, DeLong ER, Peterson ED, et al. Outcome of acute myocardial infarction according to the specialty of the admitting physician. *N Engl J Med* 1996;335:1880–1887.
89. Ayanian JZ, Guadagnoli E, McNeil BJ, et al. Treatment and outcomes of acute myocardial infarction among patients of cardiologists and generalist physicians. *Arch Intern Med* 1997;157:2570–2576.
90. Jong P, Gong Y, Liu PP, et al. Care and outcomes of patients newly hospitalized for heart failure in the community treated by cardiologists compared with other specialists. *Circulation* 2003;108:184–191.
91. Peterson ED, Roe MT, Li Y, et al. Influence of physician specialty on care and outcomes of acute coronary syndrome patients: results from CRUSADE. *J Am Coll Cardiol* 2003;41:534A(abst).
92. Cheitlin MD, Gerstenblith G, Hazzard WR, et al. AHA Conference Proceedings: do existing databases hold the answers to clinical questions in geriatric cardiovascular disease and stroke? Executive Summary. Database Conference, January 27–30, 2000. Washington, DC, USA. *Circulation* 2001; 104:E39.
93. Alexander KP, Roe MT, Chen AY, et al. Evolution in cardiovascular care for elderly patients with non–ST-segment elevation acute coronary syndromes: results from CRUSADE. *J Am Coll Cardiol* 2005;46:1479–1487.
94. Sonel AF, Good CB, Mulgund J, et al., for the CRUSADE Investigators. Racial variations in treatment and outcomes of black and white patients with high risk non–ST-elevation acute coronary syndromes: insights from CRUSADE. *Circulation* 2005;111:1225–1232.
95. Alexander KP, Peterson ED. Medical and surgical management of coronary artery disease in women. *Am J Manag Care* 2001;7:951–956.
96. Blomkalns AL, Chen AY, Hochman JS, et al., for the CRUSADE Investigators. Gender disparities in the diagnosis and treatment of non–ST-segment elevation acute coronary syndromes: large-scale observations from the CRUSADE National Quality Improvement Initiative. *J Am Coll Cardiol* 2005;45:832–837.
97. Rao SV, Kaul P, Newby LK, et al. Poverty, process of care, and outcome in acute coronary syndromes. *J Am Coll Cardiol* 2003;41:1948–1954.
98. Yang X, Alexander KP, Chen AY, et al., for the CRUSADE Investigators. The implications of blood transfusions for patients with non–ST-segment elevation acute coronary syndromes: results from CRUSADE. *J Am Coll Cardiol* 2005;46:1490–1495.
99. Alexander KP, Chen AY, Roe MT, et al., for the CRUSADE Investigators. Anti-platelet and anti-thrombin dose variation in patients with NST elevation ACS. *Circulation* 2005;111:e312.
100. Krumholz HM, Baker DW, Ashton CM, et al. Evaluating quality of care for patients with heart failure. *Circulation* 2000;101:e122–e140.
101. Masoudi FA, Rathore SS, Wang Y, et al. National patterns of use and effectiveness of angiotensin-converting enzyme inhibitors in older patients with heart failure and left ventricular systolic dysfunction. *Circulation* 2004;110:724–731.
102. Fonarow GC, for the ADHERE Scientific Advisory Committee. The Acute Decompensated Heart Failure National Registry (ADHERE): opportunities to improve care of patients hospitalized with acute decompensated heart failure. *Rev Cardiovasc Med* 2003;4(suppl 7):S21–S30.
103. Juurlink DN, Mamdani MM, Lee DS, et al. Rates of hyperkalemia after publication of the Randomized Aldactone Evaluation Study. *N Engl J Med* 2004;351:543–551.
104. Masoudi FA, Gross CP, Wang Y, et al. Adoption of spironolactone therapy for older patients with heart failure and left ventricular systolic dysfunction in the United States, 1998–2001. *Circulation* 2005;112:39–47.
105. Hannan EL, Kilburn H Jr, Racz M, et al. Improving the outcomes of coronary artery bypass surgery in New York State. *JAMA* 1994;271:761–766.
106. Ferguson TB, Hammill B, Peterson ED, et al. A decade of change: risk profiles for isolated CABG procedures, 1990-1999. A report from the STS National Database Committee and the Duke Clinical Research Institute. *Ann Thorac Surg* 2002;73:480–490.
107. Ferguson TB Jr, Coombs LP, Peterson ED. Internal thoracic artery grafting in the elderly patient undergoing coronary artery bypass grafting: room for process improvement? *J Thorac Cardiovasc Surg* 2002;123:869–880.
108. Ferguson TB Jr, Coombs LP, Peterson ED. Preoperative β-blocker use and mortality and morbidity following CABG surgery in North America. *JAMA* 2002;287:2221–2227.
109. Foody JM, Ferdinand FD, Galusha D, et al. Patterns of secondary prevention in older patients undergoing coronary artery bypass grafting during hospitalization for acute myocardial infarction. *Circulation* 2003; 108(suppl 1):I124–I128.
110. Brindis RG, Fitzgerald S, Anderson HV, et al., on behalf of the ACC-NCDR. The American College of Cardiology–National Cardiovascular Data Registry (ACC-NCDR): building a National Clinical Data Repository. *J Am Coll Cardiol* 2001;37:2240–2245.
111. Califf RM. Stenting or surgery: an opportunity to do it right. *J Am Coll Cardiol* 2005;46:589–591.
112. American Heart Association. Heart facts 2005. Available on line at: www.americanheart.org/presenter.jhtml?identifier=3000992.
113. Newby LK, LaPointe NM, Chen AY, et al. Long-term adherence to evidence-based secondary prevention therapies in coronary artery disease. *Circulation* 2006;113:203–212.
114. Kulkarni SP, Alexander KP, Lytle B, et al. Long-term adherence with cardiovascular drug regimens. *Am Heart J* 2006;151:185–191.
115. Kramer JM, Fetterolf D, Charde JP, et al. National evaluation of long-term adherence to beta-blocker therapy after acute myocardial infarction in patients with commercial health insurance. *J Am Coll Cardiol* 2004;43:415A.
116. Eisenberg JM. Physician utilization: the state of research about physicians' practice patterns. *Med Care* 1985;23:461–483.
117. Conroy M, Shannon W. Clinical guidelines: their implementation in general practice. *Br J Gen Pract* 1995;45:371–375.
118. Pathman DE, Konrad TR, Freed GL, et al. The awareness-to-adherence model of the steps to clinical guideline compliance: the case of pediatric vaccine recommendations. *Med Care* 1996;34:873–889.
119. Oxman AD, Thomson MA, Davis DA, et al. No magic bullets: a systemic review of 102 trials of interventions to improve professional practice. *Can Med Assoc J* 1995;153:1423–1431.
120. Cabana MD, Rand CS, Powe NR, et al. Why don't physicians follow clinical practice guidelines? A framework for improvement. *JAMA* 1999; 282:1458–1465.
121. Carruthers SG. Assimilating new therapeutic interventions into clinical practice: how does hypertension compare with other therapeutic areas? *Am Heart J* 1999;138:256–260.
122. Shekelle PG, Ortiz E, Rhodes S, et al. Validity of the Agency for Healthcare Research and Quality clinical practice guidelines: how quickly do guidelines become outdated? *JAMA* 2001;286:1461–1467.
123. Bradley, EH, Holmboe ES, Mattera JA, et al. A qualitative study of increasing beta-blocker use after myocardial infarction. *JAMA* 2001;285:2604–2611.
124. Eisenberg JM. *Doctors' decisions and the cost of medical care: the reasons for doctors' practice patterns and ways to change them.* Ann Arbor, MI: Health Administration Press, 1986.
125. Greco PJ, Eisenberg JM. Changing physicians' practices. *N Engl J Med* 1993;329:1271–1273.
126. Bero LA, Grilli R, Grimshaw JM, et al. Closing the gap between research and practice: an overview of systematic reviews of interventions to promote the implementation of research findings. *BMJ* 1998;317:465–468.
127. Thomas MA, Oxman AD, Davis DA, et al. *Audit and feedback to improve health professional practice and health care outcomes (part 2).* Oxford: Cochrane Library, 1998.
128. Thomas MA, Oxman AD, Davis DA, et al. *Outreach visits to improve professional practice and health care outcomes.* Oxford: Cochrane Library, 1998.
129. Thomas MA, Oxman AD, Davis DA, et al. *Audit and feedback to improve health professional practice and health care outcomes (part 1).* Oxford: Cochrane Library, 1998.
130. Thomas MA, Oxman AD, Haynes RB, et al. *Local opinion leaders to improve health professional practice and health care outcomes.* Oxford: Cochrane Library, 1998.
131. Miller GE. Continuing education for what? *J Med Educ* 1967;42:320–326.
132. Davis DA, Thomson MA, Oxman AD, et al. Evidence for the effectiveness of CME: a review of 50 randomized controlled trials. *JAMA* 1992; 268:1111–1117.
133. Davis DA, Thomson MA, Oxman AD, et al. Changing physician performance: a systematic review of the effect of continuing medical education strategies. *JAMA* 1995;274:700–705.
134. Soumerai SB, Avorn J. Principles of educational outreach ("academic detailing") to improve clinical decision making. *JAMA* 1990;263:549–556.
135. Soumerai SB, McLaughlin TJ, Gurwitz JH, et al. Effect of local medical opinion leaders on quality of care for acute myocardial infarction: a randomized controlled trial. *JAMA* 1998;279:1358–1363.
136. Winkens RA, Pop P, Bugter-Maessen AM, et al. Randomised controlled trial of routine individual feedback to improve rationality and reduce numbers of test requests. *Lancet* 1995;345:498–502.
137. Meyer TJ, Van Kooten D, Marsh S, et al. Reduction of polypharmacy by feedback to clinicians. *J Gen Intern Med* 1991;6:133–136.
138. Martin AR, Wolf MA, Thibodeau LA, et al. A trial of two strategies to modify the test-ordering behavior of medical residents. *N Engl J Med* 1980; 303:1330–1336.
139. Manheim LM, Feinglass J, Hughes R, et al. Training house officers to be cost conscious: effects of an educational intervention on charges and length of stay. *Med Care* 1990;28:29–42.
140. Gehlbach SH, Wilkinson WE, Hammond WE, et al. Improving drug prescribing in a primary care practice. *Med Care* 1984;22:193–201.
141. Boekeloo BO, Becker DM, Levine DM, et al. Strategies for increasing house staff management of cholesterol with inpatients. *Am J Prev Med* 1990; 6(suppl 2):51–59.
142. Classen DC. Clinical decision support systems to improve clinical practice and quality of care. *JAMA* 1998;280:1360–1361.
143. Donabedian A. *The definition of quality and approaches to its assessment (explorations in quality assessment and monitoring).* Ann Arbor, MI: Health Administration Press, 1980.
144. Donabedian A. Evaluating the quality of medical care. *Milbank Mem Fund Q* 1966;44(suppl):166–206.
145. Mehta RH, Montoye CK, Faul J, et al., for the American College of Cardiology Guidelines Applied in Practice Steering Committee. Enhancing quality of care for acute myocardial infarction: shifting the focus of improvement from key indicators to process of care and tool use. *J Am Coll Cardiol* 2004; 43:2166–2173.
146. DW Bates, AA Gawande. Error in medicine: what have we learned? *Ann Intern Med* 2000;132:763–767.

147. Johnston ME, Langton KB, Haynes RB, et al. Effects of computer-based clinical decision support systems on clinician performance and patient outcome: a critical appraisal of research. *Ann Intern Med* 1994;120:135–142.
148. Chodorow S. Educators must take the electronic revolution seriously. *Acad Med* 1996;71:221–226.
149. Masys DR. Advances in information technology: implications for medical education. *West J Med* 1998;168:341–347.
150. Bates DW, Leape LL, Cullen DJ, et al. Effect of computerized physician order entry and a team intervention on prevention of serious medication errors. *JAMA* 1998;280:1311–1316.
151. Berwick DM. Continuous improvement as an ideal in health care. *N Engl J Med* 1989;320:53–56.
152. Koppel R, Metlay JP, Cohen A, et al. Role of computerized physician order entry systems in facilitating medication errors. *JAMA* 2005;293:1197–1203.
153. Laffel G, Blumenthal D. The case for using industrial quality management science in health care organizations. *JAMA* 1989;262:2869–2873.
154. Blumenthal D, Kilo CM. A report card on continuous quality improvement. *Milbank Q* 1998;76:625–648.
155. Shortell SM, Bennett CL, Byck GR. Assessing the impact of continuous quality improvement on clinical practice: what it will take to accelerate progress. *Milbank Q* 1998;76:593–624.
156. Batalden PB, Mohr JJ. Building knowledge of health care as a system. *Qual Manag Health Care* 1997;5:1–12.
157. Fonarow GC, Gawlinski A, Moughrabi S, et al. Improved treatment of coronary heart disease by implementation of a Cardiac Hospitalization Atherosclerosis Management Program (CHAMP). *Am J Cardiol* 2001;87:819–822.
158. Mehta RH, Montoye CK, Gallogly M, et al., for the GAP Steering Committee of the American College of Cardiology. Improving quality of care for acute myocardial infarction: The Guidelines Applied in Practice (GAP) Initiative. *JAMA* 2002;287:1269–1276.
159. National Registry of Myocardial Infarction (NRMI) Web site. Available at: www.nrmi.org/index.html. Accessed September 8, 2005.
160. *Get with the guidelines* home page. American Heart Association Web site. Available at: www.americanheart.org/presenter.jhtml?identifier=1165. Accessed September 8, 2005.
161. Roe MT, Ohman EM, Pollack CV, et al. Changing the model of care for patients with acute coronary syndromes: implementing practice guidelines and altering physician behavior. *Am Heart J* 2003;146:605–612.
162. Brindis RG, Fitzgerald S, Anderson HV, et al. The American College of Cardiology-National Cardiovascular Data Registry (ACC-NCDR): building a national clinical data repository. *J Am Coll Cardiol* 2001;37:2240–2245.
163. Ferguson TB Jr, Peterson ED, Coombs LP, et al., for the Society of Thoracic Surgeons and the National Cardiac Database. Use of continuous quality improvement to increase use of process measures in patients undergoing coronary artery bypass graft surgery: a randomized controlled trial. *JAMA* 2003:290;49–56.
164. Fonarow GC, Gawlinski A, Moughrabi S, Tillisch JH. Improved treatment of coronary heart disease by implementation of a Cardiac Hospitalization Atherosclerosis Management Program (CHAMP). *Am J Cardiol* 2001;87:819–822.
165. Hoekstra JT, Pollack CV Jr, Roe MT, et al. Improving the care of patients with non–ST-elevation acute coronary syndromes in the emergency department: the CRUSADE initiative. *Acad Emerg Med* 2002;9:1146–1155.
166. Smaha LA. American Heart Association: the American Heart Association Get with the Guidelines program. *Am Heart J* 2004;148(5 Suppl):S46–S48.
167. Dehmer GJ, Elma M, Hewitt K, et al. Bringing measurement and management science to the cath laboratory: the National Cardiovascular Data Registry (ACC-NCDR) and the Cardiac Catheterization Laboratory Continuous Quality Improvement Toolkit (ACC-CathKIT). *J Cardiovasc Manag* 2004;15:20–26.
168. Schneider EC, Epstein AM. Influence of cardiac-surgery performance reports on referral practices and access to care: a survey of cardiovascular specialists. *N Engl J Med* 1996;335:251–256.
169. Naylor CD. Public profiling of clinical performance. *JAMA* 2002;287:1323–1325.
170. Hannan EL, Siu AL, Kumar D, et al. Assessment of coronary artery bypass graft surgery performance in New York: is there a bias against taking high-risk patients? *Med Care* 1997;35:49–56.
171. Landro L. Booster shot: to get doctors to do better, health plans try cash bonuses. *Wall Street Journal* September 17, 2004:A1.
172. Roland M. Linking physicians' pay to the quality of care: a major experiment in the United Kingdom. *N Engl J Med* 2004;351:1448–1454.
173. Fox E, Tulsky JA. Recommendations for the ethical conduct of quality improvement. *J Clin Ethics* 2005;16:61–71.
174. Blumenthal D, Epstein AM. Part 6: the role of physicians in the future of quality management. *N Engl J Med* 1996;335:1328–1331.
175. Teistein PS. Credentialing for coronary interventions: practice makes perfect. *Circulation* 1997;95:2467–2470.
176. Ellis SG, Weintraub W, Holmes D, et al. Relation of operator volume and experience to procedural outcome of percutaneous coronary revascularization at hospitals with high interventional volumes. *Circulation* 1997;96:2479–2484.
177. Jollis JG, Peterson ED, Nelson CL, et al. Relationship between physician and hospital coronary angioplasty volume and outcome in elderly patients. *Circulation* 1997;95:2485–2491.
178. Firshein J. US employers ignore hospital mortality data. *Lancet* 1997;349:1459.
179. Green J, Wintfeld N, Krasner M, et al. In search of America's best hospitals: the promise and reality of quality assessment. *J Am Coll Cardiol* 1997;277:1152–1155.
180. Carlsen W. Physicians' files could be unsealed: assembly considers opening records. *San Francisco Chronicle* May 5, 1997:A1.
181. Iezzoni LI. How much are we willing to pay for information about quality of care? *Ann Intern Med* 1997;126:391–393.
182. Taylor Jr DH, Whellan DJ, Sloan FA. Effects of admission to a teaching hospital on the cost and quality of care for Medicare beneficiaries. *N Engl J Med* 1999;340:293–299.
183. Iezzoni LI. The risks of risk adjustment. *JAMA* 1997;278:1600–1607.
184. Hofer TP, Hayward RA, Greenfield S, et al. The unreliability of individual physician "report cards" for assessing the costs and quality of care of a chronic disease. *JAMA* 1999;281:2098–2105.
185. Bindman AB. Can physician profiles be trusted? *JAMA* 1999;281:2142–2143.
186. Davies HTO, Marshall MN. Public disclosure of performance data: does the public get what the public wants? *Lancet* 1999;353:1639–1640.
187. Baldwin L-M, Hart LG, Oshel RE, et al. Hospital peer review and the National Practitioner Data Bank: clinical privileges action reports. *JAMA* 1999;282:349–355.
188. Epstein AM. Public release of performance data: a progress report from the front. *JAMA* 2000;283:1884–1886.
189. Schneider EC, Epstein AM. Use of public performance reports: a survey of patients undergoing cardiac surgery. *JAMA* 1998;279:1638–1642.
190. Marshall MN, Shekelle PG, Leatherman S, et al. The public release of performance data: what do we expect to gain? A review of the evidence. *JAMA* 2000;283:1866–1874.
191. Peabody JW, Luck J, Glassman P, et al. Comparison of vignettes, standardized patients, and chart abstraction: a prospective validation study of 3 methods for measuring quality. *JAMA* 2000;283:1715–1722.
192. Shine KI. Closing the gap in quality health care for Americans. *Circulation* 2000;101:2325–2327.
193. Bodenheimer T. The American health care system: the movement for improved quality in health care. *N Engl J Med* 1999;340:488–492.
194. Rawlins M. In pursuit of quality: the National Institute for Clinical Excellence. *Lancet* 1999;353:1079–1082.
195. O'Connor GT, Eagle KA. How do we know how well we are doing? *J Am Coll Cardiol* 1998;32:1000–1001.
196. Bodenheimer T. The American health care system: physicians and the changing medical marketplace. *N Engl J Med* 1999;340:584–588.
197. Bernstein SJ, Brorsson B, Åberg T, et al., on behalf of the SECOR/SBU Project Group. Appropriateness of referral of coronary angiography patients in Sweden. *Heart* 1999;81:470–477.
198. Shekelle PG. Are appropriateness criteria ready for use in clinical practice? *N Engl J Med* 2001;344:677–678.
199. Bindman AB. Can physician profiles be trusted? *JAMA* 1999;281:2142–2143.
200. Wass V, Van der Vleuten C, Shatzer J, et al. Assessment of clinical competence. *Lancet* 2001;357:945–949.
201. Casalino LP. The unintended consequences of measuring quality on the quality of medical care. *N Engl J Med* 1999;341:1147–1150.

SECTION THREE
CARDIOVASCULAR IMAGING

JAMES THOMAS, MD

CHAPTER 46 ■ PRINCIPLES OF IMAGING

JAMES D. THOMAS

OVERVIEW

Accurate imaging is essential for assessing cardiac anatomy, function, perfusion, and metabolism. Revolutionary advances have been made in the last 20 years primarily because of improvements in computer technology and digital signal processing. The heart can be imaged by using x-rays (radiography, angiography, computed tomography), γ-rays (radionuclide imaging, positron emission technology), sound waves (Doppler echocardiography), and the magnetic properties of the hydrogen nucleus (magnetic resonance imaging). Tests can be compared in terms of their ability to detect and exclude disease (sensitivity and specificity, respectively), but the predictive value of a test depends largely on the prevalence of the disorder in the population being tested (Bayesian analysis). Computer processing is important both in generating images and in enhancing the images for display (smoothing and edge enhancement); Fourier transformation is commonly used to analyze the frequency content of images and data in Doppler echocardiography, magnetic resonance imaging, and radionuclide ventriculography. Digital image storage is becoming feasible with reductions in computer costs and agreement on the Digital Imaging and Communications in Medicine (DICOM) standard for medical image exchange created by the National Electrical Manufacturers Association (NEMA). The massive storage requirements can be reduced by careful clinical editing of studies and with digital compression algorithms. All-digital storage and transmission will greatly enhance the value of cardiac studies and facilitate telemedicine.

GLOSSARY

Convolution: Altering a pixel based on the values of surrounding pixels.

DICOM: Digital Imaging and Communications in Medicine, a formatting standard to that allows the exchange of medical images.

Digital compression: Recording an image to so that it requires less storage. *Lossless* compression does not change the appearance at all but yields little compression, whereas *lossy* compression yields greater savings but with some alteration of the image.

Doppler principle: The principle according to which waves, including ultrasound signals, have their frequency shifted in proportion to the velocity of the object emitting them, in the present context, blood velocity.

Fourier analysis: Analysis of the frequency content of an image or signal.

γ-Rays: High-energy photons produced by nuclear decay.

Nuclear magnetic resonance: Spinning or precessing of certain nuclei (typically the hydrogen proton) in the presence of a magnetic field.

Photons: "Particles" of electromagnetic radiation.

Piezoelectric: A property of matter by which electricity is converted into vibration and vice versa.

Point processing: Altering an image gray scale, pixel by pixel.

Positrons: Positive electrons (antimatter); when a positron encounters an electron, both are annihilated and two 511-keV photons are emitted in opposite directions; the process is the physical basis for positron emission tomography.

x-Rays: High-energy photons produced by rearrangement of an atom's electron cloud.

INTRODUCTION

The fine structure and complex motion of the heart demands imaging modalities with higher temporal and spatial resolution than that needed for any other organ. Fortunately, research over the last 50 years has led to dramatic improvements in our ability to characterize and quantify disorders of the cardiovascular system. The chapters in this section of the book describe the clinical aspects of the major cardiovascular imaging modalities. As a prelude, this chapter describes many of the concepts common to these techniques, including image generation, computer processing, assessment of diagnostic accuracy, and the emerging area of digital storage and transmission. An understanding of the physical background of these methods will help the reader to understand better the clinical applications described in later chapters.

Here we consider four broad ways to acquire images of the heart: x-ray transmission, radionuclide emission, ultrasonic reflection, and nuclear magnetic resonance. Although these techniques share many features, together they span virtually all of classical and quantum physics. This chapter can only touch on these topics, and the reader is referred to a number of excellent texts for greater detail (1–13).

What Is Imaging?

In a broad sense, imaging displays the differential interaction of energy with matter to discern structure or function. For instance, radiography exploits the fact that more x-rays are absorbed by bone than by soft tissue, and echocardiography displays the reflection of ultrasonic energy from the border of two tissues with different acoustic impedances. Radionuclide techniques are slightly different in that they deliver an energy source (the radioactive compound) to the body, where it is concentrated in structures of interest and then localized by external detectors. Magnetic resonance imaging defines the differential distribution of weak magnetic characteristics within the body.

Basic Concepts

A number of terms and concepts are common to all imaging modalities.

Resolution

Spatial resolution refers to the smallest separation at which two objects can be distinguished. For example, spatial resolution is measured in radiography with a grid of finely spaced lines and specified as the number of line pairs per centimeter, a relatively constant number across the field of view. Echocardiography typically has greater resolution in the near field than in the far field because of the divergence of the ultrasound beam and is *anisotropic,* better in the axial direction (along a scan line) than in the lateral direction (across scan lines). One must distinguish the physical resolution of the imaging modality from the resolution of the display. The spacing of the picture elements (pixels) on the screen may be greater or lesser than the physical resolution and is stated as the number of pixels in the horizontal and vertical directions (640 × 480 is typical for echocardiography, 1024 × 1024 for high-resolution digital angiography, and 2048 × 2048 or even higher for digital radiographic and mammographic images). The functional spatial resolution is always the lesser of the physical and screen resolutions.

Temporal resolution refers to the frequency with which an image is generated, usually stated in frames per second. Plain radiographs are typically taken as single images, but temporal resolution may still be relevant because the shutter speed (the time the film is actually exposed to x-rays) determines whether rapid movements (such as prosthetic valve motion) can be "frozen" in the image. There often is a trade-off between temporal and spatial resolution. Echocardiograms can be generated more frequently at the expense of fewer scan lines per image, whereas multigated nuclear scans can be divided into shorter temporal "bins," but this reduces the amount of data available for each image, reducing the signal-to-noise ratio and spatial resolution. Velocity resolution refers to the smallest difference in velocity that can be discerned.

Dimensionality

The heart can be considered a four-dimensional (4D) structure, possessing three spatial dimensions and one temporal one. Most imaging modalities have two spatial dimensions (i.e., a picture, like a radiograph or an echocardiographic image), but some magnetic resonance, computed tomographic, nuclear, and echocardiographic studies are intrinsically three dimensional, although the display may be on a 2D screen.

Transmission versus Tomographic Imaging

Two-dimensional images of the heart can be generated by either *transmission* or *tomographic* techniques. In transmission imaging, the full thickness of the heart is projected onto a screen, whereas a tomogram displays structures lying within a single plane of the heart. For most applications, tomographic imaging (used in magnetic resonance imaging [MRI], computed tomography [CT], echocardiography, and many nuclear tests) is preferable because there is no interference from overlying structures. For angiography, however, transmission imaging is actually an advantage because the full course of the vessel can be visualized, something no single tomographic plane could do. Indeed, in MR and CT angiography, the 3D data set is projected onto a plane to generate a transmission image for easier diagnosis.

IMAGING WITH ELECTROMAGNETIC RADIATION: X-RAYS AND γ-RAYS

Although radiography uses x-rays delivered externally to image the body and nuclear imaging uses γ-rays produced inside the body, there actually is no physical difference between x-rays and γ-rays, both being forms of high-energy electromagnetic radiation. By definition, γ-rays are produced by radioactive decay within the atomic nucleus, whereas x-rays are produced by processes in the electron cloud surrounding the nucleus. Electromagnetic radiation can be thought of as a wave with frequency f and wavelength λ, the product of which is equal to the speed of light (299,792 km/sec). It can also be thought of as a stream of discrete massless particles (*photons*) propagating at the speed of light with an energy proportional to the frequency and usually expressed in units of the electron volt (eV), the energy acquired by an electron when it is accelerated by 1 volt. Figure 46.1 illustrates these concepts, and Table 46.1 shows typical values for a range of electromagnetic radiation. It is important to remember that neither the particle nor the wave nature of electromagnetic radiation is "correct." Both are correct all of the time, although in practice, one aspect or the other is typically more evident. Indeed, quantum mechanics has even taught us that particles such as the electron can have wavelike properties.

Interaction of x-Rays and γ-Rays with Matter

Radiography depends on the differential absorption and scattering of photons by various types of tissue. In nuclear imaging, by contrast, nuclide distribution in the body is the primary

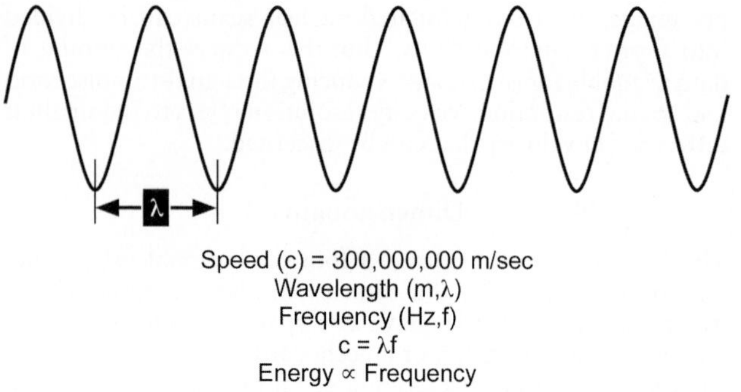

FIGURE 46.1. Parameters of electromagnetic radiation. In the wave representation of electromagnetic radiation, key parameters are the wavelength λ (in meters) and frequency f (in hertz), the product of which is the speed of light $c = 300{,}000{,}000$ m/sec. In the particle representation, the key parameter is photon energy, which is proportional to frequency.

determinant, although photon scattering is a major cause of image degradation. For photons in the 50- to 500-keV range (those of principal diagnostic importance), there are two major interactions with matter to consider: the *photoelectric effect* and *Compton scattering*. In the photoelectric effect, a photon is completely absorbed by an atom (the desired response), whereas in Compton scattering, the original photon is not completely absorbed, but rather is scattered at a lower energy and at a different angle from the original direction and thus can degrade the image, striking the x-ray film in random locations. This scattering can be partially ameliorated by a placing collimating grid in front of the film to admit only photons traveling in a straight line from the x-ray source (Fig. 46.2), but it is harder to exclude these scattered photons in nuclear imaging.

The likelihood of the photoelectric effect (PE) is inversely proportional to the third power of the photon energy E and directly proportional to the fourth power of the atomic number Z (number of protons) of the interacting atom: $PE \approx Z^4/E^3$. For soft tissue (average $Z \approx 5$), virtually all interaction is caused by Compton scattering above an energy of 80 keV (typical for a diagnostic x ray or thallium decay). By comparison, the Z dependence is exploited in iodinated contrast agents and sodium iodide detectors for nuclear medicine; because iodine has a Z of 53, the photoelectric effect is dominant up to photon energies of 300 keV.

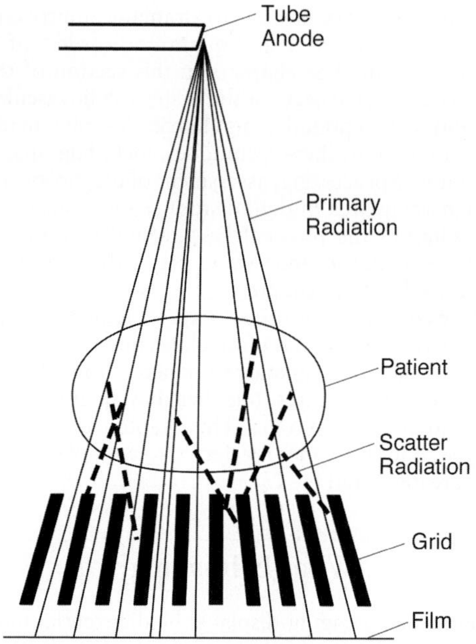

FIGURE 46.2. Exclusion of Compton-scattered photons by a collimating grid. The grid is oriented so that only photons that emanated from the x-ray tube will pass on to the film or detector, thereby excluding photons that are Compton-scattered in other directions.

Photon Attenuation

Thus, Compton scattering and the photoelectric effect remove a certain percentage of photons for each centimeter of tissue they pass through, as determined by the linear attenuation coefficient μ (cm^{-1}) of the tissue, and this causes the intensity of an x-ray beam to decrease exponentially with distance traveled through the body. The value of μ varies for different tissues in the body, being low for lung, intermediate for soft tissue, and high for bone and radiographic contrast media such as barium and iodine. The 2D image that results from the passage of x-rays thus has lost all information about the distribution of matter along the x-ray path. Computer tomographic techniques must be used to reconstruct the 3D distribution of μ.

Note that in radiography, all diagnostic information results from differential attenuation of x-rays passing through the body, whereas in nuclear medicine, attenuation degrades the image and should be minimized or compensated for.

TABLE 46.1

ELECTROMAGNETIC RADIATION

Radiation	Frequency (Hz)	Wavelength (m)	Energy (eV)
AM radio	1.00×10^6	300	4.14×10^{-9}
^{1}H in 1-T field	4.26×10^7	7.04	1.76×10^{-7}
FM radio	1.00×10^8	3.00	4.14×10^{-7}
Microwave oven	2.45×10^9	1.22×10^{-1}	1.01×10^{-5}
Infrared	4.29×10^{14}	7.00×10^{-7}	1.78
Green light	6.00×10^{14}	5.00×10^{-7}	2.48
Ultraviolet	1.00×10^{15}	3.00×10^{-7}	4.13
Diagnostic x-ray	1.45×10^{19}	2.07×10^{-11}	6.00×10^4
^{99m}Tc γ-ray	3.38×10^{19}	8.87×10^{-12}	1.40×10^5
β^+, β^- γ-ray	1.23×10^{20}	2.43×10^{-12}	5.11×10^5
Therapeutic γ-ray	4.80×10^{21}	6.25×10^{-14}	2.00×10^7
Cosmic rays	6.00×10^{21}	5.00×10^{-14}	2.49×10^7

The distinctive features of radiography and nuclear medicine will now be discussed.

Imaging with x-Rays

The signal-to-noise ratio in an x-ray image is related to the difference in attenuation coefficient between the object of interest and the background, as well as the number of photons passing through the body. How may resolution be improved? An obvious solution is to do something to increase the attenuation difference, $\Delta\mu$, such as infusing iodinated contrast medium into a vessel. Increasing the density of the incident photons (by increasing the current in the x-ray tube or lengthening the pulse) will help some but not much; it takes about a 16-fold increase in photon density to improve the resolution by a factor of 2. One may also reduce attenuation by increasing x-ray energy, but this effect must be balanced against the reduction in $\Delta\mu$, which also typically occurs with increasing photon energy.

Geometric Limits to x-Ray Image Resolution

Figure 46.3 illustrates how the second major determinant of x-ray image quality relates to the finite size of the x-ray source. Typically x-rays arise from a small spot, perhaps 1 mm^2 in area, but even this may blur the image. For a focal spot *a* centimeters in diameter positioned *A* centimeters from the patient with the film *B* centimeters from the patient, the width of blurring will be *aB*/*A*. To minimize this, one seeks as small a focal spot as possible, but heating of the x-ray tube limits this. Similarly, *B* should be as small as possible, but this is usually dictated by patient size. Finally, resolution can be improved by positioning the focal spot as far from the patient as possible (large *A*), but because x-ray density declines as $1/A^2$, a trade-off exists between signal-to-noise ratio and blurring.

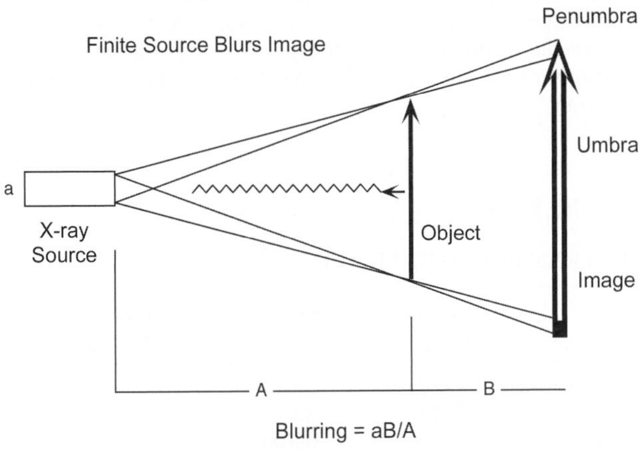

FIGURE 46.3. Geometric limits to x-ray resolution. The finite size *a* of the x-ray source leads to a penumbra around solid objects of *aB*/*A*. (Adapted from Fozzard HA, Haber E, Jennings RB, et al., eds. *The heart and cardiovascular system. Scientific foundations*, 2nd ed. New York: Raven Press, 1992:630.)

Nuclear Imaging

Nuclear imaging uses trace quantities of radioactive isotopes to produce high-energy photons inside the body. The internal distribution of the radioactive compound is based on its chemical properties, which give it an affinity for specific anatomic or pathologic structures (e.g., bone, blood, myocardium). Localization and quantification of photon production gives diagnostic information about these structures.

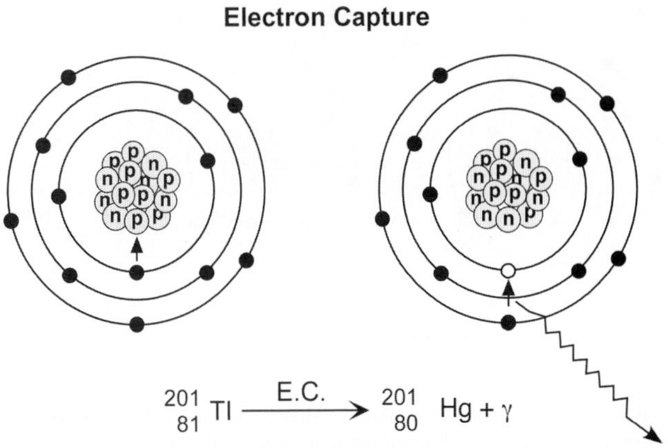

FIGURE 46.4. Photon emission by electron capture (E.C.). See text for details. (Adapted from Fozzard HA, Haber E, Jennings RB, et al., eds. *The heart and cardiovascular system. Scientific foundations*, 2nd ed. New York: Raven Press, 1992:630.)

In general, the isotopes of nuclear medicine can be divided into two broad types, those that produce single photons when they disintegrate and those that produce pairs of oppositely directed photons.

Single-Photon Production

A common way to produce single photons is electron capture (Fig. 46.4), whereby a nuclear proton captures an inner-shell electron, converting the proton to a neutron. Typical of this class of decay is thallium, ${}^{201}{}_{81}Tl$, which captures an electron and becomes mercury, ${}^{201}{}_{80}Hg$. As an outer electron falls to fill the vacancy in the lower-energy inner shell, it releases an x-ray, usually of 80 keV.

Another single-photon scheme is β-decay (Fig. 46.5), in which a nuclear neutron becomes a proton by emitting an electron (β-particle) and an antineutrino. As the nucleus "reshuffles," a γ-ray is emitted, but this may occur after some delay. This *isomeric transition* is used by the important cardiac imaging isotope technetium-99m, where the "m" stands for metastable.

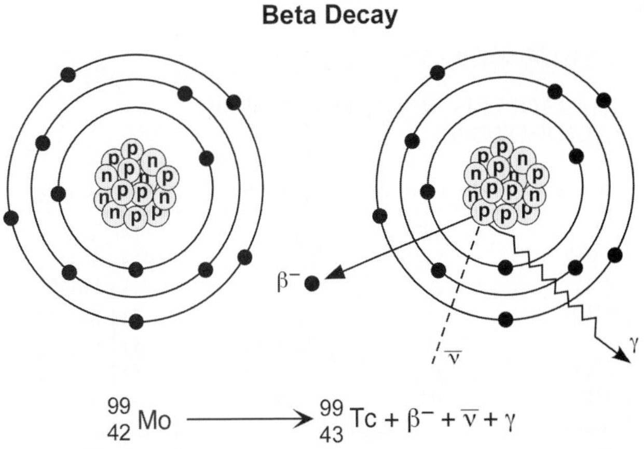

FIGURE 46.5. Photon emission by beta decay. See text for details. (Adapted from Fozzard HA, Haber E, Jennings RB, et al., eds. *The heart and cardiovascular system. Scientific foundations*, 2nd ed. New York: Raven Press, 1992:632.)

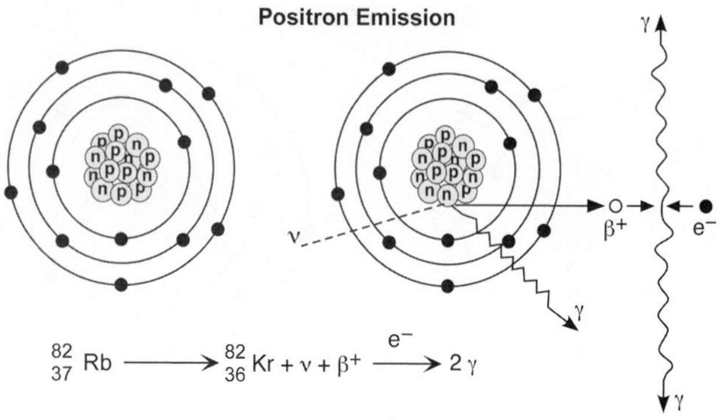

FIGURE 46.6. Positron emission. This is similar to beta decay, except that a positively charged electron is emitted, which is rapidly annihilated, producing two high-energy (511 keV) photons directed in opposite directions. See text for details. (Adapted from Fozzard HA, Haber E, Jennings RB, et al., eds. *The heart and cardiovascular system. Scientific foundations*, 2nd ed. New York: Raven Press, 1992:632.)

Dual-Photon Production

All dual-γ-ray isotopes decay by *positron emission*, in which a nuclear proton turns into a neutron and a positive electron (positron) (Fig. 46.6), which travels only a very short distance before it collides with an electron, a process that annihilates both. The mass of the two particles is completely converted into energy (in accord with $E = mc^2$), which results in two 511-keV photons being emitted in opposite directions.

Table 46.2 lists the decay mechanism and photon energy of several important isotopes.

Radioactive Decay Rates

The number of disintegrations per second in an isotope is proportional to the amount of the isotope and to a decay constant λ, the likelihood of a given atom decaying per second. Another common term is the half-time $t_{1/2}$, the time required for half of the isotope to decay, related to λ by $t_{1/2} = 0.693/\lambda$. The half-time of an isotope has important practical and safety impacts. If $t_{1/2}$ is too long, then a large dose of the isotope will be needed to get adequate images, leading to excessive long-term exposure unless the compound is cleared from the body chemically (e.g., via the kidneys). If $t_{1/2}$ is too short, however, the isotope may be impossible to transport: Many positron emitters have a $t_{1/2}$ measured in minutes and must be generated by an on-site cyclotron.

TABLE 46.2

CHARACTERISTICS OF DIAGNOSTIC RADIOISOTOPES

Isotope	Decay mode	Half-life	Photon energy
^{99m}Tc	IT	6.0 h	140 keV
^{201}Tl	EC	73.0 h	69–83 keV
^{133}Xe	β^-	5.3 d	81 keV
^{82}Rb	β^+	1.25 min	511 keV (2)
^{11}C	β^+	20.5 min	511 keV (2)
^{15}O	β^+	2.0 min	511 keV (2)
^{18}F	β^+	1.8 h	511 keV (2)

Photon energies are for the principal decay mode. There usually are other emissions of lower frequency.
IT, isomeric transition; EC, electron capture; β^-, β^-emission; β^+, positron emission.

Imaging the Emitted γ-Rays

The Anger γ-camera uses a large sodium iodide (NaI) crystal that emits light by the photoelectric effect in proportion to the energy of an impinging high-energy photon. This provides a means of not only counting the photons but also of identifying the isotopes from which they arise. When a scintillation event occurs, it is "seen" by several photomultiplier tubes behind the NaI crystal, triangulating the position of the discharge before computer storage.

To exclude the undesirable Compton-scattered photons (up to 50% of photons escaping the body) requires a collimator, such as a pin hole in a sheet of lead. Although this gives reasonable image resolution, it is extremely inefficient and may capture only 1 photon in 10,000 produced in the heart. Multihole collimators help somewhat, although with a trade-off between resolution and sensitivity.

Scattered photons may also be excluded on the basis of their energy. If the primary photon radiation from an isotope is in a narrow range, it should be possible to ignore lower-energy Compton photons, but this is more feasible for high-energy photons, as in positron emission tomography (PET) imaging, than for thallium or technetium.

Imaging positron emitters can be done more precisely because two high-energy photons are emitted simultaneously in opposite directions, aiding in localization (14). Technical aspects of this are described in Chapter 55.

IMAGING WITH ULTRASOUND

We now turn from imaging modalities that use high-energy photons to the use of high-frequency sound waves, which have a much longer wavelength and slower propagation than the photons considered previously. In addition, the speed of sound c is not constant like the speed of light, but varies with the medium through which it is passing. For typical soft tissue, this speed is about 1,540 m/sec, or 1.54 mm/μs (Table 46.3). As with electromagnetic radiation, there is an inverse relationship between wavelength λ and frequency f: $\lambda = c/f$.

Production of Ultrasound

Typical ultrasonic transducers have frequencies from 2.5 to 15 MHz, corresponding to wavelengths from 0.6 to 0.1 mm, respectively. They produce ultrasonic vibrations by the piezoelectric effect, in which a ceramic crystal vibrates when a high voltage is applied across it (Fig. 46.7). When ultrasound strikes the transducer, the opposite occurs as the induced vibrations cause an electrical signal that can be detected for imaging.

TABLE 46.3

ULTRASONIC PARAMETERS

Tissue	Velocity (m/sec)	Attenuation (cm^{-1})	Impedance (10^4 kg/m^2 s)
Blood	1580	0.0198	1.6
Bone	2240	3.01	3.8–7.4
Fat	1450	0.100	1.4
Muscle	1580	0.193	1.7
Lung			0.26
Plasma		0.0069	1.5
Water	1480		

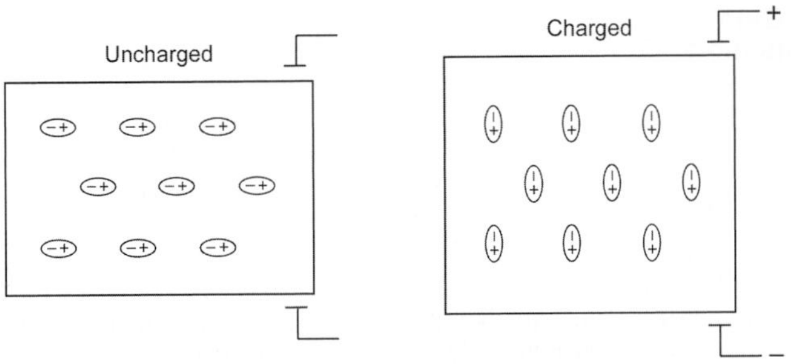

FIGURE 46.7. Piezoelectric crystal. When a voltage is applied across the crystal, the highly polarized molecular dipoles rotate, causing the crystal to thicken and produce ultrasound. Conversely, when ultrasound is received, the mechanical vibration of these structures produces an output voltage. (Adapted from Fozzard HA, Haber E, Jennings RB, et al., eds. *The heart and cardiovascular system. Scientific foundations*, 2nd ed. New York: Raven Press, 1992:635.)

Interaction of Ultrasound with Matter

The important interactions to consider are attenuation, reflection, refraction, and scattering. Like electromagnetic radiation, ultrasound suffers an exponential decrease in amplitude as it passes through homogeneous tissue. Attenuation varies with tissue type (Table 46.3) and is faster at higher frequencies, limiting the frequency that can be used clinically in echocardiography (15).

Whenever a sound wave encounters a boundary between two types of tissue, the energy is partially reflected and the remainder is transmitted into the second tissue, the proportion being determined by the difference in acoustic impedance Z of the two tissues, defined as the product of sound velocity c and tissue density ρ: $Z = \rho c$. For relatively large, flat boundaries, the amount of reflected energy I_R is given by $I_R = I_i\,[(Z_2 - Z_1)/(Z_2 + Z_1)]^2$, where I_i is the incident intensity and Z_1 and Z_2 are the respective impedances for the two tissues (16) (Table 46.3). Boundaries with a large difference in impedance reflect much more energy than those between tissues with similar acoustic properties. For instance, the heart–lung interface reflects 54% of the incident ultrasound, whereas the blood–myocardium boundary reflects less than 0.1%.

For interactions with smaller structures than the wavelength of sound, *scattering* occurs; the small object radiates sound outward as 3D spherical waves. Scattering intensity varies approximately with the sixth power of particle radius and the fourth power of ultrasound frequency, strongly favoring larger particles and higher frequency. Scattering occurs within tissue at inhomogeneities between cellular and matrix elements that are not simple point scatterers. Furthermore, these sources are so close to each other that the reflected waves interfere with each other producing a complex ultrasound pattern, *speckle*. Because speckle is relatively constant over time, it is possible to track its motion over time to detect tissue deformation and strain (16a).

Echocardiographic Imaging

In echocardiography, short pulses of ultrasound are attenuated, scattered, and refracted as they pass through tissue, with a small amount of energy reflected from deep structures to the transducer. Assuming the velocity of sound c to be constant in soft tissue (1540 m/sec), we find that the depth d of a reflector is given by the time delay Δt between transmission of the ultrasound pulse and receipt of the echo: $d = c\Delta t/2$; the factor of 2

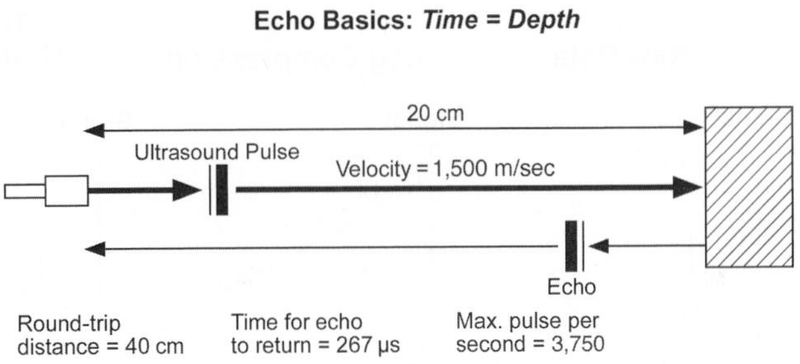

FIGURE 46.8. Basics of echocardiographic imaging. Because of the relatively fixed speed of sound in tissue, the delay in echo return can be translated into the distance to the reflection.

enters because Δt includes time *to* and *from* the object, about 13 μs per centimeter of depth (Fig. 46.8).

Echocardiographic Transducers

Although the original ultrasound transducers were single, flat crystals, most current transducers are linear arrays of 64 to 256 narrow piezoelectric crystals. By precisely timing their firing, it is possible to direct the ultrasound in any direction within a wide sector coplanar with the array (Fig. 46.9) and to adjust the focal zone both on transmission and receiving. Furthermore, by the principle of superposition of sound waves, it is possible to stimulate the array to send out (and receive) multiple ultrasound pulses simultaneously in different directions, dramatically improving ultrasound frame rate by processing multiple scan lines in parallel. Finally, transducer technology has recently been expanded to 2D arrays of crystals, allowing ultrasound pulses to be directed anywhere in a pyramid-shaped volume below the transducer, facilitating real-time 3D imaging.

Ultrasound Reception and Display

When a reflected echo strikes the transducer, the piezoelectric crystal produces a minuscule voltage in response to the vibrations from the returning ultrasound. To adjust for the significantly weaker echoes from deep structures (which vary as much as a billionfold), *logarithmic compression* and *time-gain compensation* apply greater amplification to echoes returning at longer intervals from the echo pulse (Fig. 46.10). The amplified signal is then demodulated to extract the *amplitude* and *phase* information from tissue reflections, allowing objects to be localized and displayed.

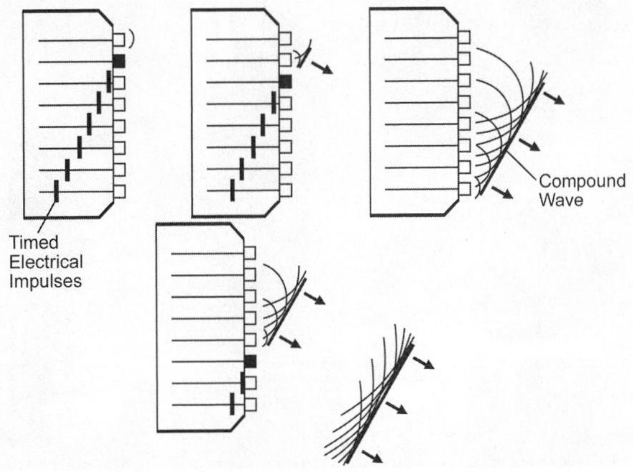

FIGURE 46.9. Phased-array echo transducer. By changing the timing of transmission from a linear array of crystals, it is possible to steer a planar ultrasound wave in different directions.

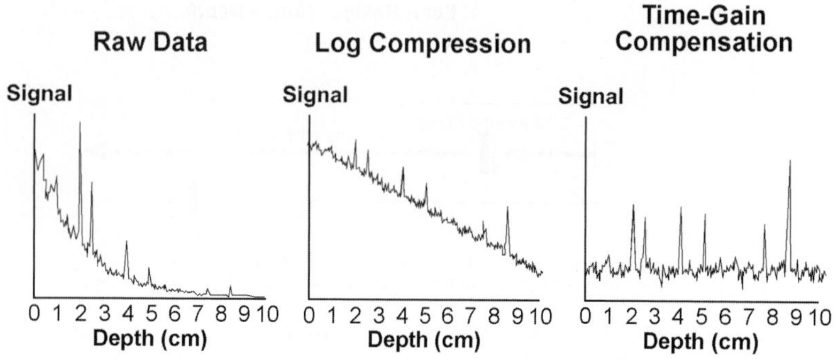

FIGURE 46.10. Scan-line processing. To normalize the billionfold variation in signal strength with depth, logarithmic compression and time-gain compensation must be applied to the returning echoes.

As discussed in the clinical echo chapter, echo signals can be displayed as *M-mode* (a time–distance sweep showing motion of structures along a single scan line) (Fig. 46.11), a *2D* or *sector* scan (moving image of a single plane through the heart), or a surface rendering of a 3D echo (Fig. 46.12).

One of the greatest advances in echocardiographic image quality in the last several years has been the development of tissue harmonic imaging. When ultrasound waves propagate through tissue, their frequency content does not remain constant, but rather shifts to increasing amounts of higher frequencies (17). By imaging the second frequency harmonic, much of the image noise is eliminated. Figure 46.13 shows the impact of harmonic imaging in a patient with mitral stenosis, demonstrating improved endocardial definition and imaging of the subvalvular apparatus. Clinical tests on this modality have shown improved contrast between the wall and cavity (18) without adverse impact on valve thickness (19).

Doppler Echocardiography

Doppler measurement of intracardiac blood velocity adds enormous value to echocardiography (20,21). When sound reflects from moving objects its frequency shifts in proportion to the ratio of object velocity v and sound velocity c: $f_D = 2vf_0/c$, where f_0 is the transducer frequency and f_D is the amount of the Doppler shift. The factor 2 occurs because the frequency is shifted when the sound hits the moving particle and again when it is reradiated by scattering. Only the component of particle velocity parallel to the ultrasound beam affects the Doppler shift. For a particle moving at an angle θ to the scan line, the Doppler shift is proportional to the cosine of θ: 30° misalignment leads to a 13% velocity underestimation.

In general, three different types of Doppler processing are available on contemporary echocardiographic equipment: continuous-wave Doppler, pulsed Doppler, and Doppler flow mapping ("color Doppler").

Continuous-Wave Doppler

In continuous-wave (CW) Doppler, the transducer contains two crystals, one to send, the other to receive ultrasound continuously (Fig. 46.14). The frequency shift is determined by quadrature demodulation and Fourier analysis. In contrast to pulsed Doppler, CW Doppler can quantify high-velocity flow, but gives no information as to where along the scan line the velocity arises.

Pulsed Doppler

In pulsed Doppler, brief (1 to 4 μs) bursts of ultrasound are transmitted with the receiver timed to "listen" to the returning signal at a specific time delay Δt after the pulse transmission, corresponding to reflections from depth $d = c\Delta t/2$ (Fig. 46.15). If the Doppler shift frequency f_D is more than twice the pulse repetition frequency ($1/\Delta t$), then *aliasing* occurs, in which the blood suddenly appears to be moving in the opposite direction. In general, at depth d (in cm) and imaging frequency f_0 (in

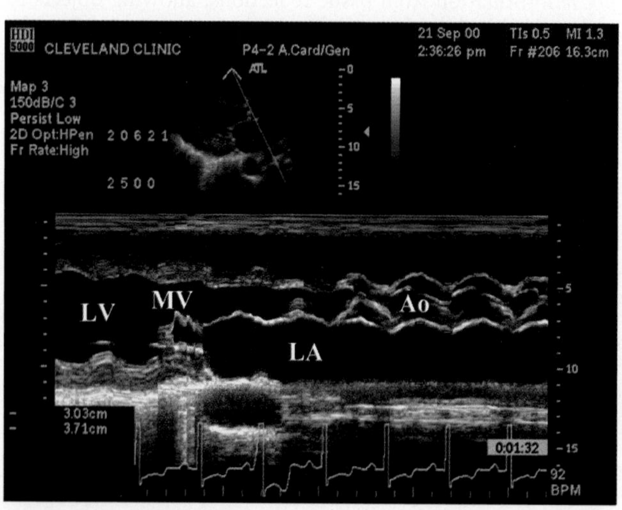

FIGURE 46.11. M-mode echocardiographic imaging. The M-mode display shows depth vertically and time horizontally. Ao, aorta; LA, left atrium; LV, left ventricle; MV, mitral valve.

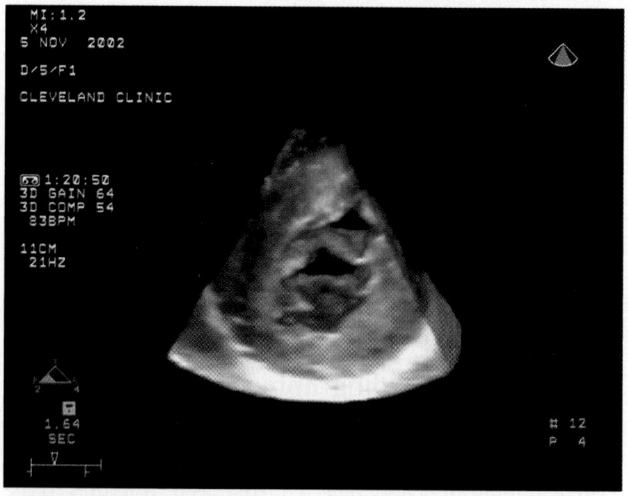

FIGURE 46.12. Three-dimensional echocardiographic imaging. Echocardiographic data can be obtained in solid pyramid of tissue at 20 to 30 volumes per second. This shows surface rendering of a patient with hypertrophic cardiomyopathy.

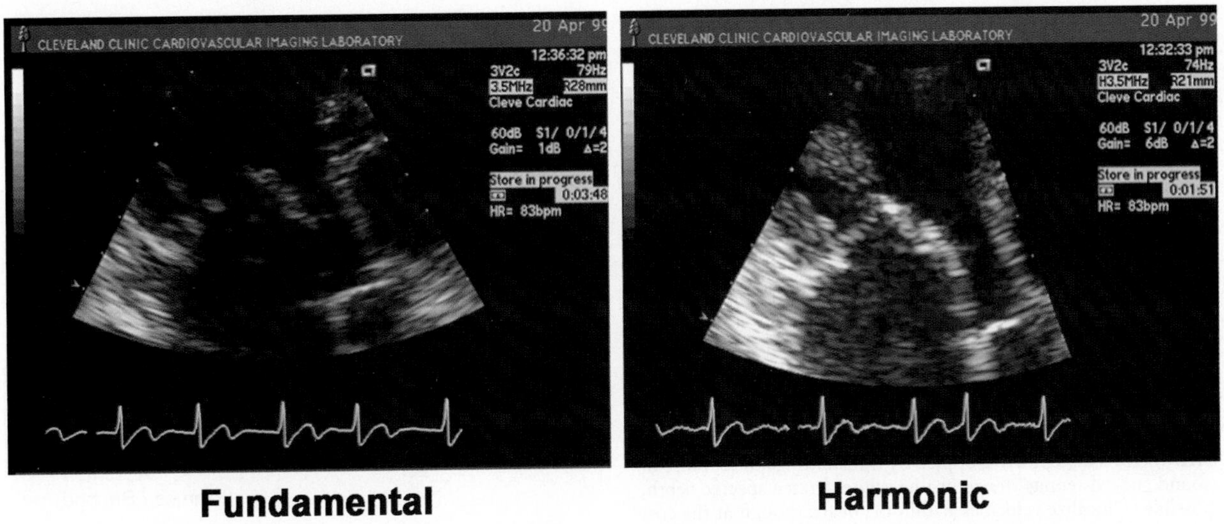

FIGURE 46.13. Harmonic imaging. In this patient with mitral stenosis, harmonic imaging (**right**) shows the endocardial definition and subvalvular apparatus with greater clarity than fundamental imaging (**left**).

MHz), the maximal velocity (in m/sec) that can be resolved unambiguously is approximately $35/df_0$. If flow is known to be in one direction, this velocity can be doubled by shifting the baseline of the display.

Doppler Velocity Mapping

Doppler velocity mapping uses pulsed Doppler to superimpose color on an echo sector scan to show blood velocity throughout the heart, with red directed toward the transducer and blue away; it is useful for imaging valvular regurgitation, stenosis, and various shunt lesions (Fig. 46.16) (22). Because multiple scan lines must be interrogated per frame, frame rate and velocity resolution are limited. Indeed the pulse repetition frequency cannot be exceeded by the product of (a) the frame rate, (b) the number of color scan lines per frame, and (c) the number of pulses per scan line (typically 4 to 10, with higher-quality color given with more pulses) (Fig. 46.17). Parallel processing allows this frame rate to be increased considerably.

MAGNETIC RESONANCE IMAGING

Nuclear magnetic resonance (NMR) is less familiar than electromagnetic and sonic radiation. The first suggestion of microscopic magnetic moments within atomic nuclei was made by

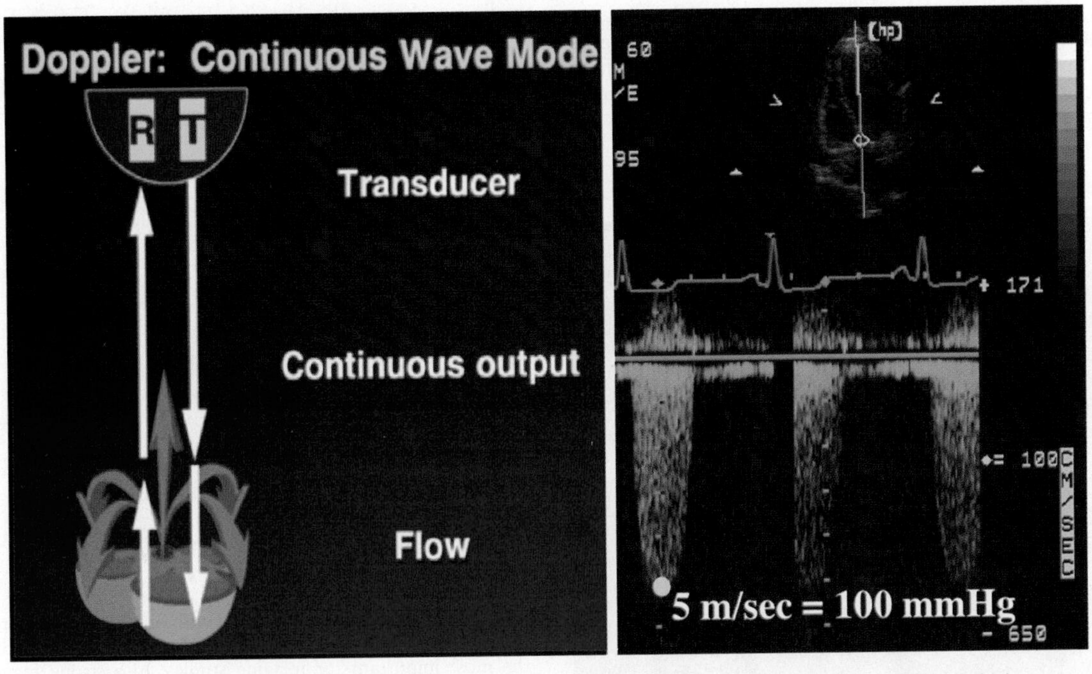

FIGURE 46.14. Continuous-wave Doppler. By continuously transmitting and receiving Doppler-shifted echoes, it is possible to quantify velocities of any magnitude, although at the cost of not having range information as to the specific depth of that velocity. A common application is quantification of aortic stenosis (**right**), using the simplified Bernoulli equation, $\Delta p = 4v^2$, where p is pressure difference in mmHg and v is velocity (m/sec).

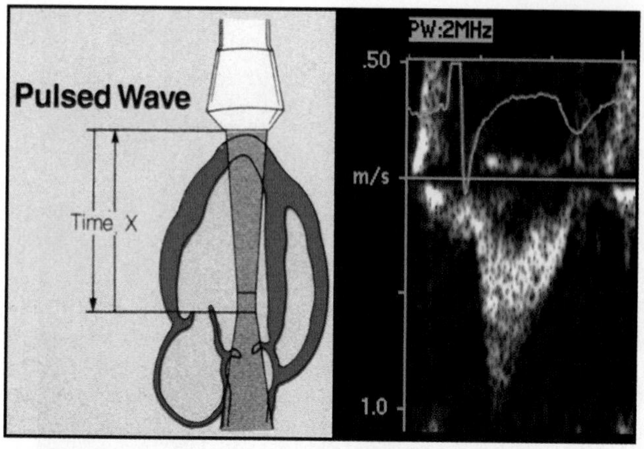

FIGURE 46.15. Pulsed-wave Doppler. By transmitting a brief pulse of ultrasound and "listening" for returning echoes from a specific depth, it is possible to localize velocities within the heart, though at the cost of not being able to quantify very high velocities.

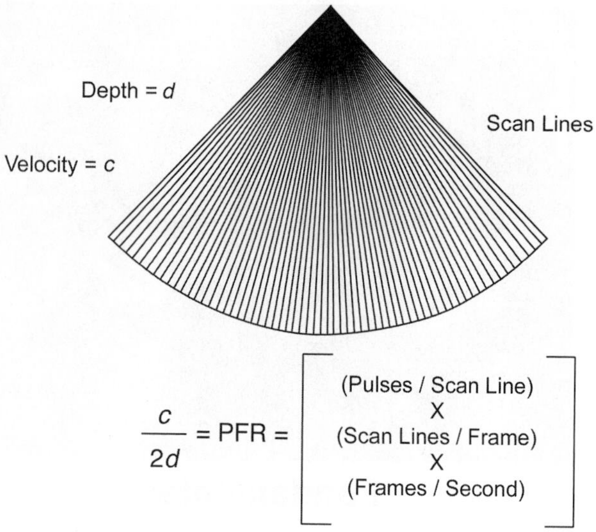

FIGURE 46.17. Temporal, spatial, and velocity trade-offs in Doppler flow mapping. The pulse repetition frequency (PRF, number of interrogations per second) is determined by the depth of imaging d and the velocity of sound c: PRF = $c/2d$. This PRF must be divided among the number of pulses per scan line (which determines velocity resolution), the number of scan lines per frame (which determines spatial extent and resolution of the flow map), and the number of frames per second (which is temporal resolution).

W. Pauli in 1924 and further elaborated in 1946 by E. Purcell and F. Bloch, who shared the Nobel Prize for Physics in 1952.

Physical Principles

Although many nuclei are magnetic, by far the most important to medical imaging is the single hydrogen proton (^{1}H). An individual proton in an external magnetic field spins or *precesses* about the magnetic field at the *Larmor frequency f*, which is proportional to the strength of the external field B_0 and the magnetogyric ratio γ, a constant specific to each nuclear species: $f = \gamma B_0/2\pi$. For the hydrogen proton, $\gamma/2\pi$ is 42.58 MHz per tesla (T) (Fig. 46.18), where the tesla is a standard unit of magnetic field strength, equivalent to 10,000 gauss (G), an older unit. Typical MRI magnets have field strengths from 0.5 to 4 T. By way of comparison, Earth's magnetic field strength is about 0.3 Gauss, or 3×10^{-5} T, and thus a proton in Earth's magnetic field will precess at about 1280 Hz.

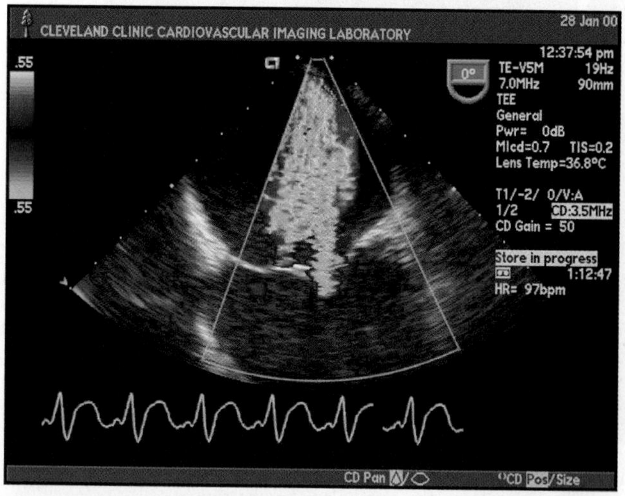

FIGURE 46.16. Color Doppler echocardiography. By processing successive ultrasound pulses with autocorrelation techniques, it is possible to map velocity throughout the imaging sector.

Production and Control of the Magnetic Moment

If a person is placed in a strong magnetic field, a small proportion (fewer than 0.001% in a 1-T field) of the protons will align with the field, setting the stage for imaging. This induced magnetic vector must next be tipped away from the direction of the main magnetic field so it will precess within that field, emitting radiation that can be detected (Fig. 46.19). This is done with a

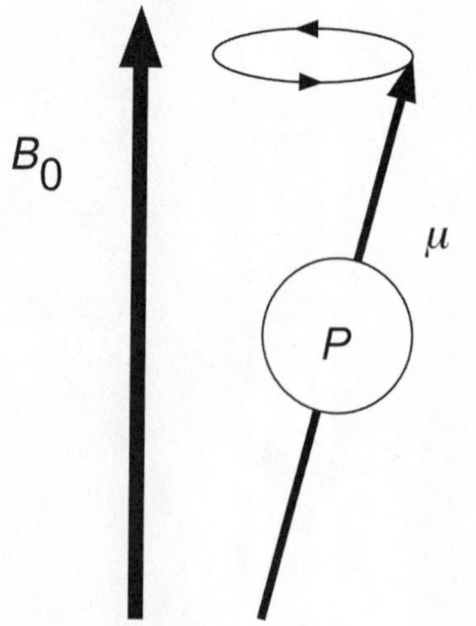

FIGURE 46.18. Precession. Nuclei with odd numbers of protons and neutrons are weakly magnetic with magnetic moment μ, with ^{1}H being the most important for imaging studies. In a strong magnetic field (strength B_0), a few protons line up; in a 1-T field (30,000 times that of Earth), <0.001% are aligned. If these "aligned" protons are tipped out of alignment, they will precess like a wobbling top at 42.6 MHz per tesla. This Larmor frequency is proportional to the magnetic field, critical to MRI.

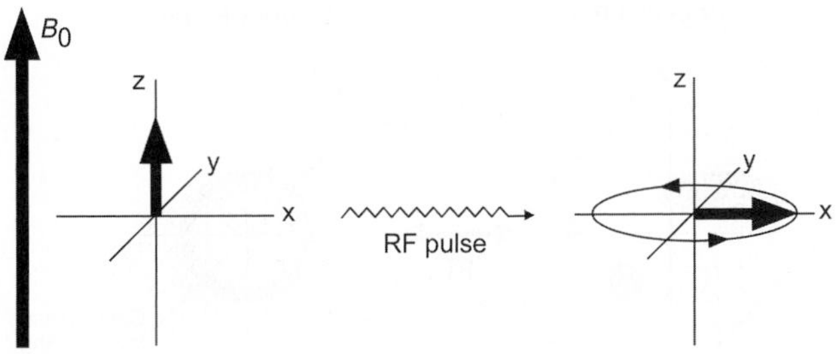

FIGURE 46.19. Delivery of radiofrequency energy at the Larmor frequency causes the mean magnetization vector to tip away from the z-axis. Precise timing of the pulse will tip the vector by precisely 90° into the x-y plane, where it will precess about B_0, emitting electromagnetic radiation (again at the Larmor frequency), which can be detected externally.

pulse of electromagnetic radiation applied at the precessional frequency (termed a radiofrequency [RF] pulse), which exerts a torque on the magnetization vector. The longer the duration of the RF pulse, the more the magnetization vector is tipped away from the main magnetic field, say 90° or 180°. When the RF pulse is removed, the tipped magnetic moment precesses about the main magnetic vector and emits electromagnetic radiation at the Larmor frequency, which can be detected externally. The initial strength of this signal depends primarily on the local proton density, but this does not vary enough within the body to give sufficient contrast to distinguish tissues. Fortunately, there are several other magnetic properties that can be exploited to enhance contrast (Fig. 46.20), the first of which is the rapidity with which the tipped magnetization vector realigns itself with the external magnetic field. This time constant, termed T1, the longitudinal relaxation time, or the spin-lattice relaxation time, typically is of the order of 200 ms to 3 seconds (Table 46.4). The second time constant, T2, refers to the rapidity with which the precessing vector loses coherence in the transverse plane because of the interaction of adjacent magnetic moments. For this reason, it is also called the transverse or spin-spin relaxation time and is always shorter than corresponding T1 values, typically 20 to 400 ms. By delaying the signal reception for a certain period after the RF pulse, it is possible to highlight either T1 or T2 differences between tissues of interest. The subject of pulse

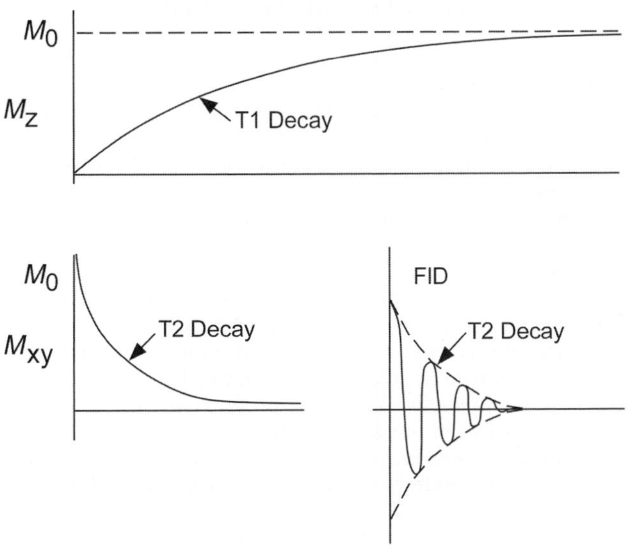

FIGURE 46.20. Relaxation parameters used in magnetic resonance imaging. T1 represents the realignment of the magnetic moment with the external field (directed along the z-axis), and T2 represents the loss of coherence in the x-y plane of the precessing protons.

TABLE 46.4

MAGNETIC RESONANCE IMAGING PARAMETERS

Tissue	^{1}H density (% H_2O)	T1 (ms)	T2 (ms)
Muscle	100	600	40
Liver	91	270	50
Renal cortex	95	360	70
Renal medulla	95	680	140
Spleen	92	480	80
Fat	98	180	90
White matter	100	390	90
Gray matter	94	520	100
Blood	90	800	180
Cerebrospinal fluid	96	2,000	300
Water	100	2,500	2,500

Adapted from Bushong SC. *Magnetic resonance imaging*. St. Louis, MO: Mosby, 1988: Tables 6-1, 6-2, 6-3.

sequencing to contrast magnetic properties is highly complex and is discussed in detail elsewhere (23,24). Cardiac imaging involves several additional difficulties because of the periodic contraction of the heart and the motion of blood within it. Gated NMR (to avoid motion artifact) and pulse sequencing to highlight blood flow are discussed in Chapter 54.

Localizing the Signal

The final issue to contend with is localizing a particular magnetic signal within the body. Because the protons precess with a same frequency proportional to the external field, if we apply a gradient that varies the field across the body, then protons on the left of the patient will "ring" at a frequency different from those on the right, allowing them to be localized just as one can tell whether the right or left end of the piano keyboard has been struck simply by listening to the pitch of the emitted note (Fig. 46.21). The mathematical technique of Fourier analysis (extracting frequency content from a time- or space-varying signal) is heavily relied on in MRI. To build up the full MR image, one must apply spatial encoding gradients in both the x- and y-directions as shown in Figure 46.22. More comprehensive discussion of this is available elsewhere (25).

The mathematical underpinnings of digital image end signal processing are beyond the scope of this chapter. However, several relevant references are listed for the interested reader (26–62).

COMPUTED TOMOGRAPHY

Fourier analysis also plays a pivotal role in the theoretical underpinnings and practical implementation of computed x-ray tomography (CT) (63–65). Similar to MRI, a CT scan is built from a series of slices, except that each slice is generated from a number of x-ray projections across the slice. The difficulty lies in obtaining information across the depth of the slice from these projections, which (as in standard radiography) blur all details along the path of the beam. However, by taking projections through the heart from many different angles, it is possible to build up the full Fourier transform of the image, from which the actual anatomy can be extracted (Fig. 46.23). In actual implementation, a related numerical approach called filtered backprojection is used, but the overall principle is the same. Recent years have seen dramatic advances in CT technology, with the development of multislice scanners in which many

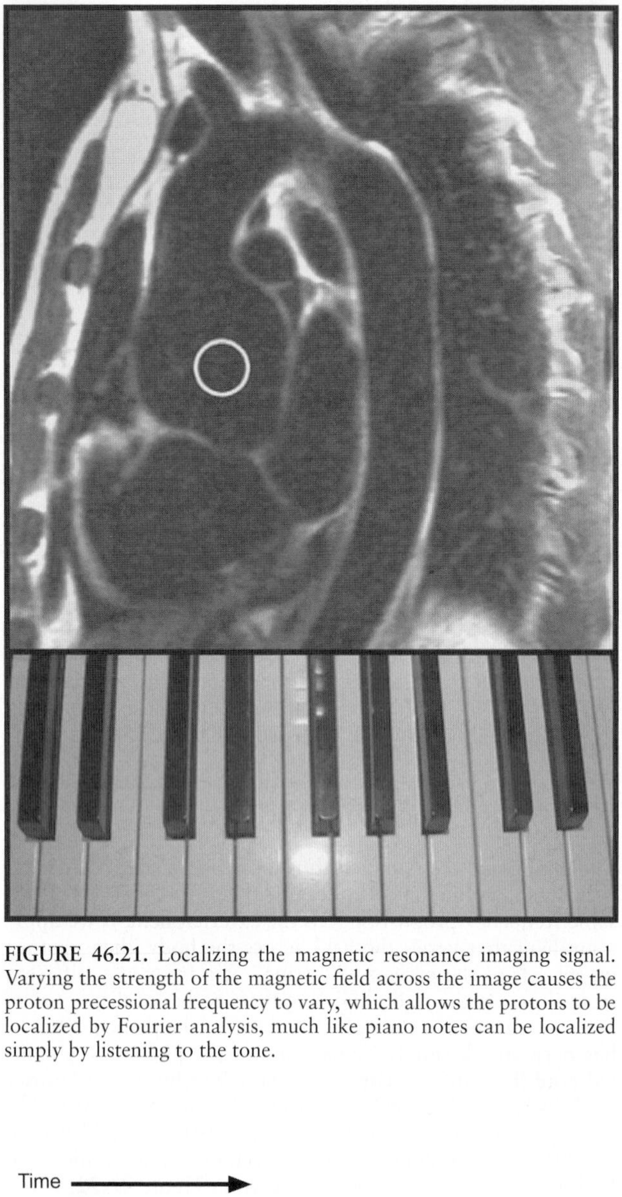

FIGURE 46.21. Localizing the magnetic resonance imaging signal. Varying the strength of the magnetic field across the image causes the proton precessional frequency to vary, which allows the protons to be localized by Fourier analysis, much like piano notes can be localized simply by listening to the tone.

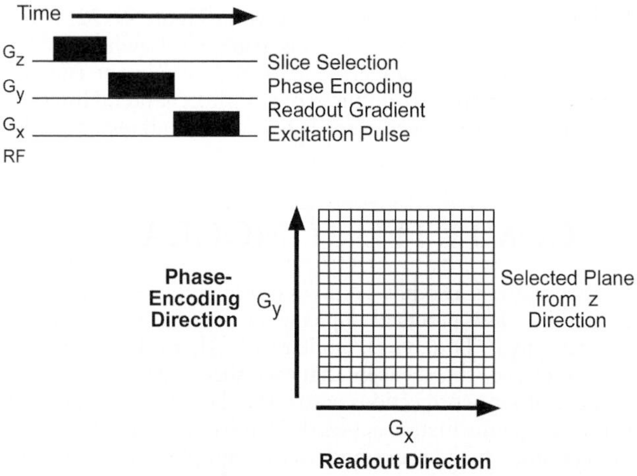

FIGURE 46.22. Building the magnetic resonance image. After selectively exciting a single slice of tissue (with the z gradient), a phase-encoding gradient is applied in the y-direction followed by a frequency-encoding x gradient during the signal readout period. By combining data from multiple phase-encoding steps (which highlight specific Fourier components in the y-direction) one is left with a two-dimensional Fourier transform of the tissue slice from which one can reconstruct the original anatomy. RF, radiofrequency.

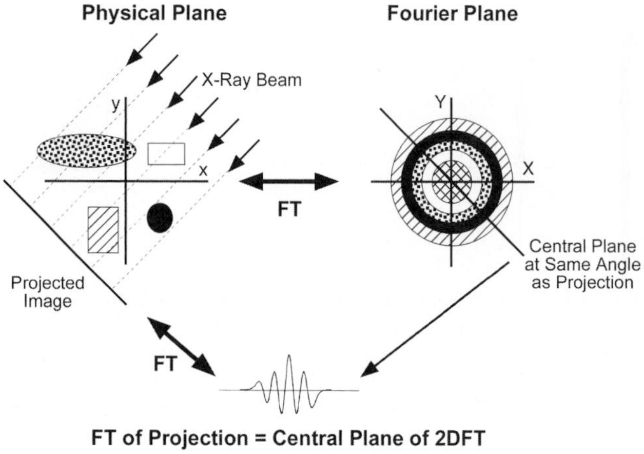

FIGURE 46.23. Image reconstruction in computed tomography. Each projected image blurs all structures along the direction of the x-ray beam (just as a standard x-ray does). By Fourier and other analysis, it is possible to use multiple such projections to extract the full three-dimensional distribution within the image. 2D, two-dimensional; FT, Fourier transform.

detectors are used to reconstruct the heart in a short enough time to freeze cardiac motion and show coronary anatomy. The number of slices has doubled approximately annually in recent years; it is currently 64 but with expectations for 128 and 256 slices in the near future. The high signal-to-noise content of contrast CT lends itself to a host of compelling 3D displays, as detailed in Chapter 56.

COMPARISON OF TECHNIQUES

The preceding physical descriptions and the subsequent chapters show that there is a host of diagnostic tests available for most cardiovascular disorders. To choose among them in the workup of a given patient, one must consider cost, safety, accuracy, and availability of the test. Also of critical importance is the likelihood that a particular disease is actually present in the patient.

Sensitivity and Specificity

Two key parameters for test accuracy are sensitivity and specificity. *Sensitivity* refers to the likelihood that a patient with a given disease will have a positive test, whereas *specificity* is the likelihood that a patient without that disease will have a negative test. We can divide patients into four general classes: true positives (TP) (those with disease who have a positive test), true negatives (TN) (those without disease who have a negative test), false positives (FP) (those without disease who have a positive test), and false negatives (FN) (those with disease who have a negative test). Sensitivity then is defined as TP/(TP + FN), whereas specificity is TN/(TN + FP). Closely related are the positive predictive value, the proportion of patients with positive tests who in fact have the disease, TP/(TP + FP), and the negative predictive value, the proportion with a negative test who are free of the disease, TN/(TN + FN). Overall accuracy of the test is given by the percentage of patients who have the proper test result: (TP + TN)/(TP + TN + FP + FN).

Bayesian Analysis

Critical to rational use of sensitivity and specificity requires applying Bayesian analysis to the known prevalence of disease in the test population. If the prevalence of a disease in some population is p, then the likelihood of being free of that disease is $1 - p$. Sensitivity (Se) and specificity (Sp) data can then be used to derive the positive and negative predictive values:

$$\text{Positive predictive value} = \text{Se}\cdot p/[\text{Se}\cdot p + (1 - \text{Sp})(1 - p)]$$
$$\text{Negative predictive value} = \text{Sp}\cdot p/[\text{Sp}\cdot p + (1 - \text{Se})(1 - p)]$$

For example, a test with a specificity of 95% sounds very accurate, but in a population in which disease prevalence is only 1 in 1,000, there will be 50 false-positive tests for every patient who actually has the disease. The "break-even point" for prevalence (equal odds of true vs. false positive) is given by $p = (1 - \text{Sp})/(1 + \text{Se} - \text{Sp})$. It is usually unwise to perform tests in populations with either a very low prevalence of disease (high proportion of false-positive tests) or a very high prevalence (most negative tests are false negatives).

Receiver/Operator Curve Analysis

A receiver/operator curve (ROC) is useful for determining the optimal test threshold as well as judging the overall value of a test that has a continuous output variable (like number of millimeters of ST depression in an exercise test). In ROC analysis (Fig. 46.24), specificity is plotted along the x-axis and sensitivity is plotted along the y-axis, with various points plotted corresponding to alternative test thresholds. A random test will produce a diagonal line between (0, 0) and (1, 1). There is always a trade-off between sensitivity and specificity of a test as the threshold is altered, but generally the optimal point is the one that is closest to the upper left-hand corner of the receiver/operator box (0, 1). The area under the ROC curve (or between the ROC curve and the line of identity) is a measure of the overall worth of the test, and tests that approach the ideal are those that are skewed strongly to the upper left-hand corner.

Economic Analysis

With the current restraints on health care expenditures, the cost of a diagnostic test must be considered in judging its overall worth. Unfortunately, determining the cost-effectiveness of a diagnostic test (in terms such as the cost per additional quality year of life) is more difficult than a therapeutic maneuver (65a). With a therapeutic intervention, there is a discrete encounter with a well-defined cost and an outcome that can be tracked from that point forward. With a diagnostic test, however, a physician must act on the test, putting a cloud of therapeutic uncertainty between the diagnostic test and the outcome. Furthermore, this evaluation does not in any way account for the significant reassurance that a patient may feel by having a negative test outcome.

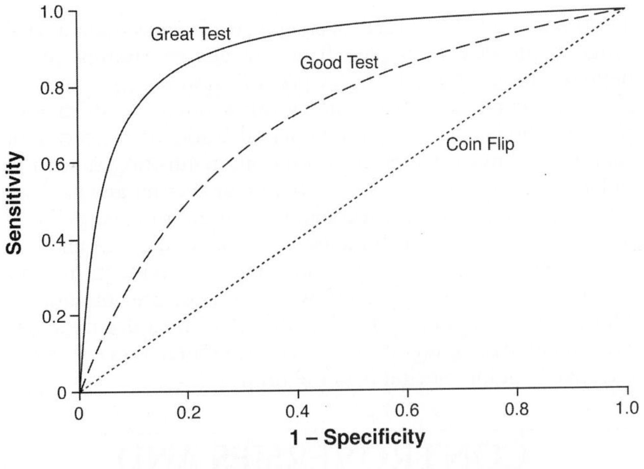

FIGURE 46.24. Receiver-operator curve analysis. For tests with continuous output parameters, there is a trade-off between sensitivity and specificity based on the choice of the cut-off to declare a test positive. The closer a test approaches the ideal of 100% sensitivity and specificity (upper left-hand corner), the better is the test.

PRACTICAL ASPECTS OF DIGITAL IMAGING

The foregoing indicates that much of contemporary cardiac imaging relies on direct digital acquisition, storage, and visualization, which has a number of advantages over analog (film and video tape) techniques. Among the advantages of digital storage are the following (66,67): (a) the examination can be efficiently reviewed without searching through the entire study for a given view; (b) prior examinations are available for comparison; (c) studies can be reviewed throughout the hospital; (d) images can be easily transferred to other institutions for consultation or referral (68,69); (e) calibration data can be stored within the study, facilitating quantitative analysis; (f) image-processing algorithms can improve visualization; (g) images can be duplicated without degradation; (h) long-term archiving can be accomplished without loss of quality; (i) costs may be lower than with analog techniques; and (j) medical education is greatly facilitated. To accomplish this goal has required agreement on formatting standards, dramatic improvement in the cost-effectiveness of computers and networks, and agreement within the clinical community as to the degree of data compression that will be allowable.

DICOM Image Format Standard

Beginning in the early 1980s the American College of Radiology (ACR) and the National Electrical Manufacturers' Association (NEMA) organized to standardize the exchange of digital images (70). This evolved by the mid-1990s with version 3 of the ACR/NEMA standard, now specified as DICOM, to emphasize its role in the general field of medical imaging as well as the inclusion of many other professional organizations (including the American College of Cardiology, the American Society of Echocardiography, and the Society for Nuclear Cardiology). It specifies standards for all modalities, including ultrasound, MRI, nuclear cardiology, CT, and x-ray angiography.

Overall Structure of DICOM

DICOM is simply a set of rules for exchanging images, specifying information on the patient, the purpose and technique of the examination, and the pixel data themselves. Each modality (echo, CT, MRI, nuclear, angiography) has specified required and optional data elements and ways in which the pixels are stored, including any possible digital compression. Images may be exchanged either by network or by disk, protocols that are defined in the standard. Note that DICOM is not an archival standard, but rather a communication and exchange standard. Within an institution, images may be stored on whatever media are most appropriate.

Modality-Specific DICOM Protocols

Each modality specifies its own standard. Angiographic studies are stored as 512 × 512 pixel images with 8 bits of grayscale information. Only the JPEG (Joint Photographic Expert

Group) lossless compression algorithm is allowed, reducing storage needs by a mere 50% to 60%, since a large trial showed that *lossy* compression is unacceptable for angiographic storage, resulting in loss of interobserver agreement (71).

Echocardiography has more diverse needs, requiring grayscale, color, and spectral Doppler storage. Calibration factors may be stored for linear, temporal, and velocity measurements and 3D registration. Images may be stored either uncompressed or with lossless or lossy JPEG compression as high as ~20:1 (72).

The DICOM nuclear standard encompasses the many complex studies of nuclear cardiology. Truly multidimensional data sets may be stored, reflecting the 4D, multistage, multinuclide nature of contemporary protocols. Because the size of the actual data sets is small in comparison to those for echocardiography and angiography, nuclear studies are stored without any compression.

Digital Compression of Images

Cardiac images are voracious consumers of disk storage and network bandwidth. An uncompressed angiographic run (512 × 512 × 8 bits × 30 frames/second) requires 7.5 MB/second, as much as 1 GB in a complex interventional study. Full-color echocardiography (640 × 480 × 24 bits × 30 frames per second) requires 30 MB/second, up to 20 GB for a typical 10-minute study. Such requirements outstrip contemporary, affordable computer systems, highlighting the need for data reduction in cardiac imaging.

Clinical Compression

Much efficiency can be obtained through judicious editing of images on clinical grounds. In echocardiography, for example, single cardiac cycle loops can be stored instead of 30 seconds on a given view. However, for both echocardiography and angiography—where such clinical editing is not advocated—storage and transfer efficiency demands further digital compression of the images.

Digital Compression

Digital compression may be *lossless* or *lossy.* Lossless algorithms allow the original image to be recovered in every detail, removing all concern that such compression might affect the clinical content of the image. A disadvantage of all lossless techniques is relatively poor compression ratios, typically 2:1 or 3:1. Further compression (often beyond 100:1) requires that lossy algorithms be employed, which distort the recovered image in a slight (and insignificant, it is hoped) fashion. The DICOM echocardiography standard allows the use of the lossy JPEG algorithm, which has shown little degradation of echocardiographic images at compression ratios as high as 20:1, whereas images stored on SVHS videotape have a degradation equivalent to 26:1 to 30:1 compression (73,74). In a blind comparison, echocardiographers overwhelmingly selected digital echocardiograms over videotape equivalents, with no impact of 20:1 JPEG compression (75). Other trials have shown the acceptability of lossy compression for computed tomography (76) and nuclear medicine (77), although these have not been codified in the DICOM standard.

Higher degrees of compression are available but have not yet been included within DICOM. The MPEG (Motion Pictures Expert Group) standard extends JPEG by exploiting redundancies between frames, achieving compression ratios beyond 100:1 with excellent fidelity. MPEG encoding has diagnostic content equivalent to videotape (78), and even higher quality can be achieved using MPEG-2 encoding (79). Also under evaluation is wavelet compression, which uses a continuum of frequencies to compress the image rather than the discrete frequencies of the Fourier transform (80).

Digital Imaging at the Cleveland Clinic Foundation

In the year 2000 digital storage became a reality in echocardiography and catheterization laboratories. Figure 46.13 shows the current architecture in use for digital echocardiography in our laboratory. All echo machines in the inpatient and outpatient labs, the operating rooms, and the regional satellite facilities are capable of digital output of still images and loops in the DICOM format using a standard TCP/IP network (100 Mbps for the local machines, 1.54 Mbps or higher-speed lines for the regional facilities). For portable studies performed outside the high-speed network, studies can be stored temporarily on the machine's hard disk for later network export or stored on a magnetooptical disk for "sneaker netting" onto the archive. Within the echo lab, all image traffic is handled over a network that is isolated by switches so as not to degrade performance of the remainder of the cardiology network. A typical study in our lab contains 30 to 80 single-cycle cine loops with an additional 10 to 20 still frames of spectral Doppler and M-mode tracings, yielding an average study size of approximately 60 MB. With 250 studies performed daily, this requires 15 GB of storage daily, or approximately 3.5 TB of storage annually. To handle this enormous storage need while providing rapid review of recent studies (access times <30 seconds), data sets are initially stored on a local hard drive with greater than 1 TB of storage, where they remain for 30 to 60 days. Simultaneously, data are also copied to a long-term digital tape archive providing over 1 PB (pedabyte, 10^{15} bytes) storage with 2- to 3-minute access time. All of this is controlled by a dedicated software program running on several viewing stations in the laboratory. A similar architecture is used in the catheterization laboratory, with a dedicated network providing access to up to 60 angiographic studies performed daily and stored using the DICOM standard and lossless JPEG encoding. All radiology imaging, including CT and MR, is handled on a dedicated network for digital manipulation and review. For communication with referring physicians, all studies are made available through an interface in our electronic medical record. Although rendered in high enough quality for review purposes, for speed of transmission they are compressed to a point that they should not be used in the actual diagnostic interpretation.

SUMMARY

The theory underlying cardiac imaging techniques spans a wide range of physical principles, from low-energy photons (magnetic resonance) to high-energy photons (radiography and nuclear medicine) to acoustic energy (ultrasound). With each of these methods, there are fundamental trade-offs in terms of spatial resolution, temporal resolution, acquisition time, and radiation exposure. Finally, combining data from any of these imaging modalities with techniques of digital image processing may provide new techniques for automated image analysis and understanding, assisted by ongoing improvements in computing power. Although the laws of physics are immutable, Moore's law continues to hold, with continued dramatic improvement in computer processing power that makes ever more effective imaging inevitable in the future.

CONTROVERSIES AND PERSONAL PERSPECTIVES

Each year brings dramatic new developments in cardiac imaging. Because the physical interaction of photons, ultrasound, and magnetism with matter has changed little, most of these improvements result from enhancement in the computer processing of these data. Extrapolating to the future, we can only expect this to continue. Moore's law states that over the last 50 years, computer processing power (per unit cost) has doubled every 18 months. Had the auto industry shown similar productivity gains, the cost of a new car would be less than 1 cent! Over the last 5 years, the trend toward all-digital acquisition and storage for radiography, angiography, and echocardiography has become reality, with practical solutions available from several vendors. Although in the past these systems were isolated from each other, the importance of combining modalities to maximize information exchange is being increasingly recognized, and users are insisting on solutions that can read multiple modalities and deliver these quickly to the practitioner's screen, allowing the easy integration of echo, nuclear, catheterization, and MRI data to guide management of the patient.

Digital storage and transmission should also make health care more economical by reducing the need for duplicate studies. Patients will carry their medical records and images with them, initially on a compact disk, but perhaps soon on a small holographic card. Images are now transmittable via telephone, satellite, or the Internet, allowing remote consultation and timely referral. Equally important is extracting as much data as we can from any given study. In this regard, several modalities tout themselves as "one-stop shopping" for cardiac structure, function, and perfusion. Of all imaging modalities, ultrasound permits the least expensive assessment of chamber size, global and regional ventricular function, and valvular stenosis and regurgitation. With the development of stress echocardiography and novel contrast agents, myocardial perfusion may similarly be measurable. Unfortunately, echocardiography has been used traditionally in a largely qualitative fashion; it is hoped that the trend toward quantitative processing of color Doppler velocities and regional wall motion will continue. Nuclear imaging has seen great improvement in the last two decades and represents the current gold standard for myocardial perfusion and metabolism. PET scanning is uniquely informative, but it is so expensive as to be confined to a few large medical centers. In this era of cost containment, dissemination of this technology may be limited. Magnetic resonance imaging provides high-resolution isotropic 3D data throughout the body without the restriction of echocardiographic windows. With improvements, the large epicardial coronary arteries may be routinely imaged, contrast may assess myocardial perfusion, and spectrographic techniques may detect ischemia. Like PET, though, the large capital investment and operating expense of MRI will likely limit it to specialized applications in major medical centers. Recently computer tomography with spiral scanning techniques has allowed rapid acquisition of gated cardiac images and excellent visualization of the aorta and coronaries at considerably lower cost and complexity than MRI. With continued improvement in image quality, one could well imagine CT replacing diagnostic catheterization as the standard assessment of coronary anatomy. Before this happens, we must demand solid data demonstrating its accuracy across all patient groups (e.g., calcified and noncalcified coronaries) and carefully balance the information provided with the risk of the considerable radiation exposure as well as invasive procedures that may result from a false reading. It is clear that all four modalities have important roles in our diagnostic armamentarium, and that used intelligently together, their whole is much greater than the sum of their individual parts.

THE FUTURE

The next decade will see continued technical progress in all cardiac imaging modalities, but economic forces will increasingly force clinicians to choose among them. Those tests that provide the most comprehensive assessment of the heart at the least cost will prosper, whereas others may see diminished use. A great challenge is the routine exchange of digital studies both within and among institutions. Vendors and professional societies have agreed on the DICOM standard for this exchange, but implementation remains incomplete. The medical community must insist on adherence to standards if global interoperability is ever to be achieved.

References

1. Collins SM, Skorton DJ, eds. *Cardiac imaging and image processing*. New York: McGraw-Hill, 1985.
2. Chandra R. *Introductory physics of nuclear medicine*. Philadelphia: Lea & Febiger, 1982.
3. Coulam CM, Erickson JJ, Rollo FD, James Jr AE, eds. *The physical basis of medical imaging*. New York: Appleton-Century-Crofts, 1981.
4. Gifford D. *A handbook of physics for radiologists and radiographers*. New York: Wiley, 1984.
5. Weyman AE. *Cross-sectional echocardiography*, 2nd ed. Philadelphia: Lea & Febiger, 1994.
6. Stark DD, Bradley Jr WG. *Magnetic resonance imaging*. St. Louis, MO: Mosby, 1988.
7. Meredeth WJ. *Fundamental physics of radiology*. Bristol: J. Wright, 1977.
8. James AE Jr, Anderson JH, Higgins CB, eds. *Digital image processing in radiology*. Baltimore: Williams & Wilkins, 1985.
9. Skorton DJ, et al., eds. *Marcus' cardiac imaging*, 2nd ed. Philadelphia: WB Saunders, 1996.
10. Saxon D. *Elementary quantum mechanics*. San Francisco: Holden-Day, 1968:1–16.
11. Curry TS III, Dowdey JE, Murry Jr RC. *Christensen's introduction to the physics of diagnostic radiology*. Philadelphia: Lea & Febiger, 1984.
12. Wachsmann F, Drexler G. *Graphs and tables for use in radiology*. New York: Springer-Verlag, 1976.
13. Ell PJ, Holman BL, eds. *Computed emission tomography*. New York: Oxford University Press, 1982.
14. Budinger TF. Time-of-flight positron emission tomography: status relative to conventional PET. *J Nucl Med* 1983;24:73–78.
15. Miller JG, Yuhus DE, Mimbs JW, et al. Ultrasonic tissue characterization: correlation between biochemical and ultrasonic indices of myocardial injury. In: *Ultrasonics symposium 1976*, New York: IEEE, 1976:33–43.
16. Wells PNT. *Biomedical ultrasonics*. New York: Academic Press, 1977.

16a. Leitman M, Lysyansky P, Sidenko S, et al. Two-dimensional strain—a novel software for real-time quantitative echocardiographic assessment of myocardial function. *J Am Soc Echocardiogr* 2004;17:1021–1029.

17. Thomas JD, Rubin DN. Tissue harmonic imaging: why does it work? *J Am Soc Echocardiogr* 1998;11:803–808.
18. Rubin DN, Yazbek N, Garcia MJ, et al. Qualitative and quantitative effects of harmonic echocardiographic imaging on endocardial edge definition and side-lobe artifacts. *J Am Soc Echocardiogr* 2000;13:1012–1018.
19. Prior DL, Jaber WA, Homa DA, et al. Impact of tissue harmonic imaging on the assessment of rheumatic mitral stenosis. *Am J Cardiol* 2000;86:573–576.
20. Hatle L, Angelsen B. *Doppler ultrasound in cardiology: physical principles and clinical applications*. Philadelphia: Lea & Febiger, 1982.
21. Goldberg SJ. *Doppler echocardiography*. Philadelphia: Lea & Febiger, 1988.
22. Kasai C, Namekawa K, Koyano A, Omoto R. Real-time two-dimensional blood flow imaging using an autocorrelation technique. *IEEE Trans Sonics Ultrasonics* 1985;SU-32:458–464.
23. Fukushima E, Roeder SBW. *Experimental pulse NMR*. Reading, MA: Addison-Wesley, 1981.
24. Bushong SC. *Magnetic resonance imaging*. St. Louis, MO: Mosby, 1988.
25. Nagel E, van Rossum AC, Fleck E, eds. *Cardiovascular magnetic resonance*. Darmstadt, Germany: Steinkopff-Verlag, 2004:3–49.
26. Pratt WK. *Digital image processing*. New York: Wiley, 1978:593–598.
27. Ophir J, Maklad NF. Digital scan converters in diagnostic ultrasound imaging. *Proc IEEE* 1979;67:654–664.
28. Leavitt SC, Hunt BF, Larsen HG. A scan conversion algorithm for displaying ultrasound images. *Hewlett-Packard J* 1983;34(10):30–34.
29. Rosenfield A, Kak AC. *Digital picture processing*, 2nd ed. New York: Academic Press, 1982.
30. Skorton DJ, McNary CA, Child JS, et al. Digital image processing of two-dimensional echocardiograms: identification of the endocardium. *Am J Cardiol* 1981;48:479.
31. Zwehl W, Levy R, Garcia E, et al. Validation of a computerized edge detection algorithm for quantitative two-dimensional echocardiography. *Circulation* 1983;68:1127.

32. Collins SM, Skorton DJ, Geiser EA, et al. Computer assisted edge detection in two-dimensional echocardiography: comparison with anatomic data. *Am J Cardiol* 1984;53:1980.
33. Delp EJ, Buda AJ, Swastek MR, et al. The analysis of two-dimensional echocardiograms using a time varying image approach. In: *Computers in cardiology*. Long Beach, CA: IEEE Computer Society, 1982:391–394.
34. Parker DL, Pryor TA, Ridges JD. Enhancement of two-dimensional echocardiographic images by lateral filtering. *Comput Biomed Res* 1979;12:265.
35. Garcia E, Gueret P, Bennett M, et al. Real-time computerization of two-dimensional echocardiography. *Am Heart J* 1981;101(6):783–792.
36. Jenkins JM, Qian G, Besozzi M, et al. Computer processing of echocardiographic images for automated edge detection of left ventricular boundaries. In: *Computers in cardiology*. Long Beach, CA: IEEE Computer Society, 1981:391–394.
37. Brennecke R, Hahne HJ, Wessel A, Heintzen PH. Computerized enhancement techniques for echocardiographic sector scans. In: *Computers in cardiology*. Long Beach, CA: IEEE Computer Society, 1981:7–11.
38. Horn BKP, Schunck BG. Determining optical flow. *Artificial Intelligence* 1981;17:185–203.
39. Mailloux GE, Bleau A, Bertrand M, Petticlerc R. Measurement of heart motion from two-dimensional echocardiograms. In *Computers in cardiology*. Long Beach, CA: IEEE Computer Society, 1986:397–400.
40. Mailloux GE, Langlois F, Bertrand M, Petticlerc R. Analysis of heart motions from two-dimensional echocardiograms by velocity field decomposition. In: *Computers in cardiology*. Long Beach, CA: IEEE Computer Society, 1987:441–444.
41. Thomas JD, Higginbotham RD, Waxman AM, et al. Real-time echocardiographic noise reduction, border extraction, and velocity derivation. In: *Computers in cardiology*. Long Beach, CA: IEEE Computer Society, 1988:129–132.
42. Fujita M, Sasayama S, Kawai C, et al. Automatic processing of cineventriculograms for analysis of regional myocardial function. *Circulation* 1981;63:1065.
43. Mancini GBJ, Norris SL, Peterson KL, et al. Quantitative assessment of segmental wall motion abnormalities at rest and after atrial pacing using digital intravenous ventriculography. *J Am Coll Cardiol* 1983;2:70.
44. Spear JR, Sandor T, Als AV, et al. Computerized image analysis for quantitative measurement of vessel diameter from cineangiograms. *Circulation* 1983;68:453.
45. Kirkeeide RL, Fung P, Smalling RW, Gould KL. Automated evaluation of vessel diameter from arteriograms. In: *Computers in cardiology*. Long Beach, CA: IEEE Computer Society, 1982:215–218.
46. Okada RD, Kirshenbaum HD, Kushner FG. Observer variance in the qualitative evaluation of left ventricular wall motion and the quantitation of left ventricular ejection fraction using rest and exercise multigated blood pool imaging. *Circulation* 1980;61:128.
47. Reiber JHC, Lie SP, Simoons ML, et al. Clinical validation of fully automated computation of ejection fraction from gated equilibrium blood-pool scintigrams. *J Nucl Med* 1983;24:1099.
48. Bacharach SL, Green MV, Vitale D, et al. Optimum Fourier filtering of cardiac data: A minimum error method. *J Nucl Med* 1983;24:1176.
49. Frais MA, Botvinick EH, Shosa DW, et al. Phase image characterization of ventricular contraction in right and left bundle branch block. *Am J Cardiol* 1982;50:95–105.
50. Ratib O, Henze E, Schon H, Schelbert HR. Phase analysis of radionuclide ventriculograms for the detection of coronary artery disease. *Am Heart J* 1982;104:1.
51. Eiho S, Matsumoto N, Kuwahara M, Matsuda T, Kawai: 3D reconstruction and display of moving heart shapes from MRI data. In: *Computers in cardiology*. Long Beach, CA: IEEE Computer Society, 1987:349–352.
52. Zhang L, Geiser EL. An approach to optimal threshold selection on a sequence of two-dimensional echocardiographic images. *IEEE Trans Biomed Eng* 1982;BME-29:577–585.
53. Buda AJ, Delp EJ, Meyer CR, et al. Automatic computer processing of 2-dimensional echocardiograms. *Am J Cardiol* 1983;52:384–349.
54. Adam D, Hareuveni O, Sideman S. Semiautomated border tracking of cine echocardiographic ventricular images. *IEEE Trans Med Imaging* 1987;MI-6:266–271.
55. Angermann CE, Hart RJ, Spes CH, et al. Computerized quantitative evaluation of the enchocardium in serial two-dimensional echocardiograms of the left ventricular short axis. In: *Computers in cardiology*, Long Beach, CA: IEEE Computer Society, 1987:437–440.
56. Brinkley JF. Knowledge driven ultrasonic three-dimensional organ modelling. *IEEE Trans Pattern Analysis Machine Intelligence* 1985;PAMI-7: 431–441.
57. Bracewell RN. *The Fourier transform and its applications*. New York: McGraw-Hill, 1978.
58. Brigham EO. *The fast Fourier transform*. Englewood Cliffs, NJ: Prentice-Hall, 1974.
59. Arfken G. *Mathematical methods for physicists*. New York: Academic Press, 1985.
60. Thomas JD, Hagege AA, Choong CY, et al. Improved accuracy of echocardiographic endocardial borders by spatiotemporal filtered Fourier reconstruction: description of the method and optimization of the cutoffs. *Circulation* 1988;77:415–428.
61. Mansfield P, Morris PG. *NMR imaging in biomedicine*. New York: Academic Press, 1982.
62. Kumar A, Welti D, Ernst RR. NMR Fourier zeugmatography. *J Magnet Res* 1975;16:69.
63. Lee JKT, Sagel SS, Stanley RJ, eds. *Computed body tomography*. New York: Raven Press, 1983.
64. Brooks RA, DiCharo G. Theory of image reconstruction in computed tomography. *Radiology* 1975;117:561–572.
65. Gordon R, Herman GT. Three-dimensional reconstruction from projections: a review of algorithms. *Int Rev Cytol* 1974;38:111–151.
65a. Doubilet P, Weinstein MC, McNeil BJ. Use and misuse of the term "cost-effective" in medicine. *N Engl J Med* 1986;314:253–256.
66. Thomas JD, Khandheria BK. Digital formatting standards in medical imaging: a primer for echocardiographers. *J Am Soc Echocardiogr* 1994;7:100–104.
67. Thomas JD, Nissen SE. Digital storage and transmission of cardiovascular images: what are the costs, benefits and timetable for conversion? *Heart* 1996;76:13–17.
68. Alboliris ET, Berdusis K, Fisher J, et al. Transmission of full-length echocardiographic images over ISDN for diagnosing congenital heart disease. *Telemedicine J* 1996;2:251–258.
69. Sobczyk WL, Solinger RE, Rees AH, Elbl F. Transtelephonic echocardiography: Successful use in a tertiary pediatric referral center. *J Pediatr* 1993;122:S84–88.
70. Nissen SE, Pepine CJ, Bashore TM, et al. Cardiac angiography without cine film: erecting a "tower of Babel" in the cardiac catheterization laboratory (American College of Cardiology position statement). *J Am Coll Cardiol* 1994;24:834–837.
71. Kerensky RA, Cusma JT, Kubilis P, et al. American College of Cardiology/European Society of Cardiology International Study of Angiographic Data Compression Phase I: the effect of lossy data compression on recognition of diagnostic features in digital coronary angiography. *J Am Coll Cardiol* 2000;35(5):1370–1379.
72. Thomas JD. The DICOM image formatting standard: what it means for echocardiographers. *J Am Soc Echocardiogr* 1995;8:319–327.
73. Karson TH, Chandra S, Morehead AJ, et al. JPEG compression of digital echocardiographic images: impact on image quality. *J Am Soc Echocardiogr* 1995;8:306–318.
74. Thomas JD, Chandra S, Karson TH, et al. Digital compression of echocardiograms: impact on quantitative interpretation of color Doppler velocity. *J Am Soc Echocardiogr* 1996;9:606–615.
75. Karson TH, Zepp RC, Chandra S, et al. Digital storage of echocardiograms offers superior image quality to analog storage even with 20:1 digital compression: results of the Digital ERA (Echo Record Access) study. *J Am Soc Echocardiogr* 1996;9:769–778.
76. Cosman PC, Davidson HC, Bergin CJ, et al. Thoracic CT images: effect of lossy image compression on diagnostic accuracy. *Radiology* 1994;190:517–524.
77. Rebolo MS, Furuie SS, Munhoz AC, et al. Lossy compression in nuclear medicine images. *Proc Annu Symp Computer Appl Med Care* 1993;824–828.
78. Soble JS, Yurow G, Brar R, et al. Comparison of MPEG digital video with super VHS tape for diagnostic echocardiographic readings. *J Am Soc Echocardiogr* 1998;11:819–825.
79. Main ML, Foltz D, Firstenberg MS, et al. Real-time transmission of full-motion echocardiography over a high-speed data network: impact of data rate and network quality of service. *J Am Soc Echocardiogr* 2000;13(8): 764–770.
80. Goldberg MA, Pivovarov M, Mayo-Smith WW, et al. Application of wavelet compression to digitized radiographs. *Am J Roentgenol* 1994;163: 463–468.

CHAPTER 48 ■ EXERCISE ELECTROCARDIOGRAPHY

PETER M. OKIN

OVERVIEW

Exercise electrocardiography (ECG) remains the most widely used method for assessment of the presence and severity of coronary artery disease. Clinical confidence in the exercise ECG has been eroded by the limited sensitivity and predictive value of standard ST-segment depression criteria and by the overapplication of bayesian principals to interpretation of the exercise ECG in comparison with other noninvasive modalities. However, the development of new approaches to analysis of the ST-segment response to exercise, including heart rate (HR) adjustment of ST-segment depression (the ST/HR slope and ST/HR index) and treadmill exercise scores, has produced a resurgence of clinical and research interest in the exercise ECG. These methods improve the accuracy of the exercise ECG for the identification and quantification of coronary disease and for risk stratification in both asymptomatic low-risk subjects and symptomatic patients with coronary disease. Application of HR-adjusted techniques has been supported by theoretic and experimental evidence relating the magnitude of ST-segment depression at peak exercise to both the area of ischemic territory and the degree of myocardial oxygen supply-demand mismatch as reflected by changing HR. Novel approaches to analysis of the ECG during exercise, including changes in QRS complex duration and high-frequency content, and assessment of HR responses during both exercise and recovery hold promise for future improvements in test performance.

GLOSSARY

Bayesian analysis: Relation of test performance to population prevalence of disease.

Chronotropic response index: Fraction of heart rate reserve achieved with exercise adjusted by the fraction of metabolic reserve achieved.

ECG: Electrocardiogram or electrocardiography.

ETT: Exercise tolerance test (or exercise electrocardiogram).

J-Point: Junction of the end of the QRS complex and beginning of the ST segment.

Rate-recovery loop: Plot of ST-segment depression as a function of heart rate during both exercise and recovery.

ST/HR index: Maximal change in ST-segment depression with exercise divided by the total change in heart rate.

ST/HR slope: Linear regression-based calculation of maximal rate of change in ST-segment depression as a function of change in heart rate during exercise.

INTRODUCTION

Exercise ECG, or the exercise tolerance test (ETT), remains the most widely used and available technique for the investigation of known or suspected coronary artery disease. It has been estimated that 6 to 8 million treadmill tests are performed annually in the United States. Nonetheless, clinical confidence in the simple ETT has been eroded by the limited sensitivity and predictive value of standard ECG criteria. However, newer approaches to analysis of the ETT have been developed since the mid-1980s that improve accuracy of the exercise ECG to levels found for more expensive and less widely available imaging methods. This chapter reviews the development of exercise ECG, gives a brief review of the pathophysiologic basis for exercise-induced ST-segment depression, provides detailed information on the performance, interpretation, and applications of the ETT, and addresses the controversies and future directions in exercise ECG.

PERFORMING AN EXERCISE ELECTROCARDIOGRAM

Indications and Contraindications

The most widely accepted indications for performing an ETT are in patients with known or suspected coronary disease, to determine the likelihood of coronary disease, to assess the likelihood of anatomic or functionally severe disease that may be of prognostic importance, to determine functional capacity, and to assess the effects of therapy (1,2). Although indications for the exercise ECG continue to evolve, a joint committee of the American College of Cardiology and American Heart Association has published categories of indications for the ETT based on the literature (Table 48.1) (1). Clinical contraindications to performing diagnostic exercise ECG include acute myocardial infarction (MI), unstable angina before a period of stabilization, uncompensated severe congestive heart failure, advanced atrioventricular (AV) block or life-threatening arrhythmias, acute myocarditis or pericarditis, severe aortic stenosis, severe resting hypertension, and any medical condition that precludes the patient from being able to walk safely on the treadmill. The presence of left bundle branch block, left ventricular hypertrophy with strain, ventricular preexcitation (Wolf-Parkinson-White syndrome), or permanent ventricular pacing on the ECG are contraindications to use of the exercise ECG for diagnostic purposes, owing to the uncertain diagnostic value of additional ST-segment changes in these settings, but these conditions do not preclude use of the ETT to assess exercise performance or evaluate the risk of arrhythmia when indicated.

Patient Preparation and Technique

The American Heart Association has published guidelines for clinical ETT laboratories that provide recommendations regarding the performance of clinical ETTs (3). A directed physical examination should be performed to exclude the presence of significant valvular or myopathic disease that could preclude exercise evaluation. The risks and benefits of the procedure should be carefully explained and informed consent obtained before beginning the study.

Attention to adequate skin preparation before electrode placement is the most important technical aspect in obtaining high-quality ECG recordings. The areas where electrodes are to be placed should first be cleaned with alcohol to remove surface oils and then abraded with a scouring pad or other rough material to remove the most superficial layer of skin. Abrasion should be performed to reduce resistance at the skin-electrode interface to 5000 ohm or less. Silver-silver chloride electrodes should be used to produce high-quality tracings.

Before exercise, a supine 12-lead ECG should be obtained with the limb electrodes on the extremities in the normal positions; this tracing should be carefully examined for any signs of active ischemia, interval MI, or abnormalities that would prohibit performance of the ETT. Limb electrodes should then be shifted to the more proximal positions recommended by Mason and Likar (4), and additional ECG tracings should be obtained in the supine and standing positions.

A 12-lead ECG should be obtained each minute during exercise, at peak exercise, and every minute during the postexercise recovery period. Blood pressure should be measured immediately before exercise in the standing position, immediately before the end of each stage of exercise, and for each minute of recovery until the blood pressure has returned to baseline. Patient position in the postexercise recovery phase varies among laboratories. Many laboratories have the patient assume the supine position immediately after peak exercise; this will increase venous return and increase end-diastolic volume, and it may augment ST-segment changes that are present at the end of exercise. In our laboratory, we have the patient remain in the upright position, if possible, and have used a cool-down phase of 3 minutes immediately after peak exercise during which the patient continues to walk at 1.7 mph at a 0% grade. This allows patients a more gradual decrease in HR after exercise and appears to decrease the incidence of postexercise vagally mediated hypotension.

TABLE 48.1

INDICATIONS FOR EXERCISE ELECTROCARDIOGRAPHY

Clearly indicated
Diagnosis of CAD in men with atypical symptoms
Patient has known CAD; assess prognosis and functional capacity
Symptomatic, recurrent, exercise-induced arrhythmias
Patient has experienced an uncomplicated myocardial infarction; evaluate prognosis and functional capacity
Patient has undergone coronary artery revascularization; evaluation recommended
Possibly indicated
Diagnosis of CAD in woman with typical or atypical angina
Diagnosis of CAD in patient taking digitalis
Diagnosis of CAD in patient with complete right bundle branch block
Patient has CAD or heart failure; evaluate functional capacity and response to therapy
Patient has variant angina; evaluation recommended
Patient has known CAD; serial evaluation recommended
Asymptomatic man who is older than 40 yr and in a high-risk occupation, who has two or more risk factors for CAD, or who is sedentary and plans to begin a vigorous exercise program; evaluation recommended
Asymptomatic patient after coronary revascularization; annual evaluation recommended
Selected patients with valvular heart disease; evaluate functional capacity
Probably not indicated
Asymptomatic patient with isolated ventricular ectopy; evaluation recommended
Patient is enrolled in a cardiac rehabilitation program; serial evaluation recommended
Diagnosis of CAD in patient with left bundle branch block or ventricular preexcitation (Wolff-Parkinson-White) syndrome on resting electrocardiography
Asymptomatic man or woman; evaluation recommended
Man or woman with chest pain of noncardiac etiology: evaluation recommended

CAD, coronary artery disease.
Adapted from Schlant RC, Blomqvist CG, Brandenburg RO, et al. Guidelines for exercise testing: a report of the American College of Cardiology/American Heart Association Task Force on Assessment of Cardiovascular Procedures (Subcommittee on Exercise Testing). *J Am Coll Cardiol* 1986;8:725, with the permission of Elsevier Science, Inc.

TABLE 48.2

COMPARISON OF STANDARD BRUCE PROTOCOL AND THE CORNELL PROTOCOL

		Bruce protocol		Cornell protocol	
Walking speed (mph)	Grade (%)	Stage	Elapsed time (min)	Stage	Elapsed time (min)
1.7	0			0	2
1.7	5			0.5	4
1.7	10	1	3	1.0	6
2.1	11			1.5	8
2.5	12	2	6	2.0	10
3.0	13			2.5	12
3.4	14	3	9	3.0	14
3.8	15			3.5	16
4.2	16	4	12	4.0	18
4.6	17			4.5	20
5.0	18	5	15	5.0	22

Equipment and Personnel

Although excellent-quality stress tests can be obtained using standard 12-lead ECGs that conform to the recommendations of the American Heart Association, most ETTs currently performed utilize equipment specifically designed for ETT. These computerized systems combine an ECG with a display monitor for continuous rhythm analysis and are capable of controlling treadmills and bicycle ergometers according to specific exercise protocols. The stress laboratory should be equipped with a defibrillator with the ability to perform synchronous cardioversion, an Ambu-bag and oxygen supply, and a cardiac arrest cart.

ETTs should be performed under the supervision of a physician who has been trained to conduct them. The degree of supervision required primarily depends on the type of patient tested, and it can range from direct performance of the test in patients who are at higher risk of complications to assigning the performance of the test to an appropriately trained exercise physiologist or specialist in patients at lower risk. In all cases, a physician should be immediately available during the ETT.

Treadmill Protocol

Although numerous excellent treadmill protocols are available for use, by far the most commonly used are the original protocol of Bruce (5) and modifications of this protocol. The Cornell protocol, originally developed in our laboratory to produce the smaller HR increments between stages necessary for calculation of the ST/HR slope (6), is a more graded modification of the Bruce protocol that divides each standard stage into 2-minute half-stages (Table 48.2).

Lead Systems

The number and type of leads used in exercise ECG vary widely, but with the advent of modern recording devices, most stress laboratories monitor and record at least three leads during the test. Although the use of all 12 conventional leads is becoming more common, almost all the useful diagnostic ST-segment information from these leads is present in limb leads II, III, aVF, and precordial leads V_3 to V_6. Bipolar lead systems that include one electrode in the V_5 position provide additional diagnostic information; bipolar lead CM_5 is the most sensitive for ST-segment changes (7) and is particularly important in optimal performance of the ST/HR slope (8). Preliminary results in 245 patients suggest that incorporation of ST-segment depression and elevation in right precordial leads may improve sensitivity of the ETT with no apparent decrease in specificity (9). Further validation of these findings will be necessary before routine use of right precordial leads can be recommended.

Indications for Test Termination

The general indications for terminating an ETT are outlined in Table 48.3. In the absence of symptoms or signs that warrant termination of the exercise ECG, patients should be exercised with 100% of age-predicted target HR as the goal. However, in general, achievement of greater than 85% of target HR provides an adequate level of stress for diagnostic exercise ECG (10). Various equations have been used to relate target HR to age, but the simplest and most commonly used are 220—age and 200—(age/2). Although angina alone is not an absolute indication for test termination, progressively worsening typical anginal symptoms should be considered a reason to stop the test, as are any other symptoms that limit further walking on the treadmill. ST-segment elevation in the absence of Q waves, which should be considered consistent with possible transmural injury, or marked ST-segment depression (>3 mm of additional ST-segment depression compared with baseline) warrants test termination in the absence of other findings.

Other Applications of Stress Testing

Performance of an ETT for indications other than routine assessment of the presence or severity of coronary disease or evaluation of functional capacity deserves comment. After uncomplicated MI, an ETT is frequently performed to assess functional capacity and to help stratify risk (11). When performed early after MI (i.e., before discharge or within 2 to 3 weeks of the infarction), submaximal symptom-limited testing is recommended (2) to a target HR of 140 beats per minute or a metabolic equivalent (MET) of 7 in patients less than 40 years old and to an upper rate of 130 beats per minute or a MET level of 5 in patients 40 years old and older. A full symptom-limited maximal test is appropriate more than 3 weeks after MI. Exercise ECGs are also commonly performed to evaluate the risk of exercise-induced tachyarrhythmias in patients with exercise-related presyncope or syncope.

Exercise ECG is also utilized after percutaneous coronary interventions to stratify risk and to aid in the assessment of restenosis, and it appears to be well tolerated (12,13). However, reports of acute stent thrombosis associated with ETT soon after stent placement (14) raise the question whether ETT should be performed in the immediate poststent period. Until further data become available, caution should be employed in the utilization of ETT soon after the stent placement, with strong consideration given to the use of pharmacologic stress if early noninvasive assessment is indicated (14).

INTERPRETATION OF THE EXERCISE ELECTROCARDIOGRAM

ST-Segment Depression Criteria

To appreciate fully the ST-segment excursions that occur during the transient ischemia associated with exercise in patients with coronary disease requires some understanding of the ST-segment changes that occur during exercise in physiologically normal subjects (Fig. 48.1). At baseline, most normal subjects have ST segments that are either at the isoelectric level or slightly elevated owing to physiologic early repolarization of the J-point. As HR increases, progressive J-point depression occurs, with resultant rapidly upsloping ST segments (15,16). After exercise is terminated, the J-point depression tends to resolve quickly (usually within the first 2 minutes), as does the rapidly upsloping ST-segment depression. In contrast, the ST-segment depression associated with subendocardial ischemia is more likely to be horizontal or downsloping, but it may also be slowly upsloping (Fig. 48.2) (10,16). With progressive exercise, increasing HR, and thus increasing myocardial oxygen demand, the magnitude of ischemic ST-segment depression will increase. Placing the patient in the supine position immediately after exercise may accentuate ischemic ST-segment depression; however, ischemic ST-segment depression may occur during exercise only; in a small percentage of cases, ischemic ST-segment depression will be seen during recovery only (17). In the rare instances of exercise-induced transmural ischemia or injury, ST-segment elevation similar to that seen during the acute injury of MI may also occur.

Differences in the patterns of ST-segment depression in normal subjects and patients with coronary disease highlight the importance of choosing the correct point on the ST segment to measure the magnitude of ST-segment depression (15,16,18). Recommendations for the measurement of ST-segment depression have varied from the J-point (19) to between 60 and 80 milliseconds after the J-point (1,10). Performance of standard ST-segment depression criteria vary with the timing of ST-segment measurement relative to the J-point, but measurements made at 60 milliseconds after the J-point have generally outperformed J-point measurements for the identification of coronary disease (15,16,18). We previously found that performance characteristics of HR-adjusted ST-segment depression criteria are optimized when ST-segment depression is measured at 60 milliseconds after the J-point, whereas use of J-point depression reduces performance of HR-adjusted criteria to the level of standard criteria (16). Thus, we currently recommend that ST-segment depression be measured at 60 milliseconds after the J-point (8).

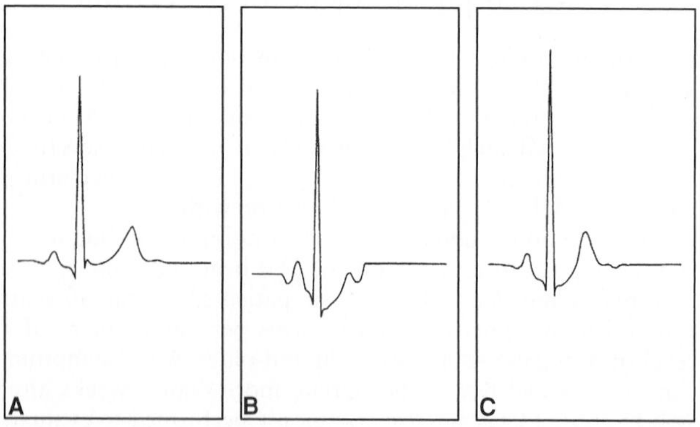

FIGURE 48.1. Progression of ST-segment changes that occur in normal subjects from isoelectric at baseline (A) to J-point depression with rapidly upsloping ST-segment depression at peak exercise (B) and rapid resolution of the ST-segment changes in recovery (C).

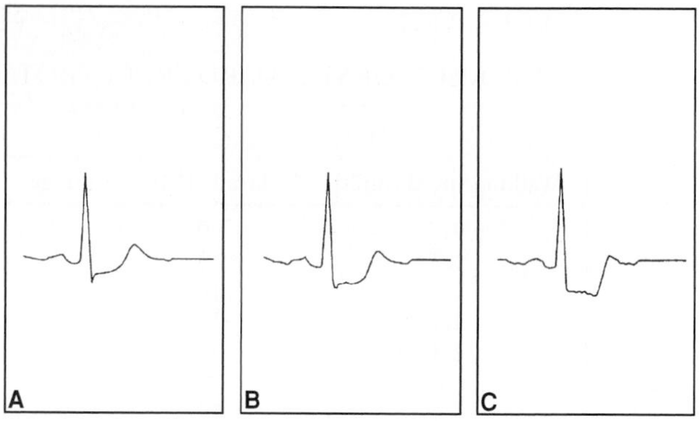

FIGURE 48.2. Comparison of the different patterns of ST depression. A: Slowly upsloping ST-segment depression. B: Horizontal ST-segment depression. C: Downsloping ST-segment depression.

The actual measurement of ST-segment deviation on the exercise ECG is most accurately performed by the computerized systems that are widely in use today, but accurate ST-segment measurements can be performed by hand with careful attention to proper selection of the correct measurement points. When measuring ST-segment deviation, the PQ segment is usually chosen as the isoelectric point, and ST-segment depression should be measured at 60 milliseconds after the J-point. Computer systems are clearly capable of accurately measuring ST-segment deviation to the nearest 10 μV, and careful hand measurements using calipers or a magnifying graticle can readily achieve a precision of 25 μV for ST-segment measurements (20). However, when using computer measurements, it is important to recognize that motion artifact, electrical interference, and changes in QRS or AV conduction can interfere with PQ-segment and J-point determinations and can introduce error into the computerized ST-segment measurements. Therefore, physicians should routinely compare the raw ECG signal with the computer-averaged or median beats used to perform ST-segment measurements before accepting the computer measurements as accurate.

Standard Test Criteria

Assessment of the magnitude and configuration of ST-segment depression on the exercise ECG provides the basis for standard ST-segment depression criteria that are commonly in use. A positive test by standard ST-segment depression criteria has been routinely defined as the achievement of $\geq$ 0.1 mV (100 μV) of horizontal or downsloping ST-segment depression at peak exercise or in early recovery compared with the baseline before exercise ECG (1,2,10). However, as discussed later, these criteria have only limited test sensitivity for the presence of coronary disease and variable performance for identification of anatomically severe disease and for risk stratification (7–10, 18,21). Additional factors that can increase the likelihood of coronary disease in the presence of traditional criteria and also make multivessel disease more likely include the magnitude, time of onset, duration, and number of leads with ST-segment depression. Although inclusion of upsloping ST-segment depression of ≥ 0.1 mV or 0.15 mV has been suggested as an additional component of standard criteria to increase sensitivity for the detection of coronary disease (22,23), the incorporation of upsloping ST-segment depression also lowers test specificity (10,21,22,24). As a consequence, we consider the presence of upsloping ST-segment depression of 1 mm (0.1 mV) or more to be an "equivocal" test response by standard criteria.

Heart Rate–Adjusted Criteria

HR adjustment of the magnitude of ST-segment depression is a rational, physiologic approach to interpretation of the ETT. Two related but distinct methods of HR adjustment of ST-segment depression during exercise have evolved: the linear regression–based ST/HR slope and the simpler ST/HR index. The ST/HR slope is calculated from the maximal rate of change of ST-segment depression relative to HR during the period of active ischemia that accompanies the end of exercise (Fig. 48.3) (6,8,16,20,24–30). The ST/HR index represents the average change of ST-segment depression relative to HR change over the entire course of exercise, which therefore underestimates the maximal ST/HR slope because it includes a large change in HR before any ischemia occurs (see Fig. 48.3). Both these methods specifically do not consider any ST-segment depression that occurs during the postexercise recovery period.

Calculations of the ST/HR slope and ST/HR index are illustrated in Figure 48.3. Measurement of the ST/HR slope is determined by linear regression analysis to relate the magnitude of ST-segment depression in each lead to the HR at the end of each stage of exercise and at peak exercise. Because the maximal rather than the average rate of change is sought, linear regression analysis is performed from the end of exercise to progressively earlier intermediate stage data points using HR as the independent variable and ST-segment depression as the dependent variable. The highest ST/HR slope with a statistically significant correlation coefficient is taken as the test finding for that lead (in μV/beats per minute). After calculation of the maximal ST/HR slope in each lead, the highest ST/HR slope among all the leads (including bipolar lead CM_5 but excluding aVR, aVL, and V_1) is taken as the final test result (8,20). The ST/HR index is derived by dividing the maximal change in ST-segment depression during exercise by the total change in HR from rest to peak effort (8,31). Initial studies from our laboratory (24) established partition values with specificities of 95% in normal subjects of more than 2.40 μV/beat per minute for the ST/HR slope and more than 1.60 μV/beat per minute for the ST/HR index for the identification of coronary disease. Partition values of more than 6.0 μV/beat per minute and more than 3.3 μV/beat per minute, respectively, have been established for the identification of three-vessel, left main, or functionally severe coronary artery disease (8).

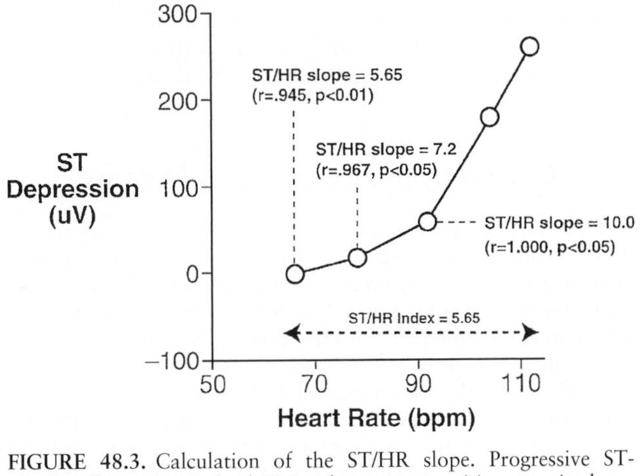

FIGURE 48.3. Calculation of the ST/HR slope. Progressive ST-segment depression in lead CM_5 (shown as a positive magnitude on the vertical axis) is plotted against exercise heart rate in a patient with three-vessel coronary artery disease. This cases illustrates the linear relation of ST-segment depression to heart rate as peak exercise is approached. As a result, the slope of the line relating the final three data points by linear regression is higher than the slope of lines incorporating earlier data points. When more than one linear correlation is statistically significant, the greatest value (in this case, 10.0) is taken as the test result for that patient. The value obtained by simply dividing the total change in ST-segment depression by the total change in heart rate (the ST/HR index) markedly underestimates the true ST/HR slope. (From Okin PM, Kligfield P. Heart rate adjustment of ST depression and performance of the exercise electrocardiogram: a critical evaluation. *J Am Coll Cardiol* 1995;25:1726, with permission of Elsevier Science, Inc.)

Analysis of the behavior of ST-segment depression as a function of HR during both exercise and recovery using the rate-recovery loop (8,25,26) can provide additional diagnostic and prognostic information from the ETT. Physiologic correlates of rate-recovery loop patterns can be found in the initial observations of Detry and Bruce (32,33), comparing myocardial ischemia during exercise and recovery. These investigators found a close linear relation of ST-segment depression during exercise to myocardial oxygen demand, as reflected by the tension-time index, in patients with coronary disease. During recovery, however, this relation was nonlinear, with similar ST-segment depressions observed at lower tension-time indexes than during exercise. Additional support for this approach is found in observations of subendocardial ischemia continuing into the recovery period with persistent ST-segment depression that remains greater relative to HR during early recovery than during the development of ischemia (34,35). Rate-recovery loops are constructed by plotting ST-segment deviation with reference to changing HR throughout treadmill exercise and recovery (Fig. 48.4). Normal subjects typically exhibit a clockwise loop of ST-segment depression as a function of HR during exercise and recovery, whereas patients with coronary disease commonly exhibit a counterclockwise loop. Quantification of the degree of abnormal rate-recovery loop behavior by integrating the difference in ST-segment depression between exercise and recovery phases from peak exercise to the end of 3 minutes of the recovery phase can further stratify the presence and severity of coronary disease (36).

Treadmill Exercise Scores

Numerous investigators have used either multivariate analyses or bayesian theory to produce clinical scores in an attempt to improve accuracy of the ETT (37–42). Two methods that have utilized data only from the ETT are the Hollenberg exercise score (37) and the Duke treadmill score (Table 48.4) (38,39). The Hollenberg exercise score quantifies the ECG response to exercise by measuring the cumulative area of ST-segment depression and ST-segment slope in leads V_5 and aVF during exercise and recovery, which is then normalized for R-wave height and workload (exercise duration and HR). The Duke treadmill score is a simple score that includes exercise duration and weighted measures of ST-segment deviation and an angina score. The prognostic value of this score has been validated in ambulatory patients (38) and in those undergoing angiography (39).

ST Integral

Originally proposed by Sheffield and colleagues (43), the time-voltage integral of ST-segment depression (the ST integral) examines the total area of repolarization abnormality from the J-point to a terminal point late in the ST segment where the ST

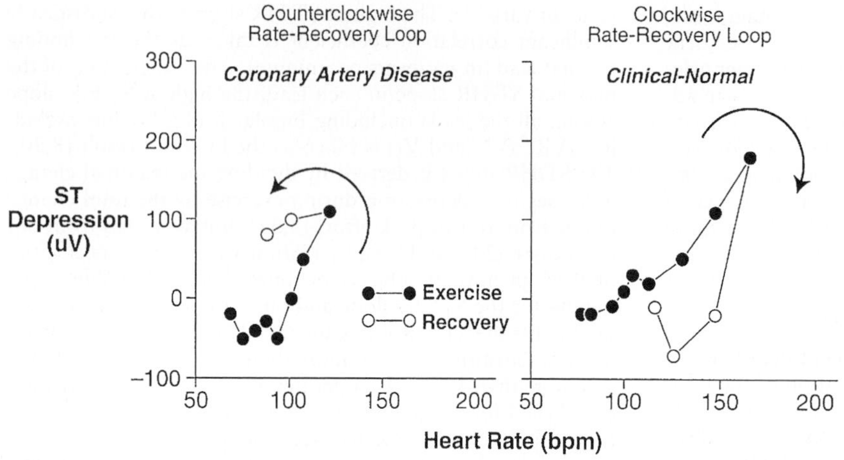

FIGURE 48.4. ST-segment deviation as a function of heart rate during exercise and recovery, with ST-segment depression shown in the upward direction and ST-segment elevation shown in the downward direction. Typical rate-recovery loops are shown for a clinically normal subject (**right**) and a patient with coronary disease (**left**). Despite a greater magnitude of ST-segment depression at peak exercise in the clinically normal subject, there is a clockwise pattern of ST-segment depression relative to heart rate during recovery; the patient with coronary disease has the opposite, counterclockwise pattern. (From Okin PM, Kligfield P. Heart rate adjustment of ST depression and performance of the exercise electrocardiogram: a critical evaluation. *J Am Coll Cardiol* 1995;25:1726, with permission of Elsevier Science, Inc.)

segment crosses the isoelectric baseline. This method has primarily been applied in a series of population-based studies to assess risk (44,45), but the need for computer measurements and the lower accuracy of this method relative to standard ST-segment depression criteria (46) have limited its general applicability.

QRS Complex Criteria

An increase in R-wave amplitude with exercise has been proposed as a possible marker of myocardial ischemia and left ventricular dysfunction in patients with coronary artery disease (47). However, subsequent studies have demonstrated that R-wave amplitude changes with exercise are highly correlated with HR and that much of the discrimination between normal subjects and patients with coronary disease thought to result from R-wave amplitude changes actually reflects differences in exercise HRs achieved (48).

Changes in QRS complex duration and in intra-QRS amplitudes have also been suggested as possible markers of ischemia (49,50). Michaelides and colleagues (49) demonstrated that normal subjects were more likely to shorten QRS duration with exercise compared with patients with coronary disease, who were on average more likely to increase QRS duration. These investigators further found that the magnitude of QRS duration prolongation in patients with disease was directly related to both the number of obstructed coronary arteries and the number of segmental wall motion abnormalities. Investigation of a more experimental nature using signal averaging of high-frequency ECGs during myocardial ischemia produced by balloon catheter inflation in the catheterization laboratory has demonstrated a reversible reduction in mid-QRS high-frequency signal strength during ischemia with a sensitivity of 88% for acute coronary occlusion, significantly greater than the 71% sensitivity of standard ST-segment elevation changes (50). These findings offer promise for increased use of QRS complex changes during exercise to improve the recognition of myocardial ischemia, but further work using computer measurements based on digital data recorded at high acquisition rates (500 to 1,000 Hz) during exercise will be necessary to clarify the role of these approaches in the diagnosis of coronary disease.

TABLE 48.3

GENERAL INDICATIONS FOR TERMINATING AN EXERCISE TEST

Achievement of target heart rate (see text for definitions)
Progressive angina
Other limiting symptoms (dyspnea, fatigue, lightheadedness, claudication)
ST-segment elevation >2 mm (in leads without a resting Q wave)
Severe ST-segment depression (see text)
Nonsustained ventricular tachycardia (three or more sequential ventricular premature contractions)
New onset of atrial fibrillation, atrial flutter, or of a supraventricular tachycardia
Development of second- or third-degree atrioventricular block
Development of a new left bundle branch block
A 10-mm Hg drop in systolic blood pressure
Extreme elevation of systolic or diastolic blood pressure
A progressive drop in heart rate with continued exercise
Equipment problems, such as loss of electrocardiographic signal

Chronotropic Response to Exercise

An attenuated HR response to exercise, a measure of chronotropic incompetence, has been associated with the presence and severity of coronary disease (28,51) and can predict coronary heart disease events and total mortality (52–54). Assessment of the adequacy of HR response to exercise includes simple measures, such as peak exercise HR, percentage of target HR achieved, and change in HR with exercise. In addition, simple and HR-adjusted ST-segment depression criteria can be corrected for an attenuated HR response to exercise by adjusting these measurements for the fraction of HR reserve achieved during exercise, which is the change in HR with exercise divided by the difference between 100% of age-predicted target HR and the HR at standing rest (28). A more complex measure is the chronotropic response index (28,52), which adjusts the fraction of HR reserve achieved for workload as measured by the fraction of metabolic reserve. HR changes during the recovery phase of the ETT have also been demonstrated to provide prognostic information. A delayed decrease in HR after exercise, or abnormal HR recovery, predicts all-cause mortality among healthy adults and in patients referred for ETT, independent of evidence of inducible ischemia and beyond that provided by exercise-phase changes in HR (55–57).

TABLE 48.4

TREADMILL EXERCISE SCORES

Hollenberg exercise score (16)

$$\text{Exercise score} = \frac{\text{area(j-point + ST slope)}V_5 \times 12/RV_5 + \text{area(j-point + ST slope)aVf}}{\text{exercise duration} \times \text{fraction of maximal predicted heart rate}}$$

(where exercise duration is in min and R-wave amplitudes are in mm)

Duke treadmill score (26)

Treadmill score = exercise duration − (5 × ST deviation) − (4 × TM angina index)
[where exercise duration is in min; ST deviation is in mm; and TM (treadmill) angina index = 0 for no angina, 1 for nonlimiting angina, or 2 for exercise-limiting angina]

Blood Pressure Changes

Among patients with coronary disease, both failure to increase systolic blood pressure to $\geq$ 120 mm Hg and a sustained decrease in systolic blood pressure of $\geq$ 10 mm Hg have been associated with an increased likelihood of anatomically extensive disease. However, other conditions can produce a blunted blood pressure response to exercise, such as obstruction to left ventricular outflow, hypovolemia, left or right ventricular dysfunction, cardioactive medications, and vigorous exercise. In contrast, an exaggerated blood pressure response to exercise is associated with an increased risk of developing hypertension at rest and with a greater prevalence of left ventricular hypertrophy (58), but the prevalence of coronary disease appears to be similar among patients with and without exercise hypertension ($\geq$ 210 mm Hg in men and $\geq$ 190 mm Hg in women) (59).

In the postexercise recovery phase, there is normally a progressive decline in systolic blood pressure. The failure of systolic pressure to decline normally during early recovery, as measured by an increased ratio (>0.90) of systolic pressure during the first 3 minutes of recovery to peak exercise systolic blood pressure, has been reported to be useful in the diagnosis of coronary artery disease (60). However, an increased ratio is also seen in patients with hypertension and no significant coronary obstructions (60), and additional studies have not substantiated a high sensitivity of this ratio for coronary disease (61). Further study of the utility of blood pressure changes to improve ETT diagnosis of coronary disease are necessary before the routine application of these criteria can be recommended.

Rhythm and Conduction Changes

The ETT can be used to evaluate the risk of significant abnormalities of cardiac rhythm and conduction under appropriate conditions. Exercise-induced ventricular premature contractions are common, increase in prevalence with age, are more frequent, and may be associated with a somewhat worse prognosis in patients with coronary disease (62). Whereas the development of frequent ventricular premature contractions during exercise and/or the postexercise recovery phase appears to convey an increased mid- to long-term mortality risk (63,64), the appearance of nonsustained ventricular tachycardia during ETT does not appear to convey an increased short-term risk (65). The development of sustained ventricular tachycardia during ETT in patients with coronary disease is most commonly the result of myocardial ischemia and can be prevented by treatment of the underlying ischemia. In patients without obvious structural heart disease, ETT can play an important adjunctive role to electrophysiologic studies in the evaluation of patients with exercise-induced ventricular tachycardia in whom the presumptive mechanisms are afterdepolarizations or enhanced automaticity. A left bundle branch block morphology and termination of ventricular tachycardia with vagal maneuvers or adenosine are highly suggestive of delayed afterdepolarizations as the cause of the tachycardia. Exercise-induced supraventricular arrhythmias occur in between 4% and 8% of patients, increase in frequency with age, and do not reflect the presence of coronary artery disease.

Changes in AV and intraventricular conduction may occur during exercise. Rarely, ETT can elicit second-degree AV block in patients with exertional fatigue or dyspnea, but more commonly AV conduction is enhanced with exercise owing to increased sympathetic tone and increased circulating catecholamines. Exercise-induced, rate-related development of right or left bundle branch block is relatively rare and is not associated with an increased incidence of underlying coronary disease in younger subjects (<40 years old), but it appears to be associated with coronary disease in older subjects. In the presence of right bundle branch block on the resting ECG, exercise-induced ST-segment depression in leads V_1 to V_4 commonly occurs and is not diagnostic for coronary disease; ST-segment depression in the inferior leads and in leads V_5 and V_6 can be considered consistent with ischemia. ST-segment changes in the presence of left bundle branch block are best considered nondiagnostic for coronary disease.

The presence of preexcitation on the ECG invalidates the use of ST-segment depression criteria for the diagnosis of coronary disease owing to abnormal repolarization that frequently occurs in the setting of the aberrant depolarization associated with anterograde conduction over an accessory pathway. Exercise ECG may play a useful adjunctive role in the assessment of accessory pathway physiology in patients with preexcitation at rest. The abrupt disappearance of a δ wave during exercise reflects a longer effective refractory period during anterograde conduction over the bypass tract and may be associated with a lower risk. Although a more gradual disappearance of preexcitation can occur when the enhancement in AV nodal conduction with increased sympathetic stimulation is greater than the increased conduction in the accessory pathway, this finding does not exclude the possibility of a shortening of accessory pathway refractory period that can be associated with an increased risk of ventricular fibrillation when atrial fibrillation is manifest. As a consequence, caution should be used in basing therapeutic decisions in patients with preexcitation solely on the results of exercise evaluation, and electrophysiologic testing should be employed where indicated (see Chapter 61).

Drugs and Hormonal Effects

Cardioactive drugs and sex hormones can significantly affect interpretation of the ETT. Drugs that blunt the HR and blood pressure response to exercise, such as β-blockers, diltiazem, and verapamil, may delay or diminish ST-segment depression with exercise and can reduce sensitivity of standard test criteria. Although sensitivity of HR-adjusted criteria appears to be less affected by these medications (8), failure to induce ischemia during exercise because of medications will limit the diagnostic accuracy of any noninvasive modality. Conversely, digitalis preparations can produce ST-segment changes in the absence of heart disease, thus significantly decreasing the specificity of all ST-segment depression criteria. Endogenous and exogenous estrogens and progesterones have been implicated in abnormal ST-segment responses in healthy women (66,67). Moreover, the administration of estrogens can increase the magnitude of ST-segment depression in men and women with ischemic disease (27,66,67), and consideration of estrogen status significantly improves the overall accuracy of the ETT in women (68). Although numerous investigators have reported lower accuracy of standard ST-segment depression criteria in women than in men, it remains controversial whether these differences are better explained by lower test sensitivity or lower specificity in women (27). Although the mechanisms of ST-segment changes in response to cyclic hormonal variations remain to be determined (27,66,67), both the ST/HR index and the ST/HR slope provide similar diagnostic accuracy in men and women despite these potential limitations (27).

APPLICATIONS AND TEST PERFORMANCE OF THE EXERCISE ELECTROCARDIOGRAM

Identification of Coronary Artery Disease

The diagnosis of coronary artery disease remains the most frequent indication for ETT with standard ST-segment depression criteria based on achievement of at least 0.1 mV of additional horizontal or downsloping ST-segment depression the most common diagnostic criterion applied. Unfortunately, utility of the standard ETT for this purpose has been limited by the relatively low sensitivity and poor predictive accuracy of standard criteria (7,8,10,21,24). Although exact performance of any test is difficult to determine as a result of issues of study design, population selection, and referral bias (8,21,69–71), a metaanalysis assessing the sensitivity and specificity of ETT in 24,074 patients evaluated in 147 consecutively published reports provides some important insights into the performance of standard ST-segment depression criteria (21). Using 50% luminal obstruction at angiography as the diagnostic standard for coronary disease, the weighted mean sensitivity was 68% (range, 23% to 100%) and the mean specificity was 77% (range, 17% to 100%); considering upsloping ST-segment depression as abnormal significantly reduced test specificity (from 80% to 73%) but increased sensitivity by a similar amount (8%). Predictably, use of these criteria for the identification of multivessel disease or left main or triple-vessel disease was associated with higher sensitivity (mean, 81% and 86%, respectively), but it was also associated with lower test specificity (mean, 66% and 53%) (72).

The results of this metaanalysis highlight the effects that differences in patient population can have on the sensitivity and specificity of standard ST-segment depression criteria. Although sensitivity has been found to vary with the severity of coronary disease in the study population, specificity will vary with the admixture of noncoronary heart disease that can produce ST-segment changes in the study population; both measures of test performance will be affected by the degree of workup or referral bias (40,69–71,73,74). These combined effects of population selection are reflected in the results of one study from our laboratory (71) in which the 54% sensitivity of standard ST-segment depression criteria in patients with clinical angina who had not undergone angiography was significantly lower than the 70% sensitivity in patients with disease defined by angiography. Similar effects of population selection were observed on standard test specificity: the 97% specificity in clinically normal subjects was significantly greater than the 74% specificity in patients referred to angiography and found to have no significant coronary luminal obstruction greater than 50% (71).

Although some controversy persists over the value of HR-adjusted criteria (see the later discussion of controversies and personal perspectives), most published studies that have adhered to prescribed requirements for ST-segment depression measurements have demonstrated that the ST/HR slope and the simple ST/HR index improve performance of the ETT for the recognition of coronary disease. Initial studies from our laboratory, using computerized ST-segment measurements at 60 milliseconds after the J-point and employing the Cornell modification of the Bruce protocol, derived criteria for the ST/HR slope and the ST/HR index with 95% specificity in clinically normal subjects, similar to the specificity of standard test criteria in the same subjects (24). Test sensitivity of these criteria in separate groups of patients with clinical angina and with angiographically proven coronary disease were 94% and 95%, respectively, for the ST/HR slope and 88% and 93% for the ST/HR index, each significantly greater than the 68% sensitivity of standard ST-segment depression criteria in these populations (24). Moreover, these new criteria maintained similar specificity to standard criteria among patients with no significant obstruction at angiography (ST/HR slope 72%, ST/HR index 61%, and standard criteria 56%). Compared with standard test criteria, rate-recovery loops have demonstrated similarly high specificity in normal subjects (95% versus 93%), similar specificity in patients with no significant coronary obstruction at angiography (71% versus 71%), and improved sensitivity for the detection of coronary disease (93% versus 74%) (25). Additional studies of the ST/HR slope from our laboratory and from investigators in Japan, Europe, and the United States have confirmed the superior performance of this method for the detection of coronary disease (8). Improved accuracy for the detection of coronary disease has also been found for the simple ST/HR index in most but not all studies from other centers (8,19,31,42).

Detection of Anatomically and Functionally Severe Coronary Disease

The poorer prognosis of patients with multivessel, and in particular three-vessel or left main, coronary disease has made recognition of these patients a clinical priority. A metaanalysis of 12,030 patients involving 60 consecutively published reports comparing the ETT with findings at coronary angiography found a weighted mean sensitivity of 81% (range, 40% to 100%) and mean specificity of 66% (range, 17% to 100%) for multivessel disease and mean sensitivity of 86% and specificity of 53% for three-vessel or left main coronary disease (72). In this metaanalysis, use of HR adjustment of ST-segment depression was independently associated with improved specificity of the ETT for the identification of three-vessel or left main coronary disease (72). Factors that have been found to improve performance of standard test criteria for these purposes include use of ≥ 2 mm horizontal or downsloping ST-segment depression, early test positivity (Stage 2 Bruce or earlier) and persistence of test positivity ≥ 8 minutes into recovery, all of which will improve test specificity. In addition, both the Duke treadmill score and a consensus score that includes clinical variables have been shown to provide useful information for the recognition of anatomically severe coronary artery disease (75,76).

Studies from multiple investigators have demonstrated that both the ST/HR slope and the ST/HR index improve performance of the ETT for the identification of multivessel coronary disease. In early studies from our laboratory, standard test criteria identified multivessel coronary disease with a sensitivity of 76%, significantly lower than the 97% sensitivity of an ST/HR slope greater than 2.4 and than the 94% sensitivity of an ST/HR index greater than 1.6, with similar differences in test sensitivity for three-vessel disease (24). Similarly, when criteria that are specifically designed for the identification of three-vessel disease are employed, the ST/HR slope significantly improves performance of the ETT for anatomically or functionally severe coronary disease compared with standard test criteria. An ST/HR slope greater than 6.0 μV/beats per minute significantly improves ETT identification of three-vessel or left main coronary disease and has been shown to be more accurate than standard criteria for assessment of the anatomic extent of coronary obstruction as alternatively defined by high Duke jeopardy scores or Gensini scores (8,77–79). Further, as a functional consequence of extensive coronary obstruction, high ST/HR slopes have been found to correlate with large decreases in left ventricular ejection fraction during exercise and with abnormal thallium imaging (78,79). However, the simple ST/HR index does not appear consistently to improve the exercise ECG identification of extensive coronary disease compared with standard test criteria (8).

Risk Stratification and Assessment of Prognosis

Although the value of screening asymptomatic subjects for coronary disease remains controversial owing to the poor predictive value of positive test findings in populations with low prevalences of disease (26,73,74,80,81), numerous studies have documented the ability of the ETT to stratify risk in low-risk populations (26,44,45,82–84). An ischemic ST-segment response to exercise by standard criteria was a significant predictor of cardiac morbidity and mortality in the overall population of the Seattle Heart Watch (83) and in a referred group of clinically normal male Air Force personnel (82). However, standard test criteria did not significantly concentrate risk among the large subset of asymptomatic healthy subjects in Seattle (83), did not concentrate risk in a nonreferred subset of normal pilots and astronauts undergoing ETT a part of routine preflight assessment (82), was not predictive of coronary events in more than 3,000 asymptomatic men and women in the Framingham Offspring Study (Fig. 48.5) (26), and was not predictive of coronary heart disease mortality in 5,940 asymptomatic men from the Usual Care arm of MRFIT (Fig. 48.6) (84).

In contrast, an ST/HR index greater than 1.60 μV/beat per minute significantly concentrated the risk of primarily nonfatal coronary events in asymptomatic men and women in the Framingham Offspring Study (see Fig. 48.5) and stratified the risk of coronary heart disease death in MRFIT (see Fig. 48.6) (26,84). In both studies, risk concentration by the ST/HR index was independent of age and additional cardiac risk factors and, in Framingham, was similar in men and women. An ST/HR index greater than 3.3 μV/beats per minute, previously demonstrated to be associated with anatomically extensive coronary disease (77,79), was associated with a nearly 10-fold increase in risk of coronary death in MRFIT (84). In addition, an abnormal rate-recovery loop, both alone and in combination with the ST/HR index, and a blunted HR response to exercise, independent of ST-segment depression findings, improved risk stratification by the ETT in the Framingham Study (26,52). Perhaps most importantly, the decreased 7-year coronary mortality in the Special Intervention group of MRFIT with an abnormal ST/HR index compared with the Usual Care group suggests that this methodology can be used to identify men at increased risk of coronary death that will benefit from an aggressive risk factor reduction program (85).

The ETT can also be used to stratify risk among symptomatic patients with known or presumed coronary artery disease (38,39,53,57,86). In 4,083 medically treated patients from the Coronary Artery Surgery Study (CASS) registry, a high-risk subset with an annual mortality in excess of 5% was identified when patients had a positive standard test and an exercise workload lower than Bruce stage 1; a low-risk subset with an annual mortality of less than 1% was identified by the ability to exercise to at least stage 3 of the Bruce protocol with a negative ST-segment response (86). The Duke treadmill exercise score (38,39,57,87) provides additional risk stratification to that provided by ST-segment depression criteria alone. Further, among 1,300 symptomatic patients with coronary disease at angiography, the ST/HR index improved risk stratification by the Duke treadmill score and clinical variables, and it was an independent predictor of cardiac death in both men and women (88).

The prognostic value of standard ST-segment depression criteria after MI has been well studied. In a metaanalysis of post-MI ETT (11), exercise-induced ST-segment depression, poor effort tolerance, and an abnormal systolic blood pressure response to exercise were associated with increased risk. The prognostic value of ST-segment changes after MI in the thrombolytic era remains uncertain because of similar outcomes in patients with and without ischemic ST-segment changes (89). However, an inability to perform a predischarge low-level ETT appears to be associated with a poor prognosis after MI, independent of the use of thrombolytic agents (11,89).

Independent of ECG, thallium imaging, or echocardiographic evidence of myocardial ischemia, attenuated HR changes, both during exercise and in the postexercise recovery phase, have been demonstrated to stratify the risk of all-cause mortality in asymptomatic subjects and in patients undergoing diagnostic ETT (52,54–57,90). An impaired chronotropic response to exercise, defined as failure to achieve 85% of target HR or a low chronotropic index, was associated with a 1.8- to 2.2-fold increased risk of all-cause mortality after adjusting for confounders (90). A delayed decrease in HR during the first minute of recovery provides similar risk concentration for overall mortality, even when exercise-phase HR responses were taken into account (55).

Test Performance in Women

Among the problems with the standard ETT is the lower overall test accuracy for the identification of coronary disease in women than in men. However, it remains unclear whether reduced test performance in women is the result of lower test sensitivity or lower specificity. In a large subgroup of men and women from CASS who were matched for age, prevalence, and severity of coronary disease (91), there was no significant difference in test sensitivity between women and men (76% versus 78%), but specificity was significantly lower in women (64% versus 73%). Barolsky and colleagues (92) reported similarly lower specificities in women than in men (68% versus 89%) with no significant gender differences in sensitivity (60% versus 65%). However, when patients taking digitalis preparations were excluded from their analyses, standard ST-segment depression criteria had identical 95% specificities, but lower sensitivity in women than in men (50% versus 64%). We have found similar differences in sensitivity of standard test criteria between women and men (51% versus 67%) with matched specificities of 96% (27). Morise and associates (68) found lower overall test accuracy in women that resulted from a

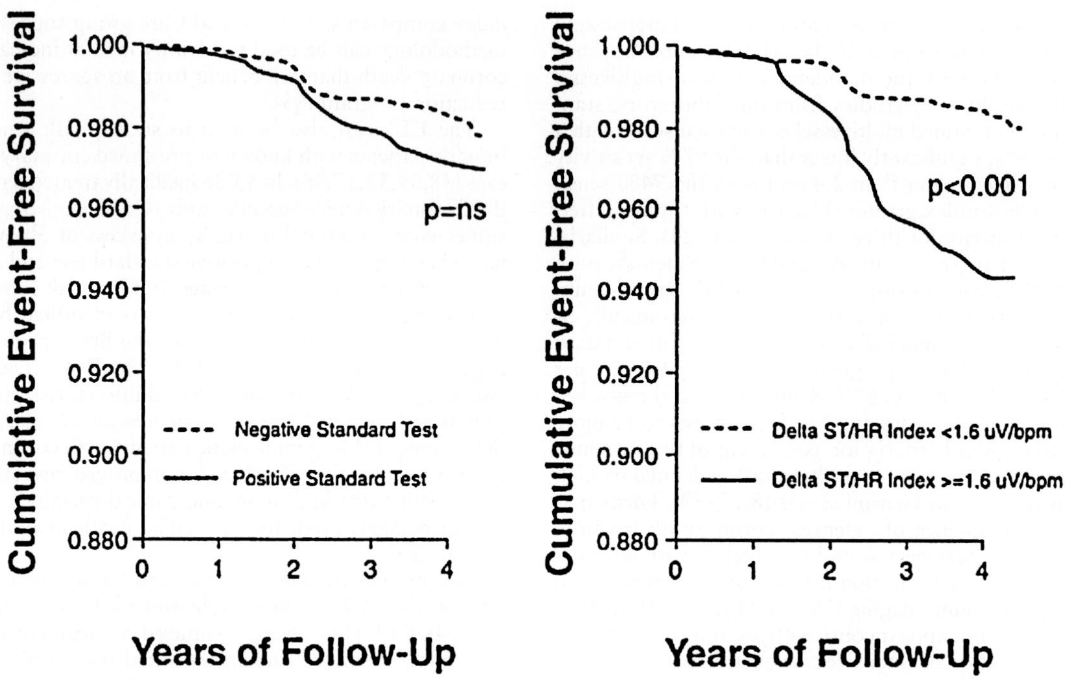

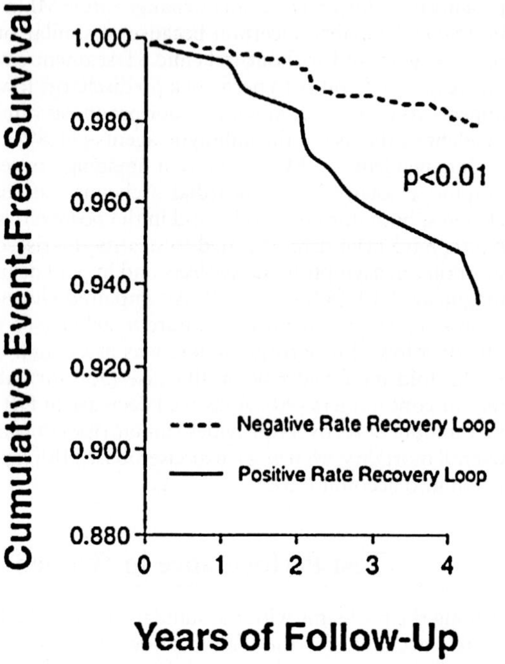

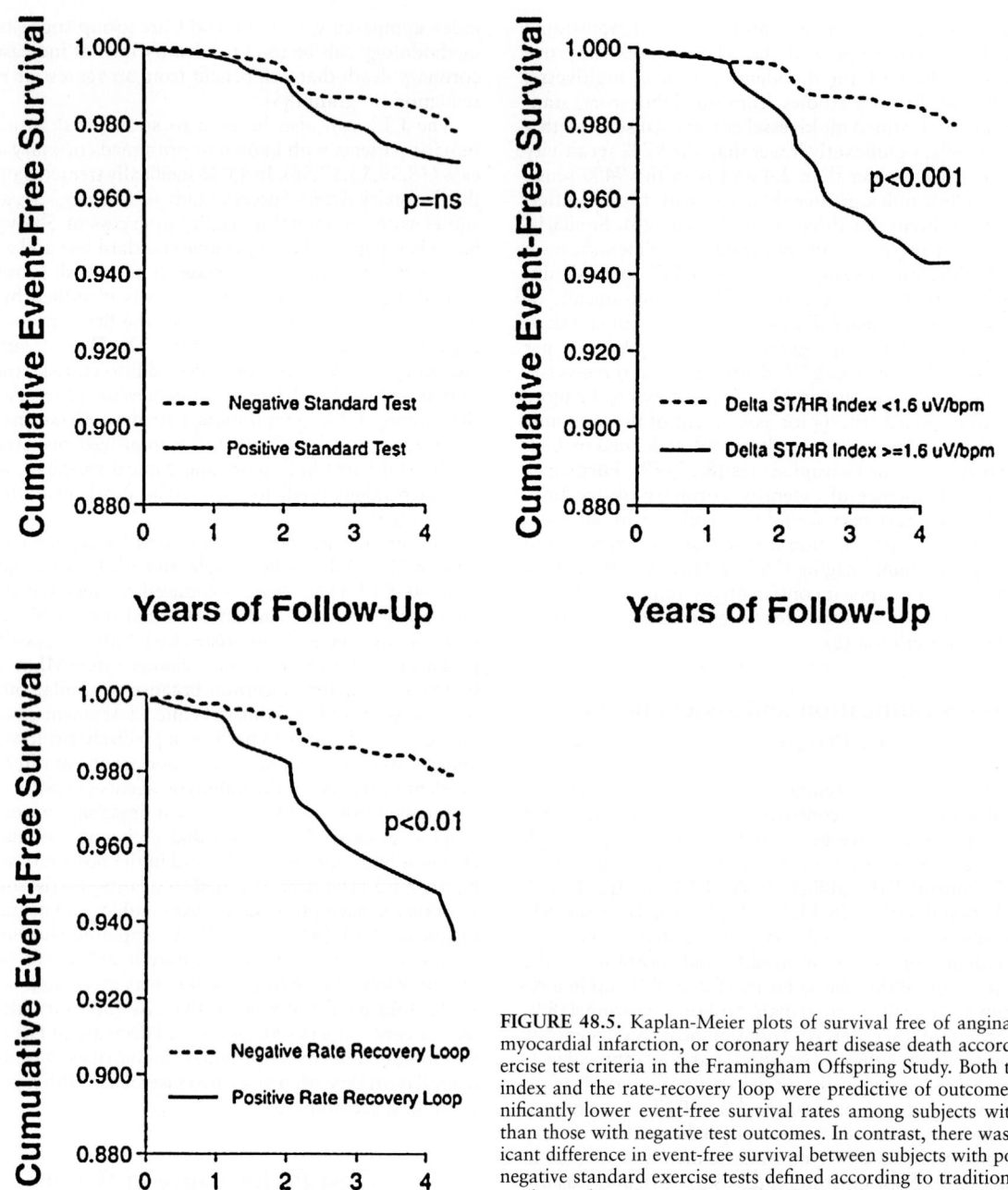

FIGURE 48.5. Kaplan-Meier plots of survival free of angina, nonfatal myocardial infarction, or coronary heart disease death according to exercise test criteria in the Framingham Offspring Study. Both the ST/HR index and the rate-recovery loop were predictive of outcome, with significantly lower event-free survival rates among subjects with positive than those with negative test outcomes. In contrast, there was no significant difference in event-free survival between subjects with positive and negative standard exercise tests defined according to traditional electrocardiographic criteria. (From Okin PM, Anderson KM, Levy D, Kligfield P. Heart rate adjustment of exercise-induced ST segment depression: Improved risk stratification in the Framingham Offspring Study. *Circulation* 1991;83:866, with the permission of the American Heart Association.)

combination of lower sensitivity and specificity in women than in men.

Differences in the magnitude of ST-segment depression between otherwise healthy men and women have been suggested as a possible explanation for gender differences in test specificity. However, we found no significant difference in either standard test specificity or in the mean values or frequency distributions of ST-segment depression between clinically normal men and women (27). In contrast, the lower sensitivity of standard ST-segment depression criteria in women in our study (27) could be directly attributed to the lower magnitude of ST-segment depression among women with coronary disease. Gender differences in the magnitude of ST-segment depression may result in part from the effects of either estrogens or progesterones on the ST-segment response to exercise in women (66–68). The observation that consideration of estrogen status significantly improves the accuracy of the ETT in women (68) further supports this possibility. Finally, solid-angle theory provides a basis for the theory that gender differences in ST-segment depression may in part reflect the effects of gender differences in left ventricular mass or chamber size on the projection of ST-segment changes to the body surface (93–95). However, this concept remains speculative.

Independent of these findings, it is clear that HR adjustment of ST-segment depression improves test performance in women (27,42,96). In a study of 620 patients (27), we found that, compared with use of non–gender-specific test criteria in both sexes, use of gender-specific test criteria with high specificity improved sensitivity of the ST/HR slope for the identification of coronary disease in women from 84% to

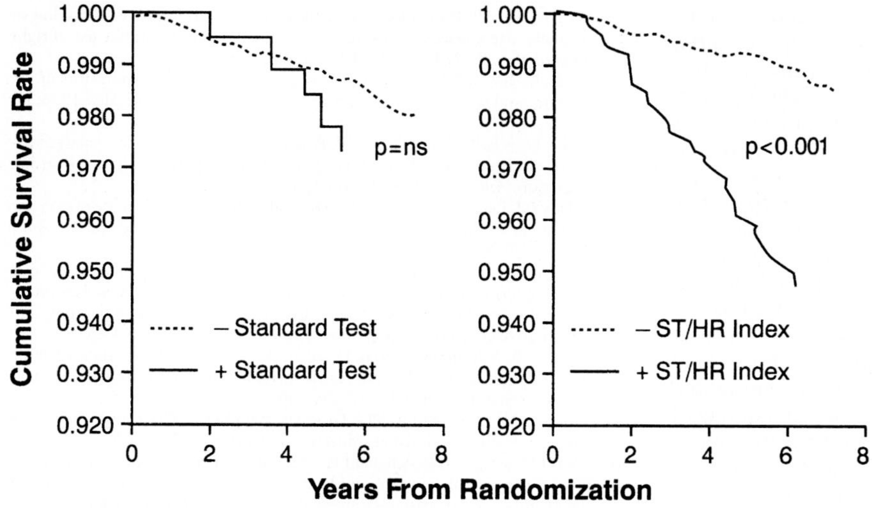

FIGURE 48.6. Kaplan-Meier plots of cumulative survival according to exercise test criteria in 5,940 asymptomatic men from the Usual Care arm of the Multiple Risk Factor Intervention Trial. An abnormal ST/HR index identified a group of men with a significantly lower 7-year survival rate. In contrast, there was no significant difference in survival rates between men with positive and negative standard exercise test responses. (From Okin PM, Grandits G, Rautaharju P, et al. Prognostic value of heart rate adjustment of exercise-induced ST segment depression in the Multiple Risk Factor Intervention Trial. *J Am Coll Cardiol* 1966;27:1437, with the permission of Elsevier Science, Inc.)

91% with no decrease in sensitivity in men. Compared with standard criteria, the increase in sensitivity provided by HR adjustment was significantly greater in women than in men both for the detection of any coronary obstruction (40% versus 21%) and for the identification of three-vessel coronary disease (50% versus 9%) (Fig. 48.7). Thus, we currently recommend the use of HR-adjusted criteria for improved test accuracy in women.

CONTROVERSIES AND PERSONAL PERSPECTIVES

Although most studies performed to date suggest that HR adjustment improves performance of ST-segment depression criteria, some controversy remains (8,19). Initial reports from England reporting perfect test accuracy for the ST/HR slope (29) were met with well-deserved skepticism. These studies and other early reports documenting the expected imperfect performance of this technique severely hindered acceptance of HR adjustment of ST-segment depression, as did more recent studies that reported no improvement in sensitivity with use of the simple ST/HR index (19). However, these studies did not reproduce the methods previously utilized, and it has subsequently been shown that improved accuracy of HR-adjusted methods is strongly dependent on exercise protocol, the number of ECG leads, the time of ST-segment measurement relative to the J-point, and the precision and accuracy of ST-segment measurement (6,8,16,20,46). Additional reports have demonstrated that HR adjustment improves risk stratification compared with standard test criteria in multiple different studies from various other centers (26,84,88), a finding further highlighting the utility of these methods. Although final acceptance of these methods will require even further study in clinically more diverse populations, no study has demonstrated *lower* sensitivity of HR-adjusted ST-segment depression criteria compared with standard test criteria, and numerous manufacturers have incorporated ST/HR slope calculation into their clinical ETT systems (20).

The diagnostic utility of the ETT in the presence of some resting ECG abnormalities and in the presence of digoxin is variable, so caution must be utilized when applying ST-segment depression criteria under these circumstances. We have found that the high sensitivity and specificity of the HR-adjusted ST-segment depression criteria appear to be maintained in patients with isolated ST-segment depression and minor intraventricular conduction delays on the resting ECG. In contrast, we have observed that digoxin can produce marked ST-segment depression during exercise, even in normal subjects with normal resting ECGs who have normal ETTs when exercised while not taking digoxin. Unfortunately, we do not have enough data to date to assess the performance of these criteria in patients with left ventricular hypertrophy (by ECG or echocardiography); ongoing studies will help to address this gap in our knowledge. As a consequence, at the present time I would advocate the use of imaging modalities in conjunction with ECG criteria in patients with left ventricular hypertrophy and in patients using digitalis preparations.

My own perspective is that exercise ECG is not optimally utilized in current practice. In large part because of limited confidence in the accuracy of the simple ETT, there has been a

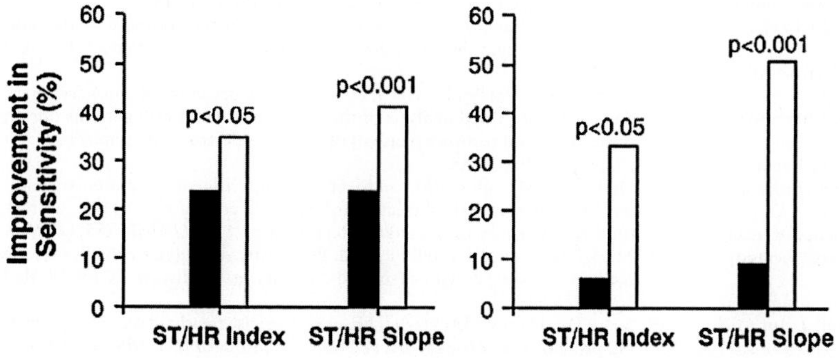

FIGURE 48.7. Bar graphs showing sex differences in the improvement in sensitivity obtained using the ST/HR index and ST/HR slope compared with standard test criteria for the identification of coronary artery disease (*left*) and for the identification of three-vessel coronary disease (*right*). Solid bars represent men; white bars, women. (Reprinted from Okin PM, Kligfield P. Gender-specific criteria and performance of the exercise electrocardiogram. *Circulation* 1995;92:1209, with the permission of the American Heart Association).

dramatic increase in the number of nuclear and echocardiographic imaging stress tests performed in this country. Although these methods provide important localizing information and are clearly indicated in situations in which performance of the exercise ECG is known to be poor, I believe that imaging stress tests are overutilized in the routine assessment of patients with known or suspected coronary disease. In addition, it is also clear that ETT in general is inappropriately applied in large numbers of low-risk patients who undergo screening stress tests as part of annual physical examinations. The appropriate application of bayesian analysis to these populations demonstrates that the large number of false-positive test responses (independent of the test employed) is a consequence of the extremely low pretest likelihood of disease and leads to further noninvasive and invasive testing at substantial cost and some risk to these patients. A better understanding of the limitations and indications of ETT in concert with application of the more accurate HR-adjusted ST-segment depression criteria hold promise to improve the utilization and accuracy of the exercise ECG in clinical practice.

THE FUTURE

Essential to the goal of improved performance of the ETT is the development of new ECG criteria with increased sensitivity at high specificity, based on precise computer-based measurements. The increased accuracy seen with incorporation of measures of chronotropic incompetence in analysis of the ETT (24,25) suggests that further improvements in test performance may be achievable with better adjustment of ST-segment depression for HR changes with exercise. Additional refinements in the ETT may be achieved by the combination of HR-adjusted ST-segment depression criteria with less expensive imaging modalities, such as stress echocardiography, to increase accuracy and to localize ischemia. Novel and interesting approaches to ETT analysis based on examination of ECG findings that are distinct from the ST segment itself also hold promise. These include measures of amplitude, duration, and frequency content of the QRS complex and measures of duration and dispersion of repolarization during exercise. Development and further refinement of computerized methods are needed before many of these new approaches can be adequately evaluated and moved into clinical practice.

References

1. Gibbons RJ, Balady GJ, Beasley JW, et al. ACC/AHA guidelines for exercise testing: executive summary. A report of the American College of Cardiology/American Heart Association Task Force on Practice Guidelines (Committee on Exercise Testing). *Circulation* 1997;96:345.
2. Fletcher GF, Balady G, Froelicher VF, et al. Exercise standards: a statement for healthcare professionals from the American Heart Association. *Circulation* 1995;91:580.
3. Pina IL, Balady GJ, Hanson P, et al. Guidelines for clinical exercise testing laboratories: a statement for healthcare professionals from the committee on exercise and rehabilitation, American Heart Association. *Circulation* 1995;91:912.
4. Mason RE, Likar I. A new system of multiple lead exercise electrocardiography. *Am Heart J* 1966;71:196.
5. Bruce RA, Blackmon JR, Jones JW, Strait G. Exercise testing in adult normal subjects and cardiac patients. *Pediatrics* 1963;32(suppl):742.
6. Okin PM, Ameisen O, Kligfield P. A modified treadmill protocol for computer-assisted analysis of the ST segment/heart rate slope: methods and reproducibility. *J Electrocardiol* 1986;19:311.
7. Chaitman BR, Bourassa MG, Wagniart P, et al. Improved efficiency of treadmill exercise testing using a multiple lead ECG system and basic hemodynamic response. *Circulation* 1978;57:71.
8. Okin PM, Kligfield P. Heart rate adjustment of ST depression and performance of the exercise electrocardiogram: a critical evaluation. *J Am Coll Cardiol* 1995;25:1726.
9. Michaelides AP, Psomadaki ZD, Dilaveris PE, et al. Improved detection of coronary artery disease by exercise electrocardiography with the use of right precordial leads. *N Engl J Med* 1999;340:340.
10. Goldschlager N, Selzer A, Cohn K. Treadmill stress tests as indicators of the presence and severity of coronary artery disease. *Ann Intern Med* 1976;85:277.
11. Froelicher VF, Perdue S, Pewen W, Risch M. Application of meta-analysis using an electronic spread sheet to exercise testing in patients after myocardial infarction. *Am J Med* 1987;83:1045.
12. Balady GJ, Leitschuh ML, Jacobs AK, et al. Safety and clinical use of exercise testing one to three days after percutaneous transluminal angioplasty. *Am J Cardiol* 1992;69:1259.
13. Laarman G, Luitjen HE, van Zeyl LG, et al. Assessment of silent restenosis and long-term follow-up after successful angioplasty in single vessel coronary artery disease: the value of quantitative exercise electrocardiography and quantitative coronary angiography. *J Am Coll Cardiol* 1990;16:578.
14. Samuels B, Schumann J, Kiat H, et al. Acute stent thrombosis associated with exercise testing after successful percutaneous transluminal coronary angioplasty. *Am Heart J* 1995;130:1120.
15. Simoons ML, Hugenholtz PG. Gradual changes of ECG waveform during and after exercise in normal subjects. *Circulation* 1975;52:570.
16. Okin PM, Bergman G, Kligfield P. Effect of ST segment measurement point on performance of standard and heart rate-adjusted ST segment criteria for the identification of coronary artery disease. *Circulation* 1991;84:57.
17. Lachterman B, Lehmann KG, Abrahamson D, Froelicher VF. Recovery only ST-segment depression and the predictive accuracy of the exercise test. *Ann Intern Med* 1990;112:11.
18. Simoons ML. Optimal measurements for detection of coronary artery disease by exercise electrocardiography. *Comput Biomed Res* 1977;10:483.
19. Lachterman B, Lehmann KG, Detrano R, et al. Comparison of ST segment/heart rate index to standard ST criteria for analysis of exercise electrocardiogram. *Circulation* 1990;82:44.
20. Okin PM, Kligfield P. Computer-based implementation of the ST segment/heart rate slope. *Am J Cardiol* 1989;64:926.
21. Gianrossi R, Detrano R, Mulvihill D, et al. Exercise-induced ST depression in the diagnosis of coronary artery disease: a meta analysis. *Circulation* 1989;80:87.
22. Rijneke RD, Ascoop CA, Talmon JL. Clinical significance of upsloping ST segments in exercise electrocardiography. *Circulation* 1980;61:671.
23. Ascoop CA, Distelbrink CA, DeLong P. Clinical value of quantitative analysis of ST slope during exercise. *Br Heart J* 1977;39:212.
24. Kligfield P, Ameisen O, Okin PM. Heart rate adjustment of ST segment depression for improved detection of coronary artery disease. *Circulation* 1989;79:245.
25. Okin PM, Ameisen O, Kligfield P. Recovery phase patterns of ST segment depression in the heart rate domain: Identification of coronary artery disease by the rate recovery loop. *Circulation* 1989;80:533.
26. Okin PM, Anderson KM, Levy D, Kligfield P. Heart rate adjustment of exercise-induced ST segment depression: improved risk stratification in the Framingham Offspring Study. *Circulation* 1991;83:866.
27. Okin PM, Kligfield P. Gender-specific criteria and performance of the exercise electrocardiogram. *Circulation* 1995;92:1209.
28. Okin PM, Lauer MS, Kligfield P. Chronotropic response to exercise: improved performance of ST segment depression criteria after adjustment for heart rate reserve. *Circulation* 1996;94:3226.
29. Elamin MS, Mary DASG, Smith DR, Linden RJ. Prediction of severity of coronary artery disease using slope of submaximal ST segment/heart rate relationship. *Cardiovasc Res* 1980;14:681.
30. Berenyi I, Hajduczki S, Baszoremenyi E. Quantitative evaluation of exercise-induced ST segment depression for estimation of degree of coronary artery disease. *Eur Heart J* 1984;5:289.
31. Detrano R, Salcedo E, Passalaqua M, Friis R. Exercise electrocardiographic variables: a critical appraisal. *J Am Coll Cardiol* 1986;8:836.
32. Detry JMR, Bruce RA. Effects of nitroglycerin on maximal oxygen intake and exercise electrocardiogram in coronary heart disease. *Circulation* 1971;43:155.
33. Detry JMR, Piette F, Brasseur LA. Hemodynamic determinants of exercise ST segment depression in coronary patients. *Circulation* 1970;42:593.
34. Parker JO, Chiong MA, West RO, Case RB. Sequential alterations in myocardial lactate metabolism, ST segments, and left ventricular function during angina induced by atrial pacing. *Circulation* 1969;40:113.
35. Tomoike H, Franklin D, McKown D, et al. Regional myocardial dysfunction and hemodynamic abnormalities during strenuous exercise in dogs. *Circ Res* 1978;42:487.
36. Lehtinen R, Sievanen H, Viik J, et al. Accurate detection of coronary artery disease by integrated analysis of the ST segment/heart rate patterns during the exercise and recovery phase of the exercise electrocardiography test. *Am J Cardiol* 1996;78:1002.
37. Hollenberg M, Zoltick JM, Go M, et al. Comparison of a quantitative treadmill score with standard electrocardiographic criteria in screening asymptomatic young men for coronary artery disease. *N Engl J Med* 1985;313:600.
38. Mark DB, Shaw L, Harrell FE, et al. Prognostic value of a treadmill exercise score in outpatients with suspected coronary artery disease. *N Engl J Med* 1991;325:849.
39. Mark DB, Hlatky MA, Harrell FE, et al. Exercise treadmill score for predicting prognosis in coronary artery disease. *Ann Intern Med* 1987;106:793.

40. Froelicher VF, Lehmann KG, Thomas R, et al. The electrocardiographic stress test in a population with reduced workup bias: diagnostic performance, computerized interpretation, and multivariable prediction. *Ann Intern Med* 1998;1:965.
41. Do D, West JA, Morise A, Froelicher V. A consensus approach to diagnosing coronary artery disease based on clinical and exercise test data. *Chest* 1997; 111:1742.
42. Robert AR, Melin JA, Detry JMR. Logistic discriminant analysis improves diagnostic accuracy of exercise testing for coronary artery disease in women. *Circulation* 1991;83:1202.
43. Sheffield LT, Holt JH, Lester FM, et al. On-line analysis of the exercise electrocardiogram. *Circulation* 1969;40:935.
44. Gordon DJ, Ekelund LG, Karon JM, et al. Predictive value of the exercise tolerance test for mortality in North American Men: the Lipid Research Clinics Mortality Follow-up Study. *Circulation* 1986;74:252.
45. Rautaharju PM, Prineas RJ, Eifler WJ, et al. Prognostic value of exercise electrocardiogram in men at high risk of future coronary heart disease: Multiple Risk Factor Intervention Trial experience. *J Am Coll Cardiol* 1986;8: 1.
46. Okin PM, Bergman G, Kligfield P. Measurement variables for optimal performance of the ST integral. *J Am Coll Cardiol* 1993;22:168.
47. Bonoris PE, Greenberg PS, Christison GW, et al. Evaluation of R wave changes vs. ST segment depression in stress testing. *Circulation* 1978;57: 904.
48. de Caprio L, Cuomo S, Vigorito C, et al. Influence of heart rate on exercise-induced R-wave amplitude changes in coronary patients and normal subjects. *Am Heart J* 1984;107:61.
49. Michaelides A, Ryan J, Van Fossen D, et al. Exercise-induced QRS prolongation in patients with coronary artery disease: a marker of myocardial ischemia. *Am Heart J* 1993;126:1320.
50. Pettersson J, Pahlm O, Edenbrandt L, et al. Changes in high-frequency QRS components are more sensitive than ST-segment deviation for detecting acute coronary occlusion. *J Am Coll Cardiol* 2000;36:1827.
51. Brenner SJ, Pashkow FJ, Harvey SA, et al. Chronotropic response to exercise predicts angiographic severity in patients with suspected or stable coronary artery disease. *Am J Cardiol* 1995;76:1228.
52. Lauer MS, Okin PM, Larson MG, et al. Impaired heart rate response to graded exercise: prognostic implications of chronotropic incompetence in the Framingham Heart Study. *Circulation* 1996;93:1520.
53. Ellestad MH, Wan MKC. Predictive implications of stress testing: follow-up of 2700 subjects after maximal treadmill stress testing. *Circulation* 1975;51: 363.
54. Lauer MS, Mehta R, Pashkow FJ, et al. Association of chronotropic incompetence with echocardiographic ischemia and prognosis. *J Am Coll Cardiol* 1998;32:1280.
55. Cole CR, Blackstone EH, Pashkow FJ, et al. Heart rate recovery immediately after exercise as a predictor of mortality. *N Engl J Med* 1999;341:1351.
56. Cole CR, Foody JM, Blackstone EH, Lauer MS. Heart rate recovery after submaximal exercise testing as a predictor of mortality in a cardiovascularly healthy cohort. *Ann Intern Med* 2000;132:552.
57. Nishime EO, Cole CR, Blackstone EH, et al. Heart rate recovery and treadmill exercise score as predictors of mortality in patients referred for exercise ECG. *JAMA* 2000;284:1392.
58. Lauer MS, Levy D, Anderson KM, Plehn JF. Is there a relationship between exercise systolic blood pressure response and left ventricular mass? The Framingham Heart Study. *Ann Intern Med* 1992;116:203.
59. Lauer MS, Pashkow FJ, Harvey SA, et al. Angiographic and prognostic implications of an exaggerated exercise systolic blood pressure response and rest systolic blood pressure in adults undergoing evaluation for suspected coronary artery disease. *J Am Coll Cardiol* 1995;26:1630.
60. Wray Amon K, Richards KL, Crawford MH. Usefulness of the postexercise response to systolic blood pressure in the diagnosis of coronary artery disease. *Circulation* 1984;70:951.
61. Acanfora D, De Caprio L, Cuomo S, et al. Diagnostic value of the ratio of recovery systolic blood pressure to peak exercise systolic blood pressure for the detection of coronary artery disease. *Circulation* 1988;77:1306.
62. Udall JA, Ellestad MH. Predictive implications of ventricular premature contractions associated with treadmill stress testing: a follow-up of 6,500 patients after maximal treadmill stress testing. *Circulation* 1977;56:985.
63. Jouven X, Zureik M, Desnos M, et al. Long-term outcome in asymptomatic men with exercise-induced premature ventricular depolarizations. *N Engl J Med* 2000;343:826.
64. Frolkis JP, Pothier CE, Blackstone EH, Lauer MS. Frequent ventricular ectopy after exercise as a predictor of death. *N Engl J Med* 2003;348:1508.
65. Yang JC, Wesley RC, Froelicher VF. Ventricular tachycardia during routine treadmill testing. *Arch Intern Med* 1991;151:349.
66. Jaffe MD. Effect of oestrogens on postexercise electrocardiograms. *Br Heart J* 1977;38:1299.
67. Clark PI, Glasser SP, Lyman GH, et al. Relation of results of exercise stress tests in young women to phases of the menstrual cycle. *Am J Cardiol* 1988; 61:197.
68. Morise AP, Dalal JN, Duval RD. Value of a simple measure of estrogen status for improving the diagnosis of coronary artery disease in women. *Am J Med* 1993;94:491.
69. Ransohoff DF, Feinstein AR. Problems of spectrum and bias in evaluating the efficacy of diagnostic test. *N Engl J Med* 1978;299:926.
70. Hlatky MA, Pryor DB, Harrell FE, et al. Factors affecting sensitivity and specificity of exercise electrocardiography. *Am J Med* 1984;77:64.
71. Okin PM, Kligfield P. Population selection and performance of the exercise ECG for the identification of coronary artery disease. *Am Heart J* 1994; 127:296.
72. Detrano R, Gianrossi R, Mulvihill D, et al. Exercise-induced ST segment depression in the diagnosis of multivessel coronary artery disease: a meta analysis. *J Am Coll Cardiol* 1989;14:1501.
73. Rifkin RD, Hood WB Jr. Bayesian analysis of electrocardiographic exercise stress testing. *N Engl J Med* 1977;297:681–686.
74. Diamond GA, Forrester JS. Analysis of probability as an aid in the clinical diagnosis of coronary artery disease. *N Engl J Med* 1979;300:1350.
75. Shaw LJ, Peterson ED, Kesler KL, et al. Use of a prognostic treadmill score in identifying coronary disease subgroups. *Circulation* 1998;98:1622.
76. Do D, Morise A, Atwood AE, Froelicher V. An agreement approach to predict severe angiographic coronary artery disease with clinical and exercise test data. *Am Heart J* 1997;134:672.
77. Okin PM, Kligfield P, Ameisen O, et al. Identification of anatomically extensive coronary artery disease by the exercise electrocardiographic ST segment/heart rate slope. *Am Heart J* 1988;115:1002.
78. Finkelhor RS, Newhouse KE, Vrobel TR, et al. The ST segment/heart rate slope as a predictor of coronary artery disease: comparison with quantitative thallium imaging and conventional ST segment criteria. *Am Heart J* 1986; 112:296.
79. Kligfield P, Okin PM, Ameisen O, et al. Correlation of the exercise ST/HR slope in stable angina pectoris with anatomic and radionuclide cineangiographic findings. *Am J Cardiol* 1985;56:418.
80. Epstein SE, Quyyumi AA, Bonow RO. Sudden cardiac death without warning: possible mechanisms and implications for screening asymptomatic populations. *N Engl J Med* 1989;321:320.
81. Detrano R, Froelicher VF. A logical approach to screening for coronary artery disease. *Ann Intern Med* 1987;106:846.
82. Froelicher VF, Thomas MM, Pillow C, Lancaster MC. Epidemiologic study of asymptomatic men screened by maximal treadmill testing for latent coronary artery disease. *Am J Cardiol* 1974;34:770.
83. Bruce RA, Hossack KF, DeRouen TA, Hofer V. Enhanced risk assessment for primary coronary heart disease events by maximal exercise testing: 10 years experience of the Seattle Heart Watch Study. *J Am Coll Cardiol* 1983;2: 565.
84. Okin PM, Grandits G, Rautaharju P, et al. Prognostic value of heart rate adjustment of exercise-induced ST segment depression in the Multiple Risk Factor Intervention Trial. *J Am Coll Cardiol* 1996;27:1437.
85. Okin PM, Prineas RJ, Grandits G, et al. Heart rate adjustment of exercise-induced ST segment depression identifies men who benefit from a risk factor reduction program. *Circulation* 1997;96:2899.
86. Weiner DA, Ryan TJ, McCabe CH, et al. Prognostic importance of a clinical profile and exercise test in medically treated patients with coronary artery disease. *J Am Coll Cardiol* 1984;3:772.
87. Kwok JM, Miller TD, Christian TF, et al. Prognostic value of a treadmill exercise score in symptomatic patients with nonspecific ST-T abnormalities on resting ECG. *JAMA* 1999;282:1047.
88. Shaw LJ, Kesler KL, DeLong ER, et al. Is the prognostic value of ST depression improved with heart rate adjustment. *Circulation* 1996;94:567.
89. Chaitman BR, McMahon RP, Terrin M, et al. Impact of treatment strategy on predischarge exercise test in the Thrombolysis in Myocardial Infarction (TIMI) II Trial. *Am J Cardiol* 1993;71:131.
90. Lauer MS, Francis GS, Okin PM, et al. Impaired chronotropic response to exercise as a predictor of mortality. *JAMA* 1999;281:524.
91. Weiner DA, Ryan TJ, McCabe CH, et al. Exercise stress testing: correlations among history of angina, ST segment response and prevalence of coronary artery disease in the Coronary Artery Surgery Study (CASS). *N Engl J Med* 1979;301:230.
92. Barolsky SM, Gilbert CA, Faruqui A, et al. Differences in electrocardiographic response to exercise of women and men: a non-Bayesian factor. *Circulation* 1979;60:1021.
93. Holland RP, Brooks H. Precordial and epicardial surface potentials during myocardial ischemia in the pig. *A theoretical and experimental analysis of the TQ and ST segments. Circ Res* 1975;37:471.
94. Holland RP, Brooks H. TQ- ST segment mapping: critical review and analysis of current concepts. *Am J Cardiol* 1977;40:110.
95. Okin PM, Kligfield P. Solid angle theory and heart rate adjustment of ST segment depression for the identification and quantification of coronary artery disease. *Am Heart J* 1994;127:658.
96. Deckers JW, Rensing BJ, Tijssen JG, et al. A comparison of methods of analysing exercise tests for diagnosis of coronary artery disease. *Br Heart J* 1989;62:438.

CHAPTER 49 ■ TRANSTHORACIC ECHOCARDIOGRAPHY

RICHARD A. GRIMM AND JAMES D. THOMAS

OVERVIEW AND HISTORY

Echocardiography (cardiac ultrasound) remains the most powerful diagnostic tool in cardiology (1). Although technically demanding, its diagnostic accuracy, cost effectiveness, availability, and noninvasive nature have made it the largest cardiovascular expense item in the Medicare budget.

MODALITIES OF ECHOCARDIOGRAPHY

M-mode echocardiography was the first form of cardiac ultrasound (Fig. 49.1), in which a single beam is directed toward the heart and reflected signals are displayed on a strip chart or oscillograph at high data rates (200 Hz in most contemporary machines). Two-dimensional echocardiography (Fig. 49.2) is created by sweeping an ultrasound beam back and forth through an arc either mechanically or by phased-array transducer.

ECHOCARDIOGRAPHIC EVALUATION OF THE VENTRICLES

Left Ventricle

Left ventricular (LV) evaluation is probably the single most important clinical application of echocardiography. A combined M-mode, two-dimensional, and Doppler evaluation of the LV can provide reliable information about overall systolic function, regional wall motion, and ventricular mass and geometry (2).

Evaluation of Global Systolic Function

Reliable determinations of LV function require the qualitative and quantitative evaluation of images taken from several standard windows. Typically, the LV is first viewed in the parasternal long-axis and short-axis planes (Fig. 49.2). From these planes, M-mode tracings are generated. If quantitation of M-mode tracings is used clinically, the American Society of Echocardiography recommends obtaining these from the parasternal short-axis view in the two-dimensional M-mode image (3,4) (Fig. 49.3).

M-Mode Evaluation

Standard M-mode measurements are shown in Figure 49.4. Fractional shortening by M-mode imaging is given by LV diameter at end diastole ($LVED_d$) minus LV diameter at end systole ($LVES_d$)/$LVED_d$ where ED_d is the LV minor axis in diastole and ES_d in systole. Normally, fractional shortening is approximately 50% and is considered clearly abnormal when it falls to less than 30% (5,6). Another M-mode measurement is the E-point septal separation (7,8), which is a marker of LV dysfunction when it exceeds 7 mm.

Apical Window Imaging

After the parasternal images, the LV is displayed along its long axis from the apical impulse location. The standard examination typically includes the apical four- and two-chamber views (orthogonal to each other, Fig. 49.2) and the apical long-axis view (9,10).

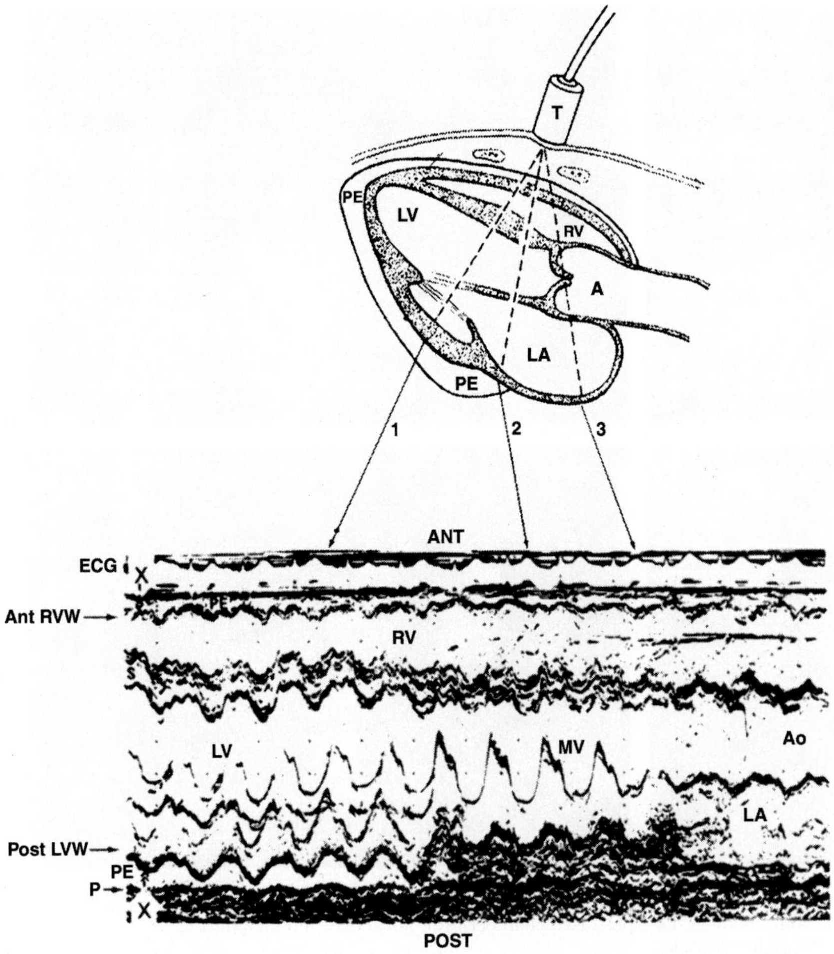

FIGURE 49.1. M-mode echocardiogram displaying motion along a single scan line within the heart. Here, the transducer (T) is swept from the left ventricular level (**left**) to the mitral valve level (**middle**) and up to the left atrial level (**right**). A, aorta; ANT, anterior; Ao, aorta; ECG, electrocardiogram; LA, left atrium; LV, left ventricle; MV, mitral valve; P, pericardium; PE, pericardial effusion; POST, posterior; RV, right ventricle; RVW, right ventricular wall. (From Cheitlin MD, Sokolow M, McIlroy MB. *Clinical cardiology*, 6th ed. Norwalk, CT: Appleton & Lange, 1993.)

The four-chamber view (9) displays the midseptum and inferolateral LV wall as well as the right ventricle (RV) at its widest point, including the moderator band. At the cardiac base, the mitral valve (MV) and the tricuspid valve (TV) are shown, with the TV displaced approximately 1 cm more apically than the MV by the membranous septum. The atria are shown partitioned by the interatrial septum. Posterior transducer angulation reveals the coronary sinus and papillary muscles. Anterior angulation shows the LV outflow tract. To enhance endocardial definition, ultrasonic contrast agents that cross the lungs intact (unlike agitated saline contrast) can be used. Contrast augmentation is gained by displaying the second harmonic of the transmitted ultrasound carrier frequency.

The shape of a healthy LV is a truncated ellipsoid with the long axis roughly twice the length of the short axis. As the heart decompensates, it assumes a more globular shape (11). Diastolic wall thickness is viewed in absolute terms (approximately 1 cm is normal, >1.2 cm is considered hypertrophied) and relative to LV cavity size, with a radius-to-thickness ratio that is typically about 2:1. The distribution of hypertrophy is important. In secondary hypertrophy (e.g., from hypertension or outflow obstruction), the increase in wall thickness is uniform or concentric, whereas it is typically confined to the septum in asymmetric hypertrophy. Regional LV function is assessed by evaluating segmental thickening and wall excursion. Myocardial texture is also informative. Scar formation results in a thin bright segment, and infiltrative disease yields increased reflectance in approximately half of such cases. Geometric uniformity is another useful feature and becomes important after infarction. LV remodeling in its extreme form involves an entire region in an aneurysm that is distinguished from simple dysfunction by deformity throughout the cardiac cycle. Generally, all endocardial segments should move inward synchronously, with incoordinate contraction suggesting at least moderate LV dysfunction. However, dyssynchronous contraction can also be seen with left bundle branch block (12) or RV apical pacing. Finally, the longitudinal motion of the heart can be observed by the descent of the cardiac base (annular plane) toward the nearly fixed cardiac apex (13). A decrease in this parameter is often the first sign of nascent cardiomyopathy.

Quantitation of Left Ventricular Function

Although automated methods of measurement have been developed for assessing LV function (14), the standard method remains manual border tracing (15–17). Ejection fraction (EF) is commonly estimated by visual inspection, but this approach is prone to error and interobserver variability.

M-mode measurements of LV function (18–21) are limited because they use a single LV short-axis dimension, generally assuming a long-axis–to–short-axis ratio of 2:1 to extrapolate information to three dimensions. Unfortunately, many pathologic states introduce regional asymmetry or alter the ratio toward unity. Because volume is a cube function of dimension, errors are compounded. In contrast, two-dimensional volumes and mass compare favorably with those that are obtained from angiography and autopsy, but only if care is taken to optimize data acquisition and analysis (3).

The best apical images are obtained with the patient lying in the left recumbent position and during unforced suspended expiration. A foreshortened ventricle can be avoided by maximizing the visualized long axis.

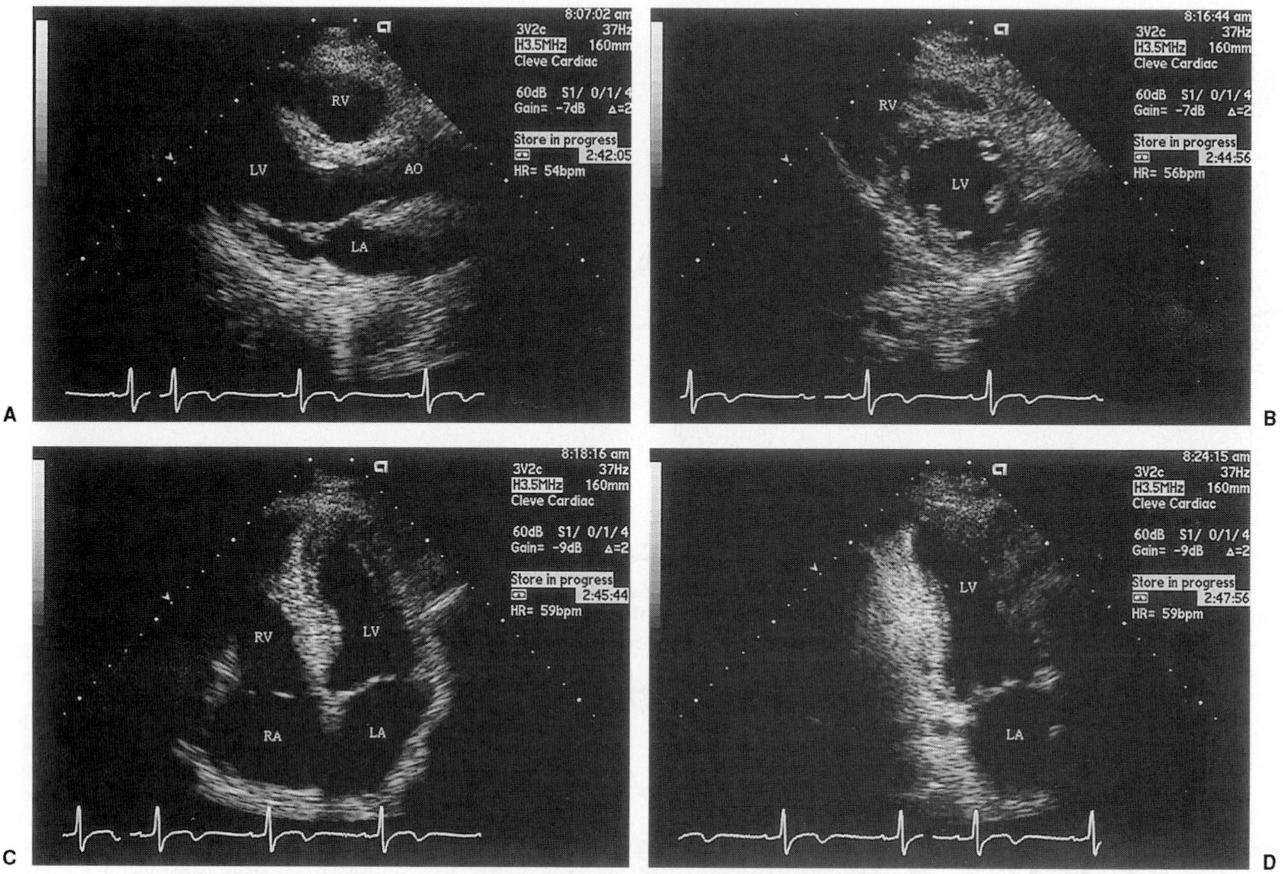

FIGURE 49.2. Two-dimensional echocardiography. Four standard views. **A:** Parasternal long axis. **B:** Parasternal short axis. **C:** Apical four chamber. **D:** Apical two chamber. AO, aorta; LA, left atrium; LV, left ventricle; RA, right atrium; RV, right ventricle.

The biplane method of disks (referred to less precisely as the *modified Simpson rule*) most closely predicts angiographic volumes (10,15–17). The single-plane area length is also suitable, provided the ventricle is symmetric (22) (Fig. 49.5). These algorithms are applied to orthogonal apical two- and four-chamber views. The apical four-chamber view (10) should display the true LV apex, by showing neither the aorta nor the coronary sinus while maximizing RV size. The two-chamber view should not include any portion of the RV, aorta, or right atrium (RA) (Fig. 49.2).

LV mass computed from two-dimensional images is more reproducible and anatomically more rational than with M-mode imaging but is still limited by relatively wide standard deviations (± 35 g for 95% confidence intervals) (23). The truncated ellipsoid and area-length methods are both recommended by the American Society of Echocardiology for mass determination (3,24).

Wall Thickness and Left Ventricular Mass

Hypertrophy is defined anatomically as an increase in the mass of the ventricular myocardium, but wall thickness often serves as its surrogate. Initially obtained from M-mode imaging (25), wall thickness is usually determined from two-dimensional images with normal values from 0.6 to 1.1 cm. Wall thickness should be measured at the onset of the QRS complex (rather than in diastasis), because atrial contraction may thin the wall considerably. Analogously, if filling volume is greatly reduced (e.g., in cardiac tamponade), the wall becomes thickened despite normal mass, and a dilated ventricle may have increased

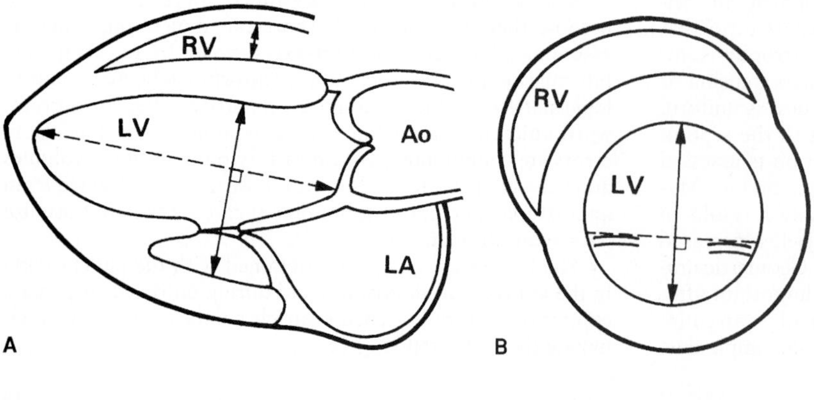

FIGURE 49.3. Quantitation of left ventricular size. Measurement sites recommended by the American Society of Echocardiography. **A:** Parasternal long-axis view. **B:** Parasternal short-axis view. Ao, aorta; LA, left atrium; LV, left ventricle; RV, right ventricle. (From reference 3.)

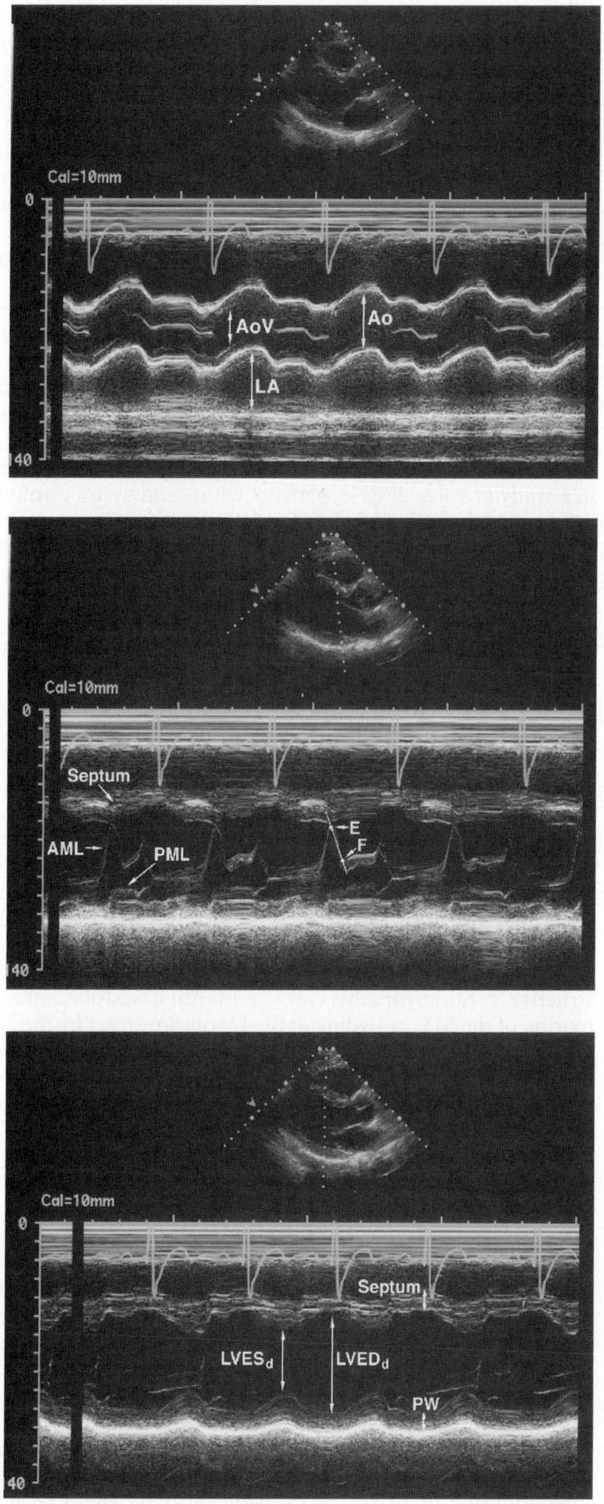

FIGURE 49.4. Standard measurements from an M-mode echocardiogram. Shown are sweeps at the aortic level (**A**), mitral valve level (**B**), and left ventricular level (**C**). AML, anterior mitral leaflet; Ao, aortic root diameter; AoV, opening of aortic valve; EF, E to F slope (rate of closure of mitral valve); LA, end-systolic left atrial diameter; LVED$_d$, left ventricular diameter at end diastole; LVES$_d$, left ventricular diameter at end systole; PML, posterior mitral leaflet; PW, posterior wall thickness; SEPTUM, septal thickness.

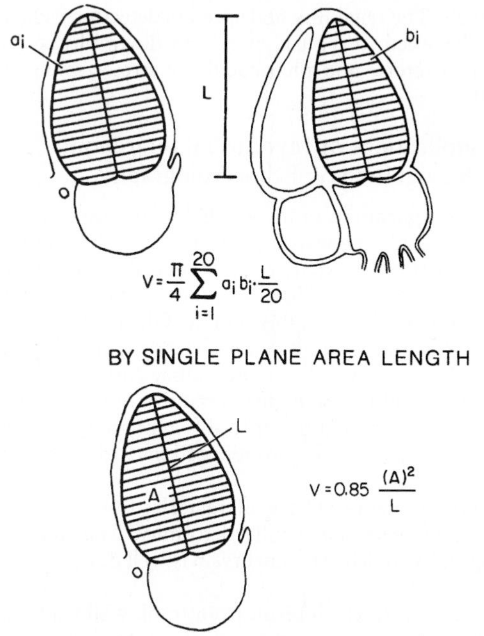

FIGURE 49.5. Left ventricular (LV) volume determination. The biplane method of disks (**top**) requires orthogonal two- and four-chamber apical views and is more accurate in asymmetric hearts than the single-plane method shown at the **bottom**. In symmetric ventricles, the single-plane method is almost as accurate as the biplane method. (From reference 3.)

mass with normal thickness. To overcome the shortcomings of simple wall thickness, actual mass can be estimated. However, M-mode formulas (18,26–28) suffer the same theoretic limitation as the cube method of estimating LV volume, especially in hearts with asymmetric thickening (29). Despite this, the Framingham Heart Study has used M-mode methods to yield valuable insight into the electrocardiographic (ECG) criteria for hypertrophy (27,30,31) and the adverse prognosis of ventricular hypertrophy (32).

Most two-dimensional methods for determining LV mass (3,23,24,33) are similar because they combine a short-axis estimation of wall thickness with an estimation of ventricular length. The difference between the endocardial and epicardial volumes multiplied by the specific gravity of myocardium (1.05 g/mL) yields myocardial mass. Even two-dimensional methods have relatively wide 95% confidence bounds (±25 g) (23,33,34).

Two-Dimensional Echocardiography in Ischemic Heart Disease

Myocardial infarction produces regional akinesis within seconds of coronary occlusion. The presence of scarring (thinning and increased brightness) indicates an old infarction. The interface between contracting and akinetic tissue forms a visually distinctive "hinge point." The diffuse hypokinesis of ischemic cardiomyopathy can be difficult to distinguish from primary myocardial disease.

To localize segmental wall motion abnormalities in a standardized format, the American Heart Association has recommended dividing the ventricle into 17 segments (35). Grading of these segments generates a wall motion score index that has been shown to have prognostic value (36). A diastolic deformity, sharply demarcated, indicates aneurysm formation. Hypokinesis without wall thinning suggests ischemia rather than completed infarction, but the specificity of this is not high.

Echocardiography is valuable in the assessment of chest pain (37–41), because a normal echocardiogram makes cardiac ischemia unlikely. The reliability and speed in detecting ischemic hypokinesis have led to the use of echocardiography in conjunction with exercise and pharmacologic stress testing (see Chapter 50).

Complications of Myocardial Infarction: Recognition by Echocardiography

Many of the complications of myocardial infarction can be diagnosed by a bedside echocardiogram. LV thrombi occur frequently in the setting of extensive anteroapical infarction and rarely in inferior infarction. They can appear within days of the infarction and typically are highly mobile. Older thrombi tend to have smooth surfaces and a texture like liver, and they may have a layered appearance. The more mobile and irregular the surface of the thrombus, the higher is the risk of embolization (42–45). Thrombi can be difficult to differentiate from apical trabeculations, which may be pronounced in cardiomyopathy (46).

Postinfarction aneurysms are characterized by a wall motion abnormality with a diastolic deformity. The ability of echocardiography to delineate aneurysm is well described (47–49).

Pseudoaneurysms, which result from frank wall rupture or cardiorrhexis, are actually composed of pericardium, which confines the rupture. Because only small ruptures in the wall are compatible with survival, pseudoaneurysms tend to have narrow necks, in contrast to the more open neck of true aneurysms (see Chapter 105). Pseudoaneurysms typically form at the inferoposterior base of the heart, are usually accompanied by pericardial effusion (50), and carry a poor prognosis if they are not repaired.

Abrupt myocardial rupture into the pericardial sac is rapidly fatal, although slower accumulations can allow time for surgery. Most postinfarction pericardial effusions are the result of either local inflammation (early) or Dressler syndrome (late). The incidence of pericardial effusions has ranged from 6% (51) to 37% (52) after infarction, and the correlation with physical signs of pericarditis is poor. Ventricular septal defect is a contained cardiorrhexis (53–57), typically at the anteroapex for left coronary infarction and the inferior base for right coronary infarction.

Mitral regurgitation (MR) is regularly encountered as a periinfarction complication (11,53). Papillary muscle rupture is always disabling and may be rapidly fatal (58,59). Because of cross support of the chordae, free motion of the liberated papillary muscle can sometimes be inapparent. Therefore, any patient with severe heart failure and unexpectedly good ventricular function after infarction should have papillary muscle rupture considered. Less severe MR is also commonly seen after myocardial infarction, typically owing to the abnormal wall motion displacing or undermining the papillary muscle (see Chapter 51).

RV infarction can be seen in approximately 40% of inferior infarctions (60,61), with injury ranging from subclinical depression to severe RV dysfunction causing a low-output state with high mortality. RV infarction is characterized by ventricular enlargement, decreased descent of the base, and inferior vena cava (IVC) plethora (60,61). Elevation of right-sided filling pressures can cause right-to-left shunting through a patent foramen ovale and can be easily documented by the passage of saline microbubbles across the interatrial septum.

Cardiomyopathies: Their Recognition by Echocardiography

Dilated, hypertrophic, and restrictive cardiomyopathies can be characterized by two-dimensional echocardiography. Congestive cardiomyopathy shows spheric cavitary dilatation (LV volume often >250 mL), normal wall thickness, and poor wall thickening and endocardial motion. M-mode echocardiography displays MV septal E-point separation, poor MV and aortic valve (AV) opening, and decreased systolic aortic root motion. Involvement of the right side of the heart is important because it implies pulmonary hypertension and RV cardiomyopathy, which independently worsen prognosis (62,63). In spite of an EF of less than 30%, cardiac output (stroke volume × heart rate) may be normal because of tachycardia and the large end-diastolic volume.

Early signs of cardiomyopathy are a decrease in the descent of the cardiac base (13), an increase in sphericity (13), and a rise in end-systolic volume index (64,65). This latter value is highly useful in detecting early cardiomyopathy because the end-systolic volume tends to be more sensitive to contractility than the preload volume (22). An end-systolic volume index that exceeds 30 mL/m^2 indicates significant global dysfunction. In a study of valve disease, patients whose end-systolic volume index exceeded 60 mL/m^2 (64) had a much poorer outcome than did other patients. Similarly, in ischemic cardiomyopathy, the value of 45 mL/m^2 segregates patients with poor outcome.

Hypertrophic Cardiomyopathies. Primary hypertrophic cardiomyopathies are characterized by increased LV mass without apparent cause, such as hypertension or aortic stenosis (AS), and they can be asymmetric or symmetric (66–69). In asymmetric septal hypertrophy (ASH), the increased wall thickness is typically localized in the basal septum (67), and although it is clearly heritable, there is variable expressivity among affected family members. An unusual variation of ASH is apical hypertrophy (so-called Yamaguchi disease) (70,71). When dynamic outflow tract obstruction accompanies ASH, hypertrophic obstructive cardiomyopathy is present (72–74). Findings that are consistent with obstruction may be noted echocardiographically at rest or with provocation by amyl nitrite, exercise, or inotropic stimulation (66). Fully developed hypertrophic obstructive cardiomyopathy consists of ASH, systolic anterior motion of the MV, crowding of the LV outflow tract by the MV apparatus and septum, partial midsystolic closure or notching of the AV, and MV annular calcification.

Secondary LV hypertrophy (LVH) is most commonly the result of hypertension and conveys a poor prognosis (32). The sensitivity of M-mode echocardiography for detecting LVH is clearly superior to that of ECG (30), but two-dimensional echocardiography has superior reproducibility.

Restrictive Cardiomyopathy. Restrictive cardiomyopathies are more difficult to diagnose than hypertrophic or congestive states, but echocardiography remains the most effective diagnostic test. The most common restrictive state is the small, stiff heart of diabetes (75). It is clinically inapparent in the majority of diabetic patients but may lead to pulmonary congestion in association with regional ischemia.

Amyloid heart disease is rare (76–78) and carries a poor prognosis (79). Amyloid infiltration is characterized echocardiographically by increased LV wall thickness and a peculiar glittering appearance of the myocardium. Superficially, amyloid heart disease can resemble typical LVH (76). Contractile function is nearly normal or mildly depressed, and the left atrium (LA) is usually enlarged. The presence of these findings along with typical clinical signs or symptoms (e.g., low ECG voltage, neuropathy) should prompt a gingival or rectal biopsy.

Unclassified Cardiomyopathy. *Ventricular noncompaction* is a rare form of ventricular dysplasia that results from intrauterine arrest in endomyocardial morphogenesis (80,81). It involves the LV or the LV and RV, most commonly in association with other congenital malformations, but occasionally in isolation (82). The myocardium is characterized by numerous prominent, excessive trabeculations with deep intertrabecular recesses. Noncompaction most commonly affects the apical, midinferior, and midlateral segments (83).

Left Ventricular Masses

Nonthrombotic LV masses are quite rare, but approximately 25% are malignant (33% angiosarcomas, 20% rhabdomyosarcomas, 10% mesotheliomas, and 11% fibrosarcomas with melanomas reported) (84). In the pediatric population, the most common tumors are rhabdomyomas associated with tuberous sclerosis. Nonmalignant lesions include myxomas and fibroelastomas, and both have considerable embolic potential. Myxomas can occur anywhere in the LV cavity, whereas fibroelastomas usually occur on the MV or valvular apparatus.

Endomyocardial fibrosis is a disease of impoverished persons living in North Africa and South America. It is associated with restriction of LV and RV filling by obliteration of one or both cardiac apices by a thrombotic fibrocalcific process (85). The disease can also occur in relation to eosinophilia and eosinophilic leukemia. In addition to the unique appearance of the apices, the atria are strikingly enlarged, with MR and TV regurgitation (TR) complicating the picture. Its recognition depends on a high degree of clinical suspicion and a characteristic echocardiographic appearance. In South America, a surgical approach has been developed that debulks fibrotic material from the apex and restores LV compliance.

Right Ventricle

RV imaging is an essential portion of a comprehensive echocardiographic evaluation, because occult right-sided heart disease may occur as a result of a left-sided pathologic process.

Right Ventricular Wall Thickness, Contractile Function, and Size

RV wall thickness, assessed from the parasternal or subcostal windows, should be only 3 to 4 mm, with 5 mm considered hypertrophied (4,25,86). It has been described as a pyramid with a triangular base. The tomographic nature of echocardiography makes imaging this irregularly shaped organ in a single plane or volumetric measurement impractical (86–91). The normal RV size is considerably less than LV size, whether imaged from the parasternal long axis, the parasternal short axis, or the apical four-chamber view (Fig. 49.2). In the last view, the LV should form the cardiac apex. If the RV even shares the apex, RV dilatation should be suspected.

RV volume and EF can be estimated by the area-length algorithm applied from the apical four-chamber or subcostal views (89–91). This correlates reasonably well ($r = 0.83$) with radionuclide scanning for EF (88), although absolute volumes are significantly underestimated. The four-chamber area-length RV-to-LV volume ratio should be approximately 0.6, but it increases to greater than 1.1 in cor pulmonale (92).

Descent of the RV base toward the fixed apex (2.0 ± 0.2 cm in normal hearts) is easily seen in the subcostal and four-chamber views and, if depressed, is a sensitive indicator of RV systolic dysfunction (91). Doppler tissue imaging has yielded similar results in normal subjects (93).

Segmental Abnormalities of the Right Ventricle

The most common segmental RV abnormality results from RV infarction, usually in the setting of inferior wall myocardial infarction (60), and it may lead to a lethal low-output syndrome even when LV damage is not extensive. In RV infarction, there is cavity enlargement (61), with midanterior and inferior wall akinesis or even aneurysm by two-dimensional imaging. The degree of RV dilatation and IVC plethora provides clues to the hemodynamic severity of RV infarction (60).

Right Ventricular Tumors and Masses

RV masses can be primary, metastatic, or embolic (94,95). Generally, the same masses that affect the LV can also involve the RV. Myxomas are the most common benign RV tumors. Primary malignant tumors are very rare and are usually angiosarcomas. Metastatic melanoma can occur, but usually very late in the course of the disease. More commonly, tumors reach the right side of the heart by propagating through the venae cavae.

The most important propagating masses are embolic thrombi from the lower extremities (96). These thrombi, which may present as a localized mobile RV mass, are generally less reflective than malignant masses. RV enlargement and pulmonary hypertension suggest multiple pulmonary emboli. These masses may remain in the right side of the heart, embolize to the lungs, or rarely cross a patent foramen ovale (97). These thrombi generally have an ominous prognosis and require aggressive medical or surgical intervention.

Conditions Associated with Right Ventricular Dilatation

RV volume overload without pulmonary hypertension is seen in atrial septal defect (ASD), TV insufficiency, and pulmonary insufficiency. RV contractile function is usually preserved, and wall thickness remains normal. In ASD, the pulmonary artery is also enlarged. If the right pulmonary artery is of normal caliber, pulmonary hypertension and left-to-right shunts of any magnitude are unlikely. Similarly, the short-axis basal precordial view is the best window for evaluating the size of the main pulmonary artery.

An ASD can be further confirmed by saline contrast injection, which shows a negative contrast jet in the RA or right-to-left shunt flow in the LA. Sometimes the defect itself can be seen, especially with color Doppler, which may also show discrepant flow through the RV and LV outflow tracts (88). Congenital absence of the pericardium may cause RV enlargement (98) as a result of rotation of the heart, but with a small pulmonary artery, low pulmonary pressure, and a normal contrast study. RV enlargement may also be caused by severe TR, most commonly the result of LV dysfunction, rheumatic disease, endocarditis, and primary pulmonary hypertension. Chronically elevated pulmonary vascular resistance leads to cor pulmonale with a dilated apex-forming RV (92), mild to moderate RV hypertrophy (RVH), and a dilated IVC that is unresponsive to respiration. A patent foramen ovale (20% to 30% of patients) may show right-to-left shunting with contrast injection. The cause usually is chronic obstructive lung disease or other primary pulmonary disease states.

Echocardiographic features of primary pulmonary hypertension are similar to those of cor pulmonale but with greater RVH and septal flattening, often preceding IVC plethora. Pulmonary hypertension from congenital heart disease (atrial or ventricular septal defect) may cause severe RVH, but right-sided heart failure may be minimal early in the disease course. In the end stage, it may be difficult to distinguish ASD/Eisenmenger complex from primary pulmonary hypertension with a patent foramen ovale.

Isolated RV dilatation may be seen in arrhythmogenic RV dysplasia (parchment ventricle or Uhl disease) (99). Features of RV dysplasia include a thin RV wall, increased epicardial fat, aneurysms of the RV free wall, and a prominent moderator band with complex attachment to the septum and RV free wall. Spontaneous fatal ventricular arrhythmias may be seen in patients with this condition. In Ebstein anomaly, the septal leaflet of the TV is displaced (>1 cm) toward the RV apex, leaving an "atrialized ventricle" behind the valve. Contraction during systole may cause right-to-left shunting across a patent foramen and cyanosis (100,101).

ECHOCARDIOGRAPHY OF THE LEFT ATRIUM

The LA serves reservoir, conduit, and booster pump functions for blood that enters the LV. It is commonly involved in pathologic processes, including dilation, thromboembolic and neoplastic disease, extrinsic compression, and fibrillation, each of which is well assessed by echocardiography.

Left Atrial Volume and Function

The standard parasternal M-mode image yields the anterior-to-posterior dimension of the LA (Fig. 49.4), typically the smallest, perhaps because of confinement between the sternum and the spine (102). This dimension is the least sensitive to enlargement but, when increased, is highly specific.

Because this single anterior-to-posterior dimension may underestimate overall LA size, volume estimates are preferred, requiring two sector scans, preferably orthogonal apical planes. The area-length formula has shown good correlation ($r = 0.82 - 0.98$) with angiography and contrast computed tomographic scanning (102,103), with some underestimation ($\leq$23%) but good reproducibility (95% confidence interval, 10 mL). In the healthy young heart, only 10 mL atrial transport occurs with atrial contraction, the rest entering by passive flow early in diastole. With aging, the amount of active atrial transport more than doubles.

Atrial fibrillation causes progressive LA enlargement (104), which may be prevented by cardioversion (105). In rheumatic disease, LA diameter is predictive of atrial fibrillation (106) and the restoration of atrial function after cardioversion (107). However, the recurrence of lone atrial fibrillation appears to be independent of atrial diameter (108).

Left Atrial Thrombi, Masses, and Tumors

LA thrombi are common but must be large to be identified by transthoracic echocardiography (TTE). This is especially true of the LA appendage, which usually requires transesophageal echocardiography (TEE) (109).

The most common LA tumor is myxoma, a benign mass that most often arises from the inferior limb of the fossa ovalis. It can present with embolism or obstruction to MV inflow. Myxomas may be encapsulated or highly mobile and amorphous, with the latter at highest risk for peripheral emboli. Encapsulated myxomas may have clear spaces (cysts) and highly reflective patches (bone). Attachment is typically by a stalk to the interatrial septum and may be biatrial. Malignant LA tumors include fibrosarcoma, liposarcoma, and osteogenic sarcoma that may metastasize through the pulmonary vein.

ECHOCARDIOGRAPHY OF THE CARDIAC VALVES

Echocardiography images the cardiac valves as does no other modality. It provides high temporal and spatial resolution while relating valve structure to surrounding structures. Doppler imaging is also critical to valve interrogation, as discussed in detail in Chapter 51.

Mitral Valve

Historically, the MV was the first structure to be identified by echocardiography (110–113). An integrated investigation of the MV includes an M-mode tracing, several two-dimensional views, a Doppler evaluation, and, if needed, TEE (109).

The anterior MV leaflet is highly mobile and quite echogenic, whereas the posterior leaflet is somewhat less apparent (Fig. 49.2). By M-mode examination, an M-shaped pattern of MV motion is seen, reflecting first passive rapid filling and second atrial contraction, with near closure during diastasis, although blood may still pass from pulmonary veins to LV using the atrium as a conduit (114). Final closure results from atrial inflow deceleration and isovolumic LV contraction (Fig. 49.4).

By two-dimensional imaging in the short-axis plane (Fig. 49.2), the MV is an ovoid orifice. In the long-axis plane, it resembles clapping hands moving freely in diastole, but forming a stable coaptation plane in systole. The MV and annulus descend with the cardiac base to assist LA filling.

Normal MV leaflets are thin (<2 mm), although somewhat thicker at points of chordal attachment to the free margin (primary chordae) and leaflet body (secondary chordae). The papillary muscles can be seen in the short-axis view at 4 and 8 o'clock with highly variable anatomy. From the apical four-chamber view, posterior angulation (typically showing the coronary sinus) is necessary to show the papillary muscles and chordae. Normal chordae appear fragmented unless they are thickened and fused by fibrosis or calcification. The mitral annulus has been shown to be saddle shaped and highly dynamic by three-dimensional imaging.

Mitral Stenosis

From the earliest days of echocardiography (111), mitral stenosis (MS) has been recognized by altered motion of the valve resulting from commissural fusion and chordal shortening. MS severity can be assessed on M-mode imaging by measuring the delay in diastolic closure (E-F slope). A normal value is greater than 60 mm per second; a slope of less than 10 mm per second indicates severe MS (115). By two-dimensional echocardiography, the leaflets dome into the ventricle throughout diastole. In short axis, the MV orifice can be reliably measured by direct planimetry (115,116), with an area of less than 1 cm^2 defining severe MS. Doppler quantitation methods are discussed in Chapter 51.

Indirect signs of MS severity include chordal shortening, leaflet calcification, LA enlargement, LV underloading, and right-sided heart involvement (pulmonary hypertension). Progression cannot be accurately predicted, although disease in patients with mild MS and aortic insufficiency progresses slightly faster (117).

Mitral Regurgitation

Regurgitant lesions may be structurally more subtle than stenotic lesions, and Doppler (see Chapter 51) plays an even more dominant role in imaging. Nevertheless, careful structural interrogation is critical to evaluating MR, particularly as it relates to feasibility of surgical repair.

Rheumatic Mitral Regurgitation. In rheumatic disease, the posterior leaflet is fixed and shortened, allowing the anterior leaflet to override it on closure and resulting in posteriorly directed MR. The degree of malcoaptation is predictive of MR severity (118).

Mitral Valve Prolapse

The original clinical, auscultatory, and angiographic descriptions of MV prolapse (MVP) (119,120) were rapidly supplemented by echocardiographic studies (121–123), which contributed to an "epidemic" of MVP by overly liberal diagnostic criteria.

Although MVP has a classic appearance on M-mode imaging (midsystolic or pansystolic posterior motion), up to 23% of healthy asymptomatic women may be diagnosed by these criteria (123). Two-dimensional echocardiography yielded a similar diagnostic prevalence until Levine et al. (124) demonstrated that the MV annulus was saddle-shaped (nonplanar). Thus, leaflets may appear to close above the annulus in the apical four-chamber view (cutting through the low points of the annulus), while being normally oriented in a long-axis view (through the high points of the annulus). Current diagnosis of MVP rests on this long-axis displacement, although anatomic variability dictates that the full anterior leaflet and each of the three posterior scallops be thoroughly interrogated.

MVP is also associated with myxomatous leaflet thickening and redundancy, with the tips sometimes being club-like, with a ground-glass appearance extending onto the chordae. The degree of MV deformity has been related to chest pain, arrhythmias, endocarditis, systemic emboli, and chordal rupture (125). Extreme MVP may be difficult to differentiate from frank chordal rupture or endocarditis.

Aortic Valve

Normal Aortic Valve

M-mode echocardiography of the AV and root demonstrates leaflet closure at the midpoint of the aortic root and opening throughout systole to the walls of the aortic root, producing a box-like M-mode waveform. Fine systolic vibrations can be seen and correspond to a normal flow murmur. Failure to achieve or sustain full opening implies decreased stroke volume. Abrupt early closure may be caused by fixed subvalvular stenosis, and subsequent reopening in later systole may imply dynamic subvalvular obstruction. The coapted leaflets move parallel to the aortic root in diastole, with vibrations suggesting valve disruption or endocarditis. Eccentricity on closure typically indicates a congenital bicuspid valve.

Two-dimensional imaging of the normal AV demonstrates three thin leaflets, opening as a circular orifice and closing as a three-pointed star with slight central thickening. The left coronary cusp is adjacent to the LA appendage, the left main coronary artery, and the pulmonary valve and artery. The right lies just posterior to the RV outflow tract, close to the septal attachment of the TV. The noncoronary cusp sits above the RA and the interatrial septum. Aortic diameter is largest at the sinuses of Valsalva and should not exceed 3.5 cm.

Aortic Stenosis

In severe AS, the M-mode image shows dense persistent echoes with little systolic separation (126). Aortic sclerosis without AS shows dense echoes, but at least one leaflet will move rapidly or will vibrate, indicating a peak systolic gradient of less than 50 mm Hg.

Cusp separation by two-dimensional imaging is helpful if it is less than 8 mm or more than 12 mm, but it is poorly predictive between 8 and 12 mm (127). Leaflet doming, poststenotic aortic dilatation, and LVH predict significant AS, although none approaches the utility of Doppler-derived pressure gradient and valve area (127–130).

The severe calcification of senile AS is nonspecific regarding the underlying disease. In younger patients, bicuspid valves show eccentric opening and only two moving leaflets. On closure of the valve, three commissures may be seen as a result of raphe formation between two leaflets, usually the left and right. Patients with rheumatic AS show commissural fusion and leaflet retraction, generally associated with rheumatic MV disease.

Subvalvular and Supravalvular Stenosis. Fixed subvalvular stenosis is occasionally encountered in the adult population (131–133), often with prior ventricular septal defect. The subvalvular membrane is a narrow ridge in the distal septum. Because the narrowing may be difficult to appreciate by inspection, Doppler imaging remains the definitive quantitative modality. Dynamic subvalvular stenosis is discussed earlier in relation to the normal aortic valve. Supravalvular AS is rarely seen in adults. Features include narrowing above and affixed to the valve leaflets, aortic insufficiency, enlarged coronary arteries (sometimes obstructed), and severe hypertrophy (134).

Aortic Regurgitation

Aortic regurgitation (AR) can be seen with diastolic fluttering of the anterior MV leaflet by M-mode echocardiography (135), a sign largely supplanted by Doppler imaging. With severe acute AR, M-mode images may show early closure of the MV (136), thus indicating precarious hemodynamics and a need for urgent pharmacologic or surgical intervention (136). Henry et al. (137) suggested that an LV end-systolic dimension of greater than 55 mm predicts poor operative results, a concept challenged by Fioretti et al. (138), perhaps because of improvements in myocardial preservation at surgery. Assessment of AR severity by two-dimensional echocardiography has not been adequately studied (139). Posteriorly directed AR may reverse the diastolic curvature of the anterior mitral leaflet (140), but no two-dimensional sign replaces a quantitative Doppler examination (135,141) (see Chapter 51).

Senile calcification typically results in mild AR. Rheumatic disease causes leaflet retraction and a central AR jet. Bicuspid AVs may have significant AR as a result of leaflet prolapse, usually of a conjoined anterior leaflet. Endocarditis may cause acute severe AR, recognized as mobile echoes prolapsing into the LV outflow tract. TEE has greatly improved detection of aortic vegetations (142). AR can arise from subaortic membrane jets that undermine valve integrity. Myxomatous disease can cause AV prolapse. In Marfan disease, isolated dilation of the sinuses of Valsalva causes traction on the aortic commissures and a central jet of AR (143). Other aortic diseases that are associated with AR include dissection, sinus of Valsalva aneurysms, aortoannular ectasia, and aneurysms resulting from atherosclerosis, syphilis, and ankylosing spondylitis. As discussed in Chapter 52, TEE is preferred for emergency diagnosis (109).

Tricuspid Valve

The TV has anterior, septal, and posterior leaflets; the latter two are somewhat variable in size and position. Two-dimensional imaging can be recorded from the parasternal long- and short-axis and apical four-chamber views for anatomic and Doppler evaluation. The TV is apically displaced by the membranous septum, and this is useful in identifying the TV in congenital heart disease. TEE offers relatively little advantage, especially for measuring TR velocity (144).

Tricuspid Insufficiency

Contemporary echocardiography confirms Sir James Mackenzie's claim, made in 1908, that TR is ubiquitous. Present in 80% of normal subjects and in nearly all cardiac patients, this "abnormality" usually is just a convenient means to estimate pulmonary artery pressure (145). Pathologic TR causes RV and RA enlargement, paradoxic septal motion, and systolic IVC pulsation from retrograde flow. M-mode imaging shows paradoxic septal motion, with anterior systolic motion of the septum related to the exaggerated RV stroke volume. By two-dimensional imaging, RV dilatation can be seen, although quantitation is imprecise (92), and hyperdynamic function can be seen as a result of the augmented stroke volume (13,146). RA enlargement is common and is related to TR duration and to the severity and the presence of atrial fibrillation. With severe TR, the normal leftward bulging of the interatrial septum is reversed (147).

The most common cause of significant TR is RV failure from high LV filling pressures, with annular dilatation and failure of leaflet coaptation (148). Rheumatic TR rarely exists without MV involvement. It is characterized by leaflet thickening, commissural fusion and calcification, and chordal shortening. Myxomatous MV disease may be accompanied by TV prolapse (149), but severe TR is uncommon unless there is chordal rupture (150). RV biopsy may cause iatrogenic chordal rupture (151). Endocarditis (usually related to intravenous drug use) causes bulky prolapsing vegetations and flail leaflets (152). Metastatic liver carcinoid causes TV leaflet shortening with more regurgitation than stenosis (153). Ebstein anomaly commonly causes severe TR (100).

Tricuspid Stenosis

TV stenosis may result from rheumatic disease, carcinoid syndrome, or prolapsing RA tumors. Because two-dimensional planimetry is not reliable, Doppler imaging is the mainstay of quantitation.

Pulmonary Valve and Artery

Pulmonary valve disorders are common in congenital disease but are rarely acquired. M-mode and two-dimensional imaging are limited to leaflet inspection (often difficult) and pulmonary artery dilatation. The M-mode image in pulmonary stenosis (PS) shows an exaggerated diastolic "a wave" caused by powerful RA contraction opening or doming the pulmonary valve. By two-dimensional imaging, PS is characterized by systolic leaflet doming, variable leaflet thickening, poststenotic dilation of the main pulmonary artery with decreased pulsations, and variable RVH. PS must be distinguished from subpulmonic stenosis and double-chamber RV that results from prior ventricular septal defect.

Trivial pulmonary regurgitation (PR) is present in most healthy persons. Severe PR rarely occurs from prior tetralogy of Fallot repair, endocarditis (154), or carcinoid (153). Moderate PR can result from pulmonary hypertension (Graham Steell murmur).

Infective Endocarditis

Echocardiography is essential to the diagnosis and management of patients with infective endocarditis (IE). Early studies of echocardiography and IE used the criteria of Von Reyn et al. (155) for diagnosis. Newer echocardiographic criteria for diagnosing IE have been prospectively tested by the Duke Endocarditis Service (156,157). In these studies, echocardiography increased the sensitivity for detecting IE from 51% to 80%, although TEE was required to visualize the vegetations in 41% of cases.

Two-Dimensional Imaging

In a meta-analysis of 16 early studies (641 patients), O'Brien and Geiser (158) reported a mean sensitivity of 79% for two-dimensional detection of vegetations and 52% for M-mode imaging, with vegetations as small as 3 mm reported by two-dimensional imaging (159). More recently, however, the reported sensitivity of TTE has dropped to 62% despite equipment improvement (142,160–165), a finding reflecting less biased case selection and the fact that these studies used TEE (sensitivity of 92%).

Sanfilippo et al. (166) retrospectively studied 204 patients with IE and showed that larger (>10 mm) mobile noncalcified vegetations were predictive of antibiotic failure, congestive heart failure, embolization, surgery, and death. Size was highly predictive of complications: 10% for 6-mm vegetations, 50% at 11 mm, and almost 100% at 16 mm. DiSalvo and colleagues also reported that vegetation size (>10 mm) and mobility by TEE predicted embolic events on multivariate analysis among 178 patients with IE (167).

Transesophageal Echocardiography

TV IE (usually *Staphylococcus aureus*) typically occurs in intravenous drug users (168) and typically causes large vegetations.

PERICARDIAL DISORDERS

Echocardiography detects virtually all pericardial effusions (169), and it is the diagnostic test of choice providing important hemodynamic data as well (170). Normally, less than 20 mL pericardial fluid is present (171), and it is barely detected during systole by M-mode imaging. The high temporal resolution of M-mode imaging is valuable in assessing pericardial motion and RA and RV dynamics. The parietal pericardium is highly echogenic.

Two-Dimensional Echocardiography

Two-dimensional echocardiography and Doppler imaging are key in assessing pericardial disease, with small effusions first seen above the RA. The normal systolic torsion of the heart is lost when inflammation causes adhesions between the pericardial layers. Pericardial fat may mimic effusion (172), typically seen anterior to the heart. D'Cruz and Hoffman (173) have described an ellipsoid formula for estimating effusion size, although effusions typically are graded as small (separation seen throughout the cardiac cycle), medium, and large (typically >2 cm circumferentially). Although transudates, exudates, and blood appear similar, septations suggest chronicity.

Tamponade

Tamponade is a continuum of hemodynamic embarrassment, often associated with large effusions (174–181), although a small, rapid accumulation can be life-threatening. Characteristic echocardiographic features are listed in Table 49.1. The heart is usually small, unless previously enlarged (175), and respirophasic ventricular interdependence is seen. The RV enlarges with inspiration and the LV with expiration, the echocardiographic equivalent of pulsus paradoxus (146,175). RV diastolic collapse and RA invagination (for more than one third of the cardiac cycle) are seen (175,176,178,179). Central venous pressure (CVP) can be estimated from IVC dynamics (177). If CVP is normal, the IVC is greater than 17 mm and decreases by more than 5 mm during inspiration. With elevated CVP, typical of tamponade, the IVC exceeds 20 mm and respiratory change is blunted (177,182), a sign that is less useful with mechanical ventilation (183).

TABLE 49.1

NORMAL VALUES FOR LEFT AND RIGHT VENTRICULAR VOLUME, LEFT VENTRICULAR MASS, AND LEFT AND RIGHT ATRIAL VOLUME DERIVED FROM SEVERAL STUDIES

END-DIASTOLIC VOLUME LEFT VENTRICLE (TWO- AND FOUR-CHAMBER APICAL VIEWS/BIPLANE METHOD OF DISKS)
Male: 111 mL index 58 mL/m^2 [80 (45)]
Female: 80 mL index 50 mL/m^2 [66 (103)]
END-SYSTOLIC VOLUME LEFT VENTRICLE (TWO- AND FOUR-CHAMBER APICAL VIEWS/BIPLANE METHOD OF DISKS)
Male: 34 index 18 mL/m^2 [30 (19)]
Female: 29 index 18 mL/m^2 [32 (21)]
EJECTION FRACTION
61 ± 10%
END-DIASTOLIC VOLUME RIGHT VENTRICLE (BASED ON NORMAL RATIO OF LEFT VENTRICLE TO RIGHT VENTRICLE OF 0.6)
Male: 67 mL
Female: 48 mL
LEFT VENTRICULAR MASS (TRUNCATED ELLIPSOID)
Male: 135 g index 71 g/m^2 [96 (61)]
Female: 99 g index 62 g/m^2 [89 (54)]
Volume-to-mass ratio: 83
LEFT ATRIAL VOLUME (TWO- AND FOUR-CHAMBER APICAL VIEWS/BIPLANE METHOD OF DISKS)
Male: 38 mL index 21 mL/m^2
Female: 32 mL index 21 mL/m^2
LEFT ATRIAL VOLUME FOUR-CHAMBER VIEW (SINGLE-PLANE AREA LENGTH)
Male: 38 mL
Female: 34 mL
LEFT ATRIAL VOLUME TWO-CHAMBER VIEW (SINGLE-PLANE AREA LENGTH)
Male: 46 mL
Female: 36 mL
RIGHT ATRIAL VOLUME FOUR-CHAMBER VIEW (SINGLE-PLANE AREA LENGTH)
Male: 39 mL
Female: 27 mL

Pleural versus Pericardial Effusion

Left pleural effusions can be distinguished by their posterior location, passing behind the descending aorta. Large bilateral pleural effusions may occasionally cause tamponade that is responsive to drainage (184).

Pericardial Thickening and Constriction

Pericardial thickening is common, although constriction is rare. Thickening and adhesion are distinguished from simple effusion by the parallel (rather than damped) motion of the epicardium and visceral pericardium with the parietal pericardium. Pericardial constriction is a continuum of hemodynamic impairment, which may overlap with tamponade and (when the visceral layer is primarily involved) may have a component of restriction. By M-mode imaging, a septal notch may be seen in early diastole around the time of the pericardial knock (between S_2 and S_3) (185,186). Two-dimensional echocardiography may show extensive adhesion and a diastolic septal bounce (182), which may resemble left bundle branch block or RV pacing. One usually sees IVC plethora (177,182), unless the patient is severely dehydrated. In the four-chamber view, the ventricles appear elongated, and the atria are globally enlarged. Malignancy often causes pericardial effusions and pericardial studding, and a frank mass effect may be seen.

Congenital Abnormalities

Complete absence of the pericardium causes RV enlargement and paradoxic septal motion (187). Partial absence may cause LV herniation through the defect with coronary compression and myocardial infarction. Pericardial cysts are difficult to localize by echocardiography because of their lateral position (188).

AORTA AND GREAT VESSELS

Despite the primacy of TEE, TTE is useful in assessing the great vessels. The aortic root and ascending aorta are well seen in the parasternal long- and short-axis views. Coronary artery ostia can be visualized, sometimes allowing for diagnosis of coronary anomalies and Kawasaki disease.

Aortic Aneurysm

Symmetric sinus of Valsalva aneurysms (189,190) may be seen in Marfan syndrome. Echocardiographic enlargement of the root beyond 55 mm should generally prompt surgery. Ascending aortic dilatation may be poststenotic or atherosclerotic in origin, requiring high parasternal and right parasternal imaging to observe. The descending thoracic aorta can be seen in the long- and short-axis parasternal views posterior to the atrioventricular groove. The left and right pulmonary arteries may be seen in the short-axis view. In the apical views, posterior angulation often produces long- (two-chamber) and short- (four-chamber) axis views of the thoracic aorta. Atheroma and aneurysms of the abdominal aorta may be seen subcostally to the left of and deep to the IVC (191). Thoracic aortic dissection with effusion can also be imaged from the left paraspinal window, although TEE is the preferred method to assess the aorta (192).

Great Veins

The IVC is seen subcostally. It crosses the diaphragm just after receiving the confluence of the hepatic veins. Its size and response to respiration predict RA pressure (193,194). If the vessel loses 50% of its initial expiratory diameter during deep inspiration (while the patient is lying supine with knees bent), RA pressure is considered normal.

CONTROVERSIES AND PERSONAL PERSPECTIVES

TTE is the single most useful imaging test in cardiology. Its use has grown tremendously over the last 10 years. However,

TABLE 49.2

TWO-DIMENSIONAL ECHOCARDIOGRAPHIC FINDINGS IN TAMPONADE

Large effusion
RA expiratory collapse
RV expiratory compression or collapse
IVC plethora with diminished respiratory response
Left atrial compression
Small chamber volumes
Reciprocal size changes between right and left ventricles and excursion between mitral and tricuspid valves

Sensitivity, specificity, and positive and negative predictive values

	Sensitivity	Specificity	PPV	NPV
Size (large vs. moderate)	—	97	45	99
RV compression	48	95	38	99
RA compression	55	88	10	99
IVC plethora	97	66	7	99

IVC, inferior vena cava; NPV, negative predictive value; PPV, positive predictive value; RA, right atrial; RV, right ventricular.

this examination is not performed and interpreted uniformly, an issue that has attracted unfavorable attention to the potential overuse of echocardiography in the United States. Of particular concern is the lack of quantitation in many echocardiographic reports. Echocardiography is quantitative in nature. Calibration marks are included, and the Digital Imaging and Communications in Medicine (DICOM) standard allows them to be stored digitally. Nonetheless, echocardiograms too often are interpreted in general categoric terms.

In addition to the emerging echocardiographic technologies such as three-dimensional imaging and contrast echocardiography, newer applications such as its role in selection and device optimization for patients undergoing cardiac resynchronization therapy and guidance of interventional procedures have helped to maintain the dominance of echocardiography as a cardiac diagnostic modality. Three-dimensional reconstruction has been available commercially for several years and is a valuable tool in quantifying chamber size and in visualizing cardiac structures. Nevertheless, it has failed to penetrate the clinical arena completely, in part because of the prolonged acquisition and display times. The development of real-time three-dimensional acquisition has addressed this limitation, and examination times have become shorter as structural data can be captured in a data set from a single cardiac cycle.

Advances in echocardiography have resulted in improvements in image quality, especially for patients whose echocardiographic examination was previously suboptimal. Intravenous contrast agents are now available for LV opacification and endocardial border detection. Guidelines for the use of ultrasonic contrast in echocardiography have been published (195). Intravenous contrast agents should be used to provide additional diagnostic information for the detection of cardiac disease in patients whose hearts are difficult to image. These agents have been shown to be especially beneficial in obese patients, those with lung disease, and individuals who are receiving mechanical ventilation.

In the midst of the tremendous success of resynchronization therapy for heart failure, echocardiography has emerged as the diagnostic modality of choice for identifying potential candidates as well as for optimizing devices following pacemaker implantation (196). The unique ability of Doppler echocardiography to evaluate structure, function, and electrical mechanical event timing in real time has made cardiac ultrasound the clear-cut front runner in evaluating these patients. Furthermore, the portability (TTE, intracardiac echocardiography, or TEE) and improved image quality have made echocardiography the diagnostic modality of choice to assist with atrial fibrillation ablation procedures, percutaneous balloon MV valvuloplasty, and device closures of ASDs, patent foramen ovale, and the LA appendage, as well as for guidance of percutaneous MV repairs.

THE FUTURE

The field of echocardiography will continue to be under intense pressure as cost containment leads to decreased reimbursement. This may seem paradoxic, because the value of the test should grow enormously as contrast, three-dimensional, improved quantification methods, and digital technologies mature. Additionally, increasing applications for procedural guidance and monitoring will enhance the utility of the test. Although videotape may still be used, digital storage, which allows retrieval throughout the hospital, permits transmission anywhere in the world, and eliminates repetition of tests, will be the standard. Adherence to international formatting standards is mandatory.

References

1. Feigenbaum H. Evolution of echocardiography. *Circulation* 1996;93:1321–1327.
2. Qin JX, et al. The development of real time three-dimensional echocardiography is ideally suited for assessment of LV size and function and compares very well to cardiac MRI: validation of real time three dimensional echocardiography for quantifying left ventricular volumes in the presence of a left ventricular aneurysm: in vitro and in vivo studies. *J Am Coll Cardiol* 2000;36:900–907.
3. Schiller, N. B, et al. Recommendations for quantitation of the left ventricle by two-dimensional echocardiography: American Society of Echocardiography Committee on Standards, Subcommittee on Quantitation of Two-Dimensional Echocardiograms. *J Am Soc Echocardiogr* 1989;2:358–367.
4. Schnittger, I, et al. Standardized intracardiac measurements of two-dimensional echocardiography. *J Am Coll Cardiol* 1983;2:934–938.
5. Feigenbaum H. *Echocardiography,* 5th ed. Philadelphia: Lea & Febiger, 1994.
6. Weyman A. *Principles and practice of echocardiography,* 2nd ed. Philadelphia: Lea & Febiger, 1994.
7. Massie BM, et al. Mitral-septal separation: new echocardiographic index of left ventricular function. *Am J Cardiol* 1977;39:1008–1016.
8. Child JS, Krivokapich J, Perloff JK. Effect of left ventricular size on mitral E point to ventricular septal separation in assessment of cardiac performance. *Am Heart J* 1981;101:797–805.

9. Silverman NH, Schiller NB. Apex echocardiography: a two-dimensional technique for evaluating congenital heart disease. *Circulation* 1978;57: 503–511.
10. Silverman NH, et al. Determination of left ventricular volume in children: echocardiographic and angiographic comparisons. *Circulation* 1980;62:548–557.
11. Van Dantzig JM, et al. Pathogenesis of mitral regurgitation in acute myocardial infarction: importance of changes in left ventricular shape and regional function. *Am Heart J* 1996;131:865–871.
12. Dillon JC, Chang S, Feigenbaum H. Echocardiographic manifestations of left bundle branch block. *Circulation* 1974;49:876–880.
13. Simonson JS, Schiller NB. Descent of the base of the left ventricle: an echocardiographic index of left ventricular function. *J Am Soc Echocardiogr* 1989;2:25–35.
14. Lang RM, et al. Echocardiographic quantification of regional left ventricular wall motion with color kinesis. *Circulation* 1996;93:1877–1885.
15. Schiller NB, et al. Left ventricular volume from paired biplane two-dimensional echocardiography. *Circulation* 1979;60:547–555.
16. Folland ED, et al. Assessment of left ventricular ejection fraction and volumes by real-time, two-dimensional echocardiography: a comparison of cineangiographic and radionuclide techniques. *Circulation* 1979;60:760–766.
17. Starling MR, et al. Comparative accuracy of apical biplane cross-sectional echocardiography and gated equilibrium radionuclide angiography for estimating left ventricular size and performance. *Circulation* 1981;63:1075–1084.
18. Corya BC, et al. M-mode echocardiography in evaluating left ventricular function and surgical risk in patients with coronary artery disease. *Chest* 1977;72:181–185.
19. Fortuin NJ, Hood WP Jr, Craige E. Evaluation of left ventricular function by echocardiography. *Circulation* 1972;46:26–35.
20. Kisslo J, et al. Ultrasound assessment of left ventricular function following aortocoronary saphenous vein bypass grafting. *Circulation* 1973;48(suppl III):III156–III161.
21. McDonald IG, Feigenbaum H, Chang S. Analysis of left ventricular wall motion by reflected ultrasound: application to assessment of myocardial function. *Circulation* 1972;46:14–25.
22. Sagawa K, et al. End-systolic pressure/volume ratio: a new index of ventricular contractility. *Am J Cardiol* 1977;40:748–753.
23. Kuecherer HF, et al. Echocardiography in serial evaluation of left ventricular systolic and diastolic function: importance of image acquisition, quantitation, and physiologic variability in clinical and investigational applications. *J Am Soc Echocardiogr* 1991;4:203–214.
24. Schiller NB. Considerations in the standardization of measurement of left ventricular myocardial mass by two-dimensional echocardiography. *Hypertension* 1987;9(suppl):II33–II35.
25. Sahn DJ, et al. Recommendations regarding quantitation in M-mode echocardiography: results of a survey of echocardiographic measurements. *Circulation* 1978;58:1072–1083.
26. Troy BL, Pombo J, Rackley CE. Measurement of left ventricular wall thickness and mass by echocardiography. *Circulation* 1972;45:602–611.
27. Devereux RB, et al. Echocardiographic assessment of left ventricular hypertrophy: comparison to necropsy findings. *Am J Cardiol* 1986;57:450–458.
28. Devereux RB, et al. Standardization of M-mode echocardiographic left ventricular anatomic measurements. *J Am Coll Cardiol* 1984;4:1222–1230.
29. Teichholz LE, et al. Problems in echocardiographic volume determinations: echocardiographic-angiographic correlations in the presence of absence of asynergy. *Am J Cardiol* 1976;37:7–11.
30. Devereux RB, et al. Electrocardiographic detection of left ventricular hypertrophy using echocardiographic determination of left ventricular mass as the reference standard: comparison of standard criteria, computer diagnosis and physician interpretation. *J Am Coll Cardiol* 1984;3:82–87.
31. Casale PN, et al. Electrocardiographic detection of left ventricular hypertrophy: development and prospective validation of improved criteria. *J Am Coll Cardiol* 1985;6:572–580.
32. Levy D, et al. Prognostic implications of echocardiographically determined left ventricular mass in the Framingham Heart Study. *N Engl J Med* 1990;322:1561–1566.
33. Byrd BFD, et al. Accuracy and reproducibility of clinically acquired two-dimensional echocardiographic mass measurements. *Am Heart J* 1989;118: 133–137.
34. Collins HW, Kronenberg MW, Byrd BFD. Reproducibility of left ventricular mass measurements by two-dimensional and M-mode echocardiography. *J Am Coll Cardiol* 1989;14:672–676.
35. Cerqueira M, et al. Standardized myocardial segmentation and nomenclature for tomographic imaging of the heart. *Circulation* 2002;105:539–542.
36. Nishimura RA, et al. Prognostic value of predischarge 2-dimensional echocardiogram after acute myocardial infarction. *Am J Cardiol* 1984;53:429–432.
37. Gibson RS, et al. Value of early two dimensional echocardiography in patients with acute myocardial infarction. *Am J Cardiol* 1982;49:1110–1119.
38. Kan G, et al. Early two-dimensional echocardiographic measurement of left ventricular ejection fraction in acute myocardial infarction. *Eur Heart J* 1984;5:210–217.
39. Kumar A, Minagoe S, Chandraratna PA. Two-dimensional echocardiographic demonstration of restoration of normal wall motion after acute myocardial infarction. *Am J Cardiol* 1986;57:1232–1235.
40. Roberts CS, et al. Early and late remodeling of the left ventricle after acute myocardial infarction. *Am J Cardiol* 1984;54:407–410.
41. Stamm RB, et al. Echocardiographic detection of infarct-localized asynergy and remote asynergy during acute myocardial infarction: correlation with the extent of angiographic coronary disease. *Circulation* 1983;67:233–244.
42. Haugland JM, et al. Embolic potential of left ventricular thrombi detected by two-dimensional echocardiography. *Circulation* 1984;70:588–598.
43. Reeder GS, Tajik AJ, Seward JB. Left ventricular mural thrombus: two-dimensional echocardiographic diagnosis. *Mayo Clin Proc* 1981;56:82–86.
44. Visser CA, et al. Two dimensional echocardiography in the diagnosis of left ventricular thrombus: a prospective study of 67 patients with anatomic validation. *Chest* 1983;83:228–232.
45. Visser CA, et al. Long-term follow-up of left ventricular thrombus after acute myocardial infarction: a two-dimensional echocardiographic study in 96 patients. *Chest* 1984;86:532–536.
46. Keren A, Billingham ME, Popp RL. Echocardiographic recognition and implications of ventricular hypertrophic trabeculations and aberrant bands. *Circulation* 1984;70:836–842.
47. Arvan S, Varat MA. Persistent ST-segment elevation and left ventricular wall abnormalities: a 2-dimensional echocardiographic study. *Am J Cardiol* 1984;53:1542–1546.
48. Matsumoto M, et al. Left ventricular aneurysm and the prediction of left ventricular enlargement studied by two-dimensional echocardiography: quantitative assessment of aneurysm size in relation to clinical course. *Circulation* 1985;72:280–286.
49. Wong M, Shah PM. Accuracy of two-dimensional echocardiography in detecting left ventricular aneurysm. *Clin Cardiol* 1983;6:250–254.
50. Kaul S, et al. Atypical echocardiographic and angiographic presentation of a postoperative pseudoaneurysm of the left ventricle after repair of a true aneurysm. *J Am Coll Cardiol* 1983;2:780–784.
51. Wunderink RG. Incidence of pericardial effusions in acute myocardial infarctions. *Chest* 1984;85:494–496.
52. Kaplan K, et al. Frequency of pericardial effusion as determined by M-mode echocardiography in acute myocardial infarction. *Am J Cardiol* 1985;55: 335–337.
53. Lindower P, Embrey R, Vandenberg B. Echocardiographic diagnosis of mechanical complications in acute myocardial infarction. *Clin Intensive Care* 1993;4:276–283.
54. Drobac M, et al. Ventricular septal defect after myocardial infarction: diagnosis by two-dimensional contrast echocardiography. *Circulation* 1983;67:335–341.
55. Recusani F, et al. Ventricular septal rupture after myocardial infarction: diagnosis by two-dimensional and pulsed Doppler echocardiography. *Am J Cardiol* 1984;54:277–281.
56. Keren G, et al. Diagnosis of ventricular septal rupture from acute myocardial infarction by combined 2-dimensional and pulsed Doppler echocardiography. *Am J Cardiol* 1984;53:1202–1203.
57. Eisenberg PR, Barzilai B, Perez JE. Noninvasive detection by Doppler echocardiography of combined ventricular septal rupture and mitral regurgitation in acute myocardial infarction. *J Am Coll Cardiol* 1984;4:617–620.
58. Nishimura RA, et al. Papillary muscle rupture complicating acute myocardial infarction: analysis of 17 patients. *Am J Cardiol* 1983;51:373–377.
59. Nishimura RA, Shub C, Tajik AJ. Two dimensional echocardiographic diagnosis of partial papillary muscle rupture. *Br Heart J* 1982;48:598–600.
60. Goldberger JJ, et al. Right ventricular infarction: recognition and assessment of its hemodynamic significance by two-dimensional echocardiography. *J Am Soc Echocardiogr* 1991;4:140–146.
61. Sharpe DN, et al. The noninvasive diagnosis of right ventricular infarction. *Circulation* 1978;57:483–490.
62. Unverferth DV, et al. Factors influencing the one-year mortality of dilated cardiomyopathy. *Am J Cardiol* 1984;54:147–152.
63. Lewis JF, et al. Discordance in degree of right and left ventricular dilation in patients with dilated cardiomyopathy: recognition and clinical implications. *J Am Coll Cardiol* 1993;21:649–654.
64. Borow KM, et al. End-systolic volume as a predictor of postoperative left ventricular performance in volume overload from valvular regurgitation. *Am J Med* 1980;68:655–663.
65. White HD, et al. Left ventricular end-systolic volume as the major determinant of survival after recovery from myocardial infarction. *Circulation* 1987;76:44–51.
66. Abbasi AS, et al. Echocardiographic diagnosis of idiopathic hypertrophic cardiomyopathy without outflow obstruction. *Circulation* 1972;46:897–904.
67. Maron BJ, et al. Patterns of inheritance in hypertrophic cardiomyopathy: assessment by M-mode and two-dimensional echocardiography. *Am J Cardiol* 1984;53:1087–1094.
68. Maron BJ. Asymmetry in hypertrophic cardiomyopathy: the septal to free wall thickness ratio revisited. *Am J Cardiol* 1985;55:835–838.
69. Nair CK, et al. Echocardiographic and electrocardiographic characteristics of patients with hypertrophic cardiomyopathy with and without mitral anular calcium. *Am J Cardiol* 1987;59:1428–1430.
70. Maron BJ, et al. Hypertrophic cardiomyopathy with ventricular septal hypertrophy localized to the apical region of the left ventricle (apical hypertrophic cardiomyopathy). *Am J Cardiol* 1982;49:1838–1848.
71. Kereiakes DJ, et al. Apical hypertrophic cardiomyopathy. *Am Heart J* 1983;105:855–856.

72. Maron BJ, et al. Systolic anterior motion of the posterior mitral leaflet: a previously unrecognized cause of dynamic subaortic obstruction in patients with hypertrophic cardiomyopathy. *Circulation* 1983;68:282–293.
73. Spirito P, Maron BJ. Patterns of systolic anterior motion of the mitral valve in hypertrophic cardiomyopathy: assessment by two-dimensional echocardiography. *Am J Cardiol* 1984;54:1039–1046.
74. Yock PG, Hatle L, Popp RL. Patterns and timing of Doppler-detected intracavitary and aortic flow in hypertrophic cardiomyopathy. *J Am Coll Cardiol* 1986;8:1047–1058.
75. Bouchard A, et al. Noninvasive assessment of cardiomyopathy in normotensive diabetic patients between 20 and 50 years old. *Am J Med* 1989;87:160–166.
76. Sedlis SP, et al. Cardiac amyloidosis simulating hypertrophic cardiomyopathy. *Am J Cardiol* 1984;53:969–970.
77. Siqueira-Filho AG, et al. M-mode and two-dimensional echocardiographic features in cardiac amyloidosis. *Circulation* 1981;63:188–196.
78. Nicolosi GL, et al. Prospective identification of patients with amyloid heart disease by two-dimensional echocardiography. *Circulation* 1984;70:432–437.
79. Klein AL, et al. Prognostic significance of Doppler measures of diastolic function in cardiac amyloidosis: a Doppler echocardiography study. *Circulation* 1991;83:808–816.
80. Allenby PA, et al. Dysplastic cardiac development presenting as cardiomyopathy. *Arch Pathol Lab Med* 1988;112:1255–1258.
81. Jenni R, et al. Persisting myocardial sinusoids of both ventricles as an isolated anomaly: echocardiographic, angiographic, and pathologic anatomical findings. *Cardiovasc Intervent Radiol* 1986;9:127–131.
82. Agmon, Y, et al. Noncompaction of the ventricular myocardium. *J Am Soc Echocardiogr* 1999;12:859–863.
83. Oechslin EN, et al. Long-term follow-up of 34 adults with isolated left ventricular noncompaction: a distinct cardiomyopathy with poor prognosis. *J Am Coll Cardiol* 2000;36:493–500.
84. Ports TA, et al. Echocardiography of left ventricular masses. *Circulation* 1978;58:528–536.
85. Acquatella H, et al. Value of two-dimensional echocardiography in endomyocardial disease with and without eosinophilia: a clinical and pathologic study. *Circulation* 1983;67:1219–1226.
86. Cooper MJ, et al. Comparison of M-mode echocardiographic measurement of right ventricular wall thickness obtained by the subcostal and parasternal approach in children. *Am J Cardiol* 1984;54:835–838.
87. Jiang L, et al. Three-dimensional echocardiography: in vivo validation for right ventricular volume and function. *Circulation* 1994;89:2342–2350.
88. Silverman NH, Hudson S. Evaluation of right ventricular volume and ejection fraction in children by two-dimensional echocardiography. *Pediatr Cardiol* 1983;4:197–203.
89. Levine RA, et al. Echocardiographic measurement of right ventricular volume. *Circulation* 1984;69:497–505.
90. Starling MR, et al. A new two-dimensional echocardiographic technique for evaluating right ventricular size and performance in patients with obstructive lung disease. *Circulation* 1982;66:612–620.
91. Kaul S, et al. Assessment of right ventricular function using two-dimensional echocardiography. *Am Heart J* 1984;107:526–531.
92. Himelman RB, et al. Improved recognition of cor pulmonale in patients with severe chronic obstructive pulmonary disease. *Am J Med* 1988;84:891–898.
93. Isaaz K, et al. Quantitation of the motion of the cardiac base in normal subjects by Doppler echocardiography. *J Am Soc Echocardiogr* 1993;6:166–176.
94. Ports TA, Schiller NB, Strunk BL. Echocardiography of right ventricular tumors. *Circulation* 1977;56:439–447.
95. Lee CC, Celik C, Lajos TZ. Excision of papillary fibroelastoma arising from the septal leaflet of the tricuspid valve. *J Card Surg* 1995;10:589–591.
96. Nellessen U, et al. Impending paradoxical embolism from atrial thrombus: correct diagnosis by transesophageal echocardiography and prevention by surgery. *J Am Coll Cardiol* 1985;5:1002–1004.
97. Higgins JR, Strunk BL, Schiller NB. Diagnosis of paradoxical embolism with contrast echocardiography. *Am Heart J* 1984;107:375–377.
98. Payvandi MN, Kerber RE. Echocardiography in congenital and acquired absence of the pericardium: an echocardiographic mimic of right ventricular volume overload. *Circulation* 1976;53:86–92.
99. Marcus FI, Fontaine G. Arrhythmogenic right ventricular dysplasia/cardiomyopathy: a review. *Pacing Clin Electrophysiol* 1995;18:1298–314.
100. Ports TA, Silverman NH, Schiller NB. Two-dimensional echocardiographic assessment of Ebstein's anomaly. *Circulation* 1978;58:336–343.
101. Silverman NH, et al. Pathologic elucidation of the echocardiographic features of Ebstein's malformation of the morphologically tricuspid valve in discordant atrioventricular connections. *Am J Cardiol* 1995;76:1277–1283.
102. Schabelman S, et al. Left atrial volume estimation by two-dimensional echocardiography. *Cathet Cardiovasc Diagn* 1981;7:165–178.
103. Kircher B, et al. Left atrial volume determination by biplane two-dimensional echocardiography: validation by cine computed tomography. *Am Heart J* 1991;121:864–871.
104. Sanfilippo AJ, et al. Atrial enlargement as a consequence of atrial fibrillation: a prospective echocardiographic study. *Circulation* 1990;82:792–797.
105. Welikovitch L, et al. Change in atrial volume following restoration of sinus rhythm in patients with atrial fibrillation: a prospective echocardiographic study. *Can J Cardiol* 1994;10:993–996.
106. Diker E, et al. Prevalence and predictors of atrial fibrillation in rheumatic valvular heart disease. *Am J Cardiol* 1996;77:96–98.
107. Mattioli AV, et al. Restoration of atrial function after atrial fibrillation of different etiological origins. *Cardiology* 1996;87:205–211.
108. Rostagno C, et al. Left atrial size changes in patients with paroxysmal lone atrial fibrillation: an echocardiographic follow-up. *Angiology* 1996;47:797–801.
109. Schiller NB, Foster E, Redberg RF. Transesophageal echocardiography in the evaluation of mitral regurgitation: the twenty-four signs of severe mitral regurgitation. *Cardiol Clin* 1993;11:399–408.
110. Edler I. Ultrasound cardiogram in mitral valve disease. *Acta Chir Scand* 1956;111:230.
111. Edler I. Ultrasonic cardiogram in mitral stenosis. *Acta Med Scand* 1957;159:85.
112. Edler I. Ultrasound cardiography in mitral valve stenosis. *Am J Cardiol* 1967;19:18–31.
113. Fagard R, et al. Noninvasive assessment of seasonal variations in cardiac structure and function in cyclists. *Circulation* 1983;67:896–901.
114. Gutman J, et al. Normal left atrial function determined by 2-dimensional echocardiography. *Am J Cardiol* 1983;51:336–340.
115. Nichol PM, Gilbert BW, Kisslo JA. Two-dimensional echocardiographic assessment of mitral stenosis. *Circulation* 1977;55:120–128.
116. Wann LS, et al. Determination of mitral valve area by cross-sectional echocardiography. *Ann Intern Med* 1978;88:337–341.
117. Sagie A, et al. Doppler echocardiographic assessment of long-term progression of mitral stenosis in 103 patients: valve area and right heart disease. *J Am Coll Cardiol* 1996;28:472–479.
118. Wann LS, et al. Cross-sectional echocardiographic detection of rheumatic mitral regurgitation. *Am J Cardiol* 1978;41:1258–1263.
119. Allen H, Harris A, Leatham A. Significance and prognosis of an isolated late systolic murmur: a 9- to 22-year follow-up. *Br Heart J* 1974;36:525–532.
120. Barlow JB, Pocock WA. Mitral valve prolapse, the specific billowing mitral leaflet syndrome, or an insignificant non-ejection systolic click (editorial). *Am Heart J* 1979;97:277–285.
121. Kerber RE, Isaeff DM, Hancock EW. Echocardiographic patterns in patients with the syndrome of systolic click and late systolic murmur. *N Engl J Med* 1971;284:691–693.
122. Dillon JC, et al. Use of echocardiography in patients with prolapsed mitral valve. *Circulation* 1971;43:503–507.
123. Markiewicz W, et al. Mitral valve prolapse in one hundred presumably healthy young females. *Circulation* 1976;53:464–473.
124. Levine RA, et al. The relationship of mitral annular shape to the diagnosis of mitral valve prolapse. *Circulation* 1987;75:756–767.
125. Nishimura RA, et al. Echocardiographically documented mitral-valve prolapse: long-term follow-up of 237 patients. *N Engl J Med* 1985;313:1305–1309.
126. Chin ML, et al. Aortic valve systolic flutter as a screening test for severe aortic stenosis. *Am J Cardiol* 1983;51:981–985.
127. Godley RW, et al. Reliability of two-dimensional echocardiography in assessing the severity of valvular aortic stenosis. *Chest* 1981;79:657–662.
128. Stoddard MF, Hammons RT, Longaker RA. Doppler transesophageal echocardiographic determination of aortic valve area in adults with aortic stenosis. *Am Heart J* 1996;132:337–342.
129. Teirstein P, et al. Doppler echocardiographic measurement of aortic valve area in aortic stenosis: a noninvasive application of the Gorlin formula. *J Am Coll Cardiol* 1986;8:1059–1065.
130. Yeager M, Yock PG, Popp RL. Comparison of Doppler-derived pressure gradient to that determined at cardiac catheterization in adults with aortic valve stenosis: implications for management. *Am J Cardiol* 1986;57:644–648.
131. Choi JY, Sullivan ID. Fixed subaortic stenosis: anatomical spectrum and nature of progression. *Br Heart J* 1991;65:280–286.
132. Kitchiner D, et al. Morphology of left ventricular outflow tract structures in patients with subaortic stenosis and a ventricular septal defect. *Br Heart J* 1994;72:251–260.
133. Kleinert S, Geva T. Echocardiographic morphometry and geometry of the left ventricular outflow tract in fixed subaortic stenosis. *J Am Coll Cardiol* 1993;22:1501–1508.
134. Braunstein PW Jr, et al. Repair of supravalvar aortic stenosis: cardiovascular morphometric and hemodynamic results. *Ann Thorac Surg* 1990;50:700–707.
135. Landzberg JS, et al. Etiology of the Austin Flint murmur. *J Am Coll Cardiol* 1992;20:408–413.
136. Botvinick EH, et al. Echocardiographic demonstration of early mitral valve closure in severe aortic insufficiency: its clinical implications. *Circulation* 1975;51:836–847.
137. Henry WL, et al. Observations on the optimum time for operative intervention for aortic regurgitation. I. Evaluation of the results of aortic valve replacement in symptomatic patients. *Circulation* 1980;61:471–483.
138. Fioretti P, et al. Echocardiography in chronic aortic insufficiency: is valve replacement too late when left ventricular end-systolic dimension reaches 55 mm? *Circulation* 1983;67:216–221.
139. Vandenbossche JL, et al. Relation of left ventricular shape to volume and mass in patients with minimally symptomatic chronic aortic regurgitation. *Am Heart J* 1988;116:1022–1027.

140. Robertson WS, et al. Reverse doming of the anterior mitral leaflet with severe aortic regurgitation. *J Am Coll Cardiol* 1984;3:431–436.
141. Pflugfelder PW, et al. Comparison of cine MR imaging with Doppler echocardiography for the evaluation of aortic regurgitation. *AJR Am J Roentgenol* 1989;152:729–735.
142. Shively BK, et al. Diagnostic value of transesophageal compared with transthoracic echocardiography in infective endocarditis. *J Am Coll Cardiol* 1991;18:391–397.
143. Freed C, Schiller NB. Echocardiographic findings in Marfan's syndrome. *West J Med* 1977;126:87–90.
144. San Roman JA, et al. Transesophageal echocardiography in right-sided endocarditis. *J Am Coll Cardiol* 1993;21:1226–1230.
145. Schiller NB. Pulmonary artery pressure estimation by Doppler and two-dimensional echocardiography. *Cardiol Clin* 1990;8:277–287.
146. Ho GM, Eisenberg MJ, Schiller NB. Variation of blood flow in the thoracic aorta during cardiac tamponade. *Am Heart J* 1994;128:190–193.
147. Kusumoto FM, et al. Response of the interatrial septum to transatrial pressure gradients and its potential for predicting pulmonary capillary wedge pressure: an intraoperative study using transesophageal echocardiography in patients during mechanical ventilation. *J Am Coll Cardiol* 1993;21:721–728.
148. Sagie A, et al. Determinants of functional tricuspid regurgitation in incomplete tricuspid valve closure: Doppler color flow study of 109 patients. *J Am Coll Cardiol* 1994;24:446–453.
149. Werner JA, Schiller NB, Prasquier R. Occurrence and significance of echocardiographically demonstrated tricuspid valve prolapse. *Am Heart J* 1978;96:180–186.
150. Bonmassari R, Nicolosi GL, Disertori M. Tricuspid insufficiency with rupture of the chordae tendineae caused by closed thoracic trauma: evaluation by transesophageal echocardiography: description of a case. *G Ital Cardiol* 1994;24:763–768.
151. Tucker PA, et al. Flail tricuspid leaflet after multiple biopsies following orthotopic heart transplantation: echocardiographic and hemodynamic correlation. *J Heart Lung Transplant* 1994;13:466–472.
152. Hausen B, et al. Tricuspid valve regurgitation attributable to endomyocardial biopsies and rejection in heart transplantation. *Ann Thorac Surg* 1995;59:1134–1140.
153. Himelman RB, Schiller NB. Clinical and echocardiographic comparison of patients with the carcinoid syndrome with and without carcinoid heart disease. *Am J Cardiol* 1989;63:347–352.
154. Winslow T, et al. Pulmonary valve endocarditis: improved diagnosis with biplane transesophageal echocardiography. *J Am Soc Echocardiogr* 1992;5:206–210.
155. Von Reyn CF, et al. Infective endocarditis: an analysis based on strict case definitions. *Ann Intern Med* 1981;94:505–518.
156. Bayer AS, et al. Evaluation of new clinical criteria for the diagnosis of infective endocarditis. *Am J Med* 1994;96:211–219.
157. Durack DT, Lukes AS, Bright DK. New criteria for diagnosis of infective endocarditis: utilization of specific echocardiographic findings: Duke Endocarditis Service. *Am J Med* 1994;96:200–209.
158. O'Brien JT, Geiser EA. Infective endocarditis and echocardiography. *Am Heart J* 1984;108:386–394.
159. Gilbert BW, et al. Two-dimensional echocardiographic assessment of vegetative endocarditis. *Circulation* 1977;55:346–353.
160. Mugge A, et al. Echocardiography in infective endocarditis: reassessment of prognostic implications of vegetation size determined by the transthoracic and the transesophageal approach. *J Am Coll Cardiol* 1989;14:631–638.
161. Jaffe WM, et al. Infective endocarditis, 1983–1988: echocardiographic findings and factors influencing morbidity and mortality. *J Am Coll Cardiol* 1990;15:1227–1233.
162. Burger AJ, et al. The role of two-dimensional echocardiology in the diagnosis of infective endocarditis (published erratum appears in *Angiology* 1991;42:765). *Angiology* 1991;42:552–560.
163. Daniel WG, et al. Improvement in the diagnosis of abscesses associated with endocarditis by transesophageal echocardiography. *N Engl J Med* 1991;324:795–800.
164. Sochowski RA, Chan KL. Implication of negative results on a monoplane transesophageal echocardiographic study in patients with suspected infective endocarditis. *J Am Coll Cardiol* 1993;21:216–221.
165. Shapiro SM, et al. Transesophageal echocardiography in diagnosis of infective endocarditis. *Chest* 1994;105:377–382.
166. Sanfilippo AJ, et al. Echocardiographic assessment of patients with infectious endocarditis: prediction of risk for complications. *J Am Coll Cardiol* 1991;18:1191–1199.
167. DiSalvo G, et al. Echocardiography predicts embolic events in the infective endocarditis. *J Am Coll Cardiol* 2001;37:1069–1076.
168. Hecht SR, Berger M. Right-sided endocarditis in intravenous drug users: prognostic features in 102 episodes. *Ann Intern Med* 1992;117:560–566.
169. Feigenbaum H, Zaky A, Grabhorn LL. Cardiac motion in patients with pericardial effusion: a study using reflected ultrasound. *Circulation* 1966;34:611–619.
170. Eisenberg MJ, et al. Diagnostic value of chest radiography for pericardial effusion. *J Am Coll Cardiol* 1993;22:588–593.
171. Horowitz MS, et al. Sensitivity and specificity of echocardiographic diagnosis of pericardial effusion. *Circulation* 1974;50:239–247.
172. Rifkin RD, et al. Combined posteroanterior subepicardial fat simulating the echocardiographic diagnosis of pericardial effusion. *J Am Coll Cardiol* 1984;3:1333–1339.
173. D'Cruz IA, Hoffman PK. A new cross sectional echocardiographic method for estimating the volume of large pericardial effusions. *Br Heart J* 1991;66:448–451.
174. Eisenberg MJ, et al. Prognostic value of echocardiography in hospitalized patients with pericardial effusion. *Am J Cardiol* 1992;70:934–939.
175. Schiller NB, Botvinick EH. Right ventricular compression as a sign of cardiac tamponade: an analysis of echocardiographic ventricular dimensions and their clinical implications. *Circulation* 1977;56:774–779.
176. Schiller NB. Echocardiography in pericardial disease. *Med Clin North Am* 1980;64:253–282.
177. Himelman RB, et al. Inferior vena cava plethora with blunted respiratory response: a sensitive echocardiographic sign of cardiac tamponade. *J Am Coll Cardiol* 1988;12:1470–1477.
178. Armstrong WF, et al. Diastolic collapse of the right ventricle with cardiac tamponade: an echocardiographic study. *Circulation* 1982;65:1491–1496.
179. Singh S, et al. Right ventricular and right atrial collapse in patients with cardiac tamponade: a combined echocardiographic and hemodynamic study. *Circulation* 1984;70:966–971.
180. Kronzon I, Cohen ML, Winer HE. Diastolic atrial compression: a sensitive echocardiographic sign of cardiac tamponade. *J Am Coll Cardiol* 1983;2:770–775.
181. D'Cruz IA, Constantine A. Problems and pitfalls in the echocardiographic assessment of pericardial effusion. *Echocardiography* 1993;10:151–166.
182. Himelman RB, Lee E, Schiller NB. Septal bounce, vena cava plethora, and pericardial adhesion: informative two-dimensional echocardiographic signs in the diagnosis of pericardial constriction. *J Am Soc Echocardiogr* 1988;1:333–340.
183. Jue J, Chung W, Schiller NB. Does inferior vena cava size predict right atrial pressures in patients receiving mechanical ventilation? *J Am Soc Echocardiogr* 1992;5:613–619.
184. Klopfenstein HS, Wann LS. Can pleural effusions cause tamponade-like effects? *Echocardiography* 1994;11:489–492.
185. Tei C, et al. Atrial systolic notch on the interventricular septal echogram: an echocardiographic sign of constrictive pericarditis. *J Am Coll Cardiol* 1983;1:907–912.
186. Gibson TC, et al. An echocardiographic study of the interventricular septum in constrictive pericarditis. *Br Heart J* 1976;38:738–743.
187. Felner JM, Churchwell AL, Murphy DA. Right atrial thromboemboli: clinical, echocardiographic and pathophysiologic manifestations. *J Am Coll Cardiol* 1984;4:1041–1051.
188. Hynes JK, et al. Two-dimensional echocardiographic diagnosis of pericardial cyst. *Mayo Clin Proc* 1983;58:60–63.
189. Eisenberg MJ, et al. The clinical spectrum of patients with aneurysms of the ascending aorta. *Am Heart J* 1993;125:1380–1385.
190. Dev V, et al. Echocardiographic diagnosis of aneurysm of the sinus of Valsalva. *Am Heart J* 1993;126:930–936.
191. Eisenberg MJ, Geraci SJ, Schiller NB. Screening for abdominal aortic aneurysms during transthoracic echocardiography. *Am Heart J* 1995;130:109–115.
192. Banning AP, et al. Transoesophageal echocardiography as the sole diagnostic investigation in patients with suspected thoracic aortic dissection. *Br Heart J* 1994;72:461–465.
193. Popp RL, Yock PG. Noninvasive intracardiac pressure measurement using Doppler ultrasound (editorial). *J Am Coll Cardiol* 1985;6:757–758.
194. Simonson JS, Schiller NB. Sonospirometry: a new method for noninvasive estimation of mean right atrial pressure based on two-dimensional echographic measurements of the inferior vena cava during measured inspiration. *J Am Coll Cardiol* 1988;11:557–564.
195. Mulvagh SL, et al. Contrast echocardiography: current and future applications. *J Am Soc Echocardiogr* 2000;13:331–342.
196. Bax J, et al. Echocardiographic evaluation of cardiac resynchronization therapy: ready for routine clinical use? *J Am Coll Cardiol* 2004;44:1–9.

CHAPTER 50 ■ STRESS ECHOCARDIOGRAPHY

THOMAS H. MARWICK

OVERVIEW

Stress echocardiography uses stress-induced changes in wall thickening, wall motion, and left ventricular (LV) volumes to infer the presence of myocardial ischemia and viability. The attraction of echocardiography is that it may be combined with various stressors and used in a variety of environments. The test is patient friendly because it is rapidly performed and inexpensive.

The accuracy of stress echocardiography in detecting significant coronary artery disease (CAD) ranges from 80% to 90%, exceeding that of exercise electrocardiography (ECG), especially in subgroups among whom the latter is unreliable (e.g., women and patients with LV hypertrophy). Its accuracy is comparable to that of stress myocardial perfusion scintigraphy, even though the underlying physiology of the test mandates the development of myocardial ischemia rather than perfusion heterogeneity, and this limits its sensitivity in patients who exercise submaximally or who are receiving antianginal therapy. In addition to its diagnostic role, the prognostic information provided by stress echocardiography makes it a valuable guide to management in chronic CAD, after infarction, and before major noncardiac surgery. Similarly, the presence and extent of viable myocardium are adjuncts to decision making in the management of ischemic LV dysfunction, and the detection of contractile reserve may be useful in assessing valvular and primary myocardial disease.

Several new advances are promising. Feasibility has been improved by LV opacification. Quantitative interpretation is possible with tissue Doppler and strain imaging and acoustic quantification. Evaluation of both function and perfusion is possible with echo-contrast agents. Three-dimensional imaging permits comparison of the same tissue planes before and after stress.

GLOSSARY

Coronary steal: A situation in which a vasodilator increases runoff to a normal branch, thus reducing the driving pressure in an artery proximal to a stenosis and causing ischemia because of reduced blood flow across the stenosis.

Echocardiographic contrast agents: Injectable compounds comprising gas-filled microbubbles that increase the reflected signal of the cardiac structures in which they are located.

Myocardial strain imaging: Quantification of regional shortening using either tissue Doppler or gray-scale imaging.

Sensitivity: Proportion of patients with CAD correctly identified as abnormal.

Single-photon emission computed tomography (SPECT): A means of acquiring and portraying scintigraphic data in a tomographic fashion.

Specificity: Proportion of patients without CAD correctly identified as normal.

Viable myocardium: Myocardial segments characterized by reduced function at rest but potentially recoverable either spontaneously (*stunned*) or with revascularization, usually associated with reduced myocardial perfusion (i.e., *hibernating myocardium*).

INTRODUCTION

The exercise ECG has been the most commonly accepted functional test, but in certain situations it is inappropriate. First, patients who either cannot exercise or who exercise submaximally account for 30% to 40% of those presenting for functional testing (1). These patients are best studied using the combination of pharmacologic stress with an imaging technique. Second, even if the patient is able to exercise, the ECG may be uninterpretable because of repolarization abnormalities. In these circumstances, the ability of the patient to exercise is exploited by the combination of exercise testing with imaging. Third, imaging is needed if clinical decision making requires the localization of ischemic or viable tissue.

The use of stress imaging tests is not restricted to the diagnosis of CAD. In patients with known coronary anatomy, a functional evaluation may help understand the site of ischemia (and thereby the culprit lesion) and distinguish among ischemic, infarcted, and viable myocardium. Similarly, the functional responses to stress may guide the management of valvular heart disease, primary myocardial disease, and some obstructive lesions.

PATHOPHYSIOLOGY

Detection of Ischemia by Echocardiography

The normal responses of the LV to increasing workload are a uniform increase of regional wall motion, thickening, and a reduction of end-systolic LV cavity size (2). These changes return to baseline shortly after the test (3).

Although cardiomyopathic processes may be regional rather than global, the diagnostic algorithm for stress echocardiography (Table 50.1) assumes that regional systolic dysfunction is usually caused by CAD. In addition to reduction in the extent of thickening (Fig. 50.1) (4,5), ischemia may be identified by its timing (6). LV enlargement after stress is a marker of severe ischemia or other serious heart muscle diseases. Wall motion abnormalities may rapidly recover following the cessation of stress (7,8), but they may also persist for 30 minutes or longer (9); the time course of recovery probably reflects the severity and duration of ischemia.

Resting wall motion abnormalities may be caused by transmural infarction, nontransmural infarction or viable, noninfarcted tissue (10), which may recover spontaneously (if the tissue is stunned) or following revascularization (if the myocardium is hibernating) (11,12). Probably, both stunned tissue and hibernating tissue contribute to chronic LV dysfunction resulting from CAD. Residual viable tissue is more common in hypokinetic than akinetic segments and is least common in dyskinetic segments (13). The augmentation of viable myocardium in response to inotropic stimulation may be detected using echocardiography with low doses of stressors (see Table 50.1). This may be combined with deterioration of function at peak dose (Fig. 50.2).

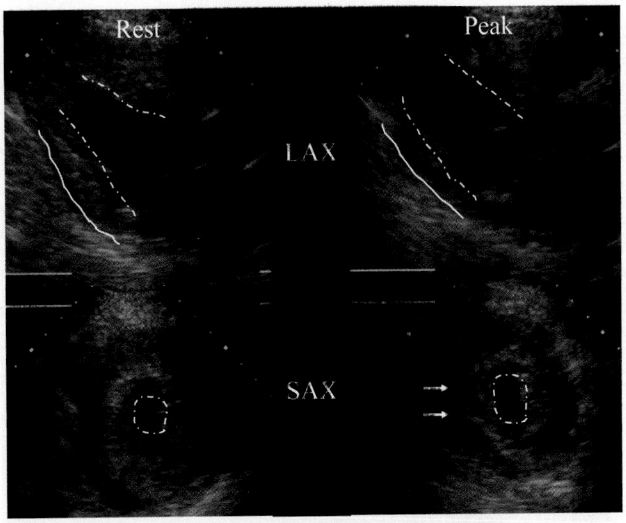

FIGURE 50.1. End-systolic frames showing myocardial ischemia at exercise echocardiography in parasternal long-axis (LAX) and short-axis (SAX) views. The middle and basal posterior wall become akinetic after stress, with change of shape and reduced thickening consistent with left circumflex disease. Dotted lines mark endocardium and solid lines mark epicardium. Epicardium may be difficult to identify (*arrows*). This suggests left circumflex disease.

METHODOLOGY OF STRESS ECHOCARDIOGRAPHY

Stress Testing Modalities

Exercise Stress

The performance of stress echocardiography in patients with known or suspected CAD *who are able to exercise* incorporates either treadmill stress or upright or supine cycle ergometry. In general, treadmill exercise is more widely accepted among

TABLE 50.1

INTERPRETATION OF EXERCISE AND PHARMACOLOGIC STRESS ECHOCARDIOGRAPHY

Characterization of tissue	Resting function	Low-dose	Peak/poststress function
Normal	Normal	Normal	Hyperkinetic
Ischemic	Normal	Normal (ischemic with severe coronary artery disease)	Reduction versus rest Reduction versus adjacent segments Delayed contraction
Viable, nonischemic	Rest WMA	Improvement	Sustained improvement
Viable, ischemic	Rest WMA	Improvement	Reduction (compared with low-dose)
Infarction	Rest WMA	No change	No change

WMA, wall motion abnormalities (severe hypokinesis, akinesis, dyskinesis).

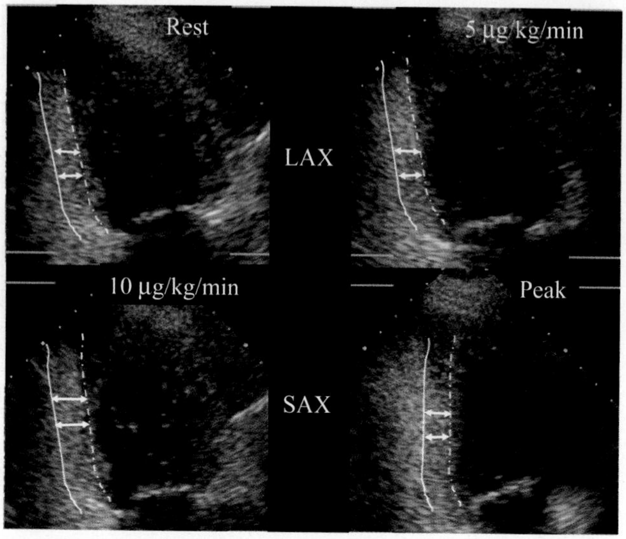

FIGURE 50.2. Dobutamine stress echocardiogram showing a biphasic response. The quad-screen display shows resting images in the **upper left,** low-dose (5 and 10 μg/kg per minute) in **upper right** and **lower left,** and peak stress images in the **lower right,** in the apical two-chamber view. A resting wall motion abnormality of the basal and midinferior segments improves to normal at 10 μg/kg per minute but deteriorates at peak stress. Endocardial (dotted line) and epicardial (solid line) lines show reduced thickening (*arrows*).

patients and physicians in the United States, and patients are more likely to stress maximally, although the disadvantage is that imaging is performed after stress. During exercise, heart rate, blood pressure, and inotropic state increase in proportion to the increase of cardiac work, and preload is relatively reduced during upright exercise, although this may not occur during supine exercise. The lower attainable workload with bicycle than treadmill exercise is compensated by avoiding the gap between completion of stress and the initiation of imaging. Neither bicycle nor treadmill exercise is clearly superior, so the choice depends on local expertise and familiarity. Imaging at peak stress is attractive for making assessments of the functional severity of coronary stenoses and for the assessment of valvular lesions. Moreover, the performance of imaging during stress may facilitate definition of the ischemic threshold.

Sympathomimetic Stressors

Hemodynamic Response. The attainable peak heart rates with dobutamine—from 120 to 140 beats per minute (14)—correspond to at least 85% of age-predicted heart rate in most patients. The systolic blood pressure usually increases by 30 to 40 mm Hg, with peak pressures of 170 to 180 mm Hg, and peak rate-pressure products of approximately 20,000. However, considerable variability occurs among patients with respect to both the extent and the speed of these hemodynamic responses.

Side Effects. Many patients requiring dobutamine stress are elderly and have serious noncardiac diseases or even severe CAD and LV dysfunction. Despite the use of high doses of these agents, serious complications occur in approximately 3 in 1,000 (15).

Administration Protocol. The protocol for dobutamine administration is empiric. Most centers now use a high-dose protocol (to 40 μg/kg per minute) (14,16), although low-dose protocols provide adequate stress if the duration of each stage is longer (e.g., 5 rather than 3 minutes) (17). Atropine has been combined with dobutamine at peak dose if the heart-rate target is not attained (18), and more recently it has been administered earlier in an attempt to shorten test duration (19). When evidence of myocardial viability is being sought, augmentation of function may occur only at very low doses of dobutamine, and some authors have suggested specific low-dose protocols (e.g., to 12.5 μg/kg per minute in 2.5-μg increments) for this purpose. Our practice is to use a single standard protocol with 3-minute increments, involving low-dose imaging at 5 and 10 μg/kg per minute, and proceeding in 10 μg/kg per minute increments to 40 μg/kg per minute unless this is considered unsafe, for example, because of hemodynamic instability. This offers the versatility of identifying both viability and ischemia while at the same time providing a study of acceptable length. Although caution should be exercised, the high-dose protocol appears safe for studying patients with severe LV dysfunction (20–22), and this gives the benefit of detecting a biphasic response, which is the most reliable marker of recovery of LV function. At present, none of the dobutamine protocols is clearly superior, and the main consideration should be to ensure the adequacy of stress.

Vasodilator Stress

Hemodynamic Response. These stressors exert minor hemodynamic effects. Blood pressure is usually little altered, and heart rate increments are small and may be attributable to various side effects.

Side Effects. Serious side effects occur in approximately 1 in 1,000 patients. The most common side effects of dipyridamole and adenosine are headache and dyspnea, respectively (23,24). The speed of onset and potency of adenosine render its side effects less well tolerated, but these effects resolve rapidly with cessation of the drug. Both techniques are contraindicated in patients with untreated atrioventricular block and bronchospastic disorders, and abstinence from xanthene-containing foods and drugs is required before either stress.

Administration Protocol. The standard dipyridamole dose for myocardial perfusion imaging is 0.56 mg/kg administered over 4 minutes. For stress echocardiography, this dose induces ischemia only in patients with severe CAD, so if ischemia is not induced, an additional 0.28 mg/kg is administered over 2 minutes, followed if necessary by atropine (25), with imaging continued over 16 minutes. Although reversal of dipyridamole with aminophylline is not usually necessary, it may be useful in the presence of significant side effects. If aminophylline is needed, the supervising physician should be aware that the effect of dipyridamole may last longer than that of aminophylline, thus leading patients to become ischemic after they have left the stress laboratory.

The standard dose of adenosine for myocardial perfusion imaging is 0.14 mg/kg per minute intravenously over 4 minutes. This is also the most widely used dose for stress echocardiography, although both higher and lower doses have been studied. Although analogous to the dose of dipyridamole, higher-dose protocols are constrained by dose-limiting side effects.

Selection of the Optimal Stress Agent

Pharmacologic stressors enhance the feasibility of imaging, but they have a number of important disadvantages (Table 50.2), and exercise stress is preferable in an active patient unless the test has been performed for other reasons than the

TABLE 50.2

BENEFITS OF EXERCISE OVER PHARMACOLOGIC STRESS

Evaluates exercise capacity
Correlates symptoms with physical workload
ST-segment evaluation
Cardiac workload is greater with exercise
Prognostic information
Probably greater sensitivity for ischemia

detection of myocardial ischemia (e.g., identification of viability or coronary spasm). Although comparable levels of sensitivity are obtainable, the performance of submaximal stress owing to drug side effects is an important limitation. The development of new technologies such as strain rate imaging has made pharmacologic stressors more attractive, but whether the incremental data offered by the addition of these features justify the disadvantages of using a pharmacologic stressor in all patients remains to be established. The feasibility of perfusion assessment with myocardial contrast echocardiography is optimized by vasodilator stress, although this may be at the cost of lower sensitivity for inducible wall motion abnormalities. The combination of inotropic and vasodilator stressors was used in the past, and the desire to use vasodilators with contrast may lead these combinations to undergo a renaissance.

The type of pharmacologic stress may also be the source of debate. Serious side effects are rare with either stress, and the frequency of all side effects with dipyridamole and dobutamine stress is comparable, but the contraindications to each test are different. Patients with asthma or untreated conduction system disease may be better tested using dobutamine echocardiography, whereas dipyridamole stress would be preferable in those with serious arrhythmias or severe hypertension. In the majority of patients, who do not fall into these categories, either stressor may be used, and the choice may be based on physician preference, cost, and the clinical situation. If the question relates to the diagnosis of CAD in a patient with chest pain, the sensitivity of dobutamine echocardiography is somewhat greater than that of dipyridamole echocardiography, especially in patients with single-vessel disease. If the main interest is in prognostic evaluation, the agents are both attractive, and certainly a wealth of information is available regarding dipyridamole echocardiography as a prognostic test (see the section on prognostic considerations in CAD).

Imaging Techniques

Stress echocardiography is almost universally performed using transthoracic echocardiography, although transesophageal imaging is sometimes used in the setting of poor image quality. The procedure brings together facilities for stress testing, echocardiography, and at least two and sometimes three staff members including physician, sonographer, and nurse. The commitment of so many resources limits the feasibility of performing an exhaustive echocardiographic examination in the context of stress echocardiography, but we perform a screening M-mode and color Doppler examination at the beginning of every study. If more complex (e.g., valvular) problems are identified, these issues should be analyzed by echocardiography at another time.

Analysis of digital loops is beneficial for the interpretation of all forms of stress echocardiography. Side-by-side comparison of cine loops in a split-screen display permits easy comparison of regional wall motion at rest and stress, and frame-by-frame review facilitates definition of the endocardium as well as evaluation of the temporal sequence of contraction. The disadvantages of this approach, however, are the finite number of views that can be compared using the quad-screen display and the presentation of a limited number of cardiac cycles. Despite the advantages and ubiquity of digital storage, review of the videotape remains an important and underutilized part of stress echocardiographic interpretation, especially in difficult studies (26).

Interpretation of Stress Echocardiography

Qualitative Approaches

The interpretation of stress echocardiography using the standard, qualitative approach is centered on comparison of each LV segment is before, during, and after stress. Myocardial thickening (see Fig. 50.1) should be examined in preference to myocardial motion, which may result from translational movement, or tethering. The standard criteria used to identify ischemia, myocardial viability, and myocardial scar have been summarized earlier (see Table 50.1). Delayed contraction is a subtle index of ischemia that may be difficult to identify in continuous-loop playback but can be appreciated by stepping through individual freeze-frame images. Stress-induced LV enlargement is often a marker of multivessel CAD, and changes of ventricular shape as well as size are useful diagnostic clues to ischemia. Myocardial viability is characterized by improvement of a dyssynergic zone in response to *low-dose* dobutamine. The "biphasic" response, an association of this finding with ischemia at peak doses of dobutamine (see Fig. 50.2), is an indicator of myocardial viability in the setting of a stenosed vessel (27). An improvement without subsequent deterioration is an ambiguous finding that may signify viability or nontransmural infarction. The presence of augmentation at *peak doses* of dobutamine is a nonspecific response, poorly predictive of myocardial viability.

The subjectivity of current approach to the interpretation of stress echocardiography is the greatest shortcoming of this technique. This has two major manifestations: first, the need for training, and, second, the problems posed for reproducibility. Despite technical advances, repeated studies since the mid-1980's have confirmed the need for specific training in stress echocardiography (28). The exact characteristics of this training period are not well defined, but evidence has been gathered to show improvement to expert level with 100 studies (Fig. 50.3), and some improvement has been documented even with short courses (29). However, once this level of skill is attained, we believe that a regular workload is required to prevent it from attenuating. Finally, even among expert readers, although the concordance of interpretations within the same center is high (30), concordance among different centers may be less than 80% (31), even when uniform interpretive criteria are used (32). Poor concordance is particularly a problem in studies of poor technical quality, and the problem has been reduced by technical advances including harmonic imaging and digital display (33). Nonetheless, interpretive disagreements remain common, especially in patients with subtle abnormalities resulting from mild CAD.

To control issues related to subjectivity and concordance among observers, we review stress echocardiograms systematically. Quad-screen displays are first examined to assess their quality and the presence of technical limitations (e.g., gating problems); in technically limited studies, more reliance will need to be based on analysis of the videotape. Resting images

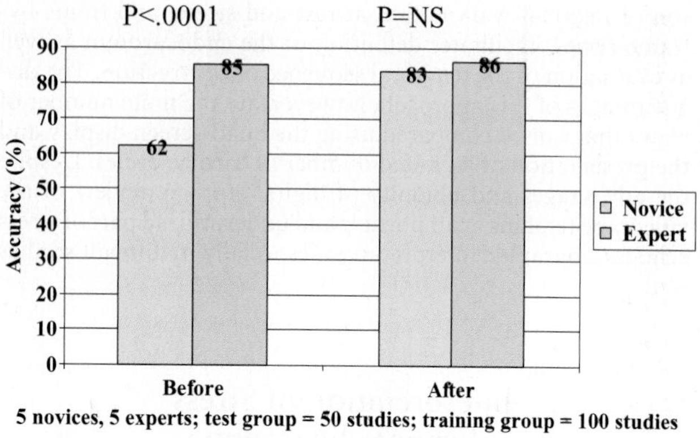

FIGURE 50.3. The learning curve of stress echocardiography. Over 6 months and 100 supervised echocardiograms, trainees (*hatched bars*) increased their accuracy from approximately 60% to 80%. (From Picano E, Lattanzi F, Orlandini A, et al. Stress echocardiography and the human factor: the importance of being expert. *J Am Coll Cardiol* 1991;17:666–669.)

are then examined in each view, using a segmental model to score regional wall motion (Fig. 50.4). Global function may be assessed subjectively by calculation of a wall motion scoring index or by measurement of the ejection fraction. The rest and stress images are then compared. The first step is to check for the presence of LV enlargement and shape changes, which are global indicators of ischemia, and in the case of the former, of multivessel disease. Each segment is then scored and compared with the equivalent segment at rest to identify the site, extent, and severity of abnormal function. If a bicycle or dobutamine stress study is used, the ischemic threshold is an important clue to the severity of ischemia. The report should therefore describe the site, extent, and severity of scar and ischemia, the global LV function before and after stress, and the presence of other abnormalities.

Quantitative Approaches

Quantitative techniques may be used for the measurement of radial or longitudinal function (Table 50.3). Myocardial displacement may be measured in the short- or long-axis dimension. The centerline approach is well established for measuring regional radial function, which has been applied to the interpretation of stress echocardiograms (34). Using this technique, radial excursion is measured by tracing of the endocardial surface (thickening is sometimes possible to measure by tracing of endocardial and epicardial surfaces) at peak diastole and peak systole, and it is compared with a normal range. This technique has three major limitations. First, many stress echocardiograms are not of satisfactory quality to provide excellent border definition. Second, the approach requires compensation for translational or rotational cardiac movement, and methodologies for compensating for these technical issues are not well defined. Third, the process of tracing the wall is time consuming and is not applicable in a busy clinical laboratory.

TABLE 50.3

QUANTITATIVE TECHNIQUES FOR THE EVALUATION OF STRESS ECHOCARDIOGRAPHY

	Radial	Longitudinal
Displacement	Centerline Acoustic quantification	M-mode
Thickening	Anatomic M-mode	Backscatter
Velocity (including velocity gradient)	Tissue Doppler	Tissue Doppler, strain
Timing	Tissue Doppler	Tissue Doppler

Because of these limitations, efforts to quantify stress echocardiography have moved more to the measurement of longitudinal function using strain and strain rate imaging. Currently, this is performed using tissue Doppler imaging (Fig. 50.5), although recent developments have focused on obtaining these data from speckle-tacking from standard two-dimensional echocardiography.

DIAGNOSIS OF CORONARY ARTERY DISEASE

Influences on Accuracy of Stress Echocardiography

Adequacy of Stress

Failure to stress the heart maximally will not engender either maximal coronary hyperemia (used for myocardial perfusion

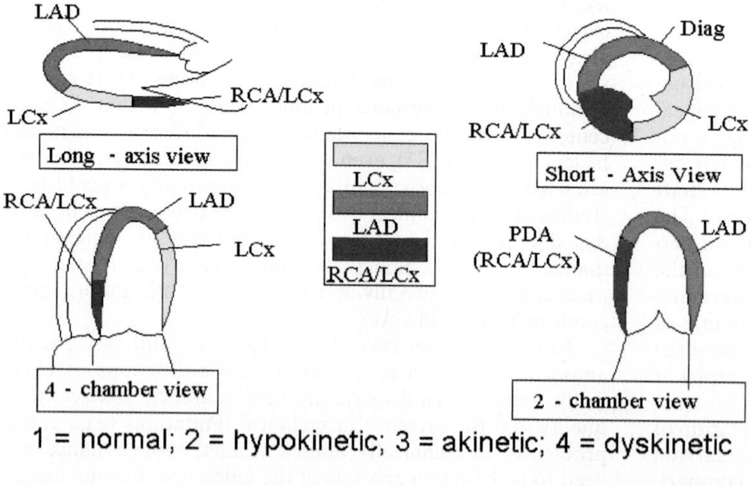

FIGURE 50.4. Systematic evaluation of the left ventricle using a 16-segment model. Each segment must be scored individually at rest and during and/or after stress. The American Society of Echocardiography now recommends a 17-segment model (including a seventeenth segment in the apical cap), to facilitate concordance with other imaging modalities, but foreshortening of the apex is common during stress echocardiography. LAD, left anterior descending coronary artery; LCx, left circumflex artery; PDA, posterior descending coronary artery; RCA, right coronary artery.

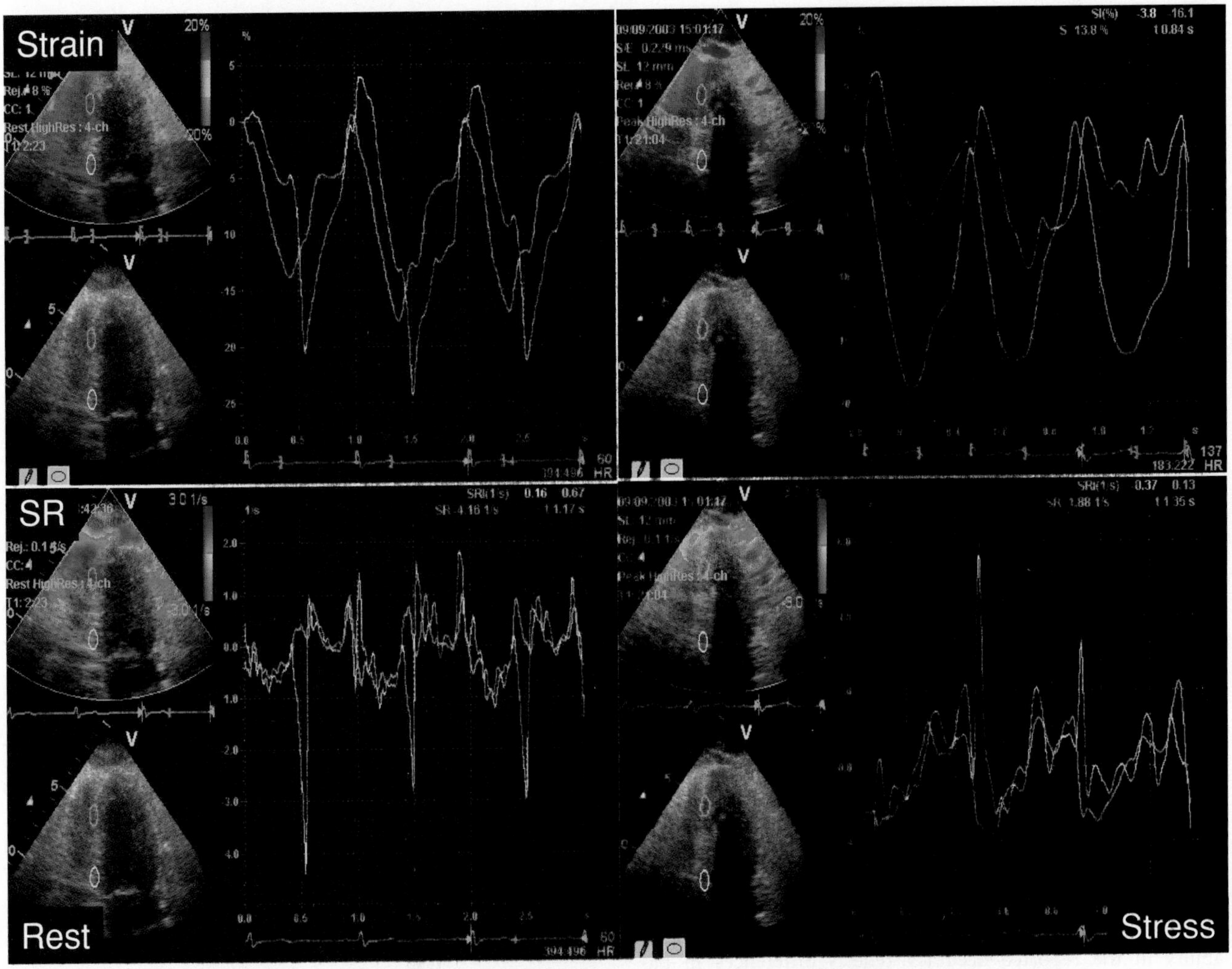

FIGURE 50.5. Application of strain (**above**) and strain rate (SR) (**below**) imaging to quantification of stress echocardiography. Curves obtained at baseline show similar degrees of strain rate and strain in the basal (yellow) and midseptal segments (green), although contraction is slightly delayed in the basal septum. After stress (**right**), the magnitude of both strain and strain rate is reduced, and delay is increased.

imaging) or ischemia (used for stress echocardiography and ECG analysis). Thus, failure to stress the patient maximally will be associated with reduced sensitivity, especially for milder CAD. Indeed, in our experience of exercise echocardiography, apart from the number and severity of coronary stenoses, the only predictor of false-negative results was failure to obtain 85% of age-predicted maximum heart rate (35). As discussed previously, patients who are unable to exercise or who are likely to exercise submaximally should undergo pharmacologic stress testing.

The use of pharmacologic stress testing may be particularly useful in patients with previous myocardial infarction and resting wall motion abnormalities. In these situations, the identification of ischemia may be facilitated by the availability of low-dose augmentation in viable tissue (36), which may not be appreciated during exercise testing. This topic is discussed further in a later section on identification of myocardial viability.

Echocardiographic Considerations

Poor image quality reduces concordance among expert observers (31), and it likely reduces the accuracy of the test, if not for the identification of CAD (35) then at least for the ability to recognize multivessel disease. Not all segments of the myocardium are equally well visualized; the lateral wall is usually parallel to the ultrasound beam in the apical four-chamber view, and the endocardium may be poorly defined, with consequent effects on the sensitivity for left circumflex disease. Fortunately, this problem has been improved by the development of lateral gain correction, harmonic imaging, and LV opacification. The basal inferoposterior walls are particularly difficult to interpret owing to tethering to the plane of the mitral valve and poor endocardial definition. Wall motion abnormalities involving the latter segments should be identified only if adjacent segments are abnormal.

Several interpretive factors may also influence the accuracy of the data. First, a low threshold for identifying wall motion abnormalities (e.g., identification of minor stress-induced wall motion abnormalities as ischemic or identification of failure to enhance function as being indicative of ischemia) is attended by a high sensitivity, but a correspondingly low specificity. Interpreter bias may also be an important source of inaccuracy. It is important to interpret the echocardiographic data independent of the clinical and stress testing data; failure to do so may compromise accuracy (particularly the specificity). The experience of the reader is obviously an important determinant of

TABLE 50.4

CAUSES OF FALSE-NEGATIVE AND FALSE-POSITIVE STRESS ECHOCARDIOGRAM RESULTS

False-negative results	False-positive results
Inadequate stress	Overinterpretation, interpreter bias
Antianginal therapy	Localized basal inferior wall abnormalities
Mild coronary artery disease	Abnormal septal motion (left bundle branch block, post–coronary artery bypass grafting)
Left circumflex disease	
Poor image quality	Cardiomyopathies
Delayed images poststress	Hypertensive responses to stress

accuracy during stress echocardiography. Factors responsible for false-negative and false-positive results are summarized in Table 50.4.

Exercise Echocardiography

With appropriate patient selection according to exercise capacity, and with an expert sonographer, exercise echocardiography is feasible in almost all patients. A recent metaanalysis (37) identified 41 studies of exercise echocardiography, with an average sensitivity of 83% and specificity of 84% (Fig. 50.6). Important landmarks in developing the evidence base have been the initial validation of treadmill exercise echocardiography (38), its application in standard clinical practice (35), and the initial major bicycle stress study (39). Generally, variability in the reported accuracy reflects differences in patient mix among studies, although some differences arise because of different criteria for significant stenoses (9). Quantitative angiography has been used in a few studies; Sheikh and associates (40) reported that inducible wall motion abnormalities were associated with a stenosis diameter of 1.0 mm, compared with patients without inducible ischemia in spite of detectable stenoses, among whom the diameter was 1.7 mm. Agati and colleagues (41) identified an absolute lumen diameter of 0.7 mm, corresponding to an 85% diameter stenosis, as best predictive of inducible wall motion abnormalities.

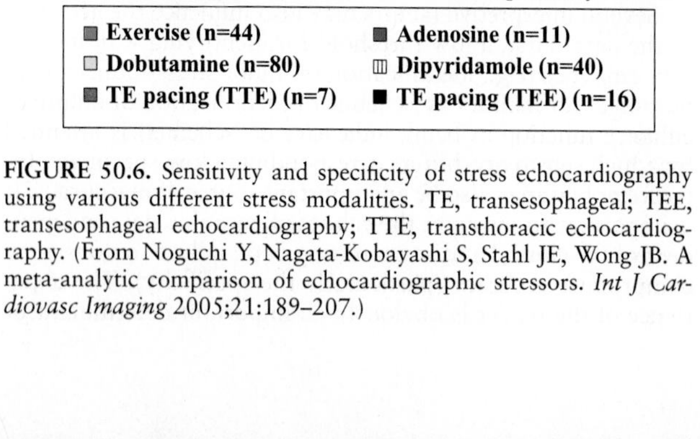

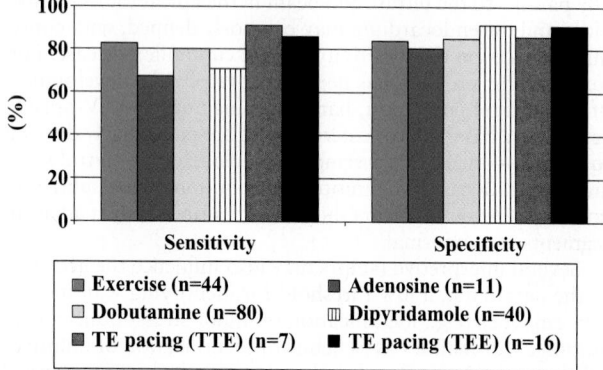

FIGURE 50.6. Sensitivity and specificity of stress echocardiography using various different stress modalities. TE, transesophageal; TEE, transesophageal echocardiography; TTE, transthoracic echocardiography. (From Noguchi Y, Nagata-Kobayashi S, Stahl JE, Wong JB. A meta-analytic comparison of echocardiographic stressors. *Int J Cardiovasc Imaging* 2005;21:189–207.)

Pharmacologic Stress Echocardiography

Dobutamine Stress Echocardiography

The metaanalysis (37) identified 80 studies of dobutamine echocardiography, with an average sensitivity of 80% and specificity of 85% (see Fig. 50.6). Variability in the reported accuracy of the test arises from reasons related to the test and study population. The addition of atropine increases sensitivity (18), as does the use of transesophageal echocardiography (42), although the feasibility of the latter is limited.

At quantitative coronary angiography (43–45), the optimal correlates of a positive dobutamine test result are a lumen diameter of 1.07 mm, percent diameter stenosis of 52%, and percent area stenosis of 75%; minimal lumen diameter has the best predictive value for a positive dobutamine stress test result (sensitivity, 94%; specificity, 75%; odds ratio, 51) (43). Stenoses less than 1 mm in diameter can be identified with a sensitivity of 86% (44,45). However, although quantitative angiography deals with the problem of reproducibility of angiographic interpretation, it still has the limitation of being an anatomic measure of disease severity, which may not necessarily correlate with functional indices. One such parameter that takes into account collateral flow is myocardial fractional flow reserve, which is calculated as the ratio of mean hyperemic distal coronary to aortic pressure. The magnitude of wall motion abnormalities correlated more closely with functional than anatomic markers of lesion severity, and dobutamine echocardiography was found to be a more sensitive marker of ischemia in lesions involving larger (>2.6 mm in diameter) vessels than smaller vessels (44).

Some of the earlier studies of dobutamine echocardiography (16,46) show a sensitivity above the usual level, suggesting a decrement in the accuracy of dobutamine stress since its inception and reflecting clinical application of the test. Because the technique is applied for clinical decision making, referral bias to angiography may inflate sensitivity but produce more adverse findings for specificity (47). Moreover, dobutamine is not a very robust stress, and sensitivity is likely to be compromised if the cardiac workload is reduced by medical therapy or dose-limiting side effects. Comparison of the quoted ranges (see Fig. 50.6) suggests that the sensitivity of dobutamine echocardiography is somewhat less than that of exercise echocardiography, but its specificity is slightly greater. In studies in which exercise and pharmacologic stress echocardiography were performed in the same patients, the accuracy of stress echocardiography was comparable with either stressor (48–53). In situations in which stress is submaximal because of side effects with pharmacologic agents, exercise is superior. Clearly, the converse is true when patients are unable to exercise maximally and a pharmacologic agent is more desirable. Nonetheless, the hemodynamic effects of the agents are different, so the markers of severe (including left main) disease including LV cavity dilation and marked ST-segment depression occur more often with exercise than with dobutamine echocardiography (54). Because exercise is a more potent stress on the heart, a greater extent of abnormal wall motion may be induced, and this may compensate for the more difficult imaging with exercise (51,53). As discussed previously, numerous features favor the use of exercise testing over pharmacologic techniques, provided the patient can exercise maximally.

Vasodilator Stress Echocardiography

The metaanalysis described earlier (37) identified 40 studies of dipyridamole and 11 studies of adenosine echocardiography, with an average sensitivity of 71% and a specificity of 92% for dipyridamole and 68% and 81% for adenosine (see Fig. 50.6). The low-dose dipyridamole protocol (0.56 mg/kg) is associated with low sensitivity. For the high-dose and adenosine protocols, more variability is present than for any of the other stressors, reflecting variations in the populations studied. The inclusion in some studies of patients with prior myocardial infarction has inflated the sensitivity of adenosine echocardiography, but the sensitivity of patients without prior infarction is only approximately 60% (55,56). Likewise, populations with a high prevalence of extensive CAD are associated with a high sensitivity, but single-vessel disease is more difficult to detect using this technique (56).

The type of pharmacologic agent to select in a patient who is unable to exercise maximally remains a source of debate. Studies comparing dobutamine and vasodilator agents in the same patients have shown that the sensitivity of dobutamine is somewhat higher than that of dipyridamole echocardiography, this difference being mainly attributable to patients with single-vessel disease (Table 50.5) (48,49,52,56–62). In an environment in which most of the studies are being performed for diagnostic purposes, dobutamine is probably more attractive because some patients may have single-vessel disease. When the main interest is prognostic evaluation, both agents are attractive, and certainly a wealth of information is available regarding dipyridamole echocardiography as a prognostic test (see the section on prognostic considerations in CAD). Other factors influencing this decision, such as side effects and cost, have been discussed earlier in the section on the selection of the optimal stress agent.

Important Limitations in the Diagnostic Use of Stress Echocardiography

Extent and Severity of Disease

Stress echocardiography is effective for the detection of severe coronary stenoses, because these lesions are usually associated with more extensive wall motion abnormalities (44). Extensive CAD is also marked by an early onset of ischemia, at a low heart rate and rate-pressure product, or at a low dose of pharmacologic stressor. However, the sensitivity of stress echocardiography for single-vessel CAD has been quite limited in several studies and is probably less than that of myocardial perfusion scintigraphy. This reflects the need for ischemia to involve a significant extent of myocardium for the stress echocardiogram to be positive, which may not be fulfilled if the involved vessel is small or distal or if the stenosis is only mildly flow limiting.

The presence of extensive areas of ischemia, the development of global ventricular dysfunction (reduction of ejection fraction or LV enlargement), or both, indicate the presence of multivessel disease (Fig. 50.7). However, although the predictive value of these findings is high (63), the predictive value of their absence is dependent on the resting LV function. In patients with a history of previous myocardial infarction, the sensitivity of stress echocardiography for recognition of multivessel disease (effectively, "ischemia at a distance") is approximately 80% to 85%. In contrast, the sensitivity for multivessel disease in patients without previous infarction is approximately 50% (64). These data contrast with a sensitivity greater than 70% in this situation when myocardial perfusion scintigraphy is used (65). However, when the extent of ischemia defined by dobutamine echocardiography and perfusion scintigraphy was compared with the angiographic extent of disease (a modified Gensini score), the extent was comparable, and both underestimated the disease extent (56).

The identification of ischemia within areas of resting wall motion abnormalities is difficult, because of the problems posed by identification of minor gradations of wall motion in the setting of abnormal function. Comparison of the regional findings of exercise echocardiography and SPECT have shown this to be an important cause of discordant diagnoses (66). The problem is probably less during dobutamine stress because ischemic segments with abnormal resting function often show a biphasic response (36).

These aspects represent a fundamental limitation of an ischemia-based technique. Their solution will require either a more sensitive tool for assessment of wall motion or combination with a perfusion marker such as contrast echocardiography.

Site of Disease

Although the extent of CAD has an important influence on the accuracy of functional testing in general, the location of CAD may have important implications for the sensitivity of stress echocardiography in particular. The allocation of segments to particular vascular territories is ambiguous, especially in the apex (usually assumed to be within the territory of the left anterior descending coronary artery) and the posterior wall (usually assumed to be supplied by the left circumflex). The sensitivity for circumflex disease may be limited by difficulties in the evaluation of the lateral wall owing to unfavorable imaging characteristics.

COMPARISON WITH OTHER TECHNIQUES

Comparison with Stress Electrocardiography

The presence of ST-segment depression in response to exercise remains the simplest and most widely used test for the documentation of myocardial ischemia. However, the proportion of patients who cannot perform adequate exercise or in whom the ST segment is uninterpretable exceeds 50% in many tertiary referral centers. In patients who are unable to exercise maximally, exercise testing is attended by inadequate sensitivity (67). Even if pharmacologic stress testing is performed, the combination of these stresses with ECG alone has limitations with respect to sensitivity (68–70). Even in patients who can exercise and who have an interpretable ECG, exercise echocardiography has benefits in both sensitivity and specificity (35,66,71,72). This greater sensitivity of exercise echocardiography over the exercise ECG is not surprising in view of the earlier occurrence of wall motion abnormalities than ST-segment changes during stress; these data are analogous to those reported for thallium imaging. Indeed, some provocative analyses have shown that the additional cost of stress echocardiography is outweighed by lesser costs of subsequent investigation because the referring clinician responds more appropriately to echocardiographic than ECG assessment of risk (73). However, because of the logistic problems posed by replacement of diagnostic exercise testing with imaging, we have sought subgroups in whom the standard stress test is unreliable, despite an interpretable ECG. These groups may include women and patients with LV hypertrophy.

The accuracy of exercise ECG in women has been extensively debated. Depending on the population studied, either

TABLE 50.5

STUDIES COMPARING SENSITIVITY AND SPECIFICITY OF DOBUTAMINE AND VASODILATOR STRESS ECHOCARDIOGRAPHY IN GREATER THAN 100 PATIENTS

Author	No.	No. (% CAD)	Multivessel (% all CAD)	Myocardial infarction (% all CAD)	Sensitivity, dobutamine (%)	Sensitivity, dipyridamole (%)	Sensitivity, single-vessel disease, dobutamine (%)	Sensitivity, single-vessel disease, dipyridamole (%)	Specificity, dobutamine (%)	Specificity, dipyridamole (%)
Ostojic, et al. (57)	150	131 (87)	16 (12)	38 (29)	75	71	—	—	79	89
Beleslin, et al. (48)	136	119 (88)	11 (9)	41 (34)	82	74	82	72	77	94
Anthopoulos[a], et al. (58)	120	89 (74)	48 (40)	38 (30)	87	66	—	—	84	90
San Roman, et al. (59)	102	63 (62)	34 (54)	0 (0)	77	77	69	62	95	97
Fragasso, et al. (60)	101	56 (56)	—	—	88	61	88	61	80	91

CAD, coronary artery disease.
[a]Adenosine used instead of dipyridamole.

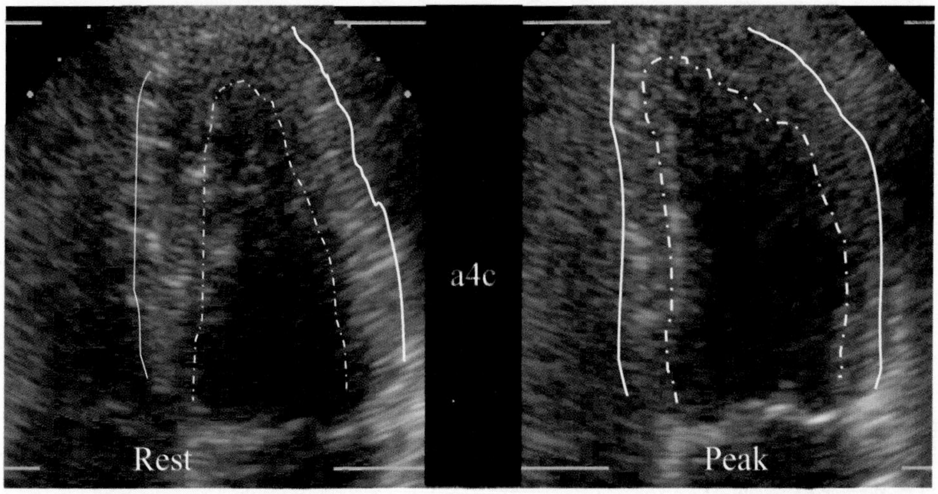

FIGURE 50.7. Diagnostic information from changes in left ventricular (LV) shape and size at exercise echocardiography in a patient with left anterior descending coronary artery and left circumflex artery disease. The apical four-chamber (a4c) view shows development of akinesis in the midseptum and apical septum after stress. The development of LV cavity enlargement draws attention to a lateral wall motion abnormality after stress.

the sensitivity or the specificity may be compromised (74–77). Although some of the differences from stress testing in men may be caused by lower disease prevalence, these results are influenced by nonbayesian factors, including the presence of milder CAD in women than men, the likelihood of submaximal stress, and intrinsic gender-based differences in the ST-segment response. Numerous large studies have now shown that the accuracy of stress echocardiography is not compromised in women (78–81), and these results are superior to those of the exercise ECG, even after correction for referral bias. A cost analysis suggested that the use of exercise echocardiography as an initial test caused more initial expense but was cheaper in the long run because of the avoidance of unnecessary angiograms in patients with false-positive ECG responses (78).

Comparison with Stress Perfusion Imaging

Despite competition from echocardiography, perfusion scintigraphy remains the most widely performed stress imaging test in the United States, and its use continues to increase.

Studies of the accuracy of SPECT myocardial perfusion scintigraphy have shown that this technique has a sensitivity greater than 90% for the detection of CAD (82). However, these studies also show that the specificity is approximately 70%, partly reflecting the phenomenon of posttest referral bias (47), as well as the problems of false-positive results related to image artifacts. In a metaanalysis, the superior sensitivity of SPECT was balanced by a greater specificity with echocardiography, so the accuracy of the techniques was comparable (83). The same findings have been reported in direct comparison in the same patients (Table 50.6) (56,66,84–89). The slightly lower sensitivity of stress echocardiography than perfusion scintigraphy may reflect superiority of perfusion imaging (which does not require the development of ischemia in a metabolic or functional sense) for the identification of patients with single-vessel disease. Similarly, patients receiving therapy with antianginal agents may be better studied using perfusion scintigraphy (because ischemia does not need to be induced for the test result to be positive). Perfusion scintigraphy also appears to be more sensitive for the recognition of multivessel disease (65) and may be superior for the detection of ischemia in the setting of resting wall motion abnormalities (66), although this benefit cannot be appreciated by consideration of sensitivity and specificity. Finally, scintigraphy is superior in patients with poor echocardiographic windows (e.g., resulting from pulmonary disease).

There appears to be a particular benefit of echocardiography over perfusion scintigraphy with respect to specificity. This difference is most marked in patients with LV hypertrophy and left bundle branch block. Breast attenuation artifacts and other issues have led to lower reported levels of accuracy of perfusion imaging in women, and the results of a metaanalysis suggest this may be a group better studied with stress echocardiography (90). Finally, stress echocardiography is versatile, rapidly performed, and less expensive than perfusion imaging. In situations in which other cardiac problems are present as well as ischemia (e.g., valvular and pericardial diseases), the selection of stress echocardiography avoids duplicate testing.

Practical Considerations

The choice between SPECT and stress echocardiography is influenced by numerous factors, some of which are summarized in Table 50.7. Of these, the most important is local expertise. Thus, at a center with an excellent nuclear laboratory and an echocardiographer inexperienced in stress echocardiography, the selection of the latter test would likely engender unfavorable results. The converse is true of facilities without the requisite nuclear experience.

Comparison with Magnetic Resonance Imaging

Modern MRI protocols promise to deliver information of gross cardiac anatomy, details of structure, function, and perfusion, all of which are of value in the diagnosis and evaluation of ischemic heart disease and are discussed in Chapter 54. There is no question that MRI can provide information as accurate as that furnished by echocardiography during stress, both for identification of ischemia (91) and for assessment of viable myocardium (92). The problems with the widespread application of this technology relate to issues of feasibility, access, and cost. It seems most likely that in the future, technically difficult studies will be performed using MRI, and this modality will be especially useful for evaluation of complex problems such as detection of viable myocardium in severe LV dysfunction.

TABLE 50.6

SENSITIVITY AND SPECIFICITY OF STRESS ECHOCARDIOGRAPHY AND MYOCARDIAL PERFUSION IMAGING FOR DIAGNOSIS OF CORONARY ARTERY DISEASE (STUDIES GREATER THAN 75 PATIENTS)

Author	No.	Significant stenosis (%)	Patients with CAD	Multivessel CAD	Stress methodology	Nuclear methodology	Sensitivity, echocardiography (%)	Sensitivity, nuclear (%)	Sensitivity, single-vessel disease, echocardiography (%)	Sensitivity, single-vessel disease, nuclear (%)	Specificity, echocardiography (%)	Specificity, nuclear (%)
Marwick, et al. (84)	217	>50	142	74 (52%)	Db 40 μg/kg/min	SPECT-MIBI	72	76	66	74	83	67
Smart, et al. (99)	183	>50	119	58 (49%)	Db 40 μg + atro	SPECT-MIBI	87	80	84	71	91	73
Takeuchi, et al. (86)	120	>50	74	37 (50%)	Db 30 μg/kg/min	SPECT-Tl	85	89	—	—	93	85
Quinones, et al. (66)	112	>50	86	45 (52%)	Treadmill	SPECT-Tl	74	76	58	61	88	81
San Roman, et al. (87)	102	>50	49	—	Db 40 μg + atro	SPECT-MIBI	78	87	—	—	88	70
San Roman, et al. (87)	102	>50	49	—	Dipy 0.84 mg/kg	SPECT-MIBI	81	87	—	—	94	70
Marwick, et al. (56)	97	>50	59	28 (47%)	Ad 0.18 mg/kg/min	SPECT-MIBI	58	86	52	81	87	71
Huang, et al. (88)	93	>50	67	—	Db 40 μg	SPECT-Tl	93	90	—	—	77	81
Pozzoli, et al. (89)	75	>50	49	16 (33%)	Upright bike	SPECT-MIBI	71	84	60	82	96	88

atro, atropine; CAD, coronary artery disease; Db, dobutamine; Dipy, dipyridamole; SPECT-MIBI, single-photon emission computed tomography, methyl isobutyl isonitrile; SPECT-Tl, single-photon emission computed tomography, thallium.

TABLE 50.7

ADVANTAGES AND DISADVANTAGES OF STRESS ECHOCARDIOGRAPHY AND MYOCARDIAL PERFUSION SCINTIGRAPHY

Consideration		Stress echocardiography	Myocardial perfusion imaging
Application	Versatility	++	–
	Cost	++	–
	Credentialing	–	++ (Nuclear Regulatory Commission)
Interpretation	Training/quality control	±	±
	Artifacts	+ (better with contrast?)	+ (better with sestamibi?)
	Quantitation	–	++
Clinical value	Sensitivity	80–85%	90%
	Specificity	85%	70%
	Prognostic value	+	++ (established role)
	Familiarity	±	++
	Ancillary data	++	–

USE OF STRESS ECHOCARDIOGRAPHY IN MANAGEMENT DECISIONS

Evaluation of Patients undergoing Myocardial Revascularization

Patients undergoing myocardial revascularization procedures should have some documentation of the presence and site of ischemia (93). Although stress echocardiography can accurately localize disease, the assumptions inherent in allocating myocardial regions to individual coronary vessels may compromise its ability to designate a "culprit" lesion. This is particularly problematic if multivessel disease is present, in which case the most ischemic territory is most commonly detected. Following both surgical (94,95) and percutaneous revascularization (96), stress echocardiography appears to have similar accuracy to its use in patients with native disease. However, its use in asymptomatic patients may be limited by bayesian considerations.

Identification of Myocardial Viability

Background

Sympathomimetic amines such as isoproterenol and dobutamine have been shown to reverse regional LV dysfunction in acute animal models of myocardial stunning (97). The same response appears to be applicable to chronic ischemic LV dysfunction. In the presence of dysfunctional but viable myocardium, regional function is enhanced by the inotropic effect of dobutamine at a low dose (usually 5 to 10 μg/kg per minute), whereas at higher doses, dobutamine-induced tachycardia increases oxygen consumption and leads to ischemia. Dipyridamole also exerts similar effects at a low dose, the mechanism of which is ill defined. Viable myocardium supplied by a patent infarct-related vessel (generally corresponding to stunned myocardium) demonstrates a sustained improvement during the infusion. Viable tissue supplied by a stenosed infarct-related artery (which may involve stunned or hibernating tissue) is characterized by an initial improvement, followed by deterioration of regional function as the chronotropic effect becomes more prominent and myocardial work increases (see Table 50.1).

Accuracy for Detection of Improvement after Revascularization

Dobutamine echocardiography has been effective for the prediction of myocardial viability in patients after infarction and chronic ischemic LV dysfunction. In these studies, the sensitivity of dobutamine stress to identify an improvement of systolic function in response to revascularization ranged from 69% to 86%, with a range of specificity from 57% to 100% (98–104).

Comparison of Stress Echocardiography with Other Techniques for Identification of Viable Myocardium

The ability of dobutamine echocardiography and other techniques to predict recovery of regional function (Fig. 50.8) has been compared in metaanalyses (105,106) and in direct comparison in individual patients. Both analyses suggest that

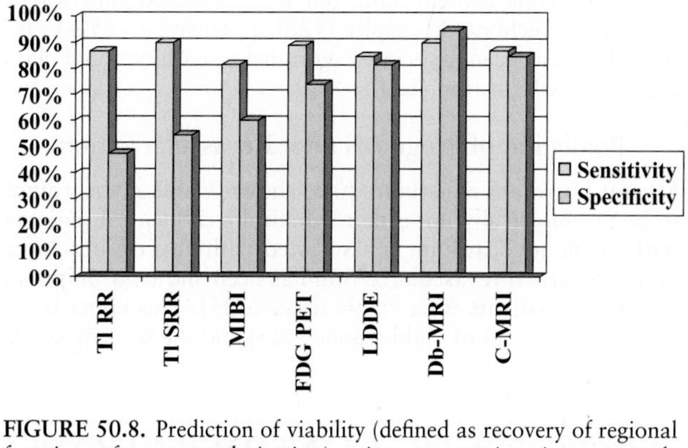

FIGURE 50.8. Prediction of viability (defined as recovery of regional function after revascularization) using current imaging protocols for the detection of viable myocardium. C, contrast; Db, dobutamine; FDG PET, fluorodeoxyglucose positron emission tomography; LDDE, low dose dobutamine echo; MIBI, methoxyl isobutyl isonitrile; MRI, magnetic resonance imaging; RR, rest redistribution; SRR, stress-reinjection-redistribution; Tl, thallium. (Adapted from Bax JJ, Cornel JH, Visser FC, et al. Prediction of recovery of myocardial dysfunction after revascularization: comparison of fluorine-18 fluorodeoxyglucose/thallium-201 SPECT, thallium-201 stress-reinjection SPECT and dobutamine echocardiography. *J Am Coll Cardiol* 1996;28:558–564.)

the accuracy of dobutamine echocardiography for identification of viable myocardium is equivalent to that of thallium-201 reinjection imaging (107–118). In comparison with thallium imaging, dobutamine echocardiography was similarly somewhat less sensitive but substantially more specific. The prediction of myocardial viability using low-dose dobutamine echocardiography correlates with positron emission tomography (PET) in about 80% of segments (98,119); although dobutamine echocardiography is less sensitive than PET, it is more specific (120). Finally, as mentioned previously, the accuracy of dobutamine echocardiography and of MRI is similar, especially if good echocardiographic images are obtained (92).

Prediction of Recovery of Functional Capacity

The evidence base regarding the accuracy of tests for prediction of myocardial viability is based on comparison with recovery of regional LV function. However, decision making regarding revascularization in patients with LV dysfunction is more strongly influenced by the likelihood of improving ejection fraction, functional capacity, and quality of life.

Although ejection fraction is the most widely used index of global LV function and is an important predictor of outcome, it is not a good marker for recovery of viable tissue because it is load dependent and is influenced by changes elsewhere in the heart. Hypercontractility in uninvolved regions of the myocardium may compensate for regional dysfunction; when these dysfunctional segments improve after revascularization, the compensating segments may resume normal function and the ejection fraction may remain unchanged. Nonetheless, improvement of ejection fraction can be expected if sufficient viable tissue is identified before revascularization; if more than 25% of segments are viable (121) or if there is an improvement of ejection fraction with low-dose dobutamine (122), a significant (5%) improvement in ejection fraction can be predicted with an accuracy greater than 80%. Clearly, the response to revascularization also depends on other variables, including the adequacy of revascularization target vessels, the overall status of the ventricle (very large ventricles are unlikely to recover dramatically), and the extent of scar tissue (thinned tissue is unlikely to recover). The extent of data regarding the ability to predict global functional recovery with dobutamine echocardiography is still limited. In patients with severe LV dysfunction, improvement in exercise capacity was predicted by the extent of viable myocardium, but PET appeared superior to dobutamine echocardiography (123). Extensive (>25%) viability has also been associated with increased functional class after revascularization (124).

Prediction of Prognosis after Revascularization

Several observational studies have shown viable myocardium to be prognostically important. Medical treatment of patients with viable myocardium is associated with adverse outcome, and myocardial revascularization has been shown to improve survival in patients with viable tissue (125). This effect is related to the extent of viable tissue (126) and the severity of LV dysfunction (127).

PROGNOSTIC CONSIDERATIONS IN CORONARY ARTERY DISEASE

Stable Chronic Coronary Artery Disease

In addition to information regarding the presence of ischemia and scar, exercise and pharmacologic stress testing techniques offer adjunctive information that may be of prognostic significance. With exercise, these include exercise capacity, hemodynamic responses to exercise, and the ST-segment response. Although ECG evidence of ischemia carries prognostic value, most prognostic information derives from echocardiographic evidence of ischemia. Similarly, although reduced exercise capacity appears to be a strong predictor of adverse outcome, the presence of ischemia at stress echocardiography adds significant prognostic information. With dobutamine, the rate pressure product at the onset of ischemia is important (128), and the equivalent measure using dipyridamole stress testing (dipyridamole time) is also of prognostic value. However, as discussed previously, the ECG component of both dipyridamole and dobutamine stress testing is insensitive, and the development of hypotension during these tests is not meaningful prognostically.

Many patients who present for exercise testing are either unable to exercise or exercise submaximally, and these individuals have a high cardiac event rate (129). From the prognostic standpoint, the detection of ischemia during either dobutamine or dipyridamole stress is analogous to its development during exercise stress. Likewise, the detection of ischemia during dobutamine stress (relative risk, 5.6) was a stronger predictor of outcome than most clinical variables and was superior to the prognostic significance of significant coronary stenoses (130). Although ejection fraction is recognized as an important predictor of cardiac events, the change of ejection fraction in response to dobutamine does not appear to be predictive of outcome (131). Similar findings have been reported using dipyridamole echocardiography; in the largest reported study, death and hard events were predicted by the presence of a positive dipyridamole echocardiographic test result, together with ECG positivity and angina (79,132). In particular, the degree of stress required to induce ischemia (evidenced by the dipyridamole time) was most predictive of hard events, whereas total events were predicted by the wall motion score at peak stress, reflecting the extent of both ischemia and infarction. Moreover, some studies have reported that the stress data are not only independent of other variables, but also incremental to the information obtained clinically (79,133,134).

Stress echocardiography offers important prognostic information in patients with chronic stable CAD (Fig. 50.9) (130,132–140). The presence and time of onset of ischemia are clearly associated with increased events, and these data are adjunctive to exercise capacity and ST-segment changes. Unfortunately, only limited comparisons are available between stress echocardiography and perfusion scintigraphy in terms of the ability to predict events; these data suggest that the techniques are comparable (141).

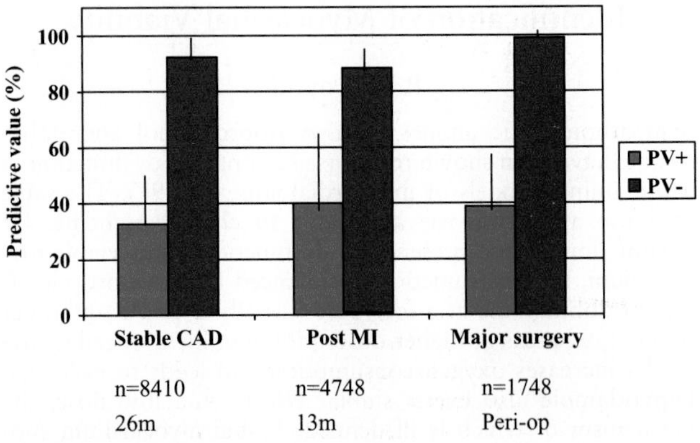

FIGURE 50.9. Predictive value (PV) of positive and negative stress echocardiography (prediction of composite events) in large prognostic studies in patients with stable (known or suspected) coronary artery disease (CAD), after myocardial infarction (MI), and before major noncardiac surgery (see text). The number of patients and average duration of follow-up are shown for each category.

Postinfarct Risk Stratification

The adoption of progressively more aggressive strategies for angiography and percutaneous intervention has reduced the use of stress echocardiography to stratify risk after infarction. Nonetheless, when intervention is less desirable, stress echocardiography provides evidence about the factors that are most predictive of outcome: ejection fraction and the presence and extent of ischemic and viable myocardium. Numerous large studies have gathered prognostic data using stress echocardiography in patients after myocardial infarction (142–148) (see Fig. 50.9). Most of these data have been obtained with pharmacologic stress, with only two small studies using exercise echocardiography (149,150). This finding may reflect a reluctance to perform exercise stress in the early postinfarct period. In contrast to patients with chronic stable CAD, cardiac events more commonly occur than in patients without evidence of ischemia (reflecting the risk associated with LV dysfunction), but hard events occur in more than 50% of those with positive stress echocardiographic results.

The timing of postinfarct risk stratification is a critical consideration, given than recurrent cardiac events may occur early after infarction. Because dipyridamole leads to a negligible increment of cardiac workload, this stress is attractive for early stress testing; as early as 3 days following myocardial infarction (144), ischemia at dipyridamole stress testing was predictive of both total and hard events. Echocardiographic signs of ischemia and angina are the strongest independent predictors of subsequent events, followed by ischemia alone, and anterior infarction. Hibernating myocardium may be identified by dobutamine echocardiography (see Table 50.6), and it may have a significant prognostic effect, especially if it is left unrevascularized (127). The influence of resting wall motion abnormalities on the identification of ischemia is an important limitation of the interpretation of stress echocardiography in the evaluation of patients following myocardial infarction. However, this problem concerns homozonal ischemia, and the presence of previous infarction does not compromise the ability to recognize ischemia in another zone. The ability of stress echocardiography to recognize heterozonal ischemia may explain the ability of stress echocardiography to predict events in postinfarction patients.

Peripheral Vascular Disease

Anatomic evidence of CAD is present in more than 80% of patients with aortic, lower limb, and cerebral vascular disease (151). However, the challenge of preoperative risk stratification is that although *anatomic* CAD is highly prevalent, serious perioperative cardiac complications are infrequent; cardiac death and myocardial infarction occur in 5% of unselected patients who undergo vascular surgery (152). The identification of this small subgroup is a major challenge on bayesian grounds, because the low pretest probability of an event influences the posttest probability, irrespective of the results of testing. This problem may at least in part be addressed by clinical evaluation (e.g., using the Eagle criteria for assigning the risk of a cardiac event). Patients with none of these factors (diabetes, age >70 years, angina, myocardial infarction, or heart failure) have a negligible risk of cardiac complications, irrespective of the results of stress testing (153).

The inability of most of these patients to exercise maximally necessitates the use of pharmacologic stress testing. Dipyridamole and dobutamine echocardiography is predictive of perioperative cardiac events (see Fig. 50.9) (154–161), and echocardiographic test results appear to be at least as predictive as those performed with nuclear imaging (162). As in many studies of risk stratification, although a negative test result renders a cardiac complication unlikely, a positive result generally confers 20% to 30% risk of a cardiac complication. Risk stratification may be enhanced by considering the ischemic threshold (i.e., the cardiac workload necessary to induce myocardial ischemia) (160) or the extent of ischemia (155). The combination of clinical evaluation and the presence and threshold of ischemia may be integrated into a patient care algorithm as illustrated in Figure 50.10. No single management strategy seems to address the risk of patients with a positive test adequately. Prophylactic β-blockade avoids events in low- to intermediate-risk patients, but not in those at high risk (163,164). Possibly, these high-risk patients may be helped by coronary revascularization (165), but generally this strategy has been disappointing (166).

In summary, stress echocardiography offers useful prognostic data. More material needs to be obtained for the comparison between stress echocardiography and perfusion scintigraphy for prognostic purposes, with respect to both accuracy and cost effectiveness.

CONTROVERSIES AND PERSONAL PERSPECTIVES

The use of stress echocardiography as a diagnostic tool is supported by a large evidence base. Although studies of the learning curve have been presented, limited data reflect the accuracy of this technique outside of the hands of experts. However, the future of this technique is likely to be influenced by the balance

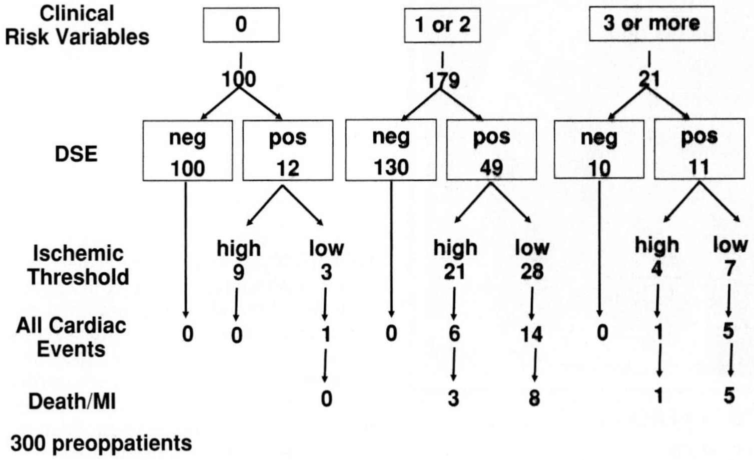

FIGURE 50.10. Integration of clinical data with ischemic threshold to dobutamine to predict events in patients undergoing vascular surgery. DSE, dobutamine stress echocardiography; MI, myocardial infarction; neg, negative. (From Poldermans D, Arnese M, Fioretti PM, et al. Improved cardiac risk stratification in major vascular surgery with dobutamine-atropine stress echocardiography. *J Am Coll Cardiol* 1995;26:648–653.)

between the training requirements of this methodology and technical developments. The growth of this methodology has been so dramatic that many studies are likely being performed by individuals with limited training in this discipline. The need for training and quality control in this, as in other, diagnostic techniques warrants attention. However, the development of new quantitative approaches may improve the reproducibility and robustness of this technique. Of the new technologies, myocardial Doppler and contrast echocardiography are most likely to offer lasting contributions.

Apart from the impetus of technologic development, the driving forces behind the growth of stress echocardiography have been practical. In comparison with nuclear imaging, stress echocardiography is relatively inexpensive to perform; there are no disposables, equipment is cheaper, and less processing is required. A less costly test was attractive to the patient and insurer in the conventional fee-for-service model of care, but it is even more so for the physician and hospital in the current era of managed care and capitation. Finally, although the new dual-isotope techniques are shorter to perform than the older thallium techniques, stress echocardiography is versatile and patient friendly. The results are available immediately after testing, and the equipment is relatively inexpensive and portable, thereby enabling the service to be offered in the physician's office or at a satellite clinic.

As in other fields of medicine, the challenge of the future will be to balance the technologic and financial forces supporting the growth of stress echocardiography with the need to maintain simplicity and cost-effectiveness.

THE FUTURE

Quantitative Techniques for Interpretation of Stress Echocardiography

Although suboptimal imaging remains a problem in some patients, despite the advances of harmonic imaging and contrast echocardiography, the issues of training and expertise remain the most pressing problems for stress echocardiography. A feasible quantitative approach to interpretation is needed. However, despite developments in myocardial imaging of longitudinal motion and integrated backscatter-based approaches, further advances will be needed before quantitation becomes a routine component of the interpretation of stress echocardiography.

Ancillary Techniques for Detecting Ischemia

The detection of myocardial ischemia is currently dependent on the detection of stress-induced wall motion abnormalities. As discussed in the section on limitations, this may cause problems with the recognition of multivessel disease, the detection of single-vessel CAD, and the distinction of ischemia and scar. Techniques that detect more subtle evidence of ischemia, such as myocardial contrast echocardiography, may supplement these findings and may indeed exceed the sensitivity of two-dimensional echocardiography alone for the detection of CAD.

Echocardiographic contrast agents traverse the lungs to reach a high concentration in the left-sided heart chambers and thereby may enhance the reflectivity of the myocardium. Although the degree of myocardial opacification (i.e., the concentration of tracer) is a reflection of myocardial blood volume, a more accurate marker of myocardial blood flow is the rate of refill after bubble destruction, which can be assessed either qualitatively or quantitatively. Myocardial contrast echocardiography has already been successfully applied during stress by several authors (167), and it has been shown to improve the sensitivity of stress echocardiography for single-vessel disease and to improve the recognition of multiple involved vascular territories in patients with multivessel disease (168,169). Thus, it seems likely that the use of myocardial contrast will facilitate detection of CAD by examination of both wall motion and perfusion at stress echocardiography.

The second group of ancillary techniques consists of quantitative parameters of myocardial deformation, although these may be more useful to assist in the detection of myocardial viability than in the detection of ischemia. A strain rate at low dose of more than 0.7 per second or an increment of more than 0.25 per second is predictive of viability, either defined as PET evidence (170) or functional recovery (171). Although the backscatter profile of myocardium is altered during ischemia, strain rate imaging has been shown to improve the accuracy of stress echocardiography in only a single study (172). Other work suggests that "false-negative" segments (i.e., no ischemia despite significant disease) lack evidence of ischemia with these markers, and they occur because of failure to

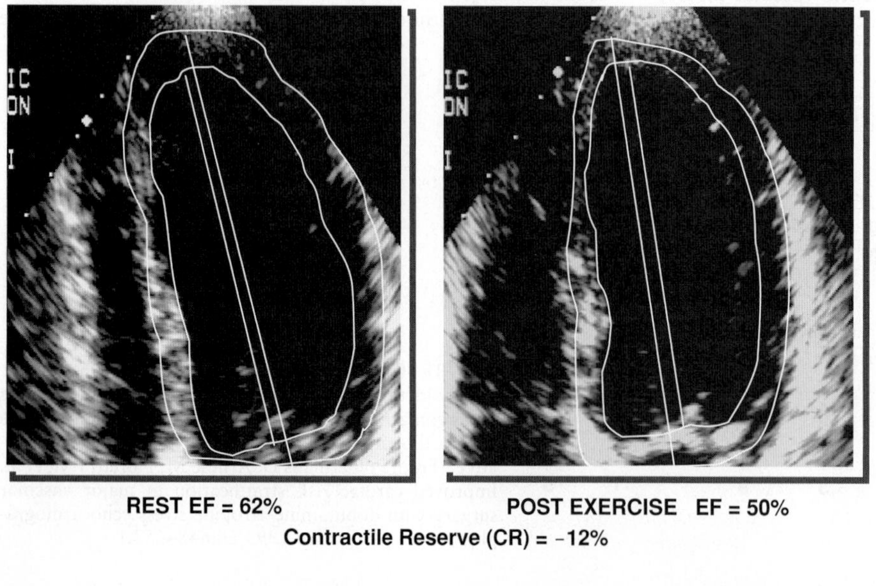

FIGURE 50.11. Determination of left ventricular (LV) contractile reserve in a patient with severe mitral regurgitation and preserved resting function (**left**). After exercise (**right**), the LV cavity increases and ejection fraction (EF) falls, as seen on echocardiography. Despite normal LV size and function at rest, this response implies that the ventricle is becoming compromised.

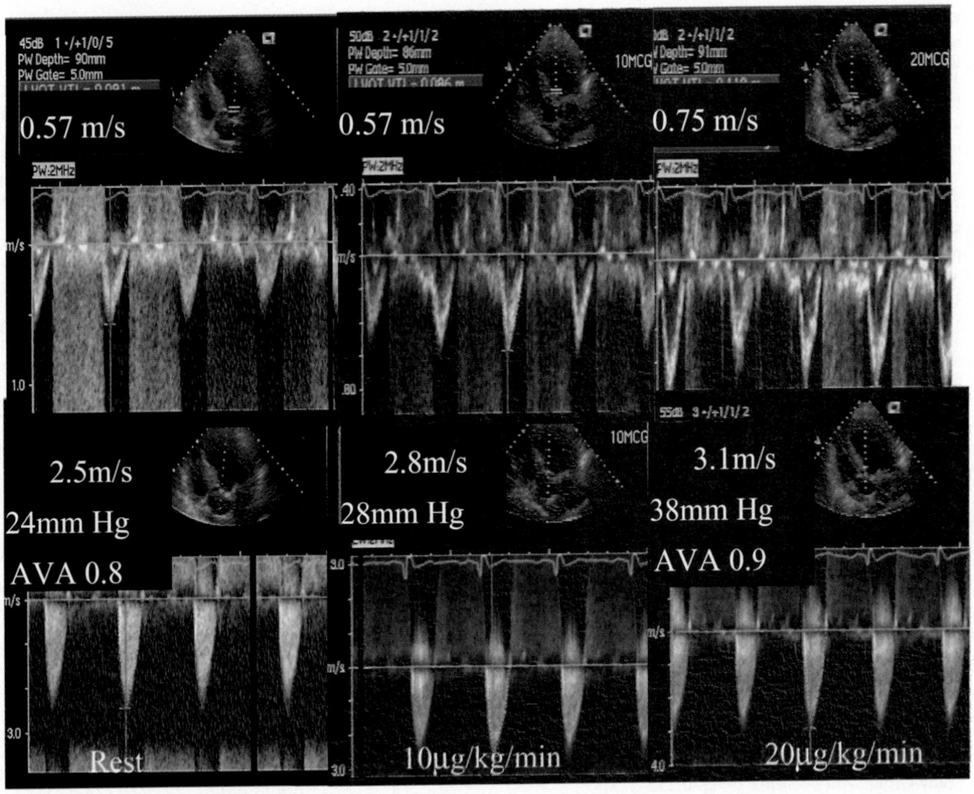

FIGURE 50.12. Application of dobutamine echocardiography to low-output aortic stenosis. Resting Doppler measurements show a low gradient in the setting of left ventricular (LV) dysfunction. The increment of the valvular gradient (which exceeds that of the LV outflow tract velocity) signifies a primary valvular problem. AVA, aortic valve area.

provoke ischemia rather than failure to recognize the problem (173). It seems likely that the main benefit of these quantitative techniques will be to enhance agreement among observers more than to improve accuracy.

Use in Noncoronary Heart Diseases

The stress echocardiography literature mostly pertains to the detection of myocardial ischemia. However, the functional response to stress is important in the evaluation of myocardial and valvular heart diseases, and the importance of stress echocardiography for this purpose is likely to grow. Patients at risk for anthracycline toxicity may be detected using stress echocardiography (174,175). Similarly, loss of contractile reserve in response to stress also appears to be a marker of impending contractile dysfunction in patients with LV volume loading related to mitral regurgitation (Fig. 50.11) (176).

In patients with valvular stenosis, the response to stress may differentiate the interrelated influences of ventricular function and valvular disease on the production of gradients. The finding of a low gradient in a patient with aortic stenosis may reflect the influence of reduced ventricular function. In these patients, lack of contractile reserve at low-dose dobutamine echocardiography identifies severe myocardial disease, in which case the outcome is poor (177). The optimal situation is one in which the LV improves and gradients increase, signifying tight aortic stenosis (Fig. 50.12). Similarly, patients with latent LV outflow tract obstruction may demonstrate exercise-induced outflow tract obstruction in response to exercise or amyl nitrite (178).

Finally, measurement of tricuspid regurgitant velocity may be used to calculate pulmonary artery pressure after exercise. Exercise-induced pulmonary hypertension is a common pathway of cardiac decompensation following stress and may be a particularly useful measurement in patients with apparently moderate mitral stenosis at rest but marked decompensation with stress. The development of this response may correlate with a marked increment of diastolic gradient with exercise.

References

1. Marwick TH. Current status of non-invasive techniques for the diagnosis of myocardial ischemia. *Acta Clin Belg* 1992;47:1–5.
2. Kraunz RF, Kennedy JW. Ultrasonic determination of left ventricular wall motion in normal man: studies at rest and after exercise. *Am Heart J* 1970; 79:36–43.
3. Koike A, Itoh H, Doi M, et al. Beat-to-beat evaluation of cardiac function during recovery from upright bicycle exercise in patients with coronary artery disease. *Am Heart J* 1990;120:316–323.
4. Tennant R, Wiggers CJ. The effect of coronary occlusion on myocardial contraction. *Am J Physiol* 1935;112:351–361.
5. Kerber RE, Martins JB, Marcus ML. Effect of acute ischemia, nitroglycerin and nitroprusside on regional myocardial thickening, stress and perfusion: experimental echocardiographic studies. *Circulation* 1979;60:121–129.
6. Takayama M, Norris RM, Brown MA, et al. Postsystolic shortening of acutely ischemic canine myocardium predicts early and late recovery of function after coronary artery reperfusion. *Circulation* 1988;78:994–1007.
7. Presti CF, Armstrong WF, Feigenbaum H. Comparison of echocardiography at peak exercise and after bicycle exercise in evaluation of patients with known or suspected coronary artery disease. *J Am Soc Echocardiogr* 1988; 1:119–126.
8. Ryan T, Segar DS, Sawada SG, et al. Detection of coronary artery disease with upright bicycle exercise echocardiography. *J Am Soc Echocardiogr* 1993;6:186–197.
9. Robertson WS, Feigenbaum H, Armstrong WF, et al. Exercise echocardiography: a clinically practical addition in the evaluation of coronary artery disease. *J Am Coll Cardiol* 1983;2:1085–10891.
10. Armstrong WF. "Hibernating" myocardium: asleep or part dead? *J Am Coll Cardiol* 1996;28:530–535.

11. Kloner RA, Przyklenk K, Patel B. Altered myocardial states: the stunned and hibernating myocardium. *Am J Med* 1986;86(suppl 1A):14–17.
12. Rahimtoola SH. The hibernating myocardium. *Am Heart J* 1989;117: 2113–2115.
13. Fudo T, Kambara H, Hashimoto T, et al. F-18 deoxyglucose and stress N-13 ammonia positron emission tomography in anterior wall healed myocardial infarction. *Am J Cardiol* 1988;61:1191–1197.
14. Cohen JL, Greene TO, Ottenweller J, et al. Dobutamine digital echocardiography for detecting coronary artery disease. *Am J Cardiol* 1991;67:1311–1318.
15. Secknus MA, Marwick TH. Evolution of dobutamine echocardiography protocols and indications: safety and side effects in 3,011 studies over 5 years. *J Am Coll Cardiol* 1997;29:1234–1240.
16. Sawada SG, Segar DS, Ryan T, et al. Echocardiographic detection of coronary artery disease during dobutamine infusion. *Circulation* 1991;83: 1605–1614.
17. Weissman NJ, Nidorf SM, Guerrero JL, et al. Optimal stage duration in dobutamine stress echocardiography. *J Am Coll Cardiol* 1995;25:605–609.
18. McNeill AJ, Fioretti PM, el-Said SM, et al. Enhanced sensitivity for detection of coronary artery disease by addition of atropine to dobutamine stress echocardiography. *Am J Cardiol* 1992;70:41–46.
19. Lewandowski TJ, Armstrong WF, Bach DS. Reduced test time by early identification of patients requiring atropine during dobutamine stress echocardiography. *J Am Soc Echocardiogr* 1998;11:236–242.
20. Cornel JH, Balk AH, Boersma E, et al. Safety and feasibility of dobutamine-atropine stress echocardiography in patients with ischemic left ventricular dysfunction. *J Am Soc Echocardiogr* 1996;9:27–32.
21. Williams MJ, Odabashian J, Lauer MS, et al. Prognostic value of dobutamine echocardiography in patients with left ventricular dysfunction. *J Am Coll Cardiol* 1996;27:132–139.
22. Poldermans D, Rambaldi R, Bax JJ, et al. Safety and utility of atropine addition during dobutamine stress echocardiography for the assessment of viable myocardium in patients with severe left ventricular dysfunction. *Eur Heart J* 1998;19:1712–1718.
23. Picano E, Marini C, Pirelli S, et al. Safety of intravenous high-dose dipyridamole echocardiography: the Echo-Persantine International Cooperative Study Group. *Am J Cardiol* 1992;70:252–258.
24. Cerqueira MD, Verani MS, Schwaiger M, et al. Safety profile of adenosine stress perfusion imaging: results from the Adenoscan Multicenter Trial Registry. *J Am Coll Cardiol* 1994;23:384–389.
25. Picano E, Pingitore A, Conti U, et al. Enhanced sensitivity for detection of coronary artery disease by addition of atropine to dipyridamole echocardiography. *Eur Heart J* 1993;14:1216–1222.
26. Attenhofer CH, Pellikka PA, Oh JK, et al. Is review of videotape necessary after review of digitized cine-loop images in stress echocardiography? A prospective study in 306 patients. *J Am Soc Echocardiogr* 1997;10:179–184.
27. Afridi I, Kleiman NS, Raizner AE, Zoghbi WA. Dobutamine echocardiography in myocardial hibernation: optimal dose and accuracy in predicting recovery of ventricular function after coronary angioplasty. *Circulation* 1995;91:663–670.
28. Picano E, Lattanzi F, Orlandini A, et al. Stress echocardiography and the human factor: the importance of being expert. *J Am Coll Cardiol* 1991;17: 666–669.
29. Varga A, Picano E, Dodi C, et al. Madness and method in stress echo reading. *Eur Heart J* 1999;20:1271–1275.
30. Oberman A, Fan PH, Nanda NC, et al. Reproducibility of two-dimensional exercise echocardiography. *J Am Coll Cardiol* 1989;14:923–928.
31. Hoffmann R, Lethen H, Marwick T, et al. Analysis of interinstitutional observer agreement in interpretation of dobutamine stress echocardiograms. *J Am Coll Cardiol* 1996;27:330–336.
32. Hoffmann R, Lethen H, Marwick T, et al. Standardized guidelines for the interpretation of dobutamine echocardiography reduce interinstitutional variance in interpretation. *Am J Cardiol* 1998;82:1520–1524.
33. Hoffmann R, Poldermans D, van der Meer, P, et al. The maturing of stress echocardiography: improved intercenter agreement in interpretation of dobutamine stress echocardiograms using new techniques. *Eur Heart J* 2002;23:321–329.
34. Ginzton LE, Conant R, Brizendine M, et al. Quantitative analysis of segmental wall motion during maximal upright dynamic exercise: variability in normal adults. *Circulation* 1986;73:268–275.
35. Marwick TH, Nemec JJ, Pashkow FJ, et al. Accuracy and limitations of exercise echocardiography in a routine clinical setting. *J Am Coll Cardiol* 1992;19:74–81.
36. Senior R, Lahiri A. Enhanced detection of myocardial ischemia by stress dobutamine echocardiography utilizing the "biphasic" response of wall thickening during low and high dose dobutamine infusion. *J Am Coll Cardiol* 1995;26:26–32.
37. Noguchi Y, Nagata-Kobayashi S, Stahl JE, Wong JB. A meta-analytic comparison of echocardiographic stressors. *Int J Cardiovasc Imaging* 2005;21: 189–207.
38. Armstrong WF, O'Donnell J, Ryan T, Feigenbaum H. Effect of prior myocardial infarction and extent and location of coronary disease on accuracy of exercise echocardiography. *J Am Coll Cardiol* 1987;10:531–538.
39. Hecht HS, DeBord L, Sotomayor N, et al. Supine bicycle stress echocardiography: peak exercise imaging is superior to postexercise imaging. *J Am Soc Echocardiogr* 1993;6:265–271.
40. Sheikh KH, Bengtson JR, Helmy S, et al. Relation of quantitative coronary lesion measurements to the development of exercise-induced ischemia assessed by exercise echocardiography. *J Am Coll Cardiol* 1990;15:1043–1051.
41. Agati L, Arata L, Luongo R, et al. Assessment of severity of coronary narrowings by quantitative exercise echocardiography and comparison with quantitative arteriography. *Am J Cardiol* 1991;67:1201–1207.
42. Prince CR, Stoddard MF, Morris GT, et al. Dobutamine two-dimensional transesophageal echocardiographic stress testing for detection of coronary artery disease. *Am Heart J* 1994;128:36–41.
43. Baptista J, Arnese M, Roelandt JR, et al. Quantitative coronary angiography in the estimation of the functional significance of coronary stenosis: correlations with dobutamine-atropine stress test. *J Am Coll Cardiol* 1994;23:1434–1439.
44. Bartunek J, Marwick TH, Rodrigues AC, et al. Dobutamine-induced wall motion abnormalities: correlations with myocardial fractional flow reserve and quantitative coronary angiography. *J Am Coll Cardiol* 1996;27:1429–1436.
45. Segar DS, Brown SE, Sawada SG, et al. Dobutamine stress echocardiography: correlation with coronary lesion severity as determined by quantitative angiography. *J Am Coll Cardiol* 1992;19:1197–1202.
46. Marcovitz PA, Armstrong WF. Accuracy of dobutamine stress echocardiography in detecting coronary artery disease. *Am J Cardiol* 1992;69:1269–1273.
47. Roger VL, Pellikka PA, Bell MR, et al. Sex and test verification bias: impact on the diagnostic value of exercise echocardiography. *Circulation* 1997;95:405–410.
48. Beleslin BD, Ostojic M, Stepanovic J, et al. Stress echocardiography in the detection of myocardial ischemia: head-to-head comparison of exercise, dobutamine, and dipyridamole tests. *Circulation* 1994;90:1168–1176.
49. Previtali M, Lanzarini L, Fetiveau R, et al. Comparison of dobutamine stress echocardiography, dipyridamole stress echocardiography and exercise stress testing for diagnosis of coronary artery disease. *Am J Cardiol* 1993;72:865–870.
50. Cohen JL, Ottenweller JE, George AK, Duvvuri S. Comparison of dobutamine and exercise echocardiography for detecting coronary artery disease. *Am J Cardiol* 1993;72:1226–1231.
51. Marwick TH, D'Hondt AM, Mairesse GH, et al. Comparative ability of dobutamine and exercise stress in inducing myocardial ischaemia in active patients. *Br Heart J* 1994;72:31–38.
52. Dagianti A, Penco M, Agati L, et al. Stress echocardiography: comparison of exercise, dipyridamole and dobutamine in detecting and predicting the extent of coronary artery disease. *J Am Coll Cardiol* 1995;26:18–25.
53. Rallidis L, Cokkinos P, Tousoulis D, Nihoyannopoulos P. Comparison of dobutamine and treadmill exercise echocardiography in inducing ischemia in patients with coronary artery disease. *J Am Coll Cardiol* 1997;30:1660–1668.
54. Attenhoffer CH, Pellikka PA, Oh JK, et al. Comparison of ischemic response during exercise and dobutamine echocardiography in patients with left main coronary artery disease. *J Am Coll Cardiol* 1996;27:1171–1177.
55. Zoghbi WA, Cheirif J, Kleiman NS, et al. Diagnosis of ischemic heart disease with adenosine echocardiography. *J Am Coll Cardiol* 1991;18:1271–1279.
56. Marwick T, Willemart B, D'Hondt AM, et al. Selection of the optimal nonexercise stress for the evaluation of ischemic regional myocardial dysfunction and malperfusion: comparison of dobutamine and adenosine using echocardiography and 99mTc-MIBI single photon emission computed tomography. *Circulation* 1993;87:345–354.
57. Ostojic M, Picano E, Beleslin B, et al. Dipyridamole-dobutamine echocardiography: a novel test for the detection of milder forms of coronary artery disease. *J Am Coll Cardiol* 1994;23:1115–1122.
58. Anthopoulos LP, Bonou MS, Kardaras FG, et al. Stress echocardiography in elderly patients with coronary artery disease: applicability, safety and prognostic value of dobutamine and adenosine echocardiography in elderly patients. *J Am Coll Cardiol* 1996;28:52–59.
59. San Roman JA, Vilacosta I, Castillo JA, et al. Dipyridamole and dobutamine-atropine stress echocardiography in the diagnosis of coronary artery disease: comparison with exercise stress test, analysis of agreement, and impact of antianginal treatment. *Chest* 1996;110:1248–1254.
60. Fragasso G, Lu C, Dabrowski P, et al. Comparison of stress/rest myocardial perfusion tomography, dipyridamole and dobutamine stress echocardiography for the detection of coronary disease in hypertensive patients with chest pain and positive exercise test. *J Am Coll Cardiol* 1999;34:441–447.
61. Santoro GM, Sciagra R, Buonamici P, et al. Head-to-head comparison of exercise stress testing, pharmacologic stress echocardiography, and perfusion tomography as first-line examination for chest pain in patients without history of coronary artery disease. *J Nucl Cardiol* 1998;5:19–27.
62. Loimaala A, Groundstroem K, Pasanen M, et al. Comparison of bicycle, heavy isometric, dipyridamole-atropine and dobutamine stress echocardiography for diagnosis of myocardial ischemia. *Am J Cardiol* 1999;84:1396–1400.
63. Olson CE, Porter TR, Deligonul U, et al. Left ventricular volume changes during dobutamine stress echocardiography identify patients with more extensive coronary artery disease. *J Am Coll Cardiol* 1994;24:1268–1273.
64. Marwick TH, Nemec JJ, Stewart WJ, Salcedo EE. Diagnosis of coronary artery disease using exercise echocardiography and positron emission

tomography: comparison and analysis of discrepant results. *J Am Soc Echocardiogr* 1992;5:231–238.
65. O'Keefe JH Jr, Barnhart CS, Bateman TM. Comparison of stress echocardiography and stress myocardial perfusion scintigraphy for diagnosing coronary artery disease and assessing its severity. *Am J Cardiol* 1995;75:25D–34D.
66. Quinones MA, Verani MS, Haichin RM, et al. Exercise echocardiography versus 201Tl single-photon emission computed tomography in evaluation of coronary artery disease: analysis of 292 patients. *Circulation* 1992;85:1026–1031.
67. Cumming GR. Yield of ischemic exercise electrocardiograms in relation to exercise intensity in a normal population. *Br Heart J* 1972;34:919–923.
68. Mairesse GH, Marwick TH, Vanoverschelde JL, et al. How accurate is dobutamine stress electrocardiography for detection of coronary artery disease? Comparison with two-dimensional echocardiography and technetium-99m methoxyl isobutyl isonitrile (MIBI) perfusion scintigraphy. *J Am Coll Cardiol* 1994;24:920–927.
69. Chambers CE, Brown KA. Dipyridamole-induced ST segment depression during thallium-201 imaging in patients with coronary artery disease: angiographic and hemodynamic determinants. *J Am Coll Cardiol* 1988;12:37–41.
70. Villanueva FS, Smith WH, Watson DD, Beller GA. ST-segment depression during dipyridamole infusion, and its clinical, scintigraphic and hemodynamic correlates. *Am J Cardiol* 1992;69:445–448.
71. Armstrong WF, O'Donnell J, Dillon JC, et al. Complementary value of two-dimensional exercise echocardiography to routine treadmill exercise testing. *Ann Intern Med* 1986;105:829–835.
72. Ryan T, Vasey CG, Presti CF, et al. Exercise echocardiography: detection of coronary artery disease in patients with normal left ventricular wall motion at rest. *J Am Coll Cardiol* 1988;11:993–999.
73. Marwick TH, Shaw L, Case C, et al. Clinical and economic impact of exercise electrocardiography and exercise echocardiography in clinical practice. *Eur Heart J* 2003;24:1153–1163.
74. Hung J, Chaitman BR, Lam J, et al. Noninvasive diagnostic test choices for the evaluation of coronary artery disease in women: a multivariate comparison of cardiac fluoroscopy, exercise electrocardiography and exercise thallium myocardial perfusion scintigraphy. *J Am Coll Cardiol* 1984;4:8–16.
75. Okin PM, Kligfield P. Gender-specific criteria and performance of the exercise electrocardiogram. *Circulation* 1995;92:1209–1216.
76. Cumming GR, Dufresne C, Kich L, Samm J. Exercise electrocardiogram patterns in normal women. *Br Heart J* 1973;35:1055–1061.
77. Sketch MH, Mohiuddin SM, Lynch JD, et al. Significant sex differences in the correlation of electrocardiographic exercise testing and coronary arteriograms. *Am J Cardiol* 1975;36:169–173.
78. Marwick TH, Anderson T, Williams MJ, et al. Exercise echocardiography is an accurate and cost-efficient technique for the detection of coronary artery disease in women. *J Am Coll Cardiol* 1995;26:335–341.
79. Severi S, Picano E, Michelassi C, et al. Diagnostic and prognostic value of dipyridamole echocardiography in patients with suspected coronary artery disease: comparison with exercise electrocardiography. *Circulation* 1994;89:1160–1173.
80. Dionisopoulos PN, Collins JD, Smart SC, et al. The value of dobutamine stress echocardiography for the detection of coronary artery disease in women. *J Am Soc Echocardiogr* 1997;10:811–817.
81. Secknus MA, Marwick TH. Influence of gender on physiologic response and accuracy of dobutamine echocardiography. *Am J Cardiol* 1997;80:721–724.
82. Mahmarian J, Boyce T, Goldberg R, et al. Quantitative exercise thallium-201 single photon emission computed tomography for the enhanced diagnosis of ischemic heart disease. *J Am Coll Cardiol* 1990;15:318–325.
83. Fleischmann KE, Hunink MG, Kuntz KM, Douglas PS. Exercise echocardiography or exercise SPECT imaging? A meta-analysis of diagnostic test performance. *JAMA* 1998;280:913–920.
84. Marwick T, D'Hondt AM, Baudhuin T, et al. Optimal use of dobutamine stress for the detection and evaluation of coronary artery disease: combination with echocardiography or scintigraphy, or both? *J Am Coll Cardiol* 1993;22:159–167.
85. Oosterhuis WP, Breeman A, Niemeyer MG, et al. Patients with a normal exercise thallium-201 myocardial scintigram: always a good prognosis? *Eur J Nucl Med* 1993;20:151–158.
86. Takeuchi M, Araki M, Nakashima Y, Kuroiwa A. Comparison of dobutamine stress echocardiography and stress thallium-201 single-photon emission computed tomography for detecting coronary artery disease. *J Am Soc Echocardiogr* 1993;6:593–602.
87. San Roman JA, Rollan MJ, Vilacosta I, et al. [Echocardiography and MIBI-SPECT scintigraphy during dobutamine infusion in the diagnosis of coronary disease]. *Rev Esp Cardiol* 1995;48:606–614.
88. Huang PJ, Ho YL, Wu CC, et al. Simultaneous dobutamine stress echocardiography and thallium-201 perfusion imaging for the detection of coronary artery disease. *Cardiology* 1997;88:556–562.
89. Pozzoli MM, Fioretti PM, Salustri A, et al. Exercise echocardiography and technetium 99m MIBI single photon emission computed tomography in the detection of coronary artery disease. *Am J Cardiol* 1991;67:350–355.
90. Kwok Y, Kim C, Grady D, et al. Meta-analysis of exercise testing to detect coronary artery disease in women. *Am J Cardiol* 1999;83:660–666.
91. Nagel E, Lehmkuhl HB, Bocksch W, et al. Noninvasive diagnosis of ischemia-induced wall motion abnormalities with the use of high-dose dobutamine stress MRI: comparison with dobutamine stress echocardiography. *Circulation* 1999;99:763–770.
92. Baer FM, Theissen P, Crnac J, et al. Head to head comparison of dobutamine-transoesophageal echocardiography and dobutamine-magnetic resonance imaging for the prediction of left ventricular functional recovery in patients with chronic coronary artery disease. *Eur Heart J* 2000;21:981–991.
93. Topol EJ, Ellis SG, Cosgrove DM, et al. Analysis of coronary angioplasty practice in the United States with an insurance-claims data base. *Circulation* 1993;87:1489–1497.
94. Sawada SG, Judson WE, Ryan T, et al. Upright bicycle exercise echocardiography after coronary artery bypass grafting. *Am J Cardiol* 1989;64:1123–1129.
95. Elhendly A, Geleijnse ML, Roelandt JR, et al. Assessment of patients after coronary artery bypass grafting by dobutamine stress echocardiography. *Am J Cardiol* 1996;77:1234–1236.
96. Hecht HS, DeBord L, Shaw R, et al. Usefulness of supine bicycle stress echocardiography for detection of restenosis after percutaneous transluminal coronary angioplasty. *Am J Cardiol* 1993;71:293–296.
97. Ellis SG, Wynne J, Braunwald E, et al. Response of reperfusion-salvaged, stunned myocardium to inotropic stimulation. *Am Heart J* 1984;107:13–19.
98. Pierard LA, De Landsheere CM, Berthe C, et al. Identification of viable myocardium by echocardiography during dobutamine infusion in patients with myocardial infarction after thrombolytic therapy: comparison with positron emission tomography. *J Am Coll Cardiol* 1990;15:1021–1031.
99. Smart SC, Sawada S, Ryan T, et al. Low-dose dobutamine echocardiography detects reversible dysfunction after thrombolytic therapy of acute myocardial infarction. *Circulation* 1993;88:405–415.
100. Previtali M, Poli A, Lanzarini L, et al. Dobutamine stress echocardiography for assessment of myocardial viability and ischemia in acute myocardial infarction treated with thrombolysis. *Am J Cardiol* 1993;72:124G–130G.
101. Watada H, Ito H, Oh H, et al. Dobutamine stress echocardiography predicts reversible dysfunction and quantitates the extent of irreversibly damaged myocardium after reperfusion of anterior myocardial infarction. *J Am Coll Cardiol* 1994;24:624–630.
102. Bolognese L, Antoniucci D, Rovai D, et al. Myocardial contrast echocardiography versus dobutamine echocardiography for predicting functional recovery after acute myocardial infarction treated with primary coronary angioplasty. *J Am Coll Cardiol* 1996;28:1677–1683.
103. Poli A, Previtali M, Lanzarini L, et al. Comparison of dobutamine stress echocardiography with dipyridamole stress echocardiography for detection of viable myocardium after myocardial infarction treated with thrombolysis. *Heart* 1996;75:240–246.
104. Varga A, Ostojic M, Djordjevic-Dikic A, et al. Infra-low dose dipyridamole test: a novel dose regimen for selective assessment of myocardial viability by vasodilator stress echocardiography. *Eur Heart J* 1996;17:629–634.
105. Stewart S. Current theories and therapies relating to acute myocardial infarction and reperfusion injury. *Intensive Crit Care Nurs* 1992;8:104–112.
106. Bonow RO. Identification of viable myocardium. *Circulation* 1996;94:2674–2680.
107. Marzullo P, Parodi O, Reisenhofer B, et al. Value of rest thallium-201/technetium-99m sestamibi scans and dobutamine echocardiography for detecting myocardial viability. *Am J Cardiol* 1993;71:166–172.
108. Charney R, Schwinger ME, Chun J, et al. Dobutamine echocardiography and resting-redistribution thallium-201 scintigraphy predicts recovery of hibernating myocardium after coronary revascularization. *Am Heart J* 1994;128:864–869.
109. Kostopoulos KG, Kranidis AI, Bouki KP, et al. Detection of myocardial viability in the prediction of improvement in left ventricular function after successful coronary revascularization by using the dobutamine stress echocardiography and quantitative SPECT rest-redistribution-reinjection 201Tl imaging after dipyridamole infusion. *Angiology* 1996;47:1039–1046.
110. Qureshi U, Nagueh SF, Afridi I, et al. Dobutamine echocardiography and quantitative rest-redistribution 201Tl tomography in myocardial hibernation: relation of contractile reserve to 201Tl uptake and comparative prediction of recovery of function. *Circulation* 1997;95:626–635.
111. Nagueh SF, Vaduganathan P, Ali N, et al. Identification of hibernating myocardium: comparative accuracy of myocardial contrast echocardiography, rest-redistribution thallium-201 tomography and dobutamine echocardiography. *J Am Coll Cardiol* 1997;29:985–993.
112. Senior R, Glenville B, Basu S, et al. Dobutamine echocardiography and thallium-201 imaging predict functional improvement after revascularisation in severe ischaemic left ventricular dysfunction. *Br Heart J* 1995;74:358–364.
113. Arnese M, Cornel JH, Salustri A, et al. Prediction of improvement of regional left ventricular function after surgical revascularization: a comparison of low-dose dobutamine echocardiography with 201Tl single-photon emission computed tomography. *Circulation* 1995;91:2748–2752.
114. Perrone-Filardi P, Pace L, Prastaro M, et al. Assessment of myocardial viability in patients with chronic coronary artery disease: rest-4-hour-24-hour 201-Tl tomography versus dobutamine echocardiography. *Circulation* 1996;94:2712–2719.

115. Bax JJ, Cornel JH, Visser FC, et al. Prediction of recovery of myocardial dysfunction after revascularization: comparison of fluorine-18 fluorodeoxyglucose/thallium-201 SPECT, thallium-201 stress-reinjection SPECT and dobutamine echocardiography. *J Am Coll Cardiol* 1996;28:558–564.
116. Haque T, Furukawa T, Takahashi M, Kinoshita M. Identification of hibernating myocardium by dobutamine stress echocardiography: comparison with thallium-201 reinjection imaging. *Am Heart J* 1995;130:553–563.
117. Vanoverschelde JL, D'Hondt AM, Marwick T, et al. Head-to-head comparison of exercise-redistribution-reinjection thallium single-photon emission computed tomography and low dose dobutamine echocardiography for prediction of reversibility of chronic left ventricular ischemic dysfunction. *J Am Coll Cardiol* 1996;28:432–442.
118. Elsasser A, Muller KD, Vogt A, et al. Assessment of myocardial viability: dobutamine echocardiography and thallium-201 single-photon emission computed tomographic imaging predict the postoperative improvement of left ventricular function after bypass surgery. *Am Heart J* 1998;135:463–475.
119. Chan RKM, Lee KJ, Calafiore P, et al. Comparison of dobutamine echocardiography and positron emission tomography in patients with chronic ischemic left ventricular dysfunction. *J Am Coll Cardiol* 1996;27:1601–1607.
120. Pasquet A, Williams MJ, Secknus MA, et al. Correlation of preoperative myocardial function, perfusion, and metabolism with postoperative function at rest and stress after bypass surgery in severe left ventricular dysfunction. *Am J Cardiol* 1999;84:58–64.
121. Cornel JH, Bax JJ, Elhendy A, et al. Biphasic response to dobutamine predicts improvement of global left ventricular function after surgical revascularization in patients with stable coronary artery disease: implications of time course of recovery on diagnostic accuracy. *J Am Coll Cardiol* 1998;31:1002–1010.
122. Pasquet A, Lauer MS, Williams MJ, et al. Prediction of global left ventricular function after bypass surgery in patients with severe left ventricular dysfunction: impact of pre-operative myocardial function, perfusion, and metabolism. *Eur Heart J* 2000;21:125–136.
123. Marwick TH, Zuchowski C, Lauer MS, et al. Functional status and quality of life in patients with heart failure undergoing coronary bypass surgery after assessment of myocardial viability. *J Am Coll Cardiol* 1999;33:750–758.
124. Bax JJ, Poldermans D, Elhendy A, et al. Improvement of left ventricular ejection fraction, heart failure symptoms and prognosis after revascularization in patients with chronic coronary artery disease and viable myocardium detected by dobutamine stress echocardiography. *J Am Coll Cardiol* 1999;34:163–169.
125. Afridi I, Grayburn PA, Panza JA, et al. Myocardial viability during dobutamine echocardiography predicts survival in patients with coronary artery disease and severe left ventricular systolic dysfunction. *J Am Coll Cardiol* 1998;32:921–926.
126. Meluzin J, Cerny J, Frelich MS, et al. Prognostic value of the amount of dysfunctional but viable myocardium in revascularized patients with coronary artery disease and left ventricular dysfunction. *J Am Coll Cardiol* 1998;32:912–920.
127. Allman KC, Shaw LJ, Hachamovitch R, Udelson JE. Myocardial viability testing and impact of revascularization on prognosis in patients with coronary artery disease and left ventricular dysfunction: a meta-analysis. *J Am Coll Cardiol* 2002;39:1151–1158.
128. Marwick TH, Case C, Poldermans D, et al. A clinical and echocardiographic score for assigning risk of major events after dobutamine echocardiograms. *J Am Coll Cardiol* 2004;43:2102–2107.
129. Krone RJ, Gillespie JA, Weld FM, et al. Low-level exercise testing after myocardial infarction: usefulness in enhancing clinical risk stratification. *Circulation* 1985;71:80–89.
130. Poldermans D, Fioretti PM, Boersma E, et al. Dobutamine-atropine stress echocardiography and clinical data for predicting late cardiac events in patients with suspected coronary artery disease. *Am J Med* 1994;97:119–125.
131. Mazeika PK, Nadazdin A, Oakley CM. Prognostic value of dobutamine echocardiography in patients with high pretest likelihood of coronary artery disease. *Am J Cardiol* 1993;71:33–39.
132. Picano E, Severi S, Michelassi C, et al. Prognostic importance of dipyridamole-echocardiography test in coronary artery disease. *Circulation* 1989;80:450–457.
133. Krivokapich J, Child JS, Gerber RS, et al. Prognostic usefulness of positive or negative exercise stress echocardiography for predicting coronary events in ensuing twelve months. *Am J Cardiol* 1993;71:646–651.
134. Marwick TH, Mehta R, Arheart K, Lauer MS. Use of exercise echocardiography for prognostic evaluation of patients with known or suspected coronary artery disease. *J Am Coll Cardiol* 1997;30:83–90.
135. McCully RB, Roger VL, Mahoney DW, et al. Outcome after normal exercise echocardiography and predictors of subsequent cardiac events: follow-up of 1,325 patients. *J Am Coll Cardiol* 1998;31:144–149.
136. Syed MA, Al Malki Q, Kazmouz G, et al. Usefulness of exercise echocardiography in predicting cardiac events in an outpatient population. *Am J Cardiol* 1998;82:569–573.
137. Kamaran M, Teague SM, Finkelhor RS, et al. Prognostic value of dobutamine stress echocardiography in patients referred because of suspected coronary artery disease. *Am J Cardiol* 1995;76:887–891.
138. Marcovitz PA, Shayna V, Horn RA, et al. Value of dobutamine stress echocardiography in determining the prognosis of patients with known or suspected coronary artery disease. *Am J Cardiol* 1996;78:404–408.
139. Chuah SC, Pellikka PA, Roger VL, et al. Role of dobutamine stress echocardiography in predicting outcome in 860 patients with known or suspected coronary artery disease. *Circulation* 1998;97:1474–1480.
140. Poldermans D, Fioretti PM, Boersma E, et al. Long-term prognostic value of dobutamine-atropine stress echocardiography in 1737 patients with known or suspected coronary artery disease: a single-center experience. *Circulation* 1999;99:757–762.
141. Olmos LI, Dakik H, Gordon R, et al. Long-term prognostic value of exercise echocardiography compared with exercise 201Tl, ECG, and clinical variables in patients evaluated for coronary artery disease. *Circulation* 1998;98:2679–2686.
142. Bolognese L, Rossi L, Sarasso G, et al. Silent versus symptomatic dipyridamole-induced ischemia after myocardial infarction: clinical and prognostic significance. *J Am Coll Cardiol* 1992;19:953–959.
143. Picano E, Landi P, Bolognese L, et al. Prognostic value of dipyridamole echocardiography early after uncomplicated myocardial infarction: a large-scale, multicenter trial: the EPIC Study Group. *Am J Med* 1993;95:608–618.
144. Chiarella F, Domenicucci S, Bellotti P, et al. Dipyridamole echocardiographic test performed 3 days after an acute myocardial infarction: feasibility, tolerability, safety and in-hospital prognostic value. *Eur Heart J* 1994;15:842–850.
145. Picano E, Pingitore A, Sicari R, et al. Stress echocardiographic results predict risk of reinfarction early after uncomplicated acute myocardial infarction: large-scale multicenter study. Echo Persantine International Cooperative (EPIC) Study Group. *J Am Coll Cardiol* 1995;26:908–913.
146. Carlos ME, Smart SC, Wynsen JC, Sagar KB. Dobutamine stress echocardiography for risk stratification after myocardial infarction. *Circulation* 1997;95:1402–1410.
147. Sicari R, Picano E, Landi P, et al. Prognostic value of dobutamine-atropine stress echocardiography early after acute myocardial infarction: Echo Dobutamine International Cooperative (EDIC) Study. *J Am Coll Cardiol* 1997;29:254–260.
148. Picano E, Sicari R, Landi P, et al. Prognostic value of myocardial viability in medically-treated patients with global left ventricular dysfunction early after acute uncomplicated myocardial infarction: a dobutamine stress echocardiographic study. *Circulation* 1998;98:1078–1084.
149. Applegate RJ, Dell'Italia LJ, Crawford MH. Usefulness of two-dimensional echocardiography during low-level exercise testing early after uncomplicated acute myocardial infarction. *Am J Cardiol* 1987;60:10–14.
150. Ryan T, Armstrong WF, O'Donnell JA, Feigenbaum H. Risk stratification after acute myocardial infarction by means of exercise two-dimensional echocardiography. *Am Heart J* 1987;114:1305–1316.
151. Hertzer NR, Beven EG, Young JR, et al. Coronary artery disease in peripheral vascular patients: a classification of 1000 coronary angiograms and results of surgical management. *Ann Surg* 1984;199:223–233.
152. Mangano DT, London MJ, Tubau JF, et al. Dipyridamole thallium-201 scintigraphy as a preoperative screening test: a reexamination of its predictive capacity. *Circulation* 1991;84:493–502.
153. Eagle KA, Brundage BH, Chaitman BR, et al. Guidelines for perioperative cardiovascular evaluation for noncardiac surgery: report of the ACC/AHA Task Force on Practice Guidelines. *J Am Coll Cardiol* 1996;27:910–948.
154. Tischler MD, Lee TH, Hirsch AT. Prediction of major cardiac events after peripheral vascular surgery using dipyridamole echocardiography. *Am J Cardiol* 1991;68:593–599.
155. Sicari R, Picano E, Lusa AM, et al. The value of dipyridamole echocardiography in risk stratification before vascular surgery: a multicenter study. *Eur Heart J* 1995;16:842–847.
156. Miyazono Y, Kisanuki A, Toyonaga K, et al. Usefulness of adenosine triphosphate-atropine stress echocardiography for detecting coronary artery stenosis. *Am J Cardiol* 1998;82:290–294.
157. Pasquet A, D'Hondt AM, Verhelst R, et al. Comparison of dipyridamole stress echocardiography and perfusion scintigraphy for cardiac risk stratification in vascular surgery patients. *Am J Cardiol* 1998;82:1468–1474.
158. Poldermans D, Fioretti PM, Forster T, et al. Dobutamine stress echocardiography for assessment of perioperative cardiac risk in patients undergoing major vascular surgery. *Circulation* 1993;87:1506–1512.
159. Poldermans D, Fioretti PM, Forster T, et al. Dobutamine-atropine stress echocardiography for assessment of perioperative and late cardiac risk in patients undergoing major vascular surgery. *Eur J Vasc Surg* 1994;8:286–293.
160. Poldermans D, Arnese M, Fioretti PM, et al. Improved cardiac risk stratification in major vascular surgery with dobutamine-atropine stress echocardiography. *J Am Coll Cardiol* 1995;26:648–653.
161. Ballal RS, Kapadia S, Secknus MA, et al. Prognosis of patients with vascular disease after clinical evaluation and dobutamine stress echocardiography. *Am Heart J* 1999;137:469–475.
162. Shaw LJ, Eagle KA, Gersh BJ, Miller DD. Meta-analysis of intravenous dipyridamole-thallium-201 imaging (1985 to 1994) and dobutamine echocardiography (1991 to 1994) for risk stratification before vascular surgery. *J Am Coll Cardiol* 1996;27:787–798.
163. Poldermans D, Boersma E, Bax JJ, et al. The effect of bisoprolol on perioperative mortality and myocardial infarction in high-risk patients undergoing

vascular surgery: Dutch Echocardiographic Cardiac Risk Evaluation Applying Stress Echocardiography Study Group. *N Engl J Med* 1999;341:1789–1794.
164. Boersma E, Poldermans D, Bax JJ, et al. Predictors of cardiac events after major vascular surgery: Role of clinical characteristics, dobutamine echocardiography, and beta-blocker therapy. *JAMA* 2001;285:1865–1873.
165. Landesberg G, Mosseri M, Wolf YG, et al. Preoperative thallium scanning, selective coronary revascularization, and long-term survival after major vascular surgery. *Circulation* 2003;108:177–183.
166. McFalls EO, Ward HB, Moritz TE, et al. Coronary-artery revascularization before elective major vascular surgery. *N Engl J Med* 2004;351:2795–2804.
167. Porter TR, Xie F, Kilzer K, Deligonul U. Detection of myocardial perfusion abnormalities during dobutamine and adenosine stress echocardiography with transient myocardial contrast imaging after minute quantities of intravenous perfluorocarbon-exposed sonicated dextrose albumin. *J Am Soc Echocardiogr* 1996;9:779–786.
168. Moir S, Haluska BA, Jenkins C, et al. Incremental benefit of myocardial contrast to combined dipyridamole-exercise stress echocardiography for the assessment of coronary artery disease. *Circulation* 2004;110:1108–1113.
169. Elhendy A, O'Leary EL, Xie F, et al. Comparative accuracy of real-time myocardial contrast perfusion imaging and wall motion analysis during dobutamine stress echocardiography for the diagnosis of coronary artery disease. *J Am Coll Cardiol* 2004;44:2185–2191.
170. Hoffmann R, Altiok E, Nowak B, et al. Strain rate measurement by Doppler echocardiography allows improved assessment of myocardial viability in patients with depressed left ventricular function. *J Am Coll Cardiol* 2002;39:443–449.
171. Hanekom L, Jenkins C, Short L, Marwick TH. Accuracy of strain rate techniques for identification of viability at dobutamine stress echo: a follow-up study after revascularization. *J Am Coll Cardiol* 2004;43:360A.
172. Voigt JU, Exner B, Schmiedehausen K, et al. Strain-rate imaging during dobutamine stress echocardiography provides objective evidence of inducible ischemia. *Circulation* 2003;107:2120–2126.
173. Yuda S, Fang ZY, Leano R, Marwick TH. Is quantitative interpretation likely to increase sensitivity of dobutamine stress echocardiography? A study of false-negative results. *J Am Soc Echocardiogr* 2004;17:448–453.
174. Weesner KM, Bledsoe M, Chauvenet A, Wofford M. Exercise echocardiography in the detection of anthracycline cardiotoxicity. *Cancer* 1991;68: 435–438.
175. Fukazawa R, Ogawa S, Hirayama T. Early detection of anthracycline cardiotoxicity in children with acute leukemia using exercise-based echocardiography and Doppler echocardiography. *Jpn Circ J* 1994;58:625–634.
176. Leung DY, Griffin BP, Stewart WJ, et al. Left ventricular function after valve repair for chronic mitral regurgitation: Predictive value of preoperative assessment of contractile reserve by exercise echocardiography. *J Am Coll Cardiol* 1996;28:1198–1205.
177. Monin JL, Monchi M, Gest V, et al. Aortic stenosis with severe left ventricular dysfunction and low transvalvular pressure gradients: risk stratification by low-dose dobutamine echocardiography. *J Am Coll Cardiol* 2001;37:2101–2107.
178. Marwick TH, Nakatani S, Haluska B, et al. Provocation of left ventricular outflow tract gradients with amyl nitrite and exercise in hypertrophic cardiomyopathy. *Am J Cardiol* 1995;75:805–809.

CHAPTER 51 ■ DOPPLER ECHOCARDIOGRAPHY

FRANK A. FLACHSKAMPF

OVERVIEW

Doppler echocardiography (DE), an ultrasound-based noninvasive diagnostic technique, measures velocities of blood or solid tissue relative to the transducer. From blood flow velocities, pressure gradients across stenotic, regurgitant, or shunt lesions can be calculated. Estimates of cardiac output, severity of regurgitation, shunt magnitude, and systolic pulmonary artery pressure are obtainable. Tissue DE, together with blood flow DE, allows assessment of global systolic and diastolic myocardial function, detection of myocardial diseases in early stages, assessment of synchronicity of myocardial contraction, and identification of regional ischemia. Thus, DE is an integral and mandatory part of every complete echocardiographic examination.

GLOSSARY

Aliasing: The maximal velocity unambiguously identifiable by pulsed (and color) DE is the aliasing velocity, which depends on the pulse repetition frequency, the frame rate, the sampling depth, and the carrier frequency.

Color Doppler flow mapping: A Doppler display that codes blood flow velocities by colors (red toward the transducer, and blue away from the transducer) and superimposes this color map on the 2D image. Thus, a cross-sectional display of blood flow velocities is created. Color Doppler is a way of simultaneously displaying Doppler data from multiple sites in an easily interpretable way. This modality serves for quick orientation about pathologic blood flow (turbulence, regurgitation, shunt flows) and for analysis of valvular regurgitation.

Continuous wave Doppler: A Doppler modality that measures velocities along one scan line. Any velocities are measured unequivocally, but along the scan line there is no spatial resolution. This modality serves to measure the high velocities encountered in valvular stenosis or regurgitation.

Flow profile: The plot of flow velocities measured by pulsed or continuous wave Doppler over time (e.g., diastole for the mitral valve). Essentially synonymous with spectral Doppler display.

Gradient: Pressure drop (or difference) across a restrictive orifice (e.g., a valve).

Jet: A flow stream created by discharge from a narrow orifice (e.g., valvular regurgitation occurs as a jet).

Myocardial velocity gradient: Conceptually equivalent to strain rate.

Orifice: See *restrictive orifice*.

Pressure half-time: The time that it takes for a pressure gradient to decay to half of its peak value. The pressure half-time is used to evaluate mitral stenosis and aortic regurgitation.

Pulsed wave Doppler: A Doppler modality that measures blood flow velocity in a specific region, the "sample volume." Thus, unlike continuous wave Doppler, pulsed wave Doppler allows the choice of the site of measurement. The trade off is that the maximal unequivocally identifiable velocity is limited (see *aliasing*).

Restrictive orifice: Narrowing in the path of flow stream. Stenotic and regurgitant lesions are restrictions to forward and backward flow, respectively. Restrictive orifices have a geometrical or anatomic orifice area, which is the smallest cross-sectional area between the solid boundaries of the lesion, and an effective area, which is the smallest cross-section of the jet created by such a lesion.

Sample volume: The volume of blood or tissue from which an average velocity is measured by pulsed Doppler. Technically, the length of the sample volume depends on the pulse length (the number of ultrasound wavelengths in one pulse), and the axial position of the sample volume along the cursor depends on the range gate, which defines which time interval is allowed to elapse between transmit and receive. Spatial position and sample volume length can be chosen by the operator, and angle correction is also possible.

Spectral Doppler: Display of continuous or pulsed wave Doppler plotting blood flow velocity against time.

Strain (rate): The deformation (lengthening or shortening, thickening or thinning) of myocardium during the cardiac cycle. It is dimensionless (e.g., a strain of 0.2 means a 20% elongation). Strain rate (strain divided by corresponding time, in 1/s units) is measurable by tissue Doppler between two chosen points in the myocardium by subtracting the tissue velocities at these points and dividing by the distance between the points. From strain rate, strain is obtained by temporal integration. Strain rate and myocardial velocity gradient are conceptually equivalent.

Stroke length, stroke distance: Synonymous with *velocity–time integral*.

Tissue Doppler: Pulsed or color Doppler modality measuring the velocity of solid cardiac structures with respect to the transducer. These are low-velocity (typically <15 cm/s), high-amplitude signals, in contrast to signals from intracardiac blood flow measured by classic Doppler, which even in normals reach 1 m/s and more and have low amplitudes.

Velocity–time integral: The area enclosed by the envelope (the boundary) of the spectral pulsed or continuous wave Doppler display (unit: centimeter). This term is synonymous with *stroke length*.

Turbulence: Characteristic of flow under certain conditions (especially at high velocities) where fluid particle velocity and direction changes rapidly and chaotically.

HISTORICAL PERSPECTIVE

The Austrian physicist Christian Doppler (1803–1853) first precisely analyzed the effect of motion of the observer relative to the source of a wave on the perceived wave frequency (the *Doppler effect*) (1). Ultrasound Doppler was first used in medicine to measure intravascular blood flow (2,3). Whereas the first instruments used a continuous emission of ultrasound, pulsed Doppler devices were introduced at the end of the 1960s (4,5). The breakthrough for DE came with its success in quantifying pressure drops across valvular stenoses by means of the simplified Bernoulli equation in the late 1970s (6,7). Since then, the Doppler technique became progressively integrated into ultrasound equipment, and "duplex" instruments emerged, combining two-dimensional (2D) imaging and Doppler blood velocimetry. With the use of multigated pulsed DE, a color-encoded display or "map" of velocities could be superimposed on M-mode and later 2D echocardiographic images (8–11). Transesophageal Doppler recordings of aortic blood flow velocity were obtained as early as 1973 (12), and in the 1980s Doppler capabilities were added to transesophageal imaging probes. Finally, tissue DE was introduced in the early 1990s (13).

FROM DOPPLER SIGNALS TO HEMODYNAMICS: BASIC CONCEPTS

The Doppler Signal

The Doppler signal contains the following data:

1. The Doppler frequency shift (between transmitted and received ultrasound) quantifies the instantaneous velocity component of the moving reflectors (blood cells or tissue) toward or away from the transducer at a site determined by the sample volume of the pulsed Doppler, or along the scan line in continuous wave Doppler. The display of this instantaneous velocity over time is called the spectral Doppler display (Fig. 51.1). If velocities are integrated over time, the time velocity integral (in centimeters) is obtained. With color Doppler, multiple measurements at different sites in the heart cavities are made simultaneously and represented qualitatively in colors (see Fig. 51.1). Velocities toward the transducer typically are represented in shades of red, and away from the transducer in shades of blue. Rapid variations in velocity, as in turbulent flow, can be characterized by an admixture of other colors. It is crucial to understand that any velocity at an angle α with the Doppler scan line will be underestimated by the factor cos α. This angle error occurs regardless of the modality, that is, with pulsed, continuous, color, or tissue DE.
2. The intensity (amplitude) of the signal is represented in shades of grey in the spectral display. It is related to the number of scatterers (red blood cells or tissue reflectors) found within the sample volume moving with the measured velocity. The width of the signal reflects the variation in velocity within the sample volume. The brightest line is the "modal" velocity, which is the velocity most frequently measured by the Doppler device in the sample volume (Fig. 51.1). This is important when calculating flow rates from cross-sectional areas and blood flow velocities. In contrast, continuous wave spectral displays are filled with white signals up to the maximal velocity, the envelope. The reason is that the continuous wave Doppler device measures velocities along a whole scan line, so that all flow velocities which the scan line encounters are represented.
3. The audio signal (with blood flow DE). Experienced echocardiographers use the audio signal to optimize the angulation of the transducer. The magnitude of the Doppler shift caused by blood flow velocity lies within the audible range (<20 kHz). Therefore, high pitch corresponds to high blood flow velocity, and purity of tone to a narrow range of flow velocities.
4. Tissue DE (Fig. 51.2A). This technique provides analogous information as blood flow DE, except that solid tissue velocities (usually from the myocardium) instead of blood flow velocities are measured. This is accomplished by a set of filters which largely eliminates the high-velocity, low-intensity signals from blood and retains the low-velocity, high-intensity signals from tissue. The results are displayed either as a spectral pulsed Doppler display (velocity over time) or as a color coded map. Because of the low velocities of tissue (typically <15 cm/s), neither continuous wave nor audio signals are used in tissue DE.

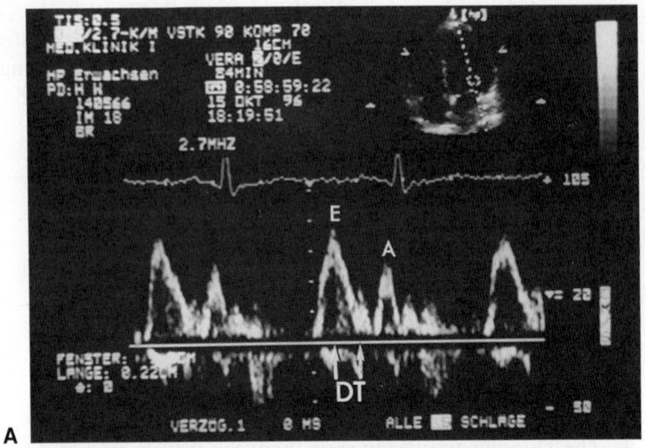

A

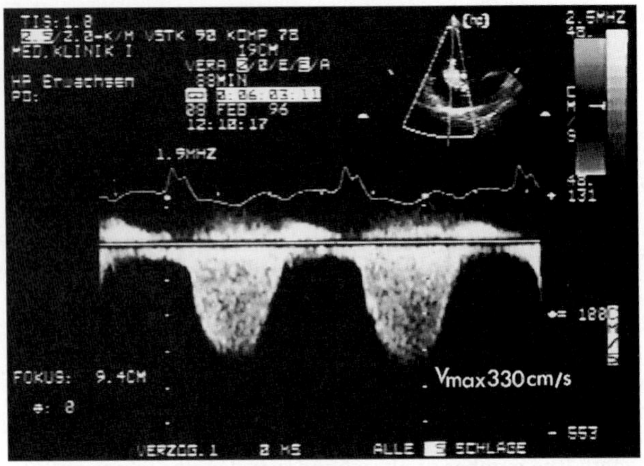

B

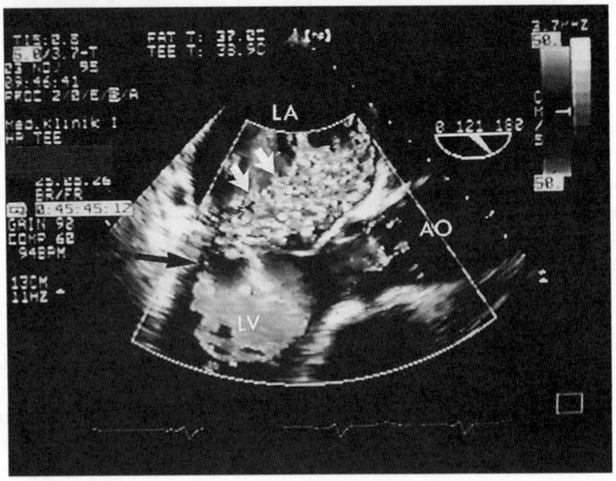

C

FIGURE 51.1. Pulsed, continuous, and color flow Doppler. (**A**) Normal diastolic transmitral flow pattern in sinus rhythm, consisting of an early, usually larger and higher E (*E*) wave, and late, usually smaller A wave (*A*). Deceleration time (*DT*; *arrows*) is the time between peak E wave velocity and cessation of E wave. (**B**) Continuous wave Doppler of tricuspid regurgitation in pulmonary hypertension. The maximal regurgitant velocity of 330 cm/s implies a maximal systolic right ventricular pressure of 44 mm Hg plus central venous pressure. (**C**) Transesophageal color Doppler flow mapping of severe mitral regurgitation owing to a flail posterior leaflet. A proximal convergence zone (*black arrow*) is seen, as well as the eccentric, anteriorly directed turbulent jet in the left atrium (*white arrows*). *Abbreviations:* LV left ventricle, LA left atrium, AO ascending aorta.

A derived modality is deformation imaging, also known as *strain* or *strain rate imaging,* which extracts the local deformation rate in the direction of the ultrasound beam (percentage elongation or shortening divided by time). Strain rate (equivalent to the myocardial velocity gradient), and its temporal integral, strain, can be calculated by subtracting the simultaneous velocities at two myocardial points along a scan line at a small distance (<1 cm) and dividing the results by the distance between the two points; its unit is Hz (s^{-1}). Integrating strain rate over time yields strain, a dimensionless number indicating the fractional elongation or shortening; for example, a strain of +30% means that the tissue has elongated in the direction of the Doppler beam by 30% compared to baseline (Fig. 51.2B–F). In contrast to tissue velocities, strain rate and strain are largely unaffected by movements of the heart as a whole with respect to the transducer or by tethering from adjacent myocardial regions and therefore are truly regional parameters.

Basic Hydrodynamic Principles

The Continuity Principle

This is an application of the law of the conservation of mass in a closed system (Fig. 51.3). In steady flow of an incompressible fluid through a tube, the volume flow rate (mL/s) is equal at any cross-section of the tube. Because flow rate is equal to the product of (mean) velocity v and cross-sectional area A,

$$v_1{}^* A_1 = v_2{}^* A_2$$

at any cross-sections 1 and 2 of the flow stream. Thus, effective orifice area A_{EFF} of a narrowed flow cross-section (e.g., a stenosis) can be calculated from the maximal flow velocity across the orifice v_{MAX}, cross-sectional area A_1, and mean flow velocity v_1 of any other cross-section by:

$$A_{EFF} = A_1{}^* v_1 / v_{MAX}.$$

This relationship is the basis for calculation of stenotic aortic valve area by continuity. The *effective* orifice area of flow is always smaller than the geometrical orifice area and is situated slightly downstream from the restrictive orifice. The ratio between effective and geometric area is called the *coefficient of contraction* and is always smaller than 1. Hence, effective orifice area by the continuity equation is smaller by a variable factor than orifice area by planimetry or by the Gorlin equation. The continuity principle is valid instantaneously, and thus effective area can be calculated both from the time–velocity integrals or the maximal instantaneous velocities at two cross-sections. Both are equal if the cross-sections are constant over time.

Restrictions to Flow: Stenotic, Regurgitant, and Shunt Lesions. Because of the continuity principle, any narrowing of the cross-sectional area of flow implies an increase in flow velocity. The "convective" flow acceleration necessary for this increase in flow velocity is the main cause of the pressure drop across cardiac restrictive lesions, whereas factors such as viscosity, pulsatile acceleration of stagnant blood, and others only play a minor role. In contrast, normal cardiac valves pose very little restriction to flow, such that the energy consumed to propel blood across native valves is largely due to pulsatile acceleration of blood mass. The general relationship between pressure difference and velocity difference between two points along a streamline is expressed by the Bernoulli equation, which is

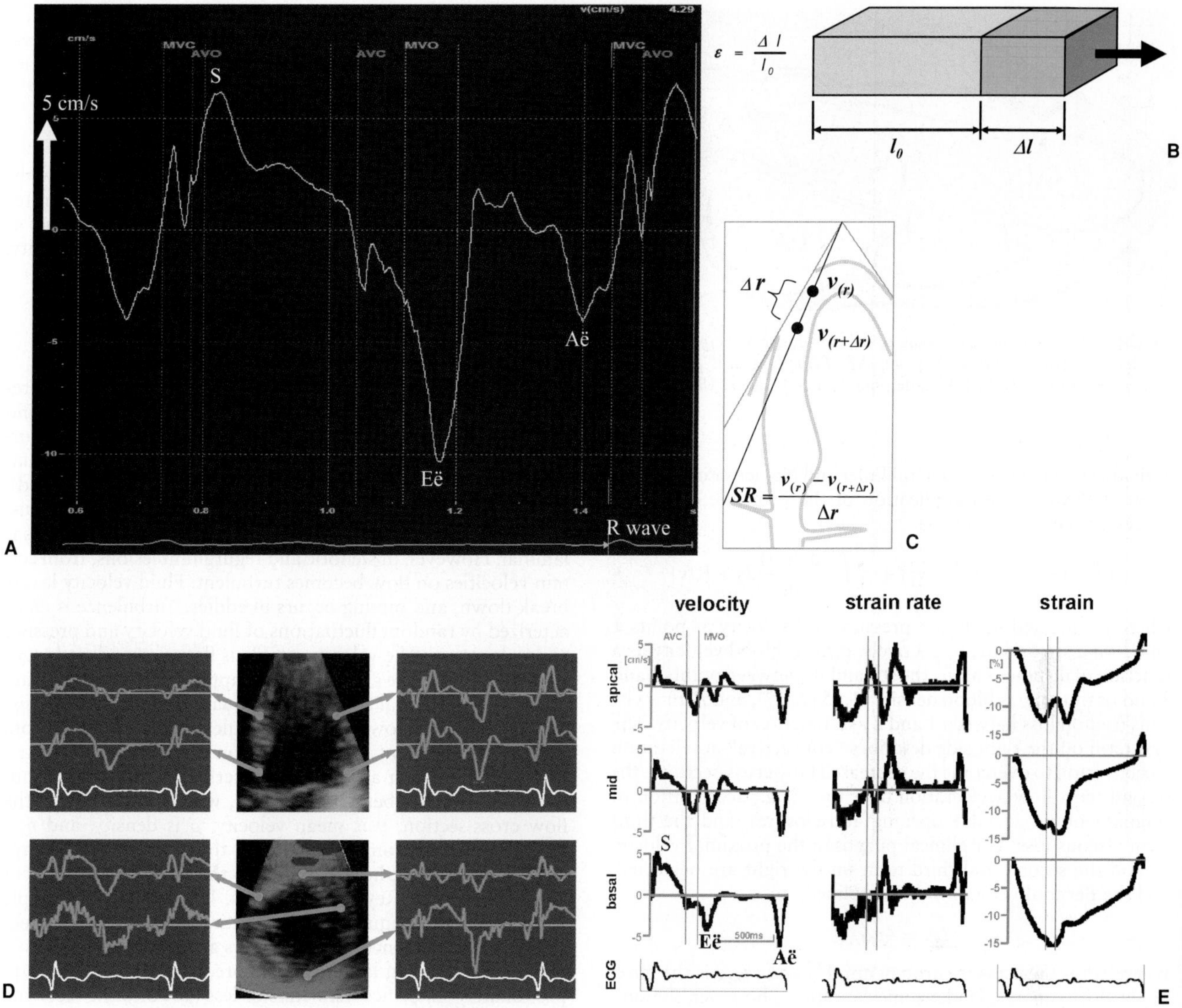

FIGURE 51.2. (A) Spectral tissue Doppler tracing. Normal tissue velocities from the basal septum. Note peak systolic (S) and early (E′) and late (A) diastolic tissue velocities. *Abbreviations:* MVO, mitral valve opening; MVC, mitral valve closure; AVO, aortic valve opening; AVC, aortic valve closure. (B) One-dimensional strain ϵ is defined as the change in length Δl relative to baseline length l_0 after a deformation (right part of the box) owing to a force (*arrow*). (*Source:* From Flachskampf FA [ed]. *Praxis der Echokardiographie.* Stuttgart: Thieme; 2002. (C) Calculation of regional strain rate from measurement of myocardial velocities $v_{(r)}$ and $v_{(r+\Delta r)}$ at two neighboring points at a small distance Δr ("offset") in the direction of the ultrasound beam. (*Source:* From Voigt JU, Flachskampf FA. Strain and strain rate: new and clinically relevant echo parameters of regional myocardial function. *Z Kardiol* 2004;93:249–258.) (D) Tissue velocity and derived parameters (strain/strain rate) depend on the imaging window; they are measured along the ultrasound beam. The central figures show color-coded tissue Doppler velocities, from which the spectral recordings are taken. *Top,* longitudinal velocities measured from apical window in the basal and midseptal (*left*) and lateral (*right*) walls. Systolic contraction leads to upward (positive) velocities (*S*), and diastolic elongation to negative velocities (*E′*). Basal velocities are higher than midwall velocities, and lateral velocities are higher than septal velocities. *Bottom,* radial and circumferential velocities measured in a parasternal short axis view. *Left,* circumferential velocities from septal and lateral wall, showing positive velocities in systole. *Right,* radial velocities from anteroseptal and inferior wall, also showing positive velocities in systole, corresponding to systolic thickening. (*Source:* From Flachskampf FA [ed]. *Praxis der Echokardiographie.* Stuttgart: Thieme; 2002, with permission.) (E) Tissue Doppler parameters of longitudinal velocity, strain rate, and strain from apical, mid, and basal segments in a normal subject recorded from an apical transducer position. Velocity and strain rate have a systolic peak (*S*) and an early (*E′*) and late (*A′*) diastolic wave. Direction of tissue velocity and strain rate waves is opposite; systolic contraction produces a tissue velocity toward the transducer (positive velocity), but regional myocardial shortening (strain/strain rate), which by convention has a negative sign. Strain shows a single wave peaking in late systole or early diastole. Amplitudes decrease from base to apex for tissue velocity, whereas strain and strain rate amplitudes are similar in all three segments. *Abbreviations:* AVC, aortic valve closure; MVO, mitral valve opening. (*Source:* Modified, from Voigt JU, Nixdorff U, Bogdan R, et al. Comparison of deformation imaging and velocity imaging for detecting regional inducible ischaemia during dobutamine stress echocardiography. *Eur Heart J* 2004;25,1517–1525.)

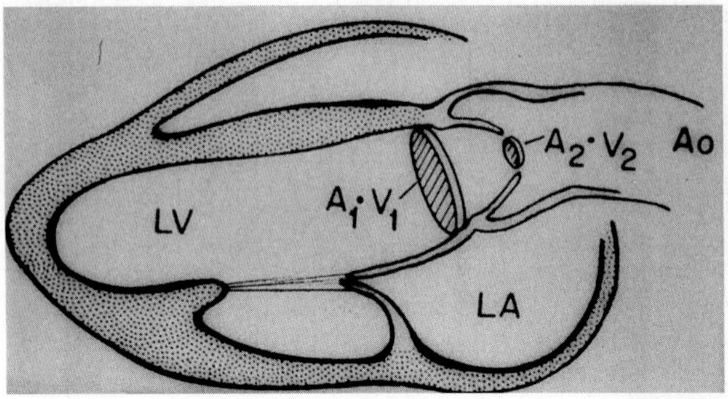

FIGURE 51.3. Schematic drawing of the continuity principle. See text for details. (*Source:* From Weyman AE. *Principles and practice of echocardiography*. 2nd ed. Philadelphia: Lea & Febiger; 1994.)

derivable from the more general Euler and Navier–Stokes equations of flow. It is an application of the principle of energy conservation:

$$p_1 - p_2 = \%o\rho\left(v_2^2 - v_1^2\right) + \rho\int_1^2 \frac{dv(s,t)}{dt}ds + R(v)$$

where p_1, v_1, and p_2, v_2 are pressure and velocity at points 1 and 2 on a streamline, respectively, $v(s,t)$ is blood velocity as a function of distance s along the streamline between points 1 and 2 and of time t, ρ is blood density (1.05 g/cm^3), and $R(v)$ is viscous friction loss between 1 and 2 as a function of velocity. The first term on the right side describes "convective" acceleration (acceleration to overcome the decreased flow cross-section), the second term flow acceleration over time (e.g., acceleration of stagnant blood at valve opening and closure), and the third term viscous loss. For clinical purposes, the proximal velocity v_1 and the second and third term on the right are neglected, and the Bernoulli equation is "simplified" to

$$\Delta p = 4{v_{MAX}}^2$$

where Δp is the pressure drop in mm Hg and v_{MAX} is the maximal velocity in m/s. Under some conditions, however, the simplified version does not apply:

1. In normal native valves. Proximal velocity is not negligible in relation to maximal transvalvular velocity, and time dependent, "pulsatile" flow acceleration is not negligible compared to convective acceleration.
2. In the presence of high prestenotic velocities, as in subaortic obstruction or significant regurgitation coexisting with stenosis. Here, the proximal velocity v_{PROX} has to be taken into account

$$\Delta p = 4({v_{MAX}}^2 - {v_{PROX}}^2)$$

3. If pressure recovery occurs, the kinetic energy present at the effective orifice area of restrictive cardiac lesions is partly dissipated in turbulent eddies and, ultimately, heat. This energy is lost irretrievably. However, restriction geometries that allow the jet to expand gradually until reaching the boundaries of the receiving chamber minimize eddy formation and allow some of the kinetic energy to be reconverted into static pressure energy downstream. The most prominent example of this is seen in bileaflet prostheses in the aortic position (see below and Chapter 25). The amount of pressure recovery depends on the morphology of the obstruction and the receiving chamber, being large in gradually tapering and flaring obstructions and in narrow receiving chambers (e.g., a narrow ascending aorta) and low in abrupt narrowings and wide receiving chambers (e.g., the left ventricle).
4. In tunnel-like lesions, where the length of the obstruction is not negligible, as in some forms of congenital subaortic stenosis. Here, Poiseuille's law (see next section) is more appropriate.

Laminar and Turbulent Flow

Laminar flow ideally occurs in separate layers of velocity without mixing between the layers. In a tube, laminar flow generates a parabolic flow profile, where the maximal velocity occurs at the central axis and is approximately twice the mean velocity. Poiseuille's law applies:

$$\Delta p = Q^*8^*\eta^*L/(\pi^*r^4) = v^*8^*\eta^*L/r^2 \text{ and/or}$$
$$R = 8^*\eta^*L/(\pi^*r^4)$$

where Δp is pressure drop, Q is volume flow, R is vascular resistance, v is mean velocity, η is viscosity, L is tube length, and r is tube radius. Pressure drop is directly and linearly proportional to flow rate (as opposed to the simplified Bernoulli equation, where pressure drop is proportional to flow rate squared), and inversely proportional to the fourth power of tube radius. Flow in the heart chambers and through normal heart valves is laminar. However, in stenotic and regurgitant lesions, from certain velocities on flow becomes turbulent. Fluid velocity layers break down, and mixing occurs in eddies. Turbulence is characterized by random fluctuations of fluid velocity and pressure at any location. The velocity profile is flattened and no longer parabolic. Poiseuille's law no longer applies; turbulent pressure drop is proportional to flow rate squared. Hence, flow resistance increases if flow becomes turbulent. The transition from laminar to turbulent flow depends on the relation of inertial to viscous forces in a flow field, described by the dimensionless Reynolds number ($2r * v * \rho/\eta$), where r is radius of the flow cross-section, v is mean velocity, ρ is density, and η is viscosity. Flow becomes turbulent if this number exceeds approximately 2,300; however, in vivo the transition may occur at lower or higher Reynolds numbers. The continuity principle and the Bernoulli equation are valid independently of the occurrence of turbulence. Turbulent jets at their orifice contain a very small, tapering laminar flow core, which extends for approximately six orifice diameters or less (14) into the receiving chamber, from where on the jet is fully turbulent. The jet maintains the maximal velocity in the laminar core; after becoming fully turbulent, flow velocity decays inversely proportional to the distance from the orifice.

The Proximal Convergence Zone Concept

This is a continuity-based approach to measure flow rate through an orifice (usually in regurgitant lesions) by analysis of the flow velocity field proximal of the orifice (15) (Fig. 51.4). For this purpose, it is assumed that concentric hemispheric layers of fluid particles of the same velocity centered at the orifice are formed at each moment in time (hence, this concept is also called *proximal isovelocity surface area*). The smaller the radius of the hemisphere, the higher the flow velocity toward the orifice. Because of the continuity principle, flow rate through the orifice is equal to flow rate across each hemisphere, which is the product of hemisphere surface area and corresponding flow velocity. If the radius r of a hemisphere and the corresponding velocity v are known, instantaneous flow rate Q can be calculated as

$$Q = 2\pi^*r^{2*}v.$$

Color DE can be used to measure r and v. This concept can in principle be applied to restrictive as well as stenotic and shunt lesions. The assumption of hemispheric isovelocity surfaces is a simplification neglecting irregular orifices, solid boundaries, simultaneous other intracardiac flows and so on.

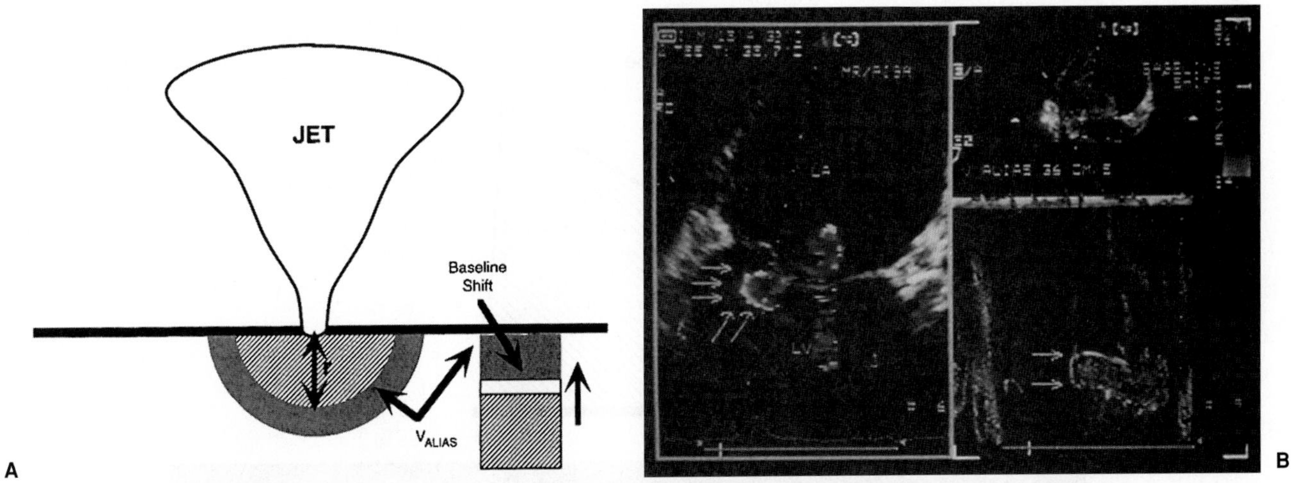

FIGURE 51.4. (A) Schematic drawing of the proximal flow convergence concept. Flow through a restrictive orifice is shown as imaged by color Doppler. Upstream from the orifice, concentric isovelocity shells of hemispheric shape develop. At the distance r to the orifice, the aliasing velocity v_{ALIAS} occurs. Flow rate is calculated by multiplying the surface of the shell with radius r by v_{ALIAS}. (B) Example of proximal convergence zone analysis by transesophageal color DE of mitral regurgitation. The proximal convergence zone (*arrows*) is seen on the ventricular side of the mitral valve. To increase the aliasing radius, the color bar baseline was shifted upward. The radius can also be measured from color M-mode (*lower right*). Maximal instantaneous regurgitant flow rate was $2\pi * (1.1 \text{ cm})^2 * 36 \text{ cm/s} = 274 \text{ cm}^3/\text{s}$, corresponding to severe mitral regurgitation.

Evaluation of Stenotic Lesions

A *stenosis* is a restriction to flow and thus characterized by a reduction in the geometrical cross-section of flow, a pressure drop, and an increase in local flow velocity. The maximal instantaneous pressure drop can be calculated from the maximal instantaneous blood flow velocity by the *simplified Bernoulli equation*:

$$\Delta p = 4v^2$$

where Δp is pressure drop in mm Hg, and v is velocity in m/s. For calculating mean pressure drop, the instantaneous pressure drops are averaged over the duration of flow.

Another way to quantify stenoses is the calculation of stenotic orifice area, which is usually accomplished by the continuity equation (see Fig. 51.3):

$$A_2 = A_1{}^*TVI_1/TVI_2$$

where A_2 is the stenotic orifice area, A_1 is the area of a nonstenotic flow cross-section (usually calculated as $\pi * d^2/4$ where d is the left ventricular outflow tract diameter), TVI_1 is the time velocity integral at the nonstenotic flow cross-section by pulsed wave DE, usually in the left ventricular outflow tract, and TVI_2 is the transstenotic time velocity integral (by continuous wave DE). Instead of time velocity integrals, the maximal transstenotic velocity and the maximal velocity in the outflow tract can also be used.

From the instantaneous pressure drop calculated by the simplified Bernoulli equation maximal and mean pressure drops, or "gradients" in cardiology parlance, can be calculated and are in principle identical to invasively measured maximal instantaneous and mean gradients (but not to "peak-to-peak" gradients) (Fig. 51.5). Note that the mean gradient is the mean of $4v_1{}^2$, $4v_2{}^2 \ldots$, where v_1, $v_2 \ldots$ are the maximal instantaneous velocities, which is not identical to $4v_{\text{MEAN}}{}^2$. Clinically, the pressure drop depends not only on the stenotic orifice area, but also on other factors, most prominently stroke volume. Orifice area can be measured directly by planimetry from 2D images in mitral and, transesophageally, in aortic stenosis. Alternatively, the continuity principle can be used, and stroke volume from another valve is divided by time–velocity integral of the stenotic valve to yield effective orifice area (if both valves are competent). It must be kept in mind, however, that the orifice area calculated by continuity is smaller than planimetric or (invasively obtained) Gorlin orifice area. Native mitral stenosis can also be estimated using the pressure half-time concept (Fig. 51.6). This concept, derived from hemodynamics, uses the time in which the pressure drop falls to one half of its initial value as an estimate of the severity of obstruction, which is less flow dependent than the pressure drop itself. Additionally, resistance of a stenosis can be calculated by dividing the mean pressure gradient (from the simplified Bernoulli equation) by the stroke volume. However, resistance appears to have no clear advantage over pressure drop and orifice area (16,17) in characterizing stenosis.

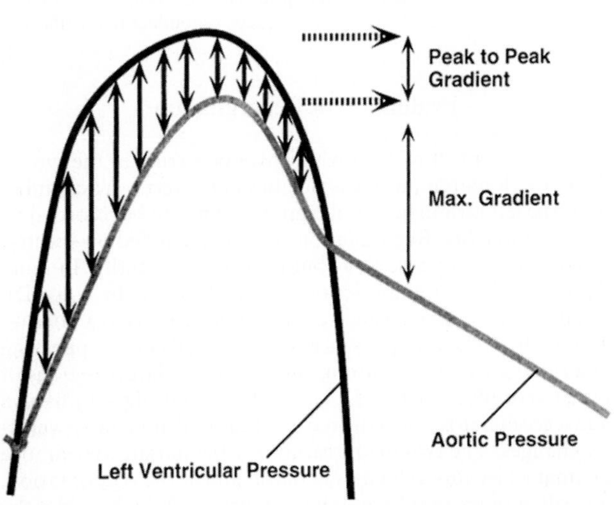

FIGURE 51.5. Schematic drawing of pressure gradients in aortic stenosis. Mean gradient is the average of the *red arrows*. Peak to peak gradient is neither identical with maximal nor mean pressure gradient.

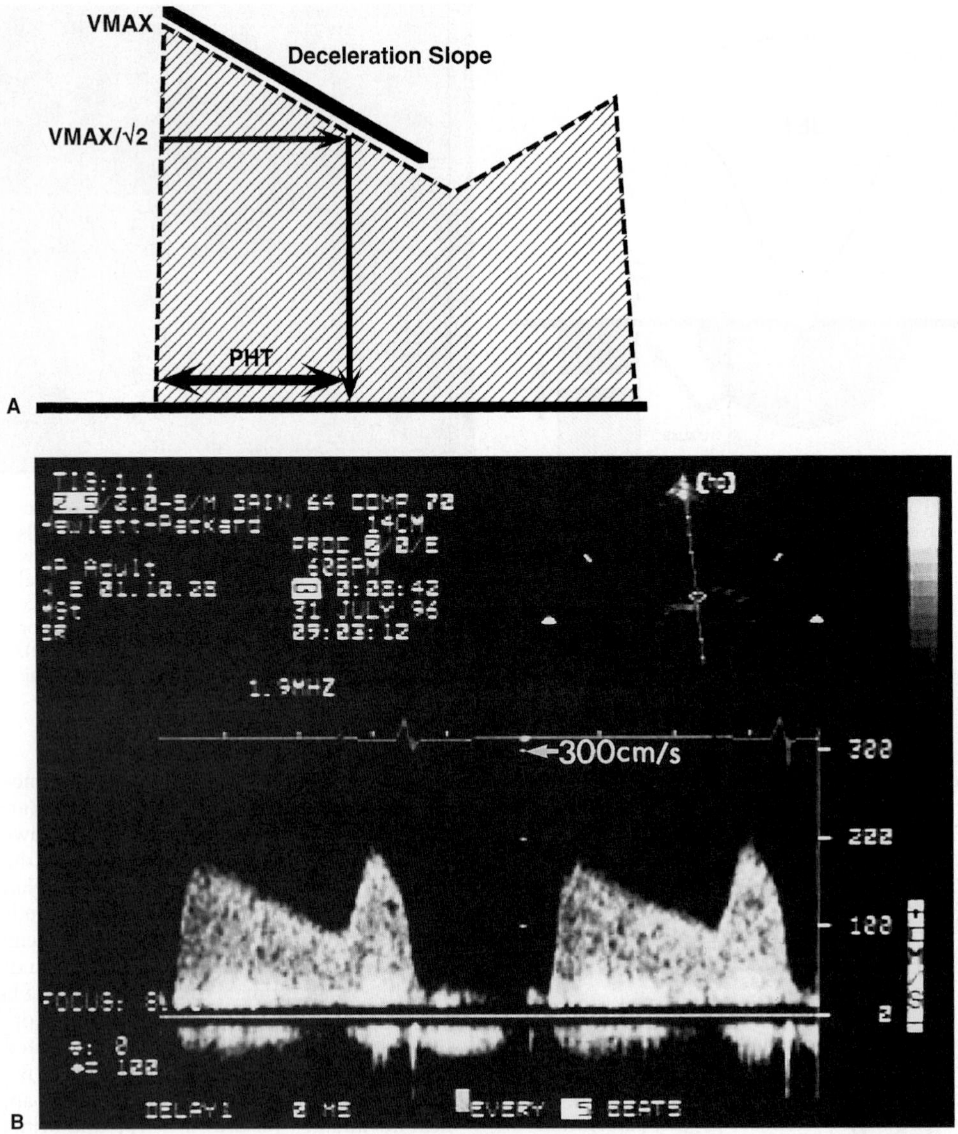

FIGURE 51.6. (A) Measurement of time–velocity integral and pressure half-time (PHT) in mitral stenosis. VMAX is the maximal early diastolic velocity. The area surrounded by the *dotted line* is the time–velocity integral. See text for details. (B) Transmitral flow by apical continuous wave Doppler in mitral stenosis with preserved sinus rhythm. Peak gradient is 15 mm Hg, mean gradient is 9 mm Hg, and pressure half-time is 228 ms, corresponding to a orifice area of 1 cm^2.

Evaluation of Regurgitation

Regurgitation is flow through a valve occurring in the wrong direction. Regurgitant flow velocities in the receiving chamber (e.g., the left atrium in mitral regurgitation) can be recorded by any DE modality. Regurgitation is easily identified on spectral or color DE as reverse flow, but difficult to quantify. In more than "trace" regurgitant lesions, regurgitant jets by color DE usually do not have a single color, but instead have a core region with a mosaic appearance containing all colors appearing in a rapidly changing pattern, surrounded by larger regions of pure red or blue (see Fig. 51.1). Most color DE algorithms also add a green hue to the basic red and blue to denote rapid velocity changes. The two main reasons for the mosaic appearance are that (i) jet core velocities in mitral and aortic regurgitation, and often in tricuspid regurgitation, are much higher than the aliasing velocity of the color map and thus, multiple aliasing occurs; and (ii) regurgitant jets almost always are truly turbulent, so that flow velocities in all directions occur in random fashion. Note that the color mosaic appearance does not necessarily denote true turbulence, and, on the other hand, in very severe regurgitation, when there is nearly pressure equalization between issuing and receiving chamber, the driving pressure difference between the chambers may become so small that a typical "turbulent jet" is absent.

The easiest way to grade regurgitation severity is by eyeballing or measuring the maximal color jet area of the regurgitant jet in the frame and the cross-section where it appears largest. Although a rough estimate of severity, it is more strongly related to the square of regurgitant flow velocity than to flow rate and therefore is highly load dependent. Specifically, color jet area is proportional to the transfer of momentum (the product of mass and velocity) over time in the regurgitant jet (18). Because color jet area is proportional to jet momentum flux, it is quadratically related to regurgitant flow velocity, whereas regurgitant volume or regurgitant fraction are linearly related to regurgitant velocity. In other words, a volume of blood regurgitating at a high velocity owing to a

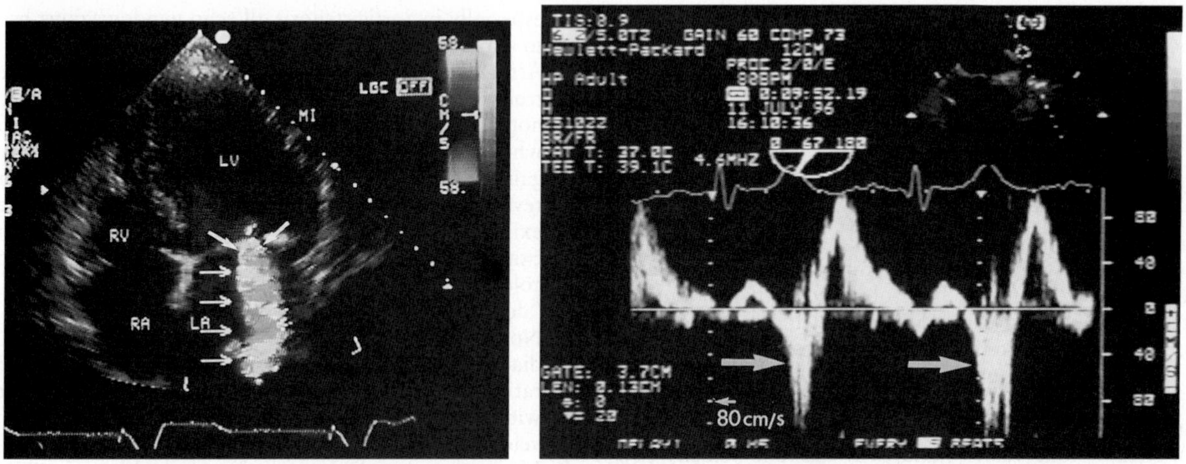

A B

FIGURE 51.7. (A) Measurement of proximal diameter of a severe mitral regurgitant jet (*horizontal arrows*). The proximal diameter is marked by the oblique arrows. Apical four-chamber view. *Abbreviations:* LV, left ventricle; LA, left atrium; RA, right atrium; RV, right ventricle. (B) Left upper pulmonary venous flow in severe mitral regurgitation by transesophageal pulsed DE. Small positive systolic wave, followed by reversed systolic flow (*arrows*). Diastolic velocities are increased.

high pressure difference has a larger color jet area than the same amount of blood regurgitating at a lower velocity owing to a lower pressure difference. Another important problem is that jets often are eccentric and may spread out on an adjacent wall (in the left atrium) or hug the anterior mitral leaflet (in aortic regurgitation). Eccentric jets are therefore substantially underestimated by color area (19). Finally, instrument settings, carrier frequency, and other factors influence the area of a regurgitant jet. Assessment of color jet size reliably discriminates mild from more severe regurgitation, but is unreliable to distinguish moderate and severe degrees of regurgitation. Several other methods are available to assess the severity of regurgitant lesions (20):

1. The proximal jet diameter (Fig. 51.7A). This parameter, measured as the smallest diameter immediately downstream of the jet's anatomic orifice, ideally represents the diameter of the regurgitant orifice area (ROA). Since this area is not necessarily circular, it can also be planimetered or two orthogonal diameters can be measured to calculate an ellipse area. Cut-off values with good discriminating power have been reported especially for mitral regurgitation, with diameters of more than 7 mm indicating severe regurgitation. The limiting factors are image quality, influence of gain, and measurement error.
2. Comparison of the stroke volume of different valves, if only one of them is insufficient. In mitral regurgitation, regurgitant volume is calculated by subtracting aortic stroke volume from total stroke volume, which is obtained either as mitral stroke volume or as the difference of diastolic and systolic left ventricular volumes. Aortic regurgitant volume can be calculated analogously. From the regurgitant volumes, ROA can be calculated by dividing regurgitant volume by the continuous wave time velocity integral of regurgitation. A ROA of more than 0.3 cm^2 indicates severe mitral or aortic regurgitation. Although validated in dedicated hands, its accuracy depends on the reliability of all the stroke volume calculations and therefore is prone to errors.
3. The proximal convergence zone method (see Fig. 51.4). The concept is outlined above. Several derived parameters can be calculated from the maximal regurgitant flow rate Q_{max}:
   a. ROA, for which maximal regurgitant flow velocity (v_{max}) must be additionally measured (by continuous wave DE): ROA $= Q_{max}/v_{max}$; for cut-off points see above. ROA can vary over the duration of regurgitation (21,22), but is less load dependent than maximal regurgitant flow rate.
   b. Regurgitant volume (RV), which is the product of the regurgitant time velocity integral from continuous wave DE (TVI) and ROA: RV = TVI * ROA. Application of the proximal convergence zone method requires good image quality and works best for severe regurgitation because of the better delineation of the proximal convergence zone (see Fig. 51.4). Although applicable to any flow through a restrictive orifice, the method has been clinically validated for mitral regurgitation and stenosis (23). Its application to aortic regurgitation is less well validated than for mitral regurgitation (24).

Another useful approach is to search for reverse flow patterns upstream of the lesion (e.g., pulmonary or hepatic venous flow reversal in mitral and tricuspid regurgitation).

Flow Rates and Cardiac Output

Stroke volume across any flow cross-section and thus across any valve can in theory be calculated by multiplying the time–velocity integral across that valve by the corresponding valve orifice area. Usually, stroke volume (and hence, by multiplication with heart rate, cardiac output) is measured by multiplying the time–velocity integral of the pulsed DE signal of systolic transaortic flow by the aortic annular area (calculated by $\pi * d^2/4$ where d is the aortic annulus diameter). An apical long axis view is used to acquire the pulsed DE recording, with the sample volume positioned at the annulus or, in the presence of aortic stenosis, in the outflow tract directly below the aortic valve (25). Stroke volume clinically is also frequently measured across the mitral and pulmonary valves. For mitral stroke volume, diameter of the annulus is measured in early diastole in the four-chamber view, a circular orifice is assumed, and area is multiplied with the time–velocity integral from pulsed DE at the annulus level. From such calculations, regurgitant volumes or shunt ratios (Q_P/Q_S) are derived (as the ratio of pulmonary stroke volume and left ventricular outflow tract stroke volume, if no pulmonary or aortic regurgitation is present). It should be noted that considerable errors may occur, mainly because of angle errors, skewed flow profiles, and irregular flow cross-sections. Techniques for automated integration of color DE velocities are becoming available, which in principle take into account true flow profiles and compensate for angle errors.

TISSUE DOPPLER ECHOCARDIOGRAPHY AND DEFORMATION IMAGING

These techniques provide information on global and regional left ventricular systolic and diastolic function. The largest clinical experience to date has been obtained with longitudinal shortening and elongation velocities of the left ventricular walls assessed by tissue DE in the three apical views. There is a systolic longitudinal shortening wave, leading to positive velocities toward the transducer, and two diastolic elongation waves, leading to negative velocities away from the transducer (see Fig. 51.2). Peak systolic velocity and early diastolic velocity (*E′*) are closely related to myocardial contraction and relaxation, and measurement of these velocities at the base of the left ventricular walls, for example, at the base of the septum and the lateral wall, give useful estimates of global systolic and diastolic function. Regional wall motion abnormalities, for example, in ischemic, stunned, hibernating, or scarred myocardium, exhibit lower than normal velocities (26). Furthermore, in ischemia, shortening in systole is delayed and reduced and extends past aortic valve closure into early diastole ("postsystolic shortening"). From the parasternal window, radial myocardial velocities (thickening and thinning) of posterior and anterior segments can be evaluated. Some instruments provide an angle correction to enable assessment of other short axis segments as well.

Unfortunately, discrimination of normal and abnormal velocities is not easy; longitudinal contraction velocities decrease from base to apex, are age and heart rate dependent, vary by segment, and are subject to tethering by the physical continuity between wall segments. Therefore, measurement of deformation (strain and strain rate) is theoretically better suited to regional analysis, because it largely eliminates tethering and translational effects (see Figs. 51.2B–F). However, deformation parameters are noisier than tissue velocities and prone to artifacts and thus often difficult to interpret.

THE CLINICAL BLOOD FLOW DOPPLER EXAMINATION

DE is performed via the same transducer used for 2D imaging. The position of the continuous wave cursor or the pulsed wave sample volume is displayed in the 2D image, and color DE maps are superimposed on the 2D image. The following practical points should be observed:

1. The interrogating beam should be aligned as well as possible with the direction of the flow interrogated. It is better to optimize the transducer position to enable optimal alignment than to use the angle correction option.
2. Several heart cycles should be recorded, especially in atrial fibrillation. Measuring only the highest velocities in a patient with atrial fibrillation leads to overestimation of gradients.
3. Both visual and audio output should be used to optimize the signal.
4. Attention should be paid to the timing of Doppler signals. For example, the mitral regurgitation signal, which may be mistaken for an aortic stenosis signal, begins earlier (immediately after mitral valve closure) than the aortic ejection signal.
5. There is no formal proof that the recorded velocities are truly the highest ones, because there is always the possibility of false placement or malalignment of the echo beam. Thus, especially in aortic stenosis all echo windows must be used to search for the highest velocities.
6. Artifacts: Clear flow velocity recordings by DE represent true blood velocities, but they can represent a flow that was not intended to record. An exception are mirror artifacts, which are created by very high amplitude signals (or too high gain) and duplicate an existing signal with inverse sign, or reverberations of color DE signals, which also duplicate real existing flow at a manifold of the real depth. An important example of the latter is "phantom flow" in transesophageal color DE images of the descending aorta, resulting in a "double-barrel" descending aorta.
7. Normal values for forward flow velocities depend on cardiac output, heart rate, and other factors. For instance, the ratio of early to late velocity of transmitral flow decreases with age, and so does the ratio of diastolic to systolic peak velocity of pulmonary venous flow.
8. Minimal or "trace" regurgitation by color and pulsed DE is frequently seen in all valves without clinical evidence of heart disease. The incidence increases with age.

All 2D windows are used for DE recordings. However, the best transducer position for DE interrogation almost regularly is not the best position for imaging. DE recordings can be sufficient even if 2D image quality is impaired, because the signal to noise ratio in DE recordings is higher than for 2D echo. Right parasternal windows (for aortic stenosis, with the patient in the right lateral decubitus position) and suprasternal windows (for aortic stenosis or aortic coarctation) are often helpful, as well as epigastric windows.

Gain, scale (which in pulsed and color DE is equivalent to pulse repetition frequency), baseline, and filter settings should be individualized to obtain a well-defined signal.

The Routine Examination and Normal Findings

In the parasternal views, because the occurring left heart flows are approximately orthogonal to the echo beam, velocity measurements by spectral Doppler are not practical. However, color DE reveals occurrence and direction of mitral and aortic regurgitation. Width of these jets is well assessed in parasternal long axis views, and the minimal cross-section in appropriate basal short axis views. Subaortic obstruction and ventricular septal defects can also be detected by color DE. Short axis views at the aortic root level allow DE assessment of the right ventricular inflow and outflow tract, including tricuspid and pulmonary forward and regurgitant flow. Congenital anomalies as atrial septal defects, membranous ventricular septal defects, or a patent ductus arteriosus may also be detected. The parasternal right ventricular inflow view offers a window on the tricuspid valve. The apical views are ideally suited to record left ventricular inflow and outflow velocities. Transmitral flow is well assessed in the apical four-chamber view and should be recorded at the leaflet tips (where velocities are highest) for assessment of diastolic filling and at the mitral annulus level if stroke volume is to be calculated. The normal transmitral flow velocity signal consists of an early (E) wave, which is generated by the rapid fall in left ventricular pressure due to relaxation below the level of left atrial pressure (Fig. 51.8). E wave upslope reflects the rapid growth of the early diastolic atrioventricular pressure gradient. E wave deceleration reflects the compliance of the left ventricle and left atrium, with a steep deceleration if compliance is low and a slow deceleration if compliance is high. The E wave in sinus rhythm is followed by the late diastolic atrial (A) wave, which is the result of atrial contraction and occurs after the P wave of the ECG. It reflects atrial contraction force and elastic properties of the left ventricle and

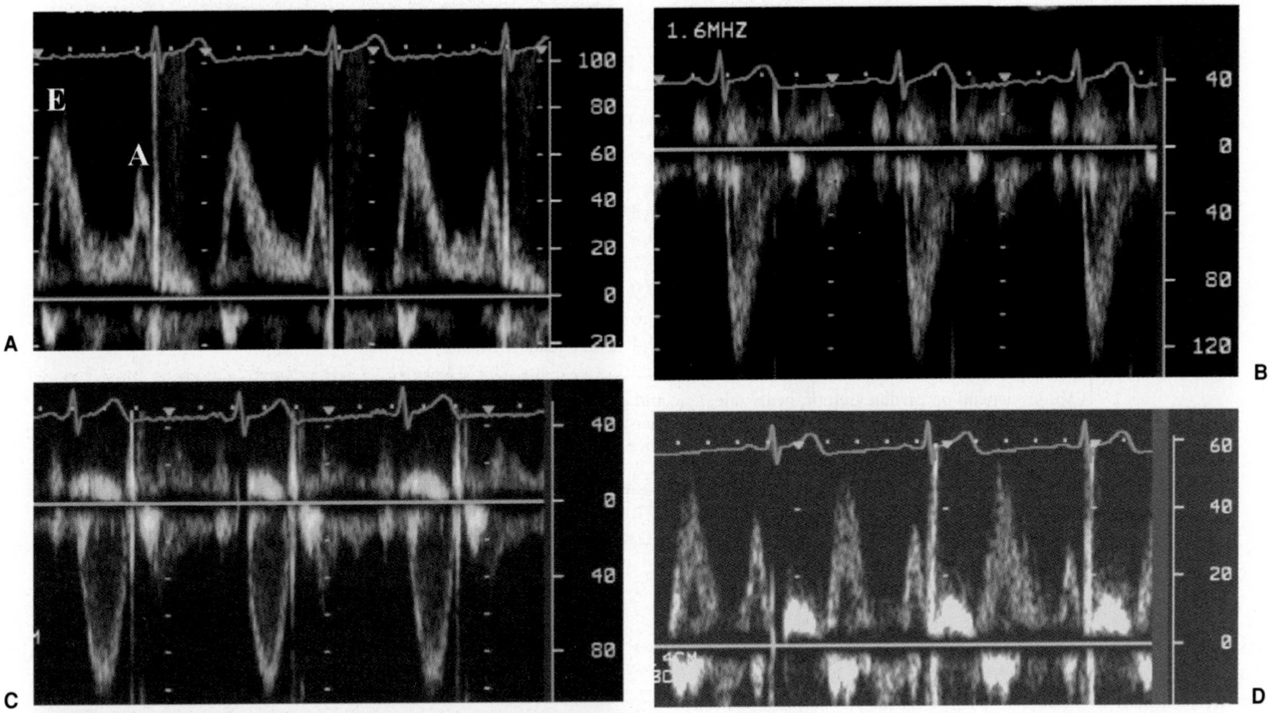

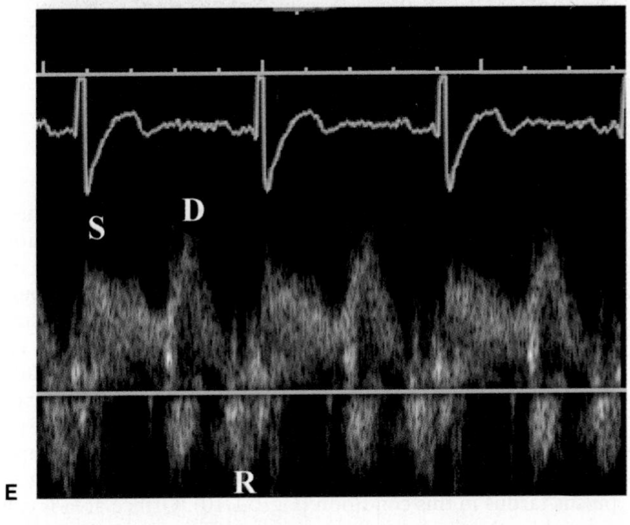

FIGURE 51.8. Normal cardiac flow velocity profiles by pulsed DE. (A) Mitral valve. *Abbreviations:* E, early inflow wave; A, late atrial wave. (B) Aortic valve. (C) Pulmonary valve. (D) Tricuspid valve. (E) Pulmonary venous inflow from right upper pulmonary vein by transthoracic DE. *Abbreviations:* S, systolic; D, diastolic inflow into the left atrium; R, reverse wave owing to atrial contraction.

atrium at end diastole. The ratio of maximal E and A velocities is multifactorial, depending on age, heart rate, left atrial pressure and function, left ventricular diastolic characteristics, and other factors.

Flow velocities in the left ventricular outflow tract and at the aortic valve level are recorded in the apical long axis view and the five-chamber view. Aortic valve flow velocities have an approximately triangular shape, with a slightly more rapid upslope than downslope (see Fig. 51.8). The slopes reflect left ventricular contraction and relaxation and aortic resistance. Aortic flow ends before mitral flow begins, and the time between aortic valve closure and mitral flow onset is the isovolumic relaxation time. Conversely, mitral valve closure is followed by isovolumic contraction time until transaortic flow begins.

The four-chamber view also allows assessment of tricuspid forward and regurgitant flow. Transtricuspid flow velocities are the lowest of all valves, because the tricuspid valve has the largest orifice area. Tricuspid forward flow velocities form an early diastolic wave and a late wave after atrial contraction, analogous to the transmitral flow pattern (see Fig. 51.8). Pulmonary forward flow is represented by an approximately triangular shaped systolic velocity signal with a symmetric upslope and deceleration. A steep upslope (short acceleration time) and a midsystolic notch are typical of pulmonary hypertension.

Atrial and ventricular septal defects (especially of the muscular type) may be detected by color DE in the apical four-chamber view. Pulmonary venous flow may be interrogated in a slightly cranially angulated four-chamber view in the right upper pulmonary vein. Mitral regurgitation is sought by color DE in all apical views. A transaortic flow profile is recorded by pulsed DE. An additional continuous wave recording of outflow tract and aortic valve is valuable to exclude an obstruction.

The subcostal views are rarely optimal windows for DE examination except for a color DE examination for atrial septal defects. The subcostal views provide a valuable alternative if more cranial windows are insufficient, for example, in aortic stenosis. Aortic coarctation and aortic stenosis should be evaluated from the suprasternal position, which in adults often is difficult to use except with a dedicated continuous wave probe.

Pulmonary venous flow velocities in sinus rhythm have a systolic and a diastolic portion directed toward the left

TABLE 51.1

NORMAL VALUES FOR INTRACARDIAC FLOW VELOCITIES IN ADULTS

	Maximal velocity (m/s)	Range
Mitral valve	0.9 (E wave) 0.5 ± 0.1 (A wave)	0.6–1.3
Aortic valve	1.35	1.0–1.7
Tricuspid valve	0.5 (E wave)	0.3–0.7
Pulmonary valve	0.75	0.6–0.9
Left ventricular outflow tract	0.9	0.7–1.1
Left upper pulmonary venous inflow	0.6 ± 0.2 (systolic wave) 0.4 ± 0.1 (diastolic wave)	

Values depend on cardiac output, heart rate, age, and other factors.
Source: Compiled from Hatle L, Angelsen B. Doppler ultrasound in cardiology. 2nd ed. Philadelphia: Lea & Febiger; 1985; Weyman AE. Principles and practice of echocardiography. 2nd ed. Philadelphia: Lea & Febiger; 1994; and Castello R, Pearson AC, Lenzen P, et al. Evaluation of pulmonary venous flow by transesophageal echocardiography in subjects with a normal heart: comparison with transthoracic echocardiography. *J Am Coll Cardiol* 1991;18:65–71.

atrium, and a short, low-velocity retrograde wave after atrial contraction (see Fig. 51.8). Systolic and diastolic inflow velocities in young individuals are approximately equal. Diastolic inflow velocities decrease with age and in general behave as the transmitral E wave; in early diastole the atrium acts as a passive conduit. Normal values for the flow velocities obtained during routine examination are given in Table 51.1.

Transesophageal Doppler Echocardiography

Transesophageal echo offers a full additional set of almost never obstructed echo windows (27). Transmitral flow can be studied under ideal conditions, and aortic regurgitation is well seen by color DE from transesophageal windows, especially in long axis views (at 130–160 degrees) of the left ventricular outflow tract. It is difficult, however, to obtain a good alignment of transvalvular aortic flow with the echo beam; this is best done from a transgastric position by rotating from the left ventricular short axis to a long axis view or using maximal anteflection of the instrument in the stomach. Tricuspid flow is also difficult to align with the transesophageal echo beam. The pulmonary valve is frequently not well visualized transesophageally. Further, emptying and filling velocities of the left atrial appendage can be measured, which are related to thromboembolic risk. Additionally, pulmonary venous flow is easily interrogated either in the left upper or right upper pulmonary vein. Given the excellent visibility of the interatrial septum, a color DE examination for an atrial septal defect should be performed. Flow velocities in the ascending and descending aorta can be visualized by color DE, and in aortic dissection, flow in the false lumen as well as entry and reentry jets can be visualized.

Contrast Doppler Echocardiography

Injection of right heart echo contrast (e.g., saline) enhances the amplitude and signal to noise ratio of the Doppler flow signal, which in rare cases helps in evaluating valvular heart disease or pulmonary venous flow. A new application of DE is power Doppler to image left heart contrast agents, which can be used as myocardial perfusion tracers. Doppler power (the square of the amplitude of the Doppler signal) is primarily related to the number of scatterers, not their velocity or direction. Contrast bubbles create power Doppler signals both by their motion and by ultrasound induced destruction of contrast bubbles, which leads to the creation of a strong Doppler shift (28).

ACQUIRED VALVULAR HEART DISEASE

Aortic Stenosis

For the assessment of aortic stenosis, three parameters are necessary: the transaortic continuous wave Doppler, the subaortic pulsed Doppler, and the left ventricular outflow tract diameter (Fig. 51.9). Continuous wave Doppler signals should be recorded from all obtainable windows (apical, subcostal, suprasternal, right parasternal) to ensure that the maximal velocities have been detected. Mean and maximal pressure gradients are calculated from the continuous wave tracing. A slowed early systolic rise in flow velocities across the aortic valve, resulting in an approximately symmetric upslope and downslope, indicates severe stenosis, analogous to the clinical finding of pulsus tardus in this condition (Fig. 51.10). Orifice area is calculated by the continuity equation and is largely independent of cardiac output and heart rate and thus particularly valuable in impaired left ventricular function, when a low pressure gradient can reflect mild obstruction, low stroke volume, or both. Typical errors in assessment of aortic stenosis are:

1. Doppler gradient "too high":
   - Misreading the mitral regurgitation signal for aortic stenosis (check timing of velocities).
   - Neglect of high proximal velocities, as in aortic regurgitation or high cardiac output.
   - Pressure recovery, which may occur to a clinically meaningful extent in native aortic stenosis if the ascending aorta has a diameter under 3 cm, leading to "overestimation" of peak and mean gradients by Doppler as compared to invasive hemodynamics. Formulae for estimating the amount of pressure recovery have been published (29,30).
   - Atrial fibrillation with high beat-to-beat variation in gradient.
2. Doppler gradient "too low":
   - Missing the maximal signal (use all available windows).

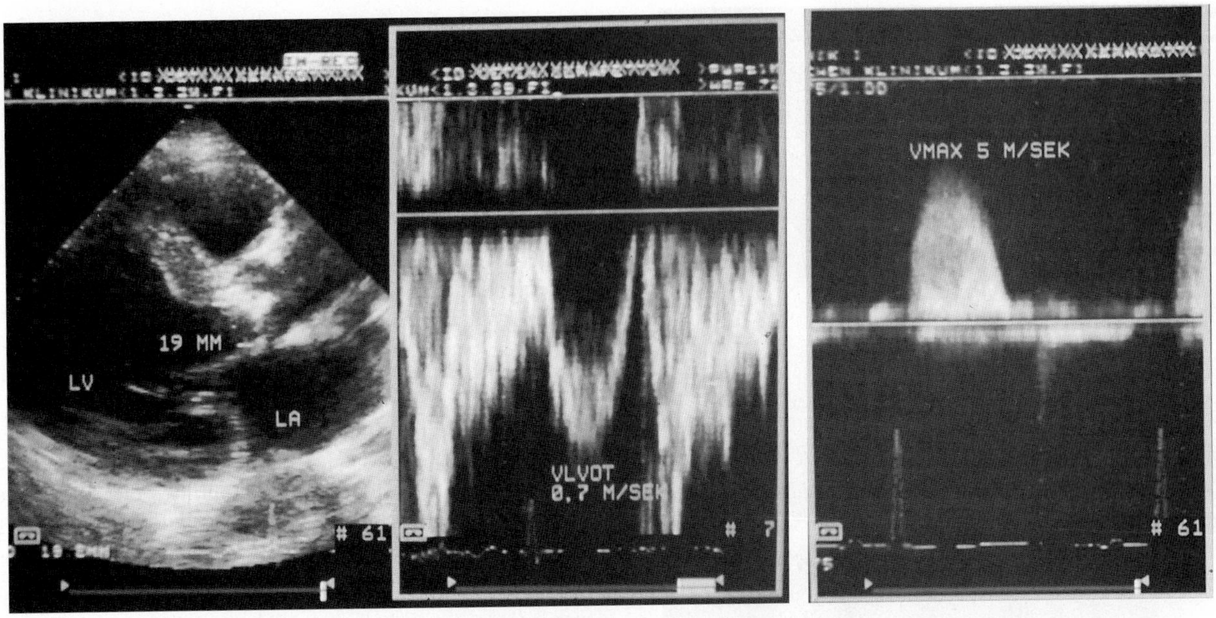

FIGURE 51.9. Aortic valve area calculation by the continuity principle. *Left upper figure:* Measurement of left ventricular outflow tract diameter in the parasternal long axis view (19 mm, corresponding to an area of 2.8 cm^2). *Middle figure:* Pulsed DE recording in the left ventricular outflow tract. *Right figure:* Continuous wave DE of transstenotic flow velocities. By the continuity equation, an aortic valve area of 0.4 cm^2 was calculated.

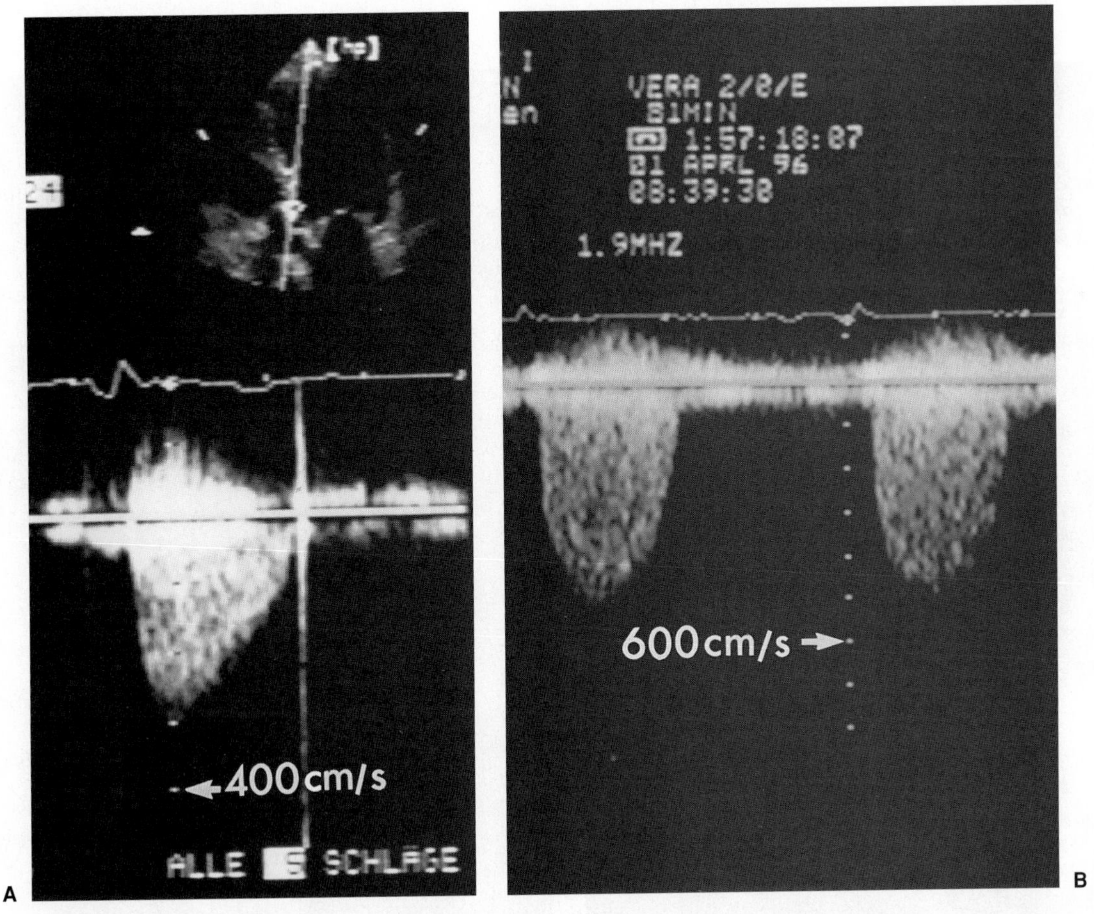

FIGURE 51.10. (A) Moderate aortic stenosis with a triangular shape and steep upslope. (B) Severe aortic stenosis with a parabolic shape and a slow upslope.

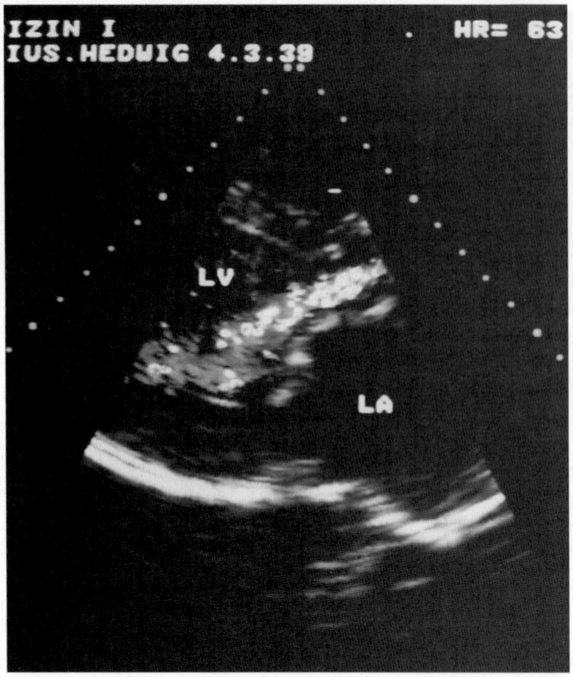

FIGURE 51.11. Aortic regurgitation. Color Doppler flow mapping in a parasternal long axis view. The regurgitant jet is depicted in the left ventricular outflow tract and left ventricle, hugging the anterior mitral leaflet. *Abbreviations:* LV, left ventricle; LA, left atrium.

The evaluation of patients with low cardiac output owing to impaired left ventricular function and aortic stenosis is difficult. Augmentation of cardiac output by 10 to 20 μg/kg per minute of intravenous dobutamine may unmask a "stretch reserve" of the stenotic orifice area in a few patients with mitral or aortic stenosis. If the stenosis "gives in" to dobutamine-increased stroke volume, it can be assumed to be less severe than apparent at baseline (31). At the same time, dobutamine stress also identifies presence or absence of a contractile reserve, which impacts postoperative survival (32).

Aortic Regurgitation

Aortic regurgitation is the most difficult valvular lesion to evaluate. Both jet height (in parasternal long axis views; Fig. 51.11) or jet area (in short axis views) are used and normalized to diameter or area of the left ventricular outflow tract, respectively. Twenty percent and 60% of left ventricular outflow tract area (25% and 65% of left ventricular outflow tract diameter) are the cut-off values for mild, moderate, and severe regurgitation (33); they are unreliable in eccentric jets. Another useful parameter is the pressure half-time of the continuous wave Doppler of regurgitant flow (Fig. 51.12). The shorter the pressure half-time, the more rapidly pressure equalizes between ascending aorta and left ventricle, and the more severe is aortic regurgitation. Values under 250 ms indicate severe aortic regurgitation. However, pressure half-time does not exclusively reflect severity of regurgitation, but also depends on left ventricular

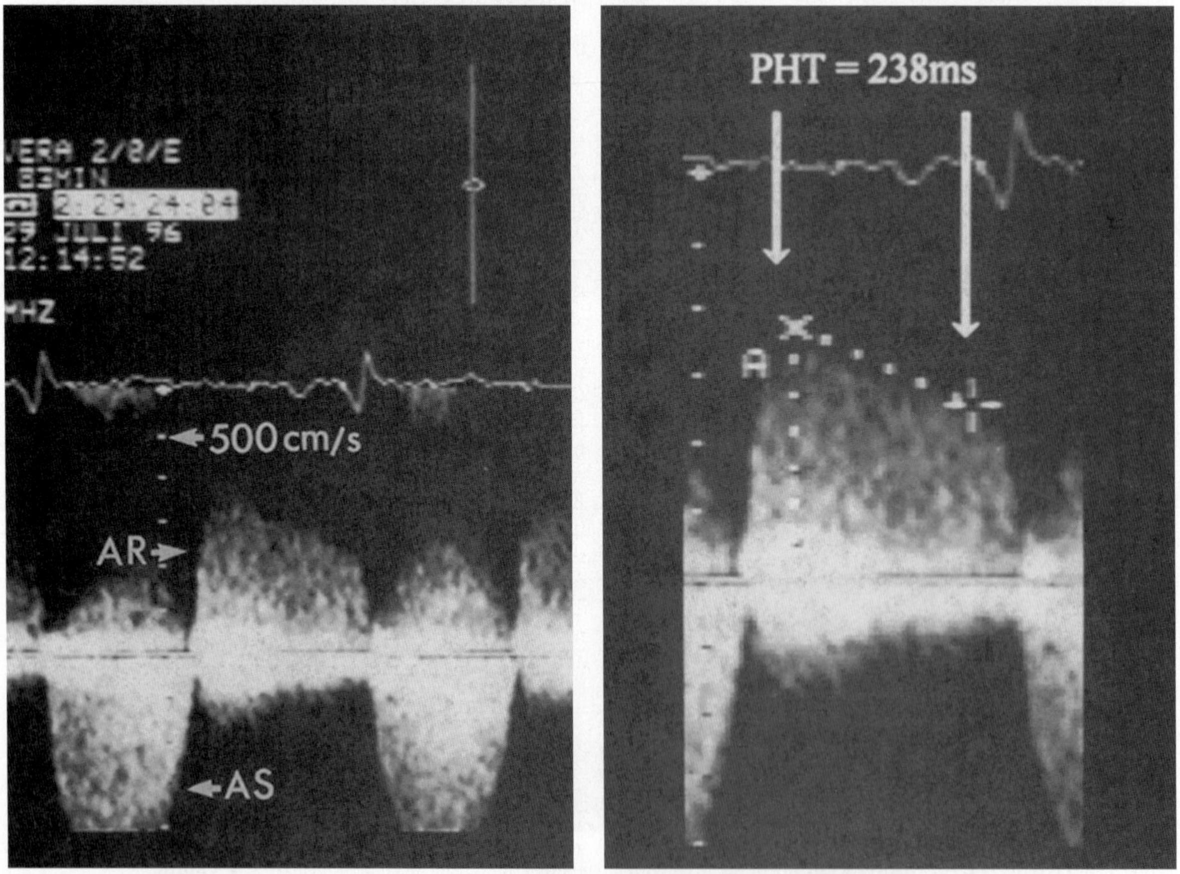

FIGURE 51.12. *Left:* Continuous wave Doppler of combined severe aortic stenosis (AS) and regurgitation (AR). *Right:* Calculation of the pressure half-time of the aortic regurgitation signal. Pressure half-time shortens with increasing severity of aortic regurgitation. The value of 238 ms indicates severe regurgitation.

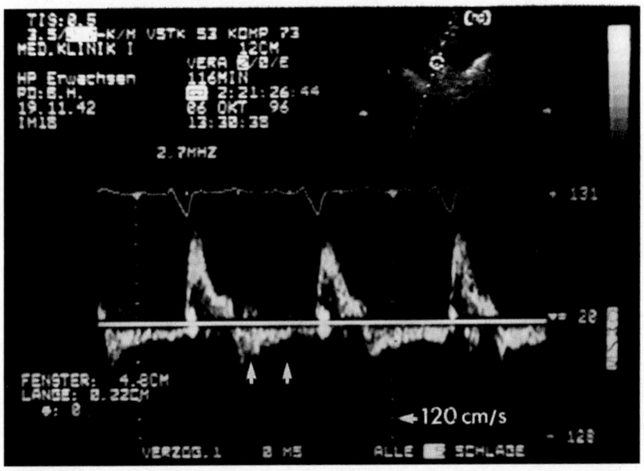

FIGURE 51.13. Holodiastolic flow reversal (*arrows*) in the descending aorta in severe aortic regurgitation. Pulsed DE from the suprasternal notch.

diastolic compliance and systemic arterial resistance. The presence of a holodiastolic flow signal on pulsed DE recordings in the descending, or abdominal aorta, or a large systemic artery, is a reliable sign of at least moderate aortic regurgitation, especially if end-diastolic retrograde velocity is 18 cm/s or more (34) (Fig. 51.13).

Mitral Regurgitation

Mitral regurgitation should be evaluated by color DE using all available windows, especially the apical views. Mitral regurgitant jets often are eccentric, hugging the atrial walls (see Fig. 51.1). Mitral valve prolapse or flail creates jets directed to the opposite side of the leaflet, whereas leaflets restricted in motion produce jets to the same side. Eyeballing of maximal color DE turbulent jet size yields a rough estimate of severity. Division by left atrial area in the same view to "normalize" jet size has been proposed and is convenient (with cut-off values of 20% and 40% of left atrial size) (35), but lacks theoretical justification. Eccentric, wall-hugging jets are underestimated by an average of 40% by the jet area method (19). Although very small and very large jets are usually well identified, the intermediate severities are impossible to reliably grade by color jet area. The pulmonary venous flow pattern and two color Doppler–based approaches have been well validated and are clinically practical (20), if image quality is good:

1. Measurement of the proximal jet diameter in the parasternal long axis or apical four-chamber view (or their transesophageal equivalents, but not in the apical two-chamber view). The smallest diameter of the jet should be measured, which is within millimeters of its origin (see Fig. 51.7A). Jet diameter or more than 7mm indicates severe regurgitation (36,37).
2. The proximal convergence zone method: Maximal regurgitant flow rates of greater than 150 mL/s and effective ROAs of greater than 0.3 cm^2 indicate 3+ or 4+ mitral regurgitation (20,38) (see Fig. 51.4).

Pulmonary venous flow recordings show a reduction in the systolic portion of pulmonary venous inflow into the left atrium. In severe mitral regurgitation, systolic pulmonary venous flow is often reversed and merges with the end-diastolic retrograde flow wave (see Fig. 51.7B). Although flow reversal is highly specific for severe regurgitation, blunting of systolic flow is not very specific and occurs also in atrial fibrillation or impaired systolic function. High saturation of the DE signals and increased diastolic transmitral velocities (>1.5 m/s) also are typically present in severe regurgitation.

Mitral Stenosis

Mitral stenosis is best assessed in the apical views. The mean gradient and the pressure half-time should be calculated (see Fig. 51.6). The latter is calculated from the downslope of the E wave or the single diastolic wave in atrial fibrillation. It is the time of decay from maximal velocity of flow (immediately after mitral valve opening) to $1/\sqrt{2}$ of the maximal velocity (the $1/\sqrt{2}$ factor is due to the quadratic relation between pressure drop and velocity in the Bernoulli equation). The pressure half-time (in milliseconds) is relatively robust against changes in cardiac output, heart rate, and the presence of mitral regurgitation; a useful empirical relationship exists with mitral valve area (MVA, in cm^2), given by MVA = 220/PHT, where PHT is the pressure half-time (the Hatle formula) (39). However, pressure half-time also depends on left atrial and left ventricular compliance, the maximal pressure gradient, concomitant aortic regurgitation (which shortens pressure half-time), the presence of an atrial septal defect, or the presence and type of a prosthetic mitral valve (40–42), and in these instances may be unreliable. In atrial fibrillation, at least a short and long diastolic period should be recorded to document the range of occurring gradients and pressure half-times. Other ways to calculate MVA from DE data are to obtain cardiac output and to divide it by the time–velocity integral of the mitral valve, or to use the diameters of the forward jet by color DE in the four-chamber view (D_{4CV}) and the two-chamber view (D_{2CV}) to approximate MVA by

$$\pi * D_{4CV} * D_{2CV}/4$$

(the ellipse formula). Alternatively, the proximal convergence zone principle may be used (23).

Tricuspid Valve Disease

The mean pressure gradient is calculated from continuous wave or pulsed wave DE recordings in analogy to transmitral gradients. The pressure half-time may be used for serial measurements, but its use to calculate orifice areas has not been validated. Tricuspid regurgitation is best detected by color DE in the apical (or subcostal) four chamber view (Fig. 51.14). On continuous wave DE, it produces a systolic regurgitant velocity spectrum of parabolic shape, similar to mitral regurgitation. The maximal regurgitant velocity is important to diagnose the presence of pulmonary hypertension. By the simplified Bernoulli equation, the maximal systolic pressure difference between right ventricle and right atrium can be calculated from the maximal tricuspid regurgitant velocity. This is an estimate of maximal right ventricular, and thus, pulmonary pressure. The pressure difference can either be reported as such, or 10 mm Hg added as an estimate of right atrial pressure, or right atrial pressure can be assessed clinically by the collapse level of the neck veins.

Pulmonary Valve Disease

This valve is best examined in the parasternal basal short axis view, or alternatively in a subcostal short axis view. Minimal pulmonary regurgitation is very frequent in individuals without clinical evidence of cardiac disease. Pulmonary stenosis is evaluated reliably by the mean transvalvular gradient from continuous wave DE.

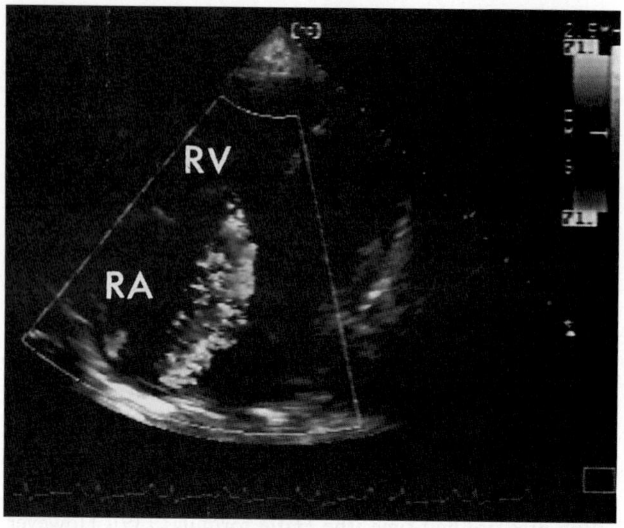

FIGURE 51.14. Moderate tricuspid regurgitation by color DE (apical four-chamber view). *Abbreviations:* RV, right ventricle; RA, right atrium.

Prosthetic Heart Valves

Obstruction

Pulsed and continuous wave measurement of forward flow velocities across valvular prostheses is usually well obtainable even if 2D image quality is impaired by prosthetic artifacts. Opening and closing clicks are seen on the spectral Doppler display as narrow, bright vertical lines (Fig. 51.15). Maximal and mean gradients should be calculated in the same way as described for native stenotic valves. Contrary to normal native valves, there is some degree of obstruction inherent in all prosthetic valves. Normal values depend on the implantation site, the type of prosthesis, and the stroke volume, and therefore limits of normalcy are rather wide (43,44) creating a grey zone where mild obstruction cannot be diagnosed with certainty unless comparison with previous recordings is possible.

Especially, but not exclusively, the bileaflet valves by their design create high local gradients and pressure recovery downstream (see section on Basic Hydrodynamic Principles) (45,46). The maximal velocities by continuous wave Doppler therefore can lead to a calculated pressure drop higher than the net pressure drop between the left ventricle and the ascending aorta a few centimeters downstream from the prostheses. Furthermore, in partial obstruction of the prosthesis, pressure recovery diminishes, thus leaving a wide grey zone between normal and pathologic gradients. Therefore it may be necessary to directly image leaflet mobility (by 2D echo or, preferably, fluoroscopy) to exclude prosthetic dysfunction. Continuity areas of prosthetic valves can be calculated analogously to native valves. Since these are effective areas, they are considerably smaller than areas predicted by sewing ring size. For example, for intact St. Jude Medical Nr. 21 aortic prostheses effective orifice areas of 1.25 ± 0.21 cm^2 have been calculated in clinical studies (47), when the inner sewing ring (1.7 cm) diameter would predict a geometric orifice area of 2.3 cm^2. Pressure recovery also affects continuity area calculations.

"Mismatch" obstruction results from the implantation of a prosthesis that is too small for the site and patient. This is mainly a problem in aortic valve replacement. For example, the effective orifice areas of ring size Nr. 21 and smaller prostheses would be considered mild-to-moderate aortic stenosis in a native valve. This type of obstruction must be differentiated from new prosthetic obstruction owing to thrombosis or pannus by comparison with earlier studies or by fluoroscopy. The possibility of pressure recovery and patient–prosthesis mismatch underline the importance of documenting baseline velocities or gradients of valvular prostheses postoperatively for later comparison. Other parameters of prosthetic obstruction have been proposed. The simplest one is the velocity index, which is based on the continuity concept and is defined as the ratio of maximal outflow and maximal transprosthetic velocity. It is theoretically independent of cardiac output and obviates the need to measure left ventricular outflow tract diameter. Values under 0.25 are considered pathologic. The problem of pressure recovery in bileaflet prostheses, however, is not avoided by using the velocity index.

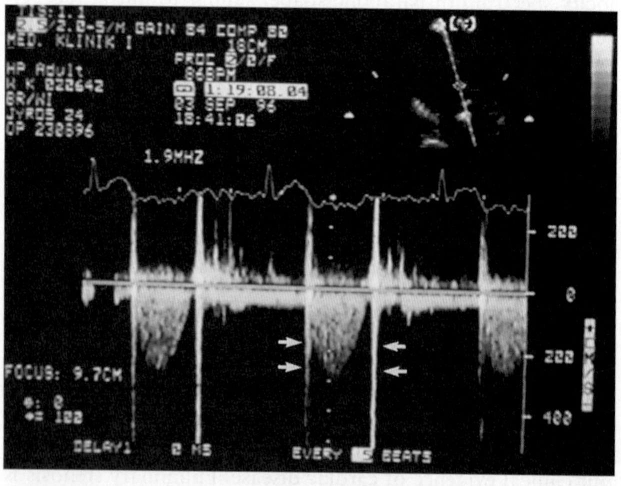

FIGURE 51.15. Aortic prosthetic flow in a normal mechanical bileaflet prosthesis, with clicks (*arrows*).

Regurgitation

All mechanical prostheses, except for the caged-ball Starr–Edwards valve, exhibit some amount of inbuilt, transvalvular leakage, which is intended to prevent the formation of microthrombi at the hinge points and to preclude sticking of the occluder in the closed position. Depending on the prosthesis type, typical spatial orientation patterns of the regurgitant jets can be visualized (48) (Fig. 51.16). Bioprostheses, too, almost invariably present some transvalvular regurgitation. Wear-and-tear lesions in bioprostheses may lead to unpredictable, sudden increases in the severity of regurgitation. In addition to transvalvular regurgitation, paravalvular leakage is frequent in prosthetic valves (Fig. 51.17). Some of these leaks close spontaneously postoperatively; others may arise during follow-up as a result of suture failure or endocarditic tissue destruction. Transesophageal echocardiography is usually better suited than transthoracic imaging to characterize and classify prosthetic regurgitation (49), in particular in mechanical mitral prostheses. The occurrence of a reproducible, large (>1 cm^2) proximal convergence zone on the ventricular side of a mitral prosthesis indicates severe regurgitation even if the atrium itself is not visualized (50) (Fig. 51.18).

Aortic Disease

From the suprasternal window, flow velocity in the ascending and descending aorta can be sampled. Aortic coarctation can be visualized by turbulency, and the gradient measured directly (Fig. 51.19). However, the simplified Bernoulli equation may overestimate the true pressure drop in long, tunnel-like

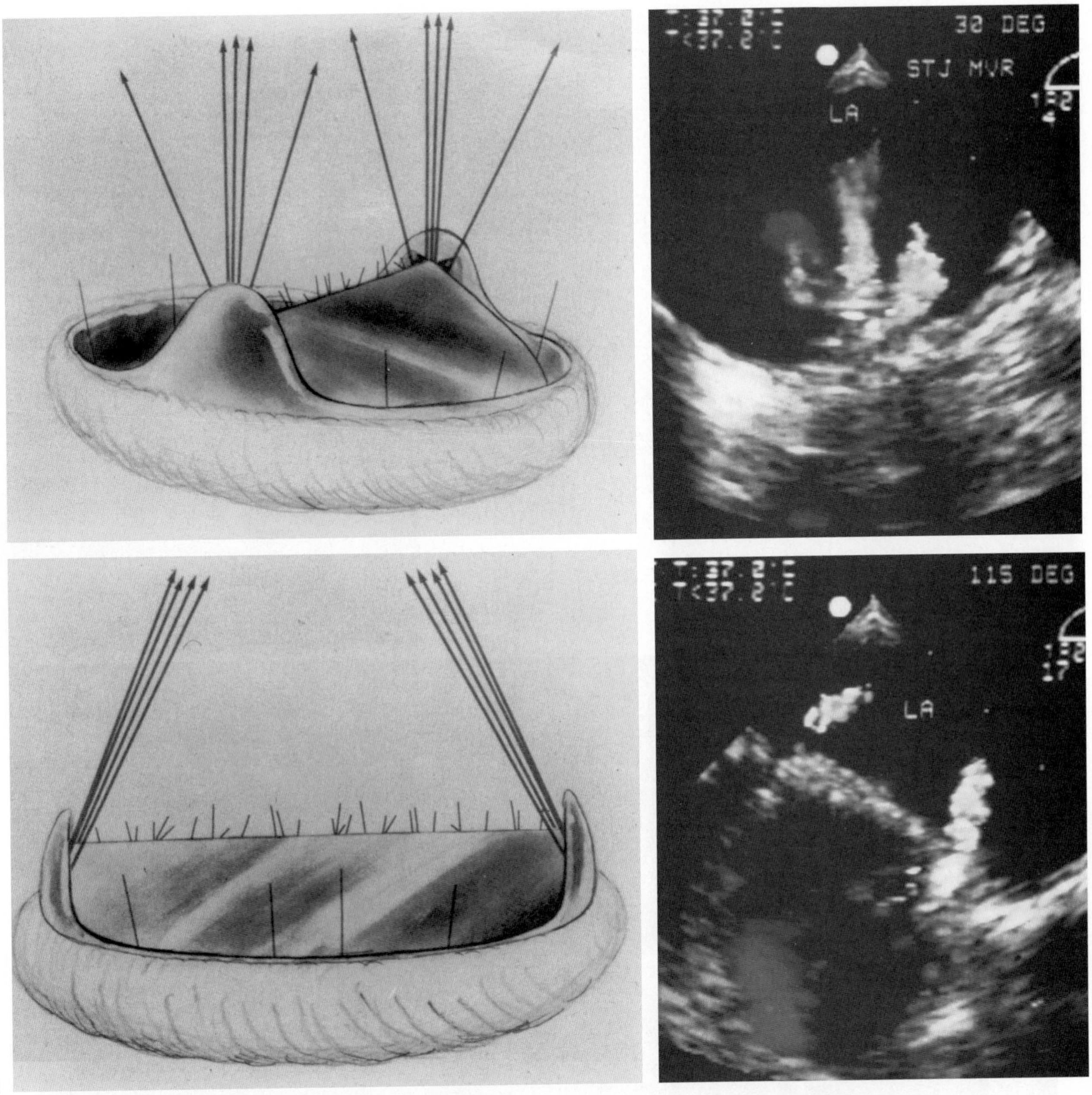

A

FIGURE 51.16. Aortic coarctation. Color DE from the suprasternal notch. *Left:* Ascending aorta is seen in *red*. *Right:* Descending aorta in *blue*. At the stenotic segment (COARC), turbulent flow is present. *Abbreviation:* AOARCH, aortic arch. (Continued)

obstructions, in the presence of high proximal velocities or downstream pressure recovery. In aortic dissection, flow in the true lumen by transesophageal color DE is usually brighter than in the false lumen, where it may be absent if stasis and thrombosis have ensued. Entry and reentry tears of the intima may also be identified by the presence of color DE jets (Fig. 51.20).

CONGENITAL HEART DISEASE

Stenotic and Regurgitant Lesions

Congenital valvular lesions are evaluated in the same way as acquired valvular disease. Except for serial or tunnel-like obstructions and aortic coarctation, the simplified Bernoulli equation is applicable.

Shunts

Atrial and ventricular septal defects mostly can be directly detected by color Doppler displaying the pathologic flow (Fig. 51.21). Atrial septal defects are best examined from the subcostal window or be transesophageal echo. Sinus venosus defects may be overlooked transthoracically. Left-to-right shunt usually shows a biphasic, midsystolic to mid-diastolic and late diastolic flow from the left to the right atrium, with a short reversal of direction (right to left) in early systole. Transtricuspid forward flow velocities are elevated and match or exceed transmitral flow velocities. Ventricular septal defects are best detected by color DE; membranous defects usually are best identified in parasternal views, and muscular defects in apical or subcostal four-chamber view (Fig. 51.22). Continuous wave Doppler tracings showing high systolic flow velocity

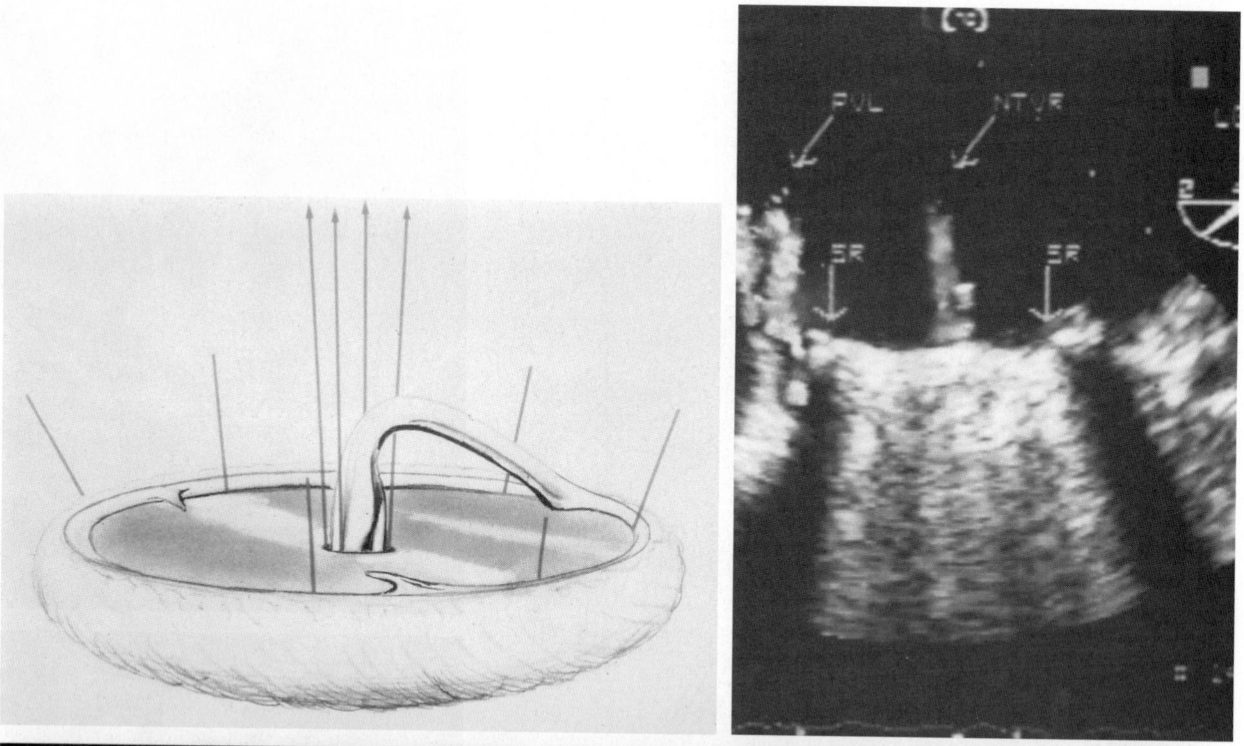

B

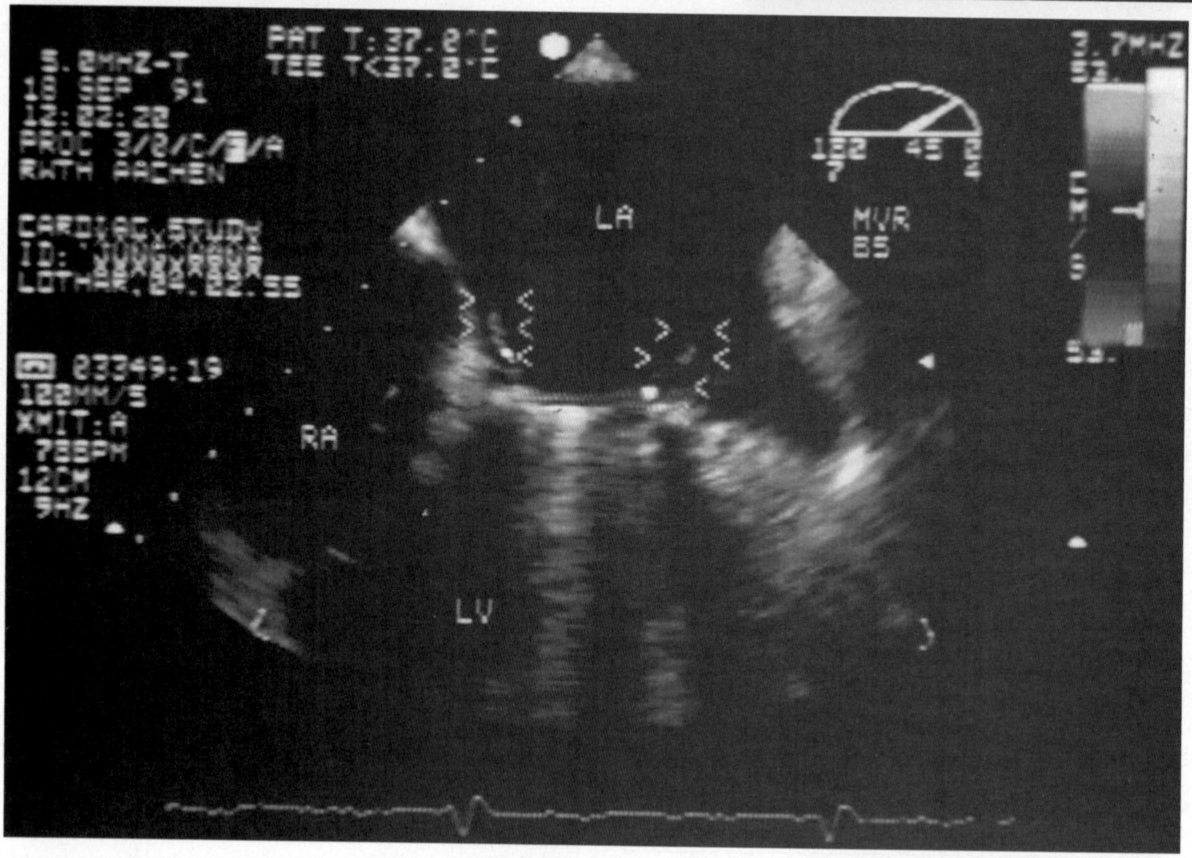

C

FIGURE 51.16. (Continued)

toward the right ventricle allow to approximate the maximal systolic pressure difference between left and right ventricle. A patent ductus arteriosus is best visualized in suprasternal, parasternal, or subcostal views displaying a long axis of the pulmonary artery. Continuous wave DE reveals the shunt pattern, which in left-to-right shunt is systolic–diastolic with a late systolic peak. By color DE, a diastolic flow convergence region in the proximal descending aorta may be seen, especially by transesophageal echo. In right-to-left shunts, maximal velocities are recorded at the aortic end of the duct, and

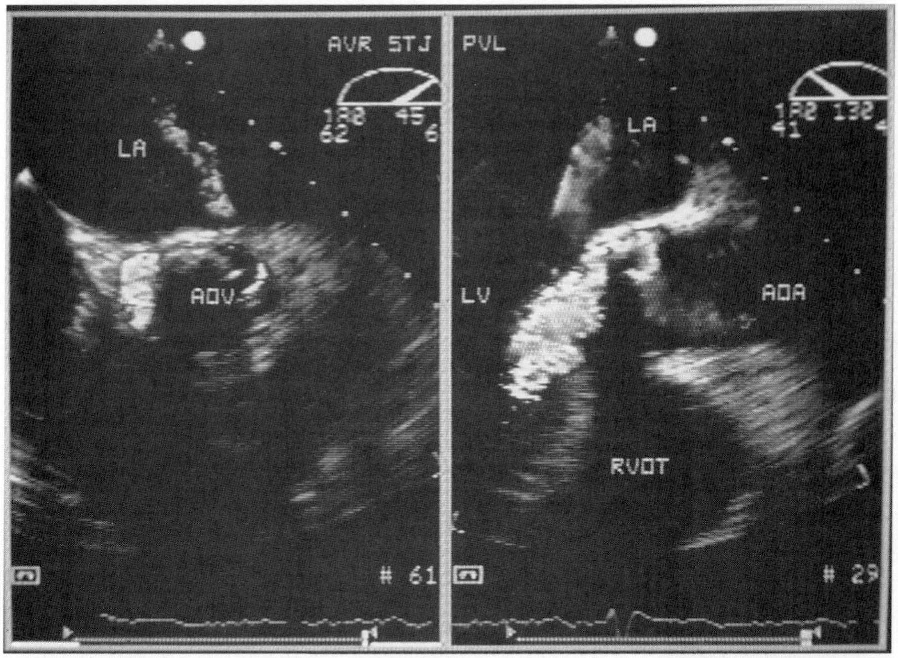

FIGURE 51.17. Aortic dissection (DeBakey Type I/Stanford Type A). Transesophageal image of the dilated ascending aorta (5 cm). An intimal flap is seen separating a false lumen (FL) from the true lumen (TL). A small entry jet is seen by color Doppler (ENTRY). *Abbreviation:* LA, left atrium.

retrograde flow in the descending aorta may be seen. To calculate the left-to-right shunt ratio, the ratio of cardiac output at the aortic and the pulmonary valve level has been used, but has considerable error margins. Maximal systolic pulmonary pressure can be estimated from maximal tricuspid regurgitant velocity.

EVALUATION OF CARDIAC FUNCTION

Systolic Left Ventricular Function

A fundamental parameter of overall left ventricular function is cardiac output. A further parameter of systolic function obtainable in the presence of mitral regurgitation is the rate of systolic left ventricular pressure increase (d_p/d_t), which is calculated from the rise of regurgitant velocities in early systole. For example, the time interval between the points where regurgitant velocity reaches 1 m/s and 3 m/s is measured and the corresponding pressure drops (4 and 36 mm Hg) are used to calculate early systolic pressure rise as 32 mm Hg/Δt (51). However, because the pressure in the left atrium is not known, these values are an approximation and they do not necessarily represent the maximal rate of pressure increase.

The peak systolic tissue Doppler velocity at the annular level (septal or lateral basal segment) reflects overall longitudinal left ventricular contraction and correlates well with ejection fraction. It is a robust parameter which can be used even in difficult to image patients. Values are slightly lower at the basal septum and decline with age (see Table 51.2 for normal values). It has been shown that peak systolic annular velocities can detect subtle deterioration of myocardial function, even if the ejection fraction remains in the normal range. This is the case in early cardiomyopathies, left ventricular hypertrophy

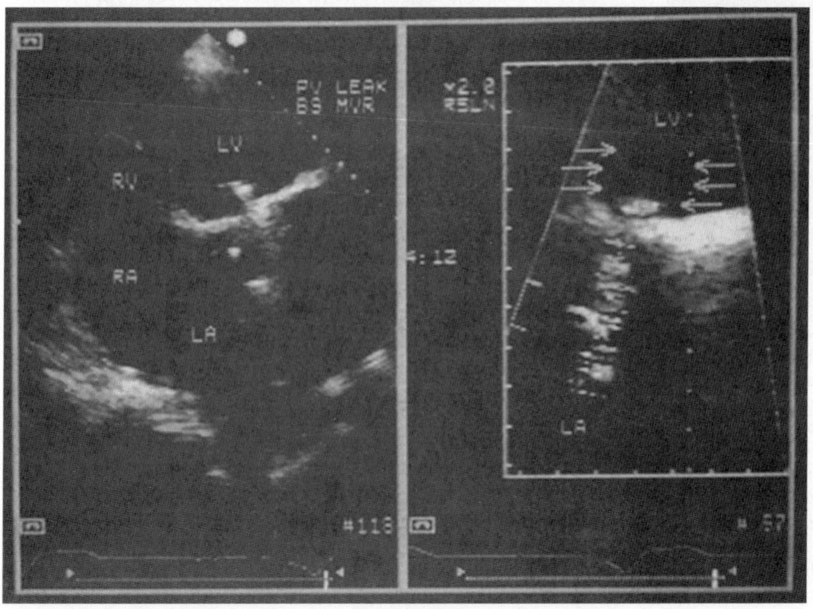

FIGURE 51.18. Atrial septal defect, secundum type. *Left:* Subcostal color DE. *Right:* Transesophageal color and pulsed DE of atrial septal defect (*arrow*). Left-to-right flow velocities in late systole and early diastole, followed by a smaller late diastolic wave. *Abbreviation:* RA, right atrium.

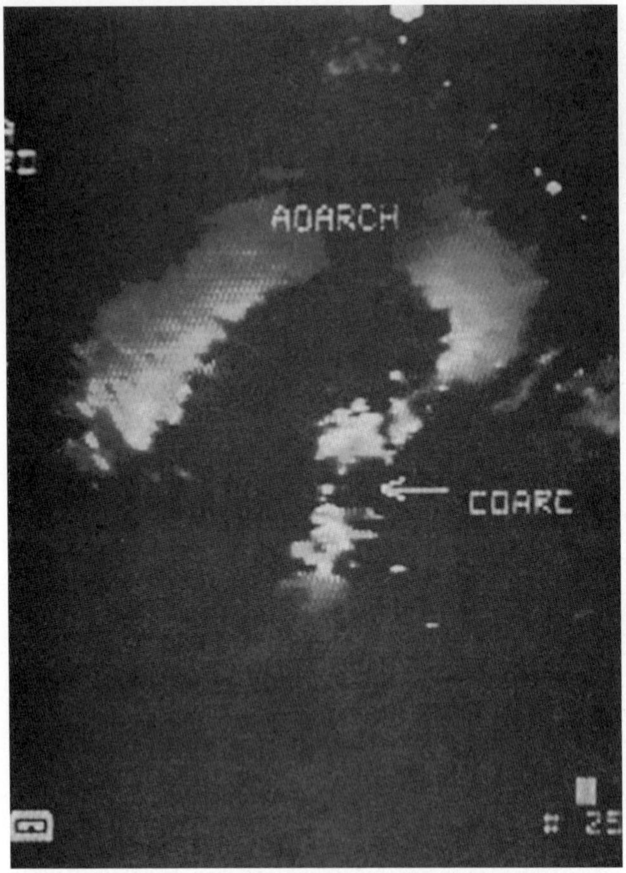

FIGURE 51.19. Ventricular septal defect. (A) Parasternal long axis view with color DE of a small congenital ventricular septal defect immediately below the aortic valve. Note the proximal convergence zone on the left ventricular side. (B) Ventricular septal defect complicating anterior myocardial infarction. Color DE in the apical four-chamber view shows septal rupture in the apex with a turbulent jet in the right ventricle.

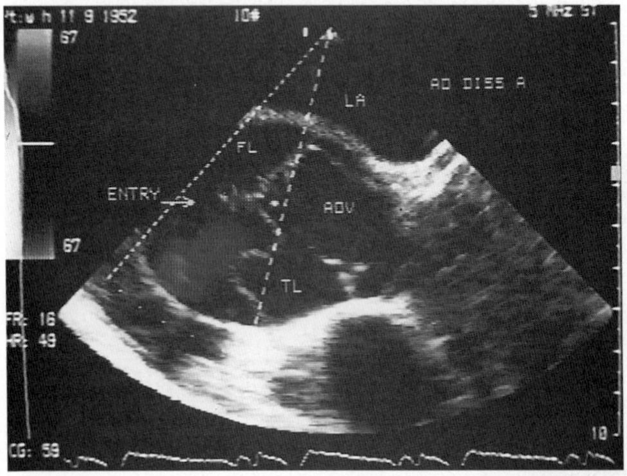

FIGURE 51.20. Typical tissue velocity curves at basal septal segment in a normal control subject, in an asymptomatic patient with DE signs of diastolic dysfunction with preserved ejection fraction (DD), in a patient with diastolic heart failure, but preserved ejection fraction (DHF), and a patient with systolic heart failure and reduced ejection fraction (SHF). Note progressive decrease in peak myocardial sustained systolic velocities (*arrows*) and early diastolic velocities (*arrowheads*) from DD to SHF, all of which were lower than in control subjects. (*Source:* From Yu CM, Lin H, Yang H, et al. Progression of systolic abnormalities in patients with "isolated" diastolic heart failure and diastolic dysfunction. *Circulation* 2002 Mar 12;105:1195–1201, with permission.)

owing to hypertension or aortic stenosis, and other diseases. Thus, assessment of peak systolic tissue velocity, together with E', provides useful objective evidence of myocardial contractile impairment. There is a continuous and progressive reduction in absolute values from normals to patients with preserved ejection fraction, but increased diastolic filling pressures, and further to combined systolic and diastolic dysfunction (Figs. 51.23 and 51.24), hence indicating that systolic and diastolic function are not two separate entities but rather two aspects of myocardial function whose manifestations depend on the severity of myocardial disease.

Diastolic Left Ventricular Function

Diastolic left ventricular function is in itself heterogeneous, comprising active (relaxation) and passive (chamber stiffness) characteristics of the left ventricle, among other factors. It is characterized in classic hemodynamics by the diastolic time course of left ventricular pressure and volume. Several parameters obtainable by DE are used to evaluate left ventricular diastolic function (52):

- *Isovolumic relaxation time* (IVRT; the time from aortic valve closure to mitral valve opening), which depends on the velocity of myocardial relaxation, the end-systolic pressure level of the aorta, and the early diastolic pressure level of the left atrium. Positioning the Doppler beam in an apical long axis or five-chamber view between left ventricular inflow and outflow, the end of outflow and the onset of inflow can be read from the spectral display. Slowed relaxation and acute ischemia lengthen IVRT, whereas elevated left atrial pressures tend to shorten it.
- *The transmitral flow profile:* The ratio of peak E and A wave has been studied extensively. In young healthy persons, maximal E velocity is higher than A wave velocity. The following factors decrease the E wave: age, heart rate (in heart rates over 100/minute, there is generally E and A wave fusion), slowed left ventricular relaxation, preload reduction (decreased left atrial pressure; Fig. 51.25A). The site of measurement is important (E/A ratio is lower at the mitral annulus than at the leaflet tips). Maximal A wave velocity depends on left atrial contraction and late diastolic left ventricular compliance. Because the E/A ratio is multifactorial, "filling is not function." With impaired early filling owing to hypertrophy, acute ischemia (Fig. 51.25B), or other causes, E/A decreases, together with increased IVRT (impaired relaxation pattern). Once left atrial pressure increases E/A rises again to normal levels (pseudonormalization pattern). With high atrial pressures and a stiff left ventricle, E/A increases further and deceleration time (from peak E wave to cessation of the E wave) shortens (restrictive pattern, E/A >2 and deceleration time <150 ms), together with a shortened IVRT (Figs. 51.25C,D). The presence of the restrictive mitral inflow pattern with short deceleration implies high pulmonary capillary pressure, impaired functional class, and bad prognosis in post-infarction patients (53,54), dilated cardiomyopathy (55,56), cardiac amyloidosis (57), and others.
- *Pulmonary venous flow:* Whereas peak diastolic flow changes in parallel to the transmitral E wave, peak velocity and duration of the reverse wave increase with left atrial pressure (58). If the reverse pulmonary venous wave exceeds transmitral A wave in duration or peak reverse flow velocity of more than 35 cm/s, increased left atrial and left ventricular end-diastolic pressures over 15 mm Hg are likely.

Other blood flow DE approaches to the evaluation of diastolic function include measurement of the velocity of flow propagation into the left ventricle during diastole (59). This velocity is less preload dependent than the E wave and can be measured as

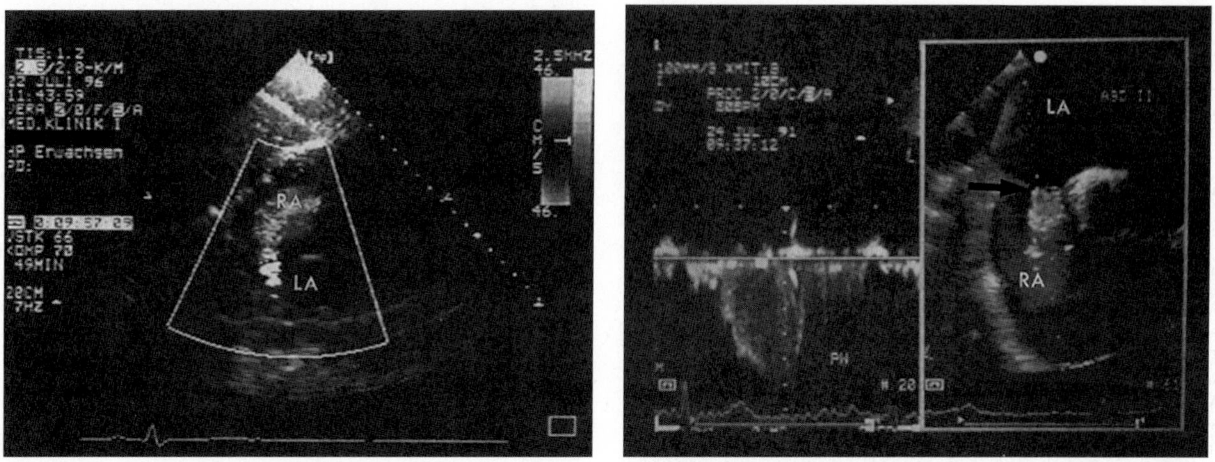

A B

FIGURE 51.21. *Left:* Normal systolic and diastolic tissue velocities *S* and *E′* from basal septum in a normal subject. *Right:* Reduced tissue velocities in a patient with impaired systolic and diastolic function.

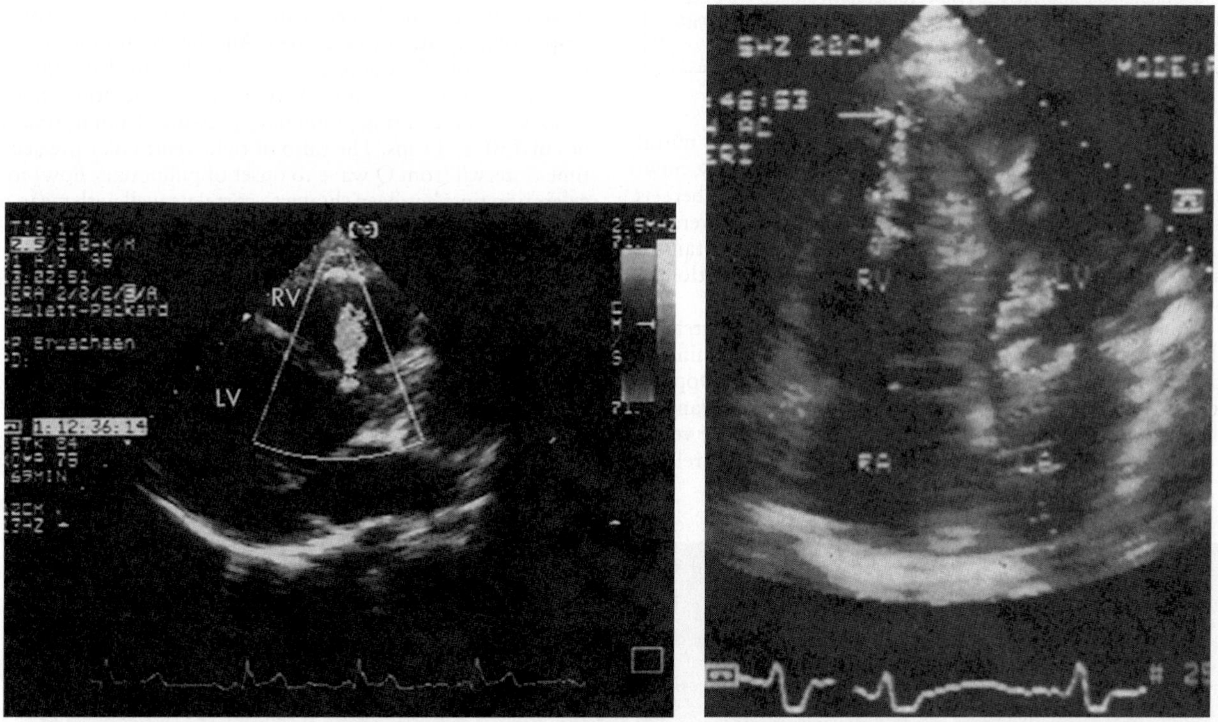

A B

FIGURE 51.22. (**A**) Transmitral flow profile changes induced by changes in preload. Example from a patient before (**A**) and after (**B**) preload reduction by nitroglycerine. Pattern B is indistinguishable from "impaired relaxation." (*Source:* From Choong CY, Herrmann HC, Weyman AE, et al. Preload dependence of Doppler-derived indexes of left ventricular diastolic function in humans. *J Am Coll Cardiol* 1987;10:800–808.) (**B**) Impaired relaxation pattern of transmitral flow during percutaneous transluminal coronary angiography of the left anterior descending artery (pulsed Doppler). At baseline and after recovery, there is a slightly decreased E:A ratio. During balloon inflation, there is a massive decrease of the E wave and some increase of the A wave, reflecting impaired relaxation by acute ischemia, also documented in the ECG. (*Source:* From Labovitz AJ, Lewen MK, Morton K, et al. Evaluation of left ventricular systolic and diastolic dysfunction during transient myocardial ischemia produced by angioplasty. *J Am Coll Cardiol* 1987:10:748–755.) (**C**) Schematic drawing of transmitral flow patterns and their relationship. Pattern I ("impaired relaxation") is characterized by a prolonged isovolumic relaxation time (IVRT), a low E and a high A wave. Pattern II ("restrictive pattern") is characterized by a short IVRT, a high and short E wave, and a small A wave. Pattern I may change to pattern II, which represents advanced stages of disease, by going through a phase of pseudonormalization indistinguishable from the normal transmitral flow pattern. (*Source:* From Appleton CP, Jensen JL, Hatle LK, et al. Doppler evaluation of left and right ventricular diastolic function: a technical guide for obtaining optimal flow velocity recordings. *J Am Soc Echocardiogr* 1997;10:271–291.) (**D**) Restrictive transmitral flow pattern with high, short E wave and diminished A waves (E: A > 2). It reflects high early diastolic filling pressure and low left ventricular compliance.

TABLE 51.2

NORMAL TISSUE DOPPLER VELOCITIES IN ADULTS

Peak systolic longitudinal contraction (cm/s)	
Basal lateral segment	10.2 ± 2.1
Basal septal segment	7.8 ± 1.1
Peak early diastolic elongation (*E'*) (cm/s)	
Basal lateral segment	14.9 ± 3.5
Basal septal segment	11.2 ± 1.9
Peak systolic longitudinal strain rate (s^{-1})	1.27 ± 0.39
Systolic longitudinal strain (%)	19 ± 6

These values depend on age, heart rate, and other factors.
Source: Compiled from Kukulski T, Voigt JU, Wilkenshoff UM, et al. A comparison of regional myocardial velocity information derived by pulsed and color Doppler techniques: an in vitro and in vivo study. *Echocardiography* 2000;17:639–651; Voigt JU, Arnold MF, Karlsson M, et al. Assessment of regional longitudinal myocardial strain rate derived from Doppler myocardial imaging indexes in normal and infarcted myocardium. *J Am Soc Echocardiogr* 2000;13: 588–598; and Davidavicius G, Kowalski M, Williams RI, et al. Can regional strain and strain rate measurement be performed during both dobutamine and exercise echocardiography, and do regional deformation responses differ with different forms of stress testing? *J Am Soc Echocardiogr* 2003;16:299–308.

the slope of an apical color M-mode through the mitral valve during diastole. Because of limited reproducibility, however, this parameter is not widely used. Further, if there is mitral regurgitation, an estimate of the rate of fall of left ventricular pressure (relaxation rate) in late systole can be obtained, analogous to calculation of positive d_p/d_t (see Evaluation of Systolic Left Ventricular Function).

Blood flow DE parameters often are difficult to interpret due to load dependence and difficult measurement. A significant addition therefore comes from measurement of tissue Doppler velocities (see Fig. 51.24). The ratio of *E*/*E'*, where *E* is transmitral peak E wave velocity and *E'* is early diastolic tissue velocity at the mitral annulus level is directly and robustly related to left atrial pressure and left ventricular end-diastolic pressure (60,61). This easy to measure parameter largely solves the problem of pseudonormalization of the transmitral flow profile and should be obtained in every case where elevated filling pressures are investigated. E′ is one of the most sensitive parameters for detecting overall myocardial dysfunction. In hypertrophic cardiomyopathy, E′ is reduced in genetically affected, but phenotypically normal patients with normal wall thickness and ejection fraction, well before symptoms occur (62,63). Similarly, E′ is lower than normal in cardiac amyloidosis, cardiac involvement in Friedreich ataxia, or Fabry disease before these diseases become symptomatic or detectable by conventional echo (64–67).

Right Heart Function and Pulmonary Hypertension

Right heart output can be calculated at the pulmonary valve level by multiplying the pulmonary time velocity integral by the orifice area of the pulmonary valve ($\pi d^2/4$ where d is the diameter of the pulmonary annulus). The presence of chronic or acute pulmonary hypertension is easiest to assess from tricuspid regurgitation (see above). Another useful index is pulmonary systolic flow acceleration time (the time from the onset of transvalvular flow to peak velocity). Acceleration time decreases with increasing pulmonary pressures from normal values of 130 ± 15 ms. The ratio of right ventricular preejection time (interval from Q wave to onset of pulmonary flow) to acceleration time has been shown to correlate well with mean pulmonary pressure, with values above 1.2 indicating pulmonary hypertension (68). In acute severe pulmonary embolism, systolic right ventricular pressures may be only modestly elevated to right ventricular failure.

Coronary Artery Disease

In acute myocardial ischemia, impairment of left ventricular relaxation precedes systolic wall motion abnormalities. Acute

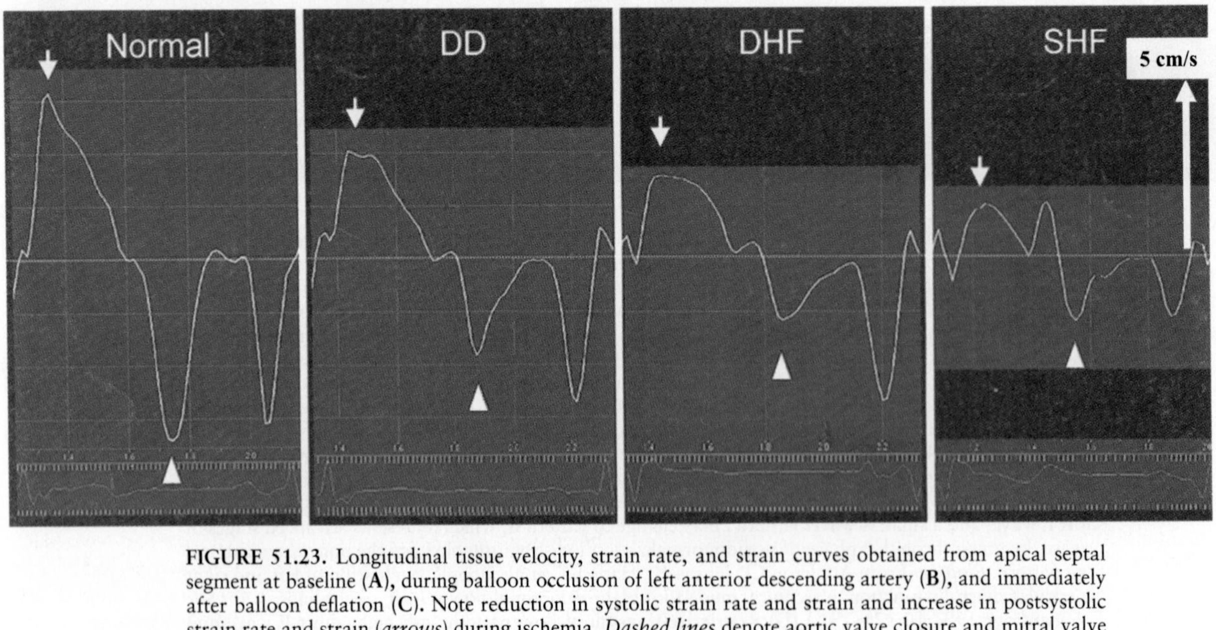

FIGURE 51.23. Longitudinal tissue velocity, strain rate, and strain curves obtained from apical septal segment at baseline (**A**), during balloon occlusion of left anterior descending artery (**B**), and immediately after balloon deflation (**C**). Note reduction in systolic strain rate and strain and increase in postsystolic strain rate and strain (*arrows*) during ischemia. *Dashed lines* denote aortic valve closure and mitral valve opening. (*Source:* From Kukulski T, Jamal F, D'Hooge J, et al. Acute changes in systolic and diastolic events during clinical coronary angioplasty: a comparison of regional velocity, strain rate and strain measurement. *J Am Soc Echocardiogr* 2002;15:1–12, with permission.)

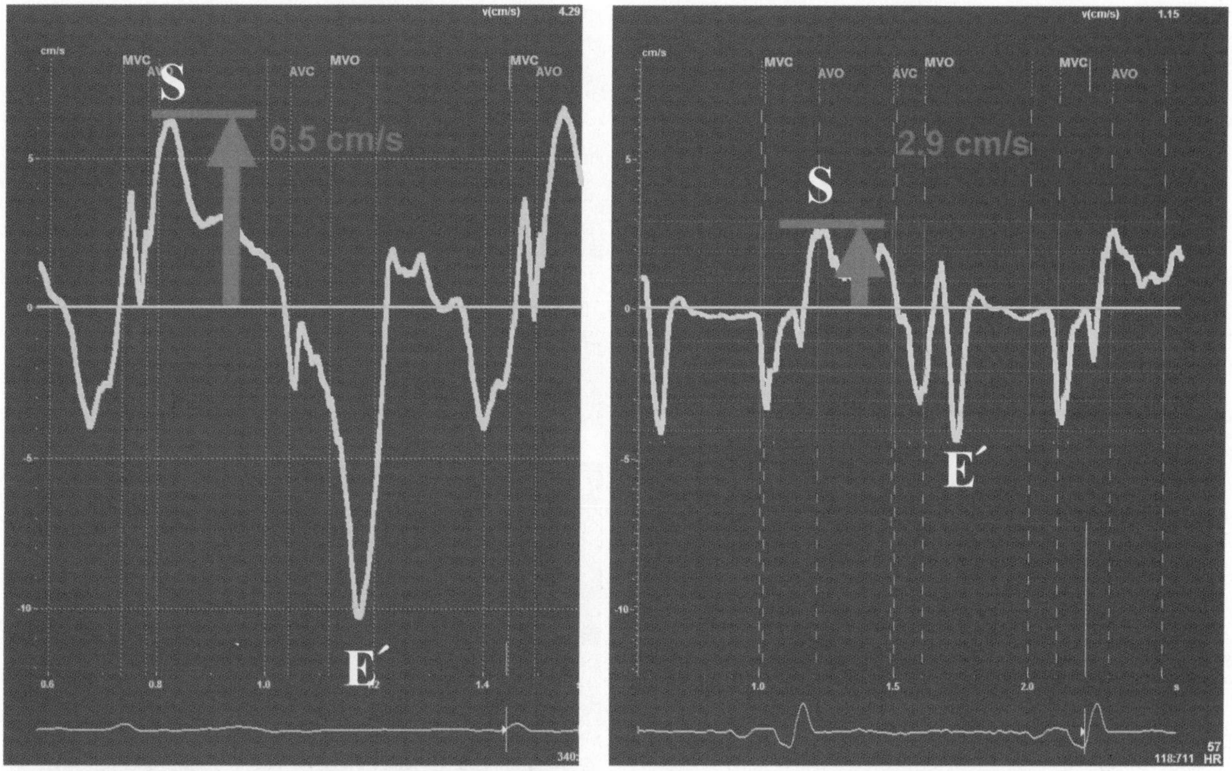

FIGURE 51.24. (**A**) Left ventricular pseudoaneurysm (*arrows*) after inferior infarction. Transgastric short axis view in systole and diastole. *Abbreviation:* LV, left ventricle. (**B**) Flow into (filling, upward, in systole) and out of the pseudoaneurysm (emptying, downward, in diastole) is recorded by pulsed Doppler.

transmitral E/A ratio decrease has been documented during percutaneous transluminal coronary angiographic balloon inflation (69) and stress-induced ischemia (70). Tissue velocities decrease during ischemia (Fig. 51.26). Because of tethering by adjacent segments, however, there is a large overlap between normal and ischemic tissue velocities, especially if ischemia is not severe. Nevertheless, tissue velocities can be used to detect inducible ischemia during stress echo (71). An attractive technique is deformation imaging, because it detects truly local changes in myocardial deformation and is largely unaffected by tethering. During ischemia, systolic strain decreases and contraction progressively lasts into early mechanical diastole (after aortic valve closure), a phenomenon called *postsystolic shortening,* which can be detected during dobutamine stress echo and aid in the detection of inducible ischemia (72) (Fig. 51.27). Although a modest percentage of postsystolic shortening can occur in normal segments, significant post-systolic shortening (>30% of total deformation) is typical for acute ischemia (73). For assessment of global systolic and diastolic function, see the corresponding sections. DE has an important role in the identification of structural complications of myocardial infarction, especially in septal rupture leading to a ventricular septal defect located mostly in the apical septum, and in acute mitral regurgitation after papillary muscle rupture. In left ventricular pseudoaneurysm, recordings at the rupture site may reveal biphasic flow, with flow into the pseudoaneurysm during both systole and after atrial contraction, and flow from the pseudoaneurysm into the ventricle during early to mid-diastole (74) (Fig. 51.28).

Direct evaluation of flow in the proximal left coronary artery is possible by transesophageal echocardiography. The proximal left anterior descending artery often can be interrogated by pulsed DE, showing the typical coronary flow signal with diastolic predominance. Transthoracic interrogation of the distal left anterior descending and right coronary artery is also feasible. Hemodynamically significant stenosis of these arteries or restenosis after intervention can be diagnosed by lack of increase in flow after adenosine (75,76). Similarly, flow in left internal mammary grafts (from the supraclavicular groove) and also venous grafts (from the second to fourth left intercostal space) has been successfully evaluated transthoracically (77).

Cardiomyopathies, Constrictive Pericarditis, and the Transplanted Heart

Dilated Cardiomyopathy

Apart from measuring a reduced cardiac output, DE examination is useful to estimate systolic pulmonary pressure by the peak tricuspid regurgitation velocity (see section on Right Heart Function and Pulmonary Hypertension), to assess mitral regurgitation, and to evaluate the transmitral filling pattern. A restrictive pattern (E/A > 1.5, E wave deceleration time <150 ms; see Fig. 51.25D) indicates high filling pressures and a reduced left ventricular compliance and is associated with a poor prognosis (55,56).

Hypertrophic Cardiomyopathy

The main task of the DE examination is to detect and assess left ventricular outflow obstruction. Hypertrophic obstructive cardiomyopathy characteristically produces a saber-shaped, late peaking systolic velocity profile in the left ventricular outflow tract well different from the (mostly also present) mitral regurgitation in the continuous wave DE examination in the apical long axis view (Fig. 51.29). The diagnosis can be confirmed by

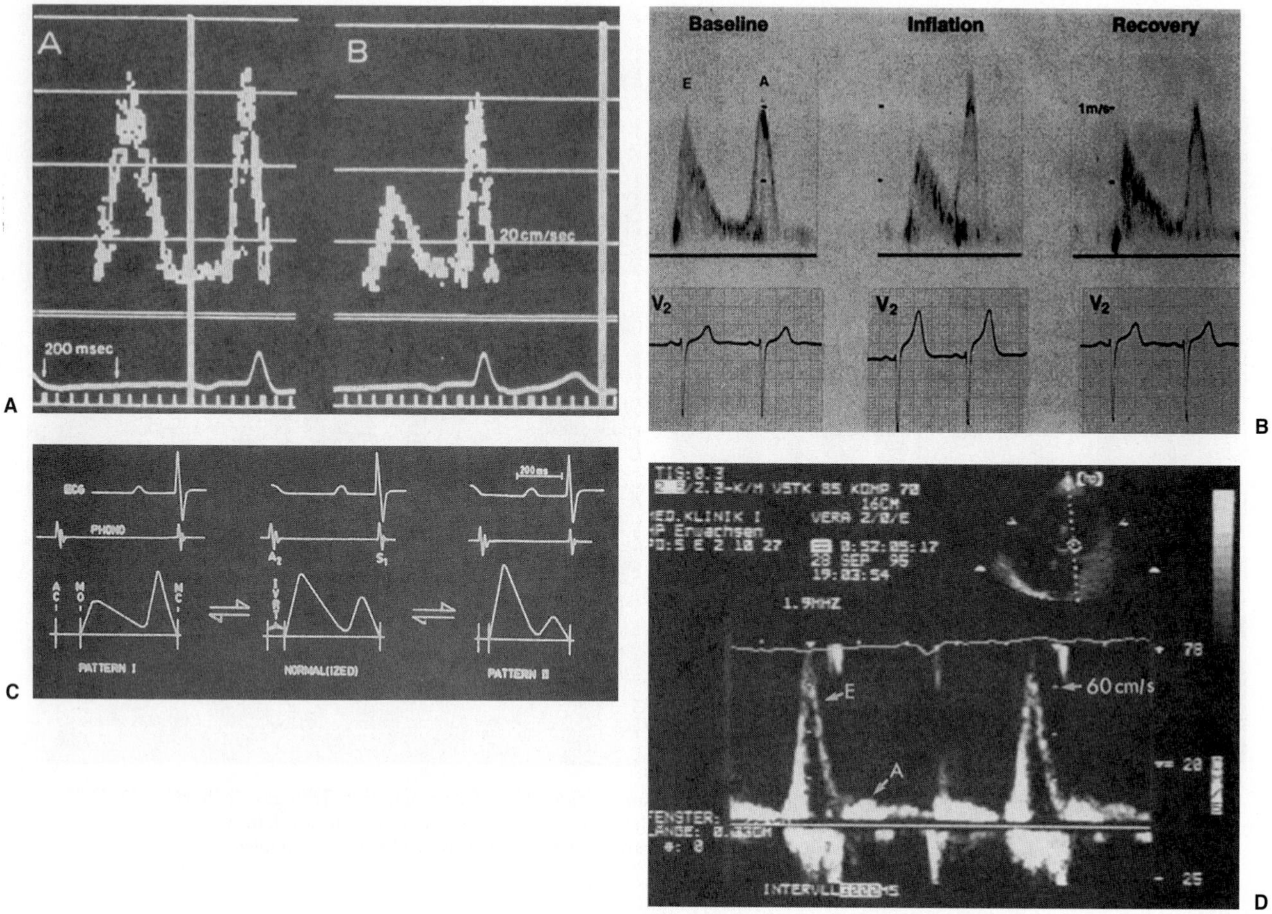

FIGURE 51.25. Examples of ischemic and nonischemic stress response. *Left,* baseline; *right,* peak stress. *Dotted vertical lines* indicate mitral and aortic valve opening and closure, aortic valve opening. (**A**) Two-chamber views with color-coded strain rate overlay and perfusion scintigraphy images in matching orientation. There is stress-induced inferoapical ischemia (*red arrow*). Markers *apical* and *basal* indicate where strain rate and strain curves (*below*) were recorded. (**B**) Strain rate. Typical nonischemic patterns at baseline and in basal curve at peak stress. In ischemic apical region, note delayed onset and end of shortening and low peak systolic strain rate at peak stress. (**C**) Strain curves. Note early systolic bulging (*arrow*) and marked PSS in inferoapical curve at peak stress. Other curves show typical nonischemic patterns. (**D**) ECG. (*Source:* From Voigt JU, Exner B, Schmiedehausen K, et al. Strain rate imaging during dobutamine stress echocardiography provides objective evidence of inducible ischemia. *Circulation* 2003;107:2120–2126, with permission.)

moving the sample volume of the pulsed Doppler systematically along the interventricular septum from the midventricle to the aortic valve to map the velocities toward the aortic valve, as well as by color Doppler evidence of turbulent flow in the outflow tract. Tissue DE can detect hypertrophic cardiomyopathies at an early stage, before hypertrophy is evident on 2D echo (62,63,66,67). The hallmark is reduced E′ and peak systolic tissue velocity in the basal segments of the left ventricular walls.

Constrictive Pericarditis and Restrictive Cardiomyopathy

The transmitral flow profile in these cardiomyopathies is characterized by tall, short E waves and small A waves (the "restrictive" pattern) and a short isovolumic relaxation time. In constrictive pericarditis, but not in restrictive cardiomyopathy, accentuated influence of respiration on cardiac flow velocities is present: during inspiration, transmitral flow velocities decrease (more than the normal approximately 10% decrease), transtricuspid flow velocities increase, and left ventricular relaxation time also increases (78) (Fig. 51.30). Profiles should be recorded at a slow sweep speed to obtain several respiration cycles on one sweep. The pulmonary venous diastolic flow in constrictive pericarditis mirrors the transmitral E wave behavior. Tissue velocities, particularly E′, are high in constrictive pericarditis, aiding in differentiating this condition from restrictive cardiomyopathy.

Restrictive cardiomyopathy (e.g., cardiac amyloidosis) exhibits no marked respiratory variation in mitral flow velocities and is characterized by particularly short mitral and tricuspid deceleration times. Often, diastolic mitral and tricuspid regurgitation are present following the E wave. There is usually at least moderate pulmonary hypertension, and ventricular walls are frequently thickened (e.g., in cardiac amyloidosis, which represents the most frequent and classical form of restrictive cardiomyopathy). Systolic and early diastolic (E′) tissue velocities are reduced early in the disease and can be utilized for diagnosis of preclinical cardiac amyloidosis (64).

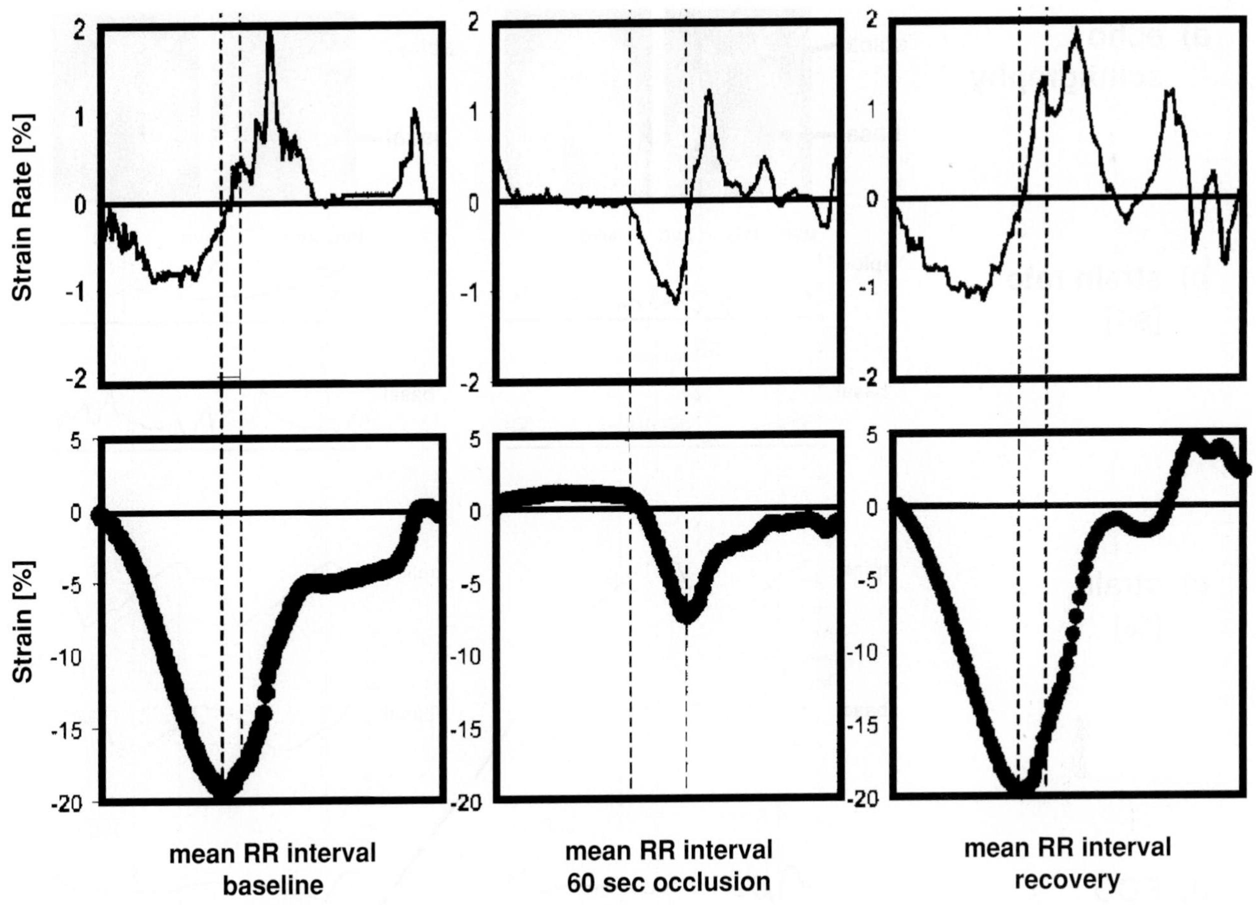

FIGURE 51.26. Left ventricular outflow tract obstruction in hypertrophic obstructive cardiomyopathy recorded by continuous wave DE. Typical profile with a late systolic peak.

The Transplanted Heart

Patients with a transplanted heart almost always present mild or moderate mitral and tricuspid regurgitation. If the residual native atria still are electrically and mechanically active, two distinct and dissociated A waves may be recorded on pulsed DE transmitral or tricuspid flow profiles. The noninvasive detection of graft rejection by DE remains a problem. Because alterations in systolic function ensue only late in the course of rejection, several diastolic parameters have been analyzed for this purpose. A decrease in isovolumic relaxation time and a decrease in E wave deceleration time have been associated with acute rejection and are reversible after treatment. In a small subset of patients, a chronic "restrictive physiology" develops. Because all of these parameters are multifactorial and especially preload dependent, there is no definitive set of values reliably identifying acute rejection, but serial follow-up in a given patient seems to allow the noninvasive detection of at least moderate acute rejection by observing changes in isovolumic relaxation time and in E wave deceleration with reasonable sensitivity and specificity. A decrease of tissue velocities has been reported to have high diagnostic sensitivity for rejection if serial measurements in individual patients are performed (79).

LEFT ATRIAL APPENDAGE FLOW

In sinus rhythm, the left atrial appendage shows four brief flow waves by transesophageal DE: a small emptying wave in early diastole and a larger one during atrial contraction after the P wave of the ECG. Both emptying waves are followed by a filling wave of similar velocity. Peak emptying and filling velocities occur immediately before and after the QRS complex. In nonvalvular atrial fibrillation, although the transmitral A wave is absent, emptying and filling velocities of the appendage are still well detectable, because the appendage encloses a very small blood volume, on which the decreased wall motion during fibrillation still imparts enough acceleration to create inward and outward flow. In patients with large atria, especially in mitral stenosis, and in rare cases of left atrial appendage standstill in sinus rhythm, these velocities are close to 0, indicating a high thromboembolic risk. Appendage flow velocities stratify the thrombo-embolic risk of patients with nonvalvular atrial fibrillation, with peak velocities of less than 25 cm/second, indicating a higher risk (80).

CARDIAC TAMPONADE

The DE characteristics of cardiac tamponade resemble those of constrictive pericarditis. There is a marked (30%–40%) inspiratory decrease of transmitral, transaortic, and diastolic pulmonary venous inflow velocities (corresponding to the clinical finding of pulsus paradoxus), and an even more pronounced (>80%) inspiratory increase in transtricuspid (and transpulmonic) flow velocities. Left ventricular isovolumic relaxation time increases in inspiration.

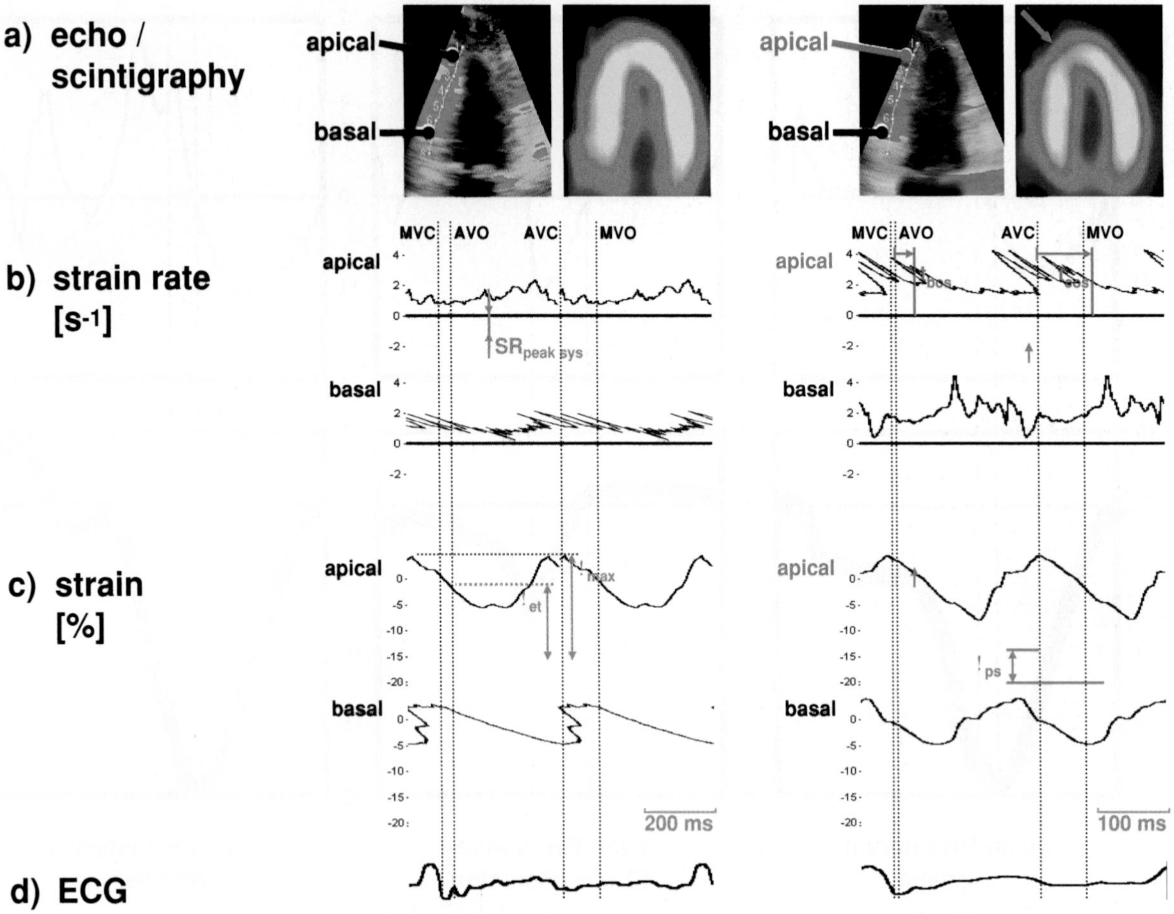

FIGURE 51.27. Transmitral flow profiles in constrictive pericarditis. A "restrictive" transmitral flow pattern with high and short E waves is seen. Peak E wave velocities show pathologic respiratory variation (>10%) with a decrease during inspiration (INSP).

ASSESSMENT OF INTERVENTRICULAR AND INTRAVENTRICULAR DYSSYNCHRONY AND SELECTION OF CANDIDATES FOR CARDIAC RESYNCHRONIZATION THERAPY

Traditionally, presence left bundle branch block and long QRS duration have defined candidates for cardiac resynchronization therapy (CRT; see Chapter 75). It is intuitively attractive, however, to assess the potential mechanical benefit from CRT (improvement in cardiac output), by echocardiographically evaluating mechanical dyssynchrony. Conceptually, dyssynchrony can be divided into

1. *Interventricular dyssynchrony.* The time delay between left and right ventricular ejection can be easily assessed by comparing the timing of flow in the right and left outflow tracts by pulsed DE. A delay of 40 ms, with the left ventricle trailing the right, is considered sufficiently large to support interventricular resynchronization by appropriate left ventricular or biventricular pacing.
2. *Intraventricular dyssynchrony.* In classic left bundle branch block, the lateral wall of the left ventricle contracts later than the septum and the other walls of the left ventricle. In advanced heart failure with asynchronously contracting left ventricles, however, regional timing of contraction often does not follow simple patterns. To evaluate whether left ventricular free wall pacing will improve mechanical efficiency, several approaches have been proposed and to some extent validated:
   a. The delay between anteroseptal wall contraction and posterior wall contraction by M-mode, with a cut-off of 130 ms (81).
   b. The standard deviation of the time to peak systolic tissue velocity at the base of all six left ventricular walls (82). A cut-off of 33 ms predicts benefit from CRT.
   c. Postsystolic (after aortic valve closure) shortening or "delayed longitudinal contraction" (83).
   d. Timing of regional left ventricular inward motion of endocardium by 3D echocardiography and semiautomated boundary detection.

At the present time, however, none of these criteria have been evaluated in a large number of patients, or with respect to clinical outcomes.

CONTROVERSIES AND PERSONAL PERSPECTIVES

Although a tremendous success story, some problems in the echo DE assessment of valvular stenosis and regurgitation remain. One fundamental limitation in the present quantitative

A
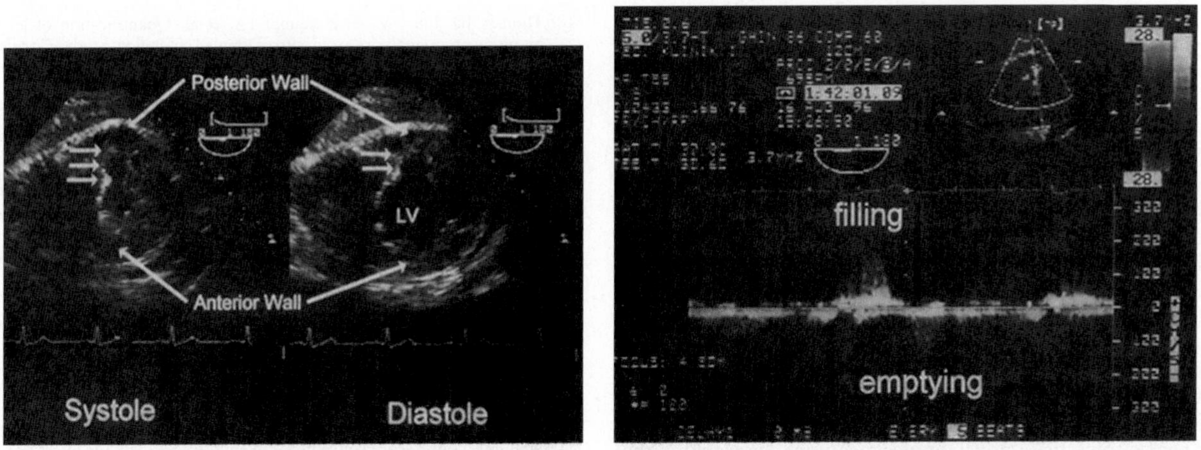

B

FIGURE 51.28. Normal regurgitant flow patterns of mechanical valves. (**A**) St. Jude Medical bileaflet prosthesis. Normal regurgitation mainly occurs at the hinge points of the leaflets. *Left:* Schematic drawing. *Right:* Flow imaging by transesophageal color Doppler. (**B**) Medtronic–Hall tilting-disc prosthesis. Normal regurgitation mainly occurs across the central orifice. *Left:* Schematic drawing. *Right:* In the closed position, a normal central transvalvular regurgitation (NTVR) and a medial small paravalvular leak (PVL) are seen. SR sewing ring. (**C**) Björk–Shiley tilting-disc prosthesis in the mitral position with small peripheral normal regurgitant jets occurring between occluder and valve ring. *Abbreviations:* LA, left atrium; LV, left ventricle; RV, right ventricle; RA, right atrium. (*Source:* From Flachskampf FA, Guerrero JL, O'Shea JP, et al. Patterns of normal transvalvular regurgitation in mechanical valve prostheses. *J Am Coll Cardiol* 1991;18:1493–1498.)

DE approaches to regurgitation is the characterization of spatially complex 3D flow velocity fields in the heart by limited, mostly 2D data. For instance, a single pulsed Doppler sample volume is used in transvalvular flow rate calculations. These problems may ultimately be overcome by real-time, 3D multigated pulsed Doppler. In the assessment of stenotic lesions, future 3D echo capabilities could help to solve the pressure recovery dilemma and reconcile the discrepancies between effective and geometric orifice areas by combining spatial morphologic and functional data. However, it is mostly the effect on myocardial function rather than the valvular lesion per se that clinically matters most, in particular in chronic regurgitant lesions. Thus, the quest for the single magic number representing the severity of a valvular lesion is misleading. The advent of tissue DE has enabled us to look at myocardial contraction and relaxation with very high time resolution, generating new insights into the effects of ischemia and cardiomyopathy. The diagnostic power of assessing myocardial mechanics will soon be potentiated by speckle-tracking techniques, which theoretically allow following myocardial structures in all three spatial dimensions. A unified diagnostic approach to the noninvasive diagnosis of myocardial function is emerging, together with the understanding of systolic and diastolic function as different aspects of one myocardial function. Early detection of cardiomyopathies and other myocardial diseases before symptoms or morphologic abnormalities occur begins to be possible, potentially affecting management of relatives of patients with manifest cardiomyopathy.

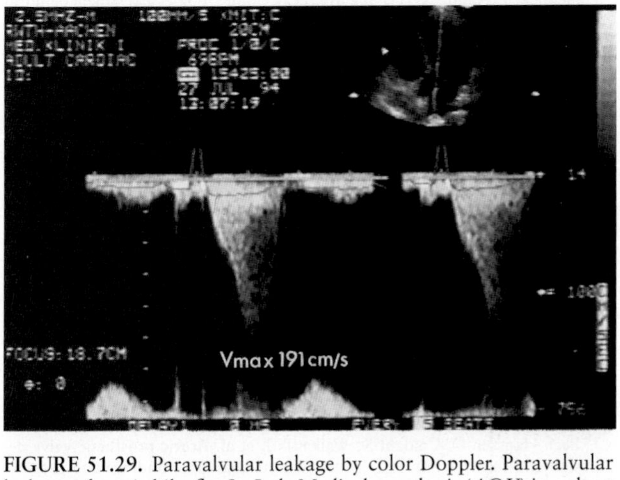

FIGURE 51.29. Paravalvular leakage by color Doppler. Paravalvular leakage of aortic bileaflet St. Jude Medical prosthesis (*AOV*) in a short axis (*left*) and long axis (*right*) transesophageal view. The leakage cross-section and the paravalvular path of the leakage are well seen. *Abbreviations:* RVOT, right ventricular outflow tract; AOA, ascending aorta. (*Source:* From Flachskampf FA, Hoffmann R, Verlande M, et al. Initial experience with a multiplane transesophageal echo-transducer: assessment of diagnostic potential. *Eur Heart J* 1992;13:1201–1206.)

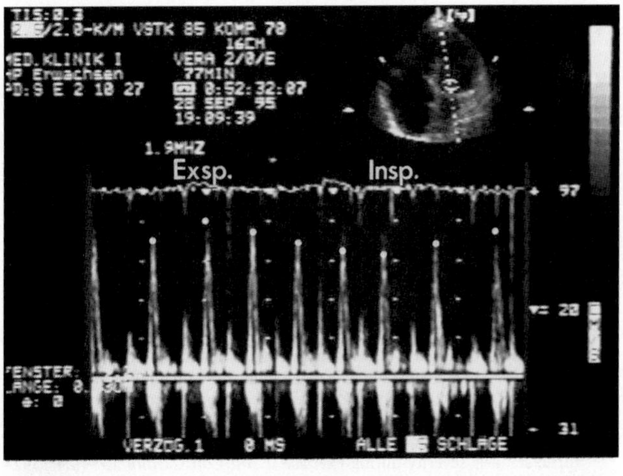

FIGURE 51.30. Proximal convergence zone in a paravalvular leak of a Björk–Shiley mitral prosthesis. The regurgitant jet in the left atrium (*right*) is obscured by prosthetic artifacts. However, the proximal convergence zone (*arrows*) is clearly visible on the ventricular side.

THE FUTURE

Several important technical improvements are on the horizon of blood flow DE, including:

1. "Unwrapping" of high velocities enabling to fully map the velocity field of regurgitant jets. Thus, jet momentum could be calculated, and because momentum is conserved in the cross-sections of a jet, flow rate at the regurgitant orifice can be derived. Moreover, measurement of the length of the jet's laminar core might allow to estimate regurgitant orifice size (14).
2. Automated integration of color Doppler velocities in two or three dimensions and 3D DE of proximal convergence zone.
3. Use of Doppler power (amplitude squared) for flow calculations (84).
4. Speckle tracking, a non-Doppler technique, by tracking the spatial path of tiny ensembles of reflectors theoretically promises angle-independent velocimetry in all dimensions.

Tissue DE so far is limited to velocities in the direction of the echo beam. Speckle tracking may enable 2D and 3D deformation imaging, thus more faithfully describing myocardial mechanics. This as well as the use of matrix arrays will enable true 3D representation of blood flow and tissue mechanics and further improve the diagnosis of ischemia and cardiomyopathy, as well as detection of the subtle abnormalities in early hypertension, diabetes, valvular heart disease, and other conditions.

References

1. Doppler C. *Über das farbige Licht der Doppelsterne und einiger anderer Gestirne des Himmels*. Abhandlungen der Königlich-Böhmischen Gesellschaft der Wissenschaften. 1842; 2.Band, 5.Folge; pp. 465–483.
2. Satomura S. Ultrasonic Doppler method for the inspection of cardiac functions. *J Acoust Soc Am* 1957;29:1181–1185.
3. Franklin DL, Schlegal WA, Rushmer RF. Blood flow measured by Doppler frequency shift of backscattered ultrasound. *Science* 1961;134:564–565.
4. Peronneau P, Deloche A, Bui-Mong-Hung, et al. Debitmetrie ultrasonore: Développements et applications expérimentales. *Eur Surg Res* 1969;1:147–156.
5. Baker DW. Pulsed ultrasonic Doppler blood-flow sensing. *IEEE Trans Sonics Ultrasonics* 1970;SU-17:170–185.
6. Holen J, Aaslid R, Landmark K, et al. Determination of pressure gradient in mitral stenosis with a non-invasive ultrasound Doppler technique. *Acta Med Scand* 1976;19:455–460.
7. Hatle L, Angelsen BA, Tromsdal A. Non-invasive assessment of aortic stenosis by Doppler ultrasound. *Br Heart J* 1980;43:284–292.
8. Brandestini MA, Howard EA, Weiler EB, et al. The synthesis of echo and Doppler in M-mode and sector scan. *Proc Annu Meet AIUM* 1979;125:704.
9. Namekawa K, Kasai C, Koyano A. Imaging of blood flow using autocorrelation. *Ultrasound Med Biol* 1982;8:138.
10. Bommer W, Miller L. Real-time two-dimensional color flow Doppler-enhanced imaging in the diagnosis of cardiovascular disease. *Am J Cardiol* 1982;49:944.
11. Kasai C, Namekawa K, Koyano A, et al. Real-time two dimensional blood flow imaging using an autocorrelation technique. *IEEE Trans Son Ultrason* 1985;32:458.
12. Side CD, Gosling RG. Non-surgical assessment of cardiac function. *Nature* 1971;232:335–336.
13. McDicken WN, Sutherland GR, Moran CM, et al. Colour Doppler velocity imaging of the myocardium. *Ultrasound Med Biol* 1992;18:651–654.
14. Diebold B, Delouche A, Delouche P, et al. A In vitro flow mapping of regurgitant jets. Systematic description of free jet with laser Doppler velocimetry. *Circulation* 1996;94:158–169.
15. Recusani F, Bargiggia GS, Yoganathan AP, et al. A new method for quantification of regurgitant flow rate using color flow imaging of the flow convergence region proximal to a discrete orifice: an in vitro study. *Circulation* 1991;83:594–604.
16. Burwash IG, Pearlman AS, Kraft CD, et al. Flow dependence of measures of aortic stenosis severity during exercise. *J Am Coll Cardiol* 1994;24:1342–1350.
17. Voelker W, Reul H, Nienhaus G, et al. Comparison of valvular resistance, stroke work loss, and Gorlin valve area for quantification of aortic stenosis. An in vitro study in a pulsatile aortic flow model. *Circulation* 1995;91:1196–1204.
18. Thomas JD, Liu CM, Flachskampf FA, et al. Quantification of jet flow by momentum analysis: an in vitro Doppler color flow study. *Circulation* 1990;81:247–259.
19. Chen C, Thomas JD, Anconina J, et al. Impact of impinging wall jet on color Doppler quantification of mitral regurgitation. *Circulation* 1991;84:712–720.
20. Zoghbi WA, Enriquez-Sarano M, Foster E, et al. Recommendations for evaluation of the severity of native valvular regurgitation with two-dimensional and Doppler echocardiography. *J Am Soc Echocardiogr* 2003;16:777–802.
21. Schwammenthal E, Chen C, Benning F, et al. Dynamics of mitral regurgitant flow and orifice area. Physiologic application of the proximal flow convergence method: clinical data and experimental testing. *Circulation* 1994;90:307–322.
22. Reimold SC, Maier SE, Fleischmann KE, et al. Dynamic nature of the aortic regurgitant orifice area during diastole in patients with chronic aortic regurgitation. *Circulation* 1994;89:2085–2092.
23. Rodriguez L, Thomas JD, Monterroso V, et al. Validation of the proximal flow convergence method: calculation of orifice area in patients with mitral stenosis. *Circulation* 1993;88:1157–1165.
24. Tribouilloy CM, Enriquez-Sarano M, Fett SL, et al. Application of the proximal flow convergence convergence method to calculate the effective regurgitant orifice area in aortic regurgitation. *J Am Coll Cardiol* 1998;32:1032–1039.
25. Quinones MA, Otto CM, Stoddard M, et al. Recommendations for quantification of Doppler echocardiography: a report from the Doppler Quantification Task Force of the Nomenclature and Standards Committee of the American Society of Echocardiography. *J Am Soc Echocardiogr* 2002;15:167–184.
26. Derumeaux G, Ovize M, Loufoua J, et al. Assessment of nonuniformity of transmural myocardial velocities by color-coded tissue Doppler imaging: characterization of normal, ischemic, and stunned myocardium. *Circulation* 2000;101:1390–1395.
27. Flachskampf FA, Decoodt P, Fraser AG, et al. Recommendations for performing transesophageal echocardiography. *Eur J Echocardiogr* 2001;2:8–21.
28. Yamada S, Komuro K, Mikami T, et al. Novel quantitative assessment of myocardial perfusion by harmonic power Doppler imaging during myocardial contrast echocardiography. *Heart* 2005;91:183–188.
29. Baumgartner H, Stefenelli T, Niederberger J, et al. "Overestimation" of catheter gradients by Doppler ultrasound in patients with aortic stenosis: a predictable manifestation of pressure recovery. *J Am Coll Cardiol* 1999;33:1655–1661.
30. Garcia D, Pibarot P, Dumesnil JG, et al. Assessment of aortic valve stenosis severity. A new index based on the energy loss concept. *Circulation* 2000;101:765–771
31. deFilippi CR, Willett DL, Brickner ME, et al. Usefulness of dobutamine echocardiography in distinguishing severe from nonsevere valvular aortic stenosis in patients with depressed left ventricular function and low transvalvular gradients. *Am J Cardiol* 1995;75:191–194.
32. Monin JL, Quéré JP, Monchi M, et al. Low-gradient aortic stenosis. Operative risk stratification and predictors for long-term outcome: a multicenter study using dobutamine stress hemodynamics. *Circulation* 2003;108:319–324.
33. Perry GJ, Helmcke F, Nanda, NC, et al. Evaluation of aortic insufficiency by Doppler color flow mapping. *J Am Coll Cardiol* 1987;9:952–959.
34. Tribouilloy C, Avinee P, Shen WF, et al. End diastolic flow velocity just beneath the aortic isthmus assessed by pulsed Doppler echocardiography: a new predictor of the aortic regurgitant fraction. *Br Heart J* 1991;65:37–40.
35. Helmcke F, Nanda NC Hsiung MC, et al. Color Doppler assessment of mitral regurgitation with orthogonal planes. *Circulation* 1987;75:175–183.
36. Tribouilloy C, Shen WF, Quéré JP, et al. Assessment of severity of mitral regurgitation by measuring regurgitant jet width at its origin with transesophageal Doppler color flow imaging. *Circulation* 1992;85:1248–1253.
37. Mele D, Vandervoort P, Palacios I, et al. Proximal jet size by Doppler color flow mapping predicts severity of mitral regurgitation. Clinical studies. *Circulation* 1995;91:746–754.
38. Rivera JM, Vandervoort PM, Thoreau DH, et al. Quantification of mitral regurgitation with the proximal flow convergence method: a clinical study. *Am Heart J* 1992;124:1289–1296.
39. Hatle L, Angelsen B, Tromsdal A. Noninvasive assessment of atrioventricular pressure half-time by Doppler ultrasound. *Circulation* 1989;6:1096–1104.
40. Flachskampf FA, Weyman AE, Gillam L, et al. Aortic regurgitation shortens Doppler pressure half-time in mitral stenosis: theoretical analysis, in vitro modelling, and clinical evidence. *J Am Coll Cardiol* 1990;16:396–404.
41. Flachskampf FA, Weyman AE, Guerrero JL, et al. Calculation of atrioventricular compliance from the mitral flow profile: analytical and in vitro study. *J Am Coll Cardiol* 1992;19:998–1004.
42. Thomas JD, Weyman AE. Doppler mitral pressure half-time: a clinical tool in search of theoretical justification. *J Am Coll Cardiol* 1987;10:923–929.
43. Bech-Hanssen O, Caidahl K, Wallentin I, et al. Aortic prosthetic valve design and size: relation to Doppler echocardiographic findings and pressure recovery—an in vitro study. *J Am Soc Echocardiogr* 2000;13:39–50.
44. Rosenhek R, Binder T, Maurer G, et al. Normal values for Doppler echocardiographic assessment of heart valve prostheses. *J Am Soc Echocardiogr* 2003;16:1116–1127.
45. Baumgartner H, Khan S, DeRobertis M, et al. Discrepancies between Doppler and catheter gradients in aortic prosthetic valves in vitro. A manifestation of localized gradients and pressure recovery. *Circulation* 1990;82:1467–1475.

46. Baumgartner H, Schima H, Kühn P. Effect of prosthetic valve malfunction on the Doppler-catheter gradient relation for bileaflet aortic valve prostheses. *Circulation* 1993;87:1320–1327.
47. Chafizadeh ER, Zoghbi WA. Doppler echocardiographic assessment of the St. Jude Medical prosthetic valve in the aortic position using the continuity equation. *Circulation* 1991;83:213–223.
48. Flachskampf FA, Guerrero JL, O'Shea JP, et al. Patterns of normal transvalvular regurgitation in mechanical valve prostheses. *J Am Coll Cardiol* 1991;18:1493–1498.
49. Flachskampf FA, Hoffmann R, Franke A, et al. Does multiplane transesophageal echocardiography improve the assessment of prosthetic valve regurgitation? *J Am Soc Echocardiogr* 1995;8:70–78.
50. Yoshida K, Yoshikawa J, Akasaka T, et al. Value of acceleration flow signals proximal to the leaking orifice in assessing the severity of prosthetic mitral valve regurgitation. *J Am Coll Cardiol* 1992;19:333–338.
51. Bargiggia GS, Bertucci C, Recusani F, et al. A new method for estimating left ventricular dP/dt by continuous wave Doppler echocardiography: validation studies at catheterization. *Circulation* 1989;80:1287–1292.
52. Oh JK, Appleton CP, Hatle LK, et al. The noninvasive assessment of left ventricular diastolic function with two-dimensional and Doppler echocardiography. *J Am Soc Echocardiogr* 1997;10:246–270.
53. Oh JK, Ding ZP, Gersh BJ, et al. Restrictive left ventricular diastolic filling identifies patients with heart failure after acute myocardial infarction. *J Am Soc Echocardiogr* 1992;5:497–503.
54. Pozzoli M, Capomolla S, Sanarico M, et al. Doppler evaluations of left ventricular diastolic filling and pulmonary wedge pressure provide similar prognostic information in patients with systolic dysfunction after myocardial infarction. *Am Heart J* 1995;129:716–725.
55. Pinamonti B, Di Lenarda A, Sinagra G, et al. Restrictive left ventricular filling pattern in dilated cardiomyopathy assessed by Doppler echocardiography: clinical, echocardiographic and hemodynamic correlations and prognostic implications. *J Am Coll Cardiol* 1993;22:808–815.
56. Vanoverschelde JLJ, Raphael DA, Robert AR, et al. Left ventricular filling in dilated cardiomyopathy: Relation to functional class and hemodynamics. *J Am Coll Cardiol* 1990;15:1288–1295.
57. Klein AL, Hatle LK, Taliercio CP, et al. Prognostic significance of Doppler measures of diastolic function in cardiac amyloidosis. A Doppler echocardiographic study. *Circulation* 1991;83:808–816.
58. Rossvoll O, Hatle L. Pulmonary venous flow velocities recorded by transthoracic Doppler ultrasound: relation to left ventricular diastolic pressures. *J Am Coll Cardiol* 1993;21:1687–1696.
59. Stugaard M, Smiseth OA, Risöe C, et al. Intraventricular early diastolic filling during acute myocardial ischemia. Assessment by multigated color M-mode Doppler echocardiography. *Circulation* 1993;88:2705–2713.
60. Nagueh SF, Middleton KJ, Kopelen HA, et al. Doppler tissue imaging: a noninvasive technique for evaluation of left ventricular relaxation and estimation of filling pressures. *J Am Coll Cardiol* 1997;30:1527–1533.
61. Nagueh SF, Mikati I, Kopelen HA, et al. Doppler estimation of left ventricular filling pressure in sinus tachycardia. A new application of tissue Doppler imaging. *Circulation* 1998;98:1644–1650.
62. Nagueh SF, Lakkis NM, Middleton KJ, et al. Doppler estimation of left ventricular filling pressures in patients with hypertrophic cardiomyopathy. *Circulation* 1999;99:254–261.
63. Ho CY, Sweitzer NK, McDonough B, et al. Assessment of diastolic function with Doppler tissue imaging to predict genotype in preclinical hypertrophic cardiomyopathy. *Circulation* 2002;105:2992–2997.
64. Koyama J, Ray-Sequin PA, Falk RH. Longitudinal myocardial function assessed by tissue velocity, strain, and strain rate tissue Doppler echocardiography in patients with AL (primary) cardiac amyloidosis. *Circulation* 2003;107:2446–2452.
65. Dutka DP, Donnelly E, Palka P, et al. Echocardiographic characterization of cardiomyopathy in Friedreich's ataxia with tissue Doppler echocardiographically derived myocardial velocity gradients. *Circulation* 2002;102:1276–1282.
66. Weidemann F, Breunig F, Beer M, et al. Improvement of cardiac function during enzyme replacement therapy in patients with Fabry disease: a prospective strain rate imaging study. *Circulation* 2003;108:1299–1301.
67. Pieroni M, Chimenti C, Ricci R, et al. Early detection of Fabry cardiomyopathy by tissue Doppler imaging. *Circulation* 2003;107:1978–1984.
68. Jiang L, Stewart WJ, King ME, et al. An improved method for estimation of pulmonary artery pressure using Doppler velocity time intervals. *J Am Coll Cardiol* 1984;3:613.
69. Labovitz AJ, Lewen MK, Morton K, et al. Evaluation of left ventricular systolic and diastolic dysfunction during transient myocardial ischemia produced by angioplasty. *J Am Coll Cardiol* 1987;10:748–755.
70. el-Said ES, Fioretti PM, Roelandt JR, et al. Dobutamine stress-Doppler echocardiography before and after coronary angioplasty. *Eur Heart J* 1993;14:1011–1021.
71. Madler CF, Payne N, Wilkenshoff U, et al. Myocardial Doppler in Stress Echocardiography (MYDISE) Study Investigators. Non-invasive diagnosis of coronary artery disease by quantitative stress echocardiography: optimal diagnostic models using off-line tissue Doppler in the MYDISE study. *Eur Heart J* 2003;24:1584–1594.
72. Voigt JU, Exner B, Schmiedehausen K, et al. Strain rate imaging during dobutamine stress echocardiography provides objective evidence of inducible ischemia. *Circulation* 2003;107:2120–2126.
73. Voigt JU, Lindenmeier G, Exner B, et al. Incidence and characteristics of segmental postsystolic longitudinal shortening in normal, acutely ischemic and scarred myocardium. *J Am Soc Echocardiogr* 2003;16:415–423.
74. Roelandt JRTC, Sutherland GR, Yoshida K, et al. Improved diagnosis and characterization of left ventricular pseudoaneurysm by Doppler color flow imaging. *J Am Coll Cardiol* 1988;807–811.
75. Lethen H, Tries HP, Brechtken J, et al. Comparison of transthoracic Doppler echocardiography to intracoronary Doppler guidewire measurements for assessment of coronary flow reserve in the left anterior descending artery for detection of restenosis after coronary angioplasty. *Am J Cardiol* 2003;91:412–417.
76. Lethen H, Tries HP, Kersting S, et al. Validation of noninvasive assessment of coronary flow velocity reserve in the right coronary artery. A comparison of transthoracic echocardiographic results with intracoronary Doppler flow wire measurements. *Eur Heart J* 2003;24:1567–1575.
77. Chirillo F, Bruni A, Balestra G, et al. Assessment of internal mammary artery and saphenous vein graft patency and flow reserve using transthoracic Doppler echocardiography. *Heart* 2001;86:424–431.
78. Hatle LK, Appleton CP, Popp RL. Differentiation of constrictive pericarditis and restrictive cardiomyopathy by Doppler echocardiography. *Circulation* 1989;79:357–370.
79. Dandel M, Hummel M, Muller J, et al. Reliability of tissue Doppler wall motion monitoring after heart transplantation for replacement of invasive routine screenings by optimally timed cardiac biopsies and catheterizations. *Circulation* 2001;104(12 Suppl 1):I184–I191.
80. Mügge A, Kühn H, Nikutta P, et al. Assessment of left atrial appendage function by biplane transesophageal echocardiography in patients with nonrheumatic atrial fibrillation: identification of a subgroup of patients at increased embolic risk. *J Am Coll Cardiol* 1994;23:599–607.
81. Pitzalis MV, Iacoviello M, Romito R, et al. Cardiac resynchronization therapy tailored by echocardiographic evaluation of ventricular asynchrony. *J Am Coll Cardiol.* 2002;40:1615–1622.
82. Yu CM, Fung WH, Lin H, et al. Predictors of left ventricular reverse remodeling after cardiac resynchronization therapy for heart failure secondary to idiopathic dilated or ischemic cardiomyopathy. *Am J Cardiol* 2003;91:684–688.
83. Sogaard P, Egeblad H, Kim WY, et al. Tissue Doppler imaging predicts improved systolic performance and reversed left ventricular remodeling during long-term cardiac resynchronization therapy. *J Am Coll Cardiol.* 2002;40:723–730.
84. Buck T, Mucci RA, Guerrero JL, et al. The power-velocity integral at the vena contracta. A new method for direct quantification of regurgitant volume flow. *Circulation* 2000;102:1053–1061.

CHAPTER 52 ■ TRANSESOPHAGEAL ECHOCARDIOGRAPHY

CHRISTIAN GRING AND BRIAN P. GRIFFIN

OVERVIEW

Transesophageal echocardiography (TEE) is a diagnostic ultrasound technique in which images of the heart are acquired from the esophagus rather than from the chest wall. The esophageal window has advantages over the transthoracic approach in that higher-resolution images, especially of posterior cardiac structures and the aorta, are possible, and acoustic shadowing from prosthetic material is less. TEE requires passage of the esophageal probe into the esophagus and stomach by using conscious sedation, and it has a finite if low risk of serious complications. It is usually performed when transthoracic echocardiography (TTE) has failed to resolve an important diagnostic question adequately. Standard planes in which to image the heart from the esophagus and stomach have been described. Multiplane transducers for adult and pediatric use with full Doppler capabilities are now widely available. TEE is frequently indicated for the evaluation of a possible cardiac source of embolism, assessment of native and prosthetic valves, endocarditis, evaluation of the left atrium and atrial septum, in disease of the thoracic aorta especially when acute dissection is suspected, and in patients with uninterpretable TTE studies. TEE is useful in the evaluation of patients with hemodynamic compromise in intensive care units, in adult congenital heart disease, in an assessment of the proximal coronary vasculature, and in interventional procedures such as balloon mitral valvuloplasty. Specific areas in which the superiority of TEE over TTE is best established and in which TEE is usually required for a complete evaluation include suspected prosthetic endocarditis, poorly characterized native or prosthetic regurgitation, aortic root abscess and other pyogenic complications of endocarditis, left atrial appendage thrombus, sinus venosus atrial septal defect, aortic dissection, and aortic atheroma.

TEE is an important tool in the evaluation of cardiac structure and function and in assessing the thoracic aorta. TEE images are acquired from an esophageal or gastric imaging window rather than from the chest wall (Table 52.1); thus, TEE usually permits higher-frequency and higher-resolution imaging than TTE. Moreover, the posterior windows avoid air-filled lung tissue and circumvent acoustic shadowing from strong reflectors of ultrasound such as prosthetic valves. Therefore, TEE is particularly powerful in imaging posterior structures such as the atria, the atrial appendages, the interatrial septum, and the aorta.

TEE is invasive and frequently requires local anesthesia and intravenous sedation. It is also more time consuming, more expensive, and less acceptable to patients than TTE. TTE can provide adequate clinical information in many instances and is therefore usually acquired first. TEE is performed if additional information is required or if transthoracic image quality is suboptimal. In most adult echocardiography laboratories, fewer than 10% of all studies are performed by the transesophageal approach (1,2). Major current indications for TEE are shown in Table 52.2.

ANATOMIC CONSIDERATIONS

The esophagus is approximately 25 cm in length and extends from the pharynx to the stomach. It descends vertically and slightly to the left, passing behind the trachea, left mainstem bronchus, left atrium, and left ventricle before passing through the diaphragm. The ascending aorta and arch lie anterior to the esophagus (Fig. 52.1). The air-filled trachea and left mainstem bronchus interpose between the esophagus and portion of the ascending aorta and ascending arch, causing a "blind spot"

TABLE 52.1

COMPARISON OF TRANSTHORACIC AND TRANSESOPHAGEAL ECHOCARDIOGRAPHY

	TTE	TEE
Imaging location	Chest wall, subcostal	Esophagus, stomach
Transducer frequency	2.0–5.0 MHz	3.5–7.0 MHz
Examination preparation	None	Sedation, anesthesia
Advantages	Widely applicable, noninvasive, multiple imaging windows, complete Doppler evaluation	High-resolution images, circumvents prosthetic shadowing, posterior structures (aorta, atria) well imaged
Disadvantages	Often suboptimal images, far-field structures (aorta, atria) and prostheses poorly imaged	Semiinvasive, imaging windows highly variable
Indications	Usually first-line cardiac ultrasound modality	When TTE fails to answer clinical question adequately

TEE, transesophageal echocardiography; TTE, transthoracic echocardiography.

in imaging the aorta from the transesophageal window. The esophagus twines around the descending aorta, and therefore the transducer must be rotated while imaging the descending aorta to keep the structure in view.

TECHNOLOGY: TRANSDUCERS AND PROBES

TEE requires the use of a special esophageal probe that interfaces with a conventional cardiac ultrasound system. The esophageal probes currently in use consist of an ultrasound transducer mounted at the end of a 100-cm flexible gastroscope from which the fiberoptic cables and suction capability have been removed. Adult transducers vary in length from 27 to 45 mm, are 14 to 17 mm wide, and are approximately 11 mm thick. The gastroscope cable is approximately 10 mm wide in adult probes, although 7-mm diameter probes are now available and allow imaging even in infants as small as 3 kg (3). Early-generation TEE systems used monoplane or biplane transducers (4,5); current systems, however, use multiplane phased arrays that allow the operator to rotate the transducer around a central axis through 180 degrees (5) (Fig. 52.2). The

TABLE 52.2

INDICATIONS FOR TRANSESOPHAGEAL ECHOCARDIOGRAPHY

1. Nondiagnostic TTE images	COPD, obesity, dressings preventing adequate TTE images
2. Atrial pathology and function	Atrial thrombus, spontaneous contrast, tumor
3. Interatrial septum	ASD, PFO, atrial septal aneurysm
4. Disease of thoracic aorta	Dissection, intramural hematoma, aortic trauma, atheroma
5. Endocarditis	Small vegetations, abscess, fistulae, prosthetic endocarditis
6. Native valve disease	Flail valves, severity of mitral regurgitation, aortic valve morphology
7. Prosthetic valves	Prosthetic regurgitation, thrombosis, suspected dysfunction
8. Source of embolus	Atrial thrombus, PFO, atrial septal aneurysm, vegetation, valve strand, aortic atheroma, tumor
9. Coronary disease	Coronary anomalies and fistulae, stenoses, flow reserve, stress imaging
10. Critical care unit	Unexplained hypotension, complications of myocardial infarction, pulmonary emboli, postsurgical tamponade
11. Congenital heart disease	Atrial situs, straddling atrioventricular valves, follow-up of Senning, Mustard, and Fontan procedures, pulmonary venous anomalies
12. Interventional procedures	PMV, ASD, or VSD closure, septostomy
13. Miscellaneous indications	Pulmonary vein pathology, assessment of hemodynamics, masses

ASD, atrial septal defect; COPD, chronic obstructive pulmonary disease; PFO, patent foramen ovale; PMV, prolapse of mitral valve; TTE, transthoracic echocardiography; VSD, ventricular septal defect.

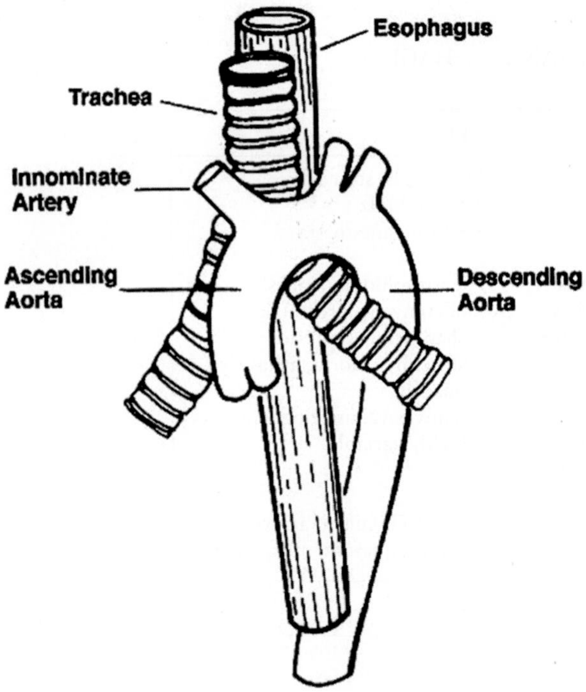

FIGURE 52.1. Intertwining of the aorta and esophagus from the diaphragm to the arch. (From Weyman AE. *Principles and practice of echocardiography,* 2nd ed. Philadelphia: JB Lippincott, 1994.)

horizontal transducer position is by convention at 0 degrees, whereas the longitudinal position is at 90 degrees. These transducers operate at multiple frequencies from 3.5 to 7.0 MHz, and they are capable of performing all Doppler modalities, M-mode, and two-dimensional imaging. Esophageal probes have the standard gastroscope controls that allow anteroflexion and retroflexion of the transducer, as well as side-to-side lateral motion.

TECHNIQUE

TEE is performed similarly to upper gastrointestinal endoscopy and requires experience in the safe intubation of the esophagus and stomach. Only operators who have adequate training in esophageal intubation and in echocardiography should perform this procedure.

TABLE 52.3

TRANSESOPHAGEAL ECHOCARDIOGRAPHY PROCEDURE

1. Appropriate indication
2. Informed consent
3. No specific contraindication or allergy to drug used in the procedure
4. Fasting >4 hours
5. Monitoring of electrocardiogram, blood pressure, and oximetry
6. Pharyngeal anesthesia with topical lidocaine
7. Intravenous sedation with meperidine and midazolam
6. Left lateral decubitus position

Patient Selection

Patients should fast for at least 4 hours before the procedure (Table 52.3). A detailed history should be obtained first, with attention paid to a history of dysphagia, esophageal problems, and drug allergies. The esophageal probe is passed blindly in TEE; thus disorders of the esophagus that may interfere with the passage of the probe or that may lead to injury by the probe are considered contraindications (Table 52.4). All oral prostheses and dentures are removed, and intravenous access is acquired. Blood pressure, electrocardiographic monitoring, and oximetry are undertaken throughout the study. Resuscitation equipment, suction, and oxygen should be readily available.

Anesthesia and Sedation

Pharyngeal anesthesia helps to reduce gagging on probe insertion. The pharynx is sprayed with lidocaine (Xylocaine) 4% or 10% Cetacaine. The patient may also gargle viscous lidocaine 2% for additional anesthetic effect. The effects of anesthesia are apparent within a few minutes and persist for 30 to 45 minutes after the procedure. Patients should not eat or drink during this period because of the risk of aspiration. At the Cleveland Clinic in Cleveland, Ohio, we use both fentanyl and a benzodiazepine (midazolam) for sedation, starting with 12.5 to 25 μg of fentanyl and 0.5 to 1.0 mg of midazolam. The sedation is titrated as necessary while one monitors the effects on heart rate, blood pressure, and oximetry. Sedation can lead

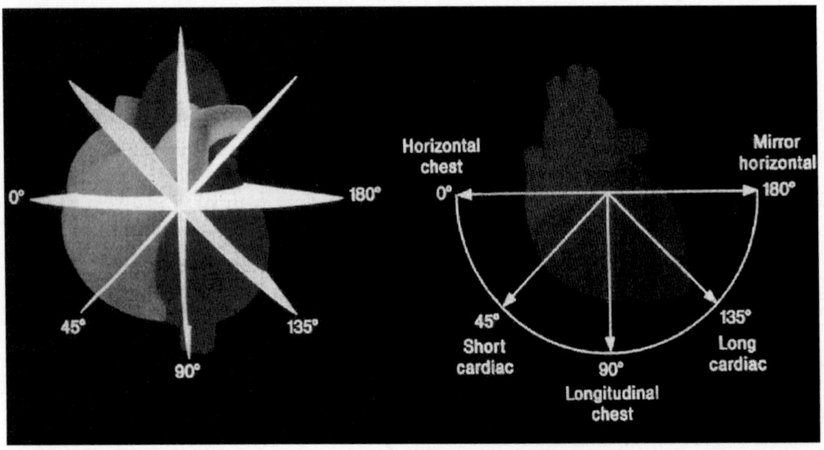

FIGURE 52.2. Scan planes of biplane and multiplane transducers. With the monoplane probe, the transducer is usually fixed and can only image in the transverse plane at 0 degrees. Biplane probes have an additional transducer mounted to image in the longitudinal orientation at 90 degrees. In multiplane imaging, the transducer may rotate so many additional imaging planes in between the transverse and longitudinal and mirror image of the transverse planes may be obtained. (From Khandheria BK. Transesophageal echocardiography in the evaluation of prosthetic valves. *Cardiol Clin* 1993;11:427–436.)

TABLE 52.4

CONTRAINDICATIONS TO TRANSESOPHAGEAL ECHOCARDIOGRAPHY

1. Significant dysphagia of unknown origin
2. Significant esophageal disorder
   - Esophageal diverticulum (Zenker)
   - Invasive esophageal tumor
   - Esophageal stricture, undilated
   - Esophageal tear, fistula, or rupture
   - Severe esophagitis or ulceration
   - Esophageal varices, especially with recent bleeding
3. Instability of the cervical vertebrae
4. Fasting <4 hours
5. Uncooperative patient

to respiratory depression or hypotension; thus, specific antagonists (e.g., flumazenil, naloxone) should be available for use if indicated. Additional sedation may be required throughout the procedure to maintain patient comfort. Ambulatory patients should be accompanied, to prevent their driving home under the influence of sedative and narcotic drugs.

Need for Antibiotic Prophylaxis

Many patients undergoing TEE have valvular or other lesions that pose a risk for endocarditis, and case reports have suggested that TEE was a causative factor in the development of endocarditis (6). However, several studies involving a total of 522 patients failed to detect significant bacteremia of oral flora associated with the TEE procedure or of clinical infection at follow-up (7–9). Therefore, the risk of endocarditis with TEE in experienced hands seems low, and routine prophylaxis is not indicated. Antibiotic coverage may be considered if the intubation is unexpectedly difficult or traumatic.

Probe Insertion

After the patient assumes a left lateral decubitus position with the neck flexed, the probe is guided into the upper esophagus. As the patient swallows, the probe is gently but firmly advanced into the distal esophagus. A bite block is inserted between the teeth to protect the probe. In ventilated patients, probe insertion is performed with the patient supine, while flexing the neck and manually retracting the tongue and anterior pharyngeal wall in an anterior direction. The probe should never be forcibly advanced because this risks causing an esophageal tear. If the probe does not pass smoothly, assistance from an endoscopist should be sought. At the end of the procedure, the patient should be monitored until vital signs have returned to baseline or at least normal values and the sedation has begun to wear off. The probe is washed and then sterilized by immersion in an antimicrobial solution (glutaral [Cidex]) for 20 minutes. The probe is rinsed and is allowed to air dry.

SAFETY AND COMPLICATIONS

Although TEE is invasive and is often performed in critically ill patients, successful intubation is possible in more than 98% of appropriately selected patients, and complications are uncommon (1,2). Inability to pass the probe is most often the result of operator inexperience, patient noncompliance, or, rarely, pathologic lesions in the esophagus. Once successful probe passage has occurred, early cessation of the procedure occurs in less than 1% of cases. The most common reason is patient intolerance of the probe, rather than the onset of a complication (1).

Major Complications

Major complications such as death, esophageal perforation, serious arrhythmia, congestive heart failure, and laryngospasm are uncommon and occur in less than 0.3% of patients (1). One death was reported out of 3,827 consecutive patients examined in one series. This was caused by arrhythmia following the procedure in a patient with autopsy-proven myocarditis (2). Another death was reported in a series of 10,419 patients and was the result of esophageal perforation in a patient with an unsuspected esophageal neoplasm (1). A third death following TEE was reported in a patient with acute aortic dissection in whom aortic rupture occurred during a bout of severe retching and nausea after probe insertion (10). Although serious esophageal injuries including perforation and tears have been reported (11), they are very rare. Laryngospasm and severe bronchospasm occasionally occur because of aspiration of anesthetic agents or lubricants used for probe insertion and rarely from inadvertent passage of the probe into the airway (12).

Minor Complications

Minor complications such as transient hypoxia, hypotension, hypertension, angina, bronchospasm, atrioventricular block, supraventricular tachycardia, and nonsustained ventricular arrhythmia occur in less than 3% of cases (2). Transient vocal cord paralysis (13), compression of anomalous vascular structures by the esophageal probe (14), and adverse reactions to the drugs used in patient preparation occur but are uncommon. The most common adverse medication reaction is methemoglobinemia in susceptible subjects receiving topical anesthesia (15). Sore throat and mild dysphagia are common following the procedure but rarely are prolonged for more than 24 hours.

IMAGING PLANES

TEE can be challenging, because the esophagus is not usually precisely aligned with the true long and short axis of the heart (Fig. 52.3). Furthermore, the relationship between the esophagus and cardiac structures is variable. Nevertheless, standard imaging planes have been described for TEE, which are greatly facilitated by multiplane technology and endoscope manipulation. The transesophageal examination is usually goal oriented, but it still is important to examine systematically all major cardiac structures and the aorta, so a complete examination is always performed.

Base of the Heart

At about 30 cm from the incisors, the probe lies behind the left atrium and the base of the heart. In the transverse plane (0 degrees) at this level, the aortic valve is seen in cross section, with portions of the left and right atrium and interatrial septum (Fig. 52.4). Withdrawing the probe slightly from this view allows imaging of the left atrial appendage, the superior vena cava, the right ventricular outflow tract, the ostia of the coronary vessels, the main pulmonary artery to its bifurcation, and a portion of the right pulmonary artery. The proximal

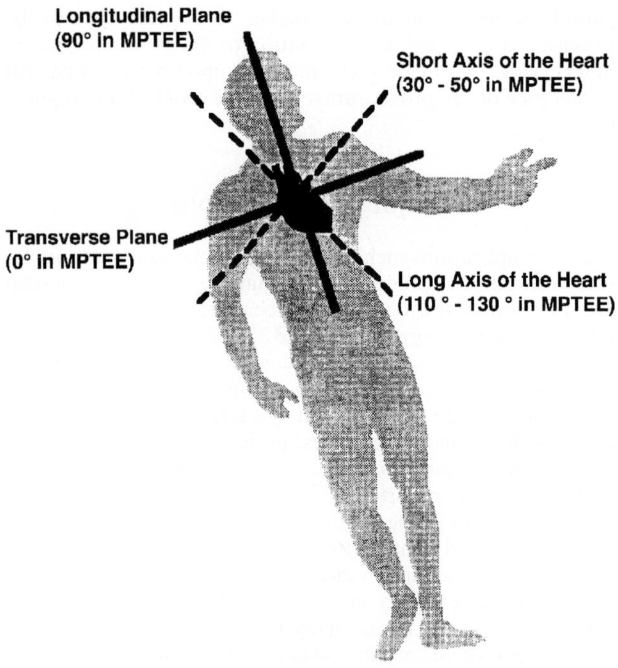

FIGURE 52.3. Relationship of horizontal and vertical vectors of the heart with those of the body and esophagus. The transverse (0 degree) and longitudinal (90 degree) esophageal imaging planes do not parallel the true short and long axis of the heart, which are imaged at 30 to 50 degrees and 110 to 130 degrees, respectively. The true short axis and long axis vary with individual habitus. MPTEE, multiplane transesophageal echocardiography. (From Schneider AT, Hsu TL, Schwartz SI, et al. Single, biplane, multiplane, and three-dimensional transesophageal echocardiography: echocardiographic-anatomic correlations. *Cardiol Clin* 1993;11:361–387.)

portion of the ascending aorta is imaged in this view, but it and the distal portions of the left pulmonary artery are difficult to image because of the interposition of air-filled large airways.

The longitudinal imaging plane (90 degrees) at this level provides important images of the great vessels, interatrial septum, left atrial appendage, and pulmonary veins. When the transducer is rotated to the left, a two-chamber view of the left atrium and left ventricle is seen. The left atrial appendage and the left pulmonary veins are often most easily imaged in this view. The mitral valve is also clearly seen in this view, and mitral regurgitation may be sought here. With clockwise rotation of the probe, the right ventricular outflow tract, pulmonary valve, and main pulmonary artery may be imaged. With additional clockwise rotation, the aortic valve and ascending aorta are seen. This view is important in the evaluation of the ascending aorta, particularly with regard to aortic dissection and in assessing aortic regurgitation. Finally, with further clockwise rotation, the right atrium, interatrial septum, and superior vena cava may be imaged. This plane is important in the detection of a communication at the atrial level and in assessing disorders of the superior vena cava. Multiplane imaging is especially useful at this level in allowing the true long and short axis of the aortic valve and ascending aorta to be obtained. Typically, the true short axis is seen at approximately 30 to 60 degrees and the true long axis at 120 to 150 degrees (Fig. 52.5).

Midesophageal Views

By advancing the probe into the midesophagus beyond the base of the heart, portions of both atria and ventricles, the interventricular septum, and the mitral and tricuspid valves are seen in the transverse imaging plane (see Fig. 52.4). A four-chamber view is acquired at this level by flexing the probe

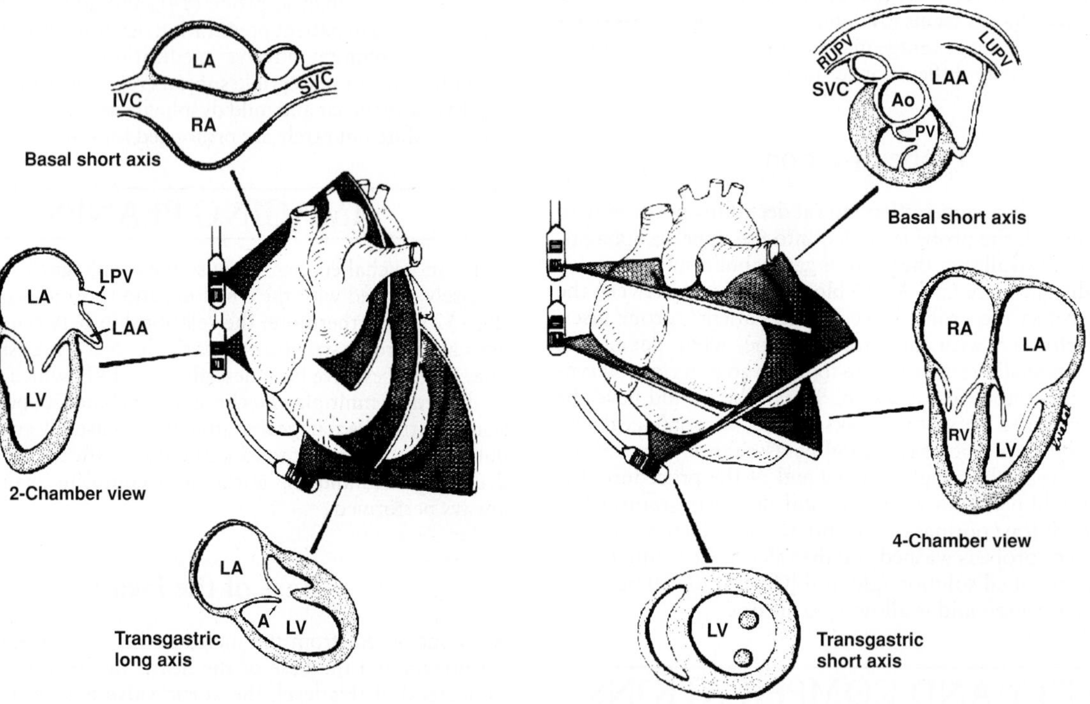

FIGURE 52.4. Transverse (**left**) and longitudinal (**right**) imaging planes at base of the heart, midesophagus, and transgastric windows. A, anterior leaflet of the mitral valve; Ao, aorta; IVC, inferior vena cava; LA, left atrium; LAA, left atrial appendage; LPV, left pulmonary vein; LUPV, left upper pulmonary vein; LV, left ventricle; PV, pulmonary valve; RA, right atrium; RUPV, right upper pulmonary vein; RV, right ventricle; SVC: superior vena cava. (From Khandheria BK. Transesophageal echocardiography in the evaluation of prosthetic valves. *Cardiol Clin* 1993;11:427–436.)

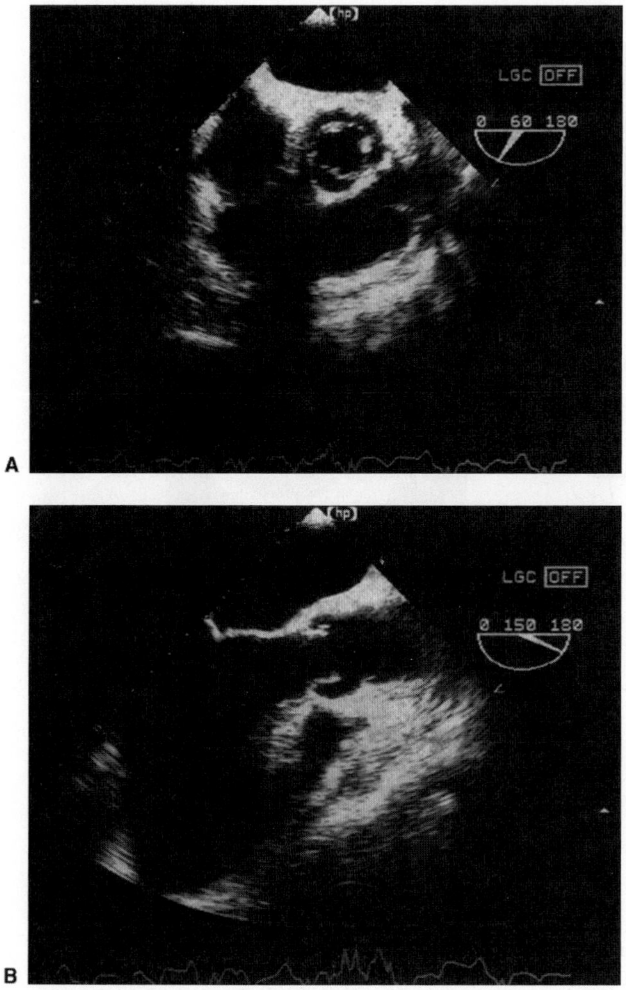

FIGURE 52.5. Multiplane images of a normal aortic valve. The true short axis was seen at 60 degrees (A) and the true long axis (B) at 150 degrees in this patient.

posteriorly. This view is similar to the apical four-chamber view acquired transthoracically, except the imaging plane does not cut through the true apex. This represents an inherent limitation of transesophageal imaging in the acquisition of ventricular volumes and in the detection of apical thrombus. This imaging plane is helpful in detecting regurgitation at the mitral and tricuspid valves and in global assessment of ventricular function. With slight counterclockwise rotation of the transducer, the left ventricular outflow tract and the proximal ascending aorta are seen. Longitudinal imaging at this level produces a two-chamber image of the heart already described. Multiplane images at this level are useful in distinguishing the individual leaflets of the mitral valve and the scallops of the posterior leaflet and in detecting eccentric jets of mitral regurgitation. Optimal differentiation between anterior and posterior mitral leaflet disorders is at about 140 degrees, whereas the full extent of the mitral closure line, from medial to lateral commissure, is at about 50 degrees.

Transgastric Views

To obtain this series of views, the probe is advanced into the stomach. Generally, the tip of the probe must be flexed to bring the transducer in contact with the mucosa of the gastric fundus. In the transverse plane, a short-axis view of the left and right ventricle is acquired (see Fig. 52.4). This view allows an assessment of regional and global left ventricular function. The mitral valve apparatus and leaflets are also well seen in this view. A longitudinal view at this level allows the mitral valve and the left ventricle to be imaged in long axis. The anterior and inferior walls are clearly seen, as are the papillary muscles and chordae. The true apex of the heart is most likely to be displayed in this view. Rotation of the probe in the long axis frequently allows the left ventricular outflow tract to be aligned with the Doppler cursor so a Doppler evaluation of the aortic valve and left ventricular outflow tract may be performed. Further rotation allows examination of the right ventricle and outflow tract. Another series of images is frequently possible by passing the probe further into the stomach and anteflexing (the deep transgastric view). In this view, the transducer is close to the apex, and the images obtained simulate those acquired in a transthoracic five-chamber or subcostal view. This view often optimizes Doppler interrogation of the aortic valve and outflow tract.

Aorta

The aorta may be examined from the ascending aorta to below the diaphragm (Fig. 52.6). The examination of the ascending aorta has already been described. The descending aorta is evaluated by rotating the probe to the left and posteriorly at the midesophageal level. The aorta is seen in cross section using the transverse transducer at this level and in the long axis using the longitudinal transducer. As the probe is withdrawn to approximately 20 to 25 cm, the transverse arch and distal portions of the ascending aorta are seen. The proximal portions of the left subclavian and other head and neck vessels may be imaged with a longitudinal or multiplane transducer.

INDICATIONS

Left and Right Atrium

Atrial Thrombus

TEE is now the technique of choice for the diagnosis of atrial thrombus (Fig. 52.7) (16,17). The sensitivity and specificity of TEE for the detection of thrombus in both the body and appendage of the left (18–20) and right (21) atria are superior to those of TTE and have exceeded 90% in a number of large series with surgical validation (22) as compared with less than 50% for TTE.

Spontaneous Contrast. TEE often identifies spontaneous echo contrast in the left atrium or appendage, especially in patients with atrial fibrillation or atrial thrombus (Fig. 52.8). This feature is reported in as many as 20% of all patients undergoing TEE but is rarely seen by TTE (23). Spontaneous contrast in the left atrium is an independent risk factor for systemic embolization in both mitral stenosis and nonvalvular atrial fibrillation (24,25). It also occurs in 2% of patients with sinus rhythm and is an independent risk factor for stroke (26). Anticoagulation has not been shown to affect the prevalence or intensity of spontaneous contrast (27,28).

TEE is now routinely used to allow early cardioversion of patients with atrial fibrillation without the standard 3 to 4 weeks of antecedent anticoagulation. The prospective, randomized Assessment of Cardioversion Using Transesophageal Echocardiography (ACUTE) study (29) convincingly demonstrated that patients who underwent early, TEE-guided cardioversion had a very low risk of embolization, similar to that

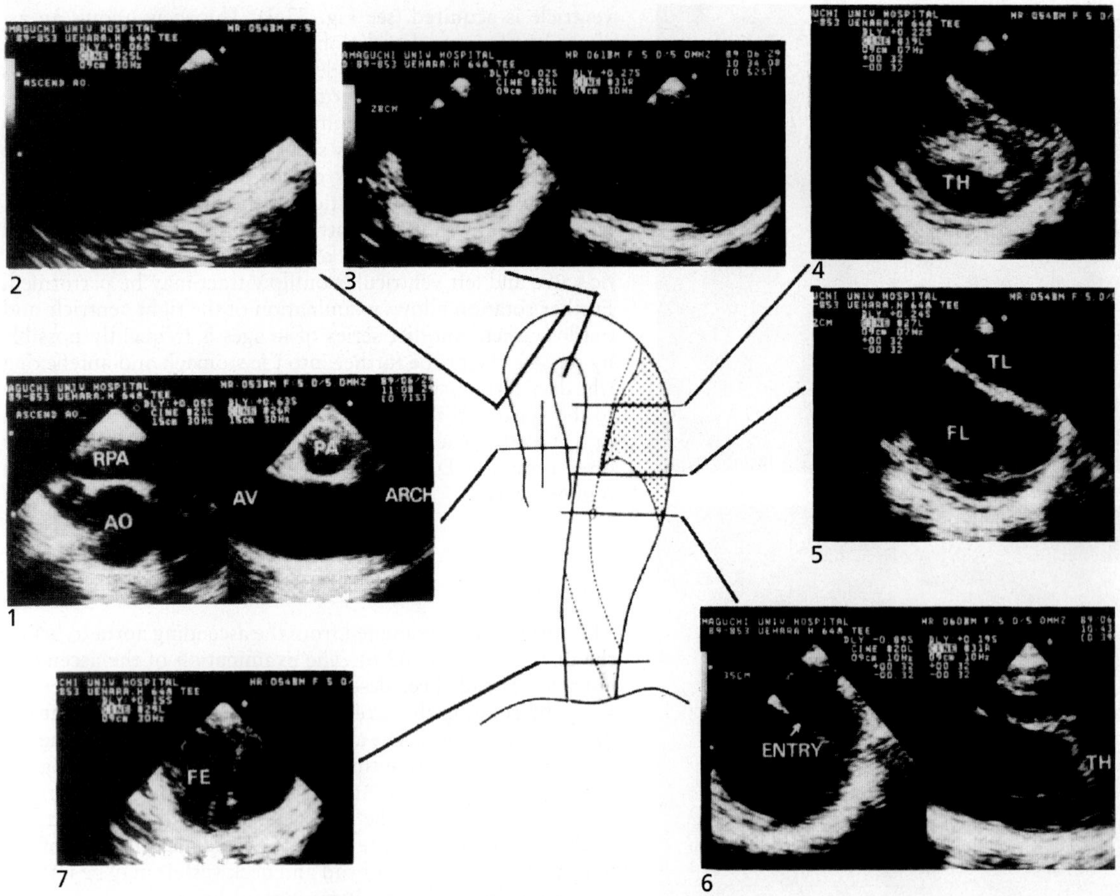

FIGURE 52.6. Imaging planes of the aorta. Biplane imaging planes of the aorta illustrated in a patient with dissection flap confined to the distal aorta. **Panel 1:** Transverse (**left**) and longitudinal plane (**right**) images of the ascending aorta. **Panel 2:** Transverse plane image of the aortic arch. **Panel 3:** Transverse (**left**) and longitudinal (**right**) plane images of the proximal descending aorta at the junction with the arch. **Panels 4 to 7:** Transverse (**panels 4 to 7**) and longitudinal (**panel 6, right**) plane images of the aortic dissection flap and its variable orientation in various portions of the descending aorta. AO, aorta; AV, aortic valve; entry, communication between the true and false lumina; FL, false lumen; PA, pulmonary artery; RPA, right pulmonary artery; TH, thrombus; TL, true lumen. (From Matsuzaki M, Toma Y, Kusukawa R. Clinical applications of transesophageal echocardiography. *Circulation* 1990;82:709–722.)

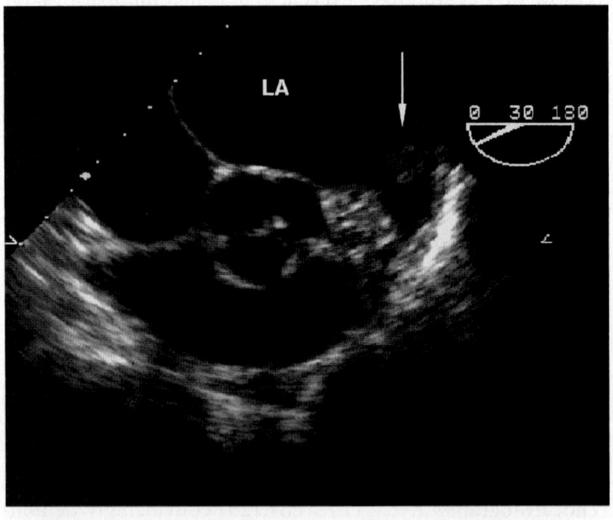

FIGURE 52.7. Left atrial appendage thrombus (*arrow*). LA, left atrium.

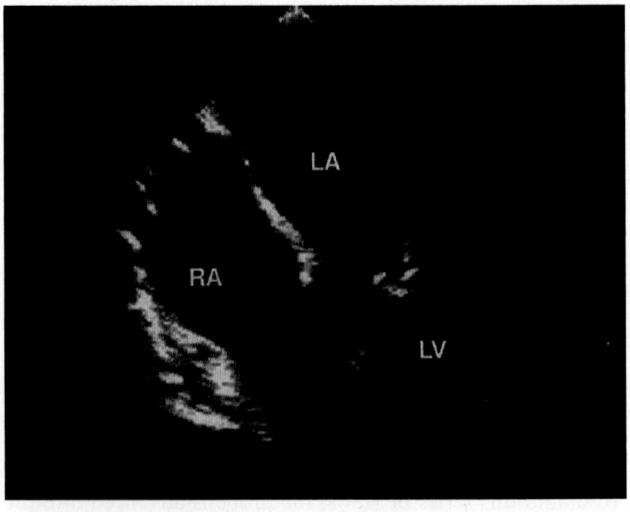

FIGURE 52.8. Swirling echoes of spontaneous contrast in the left atrium (LA) in a patient with mitral stenosis. LV, left ventricle; RA, right atrium.

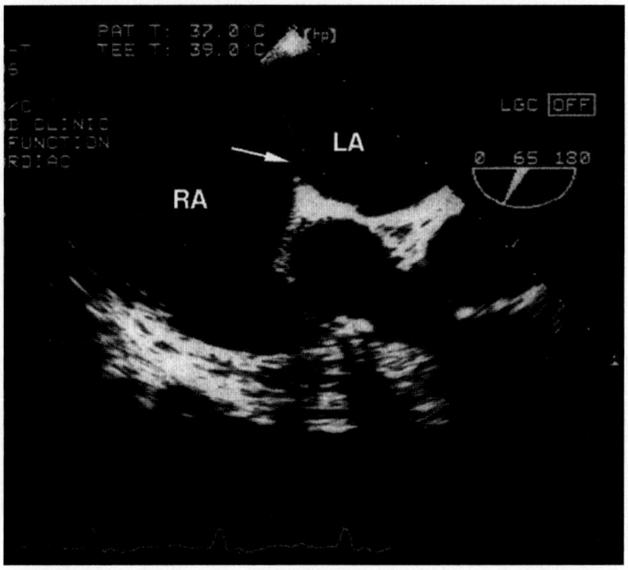

FIGURE 52.9. Patent foramen ovale by multiplane transesophageal echocardiography (*arrow*). LA, left atrium; RA, right atrium.

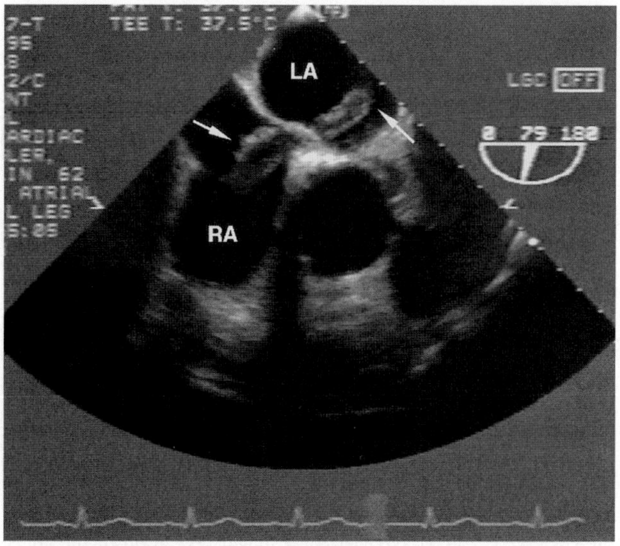

FIGURE 52.10. Embolus in transit across a patent foramen ovale (*arrows*). LA, left atrium; RA, right atrium.

of patients in the conventional therapy group. Notably, thromboembolic complications were reported in patients who were cardioverted despite a TEE negative for atrial thrombus but who were inadequately anticoagulated (27). Temporary deterioration of atrial function following return of normal sinus rhythm with subsequent thrombus formation and embolization is postulated to account for these embolic events, rather than embolization of thrombus undetected by TEE (22,23,28). Anticoagulation for a number of weeks is indicated following cardioversion even when TEE does not show atrial thrombus, to minimize the risk of embolism following the procedure.

Interatrial Septum

Atrial Septal Defect

TEE is the technique of choice in the diagnosis of abnormalities of the interatrial septum (Fig. 52.9), particularly patent foramen ovale and small or sinus venosus–type atrial septal defects (30). Anomalous drainage of pulmonary veins, which often accompanies sinus venosus–type defects, is also reliably detected by TEE (31). TEE measurements of anatomic size and shunt flow compare well with similar measurements made at the time of surgery (32).

Patent Foramen Ovale

Patent foramen ovale occurs in 25% to 30% of the physiologically normal population and is more commonly found in patients with unexplained stroke (33,34). The latter finding and the TEE demonstration of passage of a paradoxic embolus through a patent foramen ovale support a causative role in cerebral embolism (35) (Fig. 52.10). TEE is highly sensitive and specific in the detection of patent foramen ovale and is superior to TTE (36,37). Contrast venous injection is useful in the detection of right-to-left shunting, whereas color flow imaging is the method of choice in detecting left-to-right shunting (38). Both color flow and contrast techniques are performed in practice.

Atrial Septal Aneurysm

Atrial septal aneurysm (ASA) is also a risk factor for cerebral embolism and is detected more frequently by TEE than by conventional echocardiography (39). ASA occurs in 2.2% of the population and is associated with a single patent foramen ovale or rarely with multiple fenestrations (40,41). It is three times more common in patients with a history of cerebral ischemia (42) (Fig. 52.11).

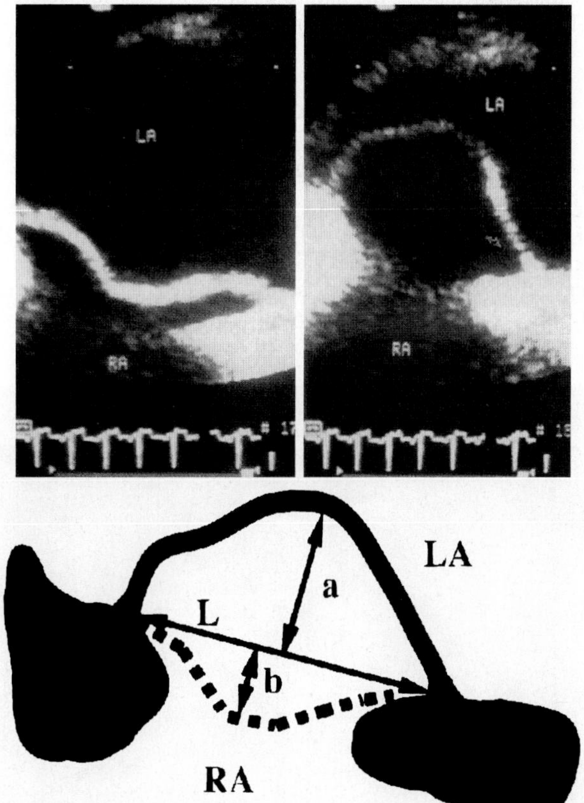

FIGURE 52.11. Mobile atrial septal aneurysm by transesophageal echocardiography. The **bottom panel** illustrates measurements. a and b, maximal extent of oscillation into the left and right atrium, respectively; L, length; LA, left atrium; RA, right atrium. (From Mugge A, Daniel WG, Angermann C, et al. Atrial septal aneurysm in adult patients: a multicenter study using transthoracic and transesophageal echocardiography. *Circulation* 1995;91:2785–2792.)

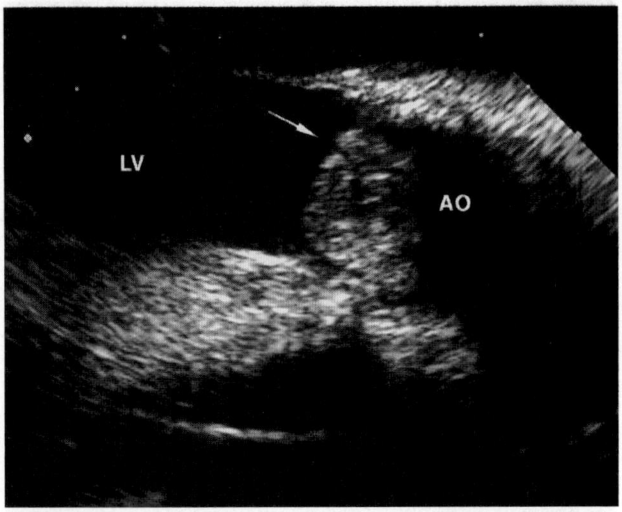

FIGURE 52.12. Long-axis view of a fungal vegetation of the aortic valve *(arrow)*. AO, aorta; LV, left ventricle.

Other Atrial Abnormalities

The membrane of cor triatriatum is particularly well delineated by TEE. Atrial tumors such as myxomas are usually clearly characterized by TTE. TEE is useful when there is diagnostic uncertainty and is superior in detecting the site of attachment to the wall and the composition of the tumor (43). It is also useful in elucidating the nature of other masses suspected by TTE and in distinguishing them from normal variants.

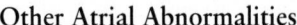

Endocarditis

Diagnosis

Echocardiography is now an integral part of the evaluation of suspected endocarditis (44). TEE is more sensitive in diagnosing endocarditis because it provides better resolution of vegetations than TTE. In one study, TTE detected 63% of vegetations, whereas TEE detected all of them (45) (Fig. 52.12).

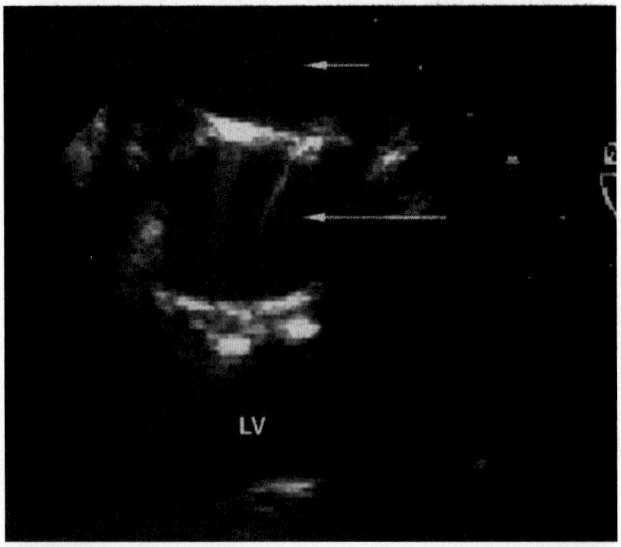

FIGURE 52.13. Vegetation (*short arrow*) on the atrial side of a mechanical mitral prosthesis (*long arrow*) detected by transesophageal echocardiography. LV, left ventricle.

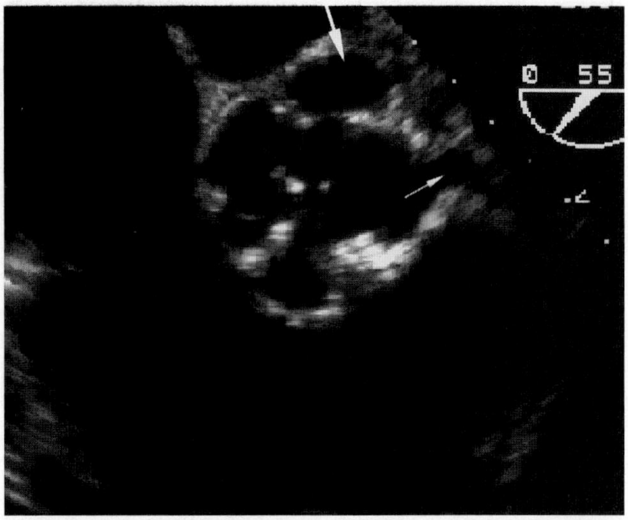

FIGURE 52.14. Short-axis view of an abscess (*wide arrow*) of a native aortic valve detected by multiplane transesophageal echocardiography. The left main coronary is shown by the *narrow arrow.*

In that study, TTE had diagnostic accuracy equivalent to that of TEE in detection of vegetations greater than 11 mm, but TTE detected only 25% of vegetations less than 5 mm and 69% of vegetations between 6 and 10 mm. Both TEE and TTE have a reported specificity in the diagnosis of vegetations of more than 90% (46). The superiority of TEE in the detection of prosthetic endocarditis is even greater than for native valve disease (Fig. 52.13); the sensitivities of TEE and TTE in this setting are greater than 80% and less than 45%, respectively (47,48). Vegetations on the tricuspid valve are detected with equal frequency by TEE and TTE (49). However, endocarditis of the pulmonary valve is more often recognized by TEE than by TTE (50), as is endocarditis at unusual sites, such as on pacemaker wires (51).

Complications

TEE is more reliable than TTE in detecting perforation of a valve leaflet in endocarditis (52). TEE can detect pyogenic complications of endocarditis such as abscess and fistula formation (Figs. 52.14 and 52.15) more readily than TTE (53,54).

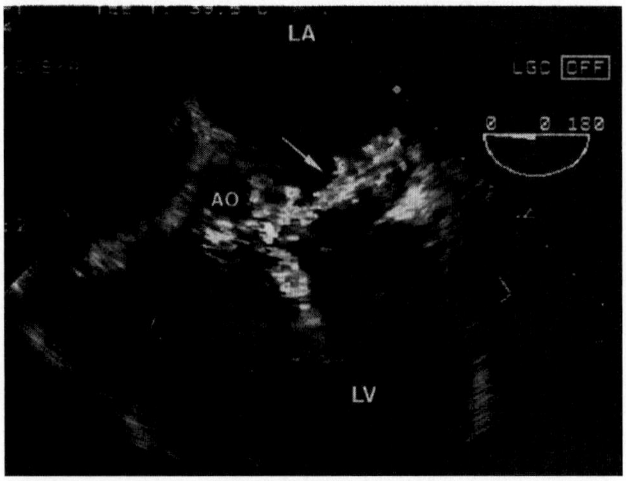

FIGURE 52.15. Fistula (*arrow*) from the aorta (Ao) to the left atrium (LA) by transesophageal echocardiography color flow imaging. LV, left ventricle.

These complications are associated with increased mortality, usually require operative intervention for successful treatment, and occur in approximately one third of endocarditis cases. Such complications occur most often in patients with staphylococcal infections of the aortic valve and in those with prosthetic endocarditis (53,55,56). The sensitivity of TEE in the detection of abscess or infected pseudoaneurysm has been reported at 87% to 100%, whereas that of TTE has varied from 28% to 43% (51,56). TEE is more reliable (100% sensitive) than TTE (32% sensitive) in the detection of endocarditis in patients with *Staphylococcus aureus* sepsis.

Predictive Value and Utility of Transesophageal Echocardiography

In patients with suspected endocarditis, TEE has a very high negative predictive value (57). However, TEE may fail to detect endocarditis early in the course of the illness or following embolization of a vegetation. Serial studies are indicated if the clinical suspicion is high despite an initially negative TEE. Many findings on native and prosthetic valves may simulate vegetations. These include degenerative change such as Lambl excrescences on the aortic valve or suture material in the case of prostheses. Comparison with prior studies is very useful in these instances. Because of the high sensitivity, specificity, and negative predictive value of TEE in the detection of endocarditis, TEE has been advocated as the technique of choice in the evaluation of this condition. In a study addressing the incremental utility of TTE and TEE over clinical criteria in the diagnosis of endocarditis (58), TEE was incrementally useful in patients with intermediate or high probability of disease based on clinical criteria and TTE and in those with suspected prosthetic endocarditis. TEE and TTE were equivalent in excluding endocarditis in patients with a low likelihood of endocarditis on clinical grounds. Recently, TEE was shown to improve the diagnosis of native valve endocarditis based on the Duke criteria and TTE in 11% of the study patients, most of whom had an intermediate likelihood of disease (59).

Disease of the Aorta

TEE has become the technique of choice in many institutions in the diagnosis of acute dissection because of its high sensitivity, portability, and the speed with which the diagnosis may be made (60). It is also used in the diagnosis of aortic trauma and aortic atheroma.

Diagnosis of Dissection

TEE has been reported to be more than 95% sensitive in the detection of aortic dissection in multiple studies (Fig. 52.16) (61,62). The detection rate reported is somewhat less for dissection involving the ascending aorta, mainly because of the blind spot in the distal ascending aorta and proximal arch, as already described (63–65). The detection rate is also lower in patients who have had prior surgery of the aorta (66), when the dissection flap is very localized, or when the false lumen is thrombosed (67,68). The reported specificity of TEE in the detection of aortic dissection has varied from 68% to 100% (63,64,69). False-positive results are most common in the ascending aorta and are often caused by reverberation simulating a dissection flap (63,70). These artifacts may be with minimized M-mode echocardiography, which is useful in timing and localizing reverberation (71), or with color flow mapping at the site of the supposed dissection flap.

Aortic dissection is most conveniently classified based on the presence (type A) or absence (type B) of a dissection flap in the ascending aorta. The accuracy of classification of dissection

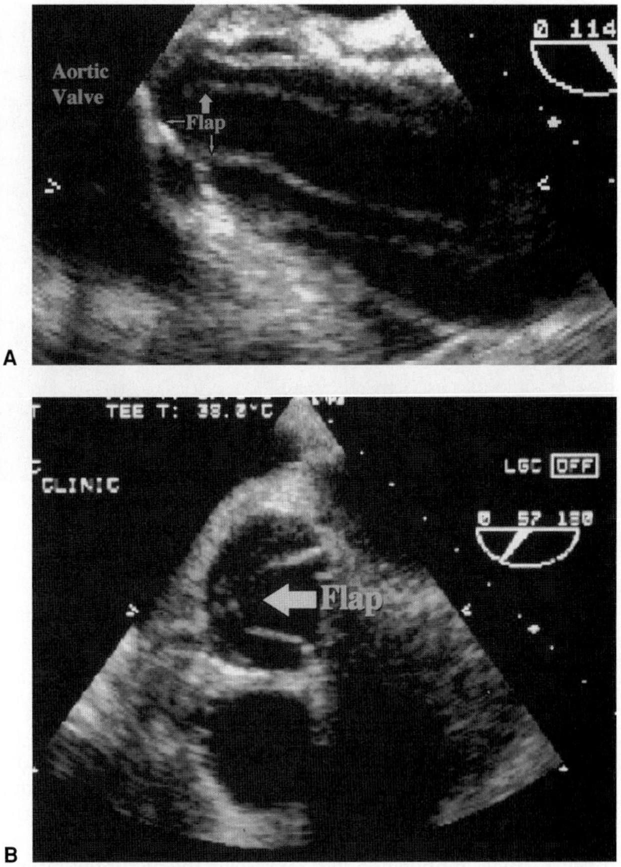

FIGURE 52.16. Aortic dissection with a flap in the ascending aorta. **A:** Long axis. **B:** Short axis.

by TEE has varied from 89% to 100% (61,69). Additionally, TEE can detect the primary tear in 73% to 89% of type A dissections (61,64), as well as thrombus in the false lumen. Important complications of dissection such as pericardial effusion, cardiac tamponade, the mechanism and severity of aortic regurgitation, and involvement of the coronary ostia are also accurately diagnosed by TEE.

Intramural Hematoma

Intramural hematoma is a contained hemorrhage within the medial layer of the aortic wall. This is distinct from a true dissection in which the media and the aortic lumen communicate through an intimal tear. The clinical presentation and prognosis of intramural hematoma are similar to those of aortic dissection. In fact, intramural hematoma may develop into a dissection over time and may involve any portion of the aorta (72,73). It is recognized by TEE as a crescentic thickening of the aortic wall that extends for a variable length (74) with displaced intimal calcium. Intramural hematoma is most often seen in elderly patients and may be difficult to differentiate from atherosclerotic changes or from thrombosis of a localized dissection.

Penetrating Atherosclerotic Ulcer of the Aorta

Penetrating ulcer is associated with hypertension and atheroma and may present with chest or back pain. It frequently coexists with intramural hematoma and a limited dissection. It is recognized by TEE as a localized outpouching of the aortic wall that may be calcified (75). Pseudoaneurysm formation may also occur. TEE was shown to detect 88% of penetrating

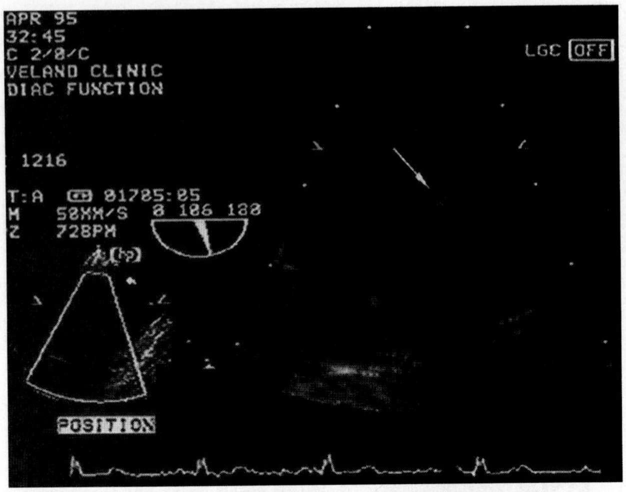

FIGURE 52.17. Mobile aortic atheroma (*arrow*).

ulcers that were confirmed at surgery or by another imaging modality (76).

Aortic Trauma

TEE has become an important tool in the rapid evaluation of aortic injury following major trauma. Aortic trauma most often involves the aortic isthmus just distal to the ligamentum arteriosum. Subadventitial disruption requires immediate surgical intervention and is recognized echocardiographically as a dense, thick, mobile flap that represents the disrupted intima and media. Asymmetric aortic enlargement is seen in this area as a result of the formation of a pseudoaneurysm. TEE can be performed rapidly and safely in trauma patients, and it has more than 90% sensitivity and specificity for the detection of significant aortic disruption (77).

Aortic Atherosclerosis

Aortic atheroma appears as echodense thickening of the intimal surface, often with superimposed thrombus or calcification. It is most commonly seen in the descending thoracic aorta, less often in the aortic arch, and least often in the ascending aorta (78) (Fig. 52.17). Aortic atheroma on TEE is a sensitive marker of significant coronary (79), peripheral vascular, and carotid disease (80). Importantly, plaque morphology and thickness predict the risk of embolic events. Complex mobile plaque confers a higher risk of embolization than sessile plaque (81). Plaque in the aortic arch that was thicker than 4 mm as shown by TEE was an independent risk factor for ischemic stroke in one study (82). Other studies indicated that aortic atheroma on TEE increases the risk of perioperative stroke in patients undergoing bypass surgery and the risk of atherogenic embolism following other procedures (83,84).

Other Aortic Conditions

TEE can characterize thoracic aneurysms involving the sinuses of Valsalva, the ascending aorta, and the descending aorta. It is useful in improving the resolution of sinus of Valsalva aneurysm and in detecting communication with individual cardiac chambers.

Native Valve Disease

TTE can usually provide a complete anatomic and hemodynamic profile of abnormal valves. TEE is used in addition when improved resolution of valve structure is needed or when the hemodynamic severity of a regurgitant lesion is in question.

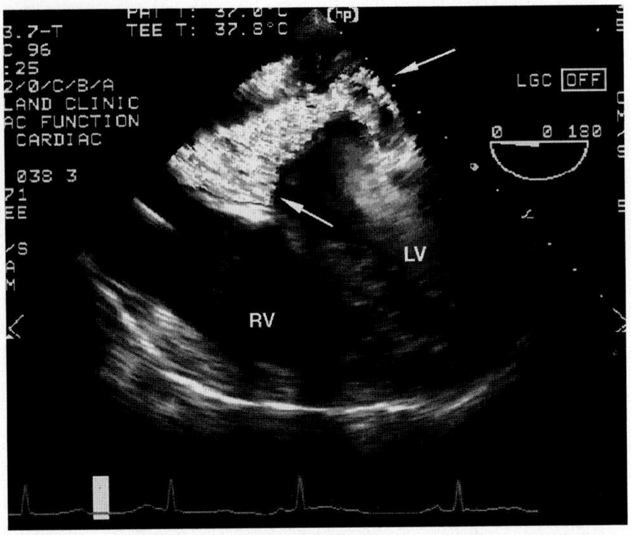

FIGURE 52.18. Severe anteriorly directed mitral regurgitation owing to a flail posterior leaflet (*arrows*) imaged in the transverse four-chamber view. LV, left ventricle; RV, right ventricle.

Mitral Valve

TEE is highly sensitive and specific in the detection of flail mitral valve leaflets and chordae and is superior to TTE in differentiating flail leaflets from vegetations (85,86) (Fig. 52.18). TEE is also superior in defining the mechanism and site of regurgitation, the likelihood of repair, and a subset of patients at greatest risk for the development of complications such as systolic motion of the mitral valve following repair for myxomatous disease (87–89). TEE is superior to TTE in the detection of papillary muscle rupture in critically ill patients (90) and in the evaluation of eccentric regurgitant jets. TEE is particularly suited to the precise assessment of regurgitation because of the excellent resolution of the vena contracta width, the proximal flow convergence area, and the pulmonary vein flow pattern.

Aortic and Other Valves

Multiplane TEE has facilitated imaging of the aortic valve and allows the true long and short axis to be acquired. High-resolution images obtained by this technique are useful in diagnosing bicuspid valves, subaortic stenosis or membranes (91), or other structural abnormalities. In a study with operative confirmation, multiplane TEE was significantly better than TTE at detection of bicuspid aortic valves and had a sensitivity of 87% and specificity of 97% (92). Interrogation of the aortic valve with continuous-wave Doppler is more difficult than with TTE, but planimetry of the aortic valve orifice is usually feasible. Aortic valve area assessed by planimetry has excellent correlation with valve areas measured at cardiac catheterization or by TTE (93).

Prosthetic Valves

TEE allows improved resolution of prosthetic leaflets and regurgitation, both in mechanical prostheses and in bioprosthesis, as compared to TTE (47,94). In one study of 148 prosthetic valves (113 bioprostheses and 35 mechanical prostheses) in which abnormality was confirmed pathologically, TEE and

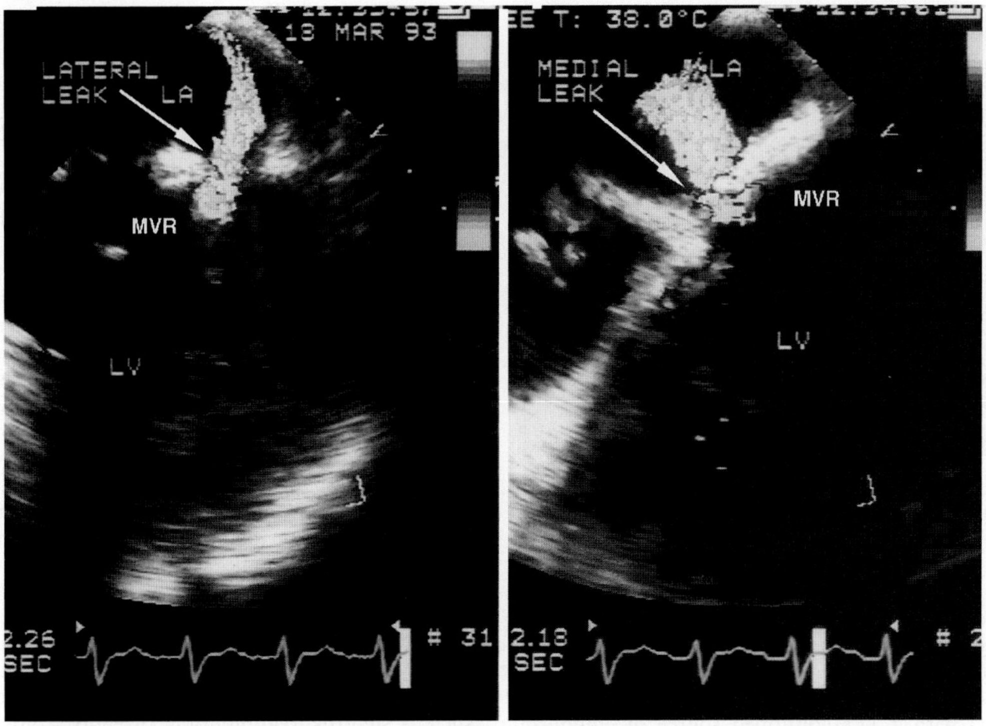

FIGURE 52.19. Two periprosthetic regurgitant leaks (lateral, A; medial, B) at a mitral mechanical prosthesis (MVR) demonstrated by multiplane transesophageal echocardiography. LA, left atrium; LV, left ventricle.

TTE were 86% and 57% sensitive, respectively, in the detection of abnormalities (47). TEE was superior to TTE in the detection of abnormalities in mechanical prostheses (83% versus 22%), bioprostheses (87% versus 65%), aortic prostheses (77% versus 50%), and mitral prostheses (97% versus 65%) (47). In patients with mechanical mitral valves, TEE may detect thrombus that is clinically unsuspected but is a risk factor for thromboembolic events (95).

Prosthetic Regurgitation

A small amount of regurgitation occurs normally in mechanical prostheses by design. This is readily detected by TEE and less often by TTE. The pattern of regurgitation is specific to individual prosthetic types and is usually easily differentiated from abnormal regurgitation by the relative low velocity, short duration, and small size of the normal jets (96). Abnormal regurgitation at mitral prostheses is more reliably detected by TEE than TTE, but its superiority in this regard is less pronounced for aortic prostheses (94,97). TEE is also more accurate than TTE in defining the origin of the prosthetic regurgitation (97,98), particularly paravalvular leaks (Fig. 52.19).

Prosthetic Stenosis

Although TTE is used to characterize the valve gradients, TEE provides significant incremental information on structural abnormalities of the valve leaflets or sewing ring once stenosis is suspected. TEE is especially useful in the detection of thrombus on the prosthetic leaflets (99) and in differentiating thrombus from pannus on mechanical valve prostheses (100,101). Thrombus may not be apparent on TTE and may occur despite normal prosthetic gradients. In one study, TEE detected thrombus on a mechanical valve in 13% of 114 patients in whom it was unsuspected by TTE (102). In another study, TEE detected all eight prosthetic thrombi (100%), whereas TTE detected only one (13%) of them (47). TEE is useful in predicting whether a thrombosed valve will respond to thrombolytic treatment; nonobstructive thrombus is more often successfully treated with lytic therapy compared with thrombus that completely occludes the prosthesis (102).

Source of Embolism

Currently, the leading indication for TEE in most medical centers is in the evaluation of source of embolism. Some studies have indicated that TEE is more likely than TTE to detect a potential cardiac source of embolism in patients with cerebral ischemia (36,103–106). These embolic sources or risk factors include left atrial thrombus, left atrial spontaneous contrast, patent foramen ovale, ASA, valvular strands, vegetations, and aortic atheroma. TEE is more likely than TTE to detect a source of embolism in patients without a prior cardiac history. In one study of 79 patients with cerebral ischemia in the absence of cerebrovascular disease, a cardiac source of embolism was detected in 15% by TTE and in 57% by TEE (36). In patients without a prior cardiac history, a potential source of embolism was detected by TEE in 39% and in 19% by TTE. In another study of 50 patients without cerebrovascular disease who had a recent stroke or transient ischemic attack, TEE detected a potential source of embolism in 52% of all patients and in 33% of those without a prior cardiac history, whereas TTE failed to detect a cardiac source of embolism in any patient (106).

Situations in which information from TEE is most likely to be of value include the following: (a) younger stroke patients (<60 years) without a history of cerebrovascular disease or obvious embolic source, (b) patients with recurrent embolic events, (c) when anticoagulation has a higher than normal risk owing to comorbidities, (d) the presence of a prosthetic valve, (e) patients with suspected endocarditis. Furthermore, the finding of a source of embolism on TEE may have prognostic value

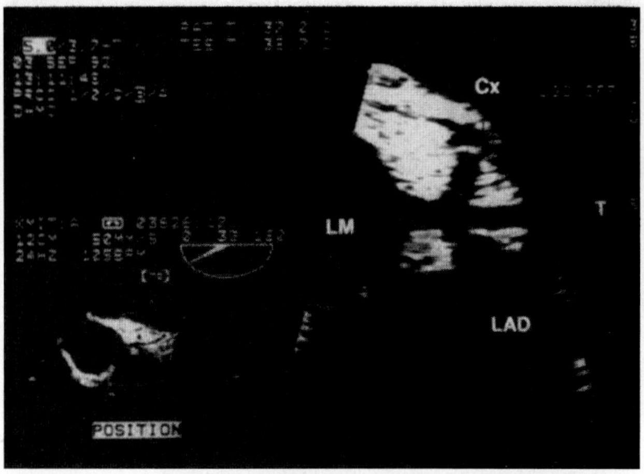

FIGURE 52.20. Coronary vessels imaged by multiplane transesophageal echocardiography. Cx, circumflex; LAD, left anterior descending; LM, left main coronary; T, trifurcation branch.

in predicting recurrent events. In a prospective study of 145 patients with cerebral ischemia, TEE detected a source of embolism in 45% of those with unexplained stroke or transient ischemic attack. Recurrent cerebral ischemia was more common in patients with a TEE-confirmed source of embolism over a follow-up period of 18 months (106a).

Coronary Disease

Although not a primary imaging modality for coronary artery disease, TEE is capable of imaging the ostia and variable portions of the coronary tree. It can identify coronary anomalies and may detect and quantify coronary stenoses. The coronary vessels, particularly the left main and proximal left anterior descending arteries, are seen in the majority of patients and are most readily imaged in the basal short-axis view (107,108). The proximal right coronary artery is more difficult to image (107). Medial and distal portions of vessels are adequately imaged only in a minority of patients, even with multiplane transducers (109) (Fig. 52.20). TEE is useful in confirming left coronary ostial stenosis when this is suspected at catheterization (110). It is also accurate in the detection and classification of anomalous coronary origin and fistula formation and of aneurysm formation (111,112).

Stress Imaging

The transesophageal imaging window has been used to perform stress echocardiography. Excellent short- and long-axis images are obtained from the transgastric window, and all three major coronary territories are represented in this view (113). Excellent endocardial resolution is usually obtained, and this facilitates detection of ischemic wall motion abnormalities. One limitation with TEE imaging is the evaluation of ischemia at the cardiac apex, which may be difficult to visualize even with multiple imaging planes. Esophageal pacing, intravenous vasodilators such as adenosine and dipyridamole (114), and inotropic agents such as dobutamine have been used to produce ischemia (115–117). Sensitivity and specificity of more than 80% in the detection of coronary disease have been reported for all these stress TEE methods (115,116,118). The increased invasiveness of stress echocardiography from the transesophageal approach has limited its widespread application. Clinical use of TEE stress echocardiography has been confined to patients in whom adequate images are not available from TTE, especially morbidly obese patients who cannot be evaluated by other methods (119).

Pediatric Cardiology and Adult Congenital Heart Disease

Excellent TTE images are usually available in children. Nevertheless, TEE may provide additional diagnostic information in specific instances. Some studies have indicated that TEE is safe in neonates and young children, although general anesthesia is usually required (120,121). TEE has represented a significant advance in the evaluation of adults with congenital heart disease with complex anatomy (122–124). TEE is more reliable than TTE in the determination of atrial situs (120), in defining abnormalities in the systemic and pulmonary venous connections (125), and in defining the morphology of the chordal apparatus of the atrioventricular valves (126).TEE long-axis imaging planes of the right and left ventricular outflow tract often provide better definition than TTE of the site and nature of obstruction in the subvalvar area and in the pulmonary artery or aorta (121,124,127). TEE is also superior to TTE in detecting abnormalities of flow or leaks across the atrial baffle following Mustard or Senning procedures (128) and in identifying complications of the Fontan procedure (129,130). Complications associated with ventriculopulmonary conduits such as stenosis, regurgitation, or endocarditis are often best detected by TEE, especially in adults (121).

Interventional Cardiology

TEE has been used as a monitoring and diagnostic tool during many types of interventional procedure, although it is not absolutely required. With the advent of intracardiac echocardiography, TEE may in fact become a secondary imaging tool to monitor these procedures. However, TEE remains a valuable tool in balloon valvuloplasty of the mitral valve (131), as well as several other procedures. TEE can optimize the site of septal puncture and balloon placement within the mitral valve. It can also determine the immediate effect of sequential balloon inflation on mitral valve structure, gradient, area, and mitral regurgitation. Periprocedural complications may be rapidly detected. These include thrombus formation on catheters or at the site of endothelial injury, valve disruption, and pericardial effusion and tamponade (132). TEE is more sensitive than either oximetry or TTE in detecting a residual atrial septal defect following the septal puncture (32). TEE is also useful in percutaneous catheter closure of septal defects and patent ductus arteriosus (133,134). The exact position of the closure device can be ascertained and positional adjustments made to minimize residual shunt flow. Other interventional techniques in which TEE has been used include endomyocardial biopsy, electrophysiologic ablation procedures, and septostomy and other procedures in the pediatric group (135–137). TEE can assess the results of balloon dilatation of coarctation and intimal dissection, which commonly occurs with this procedure (138). It may be used instead of fluoroscopy in positioning catheters or pacemakers when radiation exposure is best avoided, such as in pregnancy (139).

CONTROVERSIES AND PERSONAL PERSPECTIVES

TEE technology and expertise have matured over the years, and TEE is now an established means of cardiac diagnostic imaging. Technologic improvements in TTE and in intracardiac imaging have also occurred such that TEE remains a relatively stable proportion of the diagnostic echocardiography studies in most institutions (140–143). As a mature technology, controversies in its use have been resolved either on the basis of clinical studies or, more commonly, based on widespread clinical experience.

THE FUTURE

TEE is used in many institutions to exclude thrombus before cardioversion in those patients who have not been adequately anticoagulated. This has required two procedures, the TEE and then the cardioversion, both of which require sedation. A novel technology has been reported in an animal model of an esophageal probe capable of both diagnostic ultrasound imaging and cardiac defibrillation (144). This raises the future possibility of performing TEE cardioversion as a single procedure in human patients.

References

1. Daniel WG, Erbel R, Kasper W, et al. Safety of transesophageal echocardiography: a multicenter survey of 10,419 examinations. *Circulation* 1991; 83:817–821.
2. Seward JB, Khanderia BK, Oh JK, et al. Critical appraisal of transesophageal echocardiography: limitations, pitfalls and complications. *J Am Soc Echocardiogr* 1992;5:288–305.
3. Gentles TL, Rosenfeld HM, Sanders SP, et al. Pediatric biplane transesophageal echocardiography: preliminary experience. *Am Heart J* 1994; 128:1225–1233.
4. Seward JB, Khandheria BK, Edwards WD, et al. Biplanar transesophageal echocardiography: anatomic correlations, image orientation, and clinical applications. *Mayo Clin Proc* 1990;65:1193–1213.
5. Schneider AT, Hsu TL, Schwartz Sl, et al. Single, biplane, multiplane, and three-dimensional transesophageal echocardiography: echocardiographic-anatomic correlations. *Cardiol Clin* 1993;11:361–387.
6. Foster E, Kusumoto FM, Sobois M, et al. Streptococcal endocarditis temporarily related to transesophageal echocardiography. *J Am Soc Echocardiogr* 1990;3:424–427.
7. Nikutta P, Mantey-Steirs F, Becht I, et al. Risk of bacteremia induced by transesophageal echocardiography: analysis of 100 consecutive procedures. *J Am Soc Echocardiogr* 1992;5:168–172.
8. Pongratz G, Henneke KH, von der Grun M, et al. Risk of endocarditis in transesophageal echocardiography. *Am Heart J* 1993;125:190–193.
9. Shyu KG, Hwang JJ, Tzou SS, et al. Prospective study of blood cultures during transesophageal echocardiography. *Am Heart J* 1992;124:1541–1544.
10. Silvey SV, Stoughton TL, Pearl W, et al. Rupture of the outer partition of aortic dissection during transesophageal echocardiography. *Am J Cardiol* 1991;68:286–287.
11. Dewhirst WE, Stragand JJ, Fleming BM. Mallory-Weiss tear complicating intraoperative transesophageal echocardiography in a patient undergoing aortic valve replacement. *Anesthesiology* 1990;73:777–778.
12. Chan KL, Cohen GI, Sochowski RA, et al. Complications of transesophageal echocardiography in ambulatory adult patients. *J Am Soc Echocardiogr* 1991;4:577–582.
13. Cucchiara RF, Nugent M, Seward JB, et al. Air embolism in upright neurosurgical patients: detection and localization by two-dimensional transesophageal echocardiography. *Anesthesiology* 1984;60:353–355.
14. Frommelt PC, Stuth EA. Transesophageal echocardiography in total anomalous pulmonary venous drainage: hypotension caused by compression of the pulmonary venous confluence during probe passage. *J Am Soc Echocardiogr* 1994;76:652–654.
15. Marcovitz PA, Williamson BD, Armstrong WF. Toxic methemoglobinemia caused by topical anesthetic given before transesophageal echocardiography. *J Am Soc Echocardiogr* 1991;4:615–618.
16. Shrestha NK, Moreno FL, Narciso FV, et al. Two-dimensional echocardiographic diagnosis of left atrial thrombus in rheumatic heart disease: a clinicopathologic study. *Circulation* 1983;67:341–347.
17. Aschenberg W, Schluter M, Kremer P, et al. Transesophageal two-dimensional echocardiography for the detection of left atrial appendage thrombus. *J Am Coll Cardiol* 1986;7:163–166.
18. Brickner ME, Friedman DB, Cigarroa CG, et al. Relation of thrombus in the left atrial appendage by transesophageal echocardiography to clinical risk factors for thrombus formation. *Am J Cardiol* 1994;7:391–393.
19. Leung DY, Davidson PM, Cranney GB, et al. Thromboembolic risks of left atrial thrombus detected by transesophageal echocardiogram. *Am J Cardiol* 1997;79:626–629.
20. Manning WJ, Weintraub RM, Wakomonski CA, et al. Accuracy of transesophageal echocardiography for identifying left atrial thrombi: a prospective intraoperative study. *Ann Intern Med* 1995;123:817–822.
21. Irani WN, Grayburn PA, Afridi I. Prevalence of thrombus, spontaneous echo contrast, and atrial stunning in patients undergoing cardioversion of atrial flutter: a prospective study using transesophageal echocardiography. *Circulation* 1997;95:962–966.
22. Schwartzbard AZ, Tunick PA, Rosenzweig BP, et al. The role of transesophageal echocardiography in the diagnosis and treatment of right atrial thrombi. *J Am Soc Echocardiogr* 1999;12:64–69.
23. Daniel WG, Nellessen V, Schroder E, et al. Left atrial spontaneous contrast in mitral valve disease: an indicator for an increased thromboembolic risk. *J Am Coll Cardiol* 1988;11:1204–1211.
24. Black IW, Hopkins AP, Lee LCL, et al. Left atrial spontaneous echo contrast: a clinical and echocardiographic analysis. *J Am Coll Cardiol* 1991;18:398–404.
25. Leung DY, Black IW, Cranney GB, et al. Prognostic implications of left atrial spontaneous echo contrast in nonvalvular atrial fibrillation. *J Am Coll Cardiol* 1994;24:755–762.
26. Sadanandan S, Sherrid MV. Clinical and echocardiographic characteristics of left atrial spontaneous echo contrast in sinus rhythm. *J Am Coll Cardiol* 2000;35:1932–1938.
27. Black IW, Fatkin D, Sagar KB, et al. Exclusion of atrial thrombus by transesophageal echocardiography does not preclude embolism after cardioversion of atrial fibrillation: a multicenter study. *Circulation* 1994;89:2509–2513.
28. Grimm RA, Stewart WJ, Black IW, et al. Should all patients undergo transesophageal echocardiography before electrical cardioversion of atrial fibrillation? *J Am Coll Cardiol* 1994;23:533–541.
29. Klein AL, Grimm RA, Murray AD, et al. Assessment of cardioversion using transesophageal echocardiography investigators: use of transesophageal echocardiography to guide cardioversion in patients with atrial fibrillation. *N Engl J Med* 2001;344:1411–1420.
30. Hausmann D, Daniel WG, Mugge A, et al. Value of transesophageal color Doppler echocardiography for detection of different types of atrial septal defect in adults. *J Am Soc Echocardiogr* 1992;5:481–488.
31. Kronzon I, Tunick PA, Freedberg RS, et al. Transesophageal echocardiography is superior to transthoracic echocardiography in the diagnosis of sinus venosus atrial septal defect. *J Am Coll Cardiol* 1991;17:537–542.
32. Rittoo D, Sutherland GR, Shaw TR. Quantification of left-to-right shunting and defect size after balloon mitral commissurotomy using biplane transesophageal echocardiography, color flow Doppler mapping, and the principle of proximal flow convergence. *Circulation* 1993;87:1591–1603.
33. Hagen PT, Scholz DG, Edwards WD. Incidence and size of patent foramen ovale during the first 10 decades of life: an autopsy study of 965 normal hearts. *Mayo Clin Proc* 1984;59:17–20.
34. Lechat P, Mas JL, Lascault G, et al. Prevalence of patent foramen ovale in patients with stroke. *N Engl J Med* 1988;318:1148–1152.
35. Meacham RR 3rd, Headley AS, Bronze MS, et al. Impending paradoxical embolism. *Arch Intern Med* 1998;158:438–448.
36. Pearson AC, Labovitz AJ, Tatineni S, et al. Superiority of transesophageal echocardiography in detecting cardiac source of embolism in patients with cerebral ischemia of uncertain etiology. *J Am Coll Cardiol* 1991;17:66–72.
37. Schneider B, Zienkiewicz T, Jansen V, et al. Diagnosis of patent foramen ovale by transesophageal echocardiography and correlation with autopsy findings. *Am J Cardiol* 1996;77:1202–1209.
38. de Belder MA, Tourikis L, Griffith M, et al. Transesophageal contrast echocardiography and color flow mapping: methods of choice for the detection of shunts at the atrial level. *Am Heart J* 1992;1992:1545–1550.
39. Pearson AC, Nagelhout D, Castello R, et al. Atrial septal aneurysm and stroke: a transesophageal echocardiographic study. *J Am Coll Cardiol* 1991;18:1223–1229.
40. Agmon Y, Khandheria BK, Meissner I, et al. Frequency of atrial septal aneurysms in patients with cerebral ischemic events. *Circulation* 1999;99: 1942–1944.
41. Burstow DJ, McEniery PT, Stafford EG. Fenestrated atrial septal aneurysm: diagnosis by transesophageal echocardiography. *J Am Soc Echocardiogr* 1990;3:499–501.
42. Mugge A, Daniel WG, Angermann C, et al. Atrial septal aneurysm in adult patients: a multicenter study using transthoracic and transesophageal echocardiography. *Circulation* 1995;91:2785–2792.
43. Mugge A, Daniel WG, Haverick A, et al. Diagnosis of noninfective cardiac mass lesions by two-dimensional echocardiography: comparison of transthoracic and transesophageal approaches. *Circulation* 1991;83:70–78.
44. Durack DT, Lukes AS, Bright DK. New criteria for diagnosis of infective endocarditis: utilization of specific echocardiographic findings: Duke Endocarditis Service. *Am J Med* 1994;96:200–209.
45. Erbel R, Rohmann S, Drexler M, et al. Improved diagnostic value of echocardiography in patients with infective endocarditis by transesophageal approach: a prospective study. *Eur Heart J* 1988;9:43–53.

46. Shively BK, Gurule FT, Roldan CA, et al. Diagnostic value of transesophageal compared with transthoracic echocardiography in infective endocarditis. *J Am Coll Cardiol* 1991;18:391–397.
47. Daniel WG, Mugge A, Grote J, et al. Comparison of transthoracic and transesophageal echocardiography for detection of abnormalities of prosthetic and bioprosthetic valves in the mitral and aortic positions. *Am J Cardiol* 1993;71:210–215.
48. Zabalgoitia M, Herrera CJ, Chaudhry FA, et al. Improvement in the diagnosis of bioprosthetic valve dysfunction by transesophageal echocardiography. *J Heart Valve Dis* 1993;2:595–603.
49. San Roman JA, Vilacosta I, Zamorano JL, et al. Transesophageal echocardiography in right-sided endocarditis. *J Am Coll Cardiol* 1993;21:1226–1230.
50. Shapiro SM, Young E, Ginzton LE, et al. Pulmonic valve endocarditis as an underdiagnosed disease: role of transesophageal echocardiography. *J Am Soc Echocardiogr* 1992;5:48–51.
51. Vilacosta I, Sarria C, San Roman JA, et al. Usefulness of transesophageal echocardiography for diagnosis of infected transvenous permanent pacemakers. *Circulation* 1994;89:2684–2687.
52. De Castro S, Cartoni D, d'Amati G, et al. Diagnostic accuracy of transthoracic and multiplane transesophageal echocardiography for valvular perforation in acute infective endocarditis: correlation with anatomic findings. *Clin Infect Dis* 2000;30:825–826.
53. Daniel WG, Mugge A, Martin R, et al. Improvement in the diagnosis of abscesses associated with endocarditis by transesophageal echocardiography. *N Engl J Med* 1991;324:795–800.
54. Karalis DG, Bansal RC, Hauck AJ, et al. Transesophageal echocardiographic recognition of subaortic complication in aortic valve endocarditis: clinical and surgical implications. *Circulation* 1992;86:353–362.
55. Rohmann S, Erbel R, Mohr-Kahaly S, et al. Use of transesophageal echocardiography in the diagnosis of abscess in infective endocarditis. *Eur Heart J* 1995;16:54–62.
56. Leung DY, Cranney GB, Hopkins AP, et al. Role of transesophageal echocardiography in the diagnosis and management of aortic root abscess. *Br Heart J* 1994;72:175–181.
57. Sochowski RA, Chan KL. Implication of negative results on a monoplane transesophageal echocardiographic study in patients with suspected infective endocarditis. *J Am Coll Cardiol* 1993;21:216–221.
58. Lindner JR, Case RA, Dent JM, et al. Diagnostic value of echocardiography in suspected endocarditis: an evaluation based on the pretest probability of disease. *Circulation* 1996;93:730–736.
59. Roe MT, Abramson MA, Li J, et al. Clinical information determines the impact of transesophageal echocardiography on the diagnosis of infective endocarditis by the duke criteria. *Am Heart J* 2000;139:945–951.
60. Adachi H, Omoto R, Kyo S, et al. Emergency surgical intervention of acute aortic dissection with the rapid diagnosis by transesophageal echocardiography. *Circulation* 1991;84(suppl 3):14–19.
61. Simon P, Owen AN, Havel M, et al. Transesophageal echocardiography in the emergency surgical management of patients with aortic dissection. *J Thorac Cardiovasc Surg* 1992;103:1113–1117.
62. Cigarrao JE, Isselbacher EM, DeSanctis RW, et al. Diagnostic imaging in the evaluation of suspected aortic dissection: old standards and new directions. *N Engl J Med* 1993;328:35–43.
63. Nienaber CA, Spielman RP, Kodolitsch YV, et al. Diagnosis of thoracic aortic dissection: magnetic resonance imaging versus transesophageal echocardiography. *Circulation* 1992;85:434–447.
64. Nienaber CA, von Kodolitsch Y, Nicolas V, et al. The diagnosis of thoracic aortic dissection by noninvasive imaging procedures. *N Engl J Med* 1993;328:1–9.
65. Bansal RC, Chandrasekaran K, Ayala K, et al. Frequency and explanation of false negative diagnosis of aortic dissection by aortography and transesophageal echocardiography. *J Am Coll Cardiol* 1995;25:1393–1401.
66. Deutsch HJ, Sechtem U, Meyer H, et al. Chronic aortic dissection: comparison of MR imaging and transesophageal echocardiography. *Radiology* 1994;192:845–850.
67. Adachi H, Kyo S, Takamoto S, et al. Early diagnosis and surgical intervention of acute aortic dissection by transesophageal color flow mapping. *Circulation* 1990;82(suppl 4):19–23.
68. Svensson LG, Labib SB, Eisenhauer AC, et al. Intimal tear without hematoma: an important variant of aortic dissection that can elude current imaging techniques. *Circulation* 1999;99:1331–1336.
69. Ballal RS, Nanda NC, Gatewood R, et al. Usefulness of transesophageal echocardiography in assessment of aortic dissection. *Circulation* 1991;84:1903–1914.
70. Applebe AF, Walker PG, Yeoh JK, et al. Clinical significance and origin of artifacts in transesophageal echocardiography of the thoracic aorta. *J Am Coll Cardiol* 1993;21:754–760.
71. Evangelista A, Garcia-del-Castillo H, Gonzalez-Alujas T, et al. Diagnosis of ascending aortic dissection by transesophageal echocardiography: utility of M-mode in recognizing artifacts. *J Am Coll Cardiol* 1996;27:102–107.
72. Harris KM, Braverman AC, Gutierrez FR, et al. Transesophageal echocardiographic and clinical features of aortic intramural hematoma. *J Thorac Cardiovasc Surg* 1997;114:619–626.
73. Vilacosta I, San Roman JA, Ferreiros J, et al. Natural history and serial morphology of aortic intramural hematoma: a novel variant of aortic dissection. *Am Heart J* 1997;134:495–507.
74. Mohr-Kahaly S, Erbel R, Kearney P, et al. Aortic intramural hemorrhage visualized by transesophageal echocardiography: findings and prognostic implications. *J Am Coll Cardiol* 1994;23:658–664.
75. Atar S, Nagai T, Birnbaum Y, et al. Transesophageal echocardiographic Doppler findings in patients with penetrating aortic ulcers. *Am J Cardiol* 1999;83:133–135.
76. Vilacosta I, San Roman JA, Aragoncillo P, et al. Penetrating atherosclerotic aortic ulcer: documentation by transesophageal echocardiography. *J Am Coll Cardiol* 1998;32:83–89.
77. Smith MD, Cassidy JM, Souther S, et al. Transesophageal echocardiography in the diagnosis of traumatic rupture of the aorta. *N Engl J Med* 1995;332:356–362.
78. Tunick PA, Kronzon I. Atheromas of the thoracic aorta: clinical and therapeutic update. *J Am Coll Cardiol* 2000;35:545–554.
79. Tribouilloy C, Shen WF, Peltier M, et al. Noninvasive prediction of coronary artery disease by transesophageal echocardiographic detection of thoracic aortic plaque in valvular heart disease. *Am J Cardiol* 1994;74:258–260.
80. Nihoyannopoulos P, Joshi J, Athanasopoulos G, et al. Detection of atherosclerotic lesions in the aorta by transesophageal echocardiography. *Am J Cardiol* 1993;71:208–212.
81. Karalis DG, Chandrasekaran K, Victor MF, et al. The recognition and embolic potential of intraaortic atherosclerotic debris. *J Am Coll Cardiol* 1991;17:73–78.
82. Amarenco P, Cohen A, Tzourio C, et al. Atherosclerotic disease of the aortic arch and the risk of ischemic stroke. *N Engl J Med* 1994;331:1474–1479.
83. Katz ES, Tunick PA, Rusinek H, et al. Protruding aortic atheromas predict stroke in elderly patients undergoing cardiopulmonary bypass: experience with intraoperative transesophageal echocardiography. *J Am Coll Cardiol* 1992;20:70–77.
84. Bansal RC, Pauls GL, Shankel SW. Blue digit syndrome: transesophageal echocardiographic identification of thoracic aortic plaque-related thrombi and successful outcome with warfarin. *J Am Soc Echocardiogr* 1993;6:319–323.
85. Hozumi T, Yoshikawa J, Yoshida K, et al. Direct visualization of ruptured chordae tendineae by transesophageal two-dimensional echocardiography. *J Am Coll Cardiol* 1990;16:1315–1319.
86. Sochowski RA, Chan KL, Ascah KJ, et al. Comparison of accuracy of transesophageal versus transthoracic echocardiography for the detection of mitral valve prolapse with ruptured chordae tendineae (flail mitral leaflet). *Am J Cardiol* 1991;67:1251–1255.
87. Foster GP, Isselbacher EM, Rose GA, et al. Accurate localization of mitral regurgitant defects using multiplane transesophageal echocardiography. *Ann Thorac Surg* 1998;65:1025–1031.
88. Maslow AD, Regan MM, Haering JM, et al. Echocardiographic predictors of left ventricular outflow tract obstruction and systolic anterior motion of the mitral valve after mitral valve reconstruction for myxomatous valve disease. *J Am Coll Cardiol* 1999;34:2096–2104.
89. Enriquez-Sarano M, Freeman WK, Tribouilloy CM, et al. Functional anatomy of mitral regurgitation: accuracy and outcome implications of transesophageal echocardiography. *J Am Coll Cardiol* 1999;34:1129–1136.
90. Stoddard MF, Keedy DL, Kupersmith J. Transesophageal echocardiographic diagnosis of papillary muscle rupture complicating acute myocardial infarction. *Am Heart J* 1990;120:690–692.
91. Widimsky P, Ten Cate FJ, Vletter W, et al. Potential applications for transesophageal echocardiography in hypertrophic cardiomyopathies. *J Am Soc Echocardiogr* 1992;5:163–167.
92. Espinal M, Fuisz AR, Nanda NC, et al. Sensitivity and specificity of transesophageal echocardiography for determination of aortic valve morphology. *Am Heart J* 2000;139:1071–1076.
93. Stoddard MF, Acre J, Liddell NE, et al. Two-dimensional transesophageal echocardiographic determination of aortic valve area in adults with aortic stenosis. *Am Heart J* 1991;122:1415–1422.
94. Nellessen U, Schnittger I, Appleton CP, et al. Transesophageal two-dimensional echocardiography and color Doppler flow velocity mapping in the evaluation of cardiac valve prosthesis. *Circulation* 1988;78:848–855.
95. Laffort P, Roudaut R, Roques X, et al. Early and long-term (one-year) effects of the association of aspirin and oral anticoagulant on thrombi and morbidity after replacement of the mitral valve with the St. Jude medical prosthesis: a clinical and transesophageal echocardiographic study. *J Am Coll Cardiol* 2000;35:739–746.
96. Flachskampf FA, O' Shea JP, Griffin BP, et al. Patterns of transvalvular regurgitation in normal mechanical prosthetic valves. *J Am Coll Cardiol* 1991;18:1493–1498.
97. Chaudhry FA, Herrera C, DeFrino PF, et al. Pathologic and angiographic correlations of transesophageal echocardiography in prosthetic heart valve dysfunction. *Am Heart J* 1991;122:1057–1064.
98. Karalis DG, Chandrasekaran K, Ross JJ Jr, et al. Single-plane transesophageal echocardiography for assessing function of mechanical or

bioprosthetic valves in the aortic valve position. *Am J Cardiol* 1992;69: 1310–1315.
99. Gueret P, Vignon P, Fournier P, et al. Transesophageal echocardiography for the diagnosis and management of nonobstructive thrombosis of mechanical mitral valve prosthesis. *Circulation* 1995;91:103–110.
100. Barbetseas J, Nagueh SF, Pitsavos C, et al. Differentiating thrombus from pannus formation in obstructed mechanical prosthetic valves: an evaluation of clinical, transthoracic and transesophageal echocardiographic parameters. *J Am Coll Cardiol* 1998;32:1410–1417.
101. Lin SS, Tiong IYH, Asher CR, et al. Prediction of thrombus-related mechanical prosthetic valve dysfunction using transesophageal echocardiography. *Am J Cardiol* 2000;86:1097–1101.
102. Ozkan M, Kaymaz C, Kirma C, et al. Intravenous thrombolytic treatment of mechanical prosthetic valve thrombosis: a study using serial transesophageal echocardiography. *J Am Coll Cardiol* 2000;35:1881–1889.
103. Come PC, Riley MF, Bivas NK. Roles of echocardiography and arrhythmia monitoring in the evaluation of patients with suspected systemic embolism. *Ann Neurol* 1983;13:527–531.
104. Sansoy V, Abbott RD, Jayaweera AR, et al. Low yield of transthoracic echocardiography for cardiac source of embolism. *Am J Cardiol* 1995;75: 166–169.
105. DeRook FA, Comess KA, Albers GW, et al. Transesophageal echocardiography in the evaluation of stroke. *Ann Intern Med* 1992;117:922–932.
106. Lee RJ, Bartzokis T, Yeoh TK, et al. Enhanced detection of intracardiac sources of cerebral emboli by transesophageal echocardiography. *Stroke* 1991;22:734–739.
106a. Comess KA, DeRook FA, Beach KW, et al. Transesophageal echocardiography and carotid ultrasound in patients with cerebral ischemia: prevalence of findings and recurrent stroke risk. *J Am Coll Cardiol* 1994;23:1598–1603.
107. Tardif JC, Vannon MA, Taylor K, et al. Delineation of extended lengths of coronary arteries by multiplane transesophageal echocardiography. *J Am Coll Cardiol* 1994;24:909–919.
108. Samdarshi TE, Nanda NC, Gatewood RP Jr, et al. Usefulness and limitations of transesophageal echocardiography in the assessment of proximal coronary artery stenosis. *J Am Coll Cardiol* 1992;19:572–580.
109. Yoshida K, Yoshikawa J, Hozumi T, et al. Detection of left main coronary artery stenosis by transesophageal color Doppler and two-dimensional echocardiography. *Circulation* 1990;81:1271–1276.
110. Firstenberg MS, Greenberg NL, Lin SS, et al. Transesophageal echocardiography assessment of severe ostial left main coronary stenosis. *J Am Soc Echocardiogr* 2000;13:696–698.
111. Calafiore PA, Raymond R, Schiavone W, et al. Precise evaluation of a complex coronary arteriovenous fistula: the utility of transesophageal color Doppler. *J Am Soc Echocardiogr* 1989;2:337–341.
112. Kosar E, Chandraratna PA. Assessment of coronary artery aneurysms with multiplane transesophageal echocardiography. *Am Heart J* 1997;133:526–533.
113. Skiles JA, Griffin BP. Transesophageal echocardiographic (TEE) evaluation of ventricular function. *Cardiol Clin* 2000;18:681–697.
114. Agati L, Renzi M, Sciomer S, et al. Transesophageal dipyridamole echocardiography for diagnosis of coronary artery disease. *J Am Coll Cardiol* 1992;19:765–770.
115. Frohwein S, Klein JL, Lane A, et al. Transesophageal dobutamine stress echocardiography in the evaluation of coronary artery disease. *J Am Coll Cardiol* 1995;25:823–829.
116. Hoffmann R, Kleinhans E, Lambertz H, et al. Transesophageal pacing echocardiography for detection of restenosis after percutaneous transluminal coronary angioplasty. *Eur Heart J* 1994;15:823–831.
117. Panza JA, Laurienzo JM, Curiel RV, et al. Transesophageal dobutamine stress echocardiography for evaluation of patients with coronary artery disease. *J Am Coll Cardiol* 1994;24:1260–1267.
118. Panza JA, Curiel RV, Laurienzo JM, et al. Relation between ischemic threshold measured during dobutamine stress echocardiography and known indices of poor prognosis in patients with coronary artery disease. *Circulation* 1995;92:2095–2101.
119. Madu EC. Transesophageal dobutamine stress echocardiography in the evaluation of myocardial ischemia in morbidly obese subjects. *Chest* 2000;117:657–661.
120. Stumper OF, Elzenga NJ, Hess J, et al. Transesophageal echocardiography in children with congenital heart disease: an initial experience. *J Am Coll Cardiol* 1990;16:433–441.
121. Weintraub R, Shiota T, Elkadi T, et al. Transesophageal echocardiography in infants and children with congenital heart disease. *Circulation* 1992;86:711–722.
122. Marelli AJ, Child JS, Perloff JK. Transesophageal echocardiography in congenital heart disease in the adult. *Cardiol Clin* 1993;11:505–520.
123. Vargas-Barron J, Rijlaardsam M, Romero-Cardenas A, et al. Transesophageal echocardiography in adults with congenital cardiopathies. *Am Heart J* 1993;126:426–432.
124. Sreeram N, Sutherland GR, Geuskens R, et al. The role of transoesophageal echocardiography in adolescents and adults with congenital heart defects. *Eur Heart J* 1991;12:231–240.
125. Stumper O, Vargas-Barron J, Rijlaarsdam M, et al. Assessment of anomalous systemic and pulmonary venous connections by transesophageal echocardiography in infants and children. *Br Heart J* 1991;66:411–418.
126. Sreeram N, Stumper OF, Kaulitz R, et al. Comparative value of transthoracic and transesophageal echocardiography in the assessment of congenital abnormalities of the atrioventricular junction. *J Am Coll Cardiol* 1990;16: 1205–1214.
127. Gnanapragasam JP, Houston AB, Doig WB, et al. Transesophageal echocardiographic assessment of fixed subaortic obstruction in children. *Br Heart J* 1991;66:281–284.
128. Kaulitz R, Oliver F, Stumper W, et al. Comparative values of the precordial and transesophageal approaches in the echocardiographic evaluation of atrial baffle function after an atrial correction procedure. *J Am Coll Cardiol* 1990;16:686–694.
129. Stumper O, Sutherland GR, Geuskens R, et al. Transesophageal echocardiography in evaluation and management after a Fontan procedure. *J Am Coll Cardiol* 1991;17:1152–1160.
130. Fyfe DA, Kline CH, Sade RM, et al. Transesophageal echocardiography detects thrombus formation not identified by transthoracic echocardiography after the Fontan operation. *J Am Coll Cardiol* 1991;18:1733–1737.
131. Goldstein SA, Campbell AN. Mitral stenosis: evaluation and guidance of valvuloplasty by transesophageal echocardiography. *Cardiol Clin* 1993;11:409–425.
132. Lee KS, Tuzcu EM, Elliott JM, et al. Rapid development of left atrial thrombus associated with percutaneous mitral valvuloplasty. *Cathet Cardiovasc Diagn* 1994;33:345–348.
133. Tumbarello R, Sanna A, Cardu G, et al. Usefulness of transesophageal echocardiography in the pediatric catheterization laboratory. *Am J Cardiol* 1993;71:1321–1325.
134. Dhillon R, Thanopoulos B, Tsaousis G, et al. Transcatheter closure of atrial septal defects in adults with the Amplatzer septal occluder. *Heart* 1999;82: 559–562.
135. Rubin DC, Ziskind AA, Hawke MW, et al. Transesophageal echocardiographically guided percutaneous biopsy of a right atrial cardiac mass. *Am Heart J* 1994;127:935–936.
136. Pytlewski G, Georgeson S, Burke J, et al. Endomyocardial biopsy under transesophageal echocardiographic guidance can be safely performed in the critically ill cardiac transplant recipient. *Am J Cardiol* 1994;73:1019–1020.
137. Stumper O, Witsenburg M, Sutherland GR, et al. Transesophageal echocardiographic monitoring of interventional cardiac catheterization in children. *J Am Coll Cardiol* 1991;18:1506–1514.
138. Erbel R, Bednarczyk I, Pop T, et al. Detection of dissection of the aortic intima and media after angioplasty of coarctation of the aorta: an angiographic, computer tomographic, and echocardiographic comparative study. *Circulation* 1990;81:805–814.
139. Jordaens LJ, Vandenbogaerde JF, Van de Bruaene P, et al. Transesophageal echocardiography for insertion of a physiological pacemaker in early pregnancy. *Pacing Clin Electrophysiol* 1990;13:955–957.
140. Khandheria BK. Transesophageal echocardiography in the evaluation of prosthetic valves. *Cardiol Clin* 1993;11:427–436.
141. Fisher EA, Stahl JA, Budd JH, et al. Transesophageal echocardiography: procedures and clinical application. *J Am Coll Cardiol* 1991;18:1333–1348.
142. Matsuzaki M, Toma Y, Kusukawa R. Clinical applications of transesophageal echocardiography. *Circulation* 1990;82:709–722.
143. Weyman AE. *Principles and practice of echocardiography,* 2nd ed. Philadelphia: JB Lippincott, 1994.
144. Schimpf T, Mischke K, Plisiene J, et al. Single-step atrial thrombus exclusion and internal cardioversion of atrial fibrillation via a transesophageal echocardiography probe. *J Am Coll Cardiol* 2005;46:560–561.

CHAPTER 53 ■ IMAGING TECHNIQUES IN NUCLEAR CARDIOLOGY

MANUEL D. CERQUEIRA

Myocardial perfusion imaging (MPI) using radionuclide techniques with electrocardiographically (ECG)-gated single photon emission computed tomography (SPECT) is the most commonly performed diagnostic test for assessing the presence of critical coronary artery stenosis and determining prognosis. It provides diagnostic and prognostic clinical benefit in the initial evaluation of patients with suspected, but unproved coronary artery disease (CAD) and in those patients where a diagnosis of CAD has been established and information on prognosis or risk is required (1). Although radionuclide techniques can also be used to assess function, metabolism, innervation, and infarction, these techniques are seldom used in clinical practice. Positron emission tomography (PET) has superior imaging properties and capabilities over SPECT, but the cost and limited availability of cyclotron or generator produced radioactive radiotracers has limited widespread utilization. Currently there are more than 8 million cardiac SPECT but fewer than 50,000 cardiac PET procedures preformed annually in the United States.

Since the last publication of this textbook, new American College of Cardiology (ACC)/American Heart Association (AHA)/American Society of Nuclear Cardiology (ASNC) Guidelines for the Clinical Use of Cardiac Radionuclide Imaging have been published and are included in this section (1). In addition, a new process for assessing the appropriateness of radionuclide imaging was undertaken and published as the ACC/ASNC Appropriateness Criteria for Single-Photon Emission computed Tomography Myocardial Perfusion Imaging (SPECT MPI) (2). This chapter reviews the basic physiologic basis for SPECT MPI, radionuclides, protocols, exercise and pharmacologic stress, image interpretation, and the application of these techniques based on the guidelines in important clinical settings.

BASIS OF MYOCARDIAL PERFUSION IMAGING

During stress, blood flow increases through normal coronary arteries. In vessels with significant luminal stenosis, variously defined as anywhere from 50% to 80% luminal cross-sectional narrowing, or abnormal functional flow reserve, there is no increase, the increase is less or occasionally there may even be a decrease in coronary artery blood flow. This diminished coronary flow reserve is not an all-or-none phenomenon; rather, flow reserve decreases gradually as the severity of the coronary stenosis progresses. The most severe stenosis, greater than 85%, typically have no flow reserve. Given this framework, the use of radionuclides requires a measurement of flow in the resting state and after some maneuver, usually exercise or pharmacologic stress, that increases coronary blood flow and results in flow heterogeneity between normal vessels and those with anatomic narrowing or physiologic impairment.

RADIOTRACERS AND PROTOCOLS

The three commonly used radiotracers are thallium-201 (Tl-201) and the 2 technetium-99m (Tc-99m) labeled compounds, sestamibi, and tetrofosmin. The properties of these tracers are listed in Table 53.1.

Radiotracers

Thallium-201

Tl-201 was the first radiotracer used for clinical MPI. It is a K^+ analog that is transported across cell membranes by the Na/K ATPase system (3). It has an initial myocardial uptake that is proportional to blood flow over a wide physiologic range and depends on the presence of viable myocardial cells. Following the very rapid and high initial uptake, Tl-201 reequilibrates with the lower concentration in the blood in a time-dependent fashion. This is called *washout* or *redistribution* and, like the initial uptake of Tl-201, is directly proportional to blood flow to the area and the presence of functioning myocytes. In the typical imaging sequence using Tl-201 (Figure 53.1), the patient has a stress study with dynamic exercise or pharmacologic

TABLE 53.1

COMPARISON OF THALLIUM-201, SESTAMIBI, AND TETROFOSMIN FOR MPI

Variable	Thallium-201	Sestamibi	Tetrofosmin
Dose (mCi)	3.0–4.0	10–30	10–30
Energy (KeV)	80	140	140
Cyclotron product	Yes	No	No
Half-life (h)	73	6	6
Extraction at normal flow (%)	85	65	60
Extraction at high flow	Lower	Lower	Lower
Myocardial uptake	Adenosine triphosphatase	Unknown	Unknown
Myocardial clearance	Fast, variable	Very slow	Very slow
Hepatobiliary excretion	No	Yes	Yes
Perfusion function studies	Yes	Yes	Yes
Gated perfusion	Yes	Yes	Yes
Stress redistribution	Yes	No	No
Stress rest	No	Yes	Yes
Time between injections (hours)	NA	≥2	≥2
Time to imaging (min)	<10	15–60	15–60
Feasibility with pharmacologic stressor	Yes	Yes	Yes
Assessment of viability	Yes	Yes	Yes
Imaging protocol (days)	1	1 or 2	1 or 2

stress. Within 10 to 15 minutes of completion of stress the patient is imaged and this is followed 2.5 to 4 hours later by a redistribution set of images. Areas of myocardium supplied by normal coronary arteries have a high and uniform uptake on both the stress and redistribution images. Areas of infarction have very low or absent uptake on the initial stress images; there are a diminished number of myocytes and there is no change on the redistribution images. Following stress, there is an increase in blood flow and those areas of myocardium beyond a flow-limiting critical anatomic or physiologic coronary stenosis have low uptake of Tl-201 relative to the areas of myocardium with normal coronary blood supply. Areas of ischemia and infarction look identical on the poststress images. However, with ischemia the redistribution images show improvement in the ischemic areas and this allows the differentiation to be made between infarct and ischemic myocardium.

One of the major advantages of using Tl-201 is that it is also an excellent marker of myocardial viability (4). The high and nearly linear initial myocardial uptake following stress makes Tl-201 a marker of myocardial blood flow. The uptake and redistribution over time is a marker of the K^+ blood pool and of viable myocardium. In areas where blood flow is severely reduced following stress, there may be very low uptake of Tl-201 initially despite the presence of living myocytes. Even the 3- to 4-hour redistribution images may still be abnormal. However, over time, if there are viable myocytes with an intact Na/K ATPase system, Tl-201 is eventually taken up and these areas are clearly identified as hibernating myocardium and not infarction.

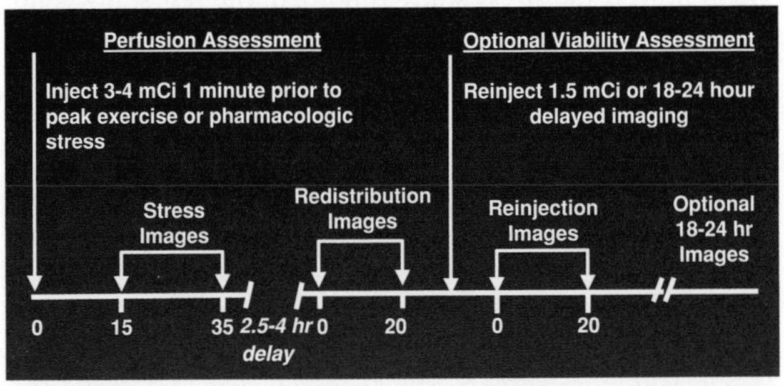

FIGURE 53.1. Time course for an exercise stress and 3- to 4-hour delayed redistribution Tl-201 imaging sequence. Reinjection of an additional 1 mCi of Tl-201 can be performed before or after redistribution imaging or repeat imaging can be performed at 24 hours for optimal identification of myocardial viability.

Assessment of viability is especially important in patients with congestive heart failure, known cardiomyopathies, or recent myocardial infarction. In patients where myocardial viability assessment is of critical clinical importance and PET is not available, several approaches using Tl-201 are shown in Figure 53.1 that can be used to further improve on the accuracy of the regular stress/redistribution sequence. These approaches include a rest injection followed 3 to 4 hours later by redistribution images; reinjection of Tl-201 before the redistribution imaging in a stress redistribution sequence; or delayed imaging at 18 to 24 hours in the typical stress/redistribution sequence.

Tc-99m Radiotracers

Tc-99m tracers were developed to overcome limitations of Tl-201. There are two Tc-99m tracers used clinically: Tc-99m sestamibi (Cardiolite) and Tc-99m tetrofosmin (Myoview). The monoenergetic140 keV higher energy of Tc-99m versus the 69-83 keV of Tl-201 results in improved resolution with less overall attenuation and scatter during imaging. Tc-99m has a half-life of 6 hours in comparison to the 72 hours of Tl-201. The shorter half-life allows administration of a higher Tc-99m dose resulting in high-count images. As an example, 4 mCi of Tl-201 are administered as compared to 30 mCi of the Tc-99m radiotracers. The higher counts obtained with a Tc-99m radiopharmaceutical and the lack of redistribution allows ECG-triggered gated acquisition, ECG-gated SPECT, for assessment of function. The minimal redistribution of Tc-99m tracers following injection allows greater flexibility as to when acquisition can be performed; as soon as 10 minutes or as long as 4 hours following stress. Patients can be injected in remote locations of the hospital, such as in the emergency department for patients presenting with chest pain and a nondiagnostic ECG. They can be safely and conveniently transported for imaging when they are stable. The improved imaging characteristics of Tc-99m tracers are especially beneficial in women and obese patients where soft tissue attenuation has been a traditional problem for Tl-201. This frequently resulted in false-positive interpretations and a low specificity.

Tc-99m Sestamibi and Tetrofosmin

Both Tc-99m sestamibi and tetrofosmin are monovalent hydrophilic cations, which makes them very lipophilic and facilitates entry into cells. Uptake depends on blood flow, plasma- and mitochondrial-derived membrane electrochemical gradients, cellular pH, and intact energy pathways (3). Chemical or structural conversion of the molecule is not required, and inhibitors of Na^+, K^+, and Ca^{2+} transport do not prevent uptake or retention in myocytes. Once inside the myocyte, they remain trapped with the greatest concentration in the mitochondria and there is minimal washout. Following intravenous injection they are cleared from blood by the liver, concentrated in the gallbladder and excreted through the common bile duct into the gastrointestinal (GI) tract. The initial high liver uptake does not allow the inferior wall to be seen clearly early postinjection and requires waiting 30 to 60 minutes following resting or pharmacologic stress injection to obtain adequate visualization. Clearance postexercise is rapid and image acquisition can be started as soon as 10 to 20 minutes following injection.

Tc-99m Radiotracer Imaging Protocol Options

The clearance characteristics of Tc-99m sestamibi and tetrofosmin are sufficiently similar that recommendations for imaging are identical with some variation between injection time and when to image owing to differences in liver clearance (5). The following wait time intervals between injection and starting imaging are recommended: 10 to 20 minutes following exercise stress and 30 to 60 minutes after rest or pharmacologic stress.

There are several protocol options for Tc-99m radiotracer imaging: a 2-day protocol, a 1-day split-dose protocol using either a stress/rest or rest/stress sequence, and a dual isotope approach using Tl-201 at rest and a Tc-99m radiotracer with exercise or pharmacologic stress. Diagnostic accuracy results reported in the literature did not report significant differences between the various protocol options or between these agents and Tl-201 (1).

Two-Day Protocol

The sequence for a 2-day imaging protocol (Figure 53.2) allows the administration of the maximal dose of Tc-99m—20 to 30 mCi—for both the rest and stress studies and results in high counts and better image quality. It is mandatory in obese patients, and allows a true rest ejection fraction (EF) to be calculated as well as poststress measurement, which provides additional value. Although this is the best way to perform Tc-99m MPI, it is inconvenient for most patients to make two visits

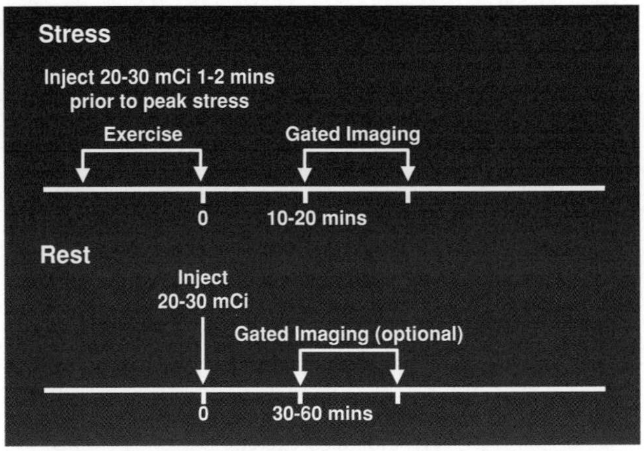

FIGURE 53.2. Time course for a 2-day stress/rest protocol using a Tc-99m radiotracer. This protocol uses high and equal doses for stress and rest and avoids contamination or residual activity from the stress dose when the rest images are acquired.

and there is a delay in providing referring physicians with the needed clinical information.

The advantage of doing the stress study on the first day is that if it is normal, the resting study is not needed. This approach minimizes delay in getting results to the referring physician, patient inconvenience is minimal, and total study cost and radiation exposure are lower. Unfortunately, in obese patients with soft tissue attenuation and low counts, there are usually enough areas in question owing to attenuation that the resting study is usually required the following day. Gating and attenuation correction improve specificity and decrease the number of patients needing to return for a rest study (6,7).

One-Day Studies

For logistical reasons, stress and rest studies are usually performed using a 1-day protocol as shown in Figures 53.3, 53.4, 53.5, and 53.6 for exercise and pharmacologic stress. This requires administration of a low dose, one third of the total dose or 8 to 12 mCi, for the first study and a larger dose, two thirds of the total dose or 20 to 30 mCi, for the second study and waiting as long as possible between studies, usually 1.5 to 2.5 hours, to allow for physical decay of Tc-99m. Using this approach, when the second set of images area are acquired, there is relatively little contamination from the first injection. The timing and sequence for a 1-day stress/rest Tc-99m radiotracer study is shown in Figure 53.3. In this sequence, the lower Tc-99m radiotracer dose is administered when myocardial blood flow is the highest, during stress, and background activity in the subdiaphragmatic area is low owing to a decrease in mesenteric blood flow. If the stress study is normal, the rest study is not needed. If the stress is abnormal, the rest study, using a higher dose, can be started almost immediately.

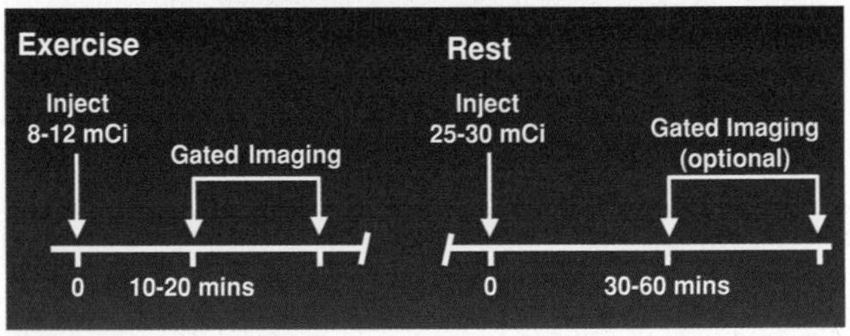

FIGURE 53.3. Time course for a 1-day exercise stress/rest protocol for use with Tc-99m radiotracers. When the initial stress study is normal, the resting study is optional.

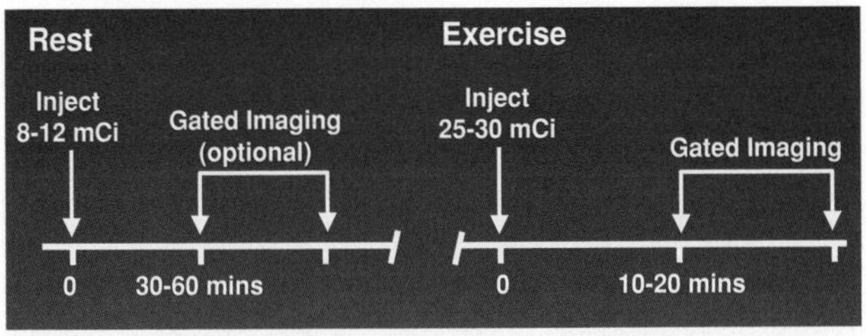

FIGURE 53.4. Time course for a 1-day rest/exercise protocol for use with Tc-99m radiotracers.

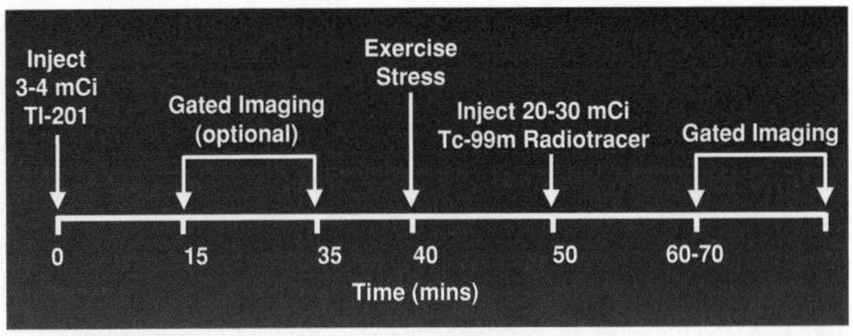

FIGURE 53.5. Time course for a separate acquisition dual isotope study using Tl-201 at rest and Tc-99m radiotracer tracer for the stress study.

The 1-day rest/stress sequence (Figure 53.4) is the most frequently performed protocol. The disadvantage of this sequence is that the low Tc-99m tracer dose is given during the rest study when blood flow is lowest and there is less myocardial uptake. The higher stress dose, administered when blood flow is maximal, gives higher counts and better quality images. The gated poststress image in patients with extensive ischemia may give a lower EF, owing to residual myocardial stunning, then a true resting EF (8). In patients with ischemia, a lower poststress EF is a better predictor of higher cardiac death and infarction rate then the size and severity of the defect alone (9,10).

Separate Acquisition Dual Isotope Thallium-201/Tc99 Radiotracer Protocol

The timing and sequence for a Tl-201/Tc-99m radiotracer dual isotope separate acquisition protocol is displayed in Figure 53.7. For the resting Tl-201 study, the patient should be fasting and a dose of 3 to 4 mCi of Tl-201 injected. Imaging should be delayed for 10 to 15 minutes. After acquiring these images, the patient is stressed and injected with 20 to 30 mCi of a Tc-99m tracer. The separate acquisition approach takes advantage of the two distinct and separate energy levels of Tl-201 and Tc-99m. During the second acquisition, the γ-camera selectively acquires data centering on the higher energy Tc-99m window. Although, there is residual Tl-201 present from the resting study, the lower energy Tl-201 photons are excluded by the higher Tc-99m window. The small amount of higher energy Tl-201 decay that is incorrectly registered in the Tc-99m window has a negligible effect on the images.

In situations where critical management decisions need to be made regarding myocardial hibernation, a rest–4 hour redistribution Tl-201 study should be performed prior to performing the stress study (11). Patients can also be injected with Tl-201 the evening before imaging to give an approximate 12-hour Tl-201 acquisition the following morning. This is an excellent method for the identification of myocardial viability. When the stress study has already been performed and questions of viability remain, delayed Tl-201 imaging cannot be performed on the same day because of the downscatter of the Tc-99m into the Tl-201 energy window. Patients can return the next day for imaging when decay of the Tc-99m has occurred and the distribution of Tl-201 can be imaged to assess viability.

Pharmacologic Stress Agents and Protocols

All MPI studies should be done using dynamic exercise stress whenever possible (12). Dynamic exercise stress provides important information for diagnosis and management that is not available from pharmacologic stress agents. Pharmacologic stress is reserved for patients who are unable to exercise or are unable to achieve maximal exercise as determined by the age-adjusted heart rate or by reaching an ischemic endpoint on the bases of symptoms or ECG changes. Sensitivity of MPI decreases in patients who achieve less than 85% of the predicted heart rate (13). If the myocardial perfusion images are normal, it cannot be certain if they are truly normal or owing to an inadequate level of stress achieved during submaximal exercise. Alternatively, if there is ischemia, it is never certain if the full extent of ischemia was detected or only the most severe areas of coronary artery obstruction. Either way, uncertainty remains and a second stress test using a pharmacologic agent must be performed.

The pharmacologic stress agents and their characteristics are listed in Table 53.2. They can be classified into two categories: adenosine and dipyridamole, which are vasodilators, and dobutamine, which is an adrenergic stimulant. The vasodilators produce maximal coronary hyperemia creating flow heterogeneity by causing a greater increase in blood flow in normal coronary arteries then in arteries with flow-limiting stenosis. Dobutamine increases blood flow, heart rate, and blood pressure and may create true ischemia.

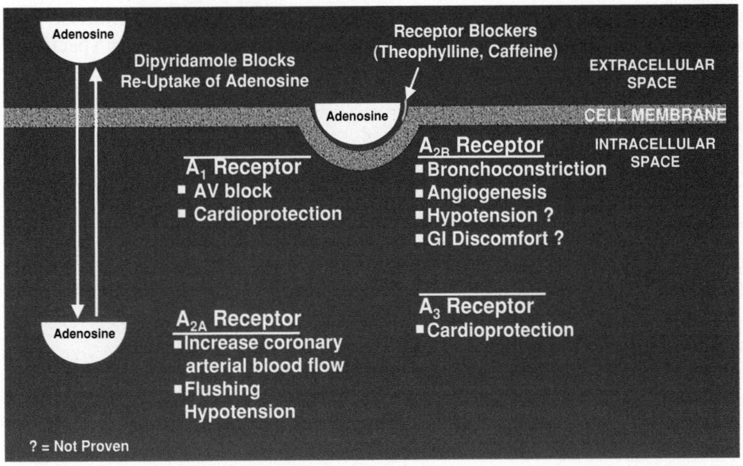

FIGURE 53.6. Mechanism of action of adenosine and dipyridamole at the cellular level.

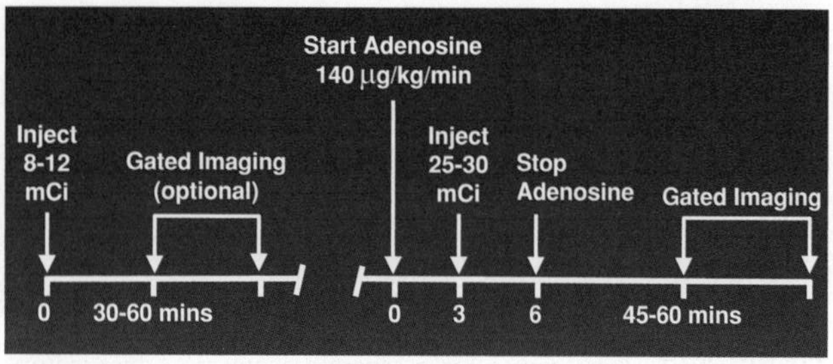

FIGURE 53.7. Protocol for adenosine pharmacologic stress testing using a 1-day Tc-99m imaging sequence.

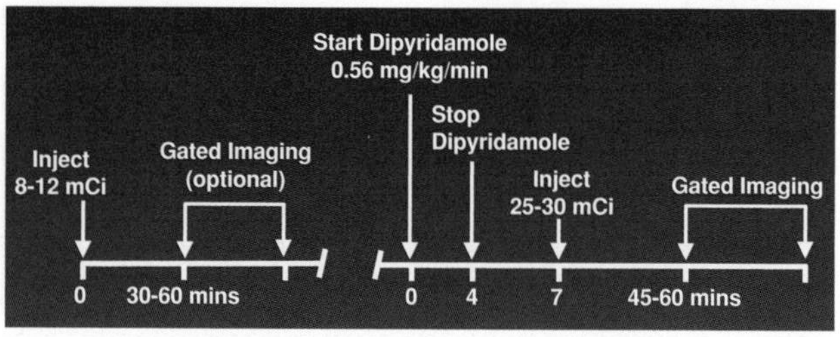

FIGURE 53.8. Protocol for dipyridamole pharmacologic stress testing using a 1-day Tc-99m imaging sequence.

Vasodilators

Mechanism of Action. As shown in Figure 53.8, adenosine is produced inside many cell types where it has no effect on blood flow. It is actively transported into the extracellular space, where it is capable of binding and stimulating a series of adenosine (A) receptors. Inactivation of extracellular adenosine is less than 10 seconds via reuptake by the same transport system and active metabolism. Dipyridamole blocks this reuptake mechanism and increases extracellular concentration of endogenously produced adenosine. Adenosine nonselectively stimulates all A receptors. The A_{2a} receptors, present on vascular smooth muscle and endothelial cells, enhances arterial wall smooth muscle dilation, and increases coronary blood flow. Adenosine also stimulates the A1, A2b, and A3 receptors, which cause other responses that in the context of inducing hyperemia for radionuclide imaging, are considered side effects.

Caffeine and methyl xanthenes bind to the adenosine receptors without causing stimulatory or inhibitory effects, but effectively block binding and stimulation by adenosine. If they are present when adenosine is administered, the vasodilatory effects are blocked; flow heterogeneity is not created and in patients with CAD results in a false-negative test. This blocking effect, however, is helpful when side effects are present and administration of aminophylline blocks the adenosine receptors and reverses the effects.

Side Effects. Following adenosine or dipyridamole infusion, there is a 10-mm Hg decrease in systolic and diastolic blood pressure (14,15). The most common cardiac side effects with dipyridamole include chest pain (20%), ECG changes (16%), and ST depression (7.5%). With adenosine, the cardiac side effects included chest pain (35%), atrioventricular (AV) nodal block (7.6%), and ST-T wave changes (5.7%). The AV nodal block was transient in all patients. The majority of reported chest pain is not ischemic, but due to nonselective stimulation of bradykinin pain receptors by adenosine. Patients with ECG changes consistent with ischemia are felt to have a higher dependence on collateral vessel blood flow, which may be decreased owing to coronary steal associated with a marked increase in coronary flow in normal vessels during vasodilation and a resultant decrease in collateral flow. Side effects occurred in 50% of patients receiving dipyridamole and aminophylline reversal was required in 12% (16). At some institutions, it is standard practice to reverse the effects of dipyridamole in all patients using aminophylline. The effective half-life of dipyridamole is 30 minutes, which is longer than the half-life of aminophylline and this means additional doses may be required to prevent recurrence of side effects. During adenosine infusion, side effects included flushing in 36.5%, shortness of breath or dyspnea in 35.2%, GI discomfort in 14.6%, headache in 14.2%, and neck discomfort in 11.6%. The number of patients reporting any side effect was 80% (14). Aminophylline was seldom required (0.8%) following adenosine administration because of the ultrashort half-life of less than 10 seconds, which means side effects resolve almost immediately following termination of infusion.

Safety of Pharmacologic Stress Testing. Dipyridamole and adenosine have been used extensively in the United States and have an excellent overall safety record. Although general side effects are common, cardiac and severe adverse events are rare. When considering that patients referred for pharmacologic stress testing are generally more debilitated, overall safety is comparable to that reported for conventional dynamic exercise stress testing (14,15). Severe adverse complications such as death and myocardial infarction in association with pharmacologic stress testing are uncommon. In a retrospective review of 73,806 patients from 59 centers in 19 countries, there were 9 reported cardiac deaths and 13 nonfatal myocardial infarctions using intravenous dipyridamole (15). In a prospective registry that included 9,256 patients receiving intravenous adenosine, there were no deaths; 1 patient had a myocardial infarction (14).

Efficacy. The reported diagnostic accuracy using adenosine or dipyridamole has been shown to be comparable to exercise. In early studies performed mostly using planar Tl-201 imaging in which each patient was studied twice with exercise and dipyridamole, sensitivity was in the 80% range and specificity

TABLE 53.2

PHYSICAL PROPERTIES OF ADENOSINE, DIPYRIDAMOLE, AND DOBUTAMINE

	Adenosine	Dipyridamole	Dobutamine
Half-life	<10 sec	33–62 min	2 min
Mean time to peak coronary flow velocity	55 sec	6.5 min	≤10 min
Onset of action	seconds	2 min	1–2 min
Mechanism of action	Direct	Indirect	Indirect
Patients with side effects requiring medical intervention (%)	0.6	16	NA

in the range of 90%. There were no differences between the two forms of stress (17). The published studies looking at the accuracy of adenosine stress did not in general perform stress twice and used predominately SPECT imaging with Tl-201 or the Tc-99m tracers. The average sensitivity for pharmacologic stress with vasodilators was 87% and the specificity was 74% (17). Based on extensive publications and practical clinical experience in everyday use, the accuracy of vasodilator pharmacologic stress is accepted as being equivalent to exercise stress.

Adenosine and Dipyridamole Pharmacologic Stress Protocols

Figures 53.5 and 53.6 demonstrate the protocols for using adenosine and pharmacologic stress in combination with a 1-day Tc-99m radiotracer. Patients should fast a minimum of 8 hours and medications and foods containing caffeine should be stopped for 12 to 24 hours before testing. Methylxanthines and dipyridamole need to be stopped for 48 hours prior to testing because they inhibit the vasodilatory effects of the adenosine and dipyridamole and patients taking dipyridamole can have a severe response to adenosine. Patients with second-degree AV nodal block (Mobitz type II) or third-degree AV nodal block without a functioning pacemaker should not receive adenosine because of the potential AV node blocking effects. Patients with a prolonged PR interval or Wenckebach can be tested safely. The use of vasodilator stress is recommended in all patients with a left bundle branch block (LBBB); the use of exercise leads to a higher rate of false-positive studies due to septal defects (5). This is felt to be mediated by a decrease in blood flow through septal perforators at high heart rates, which is not present at rest.

Adenosine is infused at a rate of 140 μg/kg for minute for 4 or 6 minutes with the radiotracer injected at minutes 2 or 3 and the infusion continued a minimum of 1 minute to allow maximal extraction, especially of the Tc-99m tracers which have a lower extraction fraction then Tl-201 across the coronary bed (Figure 53.8). If the patient has evidence of ischemia by symptoms or profound ECG changes, the radiotracer can be administered earlier, but the infusion must be maintained a minimum of 1 minute to allow radiotracer extraction at the high coronary blood flow rates. The ultrashort half-life of adenosine (<10 seconds) quickly reverses side effects and intravenous aminophylline is rarely required. Performing low-level exercise during adenosine infusion decreases side effects, improves image quality, and is recommended for all patients capable of walking on a treadmill.

Dipyridamole is infused at a rate of 0.56 mg/kg of body weight over 4 minutes to a maximum total dose of 60 mg. Tl-201 or a Tc-99m radiotracer can be administered by bolus injection 3 to 4 minutes following completion of the infusion or earlier if the patient has evidence of ischemia by symptoms or profound ECG changes. Maximal coronary hyperemia is delayed because of the need to allow endogenous adenosine levels to increase following the inhibition of the reuptake mechanism by dipyridamole. Aminophylline administration is required more often because of the longer half-life; side effects may recur because of the shorter half-life of aminophylline.

Catecholamines

Dobutamine is used infrequently for MPI. The protocol requires 3 minute stepwise infusion stages of increasing doses of dobutamine and take longer then vasodilator stress (18). Patients with hypertension, abdominal aortic aneurysms, poorly controlled supraventricular arrhythmias, or ventricular arrhythmias should not be studied. Although some nuclear cardiology laboratories use it exclusively, at most centers it is used predominately in patients with severe and poorly controlled lung disease and in patients who have ingested caffeine on the day of testing and vasodilators cannot be used.

ECG-GATED SPECT PERFUSION IMAGING

This technique of acquisition, analysis, and quantitation allows assessment of global and regional left ventricular function during the routine acquisition of the perfusion study. Since its introduction in the mid 1990s, it is now a critical element of all SPECT studies and more than 90% of all perfusion studies are performed with gating (19,20). Gating can be performed with both Tl-201 and Tc-99m agents. However, because of the higher count rates achieved with Tc-99m perfusion tracers, these are the preferred agents for ECG-gated SPECT. Viewing wall motion and thickening from gated SPECT improves recognition of artifacts and attenuation due to breast tissue and the diaphragm and improve specificity (21).

Gated SPECT Acquisition

Gated SPECT studies are acquired using 8 or 16 time frames in the heart cycle. It has been demonstrated that 16 frames are more accurate for EF calculation, but at the expense of poor image quality as each of the 16 frames only has half the counts contained in the 8-frame acquisition. EF measured using 8 frames gives values that are approximately 3 EF units lower than when 16-frame acquisition is performed. Sixteen-frame acquisition allows analysis of filling and ejection rates that can be used for assessment of diastolic function (22,23).

For arrhythmia rejection, it is best to avoid selection of parameters that compromise the perfusion information or prolong the acquisition. Thus, accepting all beats guarantees high-count perfusion images without increasing the imaging time, but this may compromise the results of the EF calculation. To guarantee optimal perfusion information, a $\pm 50\%$ acceptance window gives the most counts. Newer equipment allows separate perfusion and gated information to be acquired, in which case a tighter acceptance window can be used to get the most accurate EF without compromising the perfusion data. Patients in atrial fibrillation with a narrow RR interval give accurate EF measurements. When the RR interval is wide, EF measurements are less reliable (24). If more than one out of every six beats is an APC or premature ventricular contraction, EF measurements are not reliable.

Gated SPECT Wall Motion Analysis

Areas that have normal wall motion and thickening may be associated with normal myocardium, the majority of areas having ischemia on perfusion imaging, anatomic variants such as apical thinning, or areas with breast or diaphragm attenuation. Because gated Tc-99m studies are acquired a minimum of 15 minutes following peak exercise stress, regional wall motion in most patients with ischemia usually returns to normal by the time of imaging. If there is profound ischemia, areas of myocardium may continue to have persistent wall motion abnormalities that are detected during gated acquisition in as many as one third of cases. This has been reported in the literature for sestamibi, and is also seen with tetrofosmin (8,25). One of the most important benefits of gated SPECT acquisition is helping to differentiate attenuation due to the diaphragm or breast from areas of old myocardial infarction or scarring (26,27). Areas of scarring have absent or diminished motion and thickening whereas areas with decreased activity due to attenuation show normal motion and thickening. Patients with prior heart surgery show akinesis or hypokinesis of the septum because of the surgery in the absence of ischemia or infarction.

TABLE 53.3

STEPWISE APPROACH TO THE INTERPRETATION OF MYOCARDIAL PERFUSION IMAGES

Interpret all images on computer workstation
Perform quality control on rotating projection images
Review optimally displayed serial aligned slices
Review gated images
Reach conclusion based on images
Review clinical indications and ETT
Final conclusion based on images and clinical data

Validation of Gated SPECT Ejection Fraction With Blood Pool Imaging

In addition to improving diagnostic accuracy during subjective visual image interpretation, gated Tc-99m measurements of global EF and regional wall thickening have been validated using equilibrium blood pool imaging, cardiac catheterization, and cardiac magnetic resonance imaging (28–31). These studies found excellent agreement across EF values ranging from 12 to 88. Small hearts gave very high EF values because of the poor spatial of the SPECT systems.

Image Interpretation

As listed in Table 53.3, accurate interpretation of SPECT MPI studies involves a systematic approach that starts with technical quality control performed on the rotating projection images, rest/stress perfusion and function comparison, reaching a conclusion based on the imaging information, reviewing the clinical indications and the stress test results, and reconciling all these data to reach a final conclusion (26,32). An important part of this process is the initial quality control that must be done on an interactive workstation that allows image manipulation and modification. The items listed in Table 53.4 must be systematically examined on every study to identify technical factors that may influence the perfusion data seen on the aligned slices. False-positive SPECT MPI studies very often are due to poor quality acquisition data that in the process of filtering, reconstruction and display, perfusion defects are created and not recognized.

ACUTE CORONARY SYNDROMES

Chest Pain in the Emergency Department

Patients presenting to an emergency department within several hours of chest pain and a nondiagnostic ECG can be risk stratified based on the acute injection of a Tc-99m perfusion tracer. Patients with a perfusion abnormality are at high risk for having non–ST segment elevation myocardial infarction or unstable angina and merit aggressive medical and interventional management. Such patients have abnormal perfusion owing to occlusion or spasm of an unstable vessel and the perfusion abnormalities can be detected prior to elevation of serum enzyme markers (27,33,34). The closer to the time of chest pain the isotope is injected, the greater the sensitivity of the study. Injection 2 hours after symptoms are less reliable. Studies have a very high negative predictive value and patients discharged have a very low likelihood for having cardiac events. If the acute study is normal, it can be used as the resting image for comparison following exercise or pharmacologic stress to exclude underlying CAD in such patients. In a prospective randomized controlled study comparing imaging to conventional ED care to such care with imaging, imaging significantly lowered hospitalization rates from 52% to 42% (34).

TABLE 53.4

ESSENTIAL ITEMS TO REVIEW ON THE ROTATING PROJECTION IMAGES AS PART OF THE QUALITY CONTROL PRIOR TO INTERPRETATION OF MYOCARDIAL PERFUSION IMAGES

Patient motion
Count density
Sources of attenuation such as breast and diaphragm
Extracardiac activity: liver, gallbladder, stomach, bowel
Lung uptake
Cardiac chamber size: rest, stress and any change between them owing to transient ischemic dilation
Pathologic soft tissue uptake

STEMI

Studies have shown that injection of Tc-99m tracers at presentation or prior to treatment of STEMI identifies the area at risk and repeat studies show the extent of salvage and final infarct size which is predictive of EF and long term survival (35–38). The logistics and time demands of performing radionuclide imaging in the ED in patients with nondiagnostic chest pain or ACS have limited the widespread application of this technique. At present it is performed at limited centers. Some facilities will inject chest pain patients during regular business hours when issues of radioisotope and technologists availability and radiation safety can be conveniently handled (39). Off hour patients are treated in the conventional manner with serial enzymes and if negative, stress MPI performed during regular hours in the morning. The Guidelines recommend rest imaging in patients with possible ACS and negative initial enzymes and nondiagnostic ECGs and same day rest/stress perfusion imaging in patients with nondiagnostic ECGs, negative enzymes or a normal perfusion study when injected close to the time of chest pain (1).

Risk Assessment After Acute Coronary Syndrome

The use of radionuclide imaging after infarction has declined as most patients either have acute or delayed diagnostic and therapeutic angiography. In patients receiving thrombolytic therapy where angiography is not scheduled, MPI can be used for appropriate risk stratification and the need for angiography (40). Imaging is useful in those patients at high risk for angiography, those with equivocal lesions, or where there is a need for detecting inducible ischemia, measuring EF, or assessing the adequacy of medical treatment (41,42).

DIAGNOSIS OF CORONARY ARTERY DISEASE AND CHRONIC SYNDROMES

Diagnosis of Coronary Artery Disease

Sensitivity and specificity for MPI have been extensively reported starting with planar Tl-201 to more recent publications using the Tc-99m tracers with SPECT with quantitative analysis and the use of ECG gating (13,43–46). The accuracy is heavily influenced by the populations being studied and the influence of posttest referral bias (47). In a meta-analysis using primarily planar Tl-201 studies weighted by sample size, a sensitivity of 87% and a specificity of 64% were reported (48). In an analysis including more contemporary studies with Tc-99m SPECT and gating, the sensitivity was found to be 87% and the specificity was 73% (1). Tc-99m radiotracers provide the highest quality gated images, and are the most commonly used. Attenuation correction using transmission or computed tomography (CT) is recommended to improve specificity and overall accuracy but is not used widely (49,50). Overall sensitivity is not improved by attenuation correction (1).

Specific Patient Populations

The effects of referral bias, testing in patients with prior revascularization, and the documented occurrence of abnormal perfusion in patients without obstructive CAD but functionally abnormal flow reserve, all influence the accuracy of testing when comparing it to the gold standard, namely, coronary angiography. For that reason, accuracy of testing for the detection of disease and assessment of prognosis are discussed in the context of recognized specific patient populations that can influence the results of testing.

Ethnic and Racial Differences. Many of the published studies enrolled predominately Caucasian males capable of performing dynamic exercise. When tests are performed in other groups, MPI accuracy and prognosis results vary and usually loose accuracy and prognostic value (51–53). Many of these groups have a higher cardiovascular risk factor profile and other potential factors influencing test performance such as left ventricular hypertrophy (LVH) and arrhythmic death. African Americans have overall lower test accuracy and worse prognosis across the range of ischemia. Whereas the death and myocardial infarction rate in Caucasians is less than 1% with a normal SPECT MPI, two studies have shown it to be 2% per year in African Americans.

Women. Radionuclide MPI in women is influenced by gender differences in the prevalence of CAD and technical limitations, primarily breast attenuation, that lower study accuracy owing to lower specificity (54–57). Low specificity was a major limitation in the early studies using planar Tl-201 that was overcome with the availability of SPECT, ECG gating, and the use of attenuation correction. Using these advanced techniques, gender differences in the performance of testing for diagnosis have been minimized, but not totally eliminated, and the specificity is comparable to those reported for stress echocardiography (54). Similarly, the prognostic value of SPECT MPI has been shown to be accurate in women undergoing exercise or pharmacologic stress testing (55–57).

Normal Resting Electrocardiograph, Able to Exercise. For those patients who present with chest pain or with a high prevalence of risk factors, the exercise ECG has a higher specificity and has been shown to be the most cost-effective approach for identification of patients with left main or three-vessel CAD (58–61). As a result of these studies, it is recommended that treadmill testing be used first in a stepwise approach for patients with an intermediate risk for CAD who have a normal baseline ECG and are capable of performing dynamic exercise (62). However, SPECT MPI should be done first for patients with abnormal ST changes, LBBB, ventricular paced rhythms, preexcitation, LVH, or prior revascularization (62,63).

Intermediate-Risk Duke Treadmill Score. The Duke treadmill score has been shown to have excellent prognostic value for normal or high-risk patients, but SPECT MPI provides additional information for management, especially in the intermediate risk category (64). In a study with 4,649 intermediate Duke Score patients who had normal perfusion, the 7-year cardiac mortality was very low (1.5%) and the cumulative frequency of catheterization was 17% (65).

Normal Resting Electrocardiograph, Unable to Exercise. For patients who are unable to exercise, SPECT MPI is capable of providing diagnostic and prognostic information that cannot be gotten from treadmill testing. However, such patients have more risk factors and even if the study is normal, the occurrence of cardiac death is higher then in patients who are capable of exercising (66).

Left Bundle Branch Block/Pacemakers, Left Ventricular Hypertrophy, and Patients With Nonspecific ST-T Wave Changes. For patients in these categories, treadmill testing does not provide accurate diagnostic or prognostic information and SPECT MPI is indicated for evaluation. Patients with LBBB with exercise MPI have a low specificity in the LAD distribution owing to a septal defect caused by diminished septal blood flow at high heart rates in the absence of obstructive CAD (67–71). If there are associated defects in the apex or anterior wall, specificity is improved but the use of vasodilator stress improves diagnostic accuracy and gives prognostic information. Overall prognosis is worse in such patients, but imaging is predictive of events. In 245 patients the 3-year survival was 27% in high-risk scans and 87% in low-risk scans (71). Less well documented is the effect of pacemakers on accuracy and prognosis, but patients are treated in the same way as those with LBBB and prognostic value is retained (72).

In the presence of LVH, hypertension, or nonspecific ST-T wave changes on the resting ECG, imaging retains diagnostic and prognostic value (73,74). Well-trained athletes with LVH by echocardiography have been reported to have a higher incidence of false-positive studies owing to "hot spot" scaling problems (75).

The Elderly. Diagnostic and prognostic accuracy is retained in the elderly where the prevalence of disease is greater (76). A normal study in an intermediate risk group in the elderly still has a 3% yearly mortality rate.

Asymptomatic Patients. Although testing is not recommended in asymptomatic patients, SPECT MPI can detect the presence of disease and give prognostic information (77–80). Testing maybe appropriate in high-risk occupations such as aviators, fireman, and policeman, who have multiple risk factors but no CAD symptoms (62).

Diabetes. Patients with diabetes are at a very high risk for having critical coronary stenosis and cardiovascular events (81). Despite the diffuse nature of vessel involvement with a higher occurrence of balanced disease, SPECT MPI continues to have diagnostic and prognostic value (82–85). In a retrospective analysis, event-free survival was found to be lower in diabetics across all categories of ischemia (84). In a prospective study involving 1,123 carefully screened 50- to 75-year-old asymptomatic diabetics, 522 were randomized to SPECT imaging and 118 (22%) were found to have silent ischemia on SPECT MPI, 33 of whom (6%) had moderate or large perfusion defects. The high prevalence of silent ischemia was higher than expected. All patients in this study are being prospectively followed to determine if imaging will influence management and long-term survival.

Before and After Revascularization

Radionuclide Imaging Before Revascularization Interventions

Beyond detecting ischemia and appropriately selecting patients for coronary angiography, the ability of SPECT MPI to assess the highly variable physiologic relationship between lesion severity and coronary flow reserve, especially in the 25% to

75% lesions, has value for management postangiography (86). Even in the presence of flow-limiting stenosis, if exercise or pharmacologic stress perfusion is normal, patients are at low risk for cardiac events (87,88). Using SPECT MPI as a gatekeeper for referral to coronary angiography has been shown to not only be cost effective, but in no circumstance does it place patients at a higher risk for cardiac death or nonfatal myocardial infarction in comparison to the more expensive and invasive approach of performing angiography on all patients (89). It also has a role in determining the sequence and number of grafted vessels in high-risk coronary artery bypass grafting (CABG) patients and for identification of the culprit lesion at the time of percutaneous coronary intervention.

Radionuclide Imaging After Percutaneous Coronary Intervention

Routine testing is not indicated at any time in the first 2 years in asymptomatic patients (2). In the first few months after a procedure it has been shown that fewer than 30% of symptomatic patients have documented stenosis (90). In addition, periprocedural changes in the treated area may result in perfusion defects even in the absence of restenosis and testing in symptomatic patients the first 4 to 6 weeks following a procedure is not recommended because of the occurrence of false positives (91,92). If ischemia is detected beyond the immediate period of the procedure, the prognostic value of SPECT MPI persists and the occurrence of cardiac death and myocardial infarction is increased in patients with large amounts of ischemia (93). With the placement of drug-eluting stents to prevent restenosis, delayed healing, prolonged inflammation, and exercise-induced paradoxical coronary vasoconstriction of the adjacent segment have been reported (94,95).

Radionuclide Imaging After Coronary Artery Bypass Grafting

Even with the altered anatomy following CABG, SPECT MPI retains diagnostic and prognostic accuracy early and late for detection of flow limitations that maybe present in grafts as well as in the native vessel (96–98). Routine testing in asymptomatic patients is not recommended (2). The extent and severity of perfusion abnormalities detected by SPECT MPI is predictive of death in both symptomatic and asymptomatic patients in the first 5 years after surgical revascularization (98). Beyond 5 years, it has been shown that the presence of ischemia is the strongest predictor of mortality (97,99,100). In 9,000 asymptomatic patients, the presence of ischemia predicted a 3% annual mortality (99).

Radionuclide Imaging Before Noncardiac Surgery

Risk assessment prior to noncardiac surgery requires a thorough review of the clinical, demographic, and surgical indications of risk rather then nonselective use of noninvasive imaging techniques (101). Major predictors of increased perioperative risk include recent acute myocardial infarction, unstable angina pectoris, decompensated congestive heart failure, significant arrhythmias, high degree of AV block, and severe valvular disease. Intermediate predictors include mild angina pectoris, prior myocardial infarction, compensated or prior congestive heart failure, and diabetes mellitus.

In addition to the clinical risk the patient brings to the operation, surgery itself may be classified into risk categories. High-risk surgical procedures include a major emergency operation, such as aortic and other major vascular surgery, and peripheral vascular surgery, especially in elderly patients. Intermediate-risk procedures include carotid endarterectomy, head and neck surgery, and intraperitoneal, intrathoracic, orthopedic, and prostate surgery. Low-risk procedures include endoscopic procedures, superficial procedures, cataract removal, and breast surgery.

Patients who are at low risk for CAD, especially if they are undergoing a low-risk surgical procedure, may not need preoperative stress testing. Surgery should be avoided, whenever possible, in patients who recently experienced a myocardial infarction or with unstable angina pectoris, until the clinical condition has been stabilized; if surgery must be performed, then coronary angiography is recommended. However, with the use of drug-eluting stents, prolonged platelet inhibition is required to prevent thrombosis and if surgery cannot be delayed, bare metal stents and 4 weeks of aggressive anitplatelet drugs should be considered. It is in patients with an intermediate risk who are going for intermediate- or high-risk surgery that noninvasive imaging is indicated. The greatest amount of experience by far is in the use of pharmacologic perfusion imaging with dipyridamole or adenosine (1,102). The negative predicative value in both vascular and nonvascular surgery cases was 96% to 100%, but the positive predictive value of any ischemia ranged from 4% to 20% in vascular patients. Perfusion markers of high risk include a large area of ischemia, perfusion defects in multiple vascular territories, left ventricular dilatation, or increased lung Tl-201 uptake and such patients are candidates for angiography. The ACC/AHA guidelines recommend coronary angiography should be performed in patients for whom the results of noninvasive testing indicate a high risk of cardiac events or who have angina pectoris that is unresponsive to medical therapy. However, it has not been conclusively shown that angiography and revascularization improves the outcomes in these patients in the perioperative period or long term.

To further complicate matters, it has been shown in a randomized trial that high-risk patients identified by dobutamine echocardiography going for high-risk vascular surgery had a lower death and myocardial infarction rate (3.4% versus 34%) in the control group, when placed on β-blockers (103).

Heart Failure

For patients with heart failure owing to ischemic or nonischemic causes, hypertrophic cardiomyopathy, hypertensive heart disease, or valvular heart disease, radionuclide techniques have proven value. These techniques are useful for initial assessment of left and right ventricular systolic and diastolic function and for the assessment of myocardial viability and/or underlying ischemia in those patients being considered for revascularization who do not have angina (1).

Assessment of Function

Although ERNA can be used to reproducibly and quantitatively assess left ventricular systolic and diastolic function, the additional information provided by echocardiography makes it the best test for evaluation. The one area where ERNA continues to have a role is for the serial monitoring of patients receiving anthracyclines or trastuzumab for the treatment of malignancies (104–106). This approach allows patients to receive the highest possible doses of these drugs for effective tumor treatment at the lowest possible risk of developing cardiotoxicity, which in early studies could be as deadly as the tumor. Attempts to develop less toxic drugs or to pretreat patients with agents to lower cardiotoxicity have been unsuccessful and serial monitoring is still required. In this setting the reproducibility and quantitative nature of the technique offers advantages over echocardiography (107). EF measurements by ECG-gated SPECT MPI are usually not obtained as the primary method to assess function, but when there is a need to assess perfusion, the information is valuable.

Assessment of Viability

Resting Perfusion. Regions of myocardial dysfunction may consist of scar, hibernating, stunned, ischemic, or infiltrated myocardium. As shown by histologic analysis, many times there is a continuum of all of these states and radionuclide perfusion tracer uptake in such patients needs to have a linear relationship with the extent of viability and the probability of functional recovery after revascularization (108,109). Resting uptake of Tl-201 and the two T-99m tracers is capable of identifying areas of myocardium that will show functional recovery after revascularization, but accuracy is best when a threshold of 60% is used for Tl-201 and 55% for the Tc-99m tracers (110). There were no differences between the three tracers using these thresholds.

Assessment of Viability

Preserved Metabolic Activity. An alternative method of viability assessment measures preserved metabolic activity at rest using F-18-FDG– or C-11–labeled fatty acids (111–114). Such studies use a perfusion tracer, usually N-13 ammonia, O-15 water, or Rb-82, and compare it to the marker of viability. Areas that have a perfusion/metabolism mismatch—severely diminished or absent perfusion but preserved or enhanced metabolic activity—have a high probability of regaining function after revascularization and improving long-term survival (88% versus 50%) with medical treatment. Not only was survival improved, but heart failure symptoms were fewer after revascularization (115). The benefits of revascularization was shown a larger group of patients who benefited from revascularization regardless of the amount of viability.

CONTROVERSIES AND PERSONAL PERSPECTIVES

The future for nuclear cardiology can be viewed in terms of the things that have been aggressively promoted in the past by academia and industry, but for whatever reason have not delivered, and the swing toward keeping things simple and efficient. Eventually, we are going to need both to move the field forward.

The promise of new perfusion tracers with linear uptake over a wide flow range and a method of extraction that does not cause liver or GI interference has not been fulfilled. New agents to image hypoxia, apoptosis, vulnerable plaque, innervation, gene expression, and so on have not materialized after many years of promise. Attenuation correction has not gained widespread utilization because of problems with implementation, lack of reimbursement, and an old camera base that cannot be readily converted. New hybrid systems combining 1- to 64-slice CT systems combined with PET or SPECT systems are now available, but their role in improving accuracy has not been demonstrated. They are also much more expensive, take up 40% to 60% more space, and diminish efficiency by doing two types of imaging in the same setting.

The reason SPECT MPI has such an important role in patient management is because of the excellent quality control and standardization that has developed over the years and the ability to get smaller imaging systems into an office-based setting for easier patient access and involvement by clinicians well trained in image processing and interpretation. We need to stay close to this model of success and make every effort to develop small imaging systems capable of acquiring studies in a much shorter time period to improve quality and increase throughput. If these systems could be equipped with accurate methods for attenuation correction using CT, there would be greater penetration into the marketplace and a further increase in quality.

We still need new tracers and perhaps what is needed is to move forward a tracer with which we have some experience, I-123 MIBG for imaging of cardiac innervation (116). This agent could be extremely useful for the management of heart failure patients with regard to medical management as well as with the selection for expensive interventions such as implantable cardioverter defibrillator placement (117). To make I-123 MIBG widely available, new sources of I-123 production need to be developed; this will open up the possibility of developing new agents that are iodinated rather then Tc-99m or positron labeled. This makes the chemistry easier and could overcome many of the limitations we have faced using Tc-99m.

The development of new A2a agents for performing pharmacologic stress will not only reduce the side effect profile of adenosine but allow the administration of a bolus of activity rather than continuous pump infusion (118,119). These agents have been carefully designed to obtain an adequate increase in coronary blood flow without reaching the roll off point at which uptake becomes nonlinear. On going Phase III clinical trials will give results in the very near future on the efficacy and side effect profile for these agents.

The other area that is important for the future of the field is to show that studies are being performed in a responsible and appropriate manner. This requires documentation of training and a minimal level of competence for physicians and technologists. Physician certification by the Certification Board of Nuclear Cardiology has received recognition by the private payers and regulatory agencies such as the Nuclear Regulatory Commission. The laboratory accreditation process developed by the Intersocietal Commission for the Accreditation of Nuclear Laboratories has also been recognized by payers and it will be incumbent upon all laboratories providing nuclear cardiology services to meet the established standards.

Another area under great scrutiny is overutilization of procedures. This approach was initially piloted in nuclear but will be used in all other cardiac imaging modalities. Appropriateness criteria for nuclear cardiology were developed using the evidence guidelines as the basis, but trying to factor into the equation the uncertainty that exists in everyday clinical practice (2). There were 52 indications selected reflecting common clinical presentations and scenarios in which nuclear cardiology studies might be appropriate. A panel of 11 diverse experts used the Rand/UCLA methodology to rate them, had a face-to-face discussion and rated them a second time on a scale of 1 to 9 with a median score of 7 to 9 being appropriate, 4 to 6 being uncertain or possibly appropriate for that indication, and 1 to 3 being an inappropriate indication. Thirteen indications (25%) were inappropriate, 27 (52%) were appropriate, and 12 (23%) were uncertain. The majority of inappropriate indications addressed issues of routine repeat testing or testing in asymptomatic patients.

Another area in which the field will have to demonstrate self-scrutiny is the development of quantifiable measures of quality and outcome in imaging. This is being required by payers who want to see development of performance standards that must be met by physicians and laboratories. These are more specific and require accuracy of interpretation in comparison to a "gold standard" or outcomes that influence management and survival. In some ways, SPECT MPI is ahead of the other imaging modalities in developing and implementing these requirements, but they will become more widespread and enforced over the next several years and will likely by linked to pay-for-performance criteria.

The field of nuclear cardiology is in a position to continue widespread utilization, but external pressures from payers and regulatory bodies will slow the double-digit growth it has experienced. There is also the need to develop new tracers and instrumentation that are practical, efficient, cost effective, and capable of documenting that it is appropriate and high quality exists in the final product.

References

1. Klocke FJ, Baird MG, Lorell BH, et al. ACC/AHA/ASNC guidelines for the clinical use of cardiac radionuclide imaging—executive summary: a report of the American College of Cardiology/American Heart Association Task Force on Practice Guidelines (ACC/AHA/ASNC Committee to Revise the 1995 Guidelines for the Clinical Use of Cardiac Radionuclide Imaging). *J Am Coll Cardiol* 2003;42:1318–1333.
2. Brindis RG, Douglas PS, Hendel RC, et al. ACCF/ASNC appropriateness criteria for single-photon emission computed tomography myocardial perfusion imaging (SPECT MPI): a report of the American College of Cardiology Foundation Quality Strategic Directions Committee Appropriateness Criteria Working Group and the American Society of Nuclear Cardiology endorsed by the American Heart Association. *J Am Coll Cardiol* 2005;46: 1587–1605.
3. Taillefer R. Kinetics of Myocardial Perfusion Imaging Radiotracers. In: Iskandarian A, Verani MS, eds. *Nuclear Cardiac Imaging*. 3 ed. New York: Oxford; 2003:51–73.
4. Udelson JE, Bonow RO, Dilsizian V. The historical and conceptual evolution of radionuclide assessment of myocardial viability. *J Nucl Cardiol* 2004;11:318–334.
5. Updated imaging guidelines for nuclear cardiology procedures, part 1. *J Nucl Cardiol* 2001;8:G5–G58.
6. Heller GV, Bateman TM, Johnson LL, et al. Clinical value of attenuation correction in stress-only Tc-99m sestamibi SPECT imaging. *J Nucl Cardiol* 2004;11:273–281.
7. Thompson RC, Heller GV, Johnson LL, et al. Value of attenuation correction on ECG-gated SPECT myocardial perfusion imaging related to body mass index. *J Nucl Cardiol* 2005;12:195–202.
8. Johnson LL, Verdesca SA, Aude WY, et al. Postischemic stunning can affect left ventricular ejection fraction and regional wall motion on post-stress gated sestamibi tomograms. *J Am Coll Cardiol* 1997;30:1641–1648.
9. Sharir T, Germano G, Kang X, et al. Prediction of myocardial infarction versus cardiac death by gated myocardial perfusion SPECT: risk stratification by the amount of stress-induced ischemia and the poststress ejection fraction. *J Nucl Med* 2001;42:831–837.
10. Sharir T, Germano G, Kavanagh PB, et al. Incremental prognostic value of post-stress left ventricular ejection fraction and volume by gated myocardial perfusion single photon emission computed tomography. *Circulation* 1999;100:1035–1042.
11. Dilsizian V, Bonow RO. Current diagnostic techniques of assessing myocardial viability in patients with hibernating and stunned myocardium. *Circulation* 1993;87:1–20.
12. Cerqueira MD. Pharmacologic stress versus maximal-exercise stress for perfusion imaging: which, when, and why? *J Nucl Cardiol* 1996;3:S10–S14.
13. Iskandrian AS, Heo J, Kong B, et al. Effect of exercise level on the ability of thallium-201 tomographic imaging in detecting coronary artery disease: analysis of 461 patients. *J Am Coll Cardiol* 1989;14:1477–1486.
14. Cerqueira MD, Verani MS, Schwaiger M, et al. Safety profile of adenosine stress perfusion imaging: results from the Adenoscan Multicenter Trial Registry. *J Am Coll Cardiol* 1994;23:384–389.
15. Lette J, Tatum J, Fraser S, et al. Safety of dipyridamole testing in 73,806 patients: the Multicenter Dipyridamole Safety Study. *J Nucl Cardiol* 1995;2: 3–17.
16. Ranhosky A, Kempthorne-Rawson J. The safety of intravenous dipyridamole thallium myocardial perfusion imaging. Intravenous Dipyridamole Thallium Imaging Study Group. *Circulation* 1990;81:1205–1209.
17. Leppo JA. Comparison of pharmacologic stress agents. *J Nucl Cardiol* 1996;3:S22–S26.
18. Hays JT, Mahmarian JJ, Cochran AJ, et al. Dobutamine thallium-201 tomography for evaluating patients with suspected coronary artery disease unable to undergo exercise or vasodilator pharmacologic stress testing. *J Am Coll Cardiol* 1993;21:1583–1590.
19. Germano G, Kiat H, Kavanagh PB, et al. Automatic quantification of ejection fraction from gated myocardial perfusion SPECT. *J Nucl Med* 1995; 36:2138–2147.
20. Bateman TM, Berman DS, Heller GV, et al. American Society of Nuclear Cardiology position statement on electrocardiographic gating of myocardial perfusion SPECT scintigrams. *J Nucl Cardiol* 1999;6:470–471.
21. Choi JY, Lee KH, Kim SJ, et al. Gating provides improved accuracy for differentiating artifacts from true lesions in equivocal fixed defects on technetium 99m tetrofosmin perfusion SPECT. *J Nucl Cardiol* 1998;5:395–401.
22. Germano G, Berman DS. On the accuracy and reproducibility of quantitative gated myocardial perfusion SPECT. *J Nucl Med* 1999;40:810–813.
23. Akincioglu C, Berman DS, Nishina H, et al. Assessment of diastolic function using 16-frame 99mTc-sestamibi gated myocardial perfusion SPECT: normal values. *J Nucl Med* 2005;46:1102–1108.
24. Cullom SJ, Case JA, Bateman TM. Electrocardiographically gated myocardial perfusion SPECT: technical principles and quality control considerations. *J Nucl Cardiol* 1998;5:418–425.
25. Everaert H, Vanhove C, Franken PR. Assessment of perfusion, function, and myocardial metabolism after infarction with a combination of low-dose dobutamine tetrofosmin gated SPECT perfusion scintigraphy and BMIPP SPECT imaging. *J Nucl Cardiol* 2000;7:29–36.
26. Hendel RC, Wackers FJ, Berman DS, et al. American society of nuclear cardiology consensus statement: reporting of radionuclide myocardial perfusion imaging studies. *J Nucl Cardiol* 2003;10:705–708.
27. Heller GV, Stowers SA, Hendel RC, et al. Clinical value of acute rest technetium-99m tetrofosmin tomographic myocardial perfusion imaging in patients with acute chest pain and nondiagnostic electrocardiograms. *J Am Coll Cardiol* 1998;31:1011–1017.
28. Everaert H, Franken PR, Flamen P, et al. Left ventricular ejection fraction from gated SPET myocardial perfusion studies: a method based on the radial distribution of count rate density across the myocardial wall. *Eur J Nucl Med* 1996;23:1628–1633.
29. Everaert H, Vanhove C, Franken PR. Gated SPET myocardial perfusion acquisition within 5 minutes using focussing collimators and a three-head gamma camera. *Eur J Nucl Med* 1998;25:587–593.
30. Gunning MG, Anagnostopoulos C, Davies G, et al. Gated technetium-99m-tetrofosmin SPECT and cine MRI to assess left ventricular contraction. *J Nucl Med* 1997;38:438–442.
31. Mochizuki T, Murase K, Tanaka H, et al. Assessment of left ventricular volume using ECG-gated SPECT with technetium-99m-MIBI and technetium-99m-tetrofosmin. *J Nucl Med* 1997;38:53–57.
32. Cerqueira MD. The user-friendly nuclear cardiology report: what needs to be considered and what is included. *J Nucl Cardiol* 1996;3:350–355.
33. Tatum JL, Jesse RL, Kontos MC, et al. Comprehensive strategy for the evaluation and triage of the chest pain patient. *Ann Emerg Med* 1997;29:116–125.
34. Udelson JE, Beshansky JR, Ballin DS, et al. Myocardial perfusion imaging for evaluation and triage of patients with suspected acute cardiac ischemia: a randomized controlled trial. *JAMA* 2002;288:2693–2700.
35. Cerqueira MD, Maynard C, Ritchie JL, et al. Long-term survival in 618 patients from the Western Washington Streptokinase in Myocardial Infarction trials. *J Am Coll Cardiol* 1992;20:1452–1459.
36. Christian TF, Clements IP, Gibbons RJ. Noninvasive identification of myocardium at risk in patients with acute myocardial infarction and nondiagnostic electrocardiograms with technetium-99m-sestamibi. *Circulation* 1991;83:1615–1620.
37. Christian TF, Schwartz RS, Gibbons RJ. Determinants of infarct size in reperfusion therapy for acute myocardial infarction. *Circulation* 1992;86: 81–90.
38. Miller TD, Christian TF, Hopfenspirger MR, et al. Infarct size after acute myocardial infarction measured by quantitative tomographic 99mTc sestamibi imaging predicts subsequent mortality. *Circulation* 1995;92:334–341.
39. Wackers FJ, Brown KA, Heller GV, et al. American Society of Nuclear Cardiology position statement on radionuclide imaging in patients with suspected acute ischemic syndromes in the emergency department or chest pain center. *J Nucl Cardiol* 2002;9:246–250.
40. Dakik HA, Mahmarian JJ, Kimball KT, et al. Prognostic value of exercise 201Tl tomography in patients treated with thrombolytic therapy during acute myocardial infarction. *Circulation* 1996;94:2735–2742.
41. Amanullah AM, Lindvall K. Prevalence and significance of transient—predominantly asymptomatic—myocardial ischemia on Holter monitoring in unstable angina pectoris, and correlation with exercise test and thallium-201 myocardial perfusion imaging. *Am J Cardiol* 1993;72:144–148.
42. Verani MS. Risk stratifying patients who survive an acute myocardial infarction. *J Nucl Cardiol* 1998;5:96–108.
43. Azzarelli S, Galassi AR, Foti R, et al. Accuracy of 99mTc-tetrofosmin myocardial tomography in the evaluation of coronary artery disease. *J Nucl Cardiol* 1999;6:183–189.
44. Iskandrian AE, Heo J, Nallamothu N. Detection of coronary artery disease in women with use of stress single-photon emission computed tomography myocardial perfusion imaging. *J Nucl Cardiol* 1997;4:329–335.
45. Mahmarian JJ, Boyce TM, Goldberg RK, et al. Quantitative exercise thallium-201 single photon emission computed tomography for the enhanced diagnosis of ischemic heart disease. *J Am Coll Cardiol* 1990;15:318–329.
46. Van Train KF, Garcia EV, Maddahi J, et al. Multicenter trial validation for quantitative analysis of same-day rest-stress technetium-99m-sestamibi myocardial tomograms. *J Nucl Med* 1994;35:609–618.
47. Rozanski A, Diamond GA, Forrester JS, et al. Alternative referent standards for cardiac normality. Implications for diagnostic testing. *Ann Intern Med* 1984;101:164–171.
48. Fleischmann KE, Hunink MG, Kuntz KM, et al. Exercise echocardiography or exercise SPECT imaging? A meta-analysis of diagnostic test performance. *JAMA* 1998;280:913–920.
49. Heller GV, Links J, Bateman TM, et al. American Society of Nuclear Cardiology and Society of Nuclear Medicine joint position statement: attenuation correction of myocardial perfusion SPECT scintigraphy. *J Nucl Cardiol* 2004;11:229–230.

50. Masood Y, Liu YH, Depuey G, et al. Clinical validation of SPECT attenuation correction using x-ray computed tomography-derived attenuation maps: multicenter clinical trial with angiographic correlation. *J Nucl Cardiol* 2005;12:676–686.
51. Akinboboye OO, Idris O, Onwuanyi A, et al. Incidence of major cardiovascular events in black patients with normal myocardial stress perfusion study results. *J Nucl Cardiol* 2001;8:541–547.
52. Alkeylani A, Miller DD, Shaw LJ, et al. Influence of race on the prediction of cardiac events with stress technetium-99m sestamibi tomographic imaging in patients with stable angina pectoris. *Am J Cardiol* 1998;81:293–297.
53. Shaw LJ, Hendel RC, Cerquiera M, et al. Ethnic differences in the prognostic value of stress technetium-99m tetrofosmin gated single-photon emission computed tomography myocardial perfusion imaging. *J Am Coll Cardiol* 2005;45:1494–1504.
54. Taillefer R, DePuey EG, Udelson JE, et al. Comparative diagnostic accuracy of Tl-201 and Tc-99m sestamibi SPECT imaging (perfusion and ECG-gated SPECT) in detecting coronary artery disease in women. *J Am Coll Cardiol* 1997;29:69–77.
55. Marwick TH, Shaw LJ, Lauer MS, et al. The noninvasive prediction of cardiac mortality in men and women with known or suspected coronary artery disease. Economics of Noninvasive Diagnosis (END) Study Group. *Am J Med* 1999;106:172–178.
56. Hachamovitch R, Berman DS, Kiat H, et al. Gender-related differences in clinical management after exercise nuclear testing. *J Am Coll Cardiol* 1995;26:1457–1464.
57. Amanullah AM, Kiat H, Friedman JD, et al. Adenosine technetium-99m sestamibi myocardial perfusion SPECT in women: diagnostic efficacy in detection of coronary artery disease. *J Am Coll Cardiol* 1996;27:803–809.
58. Christian TF, Miller TD, Bailey KR, et al. Exercise tomographic thallium-201 imaging in patients with severe coronary artery disease and normal electrocardiograms. *Ann Intern Med* 1994;121:825–832.
59. Hachamovitch R, Berman DS, Kiat H, et al. Value of stress myocardial perfusion single photon emission computed tomography in patients with normal resting electrocardiograms: an evaluation of incremental prognostic value and cost-effectiveness. *Circulation* 2002;105:823–829.
60. Mattera JA, Arain SA, Sinusas AJ, et al. Exercise testing with myocardial perfusion imaging in patients with normal baseline electrocardiograms: cost savings with a stepwise diagnostic strategy. *J Nucl Cardiol* 1998;5:498–506.
61. Nallamothu N, Ghods M, Heo J, et al. Comparison of thallium-201 single-photon emission computed tomography and electrocardiographic response during exercise in patients with normal rest electrocardiographic results. *J Am Coll Cardiol* 1995;25:830–836.
62. Gibbons RJ, Balady GJ, Bricker JT, et al. ACC/AHA 2002 guideline update for exercise testing: summary article. A report of the American College of Cardiology/American Heart Association Task Force on Practice Guidelines (Committee to Update the 1997 Exercise Testing Guidelines). *J Am Coll Cardiol* 2002;40:1531–1540.
63. Gibbons RJ, Abrams J, Chatterjee K, et al. ACC/AHA 2002 guideline update for the management of patients with chronic stable angina—summary article: a report of the American College of Cardiology/American Heart Association Task Force on practice guidelines (Committee on the Management of Patients With Chronic Stable Angina). *J Am Coll Cardiol* 2003;41:159–168.
64. Shaw LJ, Hachamovitch R, Peterson ED, et al. Using an outcomes-based approach to identify candidates for risk stratification after exercise treadmill testing. *J Gen Intern Med* 1999;14:1–9.
65. Gibbons RJ, Hodge DO, Berman DS, et al. Long-term outcome of patients with intermediate-risk exercise electrocardiograms who do not have myocardial perfusion defects on radionuclide imaging. *Circulation* 1999;100:2140–2145.
66. Hachamovitch R, Berman DS, Shaw LJ, et al. Incremental prognostic value of myocardial perfusion single photon emission computed tomography for the prediction of cardiac death: differential stratification for risk of cardiac death and myocardial infarction. *Circulation* 1998;97:535–543.
67. Burns RJ, Galligan L, Wright LM, et al. Improved specificity of myocardial thallium-201 single-photon emission computed tomography in patients with left bundle branch block by dipyridamole. *Am J Cardiol* 1991;68:504–508.
68. Nallamothu N, Bagheri B, Acio ER, et al. Prognostic value of stress myocardial perfusion single photon emission computed tomography imaging in patients with left ventricular bundle branch block. *J Nucl Cardiol* 1997;4:487–493.
69. O'Keefe JH, Jr., Bateman TM, Silvestri R, et al. Safety and diagnostic accuracy of adenosine thallium-201 scintigraphy in patients unable to exercise and those with left bundle branch block. *Am Heart J* 1992;124:614–621.
70. Vaduganathan P, He ZX, Raghavan C, et al. Detection of left anterior descending coronary artery stenosis in patients with left bundle branch block: exercise, adenosine or dobutamine imaging? *J Am Coll Cardiol* 1996; 28:543–550.
71. Wagdy HM, Hodge D, Christian TF, et al. Prognostic value of vasodilator myocardial perfusion imaging in patients with left bundle-branch block. *Circulation* 1998;97:1563–1570.
72. Gioia G, Bagheri B, Gottlieb CD, et al. Prediction of outcome of patients with life-threatening ventricular arrhythmias treated with automatic implantable cardioverter-defibrillators using SPECT perfusion imaging. *Circulation* 1997;95:390–394.
73. Amanullah AM, Berman DS, Kang X, et al. Enhanced prognostic stratification of patients with left ventricular hypertrophy with the use of single-photon emission computed tomography. *Am Heart J* 2000;140:456–462.
74. Elhendy A, van Domburg RT, Sozzi FB, et al. Impact of hypertension on the accuracy of exercise stress myocardial perfusion imaging for the diagnosis of coronary artery disease. *Heart* 2001;85:655–661.
75. Bartram P, Toft J, Hanel B, et al. False-positive defects in technetium-99m sestamibi myocardial single-photon emission tomography in healthy athletes with left ventricular hypertrophy. *Eur J Nucl Med* 1998;25:1308–1312.
76. Hilton TC, Shaw LJ, Chaitman BR, et al. Prognostic significance of exercise thallium-201 testing in patients aged greater than or equal to 70 years with known or suspected coronary artery disease. *Am J Cardiol* 1992;69:45–50.
77. Blumenthal RS, Becker DM, Moy TF, et al. Exercise thallium tomography predicts future clinically manifest coronary heart disease in a high-risk asymptomatic population. *Circulation* 1996;93:915–923.
78. Blumenthal RS, Becker DM, Yanek LR, et al. Detecting occult coronary disease in a high-risk asymptomatic population. *Circulation* 2003;107:702–707.
79. Fleg JL, Gerstenblith G, Zonderman AB, et al. Prevalence and prognostic significance of exercise-induced silent myocardial ischemia detected by thallium scintigraphy and electrocardiography in asymptomatic volunteers. *Circulation* 1990;81:428–436.
80. Schwartz RS, Jackson WG, Celio PV, et al. Accuracy of exercise 201Tl myocardial scintigraphy in asymptomatic young men. *Circulation* 1993;87: 165–172.
81. Diabetes mellitus: a major risk factor for cardiovascular disease. A joint editorial statement by the American Diabetes Association; The National Heart, Lung, and Blood Institute; The Juvenile Diabetes Foundation International; The National Institute of Diabetes and Digestive and Kidney Diseases; and The American Heart Association. *Circulation* 1999;100:1132–1133.
82. Giri S, Shaw LJ, Murthy DR, et al. Impact of diabetes on the risk stratification using stress single-photon emission computed tomography myocardial perfusion imaging in patients with symptoms suggestive of coronary artery disease. *Circulation* 2002;105:32–40.
83. Kang X, Berman DS, Lewin H, et al. Comparative ability of myocardial perfusion single-photon emission computed tomography to detect coronary artery disease in patients with and without diabetes mellitus. *Am Heart J* 1999;137:949–957.
84. Kang X, Berman DS, Lewin HC, et al. Incremental prognostic value of myocardial perfusion single photon emission computed tomography in patients with diabetes mellitus. *Am Heart J* 1999;138:1025–1032.
85. Wackers FJ, Young LH, Inzucchi SE, et al. Detection of silent myocardial ischemia in asymptomatic diabetic subjects: the DIAD study. *Diabetes Care* 2004;27:1954–1961.
86. White CW, Wright CB, Doty DB, et al. Does visual interpretation of the coronary arteriogram predict the physiologic importance of a coronary stenosis? *N Engl J Med* 1984;310:819–824.
87. Abdel Fattah A, Kamal AM, Pancholy S, et al. Prognostic implications of normal exercise tomographic thallium images in patients with angiographic evidence of significant coronary artery disease. *Am J Cardiol* 1994;74:769–771.
88. Brown KA, Rowen M. Prognostic value of a normal exercise myocardial perfusion imaging study in patients with angiographically significant coronary artery disease. *Am J Cardiol* 1993;71:865–867.
89. Shaw LJ, Hachamovitch R, Berman DS, et al. The economic consequences of available diagnostic and prognostic strategies for the evaluation of stable angina patients: an observational assessment of the value of precatheterization ischemia. Economics of Noninvasive Diagnosis (END) Multicenter Study Group. *J Am Coll Cardiol* 1999;33:661–669.
90. McPherson JA, Robinson PS, Powers ER, et al. Angiographic findings in patients undergoing catheterization for recurrent symptoms within 30 days of successful coronary intervention. *Am J Cardiol* 1999;84:589–592, A588.
91. Jain A, Mahmarian JJ, Borges-Neto S, et al. Clinical significance of perfusion defects by thallium-201 single photon emission tomography following oral dipyridamole early after coronary angioplasty. *J Am Coll Cardiol* 1988;11:970–976.
92. Manyari DE, Knudtson M, Kloiber R, et al. Sequential thallium-201 myocardial perfusion studies after successful percutaneous transluminal coronary artery angioplasty: delayed resolution of exercise-induced scintigraphic abnormalities. *Circulation* 1988;77:86–95.
93. Ho KT, Miller TD, Holmes DR, et al. Long-term prognostic value of Duke treadmill score and exercise thallium-201 imaging performed one to three years after percutaneous transluminal coronary angioplasty. *Am J Cardiol* 1999;84:1323–1327.
94. Finn AV, Kolodgie FD, Harnek J, et al. Differential response of delayed healing and persistent inflammation at sites of overlapping sirolimus- or paclitaxel-eluting stents. *Circulation* 2005;112:270–278.
95. Togni M, Windecker S, Cocchia R, et al. Sirolimus-eluting stents associated with paradoxic coronary vasoconstriction. *J Am Coll Cardiol* 2005;46:231–236.
96. Miller TD, Christian TF, Hodge DO, et al. Prognostic value of exercise thallium-201 imaging performed within 2 years of coronary artery bypass graft surgery. *J Am Coll Cardiol* 1998;31:848–854.

97. Palmas W, Bingham S, Diamond GA, et al. Incremental prognostic value of exercise thallium-201 myocardial single-photon emission computed tomography late after coronary artery bypass surgery. *J Am Coll Cardiol* 1995;25:403–409.
98. Zellweger MJ, Lewin HC, Lai S, et al. When to stress patients after coronary artery bypass surgery? Risk stratification in patients early and late post-CABG using stress myocardial perfusion SPECT: implications of appropriate clinical strategies. *J Am Coll Cardiol* 2001;37:144–152.
99. Lauer MS, Lytle B, Pashkow F, et al. Prediction of death and myocardial infarction by screening with exercise-thallium testing after coronary-artery-bypass grafting. *Lancet* 1998;351:615–622.
100. Nallamothu N, Johnson JH, Bagheri B, et al. Utility of stress single-photon emission computed tomography (SPECT) perfusion imaging in predicting outcome after coronary artery bypass grafting. *Am J Cardiol* 1997;80: 1517–1521.
101. Eagle KA, Berger PB, Calkins H, et al. ACC/AHA guideline update for perioperative cardiovascular evaluation for noncardiac surgery—executive summary: a report of the American College of Cardiology/American Heart Association Task Force on Practice Guidelines (Committee to Update the 1996 Guidelines on Perioperative Cardiovascular Evaluation for Noncardiac Surgery). *J Am Coll Cardiol* 2002;39:542–553.
102. Mangano DT, Goldman L. Preoperative assessment of patients with known or suspected coronary disease. *N Engl J Med* 1995;333:1750–1756.
103. Poldermans D, Boersma E, Bax JJ, et al. The effect of bisoprolol on perioperative mortality and myocardial infarction in high-risk patients undergoing vascular surgery. Dutch Echocardiographic Cardiac Risk Evaluation Applying Stress Echocardiography Study Group. *N Engl J Med* 1999;341:1789–1794.
104. Alexander J, Dainiak N, Berger HJ, et al. Serial assessment of doxorubicin cardiotoxicity with quantitative radionuclide angiocardiography. *N Engl J Med* 1979;300:278–283.
105. Feldman AM, Lorell BH, Reis SE. Trastuzumab in the treatment of metastatic breast cancer: anticancer therapy versus cardiotoxicity. *Circulation* 2000;102:272–274.
106. Schwartz RS. Overview of the biochemistry and safety of a new native intravenous gamma globulin, IGIV, pH 4.25. *Am J Med* 1987;83:46–51.
107. van Royen N, Jaffe CC, Krumholz HM, et al. Comparison and reproducibility of visual echocardiographic and quantitative radionuclide left ventricular ejection fractions. *Am J Cardiol* 1996;77:843–850.
108. Perrone-Filardi P, Pace L, Prastaro M, et al. Dobutamine echocardiography predicts improvement of hypoperfused dysfunctional myocardium after revascularization in patients with coronary artery disease. *Circulation* 1995;91:2556–2565.
109. Udelson JE, Coleman PS, Metherall J, et al. Predicting recovery of severe regional ventricular dysfunction. Comparison of resting scintigraphy with 201Tl and 99mTc-sestamibi. *Circulation* 1994;89:2552–2561.
110. Acampa W, Cuocolo A, Petretta M, et al. Tetrofosmin imaging in the detection of myocardial viability in patients with previous myocardial infarction: comparison with sestamibi and Tl-201 scintigraphy. *J Nucl Cardiol* 2002;9:33–40.
111. Allman KC, Shaw LJ, Hachamovitch R, et al. Myocardial viability testing and impact of revascularization on prognosis in patients with coronary artery disease and left ventricular dysfunction: a meta-analysis. *J Am Coll Cardiol* 2002;39:1151–1158.
112. Bonow RO. Identification of viable myocardium. *Circulation* 1996;94: 2674–2680.
113. Di Carli MF, Asgarzadie F, Schelbert HR, et al. Quantitative relation between myocardial viability and improvement in heart failure symptoms after revascularization in patients with ischemic cardiomyopathy. *Circulation* 1995;92:3436–3444.
114. Tarakji KG, Brunken R, McCarthy PM, et al. Myocardial viability testing and the effect of early intervention in patients with advanced left ventricular systolic dysfunction. *Circulation* 2006;113:230–237.
115. Di Carli MF, Davidson M, Little R, et al. Value of metabolic imaging with positron emission tomography for evaluating prognosis in patients with coronary artery disease and left ventricular dysfunction. *Am J Cardiol* 1994;73:527–533.
116. Arora R, Ferrick KJ, Nakata T, et al. I-123 MIBG imaging and heart rate variability analysis to predict the need for an implantable cardioverter defibrillator. *J Nucl Cardiol* 2003;10:121–131.
117. Chambers MG, Narula J, Cerqueira MD. The economic burden of heart failure and implantable cardioverter defibrillators: The value of noninvasive imaging of high-risk patients. *J Nucl Cardiol* 2002;9(5 Suppl):71S–80S.
118. Hendel RC, Bateman TM, Cerqueira MD, et al. Initial clinical experience with regadenoson, a novel selective A2A agonist for pharmacologic stress single-photon emission computed tomography myocardial perfusion imaging. *J Am Coll Cardiol* 2005;46:2069–2075.
119. Udelson JE, Heller GV, Wackers FJ, et al. Randomized, controlled dose-ranging study of the selective adenosine A2A receptor agonist binodenoson for pharmacological stress as an adjunct to myocardial perfusion imaging. *Circulation* 2004;109:457–464.

CHAPTER 54 ■ CARDIOVASCULAR MAGNETIC RESONANCE IMAGING

MILIND Y. DESAI, RICHARD D. WHITE, DAVID A. BLUEMKE, AND JOAO A. C. LIMA

INTRODUCTION

Cardiovascular magnetic resonance imaging (MRI) is a rapidly evolving technology that is very well suited for the morphologic and physiologic evaluation of a wide range of acquired and congenital disease processes affecting the heart, pericardium, and great arteries and veins of the thorax. MRI is unique in its ability to provide four-dimensional (three spatial dimensions over the dimension of time) imaging of the cardiovascular system based on definition of high-detail anatomy, histologic characterization, intracardiac or intravascular blood flow, cardiac chamber contraction and filling, regional myocardial mechanics, and tissue perfusion. Hence, MRI is playing a major role as a diagnostic modality in all facets of cardiovascular medicine. Furthermore, its potential is clearly becoming evident in the fields of atherosclerosis imaging, molecular imaging, and interventional cardiovascular medicine.

PRINCIPLES AND TECHNIQUES

Brief History

Nuclear magnetic resonance is a phenomenon exhibited by certain atomic nuclei. It was introduced by Block et al. (1) and Purcell et al. (2) in 1946. In 1973, Lauterbur (3) first described a method for producing images using related techniques, and as early as 1977 human whole-body images were already being produced by MRI (4). By the early 1980s (5,6), high-quality static anatomic imaging of the cardiovascular structures was being accomplished by electrocardiogram (ECG)-gated MRI. The mid to late 1980s saw the development and clinical implementation of dynamic MRI techniques allowing physiologic assessment of cardiac function and blood flow (7,8); this was promoted by the use of the more rapid acquisition techniques (9). Since then, MRI has profited from technical advances allowing the following capabilities: near-real-time imaging (10,11), tissue tagging-tracking (12), and three-dimensional (3D) acquisition and display (13); the result has been improvement in the assessment of myocardial physiology and complex and/or fine-detail anatomy of the cardiovascular system.

Magnetic Resonance Imaging Principles

A detailed discussion of MRI principles is beyond the scope of this book. A brief discussion follows. Atomic nuclei with odd numbers of protons or neutrons spin about an axis and can be aligned along the direction of a magnetic field. This characteristic is vital because it causes nuclei to precess when tipped from alignment with the main magnetic field. The ^1H proton has been most widely applied in MRI because of its natural abundance; therefore, this discussion will refer to hydrogen-based MRI. The MRI signal originates primarily from the hydrogen of water and less so from the small hydrogen content of lipids. The actual appearance of the image is affected by a variety of physical parameters. Some of these parameters are characteristic of the tissue sampled and others relate to the MRI sequences. An essential difference between MRI and other modalities is the control that the user has over how data are generated and utilized. The agent of this control is *k*-space (Fourier space), the platform onto which data are acquired, positioned, and then transformed into the desired image (14). Raw image data are obtained during sampling through *k*-space, which depicts the spatial frequency domain. High spatial frequencies encode fine details, whereas overall contrast is encoded in the lower frequencies. Data are acquired at discrete intervals to fill *k*-space as signal amplitude is stored as a function of the spatial frequencies along the read-out and phase-encoding directions. An image is simply the inverse Fourier transform of the sampled *k*-space (15).

MRI uses high-power static magnetic fields and radiofrequency (RF) pulses to generate tomographic images. Application of weak RF-modulated pulses of a specific frequency will partially align the magnetic moments of protons within the tissue sample against the magnetic field and will induce their resonance; the effect of this RF field is maximal when the nuclei have been deflected by 90°. When the RF pulse ceases, the protons return to equilibrium. During this process, they emit the RF energy of the same frequency, which is then Fourier transformed by a computer into a spatially accurate image whereby differences in signal intensity result in differences in gray levels. The signal intensity depends not only on hydrogen density, but also on the longitudinal relaxation time (T1), reflecting the rate of realignment with the external magnetic field (enhancing the signal), and on the transverse relaxation time (T2), indicating the rate at which nuclei lose coherence with each other (degrading the signal). In normal myocardium, T2 is much shorter (i.e., 60 msec at 1.5 T) than T1 (i.e., 500 msec). The characteristic T1 and T2 relaxation times are exploited to distinguish between normal tissues and to characterize disease processes. In general, MRI contrast improves with increasing hydrogen density, shortening of T1, and lengthening of T2.

Basically, an MRI scanner consists of five major parts: magnet, transmitter, antenna, receiver, and computer. Most modern clinical MRI scanners have magnets consisting of liquid helium–cooled superconducting solenoids operating at a field strength of 0.1 to 3.0 T and with a bore size of approximately 1 m; MRI is best performed with a magnet with higher field strength and homogeneity to improve the signal-to-noise ratio. The transmitter is used for transmitting RF pulses to an antenna or coil, which in turn transmits RF power to the patient and also receives the returning signal. The coil usually surrounds the patient or may be placed directly on the patient's surface, depending on whether information is required from the whole body or from a selected organ of interest; although surface coils provide higher sensitivity and, therefore, excellent spatial localization of signal, they have the disadvantage of an inhomogeneous RF field, which produces an inhomogeneous signal intensity distribution on images. The receiver amplifies the signal picked up by the coil, and the signal is processed by a computer, which is also needed to operate the entire MRI system.

Specific Magnetic Resonance Imaging Techniques

A detailed discussion of MRI physics is beyond the scope of this chapter, but can be studied from many dedicated textbooks. We briefly discuss some features, including the commonly used imaging sequences in cardiac imaging.

Spin-Echo Sequence

Conventional spin-echo (SE) imaging was for a long time the workhorse of cardiac MRI studies. It has been supplanted by more modern techniques that allow for faster imaging. Nonetheless, spin-echo is still frequently performed with T1 weighting; T2-weighted sequences can be used to demonstrate tumors, inflammation, or myocardial tissue abnormalities. A typical cardiac MRI study is initiated by acquiring scout views through the chest. This is accomplished in a very short time interval, using a fast MRI pulse sequence that has a moderate spatial resolution. The scout views are used to prescribe a volume of interest that is studied with subsequent stacks of SE slices. Each stack has a different orientation (often the three orthogonal planes: coronal, sagittal, and axial) and is acquired in 3 to 5 minutes. Image (slice) thickness, gap, and orientation can be freely chosen. With SE MRI, flowing blood usually generates no signal, whereas myocardium and fatty tissue produce intermediate and high signal intensity. SE MRI is ideal for visualizing morphology, but its limited time resolution does not easily allow functional analysis. The turbo (fast)-spin-echo sequence (TSE) is a faster version of the spin-echo sequence. Instead of one spin-echo pulse, the 90° excitation pulse is followed by a series of 180° pulses that produce several echo signals, each with a different phase encoding. This means that instead of one *k*-line, several *k*-lines are measured. The number of 180° pulses is also referred to as the turbo factor. The acquisition time can be shortened with respect to spin-echo imaging by the turbo factor. The most frequent application of TSE sequences is in acquisitions with T2 contrast, in which high turbo factors can be used and the greatest reduction in measuring time can be achieved.

Gradient-Echo Sequence

Gradient-echo (GRE) imaging is a faster technique. In contrast to SE, orderly blood flow generates high signal intensities in GRE imaging. GRE is fast enough to "catch" the signal from previously excited magnetic spins in the blood volume of the image section under study before the blood flow has moved the spins out of the image section. With GRE, the same section can be measured with high repetition rate, enabling the reconstruction of a cine loop of that particular section. This can be achieved in the axial, long axis, short axis, or any desired plane, with a time frame interval of less than 25 msec. GRE can thus be used to detect turbulent blood flow occurring in stenosis, regurgitation, or shunts. Such lesions become particularly obvious when viewing the tomographic section in a cine loop. Turbulent blood flow causes loss of the signal, so stenosis, regurgitation, or shunt flow is detected by a jet of signal void. Cine GRE MRI can be used to assess left (LV) and right (RV) ventricular function in terms of volumes and myocardial mass without geometric assumptions regarding the shape of the ventricles (16). A complete stack that encompasses the heart consists of 10 to 12 adjacent GRE images (typically of 10 mm thickness), each with its own set of time frames, and can be acquired in 10 to 15 minutes. End-diastolic and end-systolic volumes can be measured, or if desired a complete ventricular time–volume curve can be obtained. Another modification of the gradient-echo sequence is the segmented (multishot) gradient-echo sequence, in which only a segment of the image is acquired. In order to achieve all segments, measurements must be made over several RR intervals. Each segment (sometimes also referred to as a "shot") comprises a certain number of slice-selective RF pulses followed by phase encoding and signal measurement. The segments are distinguished from each other by different values of the phase-encoding gradients (k_y values) and consequently provide different *k*-lines. The newer balanced steady-state free-precession sequences give the best image quality, particularly if the repetition and echo times are kept very short and there has been adequate shimming of the static magnetic field to the region of the heart (17).

Magnetic Resonance Imaging Prepulses

All of the basic pulse sequences (SE, GRE, TSE) can be extended by a prepulse that is transmitted before the actual excitation pulse. The prepulse can consist of one or more RF pulses, sometimes in combination with gradient switching (slice selection, dephasing, etc.). Prepulses can be used for various purposes, such as influencing the contrast and suppressing fat or blood signals. A 180° pulse (inversion pulse) can be used to increase the T1 contrast. The longitudinal magnetization is inverted, and the T1 relaxation does not start at zero, as in the case of a 90° pulse, but at –1. In other words, the contrast range is doubled. The strength of the T1 contrast can be controlled by the interval between the inversion pulse and the excitation pulse, known as the inversion time (TI). In addition, TI can be chosen in such a way that the magnetization of a tissue during excitation is equal to zero, so that the signal from the corresponding tissue disappears. In this way, the fat signal can be suppressed by using a short TI (e.g., short inversion time inversion recovery [STIR] sequence), or a longer TI can be used to suppress the fluid signal (e.g., fluid-attenuated inversion recovery [FLAIR] sequence). An inversion pulse can be combined with all of the basic pulse sequences. In segmented gradient-echo sequences, the interval between the inversion pulse and the *k*-line determining the contrast of the shots ($k_y = 0$) is also referred to as the prepulse delay (pp delay). Similarly, a 90° pulse can be used to increase the T1 contrast. In ECG-triggered acquisitions, the relaxation state of the longitudinal magnetization depends on the RR interval. It can therefore have varying values in arrhythmic patients with RR intervals of differing length. If a 90° pulse is transmitted by systole, so that the longitudinal magnetization is reduced to zero, the same T1 relaxation state is ensured after the pp delay, regardless of arrhythmias.

Another prepulse that is applied in cardiovascular diagnosis is the black-blood pulse, which is used to suppress the blood signal. The black-blood pulse consists of a series of two 180° pulses. The first pulse is non–slide selective (so-called block pulse). It inverts the magnetism in the total range of the transmission coil (in heart examinations, this can be the whole chest). The second 180° pulse, which is transmitted after the first, is slice selective, and returns the magnetization in the acquisition slice back to its original value. The magnetization of blood flowing into the acquisition slice begins to relax and, after a delay dependent on TR (or the heart frequency), is equal to zero. If the contrast-relevant values of the sequence are measured at this point, the blood signal will be suppressed. The black-blood pulse is often used with TSE sequences (T1 and T2 contrast).

Myocardial Tagging

Regional myocardial function is best assessed using a unique MR technique called myocardial tagging (12), commonly acquired by spatial modulation of magnetization (18). Spatial modulation of magnetization is obtained by applying a radiofrequency prepulse perpendicular to the imaging plane. This prepulse induces local changes in saturation within their planes that label the heart muscle with a dark grid and enables three-dimensional analysis of cardiac rotation, strain (in the subendocardial, mid-wall, and subepicardial layers), displacement, and deformation of different myocardial layers during the cardiac cycle (19). The tags can be applied immediately after the R wave on the electrocardiogram to image systolic function or in late systole to image diastolic function. However, until recently it had not been widely used in clinical cardiac imaging, mainly because of the extensive postprocessing that is required because of the vast amount of information produced by MR tagging series. Recently developed postprocessing software has significantly reduced the time it takes to analyze these tags, making the technique clinically viable (20).

Conventional Magnetic Resonance Angiography and Blood Flow Quantification

MR angiography (MRA) techniques can be divided in time-of-flight (TOF) MRA, phase-contrast angiography (PCA), and contrast-enhanced MRA.

Time-of-Flight Magnetic Resonance Angiography. This is an older technique, which has been used less frequently since the emergence of contrast MRA. In gradient-echo sequences, the longitudinal magnetization of stationary tissue is reduced by repeated excitations. Due to the saturation of the longitudinal magnetization, the signal from the stationary tissue is low. When the blood vessel runs perpendicularly through the slice, "fresh" unsaturated blood (not previously excited, with full longitudinal magnetization) will produce the maximum signal in the excited slice. The overall result is higher contrast between the flowing blood and the saturated stationary tissue. If many overlapping slices are combined, or if 3D techniques are used, inflow MRA can also be used to cover larger volumes.

Phase-Contrast Angiography. With the use of this technique, blood flow velocity is encoded in the phase of the MRI signal and phase changes occur linearly with changes in velocity. An image displaying the phase values across a vessel lumen can therefore be regarded as a velocity map. The signal intensity on quantitative PCA images increases toward bright or dark, depending on the direction of the flow, linearly with the velocity. PCA can be performed across a perpendicular vascular cross section, which allows assessment of instantaneous peak velocity and (spatial) average velocity at frequent time points during a cardiac cycle. Alternatively, to study the jet across a stenotic lesion, the image plane can also be chosen along the longitudinal axis of a vessel. Because true spatial average velocity can be measured, volumetric flow (mL/second) can be calculated by multiplication with the corresponding vascular cross-sectional area. This unique feature of MRI is superior to deriving mean velocity from a sample volume as in Doppler echocardiography. The contour of a vascular cross section is traced by hand, or preferably automatically, using commercially available computer software. The contour is adjusted, if necessary, for changes in position and diameter in every time frame. From these data, velocity and volume of flow can be plotted against time, and stroke volume can be calculated. This technique is being used as an elegant and reliable method for quantifying aortic and pulmonary blood flow because it enables quantification of intracardiac shunts, valvular regurgitation, or differential pulmonary blood flow (21,22). It has also been used to assess endothelial function not only by measuring vessel diameter, as by ultrasound, but also by integrating anatomic and flow velocity data to quantify endothelial shear stress (23,24).

Contrast-Enhanced Magnetic Resonance Angiography

Gadolinium-diethylenetriamine pentaacetic acid (Gd-DPTA) is a contrast agent with no known nephrotoxicity that alters the magnetic properties of blood, allowing measurements of a volume of interest with short repetition time (25). Gd-enhanced MRA is now being used in a rapid 3D fashion.

Within one breath-hold, a tissue volume encompassing the entire thoracic aorta or pulmonary artery with their respective branches is imaged. Imaging is timed to the arrival of a Gd bolus (generally 30 mL) in the area of interest. If it is so desired, acquisition can be rapidly repeated to visualize early and late venous phases. This technique has proven to be very valuable in (postoperative) coarctation, pulmonary stenosis, and preoperative evaluation of pulmonary atresia. In particular, the use of maximum-intensity-projection (MIP) reconstructions allows visualization of the aortic and pulmonary branches from any desired angle. Three-dimensional views display complex spatial information to clinicians who are less trained in image interpretation.

Delayed Postcontrast Imaging for Myocardial Viability

The current technique involves the rapid infusion of a gadolinium chelate (doses are typically in the range of 0.1 to

0.2 mmol/kg) followed approximately 5 to 30 minutes later by a high-resolution, cardiac-gated, multishot, inversion-recovery–prepared, T1-weighted gradient-echo sequence (26). Images are acquired 5 to 30 minutes after contrast agent infusion (27). Choice of the appropriate inversion time (approximately 200 msec) to null the signal intensity of normal myocardium is critical for accurate delineation of the infarcted region. The healthy myocardium appears dark, whereas the enhancing myocardium appears bright. However, the optimal inversion time will lengthen over time as the concentration of gadolinium in the blood and myocardium gradually diminishes. Phase-sensitive reconstructions render the technique less sensitive to the choice of inversion time and reduce the variation in apparent infarct size (28). Imaging too early (e.g., <5 minutes after contrast agent infusion) may result in an underestimation of the infarcted region, whereas imaging too late (e.g., after >30 minutes) may result in excessive washout of the contrast agent and a poor signal-to-noise ratio (SNR). Findings in acute myocardial infarction showed a substantial change in the portion of left ventricle that enhanced depending on the timing of the acquisition with respect to the contrast agent infusion, with overestimation of infarct size if imaging was performed too early (29).

Image Planes

The orientations traditionally used for cardiovascular MRI are the transaxial, sagittal, and coronal planes; they are orthogonal to the thorax but oblique to the heart and great vessels. Complete sets of these images are most useful in gaining a global perspective of the relationships of the cardiac chambers, great vessels, and adjacent structures. They also serve as important localizing images for oblique imaging along the natural axes of the cardiovascular structures, such as with the long axis of the thoracic aorta. With further axial rotation, double-oblique imaging also can be performed to acquire images of the heart equivalent to the 2D echo short-axis and long-axis orientations (e.g., two-chamber, four-chamber, LV outflow) (30). The limitations of orthogonal imaging relate to deficiencies in the MRI evaluation of some regions of the cardiac chambers for anatomic or physiologic abnormalities. In transaxial imaging, for example, the undersurface of the LV may be obscured due to volume averaging with the adjacent diaphragm, or its wall may have the appearance of being abnormally thickened because it is sliced tangentially (31). This problem with orthogonal MRI of the heart can be overcome by using either another orthogonal (e.g., coronal) or an appropriate oblique (e.g., short-axis) orientation.

Compensation of Cardiac Motion

The formation of an MRI image requires a number of measurements, typically 128 or 256 or a fraction of that. In stationary tissue, these measurements can be done continuously. The heart, however, requires a different approach. To compensate for cardiac motion, every measurement is performed at a fixed time delay after a trigger signal from the R wave of the ECG. An image (slice) can thus be reconstructed after acquiring data during several consecutive cardiac cycles. The remaining slices of the selected volume are measured simultaneously, all with a slightly different time delay after the ECG trigger. Thus, a stack of slices is obtained in several minutes, each slice representing a different time point of the cardiac cycle. With prospective ECG triggering, no measurements can be performed in a certain time interval before the next QRS complex to allow for variations in heart rate. This means that no data can be collected during end-diastole, a drawback when studying diastolic phenomena. With retrospective gating, measurements are being made continuously, with simultaneous registration of the ECG signal. After acquisition, the data are attributed to the corresponding time frame and a complete cine loop is reconstructed that displays the full cardiac cycle. Another problem with ECG gating occurs under the influence of a strong static magnetic field, the enhancement of the so-called magnetohydrodynamic effect. It leads to artifactual augmentation of the T wave and may frequently mislead the R-wave detection algorithm so that triggering is performed on the T wave instead of the R wave. Because this artifact increases with field strength, this presents a major challenge for 3T. However, by analyzing the ECG vector in 3D space using the vector ECG approach (32), the true T wave can be separated from the artifactual T-wave augmentation, and reliable R-wave detection has shown to be feasible even at higher field strength (33). In general, severe arrhythmias will cause image quality degradation and unreliable quantitative MRI studies.

Compensation of Respiratory Motion

The second major impediment to MRI is respiratory motion. To compensate for respiratory motion, breath-holding was implemented early to allow for suppression of respiratory motion. Breath-hold approaches offer the advantage of rapid imaging and are technically easy to implement in compliant subjects. However, breath-holding strategies have several limitations. Some patients may have difficulty sustaining adequate breath-holds, particularly when the duration exceeds a few seconds. In addition, it has been shown that during a sustained breath-hold there is cranial diaphragmatic drift (34), which is substantial in many cases (~1 cm). Among serial breath-holds, the diaphragmatic and cardiac positions frequently vary by up to 1 cm, resulting in registration errors (35,36). To overcome limitations associated with breath-holding, different methods such as MR navigators (37) have been developed to allow for free-breathing coronary MRA. With vertical positioning of the navigator at the dome of the right hemidiaphragm (lung–liver interface), the diaphragmatic craniocaudal displacement can be monitored. Although navigator approaches greatly improve patient comfort and do not require significant subject motivation, their use prolongs MRI data acquisition, commonly collected during 50% of typical RR intervals (38).

Safety Concerns During a Magnetic Resonance Imaging Examination

MRI should not be performed in patients with vascular clips used for cerebral aneurysm surgery due to the potential risk of dislodgement from the vessel (39). Implanted cardiac pacemakers, cardiac defibrillators, and neurologic stimulators represent contraindications, and patients with these electronic implants should not undergo MRI due to the risks from malfunctioning of the device or current induction (39). However there are emerging data about the feasibility and safety of performing MRI in patients with modern pacemakers at 1.5 T (40,41). On the other hand, the vast majority of prosthetic heart valves are compatible with MRI. Only a few high-profile prosthetic valves containing large amounts of alloy (e.g., Starr-Edwards pre-6000 series) should be avoided (42). Hemostatic clips, metallic sternal suture wires, and retained surgical epicardial pacing wires are not known to lead to complications from MRI, aside from local imaging artifacts (39). Critically ill patients are less-than-optimal candidates for MRI because either they are dependent on life-support or continuous-monitoring systems that cannot be brought near the scanner or their clinical condition is too fragile for the limited monitoring that is compatible with the MRI environment. Nevertheless, such patients can be safely evaluated if physiologic monitoring is supplemented during close observation by trained personnel. Claustrophobia may impede MRI in up to 5% of patients. This problem can be controlled by premedication with sedatives. Finally, the use of gadolinium contrast agent might be associated with metallic taste in the mouth, tingling in the arm, nausea, or headache. These symptoms occur in less than 1% (<1 in 100) of patients undergoing MRI and subside quickly. Very rarely, there may be an allergic reaction, but there is less than a 1 in 300,000 chance that such reaction would be severe.

SPECIFIC CLINICAL APPLICATIONS

Here we focus on the application of MRI to cardiovascular diseases (Table 54.1). We also discuss some emerging applications of MRI.

Evaluation of Ischemic Heart Disease

Evaluation of ischemic heart disease is one of the most important indications for cardiac MRI. Following is a brief description of the different aspects of MR evaluation for ischemic heart disease (IHD).

Assessment of Global Ventricular Function

MRI techniques have been used to estimate impaired ejection fraction (EF) as a result of ischemic heart disease. EF is obtained from the end-diastolic and end-systolic images of the LV, and the resulting values derived, using the area-length method, correlate well with those obtained by single-plane and biplane LV ventriculography (e.g., $R = .79$ and $R = .95$ for parallel and perpendicular to the interventricular septum, respectively) (43,44). EF determination in patients with IHD can be performed more efficiently and with better temporal resolution using multilevel-cine MRI (45,46). In patients imaged within 7 days of acute MI using cine, LVEF by MRI has been shown to correlate better with EF by contrast ventriculography (e.g., $R = .94$) than with EF by radionuclide ventriculography (e.g., $R = .82$) (47). Cine images show the motion of the heart and blood over multiple phases of the cardiac cycle (48,49) by using some form of a multishot ("segmented") gradient echo. Use of a small number of phase-encoding steps in each breath-hold (encompassing a small portion of the cardiac cycle, e.g., 20 to 60 msec) minimizes blurring from cardiac motion. Accumulation of multiple segments over a typical breath-hold period of 10 to 20 heart beats results in a complete cine examination (10). The newer balanced steady-state free-precession sequences give the best image quality (17). Because of these, MRI has become a gold standard in assessing LVEF and LV volumes.

TABLE 54.1

CLINICAL UTILITY OF MAGNETIC RESONANCE IMAGING: CURRENT APPLICATIONS

Ischemic heart disease	
Reversible	
Induced	++++
Stunned/hibernating	++++
Irreversible	
Acute (e.g., acute myocardial infarction)	++++
Chronic (e.g., post–myocardial infarction aneurysm)	++++
Coronary artery disease	
Anomalous coronary arteries	+++
Atherosclerotic coronary artery disease	++
Valvular heart disease	
Stenosis	+++
Regurgitation	+++
Myocardial disease	
Dilated cardiomyopathy	++++
Hypertrophic cardiomyopathy	++++
Restrictive cardiomyopathy (primary and secondary)	++++
Right ventricular cardiomyopathy	++++
Pericardial disease	
Pericarditis and constriction	++++
Pericardial masses	
Aortic disease	++++
Aneurysm (true, pseudo, and mycotic)	++++
Dissection	
Acute dissection	++++
Nonacute	++++
Intramural hematoma	++++
Pulmonary artery disease	++++
Pulmonary emboli	+
Pulmonary hypertension	++
Thrombi	
Ventricular thrombi	++++
Atrial thrombi	++
Cardiac masses	
Intracardiac (benign and malignant)	++++
Extracardiac (benign and malignant)	++++
Adult congenital heart disease	
Simple cardiac abnormality	++++
Complex cardiac abnormality	++++
Great vessel abnormality	++++

+, minimal utility; ++++, maximal utility.

Assessment of Regional Ventricular Function

Regional myocardial function relates to the amplitude and rapidity of contractile deformation of a segment of the left ventricular wall in the face of a given load or stress. The assessment of regional function is crucial to the complete evaluation of patients with most types of cardiac disease. For example, the demonstration of functional recovery in injured segments or those partially involved by necrosis is important as parameters of viability, and the study of regional function is important to quantify the development or progression of left ventricular remodeling after ischemic and other types of myocardial injury.

Visual assessment of systolic endocardial motion and wall thickening have been used most frequently in previous acute and chronic studies of regional myocardial function. These studies have reported varying levels of intra- and interobserver variability, which may be acceptable in certain situations when the assessment is performed in a before-and-after setting by very well trained observers. Ideally, however, myocardial functional studies should be objectively quantified to allow for less biased comparisons. Commonly, endocardial motion is obtained from cine MRI studies by endo- and epicardial border delineation. These measurements are unfortunately also quite variable due to technical and geometric factors intrinsic to left ventricular architecture and function. More recently, MRI methods for measuring myocardial deformation objectively in multiple orientations have become available (12,18,50–54). These novel techniques have virtually eliminated the use of experimental sonomicrometer implantation for assessing local myocardial function in basic research and have more recently revolutionized the use of imaging methods for assessing left ventricular performance in clinical (50) and population-based research (50).

Moreover, it is very important to emphasize the importance of local load or stress for the adequate interpretation of functional parameters based on myocardial deformation assessed as endocardial motion, systolic thickening, or myocardial strain by MRI. This local load or stress dependence is particularly complex in the regionally ischemic or infarcted left ventricle, where the interaction between infarcted subendocardial layers and preserved subepicardial tissue occurs frequently (55,56). Similarly, the interaction between preserved myocardium located adjacent to acute or chronically infarcted regions depends not only on its own contractile reserve, but also on the mechanical behavior of remote noninfarcted regions and global loading conditions (51,57–59). For these reasons, load interdependence at both the global and regional levels is frequently overlooked or completely ignored in clinical studies as parameters that are difficult or impossible to quantify. Their existence highlights the limitations of functional parameters as indices of myocardial viability, but on the other hand, it is also important to have in mind that the heart's ultimate function is to develop tension and contract in order to eject blood at adequate circulatory pressures. For that reason, functional indices of systolic and diastolic performance will always remain crucial parameters in the evaluation of the heart in health and disease.

Regional myocardial wall thickening abnormalities are frequently observed on MRI in association with ischemic heart disease, starting as early as 5 minutes after coronary artery occlusion (60). Regional wall-motion abnormality appears to be the most predictive and specific MRI finding associated with either a recent or remote myocardial infarction (MI) (61). Cine MRI is suited for evaluation of regional ventricular function in patients with ischemic heart disease (47,49,62). Compared with contrast ventriculography, the concordance in regional wall motion has been similar for cine (e.g., 69%) and radionuclide ventriculography (65%) (47). Although a multilevel cine series gives the advantage of full representation of the ventricles, when patients with suspected coronary artery disease (CAD) have been studied using only biplane cine and biplane LV ventriculography, 96% agreement in the right anterior oblique view and 92% agreement in the left anterior oblique view have been demonstrated (63). Cine has been found to be more accurate than echo in the measurement of LV systolic wall thickening (64).

The ability to perform MRI tissue tagging is particularly advantageous because it can quantify local myocardial segmental shortening throughout the LV at sites across the LV wall (12,18). Tagging uses selective radiofrequency excitation to saturate the magnetization in a thin planar region perpendicular to the imaging plane before acquiring image data. The altered magnetization in the tagged region appears as a dark line in the subsequent image where it intersects the imaging plane, persisting during systole and most of diastole. If the underlying tissue moves between the times of tagging and imaging, the altered magnetization of the tag line deforms with it. Hence, motion of the tag line faithfully follows underlying tissue motion. In the assessment of postinfarct remodeling, myocardial tagging has been used to provide unique functional information about regions of MI and compensatory changes of noninfarcted portions of the LV (51). In patients with one-vessel disease leading to an acute MI, reduced intramyocardial circumferential shortening has been noted throughout the LV, including remote noninfarcted regions (65). Based on the use of tagging, LV dilation and eccentric hypertrophy from remodeling have been shown to be associated with persistent differences in segmental function and wall stress between adjacent and remote noninfarcted myocardium (65).

Similarly, in the assessment of myocardial viability, MRI with tissue tagging has provided important diagnostic information. The improved predictive value of dobutamine-tagged MRI in detecting chronic hibernation, for example, was examined in 10 patients with ischemic cardiomyopathy studied before and 4 to 8 weeks after revascularization (66). The presence of contractile reserve by dobutamine MRI was 89% sensitive and 93% specific for functional recovery. The detection of stunning was reported in a cohort of 20 patients with first acute reperfused MI who were studied with tagged MRI at 4 days and 8 weeks postinfarct (67). Tagged MRI had a sensitivity of 89%. Moreover, because of the spatial resolution of MRI, contractile reserve in the different layers across the myocardial wall could be assessed. A recent study directly compared quantitative stress tagged MRI to qualitative assessment of echocardiographic contractile reserve in 22 patients 3 days after acute reperfused MI (68). The outcome variable was 8-week postinfarct functional improvement by echocardiography. Echocardiography and MRI were concordant in 76% of the segments. Compared to echo, MRI had similar sensitivity (82% vs. 86%) but lower specificity (69% vs. 87%). However, the overall accuracy of MRI and echo was 76% and 85%, respectively, which was not statistically different. One reason for the lower specificity includes difficulties in cross-registering locations between the two imaging modalities. In addition, the subendocardial response to dobutamine by MRI is known to be lower (67). To more directly compare with echo, this study averaged the MRI response across the three transmural layers, which likely contributed to the difference.

In addition to assessing two-dimensional shortening, tagged MRI can be applied in three dimensions to assess regional function not only in the circumferential, but also in the radial and longitudinal directions (69,70). The sequential tag positions during the cardiac cycle can be fitted to a finite-element model of heart wall deformation. The components of strain (deformation) can then be separated from rigid-body motion (translation and rotation). This approach is an accurate and precise measure of mechanical function (52,69,71). In particular, it accounts for conformational changes of the heart during systole such as the base-to-apex shortening and twist.

Widespread clinical application of stress MRI, particularly with tagging, has been limited by relatively long imaging times and requirements for time-consuming postprocessing and off-line analysis. New approaches are available that decrease imaging and postprocessing time and potentially provide online quantitative assessment of wall motion in near real time (53,54,72,73). This may prove beneficial in detecting ischemia with higher sensitivity and at an earlier point in the stress protocol, improving both accuracy and patient safety.

Assessment of Myocardial Perfusion Using Magnetic Resonance Imaging

Myocardial perfusion by has been assessed in the following ways using MRI methods.

Dynamic First-Pass Imaging. This is a very practical method for evaluating myocardial perfusion (74–78) and is achieved with use of extravascular agents that are widely available (e.g., gadolinium-based agents), even though 30% to 50% of the agent leaks out of the vascular bed during the first pass (79). In patients, there is good correlation between the perfusion reserve with MRI and the coronary flow reserve with Doppler ultrasonography ($R = .80$) (80). From a theoretical point of view, the use of an intravascular contrast agent simplifies the modeling of tissue perfusion because one does not need to model tissue extravasation, but such agents are not yet available for routine clinical use. For quantification of myocardial perfusion, qualitative measures such as the maximum myocardial enhancement, transit time, or upslope of myocardial enhancement (i.e., slope of the initial portion of the signal intensity versus time curve after gadolinium administration) (81) have been implemented. In one study of 104 patients, MR imaging had a 90% sensitivity for depicting at least one coronary artery with significant stenosis and an 85% specificity in identification of patients with significant coronary artery stenoses (82). The authors found that stress enhancement at dynamic MR imaging correlated more closely with quantitative coronary angiography results than did stress enhancement at single-photon-emission computed tomography (SPECT).

Resting Perfusion. Imaging of resting perfusion is only moderately sensitive in CAD. For instance, a study of 12 patients with significant stenoses of major epicardial vessels demonstrated a sensitivity of only 77% (83). Early after acute myocardial infarction, the resting perfusion deficit correlates with the long-term severity of left ventricular functional abnormality, and one finds higher perfusion in segments that have a residual contractile reserve at stress echocardiography (84).

Stress Perfusion. To detect significant stenoses of the epicardial coronary arteries, it is helpful to stress the patient so that a measure of the coronary flow reserve, or similar other measures such as the myocardial perfusion reserve index, can be obtained. Although it is technically possible, it is awkward to perform a physiologic exercise stress test within the confined bore of an MR imager. Instead, a pharmaceutical agent, such as dipyridamole (typical dose, 0.56 mg/kg of body weight) or shorter-acting adenosine (typical dose, 140 μg/kg/minute), may be administered to induce coronary vasodilation. The safety profile and more consistent course of action make adenosine the preferred agent for stress perfusion MR imaging. An abnormal perfusion reserve at MR imaging helps distinguish patients with CAD from normal individuals (85). In a study of 34 patients with a stenosis of an epicardial coronary artery of at least 75%, a cutoff value of 1.5 for MR imaging perfusion reserve helped differentiate normal from ischemic myocardial segments (86). This cutoff value yielded high sensitivity (90%), specificity (83%), and diagnostic accuracy (87%) for CAD, with excellent inter- and intraobserver agreement. Perfusion MR imaging also demonstrates the effectiveness of coronary interventions. In a study of 35 patients with single- and multivessel CAD imaged within 24 hours of coronary revascularization, a myocardial perfusion reserve index (upslope index) was calculated from resting and stress perfusion MR imaging (87). The perfusion reserve index improved but did not normalize after successful revascularization. The improvement was greater in patients receiving stents than in those only undergoing angioplasty. The coronary flow reserve determined at contrast-enhanced MR imaging correlates well with that at nitrogen-13 ammonia positron emission tomography (PET) (88). Flow reserve values at MR imaging are lower than those at PET, in part owing to a low extraction fraction for extracellular agents such as gadopentetate dimeglumine. Findings of several studies have confirmed the sensitivity and specificity of stress perfusion MR imaging as equivalent or superior to those of SPECT. In the literature, sensitivity and specificity values of MR imaging range from 64% to 92% and from 71% to 100%, respectively (89–94). MRI would therefore appear to be a reasonable alternative to SPECT for the evaluation of patients suspected of having CAD, with the additional advantages of better depiction of wall motion, cardiac morphology, and myocardial viability, in addition to the lack of radiation intrinsic to nuclear methods. Nonetheless, MR imaging has yet to make much impact on routine clinical practice, in part because SPECT or dobutamine stress echocardiography can generally provide the needed diagnostic information and because of a lack of the large-scale multicenter trials that would validate any potential superiority of MRI.

Postinfarct Microcirculatory Function and Microvascular Obstruction by Magnetic Resonance Imaging

During routine coronary angiography, it is not possible to adequately assess the microvasculature (arterioles, capillaries, and venules). There are many instances of coronary arterial beds in which, despite the recanalization of the epicardial artery, there is persistently diminished blood flow because the microvasculature remains plugged by red blood cell stasis (95), myocardial edema, or endothelial cell damage from free radical formation. This is known as the "no-reflow" phenomenon, which indicates lack of reperfusion from microvascular impairment at the core of a reperfused infarct. In a study of 22 patients with acute myocardial infarction, contrast-enhanced imaging performed a few minutes after contrast agent infusion showed subendocardial hypoenhancement inside hyperenhancing myocardium in nearly 50% of the cases, which is consistent with no reflow and microvascular obstruction (96). Microvascular obstruction has been demonstrated to indicate a worsened prognosis (97) and may predict a larger amount of adverse left ventricular remodeling (98). Microvascular obstruction is also associated with an increased incidence of intramyocardial hemorrhage (99) and is more common after angioplasty than thrombolysis with or without angioplasty (100).

Assessment of Myocardial Viability by Magnetic Resonance Imaging

MRI has emerged as a powerful modality for assessing myocardial viability (Fig. 54.1), with a significant role in patients being considered for coronary revascularization. The following are the MR techniques that help assess myocardial viability.

Low-Dobutamine Stress Magnetic Resonance Imaging. Viability can be assessed without the need for contrast media by performing cine MR imaging during a low-dose infusion (5 to 10 μg/kg/minute) of dobutamine, which is comparable to dobutamine stress echocardiography. Improved left ventricular wall thickening with stress in a segment that functions poorly at rest indicates viability (101). In addition to the studies using MRI tagging cited previously, comparisons among dobutamine stress transesophageal echocardiography, dobutamine cine MRI, and fluorine-18 (^{18}F)-fluorodeoxyglucose PET in 43 patients with chronic infarction and wall-motion abnormalities resulted in a respective sensitivity and specificity of 77% and 81% for echocardiography and 94% and 100% for MRI (102). Criteria for viability were a resting wall thickness greater than 5.5 mm or wall thickening of at least 1 mm with stress. Dobutamine stress MRI can also be used to detect ischemic myocardium (103). In patients with nondiagnostic echocardiograms, dobutamine stress cardiac MRI may have prognostic value (104). The presence of inducible ischemia or left ventricular ejection fraction of less than 40% was associated with future myocardial infarction or cardiac death, independent of the presence of risk factors for coronary arteriosclerosis.

Delayed Enhancement. Postcontrast myocardial delayed enhancement detected by MRI is the most accurate means of detecting myocardial infarction. Cellular degradation in the infarcted region results in an increase in the permeability and enlargement of the extravascular space and hence an increased distribution volume for the extracellular contrast agent. Gadolinium chelates wash out of infarcted tissue more slowly than out of healthy myocardium. The net result is that infarcted regions appear bright on delayed contrast-enhanced T1-weighted images. The size and location of the infarcted region, as demonstrated histochemically in animal models, correlate with the size and location of myocardial delayed

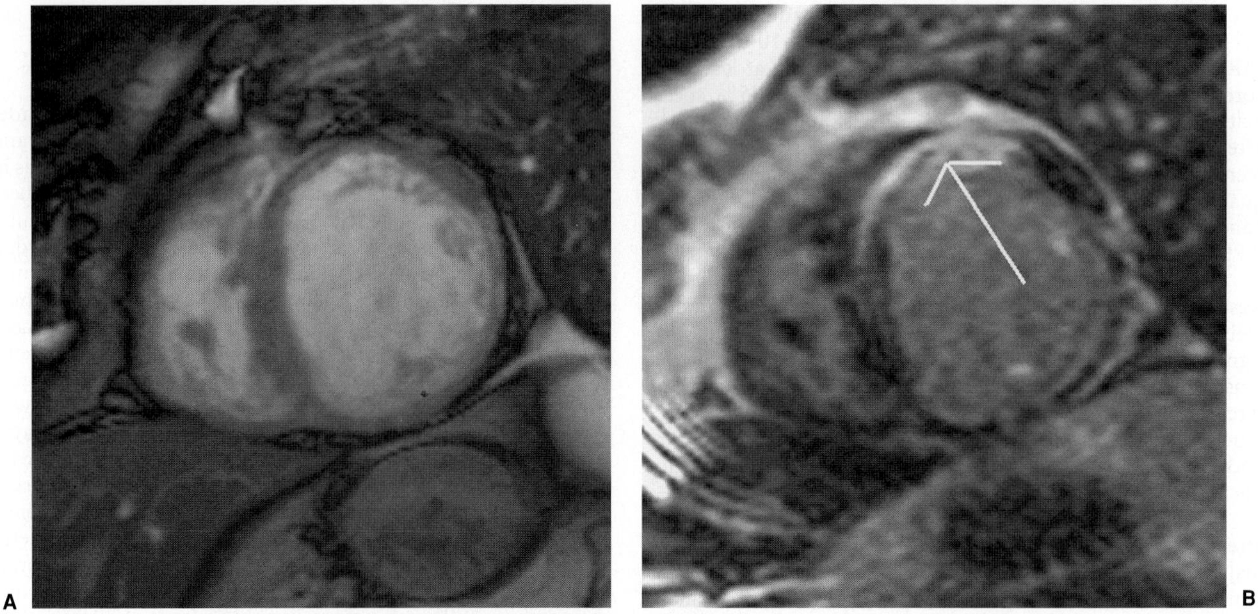

FIGURE 54.1. Patient with a diagnosis of ischemic cardiomyopathy. **A:** Short-axis gradient-echo image demonstrating a dilated left ventricle with prominent thinning (infarction) in the left anterior descending territory. **B:** Delayed gadolinium-enhanced short-axis image of the heart showing areas of hyperenhancement suggestive of myocardial fibrosis (infarction) in left anterior descending territory (*arrow*).

enhancement. Delayed hyperenhancement correlates well with dobutamine stress echocardiography (105) and with areas of decreased flow and metabolism at PET (106). However, MRI appears to be more sensitive (in one study, 11% of segments called viable with PET showed delayed enhancement with MRI). Another study of 26 patients demonstrated a 96% sensitivity and 84% specificity for myocardial delayed enhancement, with ^{18}F-fluorodeoxyglucose PET as the standard (107). MRI is superior in detecting subendocardial infarction. There is also good agreement with SPECT, but myocardial delayed-enhancement MRI has the major advantage of superior spatial resolution by an order of magnitude and the capability of incorporating anatomic and cine imaging in the same imaging session. In a study of 91 patients, SPECT depicted all of the nearly transmural infarctions but missed 47% of subendocardial infarctions that were seen at myocardial delayed-enhancement MRI (108). Another study of 20 patients with equivocal stress-rest sestamibi SPECT examination findings found the presence of subendocardial infarction at myocardial delayed-enhancement MR imaging in 40% of the patients (109).

Studies have shown that the amount of delayed transmural enhancement predicts the degree of functional recovery after acute myocardial infarction. Extensive transmural myocardial delayed enhancement is highly predictive of a lack of functional improvement after revascularization; conversely, absence of myocardial delayed enhancement correlates with a likelihood of functional recovery (110). The presence of a high-grade perfusion deficit or delayed enhancement in the early-phase MR imaging study is highly predictive of scar formation and lack of functional recovery at 1 year. Increased signal intensity on T2-weighted images indicates myocardial edema but does not always indicate infarction (111). That distinction requires the additional use of myocardial delayed enhancement. In another study of acute myocardial infarction, 20 patients were imaged within 1 week of the acute event and 7 months later (50). Enhancement patterns correlated with regional circumferential shortening strain (a measure of myocardial function) as determined with the harmonic phase imaging technique. Absence of myocardial delayed enhancement had a positive predictive value of 77% for functional recovery, whereas presence of myocardial delayed enhancement had a negative predictive value of 66%. It was concluded that, compared with the lack of early hypoenhancement, lack of delayed hyperenhancement is more accurate in predicting functional improvement in dysfunctional segments. The early hypoenhanced regions, corresponding to regions with microvascular obstruction, resulted in substantial underestimation of the amount of irreversibly injured myocardium after acute myocardial ischemia. History of myocardial infarction greatly increases the mortality rate compared with that of the general population. MRI may be useful in detection of unsuspected myocardial infarcts. In a study of 82 subjects, myocardial delayed enhancement helped to predict the presence, location, and transmural extent of healed Q-wave and non–Q-wave myocardial infarction (112).

Myocardial Delayed Enhancement and Myocardial Stunning. Transient hypoperfusion can cause myocardial stunning, which is associated with wall-motion abnormalities in the clinical setting of suspected acute myocardial infarction. Myocardial delayed enhancement in combination with cine MRI helps to differentiate wall-motion abnormalities of myocardial stunning, which are reversible, from those of myocardial infarction, which are often irreversible, depending on the severity of the injury. Either condition may cause a wall-motion abnormality, but delayed enhancement occurs only with infarcts. Lack of delayed enhancement indicates stunning rather than infarction and a high likelihood that left ventricular function will fully recover (113). In a study of 30 patients imaged approximately 1 week and 13 weeks after a reperfused myocardial infarction, the likelihood of functional improvement of segments without hyperenhancement was 3, 14, and 20 times higher than that of segments with 26% to 50%, 51% to 75%, and more than 75% hyperenhancement, respectively. The likelihood of complete functional recovery of segments without hyperenhancement was 3.8, 11.1, and 50.0 times higher than that of segments with 26% to 50%, 51% to 75%, and more than 75% hyperenhancement, respectively (114). Thus, functional improvement of stunned myocardium is predicted with myocardial delayed-enhancement MRI.

Triage of Patients with Chest Pain. A study of 161 patients with more than 30 minutes of chest pain but a nondiagnostic electrocardiogram found that the combination of myocardial delayed-enhancement, cine, and perfusion MR imaging was the strongest predictor of CAD and added diagnostic value over clinical parameters (115).

Diagnosis of Ventricular Aneurysms. In addition to impairment of left ventricular function and arrhythmias, complications of myocardial infarction include true and false aneurysms. True aneurysms, which are composed of pericardium adherent to underlying epicardium and scar tissue from infarcted myocardium, do not usually rupture. However, false aneurysms, which consist of pericardium that contains a ruptured left ventricle, may enlarge over time and require surgical resection. MR imaging can help make this distinction based on morphologic criteria (e.g., a wide mouth and anterior location for true aneurysm) (116) but also through the detection of a typical scar in patients with a true aneurysm (117).

Right Ventricular Infarction. Right ventricular infarction occurs commonly in patients with ostial right coronary artery occlusion, but the diagnosis is elusive. Delayed-enhancement MRI is likely the best technique for the noninvasive identification of patients with this syndrome (118).

Evaluation of Coronary Arteries

The current gold standard for the diagnosis of coronary artery disease is x-ray coronary angiography. Approximately 1 million cardiac catheterizations are performed each year in the Western world. However, x-ray coronary angiography is expensive and invasive, exposing patients and operators to ionizing radiation, and a small but finite risk of serious complications exists. A more cost-effective, noninvasive, and patient-friendlier imaging modality like coronary magnetic resonance angiography (MRA) overcomes many of these problems. Therefore, the utility of coronary MRA has been investigated since the late 1980s (119,120). For successful coronary MRI, a series of major obstacles has to be overcome. The heart is subject to intrinsic and extrinsic motion due to its natural periodic contraction and due to breathing. Both of these motion components exceed the coronary artery dimensions by a multiple, and therefore coronary MR data acquisition in the submillimeter range is technically very challenging, and efficient motion suppression strategies need to be applied. In addition, an enhanced contrast between the coronary lumen and the surrounding tissue is crucial for a successful visualization of both coronary lumen and the coronary vessel wall. The details of cardiac and respiratory motion compensations were discussed earlier. Even though great progress has been made in motion suppression and MRI hardware, software, scanning protocols, and contrast agents, the spatial resolution obtained by MRI remains to be further improved to approach that of x-ray coronary angiography ($<300\ \mu$m). Although an enhancement in spatial resolution is always accompanied by a penalty in SNR, this may partly be overcome by the use of high-field systems (33) and contrast agents (121).

Contrast Enhancement in Coronary Magnetic Resonance Angiography. Using MRI, one can manipulate the contrast between the coronary blood pool and the surrounding tissue using the in-flow effect (122) or by the application of MR prepulses. Nonexogenous contrast enhancement between the coronary arteries and the surrounding tissue has been obtained by the use of fat-saturation prepulses (122), magnetization transfer contrast prepulses (MTC) (123), or, more recently, T2 preparatory pulses (T2Prep) (124,125) that take advantage of natural T2 differences between blood and surrounding myocardium. With these techniques, the coronary lumen appears bright and the surrounding myocardium appears with reduced signal intensity. An alternative to the bright-blood visualization of the coronary arteries is black-blood coronary MRA, in which the coronary lumen appears signal attenuated and the surrounding tissue displays with high signal intensity (126).

With the use of MR contrast agents, the T1 relaxation of blood can be shortened, allowing for increased contrast-to-noise ratio (CNR) during coronary MRA (127,128). Examples of extracellular agents include gadopentetate dimeglumine (Magnevist; Berlex Laboratories, Wayne, NJ), gadodiamide (Omniscan; Nycomed-Amersham, Buckinghamshire, UK), and gadotetriol (Prohance; Bracco Diagnostics, Princeton, NJ) and intravascular agents such as iron oxide (AMI 227; Advanced Magnetics, Cambridge, MA), MS-325 (Angiomark; EPIX Medical, Cambridge, MA/Mallinkrodt, St. Louis, MO), NC100150 (Clariscan; Nycomed-Amersham, Buckinghamshire, UK) (127–131), and B-22956 (gadocoletic acid; Bracco Imaging SpA, Milan, Italy). Because extracellular agents quickly extravasate into the extravascular space, their use requires rapid first-pass imaging and thus necessitates breath-holding (132). First-pass coronary MRA with extravascular contrast agents is also limited by the need for repeated contrast injections when more than one slab is imaged. With each subsequent injection, the CNR will be lower because the signal from the extracellular space continuously increases after initial contrast administration. The use of intravascular agents has the inherent advantage of allowing image acquisition over longer time periods after intravenous administration of the contrast agent. Thus, non–breath-hold schemes can be used, and repeated scans have similar CNRs without the need for repeated injections (127). With the use of the intravascular contrast agent B-22956, a substantial (50%) SNR enhancement was accompanied by a 160% CNR improvement when compared to the non–contrast-enhanced technique used in previous international coronary MRA multicenter trials (121,127,133). Similar results were found in a parallel volunteer study using the contrast agent SH L 643A (Schering, Berlin, Germany) (134).

Identification of Coronary Stenosis. Although current breath-hold coronary MRA techniques have relatively limited in-plane spatial resolution, the technique has been shown to identify proximal coronary stenoses in several clinical series. Gradient-echo techniques depict focal stenoses as signal voids. In one of the earliest prospective patient studies comparing x-ray coronary angiography and coronary MRA (135), a segmented *k*-space, 2D, breath-hold, ECG-gated gradient-echo pulse sequence was used. Overall sensitivity and specificity of the 2D coronary MRA technique for correctly classifying individual vessels as having or not having significant CAD (50% diameter on conventional contrast angiography) were 90% and 92%, respectively. Subsequent studies (136–140) have reported variable sensitivity and specificity values for the detection of significant CAD. Explanations for this variability in these single-center studies include differences in the MR sequences used, inadequate patient cooperation with breath-holding, and irregular rhythms, all of which contribute to image degradation. Newer breath-hold (141) and non–breath-hold approaches for 3D coronary MRA have also demonstrated the ability of this technique to detect coronary stenoses. Previous multicenter trials that prospectively compared coronary MRA to the gold-standard x-ray coronary angiography demonstrated that free-breathing submillimeter 3D coronary MRA accurately identifies significant proximal and midcoronary disease, whereas nonsignificant coronary disease can be excluded with high confidence. The specificity (false-positive readings) remains to be improved, and quantitative stenosis *grading* remains to be investigated.

Evaluation of Valvular Heart Disease

MRI is generally considered second in line after echocardiography for evaluation of valvular diseases. However, MRI has the following advantages: Its 3D nature makes it operator independent; it may be less susceptible to missing or underestimating eccentrically directed flow through a diseased valve; and it is free from geometric assumptions if cardiac chamber volumes are to be calculated (142). Using a combination of cine images (for valve excursion, semiquantitative assessment of regurgitation), velocity-encoded phase-contrast techniques (for a more accurate determination of regurgitant fraction/volumes, pressure gradients, and valve areas), and standard anatomic imaging, MRI can provide much valuable information in evaluation of patients with valvular heart disease. Abnormalities of the adjacent chambers are easily detected with MRI. In the presence of stenosis, dilation of the recipient chamber, concentric hypertrophy of a proximal ventricle, and generalized dilation of a proximal atrium have been described; and with regurgitation present (142,143), generalized dilation of the proximal and distal chambers and eccentric hypertrophy of an associated ventricle have been noted.

Mitral Valve

Mitral Stenosis. The following anatomic abnormalities of mitral stenosis (MS) have been described by MRI: thickened leaflets with reduced diastolic opening, enlarged left atrium, abnormal left atrial signal, and abnormal diastolic transmitral signal (144). A signal-void jet begins at the site of the mitral valve level and extends into the cavity of the LV during diastole on cine (142,143). Cine MRI has demonstrated the ability to quantitatively evaluate the following physiologic abnormalities associated with MS: valve leaflet separation (R = .81 vs. area by Doppler by pressure half-time method) (144), relative distal signal-void jet area (R = .77 vs. peak transvalve gradient by catheterization) (145), and peak transvalve gradient (R = .89 vs. gradient by Doppler) (146). In a recent study of 17 patients with documented MS, velocity-encoded MRI was used to determine E wave, A wave, and pressure half-time, similar to Doppler echocardiography (147). There was highly significant correlation for valve size estimates, peak E, peak A, and pressure half-time measurements between MRI and Doppler echocardiography (R = .94, .99, .99, and .83, respectively; all $p < .01$).

Mitral Regurgitation. Mitral regurgitation is readily identified on cine because of the signal-void jet of turbulent flow extending from the mitral valve level into the left atrial cavity during systole. Based on the detection of a jet, mitral regurgitation is identified with a high degree of accuracy (94% to 100% sensitivity and 95% to 100% specificity vs. color Doppler) (148,149). Quantitative physiologic assessment by cine MRI has included the following: distal signal-void jet grade [70% concordance vs. grade by color Doppler (150) and R = .77 vs. ventriculography (151)]; distal signal-void jet size [length, R = .74 vs. color Doppler (151); absolute area, R = .71 vs. color Doppler (151); relative area, R = .74 to .87 vs. color Doppler (149,151); volume, R = .84 vs. regurgitant volume by cine volumetric analysis (148)]; volumetric regurgitant fraction [R = .84 vs. ventriculography (150)]; volume-flow regurgitant fraction [R = .87 to 0.96 vs. grading by color Doppler (152,153)]; and combined volumetric and volume-flow regurgitant fraction [R = .96 vs. ventriculography (153)].

Aortic Valve

Aortic Stenosis. The anatomic abnormalities of aortic stenosis (AS) evaluated by MRI have included concentric LV hypertrophy, dilation of the ascending aorta, reduced aortic valve area [R = .75 by SE vs. catheterization or Doppler (154)], and mean difference by velocity mapping of 0.2 cm^2 versus catheterization by the Gorlin formula and of 0.1 cm^2 versus Doppler by the continuity equation (155). A double-oblique cine image taken through the aortic valve plane best demonstrates the cusps and their coaptation and serves to differentiate acquired AS from congenital AS with a bicuspid aortic valve. Cine MRI has proved its ability to quantitatively evaluate physiologic abnormalities associated with AS. The following have been assessed: absolute distal signal-void jet length [R = .86 vs. peak transvalve gradient by catheterization (145)] and peak transvalve gradient [R = .96 vs. gradient by Doppler (155) and R = .67 to .97 vs. catheterization (155,156)]. In a recent study of 24 patients with documented AS, velocity-encoded MRI was used to obtain velocity information in the aorta and LV outflow tract; pressure gradients were estimated using the Bernoulli equation, followed by calculation of aortic valve area, similar to Doppler echocardiography (157). There was highly significant correlation for valve size estimates, peak pressure gradient, and mean pressure gradient between MRI and Doppler echocardiography (R = .83, .83, .99, and .87, respectively; all $p < .01$).

Aortic Regurgitation. The signal-void jet of aortic regurgitation (AR) on cine has been fully described and evaluated for its potential to stage the severity of disease (142,143,145). Qualitative assessment by cine has also involved proximal flow convergence detection (158) (87% sensitivity and 100% specificity vs. aortography) (159) and distal signal-void jet detection (89% to 92% sensitivity and 93% to 98% specificity vs. Doppler) (148). For quantitative physiologic assessment, cine MRI has been used for proximal convergent flow signal-void area (significantly greater than for all grades by echo) (159); distal signal-void jet grade (93% concordance vs. grade by aortography) (160); distal signal-void jet size [area significantly greater than for moderate to severe vs. normal to mild 2D echo grades (161); volume, R = .84 vs. regurgitant volume by cine volumetrics (148), significantly greater than for moderate versus mild and for severe versus moderate 2D echo grades (148)]; volumetric regurgitant fraction (significantly greater than for moderate to severe versus normal to mild 2D echo grades) (162); and volume-flow regurgitant fraction [R = .97 to .98 vs. cine volumetrics (216,229); R = .80 vs. grading by aortography (163)].

Tricuspid and Pulmonic Valves

The value of MRI in assessing the presence and severity of congenital tricuspid abnormalities, including Ebstein's anomaly or pulmonic valve disease, has been well established (164). The techniques are similar to those used for assessment of left-sided valvular heart disease. Volume-flow regurgitant fraction of pulmonic regurgitation has been validated (R = .93 vs. cine volumetrics) (165).

Prosthetic Valves

Studies in vitro and in vivo have shown that patients with artificial heart valves can be safely examined in high-field magnets (39,42). On MRI, little image distortion outside the immediate area of the prosthetic valve and no patient discomfort have been observed in related studies (166). When the diagnostic value of cine for detecting regurgitation in prosthetic valves was compared with that of transesophageal color Doppler echo, excellent (e.g., 96%) agreement between the methods in distinguishing physiologic from pathologic regurgitation was observed (167). In addition, quantitative physiologic evaluation of the severity of regurgitation has been quite promising [75% concordance of grade vs. grade by Doppler (234); $R = .85$ distal signal-void jet length, and $R = .91$ distal signal-void jet vs. Doppler (167)].

Evaluation of Cardiomyopathies

Cardiomyopathies (CMPs) are chronic progressive myocardial diseases with distinct morphologic, functional and electrophysiologic characteristics. According to the classification issued by the International Society and Federation of Cardiology Task Force (1996), they are divided into dilated, restrictive, hypertrophic, and arrhythmogenic right ventricular dysplasia (1,168). MRI, because of a high degree of accuracy and reproducibility in visualization of LV and RV morphology and function, is superior to all other imaging modalities in determination of the left ventricular mass and volumes (169) and is fast becoming the gold standard for in vivo identification of CMPs. For delineating cardiac anatomy, "black-blood" T1-weighted spin-echo techniques provide excellent contrast between the myocardium and adjacent structures. Gadolinium administration followed by a repeat T1 study helps in defining infiltrative and inflammatory myocardial disease. Fluid accumulation in inflammatory and malignant diseases can be more easily identified because of the improved T2-weighted image quality due to shorter T1 inversion recovery techniques (170). Contrast-enhanced MRI is also being recognized as useful in intramyocardial fibrosis (171). MR spectroscopy using ^{1}H and ^{31}P has also been applied in several studies of CMP, particularly those involving ^{31}P in dilated CMP (172) and hypertrophic cardiomyopathy (173). Although the technique is still experimental, there is growing evidence to support its utility.

Dilated Cardiomyopathy

The histologic hallmark of dilated CMP (DCM) is progressive interstitial fibrosis, decreased myocardial contractility. and relative wall thinning in the late disease stages (174). In DCM, MRI is useful in the study of LV morphology and function, using different MRI sequences with low inter- and intraobserver variability of LV mass and volumes (175). It is also useful for analyzing wall thickening (176), impaired fiber shortening (55) and end-systolic wall stress (which is a very sensitive parameter of changes in LV systolic function) (177). It can also accurately assess the morphology and function of the RV, which is also frequently affected in DCM (178). MRI is rapidly becoming the method of choice for longitudinal follow-up in patients with DCM who are undergoing therapeutic interventions (179). From a research perspective, the sample size needed to detect LV parameter changes in a clinical trial is far less, on the range of one order of magnitude, with MRI than with 2D echocardiography, which markedly reduces the time and cost of patient care and pharmaceutical trials (180). MR spectroscopy has also revealed changes in phosphate metabolism in patients with DCM (172). A ratio of phosphocreatine to ATP has some prognostic value in DCM. Use of contrast-enhanced T1-weighted images is also helpful in detecting changes of acute myocarditis (increased gadolinium accumulation is thought to be due to inflammatory hyperemia–related increased flow, slow wash-in/wash-out kinetics, and diffusion into necrotic cells). There is also evidence of similar changes in chronic DCM (181). Contrast-enhanced MRI could also increase the sensitivity of endomyocardial biopsy by visualization of inflamed areas, which would aid in determining biopsy site (182). Thus, MRI is very helpful in the diagnosis and follow-up of patients with inflammatory myocardial diseases presenting as DCM. However, further studies with improved imaging techniques are needed to augment the specificity of contrast-enhanced MRI.

Hypertrophic Cardiomyopathy

Hypertrophic cardiomyopathy (HCM) is characterized by inappropriate myocardial hypertrophy, loss of diastolic function, and, in many instances, the development of an LV outflow tract gradient. Histologically, the hypertrophic areas reveal myofibrillar disarray and areas of patchy necrosis (170) (Fig. 54.2). Due to its high accuracy, MRI is becoming useful for assessing morphology, function, tissue characterization, and degree of LV outflow tract (LVOT) obstruction in patients with hypertrophic cardiomyopathy. MRI is very accurate in assessing LV mass, regional hypertrophy patterns, and different phenotypes of the disease (e.g., apical HCM) (169). Similarly, postsurgical changes after myomectomy can also be reliably monitored (183). The turbulent jet during systolic LVOT obstruction is also easily detected by using suitable echo times (about 4 msec). MRI can also detect the systolic anterior motion of the mitral valve in the four-chamber view or a short-axis view at the valvular plane (184). Mitral regurgitation can also be well documented and quantified by MRI (170). MRI spectroscopy also reveals changes in the phosphate metabolism in patients with HCM (173). In addition, analysis of blood flow in the coronary sinus using MRI can be helpful in determining the alterations in coronary flow reserve in patients with HCM (185). A relatively newer technique relies on measurements of the effective LVOT area by MRI planimetry during systole. This method has the potential to overcome the problem of interstudy variability of the LVOT gradient due to its independence from the hemodynamic status (186). There are preliminary data indicating that assessment of diastolic function using MRI may be superior to conventional parameters using echocardiography (187). Analysis of early untwisting motion of the myocardium could be helpful in assessing diastolic function (188). Other functional changes using myocardial tagging include a reduction in posterior rotation, reduced radial displacement of the inferoseptal myocardium, reduced 3D myocardial shortening, and heterogeneity of regional function (170). MRI is also very useful in the follow-up of patients after surgical or pharmacologic interventions (184). MRI also easily detects the acute and chronic changes after septal artery ablation (189). MRI not only quantifies alcohol-induced endothelial and myocardial necrosis, but also easily detects the acute and chronic changes in left ventricular structure and function caused by septal artery ablation (189). Delayed postcontrast enhancement occurs with HCM, probably reflecting the presence of abundant connective tissue or foci of necrosis (190). When myocardial scar is visualized, it is generally present in hypertrophied regions as patchy and with multiple foci, predominantly involving the middle third of the left ventricular wall. It is correlated positively with regional hypertrophy and inversely with regional contraction. In this regard, the extent of hyperenhancement may have prognostic implications for the risk of progressive ventricular dilation and sudden death (191).

Arrhythmogenic Right Ventricular Dysplasia

Arrhythmogenic right ventricular dysplasia (ARVD) is characterized by a progressive degeneration of the RV, morphologically leading to fibrous/fatty replacement of myocardial tissue, significant wall thinning, and atypical arrangement of trabecular muscles. These fibromuscular bundles, which are separated by fatty tissues, lead to reentry phenomena and ventricular arrhythmias, syncope, and sudden death (55).

MRI has become very useful in arriving at the diagnosis of ARVD (Fig. 54.3). In fact, it is rapidly becoming the diagnostic

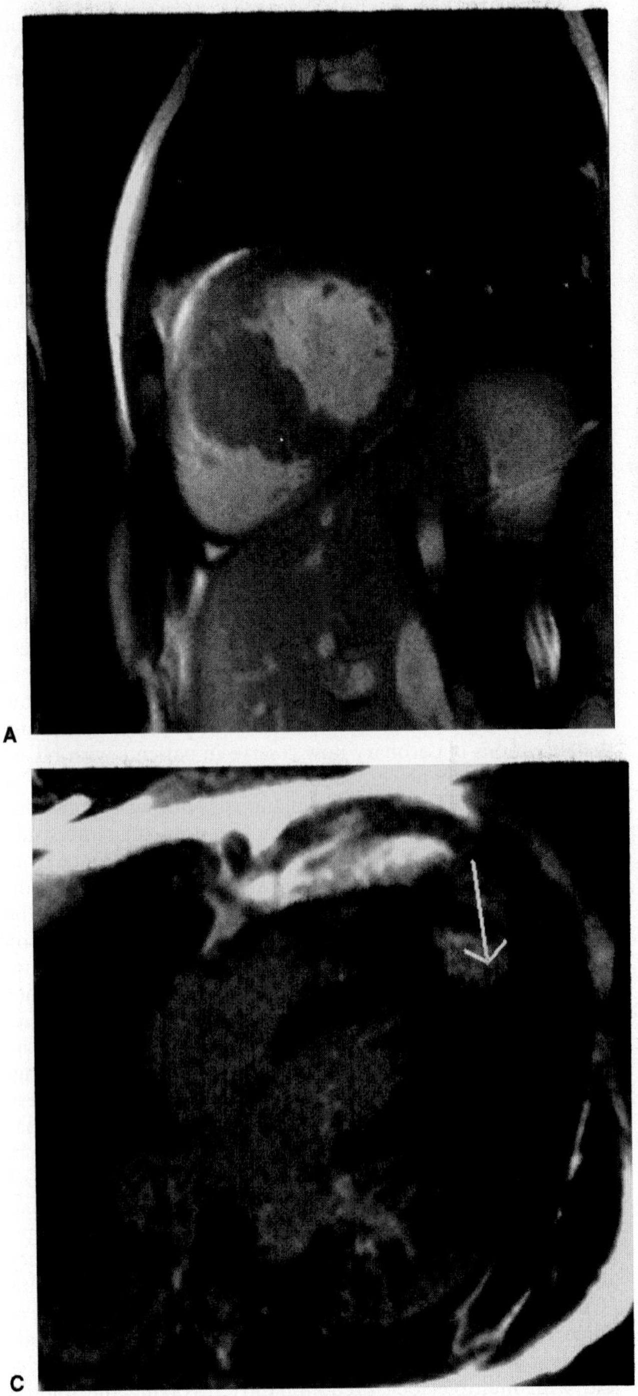

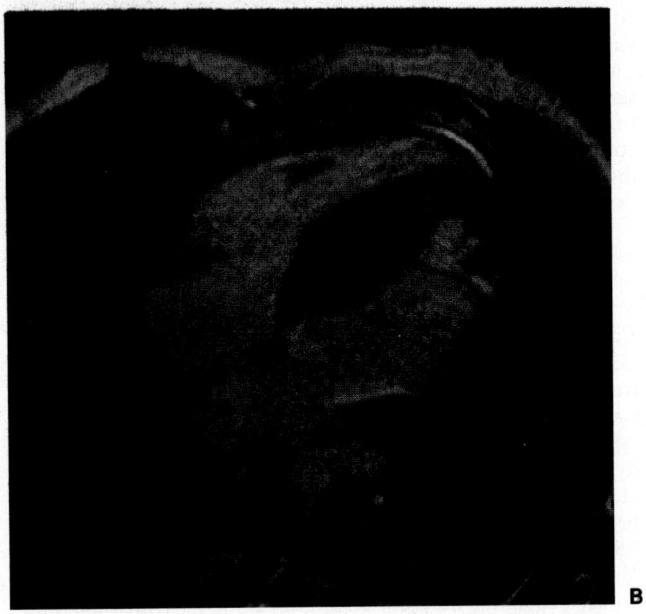

FIGURE 54.2. Patient with a diagnosis of hypertrophic cardiomyopathy. **A:** Short-axis gradient-echo image demonstrating severe thickening of the interventricular septum. **B:** Delayed gadolinium-enhanced four-chamber view of the heart of the same patient as in panel A showing areas of hyperenhancement suggestive of myocardial fibrosis in the distal septum (*arrow*). **C:** Delayed gadolinium-enhanced four-chamber view of the heart of another patient with apical hypertrophic cardiomyopathy showing areas of hyperenhancement suggestive of myocardial fibrosis in the apex.

technique of choice for ARVD. T1-weighted SE images reveal an increased signal intensity due to fatty infiltration, thinned walls, and dysplastic trabecular structures. To differentiate the normal fat surrounding the heart from the fatty infiltration of the RV free wall, some authors have proposed imaging in prone position using phased-array coils (192). Axial, sagittal, and short-axis views are usually recommended for optimal results (170). Standard gradient field echo (GRE) or the newer steady-state free-precession (SSFP) techniques reveal characteristic regional wall-motion changes, localized early diastolic bulging, wall thinning, and saccular aneurysmal outpouchings (192,193). The working group classification proposed by Corrado et al. is the recognized standard for arriving at the diagnosis (194). Table 54.2 shows the major and minor MRI criteria for the diagnosis of ARVD. ARVD needs to be differentiated from RV outflow tract (RVOT) tachycardia. This disease is commonly associated with fixed focal wall thinning, regional decreased systolic wall thickening, and areas of wall-motion abnormalities during systole, usually located above the crista supraventricularis and in the anterior and lateral RVOT (195).

Restrictive Cardiomyopathy

Primary infiltration of the myocardium by fibrosis or other types of tissues leads to the development of restrictive CMP, characterized by normal LV size and systolic function, severe diastolic dysfunction, and biatrial enlargement. It frequently requires differentiation from constrictive pericarditis, which can be done very effectively using T1-weighted spin-echo techniques by MRI. LV size and thickness are quantified using

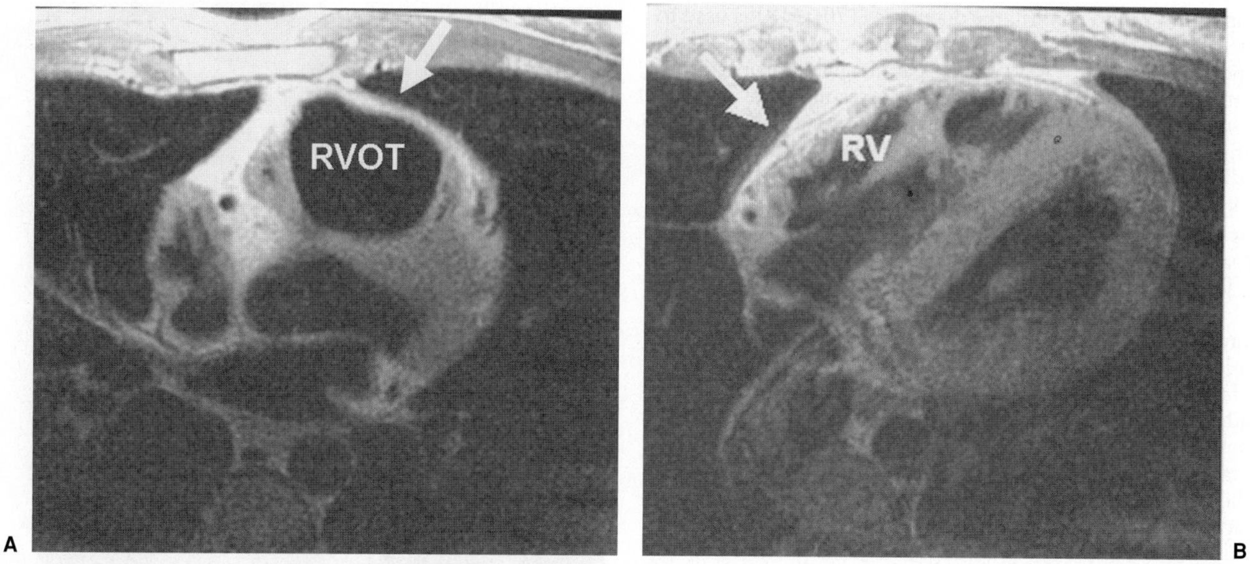

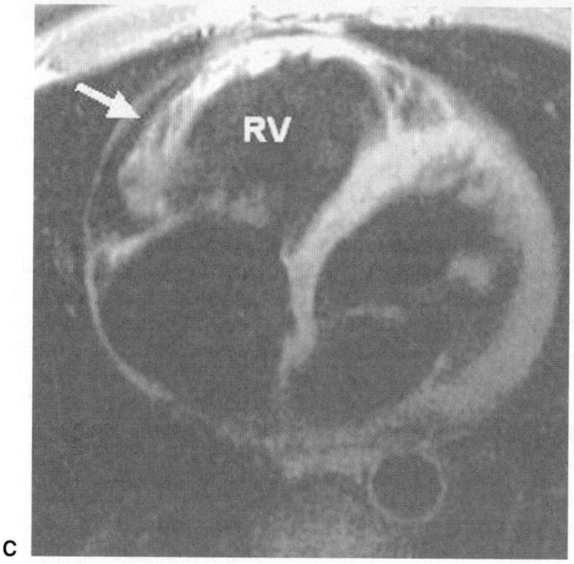

FIGURE 54.3. Patient with a diagnosis of arrhythmogenic right ventricle cardiomyopathy. **A:** Fast spin-echo T1 axial image of the heart showing the right ventricle outflow tract (RVOT) dilation with increased T1 signal (*arrow*). **B:** Fast spin-echo T1 axial image of the heart showing dilation of the right ventricle (RV) with signal abnormality (*arrow*). **C:** Fast spin-echo T1 with fat saturation axial image of the heart confirming fat infiltration of the RV wall (*arrow*).

gradient-echo sequences. Atrial enlargement is assessed in a four-chamber view. Velocity-encoded cine-MR imaging can also be used to quantify and monitor the restrictive filling pattern of the ventricles during therapy in restrictive cardiomyopathy (RCM) patients by measuring diastolic flow across the mitral and tricuspid valves (196). Moreover, mitral or tricuspid regurgitation can likewise be demonstrated and quantified with cine-MR imaging.

The following different secondary CMPs can also be effectively assessed using MRI.

TABLE 54.2

MAGNETIC RESONANCE FINDINGS OF ARRHYTHMOGENIC RIGHT VENTRICULAR DYSPLASIA

Major criteria	Minor criteria
High signal intensity of RV on T1-weighted images	Mild RVOT dilation
Diffuse myocardial thinning of the RV	Mild RV dilation
Severe dilation of the RVOT	Regional contraction abnormalities
Severe dilation of the RV with systolic dysfunction	Global diastolic dysfunction
Aneurysms of the RV and RVOT	

RV, right ventricle; RVOT, right ventricular outflow tract.

Sarcoidosis. The incidence of myocardial involvement in systemic sarcoidosis is 20% to 30% (197), and up to 50% (198) of the deaths in sarcoidosis may be due to cardiac involvement. MRI is becoming a useful tool in the assessment of sarcoidosis. Sarcoid lesions may lead to different signal intensities, most likely due to different stages of the disease. Previous studies have reported high-intensity areas in T2-weighted MRI, whereas other studies have reported a central low-intensity area on T1- and T2-weighted imaging surrounded by a high-signal ring (199). In a study of 16 patients with cardiac sarcoidosis, postcontrast images revealed enhancement in half of the cases, which diminished after steroid therapy (200). Occasionally, MRI may be useful in guiding endomyocardial biopsy 170.

Hemochromatosis. Extensive iron deposits leading to wall thickening, ventricular dilation, congestive heart failure (CHF), and death characterize cardiac hemochromatosis. Usually the iron deposits are subepicardial, and hence the endomyocardial biopsy may fail to confirm the diagnosis (170). MRI is used to detect iron deposits associated with hemochromatosis, which is possible due to the very strong paramagnetic properties of iron, which leads to extensive signal losses in native T1- and T2-weighted images (201). The pattern of focal signal loss within dysfunctional myocardium associated with an abnormally "dark" liver might be sufficient to confirm the diagnosis of systemic hemochromatosis. LV function can also be accurately assessed using MRI, which is also useful in the follow-up of these patients as they undergo intensified medical therapy (170).

Amyloidosis. Infiltration of the heart by amyloid deposits is found in almost all cases of primary amyloidosis and in 25% of familial amyloidosis. MRI can be useful in detection of amyloidosis and its differentiation from HCM. Interatrial septal thickening or right atrial posterior wall greater than 6 mm is fairly specific for amyloid infiltration and consistent with echocardiographic data (202). Tissue characterization in cardiac amyloidosis has not been well studied and few data are available.

Endomyocardial Fibrosis. Endomyocardial fibrosis (also termed Loeffler endocarditis) leads to posterobasal concentric wall thickening, followed by extensive subendocardial fibrosis, apical thrombus formation, with progressive obliteration of both apices, diastolic dysfunction, and reduced stroke volume (170). The morphologic and functional features of endomyocardial fibrosis and the mitral and tricuspid insufficiencies that can be associated with this condition are well quantified by MRI. The fibrosis may be visible as a dark, thick apical rim in bright-blood–prepared gradient-echo sequences. Delayed imaging after administration of gadolinium-DTPA might have a role in the detection of associated fibrosis.

Evaluation of Pericardial Disease

The pericardium is a two-layered membrane that envelops all four cardiac chambers and the origins of the great vessels. The parietal and visceral layers are separated by a small amount of serous fluid—normally, about 15 to 50 mL—that is mainly an ultrafiltrate of plasma. Many disease processes can affect the pericardium, including infection, neoplasm, trauma, primary myocardial disease, and congenital disease. The pericardial sac responds to an acute injury with (a) congestion, (b) increased exudation of fluid into the sac, (c) exudation of both fibrin and acute inflammatory cells into the sac, or (d) a combination of these reactions. Echocardiography is the imaging modality most often used for the initial evaluation of pericardial disease, especially in patients suspected of having pericardial effusion or tamponade. However, MRI (along with CT) offers distinct advantages in the imaging of the pericardium. They provide a larger field of view than echocardiography, thus allowing the examination of the entire chest and detection of associated abnormalities in the mediastinum and lungs. MRI provides excellent anatomic delineation and enables precise localization of pericardial masses. In addition, MRI is performed in standard imaging planes and does not require use of a transducer; therefore, it is less operator dependent than echocardiography. The thickness of the normal pericardium, as measured on CT scans and MR images, is less than 2 mm.

Effusion and Tamponade

Pericardial effusion originates in the obstruction of venous or lymphatic drainage from the heart. MRI is indicated when a complex effusion or pericardial thickening is suspected (203,204) or when findings at echocardiography are inconclusive. The appearance of pericardial fluid is different on SE and GRE cine MR images. Nonhemorrhagic fluid has low signal intensity on T1-weighted SE images and high intensity on GRE cine images (205), whereas hemorrhagic effusion is characterized by high signal intensity on T1-weighted SE images and low intensity on GRE cine images (205). When an effusion is secondary to malignancy, an irregularly thickened pericardium or pericardial nodularity may be depicted on MRI.

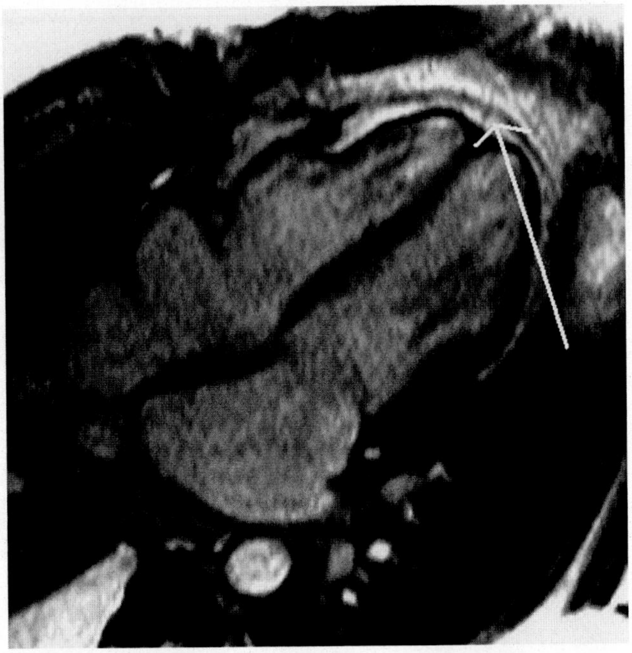

FIGURE 54.4. Patient with a diagnosis of constrictive pericarditis. Four-chamber gradient-echo images showing diffuse thickening of the pericardium, with a conical appearance of the heart and dilated atria.

Pericarditis and Constriction

Clinically, it is difficult to differentiate between constrictive pericarditis and restrictive cardiomyopathy. In both conditions, ventricular filling is restricted, leading to an increase in diastolic pressure in all four cardiac chambers. It is important, however, to distinguish between constrictive pericarditis (Fig. 54.4) and restrictive cardiomyopathy because patients with constrictive pericarditis might benefit from pericardial stripping, whereas those with restrictive disease would not. MRI provides crucial information on the differential diagnosis of constrictive pericarditis versus restrictive cardiomyopathy. Normal pericardial thickness is less than 2 mm (203,206). Pericardial thickness of 4 mm or more indicates abnormal thickening, and, when it is accompanied by clinical findings of heart failure, is highly suggestive of constrictive pericarditis. MRI has a reported accuracy of 93% for differentiation between constrictive pericarditis and restrictive cardiomyopathy on the basis of depiction of thickened pericardium (4 mm) (207). Pericardial thickening may be limited to the right side of the heart or to an even smaller area, such as the right atrioventricular groove. A disadvantage of MRI is its limited ability to detect pericardial calcification. It is important to remember, however, that neither pericardial thickening nor calcification is diagnostic of constrictive pericarditis unless the patient also has symptoms of physiologic constriction or restriction. The central cardiovascular structures may show a characteristic morphology in constrictive pericarditis. The right ventricle tends to have a narrow tubular configuration. In some patients, a sigmoid-shaped ventricular septum or prominent leftward convexity in the septum can be observed.

Because of the higher temporal resolution provided with cine MRI, the abrupt limitation of late diastolic filling of the ventricles because of the abnormally thickened and confining pericardium in constrictive pericarditis is distinguishable from the delayed diastolic filling patterns of the ventricles caused by restrictive CM in the absence of significant pericardial thickening.

Pericarditis without Constriction

Pericardial thickening may occur in the absence of constrictive pericarditis. Pericardial thickening may result from inflammation caused by a variety of conditions, including acute pericarditis, uremia, rheumatic heart disease, rheumatoid arthritis, sarcoidosis, and mediastinal irradiation. Normal pericardium is composed primarily of fibrous tissue and has a low signal intensity on both T1- and T2-weighted MR images. The purely fibrous or calcified pericardium in chronic pericardial disease also has low signal intensity. However, in subacute forms of pericarditis, the thickened pericardium has moderate to high signal intensity on SE images. Enhancement of the thickened pericardium after the administration of gadolinium-based contrast material also suggests inflammation. The effusive-constrictive form of pericarditis involves both pericardial thickening and pericardial effusion.

Pericardial Masses

The differential diagnosis of pericardial masses includes pericardial cyst, hematoma, and neoplasm. Although pericardial masses are often detected initially with echocardiography, MRI is useful for the further evaluation of these masses. MR signal intensity characteristics, degree of contrast enhancement, and presence or absence of blood flow on cine MR images can help to differentiate among pericardial masses.

Cysts. Congenital pericardial cysts are formed when a portion of the pericardium is pinched off during early development. Pericardial cysts usually have thin, smooth walls without internal septa. On MRI, they typically have low or intermediate signal intensity on T1-weighted images and homogeneous high intensity on T2-weighted images. They are not enhanced with the administration of gadolinium chelates (208). Occasionally, a cyst may contain highly proteinaceous fluid, which may have a high signal intensity on T1-weighted images. Pericardial cysts may occur anywhere in the mediastinum, although they usually are found in the right cardiophrenic angle. A pericardial cyst in an unusual location may be indistinguishable from a bronchogenic cyst or thymic cyst.

Hematomas. MRI is particularly useful for the diagnosis of pericardial hematomas, which have a characteristic signal intensity on T1-weighted and T2-weighted MR images: Acute hematomas demonstrate homogeneous high signal intensity (209,210), whereas subacute hematomas that are 1 to 4 weeks old typically show heterogeneous signal intensity, with areas of high signal intensity on both T1-weighted and T2-weighted images (209,211). On T1-weighted and gradient-echo images, chronic organized hematomas may show a dark peripheral rim and low-signal-intensity internal foci that may represent calcification, fibrosis, or hemosiderin deposition (212,213). High-signal-intensity areas on T1-weighted or T2-weighted images often correspond to hemorrhagic fluid (214). Coronary or ventricular pseudoaneurysms or neoplasms may resemble hematomas on MR images. However, the administration of gadolinium chelates allows the differentiation of these entities because hematomas do not become enhanced. In addition, velocity-encoded cine MR imaging may be used to detect internal flow in pseudoaneurysms (215) and thus to differentiate pseudoaneurysms from hematomas.

Neoplasms. Pericardial metastases are much more common than primary pericardial tumors and are discovered at autopsy in 10% to 12% of all patients with malignancy (216,217). Tumors may seed the pericardium via the lymph system or the blood stream or may invade directly from the lung or mediastinum (218). Breast and lung cancers are the most common sources of metastases in the pericardium, followed by lymphomas and melanomas (217). On MRI, an intact pericardial line may be observed if an adjacent tumor extends to the pericardium but not through it. Tumors that have invaded the pericardium may be recognized by focal obliteration of the pericardial line and the presence of pericardial effusion. Hemorrhagic pericardial effusions secondary to metastases usually have high signal intensity on SE images (205). Most neoplasms have low signal intensity on T1-weighted images and high signal intensity on T2-weighted images (219). Metastatic melanoma is an exception; it may have high signal intensity on T1-weighted images because of the paramagnetic metals bound by melanin (220,221). Sites of malignant disease usually become significantly enhanced after the administration of contrast material (222). Primary neoplasms of the pericardium are rare. Benign pericardial tumors include lipoma, teratoma, fibroma, and hemangioma; malignant tumors include mesothelioma, lymphoma, sarcoma, and liposarcoma. Lipoma typically has high signal intensity on T1-weighted SE images. Fibroma characteristically has low signal intensity on T2-weighted images and often shows either no enhancement or heterogeneous enhancement because of poor vascularization (222,223). Primary malignant mesothelioma of the pericardium may manifest as pericardial effusion, occasionally accompanied by pericardial nodules or plaques. Malignant pleural mesothelioma also may invade the pericardium directly. Lymphoma, sarcoma, and liposarcoma typically appear as large heterogeneous masses frequently associated with serosanguineous pericardial effusion. Biopsy and histopathologic analysis are necessary to achieve a definitive diagnosis of most pericardial tumors.

Evaluation of Aortic Disease

MRI has come to play a significant role in the initial evaluation of diseases of the thoracic aorta (224), as well as for detecting postoperative complications from thoracic aortic surgery (225,226). Designing an MR imaging strategy for evaluating the thoracic aorta typically requires a combination of black-blood and bright-blood techniques along with contrast MR angiography (Fig. 54.5) and cine techniques. In addition, the protocol must be targeted for the primary regions of disease involvement, include proper imaging of the disease's extent and pattern, and provide proper visualization of associated extravascular findings. Beginning at the aortic valve, the thoracic aorta can be divided into three distinct regions in the proximal-to-distal direction, namely, the aortic root, ascending aorta, aortic arch, and descending aorta.

Aortic Root

Sinuses of Valsalva. Discrete aneurysms involving one or more sinuses of Valsalva occur below the sinotubular ridge (227). In a nonacute setting, MRI may be used in the imaging evaluation to demonstrate the aneurysm, the donor sinus, and the recipient chamber of a small fistula. Bright-blood techniques are particularly well suited for these evaluations (227). Cine imaging might be useful in demonstrating a fistula.

Sinotubular Junction. Diseases involving the tubular portion of the ascending aorta typically spare the sinotubular junction with the exception of annuloaortic ectasia (228). Cystic medial necrosis is characterized histologically as myxomatous change

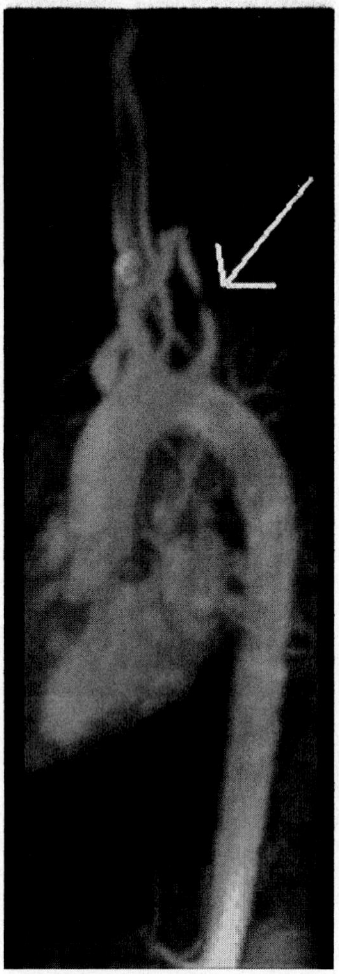

FIGURE 54.5. Contrast-enhanced MR angiogram in a patient demonstrating severe left subclavian artery stenosis.

of cardiac valves, with enlargement of the sinuses of Valsalva and annular dilation of the ascending aorta with a return to normal caliber by the innominate artery origin. Effacement of the sinotubular ridge and dilation of all three sinuses of Valsalva create the spring "onion bulb" appearance.

Ascending Aorta

The ascending thoracic aorta extends from the sinotubular ridge to immediately proximal to the innominate artery origin. A serious and potentially life-threatening conditions involving the aortic root and ascending aorta is aortic dissection (229,230). The DeBakey and Stanford criteria divide aortic dissections into those that involve the ascending aorta or aortic arch (Stanford type A or DeBakey I and II) and those that are delimited to only the descending thoracic aorta beyond the left subclavian artery origin (Stanford type B or DeBakey III) (230). This distinction is important for deciding between a surgical or medical approach. The first goal is to determine the most proximal site of involvement. Dissection may be fatal if it extends proximally into the aortic root, the aortic valve, and the coronary arteries, potentially resulting in intrapericardial hemorrhage and cardiac tamponade, acute aortic insufficiency, and myocardial ischemia, respectively. In addition, extension of the intimal flap into one or more of the aortic arch vessels may produce cerebral ischemia or infarction. For this reason, Stanford type A dissections typically warrant acute surgical repair. Type B aortic dissections tend to be more stable and can be managed medically. Intramural hematoma results from bleeding from vasa vasorum of the aortic media (231,232). Subacute hemorrhage (methemoglobin) appears as crescentic or lentiform high intramural signal with adjacent normal signal void on non-contrast-enhanced T1-weighted sequences. The goals of MRI in aortic dissections, both acute and chronic, are to identify the intimal flap (by different imaging sequences), its extent, orientation, and involvement with aortic arch branch vessels and coronary arteries, and the location of entry and reentry tears of the intima and to assess for areas of flow and thrombus within the false channel (224,233,234). In addition, potential complications such as pleural effusion, pericardial tamponade, and aortic regurgitation must be assessed. A common hurdle is the distinction between a thrombosed false channel within a chronic dissection and an intraluminal thrombus adherent to the wall of an aneurysm. These are not always possible to differentiate because a chronic intraluminal thrombus may neoepithelialize, giving the appearance of an intimal flap overlying the chronic thrombus (224, 235). Signs that have been reported to be more consistent with a diagnosis of thrombosed false channel associated with dissection are a compressed or eccentric patent channel and extensive thrombus with associated wall thickening over a length greater than 7 cm; these signs are easily appreciated on MRI (235).

MRI is a highly sensitive and specific technique for the detection of aortic dissection that has proven to be superior to conventional angiography, computed tomography (CT), and transthoracic echo studies (233). It also has been compared with transesophageal echocardiography; they have demonstrated a similar high sensitivity (e.g., 98% to 100%), but MRI has a significantly higher specificity (e.g., 98% to 100%) than transesophageal echocardiography (e.g., 68% to 77%) in high-risk populations (233). The advantages of MRI include an ability to evaluate not just the intravascular space and walls of the aorta, but also the extravascular space, which may yield further information, particularly with regard to more serious complications of aortic dissection (224). However, artifacts may erroneously lead to the appearance of an intimal tear or, conversely, obscure it. Artifacts occur due to a number of reasons, such as the normal pulsatility of aortic blood flow, the movement of the aortic valve leaflets, and cardiac motion. The use of current bright-blood techniques, namely SSFP and 3D contrast-enhanced MRA, generally results in an accurate diagnosis. One additional aid in the recognition of an intimal flap is its configuration. Type A dissections typically spiral along the outer greater curvature of the aorta, with the false channel usually rightward in the ascending aorta and posterolateral in the descending aorta. When performing 3D contrast-enhanced MR angiography, the upper abdominal aorta should be included in the field of view. An oblique sagittal acquisition using a large field of view will usually enable reasonable coverage of the upper abdominal aorta, including the renal arteries.

Another common indication for thoracic MRI is the evaluation of a suspected or known aortic aneurysm (236–238). The normal aortic diameter on ECG-gated black-blood images has been reported (228) to be as follows: aortic root, 3.3 cm; midascending aorta, 3.0 cm; aortic arch, 2.7 cm; and descending aorta, 2.4 cm. Aneurysms that measure greater than 5 cm, that are expanding rapidly, or that are symptomatic will generally be repaired. Care must be taken to obtain aortic diameter measurements in a plane perpendicular to the aorta. On an axial image, measurement at the level of the horizontal portion of the right pulmonary artery will ensure that the aorta is generally vertical, and that diameter measurements accurately reflect the aorta's cross-sectional size. In children, the ascending aorta is aneurysmal if the ratio of the ascending-aorta to the descending-aorta diameter is greater than 1.5 (239). Dilation of the ascending thoracic aorta can occur from intrinsic pathology that is acquired, such as atherosclerotic disease, or congenital, such as connective tissue disorders such as

Marfan syndrome. Dilation of the ascending aorta can also occur owing to aortic valve disease.

Thoracic aortic aneurysms are classified as true aneurysms, meaning that all three mural layers of the aortic wall are involved, or as pseudoaneurysms, in which there has been a break in the intima and possibly media, leaving only the remaining wall to contain the intraaortic blood pool. These forms of aneurysm are characteristically represented by fusiform (i.e., circumferential enlargement of the involved segment) or saccular (i.e., asymmetric or focal outpouching of the involved segment) dilations, respectively. The saccular configuration connotes a less stable condition than the other configuration. These characteristics of a thoracic aortic aneurysm can be easily delineated with MRI for planning of therapy or for clinical monitoring (224). In addition, because of the abilities of MRI to depict the configuration and associated mural changes, it is critical in differentiating the various etiologies of thoracic aortic aneurysms (240). On MRI, the aortic wall is thickened and irregular, secondary to atherosclerotic plaque (241). Mural calcification is common and is manifested by areas of focal signal absence on both SE and cine, although it is better seen on CT. Intraluminal thrombus also is common and may be difficult to distinguish from atherosclerotic plaque, although thrombus usually has a smooth internal border, as opposed to atherosclerosis, which typically is irregular (224). In atherosclerotic aneurysms involving the ascending portion, the sinotubular junction and aortic valve function usually are preserved, which are important characteristics appreciated on MRI. Aortic aneurysms that may occur secondary to aortic valvular disease are also characterized by relative preservation of the aortic root and sinotubular junction on MRI (224). In cases of AS, the aneurysmal dilation usually is limited to the midascending aorta, where the poststenotic flow effects are most prominent (156). In AR, aneurysmal dilation of the thoracic aorta typically involves the ascending aorta but extends into the transverse arch because of the "water hammer" effect and, in long-standing cases, also may involve the descending thoracic aorta; often there is slight effacement of the sinotubular junction and dilation of the aortic root in primary AR because of their relationship (160). Another configuration of thoracic aortic aneurysms that is important to identify on MRI is saccular dilation from a mycotic or pseudoaneurysm. Mycotic aneurysms result from weakening of the aortic wall by infection (240), although pseudoaneurysms typically are caused by trauma (e.g., automobile accidents) and occur most commonly at the level of the ligamentum arteriosum or after surgery at anastomotic or cannulation sites (242).

The entity of noncommunicating dissecting intramural hematoma is being detected with increasing frequency with the development of tomographic imaging, including MRI. Technically, this may be described as dissection of the aortic wall without intimal rupture or tear; the etiology is unknown, but presumably it is related to a weakening of the media. Clinically, the presentation is almost always similar to that of aortic dissection; the diagnosis of an intramural hematoma is entertained once communicating aortic dissection has been excluded. On MRI designed to exclude communicating aortic dissection, an intramural hematoma is identified as a smooth crescentic to circumferential area of thickened aortic wall without evidence of blood flow in the false channel. Depending on the age of the hematoma, the area of thickening may be isointense or hyperintense relative to skeletal muscle on SE MRI; the signal intensity is relatively isointense in the acute phase and then becomes greatest in the subacute stage (232). If intramural bleeding stops, the intramural hematoma resolves with decreasing thickness and returns to SE isointensity in the more chronic stages. Knowledge is limited regarding the natural course of an intramural hematoma. However, complete resolution and evolution to dissection have been demonstrated on MRI (232,243). Involvement of the ascending aorta by intramural hematoma has been shown to predispose the development of communicating aortic dissection in most cases; rebleeding before development of communicating dissection has been detected based on SE intensity changes (232,243).

Aortic Arch

The aortic arch begins at the brachiocephalic, or innominate, artery and extends to the ligamentum arteriosus. The classic configuration of three aortic arch vessels, namely, the innominate artery, the left common carotid artery, and the left subclavian artery, in the proximal-to-distal direction is found in about two thirds to three fourths of individuals. Variant anatomy is common, particularly a common origin of the innominate and left common carotid arteries (so-called "bovine arch"), which has been reported in up to 22% of the population. Other variants to consider are a separate origin of the left vertebral artery from the arch.

Failure of the primitive aortic arches to fuse or regress can result in anomalous arch configurations called vascular rings that can encircle the trachea of esophagus and result in stridor, wheezing, or dysphagia (244,245). The most common vascular rings are a left aortic arch with an aberrant right subclavian artery, a right aortic arch with an aberrant left subclavian artery, and a double aortic arch. Aberrant subclavian arteries may also be associated with a diverticulum of Kommerell and are typically retroesophageal. Vascular rings are usually well demonstrated on black-blood imaging with supplemental cine MR. Three-dimensional contrast-enhanced MR angiography is often not necessary for diagnosing vascular rings but may be helpful for surgical planning.

Entities that involve the ascending aorta may also affect the arch and its branches, either as an extension with type A dissection or a large ascending aortic aneurysm or as its primary location. Atherosclerosis is a systemic process that can commonly result in aneurysms or branch vessel stenosis.

Ligamentum Arteriosum. The ligamentum arteriosum is the remnant of the fetal ductus arteriosus and approximates a boundary between the aortic arch and descending thoracic aorta. One of the most common entities that involve this region is coarctation of the aorta (see the section on congenital diseases). Pseudoaneurysms are typically posttraumatic and affect the lesser curvature of the aorta at the fixed point of attachment to the left pulmonary artery by the ligamentum arteriosum, the vestigial remnant of the ductus arteriosus (246). The risk of delayed rupture remains high even in stable patients with remote trauma. Pseudoaneurysms are typically saccular and can be well evaluated using 3D contrast-enhanced MR angiography.

Descending Aorta

The descending thoracic aorta extends from the ligamentum to the aortic hiatus of the diaphragm. True aortic aneurysms involve all three layers (intima, media, and adventitia) of the aortic wall and are typically atherosclerotic in nature or related to connective tissue disorders. Atherosclerotic aneurysms occur most typically in the descending thoracic aorta and may be fusiform or saccular in morphology (237,238,246). A penetrating aortic ulcer (246,247) is another entity that tends to present in the descending aorta where the bulk of atherosclerosis occurs. The natural history of penetrating atherosclerotic ulcers remains controversial, and its treatment generally parallels that of dissection. Penetrating atherosclerotic ulcers need to be differentiated from focal saccular aneurysm and intramural hematoma. In patients with a suspicion of a penetrating ulcer and aortic dissection, it is generally advisable that precontrast T1-weighted images be performed. Intramural hematomas (also called aortic dissection without an intimal flap) are often subtle and may only be evident on precontrast images as hemorrhages within thickened regions of the aortic wall.

Evaluation of Pulmonary Artery Disease

MRI can be used to detect intrinsic pulmonary artery disease and to evaluate the secondary effects of adjacent extravascular disease.

Pulmonary Emboli

Because of the signal void of normally flowing blood, thrombus within a pulmonary artery can usually be readily discerned on systolic SE images; the intensity of thrombus is variable, depending on its age. Recent reports have successfully demonstrated the potential of molecular targeted MRI of pulmonary emboli using low-dose application of a fibrin-specific contrast agent (EP-2104R; Epix Pharmaceuticals, Cambridge, MA) in a swine model (248,249).

Pulmonary Hypertension

The primary use of MRI in evaluation of pulmonary arterial hypertension (PAH) is the description of secondary changes (250). Anatomic findings include RV hypertrophy in proportion to the pulmonary artery pressures, reversal of septal curvature when pulmonary artery pressures approximate systemic pressures, and pulmonary artery dilation. The utility of MRI is clearly evident in the assessment of patients undergoing evaluation for possible lung transplantation or for monitoring after this surgery. Improved RV function and enhanced pulmonary artery flow in transplanted lungs have been shown (251).

Evaluation of Thrombi and Masses

MRI (252–254) plays an important role in the evaluation of patients with masses in the central cardiovascular system, not only for the primary diagnosis, but also for planning therapy. It also evaluates the paracardiac regions of the lungs and mediastinum with extreme accuracy. MRI is excellent in terms of soft-tissue contrast resolution, permitting better depiction of the morphologic details of a mass, including its extent, site of origin, and secondary effects on adjacent structures. Dynamic MRI (cine and tagging) also have the ability to provide functional images of the heart that can be used to study the pathophysiologic consequences of cardiac masses; another advantage of MRI is the depiction of cardiovascular structures without the use of contrast material, although use of MRI contrast (e.g., gadolinium-DTPA) for angiographic or ultrafast-tissue perfusion studies is becoming more commonplace. Because tumor hypervascularity due to angiogenesis can be detected, tissue studies have become commonplace in the assessment of masses and thrombi. The use of tissue-perfusion imaging is particularly helpful in distinguishing neoplasms from thrombi and in evaluating the extent of tumor (255,256). However, one disadvantage of MRI is its inability to detect calcification.

Cardiac and Paracardiac Masses

Primary cardiac tumors are rare. The cumulative prevalence is estimated to be between 0.002% and 0.3% in autopsy series (257). Approximately 75% of primary cardiac tumors are benign. The most common benign tumor is the myxoma, which accounts for approximately 30% of all primary tumors and 50% of benign tumors (257,258). Almost all primary malignant tumors of the heart are sarcomas; the most common are angiosarcomas and rhabdomyosarcomas. These tumors are clinically silent at first and produce symptoms only when blood flow becomes obstructed or valvular function is disrupted. Even then, symptoms are frequently nonspecific and may include chest pain and dyspnea (259). Primary malignant pericardial tumors are very rare and are mostly mesotheliomas. Metastatic cardiac and pericardial tumors are much more common, occurring in 1.5% to 0.6% of patients with malignant disease (260). Metastases usually involve the pericardium and myocardium, but rarely involve the valves and the endocardium. In addition, the right side of the heart is more frequently involved than the left side. Metastases may involve the heart via direct extension, hematogenous dissemination, or lymphatic spread. The most frequent primary malignancy that metastasizes to the heart is bronchogenic carcinoma followed by breast carcinoma, malignant melanoma, lymphoma, and leukemia (261).

Cardiac MRI does not unequivocally differentiate benign from malignant tumors; however, there are certain findings that suggest malignancy. Involvement of the right side of the heart, masses in the ventricles that infiltrate the myocardium, and associated hemopericardium support the diagnosis of malignant tumors. Conversely, benign tumors tend to occur on the left side of the heart along the interatrial septum and rarely cause pericardial effusion (262). MRI is capable of differentiating adipose from soft tissue and both from cystic fluid collections. Because myocardial tumors may be infiltrative, there may be difficulty in visualizing them. Contrast-enhanced MRI increases the sensitivity of tumor detection due to appreciation of vascularized areas in the areas of malignancy; generally, tumors become enhanced more intensely than the surrounding myocardium (263). However, the variable enhancement pattern of myocardial tumors complicates differentiating benign from malignant masses.

Cardiac Masses: Intracavitary. Myxomas are the most common benign primary cardiac tumor. Seventy percent of myxomas occur in middle-aged men and women. Myxomas are located within the cavity of the left atrium, attached to the interatrial septum at the border of the fossa ovalis in 85% of the cases. They originate from the posterior and anterior atrial walls, as well as from the atrial appendage (258). Usually myxomata are solitary tumors and are polypoid or pedunculated. Most patients present with one or more of the triad of embolism, obstruction, and constitutional symptoms (264). On MRI, variability in the appearance of myxomas may reflect their variable composition of water-rich myxomatous tissue versus fibrous tissue and calcification. Myxomata tend to have higher signal intensity than myocardium on T2-weighted imaging (T2WI) (265). Cine-MRI may show the characteristic mobility of the pedunculated tumor (223).

Lipomas are the second-most-common benign tumor of the heart, accounting for 10% of all cardiac tumors (223,266). There is no sex or age predisposition. About 50% arise subendocardially, 25% subepicardially, and 25% from the wall of a cardiac chamber to extend intracavitary (223). On MRI, lipomatous tissue has a uniquely short T1, and the signal intensity is similar that of subcutaneous fat, having a relatively high signal intensity on spin-echo T1-weighted imaging and a moderate signal intensity on T2-weighted imaging. A decrease in signal intensity using a fat presaturation technique verifies the diagnosis (223).

Overall, thrombi are the most common of intracardiac masses and typically occur along the posterolateral wall of the left atrial cavity or within the left atrial appendage (Fig. 54.6). Usually, a predisposing condition such as atrial fibrillation is present to promote the formation of the thrombus at these locations. Thrombus is also frequently observed in the apex of the impaired left ventricle due to slow blood flow in the region. On MRI, fresh thrombus often has higher signal intensity than

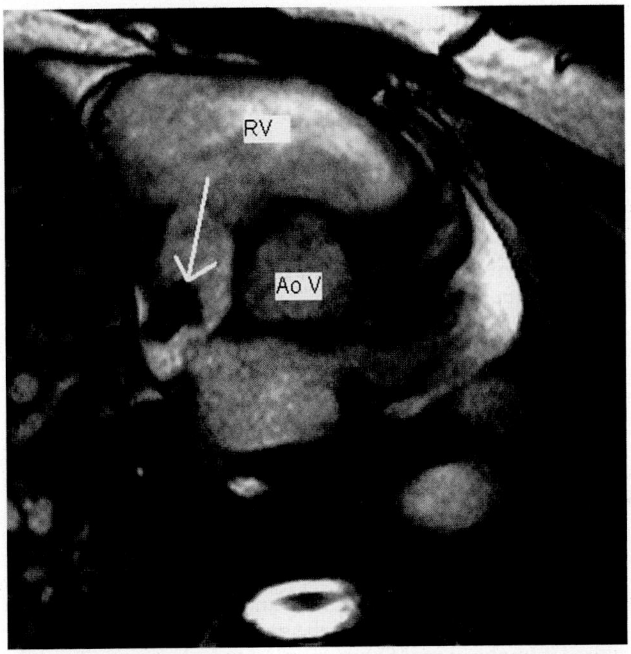

FIGURE 54.6. Gradient-echo image demonstrating the presence of a thrombus in the right atrium. AoV, aortic valve; RV, right ventricle.

myocardium on T1-weighted images. However, depending on the age of the thrombus, alterations in signal intensity are possible. After 1 or 2 weeks, paramagnetic compounds of the organizing thrombus such as deoxyhemoglobin and methemoglobin cause T1 and T2 shortening that may result in increased signal intensity on T1-weighted and decreased intensity on T2-weighted images (223,267).

Intramyocardial Cardiac Masses: Malignant. Angiosarcomas, rhabdomyosarcomas, and fibrosarcomas are the most frequent primary malignant tumors of the heart. Angiosarcomas are the most common primary malignant tumor of myocardium in adults, accounting for approximately 33% of primary malignant cardiac tumors. They are typically found in patients between the ages of 20 and 50 years (259,268). Patients usually present with right-sided right failure and tamponade because this tumor exhibits a striking predilection for the right side of the heart, especially the right atrium. They also have a propensity to involve the pericardium, resulting in bloody pericardial effusion (268). Metastases occur in 66% to 89% of the cases, with the lungs being the most frequent site of spread (269).MRI of cardiac angiosarcoma most often reveals a mass arising from the right atrium accompanied by significant hemopericardium. MRI demonstrates a nonhomogeneous mass with hyperintense areas on T1-weighted images corresponding to hemorrhage (254,270). After the administration of gadolinium-DTPA, T1-weighted images typically show nonhomogeneous enhancement, especially in the periphery of the lesion (254). Rhabdomyosarcomas are malignant tumor of striate muscle. Rhabdomyosarcomas are the most common malignant tumors of infants and children, although they account for only 4% to 7% of all cardiac sarcomas. Frequently rhabdomyosarcomas extend beyond myocardium, causing a polypoid extension into a chamber cavity, simulating a myxoma (271). Although some reports suggest a predisposition for right-sided cavities (272), rhabdomyosarcomas have no strong predilection for a specific chamber, and multiple locations are frequently found (60%). A rhabdomyosarcoma is more likely than other sarcomas to involve or arise from cardiac valves (270). Pericardial involvement is also frequent (273). MRI signal intensity is intermediate on precontrast T1-weighted images, similar to that of adjacent myocardial tissue, but shows enhancement of the lesion after administration of contrast (273). Fibrosarcoma is another malignancy that diffusely infiltrates the myocardium. It often involves the left atrium and usually manifests as congestive heart failure due to blood flow obstruction. On MRI, a fibrosarcoma may be heterogeneous or isointense relative to myocardium on T1-weighted images (270), although the malignant nature can be depicted with T2-weighted images or contrast-based imaging.

Intramyocardial Cardiac Masses: Benign. Rhabdomyomas are the most common cardiac tumors of infants and children, with the majority occurring in newborns (274); they are associated with tuberous sclerosis in 50% of the cases. These benign tumors nearly always involve the myocardium or the ventricles, affecting both ventricles with equal frequency. At least half of the lesions are large enough to cause obstruction of a valve or cardiac chamber. There are multiple sites involved in 90% of cases; the atria are involved in 30% of cases of rhabdomyomas (274). On MRI, a rhabdomyoma may be slightly hypointense to slightly hyperintense to the myocardium on T1-weighted images and slightly hyperintense on T2-weighted images (219,223). Fibromas are a benign tumor primarily affecting children and are usually discovered before the age of 10 years. Almost all involve the myocardium, with a predilection for the anterior free wall and interventricular septum (223). These tumors usually cause blood flow obstruction, ventricular dysfunction, or conduction abnormalities (275). On MRI, fibromas are hypointense to slightly hyperintense on T1-weighted images when compared to skeletal muscle, but they have lower signal intensity than myocardium on T2-weighted images. This is because of their fibrous nature or due to deposits of calcium related to necrosis (252).

Paracardiac Masses. Many different sources of paracardiac masses, frequently unrelated to the heart (e.g., hiatal hernia) can be easily identified by MRI. The identification of such mass lesions potentially influencing the central cardiovascular structures is important. The relationship to the pericardium is a key issue. Metastases are by far the leading cause of pericardial masses. From 5% to 15% of patients with malignant neoplasm have pericardial metastases. Bronchogenic carcinoma, breast cancer, leukemia, and lymphoma account for 80% of pericardial metastases (276). Metastases may result in nodular deposits or local or diffuse pericardial thickening. Metastatic involvement may lead to hemorrhagic or serosanguineous pericardial effusions.

Evaluation of Congenital Heart Disease

MRI is a powerful modality for assessing the morphology and physiology of simple and complex congenital cardiac conditions (both before and after corrective/palliative interventions). With a growing adult congenital heart disease population, the requirements are likely to grow in the near future. Because of the wide range of anatomic and functional problems, a successful MRI study of a congenitally malformed heart requires a cardiovascular radiologist or cardiologist who has knowledge of the range of available MR pulse sequences (including standard spin-echo and gradient-echo sequences, cine sequences, and phase-contrast techniques) and also good expertise with regard to congenital heart disease. His or her presence near the scanner during the study is often necessary because imaging protocols often have to be tailored to the individual patient and adjustments are frequently made during the imaging session. The physician in charge of MRI needs to be in close contact with the referring physician and has to be informed about prior surgical or percutaneous intervention, and previous imaging studies should be available. The evaluation of various congenital diseases is discussed later.

Sequential analysis is the generally approved strategy for morphologic description of a congenital cardiac malformation. The first step in this approach is the determination of atriovisceral situs by reviewing the localization of inferior vena cava, abdominal aorta, liver, spleen and stomach, and the morphology of the atrial appendages and mainstem bronchi. This is followed by determining ventricular morphology, using the muscular outflow tract and the moderator band as landmarks of the anatomic RV. The aortic arch and the pulmonary bifurcation identify the great vessels. Then atrioventricular and ventriculoarterial connections are assessed to be either concordant or discordant. A concordant atrioventricular connection means that the anatomic right atrium is connected to an anatomic left ventricle. A discordant ventriculoarterial connection means that the anatomic right ventricle is connected to the ascending aorta (as in classic D-transposition of the great arteries [TGA]). Combined atrioventricular and ventriculoarterial discordance is the hallmark L-transposition. Finally, associated lesions such as septal defects or aortic arch coarctation are evaluated.

Aortic Anomalies

Bicuspid Aortic Valve. Congenital bicuspid aortic valve occurs in between 0.9% and 2% of all individuals in autopsy series. Although valve area may be reduced at birth, it is usually not responsible for severe stenosis until later in adulthood. About one third of patients with bicuspid aortic valves develop aortic regurgitation on the basis of organic structural abnormality or after a bout of acute bacterial endocarditis. MRI will demonstrate decreased aortic annular caliber, thickened valve leaflets, maldistribution of the three aortic sinuses of Valsalva by the unseparated valvular commissures, and aortic valve leaflet doming. In cases with mixed valvular stenosis and regurgitation, both the ascending aorta and left ventricle are dilated.

Coarctation of the Aorta. Coarctation of the presents with hypoplasia of the distal aortic arch and focal narrowing of the proximal descending aorta, most commonly at the junction of the ductus arteriosus and aorta. MRI demonstrates the location and length of the coarctation segment, the status of the aortic isthmus, and the degree of arterial collateralization present. It may be useful in delineating dilated intercostal arteries traveling along the underside of the posterior upper ribs or dilated internal mammary arteries running along the inner aspect of the anterior chest wall. MRI is useful for following the results of balloon dilation and surgical repair of coarctation (277). Serial examination allows close follow-up and assessment of residual stenosis and early demonstration of aneurysmal dilation.

Marfan Syndrome. MRI is very suitable for imaging the aorta in Marfan syndrome (228,278–283). The characteristically pear-shaped dilatation of the aortic root is well demonstrated with MRI, and its diameter can be accurately measured using only conventional SE techniques. The aortic root diameter is an important criterion in surgical decision-making. Associated dissection can be detected and aortic valve incompetence quantified with MRI. Furthermore, MR studies have looked at the compliance of the aortic wall, either by using conventional pulse sequences (284) or by measuring the velocity of the flow wave along the descending aorta (285). This can be used to monitor the effect of β-blocker medication that may slow down the loss of elasticity in Marfan patients (286). Very recently, MRI was reported to demonstrate dural ectasia, one of the rare diagnostic criteria, which occurs in 92% of Marfan patients, and therefore this is potentially very important.

Pulmonary Artery Anomalies

The preoperative evaluation of pulmonary atresia has been difficult with noninvasive imaging techniques predominantly because the patients of concern are mostly infants. MRI was successful and reported to be superior to echocardiography in demonstration of pulmonary artery branch anomalies (280,287–291). However, MRI is not easily performed in very young children, who often require sedation or anesthesia. Pulmonary artery stenosis can occur at the infundibular, valvular, or supravalvular level or in the peripheral branches, for instance, after previous systemic-to-pulmonary artery shunt. Obstructive hypertrophy of the RV infundibulum is adequately visualized with MRI. The pulmonary valve itself is difficult to demonstrate, although cusp movements are clearly shown on conventional cine sequences. A stenotic pulmonary valve, however, can be recognized by its doming configuration and by poststenotic dilation of the central pulmonary artery, a phenomenon not seen with infundibular obstruction.

Intracardiac Shunts

In addition to demonstrating the intracardiac defect, MRI also defines specific chamber dilation and hypertrophy, which is useful for characterization of the severity of the shunt and acquired complications. Shunt fraction calculation is generally performed using volume-flow analysis of great artery flow with velocity mapping. With this approach, quantitation of shunt size can be accomplished by measuring net blood flow volumes within the main pulmonary artery and ascending aorta over a cardiac cycle. Shunts produce discrepant pulmonary and systemic arterial flows, with the former exceeding the latter in left-to-right shunts, and conversely in right-to-left shunts (292). This difference can be expressed either in absolute terms (e.g., shunt volume) or in relative terms (e.g., pulmonary-to-systemic blood flow ratio, Qp/Qs). Values for shunting derived by volume-flow analysis have correlated well with the results from cardiac catheterization or nuclear first-pass ventriculography (292).

Atrial Septal Defects. Using a combination of various sequences (cine, spin-echo, gradient-echo, and phase-contrast), MRI can be used to classify atrial septal defects (ASDs). Secundum defect, the most common form of ASD, is usually large and centrally located in the septum. Primum ASDs are medially and inferiorly located, immediately superior to the atrioventricular (AV) valves. Sinus venosus defects are actually defects between the posterior inferior border of the inferior vena cava and the left atrium. These defects are almost always associated with anomalous drainage of the right upper-lobe pulmonary vein to the superior vena cava. Right ventricular myocardium in simple ASD is not hypertrophied. With imaging in the axial plane, MRI has an overall 97% sensitivity and 90% specificity for the detection of ASDs (293). MRI is excellent in detecting concomitant anomalous pulmonary venous return. It might be to the right atrium or coronary sinus, to the inferior vena cava or portal vein systemic veins, or to the innominate vein or superior vena cava. In a series of 56 patients with various types of congenital heart disease but normal pulmonary venous connection, axial spin-echo MRI showed the sites of connection of all four pulmonary veins in 88% of cases; in a parallel series of 22 patients with partial or total anomalous pulmonary venous return, pulmonary venous anomalies were identified in 95% of cases (294).

Ventricular Septal Defect. MRI can be used to diagnose the presence and characterize the size of ventricular septal defects (VSDs) (295,296). Large subaortic VSDs are readily demonstrated on axial MR spin-echo or double-inversion recovery images as a break in the interventricular septum to the left of the AV rings and to the right of the crest of the muscular interventricular septum. Visual separation of the actual defect from the inferior extension of an aortic sinus of Valsalva can be improved by obtaining images in oblique sagittal section. Membranous VSDs are identified by the absence of signal (or a break in the interventricular septum) in the posterior superiormost aspect of the interventricular septum, immediately below the aortic valve, and adjacent to the septal leaflet of the tricuspid valve. Cine MRI identifies left-to-right, right-to-left, and bidirectional shunts. AV septal defects (endocardial cushion defects) involve the AV septum and primum portion of the interatrial septum and may involve the anterior mitral and septal tricuspid leaflets and the membranous interventricular septum. MRI may be used to determine the size of the ventricular component of the defect as well as the presence of ventricular hypoplasia.

Evaluation of Complex Congenital Malformations

Tetralogy of Fallot. Tetralogy of Fallot is the most common cyanotic form of congenital heart disease, and surgical correction in early infancy has significantly improved survival. After repair, however, patients have residual defects or sequelae, and a comprehensive analysis of the postoperative status can be made with MRI (Fig. 54.7) (297). Residual or recurrent pulmonary stenosis, at either the infundibular or valvular level, frequently occurs. When clinically significant stenosis is relieved by placement of a transannular outflow patch, pulmonary regurgitation occurs. The RV is subsequently subjected to volume overload of varying severity, and the importance of detecting and measuring pulmonary regurgitation is increasingly being recognized. MRI, including phase-contrast techniques, has been shown useful and accurate for this purpose (165). Occasionally, residual ventricular septal defect requires quantitative analysis that is easily performed with MRI. The morphology of the central pulmonary arteries is crucial. After Fallot repair, for instance, after previous Blalock-Taussig anastomosis, patients often suffer from pulmonary artery branch stenosis, which is well visualized by SE MRI (289,298) or Gd-enhanced MRA. Finally, LV and RV systolic and diastolic function can be measured from a stack of cine images. Both LV and RV functional deteriorations were shown to be associated with pulmonary regurgitation (165,299,300).

Functional Single Ventricle: Tricuspid Atresia and Double Inlet Left Ventricle. Patients with tricuspid atresia or double inlet LV have functionally a single ventricle. Several surgical options have been developed to redirect the systemic venous blood to the pulmonary arteries. Some of these surgical procedures have already been abandoned, and others are still being modified. The Fontan procedure and all its variants have had a major impact on the treatment of single ventricle, but long-term outcome remains uncertain. The classic Fontan operation consisted of a conduit from the right atrium to the central pulmonary arteries. In particular, a valved conduit was prone to become stenotic. Sometimes the conduit only connected to the left pulmonary artery in combination with a Glenn procedure, a separate anastomosis of the superior vena cava to the right pulmonary artery. Occasionally, a conduit from the right atrium to a hypoplastic RV outflow tract was used, a mostly abandoned modification aiming at the development of a physiologic arterial type of pulmonary blood flow. Nowadays, the right atrium is mostly excluded by performing a bidirectional Glenn procedure (also named a hemi-Fontan), with secondary completion of the Fontan procedure (a complete cavopulmonary anastomosis) by establishing also a connection (sometimes a fenestrated baffle) between the inferior vena cava and the pulmonary arteries. MRI flow studies demonstrated that the success of RV incorporation could not be reliably determined on the basis of flow velocity measurements alone, but that volumetric flow also had to be taken into account. Furthermore, the ratio of left-to-right pulmonary artery flow was found to

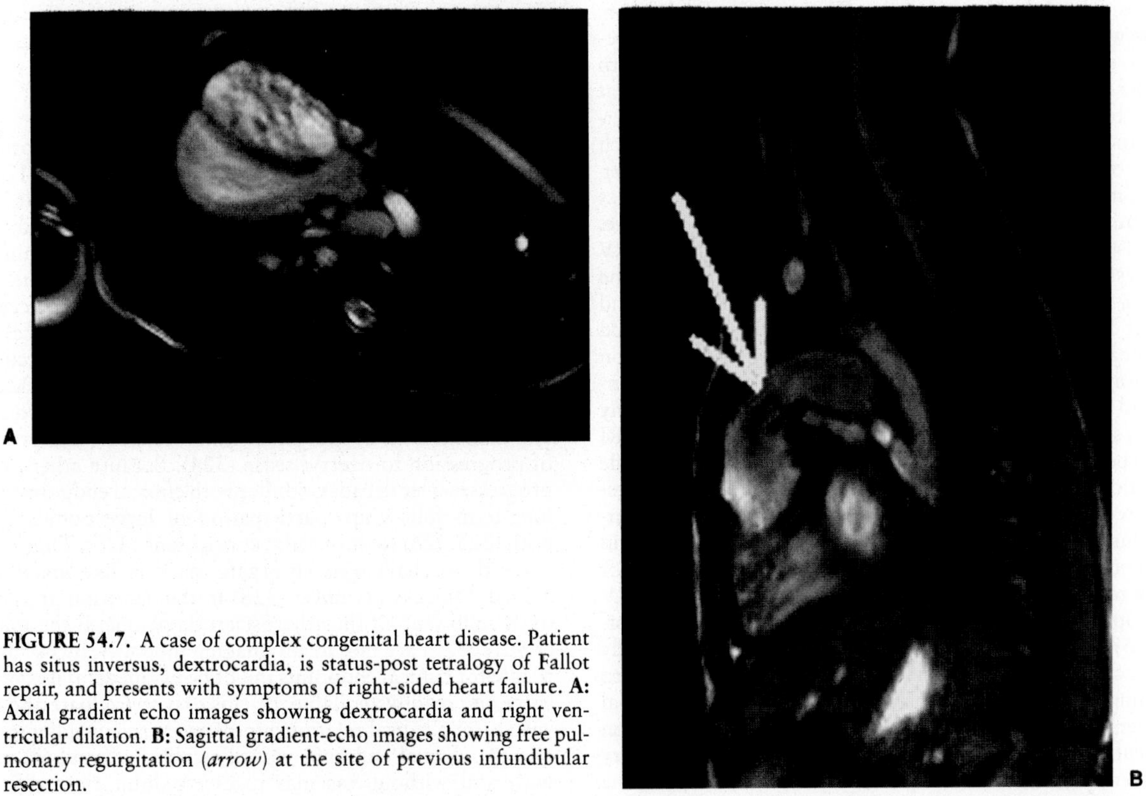

FIGURE 54.7. A case of complex congenital heart disease. Patient has situs inversus, dextrocardia, is status-post tetralogy of Fallot repair, and presents with symptoms of right-sided heart failure. **A:** Axial gradient echo images showing dextrocardia and right ventricular dilation. **B:** Sagittal gradient-echo images showing free pulmonary regurgitation (*arrow*) at the site of previous infundibular resection.

be reversed after Fontan surgery (301). The hypothesis of constant total heart volume and center of mass, promoting efficient use of cardiac energy, was tested in a cohort of patients during staged Fontan surgery. It was shown that total heart volume and mass center did not remain constant during the sequence of operations (302,303). Pulmonary artery size and confluence of the central pulmonary artery branches are crucial determinants of outcome after Fontan surgery, and MRI was shown to be superior to echocardiography in evaluating these parameters (304). Ventriculoventricular interaction has been studied with an MR myocardial tagging technique. This particular study showed differences in strain and motion of the RV in the systemic position after Fontan surgery when compared to a systemic RV that has an LV to support it, as in patients after Mustard or Senning repair for TGA (305). It was also demonstrated with MRI that a hemi-Fontan operation posed no significant changes in ventricular geometry or performance; however, a significant decrease of ventricular volume, mass, and performance was found 1 to 2 years after completion of the Fontan procedure (306). The relative cardiac and respiratory contribution to pulmonary blood flow after total cavopulmonary anastomosis has been studied using an MR blood-tagging technique (307). Fairly recently, also using an MR blood-labeling technique, it was elegantly demonstrated that after total cavopulmonary anastomosis, inferior vena cava blood is directed more toward the left pulmonary artery and superior vena cava blood more toward the right pulmonary artery (308). Others have used multidimensional quadratic principal component analysis (Q-PCA) to study pulmonary blood flow patterns after total cavopulmonary anastomosis and classic atriopulmonary Fontan connection. In the former category, pulmonary flow is more organized and uniform, suggesting that it is more hemodynamically efficient (309). A similar study showed reduced total pulmonary blood flow after both types of Fontan surgery compared to normal, attributable to the smaller size of the pulmonary arteries. In addition, swirling pulmonary artery flow patterns indicated increased shear stress in both categories (310).

Transposition of the Great Arteries: Postoperative Evaluation. Patients with D-type TGA (discordant atrioventricular connection) have to be separated into those who were treated with the older and nowadays mostly abandoned techniques that redirect blood at the atrial level (Mustard or Senning operation) and those who were treated with the arterial switch (Jatene) operation. The latter patients are generally younger, with the majority now reaching adulthood. The two categories have significantly different postoperative residua and sequelae. The Mustard or Senning procedures leave the anatomic RV in the systemic position, and we now know that this is at the base of a range of problems, with late sudden RV failure and death at the end of the spectrum. Other often-encountered hemodynamic problems are arrhythmias, (baffle) obstruction to pulmonary or systemic venous return, pulmonary hypertension, and tricuspid regurgitation. The post-Mustard anatomy has been successfully demonstrated with MRI (311–313). MRI has also been used for follow-up after stent placement for baffle obstruction (314). The function of the anatomic RV in the systemic circulation appears to be of particular interest. Late cardiac failure is a serious matter of concern in these patients, and diastolic dysfunction may be an early sign. After Mustard or Senning repair, cine MRI techniques were used to quantify RV hypertrophy, but RV volumes and ejection fraction were normal (315). Phase-contrast techniques have been used to study diastolic characteristics by measuring tricuspid flow in Mustard or Senning patients and demonstrating differences from normal volunteers (316). After the arterial switch procedure, common complications are RV outflow tract obstruction and pulmonary artery stenosis, either at the supravalvular or branch level. The postoperative status of the great vessels has been adequately assessed with SE MRI (298,317,318). The morphology of congenitally corrected TGA (CCTGA, combined atrioventricular and ventriculoarterial discordance) has been studied with conventional MRI techniques (319,320). This is a small category of patients, often detected at a later age. Furthermore, some patients with CCTGA suffer from arrhythmias or carry a pacemaker, making them unsuitable for MRI.

CONTROVERSIES AND PERSONAL PERSPECTIVES

MRI is a rapidly emerging and complex noninvasive test of choice for patients with a multitude of cardiovascular problems. Its emerging role as one of the dominant imaging modalities in most facets of clinical cardiology cannot be understated. It has entered an important phase in its evolution, with an anticipated exponential growth in its current clinical applications and through the development of newer targeted molecular imaging and interventional applications. Furthermore, the availability of magnets with higher field strengths (e.g., 3 T and higher), improvements in coil design, and newer pulse sequences will be extremely important in enabling the success of this technology. For this potential to be realized, however, several types of obstacles must be overcome.

One of the biggest obstacles is the current medical environment with its increasing emphasis on cost containment and capitated reimbursement. Other obstacles include increasing demands on physicians involved in cardiac MRI to pursue clinical productivity in more basic diagnostic imaging areas, where reimbursement may be better established, and greater limitations on research time and institutional support for needed clinical investigation in cardiac MRI. Finally, for this technology to evolve further and flourish, a solid collaboration between cardiology and radiology, like the one that exists in our respective institutions, is the primary prerequisite.

THE FUTURE

Atherosclerosis Imaging

Atherosclerosis, a leading cause of morbidity and mortality in the Western world, is responsible for an estimated $112 billion in socioeconomic burden in the United States alone. It consists of a gradual process that begins as early as the second or third decade in the vessel wall as outward arterial thickening (positive arterial remodelling with a normal vessel lumen); significant obstruction to the arterial blood flow does not occur until the later stages of disease (321). Indeed, acute clinical events from atherosclerotic lesions have been shown to occur more often in mild to moderate than in severe stenoses (322,323). Therefore, focus is now beginning to shift toward the diagnosis and management of subclinical atherosclerosis and prevention of progression to overt disease (324). Because atherosclerosis progresses over decades, studies with clinical endpoints require long-term follow-up, participation of large populations, or both (325,326) to draw valid conclusions (327). Thus, to overcome these challenges, surrogate markers like imaging have gained immense attention (328) in the detection and longitudinal follow-up of the atherosclerotic plaque. If the following criteria (329) are met by an imaging modality, its use as a surrogate for clinical endpoints might be justified: (a) it is very sensitive and readily available, (b) it is easy to evaluate and noninvasive, (c) a causal relationship between the imaging modality and the clinical endpoint is well established, and (d) patients with and without vascular disease exhibit clear differences in surrogate marker measurements. The characterization of the different stages of atherosclerosis (from early positive arterial remodelling to overt atherosclerosis) can be made in vivo in humans using various invasive and noninvasive techniques [carotid ultrasound (330), electron beam or multislice computed tomography (331,332), intravascular ultrasound (333)].

MRI, because of its high resolution, 3D capabilities, truly noninvasive nature, and capacity for soft tissue characterization, has emerged as a powerful modality for assessing subclinical and overt atherosclerotic changes in different vascular beds (334,335). With regard to atherosclerosis, the surrogate criteria just described (329) appear to be fulfilled by MRI in a truly noninvasive fashion. However, there are many technical considerations, and the following factors need to be taken into consideration to accurately visualize the atherosclerotic plaque by MRI.

Technical Considerations of Magnetic Resonance–Based Atherosclerosis Imaging

A normal artery wall is extremely thin (around 1 mm for the coronaries and thicker for the aorta and carotids), but with progressive arterial remodeling, this thickness can vary from a few millimeters to greater than 1 cm. Using sophisticated receiver coils and improvements in hardware, it is now possible to achieve submillimeter in-plane spatial resolution on the order of $0.25 \times 0.25\ mm^2$ in the carotids, $0.8 \times 0.8\ mm^2$ in the aorta, and $0.46 \times 0.46\ mm^2$ in the coronaries, with a 2- to 5-mm slice thickness (336–338), using a 1.5-T magnet. The use of phased-array surface coil techniques has proven to be very effective in improving the signal to-noise-ratio (SNR) (339,340). The widespread availability of 3-T magnets will likely help to improve the SNR, which can be partially traded for an improved spatial resolution.

The next technical issue to consider is the presence of artefacts, including cardiac contraction, breathing, blood flow, and random motion as with swallowing or tremors, all of which can significantly degrade image quality. To counter that, cardiac gating is used to improve the quality of the scan. For aortic and coronary imaging, along with cardiac gating, breathing is also an issue, which is countered by breath-holding or use of respiratory navigators (337,338,341). In addition, perivascular fat, which can obscure signal from the vessel wall and lead to chemical-shift artifacts, can be suppressed using advanced fat-saturation techniques (123). Two other major steps in imaging atherosclerosis by MR include the quantitative analysis and the characterization of the atherosclerotic plaque: Accurate quantification of vessel wall dimensions depends on the ability to discern the inner and outer boundaries of the vessel wall. Use of techniques to suppress the blood-flow signal [e.g., double inversion recovery (342) combined with fast spin-echo) enhances the conspicuity of the vessel wall and its components against the backdrop of a hypointense lumen (336–338,343). Several semi-automatic image processing tools have been proposed for vessel boundary detection (344,345). In general, dimension measurement is preferred in continuous rather than categorical form to enable inferences about longitudinal regression/progression of plaque because atherosclerosis is generally not a uniform process, and accurate and reproducible determination of vessel wall dimensions is extremely important for valid conclusions to be drawn longitudinally. Arterial wall dimension assessment using MRI has been found to be highly reproducible in the carotid arteries (346,347), aorta (348), and the coronaries (349).

Another consideration is the ability to discern different plaque components including fibrous cap, lipid core, hemorrhage, and calcification. Based on histologic studies, it is known that different plaque components coexist, and these different components produce differences in the MR signal based on their physical properties (350). Thus, to achieve tissue contrast and hence plaque characterization, images obtained using different weightings are necessary (337,351). Different plaque components have been characterized by different (T1, T2, and proton density [PD]) weightings in animals (352,353), ex vivo specimens (354,355), in vivo carotids (354,356), in vivo aortas (337), and, more recently, the coronaries (338,340). The characteristic appearance of different plaque components by MRI has been previously validated (336,350,354). Generally, lipid components appear as isointense regions within the plaque on T1- and PD-weighted images but as hypointense on T2-weighted images. On the other hand, the fibrous cap appears bright, whereas calcium appears very hypointense on all three weightings. Thrombus appears hyperintense (albeit less than fibrous cap) on all three weightings. Perivascular fat, which predominantly has triglycerides, has a different MR appearance than lipid core, which generally consists of unesterified cholesterol and cholesterol esters (350,355). Recent studies have demonstrated that the use of paramagnetic contrast agents such as gadolinium would enable subtle distinctions among different plaque components. Increases in T1 relaxation by gadolinium leads to increased contrast enhancement on T1-weighted pulse sequences. There is evidence of neovascularization and inflammation in atherosclerotic plaque (357), and it has been proposed that contrast-enhanced MRI can further aid in plaque characterization by helping to detect these changes (358,359). In these studies, it was demonstrated that pre- and postcontrast MRI helped differentiate between the necrotic core and fibrous tissue. In another study, it was also demonstrated that postcontrast signal enhancement in carotid arteries and aorta was associated with elevated serum levels of interleukin-6, C-reactive protein, and cell adhesion molecules (360). Another interesting development in this field is the use of contrast agents to enhance plaque components, which generally involve gadolinium-based agents (358,359). The latter agents have proven usefulness in the assessment of plaque size and composition. Newer data, with the use of novel contrast agents like ultrasmall paramagnetic particles of iron oxide (USPIOs) or fibrin-specific agents, are emerging in this field at a rapid pace (361–363). USPIOs alter the relaxation times of adjacent tissue and are avidly taken up by macrophages. It has been demonstrated that that injection of USPIO into hyperlipidemic rabbits was associated with appearance of signal voids on the luminal surface of the aorta (364). Another active area of research is that of detection of thrombus or fibrin, which has been demonstrated to play a role in the progression of atherosclerotic plaque (365). Contrast agents that can detect and characterize thrombi have been developed, and fibrin has been identified by lipid-encapsulated perfluorocarbon paramagnetic nanoparticles in vitro (362,366) as well as in vivo (362).

Magnetic Resonance Imaging of Carotid Atherosclerosis

The carotid artery has become the most common target vessel for MR imaging of atherosclerosis. Reasons for this include the use of phased-array coils, well-validated multicontrast imaging protocols (336,354), and the existence of a reference based on histologic examination of atherosclerotic lesions obtained surgically during carotid endarterectomy (367). MRI has been used to demonstrate the state of carotid plaque substructure, including the fibrous cap (Fig. 54.8). In one study, the in vivo state of the fibrous cap was characterized based on its appearance on MR images (intact and thin, intact and thick or ruptured), and there was a high level of agreement between MR images and the histologic state of the fibrous cap (356). When multicontrast MR imaging was compared to histology, a sensitivity of 81% and a specificity of 90% were demonstrated for

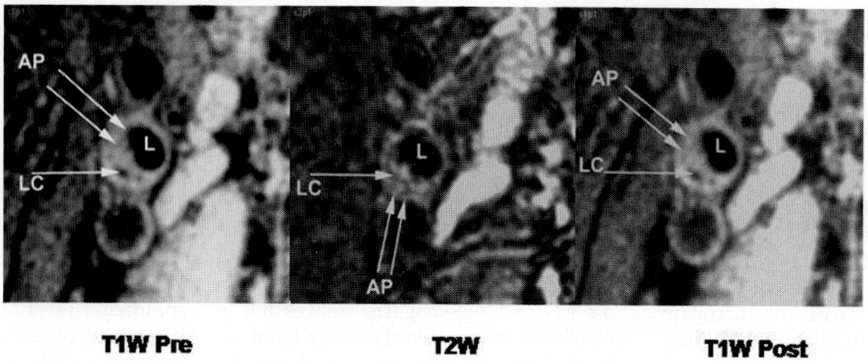

FIGURE 54.8. Carotid MRI in an atherosclerotic patient. **Left:** Precontrast T1-weighted image showing atherosclerotic plaque (AP) with lipid core (LC). L, lumen. **Middle:** Precontrast T2-weighted image showing atherosclerotic plaque with lipid core and lumen. **Right:** Postcontrast T1-weighted image showing atherosclerotic plaque with lipid core.

identification of an unstable fibrous cap (368). A ruptured fibrous cap identified on MR imaging was highly associated with a stroke or transient ischemic attack (369). MRI also has a high sensitivity and specificity in detecting lipid core, hemorrhage, and calcification in ex vivo imaging (90% to 100%) (370) and in vivo study (85% to 92%) (351) of endarterectomy specimens. Studies have demonstrated the ability of MRI to detect longitudinal changes in plaque size after aggressive therapeutic intervention using statins. A recent study compared the effects of aggressive and conventional lipid lowering by two different doses of simvastatin on early human atherosclerotic lesions using serial carotid and aortic (see subsequent discussion) MRI (371). Post hoc analysis showed that patients reaching a mean on-treatment low-density-lipoprotein cholesterol of 100 mg/dL or less had larger decreases in plaque size. In another study of 21 asymptomatic hypercholesterolemic patients, use of simvastatin resulted in 8% reduction in carotid wall thickness (372). In a recent study, we demonstrated the ability of MRI to show associations between cholesterol subfractions and atherosclerotic plaque components of carotid artery (347).

Magnetic Resonance Imaging of Aortic Atherosclerosis

Aortic atherosclerosis can be accurately detected using surface MRI when compared to histopathology (373) and transesophageal echocardiography (TEE) as a reference (337). It has been demonstrated that MR assessment of the aorta correlated well with TEE for the assessment of plaque thickness, extent, and composition. This technique has been found to be highly reproducible (343). In participants in the Framingham Heart Study, aortic plaque burden increases with age (374). MRI of the aorta demonstrated plaque regression by 8% after 1 year of lipid-lowering therapy using simvastatin without a change in the cross-sectional area of the arterial lumen (372,375). In another study of aortic atherosclerosis, the effects of 20-mg versus 5-mg atorvastatin was investigated on thoracic and abdominal aortic plaques in 40 hypercholesterolemic patients (376). The 20-mg dose reduced vessel wall thickness and area of thoracic aortic plaques (−12% and −18%, respectively; $p < .001$), whereas the 5-mg dose did not (+1% and +4%, respectively). In abdominal aortic plaques, even 20 mg could not reduce the vessel wall thickness or area (−1% and +3%, respectively), but instead progression was observed with the 5-mg treatment (+5% and +12%, respectively; $p < .01$). Another technique, transesophageal MRI (TEMRI), using a loopless antenna coil, has been developed for improved aortic MRI. The feasibility and utility of this technique were demonstrated in patients with aortic atherosclerosis (377). It was recently demonstrated that the addition of the TEMRI coil increased the signal by 157% to 225% in the aortic arch and descending aorta, respectively, above that attained by surface coils alone (348). Furthermore, using the combined surface MRI and TEMRI, it was recently demonstrated that aortic plaque regression of about 12% can be detected as early as 6 months (as compared to 1 year or longer) after lipid-lowering therapy (378).

Magnetic Resonance Imaging of Coronary Atherosclerosis

To successfully image coronary artery vessel wall and the atherosclerotic changes associated with it, a high contrast between the coronary lumen blood pool and the surrounding coronary vessel wall is mandatory. The first successful implementations of coronary vessel wall imaging in humans included the use of a dual-inversion fast spin-echo sequence. Using this method, single slices of the coronary artery vessel wall could be acquired during a prolonged breath-hold period, and relative thickening of the coronary arterial vessel wall could successfully be demonstrated in selected cases (338). Subsequently, and to remove the limitations associated with breath-holding, this technique was extended with the use of navigators for free-breathing data acquisition (379). More recently, the free-breathing navigator approach was combined with 3D spiral imaging in conjunction with a "local inversion" technique (380). This enables a larger anatomic coverage with reconstructed slices that are much thinner than those of the earlier 2D approaches. Therefore, it is now possible to visualize long, contiguous sections of the coronary artery vessel wall in a highly reproducible manner (381). This local-inversion 3D spiral technique was used to demonstrate positive arterial remodeling of the coronary vessel wall was (341). This novel approach has the potential of quantifying subclinical disease as well as following changes in the coronary vessel wall longitudinally.

Future developments will include the use of higher magnetic field strengths, contrast agents for plaque characterizations (358,359), and longitudinal studies of vessel wall thickness after interventions (382). Other potential applications include individually tailored therapy in patients based on their plaque characteristics and plaque burden, use as a screening tool to stratify patients based on their cardiovascular risk, and in vivo molecular imaging of the atherosclerotic plaque.

Molecular Imaging Using Magnetic Resonance Imaging

Technological advances in genomics, proteomics, and molecular biology are creating an unprecedented opportunity to change the current reactive medical paradigm of "see and treat" to an early "detect and prevent" strategy. Among these personal-medicine technologies, MRI is proving to be particularly advantageous, given its abilities to simultaneously elicit both anatomic and physiologic information with high spatial resolution as well as extract quantitative data from targeted contrast agents. Molecular imaging contrast agents take many forms, including the successful emergence of nanoparticulate systems. These contrast agents passively accumulate in clearance organ/cells or preferentially target biochemical signatures of disease via homing ligands. Nanoparticulate agents can be used to track cellular migration and tissue integration after local implantation or systemic injection. Contrast agents concentrate within a site by either passive or active targeting mechanisms. Passive targeting agents primarily highlight phagocytic cells and organs naturally responsible for particle clearance within the body, and are removed from the circulation in a size-dependent hierarchy by the lung (largest), spleen, liver, and bone marrow (smallest). Active targeting refers to ligand-directed, site-specific accumulation of contrast and/or therapeutic agents. A wide variety of ligands, including antibodies, peptides, polysaccharides, aptamers, and drugs, may be utilized to specifically home agents to cellular biomarkers. These ligands may be attached covalently (i.e., chemical conjugation) or noncovalently (e.g., avidin-biotin interactions) to the contrast agent.

Superparamagnetic Nanoparticles

In general terms, iron oxide particles are categorized based on their nominal diameter into superparamagnetic iron oxides (SPIOs; 50 to 500 nm) and ultrasmall SPIOs (USPIOs; <50 nm), which dictates their physicochemical and pharmacokinetic properties. SPIOs have been investigated with MRI for detection of atherosclerosis in ApoE−/− mice (383), and findings have been corroborated with histology. In these studies, SPIO particles were phagocytosed by macrophages and superficially restricted to the subendothelium of atherosclerotic plaques. Newly recruited macrophages represented most of the iron-laden cells, which explains the preferential targeting of superficial aspects of atherosclerotic lesions. The creation of USPIOs with a mean diameter of 10 to 50 μm (384) has resulted in increased intravascular half-life because these particles are not immediately recognized by the mononuclear phagocytic system in the liver and spleen. Although the concentration of USPIOs in macrophages has been confirmed histologically in atherosclerotic plaque, the particles are small enough to migrate through interendothelial junctions and capillary pores or fissures (385,386) and then potentially accumulate in the vascular wall. USPIOs are phagocytosed by macrophages in atherosclerotic plaque of Watanabe heritable hyperlipidemic (WHHL) rabbits (as confirmed by histology) in quantities sufficient to be detected by MRI (364), and accumulation of USPIOs in rat macrophages has been associated with cardiac allograft rejection (387). Recently, USPIOs have been used in humans to detect atherosclerotic plaques in vivo (361). Atherosclerotic lesions with high macrophage content in carotid arteries caused significant MR signal decreases in vivo. This finding correlated with histologic analysis after carotid endarterectomy.

Cell Tracking of Iron Oxides. The concept of cellular tracking takes advantage of the strong effects of iron oxide on T2 relaxation and the high spatial resolution that results from diminished background disturbance when individual cells are magnetically labeled before reaching their target location. MRI tracking of mesenchymal stem cell (MSC) implantation and engraftment into injured myocardium has been reported in a porcine myocardial infarction model (388). In these injured animals, magnetically labeled mesenchymal stem cells were injected into the myocardium via a catheter under x-ray fluoroscopy guidance, and conventional 1.5-T MRI was used to visualize the MR-MSCs over the next 3 weeks. MRI location of the superparamagnetic cells at 3 weeks was corroborated by histology. A recently developed MR-trackable intramyocardial injection catheter for implantation of MR-MSC has been successfully tested in two canine and one porcine closed-chest myocardial infarction models (389) and offers the possibility of a simpler, MR-based-only cell delivery technique.

Paramagnetic Nanoparticles

Although SPIOs produce dark or negative contrast effects that obscure image detail immediately around the particle, paramagnetic agents offer bright contrast in T1-weighted images.

Perfluorocarbon Nanoparticles. Liquid perfluorocarbon nanoparticle (PFC) emulsions provide a lipid surface area that can be functionalized with homing ligands, magnetic labels, and hydophobic drugs. The larger size of PFC nanoparticles (250 nm nominal diameter) focuses their utility toward vascular-accessible targets, such as thrombosis, atherosclerosis, restenosis, and other angiogenic-dependent diseases. Each bound paramagnetic nanoparticle delivers 50,000 to 90,000 or more gadolinium ions (362,390), which can be detected with low-resolution scans. PFC nanoparticles have been targeted to a variety of molecular epitopes, including high-density epitopes, such as fibrin in thrombi, and very sparse biomarkers, such as integrins in neovascular beds. One molecular signature, $\alpha v\beta 3$-integrin, is expressed on the luminal surface of activated endothelial and smooth muscle cells in injured media but not on mature quiescent cells. In New Zealand White (NZW) rabbits bearing 12d Vx-2 tumors (<1.0 cm), $\alpha v\beta 3$-integrin-targeted nanoparticles sensitively detect angiogenic endothelium at 1.5 T (391). Molecular images of $\alpha v\beta 3$-integrin expression obtained with MRI paralleled those obtained with immunohistochemical staining, which revealed an asymmetric distribution along the border of the tumor capsule. The MRI signal from tumor neovasculature was enhanced by 126% within 2 hours of injection by $\alpha v\beta 3$-integrin-targeted nanoparticles. Moreover, in vivo competition-blockade studies diminished targeted signal enhancement by more than 50%, which supports the specificity of the $\alpha v\beta 3$-integrin-targeted paramagnetic agent. Angiogenesis is also central to the progression of atherosclerotic plaque development. Noninvasive, specific recognition of angiogenesis in early vascular disease is not possible with current medical imaging techniques. However, $\alpha v\beta 3$-integrin-targeted paramagnetic nanoparticles have been demonstrated to spatially localize and quantify early atherosclerotic burdens in hyperlipidemic NZW rabbits (392). In addition, recent studies have demonstrated the unique capability of these agents to locally deliver antiangiogenic therapy via a process termed contact-facilitated drug delivery.

Interventional Cardiovascular Magnetic Resonance Imaging

In recent years, with the improvements in MR-scanner hardware, superfast interactive MRI, and development of miniature MR-compatible internal catheters, guidewires, and ablation catheters, the field of interventional and therapeutic MRI has been expanding at a very rapid rate. Furthermore, because of radiation-related issues, which are generally compounded in children, pediatric interventional MRI appears promising. The biggest stumbling block for real-time MR techniques was the inability of the imaging hardware to perform these tasks because they were not designed for this purpose. One of the most important developments has been that of real-time MRI.

Real-Time Magnetic Resonance Imaging

Advances in MR gradient hardware have made it possible to rapidly encode spatial information of the imaging data required to produce a 256 × 256 image of a 24-cm field of view (about

1 mm spatial resolution) in about 120 msec. If the spatial resolution is reduced to 128 × 128, this time is further reduced to 50 msec (20 frames/second). The next important development in this field was the ability to perform real-time interactive manipulations of the imaging data utilizing a user interface in conjunction with a short-bore cardiovascular scanner and fast spiral imaging. Such developments lead to (a) rapid data acquisition, data transfer, image reconstruction, and real-time display, (b) interactive real-time control of the image slice, and (c) high-quality images without cardiac or respiratory gating. The real-time MR-hardware platform consists of a workstation and a bus adapter and can be adapted onto a conventional scanner at a reasonable cost.

Accurate visualization and positioning of the interventional devices in relation to the surrounding anatomy is critical for a successful and safe image-guided interventional procedure. There are primarily two methods that have evolved over the years to aid in navigation of endovascular navigation of the interventional devices: passive and active MR tracking (393,394). Passive MR tracking techniques are based on visualization of the signal void and susceptibility artifacts caused by the interventional instruments themselves due to displacement of the protons. This form of tracking constitutes the normal imaging process and does not require any extra postprocessing or hardware. The artifact generated by a particular material depends on a multitude of factors including the magnetic field strength, the spatial orientation of the device with respect to the magnetic field, the physical cross section of the device, the pulse sequence, and the imaging parameters. Active tracking requires the creation of a signal that is actively detected or emitted by the device to identify its location. This can be achieved by visualizing a signal from a miniature radiofrequency (RF) coil that is incorporated into the commercially available interventional devices such as embolization catheters and balloon catheters (394–397). The miniature coils are connected, through a fully insulated coaxial cable embedded in the catheter wall, onto the surface coil reception port for signal reception. A coil-tipped catheter is made by winding the miniature coil, which is a copper wire spiral, for 16 to 20 turns around the tips of interventional devices to actively identify their position (394,396). In the active tracking technique, the position of the device is derived from the signal received by a miniature RF coil that is attached to the instrument itself (394,398,399). Three-dimensional coordinates of the coil can be tracked in real time at 20 frames/second with a spatial resolution of 1 mm. The position of the coil is used to control the motion of a cursor over a scout (road map) image. Another technique in active tracking uses a loopless antenna (400) consisting of a conducting wire that is an extended inner conductor from a coaxial cable. A loopless antenna is particularly useful because it provides a superior field of view when compared to internal coils. In this regard, although it was first developed to guide endovascular procedures (400), it was adapted to support transesophageal MRI (401) and later the entire development of MR-guided electrophysiology (also see later discussion) (402). The entire body of the loopless antenna can be observed under MR imaging. This antenna can be either directly inserted into small or tortuous vessels or placed into the central channel of interventional devices. Because the loopless antenna is expected to function not only as an intravascular MR receiver probe for intravascular MR imaging and for creation of intravascular MR fluoroscopy, but also as a conventional guidewire for interventional MR imaging, it is called an MR imaging-guidewire (MRIG) (403). Indeed, for reasons of safety and for technical purposes, such as torque control and subselective placement as well as negotiation of hard atherosclerotic lesions, this antenna/guidewire must also function as an imaging receiver probe intravascular MR-guided interventional procedures are performed. The MRIG has been tested in vivo and found to be useful for both intravascular MR imaging and cardiovascular interventional MR imaging (404).

Applications of Interventional Cardiovascular Magnetic Resonance Imaging

Magnetic Resonance Imaging–Guided Balloon Angioplasty. The notion that endovascular procedures could be performed under MRI guidance stemmed from studies that tested (395,405,406) and validated (407) the use of intravascular coils. With the development of newer active and passive tracking techniques, ultrafast imaging, gadolinium-filled balloons, and small-diameter coils, performance and monitoring of balloon angioplasty using MRI has become technically feasible. A cable-tie created stenotic model has been used to test the monitoring of the inflation/deflation of an angioplasty balloon catheter of a rabbit aorta (403,404). In this study, a 1.5-F loopless antenna was used as a guidewire with a standard 4-cm, 4-F balloon angioplasty catheter. The intravascular antenna was also used as a high-resolution imaging probe to monitor vessel dilation using an MR fluoroscopy sequence. A subsequent study with the same stenotic model demonstrated the feasibility of performing intravascular MR-guided balloon angioplasty in vivo. Recently, the feasibility of using MR imaging to guide balloon angioplasty of renal artery stenosis generated by a constrictor has been demonstrated using a passive tracking approach with MR angiography (408). In addition, the success of MRI-guided percutaneous transluminal coronary angioplasty (PTCA) in living animals has been reported. Using active tracking methods, investigators performed the entire process, including (a) catheterization of the targeted coronary artery, (b) generation of selective coronary MR angiography, (c) creation of high-resolution MR images of the target coronary arterial wall, and (d) positioning and inflation/deflation of an angioplasty balloon under MRI guidance (409).

Magnetic Resonance Imaging–Guided Stent Imaging and Placement. The feasibility of stent deployment in coronary and peripheral vasculature using MRI has also been tested in both animals and humans. Buecker et al. demonstrated the feasibility of MRI-guided iliac Nitinol stent placement in pigs using radial scanning together with a sliding window reconstruction technique (410). Stainless steel balloon-expandable coronary stents have recently been placed in animals under real-time MRI guidance using a newly developed real-time steady-state free-procession sequence with radial *k*-space sampling (411). In a porcine model, 10 of 11 stents were successfully placed in the left main coronary artery without complication. Manke et al. described the first human MRI-guided Nitinol stent placement study in 13 patients with iliac artery stenosis (412).

Magnetic Resonance Imaging–Guided Interventional Electrophysiology. Ablation procedures in electrophysiology are typically very long, with significant radiation exposure. MRI could be a logical alternative to x-ray fluoroscopic techniques with the following advantages: (a) real-time catheter placement with detailed endocardial anatomic information, (b) rapid high-resolution three-dimensional visualization of cardiac chambers, (c) high-resolution functional atrial imaging for evaluating atrial function and flow dynamics during therapy, (d) the potential for real-time spatial and temporal lesion monitoring during therapy, and (e) elimination of patient and physician radiation exposure. Using a standard external surface coil, it has been shown that (a) MR images and intracardiac electrograms could be acquired *during* radiofrequency ablation therapy using special filtering techniques, (b) nonmagnetic, MR-compatible catheters could be successfully visualized and placed at right atrial and right ventricular targets using real-time MR imaging sequences with interactive scan-plane modification, and (c) regional changes in ablated cardiac tissue can be detected (413). Intracardiac spectroscopic measurements made at least two decades ago (414) were the foundations for applying developments originally conceived to enable endovascular procedures (see prior discussion) for the purposes of guiding electrophysiologic studies (402). MRI-guided ablation therapy can visualize and monitor lesion formation with high temporal and spatial resolution. Lesions appear as elliptical hyperintense regions (most likely due to interstitial edema) directly adjacent to the catheter tip on T2-weighted turbo spin-echo images. MRI can detect changes due to heat-induced biophysical changes in cardiac tissue, such as interstitial edema, hyperemia, conformational changes, cellular shrinkage, and tissue coagulation. In addition, lesion detection 1 to 2 minutes after ablation with subsequent formation over 10 to 15 minutes is consistent with the temporal physiologic response of local acute interstitial edema.

In Vivo Magnetic Resonance Imaging of Vascular Gene Therapy. Gene therapy is rapidly emerging as a viable modality and has shown a tremendous potential in the treatment of atherosclerotic diseases. Recently, MRI has been tested for monitoring and guiding vascular gene delivery, tracking vascular gene expression, and enhancing vascular gene transfection/transduction (415). Gene transfer into a target-specific cell is a major challenge in this field and has a very low success rate (1%). Several studies have shown that gene transfection or expression can be significantly enhanced one- to fourfold with heating (416,417). Local heat generation at the target site using an easily placed internal heating source could be a logical way of achieving that. An MRI guidewire called an MR imaging-heating-guidewire (MRIHG) (400) can be used to deliver external thermal energy into the target vessels, and has the following functions: (a) as a receiver antenna to generate intravascular high-resolution MR imaging of atherosclerotic plaques of the vessel wall (418), (2) as a conventional guidewire to guide endovascular interventions under MRI (28,403), and (c) as an intravascular heating source to deliver external thermal energy into the target vessel wall during MRI of vascular gene delivery and thereby enhance vascular gene transfection.

Tracking gene expression involves the use of imaging methods to assess gene function by detecting functional transgene-encoding proteins (referred to as "imaging downstream") at the targets over time. MRI can be used to track overexpression of the transferrin gene, which produces a cell-surface transferrin receptor. The transferrin receptor is then probed specifically by a superparamagnetic transferrin that can be subsequently detected under MRI (419).

Safety of Interventional Magnetic Resonance Imaging

The obvious concerns with interventional MRI include electromagnetic exposure and internal heating in addition to intervention-related issues. Studies have found that conventional MRI is safe in this regard (420). Interventional procedures present new challenges, however, including the placement of monitoring equipment and surgical instruments in close proximity to a high magnetic field and in vivo placement of long conductive wires and electrical components in rapidly changing magnetic fields, all of which can lead to local heating (397). Such heating effects can be minimized by using a decoupling circuitry into the device, thus limiting the transfer of energy through the probe/wire by the transmit coil. In addition, the careful use of imaging sequences that limit RF power disposition and duration also helps to reduce the possibility of excessive heating. Existing studies do point toward the safety of this technology, but further comprehensive studies are required to further ascertain this.

References

1. Bloch F, Hansen WW, Packard ME. Nuclear induction. *Phys Rev* 1946;69:127.
2. Purcell EM, Torrey HC, Pound RV. Resonance absorption by nuclear magnetic movements in a solid. *Phys Rev* 1946;69:37.
3. Lauterbur P. Image formation by induced local interactions: examples employing nuclear magnetic resonance. *Nature* 1973;242:190.
4. Damadian R, Goldsmith M, Minkoff L. NMR in cancer: XVI. FONAR image of the live human body. *Physiol Chem Phys* 1977;9(1):97–100, 108.
5. Alfidi RJ, Haaga JR, El-Yousef SJ, et al. Preliminary experimental results in humans and animals with a superconducting, whole-body, nuclear magnetic resonance scanner. *Radiology* 1982;143(1):175–181.
6. Herfkens RJ, Higgins CB, Hricak H, et al. Nuclear magnetic resonance imaging of the cardiovascular system: normal and pathologic findings. *Radiology* 1983;147(3):749–759.
7. Sechtem U, Pflugfelder PW, White RD, et al. Cine MR imaging: potential for the evaluation of cardiovascular function. *AJR Am J Roentgenol* 1987;148(2):239–246.
8. Firmin DN, Nayler GL, Klipstein RH, et al. In vivo validation of MR velocity imaging. *J Comput Assist Tomogr* 1987;11(5):751–756.
9. Frahm J, Haase A, Matthaei D. Rapid NMR imaging of dynamic processes using the FLASH technique. *Magn Reson Med* 1986;3(2):321–327.
10. Atkinson DJ, Edelman RR. Cineangiography of the heart in a single breath hold with a segmented turboFLASH sequence. *Radiology* 1991;178(2):357–360.
11. Rzedzian RR, Pykett IL. Instant images of the human heart using a new, whole-body MR imaging system. *AJR Am J Roentgenol* 1987;149(2):245–250.
12. Zerhouni EA, Parish DM, Rogers WJ, et al. Human heart: tagging with MR imaging—a method for noninvasive assessment of myocardial motion. *Radiology* 1988;169(1):59–63.
13. Edelman RR, Mattle HP, Atkinson DJ, et al. MR angiography. *AJR Am J Roentgenol* 1990;154(5):937–946.
14. Mezrich R. A perspective on K-space. *Radiology* 1995;195(2):297–315.
15. Chien D, Edelman RR. Ultrafast imaging using gradient echoes. *Magn Reson Q* 1991;7(1):31–56.
16. Boxt LM. Radiology of the right ventricle. *Radiol Clin North Am* 1999;37(2):379–400.
17. Carr JC, Simonetti O, Bundy J, et al. Cine MR angiography of the heart with segmented true fast imaging with steady-state precession. *Radiology* 2001;219(3):828–834.
18. Axel L, Dougherty L. MR imaging of motion with spatial modulation of magnetization. *Radiology* 1989;171(3):841–845.
19. Reichek N. MRI myocardial tagging. *J Magn Reson Imaging* 1999;10(5):609–616.
20. Pan L, Lima JA, Osman NF. Fast tracking of cardiac motion using 3D-HARP. *Inf Process Med Imaging* 2003;18:611–622.
21. Rebergen SA, Niezen RA, Helbing WA, et al. Cine gradient-echo MR imaging and MR velocity mapping in the evaluation of congenital heart disease. *Radiographics* 1996;16(3):467–481.
22. Rebergen SA, van der Wall EE, Doornbos J, et al. Magnetic resonance measurement of velocity and flow: technique, validation, and cardiovascular applications. *Am Heart J* 1993;126(6):1439–1456.
23. Silber HA, Ouyang P, Bluemke DA, et al. A novel method for assessing arterial endothelial function using phase contrast magnetic resonance imaging: vasoconstriction during reduced shear. *J Cardiovasc Magn Reson* 2005;7(4):615–621.
24. Silber HA, Bluemke DA, Ouyang P, et al. The relationship between vascular wall shear stress and flow-mediated dilation: endothelial function assessed by phase-contrast magnetic resonance angiography. *J Am Coll Cardiol* 2001;38(7):1859–1865.
25. Prince MR. Gadolinium-enhanced MR aortography. *Radiology* 1994;191(1):155–164.
26. Kim RJ, Shah DJ, Judd RM. How we perform delayed enhancement imaging. *J Cardiovasc Magn Reson* 2003;5(3):505–514.
27. Simonetti OP, Kim RJ, Fieno DS, et al. An improved MR imaging technique for the visualization of myocardial infarction. *Radiology* 2001;218(1):215–223.
28. Kellman P, Arai AE, McVeigh ER, et al. Phase-sensitive inversion recovery for detecting myocardial infarction using gadolinium-delayed hyperenhancement. *Magn Reson Med* 2002;47(2):372–383.
29. Oshinski JN, Yang Z, Jones JR, et al. Imaging time after Gd-DTPA injection is critical in using delayed enhancement to determine infarct size accurately with magnetic resonance imaging. *Circulation* 2001;104(23):2838–2842.
30. Dinsmore RE, Wismer GL, Levine RA, et al. Magnetic resonance imaging of the heart: positioning and gradient angle selection for optimal imaging planes. *AJR Am J Roentgenol* 1984;143(6):1135–1142.
31. White RD, Cassidy MM, Cheitlin MD, et al. Segmental evaluation of left ventricular wall motion after myocardial infarction: magnetic resonance imaging versus echocardiography. *Am Heart J* 1988;115(1 Pt 1):166–175.
32. Fischer SE, Wickline SA, Lorenz CH. Novel real-time R-wave detection algorithm based on the vectorcardiogram for accurate gated magnetic resonance acquisitions. *Magn Reson Med* 1999;42(2):361–370.

33. Stuber M, Botnar RM, Fischer SE, et al. Preliminary report on in vivo coronary MRA at 3 Tesla in humans. *Magn Reson Med* 2002;48(3):425–429.
34. Danias PG, Stuber M, Botnar RM, et al. Navigator assessment of breath-hold duration: impact of supplemental oxygen and hyperventilation. *AJR Am J Roentgenol* 1998;171(2):395–397.
35. Liu YL, Riederer SJ, Rossman PJ, et al. A monitoring, feedback, and triggering system for reproducible breath-hold MR imaging. *Magn Reson Med* 1993;30(4):507–511.
36. Wang Y, Grimm RC, Rossman PJ, et al. 3D coronary MR angiography in multiple breath-holds using a respiratory feedback monitor. *Magn Reson Med* 1995;34(1):11–16.
37. Ehman RL, Felmlee JP. Adaptive technique for high-definition MR imaging of moving structures *Radiology* 1989;173(1):255–263.
38. Stuber M, Botnar RM, Danias PG, et al. Double-oblique free-breathing high resolution three-dimensional coronary magnetic resonance angiography. *J Am Coll Cardiol* 1999;34(2):524–531.
39. Shellock FG, Kanal E. Guidelines and recommendations for MR imaging safety and patient management. III. Questionnaire for screening patients before MR procedures The SMRI Safety Committee. *J Magn Reson Imaging* 1994;4(5):749–751.
40. Roguin A, Zviman MM, Meininger GR, et al. Modern pacemaker and implantable cardioverter/defibrillator systems can be magnetic resonance imaging safe: in vitro and in vivo assessment of safety and function at 1.5 T. *Circulation* 2004;110(5):475–482.
41. Martin ET, Coman JA, Shellock FG, et al. Magnetic resonance imaging and cardiac pacemaker safety at 1.5-Tesla. *J Am Coll Cardiol* 2004;43(7):1315–1324.
42. Edwards MB, Taylor KM, Shellock FG. Prosthetic heart valves: evaluation of magnetic field interactions, heating, and artifacts at 1.5 T. *J Magn Reson Imaging* 2000;12(2):363–369.
43. Stratemeier EJ, Thompson R, Brady TJ, et al. Ejection fraction determination by MR imaging: comparison with left ventricular angiography. *Radiology* 1986;158(3):775–777.
44. van Rossum AC, Visser FC, van Eenige MJ, et al. Magnetic resonance imaging of the heart for determination of ejection fraction. *Int J Cardiol* Jan 1988;18(1):53–63.
45. Sakuma H, Fujita N, Foo TK, et al. Evaluation of left ventricular volume and mass with breath-hold cine MR imaging. *Radiology* 1993;188(2):377–380.
46. Van Rossum AC, Visser FC, Sprenger M, et al. Evaluation of magnetic resonance imaging for determination of left ventricular ejection fraction and comparison with angiography. *Am J Cardiol* 1988;62(9):628–633.
47. Meese RB, Spritzer CE, Negro-Vilar R, et al. Detection, characterization and functional assessment of reperfused Q-wave acute myocardial infarction by cine magnetic resonance imaging. *Am J Cardiol* 1990;66(1):1–9.
48. Pettigrew RI. Dynamic cardiac MR imaging. Techniques and applications. *Radiol Clin North Am* 1989;27(6):1183–1203.
49. Higgins CB, Holt W, Pflugfelder P, et al. Functional evaluation of the heart with magnetic resonance imaging. *Magn Reson Med* 1988;6(2):121–139.
50. Gerber BL, Garot J, Bluemke DA, et al. Accuracy of contrast-enhanced magnetic resonance imaging in predicting improvement of regional myocardial function in patients after acute myocardial infarction. *Circulation* 2002;106(9):1083–1089.
51. Kramer CM, Lima JA, Reichek N, et al. Regional differences in function within noninfarcted myocardium during left ventricular remodeling. *Circulation* 1993;88(3):1279–1288.
52. Lima JA, Jeremy R, Guier W, et al. Accurate systolic wall thickening by nuclear magnetic resonance imaging with tissue tagging: correlation with sonomicrometers in normal and ischemic myocardium. *J Am Coll Cardiol* 1993;21(7):1741–1751.
53. Aletras AH, Balaban RS, Wen H. High-resolution strain analysis of the human heart with fast-DENSE. *J Magn Reson* 1999;140(1):41–57.
54. Osman NF, Sampath S, Atalar E, et al. Imaging longitudinal cardiac strain on short-axis images using strain-encoded MRI. *Magn Reson Med* 2001; 46(2):324–334.
55. MacGowan GA, Shapiro EP, Azhari H, et al. Noninvasive measurement of shortening in the fiber and cross-fiber directions in the normal human left ventricle and in idiopathic dilated cardiomyopathy. *Circulation* 1997;96(2):535–541.
56. Garot J, Bluemke DA, Osman NF, et al. Transmural contractile reserve after reperfused myocardial infarction in dogs. *J Am Coll Cardiol* 2000;36(7): 2339–2346.
57. Melillo G, Lima JA, Judd RM, et al. Intrinsic myocyte dysfunction and tyrosine kinase pathway activation underlie the impaired wall thickening of adjacent regions during postinfarct left ventricular remodeling. *Circulation* 1996;93(7):1447–1458.
58. Lima JA, Becker LC, Melin JA, et al. Impaired thickening of nonischemic myocardium during acute regional ischemia in the dog. *Circulation* 1985;71(5):1048–1059.
59. Smalling RW, Ekas RD, Felli PR, et al. Reciprocal functional interaction of adjacent myocardial segments during regional ischemia: an intraventricular loading phenomenon affecting apparent regional contractile function in the intact heart. *J Am Coll Cardiol* 1986;7(6):1335–1346.
60. Tscholakoff D, Higgins CB, McNamara MT, et al. Early-phase myocardial infarction: evaluation by MR imaging. *Radiology* 1986;159(3):667–672.
61. Filipchuk NG, Peshock RM, Malloy CR, et al. Detection and localization of recent myocardial infarction by magnetic resonance imaging. *Am J Cardiol* 1986;58(3):214–219.
62. Pflugfelder PW, Sechtem UP, White RD, et al. Quantification of regional myocardial function by rapid cine MR imaging. *AJR Am J Roentgenol* 1988;150(3):523–529.
63. Lotan CS, Cranney GB, Bouchard A, et al. The value of cine nuclear magnetic resonance imaging for assessing regional ventricular function. *J Am Coll Cardiol* 1989;14(7):1721–1729.
64. Fedele F, Scopinaro F, Montesano T, et al. Characterization of reversible myocardial dysfunction by magnetic resonance imaging. *Herz* 1994;19(4): 210–220.
65. Kramer CM, Rogers WJ, Theobald TM, et al. Remote noninfarcted region dysfunction soon after first anterior myocardial infarction. A magnetic resonance tagging study. *Circulation* 1996;94(4):660–666.
66. Sayad DE, Willett DL, Hundley WG, et al. Dobutamine magnetic resonance imaging with myocardial tagging quantitatively predicts improvement in regional function after revascularization. *Am J Cardiol* 1998;82(9):1149–1151, A1110.
67. Geskin G, Kramer CM, Rogers WJ, et al. Quantitative assessment of myocardial viability after infarction by dobutamine magnetic resonance tagging. *Circulation* 1998;98(3):217–223.
68. Kramer CM, Malkowski MJ, Mankad S, et al. Magnetic resonance tagging and echocardiographic response to dobutamine and functional improvement after reperfused myocardial infarction. *Am Heart J* 2002;143(6): 1046–1051.
69. Moore CC, O'Dell WG, McVeigh ER, et al. Calculation of three-dimensional left ventricular strains from biplanar tagged MR images. *J Magn Reson Imaging* 1992;2(2):165–175.
70. O'Dell WG, Moore CC, Hunter WC, et al. Three-dimensional myocardial deformations: calculation with displacement field fitting to tagged MR images. *Radiology* 1995;195(3):829–835.
71. Young AA, Axel L, Dougherty L, et al. Validation of tagging with MR imaging to estimate material deformation. *Radiology* 1993;188(1):101–108.
72. Kraitchman DL, Sampath S, Castillo E, et al. Quantitative ischemia detection during cardiac magnetic resonance stress testing by use of FastHARP. *Circulation* 2003;107(15):2025–2030.
73. Osman NF, Kerwin WS, McVeigh ER, et al. Cardiac motion tracking using CINE harmonic phase (HARP) magnetic resonance imaging. *Magn Reson Med* 1999;42(6):1048–1060.
74. Keijer JT, Bax JJ, van Rossum AC, et al. Myocardial perfusion imaging: clinical experience and recent progress in radionuclide scintigraphy and magnetic resonance imaging. *Int J Card Imaging* 1997;13(5):415–431.
75. Nagel E, al-Saadi N, Fleck E. Cardiovascular magnetic resonance: myocardial perfusion. *Herz* 2000;25(4):409–416.
76. Laddis T, Manning WJ, Danias PG. Cardiac MRI for assessment of myocardial perfusion: current status and future perspectives. *J Nucl Cardiol* 2001;8(2):207–214.
77. Arai AE. Magnetic resonance first-pass myocardial perfusion imaging. *Top Magn Reson Imaging* 2000;11(6):383–398.
78. Wagner A, Mahrholdt H, Sechtem U, et al. MR imaging of myocardial perfusion and viability. *Magn Reson Imaging Clin North Am* 2003;11(1):49–66.
79. Tong CY, Prato FS, Wisenberg G, et al. Techniques for the measurement of the local myocardial extraction efficiency for inert diffusible contrast agents such as gadopentate dimeglumine. *Magn Reson Med* 1993;30(3): 332–336.
80. Wilke N, Jerosch-Herold M, Wang Y, et al. Myocardial perfusion reserve: assessment with multisection, quantitative, first-pass MR imaging. *Radiology* 1997;204(2):373–384.
81. Eichenberger AC, Schuiki E, Kochli VD, et al. Ischemic heart disease: assessment with gadolinium-enhanced ultrafast MR imaging and dipyridamole stress. *J Magn Reson Imaging* 1994;4(3):425–431.
82. Ishida N, Sakuma H, Motoyasu M, et al. Noninfarcted myocardium: correlation between dynamic first-pass contrast-enhanced myocardial MR imaging and quantitative coronary angiography. *Radiology* 2003;229(1): 209–216.
83. Penzkofer H, Wintersperger BJ, Knez A, et al. Assessment of myocardial perfusion using multisection first-pass MRI and color-coded parameter maps: a comparison to 99mTc Sesta MIBI SPECT and systolic myocardial wall thickening analysis. *Magn Reson Imaging* 1999;17(2):161–170.
84. Lombardi M, Kvaerness J, Torheim G, et al. Relationship between function and perfusion early after acute myocardial infarction. *Int J Cardiovasc Imaging* 2001;17(5):383–393.
85. Cullen JH, Horsfield MA, Reek CR, et al. A myocardial perfusion reserve index in humans using first-pass contrast-enhanced magnetic resonance imaging. *J Am Coll Cardiol* 1999;33(5):1386–1394.
86. Al-Saadi N, Nagel E, Gross M, et al. Noninvasive detection of myocardial ischemia from perfusion reserve based on cardiovascular magnetic resonance. *Circulation* 2000;101(12):1379–1383.
87. Al-Saadi N, Nagel E, Gross M, et al. Improvement of myocardial perfusion reserve early after coronary intervention: assessment with cardiac magnetic resonance imaging. *J Am Coll Cardiol* 2000;36(5):1557–1564.
88. Ibrahim T, Nekolla SG, Schreiber K, et al. Assessment of coronary flow reserve: comparison between contrast-enhanced magnetic resonance imaging

and positron emission tomography. *J Am Coll Cardiol* 2002;39(5):864–870.
89. Hartnell G, Cerel A, Kamalesh M, et al. Detection of myocardial ischemia: value of combined myocardial perfusion and cineangiographic MR imaging. *AJR Am J Roentgenol* 1994;163(5):1061–1067.
90. Lauerma K, Virtanen KS, Sipila LM, et al. Multislice MRI in assessment of myocardial perfusion in patients with single-vessel proximal left anterior descending coronary artery disease before and after revascularization. *Circulation* 1997;96(9):2859–2867.
91. Walsh EG, Doyle M, Lawson MA, et al. Multislice first-pass myocardial perfusion imaging on a conventional clinical scanner. *Magn Reson Med* 1995;34(1):39–47.
92. Panting JR, Gatehouse PD, Yang GZ, et al. Echo-planar magnetic resonance myocardial perfusion imaging: parametric map analysis and comparison with thallium SPECT. *J Magn Reson Imaging* 2001;13(2):192–200.
93. Keijer JT, van Rossum AC, van Eenige MJ, et al. Magnetic resonance imaging of regional myocardial perfusion in patients with single-vessel coronary artery disease: quantitative comparison with (201)thallium-SPECT and coronary angiography. *J Magn Reson Imaging* 2000;11(6):607–615.
94. Wilke NM, Jerosch-Herold M, Zenovich A, et al. Magnetic resonance first-pass myocardial perfusion imaging: clinical validation and future applications. *J Magn Reson Imaging* 1999;10(5):676–685.
95. Ambrosio G, Weisman HF, Mannisi JA, et al. Progressive impairment of regional myocardial perfusion after initial restoration of postischemic blood flow. *Circulation* 1989;80(6):1846–1861.
96. Lima JA, Judd RM, Bazille A, et al. Regional heterogeneity of human myocardial infarcts demonstrated by contrast—enhanced MRI. Potential mechanisms. *Circulation* 1995;92(5):1117–1125.
97. Wu KC, Zerhouni EA, Judd RM, et al. Prognostic significance of microvascular obstruction by magnetic resonance imaging in patients with acute myocardial infarction. *Circulation* 1998;97(8):765–772.
98. Ito H, Maruyama A, Iwakura K, et al. Clinical implications of the 'no reflow' phenomenon. A predictor of complications and left ventricular remodeling in reperfused anterior wall myocardial infarction. *Circulation* 1996;93(2):223–228.
99. Asanuma T, Tanabe K, Ochiai K, et al. Relationship between progressive microvascular damage and intramyocardial hemorrhage in patients with reperfused anterior myocardial infarction: myocardial contrast echocardiographic study. *Circulation* 1997;96(2):448–453.
100. Motoyama S, Kondo T, Anno H, et al. Relationship between thrombolytic therapy and perfusion defect detected by Gd-DTPA-enhanced fast magnetic resonance imaging in acute myocardial infarction. *J Cardiovasc Magn Reson* 2001;3(3):237–245.
101. Dendale PA, Franken PR, Waldman GJ, et al. Low-dosage dobutamine magnetic resonance imaging as an alternative to echocardiography in the detection of viable myocardium after acute infarction. *Am Heart J* 1995;130(1):134–140.
102. Baer FM, Voth E, LaRosee K, et al. Comparison of dobutamine transesophageal echocardiography and dobutamine magnetic resonance imaging for detection of residual myocardial viability. *Am J Cardiol* 1996;78(4):415–419.
103. Nagel E, Lehmkuhl HB, Bocksch W, et al. Noninvasive diagnosis of ischemia-induced wall motion abnormalities with the use of high-dose dobutamine stress MRI: comparison with dobutamine stress echocardiography. *Circulation* 1999;99(6):763–770.
104. Hundley WG, Morgan TM, Neagle CM, et al. Magnetic resonance imaging determination of cardiac prognosis. *Circulation* 2002;106(18):2328–2333.
105. Zamorano J, Delgado J, Almeria C, et al. Reason for discrepancies in identifying myocardial viability by thallium-201 redistribution, magnetic resonance imaging, and dobutamine echocardiography. *Am J Cardiol* 2002;90(5):455–459.
106. Klein C, Nekolla SG, Bengel FM, et al. Assessment of myocardial viability with contrast-enhanced magnetic resonance imaging: comparison with positron emission tomography. *Circulation* 2002;105(2):162–167.
107. Kuhl HP, Beek AM, van der Weerdt AP, et al. Myocardial viability in chronic ischemic heart disease: comparison of contrast-enhanced magnetic resonance imaging with (18)F-fluorodeoxyglucose positron emission tomography. *J Am Coll Cardiol* 2003;41(8):1341–1348.
108. Wagner A, Mahrholdt H, Holly TA, et al. Contrast-enhanced MRI and routine single photon emission computed tomography (SPECT) perfusion imaging for detection of subendocardial myocardial infarcts: an imaging study. *Lancet* 2003;361(9355):374–379.
109. Lee VS, Resnick D, Tiu SS, et al. MR imaging evaluation of myocardial viability in the setting of equivocal SPECT results with (99m)Tc sestamibi. *Radiology* 2004;230(1):191–197.
110. Kim RJ, Wu E, Rafael A, et al. The use of contrast-enhanced magnetic resonance imaging to identify reversible myocardial dysfunction. *N Engl J Med* 2000;343(20):1445–1453.
111. de Roos A, van der Wall EE, Bruschke AV, et al. Magnetic resonance imaging in the diagnosis and evaluation of myocardial infarction. *Magn Reson Q* 1991;7(3):191–207.
112. Wu E, Judd RM, Vargas JD, et al. Visualisation of presence, location, and transmural extent of healed Q-wave and non-Q-wave myocardial infarction. *Lancet* 2001;357(9249):21–28.
113. Weiss CR, Aletras AH, London JF, et al. Stunned, infarcted, and normal myocardium in dogs: simultaneous differentiation by using gadolinium-enhanced cine MR imaging with magnetization transfer contrast. *Radiology* 2003;226(3):723–730.
114. Beek AM, Kuhl HP, Bondarenko O, et al. Delayed contrast-enhanced magnetic resonance imaging for the prediction of regional functional improvement after acute myocardial infarction. *J Am Coll Cardiol* 2003;42(5):895–901.
115. Kwong RY, Schussheim AE, Rekhraj S, et al. Detecting acute coronary syndrome in the emergency department with cardiac magnetic resonance imaging. *Circulation* 2003;107(4):531–537.
116. Harrity P, Patel A, Bianco J, et al. Improved diagnosis and characterization of postinfarction left ventricular pseudoaneurysm by cardiac magnetic resonance imaging. *Clin Cardiol* 1991;14(7):603–606.
117. Kumbasar B, Wu KC, Kamel IR, et al. Left ventricular true aneurysm: diagnosis of myocardial viability shown on MR imaging. *AJR Am J Roentgenol* 2002;179(2):472–474.
118. Finn AV, Antman EM. Images in clinical medicine. Isolated right ventricular infarction. *N Engl J Med* 2003;349(17):1636.
119. Lieberman JM, Botti RE, Nelson AD. Magnetic resonance imaging of the heart. *Radiol Clin North Am* 1984;22(4):847–858.
120. Paulin S, von Schulthess GK, Fossel E, et al. MR imaging of the aortic root and proximal coronary arteries. *AJR Am J Roentgenol* 1987;148(4):665–670.
121. Huber ME, Paetsch I, Schnackenburg B, et al. Performance of a new gadolinium-based intravascular contrast agent in free-breathing inversion-recovery 3D coronary MRA. *Magn Reson Med* 2003;49(1):115–121.
122. Edelman RR, Manning WJ, Burstein D, et al. Coronary arteries: breath-hold MR angiography. *Radiology* 1991;181(3):641–643.
123. Li D, Paschal CB, Haacke EM, et al. Coronary arteries: three-dimensional MR imaging with fat saturation and magnetization transfer contrast. *Radiology*. 1993;187(2):401–406.
124. Brittain JH, Hu BS, Wright GA, et al. Coronary angiography with magnetization-prepared T2 contrast. *Magn Reson Med* 1995;33(5):689–696.
125. Botnar RM, Stuber M, Danias PG, et al. Improved coronary artery definition with T2-weighted, free-breathing, three-dimensional coronary MRA. *Circulation* 1999;99(24):3139–3148.
126. Stuber M, Botnar RM, Kissinger KV, et al. Free-breathing black-blood coronary MR angiography: initial results. *Radiology* 2001;219(1):278–283.
127. Stuber M, Botnar RM, Danias PG, et al. Contrast agent-enhanced, free-breathing, three-dimensional coronary magnetic resonance angiography. *J Magn Reson Imaging* 1999;10(5):790–799.
128. Hofman MBM, Henson RE, Kovacs SJ, et al. Blood pool agent strongly improves 3D magnetic resonance coronary angiography using an inversion pre-pulse. *Magn Reson Med* 1999;41(2):360–367.
129. Li D, Dolan RP, Walovitch RC, et al. Three-dimensional MRI of coronary arteries using an intravascular contrast agent. *Magn Reson Med* 1998;39:1014–1018.
130. Stillman AE, Wilke N, Jerosch-Herold M. Use of an intravascular T1 contrast agent to improve MR cine myocardial-blood pool definition in man. *J Magn Reson Imaging* 1997;7(4):765–767.
131. Taylor AM, Panting JR, Keegan J, et al. Safety and preliminary findings with the intravascular contrast agent NC100150 injection for MR coronary angiography. *J Magn Reson Imaging* 1999;9(2):220–227.
132. Goldfarb JW, Edelman RR. Coronary arteries: breath-hold, gadolinium-enhanced, three-dimensional MR angiography. *Radiology* 1998;206(3):830–834.
133. Kim WY, Danias PG, Stuber M, et al. Coronary magnetic resonance angiography for the detection of coronary stenoses. *N Engl J Med* 2001;345(26):1863–1869.
134. Herborn CU, Barkhausen J, Paetsch I, et al. Coronary arteries: contrast-enhanced MR imaging with SH L 643A—experience in 12 volunteers. *Radiology* 2003;229(1):217–223.
135. Manning WJ, Li W, Edelman RR. A preliminary report comparing magnetic resonance coronary angiography with conventional angiography. *N Engl J Med* 1993;328(12):828–832.
136. Duerinckx AJ, Urman MK. Two-dimensional coronary MR angiography: analysis of initial clinical results. *Radiology* 1994;193(3):731–738.
137. Post JC, van Rossum AC, Hofman MB, et al. Three-dimensional respiratory-gated MR angiography of coronary arteries: comparison with conventional coronary angiography. *AJR Am J Roentgenol* 1996;166(6):1399–1404.
138. Müller MF, Fleisch M, Kroeker R, et al. Proximal coronary artery stenosis: three-dimensional MRI with fat saturation and navigator echo. *J Magn Reson Imaging* 1997;7(4):644–651.
139. Post JC, van Rossum AC, Hofman MB, et al. Clinical utility of two-dimensional magnetic resonance angiography in detecting coronary artery disease. *Eur Heart J* 1997;18(3):426–433.
140. Pennell DJ, Bogren HG, Keegan J, et al. Assessment of coronary artery stenosis by magnetic resonance imaging. *Heart* 1996;75(2):127–133.
141. van Geuns RJ, Wielopolski PA, de Bruin HG, et al. MR coronary angiography with breath-hold targeted volumes: preliminary clinical results. *Radiology* 2000;217(1):270–277.
142. Globits S, Higgins CB. Assessment of valvular heart disease by magnetic resonance imaging. *Am Heart J* 1995;129(2):369–381.
143. Underwood SR, Klipstein RH, Firmin DN, et al. Magnetic resonance assessment of aortic and mitral regurgitation. *Br Heart J* 1986;56(5):455–462.

144. Casolo GC, Zampa V, Rega L, et al. Evaluation of mitral stenosis by cine magnetic resonance imaging. *Am Heart J* 1992;123(5):1252–1260.
145. Mitchell L, Jenkins JP, Watson Y, et al. Diagnosis and assessment of mitral and aortic valve disease by cine-flow magnetic resonance imaging. *Magn Reson Med* 1989;12(2):181–197.
146. Heidenreich PA, Steffens J, Fujita N, et al. Evaluation of mitral stenosis with velocity-encoded cine-magnetic resonance imaging. *Am J Cardiol* 1995;75(5):365–369.
147. Lin SJ, Brown PA, Watkins MP, et al. Quantification of stenotic mitral valve area with magnetic resonance imaging and comparison with Doppler ultrasound. *J Am Coll Cardiol* 2004;44(1):133–137.
148. Wagner S, Auffermann W, Buser P, et al. Diagnostic accuracy and estimation of the severity of valvular regurgitation from the signal void on cine magnetic resonance images. *Am Heart J* 1989;118(4):760–767.
149. Aurigemma G, Reichek N, Schiebler M, et al. Evaluation of mitral regurgitation by cine magnetic resonance imaging. *Am J Cardiol* 1990;66(5):621–625.
150. Nishimura T, Yamada N, Itoh A, et al. Cine MR imaging in mitral regurgitation: comparison with color Doppler flow imaging. *AJR Am J Roentgenol* 1989;153(4):721–724.
151. Glogar D, Globits S, Neuhold A, et al. Assessment of mitral regurgitation by magnetic resonance imaging. *Magn Reson Imaging* 1989;7(6):611–617.
152. Fujita N, Chazouilleres AF, Hartiala JJ, et al. Quantification of mitral regurgitation by velocity-encoded cine nuclear magnetic resonance imaging. *J Am Coll Cardiol* 1994;23(4):951–958.
153. Hundley WG, Li HF, Willard JE, et al. Magnetic resonance imaging assessment of the severity of mitral regurgitation. Comparison with invasive techniques. *Circulation* 1995;92(5):1151–1158.
154. Kupari M, Hekali P, Keto P, et al. Assessment of aortic valve area in aortic stenosis by magnetic resonance imaging. *Am J Cardiol* 1992;70(9):952–955.
155. Sondergaard L, Hildebrandt P, Lindvig K, et al. Valve area and cardiac output in aortic stenosis: quantification by magnetic resonance velocity mapping. *Am Heart J* 1993;126(5):1156–1164.
156. Eichenberger AC, Jenni R, von Schulthess GK. Aortic valve pressure gradients in patients with aortic valve stenosis: quantification with velocity-encoded cine MR imaging. *AJR Am J Roentgenol* 1993;160(5):971–977.
157. Caruthers SD, Lin SJ, Brown P, et al. Practical value of cardiac magnetic resonance imaging for clinical quantification of aortic valve stenosis: comparison with echocardiography. *Circulation* 2003;108(18):2236–2243.
158. Cranney GB, Benjelloun H, Perry GJ, et al. Rapid assessment of aortic regurgitation and left ventricular function using cine nuclear magnetic resonance imaging and the proximal convergence zone. *Am J Cardiol* 1993; 71(12):1074–1081.
159. Yoshida K, Yoshikawa J, Hozumi T, et al. Assessment of aortic regurgitation by the acceleration flow signal void proximal to the leaking orifice in cinemagnetic resonance imaging. *Circulation* 1991;83(6):1951–1955.
160. Nishimura F. Oblique cine MRI for the evaluation of aortic regurgitation: comparison with cineangiography. *Clin Cardiol* 1992;15(2):73–78.
161. Honda N, Machida K, Hashimoto M, et al. Aortic regurgitation: quantitation with MR imaging velocity mapping. *Radiology* 1993;186(1):189–194.
162. Pflugfelder PW, Landzberg JS, Cassidy MM, et al. Comparison of cine MR imaging with Doppler echocardiography for the evaluation of aortic regurgitation. *AJR Am J Roentgenol* 1989;152(4):729–735.
163. Sondergaard L, Lindvig K, Hildebrandt P, et al. Quantification of aortic regurgitation by magnetic resonance velocity mapping. *Am Heart J* 1993;125(4):1081–1090.
164. Wexler L, Higgins CB. The use of magnetic resonance imaging in adult congenital heart disease. *Am J Card Imaging* 1995;9(1):15–28.
165. Rebergen SA, Chin JG, Ottenkamp J, et al. Pulmonary regurgitation in the late postoperative follow-up of tetralogy of Fallot. Volumetric quantitation by nuclear magnetic resonance velocity mapping. *Circulation* 1993;88 (5 Pt 1):2257–2266.
166. Randall PA, Kohman LJ, Scalzetti EM, et al. Magnetic resonance imaging of prosthetic cardiac valves in vitro and in vivo. *Am J Cardiol* 1988;62(13): 973–976.
167. Deutsch HJ, Bachmann R, Sechtem U, et al. Regurgitant flow in cardiac valve prostheses: diagnostic value of gradient echo nuclear magnetic resonance imaging in reference to transesophageal two-dimensional color Doppler echocardiography. *J Am Coll Cardiol* 1992;19(7):1500–1507.
168. Richardson P, McKenna W, Bristow M, et al. Report of the 1995 World Health Organization/International Society and Federation of Cardiology Task Force on the Definition and Classification of Cardiomyopathies. *Circulation* 1996;93(5):841–842.
169. Bottini PB, Carr AA, Prisant LM, et al. Magnetic resonance imaging compared to echocardiography to assess left ventricular mass in the hypertensive patient. *Am J Hypertens* 1995;8(3):221–228.
170. Friedrich MG. Magnetic resonance imaging in cardiomyopathies. *J Cardiovasc Magn Reson.* 2000;2(1):67–82.
171. Aso H, Takeda K, Ito T, et al. Assessment of myocardial fibrosis in cardiomyopathic hamsters with gadolinium-DTPA enhanced magnetic resonance imaging. *Invest Radiol* 1998;33(1):22–32.
172. Neubauer S, Krahe T, Schindler R, et al. 31P magnetic resonance spectroscopy in dilated cardiomyopathy and coronary artery disease. Altered cardiac high-energy phosphate metabolism in heart failure. *Circulation* 1992;86(6):1810–1818.
173. Jung WI, Sieverding L, Breuer J, et al. 31P NMR spectroscopy detects metabolic abnormalities in asymptomatic patients with hypertrophic cardiomyopathy. *Circulation* 1998;97(25):2536–2542.
174. Kasper EK, Agema WR, Hutchins GM, et al. The causes of dilated cardiomyopathy: a clinicopathologic review of 673 consecutive patients. *J Am Coll Cardiol* 1994;23(3):586–590.
175. Benjelloun H, Cranney GB, Kirk KA, et al. Interstudy reproducibility of biplane cine nuclear magnetic resonance measurements of left ventricular function. *Am J Cardiol 15* 1991;67(16):1413–1420.
176. Buser PT, Auffermann W, Holt WW, et al. Noninvasive evaluation of global left ventricular function with use of cine nuclear magnetic resonance. *J Am Coll Cardiol* 1989;13(6):1294–1300.
177. Fujita N, Duerinekx AJ, Higgins CB. Variation in left ventricular regional wall stress with cine magnetic resonance imaging: normal subjects versus dilated cardiomyopathy. *Am Heart J* 1993;125(5 Pt 1):1337–1345.
178. Sechtem U, Pflugfelder PW, Gould RG, et al. Measurement of right and left ventricular volumes in healthy individuals with cine MR imaging. *Radiology* 1987;163(3):697–702.
179. Doherty 3rd NE, Seelos KC, Suzuki J, et al. Application of cine nuclear magnetic resonance imaging for sequential evaluation of response to angiotensin-converting enzyme inhibitor therapy in dilated cardiomyopathy. *J Am Coll Cardiol* 1992;19(6):1294–1302.
180. Semelka RC, Tomei E, Wagner S, et al. Normal left ventricular dimensions and function: interstudy reproducibility of measurements with cine MR imaging. *Radiology* 1990;174(3 Pt 1):763–768.
181. Friedrich MG, Strohm O, Schulz-Menger J, et al. Contrast media-enhanced magnetic resonance imaging visualizes myocardial changes in the course of viral myocarditis. *Circulation* 1998;97(18):1802–1809.
182. Bellotti G, Bocchi EA, de Moraes AV, et al. In vivo detection of *Trypanosoma cruzi* antigens in hearts of patients with chronic Chagas' heart disease. *Am Heart J* 1996;131(2):301–307.
183. Franke A, Schondube FA, Kuhl HP, et al. Quantitative assessment of the operative results after extended myectomy and surgical reconstruction of the subvalvular mitral apparatus in hypertrophic obstructive cardiomyopathy using dynamic three-dimensional transesophageal echocardiography. *J Am Coll Cardiol* 1998;31(7):1641–1649.
184. White RD, Obuchowski NA, Gunawardena S, et al. Left ventricular outflow tract obstruction in hypertrophic cardiomyopathy: presurgical and postsurgical evaluation by computed tomography magnetic resonance imaging. *Am J Card Imaging* 1996;10(1):1–13.
185. Kawada N, Sakuma H, Yamakado T, et al. Hypertrophic cardiomyopathy: MR measurement of coronary blood flow and vasodilator flow reserve in patients and healthy subjects. *Radiology* 1999;211(1):129–135.
186. Schulz-Menger J, Strohm O, Waigand J, et al. The value of magnetic resonance imaging of the left ventricular outflow tract in patients with hypertrophic obstructive cardiomyopathy after septal artery embolization. *Circulation* 2000;101(15):1764–1766.
187. Rosen BD, Gerber BL, Edvardsen T, et al. Late systolic onset of regional LV relaxation demonstrated in three-dimensional space by MRI tissue tagging. *Am J Physiol Heart Circ Physiol* 2004;287(4):H1740–H1746.
188. Stuber M, Scheidegger MB, Fischer SE, et al. Alterations in the local myocardial motion pattern in patients suffering from pressure overload due to aortic stenosis. *Circulation* 1999;100(4):361–368.
189. Suzuki J, Shimamoto R, Nishikawa J, et al. Morphological onset and early diagnosis in apical hypertrophic cardiomyopathy: a long term analysis with nuclear magnetic resonance imaging. *J Am Coll Cardiol* 1999;33(1):146–151.
190. Bogaert J, Goldstein M, Tannouri F, et al. Original report. Late myocardial enhancement in hypertrophic cardiomyopathy with contrast-enhanced MR imaging. *AJR Am J Roentgenol* 2003;180(4):981–985.
191. Moon JC, McKenna WJ, McCrohon JA, et al. Toward clinical risk assessment in hypertrophic cardiomyopathy with gadolinium cardiovascular magnetic resonance. *J Am Coll Cardiol* 2003;41(9):1561–1567.
192. Ricci C, Longo R, Pagnan L, et al. Magnetic resonance imaging in right ventricular dysplasia. *Am J Cardiol* 1992;70(20):1589–1595.
193. Blake LM, Scheinman MM, Higgins CB. MR features of arrhythmogenic right ventricular dysplasia. *AJR Am J Roentgenol* 1994;162(4):809–812.
194. Corrado D, Fontaine G, Marcus FI, et al. Arrhythmogenic right ventricular dysplasia/cardiomyopathy: need for an international registry. Study Group on Arrhythmogenic Right Ventricular Dysplasia/Cardiomyopathy of the Working Groups on Myocardial and Pericardial Disease and Arrhythmias of the European Society of Cardiology and of the Scientific Council on Cardiomyopathies of the World Heart Federation. *Circulation* 2000;101(11):E101–E106.
195. Carlson MD, White RD, Trohman RG, et al. Right ventricular outflow tract ventricular tachycardia: detection of previously unrecognized anatomic abnormalities using cine magnetic resonance imaging. *J Am Coll Cardiol* 1994;24(3):720–727.
196. Hartiala JJ, Mostbeck GH, Foster E, et al. Velocity-encoded cine MRI in the evaluation of left ventricular diastolic function: measurement of mitral valve and pulmonary vein flow velocities and flow volume across the mitral valve. *Am Heart J* 1993;125(4):1054–1066.
197. Flora GS, Sharma OP. Myocardial sarcoidosis: a review. *Sarcoidosis* 1989; 6(2):97–106.
198. Perry A, Vuitch F. Causes of death in patients with sarcoidosis. A morphologic study of 38 autopsies with clinicopathologic correlations. *Arch Pathol Lab Med* 1995;119(2):167–172.

199. Otake S, Banno T, Ohba S, et al. Muscular sarcoidosis: findings at MR imaging. *Radiology* 1990;176(1):145–148.
200. Shimada T, Shimada K, Sakane T, et al. Diagnosis of cardiac sarcoidosis and evaluation of the effects of steroid therapy by gadolinium-DTPA-enhanced magnetic resonance imaging. *Am J Med* 2001;110(7):520–527.
201. Siegelman ES, Mitchell DG, Semelka RC. Abdominal iron deposition: metabolism, MR findings, and clinical importance. *Radiology* 1996;199(1): 13–22.
202. Fattori R, Rocchi G, Celletti F, et al. Contribution of magnetic resonance imaging in the differential diagnosis of cardiac amyloidosis and symmetric hypertrophic cardiomyopathy. *Am Heart J* 1998;136(5):824–830.
203. Bull RK, Edwards PD, Dixon AK. CT dimensions of the normal pericardium. *Br J Radiol* 1998;71(849):923–925.
204. Isner JM, Carter BL, Bankoff MS, et al. Computed tomography in the diagnosis of pericardial heart disease. *Ann Intern Med* 1982;97(4):473–479.
205. Mulvagh SL, Rokey R, Vick 3rd GW, et al. Usefulness of nuclear magnetic resonance imaging for evaluation of pericardial effusions, and comparison with two-dimensional echocardiography. *Am J Cardiol* 1989;64(16):1002–1009.
206. Sechtem U, Tscholakoff D, Higgins CB. MRI of the abnormal pericardium. *AJR Am J Roentgenol* 1986;147(2):245–252.
207. Masui T, Finck S, Higgins CB. Constrictive pericarditis and restrictive cardiomyopathy: evaluation with MR imaging. *Radiology* 1992;182(2):369–373.
208. White CS. MR evaluation of the pericardium. *Top Magn Reson Imaging* 1995;7(4):258–266.
209. Seelos KC, Funari M, Chang JM, et al. Magnetic resonance imaging in acute and subacute mediastinal bleeding. *Am Heart J* 1992;123(5):1269–1272.
210. Vilacosta I, Gomez J, Dominguez J, et al. Massive pericardiac hematoma with severe constrictive pathophysiologic complications after insertion of an epicardial pacemaker. *Am Heart J* 1995;130(6):1298–1300.
211. Meleca MJ, Hoit BD. Previously unrecognized intrapericardial hematoma leading to refractory abdominal ascites. *Chest* 1995;108(6):1747–1748.
212. Brown DL, Ivey TD. Giant organized pericardial hematoma producing constrictive pericarditis: a case report and review of the literature. *J Trauma* 1996;41(3):558–560.
213. Ferguson ER, Blackwell GG, Murrah CP, et al. Evaluation of complex mediastinal masses by magnetic resonance imaging. *J Cardiovasc Surg (Torino)* 1998;39(1):117–119.
214. Isobe M, Yamaoki K, Sugiyama T, et al. Right ventricular inflow obstruction due to giant hematoma formed by chronic constrictive pericarditis. *Intern Med* 1993;32(4):346–349.
215. Higgins CB, Sakuma H. Heart disease: functional evaluation with MR imaging. *Radiology* 1996;199(2):307–315.
216. Abraham KP, Reddy V, Gattuso P. Neoplasms metastatic to the heart: review of 3314 consecutive autopsies. *Am J Cardiovasc Pathol* 1990;3(3):195–198.
217. Klatt EC, Heitz DR. Cardiac metastases. *Cancer* 1990;65(6):1456–1459.
218. Schoen FJ, Berger BM, Guerina NG. Cardiac effects of noncardiac neoplasms. *Cardiol Clin* 1984;2(4):657–670.
219. Fujita N, Caputo GR, Higgins CB. Diagnosis and characterization of intracardiac masses by magnetic resonance imaging. *Am J Card Imaging* 1994;8(1):69–80.
220. Enochs WS, Petherick P, Bogdanova A, et al. Paramagnetic metal scavenging by melanin: MR imaging. *Radiology* 1997;204(2):417–423.
221. Mousseaux E, Meunier P, Azancott S, et al. Cardiac metastatic melanoma investigated by magnetic resonance imaging. *Magn Reson Imaging* 1998; 16(1):91–95.
222. Funari M, Fujita N, Peck WW, et al. Cardiac tumors: assessment with Gd-DTPA enhanced MR imaging. *J Comput Assist Tomogr* 1991;15(6):953–958.
223. Hoffmann U, Globits S, Frank H. Cardiac and paracardiac masses. Current opinion on diagnostic evaluation by magnetic resonance imaging. *Eur Heart J* 1998;19(4):553–563.
224. Link KM, Loehr SP, Baker DM, et al. Magnetic resonance imaging of the thoracic aorta. *Semin Ultrasound CT MR* 1993;14(2):91–105.
225. White RD, Higgins CB. Magnetic resonance imaging of thoracic vascular disease. *J Thorac Imaging* 1989;4(2):34–50.
226. Auffermann W, Olofsson P, Stoney R, et al. MR imaging of complications of aortic surgery. *J Comput Assist Tomogr* 1987;11(6):982–989.
227. Ho VB, Kinney JB, Sahn DJ Ruptured sinus of Valsalva aneurysm: cine phase-contrast MR characterization. *J Comput Assist Tomogr* 1995;19(4): 652–656.
228. Kersting-Sommerhoff BA, Sechtem UP, Schiller NB, et al. MR imaging of the thoracic aorta in Marfan patients. *J Comput Assist Tomogr* 1987; 11(4):633–639.
229. Amparo EG, Higgins CB, Hricak H, et al. Aortic dissection: magnetic resonance imaging. *Radiology* 1985;155(2):399–406.
230. Debakey ME, Henly WS, Cooley DA, et al. Surgical management of dissecting aneurysms of the aorta. *J Thorac Cardiovasc Surg* 1965;49:130–149.
231. Yamada T, Tada S, Harada J. Aortic dissection without intimal rupture: diagnosis with MR imaging and CT. *Radiology* 1988;168(2):347–352.
232. Murray JG, Manisali M, Flamm SD, et al. Intramural hematoma of the thoracic aorta: MR image findings and their prognostic implications. *Radiology* 1997;204(2):349–355.
233. Nienaber CA, von Kodolitsch Y, Nicolas V, et al. The diagnosis of thoracic aortic dissection by noninvasive imaging procedures. *N Engl J Med* 1993;328(1):1–9.
234. Nienaber CA, Spielmann RP, von Kodolitsch Y, et al. Diagnosis of thoracic aortic dissection. Magnetic resonance imaging versus transesophageal echocardiography. *Circulation* 1992;85(2):434–447.
235. Flamm SD, VanDyke CW, White RD. MR imaging of the thoracic aorta. *Magn Reson Imaging Clin North Am* 1996;4(2):217–235.
236. Prince MR, Narasimham DL, Jacoby WT, et al. Three-dimensional gadolinium-enhanced MR angiography of the thoracic aorta. *AJR Am J Roentgenol* 1996;166(6):1387–1397.
237. Krinsky GA, Rofsky NM, DeCorato DR, et al. Thoracic aorta: comparison of gadolinium-enhanced three-dimensional MR angiography with conventional MR imaging. *Radiology* 1997;202(1):183–193.
238. Link KM, Lesko NM. The role of MR imaging in the evaluation of acquired diseases of the thoracic aorta. *AJR Am J Roentgenol* 1992;158(5):1115–1125.
239. Bank ER. Magnetic resonance of congenital cardiovascular disease. An update. *Radiol Clin North Am* 1993;31(3):553–572.
240. Tennant WG, Hartnell GG, Baird RN, et al. Inflammatory aortic aneurysms: characteristic appearance on magnetic resonance imaging. *Eur J Vasc Surg* 1992;6(4):399–402.
241. Yucel EK, Steinberg FL, Egglin TK, et al. Penetrating aortic ulcers: diagnosis with MR imaging. *Radiology* 1990;177(3):779–781.
242. Woodard PK, Patz EF, Sostman HD. Pseudoaneurysms at aortic cannulation site after coronary artery bypass graft: MR findings. *J Comput Assist Tomogr* 1992;16(6):883–887.
243. Nienaber CA, von Kodolitsch Y, Petersen B, et al. Intramural hemorrhage of the thoracic aorta. Diagnostic and therapeutic implications. *Circulation* 1995;92(6):1465–1472.
244. Ho VB, Kinney JB, Sahn DJ. Contributions of newer MR imaging strategies for congenital heart disease. *Radiographics* 1996;16(1):43–60; discussion 61.
245. Bisset 3rd GS, Strife JL, Kirks DR, et al. Vascular rings: MR imaging. *AJR Am J Roentgenol* 1987;149(2):251–256.
246. Ho VB, Prince MR. Thoracic MR aortography: imaging techniques and strategies. *Radiographics* 1998;18(2):287–309.
247. Welch TJ, Stanson AW, Sheedy 2nd PF, et al. Radiologic evaluation of penetrating aortic atherosclerotic ulcer. *Radiographics* 1990;10(4):675–685.
248. Spuentrup E, Buecker A, Katoh M, et al. Molecular magnetic resonance imaging of coronary thrombosis and pulmonary emboli with a novel fibrin-targeted contrast agent. *Circulation* 2005;111(11):1377–1382.
249. Spuentrup E, Katoh M, Wiethoff AJ, et al. Molecular magnetic resonance imaging of pulmonary emboli with a fibrin-specific contrast agent. *Am J Respir Crit Care Med 15* 2005;172(4):494–500.
250. Bouchard A, Higgins CB, Byrd 3rd BF, et al. Magnetic resonance imaging in pulmonary arterial hypertension. *Am J Cardiol* 1985;56(15):938–942.
251. Mohiaddin RH, Paz R, Theodoropoulos S, et al. Magnetic resonance characterization of pulmonary arterial blood flow after single lung transplantation. *J Thorac Cardiovasc Surg* 1991;101(6):1016–1023.
252. Winkler M, Higgins CB. Suspected intracardiac masses: evaluation with MR imaging. *Radiology* 1987;165(1):117–122.
253. Lund JT, Ehman RL, Julsrud PR, et al. Cardiac masses: assessment by MR imaging. *AJR Am J Roentgenol* 1989;152(3):469–473.
254. Bruna J, Lockwood M. Primary heart angiosarcoma detected by computed tomography and magnetic resonance imaging. *Eur Radiol* 1998;8(1):66–68.
255. Bhujwalla ZM, Artemov D, Glockner J. Tumor angiogenesis, vascularization, and contrast-enhanced magnetic resonance imaging. *Top Magn Reson Imaging* 1999;10(2):92–103.
256. Gulbins H, Reichenspurner H, Wintersperger BJ, et al. Minimally invasive extirpation of a left-ventricular myxoma. *Thorac Cardiovasc Surg* 1999; 47(2):129–130.
257. Urba W, Longo DL. Primary solid tumors of the heart. In: Kapoor A, ed. *Cancer of the heart.* New York: Springer-Verlag, 1986.
258. Reynen K. Cardiac myxomas. *N Engl J Med* 1995;333(24):1610–1617.
259. Mader MT, Poulton TB, White RD. Malignant tumors of the heart and great vessels: MR imaging appearance. *Radiographics* 1997;17(1):145–153.
260. Israeli A, Rein AJ, Krivisky M, et al. Right ventricular outflow tract obstruction due to extracardiac tumors. A report of three cases diagnosed and followed up by echocardiographic studies. *Arch Intern Med* 1989;149(9): 2105–2106.
261. Roberts WC, Glancy DL, DeVita VT, Jr. Heart in malignant lymphoma (Hodgkin's disease, lymphosarcoma, reticulum cell sarcoma and mycosis fungoides). A study of 196 autopsy cases. *Am J Cardiol* 1968;22(1):85–107.
262. Verkkala K, Kupari M, Maamies T, et al. Primary cardiac tumours—operative treatment of 20 patients. *Thorac Cardiovasc Surg* 1989;37(6): 361–364.
263. Niwa K, Tashima K, Terai M, et al. Contrast-enhanced magnetic resonance imaging of cardiac tumors in children. *Am Heart J* 1989;118(2):424–425.
264. Peters MN, Hall RJ, Cooley DA, et al. The clinical syndrome of atrial myxoma. *JAMA* 1974;230(5):695–701.
265. Amparo EG, Higgins CB, Farmer D, et al. Gated MRI of cardiac and paracardiac masses: initial experience. *AJR Am J Roentgenol* 1984;143(6): 1151–1156.

266. Vanderheyden M, De Sutter J, Wellens F, et al. Left atrial lipoma: case report and review of the literature. *Acta Cardiol* 1998;53(1):31–32.
267. Dooms GC, Higgins CB. MR imaging of cardiac thrombi. *J Comput Assist Tomogr* 1986;10(3):415–420.
268. Kim EE, Wallace S, Abello R, et al. Malignant cardiac fibrous histiocytomas and angiosarcomas: MR features. *J Comput Assist Tomogr* 1989;13(4): 627–632.
269. Janigan DT, Husain A, Robinson NA. Cardiac angiosarcomas. A review and a case report. *Cancer* 1986;57(4):852–859.
270. Araoz PA, Eklund HE, Welch TJ, et al. CT and MR imaging of primary cardiac malignancies. *Radiographics* 1999;19(6):1421–1434.
271. Teixeira A, Cachulo MC, Miranda O, et al. Rhabdomyosarcoma mimicking left atrial myxoma. Report of a clinical case. *Rev Port Cardiol* 1995;14(4): 325–327.
272. Putnam Jr JB, Sweeney MS, Colon R, et al. Primary cardiac sarcomas. *Ann Thorac Surg* 1991;51(6):906–910.
273. Villacampa VM, Villarreal M, Ros LH, et al. Cardiac rhabdomyosarcoma: diagnosis by MR imaging. *Eur Radiol* 1999;9(4):634–637.
274. Fenoglio Jr JJ, McAllister HA, Ferrans VJ. Cardiac rhabdomyoma: a clinicopathologic and electron microscopic study. *Am J Cardiol* 1976;38(2):241–251.
275. Van der Hauwaert LG. Cardiac tumours in infancy and childhood. *Br Heart J* 1971;33(1):125–132.
276. Posner MR, Cohen GI, Skarin AT. Pericardial disease in patients with cancer. The differentiation of malignant from idiopathic and radiation-induced pericarditis. *Am J Med* Sep 1981;71(3):407–413.
277. Soulen RL, Kan J, Mitchell S, et al. Evaluation of balloon angioplasty of coarctation restenosis by magnetic resonance imaging. *Am J Cardiol* 1987; 60(4):343–345.
278. Banki JH, Meiners LC, Barentsz JO, et al. Detection of aortic dissection by magnetic resonance imaging in adults with Marfan's syndrome. *Int J Card Imaging* 1992;8(4):249–254.
279. Boxer RA, LaCorte MA, Singh S, et al. Evaluation of the aorta in the Marfan syndrome by magnetic resonance imaging. *Am Heart J* 1986;111(5):1001–1002.
280. Fletcher BD, Jacobstein MD. MRI of congenital abnormalities of the great arteries. *AJR Am J Roentgenol* 1986;146(5):941–948.
281. Roman MJ, Rosen SE, Kramer-Fox R, et al. Prognostic significance of the pattern of aortic root dilation in the Marfan syndrome. *J Am Coll Cardiol* 1993;22(5):1470–1476.
282. Schaefer S, Peshock RM, Malloy CR, et al. Nuclear magnetic resonance imaging in Marfan's syndrome. *J Am Coll Cardiol* 1987;9(1):70–74.
283. Soulen RL, Fishman EK, Pyeritz RE, et al. Marfan syndrome: evaluation with MR imaging versus CT. *Radiology* 1987;165(3):697–701.
284. Rees S, Somerville J, Ward C, et al. Coarctation of the aorta: MR imaging in late postoperative assessment. *Radiology* 1989;173(2):499–502.
285. Mohiaddin RH, Longmore DB. MRI studies of atherosclerotic vascular disease: structural evaluation and physiological measurements. *Br Med Bull* 1989;45(4):968–990.
286. Groenink M, de Roos A, Mulder BJ, et al. Changes in aortic distensibility and pulse wave velocity assessed with magnetic resonance imaging following beta-blocker therapy in the Marfan syndrome. *Am J Cardiol* 1998; 82(2):203–208.
287. Canter CE, Gutierrez FR, Mirowitz SA, et al. Evaluation of pulmonary arterial morphology in cyanotic congenital heart disease by magnetic resonance imaging. *Am Heart J* 1989;118(2):347–354.
288. Duerinckx AJ, Wexler L, Banerjee A, et al. Postoperative evaluation of pulmonary arteries in congenital heart surgery by magnetic resonance imaging: comparison with echocardiography. *Am Heart J* 1994;128(6 Pt 1):1139–1146.
289. Greenberg SB, Crisci KL, Koenig P, et al. Magnetic resonance imaging compared with echocardiography in the evaluation of pulmonary artery abnormalities in children with tetralogy of Fallot following palliative and corrective surgery. *Pediatr Radiol* 1997;27(12):932–935.
290. Vick 3rd GW, Rokey R, Huhta JC, et al. Nuclear magnetic resonance imaging of the pulmonary arteries, subpulmonary region, and aorticopulmonary shunts: a comparative study with two-dimensional echocardiography and angiography. *Am Heart J* 1990;119(5):1103–1110.
291. Weinberg PM, Hubbard AM, Fogel MA. Aortic arch and pulmonary artery anomalies in children. *Semin Roentgenol* 1998;33(3):262–280.
292. Rees S, Firmin D, Mohiaddin R, et al. Application of flow measurements by magnetic resonance velocity mapping to congenital heart disease. *Am J Cardiol* 1989;64(14):953–956.
293. Diethelm L, Dery R, Lipton MJ, et al. Atrial-level shunts: sensitivity and specificity of MR in diagnosis. *Radiology* 1987;162(1 Pt 1):181–186.
294. Masui T, Seelos KC, Kersting-Sommerhoff BA, et al. Abnormalities of the pulmonary veins: evaluation with MR imaging and comparison with cardiac angiography and echocardiography. *Radiology* 1991;181(3):645–649.
295. Didier D, Higgins CB. Identification and localization of ventricular septal defect by gated magnetic resonance imaging. *Am J Cardiol* 1986;57(15): 1363–1368.
296. Yoo SJ, Lim TH, Park IS, et al. MR anatomy of ventricular septal defect in double-outlet right ventricle with situs solitus and atrioventricular concordance. *Radiology* 1991;181(2):501–505.
297. Hubbard AM, Fellows KE, Weinberg PM, et al. Preoperative and postoperative MRI of congenital heart disease. *Semin Roentgenol* 1998;33(3):218–227.
298. Kersting-Sommerhoff BA, Seelos KC, Hardy C, et al. Evaluation of surgical procedures for cyanotic congenital heart disease by using MR imaging. *AJR Am J Roentgenol* 1990;155(2):259–266.
299. Helbing WA, Niezen RA, Le Cessie S, et al. Right ventricular diastolic function in children with pulmonary regurgitation after repair of tetralogy of Fallot: volumetric evaluation by magnetic resonance velocity mapping. *J Am Coll Cardiol* 1996;28(7):1827–1835.
300. Niezen RA, Helbing WA, van der Wall EE, et al. Biventricular systolic function and mass studied with MR imaging in children with pulmonary regurgitation after repair for tetralogy of Fallot. *Radiology* 1996;201(1): 135–140.
301. Rebergen SA, Ottenkamp J, Doornbos J, et al. Postoperative pulmonary flow dynamics after Fontan surgery: assessment with nuclear magnetic resonance velocity mapping. *J Am Coll Cardiol* 1993;21(1):123–131.
302. Fellows KE, Fogel MA. MR imaging and heart function in patients pre- and post-Fontan surgery. *Acta Paediatr Suppl* 1995;410:57–59.
303. Fogel MA, Weinberg PM, Fellows KE, et al. Magnetic resonance imaging of constant total heart volume and center of mass in patients with functional single ventricle before and after staged Fontan procedure. *Am J Cardiol* 1993;72(18):1435–1443.
304. Fogel MA, Donofrio MT, Ramaciotti C, et al. Magnetic resonance and echocardiographic imaging of pulmonary artery size throughout stages of Fontan reconstruction. *Circulation* 1994;90(6):2927–2936.
305. Fogel MA, Weinberg PM, Fellows KE, et al. A study in ventricular–ventricular interaction. Single right ventricles compared with systemic right ventricles in a dual-chamber circulation. *Circulation* 1995;92(2):219–230.
306. Fogel MA, Weinberg PM, Chin AJ, et al. Late ventricular geometry and performance changes of functional single ventricle throughout staged Fontan reconstruction assessed by magnetic resonance imaging. *J Am Coll Cardiol* 1996;28(1):212–221.
307. Fogel MA, Weinberg PM, Hoydu A, et al. The nature of flow in the systemic venous pathway measured by magnetic resonance blood tagging in patients having the Fontan operation. *J Thorac Cardiovasc Surg* 1997;114(6):1032–1041.
308. Fogel MA, Weinberg PM, Rychik J, et al. Caval contribution to flow in the branch pulmonary arteries of Fontan patients with a novel application of magnetic resonance presaturation pulse. *Circulation* 1999;99(9):1215–1221.
309. Be'eri E, Maier SE, Landzberg MJ, et al. In vivo evaluation of Fontan pathway flow dynamics by multidimensional phase-velocity magnetic resonance imaging. *Circulation* 1998;98(25):2873–2882.
310. Morgan VL, Graham Jr TP, Roselli RJ, et al. Alterations in pulmonary artery flow patterns and shear stress determined with three-dimensional phase-contrast magnetic resonance imaging in Fontan patients. *J Thorac Cardiovasc Surg* 1998;116(2):294–304.
311. Chung KJ, Simpson IA, Glass RF, et al. Cine magnetic resonance imaging after surgical repair in patients with transposition of the great arteries. *Circulation* 1988;77(1):104–109.
312. Rees S, Somerville J, Warnes C, et al. Comparison of magnetic resonance imaging with echocardiography and radionuclide angiography in assessing cardiac function and anatomy following Mustard's operation for transposition of the great arteries. *Am J Cardiol* 1988;61(15):1316–1322.
313. Sampson C, Kilner PJ, Hirsch R, et al. Venoatrial pathways after the Mustard operation for transposition of the great arteries: anatomic and functional MR imaging. *Radiology* 1994;193(1):211–217.
314. Ward CJ, Mullins CE, Nihill MR, et al. Use of intravascular stents in systemic venous and systemic venous baffle obstructions. Short-term follow-up results. *Circulation* 1995;91(12):2948–2954.
315. Lorenz CH, Walker ES, Graham Jr TP, et al. Right ventricular performance and mass by use of cine MRI late after atrial repair of transposition of the great arteries. *Circulation* 1995;92(9 Suppl):II233–II239.
316. Rebergen SA, Helbing WA, van der Wall EE, et al. MR velocity mapping of tricuspid flow in healthy children and in patients who have undergone Mustard or Senning repair. *Radiology* 1995;194(2):505–512.
317. Beek FJ, Beekman RP, Dillon EH, et al. MRI of the pulmonary artery after arterial switch operation for transposition of the great arteries. *Pediatr Radiol* 1993;23(5):335–340.
318. Hardy CE, Helton GJ, Kondo C, et al. Usefulness of magnetic resonance imaging for evaluating great-vessel anatomy after arterial switch operation for D-transposition of the great arteries. *Am Heart J* 1994;128(2):326–332.
319. Guit GL, Bluemm R, Rohmer J, et al. Levotransposition of the aorta: identification of segmental cardiac anatomy using MR imaging. *Radiology* 1986;161(3):673–679.
320. Park JH, Han MC, Kim CW. MR imaging of congenitally corrected transposition of the great vessels in adults. *AJR Am J Roentgenol* 1989;153(3):491–494.
321. Glagov S, Weisenberg E, Zarins CK, et al. Compensatory enlargement of human atherosclerotic coronary arteries. *N Engl J Med* 1987;316(22):1371–1375.
322. Ambrose JA, Tannenbaum MA, Alexopoulos D, et al. Angiographic progression of coronary artery disease and the development of myocardial infarction. *J Am Coll Cardiol* 1988;12(1):56–62.
323. Little WC, Constantinescu M, Applegate RJ, et al. Can coronary angiography predict the site of a subsequent myocardial infarction in patients with mild-to-moderate coronary artery disease? *Circulation* 1988;78(5 Pt 1): 1157–1166.

324. George BS. Combined coronary and peripheral intervention: the oculo-stenotic-dilatory reflex or good medicine? *Catheter Cardiovasc Interv* 2001; 52(1):105.
325. Solberg LA, Strong JP. Risk factors and atherosclerotic lesions. A review of autopsy studies. *Arteriosclerosis* 1983;3(3):187–198.
326. Murray CJ, Lopez AD. Mortality by cause for eight regions of the world: Global Burden of Disease Study. *Lancet* 1997;349(9061):1269–1276.
327. Prentice RL. Surrogate endpoints in clinical trials: definition and operational criteria. *Stat Med* 1989;8(4):431–440.
328. Wittes J, Lakatos E, Probstfield J. Surrogate endpoints in clinical trials: cardiovascular diseases. *Stat Med* 1989;8(4):415–425.
329. Boissel JP, Collet JP, Moleur P, et al. Surrogate endpoints: a basis for a rational approach. *Eur J Clin Pharmacol* 1992;43(3):235–244.
330. O'Leary DH, Polak JF. Intima-media thickness: a tool for atherosclerosis imaging and event prediction. *Am J Cardiol* 2002;90(10C):18L–21L.
331. Greenland P, LaBree L, Azen SP, et al. Coronary artery calcium score combined with Framingham score for risk prediction in asymptomatic individuals. *JAMA* 2004;291(2):210–215.
332. Achenbach S, Ropers D, Hoffmann U, et al. Assessment of coronary remodeling in stenotic and nonstenotic coronary atherosclerotic lesions by multidetector spiral computed tomography. *J Am Coll Cardiol* 2004;43(5):842–847.
333. Nissen SE, Yock P. Intravascular ultrasound: novel pathophysiological insights and current clinical applications. *Circulation* 2001;103(4):604–616.
334. Desai MY, Bluemke DA. Atherosclerosis imaging using MR imaging: current and emerging applications. *Magn Reson Imaging Clin North Am* 2005;13(1):171–180, vii.
335. Choudhury RP, Fuster V, Badimon JJ, et al. MRI and characterization of atherosclerotic plaque: emerging applications and molecular imaging. *Arterioscler Thromb Vasc Biol* 2002;22(7):1065–1074.
336. Yuan C, Mitsumori LM, Beach KW, et al. Carotid atherosclerotic plaque: noninvasive MR characterization and identification of vulnerable lesions. *Radiology* 2001;221(2):285–299.
337. Fayad ZA, Nahar T, Fallon JT, et al. In vivo magnetic resonance evaluation of atherosclerotic plaques in the human thoracic aorta: a comparison with transesophageal echocardiography. *Circulation* 2000;101(21): 2503–2509.
338. Fayad ZA, Fuster V, Fallon JT, et al. Noninvasive in vivo human coronary artery lumen and wall imaging using black-blood magnetic resonance imaging. *Circulation* Aug 1, 2000;102(5):506–510.
339. Hayes CE, Mathis CM, Yuan C. Surface coil phased arrays for high-resolution imaging of the carotid arteries. *J Magn Reson Imaging* 1996; 6(1):109–112.
340. Botnar RM, Stuber M, Kim WY, et al. Magnetic resonance coronary lumen and vessel wall imaging. *Rays* 2001;26(4):291–303.
341. Kim WY, Stuber M, Bornert P, et al. Three-dimensional black-blood cardiac magnetic resonance coronary vessel wall imaging detects positive arterial remodeling in patients with nonsignificant coronary artery disease. *Circulation* 2002;106(3):296–299.
342. Edelman RR, Chien D, Kim D. Fast selective black blood MR imaging. *Radiology* 1991;181(3):655–660.
343. Chan SK, Jaffer FA, Botnar RM, et al. Scan reproducibility of magnetic resonance imaging assessment of aortic atherosclerosis burden. *J Cardiovasc Magn Reson* 2001;3(4):331–338.
344. Yuan C, Lin E, Millard J, et al. Closed contour edge detection of blood vessel lumen and outer wall boundaries in black-blood MR images. *Magn Reson Imaging* 1999;17(2):257–266.
345. Ladak HM, Thomas JB, Mitchell JR, et al. A semi-automatic technique for measurement of arterial wall from black blood MRI. *Med Phys* 2001; 28(6):1098–1107.
346. Zhang S, Hatsukami TS, Polissar NL, et al. Comparison of carotid vessel wall area measurements using three different contrast-weighted black blood MR imaging techniques. *Magn Reson Imaging* 2001;19(6):795–802.
347. Desai MY, Rodriguez A, Wasserman BA, et al. Association of cholesterol sub-fractions and carotid lipid core measured by MRI. *Arterioscler Thromb Vasc Biol* 2005;25:e110–e111.
348. Steen H, Warren WP, Desai M, et al. Combined transesophageal and surface MRI provides optimal imaging in aortic atherosclerosis. *J Cardiovasc Magn Reson* 2004;6(4):909–916.
349. Desai MY, Lai S, Weiss RG, et al. Reproducibility of coronary vessel wall dimension measurement obtained using 3D free breathing black blood MRI [Abstract]. *J Cardiovasc Magn Reson* 2005;7(1):196–197.
350. Yuan C, Petty C, O'Brien KD, et al. In vitro and in situ magnetic resonance imaging signal features of atherosclerotic plaque-associated lipids. *Arterioscler Thromb Vasc Biol* 1997;17(8):1496–1503.
351. Yuan C, Mitsumori LM, Ferguson MS, et al. In vivo accuracy of multispectral magnetic resonance imaging for identifying lipid-rich necrotic cores and intraplaque hemorrhage in advanced human carotid plaques. *Circulation* 2001;104(17):2051–2056.
352. Skinner MP, Yuan C, Mitsumori L, et al. Serial magnetic resonance imaging of experimental atherosclerosis detects lesion fine structure, progression and complications in vivo. *Nat Med* 1995;1(1):69–73.
353. Helft G, Worthley SG, Fuster V, et al. Atherosclerotic aortic component quantification by noninvasive magnetic resonance imaging: an in vivo study in rabbits. *J Am Coll Cardiol 15* 2001;37(4):1149–1154.
354. Toussaint JF, LaMuraglia GM, Southern JF, et al. Magnetic resonance images lipid, fibrous, calcified, hemorrhagic, and thrombotic components of human atherosclerosis in vivo. *Circulation* 1996;94(5):932–938.
355. Toussaint JF, Southern JF, Fuster V, et al. T2-weighted contrast for NMR characterization of human atherosclerosis. *Arterioscler Thromb Vasc Biol* 1995;15(10):1533–1542.
356. Hatsukami TS, Ross R, Polissar NL, et al. Visualization of fibrous cap thickness and rupture in human atherosclerotic carotid plaque in vivo with high-resolution magnetic resonance imaging. *Circulation* 2000;102(9):959–964.
357. de Boer OJ, van der Wal AC, Teeling P, et al. Leucocyte recruitment in rupture prone regions of lipid-rich plaques: a prominent role for neovascularization? *Cardiovasc Res* 1999;41(2):443–449.
358. Yuan C, Kerwin WS, Ferguson MS, et al. Contrast-enhanced high resolution MRI for atherosclerotic carotid artery tissue characterization. *J Magn Reson Imaging* 2002;15(1):62–67.
359. Wasserman BA, Smith WI, Trout 3rd HH, et al. Carotid artery atherosclerosis: in vivo morphologic characterization with gadolinium-enhanced double-oblique MR imaging initial results. *Radiology* 2002;223(2):566–573.
360. Weiss CR, Arai AE, Bui MN, et al. Arterial wall MRI characteristics are associated with elevated serum markers of inflammation in humans. *J Magn Reson Imaging* 2001;14(6):698–704.
361. Kooi ME, Cappendijk VC, Cleutjens KB, et al. Accumulation of ultrasmall superparamagnetic particles of iron oxide in human atherosclerotic plaques can be detected by in vivo magnetic resonance imaging. *Circulation* 2003;107(19):2453–2458.
362. Flacke S, Fischer S, Scott MJ, et al. Novel MRI contrast agent for molecular imaging of fibrin: implications for detecting vulnerable plaques. *Circulation* 2001;104(11):1280–1285.
363. Botnar RM, Buecker A, Wiethoff AJ, et al. In vivo magnetic resonance imaging of coronary thrombosis using a fibrin-binding molecular magnetic resonance contrast agent. *Circulation* 2004;110:1463–1466.
364. Ruehm SG, Corot C, Vogt P, et al. Magnetic resonance imaging of atherosclerotic plaque with ultrasmall superparamagnetic particles of iron oxide in hyperlipidemic rabbits. *Circulation* 2001;103(3):415–422.
365. Virmani R, Kolodgie FD, Burke AP, et al. Lessons from sudden coronary death: a comprehensive morphological classification scheme for atherosclerotic lesions. *Arterioscler Thromb Vasc Biol* 2000;20(5):1262–1275.
366. Yu X, Song SK, Chen J, et al. High-resolution MRI characterization of human thrombus using a novel fibrin-targeted paramagnetic nanoparticle contrast agent. *Magn Reson Med* 2000;44(6):867–872.
367. Thackray BD, Burns DH, Ferguson MS, et al. A new method for studying plaque morphology. *Am J Card Imaging* 1995;9(3):149–156.
368. Mitsumori LM, Hatsukami TS, Ferguson MS, et al. In vivo accuracy of multisequence MR imaging for identifying unstable fibrous caps in advanced human carotid plaques. *J Magn Reson Imaging* 2003;17(4):410–420.
369. Yuan C, Zhang SX, Polissar NL, et al. Identification of fibrous cap rupture with magnetic resonance imaging is highly associated with recent transient ischemic attack or stroke. *Circulation* 2002;105(2):181–185.
370. Shinnar M, Fallon JT, Wehrli S, et al. The diagnostic accuracy of ex vivo MRI for human atherosclerotic plaque characterization. *Arterioscler Thromb Vasc Biol* 1999;19(11):2756–2761.
371. Corti R, Fuster V, Fayad ZA, et al. Effects of aggressive versus conventional lipid-lowering therapy by simvastatin on human atherosclerotic lesions: a prospective, randomized, double-blind trial with high-resolution magnetic resonance imaging. *J Am Coll Cardiol.* 2005;46(1):106–112.
372. Corti R, Fuster V, Fayad ZA, et al. Lipid lowering by simvastatin induces regression of human atherosclerotic lesions: two years' follow-up by high-resolution noninvasive magnetic resonance imaging. *Circulation* 2002;106(23):2884–2887.
373. Correia LC, Atalar E, Kelemen MD, et al. Intravascular magnetic resonance imaging of aortic atherosclerotic plaque composition. *Arterioscler Thromb Vasc Biol* 1997;17(12):3626–3632.
374. Jaffer FA, O'Donnell CJ, Larson MG, et al. Age and sex distribution of subclinical aortic atherosclerosis: a magnetic resonance imaging examination of the Framingham Heart Study. *Arterioscler Thromb Vasc Biol* 2002; 22(5):849–854.
375. Corti R, Fayad ZA, Fuster V, et al. Effects of lipid-lowering by simvastatin on human atherosclerotic lesions: a longitudinal study by high-resolution, noninvasive magnetic resonance imaging. *Circulation* 2001;104(3):249–252.
376. Yonemura A, Momiyama Y, Fayad ZA, et al. Effect of lipid-lowering therapy with atorvastatin on atherosclerotic aortic plaques detected by noninvasive magnetic resonance imaging. *J Am Coll Cardiol* 2005;45(5):733–742.
377. Shunk KA, Garot J, Atalar E, et al. Transesophageal magnetic resonance imaging of the aortic arch and descending thoracic aorta in patients with aortic atherosclerosis. *J Am Coll Cardiol* 2001;37(8):2031–2035.
378. Lima JA, Desai MY, Steen H, et al. Statin-induced cholesterol lowering and plaque regression after 6 months of magnetic resonance imaging–monitored therapy. *Circulation* 2004;110(16):2336–2341.
379. Botnar RM, Stuber M, Kissinger KV, et al. Noninvasive coronary vessel wall and plaque imaging with magnetic resonance imaging. *Circulation* 2000;102(21):2582–2587.
380. Botnar RM, Kim WY, Bornert P, et al. 3D coronary vessel wall imaging utilizing a local inversion technique with spiral image acquisition. *Magn Reson Med* 2001;46(5):848–854.

381. Desai MY, Lai S, Barmet C, et al. Reproducibility of 3D free-breathing magnetic resonance coronary vessel wall imaging. *Eur Heart J* 2005;26:2320–2324.
382. Nissen SE, Tsunoda T, Tuzcu EM, et al. Effect of recombinant ApoA-I Milano on coronary atherosclerosis in patients with acute coronary syndromes: a randomized controlled trial. *JAMA* 2003;290(17):2292–2300.
383. Litovsky S, Madjid M, Zarrabi A, et al. Superparamagnetic iron oxide-based method for quantifying recruitment of monocytes to mouse atherosclerotic lesions in vivo: enhancement by tissue necrosis factor-alpha, interleukin-1beta, and interferon-gamma. *Circulation* 2003;107(11):1545–1549.
384. Weissleder R, Elizondo G, Wittenberg J, et al. Ultrasmall superparamagnetic iron oxide: characterization of a new class of contrast agents for MR imaging. *Radiology* 1990;175(2):489–493.
385. Renkin EM. Multiple pathways of capillary permeability. *Circ Res* 1977; 41(6):735–743.
386. van Hinsbergh WM. Endothelial permeability for macromolecules. Mechanistic aspects of pathophysiological modulation. *Arterioscler Thromb Vasc Biol* 1997;17(6):1018–1023.
387. Kanno S, Wu YJ, Lee PC, et al. Macrophage accumulation associated with rat cardiac allograft rejection detected by magnetic resonance imaging with ultrasmall superparamagnetic iron oxide particles. *Circulation* 2001; 104(8):934–938.
388. Kraitchman DL, Heldman AW, Atalar E, et al. In vivo magnetic resonance imaging of mesenchymal stem cells in myocardial infarction. *Circulation* 2003;107(18):2290–2293.
389. Karmarkar PV, Kraitchman DL, Izbudak I, et al. MR-trackable intramyocardial injection catheter. *Magn Reson Med* 2004;51(6):1163–1172.
390. Lanza GM, Lorenz CH, Fischer SE, et al. Enhanced detection of thrombi with a novel fibrin-targeted magnetic resonance imaging agent. *Acad Radiol* 1998;5(Suppl 1):S173–S176; discussion, S183–S174.
391. Winter PM, Caruthers SD, Kassner A, et al. Molecular imaging of angiogenesis in nascent Vx-2 rabbit tumors using a novel alpha(nu)beta3-targeted nanoparticle and 1.5 tesla magnetic resonance imaging. *Cancer Res* 2003;63(18):5838–5843.
392. Winter PM, Morawski AM, Caruthers SD, et al. Molecular imaging of angiogenesis in early-stage atherosclerosis with alpha(v)beta3-integrin-targeted nanoparticles. *Circulation* 2003;108(18):2270–2274.
393. Bakker CJ, Hoogeveen RM, Hurtak WF, et al. MR-guided endovascular interventions: susceptibility-based catheter and near-real-time imaging technique. *Radiology* 1997;202(1):273–276.
394. Leung DA, Debatin JF, Wildermuth S, et al. Intravascular MR tracking catheter: preliminary experimental evaluation. *AJR Am J Roentgenol* 1995; 164(5):1265–1270.
395. Kandarpa K, Jakab P, Patz S, et al. Prototype miniature endoluminal MR imaging catheter. *J Vasc Interv Radiol* 1993;4(3):419–427.
396. Aoki S, Nanbu A, Araki T, et al. Active MR tracking on a 0.2 Tesla MR imager. *Radiat Med* 1999;17(3):251–257.
397. Wildermuth S, Dumoulin CL, Pfammatter T, et al. MR-guided percutaneous angioplasty: assessment of tracking safety, catheter handling and functionality. *Cardiovasc Interv Radiol* 1998;21(5):404–410.
398. Ladd ME, Erhart P, Debatin JF, et al. Guidewire antennas for MR fluoroscopy. *Magn Reson Med* 1997;37(6):891–897.
399. Wendt M, Busch M, Wetzler R, et al. Shifted rotated keyhole imaging and active tip-tracking for interventional procedure guidance. *J Magn Reson Imaging* 1998;8(1):258–261.
400. Ocali O, Atalar E. Intravascular magnetic resonance imaging using a loopless catheter antenna. *Magn Reson Med* 1997;37(1):112–118.
401. Shunk KA, Lima JA, Heldman AW, et al. Transesophageal magnetic resonance imaging. *Magn Reson Med* 1999;41(4):722–726.
402. Lardo AC, McVeigh ER, Jumrussirikul P, et al. Visualization and temporal/spatial characterization of cardiac radiofrequency ablation lesions using magnetic resonance imaging. *Circulation* 2000;102(6):698–705.
403. Yang X, Atalar E. Intravascular MR imaging–guided balloon angioplasty with an MR imaging guide wire: feasibility study in rabbits. *Radiology* 2000;217(2):501–506.
404. Yang X, Bolster Jr BD, Kraitchman DL, et al. Intravascular MR-monitored balloon angioplasty: an in vivo feasibility study. *J Vasc Interv Radiol* 1998; 9(6):953–959.
405. Martin AJ, Plewes DB, Henkelman RM. MR imaging of blood vessels with an intravascular coil. *J Magn Reson Imaging* 1992;2(4):421–429.
406. Hurst GC, Hua J, Duerk JL, et al. Intravascular (catheter) NMR receiver probe: preliminary design analysis and application to canine iliofemoral imaging. *Magn Reson Med* 1992;24(2):343–357.
407. Atalar E, Bottomley PA, Ocali O, et al. High resolution intravascular MRI and MRS by using a catheter receiver coil. *Magn Reson Med* 1996; 36(4):596–605.
408. Omary RA, Frayne R, Unal O, et al. MR-guided angioplasty of renal artery stenosis in a pig model: a feasibility study. *J Vasc Interv Radiol* 2000; 11(3):373–381.
409. Serfaty JM, Yang X, Foo TK, et al. MRI-guided coronary catheterization and PTCA: a feasibility study on a dog model. *Magn Reson Med* 2003; 49(2):258–263.
410. Buecker A, Neuerburg JM, Adam GB, et al. Real-time MR fluoroscopy for MR-guided iliac artery stent placement. *J Magn Reson Imaging* 2000; 12(4):616–622.
411. Spuentrup E, Ruebben A, Schaeffter T, et al. Magnetic resonance–guided coronary artery stent placement in a swine model. *Circulation* 2002;105(7): 874–879.
412. Manke C, Nitz WR, Djavidani B, et al. MR imaging–guided stent placement in iliac arterial stenoses: a feasibility study. *Radiology* 2001;219(2):527–534.
413. Dickfeld T, Calkins H, Zviman M, et al. Stereotactic magnetic resonance guidance for anatomically targeted ablations of the fossa ovalis and the left atrium. *J Interv Card Electrophysiol* 2004;11(2):105–115.
414. Kantor HL, Briggs RW, Balaban RS. In vivo 31P nuclear magnetic resonance measurements in canine heart using a catheter-coil. *Circ Res* 1984; 55(2):261–266.
415. Yang X, Atalar E, Li D, et al. Magnetic resonance imaging permits in vivo monitoring of catheter-based vascular gene delivery. *Circulation* 2001; 104(14):1588–1590.
416. Takai T, Ohmori H. Enhancement of DNA transfection efficiency by heat treatment of cultured mammalian cells. *Biochim Biophys Acta* 1992; 1129(2):161–165.
417. Blackburn RV, Galoforo SS, Corry PM, et al. Adenoviral-mediated transfer of a heat-inducible double suicide gene into prostate carcinoma cells. *Cancer Res* 1998;58(7):1358–1362.
418. Yang X, Atalar E, Zerhouni EA. Intravascular MR imaging and intravascular MR-guided interventions. *Int J Cardiovasc Interv* 1999;2(2):85–96.
419. Weissleder R, Moore A, Mahmood U, et al. In vivo magnetic resonance imaging of transgene expression. *Nat Med Mar* 2000;6(3):351–355.
420. Budinger TF. Nuclear magnetic resonance (NMR) in vivo studies: known thresholds for health effects. *J Comput Assist Tomogr Dec* 1981;5(6):800–811.

CHAPTER 55 ■ POSITRON EMISSION TOMOGRAPHY

MARKUS SCHWAIGER AND SIBYLLE ZIEGLER

OVERVIEW

Positron emission tomography (PET) and PET in combination with computed tomography (PET/CT) represent the most advanced scintigraphic imaging technique developed for in vivo quantification of cardiac physiology and biochemistry. The state-of-the-art PET instrumentation allows delineation of regional tracer activity with high spatial (4–8 mm) and temporal resolution (few seconds per image). The combination of PET and multidetector CT integrates structural and biological imaging for a comprehensive evaluation of cardiac disease. A large number of radiopharmaceuticals have been developed to study myocardial perfusion, energy metabolism, and autonomic innervation of the heart. Initial research applications included assessment of fatty acid and glucose metabolism, followed by the quantification of regional myocardial perfusion in patients with coronary artery disease (CAD). More recently, newer tracers such as radiolabeled β receptor antagonists allow the pre- and postsynaptic evaluation of sympathetic cardiac innervation. Metabolic imaging with F-18 deoxyglucose has emerged as important clinical application for the assessment of tissue viability in patients with impaired left ventricular function with well-validated diagnostic and prognostic information. PET/CT in combination with short-lived perfusion tracers provides accurate diagnosis and localization of CAD and in the future plaque imaging. The development of new radiopharmaceuticals for molecular tissue characterization is expected to ensure that PET and PET/CT remain competitive clinical and research tools in cardiology.

GLOSSARY

PET: Positron emission tomography.
CT: X-ray computed tomography.
SPECT: Single photon emission computerized tomography.
Transmission scan: Measurement of photon attenuation using external sources. Data are used for correction of emission data.
Polar map: Planar representation of tracer accumulation in the left ventricular myocardium, determined by volumetric sampling of the scintigraphic data.
Tracer: Very small amount of substance, labeled with a radioactive isotope, and the decay can be detected externally.
F-18: Fluorine-18.
C-11: Carbon-11.
N-13: Nitrogen-13.
O-15: Oxygen-15.
Rb-82: Rubidium-82.
FDG: Fluorodeoxyglucose can be labeled with F-18.
HED: Hydroxyephedrine, can be labeled with C-11.

HISTORICAL PERSPECTIVE

PET was developed as a noninvasive method for quantitative imaging of tissue tracer distribution in vivo. Three important technical requirements contribute to this method: the labeling of a biological substance with short-lived positron emitters, the detection of the annihilation radiation, and the reconstruction of 3-dimensional tracer distribution in the body. Radiopharmacy, instrumentation, and data processing have evolved over the last 70 years since the discovery of artificial radioactivity by Curie and Joliot in 1934. Radioactive isotopes such as C-11, N-13, or F-18 became available in the late 1930s and early 1940s after the development of the cyclotron by Lawrence and were used in biological (1) and first human studies (2). The advantage of using coincidence measurements for collimation became apparent and was implemented for the first time in a positron probe by Brownell and Sweet (3) and in a positron scanner for brain studies by Aronow (4). With the tomographic imaging of single photon emitters, Kuhl and Edwards introduced transverse section scanning using a backprojection algorithm in 1963 (5). These advances in reconstruction also promoted the development of tomographs for positron imaging in the early 1970s, when the research group of Hoffman, Phelps, and Ter Pogossian at Washington University built the first positron emission tomograph for brain imaging (6,7).

PET was introduced in the 1970s as a new imaging modality in cardiology by investigators at Washington University in St. Louis (8). Initial studies employed metabolic tracers such as F-18 deoxyglucose and C-11 palmitate for the noninvasive characterization of myocardial substrate metabolism. With the introduction of flow markers such as N-13 ammonia and O-15 water, the application of PET shifted toward the evaluation of myocardial perfusion primarily in patients with CAD.

Quantitative PET requires a transmission measurement for the correction of photon attenuation. Thus, the combination of CT with PET in one device not only offered the combination of functional and anatomical information, but also the potential of reducing total scanning time. Townsend and his group at the University of Pittsburgh first realized the combination of both imaging modalities in the late 1990s (9,10). PET/CT imaging has rapidly gained acceptance in the oncology community by providing not only efficient measurements of attenuation, but also by allowing the integration of morphologic and metabolic information for detection, staging, and therapy control (11). The intention of using multidetector CT exclusively for attenuation correction is being increasingly replaced by the concept of applying both, PET and CT, at their fullest diagnostic potential, which opens new diagnostic strategies in cardiology.

This chapter reviews the current role of PET and PET/CT in the functional evaluation of CAD, and other cardiovascular disorders. Established clinical applications, as well as experimental concepts, are discussed. Finally, the results obtained with PET and PET/CT are compared with those derived from other imaging modalities to define the clinical role of PET in cardiology.

IMAGING PRINCIPLES

After emission from the nucleus, positrons travel a short distance and quickly decay by annihilation with an electron. Positron and electron mass are converted into energy and a pair of γ rays is generated. Conservation of energy and momentum require the γ rays to travel in nearly opposite directions (180 degrees apart) with an energy of 511 keV each (Fig. 55.1). They can be detected by using pairs of collinearly aligned detectors. The detector pairs of a PET system are installed in a ringlike pattern, which allows measurement of radioactivity along lines through the organ of interest at a series of angles and radial distances. This angular information is used to reconstruct tomographic images of regional radioactivity distribution.

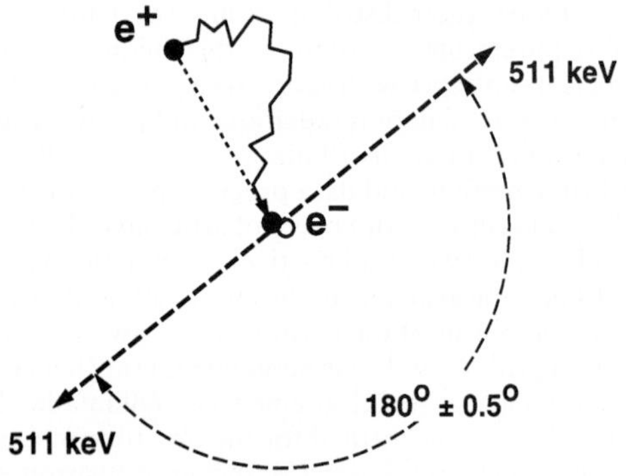

FIGURE 55.1. Positron emission and decay. The energetic positron (e^+) travels several millimeters on the tissue before it combines with an electron (e^-). The positron and electron annihilate, resulting in two opposing γ rays with 511 keV each. See text for details.

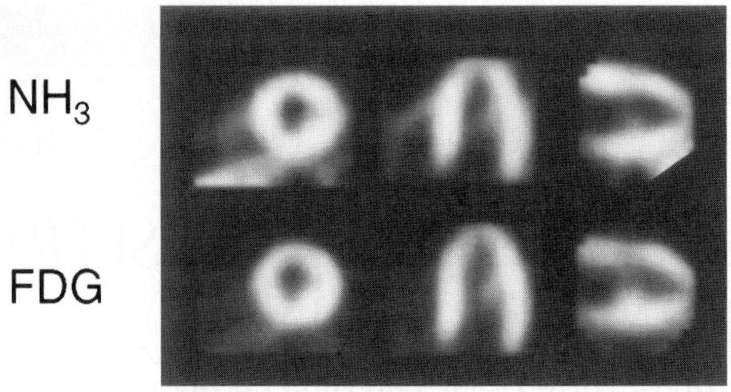

FIGURE 55.2. Positron emission tomographic images of normal volunteer with nitrogen-13 ammonia (NH_3) and fluorine-18 fluorodeoxyglucose (FDG).

Because the left ventricular wall is about 10 mm thick, high spatial resolution is necessary for the quantitative analysis of tissue tracer concentration (Fig. 55.2). The spatial resolution of PET approaches 5 to 7 mm in all axes and is expected to improve to about 2 to 3 mm in the future. High spatial resolution is of utmost importance for the detection of activity within small structures such as the coronary vessel wall. Based on a vessel wall thickness of about 1 to 2 mm, the recovery of activity information requires a high biological contrast, even when a system resolution of 3 mm can be reached: Myocardial movement and change in wall thickness during the cardiac cycle also affect the image resolution. Thus, PET data quality can be improved by ECG gated acquisitions, providing not only motion correction but also measurements of regional and global left ventricular function (12).

The PET detector system has to perform linearly over a wide range of count rates, and allow for short scan time intervals to monitor the rapid uptake and release of tracers. Most of the current commercial tomographs employ block detectors made of scintillation crystals (bismuth germanate) and photomultiplyer tubes (13). New detector materials such as lutetium oxyorthosilicate and gadolinium oxyorthosilicate improve imaging performance at a reasonable cost (14).

Correction of photon attenuation is a prerequisite for tracer distribution measurements in the heart to avoid artifacts caused by tissue surrounding the heart. External sources are used to perform a transmission scan, which allows estimates of regional attenuation factors. Rotating rod sources made of positron emitters are used for this purpose (15,16). With PET/CT the CT information can be used for attenuation correction in PET. CT images of the chest require only a few seconds using multidetector CT instrumentation and low-dose CT images can be generated with good spatial resolution while minimizing radiation exposure to less than 1 mSv. However, as the attenuation factors for 511 keV have to be extrapolated from low-energy x-ray measurements conversion factors have to be employed for different tissue densities (e.g., heart, lung, and bone) (17). In addition, coregistration of data becomes an important part of attenuation correction using CT because transmission and PET emission data acquisition are performed separately. The CT acquisition is completed within few seconds; PET data are collected over several minutes. Ongoing methodologic research is concerned with optimizing CT-based PET attenuation correction.

PRINCIPLES OF RADIONUCLIDE PRODUCTION AND RADIOCHEMISTRY

Carbon-11, nitrogen-13, oxygen-15, and fluorine-18 are the most common positron-emitting radionuclides, all of which

TABLE 55.1

TRACERS COMMONLY AVAILABLE FOR CARDIAC PET APPLICATIONS

Radionuclide	$t_{1/2}$	Radiopharmaceutical	Application
Rb-82	76 sec	Rubidium	Flow
O-15	120 sec	Water	Flow
N-13	10 min	Ammonia	Flow
C-11	20 min	Palmitate	Fatty acid metabolism
F-18	110 min	Acetate	Oxygen consumption
		Hydroxyephedrine	Catecholamine uptake
		CGP-12177	Beta-receptor density
		Deoxyglucose	Glucose metabolism
		Misonidazole	Hypoxia
		FTHA	Fatty acid metabolism

Abbreviation: $t_{1/2}$, physical half life.

have a short physical half-life ranging from 122 seconds for oxygen-15 to 110 minutes for fluorine-18 (Table 55.1).

The predominant and most efficient production method of these isotopes is to modify the nuclear structure of specific stable radionuclides by accelerated particle bombardment with either protons or deuterons. A cyclotron is a particle accelerator employed most often for radioisotope production in PET imaging (18,19). Few positron-emitting radionuclides such as rubidium-82 are generator produced. A generator consists of a parent–daughter radionuclide pair in an apparatus, which permits a separation and extraction of the daughter compound from the parent.

Because there are positron-emitting radionuclides of oxygen, carbon, and nitrogen, it is theoretically possible to label any organic compound of interest, whether it is a natural substance or a synthetic drug. Fluorine, although not often found in naturally occurring molecules, can be readily substituted for a hydrogen or hydroxyl group, and is a favorite of radiochemists designing new pharmaceuticals. With these four radionuclides, a large number of positron-emitting tracers can be synthesized and used in clinical studies (20).

ASSESSMENT OF MYOCARDIAL BLOOD FLOW

Flow Tracer

Blood flow tracers can be classified based on their physiologic behavior. Oxygen-15 water, for example, represents a freely diffusible tracer, which washes in and out of myocardial tissue as a function of blood flow. The first pass extraction of O-15 water in the heart is neither diffusion limited, nor is O-15 water tissue extraction affected by any metabolic pathways (21–23) (Fig. 55.3).

The second group of flow markers are radiotracers, which are retained in myocardial tissue proportional to myocardial blood flow. For these radiopharmaceuticals, the initial tracer extraction (first-pass extraction) and their tissue retention are important factors defining their suitability as blood flow tracers. N-13 ammonia is highly extracted by myocardial tissue in the form of N-13 ammonia (24–26). Within the tissue, the tracer can either back diffuse into the vascular space or be trapped in the form of N-13 glutamine.

Ionic tracers such as rubidium-82, rubidium-81, or potassium-38 display similar tracer kinetics to thallium-201 (27–29). Initial extraction of these compounds ranges between 50% and 70%. For both N-13 ammonia retention and ionic tracer extraction, a nonlinear relationship exists between blood flow and tissue tracer extraction (27,30). For methodologic details of myocardial flow measurements by PET please refer to an excellent recent review by Kaufmann (31).

Clinical Application

Qualitative Assessment of Regional Myocardial Blood Flow

Initial applications of PET for the detection of CAD consisted of the visual assessment of regional myocardial tracer distribution under rest and stress conditions (32–37). In most studies, pharmacologic stress testing with adenosine or dipyridamole has been employed to assess coronary reserve (32). The advantage of this approach is the standardized stress procedure, which can be performed in the PET gantry without moving the patient between rest and stress imaging (38).

The most commonly used tracers are rubidium-82 and N-13 ammonia (24,36). With rubidium-82, the rest/stress

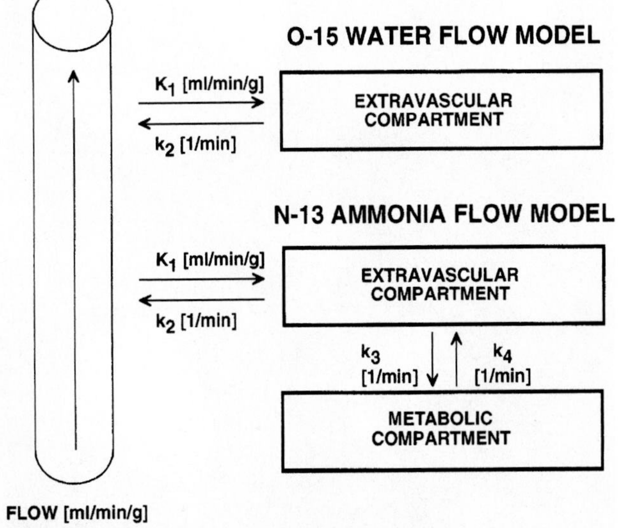

FIGURE 55.3. Diagram illustrating the compartment models for oxygen-15 water (*top*) and nitrogen-13 ammonia (*bottom*).

TABLE 55.2

DIAGNOSTIC PERFORMANCE OF POSITRON EMISSION TOMOGRAPHY FLOW DETERMINATIONS

	n	Sensitivity (%)	Specificity (%)
N-13 ammonia			
Schelbert (254)	45	98	100
Tamaki (363)	51	98	100
Muzik (41)	35	87	96
Rubidium-82			
Go (275)	202	93	78
Stewart (110)	81	83	86
Grover McKay (421)	31	100	13
Marwick (420)	74	90	100

protocol can be completed in about 1 hour, whereas N-13 ammonia blood flow studies require about 2 hours. Extensive clinical data exist with both radiopharmaceuticals to document the high diagnostic accuracy with sensitivity and specificity values ranging from 83% to 95% (Table 55.2). Most studies employed visual data analysis similar to the methods used routinely for thallium-201 or technetium-99m sestamibi single photon emission computerized tomography (SPECT) imaging (25,33,34,39). Automated techniques for semiquantitative data analysis, similar to those used for SPECT imaging, have also been developed for PET flow studies (40,41) (Fig 55.4). A number of studies have demonstrated the superiority of PET-Rb-82 compared to SPECT imaging (33,34,39,42). Combining the perfusion pattern with CT assessment of coronary calcification or CT angiography—as now possible with PET/CT—provides a comprehensive examination addressing structural and functional aspects of CAD (Fig. 55.5) (43,44). Future studies have to define the diagnostic and prognostic gain of the combined evaluation of coronary calcification, coronary angiography and myocardial perfusion.

Demer et al. (37) demonstrated that the severity of perfusion abnormalities determined by PET imaging correlated with the angiographically predicted coronary reserve measurements for a given vascular territory. Gould et al. (45) reported a significant gradient in regional perfusion from base to apex in patients with mild but diffuse arteriographic disease, suggesting greater downstream flow abnormalities in the absence of regional limiting stenoses.

In addition to the diagnosis of CAD, the follow-up of patients with CAD by noninvasive means is of clinical interest (46). Longitudinal studies evaluating the effect of therapeutic or life-style interventions provide objective outcome criteria and are especially important in patients considered at high risk for progression of disease severity (47).

Quantitative Assessment of Myocardial Blood Flow

The potential of PET for the quantitative assessment of myocardial blood flow represents a major advantage over SPECT and magnetic resonance (MR) imaging. Such measurements provide flow estimates in milliliters per minute per 100 g of tissue, which can be used to assess myocardial microcirculation under resting and stress conditions as well as before and after pharmacologic interventions. For such flow measurements dynamic data acquisition is necessary to describe arterial input function as well as tissue response.

O-15 Water. Oxygen-15 water can be administered either as bolus injection or O-15 labeled CO_2 inhalation (22,23,48,49). Radiolabeled CO_2 is rapidly converted to water in lung tissue and transported to the heart as O-15 water. Both approaches

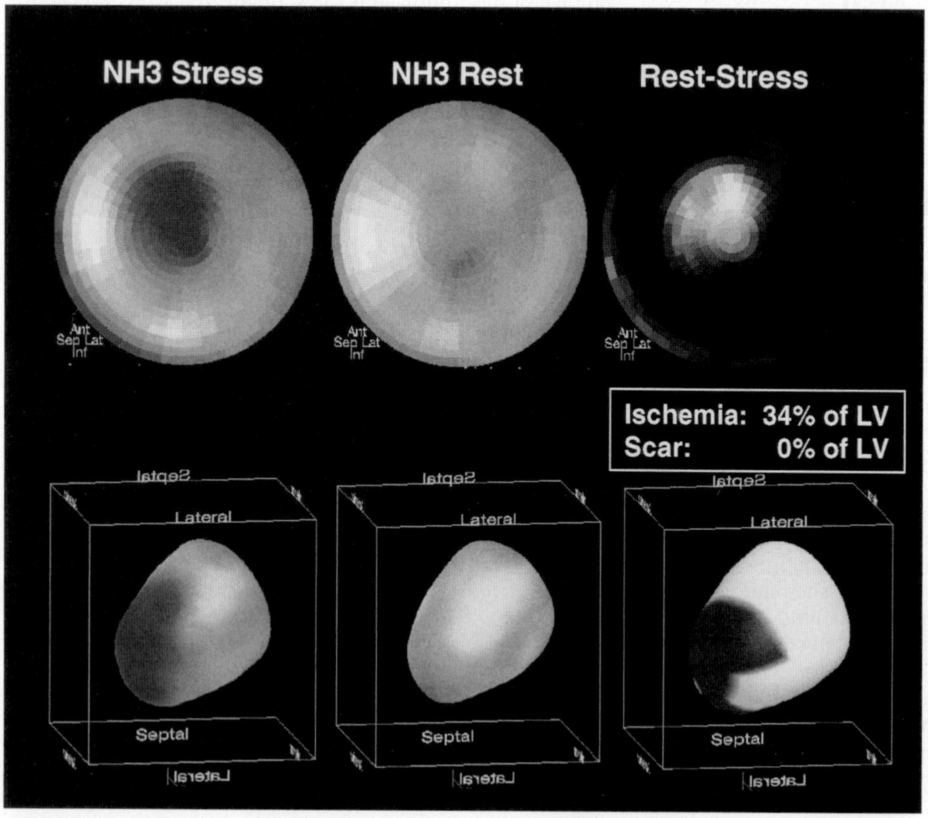

FIGURE 55.4. Polar maps (*top*) and three-dimensional visualization (*bottom*) of nitrogen-13 ammonia (NH_3) uptake in patient with a stress-induced defect. Results provide semiquantitative assessment if ischemic and scar tissue. *Abbreviation:* LV, left ventricle.

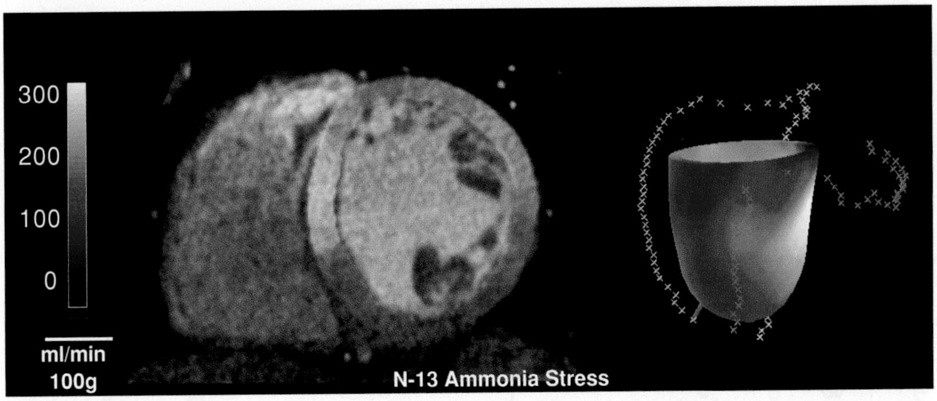

FIGURE 55.5. Coregistered CTA and PET provide excellent correlation of structural and functional aspects of CAD. Myocardial blood flow under stress conditions was calculated using dynamic data with a three-compartment model. Regional flow values were mapped onto the segmented wall from the CTA study. Additionally, the coronary tree was manually extracted and superimposed on the three-dimensional polar map of myocardial blood flow.

use the uptake as well as washout of radioactivity from the myocardium assuming a constant partition coefficient (0.80–0.90) of water between vascular and tissue space (Fig. 55.3). The water method also assumes homogeneous tissue within the region of interest used for quantitation of myocardial blood flow. To delineate myocardial tissue boundaries, the blood pool contribution has to be removed from O-15 water studies. For this purpose, a separate inhalation of O-15 labeled CO is commonly employed (23). More recently, factor analysis of dynamic O-15 water has been shown to allow for delineation of myocardial structures (50,51). The tracer kinetic model approach for O-15 water flow measurement includes a term correcting for the geometric distortion due to limited image resolution provided by PET (partial volume effect, activity cross-contamination) (21,23,52). The use of O-15 water (as a blood flow marker) has been validated in various animal models, and has demonstrated close agreement with microsphere flow measurements (52–54). Correction of flow values with the perfused tissue fraction leads to a determination of an index describing the relative amount of perfused tissue within a myocardial segment (55). In addition, methods have been developed to quantify not only flow, but also oxygen metabolism using O-15 tracer (56).

N-13 Ammonia. Several approaches have been introduced to describe the myocardial kinetics of N-13 ammonia using a compartmental model, which relates the N-13 activity in the vascular, the free intracellular, and the metabolic space (57–59) (Fig. 55.3). Assuming the first transit extraction of N-13 ammonia is approximately 100%, the model estimate serves as a quantitative index of perfusion ($F = K_1 \times \text{EF}$) (24). These methods have been validated in the animal laboratory comparing N-13 ammonia perfusion measurements with microsphere measurements as a gold standard, or with O-15 reference PET measurements (53,59,60).

Other Tracers (Rubidium-82, Copper-62 PTSM, Potassium-38). Rubidium-82 has been proposed for quantitative flow measurements (61,62). Data in the animal model and preliminary clinical results demonstrate the feasibility of using this radiopharmaceutical for quantitative flow measurements. Copper-62 PTSM has also been employed for the assessment of myocardial blood flow (63).

Clinical Application

The quantitation of regional coronary flow reserve (CFR) has been advocated by Gould et al. (64) for the functional assessment of the severity of coronary artery stenosis in patients with CAD. The parameter flow reserve describes not only the functional significance of a given coronary lesion but also vascular reactivity and collateral blood flow in the poststenotic vascular territories. Such functional measurements complement the anatomic description of CAD and link the morphologic alterations of epicardial arteries with perfusion patterns assessed at the level of microcirculation. Limitations of angiographic characterization of CAD are widely appreciated owing to the complex three-dimensional nature of atherosclerotic plaques as well as considerable interobserver variability in angiographic data interpretation (46,64–66).

PET blood flow measurements have been extensively validated in animals and in healthy volunteers. There is good reproducibility of blood flow measurements under resting as well as stress conditions in volunteers and patients with CAD, as shown by the consistent measurements of coronary reserve values (67,68). In patients with CAD, CFR measurements are reduced (69–73). A correlation between the severity of CAD and severity of flow reserve impairment has been documented in several studies (69,72–75) (Fig. 55.6).

CFR over 2.5 times resting flow must be considered "normal" based on the standard deviation of measurements in individuals at low likelihood of CAD (69,76).

A relationship between coronary reserve measurements and age in subjects without CAD has been demonstrated (77–79). However, there are other factors, such as left ventricular hypertrophy, hypertension, as well as syndrome X that may affect coronary reserve measurements in the absence of vascular abnormalities defined by angiography (31,80). Animal and clinical data have indicated that arterial hypertension leads to reduced CFR. It also has been shown, using PET, that therapy of patients with arterial hypertension may improve regional coronary reserve measurements (81). Therefore, quantitative regional flow measurements may be useful monitor pharmacologic interventions as well as to assess the effect of regional revascularization by PCI and surgery (82–90).

Detection of Early Coronary Artery Disease by Flow Measurements. Comparing the incidence of abnormal CFR with the severity of stenosis, as defined by quantitative angiography, reveals a very high sensitivity of CFR measurements for the detection of severe coronary artery stenosis (>95%) (91,92). The high incidence (about 30%) of abnormal CFR in territories with only mild CAD is surprising as defined by angiography (76). These data have been confirmed by several laboratories, indicating that CFR with pharmacologic stress agents may provide more sensitive means to detect early CAD than angiographic criteria alone (69,93). This hypothesis has been addressed by several investigators (94–97) who have demonstrated that CFR in asymptomatic male patients without clinical evidence of myocardial ischemia, but at high risk for the development of CAD based on risk factor profile

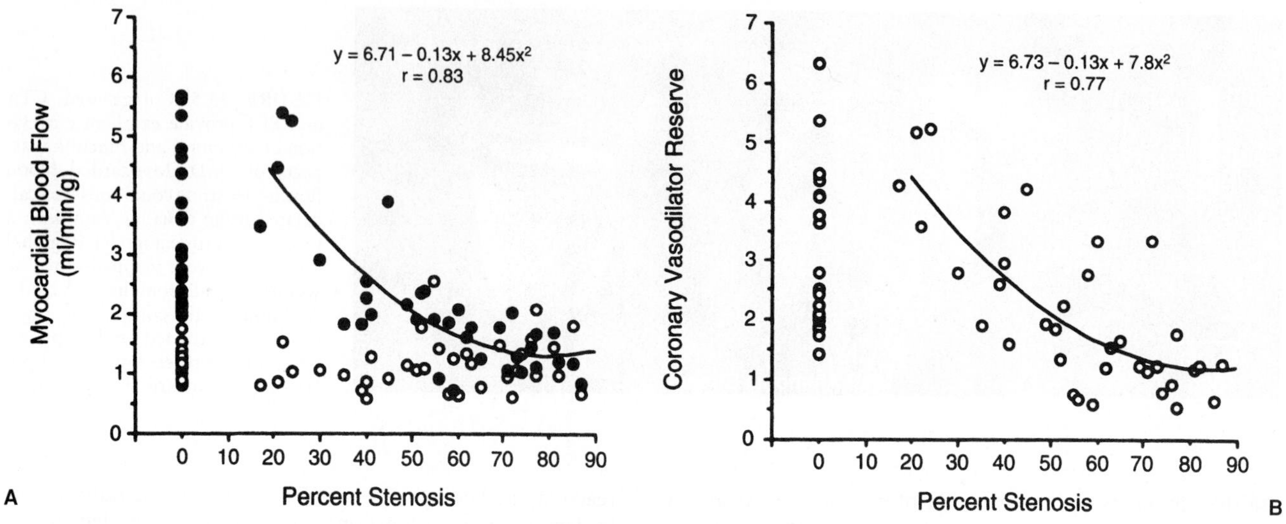

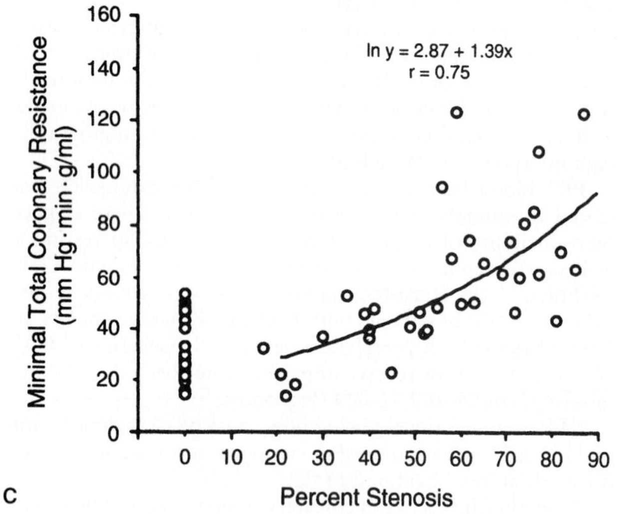

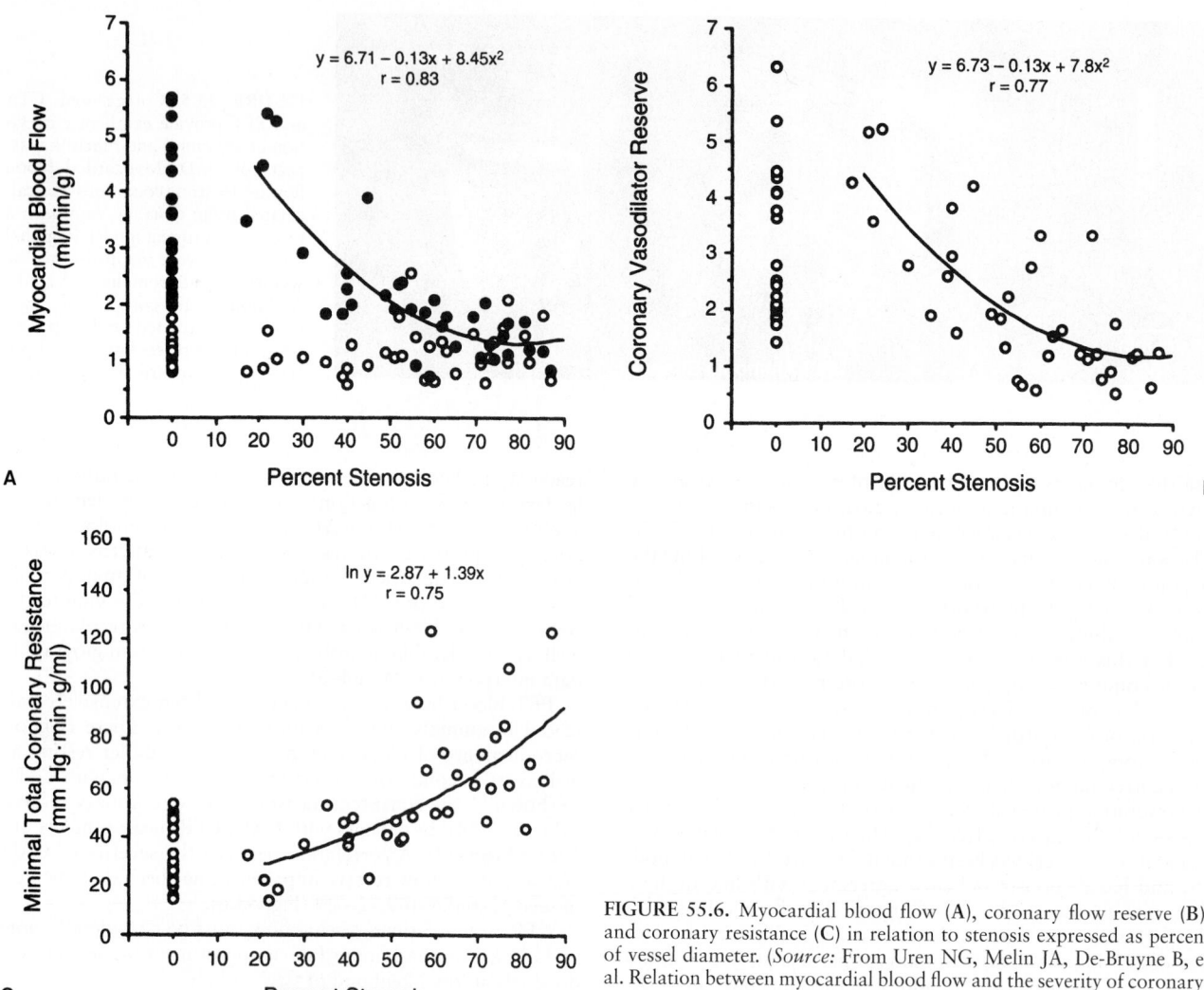

FIGURE 55.6. Myocardial blood flow (A), coronary flow reserve (B), and coronary resistance (C) in relation to stenosis expressed as percent of vessel diameter. (*Source:* From Uren NG, Melin JA, De-Bruyne B, et al. Relation between myocardial blood flow and the severity of coronary-artery stenosis. *N Engl J Med* 1994;330:1782–1788.)

was abnormal. A significant relationship between the impairment of CFR and plasma cholesterol, low-density lipoproteins, high-density lipoprotein, and oxidized low-density lipoprotein (oxLDL) has been reported. CFR has been shown to be reduced in young men with familial hyperlipidemia, especially with combined abnormalities in cholesterol and triglyceride serum levels (phenotype IIB) (98). Furthermore, reduction of flow reserve has been observed in asymptomatic patients with insulin-dependent and non–insulin-dependent diabetes mellitus (94). The pathophysiologic mechanism of the reduced CFR in territories with no or only mild angiographic evidence of stenoses is not yet known, but may represent complex interplay of vascular alterations, as well as endothelial dysfunction (99).

Most recently, Mauriello et al. (100) demonstrated that inflammatory processes involve larger segments of the coronary tree than appreciated by the structural changes occurring in coronary plaques. Plaque rupture may be a regional appearance of an inflammatory process affecting the entire coronary artery. Endothelial dysfunction may be a sensitive marker for vascular inflammation. This hypothesis is supported by the observation that CFR is reduced in remote vascular territories of patients suffering acute myocardial infarction (101).

The hemodynamic response to dipyridamole or adenosine can be modified by α- or β-receptor blockade, enhancing the range of coronary flow measurements (102,103). First results employing cold pressor stress testing in combination with PET confirm the results obtained in the catheterization laboratory using intracoronary acetylcholine infusion (104,105). Several investigators have observed a relationship between vascular reactivity to acetylcholine and prognosis in patients with CAD (106,107). Most recently, Schindler et al. (108) demonstrated that a reduced PET flow response to sympathetic stimulation is associated with impaired prognosis. In addition, mental stress has been used to investigate coronary vascular reactivity in normal and CAD patients, which demonstrated reduced flow response in this patient group (109).

PET measurements have been employed to assess the acute and chronic effects of smoking on dipyridamole-induced flow changes. Smoking during the PET study decreased the dipyridamole-induced hyperemia and coronary reserve (97). The effects of smoking on coronary vascular reactivity can be reversed by intravenous L-arginine (104) or administration of the antioxidant vitamin C (97).

Cardiovascular conditioning is thought to alter favorably the natural history of CAD. Czernin et al. (110) investigated patients undergoing a short-term exercise/diet program. The beneficial effect of this program on heart rate, blood pressure, and cholesterol was associated with a significant increase of flow reserve. Pharmacologic therapy with lipid-lowering drugs (simvastatin, fluvastatin) is associated with improvement of CFR (111–115). Guethlin et al. (112) reported a delayed response when flow measurements at 2 months were compared

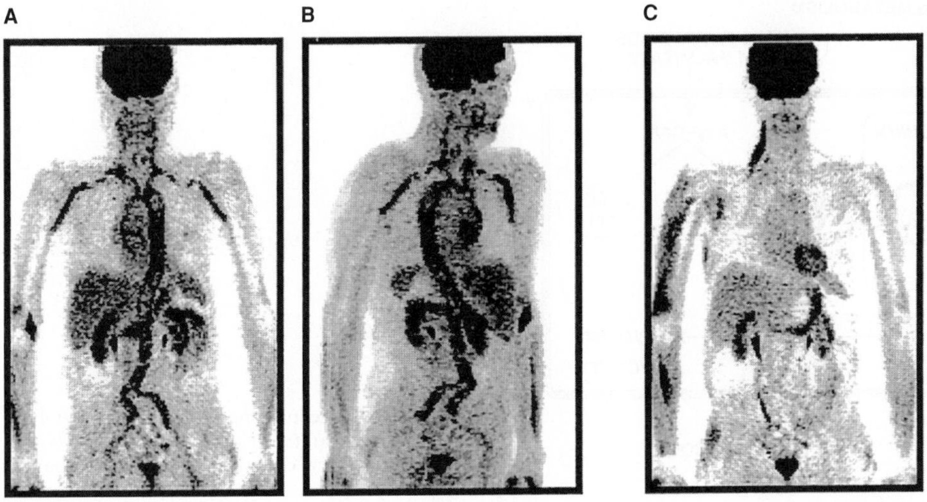

FIGURE 55.7. 18F-FDG-PET studies show increased 18F-FDG uptake along the large vessel walls before, but not after, corticosteroid treatment. Pretreatment images with anterior view and right posterior oblique position are shown in **A** and **B**. (**C**) Posttreatment control with anterior view.

to those obtained at 6 months after initiation of lipid-lowering therapy. These data suggest that other factors (i.e., control of inflammation, remodeling) than only lipid serum levels may be responsible for the beneficial effects of statins on vascular reactivity.

PET/CT application provides further diagnostic strategies by combining functional measurements of myocardial perfusion and extent of calcification (43). Both measurements have shown prognostic value, although the combined prognostic information remains to be defined. With increasing appreciation of inflammation as an important contributor to ischemic syndromes, imaging will play a role identifying the active inflammatory process by imaging markers (116). Rudd et al. (117) demonstrated an increased fluorodeoxyglucose (FDG) uptake in unstable carotid plaques. Acute vasculitis is associated with increased FDG uptake in the vessel wall (Fig. 55.7).

A number of preclinical studies address the possible role of imaging to identify the atherosclerotic process by molecular biomarkers such as overexpression of matrix metalloproteinases (MMPs) (118), integrins (119), adhesion molecules (120), apoptosis (121,122), or collagen exposure (123). Future clinical and experimental studies have to define the role of PET/CT, combining structural and molecular imaging in the characterization of the atherosclerotic disease process.

Other Cardiovascular Diseases. Quantitative flow measurements with PET have been employed in patients with cardiac transplantation to study coronary physiology in this patient population. Several studies have indicated that coronary reserve is maintained in the cardiac transplant (71,124). Wolpers et al. (125) also demonstrated a relationship between angiographic evidence of vasculopathy and PET flow reserve. Quantitative PET flow measurements were also performed in patients with cardiomyopathy (126,127). Patients with hypertrophic cardiomyopathy display a reduced coronary reserve, which not only affects the hypertrophied interventricular septum, but also the free lateral wall (70). These findings indicate that the pathophysiologic process involving the myocardium of patients with hypertrophic cardiomyopathy may not be limited to the hypertrophied interventricular septum (70). In patients with dilated cardiomyopathy, there appears to be a reduction in CFR, which may provide prognostic information (128–130). Data from Parodi et al. (131) show that the flow response to pacing and dipyridamole is altered in patients with dilated cardiomyopathy, suggesting endothelial dysfunction (132). This hypothesis is supported by data reporting decreased flow response to cold pressor testing in this patient population (133).

ASSESSMENT OF SUBSTRATE METABOLISM

Several PET radiopharmaceuticals have been developed to investigate the myocardial energy metabolism, which depends on the oxidation of various substrates (see Table 55.1). Under fasting conditions, the majority of cardiac ATP production relies on the oxidation of free fatty acids (134,135). Free fatty acids are avidly extracted by the myocardium where long-chain acetyl-coenzyme A (CoA) is rapidly formed. Activated fatty acids are used in the synthesis of triglycerides or phospholipids. The majority of acyl-CoA, however, is transported via the carnitine shuttle into the mitochondria where β-oxidation takes place (Fig. 55.8). The end product of β-oxidation is acetyl-CoA, which enters the tricarboxylic acid cycle (TCA) cycle, the final pathway of oxidative metabolism of all substrates. In the presence of high free fatty acid and low insulin plasma levels, only a small amount of glucose is extracted by the myocardium. However, in the postprandial state, glucose transport into the cell is enhanced and glycolytic rate is increased. But even after carbohydrate loading, only about 30% to 50% of overall cardiac substrate metabolism depends on oxidative metabolism of glucose (136). During physical exercise, plasma lactate levels increase and contribute to myocardial energy metabolism (137).

During heart failure, distinct changes in substrate metabolism occur with downregulation of fatty acid metabolism, reduced respiratory chain activity and impaired reserve for mitochondrial oxidative flux (138).

Fatty Acid Metabolism

The first radiopharmaceutical used in combination with PET for the assessment of regional cardiac metabolism was C-11 palmitate. Experimental studies changing cardiac workload or cardiac substrate availability demonstrated changes in C-11 palmitate kinetics (139,140).

To avoid the complexity of substrate interaction defining the relative contribution of long-chain fatty acids and carbohydrates to overall oxidative metabolism, C-11 acetate has been proposed as an alternative probe to describe oxidative metabolism. C-11 acetate is converted to C-11 acetyl-CoA in the mitochondria and enters the TCA cycle. C-11 activity equilibrates within TCA cycle intermediates and C-11 activity clears from the myocardium in the form of C-11-CO_2 (Fig. 55.8). Several studies have indicated that C-11 acetate kinetics, as

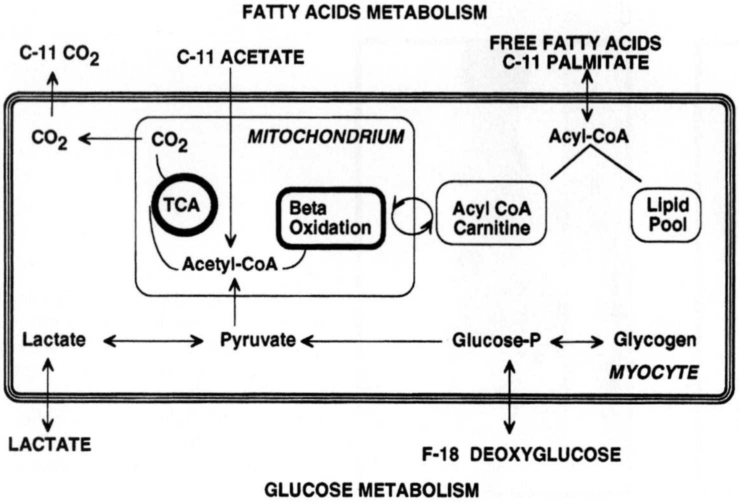

FIGURE 55.8. Conceptual model illustrating metabolic fate of various substrates in the myocardium. *Abbreviations:* Acyl-CoA, acyl-coenzyme A; TCA, tricarboxylic acid cycle.

assessed by dynamic PET imaging, correlate closely with myocardial oxygen consumption. Kinetics of C-11 acetate are only sparsely affected by substrate interactions, and thus allow quantification of myocardial oxygen consumption yielding parameters of oxidative metabolism as well as blood flow (141–145).

Glucose Metabolism

F-18 deoxyglucose traces transmembranous transport, as well as phosphorylation of exogenous glucose (146,147). F-18 deoxyglucose-6-phosphate does not enter any further metabolic pathways, but accumulates in myocardium proportional to glucose transport and phosphorylation (148,149). Exogenous glucose utilization can be quantified using a simple fitting procedure of FDG myocardial kinetics, and parametric display of regional metabolic data (150). The comparison of C-11 acetate uptake and clearance with regional FDG kinetics in normal volunteers demonstrated an inhomogeneity of regional glucose utilization in the heart (151). Regional FDG uptake is increased in the lateral wall of the left ventricle and slightly decreased in the area of intraventricular septum (152). FDG measurements have been performed to evaluate cardiac glucose metabolism in patients with insulin-dependent and non–insulin-dependent diabetes mellitus. In patients with insulin-dependent diabetes, there was no significant difference in overall glucose utilization as compared to a control population, when insulin was substituted by a euglycemic-insulin clamp (153–155). The quantitative nature of the PET measurements allow for in vivo studies under varying conditions to study the relationship of insulin and glucose metabolism in heart and skeletal muscle (156).

Clinical Applications of Metabolic Imaging

Ischemic Heart Disease

Specific changes in regional substrate utilization can occur during acute myocardial ischemia and in patients with chronic ischemic heart disease as demonstrated by PET imaging (157–160). Myocardial ischemia results in impaired oxidative metabolism of fatty acids and increased myocardial glucose utilization (161). Comparing regional myocardial FDG uptake and myocardial blood flow, as assessed by microspheres during acute myocardial ischemia, showed a dissociation of myocardial blood flow and glucose utilization (161). In severe ischemia, however, both blood flow and glucose utilization are reduced, although there is evidence for increased FDG uptake during moderate ischemia.

Experimental studies have shown that myocardial glucose transport and metabolism is upregulated during myocardial ischemia with production and release of lactate (161,162). However, following ischemic episodes, glycolysis remains enhanced with evidence of oxidative and nonoxidative utilization of exogenous glucose. There is evidence that enhanced myocardial oxidative glucose metabolism persists after an ischemic episode, most likely owing to an upregulation of glucose transport (163–165). Biopsy studies in patients with severe CAD and chronic dysfunction of left ventricular segments have shown increased glycogen storage, as evidence of chronic alterations of glucose metabolism in hibernating myocardium (166). Such a metabolic pattern may reflect cell dedifferentiation and altered gene expression profiles in repetitively ischemic myocardium with predominant glycolytic metabolism (167) as protective mechanism to avoid cell death in form of apoptosis or acute necrosis (168–171).

Metabolic Evaluation of Dysfunctioning Myocardium. Animal and clinical studies using FDG as metabolic tracer have shown that reversible left ventricular dysfunction (stunned, hibernating myocardium) is associated with maintained or even increased tissue FDG uptake (157,160,172). Experimental data support the notion that reversible chronic left ventricular dysfunction in patients with advanced CAD does not represent ongoing ischemia, but downregulation of function (168,173). There are two experimental conditions that may serve as a model for the clinical presentation of reversible dysfunction in ischemic heart disease. First, transient ischemia with restoration of blood flow leads to slow functional recovery on the basis of "stunning" (174). Second, chronic reduction of blood flow in the animal model is associated with metabolic adaptive changes, which minimize the imbalance of oxygen supply and demand, limiting the development of irreversible cell injury (hibernation) (175,176). There is increasing evidence that similar mechanisms are involved in the pathophysiology of reversible chronic dysfunction in patients with advanced CAD (177,178). Rahimtoola (177) first described this condition as *hibernating myocardium.* His definition included chronic reduction of blood flow as a culprit for the observed dysfunction, implying chronic ischemia. However, subsequent studies with PET have shown that blood flow can either be normal or only slightly decreased in dysfunctioning viable myocardium (55,179). Based on these results, there is ongoing discussion as to whether reversible left ventricular dysfunction in severe ischemic heart

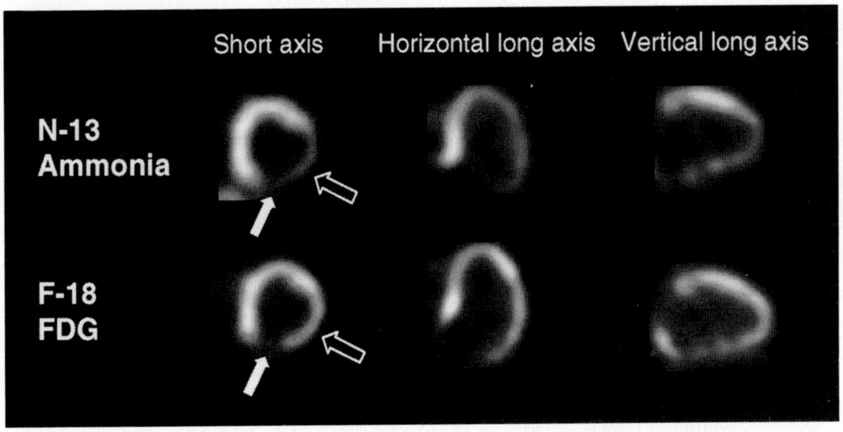

FIGURE 55.9. Positron emission tomographic images using nitrogen-13 ammonia and fluorine-18-fluorodeoxyglucose (F-18-FDG) of a patient with a perfusion to metabolism mismatch pattern (hibernating myocardium, *open arrows*) and scar (*filled arrows*).

disease reflects "repetitive stunning" or "hibernation" (180). The clinical situation in most patients is characterized by a heterogeneous ischemic injury, consisting of necrosis/scar tissue in the subendocardium surrounded by viable but compromised tissue. The dynamic nature of ischemic heart disease renders these segments ischemic during daily life activities, which may lead to repetitive stunning. On the other hand, severe flow restriction may result in chronic hypoperfusion, fulfilling the original criteria of hibernation. PET flow studies demonstrated decreased N-13 ammonia and increased FDG uptake (mismatch) in viable myocardium, which has been considered the scintigraphic hallmark of hibernation (160) (Fig. 55.9). Although such a pattern suggests reduced blood flow, the intensity of tracer uptake depends not only on flow, but also on left ventricular wall thickness (partial volume effect). Therefore, reduction of N-13 ammonia uptake may reflect wall thinning or admixture of viable and scarred myocardium (181). Flow measurements with 0-15 water are less sensitive to partial volume effect, but may overestimate transmural flow (182). In contrast, the FDG signal indicates a relatively higher FDG extraction compared to N-13 ammonia. Using information on both blood flow and glucose metabolism, sensitive specific identification of viable myocardium can be performed. This was first shown by Tillisch et al. (160), who compared relative FDG uptake in patients with advanced CAD and impaired regional and global function before and after revascularization. This study demonstrated that maintained FDG uptake in dysfunctioning segments with reduced flow is associated with functional recovery after revascularization, whereas segments with concordantly decreased flow and metabolism did not recover after restoration of blood flow. Subsequently, a large number of similar studies confirmed the predictive value of FDG imaging. Table 55.3 summarizes clinical PET results, which were collected from several laboratories documenting the high predictive value of PET metabolic imaging for tissue recovery following revascularization. In all studies, recovery of regional function after revascularization served as the gold standard for tissue viability. It has been shown that functional recovery of hibernating myocardium may require several months (183,184).

The degree of functional recovery of patients after revascularization can be predicted based on the scintigraphic pattern, as well as extent of mismatch (181,185). DiCarli reported an 80% likelihood of functional improvement in the presence of mismatch exceeding 18% of the left ventricle. Pagano et al. (185) indicated that the extent of viability correlates not only with functional recovery, but also survival.

Comparison With Other Imaging Modalities. Numerous investigations exist comparing regional FDG uptake with electrocardiographic criteria, standard thallium-201 and Tc-99m flow agents imaging stress echocardiography and MR imaging (187,188). Early observations of discrepant results between FDG distribution and thallium-201 redistribution pattern emphasized the limitations of thallium-201 redistribution imaging for assessment of tissue viability, which are partly overcome by reinjection techniques (189). The use of Tc-99m sestamibi also provides clinically useful information on tissue viability. In combination with nitrate application, the predictive value of Tc-99m sestamibi imaging can be enhanced. Comparing scintigraphic data with those obtained after positive inotropic interventions, it appears that tracer retention provides more sensitive markers of viable myocardium, and assessment of contractile reserve is associated with higher specificity for reversible myocardial dysfunction (189,190).

Late enhancement of the MR signal after intravenous injection of Gadolinium Diethylene triamine acid (Gd DTPA)

TABLE 55.3

PREDICTIVE VALUE OF VIABILITY ASSESSMENT

Reference	Patients	Dysfunctional segments	Predictive accuracy (%)	Positive predictive accuracy (%)	Negative predictive accuracy (%)
Tillish (185)	17	67	88	85	92
Tamaki (256)	22	46	78	78	78
Tamaki (257)	11	56	82	80	100
Marwick (258)	16	85	74	68	79
Lucignani (259)	14	54	91	95	80
Carrel (260)	21	23	83	84	75
Gropler (216)	16	53	81	79	83
Vom Dahl (196)	37	45	80	69	84
Total	154	429	82	82	83

TABLE 55.4

PROGNOSIS OF POSITRON EMISSION TOMOGRAPHY

			n	LVEF (%)	Complications
Hibernating	Drug therapy	Tamaki (208)	31	—	12 (39%)
		Eitzman (207)	18	33	9 (50%)
		Maddahi (302)	17	24	7 (41%)
Scarred	Drug therapy	Tamaki (208)	17	—	1 (6%)
		Eitzman (207)	24	32	3 (13%)
		Maddahi (302)	33	24	3 (9%)
Hibernating	PTCA or CABG	Eitzman (207)	26	36	3 (12%)
		Maddahi (302)	26	25	3 (12%)
Scarred	PTCA or CABG	Eitzman (207)	14	37	1 (7%)
		Maddahi (302)	17	25	1 (6%)

Abbreviations: CABG, coronary artery bypass grafting; LVEF, left ventricular ejection fraction; PTCA, percutaneous transluminal coronary angiography.

has been shown experimentally and clinically to identify irreversible tissue injury (191). Acute myocardial infarction as well as chronic scar formation can be identified with high spatial resolution (192). However, the accurate differentiation of the transmural extent may be difficult. There are several studies comparing PET and MR imaging demonstrating good agreement delineating the area of scar, although the predictive value for tissue recovery and cardiac complications of MR imaging is not yet defined (193–195).

Prognostic Significance of Metabolic Imaging. Aside from the predictive value of FDG for tissue recovery, the prognostic information provided by FDG uptake in segments with reduced perfusion as assessed by N-13 ammonia, PET has been emphasized by several groups (Table 55.4). Retrospective data analysis revealed a high incidence of cardiovascular complications in patients with decreased blood flow, but maintained FDG uptake in patients who did not undergo revascularization (196–198). In contrast, the incidence of cardiovascular complications was similar in groups with scintigraphic evidence of scar or normal myocardium, regardless of whether or not they were revascularized. These data indicate that the mismatch pattern identifies a subgroup of patients at increased risk for cardiovascular complications. The prognostic information appears independent of the traditional markers such as left ventricular ejection fraction or New York Heart Association classification, which were not different among the investigated subgroups. Survival was significantly higher in revascularized patients with mismatch, as demonstrated by DiCarli et al. (185,199).

Furthermore, delay of revascularization in these patients is associated with increased mortality, confirming the prognostic significance of the identification of viable, but jeopardized myocardium (200). Patients with severe left ventricular dysfunction are at higher risk for complications associated with revascularization. Dreyfus et al. (201) reported that assessment of tissue viability in such patients prior to surgery improves the selection process for revascularization with low perioperative mortality. Haas et al. (202) confirmed this prognostic role of PET by comparing short-term and midterm survival following surgical revascularization in two groups of patients with three-vessel disease and impaired left ventricular function.

Metabolic Imaging in Patients With Other Cardiovascular Diseases

Dilated Cardiomyopathy. C-11 palmitate has been employed to study fatty acid metabolism in patients with dilated cardiomyopathy. Observations by Geltman et al. (203) revealed a heterogeneous fatty acid metabolism in patients with dilated cardiomyopathy in the presence of relatively homogeneous perfusion, as measured with thallium-201 scintigraphy. Kelly et al. (204) addressed the role of C-11 palmitate in probing mitochondrial enzyme defects resulting in an impairment of β-oxidation. These investigators were able to demonstrate that oxidation of C-11 acetate was dissociated from that of C-11 palmitate in patients affected with this enzyme disorder. As discussed above, C-11 acetate allows the noninvasive assessment of myocardial oxygen consumption (205). This tracer approach can be used to probe myocardial oxygen consumption in the normal as well as diseased cardiac muscle. In addition, this technique can be used to assess right ventricular oxygen consumption, as demonstrated by Hicks et al. (206), who described a close relationship between right ventricular acetate kinetics in patients and pulmonary artery pressure. Wolpers et al. (207) first introduced the concept of noninvasively assessing myocardial efficiency by PET as defined by external work of the left ventricle divided by oxygen consumption. Such a parameter allows the assessment of the link between mechanical performance and metabolic demand under various pathophysiologic conditions as well as after therapeutic interventions (143,208).

Beanlands et al. (209) applied this method in patients with cardiomyopathy before and after therapy with dobutamine and nitroprusside. Myocardial efficiency increased following both pharmacologic interventions. In both instances, the improvement in cardiac efficiency was most related to changes in left ventricular afterload. More recently, Beanlands et al. (143) demonstrated the beneficial effect of β-blockade (metoprolol) on metabolic left ventricular performance in heart failure patients using C-11 acetate.

ASSESSMENT OF AUTONOMIC INNERVATION

Tracer approaches are uniquely suited to the assessment of specific tissue function. Although tracers have been developed for the parasympathetic nervous system, the sparse cholinergic innervation of the left ventricle limits the presynaptic evaluation of this system in vivo. Therefore, most imaging approaches focus on the scintigraphic delineation of the pre- and postsynaptic sympathetic nervous systems because the left and right ventricles are densely innervated by sympathetic fibers. Figure 55.10 displays the nerve terminal, which is an important functional unit of the sympathetic nervous system.

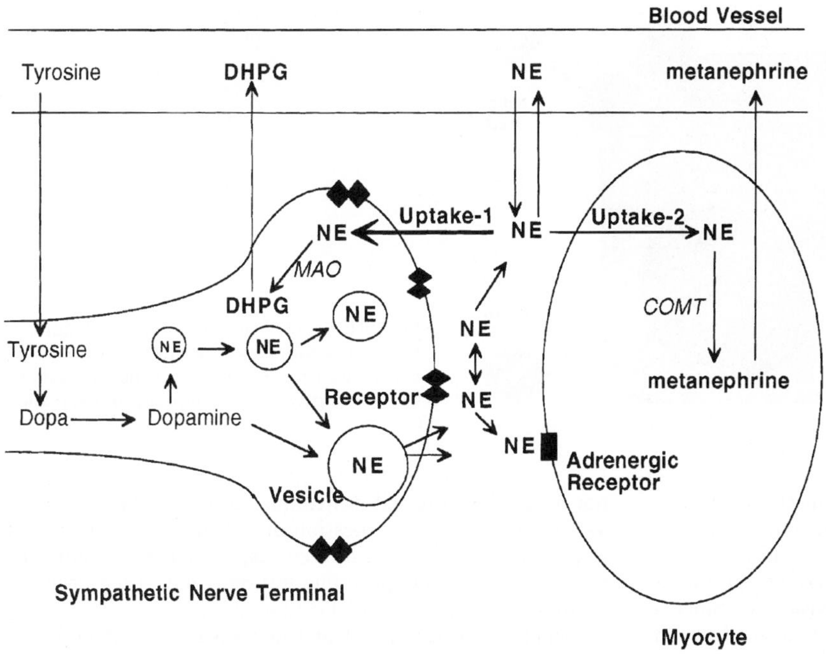

FIGURE 55.10. Conceptual model of a sympathetic nerve terminal. *Abbreviations:* COMT, catechol-O-methyl transferase; DHPG, 3,4-dihydroxyphenylglycol; MAO, monoamine oxidase; NE, norepinephrine.

Imaging of Presynaptic Nerve Terminals

The use of radiolabeled norepinephrine or analogs appears to be most promising for the visualization of the sympathetic nerve terminals, because norepinephrine is the predominant cardiac neurotransmitter and undergoes a rapid reuptake in the nerve terminal via uptake 1. C-11 hydroxyephedrine (HED) has been synthesized at the University of Michigan (Fig 55.10) (210). This norepinephrine analog is taken up by the nerve terminal, but is not metabolized by the intraneuronal enzyme systems. The myocardial retention of this tracer reflects the activity of uptake 1 mechanism and, to a lesser degree, the storage of norepinephrine in nerve terminals (211). In contrast, the more recently introduced compound C-11 epinephrine is not only taken up by the nerve terminal, but also stored in the vesicles of nerve terminals (212). A further analog of epinephrine is phenylephrine, which enters the nerve terminal via uptake 1, but is primarily metabolized by the MAO enzyme system (213). Other radiopharmaceuticals for the characterization of the presynaptic nerve terminal include F-18 dopamine and F-18 norepinephrine, as well as metabromobenzylguanidine (MBBG) (214–216).

Clinical Application

Initial clinical applications of C-11 HED show excellent image quality with high contrast between myocardial tracer activity and blood pool, as well as lung tissue surrounding the heart (Fig. 55.9). The specificity of the tracer approach for neuronal tissue has been well-documented by studies in cardiac transplant patients, which showed a marked reduction of tracer uptake, suggesting only little nonspecific binding of this tracer (211), which allows for quantitative image analysis (217). Studies in transplant patients at various time points following surgery indicate partial reinnervation of transplanted myocardium by retention of C-11 HED in the anterior septal segments of the left ventricle in transplant recipients several years after operation (218). Comparison of this scintigraphic pattern with heart rate variability suggests that the partial reinnervation of left ventricle is associated with evidence of functional reinnervation (219–221), yielding better hemodynamic adaptation to exercise as assessed by left ventricular ejection fraction and regional wall motion (222).

Allman et al. (223) employed C-11 HED in the assessment of patients with acute myocardial infarction undergoing thrombolytic therapy. Experimental data indicated that the extent of neuronal damage following transient ischemia is larger than the area of tissue necrosis. Wolpers et al. (224) demonstrated a decreased retention fraction of C-11 HED in reperfused canine myocardium, suggesting a high sensitivity of neurons to ischemic injury. Similar data have been observed in the clinical setting (224). The area of neuronal dysfunction, as evidenced by C-11 HED defects, was significantly larger than the area of perfusion abnormalities in patients with acute myocardial infarction and correlated closely with the area of risk as assessed by Tc-99m sestamibi imaging in the same patients confirming the experimental data (225). C-11 HED PET studies were also performed in patients with diabetic neuropathy. These studies revealed a correlation between the results of autonomic nervous system testing and the abnormalities of HED distribution. Surprising was the finding that regional cardiac denervation represents a heterogeneous process in patients with diabetic neuropathy. C-11 HED defects were most severe in the apical segments of the left ventricle and least severe in the proximal segments of the left ventricle (226–228). Comparison of neuronal dysfunction and blood flow measurements by PET revealed impaired vasodilator response in diabetic patients (229).

Preliminary studies suggest the prognostic possible role of HED imaging in patients with congestive heart failure (230). Several investigators demonstrated decreased HED uptake in patients with severely impaired left ventricular function, suggesting neuronal damage in this patient population (231, 232). Again, this process appears to be heterogeneous with pronounced abnormalities in the apical segments of the left ventricle.

Postsynaptic Receptor Sites

The development of radiotracers and the initial clinical validation of tracer methods for the visualization of the adrenergic receptor system has been initiated by the group of Syrota et al. (233). The specific visualization of cardiac β-receptors became possible by the successful radiosynthesis of a more hydrophilic

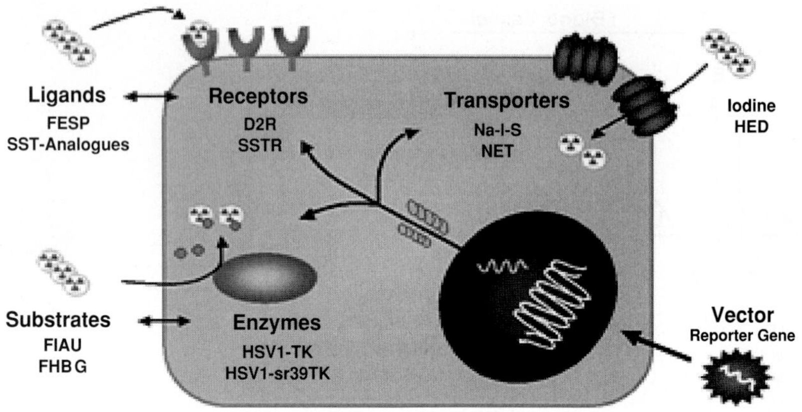

FIGURE 55.11. Schematic display of different types of reporter gene products and their specific labeled reporter probes, which are suitable for noninvasive imaging of transgene expression.

β-receptor antagonist (CGP-12177). This nonselective C-11–labeled β-receptor antagonist provided excellent image quality of the postsynaptic binding sites in the heart (233). A tracer kinetic model approach has yielded estimates of receptor densities in agreement with in vitro β-receptor density assessments (234). Clinical validation of this approach confirmed the in vitro demonstrated reduction of β-receptor density in patients with congestive heart failure. This approach has also been adapted by Camici et al. and used in patients with hypertrophic cardiomyopathy, arrhythmogenic right ventricular cardiomyopathy and syndrome X (235–238).

IMAGING OF GENE EXPRESSION

Receptor gene imaging has been introduced to follow gene or cell therapy strategies (239,240). This technology has emerged as an attractive tool in experimental medicine to monitor specific gene expression based on reporter protein synthesis, which can be linked to tissue- and/or pathway-specific promoters (241). It is also expected that reporter gene imaging may help to identify stem cells in cardiac tissue and to follow protein expression patterns based on cell differentiation (242). Several gene products have been proposed to serve as reporter signals (Fig. 55.11). Initially, the herpes simplex virus thymidine kinase (HSV1-Tk) was used as gene products, which can be targeted by radiolabeled substrates such as pyrimidine or acyloguanosine analogues (243–245). Animal studies have shown that the scintigraphic signal quantitatively correlates with the protein expression providing a high biological contrast; this protein is not naturally expressed in mammalian tissue (246). As alternative approach, the expression of cell-surface receptors such as dopamine, somatostatin receptors, as well as transport proteins, such as iodine, or amine transport have been proposed as imaging targets (Fig. 55.11) (246–248).

Bengel et al. (239,245) first demonstrated that HSV1-Tk reporter gene imaging cannot only be applied in tumor tissue, but is also suitable to monitor cardiac gene expression. Most recently, the human sodium/iodide symporter gene (*hNIS*) symporter gene has been shown to be highly effective for reporter gene imaging in cardiac tissue (247). In comparison to the HSV1-Tk gene, the imaging contrast was significantly higher with *hNIS* as reporter gene (Fig. 55.12). Despite impressive first results, the limitations of reporter gene imaging concerning vector systems, local delivery, and immune response to virus and protein, limiting the time period of expression have to be overcome before these techniques can be transferred to clinical application (240). Newer approaches include vector constructs, which include therapeutic (VEGF) as well as reporter (HSVTK) gene expression. Anton et al. (249) demonstrated a close correlation of VEGF expression and reporter gene imaging signal in cell culture as well in an in vivo pig model. First experimental applications in combination with cardiac myoblasts injected directly into cardiac tissue suggest the feasibility of imaging transfected cells yielding new means to monitor cell migration and differentiation (242). Future experimental studies have to address the question of whether the sensitivity of PET imaging compared to optical imaging is high enough to noninvasively follow individual cell clusters by in vivo imaging (242).

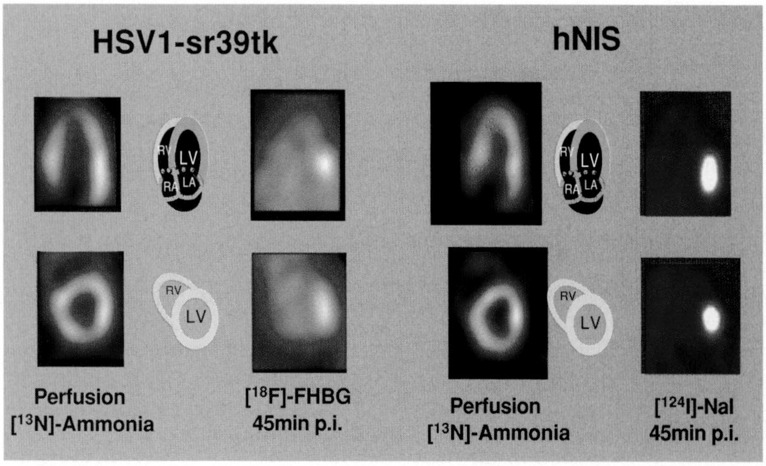

FIGURE 55.12. PET imaging of cardiac reporter gene expression. Shown are tomographic images of pig hearts 2 days after regional adenoviral transfer of a mutant herpes viral thymidine kinase gene (HSV1-sr39tk, left) or the human sodium-iodide symporter gene (hNIS, *right*), into basal anterolateral wall. Perfusion, assessed by 13N-ammonia, is regionally homogeneous in both cases. Accumulation of specific reporter probes (18F-FHBG for HSV1-sr39tk and 124I-NaI for hNIS) is used to successfully identify regional reporter gene expression. Note the stronger imaging signal derived from hNIS and 124I, indicating a potential advantage when using this reporter gene for imaging of transfected stem cells or coexpressed therapeutic genes.

It is expected that molecular PET imaging will play an important and unique role in translating new biological imaging signals—validated in the animal model—to clinical research to evaluate new cell- or gene-based therapies.

SUMMARY OF CURRENT STATUS

The improved imaging technology of PET and especially PET/CT allows for the highly accurate characterization of CAD. Coronary reserve measurements together with vascular CT imaging may be useful in the early detection of vascular abnormalities and follow-up of therapeutic interventions designed to stop or reverse CAD. Molecular targets accessible by imaging may be helpful to visualize plaque biology. Finally, such measurements may serve as endpoints in the evaluation of new drugs altering the atherosclerotic process.

Assessment of tissue viability has become an important application for PET in cardiology. Metabolic imaging documented the high incidence of reversible dysfunction in patients with severe CAD. These PET findings resulted in increasing diagnostic efforts to identify viable myocardium by various methods. Currently, PET must still be considered the reference method for identification of tissue viability with established diagnostic and—more importantly—prognostic value. Finally, new tracer approaches designed to map cardiac innervation and molecular processes, such as angiogenesis and apoptosis may not only prove useful in clinical and experimental research, but also provide important prognostic information in patients with heart failure and primary myocardial disease.

CONTROVERSIES AND PERSONAL PERSPECTIVES

Cardiovascular imaging has witnessed an impressive growth in recent years. Competing modalities have advanced rapidly driven by the large market "coronary artery disease." Noninvasive coronary angiography is around the corner, which will change established diagnostic strategies and challenge organizational aspects of in- and outpatient care. However, aside from the noninvasive detection of coronary stenoses, the diagnostic quality in CAD needs to be improved by introducing new biomarkers, which reflect the increasing pathophysiologic understanding of the atherosclerotic disease process. The structural description of coronary artery stenosis will increasingly be replaced by signals, which biologically characterize the vessel wall allowing early and specific delineation of atherosclerosis and inflammation. For this purpose, multimodality imaging such as PET/CT and MR/PET will combine the high spatial resolution necessary for structural imaging of vascular structures with the high sensitivity of tracer techniques necessary to visualize biological targets.

Future applications of optical techniques may provide both spatial resolution and sensitivity, but the difficult detection of the light signal by noninvasive imaging may restrict the clinical application of optical methods to intravascular probes. Not only CAD will benefit from molecular imaging, but also myocardial diseases will be characterized and followed by imaging techniques, which define function, biochemistry, and molecular biology of myocardial tissue and describe changes induced by therapy. Identification of therapeutic targets such as apoptosis, angiogenesis, and inflammation may provide guidance of individual therapies and can be used as surrogate endpoints for the efficient evaluation of new drugs.

Despite increasing complexity, I strongly believe in the future of multimodality imaging combining the strengths of each modality in an interdisciplinary effort to improve patient care and clinical research.

ACKNOWLEDGMENTS

The authors thank Gabriele Sonoda for her excellent and untiring secretarial support for this project.

References

1. Buchanan J, Hastings A. The use of isotopically marked carbon in the study of intermediary metabolism. *Physiol Rev* 1946;26:120–155.
2. Tobias C, Lawrence J, Roughton F. The elimination of carbon monoxide from human body with reference to the possible conversion of carbon monoxide to carbon dioxide. *Am J Physiol* 1945;145:253–263.
3. Brownell G, Sweet W. Localization of brain tumors with positron-emitters. *Nucleonics* 1953;11:40–45.
4. Aronow S. Positron scanning. In: Hine G, ed. *Instrumentation in nuclear medicine*. New York: Academic Press; 1967:461–483.
5. Kuhl D, Edwards R. Image separation radioisotope scanning. *Radiology* 1963;80:653–661.
6. Phelps M, Hoffman E, Mullani N, Ter-Pogossian M. Application of annihilation coincidence detection to transaxial reconstruction tomography. *J Nucl Med* 1975;16:210–224.
7. Ter Pogossian M, Phelps M, Hoffman E. A positron emission transaxial tomograph for nuclear medicine imaging (PETT). *Radiology* 1975;114:89–98.
8. Hoffman EJ, Phelps ME, Weiss ES, Welch MJ, et al. Transaxial tomographic imaging of canine myocardium with 11C-palmitic acid. *J Nucl Med* 1977;18:57–61.
9. Beyer T, Townsend DW, Brun T, et al. A combined PET/CT scanner for clinical oncology. *J Nucl Med* 2000;41:1369–1379.
10. Townsend DW, Cherry SR. Combining anatomy and function: the path to true image fusion. *Eur Radiol* 2001;11:1857–1858.
11. Lardinois D, Weder W, Hany TF, et al. Staging of non-small-cell lung cancer with integrated positron-emission tomography and computed tomography. *N Engl J Med* 2003;348:2500–2507.
12. Porenta G, Kuhle W, Sinha S, et al. Parameter estimation of cardiac geometry by ECG-gated PET imaging: validation using magnetic resonance imaging and echocardiography. *J Nucl Med* 1995;36:1123–1129.
13. Casey M, Nutt R. Multi-crysta two-dimensional BGO detector system for positron emission tomography. *IEEE Trans Nucl Sci* 1986;33:460–463.
14. Humm JL, Rosenfeld A, Del Guerra A. From PET detectors to PET scanners. *Eur J Nucl Med Mol Imaging* 2003;30:1574–1597.
15. Meikle S, Dahlbom M, Cherry S. Attenuation correction using count-limited transmission data in positron emission tomography. *J Nucl Med* 1993;34:143–150.
16. Thompson CJ, Ranger N, Evans AC, Gjedde A. Validation of simultaneous PET emission and transmission scans. *J Nucl Med* 1991;32:154–160.
17. Kinahan PE, Townsend DW, Beyer T, Sashin D. Attenuation correction for a combined 3D PET/CT scanner. *Med Phys* 1998;25:2046–2053.
18. Hoop B, Laughlin JS, Tilbury RS. Cyclotrons in nuclear medicine. In: Hine GJ, Sorensen JA, eds. *Instrumentation in nuclear medicine*. New York: Academic Press; 1974:407.
19. Fowler JS, Wolf AP. Positron emitter-labeled compounds: priorities and problems. In: Phelps ME, Mazziotta JC, Schelbert HR, eds. *Positron emission tomography and autoradiography: Principles and applications for the brain and heart*. New York: Raven Press; 1986:391.
20. *Handbook of Radiopharmaceuticals*. Chichester: John Wiley & Sons Ltd; 2003.
21. Iida H, Kanno I, Takahashi A, et al. Measurement of absolute myocardial blood flow with $H_2{}^{15}O$ and dynamic positron emission tomography. Strategy for quantification in relation to the partial-volume effect. *Circulation* 1988;78:104–115.
22. Araujo LI, Lammertsma AA, Rhodes CG, et al. Noninvasive quantification of regional myocardial blood flow in coronary artery disease with oxygen-15-labeled carbon dioxide inhalation and positron emission tomography. *Circulation* 1991;83:875–885.
23. Bergmann S, Herrero P, Markham J, et al. Non-invasive quantitation of myocardial blood flow in human subjects with oxygen-15 labeled water and positron emission tomography. *J Am Coll Cardiol* 1989;14:639–652.
24. Schelbert HR, Phelps ME, Huang S-C, et al. N-13 Ammonia as an indicator of myocardial blood flow. *Circulation* 1981;63:1259–1272.
25. Schelbert H, Phelps M, Hoffman E, et al. Regional myocardial perfusion assessed with N-13 labeled ammonia and positron emission computerized axial tomography. *Am J Cardiol* 1979;43:209–218.
26. Bergmann SR, Hack S, Tewson T, et al. The dependence of accumulation of 13NH3 by myocardium on metabolic factors and its implications for quantitative assessment of perfusion. *Circulation* 1980;61:34–43.
27. Mullani NA, Goldstein RA, Gould KL, et al. Myocardial perfusion with rubidium-82. I. Measurement of extraction fraction and flow with external detectors. *J Nucl Med* 1983;24:898–906.
28. Melon P, Brihaye C, Degueldre C, et al. Myocardial kinetics of potassium-38 in man and comparison with copper-62-PTSM. *J Nucl Med* 1994;35:1122–1124.

29. Beller GA, Cochavi S, Smith TW, Brownell GL. Positron emission tomographic imaging of the myocardium with Rb-81. *J Comput Assist Tomogr* 1982;6:341–349.
30. Krivokapich J, Huang S, Phelps M, et al. Dependence of $^{13}NH_3$ myocardial extraction and clearance on flow and metabolism. *Am J Physiol* 1982;242:H536–542.
31. Kaufmann PA, Camici PG. Myocardial blood flow measurement by PET: technical aspects and clinical applications. *J Nucl Med* 2005;46:75–88.
32. Gould K. Assessment of coronary stenoses with myocardial perfusion imaging during pharmacologic coronary vasodilation. *Am J Cardiol* 1978;42:761–768.
33. Go RT, Marwick TH, MacIntyre WJ, et al. A prospective comparison of rubidium-82 PET and thallium-201 SPECT myocardial perfusion imaging utilizing a single dipyridamole stress in the diagnosis of coronary artery disease [see comments]. *J Nucl Med* 1990;31:1899–1905.
34. Stewart RE, Schwaiger M, Molina E, et al. Comparison of Rubidium-82 positron emission tomography and thallium-201 SPECT imaging for detection of coronary artery disease. *Am J Cardiol* 1991;67:1303–1310.
35. Tamaki N, Yonekura Y, Senda M, et al. Myocardial positron computed tomography with 13N-ammonia at rest and during exercise. *Eur J Nucl Med* 1985;11:246–251.
36. Gould KL, Goldstein RA, Mullani NA, et al. Noninvasive assessment of coronary stenoses by myocardial perfusion imaging during pharmacologic coronary vasodilation. VIII. Clinical feasibility of positron cardiac imaging without a cyclotron using generator-produced rubidium-82. *J Am Coll Cardiol* 1986;7:775–789.
37. Demer LL, Gould KL, Goldstein RA, et al. Assessment of coronary artery disease severity by positron emission tomography. Comparison with quantitative arteriography in 193 patients. *Circulation* 1989;79:825–835.
38. Chan SY, Brunken RC, Czernin J, et al. Comparison of maximal myocardial blood flow during adenosine infusion with that of intravenous dipyridamole in normal men. *J Am Coll Cardiol* 1992;20:979–985.
39. Tamaki N, Yonehura Y, Senda M, et al. Value and limitation of stress thallium-201 single photon positron emission computed tomography: comparison with nitrogen-13 ammonia positron tomography. *J Nucl Med* 1988;29:1181–1188.
40. Porenta G, Kuhle W, Czernin J, et al. Semiquantitative assessment of myocardial blood flow and viability using polar map displays of cardiac PET images. *J Nucl Med* 1992;33:1628–1636.
41. Laubenbacher C, Rothley J, Sitomer J, et al. An automated analysis program for the evaluation of cardiac PET studies: initial results in the detection and localization of coronary artery disease using nitrogen-13-ammonia. *J Nucl Med* 1993;34:968–978.
42. Yoshinaga K, Katoh C, Noriyasu K, et al. Reduction of coronary flow reserve in areas with and without ischemia on stress perfusion imaging in patients with coronary artery disease: a study using oxygen 15-labeled water PET. *J Nucl Cardiol* 2003;10:275–283.
43. Pirich C, Leber A, Knez A, et al. Relation of coronary vasoreactivity and coronary calcification in asymptomatic subjects with a family history of premature coronary artery disease. *Eur J Nucl Med Mol Imaging* 2004;31:663–670.
44. Berman DS, Wong ND, Gransar H, et al. Relationship between stress-induced myocardial ischemia and atherosclerosis measured by coronary calcium tomography. *J Am Coll Cardiol* 2004;44:923–930.
45. Gould KL, Nakagawa Y, Nakagawa K, et al. Frequency and clinical implications of fluid dynamically significant diffuse CAD manifest as graded, longitudinal, base-to-apex myocardial perfusion abnormalities by noninvasive PET. *Circulation* 2000;101:1931–1939.
46. Gould KL, Martucci JP, Goldberg DI, et al. Short-term cholesterol lowering decreases size and severity of perfusion abnormalities by positron emission tomography after dipyridamole in patients with coronary artery disease: a potential noninvasive marker of healing coronary endothelium. *Circulation* 1994;89:1530–1538.
47. Gould KL, Ornish D, Scherwitz L, et al. Changes in myocardial perfusion abnormalities by positron emission tomography after long-term, intense risk factor modification. *JAMA* 1995;274:894–901.
48. Iida H, Takahashi A, Ono Y, et al. Quantitative and noninvasive measurement of myocardial blood flow using H2-15O and dynamic positron emission tomography. *J Nucl Med* 1986;27.
49. Hermansen F, Rosen S, Fath-Ordoubadi F, et al. Measurement of myocardial blood flow with oxygen-15 labelled water: comparison of different administration protocols. *Eur J Nucl Med* 1998;25:751–759.
50. Ahn J, Lee D, Lee J, et al. Quantification of regional myocardial blood flow using dynamic H2(15)O PET and factor analysis. *J Nucl Med* 2001;42:782–787.
51. Schafers KP, Spinks TJ, Camici PG, et al. Absolute quantification of myocardial blood flow with H(2)(15)O and 3-dimensional PET: an experimental validation. *J Nucl Med* 2002;43:1031–1040.
52. Bergmann SR, Fox K, Rand A, et al. Quantification of regional myocardial blood flow with H215-0. *Circulation* 1984;70:724–733.
53. Muzik O, Beanlands RS, Hutchins GD, et al. Validation of nitrogen-13-ammonia tracer kinetic model for quantification of myocardial blood flow using PET. *J Nucl Med* 1993;34:83–91.
54. Bol A, Melin JA, Vanoverschelde JL, et al. Direct comparison of [13N]ammonia and [15O]water estimates of perfusion with quantification of regional myocardial blood flow by microspheres. *Circulation* 1993;87:512–525.
55. Iida H, Tamura Y, Kitamura K, et al. Histochemical correlates of 15O-water-perfusable tissue fraction in experimental canine studies of old myocardial infarction. *J Nucl Med* 2000;41:1737–1745.
56. Katoh C, Ruotsalainen U, Laine H, et al. Iterative reconstruction based on median root prior in quantification of myocardial blood flow and oxygen metabolism. *J Nucl Med* 1999;40:862–867.
57. Krivokapich J, Smith GT, Huang S-C, et al. 13N ammonia myocardial imaging at rest and with exercise in normal volunteers: quantification of absolute myocardial perfusion with dynamic positron emission tomography. *Circulation* 1989;80:1328–1337.
58. Hutchins G, Schwaiger M, Rosenspire K, et al. Noninvasive quantification of regional myocardial blood flow in the human heart using N-13 ammonia and dynamic positron emission tomographic imaging. *J Am Coll Cardiol* 1990;15:1032.
59. Choi Y, Huang SC, Hawkins RA, et al. A simplified method for quantification of myocardial blood flow using nitrogen-13-ammonia and dynamic PET. *J Nucl Med* 1993;34:488–497.
60. Choi Y, Huang SC, Hawkins RA, et al. Quantification of myocardial blood flow using 13N-ammonia and PET: comparison of tracer models. *J Nucl Med* 1999;40:1045–1055.
61. Herrero P, Markham J, Shelton ME, et al. Noninvasive quantification of regional myocardial perfusion with rubidium-82 and positron emission tomography. *Circulation* 1990;82:1377–1386.
62. deKemp RA, Ruddy TD, Hewitt T, et al. Detection of serial changes in absolute myocardial perfusion with 82Rb PET. *J Nucl Med* 2000;41:1426–1435.
63. Herrero P, Markham J, Weinheimer CJ, et al. Quantification of regional myocardial perfusion with generator-produced 62Cu-PTSM and positron emission tomography. *Circulation* 1993;87:173–183.
64. Gould K, Kirkeeide R, Buchi M. Coronary flow reserve as a physiologic measure of stenosis severity. *J Am Coll Cardiol* 1990;15:459–474.
65. Mancini JGB, Williamson PR, DeBoe SF. Effect of coronary stenosis severity on variability of quantitative arteriography and implications for interventional trials. *Am J Cardiol* 1992;69:806–807.
66. Wilson RF, Marcus ML, White CW. Prediction of the physiologic significance of coronary arterial lesions by quantitative lesion geometry in patients with limited coronary artery disease. *Circulation* 1987;75:723–732.
67. Sawada S, Muzik O, Beanlands RSB, et al. Interobserver and interstudy variability of myocardial blood flow and flow-reserve measurements with nitrogen 13 ammonia-labeled positron emission tomography. *J Nucl Cardiol* 1995;2:413–422.
68. Kaufmann PA, Gnecchi-Ruscone T, Yap JT, et al. Assessment of the reproducibility of baseline and hyperemic myocardial blood flow measurements with 15O-labeld water PET. *J Nucl Med* 1999;40:1848–1856.
69. Beanlands RS, Muzik O, Melon P, et al. Noninvasive quantification of regional myocardial flow reserve in patients with coronary atherosclerosis using nitrogen-13 ammonia positron emission tomography. Determination of extent of altered vascular reactivity. *J Am Coll Cardiol* 1995;26:1465–1475.
70. Camici P, Chiriatti G, Lorenzoni R, et al. Coronary vasodilation is impaired in both hypertrophied and nonhypertrophied myocardium of patients with hypertrophic cardiomyopathy: a study with nitrogen-13 ammonia and positron emission tomography. *J Am Coll Cardiol* 1991;17:879–886.
71. Krivokapich J, Stevenson LW, Kobashigawa J, et al. Quantification of absolute myocardial perfusion at rest and during exercise with positron emission tomography after human cardiac transplantation. *J Am Coll Cardiol* 1991;18:512–517.
72. Uren NG, Melin JA, De-Bruyne B, et al. Relation between myocardial blood flow and the severity of coronary-artery stenosis. *N Engl J Med* 1994;330:1782–1788.
73. DiCarli M, Czernin J, Hoh CK, et al. Relation among stenosis severity, myocardial blood flow, and flow reserve in patients with coronary artery disease. *Circulation* 1995;91:1944–1951.
74. Araujo LI. Myocardial perfusion and metabolic changes associated with transient episodes of ischemia in patients with coronary artery disease as assessed by positron emission tomography. *Coron Artery Dis* 1990;1:54106 (abstract).
75. Picano E, Parodi O, Lattanzi F, et al. Assessment of anatomic and physiological severity of single-vessel coronary artery lesions by dipyridamole echocardiography. Comparison with positron emission tomography and quantitative angiography. *Circulation* 1994;89:753–761.
76. Muzik O, Duvernoy C, Beanlands R, et al. Assessment of diagnostic performance of quantitative flow measurements in normal subjects and patients with angiographically documented CAD by means of nitrogen-13 ammonia and using PET. *J Am Coll Cardiol* 1998;31:534–540.
77. Czernin J, Muller P, Chan S, Brunken R, et al. Influence of age and hemodynamics on myocardial blood flow and flow reserve. *Circulation* 1993;88:62–69.
78. Uren NG, Camici PG, Melin JA, et al. Effect of aging on myocardial perfusion reserve. *J Nucl Med* 1995;36:2032–2036.
79. Chareonthaitawee P, Kaufmann PA, Rimoldi O, Camici PG. Heterogeneity of resting and hyperemic myocardial blood flow in healthy humans. *Cardiovasc Res* 2001;50:151–161.

80. Rosen SD, Uren NG, Kaski JC, et al. Coronary vasodilator reserve, pain perception, and sex in patients with syndrome X. *Circulation* 1994;90:50–60.
81. Parodi O, Neglia D, Sambuceti G, et al. Regional myocardial blood flow and coronary reserve in hypertensive patients. The effect of therapy. *Drugs* 1992;1:48–55.
82. Kitsiou AN, Bacharach SL, Bartlett ML, et al. 13N-ammonia myocardial blood flow and uptake: relation to functional outcome of asynergic regions after revascularization. *J Am Coll Cardiol* 1999;33:678–686.
83. Bogaert J, Maes A, Van der Werf F, et al. Functional recovery of subepicardial myocardial tissue in transmural myocardial infarction after successful reperfusion: an important contribution to the improvement of regional and global left ventricular function. *Circulation* 1999;99:36–43.
84. Rimoldi O, Burns SM, Rosen SD, et al. Measurement of myocardial blood flow with positron emission tomography before and after transmyocardial laser revascularization. *Circulation* 1999;100:134–138.
85. Hughes GC, Kypson AP, St. Louis JD, et al. Improved perfusion and contractile reserve after transmural laser revascularization in a model of hibernating myocardium. *Ann Thorac Surg* 1999;67:1714–1720.
86. Schneider CA, Voth E, Moka D, et al. Improvement of myocardial blood flow to ischemic regions by angiotensin-converting enzyme inhibition with quinaprilat IV: a study using [15O] water dobutamine stress positron emission tomography. *J Am Coll Cardiol* 1999;34:1005–1011.
87. Kosa I, Blasini R, Schneider-Eicke J, et al. Early recovery of coronary flow reserve after stent implantation as assessed by PET. *J Am Coll Cardiol* 1999;34:1036–1041.
88. Spyrou N, Khan MA, Rosen SD, et al. Persistent but reversible coronary microvascular dysfunction after bypass grafting. *Am J Physiol Heart Circ Physiol* 2000;279:H2634–H2640.
89. Campisi R, Czernin J, Schoder H, et al. Effects of long-term smoking on myocardial blood flow, coronary vasomotion, and vasodilator capacity. *Circulation* 1998;98:119–125.
90. Gnecchi-Ruscone T, Bernard X, Pierre P, et al. Effect of naratriptan on myocardial blood flow and coronary vasodilator reserve in migraineurs. *Neurology* 2000;55:95–99.
91. Muzik O, Duvernoy C, Beanlands RS, et al. Assessment of diagnostic performance of quantitative flow measurements in normal subjects and patients with angiographically documented coronary artery disease by means of nitrogen-13 ammonia and positron emission tomography. *J Am Coll Cardiol* 1998;31:534–540.
92. Kuhle WG, Porenta G, Huang SC, et al. Quantification of regional myocardial blood flow using 13N-ammonia and reoriented dynamic positron emission tomographic imaging. *Circulation* 1992;86:1004–1017.
93. Uren NG, Marraccini P, Gistri R, et al. Altered coronary vasodilator reserve and metabolism in myocardium subtended by normal arteries in patients with coronary artery disease. *J Am Coll Cardiol* 1993;22:650–658.
94. Pitkanen OP, Nuutila P, Raitakari OT, et al. Coronary flow reserve is reduced in young men with IDDM. *Diabetes* 1998;47:248–254.
95. Raitakari O, Pitkänen O-P, Lehtimäki T, et al. In vivo low density lipoprotein oxidation relates to coronary reactivity in young men. *J Am Coll Cardiol* 1997;30.
96. Duvernoy C, Meyer C, Seifert-Klauss V, et al. Gender differences in myocardial blood flow dynamics: lipid profile and hemodynamic effects. *J Am Coll Cardiol* 1999;33:463–470.
97. Kaufmann PA, Gnecchi-Ruscone T, di Terlizzi M, et al. Coronary heart disease in smokers: vitamin C restores coronary microcirculatory function. *Circulation* 2000;102:1233–1238.
98. Pitkanen OP, Nuutila P, Raitakari OT, et al. Coronary flow reserve in young men with familial combined hyperlipidemia. *Circulation* 1999;99:1678–1684.
99. Maseri A, Crea F, Cianflone D. Myocardial ischemia caused by distal coronary vasoconstriction [editorial]. *Am J Cardiol* 1992;70:1602–1605.
100. Mauriello A, Sangiorgi G, Fratoni S, et al. Diffuse and active inflammation occurs in both vulnerable and stable plaques of the entire coronary tree: a histopathologic study of patients dying of acute myocardial infarction. *J Am Coll Cardiol* 2005;45:1585–1593.
101. Uren NG, Crake T, Lefroy DC, et al. Reduced coronary vasodilator function in infarcted and normal myocardium after myocardial infarction. *N Engl J Med* 1994;331:222–227.
102. Bottcher M, Czernin J, Sun K, et al. Effect of beta 1 adrenergic receptor blockade on myocardial blood flow and vasodilatory capacity. *J Nucl Med* 1997;38:442–446.
103. Rosen SD, Lorenzoni R, Kaski JC, et al. Effect of alpha1-adrenoceptor blockade on coronary vasodilator reserve in cardiac syndrome X. *J Cardiovasc Pharmacol* 1999;34:554–560.
104. Campisi R, Czernin J, Schoder H, et al. L-Arginine normalizes coronary vasomotion in long-term smokers. *Circulation* 1999;99:491–497.
105. Bottcher M, Botker HE, Sonne H, et al. Endothelium-dependent and -independent perfusion reserve and the effect of L-arginine on myocardial perfusion in patients with syndrome X. *Circulation* 1999;99:1795–1801.
106. Schachinger V, Zeiher AM. Prognostic implications of endothelial dysfunction: does it mean anything? *Coron Artery Dis* 2001;12:435–443.
107. Halcox JP, Schenke WH, Zalos G, et al. Prognostic value of coronary vascular endothelial dysfunction. *Circulation* 2002;106:653–658.
108. Schindler TH, Nitzsche EU, Schelbert HR, et al. Positron emission tomography-measured abnormal responses of myocardial blood flow to sympathetic stimulation are associated with the risk of developing cardiovascular events. *J Am Coll Cardiol* 2005;45:1505–1512.
109. Schoder H, Silverman DH, Campisi R, et al. Effect of mental stress on myocardial blood flow and vasomotion in patients with coronary artery disease. *J Nucl Med* 2000;41:11–16.
110. Czernin J, Barnard RJ, Sun KT, et al. Effect of short-term cardiovascular conditioning and low-fat diet on myocardial blood flow and flow reserve. *Circulation* 1995;92:197–204.
111. Huggins G, Pasternack R, Alpert N, et al. Effects of short-term treatment of hyperlipidemia on coronary vasodilator function and myocardial perfusion in regions having substantial impairment of baseline dilator reverse. *Circulation* 1998;98:1291–1296.
112. Guethlin M, Kasel AM, Coppenrath K, et al. Delayed response of myocardial flow reserve to lipid-lowering therapy with fluvastatin. *Circulation* 1999;99:475–481.
113. Baller D, Notohamiprodjo G, Gleichmann U, et al. Improvement in coronary flow reserve determined by positron emission tomography after 6 months of cholesterol-lowering therapy in patients with early stages of coronary atherosclerosis. *Circulation* 1999;99:2871–2875.
114. Yokoyama I, Yonekura K, Inoue Y, et al. Long-term effect of simvastatin on the improvement of impaired myocardial flow reserve in patients with familial hypercholesterolemia without gender variance. *J Nucl Cardiol* 2001;8:445–451.
115. Janatuinen T, Laaksonen R, Vesalainen R, et al. Effect of lipid-lowering therapy with pravastatin on myocardial blood flow in young mildly hypercholesterolemic adults. *J Cardiovasc Pharmacol* 2001;38:561–568.
116. Narula J, Finn AV, Demaria AN. Picking plaques that pop. *J Am Coll Cardiol* 2005;45:1970–1973.
117. Rudd JH, Warburton EA, Fryer TD, et al. Imaging atherosclerotic plaque inflammation with [18F]-fluorodeoxyglucose positron emission tomography. *Circulation* 2002;105:2708–2711.
118. Schafers M, Riemann B, Kopka K, et al. Scintigraphic imaging of matrix metalloproteinase activity in the arterial wall in vivo. *Circulation* 2004;109:2554–2559.
119. Haubner R, Weber WA, Beer AJ, et al. Noninvasive visualization of the activated alphavbeta3 integrin in cancer patients by positron emission tomography and [18F]Galacto-RGD. *PLoS Med* 2005;2:e70.
120. Narula J, Strauss HW. Imaging of unstable atherosclerotic lesions. *Eur J Nucl Med Mol Imaging* 2005;32:1–5.
121. Blankenberg FG, Strauss HW. Will imaging of apoptosis play a role in clinical care? A tale of mice and men. *Apoptosis* 2001;6:117–123.
122. Kolodgie FD, Petrov A, Virmani R, et al. Targeting of apoptotic macrophages and experimental atheroma with radiolabeled annexin V: a technique with potential for noninvasive imaging of vulnerable plaque. *Circulation* 2003;108:3134–3139.
123. Gawaz M, Konrad I, Hauser AI, et al. Non-invasive imaging of glycoprotein VI binding to injured arterial lesions. *Thromb Haemost* 2005;93:910–913.
124. Senneff MJ, Hartman J, Sobel BE, et al. Persistence of coronary vasodilator responsivity after cardiac transplantation. *Am J Cardiol* 1993;71:333–338.
125. Wolpers HG, Koster C, Burchert W, et al. Coronary reserve after orthotopic heart transplantation: quantification with N-13 ammonia and positron emission tomography. *Z Kardiol* 1995;84:112–120.
126. Tadamura E, Yoshibayashi M, Yonemura T, et al. Significant regional heterogeneity of coronary flow reserve in paediatric hypertrophic cardiomyopathy. *Eur J Nucl Med* 2000;27:1340–1348.
127. Choudhury L, Elliott P, Rimoldi O, et al. Transmural myocardial blood flow distribution in hypertrophic cardiomyopathy and effect of treatment. *Basic Res Cardiol* 1999;94:49–59.
128. van den Heuvel AF, van Veldhuisen DJ, van der Wall EE, et al. Regional myocardial blood flow reserve impairment and metabolic changes suggesting myocardial ischemia in patients with idiopathic dilated myopathy. *J Am Coll Cardiol* 2000;35:19–28.
129. Shikama N, Himi T, Yoshida K, et al. Prognostic utility of myocardial blood flow assessed by N-13 ammonia positron emission tomography in patients with idiopathic cardiomyopathy. *Am J Cardiol* 1999;84:434–439.
130. Neglia D, Michelassi C, Trivieri MG, et al. Prognostic role of myocardial blood flow impairment in idiopathic left ventricular dysfunction. *Circulation* 2002;105:186–193.
131. Parodi O, De-Maria R, Oltrona L, et al. Myocardial blood flow distribution in patients with ischemic heart disease or dilated cardiomyopathy undergoing heart transplantation. *Circulation* 1993;88:509–522.
132. Stolen KQ, Kemppainen J, Kalliokoski KK, et al. Myocardial perfusion reserve and peripheral endothelial function in patients with idiopathic dilated cardiomyopathy. *Am J Cardiol* 2004;93:64–68.
133. Drzezga A, Blasini R, Ziegler S, et al. Coronary microvascular reactivity to sympathetic stimulation in patients with idiopathic dilated cardiomyopathy. *J Nucl Med* 2000;41:837–844.
134. Liedtke AJ. Alterations of carbohydrate and lipid metabolism in the acutely ischemic heart. *Prog Cardiovasc Dis* 1981;23:321–336.
135. Taegtmeyer H. Myocardial metabolism. In: Phelps M, Mazziotta J, Schelbert H, eds. *Positron emission tomography and autoradiography: Principles and applications for the brain and heart.* New York: Raven Press; 1986:149–195.
136. Depre C, Vanoverschelde JL, Taegtmeyer H. Glucose for the heart. *Circulation* 1999;99:578–588.

137. Gertz EW, Wisneski JA, Stanley WC, Neese RA. Myocardial substrate utilization during exercise in humans. Dual carbon-labeled carbohydrate isotope experiments. *J Clin Invest* 1988;82:2017–2025.
138. Stanley WC, Recchia FA, Lopaschuk GD. Myocardial substrate metabolism in the normal and failing heart. *Physiol Rev* 2005;85:1093–1129.
139. Schelbert H, Henze E, Schon H, et al. C-11 palmitic acid for the non-invasive evaluation of regional myocardial fatty acid metabolism with positron computed tomography. IV. In vivo demonstration of impaired fatty acid oxidation in acute myocardial ischemia. *Am Heart J* 1983;106:736–750.
140. Schelbert HR, Henze E, Sochor H, et al. Effects of substrate availability on myocardial C-11 palmitate kinetics by positron emission tomography in normal subjects and patients with ventricular dysfunction. *Am Heart J* 1986;111:1055–1064.
141. Buxton DB, Schwaiger M, Nguyen A, et al. Radiolabeled acetate as a tracer of myocardial tricarboxylic acid cycle flux. *Circ Res* 1988;63:628–634.
142. Brown MA, Marshall DR, Sobel BE, Bergmann SR. Delineation of myocardial oxygen utilization with carbon-11 labeled acetate. *Circulation* 1987;76:687–696.
143. Beanlands RS, Nahmias C, Gordon E, et al. The effects of beta(1)-blockade on oxidative metabolism and the metabolic cost of ventricular work in patients with left ventricular dysfunction: a double-blind, placebo controlled, positron emission tomography study. *Circulation* 2000;102:2070–2075.
144. Buck A, Wolpers HG, Hutchins GD, et al. Effect of carbon-11-acetate recirculation on estimates of myocardial oxygen consumption by PET [see comments]. *J Nucl Med* 1991;32:1950–1957.
145. Gropler RJ, Siegel BA, Geltman EM. Myocardial uptake of carbon-11-acetate as an indirect estimate of regional myocardial blood flow. *J Nucl Med* 1991;32:245–251.
146. Sokoloff L, Reivich M, Kennedy C, et al. The (14C) deoxyglucose method for the measurement local cerebral glucose utilization: theory, procedure and normal values in the conscious and anesthetized albino rat. *J Neurochem* 1977;28:897–916.
147. Phelps ME, Huang SC, Hoffman EJ, et al. Tomographic measurement of local cerebral glucose metabolic rate in humans with (F-18)2-fluoro-2-deoxy-D-glucose: validation of method. *Ann Neurol* 1979;6:371–388.
148. Krivokapich J, Huang SC, Phelps ME, et al. Estimation of rabbit myocardial metabolic rate for glucose using fluorodeoxyglucose. *Am J Physiol* 1982;243:H884–H894.
149. Krivokapich J, Huang SC, Selin CE, Phelps ME. Fluorodeoxyglucose rate constants, lumped constant, and glucose metabolic rate in rabbit heart. *Am J Physiol* 1987;252:H777–787.
150. Patlak CS, Blasberg RG. Graphical evaluation of blood-to-brain transfer constants from multiple-time uptake data. Generalizations. *J Cereb Blood Flow Metab* 1985;5:584–590.
151. Hicks RJ, Herman WH, Wolfe E, et al. Regional variation in oxidative and glucose metabolism in the normal heart: comparison of PET-derived C-11 acetate and FDG kinetics. *J Nucl Med* 1990;31:774.
152. Gropler RJ, Lee KJ, Moerlein SM, et al. Regional variation in myocardial accumulation of 18F-fluorodeoxyglucose in fasted normal subjects. *J Am Coll Cardiol* 1990;15:81A.
153. vom Dahl J, Herman WH, Hicks RJ, et al. Myocardial glucose uptake in patients with insulin-dependent diabetes mellitus assessed quantitatively by dynamic positron emission tomography. *Circulation* 1993;88:395–404.
154. Ohtake T, Yokoyama I, Watanabe T, et al. Myocardial glucose metabolism in noninsulin-dependent diabetes mellitus patients evaluated by FDG-PET. *J Nucl Med* 1995;36:456–463.
155. Knuuti MJ, Nuutila P, Ruotsalainen U, et al. Euglycemic hyperinsulinemic clamp and oral glucose load in stimulating myocardial glucose utilization during positron emission tomography. *J Nucl Med* 1992;33:1255–1262.
156. Takala TO, Nuutila P, Knuuti J, et al. Insulin action on heart and skeletal muscle glucose uptake in weight lifters and endurance athletes. *Am J Physiol* 1999;27:E706–711.
157. Schwaiger M, Fishbein MC, Block M, et al. Metabolic and ultrastructural abnormalities during ischemia in canine myocardium: non-invasive assessment by positron emission tomography. *J Mol Cell Cardiol* 1987;19:259–269.
158. Marshall RC, Huang SC, Nash WW, Phelps ME. Assessment of the (18F)fluorodeoxyglucose kinetic model in calculations of myocardial glucose metabolism during ischemia. *J Nucl Med* 1983;24:1060–1064.
159. Schelbert HR, Henze E, Phelps ME, Kuhl DE. Assessment of regional myocardial ischemia by positron-emission computed tomography. *Am Heart J* 1982;103:588–597.
160. Tillisch J, Brunken R, Marshall R, et al. Reversibility of cardiac wall motion abnormalities predicted by positron tomography. *N Engl J Med* 1986;314:884–888.
161. Kalff V, Schwaiger M, Nguyen N, et al. The relationship between myocardial blood flow and glucose uptake in ischemic canine myocardium determined with fluorine-18-deoxyglucose. *J Nucl Med* 1992;33:1346–1353.
162. Opie LH. Effects of regional ischemia on metabolism of glucose and fatty acids. Relative rates of aerobic and anaerobic energy production during myocardial infarction and comparison with effects of anoxia. *Circ Res* 1976;38:I52–74.
163. Sun DQ, Nguyen N, DeGrado TR, et al. Ischemia induces translocation of the insulin-responsive glucose transporter GLUT4 to the plasma membrane of cardiac myocytes. *Circulation* 1994;89:793–798.
164. Young LH, Russell RR 3rd, Yin R, et al. Regulation of myocardial glucose uptake and transport during ischemia and energetic stress. *Am J Cardiol* 1999;83:24H–30H.
165. Egert S, Nguyen N, Schwaiger M. The contribution of alpha-adrenergic and beta-adrenergic stimulation on ischemia-induced GLUT4 and GLUT1 translocation in the isolated perfused rat heart. *Circ Res* 1999;84:1407–1415.
166. Borgers M, Thoné F, Wouters L, et al. Structural correlates of regional myocardial dysfunction in patients with critical coronary artery stenosis: chronic hibernation? *Cardiovasc Pathol* 1993;2:237–245.
167. Ausma J, Schaart G, Thone F, et al. Chronic ischemic viable myocardium in man: aspects of dedifferentiation. *Cardiovasc Pathol* 1995;4:29–37.
168. Depre C, Taegtmeyer H. Metabolic aspects of programmed cell survival and cell death in the heart. *Cardiovasc Res* 2000;45:538–548.
169. Thijssen VL, Borgers M, Lenders MH, et al. Temporal and spatial variations in structural protein expression during the progression from stunned to hibernating myocardium. *Circulation* 2004;110:3313–3321.
170. Depre C, Kim SJ, John AS, et al. Program of cell survival underlying human and experimental hibernating myocardium. *Circ Res* 2004;95:433–440.
171. Kim SJ, Depre C, Vatner SF. Novel mechanisms mediating stunned myocardium. *Heart Fail Rev* 2003;8:143–153.
172. Vanoverschelde JL, Wijns W, Depre C, et al. Mechanisms of chronic regional postischemic dysfunction in humans. New insights from the study of noninfarcted collateral-dependent myocardium. *Circulation* 1993;87:1513–1523.
173. Wijns W, Vatner SF, Camici PG. Hibernating myocardium. *N Engl J Med* 1998;339:173–181.
174. Camici PG, Wijns W, Borgers M, et al. Pathophysiological mechanisms of chronic reversible left ventricular dysfunction due to coronary artery disease (hibernating myocardium). *Circulation* 1997;96:3205–3214.
175. Pantely GA, Malone SA, Rhen WS, et al. Regeneration of myocardial phosphocreatine in pigs despite continued moderate ischemia. *Circ Res* 1990;67:1481–1493.
176. Schulz R, Heusch G. Hibernating myocardium. *Heart* 2000;84:587–594.
177. Rahimtoola SH. The hibernating myocardium. *Am Heart J* 1989;117:211–221.
178. Braunwald E, Kloner R. The stunned myocardium: prolonged, postischemic ventricular dysfunction. *Circulation* 1982;66:1146–1149.
179. Yamamoto Y, de Silva R, Rhodes C, et al. A new strategy for the assessment of viable myocardium and regional myocardial blood flow using 15O-water and dynamic positron emission tomography. *Circulation* 1992;86:167–178.
180. Heusch G, Schulz R, Rahimtoola SH. Myocardial hibernation: a delicate balance. *Am J Physiol Heart Circ Physiol* 2005;288:H984–999.
181. vom Dahl J, Eitzman DT, al-Aouar ZR, et al. Relation of regional function, perfusion, and metabolism in patients with advanced coronary artery disease undergoing surgical revascularization. *Circulation* 1994;90:2356–2366.
182. Gerber BL, Melin JA, Bol A, et al. Nitrogen-13-ammonia and oxygen-15-water estimates of absolute myocardial perfusion in left ventricular ischemic dysfunction. *J Nucl Med* 1998;39:1655–1662.
183. Haas F, Augustin N, Holper K, et al. Time course and extent of improvement of dysfunctioning myocardium in patients with coronary artery disease and severely depressed left ventricular function after revascularization: correlation with positron emission tomographic findings. *J Am Coll Cardiol* 2000;36:1927–1934.
184. Vanoverschelde JL, Depre C, Gerber BL, et al. Time course of functional recovery after coronary artery bypass graft surgery in patients with chronic left ventricular ischemic dysfunction. *Am J Cardiol* 2000;85:1432–1439.
185. DiCarli MF, Asgarzadie F, Schelbert HR, et al. Quantitative relation between myocardial viability and improvement in heart failure symptoms after revascularization in patients with ischemic cardiomyopathy. *Circulation* 1995;92:3436–3444.
186. Pagano D, Lewis ME, Townend JN, et al. Coronary revascularization for postischaemic heart failure: how myocardial viability affects survival. *Heart* 1999;82:684–688.
187. Baer FM, Voth E, Schneider CA, et al. Comparison of low-dose dobutamine-gradient-echo magnetic resonance imaging and positron emission tomography with [18F]fluorodeoxyglucose in patients with chronic coronary artery disease. A functional and morphological approach to the detection of residual myocardial viability. *Circulation* 1995;91:1006–1015.
188. Bax JJ, Wijns W, Cornel JH, et al. Accuracy of currently available techniques for prediction of functional recovery after revascularization in patients with left ventricular dysfunction due to chronic coronary artery disease: comparison of pooled data. *J Am Coll Cardiol* 1997;30:1451–1460.
189. Dilsizian V, Rocco TP, Freedman NM, et al. Enhanced detection of ischemic but viable myocardium by the reinjection of thallium after stress-redistribution imaging [see comments]. *N Engl J Med* 1990;323:141–146.
190. Bax JJ, Patton JA, Poldermans D, et al. 18-Fluorodeoxyglucose imaging with positron emission tomography and single photon emission computed tomography: cardiac applications. *Semin Nucl Med* 2000;30:281–298.
191. Kim RJ, Wu E, Rafael A, et al. The use of contrast-enhanced magnetic resonance imaging to identify reversible myocardial dysfunction. *N Engl J Med* 2000;343:1445–1453.
192. Ibrahim T, Nekolla SG, Hornke M, et al. Quantitative measurement of infarct size by contrast-enhanced magnetic resonance imaging early after

acute myocardial infarction: comparison with single-photon emission tomography using Tc99m-sestamibi. *J Am Coll Cardiol* 2005;45:544–552.
193. Klein C, Nekolla SG, Bengel FM, et al. Assessment of myocardial viability with contrast-enhanced magnetic resonance imaging: comparison with positron emission tomography. *Circulation* 2002;105:162–167.
194. Knuesel PR, Nanz D, Wyss C, et al. Characterization of dysfunctional myocardium by positron emission tomography and magnetic resonance: relation to functional outcome after revascularization. *Circulation* 2003;108:1095–1100.
195. Kuhl HP, Beek AM, van der Weerdt AP, et al. Myocardial viability in chronic ischemic heart disease: comparison of contrast-enhanced magnetic resonance imaging with (18)F-fluorodeoxyglucose positron emission tomography. *J Am Coll Cardiol* 2003;41:1341–1348.
196. Eitzman D, Al-Aouar Z, Kanter H, et al. Clinical outcome of patients with advanced coronary artery disease following positron emission tomography viability studies. *J Am Coll Cardiol* 1992;20:559–565.
197. Tamaki N, Yonekura Y, Yamashita K, et al. Prognostic value of an increase in fluorine-18 deoxyglucose uptake in patients with myocardial infarction: comparison with stress thallium imaging. *J Am Coll Cardiol* 1993;22:1621–1627.
198. Maddahi J, DiCarli M, Davidson M, et al. Prognostic significance of PET assessment of myocardial viability in patients with left ventricular dysfunction. *J Am Coll Cardiol* 1992;19:142A.
199. DiCarli MF, Davidson M, Little R, et al. Value of metabolic imaging with positron emission tomography for evaluating prognosis in patients with coronary artery disease and left ventricular dysfunction. *Am J Cardiol* 1994;73:527–533.
200. Beanlands R, Hendry P, Masters R, et al. Delay in revascularization is associated with increased mortality rate in patients with severe left ventricular dysfunction and viable myocardium on fluorine 18-fluorodeoxyglucose positron emission tomography imaging. *Circulation* 1998;98(19 Suppl):II51–56.
201. Dreyfus GD, Duboc D, Blasco A, et al. Myocardial viability assessment in ischemic cardiomyopathy: benefits of coronary revascularization. *Ann Thorac Surg* 1994;57:1402–1407.
202. Haas F, Hähnel C, Sebening F, et al. Effect of preoperative PET viability on peri- and postoperative risk. *J Am Coll Cardiol* 1996;27:300A.
203. Geltman E. Metabolic findings in cardiomyopathies. In: Marcus ME, Schelbert HR, Skorton MD, Wolf G, eds. *Cardiac imaging: a companion to Braunwald's heart disease*. Philadelphia: W.B. Saunders; 1991:1244–1255.
204. Kelly D, Mendelsohn N, Sobel B, Bergmann S. Detection and assessment by positron emission tomography of a genetically determined defect in myocardial fatty acid utilization (long-chain acyl-CoA dehydrogenase deficiency). *Am J Cardiol* 1993;71:738–744.
205. Buxton DB, Nienaber CA, Luxen A, et al. Noninvasive quantitation of regional myocardial oxygen consumption in vivo with [1-11C]acetate and dynamic positron emission tomography. *Circulation* 1989;79:134–142.
206. Hicks RJ, Kalff V, Savas V, et al. Assessment of right ventricular oxidative metabolism by positron emission tomography with C-11 acetate in aortic valve disease. *Am J Cardiol* 1991;67:753–757.
207. Wolpers GH, Buck A, Nguyen N, et al. An approach to ventricular efficiency by use of carbon-11 labeled acetate and positron emission tomography. *J Nucl Cardiol* 1994;1:262–269.
208. Bengel FM, Permanetter B, Ungerer M, et al. Non-invasive estimation of myocardial efficiency using positron emission tomography and carbon-11 acetate—comparison between the normal and failing human heart. *J Nucl Med* 2000;41:837–844.
209. Beanlands RS, Bach DS, Raylman R, et al. Acute effects of dobutamine on myocardial oxygen consumption and cardiac efficiency measured using carbon-11 acetate kinetics in patients with dilated cardiomyopathy. *J Am Coll Cardiol* 1993;22:1389–1398.
210. Rosenspire K, Haka M, Jewett D, et al. Synthesis and preliminary evaluation of 11C-meta-hydroxyephedrine: a false transmitter agent for heart neuronal imaging. *J Nucl Med* 1990;31:1328–1334.
211. Schwaiger M, Kalff V, Rosenspire K, et al. The noninvasive evaluation of the sympathetic nervous system in the human heart by PET. *Circulation* 1990;82:457–464.
212. Munch G, Nguyen N, Nekolla S, et al. Evaluation of sympathetic nerve terminals using C-11 Epinephrine and C-11 Hydroxyephedrine and PET. *Circulation* 2000;101:516–523.
213. Corbett J, Chiao P-C, del Rosario R, et al. Mapping neuronal enzyme function of the human heart with C-11 phenylephrine. *J Nucl Med* 1994;35:109P.
214. Goldstein D, Eisenhofer G, Dunn B, et al. Positron emission tomographic imaging of cardiac sympathetic innervation using 6-18F-fluorodopamine: initial findings in humans. *J Am Coll Cardiol* 1993;22:1961–1971.
215. Ding Y, Fowler J, Dewey S, et al. Comparison of high specific activity (−) and (+)-6-18F-fluoronorepinephrine and 6-18F-fluorodopamine in baboons: heart uptake, metabolism and the effect of desipramine. *J Nucl Med* 1993;34:619–629.
216. Valette H, Loc'h C, Mardon K, et al. Bromine-76-metabromobenzylguanidine: a PET radiotracer for mapping sympathetic nerves of the heart. *J Nucl Med* 1993;34:1739–1744.
217. Caldwell JH, Kroll K, Li Z, et al. Quantitation of presynaptic cardiac sympathetic function with carbon-11-meta-hydroxyephedrine. *J Nucl Med* 1998;39:1327–1334.
218. Schwaiger M, Hutchins GD, Kalff V, et al. Evidence for regional catecholamine uptake and storage sites in the transplanted human heart by positron emission tomography. *J Clin Invest* 1991;87:1681–1690.
219. Ziegler S, Frey A, Uberfuhr P, et al. Assessment of myocardial reinnervation in cardiac transplants by positron emission tomography: functional significance tested by heart rate variability. *Clin Sci* 1996;91(Suppl):126–128.
220. Uberfuhr P, Frey AW, Ziegler S, et al. Sympathetic reinnervation of sinus node and left ventricle after heart transplantation in humans: regional differences assessed by heart rate variability and positron emission tomography. *J Heart Lung Transplant* 2000;19:317–323.
221. Bengel FM, Ueberfuhr P, Ziegler SI, et al. Serial assessment of sympathetic reinnervation after orthotopic heart transplantation. A longitudinal study using PET and C-11 hydroxyephedrine. *Circulation* 1999;99:1866–1871.
222. Bengel FM, Ueberfuhr P, Schiepel N, et al. Effect of sympathetic reinnervation on cardiac performance after heart transplantation. *N Engl J Med* 2001;345:731–738.
223. Allman KC, Wieland DM, Muzik O, et al. Carbon-11 hydroxyephedrine with positron emission tomography for serial assessment of cardiac adrenergic neuronal function after acute myocardial infarction in humans. *J Am Coll Cardiol* 1993;22:368–375.
224. Wolpers H, Nguyen N, Rosenspire K, et al. C-11 hydroxyephedrine as marker for neuronal dysfunction in reperfused canine myocardium. *Coron Artery Dis* 1991;2:923–929.
225. Matsunari I, Schricke U, Bengel FM, et al. Extent of cardiac sympathetic neuronal damage is determined by the area of ischemia in patients with acute coronary syndromes. *Circulation* 2000;101:2579–2585.
226. Stevens MJ, Raffel DM, Allman KC, et al. Cardiac sympathetic dysinnervation in diabetes: implications for enhanced cardiovascular risk. *Circulation* 1998;98:961–968.
227. Stevens M, Dayanikli F, Raffel D, et al. Scintigraphic assessment of regionalized defects in myocardial sympathetic innervation and blood flow regulation in diabetic patients with autonomic neuropathy. *J Am Coll Cardiol* 1998;31:1575–1584.
228. Stevens MJ, Raffel DM, Allman KC, et al. Regression and progression of cardiac sympathetic dysinnervation complicating diabetes: an assessment by C-11 hydroxyephedrine and positron emission tomography. *Metabolism* 1999;48:92–101.
229. DiCarli MF, Bianco-Batlles D, Landa ME, et al. Effects of autonomic neuropathy on coronary blood flow in patients with diabetes mellitus. *Circulation* 1999;100:813–819.
230. Pietila M, Malminiemi K, Ukkonen H, et al. Reduced myocardial carbon-11 hydroxyephedrine retention is associated with poor prognosis in chronic heart failure. *Eur J Nucl Med* 2001;28:373–376.
231. Ungerer M, Hartmann F, Karoglan M, et al. Regional in vivo and in vitro characterization of autonomic innervation in cardiomyopathic human heart. *Circulation* 1998;97:174–180.
232. Hartmann F, Ziegler S, Nekolla S, et al. Regional patterns of myocardial sympathetic denervation in dilated cardiomyopathy: an analysis using carbon-11 hydroxyephedrine and positron emission tomography. *Heart* 1999;81:262–270.
233. Syrota A. Positron emission tomography: evaluation of cardiac receptors. In: Marcus ML, Skorton DJ, Schelbert HR, et al., eds. *Cardiac imaging principles and practice: a companion of Braunwald's heart disease*. 3rd ed. Philadelphia: W.B. Saunders Company, Harcourt Brace Jovanovich, Inc.; 1991:1256–1270.
234. Valette H, Syrota A, Merlet P. Use of PET radiopharmaceuticals to probe cardiac receptors. In: Schwaiger M, ed. *Cardiac positron emission tomography*. Boston: Kluwer; 1996:331–351.
235. Rosen SD, Boyd H, Rhodes CG, et al. Is overactivity of the sympathetic nervous system demonstrable in patients with syndrome X? *Circulation* 1995;92:I-652.
236. Wichter T, Schafers M, Rhodes CG, et al. Abnormalities of cardiac sympathetic innervation in arrhythmogenic right ventricular cardiomyopathy: quantitative assessment of presynaptic norepinephrine reuptake and postsynaptic beta-adrenergic receptor density with positron emission tomography. *Circulation* 2000;101:1552–1558.
237. Schafers M, Lerch H, Wichter T, et al. Cardiac sympathetic innervation in patients with idiopathic right ventricular outflow tract tachycardia. *J Am Coll Cardiol* 1998;32:181–186.
238. Schafers M, Dutka D, Rhodes CG, et al. Myocardial presynaptic and postsynaptic autonomic dysfunction in hypertrophic cardiomyopathy. *Circ Res* 1998;82:57–62.
239. Bengel FM. Noninvasive imaging of cardiac gene expression and its future implications for molecular therapy. *Mol Imaging Biol* 2005;7:22–29.
240. Wu JC, Tseng JR, Gambhir SS. Molecular imaging of cardiovascular gene products. *J Nucl Cardiol* 2004;11:491–505.
241. Iyer M, Salazar FB, Lewis X, et al. Non-invasive imaging of a transgenic mouse model using a prostate-specific two-step transcriptional amplification strategy. *Transgenic Res* 2005;14:47–55.
242. Wu JC, Chen IY, Sundaresan G, et al. Molecular imaging of cardiac cell transplantation in living animals using optical bioluminescence and positron emission tomography. *Circulation* 2003;108:1302–1305.
243. Blasberg RG, Tjuvajev JG. Molecular-genetic imaging: current and future perspectives. *J Clin Invest* 2003;111:1620–1629.

244. Inubushi M, Wu JC, Gambhir SS, et al. Positron-emission tomography reporter gene expression imaging in rat myocardium. *Circulation* 2003;107:326–332.
245. Bengel FM, Anton M, Avril N, et al. Uptake of radiolabeled 2′-Fluoro-2′Deoxy-5-Iodo-1-beta-D-Arabinofuranosyluracil in cardiac cells after adenoviral transfer of the herpes virus thymidine kinase gene (the cellular basis for cardiac gene imaging). *Circulation* 2000;102:948–950.
246. Blasberg RG, Gelovani J. Molecular-genetic imaging: a nuclear medicine-based perspective. *Mol Imaging* 2002;1:280–300.
247. Miyagawa M, Anton M, Wagner B, et al. Non-invasive imaging of cardiac transgene expression with PET: comparison of the human sodium/iodide symporter gene and HSV1-tk as the reporter gene. *Eur J Nucl Med Mol Imaging* 2005.
248. Jaffer FA, Weissleder R. Molecular imaging in the clinical arena. *JAMA* 2005;293:855–862.
249. Anton M, Wittermann C, Haubner R, et al. Coexpression of herpes viral thymidine kinase reporter gene and VEGF gene for noninvasive monitoring of therapeutic gene transfer: an in vitro evaluation. *J Nucl Med* 2004;45:1743–1746.

CHAPTER 56 ■ COMPUTED TOMOGRAPHY OF THE HEART

ROSS T. MURPHY AND MARIO J. GARCIA

HISTORICAL PERSPECTIVE

The ability to rapidly obtain cross-sectional images of the body with x-ray computed tomography (CT) has revolutionized medicine since its introduction as a clinical tool in 1972. Although the physical principles behind CT were described as early as 1917 by Radon, credit for the technical development is owed to Hounsfield and Cormack, who received the Nobel Prize in Physiology or Medicine in 1979. More recent advances have led to the development of electron-beam CT (EBCT) and multidetector CT (MDCT), which make it possible to obtain electrocardiogram (ECG)-gated images with sufficient temporal and spatial resolution to visualize the beating heart. The first clinical applications of cardiac EBCT in the 1980s were focused on the evaluation of cardiac volumes and function, the pericardium, and the great vessels. Subsequently, this technology gained popularity for the detection and quantification of coronary calcifications. The first cardiac application of MDCT followed the introduction of four-detector scanners in the late 1990s. In addition to evaluating coronary calcifications, both EBCT and MDCT have demonstrated the capability of performing contrast-enhanced coronary angiography (1–7). The evolution of MDCT technology has occurred much faster than that of EBCT over the last decade. State-of-the-art MDCT technology represents the seventh generation of CT scanners and has overcome many of its previous limitations. Image quality is undergoing constant refinement, and the number of uninterpretable coronary studies has gradually decreased from 20% to 40% using 4-detector systems, to 15% to 25% with 16-detector systems, to as low as 3% to 10% with 64-detector systems.

PHYSICAL PRINCIPLES OF COMPUTED TOMOGRAPHY

Image Acquisition

The clinical value of cardiac CT was quite limited prior to current iterations of CT technology. Cardiac imaging demands a very high temporal resolution because the heart is in constant, rapid phasic motion with translational movement and torsion, which have been difficult to capture even with high-frame-rate echocardiography until recently. For the purpose of coronary imaging, submillimeter spatial resolution is also needed because of the diameter of the coronary vessels.

The physics of EBCT and MDCT differ significantly, but they share some common principles: (a) an x-ray source is required to produce the images, (b) a detector crystal receives the x-rays after they travel through the imaging target and converts photons into electrical impulses, (c) x-ray data need to be collected for a minimum of 180° to form a cross-sectional image, (d) the in-plane pixel dimensions define the x- and y-axis resolution, but the slice thickness determines the z-axis resolution, (e) multiple cross-sectional images need to be acquired to form a three-dimensional volume, and (f) advanced computing power is used to reconstruct a three-dimensional data set with a unique set of x, y, and z locations corresponding to each target of information collected, using a standard technique called filtered backprojection. In addition, cardiac CT requires temporal registration to match data collected at the same time of the cardiac cycle because of the continuous motion and deformation of the heart.

With EBCT, a rapidly rotating electron beam generates x-rays without the need for mechanical rotating parts. This technology was developed specifically with cardiac imaging in mind. A stationary high-voltage electron gun produces a beam of electrons, which is rapidly steered to sweep over tungsten targets arranged in a semicircular array under the patient table. Thus a fan of x-rays is created that penetrates the patient. Stationary detector arrays receive the attenuated signal. Cross-sectional images thus can be rapidly acquired without the constraints of mechanical motion: The electron beam can sweep across the target rings very rapidly in one rotation providing temporal resolution as fast as 33 to 50 msec. A limitation of EBCT technology is its relatively slow speed of data collection in the z-axis because only one slice of data can be collected at a time. This results in limited spatial resolution in the z-axis and/or prolonged scan acquisition time. In addition, x-ray power delivery is fixed and limited, resulting in noisier images, in particular when imaging obese patients.

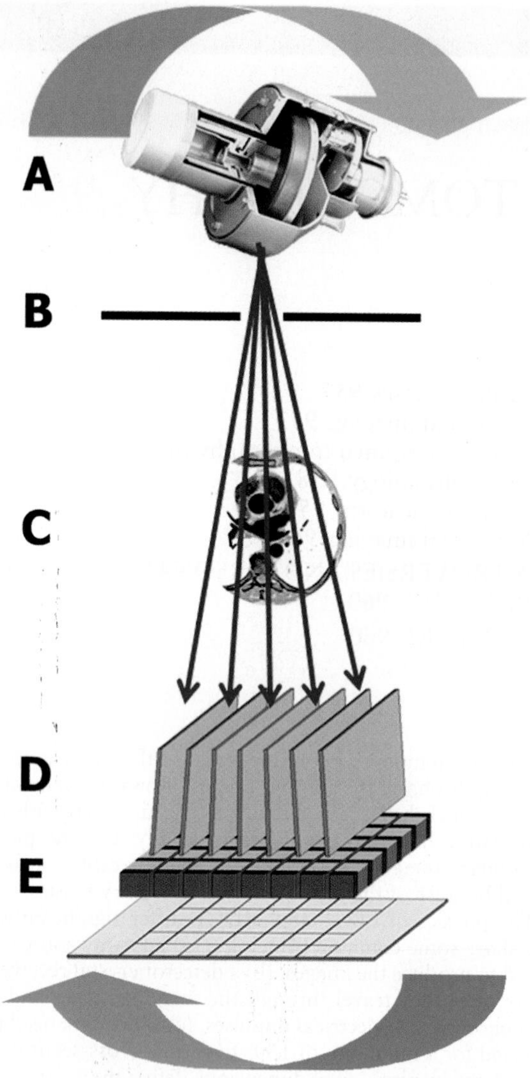

FIGURE 56.1. Diagram of the rotating gantry of a multidetector computed tomographic system. **A:** X-ray tube. **B:** Precollimator. **C:** Target (body). **D:** Postcollimator. **E:** Multidetector array.

MDCT imaging involves an x-ray source that rotates around the patient and emits a fan-shaped beam of x-rays that passes through the body at many angles (Fig. 56.1). Collimators are used to confine the x-ray beam to the slice to be imaged. Current-generation MDCT scanners use a spiral or helical scanning mode that offers faster coverage of larger volumes than older "stop and shoot" scanning, but they require that the x-ray tube and the detector array be rapidly rotated around the body. While the gantry (with x-ray tube and detectors) is rotating and data are being acquired continuously, the table where the patient lies supine is advanced at a constant speed. After the x-ray data set has been collected, images can be reconstructed retrospectively. To reconstruct an image at a given level, a set of projections from numerous angles needs to be acquired at that level. Because the tube does not perform a full rotation in any given plane, x-ray data for every projection angle are "interpolated" with data from the rotation before and after. Recent advances include a "slip ring" so gantry rotation is wireless, mathematical filtering of the acquired data with a filter or "kernel," and complex algorithms for digital image display. Multiple-detector arrays have been introduced to clinical practice. Commercially available state-of-the-art MDCT scanners have up to 64-detector arrays, but 128- and 256-detector scanners are already in use in a research setting. The simultaneous acquisition of multiple cross-sectional images makes it possible to do a complete acquisition of the heart in a single 8- to 12-second breath-hold. One limitation of MDCT is its lower temporal resolution (175 to 220 msec), which is determined by the rotational speed of the gantry. This can result in motion artifacts when imaging the coronary arteries. Thus, most studies require the administration of β-blockers to reduce the patient's heart rate during acquisition. However, a novel algorithm can be implemented to collect data from different detector arrays to form a single slice. These multicycle reconstruction algorithms can often improve temporal resolution to 80 to 120 msec but require a very steady heart rate and rhythm.

Image Reconstruction

Although cardiac CT provides continuous cross-sectional images of the heart, every displayed image must be synchronous with and constructed from the same phase of the cardiac cycle. If this is not done, gaps in the data set and/or temporal misregistration artifacts may render the study useless. Data acquisition can be prospectively triggered by the patient's ECG. In this mode, the data are acquired intermittently at a time determined by the position of the QRS. Prospective ECG gating is mostly used during EBCT scanning. Alternatively, data can be acquired continuously together with the ECG signal, and then portions of the data set corresponding to specific phases of the cardiac cycle can be reconstructed to form a static three-dimensional image. This method, referred as retrospective ECG gating, involves greater radiation exposure because the x-ray tube is being used continuously, but it provides more-consistent image quality if irregularities in the heart rhythm occur. As a general rule, however, imaging of the coronary arteries is unreliable in patients with irregular rhythms. To reconstruct a complete cross-sectional image, data collected from projections over 180° plus the width of the fan angle emitted by the x-ray tube (approximately 50°) are required. Image reconstruction algorithms that use projections covering less than 360° are called *partial scan reconstruction algorithms*. With this reconstruction technique, a temporal resolution of about one half of the gantry rotation time can be achieved in the center of the scan field. To fill gaps and provide missing projection angles for reconstruction of an image at a given level, data are used that are acquired during a later heart beat by another detector and assigned to the correct heart phase by means of the simultaneously recorded ECG.

Image Display

Each pixel of the image to be reconstructed is assigned an x-ray attenuation value expressed in Hounsfield units (HU). The Hounsfield scale is a prespecified score with values of 0 HU for water, –1,000 HU for air, and approximately +1,000 HU for bony cortex, with a range from –1,024 to 3,071 HU. Because the human eye cannot distinguish gray scale over such a wide range, adjustments (window "width" and window "level" or "center") are made to analyze the reconstructed images. The "width" value is the range of gray-scale CT numbers to be displayed. Each value below that range is shown black; each value above the range is shown white. The "level" or "center" value determines the CT number on either side of which the "window" is fixed (thus in an image display with a center of 600 HU and width of 400 HU—i.e., ±200, each pixel with a density of <400 HU will displayed black and each pixel with a density of >800 HU will be displayed white). Soft tissue, including muscle, and nonenhanced blood have a score ranging from −100 to +200, but arterial blood with contrast has a score of +200 to +400.

Once transformed and reconstructed, the CT data set can be displayed in a number of different ways. These postprocessing protocols include the following:

1. Axial image assessment. This should be the first step in any assessment of acquired study. Scrolling up and down though the originally acquired cross-sectional images is useful to assess for normal anatomy, chamber, and vessel relationships.
2. Multiplanar reconstruction (MPR) images are reconstructed from the three-dimensional data set in any coronal, sagittal, or oblique orientation. This is relatively simple with the new-generation MDCT scanners because they provide isotropic resolution.
3. Curved multiplanar images are on a plane reformatted to fit a curve (usually following a coronary artery) and allow the display of the entire structure in a single image. Although this creates some distortion, it is a useful way to analyze a tortuous vessel. Careful adjustment of image center and window levels is useful to differentiate the contrast-enhanced lumen from calcified and noncalcified coronary plaques. This procedure is repeated for each vessel and its branches.
4. Maximum intensity projection (MIP) images smooth out the projection of three-dimensional images and assign the maximum detected value to that portion of the image, thus projecting the highest attenuation values in that two-dimensional direction, a little like conventional coronary angiography. Obscuring lower-density structures highlights contrast-filled vessels over other structures. The "slab" image may thickened at will to smooth out planes, and is also useful for displaying long segments of vessels.
5. Volume-rendered images. These images use all the volumetric data acquired in the scan and combine the "voxels" (volume elements) into a three-dimensional image. These images are useful for assessing the relationships between different structures. Coloring the image often provides a "realistic" anatomic view.
6. Reconstructions combining set fixed points in the cardiac cycle (0% of the RR interval + 10% + 20%...) can generate a cine film. Atrial and ventricular volumes and ejection fraction can be then quantified from the four-dimensional data set.

Radiation Dose and Patient Safety

Cardiac CT, like invasive angiography, involves radiation exposure. The "effective dose," expressed in millisieverts (mSv), depends on multiple factors including volume of acquisition required, duration of the scan, and radiation energy level. The volume of acquisition is typically 12 to 16 cm for coronary angiography and 18 to 25 cm for angiography for coronary bypass conduits. The radiation energy level required to obtain adequate image quality also depends on the weight of the patient. Obese individuals require larger amount of energy due to scattering and attenuation. Current-generation systems with 64 detectors provide a typical dose range in the order of 4 to 12 mSv for MDCT coronary angiography. This compares to 2 to 6 mSv for invasive angiography, 10 to 20 mSv for nuclear stress tests involving thallium, and 3.6 mSv from yearly background radiation exposure. EBCT examinations result in an effective dose of about 1.1 to 2.0 mSv. Strategies to minimize the effective dose in MDCT include dose modulation, in which the x-ray dose is stepped up in the ECG-gated target area in mid-diastole and stepped down in the rest of the cardiac cycle. This can reduce total radiation exposure by up to 50% and should be used whenever possible in coronary MDCT. The estimated risk of cancer increases by 1:2000 MDCT coronary studies. Studies suggest that the longitudinal risk of cancer secondary to radiation exposure decreases with age and is significantly higher in pediatric patients and lower in older adults. Because of these concerns, the indiscriminate use of MDCT as a screening test is not warranted at present, and professional society guidelines for the appropriate use of this technology are awaited.

CLINICAL APPLICATIONS

Calcium Scoring

Electron-beam computed tomography scanners have been in clinical use for more than a decade and are used to detect and quantify coronary artery calcifications. Designed with cardiac motion in mind, they can acquire a full data set in as little as 50 msec. The most widely used measure of calcium burden is the calcium score, based on a radiographic density-weighted volume of plaques with pixel numbers of a least 130 HU. The prognostic value of calcification scores has been established (8). Coronary calcification is a robust predictor (the relative risk [RR] for a calcium score of >100 is 1.88) of hard cardiovascular outcomes (death and nonfatal myocardial infarction) at 7 years follow-up. Although very high calcium scores impart an approximate 10-fold increased risk, they do not always imply a tight coronary stenosis. The role of EBCT screening of asymptomatic individuals is controversial, and a study of the incorporation of this type of investigation into a comprehensive risk screening with CRP and cholesterol measurements is ongoing. There is some evidence to support the incorporation of calcium scores into an overall risk stratification of older individuals using clinical algorithms such as the Framingham Risk Score. In the South Bay Heart Watch study (9), a calcium score of greater than 300 was associated with a significant increase in coronary heart disease (CHD) event risk compared with that determined by clinical score alone. These data support the hypothesis that high coronary artery calcium score (CACS) can modify predicted risk, especially among patients in the intermediate-risk category in whom clinical decision-making is most difficult. Those at low risk by clinical score derived no additional benefit from calcium scoring. However, the use of EBCT to improve cardiovascular risk prediction in a population with no cardiac symptoms who are at low absolute risk is very expensive. Some authorities (10) even suggest that EBCT may in aggregate have a detrimental effect on the quality of life of screening populations.

Computed Tomography Coronary Angiography

Without doubt, the ability of providing anatomic information about the coronary arteries is one of the most exciting and potentially important applications in cardiac CT. Adequate training for conducting and interpreting CT coronary studies is absolutely essential to obtain adequate results. Guidelines for training were recently issued by the American College of Cardiology and American Heart Association (11). Neither experience in computed tomography nor that in invasive coronary angiography alone is sufficient to provide the required training. Accordingly, the best results are obtained by the joint effort of cardiologists and radiologists providing complementary expertise.

Contrast-enhanced EBCT can define the coronary anatomy and quantification of stenosis but is limited by poor visualization of distal vessels, and excess calcification can obscure lumen definition. A meta-analysis (12) of the 10 published studies comparing EBA to coronary angiography shows a sensitivity and specificity of 87% and 91%, respectively, for the detection of obstructive coronary atherosclerosis. An important number (8% to 25%) of the coronary segments, however, were deemed uninterpretable in these studies.

Appropriate patient selection is important for obtaining adequate results (13). A careful review of the medical history is important before performing each procedure, including knowledge about prior allergy to iodine contrast, renal function, heart rate, and regularity of rhythm. Adequate oral hydration is encouraged before and after performing the study. A stable, low heart rate is most important during scanning because this determines the target for ECG-gated image reconstruction and sometimes the target for dose modulation (see later discussion). We use intravenous β-blockers administered just before the study and aim for a resting regular heart rate of 50 to 55 beats per minute. In most patients with a heat rate below 60 beats per minute, the time of least coronary artery motion is centered on 75% of the RR interval, corresponding to the diastasis phase of diastole. At higher rates, from 80 to 90 beats per minute, diastasis disappears; therefore image reconstruction at about 40% of the cardiac cycle is preferred. These phases are not merely coincidental with cardiac stasis but also represent the optimal multiple of the gantry rotation plus fan angle for each manufacturer, using reconstruction algorithms. Thus in scanners capable of performing multicycle reconstruction, which provide effective temporal resolution of 100 to 120 msec, adequate coronary visualization may be obtained in many patients with stable heart rates up to 80 to 95 beats per minute (14). Nevertheless, there is significant patient-to-patient variability, and examination of several phases reconstructed at 5% to 10% intervals from 40% to 90% of the RR is sometimes needed. Some centers administer oral β-blockers the night before the procedure. β-Blockers also reduce heart rate variability during the scan, and for that reason we recommend their administration almost routinely unless contraindicated.

Once adequate heart rate is achieved and sublingual nitrates are given, data acquisition is started. In many centers, a calcium-score scan (with no contrast and low radiation of 1 to 2 mSv) is performed first. This is followed by a scout scan (planar x-ray mode), which will be used to select the region of interest (usually from the carina to slightly below the diaphragm, but from the subclavian artery down if an internal thoracic graft is be assessed). The survey scan should be acquired during a brief inspiratory breath-hold.

An iodinated contrast agent is injected to increase the CT attenuation of the blood pool (CT imaging of the heart can be performed without injection of a contrast agent, usually to assess calcified structures within the heart, most notably coronary artery calcification). A remotely controlled dual-injection system capable of administering iodine contrast and saline separately is used. Correct timing of the actual CT scan relative to contrast injection is important. CT scanning can start when the contrast agent reaches a prespecified threshold density in the descending aorta. This is usually 15 to 25 seconds after the start of contrast injection into a peripheral vein. If only arterial structures (left ventricle, coronary arteries) are to be investigated, acquisition can occur 6 seconds after threshold. If structures of the right heart and pulmonary circulation are also to be analyzed, acquisition is adjusted to start later.

Figures 56.2 and 56.3 demonstrate examples of normal and severely stenosed coronary artery. It is important to understand from the outset that MDCT gives a qualitatively different view of the coronary arteries than invasive angiography because the images show Glagovian remodeling and extraluminal atherosclerosis. It is thus facile to expect exact equivalence

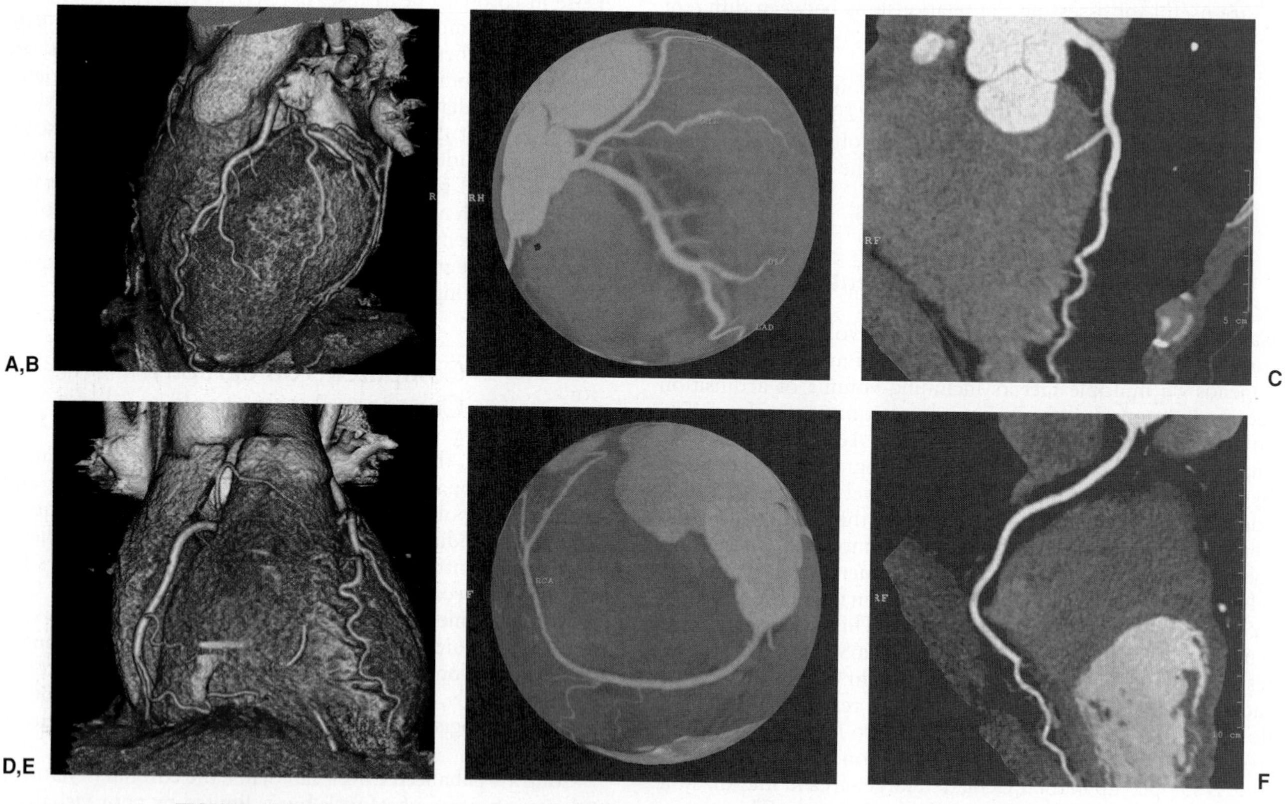

FIGURE 56.2. Normal coronary arteries. **A:** Volume-rendered image oriented to show the left anterior descending (LAD) coronary system. **B:** Three-dimensional multiplanar reconstruction (MPR) of the LAD and circumflex (LCx). **C:** Two-dimensional curved MPR of the right coronary artery (RCA). **D:** Three-dimensional MPR of the RCA. **E:** Two-dimensional curved MPR of the RCA.

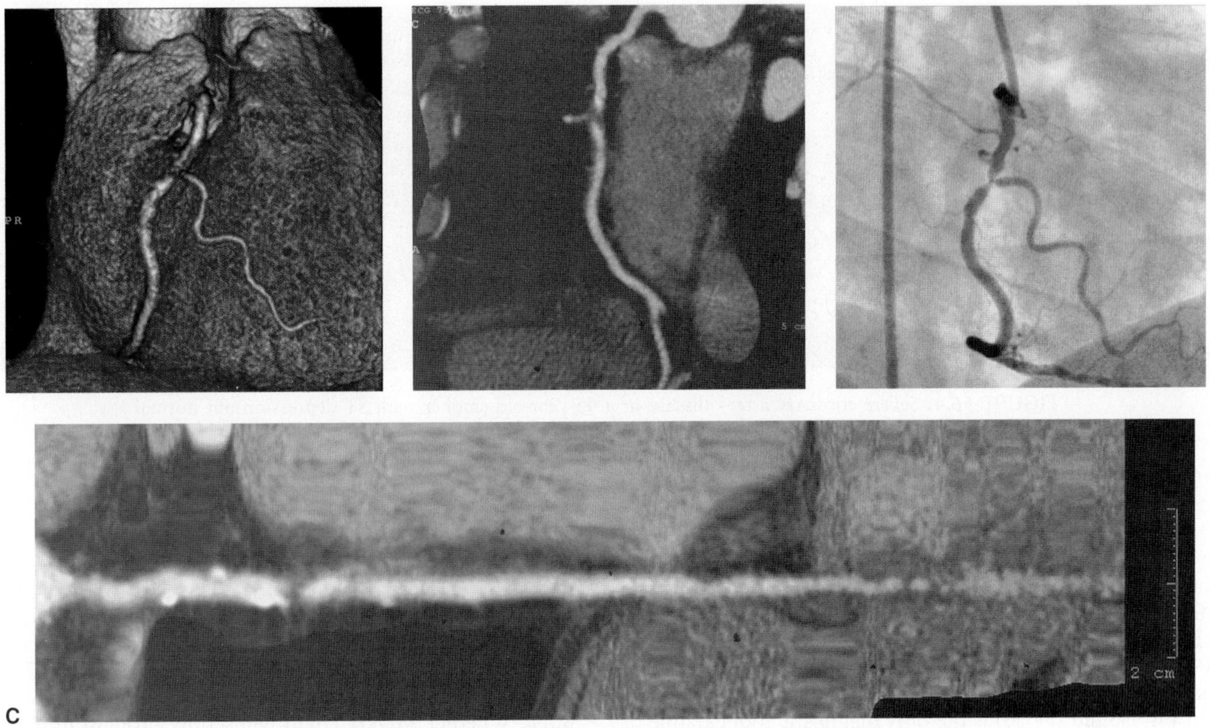

FIGURE 56.3. Proximal right coronary artery (RCA) stenosis caused by a noncalcified plaque. **A:** Volume-rendered image. **B:** Two-dimensional curved multiplanar reconstruction (MPR). **C:** "Stretched-vessel" MPR. **D:** Fluoroscopic image obtained during invasive coronary angiography.

between the two imaging modalities. A number of important studies (15–24) investigated the accuracy of 16- and 64-slice MDCT coronary angiography for the detection of coronary artery stenosis in patients with known or suspected coronary artery disease (CAD) referred for invasive coronary angiography (Table 56.1). In all these studies, analysis of the MDCT data was performed by investigators blinded to the results of invasive angiography, and in all but two, the study was limited to coronary segments of greater than 1.5 or 2 mm in diameter. In most cases, significant coronary artery stenosis was defined as a lesion of 50% or greater, and sensitivity, specificity, and positive and negative predictive values were calculated. The prevalence of significant CAD in patients enrolled in these studies ranged from 42% to 83%. It is important to note that about 5% to 20% of all analyzable segments were considered nonevaluable due to motion, severe calcified plaques, and other imaging artifacts. In addition, most of these studies did not enroll a clinical series of truly consecutive patients, and only a few reported the accuracy of MDCT using each patient as the unit of analysis. Moreover, these studies were performed in few selected single centers.

Based on published data, the sensitivity of MDCT coronary angiography ranges between 72% and 95% per coronary segment and between 85% and 100% when using each patient as the denominator unit. The specificity per segment has been reported as between 86% and 98% per coronary segment and between 78% and 86% per patient. Positive predictive values have ranged between 72% and 90% per segment and between 81% and 97% per patient (the important denominator) and negative predictive values between 97% and 99% and between 82% and 100%, respectively. As expected, sensitivity was higher in those studies that excluded small vessel segments and was lower in populations with significant obesity. In 10 patients with a body mass index (BMI) of less than 25 kg/m^2, sensitivity was 100% for the detection of significant coronary disease (24). Nonetheless, the most recent analysis of 64-slice MDCT with state-of-the-art scanning and analysis of all segments identified 19 of 21 severe lesions requiring

TABLE 56.1

ACCURACY OF MULTI-DETECTOR COMPUTED TOMOGRAPHY COMPARED TO INVASIVE ANGIOGRAPHY FOR DETECTING >50% CORONARY STENOSIS USING SEGMENT UNIT ANALYSIS

Author (year)	No. detectors	No. subjects	No. segments	Sensitivity (%)	Specificity (%)	NPV (%)	PPV (%)
Raff (2005)	64	70	1,065	86	95	98	66
Leber (2005)	64	59	825	73	97	—	—
Kuettner (2005)	16	72	936	82	98	97	87
Mollet (2005)	16	51	610	95	98	99	87
Mollet (2004)	16	128	1,384	92	95	98	79
Martuscelli (2004)	16	64	729	89	98	98	90
Kuettner (2004)	16	58	763	72	97	97	72

A,B 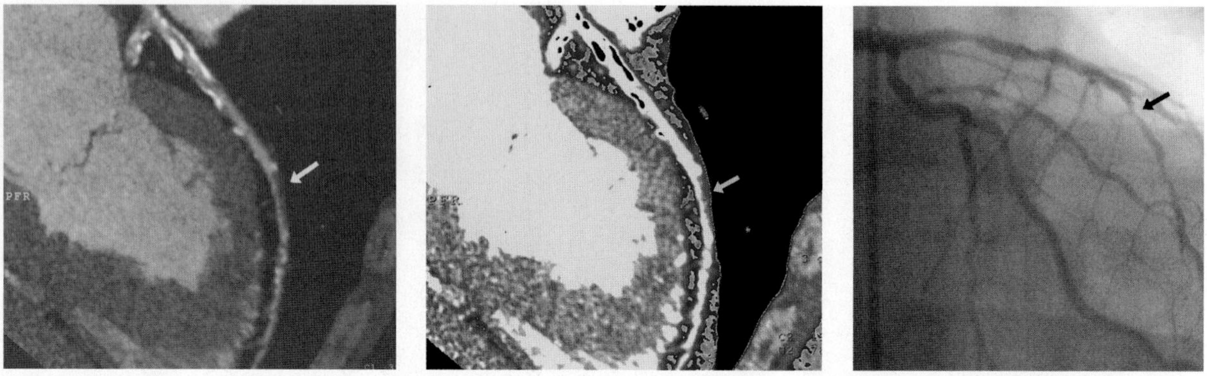 C

FIGURE 56.4. Severe coronary artery disease in a 45-year-old smoker with ST depression but normal nuclear perfusion scan. **A:** Severe tubular stenosis in distal left anterior descending artery caused by noncalcified plaque (*arrow*). **B:** Color-encoded image representing calcified plaques in black, normal lumen in white, and noncalcified plaques in red. **C:** Fluoroscopic image obtained during invasive coronary angiography.

revascularization at subsequent catheterization. False-positive results remain a problem.

Figure 56.4 shows a curved multiplanar reconstructed image of a severely stenosed left anterior descending artery with mixed calcified and noncalcified plaques. Currently, intravascular ultrasound (IVUS) is the only diagnostic tool capable of detecting the presence and make-up of these plaques in the coronary arteries in vivo (25,26). Clearly the widespread use of IVUS as a screening tool for risk assessment is impractical due to the high cost and invasive nature of cardiac catheterization. However, MDCT angiography has a unique potential for imaging the vessel wall as well as defining the lumen (27,28). Recent studies have shown the accuracy of MDCT in visualizing atherosclerotic coronary plaques and differentiating calcified from noncalcified lesions based on Hounsfield unit values. In a series of 22 patients clinically referred for IVUS (29), MDCT correctly identified the presence of coronary atherosclerotic plaques in 41 of 50 affected segments. The sensitivity of MDCT is greater for calcified (94%) than for mixed (78%) or soft (53%) plaques, and is limited for small-caliber vessels. Plaque volume tends to be systematically underestimated by MDCT compared to IVUS, and luminal calcified plaque tends to be overestimated. In a recent study (23) using 64-slice MDCT, there was reasonable correlation between mean plaque area defined by IVUS and MDCT ($r = 0.73$), but sensitivity for detection of greater-than-75% stenosis was only 80%. Whether MDCT could be usefully brought into clinical practice as a screening test remains to be proven, but in selected patients at intermediate risk, it could potentially help to justify lifelong aggressive preventive intervention. MDCT plaque characterization could also potentially serve to guide revascularization strategies and device selection.

MDCT coronary angiography is very useful in assessing the origin and course of congenitally anomalous coronary arteries (30,31). Compared to conventional angiography, MDCT can easily determine the three-dimensional relationship of anomalous coronary arteries with the aorta and pulmonary arterial trunk. Figure 56.5 illustrates the most malignant of these anomalies—a left coronary artery arising from the right coronary cusp and then running between pulmonary artery and aortic root, associated with sudden death in adults and with infantile heart failure. Table 56.2 lists the types and relative

A 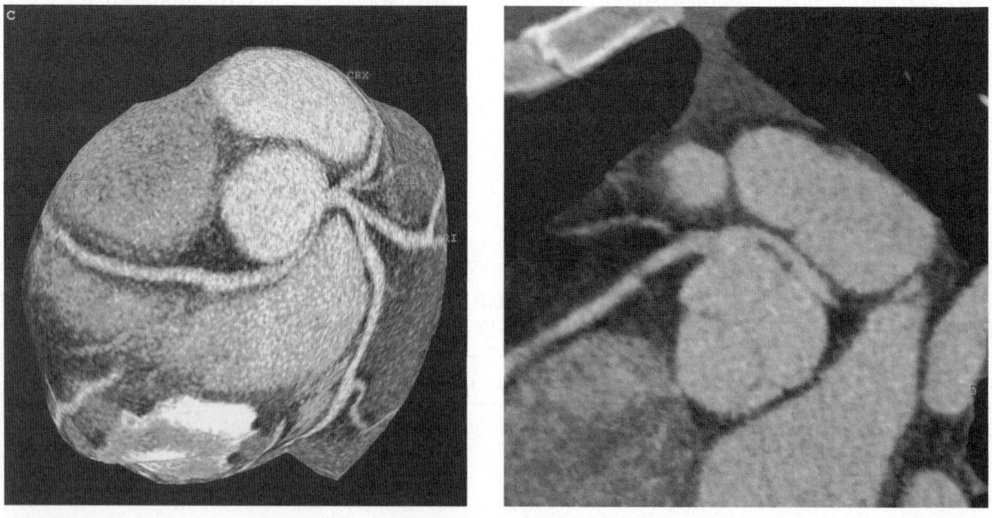 B

FIGURE 56.5. Coronary anomalies. **A:** Left main stem coronary (LM) anomaly in a 16-year-old with syncope. The LM arises from the right coronary cusp and runs between the aorta and the pulmonary trunk. **B:** Similar lesion in a 27-year-old with atypical chest pain and a positive nuclear stress test for anterior ischemia.

TABLE 56.2

CONGENITAL CORONARY ANOMALIES READILY IDENTIFIABLE BY MDCT

1. Anomalous origin of left main (LM) or left anterior descending (LAD) artery from pulmonary artery
2. Anomalous origin of LM or LAD from right coronary cusp with interarterial course
3. Anomalous origin of right coronary artery (RCA) from left coronary cusp
4. Single ostium from right or left coronary cusp
5. RCA and left circumflex artery from RCC
6. RCA and/or LMS from non-coronary cusp
7. Coronary artery fistulae

frequency of coronary anomalies. Arteriovenous fistulae can also be well visualized by MDCT, and Figure 56.6 shows a circumflex arteriovenous fistula draining to a persistent left superior vena cava. In addition, MDCT can also detect myocardial bridges and aneurysmal dilation of the coronary vessels in patients with symptoms of chest pain. EBCT has also been used successfully to evaluate the origin and course of coronary anomalies and, by using axial source images and three-dimensional volume-rendered images, has performed favorably compared to invasive angiography (32).

Accurate assessment of previously stented coronary vessels remains an important limitation to MDCT coronary angiography (33). A noninvasive, accurate test for in-stent restenosis would be invaluable in patients with postintervention chest pain. This is particularly true because the widespread use of drug-eluting stents reduces the incidence of in-stent restenosis, thus reducing the yield from repeat invasive coronary angiography. In a recent study using 16-slice MDCT (34), however, MDCT yielded valuable lumen images for only 126 of 232 stents (64%). Smaller stents in vessels of less than 3 mm were harder accurately to evaluate. Internal luminal diameter is often underestimated. In another study (23), 13 stented segments were assessed with a 64-slice MDCT. Two stents (of 2) with severe stenosis were accurately identified, 2 other stents (of 2) with moderate stenosis were called normal by MDCT, and 4 (of 9) stents with no angiographic restenosis were thought stenotic by MDCT. The ability to evaluate the lumen of stented vessels depends on the type and the diameter of the stent. Practical delineation of in-stent stenosis remains difficult in lumens smaller than 3 mm in diameter. Dedicated postprocessing "kernels' or filters may improve the resolution of stent lumen in the future (35). Figure 56.7 shows a patent stent in a large proximal right coronary artery.

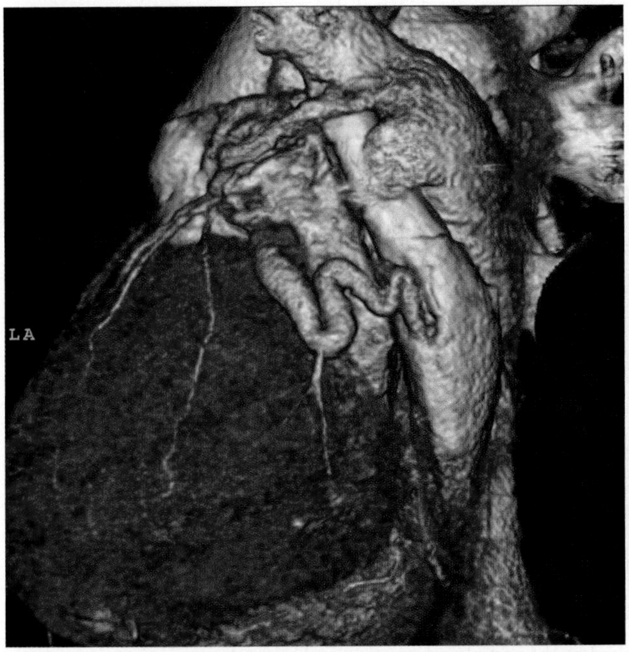

FIGURE 56.6. Congenital arteriovenous fistula in a 52-year-old with ischemia on stress testing. The markedly dilated and tortuous circumflex coronary artery feeds into a persistent left superior vena cava.

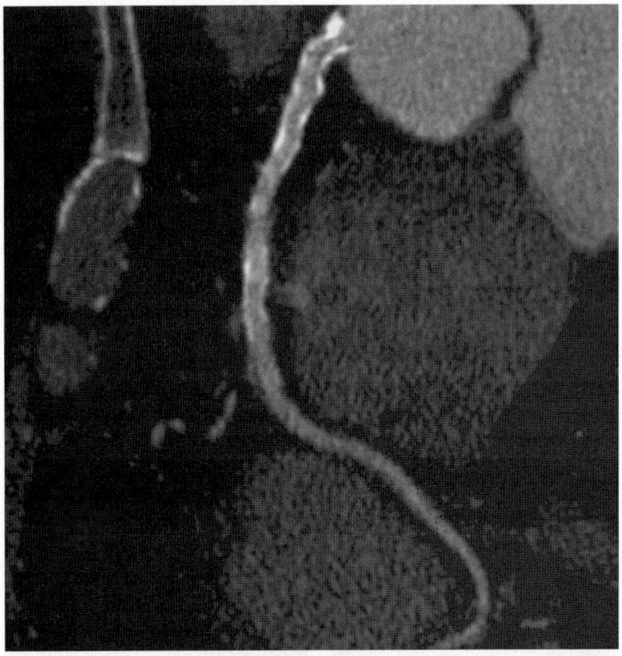

FIGURE 56.7. Curved multiplanar reconstruction of a patent coronary stent in the proximal right coronary artery.

CT has been proposed for the evaluation of coronary artery bypass grafts (CABGs) (Fig. 56.8). Exact delineation of vein graft lumen can be a technical challenge with MDCT. Studies using 16-slice MDCT have investigated the accuracy in identifying stenosis in coronary bypass conduits (36). This study reported successful visualization in all bypass conduits after excluding 3 subjects due to poor overall image quality. The reported sensitivity, specificity, and positive and negative predictive values for detecting total graft occlusion were 96%, 95%, 81%, and 99%, respectively. Imaging of the distal anastomosis site was possible in almost 75% of patients. Thus, determining total vein graft occlusion is quite straightforward, but quantifying moderate stenoses can be difficult. Figure 56.8B shows a volume-rendered image of an occluded vein graft to the right coronary artery arising from the ascending aorta. Motion artifacts and interference by surgical clips often limit the assessment of vessel anastomosis. Although graft position is easily visualized in patients following CABG, analysis of the native vessels is often more difficult in these patients due to poor run-off, more extensive calcification, and smaller lumen size. This can potentially limit the diagnostic utility of MDCT angiography in this setting. MDCT angiography may also help to characterize the three-dimensional location of preexisting coronary grafts in relationship to each other and to the chest wall in patients undergoing repeat sternotomy. EBCT analysis of coronary bypass grafts also shows some promise, with sensitivities of 93% to 96% for graft patency.

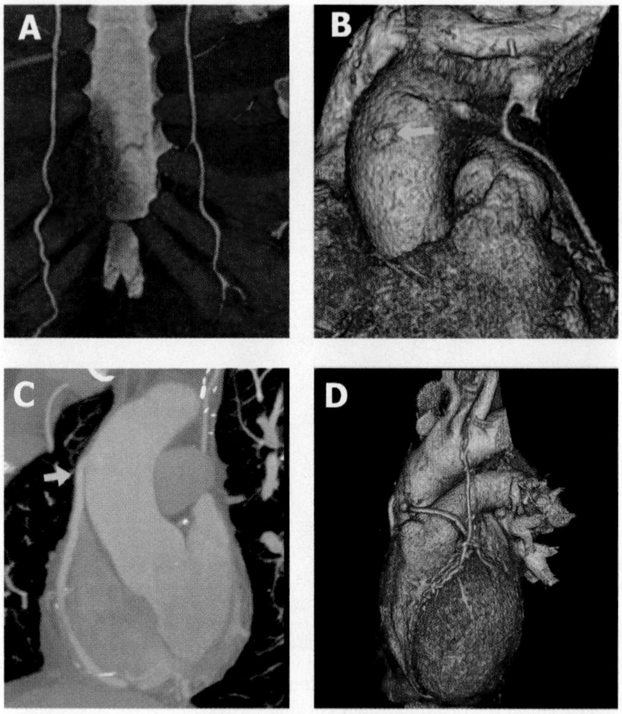

FIGURE 56.8. Computed tomography in coronary artery bypass surgery (CABG). **A:** Volume-rendered image of patent in situ bilateral internal thoracic arteries (ITA) prior to CABG. **B:** Volume-rendered image of occluded saphenous bypass grafts (SVG) and a left ITA graft. **C:** Curved multiplanar reconstruction showing patent SVG graft to right coronary artery (RCA). **D:** Volume-rendered image of patent left ITA graft from subclavian artery to left anterior descending (LAD).

There are four areas where specific problems, if identified before scanning, should give consideration for aborting the procedure because the diagnostic yield will be lower than acceptable:

1. Severe calcification can cause problems. Calcium has a Hounsfield Unit score of greater than +1,000, and reconstructions involving calcified structures tend to overestimate the volume set representing calcium ("blooming") because of "partial volume averaging," by which much of the coronary lumen is apparently occupied by calcified plaque, and "beam hardening," in which the calcium shields the true lumen and suggests more soft plaque than is truly there. Altering the window and level or rotating the curved multiplanar reconstructions may allow fuller characterization of the lumen. Figure 56.9 shows the same lumen with calcium blooming at two different levels, as compared to lumen from invasive angiography. One recent study (17) analyzed the performance of MDCT after excluding patients with very high calcium score. In that series the respective sensitivity and specificity were 77% and 97% for all patients (n = 60) versus 98% and 98% when only those patients with a score of less than 1,000 were included (n = 46). Because symptomatic patients with very high calcium scores have a very high probability of having obstructive coronary artery disease, it is reasonable to avoid MDCT angiography and proceed directly to invasive catheterization in these patients.
2. Stents/surgical clips artifacts remain a significant obstacle to image quality. This is a particular problem at sites of surgical graft clips for the internal thoracic grafts, where the vessel lumen becomes essentially uninterpretable at that point. The only likely solution to this problem is the introduction of nonmetallic clips to surgical practice (Fig. 56.10).
3. Atrial fibrillation/multiple ectopics undermine the basis of recent advances in MDCT, in that the ability to reconstruct images from five to eight consecutive cardiac cycles is totally dependent on ECG gating of predictable, stable RR intervals. Image quality of the coronary arteries is often suboptimal in patients with atrial fibrillation, and scanning is not recommended unless there happen to be relatively stable RR intervals. Similarly, if frequent premature beats are detected prior to scan acquisition, strong consideration should be given to not proceeding with the procedure. The gating artifact thus produced appears as a motion artifact but is localized to a specific block of data.
4. Morbid obesity is sometimes used a pretext for avoiding invasive angiography, and this represents a serious challenge to MDCT as well. Strategies for improving image quality include increasing tube current (often using >850 mA) at the cost of a significant increase in effective dose of radiation, even with careful use of dose modulation.

CT imaging of the moving heart is based on a combination of multiple technical advances and stretches the temporal and spatial resolution of CT scanners to their limits. Imaging

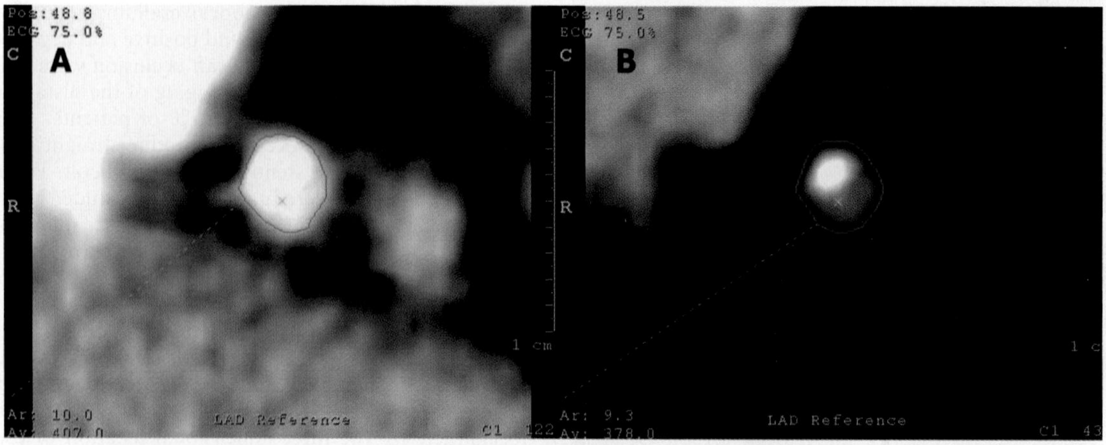

FIGURE 56.9. The "Blooming effect" of calcium is caused by the partial volume effect and interpolation in computed tomography. In these "virtual intravascular" cross-sectional images, changing the window width and center levels can exaggerate the "blooming effect" volume of calcified plaque in this mid left anterior descending (LAD) lesion in panel A compared to panel B.

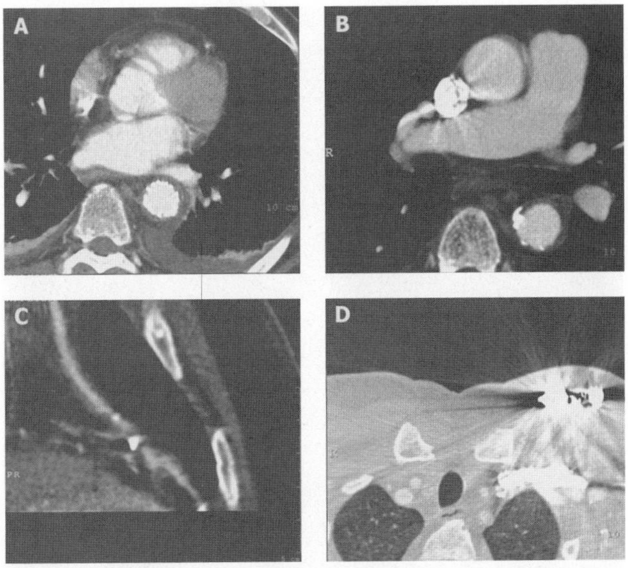

FIGURE 56.10. Imaging artifacts in computed tomography. **A:** A typical motion artifact at the ascending aorta in a nongated study. **B:** Contrast in the superior vena cava causing a radial streaking artifact. **C:** Surgical clips adjacent to a left internal thoracic artery bypass graft obscuring the anastomosis site to the left anterior descending artery. **D:** Pacemaker causing severe flash artifact.

artifacts from any of these technical algorithms can render studies partially or completely uninterpretable or even produce false-positive findings. Recognition of these artifacts is thus vital to a clinical service. Motion or breathing artifacts will typically blur the contours of the heart, the coronary arteries, and the ascending aorta (Fig. 56.10A). Inconsistent triggering or arrhythmias may cause misalignment of adjacent slices. In combination with motion, partial scan reconstruction can cause streaks and low-density artifacts especially beside metal or calcium. Contrast in the superior vena cava can cause streaking artifacts (Fig. 56.10B). Edge-enhancing reconstruction filters can lead to artifacts along borders between very low and high density (e.g., the interface between lung and cardiac tissue) by smoothing out boundaries and assigning artificially high CT numbers to pixels along the edge zone. Finally, the "partial volume effect" is common in CT imaging: if an image pixel is only partially filled by a structure of very high attenuation (e.g., metal), the highest CT number will be assigned to the complete pixel, which will thus appear bright on the image. This will exaggerate the dimensions of high-intensity objects such as calcified plaque and cause significant difficulties in image analysis.

Cardiac Masses

Although cardiac magnetic resonance imagining (MRI) has superior tissue characterization, MDCT can be utilized in certain circumstances to determine localization and anatomic relationships of tumors (37). Although rare, benign tumors outnumber their primary malignant counterparts three to one. In adults and children, myxomas and rhabdomyomas, respectively, represent the most common benign tumors, which can be grouped into tissue-specific subtypes, such as rhabdomyomas, fibromas, lipomas, teratomas, and so on. In malignant disease, CT provides additional physical, spatial, and functional information that further aids in the evaluation of metastases. For instance, CT provides superior resolution for detecting calcification, evaluating perfusion, and determining relationship to other structures given its three-dimensional nature. Figure 56.11 describes a multilobulated cardiac tumor picked up incidentally by MDCT, which subsequently proved to be a malignant sarcoma. In addition, intracardiac thrombus may be seen by MDCT. Figure 56.12 shows left atrial appendage thrombus in a patient awaiting a pulmonary vein isolation procedure. This was missed on transesophageal echocardiography. However, the relative sensitivity of MDCT in identifying thrombus has not been firmly established.

Functional Imaging

MRI provides a better assessment of real-time left ventricular (LV) volumes and ejection fraction (EF) than MDCT, but the ability to combine retrospectively gated phases of the cardiac cycle now allows for accurate quantification of LV mass and volumes and EF (38,39). These methods create a 17-segment model, perform favorably in comparison to invasive ventriculography, and may be used to quantify regional LV dysfunction. The data are acquired at the time of the coronary study and require no additional contrast or radiation. Commercial packages that automatically segment cardiac chambers and calculate volumes/ejection fraction are becoming available. Furthermore, there is growing interest in the potential ability to define myocardial perfusion by CT (40) with and without a "hybrid" approach with positron emission tomography (PET) scanning. The potential of being able to assess simultaneously coronary anatomy/stenosis and local tissue perfusion represents one of the more exciting aspects of current MDCT development.

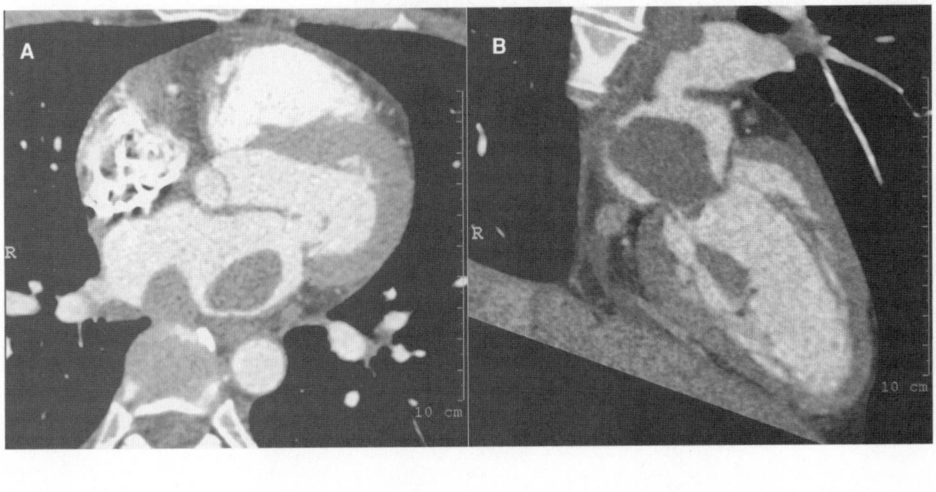

FIGURE 56.11. (**A**) Coronal axial and (**B**) multiplanar reconstructed images of multiple lobulated masses in the left atrium consistent with neoplastic tumor (spindle cell sarcoma).

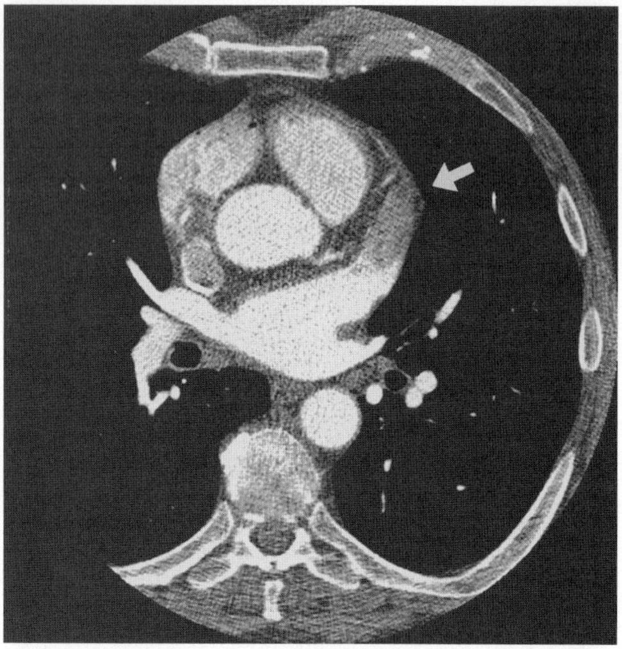

FIGURE 56.12. Filling defect consistent with thrombus in the left atrial appendage in a patient in atrial fibrillation.

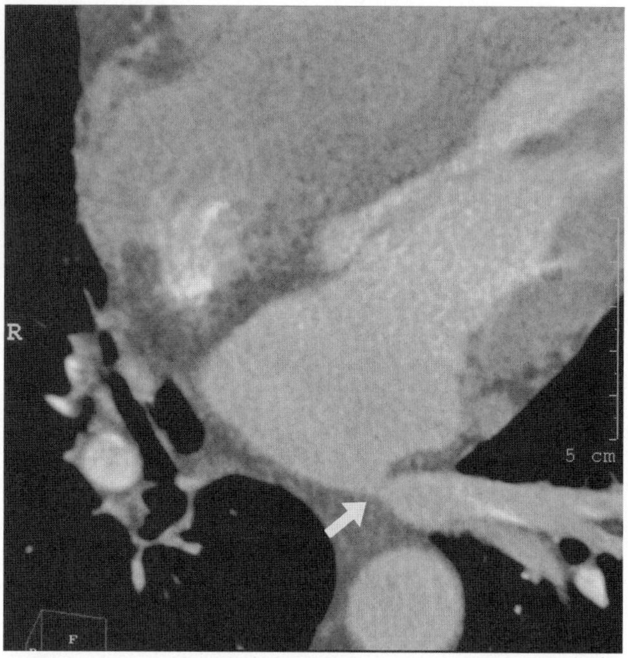

FIGURE 56.13. Pulmonary vein stenosis 6 months after radiofrequency ablation for atrial fibrillation in a 63-year-old patient with progressive exertional dyspnea.

Cardiac Computed Tomography in Electrophysiology

With the widespread utilization of pulmonary vein isolation procedures for atrial fibrillation, noninvasive analysis of left atrial and pulmonary vein anatomy is becoming desirable prior to invasive catheter ablation. Complications such as esophageal perforation and pulmonary vein stenosis, although uncommon, can be difficult to treat and are often fatal. The incidence of pulmonary vein stenosis varies according to the experience of the operator and the technique but can be as high as 20% (41) as detected by MDCT. Figure 56.13 shows a patient with left lower pulmonary vein stenosis and right upper pulmonary vein occlusion 6 months after a technically successful ablation for chronic atrial fibrillation. The pulmonary veins have a complex anatomy, differing from patient to patient. Both EBCT and MDCT can provide excellent three-dimensional visualization of the left atrium, pulmonary veins, and their relationship with surrounding structures (Fig. 56.14). MDCT images can be registered with the catheter system to provide virtual three-dimensional navigation during the procedure (Fig. 56.15) (42).

Contrast MDCT studies can also delineate the coronary sinus and its tributaries prior to cardiac resynchronization therapy, and they allow the electrophysiologist to plan a two-stage procedure with epicardial lead implantation where the coronary sinus anatomy is unfavorable (Figs. 56.16, 56.17) (43).

The Thoracic Aorta

CT been used for many years to define aortic pathology and is a mainstay of diagnosis for aortic dissection and aneurysm and the definition of aortic atheroma. Recent developments have allowed imaging of these pathologies along with coronary artery disease, thus bringing the possibility of a complete noninvasive vascular workup closer to reality. Thus a preoperative

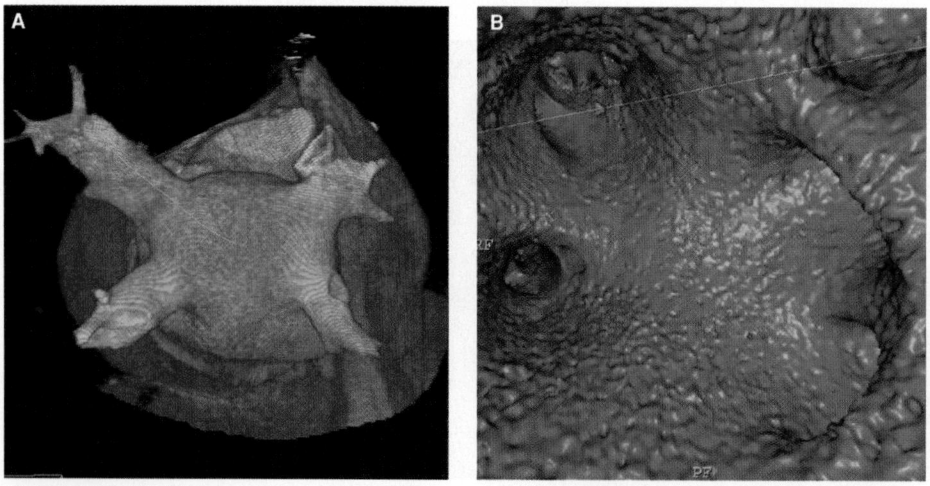

FIGURE 56.14. Volume-rendered exterior and virtual interior views of the left atrium and pulmonary veins by computed tomography.

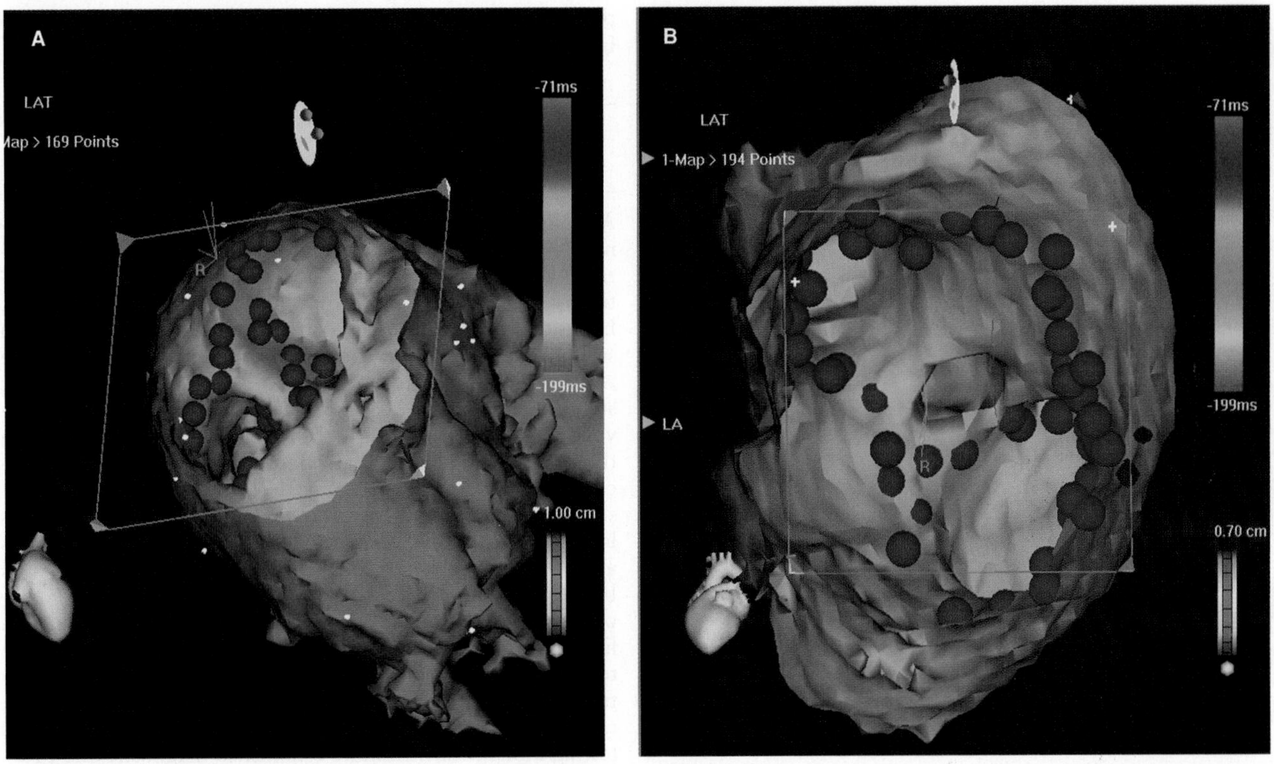

FIGURE 56.15. Co-registration of catheter radiofrequency ablation lesions and three-dimensional CT images of (**A**) the left and (**B**) the right pulmonary vein ostia in a patient undergoing ablation for atrial fibrillation.

approach to a patient with suspected aortic dissection routinely includes MDCT to delineate the aortic dissection and the coronary arteries and the presence of pericardial effusions, mediastinal leaks, and pseudoaneurysm formation. Many of these disorders are interrelated, and the common occurrence of cystic medial necrosis in the ascending aorta of patients with bicuspid aortic valves confirms the need to consider the aortopathies and the connective tissue disorders as a spectrum of disease, many of which need serial studies of aortic dimensions by tomographic methods (44). Figure 56.18 shows an aortic arch pseudoaneurysm in a patient with extensive atherosclerosis and a prior descending aortic stent graft. Patients with Marfan disorder may be reliably followed by serial MDCT studies to monitor expansion of an aneurysmal aorta.

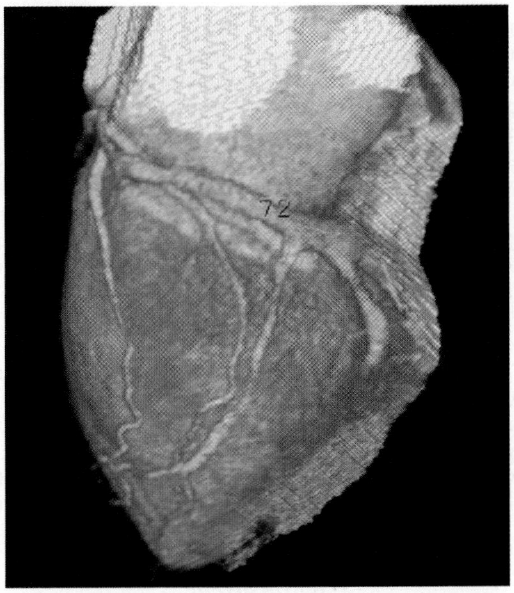

FIGURE 56.16. Contrast-enhanced volume-rendered imaged of the cardiac venous anatomy. Measurement of the take-off angle of the posterolateral cardiac vein.

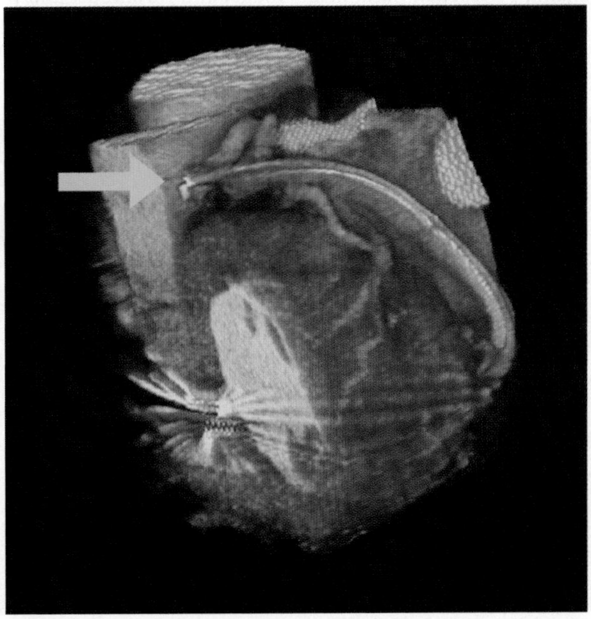

FIGURE 56.17. Images of the pacing leads after implantation for cardiac resynchronization therapy in a heart failure patient. The left lead is incorrectly placed in the anterior cardiac vein.

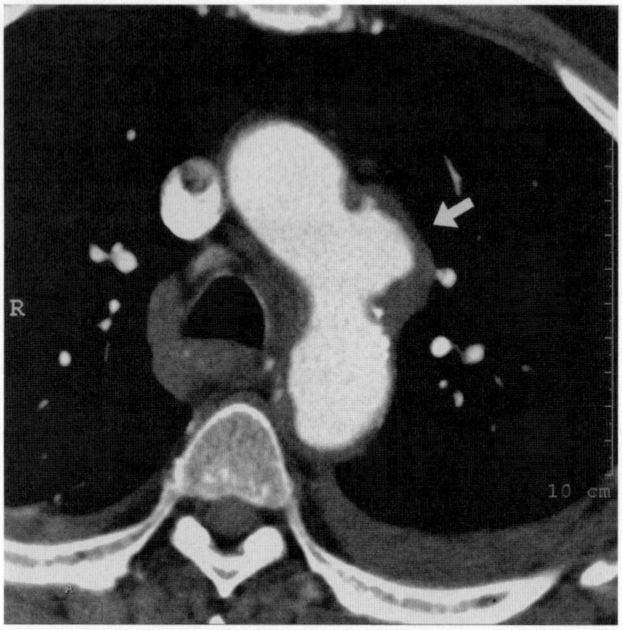

FIGURE 56.18. Large atheromatous pseudoaneurysm in the aortic arch of a 75-year-old patient with extensive atherosclerosis.

Pericardial Imaging

The pericardium is well visualized by MDCT and is usually surrounded by clearly delineated fat. Pericardial cysts can be visualized and infiltrative tumor characterized. Primary pericardial tumors such as mesothelioma are rare, but pericardium is a frequent site of late metastasis from other sites, often accompanied by bloody effusions (37). Thickening (>2 mm) and calcification of the pericardium can suggest constriction, but MDCT does not give the physiologic information needed to establish a diagnosis of pericardial constriction; thus echocardiography and MRI are superior in this regard. In the postoperative patient, MDCT is a robust tool for identifying and localizing pericardial fluid, hemorrhage, and thrombus, and the Hounsfield score can be used to help differentiate thrombus from free fluid. Figure 56.19 shows longstanding pericardial thickening and calcification with hematoma between the two layers of pericardium.

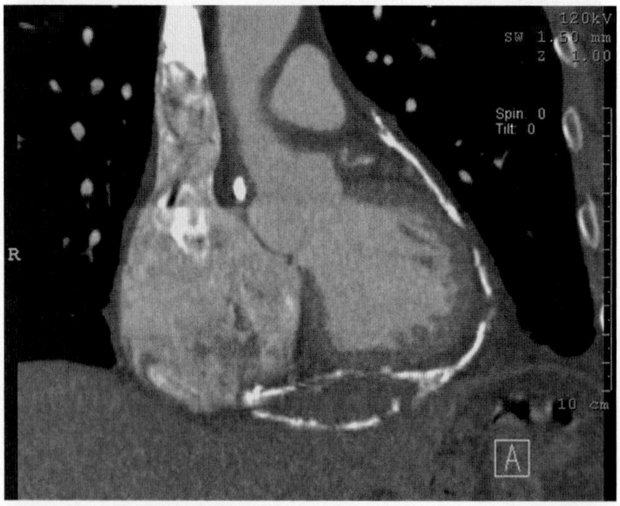

FIGURE 56.19. Pericardial calcification and intrapericardial hematoma in a 62-year-old man with a 9-year history of constrictive pericarditis.

CONTROVERSIES AND PERSONAL PERSPECTIVE

Although there is growing enthusiasm for the use of CT coronary angiography, there are many doubts regarding the accuracy of the technique and its clinical utility. It is evident that patient selection is very important to achieving adequate results. Image quality is compromised in very obese patients, those with severe coronary calcifications or coronary stents, and those with rapid or irregular heart rates. In addition, MDCT requires significant radiation exposure, a concern for patients of very young age and for those who may require repetitive use. In those patients with typical anginal symptoms and/or unequivocally abnormal stress test results, the likelihood of a negative result is low. Proceeding directly to invasive catheterization seems logical because MDCT can only used for diagnostic purposes at this time. Accordingly, MDCT coronary angiography should be most useful for evaluating symptomatic patients with equivocal stress test results or asymptomatic patients with borderline abnormal tests who are at an intermediate risk according to clinical history and risk factors. In addition, the information derived from MDCT should be seen as complementary, not as a replacement for that derived from other diagnostic testing modalities with more established diagnostic and prognostic value.

The role of the CT calcium score for risk stratification, although still controversial, appears to be justified in asymptomatic patients with intermediate risk for developing coronary artery disease and who do clearly meet criteria for pharmacologic intervention. The use of CT angiography in this setting is interesting from a research perspective. CT coronary angiography can establish the presence and burden of noncalcified plaque even in the absence of coronary calcifications. Clinical application of this test in this setting, however, is even more controversial in the absence of prognostic data.

THE FUTURE

The advances in CT technology are occurring so fast that clinical results often apply to obsolete technology by the time they reach publication. Most CT manufacturers and investigators recognize that there are advances that need to be made to reduce the number of poor-quality studies and decrease radiation exposure. There are many approaches that are being considered that will require faster scan rotational speeds and more efficient x-ray sources and detection systems. Technically, it is conceivably possible to perform an entire study in a single heartbeat and/or with temporal resolutions below 100 msec. This would dramatically reduce the number of artifacts and reduce contrast dose required, and could reduce radiation exposure by 50% to 75%.

In addition to improving accuracy, clinical trials should be conducted to determine whether the use of CT as a diagnostic or a screening test could result in improve outcomes and cost savings. In an era when diagnostic medical imaging is under intense scrutiny and health care costs continue to rise faster than funding, these data will need to be rigorously collected.

References

1. Garcia MJ. Noninvasive coronary angiography: hype or new paradigm? *JAMA* 2005;293:2531–2533.

2. Schoenhagen P, Stillman AE, Halliburton SS, et al. Non-invasive coronary angiography with multi-detector computed tomography: comparison to conventional X-ray angiography. *Int J Cardiovasc Imaging* 2005;21:63–72.
3. Schoenhagen P, Stillman AE, Halliburton SS, White RD. CT of the heart: principles, advances, clinical uses. *Cleve Clin J Med* 2005;72:127–138.
4. Stillman A. Cardiovascular CT techniques. *Int J Cardiovasc Imaging* 2001; 17:445–446.
5. Achenbach S, Moshage W, Ropers D, et al. Value of electron-beam computed tomography for the noninvasive detection of high-grade coronary-artery stenoses and occlusions. *N Engl J Med* 1998;339:1964–1970.
6. Hoffmann MHK, Shi H, Manzke R, et al. Noninvasive coronary angiography with 16-detector row CT: effect of heart rate. *Radiology* 2005;234:86–97.
7. White RD. MR and CT assessment for ischemic cardiac disease. *J Magn Reson Imaging* 2004;19:659–675.
8. Keelan PC, Bielak LF, Ashai K, et al. Long-term prognostic value of coronary calcification detected by electron-beam computed tomography in patients undergoing coronary angiography. *Circulation* 2001;104:412–417.
9. Greenland P, LaBree L, Azen SP, et al. Coronary artery calcium score combined with Framingham score for risk prediction in asymptomatic individuals. *JAMA* 2004;291:210–215.
10. O'Malley PG, Greenberg BA, Taylor AJ. Cost-effectiveness of using electron beam computed tomography to identify patients at risk for clinical coronary artery disease. *Am Heart J* 2004;148:106–113.
11. Budoff MJ, Cohen MC, Garcia MJ, et al. ACCF/AHA clinical competence statement on cardiac imaging with computed tomography and magnetic resonance. *Circulation* 2005;112:598–617.
12. Budoff MJ, Achenbach S, Duerinckx A. Clinical utility of computed tomography and magnetic resonance techniques for noninvasive coronary angiography. *J Am Coll Cardiol* 2003;42:1867–1878.
13. Garcia MJ. Could cardiac CT revolutionize the practice of cardiology? *Cleve Clin J Med* 2005;72:88–89.
14. Vembar M, Garcia M, Heuscher DJ, et al. Dynamic approach to identifying desired physiological phases for cardiac imaging using multislice spiral CT. *Med Phys* 2003;30:1683–1693.
15. Nieman K, Cademartiri F, Lemos PA, et al. Reliable noninvasive coronary angiography with fast submillimeter multislice spiral computed tomography. *Circulation* 2002;106:2051–2054.
16. Ropers D, Baum U, Pohle K, et al. Detection of coronary artery stenoses with thin-slice multi-detector row spiral computed tomography and multiplanar reconstruction. *Circulation* 2003;107:664–666.
17. Kuettner A, Beck T, Drosch T, et al. Diagnostic accuracy of noninvasive coronary imaging using 16-detector slice spiral computed tomography with 188 ms temporal resolution. *J Am Coll Cardiol* 2005;45:123–127.
18. Dewey M, Laule M, Krug L, et al. Multisegment and halfscan reconstruction of 16-slice computed tomography for detection of coronary artery stenoses. *Invest Radiol* 2004;39:223–229.
19. Kuettner A, Trabold T, Schroeder S, et al. Noninvasive detection of coronary lesions using 16-detector multislice spiral computed tomography technology—initial clinical results. *J Am Coll Cardiol* 2004;44:1230–1237.
20. Mollet NR, Cademartiri F, Krestin GP, et al. Improved diagnostic accuracy with 16-row multi-slice computed tomography coronary angiography. *J Am Coll Cardiol* 2005;45:128–132.
21. Mollet NR, Cademartiri F, Nieman K, et al. Multislice spiral computed tomography coronary angiography in patients with stable angina pectoris. *J Am Coll Cardiol* 2004;43:2265–2270.
22. Martuscelli E, Romagnoli A, D'Eliseo A, et al. Accuracy of thin-slice computed tomography in the detection of coronary stenoses. *Eur Heart J* 2004; 25:1043–1048.
23. Leber AW, Knez A, von Ziegler F, et al. Quantification of obstructive and nonobstructive coronary lesions by 64-slice computed tomography: a comparative study with quantitative coronary angiography and intravascular ultrasound. *J Am Coll Cardiol* 2005;46:147–154.
24. Raff GL, Gallagher MJ, O'Neill WW, Goldstein JA. Diagnostic accuracy of noninvasive coronary angiography using 64-slice spiral computed tomography. *J Am Coll Cardiol* 2005;46:552–557.
25. Nissen SE, Grinses CL, Gurley JC, et al. Application of a new phased-away ultrasound imaging catheter in the assessment of vascular dimensions: in vivo comparison to cine angiography. *Circulation* 1980;81:660–666.
26. Vince D, Dixon K, Cothern R, et al. Comparison of texture analysis methods for the characterization of coronary plaques in intravascular ultrasound images. *Comput Med Imag Graph* 2000;24:221–229.
27. Kopp A, Schroeder S, Baumbach A, et al. Non-invasive characterization of lesion morphology and composition by multislice CT: results in comparison with intracoronary ultrasound. *Eur Radiol* 2001;11:1607–1611.
28. Schoenhagen P, Tuzcu EM, Stillman AE, et al. Non-invasive assessment of plaque morphology and remodeling in mildly stenotic coronary segments: comparison of 16-slice computed tomography and intravascular ultrasound. *Coron Artery Dis* 2003;14:459–462.
29. Achenbach S, Moselewski F, Ropers D, et al. Detection of calcified and noncalcified coronary atherosclerotic plaque by contrast-enhanced, submillimeter multidetector spiral computed tomography. A segment-based comparison with intravascular ultrasound. *Circulation* 2004;109:14–17.
30. Taylor AJ, Byers JP, Cheitlin MD, Virmani R. Anomalous right or left coronary artery from the contralateral coronary sinus: "high-risk" abnormalities in the initial coronary artery course and heterogeneous clinical outcomes. *Am Heart J* 1997;133:428–435.
31. Shi H, Aschoff AJ, Brambs HJ, et al. Multislice CT imaging of anomalous coronary arteries. *Eur Radiol* 2004;14:2172–2181.
32. Memisoglu E, Hobikoglu G, Tepe MS, et al. Congenital coronary anomalies in adults: comparison of anatomic course visualization by catheter angiography and electron beam CT. *Catheter Cardiovasc Interv* 2005;66:34–42.
33. Gilard M, Cornily JC, Rioufol G, et al. Noninvasive assessment of left main coronary stent patency with 16-slice computed tomography. *Am J Cardiol* 2005;95:110–112.
34. Hong C, Chrysant GS, Woodard PK, et al. Coronary artery stent patency assessed with in-stent contrast enhancement measured at multi-detector row CT angiography: initial experience. *Radiology* 2004;233:286–291.
35. Seifarth H, Raupach R, Schaller S, et al. Assessment of coronary artery stents using 16-slice MDCT angiography: evaluation of a dedicated reconstruction kernel and a noise reduction filter. *Eur Radiol* 2005;15:721–726.
36. Schlosser T, Konorza T, Hunold P, et al. Noninvasive visualization of coronary artery bypass grafts using 16-detector row computed tomography. *J Am Coll Cardiol* 2004;44:1224–1229.
37. Restrepo CS, Largoza A, Lemos DF, et al. CT and MR imaging findings of malignant cardiac tumors. *Curr Probl Diagn Radiol* 2005;34:1–11.
38. Hundt W, Siebert K, Wintersperger BJ, et al. Assessment of global left ventricular function: comparison of cardiac multidetector-row computed tomography with angiocardiography. *J Comput Assist Tomogr* 2005;29:373–381.
39. Salm LP, Schuijf JD, de Roos A, et al. Global and regional left ventricular function assessment with 16-detector row CT: comparison with echocardiography and cardiovascular magnetic resonance. *Eur J Echocardiogr* 2005.
40. Raggi P, Berman DS. Computed tomography coronary calcium screening and myocardial perfusion imaging. *J Nucl Cardiol* 2005;12:96–103.
41. Saad EB, Rossillo A, Saad C, et al. Pulmonary vein stenosis after radiofrequency ablation of atrial fibrillation: functional characterization, evolution, and influence of the ablation strategy. *Circulation* 2003;108:3102–3107.
42. Verma A, Marrouche N, Natale A. Novel method to integrate three-dimensional computed tomographic images of the left atrium with real-time electroanatomic mapping. *J Cardiovasc Electrophysiol* 2004;15:968.
43. Shinbane JS, Girsky MJ, Mao S, Budoff MJ. Thebesian valve imaging with electron beam CT angiography: implications for resynchronization therapy. *Pacing Clin Electrophysiol* 2004;27:1566–1567.
44. Isselbacher EM. Thoracic and abdominal aortic aneurysms. *Circulation* 2005;111:816–28.

[illegible]

[redacted]

[illegible]

SECTION FOUR
ELECTROPHYSIOLOGY AND PACING

ERIC N. PRYSTOWSKY, MD

CHAPTER 58 ■ GENETICS OF ARRHYTHMIAS

MARK E ANDERSON, DAWOOD DARBAR, AND PRINCE KANNANKERIL

OVERVIEW

In recent years, the identification of gene defects in a vast array of monogenic disorders has revolutionized our understanding of the basic mechanisms underlying numerous disease processes. Mutations in cardiac ion channels have been identified as the basis of a wide range of inherited arrhythmia syndromes, including the congenital long QT syndromes (LQTSs), Brugada syndrome, Lenegre syndrome, Andersen syndrome, and familial atrial fibrillation (AF). More recently, it has been observed that not only transmembrane cardiac ion channels cause cardiac arrhythmias, but also intracellular channel and non–ion conduction proteins that may be pathophysiologically linked to inherited arrhythmias. The identification of genes underlying the inherited arrhythmia syndromes has greatly contributed to our understanding of the substrates for arrhythmia development, but an unexpected complexity has emerged in the genotype-phenotype relationship. Phenotypic expression of a given mutation does not always appear to be uniform in human patients, a finding implying a contribution from environmental factors and/or the presence of other genetically encoded modifiers. Accumulating evidence suggests that "multiple hits" affecting the interaction and integrity of signaling pathways may be responsible for many forms of arrhythmias.

Although we have witnessed significant strides in our understanding of the genetic basis of inherited arrhythmia disorders in the past decade, many challenging issues still need to be addressed. Developments are likely to come from studies using new model systems that assess the function of mutant proteins in preparations that are more closely allied to the physiologic environment in which these proteins are distributed. These more physiologic expression systems will be useful not only to characterize individual mutations, but also to elucidate the effects of mutations on the complex physiology of cardiac cells. In this chapter, we first summarize our present understanding of the molecular basis for cardiac arrhythmias by using the congenital LQTS as a case study in monogenic diseases. Second, ion channel and non–ion channel inherited arrhythmia syndromes are reviewed. Finally, we briefly discuss the use of arrhythmia models that may be used to understand inherited arrhythmia syndromes better.

GENETICS GLOSSARY

Allele: Alternate form of a gene.

Alternative splicing: A regulatory mechanism by which variations in the incorporation of a gene's exons, or coding regions, into mRNA lead to the production of more than one related protein, or isoform.

Codon: A three-base sequence of DNA or RNA that specifies a single amino acid.

Complex disease: Combing the effects of several genes and the environment, also referred to as multifactorial or polygenic.

Compound heterozygote: Carrying two different mutations for one gene, each provided by a different parent.

Conservative mutation: A change in a DNA or RNA sequence that leads to the replacement of one amino acid with a biochemically similar one.

Exon: A region of a gene that codes for a protein.

Frame-shift mutation: The addition or deletion of a number of DNA bases that is not a multiple of three, thus causing a shift in the reading frame of the gene. This shift produces a change in the reading frame of all parts of the gene that are downstream from the mutation, often leading to a premature stop codon and, ultimately, to a truncated protein.

Gain-of-function mutation: A mutation that produces a protein that takes on a new or enhanced function.

Gene dose effect: A relationship between the number of diseased alleles and phenotype severity.

Genetic heterogeneity: Mutations in several genes causing similar phenotype.

Genomics: The study of a functions and interactions of all the genes in the genome, including their interactions with environmental factors.

Genotype: The genetic makeup of an individual; it also refers to the alleles at a given locus.

Haplotype: A group of nearby alleles that are inherited together.

Heterozygous: Carrying two different alleles of a given gene.

Homozygous: Carrying two identical alleles of a given gene.

Intron: A region of a gene that does not code for a protein.

Locus: Location of a gene on a chromosome.

Loss-of-function mutation: A mutation that decreases the production or function of a protein (or does both).

Missense mutation: Substitution of a single DNA base that results in a codon that specifies an alternative amino acid.

Modifier genes: Genes that are not primarily responsible for a trait but that can alter a trait's expression or severity.

Monogenic: Caused by a mutation in a single gene.

Nonsense mutation: Substitution of a single DNA base that results in a stop codon, thus leading to truncation of a protein.

Penetrance: The likelihood that a person carrying a particular mutant gene will have an altered phenotype.

Phenotype: The observable physical or biochemical characteristics of an organism.

Point mutation: The substitution of a single DNA base in the normal DNA sequence.

BASIC GENETIC PRINCIPLES

Hereditary information is encoded in DNA via a sequence of purine (adenine, guanine) and pyrimidine (cytosine, thymine) bases. The hereditary unit is called a gene and consists of a segment of DNA that encodes for a specific protein. There are 30,000 to 35,000 genes in the human genome, and each individual has two copies of each gene called *alleles*. The human genome has 23 pairs of chromosomes (44 autosomal and 2 sex chromosomes) containing approximately 3 billion base pairs of DNA. Each parent contributes one-half of each chromosome pair and thus one copy of each gene. The site at which a gene is located on a particular chromosome is called the *genetic locus*. The genetic information on DNA is translated into protein through a translational code passed through messenger RNA (mRNA), in which three bases, referred as a *codon*, encode for an amino acid. The transcribed mRNA serves as the template that determines the sequence of amino acids in the resulting protein.

DNA nucleotide sequences generally remain constant when passed from parent to child. Base sequence changes are referred to as *mutations*. Mutations can be the result of environmental factors, including radiation, chemicals, drugs, and errors introduced by the DNA synthetic and editing enzymes. There are several ways to categorize mutations. One is according to the causative mechanism, whereas another is according to their functional effect. When classified according to the genetic cause, point mutations (i.e., a change in a single DNA base in the sequence) are the most common. Many types of point mutations are recognized. One type is a missense mutation, a substitution that leads to an alternative amino acid because of the way in which it changes the codon. Nonsense mutations are a more dramatically deleterious type of point mutations that change the codon to a "stop" codon, a codon that causes the termination of the protein instead of producing an amino acid. Another type of mutation is the frameshift mutation, which changes the reading frame of the gene downstream from it, often leading to a premature stop codon. Many variants in the human genome sequence have no phenotypic effect. Among these are silent mutations, which replace one base with another, so the resultant codon still codes for the same amino acid. This is a conservative mutation and can occur because codons are redundantly formatted so multiple base pair triplets (codons) can specify the same amino acid. Moreover, mutations may not change the phenotype if the altered codon encodes for an amino acid with similar properties. Nonconservative mutations replace an amino acid with a very different one and are more likely to affect phenotype.

Hereditary diseases are generally classified into three broad categories: (a) chromosomal duplication or deletions, (b) single gene or monogenic disorders, and (c) polygenic or complex traits that are the result of interactions between defects in multiple genes. Our discussion focuses on monogenic and polygenic disorders. Diseases caused by a single genetic defect are referred to as monogenic disorders; they follow mendelian inheritance and are classified as autosomal dominant, autosomal recessive, or X-linked (dominant or recessive). Approximately 5,000 monogenic diseases have been identified, and more than 1,000 genes responsible for these disorders are known. Most single-gene diseases display an autosomal dominant mode of inheritance, in which case approximately half of family members are affected. Monogenic disorders with an autosomal recessive inheritance are secondary to mutations in both copies of the gene; in which case only 25% of children exhibit the phenotype, 50% carry the mutation, and 25% are normal. With X-linked inheritance, only males generally exhibit the disease, whereas females do not show the phenotype, unless the mutation involves a major protein, in which case the females could exhibit the clinical phenotype. In diseases secondary to mitochondrial DNA mutations, inheritance is from the mother, because mitochondrial DNA is primarily inherited from the ovum. In cardiology, there are two major clusters of monogenic disorders: (a) the cardiomyopathies resulting from alterations in sarcomeric and in cytoskeletal proteins and (b) the arrhythmogenic diseases caused by mutations in ion channels and ion channel–controlling proteins such as the LQTS, Brugada syndrome, the short QT syndrome, catecholaminergic polymorphic ventricular tachycardia (CPVT), familial AF, and Andersen syndrome. Polygenic disorders are caused by mutations in multiple genes. Single nucleotide alterations, referred to as single nucleotide polymorphisms, occur with a frequency of approximately 1 per 600 base pair and can account for morphologic distinctions, susceptibility to disease, and response to drugs and therapeutic agents. Polygenic disorders underlie the majority of cardiovascular diseases and are inherently more difficult for assigning genetic causation than is the case for monogenic diseases.

Genetic heterogeneity refers to the observation that different mutations in the same (allele heterogeneity) or different genes (locus heterogeneity) can cause the same phenotype. Within a given family, a single mutation is usually responsible for the disorder in all affected family members. The congenital LQTS provides an example for both types of heterogeneity because they have been mapped to seven different genes (locus heterogeneity), and multiple mutations in each of these genes give rise to disease phenotypes (allelic heterogeneity). Currently, eight genes can cause the phenotype of the congenital LQTS and are responsible for 50% to 60% of clinically diagnosed cases. In contrast, only *SCN5A*, the primary cardiac sodium (Na) channel gene, is known to cause Brugada syndrome, but several other genes are likely to be implicated in this disease because only 20% of the clinical diagnoses result in positive tests at genetic screening. It is possible that the overlapping phenotypes may necessitate classifying each genetic variant as a separate disease entity based on the specific defect, particularly because emerging data suggest that the genetic substrate may be a major determinant of prognosis in patients harboring different genetic defects.

Numerous genetic and environmental factors can affect expression of a gene mutation. When these factors mask the phenotype, penetrance is said to be low. Hence, the penetrance of a monogenic disease is defined as the percentage of individuals with a mutant allele who develop the phenotype of the related disease. Penetrance can vary from 10% to 100%. The expressivity of a disease refers to different phenotypic manifestations that can be observed among carriers of the same genetic defect. Variation in penetrance and expressivity of genetic mutations suggests that many factors, including environment and modifier genes, can influence the phenotype of patients with monogenic diseases.

COMPLEXITY BEYOND MONOGENIC ARRHYTHMIA SYNDROMES

The first genetic defects causing the congenital LQTS were identified in 1995 by Keating and colleagues (1,2). Since then, hundreds of mutations have been identified in various ion channel subunits and in proteins important for the proper functioning of cardiac ion channels. Although it was initially assumed that all carriers of pathogenic mutations would manifest the corresponding phenotype, it soon became apparent that the clinical consequences of genetic defects are far more variable than expected. However, when variable penetrance and expressivity of the disease are taken into consideration, it is not a surprise that carriers of a DNA mutation may manifest a very wide range of phenotypes.

The genotype and phenotype connection is further complicated by mutations in one gene leading not only to variable phenotypes within the same disease, but also to profoundly different diseases. This diversity is well exemplified by mutations in the lamin *A/C* gene, which are known to cause at least eight phenotypes (allelic diseases) as varied as dilated cardiomyopathy, Emery-Dreifuss muscular dystrophy, familial partial lipodystrophy, Charcot-Marie-Tooth disease, mandibuloacral dysplasia, Hutchinson-Gilford progeria, lipoatrophy with diabetes, hypertrophic cardiomyopathy, and limb girdle muscular dystrophy. In inherited arrhythmia syndromes, mutations of the cardiac Na channel gene are associated with three diseases (the congenital LQTS, Brugada syndrome, and progressive conduction disease). Similarly, mutations in the *KCNQ1* gene encoding the a-subunit of the potassium (K) channel conducting the slow component of the delayed rectifier (I_{Ks}) are associated with three distinct diseases (the LQTS, the short QT syndrome, and familial AF). It is therefore clear that the identification of a mutation in a given gene is often insufficient to diagnose a single disease, and the identification of a mutation in an individual with a known disease is not enough to predict the phenotype of that individual.

GENETIC MODIFIERS

Our inability to predict clinical phenotype completely based on in vitro studies is not wholly unexpected especially because the characterization of a mutation is performed in the artificial settings of a noncardiac expression system. These cellular models systems typically utilize an approach based upon overexpression of a disease candidate gene in an immortalized nonmuscle cell line. These cells are very different from cardiac myocytes and do not incorporate key elements such as calcium (Ca) homeostasis, intercellular coupling, second messengers, membrane receptors, and other key proteins essential for phenotypic expression. Thus, improved systems biology approaches are needed to understand and evaluate genotype-phenotype connections in genetic arrhythmia syndromes.

MOLECULAR BASIS OF INHERITED ARRHYTHMIA SYNDROMES

Cardiac arrhythmias generally result from abnormalities in four classes of protein: (a) ion channels, exchangers, and their modulators (primary electrical disease); (b) cell-to-cell junction proteins, such as those responsible for arrhythmogenic right ventricular cardiomyopathy; (c) contractile sarcomeric proteins, such as those responsible for hypertrophic cardiomyopathy; and (d) cytoskeletal proteins, which are responsible for dilated cardiomyopathy. Tables 58.1 to 58.4 present a list of known genetic disorders based on phenotypic characteristics.

Congenital Long QT Syndrome: A Case Study of Monogenic Arrhythmia Syndromes

Since the initial description of congenital deafness, prolongation of the QT interval, and sudden death by Jervell and Lange-Nielsen in 1957 (3), our understanding of the genetic basis of the congenital LQTS has progressed significantly. Shortly after the autosomal recessive Jervell-Lange-Nielsen syndrome was described, Romano and Ward each independently described an "autosomal dominant" form without congenital deafness (4,5). The findings that the QT interval could be prolonged by right stellectomy and the successful treatment of a medically refractory young patient with the LQTS by left stellectomy led to the hypothesis that the disease was primarily a disorder of cardiac sympathetic innervation (6). Although we now know that this is not the primary cause of the LQTS, the importance of these early observations is evident in that autonomic modulation remains an important therapeutic approach in patients with this syndrome.

The subsequent theory that the underlying cause of the LQTS was an alteration of one of the repolarizing K currents was proposed nearly 10 years before the identification of the first LQTS genes in 1995 (1,2,7,8). Indeed, four forms of the LQTS, and the two most common forms (LQT1 and LQT2), are caused by mutations in genes that encode proteins that form repolarizing K channels. In the late 1990s, the first five LQTS genes were identified (see Table 58.1), all of which encoded proteins that form ion channels underlying the cardiac action potential (Fig. 58.1). The most commonly identified genes, *KCNQ1* and *KCNH2*, encode proteins that form the α-subunits of two major repolarizing K currents, I_{Ks} and I_{Kr}. Two other LQTS genes encode for the corresponding β-subunits (*KCNE1* and *KCNE2*). The other major LQTS gene, *SCN5A*, encodes the α-subunit of the cardiac Na channel. Either loss-of-function mutations in K channel genes or gain-of-function mutations in the cardiac Na or Ca channels lead to prolongation of ventricular repolarization and therefore a prolonged QT interval. Furthermore, we now know that the Jervell-Lange-Nielsen syndrome is simply a more severe form of the LQTS, because patients with Romano-Ward syndrome carry a single mutation, whereas it is now accepted that homozygous mutations of *KCNQ1* or *KCNE1* cause Jervell-Lange-Nielsen syndrome (Fig. 58.2) (9,10). The extracardiac finding of congenital deafness requires the presence of two mutant alleles and results from lack of functioning I_{Ks} in the inner ear (11). Patients with Jervell-Lange-Nielsen syndrome are also thought to be highly susceptible to arrhythmias; thus, arrhythmia risk seems partly dependent on "gene dosage." These first five forms of the LQTS represent classic LQTS, in that single mutations in ion channel genes resulted in action potential prolongation and prolonged QT intervals, with an increased risk for torsades de pointes and sudden death, without significant extracardiac manifestations.

TABLE 58.1

INHERITED ARRHYTHMIA SYNDROMES

Phenotype	Rhythm	Inheritance	Locus	Ion channel	Gene
VENTRICULAR					
LQTS (RW)	TdP	AD			
LQT1			11p15	I_{Ks}	*KCNQ1, KvLQT1*
LQT2			7q35	I_{Kr}	*KCNH2, HERG*
LQT3			3p21	I_{Na}	*SCN5A*
LQT4			4q25		*ANKB, ANK2*
LQT5			21q22	I_{Ks}	*KCNE1, minK*
LQT6			21q22	I_{Kr}	*KCNE2, MiRP1*
LQT7			17q23	I_{K1}	*KCNJ2, Kir2.1*
LQT8			12p13.3	$I_{Ca\text{-}L}$	*CACNA1C*
LQTS (JLN)	TdP	AR	11p15	I_{Ks}	*KCNQ1, KvLQT1*
			21q22	I_{Kr}	*minK*
Catecholaminergic VT	VT	AD	1q42		*RYR2*
		AR	1p13-p11		*CASQ2*
Brugada syndrome	VT/VF	AD	3p21	I_{Na}	*SCN5A*
			3p22-25		
Short QT syndrome	AF/VF	AD	21q22	I_{Kr}	*KCNH2*
			21q22	I_{Ks}	*KCNQ1, KvLQT1*
			17q23	I_{K1}	*KCNJ2, Kir2.1*
SUPRAVENTRICULAR					
AF	AF	AD	10q22-24		—
			11p15	I_{Ks}	*KCNQ1, KvLQT1*
			6q14-16		—
			21q22	I_{Ks}	*KCNE2, MiRP*
			17q23	I_{K1}	*KCNJ2, Kir2.1*
Atrial standstill	SND, AF	AD	3q21	I_{Na}	*SCN5A*
Absent sinus rhyhm	SND, AF	AD	—		—
WPW syndrome	AVRT	AD	—		*PRKAG2*
CONDUCTION DISORDER					
Progressive conduction disease	AVB	AD	19q13	I_{Na}	*SCN5A*
			3q21		

AD, autosomal dominant; AF, atrial fibrillation; AR, autosomal recessive; AVB, atrioventricular block; AVRT, atrioventricular reentrant tachycardia; JLN, Jervell and Lange-Nielsen; LQTS, long QT syndrome; RW, Romano-Ward; SND, sinus node dysfunction; TdP, torsades de pointes; VF, ventricular fibrillation; VT, ventricular tachycardia; WPW, Wolff-Parkinson-White syndrome.

TABLE 58.2

GENETIC CAUSES FOR ARRHYTHMOGENIC RIGHT VENTRICULAR CARDIOMYOPATHY

	Inheritance	Protein	Locus	Gene	Function
ARVC1	AD		14q24.3		
ARVC2	AD	Ryanodine receptor 2	1q42	*RYR2*	Calcium release channel
ARVC3	AD		14q11-q12		
ARVC4	AD		2q32		
ARVC5	AD		3p23		
ARVC6	AD		10p12-p14		
ARVC7	AD		10q22		
ARVC8	AD	Desmoplakin	*6p28*	*DSP*	Adherens junction protein
ARVC9	AD	Plakophilin 2	*12p11*	*PKP2*	
Naxos disease	AR	Plakoglobin	17q21	*JUP*	Cell junction

AD, autosomal dominant; AR, autosomal recessive; ARVC, arrhythmogenic right ventricular cardiomyopathy.

TABLE 58.3

GENETIC CAUSES FOR HYPERTROPHIC CARDIOMYOPATHY

Protein	Locus	Gene	Inheritance
β-Myosin heavy chain	14q12	*MYH7*	AD
Myosin binding protein-C	11p11.2	*MYBPC3*	AD
Cardiac troponin T	1q32	*TNNT2*	AD
Cardiac troponin I	19p13.2	*TNN13*	AD
α-Tropomyosin	15q22.1	*TPM1*	AD
Essential myosin light chain	3p21.3	*MYL3*	AD
Regulatory myosin light chain	12q23-24.3	*MYL2*	AD
Cardiac α-actin	15q11	*ACTC*	AD
Titin	2q24.1	*TTN*	AD
α-Myosin heavy chain	14q1	*MYH6*	AD
Cardiac troponin C	3p21.3-3p14.3	*TNNC1*	AD

AD, autosomal dominant.

With the finding of *ANK2* mutations underlying LQT4 (12), we find that the spectrum of LQTS genes is not limited to genes that encode ion channel proteins. *ANK2* encodes ankyrin-B, one isoform of a ubiquitously expressed family of proteins originally identified in the erythrocyte as a link between membrane proteins. Cardiomyocytes heterozygous for a null mutation in ankyrin-B display reduced expression and abnormal localization of the Na/Ca exchanger, Na/K adenosine triphosphatase, and $InsP_3$ receptor, but normal expression and localization of other cardiac proteins, including the L-type Ca^{2+} channel and the cardiac Na^+ channel (13). Action potential duration is normal, but myocytes display abnormalities in Ca homeostasis leading to early and delayed afterdepolarizations (12). Further clinical characterization of patients with *ANK2* mutations reveals that although these patients are at risk for sudden death, they do not uniformly display prolonged QT intervals (13), a finding suggesting that ankyrin-B diseases are distinct from the LQTS (14). Andersen-Tawil syndrome (ATS), termed by some as LQT7 (15), is the result of mutations in *KCNJ2* and is associated with significant extracardiac findings, including periodic

TABLE 58.4

GENETIC CAUSES FOR DILATED CARDIOMYOPATHY

Locus	Gene	Protein	Inheritance
DCM only			
1q32	*TNNT2*	Cardiac troponin T	AD
2q31	*TTN*	Titin	AD
2q35	*DES*	Desmin	AD
5q33	*SGCD*	δ-Sarcoglycan	AD
6q12-q16	—	—	AD
9q13-q22	—	—	AD
9q22-q31	—	—	AD
10q22-q23	*VCL*	Metavinculin	AD
11p11	*MYBPC3*	Cardiac myosin binding	AD
14q12	*MYH7*	Protein C	AD
15q14	*ACTC*	β-Myosin heavy chain	AD
15q22	*TPM1*	Cardiac actin	AD
		α-tropomyosin	
DCM + conduction system disease			
1p1-q21	*LMNA*	Lamins A and C	AD
2q14-q22	—		AD
3p22-p25	—		AD
DCM + skeletal myopathy ± conduction system disease			
1p1-q21	*LMNA*	Lamins A and C	AD
6q23	—	—	AD
DCM + sensorineural deafness			
6q23-q24	—	—	AD
Xp21 (DCM)	*DMD*	Dystrophin	X-linked
Xq28 (infantile DCM)	*G4.5*	Tafazzin	X-linked

AD, autosomal dominant; DCM, dilated cardiomyopathy.

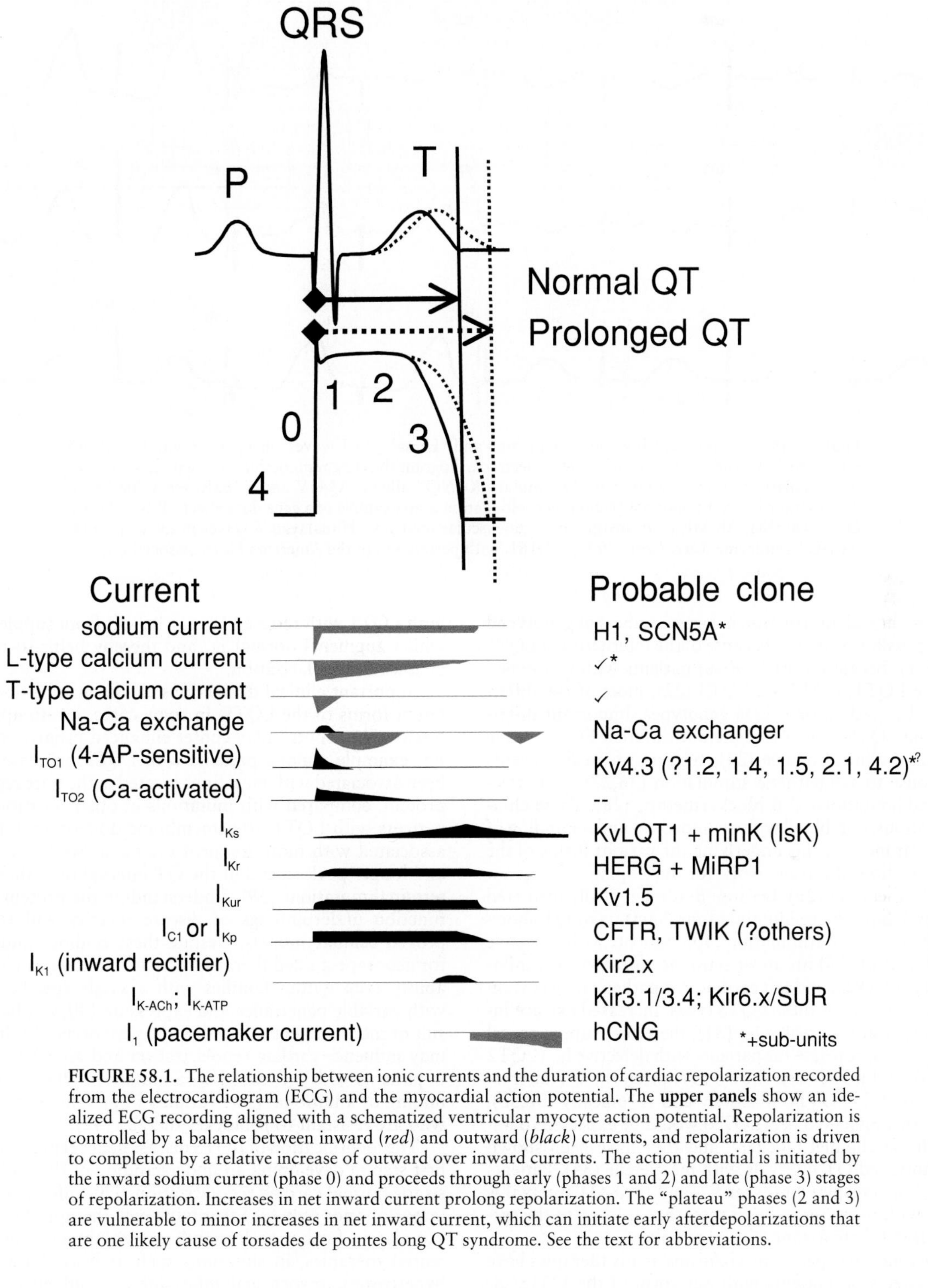

Current		Probable clone
sodium current		H1, SCN5A*
L-type calcium current		✓*
T-type calcium current		✓
Na-Ca exchange		Na-Ca exchanger
I_{TO1} (4-AP-sensitive)		Kv4.3 (?1.2, 1.4, 1.5, 2.1, 4.2)*?
I_{TO2} (Ca-activated)		--
I_{Ks}		KvLQT1 + minK (IsK)
I_{Kr}		HERG + MiRP1
I_{Kur}		Kv1.5
I_{C1} or I_{Kp}		CFTR, TWIK (?others)
I_{K1} (inward rectifier)		Kir2.x
I_{K-ACh}; I_{K-ATP}		Kir3.1/3.4; Kir6.x/SUR
I_1 (pacemaker current)		hCNG *+sub-units

FIGURE 58.1. The relationship between ionic currents and the duration of cardiac repolarization recorded from the electrocardiogram (ECG) and the myocardial action potential. The **upper panels** show an idealized ECG recording aligned with a schematized ventricular myocyte action potential. Repolarization is controlled by a balance between inward (*red*) and outward (*black*) currents, and repolarization is driven to completion by a relative increase of outward over inward currents. The action potential is initiated by the inward sodium current (phase 0) and proceeds through early (phases 1 and 2) and late (phase 3) stages of repolarization. Increases in net inward current prolong repolarization. The "plateau" phases (2 and 3) are vulnerable to minor increases in net inward current, which can initiate early afterdepolarizations that are one likely cause of torsades de pointes long QT syndrome. See the text for abbreviations.

paralysis, hypertelorism, and clinodactyly (16). Because many patients with ATS have mild or no prolongation of the QT interval, and the clinical manifestations, electrocardiographic (ECG) characteristics, and outcomes are quite different from those of the LQTS, it seems that ATS is not a subtype of the LQTS, and it has been recommended that the annotation of *KCNJ2*-positive ATS individuals should be ATS1 rather than LQT7 (17). Recently, mutations in the gene encoding the L-type Ca channel have been found to underlie Timothy syndrome, a rare multisystem disorder characterized by QT prolongation as well as syndactyly, autism, and immune deficiencies (18). This has been termed LQT8 (19), and it does cause a gain

of function of I_{Ca} due to slowed inactivation, which directly prolongs the QT interval (see Fig. 58.1), similar to the other forms of the LQTS. However, the first described case of Timothy syndrome differs from classic forms of the LQTS in that it is associated with significant extracardiac manifestations. More recently, other Ca^{2+} channel gene (*CACNA1C*) mutations have been identified that increase the QT interval but result in less severe extracardiac manifestations (20).

Even when limited to "classic" forms of the LQTS, important clinical differences among affected patients depending on the specific gene (and in some cases the specific mutation) have been observed, so called genotype-phenotype correlation.

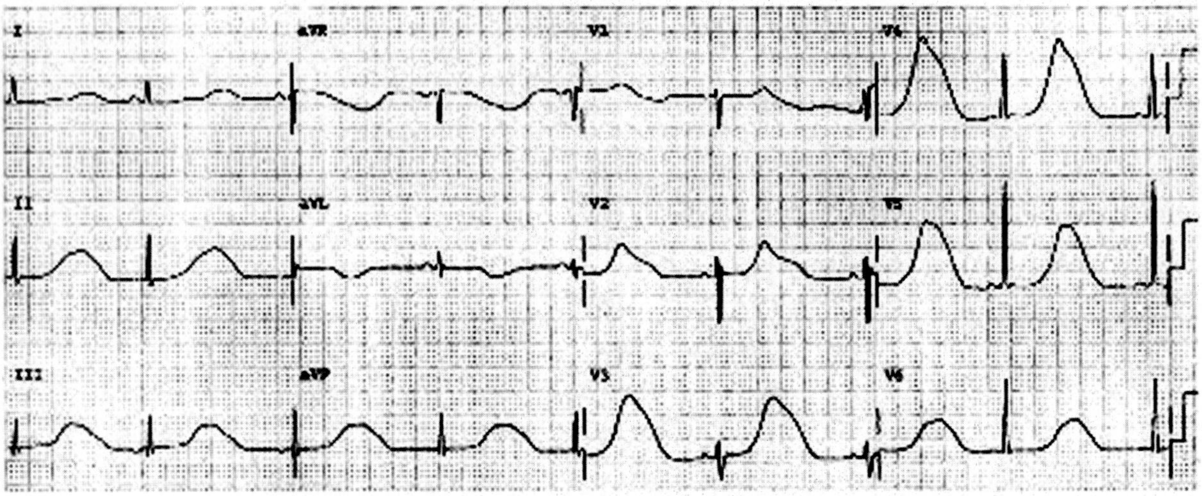

FIGURE 58.2. Extreme QT interval prolongation and "Himalayan T waves" in a patient with Jervell and Lange-Nielsen syndrome. This is a 12-lead electrocardiogram showing remarkable lengthening of ventricular repolarization in a patient with two mutant *KCNQ1* alleles (A341V and K362R, see Table 58.1). This extraordinary amount of QT interval prolongation is an example of a gene dose effect. (From Darbar D, Roden DM, Ali MF, et al. Images in cardiovascular medicine: Himalayan T waves in the congenital long-QT syndrome. *Circulation* 2005;111:161, with permission of the American Heart Association).

Much of the clinical information in large numbers of genotyped patients is possible primarily because of the International LQTS Registry (21). Because most (>90%) patients with genotyped LQTS have LQT1, LQT2, or LQT3 (22), most of the differences are observed among these genotypes. Important differences among LQTS types 1 to 3 include different ECG T-wave patterns (23), clinical course (24), triggers of cardiac events (25), response to sympathetic stimulation (26,27), and effectiveness and limitations of β-blockertherapy (28). These clinical observations, combined with an improved understanding of the molecular mechanisms underlying the various forms of the LQTS, have allowed a framework for developing some genotype specific therapies (29). Because β-adrenergically mediated increases in I_{Ks} are the predominant mechanisms of QT shortening with adrenergic stimulation (30), patients with defective I_{Ks} (LQT1 and LQT5) are most sensitive to autonomic influences, and β-blockers and left cardiac sympathetic denervation seem most effective for these LQTS types. Increased extracellular K paradoxically increases I_{Kr} (31); therefore, supplemental K seems most appropriate for patients with defective I_{Kr} (LQT2 and LQT6), and it has been shown to shorten the QT interval in patients with LQT2, both acutely and chronically (32,33). Patients with augmented I_{Na} (LQT3) would be expected to improve with Na channel blockers, and they have been shown to have shortened QT intervals with mexiletene (34). Patients with LQT3 also display bradycardia, and their QT interval is shortened with increases in heart rate, thus leading to the recommendation for treatment with pacemakers.

Despite genotype-specific mechanisms, many therapies have beneficial effects on patients with any form of the LQTS. β-Blockers are recommended for all patients with the LQTS, and mexiletine may have beneficial effects in LQT1 and LQT2 (35,36). This is consistent with the concept of "reduced repolarization reserve;" (37) multiple redundant mechanisms contribute to normal repolarization, and when one or more of these cause a net increase in inward current during repolarization, it manifests as QT prolongation with increased risk for torsades de pointes. A specific therapy may target the underlying defect as when an Na channel blocker normalizes the QT interval in a patient with LQT3 with an abnormally augmented Na current. Alternatively, a therapy may enhance a normal mechanism and thereby offset the diseased one. For example, a patient with LQT1 with reduced I_{Ks}may benefit from supplemental K, which augments normal I_{Kr} and thereby helps to restore the balance of repolarization.

Important clinical distinctions can be made among the different forms of the LQTS. In some cases, it also appears that disease "hot spots" may confer enhanced proarrhythmic risk. For example, among patients with LQT2, increased risk has been associated with mutations located in the pore region of the protein, compared with mutations in other locations (38). In patients with LQT1, transmembrane domain mutations were associated with more frequent events, as well as longer QTc and longer peak to end of the QT interval than those with C-terminal mutations (39). Understanding the protein structure-function underpinnings of disease severity will require improved cellular models. Despite these findings and the hope for genotype-guided therapy, there is tremendous clinical variability even within families with a single specific mutation, with variable penetrance and expression (40,41), likely the result of modifier genes that alter the phenotype. Multiple genes may influence cardiac repolarization and alter the phenotype in patients with the same LQTS mutation. One example is the finding of additional gene variants in patients with the LQTS who are resistant to β-blocker therapy (42).

The identification of LQTS disease genes represents a crucial first step in developing an understanding of the molecular basis for normal cardiac repolarization. This information will be important not only for identifying new therapies in the LQTS, but also in further understanding arrhythmias, and their potential therapies, in situations such as heart failure, cardiac hypertrophy, myocardial infarction, or sudden infant death syndrome, in which abnormal repolarization has been linked to sudden death (43). The congenital LQTS thus represents a paradigm for studying monogenic arrhythmia syndromes, but the revealed complexities have highlighted the need for more integrated systems-based approaches to understanding, modeling and predicting arrhythmia risk in patients. The congenital LQTS also shares similarities with proarrhythmic "electrical remodeling" that occurs in common forms of structural heart disease. The action potential duration is prolonged in human heart failure for a variety of causes, including myocardial infarction, hypertension, and genetic mutations. It now seems likely that arrhythmia mechanisms identified in models of the

LQTS, such as afterdepolarizations and transmural dispersion of repolarization, are also operative and contribute to sudden cardiac death in patients with common forms of structural heart disease. Thus, genetically defined arrhythmias may reveal important insights into mechanisms of arrhythmias that affect large numbers of people and represent a significant public health challenge.

Familial Atrial Fibrillation

AF, the most common cardiac arrhythmia, affects approximately 2% of the U.S. population and results in substantial morbidity and mortality. The increasing prevalence of AF is largely the result of an increasing elderly population. AF is also the most common arrhythmia requiring drug therapy. The limited success in the therapy of AF is in part the result of our poor understanding of its molecular pathophysiology. One approach to unraveling the molecular pathogenesis of AF is through the identification of a gene responsible for the familial form of the disease. Evidence for the heritability of AF has come from the following: (a) the analysis of AF kindreds in which different members of a family have the arrhythmia as a primary electrical disease, (b) the analysis of the AF presenting in the setting of another familial disease, and (c) the analysis of genetic backgrounds that may predispose to AF.

Monogenic familial AF was first reported in 1943 (44), and although it may be uncommon, there has been no attempt to determine the overall prevalence of familial AF. Recent analysis of the Framingham data, however, has shown a genetic susceptibility to AF, demonstrated by the finding that parental AF increased the risk of AF in the children (45). Furthermore, studies from our group and others indicate that 5% of the patients with AF and up to 15% of the individuals with lone AF may have a familial form of the disease (46). This finding suggests that familial AF may have a higher prevalence than previously suspected. A gene locus for AF was first reported in 1997, based on genetic mapping studies in three families from Spain who appeared to share common ancestry (47). However, the gene responsible for AF in this kindred has not yet been identified, but resides within a relatively large chromosomal region spanning 14 centimorgans. A second locus for AF on the proximal long arm of chromosome 6 was identified in 2003 (48). Taken together, these reports support the idea that familial AF is a genetically heterogeneous disease. Similar heterogeneity has been described for many other inherited arrhythmia syndromes.

Recently, the first genes for AF were identified, providing a link between ion channelopathies and the disease. In a single four-generation Chinese family in which the LQTS and early-onset AF cosegregate, a mutation (S140G) in *KCNQ1* gene on chromosome 11p15.5 has been reported (49). The *KCNQ1* gene encodes the pore-forming α-subunit of the cardiac I_{Ks} (*KCNQ1/KCNE1*), the *KCNQ1/KCNE2,* and the *KCNQ1/KCNE3* K channels. Functional analysis of the S140G mutant revealed a gain-of-function effect in the *KCNQ1/KCNE1* and *KCNQ1/KCNE2* currents, which contrasts with the dominant negative or loss-of-function effects of the *KCNQ1* mutations previously identified with the LQTS. The gain-of-function mutation is a logical explanation for the shortening of the action potential duration and effective refractory period that is linked to the mechanism of AF, but it is at odds with the loss–of-function mechanism thought to underlie the LQTS phenotype. More recently, also from the same group in China, a link between *KCNE2* and AF has been provided with the identification of the same mutation in two families with AF (50). The mutation *R27C* caused a gain of function when coexpressed with *KCNQ1* but had no effect when expressed with *HERG*. These studies firmly establish the role of K^+ channels in the pathogenesis of some cases of AF.

AF is associated with other monogenic diseases. Studies of other cardiac monogenic disorders have also provided evidence for the genetic basis for AF. These include diseases such as hypertrophic cardiomyopathy, skeletal myopathies, familial amyloidosis, and atrial myopathies. However, it is likely that AF in these cases is related at least in part to morphologic changes in the atria caused by the underlying cardiac disorder. AF can also present in other ion channelopathies such as LQT4, Brugada syndrome, and the short QT syndrome. The high incidence of atrial arrhythmias in patients with the short QT syndrome (49) and the gain-of-function mutations in I_{Ks} (51) point to an important role for shortening of the action potential in the development of AF.

Most patients with AF have one or more traditional risk factors, but many or even most patients with these risk factors do not develop AF. Thus, it is likely that genetic determinants favor AF in some individuals with traditional risk factors. Studies comparing cases of nonfamilial AF with age-related and gender-matched controls (association studies) have provided some insight into the genetic basis of acquired AF. One study evaluated a polymorphism in *KCNE1* (minK) and AF and identified an association with the 38G allele (52). Although the 38G allele appears to reduce I_{Ks} (53), mice lacking *KCNE1* are prone to AF because of an unexpected increase in I_{Ks} (54), a finding suggesting that the consequences of ion channel protein mutations are not always straightforward.

Catecholaminergic Polymorphic Ventricular Tachycardia

First reported as a single case in 1975 (55),and subsequently in a series by Coumel and associates (56), the clinical entity of CPVT may lead to syncope or sudden death in young children with normal hearts (57). The familial transmission, risk of physical or emotional stress, and benefits of β-blocker therapy were recognized since these first reports. Recently, swimming-triggered events, previously thought to be specific for LQT1, have been associated with CPVT (58). In contrast to the LQTS, the baseline ECG is normal, and exercise induces a characteristic bidirectional ventricular tachycardia (VT) (Fig. 58.3). The bidirectional VT may be asymptomatic; however, polymorphic VT and ventricular fibrillation (VF) may also occur (59). Electrophysiology study with programmed ventricular stimulation usually does not provoke any arrhythmias, and a defibrillator may be required in up to 30% of patients who are resistant to β-blocker therapy (57,59).

Linkage of CPVT to chromosome 1q42-q43 was accomplished in two unrelated families in 1999 (60), followed by identification of mutations in the cardiac ryanodine receptor (RYR2) in 2001 (61). The ryanodine receptor resides on the membrane, not of the myocyte, but on the sarcoplasmic reticulum, and it releases Ca from the sarcoplasmic reticulum in response to Ca influx from the L-type Ca channels (Ca-induced Ca release) (62). Functional assessment of mutant RYR2 revealed increased Ca release from mutant RYR2 under adrenergic stimulation (63,64). Further evidence that mutations in RYR2 underlie CPVT is found in the recent report of the characteristic phenotype of bidirectional VT and VF in a transgenic mouse with an RYR2 mutation (65). Mutations in calsequestrin 2 (*CASQ2*) have also been identified in an autosomal recessive form of CPVT (66,67).To date, functional assessment is available on only one *CASQ2* mutant (68), but abnormal Ca release from the sarcoplasmic reticulum seems to be a common finding in CPVT mutations. Experimental studies simulating adrenergic stimulation in the setting of abnormal Ca release reveal epicardial origin of ectopic beats increasing transmural dispersion of repolarization, thus providing the substrate for

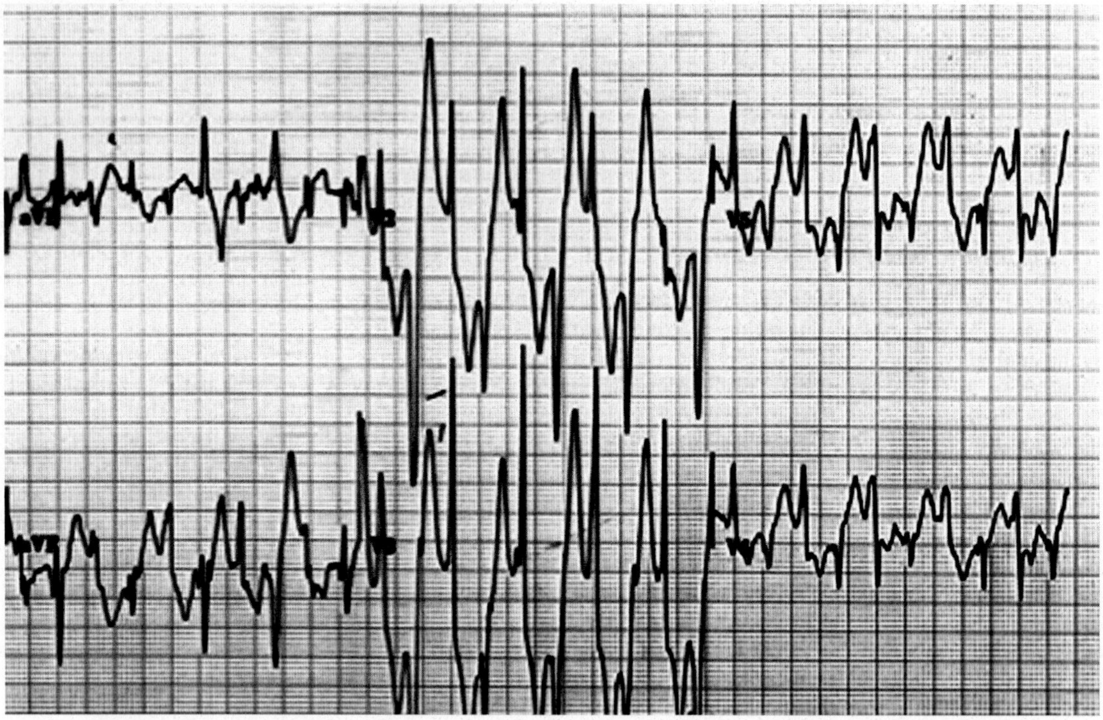

FIGURE 58.3. Bidirectional ventricular tachycardia in a patient with catecholaminergic polymorphic ventricular tachycardia. This is a 12-lead electrocardiogram showing tachycardia with alternating QRS morphologies.

catecholaminergic VT. Furthermore, bidirectional VT results as a consequence of alternation in the origin ofectopic activity between endocardial and epicardial regions (69).

Brugada Syndrome

The syndrome of a typical ECG pattern (ST-elevation in the right precordial leads; Fig. 58.4) associated with a risk of ventricular arrhythmias and sudden death, now termed Brugada syndrome, is attributed to Brugada and Brugada from their description in 1992 (70). The characteristic ECG was published in 1953 by Osher and Wolff (71), and it was associated with a risk for sudden death by Martini in 1989 (72). With improved recognition of the syndrome, it is now apparent that most, if not all, cases of sudden unexplained nocturnal death syndrome (73), and some cases of sudden infant death syndrome, are the result of Brugada syndrome (74,75). The ECG findings in Brugada syndrome are dynamic and may be concealed, but they can be unmasked by Na channel blocking drugs such asflecainide, ajmaline, or procainamide (76). In contrast to most forms of the LQTS and CPVT, cardiac events in Brugada syndrome occur during rest or sleep (77), similar to LQT3. To date, only one Brugada syndrome gene has been identified, *SCN5A*, the same gene underlying LQT3 (78), but most patients with Brugada syndrome do not have identified *SCN5A* mutations, a finding

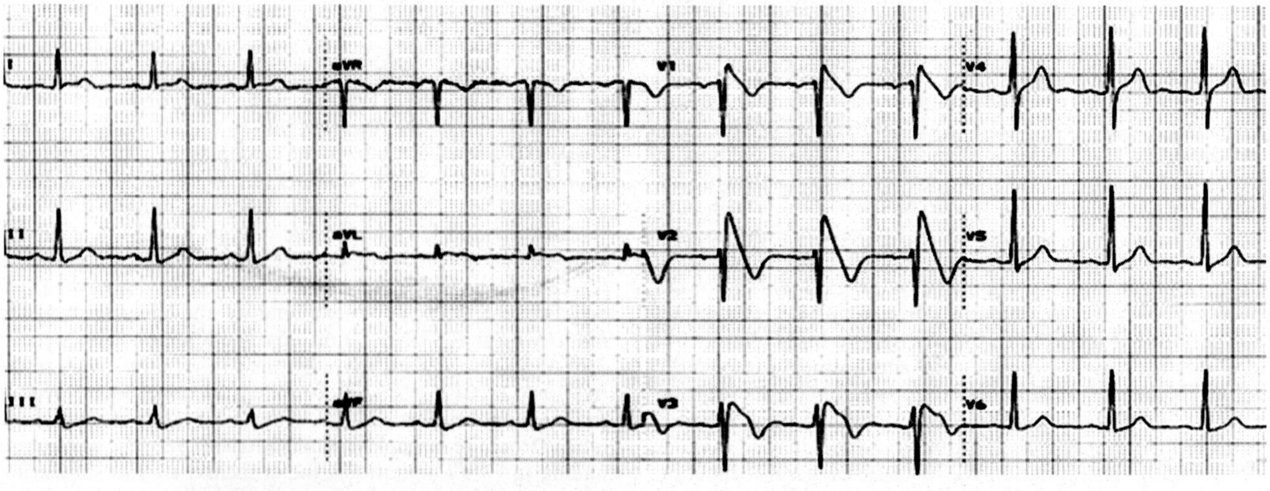

FIGURE 58.4. This 12-lead electrocardiogram (ECG) of patient with the Brugada syndrome shows the characteristic coved-type ST-segment elevation in leads V_1 and V_2. This 12-lead ECG shows sinus rhythm with marked ST-segment elevation that is characteristic of some patients with Brugada syndrome.

suggesting that other factors are also important. Brugada syndrome *SCN5A* mutations result in reduced Na current, as opposed to augmented late Na current in LQT3. Experimental studies have revealed loss of Na current leaves the transient outward current (I_{to}) unopposed, resulting in the characteristic ECG as well as an increased risk for VT and VF (79). Interestingly, fever has been reported to unmask the ECG findings and to elicit storms of VT in Brugada syndrome (80,81). Correspondingly, some mutations have temperature-dependent functional consequences (82). Although quinidine, likely by blocking I_{to}, has demonstrated some protective effects (83,84), the only proven effective therapy for Brugada syndrome is an implantable cardioverter defibrillator, which is recommended for symptomatic patients or for those with a spontaneously abnormal ECG and inducible VF with programmed stimulation (85,86).

Short QT Syndrome

Just as patients with prolonged QT intervals (whether congenital or acquired) have an increased risk of sudden death, it has been recognized since the 1990s that excessively short QT intervals are also associated with increased mortality (87). In 2000, the possibility of a new genetic arrhythmia syndrome was raised when persistently short QT intervals were noted in a family with AF and in an unrelated patient who suffered sudden death (51,88). Subsequently, two other families with short QT intervals, short atrial and ventricular effective refractory periods, and inducible VF at electrophysiology study were reported (89). The ECG in these patients reveals not only a short QT interval, but also an absence of the ST segment and abnormally high-amplitude T waves. Identification of gain-of-function mutations in *KCNH2*, *KCNQ1*, and *KCNJ2* in patients with the short QT syndrome followed only 4 to 5 years after the initial description of the syndrome (90–92). The risk for VF in the short QT syndrome may also stem from an increased transmural dispersion of repolarization (93).

As with any new syndrome, the initially recognized cases tend to be the most severe. The high incidence of sudden death in this cohort is therefore not surprising. The reported cases of the short QT syndrome have corrected QT intervals between 250 and 320 milliseconds (94). Defibrillator therapy has been recommended for these high-risk patients, but it is complicated by the potential for frequent inappropriate shocks owing to oversensing of the high-amplitude T waves in this disorder (95). As more patients with the short QT syndrome are identified, clinical heterogeneity will likely be uncovered, and risk stratification may become possible. Multiple drugs, including flecainide, sotalol, ibutilide, and quinidine, have been tested in a few patients with the short QT syndrome (96). Quinidine significantly prolonged the QT interval and ventricular refractory period and prevented inducibility of VF. Importantly, drug testing has been reported only in a few patients, all with *KCNH2* mutations. This limited experience leaves the role of pharmacologic therapy uncertain at this time.

Familial Wolf-Parkinson-White syndrome

Although it is not common for the preexcitation Wolf-Parkinson-White syndrome to be inherited, familial forms have been linked to mutations in several genes. When the syndrome is associated with hypertrophic cardiomyopathy, the genes involved include *PRKAG2, TNNI3*, or *MYBPC3* mutations (97,98). It has also been reported in patients with Pompe disease, resulting from mutations in α-1,4-glucosidase, and in Leber hereditary optic neuropathy, which is caused by mutations in mitochondrial DNA. Hereditary seems to follow an autosomal dominant pattern.

ARRHYTHMIA MODELS: PAST, PRESENT, AND FUTURE

Cellular and animal models are essential for understanding the consequences of genetic mutations for arrhythmias. Ideal models will faithfully reproduce a human biologic environment (i.e., the atrial or ventricular myocardium) in which to test the expression of mutant genes. Currently available models are far from ideal, but significant progress has been made, and major efforts in systems biology (a melding of quantification and modeling with physiologic signaling networks on the molecular, cellular, organ, and whole-animal organizational levels) are likely to lead us to more ideal models. The initial mapping of mutant ion channel genes to patients with the LQTS used biophysical characterization of mutant ion channel proteins in *Xenopus* oocytes (i.e., frog eggs) (99), which are advantageous for robust and rapid protein expression. Although these early studies provided stunning and valuable information that initiated modern understanding of the genetic basis of arrhythmias, later studies showed that *Xenopus* oocytes could provide misleading information because they also expressed multiple auxiliary proteins, they possessed highly active systems for protein phosphorylation befitting a cell geared up for growth and development but dissimilar to cardiac myocytes, and because they trafficked mutant proteins to the cell membrane that were not similarly trafficked in mammalian cells (100).

Although the number of recognized mutations in LQTS genes has grown significantly (numbering in the hundreds currently), functional characterization of new mutations is critical for a true understanding of the phenotype. Certainly, the function of many mutations in genes encoding K currents has been studied in heterologous expression systems and has been shown to reduce current (loss of function), and in some cases by more than 50% (dominant negative) (101,102). Furthermore, some mutations in *SCN5A* result in reduced inactivation, leading to augmented late Na current (103,104). However, the functional consequences of the majority of mutations have not been studied. Many variants are reported in association with the LQTS; if the mutation alters the protein and is absent in a large number of control subjects, it is considered evidence that the mutation underlies the disease (105). This approach, of course, may overemphasize the role of the identified mutation as the causative factor. Conversely, the absence of an effect on current should not immediately be interpreted as a silent mutation. Mutations that do not alter ionic current in heterologous expression systems may still cause disease by altering protein trafficking to the membrane, resulting in loss of function (100). Abnormal trafficking may be a common mechanism in the LQTS and one that is potentially amenable to pharmacologic rescue (106). The complexity of assessing functional consequences of a mutation is highlighted by the recent finding of a patient with the LQTS who had a *KCNH2* mutation that increases I_{Kr} current when coexpressed with wild-type channels, a gain of function, predicting a short QT interval. However, this mutation also resulted in defective trafficking, with retention in the endoplasmic reticulum, a loss of function that surpassed the gain of function and resulted in the LQTS (107).

Further insights into mechanisms of arrhythmia risk have been elucidated by studies in left ventricular wedge preparations (108). The presence of three cell types across the ventricular wall (endocardial, M cells, and epicardial), each with distinct electrophysiologic and pharmacologic properties, leads to heterogeneity of repolarization across the ventricular wall and transmural dispersion of repolarization. Under experimental I_{Ks} block, action potentials are prolonged in all cell types, leading to QT interval prolongation, but no increased susceptibility to torsades de pointes. With the addition of isoproterenol, epicardial and endocardial action potentials shorten, whereas M cell action potential remains long, leading to significant increase in transmural dispersion of repolarization and spontaneous and induced torsades de pointes (13). Similar studies in experimental models of LQT2 and LQT3 also suggest that arrhythmia risk may be more closely linked to transmural dispersion of repolarization than to QT prolongation itself (109). The peak to end of the QT interval on the surface ECG is a correlate of transmural dispersion of repolarization, and clinical studies have supported the role of transmural dispersion of repolarization in the LQTS (110–112). The wedge preparation is extremely useful for studying dispersion of activation and repolarization, tissue properties that can be measured only in a multicellular cardiac model. However, the wedge preparation requires tissue injury and is not tractable for genetic manipulation.

Cardiac myocytes have a highly ordered ultrastructure that is designed to optimize their function as contracting cells. Normally, expression of ion channel proteins is highly enriched at T-tubule invaginations of the cell membrane, so many ion channels critical for the LQTS are in close proximity to highly active intracellular Ca^{2+} stores that rhythmically increase the Ca^{2+} concentration by 100- to 1,000-fold over resting levels with each heart beat (113). This remarkable physiology is not recapitulated by noncardiac cells. Adult cardiac myocytes are difficult to culture and to transduce for protein overexpression or gene silencing, but recent advances have been made by several groups suggesting that these obstacles will soon be solved (12,13).

Mice have a four-chambered heart that is anatomically similar to the human heart. For this reason and because of the relative ease of genetic manipulation, mice have become important for studying arrhythmias and genetic causes of structural heart disease (114,115). Despite the power of the mouse, significant differences exist between mouse and human, including heart rates (10 times faster in mice) and ionic currents underlying repolarization (116). Despite these differences, mice do develop ventricular and atrial arrhythmias that are in many cases very similar to human counterparts (54,117–119). Recently, work has commenced on developing genetic models of rabbits and other larger animals, which have heart rates and action potentials that are more similar to human (120–122). It is likely that multiple model systems will be required for building a clinically relevant understanding of genetic arrhythmia mechanisms.

CONTROVERSIES AND PERSONAL PERSPECTIVES

Tremendous strides have been made over the past decade in defining genetic mutations linked to arrhythmias in patients. Although these mutations point to molecular substrates important for arrhythmias, by themselves they are insufficient to define arrhythmia mechanisms. For example, LQTS mutations in repolarizing K^+ currents cause action potential prolongation and loss of repolarization reserve. Conversely, additional factors caused by excessive action potential prolongation such as disordered intracellular Ca^{2+} or enhanced intramyocardial repolarization gradients may be the proximate "cause" of arrhythmias. These distinctions will become more important and more complex as the definition of genetic arrhythmias is expanded to include more common gene polymorphisms that are likely to confer arrhythmia risk by combinations of subtle changes in cellular electrophysiology.

THE FUTURE

Until recently, genetic arrhythmia syndromes were thought to be rare but interesting curiosities. However, the accelerating pace of discovery has revealed that genetically defined arrhythmias are far more common than originally recognized. Genetic arrhythmias have provided important insights into molecular arrhythmia mechanisms and have contributed to understanding of more common arrhythmias in patients with structural heart disease. Although work so far has established that single-gene mutations cause defined arrhythmia syndromes, the potential relationship of enhanced arrhythmia susceptibility to more common gene polymorphisms remains uncertain. It seems likely that identification and understanding of such polymorphisms, alone or in combination, will enable physicians to assign a profile of arrhythmia risk to individual patients. The ability to assign risk with high sensitivity and specificity will allow for individualized treatment decisions about drug use and application of device-based therapies.

ACKNOWLEDGMENTS

This work was supported in part by grants from the U.S. Public Health Service (HL076264, HL075266, HL62494, HL70250, and HL46681). Dr. Anderson is an Established Investigator of the American Heart Association. We are grateful to Ms Linda Selfridge for excellent technical assistance in preparing this manuscript.

References

1. Wang Q, Shen J, Splawski I, et al. SCN5A mutations associated with an inherited cardiac arrhythmia, long QT syndrome. *Cell* 1995;80:805–811.
2. Curran ME, Splawski I, Timothy KW, et al. A molecular basis for cardiac arrhythmia: HERG mutations cause long QT syndrome. *Cell* 1995;80:795–803.
3. Jervell A, Lange-Nielsen F. Congenital deaf-mutism, functional heart disease with prolongation of the Q-T interval and sudden death. *Am Heart J* 1957;54:59–68.
4. Romano C, Gemme G, Pongiglione R. Rare cardiac arrhythmias of the pediatric age. II. Syncopal attacks due to paroxysmal ventricular fibrillation. (Presentation of 1st case in Italian pediatric literature.) *Clin Pediatr (Bologna)* 1963;656–683.
5. Ward, OC. A new familial cardiac syndrome in children. *J Ir Med Assoc* 1964;54:103–106.
6. Schwartz PJ, Periti M, Malliani A. The long Q-T syndrome. *Am Heart J* 1975;89:378–390.
7. Moss AJ. Prolonged QT-interval syndromes. *JAMA* 1986;256:2985–2987.
8. Wang Q, Curran ME, Splawski I, et al. Positional cloning of a novel potassium channel gene: KVLQT1 mutations cause cardiac arrhythmias. *Nat Genet* 1996;12:17–23.
9. Schulze-Bahr E, Wang Q, Wedekind H, et al. KCNE1 mutations cause Jervell and Lange-Nielsen syndrome. *Nat Genet* 1997;17:267–268.
10. Tyson J, Tranebjaerg L, Bellman S, et al. IsK and KvLQT1: mutation in either of the two subunits of the slow component of the delayed rectifier potassium channel can cause Jervell and Lange-Nielsen syndrome. *Hum Mol Genet* 1997;6:2179–2185.
11. Neyroud N, Tesson F, Denjoy I, et al. A novel mutation in the potassium channel gene KVLQT1 causes the Jervell and Lange-Nielsen cardioauditory syndrome. *Nat Genet* 1997;15:186–189.
12. Mohler PJ, Schott JJ, Gramolini AO, et al. Ankyrin-B mutation causes type 4 long-QT cardiac arrhythmia and sudden cardiac death. *Nature* 2003;421:634–639.
13. Mohler PJ, Splawski I, Napolitano C, et al. A cardiac arrhythmia syndrome caused by loss of ankyrin-B function. *Proc Natl Acad Sci USA* 2004;101:9137–9142.
14. Mohler PJ, Bennett V. Ankyrin-based cardiac arrhythmias: a new class of channelopathies due to loss of cellular targeting. *Curr Opin Cardiol* 2005;20:189–193.
15. Tristani-Firouzi M, Jensen JL, Donaldson MR, et al. Functional and clinical characterization of KCNJ2 mutations associated with LQT7 (Andersen syndrome). *J Clin Invest* 2002;110:381–388.
16. Plaster NM, Tawil R, Tristani-Firouzi M, et al. Mutations in Kir2.1 cause the developmental and episodic electrical phenotypes of Andersen's syndrome. *Cell* 2001;105:511–519.

17. Zhang L, Benson DW, Tristani-Firouzi M, et al. Electrocardiographic features in Andersen-Tawil syndrome patients with KCNJ2 mutations: characteristic T-U-wave patterns predict the KCNJ2 genotype. *Circulation* 2005;111:2720–2726.
18. Splawski I, Timothy KW, Sharpe LM, et al. Ca(V)1.2 calcium channel dysfunction causes a multisystem disorder including arrhythmia and autism. *Cell* 2004;119:19–31.
19. Priori SG, Cerrone M. Genetic arrhythmias. *Ital Heart J* 2005;6:241–248.
20. Splawski I, Timothy KW, Decher N, et al. Severe arrhythmia disorder caused by cardiac L-type calcium channel mutations. *Proc Natl Acad Sci USA* 2005;102:8089–8096.
21. Moss AJ, Schwartz PJ. 25th anniversary of the International Long-QT Syndrome Registry: an ongoing quest to uncover the secrets of long-QT syndrome. *Circulation* 2005;111:1199–1201.
22. Splawski I, Shen J, Timothy KW, et al. Spectrum of mutations in long-QT syndrome genes. KVLQT1, HERG, SCN5A, KCNE1, and KCNE2. *Circulation* 2000;102:1178–1185.
23. Moss AJ, Zareba W, Benhorin J, et al. ECG T-wave patterns in genetically distinct forms of the hereditary long QT syndrome. *Circulation* 1995;92:2929–2934.
24. Zareba W, Moss AJ, Schwartz PJ, et al. Influence of genotype on the clinical course of the long-QT syndrome: International Long-QT Syndrome Registry Research Group. *N Engl J Med* 1998;339:960–965.
25. Schwartz PJ, Priori SG, Spazzolini C, et al. Genotype-phenotype correlation in the long-QT syndrome: gene-specific triggers for life-threatening arrhythmias. *Circulation* 2001;103:89–95.
26. Shimizu W, Noda T, Takaki H, et al. Diagnostic value of epinephrine test for genotyping LQT1, LQT2, and LQT3 forms of congenital long QT syndrome. *Heart Rhythm* 2004;1:276–283.
27. Noda T, Takaki H, Kurita T, et al. Gene-specific response of dynamic ventricular repolarization to sympathetic stimulation in LQT1, LQT2 and LQT3 forms of congenital long QT syndrome. *Eur Heart J* 2002;23:975–983.
28. Moss AJ, Zareba W, Hall WJ, et al. Effectiveness and limitations of beta-blocker therapy in congenital long-QT syndrome. *Circulation* 2000;101: 616–623.
29. Shimizu W. The long QT syndrome: Therapeutic implications of a genetic diagnosis. *Cardiovasc Res* 2005;67:347–356.
30. Kass RS, Wang W. Regulatory and molecular properties of delayed potassium channels in the heart: relationship to human disease. In: Zipes DP, Jalife J, eds. *Cardiac electrophysiology: from cell to bedside,* 3rd ed. Philadelphia: WB Saunders, 2000:104–112.
31. Sanguinetti MC, Jurkiewicz NK. Role of external Ca^{2+} and K^{+} in gating of cardiac delayed rectifier K^{+} currents. *Pflugers Arch* 1992;420:180–186.
32. Compton SJ, Lux RL, Ramsey MR, et al. Genetically defined therapy of inherited long-QT syndrome: correction of abnormal repolarization by potassium. *Circulation* 1996;94:1018–1022.
33. Etheridge SP, Compton SJ, Tristani-Firouzi M, et al. A new oral therapy for long QT syndrome: long-term oral potassium improves repolarization in patients with HERG mutations. *J Am Coll Cardiol* 2003;42:1777–1782.
34. Schwartz PJ, Priori SG, Locati EH, et al. Long QT syndrome patients with mutations of the SCN5A and HERG genes have differential responses to Na^{+} channel blockade and to increases in heart rate: implications for gene-specific therapy. *Circulation* 1995;92:3381–3386.
35. Shimizu W, Antzelevitch C. Sodium channel block with mexiletine is effective in reducing dispersion of repolarization and preventing torsade des pointes in LQT2 and LQT3 models of the long-QT syndrome. *Circulation* 1997;96:2038–2047.
36. Shimizu W, Antzelevitch C. Cellular basis for the ECG features of the LQT1 form of the long-QT syndrome: effects of beta-adrenergic agonists and antagonists and sodium channel blockers on transmural dispersion of repolarization and torsade de pointes. *Circulation* 1998;98:2314–2322.
37. Roden DM. Taking the "idio" out of "idiosyncratic": predicting torsades de pointes. *Pacing Clin Electrophysiol* 1998;21:1029–1034.
38. Moss AJ, Zareba W, Kaufman ES, et al. Increased risk of arrhythmic events in long-QT syndrome with mutations in the pore region of the human ether-a-go-go–related gene potassium channel. *Circulation* 2002;105:794–799.
39. Shimizu W, Horie M, Ohno S, et al. Mutation site-specific differences in arrhythmic risk and sensitivity to sympathetic stimulation in the LQT1 form of congenital long QT syndrome: multicenter study in Japan. *J Am Coll Cardiol* 2004;44:117–125.
40. Priori SG, Napolitano C, Schwartz PJ. Low penetrance in the long-QT syndrome: clinical impact. *Circulation* 1999;99:529–533.
41. Benhorin J, Moss AJ, Bak M, et al. Variable expression of long QT syndrome among gene carriers from families with five different HERG mutations. *Ann Noninvasive Electrocardiol* 2002;7:40–46.
42. Kobori A, Sarai N, Shimizu W, et al. Additional gene variants reduce effectiveness of beta-blockers in the LQT1 form of long QT syndrome. *J Cardiovasc Electrophysiol* 2004;15:190–199.
43. Schwartz PJ, Stramba-Badiale M, Segantini A, et al. Prolongation of the QT interval and the sudden infant death syndrome. *N Engl J Med* 1998; 338:1709–1714.
44. Wolf L. Familial auricular fibrillation. *N Engl J Med* 1943;229:396–397.
45. Fox CS, Parise H, D'Agostino RB Sr, et al. Parental atrial fibrillation as a risk factor for atrial fibrillation in offspring. *JAMA* 2004;291:2851–2855.
46. Darbar D, Herron KJ, Ballew JD, et al. Familial atrial fibrillation is a genetically heterogeneous disorder. *J Am Coll Cardiol* 2003;41:2185–2192.
47. Brugada R, Tapscott T, Czernuszewicz GZ, et al. Identification of a genetic locus for familial atrial fibrillation. *N Engl J Med* 1997;336:905–911.
48. Ellinor PT, Shin JT, Moore RK, et al. Locus for atrial fibrillation maps to chromosome 6q14-16. *Circulation* 2003;107:2880–2883.
49. Chen YH, Xu SJ, Bendahhou S, et al. KCNQ1 gain-of-function mutation in familial atrial fibrillation. *Science* 2003;299:251–254.
50. Yang Y, Xia M, Jin Q, et al. Identification of a KCNE2 gain-of-function mutation in patients with familial atrial fibrillation. *Am J Hum Genet* 2004;75:899–905.
51. Hong K, Bjerregaard P, Gussak I, et al. Short QT syndrome and atrial fibrillation caused by mutation in KCNH2. *J Cardiovasc Electrophysiol* 2005;16:394–396.
52. Gaborit N, Steenman M, Lamirault G, et al. Human atrial ion channel and transporter subunit gene-expression remodeling associated with valvular heart disease and atrial fibrillation. *Circulation* 2005;112:471–481.
53. Ehrlich JR, Zicha S, Coutu P, et al. Hebert TE, Nattel S. Atrial fibrillation-associated minK38G/S polymorphism modulates delayed rectifier current and membrane localization *Cardiovasc Res* 2005;67:520–528.
54. Temple J, Frias P, Rottman J, et al. Atrial fibrillation in KCNE1-null mice. *Circ Res* 2005;97:62–69.
55. Reid DS, Tynan M, Braidwood L, et al. Bidirectional tachycardia in a child: a study using His bundle electrography. *Br Heart J* 1975;37:339–344.
56. Coumel P, Fidelle J, Lucet V, et al. Catecholamine-induced severe ventricular arrhythmias with Adams-Stokes syndrome in children: report of four cases. *Br Heart J* 1978;40:28–37.
57. Leenhardt A, Lucet V, Denjoy I, et al. Catecholaminergic polymorphic ventricular tachycardia in children: a 7-year follow-up of 21 patients. *Circulation* 1995;91:1512–1519.
58. Choi G, Kopplin LJ, Tester DJ, et al. Spectrum and frequency of cardiac channel defects in swimming-triggered arrhythmia syndromes. *Circulation* 2004;110:2119–2124.
59. Priori SG, Napolitano C, Memmi M, et al. Clinical and molecular characterization of patients with catecholaminergic polymorphic ventricular tachycardia. *Circulation* 2002;106:69–74.
60. Swan H, Piippo K, Viitasalo M, et al. Arrhythmic disorder mapped to chromosome 1q42-q43 causes malignant polymorphic ventricular tachycardia in structurally normal hearts. *J Am Coll Cardiol* 1999;34:2035–2042.
61. Priori SG, Napolitano C, Tiso N, et al. Mutations in the cardiac ryanodine receptor gene (hryr2) underlie catecholaminergic polymorphic ventricular tachycardia. *Circulation* 2001;103:196–200.
62. Fabiato A, Fabiato F. Contractions induced by a calcium-triggered release of calcium from the sarcoplasmic reticulum of single skinned cardiac cells. *J Physiol (Lond)* 1975;249:469–495.
63. George CH, Higgs GV, Lai FA. Ryanodine receptor mutations associated with stress-induced ventricular tachycardia mediate increased calcium release in stimulated cardiomyocytes. *Circ Res* 2003;93:531–540.
64. Jiang D, Xiao B, Zhang L, et al. Enhanced basal activity of a cardiac Ca2+ release channel (ryanodine receptor) mutant associated with ventricular tachycardia and sudden death. *Circ Res* 2002;91:218–225.
65. Cerrone M, Colombi B, Santoro M, et al. Bidirectional ventricular tachycardia and fibrillation elicited in a knock-in mouse model carrier of a mutation in the cardiac ryanodine receptor. *Circ Res* 2005;96:e77–e82.
66. Eldar M, Pras E, Lahat H. A missense mutation in the CASQ2 gene is associated with autosomal-recessive catecholamine-induced polymorphic ventricular tachycardia. *Trends Cardiovasc Med* 2003;13:148–151.
67. Postma AV, Denjoy I, Hoorntje TM, et al. Absence of calsequestrin 2 causes severe forms of catecholaminergic polymorphic ventricular tachycardia. *Circ Res* 2002;91:e21–e26.
68. Viatchenko-Karpinski S, Terentyev D, Gyorke I, et al. Abnormal calcium signaling and sudden cardiac death associated with mutation of calsequestrin. *Circ Res* 2004;94:471–477.
69. Nam GB, Burashnikov A, Antzelevitch C. Cellular mechanisms underlying the development of catecholaminergic ventricular tachycardia. *Circulation* 2005;111:2727–2733.
70. Brugada P, Brugada J. Right bundle branch block, persistent ST segment elevation and sudden cardiac death: a distinct clinical and electrocardiographic syndrome. A multicenter report. *J Am Coll Cardiol* 1992;20:1391–1396.
71. Osher HL, Wolff L. Electrocardiographic pattern simulating acute myocardial injury. *Am J Med Sci* 1953;226:541–545.
72. Martini B, Nava A, Thiene G, et al. Ventricular fibrillation without apparent heart disease: description of six cases. *Am Heart J* 1989;118:1203–1209.
73. Vatta M, Dumaine R, Varghese G, et al. Genetic and biophysical basis of sudden unexplained nocturnal death syndrome (SUNDS), a disease allelic to Brugada syndrome. *Hum Mol Genet* 2002;11:337–345.
74. Priori SG, Napolitano C, Giordano U, et al. Brugada syndrome and sudden cardiac death in children. *Lancet* 2000;355:808–809.
75. Todd SJ, Campbell MJ, Roden DM, et al. Novel Brugada SCN5A mutation causing sudden death in children. *Heart Rhythm* 2005;2:540–543.
76. Brugada R, Brugada J, Antzelevitch C, et al. Sodium channel blockers identify risk for sudden death in patients with ST-segment elevation and right bundle branch block but structurally normal hearts. *Circulation* 2000; 101:510–515.

77. Matsuo K, Kurita T, Inagaki M, et al. The circadian pattern of the development of ventricular fibrillation in patients with Brugada syndrome. *Eur Heart J* 1999;20:465–470.
78. Chen Q, Kirsch GE, Zhang D, et al. Genetic basis and molecular mechanism for idiopathic ventricular fibrillation. *Nature* 1998;392:293–296.
79. Yan GX, Antzelevitch C. Cellular basis for the Brugada syndrome and other mechanisms of arrhythmogenesis associated with ST-segment elevation. *Circulation* 1999;100:1660–1666.
80. Saura D, Garcia-Alberola A, Carrillo P, et al. Brugada-like electrocardiographic pattern induced by fever. *Pacing Clin Electrophysiol* 2002;25:856–859.
81. Dinckal MH, Davutoglu V, Akdemir I, et al. Incessant monomorphic ventricular tachycardia during febrile illness in a patient with Brugada syndrome: fatal electrical storm. *Europace* 2003;5:257–261.
82. Dumaine R, Towbin JA, Brugada P, et al. Ionic mechanisms responsible for the electrocardiographic phenotype of the Brugada syndrome are temperature dependent. *Circ Res* 1999;85:803–809.
83. Alings M, Dekker L, Sadee A, Wilde A. Quinidine induced electrocardiographic normalization in two patients with Brugada syndrome. *Pacing Clin Electrophysiol* 2001;24:1420–1422.
84. Hermida JS, Denjoy I, Clerc J, et al. Hydroquinidine therapy in Brugada syndrome. *J Am Coll Cardiol* 2004;43:1853–1860.
85. Nademanee K, Veerakul G, Mower M, et al. Defibrillator Versus beta-Blockers for Unexplained Death in Thailand (DEBUT): a randomized clinical trial. *Circulation* 2003;07:2221–2226.
86. Antzelevitch C, Brugada P, Borggrefe M, et al. Brugada syndrome: report of the second consensus conference. *Heart Rhythm* 2005;2:429–440.
87. Algra A, Tijssen JG, Roelandt JR, et al. QT interval variables from 24 hour electrocardiography and the two year risk of sudden death. *Br Heart J* 1993;70:43–48.
88. Gussak I, Brugada P, Brugada J, et al. Idiopathic short QT interval: a new clinical syndrome? *Cardiology* 2000;94:99–102.
89. Gaita F, Giustetto C, Bianchi F, et al. Short QT Syndrome: a familial cause of sudden death. *Circulation* 2003;108:965–970.
90. Brugada R, Hong K, Dumaine R, et al. Sudden death associated with short-QT syndrome linked to mutations in HERG. *Circulation* 2004;109:30–35.
91. Bellocq C, van Ginneken AC, Bezzina CR, et al. Mutation in the KCNQ1 gene leading to the short QT-interval syndrome. *Circulation* 2004;109:2394–2397.
92. Priori SG, Pandit SV, Rivolta I, et al. A novel form of short QT syndrome (SQT3) is caused by a mutation in the KCNJ2 gene. *Circ Res* 2005;96:800–807.
93. Extramiana F, Antzelevitch C. Amplified transmural dispersion of repolarization as the basis for arrhythmogenesis in a canine ventricular-wedge model of short-QT syndrome. *Circulation* 2004;110:3661–3666.
94. Schimpf R, Wolpert C, Gaita F, et al. Short QT syndrome. *Cardiovasc Res* 2005;67:357–366.
95. Schimpf R, Wolpert C, Bianchi F, et al. Congenital short QT syndrome and implantable cardioverter defibrillator treatment: inherent risk for inappropriate shock delivery. *J Cardiovasc Electrophysiol* 2003;14:1273–1277.
96. Gaita F, Giustetto C, Bianchi F, et al. Short QT syndrome: pharmacological treatment. *J Am Coll Cardiol* 2004;43:1494–1499.
97. Gollob MH, Green MS, Tang AS, et al. Identification of a gene responsible for familial Wolff-Parkinson-White syndrome. *N Engl J Med* 2001;344:1823–1831.
98. Gollob MH, Seger JJ, Gollob TN, et al. Novel PRKAG2 mutation responsible for the genetic syndrome of ventricular preexcitation and conduction system disease with childhood onset and absence of cardiac hypertrophy. *Circulation* 2001;104:3030–3033.
99. Sanguinetti MC, Jiang C, Curran ME, et al. A mechanistic link between an inherited and an acquired cardiac arrhythmia: HERG encodes the IKr potassium channel. *Cell* 1995;81:299–307.
100. Furutani M, Trudeau MC, Hagiwara N, et al. Novel mechanism associated with an inherited cardiac arrhythmia: defective protein trafficking by the mutant HERG (G601S) potassium channel. *Circulation* 1999;99:2290–2294.
101. Hayashi K, Shimizu M, Ino H, et al. Characterization of a novel missense mutation E637K in the pore-S6 loop of HERG in a patient with long QT syndrome. *Cardiovasc Res* 2002;54:67–76.
102. Wang Z, Tristani-Firouzi M, Xu Q, et al. Functional effects of mutations in KvLQT1 that cause long QT syndrome. *J Cardiovasc Electrophysiol* 1999;10:817–826.
103. Wehrens XH, Rossenbacker T, Jongbloed RJ, et al. A novel mutation L619F in the cardiac Na^+ channel SCN5A associated with long-QT syndrome (LQT3): a role for the I-II linker in inactivation gating. *Hum Mutat* 2003;21:552.
104. Chang CC, Acharfi S, Wu MH, et al. A novel SCN5A mutation manifests as a malignant form of long QT syndrome with perinatal onset of tachycardia/bradycardia. *Cardiovasc Res* 2004;64:268–278.
105. Tester DJ, Will ML, Haglund CM, et al. Compendium of cardiac channel mutations in 541 consecutive unrelated patients referred for long QT syndrome genetic testing. *Heart Rhythm* 2005;2:507–517.
106. Rajamani S, Anderson CL, Anson BD, et al. Pharmacological rescue of human K(+) channel long-QT2 mutations: human ether-a-go-go–related gene rescue without block. *Circulation* 2002;105:2830–2835.
107. Paulussen AD, Raes A, Jongbloed RJ, et al. HERG mutation predicts short QT based on channel kinetics but causes long QT by heterotetrameric trafficking deficiency. *Cardiovasc Res* 2005;67:467–475.
108. Shimizu W, Antzelevitch C. Differential effects of beta-adrenergic agonists and antagonists in LQT1, LQT2 and LQT3 models of the long-QT syndrome. *J Am Coll Cardiol* 2000;35:778–786.
109. Antzelevitch C, Fish J. Electrical heterogeneity within the ventricular wall. *Basic Res Cardiol* 2001;96:517–527.
110. Lubinski A, Lewicka-Nowak E, Kempa M, et al. New insight into repolarization abnormalities in patients with congenital long QT syndrome: the increased transmural dispersion of repolarization. *Pacing Clin Electrophysiol* 1998;21:172–175.
111. Tanabe Y, Inagaki M, Kurita T, et al. Sympathetic stimulation produces a greater increase in both transmural and spatial dispersion of repolarization in LQT1 than LQT2 forms of congenital long QT syndrome. *J Am Coll Cardiol* 2001;37:911–919.
112. Yamaguchi M, Shimizu M, Ino H, et al. T wave peak-to-end interval and QT dispersion in acquired long QT syndrome: a new index for arrhythmogenicity. *Clin Sci (Lond)* 2003;105:671–676.
113. Bers DM. Cardiac excitation-contraction coupling. *Nature* 2002;415:198–205.
114. Molkentin JD, Lu JR, Antos CL, et al. A calcineurin-dependent transcriptional pathway for cardiac hypertrophy. *Cell* 1998;93:215–228.
115. Geisterfer-Lowrance AA, Christe M, Conner DA, et al. A mouse model of familial hypertrophic cardiomyopathy. *Science* 1996;272:731–734.
116. Nerbonne JM. Studying cardiac arrhythmias in the mouse: a reasonable model for probing mechanisms? *Trends Cardiovasc Med* 2004;14:83–93.
117. Wu Y, Temple J, Zhang R, et al Calmodulin kinase II and arrhythmias in a mouse model of cardiac hypertrophy. *Circulation* 2002;106:1288–1293.
118. Guo W, Li H, London B, et al. Functional consequences of elimination of i(to,f) and i(to,s): early afterdepolarizations, atrioventricular block, and ventricular arrhythmias in mice lacking Kv1.4 and expressing a dominant-negative Kv4 alpha subunit. *Circ Res* 2000;87:73–79.
119. Baker LC, London B, Choi BR, et al. Enhanced dispersion of repolarization and refractoriness in transgenic mouse hearts promotes reentrant ventricular tachycardia. *Circ Res* 2000;86:396–407.
120. Sanbe A, James J, Tuzcu V, et al. Transgenic rabbit model for human troponin I-based hypertrophic cardiomyopathy. *Circulation* 2005;111:2330–2338.
121. Hayase M, del MF, Kawase Y, et al. Catheter-based antegrade intracoronary viral gene delivery with coronary venous blockade. *Am J Physiol* 2005; 288:H2995–H3000.
122. Kevin DJ, Heldman AW, Fraser H, et al. Focal modification of electrical conduction in the heart by viral gene transfer. *Nat Med* 2000;6:1395–1398.

CHAPTER 59 ■ ELECTROCARDIOGRAPHY

ELENA B. SGARBOSSA AND GALEN WAGNER

HISTORICAL PERSPECTIVE

The first demonstration of the human cardiac activity was made during a congress of physiologists in London by Augustus Waller, who, in May 1887, published the first single-lead electrocardiogram (ECG) (1). Waller recorded the electrical activity of the heart from a chest lead with a capillary electrometer (a glass tube filled with mercury) (2). When the electrometer was placed on the body surface, the current was transmitted from the chest to the mercury column, which would expand or contract. This movement could be observed only through a microscope and needed to be projected onto photographic paper (Fig. 59.1).

The pioneer of clinical electrocardiography, however, was Willem Einthoven. Einthoven had a background in physics and mathematics (3). To refine Waller's concept, Einthoven worked in his laboratory in the Netherlands for years, first with the electrometer and later with the string galvanometer (2). The galvanometer was an instrument developed in 1897 by Clément Ader for telegraphic transmissions. It reduced the distortion of the electrometer because it consisted of a thin wire extended between the poles of a magnet, but it still required the use of both a microscope and photographic paper. Einthoven presented his idea of applying the galvanometer to the recording of the cardiac electrical activity in 1903 (2). He also coined the term *elektrokardiogramm* in German (the dominant language at the time for scientific publications) and labeled the recorded waveforms P, Q, R, S, T, and U to differentiate them from the original, but incomplete, A, B, C, and D described by Waller. Einthoven also described numerous abnormal findings and created the bipolar limb lead system known as the Einthoven triangle (2).

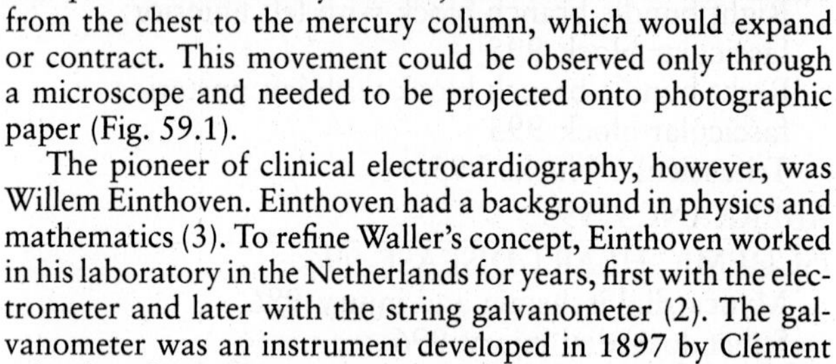

FIGURE 59.1. Reproduction of the first recording of an electrocardiogram by Waller. The electrical activity of the heart is recorded by movement on the surface of a mercury column (e). Chest wall movement is recorded by a mechanical lever (h). Time is indicated by t. (From Waller AD. A demonstration in man of electromotive changes accompanying the heart's beat. *J Physiol (Lond)* 1887;8:229–234.)

This progress was observed skeptically by Waller, who, in 1911, expressed doubts on the clinical value of electrocardiography (4). The early electrocardiograph was extremely unwieldy. It required a continuous-flow water jacket for cooling the electromagnet. The camera and the optical system were an integral part of the apparatus, and an arc lamp projected the shadow of the string onto photographic paper. The electrodes were large bowls of saline solution in which the subject immersed his or her hands or feet. The machine occupied two rooms, and five people were required to operate it (5).

It was only after many years of these initial efforts that the ECG became regarded as a potentially useful tool in clinical practice (6). Several companies in Europe and in the United States initiated the commercial manufacturing of electrocardiographs. The first table-model electrocardiograph assembled in London was leased to Sir Thomas Lewis in 1911. Lewis worked intensively in recording both normal and abnormal cardiac activity. His work was pivotal in shifting the available knowledge from the laboratory to the clinical field. Keith and Flack had reported on the existence of the sinus node in 1907, and Lewis ascribed the origin of the cardiac impulse to it. He also proved the origin of ectopic tachycardias, studied atrial fibrillation, and introduced the concept of aberrant conduction. Lewis published several books, including the first textbook of electrocardiography (2).

During World War I, Lewis had a prominent disciple named Franklin Wilson, the youngest of a group of American cardiologists selected to work in England with him. At the end of the war, Wilson returned to the University of Michigan in Ann Arbor and obtained a string galvanometer. He worked with the galvanometer under the hospital stairwells, the only space appropriate for the large apparatus, which was smaller than the original model but still needed a wheeled trolley for transportation. Wilson's investigations resulted in the theory of the ventricular gradient and in detailed descriptions of the bundle branch blocks (BBBs) (7). Perhaps Wilson's best known contribution is his creation of a unipolar chest lead system connected to a central electrode (8).

By 1920, myocardial infarction had been recognized as an entity because of the reports by Herrick (9) and Pardee (10). In 1924, Einthoven was awarded the Nobel prize for his contribution, but the relevance of electrocardiography to clinical cardiology was not yet fully appreciated. Wilson himself published an article on heartbeat disorders in 1936 with no mention of electrocardiography (11).

Subsequent improvements to the original galvanometer led to further reduction in its size and to the current electronic technology. The first portable model was introduced in 1926, and with it Lewis' vision of electrocardiography as a standard diagnostic tool became a reality (3). At that time, two distinguished electrocardiographers and investigators, Langendorf and Pick, were attending medical school in Prague. Both physicians made their main scientific contributions later in the United States by perfecting the methodology of deductive reasoning for complex cardiac arrhythmias (12).

The "post-Wilson era" which began in the mid 1950s witnessed less radical, but yet important, developments in electrocardiography. By means of ingenious clinical-pathologic-correlations, investigators from different parts of the world elucidated the ECG manifestations of the many cardiac conditions. Outstanding contributors included the following: Lepeschkin, Surawicz, and Castellanos in the United States; Sodi-Pallares and Cabrera in Mexico; Rosenbaum in Argentina; Schamroth in South Africa; and Durrer and Wellens in the Netherlands. The introduction of invasive clinical electrophysiologic studies only confirmed in most cases the deductions of these pioneers (13).

In more recent years, emphasis in ECG research has shifted to the study of dynamic patterns inherent in certain parameters (especially ventricular repolarization) with the aid of the ambulatory recordings first introduced by Holter in 1961 and then by newer, potent digital storage and analysis techniques. The advent of effective myocardial reperfusion therapies has renewed the interest in the ECG manifestations of the acute ischemic syndromes. Finally, attempts at improving the resolution of standard electrocardiography have relied on an increase in the number of recording electrodes (body surface mapping) and on an improvement in the signal-to-noise ratio of the higher frequency signals by averaging and filtering (signal-averaged electrocardiography). Initial results with these techniques are promising, but their roles in clinical practice are still unclear.

Despite the development of more sophisticated and expensive cardiac diagnostic tests, the standard 12-lead ECG remains an integral part of the clinical evaluation of all cardiac patients, particularly those with ischemic heart disease or rhythm disturbances.

ANATOMIC REFERENCES

The "view" of the electrical activity recorded from any surface ECG electrode is determined by the relative position of the heart. With the individual standing, the heart lies rather horizontally with the atria at its base and the ventricles at its apex (14). Because the heart is a conical structure rotated over its long axis, the right atrium and ventricle are more anterior than the left chambers, and the right and left sides of the heart are not aligned with the homonymous sides of the body. Thus, the interventricular septum is almost parallel to the frontal, not the sagittal, plane, and the left ventricular (LV) free wall (usually considered a lateral structure) includes nearly 300 degrees of the LV circumference and faces superiorly, posteriorly, and inferiorly (5).

ELECTROCARDIOGRAPHIC RECORDING

The 12 Leads

The cardiac electrical activity is recorded through 12 surface leads named I, II, III, aVR, aVL, aVF, V_1, V_2, V_3, V_4, V_5, and V_6. The first six points are recorded with electrodes located on the limbs, whereas leads V_1 to V_6 are recorded from the chest (Fig. 59.2).

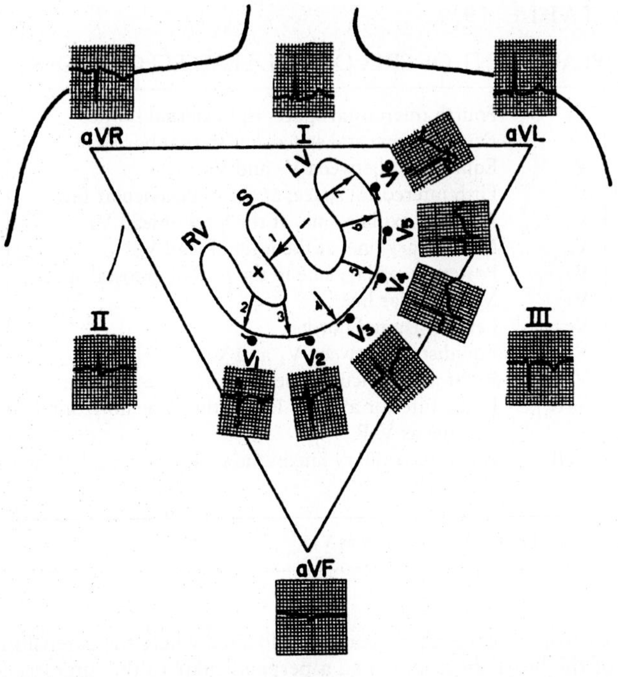

FIGURE 59.2. The standard 12 leads are shown with their recording sites. Both the frontal and the horizontal planes are depicted. Vectors 1 to 7 show the normal sequence of activation of the septum (S) and ventricles from the horizontal plane. LV, left ventricle; RV, right ventricle. (From Gazes PC, ed. *Clinical cardiology: a bedside approach.* Chicago: Year Book, 1983:39.)

Leads I, II, and III were first used when Einthoven placed recording electrodes on both arms and the left leg, to form an equilateral triangle. An additional electrode on the right leg was used for grounding. Leads I to III are bipolar because they record potential differences between two electrodes. For lead I, the left arm electrode is the positive pole, and the right arm electrode is the negative pole. Lead II has its positive pole on the left leg and its negative pole on the right arm, and it provides a view of the electrical activity along the long axis of the heart. Lead III has its positive pole on the left leg and its negative pole on the left arm. Between leads I, II, and III are 60-degree angles. These wide viewing gaps are filled with the augmented unipolar ("aV") leads aVR, aVL, and aVF, which record the electrical activity between the exploring limb electrode and a reference created connecting the other two limb electrodes together trough a 5000-ohm resistor (the Wilson central terminal) (15). Lead aVF, for example, measures the potential difference between the left leg and the average of the potentials at the right and left arms. The addition of these three aV leads to the triaxial reference system produces an hexaxial system, with the six leads separated by angles of only 30 degrees. The gap between leads II and II is filled by lead aVR, that between leads II and III by lead aVF, and that between leads III and I, by lead aVL. This provides a perspective of the frontal plane, as illustrated in Figure 59.2. The limb leads are presented in the order I, II, II, aVR, aVL, and aVF, which spatially correspond to 0, 60, 120, −150, −30, and 90 degrees, respectively.

The last set of leads introduced to clinical practice were the six unipolar precordial leads (V_1 to V_6) (3). Augmentation is not necessary because the recording electrodes are close to the heart. The Wilson central terminal provides their negative poles, whereas the sites of the exploring electrode are determined by bony landmarks on the anterior and left lateral aspects of the precordium (Table 59.1 and Fig. 59.3). The angles between these leads are slightly smaller than those between the

TABLE 59.1

PLACEMENT OF PRECORDIAL LEAD ELECTRODES

V_1	Fourth intercostal space, right sternal border
V_2	Fourth intercostal space, left sternal border
V_3	Equidistant between V_2 and V_4
V_4	Fifth intercostal space, at the midclavicular line
V_5	Anterior axillary line, at the level of lead V_4
V_6	Midaxillary line, at the level of lead V_4
V_7	Posterior axillary line in the fifth intercostal space
V_8	Midscapular line
V_9	Left paraspinal border
V_3R	Equidistant between V_1 and V_4R
V_4R	Right midclavicular line, fifth intercostal space
V_5R	Right anterior axillary line in the same horizontal plane as V_4R
V_6R	Right midaxillary line in the same horizontal plane as V_4R

Note: Lead V_2R is the same as V_1.

six frontal plane leads. Lead V_1 is located where the extension of the heart short axis (i.e., a perpendicular to the interatrial and interventricular septa) intersects with the precordial body surface. Because V_1 provides a right anterior to left posterior view, it distinguishes better between left and right cardiac electrical activity than does a lead providing a right lateral to left lateral view (e.g., lead I).

Limitations of the Current 12-Lead System

Poor Orthogonality and Redundancy

A set of three ECG leads is orthogonal if their lead vectors are at 90-degree angles with each other, thus permitting the accurate detection of the onset and offset of ECG waveforms in all spatial directions. Orthogonality in the current 12-lead system is meager because the sagittal and anteroposterior components of cardiac activity are recorded poorly by the limb leads, whereas

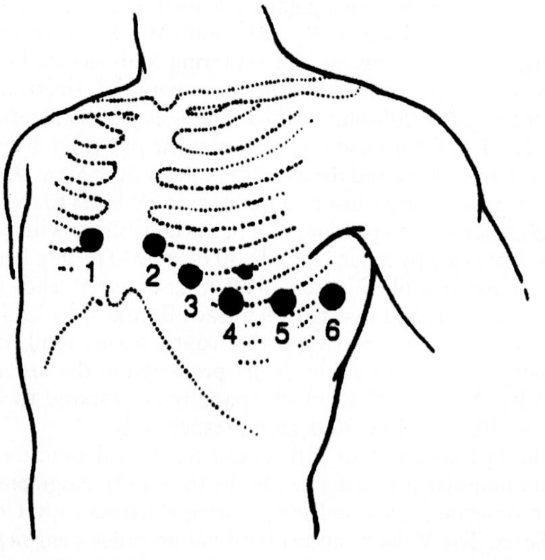

FIGURE 59.3. Location of the precordial lead electrodes. (From The electrocardiogram: fundamentals. In: Goldschlager N, Goldman MJ, eds. *Principles of clinical electrocardiography.* Stamford, CT: Appleton & Lange, 1989:1–10.)

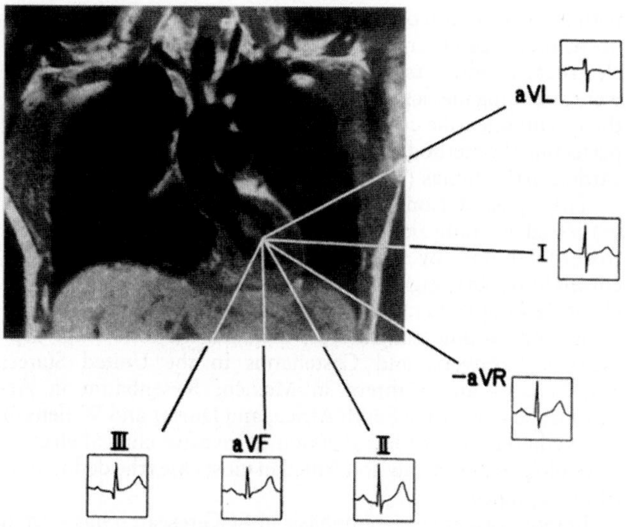

FIGURE 59.4. The panoramic display of the 12-lead electrocardiogram in an ideal sequential spatial order. (From Anderson ST, Pahlm O, Selvester RH, et al. Panoramic display of the orderly sequenced 12-lead ECG. *J Electrocardiol* 1994;27:347–352.)

the precordial leads miss the vertical components. Also, the current 12-lead system provides for superfluous recording points. Of the standard ECG, probably only eight components capture independent information on cardiac electrical activity.

Inappropriate Lead Sequencing and Gap in the Frontal Plane

In the ECG, the precordial leads are displayed to depict an orderly progression in the horizontal plane. Leads V_1 to V_6 faithfully show the spatial sequence of electrical activation (from the basal right ventricle to the midposterior LV wall). The limb leads, instead, depict a disordered spatial sequence. Leads I, II, II, aVR, aVL, and aVF correspond spatially to 0, 60, 120, −150, −30, and 90 degrees, respectively. Such array has been consecrated by usage, but it is counterintuitive. If an analogous distribution were selected for the horizontal plane, the precordial leads would be reordered as V_2, V_4, V_6, $-V_3$, V_1, and V_5 (16). This would considerably compromise the ability of the interpreter to understand the electrical phenomena in that plane rapidly. A more logical sequencing for the limb leads would be aVL, I, −aVR, II, aVF, and III (or −30, 0, 30, 60, 90, and 120 degrees); the inclusion of a negative aVR would allow to record ECG phenomena at 30° (Fig. 59.4).

Special Leads

Some leads are not considered part of the standard ECG but are useful in specific circumstances. Posterior leads (V_7, V_8, and V_9) increase the ECG sensitivity for injury in the posterior wall (17) (Table 59.1). Right precordial leads (V_{3R}, V_{4R}) are particularly useful for the diagnosis of right ventricular infarcts and of some congenital abnormalities (Table 59.1) (18). A routine use of the negative aVR (at 30 degrees) would add useful information to the standard ECG, and it would be less likely to be overlooked during routine ECG interpretation (19–21).

The P wave is not always distinctly seen in the 12-lead ECG, but it may be easily identified with special leads. Distinct P waveforms can be seen by placing the right and left arm leads in various chest positions (if possible, parallel to the vector of atrial depolarization) while recording lead I (the Lewis lead). Atrial activity can also be recorded semiinvasively from leads placed in the esophagus because the anterior wall of the esophagus lies against the left atrium. In patients with dual-chamber pacemakers, atrial electrograms can be recorded by telemetry from the pacing electrodes. In patients recovering from cardiac surgery, the placement of temporary epicardial pacing electrodes allows the direct recording of atrial activity.

Equipment

Electrocardiographers are calibrated to give a deflection of 10 mm/mV (this calibration is seen at the beginning or end of the ECG). ECG paper is graph paper divided in little squares of 1 mm each and bigger squares of 5 mm each. The paper speed is standardized to 25 mm/second. One mm equals 0.1 mV.

Commercial systems provide ECG programs with stereotyped methodologies of measurement. The only limb ECG leads that digital electrocardiographs record are leads I and II; the remaining limb leads are calculated in real time based on the Einthoven law (I + III = II) and using relationships derived from lead vectors for the aV leads. For the calculation of the electrical QRS axis, the entire QRS complex area is used. This is an advantage over the manual QRS axis estimation, based mainly on R-wave measurements.

Current electrocardiographs use digital technology. Analog data are converted into digital signals that are later processed (22). The use of compression techniques allows storage and subsequent retrieval of serial ECG recordings, as well as remote transmission of ECG data, for example, to hand-held computers for "real-time" interpretation by a cardiologist (23). After digital transmission or retrieval of serial measurements, output data can be compared with input data.

BASIC PRINCIPLES

Membrane Properties, Action Potential, and Cardiac Activation

Myocytes maintain a potential difference between the cell interior and exterior of approximately −90 mV. This electrical transmembrane gradient depends on the chemical transmembrane gradient, which exists because the concentration of negative ions is higher inside the cell than outside. Such uneven distribution of ions and their flow in and out of the cell is regulated by channels, which are complex molecular structures housed in the cell membrane (24). Electric stimuli change the resting potential inside the cell from −90 mV to about +30 mV (*depolarization*), and this electrical activity is the *action potential*. Depolarization initiates the propagation of the impulse along both the inner and outer sides of the "polarized" membrane. Thus, the electrical front, which can be represented as a vector, flows from the positively (depolarized) to the negatively (resting) charged cells. The earliest ventricular activation occurs in the left side of the septum. Then the depolarization front reaches the septum right side and the anterior wall, thus following an inside-out course. The action potential shapes differ considerably between endocardial and epicardial myocytes, secondary to differences in the distribution of currents (and channel proteins) among cardiac layers (25).

The phenomenon underlying depolarization at the cellular level is the inflow of the positive ions sodium and calcium. This inward current is at some point exceeded by an outward current of potassium ions, which ends the electrical systole and leads to *repolarization* (i.e., restitution of membrane polarity). In the atrium, repolarization proceeds in the same direction as atrial depolarization, and thus the polarity of the repolarization waveform is opposite that of depolarization. Ventricular repolarization, however, follows an inverted path. It travels from epicardium to endocardium; therefore, the repolarization waveform polarity is the same as that of depolarization. This behavior is the basis for the concept of *ventricular gradient.* The ventricular gradient measures the magnitude of the integral between the QRS complex and the T wave (i.e., between depolarization and repolarization). If all ventricular action potentials had the same magnitude and duration, the ventricular gradient would be zero. Yet repolarization forces start and end at different times within the various ventricular areas, and they also differ in duration (slope of phase 3 of the action potential). Thus, within the ventricles there is both spatial and temporal variability, or repolarization dispersion (26). To this dispersion may also contribute an additional population of cardiac cells, the intramural "M cells" (10).

Cardiac Activation: Impulse Formation, and Conduction

The heart can be considered as a dipole with a positive and a negative charge. At any given time, cardiac cells are in various stages of activation (i.e., depolarization and repolarization). The formation (i.e., pacemaking) and timely conduction of an electrical impulse depend on cardiac cells that are strategically placed and arranged in nodes, bundles, and an intraventricular network that end in *Purkinje cells.* All these specialized cells lack contractile capability, but they can act as pacemakers (i.e., spontaneously generate electrical impulses) and alter conduction speed. The intrinsic pacemaking rate is fastest in the sinus node, located in the right atrium, and is slowest in the Purkinje cells.

The intraventricular conduction network includes the common bundle of His and its right and left bundle branches, which extend along the septum toward their respective ventricles. The left bundle branch is a diffuse structure that fans broadly over the septum toward the two mitral valve papillary muscles. In the left bundle branch, two divisions can usually be distinguished; they are called anterior and posterior but are indeed superior and inferior, respectively. Because the right bundle branch remains compact until it reaches the distal interventricular septal surface (where it branches into the septum and toward the lateral right ventricular wall), many authors consider the intraventricular conduction system to be trifascicular (27,28). These intraventricular conduction pathways are composed of Purkinje cells with both pacemaking and rapid impulse conduction capabilities. Purkinje fibers branch into networks that extend just beneath the endocardial surface.

The normal activation sequence begins at the midseptum, continues in the epicardial right ventricular wall near the apex, then at the lateral and basal LV, and ends at the basal septum (Fig. 59.5). The wavefront departs from the sinus node and travels through the right and left atria in a centrifugal manner. On arrival at the atrioventricular (AV) node, the impulse is delayed, allowing for a sequential, rather than simultaneous, contraction of the ventricles after the atria. Because the Purkinje system provides a specialized path for rapid activation, the entire ventricular mass can be depolarized in a short time (similar to the depolarization timing of the much smaller atria). The impulses then proceed slowly from endocardium to epicardium throughout both ventricles (29).

Electrical Bases for Electrocardiography and Vectorcardiography

Differences in cardiac potentials of a single cardiac cell or a small group of cells do not produce enough current to be

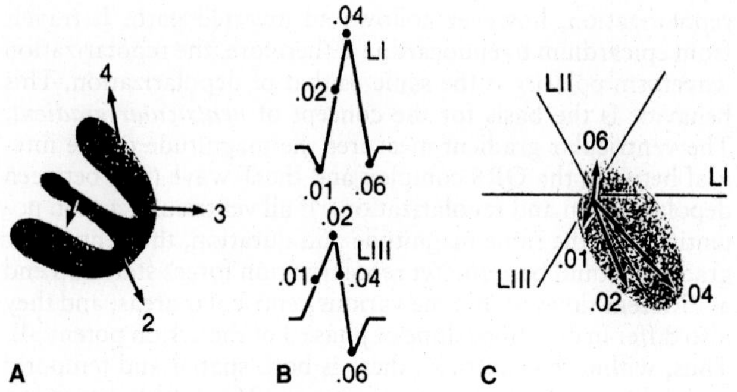

FIGURE 59.5. Correlation between the order of ventricular activation (A), scalar electrocardiogram (B), and vectorcardiogram (C). **A:** The sequence of ventricular activation is represented by four instantaneous frontal plane vectors. **B:** The four vectors plotted on leads I and III at the appropriate time during inscription of the QRS complex. **C:** Each of the four vectors is derived in the frontal plane. A line joining the ends of the vectors results in a frontal plane QRS loop. L, lead. (From Fisch C. Electrocardiography and vectorcardiography. In: Braunwald E, ed. *Heart disease: a textbook of cardiovascular medicine,* 4th ed. Philadelphia: WB Saunders, 1992:116–160.)

detected on the body surface. Electrical representation on the ECG depends on the activation of most of the atrial and ventricular masses. The depolarization process produces a relatively high-frequency ECG waveform. The earliest QRS complex is recorded in right precordial leads. While depolarization persists, the ECG recording returns to baseline. Repolarization is then represented by the ST segment and the T and U waves (10). Once the cells are in their resting state, the ECG records a flat baseline.

On the 12-lead ECG, only 10% to 15% of the ventricular activation process can be seen; the remaining activation forces cancel each other. The normal right ventricle has no ECG representation because its forces are obscured by the dipoles generated in the massive LV. The summation of all cardiac electrical forces can be represented with a single vector that originates at the center of the Einthoven triangle and whose arrowhead points to the positive pole. If all instantaneous single vectors were plotted consecutively, a vector loop would be formed in each of the three spatial planes (frontal, sagittal, and horizontal). Such recording constitutes a vectorcardiogram (Fig. 59.5). The vectorcardiogram integrates two surface leads out of three (named X, Y, and Z) in an orthogonal system and depicts a separate loop for each of the ECG components (P wave, QRS complex, T wave, and U wave). The vectorcardiogram is superior to the ECG in that it provides information not only on magnitude and direction (i.e., positive or negative) of the signals, but also on spatial orientation.

NORMAL ELECTROCARDIOGRAPHIC WAVEFORMS

Overview

The waves on the ECG represent a coincident voltage gradient generated by cellular electrical activity within the heart. The normal waveforms are depicted in Figure 59.6. The origin of the cardiac impulse in the sinus node is electrocardiographically mute; the initial recordable wave for each cardiac cycle is the P wave, which represents the spread of activation through the atria. Ventricular activation results in the QRS complex, which may appear as one (monophasic), two (diphasic), or three (triphasic) individual waveforms. Low-amplitude or narrow waves are denoted by lowercase letters (e.g., q wave) and taller, wider waves are denoted by capital letters (e.g., Q wave).

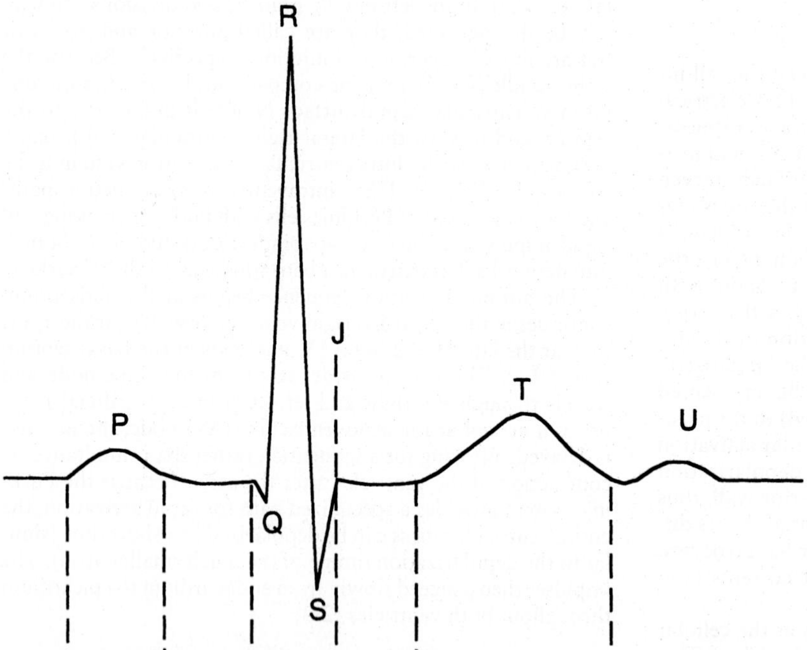

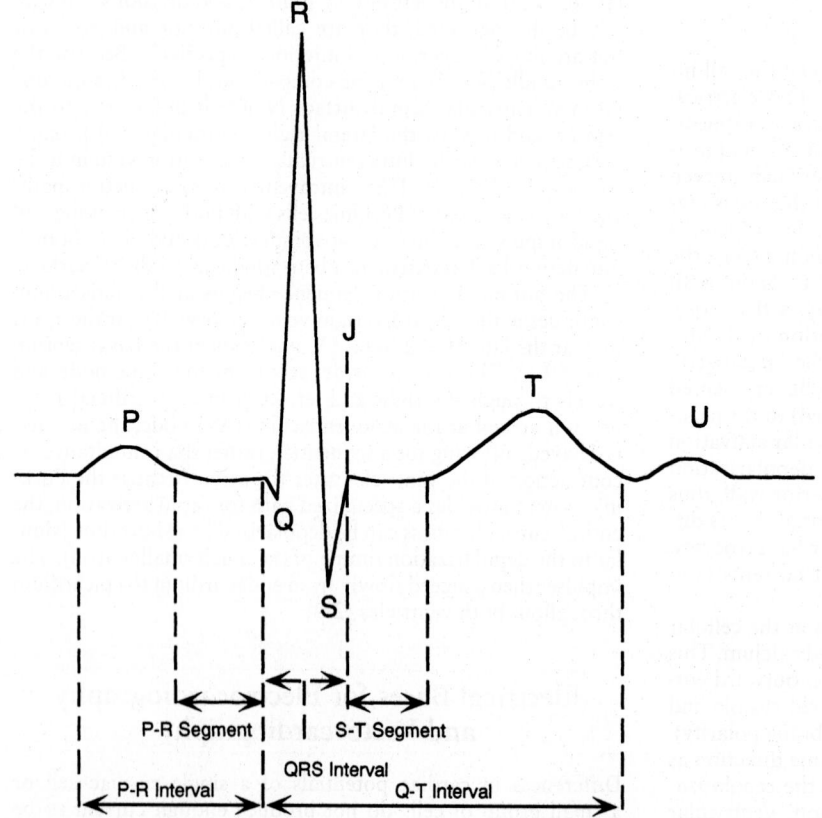

FIGURE 59.6. Waveforms and intervals of the electrocardiogram. (From Wagner GS, ed. *Marriott's practical electrocardiography,* 9th ed. Baltimore: Williams & Wilkins, 1994:13.)

The T wave represents ventricular recovery and is sometimes followed by a small upright deflection, the U wave. The ST segment is the interval between the end of ventricular activation (the plateau phase of the action potential) and the beginning of ventricular recovery. The QT interval measures the time from ventricular activation onset to end of ventricular recovery. At low heart rates the PR, ST, and TP segments are at the same horizontal level (i.e., the isoelectric line), considered the baseline for measuring various waveform amplitudes (30).

P Wave

The first part of the P wave represents the activation in the right atrium, and the middle and final sections of the P wave are recorded during left atrial activation. The normal P wave is rounded and upright in leads I and II and from V_2 to V_6. Its maximum amplitude is 0.25 mV in lead II (or 25% of the R wave), and its duration is 0.08 second. The P-wave axis is approximately 60 degrees. The intrathoracic position of the right and left atria determines that the activation front be directed first anteriorly, then posteriorly. The right atrium faces lead V_1, in which the initial portion of the P wave appears positive while its terminal part appears negative.

Ta Segment

The Ta segment (or Ta wave) represents atrial repolarization and may be seen in physiologically normal individuals, but it is more often obscured by the QRS complex and the early part of the ST segment. The Ta wave direction is opposite that of the P wave. A normal but prominent Ta wave may produce PR-segment depression and mimic a pathologic Q wave.

PR Interval

The time from onset of the P wave to onset of the QRS complex (whether its first wave is a Q or an R wave) is the PR interval. It encompasses the time between the onset of atrial depolarization in the myocardium adjacent to the sinus node and the onset of ventricular depolarization in the myocardium adjacent to the Purkinje network. A major portion of it is inscribed during the slow conduction through the AV node. The normal PR interval measures 0.12 to 0.22 second. The PR interval increases with age. It shortens as heart rates increases; this effect depends on higher sympathetic and lower vagal tones. Incremental atrial pacing at rest, however, *prolongs* the PR interval. The time from the end of the P wave to the onset of the QRS complex is called PR *segment*.

QRS Complex

The QRS complex represents ventricular activation. The contour of the QRS complex is peaked because it is composed of high-frequency signals (Fig. 59.6). The normal ventricular activation can be summarized in four vectors (Fig. 59.5): (a) initial septal activation from left to right and anteriorly (inferiorly or superiorly), producing a positive deflection (R wave) at right recording sites; (b) an overlapping wave of excitation involving both ventricles, with the vector directed inferiorly and slightly to the left, which inscribes the midportion of the QRS complex; (c) unopposed activation of the apical and central portions of the LV and of the right ventricle with a resultant vector oriented posteriorly, inferiorly, and to the left; the posteriorly positioned LV is much thicker, and its activation predominates over that of the more anterior right ventricle, with a resulting negative deflection (i.e., S wave) in aVR and in right precordial leads and in an R wave in leads I, II, III, aVL, and left precordial leads; and (d) activation of the posterior basal portion of the LV and septum with a vector directed superiorly and posteriorly, which completes the S wave in V_5 and V_6.

The QRS complex measures 0.07 to 0.10 second and increases with the subject's height (31). The QRS complex is measured from the beginning of the first appearing Q or R wave to the end of the last appearing R, S, or R′ wave. It tends to be slightly longer in male patients. The onset of the QRS complex is not recorded simultaneously in all ECG leads; this has implications when measuring QRS duration. The earliest QRS onset is recorded in right precordial leads (12). Computerized QRS measurements have the advantage of integrating information from the 12 leads.

Q Waves

A Q wave is a negative deflection at the onset of the QRS complex. It indicates that the net direction of early ventricular depolarization forces is oriented away from the positive axis of the recording lead at least by 90 degrees. Normal septal activation results in a rapid q wave in leads I, II, III, aVL, V_5, and V_6. The presence of Q waves in V_1, V_2, and V_3 or the absence of small q waves in V_5 and V_6 is abnormal (13). Positional factors may also result in the inscription of prominent but narrow Q waves. If the septal vector is horizontal, Q waves may appear in lead aVF; if the electrical axis is vertical, Q waves may appear in aVL. Precordial lead electrodes misplaced in a high position may determine the inscription of Q waves and a pseudoinfarction pattern. In right precordial leads, qr and qS complexes may be normal (32).

R Waves

The first positive wave of the QRS complex is the R wave, regardless of whether it is preceded by a Q wave. The second activation vector results in an R wave in leads II and III, and the third vector produces an R wave in leads I, II, III, aVL, aVF, V_5, and V_6. The precordial leads provide a panoramic view of the cardiac electrical activity progressing from the right ventricle to the thicker LV; consequently, the R wave increases its amplitude and duration from V_1 to V_4 or V_5. An rS pattern in leads V_{3R} and V_{4R} is normal. The R wave amplitude in V_5 and V_6 varies directly with LV dimension during exercise and with positional changes. Reversal of the normal sequence with larger R waves in V_1 and V_2 can be produced by right ventricular enlargement. When a second positive deflection occurs in any lead, it is called R′.

S Waves

A negative deflection following an R wave is an S wave. The third vector produces an S wave in leads aVr, V_1, V_2, V_3, and occasionally, V_4. The S wave in the precordial leads is large in V_1, larger in V_2, and then progressively smaller from V_3 through V_6. This sequence could be altered by ventricular enlargement. The last vector, directed superiorly and posteriorly, may result in a terminal S wave in leads I, V_5, and V_6. Leads V_{4R} and V_{3R} show an rS morphology in 80% of normal subjects (16).

Intrinsicoid Deflection

The time from the beginning of ventricular activation (onset of the QRS complex) to the point in which the impulse arrives

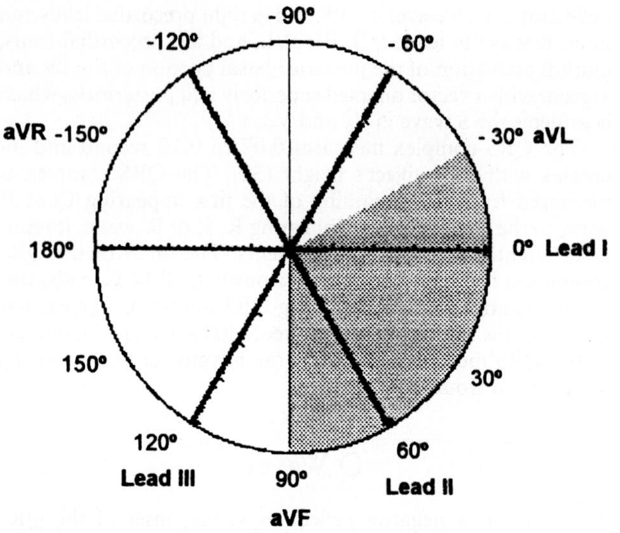

FIGURE 59.7. Frontal plane hexaxial reference system. The normal QRS axis in adults lies between –30 and +90 degrees (*area in gray*).

under a particular electrode is called the *ventricular activation time*. The downward deflection that follows is the *intrinsicoid deflection*. By definition, the intrinsicoid deflection can be measured only in precordial leads, but some authors applied this name to the turning point of the cardiac vector along the lead axis for the limb leads as well. For practical purposes, the estimate of the intrinsicoid deflection is the *R peak time*. It is measured from the onset of the QRS complex to the peak of the R wave or R′ wave. The R peak time is ≤0.04 second in V_1 and V_2, and ≤0.05 in V_5 and V_6 (33).

QRS Axis

The QRS axis can be manually determined in the frontal plane in three steps: (a) the lead with the equiphasic deflection (defined as positive and negative components of the QRS complex of similar amplitudes) is identified; (b) the lead that is perpendicular to the initial lead is identified; and (c) if in this second lead the predominant QRS polarity is positive, the axis is equal to the positive pole of this lead; if the polarity is negative, the axis is equal to the negative pole of this lead. The normal electrical axis measures between –30 and + 90 degrees (Fig. 59.7). QRS axes between 0 and –30 degrees are considered "left axis deviation."

The normal QRS complex is predominately positive in both leads I (with its positive pole at 0 degrees) and II (with its positive pole at +60 degrees). If the QRS is positive in lead I but negative in II, the axis is deviated leftward between –30 and –120 degrees. If the QRS is negative in I but positive in II, the axis is deviated rightward between +90 and ±180 degrees. The axis opposite to normal (with a predominately negative QRS orientation in both leads I and II) is rare.

The normal QRS axis is rightward in the neonate, moves during childhood to a vertical position, and then gradually moves through adulthood to a more horizontal position. In physiologically normal adults, the electrical axis is almost parallel to lead II, but it is more vertical in slender individuals and more horizontal in heavy individuals.

Because the cardiac base is firmly attached to the intrathoracic structures, true (i.e., anatomic) rotation of the heart on its long axis is limited to superior or inferior shifts of the relatively mobile cardiac apex. Most QRS axis deviations observed in the ECG in ventricular hypertrophies or fascicular blocks rather correspond to changes in the balance of epicardial versus endocardial activation forces or to different routes taken by the activation forces.

J Wave

The J wave (or Osborn wave) is a deflection that may appear on the ECG following the QRS complex as a result of electrical heterogeneities among the myocardial layers. It may be present in healthy patients with the early repolarization pattern (34).

ST Segment

The ST segment represents the time period in which the ventricular myocardium remains depolarized. The term *ST segment* is used whether the QRS complex ends in an R wave or in an S wave. At its junction with the QRS (i.e., J point), the ST segment forms a nearly 90-degree angle and then proceeds horizontally until it curves gently into the T wave. Slight upsloping (particularly in leads V_1 to V_3, and in V_{4R}–V_{3R}), downsloping, or horizontal depression of the ST segment may occur as a normal variant. The ST-segment length and appearance are influenced by factors that alter the duration of ventricular activation, such as exercise and BBB.

T Wave

The T wave represents exclusively uncanceled potential differences of ventricular repolarization (i.e., both spatial and temporal dispersion of repolarization) among the epicardium, M cells, and endocardium. The T wave accounts for 8% or less of the total time-voltage product of the heart (35). The T wave has a rounded but asymmetric shape, with the initial deflection longer than the terminal deflection. The peak of the T wave marks repolarization completion of the epicardial cells. The end of the T wave is temporally aligned with repolarization of the M cells (18). The M-cell repolarization is outlasted by that of the Purkinje cells, itself unlikely to generate an ECG wave.

The T-wave amplitude does not normally exceed 0.5 mV in limb leads or 0.10 mV in precordial leads. The T-wave vector and polarity are concordant with the R-wave vector. The T wave is always positive in lead I, nearly always positive or isoelectric in lead II, and may have any polarity in leads III and aVF (9). In precordial leads, the T wave is usually upright.

U Wave

When present, the U wave is a small, rounded wave following the T wave. It is most prominent in leads V_2 to V_3 and it usually shows the same direction as its preceding T wave, but in some patients it may be discordant (36). The U wave results from the last repolarization components. It may be generated by repolarization of the Purkinje network or by repolarization of the M cells (18,37,38).

QT Interval

The QT interval measures the time from the beginning of the QRS complex until the end of the T wave. It estimates the duration of both ventricular depolarization and repolarization, but it is used mainly as an estimate of ventricular recovery time. The term *QT* is used whether the QRS complex begins with a Q or an R wave.

Accurate QT measurements are elusive. One reason is that on a given ECG, the end of the T wave is not always obvious; its terminal portion may be isoelectric or merge with a U wave. This partially explains why the precise duration of the QT interval is notoriously difficult to determine, even by cardiologists, and to standardize (39). The problem has not been satisfactorily solved by automated programs, because of technical factors regarding acquisition of digital ECG signals.

The duration of the QT interval is affected by numerous physiologic variables. These include autonomic influences, circadian rhythms, electrolytes, and hormones. For example, the JT interval (i.e., the interval between the J point and the end of the T wave) is significantly shorter in men than in women (262 ± 31 milliseconds versus 316 ± 31 milliseconds), probably because repolarization is modulated by testosterone (40). Repolarization and the QT interval are also affected by drugs, an important reason to monitor QT-interval duration.

Another main factor influencing the QT interval is heart rate. Between the QT and the RR intervals is an inverse relationship that is nonlinear: as the heart rate increases, the QT interval initially shortens markedly and then shortens more gradually. Thus, QT-interval values require adjustment. The normal QT-interval values for a given heart rate are determined with mathematic formulas that estimate the *corrected* QT interval (QTc). Of the several QT correction formulas, that of Bazett ($QTc = QT/\sqrt{RR}$) is the most widely used. The normal value of QTc is up to 0.39 second in men and 0.44 second in women. Yet with the Bazett formula, the QTc remains undercorrected (i.e., artificially shortened) during bradycardia, whereas it paradoxically lengthens at faster rates (41). Alternative formulas to model the relationship between the RR and the QT intervals have improved the prediction of the QTc. Their adoption as part of standardization efforts at the clinical level, however, has not succeeded (42,43).

Expert guidelines for QT-interval measurement recommend measuring it manually in the lead where it is best viewed, averaging the QT-interval duration over three to five beats, and correcting the QT interval for heart rate. The best QT-interval correction formula, however, remains unclear, because none has been prospectively validated (44,45). Ethnic differences in the QT interval have not been demonstrated (46).

NORMAL ELECTROCARDIOGRAPHIC VARIANTS

ECGs as screening tests are requested worldwide daily for a number of purposes. A normal ECG is a good predictor of normal LV function, and it greatly reduces the need to request an echocardiogram to assess systolic function (47).

RSR′ Pattern in Lead V_1

An RSR′ (or rSr′) pattern in lead V1 with a QRS duration less than 0.12 second is present in 2.4% of physiologically normal persons. The R′ wave may correspond to relatively late activation of the crista supraventricularis (48). In certain patients, an rSr′ complex in V_1 may be a manifestation of a left-sided accessory pathway.

$S_1S_2S_3$ Pattern

The $S_1S_2S_3$ pattern has been observed in 20% of healthy subjects. The S waves in standard leads are inscribed when the terminal vector of the QRS complex originates in the outflow tract of the right ventricle or in the posterobasal septum and is directed rightward and superiorly. The typical $S_1S_2S_3$ pattern (with all S waves larger than their preceding R waves) is not as common as the case wherein the amplitude of the S wave in lead I is smaller than that of the R wave.

Male Pattern and Early Repolarization

In men, ST-segment elevation of 1 to 3 mm in one or more precordial leads (typically including V_2) is normal. It is called *male pattern*, and its prevalence decreases with age (49). Precordial ST-segment elevation is found instead only in 20% of healthy women, with no age variation.

Some healthy young men (particularly African Americans) have, in leads V_1 to V_3, ST-segment elevation up to 4 mm mimicking acute myocardial infarction or pericarditis (50,51) (Fig. 59.8). This pattern is called *early repolarization*. However, a premature ventricular recovery has not been demonstrated; the pattern could represent a mild intraventricular conduction delay in the right ventricle. Early repolarization appears to be an independent marker of enhanced aerobic condition (52).

Brugada Syndrome

An ECG pattern similar to that of early repolarization, the *Brugada sign,* consists of a right BBB (RBBB)–like pattern and coved ST-segment elevation in right precordial or inferior leads. The Brugada syndrome seems to be an ion channel disease similar to the long QT syndrome, inherited by an autosomal dominant pattern with variable penetrance (53,54) (Fig. 59.9). It is associated with ventricular tachyarrhythmias and sudden death (55).

The Brugada syndrome and early repolarization may have a common pathophysiologic basis (56). In both entities, ST-segment elevation is influenced by heart rate and autonomic tone.

Unusual T Waves

Negative T waves, particularly in precordial leads (from V_{6R} to V_2, and sometimes through V_6) may be seen among young, usually African American, vagotonic persons. These T waves may show intermittent changes in polarity, and in some cases they follow an elevated ST segment (early repolarization syndrome). Transient inverted T waves have been documented in physiologically normal subjects after meals or after drinking cold water (57). Bifid T waves (i.e., T waves with two peaks different from a U wave) are present in 20% of children; their incidence decreases with age. A likely mechanism producing bifid T waves is a delayed right ventricular repolarization; an asynchronous repolarization of the anterior and posterior walls would inscribe two separate peaks in the T wave.

APPROACH TO ELECTROCARDIOGRAPHIC DIAGNOSIS

Sensitivity, Specificity, and Predictive Accuracy

The ECG is a highly valuable diagnostic tool. ECG diagnoses, however, are made by inference and are therefore subject to error (58). To maximize the benefits from ECG information,

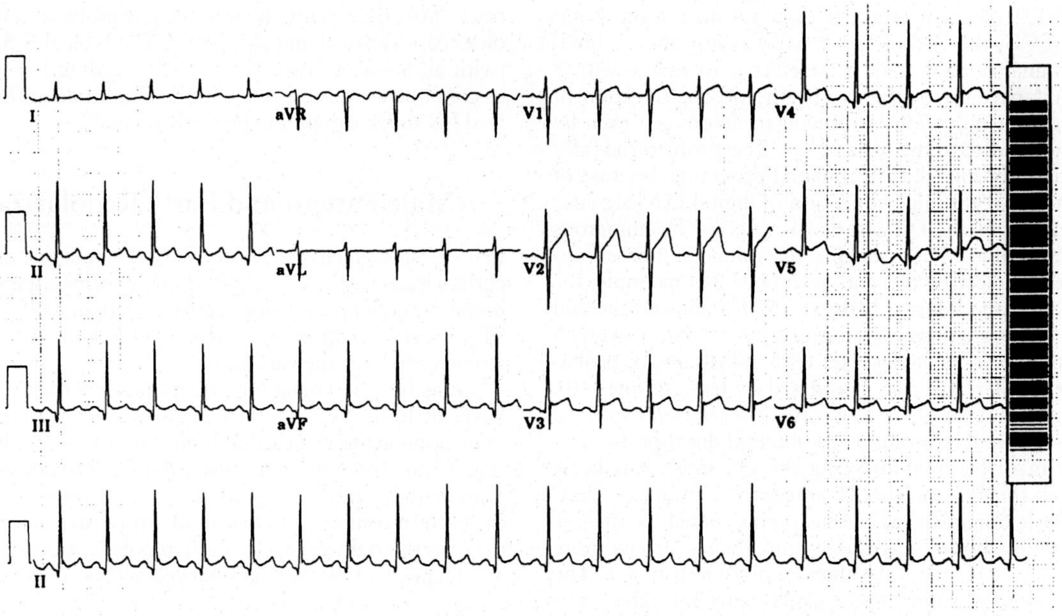

FIGURE 59.8. Electrocardiogram of patient with early repolarization and sinus tachycardia (19-year-old African American woman). ST-segment elevation is present in both inferior and precordial leads.

it is essential to apply the principles of prevalence, sensitivity, specificity, and predictive accuracy. The presence of a sign for a disorder is less informative in a clinically healthy population with a low prevalence of the disorder (59). Disorder prevalences between 40% and 60% result in the maximum drop or rise from pretest to posttest probability (60). *Sensitivity* represents the number of persons with a condition who do have a target ECG sign. A sign with perfect sensitivity will be positive in all patients with the condition; the absence of the sign rules out the condition. *Specificity* refers to the number of persons without a condition who do not have the target ECG sign. A sign with perfect specificity will be negative in all people without the condition; the presence of the sign makes a positive diagnosis. Sensitivity and specificity, however, depend on the spectrum of disease in the studied population.

At the time of requesting an ECG—when it is not known whether a particular disorder is present—a most helpful concept is that of predictive value. The *positive predictive value* is the proportion of patients with positive test results who have the condition. The *negative predictive value* is the proportion of patients with negative results who do not have the condition. Predictive values are clinically useful because they incorporate information on both the test (i.e., the ECG) and the population being tested in a particular setting (61).

Predictive accuracy is the degree to which a positive or negative ECG sign represents what it is actually intended to represent, or its ability to discriminate between two competing states. Accuracy is assessed by comparison with reference techniques ("gold standards") (62).

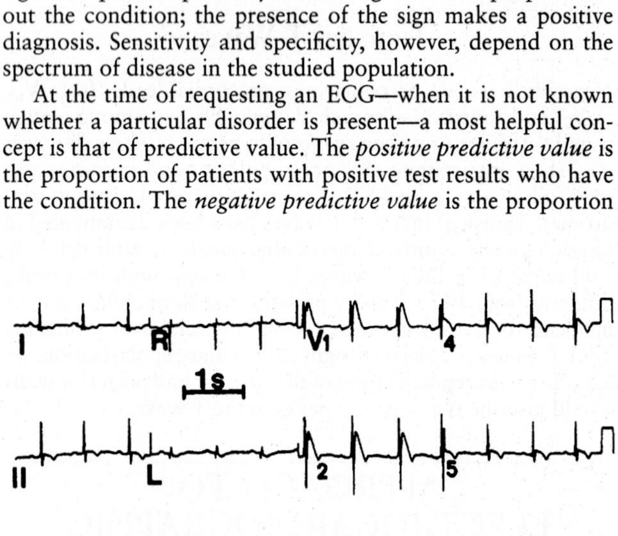

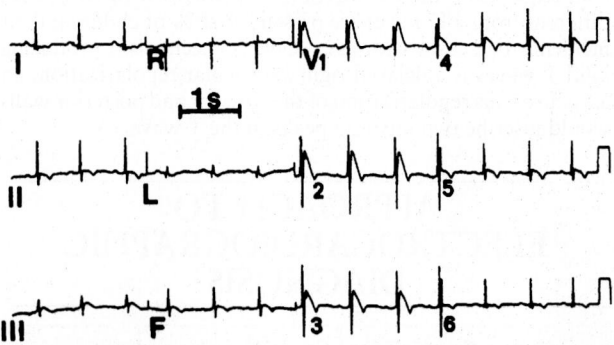

FIGURE 59.9. Electrocardiogram of patient with right bundle branch block and ST-segment elevation in leads V_1 to V_4 (Brugada syndrome). (From Brugada P, Brugada J. Right bundle branch block, persistent ST segment elevation and sudden cardiac death: a distinct clinical and electrocardiographic syndrome: a multicenter report. *J Am Coll Cardiol* 1992;20:1391–1396.)

Choice of a Cutoff Point

Most ECG information relies on continuous values, and a decision must be made about what constitutes an abnormal sign. For values that follow a normal distribution, abnormal results are defined as two standard deviations from the mean of the reference population. Thus, even 5% of normal subjects will have abnormal test results. Selecting a cutoff point involves trading a high sensitivity for a low specificity, or vice versa. The clinician must weigh the relative importance of the sensitivity and specificity of the sign selected for each patient and set the cutoff point accordingly. If false-positive results must be avoided, the cutoff point should be set to ensure high specificity. When false-negative results are undesirable, the cutoff point should be set to ensure high sensitivity. In patients with chest pain, requiring ST-segment elevation of 4 mm in two ECG limb leads would provide high specificity for acute myocardial infarction; however, it would also have poor sensitivity because many patients with acute infarction do not have as much ST-segment elevation. Setting the cutoff at 0.5 mm identifies virtually all patients with acute infarction, but many patients without infarction would also be included.

A graphic way to examine the relation between a test's sensitivity and specificity is provided by receiver-operator characteristic curves (61). The values of the test or sign are plotted along a curve, and their true-positive and false-positive rates (i.e., sensitivity and specificity, respectively) can be determined at each cutoff point. The upper left-hand corner of the curve denotes an ideal ECG sign, with a true-positive rate of 0.1 and

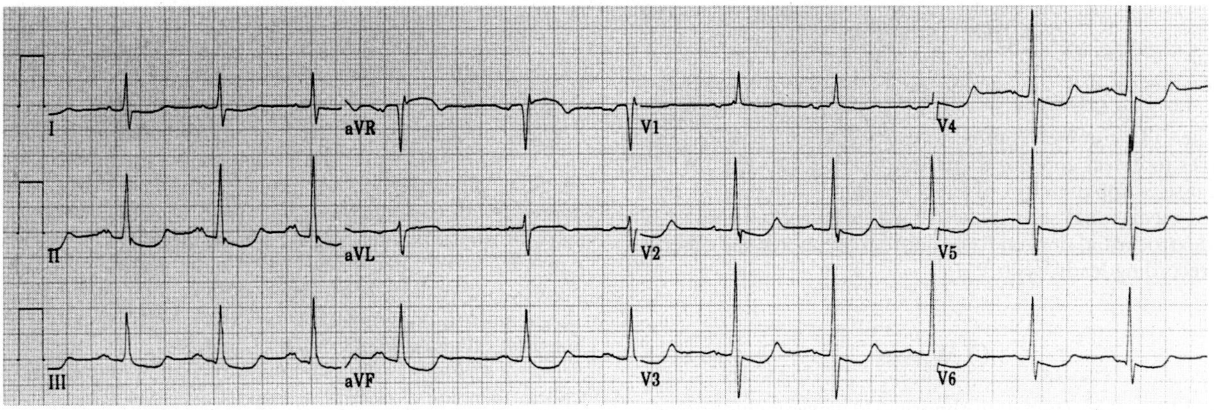

FIGURE 59.10. Left atrial abnormality. The P-wave duration is 0.125 second, and a prominent negative deflection is seen in V_1. Incomplete right bundle branch block and repolarization changes induced by digitalis are also present.

a false-positive rate of 0. The better the sign, the closer its curve will be to the upper left corner.

ABNORMAL ELECTROCARDIOGRAM

QRS Axis Deviation

Although QRS axes between 0 and –30 degrees are sometimes called left axis deviations, they are truly a normal variant. Severe left axis deviations (QRS axes between –30 and –90 degrees) are considered abnormal, but they are found in 2% of healthy adults (63).

Although the term *left axis deviation* is often used interchangeably with left anterior fascicular block (LAFB), left superior displacement of the QRS axis may occur in the absence of LAFB (in inferior myocardial infarction and other disorders). The extent of left axis deviation may vary over short periods of time, perhaps from conduction delays affecting selectively different groups of fibers in the fan-like anterior division of the left bundle branch.

P-Wave Abnormalities

Abnormalities of the P wave reflect disorders of atrial pressure or volume, or an anomalous origin of the cardiac impulse.

Right Atrial Abnormality

Right atrial enlargement has classically been diagnosed in the presence of the following: (a) tall, peaked P waves in leads II, III, and aVF ($\geq$0.25 mV in lead II) ("P pulmonale"); (b) a P-wave axis $\geq$75 degrees; and (c) a positive deflection of the P wave in V_1 or V_2 $\geq$0.15 mV (64). These ECG signs, however, correlate poorly with anatomic findings. The P-wave amplitude may paradoxically decrease as right ventricular hypertrophy progresses. Also, P-wave signs have relatively low sensitivity to detect "pure" right atrial enlargement. The most sensitive ECG manifestations of right atrial abnormality in patients with low prevalence of coronary disease, no chronic pulmonary disease, and no left-sided heart disease seem to be QRS changes in lead V_1 (R/S $\geq$1; presence of Q) (in the absence of RBBB). In addition, ST-segment depression $\geq$0.05 mV in II or aVF (probably representing a prominent atrial repolarization (Ta) wave) is highly specific.

Left Atrial Abnormality

Left atrial enlargement is characterized by the following: (a) a notched P wave with a duration $\geq$0.12 second ("P mitrale"), best observed in leads II and V_1; and (b) a wide terminal negative deflection in lead V_1 (0.1 mV amplitude per 0.4 second duration) (Fig. 59.10). The terminal force of the P wave correlates better with left atrial volume and weight than with atrial pressure (65). No characteristic of the P wave correlates with atrial size (66). The left atrial enlargement pattern signals an intraatrial conduction disturbance; thus, the term *left atrial abnormality* is preferred.

The term *pseudo-P pulmonale* denotes a prominent P wave in inferior leads that is caused by left, rather than right, atrial abnormality. The P wave revealed is enlarged only in its terminal portion, which in V_1 is markedly negative.

Biatrial Enlargement

Biatrial enlargement is characterized by tall P waves in lead II and notched and broad P waves in leads I and II, with a terminal negative deflection in V_1.

Ta Wave

Ta waves may be prominent in atrial hypertrophy or infarction and during pericarditis that has not been promptly detected. In the presence of atrial enlargement, the Ta wave is prolonged and may displace the ST segment, which appears depressed.

PR Interval

A short PR interval in the presence of a normal P-wave axis suggests an abnormally rapid conduction pathway within the AV node or its surroundings (i.e., a bundle of cardiac muscle connecting atria directly with ventricles). An impulse that bypasses the AV node leads to early activation of the ventricular myocardium (ventricular preexcitation). This creates the potential for the electrical impulse to reenter into the atria, producing a tachyarrhythmia (the Wolff-Parkinson-White [WPW] syndrome). When a short PR interval is accompanied by an abnormal P-wave direction, the site of impulse origin has moved from the sinus node to a position closer to the AV node. A prolonged PR interval with a normal P-wave axis indicates a delay in impulse transmission at some point in the pathway between the atrial and ventricular myocardium.

QRS Complex

The absence of R-wave progression from V_1 to V_5 may indicate LV necrosis. In precordial leads, the notching or slurring of the QRS complex is more sensitive than the presence of Q waves to detect anterior infarction, but it is less specific (67). A cause of apparent loss of left precordial R waves is the rightward mediastinal shift induced by a left pneumothorax (68). In dextrocardia, normal R-wave progression may be observed by recording leads V_1 to V_{5R}.

Q Waves

Conditions associated with abnormal Q waves include myocardial infarction or injury, LV hypertrophy (LVH) or dilatation, and intraventricular conduction disturbances (left BBB [LBBB], ventricular pacing and WPW syndrome). Less frequent causes of Q waves include infiltrative myocardial disease, chronic obstructive pulmonary disease (in precordial leads), acute pulmonary embolism, pneumothorax, and misplacement of precordial electrodes (69).

ST Segment

Alterations of the ST segment include elevation and depression, which depend on either of the following two cellular mechanisms, or both: (a) an injury current resulting from a difference in resting membrane potentials between injured and uninjured myocardium; and (b) a voltage gradient generated by a difference in AP plateau amplitudes.

The most important cause of ST-segment elevation is myocardial injury. Another cause is ventricular asynergy, which can produce a pseudoinfarction pattern (see later) (70). Depression of the ST segment occurs during myocardial ischemia and when ventricular repolarization is altered.

QT Interval

Long QT Interval

The malfunction of cardiac channels may lead to an intracellular excess of positive ions (sodium or potassium). This excess prolongs ventricular repolarization and, consequently, the QT interval. A prolonged QTc is a predictor of cardiovascular mortality even in the absence of overt heart disease (71). Causes of long QT interval include myocardial ischemia, cardiomyopathies, hypokalemia, hypocalcemia, autonomic influences, drug effects, hypothermia, and genetics (congenital long QT syndrome).

Ischemia. Acute myocardial ischemia may induce an initial, transient QT shortening followed by extreme QT prolongation. Changes in the QT interval often accompany T-wave or U-wave inversion (72). The QT interval usually normalizes within 72 hours, while inverted T waves may persist.

Hypertrophic Cardiomyopathy. The QT and QTc are prolonged in patients with hypertrophic cardiomyopathy, as a consequence of the increased LV mass (73).

Hypothermia. Hypothermia (core temperatures $\leq$35°C) is associated with sinus bradycardia, which, in turn, is associated with prolongation of the QT interval. In some patients, however, the QTc interval is also abnormal.

Autonomic Dysfunction. Patients with diabetes, alcoholism, and other disorders that cause autonomic dysfunction may show prolonged QT and QTc intervals (74).

Drugs. Antiarrhythmic drugs, the antibiotics erythromycin and ketoconazole, the antihistamine agents astemizole and terfenadine, the phenothiazines, and terodiline all have been associated with prolongation of both the QT and QTc intervals, with torsade de pointes, and with sudden death (75). When new drugs are under clinical development, it is important to test for a propensity to dangerous arrhythmias such as torsade. Because this is unfeasible, regulatory agencies instead require testing for drug-related changes in the QT interval (76). Recently, the selective serotonin reuptake inhibitors and the newer antipsychotic agents (e.g. clozapine, risperidone) have been reported to be associated with arrhythmias and prolonged QTc interval (77). A list of drugs associated with QT-interval prolongation is continuously updated on the Internet (78).

Congenital Long QT Syndrome. Various mutations in ion channel genes cause congenital long QT syndrome (QTc > 0.46 seconds). Five to 10% of gene carriers for this disorder, however, have QTc durations within normal range (79). Patients with the syndrome may also have marked sinus bradycardia. The T wave is often notched or biphasic, or it alternates its morphology or polarity (T-wave alternans) (80–82). Prominent U waves may also be present. The extreme prolongation of the QT interval can result in pseudo 2:1 AV block when every other P wave falls during or before the preceding T wave (29). The long QT-3 variety seems to be caused by mutations in the *SCN5A* gene, which may also underlie the Brugada syndrome.

Short QT interval

In the short QT syndrome, QTc intervals measure less than 320 milliseconds (83). Patients (including children) have a high incidence of ventricular tachyarrhythmias, syncope, sudden cardiac death, or atrial fibrillation. The condition may be associated with missense mutations in *KCNH2 (HERG)*.

T Wave

Abnormalities of the T wave (usually consisting of inverted T waves) are seen in a number of conditions. The T wave is a sensitive detector of repolarization differences over the myocardium, but the magnitude of T-wave changes is not proportional to the extent of myocardium with repolarization abnormalities (9,84). Negative T waves have classically been classified in primary when they result from changes in the duration, shape, or amplitude of ventricular action potentials (as in ischemia, myocarditis, pericarditis, drug effects), and as secondary when changes affect not the ventricular action potential but the activation sequence (as in BBB, ventricular pacing, ventricular hypertrophy, cardiomyopathies, and WPW syndrome) (9,85). This mechanistic dichotomy, however, may be challenged in light of the phenomenon of T-wave memory and perhaps also by that of T-wave alternans, changes that could result from a combination of mechanisms or from "ventricular electrical remodeling" (86).

The term T-wave abnormality has been called into question by the finding that negative T waves that develop in infarct-related ECG leads shortly after thrombolysis are associated with improved survival (87). It appears, however, that such T waves must be dynamic (i.e., revert to positive over time, with exercise, or with dobutamine) to predict myocardial viability and favorable outcome (88,89). Abnormalities of the T wave

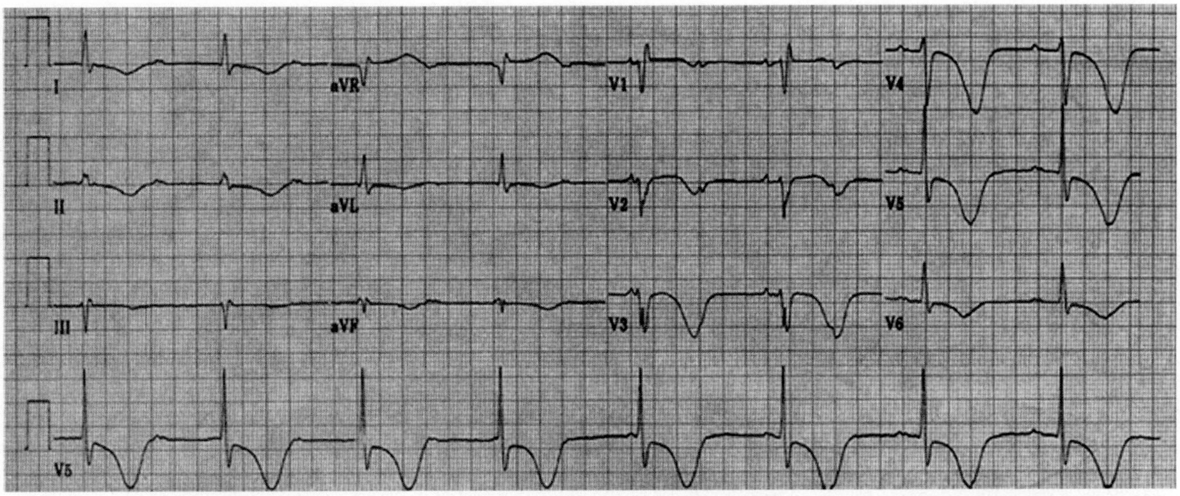

FIGURE 59.11. Memory T waves in a patient with complete atrioventricular block in whom a permanent pacemaker had been temporarily inhibited. The intrinsic rhythm shows a right bundle branch block pattern with deep, wide, negative T waves (positive in aVR) that follow the QRS morphology of the previously paced QRS complex.

on a resting ECG of male patients have been shown, conversely, to predict cardiovascular mortality (90).

Less than 1% of ECGs recorded for any reason show giant, rather permanent negative T waves. They usually correlate with LVH or coronary disease (91).

T-Wave Alternans

Electrical alternans of the T wave results from changes in the duration or the shape of the action potential. It has been documented in the congenital long QT syndrome, in hypocalcemia, and in patients treated with quinidine or amiodarone (92). It is accompanied by variable QT intervals, and it usually heralds ventricular arrhythmias (18).

T-Wave "Memory"

This term describes the aspect of the T waves that seems to "remember" an abnormal activation pattern. The T-wave polarity follows that of a preexistent ectopic QRS complex (93). After cessation of ventricular pacing or intermittent LBBB, in normally conducted beats transient abnormal T waves appear (10,31,94) (Fig. 59.11). Also, in patients with the WPW syndrome who undergo catheter ablation of the accessory pathway, the T-wave polarity is that of the former δ wave (95). Whether the *memory T waves* follow previous ectopic QRS complexes or δ waves, the magnitude and persistence of the T-wave changes are proportional to the duration of the abnormal ventricular activation.

U Waves

Positive, prominent U waves may be seen in patients taking digitalis or quinidine, as well as in the congenital long QT syndrome. Although hypokalemia has been classically associated with prominent U waves, these repolarization waves are more likely bifid or notched T waves. This is important because in hypokalemia, QT-interval measurements should include the entire T wave and should not exclude the last portion, confused with a U wave (19). Negative U waves are highly specific for the presence of heart disease, particularly hypertension, valve regurgitation, and ischemic heart disease (96).

Electrical Alternans

Electrical alternans is an alternation of the morphology of the QRS complex or of the T wave, usually in a 2:1 ratio; the PR interval and the ST segment are affected more rarely. Causes of alternans include myocardial ischemia, ventricular dysfunction, rapid tachycardias, significant pericardial effusion, and acute pulmonary embolism (97,98).

The significance of electrical alternans varies with the underlying condition. The QRS alternans seen during pericardial effusion is a manifestation of mechanical alternans and suggests imminent tamponade. Alternans of the ST segment indicates transmural injury and probable coronary spasm. Overt repolarization alternans (affecting the ST segment, the QT interval, or the T wave) has been associated with ventricular arrhythmias and is relatively common in the congenital long QT syndrome.

VENTRICULAR HYPERTROPHY

Left Ventricular Hypertrophy

LVH develops in response to a pressure or volume overload. Through the increased myocardial mass, a longer time is required for the spread of electrical activation. The thickness of the ventricular muscle correlates with the magnitude of the depolarization front, and so LVH exaggerates the normal ECG pattern of LV predominance. An augmented mean QRS vector is oriented toward the left, posteriorly and superiorly, thereby causing a positive deflection in leads I, II, aVL, V_5, and V_6. The intrinsicoid deflection, the R peak time, and the overall QRS duration are all prolonged (Fig. 59.12). The precordial transitional zone is shifted to the left. An rS pattern is usually observed in V_1 and V_2, although sometimes the initial r wave disappears.

Repolarization of the LV is also delayed. The epicardial cells no longer repolarize early, thus causing the spread of recovery to proceed from endocardium to epicardium. The reversal of the direction of recovery produces negative ST segments and T waves in leads with leftward or posterior orientation. This is

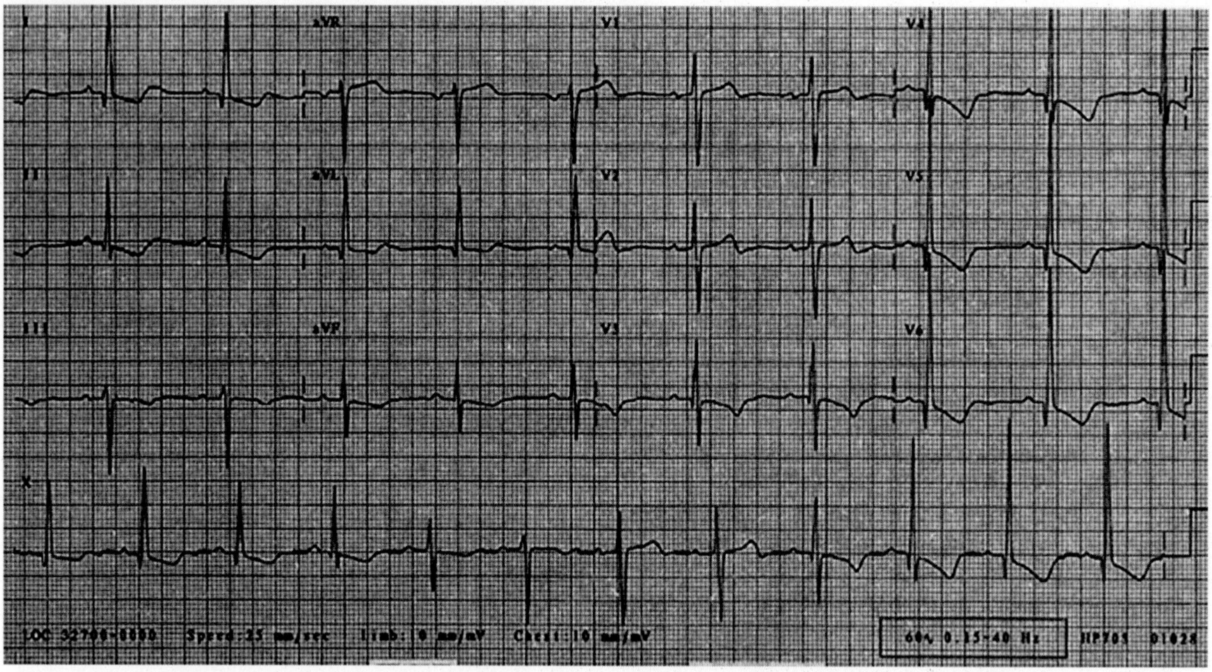

FIGURE 59.12. Left ventricular hypertrophy. Electrocardiogram recorded in an elderly woman with left ventricular pressure overload resulting from aortic stenosis. Note the LV strain. (From Wagner GS, ed. *Marriott's practical electrocardiography*, 9th ed. Baltimore: Williams & Wilkins, 1994:69.)

called *ventricular strain* (99). The development of strain correlates well with LV mass by echocardiography (100), although myocardial ischemia and intraventricular conduction delays may also contribute.

Electrocardiographic Diagnosis

Classic ECG criteria for the detection of LVH are listed in Table 59.2. These criteria are specific but not sensitive (101,102). The criterion with the highest sensitivity is high QRS voltage in precordial leads (103). The product of QRS duration and gender-specific Cornell voltage (the *Cornell product*) seems to provide the best overall accuracy and is not significantly affected by the presence of BBB (104). A strong independent predictor of increased LV mass is left atrial abnormality: each increase of 0.1 mV per second predicts a 30-g increase in LV mass (105). The ECG diagnosis of LVH is difficult, regardless of physician training and testing conditions (15).

Left Ventricular Hypertrophy with Left Bundle Branch Block

Most patients with LBBB also have anatomic LVH, and both entities increase the QRS duration. The best correlation between QRS duration and ventricular mass occurs at QRS widths of up to 135 milliseconds (106). In the presence of LBBB, increased LV mass is strongly predicted by concomitant left atrial abnormality (33). The sum of the amplitudes of the S wave in V_2 and the R wave in V_6 of 4.5 mV or more has a sensitivity of 86% and a specificity of 100% to detect LVH (107).

Left Ventricular Hypertrophy with Left Anterior Fascicular Block

LVH superimposed on LAFB increases the S wave in lead III and the R or S wave (or both) in precordial leads. An index that includes these changes (i.e., (R + S) maximal precordial ≥30 mm + SIII) has 87% specificity and 96% sensitivity for LVH, with a positive predictive value of 89% and a negative predictive value of 95% (108).

Left Ventricular Hypertrophy with Right Bundle Branch Block

The presence of RBBB decreases the sensitivity of the ECG criteria for LVH, particularly for precordial signs. In nonobese patients with RBBB, a Sokolow index ≥35 mm is 100% specific for LVH (109); another useful sign is left atrial abnormality. In lead V_1, each 0.1 mV of increase in the terminal force of the P wave is associated with approximately 25 g of increase in LV mass (110).

Right Ventricular Hypertrophy

The right ventricle dilates either during compensation for a volume overload or after hypertrophy eventually fails to compensate for a pressure overload. This dilation causes stretching of the right bundle branch, which courses from base to apex on the endocardial surface of the right side of the interventricular septum. The impulse conduction is progressively slower, and RBBB develops.

Electrocardiographic Diagnosis

Right ventricular hypertrophy is normal during the first months of life. The QRS axis measures 100 degrees or more, and the QRS complex is predominantly positive in lead V_1 and predominantly negative in V_6. This highly specific pattern for neonatal right ventricular hypertrophy can rarely be found later in life. In adults, ECG changes in response to right pressure overload are not conspicuous because the right ventricular forces must first overcome the left forces (111). Initially, the QRS complex in lead V_1 loses its negative predominance, and a late positive R′ wave may appear. Then, the initial QRS forces move anteriorly (increased R wave in V_1), and the terminal QRS forces move rightward (increased S wave in lead I), with right axis deviation. Marked hypertrophy results in a predominantly positive QRS complex in V_1; the R wave is greater than 0.7 mV, the R/S ratio is greater than 1, and the S wave is less than 0.2 mV (112,113). Repolarization of the right ventricle

TABLE 59.2

CRITERIA FOR THE DIAGNOSIS OF LEFT VENTRICULAR HYPERTROPHY

ROMHILT-ESTES SCORING SYSTEM	
1. R or S in any limb lead ≥0.20 mV or S in lead V_1 or V_2 or R in lead V_5 or V_6 ≥0.30 mV	3 points[a]
2. Left ventricular strain	
ST segment and T wave in opposite direction to QRS complex	
Without digitalis	3 points
With digitalis	1 point
3. Left atrial enlargement	
Terminal negativity of the P wave in lead V_1 is ≥0.10 mV in depth and ≥0.04 s in duration	3 points
4. Left-axis deviation of ≥−30 degrees	2 points
5. QRS duration ≥0.09 s	1 point
6. Intrinsicoid deflection in lead V_5 or V_6 ≥ 0.05 s	1 point
Total	13 points
SOKOLOW-LYON CRITERIA	
S wave in lead V_1 + R wave in lead V_5 or V_6 > 3.50 mV Or R wave in lead V_5 or V_6 > 2.60 mV	
CORNELL VOLTAGE CRITERIA	
Women, R wave in lead aVL + S wave in lead V_3 > 2.00 mV	
Men, R wave in lead aVL + S wave in lead V_3 > 2.80 mV	

[a]Left ventricular hypertrophy, 5 points; probable left ventricular hypertrophy, 4 points.
Data from Romhilt DW, Bove KE, Norris RJ, et al. A critical appraisal of the electrocardiographic criteria for the diagnosis of left ventricular hypertrophy. *Circulation* 1969;40:185; Sokolow M, Lyon TP. The ventricular complex in left ventricular hypertrophy as obtained by unipolar precordial and limb leads. *Am Heart J* 1949;37:161; and Casale PN, Devereux RB, Alonso DR, et al. Improved sex-specific criteria of left ventricular hypertrophy for clinical and computer interpretation of electrocardiograms: validation with autopsy findings. *Circulation* 1987;75:565.

is delayed, producing negativity of both the ST segment and the T wave (ventricular strain). The ECG criteria for right ventricular hypertrophy have poor sensitivity and moderate specificity (114).

Biventricular Hypertrophy

Enlargement of both ventricles may lead to cancellation of opposite forces and can result in a normal ECG. In some patients, tall R waves develop in all precordial leads with prominent, biphasic QRS complexes in midprecordial leads.

BUNDLE BRANCH AND FASCICULAR BLOCKS

An isolated conduction delay in the common His bundle affects the activation of both ventricles; therefore, it does not alter the appearance of the QRS complex. *Unifascicular blocks* occur in RBBB, LAFB, or left posterior fascicle block (LPFB). The mildest manifestation of intraventricular conduction defects is left axis deviation. The conduction time, estimated at baseline with the QRS axis at +90 degrees, increases linearly by a few milliseconds for each left shift of the QRS axis (up to −90 degrees). At −30 degrees, there is an increase of 25 milliseconds (115).

In *bifascicular blocks* the conduction is interrupted in two fascicles (i.e., LBBB, RBBB with LAFB, RBBB with LPFB). These blocks must be detected indirectly by their effects on myocardial activation and the QRS complex because the Purkinje system is not represented on the surface ECG. ECG criteria for bundle branch and fascicular blocks are listed in Table 59.3.

Right Bundle Branch Block

The right ventricle contributes minimally to the normal QRS complex. Thus, RBBB produces little distortion during the time required for LV activation. Figure 59.13 illustrates the slight changes of the early portion of the QRS complex contrasting with the marked distortion of its late portion. Late activation of the normal right ventricular myocardium via the spread of impulses from the LV produces a late prominent R′ wave in lead V_1 that follows the R wave produced by normal left to right activation of the septum. The presence of an RSR′ configuration of the QRS complex is pivotal for the diagnosis of RBBB. This pattern, however, may also be produced by a terminal conduction delay, vectorcardiographically dissimilar to either RBBB or LBBB, that is a manifestation of chronic posterior infarction (116). RSR′ patterns with QRS durations less than 0.120 seconds may correspond to incomplete RBBB or to a normal variant.

Fascicular Blocks

The anterior fascicle activates a portion of the LV that is superior and to the left of that activated by the posterior fascicle. When both fascicles are intact, the impulse travels through them at the same time to depolarize the myocardium. A delay

TABLE 59.3

CRITERIA FOR THE DIAGNOSIS OF BUNDLE BRANCH AND FASCICULAR BLOCKS

DEFINITION OF VENTRICULAR CONDUCTION DELAYS

A. Complete bundle branch blocks
- Qualifying statements:
  - S_1) QRS duration ≥0.120 s (adults)
  - S_2) Supraventricular rhythm
  - S_3) Absence of WPW pattern
- Criteria for a complete bundle branch block:
  - a) S_1 and S_2 and S_3
- 1. Complete RBBB
  - Qualifying statements:
    - S_1) R′ or r′ in V_1 or V_2
    - S_2) S duration >R duration in I and V_6
    - S_3) S duration >0.040 s in I and V_6
    - S_4) R peak time >0.050 s in V_1 or V_2
  - Criteria for RBBB:
    - a) S_1 and S_2 or
    - b) S_1 and S_3 or
    - c) S_4 and (S_2 or S_3)
- 2. Complete LBBB
  - Qualifying statements:
    - S_1) Broad and notched or slurred R in I and V_5 or V_6
    - S_2) Absence of Q wave in I and V_5 and V_6
    - S_3) R peak times ≥0.060 s in V_5 or V_6
    - Criteria for LBBB:
    - a) S_1 and S_2 and S_3
- 3. Nonspecific (unspecified) intraventricular block
  - All cases with QRS duration >0.12 s that do not meet the criteria for LBBB or RBBB

B. Incomplete bundle branch blocks
- 1. Incomplete LBBB
  - Qualifying statements:
    - S_1) QRS duration ≥0.100 s and QRS duration <0.120 s
    - S_2) Absence of Q waves in I and V_5 or V_6
    - S_3) R peak time >0.060 s in V_5 or V_6
  - Criteria for incomplete LBBB:
    - a) S_1 and S_2 and S_3
- 2. Incomplete RBBB
  - Qualifying statements:
    - S_1) QRS duration <0.120 s
    - S_2) r′ or R′ in V_1 or V_2
    - S_3) R′ > R in V_1 or V_2
    - S_4) R peak time >0.050 s in V_1 or V_2
  - Criteria for incomplete RBBB:
    - a) S_1 and S_2 and S_3 or
    - b) S_1 and S_4

C. Fascicular blocks
- 1. LAFB
  - Qualifying statements:
    - S_1) QRS duration <0.120 s
    - S_2) QRS axis ≤−45 degrees
    - S_3) QRS axis ≤−30 degrees and QRS axis >−45 degrees
    - S_4) rS pattern in II and III and aVF
    - S_5) qR pattern in aVL
    - S_6) R peak time ≥0.045 s in aVL
    - S_7) Slurred R downstroke in aVL
    - S_8) Slurred S in V_5 or V_6
  - Criteria for uncomplicated LAFB:
    - a) S_1 and S_2 and S_4 and S_5 and S_6 or
    - b) S_1 and S_2 and S_4 and S_5 and S_7 or
    - c) S_1 and S_2 and S_4 and S_5 and S_8

(Continued)

TABLE 59.3

CRITERIA FOR THE DIAGNOSIS OF BUNDLE BRANCH AND FASCICULAR BLOCKS (CONTINUED)

Qualifying statement:
S_4 is usually present with criteria a, b, and c above. If there is a QS in lead II, LAFB cannot be differentiated from interior myocardial infarction.
Criteria for possible uncomplicated LAFB:
a) S_1 and S_3 and S_4 and S_5 and S_6 or
b) S_1 and S_3 and S_4 and S_5 and S_7 or
c) S_1 and S_3 and S_4 and S_5 and S_8

2. LPFB
Qualifying statements:
S_1) QRS duration <0.120 s
S_2) QRS axis >90 degrees and QRS axis <180 degrees
S_3) R in III > R in II (S_3 is a consequence of S_2)
S_4) qR pattern in III and aVF with Q duration ≤0.040 s
S_5) absence of other causes of right-axis deviation
Criteria for LPFB:
a) S_1 and S_2 and S_3 and S_4 and S_5

LAFB, left anterior fascicular block; LBBB, left bundle branch block; LPFB, left posterior fascicular block; RBBB, right bundle branch block; WPW, Wolff-Parkinson-White syndrome.
From Willems JL, Robles Da Medina EO, Bernard R, et al. Criteria for intraventricular conduction disturbances and pre-excitation. *J Am Coll Cardiol* 1985;5:1261–1275.

of impulse conduction in one fascicle results in asynchronous activation of the LV.

LAFB is common and benign; LPFB is rare (117). Fascicular blocks are often associated with coronary artery disease. In autopsy studies, LAFB is most frequently associated with anterior infarction from proximal left anterior descending (LAD) artery occlusion. Posterior infarction, however, is not usually associated with LPFB; in LPFB, autopsies show massive infarct of the septum (compromising both the anterior and posterior areas) and widespread damage of the left bundle branch (118).

Left Anterior Fascicular Block

In epidemiologic surveys, LAFB is the most common conduction abnormality, perhaps because the left anterior fascicle is located in the outflow tract and in apposition to the aortic ring, which makes it susceptible to increases in intraventricular pressure and disorders of the aortic valve. The initial ventricular activation in LAFB spreads inferiorly and rightward via the left posterior fascicle (4). Block in the anterior fascicle removes the competition from activation directed superiorly and leftward, and Q waves appear in leads with their positive electrode on the left arm (I and aVL) (Fig. 59.14). The impulse arrives at the inferior and apical myocardium in retrograde fashion from the posterior fascicle with a minimal delay that prolongs the QRS by 0.02 second. The remainder of the left anterior ventricular wall is activated in a superior, leftward, and counterclockwise direction. These terminal forces are first represented in lead aVL and then in aVR. Thus, the peak of the terminal R in lead aVL precedes the peak of the terminal R wave in a simultaneously recorded lead aVR (119). The R waves in leads I and aVL are prominent, and the large amplitude of the R wave in aVL may mimic LVH. Prominent S waves are seen in leads II, III and aVF, causing a leftward shift of the QRS axis. This QRS axis deviation is the major criterion for the diagnosis of LAFB (17).

Left Posterior Fascicular Block

LPFB is usually associated with RBBB; its isolated form is rare. The reason for the low incidence of LPFB may be that the posterior fascicle is short and thick, lies in the less turbulent LV inflow tract, and may be "protected" by its dual blood supply from the anterior and posterior descending coronary arteries (4). LPFB occurs in coronary disease, cardiomyopathies, aortic valve disease, and calcification of the LV skeleton (120).

When the left posterior fascicle is blocked, the initial activation of the LV free wall occurs via the left anterior fascicle (4). The excitation front is directed superiorly and leftward. No

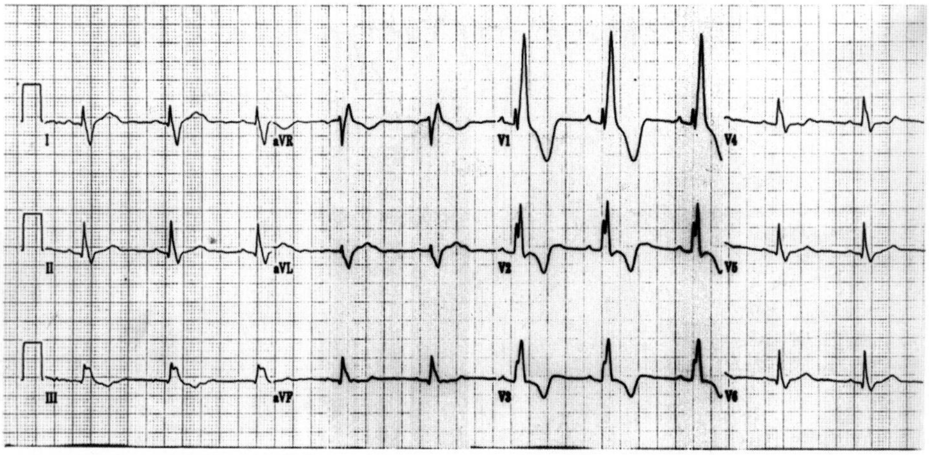

FIGURE 59.13. Right bundle branch block. The patient may also have right ventricular hypertrophy.

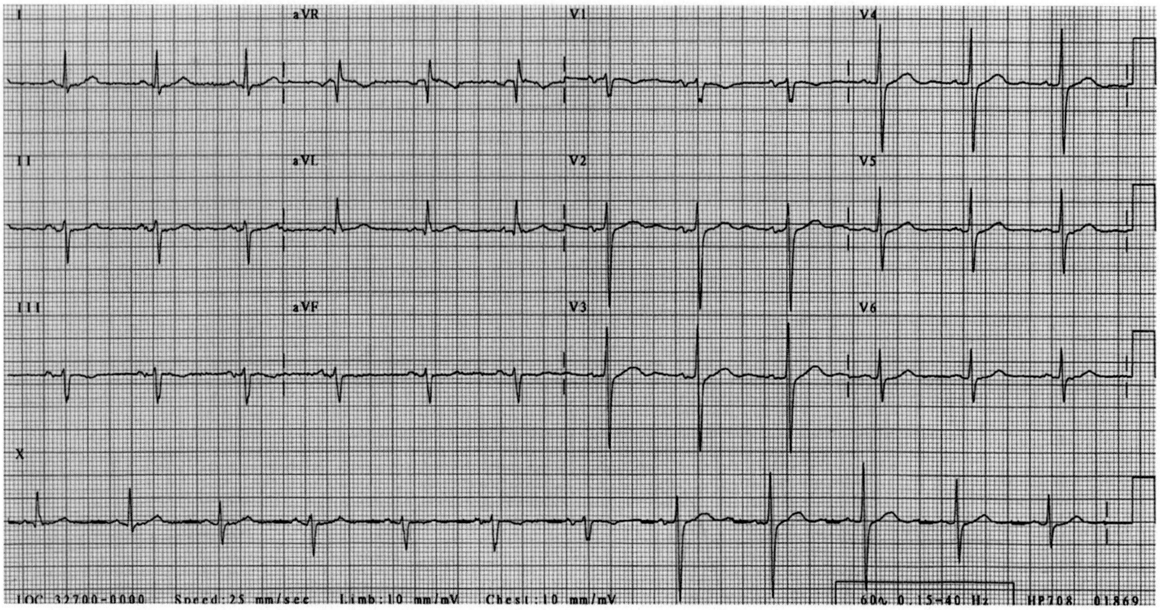

FIGURE 59.14. Left anterosuperior fascicular block. (From Wagner GS, ed. *Marriott's practical electrocardiography,* 9th ed. Baltimore: Williams & Wilkins, 1994:89.)

forces travel inferiorly or rightward, and thus Q waves appear in leads with their positive electrode on the left leg (leads II, III and aVF). Next, the activation wave spreads over the remainder of the LV free wall in an inferior and rightward direction. This produces prominent R waves in leads II, III, and aVF and prominent S waves in leads I and aVL causing a rightward shift of the QRS axis to at least +90 degrees (121). The diagnosis of LPFB is made only in the absence of right ventricular hypertrophy because this condition itself can produce the same ECG pattern as LPFB.

Left Septal Fascicle and Left Septal Fascicular Block

Between the anterior and posterior fascicles of the His bundle are discrete fibers that form a left septal fascicle. This fascicle is subject to great anatomic variation but contributes to the propagation of the cardiac impulse (122,123). The existence of left septal fascicular block is controversial. Proposed ECG criteria for left septal fascicular block include loss of septal q waves (in the absence of other causes of abnormal septal activation) and a QRS duration of 100 milliseconds or more (124).

Left Bundle Branch Block

LBBB may be caused by disease in the main left bundle branch (predivisional) or in its fascicles (postdivisional). In either case, it produces marked distortion of the QRS complex (Fig. 59.15). In a screening ECG, the presence of LBBB correlates well with LV systolic dysfunction (21).

Normally, the interventricular septum is activated from left to right. This inscribes an initial R wave in the right precordial

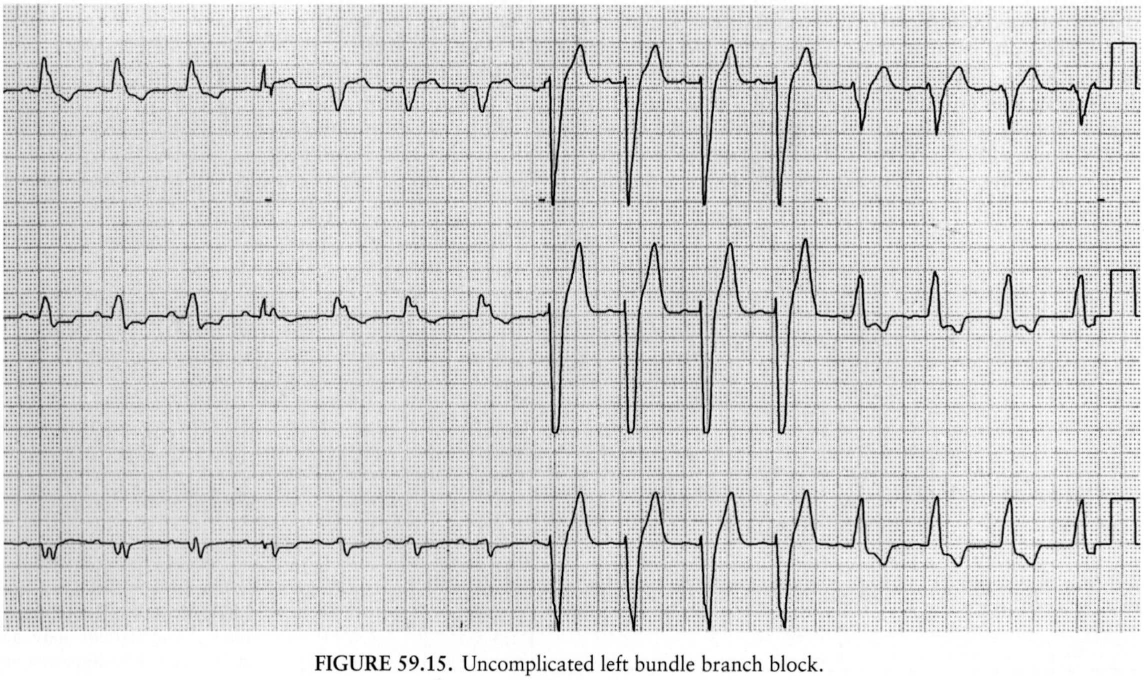

FIGURE 59.15. Uncomplicated left bundle branch block.

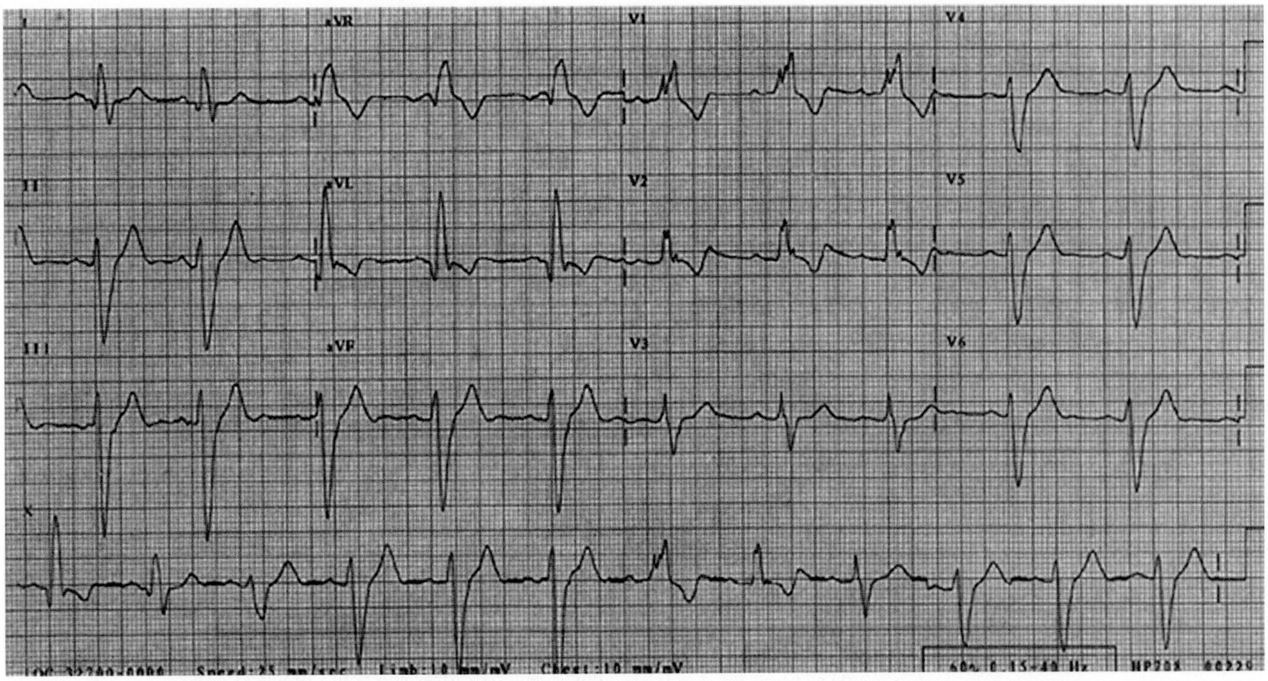

FIGURE 59.16. Right bundle branch block and left anterior fascicular block. The patient is a 66-year-old man with fibrosis of the conduction system. The markedly prolonged QRS duration (0.20 second) suggests underlying left ventricular hypertrophy. (From Wagner GS, ed. *Marriott's practical electrocardiography,* 9th ed. Baltimore: Williams & Wilkins, 1994:94.)

leads and a q wave in leads I and aVL and in left precordial leads. During LBBB, the septum is activated instead from right to left. This produces initial Q waves in right precordial leads, whereas the q waves in V_5 and V_6 disappear. The ventricular activation front then proceeds from the left interventricular septum to the adjacent anterior superior and inferior walls and then to the posterolateral free wall. This sequence of activation tends to produce monophasic QRS complexes: QS in lead V_1 and R in leads I, aVL, and V_6.

LBBB is characterized by secondary repolarization changes of opposing polarity to that of the main QRS deflection. For leads with a predominantly negative QRS complex, this results in an ECG pattern of ST-segment elevation with positive T waves, similar to the current of injury observed during acute coronary occlusion. Uncomplicated LBBB thus resembles anterior wall myocardial infarction (Fig. 59.15), and when left axis deviation is also present, the repolarization pattern mimics that of inferior infarct. The most important differential diagnosis of LBBB is the ECG pattern of the "corrected" transposition of the great vessels. In this condition, propagation of the impulse is reversed, and the initial QRS force shows the same direction as in LBBB, but QRS duration is normal.

Nonspecific Intraventricular Block

A QRS duration of 0.11 second or greater that does not satisfy the criteria for either RBBB or LBBB is considered a nonspecific intraventricular block (17).

Right Bundle Branch Block with Left Anterior Fascicular Block

LAFB often accompanies RBBB. The diagnosis is made by the late prominent R or R′ wave in V_1 typical of RBBB and by the initial R waves and prominent S waves in leads II, III, and aVF seen in LAFB. The QRS duration should be at least 0.12 second, and the frontal plane axis should be between −45 and −120 degrees (Fig. 59.16).

Right Bundle Branch Block with Left Posterior Fascicular Block

This combination is less common. The diagnosis can be made only if there is no clinical evidence of right ventricular hypertrophy. The diagnosis of RBBB with LPFB should be considered when in V_1 there is typical RBBB, and leads I and aVL show the initial R waves and prominent S waves of LPFB. The QRS duration should be 0.12 second or greater, and the frontal plane axis should measure 90 degrees or more.

Trifascicular Blocks

ECG documentation of trifascicular block during 1:1 AV conduction is rare and requires the presence of alternating RBBB and LBBB or fixed RBBB with alternating LAFB or LPFB (4). When both bundle branches are simultaneously affected by block, the ECG shows complete AV block. When the degree of block differs between the two bundle branches, ECG manifestations vary and include, for example, a shorter PR interval preceding either RBBB or LBBB or a complete BBB with a prolonged PR interval (9).

ABERRANCY

Aberrant intraventricular conduction is the abnormal, asynchronous propagation of an impulse through the His-Purkinje system resulting in an altered QRS complex. This definition excludes conduction of supraventricular impulses via accessory pathways that bypass the AV node. Changes in the QRS complex may affect its duration, axis, or amplitude; successive aberrant beats may mimic ventricular tachycardia (125).

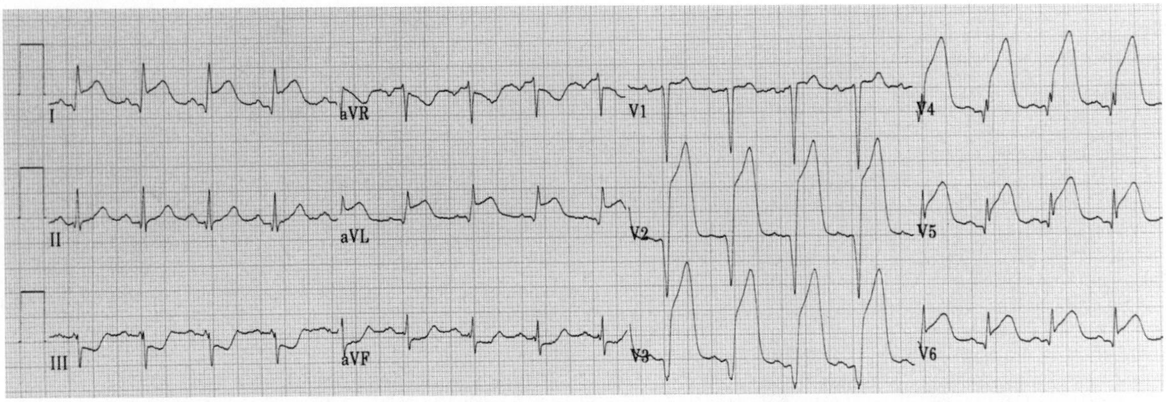

FIGURE 59.17. Acute anterior myocardial infarction, with ST-segment elevation in precordial leads (day 1). The presence of ST-segment elevation in leads I and aVL, in addition to ST-segment depression in leads III and aVF, suggests proximal left anterior descending artery occlusion.

ISCHEMIC HEART DISEASE

Myocardial Ischemia and Injury

Occlusion of a coronary artery or one of their branches leads to interruption of the blood supply and causes myocardial ischemia and injury. During myocardial ischemia, myocytes partially depolarize, and their membrane resting potential is reduced (i.e., becomes less negative). The action potential duration and amplitude then decrease. Local injury currents develop between ischemic and nonischemic cells that manifest in the ECG as ST-segment deviation toward the specifically involved area.

The first ECG change is the development of peaked, tall T waves, followed by elevation of the ST segment (126). The ischemic zone is electrically more negative than its surrounding myocardial area during the recovery phase. Thus, while ST-segment elevation is still present or after it has subsided, the T waves become inverted in relation to the QRS complexes. The T-wave inversion may regress within minutes or may persist for several months (9). These T-wave changes are not specific or sensitive for the diagnosis of myocardial ischemia (40). Factors other than ischemia (e.g., reperfusion, sympathetic denervation) may conceivably have a role in the genesis of negative T waves (40).

For the diagnosis of myocardial injury, one of the following criteria is required: (a) elevation of the origin of the ST segment at the J point of $\geq$0.10 mV in two or more limb or precordial leads V_4 to V_6 or $\geq$0.20 mV in two or more precordial leads V_1 to V_3 (Figs. 59.17 to 59.19) or (b) depression of the origin of the ST segment at the J point of $\geq$0.10 mV in two or more leads V_1 to V_3 or ST-segment elevation greater than 0.10 mV in two or more leads V_7 to V_9. Severe degrees of ischemia are associated with distortion of the later part of the QRS complex, which reverses after the acute phase (127).

A highly specific marker of myocardial injury is alternans of the ST segment. Electrical alternans consists of alternans of the degree of ST-segment elevation, and it is secondary to variations in action potential duration or amplitude. Alternating ST-segment elevation and depression have not been reported (31). The classic notion that transmural injury is characterized by ST-segment elevation while nontransmural ("subendocardial") injury is characterized by ST-segment depression has not been confirmed with imaging studies (128).

When insufficient coronary blood flow persists after the myocardial metabolic reserves have been depleted, the process of necrosis or myocardial infarction begins (129). Permanent new Q waves develop at some point after ST-segment elevation or depression has occurred. In ECG leads in which rapid q waves are normally present (Table 59.4), these waves may become pathologically wide.

Subendocardial Injury

Ischemia secondary to an increased metabolic demand (e.g., exercise) initially affects the subendocardium. Myocytes are less susceptible to ischemia during electrical depolarization than during electrical recovery; this is why the ECG changes involve

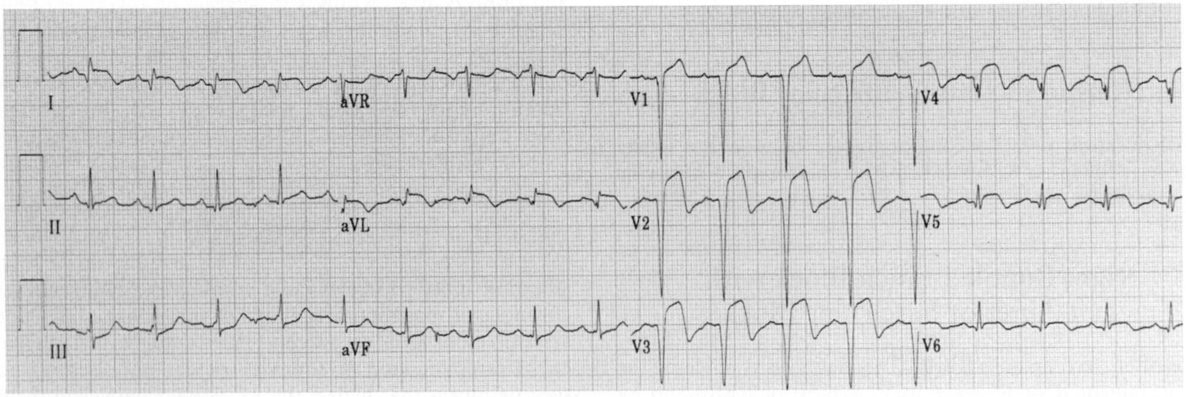

FIGURE 59.18. Subacute anterior myocardial infarction (day 2). ST-segment elevation is regressing, and negative T waves and new Q waves are developing.

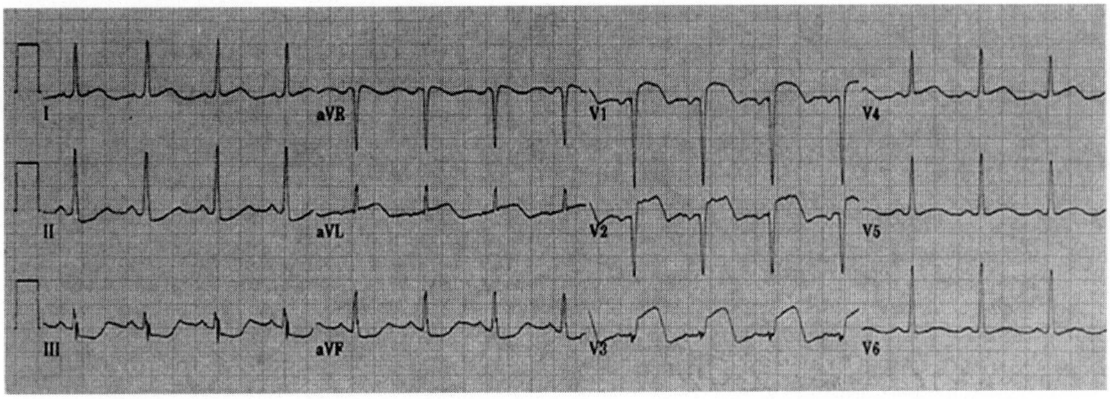

FIGURE 59.19. Acute anterior myocardial infarction. Transmural injury is manifested by ST-segment elevation of greater than 0.2 mV in leads V_1 to V_3.

mainly the ST-T waveforms (and much less the QRS complex). Initial changes include a depression of the J point of at least 0.10 mV and a horizontal or downward sloping of the ST segment toward the T wave. The T wave may or may not be altered in the same direction as the ST segment. T-wave inversion may be secondary to ST-segment depression (i.e., the T wave is "dragged" by the ST segment), or it may change as a direct manifestation of delayed repolarization in the ischemic myocardium. The ST-segment depression of subendocardial injury resolves rapidly after removal of the cardiovascular stress. When the ST-segment depression persists in the absence of increased LV workload, the diagnosis of subendocardial infarction should be considered. Ischemia-related ST-segment depression may also occur as a mirror phenomenon of injury that has induced ST-segment elevation in the myocardial area opposite the surface electrode.

Acute ST-Segment Elevation Myocardial Infarction

The evolutionary changes during acute infarction include (a) ST-segment elevation often preceded by tall T waves, (b) abnormal Q waves, and (c) return of ST-segment elevation to baseline with T wave inversion. The most typical change involves ST-segment elevation, which decreases significantly after the first 12 hours of chest pain (130) (Figs. 59.17 and 59.18). In some patients, multiple episodes of ST-segment elevation and resolution occur after thrombolytic therapy. Moderate ST-segment elevation usually persists for several days; its persistence beyond 2 weeks suggests ventricular aneurysm. If coronary reperfusion is rapidly achieved, Q waves may not develop.

TABLE 59.4

NORMAL VALUES OF THE Q WAVE

Limb leads		Precordial leads	
Lead	Upper limit (s)	Lead	Upper limit (s)
I	<0.03	V_1	0
II	<0.03	V_2	0
III	—	V_3	0
aVR	—	V_4	<0.02
aVL	<0.03	V_5	<0.03
aVF	<0.03	V_6	<0.03

Modified from Wagner GS, Freye CJ, Palmen ST, et al. Evaluation of a QRS scoring system for estimating myocardial infarct size. I: Specificity and observor agreement. *Circulation* 1982;65:345.

CLINICAL VALUE OF THE ELECTROCARDIOGRAM DURING ACUTE MYOCARDIAL INFARCTION

In general, the 12-lead ECG is specific but only moderately sensitive to detect acute myocardial injury (131,132). Systematically recording leads V_{4R}, V_8, and V_9 (i.e., a 15-lead ECG) increases the probability of detecting ST-segment elevation, with no decrease in specificity (8). The infarction descriptors "anterior," "inferior," and "lateral" have classically been attributed to occlusions of the LAD, right coronary artery (RCA), and left circumflex artery (LCX), respectively. Other terms such as "apical," "septal," "high lateral," and "posterior" are also in use. However, the 12-lead ECG is only moderately accurate to determine the anatomic location of acute infarction, and the correspondence of some ECG terms with the pertinent site of infarction is rather poor. The ECG is most sensitive to detect acute occlusion of the LAD and is least sensitive for involvement of the circumflex artery. Automated diagnoses (i.e., provided by the electrocardiographer) are specific but not sensitive; their most promising application is in the prehospital setting (133–135). Among patients presenting to the emergency department with chest pain and ST-segment elevation in the 12-lead ECG, the cause of ST-segment elevation is often uncomplicated LVH (136).

Acute Anterior/Anteroseptal/Anterolateral Infarction (Left Anterior Descending Coronary Artery Occlusion)

During acute anterior injury, the maximal ST-segment elevation is best recorded in V_2 or V_3 (137) (Figs. 59.17 and 59.18); V_2 is the most sensitive lead to record ST-segment elevation (sensitivity: 99%) and to identify the culprit lesion at the LAD. The most powerful predictors of *proximal* LAD occlusion include ST-segment elevation in aVL or aVR, concomitant ST-segment depression in inferior leads, ST-segment depression in V_5, and disappearance of preexistent septal Q waves in lateral leads (138–143).

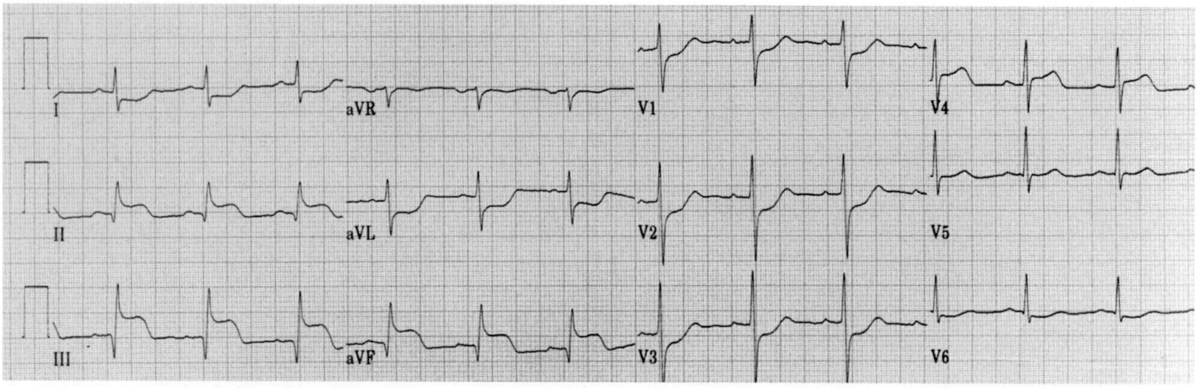

FIGURE 59.20. Acute inferior myocardial infarction. Transmural inferior injury is accompanied by ST-segment depression in leads I, aVL, and V_1 to V_3.

Lead V_1 captures electrical phenomena from the right paraseptal area, which is supplied by the septal branches of the LAD and by a conal branch of the RCA (double circulation). This explains why patients with anterior myocardial infarction usually have no ST-segment elevation in V_1 (43) (Fig. 59.19). The presence of ST-segment elevation in V_1 correlates strongly with ST-segment elevation in V_3R and predicts the less common anatomic scenario in which a small conal branch of the RCA does not reach the interventricular septum (144).

Acute Inferior Infarction (Right Coronary or Circumflex Artery Occlusion)

The typical ECG pattern of inferior infarction consists of ST-segment elevation in leads II, III, and aVF (Fig. 59.20). In 80% to 90% of patients, the culprit lesion is in the RCA (145); in the remainder, the lesion is in the LCX. Occlusion of the RCA is more likely if the ST-segment elevation in lead III is higher than in lead II (146,147), or if ST-segment depression is present in aVL (148), because lead aVL directly opposes the inferior wall. Inferior ST-segment elevation accompanied by anterior ST-segment depression instead is more likely to indicate LCX occlusion (Fig. 59.21). Horizontal ST-segment depression in V_1 to V_3/V_4 (Fig. 59.21) signals posterior wall motion abnormalities (149).

A seemingly alarming ECG is that with a combined anterior and inferior ST-segment elevation. These patients, however, have occlusion of either the proximal RCA or the medial to distal LAD. Their infarct size is limited (150).

Acute Lateral and Posterior Infarctions (Left Circumflex Artery Occlusion)

The LCX supplies a rather small ventricular area. Thus, during LCX occlusion, fewer than half the patients will have ST-segment elevation. This ST-segment elevation is usually seen in leads II, III, and aVF, followed by leads V_5, V_6, and aVL (151). There may be concomitant ST-segment depression in leads V_1 to V_3 (Fig. 59.21).

Of all patients with chest pain from LCX occlusion, one third present with isolated ST-segment depression; ST-segment depression in V_1 to V_2 is a sensitive sign (44). Another third of patients present without any ECG changes. This applies only to the 12-lead ECG; in posterior leads (V_7 through V_9), ST-segment elevation is usually detected and is associated with posterior wall motion abnormalities. For posterior infarction, leads V_7 to V_9 are more specific than precordial leads (84% versus 57%) (152). When ST-segment elevation is present in leads V_5 and V_6, posterolateral injury, triggered by either LCX or RCA occlusion, can be suspected (153).

Acute Right Ventricular Infarction

Right ventricular infarction is usually concurrent with infarction of the inferior wall (Fig. 59.22). At least half of patients

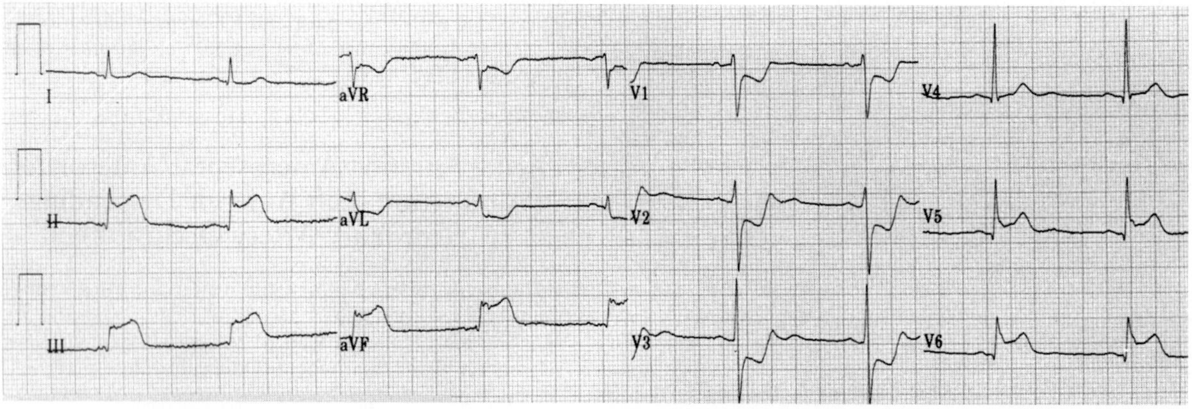

FIGURE 59.21. Acute inferior myocardial infarction produced by circumflex artery occlusion. ST-segment elevation is present in leads V_5 and V_6 (suggesting "megaartery" occlusion), and ST-segment depression with prominent U waves is seen in leads V_1 to V_3. The ST-segment depression in aVL is unusual.

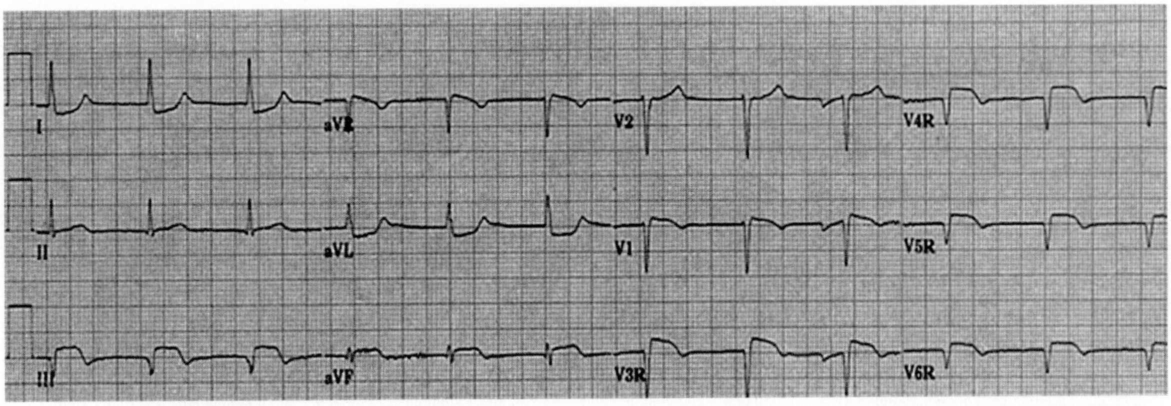

FIGURE 59.22. Inferior infarct with right ventricular compromise. Right-sided precordial leads V_2R to V_6R show ST-segment elevation.

with inferior injury have ST-segment elevation in V_4R; sensitivity and predictive accuracy for right ventricular infarction are both 93% (154). Right ventricular injury may also result in ST-segment depression in lead aVL (high sensitivity and specificity) (155) and ST-segment elevation in precordial leads, whereas ST-segment elevation in V_1 is highly specific for proximal RCA occlusion (44). The ST-segment elevation rarely extends to lead V_5. Anterior injury can be ruled out because, toward V_4, the ST-segment elevation of right ventricular injury does not increase but rather decreases. Isolated right ventricular infarction is rare and occurs mainly in patients with right ventricular hypertrophy (156).

ST-Segment Depression in Patients with Acute Coronary Syndromes

Isolated ST-Segment Depression

Approximately half of patients presenting with isolated ST-segment depression in the 12-lead ECG will develop infarction. Whether patients with ST-segment depression develop infarction or not, their 1-year mortality is high (157). ST-segment depression is associated with older age, multivessel disease, multiple infarctions, or poor LV function. A common cause of ST-segment depression is subocclusion of the left main coronary artery; the ECG shows ST-segment depression in leads I, II, or aVF with LAFB (158). When the isolated ST-segment depression is maximum in leads V_2 to V_3, it indicates LCX occlusion instead. Recognizing it is important because such patients may benefit from reperfusion therapies (159).

ST-Segment Depression Concomitant with ST-Segment Elevation

Many patients with acute chest pain present with "reciprocal" ST-segment depression, i.e., ST-segment depression concomitant with ST-segment elevation in a different lead group. Such ST-segment depression is assumed to represent mirroring, a phenomenon of electrical reflection of the transmural injury onto the opposite ventricular wall. The ST-segment depression is captured by a lead placed at 180 degrees of the lead recording ST-segment elevation, but the terms *reciprocal* and *mirror* are also loosely applied to other recording points (160). For example, a maximal ST-segment depression in V_5 to V_6 is the reciprocal of ST-segment elevation in V_{3R} (i.e., right ventricular injury) (40).

Another possible mechanism for ST-segment depression is regional subendocardial ischemia or infarction. Although strictly speaking mirroring is also involved in the ST-segment depression of subendocardial ischemia (because the ST-segment elevation in the subendocardial layer is reflected onto the epicardial layer), most clinicians consider this ST-segment depression "nonmirror" because it is a primary manifestation of artery occlusion, not secondary to ST-segment elevation in a different territory (161). In patients with chest pain and predominant ST-segment depression in any lead except aVR, ST-segment depression of at least 0.4 mV is 97% specific for acute infarction (45). Several investigators have found that inferior ST-segment depression during anterior injury is not accompanied by inferior ischemia (as assessed by perfusion imaging), a finding suggesting that mirroring, rather than inferior subendocardial ischemia, is responsible for the ST-segment depression (46). More than 85% of patients with ST-segment depression in lead aVF have a culprit lesion in the proximal LAD. Conversely, the significance of anterior ST-segment depression accompanying inferior injury may depend on the leads involved. The ST-segment depression of leads V_1 to V_3 or I to aVL seems to correspond to mere mirroring, often from LCX occlusion. An ST-segment depression deeper in V_4 to V_6 than in V_1 to V_3 is associated with anterolateral or septal subendocardial injury from a severe lesion in the LAD or in the left main coronary artery (Fig. 59.23) (162). In patients with acute ST-segment elevation and no confounding ECG factors, ST-segment depression has a specificity and positive predictive value of 93% for the diagnosis of acute myocardial infarction (163).

Nonischemic ST-Segment Depression

The most important differential diagnosis in patients with ST-segment depression and chest pain (with or without abnormal levels of creatine kinase) is aortic dissection (164). As many as 50% of patients with dissection of the thoracic aorta may present with ECG abnormalities, mainly ST-segment depression (165). When the origin of a coronary artery is involved in the dissection, signs of transmural injury develop.

Diagnosis of Acute Myocardial Infarction in the Presence of Confounding Factors and the Nondiagnostic Electrocardiogram

Diagnosis of Evolving Acute Myocardial Infarction in the Presence of Right Bundle Branch Block

The diagnosis of acute anterior infarction in patients with RBBB can be suspected when T waves of opposite polarity to the QRS complex in leads V_1 to V_3, or V_4 are replaced by QRS-concordant T waves ("pseudonormalization"). ST-segment elevation is usually easily detected.

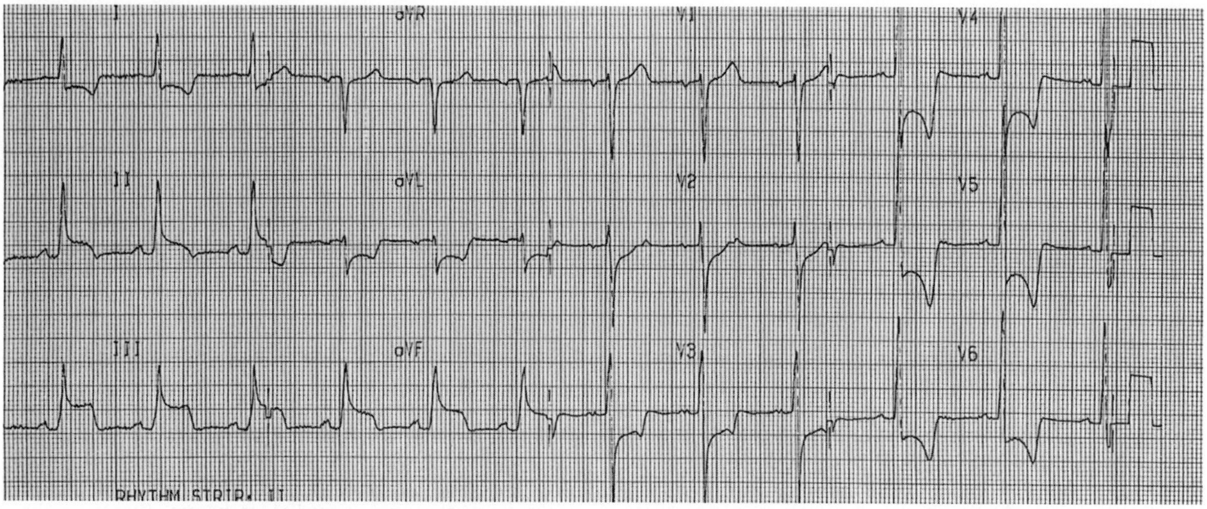

FIGURE 59.23. Electrocardiogram recorded in a patient with ST-segment elevation in inferior leads from acute right coronary thrombosis. The concomitant precordial ST-segment depression, maximum in V_3 to V_6, probably corresponds to concurrent subendocardial injury. (From Wagner GS, ed. *Marriott's practical electrocardiography,* 9th ed. Baltimore: Williams & Wilkins, 1994:140.)

Diagnosis of Evolving Acute Myocardial Infarction in the Presence of Left Bundle Branch Block

In patients who present with acute chest pain and LBBB, the changes in the normal sequence of ventricular activation by both LBBB and acute injury make ECG interpretation difficult. This may result in unnecessary hospital admissions (166). Careful examination of the ECG in a patient with LBBB reveals that during acute myocardial injury, further ST-segment elevation does occur (167–169) (Table 59.5; Fig. 59.24). The presence of ST-segment elevation $\geq$0.1 mV concordant with the QRS polarity is the most specific sign (170,171).

Diagnosis of Evolving Acute Myocardial Infarction in the Presence of Ventricular Pacing

In patients with permanent pacemakers and chest pain, ST-segment elevation $\geq$0.5 mV in leads with a negative QRS complex has a high specificity for the diagnosis of acute infarction. Also highly specific is ST-segment elevation $\geq$0.1 mV in leads with concordant QRS polarity (172).

Nondiagnostic and Nonspecific Electrocardiograms

The initial ECG of patients presenting with acute infarction is nondiagnostic in about 4% of cases, and it shows nonspecific changes in 21% of cases (173). Recording serial ECGs increases the probability of detecting acute infarction (174). However, it is ideal to maximize the information provided by the *admission* ECG because reperfusion therapies are more effective when they are administered early. In all patients with a nondiagnostic 12-lead ECG, a 15-lead ECG should be obtained; the addition of leads V_{4R}, V_8, and V_9 increases the detection rate of ST-segment elevation.

Among patients with a normal admission ECG who then develop acute infarction and survive hospitalization, the frequency of involvement of the infarct-related artery is similar for the three major arteries. Patients who never develop ECG changes have lesions in branch vessels (175). Among patients with nondiagnostic ECG changes, the most frequent culprit artery is the circumflex (45). In the absence of confounding factors, nondiagnostic ECGs are associated with an incidence of in-hospital events and mortality that is lower than that for patients with diagnostic ECGs, but it is still considerable (48).

Patients who present to the emergency department with chest pain and LVH in the ECG may pose a particular

TABLE 59.5

CRITERIA FOR THE DIAGNOSIS OF ACUTE MYOCARDIAL INFARCTION IN THE PRESENCE OF LEFT BUNDLE BRANCH BLOCK

Electrocardiographic criterion	Score
↑ST $\geq$1 mm concordant with QRSpolarity	5
↓ST $\geq$1 mm in V_1, V_2, or V_3	3
↑ST $\geq$5 mm discordant with QRS polarity	2

↑ elevated: ↓, depressed.
From Sgarbossa EB, Pinski SL, Barbagelata A, et al. Electrocardiographic diagnosis of evolving acute myocardial infarction in the presence of left bundle branch block. *N Engl J Med* 1996;334:481–487.

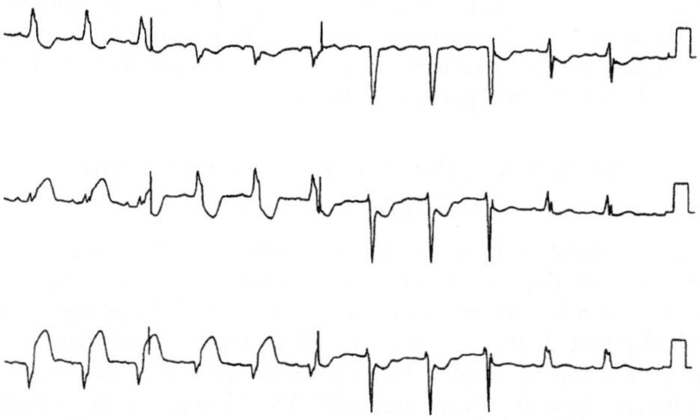

FIGURE 59.24. Electrocardiogram recorded in a patient with left bundle branch block and acute myocardial infarction. ST-segment elevation greater than 0.3 mV is present in lead II (with concordant QRS polarity), ST-segment elevation greater than 0.4 mV is present in leads III and aVF (with discordant QRS polarity), and ST-segment depression is present in leads V_2 and V_3. (From Sgarbossa EB, Pinski SL, Barbagelata A, et al. Electrocardiographic diagnosis of evolving acute myocardial infarction in the presence of left bundle branch block. *N Engl J Med* 1996;334:481–487.)

diagnostic challenge because of the repolarization changes that act as confounders. Patients with acute chest pain and LVH in the ECG, however, are significantly less likely to have an acute coronary event than patients without ECG signs of LVH (176).

ESTABLISHED MYOCARDIAL INFARCTION

Most infarctions consist of areas of both transmural and non-transmural necrosis that change quantitatively over time and whose correlation with the development of Q waves or their absence, respectively, is poor (41). The classification of Q-wave versus non–Q-wave infarcts discriminates between larger and smaller infarcts (177).

During acute myocardial injury and while the ST segment is still elevated, abnormal Q waves begin to develop as a consequence of both the loss of electrical forces in the necrotic area and the effect of the resultant force directed away from the area (Figs. 59.17 and 59.18). Pathologic Q waves can be recorded from all myocardial regions that depolarize early during the cardiac cycle. The posterobasal area depolarizes late, thereby producing positive QRS waveforms in the precordial leads opposing this zone (i.e., V_1 and V_2).

The Q waves of infarction correlate with percent scar tissue (178). Although in most patients Q waves persist indefinitely, in 15% to 30% of cases they disappear or regress. Small, rapid r waves may also result from postreperfusion recovery of electrical activity. Other patients presenting with chest pain accompanied by biologic markers of cardiac necrosis develop repolarization changes followed by nonpathologic, small q waves or r waves of diminished amplitude. Some of these non–Q-wave infarctions result from injury of the left inferoposterior wall. In these cases, in leads V_1 to V_4 of the initial ECG, there is usually horizontal ST-segment depression, as opposed to the downsloping ST-segment depression of anterior infarcts (40). For many patients with non–Q-wave infarction, the underlying angiographic finding is a recanalized vessel (179). The prognosis of non–Q-wave infarction is markedly predicted by the admission ECG (180).

Electrocardiogram During and After Reperfusion Therapy

Approximately half of patients arriving to a medical center within 1 hour of chest pain present with abnormal Q waves. These Q waves predict a larger infarct size but do not offset the benefits of reperfusion therapy (181). Thrombolytic therapy and primary percutaneous coronary intervention, when successful, accelerate the ECG evolutionary changes of acute infarction. The early appearance of T-wave inversion and rapid, complete resolution of ST-segment elevation (even in one single ECG lead) have been associated with patency of the infarct-related artery and with improved survival (182–184). Conversely, incomplete resolution of either the ST-segment elevation or a concomitant ST-segment depression predicts increased mortality (50,185).

Clinical Value of the Electrocardiogram in Established Myocardial Infarction

Autopsy, echocardiographic, and angiographic studies have shown that the 12-lead ECG has a limited capability to diagnose established myocardial infarction (186,187). The accuracy of the ECG depends on both the infarct location and size, and it may be hampered by the presence of intraventricular conduction defects, LAFB, Q-wave regression, multiple infarctions (e.g., an anterior infarct may reduce tall R waves in V_1 to V_2 from a previous posterior infarct), and LVH.

Infarct Location

The presence of abnormal Q waves in two or more leads of the same group has been classically associated to infarct areas that, anatomically, may not be accurately correlated. For example, in ventriculograms, abnormal Q waves in leads I, aVL, V_5, and V_6 are often associated with apical, rather than lateral, wall motion abnormalities. Anteroseptal infarct has classically been defined by the presence of Q waves in leads V_1 to V_3 (188), yet in patients with ST-segment elevation in V_1 to V_3, echocardiographic and angiographic data have shown anteroapical infarcts and normal septa (189,190). Anatomically defined septal infarcts result instead in disappearance of septal Q waves in inferior leads and in I, V_5, and V_6. These changes are preceded by ST-segment depression in the same leads during the acute phase or, if the infarction was inferoseptal, by precordial ST-segment depression. Initial R waves may be reduced in V_1 to V_3 (191,192).

Prominent right precordial R waves have been classically attributed to posterior infarct, but this may be a misnomer (Fig. 59.25). The term *posterior* may apply better to the thoracic wall facing these areas of the LV than to the LV itself. Prominent R waves in V_1 (duration $\geq$0.04 second, R/S $>$1) are highly specific and have a high positive predictive value for basal *lateral* asynergy of the LV (193). Specificity and positive predictive value drop slightly for prominent R waves in V_2. Abnormal R waves in V_1 in patients with chest pain are 96% specific for

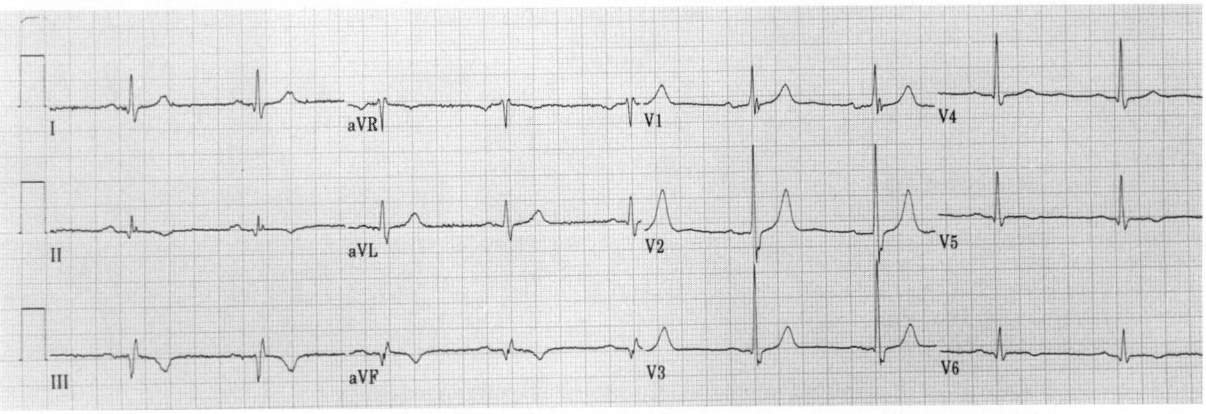

FIGURE 59.25. Inferoposterior infarction.

circumflex occlusion (194). In both posterior and inferoposterior infarcts, the culprit artery is usually the circumflex (195). In some patients, a taller R wave in V_1 and prominent R waves in V_2 to V_3 may develop after LAD occlusion (196).

The R-wave amplitude and duration may also be used for the diagnosis of established infarction (197). Because the electrical activation of the right ventricular free wall is insignificant in comparison with that of the LV myocardium, infarction of the right ventricle rarely alters the QRS complex beyond a slight voltage reduction (198). When present, Q waves in both V_{3R} and V_{4R} are highly specific markers for right ventricular infarction.

Infarct Size

Several methods have been developed to estimate the area of damaged myocardium after an acute coronary event. It appears that, in terms of prognosis, the most accurate scoring system is the Cardiac Infarction Injury Score (CIIS) (199).

ATRIAL INFARCTION

Atrial infarction is rarely recognized in the ECG; however, it may occur in 1% to 17% of patients with acute myocardial infarction (200). The injury current affects atrial repolarization and results in elevation of the Ta wave with reciprocal changes in opposite leads. This produces displacement of the PR segment, better appreciated in patients with AV block (201).

PSEUDOINFARCTION PATTERNS

Aside from the setting of acute myocardial injury, in some conditions the ECG shows ST-segment elevation, usually with a concave pattern. These conditions include severe hyperkalemia (Fig. 59.25), pericarditis, uncomplicated LBBB (Fig. 59.15), primary and secondary cardiac tumors, acute pulmonary embolism, early repolarization, ventricular aneurysm, and implantable defibrillator shocks (21,202–205).

Pathologic Q waves or decreased R-wave amplitude mimicking myocardial necrosis may occur in LVH, fascicular blocks, ventricular preexcitation, infiltrative heart disease, lead misplacement, acute pulmonary embolism, pulmonary emphysema, pleural effusion, and epicardial implantable defibrillator systems (206,207). LBBB and ventricular pacing may present the ECG appearance of acute or remote myocardial infarction (208).

MISCELLANEOUS CAUSES OF ELECTROCARDIOGRAPHIC ABNORMALITIES

Acute Pericarditis

During acute pericarditis, the myocardial area injured by inflammation is only partially depolarized. Thus, new ST vectors develop that are directed away from the ventricular cavity and toward the apical epicardium. This process results in diffuse ST-segment elevation and upright T waves (stage I), although ST-segment depression may be seen in aVR and in V_1, which faces the right atrium. There may be also PR (STa)-segment depression (209).

Acute pericarditis persists for 3 or 4 weeks. Once the ST segment and PR interval return to baseline (stage II), the T waves become inverted (stage III) and eventually normalize (stage IV). These sequential ECG changes may be interrupted by proper antiinflammatory treatment and not progress beyond stage I (53). The ECG changes of pericarditis may need to be differentiated from those of acute myocardial infarction, myocarditis, early repolarization syndrome, acute pulmonary embolism, pneumothorax, and pneumomediastinum. Pericarditis can complicate both acute myocardial infarction and myocarditis (53).

Myocardial Stunning from Sudden Emotional Stress (Stress Cardiomyopathy or Takotsubo Syndrome)

Emotional stress can induce clinical manifestations similar to those of an acute coronary event. This entity has been called *stress cardiomyopathy*, *Takotsubo syndrome*, and *broken heart syndrome* (210,211). It affects mainly postmenopausal women. Patients present with chest pain, sometimes accompanied by

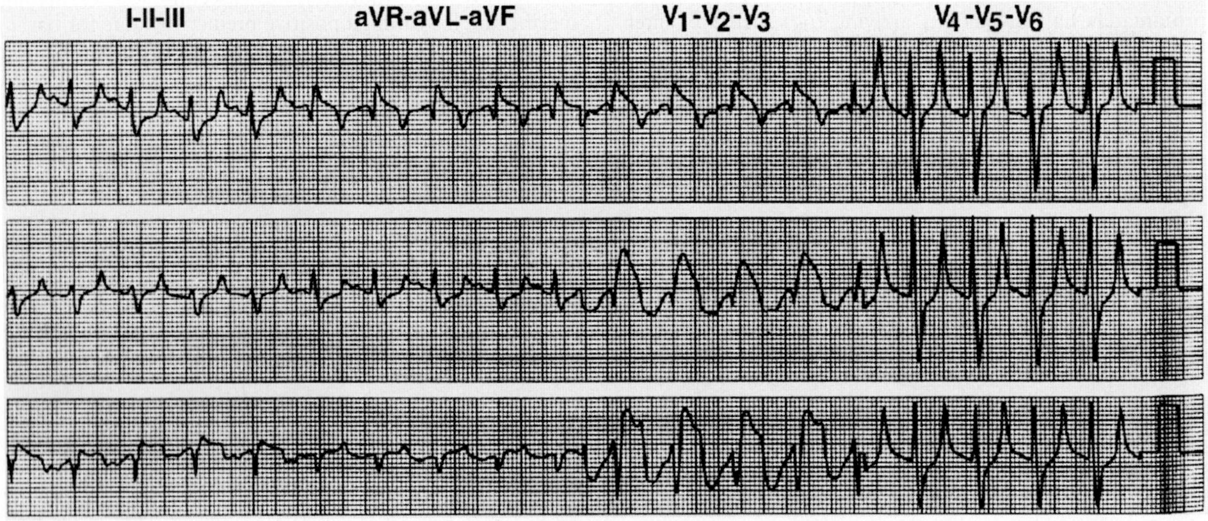

FIGURE 59.26. Pseudo–acute myocardial infarction mimicked by hyperkalemia. Peaked T waves are best seen in this case in leads V_4 to V_6. (From Kamimura M, Hancock W. Acute myocardial infarction in diabetic ketoacidosis. *Hosp Pract* 1992;27:28–30.)

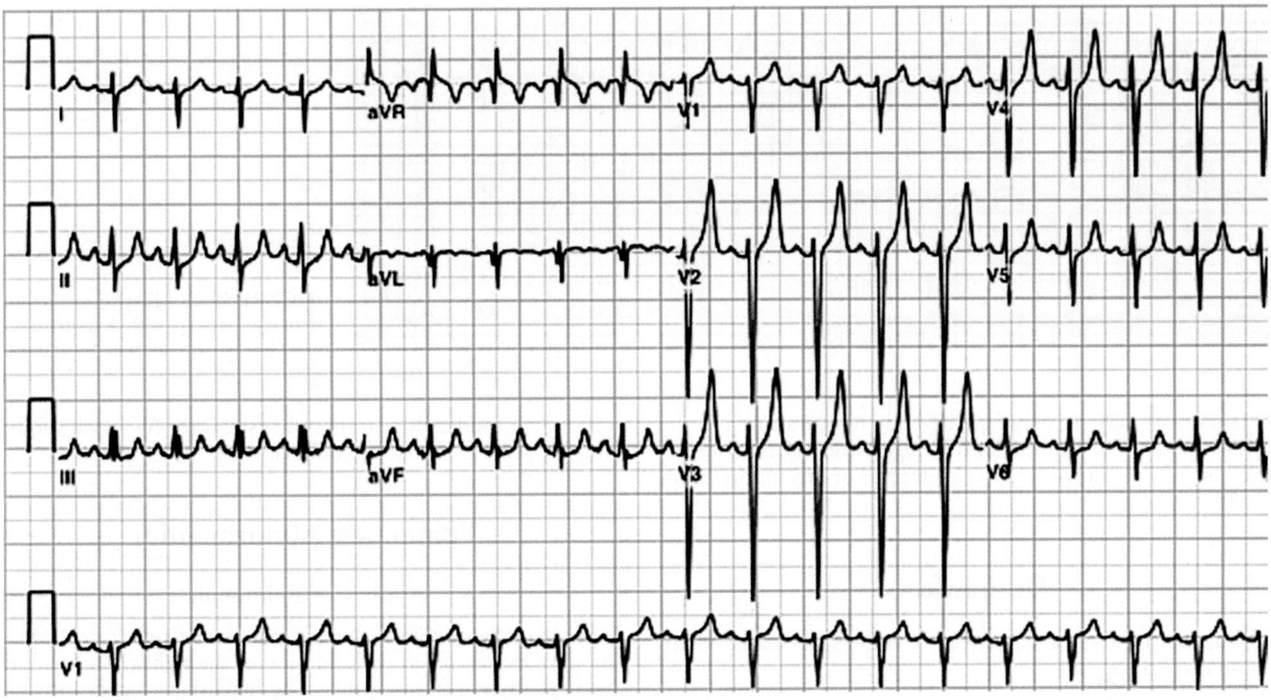

FIGURE 59.27. A 41-year-old patient with hyperkalemia.

ST-segment elevation, negative T waves, QT prolongation, pathologic Q waves, relatively minor elevation of cardiac enzyme and biomarker levels, and reversible LV dysfunction despite the absence of epicardial coronary disease. Plasma levels of catecholamines and stress-related neuropeptides are increased. Prognosis is good.

Electrolyte Abnormalities

Changes in electrolyte concentration may alter cardiac depolarization, repolarization, and conduction properties.

Hyperkalemia

Hyperkalemia may occur in patients with renal insufficiency and in patients with heart failure who are receiving angiotensin-converting enzyme inhibitors, spironolactone, or both. Potassium is a depressant of cardiac activation. The correlation between serum potassium levels and ECG changes is poor. The earliest manifestation of hyperkalemia consists of symmetric, peaked ("tented") T waves, best seen in leads II, III, and V_2 to V_4 (Fig. 59.27). This typical change, however, is only seen in 22% of patients. As potassium levels increase, the P wave decreases its amplitude and increases its duration. The PR interval is also prolonged, reflecting AV conduction delay. More severe hyperkalemia induces P-wave flattening and QRS widening. A pattern resembling RBBB, LBBB, or nonspecific conduction defects may develop. Although some patients develop typical BBB, the QRS complex in hyperkalemia is uniformly wide, and thus it differs from the BBB or preexcitation patterns (9). Sinoatrial block (either Wenckebach or Mobitz II) is not uncommon. Sometimes, ST-segment deviation mimics acute infarction. If hyperkalemia remains untreated, sinoventricular conduction, AV block, or ventricular fibrillation will occur.

Hypokalemia

Low plasma potassium levels are common in patients with acute myocardial infarction, after out-of-hospital cardiac arrest, and in patients treated with diuretics. Hypokalemia prolongs repolarization; the initial ECG signs are T-wave flattening or inversion and ST-segment depression. A typical change is prominent U waves. These waves, however, may be indeed bifid T waves. This possibility should be considered when measuring QT intervals, which should include the entire T wave, and one should not disregard its last "U" portion (9,18).

More severe hypokalemia results in a slight increase in the QRS complex and P-wave amplitudes, as well as in prolongation of the PR interval. Ectopic atrial and ventricular beats are not unusual at potassium concentrations lower than 3.3 mEq/L because automaticity increases. Severe hypokalemia is associated with atrial tachycardia with block, with AV dissociation, and, finally, with ventricular arrhythmias (torsade de pointes). Hypokalemia renders patients taking digitalis especially prone to arrhythmias.

Hypercalcemia

A high concentration of calcium increases the excitability threshold and has an inotropic effect. Hypercalcemia shortens both the ST segment and the QT interval and prolongs the PR interval and the QRS complex. Severe hypercalcemia may be associated with second- or third-degree AV block (9).

Hypocalcemia

Hypocalcemia prolongs the ST segment and the QT interval. The ST-segment duration is inversely related to the calcium blood level. The T wave remains relatively normal (9).

Hypothermia

The ECG changes of hypothermia include bradycardia, flattening of P waves, and prolongation of the PR, QRS, and QT. A typical sign, observed in approximately 80% of patients with hypothermia, is the appearance of a J wave. The J (or Osborn) wave is a deflection that distorts the QRS-ST junction and is more common in leads II, III, aVF, V_5, and V_6 (Fig. 59.28). Although the J wave disappears with normothermia, prolonged

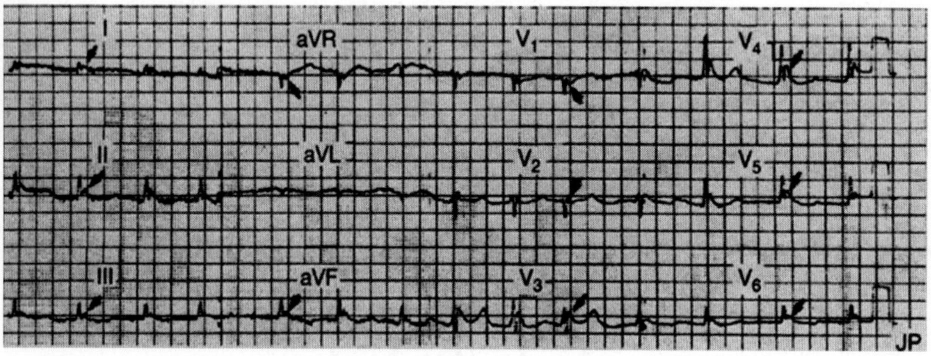

FIGURE 59.28. Electrocardiogram from a patient with hypothermia. The J-waves are marked by arrows.

QT intervals may persist after the body temperature and the QRS complex have normalized. Irregularities of the isoelectric line may result from muscular tremor or atrial fibrillation (212).

Drug Effects

Therapeutic or toxic cardiac effects of various medications may cause ECG changes.

Digitalis

Digitalis accelerates ventricular repolarization, particularly in the subendocardium. This is first represented on the ECG by flattening of the T wave and prominent U waves with shortening of the QT interval. The most typical change, however, consists of a "coved" ST-segment depression. The T wave appears biphasic, with its first portion negative and merging with the ST segment. These repolarization changes do not correlate well with therapeutic or toxic blood levels of the drug.

Digitalis intoxication is often manifested by arrhythmias similar to those of severe hypokalemia (i.e., atrial tachycardia with block and AV dissociation). Characteristics of digitalis-induced atrial tachycardia include atrial rate between 140 and 250 beats per minute, inferior-to-superior direction of atrial activation, and 2:1 AV block.

Propafenone and Class Ic Antiarrhythmic Drugs

Propafenone, flecainide, and encainide prolong the AH and HV intervals and the atrial and ventricular refractory periods. The QRS duration is increased. All class Ic drugs may induce ventricular arrhythmias (proarrhythmic effect). The JT interval is not prolonged.

Class III Antiarrhythmic Drugs

Dofetilide is pure class III antiarrhythmic agent that prolongs the refractory period and action potential duration. Dofetilide can also prolong the QT interval. *Sotalol* is a β-blocker with class III antiarrhythmic action that prolongs the QT interval.

Transplanted Hearts

In transplant recipients, the most prevalent abnormality is incomplete or complete RBBB (213). The PR and QT intervals are shorter, and the precordial transitional zone is displaced to the left. The shift in the transitional zone and the conduction delay of the right bundle would indicate a clockwise rotation of the heart on its vertical axis. The increased prevalence of RBBB during follow-up, however, may be associated with mildly increased pulmonary pressures. After heart transplantation, the sudden appearance of first-degree AV block should suggest acute graft rejection (214).

Pulmonary Abnormalities

Acute Cor Pulmonale

The ECG changes in acute cor pulmonale reflect acute pulmonary hypertension with dilation of the right chambers and perhaps myocardial ischemia. The ECG signs significantly associated with pulmonary embolism include sinus tachycardia, the classic "right heart strain" pattern $S_I Q_{III} T_{III}$, and atrial tachyarrhythmias (215). Also common are right QRS axis deviation and complete or incomplete RBBB, signs that correlate with the extent of embolization (216).

Pulmonary Emphysema

The overinflated lungs of pulmonary emphysema lower the diaphragm. The heart and the cardiac electrical axis become more vertical and rotate clockwise, with the QRS axis at $\geq$90 degrees in the frontal plane. Other changes include the following: prominent P waves (>0.25 mV; indeed, a P pulmonale is a better predictor of pulmonary emphysema or low diaphragm position than of right atrial enlargement) (34); exaggerated atrial repolarization with Ta waves producing ST-segment depression in inferior leads; decreased progression of R-wave amplitudes in precordial leads; and low voltage of the QRS complexes, especially in the left precordial leads.

Neurogenic Manifestations

Patients with acute or chronic diseases of the nervous system may show repolarization changes in the ECG. Negative T and U waves, ST-segment changes, and QT prolongation may appear during subarachnoid hemorrhage (Fig. 59.29), ischemic stroke, radical neck dissection, spinal cord trauma, electroconvulsive therapy, deep brain stimulation, and emotional stress (22,53,55,217–220).

Misplacement of Electrocardiographic Leads

Misplacement of ECG leads is common. A study of 11,432 ECGs detected reversals involving the left arm and foot or adjacent precordial electrodes in 2% of the recordings (221).

Reversal of the Right and Left Arm Cables

When the electrodes attached to the arm cables are reversed, "lead I" shows negative P and T waves and a predominantly negative QRS complex. "Lead II" is indeed lead III, and "lead aVR" is indeed lead aVL, and vice versa (222). Thus, the

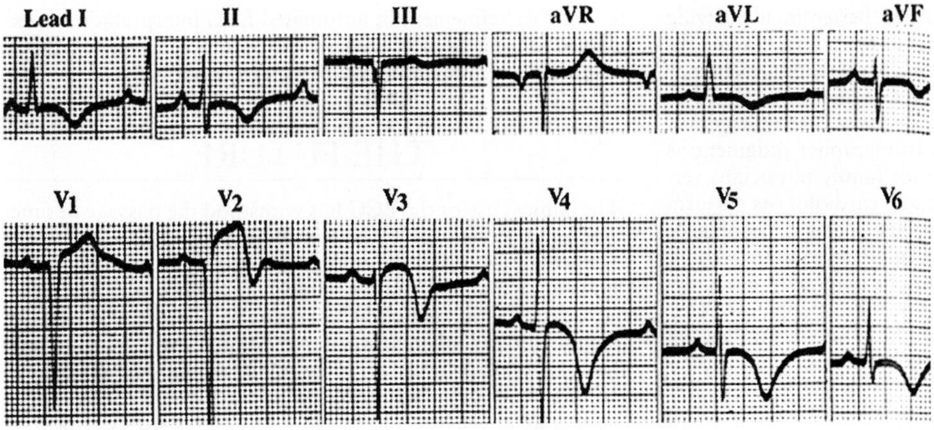

FIGURE 59.29. Electrocardiogram recorded in a patient with subarachnoid hemorrhage showing T-wave changes mimicking myocardial ischemia. (From Chou TC, Susilavorn B. Electrocardiographic-pathological conference: electrocardiographic changes in intracranial hemorrhage. *J Electrocardiol* 1969; 2:193–196.)

limb leads suggest the diagnosis of dextrocardia. The precordial leads, however, show the normal progression of R wave through V_6.

Reversal of Each Arm Cable with The Corresponding Leg Cable

When the arm cables are switched with the leg cables, "lead I" shows a flat line that records the potential difference between both legs; "lead II" is an inverted (upside-down) lead III because the positive electrode is now in the left arm. "Lead III" mirrors its image, because the polarity of its two components is inverted. "Lead aVR" is a replica of "lead aVL," because both leads now record potentials derived from comparing each leg (aVF) with the same central terminal.

Misplacement of Precordial Lead Electrodes

In a prospective study using deliberate precordial lead misplacement, 2-cm changes in electrode position (too high or too low) resulted in significant ECG abnormalities (223). Variations included changes in R-wave amplitude, ST segments, Q waves, and in the transition zone. When precordial electrodes are misplaced in a high position, QS complexes or low-voltage R waves may appear, and a differential diagnosis with anterior infarction must be made. The use of device-guided lead placement improves accuracy and reproducibility in interpretation of precordial waveforms (58).

HIGH-RESOLUTION ELECTROCARDIOGRAPHY AND BODY SURFACE MAPPING

High-Resolution Electrocardiography

Potentials generated by the His-Purkinje system and by depressed ventricular myocardium ("late potentials") produce a very small signal that is not detected by standard recording techniques (224). This finding prompted the development of special techniques: (a) temporal averaging (usually referred to as *signal averaging*), applicable only to repetitive ECG signals; and (b) spatial averaging, which can record the His-Purkinje signal and late potentials on a beat-to-beat basis. Signal averaging (the most often utilized technique) can analyze potentials in time domain, frequency domain, or a combination of both. An increased incidence of low-amplitude, high-frequency components within the QRS complex is common in patients with acute or remote myocardial infarction. Signal-averaged ECG is an interesting research tool with limited clinical applications.

Body Surface Mapping

Body surface mapping records cardiac electric events with numerous electrodes (from 16 to 200), thus adding information to that of the standard ECG. Cardiac field mapping provides details on the spatial and temporal sequence of cardiac excitation and recovery. Local intraventricular conduction disturbances, preexcitation, premature ventricular beats, and repolarization disorders can be precisely located (225). Visual inspection of the ECG maps does not suffice for diagnostic purposes; sophisticated statistical and deterministic models are necessary, and these requirements limit this technique's clinical usefulness.

CONTROVERSIES AND PERSONAL PERSPECTIVES

Proficiency and Accuracy in Recording and Interpretation

Perhaps because the ECG is widely available and easy to obtain, its recording and interpretation are regarded as minor tasks (23). Cardiologists are rarely present at the time of a patient's initial evaluation. The responsibility of ECG recording lies in nurses, technicians, and medical students. This situation is conducive to suboptimal ECG data collection. Lead misplacements and noise are common (226). In most acute clinical settings, only 12 ECG leads with few QRS complexes per lead are obtained. Special ECG leads and prolonged rhythm strips (other than in lead II) are underutilized (227). Thus, acute myocardial infarctions, arrhythmias, and intermittent BBB may remain inadequately documented.

Aside from these shortcomings in ECG recording, interpretation may also be limited. Young physicians rarely acquire a high level of individual competence in ECG principles and diagnosis (23). Even experienced physicians usually examine only 11 leads of the 12 available; lead aVR (and the information it may provide) is ignored (228).

The self-perception of proficiency in ECG interpretation, conversely, may be overoptimistic. Almost half of consecutive cases of fatal myocardial infarction may be undetected in the emergency department (229). In family practice programs, residents interpreting ECGs regularly miss acute infarctions, and their expertise may not improve with the year of residence

(230). General practitioners performed better in identifying normal ECGs (82% specificity) than in recognizing acute infarction (33% to 61% sensitivity) (231). Among emergency physicians, misreading of abnormal ST segments is related to suboptimal triage and unnecessary coronary care unit admissions (232). A study using electrocardiographer judgment as gold standard found 67% accuracy for family physicians versus 91% for cardiologists (233). Because cardiologists perform better than internists (234), the specific medical training of the interpreter may have a role in diagnostic accuracy. About one fourth of missed infarctions could be diagnosed with adequate competence in ECG reading (235). Fisch suggested that the inevitable use of automated diagnoses "may be, in fact, an obstacle to the acquisition of ECG skills" (236).

Reproducibility

The validity of ECG analyses may be questioned by high variability within or among ECG readers. Intraobserver and interobserver agreement rates are seldom tested or reported, but studies that evaluated reproducibility of ECG interpretations found an approximate 80% intraobserver rate and a 30% interobserver agreement rate (237). Discrepancies in ECG interpretation are related to the ECG waveform or interval under analysis, to variability in consecutive ECG recordings, and to the interpreter. For example, measurements of the ST segment are highly reproducible from beat to beat, but those of QT interval are not (48). Most intraobserver variation in the diagnosis of established infarction relates to leads III, aVF, and aVL. In precordial recordings, variability is often a consequence of differences in lead placement (238). There is also a day-to-day variability inherent in the 12-lead ECG of healthy people, influenced by circadian rhythms and meals.

The role of expertise in reproducibility in ECG interpretation is uncertain. At least among internal medicine residents, experience may influence more intraobserver than interobserver agreement; the latter rates may not improve after training programs in electrocardiography (61). Comparative reproducibility between cardiologists and other physicians has been scrutinized only in limited settings and has been found acceptable (239).

Role of Computerized Interpretation

Computer-assisted ECG interpretation is now widely available. Ideally, automated measurements of ECG waveforms and intervals can significantly reduce physician time in ECG analysis while providing readings that are precise at the microvolt and millisecond level. In general, however, computer-derived intervals are longer than those visually determined. Manual measurements performed with an amplification factor of 10 or 20 produce significantly wider intervals, similar to computer-derived results (17). Many computer programs apply longer-than-standard upper and lower normal limits for ECG intervals (e.g., minimum PR of 130 milliseconds and maximum QRS complex of 0.126 millisecond) (240). Additional limitations of computerized readings include minute-to-minute variability, inability to determine the anteroposterior direction of electrical forces, and discrepant measurements between programs (62,241). Automated diagnoses (e.g., "LVH") may be less reliable and accurate than automated raw measurements. Many diagnostic programs in electrocardiographs are now 25 years old (242). An investigation on commonly used ECG software found a variety of systematic errors; clinically validated ECG diagnoses of myocardial infarction or LVH had an accuracy rate of 70%, versus 76% for visual readings by cardiologists (62,243).

Further refinement in automated ECG interpretation is expected in the near future. At present, computer-analyzed ECGs require overreading by an experienced cardiologist.

THE FUTURE

The clinical use of the ECG has withstood the passage of time. The ECG is often the initial test demonstrating cardiovascular abnormalities, a role now expanded with the use of ECG in prehospital diagnosis and telemedicine (244).

Current emphasis in ECG research is on the study of dynamic patterns inherent in certain parameters (especially ventricular repolarization) with the aid of ambulatory recordings and newer, potent digital storage and analysis techniques. Attempts at improving the resolution of standard electrocardiography have relied on an increase in the number of recording electrodes (body surface mapping) and on an improvement in the signal-to-noise ratio of the higher-frequency signals by averaging and filtering (signal-averaged ECG). These techniques are promising, but their roles in clinical practice are still unclear.

E-Health and Teleconsultation

In electrocardiography, teleconsultation has become commonplace. Several systems provide for remote clinical assessment (245). In the triage of patients with chest pain, reliance on teleconsultation allows general practitioners to manage most cases by themselves (246). In the prehospital setting, paramedics can utilize telecardiology and remote ECG evaluation to reduce the time to reperfusion therapy (247).

Remote monitoring can also be used for patients with chronic conditions. Their ECG data can be first uploaded with special software and then examined by authorized consultants who, in turn, submit a diagnosis or prescription to the referring site. With some systems, the consultant can interact with the patient through a "chat" facility (248).

Patients can also use a personal digital assistant (PDA) to record their ECG actively, view it, and transmit it via a wireless connection. The ECG is reviewed by a physician and, if necessary, forwarded to a cardiologist's PDA. All these activities are logged and stored in a central database (63). Other PDA patient systems can analyze the ECG signals locally and, in the presence of arrhythmias, can remotely activate alarms (249). High-risk patients can have a cardiac monitor implanted subcutaneously. The monitor can detect ST-segment changes and can also alert companions or bystanders if cardiac arrest occurs (250).

Remote ECG interpretation and risk alerts are likely to become widely adopted and to contribute to improve survival in patients with acute myocardial infarction or complex arrhythmias. It is important, however, for medical education to emphasize the value of the ECG. Systematic instruction and supervised practice in ECG diagnosis are fundamental to maintain proficiency in ECG interpretation.

Overall, we believe that the standard 12-lead ECG will continue to expand in clinical importance and will remain an integral part of the evaluation of all cardiac patients, particularly those with ischemic heart disease or rhythm disturbances.

References

1. Waller AD. A demonstration in man of electromotive changes accompanying the heart's beat. *J Physiol (Lond)* 1887;8:229–234.
2. Cooper JK. Electrocardiography 100 years ago: origins, pioneers, and contributors. *N Engl J Med* 1986;315:461–464.

3. Shapiro E. The first textbook of electrocardiography. Thomas Lewis: clinical electrocardiography. *J Am Coll Cardiol* 1983;1:1160–1161.
4. Barker LF. Electrocardiography and phonocardiography: a collective review. *Bull Johns Hopkins Hosp* 1910;21:358–389.
5. Fleckenstein K. The early ECG in medical practice. *Med Instrument* 1984; 18:191–192.
6. Surawicz B. Introduction: historical outline. In: *Electrophysiologic basis of ECG and cardiac arrhythmias.* Baltimore: Williams & Wilkins, 1995:3–12.
7. Kyle RA, Sampo MA. Frank Wilson. *JAMA* 1983;250:2680.
8. Wilson FN, Johnston FD, Rosenbaum F, et al. The precordial electrocardiogram. *Am Heart J* 1944;27:19–85.
9. Herrick JB. An intimate account of my early experience with coronary thrombosis. *Am Heart J* 1944;27:1–18.
10. Pardee HEB. An electrocardiographic sign of coronary artery obstruction. *Arch Intern Med* 1920;26:244–257.
11. Wilson FN. Disorders of the heartbeat and cardiac failure. *South Med J* 1936;29:397–400.
12. Barold SS, Fisch C, Schamroth L, Wellens HJJ. Richard Langendorf: 1908–1987. *Pacing Clin Electrophysiol* 1988;11:1242–1247.
13. Rosenbaum MB, Elizari MV, eds. *Frontiers of cardiac electrophysiology.* Boston: Martinus Nijhoff, 1983.
14. Grant RP. The relationship between the anatomic position of the heart and the electro cardiogram: a criticism of "unipolar" electrocardiography. *Circulation* 1953;7:890–902.
15. Goldberger E. A simple indifferent, electrocardiographic electrode of zero potential and a technique of obtaining augmented, unipolar, extremity leads. *Am Heart J* 1942;23:483.
16. Anderson ST, Pahlm O, Selvester RH, et al. Panoramic display of the orderly sequenced 12-lead ECG. *J Electrocardiol* 1994;27:347–352.
17. Khaw K, Moreyra AE, Tannenbaum AK, et al. Improved detection of posterior myocardial ischemia with the 15-lead electrocardiogram. *Am Heart J* 1999;138:934–940.
18. Zalenski RJ, Rydman RJ, Sloan EP, et al. Value of posterior and right ventricular leads in comparison to the standard 12-lead electrocardiogram in evaluation of ST-segment elevation in suspected acute myocardial infarction. *Am J Cardiol* 1997;79:1579–1585.
19. Menown IBA, Adgey AAJ. Improving the ECG classification of inferior and lateral myocardial infarction by inversion of lead aVR. *Heart* 2000;83:657–660.
20. Pahlm US, Pahlm O, Wagner GS. The standard 11-lead ECG: neglect of lead aVR in the classical limb lead display. *J Electrocardiol* 1996;29:270–274.
21. Sgarbossa EB, Barold SS, Pinski SL, et al. Twelve-lead electrocardiogram: the advantages of an orderly frontal lead display including lead -aVR. *J Electrocardiol* 2004;37:141–147.
22. Bailey JJ, Berson AS, Garson Jr A, et al. Recommendations for standardization and specifications in automated electrocardiography: bandwidth and digital signal processing: a report for health professionals by an ad hoc writing group of the Committee on Electrocardiography and Cardiac Electrophysiology of the Council on Clinical Cardiology, American Heart Association. *Circulation* 1990;81:730–739.
23. Pettis KS, Savona MR, Leibrandt PN, et al. Evaluation of the efficacy of hand-held computer screens for cardiologists' interpretations of 12-lead electrocardiograms. *Am Heart J* 1999;138:765–770.
24. Surawicz B. *Electrophysiologic basis of ECG and cardiac arrhythmias.* Baltimore: Williams & Wilkins, 1995.
25. Antzelevitch C, Sicouri S, Lukas A, et al. Regional differences in the electrophysiology of ventricular cells: physiological and clinical implications. In: Zipes DP, Jalife J, eds. *Cardiac electrophysiology: from cell to bedside,* 2nd ed. Philadelphia: WB Saunders, 1995:228–245.
26. Franz M R, Ventricular repolarization, T-wave genesis, and risk prediction. *Ann Noninvasive Electrocardiol* 2001;6:1–4.
27. Rosenbaum MB, Elizari MV, Lazzari JO. *Los hemibloqueos.* Buenos Aires: Paidos, 1968:442–464.
28. Anderson RH, Ho SY, Wharton J, Becker AE. Gross anatomy and microscopy of the conducting system. In: Mandel WJ, ed. *Cardiac arrhythmias: their mechanisms, diagnosis, and management.* Philadelphia: JB Lippincott, 1995:13–54.
29. Olson CW, Warner RA, Wagner GS, Selvester RH. A dynamic three-dimensional display of ventricular excitation and the generation of the vector and electrocardiogram. *J Electrocardiol* 2001;34(suppl):7–15.
30. Macfarlane PW, Lawrie TD, eds. *Comprehensive electrocardiology: theory and practice in health and disease.* New York: Pergamon Press, 1989.
31. Surawicz B. Stretching the limits of the electrocardiogram's diagnostic utility. *J Am Coll Cardiol* 1998;32:483–485.
32. Feola M, Ribichini F, Gallone G, et al. Analysis of right electrocardiographic leads in 195 normal subjects. *G Ital Cardiol* 1994;24:375–379.
33. Willems JL, Robles De Medina EO, et al. Criteria for intraventricular conduction disturbances and pre-excitation. *J Am Coll Cardiol* 1985;5:1261–1275.
34. Yan GX, Lankipalli RS, Burke JF, et al. Ventricular repolarization components on the electrocardiogram: cellular basis and clinical significance. *J Am Coll Cardiol* 2003;42:401–409.
35. Burgess MJ, Millar K, Abildskov JA. Cancellation of electrocardiographic effects during ventricular recovery. *J Electrocardiol* 1969;2:101–107.
36. Reinig MG, Harizi R, Spodick DH. Electrocardiographic T- and U-wave discordance. *Ann Noninvasive Electrocardiol* 2005;10:41–46.
37. Surawicz B. U wave: facts, hypotheses, misconceptions, and misnomers. *J Cardiovasc Electrophysiol* 1998;9:1117–1128.
38. Antzelevitch C, Shimizu W, Yan GX, et al. The M cell: its contribution to the ECG and to normal and abnormal electrical function of the heart. *J Cardiovasc Electrophysiol* 1999;10:1124–1152.
39. Viskin S, Rosovski U, Sands AJ, et al. Inaccurate electrocardiographic interpretation of long QT: the majority of physicians cannot recognize a long QT when they see one. *Heart Rhythm* 2005;2:569–574.
40. Bidoggia H, Maciel JP, Capalozza N, et al. Sex differences on the electrocardiographic pattern of cardiac repolarization: possible role of testosterone. *Am Heart J* 2000;140:678–683.
41. Sarma JSM, Sarma RJ, Bilitch M, et al. An exponential formula for heart rate dependence of QT interval during exercise and cardiac pacing in humans: reevaluation of Bazett's formula. *Am J Cardiol* 1984;54:103–108.
42. Rautaharju PM, Zhou SH, Wong S, et al. Functional characteristics of QT prediction formulas: the concepts of QTmax and QT rate sensitivity. *Comput Biomed Res* 1993;26:188–204.
43. Spodick DH, Rifkin R, Rajasingh MC. Effect of self-correlation on the relation between QT interval and cardiac cycle length. *Am Heart J* 1990;120: 157–160.
44. Anderson ME, Al-Khatib SM, Roden DM, Califf RM. Duke Clinical Research Institute/American Heart Journal Expert Meeting on Repolarization Changes. Cardiac repolarization: current knowledge, critical gaps, and new approaches to drug development and patient management. *Am Heart J* 2002;144:769–781.
45. Al-Khatib SM, LaPointe NM, Kramer JM, Califf RM. What clinicians should know about the QT interval. *JAMA* 2003;289:2120–2127.
46. Sgarbossa EB, Pinski SL, Williams D, et al. Comparison of QT intervals in African-Americans versus Caucasians. *Am J Cardiol* 2000;86:880–882.
47. Talreja D, Gruver C, Sklenar J, et al. Efficient utilization of echocardiography for the assessment of left ventricular systolic function. *Am Heart J* 2000;l39:394–398.
48. Chou TC. Normal electrocardiogram. In: Chou TE, ed. *Electrocardiography in clinical practice: adult and pediatric.* Philadelphia: WB Saunders, 1996:3–22.
49. Surawicz B, Parikh SR. Prevalence of male and female patterns of early ventricular repolarization in the normal ECG of males and females from childhood to old age. *J Am Coll Cardiol* 2002;40:1870–1876.
50. Klatsky AL, Oehm R, Cooper RA, et al. The early repolarization normal variant electrocardiogram: correlates and consequences. *Am J Med* 2003; 115:171–177.
51. Wang K, Asinger RW, Marriott HJ. ST-segment elevation in conditions other than acute myocardial infarction. *N Engl J Med* 2003;349:2128–2135.
52. Haydar ZR, Brantley DA, Gittings NS, et al. Early repolarization: an electrocardiographic predictor of enhanced aerobic fitness. *Am J Cardiol* 2000; 85:264–266.
53. Khan IA, Nair CK. Brugada and long QT-3 syndromes: two phenotypes of the sodium channel disease. *Ann Noninvasive Electrocardiol* 2004;9:280–289.
54. Littmann L, Monroe MH, Kerns WP 2nd, et al. Brugada syndrome and "Brugada sign": clinical spectrum with a guide for the clinician. *Am Heart J* 2003;145:768–778.
55. Antzelevitch C, Brugada P, Borggrefe M, et al. Brugada syndrome: report of the second consensus conference. *Heart Rhythm* 2005;2:429–440.
56. Gussak I, Antzelevitch C. Early repolarization syndrome: clinical characteristics and possible cellular and ionic mechanisms. *J Electrocardiol* 2000; 33:299–309.
57. Surawicz B. T wave abnormalities. In: Rosenbaum M, Elizari MV, eds. *Frontiers of electrocardiography.* Boston: Martinus Nijhoff, 1983:40–66.
58. Fisch C. Evolution of clinical electrocardiogram. *J Am Coll Cardiol* 1989; 14:1127–1138.
59. Rose G, Baxter PJ, Reid DD, McCartney P. Prevalence and prognosis of electrocardiographic findings in middle aged men. *Br Heart J* 1978;40:636–643.
60. Sackett DL, Haynes RB, Guyatt GH, Tugwell P. The interpretation of diagnostic data. In: *Clinical epidemiology. a basic science for clinical medicine,* 2nd ed. Boston: Little, Brown, 1991:69–152.
61. Hulley SB, Cummings SR. Planning the measurements: precision and accuracy. In: Hulley SB, Cummings SR, eds. *Designing clinical research.* Baltimore: Williams & Wilkins, 1988:31–41.
62. Sackett DL, Haynes RB, Guyatt GH, Tugwell P. The selection of diagnostic tests. In: *Clinical epidemiology: a basic science for clinical medicine,* 2nd ed. Boston: Little, Brown, 1991:51–68.
63. Ostrander LD, Jr. Left axis deviation: prevalence, associated conditions, and prognosis. An epidemiologic study. *Ann Intern Med* 1971;75:23–28.
64. Kaplan JD, Evans T Jr, Foster E, et al. Evaluation of electrocardiographic criteria for right atrial enlargement by quantitative two-dimensional echocardiography. *J Am Coll Cardiol* 1994;23:747–752.
65. Romhilt DW, Bove KE, Conradi S, Scott RC. Morphologic significance of left atrial involvement. *Am Heart J* 1972;83:322–327.

66. Scott CC, Leier CV, Kilman JW, et al. The effect of atrial histology and dimension on P wave morphology. *J Electrocardiol* 1983;16:363–366.
67. Alpman A, Güldal M, Berkalp B, et al. Importance of notching and slurring of the resting QRS complex in the diagnosis of coronary artery disease. *J Electrocardiol* 1995;28:199–208.
68. Walston A, Brewer DL, Kitchens CS, Krook JE. The electrocardiographic manifestations of spontaneous left pneumothorax. *Ann Intern Med* 1974; 80:375–379.
69. Goldberger A. Normal and noninfarct Q waves. *Cardiol Clin* 1987;5:357–366.
70. Bär FW, Brugada P, Dassen WR, et al. Prognostic value of Q waves, R/S ratio, loss of R wave voltage, ST-T segment abnormalities, electrical axis, low voltage and notching: correlation of electrocardiogram and left ventriculogram. *J Am Coll Cardiol* 1984;4:17–27.
71. Schouten EG, Dekker JM, Meppelink P, et al. QT interval prolongation predicts cardiovascular mortality in an apparently healthy population. *Circulation* 1991;84:1516–1523.
72. Bijl M, Verheugt FW. Extreme QT prolongation solely due to reversible myocardial ischemia in single-vessel coronary disease. *Am Heart J* 1992; 123:524–526.
73. Barletta G, Lazzeri C, Franchi F, et al. Hypertrophic cardiomyopathy: electrical abnormalities detected by the extended-length ECG and their relation to syncope. *Int J Cardiol* 2004;97:43–48.
74. Oka H, Mochio S, Sato K, Isogai Y. Correlation of altered QT interval and sympathetic nervous system dysfunction in diabetic autonomic neuropathy. *Eur Neurol* 1994;34:23–29.
75. Hanrahan JP, Choo PW, Carlson W, et al. Terfenadine-associated ventricular arrhythmias and QTc interval prolongation. A retrospective cohort comparison with other antihistamines among members of a health maintenance organization. *Ann Epidemiol* 1995;5:201–209.
76. Malik M. Errors and misconceptions in ECG measurement used for the detection of drug induced QT interval prolongation. *J Electrocardiol* 2004; 37(suppl):25–33.
77. Pacher P, Kecskemeti V. Cardiovascular side effects of new antidepressants and antipsychotics: new drugs, old concerns? *Curr Pharm Des* 2004; 10:2463–2475.
78. Drugs that prolong the QT interval and/or induce torsade de pointes. www.torsades.org.
79. Moss AJ, Zareba W, Benhorin J, et al. ECG T-wave patterns in genetically distinct forms of the hereditary long QT syndrome. *Circulation* 1995;92: 2929–2934.
80. Malfatto G, Beria G, Sala S, et al. Quantitative analysis of T wave abnormalities and their prognostic implications in the idiopathic QT syndrome. *J Am Coll Cardiol* 1994;23:296–301.
81. Rosenbaum MB, Acunzo RS. Pseudo 2:1 atrioventricular block and T wave alternans in long QT syndromes. *J Am Coll Cardiol* 1991;18:1363–1366.
82. Zareba W, Moss AJ, le Cessie S, Hall WJ. T wave alternans in idiopathic long QT syndrome. *J Am Coll Cardiol* 1994;23:1541–1546.
83. Schimpf R, Wolpert C, Gaita F, et al. Short QT syndrome. *Cardiovasc Res* 2005;67:357–366.
84. Franz MR, Bargheer K, Costard-Jäckle A, et al. Human ventricular repolarization and T wave genesis. *Prog Cardiovasc Dis* 1991;33:369–384.
85. Alfonso F, Nihoyannopoulos P, Stewart J, et al. Clinical significance of giant negative T waves in hypertrophic cardiomyopathy. *J Am Coll Cardiol* 1990;15:965–971.
86. Libbus I, Rosenbaum DS. Remodeling of cardiac repolarization: mechanisms and implications of memory. *Card Electrophysiol Rev* 2002;6:302–310.
87. Sgarbossa EB, Meyer PM, Pinski SL, et al. Negative T waves shortly after ST-elevation acute myocardial infarction are a powerful marker for improved survival. *Am Heart J* 2000;140:385–394.
88. Tamura A, Nagase K, Mikuriya Y, Nasu M. Significance of spontaneous normalization of negative T waves in infarct-related leads during healing of anterior wall acute myocardial infarction. *Am J Cardiol* 1999;84;1341–1344.
89. Lancellotti P, Gerard PL, Kulbertus HE, Pierard LA. Persistent negative T waves in the infarct-related leads as an independent predictor of poor long-term prognosis after acute myocardial infarction. *Am J Cardiol* 2002;90: 833–837.
90. Beckerman J, Yamazaki T, Myers J, et al. T-wave abnormalities are a better predictor of cardiovascular mortality than ST depression on the resting electrocardiogram. *Ann Noninvasive Electrocardiol* 2005;10:146–151.
91. Otrusinik R, Alpert M, Hamm CR, et al. Factors predicting coronary artery disease in patients with giant negative T waves. *Am J Cardiol* 2000;85:873–875.
92. Bardají A, Vidal F, Richart C. T wave alternans associated with amiodarone. *J Electrocardiol* 1993;26:155–157.
93. Rosenbaum MB, Blanco HH, Elizari MV, et al. Electrotonic modulation of the T wave and cardiac memory. *Am J Cardiol* 1982;50:213–222.
94. Kolb JC. Cardiac memory-persistent T wave changes after ventricular pacing. *J Emerg Med* 2002;23:191–197.
95. Helguera ME, Pinski SL, Sterba R, Trohman RG. Memory T waves after radiofrequency ablation of accessory atrioventricular connections in the WPW syndrome. *J Electrocardiol* 1994;27:243–249.
96. Kishida H, Cole JS, Surawicz B. Negative U wave: a highly specific but poorly understood sign of heart disease. *Am J Cardiol* 1982;49:2030–2036.
97. Surawicz B, Fisch C. Cardiac alternans: diverse mechanisms and clinical manifestations. *J Am Coll Cardiol* 1992;20:483–499.
98. Tighe DA, Chung EK, Park CH. Electric alternans associated with acute pulmonary embolism. *Am Heart J* 1994;128:188–190.
99. Devereux RB, Reichek N. Repolarization abnormalities of left ventricular hypertrophy. *J Electrocardiol* 1982;15:47.
100. Casale PN, Devereux RB, Kligfield P, et al. Electrocardiographic detection of left ventricular hypertrophy: development and prospective validation of improved criteria. *J Am Coll Cardiol* 1985;6:572–589.
101. Romhilt DW, Bove KE, Norris RJ, et al. A critical appraisal of the electrocardiographic criteria for the diagnosis of left ventricular hypertrophy. *Circulation* 1969;40:185–195.
102. Okin PM, Roman MJ, Devereux RB, Kligfield P. Electrocardiographic identification of left ventricular mass by simple voltage-duration products. *J Am Coll Cardiol* 1995;25:417–423.
103. Schillaci G, Verdecchia P, Borgioni C, et al. Improved electrocardiographic diagnosis of left ventricular hypertrophy. *Am J Cardiol* 1994;74:714–719.
104. Okin PM, Roman MJ, Devereux RB, Kligfield P. Electrocardiographic identification of left ventricular hypertrophy: test performance in relation to definition of hypertrophy and presence of obesity. *J Am Coll Cardiol* 1996;27:124–131.
105. Mehta A, Jain AC, Mehta MC, Billie M. Usefulness of left atrial abnormality for predicting left ventricular hypertrophy in the presence of left bundle branch block. *Am J Cardiol* 2000;85:354–359.
106. Xiao HB, Brecker SJD, Gibson DG. Relative effects of left ventricular mass and conduction disturbance on activation in patients with pathological left ventricular hypertrophy. *Br Heart J* 1994;71:548–553.
107. Klein RC, Vera Z, De Maria AN, Mason DT. Electrocardiographic diagnosis of left ventricular hypertrophy in the presence of left bundle branch block. *Am Heart J* 1984;108:502–506.
108. Gertsch M, Theler A, Foglia E. Electrocardiographic detection of left ventricular hypertrophy in the presence of left anterior fascicular block. *Am J Cardiol* 1988;61:1098–1101.
109. Vandenberg B, Sagar K, Paulsen W, Romhilt D. Electrocardiographic criteria for diagnosis of left ventricular hypertrophy in the presence of complete right bundle branch block. *Am J Cardiol* 1989;63:1080–1084.
110. Mehta A, Jain AC, Morise AP, et al. Left atrial abnormality by electrocardiogram predicts left ventricular hypertrophy by echocardiography in the presence of right bundle branch block. *Clin Cardiol* 1998;21:109–114.
111. Selzer A. Approach to diagnosis. In: *Principles and practice of clinical cardiology.* Philadelphia: WB Saunders, 1983:7–13.
112. Sokolow M, Lyon TP. The ventricular complex in right ventricular hypertrophy as obtained by unipolar precordial and limb leads. *Am Heart J* 1949; 38:273.
113. Myers GB, Klein HA, Stoffer BE. The electrocardiographic diagnosis of right ventricular hypertrophy. *Am Heart J* 1948;35:1.
114. Surawicz B. Electrocardiographic diagnosis of chamber enlargement. *J Am Coll Cardiol* 1986;8:711–724.
115. Das G. Left axis deviation: a spectrum of intraventricular conduction block. *Circulation* 1976;53:917–919.
116. Varriale P, Chryssos BE. The RSR′ complex not related to right bundle branch block: diagnostic value as a sign of myocardial infarction scar. *Am Heart J* 1992;123:369–376.
117. Rosembaum MB, Elizari MV, Lazzari JO. *The hemiblocks.* Oldsmar: Tampa Tracings, 1970.
118. Davies MJ, Anderson RH, Becker AE. Pathology of bundle branch block. In: *The conduction system of the heart.* Boston: Butterworths, 1983:281–300.
119. Warner RA, Hill NE, Mookherjee S, Smulyan H. Improved electrocardiographic criteria for the diagnosis of left anterior hemiblock. *Am J Cardiol* 1983;51:718–722.
120. Demoulin JC, Kulbertus HE. Histopathologic correlates of left posterior fascicular block. *Am J Cardiol* 1979;44:1083–1088.
121. Rosenbaum MB. The Hemiblocks: diagnostic criteria and clinical significance. *Mod Concepts Cardiovasc Dis* 1970;39:141–146.
122. Demoulin JC, Kulbertus HE. Histopathological examination of concept of left hemiblock. *Br Heart J* 1972;34:807–814.
123. Nakaya Y, Hiasa Y, Murayama Y, et al. Prominent anterior QRS force as a manifestation of left septal fascicular block. *J Electrocardiol* 1978;11:39–46.
124. MacAlpin RN. In search of left septal fascicular block. *Am Heart J* 2002; 144:948–956.
125. Chen CM, Damato AN. Contribution of His bundle recordings to aberrant intraventricular conduction. In: *Frontiers of cardiac electrophysiology.* Boston: Martinus Nijhoff, 1983:627–656.
126. Sclarovsky S, ed. *Electrocardiography of acute myocardial ischemic syndromes.* London: Martin Dunitz, 1999.
127. Birnbaum Y, Maynard C, Wolfe S, et al. Terminal QRS distortion on admission is better than ST-segment measurements in predicting final infarct size and assessing the potential effect of thrombolytic therapy in anterior wall acute myocardial infarction. *Am J Cardiol* 1999;84:530–534.
128. Sievers B, John B, Brandts B, et al. How reliable is electrocardiography in differentiating transmural from non-transmural myocardial infarction? A study with contrast magnetic resonance imaging as gold standard. *Int J Cardiol* 2004;97:417–423.

129. Reimer KA, Ideker RE. Myocardial ischemia and infarction: anatomic and biochemical substrates for ischemic cell death and ventricular arrhythmias. *Hum Pathol* 1987;18:462–475.
130. Essen RV, Merx W, Effert S. Spontaneous course of ST-segment elevation in acute myocardial infarction. *Circulation* 1979;59:105–112.
131. Bren GB, Wasserman AG, Ross AM. The electrocardiogram in patients undergoing thrombolysis for myocardial infarction. *Circulation* 1987; 76(suppl II):II18–II24.
132. Justis DL, Hession WT. Accuracy of 22-lead ECG analysis for diagnosis of acute myocardial infarction and coronary artery disease in the emergency department: a comparison with 12-lead ECG. *Ann Emerg Med* 1992;21:1–9.
133. Elko PP, Weaver WD, Kudenchuk P, Rowlandson I. The dilemma of sensitivity versus specificity in computer-interpreted acute myocardial infarction. *J Electrocardiol* 1992;24(suppl):2–7.
134. Cairns CB, Niemann JT, Selker HP, Laks MM. Computerized version of the time-insensitive predictive instrument. *J Electrocardiol* 1992;24(suppl):46–49.
135. O'Rourke MF, Cook A, Carroll G, et al. Accuracy of a portable interpretive ECG machine in diagnosis of acute evolving myocardial infarction. *Aust NZ J Med* 1992;22:9–13.
136. Brady WJ, Perron AD, Martin ML, et al. Cause of ST segment abnormality in ED chest pain patients. *Am J Emerg Med* 2001;19:25–28.
137. Aldrich HR, Hindman NB, Hinoara T, et al. Identification of optimal electrocardiographic leads for detecting acute epicardial injury in acute myocardial infarction. *Am J Cardiol* 1987;59:20–23.
138. Engelen DJ, Gorgels AP, Cheriex EC, et al. Value of the electrocardiogram in localizing the occlusion site in the left anterior descending coronary artery in acute myocardial infarction. *J Am Coll Cardiol* 1999;34:389–395.
139. Birnbaum Y, Sclarovsky S, Solodky A, et al. Prediction of the level of left anterior descending coronary artery obstruction during anterior wall acute myocardial infarction by the admission electrocardiogram. *Am J Cardiol* 1993;72:823–826.
140. Yotsukura M, Toyofuku M, Tajino K, et al. Clinical significance of the disappearance of septal Q waves after the onset of myocardial infarction: correlation with l location of responsible coronary lesions. *J Electrocardiol* 1999;32:15–20.
141. Tamura A, Kataoka H, Mikuriya Y. Electrocardiographic findings in a patient with pure septal infarction. *Br Heart J* 1991;65:166–167.
142. Tamura A, Kataoka H, Mikuriya Y, Nasu M. Inferior ST-segment depression as a useful marker for identifying proximal left anterior descending coronary artery occlusion during acute myocardial infarction. *Eur Heart J* 1995;16:1795–1799.
143. Vasudevan K, Manjunath CN, Srinivas KH, et al. Electrocardiographic localization of the occlusion site in left anterior descending coronary artery in acute anterior myocardial infarction. *Indian Heart J* 2004;56:315–319.
144. Ben-Gal T, Sclarovsky S, Herz I, et al. Importance of the conal branch of the right coronary artery in patients with acute anterior wall myocardial infarction: electrocardiographic and angiographic correlation. *J Am Coll Cardiol* 1997;29:506–511.
145. Braat SH, Brugada P, Den Dulk K, et al. Value of lead V_{4R} for recognition of the infarct coronary in acute inferior myocardial infarction. *Am J Cardiol* 1984;53:1538–1541.
146. Herz I, Assali AR, Adler Y, et al. New electrocardiographic criteria for predicting either the right or left circumflex artery as the culprit coronary artery in inferior wall acute myocardial infarction. *Am J Cardiol* 1997;80:1343–1345.
147. Fiol M, Cygankiewicz I, Carrillo A, et al. Value of electrocardiographic algorithm based on "ups and downs" of ST in assessment of a culprit artery in evolving inferior wall acute myocardial infarction. *Am J Cardiol* 2004;94:709–714.
148. Hasdai D, Birnbaum Y, Herz I, et al. ST segment depression in lateral limb leads in inferior wall acute myocardial infarction: implications regarding the culprit artery and the site of obstruction. *Eur Heart J* 1995;16:1549–1553.
149. Porter A, Vaturi M, Adler Y, et al. Are there differences among patients with inferior acute myocardial infarction with ST depression in leads V_2 and V_3 and positive versus negative T waves in these leads on admission? *Cardiology* 1998;90:295–298.
150. Sadanandan S, Hochman JS, Kolodziej A, et al. Clinical and angiographic characteristics of patients with combined anterior and inferior ST-segment elevation on the initial electrocardiogram during acute myocardial infarction. *Am Heart J* 2003;146:653–661.
151. Huey BL, Beller GA, Kaiser DL, Gibson RS. A comprehensive analysis of myocardial infarction due to left circumflex artery occlusion: comparison with infarction due to right coronary artery and left posterior descending artery occlusion. *J Am Coll Cardiol* 1988;12:1156–1166.
152. Matetzky S, Freimark D, Feinberg MS, et al. Acute myocardial infarction with isolated ST-segment elevation in posterior chest leads V7-9: "hidden" ST-segment elevations revealing acute posterior infarction. *J Am Coll Cardiol* 1999;34:748–753.
153. Assali AR, Sclarovsky S, Herz I, et al. Comparison of patients with inferior wall acute myocardial infarction with versus without ST-segment elevation in leads V_5 and V_6. *Am J Cardiol* 1998;81:81–83.
154. Zehender M, Kasper W, Kauder E, et al. Right ventricular infarction as an independent predictor of prognosis after acute inferior myocardial infarction. *N Engl J Med* 1993;328:981–988.
155. Turhan H, Yilmaz MB, Yetkin E, et al. Diagnostic value of aVL derivation for right ventricular involvement in patients with acute inferior myocardial infarction. *Ann Noninvasive Electrocardiol* 2003;8:185–188.
156. Kopelman HA, Forman MB, Wilson H, et al. Right ventricular myocardial infarction in patients with chronic lung disease: possible role of right ventricular hypertrophy. *J Am Coll Cardiol* 1985;5:1302–1307.
157. Terkelsen CJ, Lassen JF, Norgaard BL, et al. Mortality rates in patients with ST-elevation vs. non—ST-elevation acute myocardial infarction: observations from an unselected cohort. *Eur Heart J* 2005;26:18–26.
158. Kurisu S, Inoue I, Kawagoe T, et al. Electrocardiographic features in patients with acute myocardial infarction associated with left main coronary artery occlusion. *Heart* 2004;90:1059–1060.
159. O'Keefe JH, Sayed-Taha K, Gibson W, et al. Do patients with left circumflex coronary artery-related acute myocardial infarction without ST-segment elevation benefit from reperfusion therapy? *Am J Cardiol* 1995;75:718–720.
160. Camara EJN, Chandra N, Ouyang P, et al. Reciprocal ST change in acute myocardial infarction: assessment by electrocardiography and echocardiography. *J Am Coll Cardiol* 1983;2:251–257.
161. Tabbalat RA, Haft JI. Are reciprocal changes a consequence of "ischemia at a distance" or merely a benign electric phenomenon? A PTCA study. *Am Heart J* 1993;126:95–103.
162. Birnbaum Y, Wagner GS, Barbash GI, et al. Correlation of angiographic findings and right (V_1 to V_3) versus left (V_4 to V_6) precordial ST-segment depression in inferior wall acute myocardial infarction. *Am J Cardiol* 1999; 15:83:143–148.
163. Brady WJ, Perron AD, Syverud SA, et al. Reciprocal ST segment depression: impact on the electrocardiographic diagnosis of ST segment elevation acute myocardial infarction. *Am J Emerg Med* 2002;20:35–38.
164. Davidson E, Weinberger I, Rotenberg Z, et al. Elevated serum creatine kinase levels: an early diagnostic sign of acute dissection of the aorta. *Arch Intern Med* 1988;148:2184–2186.
165. Weiss P, Weiss I, Zuber M, Ritz R. How many patients with acute dissection of the thoracic aorta would erroneously receive thrombolytic therapy based on the electrocardiographic findings on admission? *Am J Cardiol* 1993;72:1329–1330.
166. Pope JH, Ruthazer R, Kontos MC, et al. The impact of electrocardiographic left ventricular hypertrophy and bundle branch block on the triage and outcome of ED patients with a suspected acute coronary syndrome: a multicenter study. *Am J Emerg Med* 2004;22:156–163.
167. Cannon A, Freedman B, Bailey BP, Bernstein L. ST-segment changes during transmural myocardial ischemia in chronic left bundle branch block. *Am J Cardiol* 1989;64:1216–1217.
168. Stark KS, Krucoff MW, Schryver B, Kent KM. Quantification of ST-segment changes during coronary angioplasty in patients with left bundle branch block. *Am J Cardiol* 1991;67:1219–1222.
169. Wackers FJ. Complete left bundle branch block: is the diagnosis of myocardial infarction possible? *Int J Cardiol* 1983;2:521–529.
170. Sgarbossa EB. Value of the ECG in suspected acute myocardial infarction with left bundle branch block. *J Electrocardiol* 2000;33(suppl):87–92.
171. Sgarbossa EB, Pinski SL, Barbagelata A, et al. , for the GUSTO-I Investigators. Electrocardiographic diagnosis of evolving acute myocardial infarction in the presence of left bundle branch block. *N Engl J Med* 1996; 334:481–487.
172. Sgarbossa EB, Pinski SL, Gates KB, Wagner GS, for the GUSTO-I Investigators. Electrocardiographic diagnosis of acute myocardial infarction in the presence of ventricular paced rhythm. *Am J Cardiol* 1996;77:423–424.
173. Welch RD, Zalenski RJ, Frederick PD, et al. Prognostic value of a normal or nonspecific initial electrocardiogram in acute myocardial infarction. *JAMA* 2001;286:1977–1984.
174. Gibler WB, Sayre MR, Levy RC, et al. Serial 12-lead electrocardiographic monitoring in patients presenting to the emergency department with chest pain. *J Electrocardiol* 1993;26(suppl):238–243.
175. Caceres L, Cooke D, Zalenski R, et al. Myocardial infarction with an initially normal electrocardiogram. Angiographic findings. *Clin Cardiol* 1995; 18:563–568.
176. Larsen GC, Griffith JL, Beshansky JR, et al. Electrocardiographic left ventricular hypertrophy in patients with suspected acute cardiac ischemia: its influence on diagnosis, triage, and short-term prognosis. *J Gen Intern Med* 1994;9:666–673.
177. Moon JC, De Arenaza DP, Elkington AG, et al. The pathologic basis of Q-wave and non-Q-wave myocardial infarction: a cardiovascular magnetic resonance study. *J Am Coll Cardiol* 2004;44:554–560.
178. Kaandorp TA, Bax JJ, Lamb HJ, et al. Which parameters on magnetic resonance imaging determine Q waves on the electrocardiogram? *Am J Cardiol* 2005;95:925–929.
179. Park SE, Tani A, Minamino T, et al. Coronary angiographic features within 48 hours from onset of non–Q wave myocardial infarction with R wave regression and no ST segment depression. *Cardiology* 1990;77:121–129.
180. Barbagelata A, Califf RM, Sgarbossa EB, et al. Thrombolysis and Q-wave versus non–Q-wave first acute myocardial infarction: a GUSTO-I substudy. *J Am Coll Cardiol* 1997;29:770–777.
181. Raitt MH, Maynard C, Wagner GS, et al. Appearance of abnormal Q waves early in the course of acute myocardial infarction: implications for efficacy of thrombolytic therapy. *J Am Coll Cardiol* 1995;25:1084–1088.

182. Krucoff MW, Green CE, Satler LF, et al. Noninvasive detection of coronary artery patency using continuous ST-segment monitoring. *Am J Cardiol* 1996;57:916–921.
183. Brodie BR, Stuckey TD, Hansen C, et al. Relation between electrocardiographic ST-segment resolution and early and late outcomes after primary percutaneous coronary intervention for acute myocardial infarction. *Am J Cardiol* 2005;95:343–348.
184. Zeymer U, Schroder K, Wegscheider K, et al. ST resolution in a single electrocardiographic lead: a simple and accurate predictor of cardiac mortality in patients with fibrinolytic therapy for acute ST-elevation myocardial infarction. *Am Heart J* 2005;149:91–97.
185. De Luca G, Maas AC, van't Hof AW, et al. Impact of ST-segment depression resolution on mortality after successful mechanical reperfusion in patients with ST-segment elevation acute myocardial infarction. *Am J Cardiol* 2005;95:234–236.
186. Chou TC. Myocardial infarction, myocardial injury, and myocardial ischemia. In: Chou TE, ed. *Electrocardiography in clinical practice: adult and pediatric*. Philadelphia: WB Saunders, 1996:121–213.
187. Sgarbossa EB, Birnbaum Y, Parrillo JE. ECG diagnosis of acute myocardial infarction: current concepts for the clinician. *Am Heart J* 2001,141:507–517.
188. Rodriguez MI, Anselmi CA, Sodi-Pallares D. The electrocardiographic diagnosis of septal infarctions. *Am Heart J* 1953;45:524–544.
189. Shalev Y, Fogelman R, Oettinger M, Caspi A. Does the electrocardiographic pattern of "anteroseptal" myocardial infarction correlate with the anatomic location of myocardial injury? *Am J Cardiol* 1995;75:763–766.
190. Dwyer EM Jr. The predictive accuracy of the electrocardiogram in identifying the presence and location of myocardial infarction and coronary artery disease. *Ann NY Acad Sci* 1990;601:67–76.
191. Boden WE, Bough EW, Korr KS, et al. Inferoseptal myocardial infarction: another cause of precordial ST-segment depression in transmural inferior wall myocardial infarction? *Am J Cardiol* 1984;54:1216–1223.
192. Tamura A, Kataoka H, Mikuriya Y. Electrocardiographic findings in a patient with pure septal infarction. *Br Heart J* 1991;65:166–167.
193. Bough EW, Boden WE, Korr KS, Gandsman EJ. Left ventricular asynergy in electrocardiographic "posterior" myocardial infarction. *J Am Coll Cardiol* 1984;4:209–215.
194. Ward RM, White RD, Ideker RE. Evaluation of a QRS scoring system for estimating myocardial infarct size. IV. Correlation with quantitative anatomic finds for posterolateral infarcts. *Am J Cardiol* 1984;53:706–714.
195. Huey BL, Beller GA, Kaiser DL, Gibson RS. A comprehensive analysis of myocardial infarction due to left circumflex artery occlusion: comparison with infarction due to right coronary and left anterior descending artery occlusion. *J Am Coll Cardiol* 1988;12:1156–1166.
196. Hoffman I, Mehta J, Helsenrath J, Hamby RI. Anterior conduction delay: a possible cause for prominent anterior QRS forces. *J Electrocardiol* 1976;9:15–21.
197. Warner RA. Recent advances in the diagnosis of myocardial infarction. *Cardiol Clin* 1987;5:381–392.
198. Cárdenas M, Díaz del Río A, González Hermosillo JA, et al. El infarto agudo de miocardio del ventrículo derecho: en memoria de Ignacio Chávez. *Arch Inst Cardiol Mex* 1980;50:295–312.
199. Richardson K, Engel G, Yamazaki T, et al. Electrocardiographic damage scores and cardiovascular mortality. *Am Heart J* 2005;149:458–463.
200. Gardin JM, Singer DH. Atrial infarction. Importance, diagnosis and localization. *Arch Intern Med* 1981;141:1345–1348.
201. Fisch C. Electrocardiography and vectorcardiography. In: Braunwald E, ed. *Heart disease: a textbook of cardiovascular medicine*. Philadelphia: WB Saunders, 1992:116–160.
202. Sweterlitsch EM, Murphy GW. Acute electrocardiographic pseudoinfarction pattern in the setting of diabetic ketoacidosis and severe hyperkalemia. *Am Heart J* 1996;132:1086–1089.
203. Houghton JL, Sinden JR, Gross CM. Acute presentation of pseudo myocardial infarction secondary to metastatic cancer. *Am J Med Sci* 1992;303: 170–173.
204. Gurevitz O, Lipchenca I, Yaacoby E, et al. ST-segment deviation following implantable cardioverter defibrillator shocks: incidence, timing, and clinical significance. *Pacing Clin Electrophysiol* 2002;25:1429–1432.
205. Geibel A, Zehender M, Kasper W, et al. Prognostic value of the ECG on admission in patients with acute major pulmonary embolism. *Eur Respir J* 2005;25:843–848.
206. Manthous CA, Schmidt GA. Pleural effusion masquerading as myocardial infarction. *Chest* 1993;103:1619–1621.
207. Osswald S, Roelke M, O'Nunain SS, et al. Electrocardiographic pseudoinfarct patterns after implantation of cardioverter-defibrillators. *Am Heart J* 1995;129:265–272.
208. Sgarbossa EB. Recent advances in the electrocardiographic diagnosis of myocardial infarction: left bundle branch block and pacing. *Pacing Clin Electrophysiol* 1996;19:1370–1379.
209. Spodick DH. Acute pericarditis: current concepts and practice. *JAMA* 2003;289:1150–1153.
210. Bybee KA, Kara T, Prasad A, et al. Systematic review: transient left ventricular apical ballooning: a syndrome that mimics ST-segment elevation myocardial infarction. *Ann Intern Med* 2004;141:858–865.
211. Wittstein IS, Thiemann DR, Lima JA, et al. Neurohumoral features of myocardial stunning due to sudden emotional stress. *N Engl J Med* 2005; 352:539–548.
212. Mattu A, Brady WJ, Perron AD. Electrocardiographic manifestations of hypothermia. *Am J Emerg Med* 2002;20:314–326.
213. Golshayan D, Seydoux C, Berguer DG, et al. Incidence and prognostic value of electrocardiographic abnormalities after heart transplantation. *Clin Cardiol* 1998;21:680–684.
214. Calzolari V, Angelini A, Basso C, et al. Histologic findings in the conduction system after cardiac transplantation and correlation with electrocardiographic findings. *Am J Cardiol* 1999;84:756–759.
215. Sinha N, Yalamanchili K, Sukhija R, et al. Role of the 12-lead electrocardiogram in diagnosing pulmonary embolism. *Cardiol Rev* 2005;13:46–49.
216. Rodger M, Makropoulos D, Turek M, et al. Diagnostic value of the electrocardiogram in suspected pulmonary embolism. *Am J Cardiol* 2000;86: 807–809.
217. Yamour BJ, Sridharan MR, Rice JF, Flowers NC. Electrocardiographic changes in cerebrovascular hemorrhage. *Am Heart J* 1980;99:294–300.
218. Hugenholtz PG. Electrocardiographic changes typical for central nervous system after right radical neck dissection. *Am Heart J* 1967;74:438–441.
219. Gould L, Gopalaswami C, Chandy F, Kim B. Electroconvulsive therapy-induced ECG changes simulating a myocardial infarction. *Arch Intern Med* 1983;143:1786–1787.
220. Koepp M, Schmidt D, Kern A. Electrocardiographic changes in patients with brain tumors. *Arch Neurol* 1995;52:152–155.
221. Hedén B, Ohlsson M, Holst H, et al. Detection of frequently overlooked electrocardiographic lead reversals using artificial neural networks. *Am J Cardiol* 1996;78:600–604.
222. Abdollah H, Milliken JA. Recognition of electrocardiographic left arm/left leg lead reversal. *Am J Cardiol* 1997;80:1247–1249.
223. Herman MV, Ingram DA, Levy JA, et al. Variability of electrocardiographic precordial lead placement: a method to improve accuracy and reliability. *Clin Cardiol* 1991;14:469–476.
224. El-Sheriff N. High-resolution electrocardiography. In: Moss AJ, Stern S, eds. *Noninvasive electrocardiology: clinical aspects of Holter monitoring*. Philadelphia: WB Saunders, 1996:249–254.
225. Mirvis DM, ed. *Body surface electrocardiographic mapping*. Boston: Kluwer Academic, 1988.
226. Laks M. The ECG bridge to the twenty-first century: progress report for 1997 and future directions. *J Electrocardiol* 1998;30(suppl):96–197.
227. Brady WJ, Hwang V, Sullivan R, et al. A comparison of 12- and 15-lead ECGS in ED chest pain patients pain patients: impact on diagnosis, therapy, and disposition. *Am J Emerg Med* 2000;18:239–243.
228. Pahlm US, Pahlm O, Wagner GS. The standard 11-lead ECG: neglect of lead aVR in the classical limb lead display. *J Electrocardiol* 1996;29:270–274.
229. McCarthy BD, Beshansky JR, D'Agostino RB, Selker HP. Missed diagnoses of acute myocardial infarction in the emergency department: results from a multicenter study. *Ann Emerg Med* 1993;22:579–582.
230. Sur DK, Kaye L, Mikus M, et al. Accuracy of electrocardiogram reading by family practice residents. *Fam Med* 2000;32:315–319.
231. McCrea WA, Saltisi S. Electrocardiogram interpretation in general practice: relevance to prehospital thrombolysis. *Br Heart J* 1993;70:219–225.
232. Jayes RL, Larsen GC, Beshansky JR, et al. Physician electrocardiogram reading in the emergency department: accuracy and effect on triage decisions: findings form a multicenter study. *J Gen Intern Med* 1992;7:387–392.
233. Woolley D, Henck M, Luck J. Comparison of electrocardiogram interpretations by family physicians, a computer, and a cardiology service. *J Fam Pract* 1992;34:428–432.
234. Berger A, Meier JM, Stauffer JC, et al. ECG interpretation during the acute phase of coronary syndromes: in need of improvement? *Swiss Med Wkly* 2004;134:695–699.
235. Lee TH, Rouan GW, Weisberg MC, et al. Clinical characteristics and natural history of patients with acute myocardial infarction sent home from the emergency room. *Am J Cardiol* 1987;60:219–224.
236. Fisch C. Centennial of the string galvanometer and the electrocardiogram. *J Am Coll Cardiol* 2000;36:1737–1745.
237. Gjrup T, Helbæk H, Nielsen D, et al. Interpretation of the electrocardiogram in suspected myocardial infarction: a randomized controlled study of the effect of a training programme to reduce interobserver variation. *J Intern Med* 1992;231:407–412.
238. Herman MV, Ingram DA, Levy JA, et al. Variability of electrocardiographic precordial lead placement: a method to improve accuracy and reliability. *Clin Cardiol* 1991;14:469–476.
239. Sokolove PE, Sgarbossa EB, Wagner GS, et al. Interobserver agreement in the ECG diagnosis of acute myocardial infarction in the presence of left bundle branch block. *Acad Emerg Med* 1999;6:452–453.
240. Willems JL, Abreu-Lima C, Arnaud P, et al. The diagnostic performance of computer programs for the interpretation of electrocardiograms. *N Engl J Med* 1991;325:1767–1773.
241. McLaughlin SC, Aitchison TC, Macfarlane PW. Improved repeatability of 12-lead ECG analysis using continuous scoring techniques. *J Electrocardiol* 1993;26(suppl):101–107.
242. Hurst JW. Computers are of limited value in the interpretation of electrocardiograms. *Medscape Cardiol* 2000. www.medscape.com.

243. Willems JL, Arnaud P, vanBemmel JH, et al. Assessment of the performance of electrocardiography computer programs with the use of a reference database. *Circulation* 1985;71:523–534.
244. Svensson L, Axelsson C, Nordlander R, Herlitz J. Prehospital identification of acute coronary syndrome/myocardial infarction in relation to ST elevation. *Int J Cardiol* 2005;98:237–244.
245. Marozas V, Jurkonis R, Kazla A, et al. Development of teleconsultations systems for e-health. *Stud Health Technol Inform* 2004;105:337–348.
246. Scalvini S, Zanelli E, Conti C, et al. Assessment of prehospital chest pain using telecardiology. *J Telemed Telecare* 2002;8:231–236.
247. Ferguson JD, Brady WJ, Perron AD, et al. The prehospital 12-lead electrocardiogram: impact on management of the out-of-hospital acute coronary syndrome patient. *Am J Emerg Med* 2003;21:136–142.
248. Saxena SC, Kumar V, Giri VK. Telecardiology for effective healthcare services. *J Med Eng Technol* 2003;27:149–159.
249. Rodriguez J, Dranca L, Goni A, Illarramendi A. Web access to data in a mobile ECG monitoring system. *Stud Health Technol Inform* 2004;105:100–11.
250. Song Z, Jenkins J, Burke M, Arzbaecher R. The feasibility of ST-segment monitoring with a subcutaneous device. *J Electrocardiol* 2004;37:174–179.

CHAPTER 61 ■ ELECTROPHYSIOLOGIC TESTING

ANDREW KRUMERMAN AND JOHN D. FISHER

OVERVIEW

An electrophysiologic study (EPS) provides a safe and effective method for evaluation, risk stratification, and treatment of known and suspected arrhythmias. This chapter emphasizes EPS indications, techniques and normal findings.

An EPS permits assessment of individual portions of the cardiac electrical system. These assessments include evaluation of spontaneous function, responses to stresses, and vulnerability to induced tachyarrhythmias. Indications and guidelines for EPS have been established for a broad range of situations and clinical problems (1) (Table 61.1).

GLOSSARY

AH interval: The interval from the first rapid deflection of the atrial electrogram on the His bundle lead to the first inscription of the His bundle depolarization.

Cycle length (CL): Interval in milliseconds. During EPS, cycle lengths or intervals often change from beat to beat, so that these measures are more relevant than an overall rate, which is expressed in beats per minute. The use of rates in beats per minute is retained mostly to facilitate communications with physicians who are more comfortable with this terminology.

Effective and functional refractory periods: Measurements of impulse propagation at various levels in the heart (see text for detailed definitions).

Effective and functional conduction periods: Measurements of impulse propagation at various levels in the heart (see text for detailed definitions).

HV interval: The interval from the first inscription of the His bundle potential to the first evidence of ventricular depolarization on the surface ECG or the His bundle lead.

PA interval: The interval from the first evidence of sinus node depolarization, whether on the intracardiac or surface ECG, to the atrial deflection as recorded in the His bundle lead.

S1, S2, . . . , S*N*: S1 refers to the baseline or drive stimulus in a series, with each of the series of S1s being of equal intervals. S2 is the first extrastimulus, with the S1S2 interval almost always shorter than the S1S1 interval. The S3, S4, and S*N* stimuli are the second, third, and *N*th extrastimuli, respectively. See text for details.

HISTORICAL PERSPECTIVE

The leap from the experimental animal laboratory to the clinical arena and clinical cardiac electrophysiology was made possible by the development of cardiac catheterization and transvenous pacing techniques. Intracardiac recordings from

TABLE 61.1

MAJOR INDICATIONS FOR ELECTROPHYSIOLOGIC TESTING

ACC/AHA/ NASPE 1995	Class I	Class II	Class III
Sinus node function	Symptomatic patients: sinus node dysfunction is suspected but unproved	Patients with documented sinus node dysfunction in whom evaluation of AV or ventriculoatrial conduction may aid choice of pacer Sinus brady: intrinsic vs. autonomic or drug effects Symptomatic patients with sinus brady, to rule out other causes	Symptomatic patients with documented association between rhythm and symptoms, therapy would not change with EPS Asymptomatic sinus brady only with sleep, including sleep apnea
Acquired AV block	Symptomatic patients with HV block suspected but unproved	Patients with second- or third-degree AV block where site of block or response to measures (e.g., drugs) could affect therapy	Symptomatic patients with symptoms and AV block correlated with ECG
	Paced patients with AV block who are still symptomatic	Suspected concealed junctional depolarizations causing pseudo-AV block	Asymptomatic patients with transient AV block associated with sinus slowing (e.g., nocturnal type I second-degree AV block)
Chronic intraventricular conduction defects	Symptomatic patients, cause unknown	Asymptomatic patients with bundle branch block in whom pharmacologic therapy that could cause block is contemplated	Asymptomatic patients with intraventricular conduction defects Symptomatic patients in whom symptoms correlate with or are excluded by ECG
Narrow-QRS-complex tachycardia	To choose treatment for patients with poorly tolerated tachy that does not respond adequately to drugs Patients who prefer ablation	Patients with frequent episodes to be treated with drugs, but there is concern about proarrhythmia, or drug effects on sinoatrial node or AV conduction	Patients well controlled by vagal maneuvers or drugs and not candidates for nonpharmacologic treatment
Wide-QRS-complex tachycardias	Correct diagnosis is needed for treatment, but is unclear on ECG	None	Diagnosis of supraventricular tachycardia or VT certain from ECG However, EPS data may be useful in guiding subsequent treatment
Prolonged QT intervals	None	To identify proarrhythmic effects of a drug in a patient with cardiac arrest on the drug Patients with syncope and with or without long QT or TU waves, to unmask abnormal QT, e.g., with a catecholamine	Manifest long QT, with or without arrhythmias Acquired long QT syndrome with identifiable cause
Wolff-Parkinson-White syndrome	Patients being evaluated for catheter ablation Patients with deltas who have had arrest or SUO Symptomatic patients in whom EPS data could affect treatment	Asymptomatic patients with family history of sudden death, or who engage in high-risk activities (insurance?) Patients with deltas undergoing other cardiac surgery Asymptomatic patients not covered above	Asymptomatic patients not covered above
Ventricular premature contractions, couplets, and VT-NS	None	Patients with other risk factors (e.g., low ejection fraction, abnormal sinoatrial ECG, VT-NS on Holter, if EPS will be used to guide treatment if sustained VT is induced Highly symptomatic patients considered for catheter ablation	Patients with syncope of known cause whose treatment will not be altered by EPS findings

(Continued)

TABLE 61.1

(CONTINUED) MAJOR INDICATIONS FOR ELECTROPHYSIOLOGIC TESTING

ACC/AHA/ NASPE 1995	Class I	Class II	Class III
SUO	Patients with suspected structural heart disease and SUO	Patients with recurrent SUO, without structural heart disease, and with a negative tilt-test result	Patients with syncope of known cause whose treatment will not be altered by EPS findings
Cardiac arrest survivors	Survivors without new Q-wave MI Arrest >48 h after acute MI	Arrest caused by bradyarrhythmia Arrest possibly due to congenital long-QT syndrome	Arrest in first 48 h after acute MI Arrest from clear cause (e.g., acute ischemia, aortic stenosis, or long-QT syndrome)
Unexplained palpitations	Rapid pulse felt by medical personnel, without ECG Palpitations followed by syncope	"Significant" palpitations where EPS may help in diagnosis, risk assessment, or treatment	Palpitations documented to be due to noncardiac cause (e.g., hyperthyroidism)
Guiding drug therapy	Patients with sustained VT or arrest, especially if prior MI Patients with AV nodal reentry tachycardia, AV reentrant tachycardia, or atrial fibrillation with an accessory pathway in whom drug therapy is planned	Sinoatrial node reentry tachycardia, AT, atrial fibrillation, or atrial flutter, without deltas Patients with arrhythmias not inducible at baseline EPS	Isolated atrial premature contractions or ventricular premature contractions Ventricular fibrillation with a clearly identified reversible cause
Related to implantable devices	Before and during implant, and before discharge to confirm performance After implant to determine if a factor has altered the performance of the device Test interactions if two devices are to be used	In patients with documented indications for pacing, to optimize pacing mode and sites	Patients who are not device therapy candidates

ACC/AHA/NASPE, American College of Cardiology/American Heart Association/North American Society for Pacing and Electrophysiology; AT, atrial tachycardia; AV, atrioventricular; brady, bradycardia; ECG, electrocardiography; EPS, electrophysiologic study; MI, myocardial infarction; NS, nonsustained; SUO, syncope of undetermined origin; tachy, tachycardia; VT, ventricular tachycardia.

From Zipes DP, DiMarco JP, Gillette PC, et al., with Fisher JD for ablation section. Guidelines for clinical intracardiac electrophysiological and catheter ablation procedures. A report of the ACC/AHA Task Force on Practice Guidelines (Committee on Clinical Intracardiac Electrophysiological and Catheter Ablation Procedures), developed in collaboration with NASPE. *J Am Coll Cardiol* 1995;26:555–573; *Circulation* 1995;92:675–691; *J Cardiovasc Electrophysiol* 1995;6:652–679.

the right atrium, His bundle region, and right ventricle allowed direct rather than inferential analysis of normal and abnormal rhythms (2,3). Electrophysiologic testing was quickly established as the definitive method for diagnosis and subsequently for treatment of cardiac rhythm disorders.

INTRODUCTION

A complete EPS consists of a series of tests that are designed to evaluate the heart from top to bottom, that is, from the sinus node to the ventricle with steps in between. Depending on the purpose of the EPS for a given patient, all or only some of these regions may be tested, in an à la carte fashion.

The testing techniques used to evaluate each region are remarkably similar. Pacing at increasing rates and programmed electrical stimulation (PES) form the core of testing at each level, supplemented by various pharmacologic probes and physical maneuvers.

This chapter emphasizes the indications for EPS, matters related to patient preparation, vascular access, stimulation and recording techniques, and an outline of EPS related to the major parts of the heart's electrical system. Other chapters cover the details of specific arrhythmias.

Indications for Electrophysiologic Study

The earliest practical application of EPS was for assessment of the conduction system. This was followed in rapid succession by EPS for characterization of various tachycardias; as a guide for antiarrhythmic drug efficacy; identification of the cause of syncope of undetermined origin (SUO); arrhythmia mapping before and during open heart surgery; and as an integral part of the procedure for catheter ablation of tachycardias. Guidelines on the indications for EPS have been published by the American College of Cardiology (ACC) together with the American Heart Association (AHA) and by the Heart Rhythm

Society (HRS), but they have not been recently updated (1) (Table 61.1).

Patient Preparation

Education and Consent

Patients are often quite anxious about the prospect of an invasive study. Most diagnostic EP studies involve only venous access, and they are therefore safer than coronary angiography. The latter is a procedure that many patients are familiar with and tend to take for granted. Electrophysiologists often have patients referred to them who have been told by the referring physician that EPS is a minor, low-risk procedure. These patients may be alarmed to learn that no procedure is risk free and that EPS may require several hours. It is therefore important for realistic patient education to begin with the referring physician. The electrophysiologist should put the various risks in context. Patients can understand analogies, such as the risks versus the benefits of walking across a busy street. Patients should also have a realistic idea of the benefit they may derive from undergoing EPS, including the possibility that the study may be negative or equivocal.

Preprocedure Preparations

Traditionally, diagnostic EPS was performed in the "postabsorptive, nonsedated state." There are of course some problems with this idea. There is great variation among patients in the anxiety that they experience during invasive procedures. As EP procedures became longer and more complex, it became clear that sedation would be required for many of these individuals.

Twelve-Lead Electrocardiogram

It is helpful to have a 12-lead ECG available, particularly when tachyarrhythmias are expected during the procedure or for patients for whom ischemia is an issue. It is desirable for the 12 leads to be recorded simultaneously or in just a few seconds in case the arrhythmia is fast, slow, or transient.

Defibrillator Pads

Using preapplied adhesive defibrillator pads avoids the need to disrupt the sterile field in the event that electrical defibrillation/cardioversion is needed during the procedure.

Arterial Lines

Arterial lines are used routinely in a *minority* of EP labs, except in unstable patients or for certain ablation procedures. Automated/cuff blood pressure devices are usually adequate.

Sedation

Many patients benefit from minimal sedation. Longer procedures and ablations are now routinely performed using intravenous "conscious" sedation. Guidelines are published by the HRS (4).

Urinary Problems

Urinary retention may occur in individuals of either gender during lengthy EP studies, particularly if the study is combined with sedation and a tachycardia-related diuresis. When this situation is anticipated, it is useful to insert a Foley catheter *prior* to the procedure. Lubrication and topical anesthesia of the urethra using a commercially available lidocaine jelly injector system makes catheterization both acceptable and well tolerated by the patient.

Oxygen and Carbon Dioxide Monitoring

Monitoring of O_2 saturation has become virtually routine in many laboratories and is of particular value in sedated patients. If patients are receiving supplemental oxygen, the O_2 saturation may be misleadingly high. Expired CO_2 monitors are useful in preventing hypercapnia in such situations and are recommended in the guidelines for conscious sedation.

Universality of Stimulation Techniques

There is a relatively small menu of stimulation techniques useful in the study of both bradycardias and tachycardias.

Stimulus Amplitude and Pulse Duration (Pulse Width)

Most EP labs use outputs at two to four times the diastolic threshold. Twice the threshold is more common. In general, refractory periods (see later discussion) are somewhat longer when determined using twice the threshold, and this may reduce the incidence of induction of "nonclinical" tachyarrhythmias. At four times the threshold, one is at the beginning of the more vertical portion of a strength–interval curve, which may have several advantages (5,6).

A pulse duration of 1 or 2 msec is most commonly used. This dates from the early days of clinical EP when implanted pacemakers had similar pulse durations, as do current temporary pacemakers. This pulse duration is now out of synchrony with those used in implantable devices, but it has been retained for the sake of consistency in EP protocols done over long periods of time.

Most commercial EP stimulators emit constant-current pulses. Initially this too was in keeping with the norm for implantable pacemakers. The latter are now nearly universally constant-voltage devices. Testing of patients with and without clinical tachycardias with both constant-voltage and constant-current stimulation, all at four times the diastolic threshold, produced no significant difference in any of the results.

Incremental versus Decremental

Both terms are in regular use and have opposite meaning depending on whether one is considering *rate* in beats per minute or *cycle length* (CL) in milliseconds. The paragraphs that follow employ the most conventional usage.

Straight Pacing

The pacing rate or cycle length is maintained throughout the duration of the stimulation. There are several common applications for straight pacing.

(Rate) Incremental Pacing. After pacing at a given rate for a predetermined number of stimuli or seconds, the rate is then increased (with or without intervening pauses) in a series of steps until predetermined endpoints are reached. The terminology of rate incremental pacing is derived from the use of stimulators controlled by an analogue dial. Digitally controlled devices often increase the rate by choosing a sequence of cycle length *decrements*, but the term "incremental pacing" may still be used.

S1S1 Drive Stimuli. The heart is paced, or driven, at a specified rate and duration (typically 8 beats), after which a premature extrastimulus is delivered (see later discussion). The eight drive beats are each termed S1 stimuli. These S1s may be followed by first, second, third, and *N*th premature extrastimuli, which are designated S2, S3, S4, and S*N*, respectively. When extrastimuli follow a series of sinus beats, the latter may also be designated as S1s. S1S1 drive stimuli are sometimes called "trains," but this can be confused with ultrarapid train stimulation (see later discussion), which is also referred to as "trains."

Burst Pacing for Tachycardia Induction. Stimuli are delivered at a constant rate for a relatively short duration but at successively faster rates with each burst until a predetermined maximum rate (or minimum interval, i.e., CL) has been reached.

Bursts for Termination of Tachycardia. This procedure is similar to the technique used for induction. The initial pacing rate is faster than that of the tachycardia.

Underdrive Pacing for Tachycardia Termination. This refers to pacing at a rate slower than the tachycardia at a constant rate. Stimuli will therefore fall at differing points in the tachycardia cycle.

Ramps

Ramp pacing implies a smooth change in the interval between successive stimuli. Ramps too can be incremental or decremental as defined by either rate or cycle length. Ramps have several applications:

1. As a test for conduction, long ramps with small cycle-length decrements between successive stimuli provide results comparable to stepwise rate incremental pacing (7).
2. For tachycardia induction, the ramp is decreased in duration but the steepness of the slope is increased (i.e., interstimulus intervals are decreased more rapidly). Successive ramps go to higher and higher rates (shorter intervals) up to a predetermined limit.
3. For tachycardia termination, the procedure is somewhat similar to the previous one. It is commonly used in antitachycardia pacing algorithms in implantable cardioverter-defibrillators (ICDs). Programmed rate incremental ramps are also known as autodecremental pacing.

Extrastimulus Technique

One or more extrastimuli, (designated S2, S3, S*N*) are introduced at specific coupling intervals based on previous drive S1s, or spontaneous beats. Thereafter the S1S2 interval is altered, usually in 10- to 20-msec steps, until an endpoint is reached, such as tissue refractoriness or termination or induction of a tachycardia. It is usual to begin late in diastole and successively decrement the S1S2 interval. When the physician is satisfied with the results of S1S2 testing, a second extrastimulus (S3) may then be introduced with the S2S3 interval altered in a fashion similar to that used for S1S2.

Two methods are in common clinical use for decrementing the S1S2S3S4 intervals (8,9). In the *tandem method* the S1S2 is decremented until S2 does not capture, and then the S1S2 interval is increased by 40 to 50 msec and held there. S3 is then introduced, and the S2S3 interval is decremented until S3 fails to capture. At that point, the S1S2 interval is decremented, and S3 is retested to see whether it captures. From that point on, the S1S2 and S2S3 are decremented in tandem until refractory, so that both they and the S3S4 interval are altered in a fashion similar to that used for S2S3. In the *simple sequential method*, the S1S2 interval is decremented until it no longer captures, and then it is incremented until it does (usually 10 msec). The S1S2 interval is then held constant while the S2S3 interval is decremented in a similar fashion to that used for S1, and then the same for S3S4. The tandem method can be looked on as more conservative because it favors relatively longer intervals and gives a larger number of stimulation runs before moving on to the next extrastimulus. Prospective studies comparing the two methods have shown no differences between the two methods in any of the outcomes assessed (8). The choice of the simple sequential or tandem method therefore remains a matter of the investigator's choice.

Ultrarapid Train Stimulation

Stimuli are delivered at very short intervals (10 to 50 msec) for a duration sufficient to result in a desired number of captures. The technique has long been used experimentally (with sequentially increasing stimulus amplitudes) for induction of ventricular fibrillation (VF). It is now used clinically for that purpose with ICDs. Shorter trains have also proved useful in termination of tachycardias (10) and in induction of monomorphic tachycardias (11). Of all the techniques described, ultrarapid trains are the least universally employed except for VF induction with ICDs.

Stimulation Protocols

Adequacy is more important than universality. Bodies such as the Heart Rhythm Society have published guidelines on the minimum standards for an acceptable protocol (12). In addition to suggesting reasonable ranges of stimulation sites, drive cycle lengths, numbers of extrastimuli, and amplitudes and pulse durations of the extrastimuli, the guidelines also suggest outcome criteria. For example, the protocol used should be able to induce sustained monomorphic ventricular tachycardia (VT) in at least 90% of patients with coronary artery disease who present with such a rhythm.

Signal Filtering and Interelectrode Distance

The surface ECG is usually filtered at 0.1 to 100 Hz. The bulk of the energy is in the 0.1–20-Hz range. Because of interference from alternating current (AC), muscle twitches, and similar relatively high frequency interference, it is sometimes necessary to record the surface ECG over a lower frequency range or to use notch filters. Timing of events with respect to QRS onset is often important during EPS, but it is cumbersome to display all 12 leads of the regular surface ECG. Orthogonal lead systems (XYZ) are logical but not commonly used. It is more typical to use mutually perpendicular leads (I, AVF, and V1), often supplemented by lead II, which gives an indication as to the presence of abnormal left-axis deviation. Many electrophysiologists have their own favorite lead selections.

Intracardiac leads can be placed strategically at various positions within the heart. It is therefore desirable to record *local* events in the region of the lead rather than far-field events. This is accomplished by filtering intracardiac electrograms, typically at 30 or 40 to 500 Hz. Note that this eliminates the spectrum with the greatest energy that reaches the surface ECG. The higher-frequency waves carry much less energy and may be difficult to detect more than 1 cm away from the recording lead. Bipolar electrograms are generally used, and smaller interelectrode distances record increasingly local events.

Timing of Local Events

With an "unfiltered" bipolar lead, an approaching wavefront creates a positive deflection that quickly reverses itself as the lead passes directly under the electrode. This rapid reversal constitutes the "intrinsic deflection" of the electrogram and represents the timing of the most local event, that is, at the site of the bipole (13). Electrograms are filtered at 30 or 40 to 500 Hz, have a much more jagged appearance. When recorded simultaneously with an unfiltered electrogram, the midpoint of the intrinsic deflection of the unfiltered electrogram occurs at the same time as a similar deflection on the filtered electrogram, or at the peak positive or negative deflection of the filtered electrogram. The slew rate or *dV/dt* of the filtered electrogram is so rapid in normal heart tissue that the difference between the peak and the nadir of the deflection is 5 msec or less. Identification of the local event is therefore easy with either filtered or unfiltered electrograms in normal tissue. However, diseased myocardium may conduct very slowly with fractionated electrograms that make local events harder to identify. The electrophysiologist must then decide whether to use onset rather than local criteria for timing of events. Even in normal tissue, onset deflections are usually less crisp than the local deflection. Tradition plays a large role in the choices of deflections used for timing of events (see the section to follow on baseline intervals). At times there may be a deflection that is of particular interest, such as a His or bundle branch deflection, that is very small relative to the size of surrounding electrograms. This is particularly true when the gain must be markedly increased to produce a measurable deflection. In such instances, a "limiter" or "clipper" option on the amplifier/recorder system can eliminate the very highly amplified surrounding signals to allow concentration on the deflection of interest. However, limiters also eliminate the ability to determine the timing of the intrinsic deflection (local timing) of the signals being limited.

Catheterization Techniques

The percutaneous technique is used almost exclusively. The His bundle electrogram (HBE) is most commonly recorded using a lead inserted via a femoral vein and advanced through the right atrium across the tricuspid into the right ventricular inflow area. Some other areas are more easily reached through the superior vena cava. Insertion sites can also include the antecubital, jugular, and subclavian veins.

Choices of Surface and Intracardiac Signals

A classic display would include three or four surface ECGs; a recording from the high right atrium (HRA); the HBE, which includes the low medial right atrium, the His bundle deflection, and the right ventricular inflow deflection; and a recording from the right ventricular apex (RVA). Depending on the type of study and the information sought, stimulation and recording from other sites may be appropriate (Fig. 61.1).

THE ELECTROPHYSIOLOGIC STUDY

Baseline Intervals

The PR interval of the surface ECG can be further subdivided based on intracardiac electrogram (Fig. 61.1). During sinus rhythm, the earliest atrial activity is identified using the high right atrial electrogram (HRA) from the sinus node region at

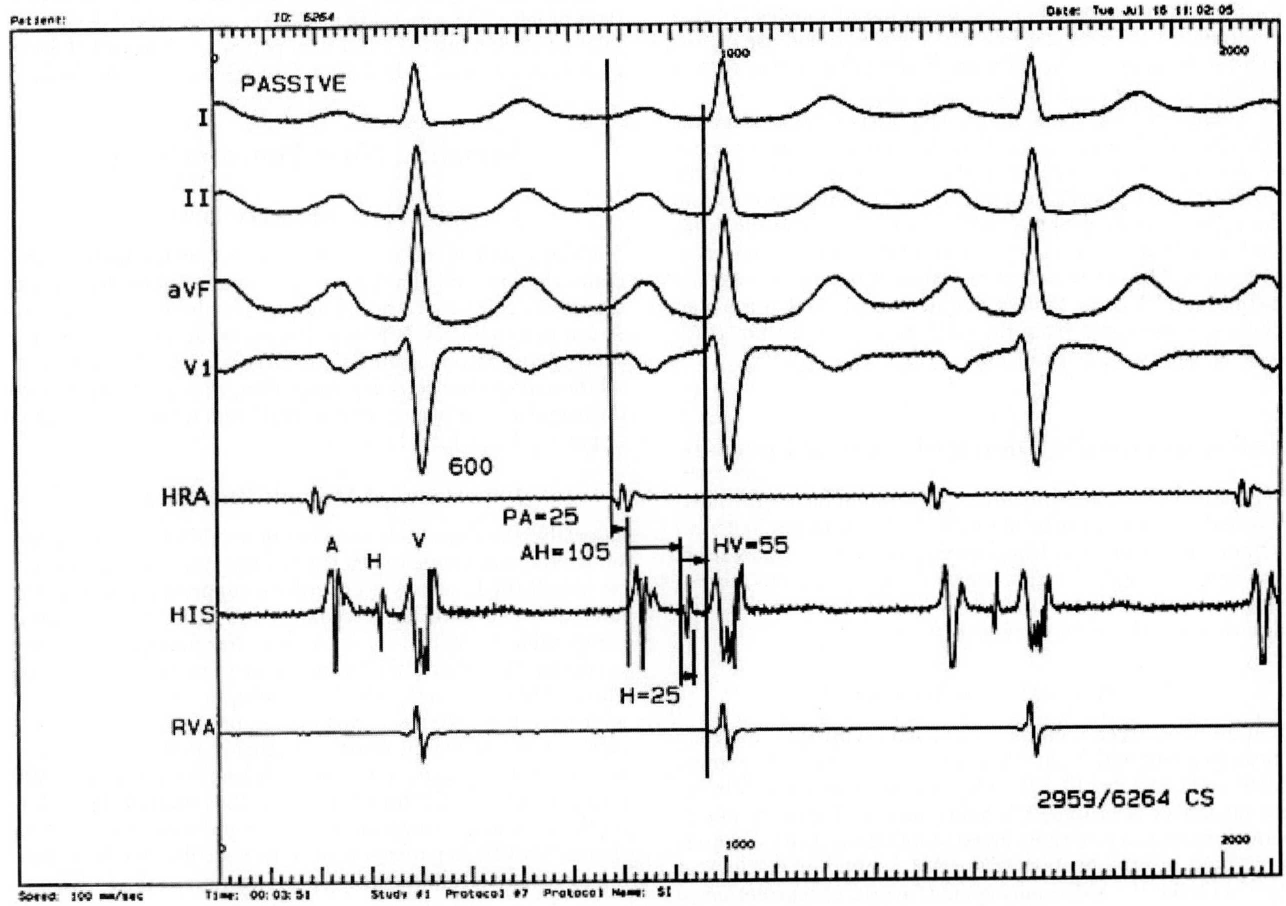

FIGURE 61.1. Normal intracardiac electrograms. This is a "passive His bundle electrogram," that is, a His bundle electrogram and accompanying recordings during sinus rhythm with no ongoing manipulations, stimuli, or intentional stresses. Semiorthogonal leads 1, AVF, and V1 are used together with lead 2, which is helpful in determining the QRS axis. The measurement of intervals is demonstrated. Definitions are provided in the text.

TABLE 61.2

NORMAL CONDUCTION INTERVALS (±2 STANDARD DEVIATIONS)

	PA intraatrial	AH AV node	H His	HV His to V	P-LA interatrial
Passive/baseline	10–45	55–130	<25	30–55	40–130
Atrial paced	10–75	[a]	<25	30–55	65–150

AV, atrioventricular; LA, left atrium.
[a]Progressive prolongation.
Based on a compilation of sources (14–22).

the junction of the superior vena cava and the right atrium. The P wave is then timed from the earliest evidence of such atrial activity, whether first seen in the HRA lead or in the surface ECG. Next, conduction through the right atrium to the region of the atrioventricular (AV) node and His bundle is then measured as the PA interval. This is defined as the interval from the P wave as just defined to the *first rapid* depolarization of the atrium recorded on the HBE lead. AV node conduction is measured by the interval from the *first rapid* deflection of the A wave in the HBE lead to the *first evidence* of His bundle depolarization on the HBE lead; this is designated the AH interval. Conduction through the His bundle and bundle branches is then measured as the timing from the *first evidence* of the His bundle deflection to the *first evidence* of ventricular deflection on the HBE lead *or* on the surface ECG, whichever comes first. Normal values for these intervals based on a compilation of sources (14–22) are found in Table 61.2. Note that the traditional use of *first rapid* deflections can be quite subjective compared with *first evidence* or the local or *intrinsic deflection.*

A minority of authors use the HQ interval rather than the HV interval. The HQ interval is the interval from the onset of the His bundle potential to the onset of the QRS and the surface ECG. Logically, one might also use information from the right ventricular apical (RVA) lead or other intracardiac leads (23,24), but these are not part of the conventional measurements. The His bundle potential itself should be crisp and distinct and less than 25 msec in duration. The *inter*atrial conduction is measured from the HRA to the left atrium (LA). Normal values are given in Table 61.2.

Influences on the Timing of Cardiac Intervals

Sympathetic and parasympathetic tone can influence the heart rate and timing of cardiac intervals (25,26). Changes in neurohumoral tone can result from anxiety, sedation, exercise, sleep, ischemia, metabolic state, pharmacologic agents, and maneuvers such as carotid sinus massage (CSM). Some of these are discussed further in the relevant sections.

Carotid Sinus Massage

In most patients, cardioinhibitory effects on the sinus node are most apparent with right CSM, whereas the AV node is more likely to be affected by left CSM, but this distinction is by no means universal (15,28–33). Sinus node inhibition results in sinus bradycardia or sinus arrest. Inhibition of the AV node can result in prolongation of the AH interval or in block at the AH level. If CSM results in sinus arrest, concurrent *atrial* pacing will determine whether there is block at the AV node level as well.

CSM may be particularly revealing in patients who have the Wenckebach phenomenon at the time of their EPS. In one of those "paradoxical responses" of medical lore, the Wenckebach phenomenon at the HV level will sometimes seem to improve with CSM. This is because the sinus node may be slowed, giving the His bundle and bundle branches (which are much less affected by vagal tone) time to recover and resume conduction. In a patient with the Wenckebach phenomenon, therefore, CSM that produces worsening of the block is "good" because such block is usually at the AV node level. This is more benign than block at the HV level, which leaves the patient with an idioventricular escape rhythm. Improvement of block with CSM may therefore be "bad."

Carotid Sinus Massage: Normal Values. Sinus pauses of 3 seconds or more in response to CSM are considered abnormal. In a control group of 98 patients without a history of AV block, bradycardia, or syncope (33), the mean sinus interval with firm right or left CSM was 1,252 msec, and +2 standard deviations (SD) was 2,364 msec. Only 1% of patients had pauses of 3 seconds or more, and 2% had second- or third-degree AV block.

Sinoatrial Node Function Tests

Sinus Node Recovery Times

The sinus node is the archetype of an automatic focus. Automatic rhythms are characterized by spontaneous depolarization, overdrive suppression, and postoverdrive "warm-up" or return to baseline cycle length. Pacing at rates in excess of the spontaneous rate of an automatic focus results in temporary inhibition of spontaneous depolarization, with gradual return to the original cycle length over several beats following cessation of pacing (Fig. 61.2) (15,32–61).

Importance of Multiple Pacing Rates

Clinically, the sinus node recovery time (SNRT) is used to test sinus node automaticity. Pacing at rates near the baseline cycle length (BCL) causes no overdrive suppression, so that the interval between the last paced beat and the next sinus beat is comparable to the BCL. If the SNRT after pacing at 500 msec is shorter than that after 600 msec or there is marked variation (>250 msec) in the SNRTs if multiple tests are performed after pacing at 500 msec, this may imply that some impulses have not penetrated the sinus node, that is, that some degree of sinoatrial block exists. At pacing cycle lengths shorter than 500 msec, there is usually little further prolongation of the SNRT; on the contrary, changes in neurohumoral tone may result in shorter SNRTs. In patients with sinus node disease, faster pacing rates may result in marked prolongation of the SNRT.

Pacing Duration

Pacing durations beyond 15 seconds usually have little effect on the SNRT in *normal* individuals. Patients with sinus node disease may have marked suppression after longer pacing

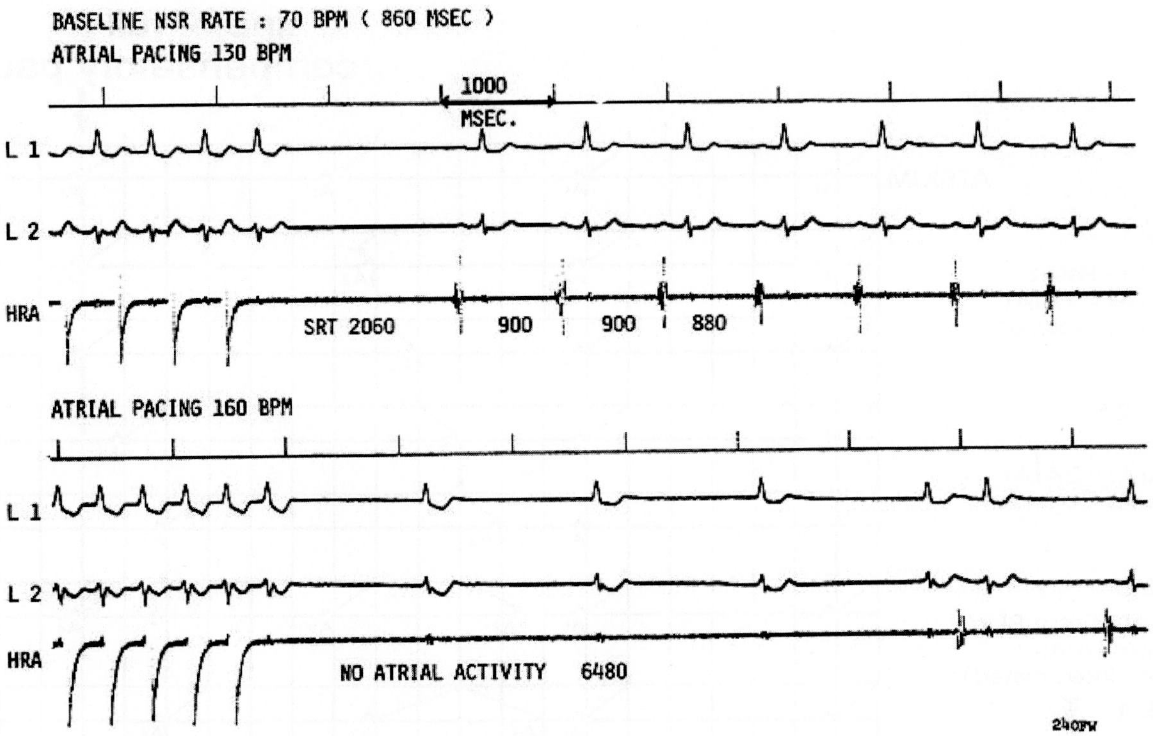

FIGURE 61.2. Prolonged sinus node recovery times. This patient had a baseline sinus rate of 70 bpm (860 msec). After pacing the high right atrium (HRA) at 130 beats per minute (bpm), the sinus recovery time (SRT) was 2,060 msec, which is markedly prolonged. In the bottom panel, after pacing at rate 160 beats per minute, there is no SRT for 6,480 msec, although there is a junctional escape rhythm at about 40 beats per minute.

durations. It is best to perform multiple SNRTs at multiple paced cycle lengths and to use pacing durations of 1 to 2 minutes in some of these trials.

Corrected Sinus Node Recovery Time

Normally, the SNRT is less than 1,500 msec, with a scatter on multiple tests of less than 250 msec. SNRTs tend to be shorter with shorter sinus cycle lengths, and therefore a variety of "corrections" have been introduced. Values derived from such tests are then called the SNRTC or CSNRT.

1. CSNRT = SNRT − sinus cycle length. This is the most common correction. Normal values have been reported from 350 to 550 msec, with 500 msec being most commonly used.
2. CSNRT = X% of sinus cycle length. Normal values range up to 160%.
3. CSNRT = 1.3 × (mean sinus cycle length in msec) + 101 msec.

Beware: The use of corrections at slow sinus rates can lead to absurd results. For example, a patient with symptomatic bradycardia at a 1,400-msec cycle length and an SNRT of 1,800 msec would have a CSNRT of 400 msec with method 1. In this case the abnormal uncorrected SNRT of 1,800 is more accurate; in fact, one does not need a value of SNRT to make the clinical diagnosis.

Recovery Beats; Total Recovery Time

After the SNRT, the pattern of subsequent beats returning to the basic sinus cycle length should also be analyzed. A variety of such patterns exists. One helpful measure is the total recovery time (TRT), that is, how long it takes to return to the basic sinus cycle length (15,58,62,63).

Secondary Pauses

Secondary pauses are identified when there is an initial shortening of the cycle length after the SNRT followed by an unexpected lengthening of the cycle length (45). In some instances, this is a sign of sinus node disease. In other cases, it can be a normal reflex following hypotension induced by pacing at rapid rates or in response to pressure overshoot in the first recovery beat because of the prolonged filling time.

The previous discussion should make it clear that a phrase such as "the SNRT was normal" is too simplistic. The number provided for the SNRT is most often the maximum or longest SNRT of several runs. Others may report the average SNRT. Sometimes only a single SNRT indicates a very superficial study. The sensitivity of a *single* SNRT is about 35% in patients with sinus node disease. This rises to greater than 85% when multiple SNRTs at different rates are recorded along with scatter and TRT, with a specificity of greater than 90%.

Sinoatrial Conduction Time

Direct Recordings. The sinus node atrial depolarization can be recorded directly in some patients using high-gain "unfiltered" electrograms (56,57,64–69). Signal-averaging techniques have also been used to measure the sinoatrial conduction time (SACT) noninvasively (70).

The Strauss Technique. This technique (15,40,42,51,53–57, 61,68,71–75) uses the extrastimulus technique to assess SACT (Fig. 61.3). Baseline sinus beats are designated A1. The premature beats (A2) are delivered after every eighth A1, and the timing of the recovery beat (A3) is measured. Very long A1A2 intervals generally do not affect the timing of the A3; that is, A1A3 = 2 A1A1, or a complete compensatory pause (designated zone 1). Shorter A1A2 intervals result in penetration of

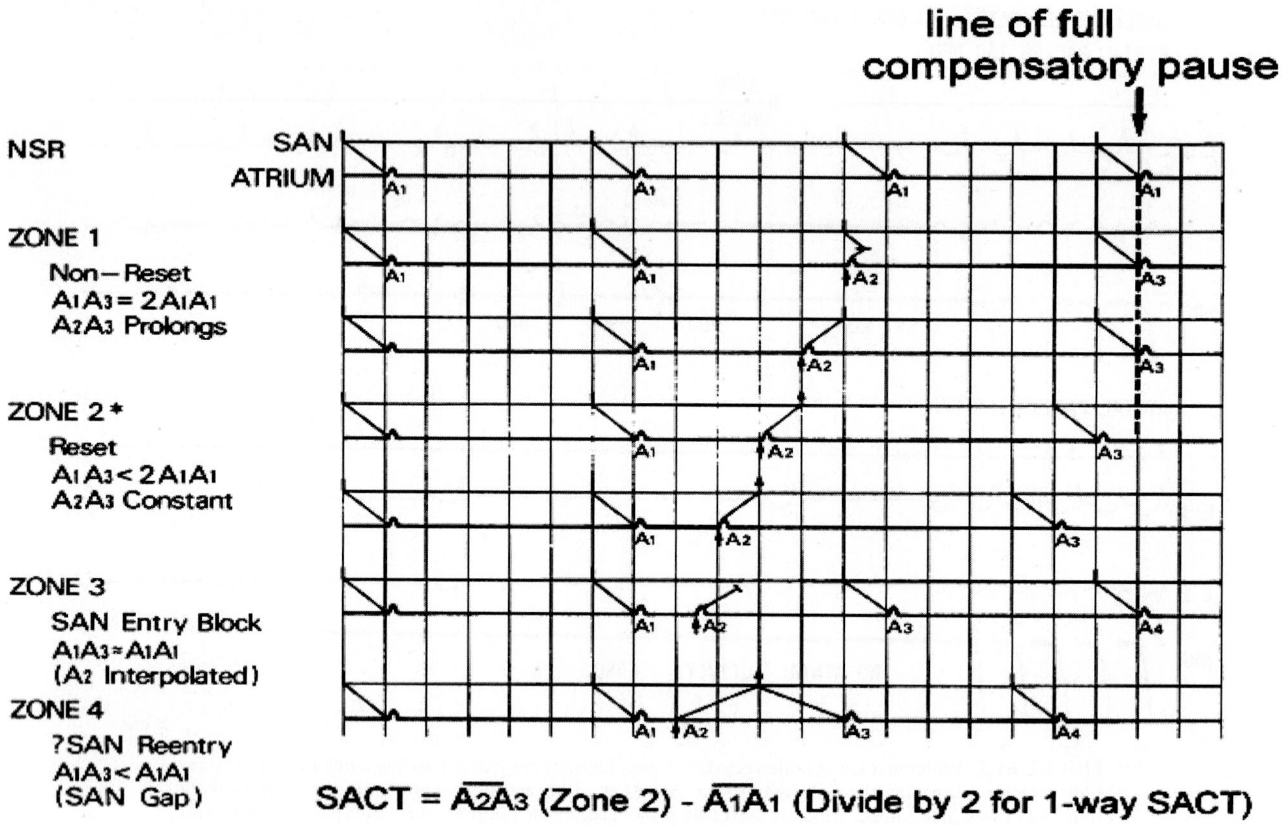

FIGURE 61.3. Sinoatrial conduction time: Strauss method. See text. The sinoatrial node (SAN) depolarizes unseen and results ultimately in atrial depolarization, designated here as A1. Premature atrial beats (A2) are introduced with increasing prematurity, and the timing of the return cycle (A3) is analyzed. The dashed line to the right indicates the line of complete compensatory pause. The sinoatrial conduction time (SACT) is calculated from zone 2 responses. (From Fisher JD. *Primer of Cardiac Electrophysiology.* Armonk: Futura. In press, with permission. Modified from Fisher JD. Role of electrophysiologic testing in the diagnosis and treatment of patients with known and suspected bradycardias and tachycardias. *Prog Cardiovasc Dis* 1981;24:25, with permission.)

the sinus node with resetting so that the resulting pause is less than compensatory. This is termed zone 2. The SACT is calculated as the mean of several zone 2 A2A3 intervals minus the corresponding mean of A1A1 intervals (SACT = A2A3 – A1A1). This value is often divided by 2 to estimate the one-way SACT, although it is understood that conduction times into and out of the SA node may be different. The upper limit of normal (one-way) SACT is about 145 msec. Reducing the A1A2 interval further will result in peculiar responses (Fig. 61.3), indicating sinus node entry block (zone 3) or reentry (zone 4). This technique was anticipated in analyses of ECGs (76) and earlier clinical electrophysiologic studies (77).

The Narula Method. This is a simpler technique for measuring the SACT (78). This assumes that pacing the atrium at rates of 10 beats per minute or less above the sinus rate will not result in significant overdrive suppression of the sinus node but that the pacing beats will gradually penetrate and reset the sinus node (Fig. 61.4). The calculation of the SACT is the same as for the Strauss method.

Kirkorian-Touboul Method. Kirkorian, Touboul, and their colleagues developed a method for determining the SACT independent of baseline sinus cycle length, which can normally be somewhat variable (79). It is less widely used than the other methods.

Comments on Sinoatrial Conduction Time Methods. The Strauss method is useful as part of an overall EPS when information is also sought on conduction system refractoriness or possible dual or accessory pathways during sinus rhythm. The Narula method is the quickest and easiest to perform but gives only the SACT. The Kirkorian-Touboul method may have several advantages but has not yet reached the level of use of the other methods. The SA node conduction time appears to be *directly* related to sinus cycle length (57,68), and the SA node refractory period is *directly* related to drive cycle length (79).

Autonomic Effects and Manipulations; Intrinsic Heart Rate

The sinus node is the archetype of the automatic rhythm, but it is subject to a wide variety of neurohumoral influences (39,51,54,56,80,81). To eliminate these, chemical denervation of the sinus node on a temporary basis can be achieved by injection of 0.2 mg/kg of propranolol (or 0.22 mg/kg of atenolol) in divided doses followed by 0.04 mg/kg of atropine (39,51,56,80,81). The intrinsic heart rate (IHR) is related to age according to the following formula: IHR (in beats per minute) = 118.1 – (0.57 × age [in years]); normal values are within 14% of this calculation for age less than 45 years and within 18% for age greater than 45 years.

Testing of SNRTs and SACT may yield improved results after autonomic blockade (37,51,53,54,56).

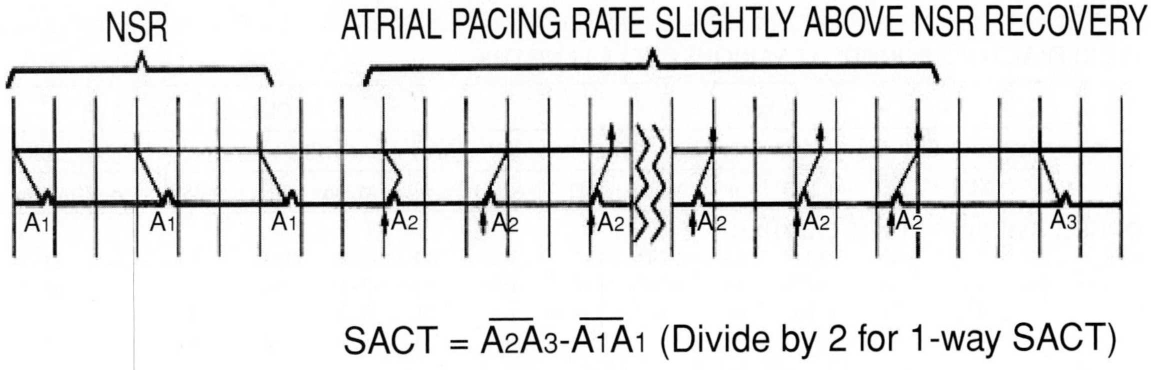

FIGURE 61.4. Determination of the sinoatrial conduction time (SACT) by the Narula method. As in the Fig. 61.3, the sinoatrial node (SAN) depolarizes unseen and ultimately results in atrial depolarization (A1). Instead of premature beats, atrial pacing at a rate slightly above that of the sinus rate is used as A2. It is assumed that such atrial pacing will depolarize the sinus node without significant overdrive suppression. The SACT is then calculated using the same formula as in the Strauss method. (From Fisher JD. *Primer of Cardiac Electrophysiology*. Armonk: Futura. In press, with permission. Modified from Fisher JD. Role of electrophysiologic testing in the diagnosis and treatment of patients with known and suspected bradycardias and tachycardias. *Prog Cardiovasc Dis* 1981;24:25, with permission.)

Atrioventricular Conduction and Refractoriness

Impulses traveling from the atrium to the ventricle must traverse the atrium, the AV node, the His bundle, and the bundle branches (His-Purkinje system). The AV node and the His Purkinje system will be considered separately. The discussion of the sinus node touched briefly on the concepts of conduction and refractoriness. These concepts require further attention for understanding impulse propagation from atrium to ventricle.

Conduction and Refractory Periods

Capture of the heart by a pacer stimulus and propagation of the wavefront to other points can be assessed using tests of conduction and refractoriness (7,82–92). *Conduction* is assessed by observing the propagation of wavefronts during pacing at progressively incremental rates (decremental cycle lengths). *Refractoriness* is tested by pacing at designated cycle lengths followed by introduction of increasingly premature extrastimuli. Results from the two methods are closely correlated but not interchangeable. For example, with incremental pacing, block usually occurs at the AV node level, whereas the extrastimulus method may result in block at any of several different levels or noncapture at the site of stimulation.

Conduction. Rate incremental pacing is delivered to a selected site in the heart, and propagation to a selected distal point is assessed. During tests of conduction, it is usual for capture to be maintained at the site of stimulation and block to occur at a distal point (7,84). As an example, stimulation of the high right atrium may be used for assessment of AV conduction. The stimulated wavefront traverses the right atrium and passes through the AV node, the His bundle, and the bundle branches. As the pacing rate increases, there is normally a slight increase in the intraatrial conduction time, a progressive increase in the AV node conduction time (the AH interval), and little change in the HV interval, with block usually at the AV node level.

The following examples continue with the model of high right atrial pacing in the assessment of AV conduction.

Stepwise Rate Incremental (Cycle Length Decremental) Pacing (Straight Pacing). Pacing is delivered to the high right atrium at a constant rate. The ability of tissue to conduct is affected by the baseline rate or cycle length of the preceding beats. Therefore the initial stimuli at any given rate may produce different effects from those observed several seconds later. This is called the period of *accommodation* (93), and may last up to 45 seconds, although 10 seconds is usually sufficient. For clinical testing, 15 seconds at any given rate is the minimum time at which intervals should be analyzed; 45 to 60 seconds is preferable, and mandatory if intervals have not stabilized by 15 seconds.

The stepwise/straight pacing method can be used simultaneously for the assessment of sinus node recovery times as described earlier.

During straight atrial pacing at a constant rate, one should look for block at the HV level at a point when the AH interval is not prolonging at that paced rate (i.e., before the development of the AV nodal Wenckebach phenomenon). This is an abnormal finding, except in some children and adults with very short AH intervals or others able to conduct through the AV node at higher rates than usual.

There are disadvantages to the straight pacing method. The prolonged pacing required at each rate is time consuming. Rapid pacing may provoke sensations or hypotension in patients that produce neurohumoral responses that can alter results.

Rate Incremental Ramp Pacing. Ramps for assessment of conduction are often an attractive alternative to the stepwise method (7,90–92). The pacing rate is slowly increased at 2 to 4 beats per minute per second, or 10 msec per cycle, until block occurs. This method avoids prolonged rapid pacing and is particularly suitable when multiple assessments of conduction are planned (e.g., after therapeutic interventions) and in the assessment of retrograde conduction. Because each successive paced interval differs from its predecessor by only a few milliseconds, the interval at which block occurs can be determined more precisely using the ramp method.

Comparative studies of the ramp and stepwise incremental pacing methods in assessment of anterograde and retrograde conduction have shown them to be comparable (7,90,92).

Conduction Periods. At pacing rates below those causing conduction block, there is a 1:1 relationship between stimulus and response at a distant site. Conduction time may be prolonged, so that the stimulus to response time is prolonged. For symmetry with the terminology used for refractory period

TABLE 61.3

NORMAL REFRACTORY PERIODS AT VARIOUS CYCLE LENGTHS

	Adults								Children (7 mo–15 yr)						
	ERP				FRP				ERP				FRP		
	n	Mean	SD	+2SD	*n*	Mean	SD	+2SD	*n*	Mean	SD	+2SD	*n*	Mean	SD
CL: LONGEST ASSURING ATRIAL CAPTURE															
Atrium	26	236*	49	334	26	274*	47	368	40	187*	53	293	35	217*	45
A V node	46	289*	44	377	45	406*	46	498	40	241*	56	353	38	345*	71
RBB	5	412*	72	(556)	—	—	—	—	11	323*	39	401	—	—	—
LBB	2	473*	67	(607)	—	—	—	—	9	361	52	(465)	—	—	—
CL: 850–600															
Atrium	28	232	80	392	28	275	49	373	10	206	80	366	6	247	53
A V node	28	290	50	390	26	401	48	497	8	303	81	(465)	8	427	74
RBB	4	443	42	(525)	—	—	—	—	1	390	—	—	—	—	—
LBB	4	434	59	(552)	—	—	—	—	6	404	31	(466)	—	—	—
CL: 599–460															
Atrium	30	232*	54	340	30	271*	49	369	37	199*	43	285	34	234*	43
A V node	30	328*	56	440	29	406*	57	520	37	260*	55	370	37	354*	66
RBB	6	367	28	423*	—	—	—	—	10	365	35	435	—	—	—
LBB	1	365	—	—	—	—	—	—	6	370	61	(492)	—	—	—
CL: 459–280															
Atrium	23	199*	28	255	23	252*	34	320	57	165*	37	239	54	200*	35
A V node	16	280*	52	384	13	345*	27	399	55	219*	45	309	49	299*	46
RBB	4	328	16	(360)	—	—	—	—	22	298	28	354	—	—	—
LBB	0	—	—	—	—	—	—	—	12	330	34	398	—	—	—

n = Number of subjects contributing; CL = Cycle Length msec; ERP = Effective Refractory Period; FRP = Functional Refractory Period.
Atrium, recording in His bundle area after high right atrial stimulation. Numbers in parentheses emphasize small sample.
H = Longest CL assuring atrial capture: 698 ± 107 for adults, 535 ± 89 for children.
*$p < 0.05$ between adult and pediatric values.

testing, the comparable terminology has sometimes been used (84).

Refractory Periods

Refractory periods are determined by assessing the effects of extrastimuli (S2, S3, S*N*) delivered decrementally after a series of spontaneous or paced beats (S1). Many variables are considered in the assessment of refractory periods. These include the stimulus amplitude and the drive rate or cycle length. Longer cycle lengths are generally associated with longer refractory periods, but refractory periods of different parts of the conducting system do not respond comparably to changes in drive cycle lengths (94). The following refractory periods exist (see Table 61.3) (15,82):

1. The *relative refractory period* is the drive to extrastimulus interval (S1S2) that produces slowing in conduction (an increase in stimulus to distal response time). Conduction is slowed when a wavefront encounters tissue that is not completely repolarized.
2. During the *absolute refractory period* the tissue cannot be depolarized, even by an extrastimulus of great amplitude.
3. The *effective refractory period* (ERP) is the longest S1S2 at a *designated stimulus amplitude* (usually two to four times the diastolic threshold) that fails to capture.
4. The *functional refractory period* (FRP) is the shortest interval at which a specified (usually distal) site can be depolarized by any S1S2 interval.

It is helpful to think of the ERP as a stimulus-to-stimulus measurement and the FRP as a response-to-response measurement (94).

The anterograde ERP and FRP of the AV conduction system are defined as follows:

1. The *atrial ERP* is the longest S1S2 interval that fails to achieve atrial capture.
2. The *atrial FRP* is the shortest A1A2 interval recorded at a designated site (often the His bundle region) prior to failure of S1S2 to capture the atrium.
3. The *AV node ERP* is the longest A1A2 not propagating to the His bundle. Although it is often based on high right atrial stimulation, the A1A2 *should* be measured at the His region to avoid the confounding effects of changes in atrial conduction times.
4. The *AV node FRP* is the shortest H1H2 in response to any A1A2. Patterns of AV nodal conduction/refractoriness are often complex (94), based on Wit et al. (85).
5. The *His-Purkinje system ERP* is the longest H1H2 not propagating to the ventricles.
6. The *His-Purkinje system FRP* is the shortest V1V2 interval prior to reaching the ERP of the His-Purkinje system.
7. The *bundle branch ERP and FRP* are as for the His-Purkinje system, but are based on production of right- or left-bundle-branch block or fascicular block.

It is important to note that atrial conduction may materially affect the determination of refractory periods. Note that *refractory periods should not be timed from the site of stimulation, but from the point in the conduction cascade that is being assessed.* For example, if the high right atrium is stimulated in a patient with a left lateral Kent bundle, an early extrastimulus may encounter the relative refractory period of the atrium, so that intraatrial conduction time is prolonged. Thus the timing of the S1S2 stimuli in the high right atrium would be shorter than the timing of the propagated impulse when it arrives at the region of the Kent bundle as the local A1A2 interval.

Limitations of Tests of Conduction and Refractoriness

It is *unusual* to be able to collect a complete set of numbers (84–88).

With conduction testing, block most commonly occurs at the AV node level. With refractory period testing, the ERP of the atrium is often longer than the ERP of the AV node so that one encounters atrial refractoriness prior to AV nodal refractoriness, precluding the possibility of assessing the latter (84–88).

An atrial stimulus cannot be used to test the His-Purkinje system if the impulse is blocked at the AV node level. This is a limitation that applies to the *majority* of patients undergoing either conduction or refractory period testing. One implication is that patients whose His-Purkinje system conduction periods or refractory periods *can* be tested are unusual, and therefore the data may be suspect. This should be kept in mind when reading literature or protocols that involve reporting of refractory periods at various levels of the conduction system.

It is possible to assess anterograde conduction and refractoriness distal to the AV node by direct pacing of the His bundle (95,96). This is not part of the routine EP evaluation, however, and is reserved for instances in which the information is particularly desired.

The Atrium (18,21,97–111)

Passive Recordings

During normal sinus rhythm, earliest atrial depolarization occurs in the region of the sinus node at the junction of the superior vena cava and the high lateral right atrium. Normal *intraatrial* conduction (PA interval) and *interatrial* conduction intervals are given in Table 61.2.

Histologically distinct pathways comparable to bundle branches do not occur in the atrium. The "internodal pathways" are physiologic manifestations related to fiber orientation and thickness (97–100). Intraatrial conduction may be very slow, but block rarely occurs (103,106–108).

Rate Incremental Atrial Pacing (Stepwise or Ramp)

The PA interval may be prolonged gradually, as may the interatrial conduction time (Table 62.2). It is usually possible to maintain 1:1 capture with incremental pacing techniques to 250 to 300 beats per minute. At such pacing rates, precipitation of atrial fibrillation is not rare and is not necessarily an abnormal response. Pacing threshold normally tends to increase at faster rates (21).

Extrastimulus Testing

This technique is used for assessment of atrial refractory periods and for induction of arrhythmias. As with incremental pacing, there is prolongation of intra- and interatrial conduction, which is more pronounced in patients with a history of atrial arrhythmias (19,104,105). Development of a fractionated atrial electrogram is more often seen in patients who have a history of atrial fibrillation (104,105,110,111). Intraatrial blocks in response to extrastimuli are unusual (106).

Occasionally double or extra stimuli induce atrial fibrillation in patients with no history of atrial rhythm disorders. Such episodes usually terminate spontaneously and are not clinically relevant in the absence of a history of known or suspected atrial arrhythmias.

Autonomic and Pharmacologic Effects

Vagal tone and medications such as adenosine and edrophonium may slow the sinus rate, but they tend to shorten the refractory period of the atrium. This makes the atrium more vulnerable to induction of atrial fibrillation. Patients with vagal-dependent atrial fibrillation typically have episodes during sleep and may be worsened by the vagotonic effects of digitalis therapy.

Atrioventricular Junction

The AV junction is not synonymous with the AV node. The junction is defined as that portion of the conduction system from the proximal portion of the AV node to the distal portion of the His bundle before its bifurcation.

Junctional Recovery Times (JRT)

Some individuals have what appears to be a stable junctional rhythm in the absence of a conducted atrial rhythm (112,113). If these patients are asymptomatic, the question of the need for pacing arises, and the junctional recovery time (JRT) (analogous to the SNRT) helps in the assessment. After atrial or ventricular pacing, a corrected JRT (CJRT = JRT − basic cycle length) of 200 msec or less, either in the baseline state or after 2 to 2.5 mg of atropine, is typical in asymptomatic patients with junctional pacemakers located *either* in the AV node or the His bundle. Patients with longer CJRTs, if symptomatic, may require pacing (Fig. 61.5).

Atrioventricular Node

Normal ranges for the AH interval, which reflects AV nodal conduction times, are shown in Table 61.2 and Figure 61.6.

AV nodal anatomy and physiology are too complex to review here in detail (114). From the clinical electrophysiologist's viewpoint the node has several pathways entering from the atrium, whose characteristics have been estimated by subtraction, that is, by assessing function after catheter ablation of alternative pathways (115,116). A *slow posterior pathway* arises near the coronary sinus ostium and proceeds anteriorly near the tricuspid annulus to the compact node. Use of this pathway is associated with slow conduction velocity (long AH and PR intervals) but ability to conduct at rapid rates in beats per minute (shorter ERP and conduction limit). The *fast anterior pathway* is near the His recording site and has properties that are the opposite of the slow pathway. There is also a presumed transseptal or left-sided input and many variations on all of these. Within the node itself there is a network of many potential pathways that normally merge to cause synchronous input at the nodal-His bundle (NH) junction (117). It is clear that there is a wide spectrum of normal AV nodal physiology (118–120).

Rate Incremental Atrial Pacing

The AH interval normally is prolonged smoothly with incremental pacing until just before block when there may be a marked increase (15) (Fig. 61.6), that can be graphed as a smooth curve. AV block at the AV node level occurs normally over a very broad range of pacing rates, from approximately 100 to 200 beats per minute (15). This range encompasses two standard deviations, but there is a continuum of possible normality that may extend somewhat below 100 or above 200 beats per minute. *Age* is also a factor, with younger individuals often having shorter AH intervals at a given pacing rate and the Wenckebach phenomenon at higher rates.

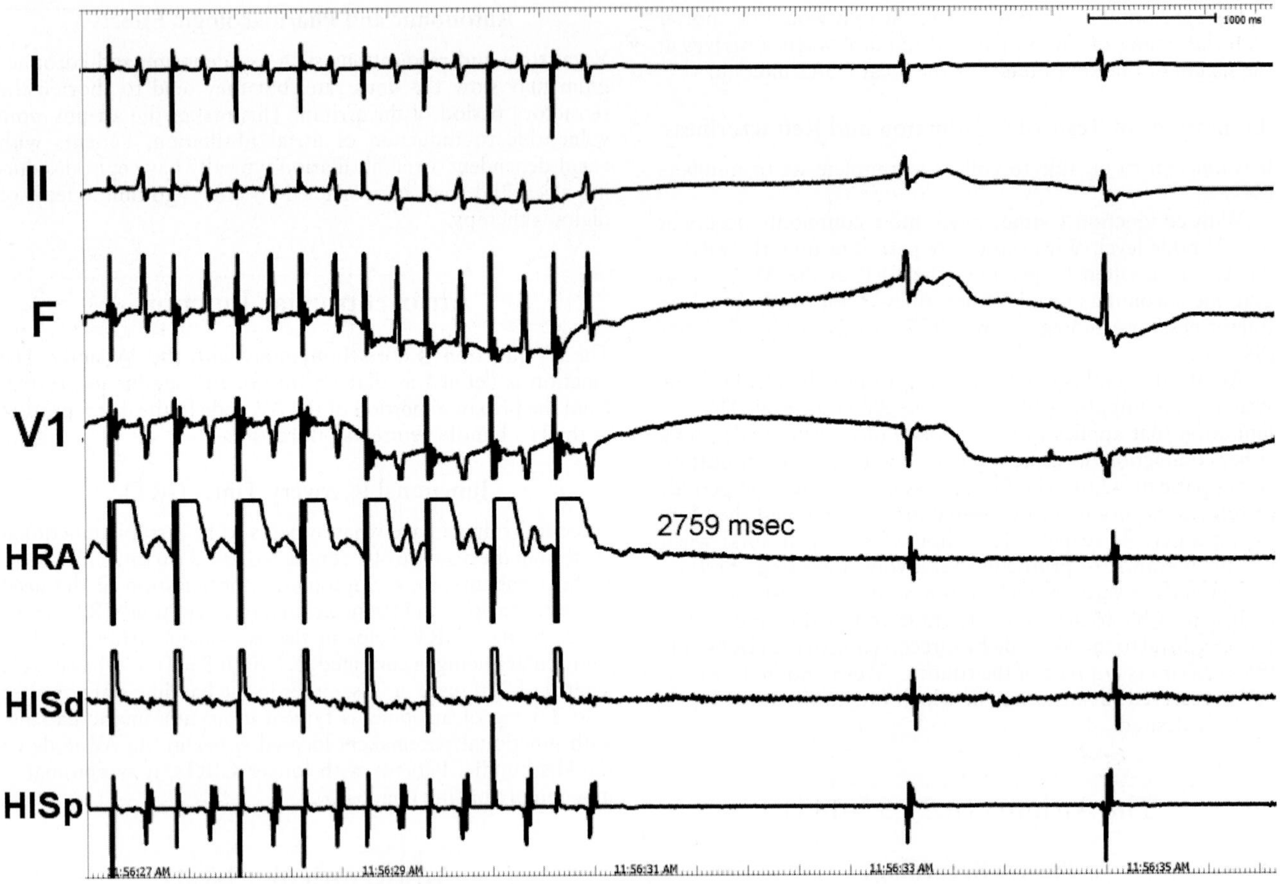

FIGURE 61.5. A prolonged junctional recovery time is demonstrated after cessation of high right atrial pacing.

Atrioventricular Node: Extrastimulus Testing and Refractoriness

Extrastimulus testing may produce evidence of *longer* refractory periods at *shorter* pacing cycle lengths (Table 61.3). However, this may hold true only for adults (83) and at relatively low pacing rates. Patterns of AH and AV curves in response to increasingly premature extrastimuli can be complex (85).

The alternative *Rosenbleuth hypothesis* is that there is a one-step delay in a refractory barrier (121–123) and that AV nodal refractoriness actually shortens with shorter drive cycle lengths if calculations are made based *not* on overall conduction delay, but at a single layer in the AV node.

The site of atrial pacing may also affect AV nodal conduction, with shorter AH intervals associated with pacing from the coronary sinus (123–127). The AH interval is similar with high and low right atrial pacing (127,128).

Echo Beats

The AV node is not a single pipeline from the atrium to the His bundle, but rather is a network of many potential pathways with mostly similar conduction and refractory characteristics. Even in normal individuals, a premature beat or extrastimulus may encounter refractoriness in one pathway. Conduction in one pathway may allow recovery of the previously refractory pathway, so that it is then able to conduct in a retrograde direction. This then emerges into the atrium as an AV nodal echo beat.

Dual Atrioventricular Node Physiology

Rate incremental pacing, or the extrastimulus technique, generally results in a smooth prolongation of the AH curve (129–131). If shortening of the paced cycle length by 10 msec (131) or shortening of the S1S2 extrastimulus interval by 10 msec (130,131) results in an increase of 50 msec or more in the AH interval, this is diagnostic of dual-AV-node-pathway physiology (Fig. 61.7). Dual-pathway physiology is the hallmark of AV node reentry tachycardia (AVNRT), but it can also be encountered in some patients with no history of such an arrhythmia. Sometimes, there will be evidence of multiple AH jumps, indicating triple- or quadruple-pathway physiology.

Atrioventricular Node Responses to Exercise versus Pacing

The PR and AH intervals change little in response to exercise and may decrease somewhat due to decrease in parasympathetic tone and increase in circulating catecholamines. With incremental atrial pacing in a recumbent patient, autonomic tone is changed only indirectly in response to factors such as anxiety or hypotension. The AH interval therefore is prolonged markedly with atrial pacing (Fig. 61.6), and this is *normal.*

His-Purkinje System (Infranodal Conduction; HV Interval)

Measurement of the HV interval was discussed in a previous section. Complete heart block at the HV level leaves the patient with an idioventricular rhythm. This may be slow enough to cause syncope or worse. Block at the infranodal/HV level is an important diagnosis to make in a patient with unexplained syncope or heart block at a previously undetermined level (3).

Beware the conventional rule of thumb that AV block in the presence of a narrow QRS implies disease at the AV node level and block in patients with a wide QRS complex or bundle

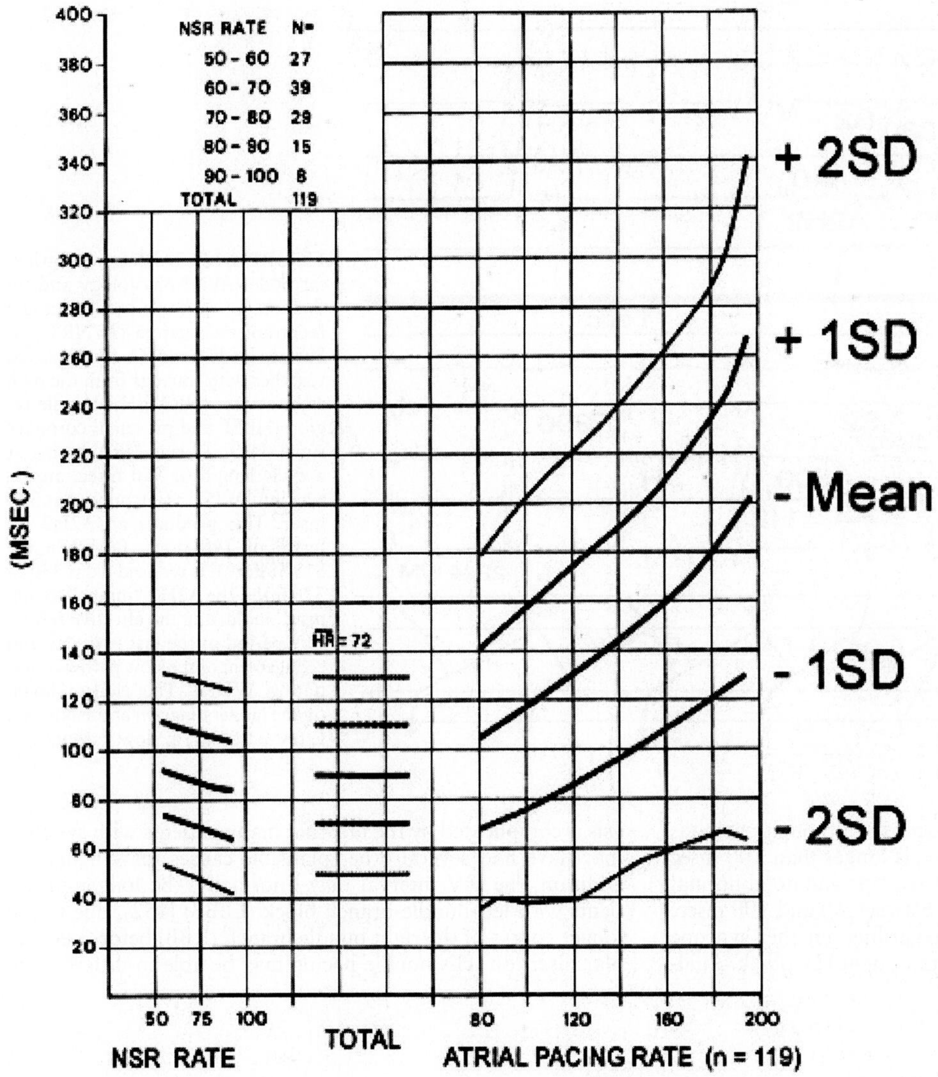

FIGURE 61.6. The AH interval during normal sinus rhythm (NSR) and during high right atrial pacing. Mean and standard deviations (SD) are shown for individuals without evidence of AV nodal disease. (From Fisher JD. *Primer of Cardiac Electrophysiology*. Armonk: Futura. In press, with permission. Modified from Fisher JD. Role of electrophysiologic testing in the diagnosis and treatment of patients with known and suspected bradycardias and tachycardias. *Prog Cardiovasc Dis* 1981;24:25, with permission.)

branch block implies that the block is at the His-Purkinje level. The rule of thumb is about 85% accurate. It may not matter if one does not pace a patient with a wide QRS who has block at the AV node level (132); but it may be quite important if one does not pace a patient with block at the HV level because the QRS complex is narrow (133). The latter situation can occur with intra-Hissian block or with balanced first-degree bundle branch block (132–134) (Figs. 61.8 to 61.11).

Incremental Atrial Pacing/Conduction Analysis

The HV interval normally remains constant at all paced rates (Table 61.2). HV block that occurs unexpectedly during straight pacing at a rate not producing AV-node Wenckebach is usually abnormal (135) and may be grounds for implantation of a permanent pacemaker (136). HV block and bundle branch block can be observed or induced by a myriad of mechanisms (137,138) summarized earlier and subsequently in this section. The physician must differentiate abnormal from physiologic responses.

Programmed Extrastimuli/Refractory Periods

The HV interval usually remains constant with increasingly premature extrastimuli because the refractory period of the AV node is usually longer than that of the His-Purkinje system. However, with closely coupled extrastimuli that are conducted through the AV node, refractoriness may be encountered in the His bundle or the right or left bundle branch. In such cases, determination of the ERP and FRP of these structures is possible. At times, extrastimulus testing will produce block that disappears with further prematurity of the extrastimuli. This "gap phenomenon" will be discussed later.

Pharmacologic Agents

Lidocaine (139,140), procainamide (140–142), and ajmaline (143,144) have all been used as pharmacologic stressors to the His-Purkinje system. Typical doses of lidocaine (75-mg bolus given twice at 30- to 45-second intervals) produce very little alteration of the HV interval. Block within or below the His is an abnormal finding (Fig. 61.10). Procainamide (140–142) 10 mg/kg over 15 to 20 minutes can normally prolong the HV interval by up to 30%. Prolongation beyond that point or block in response to pacing is an abnormal response. HV block in response to lidocaine or procainamide is very unusual in patients without suspected conduction disease and even in patients with bifasicular block who do not have a history of AV block or unexplained syncope (139–142).

Clinical Significance of the HV Interval

After three decades, this remains a matter of lively dispute (145– 151). Asymptomatic patients with prolonged HV

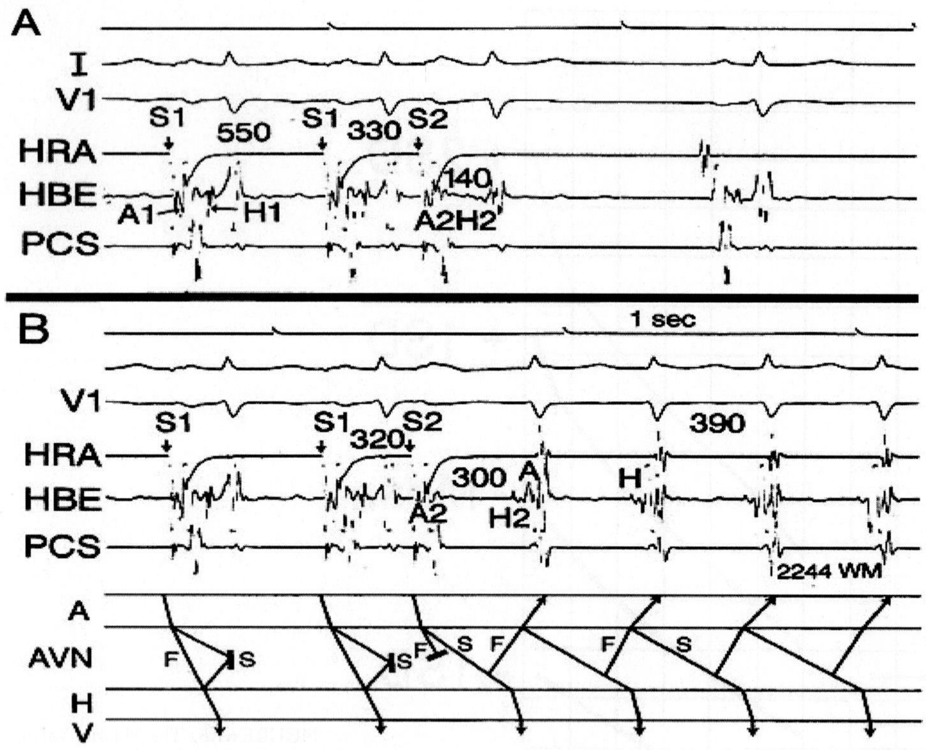

FIGURE 61.7. Dual atrioventricular node (AVN) physiology and induction of atrioventricular nodal reentrant tachycardia (AVNRT). **A:** Surface leads 1 and V1 are displayed together with tracings from the high right atrium (HRA), His bundle region (HBE), and proximal coronary sinus (PCS). During HRA pacing at a cycle length of 550 msec, an extrastimulus (S2) is introduced at 330 msec. This produces an A2H2 interval of 140 msec. **B:** When the S1S2 interval is reduced from 330 to 320 msec, the A2H2 "jumps" to 300 msec, indicating the effective refractory period of the fast pathway and engagement of the slow pathway, initiating AVNRT. This is also shown on the ladder diagram at the bottom. F, fast pathway; S, slow pathway.

intervals may enjoy a favorable prognosis, although pacing is usually recommended for HV intervals longer than 100 msec (136). In patients with unexplained syncope and no abnormal findings other than an HV interval between 60 and 100 msec, there is a broad range of opinion regarding whether syncope should be attributed to probably intermittent HV block. Analysis is complicated by the fact that many patients with syncope may have had several other plausible causes for syncope. In addition, the HV interval may "normally" be longer in patients with left-bundle-branch block (LBBB) (152), due to the longer course of the right bundle branch (RBB) before ventricular insertion. His bundle pacing may be able to differentiate

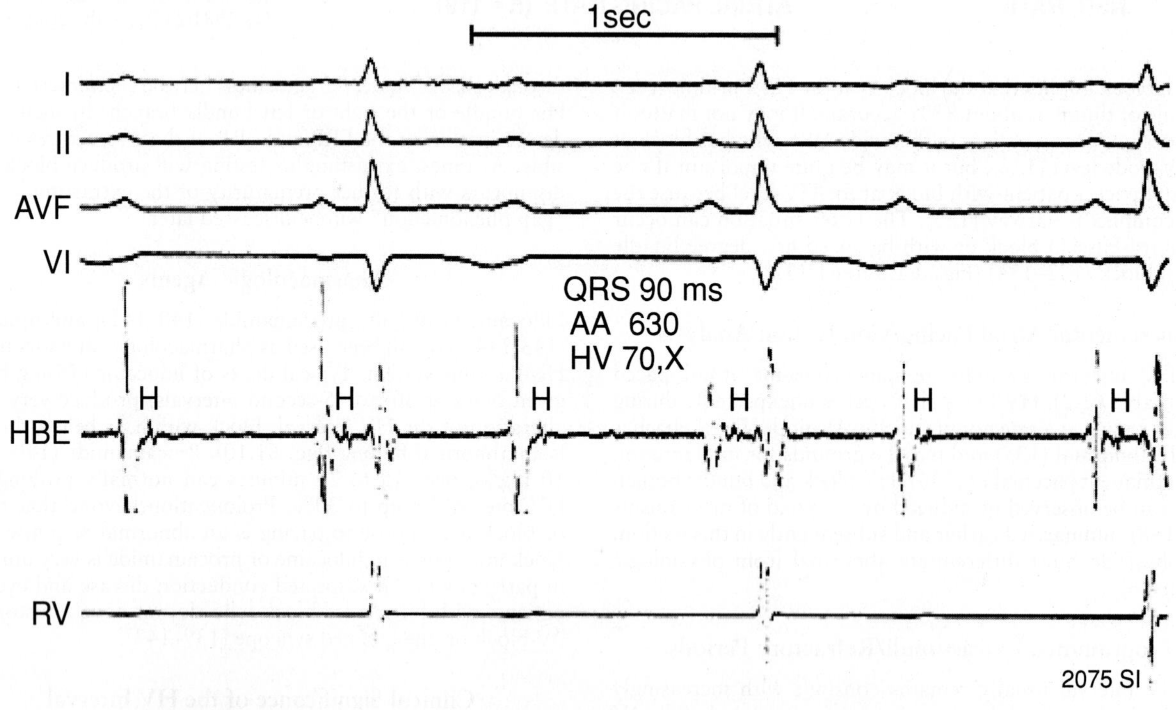

FIGURE 61.8. HV block in a patient with a narrow QRS interval. There is 2:1 HV block, with conducted HV intervals prolonged at 70 msec. The prolonged HV interval together with a narrow QRS may indicate balanced bilateral first-degree HV block (see Fig. 61.9).

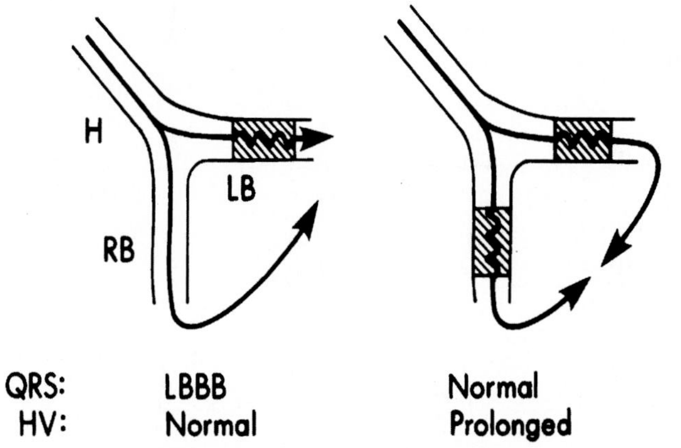

FIGURE 61.9. Balanced bundle branch block. The two panels illustrate findings on surface ECG and intracardiac His bundle recording in a patient with slow conduction velocity along the left bundle branch (LB) (**left**) and simultaneous slow conduction velocity along both right (RB) and left bundle branches (**right**). When there is simultaneous slow conduction down both bundle branches the QRS complex on the surface ECG appears narrow and there is a prolonged PR interval. H, bundle of His; LBBB, left bundle branch block.

proximal from peripheral LBBB (153,54), which may have different prognostic implications.

Catheter Bumping

The right bundle is particularly vulnerable to block due to mild trauma from the His bundle–recording catheter. This can produce an RBBB pattern or (in patients with LBBB) marked prolongation of the HV interval or even complete block at the HV level. Such blocks are almost always transient.

Conduction System in Acute Myocardial Infarction

High-degree AV block, new bundle branch block, and a prolonged HV interval are all associated with an unfavorable prognosis (155–160). Many such patients succumb to tachyarrhythmias or pump failure rather than AV block, so that the role of permanent pacing remains uncertain, unless the patient has had transient or sustained complete heart block associated with bifascicular or trifascicular disease (136,157). EP studies performed during the course of hospitalization for acute myocardial infarction often reveal disease that is more widespread or even in a different location than suggested by the ECG (160,161). Serial changes in the HV interval during the course of hospitalization for an acute infarction suggest that the outcome is more favorable when initially prolonged HV intervals subsequently normalize (158). These studies, together with prospective trials such as the Multicenter Automatic Defibrillator Implantation Trial (MADIT) and the Multicenter Unsustained Tachycardia Trial (MUSTT), underscore the value of EP studies for risk stratification in high-risk postinfarction patients.

Retrograde Conduction (Ventriculoatrial Conduction)

Absence of ventriculoatrial (VA) conduction at any paced rate is both common and normal (162–167). When present, normal VA conduction uses the normal AV conduction system, with the first atrial depolarization usually in the septal region in proximity to the AV node. In some instances, the slow posterior pathway will be preferentially engaged so that first atrial depolarization will be somewhat posterior to the AV node.

With rate incremental ventricular pacing or with ventricular extrastimulus testing, the VA interval is prolonged smoothly in a manner analogous to that for AV conduction. Dual physiology can be diagnosed in the VA direction in some patients.

To rule out (nondecremental) accessory pathways, the extrastimulus technique is usually more effective than rate incremental ventricular pacing at demonstrating normal prolongation of the VA interval. If uncertainty continues to exist, adenosine can be extremely helpful. This drug is much more likely to block AV nodal conduction than an accessory pathway.

Retrograde conduction of ventricular extrastimuli can be affected by the baseline sequence of cardiac activation, for

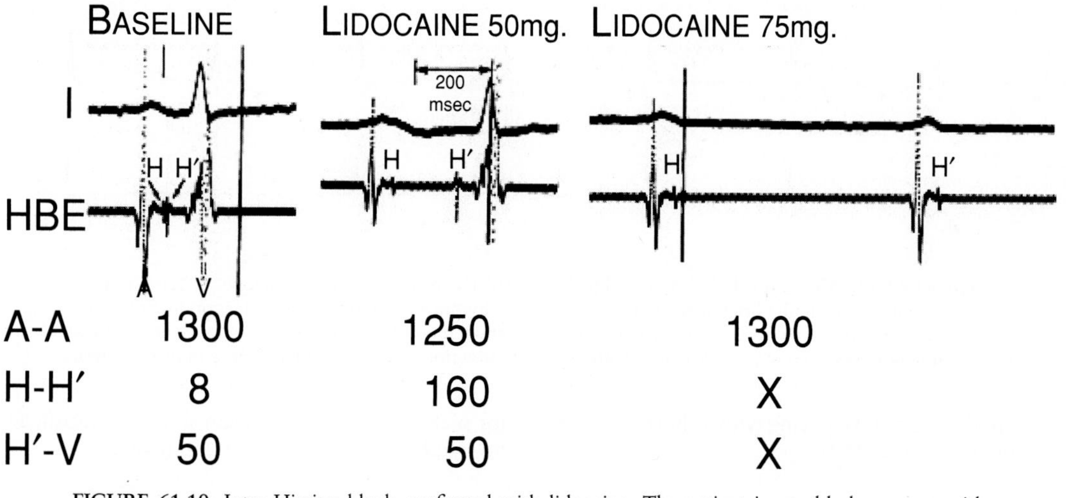

FIGURE 61.10. Intra-Hissian block confirmed with lidocaine. The patient is an elderly woman with recurrent syncope and a normal 12-lead electrocardiogram. Brief periods of complete heart block were documented but without accompanying symptoms. The baseline His bundle electrogram (HBE) revealed a multiphasic or ragged His bundle potential. After administration of 50 mg of lidocaine (**middle**), there was little change in the heart rate but the multiphasic His bundle potential split into two deflections labeled H and H′. After an additional 25 mg of lidocaine, there was complete atrioventricular block following the proximal component of the His bundle potential. (Modified from Fisher JD. Role of electrophysiologic testing in the diagnosis and treatment of patients with known and suspected bradycardias and tachycardias. *Prog Cardiovascular Dis* 1981;24:25, with permission.)

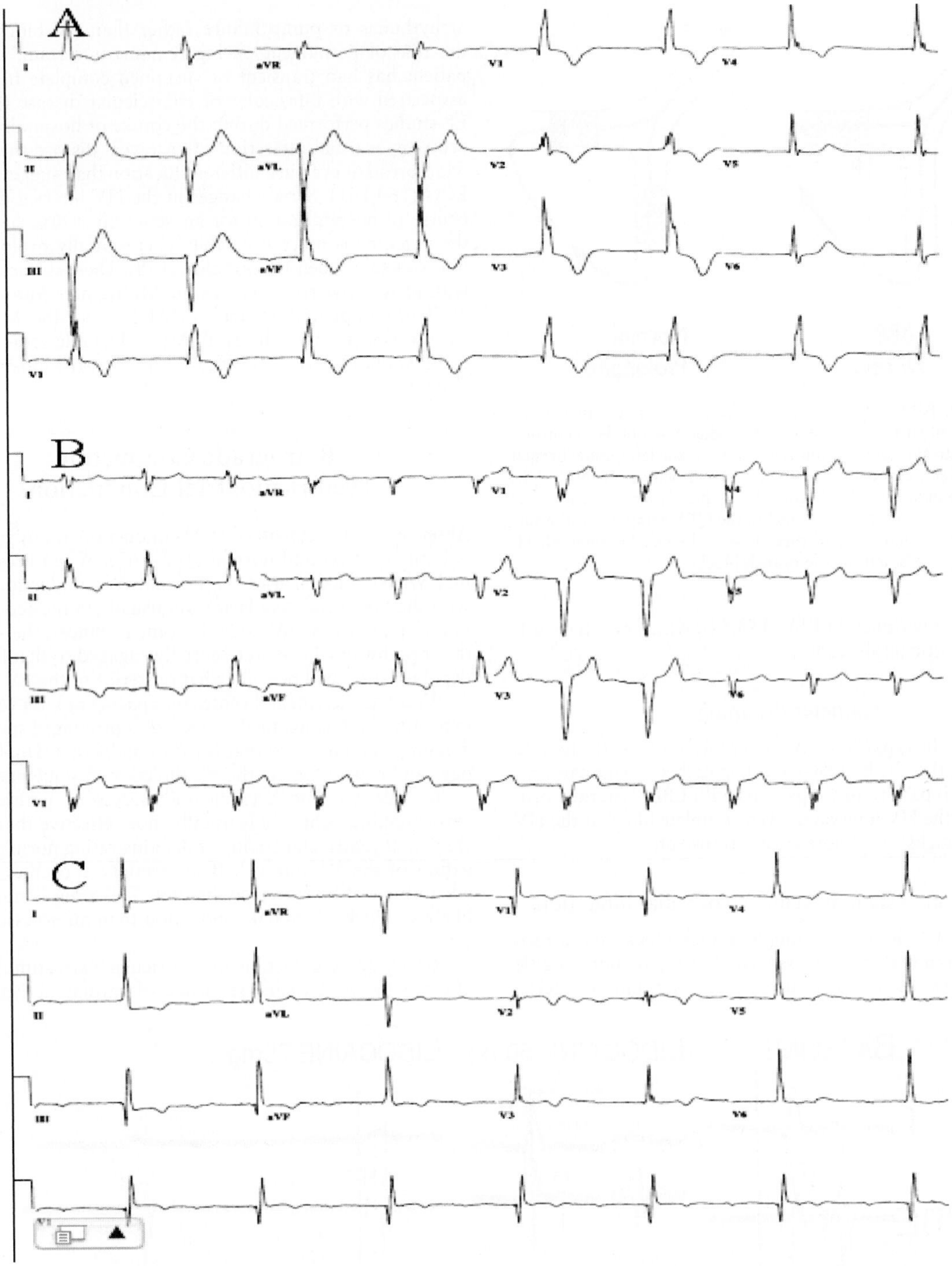

FIGURE 61.11. Alternating bundle branch block in an elderly woman with near-syncope. **A:** Ectopic atrial rhythm with right-bundle-branch block. **B:** Ectopic atrial rhythm with an intraventricular conduction delay demonstrating delayed conduction down both the right and left bundle branches. **C:** Complete heart block with junctional escape complexes demonstrating slow conduction along the right and left bundle branches.

example, sinus rhythm versus AV pacing with a short AV interval versus ventricular pacing (164).

Multilevel Disease

Many patients with heart disease have prolongation at multiple levels in the conduction system (103,106–108,169,170). It is not rare to see prolongations of the PA, AH, and HV intervals. Conversely, some patients with sick sinus syndrome have impaired AV conduction. Before permanent atrial pacing is used for such patients, the physician should be satisfied that there is no significant conduction system disease.

The Ventricle

Ventricular stimulation is used to assess retrograde (VA) conduction and refractory periods, retrograde activation patterns including sequences that may indicate an accessory pathway, and vulnerability to inducible ventricular arrhythmias. Details of ventricular stimulation for specific arrhythmias are provided in other chapters. What follows is a more general discussion of ventricular stimulation protocols supplementing the information presented earlier in this chapter.

Rate Incremental Ventricular Pacing

Straight/stepwise incremental pacing or ramp pacing increasing at 2 to 4 beats per minute per second are used in the assessment of retrograde conduction (7). It is unusual to provoke arrhythmias with these tests, even in patients with known ventricular arrhythmia (7,9,171).

Burst Pacing

The burst protocol is more aggressive than that used for assessment of retrograde conduction (9,171,172). A typical example is the use of stimuli resulting in 10 to 15 captures beginning at 150 beats per minute (400 msec) with repeated bursts in incremental steps of 25 beats per minute until a specified upper rate (commonly 300 beats per minute/200 msec) is achieved or 1:1 capture is lost.

(Steep) Ramp Pacing

In contrast to ramps used for assessment of conduction, this is a steep ramp somewhat analogous to the burst technique just described (9,171,172). Stimuli resulting in 10 to 20 captures are delivered initially at a rate range beginning at 150 beats per minute and ramping up quickly (20 msec per cycle) to 200 beats per minute (400 to 300 msec); repeat ramps are delivered to incremental maximum rates in steps, again with a typical upper limit of 300 beats per minute/200 msec or failure to maintain 1:1 capture. Because myocardial refractoriness is set by the prior interstimulus interval, it is usually possible to capture at faster rates with the ramp technique than with bursts.

The Extrastimulus Technique/Programmed Electrical Stimulation

Refractory Periods. The extrastimulus technique/programmed electrical stimulation (PES) is used for establishment of refractory periods as described earlier. In the ventricle, the effective refractory period (ERP) is the longest S1S2 interval that fails to capture. The functional refractory period (FRP) depends on investigator definitions of the site at which the resulting wavefront is measured. The FRP is the shortest coupling interval between depolarizations arriving at the designated site in response to any S1S2 interval.

In the study of ventricular arrhythmias (and this applies to atrial stimulation protocols as well), double and triple extrastimuli are often delivered. The refractory periods in response to double and triple extrastimuli must be described in somewhat altered terminology (173). For example, the ERP is usually described as the longest S1S2 interval that *fails* to capture. If extrastimuli are given in 10-msec decrements, the shortest S1S2 interval that *does* capture is thus only 10 msec longer than the classical ERP. If one is to measure refractory periods of the second and third extrastimuli (S3 and S4, respectively), then S1 must continue to capture. Therefore the terminology is slightly adjusted, with the ERPs being the shortest S1S2, S2S3, and S3S4 intervals that *do* capture.

Standard Protocols. There is no universally accepted standard protocol, but there is an agreement that an acceptable protocol should meet minimum standards, such as those established by the Heart Rhythm Society (12) (Figs. 61.12 and 61.13). Major variations are the tandem versus simple sequential method (8,9) of delivering sequential extrastimuli and the sequence for delivery of single, double, and triple extrastimuli (Fig. 61.12) (8,171,173). Comparative studies of these methods have shown the results to be comparable (8,9).

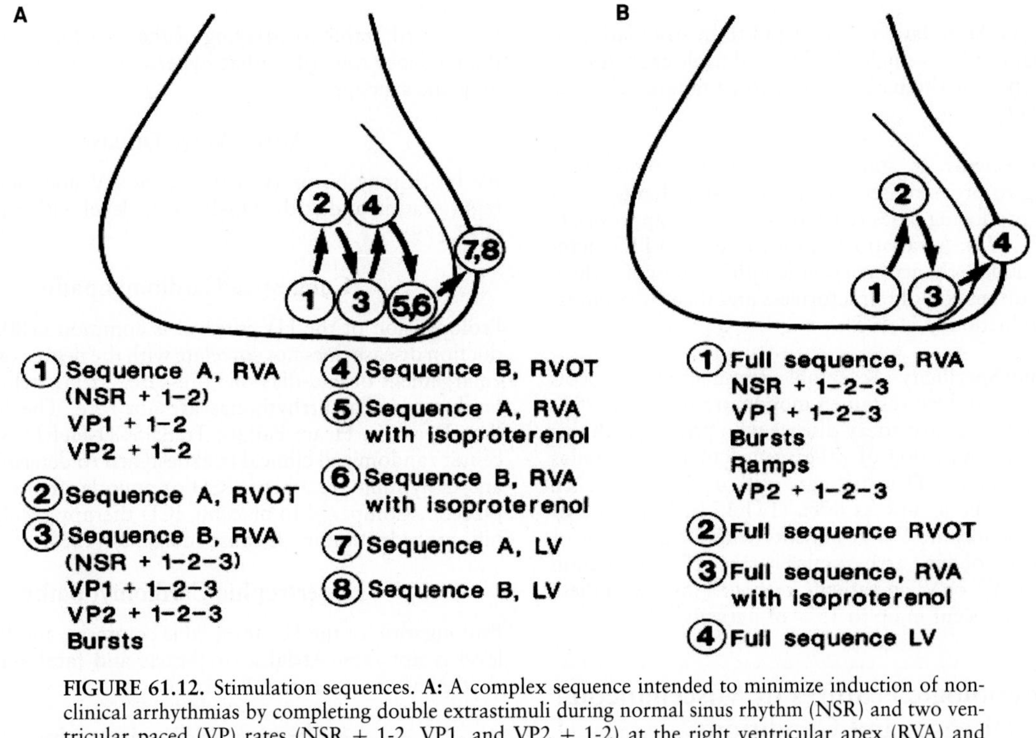

FIGURE 61.12. Stimulation sequences. **A:** A complex sequence intended to minimize induction of nonclinical arrhythmias by completing double extrastimuli during normal sinus rhythm (NSR) and two ventricular paced (VP) rates (NSR + 1-2, VP1, and VP2 + 1-2) at the right ventricular apex (RVA) and outflow tract (RVOT) before moving to triple extrastimuli. Some variations complete single extrastimuli at the RVA and RVOT before moving to doubles; this is very conservative and very time-consuming. **B:** A simpler but still effective sequence. LV, left ventricle. (From Fisher JD, Kim SG, Ferrick KJ, Roth JA. Programmed ventricular stimulation using tandem vs. simple sequential protocols. *Pacing Clin Electrophysiol* 1994;17:286–294.)

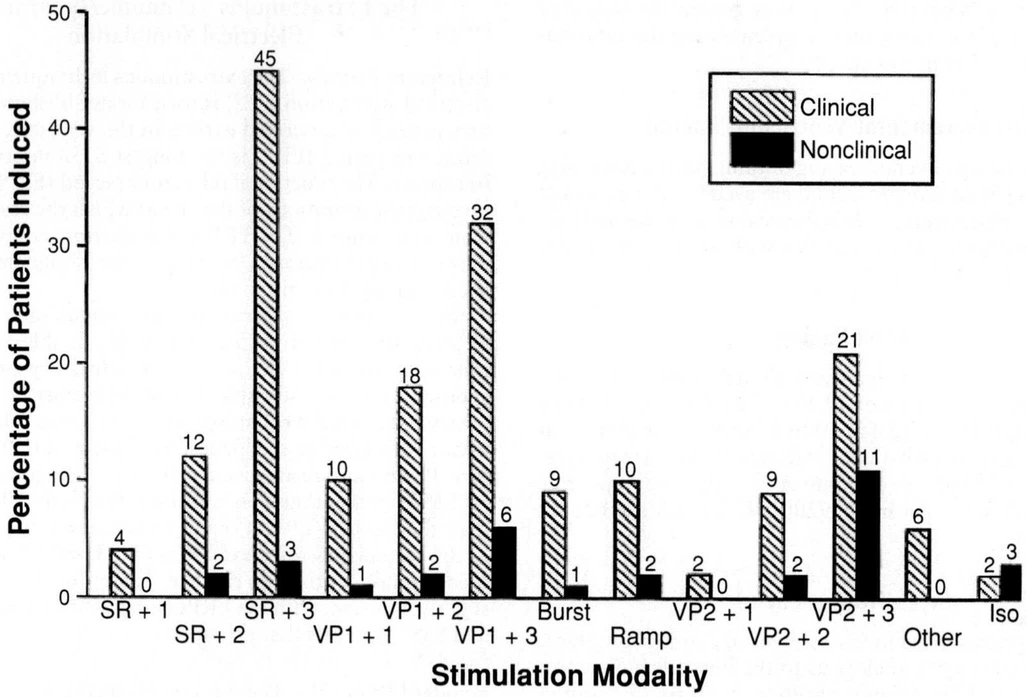

FIGURE 61.13. Frequency of induced clinical and nonclinical arrhythmia with each stimulating modality (protocol step) in a consecutive series of patients with inducible ventricular tachycardia. All patients received *all* steps. The sequence actually used is displayed on the abscissa. The ordinate indicates the percentage of uses of each modality that resulted in a clinical (*hatched*) or nonclinical (*solid*) arrhythmia. Each of the bar graphs is capped by a number indicating more precisely the percentage of arrhythmias induced. SR, sinus rhythm; VP1, the slower paced drive rate; VP2; the faster rate. Numerals 0, 1, 2, and 3 indicate the number of extrastimuli. Note that SR + 3 was more efficacious than either VP1 + 2 or VP2 + 2, and that VP1 + 3 was superior to VP2 + 2. In addition to the *p* values indicated, VP2 + 3 was more likely to induce nonclinical arrhythmias than NSR + 3 or VP1 + 3 ($p < .05$). (From Kosowsky BD, Latif P, Radoff AM. Multilevel atrioventricular block. *Circulation* 1976;54:914–921.)

Ultrarapid Train Stimulation. Ultrarapid train stimulation of a duration that produces single, double, and triple captures can be used as an efficient alternative to the extrastimulus technique (Fig. 61.14) (11).

Other Enhancements. In some patients isoproterenol, prolonged pacing to provoke ischemia, or postural changes may be helpful in producing a desired arrhythmia (see appropriate chapters) (171,173). A variation on the more usual PES methods is the "sudden change in cycle length" protocol, which may enhance dispersion of refractoriness and thereby promote arrhythmia induction (171,175).

Sensitivity and Specificity. Acceptable stimulation protocols should be able to induce sustained monomorphic VT in 90% of patients with coronary artery disease who present with this arrhythmia (12). Induction of other ventricular arrhythmias (VF or polymorphic VT) in patients *with* a history of such arrhythmias may be as low as 60% (171,174). Induction of sustained monomorphic VT in patients without a known or suspected history of such arrhythmias is rare (171). Induction of polymorphic VT or VF in patients *without* a history of these arrhythmias may occur in up to 15% of patients (171).

Electrophysiologic Features of Miscellaneous Diseases and Conditions

Mitral Valve Prolapse

Mitral valve prolapse (175–177) is associated with a variety of sinus node, atrial, and ventricular arrhythmias, the latter sometimes attributable to stressing of the papillary muscles. There is a tendency toward cardiac hyperreflexia including neurocardiogenic syncope.

Aortic Valve Disease

AV block may occur, typically at the AV node level in aortic regurgitation and at the His-Purkinje level with aortic stenosis (177,179).

Congestive Cardiomyopathy

Prolongation of the HV interval is common (180,182). Conduction disease does not correlate with the degree of ventricular enlargement or end-diastolic pressure. Atrial arrhythmias and fatal ventricular arrhythmias are not rare. The Sudden Cardiac Death in Heart Failure Trial (SCD-HeFT) was a multicenter randomized clinical trial designed to determine whether antiarrhythmic treatment (ICD or amiodarone) is better than placebo. Compared to placebo, ICD therapy resulted in a significant reduction in all-cause mortality (183).

Hypertrophic Cardiomyopathy

Prolongation of the HV interval is common, and block at that level is not rare. Atrial arrhythmias and fatal ventricular arrhythmias are not rare (184–187).

Infiltrative Cardiomyopathy

Sarcoidosis, amyloidosis, hemochromatosis, microfibrillar cardiomyopathy, atrial and ventricular tachycardias, sinus node disease, and AV block occur all too commonly (188–190). Recently described microfibrillar cardiomyopathy (190) is

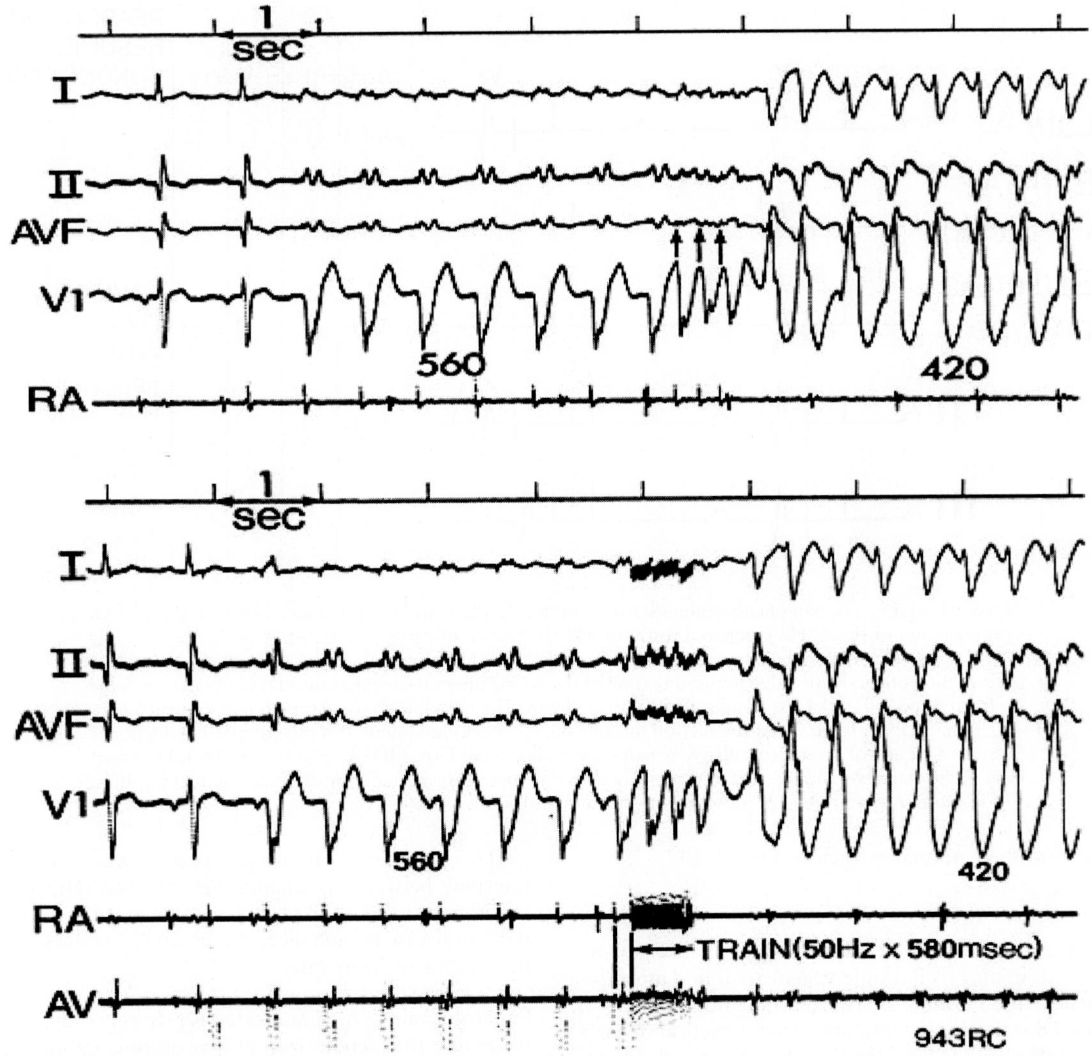

FIGURE 61.14. Conventional programmed electrical stimulation (PES) and ultrarapid train stimulation. **A:** Surface leads 1, 2, AVF, and V1 are displayed together with intracardiac recordings from the right atrium (RA) and the atrioventricular junction (AV). After two sinus beats, eight drive stimuli are delivered at a cycle length of 560 msec, resulting in seven captures. These are followed by triple programmed extrastimuli, which result in induction of ventricular tachycardia with a right-bundle-branch block morphology and a cycle length of 420 msec. **B:** In the same patient, after ventricular drive pacing at 560 msec, 50-Hz (20-msec) trains produce three captures and ventricular tachycardia of the same morphology and rate produced by conventional PES. (From Fisher JD, Ostrow E, Kim SG, Matos JA: Ultrarapid single-capture train stimulation for termination of ventricular tachycardia. *Am J Cardiol* 1983;51:1334–1338.)

associated with atrial or ventricular arrhythmias but preservation of ventricular function and a prognosis that appears to be more benign than the other conditions.

Collagen Vascular Diseases

Arrhythmias and block may occur, and are an adverse prognostic sign. Congenital complete heart block is common in offspring of mothers with connective tissue diseases (191–193).

Infectious Processes

Viral myocarditis may be associated with ventricular arrhythmias, either acutely or as a result of the subsequent development of dilated cardiomyopathy. Varicella myocarditis is associated with malignant ventricular arrhythmias and a poor prognosis. Bacterial infections may result in heart block. In South America, Chagas disease is a common cause of heart block and tachycardias (194–196).

Thyroid Disease

Thyrotoxicosis has been associated with sudden death, ventricular arrhythmias, heart block, and myocardial infarction. Hyperthyroidism has been reported to cause AV block, but facilitation of AV conduction and sinus tachycardias are more common. Hypothyroidism may cause AV block at the AV node and His-Purkinje levels, and there is prolongation of myocardial action potentials (198,199).

Other Phenomena

Phase 3 Block (Tachycardia-Dependent Block). This occurs when an impulse arrives at tissues that are still refractory (Table 61.3) due to incomplete repolarization. Manifestations include bundle branch block and fascicular block as well as complete AV block (82,83,200–203).

Phase 4 Block (Bradycardia-Dependent Block). This occurs when conduction of an impulse is blocked in tissues that

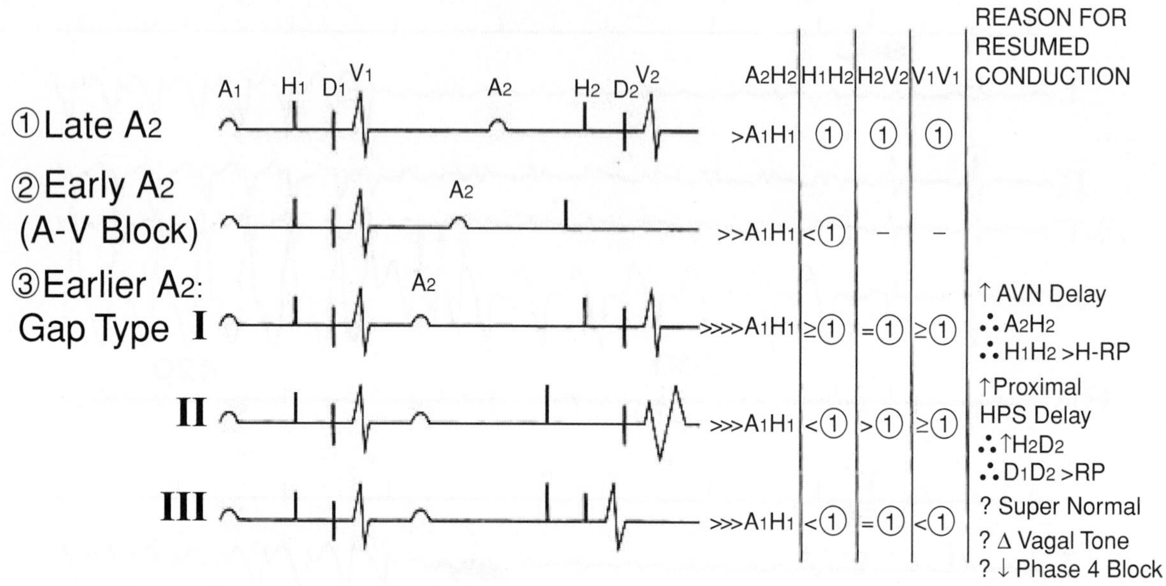

FIGURE 61.15. The gap phenomenon. See text. In line 1, a late atrial extrastimulus (A2) conducts with prolongation of the A2H2 compared to the A1H1. In line 2, an earlier A2 fails to conduct because the H1H2 interval is within the effective refractory period of the His bundle. In line 3, an earlier A2 results in resumption of conduction due to prolongation of the A2H2 interval such that the H1H2 now exceeds the refractory period of the His bundle. This is a type I gap. The next line shows a type II gap, in which conduction resumes after delayed conduction through the His-Purkinje system. In a type III gap, conduction is resumed for any of several speculative reasons. (Modified from Fisher JD. Role of electrophysiologic testing in the diagnosis and treatment of patients with known and suspected bradycardias and tachycardias. *Prog Cardiovascular Dis* 1981;24:25, with permission.)

are well beyond their normal refractory periods (82,83,200–205).

The Distal Gate and Bundle Branch Reentry. The longest refractory periods in the His-Purkinje system are found most distally, at or near the Purkinje–myocardial junction (206,207). This creates a distal gate that inhibits retroconduction of early ventricular extrasystoles. Thus when early extrastimuli are delivered to the right ventricular apex, the nearby distal gates of the RBB may still be refractory, preventing retroconduction. However, the impulse may propagate to the left ventricle, and by that time retroconduction up the LBB may be possible (208). In as many as 50% of normal individuals, the impulse propagated up the LBB may then proceed in an anterograde direction through the RBB to create a bundle branch reentry (BBRE) repetitive response (207). Such BBREs rarely last more than one or two beats in normal individuals but are an occasional cause of sustained tachycardia particularly, in dilated hearts (208,209).

Gap Phenomenon. When the extrastimulus (A2) technique is used in the atrium, AV block or bundle branch block may occur at a certain S1S2 interval, and yet, with further prematurity, conduction resumes (106,210–220). This "gap" in conduction occurs for many reasons, the most common of which are summarized in Figure 61.15.

Type I gap is most common. An atrial extrastimulus conducted with modest delay through the AV node finds the His bundle still refractory, causing block. With increasing prematurity of the atrial extrastimulus A2, the A2H2 interval prolongs further so that the H1H2 interval now exceeds the refractory period of the His bundle and conduction resumes. The same principle applies to all levels of the atrium, the AV conduction system, and the ventricle, so that there are virtually endless possibilities for gaps in both the anterograde and retrograde directions.

The gap phenomenon is *not an abnormality* but reflects the interplay between conduction velocity and refractory periods in different parts of the heart. Demonstration of the gap phenomenon can be enhanced by creating changes in neurohumoral tone or heart rate.

Supernormality. A stimulus that is precisely timed to occur immediately after repolarization may produce capture at a stimulus amplitude that fails to capture if delivered slightly earlier or later (221,222). This supernormal excitability can be seen clinically, for example, when a failing pacemaker captures just at the end of the T wave but not elsewhere in the cardiac cycle. Supernormality has been demonstrated in the His-Purkinje system, Bachmann's bundle in the dog, and working myocardium of the atrium and ventricle but not in the AV node. In a somewhat comparable fashion, supernormal *conduction* exists when a precisely timed beat results in restoration or improvement of conduction in a previously depressed or blocked area.

COMPLETE, SCREENING, AND TARGETED ELECTROPHYSIOLOGIC STUDIES

Philosophical, practical, and ethical considerations materially affect not only the decision to perform an EPS, but also the thoroughness of the study.

The Complete Diagnostic Electrophysiologic Study

The complexity and number of possible maneuvers that can be performed during an EPS make it virtually impossible to do a truly complete study. For example, one pharmacologic stress could interfere with other portions of the EPS, so that a second session would be needed to complete a thorough evaluation. In addition to the many tests and maneuvers outlined in this chapter, there are many other variations that can be applied for specific indications related to patients with known or suspected bradycardias or tachycardias (see appropriate chapters). A more complete evaluation is needed when an EPS is performed for evaluation of a patient with syncope of undetermined origin (SUO) compared with an EPS performed to assess the efficacy of a drug given to prevent induction of an arrhythmia that has previously been characterized.

Ethical Considerations

These arise on many levels: Is there a true indication for the EPS? How thorough an examination must be done before billing for a "complete diagnostic EPS"?

CONCLUSION

Electrophysiologic studies are appropriate and necessary for a broad range of indications (3). EPS has become indispensable not only for diagnosis and risk stratification, but also for selection and assessment of therapies such as pacemakers and drugs and for interventional procedures such as radiofrequency catheter ablation (224). EPS is associated with low levels of risk compared with diagnostic interventional cardiac angiographic procedures.

CONTROVERSIES AND PERSONAL PERSPECTIVES

Comprehensive or Targeted Electrophysiologic Studies?

Years ago, it was unusual to find EPS performed outside of teaching institutions. Part of the attending physician's task was to ensure that the trainees became familiar with all aspects of an EPS assessment. These assessments included tests of automaticity, refractoriness, conduction, and ability to induce tachycardias or bradycardia at each of the various levels of the heart from the sinus node to the ventricle. As workloads have increased and reimbursements have declined, it has become common in both teaching and nonteaching centers to shift to a "targeted" EPS. The most common of these are studies to determine whether VT is inducible or to locate and ablate the pathway responsible for a supraventricular tachycardia (SVT). There is nothing intrinsically bad about either approach. The extremes of a comprehensive test are impractical if applied to all patients, just as the extremes of targeted procedures may be too superficial.

Judgment is necessary. Also needed is attention to the "15–20% rule," which applies to the likelihood of finding conduction disease in patients with sinus node disease or the reverse and to the likelihood of finding an additional clinically relevant SVT in a patient in whom one has been documented.

Empathy also plays a role. I would not like to have my Wolff-Parkinson-White condition ablated, only to find that I had to return for another procedure to ablate a "recurrent" SVT that turns out to be due to AV nodal reentry tachycardia that was not screened for at the initial procedure. I would not like to return for an additional pacemaker wire because it was not realized that my sinus node function was not actually normal. I would be happy with a single-chamber defibrillator if EPS together with consideration of my underlying heart condition and my potential need for bradycardia-inducing medications all suggested that the added features and wires of a dual-chamber defibrillator would not be likely to help me in the foreseeable future.

Not Everybody Needs an Electrophysiologic Study

The indications for EPS are generally quite clear. Indications are developing and expanding, but many of the reasons for referral for an EPS are in the class II ("probable") or class III ("not indicated") categories. The indications are really guidelines in recognition of the gray zones and borderline cases that will always exist in clinical medicine. Electrophysiologists would do well to add some additional class III (not indicated) items as a kind of internal check. Some suggested class III items are (a) exceeding a certain percentage of the overall number of cases with borderline or subjective indications, (b) adding cases to meet volume expectations or quotas, (c) doing an EPS primarily to satisfy the expectations or desires of a referring physician who is not an electrophysiologist.

More Patients Need to Have an Electrophysiologic Study

Fewer patients receiving ICDs are referred for EPS before implant. Since the publication of the MADIT II and SCD-HeFT studies, most patients receiving ICD implants have bypassed an EPS. This practice ignores the importance of detecting treatable supraventricular arrhythmia as well as sinus node and conduction system disease. Patients with "undiscovered" SVT are likely receive multiple shocks. In addition, there will be numerous patients who will receive single-chamber ICDs and present with sinus node or His-Purkinje conduction system disease shortly thereafter.

We have not done a good enough job at getting the word out. EPS is a safe and effective diagnostic tool. Results can help to determine whether a device is needed, and if one is needed, it can help to optimize the choice. "Interventional" or "therapeutic" EPS in the form of ablation is now the recommended first choice for many arrhythmias. Nevertheless, there are still many physicians who think nothing of sending patients for coronary angiography, stenting, and bypass surgery but are leery about sending patients with straightforward indications for an EPS. Too many patients finally come to the electrophysiologist after years of taking a variety of medications for recurrent symptomatic SVT. More tragically, too many physicians continue to believe that revascularization is sufficient therapy for the majority of patients with cardiac arrest due to VT or VF.

Homogenize the Guidelines!

Remarkably enough, at the time of this writing the ACC/AHA guidelines for pacemaker implantation are not coordinated with the ACC/AHA guidelines for EPS. For example, in a patient referred for syncope of undetermined origin (SUO), EPS may reveal a sinus node recovery time of 5 or 10 seconds, yet there is no indication corresponding to a prolonged sinus node recovery time in the guidelines for pacemaker implantation. There are many obvious reasons why this should be rectified.

THE FUTURE

It is still too soon to tell whether molecular biology and genetics or immunology will develop probes that will help to identify the majority of patients with abnormalities of each of the various electrical generators and circuits in the heart that can lead to arrhythmias. Certainly there has been some advance, most notably in patients with conditions such as the long-QT interval syndromes, hypertrophic cardiomyopathy, and others. However, these account for only a small fraction of patients with clinical arrhythmias.

There is widespread interest in ablative techniques for atrial fibrillation. This has led to intensive efforts to develop better catheter systems, ablative energy delivery systems, and mapping systems. As these develop, they will no doubt be directed at the identification of other arrhythmias or abnormalities. Pharmacologic probes have been used (e.g., procainamide to suppress accessory pathway conduction, adenosine to suppress normal and thereby expose accessory pathway conduction, etc.). The development of more specific pharmacologic probes would be of great help. Using present methodologies, EPS enjoys sensitivities and specificities in perhaps the 80% range for detecting conditions such as sick sinus syndrome and AV conduction disease at the various levels. Thus there are patients who "pass" a comprehensive EPS only to come to the emergency room some time later with profound symptomatic bradycardia. Pharmacologic probes that would increase the sensitivity and specificity of the testing substantially would be of great clinical importance.

References

1. Zipes DP, DiMarco JP, Gillette PC, et al. ACC/AHA Task Force Report—Guidelines for clinical intracardiac electrophysiological and catheter ablation procedures. A report of the ACC/AHA Task Force on Practice Guidelines (Committee on Clinical Intracardiac Electrophysiological and Catheter Ablation Procedures), developed in collaboration with NASPE. *J Am Coll Cardiol* 1995;26:555.
2. Damato AN, Lau SH, Helfant RH, et al. Study of atrioventricular conduction in man using electrode catheter recordings of His bundle activity. *Circulation* 1969;39:287–296.
3. Damato AN, Lau SH, Helfant RH, et al. A study of heart block in man using His bundle recordings. *Circulation* 1969;39:297–305.
4. Bubien RS, Fisher JD, Gentzel JA, et al. NASPE Expert Consensus Document: use of IV (conscious) sedation/analgesia by nonanesthesia personnel in patients undergoing arrhythmia: specific diagnostic, therapeutic, and surgical procedures. *Pacing Clin Electrophysiol* 1998;21:375–385.
5. Mehra R, Furman S. Comparison of cathodal, anodal, and bipolar strength–interval curves with temporary and permanent pacing electrodes. *Br Heart J* 1979;41:468–476.
6. Roth BJ. Strength–interval curves for cardiac tissue predicted using the bidomain model. *J Cardiovasc Electrophysiol* 1996;7:722–737.
7. Zhang X, Fisher JD, Kim SG, et al. Comparison of ramp and stepwise incremental pacing in assessment of antegrade and retrograde conduction. *Pacing Clin Electrophysiol* 1986;9:42.
8. Fisher JD, Kim SG, Ferrick KJ, et al. Programmed ventricular stimulation using tandem vs. simple sequential protocols. *Pacing Clin Electrophysiol* 1994;17:286–294.
9. Fisher JD, Kim SG, Ferrick KJ, et al. Programmed electrical stimulation of the ventricle: An efficient, sensitive, and specific protocol. *Pacing Clin Electrophysiol* 1992;15:435–450.
10. Fisher JD, Ostrow E, Kim SG, et al. Ultrarapid single-capture train stimulation for termination of ventricular tachycardia. *Am J Cardiol* 1983; 51: 1334–1338.
11. Fisher JD, Platt SB, Cua MC, et al. Ultrarapid train stimulation: an efficient alternative to conventional programmed electrical stimulation for induction of ventricular arrhythmias. *J Interv Cardiac Electrophysiol* 1997;1: 15–21.
12. Zipes DP, DiMarco JP, Gillette PC, et al., with Fisher JD for ablation section. Guidelines for clinical intracardiac electrophysiological and catheter ablation procedures. A report of the ACC/AHA Task Force on Practice Guidelines (Committee on Clinical Intracardiac Electrophysiological and Catheter Ablation Procedures). *J Am Coll Cardiol* 1995;26:555–573.
13. Fisher JD, Baker J, Ferrick KJ, et al. The atrial electrogram during clinical electrophysiologic studies: onset versus the local/intrinsic deflection. *J Cardiovasc Electrophysiol* 1991;2:398–407.
14. Josephson ME. *Clinical cardiac electrophysiology, techniques and interpretations,* 2nd ed. Philadelphia: Lea & Febiger, 1993:27.
15. Fisher JD. Role of electrophysiologic testing in the diagnosis and treatment of patients with known and suspected bradycardias and tachycardias. *Prog Cardiovasc Dis* 1981;24:25.
16. Narula OS, Cohen LS, Samet P, et al. Localization of AV conduction defects in man by recording of the His bundle electrogram. *Am J Cardiol* 1970;25:228.
17. Josephson ME, Seides SF. Electrophysiologic investigation: technical aspects. In: Josephson ME, Seides SF, eds. *Clinical cardiac electrophysiology: techniques and interpretations.* Philadelphia: Lea & Febiger, 1979:17–18.
18. Ausubel K, Klementowica P, Furman S. Interatrial conduction during cardiac pacing. *Pacing Clin Electrophysiol* 1986;9:1026.
19. Buxton AE, Waxman HL, Marchlinski FE, et al. Atrial conduction: effects of extrastimuli with and without atrial dysrhythmias. *Am J Cardiol* 1984;54:755.
20. Camous JP, Raybaud F, Dolisi C, et al. Interatrial conduction in patients undergoing AV stimulation: effects of increasing right atrial stimulation rate. *Pacing Clin Electrophysiol* 1993;16:2082.
21. Plumb VJ, Karp RB, James TN, et al. Atrial excitability and conduction during rapid atrial pacing. *Circulation* 1981;63:1140.
22. Dhingra RC, Rosen KM, Rahimtoola SH. Normal conduction intervals and responses in sixty-one patients using His bundle recording and atrial pacing. *Chest* 1973;64:55.
23. Josephson ME. *Clinical cardiac electrophysiology, techniques and interpretations,* 2nd ed. Philadelphia: Lea & Febiger, 1993:28.
24. Fisher JD, Kay M, Mehra R. Increased accuracy of the corrected H-V time. In: Meere C, ed. *Proceedings of the VI World Symposium on Cardiac Pacing.* Montreal: PACE Symposium, 1979.
25. Moore EN, Spear JF. Effect of autonomic activity on pacemaker function and conduction. In: Wellens HJJ, Lie KI, Janse MJ, eds. *The conduction system of the heart.* Philadelphia: Lea & Febiger, 1976:1–10.
26. Martin P. The influence of the parasympathetic nervous system on atrioventricular conduction. *Circ Res* 1977;41:593.
27. Jewell GM, Magorien RD, Schaael SF. Autonomonic tone of patients during an electrophysiological catheterization. *Am Heart J* 1980;99:51.
28. Sigler LH. Clinical observations on the carotid sinus reflex I. The frequency and the degree of response to carotid sinus pressure under various diseased states. *Am J Med Sci* 1933;186;110.
29. Sigler LH. Further observation on the carotid sinus reflex. *Ann Intern Med* 1936;9:1380.
30. Heidorn GH, McNamara AP. Effect of carotid sinus stimulation on the electrocardiograms of clinically normal individuals. *Circulation* 1956;14:1104.
31. Hartzler GO, Maloney JD. Cardioinhibitory carotid sinus hypersensitivity. Intracardiac recordings and clinical assessment. *Arch Intern Med* 1977; 137:727.
32. Narula OS. Disorders of sinus node function. In: Narula OS, ed. *Electrophysiologic evaluation. His bundle electrocardiography and clinical electrophysiology.* Philadelphia: FA Davis, 1975:275–311.
33. Fisher JD, Katz G, Furman S, et al. Differential responses to carotid sinus massage in cardiac patients with and without syncope. In: Feruglio GA, ed. *Cardiac pacing, electrophysiology and pacemaker technology.* Florence: Piccin Medical Books, 1982:521–522.
34. Narula OS. Sick sinus syndrome: key references. *Circulation* 1979;60:1422.
35. Scarpa WJ. The sick sinus syndrome. *Am Heart J* 1976;92:648.
36. Seinfeld D, Altschuler H, Yipintsoi T, et al. Pathogenetic locus of the sick sinus syndrome. *Clin Res* 1978;26:270A.
37. Jordan JL, Yamaguchi I, Mandel WJ. Studies on the mechanism of sinus node dysfunction in the sick sinus syndrome. *Circulation* 1978;57:217.
38. Mandel W, Hayakawa H, Danzig R, et al. Evaluation of sinoatrial node function in man by overdrive suppression. *Circulation* 1971;44:59.
39. Mandel WJ, Laks MM, Orayashi K. Sinus node function. Evaluation in patients with and without sinus node disease. *Arch Intern Med* 1975;135:388.
40. Strauss HC, Bigger Jr JT, Saroff AL. Electrophysiologic evaluation of sinus node function in patients with sinus node dysfunction. *Circulation* 1976;53:763.
41. Kulbertus HE, DeLeval-Rutten D, Mary L, et al. Sinus node recovery time in the elderly. *Br Heart J* 1975;37:420.
42. Breithardt G, Seipel L, Loogen F. Sinus node recovery time and calculated sinoatrial conduction time in normal subjects and patients with sinus node dysfunction. *Circulation* 1977;56:43.
43. Gupta PK, Lichstein F, Chada KD, et al. Appraisal of sinus nodal recovery time in patients with sick sinus syndrome. *Am J Cardiol* 1974;34:265.
44. Altschuler H, Fisher JD. Increasing the yield of the sinus recovery time in the sick sinus syndrome. *Clin Res* 1976;24:205A.
45. Benditt DG, Strauss HC, Scheinman MM, et al. Analysis of secondary pauses following termination of rapid pacing in man. *Circulation* 1976; 54:436.
46. Dhingra RC, Amat-Y-Leon F, Wyndham C, et al. Electrophysiologic effects of atropine on sinus node and atrium in patients with sinus node dysfunction. *Am J Cardiol* 1976;38:848.
47. Reiffel JA, Bigger Jr JT, Giardina EGV. "Paradoxical" prolongation of sinus nodal recovery time after atropine in the sick sinus syndrome. *Am J Cardiol* 1975;36:98.
48. Dhingra RC, Deedwania PC, Cummings JM, et al. Electrophysiologic effects of lidocaine on sinus node and atrium in patients with and without sinoatrial dysfunction. *Circulation* 1978;57:448.
49. Evans TR, Callowhill EA, Krikler DM: Clinical value of tests of sino-atrial function. *Pacing Clin Electrophysiol* 1978;1:2.
50. Josephson ME. *Clinical cardiac electrophysiology, techniques and interpretations,* 2nd ed. Philadelphia: Lea & Febiger, 1993: 71–95.

51. Alboni P, Malcarne C, Pedroni P, et al. Electrophysiology of normal sinus node with and without autonomic blockade. *Circulation* 1982;65:1236.
52. Nalos PC, Deng Z, Rosenthal ME, et al. Hemodynamic influences on sinus node recovery time: effects of autonomic blockade. *J Am Coll Cardiol* 1986;7:1079.
53. Karagueuzian HS, Jordan JL, Sugi K, et al. Appropriate diagnostic studies for sinus node dysfunction. *Pacing Clin Electrophysiol* 1985;8:242.
54. Tonkin AM, Heddle WF. Electrophysiological testing of sinus node function. *Pacing Clin Electrophysiol* 1984;7:735.
55. De Marneffe M, Jacobs P, Englert M. Reproducibility of electrophysiologic parameters of extrinsic sinus node function in patients with and without sick sinus syndrome. *Pacing Clin Electrophysiol* 1986;9:482.
56. De Marneffe M, Waterschoot P, Melot C, et al. Electrophysiology of the normal sinus node. *J Electrophysiol* 1988;2:155.
57. Reiffel JA, Kuehnert MJ. Electrophysiological testing of sinus node function: diagnostic and prognostic application—including updated information from sinus node electrograms. *Pacing Clin Electrophysiol* 1994;17:349.
58. Narula OS, Shantha N, Narula LK, et al. Clinical and electrophysiological evaluation of sinus node function. In: Narula OS, ed. *Cardiac arrhythmias: electrophysiology, diagnosis and management*. Baltimore: Williams & Wilkins, 1979:176–206.
59. Engel TR, Schaal SF. Digitalis in the sick sinus syndrome: the effects of digitalis on sinoatrial automaticity and atrioventricular conduction. *Circulation* 1973;48:1201–1207.
60. Dhingra RC, Amat-Y-Leon F, Wyndham C, et al. Clinical significance of prolonged sinoatrial conduction time. *Circulation* 1977;55:8.
61. Crook B, Kitson D, McComish M, et al. Indirect measurement of sinoatrial conduction time in patients with sinoatrial disease and in controls. *Br Heart J* 1977;39:771.
62. Delius W, Wirtzfeld A. The significance of the sinus node recovery time in the sick sinus syndrome. In: Luderitz B, ed. *Cardiac pacing, diagnostic and therapeutic tools*. Berlin, Springer-Verlag, 1976:25–32.
63. Josephson ME. Clinical cardiac electrophysiology, techniques and interpretations, 2nd ed. Philadelphia: Lea & Febiger, 1993:83.
64. Reiffel JA, Zimmerman G. The duration of the sinus node depolarization on transvenous sinus node electrograms can identify sinus node dysfunction and can suggest its severity. *Pacing Clin Electrophysiol* 1989;12:1746.
65. Juillard A, Guillerm F, Van Chuong H, et al. Sinus node electrogram recording in 59 patients. Comparison with simultaneous estimation of sinoatrial conduction using premature atrial stimulation. *Br Heart J* 1983;50:75.
66. Gomes JAC, Kang PS, El-Sherif N. The sinus node electrogram in patients with and without sick sinus syndrome: techniques and correlation between directly measured and indirectly estimated sinoatrial conduction time. *Circulation* 1982;66:864.
67. Reiffel JA, Gang E, Gliklich J, et al. The human sinus node electrogram: a transvenous catheter technique and a comparison of directly measured and indirectly estimated sinoatrial conduction time in adults. *Circulation* 1980;62:1324.
68. Reiffel JA, Bigger Jr JT. The relationship between sinoatrial conduction time and sinus cycle length revisited. *J Electrophysiol* 1987;1:290.
69. Centurion OA, Fukatani M, Konoe A, et al. Different distribution of abnormal endocardial electrograms within the right atrium in patients with sick sinus syndrome. *Br Heart J* 1992;68:596.
70. Mackintosh AF, English MJ, Vincent R, et al. Low voltage electrical activity preceding right atrial depolarization in man. *Br Heart J* 1979;42:117.
71. Miller HC, Strauss HC. Measurement of sinoatrial conduction time by premature atrial stimulation in the rabbit. *Circ Res* 1974;35:935.
72. Breithardt G, Seipel L. Effect of premature atrial depolarizations on sinus node automaticity in man. *Circulation* 1976;53:920.
73. Steinbeck G, Luderitz B. Sinoatrial pacemaker shift following atrial stimulation in man. *Circulation* 1977;56:402.
74. Breithardt G, Siepel L. Comparative study of two methods of estimating sinoatrial conduction time in man. *Am J Cardiol* 1978;42:965.
75. Dhingra RC, Wyndham C, Amat-Y-Leon F, et al. Sinus nodal responses to atrial extrastimuli in patients without apparent sinus node disease. *Am J Cardiol* 1975;36:445.
76. Langendorf R, Lesser ME, Plotkin P, et al. Atrial parasystole with interpolation: observations on prolonged sinoatrial conduction. *Am Heart J* 1962;63:649–658.
77. Goldreyer BN, Damato AN. Sinoatrial node entrance block. *Circulation* 1971;44:789–802.
78. Narula OS, Shantha N, Vasquez M, et al. A new method for measurement of sinoatrial conduction time. *Circulation* 1978;58:706.
79. Kirkorian G, Touboul P, Atallah G, et al. Premature atrial stimulation during regular atrial pacing: a new approach to the study of the sinus node. *Am J Cardiol* 1984;54:109.
80. Jose AD. Effect of combined sympathetic and parasympathetic blockade on heart rate and cardiac function in man. *Am J Cardiol* 1966;18:476.
81. Jose AD, Collison D. The normal range and determinants of the intrinsic heart rate in man. *Cardiovasc Res* 1970;4:160.
82. Denes P, Wu D, Dhingra R, et al. The effects of cycle length on cardiac refractory periods in man. *Circulation* 1974;49:32.
83. Dubrow IW, Fisher EA, Amat-Y-Leon F, et al. Comparison of cardiac refractory periods in children and adults. *Circulation* 1975;51:485.
84. Fisher JD, Zhang X, Waspe LE, et al. Tests of refractoriness and conduction during clinical electrophysiologic studies: yields and roles. *J Electrophysiol* 1988;2:175.
85. Wit AL, Weiss MB, Berkowitz WD, et al. Patterns of atrioventricular conduction in the human heart. *Circ Res* 1970;27:345.
86. Akhtar M, Damato AN, Batsford WP, et al. A comparative analysis of antegrade conduction patterns in man. *Circulation* 1975;52:766.
87. Bisset JK, Kane JJ, DeSoyza N, et al. Electrophysiological significance of rapid atrial pacing as a test of atrioventricular conduction. *Cardiovasc Res* 1975;9:593.
88. Denes P. The effect of cycle length on the atrial refractory period. *Pacing Clin Electrophysiol* 1984;7:1108.
89. Ferrier GR, Dresel PE. Relationship of the functional refractory period of conduction in the atrioventricular node. *Circ Res* 1974;35:204–214.
90. Loeb JM, deTarnowsky JM, Warner MR, et al. Dynamic interactions between heart rate and atrioventricular conduction. *Am J Physiol* 1985;249:H505.
91. Warner MR, Loeb JM. Beat-by-beat modulation of AV conduction. I. Heart rate and respiratory influences. *Am J Physiol* 1986;251:H1126.
92. Warner MR, Loeb JM. Beat-by-beat modulation of AV conduction. II. Autonomic neural mechanisms. *Am J Physiol* 1986;251:H1134.
93. Lehmann MH, Denker S, Mahmud R, et al. Patterns of human atrioventricular nodal accommodation to a sudden acceleration of atrial rate. *Am J Cardiol* 1984;53:71.
94. Fisher JD. *Primer of cardiac electrophysiology*. Armonk, NY: Futura, in press.
95. Narula OS, Scherlag BJ, Samet P. Perivenous pacing of the specialized conducting system in man. *Circulation* 1970;41:77.
96. Narula OS. Validation of His bundle recordings: limitations of the catheter technique. In: Narula OS, ed. *His Bundle electrocardiography and clinical electrophysiology*. Philadelphia: FA Davis, 1975:65–93.
97. Josephson ME, Scharf DL, Kastor JA, et al. Atrial endocardial activation in man: electrode catheter technique for endocardial mapping. *Am J Cardiol* 1977;39:972.
98. James TN. The connecting pathways between the sinus node and AV node and between the right and left atrium in the human heart. *Am Heart J* 1963;66:498.
99. Sherf L. The atrial conduction system: clinical implications. *Am J Cardiol* 1976;37:814.
100. Ross AM, Proper MC, Aronson AL. Sinoventricular conduction in atrial standstill. *J Electrocardiol* 1976;9:161.
101. Giusti RP, Fisher JD. Prolongation of intra-atrial conduction time in response to atrial pacing. *Clin Res* 1976;24:218A.
102. Millar RNS, Mauer BJ, Rei DS, et al. Studies of intra-atrial conduction with bipolar atrial and His electrograms. *Br Heart J* 1973;35:604.
103. Fisher JD, Lehmann MH. Marked intra-atrial conduction delay with split atrial electrograms: substrate for reentrant supraventricular tachycardia. *Am Heart J* 1986;111:781.
104. Simpson Jr RJ, Foster JR, Gettes LS. Atrial excitability and conduction in patients with interatrial conduction defects. *Am J Cardiol* 1982;50:1331.
105. Simpson Jr RJ, Amara I, Foster JR, et al. Thresholds, refractory periods, and conduction times of the normal and diseased human atrium. *Am Heart J* 1988;116:1080.
106. Akhtar M, Caracta AR, Lau SH, et al. Demonstration of intra-atrial conduction delay, block, gap and reentry: a report of two cases. *Circulation* 1978;58:947.
107. Narula OS, Runge M, Samet P. Second-degree Wenckebach type AV block due to block within the atrium. *Br Heart J* 1972;34:1127.
108. Castellanos Jr A, Iyengar R, Agha AS, et al. Wenckebach phenomenon within the atria. *Br Heart J* 1972;34:1121.
109. Calkins H, El-Atassi R, Kalbfleisch S, et al. Effects of an acute increase in atrial pressure on atrial refractoriness in humans. *Pacing Clin Electrophysiol* 1992;15:1674.
110. Niwano S, Aizawa Y. Fragmented atrial activity in patients with transient atrial fibrillation. *Am Heart J* 1991;121:62.
111. Tanigawa M, Fukatani M, Konow A, et al. Prolonged and fractionated right atrial electrograms during sinus rhythm in patients with paroxysmal atrial fibrillation and sick sinus node syndrome. *J Am Coll Cardiol* 1991;17:403.
112. Narula OS, Narula JT. Junctional pacemakers in man: response to overdrive suppression with and without parasympathetic blockade. *Circulation* 1978;57:880.
113. Narula OS, Narula JT. Junctional pacemakers in man: response to overdrive suppression with and without parasympathetic blockade. *Circulation* 1978;57:880.
114. Mazgalev TN, Tchou PJ, eds. *Atrial–AV nodal electrophysiology*. Armonk, NY: Futura, 2000.
115. Jackman WM, Beckman KJ, McClelland JH, et al. Treatment of supraventricular tachycardia due to atrioventricular nodal reentry by radiofrequency catheter ablation of slow-pathway conduction. *N Engl J Med* 1992;327:313–318.
116. Mitrani RD, Klein LS, Hackett FK, et al. Radiofrequency ablation for atrioventricular node reentrant tachycardia: comparison between fast (anterior) and slow (posterior) pathway ablation. *J Am Coll Cardiol* 1993;21:432–441.
117. Janse MJ, Van Capelle FJL, Anderson RH, et al. Electrophysiology and structure of the atrioventricular node of the isolated rabbit heart. In: Wellens

HJJ, Lie KI, Janse MJ, eds. *The conduction system of the heart: structure, function and clinical implications*. Philadelphia: Lea & Febiger, 1976.
118. Jackman WM, Prystowsky EN, Naccarelli GV, et al. Reevaluation of enhanced atrioventricular nodal conduction: evidence to suggest a continuum of normal atrioventricular nodal physiology. *Circulation* 1983;67:441.
119. Billette J, Bonin JP. Rate-induced shortenings in refractory periods and conduction time in the dog atrioventricular node. In: Meere C, ed. *Proceedings of the VIth World Symposium on Cardiac Pacing*. Montreal: PACE Symposium, 1979:Chapter 11–4.
120. Billette J, Nattel S. Dynamic behavior of the atrioventricular node: a functional model of interaction between recovery, facilitation, and fatigue. *J Cardiovasc Electrophysiol* 1994;5:90.
121. Rosenblueth A. Mechanism of Wenckebach-Luciani cycles. *Am J Physiol* 1958;194:491–494.
122. Young ML, Wolff GS, Castellanos A, et al. Application of the Rosenblueth hypothesis to assess cycle length effects on the refractoriness of the atrioventricular node. *Am J Cardiol* 1986;57:142.
123. Malik M, Ward D, Camm AJ. Theoretical evaluation of the Rosenblueth hypothesis. *Pacing Clin Electrophysiol* 1988;11:1250.
124. Aranda J, Castellanos A, Moleiro F, et al. Effects of the pacing site on A-H conduction and refractoriness in patients with short P-R intervals. *Circulation* 1976;53:33.
125. Batsford WP, Akhtar M, Caracta AR, et al. Effect of atrial stimulation site on the electrophysiological properties of the atrioventricular node in man. *Circulation* 1974;50:283.
126. Iinuma H, Dreifus LS, Price R, et al. Influence of the site of stimulation on atrioventricular nodal refractory periods and the effect of verapamil. *Am J Cardiol* 1986;57:1167.
127. Amat y Leon F, Denes P, Wu D, et al. Effects of atrial pacing site on atrial and atrioventricular nodal function. *Br Heart J* 1975;37:576.
128. Fisher JD. Pullout His bundle/electrophysiologic studies using leads previously inserted via the subclavian vein. *Pacing Clin Electrophysiol* 1985;8: 671–677.
129. Mae GK, Preston JD, Burlington H. Physiologic evidence of a dual AV transmission system. *Circ Res* 1956;4:357–375.
130. Prystowsky EN, Klein GJ. *Cardiac arrhythmias, an integrated approach for the clinician*. New York: McGraw–Hill, 1994:120.
131. Josephson ME. Clinical cardiac electrophysiology, techniques and interpretations, 2nd ed. Philadelphia: Lea & Febiger, 1993:191.
132. Dhingra RC, Wyndham C, Amat-Y-Leon F, et al. Significance of A-H interval in patients with chronic bundle branch block: clinical, electrophysiologic and follow-up observations. *Am J Cardiol* 1976;37:231.
133. Narula OS, Samet P. Predilection of elderly females for intra-His bundle (BH) blocks. *Circulation* 1974;49–50(Suppl III):195.
134. Narula OS, Samet P. Wenckebach and Mobitz type II A-V block due to block within the His bundle and bundle branches. *Circulation* 1970;41:947.
135. Dhingra RC, Wyndham C, Bauernfeind R, et al. Significance of block distal to the His bundle induced by atrial pacing in patients with chronic bifascicular block. *Circulation* 1979;60:1455.
136. Dreifus LS, Fisch C, Griffin JC, et al. Guidelines for implantation of cardiac pacemakers and antiarrhythmia devices. A report of the American College of Cardiology/American Heart Association Task Force on Assessment of Diagnostic and Therapeutic Cardiovascular Procedures (Committee on Pacemaker Implantation). *J Am Coll Cardiol* 1991;18:1–13.
137. Prystowsky EN, Klein GJ. *Cardiac arrhythmias, an integrated approach for the clinician*. New York: McGraw-Hill, 1994:47–70.
138. Josephson ME. Clinical cardiac electrophysiology, techniques and interpretations, 2nd ed. Philadelphia: Lea & Febiger, 1993:96–149.
139. Gupta PK, Lichstein E, Chauda KD. Lidocaine-induced heart block in patients with bundle branch block. *Am J Cardiol* 1974;33:487.
140. Fisher JD, Zilo P, Kim SG. Procainamide and lidocaine as electrophysiologic stress tests. In: Feruglio GA, ed. *Cardiac pacing: electrophysiology and pacemaker technology*. Florence: Piccin Medical Books, 1982;125–126.
141. Josephson ME, Caracta AR, Ricciutti MA, et al. Electrophysiologic properties of procainamide in man. *Am J Cardiol* 1974;33:596.
142. Cannom DS. The effects of procainamide in left bundle branch block. *Circulation* 1975;51–52(Suppl II):137.
143. McKenna WJ, Rowland E, Davies J, et al. Failure to predict development atrioventricular block with electrophysiological testing supplemented by ajmaline. *Pacing Clin Electrophysiol* 1980;3:666–669.
144. Kaul U, Dev V, Narula J, et al. Evaluation of patients with bundle branch block and "unexplained" syncope: a study based on comprehensive electrophysiologic testing and ajmaline stress. *Pacing Clin Electrophysiol* 1988; 11:289.
145. Dhingra RC, Denes P, Wu D, et al. Prospective observations in patients with chronic bundle branch block and marked H-V prolongation. *Circulation* 1976;53:600.
146. Rosen KM, Dhingra RC, Wyndham C, et al. Significance of HV interval in 515 patients with chronic bifascicular block. *Am J Cardiol* 1980;45:405.
147. Scheinman MM, Peters RW, Modin G, et al. Prognostic value of infranodal conduction time in patients with chronic bundle branch block. *Circulation* 1977;56:240–244.
148. Gupta PK, Lichstein E, Chadda KD. Follow-up studies in patients with right bundle branch block and left anterior hemiblock: Significance of H-V interval. *J Electrocardiol* 1977;10:221.
149. McAnulty JH, Rahimtoola SH, Murphy ES, et al. A prospective study of sudden death in "high-risk" bundle branch block. *N Engl J Med* 1978;299: 209.
150. Vera Z, Mason DT, Fletcher RD, et al. Prolonged His-Q interval in chronic bifascicular block. Relation to impending complete heart block. *Circulation* 1976;53:46.
151. Altschuler H, Fisher JD, Furman S. Significance of isolated H-V interval prolongation in symptomatic patients without documented heart block. *Am Heart J* 1979;97:19.
152. Castellanos Jr A. H-V intervals in LBBB [Letter]. *Circulation* 1973;47:1133.
153. Narula OS. Longitudinal dissociation in the His bundle. Bundle branch block due to asynchronous conduction within the His bundle in man. *Circulation* 1977;56:996.
154. El-Sherif N, Amat-Y-Leon F, Schonfield C. Normalization of BBB patterns by distal His bundle pacing: clinical and experimental evidence of longitudinal dissociation in the pathologic His bundle. *Circulation* 1978;57: 473.
155. Hindham MC, Wagner GS, Jaro M. The clinical significance of bundle branch block complicating acute myocardial infarction. I. Clinical characteristics, hospital mortality, and one-year follow-up. *Circulation* 1978;58: 679.
156. Hindham MC, Wagner GS, Jaro M. The clinical significance of bundle branch block complicating acute myocardial infarction. II. Indications for temporary and permanent pacemaker insertion. *Circulation* 1978;58:689.
157. Ritter WS, Atkins JM, Blumqvist CG, et al. Permanent pacing in patient with transient trifascicular block during acute myocardial infarction. *Am J Cardiol* 1976;38:205.
158. Lichstein E, Gupta PK, Chadda KD. Long-term survival of patients with incomplete bundle-branch block complicating acute myocardial infarction. *Br Heart J* 1975;83:924.
159. Lie KI, Wellens HJ, Schuilenburg RM, et al. Factors influencing prognosis of bundle branch block complicating acute antero-septal infarction. The value of His bundle recordings. *Circulation* 1974;50:935.
160. Harper R, Hunt D, Vohra J, et al. His bundle electrogram in patients with acute myocardial infarction complicated by atrioventricular or intraventricular conduction disturbances. *Br Heart J* 1975;37:705.
161. Seinfeld D, Fisher JD. Unpredictability of site of conduction system injury due to acute myocardial infarction. *Clin Prog EP Pacing* 1985;3:202–206.
162. Akhtar M, Damato AN, Batsford WP, et al. A comparative analysis of antegrade and retrograde conduction patterns in man. *Circulation* 1975; 52:766–778.
163. Akhtar M, Gilbert C, Wolf FG, et al. Retrograde conduction in the His-Purkinje system: analysis of the routes of impulse propagation using His and right bundle branch recordings. *Circulation* 1979;59:1252.
164. Mahmud R, Lehmann M, Denker S, et al. Atrioventricular sequential pacing: differential effect on retrograde conduction related to level of impulse collision. *Circulation* 1983;68:23–32.
165. Akhtar M. Retrograde conduction in man. *Pacing Clin Electrophysiol* 1981;4:548.
166. Josephson ME, Kastor JA. His-Purkinje conduction during retrograde stress. *J Clin Invest* 1978;61:171.
167. Mann DE, Sensecqua JE, Easley AR, et al. Effects of upright posture on anterograde and retrograde atrioventricular conduction in patients with coronary artery disease, mitral valve prolapse or no structural heart disease. *Am J Cardiol* 1987;60:625–629.
168. Akhtar M, Gilbert C, Wolf FG, et al. Reentry within the His-Purkinje system. Elucidation of reentrant circuit utilizing right bundle branch and His bundle recordings. *Circulation* 1978;58:295.
169. Narula OS. *His bundle electrocardiography and clinical electrophysiology*. Philadelphia: FA Davis, 1975:39–175.
170. Kosowsky BD, Latif P, Radoff AM. Multilevel atrioventricular block. *Circulation* 1976;54:914–921.
171. Fisher JD, Kim SG, Ferrick KJ, et al. Programmed electrical stimulation protocols: variations on a theme. *Pacing Clin Electrophysiol* 1992;15: 2180–2187.
172. Artoul SG, Fisher JD, Kim SG, et al. Stimulation hierarchy: optimal sequence for double and triple extrastimuli during electrophysiological studies. *Pacing Clin Electrophysiol* 1992;15:790–800.
173. Strobel RE, Fisher JD, Katz G, et al. Time dependence of ventricular refractory periods: implications for electrophysiologic protocols. *J Am Coll Cardiol* 1990;15:402–411.
174. Josephson ME. Clinical cardiac electrophysiology, techniques and interpretations, 2nd ed. Philadelphia: Lea & Febiger, 1993:436–449.
175. Denker S, Lehmann M, Mahmud R, et al. Facilitation of ventricular tachycardia induction with abrupt changes in ventricular cycle length. *Am J Cardiol* 1984;53:508–515.
176. Wei JY, Bulkley BH, Schaeffer AH, et al. Mitral valve prolapse syndrome and recurrent ventricular tachyarrhythmias: a malignant variant refractory to conventional drug therapy. *Ann Intern Med* 1978;89:6–9.
177. Ware JA, Magro SA, Luck JC, et al. Conduction system abnormalities in symptomatic mitral valve prolapse: an electrophysiologic analysis of 60 patients. *Am J Cardiol* 1984;53:1075–1078.
178. Friedman HS, Zaman Q, Haft JI, et al. Assessment of A-V conduction in aortic valve disease [Abstract]. *Am J Cardiol* 1977;39:314.
179. Dhingra RC, Amat-Y-Leon F, Pietras RJ, et al. Sites of conduction disease in aortic stenosis. Significance of valve gradient and calcification. *Ann Intern Med* 1977;87:275.

180. Probst P, Pachinger O, Murad AA, et al. The HQ time in congestive cardiomyopathies. *Am Heart J* 1979;97:436.
181. Turitto G, Ahuja RK, Bekheit S, et al. Incidence and prediction of induced ventricular tachyarrhythmias in idiopathic dilated cardiomyopathy. *Am J Cardiol* 1994;73:770–773.
182. Luca C. Electrophysiological properties of right heart and atrioventricular conducting system in patients with alcoholic cardiomyopathy. *Br Heart J* 1979;42:274–281.
183. Bardy GH, Lee KL, Mark DB, et al. Amiodarone or an implantable cardioverter-defibrillator for congestive heart failure. *N Engl J Med* 2005; 352:225–237.
184. Cosio FG, Moro C, Alonso M, et al. The Q waves of hypertrophic cardiomyopathy. An electrophysiologic study. *N Engl J Med* 1980;302:96–99.
185. Johnson AD, Daily PO. Hypertrophic subaortic stenosis complicated by high degree heart block: successful treatment with an atrial synchronous ventricular pacemaker. *Chest* 1975;67:491–494.
186. McKenna WJ, Camm AJ. Sudden death in hypertrophic cardiomyopathy. Assessment of patients at high risk. *Circulation* 1989;80:1489–1492.
187. Fananapazir L, Tracy C, Leon MB, et al. Electrophysiologic abnormalities in patients with hypertrophic cardiomyopathy: a consecutive analysis of 155 patients. *Circulation* 1989;80:1259–1268.
188. Bharati S, Lev M, Denes P. Infiltrative cardiomyopathy with conduction disease and ventricular arrhythmia. Electrophysiologic and pathologic correlations. *J Cardiol* 1980;45:163.
189. Vigorita VJ, Hutchins GM. Cardiac conduction system in hemochromatosis: clinical and pathologic features of six patients. *Am J Cardiol* 1979;44:418.
190. Factor SM, Menegus MA, Kress Y, et al. Microfibrillar cardiomyopathy: an infiltrative heart disease resembling but distinct from cardiac amyloidosis. *Cardiovasc Pathol* 1992;1:307–316.
191. Wray R, Iveson M. Complete heart block and systemic lupus erythematosus. *Br Heart J* 1975;37:982.
192. McCue CM, Mantakas ME, Tingelstad JB, et al. Congenital heart block in newborns of mothers with connective tissue disease. *Circulation* 1977; 56:82–90.
193. Winkler RB, Nora AH, Nora JJ. Familial congenital complete heart block and maternal systemic lupus erythematosus. *Circulation* 1977;56:1103.
194. Fiddler GI, Campbell RWF, Pottage A, et al. Varicella myocarditis presenting with unusual ventricular arrhythmias. *Br Heart J* 1977;39:1150–1153.
195. Gann D, Narula OS, Kaplan S, et al. Complete heart block with gonococcal septicemia. *An Intern Med* 1977;86:749–750.
196. Hernandez-Pieretti O, Morales-Rocha J, Acquatella H, et al. Pacemaker implantation in chronic Chagas' heart disease complicated by Adams-Stokes syndrome. *Am J Cardiol* 1965;46:114–117.
197. Rosenbaum MB, Alvarez AJ. The electrocardiogram in chronic chagesic myocarditis. *Am Heart J* 1955;50:492.
198. Wei JY, Genecin A, Greene HL, et al. Coronary spasm with ventricular fibrillation during thyrotoxicosis: response to attaining euthyroid state. *Am J Cardiol* 1979;43:335–339.
199. Gavrilescu S, Luca C, Streian C, et al. Monophasic action potentials of right atrium and electrophysiological properties of AV conducting system in patients with hypothyroidism. *Br Heart J* 1976;38:1350–1354.
200. Watanabe Y, Nishimura M. Terminology and electrophysiologic concepts in cardiac arrhythmias. V. Phase 3 block and phase 4 block. *Pacing Clin Electrophysiol* 1979;2(Pt 1):335.
201. Watanabe Y, Nishimura M. Terminology and electrophysiologic concepts in cardiac arrhythmias. VI. Phase 3 block and phase 4 block. *Pacing Clin Electrophysiol* 1979;2(Pt 2):624.
202. El-Sherif N, Scherlag BJ, Lazarra R, et al. Pathophysiology of tachycardia- and bradycardia-dependent block in the canine proximal His-Purkinje system after acute myocardial ischemia. *Am J Cardiol* 1974;33: 540.
203. Fisher JD, Aronson RS. Rate-dependent bundle branch block: occurrence, causes and clinical correlations. *J Am Coll Cardiol* 1990;16:240–243.
204. Castellanos A, Khuddus SA, Sommer LS, et al. His bundle recordings in bradycardia-dependent AV block induced by premature beats. *Br Heart J* 1975;37:570–575.
205. Watanabe Y. Terminology and electrophysiology concepts in cardiac arrhythmias. III. Exit block, entrance block and protection block. *Pacing Clin Electrophysiol* 1978;1:498.
206. Myerburg RJ. The gating mechanism in the distal atrioventricular conducting system. *Circulation* 1971;43;955.
207. Gallagher JJ, Damato AN, Varghese PJ, et al. Localization of an area of maximum refractoriness or "gate" in the ventricular specialized conduction system in man. *Am Heart J* 1972;84:310.
208. Akhtar M, Denker S, Lehmann MH, et al. Macro-reentry within the His-Purkinje system. *Pacing Clin Electrophysiol* 1983;6:1010.
209. Fisher JD. Bundle branch reentry tachycardia: why is the HV interval often longer than in sinus rhythm? The critical role of anisotropic conduction. *J Interv Card Electrophysiol* 2001;5(2):173–176.
210. Casceres J, Jazayeri M, McKinnie J, et al. Sustained bundle branch reentry as a mechanism for clinical tachycardia. *Circulation* 1989;79:256.
211. Agha AS, Castellanos Jr A, Wells D, et al. Type I, type II, and type III gaps in bundle-branch conduction. *Circulation* 1973;47:325.
212. Wu D, Denes P, Dhingra R. Nature of the gap phenomenon in man. *Circ Res* 1974;34:682.
213. Akhtar M, Damato AN, Batsford WP, et al. Unmasking and conversion of gap phenomenon in the human heart. *Circulation* 1974;49:624.
214. Akhtar M, Damato AN, Caracta AR, et al. The gap phenomena during retrograde conduction in man. *Circulation* 1974;49:811.
215. Waleffe A, Bruninx P, Demoulin JC, et al. Two unusual cases of intra-atrial gap. *Br Heart J* 1977;39:451–455.
216. Mazgalev T, Dreifus LS, Michelson EL. A new mechanism for atrioventricular nodal-vagal modulation of conduction. *Circulation* 1989;79:417.
217. Mazgalev T, Tchou P. Atrioventricular nodal conduction gap and dual pathway electrophysiology. *Circulation* 1995;92:2705.
218. Reddy CP, Harris B. Gap phenomenon in "the right and left bundle branch systems" during retrograde conduction in man. *Am Heart J* 1979;97: 216.
219. Bexton RS, Hellestrand KJ, Nathan AW, et al. Retrograde gap in fast pathway conduction accentuated by the class I antiarrhythmic agent, flecainide. *Pacing Clin Electrophysiol* 1983;6:1273.
220. Weiss J, Stevenson WG. A new type of ventriculo-atrial gap phenomenon in man. *Pacing Clin Electrophysiol* 1984;7:46.
221. Puech P, Guimond C, Nadeau R, et al. Supernormal conduction in the intact heart. In: Narula OS, ed. Cardiac arrhythmias: electrophysiology, diagnosis and management. Baltimore: Williams & Wilkins Publishers, 1979:40–56.
222. Childers RW. Supernormality. In: *Complex electrocardiography I*. Philadelphia: FA Davis, 1973:136–158.
223. Fisher JD, Johnston DR, Kim SG, et al. Implantable pacers for tachycardia termination: stimulation techniques and long-term efficacy. *Pacing Clin Electrophysiol* 1986;9:1325–1333.
224. Buxton A, Hafley G, Lee K, et al. Relation of ejection fraction and inducible ventricular tachycardia to mode of death in patients with coronary artery disease: an analysis of patients enrolled in the Multicenter Unsustained Tachycardia Trial. *Circulation* 2002;106:2466–2472.

CHAPTER 62 ■ BRADYCARDIAS: SINUS NODAL DYSFUNCTION AND ATRIOVENTRICULAR CONDUCTION DISTURBANCES

DEBORAH L. WOLBRETTE AND GERALD V. NACCARELLI

OVERVIEW

Sinus nodal dysfunction and atrioventricular (AV) block account for the majority of significant bradyarrhythmias. In addition to structural abnormalities, drug effects and autonomic influences can cause sinus nodal dysfunction. Acquired AV block is most commonly caused by idiopathic fibrosis, acute myocardial infarction, or drug effects. Patients with asymptomatic sinus bradycardia or sinus pauses have a good prognosis and do not require treatment. On the other hand, those with tachycardia-bradycardia syndrome have a much worse prognosis because of their risk of thromboembolic complications. Therefore, the aim of therapy is prevention of atrial fibrillation. Atrial pacing and anticoagulation can greatly reduce the incidence of stroke in this high-risk group. Once appropriate pacing has been established for AV block, the prognosis is primarily dependent on the extent of the associated heart disease.

SINUS NODAL DYSFUNCTION

Anatomy and Physiology of the Sinus Node

The normal heartbeat arises from the sinus node, which is located laterally in the epicardial groove of the sulcus terminalis, near the junction of the superior vena cava and right atrium. The sinus node comprises of "nests" of principal pacemaker cells, which spontaneously depolarize and are situated within a fibrous tissue matrix. However, instead of a discreet point of impulse initiation, the sinus node is in reality a "region" (1). In addition to the nest of principal pacemaker cells, other nests contain cells with slower intrinsic depolarization rates and serve as backup pacemakers in response to changing physiologic and pathologic conditions. Therefore, the principal pacemaker site shifts within the sinus nodal region, resulting in subtle changes in P-wave morphology (2). Although blood supply to this region predominantly comes from the sinus nodal artery, which is a branch of the right coronary artery in 65% of patients, the variability of coronary anatomy and blood supply to the region makes the sinus node more vulnerable to damage during operative procedures (3).

Normal conduction velocities within the sinus node are slow, on the order of 2 to 5 cm/sec, increasing the likelihood of intranodal conduction block (4). Both parasympathetic and sympathetic mediators influence the rate of spontaneous depolarization in pacemaker cells and may cause a shift in the principal pacemaker site within the sinus nodal region (4,5). Acetylcholine, from parasympathetic nerve endings, reduces the rate of cell depolarization and prolongs cell refractoriness. Therefore, increased parasympathetic activity can produce sinus bradycardia, sinus arrest, and sinoatrial exit blocks (6). On the other hand, sympathetic mediators, such as norepinephrine and epinephrine, can increase the sinus rate and reverse sinus arrest and sinoatrial exit block (7).

Electrocardiographic Features of Sinus Nodal Dysfunction

Inappropriate Sinus Bradycardia

Sinus bradycardia (sinus rate <60 beats per minute) is considered inappropriate when it is persistent and does not increase appropriately with exercise. This arrhythmia should be distinguished from asymptomatic resting sinus bradycardia in young athletes and in normal adults during sleep (8,9). Chronotropic incompetence is not present in these individuals, as it is in patients with sinus nodal dysfunction.

Sinus Arrest

The terms *sinus arrest* and *sinus pause* are used interchangeably and refer to the condition in which the sinus node's principal pacemaker cells fail to fire. The pause is not an exact multiple of the preceding PP interval. Pauses greater than 3 seconds are rare in normal individuals and may or may not be associated with symptoms but are usually caused by sinus nodal dysfunction (10,11). In contrast, asymptomatic pauses greater than 2 seconds (but <3 seconds) are seen in 11% of normal patients during 24-hour Holter monitoring and are especially common in trained athletes (12).

Chronic Atrial Fibrillation

The presence of chronic atrial fibrillation in a patient with a slow ventricular response not secondary to drug therapy is a sign of sinus nodal dysfunction. In some cases, cardioversion results in a long sinus pause before the appearance of sinus rhythm, or junctional escape rhythm. Although a combination of sinus nodal and AV nodal conduction disease may be present in many instances, examples of rapid ventricular responses during atrial tachyarrhythmias can frequently be found.

Tachycardia-Bradycardia Syndrome

Tachycardia-bradycardia syndrome refers to the presence of intermittent sinus or junctional bradycardia alternating with atrial tachycardia (usually paroxysmal atrial fibrillation) in the same patient. This condition, frequently referred to as *sick sinus syndrome*, is a common manifestation of sinus nodal dysfunction. The highest incidence of syncope associated with sinus nodal dysfunction probably occurs in this group. Syncope typically occurs secondary to a long sinus pause after the spontaneous termination of atrial fibrillation (Fig. 62.1).

Pathophysiology

Intrinsic Sinus Nodal Dysfunction

Idiopathic degenerative disease is probably the most common cause of intrinsic sinus nodal dysfunction. Fibrous tissue replacement with age explains some but not all cases (13,14). Coronary artery disease may be responsible for one third of cases of sinus nodal dysfunction (15). Transient slowing of the sinus rate, or sinus arrest, can complicate an acute myocardial infarction. This is usually seen with an acute inferior wall myocardial infarction, is caused by neural influences, and rarely persists (16). Cardiomyopathy, long-standing hypertension, infiltrative disorders, collagen vascular diseases, inflammatory processes, orthotopic cardiac transplantation, myotonic dystrophy or Friedreich ataxia, and surgical trauma can also result in sinus nodal dysfunction (17,18).

In the pediatric population, most cases of sinus nodal dysfunction can be attributed to surgical trauma from repairs of various congenital heart disease syndromes (19–21).

Extrinsic Sinus Nodal Dysfunction

In the absence of structural abnormalities, the predominant causes of sinus nodal dysfunction are drug effects and autonomic influences. Drugs known to depress sinus nodal function include β-blockers, calcium channel blockers, digoxin (22), and sympatholytic antihypertensives (e.g., clonidine, methyldopa, and reserpine) (23). Types IA, IC, and III antiarrhythmic drugs can depress sinus nodal function (22) and occasionally may produce proarrhythmias in patients with sick sinus syndrome. Paroxysmal primary atrial tachycardias and pause-dependent ventricular tachycardia have been described (24,25). Other drugs reported to affect sinus nodal function include lithium, cimetidine, amitriptyline, and phenytoin (22).

Sinus nodal dysfunction may sometimes result from excessive vagal tone in individuals without intrinsic sinus nodal disease. Autonomically induced asystole has been reported to occur rarely and may result in sudden death (26). Hypervagatonia can be seen in carotid sinus syndrome and vasovagal syncope (Fig. 62.2). Well-trained athletes with increased vagal tone may require some deconditioning to help prevent symptomatic bradyarrhythmias (27).

Clinical Profile

Incidence and Symptoms

The estimated incidence of sinus nodal dysfunction in patients older than 50 years of age is 3 in 5,000 (28). Syncope and presyncope are the most frequent symptoms associated with significant bradycardia. Fatigue, angina, and shortness of

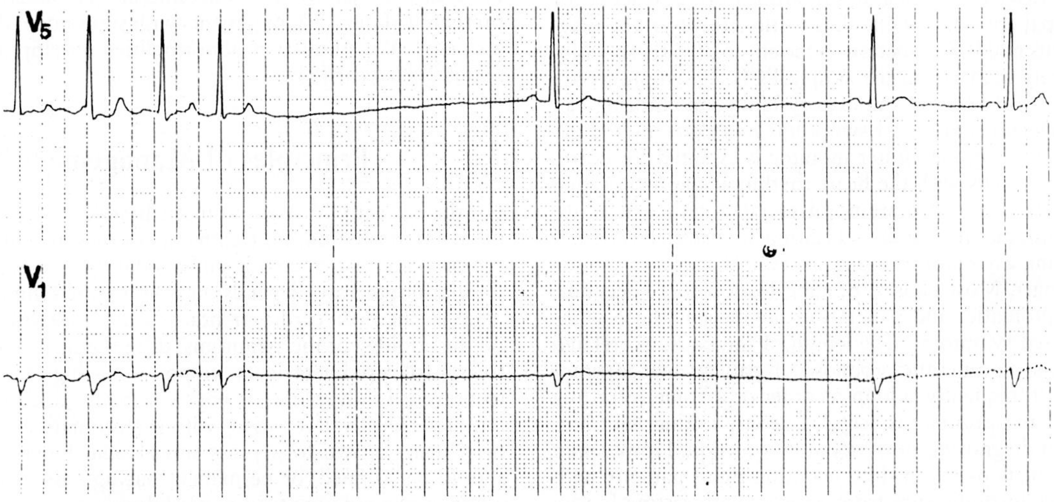

FIGURE 62.1. These rhythm strips of leads V1 and V5 were recorded simultaneously and depict sinus pauses of 3.0 and 2.8 seconds posttermination of atrial tachycardia.

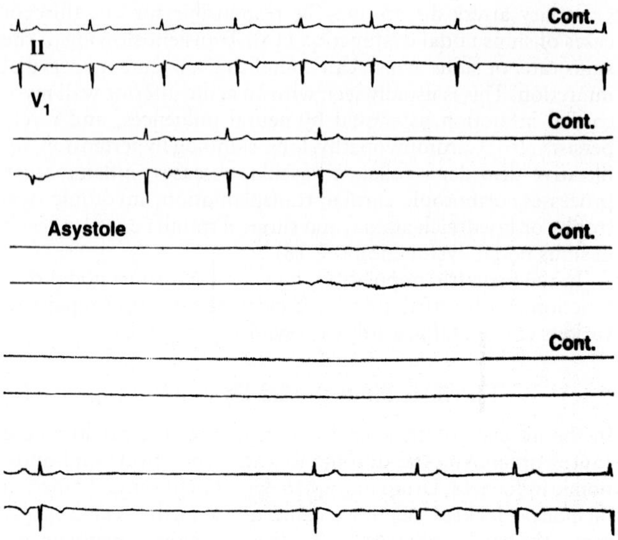

FIGURE 62.2. Example of prolonged asystole during vasovagal syncope. (Unpublished data from J. Luck.)

breath can also be seen. Elderly patients may have more subtle symptoms of gastrointestinal distress or change in mental status. Patients with tachycardia-bradycardia syndrome may only experience palpitations associated with tachycardia or embolic events. Syncope in an individual with paroxysmal atrial fibrillation is classically associated with a long sinus pause at the spontaneous termination of the tachycardia. The intermittent nature of these symptoms makes documentation of the associated rhythm disturbance difficult at times. In other cases, marked sinus bradycardia and sinus pauses may be asymptomatic (29).

Diagnostic Techniques

Both noninvasive and invasive means of diagnosing sinus nodal dysfunction are available. Generally, the noninvasive methods of electrocardiographic (ECG) monitoring, exercise testing, and autonomic testing are used first. However, if symptoms are infrequent, invasive electrophysiologic testing or an implantable monitor may be required.

Noninvasive Testing

A 12-lead ECG correlating bradycardia during syncope or near-syncopal episodes can be diagnostic. However, the diagnosis of sinus nodal dysfunction as the etiology of these symptoms is rarely made from the simple ECG. If symptoms are frequent, 24- or 48-hour ambulatory Holter monitoring can be useful. Documentation of symptoms in a diary by the patient while wearing the Holter monitor is essential for correlation of symptoms with the heart rhythm at the time. Often the sinus pauses recorded are not associated with symptoms. Several Holter monitor studies (11,30) demonstrated the futility of treating asymptomatic pauses, even if they were 3 seconds or longer. Most pauses, ranging from 2 to 15 seconds, were asymptomatic, and pacing did not benefit those without associated symptoms. The length of the pause correlated poorly with symptoms and prognosis. In patients whose symptoms occur infrequently, a loop recorder or a home recording device such as Cardionet is useful. Exercise testing is of limited value in diagnosing sinus nodal dysfunction. However, in some cases, it is useful in differentiating those patients with chronotropic incompetence from patients with resting bradycardia who demonstrate a normal heart rate increase with exercise.

Autonomic testing of the sinus node includes various pharmacologic interventions and maneuvers to test reflex responses. An abnormal response to carotid sinus massage (pause >3 seconds) may indicate sinus nodal dysfunction, but this response may also occur in asymptomatic elderly individuals (31). The most commonly used pharmacologic intervention is used to determine the intrinsic heart rate. Complete autonomic blockade is accomplished by administering atropine, 0.04 mg/kg, and propranolol, 0.20 mg/kg. The resulting intrinsic heart rate represents the sinus nodal rate without autonomic influences. The normal intrinsic heart rate is age dependent and can be calculated using the following equation: intrinsic heart rate (in beats per minute) $= 118.1 - (0.57 \times \text{age [in years]})$ (32). A low intrinsic heart rate is consistent with abnormal intrinsic sinus nodal function. A normal intrinsic heart rate in a patient with known sinus nodal dysfunction suggests abnormal autonomic regulation.

Invasive Testing

Sinus nodal function can also be evaluated invasively with an electrophysiologic study. This is usually reserved for symptomatic patients in whom sinus nodal dysfunction is suspected but cannot be documented in association with symptoms by noninvasive means. The pacing tests most commonly used are sinus nodal recovery time and sinoatrial conduction time (33). However, even when they are performed appropriately, the ability of these tests to provide a definitive diagnosis is limited (34). The reader is referred to Chapter 62 for further information on sinus nodal function tests.

Natural History

The natural history of sinus nodal dysfunction depends largely on the type of dysfunction and the presence of concomitant cardiovascular disease. The worst prognosis is associated with the tachycardia-bradycardia syndrome. Because stroke is associated with atrial fibrillation, patients with sinus nodal dysfunction complicated by chronic or intermittent atrial fibrillation have an increased risk of embolization.

Literature reviews (35,36) have revealed a significantly lower incidence of atrial fibrillation and thromboembolic events in atrially paced patients compared with those only ventricularly paced. In the future, increased use of atrial pacing and anticoagulation therapy should significantly reduce the incidence of stroke in high-risk patients with tachycardia-bradycardia syndrome. Concomitant AV nodal disease is present in about 17% of patients with sinus nodal dysfunction, and new AV conduction abnormalities develop at a rate of about 2.7%/year (35).

Principles of Management

For the patient with asymptomatic bradycardia or pauses and no atrial fibrillation, no treatment is necessary. In the case of symptomatic patients with sinus nodal dysfunction and atrial fibrillation, therapy depends on whether the symptoms are related to the tachycardia or bradycardia episodes. Depending on the etiology of the symptoms, drug therapy may be needed to control rapid ventricular response, pacing may be advised to prevent bradycardia, or both treatment modalities may be required. Ideally, if a patient with symptomatic bradycardia is on a drug known to depress sinus nodal function, the drug should be stopped, or permanent pacing may be required to allow continued use of the needed drug.

Sinus nodal dysfunction is the most commonly reported diagnosis for pacemaker implantation. However, once the decision to pace is made, choosing the optimal pacemaker prescription is essential to decrease stroke risk and improve quality of life. Atrial pacing has been shown to greatly decrease the incidence of atrial fibrillation and thromboembolism in this population, whereas patients who are ventricularly paced have not seen a similar benefit (35). Therefore, the majority of patients with symptomatic sinus nodal dysfunction should receive a dual-chamber pacemaker. Single-chamber ventricular pacing is reserved for use in patients with chronic atrial fibrillation. For patients with sinus nodal dysfunction who have normal AV conduction, a single-chamber atrial pacemaker is a reasonable choice. Rate-adaptive pacing and mode switching are important for most patients with sinus nodal dysfunction, and are generally standard features in currently available pacemakers. Guidelines for implantation of pacemakers in patients with sinus nodal dysfunction have been established by a task force from the American College of Cardiology and American Heart Association (37). Because of the high risk of thromboembolic events in patients with sinus nodal dysfunction and atrial fibrillation, anticoagulation with warfarin should be considered in these patients.

ATRIOVENTRICULAR NODAL DYSFUNCTION

Anatomic Considerations

The AV node lies directly above the insertion of the septal leaflet of the tricuspid valve and anterior to the ostium of the coronary sinus. It is part of the AV junction area, which is divided into three regions. The transitional cells, or nodal approaches, connect the atrial myocardium to the compact portion of the AV node. At its distal end, the compact portion of the AV node enters the central fibrous body, becoming the penetrating portion, or His bundle (38). The slowest conduction time (0.03 m/second) occurs within the AV node (39). The blood supply to the AV node is via the AV nodal artery, a branch of the right coronary artery in 90% of hearts, with the remaining 10% arising from the circumflex artery (40). The His bundle has a dual blood supply from branches of the anterior and posterior descending coronary arteries (41).

Like the sinus node, the AV node is richly innervated, and both are influenced by the right and left vagus nerves and stellate ganglia. However, stimulation of the nerves on the right has less affect on AV nodal conduction than on sinus rate. Conversely, left-sided autonomic stimulation exerts stronger influence on AV nodal conduction than on sinus rate (42,43).

Electrocardiographic and Electrophysiologic Findings

Normal Atrioventricular Conduction

On the surface ECG, the PR interval is normally between 120 and 200 msec in duration. This interval reflects the conduction time from the high right atrium to the point of ventricular activation. To measure the different components of the conduction system that the PR interval includes, intracardiac tracings from the high right atrium and bundle of His region are needed. The PA interval, measured from the high right atrial electrogram to the low right atrial deflection in the bundle of His electrogram, gives an indirect approximation of the right atrial conduction time. The AH interval, measured from the low atrial to the bundle of His deflection, reflects conduction time through the AV node. The HV interval, measured from the bundle of His deflection to the earliest ventricular depolarization on the surface electrogram, represents the conduction time from the proximal bundle of His to the ventricular myocardium (44) (Table 62.1).

TABLE 62.1

NORMAL CONDUCTION INTERVALS IN ADULTS

Type	Interval (ms)
PA	20–50
AH	50–140
HV	35–55
H	10–25

First-Degree Atrioventricular Block

First-degree AV block on the surface ECG is seen as a PR interval greater than 0.20 second. Each P wave is followed by a QRS complex with a constant, prolonged interval. Although the conduction delay can be anywhere along the system, the PR prolongation is usually caused by delay within the AV node (87% when the QRS complex is narrow). On the bundle of His electrogram, this would be seen as an AH interval greater than 130 msec with a normal HV interval. In cases in which first-degree AV block is seen in the presence of a bundle branch block, a bundle of His electrogram is necessary to localize the site of block (45–47). Infranodal conduction delay is present in 45% of these cases. A combination of delay within the AV node and in the His-Purkinje system must also be considered (48). In certain cases of congenital structural heart disease, such as Ebstein anomaly of the tricuspid valve or endocardial cushion defects, intraatrial conduction delay can cause first-degree AV block. In addition, intra-Hisian conduction delay can cause first-degree AV block. On the bundle of His electrogram, a split His potential can be seen, resulting in a prolonged His potential, HV, and PR intervals (52). Dual-AV-nodal physiology can produce transient, abrupt, or alternating first-degree block caused by block in the fast AV nodal pathway (which is normally used), with conduction down the slow pathway instead.

Second-Degree Atrioventricular Block

Type I. Type I second-degree AV block, or Wenckebach block, manifests on the surface electrogram as progressive prolongation of the PR interval before failure of an atrial impulse to be conducted to the ventricles. The PR interval immediately postblock returns to its baseline interval, and the sequence begins again. Features of typical Wenckebach periodicity include the following:

- Progressive lengthening of the PR interval throughout the Wenckebach cycle.
- Lengthening of the RR interval occurring at progressively decreasing increments, resulting in progressive shortening of the RR intervals.
- A pause including the nonconducted P wave that is less than the sum of any two consecutively conducted beats.
- Shortening of the PR interval postblock compared with the PR interval just preceding the blocked cycle.

Wenckebach block is almost always within the AV node when a narrow QRS complex is present (49). Intra-Hisian block is the rare exception (50). When type I block is seen with a bundle branch block, the block is still more likely to be in the AV node, but it could also be localized below the bundle of His. A bundle of His electrogram would be needed to accurately identify the level of block. Wenckebach block in the AV node is characterized by progressive prolongation of the AH interval until an atrial deflection is not followed by a bundle of His or ventricular deflection. In type I block secondary to block below the bundle of His, progressive prolongation of the HV interval is followed by an H deflection without an associated ventricular depolarization.

Type II. Type II, or Mobitz II, second-degree AV block is characterized on the surface electrogram by a constant PR interval followed by sudden failure of a P wave to be conducted to the ventricles. The PP intervals remain constant and the pause including the blocked P wave equals two PP intervals. Therefore, Mobitz II block should not be confused with a nonconducted premature atrial complex. Mobitz II block is usually associated with bundle branch block or bifascicular block. In a majority of these cases, the site of block is within or below the bundle of His (Fig. 62.3) (46,48). When presumed Mobitz II block is seen in conjunction with a narrow QRS complex, Mobitz I with only minimal PR variation should be suspected. Only rarely is Mobitz II found with a narrow QRS complex and is caused by intra-Hisian block (51). The bundle of His electrogram is useful in verifying the site of the Mobitz II block. The blocked cycle features atrial and bundle of His deflections without a ventricular depolarization. The conducted beats usually show evidence of infranodal conduction system disease, with a prolonged HV interval, or even a split bundle of His potential (48).

2:1 Atrioventricular Block. Fixed 2:1 AV block poses a diagnostic dilemma because it is usually impossible to classify as type I or II block by a surface electrogram alone. A narrow QRS complex and recently seen Wenckebach block is highly suggestive of block at the AV nodal level. A 2:1 block associated with a wide QRS complex is likely infranodal, but it could still be at the level of the AV node. A definitive diagnosis can only be made with an intracardiac recording at the bundle of His region.

Nonconduction of two or more consecutive P waves when AV synchrony is otherwise maintained is sometimes termed *high-degree AV block*. The level of block can be at the AV node or the His-Purkinje system. When high-degree AV block is caused by block in the AV node, QRS complexes of the conducted beats are usually narrow. Wenckebach periodicity is also seen, and atropine administration produces 1:1 conduction. Features pointing toward block in the His-Purkinje system are conducted beats with bundle branch block and no improvement in block with atropine. Bundle of His recordings are sometimes needed to confirm the site of block.

Third-Degree Atrioventricular Block

Third-degree, or complete, AV block is seen on the surface electrogram as completely dissociated P waves and QRS complexes, each firing at its own pacemaker rate. The atrial impulse is never conducted to the ventricles, but different levels of block are possible. The level of block determines the QRS morphology along with the site and rate of the escape rhythm. Congenital complete heart block is characterized by a narrow QRS complex with an escape rate between 40 and 60 beats per minute, which tends to increase with exercise or atropine. This is consistent with block within the AV node. Acquired complete heart block is usually associated with block in the His-Purkinje system, resulting in a wide QRS complex with an escape rate between 20 and 40 beats per minute. The intracardiac electrogram shows bundle of His deflections consistently following the atrial electrograms, but the ventricular

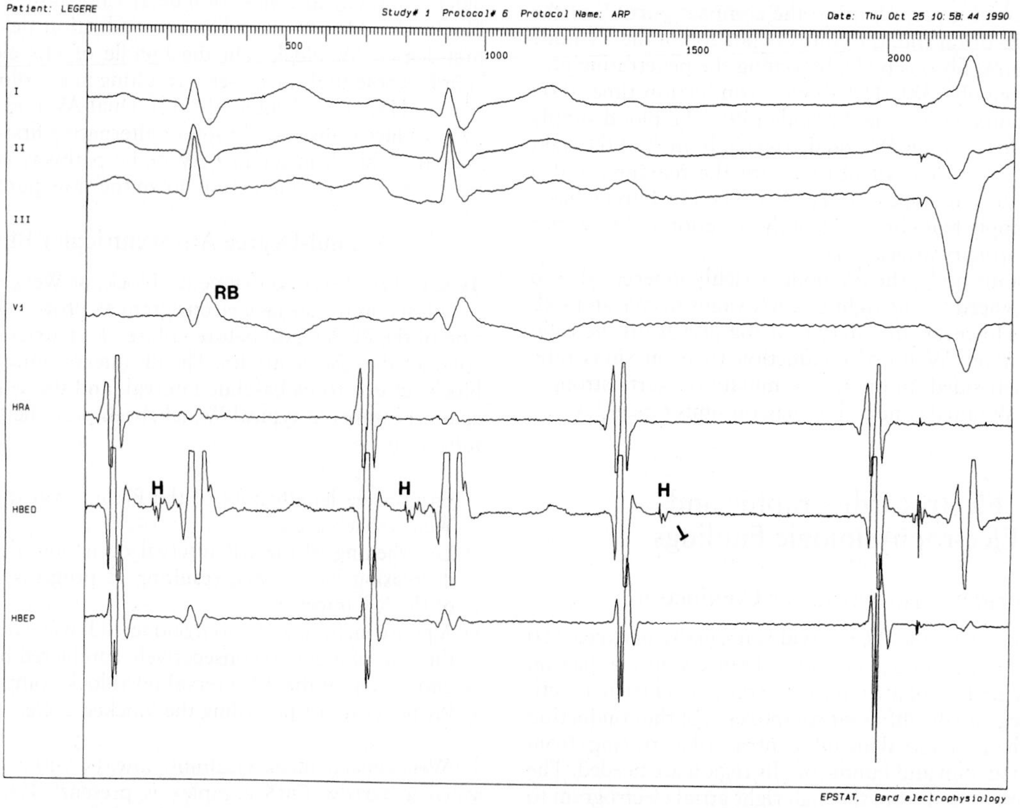

FIGURE 62.3. The surface leads I, II, III, and V1 show first-degree atrioventricular block and right-bundle-branch block (RB). The third P wave is not followed by a QRS complex. The intracardiac tracings [HRA, high right atrial recording; proximal (HBEP) and distal bundle of His electrograms (HBED)] reveal the diagnosis of block within the bundle of His. The His deflection (H) is fractionated. The third beat shows only the first half of the His, and no ventricular electrogram follows.

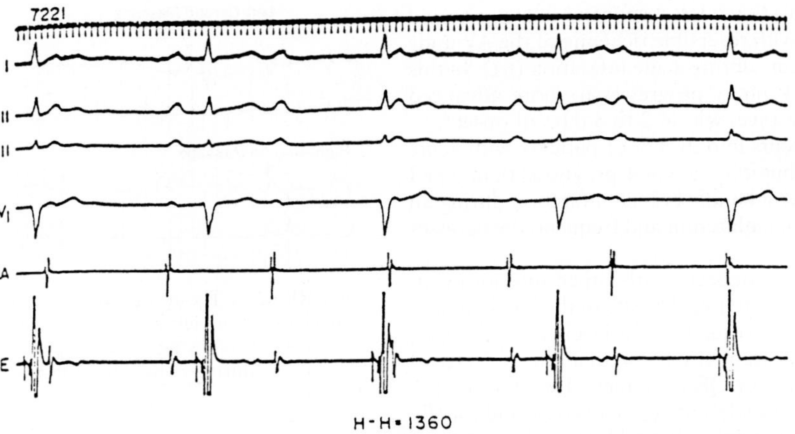

FIGURE 62.4. Congenital complete heart block located within the atrioventricular (AV) node. Sinus arrhythmia with a cycle length of approximately 860 msec is completely dissociated from a regular junctional escape rhythm with a cycle length of 1,360 msec. There is no relationship between atrial and ventricular depolarizations. There is no bundle of His deflection after any atrial depolarization. A bundle of His electrogram with a normal HV interval precedes each junctional escape complex in the bundle of His lead. Therefore, the site of AV block is within the AV node. Note the normal (narrow) morphology of the junctional escape QRS complexes. HBE, bundle of His electrogram; HRA, high right atrial recording. (From Miles MM, Klein LS. Sinus nodal dysfunction and atrioventricular conduction disturbances. In: Naccarelli GV, ed. *Cardiac arrhythmias: a practical approach*. Mount Kisco, NY: Futura, 1991:269.)

depolarization is completely dissociated from these. Block below the bundle of His is thus demonstrated. In contrast, complete heart block at the AV nodal level is seen on the intracardiac tracings as bundle of His potentials consistently preceding each ventricular depolarization. The atrial electrograms are dissociated from the HV complexes (Fig. 62.4). The sinus rate is faster than the ventricular rate in patients with complete heart block. Data collected from patients with congenital complete heart block have shown the atrial rate to usually be age appropriate (52). It is important to note that complete antegrade AV block does not always predict retrograde (VA) conduction. Retrograde conduction may be intact in an individual with complete antegrade AV block (Fig. 62.5).

Atrioventricular Dissociation. AV dissociation is a secondary phenomenon that results from a primary conduction disorder. It is characterized by the atria and ventricles depolarizing independently of each other. By definition, there is no retrograde conduction from the ventricles to the atria. AV dissociation may be complete or incomplete (53). In complete AV dissociation, both the atrial and ventricular rates remain constant, and therefore the PR interval varies with none of the atrial complexes conducted to the ventricles. In incomplete AV dissociation

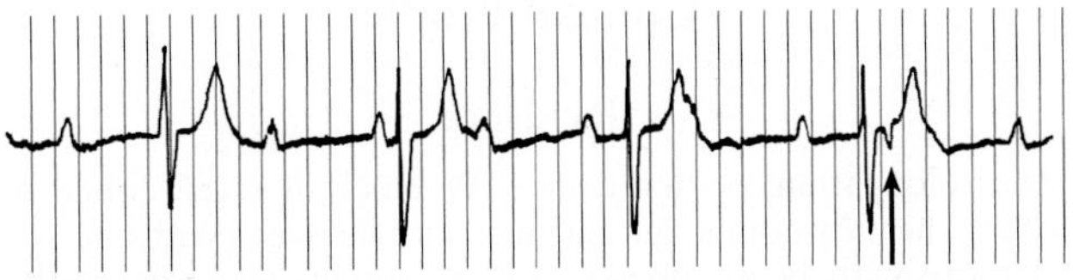

FIGURE 62.5. Electrogram of acquired complete atrioventricular block. The P-wave cycle length is 840 msec and is independent of the regular wide QRS escape mechanism at 1,800 msec (<40 per minute). There is no relationship between the P waves and the QRS complexes at any time during the recording until the next to the last P wave (*arrow*), where there is early retrograde atrial activation representing ventriculoatrial conduction despite complete anterograde atrioventricular block. Therefore, in some patients, retrograde conduction may be intact, even though anterograde conduction is not, or vice versa. (From Miles MM, Klein LS. Sinus nodal dysfunction and atrioventricular conduction disturbances. In: Naccarelli GV, ed. *Cardiac arrhythmias: a practical approach*. Mount Kisco, NY: Futura, 1991:269.)

(interference dissociation), ventricular capture beats occur because some of the atrial impulses arrive at the AV junction when the AV junction is no longer refractory. This phenomenon is common in advanced AV block with periodic capture beats.

Pathophysiology

The term *AV block* denotes a delay or nonconduction of an atrial impulse to the ventricles when the AV junction is not physiologically refractory. Drug effects are a common cause of acquired AV block in adults. Digoxin and β-blocking agents act indirectly on the AV node through their effect on the autonomic nervous system. Calcium channel blockers and other antiarrhythmic drugs, such as amiodarone, act directly to slow conduction in the AV node. Type I and III antiarrhythmic drugs can also affect conduction in the His-Purkinje system, resulting in infranodal block. Drugs that have a significant effect on blocking the sodium channels, such as flecainide, have the most effect on slowing conduction in the His-Purkinje system. When AV block occurs secondary to antiarrhythmic therapy, it is usually in cardiac patients with preexisting conduction abnormalities. Patients with normal conduction system function rarely develop complete heart block as a result of using antiarrhythmic agents.

Acute myocardial infarction is associated with varying degrees of AV block and is the most common cause of acquired complete AV block. Second- and third-degree AV blocks occur in up to 30% of patients presenting with acute myocardial infarction (54,55). Abnormalities in AV nodal conduction are seen in 20% of patients hospitalized for acute inferior myocardial infarction (56), with the onset of block falling in a bimodal distribution (57,58). Eleven percent of those presenting in the first hour of symptoms are found to have second- or third-degree AV block (57). In contrast, the incidence of heart block is low in the second hour of symptoms. The majority of conduction abnormalities occur between 2 and 72 hours (56,59). Because of the short duration of the early conduction abnormalities and their favorable response to atropine, an increase in vagal tone associated with acute inferior myocardial infarction is the probable etiology of this early phenomenon (60). Type I AV block occurring later in the course of an acute inferior myocardial infarction is less responsive to atropine and probably is associated with reversible ischemia of the AV node or the release of adenosine during acute infarction (61). In this setting, type I AV block rarely progresses to more advanced block and commonly resolves within 2 to 3 days of onset.

Type II AV block occurs in only 1% of patients with acute myocardial infarction, but it has a worse prognosis than type I block. It is associated with bundle branch infarction during an acute anterior myocardial infarction and frequently progresses to complete heart block.

Complete heart block can occur with either anterior or inferior acute myocardial infarction. The site of the block in inferior myocardial infarction is usually at the level of the AV node, resulting in a junctional escape rhythm with a rate of 50 to 60 beats per minute and narrow QRS complex. The abnormality tends to be reversed with vagolytic drugs or exercise and usually resolves in several days. Complete heart block in the setting of acute anterior myocardial infarction is usually associated with infarction of the bundle branches (62,63). The escape rhythm is approximately 40 beats per minute, with a wide QRS complex originating from the bundle branch and Purkinje system. It is less likely to be reversible. In general, patients who develop either transient or irreversible AV block are older and have a larger area of damage associated with their acute myocardial infarction. Other markers seen in this group include high levels of cardiac enzymes, bundle branch block, right ventricular infarction, and left ventricular failure (54,64–67).

The most common cause of acquired conduction system disease is progressive idiopathic fibrosis. Lev disease (68) is a result of proximal bundle branch fibrosis. It is postulated to be a hastening of the aging process by hypertension and arteriosclerosis of the blood vessels supplying the conduction system. Lenègre disease (69) is a degenerative process occurring in a younger population and involving the more distal portions of the bundle branches.

Calcification of the aortic or mitral valve annulus can extend to the nearby conduction system and produce AV block (70,71). The incidence is more frequent with aortic than mitral stenosis. AV block can also result from a stenotic bicuspid aortic valve (72,73). Other causes of AV block include infiltrative cardiomyopathies such as amyloidosis (74), sarcoidosis (74,75), and hemochromatosis (76,77), as well as the collagen vascular diseases of scleroderma (78), rheumatoid arthritis (79), Reiter syndrome (80), systemic lupus erythematosus (81), ankylosing spondylitis (82), and polymyositis (83).

Complete heart block occurs in 3% of cases of infective endocarditis, with the aortic valve being involved more frequently than the mitral valve (84). A variety of viral, bacterial, and parasitic etiologies of myocarditis result in varying degrees of AV block and include Lyme disease, rheumatic fever, Chagas disease (85), tuberculosis, measles, and mumps. Transient AV block is the most frequently seen cardiac abnormality associated with Lyme disease. First-degree block is almost always observed in these cases, representing up to 8% of those infected. Complete heart block can develop in 50% of those with first-degree block, especially if the PR interval exceeds 0.30 second (86). Acute rheumatic fever almost invariably results in PR prolongation when carditis is present (87,88). Second-degree block occurs only occasionally, and progression to complete heart block is rare (89).

Cardiac surgery can be complicated by varying degrees of AV block caused by trauma and ischemic damage to the conduction system. Block is most frequently associated with aortic valve replacement (90). In the absence of myocardial infarction or a long ischemic time, block is rarely seen post–coronary artery bypass grafting. Repair of congenital heart defects in the region of the conduction system—such as endocardial cushion malformations, ventricular septal defects, and tricuspid valve abnormalities—can lead to transient or persistent AV block.

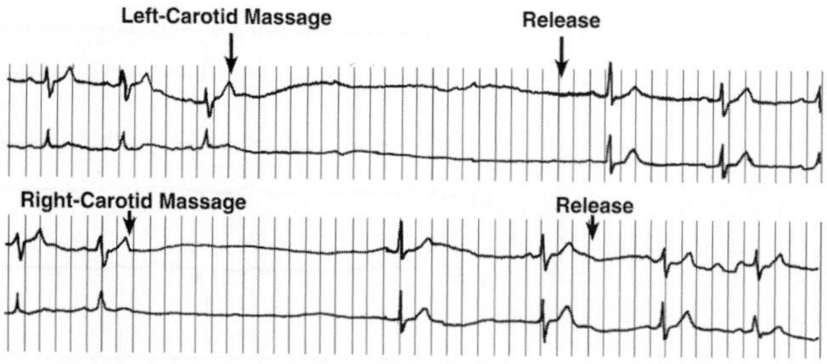

FIGURE 62.6. The top tracing demonstrates advanced atrioventricular block during left carotid massage. Two consecutive P waves are seen without following QRS complexes. The bottom tracing shows a sinus pause during right carotid massage. (Unpublished data from J. Luck.)

The block is usually temporary and thought to be secondary to postoperative local inflammation. However, block can appear years later, usually in those who had transient block just after the operation (91).

Intracardiac catheter manipulation can inadvertently produce complete heart block, which is usually temporary. This can occur during a right-sided heart catheterization in a patient with preexisting left-bundle-branch block, or even during left ventricular angiography in a patient with previous right-bundle-branch block (92–94). Radiofrequency catheter ablation techniques are used to modify the AV nodal junction or to produce complete heart block in patients with supraventricular tachyarrhythmias that cannot be controlled by medical therapy alone (95). AV block can also complicate radiofrequency catheter ablation used to treat AV nodal reentrant tachycardia or AV reentrant tachycardia. The incidence of complete heart block complicating this procedure is low when performed by experienced operators and when the bundle of His region is avoided (96,97).

Other causes of acquired AV block include hyperkalemia (98), hypermagnesemia, Addison disease (99), tumors that infiltrate the heart (100), and neuromyopathic disorders (101–103). In additional, transient AV block can be seen with carotid sinus syndrome (Fig. 62.6) (104) and vasovagal syncope (105).

Congenital complete AV block is thought to result from abnormal embryonic development of the AV node (106) and is believed to occur in 1 in 25,000 live births (107). Because the defect usually occurs proximal to the bundle of His, the QRS complex is narrow. This abnormality is found in otherwise structurally normal hearts in 50% of cases, whereas the rest have concurrent congenital heart disease (108).

Clinical Profile

Incidence

PR prolongation, or first-degree AV block, is rarely found in young, healthy adults, but the incidence increases with age and in those with heart disease. An epidemiologic study involving a large population of asymptomatic male pilots revealed PR intervals greater than 0.2 second in only 0.52% (109). Two percent of adults older than 20 years of age in Tecumseh, Michigan, were found to have a PR greater than or equal to 0.22 second (110). Both studies noted that the PR interval varied over time in young, healthy adults. Frequently in this population, the PR shortens with an increase in heart rate, suggesting vagal influence (109,110). Other epidemiologic surveys showed a 5% incidence of first-degree AV block in men older than 60 years of age and as high as 10% in older patients with cardiac disease (111,112).

In the large study of a population of healthy pilots, type II second-degree block was found to be extremely rare. In contrast, type I (Wenckebach) block can be seen in young athletes at rest and has been documented by ambulatory Holter monitoring in healthy teenagers during rest or sleep (113). Wenckebach periodicity in these settings disappears with exercise and should be considered a normal variant. On the other hand, in a population of patients with heart disease, the incidence of second-degree AV block (types I and II) was 2.7% (114).

Congenital complete heart block is estimated to occur in 1 of 15,000 to 25,000 live births, with a 60% female predominance (115,116). Acquired complete heart block is rarely seen in young individuals without heart disease (109). The highest incidence occurs in the seventh decade, and there is a 60% male predominance (117,118).

Symptoms

Individuals with first-degree AV block are asymptomatic. Symptoms of dizziness or syncope usually occur with acquired high-grade or complete AV block. With time, the majority of these patients experience a Stokes-Adams attack. Other symptoms can occur as a result of low cardiac output, including fatigue, congestive heart failure, dyspnea on exertion, angina, or even mental status changes (119).

Most children and adolescents with congenital complete heart block are asymptomatic, but some go on to develop symptoms later as adults. Those with concomitant structural heart disease, a wide QRS complex, long QT, or complete heart block discovered at an early age have an increased risk of developing symptoms, and some may die suddenly (120–122).

Diagnostic Techniques

Because the prognosis and the treatment differ in AV block depending on whether block is within the AV node or infranodal, determining the site of block is important. In many cases, this can be done noninvasively. As described previously, the QRS duration, PR intervals, and ventricular rate on the surface electrogram can provide important clues in localizing the level of block. Several noninvasive interventions may also prove helpful, such as vagal maneuvers, exercise, or administration of atropine. These methods take advantage of the differences in autonomic innervation of the AV node and His-Purkinje system. Whereas the AV node is richly innervated and highly responsive to both sympathetic and vagal stimuli, the His-Purkinje system is influenced minimally by the autonomic nervous system. Carotid sinus massage increases vagal tone and worsens AV nodal block. Exercise or atropine improves AV nodal conduction because of sympathetic stimulation. In contrast, carotid sinus massage improves infranodal block, whereas exercise and atropine worsen infranodal block because of the change in the rate of the impulses being conducted through the AV node.

Exercise testing is a useful tool for helping to confirm the level of block already suspected in second- or third-degree block caused by a narrow or wide QRS complex. Patients with presumed type I block or congenital complete heart block and a normal QRS complex usually enjoy an increased ventricular rate with exercise. On the other hand, patients with acquired complete heart block and a wide QRS complex usually show minimal or no increase in ventricular rate.

An electrophysiologic study is indicated in a patient with suspected high-grade AV block as the cause of syncope or presyncope when documentation cannot be obtained noninvasively. In patients with coronary artery disease, it may be unclear whether symptoms are secondary to AV block or ventricular tachycardia; therefore, an electrophysiologic study can be useful in establishing the diagnosis. Some patients with known second- or third-degree block may benefit from an invasive study to localize the site of AV block to help determine therapy or assess prognosis. Once symptoms and AV block are correlated by ECG, further documentation by invasive studies is not required unless additional information, as discussed previously, is needed. Others who should not undergo electrophysiologic studies are asymptomatic patients with transient Wenckebach block associated with increased vagal tone.

The electrophysiology study allows analysis of the bundle of His electrogram, as well as atrial and ventricular pacing to look for conduction abnormalities and inducible ventricular tachycardia. The AH and HV intervals are measured from the bundle of His electrogram. A markedly prolonged HV interval greater than or equal to 100 msec is associated with a high incidence of progression to complete heart block (123). See Chapter 62 for a discussion of intracardiac evaluation of AV nodal and His-Purkinje system function.

Natural History of Atrioventricular Blocks

The prognosis of any AV block is primarily dependent on the extent of the associated heart disease. First-degree AV block is usually benign and carries no increased mortality risk when seen as an isolated finding (110). Type I second-degree, or Wenckebach, AV block is also generally benign, and is usually transiently observed in the setting of acute inferior myocardial infarction or associated with increased vagal tone in healthy, athletic individuals. On the other hand, type II second-degree AV block is usually seen with bundle branch block or associated with acute anterior myocardial infarction and carries a high risk of progression to advanced or complete AV block. The prognosis of 2:1 AV block depends on whether the site of block is within or below the AV node.

Before the availability of pacemakers, the prognosis for patients with symptomatic complete heart block was dismal, regardless of the extent of underlying heart disease. The 1-year survival rate after the first Adams-Stokes attack was less than 50% (124). Nowadays, once appropriate pacing therapy has been established, the prognosis depends on the underlying disease process (125). Patients who develop complete heart block as a result of an anterior myocardial infarction have a poor prognosis because of extensive cardiac damage. In contrast, those who develop complete heart block from idiopathic bundle branch fibrosis and who have no additional cardiac disease have a prognosis similar to those of similar age without heart block.

Congenital complete heart block generally carries a more favorable diagnosis than the acquired form when not associated with underlying heart disease. However, data have shown a significant risk of syncope, sudden death, and acquired mitral insufficiency in this group (126).

Principles of Management

Pacing is now the mainstay of treatment for symptomatic heart block. Medical therapy is only effective as a short-term emergency measure, until pacing can be accomplished.

Before instituting permanent pacing, the possibility of a reversible cause of the heart block should be investigated. Any offending drugs, such as digoxin, calcium channel blockers, or membrane-active antiarrhythmic drugs, should be withdrawn, if possible, to see whether the block improves. Electrolyte abnormalities should also be looked for and corrected. The possibility of infectious processes should be considered and treated.

The key point in the decision to provide permanent pacing in AV block is the presence of symptoms. However, intermittent block may make correlating bradycardia with symptoms difficult. Patients with complete heart block and syncope have clearly been shown to have improved survival with permanent pacing (127). Most patients with acquired complete heart block are symptomatic and require pacing. Patients with congenital complete heart block are more likely to be asymptomatic, but prophylactic pacemaker implantation is an appropriate consideration (126). Block in the AV node is less likely to be associated with slow ventricular rates, progression to complete heart block, and symptoms than is infranodal block.

The decision to pace is not always clear when dealing with the asymptomatic patient. However, investigational data and the American College of Cardiology/American Heart Association task force report (37) are helpful in providing some general guidelines. Permanent pacing is recommended in asymptomatic awake patients with documented pauses of greater than 3.0 seconds or a ventricular escape rhythm of less than 40 beats per minute. When type II second-degree heart block is found in an asymptomatic individual, an electrophysiologic study is warranted to determine whether the block is infranodal. If this is the case, prophylactic pacing may be considered because of the high risk of progression to complete heart block (128). Permanent pacing is recommended in asymptomatic children with congenital heart block when found in association with a wide complex escape rhythm, complex congenital heart disease, ventricular dysfunction, or a long QT interval. In addition, exercise intolerance, abrupt pauses in the intrinsic rate, and average ventricular rate inappropriate for the child's age are criteria for pacing in this population (129–131). It is now recognized that dual-chamber pacing can be beneficial in some patients with marked first-degree AV block (> 0.3 sec) to reduce symptoms similar to pacemaker syndrome (132).

The need for permanent pacing because of advanced or complete AV block post–myocardial infarction appears to be significantly reduced by reperfusion therapy. The anticipated result of early reperfusion would be greater myocardial salvage, making damage to the conduction system less likely. Although few data are available to confirm this hypothesis, an analysis of a large series of patients with acute myocardial infarction treated with thrombolytic therapy who also underwent continuous 12-lead ECG monitoring for 36 to 72 hours shows the occurrence of persistent bundle branch block to be reduced in this group (5.3%, compared with 8% to 18% reported in the prethrombolytic era) (133). In this study population, patients with persistent bundle branch block had lower ejection fractions and most had left anterior descending artery infarcts. The higher mortality associated with bundle branch block is caused by the associated increased risk of complete heart block and sudden death in this group. Despite thrombolytic therapy, the occurrence of persistent bundle branch block still identifies a subset of patients with higher mortality than those with either transient or no bundle branch block.

CONTROVERSIES AND PERSONAL PERSPECTIVES

The proper choice of the most appropriate pacemaker is often straightforward. A patient with chronic atrial fibrillation who needs pacing should be prescribed a VVI or VVIR device. In chronotropic incompetent patients, a rate-responsive device is needed. However, choosing the optimal pacing mode for patients with sinus node dysfunction and intact AV nodal function has become more controversial. In this population, atrial pacing has been shown to be superior to ventricular pacing in reducing the risks of atrial fibrillation and congestive heart failure (134). On the other hand, no clear advantage of dual-chamber pacing over ventricular-only pacing has been proven (135). This can most likely be explained by ventricular desynchrony from right ventricular apex pacing. Analysis of the Mode Selection Trial (MOST) data revealed heart failure and atrial fibrillation risk increased with the percentage of ventricular pacing (136). In addition, defibrillator trials involving implantation of single- or dual-chamber devices in patients with left ventricular dysfunction have shown the risk of heart failure to increase with the percentage of ventricular pacing (137,138).

Based on these data, avoidance of unnecessary right ventricular pacing appears prudent. In patients with isolated sinus node dysfunction, the risk of development of AV block is low (139), and AAI or AAIR pacing should be considered. However, if AV block is still a concern, the dual-chamber device should be programmed to minimize ventricular pacing. Programming a fixed, long AV delay (140), or use of a dynamic AV interval algorithm can be effective (141). However, more effective is a new minimal ventricular pacing mode shown to decrease the percentage of ventricular pacing to 4% compared to 80% in the DDD/R mode (142).

Another topic of debate is whether all patients with AV block and in sinus rhythm should receive dual-chamber pacemakers. The United Kingdom and Cardiovascular Events (UKPACE) Trial showed no difference in the rate of death, stroke, atrial fibrillation, or heart failure in patients older than 70 years of age with high-grade AV block when randomized to single- versus dual-chamber pacemakers. Only 3% of patients crossed over from single- to dual-chamber pacing, indicating a low incidence of pacemaker syndrome in VVI/R mode. Procedural complications in the dual-chamber group were double that of the single-chamber group, secondary to problems with atrial lead placement or stability (143). Therefore, single-chamber ventricular pacing is acceptable in elderly patients with high-grade AV block.

The Canadian Trial of Physiologic Pacing (CTOPP) included a younger population and those with sinus node dysfunction. After an extended follow-up of 6.4 years, the only benefit from dual-chamber pacing (over single-chamber ventricular pacing) was a 20% reduction in the relative risk of atrial fibrillation (144). In selected younger individuals dual-chamber pacing may be worthwhile to gain the benefit of this reduced risk of atrial fibrillation.

THE FUTURE

Strategies for minimizing right ventricular apical pacing in patients with sinus node dysfunction will include more use of single-chamber atrial pacemakers and the development of algorithms to reduce unnecessary ventricular pacing in dual-chamber devices. In patients with AV block, the use of alternative ventricular pacing sites (right ventricular septum and coronary sinus) will decrease problems with ventricular desynchrony from right ventricular apical pacing.

References

1. Benditt DG, Sakaguchi S, Goldstein MA, et al. Sinus node dysfunction, pathophysiology, clinical features, evaluation, and treatment. In: Zipes DP, Jalife J, eds. *Cardiac electrophysiology: from cell to bedside.* 2nd ed. Philadelphia: WB Saunders, 1995:1215–1247.
2. Gomes JA, Winters SL. The origins of the sinus node pacemaker complex in man: demonstration of dominant and subsidiary foci. *J Am Coll Cardiol* 1987;9:45–52.
3. Becker AE. Relation between structure and function of the sinus node: general comments. In: Bonke FI, ed. *The sinus node.* The Hague: Martinus Nijhoff, 1978:212–222.
4. Strauss HC, Prystowsky EN, Scheinman MM. Sino-atrial and atrial electrogenesis. *Prog Cardiovasc Dis* 1977;19:385–404.
5. Bouman LN, Mackaay A, Bleeker WK, et al. Pacemaker shifts in the sinus node: effects of vagal stimulation, temperature and reduction of extracellular calcium. In: Bonke FI, ed. *The sinus node.* The Hague: Nijhoff Medical Division, 1978:245–257.

6. Prystowsky EN, Grant AO, Wallace AG, et al. An analysis of the effects of acetylcholine on conduction and refractoriness in the rabbit sinus node. *Circ Res* 1979;44:112–120.
7. Asseman P, Reade R, Thery C. Catecholamine modulation of sinus node automaticity during complete sinoatrial block: demonstration by direct recording. *Am Heart J* 1992;124:780–781.
8. Brodksy M, Wu D, Denes P, et al. Arrhythmias documented by 24 hour continuous electrocardiographic monitoring in 50 male medical students without apparent heart disease. *Am J Cardiol* 1977;39:390–395.
9. Romano M, Clarizia M, Onofrio E, et al. Heart rate, PR, and QT intervals in normal children: a 24-hour Holter monitoring study. *Clin Cardiol* 1988;11:839–842.
10. Ector H, Rolies L, De Geest H. Dynamic electrocardiography and ventricular pauses of 3 seconds and more: etiology and therapeutic implications. *Pacing Clin Electrophysiol* 1983;6:548–551.
11. Hilgard J, Ezri MD, Denes P. Significance of ventricular pauses of three seconds or more detected on twenty-four-hour Holter recordings. *Am J Cardiol* 1985;55:1005–1008.
12. Viitasalo MT, Kala R, Eisalo A. Ambulatory electrocardiographic recording in endurance athletes. *Br Heart J* 1982;47:213–220.
13. Lev M. Aging changes in the human sinoatrial node. *J Gerontol* 1954;9:1–9.
14. Davies MJ, Pomerance A. Quantitative study of ageing changes in the human sinoatrial node and internodal tracts. *Br Heart J* 1972;34:150–152.
15. Shaw DB, Linker NJ, Heaver PA, et al. Chronic sinoatrial disorder (sick sinus syndrome): a possible result of cardiac ischaemia. *Br Heart J* 1987; 58:598–607.
16. Rokseth R, Hatle L. Sinus arrest in acute myocardial infarction. *Br Heart J* 1971;33:639–642.
17. Heinz G, Hirschl M, Buxbaum P, et al. Sinus node dysfunction after orthotopic cardiac transplantation: postoperative incidence and long-term implications. *Pacing Clin Electrophysiol* 1992;15:731–737.
18. Caralis DG, Varghese PJ. Familial sinoatrial node dysfunction. Increased vagal tone a possible aetiology. *Br Heart J* 1976;38:951–956.
19. Gillette PC, Kugler JD, Garson Jr A, et al. Mechanisms of cardiac arrhythmias after the Mustard operation for transposition of the great arteries. *Am J Cardiol* 1980;45:1225–1230.
20. Young D. Later results of closure of secundum atrial septal defect in children. *Am J Cardiol* 1973;31:14–22.
21. Clark EB, Kugler JD. Preoperative secundum atrial septal defect with coexisting sinus node and atrioventricular node dysfunction. *Circulation* 1982; 65:976–980.
22. Benditt DG, Benson Jr DW, Dunnigan A, et al. Drug therapy in sinus node dysfunction. In: Rapaport E, ed. *Cardiology update.* New York: Elsevier, 1984:79–101.
23. Scheinman MM, Strauss HC, Evans GT, et al. Adverse effects of sympatholytic agents in patients with hypertension and sinus node dysfunction. *Am J Med* 1978;64:1013–1020.
24. Berns E, Rinkenberger RL, Jeang MK, et al. Efficacy and safety of flecainide acetate for atrial tachycardia or fibrillation. *Am J Cardiol* 1987;59:1337–1341.
25. Naccarelli GV, Dougherty AH, Berns E, et al. Assessment of antiarrhythmic drug efficacy in the treatment of supraventricular arrhythmias. *Am J Cardiol* 1986;58:31C–36C.
26. Milstein S, Buetikofer J, Lesser J, et al. Cardiac asystole: a manifestation of neurally mediated hypotension-bradycardia. *J Am Coll Cardiol* 1989;14: 1626–1632.
27. Abdon NJ, Landin K, Johansson BW. Athlete's bradycardia as an embolising disorder? Symptomatic arrhythmias in patients aged less than 50 years. *Br Heart J* 1984;52:660–666.
28. Kulbertus HE, Leval-Rutten F, Mary L, et al. Sinus node recovery time in the elderly. *Br Heart J* 1975;37:420–425.
29. Kaplan BM, Langendorf R, Lev M, et al. Tachycardia-bradycardia syndrome (so-called "sick sinus syndrome"): pathology, mechanisms and treatment. *Am J Cardiol* 1973;31:497–508.
30. Mazuz M, Friedman HS. Significance of prolonged electrocardiographic pauses in sinoatrial disease: sick sinus syndrome. *Am J Cardiol* 1983;52: 485–489.
31. Peretz DI, Abdulla A. Management of cardioinhibitory hypersensitive carotid sinus syncope with permanent cardiac pacing—a 17-year prospective study. *Can J Cardiol* 1985;1:86–91.
32. Jose AD, Collison D. The normal range and determinants of the intrinsic heart rate in man. *Cardiovasc Res* 1970;4:160–167.
33. Josephson ME. Sinus node function. In: Josephson ME, ed. *Clinical cardiac electrophysiology,* 2nd ed. Philadelphia: Lea & Febiger, 1993:83–84.
34. Zipes DP, DiMarco JP, Gillette PC, et al. Guidelines for clinical intracardiac electrophysiological and catheter ablation procedures. A report of the American College of Cardiology/American Heart Association Task Force on Practice Guidelines (Committee on Clinical Intracardiac Electrophysiologic and Catheter Ablation Procedures). *J Am Coll Cardiol* 1995;26:555–573.
35. Sutton R, Kenny RA. The natural history of sick sinus syndrome. *Pacing Clin Electrophysiol* 1986;9:1110–1114.
36. Connolly SJ, Kerr C, Gent M, et al. Dual-chamber versus ventricular pacing: critical appraisal of current data. *Circulation* 1996;94:578–583.
37. Cheitlin MD, Conill A, Epstein AE, et al. ACC/AHA guidelines for implantation of cardiac pacemakers and antiarrhythmia devices. A report of the American College of Cardiology/American Heart Association task force on practice guidelines (Committee on Pacemaker Implantation). *J Am Coll Cardiol* 1998;31:1175–1209.
38. Hecht HH, Kossmann CE, Childers RW, et al. Atrioventricular and intraventricular conduction. Revised nomenclature and concepts. *Am J Cardiol* 1973;31:232–244.
39. Scherlag BJ, Lazzara R, Helfant RH. Differentiation of "A-V junctional rhythms." *Circulation* 1973;48:304–312.
40. James TN. *Anatomy of the coronary arteries.* New York: Hoeber, Harper & Row, 1961.
41. Frink RJ, James TN. Normal blood supply to the human His bundle and proximal bundle branches. *Circulation* 1973;47:8–18.
42. James TN. Cardiac innervation: anatomic and pharmacologic relations. *Bull N Y Acad Sci* 1967;43:1041–1086.
43. Imaizumi S, Mazgalev T, Dreifus LS, et al. Morphological and electrophysiological correlates of atrioventricular nodal response to increased vagal activity. *Circulation* 1990;82:951–964.
44. Josephson ME. Electrophysiologic investigation: general concepts. In: Josephson ME, ed. *Clinical cardiac electrophysiology.* 2nd ed. Philadelphia: Lea & Febiger, 1993:26–30.
45. Rosen KM, Rahimtoola SH, Chuquimia R, et al. Electrophysiological significance of first degree atrioventricular block with intraventricular conduction disturbance. *Circulation* 1971;43:491–502.
46. Damato AN, Lau SH, Patton RD. A study of atrioventricular conduction in man using premature atrial stimulation and His bundle recordings. *Circulation* 1969;40:61–69.
47. Ranganathan N, Dhurandhar R, Phillips JH, et al. His bundle electrogram in bundle-branch block. *Circulation* 1972;45:282–294.
48. Pueck P, Grolleau R, Guimond C. Incidence of different types of AV block and their localization by His bundle recordings. In: Wellens HJJ, Lie KI, Janse NJ, eds. *The conduction system of the heart: structure, function and clinical implications.* Philadelphia: Lea & Febiger, 1976: 467–484.
49. Denes P, Levy L, Pick A, et al. The incidence of typical and atypical A-V Wenckebach periodicity. *Am Heart J* 1975;89:26–31.
50. Narula OS, Samet P. Wenckebach and Mobitz type II A-V block due to block within the His bundle and bundle branches. *Circulation* 1970;41:947–965.
51. Rosen KM. The contribution of His bundle recording to the understanding of cardiac conduction in man. *Circulation* 1971;43:961–966.
52. Kangos JJ, Griffiths SP, Blumenthal S. Congenital complete heart block. A classification and experience with 18 patients. *Am J Cardiol* 1967;20:632–638.
53. Pick A. AV dissociation: a proposal for a comprehensive classification and consistent terminology. *Am Heart J* 1963;66:147.
54. Tans AC, Lie KI, Durrer D. Clinical setting and prognostic significance of high degree atrioventricular block in acute inferior myocardial infarction: a study of 144 patients. *Am Heart J* 1980;99:4–8.
55. Berger PB, Ryan TJ. Inferior myocardial infarction. High-risk subgroups. *Circulation* 1990;81:401–411.
56. Meltzer LE, Cohen HE. The incidence of arrhythmias associated with acute myocardial infarction. In: Meltzer LE, Dunning AJ, eds. *Textbook of coronary care.* Amsterdam: Excerta Medica, 1972:197.
57. Adgey AA, Allen JD, Geddes JS, et al. Acute phase of myocardial infarction. *Lancet* 1971;2:501–504.
58. Sclarovsky S, Strasberg B, Hirshberg A, et al. Advanced early and late atrioventricular block in acute inferior wall myocardial infarction. *Am Heart J* 1984;108:19–24.
59. Lie KI, Duner D. Atrioventricular and intraventricular conduction disturbances in acute myocardial infarction: clinical aspects. In: Samet P, El-Sherif N, eds. *Cardiac pacing.* New York: Grune & Stratton, 1980:439.
60. Feigl D, Ashkenazy J, Kishon Y. Early and late atrioventricular block in acute inferior myocardial infarction. *J Am Coll Cardiol* 1984;4:35–38.
61. Clemo HF, Belardinelli L. Effect of adenosine on atrioventricular conduction. I: Site and characterization of adenosine action in the guinea pig atrioventricular node. *Circ Res* 1986;59:427–436.
62. Sutton R, Davies M. The conduction system in acute myocardial infarction complicated by heart block. *Circulation* 1968;38:987–992.
63. Hackel DB, Wagner G, Ratliff NB, et al. Anatomic studies of the cardiac conducting system in acute myocardial infarction. *Am Heart J* 1972;83:77–81.
64. Nicod P, Gilpin E, Dittrich H, et al. Long-term outcome in patients with inferior myocardial infarction and complete atrioventricular block. *J Am Coll Cardiol* 1988;12:589–594.
65. Mavric Z, Zaputovic L, Matana A, et al. Prognostic significance of complete atrioventricular block in patients with acute inferior myocardial infarction with and without right ventricular involvement. *Am Heart J* 1990;119:823–828.
66. Braat SH, de Zwaan C, Brugada P, et al. Right ventricular involvement with acute inferior wall myocardial infarction identifies high risk of developing atrioventricular nodal conduction disturbances. *Am Heart J* 1984;107: 1183–1187.
67. Strasberg B, Pinchas A, Arditti A, et al. Left and right ventricular function in inferior acute myocardial infarction and significance of advanced atrioventricular block. *Am J Cardiol* 1984;54:985–987.
68. Lev M. The pathology of complete AV block. *Prog Cardiovasc Dis* 1964;6: 317.

69. Lenegre J. Etiology and pathology of bilateral bundle block fibrosis in relation to complete heart block. *Prog Cardiovasc Dis* 1964;6: 409.
70. Rytand DA, Lipsitch LS. Clinical aspects of calcification of mitral annulus. *Arch Intern Med* 1946;78:544.
71. Narula OS, Samet P. Predilection of elderly females for intra-His bundle (BH) blocks. *Circulation* 1974;50(Suppl):195.
72. Ablaza SG, Blanco G, Maranhao V, et al. Calcific aortic valvular disease associated with complete heart block: case reports of successful correction. *Dis Chest* 1968;54:457–460.
73. Harris A, Sleight P, Drew CE. The diagnosis and treatment of aortic stenosis complicated by AV block. *Br Heart J* 1965;27:560.
74. Bharati S, Lev M, Denes P, et al. Infiltrative cardiomyopathy with conduction disease and ventricular arrhythmia: electrophysiologic and pathologic correlations. *Am J Cardiol* 1980;45:163–173.
75. Fawcett FJ, Goldberg MJ. Heart block resulting from myocardial sarcoidosis. *Br Heart J* 1974;36:220–223.
76. Schellhammer PF, Engle MA, Hagstrom JW. Histochemical studies of the myocardium and conduction system in acquired iron-storage disease. *Circulation* 1967;35:631–637.
77. Aronow WS, Meister L, Kent JR. Atrioventricular block in familial hemochromatosis treated by permanent synchronous pacemaker. *Arch Intern Med* 1969;123:433–435.
78. Kostis JB, Seibold JR, Turkevich D, et al. Prognostic importance of cardiac arrhythmias in systemic sclerosis. *Am J Med* 1988;84:1007–1015.
79. Ahern M, Lever JV, Cosh J. Complete heart block in rheumatoid arthritis. *Ann Rheum Dis* 1983;42:389–397.
80. Ruppert GB, Lindsay J, Barth WF. Cardiac conduction abnormalities in Reiter's syndrome. *Am J Med* 1982;73:335–340.
81. Bilazarian SD, Taylor AJ, Brezinski D, et al. High-grade atrioventricular heart block in an adult with systemic lupus erythematosus: the association of nuclear RNP (U1 RNP) antibodies, a case report, and review of the literature. *Arthritis Rheum* 1989;32:1170–1174.
82. Bergfeldt L. HLA-B27-associated rheumatic diseases with severe cardiac bradyarrhythmias: clinical features and prevalence in 223 men with permanent pacemakers. *Am J Med* 1983;75:210–215.
83. Kehoe RF, Bauernfeind R, Tommaso C, et al. Cardiac conduction defects in polymyositis: electrophysiologic studies in four patients. *Ann Intern Med* 1981;94:41–43.
84. DiNubile MJ, Calderwood SB, Steinhaus DM, et al. Cardiac conduction abnormalities complicating native valve active infective endocarditis. *Am J Cardiol* 1986;58:1213–1217.
85. Hagar JM, Rahimtoola SH. Chagas' heart disease in the United States. *N Engl J Med* 1991;325:763–768.
86. van der Linde MR, Crijns HJ, de Koning J, et al. Range of atrioventricular conduction disturbances in Lyme borreliosis: a report of four cases and review of other published reports. *Br Heart J* 1990;63:162–168.
87. Bland EF, Jones TD. Rheumatic fever and rheumatic heart disease. A twenty year report on 1000 patients followed since childhood. *Circulation* 1951;4:836–843.
88. Mirowski M, Rosenstein BJ, Marbowitz M. A comparison of atrioventricular conduction in normal children and in patients with rheumatic fever, glomerulonephritis, and acute febrile illnesses. *Pediatrics* 1964;33:334–340.
89. Wood P. *Diseases of the heart and circulation,* 3rd ed. Philadelphia: Lippincott, 1968:588.
90. Williams JF, Morrow AG, Braunwald E. The incidence and management of "medical" complications following cardiac operations. *Circulation* 1965;32:608–619.
91. Stevenson WG, Klitzmer T, Perloff JK. Electrophysiologic abnormalities; natural occurrence and postoperative residua and sequelae. In: Perloff JK, Child JS, eds. *Congenital heart disease in adults.* Philadelphia: WB Saunders, 1991:259–295.
92. Thomas IR, Dalton BC, Lappas DG, et al. Right bundle-branch block and complete heart block caused by the Swan-Ganz catheter. *Anesthesiology* 1979;51:359–362.
93. Jacobson LB, Scheinman M. Catheter-induced intra-Hisian and intrafascicular block during recording of His bundle electrograms. *Circulation* 1974;49:579–584.
94. Kimbiris D, Dreifus LS, Linhart JW. Complete heart block occurring during cardiac catheterization in patients with preexisting bundle branch block. *Chest* 1974;65:95–97.
95. Williamson BD, Man KC, Daoud E, et al. Radiofrequency catheter modification of atrioventricular conduction to control the ventricular rate during atrial fibrillation. *N Engl J Med* 1994;331:944–945.
96. Hindricks G. The Multicentre European Radiofrequency Survey (MERFS): complications of radiofrequency catheter ablation of arrhythmias. *Eur Heart J* 1993;14:1644–1653.
97. Mitrani RD, Klein LS, Hackett FK, et al. Radiofrequency ablation for atrioventricular node reentrant tachycardia: comparison between fast (anterior) and slow (posterior) pathway ablation. *J Am Coll Cardiol* 1993; 21:432–441.
98. Fisch C, Greenspan K, Edmands RE. Complete atrioventricular block due to potassium. *Circ Res* 1966;19:373–377.
99. Lown B, Arons WL, Ganong WF, et al. Adrenal steroids and auriculoventricular conduction. *Am Heart J* 1955;50:760–769.
100. Harvey WP. Clinical aspects of cardiac tumors. *Am J Cardiol* 1968;21:328–343.
101. Prystowsky EN, Pritchett EL, Roses AD, et al. The natural history of conduction system disease in myotonic muscular dystrophy as determined by serial electrophysiologic studies. *Circulation* 1979;60:1360–1364.
102. Perloff JK. Cardiac rhythm and conduction in Duchenne's muscular dystrophy: a prospective study of 20 patients. *J Am Coll Cardiol* 1984;3:1263–1268.
103. Zubair ul Hassan, Fastabend CP, Mohanty PK, et al. Atrioventricular block and supraventricular arrhythmias with X-linked muscular dystrophy. *Circulation* 1979;60:1365–1369.
104. Almquist A, Gornick C, Benson Jr W, et al. Carotid sinus hypersensitivity: evaluation of the vasodepressor component. *Circulation* 1985;71:927–936.
105. Benditt DG, Goldstein MA, Adler S, et al. Neurally mediated syncopal syndromes: pathophysiology and clinical evaluation. In: Mandel WJ, ed. *Cardiac arrhythmias. Their mechanisms, diagnosis, and management.* Philadelphia: Lippincott, 1995:879–906.
106. Lev M. Pathogenesis of congenital atrioventricular block. *Prog Cardiovasc Dis* 1972;15:145–157.
107. McHenry MM, Cayler GC. Congenital complete heart block in newborns, infants, children and adults. *Med Times* 1969;97:113–123.
108. Nakamura FF, Nadas AS. Complete heart block in infants and children. *N Engl J Med* 1964;270:1261.
109. Johnson RL, Averill KH, Lamb LE. Electrocardiographic findings in 67,375 asymptomatic subjects. *Am J Cardiol* 1960;6:153–177.
110. Perlman LV, Ostrander Jr LD, Keller JB, et al. An epidemiologic study of first degree atrioventricular block in Tecumseh, Michigan. *Chest* 1971;59:40–46.
111. Fox TT, Weaver JC, Francis RL. Further studies on electro-cardiographic changes in old age. *Geriatrics* 1948;3:35–41.
112. Rodstein M, Brown M, Wolloch L. First-degree atrioventricular heart block in the aged. *Geriatrics* 1968;23:159–165.
113. Dickinson DF, Scott O. Ambulatory electrocardiographic monitoring in 100 healthy teenage boys. *Br Heart J* 1984;51:179–183.
114. White PD. In: MacMillan D, ed. *Heart disease.* New York: Macmillan, 1951:933.
115. Michaelsson M, Engle MA. Congenital complete heart block: an international study of the natural history. *Cardiovasc Clin* 1972;4:85–101.
116. Perloff JK. The clinical recognition of congenital heart disease. In: Perloff JK, ed. *Congenital complete heart block.* Philadelphia: WB Saunders, 1987: 49.
117. Penton GB, Miller H, Levine SA. Some clinical features of complete heart block. *Circulation* 1956;13:801–824.
118. Ide LW. The clinical aspects of complete auriculoventricular heart block: a clinical analysis of 71 cases. *Ann Intern Med* 1952;32:510–523.
119. Friedberg CK, Donoso E, Stein WG. Nonsurgical acquired heart block. *Ann N Y Acad Sci* 1964;111:835–847.
120. Esscher EB. Congenital complete heart block in adolescence and adult life: a follow-up study. *Eur Heart J* 1981;2:281–288.
121. Karpawich PP, Gillette PC, Garson Jr A, et al. Congenital complete atrioventricular block: clinical and electrophysiologic predictors of need for pacemaker insertion. *Am J Cardiol* 1981;48:1098–1102.
122. Camm AJ, Bexton RS. Congenital complete heart block. *Eur Heart J* 1984; 5:115–117.
123. Scheinman MM, Peters RW, Sauve MJ, et al. Value of the H-Q interval in patients with bundle branch block and the role of prophylactic permanent pacing. *Am J Cardiol* 1982;50:1316–1322.
124. Katz LN, Pick A. Part I: The arrhythmias. In: *Clinical electrocardiography.* Philadelphia: Lea & Febiger, 1956:545.
125. Ginks W, Leatham A, Siddons H. Prognosis of patients paced for chronic atrioventricular block. *Br Heart J* 1979;41:633–636.
126. Michaelsson M, Jonzon A, Riesenfeld T. Isolated congenital complete atrioventricular block in adult life: a prospective study. *Circulation* 1995; 92:442–449.
127. Donmoyer TL, DeSanctis RW, Austen WG. Experience with implantable pacemakers using myocardial electrodes in the management of heart block. *Ann Thorac Surg* 1967;3:218–227.
128. Dhingra RC, Denes P, Wu D, et al. The significance of second degree atrioventricular block and bundle branch block. Observations regarding site and type of block. *Circulation* 1974;49:638–646.
129. Pinsky WW, Gillette PC, Garson Jr A, et al. Diagnosis, management, and long-term results of patients with congenital complete atrioventricular block. *Pediatrics* 1982;69:728–733.
130. Dewey RC, Capeless MA, Levy AM. Use of ambulatory electrocardiographic monitoring to identify high-risk patients with congenital complete heart block. *N Engl J Med* 1987;316:835–839.
131. Serwer GA, Dorostkar PC. Pediatric pacing. In: Ellenbogen KA, Kay GN, Wilkoff BL, eds. *Clinical cardiac pacing.* Philadelphia: WB Saunders, 1995: 706–731.
132. Barold SS. Indications for permanent cardiac pacing in first-degree AV block: class I, II, or III? *Pacing Clin Electrophysiol* 1996;19:747–751.
133. Newby KH, Pisan E, Krucoff MW, et al. Incidence and clinical relevance of the occurrence of bundle-branch blocks in patients treated with thrombolytic therapy. *Circulation* 1996;94:2424–2428.
134. Andersen HR, Nielsen JC, Thomsen PEB, et al. Long-term follow-up of

patients from a randomized trial of atrial versus ventricular pacing for sick-sinus syndrome. *Lancet* 1997;350:1210–1216.
135. Lamas GA, Lee KL, Sweeney MD, et al. for the MOST Investigators. Ventricular pacing or dual chamber pacing for sinus node dysfunction. *N Engl J Med* 2002;346:1854–1862.
136. Sweeney MO, Hellkamp AS, Ellenbogen KA, et al. Adverse effect of ventricular pacing on heart failure and atrial fibrillation among patients with normal baseline QRS duration in a clinical trail of pacemaker therapy for sinus node dysfunction. *Circulation* 2003;23:2932–2937.
137. Wilkoff BL, Cook JR, Epstein AE, et al. Dual-chamber pacing or ventricular backup pacing in patients with an implantable defibrillator: the Dual Chamber and VVI Implantable Defibrillator (DAVID) Trial. *JAMA* 2002; 288:3115–3125.
138. Steinberg JS, Fischer A, Wang P, et al. The clinical implications of cumulative right ventricular pacing in the Multicenter Automatic Defibrillator Trial II. *J Cardiovasc Electrophysiol* 2005;16(4):359–365.
139. Kristensen L, Nielsen JC, Pedersen AK, et al. AV block and changes in pacing mode during long-term follow-up of 339 consecutive patients with sick sinus syndrome treated with AAI/AAIR pacemaker. *Pacing Clin Electrophysiol* 2001;24:358–365.
140. Nielsen JC, Pedersen AK, Mortensen PT, et al. Programming a fixed long atrioventricular delay is not effective in preventing ventricular pacing in patients with sick sinus syndrome. *Europace* 1999;1:113–120.
141. Deering TF, Wilensky M, Tondato F, et al. Auto intrinsic conduction search algorithm: a prospective analysis [Abstract]. *Pacing Clin Electrophysiol* 2003;26:1080.
142. Sweeney MO, Shea JB, Fox V, et al. Randomized trial of a new atrial-based minimal ventricular pacing mode in dual chamber implantable cardioverter-defibrillators. *Heart Rhythm* 2004;1:160–167.
143. Toff WD, Camm AJ, Skehan JD, for the United Kingdom Pacing and Cardiovascular Events (UKPACE) Trial Investigators. Single-chamber versus dual-chamber pacing for high-grade atrioventricular block. *N Engl J Med* 2005;353:145–155.
144. Kerr CR, Connolly SJ, Abdollah H, et al. Canadian Trial of Physiological Pacing: effects of physiological pacing during long-term follow-up. *Circulation* 2004;109:357–362.

CHAPTER 63 ■ ATRIAL FIBRILLATION

ERIC N. PRYSTOWSKY AND AMOS KATZ

OVERVIEW

Atrial fibrillation (AF) is the most common sustained arrhythmia affecting humans. Pathology studies have found loss of atrial myocardium with fibrosis and fatty infiltration, but many similar changes can occur as a result of aging alone. Maintenance of AF may depend on reentry, with multiple wavelets occurring simultaneously, continuous triggers, or both. The initiation of AF in many patients may be caused by rapidly firing foci, typically in the pulmonary vein(s). Although the atrial rate is rapid, usually greater than 300 beats per minute, the ventricular response depends on atrioventricular (AV) node conduction properties and the level of autonomic tone. AV node conduction is facilitated by sympathetic tone and inhibited by parasympathetic tone. A variety of medical conditions are associated with AF, most frequently hypertension, coronary artery disease, and valvular heart disease. Many patients have idiopathic, or lone, AF. There are three major tenets of therapy: (a) restoration and maintenance of sinus rhythm, (b) ventricular rate control, and (c) prevention of thromboembolism. One or more of these may be indicated in a particular patient. Several antiarrhythmic agents are effective for restoring and maintaining sinus rhythm, and selection of a particular drug depends on many factors, including the presence and type of underlying heart disease, concomitant illnesses, and renal or hepatic dysfunction. Radiofrequency catheter ablation is being used more frequently to cure AF in patients failing drug therapy. β-Adrenergic blockers and calcium channel blockers are more effective than digoxin in controlling ventricular response, although digoxin is the first-line treatment for patients who have congestive heart failure. In patients who have Wolff-Parkinson-White syndrome (WPW), intravenous procainamide or ibutilide is the preferred therapy for blocking conduction over the accessory pathway during AF, and digoxin, adenosine, β-adrenergic blockers, and calcium channel blockers are contraindicated. In patients at high risk for thromboembolism, anticoagulation therapy using warfarin is recommended, aiming for an international normalized ratio (INR) of 2.0 to 3.0. Anticoagulation is also recommended for patients who are undergoing pharmacologic or electrical cardioversion if AF has been present for at least 48 hours.

HISTORICAL PERSPECTIVE

Atrial fibrillation is the most common sustained arrhythmia affecting humans. Interest in it has waxed and waned for decades, and recently it has taken a back seat to research into arrhythmias such as AV reentry (WPW), AV node reentry, sustained ventricular tachycardia, and ventricular fibrillation. However, there has been a resurgence in interest in the mechanisms and treatment of patients with atrial fibrillation, especially in the potential for curing this arrhythmia using intracardiac

TABLE 63.1

ETIOLOGY OF ATRIAL FIBRILLATION

Author	Year	Country	Number of patients	RHD (%)	HHD (%)	CHD (%)	Hyperthyroidism (%)	No heart disease (%)
Lewis (7)	1910	England	73	64	—	—	—	—
Parkinson and Campbell (11)	1930	England	200	22	24	—	14	9
Kannel et al. (12)[a]	1982	United States	98	18	48	10	—	31
Davidson et al. (13)[b]	1989	Israel	704	23	—	55	4	5
Lok and Lau (14)	1995	Hong Kong	291	11	29	25	6	29
Prystowsky et al. (15)[c]	1996	United States	285	4	56	19	11	35

[a]Some patients with no heart disease had cardiac stigmata.
[b]Atherosclerotic cardiovascular disease included hypertension.
[c]Consecutive series of outpatients only.
CHD, coronary heart disease; HHD, hypertensive heart disease; RHD, rheumatic heart disease.

catheter ablation techniques. The following is a brief summary of significant individuals who have made important observations concerning atrial fibrillation.

Evaluation of the peripheral pulse has fascinated physicians for centuries. In approximately 1187, Moses Maimonides presented aphorisms pertaining to the pulse. He described an irregular pulse that was regularly irregular and one that becomes completely irregular (1). He was at least partially correct when he mentioned, with regard to the origin of the regularity, "all types of pulses which are irregular in more than one beat are a direct result of an abnormal constitution of the heart which is also irregular or due to an affliction arising in the stomach or in one's strength". Before the electrocardiographic confirmation of atrial fibrillation, many observant physicians commented on grossly irregular pulses that, in at least some cases, were likely atrial fibrillation. William Stokes (2), in his classic text on heart disease, stated, "It has happened often to me to find the action of the heart, which, for many months together, had been in the highest degree irregular, suddenly restored to a condition in which the rhythm and sounds were perfectly natural." In 1904, Wenckebach (3) published a monograph on cardiac arrhythmias. He described cases of excessive irregularity, or "delirium cordis." One such example is accompanied by a pulse tracing that demonstrates a very irregular rhythm, likely atrial fibrillation.

Cushny (4), Mackenzie (5), Rothberger and Winterberg (6), and especially Lewis (7) made significant early observations concerning atrial fibrillation. The magnum opus of Sir Thomas Lewis is a must-read for any student of atrial fibrillation. The pioneering work of Einthoven (8) enabled clinical investigators to record the electrocardiographic representation of the clinical observations of atrial fibrillation.

EPIDEMIOLOGY

AF has a profound effect on morbidity and mortality among hundreds of thousands of patients and on health care costs in the United States (9). One report analyzed 3,806,000 patient hospital discharges in 1990 from 678 hospitals to determine the frequency with which arrhythmia was the principal diagnosis (10). Approximately 1.5% of all hospital discharges listed arrhythmia as a principal diagnosis, and AF accounted for nearly 35% of the arrhythmias noted. The epidemiology of AF has changed substantially since the early part of the twentieth century primarily because of the dramatic decrease in rheumatic fever and the longer life span of the population (Table 63.1) (11–16). The patient populations evaluated in Table 63.1 differ substantially. For example, two studies included patients admitted through the emergency department (13,14) and one evaluated only outpatients (15). Nonetheless, it is obvious that rheumatic heart disease plays a relatively minor role in the current etiology of atrial fibrillation in the Western world, whereas hypertension and, to a lesser extent, coronary artery disease currently are major etiologic factors in AF. The incidence of lone AF is quite variable and is influenced by the intensity of the diagnostic workup, the definition of *lone atrial fibrillation* used, and the patient population studied. Kannel and associates (12) reported a 31% incidence of lone AF, but some of their patients had obvious heart disease identified by an enlarged heart on chest radiography. Thus, these data are problematic. In contrast, Prystowsky and colleagues (15) studied only patients who had no known etiologic factors for AF and normal ventricular function identified by echocardiography. However, in their study, only outpatients were evaluated. It is clear that the prevalence and types of etiologic factors for AF depend on the setting in which AF is evaluated, including the country of origin.

Changes in etiology of atrial fibrillation may affect its course, especially the evolution of paroxysmal atrial fibrillation into established atrial fibrillation. In a study involving 1,212 patients from Denmark, three time periods, 1940 through 1948, 1949 through 1957, and 1958 through 1967, were evaluated (8). Atherosclerotic heart disease was present in 23%, 37%, and 38% of patients, respectively; hypertensive heart disease was present in 8%, 7%, and 10% of patients, respectively; and rheumatic heart disease occurred in 27%, 17%, and 15% of patients, respectively. During follow-up, the transition rate from paroxysmal to established or permanent atrial fibrillation varied according to the etiology of the disease and was 27% among patients with atherosclerotic heart disease, 40% among patients with hypertensive heart disease, and 66% among patients with rheumatic heart disease. Few data are given on the use of antiarrhythmic drugs to prevent transition to established atrial fibrillation. However, given the dates of the study, only quinidine would have been used with any frequency. These data suggest that the transition from paroxysmal to established atrial fibrillation is not inevitable, especially among patients without rheumatic heart disease. It is quite possible that antiarrhythmic therapy may further decrease the number of patients with established atrial fibrillation. This issue is discussed in more detail in the section entitled Therapy of Atrial Fibrillation.

Effect of Age and Gender

The prevalence of AF increases with age and is 0.5% for patients aged 50 to 59 years and 8.8% for those aged 80 to

89 years (17). Men are affected slightly more often than women. In the Framingham data, excluding individuals with rheumatic heart disease, the 2-year incidence of development of AF was 0.04% and 0.00% for men and women, respectively, aged 30 to 39 years, and 4.6% and 3.6%, respectively, for men and women aged 80 to 89 years (18). Thus, the number of patients who have AF will rise pari passu with the aging of the population. In the first two decades of life, AF is relatively rare (9). When it is found in patients in this age group, it is usually associated with heart disease or the presence of an accessory pathway.

PATHOLOGY

Changes Associated with Aging

The incidence of atrial fibrillation increases with age, and the condition is especially prevalent among individuals aged 60 years or older. Thus, it is important, in attempts to identify the pathologic changes associated with atrial fibrillation, to consider changes that are associated with the aging process in and of itself. Macroscopic and microscopic alterations in atrial tissue begin in the first year of life (19). By the fourth and fifth decades, small fat spots appear in the right atrium in the region of the AV node and septum. There is accentuation of the thickening of the plaques in later decades. In the left atrium, the endocardial thickening is diffuse. With aging, increased thickening occurs, especially at the mitral valve annulus. Calcification and fatty infiltration may be present in the annulus. Histologic examination reveals an endothelial lining, beneath which is a fibroelastic core. With aging, there is focal or diffuse proliferation of smooth muscle cells, elastic fibers, or both and, in some cases, collagen fibers. This process has been termed *endocardial hypertrophy* (19). In the fourth decade, hypertrophic and sclerotic changes occur in previously uninvolved portions of the right atrium, and in the fifth decade, atrophy of smooth muscle layers can be seen. Increased sclerotic changes occur in the sixth decade. By the fourth decade, the entire left atrium appears to be affected by hypertrophy and sclerosis, and collagen replacement is frequent. The changes associated with aging result in eventual loss of myocardial fibers and an increase in fatty metamorphosis and connective tissue in the sinus node, the AV node, and the atrial approaches to these structures (19).

Pathology of the Atrium in Atrial Fibrillation

One study analyzed pathologic changes in the atria in 145 patients with AF and control patients (19). Etiologies were diverse and included conditions such as rheumatic fever, hypertension, hyperthyroidism, and coronary artery disease. The author speculated that no specific histologic syndrome is associated with AF. In another study, lesions of the sinus node were evaluated in the hearts of 65 patients (20). The anatomy of the sinus node was compared with clinical data in a blinded manner. The sinus node was obviously damaged in 15 patients, and an established arrhythmia, usually AF, was seen in 14 patients. The sinus node was normal in 49 patients, and AF had been present in 5 patients. The common association in this study between sinus nodal damage and a clinical history of AF supports the idea that sick sinus syndrome is a panatrial disorder in many patients.

One of the most important pathologic studies of the atria of patients with AF was done by Davies and Pomerance (21). These authors analyzed the hearts of 100 patients with AF and grouped them into patients who had AF for less than 2 weeks before death and those who had AF for more than 1 month before death. Among patients who had the longer-term AF, cor pulmonale, rheumatic heart disease, and ischemic heart disease were the most frequently associated clinical conditions. In nearly 75% of cases of chronic AF, sinus node muscle loss, internodal tract muscle loss, and atrial dilation of some degree were present. Notably, left atrial appendage thrombosis was identified in 46 patients with long-term AF and cerebral infarction was identified in 19. However, only 3 of 19 patients with short-term AF had left atrial thrombus and only 1 patient had cerebral infarction. These authors offered an important hypothesis concerning the origin of pathologic changes in the atria. They stated that "while it is conventional to regard the fibrotic changes in the node and atria as the cause of atrial fibrillation, it is also possible that they result from the arrhythmia and consequent disordered function of the chamber" (13). This prescient observation supports the current belief that AF begets AF, therefore making it possible to retard or even prevent the development of permanent AF in some patients by maintaining sinus rhythm, which may beget sinus rhythm.

Some studies involving patients with lone AF have shown histologic changes on atrial biopsies consistent with myocarditis (22), and high serum levels of antibodies against myosin heavy chains have been found (23). The pathophysiologic significance of these findings is unclear.

PATHOPHYSIOLOGY

Electrophysiologic Mechanism of Atrial Fibrillation

Arrhythmias require an initiating event, for example, a premature atrial or ventricular complex, and a sustaining substrate, for example, one or more reentrant circuits. The initiating event and sustaining substrate may be all due to automaticity such as a rapidly firing atrial focus. In AF, both automaticity and reentry appear to play a role.

Automatic Focus Theory of Atrial Fibrillation

The ectopic focus theory of AF was championed by Scherf and coworkers (24,25). Topical application of aconitine to the appendix of the right or left atrium yielded arrhythmias that were similar in appearance to AF. Clamping off the area of application from the rest of the atrium allowed the arrhythmia to continue in the area that was clamped off, but not in the rest of the atria. The experiments with aconitine suggested that AF depended on a single focus.

The ectopic focus theory for AF was essentially smothered by the overwhelming weight of observations indicating that reentry was the mechanism of AF. However, observations made during intracardiac radiofrequency catheter ablation of AF have rekindled interest in the ectopic focus theory (26–28). These authors (26,27) were able to terminate AF with discrete applications of radiofrequency energy, primarily in the area of the pulmonary veins (PVs) in the left atrium, although other atrial sites including the superior vena cava, ligament of Marshall, crista terminalis, coronary sinus, and left posterior free wall, have also been identified (28–32). The PVs are most frequently the origin of these rapid atrial foci, and studies have confirmed that cardiac muscle extends onto the PVs in humans (33), and PVs have automaticity in an experimental model (34).

In patients with AF, PVs have shorter refractory periods than in control patients, and refractory periods are also shorter in the left atrium outside of the PVs (35). Decremental conduction in PVs can occur, and the heterogeneity of conduction could promote reentry in the PV or PV–left atrial juncture (36). The rapid local left atrial activation cannot be conducted in an organized way to the right atrium. Experiments in sheep hearts demonstrated a dominant fibrillation frequency in the left atrium, and this decreased with activation to the right atrium (37). This fibrillatory conduction likely explains the chaotic atrial rhythm typically noted in the electrocardiogram (ECG). However, it is often possible to observe in ECG lead V_1 well-defined P waves with a short cycle length that is irregular.

Multiple-Wavelet Reentry Theory of Atrial Fibrillation

A key development in our understanding of the mechanism of AF was the multiple wavelet hypothesis proposed by Moe and coauthors (38,39). They noted, "the grossly irregular wave front becomes fractionated as it divides about islets or strands of refractory tissue, and each of the daughter wavelets may now be considered as independent offspring. Such a wavelet may accelerate or decelerate as it encounters tissue in a more or less advanced state of recovery" (38). Thus, the larger the number of wavelets that present, the more likely it is that the arrhythmia will sustain. The number of wavelets depends on the atrial mass, the refractory period, and the conduction velocity of various areas of the atria. In essence, a large atrial mass with short refractory periods and conduction delay would yield increased wavelets and would present the most favorable situation for AF to be sustained.

Experimental validation of the multiple-wavelet hypothesis was demonstrated by Allessie and colleagues (40). They analyzed the excitation of canine atria during induced AF with two egg-shaped multiple electrodes inserted into the cavities of the atria. Each electrode contained 480 recording electrodes, with an interelectrode distance of 3 mm. This enabled the first highly detailed activation sequencing of AF. Figure 63.1 demonstrates an arbitrary moment during AF and reveals seven wavelets (40). These reentrant wavelets were not stable, and over the course of time, various pathways of reentry could be demonstrated. When only three wavelets existed, there was a high chance that all would cease to exist, but when six wavelets were present, spontaneous termination of AF did not occur.

The mechanism of initiation of AF is not certain in most cases and likely is multifactorial. For example, it may occur secondarily from another arrhythmia, so called tachycardia-induced tachycardia (41) (Fig. 63.2). In such circumstances, the initial tachycardia is the actual mechanism for induction of AF, and might be related to the tachycardia cycle length, intrinsic atrial vulnerability, contraction-excitation feedback, or a combination of these factors (41). If reentry is assumed to be the mechanism of AF, initiation would require an area of conduction block and a wavelength of activation that is short

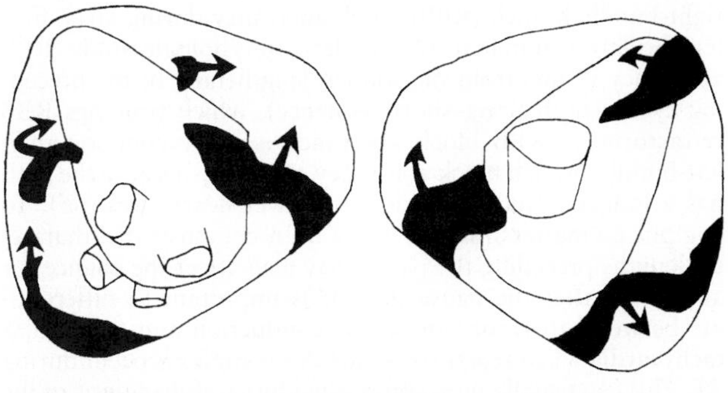

FIGURE 63.1. Canine atria with multiple propagating wavelets during sustained atrial fibrillation. Seven wavelets are present, three in the right atrium and four in the left atrium. The black contours mark the atrium that has been excited during the last 10 ms. (From Allessie MA, Lammers WJEP, Bonke FIM, et al. Experimental evaluation of Moe's multiple wavelet hypothesis of atrial fibrillation. In: Zipes DP, Jalife J, eds. *Cardiac arrhythmias*. New York: Grune & Stratton, 1985:265–276.)

enough to allow the reentrant circuit in the myocardium. The normal aging process results in anatomic changes likely to yield inhomogeneity in conduction that may create the milieu necessary for the development of reentry (42,43). These changes are likely magnified by the presence of certain disease processes, for example, those of coronary artery disease. Clearly autonomic tone influences AF initiation, especially enhanced vagal activity. The roles of increased atrial pressure and volume and activation of stretch-induced ionic channels require further study.

Tachycardia-Induced Atrial Cardiomyopathy

It has been recognized for several decades that a persistently fast ventricular rate secondary to supraventricular tachycardia can lead to ventricular cardiomyopathy, which is reversible if recognized in time. In fact, this is not an uncommon phenomenon in patients who present with AF and dilated cardiomyopathy, especially in those patients without palpitations. A tachycardia-induced atrial cardiomyopathy can also occur (44). The effect of persistent AF on changes in atrial size was investigated in 15 patients who showed no evidence of significant structural or functional cardiac abnormalities other than AF (45). During an average follow-up period of 20.6 months, mean left atrial volume increased from 45.2 to 64.1 cm^3 and right atrial volume significantly increased from 49.2 to 66.2 cm^3. In contrast, after cardioversion of AF at 6 months' follow-up, in 28 patients in whom sinus rhythm was maintained the left atrial volume decreased from 72.6 ± 15.1 to 58.5 ± 13.8 cm^3 and right atrial volume decreased from 68.7 ± 14.6 to $58. \pm 11.6$ cm^3 ($p < .05$), but atrial size did not change in patients in whom AF recurred (46).

Evidence for a tachycardia-induced atrial cardiomyopathy is supported further by echocardiographic observations before and after cardioversion (47,48). Based on the use of transesophageal echocardiography, left atrial appendage blood flow velocity and contractile function were assessed in patients with AF (48). There was an inverse correlation between the duration of AF and left atrial appendage peak outflow velocities. Patients who spontaneously cardioverted to sinus rhythm had significantly greater left atrial appendage outflow velocities. The course of recovery of atrial systolic function after cardioversion was evaluated using transthoracic Doppler echocardiography (47). Within the first week after cardioversion, atrial mechanical function was greater in patients with AF of 2 weeks or less compared with those patients who had AF greater than 6 weeks in duration. Over the course of time, atrial mechanical function improved in all groups of patients.

Electrical atrial remodeling also occurs with AF (49–51). In a goat model of repetitively induced AF, episodes of AF became progressively more sustained over time until sustained AF occurred with a rapid atrial cycle length (49). This was associated with progressive shortening of atrial refractoriness. The rapid atrial rate results in intracellular calcium loading and subsequent voltage-dependent inactivation of the calcium current (51,52). A reduction of calcium current shortens atrial action potential duration and refractoriness that favor AF maintenance. The role of potassium currents in atrial electrical remodeling remains unclear (52).

In summary, persistence of AF results in a cascade of electrical and anatomic changes in the atria that promote the persistence of AF. The result is perpetuation of AF and a decrease in atrial mechanical function secondary to tachycardia-induced atrial cardiomyopathy. If sinus rhythm is restored within a reasonable period of time, electrophysiologic changes appear to normalize, atrial size decreases, and restoration of atrial mechanical function occurs. These observations lend support to the idea that the negative downhill spiral in which AF begets AF can be arrested with sinus rhythm that perpetuates sinus rhythm.

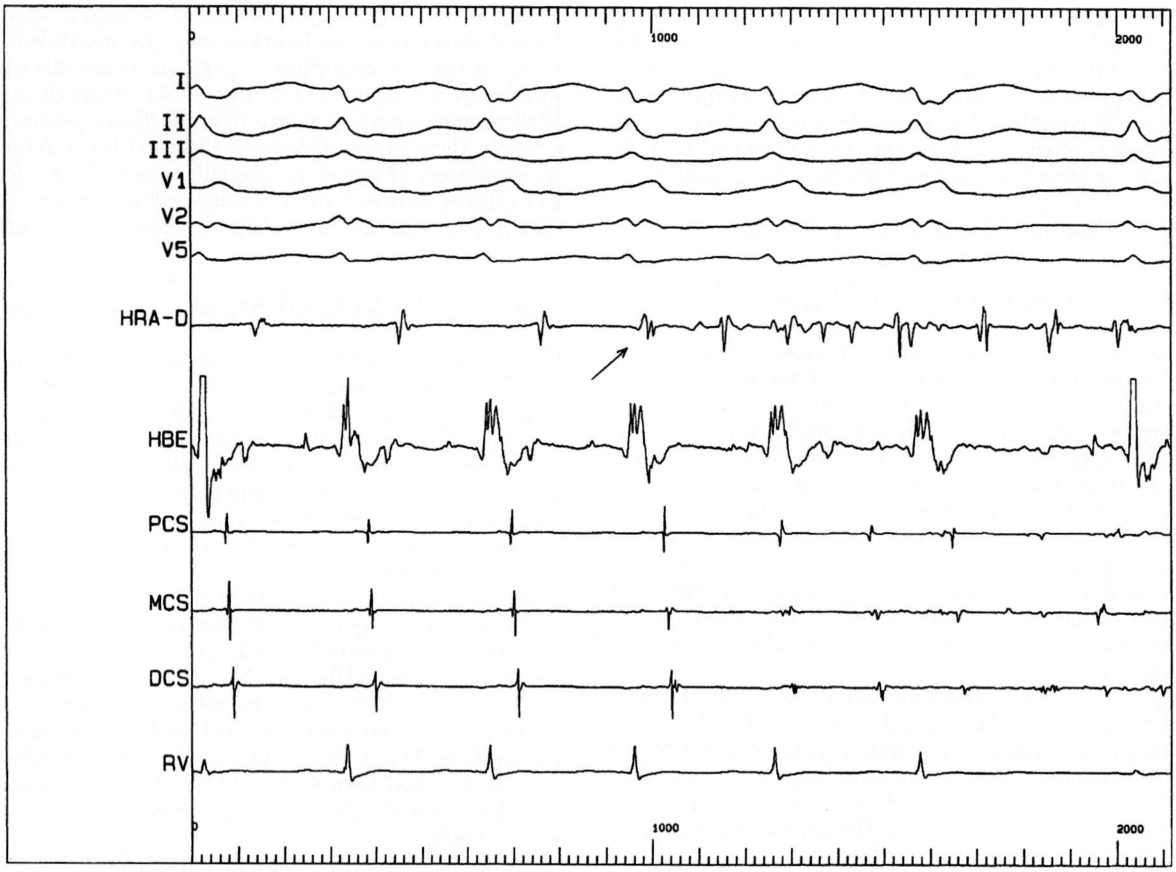

FIGURE 63.2. Patient with atrioventricular reentry using a left-sided accessory pathway in which atrioventricular reentry degenerates to atrial fibrillation. The arrow shows the earliest disorganization in the high right atrial electrogram, positioned near the junction of the right atrium and the superior vena cava. DCS, distal coronary sinus; HBE, bundle of His electrogram; HRA-D, high right atrium-distal; MCS, midcoronary sinus; PCS, proximal coronary sinus; RV, right ventricle.

Atrioventricular Conduction

In the absence of an accessory pathway, AV conduction occurs over the AV node during atrial fibrillation. The resultant ventricular rate depends on the intrinsic conduction and refractoriness of the AV node, the rate and organization of atrial inputs to the AV node, and the state of autonomic tone (53). There are two distinct atrial inputs to the AV node, anteriorly via the interatrial septum and posteriorly via the crista terminalis. Experiments in a rabbit AV nodal preparation demonstrated that propagation of impulses during AF through the AV node to the bundle of His is critically dependent on the relative timing of activation of septal inputs to the AV node at the crista terminalis and interatrial septum (54). Other investigators showed that the ventricular response also depended on atrial input frequency (55,56). Concealed AV node conduction likely plays the predominant role in determining ventricular response during AF (55,57).

Alterations of autonomic tone can have profound effects on AV nodal conduction (58–60). Enhanced parasympathetic and sympathetic tone have negative and positive dromotropic effects, respectively, on AV nodal conduction. This can be seen in Figure 63.3, in which shows recordings of AF during the awake state and during sleep. Note the substantial slowing of ventricular response, even with pauses, during sleep, a state in which there is heightened parasympathetic and decreased sympathetic tone.

Aberrant ventricular conduction commonly occurs during AF. It is important to distinguish aberrant conduction from ventricular ectopy, especially when repetitive wide QRS complexes occur. The refractoriness of the His-Purkinje tissue decreases as the heart rate increases (61). Thus, slower heart rates favor aberrancy. The gross irregularity of ventricular response during AF yields an abundance of RR cycle lengths, which statistically increases the chance for a long-short cycle length combination that will produce aberrant conduction. This phenomenon was described well by Gouaux and Ashman ("Ashman phenomenon") (62) and Lewis (63) and confirmed experimentally by Moe and coworkers (64). Figure 63.4 shows an example of right-bundle-branch (RBB) block aberrancy during atrial flutter/fibrillation initiated during electrophysiologic study. RBB aberrancy results from the sudden lengthening of the preceding cycle length (long–short sequence), which prolongs RBB refractoriness. RBB block aberrancy is more common than left-bundle-branch block aberrancy, probably because the RBB has a longer refractory period at slower heart rates (65). To complicate matters further, it has been demonstrated that cycle lengths preceding the pause may also affect the chance for aberrancy after the pause (66). It is important to differentiate between aberrant ventricular conduction and ventricular tachycardia when repetitive wide QRS complexes occur during AF. This can usually be accomplished by careful analysis of the rhythm strip and application of certain guidelines (Table 63.2) (61,67–69).

The presence of a grossly irregular, very rapid, wide QRS complex ventricular response during AF with rare exceptions is diagnostic of conduction over an accessory pathway (Fig. 63.5). At very fast heart rates, a tendency toward regularization

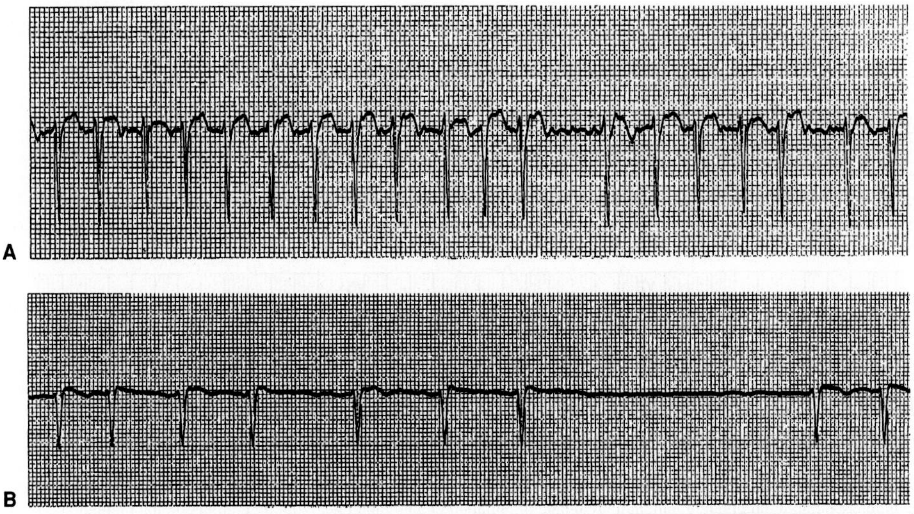

FIGURE 63.3. Effect of autonomic tone on atrioventricular node conduction during atrial fibrillation. **Top:** Relatively rapid ventricular response during the awake state. **Bottom:** Slow ventricular response recorded during sleep.

of the RR intervals is present, but careful measurement always discloses definite irregularities. It would be rare for such rapid responses to result from conduction over the AV node, and the only other alternative is ventricular tachycardia. It is axiomatic that rapid, irregular ventricular tachycardia is unstable and quickly degenerates into ventricular fibrillation. Thus, when a rapid, irregular, wide QRS complex tachycardia is noted in a patient who has a reasonably stable hemodynamic state, preexcitation is the most likely diagnosis. The ability to conduct rapidly over an accessory pathway is determined primarily by the intrinsic conduction and refractory properties of the accessory pathway. However, as with AV node conduction, factors such as spatial and temporal characteristics of atrial wavefronts during atrial fibrillation, autonomic tone, and concealed conduction influence activation over the accessory pathway (70–72).

TABLE 63.2

FACTORS FAVORING ABERRANT VENTRICULAR CONDUCTION

Long–short cycle length sequence
Typical right-bundle-branch block
Relatively rapid ventricular rate
Lack of compensatory pause
Absence of bundle branch block with shorter cycle length without preceding pause
Normalization of QRS complexes with minimal change in cycle length

CLINICAL PROFILE

Associated Disease States

AF has been reported to occur in patients with a wide variety of diseases, many of which are listed in Table 63.3. Why a particular disease results in AF is often unclear. In some cases—for example, hypertension—both occur with increased frequency in the elderly, and it is possible that a cause-and-effect relationship does not always exist. However, echocardiographic studies of left atrial function in patients who have hypertension have demonstrated that patients with paroxysmal AF had left atrial enlargement and depression of atrial contractile function associated with an increased ventricular inflow during early diastole (73). Hypertension is also associated with PV dilation (74). In patients with mitral valve disease with progressive enlargement of the atria, a pathophysiologic link between the disease state and the onset of AF is more obvious.

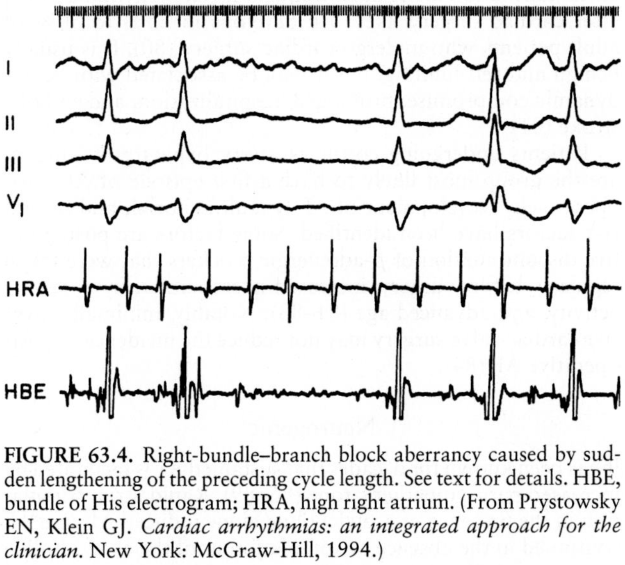

FIGURE 63.4. Right-bundle–branch block aberrancy caused by sudden lengthening of the preceding cycle length. See text for details. HBE, bundle of His electrogram; HRA, high right atrium. (From Prystowsky EN, Klein GJ. *Cardiac arrhythmias: an integrated approach for the clinician.* New York: McGraw-Hill, 1994.)

Thyrotoxicosis

Thyroid hormone affects the circulatory system and myocardium (75). There is an increase in sinus rate and a reduction in the electrical threshold for excitation of the atrium. AF is not uncommonly associated with thyrotoxicosis, is more frequent among men than among women, and increases with age, being rare in patients younger than 40 years. Although exclusion of occult thyrotoxicosis as a cause for AF is recommended, situations in which it is the cause are very uncommon (76). An increased risk of arterial thromboembolism is seen in association with thyrotoxicosis, mandating use of warfarin in patients with AF until a euthyroid state and sinus rhythm are achieved. The dose of warfarin necessary to maintain an INR of 2.0 to 3.0 may be smaller initially because of increased plasma clearance of vitamin K–dependent clotting factors, and a higher dose may be necessary as the thyroid hormone concentration decreases (75).

Congenital Heart Disease

Atrial fibrillation is relatively common in two forms of congenital heart disease, atrial septal defect and Ebstein's anomaly. In

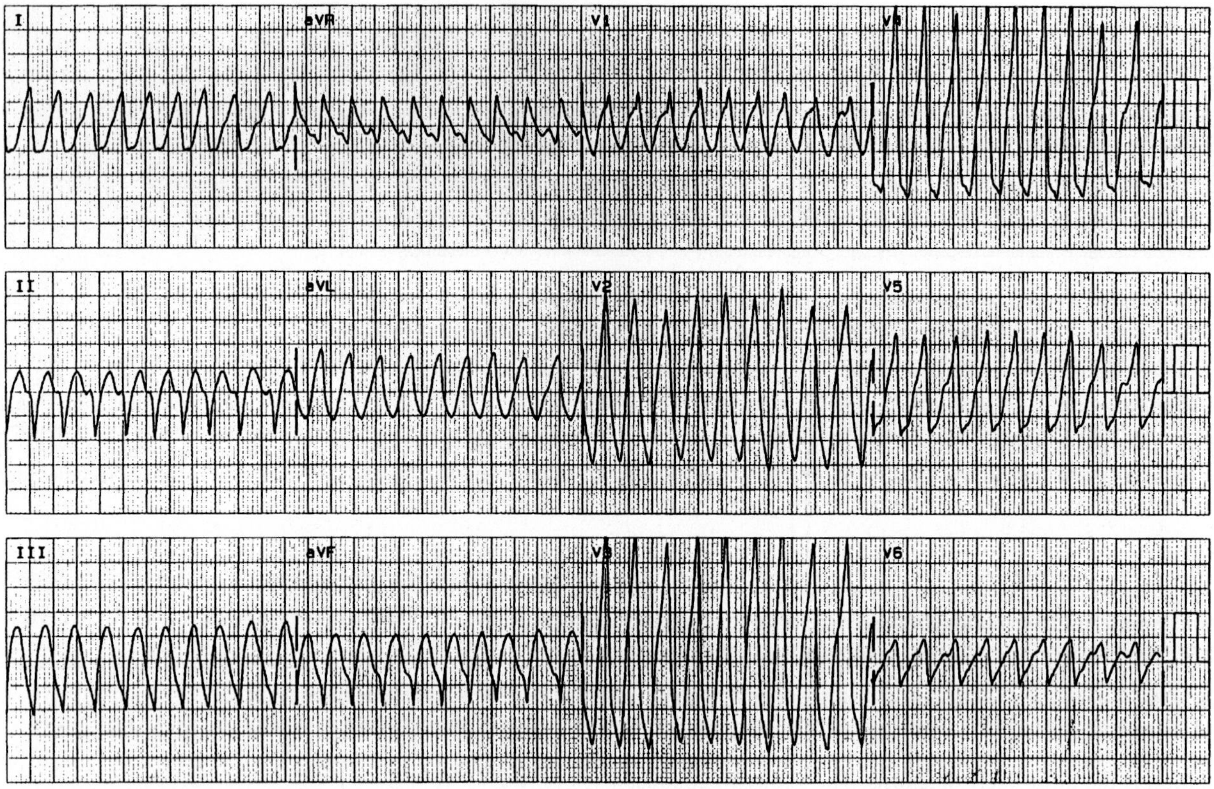

FIGURE 63.5. Twelve-lead electrocardiogram in a patient with ventricular preexcitation during atrial fibrillation who had a rapid preexcited ventricular response.

patients with atrial septal defect, the incidence of AF is greater as patients age and has been reported to be more than 50% in a study involving patients aged 60 years or older (77). In general, the incidence of AF begins to increase in the fourth decade of life.

Ebstein's anomaly is commonly associated with AF, often at an early age (78). Atrial fibrillation may be caused by the underlying atrial dysfunction or, more commonly, may be a consequence of concomitant WPW. In patients who have WPW and AV reentry, atrial fibrillation is relatively common and most often secondary to degeneration of AV reentry into atrial fibrillation (41). Among patients who underwent surgical ablation of the accessory pathway and were followed up for 6.2 years, AF was documented in 42% of the patients before surgery, and this was reduced to 9% postoperatively (79). Thus, in patients with Ebstein's anomaly, the most significant etiologic factor for AF appears to be concomitant WPW.

TABLE 63.3

FACTORS ASSOCIATED WITH ATRIAL FIBRILLATION

Hypertension
Coronary heart disease
Cardiomyopathy
Dilated
Hypertrophic
Mitral valve disease
Stenosis
Regurgitation
Thyrotoxicosis
Sick sinus syndrome
Congenital heart disease
Atrial septal defect
Ebstein's anomaly
Cardiac surgery
Pericarditis
Tumors
Alcohol
Lung disease
Neurogenic
Tachycardia-induced tachycardia
Lone (idiopathic)

Cardiac Surgery

Atrial fibrillation is the most frequent atrial arrhythmia noted after cardiac surgery. New AF develops in 25% to 50% of adult patients who undergo cardiac surgery (80). It is usually benign and self-limiting, but it may be associated with hemodynamic compromise, prolonged hospitalization, and embolic stroke (81).

Patients undergoing coronary artery bypass graft surgery are the group most likely to have a first episode of AF postoperatively. Development of AF is multifactorial, and several risk factors have been identified. Some factors are postoperative discontinuation of β-adrenergic blockers that were taken regularly before surgery, increased postoperative sympathetic activity, and advanced age (81–83). Notably, minimally invasive cardiac valve surgery may not reduce the incidence of postoperative AF (84).

Neurogenic

It has been known for decades that sustained AF is facilitated by increased parasympathetic tone (85–89). Rapid atrial stimulation in the presence of acetylcholine alone induced AF, and AF continued in the absence of stimulation until the acetylcholine infusion was discontinued (88). A nonuniform distribution of vagal effects on atrial refractoriness was found in another study (90). In the control state, right atrial refractoriness differed by no more than 40 ms between various sites, but during vagal stimulation there was marked shortening of atrial refractoriness at some sites and minimal change at others. Because dispersion of refractoriness can increase the likelihood of reentry, this may be one mechanism by which heightened vagal tone facilitates the initiation of AF.

In some patients, AF occurs during periods of enhanced vagal tone. The patient's clinical history usually provides clues for this mechanism. For example, onset of AF during swallowing of a cold substance (e.g., ice cream or an ice cube) indicates that a vagal reflex may initiate AF. A specific syndrome of vagal AF has also been described (91), with occurrence at time of heightened vagal tone such as at night, during rest, or after consumption of food or alcohol. Reportedly, patients with vagal AF have an increased number of attacks during therapy involving β-blockers and digitalis (91), although this is not well substantiated. Although many patients relate a tendency toward more episodes of AF during periods of presumed increased vagal tone, in our experience, it is rare for patients to have AF only during times of enhanced parasympathetic tone.

An adrenergic form of AF has also been described (91), with onset exclusively during the daytime hours and often preceded by emotional stress or exercise. In contrast to vagal AF, β-adrenergic blockers are the treatment of choice.

Tachycardia-Induced Tachycardia

Tachycardia-induced tachycardia is a phenomenon in which one tachycardia degenerates into another tachycardia (41). A relatively common example is rapid ventricular tachycardia that degenerates into ventricular fibrillation. Several different tachycardias can degenerate into AF (41). Atrial flutter and atrial tachycardia are likely the most common causes of tachycardia-induced tachycardia that result in AF, but arrhythmias as diverse as ventricular tachycardia, AV node reentry, and AV reentry may also initiate atrial fibrillation (Fig. 63.2) (41,92–94). In WPW, transition of AV reentry into AF can produce dire consequences, with a rapid preexcited ventricular response that degenerates into ventricular fibrillation leading to sudden death (Fig. 63.6) (61,95–98).

Identification of the role of tachycardia-induced tachycardia as a mechanism for AF has important therapeutic implications. It presents an opportunity for the clinician to prevent further episodes of AF, not by treating AF itself, but by directing therapy at the initiating arrhythmia. The paradigm for this is ablation of an accessory pathway in a patient with AV reentry.

Lone (Idiopathic) Atrial Fibrillation

Certain patients have no clear etiologic factors that explain the presence of AF; in such patients, the condition is called *idiopathic* or *lone atrial fibrillation*. Our definition for lone AF is the absence of any potential etiologic factor and the lack of evidence of ventricular dysfunction on echocardiography (15). We do not use an age cutoff point to designate lone AF. The prevalence of lone AF depends on the population of patients studied, as demonstrated in Table 63.1.

Awareness of lone AF has existed for decades (11,99–102). Because normal atria should not spontaneously fibrillate, some anatomic or electrophysiologic milieu must allow emergence of AF in these patients. In some cases, autonomic perturbations may be the etiology and likely are transient in nature. In other patients, left atrial size is increased, even though ventricular function is normal, and these patients may have some unidentified anatomic pathophysiologic basis for AF.

Familial Atrial Fibrillation

Lone AF can be familial, but the ionic mechanisms underlying this are not well understood (103). In a series from Spain, 50 of 132 family members presented with AF (103). The majority of the individuals were asymptomatic. Linkage analysis identified the locus of chromosome 10q22 (104). Two defects with a gain in function in the potassium channel were found in Chinese families (105,106). This could explain the shortened atrial refractoriness. Another locus on chromosome 6q14 to 6q16 has been identified (107).

Definition of Atrial Fibrillation

Traditionally, AF has been termed *paroxysmal* or *chronic atrial fibrillation*. However, no standardization regarding these

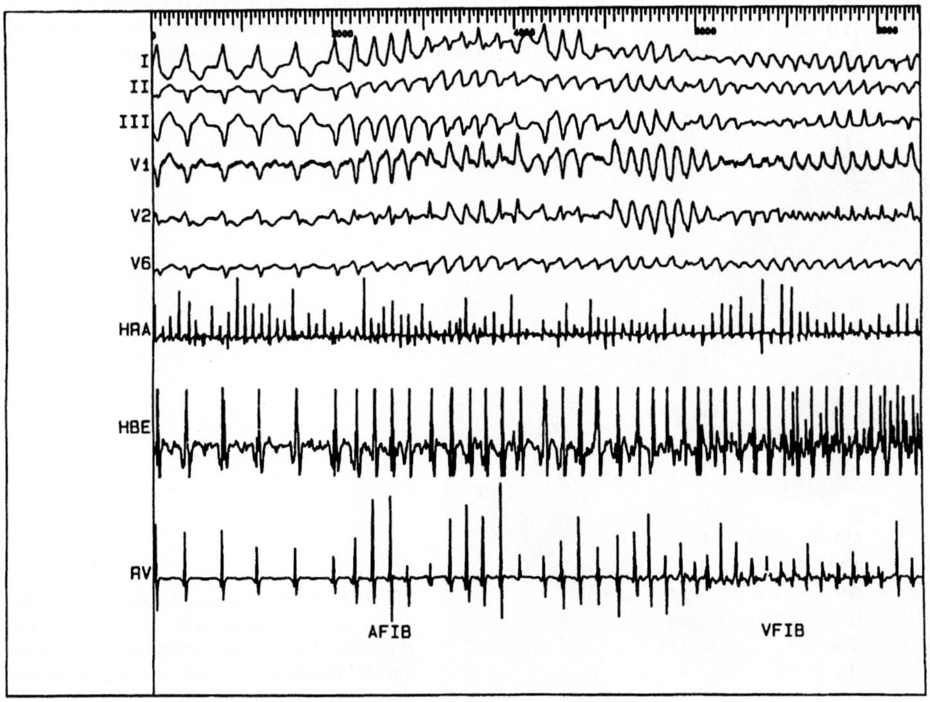

FIGURE 63.6. Atrial fibrillation in a patient with Wolff-Parkinson-White syndrome with degeneration from atrial fibrillation to ventricular fibrillation. AFIB, atrial fibrillation; HBE, bundle of His electrogram; HRA, high right atrium; RV, right ventricle; VFIB, ventricular fibrillation. (From Prystowsky EN, Knilans TK, Evans JJ. Diagnostic evaluation and treatment strategies for patients at risk for serious cardiac arrhythmias. II. Ventricular tachyarrhythmias and Wolff-Parkinson-White syndrome. *Mod Concepts Cardiovasc Dis* 1991;60:55.)

terms has been achieved, and quite disparate time frames have been proposed for each category. A new classification has been proposed by the American College of Cardiology (ACC)/American Heart Association (AHA)/European Society of Cardiology (ESC) guidelines for the management of patients with atrial fibrillation (100). Paroxysmal AF is self-terminating; persistent AF requires treatment for termination; in permanent AF, sinus rhythm cannot be restored, or the decision to avoid cardioversion has been made. Obviously, this system is not exact because there are often patients with paroxysmal AF who may have an occasional episode of persistent AF.

Symptoms of Atrial Fibrillation

Atrial fibrillation is associated with a diverse group of symptoms, palpitation being the most common (15,109). In one study that compared symptoms in patients with and without heart disease, palpitations occurred in 59% of patients with heart disease and in 77% of those with no heart disease ($p <$ .002) (15). Other frequent symptoms were presyncope, fatigue, and dyspnea, and less common symptoms were chest pain and syncope. AF often results in no symptoms, and patients with symptomatic AF typically have episodes without symptoms. Care should be taken in ascribing a specific symptom to the actual occurrence of AF because it is well documented that patients may have similar symptoms in the presence of sinus rhythm (109,110). Patients who experience dizziness, presyncope, or syncope may have associated carotid sinus hypersensitivity or neurally mediated syncope (111,112).

Why AF occurs at a particular point in time is unclear. In some patients, the onset may be related to a relative increase in parasympathetic tone, as demonstrated by an increased prevalence at night (113). Because patients with AF can have asymptomatic recurrences (114), it is possible that AF occurs even more frequently at night. In certain individuals, the reason for onset of AF is more obvious, for example, an alcoholic binge. For the majority of patients, no specific time of day, level of activity, or obvious inciting factor underlies each occurrence of AF, and initiation is likely multifactorial.

Electrocardiography of Atrial Fibrillation

During atrial fibrillation, electrocardiography demonstrates a lack of clearly defined P waves, with an undulating baseline that may alternate between recognizable atrial activity and a nearly flat line (Fig. 63.3). The ventricular response is irregular, and the rate depends on multiple factors, including intrinsic AV nodal conduction properties, level of parasympathetic and sympathetic tone, and the presence of negative dromotropic drugs such as β-adrenergic blockers, calcium channel blockers, and digitalis. The underlying atrial rate is typically greater than 300 beats per minute, but it may vary considerably at different sites in the atria. The electrocardiographic appearance at any moment depends on the predominant underlying atrial activation, which is often protean.

Echocardiography

An echocardiogram is an important test to obtain in patients with AF. It allows evaluation of atrial size, right and left ventricular function, and the presence of valvular lesions. Echocardiography, especially transesophageal echocardiography, has been valuable in investigating atrial function in patients with atrial fibrillation (44,47,48). Transesophageal echocardiography, but not transthoracic echocardiography, can provide valuable information on the presence of atrial thrombi, typically in the left atrial appendage (Fig. 63.7) (115–118). Atrial thrombi have been detected in as many as 15% of patients before cardioversion. It is important to noted new thrombi can occur after successful cardioversion and may cause embolic events (116). Thus, at least two mechanisms are possible for thromboembolism after cardioversion: dislodgment of a preexisting thrombus and formation of a new thrombus after cardioversion.

Wolff-Parkinson-White Syndrome

Atrial fibrillation in patients who have preexcitation can result in ventricular fibrillation and sudden cardiac death. This sequence of events occurs most commonly when a rapid preexcited ventricular response is present (Fig. 63.5), and degeneration to ventricular fibrillation may follow (Fig. 63.6). In our opinion, patients with ventricular preexcitation who have symptoms suggestive of tachycardia or documented arrhythmias should undergo electrophysiologic evaluation and, if indicated, endocardial catheter ablation of the accessory pathway. A more difficult situation exists for asymptomatic patients who have ventricular preexcitation during sinus rhythm (119).

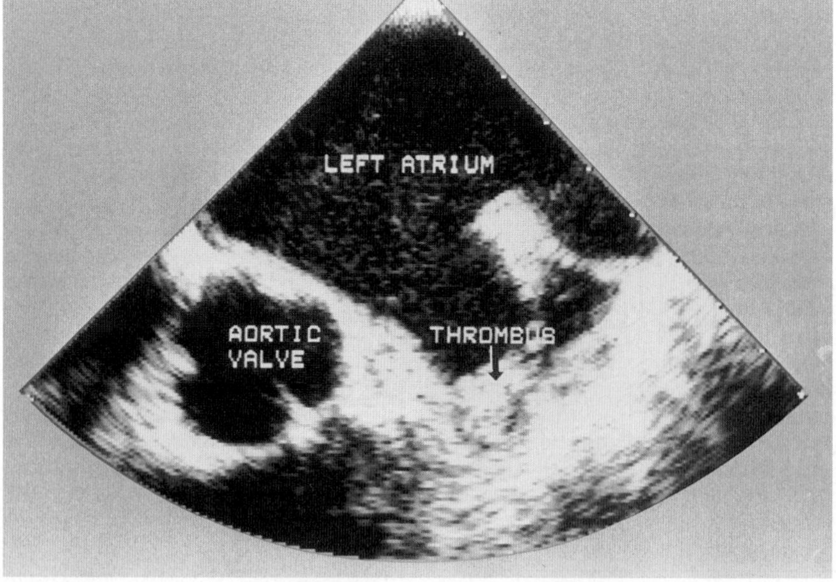

FIGURE 63.7. Transesophageal echocardiogram demonstrating left atrial appendage thrombus (*arrow*). (Courtesy of Drs. J. Bates and J. Steinmetz, the Care Group, St. Vincent Hospital, Indianapolis, IN.)

Some of these patients may be at risk for sudden cardiac death, although this is rarely the initial presentation of WPW. Because patients resuscitated from ventricular fibrillation invariably have a preexcited RR interval seen on electrophysiologic study during induced AF that is, at its shortest, less than 250 ms, the possibility for screening asymptomatic patients to detect those at risk for ventricular fibrillation exists (119). In general, we do not favor mass screening of asymptomatic patients who have ventricular preexcitation. Instead, we tend to screen patients who have a familial history of sudden death or tachycardia, patients who are considering competitive athletics, or individuals who are in certain occupations (e.g., airline pilots).

Hypertrophic Cardiomyopathy

Approximately 15% of patients with hypertrophic cardiomyopathy develop AF (120). In these individuals, AF can result in profound hemodynamic deterioration, leading to chest pain, presyncope, syncope, and even sudden cardiac death (120–122). In one retrospective study, the acute onset of AF resulted in deterioration by at least one New York Heart Association functional class in the majority of patients (120). It is important to note that the mean values for maximal left ventricular wall thickness may be lower among patients with AF than in patients with sinus rhythm (123). Thus, prediction of which patients are most likely to develop AF using analysis of ventricular wall thickness may not be possible. The weight of clinical data strongly suggests that efforts should be directed at maintaining sinus rhythm in these individuals to avoid functional deterioration and the possibility of sudden cardiac death.

THERAPY OF ATRIAL FIBRILLATION: GENERAL PRINCIPLES

There are three potential therapeutic goals of treatment for patients with AF (124). These include restoration and maintenance of sinus rhythm, rate control during AF, and prevention of thromboembolism. The decision to try to maintain sinus rhythm rather than use ventricular rate control should be individual to each patient, based on analysis of the risk–benefit ratio for that individual. Factors to consider are the severity of symptoms, type and duration of AF, patient age, presence of cardiovascular disease or other medical conditions, projected duration of therapy, and pharmacologic and nonpharmacologic options. For example, an elderly patient with minimal symptoms and years of persistent AF is an ideal candidate for a rate control and anticoagulation treatment strategy. Alternatively, a young patient with very symptomatic episodes of paroxysmal AF should be considered initially for a rhythm control treatment strategy (125).

Although maintenance of sinus rhythm may be desirable in many patients, it is not always easy to achieve and can be associated with proarrhythmia (126). The increasing success of catheter ablation to cure AF has added substantially to our armamentarium of therapies to maintain sinus rhythm (127). Nontraditional antiarrhythmic drugs may also be useful to maintain sinus rhythm, particularly those modulating the renin–angiotensin system (128–132). This is an exciting area of research with encouraging preliminary data, but large randomized trial data are not yet available. Statin-type cholesterol-lowering drugs also appear to be useful in the treatment of AF (108), but the evidence is very preliminary and not as strong as the data on angiotensin-converting-enzyme inhibitors or angiotensin-receptor blockers.

Rate versus Rhythm Control

Several randomized controlled trials have compared rate versus rhythm control treatment strategies for patients with AF (125,135–139). One important observation is that in patients at high risk for stroke, long-term anticoagulation is required regardless of whether a rhythm or rate control strategy is selected (125). Many asymptomatic patients receiving antiarrhythmic drugs to maintain sinus rhythm have recurrent unrecognized episodes of AF, which could lead to left atrial thrombus development and stroke in the absence of anticoagulation treatment.

There was no difference in mortality between the rhythm and rate control strategies (125,135–139). The Atrial Fibrillation Follow-Up Investigation of Rhythm Management (AFFIRM) trial was the largest study and contributed about 78% of the total number of patients enrolled in the five studies. The mean follow-up in AFFIRM was 3.5 years; thus, only short-term follow-up data are available. Most of the patients were in their late 60s, and persistent AF predominated. Few patients had lone AF. Although primary endpoints varied substantially among the studies, only the AFFIRM trial was sufficiently powered to evaluate all-cause mortality. Amiodarone was the only drug used in all five studies, and a variety of other drugs were used in different trials. In the rate control group β-blockers, calcium channel blockers, and digoxin, alone and in combination, were typically used. In total, these studies highlighted a lack of any advantage for rhythm control versus rate control in terms of quality of life, mortality, hospitalizations, or other endpoints. Thus, clinicians should individualize their approach and select the treatment strategy that is best for each patient.

Pharmacologic Therapy

Use of Intravenous Agents to Restore Sinus Rhythm

Intravenous verapamil, digitalis, esmolol, and propranolol are not useful for terminating AF (9,140–142). An exception might be the use of (β-adrenergic blockers in patients after cardiac surgery. In general, drugs that alter atrial electrophysiologic properties are useful for terminating AF (Table 63.4).

Procainamide

In one study, 9 of 21 patients converted to sinus rhythm while receiving procainamide at a mean dose of 13.3 ± 3.6 mg/kg (143). The range of duration of AF among patients who converted was 2 hours to 1 day. In another investigation, patients who converted to sinus rhythm had a shorter mean duration of AF than did patients who did not convert (6 ± 7 days vs. 79 ± 88 days; $p < .01$) (144). Among patients with AF of less than 24 hours' duration, 92% were converted to sinus rhythm when intravenous flecainide was administered, compared with 65% who converted when intravenous procainamide was administered (145).

Ibutilide

Ibutilide prolongs refractoriness by enhancing an inward sodium current during the plateau, although it also may block outward potassium current (146). It may increase the QT interval, and torsades de pointes can occur with its use. It is effective for converting AF to sinus rhythm (147–149). The typical recommended dose is 1.0 mg administered over 10 minutes, which can be repeated if AF does not terminate during or within 10 minutes after the end of the initial infusion. The dose can be adjusted downward for patients who weigh less than 60 kg.

TABLE 63.4

ACUTE DRUG THERAPY (INTRAVENOUS [IV]) FOR ATRIAL FIBRILLATION

Drug	Dosage
To decrease ventricular response[a]	
Verapamil	5–10 mg IV over the course of 2 min; additional 3–10 mg IV every 4–6 h for rate control
Diltiazem	0.25 mg/kg IV over the course of 2 min; if response is inadequate, a second dose of 0.35 mg/kg over the course of 2 min may be given 15 min later; bolus may be followed with constant infusion of ≤ 10 mg/h for rate control.
Propranolol	1 mg/min IV to total dose of 0.15 mg/kg or 12 mg total; additional 1-mg doses as needed for control of heart rate
Esmolol	Initial load of 500 μg/kg/min IV for 1 min followed by 50 μg/kg/min for 4 min; if response is inadequate, then repeat in 5 min with 500 μg/kg/min for 1 min and 100 μg/kg/min for 4 min; continue to titrate every 5 min until desired heart rate is reached; 50–200 μg/kg/min is usual maintenance dose
Digoxin	0.5–1.0 mg IV followed by 0.25 mg every 2–4 h, with total 24-h dose <1.5 mg
For pharmacologic conversion to sinus rhythm	
Procainamide	50 mg/min IV to total dose of 10–14 mg/kg
Ibutilide	1 mg IV over the course of 10 min; may repeat if atrial fibrillation is present after 20 min

[a] Avoid use of this agent in patients with ventricular preexcitation.

The conversion rate for AF in one study was 31%, and the success rate was higher among patients with shorter duration of AF (10 ± 13 days vs. 18 ± 15 days) (148). Torsades de pointes may be associated with ibutilide infusion, but typically occurs either during infusion or within a few hours after termination of the final ibutilide infusion. Thus, administration of ibutilide, as well as procainamide, should be performed under circumstances in which resuscitative measures can be readily performed.

Amiodarone

In some studies, the effectiveness of intravenous amiodarone was similar to that of placebo in restoring sinus rhythm (150,151), whereas other studies suggested that amiodarone has a more beneficial effect (152). Meta-analyses of the effectiveness of intravenous amiodarone in converting AF to sinus rhythm have given mixed results (153,154). Even if successful, it takes hours to work, and one should not expect success in the first few hours of administration. Intravenous amiodarone has the added effect of significantly slowing ventricular response. This can prove very useful when other agents, such as β-adrenergic blockers and slow calcium channel blockers, are relatively contraindicated.

Flecainide, Propafenone, Sotalol, and Dofetilide

Intravenous flecainide, propafenone, and sotalol are not available for use in the United States. Intravenous flecainide is very effective in converting AF to sinus rhythm (145,151,155,156). Intravenous propafenone is useful in converting recent-onset AF to sinus rhythm, but it is ineffective in patients in whom AF has lasted many months (157,158). Intravenous sotalol is minimally effective in converting AF to sinus rhythm (159). Intravenous dofetilide, which prolongs atrial refractoriness, appears to be useful in terminating AF (160–162).

Use of Oral Antiarrhythmic Agents for Restoration and Maintenance of Sinus Rhythm

A variety of antiarrhythmic drugs with disparate electrophysiologic actions can terminate or prevent AF. These include disopyramide, quinidine, procainamide, propafenone, flecainide, sotalol, dofetilide, amiodarone, and morizicine (163–187). The class IA agents quinidine, procainamide, and disopyramide have fallen out of favor and largely have been replaced by class IC and class III drugs. A single oral loading dose of 300 to 600 mg of propafenone or 200 to 300 mg of flecainide is successful in restoring sinus rhythm in more than 50% of selected patients with recent-onset atrial fibrillation (164,165). Recent data support a "pill in the pocket" treatment approach for oral propafenone and flecainide for terminating AF of recent onset outside the hospital after inpatient safety using these drugs has been demonstrated (188). Few comparative studies have assessed the efficacy of various agents in maintaining sinus rhythm during long-term follow-up. Overall, approximately 50% of patients maintain sinus rhythm for at least 6 months during antiarrhythmic therapy. Amiodarone is considered by some to be the most effective agent for drug-refractory recurrent AF, although few prospective comparative data are available (185). Amiodarone maintains sinus rhythm in nearly two thirds of patients for up to 1 year follow-up (177–180). Typically, amiodarone has been associated with frequent side effects, some life-threatening (e.g., pulmonary toxicity). However, lower doses likely will decrease the risk of nuisance and serious side effects. In a study in which amiodarone was administered at 600 mg daily for 4 weeks, approximately 16% of patients converted to sinus rhythm (180). During long-term therapy, the mean dose was 204 mg, and sinus rhythm was maintained in 53% of patients after 3 years with minimal serious side effects (180).

The efficacy of antiarrhythmic drug therapy should not be judged solely on the basis of whether AF recurs during follow-up (124). Preventing all episodes of AF over the course of years of treatment is exceedingly difficult, and asymptomatic episodes occur in many patients. Therapeutic success should be based on the reduction in frequency and duration of symptomatic episodes of AF and whether the patient feels markedly better with drug therapy. Recurrence of AF should not be equated with arrhythmias such as sustained ventricular tachycardia or ventricular fibrillation. An analogy can be made with treatment for angina or congestive heart failure. In both conditions, the need for occasional nitroglycerin use or an increase in diuretics, respectively, in patients who otherwise are well compensated is readily accepted.

Proarrhythmia

Proarrhythmia is the most serious side effect of antiarrhythmic drug therapy (9,126). Proarrhythmic events can be caused by tachyarrhythmias or bradyarrhythmias. Proarrhythmia caused by tachyarrhythmia is the most dangerous and life threatening, and torsades de pointes is the most frequently observed proarrhythmic event in this category (126). Torsade de pointes can occur during use of any drug that prolongs QT interval; amiodarone appears to have the lowest incidence among such agents. It has been postulated that early afterdepolarizations initiate torsades de pointes (126). Conditions that favor early afterdepolarizations are ventricular hypertrophy, slow heart rate, hypokalemia, and the presence of potassium channel blocking drugs, which commonly occur in patients with AF. Torsade de pointes is uncommon during AF in patients who have a relatively rapid ventricular response. It is more likely to emerge after restoration of sinus rhythm, with a resultant slower heart rate (126), which has been referred to as the "paradoxical risk of sinus rhythm for sudden cardiac death" (126). Other types of malignant ventricular arrhythmias can occur. Use of flecainide should be avoided in patients who have experienced myocardial infarction (189). Amiodarone and dofetilide do not appear to increase mortality in patients with congestive heart failure (184,190,191).

Bradyarrhythmias, including sinus nodal dysfunction and AV conduction disturbances, may also complicate antiarrhythmic drug therapy. One type of proarrhythmia, 1:1 AV conduction with conversion of AF to atrial flutter or tachycardia, is clearly preventable. This more frequently occurs with drugs such as propafenone and flecainide, which can markedly slow atrial tachycardia rates. It is important to prescribe concomitant AV nodal blocking agents to avoid this complication, especially for patients who are receiving propafenone or flecainide (124). Administration of concomitant AV nodal blocking agents is not necessary when sotalol or amiodarone is used because these agents substantially decrease conduction through the AV node.

Antiarrhythmic Drug Selection

Reversible causes of AF (e.g., excess alcohol intake) should be considered and treated if possible. Correction of electrolyte abnormalities and cardiovascular problems such as heart failure need to be addressed before an antiarrhythmic agent is administered. Prophylactic drug therapy typically is not necessary for patients who have experienced a single detected episode of AF or for patients who have infrequent, transient, and well-tolerated paroxysmal AF.

Every effort should be made to minimize the chance for proarrhythmia and other drug side effects. Antiarrhythmic drug therapy should be initiated in the hospital for patients who have heart disease, especially for patients with a history of congestive heart failure (9,124). Outpatient initiation of therapy appears to be reasonable for individuals who have normal QT intervals and no or minimal heart disease. Because no antiarrhythmic drug has been shown conclusively to be superior to other agents, selection of initial drug therapy is based more on avoidance of serious side effects than on predicted efficacy. Figure 63.7 shows a slight modification of the ACC/AHA/ESC management guideline scheme (108) for choosing initial and subsequent antiarrhythmic agents to prevent AF. For patients who have lone AF, we prefer to use drugs that have minimal organ toxicity; initial choices are flecainide, propafenone, and sotalol. For patients who have congestive heart failure, amiodarone and dofetilide are our treatments of choice. Sotalol, dofetilide, and amiodarone are our initial selections for patients who have coronary artery disease (192–194). Patients with hypertension and left ventricular hypertrophy may be at increased risk for torsades de pointes because hypertrophied ventricles appear more prone to develop early afterdepolarizations (126). Thus, we prefer to start with flecainide or propafenone. If a patient has substantial left ventricular hypertrophy, use of flecainide and propafenone carries concerns about an increased proarrhythmic risk, and we prefer to use amiodarone. Noteworthy is the use of catheter ablation as second-line treatment in all categories, as discussed in more detail later (108).

Use of Drug Therapy to Control Ventricular Rate

In the absence of ventricular preexcitation, drugs that decrease conduction in the AV node are useful in controlling ventricular rate in patients who have AF (Table 63.4). It is very important to control ventricular rate, not only to decrease symptoms, but also to prevent tachycardia-mediated ventricular cardiomyopathy. Drugs that depress conduction and prolong refractoriness in the AV node include digoxin, β-adrenergic antagonists, and calcium channel blockers (9,141,142,195–199). It is notable that the electrophysiologic effects of digoxin on the AV node are indirect and depend on an intact autonomic nervous system (200). Thus, whereas digoxin may slow ventricular response at rest, it is relatively ineffective in controlling the ventricular rate during exercise (201). β-Adrenergic blockers and calcium channel blockers are preferred over digoxin for rate control in patients who have not experienced heart failure (9). β-Adrenergic blockers are also recommended in situations in which sympathetic tone is increased, such as thyrotoxicosis (9). In patients who have congestive heart failure, digitalis is the first-line treatment (9). As noted previously, both sotalol and amiodarone may be used as monotherapy because they depress conduction through the AV node. In some patients, control of ventricular response can be facilitated with the use of combination drug therapy, for example, digoxin and a calcium channel blocker or a β-adrenergic blocker. In this situation, rate control may be achieved without undue side effects.

In patients who have WPW, control of the rapid preexcited ventricular response requires the use of agents that depress conduction over the accessory pathway. In the acute setting, intravenous procainamide and ibutilide are the treatments of choice, unless the patient is unstable and requires urgent electrical cardioversion. The use of drugs such as digoxin, calcium channel blockers, β-adrenergic blockers, and adenosine are contraindicated in this situation. They do not block conduction over the accessory pathway and may accelerate the ventricular response, resulting in a potentially very unstable clinical situation.

Treatment of Atrial Fibrillation after Cardiac Surgery

Drugs with antisympathetic activity such as sotalol, amiodarone, and β-adrenergic blockers are the best treatments

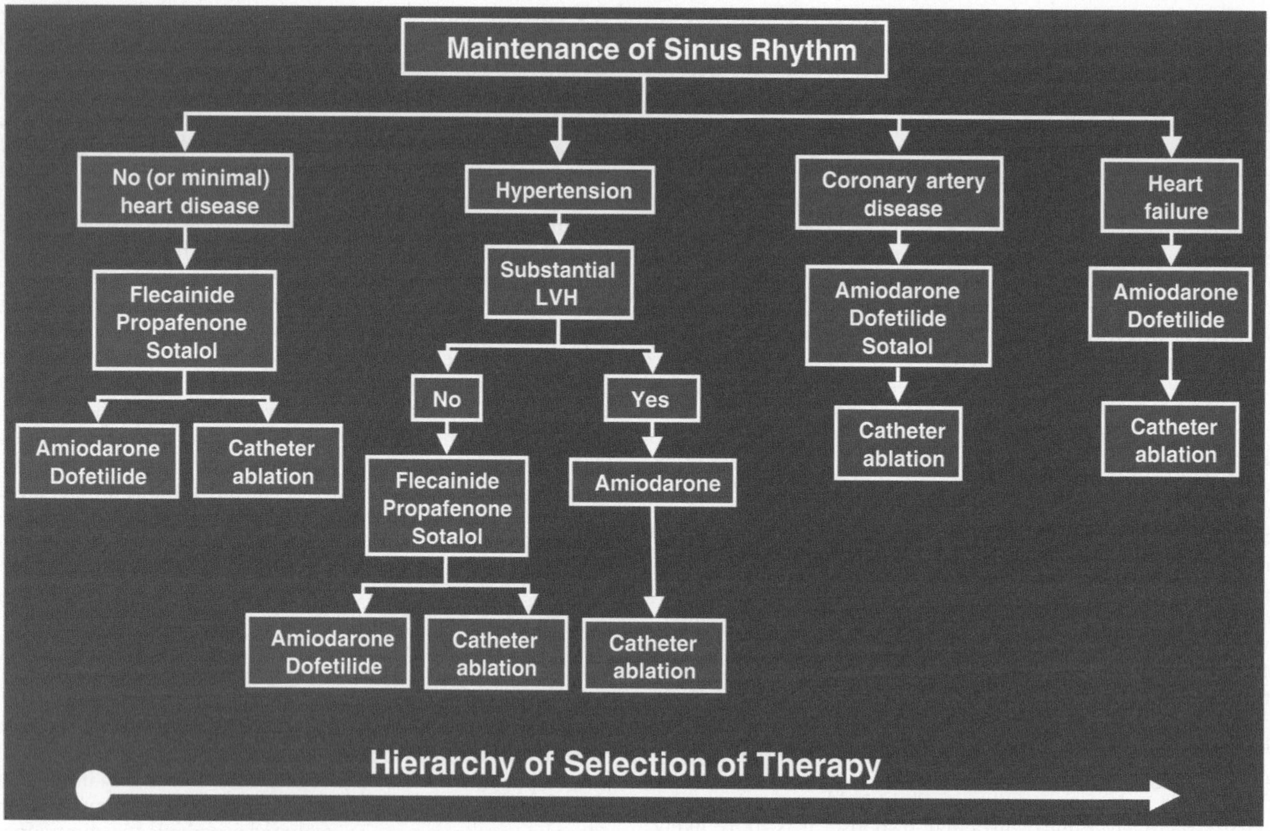

FIGURE 63.8. Therapeutic options for maintenance of sinus rhythm in patients with atrial fibrillation. See text for details. LVH, left ventricular hypertrophy. (Modified from Fuster V, Ryden LE, et al. ACC/AHA/ESC guidelines for the management of patients with atrial fibrillation. In press.)

available for prevention of AF after cardiac surgery, with β-blockers being initial therapy if possible (81,201–205). In a randomized, controlled study, sotalol demonstrated superiority to placebo in prevention of AF (206). Administration of intravenous amiodarone 1 g/day for 2 days starting immediately after cardiac surgery reduced the incidence of postoperative AF compared with placebo (207). Administration of oral amiodarone starting at least 1 week before surgery may also decrease postoperative AF (208).

The optimum approach to treating AF in the postoperative period is unclear. In most patients who experienced no preoperative AF, AF is a transient arrhythmia and typically is not a long-term problem (209). If simple measures such as administration of β-adrenergic blockers do not prevent AF, additional therapy can be pursued to restore and maintain sinus rhythm or merely to control the ventricular response. In the latter situation, the use of anticoagulation therapy should be based on established therapy for nonsurgical situations because no randomized, controlled clinical trial data are available for the postoperative AF patient (210). The patient should be reevaluated 4 to 6 weeks after surgery.

PREVENTION OF THROMBOEMBOLISM

Prevention of stroke is key to the management of the condition of patients with AF. A hypercoagulable state appears to exist in patients with AF (211,212). A high stroke risk has been well described for years in patients with AF and mitral stenosis or prosthetic mitral valves. Several prospective multicenter, randomized clinical trials have conclusively demonstrated that warfarin is highly effective in reducing the incidence of ischemic stroke among patients with AF (108). Overall, a combined risk reduction of 68% is seen.

Independent predictors of thromboembolic risk have been identified (100). High-risk patients have a 5% to 7% or greater yearly risk of thromboembolism. Highest-risk variables from prospective trials include a history of hypertension, prior stroke or transient ischemic attack, recent heart failure or ejection fraction less than 35%, and age greater than 75 years (108). It is notable that paroxysmal AF has not been found to be an independent predictor of thromboembolic risk. Other studies have considered coronary artery disease, diabetes, as well as age older than 65 years to place a patient at moderate to high risk for stroke. At present, highest-risk patients who can receive anticoagulation therapy should be treated with warfarin, with the INR adjusted to between 2.0 and 3.0. Similar therapy is recommended for patients with accumulation of moderate risk factors (108). Patients older than 75 years should be observed carefully because bleeding complications increase in elderly patients. Anticoagulation should not be discontinued because of apparent lack of AF recurrence—most patients have asymptomatic AF episodes and they are still at risk for thromboembolism. Patients with AF who have low risk for stroke may be treated with aspirin daily (108). Patients with lone atrial fibrillation who are younger than 60 years do not require specific therapy for prevention of thromboembolism. Some physicians prescribe aspirin to this group of patients, but few data are available to support this approach. Recent guidelines offer more detailed information (108).

Anticoagulation for Cardioversion

Electrical and pharmacologic cardioversion can result in thromboembolism (9). Prior anticoagulation appears to decrease the risk of emboli (9,44,108,213,214). In patients who have AF of unknown duration or duration greater than 48 hours, current recommendations are to administer warfarin for 3 weeks before and 4 weeks after cardioversion, maintaining an INR of 2.0 to 3.0 (108). In high-risk patients, warfarin therapy should be continued on a long-term basis after cardioversion. In an alternative approach, transesophageal echocardiography (TEE) is used (108,115,118) (Figure 63.7). The use of TEE appears to offer an advantage to patients who are already hospitalized or in whom restoration of sinus rhythm is more urgent. Either approach is acceptable, and the one selected should be dictated by the clinical circumstances.

NONPHARMACOLOGIC THERAPY

Pharmacologic treatment has been used for decades for cardioversion and prevention of recurrent AF. Use of antiarrhythmic drugs is associated with substantial side effects and mortality in some groups of patients. Accordingly, it is not surprising that nonpharmacologic techniques for managing AF have been developed, including electrical cardioversion, radiofrequency catheter ablation procedures, atrial pacing methods to prevent AF, and surgery.

Electrical Cardioversion

Transthoracic Electrical Cardioversion

The technique of transthoracic direct current (DC) electrical cardioversion of atrial fibrillation was developed by Lown and associates (215). Although any patient who has AF may be a candidate for transthoracic DC cardioversion, certain characteristics predict immediate success and long-term maintenance of sinus rhythm. The best candidates are patients without mitral valve disease or a very large left atrium and patients who have AF of relatively short duration. Early echocardiographic studies suggested that there was minimal possibility of achieving or maintaining sinus rhythm when the anterior–posterior diameter of the left atrium was greater than 4.5 cm (216). In contrast, a randomized study showed that the size of the left atrium was not related to the success of cardioversion or to recurrence of AF (217). No universally accepted threshold value exists for left atrial size or severity of mitral stenosis that would preclude attempts at cardioversion. It is our policy to attempt cardioversion at least once in most patients with AF in whom we think sinus rhythm would be preferable. Exceptions might be individuals known to have had AF for many years or elderly patients with no or minimal symptoms with AF.

Antiarrhythmic drugs are frequently used to maintain sinus rhythm in patients undergoing transthoracic direct current (DC) cardioversion. Drug therapy should be considered before use of cardioversion in patients with long-standing AF (e.g., >3 months), to lessen the chance of early recurrence of AF in the first few days after cardioversion. Digitalis therapy is not a contraindication to elective cardioversion, although it is customary to withhold digoxin on the day of cardioversion, a custom that is based on few scientific data. On the other hand, attempts to cardiovert arrhythmias associated with digitalis toxicity are hazardous and should be avoided (218). Concomitant antiarrhythmic drug therapy may increase energy requirements for successful cardioversion (219).

Success of transthoracic DC cardioversion in restoring sinus rhythm depends on several technical factors (220). The optimal electrode size is 12 to 13 cm in diameter. Initial electrode placement is right anterior–left posterior or left anterior–left posterior. If cardioversion with these electrode orientations is unsuccessful, a right anterior–apical electrode position can be tried. The clinician must be flexible and willing to try several electrode orientations. Application of firm pressure to the anterior electrode during full expiration may facilitate delivery of current to the heart. The use of biphasic shocks (221) has led to few failures to restore sinus rhythm in our experience. Appropriate anesthesia is mandatory before shock delivery.

Catheter Ablation

Atrioventricular Block

For some patients who have permanent AF, drug therapy used to control ventricular response is either ineffective or not tolerated. An alternative approach is endocardial catheter ablation of the AV junction that results in complete heart block (222,223). Such patients require a permanent rate-responsive pacemaker. This technique can also be used for treatment of patients who have transient or persistent AF in lieu of drugs that suppress AV node conduction. Improvement in exercise tolerance and quality of life has been demonstrated with this procedure (224). The recent demonstration of left ventricular dysfunction in some patients with long-term right ventricular pacing has dampened our enthusiasm for this therapy of "ablate and pace."

Maintenance of Sinus Rhythm

Based on the concept of multiple reentrant circuits and the success of the surgical maze procedure, the initial catheter ablation approach attempted to create a series of linear ablation lines in the right and left atrium to mimic the surgical maze approach (127,225). This technique had limited success and unacceptable complication rates. The seminal observation of Haissaguerre and colleagues (27) on the existence of pulmonary vein ectopy as a cause of AF switched the ablation approach to attempts to eliminate/isolate ectopic foci. Although the majority of focal sources of AF have been found within the pulmonary veins, other areas described are the left atrial posterior wall, superior vena cava, crista terminalis, vein of Marshall, coronary sinus, and interatrial septum (28,127,226).

Several left-atrial ablation techniques have been proposed to cure AF (227–230). Experienced operators are achieving about 80% success rates without drugs, but often more than one ablation attempt is needed. The highest success is with patients who have minimal heart disease and paroxysmal AF (127). Several serious and even life-threatening complications can occur with ablation of AF including stroke, cardiac perforation with tamponade, pulmonary vein stenosis, and atrioesophageal fistula (127). Nonetheless, in experienced hands the use of catheter ablation to cure AF has opened up new therapeutic vistas for patients with very symptomatic AF, and it is currently second-line therapy for patients with and without structural heart disease (108).

Surgery

The maze surgical procedure for treatment of AF was developed by Cox and associates (231). Multiple atrial incisions are made to direct sinus impulses through a path, or a "maze," to reach the AV node. The idea is to prevent formation of a critical mass of contiguous atrial tissue that would sustain AF. Furthermore, at least some atrial contractility is maintained. The maze operation is often successful. Alternative operations are the left atrial isolation technique, the "corridor" operation, and simple encircling of the pulmonary veins (232–234). However, surgery for AF as a primary indication is infrequently used. We have found it useful for patients with AF who are undergoing other cardiac surgery. Because the left atrial appendage is the usual site of thrombus, we recommend removal of this structure in patients undergoing other cardiac surgery, especially if the patient has a history of AF.

Cardiac Pacing

Cardiac pacing in AF has been prescribed in the past for patients with concomitant bradycardia. Two other important issues should be considered: the impact of pacing mode on development of AF and the role of permanent pacing in preventing AF.

Antibradycardia Pacing

Ventricular pacing, with or without rate-adaptive mode, is used in patients with permanent AF who have symptomatic bradycardia. Patients with sick sinus syndrome commonly develop AF, and there has been much debate on whether atrial-based or ventricular-based pacing is preferred for these patients. Two large, randomized clinical trials compared dual-chamber atrial-based pacing with single-chamber ventricular pacing (235–237). The combined enrollment was more than 4,500 patients, and atrial-based pacing showed a relative reduction in the risk of AF that ranged from 18% to 23%. The difference in the incidence of AF emerged only at 2 years. No difference in total mortality, mortality from cardiovascular causes, or stroke was observed.

A randomized, prospective study of 225 consecutive patients with sick sinus syndrome compared atrial pacing (AAI) to ventricular pacing (VVI) (238). After a follow up of 8 years, atrial pacing was associated with less AF, 14% in the AAI group versus 23% in the VVI group ($p = .012$).

A randomized, prospective study compared single-chamber pacing with dual-chamber pacing in elderly patients (mean age 80 years) with high-grade atrioventricular block (239). Dual-chamber pacing did not reduce the rate of death from all causes or from cardiovascular causes, not did it decrease the incidence of AF, myocardial infarction, congestive heart failure, stroke, transient ischemic attack, or other thromboembolism.

In summary, we feel that the data support physiologic pacing for patients with AF and sick sinus syndrome. Efforts should be made to program the device to minimize the amount of ventricular pacing when atrioventricular conduction is intact.

Role of Permanent Pacing in Preventing Atrial Fibrillation

Many pacemakers and implantable defibrillators have features designed to prevent AF and to try to terminate AF with rapid atrial pacing. The evidence to support their use is limited, although these algorithms appear to be safe and usually add little additional cost. For patients who have a bradycardia indication for pacing and also have AF, no consistent data from large randomized trials support the use of alternative single-site atrial pacing, multisite right atrial pacing, biatrial pacing, overdrive pacing, or antitachycardia atrial pacing. Even fewer data support the use of atrial pacing in the management of AF in patients without symptomatic bradycardia. At present, permanent pacing to prevent AF is not a stand-alone indication for pacing (240).

CONTROVERSIES AND PERSONAL PERSPECTIVES

Sinus Rhythm versus Rate Control

Since the publication of the AFFIRM trial, many physicians feel that it is fine, and even preferable, to start with a rate control strategy for AF therapy in lieu of attempting to restore sinus rhythm. We do not agree with this concept, and the data from AFFIRM do not address this for many patients. The AFFIRM patient population was nearly 70 years old and had risk factors for stroke. Many screened patients were excluded because either the patient or physician thought sinus rhythm was needed. Thus, for younger patients data on relative benefits or risks of rate versus rhythm treatment strategies are meager. For this reason, it is very important to decide which treatment method is best for each patient and not depend on data gathered for a very different patient group.

First-Line Therapy for Catheter Ablation for Curing Atrial Fibrillation

Remarkable advances have been made in the technique of radiofrequency catheter ablation for curing AF. Very experienced operators have very good success rates, often requiring more than one procedure. Major complications have lessened in the hands of such electrophysiologists, to about 1% to 2%. We agree with not listing ablation as first-line therapy in the 2006 ACC/AHA/ESC AF management guidelines. One important reason is that the more numerous less-experienced ablators have far less ablation success and more frequent serious complications. Guidelines need to consider the overall community of electrophysiologists, and until the technique enjoys excellent success rates with minimal complications for a wide range of ablators, it will remain a second-line treatment option. However, we feel that this is relative, and there will be patients in whom catheter ablation is preferable to drug therapy, for example, in a patient in whom the only drug option is long-term amiodarone therapy.

THE FUTURE

In the next few years there will be advances in the technique for catheter ablation for curing AF, and this will enable ablation to gain a foothold as a first-line treatment option. There could be large-scale clinical trials testing the effectiveness of atrial-selective drugs in maintaining sinus rhythm. The usefulness of left atrial appendage occlusive devices in preventing stroke and avoiding warfarin therapy should be better understood. Randomized trial data on the value of antagonists of the renin–angiotensin system in minimizing AF episodes will be available. More therapeutic approaches may be discovered as one travels further into the future. For example, the ionic mechanism for AF may become known in familial AF, and this could lead to tailored molecular-based treatments. The role of the autonomic nervous system in the genesis of AF will be uncovered, and this could lead to more treatment strategies.

ACKNOWLEDGMENTS

The authors thank Mary Kay Franklin for her superb secretarial assistance in the preparation of this chapter and Jane Gilmore for her superb artwork.

References

1. Rosner F, trans. and ed. *Maimonides' medical writings*. Haifa, Israel: The Maimonides Research Institute, 1989.
2. Stokes W. *The Diseases of the heart and the aorta*. Dublin: Hodges and Smith, 1854.
3. Wenckebach KF. *Arrhythmia of the heart: a physiological and clinical study*. Edinburgh: William Green and Sons, 1904.
4. Cushny AR. On the interpretation of pulse-tracings. *J Exp Med* 1899;4:327–347.
5. MacKenzie J. The interpretation of the pulsations in the jugular veins. *Am J Med Sci* 1907;134:12–34.
6. Rothberger CJ, Winterberg H. Vorhofflimmern and arrhythmia perpetua. Wein Klin Wochenschr 1909;22:839–844.

7. Lewis T. Auricular fibrillation and its relationship to clinical irregularity of the heart. *Heart* 1910;1:306–372.
8. Einthoven W. Le telecardiogramme, *Arch Internat Physiol* 1908;4:132–164.
9. Prystowsky EN, Benson DW, Fuster V, et al. Management of patients with atrial fibrillation: a statement for healthcare professionals from the Subcommittee on Electrocardiography and Electrophysiology, American Heart Association. *Circulation* 1996;93:1262–1277.
10. Bialy D, Lehmann MH, Schumacher DN, et al. Hospitalization for arrhythmias in the United States: importance of atrial fibrillation. *J Am Coll Cardiol* 1992;19:41A.
11. Parkinson J, Campbell M. Paroxysmal auricular fibrillation: a record of two hundred patients. *QJM* 1930;67–100.
12. Kannel WB, Abbott RD, Savage DD, et al. Epidemiologic features of chronic atrial fibrillation: the Framingham study. *N Engl J Med* 1982;306:1018–1022.
13. Davidson E, Weinberger I, Rotenberg Z, et al. Atrial fibrillation: cause and time of onset. *Arch Intern Med* 1989;149:457–459.
14. Lok NS, Lau CP. Presentation and management of patients admitted with atrial fibrillation: a review of 291 cases in a regional hospital. *Int J Cardiol* 1995;48:271–278.
15. Prystowsky EN, Margiotti R, Fogel RI, et al. Atrial fibrillation with and without heart disease: clinical characteristics and proarrhythmia risk. *Circulation* 1996;94(8):I:191.
16. Godtfresen J. Atrial fibrillation: cause and prognosis—a follow-up study of 1212 cases. In: Kulbertus HE, Olsson SB, Schlepper M, eds. *Atrial fibrillation*. Sweden: AB Hassle, 1982.
17. Wolf PA, Abbott RD, Kannel WB. Atrial fibrillation as an independent risk factor for stroke: the Framingham Study. *Stroke* 1991;22:983–988.
18. Wolf PA, Abbott RD, Kannel WB: Atrial fibrillation: a major contributor to stroke in the elderly. The Framingham Study. *Arch Intern Med* 1987; 147:1561–1564.
19. Yater WM. Pathologic changes in auricular fibrillation and in allied arrhythmias. *Arch Intern Med* 1929;43:808–838.
20. Hudson REB. The human pacemaker and its pathology. *Br Heart J* 1960;22: 153–167.
21. Davies MJ, Pomerance A. Pathology of atrial fibrillation in man. *Br Heart J* 1972;34:520–525.
22. Frustaci A, Chimenti C, Bellocci F, et al. Histological substrate of atrial biopsies in patients with lone atrial fibrillation. *Circulation* 1997;96:1180–1184.
23. Maixent JM, Paganelli F, Scaglione J, et al. Antibodies against myosin in sera of patients with idiopathic paroxysmal atrial fibrillation. *J Cardiovasc Electrophysiol* 1998;9:612–617.
24. Scherf D, Romano FJ, Terranova R. Experimental studies on auricular flutter and auricular fibrillation. *Am Heart J* 1948;36:241.
25. Scherf D, Schaffer AI, Blumenfeld S. Mechanism of flutter and fibrillation. *Arch Intern Med* 1953;91:333–352.
26. Jais P, Haissaguerre M, Shah DC. A focal source of atrial fibrillation treated by discrete radiofrequency ablation. *Circulation* 1997;95:572–576.
27. Haissaguerre M, Jais P, Shah DC, et al. Spontaneous initiation of atrial fibrillation by ectopic beats originating in the pulmonary veins. *N Engl J Med* 1998;339:659–666.
28. Chen SA, Tai CT, Yu WC, et al. Right atrial focal atrial fibrillation: electrophysiologic characteristics and radiofrequency catheter ablation. *J Cardiovasc Electrophysiol* 1999;10:328–335.
29. Tsai CF, Tai CT, Hsieh MH, et al. Initiation of atrial fibrillation by ectopic beats originating from the superior vena cava: electrophysiological characteristics and results of radiofrequency ablation. *Circulation* 2000;102:67–74.
30. Hsu LF, Jais P, Keane D, et al. Atrial fibrillation originating from persistent left superior vena cava. *Circulation* 2004;109:828–832.
31. Lin WS, Tai CT, Hsieh MH, et al. Catheter ablation of paroxysmal atrial fibrillation initiated by non–pulmonary vein ectopy. *Circulation* 2003;107: 3176–3183.
32. Schmitt C, Ndrepepa G, Weber S, et al. Biatrial multisite mapping of atrial premature complexes triggering onset of atrial fibrillation. *Am J Cardiol* 202;89:1381–1387.
33. Nathan H, Eliakim M. The junction between the left atrium and the pulmonary veins: an anatomic study of human hearts. *Circulation* 1966;34: 412–422.
34. Cheung DW. Pulmonary vein as an ectopic focus in digitalis-induced arrhythmia. *Nature* 1981;294:582–584.
35. Jais P, Hocini M, Macle L, et al. Distinctive electrophysiological properties of pulmonary veins in patients with atrial fibrillation. *Circulation* 2002; 106:2479–2485.
36. Takahashi Y, Iesake Y, Takahashi A, et al. Reentrant tachycardia in pulmonary veins of patients with paroxysmal atrial fibrillation. *J Cardiovasc Electrophysiol* 2003;14:927–932.
37. Mansour M, Mandapati R, Berenfeld O, et al. Left-to-right gradient of atrial frequencies during acute atrial fibrillation in the isolated sheep heart. *Circulation* 2001;103:2631–2636.
38. Moe GK, Abildskov JA. Atrial fibrillation as a self-sustaining arrhythmia independent of focal discharge. *Am Heart J* 1959;58:59–70.
39. Moe GK, Rheinboldt WC, Abildskov JA. A computer model of atrial fibrillation. *Am Heart J* 1964;67:200–220.
40. Allessie MA, Lammers WJEP, Bonke FIM, et al. Experimental evaluation of Moe's multiple wavelet hypothesis of atrial fibrillation. In: Zipes DP, Jalife J, eds. *Cardiac arrhythmias*. New York: Grune & Stratton, 1985:p.265–276.
41. Prystowsky EN. Tachycardia-induced tachycardia: a mechanism of initiation of atrial fibrillation. In: DiMarco JP, Prystowsky EN, eds. *Atrial arrhythmias: state of the art*. Armonk, NY: Futura, 1995.
42. Bharati S, Lev M. Histology of the normal and diseased atrium. In: Falk RH, Podrid PJ, eds. *Atrial fibrillation: mechanisms and management*. New York: Raven Press, 1992.
43. Spach MS, Boineau JP. Microfibrosis produces electrical load variations due to loss of side-to-side cell connections: a major mechanism of structural heart disease arrhythmias. *Pacing Clin Electrophysiol* 1997;20(Pt II):397–413.
44. Prystowsky EN. Management of atrial fibrillation: simplicity surrounded by controversy. *Ann Intern Med* 1997;126:244–246.
45. Sanfilippo AJ, Abascal VM, Sheehan M, et al. Atrial enlargement as a consequence of atrial fibrillation. *Circulation* 1990;82:792–797.
46. Gosselink AT, Grijns HJ, Hamer HPM, et al. Changes in left and right atrial size after cardioversion of atrial fibrillation: role of mitral valve disease. *J Am Coll Cardiol* 1993;22:1666–1672.
47. Manning WJ, Silverman DI, Katz SE, et al. Impaired left atrial mechanical function after cardioversion: relation to the duration of atrial fibrillation. *J Am Coll Cardiol* 1994;23:1535–1540.
48. Mitusch R, Garbe M, Schmucker G, et al. Relation of left atrial appendage function to the duration and reversibility of nonvalvular atrial fibrillation. *Am J Cardiol* 1995;75:944–947.
49. Wijiffels MC, Kirchhof CJ, Dorland R, et al. Atrial fibrillation begets atrial fibrillation: a study in awake chronically instrumented goats. *Circulation* 1995;92:1954–1968.
50. Daoud EG, Bogun F, Goyal R, et al. Effect of atrial fibrillation on atrial refractoriness in humans. *Circulation* 1996;94:1600–1606.
51. Yue L, Feng J, Gaspo R, et al. Ionic remodeling underlying action potential changes in a canine model of atrial fibrillation. *Circ Res* 1997;81:512–525.
52. Nattel S. New ideas about atrial fibrillation 50 years on. *Nature* 202;415: 219–226.
53. Prystowsky EN. Atrioventricular node reentry: physiology and radiofrequency ablation. *Pacing Clin Electrophysiol* 1997;20(Pt II)):552–571.
54. Mazgalev T, Dreifus LS, Bianchi J, et al. Atrioventricular nodal conduction during atrial fibrillation in rabbit heart. *Am J Physiol* 1982;243:H754–H760.
55. Moe GK, Abildskov JA. Observations on the ventricular dysrhythmia associated with atrial fibrillation in the dog heart. *Circ Res* 1964;14:447–460.
56. Chorro FJ, Kirchhof CJ, Brugada J, et al. Ventricular response during irregular atrial pacing and atrial fibrillation. *Am J Physiol* 1990;259:H1015–H1021.
57. Langendorf R, Pick AL, Katz LN. Ventricular response in atrial fibrillation: role of concealed conduction in the AV junction. *Circulation* 1965;32:69–75.
58. Prystowsky EN, Page RL. Electrophysiology and autonomic influences of the human atrioventricular node. In: LS Dreifus, T Mazgalev, EL Michaelson, eds. *Electrophysiology of the sino-atrial and atrioventricular nodes*. New York: Alan R. Liss, 1988:259–277.
59. Page RL, Tang ASL, Prystowsky EN. Effect of continuous enhanced vagal tone on atrioventricular nodal and sinoatrial nodal function in humans. *Circ Res* 1991;68:1614–1620.
60. Page RL, Wharton JM, Prystowsky EN. Effect of continuous vagal enhancement on concealed conduction and refractoriness within the atrioventricular node. *Am J Cardiol* 1996;77:260–265.
61. Prystowsky EN, Klein GJ. *Cardiac arrhythmias: an integrated approach for the clinician*. New York: McGraw-Hill, 1994.
62. Gouaux JL, Ashman R. Auricular fibrillation with aberration simulating ventricular paroxysmal tachycardia. *Am Heart J* 1947;34:366–373.
63. Lewis T. *The mechanism and graphic registration of the heart beat*, 3rd ed. London: Shaw & Sons, 1925:256.
64. Moe GK, Mendez C, Han J. Aberrant A-V impulse propagation in the dog heart: a study of functional bundle branch block. *Circ Res* 1965;16:261.
65. Chilson DA, Zipes DP, Heger JJ, et al. Functional bundle branch block: discordant response of right and left bundle branches to changes in heart rate. *Am J Cardiol* 1984;54(3):313–316.
66. Denker S, Shenasa M, Gilbert CJ, et al. Effects of abrupt changes in cycle length on refractoriness of the His-Purkinje system in man. *Circulation* 1983;67:60.
67. Pick A, Langendorf R. *Interpretation of complex arrhythmias*. Philadelphia: Lea & Febiger, 1979.
68. Pritchett ELC, Smith WM, Klein GJ, et al. The "compensatory pause" of atrial fibrillation. *Circulation* 1980;62:1021–1025.
69. Miles WM, Prystowsky EN. Alteration of human right bundle branch refractoriness by changes in atrial drive train duration. *Circulation* 1986;73: 244–248.
70. Ong JJC, Cha YM, Kriett JM, et al. The relation between atrial fibrillation wavefront characteristics and accessory pathway conduction. *J Clin Invest* 1995;96:2284–2296.
71. Prystowsky EN, Pritchett ELC, Gallagher JJ. Concealed conduction preventing anterograde preexcitation syndrome. *Am J Cardiol* 1991;53:960–961.

72. Chen PS, Prystowsky EN. Role of concealed and supernormal conduction during atrial fibrillation in the preexcitation syndrome. *Am J Cardiol* 1991;68:1329–1334.
73. Barbier P, Alioto G, Guazzi MD. Left atrial function and ventricular filling in hypertensive patients with paroxysmal atrial fibrillation. *J Am Coll Cardiol* 1994;24:165–170.
74. Herweg B, Sichrovsky T, Polosajian L, et al. Hypertension and hypertensive heart disease are associated with increased ostial pulmonary vein diameter. *J Cardiovasc Electrophysiol* 2005;16:2–5.
75. Woeber KA. Thyrotoxicosis and the heart. *N Engl J Med* 1992;327:94–98.
76. Sawin CT, Geller A, Wolf PA, et al. Low serum thyrotropin concentrations as a risk factor for atrial fibrillation in older persons. *N Engl J Med* 1994; 331:1249–1252.
77. St John Sutton MG, Tajik AJ, McGoon DC. Atrial septal defect in patients ages 60 years or older: operative results and long-term postoperative follow-up. *Circulation* 1981;64:402–409.
78. Smith WM, Gallagher JJ, Ker CR, et al. The electrophysiologic basis and management of symptomatic recurrent tachycardia in patients with Ebstein's anomaly of the tricuspid valve. *Am J Cardiol* 1982;49:1223–1234.
79. Pressley JC, Wharton JM, Tang ASL, et al. Effect of Ebstein's anomaly outcome of surgically treated patients with Wolff-Parkinson-White syndrome. *Circulation* 1992;86:1147–1155.
80. Leitch JW, Thomason D, Baired DK, et al. The importance of age as a predictor of atrial fibrillation and flutter after coronary artery bypass grafting. *J Thorac Cardiovasc Surg* 1990;100:338–342.
81. Matangi MF, Neutze JM, Graham KJ, et al. Arrhythmia prophylaxis after aorta–coronary bypass: the effect of minidose propranolol. *J Thorac Cardiovasc Surg* 1985;89:439.
82. Kalman JM, Munawar M, Howes LG, et al. Atrial fibrillation after coronary bypass grafting is associated with sympathetic activity. *Ann Thorac Surg* 1995;60:1709–1715.
83. Matthew JP, Parks R, Savino JS, et al. Atrial fibrillation following coronary artery bypass graft surgery: predictors, outcome and resources utilization. Multicenter study of perioperative research group. *JAMA* 1996;276:300–306.
84. Asher CR, Chung K, Grimm RA, et al. Is the incidence of postoperative atrial fibrillation following cardiac valve surgery reduced by minimally invasive surgery? *Circulation* 1996;94(Pt I):380.
85. Lewis T, Drury AN, Bulger HA. Observations upon flutter and fibrillation. Part VII. The effects of vagal stimulation. *Heart* 1921;8:141–170.
86. Nahum LH, Hoff HE. Production of auricular fibrillation by application of acetyl-B-methylcholine chloride to localized regions on the auricular surface. *Am J Physiol* 1940;129:428.
87. Scherf D, Chick FB. Abnormal cardiac rhythms caused by acetylcholine. *Circulation* 1951;3:764–769.
88. Burn JH, Williams EMV, Walker JM. The effects of acetylcholine in the heart-lung preparation including the production of auricular fibrillation. *J Physiol* 1995;128:277–293.
89. Loomis TA, Krop S. Auricular fibrillation induced and maintained in animals by acetylcholine or vagal stimulation. *Circ Res* 1955;3:390–396.
90. Alessi R, Nusynowitz M, Abildskov JA, et al. Nonuniform distribution of vagal effects on the atrial refractory period. *Am J Physiol* 1958;194:406–410.
91. Coumel P. Neurogenic and humoral influences of the autonomic nervous system in the determination of paroxysmal atrial fibrillation. In: Atteul P, Coumel P, Janse MJ, eds. *The atrium in health and disease*. Mount Kisco, NY: Futura, 1989:213–232.
92. Hurwitz JL, German LD, Packer DL, et al. Occurrence of atrial fibrillation in patients with paroxysmal supraventricular tachycardia due to atrioventricular nodal entry. *Pacing Clin Electrophysiol* 1990;13:705–710.
93. Campbell RWF, Smith RA, Gallagher JJ, et al. Atrial fibrillation in the preexcitation syndrome. *Am J Cardiol* 1977;40:515–520.
94. Sung RJ, Castellanos A, Mallon SM, et al. Mechanisms of spontaneous alteration between reciprocating tachycardia and atrial flutter-fibrillation in the Wolff-Parkinson-White syndrome. *Circulation* 1977;56:409–416.
95. Klein GJ, Bashore TM, Sellers TD, et al. Ventricular fibrillation in the Wolff-Parkinson-White syndrome. *N Engl J Med* 1979;301:1080–1085.
96. Fananapazir L, Packer DL, German LD, et al. Procainamide infusion test: inability to identify patients with Wolff-Parkinson-White syndrome who are potentially at risk of sudden death. *Circulation* 1988;77:1291–1296.
97. Dreifus LS, Haiat R, Watanabe T, et al. Ventricular fibrillation: a possible mechanism of sudden death in patients with Wolff-Parkinson-White syndrome. *Circulation* 1971;43:520.
98. Prystowsky EN, Knilans TK, Evans JJ. Diagnostic evaluation and treatment strategies for patients at risk for serious cardiac arrhythmias. II. Ventricular tachyarrhythmias and Wolff-Parkinson-White syndrome. *Mod Concepts Cardiovasc Dis* 1991;60:55.
99. Lewis T. Auricular fibrillation and its relationship to clinical irregularity of the heart. *Heart* 1910;1:306–372.
100. Friedlander RD, Levine SA. Auricular fibrillation and flutter without evidence of organic heart disease. *N Engl J Med* 1934;211:624–629.
101. Hanson HH, Rutledge DI. Auricular fibrillation in normal hearts. *N Engl J Med* 1949;240:947–953.
102. Evans W, Swann P. Lone auricular fibrillation. *Br Heart J* 1954;16:189–194.
103. Brugada R. Is atrial fibrillation a genetic disease?. *J Cardiovasc Electrophysiol* 205;16:553–556.
104. Brugada R, Tapscott T, Czernuszewicz GZ, et al. Identification of a genetic locus for familial atrial fibrillation. *N Engl J Med* 1997;336:905–911.
105. Chen YH, Xu SJ, Bendahhou S, et al. KCNQ1 gain-of-function mutation in familial atrial fibrillation. *Science* 2003;299:251–254.
106. Yang Y, Xia M, Jin Q, et al. Identification of a KCNE2 gain-of-function mutation in patients with familial atrial fibrillation. *Am J Hum Genet* 2004; 75:899–905.
107. Ellinor PT, Shin JT, Moore RK, et al. Locus for atrial fibrillation maps to chromosome 6q14–16. *Circulation* 2003;107:2880–2883.
108. Fuster V, Ryden LE, et al. ACC/AHA/ESC guidelines for the management of patients with atrial fibrillation. In press.
109. Bhandari AK, Anderson JL, Gilbert EM, et al. Correlation of symptoms with occurrence of paroxysmal supraventricular tachycardia or atrial fibrillation: a transtelephonic monitoring study. Flecainide Supraventricular Tachycardia Study Group. *Am Heart J* 1992;124:381–386.
110. Fogel RI, Evans JJ, Prystowsky EN. Utility and cost of event recorders in the diagnosis of palpitations, presyncope and syncope. *Am J Cardiol* 1997;79:207–208.
111. Cicogna R, Mascioli G, Bonomi FG, et al. Carotid sinus hypersensitivity and syndrome in patients with chronic atrial fibrillation. *Pacing Clin Electrophysiol* 1994;17:1635–1640.
112. Brignole M, Gianfranchi L, Menozzi C, et al. Role of autonomic reflexes in syncope associated with paroxysmal atrial fibrillation. *J Am Coll Cardiol* 1993;22:1123–1129.
113. Rostagno C, Taddei T, Paladini B, et al. The onset of symptomatic atrial fibrillation and paroxysmal supraventricular tachycardia is characterized by different circadian rhythms. *Am J Cardiol* 1993;71:453–455.
114. Page RL, Wilkinson WE, Clair WK, et al. Asymptomatic arrhythmias in patients with symptomatic paroxysmal atrial fibrillation and paroxysmal supraventricular tachycardia. *Circulation* 1994;89:224–227.
115. Manning WJ, Silverman DI, Keighley CS, et al. Transesophageal echocardiographically facilitated early cardioversion from atrial fibrillation using short-term anticoagulation: final results of a prospective 4.5-year study. *J Am Coll Cardiol* 1995;25:1354–1361.
116. Fatkin D, Kuchar DL, Thorburn CW, et al. Transesophageal echocardiography before and during direct current cardioversion of atrial fibrillation: evidence for "atrial stunning" as a mechanism of thromboembolic complications. *J Am Coll Cardiol* 1994;23:307–316.
117. Grimm RA, Stewart WJ, Maloney JD, et al. Impact of electrical cardioversion for atrial fibrillation on left atrial appendage function and spontaneous echo contrast: characterization by simultaneous transesophageal echocardiography. *J Am Coll Cardiol* 1993;22:1359–1366.
118. Klein AL, Grimm RA, Murray RD, et al. Use of transesophageal echocardiography to guide cardioversion in patients with atrial fibrillation. *N Engl J Med* 2001;344:1411–1420.
119. Klein GJ, Prystowsky EN, Yee R, et al. Asymptomatic Wolff-Parkinson-White: should we intervene? *Circulation* 1989;80:1902–1905.
120. Robinson K, Frenneaux MP, Stockins B, et al. Atrial fibrillation in hypertrophic cardiomyopathy: a longitudinal study. *J Am Coll Cardiol* 1990;15: 1279–1285.
121. Stafford WJ, Trohman RG, Bilsker M, et al. Cardiac arrest in an adolescent with atrial fibrillation and hypertrophic cardiomyopathy. *J Am Coll Cardiol* 1986;7:701–704.
122. Madariaga I, Carmona JR, Mateas FR, et al. Supraventricular arrhythmias as the cause of sudden death in hypertrophic cardiomyopathy. *Eur Heart J* 1994;15:134–137.
123. Spirito P, Lakatos E, Maron BJ. Degree of left ventricular hypertrophy in patients with hypertrophic cardiomyopathy and chronic atrial fibrillation. *Am J Cardiol* 1992;69:1217–1222.
124. Prystowsky EN. Management of atrial fibrillation: therapeutic options and clinical decisions. *Am J Cardiol* 2000;85:3D–11D.
125. Pelargonio G, Prystowsky EN: Rate versus rhythm control in the management of patients with atrial fibrillation. *Nat Clin Pract* 2005;2(10):514–521.
126. Prystowsky EN. Proarrhythmia during drug treatment of supraventricular tachycardia: paradoxical risk of sinus rhythm for sudden death. *Am J Cardiol* 1996;78(8A):35–41.
127. Padanilam BJ, Prystowsky EN: Atrial fibrillation–should ablation be first-line therapy and for whom: antagonist position. *Circulation* 2005;112(8): 1223–1229.
128. Madrid AH, Bueno MG, Rebollo JM, et al. Use of irbesartan to maintain sinus rhythm in patients with long-lasting persistent atrial fibrillation: a prospective and randomized study. *Circulation* 2002;106:331–336.
129. Webster MW, Fitzpatrick MA, Nicholls MG, et al. Effect of enalapril on ventricular arrhythmias in congestive heart failure. *Am J Cardiol* 1985;56: 566–569.
130. Zamen AG, Kearney MT, Schecter C, et al. Angiotensin-converting enzyme inhibitors as adjunctive therapy in patients with persistent atrial fibrillation. *Am Heart J* 2004;147:823–827.
131. Wachtell K, Lehto M, Gerdts E, et al. Angiotensin II receptor blockade reduces new-onset atrial fibrillation and subsequent stroke compared to atenolol: the Losartan Intervention For End Point Reduction in Hypertension (LIFE) study. *J Am Coll Cardiol* 2005;45:712–719.
132. Ueng KC, Tsai TP, Yu WC, et al. Use of enalapril to facilitate sinus rhythm

maintenance after external cardioversion of long-standing persistent atrial fibrillation. Results of a prospective and controlled study. *Eur Heart J* 2003; 24:2090–2098.
133. Siu CW, Lau CP, Tse HF. Prevention of atrial fibrillation recurrence by statin therapy in patients with lone atrial fibrillation after successful cardioversion. *Am J Cardiol* 2003;92:1343–1345.
134. Young-Xu Y, Jabbour S, Goldberg R, et al. Usefulness of statin drugs in protecting against atrial fibrillation in patients with coronary artery disease. *Am J Cardiol* 2003;92:1379–1383.
135. Hohnloser SH, Kuck KH, Lilienthal J, for the PIAF Investigators. Rhythm or rate control in atrial fibrillation—pharmacological intervention in atrial fibrillation (PIAF): a randomized trial. *Lancet* 2000;356:1789–1794.
136. The Atrial Fibrillation Follow Up Investigation of Rhythm Management (AFFIRM) Investigators. A comparison of rate control and rhythm control in patients with atrial fibrillation. *N Engl J Med* 2002;347:1825–1833.
137. Van Gelder IC, Hagen V, Bosker HA, et al., for the Rate Control Versus Electrical Cardioversion for Persistent Atrial Fibrillation Study Group. *N Engl J Med* 202;347:1834–1840.
138. Carlsson J, Miketic S, Windeler J, et al., for the STAF Investigators: Randomized trial of rate-control versus rhythm-control in persistent atrial fibrillation. The strategies of treatment of atrial fibrillation (STAF). *J Am Coll Cardiol* 2003;41:1690–1696.
139. Opolski G, Torbicki A, Kosior DA, et al., for the Investigators of the Polish HOT CAFE Trial. *Chest* 2004;126:476–486.
140. Falk RH, Knowlton AA, Bernard SA, et al. Digoxin for converting recent-onset atrial fibrillation to sinus rhythm: a randomized, double-blinded trial. *Ann Intern Med* 1987;106:503–506.
141. Salerno DM, Dias VC, Kleiger RE, et al. Efficacy and safety of intravenous diltiazem for treatment of atrial fibrillation and atrial flutter: the Diltiazem-Atrial Fibrillation/Flutter Study Group. *Am J Cardiol* 1989;63:1046–1051.
142. Rinkenberger RL, Prystowsky EN, Heger JJ, et al. Effects of intravenous and chronic oral verapamil administration in patients with supraventricular tachyarrhythmias. *Circulation* 1980;62:996–1010.
143. Halpern SW, Ellrodt G, Singh BN, et al. Efficacy of intravenous procainamide infusion in converting atrial fibrillation to sinus rhythm: relation to left atrial size. *Br Heart J* 1980;44:589–595.
144. Fenster PE, Comess KA, Marsh R, et al. Conversion of atrial fibrillation to sinus rhythm by acute intravenous procainamide infusion. *Am Heart J* 1983;106:501–504.
145. Madrid AH, Moro C, Marin–Huerta E, et al. Comparison of flecainide and procainamide in cardioversion of atrial fibrillation. *Eur Heart J* 1993;14: 1127–1131.
146. Roden DM. Ibutilide and the treatment of atrial arrhythmias. *Circulation* 1996;94:1499–1502.
147. Ellenbogen KA, Stambler BS, Wood MA, et al. Efficacy of intravenous ibutilide for rapid termination of atrial fibrillation and atrial flutter: a dose–response study. *J Am Coll Cardiol* 1996;28:130–136.
148. Stambler BS, Wood MA, Ellenbogen KA, et al. Efficacy and safety of repeated intravenous doses of ibutilide for rapid conversion of atrial flutter or fibrillation. Ibutilide Repeat Dose Study Investigators. *Circulation* 1996;94: 1613–1621.
149. Volgman AS, Carberry PA, Stambler B, et al. Conversion efficacy and safety of intravenous ibutilide compared with intravenous procainamide in patients with atrial flutter or fibrillation. *J Am Coll Cardiol* 1998;31:1414–1419.
150. Galve E, Rius T, Ballester R, et al. Intravenous amiodarone in treatment of recent-onset atrial fibrillation: results of a randomized, controlled study. *J Am Coll Cardiol* 1996;27:1079–1082.
151. Donovan KD, Power BM, Hockings BEF, et al. Intravenous flecainide versus amiodarone for recent–onset atrial fibrillation. *Am J Cardiol* 1995;75:693–697.
152. Faniel R, Schoenfeld PH. Efficacy of i.v. amiodarone in converting rapid atrial fibrillation and flutter to sinus rhythm in intensive care patients. *Eur Heart J* 1983;4:180–185.
153. Hilleman DE, Spinler SA. Conversion of recent-onset atrial fibrillation with intravenous amiodarone: a meta-analysis of randomized controlled trials. *Pharmacotherapy* 2002;22:66–74.
154. Miller MR, McNamara RL, Segal JB, et al. Efficacy of agents for pharmacologic conversion of atrial fibrillation and subsequent maintenance of sinus rhythm: a meta-analysis of clinical trials. *J Fam Pract* 2000;49:1033–1046.
155. Borgeat A, Goy JJ, Maendly R, et al. Flecainide versus quinidine for conversion of atrial fibrillation to sinus rhythm. *Am J Cardiol* 1986;58:496–498.
156. Suttorp MJ, Kingma JH, Jessurun ER, et al. The value of class IC antiarrhythmic drugs for acute conversion of paroxysmal atrial fibrillation or flutter to sinus rhythm. *J Am Coll Cardiol* 1990;16:1722–1727.
157. Bianconi L, Boccadamo R, Pappalardo A, et al. Effectiveness of intravenous propafenone for conversion of atrial fibrillation and flutter of recent onset. *Am J Cardiol* 1989;64:335–338.
158. Vita JA, Friedman PL, Cantillon C, et al. Efficacy of intravenous propafenone for the acute management of atrial fibrillation. *Am J Cardiol* 1989; 63:1275–1278.
159. Sung RJ, Tan HL, Karagounis L, et al. Intravenous sotalol for the termination of supraventricular tachycardia and atrial fibrillation and flutter: a multicenter, randomized, double-blind, placebo-controlled study. The Sotalol Multicenter Study Group. *Am Heart J* 1995;129:739–748.
160. Falk RH, Pollak A, Singh SN, et al. Intravenous dofetilide, a class III antiarrhythmic agent, for the termination of sustained atrial fibrillation or flutter. *J Am Coll Cardiol* 1997;29:385–390.
161. Norgaard BL, Wachtell K, Christensen PD, et al. Efficacy and safety of intravenously administered dofetilide in acute termination of atrial fibrillation and flutter: a multicenter, randomized, double-blind, placebo-controlled trial. Danish Dofetilide in Atrial Fibrillation and Flutter Study Group. *Am Heart J* 1999;137:1062–1069.
162. Lindeboom JE, Kingma JH, Crijns HJ, et al. Efficacy and safety of intravenous dofetilide for rapid termination of atrial fibrillation and atrial flutter. *Am J Cardiol* 2000;85:1031–1033.
163. Sokolow M, Ball RE. Factors influencing conversion of chronic atrial fibrillation with special reference to serum quinidine concentration. *Circulation* 1956;14:568–583.
164. Capucci A, Boriani G, Botto GL, et al. Conversion of recent-onset atrial fibrillation by a single oral loading dose of propafenone or flecainide. *Am J Cardiol* 1994;74:503–505.
165. Botto GL, Bonini W, Broffoni T, et al. Conversion of recent onset atrial fibrillation with single loading oral dose of propafenone: is in-hospital admission absolutely necessary? *Pacing Clin Electrophysiol* 1996;19:1939–1943.
166. Coplen SE, Antman EM, Berline JA, et al. Efficacy and safety of quinidine therapy for maintenance of sinus rhythm after cardioversion: a meta-analysis of randomized control trials. *Circulation* 1990;82:1106–1116.
167. Hartel G, Louhija A, Konttinen A. Disopyramide in the prevention of recurrence of atrial fibrillation after electroconversion. *Clin Pharmacol Ther* 1974;15:551–555.
168. Anderson JL, Gilbert EM, Alpert BL, et al. Prevention of symptomatic recurrences of paroxysmal atrial fibrillation in patients initially tolerating antiarrhythmic therapy: a multicenter, double blind, crossover study of flecainide and placebo with transtelephonic monitoring. Flecainide Supraventricular Tachycardia Study Group. *Circulation* 1989;80:1157–1570.
169. Pritchett ELC, DaTorre SD, Platt ML, et al. Flecainide acetate treatment of paroxysmal supraventricular tachycardia and paroxysmal atrial fibrillation: dose–response studies.The Flecainide Supraventricular Tachycardia Study Group. *J Am Coll Cardiol* 1991;17:197–303.
170. Aliot E, Denjoy I. Comparison of the safety and efficacy of flecainide versus propafenone in hospital out-patients with symptomatic paroxysmal atrial fibrillation/flutter. *Am J Cardiol* 1996;77:66A–71A.
171. Antman EM, Beamer AD, Cantillon C, et al. Long-term oral propafenone therapy for suppression of refractory symptomatic atrial fibrillation and atrial flutter. *J Am Coll Cardiol* 1989;12:1005–1011.
172. Connoly SJ, Hoffert DL. Usefulness of propafenone for recurrent paroxysmal atrial fibrillation. *Am J Cardiol* 1989;63:817–819.
173. Reimold SC, Cantillon CO, Friedman PL, et al. Propafenone versus sotalol for suppression of recurrent symptomatic atrial fibrillation. *Am J Cardiol* 1993;71:558–563.
174. Juul-Moller S, Edvardsson N, Rehnqvist-Ahlberg N. Sotalol versus quinidine for the maintenance of sinus rhythm after direct current conversion of atrial fibrillation. *Circulation* 1990;82:1932–1939.
175. Hohnloser SF, Van de Loo A, Baedeker F. Efficacy and proarrhythmic hazards of pharmacologic cardioversion of atrial fibrillation: prospective comparison of sotalol versus quinidine. *J Am Coll Cardiol* 1995;26:852–858.
176. Bellandi F, Dabizzi RP, Niccoli L, et al. Propafenone and sotalol in the prevention of paroxysmal atrial fibrillation: long-term safety and efficacy study. *Curr Ther Res* 1995;56:1154–1168.
177. Horowitz LN, Spielman SR, Greenspan AM, et al. Use of amiodarone in the treatment of persistent and paroxysmal atrial fibrillation resistant to quinidine therapy. *J Am Coll Cardiol* 1985;6:1402–1407.
178. Gold RL, Haffajee CI, Chros G, et al. Amiodarone for refractory atrial fibrillation. *Am J Cardiol* 1986;57:124–127.
179. Brodsky MA, Allen BJ, Walker CJ, et al. Amiodarone for maintenance of sinus rhythm after conversion of atrial fibrillation in the setting of a dilated left atrium. *Am J Cardiol* 1987;60:572–574.
180. Gosselink AT, Crijns HJ, VanGelder IC, et al. Low-dose amiodarone for maintenance of sinus rhythm after cardioversion of atrial fibrillation or flutter. *JAMA* 1992;267:3289–3293.
181. Vitolo E, Tronci M, Larovere MT, et al. Amiodarone versus quinidine in the prophylaxis of atrial fibrillation. *Acta Cardiol* 1981;36:431–444.
182. Blevins RD, Kerin NZ, Benederet D, et al. Amiodarone in the management of refractory atrial fibrillation. *Arch Intern Med* 1987;147:1401–1404.
183. Geller JC, Geller M, Lott J, et al. Moricizine is effective and safe in patients with atrial fibrillation. *Circulation* 1995;92:I–774.
184. Torp-Pedersen C, Moller M, Bloch-Thomsen PE, et al. Dofetilide in patients with congestive heart failure and left ventricular dysfunction. Danish Investigations of Arrhythmia and Mortality on Dofetilide Study Group. *N Engl J Med* 1999;341:857–865.
185. Roy D, Talajic M, Dorian P, et al. Amiodarone to prevent recurrence of atrial fibrillation. Canadian Trial of Atrial Fibrillation Investigators. *N Engl J Med* 2000;342:913–920.
186. Singh S, Zoble RG, Yellen L, et al. Efficacy and safety of oral dofetilide in converting to and maintaining sinus rhythm in patients with chronic atrial fibrillation or atrial flutter: the symptomatic atrial fibrillation investigative research on dofetilide (SAFIRE–D) study. *Circulation* 2000;102;2385–2390.
187. Prystowsky EN, Freeland SA, Branyas NA, et al. Clinical experience with dofetilide in the treatment of patients with atrial fibrillation. *J Cardiovasc Electrophysiol* 2003;14:S287–S290.

188. Alboni P, Botto GL, Baldi N, et al. Outpatient treatment of recent onset atrial fibrillation with the "pill in the pocket" approach. *N Engl J Med* 2004; 351:2384–2391.
189. Echt DS, Leibson PR, Mitchell LB, et al. Mortality and morbidity in patients receiving encainide, flecainide or placebo. The Cardiac Arrhythmia Suppression Trial. *N Engl J Med* 1991;324:781–788.
190. Singh SN, Fletcher RD, Fisher SG, et al. Amiodarone in patients with congestive heart failure and asymptomatic ventricular arrhythmia. The Survival Trial of Antiarrhythmic Therapy in Congestive Heart Failure. *N Engl J Med* 1995;333:77–82.
191. Doval HC, Nul DR, Grancelli HO, et al. Randomized trial of low-dose amiodarone in severe congestive heart failure. *Lancet* 1994;344:493–498.
192. Julian DG, Camm AJ, Frangin G, et al. Randomised trial of effect of amiodarone on mortality in patients with left ventricular dysfunction after recent myocardial infarction: EMIAT European Myocardial Infarct Amiodarone Trial Investigators. *Lancet* 1997;349:667–674. [Errata, *Lancet* 1997;349: 1180, 1776.]
193. Cairns JA, Connolly SJ, Roberts R, et al. Randomised trial of outcome after myocardial infarction in patients with frequent or repetitive ventricular premature depolarisations: CAMIAT Canadian Amiodarone Myocardial Infarction Arrhythmia Trial Investigators. *Lancet* 1997;349:675–682. [Erratum, *Lancet* 1997;349:1776.]
194. Kober L, Bloch Thomsen PE, Moller M, et al. Effect of dofetilide in patients with recent myocardial infarction and left-ventricular dysfunction: a randomised trial. *Lancet* 2000;356:2052–2058.
195. Ellenbogen KA, Dias VC, Plumb VJ, et al. A placebo-controlled trial of continuous intravenous diltiazem infusion for 24-hour heart rate control during atrial fibrillation and atrial flutter: a multicenter study. *J Am Coll Cardiol* 1991;18:891–897.
196. Waxman JL, Myerburg RJ, Appel R, et al. Verapamil for control of ventricular rate in paroxysmal supraventricular tachycardia and atrial fibrillation or flutter: a double-blind randomized cross-over study. *Ann Intern Med* 1981;94:1–6.
197. Rinkenberger RL, Prystowsky EN, Heger JJ, et al. Effect of IV and chronic oral verapamil administration in patients with a variety of supraventricular tachyarrhythmias. *Circulation* 1980;62:996–1010.
198. Anderson S, Blanski L, Byrd RC, et al. Comparison of the efficacy and safety of esmolol, a short-acting beta blocker, with placebo in the treatment of supraventricular tachyarrhythmias: the Esmolol vs. Placebo Multicenter Study Group. *Am Heart J* 1986;111:42–48.
199. David D, Segni ED, Klein HO, et al. Inefficacy of digitalis in the control of heart rate in patients with chronic atrial fibrillation: beneficial effect of an added beta adrenergic blocking agent. *Am J Cardiol* 1979;44:1378–1382.
200. Goodman DJ, Rossen RM, Cannom DS, et al. Effect of digoxin on atrioventricular conduction: studies in patients with and without cardiac autonomic innervation. *Circulation* 1975;51:251–256.
201. Rubin DA, Nieminiski KE, Reed GE, et al. Predictors, prevention, and long term prognosis of atrial fibrillation after coronary bypass graft operation. *J Thorac Cardiovasc Surg* 1987;94:331–339.
202. Silverman NA, Eright R, Levitsky S. Efficacy of low dose propranolol in preventing postoperative supraventricular tachyarrhythmias: a prospective, randomized study. *Ann Surg* 1982;196:194–200.
203. White HD, Elliott ChB, Antman MD, et al. Efficacy and safety of timolol for prevention of supraventricular tachyarrhythmias after coronary artery bypass surgery. *Circulation* 1984;70(3):479–484.
204. Daudon P, Corcos T, Gandjbakhch I, et al. Prevention of atrial fibrillation or flutter by acebutolol after coronary bypass grafting. *Am J Cardiol* 1986;58: 933–936.
205. Bradley D, Creswell LL, Hogue CW, et al. ACCP Guidelines for the prevention and management of postoperative atrial fibrillation after cardiac surgery. Pharmacological prophylaxis. *Chest* 2005;128:395–475.
206. Gomes JA, Ip J, Santoni-Rugiu F, et al. Oral d,1 sotalol reduces the incidence of postoperative atrial fibrillation in coronary artery bypass surgery patients: a randomized, double-blind, placebo controlled study. *J Am Coll Cardiol* 1999;34:334–339.
207. Guarnieri T, Nolan S, Gottlieb SO, et al. Intravenous amiodarone for the prevention of atrial fibrillation after open heart surgery: the Amiodarone Reduction in Coronary Heart (ARCH) Trial. *J Am Coll Cardiol* 1999; 34:343–347.
208. Daoud EG, Strickberger SA, Man KC, et al. Preoperative amiodarone as prophylaxis against atrial fibrillation after heart surgery. *N Engl J Med* 1997;337:1785–1791.
209. Kowey PR, Stebbins D, Igidbashian L, et al. Clinical outcome of patients who develop PAF after CABG surgery. *Pacing Clin Electrophysiol* 2001; 24:191–193.
210. Epstein AE, Alexander JC, Gutterman DD, et al. American College of Chest Physicians guidelines for the prevention and management of postoperative atrial fibrillation after cardiac surgery. *Chest* 2005;128:245–275.
211. Heppell RM, Berkin KE, McLenachan JM, et al. Haemostatic and haemodynamic abnormalities associated with left atrial thrombosis in nonrheumatic atrial fibrillation. *Heart* 1997;77:407–411.
212. Sohara H, Amitani S, Kurose M, et al. Atrial fibrillation activates platelets and coagulation in a time-dependent manner; a study in patients with paroxysmal atrial fibrillation. *J Am Coll Cardiol* 1977;29:106–112.
213. Bjerkelund CJ, Orning OM. The efficacy of anticoagulant therapy in preventing embolism related to D.C. electrical conversion of atrial fibrillation. *Am J Cardiol* 1969;23:208–216.
214. Weinberg DM, Mancini J. Anticoagulation for cardioversion of atrial fibrillation. *Am J Cardiol* 1989;63:745–746.
215. Lown B, Amarasingham R, Neuman J. New method for terminating cardiac arrhythmias: use of synchronized capacitor discharge. *JAMA* 1962;182: 548.
216. Henry WL, Morganroth J, Pearlman AS, et al. Relation between echocardiographically determined left atrial size and atrial fibrillation. *Circulation* 1976;53:273–279.
217. VanGelder IC, Crijns HJ, VanGilst WH, et al. Prediction of uneventful cardioversion and maintenance of sinus rhythm from direct-current electrical cardioversion of chronic atrial fibrillation and flutter. *Am J Cardiol* 1991;68:335–341.
218. Lown B, Krieger R, Williams J. Cardioversion and digitalis drugs: changed threshold to electrical shock in digitalized animals. *Circ Res* 1965;17:519–531.
219. Guarnieri T, Tomaselli G, Griffith LSC, et al. The interaction of antiarrhythmic drugs and the energy for cardioversion of chronic atrial fibrillation. *Pacing Clin Electrophysiol* 1991;14:1007–1012.
220. Prystowsky EN. Cardioversion of atrial fibrillation to sinus rhythm: who, when, how, and why? *Am J Cardiol* 2000;86:326–327.
221. Mittal S, Ayati S, Stein KM, et al. Transthoracic cardioversion of atrial fibrillation: comparison of rectilinear biphasic versus damped sine wave monophasic shocks. *Circulation* 2000;101:1282–1287.
222. Scheinman MM, Morady F, Hess DS, et al. Catheter induced ablation of the atrioventricular junction to control refractory supraventricular arrhythmias. *JAMA* 1982;248:851–855.
223. Gallagher JJ, Svenson RH, Kasell JH, et al. Catheter technique for closed-chest ablation of the atrioventricular conduction system: a therapeutic alternative for the treatment of refractory supraventricular tachycardia. *N Engl J Med* 1982;306:194–200.
224. Kay GN, Bubien RS, Epstein AE, et al. Effect of catheter ablation of the atrioventricular junction on quality of life and exercise tolerance in paroxysmal atrial fibrillation. *Am J Cardiol* 1988;62:741–744.
225. Packer D, Asirvatham S, Munger T. Progress in non-pharmacologic therapy of atrial fibrillation. *J Cardiovasc Electrophysiol* 2003;14:S296–S309.
226. Lin WS, Tai CT, Hsieh MH, et al. Catheter ablation of paroxysmal atrial fibrillation initiated by non-pulmonary vein ectopy. *Circulation* 2003;107 (25):3176–3183.
227. Pappone C, Santinelli V. The who, what, why and how-to guide for circumferential pulmonary vein ablation. *J Cardiovasc Electrophysiol* 2004;15: 1226–1230.
228. Hocini M, Sanders P, Jais P, et al. Techniques for curative treatment of atrial fibrillation. *J Cardiovasc Electrophysiol* 204;15:1467–1471.
229. Verma A, Marrouche NF, Natale A. Pulmonary vein antrum isolation: intracardiac echocardiography-guided technique. *J Cardiovasc Electrophysiol* 2004;15:1335–1340.
230. Nademanee K, McKenzie J, Kosar E, et al. A new approach for catheter ablation of atrial fibrillation: mapping of the electrophysiologic substrate. *J Am Coll Cardiol* 2004;43:2044–2053.
231. Cox JL, Canavan TE, Schuessler RB, et al. The surgical treatment of atrial fibrillation. II. Intraoperative electrophysiology mapping and description of the electrophysiologic basis of atrial flutter and atrial fibrillation. *J Thorac Cardiovasc Surg* 1991;101:406–426.
232. Williams JM, Ungerleider RM, Lofland GK, et al. Left atrial isolation: new technique for the treatment of supraventricular arrhythmias. *J Thorac Cardiovasc Surg* 1980;80:373–380.
233. Defauw JJ, Guiraudon GM, vanHemel NM, et al. Surgical therapy of paroxysmal atrial fibrillation with the corridor operation. *Ann Thorac Surg* 1992;53:564–571.
234. Hioki M, Ikeshita M, Iedokoro Y, et al. Successful combined operation for mitral stenosis and atrial fibrillation. *Ann Thorac Surg* 1993;55:776–778.
235. Lamas GA, Lee KL, Sweeney MO, et al. Mode Selection Trial in Sinus-Node Dysfunction. Ventricular pacing or dual-chamber pacing for sinus-node dysfunction (MOST). *N Engl J Med* 2002;346:1854–1862.
236. Connolly SJ, Kerr CR, Gent M, et al. Effects of physiologic pacing versus ventricular pacing on the risk of stroke and death due to cardiovascular causes. *N Engl J Med* 2000;342:1385–1391.
237. Kerr CR, Connolly SJ, Abdollah H, et al. Canadian Trial of Physiological Pacing: Effects of physiological pacing during long-term follow-up (CTOPP). *Circulation* 2004;109:357–362.
238. Andersen HR, Nielsen JC, Thomsen PEB, et al. Long-term follow-up of patients from a randomised trial of atrial versus ventricular pacing for sick-sinus syndrome. *Lancet* 1997;350:1210–1216.
239. Toff WD, Camm AJ, Skehan JD. United Kingdom Pacing and Cardiovascular Events Trial Investigators. Single-chamber versus dual-chamber pacing for high-grade atrioventricular block (UKPACE). *N Engl J Med* 2005; 353:145–155.
240. Knight BP, Gersh BJ, Carlson MD, et al. Role of permanent pacing to prevent atrial fibrillation: science advisory from the American Heart Association Council on Clinical Cardiology (Subcommittee on Electrocardiography and Arrhythmias) and the quality of Care and Outcomes Research Interdisciplinary Working Group, in collaboration with the Heart Rhythm Society. *Circulation* 2005;111:240–243.

CHAPTER 64 ■ ATRIAL FLUTTER

PATRICK TCHOU

INTRODUCTION

The term atrial flutter has traditionally referred to an atrial tachycardia with monomorphic P waves, sometimes referred to as flutter waves, without an isoelectric baseline, having rates in the range of 240 to 300 beats per minute. The term atrial tachycardia has frequently been used for atrial rates less than 240 beats per minute because these tend to have an isoelectric baseline between individual P waves. However, with increasing understanding of the mechanisms of atrial reentrant rhythms, the modern use of the term atrial flutter refers to a regular reentrant tachycardia within the atria having a definable reentrant circuit by our current mapping techniques, also called a macro reentrant atrial tachycardia. The term atrial tachycardia or focal atrial tachycardia tends to be used to describe a tachycardia with an automatic mechanism arising from a narrow focus or, perhaps, a reentrant mechanism confined to a narrow region too limited for current mapping systems to resolve (1). Although atrial flutter as a phenomenon was described around a century ago (2), the mechanisms of this arrhythmia in the human heart have only relatively recently been elucidated with the development of activation mapping systems capable of displaying the reentrant activation wavefront.

MECHANISM OF ATRIAL FLUTTER: THE REENTRANT CIRCUIT

For a reentrant tachycardia to exist, it must have a reentrant pathway within the myocardium that is formed by conducting tissue around a barrier. Two types of barriers are thought to be involved in demarcating the reentrant circuit of atrial flutter, anatomic barriers and functional barriers. Anatomic barriers can be structures such as the atrioventricular valves, the venous openings into the atria, or scars from surgical incisions or other degenerative/inflammatory conditions affecting the myocardium. The anatomy of the coronary sinus can be considered a barrier because this venous structure has its own myocardial lining with varying connections to the left atrium (3). Functional barriers, on the other hand, consist of conducting myocardium, which under the proper circumstances, such as rapid rates or premature beats, will develop conduction block that forms the barrier around which the reentrant wavefront circulates. The crista terminalis, for example, is a thickened part of the right atrium extending from the superior vena cava down along the anterolateral portion of the right atrium near the lateral border of the tricuspid valve and then extending into the cavotricuspid isthmus. This tissue has preferential conduction in the superior-inferior direction mostly due to fiber orientation. Transverse conduction across this structure occurs during normal heart rates, but with rapid rates, transverse conduction blocks, resulting in the crista forming a linear barrier to conduction (4).

The most common form of atrial flutter is the so-called typical form of atrial flutter. The reentrant circuit involves cranial-caudal conduction over the crista terminalis, continuing across the cavotricuspid isthmus, breaking out onto the interatrial septum and posterior atrial wall, conducting up to the roof of the right atrium anterior to the superior vena cava opening, and then entering the superior end of the crista again. When viewed from the ventricular side of the tricuspid annulus, the reentrant waveform rotates around the tricuspid annulus in a counterclockwise direction. Thus, this common form of typical flutter is sometimes called counterclockwise flutter. Early mapping studies of this type of flutter demonstrated that the wavefront propagated craniocaudally along the lateral right atrium and caudocranially along the septal portion of the right atrium, with slow conduction occurring along the inferior portions of the right atrium (5). This reentrant pathway in the human heart was also described by Feld and colleagues in their report on the use of radiofrequency ablation to interrupt the tachycardia circuit (6). The slow area of conduction in the low right atrium was identified to be the isthmus of atrial myocardium located between the tricuspid valve and the inferior vena cava. Figure 64.1 shows a schematic representation of a typical atrial flutter circuit and an actual electroanatomic map of this type of atrial flutter. Figure 64.2 shows a representative electrocardiogram (ECG) of this type of atrial flutter. Several barriers help to shape this reentrant circuit. The tricuspid valve forms the end of the atrial tissue anteriorly. The crista terminalis laterally form both a barrier and a path of conduction. The inferior vena cava provides the posterior barrier of the cavotricuspid isthmus. Although only one reentrant path is necessary for a tachycardia to exist, often there are two paths forming a figure-of-eight reentry (7). In the case of the typical flutter circuit, the reentrant loop around the tricuspid valve can be accompanied by a lower loop circulating around the inferior vena cava. The common path of the two loops forming the "waist" of the figure-of-eight is the cavotricuspid isthmus. Although less often seen clinically, the same circuits can also rotate in the opposite direction, creating the so-called clockwise typical flutter (8). The two types of circuit rotation result in different atrial activation patterns, generating somewhat different ECG morphologies of the flutter

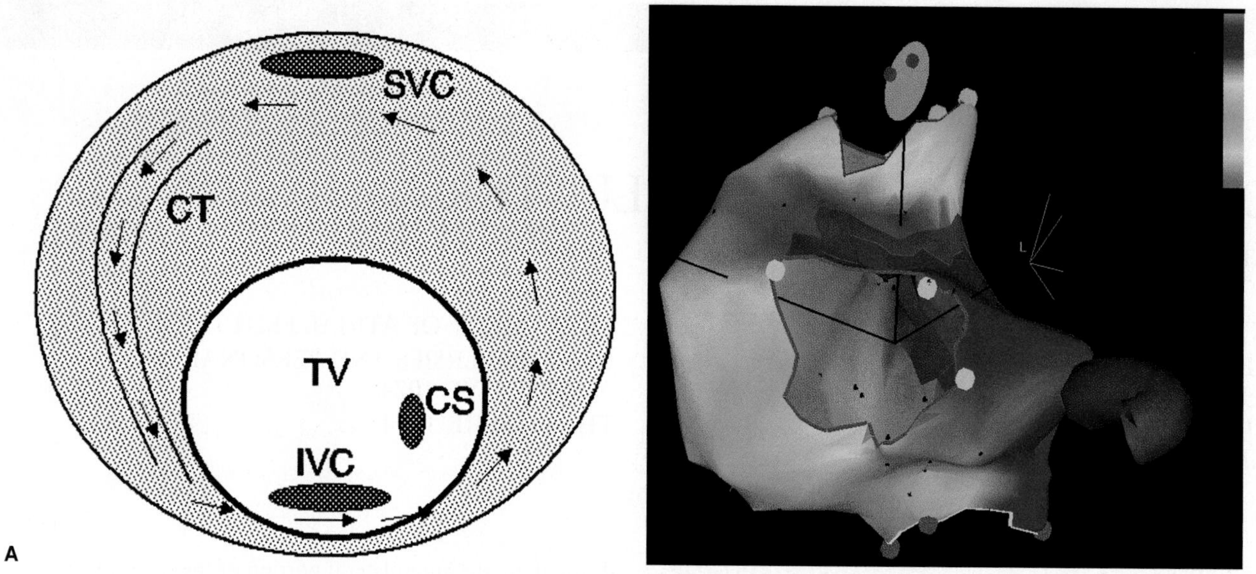

FIGURE 64.1. A: Schematic representation of a typical counterclockwise atrial flutter circuit. Arrows indicate direction of wavefront propagation. The right atrium is viewed facing the tricuspid valve (TV) from the ventricular side. Impulse propagation proceeds down the crista terminalis (CT) along the right free wall, across the cavotricuspid isthmus, and up the septum and renters the crista. Propagation of the wavefront posteriorly blocks at the crista, forcing the reentrant wavefront to enter the descending limb at the cranial end of the crista near the superior vena cava (SVC). The cavotricuspid isthmus provides a narrowed region conduction suitable for interruption of the reentrant circuit by catheter ablation. CS, coronary sinus; IVC, inferior vena cava. B: An actual map of the right atrial reentrant circuit in a patient with typical atrial flutter, obtained using an electroanatomic mapping system (Biosense Webster CARTO). The image is a left anterior oblique view with a caudal angulation. The map shows the tricuspid valve anteriorly, the superior vena cava superiorly, the coronary sinus as represented by a red tube, and the inferior vena cava opening below the tricuspid valve. The color scale on the right shows relative activation time, with red at the early end and purple at the late end. The wavefront circulates in a counterclockwise direction around the tricuspid valve, with "late" activation meeting "early" activation at around the 2 o'clock position of the valve and completing the reentrant circuit in this map. Catheter ablation aims at interrupting the wavefront by creating a line of block from the inferior end of the tricuspid valve to the inferior vena cava.

wave. With the typical pattern, atrial activation starts with septal breakout of the waveform emanating from the cavotricuspid isthmus. The remainder of the right and left atria tends to be activated more or less simultaneously. This results in the flutter wave having a superiorly directed vector on the surface ECG. In the less common clockwise version, wavefront breakout occurs at the lateral portion of the tricuspid annulus. It then spreads cranially and then across the right atrial roof before propagating across to the left atrium. A schematic view of the reentrant circuit in the right atrium is shown in Figure 64.3. This propagation pattern generates a more horizontal or inferiorly directed vector that points toward the patient's left (9). The leftward ECG leads (lead I and lead aVL) generally show a positive flutter wave. Catheter ablation of these

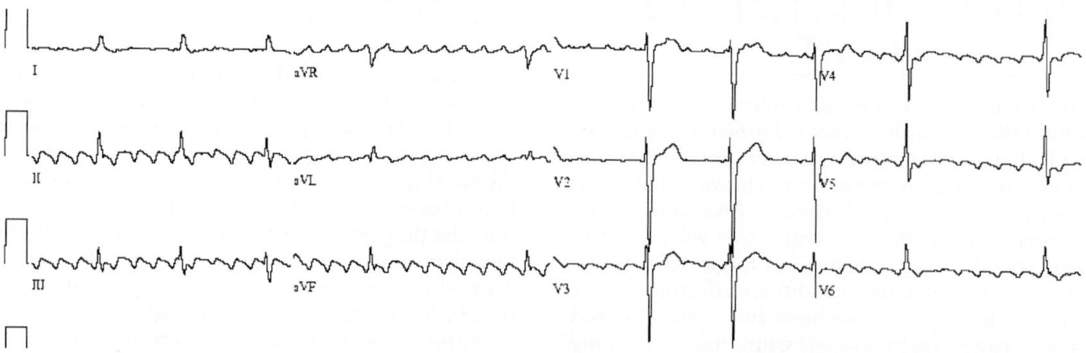

FIGURE 64.2. Electrocardiogram (ECG) of a typical form of atrial flutter. This ECG shows typical flutter wave morphology on the 12-lead ECG. The vector of the flutter wave is directed superiorly due to the breakout of the wavefront at the inferior septal portion of the right atrium. The major direction of atrial activation is from inferior septal to superior regions of both atria. Thus, the typical pattern of this type of flutter shows prominent negative flutter waves in the inferior ECG leads. The cycle lengths of the flutter can vary considerably as a function of atrial size, conduction time across the cavotricuspid isthmus, and drugs that slow overall conduction, but usually falls in the 180- to 250-msec range.

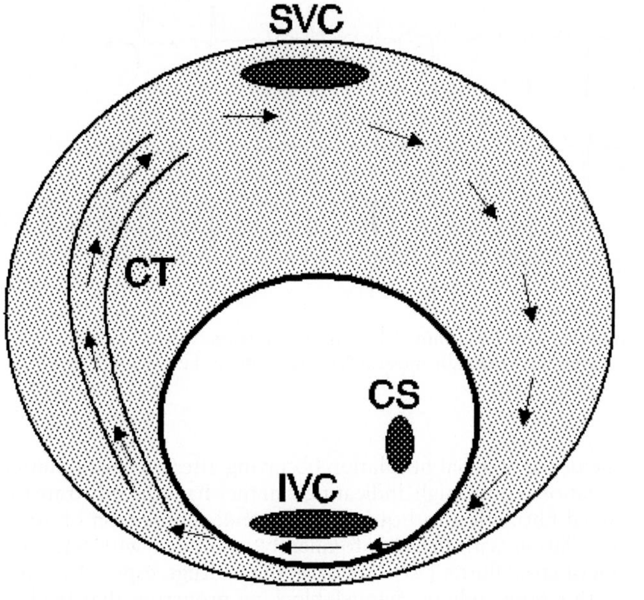

FIGURE 64.3. Schematic representation of a counterclockwise atrial flutter circuit. The reentrant pathway is essentially the reversal of the clockwise circuit seen in Figure 64.1A. CS, coronary sinus; CT, crista terminalis; IVC, inferior vena cava; SVC, superior vena cava.

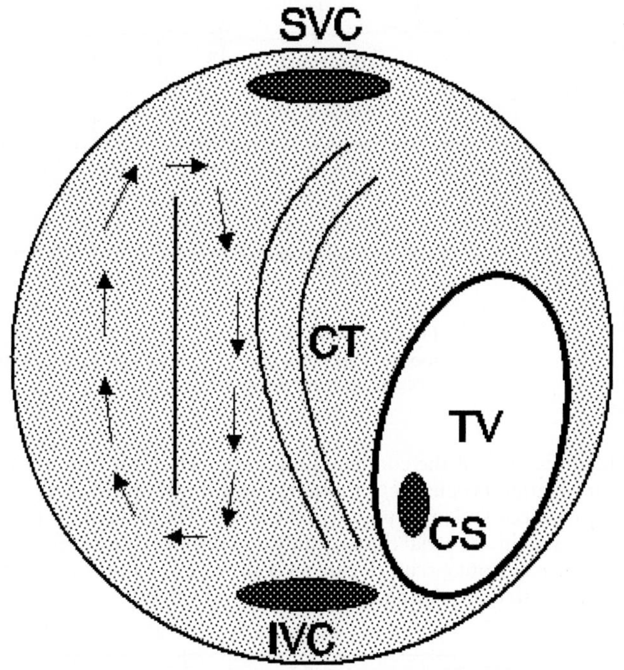

FIGURE 64.4. Atrial flutter around an incision. A surgical incision can form the barrier around which the flutter wavefront can circulate. In this schematic diagram, the right atrium is viewed anteriorly, showing the tricuspid valve (TV) pointing to the patient's left and inferiorly. The right free wall incisional scar forms the barrier around which the reentrant flutter wavefront circulates. Such a reentrant wavefront can readily exist in a dual-loop form with the typical flutter circuit illustrated in Figure 64.1A. CS, coronary sinus; CT, crista terminalis; IVC, inferior vena cava; SVC, superior vena cava.

two types of flutter is typically accomplished by interrupting the reentrant pathway within the cavotricuspid isthmus. Radiofrequency lesions are directed at the isthmus near the most inferior portion of the tricuspid annulus. If this is unsuccessful, a more septal line of lesions can also be used (10). More recently, cryoablation catheters using deep freezing as a means of ablating cardiac tissue have been successful in interrupting the flutter circuit (11,12). A possible advantage of the cryothermal approach is the lack of pain perception by the patient during the application of the cryolesion. With either approach, interruption of the flutter circuit acutely is successful more than 90% of the time. There is a recurrence rate of around 10% to 15%, however, due to which a repeat procedure may be needed.

Although the typical form of atrial flutter is the most commonly seen variety, other reentrant circuits can be the basis of an atrial flutter. These are generally referred to as atypical atrial flutters and can have a variety of mechanisms (13). Isolated reports of flutters emanating from the ostial regions of the superior vena cava (14) and reentry around the upper portions of the crista terminalis using conduction gaps in the crista have been documented (15). Probably the next-most-common type of atrial flutter after the typical flutters are those associated with incisional scars due to cardiac surgery, whether for congenital heart disease (16,17) or, more commonly in adults, valvular heart surgery (18). The incisions made to the atria for mitral and tricuspid valve surgery can form a barrier around which the flutter wavefront can circulate. Three sites of incisional scars are commonly seen. The right atrial free wall is a common site for an incision to expose the tricuspid valve as well as the interatrial septum (Fig. 64.4). With the minimally invasive approaches currently used for mitral valve surgery, access to the left atrium is obtained transseptally from the right atrium. Thus, the septal incision can also form a substrate for atrial flutter. Last, incision in the posterior portions of the left atrium, septally or between the two sets of pulmonary veins, may provide the substrate for a reentrant circuit.

Catheter ablation of flutters associated with surgical incisions are more challenging and generally require the use of an electroanatomic mapping system to adequately define the reentrant circuit as well as the optimal sites for ablation. Multiple reentrant circuits may be present such as those related to the incision and those of the more typical type (19).

Nonsurgical scars can also form the substrate for atrial flutters. These may occur secondary to a cardiomyopathic process. The scarring process can form both the barrier and the slow conduction regions needed to establish the reentrant circuit. Again, catheter ablation of this type of flutter requires the use of a mapping system to achieve a high degree of success. With the advent of pulmonary vein isolation and atrial ablation procedures aimed at eliminating atrial fibrillation, postprocedure atrial flutter has been reported. This has been associated with the regions of ablation near the pulmonary venous ostia or with linear ablations having conduction gaps (20). With the increasing use of ablation for atrial fibrillation, these types of flutters are seen more frequently. Repeat ablations aimed at eliminating the conduction gaps are usually successful in preventing recurrence of these flutters. Surgical approaches to treatment of atrial fibrillation such as the Maze surgery may also generate atypical types of flutter (21,22).

Similar to the right atrial anatomy, the left atrium also has some natural barriers that may form the substrate for a reentrant circuit. The pulmonary veins and the mitral annulus can serve as barriers around which the reentrant wavefront may circulate. An atypical form of atrial flutter has been described involving a reentrant wavefront circulating around the right pulmonary veins using the septal tissue between the veins and the mitral annulus (23,24). Other forms of left atrial flutter can circulate around the mitral annulus and possibly use the coronary sinus as part of the reentrant pathway along the inferior portions of the mitral annulus (25). Dual-loop reentry (the so-called figure-of-eight reentry) can be seen in both atria.

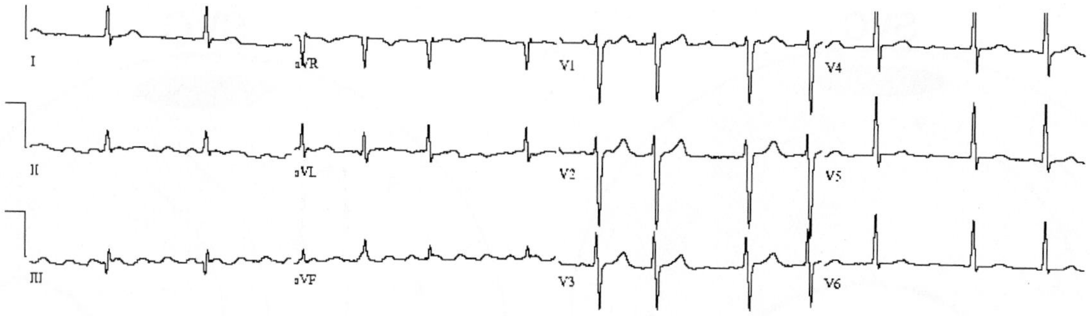

FIGURE 64.5. Electrocardiogram (ECG) of a left atrial flutter. This ECG shows the unusual flutter wave morphology seen in a patient in whom the flutter was identified through intracardiac mapping to be circulating around the mitral annulus.

Identification of the common limb in this circuit is important for ablation because interruption at this limb is most likely to create successful interruption of the flutter. The ECG of the flutter waves in left atrial flutters can vary considerably depending on the reentrant circuit. Figure 64.5 shows an example of a left atrial flutter circulating around the mitral valve.

MECHANISMS OF ATRIAL FLUTTER: INITIATION OF REENTRY

Although it is possible that many human hearts may have the potential reentrant circuit to support atrial flutter at least on a transient basis, the triggering mechanism necessary to initiate the flutter reentrant wavefront may be quite difficult to achieve. In the clinical electrophysiology laboratory, initiation of atrial flutter generally requires burst pacing at a rapid rate for many seconds before a flutter can be established. For the reentrant circuit to establish a reentrant wave front, unidirectional block needs to be established before the first reentrant beat. This block within the reentrant circuit of typical atrial flutter generally occurs within the cavotricuspid isthmus region. Clinical studies have demonstrated that initiation of typical atrial flutters with burst pacing from the coronary sinus region can generate block within this isthmus (26). This area may have good conduction capacities, however, such that block may not occur readily. Thus, long trains of rapid beats may be needed to act as a triggering mechanism to generate one blocked beat. A second requirement is that the nonblocked limb of the reentrant circuit must have enough conduction delay to permit reentrant conduction at the site of the blocked limb. In the typical flutter scenario, the "delayed" arm of the reentrant circuit is generally achieved by conduction block across the crista terminalis, forcing the wavefront to propagate to the roof of the right atrium, where it can enter the crista and propagate downward towards the isthmus. All of these requirements for initiation of typical atrial flutter are needed: a rapid triggering source of atrial beats, block in the isthmus, and transverse conduction block in the crista. Clinically, it is thus not surprising that atrial flutter is commonly seen as a companion to paroxysmal atrial fibrillation. The rapid and irregular beats associated with atrial fibrillation, at least a short episode of it, can readily provide the triggering mechanism needed to initiate flutter. Two lines of clinical evidence suggest that this may well be the dominant triggering mechanism for atrial flutter. First, longer-term follow-up studies of patients who have undergone atrial flutter ablation have shown that the incidence of clinically significant atrial fibrillation occurrences increases with time and reaches around 50% to 60% within 3 to 4 years (27,28). Thus, even in patients with only atrial flutter documented clinically, the incidence of atrial fibrillation occurring after successful flutter ablation is quite high, indicating that they have the substrate for atrial fibrillation to begin with. Second, suppression of atrial fibrillation with drugs is frequently associated with later onset of atrial flutter (29). Antiarrhythmic drugs, especially those with strong sodium channel–blocking properties that tend to slow conduction, may have a proarrhythmic potential by slowing conduction and stabilizing a flutter reentrant circuit. This proarrhythmic property may allow more ready initiation and sustainment of atrial flutter even with a short episode of atrial fibrillation. Thus, the drug may work well to suppress clinically noticeable atrial fibrillation, but even a short episode lasting a matter of seconds may be adequate for triggering a sustained atrial flutter in the presence of such antiarrhythmic medications. The type Ic agents are particularly prone to this type of proarrhythmia due to their strong sodium channel–blocking properties. These clinical observations strongly suggest that most atrial flutters, at least of the typical type, are initiated by bursts of rapid atrial tachycardia or atrial fibrillation.

TREATMENT OF ATRIAL FLUTTER

Atrial flutters tend to conduct to the ventricle at a more rapid rate than atrial fibrillation. The more rapid penetration of the atrioventricular node during atrial fibrillation may actually serve to slow throughput of impulses to the ventricle because impulses that block in the atrioventricular node can leave a residual refractoriness that interferes with conduction of subsequent impulses. It is not surprising to see a patient with relatively controlled ventricular rates during atrial fibrillation develop more rapid ventricular rates when the fibrillation changes to flutter. Thus, control of ventricular rate during atrial flutter may be more difficult, requiring treatment aimed at suppressing the rhythm in order to treat symptoms. As discussed previously, use of type Ic antiarrhythmic drugs may have a proarrhythmic effect unless they are capable of suppressing the triggering mechanism. By slowing the tachycardia, such drugs may make the reentrant rhythm more stable and less likely to break spontaneously. Another "proarrhythmic" effect of type Ic antiarrhythmic drugs can manifest as increased ventricular rate due to slowing of the atrial rate. In some circumstances, the atrial flutter rate can slow to the range of 200 beats per minute, and one-to-one atrioventricular conduction can occur in patients with good atrioventricular nodal conduction capabilities. With the rate-dependent nature of sodium channel blockade by type Ic medications, the QRS during such a slow flutter may be quite wide, mimicking the appearance of a ventricular tachycardia. Figure 64.6 shows an example of a wide-complex tachycardia that occurred in a patient treated with a type Ic antiarrhythmic

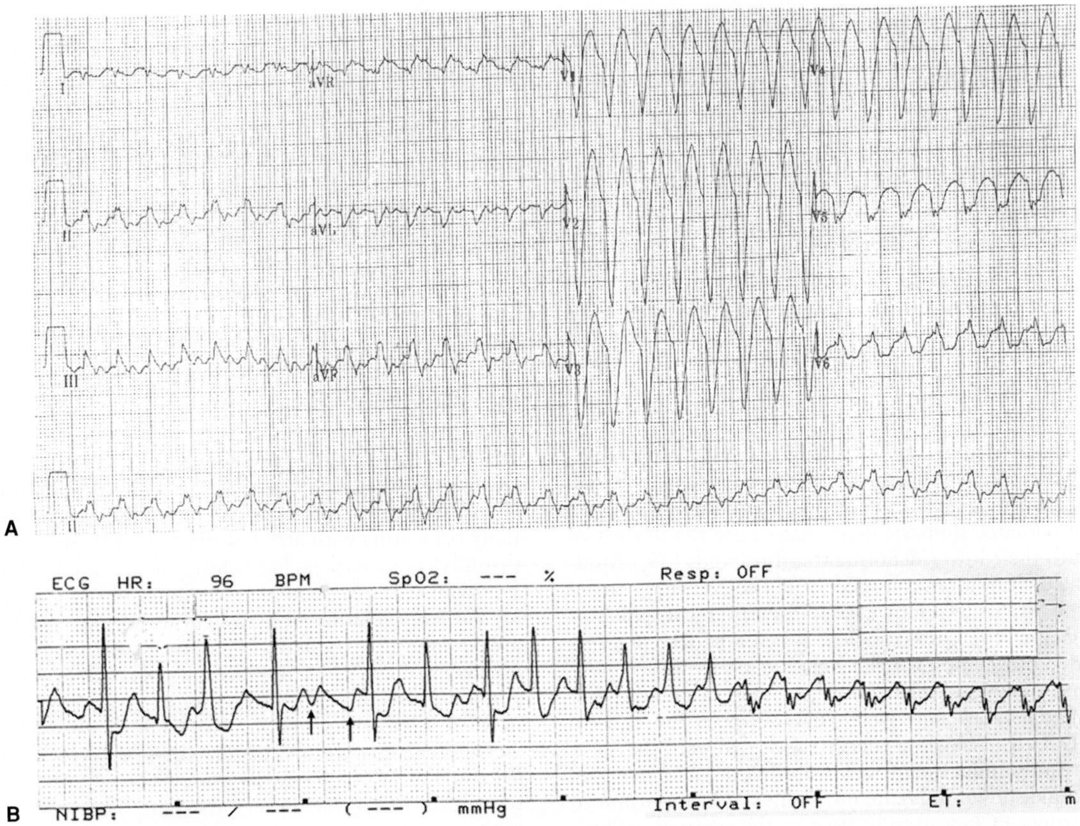

FIGURE 64.6. Atrial flutter presenting as wide-QRS tachycardia. **A:** A 12-lead electrocardiogram (ECG) from a patient presenting to the emergency room with palpitations. This patient had clinical atrial fibrillation treated with a type Ic antiarrhythmic medication. The patient also had relatively robust atrioventricular nodal conduction. The wide-QRS tachycardia had a rate of approximately 180 beats per minute. **B:** Transient slowing of atrioventricular conduction resulting in narrowing of the QRS and identifiable flutter waves (*arrows*). The flutter had the same rate as the wide-QRS tachycardia. With resumption of 1:1 atrioventricular conduction in the second half of this rhythm strip, the QRS again widens due to the strong rate-dependent effects of sodium channel blockade with type Ic medications.

medication for atrial fibrillation. Patients may also be quite symptomatic due to the rapid ventricular rate (30). Nevertheless, type Ic medications may be quite effective in suppressing the triggering atrial tachyarrhythmias of atrial flutter. This therapy, however, should be accompanied by some atrioventricular nodal blocking medications such as a β-blocker whenever possible. Furthermore, use of type Ic medications should be reserved for those patients with normal cardiac function and no evidence of ischemia.

Sotalol, dofetilide, and amiodarone are type III antiarrhythmic medications that may be quite effective. These drugs have been studied for the treatment of atrial fibrillation, but some studies have included use in atrial flutter (31). Due to its potential long-term toxicities, amiodarone is generally used as a last resort when needed.

Ibutelide is an intravenous type III antiarrhythmic drug that can be used in a bolus fashion to attempt conversion of atrial flutter to sinus rhythm. Success rates in converting atrial flutter ranged from 50% to 90% in various reports (32,33,34). After this drug is given, patients should be observed closely for the potential of developing torsades de pointes immediately after conversion, especially if they have relative sinus bradycardia. Because of this propensity toward torsades de pointes, ibutelide should not be used in a patient who is concurrently taking another type III antiarrhythmic medication. Whereas use of ibutelide is problematic in patients who are already on oral amiodarone, amiodarone may be useful given intravenously to patients who have failed cardioversion with ibutelide (35). Short-term amiodarone intravenously while the ibutelide effect is waning appears to be safe and can add additional efficacy in converting atrial flutter. Ibutelide appears to be safe and as efficacious when used in patients being treated with type Ic antiarrhythmic medications (36). Pretreatment of patients with intravenous magnesium may provide increased efficacy of ibutelide in converting atrial flutter (37).

Nonpharmacologic means of converting atrial flutter include overdrive pacing of the atria and direct current cardioversion. Overdrive pacing can be accomplished by several different approaches. In post–cardiac surgery patients, temporary epicardial pacing wires are frequently available for this purpose. Special high-rate atrial pacers may be needed, or, in some external pacers, a special atrial overdrive function is available for this purpose. Esophageal or transvenous pacing catheters can also be used when available. Success of overdrive pacing is usually in the 30% to 50% range (38). Overdrive pacing is usually started at a rate slightly higher than the atrial flutter rate (e.g., 10- to 20-msec-shorter cycle length) in bursts of pulses starting from short bursts (5 to 8 beats) to longer ones (10 to 20 beats). The rate of the burst pacing can then be increased and the bursts repeated. The ECG or intracardiac electrograms should be observed during the bursts to verify atrial capture. After each burst, the ECG is observed for termination of flutter or acceleration to another rhythm such as atrial fibrillation. Cycle length of pacing below 200 msec (300 beats per minute) may be needed but are more likely to induce atrial fibrillation.

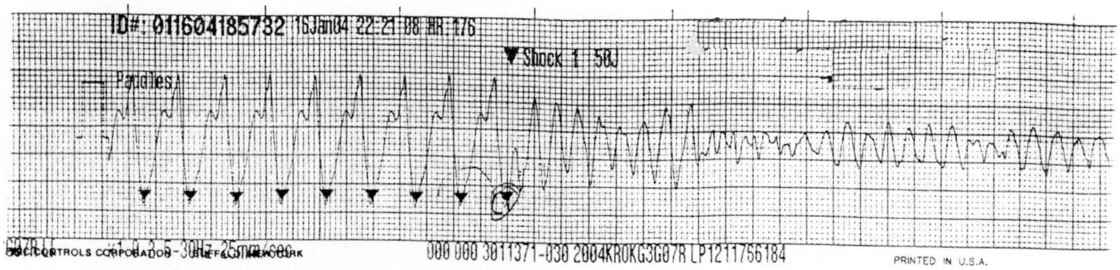

FIGURE 64.7. Inappropriate synchronization of direct current shock during wide-QRS tachycardia. This rhythm strip shows the inappropriate synchronization of the direct current shock on the T wave. Although 50 J can convert most atrial flutter, it readily induces ventricular fibrillation when synchronized to the T wave. Care should be taken to select the proper electrocardiogram lead for defibrillator synchronization so as to avoid this scenario.

Direct current cardioversion is highly successful in terminating atrial flutter. Using a short-acting intravenous sedative, one can use direct current cardioversion quickly and safely in a vast majority of patients. Biphasic defibrillators are the devices of choice due to their lower defibrillation thresholds (39). Modern biphasic defibrillators can successfully convert most atrial flutters using 50 J or less. However, it is important to synchronize the shock to the QRS complex. When a patient presents with a wide-QRS-complex atrial flutter, such as those under the influence of type Ic medications, as seen in Figure 64.6, the defibrillator shock may well synchronize on the T wave in certain ECG leads. A low-energy shock delivered on the T wave can readily induce ventricular fibrillation, as illustrated by the example shown in Figure 64.7. Thus, it is important to select the proper ECG lead to be used by the external defibrillator for appropriate synchronization. When converting such a wide-QRS tachycardia, it may be best to use the full output of the external defibrillator. A high-output shock is much less likely to induce ventricular fibrillation even if it should deliver on the T wave because the shock would probably be above the upper limit of vulnerability for fibrillation induction.

Catheter ablation of typical atrial flutter can be routinely done in most experienced electrophysiology laboratories. The ablation technique was briefly discussed in the section on mechanism. Short-term success rates are generally around 90% or greater (40). However, recurrences can occur in as many as 30% of cases and may require repeat ablations. Clearly, this procedure should be performed by physicians who have achieved competency in catheter ablation techniques. A combination approach of drug therapy for atrial fibrillation and catheter ablation for atrial flutter can be quite successful in the appropriate patient. As mentioned earlier, antiarrhythmic medication treatment of atrial fibrillation may "convert" the fibrillation to flutter. Clinically, the antiarrhythmic medication may suppress most atrial fibrillation. However, it may actually promote and stabilize the flutter circuit, thereby converting the clinical arrhythmia to the flutter. In this scenario, ablation of the flutter circuit while continuing with the antiarrhythmic medication to suppress the atrial fibrillation may work quite well (41).

CONTROVERSIES AND PERSONAL PERSPECTIVE

A discussion of treating atrial flutter would be incomplete without discussing the role of anticoagulation for the prevention of embolic stroke. Although the evidence for embolic risks in patients with atrial flutter is not as extensive as that for atrial fibrillation, there is a significant body of evidence that most atrial flutters, typically with atrial rates greater than 200 beats per minute, have similar thrombogenic potential to atrial fibrillation. Patients presenting with atrial flutter have a high incidence of subsequently having atrial fibrillation documented clinically and have the same risk for embolic events as those initially presenting with atrial fibrillation (42). Studies looking at thrombogenic markers have shown an elevated risk in patients following cardioversion of atrial flutter (43). Patients undergoing catheter ablation of persistent atrial flutter who were not adequately anticoagulated before the procedure have increased incidence of embolic complication postablation (44). Embolic complications after cardioversion of atrial flutter are similar to those after cardioversion of atrial fibrillation when patients were not adequately anticoagulated (45). Atypical flutters have the same or even greater risk for embolic events, possibly due to the fact that these flutters are more likely to be associated with scarred atria accompanied by decreased atrial mechanical function (46). Thus, it is prudent to consider anticoagulation for patients with atrial flutter in the same manner as for patients with atrial fibrillation (47).

THE FUTURE

Since the first description of atrial flutter a century ago, our understanding of atrial macro reentrant rhythms has advanced significantly. Most of these advances have been fueled by catheter ablation technologies and the ability to map electrical activation of the heart using complex computerized mapping systems. We now have some understanding of the roles that various atrial structures play in different types of flutter. Mapping systems have allowed us to appreciate the role of surgical scars and nonsurgical fibrosis in the generation of reentrant pathways that are integral to atrial flutters. We also have an understanding of the relationship between atrial fibrillation and atrial flutter and how one may be the trigger of the other in a large majority of cases. Most atrial flutters are now treatable or at least controlled clinically with medications, cardioversion, or catheter ablation approaches.

References

1. Saoudi N, Cosio F, Waldo A, et al. Classification of atrial flutter and regular atrial tachycardia according to electrophysiologic mechanism and anatomic bases: a statement from a joint expert group from the Working Group of Arrhythmias of the European Society of Cardiology and the North American Society of Pacing and Electrophysiology. *J Cardiovasc Electrophysiol* 2001;12(7):852–866.
2. Jolly WA, Richie WJ. Auricular flutter and fibrillation. *Heart* 1911;2:177–221.
3. Kasai A, Anselme F, Saoudi N. Myocardial connections between left atrial myocardium and coronary sinus musculature in man. *J Cardiovasc Electrophysiol* 2001;12(9):981–985.
4. Tai CT, Chen SA, Chen YJ, et al. Conduction properties of the crista terminalis in patients with typical atrial flutter: basis for a line of block in the reentrant circuit. *J Cardiovasc Electrophysiol* 1998;9(8):811–819.

5. Olshansky B, Okumura K, Hess PG, et al. Demonstration of an area of slow conduction in human atrial flutter. *J Am Coll Cardiol* 1990;16(7): 1639–1648.
6. Feld GK, Fleck RP, Chen PS, et al. Radiofrequency catheter ablation for the treatment of human type 1 atrial flutter. Identification of a critical zone in the reentrant circuit by endocardial mapping techniques. *Circulation* 1992;86(4):1233–1140.
7. Fujiki A, Nishida K, Sakabe M, et al. Entrainment mapping of dual-loop macroreentry in common atrial flutter: new insights into the atrial flutter circuit. *J Cardiovasc Electrophysiol* 2004;15(6):679–685.
8. Zhang S, Younis G, Hariharan R, et al. Lower loop reentry as a mechanism of clockwise right atrial flutter. *Circulation* 2004;109(13):1630–1635.
9. Lai LP, Lin JL, Lin LJ, et al. New electrocardiographic criteria for the differentiation between counterclockwise and clockwise atrial flutter: correlation with electrophysiological study and radiofrequency catheter ablation. *Heart (Br Cardiac Soc)* 1998;80(1):80–85.
10. Passman RS, Kadish AH, Dibs SR, et al. Radiofrequency ablation of atrial flutter: a randomized controlled study of two anatomic approaches. *Pacing Clin Electrophysiol* 2004;27(1):83–88.
11. Montenero AS, Bruno N, Zumbo F, et al. Cryothermal ablation treatment of atrial flutter—experience with a new 9 French 8 mm tip catheter. *J Interv Cardiac Electrophysiol* 2005;12(1):45–54.
12. Daubert JP, Hoyt RH, John R, et al., CryoCor Atrial Flutter Investigators. Performance of a new cardiac cryoablation system in the treatment of cavotricuspid valve isthmus-dependent atrial flutter. *Pacing Clin Electrophysiol* 2005;28(Suppl 1):S142–S145.
13. Della BP, Fraticelli A, Tondo C, et al. Atypical atrial flutter: clinical features, electrophysiological characteristics and response to radiofrequency catheter ablation. *Europace* 2002;4(3):241–253.
14. Merino JL, Peinado R, Abello M, et al. Superior vena cava flutter: electrophysiology and ablation. *J Cardiovasc Electrophysiol* 2005;16(6):568–575.
15. Tai CT, Huang JL, Lin YK, et al. Noncontact three-dimensional mapping and ablation of upper loop re-entry originating in the right atrium. *J Am Coll Cardiol* 2002;40(4):746–753.
16. Tanner H, Lukac P, Schwick N, et al. Irrigated-tip catheter ablation of intraatrial reentrant tachycardia in patients late after surgery of congenital heart disease. *Heart Rhythm* 2004;1(3):268–275.
17. Lukac P, Pedersen AK, Mortensen PT, et al. Ablation of atrial tachycardia after surgery for congenital and acquired heart disease using an electroanatomic mapping system: Which circuits to expect in which substrate? *Heart Rhythm* 2005;2(1):64–72.
18. Tai CT, Liu TY, Lee PC, et al. Non-contact mapping to guide radiofrequency ablation of atypical right atrial flutter. *J Am Coll Cardiol* 2004; 44(5):1080–1086.
19. Verma A, Marrouche NF, Seshadri N, et al. Importance of ablating all potential right atrial flutter circuits in postcardiac surgery patients. *J Am Coll Cardiol* 2004;44(2):409–414.
20. Gerstenfeld EP, Callans DJ, Dixit S, et al. Mechanisms of organized left atrial tachycardias occurring after pulmonary vein isolation. *Circulation* 2004;110(11):1351–1357.
21. Golovchiner G, Mazur A, Kogan A, et al. Atrial flutter after surgical radiofrequency ablation of the left atrium for atrial fibrillation. *Ann Thorac Surg* 2005;79(1):108–112.
22. Ishii Y, Gleva MJ, Gamache MC, et al. Atrial tachyarrhythmias after the maze procedure: incidence and prognosis. *Circulation* 2004;110(11 Suppl 1):II164–II168.
23. Tai CT, Lin YK, Chen SA. Atypical atrial flutter involving the isthmus between the right pulmonary veins and fossa ovalis. *Pacing Clin Electrophysiol* 2001;24(3):384–387.
24. Marrouche NF, Natale A, Wazni OM, et al. Left septal atrial flutter: electrophysiology, anatomy, and results of ablation. *Circulation* 2004;109(20): 2440–2447.
25. Olgin JE, Jayachandran JV, Engesstein E, et al. Atrial macroreentry involving the myocardium of the coronary sinus: a unique mechanism for atypical flutter. *J Cardiovasc Electrophysiol* 1998;9(10):1094–1099.
26. Poty H, Anselme F, Saoudi N. Inferior vena cava-tricuspid annulus isthmus is a critical site of unidirectional block during the induction of common atrial flutter. *J Interv Cardiac Electrophysiol* 1998;2(1):57–69.
27. Bertaglia E, Zoppo F, Bonso A, et al. Northeastern Italian Study on Atrial Flutter Ablation Investigators. Long term follow up of radiofrequency catheter ablation of atrial flutter: clinical course and predictors of atrial fibrillation occurrence. *Heart (Br Cardiac Soc)* 2004;90(1):59–63.
28. Bertaglia E, Bonso A, Zoppo F, et al. North-Eastern Italian Study on Atrial Flutter Ablation Investigators. Different clinical courses and predictors of atrial fibrillation occurrence after transisthmic ablation in patients with preablation lone atrial flutter, coexistent atrial fibrillation, and drug induced atrial flutter. *Pacing Clin Electrophysiol* 2004;27(11):1507–1512.
29. Tai CT, Chiang CE, Lee SH, et al. Persistent atrial flutter in patients treated for atrial fibrillation with amiodarone and propafenone: electrophysiologic characteristics, radiofrequency catheter ablation, and risk prediction. *J Cardiovasc Electrophysiol* 1999;10(9):1180–1187.
30. Kawabata M, Hirao K, Horikawa T, et al. Syncope in patients with atrial flutter during treatment with class Ic antiarrhythmic drugs. *J Electrocardiol* 2001;34(1):65–72.
31. Pedersen OD, Bagger H, Keller N, et al. Efficacy of dofetilide in the treatment of atrial fibrillation-flutter in patients with reduced left ventricular function: a Danish investigation of arrhythmia and mortality on dofetilide (diamond) substudy. *Circulation* 2001;104(3):292–296.
32. Ando G, Di Rosa S, Rizzo F, et al. Ibutilide for cardioversion of atrial flutter: efficacy of a single dose in recent-onset arrhythmias. *Minerva Cardioangiol* 2004;52(1):37–42.
33. Sun JL, Guo JH, Zhang N, et al. Clinical comparison of ibutilide and propafenone for converting atrial flutter. *Cardiovasc Drugs Ther* 2005; 19(1):57–64.
34. Ando G, Di Rosa S, Rizzo F, et al. Ibutilide for cardioversion of atrial flutter: efficacy of a single dose in recent-onset arrhythmias. *Minerva Cardioangiol* 2004;52(1):37–42.
35. Dilaveris P, Synetos A, Giannopoulos G, et al. Conversion of recent-onset atrial fibrillation or flutter with amiodarone after ibutilide has failed: a rapid, efficient, and safe algorithm. *Ann Noninvasive Electrocardiol* 2005; 10(3):382–386.
36. Hongo RH, Themistoclakis S, Raviele A, et al. Use of ibutilide in cardioversion of patients with atrial fibrillation or atrial flutter treated with class IC agents. *J Am Coll Cardiol* 2004;44(4):864–868.
37. Kalus JS, Spencer AP, Tsikouris JP, et al. Impact of prophylactic i.v. magnesium on the efficacy of ibutilide for conversion of atrial fibrillation or flutter. *Am J Health Syst Pharm* 2003;60(22):2308–2312.
38. Mazza A, Fera MS, Bisceglia I, et al. Efficacy and safety of ibutilide vs. transoesophageal atrial pacing for the termination of type I atrial flutter. *Europace* 2004;6(4):301–306.
39. Niebauer MJ, Brewer JE, Chung MK, et al. Comparison of the rectilinear biphasic waveform with the monophasic damped sine waveform for external cardioversion of atrial fibrillation and flutter. *Am J Cardiol* 2004;93(12):1495–1499.
40. Fischer B, Jais P, Shah D, et al. Radiofrequency catheter ablation of common atrial flutter in 200 patients. *J Cardiovasc Electrophysiol* 1996;7(12):1225–1233.
41. Huang DT, Monahan KM, Zimetbaum P, et al. Hybrid pharmacologic and ablative therapy: a novel and effective approach for the management of atrial fibrillation. *J Cardiovasc Electrophysiol* 1998;9(5):462–469.
42. Halligan SC, Gersh BJ, Brown Jr RD, et al. The natural history of lone atrial flutter. *Ann Intern Med* 2004;140(4):265–268.
43. Sakurai K, Hirai T, Nakagawa K, et al. Prolonged activation of hemostatic markers following conversion of atrial flutter to sinus rhythm. *Circ J* 2004;68(11):1041–1044.
44. Gronefeld GC, Wegener F, Israel CW, et al. Thromboembolic risk of patients referred for radiofrequency catheter ablation of typical atrial flutter without prior appropriate anticoagulation therapy. *Pacing Clin Electrophysiol* 2003;26(1 Pt 2):323–327.
45. Gallagher MM, Hennessy BJ, Edvardsson N, et al. Embolic complications of direct current cardioversion of atrial arrhythmias: association with low intensity of anticoagulation at the time of cardioversion. *J Am Coll Cardiol* 2002;40(5):926–933.
46. Demir AD, Soylu M, Ozdemir O, et al. Do different atrial flutter types carry the same thromboembolic risk? *Angiology* 2005;56(5):593–599.
47. Singer DE, Albers GW, Dalen JE, et al. Antithrombotic therapy in atrial fibrillation: the Seventh ACCP Conference on Antithrombotic and Thrombolytic Therapy. *Chest* 2004;126(3 Suppl):429S–456S.

CHAPTER 65 ■ ATRIOVENTRICULAR NODAL–DEPENDENT TACHYCARDIAS AND PREEXCITATION

ROBERT A. SCHWEIKERT AND DOUGLAS L. PACKER

OVERVIEW

Atrioventricular (AV) nodal–dependent tachycardias comprise a specific subgroup of rapid, regular supraventricular arrhythmias that critically depend on conduction through the AV node for their perpetuation. The most common forms are AV nodal reentrant tachycardia (AVNRT) and AV reciprocating tachycardia (AVRT), the latter of which uses an accessory pathway (AP) as the retrograde limb of the circuit. The anatomic location around the mitral or tricuspid annulus of APs can be identified precisely at the time of electrophysiologic testing but can also be predicted based on the morphology of retrograde P waves during tachycardia or characteristic delta waves in those patients in whom these arrhythmias occur as a component of Wolff-Parkinson-White (WPW) syndrome. AV nodal–dependent tachycardias are typically initiated by premature atrial or ventricular complexes and have reasonably specific characteristics that allow their differentiation. Although both are short RP tachycardias, AVRT must have a ventriculoatrial (VA) or RP interval of at least 70 msec, whereas most AVNRTs have intervals of less than 60 msec, with retrograde P waves presenting as a pseudo-R wave in surface electrocardiogram (ECG) lead V_1 during tachycardia. In some patients with APs, a reverse-direction tachycardia with anterograde conduction through the AP may occur, producing a maximally preexcited QRS complex on the surface ECG. Some patients with WPW syndrome are at potential risk for atrial fibrillation (AF) degenerating into ventricular fibrillation (VF). APs with unusual conduction characteristics contribute to the occurrence of preexcitation variants, including the permanent form of junctional reciprocating tachycardia (PJRT) and atriofascicular reentry. Because of their dependence on AV nodal conduction for their maintenance, AV nodal–dependent arrhythmias may be acutely terminated by vagal maneuvers or administration of adenosine or verapamil. Wide-complex tachycardias in these patients must be carefully approached without using drugs that accelerate AP conduction, which can lead to VF. Both pharmacologic and nonpharmacologic therapies may be applied in the long term for managing patients with these arrhythmias. Drug therapy may be directed at the AV node, the AP, or the initiating atrial or ventricular extrastimuli. Ablative therapy has also emerged as the mainstay of nonpharmacologic treatment of these arrhythmias.

GLOSSARY

Anterior fibrous trigone: The region of convergent, dense, fibrous tissue of the posterior aortic and anterior mitral valve annuli.

Antidromic reciprocating tachycardia: A reverse-direction AV nodal–dependent tachycardia in which anterograde conduction occurs through the AP, whereas return retrograde atrial activation proceeds through the normal VA conduction system.

Atriofascicular Mahaim fiber: An atypical AP with AV node–like properties (or an accessory AV node) typically located in the anterior or anterolateral region of the tricuspid annulus. This pathway serves as a bridge between atrial and right bundle branch tissue.

Atriofascicular or Mahaim reentrant tachycardia: A preexcitation variant tachycardia that uses an atriofascicular fiber as its anterograde limb.

Atrioventricular nodal reentrant tachycardia (AVNRT): An AV nodal–dependent tachycardia in which both anterograde and retrograde components of the reentrant substrate are located near or within the compact portion of the AV node.

Atrioventricular nodal–dependent tachycardia: A tachycardia that critically depends on conduction through the AV node for its perpetuation.

Atrioventricular reciprocating (reentrant) tachycardia (AVRT): An AV nodal–dependent tachycardia with the AV conduction system as the anterograde and the AP as the retrograde limb of the tachycardia circuit.

Concealed accessory pathway: AP with retrograde-only conduction existing without evidence of anterograde ventricular activation through that pathway.

Discontinuous conduction: Characteristic of dual AV nodal physiology in which a more than 50-msec abrupt prolongation of AV nodal conduction time occurs with a 10-msec decrease in the coupling time of an atrial premature complex (APC), producing anterograde conduction through the AV node.

Dual atrioventricular nodal physiology: Electrophysiologic manifestation of two AV nodal pathways with different anatomic and/or physiologic properties that serve as a substrate for AV nodal reentrant tachycardia.

Koch's triangle: A triangular space in the medial portion of the right atrium formed by the septal component of the tricuspid valve annulus, the coronary sinus orifice, and the tendon of Todaro. The AV node lies in the apex of this triangle.

Long RP tachycardia: Tachycardia with a retrograde P wave describing atrial activation occurring closer to the succeeding than the preceding QRS complex. These tachycardias have an RP interval that is more than 50% of the RR interval seen during tachycardia.

Permanent junctional reciprocating tachycardia (PJRT): Preexcitation variant in which retrograde atrial activation occurs through an AP with nodelike or decremental electrical properties. These long RP tachycardias may be incessant and show negative P waves in leads II, III, and aVF.

Preexcitation: Early ventricular activation before that proceeding through the normal AV conduction system, as seen in patients with APs.

Short RP tachycardia: Tachycardia with a retrograde P wave describing atrial activation that occurs closer to the preceding than the succeeding QRS complex. These tachycardias have an RP interval that is less than 50% of the RR interval seen during tachycardia.

Ventriculoatrial interval: The VA interval beginning with the local ventricular activation and ending with earliest retrograde atrial activation. The surface ECG correlate is the RP interval from onset of the surface QRS to the onset of the retrograde P wave.

INTRODUCTION

AV nodal–dependent tachycardias comprise a specific subgroup of rapid, regular supraventricular arrhythmias that critically depend on conduction through the AV node for their perpetuation. These arrhythmias typically use the normal AV conduction system as the anterograde limb of the reentrant circuit and therefore present with a narrow QRS complex on the surface ECG, as shown in Figure 65.1. Unlike atrial flutter or atrial tachycardias, which may continue despite the presence of high-grade AV block, AV nodal–dependent tachycardias are typically

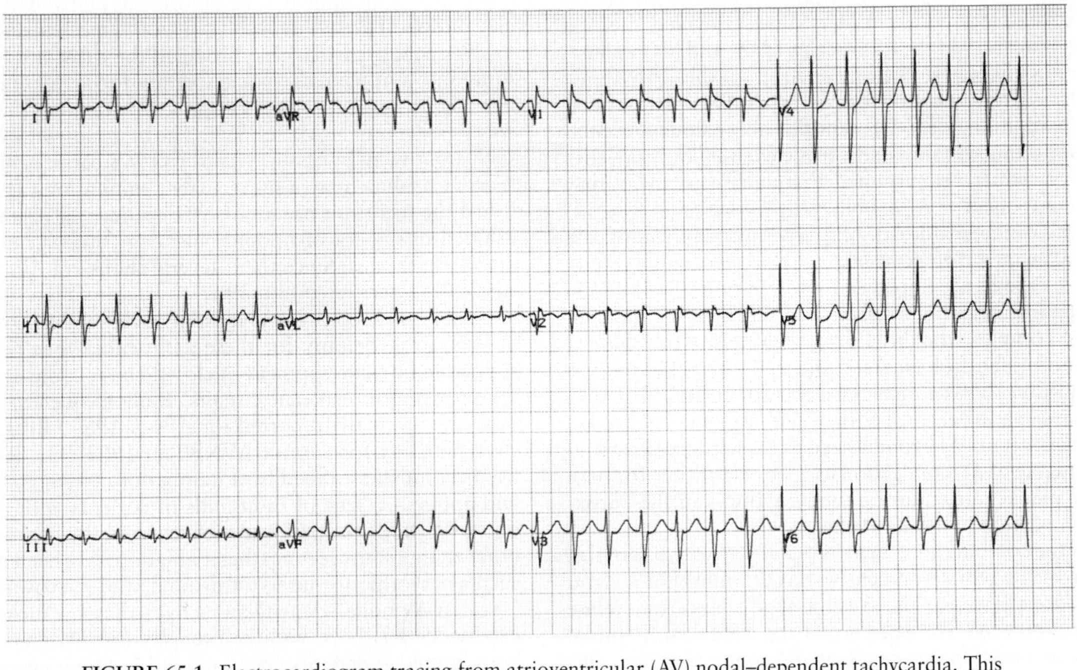

FIGURE 65.1. Electrocardiogram tracing from atrioventricular (AV) nodal–dependent tachycardia. This is a narrow-QRS-complex tachycardia with a 1:1 AV relationship in a patient with an AV nodal reentrant tachycardia.

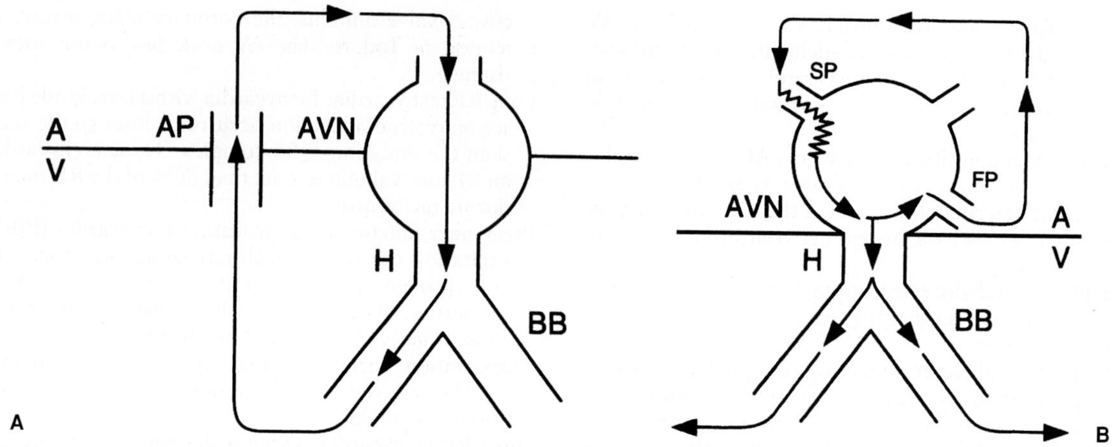

FIGURE 65.2. Mechanism of atrioventricular (AV) reentrant and AV nodal reentrant tachycardias. In both arrhythmias, the AV node serves as a mandatory component of the reentrant circuit. **A:** AV reentrant tachycardia in which the accesory pathway (AP) serves as the retrograde limb of the reentrant circuit. **B:** AV nodal reentrant tachycardia circuit with anterograde conduction through the slow pathway (SP) with return retrograde conduction through the fast pathway (FP).; AVN, atrioventricular node; BB, bundle branch; H, bundle of His; SP.

terminated by vagal, drug, or nonpharmacologic interruption of AV nodal conduction.

The most common of the AV nodal–dependent arrhythmias are AV nodal reentrant tachycardia (AVNRT) and AV reciprocating tachycardia (AVRT). AVNRT involves anterograde and retrograde components of the reentrant substrate that are near or within the compact portion of the AV node and neighboring bundle of His. AVRT involves the AV node and an AP as the limbs of the tachycardia circuit (Fig. 65.2).

HISTORICAL PERSPECTIVE

These arrhythmias have been a focus of extensive clinical interest during the last 100 years and have prompted numerous studies to clarify the underlying electrophysiology. Kent provided an early description of what we now refer to as the normal AV conduction system (1). Mines provided the first description of reentry in the AV node in 1913, and his explanation of the possible physiologic mechanism of this arrhythmia is essentially what we now refer to as "dual AV nodal physiology" (2). In addition, Kent (3) identified anomalous muscular bundles connecting the atria and ventricles. Building on Kent's observations, Mines (4) suggested that such a pathway may serve as a component of a possible reentrant circuit.

By the end of the first decade of this period, a variety of case reports documented the occurrence of relatively benign, rapid, regular tachycardias accompanied by palpitations (5–8). Wood et al. (7) reported a patient with a short PR interval and prolonged QRS complex who died during an attack of paroxysmal tachycardia. Serial histological sections of a portion of this patient's AV groove showed three muscular connections between the right auricle and ventricle at the right lateral border of the heart. Wolferth et al. (5) hypothesized that such accessory connections capable of AV conduction may be responsible for both ventricular preexcitation during sinus rhythm and the paroxysms of tachycardia in these patients.

In 1930 the combination of paroxysmal tachycardias of this type along with a bundle-branch-block QRS morphology and a short PR interval were codified as the Wolff-Parkinson-White (WPW) syndrome (8). The existence of apparent dual AV nodal physiology as additional avenues of AV conduction was further suggested by others (9–11), and in 1963 Kistin postulated the existence of multiple AV nodal pathways in humans (12). Other investigators also subsequently described the possibility of triple or multiple AV nodal pathways (13–17).

The understanding of the rhythm disorders created by these connections took a giant leap forward with the advent of catheter-based electrophysiologic studies (18–23). By positioning multiple recording electrodes within the heart and using electrical stimulation techniques, it has been possible to elucidate the roles of the AV node and AP in supraventricular tachycardias (SVTs). Furthermore, this information has also expanded our understanding of macroreentrant arrhythmias in general. In this regard, the AV nodal–dependent SVTs with their discrete anatomic components can be viewed as the "schoolmaster" of reentrant arrhythmias. Since then, volumes have been written about the preexcitation syndromes, their accompanying SVTs, and AVNRTs (24–27). More recently, the introduction of more advanced computerized and optical mapping techniques with improved resolution has allowed more precise elucidation of arrhythmia substrates and mechanisms (28–30).

These tachycardias also provided the substrate for the first foray into nonpharmacologic therapy for arrhythmias. In the late 1960s, several institutions (31,32) attempted to interrupt APs as a definitive cure for SVT. The first successful division of such a pathway by Sealy (32,33) in 1968 permanently cured a North Carolina man of his recurrent palpitations, firmly established the reentrant nature of AP-dependent arrhythmias, and ushered in the era of nonpharmacologic management of cardiac arrhythmias. Since then, several thousand APs have been surgically interrupted (34–39).

Based on lessons learned from such surgical interruption of APs, drug therapy for these arrhythmias has been largely supplanted by development of closed-chest, catheter-based ablation of these reentrant circuits. Radiofrequency (RF) ablation was originally reported for APs in 1987 (40) and for the slow pathway for cure of AVNRT in 1992 (41). RF ablation has been further refined by a number of investigators (42–48) and applied to tens of thousands of patients with AVRT and other AV nodal–dependent tachycardias. In addition to RF, other energy sources for catheter ablation have been developed, such as cryothermy, laser, ultrasound, and microwave sources (49). For AV nodal–dependent tachycardias, the most extensive experience has been with cryothermy (50,51), and there has been limited experience with lasers (52). Other energy sources for catheter ablation, such as ultrasound and microwaves, have not yet been studied extensively for AV nodal–dependent tachycardias. Because of the high success rates and low accompanying risk, catheter ablation has nearly replaced drug therapy as the mainstay of treatment for AV nodal–dependent arrhythmias. Each of these historic milestones marks important progress in both our understanding of these arrhythmias and the development of effective clinical management strategies.

ATRIOVENTRICULAR RECIPROCATING TACHYCARDIAS AND ACCESSORY PATHWAYS

Anatomic Considerations

The occurrence of an AV nodal–dependent reentrant tachycardia, like other classic reentrant arrhythmias, requires two anatomically distinct components or pathways to create the tachycardia circuit (4). By definition, the first is the AV nodal conduction system. Conduction in most AV nodal–dependent tachycardias travels anterogradely through this AV conduction system to produce the classic narrow QRS complex seen on the ECG.

APs involved as the retrograde limb of the AV reentrant tachycardia circuit are formed by minute, electrically conducting muscle bundles that transverse the AV groove. These pathways establish a nonnodal avenue for AV or VA propagation across the mitral and tricuspid annuli, which otherwise electrically isolate the atria from the ventricles. These fibers may cross the AV groove directly, proceed on an angle, or in some cases arborize with one or more branch points before insertion into either ventricular or atrial muscle (53–56).

With the exception of the region near the anterior fibrous trigone between the aortic and mitral valves, which is usually void of APs, these accessory AV connections may be distributed anywhere along the mitral or tricuspid annuli. As noted in Figure 65.3, surgical and catheter ablation studies have demonstrated that approximately 55% of these AV connections are located at the left free-wall region. Furthermore, 25% are in the posteroseptal region, 15% are in a right free-wall location, and 5% are in the anteroseptal region (35–38,43,45,47,48,57). In addition, 7% to 15% of patients may have more than one AP (23,43,45,47,48,58–61). More recently, a unique AP involving a connection between the right atrial appendage and right ventricle has been described (62–65), and due to its epicardial location, catheter ablation from an epicardial approach using percutaneous pericardial instrumentation has been necessary in

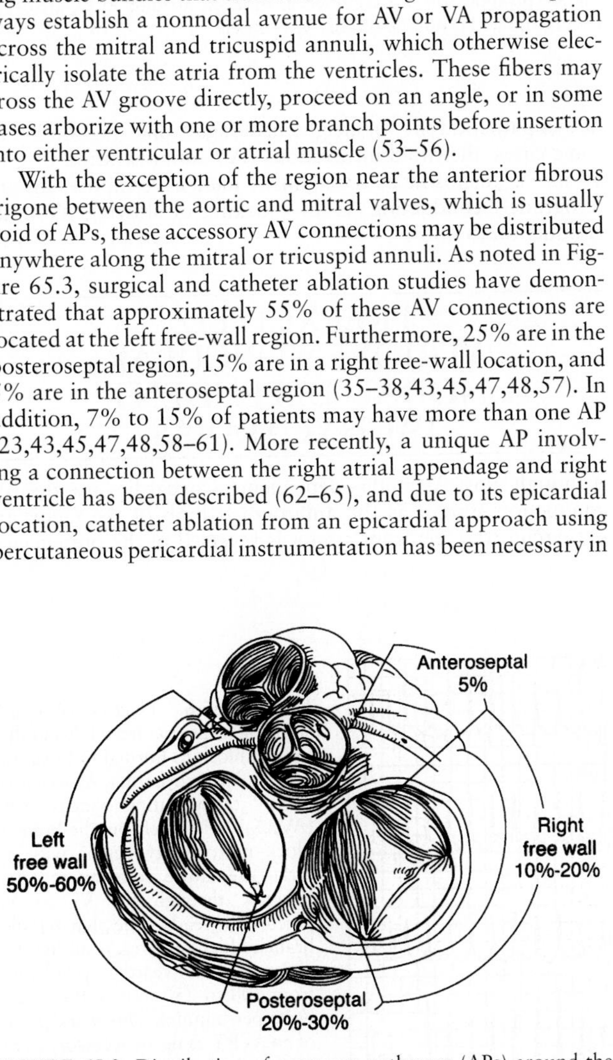

FIGURE 65.3. Distribution of accessory pathways (APs) around the mitral and tricuspid annuli. The left free-wall position is the most common AP location.

some cases (63,64). This highlights the role of interventional electrophysiology in the advancement of our understanding of arrhythmia substrates.

Of all pathways described in reports of symptomatic patients, 2% to 3% conduct in an anterograde direction only, whereas 20% to 31% conduct in the retrograde/ventricular-to-atrial direction only (43,45,47,48,66). These connections are referred to as concealed APs. The mechanism of such concealment is further related to atrial and ventricular anatomy or the characteristic electrical properties of conduction through the pathway (25,67–71).

The specific anatomic location of an AP may be inferred from a variety of clinical and electrophysiologic indicators. The most readily available of these is the delta-wave morphology inscribed on the surface ECG. Rosenbaum and colleagues (72) first described variations in anatomic location based on the precordial QRS morphology and divided the WPW syndrome into type A, with a large R wave in surface lead V_1, and type B, with S or QS morphology in this same lead. A variety of different algorithms have since been developed to predict more specifically the anatomic location of single pathways with anterograde conduction based on the surface ECG (66,73–79).

Similarly, pathway location can be discerned from the morphology of the retrograde P wave, when evident. Garcia et al. (80) showed that a positive P-wave morphology in lead V_1 during SVT is suggestive of a left free-wall pathway, whereas a negative deflection is more consistent with a right-sided pathway. Tai et al. (81) developed a stepwise algorithm for predicting AP location with an accuracy of 88% based on retrograde P-wave morphology in leads I, II, III, aVF, and V_1. The specific anatomic pathway location is more precisely identified by the earliest site of retrograde atrial activation during tachycardia or ventricular pacing on electrophysiologic testing.

Physiologic Mechanisms

The distance of the AP from the bundle of His region dictates that the time from onset of the surface QRS to the local atrial activation at the site of the pathway, referred to as the VA interval, must be at least 65 to 70 msec (66,82). For this reason, the ECG correlate of this VA interval, the "RP" interval, from the onset of the QRS complex to the P wave is usually more than 80 msec in duration. This specific VA activation time predicts that the inscription of the retrograde P wave will occur early in the ST segment or on the upslope of the T wave of the surface ECG, closer to the preceding than the succeeding QRS complex. If the RP interval is less than 50% of the RR interval from one QRS complex to the next, the tachycardia is considered to be a short RP tachycardia (Fig. 65.4).

These VA or RP intervals during AVRT are relatively constant. An important exception is the 35-msec or greater prolongation of the VA interval seen with the emergence of bundle branch block ipsilateral to the AP during the AVRT, as shown in Figure 65.5 (83,84). For example, patients with left free-wall pathways who develop left-bundle-branch block show classic prolongation of the VA interval during tachycardia. Unless this activation slowing is offset by reciprocal acceleration of conduction through the normal AV conduction system, the tachycardia in such patients is slowed. Conversely, acceleration of the tachycardia with abrupt resolution of bundle branch block, as seen on the surface ECG in Figure 65.6, is virtually pathognomonic for an AP-related tachycardia.

Physiology of Preexcitation

During "preexcited" anterograde ventricular activation through the AP during normal sinus rhythm, a delta wave and

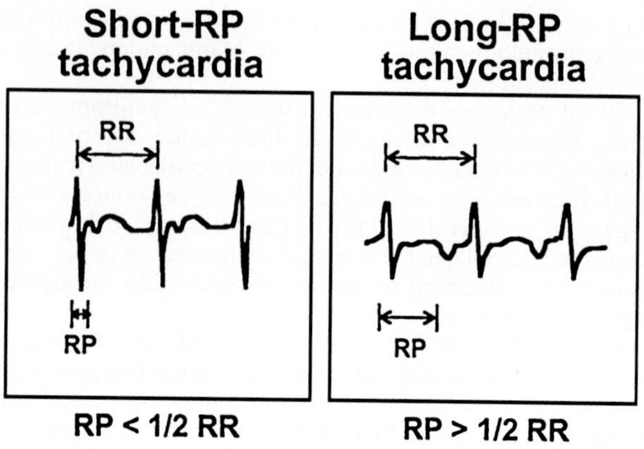

FIGURE 65.4. Classification of short- and long-RP tachycardias. **Left:** A retrograde P wave in tachycardia that occurs closer to the preceding than succeeding QRS. Supraventricular arrhythmias with such an RP interval of less than 50% of the RR interval are designated "short"-RP tachycardias. **Right:** A retrograde P wave closer to the following QRS due to prolonged retrograde conduction time. An RP interval longer than 50% of the RR cycle length qualifies as a "long"-RP tachycardia.

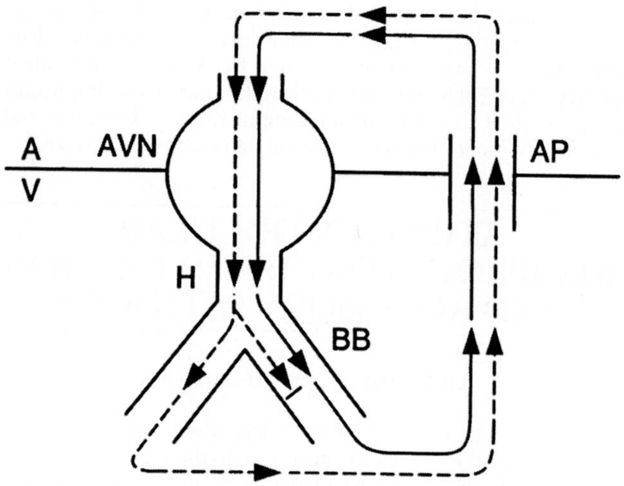

FIGURE 65.5. Change in ventriculoatrial (VA) interval with development of bundle branch (BB) aberration during orthodromic atrioventricular reciprocating tachycardia using an accessory pathway (AP). During normal conduction (*solid line*), the interval from the onset of the surface QRS to the earliest retrograde atrial activation (VA interval) is at least 70 msec because of the component conduction properties. With BB block ipsilateral to the AP, the additional conduction time due to transseptal and intramyocardial propagation (*dashed line*) to the AP prolongs the VA conduction time. A, atrium; AVN, atrioventricular node; H, bundle of His; V, ventricle.

a short PR interval are evident on the surface ECG (Fig. 65.7), and the criteria for WPW syndrome are met (8). The degree of accompanying preexcitation observed on a surface 12-lead ECG, however, depends on relative local ventricular activation proceeding through the normal AV conduction system versus that through the AP. This in turn depends on the relative time required for a propagating impulse from the sinus node to reach and traverse the AV node and His-Purkinje system or the AP (Fig. 65.8). The additional activation time required to reach an AP well removed from the sinus node along the far left lateral region of the mitral annulus decreases the likelihood of expressing ventricular preexcitation during normal sinus rhythm with this pathway location. In the setting of increased sympathoadrenergic tone such as that which accompanies exercise, ventricular activation through the normal AV conduction system is enhanced and can precede that which occurs through the AP (Fig. 65.8). During such circumstances, minimal or no ventricular preexcitation may be evident. At the other extreme, ventricular activation through the AP, yielding moderate or marked preexcitation, may be more evident with APs closer to the sinus node or in those conditions in which conduction through the AV node is slowed by intrinsic nodal factors, withdrawal of sympathetic tone, or heightened vagal tone (Fig. 65.8). In some cases, the rapid intravenous (IV) administration of 6 to 12 mg of adenosine as a diagnostic maneuver exposes an anterogradely conducting AP by blocking or slowing AV node conduction (85,86).

PREEXCITED ATRIOVENTRICULAR NODAL–DEPENDENT TACHYCARDIAS

Although most AV nodal–dependent tachycardias use the AV conduction system as the anterograde limb of the tachycardia circuit, the reentrant circuit is reversed in the presence of

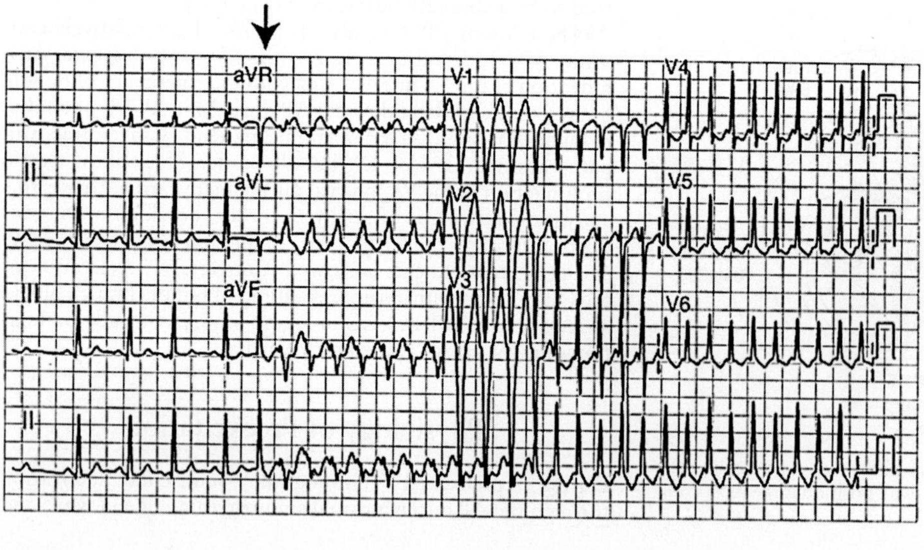

FIGURE 65.6. Electrocardiogram showing transition from left-bundle-branch block to normal QRS supraventricular tachycardia. Atrioventricular reciprocating tachycardia (AVRT) with left-bundle-branch-block morphology begins with an atrial premature complex (*arrow*). Midway through the V_1 to V_3 precordial leads, the left-bundle-branch block resolves, resulting in a decrease in tachycardia cycle length from 300 to 250 msec (200 to 240 beats per minute). This is indicative of an AVRT using an accessory pathway ipsilateral to the site of bundle branch block, which in this instance is a left free-wall accessory pathway.

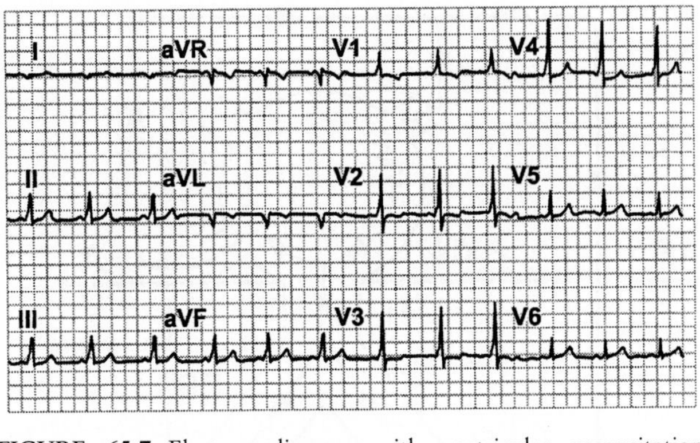

FIGURE 65.7. Electrocardiogram with ventricular preexcitation across a left free-wall accessory pathway. Note the widened QRS complex with a slurred upstroke and a shortened PR interval consistent with a diagnosis of Wolff-Parkinson-White syndrome.

antidromic AVRT, as seen in Figure 65.9. With this arrhythmia, the AV node is the requisite retrograde limb of the circuit, and ventricular activation proceeds through the AP, producing maximum QRS preexcitation. This tachycardia can be induced at electrophysiologic testing in 6% to 8% of patients with an AP (57,87–89), although only 2% to 3% of patients clinically develop this arrhythmia (57,88,89).

AVNRT with bystander conduction through a coexistent AP is a second preexcited AV nodal–dependent tachycardia. In this arrhythmia, perpetuation of the tachycardia depends on classic AVNRT using anterograde and retrograde limbs found near or within the compact portion of the AV node. The wide or preexcited QRS morphology seen on ECG is due to concomitant ventricular activation through an AP. Ablation of the AP, although it eliminates preexcitation, would not necessarily eliminate the tachycardia. Although AVNRT may be seen in 10% to 20% of patients with an AP (90–93), concurrent anterograde conduction through an AP is seen in less than 2% of patients (91). When evaluating patients with these types of AV nodal–dependent tachycardias, alternative mechanisms of preexcited tachycardias such as any atrial tachycardia or flutter with ventricular activation through an AP should be considered. Well-defined criteria for differentiating these types of tachycardias from antidromic reciprocating tachycardia have been established (89,94).

Pathophysiology of Atrial Fibrillation

Whether or not a patient has antidromic tachycardia, the greatest concern in patients with WPW is the possibility of onset of AF with a rapid ventricular response rate and further degeneration into VF. This requires both the onset of AF and the propensity for rapid conduction through the AP. Although AF may develop as an isolated or primary process in WPW patients, the disorganization of AVRT is a more likely mechanism for its occurrence in patients with an AP (95–97). Some have proposed that the presence of the rapid, pathway-dependent tachycardia produces electrophysiologic changes in the atria that facilitate the onset of AF. The role of the AP or tachycardia in this process is also inferred from the substantial reduction in clinical AF after curative surgical or catheter ablative procedures (98–101) but may nonetheless show an age-related increase in incidence (102). Evidence that AVRT is not mandatory for onset of AF, however, is the occurrence of AF in patients who do not have AVRT and in whom APs are only capable of anterograde conduction (99).

General Considerations and Clinical Presentation

The WPW pattern demonstrated by ECG has been reported to be present in 0.10% to 0.25% of the general population (103–105). There is evidence that family members of patients with WPW pattern have an increased incidence of this abnormality. In one report this incidence was a fourfold increase and appeared to be with an autosomal dominant mode of inheritance (106). Most other reports of a familial mode of inheritance described by other investigators involved "complex" WPW patients who had concomitant cardiac abnormalities such as hypertrophic cardiomyopathy (107–109). Therefore, a genetic basis for WPW abnormality in patients without concomitant cardiac abnormalities has not been firmly established.

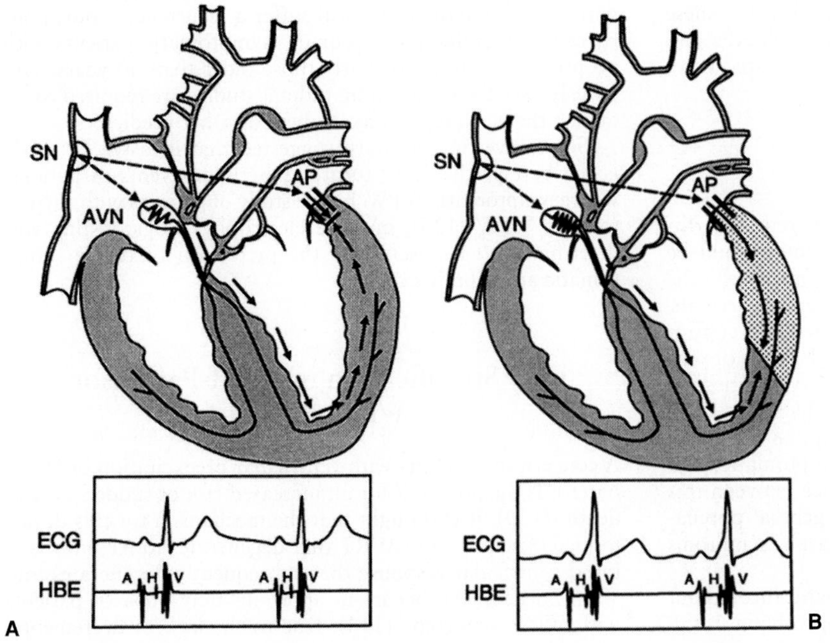

FIGURE 65.8. Variable ventricular preexcitation dependent on relative conduction through the atrioventricular node (AVN) and accessory pathway (AP). **A:** Minimal ventricular preexcitation in the setting of enhanced AV nodal conduction and an AP distant from the sinus node (SN). Prolonged conduction time to this site provides a relative advantage to ventricular activation through the AV node. Note the normal AV interval of 40 msec on the diagrammatic electrogram (*inset*). **B:** Moderate to marked ventricular preexcitation related to relatively greater ventricular activation through the AP. Here, conduction time through the AV node is prolonged, yielding a relative advantage for conduction through the AP. The His deflection occurs after the onset of ventricular activation through the AP. A, atrial electrogram; ECG, electrocardiogram; H, bundle of His; HBE, bundle of His electrogram; V, ventricular electrogram.

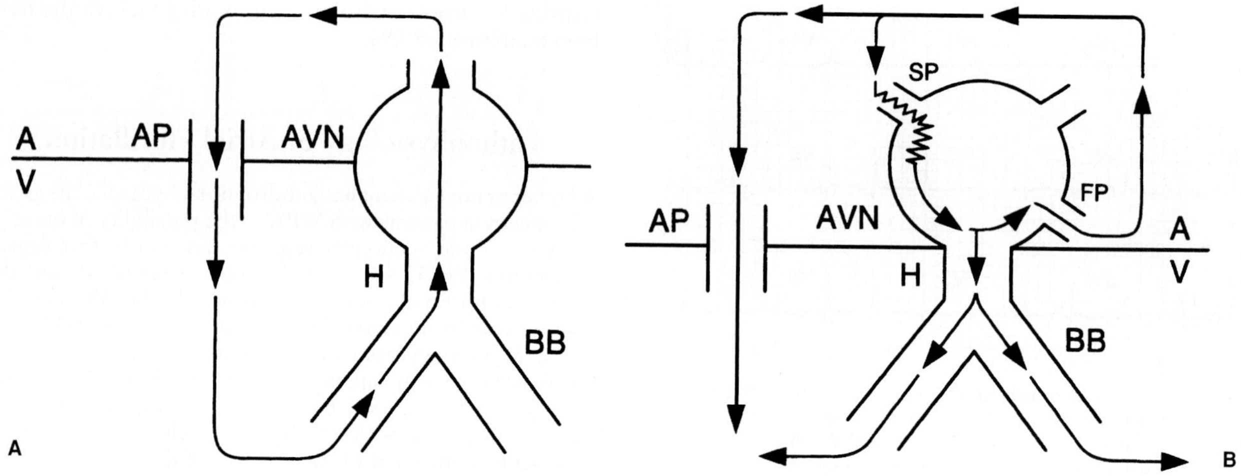

FIGURE 65.9. Mechanisms of preexcited atrioventricular (AV) nodal–dependent tachycardias. **A:** Antidromic reciprocating tachycardia with anterograde conduction through the accessory pathway (AP) and retrograde atrial activation through the normal ventriculoatrial conduction system. **B:** AV nodal reentry with a classic mechanism involving anterograde conduction through the slow pathway (SP) and retrograde or return atrial activation through the fast pathway (FP). Preexcitation occurs because of additional bystander conduction through the neighboring AP. AVN, atrioventricular node; BB, bundle branch; H, bundle of His.

Population-based studies (110) have suggested that 50% to 60% of patients with WPW pattern show symptoms ranging from palpitations to syncope. Other symptoms may include dyspnea, decreased exercise tolerance, chest discomfort or tightness, anxiety, dizziness, presyncope, or syncope. Of those patients with symptomatic arrhythmias, 85% have underlying AVRTs that use the AP as a retrograde limb (27,57,66). Only 2% to 3% of patients show clinical antidromic reciprocating tachycardia (89,111,112), whereas 30% to 40% of patients develop AF (57,66,113–116).

Unlike most ventricular tachycardias, which tend to occur in patients with cardiomyopathy, AV nodal–dependent tachycardias typically occur in the absence of any other organic heart disease. Any underlying process that does occur, such as mitral valve prolapse or hypertrophic cardiomyopathy, is therefore generally considered a chance occurrence. One exception is coexistent Ebstein malformation of the tricuspid valve and an AP (57,66,92). Of those patients with APs reported in larger studies (117,118), 7% to 10% have this coexistent structural abnormality. This finding is of clinical importance because these patients typically have a higher prevalence of multiple APs, and the success rate of RF ablation in patients with tricuspid valve abnormalities is lower.

Natural History

Predicting the likelihood and frequency of recurrent arrhythmias would be useful in deciding which patients should be treated for supraventricular arrhythmias. Unfortunately, the natural history of patients with AV nodal–dependent arrhythmias remains unestablished. The data are limited and contradictory (110,119–122). In a population-based study of 113 patients with WPW syndrome in Olmsted County, Minnesota, 60 (53%) were symptomatic at the time of first diagnosis. Over the course of 11.8 years of long-term follow-up, 28 (47%) remained symptomatic, 15 (25%) became asymptomatic, and 7 (12%) required surgery (110). The difference between this study and others reflects differences between general populations of patients and those selected by increasing symptoms requiring referral for medical evaluation.

Patients with APs may remain asymptomatic throughout life (123,124). In a population-based study involving 1,338 patient-years of follow-up, Munger et al. (110) demonstrated that only 11 of 53 (21%) patients who were asymptomatic at the time of initial diagnosis developed symptoms over time, whereas 36 (68%) remained symptom-free. Consistent with the findings of Leitch et al. (124), Munger et al. (110) also demonstrated that an asymptomatic patient older than 40 years was highly unlikely to develop progressive symptoms thereafter. In another study involving a prospective evaluation of 212 patients with asymptomatic WPW pattern by ECG, 33 (15.6%) developed symptomatic arrhythmia at a mean follow-up of 37.7 months (125).

Therefore, taken together, these data suggest several characteristics of patients likely to have recurrent tachycardias. First, the bimodal distribution of symptomatic arrhythmia predicts an initial decrease in symptoms during childhood followed by an increase in tachycardia in young adulthood. Second, the presence of anterograde conduction through an AP increases the likelihood of recurrence. Third, although 25% of patients become asymptomatic over time, more than one half of patients with an episode of AVRT will suffer a recurrence. Fourth, arrhythmia is unlikely to occur in asymptomatic patients with no preexcitation, particularly those older than 40 years. Obviously, more extensive longitudinal studies are required to establish the accuracy of any of these or other predictors.

Some investigators have suggested that invasive EP study is the best predictor of future arrhythmic events in patients with asymptomatic WPW. In one study of patients with asymptomatic WPW (125), invasive electrophysiologic testing was determined to be useful for the prediction of future symptomatic arrhythmic events.

Risk Stratification in Wolff-Parkinson-White Patients

A concern for patients with ventricular preexcitation or WPW pattern is the potential for an increased risk of sudden cardiac death (SCD). It is thought that the mechanism for this devastating consequence is AVRT that degenerates to AF with very rapid ventricular response that subsequently degenerates into VF (126,127). AF occurs in approximately 30% of patients with WPW syndrome (114). Due to the lack of decremental

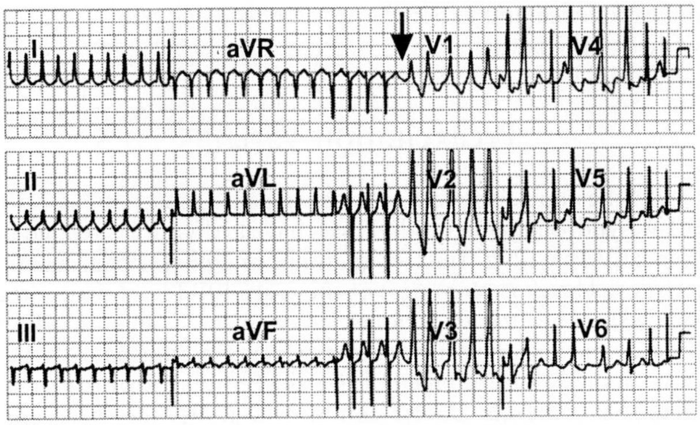

FIGURE 65.10. Atrial fibrillation with a rapid ventricular response rate during Wolff-Parkinson-White syndrome. Initial atrioventricular reentrant tachycardia degenerates into atrial fibrillation (*arrow*). The shortest RR interval in this case was 240 to 250 msec, which indicates an increased risk for sudden cardiac death.

conduction properties there is the potential for very rapid AV conduction (Fig. 65.10).

The degree of risk for SCD is related, in part, to the symptom status of the patient at the time of initial evaluation. In symptomatic patients evaluated at tertiary referral centers, the prevalence of patients with a history of aborted SCD is 2% to 11% (66,110,128). In contrast, population-based studies demonstrate a lower incidence of SCD. In one study this was found to be 0.0015 event per patient-year, or approximately 0.15% per year, occurring exclusively in previously symptomatic individuals (110). In general, several population-based studies of asymptomatic WPW patients have demonstrated a low incidence of SCD (110,129–131). Several electrophysiology-based studies (123,124,132,133) have also shown that patients who are asymptomatic at the time of diagnosis are unlikely to suffer subsequent SCD. This is related to relatively benign AP conduction capabilities in these patients.

In contrast to these studies, the study by Pappone et al. (125) involving a 5-year follow-up of 212 patients with WPW described as asymptomatic demonstrated a higher incidence of subsequent serious arrhythmias and SCD. Other investigators have reported that of patients with WPW who experience SCD, in approximately 50% it is the first manifestation of WPW syndrome (128). However, for WPW patients overall the occurrence of SCD as the first manifestation is not common (110,127,128,134).

A variety of testing methods has been proposed for stratifying the risk for SCD in WPW patients. They generally involve assessment of the propensity for extremely rapid AP conduction. Such testing includes ambulatory recordings, exercise testing, response to drugs, and invasive evaluation with electrophysiologic (EP) testing.

The most direct method of assessment is the actual induction of AF and determination of the propensity for rapid conduction as judged by the interval between consecutively preexcited QRS or "RR" complexes. This can be performed in a relatively noninvasive way with atrial pacing using an esophageal lead (85,135,136). Klein et al. (127) showed that those patients who survived a prior episode of VF had the shortest preexcited RR intervals (i.e., <250 msec in duration). Although this has been regarded as a highly sensitive marker for risk, it is of lower specificity. The positive predictive value of this finding is only 20% over short-term follow-up. On the other hand, the shortest preexcited RR interval of more than 250 msec has a negative predictive value of more than 95%. Other indicators of risk include an average RR interval during AF of 360 msec or less (137). A posteroseptal AP with accompanying rapid AV conduction capability and prior AF also suggests a higher risk (128,137).

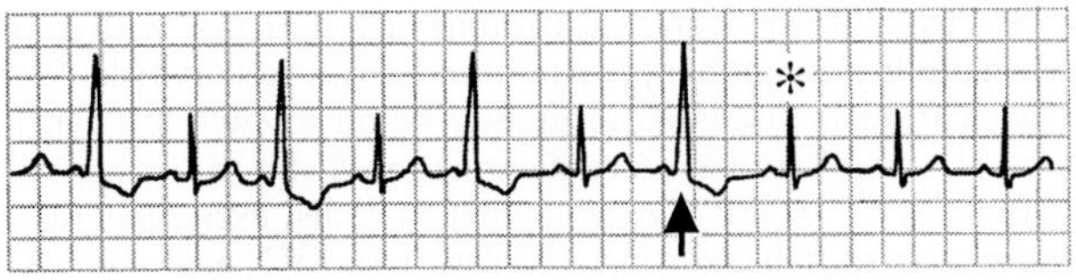

FIGURE 65.11. Rhythm strip showing intermittent preexcitation in a patient with Wolff-Parkinson-White syndrome. Both preexcited (*arrow*) and nonpreexcited (*asterisk*) QRS complexes are seen. Note the loss of QRS preexcitation from one beat to the next.

Other findings on noninvasive testing, if present, indicate a lower risk for SCD. The demonstration of intermittent preexcitation on a 12-lead ECG or ambulatory monitor strip as shown in Figure 65.11 indicates the presence of precarious conduction through an AP (138). It must be noted, however, that the term *intermittent preexcitation* specifically denotes the *abrupt* loss of preexcitation from one beat to the next on a rhythm strip or ECG; it cannot be extended to include the loss of preexcitation on an ECG from one office visit to the next. This variability is of no predictive value and is of particular concern in patients with left free-wall APs in which the distance of the AP from the sinus node decreases the chance of manifest preexcitation.

Exercise testing has also been proposed as a means of identifying patients with long AP refractoriness (139–141). Although several groups have shown that the *abrupt* loss of preexcitation during exercise indicates a low propensity for rapid conduction through an AP, this is an infrequent finding. Preexcitation more frequently disappears gradually during exercise because of enhanced conduction through the normal AV conduction system. Because of the low likelihood of an abrupt loss of preexcitation on exercise testing, persistent preexcitation during exercise testing is reasonably sensitive for identifying patients at risk for an untoward event. Unfortunately, the specificity for excluding those who are not at risk is less than 30%, which is substantially less than that of the shortest RR interval between two preexcited QRS complexes of 250 msec or less. Furthermore, the predictive accuracy of exercise testing is even lower than what is possible with the induction of AF (140).

Others have reported the use of drug-testing measures to stratify risk. This is based on the presumption that the loss of AP conduction with administration of an agent such as procainamide or ajmaline (142–144) indicates a low-risk AP. Again, however, findings using such testing maneuvers appear to be falsely reassuring (27,140,142,145).

A more invasive method of risk stratification is with EP testing. Inducibility of AVRT and AF may be assessed, and during AF, measurements of shortest and average RR intervals may be obtained. Such testing allows direct measurements of the antegrade effective refractory period of the AP, which has been shown to correlate with the ventricular rate during AF (146). One should bear in mind that all of these parameters may be assessed in a less invasive manner with an esophageal electrode (135,147,148). The presence of multiple APs has also been shown to be associated with increased risk of SCD (149). In the study by Pappone et al. (125), in which 212 patients with asymptomatic WPW pattern underwent baseline EP study, multiple APs were demonstrated in 17 (8%) patients and correlated with risk of SCD, including in all 3 patients who subsequently experienced VF.

In contrast to previous reports of electrophysiology-guided risk stratification for asymptomatic patients with WPW (123,124,132,133), in which the favorable prognosis of such patients did not justify even the small risks associated with invasive testing, Pappone et al. (125) demonstrated that EP study is very useful for risk stratification in such patients, with good predictability for patients at risk and those not at risk. Risk stratification is discussed in greater detail elsewhere (27). In general several studies have demonstrated the following risk factors for VF in WPW patients: male gender, extremely rapid ventricular response during AF, history of SVT, especially AF, and the presence of multiple APs (127,128,134,149).

At this time, practice guidelines (150,151) do not recommend invasive EP testing for patients with asymptomatic WPW pattern. This has become an area of controversy in light of the findings of Pappone et al. (125) outlined earlier, and subsequent reports from their center have recommended a reconsideration of practice guidelines to include EP testing for the routine evaluation of asymptomatic WPW patients (152). Expert opinion (153) has not agreed with this approach for all asymptomatic WPW patients. The potential harm from an invasive EP study and catheter ablation should be considered in light of the potential benefits and a decision made on an individual basis, bearing in mind the current status of practice guidelines. It bears repeating that most of the information relevant to risk stratification obtained by invasive EP study may be obtained less invasively with an esophageal lead, with the exception of the determination of multiple APs. In some patients, such as athletes or those involved in high-risk occupations, an invasive strategy for risk assessment and an ultimate goal of catheter ablation may be the best option. For other patients with asymptomatic WPW, noninvasive risk stratification appears to be the best approach until further evidence becomes available. In contrast, symptomatic patients, particularly those with a history of AF, are at higher risk for more rapid conduction through an AP during AF and warrant further evaluation (115,116,137).

Even more controversial is the matter of whether to perform catheter ablation routinely for asymptomatic WPW patients. Pappone et al. recently published two randomized studies of catheter ablation in asymptomatic WPW patients who were considered to be at high risk for future arrhythmias (154,155), one of which (154) involved asymptomatic children. Risk stratification was essentially based on the previous report (125) that demonstrated the inducibility of AVRT and/or AF as a predictor of high risk for future arrhythmias. Patients who underwent prophylactic catheter ablation had significant reduction in future arrhythmic events. The investigators suggested that such patients with asymptomatic WPW should undergo prophylactic catheter ablation.

Despite these findings, the treatment of asymptomatic WPW patients is not recommended. Practice guidelines (150,151) and expert opinion (153,156,157) stop short of advocating prophylactic catheter ablation for asymptomatic WPW patients. Regarding children in particular, according to current guidelines from the Expert Consensus Conference of the North American Society of Pacing and Electrophysiology (NASPE), now called the Heart Rhythm Society (HRS), catheter ablation of asymptomatic children older than 5 years of age is a class IIB indication (i.e., conflicting evidence or divergence of opinion about usefulness/effectiveness of the procedure with a less well established weight of evidence in favor) and a class III indication (i.e., evidence and/or general agreement that the procedure is not useful/effective and in some cases may be harmful) in younger children (158). The risks associated with any treatment, drug or ablative therapy, in these patients may be equal to or greater than the risks associated with an underlying AP. Potential exceptions to this include patients with a family history of SCD, competitive athletes, and patients with high-risk occupations whose performance may be unacceptably impaired by the unlikely occurrence of tachycardia or AF, with or without rapid ventricular response rates. As with invasive risk stratification, the decision to proceed with catheter ablation for asymptomatic patients should be made on an individual basis taking into account the potential risks and benefits, including the experience and expertise of the particular center, and the wishes of the patient.

Preexcitation Variants

Unlike the more classic presentations seen in most patients with WPW syndrome, other individuals have arrhythmias related to atypical APs with distinctive anatomic and physiologic characteristics. The most common of these are PJRT and preexcited tachycardia related to atriofascicular fibers. The hallmark of these preexcitation variants is the presence of unusual APs that show nodelike or decremental electrical conduction properties. Here, progressively slower conduction across the AP occurs with faster stimulation rates.

Permanent Junctional Reciprocating Tachycardia

Most patients with PJRT have posteroseptal APs within 1 cm of the coronary sinus orifice (24,159,160), although free-wall AP locations have been described (160,161). Like more typical APs, these connections also participate as the retrograde limb of an AV nodal–dependent tachycardia. In addition to characteristic decremental conduction properties, these pathways also have a long, circuitous route from ventricle to atrium, contributing to prolongation of retrograde conduction times (162,163). These APs also appear to conduct in the retrograde direction only, although several instances of emergent anterograde conduction and more classic ventricular preexcitation have been reported after ablation of the normal AV conduction system (164). Unlike typical reentrant tachycardias, this arrhythmia may occur spontaneously with alterations of the sinus rate without preceding APCs or VPCs. In such cases, return conduction through the AP and subsequent reactivation of the anterograde AV nodal limb of the circuit perpetuate the tachycardia (24,159).

Slow VA conduction results in inscription of the retrograde P wave in late diastole or closer to the succeeding QRS than the preceding QRS, as shown in Figure 65.12. The finding of an RP interval of more than 50% of the RR tachycardia interval invokes the descriptor “long RP” tachycardia. Because the low atrial septum is most frequently the first site of atrial activation, P waves during PJRT are typically negative in leads II, III, and aVF, indicating a low-to-high retrograde atrial activation sequence.

Many patients with this process develop rapid, nearly incessant, tachycardias, hence the designation PJRT. Because of the incessant nature of the tachycardia, the development of a tachycardia-induced cardiomyopathy that resolves after elimination of the pathway is not uncommon (165). Other patients with this type of pathway show less frequent PJRT.

Atriofascicular (Mahaim) Reentrant Tachycardias

Another type of tachycardia, referred to as atriofascicular, or Mahaim, reentrant tachycardia, is due to a decrementally conducting AP located in the right anterior or anterolateral aspect of the tricuspid annulus. When they were first described (166,167), these pathways were believed to originate in the upper portion of the AV node, with distal insertion in the ventricle or right-bundle-branch system. More recently, electrophysiologic studies (168,169) have demonstrated that the vast majority of patients with left-bundle-branch-block, left-axis-deviation Mahaim tachycardias have APs located several centimeters away from the AV node, as suggested in Figure 65.13. Local His-like potentials are usually seen when recording immediately over this pathway site.

As with the normal AV node, conduction in these pathways is strongly altered by adenosine or verapamil. This pathway, which also shows progressively longer conduction times at

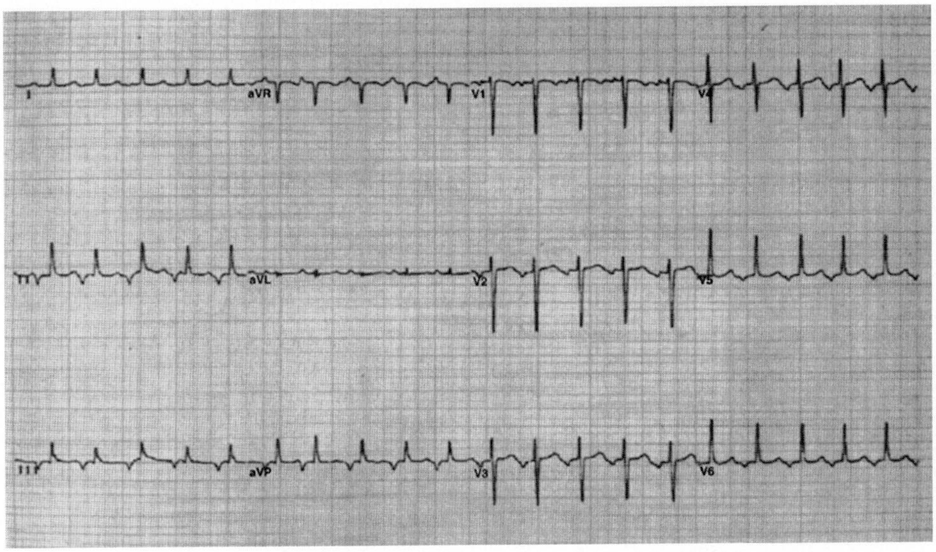

FIGURE 65.12. Twelve-lead electrocardiogram showing tachycardia in a patient with permanent junctional reciprocating tachycardia. Inspection of leads II, III, and aVF demonstrate the presence of a long-RP-interval tachycardia with negative P waves indicative of a low- to high-atrial activation sequence.

faster pacing rates, inserts into the right-bundle-branch system or right ventricular myocardium (170), giving a left-bundle-branch-block, left-axis-deviation QRS morphology on the surface ECG during tachycardia (Fig. 65.14). In addition, small, sharp R waves are typically seen in lead V_1, and the transition from negative to positive QRS morphology seen in the precordial leads typically occurs after V_4 (112). Like antidromic AVRT, the AV node serves as the retrograde limb of this circuit. Because of its left-bundle-branch-block appearance, this arrhythmia must be differentiated from other tachycardias with a left-bundle-branch-block morphology, such as any atrial or AV nodal–dependent tachycardias with bundle branch aberrancy, antidromic tachycardias using a right free-wall AP, right ventricular tachycardias as seen in patients with arrhythmogenic right ventricular dysplasia, and bundle branch reentrant ventricular tachycardias. In some cases, an atriofascicular fiber may arise near the left AV groove giving a right-bundle-branch QRS appearance (171).

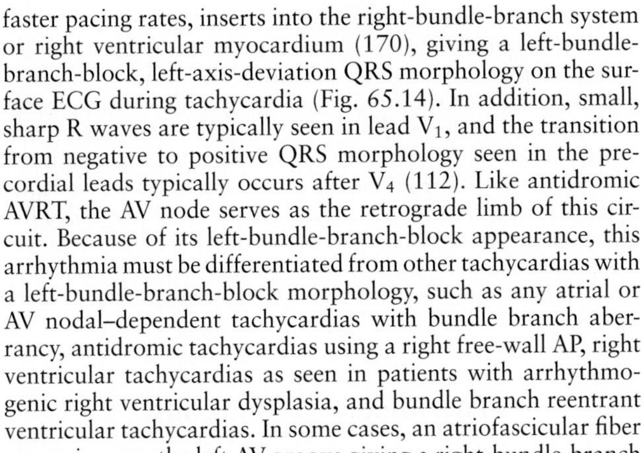

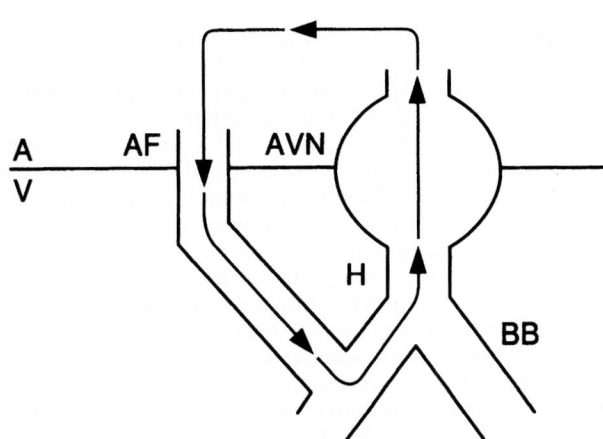

FIGURE 65.13. Mechanism of atriofascicular (AF) (Mahaim) reentrant tachycardias. Anterograde preexcitation typically occurs through a right anterolateral, decrementally conducting accessory pathway (AP) or AF pathway that inserts into the region of the right bundle branch (BB). Retrograde atrial activation occurs through the normal bundle of His (H) and atrioventricular (AV) node (AVN).

Fasciculoventricular Mahaim Fibers

A final variant of the preexcitation syndromes is created by a fasciculoventricular Mahaim fiber (66). Here, a conducting strand of tissue bypasses the distal component of the His-Purkinje system, resulting in earlier ventricular activation than expected through the normal His-Purkinje network. This is manifested at the time of electrophysiologic testing by a shortened HV interval recorded on the bundle of His electrogram. Unlike the situation with atriofascicular fibers, bundle of His pacing fails to eliminate this preexcitation because pacing at these sites is upstream from the site of the bypassing fiber.

ATRIOVENTRICULAR NODAL REENTRANT TACHYCARDIAS

Anatomic Considerations

The most common mechanism of AV nodal–dependent tachycardia is AVNRT, as shown in Figure 65.15. Approximately 60% (172–174) of all narrow-QRS-complex SVTs seen in the clinical setting are due to reentry within at least two parallel components near or within the AV nodal portion of the normal AV conduction system. The precise anatomic construct of these pathways remains a subject of controversy, with debate centering on the existence of common pathways both at the entry and exit points of the AV conduction system. It had been accepted that two pathways with differing conduction properties were confined to the compact portion of the AV node, as shown in Figure 65.15, but recently other investigators have argued successfully that at least a portion of the circuit lies outside the compact region of the AV node, as shown in Figure 65.2B (41,175–177).

In addition, early studies suggested that these functionally, if not anatomically, separate pathways joined at the upper and lower regions of the compact AV node to exit into the surrounding atrial or His-Purkinje tissue, respectively, through single, final, common pathways. This concept is supported by the uncommon occurrence of atrial dissociation from the remaining portion of the AV nodal reentrant circuit during tachycardia (173,178,179). Additional evidence for a final, lower, common pathway is found in the occurrence of dissociation of the ventricles from the tachycardia circuit. Several cases of both upper

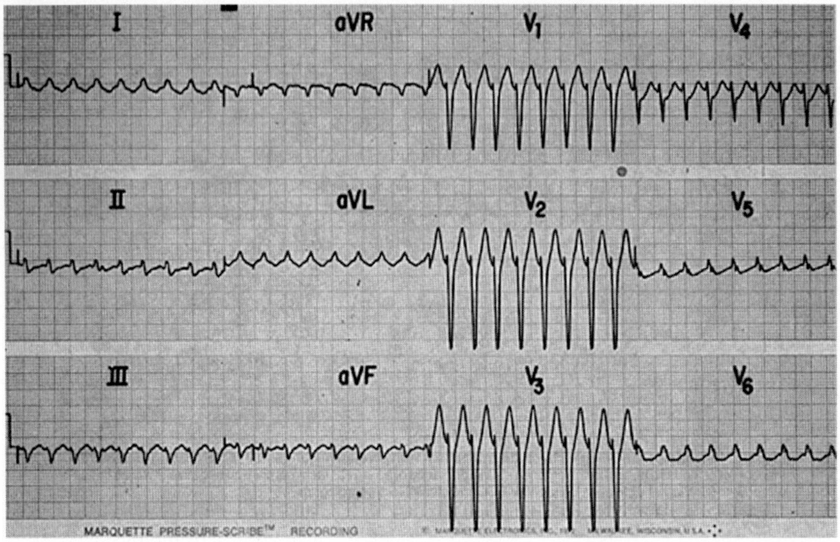

FIGURE 65.14. Wide-complex tachycardia through an atriofascicular fiber. Because of the distal insertion of the extra connection in the region of the right bundle branch, the tachycardia shows a left-bundle-branch-block, left-axis-deviation morphology with small, sharp R waves in lead V_1. Note also the characteristic late transition of QRS complexes in the precordial leads.

and lower common pathways existing in the same patient have been reported, which implies a completely intranodal reentrant circuit (180).

In contrast, other investigators (41) have argued that at least a component of the reentrant circuit lies outside the compact region of the AV node passing through atrial tissue. The presence of different retrograde atrial activation sequences with conduction through "fast" pathways (FP) versus "slow" pathways (SP) further argues against a final common upper pathway. Both surgical- and catheter-based studies have demonstrated that retrograde activation through the FP typically exits the compact portion of the AV node both anteriorly and superiorly to the distal portion of the AV node near the origin of the His bundle. In contrast, earliest retrograde activation through the SP occurs 2 to 3 cm further posteriorly along the tricuspid annulus near the coronary sinus orifice or traverses the left atrium

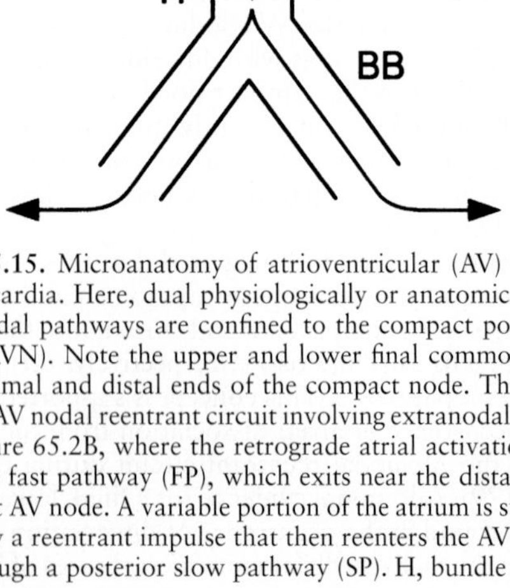

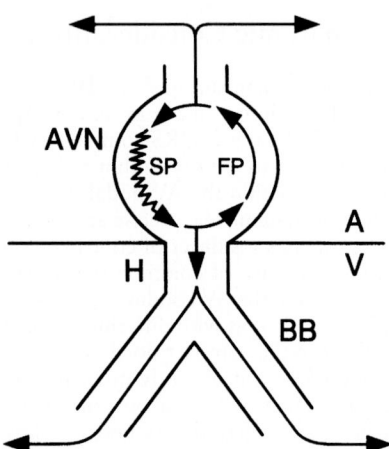

FIGURE 65.15. Microanatomy of atrioventricular (AV) nodal reentrant tachycardia. Here, dual physiologically or anatomically dissociated AV nodal pathways are confined to the compact portion of the AV node (AVN). Note the upper and lower final common pathways at the proximal and distal ends of the compact node. This is in contrast to the AV nodal reentrant circuit involving extranodal atrial tissue seen in Figure 65.2B, where the retrograde atrial activation proceeds through the fast pathway (FP), which exits near the distal portion of the compact AV node. A variable portion of the atrium is subsequently traversed by a reentrant impulse that then reenters the AV conduction system through a posterior slow pathway (SP). H, bundle of His.

(41,175–177). Investigators have described an unusual occurrence of atypical AVNRT with eccentric retrograde left-sided activation that may be confused with AVRT using a concealed left AP. It is interesting that these tachycardias can be cured with catheter ablation at the posteroseptal region of the right atrium (181). Catheter ablation of the AV nodal slow pathway for typical AVNRT from the left atrial septum via a transseptal approach when conventional right-sided techniques failed has also been described (182,183). Both left and right posterior extensions of the human compact AV node have been described from human autopsy studies and have been speculated to be involved in SP conduction (184).

Physiologic Mechanisms

Regardless of the anatomy of the circuit, pacing studies clearly demonstrate physiologically discontinuous or longitudinally separate conduction through the two or more components of the involved AV conduction system (10,11,17,175,185,186). During sinus rhythm, during slow atrial pacing, or with the introduction of late coupled APCs, AV conduction typically occurs through the faster of the dual functionally or anatomically distinct AV nodal pathways. Here, conduction times are short, and the PR interval inscribed on the surface ECG may be less than 140 msec. With faster pacing or with the introduction of progressively earlier APCs, a critical point of refractoriness or effective recovery time within the FP is reached. With subsequent decrements in the timing of the APC, AV conduction switches to the "slower" component of the dual AV conduction system, typically with a more than 50-msec prolongation of the AH interval conduction time through the AV node, as shown in Figure 65.16. This "jump" from the FP to the SP over a 10-msec decrease in the APC coupling time produces a discontinuity in the plot of the trans-AV nodal conduction time or the AH interval given as a function of the timing of the premature impulse or A_1 to A_2 interval; hence, the descriptor *discontinuous conduction*. Some patients may have several discontinuities, suggesting multiple SPs. Furthermore, the presence of such conduction may not, in and of itself, be abnormal because up to 70% of patients undergoing electrophysiologic testing who do not have clinical AVNRT reportedly have such anterograde or retrograde conduction discontinuities (187–189).

In 85% to 95% of patients, a slow/fast-type AV nodal–dependent tachycardia is seen in which the SP with the longest

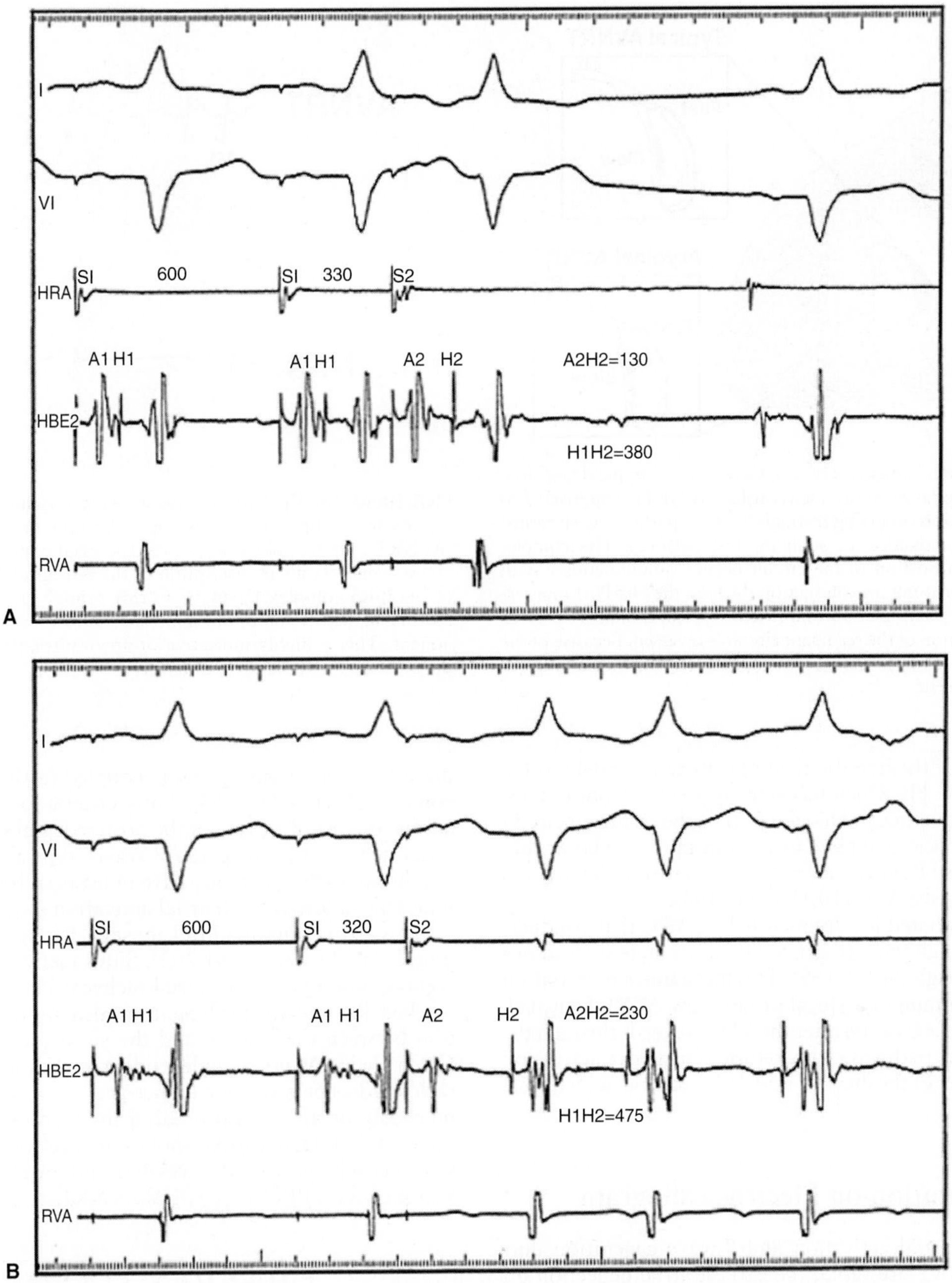

FIGURE 65.16. Intracardiac tracings showing dual atrioventricular (AV) nodal physiology and initiation of AV nodal reentrant tachycardia (AVNRT). Shown are surface leads I and V_1 as well as intracardiac leads from the high right atrium (HRA), His bundle electrogram (HBE), and right ventricular apex (RVA). **A:** An atrial premature complex introduced with an A1 to A2 interval of 330 msec conducts through the AV nodal fast pathway. **B:** With a 10-msec decrement in the A1 to A2 interval to 320 msec, block is followed by conduction through the AV nodal slow pathway and a 100-msec prolongation of the A2 to H2 interval. Thereafter, AVNRT with a ventriculoatrial interval of 40 msec is observed.

conduction time of the two AV nodal tracts comprises the anterograde limb of the reentrant circuit. This pathway is typically encountered in or near the posterior aspect of the compact portion of the AV node. Return or retrograde impulse propagation, as shown in Figure 65.17, proceeds through the FP with a shorter conduction time located in the anterior and medial aspect of the compact portion of the AV node near the origin of the bundle of His.

In 3% to 20% of patients, the tachycardia circuit direction is reversed and a fast/slow or atypical type of AVNRT is observed, as shown in Figure 65.17 (17,190–194). In this case, anterograde conduction proceeds down the faster of the two pathways, with return activation through the SP or alternative activation pathway. Given the potential of multiple SPs and therefore multiple discontinuities, the circuit involved in this atypical arrhythmia may not be the same as that involved in the slow/fast type of AVNRT seen in the same patient. Furthermore, up to 9% of individuals also display a slow/slow type of AVNRT in which both anterograde and retrograde conduction occurs through such multiple SPs (15,177,186,192,194,195).

AVNRT is most frequently initiated when a critically timed APC blocks in the FP with longer refractoriness and conducts

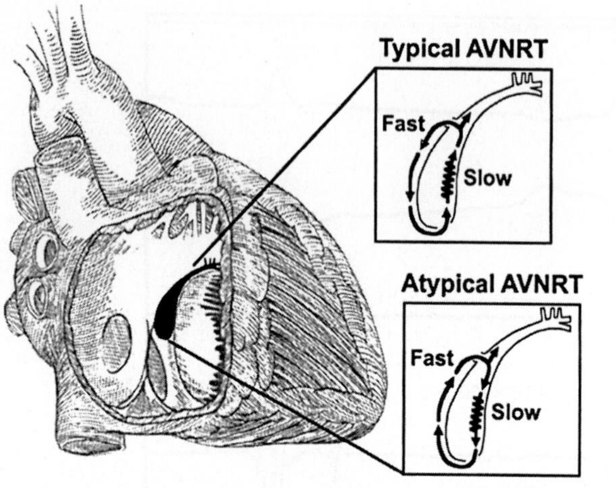

FIGURE 65.17. Mechanisms of typical slow/fast and atypical fast/slow atrioventricular nodal reentrant tachycardia (AVNRT). **Top inset:** Anterograde conduction occurring through the slow pathway with return retrograde atrial activation through the fast pathway. The completion of the return portion of the circuit occurs simultaneously with or shortly after concomitant conduction through the His-Purkinje system to activate the ventricle. **Bottom inset:** Atypical fast/slow AVNRT in which the direction of the reentrant circuit is reversed. Because of the prolonged atrial activation times through the slow pathway, a long-RP tachycardia is present.

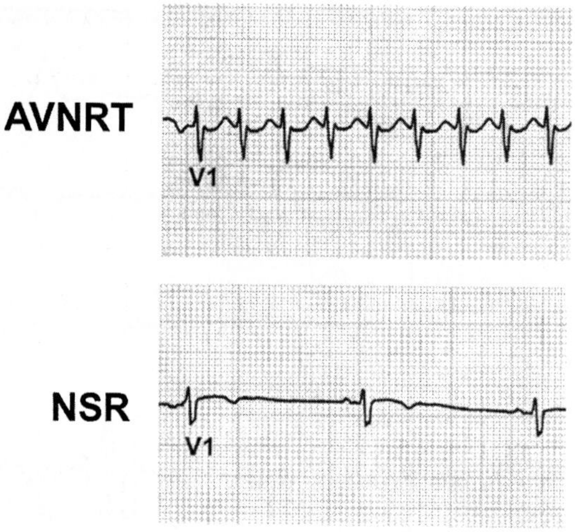

FIGURE 65.18. V_1 rhythm strips showing a pseudo-rSR′ QRS configuration in a patient with atrioventricular nodal reentrant tachycardia (AVNRT). **Upper:** The short ventriculoatrial conduction time during tachycardias results in inscription of the retrograde P wave at the end of the QRS complex, giving the "rSR prime" configuration. **Lower:** Normal sinus rhythm in the same lead shows resolution of that component. This is highly indicative of atrioventricular nodal reentry as the mechanism of the arrhythmia.

through the SP. If the impulse then returns retrogradely to the atria through the FP, which has since recovered from the anterogradely conducting and blocking APC, the reentrant circuit is completed. This is facilitated by the substantive delay within the SP, giving the FP sufficient time to recover from the original block created by the APC (10,185,196–198).

AVNRT is initiated less frequently by a VPC that conducts to the atria through the retrograde FP but reenters with return conduction through the SP (199). This mechanism of initiation is also more common in atypical or fast/slow AVNRT. In such cases, retrograde activation after the VPC proceeds through the slower AV nodal pathway, with return ventricular activation through the faster of the dual AV nodal physiologic or anatomic pathways.

Presentation on Electrocardiogram

Because return atrial activation and P-wave generation during typical AVNRT are rapid, the earliest atrial deflection on the bundle of His intracardiac electrogram during tachycardia is usually less than 60 msec (82). Although such a short VA interval excludes the possibility of a reentrant tachycardia using an AP, longer VA intervals do not eliminate the possibility of AVNRT that uses a SP as the retrograde limb of the reentrant circuit. As such, a short VA interval for diagnosing all AVNRT is not completely sensitive, although the positive predictive value is very high.

Therefore, for typical AVNRT a retrograde P wave is inscribed within or at the end of the QRS complex on the electrocardiogram. This dictates that this arrhythmia is a short-RP tachycardia (46,82,172,200,201). If the P wave occurs at the end of the QRS complex on the surface 12-lead ECG, a pseudo–R-wave deflection in V_1 not present during normal sinus rhythm may be seen, as shown in Figure 65.18 (81,200, 201). This is a highly sensitive and specific indicator of AVNRT as the mechanism for a narrow QRS complex tachycardia (81, 172,201).

In contrast, atypical AVNRT with retrograde conduction through the SP inscribes its retrograde P wave later in the RR diastolic interval, more closely coupled to the following QRS complex (41,174,193,194). Thus, criteria for a long-RP tachycardia are met. By virtue of the posteroseptal site of retrograde atrial activation, retrograde P waves typically observed during this arrhythmia are negative in leads II, III, and aVF, again indicating a low-to-high atrial activation sequence.

This arrhythmia and PJRT must be distinguished from other long-RP tachycardias (81,202). Sinus tachycardia, sinus node reentry, and a variety of atrial tachycardias in the absence of marked PR-interval prolongation also show a close association between the P wave and the subsequent QRS complex. Given their AV nodal–independent mechanisms, these atrial tachycardias persist when higher-grade AV block occurs spontaneously or after vagal or drug interventions. Furthermore, many of these tachycardias show a high-to-low atrial activation sequence with positive P waves in the inferior ECG leads, unlike that seen with PJRT or atypical AVNRT.

DIFFERENTIATING ATRIOVENTRICULAR NODE REENTRANT FROM ATRIOVENTRICULAR REENTRANT TACHYCARDIAS

Distinguishing AVRT from AVNRT is important in planning therapeutic strategies for these tachycardias. An understanding of the aforementioned mechanisms provides the needed clues for such differentiation. It was once believed that both the tachycardia rate and the presence of QRS alternans were useful in establishing a diagnosis of AVRT (172). Although AVRTs may be faster in some patients, the overlap in heart rates with these two mechanisms makes this factor unhelpful. Furthermore, the presence of QRS alternans has since been shown to be a function of heart rate and not of the specific underlying mechanism (46).

The positions of the P wave and the RP intervals in tachycardia are more useful in distinguishing these two reentrant mechanisms (46,81,200,201). P waves inscribed within the ST or T segments observed in AVRT (46,71,172,200,203,204) contrast with the even shorter RP intervals and accompanying P waves producing the r′ in lead V_1, which is highly predictive of an AVNRT mechanism (81,200,201). Obviously, in some cases the P waves are not obvious on the surface ECG, and recordings using an esophageal lead are required to determine the RP or VA interval.

Finally, it should be noted that 10% to 20% of patients with WPW syndrome also have AVNRT with a narrow QRS morphology (90,91,93,189,205,206). Therefore, the presence of a narrow-QRS SVT in a patient with WPW syndrome does not necessarily indicate AVRT. In these patients, clarification of the precise mechanisms of arrhythmia requires more detailed electrophysiologic evaluation.

PRINCIPLES OF MANAGEMENT OF ATRIOVENTRICULAR NODAL-DEPENDENT TACHYCARDIAS

Short-Term Therapy

The dependence of both AVRT and AVNRT on AV nodal conduction has important implications for the short-term management of patients with these arrhythmias. As reviewed in Figure 65.19, the simplest approach to tachycardia termination takes advantage of vagal modulation of AV nodal conduction. In many patients, a Valsalva maneuver, carotid sinus massage, or application of ice water to the face will terminate the tachycardia by increasing vagal tone. If these approaches prove unsuccessful, the use of drugs with significant negative dromotropic effects on the AV node may also readily terminate either type of SVT. Adenosine, administered in a rapid bolus at an initial dose of 6 mg IV, will terminate 62% of tachycardias, whereas 91% of these tachycardias respond to 12 mg of adenosine from a peripheral IV site (207). Alternatively, 5 to 10 mg of IV verapamil will terminate up to 90% of tachycardias (208–210). The high success rate of these IV drugs has led to their use in place of edrophonium (a short-acting cholinesterase inhibitor), phenylephrine, or β-blockers, which had been used at one time for this purpose. Although IV esmolol, a short-acting β-blocker, may also be effective, accompanying hypotension has been reported (211).

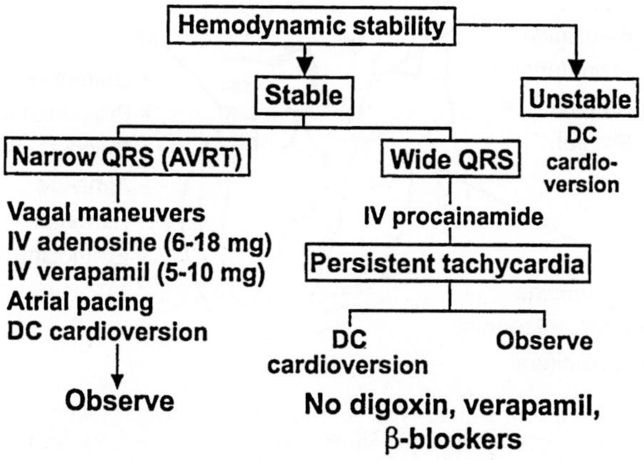

FIGURE 65.19. Algorithm for the acute management of patients with atrioventricular nodal–dependent tachycardias. Intravenous amiodarone may be used as an alternative to intravenous (IV) procainamide. AVRT, atrioventricular reciprocating tachycardia; DC, direct current.

The use of these drugs or of vagal maneuvers is also useful for the diagnosis because the development of higher-grade AV nodal block during ongoing tachycardia virtually excludes the presence of an AV nodal–dependent tachycardia. It should be noted that under rare circumstances AVNRT may show 2:1 AV block due to physiologic impairment of infra-His conduction; however, this is unlikely to occur with vagal or drug interventions.

Intravenous flecainide, propafenone, sotalol, or amiodarone may also prove effective in restoring sinus rhythm, although these drugs may take longer to produce clinically relevant effects, and of these drugs only amiodarone is available as an IV formulation in the United States. Although IV ibutilide is effective in terminating the acute onset of AF and its class III properties may effectively block AP conduction, the safety and efficacy of this agent for treating narrow-complex AV nodal–dependent tachycardia have not been established. The same is true for dofetilide and azimilide, which have been studied almost exclusively in AF and atrial flutter and are not available in IV forms in the United States.

Nonpharmacologic therapies for patients with AV nodal-dependent tachycardias are also available for restoring normal sinus rhythm. Atrial pacing using an esophageal lead positioned behind the atria proves routinely effective in terminating AV nodal–dependent tachycardia (148,212–214). Although this approach is effective, it also produces some esophageal discomfort and can initiate AF. Administration of a low-energy, synchronized direct current shock to cardiovert the tachycardia is an alternative, but it is rarely required, given the efficacy of pharmacologic and other nonpharmacologic measures.

The presence of a wide-QRS-complex tachycardia warrants careful consideration of several additional issues. Although the prolongation of the QRS complex may simply represent aberrancy accompanying an AV nodal–dependent tachycardia, the diagnosis of ventricular tachycardia should be carefully considered. The presence of underlying coronary artery disease or prior myocardial infarction has an accuracy of greater than 90% in predicting a ventricular mechanism for wide-complex arrhythmias (215). Additional mechanisms of wide-QRS tachycardia in patients with AV nodal–dependent arrhythmias include antidromic AVRT that uses an AP as its anterograde limb, AF, or other atrial tachycardias with ventricular preexcitation through the AP. Each of these arrhythmias should be manifest by their characteristic slurred upstroke delta wave seen in the first 40 msec of the wide QRS complex. During AF with a rapid ventricular response rate, however, the characteristic preexcited QRS pattern may be difficult to discern. Preexcitation may be most evident in the QRS complexes after the longest RR intervals during irregular tachycardias. Ventricular activation during AF in patients with multiple APs may proceed by several alternating avenues, thus mimicking polymorphic ventricular tachycardia or torsades de pointes on a single rhythm strip. As with evaluation of any wide-complex arrhythmias, a surface 12-lead ECG is indispensable in correctly identifying the underlying mechanism.

The short-term treatment of wide-complex tachycardia first and foremost depends on the patient's underlying hemodynamic status. In the presence of hemodynamic compromise, direct current cardioversion after appropriate anesthesia is warranted. In the presence of stable hemodynamics, several IV antiarrhythmic agents are available. Intravenous procainamide has been most widely used for this purpose. This agent not only alters propagation through the APs, but it may also directly restore normal sinus rhythm. Use of β-blockers (211,216–219) and lidocaine (216,220,221) is not effective for either purpose. Intravenous propafenone, flecainide, and sotalol are effective in both slowing the ventricular response rate during

AF and restoring normal sinus rhythm in patients with APs. Intravenous amiodarone is also effective, although the time to conversion with this agent may be longer and the overall conversion rate may be low. Intravenous ibutilide may also restore normal sinus rhythm, although its safety and efficacy in this setting have not been documented.

Several IV agents can also accelerate AV conduction through an AP, potentially causing AF to degenerate into VF. This includes digoxin (222), IV verapamil (223–227), IV but not oral diltiazem (228), and adenosine (229). This acceleration may be due to direct pathway effects, enhancement of peripheral sympathetic activity related to the precipitation of hypotension, or reduction in retrograde concealment into the AP by generation of higher-grade AV nodal block. In the presence of AF in a patient with an anterogradely conducting AP, ventricular activation proceeds through the AP or the normal AV conduction system. The latter avenue of propagation may be accompanied by impulse propagation across the ventricle in a reverse direction into the AP. This retrograde penetration or concealment blocks ventricular activation proceeding anterogradely through the AP because of impulse collision. This produces a net effect of slowing ventricular activation. Higher-grade AV nodal block can reduce this beneficial effect by withdrawing retrograde concealment.

Because of this and the potential hemodynamic deterioration of ventricular tachycardia, these drugs should not be routinely used in patients with wide-complex tachycardias. This does not mean that their use is prohibited in patients with narrow-QRS-complex tachycardias, although the possibility of degeneration of such arrhythmias into AF dictates that facilities dealing with such unlikely transitions should be available.

Long-Term Therapy

In the selection of appropriate therapy for patients with supraventricular arrhythmias, several general principles should be carefully considered. The inherent risk for untoward events accompanying the target arrhythmia as well as its impact on the patient's quality of life and the anticipated efficacy of the treatment must be carefully weighed against the accompanying risks of the therapy. Furthermore, the effectiveness and risks, including side effects, of a given treatment strategy must be carefully compared with those of other treatment options. For example, in the case of increased risk for SCD in symptomatic patients with WPW syndrome, aggressive evaluation and treatment are warranted. Here, the risks of intervention are likely to be small compared with the risks associated with the underlying arrhythmia. In fact, these patients are best treated with definitive ablative procedures. This is in part because of the relatively limited efficacy of antiarrhythmic therapy on AP conduction in those patients with the most rapid underlying conduction capabilities (230).

In contrast, in the absence of a propensity for rapid anterograde conduction through an AP during AF or of marked neurologic symptoms, such as presyncope or syncope, the majority of AV nodal–dependent tachycardias are relatively benign. As such, therapy is warranted if prevention of symptomatic arrhythmia improves quality of life and can be accomplished without undue risk to the patient. Again, the benefit of achieving such arrhythmic suppression must be weighed against possible side effects, including the proarrhythmic risk from drug therapy or complications from catheter ablation. In cases of single or infrequent tachycardia episodes with relatively mild symptoms, expectant observation without treatment or with sole use of vagal maneuvers to terminate tachycardia, where effective, may suffice. In such cases, antiarrhythmic or ablative therapy is unnecessary. Patients with frequently recurring palpitations clearly related to an AV nodal–dependent tachycardia, those with problematic, associated cardiac or central nervous system symptoms, those in whom drugs are either ineffective or accompanied by side effects, and individuals facing lifetime medical therapy are best treated with catheter ablation.

Exceptions to this approach are patients in whom the risks associated with catheter ablation may be greater than the risk of the underlying arrhythmia. For example, patients with an AP located close to the normal AV conduction system in which the risk for high-grade or complete heart block is high may be better treated with medical therapy. Obviously, if such therapy proves ineffective or if the patient is at risk for SCD, the potential complications of catheter ablation may be unavoidable to provide symptomatic relief and protection for the patient.

Other patients may benefit from the more readily available drug therapies. In the absence of anterograde preexcitation or AF, patients with AVRT may be effectively managed using calcium channel blockers, such as verapamil or diltiazem (228, 231–233), or any one of a number of β-blockers (211,218) that target the AV node, as shown in Figure 65.20. The latter may be useful in those patients with exercise-related tachycardia. These agents are also effective in modifying conduction within the SP in AVNRT and within the AP involved in PJRT or atriofascicular reentrant tachycardia. Efficacy rates of 40% to 50% in eliminating or significantly reducing the frequency of AV nodal–dependent tachyarrhythmias have been reported. Furthermore, the risk for proarrhythmia using these agents is very low, and most of these drugs can be administered in single daily doses.

In contrast, class Ia agents such as quinidine (234,235), procainamide (234–236), and disopyramide (83,237) produce beneficial effects on the AP but not on the normal AV conduction system. Other class I agents such as propafenone (238–241), flecainide (242–246), and moricizine and class III drugs such as sotalol (247–250) and amiodarone (251–255) have demonstrable effects on both the AV conduction system and the AP (Fig. 65.20). Because the FP used as the retrograde limb of AVNRT has many properties similar to those of APs, class Ic agents also produce beneficial effects on both the frequency and severity of this arrhythmia (232,256–260). Class Ic and class III drugs may also sufficiently modify the anterograde SP to reduce the occurrence of arrhythmias. These agents produce additional beneficial effects in patients with either type of AV

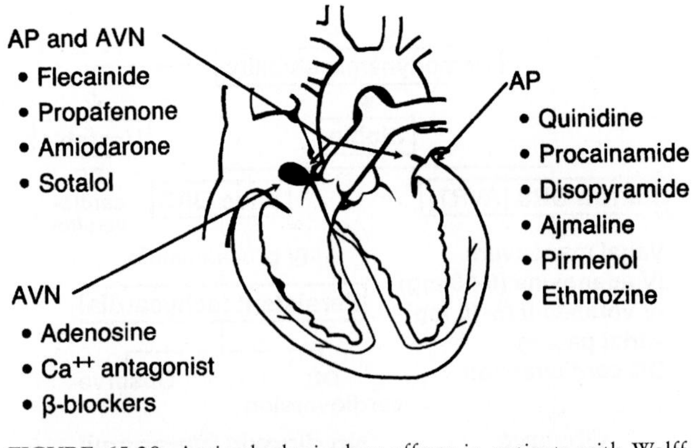

FIGURE 65.20. Antiarrhythmic drug effects in patients with Wolff-Parkinson-White syndrome. Shown here are drugs with exclusive accessory pathway (AP) effects, with exclusive atrioventricular nodal (AVN) actions, and with both AP- and AVN-modifying properties. Pharmacologic modulation of the fast pathway in AVN reentrant tachycardia is similar to that of an AP. The slow pathway behaves in a manner similar to that of AVN tissue.

nodal–dependent arrhythmia by reducing tachycardia-induced atrial or ventricular ectopy.

Regardless of the specific underlying mechanism, the efficacy of these agents in treating AV nodal–dependent arrhythmia is 60% to 80% over short-term follow-up. A new class III antiarrhythmic drug, azimilide, has been studied in patients with SVT in several randomized, double-blind, placebo-controlled trials and found to have significant dose-related efficacy for suppression of SVT with a low rate of adverse effects (261). This drug has not yet been approved by the Food and Drug Administration for use in the United States.

The choice of a specific membrane-active antiarrhythmic agent for use in patients with AVRT depends on several factors. These include (a) the presence or absence of structural heart disease or other organ system problems, (b) the presence of preexcitation, and (c) the side effect profile of a given agent, including organ toxicity, negative inotropic effects, and propensity for proarrhythmia. In the absence of underlying heart disease, any one of the class Ic, III, or Ia drugs may be effective in managing AVRT. Of these, flecainide, propafenone, and sotalol are less likely to produce organ toxicity or nuisance side effects. In this setting, the risk of a proarrhythmic event is low and ranges from 0.5% to 2.0%. In the presence of underlying heart disease, class I agents such as flecainide, propafenone, and disopyramide should not be used. In the presence of congestive heart failure or prior myocardial infarction, amiodarone is least likely to produce a proarrhythmic effect. The risk for proarrhythmia with other class I and class III drugs may be as high as 5% to 8%, particularly with the class Ia agents producing significant QT-interval prolongation in the presence of underlying heart disease. Specific drug therapy for these tachycardias and dosing strategies are reviewed in greater detail elsewhere (25–27).

Although drug therapy was the mainstay of treatment for AV nodal–dependent tachycardias for many years, the advent and improvement of surgical techniques in the 1970s ushered in an era of nonpharmacologic therapy. Patients with an AP who were at risk for SCD, patients in whom antiarrhythmic therapy had failed because of inefficacy or side effects, and patients who faced lifelong medical therapy were increasingly managed with surgical ablation. During the last decade, even this approach has been replaced by RF ablation. As described in greater detail in Chapter 73, success rates of 90% to 98% are routinely possible, although with a 5% to 8% recurrence rate of AP conduction (42,43,45,48). This ablative approach is accomplished at low risk, and the benefits to patients are achievable at lower cost and substantially less hospitalization and recovery times than are possible with surgical ablation. Hence, RF ablation is a reasonable first-line modality in patients with recurrent arrhythmias. Again, potential exceptions to this approach are patients who are at higher risk for complete heart block due to pathways in close proximity to the AV conduction system or to other factors that increase the risks of invasive procedures. In this regard, there may be an advantage of cryoablation for some APs that are near the conduction system. The ability to "cryomap" with a reversible cryolesion before delivering an irreversible lesion may minimize the development of AV block and still maintain very reasonable efficacy for procedural success (50,51).

In patients with AVNRT, excellent success rates are now possible with RF catheter ablation of the SP or atrial approaches to that pathway, which lies posteriorly along the tricuspid annulus. With RF catheter ablation, the risk for heart block in these patients is 0.5% to 3.0%, depending on the experience of the operator and on the apparent SP location. This approach has virtually supplanted the alternative ablation of the FP, which has been accompanied by heart block rates of 5% to 25% (41,42,46,262,263). Catheter ablation of the SP for AVNRT using cryoablation has been associated with slightly less efficacy (91%) but with no reports of heart block requiring implantation of a permanent pacemaker (50,51).

CONCLUSIONS

Over the last 15 to 20 years, substantial progress has been made in the treatment of AV nodal–dependent tachycardias. This has been facilitated by the development of catheter-based electrophysiology study techniques that elucidate the underlying arrhythmic mechanisms, the development of better drugs for acute and chronic management, and the refinement of nonpharmacologic therapy such as RF catheter ablation for curing these arrhythmias. This progress has not only elucidated these arrhythmias, but has also provided the foundation for extrapolating these refinements to the more complicated AV nodal–independent atrial and ventricular tachycardias. An appreciation of these issues should improve the efficacy of therapies and reduce their risk in patients with AV nodal–dependent tachycardias.

CONTROVERSIES AND PERSONAL PERSPECTIVES

Risk Stratification of Asymptomatic Wolff-Parkinson-White Patients

Although much of the physiology of the AV nodal–dependent arrhythmias has already been elucidated and management and treatment methods established, several areas of controversy remain. The prevailing weight of current practice guidelines and expert opinion suggests that risk stratification in patients with asymptomatic preexcitation is not necessary unless extenuating circumstances exist. Some clinicians, however, continue to be strong proponents of risk stratification in all patients. As discussed earlier, the likelihood of rapid conduction through an AP in the absence of symptoms is low; moreover, the risk of SCD has been shown in population-based studies to be very low. Still, the risk for an untoward event is not zero. On rare occasions, patients present with VF as the first manifestation of WPW syndrome. As such, clinicians cannot give patients blanket guarantees of freedom from untoward events over the long term. It is important that this uncertainty be discussed with patients to provide them with the necessary understanding needed to make informed decisions about proceeding with additional evaluation and treatment and any accompanying risks if they are asymptomatic. If risk stratification is to be undertaken, it should be by direct initiation of AF and assessment of the ventricular response rate. Noninvasive ECG-based methods are insufficiently predictive to be of any significant use. If rapid conduction through an AP is identified, the patient should have sufficient information to either accept the risks associated with such rapid conduction or the risks associated with ablation of the offending AP. When presented with the juxtaposition of the risks associated with no intervention versus those of catheter ablation, some patients may well opt for conservative follow-up. Others may wish to face the risks of ablation immediately rather than confront continued pathway-related risks, no matter how low, over time.

Anatomy of Atrioventricular Nodal Reentrant Tachycardias

Another area of controversy was outlined previously. Some clinicians argue that the AVNRT circuit resides within the compact portion of the AV node. Others argue that at least a component of the reentrant circuit lies outside the compact region of the AV node. In the latter case, the SP is viewed as arising from atrial tissue, with insertion into the compact AV node. Given the various considerations on both sides of this argument, it seems most likely that an appreciable component of the reentrant circuit resides outside the AV node within atrial tissue. In fact the FP and SP may even be variable manifestations of anisotropic tissue architecture in the interatrial septum. It is therefore likely that the anterograde limb of the circuit is actually composed of both the atrial tissue inputs into the posterior region of the AV node and a component of AV nodal tissue itself. Successful SP ablation may simply mean that the atrial inputs into the AV node have been sufficiently modified to make onset of tachycardias unlikely.

Radiofrequency Ablation as First-Line Therapy

Finally, in some quarters, the propriety of RF ablation as first-line treatment for AV nodal–dependent arrhythmias, or particularly for asymptomatic APs, remains controversial. Some clinicians believe that patients with AVRT in the absence of manifest preexcitation and those with AVNRT should be managed with antiarrhythmic drugs that target the AV node. Ablative therapy is reasonable first-line therapy if (a) a patient faces lifelong medical therapy, (b) there is an arrhythmia refractory to previous medical treatment, (c) the patient is at risk for an untoward event, (d) the patient resides in an area where medical therapy for tachycardia is less readily available, or (e) the pathway is located away from the AV node. Again, the risks of this therapy must be weighed against the alternative of using membrane-active antiarrhythmic drugs. Although most of these agents are reasonably tolerated when appropriately administered, constitutional side effects and the risk of potentially lethal proarrhythmia remain a reality. In the hands of experienced interventionalists, the risks associated with ablation remain very low; moreover, ablation has the added advantage of curing the arrhythmia. RF catheter ablation of SVT has been shown to be cost-effective and improve quality of life for patients with WPW who survive cardiac arrest or who experience SVT or AF (264) and for highly symptomatic patients with SVT (265). The addition of new technologies for catheter ablation, such as alternative energy sources and computerized mapping, has already provided improved safety in particular circumstances. Here again, patients should be informed of their options so they may participate in choosing an approach that best meets their needs.

THE FUTURE

Substantial progress has already been made in the area of AV nodal–dependent tachycardias. Excellent therapies are available and have been applied successfully in thousands of patients. In the future, however, we will undoubtedly better define the cost-effectiveness of the various treatment modalities through outcome-based studies. A better understanding of the natural history of AV nodal–dependent arrhythmias will be forthcoming. Technology will be developed to facilitate noninvasive substrate localization and establishment of mechanisms. Nonfluoroscopic multisite mapping for creating three-dimensional maps of specific arrhythmias and improved energy sources and delivery techniques will also be forthcoming. With the anticipated progress during the next 5 to 10 years, it would not be surprising if arrhythmogenic substrate could be eliminated through energy delivery from the body surface.

References

1. Kent A. Researches on the structure and function of the mammalian heart. *J Physiol* 1893;14:233–254.
2. Mines G. On dynamic equilibrium in the heart. *J Physiol* 1913;46:349–383.
3. Kent A. Observations on the auriculo-ventricular junction of the mammalian heart. *Q J Exp Physiol* 1913;7:193.
4. Mines G. On circulation excitation on heart muscles and their possible relation to tachycardia and fibrillation. *Trans R Soc Can* 1914;4:43.
5. Wolferth C, Wood F. The mechanism of production of short P-R intervals and prolonged QRS complexes in patients with presumably undamaged hearts: hypothesis of an accessory pathway of auriculo-ventricular conduction (bundles of Kent). *Am Heart J* 1933;8:297–311.
6. Cohn A, Fraser F. Paroxysmal tachycardia and the effect of stimulation of the vagus nerves by pressure. *Heart* 1913;5:93–107.
7. Wood F, Wolferth C, Geckler G. Histologic demonstration of accessory muscular connections between auricle and ventricle in a case of short PR interval and prolonged QRS complex. *Am Heart J* 1942: 454–462.
8. Wolff L, Parkinson J, White P. Bundle branch block with short PR interval in healthy young people prone to paroxysmal tachycardia. *Am Heart J* 1930;5:685–704.
9. Barker P, Wilson F, Johnston F. The mechanism of auricular paroxysmal tachycardia with alternation of cycle length. *Am Heart J* 1943;26:435–445.
10. Denes P, Wu D, Dhingra RC, et al. Demonstration of dual A-V nodal pathways in patients with paroxysmal supraventricular tachycardia. *Circulation* 1973;48:549–555.
11. Moe G. Physiological evidence for a dual AV nodal transmission system. *Circ Res* 1956;4:357–375.
12. Kistin A. Multiple pathways of conduction and reciprocal rhythm with interpolated ventricular premature systoles. *Am Heart J* 1963;65:162–179.
13. Dopirak MR, Schaal SF, Leier CV. Triple AV nodal pathways in man? *J Electrocardiol* 1980;13:185–188.
14. Kuck KH, Kuch B, Bleifeld W. Multiple anterograde and retrograde AV nodal pathways: demonstration by multiple discontinuities in the AV nodal conduction curves and echo time intervals. *Pacing Clin Electrophysiol* 1984;7:656–662.
15. Sebag C, Chevalier P, Davy JM, et al. Triple antegrade nodal pathway in a patient with supraventricular paroxysmal tachycardia. *J Electrocardiol* 1986;19:85–90.
16. Swiryn S, Bauernfeind RA, Palileo EA, et al. Electrophysiologic study demonstrating triple antegrade AV nodal pathways in patients with spontaneous and/or induced supraventricular tachycardia. *Am Heart J* 1982; 103:168–176.
17. Tai CT, Chen SA, Chiang CE, et al. Multiple anterograde atrioventricular node pathways in patients with atrioventricular node reentrant tachycardia. *J Am Coll Cardiol* 1996;28:725–731.
18. Durrer D, Schoo L, Schuilenburg RM, et al. The role of premature beats in the initiation and the termination of supraventricular tachycardia in the Wolff-Parkinson-White syndrome. *Circulation* 1967;36:644–662.
19. Durrer D, Roos JP. Epicardial excitation of the ventricles in a patient with Wolff-Parkinson-White syndrome (type B). *Circulation* 1967;35:15–21.
20. Wellens HJ, Schuilenberg RM, Durrer D. Electrical stimulation of the heart in patients with Wolff-Parkinson-White syndrome, type A. *Circulation* 1971;43:99–114.
21. Wellens HJ, Durrer D. Patterns of ventriculo-atrial conduction in the Wolff-Parkinson-White syndrome. *Circulation* 1974;49:22–31.
22. Tonkin AM, Dugan FA, Svenson RH, et al. Coexistence of functional Kent and Mahaim-type tracts in the pre-excitation syndrome. Demonstration by catheter techniques and epicardial mapping. *Circulation* 1975;52:193–200.
23. Gallagher JJ, Sealy WC, Kasell J, et al. Multiple accessory pathways in patients with the pre-excitation syndrome. *Circulation* 1976;54:571–591.
24. Gallagher JJ, Sealy WC. The permanent form of junctional reciprocating tachycardia: further elucidation of the underlying mechanism. *Eur J Cardiol* 1978;8:413–430.
25. Prystowsky EN, Pritchett EL, Gallagher JJ. Concealed conduction preventing anterograde preexcitation in Wolff-Parkinson-White syndrome. *Am J Cardiol* 1984;53:960–961.
26. Prystowsky EN. Diagnosis and management of the preexcitation syndromes. *Curr Probl Cardiol* 1988;13:225–310.
27. Packer D, Prystowsky E. The Wolff-Parkinson-White syndrome: further progress in evaluation and treatment. *Prog Cardiovasc Dis* 1988;1:147–187.
28. Tang D, Li Y, Wong J, et al. Characteristics of a charged-coupled-device-based optical mapping system for the study of cardiac arrhythmias. *J Biomed Opt* 2005;10:024009.
29. Wu J, Zipes DP. Mechanisms underlying atrioventricular nodal conduction and the reentrant circuit of atrioventricular nodal reentrant tachycardia using optical mapping. *J Cardiovasc Electrophysiol* 2002;13: 831–834.
30. Markides V, Davies DW. New mapping technologies: an overview with a clinical perspective. *J Interv Card Electrophysiol* 2005;13(Suppl 1):43–51.

31. Burchell HB, Frye RL, Anderson MW, et al. Atrioventricular and ventriculoatrial excitation in Wolff-Parkinson-White syndrome (type B). Temporary ablation at surgery. *Circulation* 1967;36:663–672.
32. Cobb FR, Blumenschein SD, Sealy WC. *J Biomed Opt* 2005;10:024009. Successful surgical interruption of the bundle of Kent in a patient with Wolff-Parkinson-White syndrome. *Circulation* 1968;38:1018–1029.
33. Sealy WC, Wallace AG. Surgical treatment of Wolff-Parkinson-White syndrome. *J Thorac Cardiovasc Surg* 1974;68:757–770.
34. Anselme F, Papageorgiou P, Monahan K, et al. Presence and significance of the left atrionodal connection during atrioventricular nodal reentrant tachycardia. *Am J Cardiol* 1999;83:1530–1536.
35. Cox JL, Gallagher JJ, Cain ME. Experience with 118 consecutive patients undergoing operation for the Wolff-Parkinson-White syndrome. *J Thorac Cardiovasc Surg* 1985;90:490–501.
36. Guiraudon GM, Klein GJ, Sharma AD, et al. Surgery for Wolff-Parkinson-White syndrome: further experience with an epicardial approach. *Circulation* 1986;74:525–529.
37. Iwa T, Mitsui T, Misaki T, et al. Radical surgical cure of Wolff-Parkinson-White syndrome: the Kanazawa experience. *J Thorac Cardiovasc Surg* 1986;91:225–233.
38. Ott DA, Garson A, Cooley DA, et al. Definitive operation for refractory cardiac tachyarrhythmias in children. *J Thorac Cardiovasc Surg* 1985;90:681–689.
39. Sealy WC. The Wolff-Parkinson-White syndrome and the beginnings of direct arrhythmia surgery. *Ann Thorac Surg* 1984;38:176–180.
40. Borggrefe M, Budde T, Podczeck A, et al. High frequency alternating current ablation of an accessory pathway in humans. *J Am Coll Cardiol* 1987;10:576–582.
41. Jackman WM, Beckman KJ, McClelland JH, et al. Treatment of supraventricular tachycardia due to atrioventricular nodal reentry, by radiofrequency catheter ablation of slow-pathway conduction. *N Engl J Med* 1992; 327:313–318.
42. Calkins H, Yong P, Miller JM, et al. Catheter ablation of accessory pathways, atrioventricular nodal reentrant tachycardia, and the atrioventricular junction: final results of a prospective, multicenter clinical trial. The Atakr Multicenter Investigators Group. *Circulation* 1999;99:262–270.
43. Calkins H, Langberg J, Sousa J, et al. Radiofrequency catheter ablation of accessory atrioventricular connections in 250 patients. Abbreviated therapeutic approach to Wolff-Parkinson-White syndrome. *Circulation* 1992; 85:1337–1346.
44. Calkins H, Prystowsky E, Carlson M, et al. Temperature monitoring during radiofrequency catheter ablation procedures using closed loop control. Atakr Multicenter Investigators Group. *Circulation* 1994;90:1279–1286.
45. Jackman WM, Wang XZ, Friday KJ, et al. Catheter ablation of accessory atrioventricular pathways (Wolff-Parkinson-White syndrome) by radiofrequency current. *N Engl J Med* 1991;324:1605–1611.
46. Kay GN, Epstein AE, Dailey SM, et al. Selective radiofrequency ablation of the slow pathway for the treatment of atrioventricular nodal reentrant tachycardia.Evidence for involvement of perinodal myocardium within the reentrant circuit. *Circulation* 1992;85:1675–1688.
47. Lesh MD, Van Hare GF, Schamp DJ, et al. Curative percutaneous catheter ablation using radiofrequency energy for accessory pathways in all locations: results in 100 consecutive patients. *J Am Coll Cardiol* 1992;19:1303–1309.
48. Swartz JF, Tracy CM, Fletcher RD. Radiofrequency endocardial catheter ablation of accessory atrioventricular pathway atrial insertion sites. *Circulation* 1993;87:487–499.
49. Cummings JE, Pacifico A, Drago JL, et al. Alternative energy sources for the ablation of arrhythmias. *Pacing Clin Electrophysiol* 2005;28:434–443.
50. Friedman PL, Dubuc M, Green MS, et al. Catheter cryoablation of supraventricular tachycardia: results of the multicenter prospective "frosty" trial. *Heart Rhythm* 2004;1:129–138.
51. Friedman PL. Catheter cryoablation of cardiac arrhythmias. *Curr Opin Cardiol* 2005;20:48–54.
52. Mehta D, Bharati S, Lev M, et al. Histopathological changes following laser ablation of a left-sided accessory pathway in a human. *Pacing Clin Electrophysiol* 1994;17:672–677.
53. Jackman W, Friday KJ, Yeung-Lai-Wah JA, et al. Accessory pathways: branching networks and tachycardia. *Circulation* 1985;72:III270.
54. Jackman W, Yeung-Lai-Wah JA, Friday K, et al. Tachycardias originating in accessory pathway networks mimicking atrial flutter and fibrillation. *J Am Coll Cardiol* 1986;7:6A.
55. Jackman WM, Friday KJ, Scherlag BJ, et al. Direct endocardial recording from an accessory atrioventricular pathway: localization of the site of block, effect of antiarrhythmic drugs, and attempt at nonsurgical ablation. *Circulation* 1983;68:906–916.
56. Jackman WM, Friday KJ, Yeung-Lai-Wah JA, et al. New catheter technique for recording left free-wall accessory atrioventricular pathway activation. Identification of pathway fiber orientation. *Circulation* 1988;78:598–611.
57. Gallagher JJ, Sealy WC, Cox JL, et al. Results of surgery for preexcitation caused by accessory atrioventricular pathways in 267 consecutive cases. In: Josephson ME, Wellens HJ, eds. *Tachycardia: mechanism, diagnosis and treatment.* Philadelphia: Lea & Febiger, 1984: 259–269.
58. Colavita PG, Packer DL, Pressley JC, et al. Frequency, diagnosis and clinical characteristics of patients with multiple accessory atrioventricular pathways. *Am J Cardiol* 1987;59:601–606.
59. Heddle WF, Brugada P, Wellens HJ. Multiple circus movement tachycardias with multiple accessory pathways. *J Am Coll Cardiol* 1984;4:168–175.
60. Morady F, Scheinman MM, DiCarlo Jr LA, et al. Coexistent posteroseptal and right-sided atrioventricular bypass tracts. *J Am Coll Cardiol* 1985;5:640–646.
61. Wellens HJ, Brugada P, Heddle WF. Value of the 12 lead electrocardiogram in diagnosing type and mechanism of a tachycardia: a survey among 22 cardiologists. *J Am Coll Cardiol* 1984;4:176–179.
62. Goya M, Takahashi A, Nakagawa H, et al. A case of catheter ablation of accessory atrioventricular connection between the right atrial appendage and right ventricle guided by a three-dimensional electroanatomic mapping system. *J Cardiovasc Electrophysiol* 1999;10:1112–1118.
63. Lam C, Schweikert R, Kanagaratnam L, et al. Radiofrequency ablation of a right atrial appendage-ventricular accessory pathway by transcutaneous epicardial instrumentation. *J Cardiovasc Electrophysiol* 2000;11: 1170–1173.
64. Schweikert RA, Saliba WI, Tomassoni G, et al. Percutaneous pericardial instrumentation for endo-epicardial mapping of previously failed ablations. *Circulation* 2003;108:1329–1335.
65. Soejima K, Mitamura H, Miyazaki T, et al. Catheter ablation of accessory atrioventricular connection between right atrial appendage to right ventricle: a case report. *J Cardiovasc Electrophysiol* 1998;9:523–528.
66. Gallagher JJ, Pritchett EL, Sealy WC, et al. The preexcitation syndromes. *Prog Cardiovasc Dis* 1978;20:285–327.
67. De la Fuente D, Sasyniuk B, Moe GK. Conduction through a narrow isthmus in isolated canine atrial tissue. A model of the W-P-W syndrome. *Circulation* 1971;44:803–809.
68. Inoue H, Zipes DP. Conduction over an isthmus of atrial myocardium in vivo: a possible model of Wolff-Parkinson-White syndrome. *Circulation* 1987;76:637–647.
69. Fujimura O, Kuo CS, Smith BA. Pre-excited RR intervals during atrial fibrillation in the Wolff-Parkinson-White syndrome: influence of the atrioventricular node refractory period. *J Am Coll Cardiol* 1991;18:1722–1726.
70. Klein GJ, Yee R, Sharma AD. Concealed conduction in accessory atrioventricular pathways: an important determinant of the expression of arrhythmias in patients with Wolff-Parkinson-White syndrome. *Circulation* 1984;70:402–411.
71. Prystowsky EN, Miles WM, Heger JJ, et al. Preexcitation syndromes. Mechanisms and management. *Med Clin North Am* 1984;68:831–893.
72. Rosenbaum F, Hecht H, Wilson F, et al. The potential variations of the thorax and the esophagus in anomalous atrioventricular excitation (Wolff-Parkinson-White syndrome). *Am Heart J* 1945;29:281–326.
73. Arruda MS, McClelland JH, Wang X, et al. Development and validation of an ECG algorithm for identifying accessory pathway ablation site in Wolff-Parkinson-White syndrome. *J Cardiovasc Electrophysiol* 1998;9:2–12.
74. Chiang CE, Chen SA, Teo WS, et al. An accurate stepwise electrocardiographic algorithm for localization of accessory pathways in patients with Wolff-Parkinson-White syndrome from a comprehensive analysis of delta waves and R/S ratio during sinus rhythm. *Am J Cardiol* 1995;76:40–46.
75. Fitzpatrick AP, Gonzales RP, Lesh MD, et al. New algorithm for the localization of accessory atrioventricular connections using a baseline electrocardiogram. *J Am Coll Cardiol* 1994;23:107–116.
76. Lindsay BD, Crossen KJ, Cain ME. Concordance of distinguishing electrocardiographic features during sinus rhythm with the location of accessory pathways in the Wolff-Parkinson-White syndrome. *Am J Cardiol* 1987;59:1093–1102.
77. Milstein S, Sharma AD, Guiraudon GM, et al. An algorithm for the electrocardiographic localization of accessory pathways in the Wolff-Parkinson-White syndrome. *Pacing Clin Electrophysiol* 1987;10:555–563.
78. Rodriguez LM, Smeets JL, de Chillou C, et al. The 12-lead electrocardiogram in midseptal, anteroseptal, posteroseptal and right free wall accessory pathways. *Am J Cardiol* 1993;72:1274–1280.
79. Xie B, Heald SC, Bashir Y, et al. Localization of accessory pathways from the 12-lead electrocardiogram using a new algorithm. *Am J Cardiol* 1994; 74:161–165.
80. Garcia Civera R, Ferrero JA, Sanjuan R, et al. Retrograde P wave polarity in reciprocating tachycardia utilizing lateral bypass tracts. *Eur Heart J* 1980;1:137–145.
81. Tai CT, Chen SA, Chiang CE, et al. A new electrocardiographic algorithm using retrograde P waves for differentiating atrioventricular node reentrant tachycardia from atrioventricular reciprocating tachycardia mediated by concealed accessory pathway. *J Am Coll Cardiol* 1997;29:394–402.
82. Benditt DG, Pritchett EL, Smith WM, et al. Ventriculoatrial intervals: diagnostic use in paroxysmal supraventricular tachycardia. *Ann Intern Med* 1979;91:161–166.
83. Kerr CR, Gallagher JJ, German LD. Changes in ventriculoatrial intervals with bundle branch block aberration during reciprocating tachycardia in patients with accessory atrioventricular pathways. *Circulation* 1982;66: 196–201.
84. Pritchett EL, Tonkin AM, Dugan FA, et al. Ventriculo-atrial conduction time during reciprocating tachycardia with intermittent bundle-branch block in Wolff-Parkinson-White syndrome. *Br Heart J* 1976;38:1058–1064.

85. Canby RC, Horton RP, Kessler DJ, et al. Use of transesophageal atrial pacing with adenosine infusion to evaluate ventricular preexcitation. *Am J Cardiol* 1995;75:548–550.
86. Cohen TJ, Tucker KJ, Abbott JA, et al. Usefulness of adenosine in augmenting ventricular preexcitation for noninvasive localization of accessory pathways. *Am J Cardiol* 1992;69:1178–1185.
87. Atie J, Brugada P, Brugada J, et al. Clinical and electrophysiologic characteristics of patients with antidromic circus movement tachycardia in the Wolff-Parkinson-White syndrome. *Am J Cardiol* 1990;66:1082–1091.
88. Bardy GH, Packer DL, German LD, et al. Preexcited reciprocating tachycardia in patients with Wolff-Parkinson-White syndrome: incidence and mechanisms. *Circulation* 1984;70:377–391.
89. Packer DL, Gallagher JJ, Prystowsky EN. Physiological substrate for antidromic reciprocating tachycardia. Prerequisite characteristics of the accessory pathway and atrioventricular conduction system. *Circulation* 1992;85:574–588.
90. Csanadi Z, Klein GJ, Yee R, et al. Effect of dual atrioventricular node pathways on atrioventricular reentrant tachycardia. *Circulation* 1995;91: 2614–2618.
91. Smith WM, Broughton A, Reiter MJ, et al. Bystander accessory pathway during AV node re-entrant tachycardia. *Pacing Clin Electrophysiol* 1983;6:537–547.
92. Smith WM, Gallagher JJ, Kerr CR, et al. The electrophysiologic basis and management of symptomatic recurrent tachycardia in patients with Ebstein's anomaly of the tricuspid valve. *Am J Cardiol* 1982;49:1223–1234.
93. Sung RJ, Styperek JL. Electrophysiologic identification of dual atrioventricular nodal pathway conduction in patients with reciprocating tachycardia using anomalous bypass tracts. *Circulation* 1979;60:1464–1476.
94. Packer D, Prystowsky E. Anatomical and physiological substrate for antidromic reciprocating tachycardia. In: Zipes DP, Jalife J, eds. *Cardiac electrophysiology: from cell to bedside.* Philadelphia: WB Saunders, 1995: 655–665.
95. Fujimura O, Klein GJ, Yee R, et al. Mode of onset of atrial fibrillation in the Wolff-Parkinson-White syndrome: how important is the accessory pathway? *J Am Coll Cardiol* 1990;15:1082–1086.
96. Waspe LE, Brodman R, Kim SG, et al. Susceptibility to atrial fibrillation and ventricular tachyarrhythmia in the Wolff-Parkinson-White syndrome: role of the accessory pathway. *Am Heart J* 1986;112: 1141–1152.
97. Wathen M, Klein GJ, Yee R, et al. Initiation of atrial fibrillation in the Wolff-Parkinson-White syndrome: importance of the accessory pathway. *J Am Coll Cardiol* 1992;19:227A.
98. Borggrefe M, Seidl K, Shesana M, et al. Incidence of atrial fibrillation after successful radiofrequency ablation of accessory pathways. *J Am Coll Cardiol* 1992;19:27A.
99. Chen PS, Pressley JC, Tang AS, et al. New observations on atrial fibrillation before and after surgical treatment in patients with the Wolff-Parkinson-White syndrome. *J Am Coll Cardiol* 1992;19:974–981.
100. Haissaguerre M, Fischer B, Labbe T, et al. Frequency of recurrent atrial fibrillation after catheter ablation of overt accessory pathways. *Am J Cardiol* 1992;69:493–497.
101. Sharma AD, Klein GJ, Guiraudon GM, et al. Atrial fibrillation in patients with Wolff-Parkinson-White syndrome: incidence after surgical ablation of the accessory pathway. *Circulation* 1985;72:161–169.
102. Dagres N, Clague JR, Lottkamp H, et al. Impact of radiofrequency catheter ablation of accessory pathways on the frequency of atrial fibrillation during long-term follow-up; high recurrence rate of atrial fibrillation in patients older than 50 years of age. *Eur Heart J* 2001;22:423–427.
103. Krahn AD, Manfreda J, Tate RB, et al. The natural history of electrocardiographic preexcitation in men. The Manitoba Follow-up Study. *Ann Intern Med* 1992;116:456–460.
104. Sorbo MD, Buja GF, Miorelli M, et al. [The prevalence of the Wolff-Parkinson-White syndrome in a population of 116,542 young males]. *G Ital Cardiol* 1995;25:681–687.
105. Soria R, Guize L, Fernandez F, et al. [Prevalence and electrocardiographic forms of the Wolff-Parkinson-White syndrome]. *Arch Mal Coeur Vaiss* 1982;75:1389–1399.
106. Vidaillet Jr HJ, Pressley JC, Henke E, et al. Familial occurrence of accessory atrioventricular pathways (preexcitation syndrome). *N Engl J Med* 1987;317:65–69.
107. Gollob MH, Green MS, Tang AS, et al. Identification of a gene responsible for familial Wolff-Parkinson-White syndrome. *N Engl J Med* 2001;344:1823–1831.
108. MacRae CA, Ghaisas N, Kass S, et al. Familial hypertrophic cardiomyopathy with Wolff-Parkinson-White syndrome maps to a locus on chromosome 7q3. *J Clin Invest* 1995;96:1216–1220.
109. Massumi RA. Familial Wolff-Parkinson-White syndrome with cardiomyopathy. *Am J Med* 1967;43:951–955.
110. Munger TM, Packer DL, Hammill SC, et al. A population study of the natural history of Wolff-Parkinson-White syndrome in Olmsted County, Minnesota, 1953–1989. *Circulation* 1993;87:866–873.
111. Bardy GH, Fedor JM, German LD, et al. Surface electrocardiographic clues suggesting presence of a nodofascicular Mahaim fiber. *J Am Coll Cardiol* 1984;3:1161–1168.
112. Bardy GH, Fedor JM, German LD, et al. ECG clues to the presence of a nodo-ventricular Mahaim fiber. *J Am Coll Cardiol* 1984;3:610.
113. Bauernfeind RA, Wyndham CR, Swiryn SP, et al. Paroxysmal atrial fibrillation in the Wolff-Parkinson-White syndrome. *Am J Cardiol* 1981;47:562–569.
114. Campbell RW, Smith RA, Gallagher JJ, et al. Atrial fibrillation in the preexcitation syndrome. *Am J Cardiol* 1977;40:514–520.
115. de Chillou C, Rodriguez LM, Schlapfer J, et al. Clinical characteristics and electrophysiologic properties of atrioventricular accessory pathways: importance of the accessory pathway location. *J Am Coll Cardiol* 1992;20:666–671.
116. Della Bella P, Brugada P, Talajic M, et al. Atrial fibrillation in patients with an accessory pathway: importance of the conduction properties of the accessory pathway. *J Am Coll Cardiol* 1991;17:1352–1356.
117. Cappato R, Schluter M, Weiss C, et al. Radiofrequency current catheter ablation of accessory atrioventricular pathways in Ebstein's anomaly. *Circulation* 1996;94:376–383.
118. Van Hare GF, Lesh MD, Stanger P. Radiofrequency catheter ablation of supraventricular arrhythmias in patients with congenital heart disease: results and technical considerations. *J Am Coll Cardiol* 1993;22:883–890.
119. Chen SA, Chiang CE, Tai CT, et al. Longitudinal clinical and electrophysiological assessment of patients with symptomatic Wolff-Parkinson-White syndrome and atrioventricular node reentrant tachycardia. *Circulation* 1996;93:2023–2032.
120. Clair WK, Wilkinson WE, McCarthy EA, et al. Spontaneous occurrence of symptomatic paroxysmal atrial fibrillation and paroxysmal supraventricular tachycardia in untreated patients. *Circulation* 1993;87:1114–1122.
121. Guize L, Soria R, Chaouat JC, et al. [Prevalence and course of Wolff-Parkinson-White syndrome in a population of 138,048 subjects]. *Ann Med Interne* 1985;136:474–478.
122. Lundberg A. Paroxysmal atrial tachycardia in infancy: long-term follow-up study of 49 subjects. *Pediatrics* 1982;70:638–642.
123. Klein GJ, Yee R, Sharma AD. Longitudinal electrophysiologic assessment of asymptomatic patients with the Wolff-Parkinson-White electrocardiographic pattern. *N Engl J Med* 1989;320:1229–1233.
124. Leitch JW, Klein GJ, Yee R, et al. Prognostic value of electrophysiology testing in asymptomatic patients with Wolff-Parkinson-White pattern. *Circulation* 1990;82:1718–1723.
125. Pappone C, Santinelli V, Rosanio S, et al. Usefulness of invasive electrophysiologic testing to stratify the risk of arrhythmic events in asymptomatic patients with Wolff-Parkinson-White pattern: results from a large prospective long-term follow-up study. *J Am Coll Cardiol* 2003;41: 239–244.
126. Dreifus LS, Haiat R, Watanabe Y, et al. Ventricular fibrillation. A possible mechanism of sudden death in patients and Wolff-Parkinson-White syndrome. *Circulation* 1971;43:520–527.
127. Klein GJ, Bashore TM, Sellers TD, et al. Ventricular fibrillation in the Wolff-Parkinson-White syndrome. *N Engl J Med* 1979;301:1080–1085.
128. Timmermans C, Smeets JL, Rodriguez LM, et al. Aborted sudden death in the Wolff-Parkinson-White syndrome. *Am J Cardiol* 1995;76:492–494.
129. Berkman NL, Lamb LE. The Wolff-Parkinson-White electrocardiogram. A follow-up study of five to twenty-eight years. *N Engl J Med* 1968;278:492–494.
130. Fitzsimmons PJ, McWhirter PD, Peterson DW, et al. The natural history of Wolff-Parkinson-White syndrome in 228 military aviators: a long-term follow-up of 22 years. *Am Heart J* 2001;142:530–536.
131. Goudevenos JA, Katsouras CS, Graekas G, et al. Ventricular pre-excitation in the general population: a study on the mode of presentation and clinical course. *Heart* 2000;83:29–34.
132. Satoh M, Aizawa Y, Funazaki T, et al. Electrophysiologic evaluation of asymptomatic patients with the Wolff-Parkinson-White pattern. *Pacing Clin Electrophysiol* 1989;12:413–420.
133. Milstein S, Sharma AD, Klein GJ. Electrophysiologic profile of asymptomatic Wolff-Parkinson-White pattern. *Am J Cardiol* 1986;57:1097–1100.
134. Montoya PT, Brugada P, Smeets J, et al. Ventricular fibrillation in the Wolff-Parkinson-White syndrome. *Eur Heart J* 1991;12:144–150.
135. Critelli G, Grassi G, Perticone F, et al. Transesophageal pacing for prognostic evaluation of preexcitation syndrome and assessment of protective therapy. *Am J Cardiol* 1983;51:513–518.
136. Drago F, Turchetta A, Calzolari A, et al. Detection of atrial vulnerability by transesophageal atrial pacing and the relation of symptoms in children with Wolff-Parkinson-White and in a symptomatic control group. *Am J Cardiol* 1994;74:400–401.
137. Packer D, Pressley JC, German LD, et al. Accuracy of invasive testing for direct identification of sudden death in the Wolff-Parkinson-White syndrome. *J Am Coll Cardiol* 1988;11:78A.
138. Klein GJ, Gulamhusein SS. Intermittent preexcitation in the Wolff-Parkinson-White syndrome. *Am J Cardiol* 1983;52:292–296.
139. Levy S, Broustet JP, Clementy J, et al. [Wolff-Parkinson-White syndrome. Correlation between the results of electrophysiological investigation and exercise tolerance testing on the electrical aspect of preexcitation]. *Arch Mal Coeur Vaiss* 1979;72:634–640.
140. Sharma AD, Yee R, Guiraudon G, et al. Sensitivity and specificity of invasive and noninvasive testing for risk of sudden death in Wolff-Parkinson-White syndrome. *J Am Coll Cardiol* 1987;10:373–381.
141. Strasberg B, Ashley WW, Wyndham CR, et al. Treadmill exercise testing in the Wolff-Parkinson-White syndrome. *Am J Cardiol* 1980;45:742–748.

142. Fananapazir L, Packer DL, German LD, et al. Procainamide infusion test: inability to identify patients with Wolff-Parkinson-White syndrome who are potentially at risk of sudden death. *Circulation* 1988;77:1291–1296.
143. Wellens HJ, Braat S, Brugada P, et al. Use of procainamide in patients with the Wolff-Parkinson-White syndrome to disclose a short refractory period of the accessory pathway. *Am J Cardiol* 1982;50:1087–1089.
144. Wellens HJ, Bar FW, Gorgels AP, et al. Use of ajmaline in patients with the Wolff-Parkinson-White syndrome to disclose short refractory period of the accessory pathway. *Am J Cardiol* 1980;45:130–133.
145. Cavalli A, Maggioni A, Tusa M, et al. Two false-negative responses to the ajmaline test in the Wolff-Parkinson-White syndrome. *Pacing Clin Electrophysiol* 1985;8:832–837.
146. Wellens HJ, Durrer D. Wolff-Parkinson-White syndrome and atrial fibrillation. Relation between refractory period of accessory pathway and ventricular rate during atrial fibrillation. *Am J Cardiol* 1974;34:777–782.
147. Brembilla-Perrot B, Spatz F, Khaldi E, et al. Value of esophageal pacing in evaluation of supraventricular tachycardia. *Am J Cardiol* 1990;65:322–330.
148. Gallagher JJ, Smith WM, Kasell J, et al. Use of the esophageal lead in the diagnosis of mechanisms of reciprocating supraventricular tachycardia. *Pacing Clin Electrophysiol* 1980;3:440–451.
149. Teo WS, Klein GJ, Guiraudon GM, et al. Multiple accessory pathways in the Wolff-Parkinson-White syndrome as a risk factor for ventricular fibrillation. *Am J Cardiol* 1991;67:889–891.
150. Blomstrom-Lundqvist C, Scheinman MM, Aliot EM, et al. ACC/AHA/ESC guidelines for the management of patients with supraventricular arrhythmias—executive summary. A report of the American College of Cardiology/American Heart Association Task Force on Practice Guidelines and the European Society of Cardiology Committee for Practice Guidelines (Writing Committee to Develop Guidelines for the Management of Patients with Supraventricular Arrhythmias) developed in collaboration with NASPE-Heart Rhythm Society. *J Am Coll Cardiol* 2003;42:1493–1531.
151. Zipes DP, DiMarco JP, Gillette PC, et al. Guidelines for clinical intracardiac electrophysiological and catheter ablation procedures. A report of the American College of Cardiology/American Heart Association Task Force on Practice Guidelines (Committee on Clinical Intracardiac Electrophysiologic and Catheter Ablation Procedures), developed in collaboration with the North American Society of Pacing and Electrophysiology. *J Am Coll Cardiol* 1995;26:555–573.
152. Pappone C, Santinelli V. Should catheter ablation be performed in asymptomatic patients with Wolff-Parkinson-White syndrome? Catheter ablation should be performed in asymptomatic patients with Wolff-Parkinson-White syndrome. *Circulation* 2005;112:2207–2215; discussion, 2216.
153. Todd DM, Klein GJ, Krahn AD, et al. Asymptomatic Wolff-Parkinson-White syndrome: is it time to revisit guidelines? *J Am Coll Cardiol* 2003; 41:245–248.
154. Pappone C, Manguso F, Santinelli R, et al. Radiofrequency ablation in children with asymptomatic Wolff-Parkinson-White syndrome. *N Engl J Med* 2004;351:1197–1205.
155. Pappone C, Santinelli V, Manguso F, et al. A randomized study of prophylactic catheter ablation in asymptomatic patients with the Wolff-Parkinson-White syndrome. *N Engl J Med* 2003;349:1803–1811.
156. Wellens HJ. Should catheter ablation be performed in asymptomatic patients with Wolff-Parkinson-White syndrome? When to perform catheter ablation in asymptomatic patients with a Wolff-Parkinson-White electrocardiogram. *Circulation* 2005;112:2201–2207; discussion, 2216.
157. Lerman BB, Basson CT. High-risk patients with ventricular preexcitation—a pendulum in motion. *N Engl J Med* 2003;349:1787–1789.
158. Friedman RA, Walsh EP, Silka MJ, et al. NASPE Expert Consensus Conference: radiofrequency catheter ablation in children with and without congenital heart disease. Report of the Writing Committee. North American Society of Pacing and Electrophysiology. *Pacing Clin Electrophysiol* 2002;25:1000–1017.
159. Coumel P, Cabrol C, Fabiato A. Tachycardie permanente par rhythme reciproque. *Arch Mal Coeur* 1967;60:1830–1867.
160. Gaita F, Haissaguerre M, Giustetto C, et al. Catheter ablation of permanent junctional reciprocating tachycardia with radiofrequency current. *J Am Coll Cardiol* 1995;25:648–654.
161. Ticho BS, Saul JP, Hulse JE, et al. Variable location of accessory pathways associated with the permanent form of junctional reciprocating tachycardia and confirmation with radiofrequency ablation. *Am J Cardiol* 1992;70:1559–1564.
162. Critelli G, Gallagher JJ, Monda V, et al. Anatomic and electrophysiologic substrate of the permanent form of junctional reciprocating tachycardia. *J Am Coll Cardiol* 1984;4:601–610.
163. Critelli G, Gallagher JJ, Thiene G, et al. Electrophysiologic and histopathologic correlations in a case of permanent form of reciprocating tachycardia. *Eur Heart J* 1985;6:130–137.
164. Critelli G, Perticone F, Coltorti F, et al. Antegrade slow bypass conduction after closed-chest ablation of the His bundle in permanent junctional reciprocating tachycardia. *Circulation* 1983;67:687–692.
165. Packer DL, Bardy GH, Worley SJ, et al. Tachycardia-induced cardiomyopathy: a reversible form of left ventricular dysfunction. *Am J Cardiol* 1986;57:563–570.
166. Gallagher JJ, Smith WM, Kasell JH, et al. Role of Mahaim fibers in cardiac arrhythmias in man. *Circulation* 1981;64:176–189.
167. Gillette PC, Garson Jr A, Cooley DA, et al. Prolonged and decremental antegrade conduction properties in right anterior accessory connections: Wide QRS antidromic tachycardia of left bundle branch block pattern without Wolff-Parkinson-White configuration in sinus rhythm. *Am Heart J* 1982;103:66–74.
168. Klein GJ, Guiraudon GM, Kerr CR, et al. "Nodoventricular" accessory pathway: evidence for a distinct accessory atrioventricular pathway with atrioventricular node–like properties. *J Am Coll Cardiol* 1988;11:1035–1040.
169. Tchou P, Lehmann MH, Jazayeri M, et al. Atriofascicular connection or a nodoventricular Mahaim fiber? Electrophysiologic elucidation of the pathway and associated reentrant circuit. *Circulation* 1988;77:837–848.
170. Haissaguerre M, Cauchemez B, Marcus F, et al. Characteristics of the ventricular insertion sites of accessory pathways with anterograde decremental conduction properties. *Circulation* 1995;91:1077–1085.
171. Hluchy J, Schickel S, Jorger U, et al. Electrophysiologic characteristics and radiofrequency ablation of concealed nodofascicular and left anterograde atriofascicular pathways. *J Cardiovasc Electrophysiol* 2000;11:211–217.
172. Bar FW, Brugada P, Dassen WR, et al. Differential diagnosis of tachycardia with narrow QRS complex (shorter than 0.12 second). *Am J Cardiol* 1984;54:555–560.
173. Josephson ME. Paroxysmal supraventricular tachycardia: an electrophysiologic approach. *Am J Cardiol* 1978;41:1123–1126.
174. Wu D, Denes P, Amat-y-Leon F, et al. Clinical, electrocardiographic and electrophysiologic observations in patients with paroxysmal supraventricular tachycardia. *Am J Cardiol* 1978;41:1045–1051.
175. Keim S, Werner P, Jazayeri M, et al. Localization of the fast and slow pathways in atrioventricular nodal reentrant tachycardia by intraoperative ice mapping. *Circulation* 1992;86:919–925.
176. McGuire MA, Bourke JP, Robotin MC, et al. High resolution mapping of Koch's triangle using sixty electrodes in humans with atrioventricular junctional (AV nodal) reentrant tachycardia. *Circulation* 1993;88:2315–2328.
177. Ross DL, Johnson DC, Denniss AR, et al. Curative surgery for atrioventricular junctional ("AV nodal") reentrant tachycardia. *J Am Coll Cardiol* 1985;6:1383–1392.
178. Ko PT, Naccarelli GV, Gulamhusein S, et al. Atrioventricular dissociation during paroxysmal junctional tachycardia. *Pacing Clin Electrophysiol* 1981;4:670–678.
179. Wah JA, Friday K, Sakurai M, et al. Is the His bundle part of the AV nodal reentry circuit? *Circulation* 1985;72:271.
180. Miller JM, Rosenthal ME, Vassallo JA, et al. Atrioventricular nodal reentrant tachycardia: studies on upper and lower 'common pathways'. *Circulation* 1987;75:930–940.
181. Hwang C, Martin DJ, Goodman JS, et al. Atypical atrioventricular node reciprocating tachycardia masquerading as tachycardia using a left-sided accessory pathway. *J Am Coll Cardiol* 1997;30:218–225.
182. Jais P, Haissaguerre M, Shah DC, et al. Successful radiofrequency ablation of a slow atrioventricular nodal pathway on the left posterior atrial septum. *Pacing Clin Electrophysiol* 1999;22:525–527.
183. Sorbera C, Cohen M, Woolf P, et al. Atrioventricular nodal reentry tachycardia: slow pathway ablation using the transseptal approach. *Pacing Clin Electrophysiol* 2000;23:1343–1349.
184. Inoue S, Becker AE. Posterior extensions of the human compact atrioventricular node: a neglected anatomic feature of potential clinical significance. *Circulation* 1998;97:188–193.
185. Akhtar M. Atrioventricular nodal reentrant tachycardia. *Med Clin North Am* 1984;68:819–830.
186. McGuire MA, Lau KC, Johnson DC, et al. Patients with two types of atrioventricular junctional (AV nodal) reentrant tachycardia. Evidence that a common pathway of nodal tissue is not present above the reentrant circuit. *Circulation* 1991;83:1232–1246.
187. Casta A, Wolff GS, Mehta AV, et al. Dual atrioventricular nodal pathways: a benign finding in arrhythmia-free children with heart disease. *Am J Cardiol* 1980;46:1013–1018.
188. Moulton K, Wang X, Xu Y, et al. High incidence of dual AV nodal pathway potentials in patients undergoing radiofrequency ablation of accessory pathways. *Circulation* 1990;82:III-319.
189. Hazlitt HA, McClelland J, Wang X, et al. Prevalence of slow AV nodal pathway potentials in patients without AV nodal reentrant tachycardia. *J Am Coll Cardiol* 1993;21:281A.
190. Akhtar M, Damato AN, Ruskin JN, et al. Antegrade and retrograde conduction characteristics in three patterns of paroxysmal atrioventricular junctional reentrant tachycardia. *Am Heart J* 1978;95:22–42.
191. Goldberger J, Brooks R, Kadish A. Physiology of "atypical" atrioventricular junctional reentrant tachycardia occurring following radiofrequency catheter modification of the atrioventricular node. *Pacing Clin Electrophysiol* 1992;15:2270–2282.
192. Lee MA, Morady F, Kadish A, et al. Catheter modification of the atrioventricular junction with radiofrequency energy for control of atrioventricular nodal reentry tachycardia. *Circulation* 1991;83:827–835.
193. Sung RJ, Styperek JL, Myerburg RJ, et al. Initiation of two distinct forms of atrioventricular nodal reentrant tachycardia during programmed ventricular stimulation in man. *Am J Cardiol* 1978;42:404–415.
194. Wu D, Denes P, Amat YLF, et al. An unusual variety of atrioventricular nodal re-entry due to retrograde dual atrioventricular nodal pathways. *Circulation* 1977;56:50–59.

195. Baerman JM, Wang X, Jackman W. Atrioventricular nodal reentry with an antegrade slow pathway and a retrograde slow pathway: clinical and electrophysiological properties. *J Am Coll Cardiol* 1991;17:197A.
196. Goldreyer BN, Damato AN. The essential role of atrioventricular conduction delay in the initiation of paroxysmal supraventricular tachycardia. *Circulation* 1971;43:679–687.
197. Sung RJ, Chang MS, Chiang BN. Clinical electrophysiology of supraventricular tachycardia. *Cardiol Clin* 1983;1:225–251.
198. Brugada P, Wellens HJ. Electrophysiology, mechanisms, diagnosis, and treatment of paroxysmal recurrent atrioventricular nodal reentrant tachycardia. In: Surawicz B, Reddy CP, Prystowsky E, eds. *Tachycardias*. Boston: Martinus Nijhoff, 1984.
199. Wu D, Kou HC, Yeh SJ, et al. Determinants of tachycardia induction using ventricular stimulation in dual pathway atrioventricular nodal reentrant tachycardia. *Am Heart J* 1984;108:44–55.
200. Farre J, Wellens HJ. The value of the electrocardiogram in diagnosing site or origin and mechanism of supraventricular tachycardia. In: Wellens HJ, Kulbertus HE, eds. *What's new in electrocardiography*. The Hague: Martinus Nijhoff, 1981: 131–171.
201. Kalbfleisch SJ, el-Atassi R, Calkins H, et al. Differentiation of paroxysmal narrow QRS complex tachycardias using the 12-lead electrocardiogram. *J Am Coll Cardiol* 1993;21:85–89.
202. Brugada P, Farre J, Green M, et al. Observations in patients with supraventricular tachycardia having a P-R interval shorter than the R-P interval: differentiation between atrial tachycardia and reciprocating atrioventricular tachycardia using an accessory pathway with long conduction times. *Am Heart J* 1984;107:556–570.
203. Ross DL, Uther JB. Diagnosis of concealed accessory pathways in supraventricular tachycardia. *Pacing Clin Electrophysiol* 1984;7:1069–1085.
204. Wellens HJ, Brugada P. Value of programmed stimulation of the heart in patients with the Wolff-Parkinson-White syndrome. In: Josephson ME, Wellens HJ, eds. *Tachycardias: mechanisms, diagnosis and treatment*. Philadelphia: Lea & Febiger, 1981: 199.
205. Pritchett EL, Prystowsky EN, Benditt DG, et al. "Dual atrioventricular nodal pathways" in patients with Wolff-Parkinson-White syndrome. *Br Heart J* 1980;43:7–13.
206. Jazayeri M, Dhala A, Koch K. Atrioventricular nodal reentry in patients with accessory pathway: a suitable substrate for preexcited tachycardia. *Pacing Clin Electrophysiol* 1991;14:687.
207. diMarco JP, Sellers TD, Lerman BB, et al. Diagnostic and therapeutic use of adenosine in patients with supraventricular tachyarrhythmias. *J Am Coll Cardiol* 1985;6:417–425.
208. Akhtar M. Supraventricular tachycardias: electrophysiological mechanisms, diagnosis, and pharmacologic therapy. In: Josephson ME, Wellens HJ, eds. *Tachycardias: mechanisms, diagnosis, treatment*. Philadelphia: Lea & Febiger, 1984: 137.
209. Sung RJ, Elser B, McAllister Jr RG. Intravenous verapamil for termination of re-entrant supraventricular tachycardias: intracardiac studies correlated with plasma verapamil concentrations. *Ann Intern Med* 1980;93:682–689.
210. Waxman HL, Myerburg RJ, Appel R, et al. Verapamil for control of ventricular rate in paroxysmal supraventricular tachycardia and atrial fibrillation or flutter: a double-blind randomized cross-over study. *Ann Intern Med* 1981;94:1–6.
211. Prystowsky EN, Greer S, Packer DL, et al. Beta-blocker therapy for the Wolff-Parkinson-White syndrome. *Am J Cardiol* 1987;60:46D–50D.
212. Gallagher JJ, Svenson RH, Kasell JH, et al. Catheter technique for closed-chest ablation of the atrioventricular conduction system. *N Engl J Med* 1982;306:194–200.
213. Kerr CR, Gallagher JJ, Smith WM, et al. The induction of atrial flutter and fibrillation and the termination of atrial flutter by esophageal pacing. *Pacing Clin Electrophysiol* 1983;6:60–72.
214. Rhodes LA, Walsh EP, Saul JP. Programmed atrial stimulation via the esophagus for management of supraventricular arrhythmias in infants and children. *Am J Cardiol* 1994;74:353–356.
215. Akhtar M, Shenasa M, Jazayeri M, et al. Wide QRS complex tachycardia. Reappraisal of a common clinical problem. *Ann Intern Med* 1988;109: 905–912.
216. Barrett PA, Jordan JL, Mandel WJ, et al. The electrophysiologic effects of intravenous propranolol in the Wolff-Parkinson-White syndrome. *Am Heart J* 1979;98:213–224.
217. Berkowitz WD, Wit AL, Lau SH, et al. The effects of propranolol on cardiac conduction. *Circulation* 1969;40:855–862.
218. Denes P, Cummings JM, Simpson R, et al. Effects of propranolol on anomalous pathway refractoriness and circus movement tachycardias in patients with preexcitation. *Am J Cardiol* 1978;41:1061–1067.
219. Prystowsky EN, Jackman WM, Rinkenberger RL, et al. Effect of autonomic blockade on ventricular refractoriness and atrioventricular nodal conduction in humans.Evidence supporting a direct cholinergic action on ventricular muscle refractoriness. *Circ Res* 1981;49:511–518.
220. Akhtar M, Gilbert CJ, Shenasa M. Effect of lidocaine on atrioventricular response via the accessory pathway in patients with Wolff-Parkinson-White syndrome. *Circulation* 1981;63:435–441.
221. Rosen KM, Barwolf C, Ehsani A, et al. Effects of lidocaine and propranolol on the normal and anomalous pathways in patients with preexcitation. *Am J Cardiol* 1972;30:801–809.
222. Sellers Jr TD, Bashore TM, Gallagher JJ. Digitalis in the pre-excitation syndrome.Analysis during atrial fibrillation. *Circulation* 1977;56:260–267.
223. Gulamhusein S, Ko P, Klein GJ. Ventricular fibrillation following verapamil in the Wolff-Parkinson-White syndrome. *Am Heart J* 1983;106:145–147.
224. Jacob AS, Nielsen DH, Gianelly RE. Fatal ventricular fibrillation following verapamil in Wolff-Parkinson-White syndrome with atrial fibrillation. *Ann Emerg Med* 1985;14:159–160.
225. McGovern B, Garan H, Ruskin JN. Precipitation of cardiac arrest by verapamil in patients with Wolff-Parkinson-White syndrome. *Ann Intern Med* 1986;104:791–794.
226. Rinkenberger RL, Prystowsky EN, Heger JJ, et al. Effects of intravenous and chronic oral verapamil administration in patients with supraventricular tachyarrhythmias. *Circulation* 1980;62:996–1010.
227. Rowland TW. Augmented ventricular rate following verapamil treatment for atrial fibrillation with Wolff-Parkinson-White syndrome. *Pediatrics* 1983;72:245–246.
228. Shenasa M, Fromer M, Faugere G, et al. Efficacy and safety of intravenous and oral diltiazem for Wolff-Parkinson-White syndrome. *Am J Cardiol* 1987;59:301–306.
229. Exner DV, Muzyka T, Gillis AM. Proarrhythmia in patients with the Wolff-Parkinson-White syndrome after standard doses of intravenous adenosine. *Ann Intern Med* 1995;122:351–352.
230. Wellens HJ, Bar FW, Dassen WR, et al. Effect of drugs in the Wolff-Parkinson-White syndrome. Importance of initial length of effective refractory period of the accessory pathway. *Am J Cardiol* 1980;46:665–669.
231. Harper RW, Whitford E, Middlebrook K, et al. Effects of verapamil on the electrophysiologic properties of the accessory pathway in patients with the Wolff-Parkinson-White syndrome. *Am J Cardiol* 1982;50:1323–1330.
232. Shenasa M, Gilbert CJ, Schmidt DH, et al. Procainamide and retrograde atrioventricular nodal conduction in man. *Circulation* 1982;65:355–362.
233. Wellens HJ, Tan SL, Bar FW, et al. Effect of verapamil studied by programmed electrical stimulation of the heart in patients with paroxysmal re-entrant supraventricular tachycardia. *Br Heart J* 1977;39:1058–1066.
234. Sellers Jr TD, Campbell RW, Bashore TM, et al. Effects of procainamide and quinidine sulfate in the Wolff-Parkinson-White syndrome. *Circulation* 1977;55:15–22.
235. Wellens HJ, Durrer D. Effect of procaine amide, quinidine, and ajmaline in the Wolff-Parkinson-White syndrome. *Circulation* 1974;50:114–120.
236. Mandel WJ, Laks MM, Obayashi K, et al. The Wolff-Parkinson-White syndrome: pharmacologic effects of procaine amide. *Am Heart J* 1975;90: 744–754.
237. Camm J, Ward D, Spurrell RA. The effect of intravenous disopyramide phosphate on recurrent paroxysmal tachycardias. *Br J Clin Pharmacol* 1979;8:441–449.
238. Breithardt G, Borggrefe M, Wiebringhaus E, et al. Effect of propafenone in the Wolff-Parkinson-White syndrome: electrophysiologic findings and long-term follow-up. *Am J Cardiol* 1984;54:29D–39D.
239. Hammill SC, McLaran CJ, Wood DL, et al. Double-blind study of intravenous propafenone for paroxysmal supraventricular reentrant tachycardia. *J Am Coll Cardiol* 1987;9:1364–1368.
240. Ludmer PL, McGowan NE, Antman EM, et al. Efficacy of propafenone in Wolff-Parkinson-White syndrome: electrophysiologic findings and long-term follow-up. *J Am Coll Cardiol* 1987;9:1357–1363.
241. Waleffe A, Mary-Rabine L, de Rijbel R, et al. Electrophysiological effects of propafenone studied with programmed electrical stimulation of the heart in patients with recurrent paroxysmal supraventricular tachycardia. *Eur Heart J* 1981;2:345–352.
242. Hellestrand KJ, Nathan AW, Bexton RS, et al. Cardiac electrophysiologic effects of flecainide acetate for paroxysmal reentrant junctional tachycardias. *Am J Cardiol* 1983;51:770–776.
243. Neuss H, Buss J, Schlepper M, et al. Effects of flecainide on electrophysiological properties of accessory pathways in the Wolff-Parkinson-White syndrome. *Eur Heart J* 1983;4:347–353.
244. Olsson SB, Edvardsson N. Clinical electrophysiologic study of antiarrhythmic properties of flecainide: acute intraventricular delayed conduction and prolonged repolarization in regular paced and premature beats using intracardiac monophasic action potentials with programmed stimulation. *Am Heart J* 1981;102:864–871.
245. Ward DE, Jones S, Shinebourne EA. Use of flecainide acetate for refractory junctional tachycardias in children with the Wolff-Parkinson-White syndrome. *Am J Cardiol* 1986;57:787–790.
246. Kim SS, Smith P, Ruffy R. Treatment of atrial tachyarrhythmias and preexcitation syndrome with flecainide acetate. *Am J Cardiol* 1988;62:29D–34D.
247. Kunze KP, Schluter M, Kuck KH. Sotalol in patients with Wolff-Parkinson-White syndrome. *Circulation* 1987;75:1050–1057.
248. Nathan AW, Hellestrand KJ, Bexton RS, et al. Electrophysiological effects of sotalol–just another beta blocker? *Br Heart J* 1982;47:515–520.
249. Mitchell LB, Wyse DG, Duff HJ. Electropharmacology of sotalol in patients with Wolff-Parkinson-White syndrome. *Circulation* 1987;76:810–818.
250. Touboul P, Atallah G, Kirkorian G, et al. Effects of intravenous sotalol in patients with atrioventricular accessory pathways. *Am Heart J* 1987; 114:545–550.
251. Brugada P, Wellens HJ. Effects of oral amiodarone on rate-dependent changes in refractoriness in patients with Wolff-Parkinson-White syndrome. *Am J Cardiol* 1985;56:863–866.

252. Kappenberger LJ, Fromer MA, Steinbrunn W, et al. Efficacy of amiodarone in the Wolff-Parkinson-White syndrome with rapid ventricular response via accessory pathway during atrial fibrillation. *Am J Cardiol* 1984;54:330–335.
253. Rowland E, Krikler DM. Electrophysiological assessment of amiodarone in treatment of resistant supraventricular arrhythmias. *Br Heart J* 1980;44:82–90.
254. Wellens HJ, Brugada P, Abdollah H, et al. A comparison of the electrophysiologic effects of intravenous and oral amiodarone in the same patient. *Circulation* 1984;69:120–124.
255. Wellens HJ, Lie KI, Bar FW, et al. Effect of amiodarone in the Wolff-Parkinson-White syndrome. *Am J Cardiol* 1976;38:189–194.
256. Bauernfeind RA, Wyndham CR, Dhingra RC, et al. Serial electrophysiologic testing of multiple drugs in patients with atrioventricular nodal reentrant paroxysmal tachycardia. *Circulation* 1980;62:1341–1349.
257. Naccarelli GV, Jackman WM, Akhtar M, et al. Efficacy and electrophysiologic effects of encainide for atrioventricular nodal reentrant tachycardia. *Am J Cardiol* 1988;62:31L–36L.
258. Swiryn S, Bauernfeind RA, Wyndham CR, et al. Effects of oral disopyramide phosphate on induction of paroxysmal supraventricular tachycardia. *Circulation* 1981;64:169–175.
259. Wu D, Denes P, Bauernfeind R, et al. Effects of procainamide on atrioventricular nodal re-entrant paroxysmal tachycardia. *Circulation* 1978;57:1171–1179.
260. Wu D, Hung JS, Kuo CT, et al. Effects of quinidine on atrioventricular nodal reentrant paroxysmal tachycardia. *Circulation* 1981;64:823–831.
261. Page RL, Connolly SJ, Wilkinson WE, et al. Antiarrhythmic effects of azimilide in paroxysmal supraventricular tachycardia: efficacy and dose-response. *Am Heart J* 2002;143:643–649.
262. Jazayeri MR, Hempe SL, Sra JS, et al. Selective transcatheter ablation of the fast and slow pathways using radiofrequency energy in patients with atrioventricular nodal reentrant tachycardia. *Circulation* 1992;85:1318–1328.
263. Tai CT, Chen SA, Chiang CE, et al. Electrophysiologic characteristics and radiofrequency catheter ablation in patients with multiple atrioventricular nodal reentry tachycardias. *Am J Cardiol* 1996;77:52–58.
264. Hogenhuis W, Stevens SK, Wang P, et al. Cost-effectiveness of radiofrequency ablation compared with other strategies in Wolff-Parkinson-White syndrome. *Circulation* 1993;88:II437–II446.
265. Cheng CH, Sanders GD, Hlatky MA, et al. Cost-effectiveness of radiofrequency ablation for supraventricular tachycardia. *Ann Intern Med* 2000;133:864–876.

CHAPTER 66 ■ VENTRICULAR TACHYCARDIA

DAVID WILBER

OVERVIEW

Ventricular tachycardia (VT) remains an important cause of morbidity and mortality in cardiac patients. Symptoms may be mild (palpitations and dyspnea), or they may reflect rapid and severe hemodynamic compromise (syncope, cardiac arrest). In occasional patients, congestive heart failure may be the initial presentation when VT of prolonged duration remains unrecognized. Structural heart disease (SHD) is present in 85% to 90% of patients, with healed myocardial infarction the most common cause. The specific underlying myocardial substrate has an important influence on long-term outcome and therapeutic options, and it is discussed in detail in subsequent sections.

Although rapid rates (>200 beats per minute) are more likely to produce hemodynamic compromise (1–3), autonomic compensatory mechanisms (particularly the baroreceptor reflex) play a major role independent of heart rate or pre-VT hemodynamic status (4,5). Impairment of this reflex has been associated with more rapid hemodynamic deterioration (5). Unstable VT is an important, but by no means exclusive, cause of cardiac arrest and sudden death. The exact proportion of cases in which VT is the initiating rhythm is difficult to ascertain, because it may transition rapidly to ventricular fibrillation (VF) or asystole and is thus underestimated by rhythms recorded by "first responders" at the time of arrest. Similarly, data from stored electrograms of implantable cardioverter-defibrillator (ICD) recipients may not accurately reflect rhythms at the onset of cardiac arrest, because many ICD-treated episodes may have self-terminated or been sufficiently stable to permit survival even without immediate intervention (6).

Increasing evidence indicates that the degree of hemodynamic stability at initial clinical presentation has little impact on long-term prognosis in patients with SHD. In the Antiarrhythmic vs Implantable Defibrillator (AVID) Registry (7), the mean ejection fraction was slightly higher in 440 patients presenting with stable VT (34% ± 13%) than in 1,029 patients presenting with unstable VT (31% ± 11%); congestive heart failure was also less common in patients with stable VT (34% versus 45%). Prior myocardial infarction, present in 72% of patients, and other cardiac diagnoses were similar between the two groups. Overall, increasing age, lower ejection fraction, congestive heart failure, nonuse of β-blockers, and ICDs were significant multivariate predictors of mortality. Hemodynamic stability of VT at presentation was not a predictor of mortality in univariate or multivariate analysis. These findings are corroborated by the frequent occurrence of rapid unstable VT during long-term follow-up in patients presenting with stable VT treated by an ICD (8,9).

GENERAL ASPECTS OF DIAGNOSIS AND MANAGEMENT

Electrocardiographic Recognition

VT originates from ventricular muscle, specialized conduction tissue (bundle branches and Purkinje fibers), or elements of

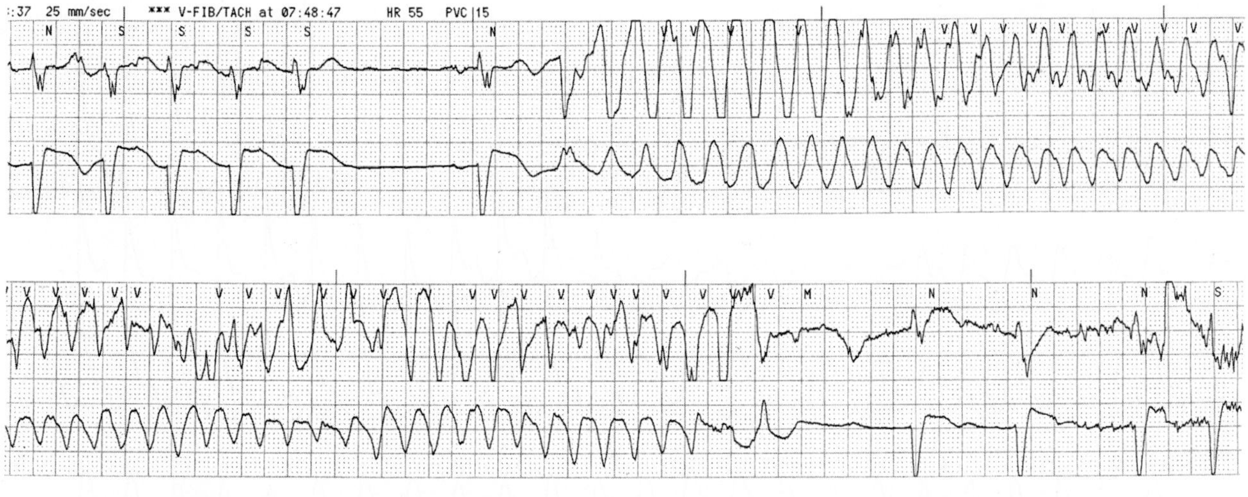

FIGURE 66.1. Polymorphic ventricular tachycardia with the features of torsade de pointes. Note the baseline QT prolongation, with abrupt lengthening of the QT interval after the pause, followed by the onset of polymorphic ventricular tachycardia, which suddenly terminates.

both. Although reentry is the most common mechanism, both normal and abnormal automaticity and triggered activity may play a role (see Chapter 57). Identification of VT begins with the recognition of three or more consecutive wide (≥120 milliseconds) complexes. Rarely, the QRS complex may be slightly narrower if the focus is within or adjacent to the proximal Purkinje system or bundle branches, with rapid early engagement of conduction over this network (10). These complexes may have a uniform appearance from beat to beat (monomorphic VT), or consecutive complexes may vary, often widely, in QRS configuration (polymorphic VT) (Fig. 66.1). A specific pattern of polymorphic VT, termed *torsade de pointes,* manifests a periodic reversal of QRS polarity associated with waxing and waning QRS amplitude. The distinction between monomorphic and polymorphic VT has important implications in terms of mechanism, underlying substrate, and prognosis that are discussed in subsequent sections. Spontaneous termination within 30 seconds is generally designated nonsustained VT, with longer durations considered sustained. Very rapid rates (>270 beats per minute) are seldom associated with discrete identifiable QRS complexes and are usually designated VF.

Most wide complex tachycardias (~80%) are ventricular in origin, particularly in the presence of known SHD, and this prior probability should influence subsequent decision making (11,12). Supraventricular tachycardia (SVT) may be associated with a wide QRS complex resulting from (a) preexisting intraventricular conduction defects, (b) aberrant conduction (from incomplete repolarization of some portion of the His-Purkinje system during tachycardia), (c) conduction over an accessory pathway, or (d) conditions associated with depressed conduction (drugs, metabolic or electrolyte abnormalities, ischemia). Rarely, ventricular pacing at rapid rates may cause diagnostic confusion because of failure to recognize the often imperceptibly small pacing artifacts on the surface electrocardiogram (ECG).

Distinction between VT and SVT with aberration can be difficult in individual patients, but several general principles are useful (Table 66.1). Capture beats and fusion beats are generally diagnostic for VT, but they are present in only a small number of cases (Fig. 66.2). Rarely, a ventricular ectopic beat during aberrantly conducted SVT can incorrectly suggest VT. Atrioventricular dissociation indicates VT with rare exceptions (Fig. 66.3). It is present in up to 70% of VTs and is more common at rapid rates. It also can be suspected if cannon A waves are observed during inspection of the jugular venous pulse during physical examination. The wider the QRS duration, the more likely the rhythm is VT. Durations of 160 milliseconds or longer during left bundle branch block patterns and of 140 milliseconds or longer during right bundle branch block patterns are useful guidelines (10). A frontal plane axis between −90 and + 180 degrees ("northwest axis") strongly favors VT. The precordial R/S criterion originally proposed by Brugada is relatively specific for VT (13). The criterion is present if either no RS complexes occur in the precordial leads, or, if R/S complexes are present, the interval from onset of the R wave to the nadir of the S wave is greater than 100 milliseconds. The absence of a typical bundle branch block pattern or rapid precordial intrinsicoid deflection favors VT. In the setting of preexisting intraventricular conduction defects, differences in QRS morphology between the baseline ECG and that of tachycardia favor a diagnosis of VT; however, similarity between the two does not exclude VT. Although numerous additional criteria have been proposed based on QRS configuration in specific leads, most have relatively low positive predictive value or are applicable only if the baseline QRS complex is normal.

Acute Therapy

Tachycardia associated with significant hypotension, heart failure, or angina should be promptly terminated by direct current cardioversion. In patients with recurring or incessant VT,

TABLE 66.1

ELECTROCARDIOGRAPHIC CRITERIA FOR THE DIAGNOSIS OF VENTRICULAR TACHYCARDIA

1. Fusion and/or capture beats
2. Atrioventricular dissociation
3. QRS width (right bundle branch block pattern ≥140 milliseconds, left bundle branch block pattern ≥160 milliseconds)
4. Frontal plane axis between −90 and +180 degrees
5. Precordial R/S criterion (absent R/S, or RS interval >100 milliseconds)
6. In the presence of baseline wide QRS, different QRS pattern during tachycardia

LBBB, left bundle branch block; RBBB, right bundle branch block.

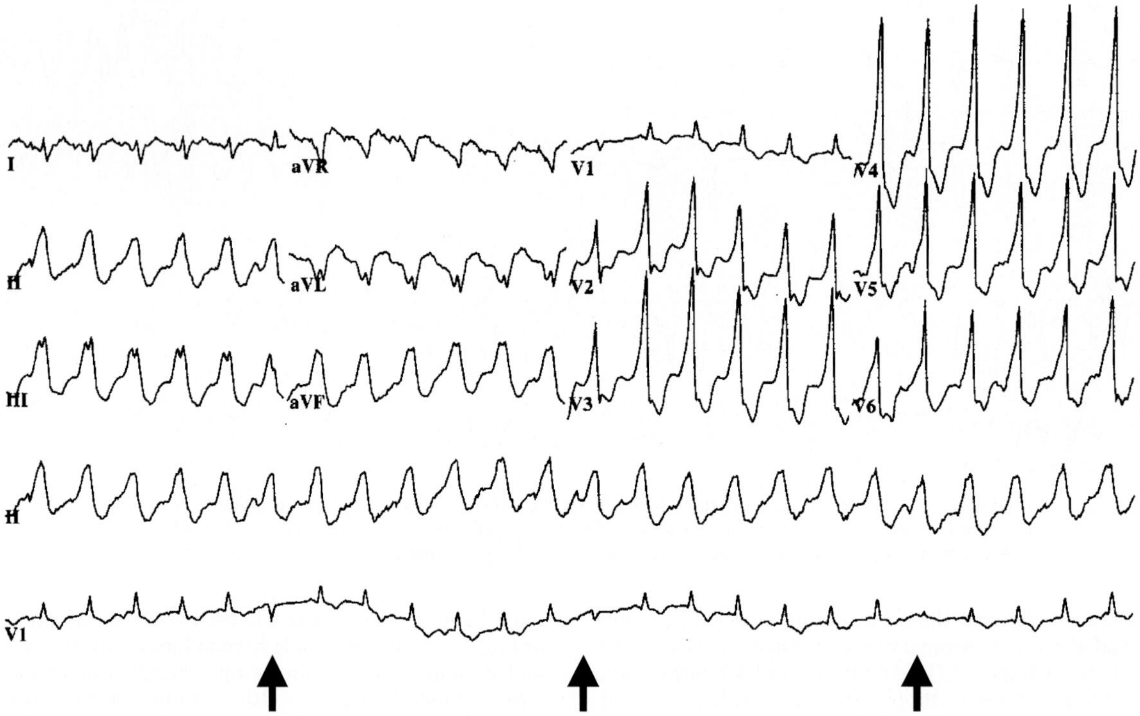

FIGURE 66.2. Wide-complex tachycardia with fusion beats indicated by the *arrows*.

evidence indicates that intravenous amiodarone leads to rapid arrhythmia control and may be superior to other antiarrhythmic therapy (14–16). In the setting of acute myocardial ischemia and unstable VT, lidocaine has potential benefits in preventing recurrences (17), although there are limited data to suggest efficacy in this setting. β-Blockers, administered intravenously if needed, are effective in treating the heightened sympathetic tone that often accompanies episodes of electrical storm (18,19). For similar reasons, sedation and occasionally general anesthesia are also useful. Angiography should be considered early in the course of management to assess the potential for ongoing myocardial ischemia. Other reversible factors, such as electrolyte abnormalities, proarrhythmic medications (including exogenous β-agonists), and hypotension should be identified and corrected. Intraaortic balloon counterpulsation may improve myocardial perfusion and hemodynamics and may ameliorate the consequences of recurring episodes (20). Rarely, ventricular assist devices and cardiac transplantation are required when other measures fail.

In patients with hemodynamically stable monomorphic VT, the reported efficacy of lidocaine for VT termination varies between 8% and 25% (21–23), although this drug continues to

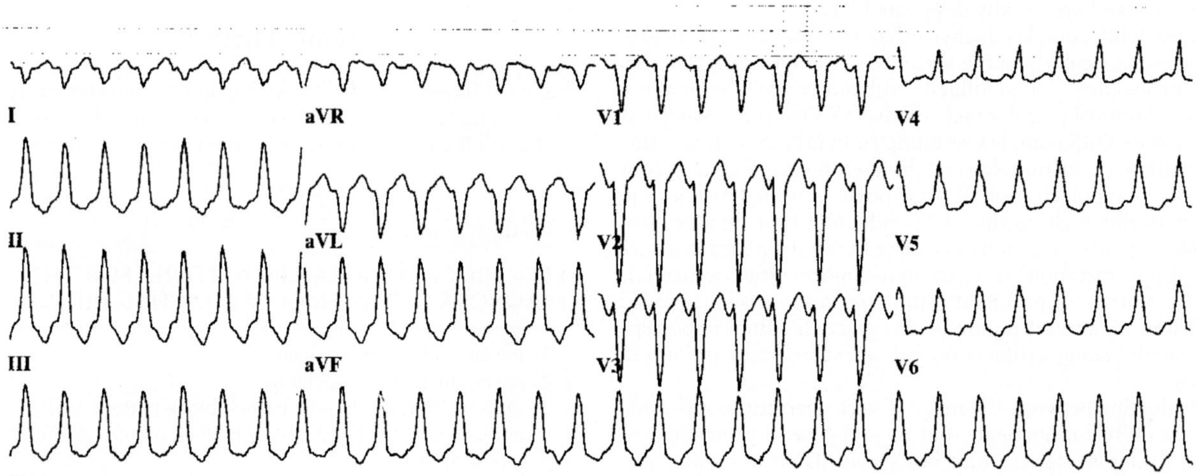

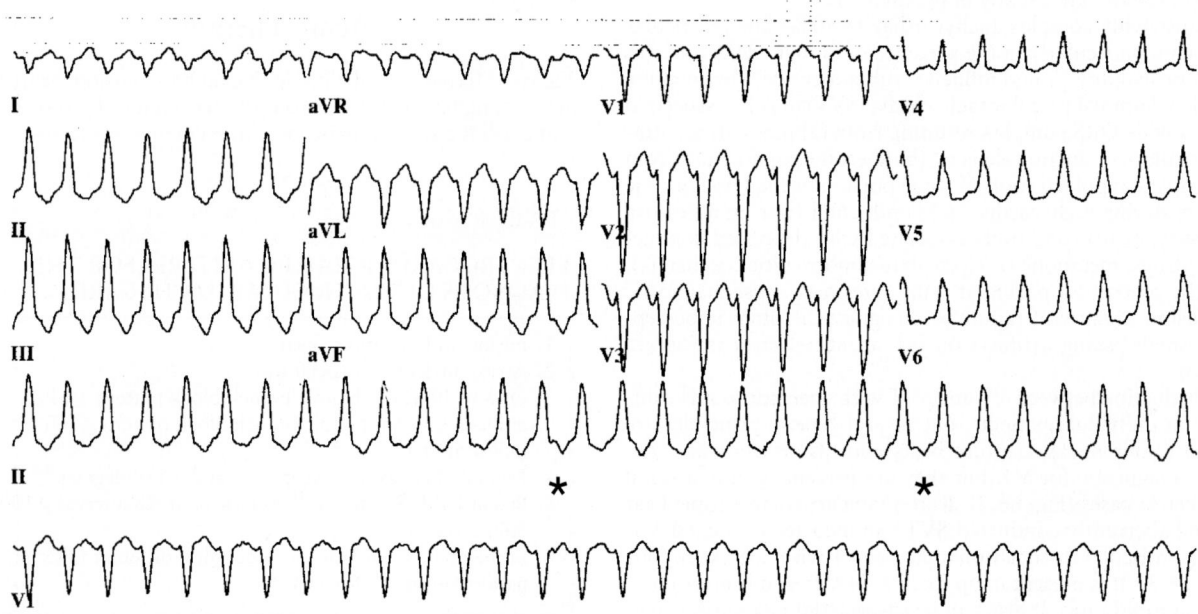

FIGURE 66.3. Wide-complex tachycardia with atrioventricular dissociation. P waves are denoted by *asterisks*.

be used because of safety and simplicity of administration. Intravenous procainamide terminates the majority of stable VTs (23), and it may result in more rapid termination in this setting. Placement of a temporary transvenous pacemaker for pace termination of VT is a useful alternative, with the advantage of allowing rapid treatment of recurring episodes. In contrast, constant pacing at modestly fast rates is rarely effective as a preventive measure for monomorphic VT. Polymorphic VTs (e.g., as seen in congenital or acquired long QT) are more likely to be pause or bradycardia dependent. In these patients, institution of pacing at physiologic rates (70 to 100 beats per minute) may dramatically reduce VT frequency.

TABLE 66.2

PRIORITIES IN THE TREATMENT OF FREQUENT VENTRICULAR TACHYCARDIA EPISODES

1. Treatment of triggering events (ischemia, heart failure, supraventricular tachycardia)
2. β-Adrenergic blockade
3. Antitachycardia pacing
4. Antiarrhythmic drugs (preferably class III)
5. Catheter ablation

Long-Term Management

Once the diagnosis of VT is established or strongly suspected, it is important to develop a detailed understanding of the underlying anatomic and physiologic substrate. This evaluation includes objective assessment of left ventricular function, evaluation of coronary artery patency, and the search for evidence of reversible myocardial ischemia. Other diagnostic testing to establish the presence and nature of underlying SHD may be appropriate in individual circumstances, as discussed in subsequent sections. Electrophysiologic testing (see Chapter 61) has played a diminishing role in the evaluation and management of patients presenting with sustained VT. It is at best a modest predictor of recurrent spontaneous VT and is of little value in the selection of antiarrhythmic therapy. Its primary applications for VT are as a means to establish a diagnosis in wide complex tachycardia of uncertain origin and as part of a potential or planned catheter ablation procedure.

The primary goal of therapy is to alleviate symptoms, to minimize or prevent recurrent VT, and to enhance long-term survival. Data from multiple clinical trials, discussed in detail in Chapter 67, indicate a significant survival benefit for ICD therapy in most patients presenting with spontaneous sustained VT and SHD, with the greatest benefit in patients with severely reduced ventricular function (24). In patients without SHD, limited data support the benefit of ICD therapy in many patients presenting with polymorphic VT and syncope, but there appear to be few ICD indications for those presenting with monomorphic VT (discussed later). However, ICD recipients with SHD remain at high risk of death over subsequent years, with a 3-year mortality of 20% to 25% (24). In patients with severe left ventricular dysfunction and prior myocardial infarction, accumulating data indicate that clinical presentation with sustained VT identifies a group of patients at higher risk for subsequent decompensated heart failure and nonarrhythmic death compared with patients with similar baseline characteristics who never develop sustained VT (25). First onset of sustained VT is often preceded by evidence of clinical deterioration (increased probability of hospitalizations for heart failure and ischemic events) compared with patients who did not develop VT (26). The extent to which current therapy of VT, including the adverse consequences of antiarrhythmic drug therapy or multiple shocks, contributes to this accelerated mortality is unclear at present. However, these data do underscore the importance of a global and comprehensive approach to long-term management, including revascularization, angiotensin-converting enzyme inhibitors, β-blockers (27), and statin therapy (28,29).

Cardiac resynchronization therapy (see Chapter 75) results in long-term improvements in left ventricular size and function, as well as survival. It could be anticipated that such positive remodeling would have a beneficial long-term impact on VT frequency. However, existing data suggest a complex relationship. Investigators have reported no change (30), reductions (30a), or increases (30b) in VT frequency in the months following institution of resynchronization therapy. In the presence of preexisting VT, the direction of this response is likely the result of certain highly patient-specific variables that remain to be elucidated.

A large majority of patients with ICDs implanted for spontaneous VT will have therapy delivered during follow-up; in 60% to 70% of patients, "appropriate" therapy will be given for recurrent ventricular arrhythmias (31). These episodes are usually recurrent VT (70% to 80%) and, much less commonly, VF (25,32). In addition, 20% to 25% of patients will have "inappropriate shocks," most commonly for rapid atrial fibrillation. The incidence of inappropriate shocks has not changed appreciably over the past decade, despite the introduction of dual-chamber devices and enhanced detection algorithms.

For these reasons, additional therapy is often required for ICD recipients (Table 66.2). Antitachycardia pacing (delivery of a programmable number and coupling interval of pacing stimuli at rates faster than the tachycardia cycle length) can terminate VT by prematurely depolarizing a portion of the reentrant circuit ahead of the advancing wavefront. Empirically programmed antitachycardia pacing has been demonstrated to reduce the need for shock therapy substantially, even for relatively fast VTs (cycle lengths, 240 to 320 milliseconds) (33–35), and it is associated with improved quality of life (35). Antiarrhythmic drug therapy may improve the response to pacing by slowing the rate and widening the window during which pacing stimuli can penetrate the reentrant circuit. In approximately 20% to 30% of patients, antitachycardia pacing is either incompletely or not effective. There is a small risk of VT acceleration requiring shocks, usually less than 5%, with current pacing protocols.

Several clinical trials have addressed the role of antiarrhythmic drug therapy in preventing first recurrent arrhythmia and ICD therapy following device implantation in patients with SHD who present predominantly with VT. Two class III drugs, sotalol (36,37) and azimilide (38), significantly reduced all-cause shocks, as well as appropriate ICD therapies compared with placebo. In the recently completed Optimal Pharmacologic Therapy in Cardioverter Defibrillator Patients (OPTIC) study, patients were randomized to β-blocker alone, β-blocker plus amiodarone, or sotalol following ICD implantation. The combination of amiodarone and β-blocker was significantly more effective in reducing all-cause shocks and ICD therapies, relative to the other two treatments, although sotalol was marginally more effective that β-blockers alone (39). An important limitation is that both amiodarone and sotalol were withdrawn because of drug intolerance in 20% to 30% of patients during the first 2 years of therapy. For this reason, routine antiarrhythmic therapy in all ICD recipients with VT cannot be recommended, and it should be selectively employed in patients with frequent VT therapies or those requiring suppression of supraventricular arrhythmias. Use of class I antiarrhythmic therapy in patients with SHD should be minimized because of their proarrhythmic potential.

Approximately 10% to 20% of patients with VT will experience at least one episode of "electrical storm," arbitrarily defined as three or more ICD therapies within a 24-hour period (40–43). Acute therapy should follow the guidelines outlined previously. Catheter ablation (discussed in detail in Chapter 73) may be an effective alternative, particularly for patients unresponsive to initial drug therapy or those who are already taking adequate doses of β-blockers and amiodarone. Some (42,43), but not all (40,41), studies indicate that survivors of electrical storm face an accelerated risk of nonarrhythmic death in the months following electrical storm despite resolution of tachycardia. Because few details of therapy were provided in these reports, such differences cannot be reconciled at present.

VENTRICULAR TACHYCARDIA ASSOCIATED WITH STRUCTURAL HEART DISEASE

Coronary Artery Disease

VT commonly arises in the setting of healed myocardial infarction, and it occurs in 1% to 2% of patients during long-term follow-up, often after an interval of several years. Early infarct revascularization has resulted in less aneurysm formation and in potentially smaller scars, but the number of at-risk patients with chronic ischemic cardiomyopathy caused by multiple infarctions and remodeling has increased owing to improvements in long-term medical care (44). The mechanism of VT is usually macroreentry, with focal nonreentrant mechanisms responsible for only 5% to 10% of tachycardias. The reentrant circuits may be several centimeters in length and typically contain at least one region of slowed conduction within the scar (45). The sites of slow conduction during VT consist of surviving muscle bundles with normal action potential characteristics, but reduced cellular coupling resulting from alterations in gap junction number, function, and distribution (46). Slow conduction regions during VT often demonstrate low-amplitude multicomponent delayed potentials detected well after the completion of the surface QRS (47,48). At least some portion of the reentrant circuit is subendocardial in a large majority of patients, but it may be intramural or epicardial as well. Multiple distinct surface ECG morphologies during different episodes of VT are common, reflecting widely separated slow conduction regions or shared areas of slow conduction with variable exits from the scar.

In patients with previous infarction and a history of VT, programmed stimulation during electrophysiologic studies results in induction of VT in 90% to 95% of cases. However, the induced rate and QRS morphology may differ from those observed during spontaneous tachycardia. The link between spontaneous and inducible VT remains incompletely understood. However, the induction of VT signifies the presence of a fixed anatomic substrate associated with an increased likelihood of future spontaneous events (25,49). Triggering factors, including acute ischemia, altered autonomic tone, acute changes in myocardial fiber stretch and wall strain, and metabolic abnormalities, provide the link between susceptibility and spontaneous occurrence of VT. However, the anatomic substrate, once present, may persist indefinitely. Even when VT appears to have transient and reversible causes, long-term risk for recurrent arrhythmias and death continues despite correction of triggering events (50).

Long-term therapy should follow the general guidelines established for patients with SHD and VT outlined previously. Patients with recurrent symptomatic VT despite ICD or drug therapy are candidates for catheter ablation. Conventional mapping techniques target a protected isthmus of slowed conduction as identified by electrogram timing and the response to pacing at various sites during tachycardia (45). This method is limited to the minority of patients in whom a stable tachycardia can be induced. Most patients have multiple stable and unstable tachycardia morphologies, so complete elimination of all VTs can be achieved in only 40% to 50%. However, for many patients this end point is not required; elimination of the clinically problematic or "target" VT is sufficient to reduce the incidence of ICD therapies dramatically and to improve quality of life. This result may be obtained in up to 80% of patients presenting with recurrent stable VT. When performed by experienced clinicians, the procedure is well tolerated, with a 1% to 2% incidence of major complications. With the increasing use of ICDs and catheter ablation, the need for surgical ablation, with its associated higher mortality (10% to 20%), has been largely eliminated. More recently, several investigators demonstrated that critical sites that maintain reentry within the borders of scar can be identified and targeted for ablation during sinus rhythm (51–53). This "substrate-based" approach extends the applicability of VT ablation to a much broader range of patients and may improve long-term outcome. Although there is continuing controversy over the need for ICD therapy following acutely successful ablation in all patients with ischemic cardiomyopathy, current consensus favors concomitant use of ICDs in most patients.

Nonischemic Dilated Cardiomyopathy

In patients with nonischemic dilated cardiomyopathy (NDC), subendocardial scarring and patchy fibrosis may occur and may contribute to decreased cellular coupling and slow conduction, thus providing an anatomic substrate for reentrant VT. However, the extent and degree of fragmented and abnormal endocardial electrograms appear to be significantly less than in patients with prior myocardial infarction (54,55). In addition, the distribution of scar is more commonly basal in NDC, contiguous with the mitral annulus. In contrast, epicardial patchy fibrosis, fractionated electrograms, and abnormal conduction may be detected in 30% to 50% of patients with DCM at the time of open heart surgery (56–58). Experimental (59) and clinical (58,60) data indicate that focal nonreentrant mechanisms (triggered activity and enhanced automaticity) may be common in patients with NDC. In this population, myocardial macroreentrant circuits may account for only 50% to 70% of VT, with focal mechanisms and bundle branch reentry comprising the remainder (60,61). Most patients have multiple distinct QRS morphologies, often with different mechanisms. Given the foregoing considerations, it is not surprising that programmed stimulation is less often successful in inducing clinical VT. In addition, early series of endocardial ablation in these patients had low success rates.

A simple and safe technique for percutaneous subxiphoid pericardial instrumentation has been introduced (62). Preliminary studies confirmed the extensive nature of epicardial scar in NCD and demonstrated successful ablation of epicardial foci or slow conduction zones not amenable to ablation from the endocardium (63,64). These techniques, combined with greater use of substrate-based approaches to ablation, have improved the overall outcome of catheter ablation in this population. The efficacy and survival benefit of ICDs for patients with sustained VT appear similar to those in patients with ischemic heart disease, and this approach recommended as primary therapy in most patients.

Right Ventricular Cardiomyopathy/Dysplasia

Right ventricular cardiomyopathy/dysplasia (ARVD) is a heart muscle disease characterized by progressive myocyte loss and fibrofatty replacement, with a predilection for the right ventricle. It is familial in 30% to 50% of cases, with a majority demonstrating an autosomal dominant pattern with incomplete penetrance. Causative mutations have been identified in plakoglobin, desmoplakin, and plakophilin, all of which encode major components of the desmosome (65). These protein complexes anchor intermediate filaments to the cytoplasmic membrane and form a three-dimensional scaffolding that provides mechanical strength. Impaired functioning of cell adhesion junctions during exposure to shear stress may lead to myocyte detachment and death, accompanied by inflammation and fibrofatty repair. In addition, disruption of cell adhesion junctions leads to gap junction remodeling and reduced cell–cell electrical coupling (66). The mechanism for VT is nearly always reentry, with surviving muscle bundles with impaired electrical coupling serving as sites of slow conduction analogous to postinfarction VT.

The process may initially be focal, preferentially affecting one or more of the anterior infundibulum, apex, and inflow tract (so-called "triangle of dysplasia"). Imaging techniques demonstrate structural and functional abnormalities including localized akinetic or dyskinetic bulges or aneurysms or more generalized akinesia and dilation (67). Global left ventricular function is generally normal, although histologic evidence of left ventricular involvement is present in up to 50% of cases. ECG abnormalities (T-wave inversion, QRS duration ≥110 milliseconds, S-wave upstroke ≥55 milliseconds in leads V_1 to V_3) are present in 80% to 90% of patients with confirmed disease (68), and they may precede functional abnormalities. Diagnostic criteria have been formulated that incorporate major clinical features and laboratory abnormalities, although the criteria may be less sensitive for early disease (69) (Table 66.3). However, excessive reliance on the nonspecific findings of imaging tests may lead to overdiagnosis (70).

Monomorphic VT is the most common sustained arrhythmia in ARVD, with peak presentation in the third and fourth decade of life (71–74). A minority of patients may present with polymorphic VT or VF. Recurrence of VT is common and often occurs in bursts with relatively long periods of quiescence. VT nearly always has a left bundle pattern, with the frontal plane axis equally divided between inferior and left superior. Multiple morphologically distinct tachycardias are present in up to 50% of patients. Consistent with a reentrant mechanism, VT can usually be induced during programmed stimulation in patients presenting with spontaneous tachycardia. Low voltage, fragmented, or delayed sinus rhythm endocardial and epicardial electrograms are often recorded from involved myocardium (75). This arrhythmogenic substrate may be detected by an abnormal signal-averaged ECG in up to 70% of patients.

Long-term prognosis is excellent in patients with ARVD and VT treated with ICDs (74,76). Device therapy also offers the potential advantage of pace termination, thus avoiding the need for long-term antiarrhythmic drugs. Drug therapy is empiric, with β-blockers, sotalol, and amiodarone all of potential utility in patients with frequent episodes. The acute success rate of catheter ablation appears is high (80%); however, there is a significant incidence of late recurrence, often the result of new foci, most likely reflecting the progressive nature of this disease (77,78). For this reason, ablation as primary therapy without ICD backup remains controversial.

TABLE 66.3

DIAGNOSTIC CRITERIA FOR RIGHT VENTRICULAR CARDIOMYOPATHY[a]

I. Functional and structural abnormalities
 A. Major
  1. Severe RV dilatation and reduced ejection fraction with no or mild left ventricular impairment
  2. Localized RV aneurysm (akinetic or dyskinetic areas with diastolic bulging)
  3. Severe segmental dilatation of the RV
 B. Minor
  1. Mild global RV dilatation and/or reduced ejection fraction
  2. Mild segmental dilatation of the RV
  3. Regional RV hypokinesis
II. Tissue characterization
 A. Major
  1. Fibrofatty replacement of myocardium on biopsy
III. Repolarization abnormalities
 B. Minor
  1. Inverted T waves in V_2 and V_3 in absence of right bundle branch block, age >12 years
IV. Depolarization abnormalities
 A. Major
  1. Epsilon waves or localized prolongation of QRS >110 ms in V_1– V_3
 B. Minor
  1. Late potentials on signal-averaged electrocardiogram
V. Arrhythmias
 A. Minor
  1. Sustained or nonsustained ventricular tachycardia with left bundle branch QRS morphology
  2. Frequent premature ventricular contractions (>1,000/24 h)
VI. Family history
 A. Major
  1. Familial disease confirmed at necropsy or surgery
 B. Minor
  1. Family history of premature sudden death (age <35 y) owing to suspected RV cardiomyopathy
  2. Family history (clinical diagnosis based on criteria)

[a] Clinical diagnosis based on the presence of two major criteria, one major and two minor criteria, or four minor criteria.
Modified from McKenna WJ, Thiene G, Nava A, et al. Diagnosis of arrhythmogenic right ventricular dysplasia/cardiomyopathy. *Br Heart J* 1994;71:215–218.

Hypertrophic Cardiomyopathy

Hypertrophic cardiomyopathy is a primary muscle disease characterized by inappropriate hypertrophy for the degree of hemodynamic loading and reflecting mutations in the genes controlling the expression and assembly of sarcomeric proteins. Fractionated electrograms and slow conduction are frequently found in regions of disordered myocardial architecture and may contribute to the arrhythmogenesis. Stable sustained monomorphic VT is unusual, and it is often associated with the secondary development of an apical aneurysm (79). However, rapid sustained VT is more commonly observed on stored electrograms from high-risk patients with ICDs, although it is often associated with rapid transition to VF (80). Nonsustained VT may be seen in 20% to 40% of patients (81,82). It is often considered one of the major risk factors for sudden death in addition to unexplained syncope, family history of sudden death, abnormal blood pressure response to exercise, and marked LV hypertrophy (>3 cm). However, isolated nonsustained VT in community-based adult populations may have a relatively benign prognosis (83,84), whereas its occurrence in young patients (≤30 years) is associated with an increased risk of sudden death (85). ICDs are recommended and effective for patients surviving an episode of sustained VT (80,86). Whether all patients presenting only with nonsustained VT should undergo ICD placement as a primary prevention measure is more controversial; risk appears to be greatest in the young and in those with other risk factors for sudden death. Management of "inappropriate" shocks, seen in 20% to 30% of patients and usually the result of rapid atrial fibrillation, presents a major clinical challenge in this population. β-Blockers should be considered routinely as initial therapy to minimize the occurrence of inappropriate shocks. Antiarrhythmic drugs have little role in this disease, except for suppression of atrial fibrillation, given the young age of these patients and the potential need for lifetime therapy.

His-Purkinje Disease

The bundle branches and the lower intraventricular septum form a potential reentrant circuit that may become manifest if fibrosis or infarction produce sufficient conduction delay in one of the branches. Not surprisingly, this form of VT, bundle branch reentry, is commonly associated with ischemic or NDC and ECG evidence of an intraventricular conduction defects (87,88). The tachycardias tend to be rapid (cycle length, <300 milliseconds) and are often associated with syncope or cardiac arrest. The most common circuit, observed in more than 95% of patients, involves antegrade conduction down the right bundle resulting in early right ventricular activation (and a left bundle branch pattern on ECG), with retrograde conduction via the left bundle. Uncommonly, the reverse circuit may occur, associated with an ECG pattern of right bundle branch block. Bundle branch reentry is responsible for approximately 2% of VT associated with SHD. It is a frequent cause of VT in patients with muscular dystrophy (89), as well as in the early months following valve surgery (90). It can occur rarely in patients without SHD who have a diseased His-Purkinje system (91). Electrophysiologic testing is required to confirm the diagnosis. Recognition of this VT mechanism is important because it can be readily cured by catheter ablation of the right bundle (88,92,93). The only significant complication is marked impairment of infranodal conduction or complete heart block in approximately 10% to 20% of patients, requiring permanent pacing. In patients with significant left ventricular dysfunction, ICD therapy should also be considered because of the high risk of VT arising elsewhere in the ventricles.

Infiltrative and Inflammatory Disease

Sarcoidosis is a systemic granulomatous disease with histopathologic evidence of cardiac involvement in 30% to 60% of patients; clinically manifest cardiac disease is far less frequent (5% to 10%) (94). Cardiac involvement is usually microscopic, consisting of focal granulomata or discrete areas of fibrosis. Because of its patchy nature, cardiac sarcoidosis may not be detected on biopsy specimens, and imaging studies may provide additional diagnostic sensitivity (95). Both VT and sudden death may occur, often associated with extensive myocardial fibrosis, but this feature correlates poorly with other measures of disease activity or overt clinical evidence of extracardiac involvement (94). Cardiac sarcoid may present with predominantly right ventricular involvement; VT in this setting may mimic that associated with ARVD (96,97). Available data support reentry as the most common mechanism for sustained VT, and low-amplitude fractionated endocardial electrograms are frequently found during electrophysiologic evaluation (55,97–99). Corticosteroid therapy is usually ineffective, a finding suggesting that fibrosis rather than active inflammation plays a more important role in arrhythmogenesis. Catheter ablation is useful in suppressing frequent VT recurrences (55,97). However, ICD therapy should be considered in most patients with sustained VT, given the uncertain and unpredictable course of the disease, and the potential risk for VF.

Ventricular arrhythmias are reported in 10% to 15% of patients with overt myocarditis caused by a variety of viral and bacterial agents, occasionally as the primary clinical manifestation (100,101). These arrhythmias are usually nonsustained, although both VF and sustained monomorphic VT may occur. The long-term outcome is strongly influenced by ventricular function and histopathologic findings; ventricular arrhythmias during the acute phase do not appear to have independent prognostic value (100,102). However, patients with sustained VT or VF may have a persistent risk of recurrences and sudden death related to residual fibrosis even if ventricular function returns to normal (102). Giant cell myocarditis is an inflammatory disease of uncertain origin that often presents with a fulminant course, including severe left ventricular dysfunction and VT (103). Evidence of myocarditis has also been reported in children with right ventricular outflow tract and apparently normal hearts (104), although the clinical significance of this finding is unclear. A distinct syndrome of focal inflammatory left ventricular microaneurysms (<1 cm in width) with preserved systolic function is associated with a high incidence of sustained and nonsustained monomorphic VT with a right bundle QRS configuration (105). Left, but not right, ventricular biopsy discloses lymphocytic myocarditis. These patients often have a benign clinical course, with frequent spontaneous resolution of VT. However, patients with apparent idiopathic small left ventricular aneurysms and drug-refractory VT have been described (106). In these patients, the VT was localized and ablated from the epicardium overlying the aneurysm (106).

Chagas disease results from infection by the protozoan *Trypanosoma cruzi* and exhibitsboth an acute and chronic phase, separated by a relatively asymptomatic period of 10 to 30 years. Approximately 30% of infected individuals ultimately develop chronic heart disease, characterized by focal segmental wall motion abnormalities and aneurysm formation, most often in the apex and lateral wall of the left ventricle, along with the frequent occurrence of conduction abnormalities and VT (107–109). Global ventricular function is often well preserved; severe systolic dysfunction is a late finding and the strongest predictor of mortality. VT originates from sites of focal myocardial involvement that often display fractionated and low-amplitude potentials. Epicardial origin of VT is common. Histopathologic studies demonstrate regions of cellular myofibrillar loss and edema, myocytolysis, and fibrosis, interspersed with normal myocytes (110). These abnormalities provide the substrate for reentry. VT is most often hemodynamically stable, and when associated with preserved ventricular function, it appears to be associated with a low risk of sudden death (111). Unstable VT and syncope carry a higher risk of arrhythmic death, and ICD therapy is recommended (112). Catheter ablation is highly effective, but it frequently requires an epicardial approach (113).

MONOMORPHIC VENTRICULAR TACHYCARDIA IN THE ABSENCE OF STRUCTURAL HEART DISEASE

Idiopathic Right Ventricular Outflow Tract Tachycardia

VT arising from the right ventricle in the absence of SHD accounts for up to 10% of VTs seen by specialized arrhythmia services. The clinical presentation is heterogenous, ranging from an asymptomatic finding during routine examination to

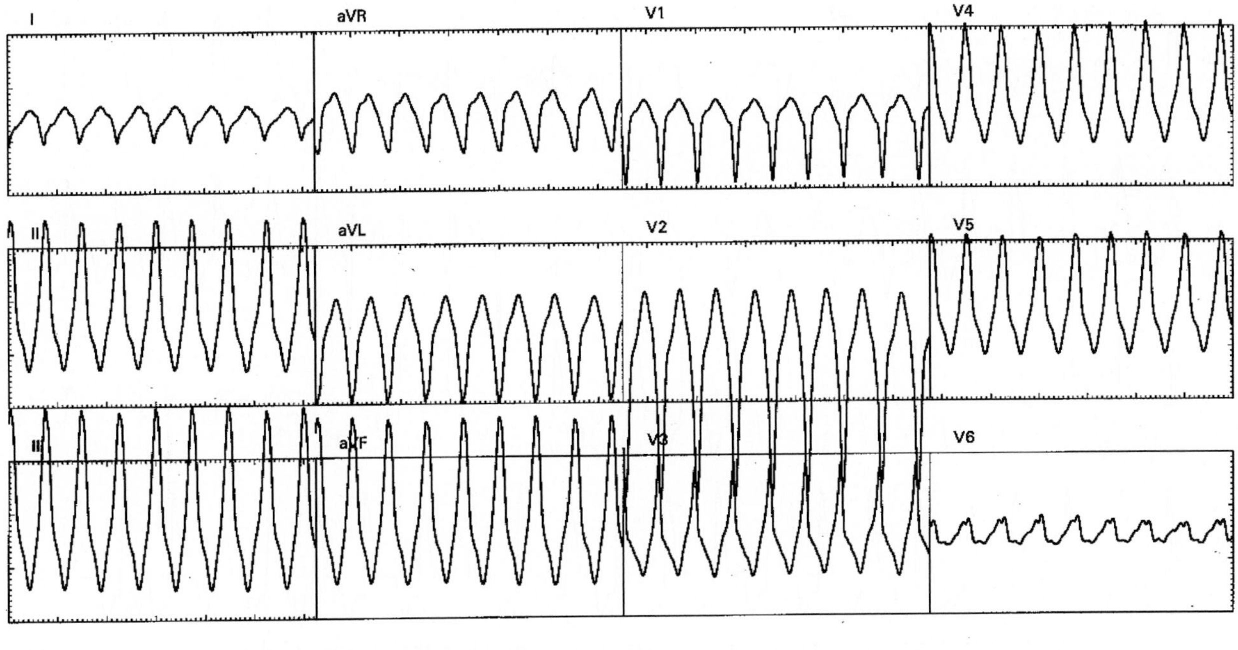

FIGURE 66.4. Electrocardiogram of right ventricular outflow tract tachycardia.

episodic palpitations, dizziness, and syncope (114–116). Typical onset is in the second to fourth decade of life, and the condition is more common in women. Nonsustained tachycardias predominate in 60% to 90% of patients, occasionally comprising a substantial proportion of the total QRS complexes during a 24-hour period. The tachycardias are monomorphic and have a characteristic left bundle inferior axis configuration (Fig. 66.4). The tachycardia is usually more frequent during exercise or catecholamine provocation, and in most patients, the mechanism appears to be triggered activity (116). Sustained VT is nearly always terminated by adenosine and often by vagal maneuvers. Consistent with triggered activity, the VT can be initiated and terminated by programmed stimulation (116,117). Catecholamine infusion is often required to provoke VT. Significant beat-to-beat changes in the QRS morphology within an episode or between different episodes is rare and should raise suspicion of occult cardiac disease. Late and fractionated endocardial electrograms are not observed during cardiac mapping, and late potentials are rarely present on the body surface signal-averaged ECG (118). VT generally arises from a focal source 1 to 2 cm below the pulmonary valve, but it may occasionally originate above the valve in the pulmonary artery (119). Minor structural abnormalities are common during magnetic resonance imaging and may cause diagnostic confusion with ARVD if they are not interpreted in the context of other clinical findings (120).

The prognosis of patients with outflow tachycardia in the absence of SHD is excellent, despite frequent recurrences of tachycardia (121). Sudden death is rare, and in such patients, occult cardiomyopathy is usually found at autopsy. Antiarrhythmic drugs may be used to provide symptomatic relief in patients with frequent or significant symptoms. Patients with a high density of VT may be at risk of tachycardia-mediated myopathy (122). β-Blockers, calcium channel blockers, sotalol, and type IC drugs as monotherapy have reported efficacies of 30% to 50% (123). Radiofrequency catheter ablation is highly effective and curative therapy, with acute success reported in more than 90% of patients (115,117,124). Inability to reproduce VT during electrophysiologic testing is a potential limitation of this approach. ICD therapy has little, if any, role in patients with idiopathic monomorphic VT irrespective of site of origin or clinical presentation.

Idiopathic Left Ventricular Outflow Tract and Epicardial Tachycardias

VT may also arise from the left ventricular outflow endocardium with an ECG morphology that in some patients resembles those arising from the right ventricular outflow tract or with a right bundle inferior QRS axis (125,126). VT may also arise from the aortic sinuses of Valsalva (most commonly left), from a crescent of ventricular epicardium underlying the base of the sinus at the aortoventricular junction (127,128). Another subgroup of idiopathic VT originates from the endocardium adjacent to the mitral annulus (129). Finally, idiopathic VT may arise from the left ventricular epicardium remote from the sinuses of Valsalva, at sites adjacent to the coronary vasculature (130).

Many of these tachycardias have a right bundle branch QRS configuration, but they may have a left bundle pattern if the origin is near the septum. In this latter group, the presence of a prominent r wave in leads V_1 and/or V_2 (r/s amplitude ratio $\geq$0.3, r wave duration $\geq$50% of total QRS duration) suggests a left ventricular origin (Fig. 66.5). Most left ventricular outflow tract and epicardial VTs have a focal pattern of activation during mapping studies. Although the mechanisms may be heterogeneous, automaticity and triggered activity are responsible for the majority. Catheter ablation is effective therapy, although care is required to avoid arterial injury at sites close to the coronary vasculature.

Fascicular Ventricular Tachycardia

Sustained monomorphic VT with a right bundle superior axis QRS configuration may be observed in patients without SHD (Fig. 66.6) (131–133). The VT can be incessant and can result in tachycardia-mediated myopathy. It occurs most commonly in male patients who are less than 40 years old, and there is

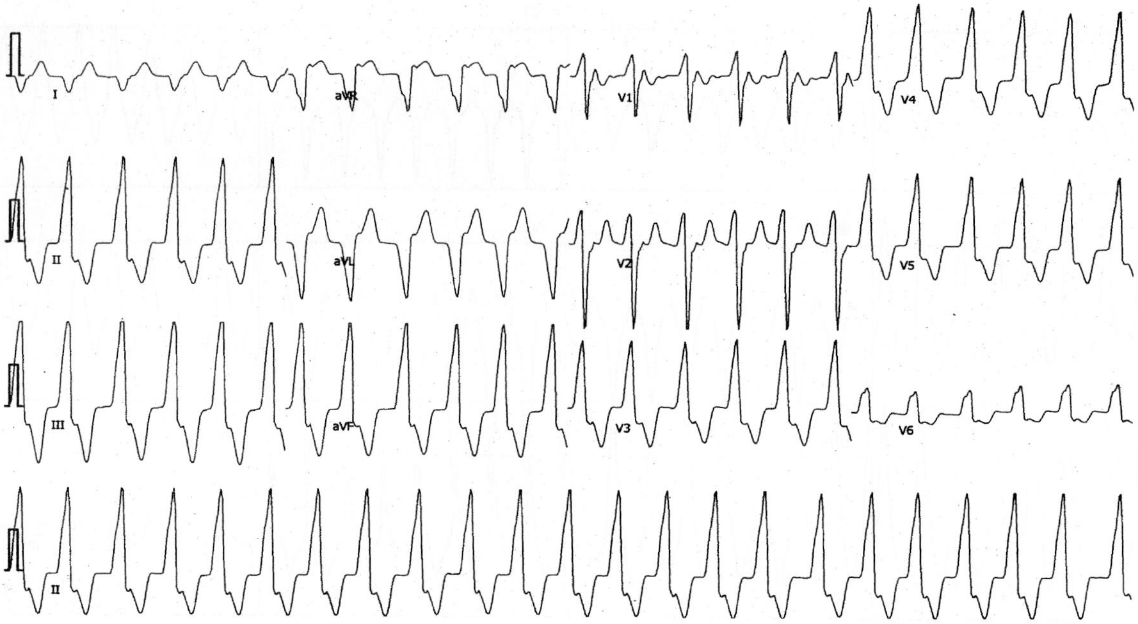

FIGURE 66.5. Electrocardiogram of ventricular tachycardia arising from the left sinus of Valsalva. Note the prominent broad R wave in leads V_1 and V_2.

geographic variability, with a higher frequency in Japan than in the United States. The mechanism is most consistent with macroreentry involving the distal Purkinje network of the posterior fascicle in the medial and apical inferior septum (133–135). A critical portion of the circuit may associated with the left ventricular fibromuscular band frequently observed during routine echocardiography (132). The tachycardia is highly sensitive to verapamil, but not to adenosine. It can be initiated and terminated by programmed stimulation, as well as by atrial pacing. In contrast to the acute response to intravenous verapamil, long-term therapy with calcium channel blockers may be less successful. Elimination of the tachycardia by radiofrequency catheter ablation is reported in approximately 85% of patients (134,135). A related verapamil-sensitive tachycardia with a right bundle inferior QRS axis is much less commonly observed. This tachycardia appears to be localized to the anterior basal or anterolateral left ventricle in the distal Purkinje fibers of the anterior fascicle (136).

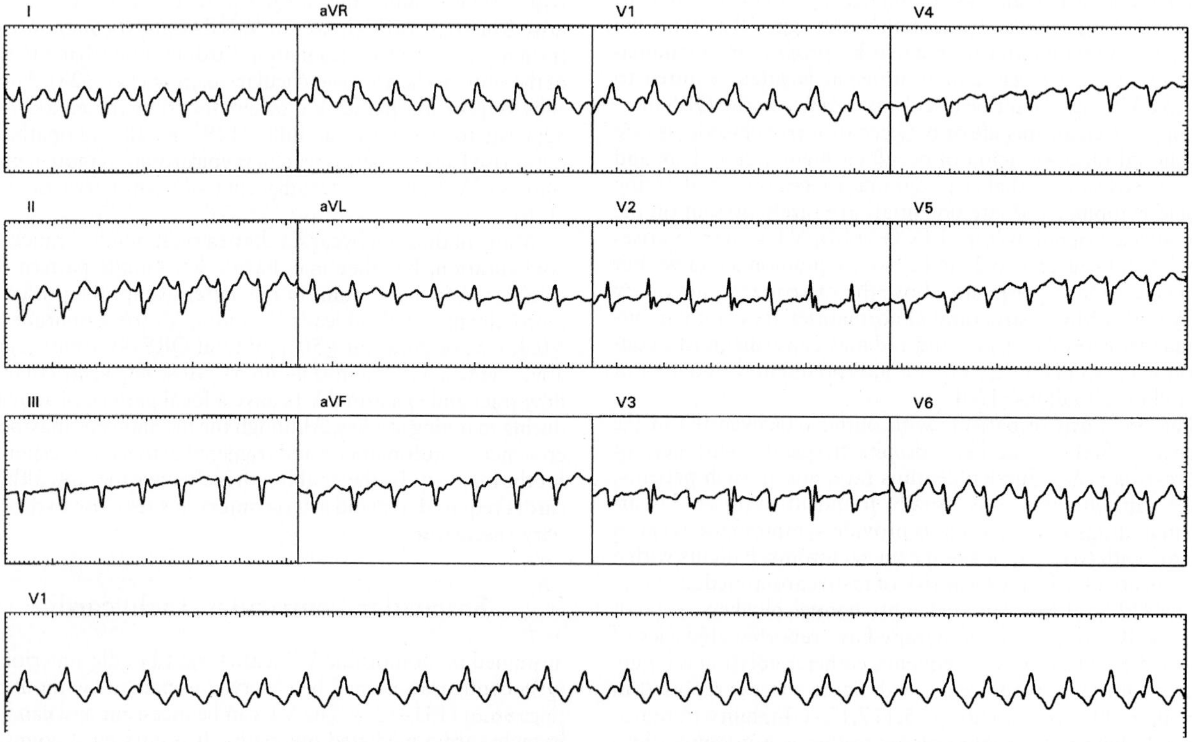

FIGURE 66.6. Electrocardiogram of posterior fascicular tachycardia.

POLYMORPHIC VENTRICULAR TACHYCARDIA IN THE ABSENCE OF STRUCTURAL HEART DISEASE

Familial Long QT Syndrome

The familial long QT syndrome is an uncommon disorder with an estimated prevalence of 1 in 3,000 to 1 in 5,000 (137–139). It is characterized by a prolonged QT interval (≥440 milliseconds in male patient and ≥460 milliseconds in female patients) associated with T-wave abnormalities and a propensity for polymorphic ventricular arrhythmias including torsade de pointes. The clinical presentation is highly variable, ranging from subclinical forms to syncope, seizures, or sudden death. These disorders are typically inherited, most commonly as an autosomal dominant pattern with variable penetrance (Romano-Ward syndrome), or less frequently as an autosomal recessive pattern (Jervell-Lange-Nielsen syndrome) associated with deafness. Sporadic cases with no prior family history are also recognized. Symptom onset is usually in the first two decades of life. The degree of QT prolongation is a robust predictor of both initial and recurrent events, with intervals longer than 500 milliseconds associated with the highest risk (140).

Molecular genetic studies have identified mutations in the genes encoding ion channel proteins that control cardiac repolarization (139). Seven genetic variants have been identified to date. Most of these mutations result in a loss or reduction in repolarizing currents. An exception is LQT3, which results in delayed inactivation of the sodium channel, leading to longer duration of depolarizing currents. The final common pathway consists of QT prolongation, reduced repolarization reserve, and a predisposition to early after depolarizations that may trigger polymorphic VT. Collectively, these variants account for only 50% to 70% of patients with long QT syndrome, and mutations in additional genes remain to be identified. Genotype-phenotype correlations with respect to clinical course and prognosis, precipitating factors for arrhythmias, ECG features, and therapeutic response are emerging (138,140,141). For example, LQT3 appears to be the most malignant form, and it is the least responsive to β-blocker therapy, with symptoms usually occurring at rest or sleep without obvious precipitants. In contrast, LQT1 typically presents with less prolonged QT intervals, a more favorable long-term prognosis, a strong association with exercise provocation (particularly swimming), and an excellent response to β-blockers.

The diagnosis of long QT syndrome may be straightforward in patients presenting with a clearly prolonged QT interval and syncope. A scoring system for the diagnosis of long QT syndrome, combining information from the ECG, clinical history, and family history, was proposed by Schwartz and associates to improve the accuracy of diagnosis (142) (Table 66.4)At least 10% to 20% of patients with confirmed mutations may have a normal QT interval on initial presentation (140,141). Provocative tests such as epinephrine infusion may be useful in disclosing occult long QT syndrome, particularly patients with the LQT1 (143). Genetic testing may be useful if a mutation is identified, but it cannot be used to exclude the diagnosis if testing reveals no abnormalities. Rapid-throughput commercial testing, focusing on known LQT variants, has recently become available.

β-Blockers remain the mainstay of treatment (144,145). Although data from randomized trials are lacking, retrospective data in symptomatic patients indicated a mortality of 9% over 15 years in patients treated with β-blockers, compared with 60% in untreated patients. In a recent analysis of data from the Long QT Registry, the 5-year incidence of sudden death or cardiac arrest during β-blocker therapy was less than 1% in asymptomatic patients, and it was approximately 3% for those presenting with syncope. Patients with a previous history of cardiac arrest are at greatest risk, 13% at 5 years, despite β-blocker therapy. These findings support the use of ICDs in this latter group of patients (146). High-risk patients with prior syncope may also benefit from ICD therapy. Cardiac pacing may be helpful, particularly in patients in whom pause dependence of the arrhythmia can be demonstrated, or in whom β-blocker therapy produces excessive bradycardia. Mexiletine may be useful in the treatment of LQT3.

TABLE 66.4

DIAGNOSTIC CRITERIA FOR CONGENITAL LONG QT SYNDROME

Clinical finding	Points
ELECTROCARDIOGRAM	
QTc >480 ms	3
QTc 460–470	2
QTc 450 (male)	1
Torsade de pointes	2
T-wave alternans	1
Notched T wave in three leads	1
Low heart rate for age (less than the second percentile)	0.5
CLINICAL HISTORY	
Syncope (exclusive of documented torsade)	
With stress	2
Without stress	1
Congenital deafness	0.5
FAMILY HISTORY	
Family member with definite long QT syndrome	1
Unexplained sudden death at <30 y in an immediate family member	0.5

>4, definite long QT syndrome; 3–4, possible long QT syndrome, <1, low probability of long QT syndrome.
From Schwartz PJ, Moss AJ, Vincent GM, Crampton RS. Diagnostic criteria for the long QT syndrome: an update. *Circulation* 1993;88: 782–784.

Acquired Long QT Syndrome

Clinical presentation similar to that observed in patients with the congenital long QT syndrome may occur in patients of any age with previously normal QT intervals who are exposed to agents or circumstances that prolong and increase the dispersion of cardiac repolarization (147,148). The diagnosis is confirmed by the characteristic pattern of torsade de pointes associated with a corrected QT interval longer than 440 milliseconds. Premature ventricular beats and torsade de pointes appear as a result of early afterdepolarizations; the occasional perpetuation of polymorphic VT and the development of VF are more likely mediated by reentry. Drug therapy is the most common initiator. The most frequently implicated drugs include class 1A and III antiarrhythmics, macrolide and fluoroquinolone antibiotics, antimalarials, imidazole antifungal agents, selected antihistamines, tricyclic antidepressants, neuroleptics, and cisapride. The sensitivity to these agents appears idiosyncratic rather than dose related. It has been hypothesized that patients prone to acquired long QT syndrome have occult abnormalities of ion channels (similar to patients with familial long QT syndrome) that are not manifest under normal conditions (149).

Several factors predispose to the development of torsade de pointes, including bradycardia, hypokalemia and hypomagnesemia, female sex, and cardiac abnormalities associated with QT prolongation (including ventricular hypertrophy and heart failure). Treatment consists of withdrawal of triggering drugs, intravenous magnesium, and correction of bradycardia by temporary pacing or isoproterenol.

Brugada Syndrome

Polymorphic VT, syncope, and sudden death may occur in patients without QT prolongation, but with a characteristic ECG appearance consisting of a right bundle branch block pattern with prominent J-point elevation ($\leq$2 mm) and a coved downsloping ST segment with T-wave inversion in the right precordial leads (type I pattern) (150–152). Referred to as the Brugada syndrome, clinical cases have become increasingly recognized and may comprise 20% to 50% of sudden deaths in persons without SHD. Symptoms typically appear between 30 and 40 years of age, with a male-to-female predominance of 4:1. Case recognition is hampered by the dynamic nature of the ECG abnormalities, which may become less specific (saddle-back or type II pattern) or may even normalize at some point during follow-up in up to 50% of patients. ECG abnormalities are enhanced by vagal stimulation, β-blockade and by potent sodium channel blockers (ajmaline, procainamide, and flecainide) and are minimized by β-adrenergic stimulation. The use of potent sodium blockers has been advocated to unmask characteristic ECG abnormalities in cases of diagnostic uncertainty (Fig. 66.7), although the sensitivity of this technique is unclear.

A familial pattern is often observed, and mutations in *SCN5A*, leading to loss of sodium channel function have been identified in 20% to 40% of patients (151,152). Reduction in sodium current exaggerates differences in transmural repolarization that are particularly prominent in the right ventricular outflow tract, leading to phase 2 reentry between the markedly shortened action potentials of the epicardium and adjacent regions with longer repolarization. The Brugada ECG pattern has been increasingly recognized in asymptomatic patients, with an estimated prevalence of 0.05% to 0.6%. There is marked geographic variability, with the highest prevalence in Southeast Asian populations. The prevalence of the type I pattern is considerably lower. Although this syndrome is considered a primary channel disorder without associated SHD, subtle alterations in right ventricular outflow tract geometry have been reported (153).

The risk of recurrent ventricular arrhythmias and sudden death appears high in patients with previous syncope or cardiac arrest associated with a spontaneous or provoked type I ECG. The ICD provides the only effective intervention for reducing mortality; β-blockers and amiodarone are ineffective. Prognosis and therapy in asymptomatic patients are controversial, as is the predictive value of induced VF during programmed stimulation (151,152). A high frequency of atrial fibrillation in these patients increases the risk of inappropriate defibrillator shocks.

Catecholaminergic Polymorphic Ventricular Tachycardia

This syndrome typically presents in childhood, although symptom onset may be delayed to the third and fourth decades of life. The clinical hallmarks are exertion or stress-related syncope, polymorphic or bidirectional VT, or cardiac arrest in a patient with a normal QT interval and no SHD (154–156). The polymorphic VT is frequently observed on routine ambulatory monitoring and can be reproduced during exercise testing or catecholamine infusion. Mutations in the cardiac ryanodine receptor gene (*RyR2*) are present in up to 50% of patients (autosomal dominant); mutations in the cardiac calsequestrin gene (*CASQ2*) have also been identified (autosomal recessive), but they occur much less frequently. The effect of both mutations is an increase in cytosolic calcium, thereby activating an inward depolarizing current through the sodium/calcium exchanger, resulting in delayed afterdepolarizations and triggered ventricular arrhythmias. Although both β-blockers and calcium channel blockers diminish the frequency of ventricular arrhythmias, the risk of recurrent symptoms and sudden death remains considerable even in treated patients (up to 40%). ICDs are increasingly employed in symptomatic patients with catecholaminergic polymorphic VT.

Short QT Syndrome

A heritable cardiac ion channel disorder associated with a high risk of recurrent syncope, polymorphic VT, and sudden death has been identified recently in several families. These patients

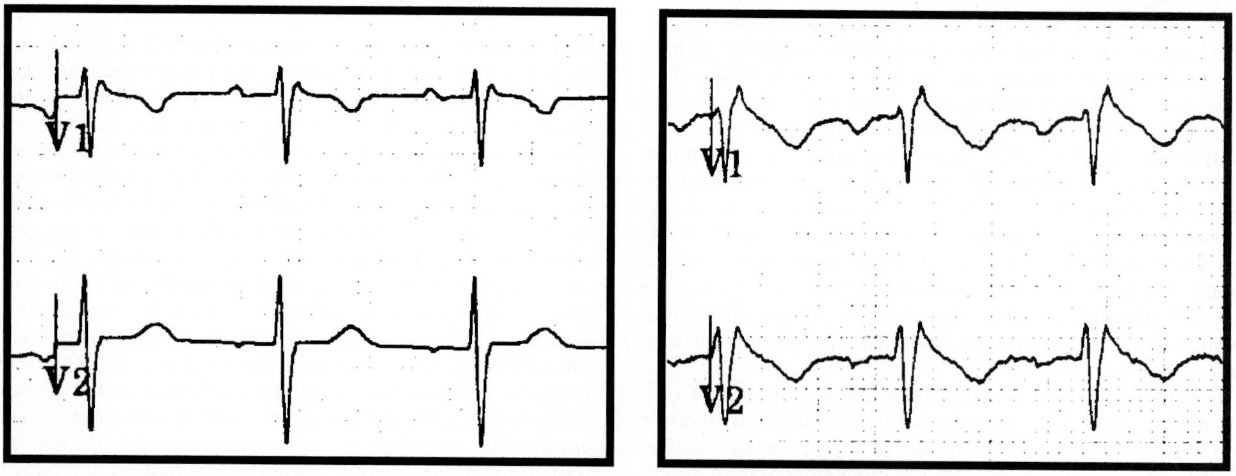

FIGURE 66.7. Dynamic nature of the electrocardiographic pattern associated with Brugada syndrome. **Left:** Nondiagnostic J point elevation in precordial leads V_1 and V_2. **Right:** Diagnostic coved ST-segment elevation in both leads following the administration of 1 g procainamide.

have extremely short QT intervals (QTc <320 milliseconds) at normal heart rates, associated with an extremely short or absent ST segment and tall peaked T waves (157–159). Mutations in the genes contributing to at least three different repolarizing currents have been identified: IKr (*KCNH2*), IKs (*KCNQ1*), and IK1 (*KCNJ2*). All these mutations result in gain of function, thus accelerating repolarization and accounting for the clinical features of the disease. Class IC and class III antiarrhythmic drugs have little effect on the QT interval, but preliminary data suggest that quinidine may be effective (160). ICDs are the most effective therapy, although the frequent coexistence of atrial fibrillation and prominent T waves that results in oversensing may increase the risk of inappropriate shocks in these patients.

Focally Triggered Polymorphic Ventricular Tachycardia

Several groups of patients have been reported characterized by episodes of syncope and polymorphic VT, not necessarily exercise related, in whom episodes are triggered by uniform morphology premature contractions, often arising from the right ventricular outflow tract or in the distal Purkinje network of the left ventricle (161–163). Clinical evaluation excluded SHD, long QT syndrome, and Brugada syndrome. Polymorphic VT may progress to VT, and there is a significant risk of sudden death. In a few patients, some episodes may also have a monomorphic appearance. Coupling intervals of the initiating beat may be short (often designated short-coupled torsade de pointes), or they may occur at the end of repolarization or later. Catheter ablation of the initiating complex is reported to eliminate subsequent episodes of polymorphic VT. It is possible that these otherwise benign extrasystoles may trigger polymorphic VT in a vulnerable substrate, analogous to that reported for Brugada syndrome and for long QT syndrome. Few of these patients have undergone molecular genetic analysis.

CONTROVERSIES AND PERSONAL PERSPECTIVES

The results of randomized ICD trials conducted over the past decade have revolutionized the clinical approach and management of patients with VT. ICD therapy provides substantial mortality benefit over a broad range patients with SHD. Appropriately, these findings have resulted in a substantial increase in the proportion of such patients receiving ICDs in contemporary practice. In the United States, ICD placement for "secondary prevention" of recurrence in patients with documented spontaneous sustained VT or VF accounts for a minority of total implants and for only a small fraction of the substantial increase in implant rate over the past few years. Justifiable concerns have been raised regarding potential overutilization of ICDs for primary prevention. Controversy continues over the annual risk for arrhythmic death that should be present to warrant implantation of prophylactic devices. However, some areas of controversy remain in patients with spontaneous VT. The survival benefit associated with ICDs in patients with only minor degrees of left ventricular dysfunction is clearly less during the short periods (2 to 3 years) of follow-up in clinical trials. It may be argued that observations extending 10 years or more would demonstrate greater benefit, and that device features not directly related to survival, such as antitachycardia pacing, improve quality of life. Alternatively, increasing effectiveness and wider use of ablation may minimize ICD benefits in this subgroup. Additional data from clinical trials will provide better answers to this question over the next few years.

Optimal care of the patient with VT frequently begins with ICD placement, but it certainly does not end there. As discussed in previous sections, the risk of death and of impaired quality of life in patients with VT and ICDs remains substantial and may partly be a result of inadequate or inappropriate therapy. There is a growing trend toward nonspecialist ICD implantation. This trend places an increasing burden on other less experienced health care providers to assume responsibility for the complexities of long-term management, including device or lead malfunction, inappropriate shocks, and frequent VT recurrences. A close working relationship between nonspecialist providers and physicians knowledgeable in managing VT remains critical. Recently, home-based remote telemetry of ICD function, therapy history, and even some clinical parameters (heart rate trends, lung impedance) has become available. These innovations are likely to enhance outcomes only if such data result in prompt, informed, and appropriate action. In addition, as information regarding disease-specific mechanisms and therapeutic alternatives expands, and as risk stratification becomes more sophisticated, the need for arrhythmia specialists, rather than implant specialists, will continue to grow.

THE FUTURE

The incidence of sustained VT early after myocardial infarction has declined as a result of improved management of acute ischemic syndromes. However, parallel improvements in the care and long-term cardiac survival of patients with SHD, and the increasingly widespread use of the ICD, suggest that the number of patients with VT is unlikely to decline in the near future. The development of new antiarrhythmic drugs that are more effective and less toxic remains an elusive goal. It is likely that the future management of VT will evolve with even less reliance on such drugs. Refinements in device-based therapy aimed at more effective treatment and prevention of VT by manipulating the timing and site of stimulation are already under way. More widespread and earlier use of catheter ablation can be expected, both in patients with VT and as a prophylactic measure. This trend will be coupled with a better understanding of how specific cardiac substrates facilitate VT, as well as with enhancements in ablation approaches and technology. Clinical trials comparing nonpharmacologic therapy with the current generation of antiarrhythmic drugs for VT suppression will be designed. It is possible that such trials will demonstrate that antiarrhythmic drug therapy contributes to the higher nonarrhythmic mortality of current patients with VT.

The spectacular success of molecular genetics in unraveling the etiology and mechanisms of polymorphic VT in patients without SHD holds promise for individualized risk stratification and tailored therapy based on specific genetic profile. In this population, initial attention has been focused on the impact of single-gene mutations. It is likely that an increasing variety of "modifier" genes with more subtle influence of cardiac electrophysiology will be discovered, thus helping to clarify the variable phenotypic expression of single mutations. This experience will help guide the exploration of genetic causes of increased arrhythmia susceptibility in the much broader population of patients with VT and SHD. It is likely that such genetic factors will help explain the differing vulnerability of these patients to environmental stress (ischemia, wall tension, autonomic fluctuations, infectious or autoimmune phenomena) both acutely, and during the chronic evolution of fixed substrate abnormalities (fibrosis and scar). Such advances hold the promise not only for better therapy, but also for an improved understanding of the factors that contribute to the maintenance of stable rhythms.

ACKNOWLEDGMENTS

This work is supported in part by a grant from the George M Eisenberg Foundation.

References

1. Hamer A, Rubin S, Peter T, et al. Factors that predict syncope during ventricular tachycardia in patients. *Am Heart J* 1984;107:997–1005.
2. Steinbach KK, Merl O, Frohner K. Hemodynamics during ventricular tachyarrhythmias. *Am Heart J* 1994;127:1102–1106.
3. Kolettis TM, Saksena S, Mathew P, et al. Right and left ventricular hemodynamic performance during sustained ventricular tachycardia. *Am J Cardiol* 1997;79:323–327.
4. Smith ML, Ellenbogen KA, Beightol LA, et al. Sympathetic neural responses to induced ventricular tachycardia. *J Am Coll Cardiol* 1991;18:1015–1024.
5. Landolina M, Mantica M, Pessano P, et al. Impaired baroreflex sensitivity is correlated with hemodynamic deterioration of sustained ventricular tachycardia. *J Am Coll Cardiol* 1997;29:568–575.
6. Raitt MH, Renfroe EG, Epstein AE, et al. "Stable" ventricular tachycardia is not a benign rhythm: insights from the Antiarrhythmics Versus Implantable Defibrillators (AVID) Registry. *Circulation* 2001;103:244–252.
7. Ellenbogen KA, Levine JH, Berger RD, et al. Defibrillators in Non-Ischemic Cardiomyopathy Treatment Evaluation (DEFINITE) Investigators: are implantable cardioverter defibrillator shocks a surrogate for sudden cardiac death in patients with nonischemic cardiomyopathy? *Circulation* 2006;113:776–782.
8. Bocker D, Block M, Isbruch F. Benefits of treatment with implantable cardioverter-defibrillators in patients with stable ventricular tachycardia without cardiac arrest. *Br Heart J* 1995;73:158–163.
9. Glikson M, Lipchenca I, Viskin S, et al. Long-term outcome of patients who received implantable cardioverter defibrillators for stable ventricular tachycardia. *J Cardiovasc Electrophysiol* 2004;15:658–664.
10. Weiss J, Stevenson WG. Narrow QRS ventricular tachycardia. *Am Heart J* 1986;112:843–847.
11. Akhtar M, Shenasa M, Jazayeri M, et al. Wide QRS tachycardia: reappraisal of a common clinical problem. *Ann Intern Med* 1988;109:905–912.
12. Griffith MJ, Garratt CJ, Mounsey P. Ventricular tachycardia as the default diagnosis in broad complex tachycardia. *Lancet* 1994;343:386–388.
13. Brugada P, Brugada J, Mont L, et al. A new approach to the differential diagnosis of a regular tachycardia with a wide QRS complex. *Circulation* 1991;83:1649–1659.
14. Scheinman MM, Levine JH, Cannom DS, et al. Dose-ranging study of intravenous amiodarone in patients with life-threatening ventricular tachyarrhythmias: the Intravenous Amiodarone Multicenter Investigators Group. *Circulation* 1995;92:3264–3272.
15. Kowey PR, Levine JH, Herre JM, et al. Randomized, double-blind comparison of intravenous amiodarone and bretylium in the treatment of patients with recurrent, hemodynamically destabilizing ventricular tachycardia or fibrillation: the Intravenous Amiodarone Multicenter Investigators Group. *Circulation* 1995;92:3255–3263.
16. Somberg JC, Bailin SJ, Haffajee CI, et al. Amio-Aqueous Investigators: intravenous lidocaine versus intravenous amiodarone. *Am J Cardiol* 2002;90:853–859.
17. Ducceschi V, Di Micco G, Sarubbi B, et al. Ionic mechanisms of ischemia-related ventricular arrhythmias. *Clin Cardiol* 1996;19:325–331.
18. Nademanee K, Taylor R, Bailey WE, et al. Treating electrical storm: sympathetic blockade versus advanced cardiac life support-guided therapy. *Circulation* 2000;102:742–747.
19. Bashir Y, Paul VE, Griffith MJ, et al. A prospective study of the efficacy and safety of adjuvant metoprolol and xamoterol in combination with amiodarone for resistant ventricular tachycardia associated with impaired left ventricular function. *Am Heart J* 1992;124:1233–1240.
20. Fotopoulos GD, Mason MJ, Walker S, et al. Stabilisation of medically refractory ventricular arrhythmia by intra-aortic balloon counterpulsation. *Heart* 1999;82:96–100.
21. Nasir N Jr, Taylor A, Doyle TK, et al. Evaluation of intravenous lidocaine for the termination of sustained monomorphic ventricular tachycardia in patients with coronary artery disease with or without healed myocardial infarction. *Am J Cardiol* 1994;74:1183–1186.
22. Marill KA, Greenberg GM, Kay D, et al. Analysis of the treatment of spontaneous sustained stable ventricular tachycardia. *Acad Emerg Med* 1997;4:1122–1128.
23. Gorgels AP, van den Dool A, Hofs A, et al. Comparison of procainamide and lidocaine in terminating sustained monomorphic ventricular tachycardia. *Am J Cardiol* 1996;78:82–83.
24. Connolly SJ, Hallstrom AP, Cappato R, et al. Meta-analysis of the implantable cardioverter defibrillator secondary prevention trials. AVID, CASH and CIDS studies. *Eur Heart J* 2000;21:2071–2078.
25. Moss AJ, Greenberg H, Case RB, et al. Multicenter Automatic Defibrillator Implantation Trial-II (MADIT-II) Research Group: long-term clinical course of patients after termination of ventricular tachyarrhythmia by an implanted defibrillator. *Circulation* 2004;110:3760–3765.
26. Singh JP, Hall WJ, McNitt S, et al. Factors influencing appropriate firing of the implanted defibrillator for ventricular tachycardia/fibrillation: findings from the Multicenter Automatic Defibrillator Implantation Trial II (MADIT-II). *J Am Coll Cardiol* 2005;46:1712–1720.
27. Brodine WN, Tung RT, Lee JK, et al. Effects of beta-blockers on implantable cardioverter defibrillator therapy and survival in the patients with ischemic cardiomyopathy (from the Multicenter Automatic Defibrillator Implantation Trial-II). *Am J Cardiol* 2005;96:691–695.
28. Mitchell LB, Powell JL, Gillis AM, et al. Are lipid-lowering drugs also antiarrhythmic drugs? An analysis of the Antiarrhythmics versus Implantable Defibrillators (AVID) trial. *J Am Coll Cardiol* 2003;42:81–87.
29. Vyas AK, Guo H, Moss AJ, et al. Reduction in ventricular tachyarrhythmias with statins in the Multicenter Automatic Defibrillator Implantation Trial (MADIT)-II. *J Am Coll Cardiol* 2006;47:769–773.
30. McSwain RL, Schwartz RA, DeLurgio DB, et al. The impact of cardiac resynchronization therapy on ventricular tachycardia/fibrillation: an analysis from the combined Contak-CD and InSync-ICD studies. *J Cardiovasc Electrophysiol* 2005;16:1168–1171.

30a. Higgins SL, Yong P, Scheck D, et al. Biventricular pacing diminishes the need for implantable cardioverter defibrillator therapy. *J Am Coll Cardiol* 2000;36:824–827.

30b. Guerra JM, Wu J, Miller JM, et al. Increase in ventricular tachycardia frequency after biventricular implantable cardioverter defibrillator upgrade. *J Cardiovasc Electrophysiol* 2003;14:1245–1247.

31. Klein RC, Raitt MH, Wilkoff BL, et al. Analysis of implantable cardioverter defibrillator therapy in the Antiarrhythmics Versus Implantable Defibrillators (AVID) Trial. *J Cardiovasc Electrophysiol* 2003;149:940–948.
32. Raitt MH, Klein RC, Wyse DG, et al. Comparison of arrhythmia recurrence in patients presenting with ventricular fibrillation versus ventricular tachycardia in the Antiarrhythmics Versus Implantable Defibrillators (AVID) Trial. *Am J Cardiol* 2003;91:812–816.
33. Schaumann A, von zur Muhlen F, Herse B, et al. Empirical versus tested antitachycardia pacing in implantable cardioverter defibrillators: a prospective study including 200 patients. *Circulation* 1998;97:66–74.
34. Wathen MS, Sweeney MO, DeGroot PJ, et al. Shock reduction using antitachycardia pacing for spontaneous rapid ventricular tachycardia in patients with coronary artery disease. *Circulation*. 2001;104:796–801.
35. Wathen MS, DeGroot PJ, Sweeney MO, et al. Prospective randomized multicenter trial of empirical antitachycardia pacing versus shocks for spontaneous rapid ventricular tachycardia in patients with implantable cardioverter-defibrillators: Pacing Fast Ventricular Tachycardia Reduces Shock Therapies (PainFREE Rx II) trial results. *Circulation* 2004;110:2591–2596.
36. Pacifico A, Hohnloser SH, Williams JH. Prevention of implantable defibrillator shocks by treatment with sotalol. *N Engl J Med* 1999;340:1855–1862.
37. Seidl K, Hauer B, Schwick NG, et al. Comparison of metoprolol and sotalol in preventing ventricular tachyarrhythmias after the implantation of a cardioverter/defibrillator. *Am J Cardiol* 1998;82:744–748.
38. Dorian P, Borggrefe M, Al-Khalidi HR, et al. SHock Inhibition Evaluation with azimiLiDe (SHIELD) Investigators: placebo-controlled, randomized clinical trial of azimilide for prevention of ventricular tachyarrhythmias in patients with an implantable cardioverter defibrillator. *Circulation* 2004;110:3646–3654.
39. Connolly SJ, Dorian P, Roberts RS, et al. Comparison of beta-blockers, amiodarone plus beta-blockers, or sotalol for prevention of shocks from implantable cardioverter defibrillators: the OPTIC Study: a randomized trial. *JAMA* 2006;295:165–171.
40. Credner SC, Klingenheben T, Mauss O, et al. Electrical storm in patients with transvenous implantable cardioverter-defibrillators: incidence, management and prognostic implications. *J Am Coll Cardiol* 1998;32:1909–1915.
41. Greene M, Newman D, Geist M, et al. Is electrical storm in ICD patients the sign of a dying heart? Outcome of patients with clusters of ventricular tachyarrhythmias. *Europace* 2000;2:263–269.
42. Exner DV, Pinski SL, Wyse DG, et al. Electrical storm presages nonsudden death: the Antiarrhythmics Versus Implantable Defibrillators (AVID) Trial. *Circulation* 2001;103:2066–2071.
43. Verma A, Kilicaslan F, Marrouche NF, et al. Prevalence, predictors, and mortality significance of the causative arrhythmia in patients with electrical storm. *J Cardiovasc Electrophysiol* 2004;15:1265–1270.
44. Wilber DJ, Zareba W, Hall WJ, et al. Time dependence of mortality risk and defibrillator benefit after myocardial infarction. *Circulation* 2004;109:1082–1084.
45. Stevenson WG, Friedman PL, Sager PT, et al. Exploring postinfarction reentrant ventricular tachycardia with entrainment mapping. *J Am Coll Cardiol* 1997;29:1180–1189.
46. Peters NS, Wit AL. Myocardial architecture and ventricular arrhythmogenesis. *Circulation* 1998;97:1746–1754.

47. de Bakker JM, van Capelle FJ, Janse MJ, et al. Slow conduction in the infarcted human heart: "zigzag" course of activation. *Circulation* 1993;88: 915–926.
48. Brunckhorst CB, Stevenson WG, Jackman WM, et al. Ventricular mapping during atrial and ventricular pacing: relationship of multipotential electrograms to ventricular tachycardia reentry circuits after myocardial infarction. *Eur Heart J* 2002;23:1131–1138.
49. Buxton AE, Lee KL, DiCarlo L, et al. Electrophysiologic testing to identify patients with coronary artery disease who are at risk for sudden death: Multicenter Unsustained Tachycardia Trial Investigators. *N Engl J Med* 2000;42:1937–1945.
50. Wyse DG, Friedman PL, Brodsky MA, et al. Life-threatening ventricular arrhythmias due to transient or correctable causes: high risk for death in follow-up. *J Am Coll Cardiol* 2001;38:1718–1724.
51. Marchlinski FE, Callans DJ, Gottlieb CD, et al. Linear ablation lesions for control of unmappable ventricular tachycardia in patients with ischemic and nonischemic cardiomyopathy. *Circulation* 2000;101:1288–1296.
52. Arenal A, del Castillo S, Gonzalez-Torrecilla E, et al. Tachycardia-related channel in the scar tissue in patients with sustained monomorphic ventricular tachycardias: influence of the voltage scar definition. *Circulation* 2004;110:2568–2574.
53. Oza S, Wilber DJ. Substrate based endocardial ablation of post infarction ventricular tachycardia. *Heart Rhythm* 2006 (in press).
54. Cassidy DM, Vassallo JA, Miller JM, et al. Endocardial catheter mapping in patients in sinus rhythm: relationship to underlying heart disease and ventricular arrhythmias. *Circulation* 1986;73:645–652.
55. Hsia HH, Callans DJ, Marchlinski FE. Characterization of endocardial electrophysiological substrate in patients with nonischemic cardiomyopathy and monomorphic ventricular tachycardia. *Circulation* 2003;108:704–710.
56. DeBakker JMT, van Capelle FJL, Janse MJ, et al. Fractionated electrograms in dilated cardiomyopathy: origin and relation to abnormal conduction. *J Am Coll Cardiol* 1996;27:1071–1078.
57. Anderson KP, Walker R, Urie P, et al. Myocardial electrical propagation in patients with idiopathic dilated cardiomyopathy. *J Clin Invest* 1993; 92:122–140.
58. Pogwizd SM, McKenzie JP, Cain ME. Mechanisms underlying spontaneous and induced ventricular arrhythmias in patients with idiopathic dilated cardiomyopathy. *Circulation* 1998;98:2404–2414.
59. Pogwizd SM. Nonreentrant mechanisms underlying spontaneous ventricular arrhythmias in a model of nonischemic heart failure in rabbits. *Circulation* 1995;92:1034–1048.
60. Wilber DJ, Burke MC, Kall JG, et al. Different mechanisms of hemodynamically stable ventricular tachycardia in patients with remote myocardial infarction and idiopathic dilated cardiomyopathy (abstract). *Pacing Clin Electrophysiol* 2000;23:174.
61. Delacretaz E, Stevenson WG, Ellison KE, et al. Mapping and radiofrequency catheter ablation of the three types of sustained monomorphic ventricular tachycardia in nonischemic heart disease. *J Cardiovasc Electrophysiol* 2000;11:11–17.
62. Sosa E, Scanavacca M, d'Avila A, et al. A new technique to perform epicardial mapping in the electrophysiology laboratory. *J Cardiovasc Electrophysiol* 1996;7:531–536.
63. Soejima K, Stevenson WG, Sapp JL, et al. Endocardial and epicardial radiofrequency ablation of ventricular tachycardia associated with dilated cardiomyopathy: the importance of low-voltage scars. *J Am Coll Cardiol* 2004;43:1834–1842.
64. Cesario DA, Vaseghi M, Boyle NG, et al. Value of high-density endocardial and epicardial mapping for catheter ablation of hemodynamically unstable ventricular tachycardia. *Heart Rhythm* 2006;3:1–10.
65. Sen Chowdhry S, Syrris P, McKenna WJ. Genetics of right ventricular cardiomyopathy. *J Cardiovasc Electrophysiol* 2005;16:927–935.
66. Saffitz JE. Adhesion molecules: why they are important to the electrophysiologist. *J Cardiovasc Electrophysiol* 2006;17:225–229.
67. Yoerger DM, Marcus F, Sherrill D, et al. Echocardiographic findings in patients meeting task force criteria for arrhythmogenic right ventricular dysplasia: new insights from the Multidisciplinary Study of Right Ventricular Dysplasia. *J Am Coll Cardiol* 2005;45:860–865.
68. Nasir K, Bomma C, Tandri H, et al. Electrocardiographic features of arrhythmogenic right ventricular dysplasia/cardiomyopathy according to disease severity: a need to broaden diagnostic criteria. *Circulation* 2004; 110:1527–1534.
69. McKenna WJ, Thiene G, Nava A, et al. Diagnosis of arrhythmogenic right ventricular dysplasia/cardiomyopathy: Task Force of the Working Group Myocardial and Pericardial Disease of the European Society of Cardiology and of the Scientific Council on Cardiomyopathies of the International Society and Federation of Cardiology. *Br Heart J* 1994;71:215–218.
70. Bomma C, Rutberg J, Tandri H, et al. Misdiagnosis of arrhythmogenic right ventricular dysplasia/cardiomyopathy. *J Cardiovasc Electrophysiol* 2004;15:300–306.
71. Sen Chowdhry S, Lowe MD, Sporton SC, et al. Arrhythmogenic right ventricular cardiomyopathy: clinical presentation, diagnosis, and management. *Am J Med* 2004;117:685–695.
72. Hulot JS, Jouven X, Empana JP, et al. Natural history and risk stratification of arrhythmogenic right ventricular dysplasia/cardiomyopathy. *Circulation* 2004;110:1879–1884.
73. Corrado D, Basso C, Thiene G. Arrhythmogenic right ventricular cardiomyopathy: diagnosis, prognosis and treatment. *Heart* 2000;83:588–595.
74. Dalal D, Nasir K, Bomma C, et al. Arrhythmogenic right ventricular dysplasia: a United States experience. *Circulation* 2005;112:3823–3832.
75. Corrado D, Basso C, Leoni L, et al. Three-dimensional electroanatomic voltage mapping increases accuracy of diagnosing arrhythmogenic right ventricular cardiomyopathy/dysplasia. *Circulation* 2005;111:3042–3050.
76. Corrado D, Leoni L, Link MS, et al. Implantable cardioverter-defibrillator therapy for prevention of sudden death in patients with arrhythmogenic right ventricular cardiomyopathy/dysplasia. *Circulation* 2003;108:3084–3091.
77. Ellison KE, Friedman PL, Ganz LI, et al. Entrainment mapping and radiofrequency catheter ablation of ventricular tachycardia in right ventricular dysplasia. *J Am Coll Cardiol* 1998;32:724–728.
78. Verma A, Kilicaslan F, Schweikert RA, et al. Short- and long-term success of substrate-based mapping and ablation of ventricular tachycardia in arrhythmogenic right ventricular dysplasia. *Circulation* 2005;111:3209–3216.
79. Alfonso F, Frenneaux MP, McKenna WJ. Clinical sustained uniform ventricular tachycardia in hypertrophic cardiomyopathy: association with left ventricular apical aneurysm. *Br Heart J* 1989;61:178–181.
80. Maron BJ, Shen WK, Link MS, et al. Efficacy of implantable cardioverter-defibrillators for the prevention of sudden death in patients with hypertrophic cardiomyopathy. *N Engl J Med* 2000;342:365–373.
81. McKenna WJ, Behr ER. Hypertrophic cardiomyopathy: management, risk stratification, and prevention of sudden death. *Heart* 2002;87:169–176.
82. Maron BJ, Estes NA, Maron MS, et al. Primary prevention of sudden death as a novel treatment strategy in hypertrophic cardiomyopathy. *Circulation* 2003;100:2872–2875.
83. Spirito P, Rapezzi C, Autore C, et al. Prognosis of asymptomatic patients with hypertrophic cardiomyopathy and nonsustained ventricular tachycardia. *Circulation* 1994;90:2743–2747.
84. Adabag AS, Casey SA, Kuskowski MA, et al. Spectrum and prognostic significance of arrhythmias on ambulatory Holter electrocardiogram in hypertrophic cardiomyopathy. *J Am Coll Cardiol* 2005;45:697–704.
85. Monserrat L, Elliott PM, Gimeno JR, et al. Nonsustained ventricular tachycardia in hypertrophic cardiomyopathy: an independent marker of sudden death risk in young patients. *J Am Coll Cardiol* 2003;42:873–879.
86. Begley DA, Mohiddin SA, Tripodi D, et al. Efficacy of implantable cardioverter defibrillator therapy for primary and secondary prevention of sudden cardiac death in hypertrophic cardiomyopathy. *Pacing Clin Electrophysiol* 2003;26:1887–1896.
87. Caceres J, Jazayeri M, McKinnie JL. Sustained bundle branch reentry as a mechanism of clinical tachycardia. *Circulation* 1989;79:256–270.
88. Blanck Z, Dhala A, Deshpande S. Bundle branch reentrant ventricular tachycardia: cumulative experience in 48 patients. *J Cardiovasc Electrophysiol* 1993;4:253–262.
89. Merino JL, Carmona JR, Fernandez-Lozano I, et al. Mechanisms of sustained ventricular tachycardia in myotonic dystrophy: implications for catheter ablation. *Circulation* 1998;98:541–546.
90. Narasimhan C, Jazayeri MR, Sra J, et al. Ventricular tachycardia in valvular heart disease: facilitation of sustained bundle-branch reentry by valve surgery. *Circulation* 1997;96:4307–4313.
91. Blanck Z, Jazayeri M, Dhala A, et al. Bundle branch reentry: a mechanism of ventricular tachycardia in the absence of myocardial or valvular dysfunction. *J Am Coll Cardiol* 1993;22:1718–1722.
92. Cohen TJ, Chien WW, Lurie KG, et al. Radiofrequency catheter ablation for treatment of bundle branch reentrant ventricular tachycardia: results and long-term follow-up. *J Am Coll Cardiol* 1991;18:1767–1773.
93. Lopera G, Stevenson WG, Soejima K, et al. Identification and ablation of three types of ventricular tachycardia involving the His-Purkinje system in patients with heart disease. *J Cardiovasc Electrophysiol* 2004;15:52–58.
94. Silverman KJ, Hutchins GM, Bulkley BH. Cardiac sarcoid: a clinicopathologic study of 84 unselected patients with systemic sarcoidosis. *Circulation* 1978;58:1204–1211.
95. Vignaux O, Dhote R, Duboc D, et al. Clinical significance of myocardial magnetic resonance abnormalities in patients with sarcoidosis: a 1-year follow-up study. *Chest* 2002;122:1895–1901.
96. Ott P, Marcus FI, Sobonya RE, et al. Cardiac sarcoidosis masquerading as right ventricular dysplasia. *Pacing Clin Electrophysiol* 2003;26:1498–1503.
97. Santucci PA, Morton JB, Picken MM, et al. Electroanatomic mapping of the right ventricle in a patient with a giant epsilon wave, ventricular tachycardia, and cardiac sarcoidosis. *J Cardiovasc Electrophysiol* 2004;15:1091–1094.
98. Winters SL, Cohen M, Greenberg S, et al. Sustained ventricular tachycardia associated with sarcoidosis: assessment of the underlying cardiac anatomy and the prospective utility of programmed ventricular stimulation, drug therapy and an implantable antitachycardia device. *J Am Coll Cardiol* 1991;18:937–943.
99. Furushima H, Chinushi M, Sugiura H, et al. Ventricular tachyarrhythmia associated with cardiac sarcoidosis: its mechanisms and outcome. *Clin Cardiol* 2004;27:217–222.
100. Magnani JW, Danik HJ, Dec GW Jr, et al. Survival in biopsy-proven myocarditis: a long-term retrospective analysis of the histopathologic,

clinical, and hemodynamic predictors. *Am Heart J* 2006; 151:463–470.

101. Bowles NE, Ni J, Kearney DL. Detection of viruses in myocardial tissues by polymerase chain reaction: evidence of adenovirus as a common cause of myocarditis in children and adults. *J Am Coll Cardiol* 2003;42:466–472.
102. D'Ambrosio A, Patti G, Manzoli A, et al. The fate of acute myocarditis between spontaneous improvement and evolution to dilated cardiomyopathy: a review. *Heart* 2001;85:499–504.
103. Cooper LT Jr, Berry GJ, Shabetai R. Idiopathic giant-cell myocarditis: natural history and treatment. Multicenter Giant Cell Myocarditis Study Group investigators. *N Engl J Med* 1997;336:1860–1866.
104. Drago F, Mazza A, Gagliardi MG, et al. Tachycardias in children originating in the right ventricular outflow tract: lack of clinical features predicting the presence and severity of the histopathological substrate. *Cardiol Young* 1999;9:273–279.
105. Chimenti C, Calabrese F, Thiene G, et al. Inflammatory left ventricular microaneurysms as a cause of apparently idiopathic ventricular tachyarrhythmias. *Circulation* 2001;104:168–173.
106. Ouyang F, Antz M, Deger FT, et al. An underrecognized subepicardial reentrant ventricular tachycardia attributable to left ventricular aneurysm in patients with normal coronary arteriograms. *Circulation* 2003;107:2702–2709.
107. Carrasco HA, Parada H, Guerrero L, et al. Prognostic implications of clinical, electrocardiographic and hemodynamic findings in chronic Chagas' disease. *Int J Cardiol* 1994;43:27–38.
108. Sarabanda AV, Sosa E, Simoes MV, et al. Ventricular tachycardia in Chagas' disease: a comparison of clinical, angiographic, electrophysiologic and myocardial perfusion disturbances between patients presenting with either sustained or nonsustained forms. *Int J Cardiol* 2005;102:9–19.
109. Viotti RJ, Vigliano C, Laucella S, et al. Value of echocardiography for diagnosis and prognosis of chronic Chagas disease cardiomyopathy without heart failure. *Heart* 2004;90:655–660.
110. Milei J, Pesce R, Valero E, et al. Electrophysiologic-structural correlations in chagasic aneurysms causing malignant arrhythmias. *Int J Cardiol* 1991;32:65–73.
111. Leite LR, Fenelon G, Simoes A Jr, et al. Clinical usefulness of electrophysiologic testing in patients with ventricular tachycardia and chronic chagasic cardiomyopathy treated with amiodarone or sotalol. *J Cardiovasc Electrophysiol* 2003;14:567–573.
112. Sternick EB, Martinelli M, Sampaio RC, et al. Sudden cardiac death in patients with Chagas heart disease and preserved left ventricular function. *J Cardiovasc Electrophysiol* 2006;17:113–118.
113. Sosa E, Scanavacca M, D'Avila A, et al. Endocardial and epicardial ablation guided by nonsurgical transthoracic epicardial mapping to treat recurrent ventricular tachycardia. *J Cardiovasc Electrophysiol* 1998;9:229–239.
114. Buxton AE, Waxman HL, Marchlinski FE, et al. Right ventricular tachycardia: clinical and electrophysiologic characteristics. *Circulation* 1983;68:917–927.
115. Joshi S, Wilber DJ. Ablation of idiopathic right ventricular outflow tract tachycardia: current perspectives. *J Cardiovasc Electrophysiol* 2005;16(suppl 1):S52–S55.
116. Lerman BB, Belardinelli L, West GA, et al. Adenosine-sensitive ventricular tachycardia evidence suggesting cyclic AMP–medicated triggered activity. *Circulation* 1986;74:270–280.
117. Wilber DJ, Baerman J, Olshansky B, et al. Adenosine-sensitive ventricular tachycardia: clinical characteristics and response to catheter ablation. *Circulation* 1993;87:126–134.
118. Kinoshita O, Kamakura S, Ohe T, et al. Frequency analysis of signal-averaged electrocardiogram in patients with right ventricular tachycardia. *J Am Coll Cardiol* 1992;20:1230–1237.
119. Sekiguchi Y, Aonuma K, Takahasi A, et al. Electrocardiographic and electrophysiologic characteristics of ventricular tachycardia originating within the pulmonary artery. *J Am Coll Cardiol* 2005;45:887–895.
120. Markowitz SM, Litvak BL, Ramirez de Arellano EA, et al. Adenosine sensitive ventricular tachycardia: right ventricular abnormalities delineated by magnetic resonance imaging. *Circulation* 1997;96:1192–2000.
121. Goy JJ, Tauxe F, Fromer M, et al. Ten-years follow-up of 20 patients with idiopathic ventricular tachycardia. *PACE* 1990;13:1142–1147.
122. Grimm W, Menz V, Hoffmann J, et al. Reversal of tachycardia induced cardiomyopathy following ablation of repetitive monomorphic right ventricular outflow tract tachycardia. *Pacing Clin Electrophysiol* 2001;24:166–171.
123. Gill JS, Mehta D, Ward DE, et al. Efficacy of flecainide, sotalol, and verapamil in the treatment of right ventricular tachycardia in patients without overt cardiac abnormality. *Br Heart J* 1992;68:392–397.
124. Ito S, Tada H, Naito S, et al. Development and validation of an ECG algorithm for identifying the optimal ablation site for idiopathic ventricular outflow tract tachycardia. *J Cardiovasc Electrophysiol* 2003;14:1280–1286.
125. Callans DJ, Menz V, Schwartzman D, et al. Repetitive monomorphic tachycardia from the left ventricular outflow tract: electrocardiographic patterns consistent with a left ventricular site of origin. *J Am Coll Cardiol* 1997;29:1023–1027.
126. Yeh SJ, Wen MS, Wang CC, et al. Adenosine-sensitive ventricular tachycardia from the anterobasal left ventricle. *J Am Coll Cardiol* 1997;30:1339–1345.
127. Kanagaratnam L, Tomassoni G, Schweikert R, et al. Ventricular tachycardia arising from the aortic sinus of Valsalva: an under-recognized variant of left outflow tract ventricular tachycardia. *J Am Coll Cardiol* 2001;37:1408–1414.
128. Ouyang F, Fotuhi P, Ho SY, et al. Repetitive monomorphic ventricular tachycardia originating from the aortic sinus cusp: electrocardiographic characterization for guiding catheter ablation. *J Am Coll Cardiol* 2002;39:500–508.
129. Tada H, Ito S, Naito S, et al. Idiopathic ventricular arrhythmia arising from the mitral annulus: a distinct subgroup of idiopathic ventricular arrhythmias. *J Am Coll Cardiol* 2005;45:877–886.
130. Daniels DV, Lu YY, Morton JB, et al. Idiopathic epicardial left ventricular tachycardia originating remote from the sinus of Valsalva: electrophysiological characteristics, catheter ablation, and identification from the 12-lead electrocardiogram. *Circulation* 2006;113:1659–1666.
131. Ohe T, Shimomura K, Aihira M, et al. Idiopathic sustained left ventricular tachycardia: clinical and electrophysiologic characteristics. *Circulation* 1988;77:560–568.
132. Thakur RK, Klein GJ, Sivaram CA, et al. Anatomic substrate for idiopathic left ventricular tachycardia. *Circulation* 1996;93:497–501.
133. Maruyama M, Terada T, Miyamoto S, et al. Demonstration of the reentrant circuit of verapamil-sensitive idiopathic left ventricular tachycardia: direct evidence for macroreentry as the underlying mechanism. *J Cardiovasc Electrophysiol* 2001;12:968–972.
134. Nogami A, Naito S, Tada H, et al. Demonstration of diastolic and presystolic Purkinje potential as critical potentials on a macroreentry circuit of verapamil-sensitive idiopathic left ventricular tachycardia. *J Am Coll Cardiol* 2000;36:811–823.
135. Ouyang F, Cappato R, Ernst S, et al. Electroanatomic substrate of idiopathic left ventricular tachycardia: unidirectional block and macroreentry within the Purkinje network. *Circulation* 2002;105:462–469.
136. Nogami A, Naito S, Tada H, et al. Verapamil-sensitive left anterior fascicular ventricular tachycardia: results of radiofrequency ablation in six patients. *J Cardiovasc Electrophysiol* 1998;9:1269–1278.
137. Moss A. Long QT syndrome. *JAMA* 2003;289:2041–2044.
138. Schwartz P. The congenital long QT syndromes from genotype to phenotype: clinical implications. *J Intern Med* 2006;259:39–47.
139. Shah M, Akar FG, Tomaselli GF. Molecular basis of arrhythmias. *Circulation* 2005;112:2517–2529.
140. Priori SG, Schwartz PJ, Napolitanto C, et al. Risk stratification in the long QT syndrome. *N Engl J Med* 2003;348:1866–1874.
141. Zareba W, Moss AJ, Schwartz PJ, et al. Influence of genotype on the clinical course of the long-QT syndrome. *N Engl J Med* 1998;339:960–965.
142. Schwartz PJ, Moss AJ, Vincent GM, et al. Diagnostic criteria for the long QT syndrome: an update. *Circulation* 1993;88:782–784.
143. Shimizu W, Noda T, Takaki H, et al. Diagnostic value of epinephrine test for genotyping LQT1, LQT2, and LQT3 forms of congenital long QT syndrome. *Heart Rhythm* 2004;1:276–283.
144. Moss AJ, Zareba W, Hall WJ, et al. Effectiveness and limitations of beta-blocker therapy in congenital long-QT syndrome. *Circulation* 2000;101:616–623.
145. Priori SG, Napolitano C, Schwartz PJ, et al. Association of long QT syndrome loci and cardiac events among patients treated with beta-blockers. *JAMA* 2005;292:1341–1344.
146. Zareba W, Moss AJ, Daubert JP, et al. Implantable cardioverter defibrillator in high-risk long QT syndrome patients. *J Cardiovasc Electrophysiol* 2003;14:337–341.
147. Yap YG, Camm AJ. Drug induced QT prolongation and torsades de pointes. *Heart* 2003;89:1363–1372.
148. Roden DM. Drug-induced prolongation of the QT interval. *N Engl J Med* 2004;350:1013–1022.
149. Roden DM, Viswanathan PC. Genetics of acquired long QT syndrome. *J Clin Invest* 2005;115:2025–2032.
150. Antzelevitch C, Brugada P, Borggrefe M, et al. Brugada syndrome: report of the second consensus conference. *Circulation* 2005;111:659–670.
151. Sarkozy A, Brugada P. Sudden cardiac death an inherited arrhythmia syndromes. *J Cardiovasc Electrophysiol* 2005;16:S8–S20.
152. Priori S, Napolitano C, Gasparini M, et al. Natural history of Brugada syndrome: insights for risk stratification and management. *Circulation* 2002;105:1342–1347.
153. Razmi R. Magnetic resonance imaging findings in patients with Brugada syndrome. *J Cardiovasc Electrophysiol* 2004;15:1139–1145.
154. Francis J, Sankar V, Nair VK, et al. Catecholaminergic polymorphic ventricular tachycardia. *Heart Rhythm* 2005;2:550–554.
155. Priori S, Napolitano C, Memmi M, et al. Clinical and molecular characterization of patients with catecholaminergic polymorphic ventricular tachycardia. *Circulation* 2002;106:69–74.
156. Sumitomo N, Harada K, Nagashima M, et al. Catecholaminergic polymorphic ventricular tachycardia: electrocardiographic characteristics and optimal therapeutic strategies to prevent sudden death. *Heart* 2003;89:66–70.
157. Gaita F, Giustetto C, Bianchi F, et al. Short QT syndrome: a familial cause of sudden death. *Circulation* 2003;108:965–970.
158. Schulze-Bahr E, Breithardt G. Short QT interval and short QT syndromes. *J Cardiovasc Electrophysiol* 2005;16:397–398.
159. Schimpf R, Wolpert C, Gaita F, et al. Short QT syndrome. *Cardiovasc Res* 2005;67:357–366.

160. Gaita F, Giustetto C, Bianchi F, et al. Short QT syndrome: pharmacological treatment. *J Am Coll Cardiol* 2004;43:1494–1499.
161. Leenhardt A, Glaser E, Burguera M, et al. Short-couples variant of torsade de pointes: a new electrocardiographic entity in the spectrum of idiopathic ventricular tachyarrhythmias. *Circulation* 1994;89:206–215.
162. Viskin S, Rosso R, Rogowski O, et al. The "short coupled" variant of right ventricular outflow ventricular tachycardia: a not-so-benign form of benign ventricular tachycardia? *J Cardiovasc Electrophysiol* 2005;16: 912–916.
163. Noda T, Shimizu W, Taguchi A, et al. Malignant entity of idiopathic ventricular fibrillation and polymorphic ventricular tachycardia initiated by premature extrasystoles originating from the right ventricular outflow tract. *J Am Coll Cardiol* 2005;46:1288–1294.

CHAPTER 69 ■ CARDIOPULMONARY RESUSCITATION

JOSEPH P. ORNATO AND MARY ANN PEBERDY

OVERVIEW

Closed-chest cardiopulmonary resuscitation (CPR), first described in 1960, circulates blood throughout the body by two different mechanisms: direct cardiac compression (the cardiac pump) and changes in intrathoracic pressure (the thoracic pump). Minimally interrupted chest compression along with a short "hands-off" interval can improve resuscitation outcome. Hyperventilation should be avoided during resuscitation.

The most common victim of sudden, unexpected cardiac arrest is a man between 50 and 75 years of age who has underlying coronary artery disease. The most common initial rhythm is pulseless ventricular tachycardia or ventricular fibrillation.

The most effective approach to resuscitation is to establish a strong chain of survival with early access to emergency care, early cardiopulmonary resuscitation, early defibrillation, and early advanced cardiac life support. Public access to defibrillation can strengthen the early-defibrillation link in the chain.

A variety of monitoring techniques can, and should, be used during clinical resuscitation.

There is little evidence that high-dose epinephrine is any better than standard 1-mg doses of epinephrine. Vasopressin, alone or alternating with epinephrine, is an alternative to epinephrine in the adult. Sodium bicarbonate is of very limited value in most cardiac arrest cases, unless hyperkalemia is present or the patient has taken an overdose of a tricyclic antidepressant or barbiturates. Intravenous amiodarone is the preferred antiarrhythmic agent for treating pulseless ventricular tachycardia or ventricular fibrillation.

Several promising new cardiopulmonary resuscitation techniques are undergoing development and clinical testing. In-hospital rapid response teams can decrease the number of cases that progress to cardiac arrest. Mild hypothermia induced after successful resuscitation appears to improve neurologically intact survival. Public access defibrillation has the potential to double survival from cardiac arrests that occur in public places.

GLOSSARY

Automated external defibrillator (AED): A defibrillator that automatically determines the cardiac rhythm and advises rescuers of the need to defibrillate using voice prompts. Fully automated devices charge and deliver the defibrillation energy with no input from the user. Semiautomated devices prompt the user to defibrillate when ventricular fibrillation is detected by the device.

Chain of survival: A coordinated system for treating victims of cardiac arrest that provides early access to emergency medical services, early cardiopulmonary resuscitation, early defibrillation, and early advanced cardiac life support.

High-dose epinephrine: Doses greater than 1.0 mg in adults (typically 3 to 15 mg).

Medical emergency team (MET): A system that identifies and treats early clinical deterioration in hospitalized patients before the development of cardiac arrest.

Public access defibrillation: The use of automated external defibrillators by laypersons.

Pulseless electrical activity (PEA): During cardiac arrest, an organized cardiac rhythm that does not generate a pulse. Previously known as electromechanical dissociation (EMD).

HISTORICAL PERSPECTIVE

Numerous and often barbaric methods for restoring life to the newly deceased have been attempted for centuries (1). It was not until about 50 years ago that the era of modern-day cardiopulmonary resuscitation (CPR) was born. The field of resuscitation is an integrated science combining chest compression, ventilation, defibrillation, and pharmacotherapeutics and has widespread use in both the prehospital and in-hospital arenas. Although it is difficult for us to imagine these elements independently, that is precisely how they began.

Artificial Ventilation

Nearly 200 years of effort and experimentation aimed at finding an effective method of artificial respiration culminated in the work of Archer Gordon in 1949. To compare various methods of artificial respiration, Gordon spent 1 year, with no salary and no funding, in Cook County Hospital, Chicago, where he was on call 24 hours/day. His experimental procedure consisted in inserting a tube into the trachea of a fresh corpse and performing multiple posturing techniques such as lifting the arms and pressing on the back or chest, lifting the hips, and rocking the deceased patient. He then observed the effects of these procedures via a respirometer connected to the tracheal tube. His results were first published in the *Journal of the American Medical Association* in 1950 (2).

In 1951, Gordon performed similar studies on medical students anesthetized with curare. Later that year he published a wealth of data (3) supporting the notion that these techniques were able to provide some degree of manual respiration. There were two limitations to Gordon's relentless efforts. The first was that he only alluded to the idea of mouth-to-mouth ventilation and did not evaluate this technique, and the second was that all of his data were collected in intubated patients in whom the airway was fully protected.

Simultaneous with these efforts, James Elam discovered that by merely using expired air one could oxygenate humans adequately. His discovery was born of a need to ventilate patients suffering from acute paralysis during a polio epidemic in 1946. His repeated experience in performing mouth-to-nose breathing over a period of several years convinced him of its value. To document his beliefs scientifically, in 1954 Elam studied intubated, anesthetized, nonbreathing postoperative patients. He merely blew into their tracheal tubes with his own exhaled air and documented that by doing this he could maintain normal arterial oxygen saturation.

It was not until 1956 that fate brought Elam and his data together with Peter Safar. Lively discussion enticed Safar to begin experiments on mouth-to-mouth artificial respiration. By 1957, Safar had proven that the mouth-to-mouth technique was clearly superior to the manual ventilation techniques that were currently employed and that it could be performed quite easily by laypersons (4). He was also able to document that tilting a person's head backward usually maintained the airway open, thus supporting previous data from patients with protected airways. By 1958, the work of Gordon, Elam, and Safar persuaded the American Medical Association and the U.S. Military to adopt the mouth-to-mouth technique as the official means of providing artificial respiration.

Defibrillation

Use of electrotherapy was a common practice for a variety of ailments ranging from paresis to death throughout much of the eighteenth and nineteenth centuries. Unfortunately, little was known about electrical forces or the ailments it purportedly treated, and there was no benefit to survival from its use. In fact, it took several decades to link electricity to the appropriate treatment for many causes of sudden death. Until the development of the electrocardiograph, ventricular fibrillation was a diagnosis that could only be made by observing the heart. It was first described in 1850 by Karl Ludwig in the dog lab (5). Ludwig noted that he could induce ventricular fibrillation by applying galvanic currents directly to a dog's heart. Although this was likely the first link between electricity and sudden death, the connection was ignored for decades. In 1889, John McWilliam refuted the notion that sudden cardiac death was caused by ventricular standstill by describing a fibrillating heart in the dog lab. He documented, as others had before him, that electricity could induce this event in the canine model (6). Unfortunately, he never attempted to use electricity to terminate the events. Although he postulated that a similar scenario might occur in humans, he did not pursue this. It was not until a decade later that two French physiologists, Frederic Battelli and Jean Louis Prevost, reported that, although a weak current passed through the heart could cause fibrillation, a stronger current was capable of terminating it (7). This singularly important discovery remained dormant for the next several decades.

In the late 1920s the Electric Company and Edison Power Company reconsidered the idea of coupling electricity with defibrillation. They commissioned William Kouwenhoven, Donald Hooker, and Orthello Langworthy at the Johns Hopkins University to research electrical effects on the heart. This group quickly documented that weak shocks could induce ventricular fibrillation and stronger shocks could eradicate it. They were the first to discover that defibrillation could be successfully performed without opening the chest (8). The group also coined the term "countershock," which was used synonymously with defibrillation. An initial shock placed the heart into ventricular fibrillation and a subsequent countershock could terminate it. None of these researchers pursued the possibility of using this countershock in humans to terminate ventricular fibrillation.

Two decades passed until Claude Beck successfully defibrillated a patient. Based on the work of Kouwenhoven, Hooker, and Langworthy, Beck constructed an alternating current (AC) internal defibrillator. Although he was successful in resuscitating a pediatric patient who had developed ventricular fibrillation during cardiac surgery, it took another 8 years for him to successfully use his device on another patient.

In 1955, Paul Zoll developed an external alternating current defibrillator. On a case- by-case basis, he documented that external defibrillation could be performed safely and effectively (9).

Defibrillators utilizing alternating current were quite heavy and cumbersome. It was very difficult to transport this equipment to needy patients in an emergency situation. In 1960, Bernard Lown developed a direct current (DC) defibrillator that was battery operated and readily transportable. This piece of equipment was the first in a long line of modern direct current defibrillators.

Closed-Chest Compressions

The first documented case of closed-chest compression for the treatment of cardiac arrest in the United States was in 1904 (10). Without the aid of defibrillation or pacing to restart the heart the concept was not particularly useful, and it never gained extensive popularity. It was not until the late 1950s that the technique of closed-chest massage was rediscovered. William Kouwenhoven and Guy Knickerbocker were studying fibrillation in their animal laboratory at the Johns Hopkins University. While performing experiments to determine how long a canine's heart could be left fibrillating and still be successfully cardioverted, Knickerbocker noted that when he placed the defibrillator paddles snugly against the closed chest of the dog there was a slight increase in arterial pressure. The investigators noted that by applying the paddles in a repetitive motion they could prolong the time that the heart could stay in fibrillation and be defibrillated successfully. James Jude joined the group, and the team began performing multiple studies using the hands to compress the chest. Through a series of trial and error experiments, it was determined that applying a downward pressure of 1 1/2 to 2 inches on the lower sternum at a rate of 60 to 80 per minute was the optimal way to perform this maneuver. The investigators published data derived from patients suffering from in-hospital cardiac arrest in 1960. Fourteen of 20 patients survived to discharge from the hospital (11). It was finally understood that closed-chest compressions could "buy time" for the patient with a fibrillating heart until an external defibrillator arrived.

Modern-Day Cardiopulmonary Resuscitation

It was not until Safar, Kouwenhoven, and Knickerbocker presented their scientific data at the Maryland Medical Society meeting on September 16, 1960, that artificial ventilation was combined with artificial circulation to create CPR. The trio lectured around the world to promote the concept of CPR. Gordon produced a training film in 1962 and coined the mnemonic ABC for airway, breathing, circulation. The popularity of this technique, which could be performed by anyone and anywhere, spread quickly.

The American Heart Association officially endorsed CPR in 1963 and developed a CPR Committee. In 1966 the National Research Council of the National Academy of Sciences brought together representatives from more than 30 organizations, including the American Red Cross, and established official recommendations regarding standardized training and performance of CPR (12). Since then, the American Heart Association has hosted special conferences in 1973, 1979, 1985, 1992, 2000, and 2005 to establish consensus recommendations for resuscitation. Each of these conferences was followed by publication of educational documents that have been used worldwide to teach the science of resuscitation.

PATHOPHYSIOLOGY

The Mechanism of Blood Flow During Cardiopulmonary Resuscitation

For 15 years after the discovery of closed-chest compression, it was generally believed that blood flow during CPR is caused by direct compression of the heart between the sternum and the spine ("cardiac pump" theory). In the 1970s, the "cardiac pump" theory was challenged by investigators who observed that increased intrathoracic pressure alone (without precordial compression) can generate blood flow. Criley et al. (13) reported that increases in intrathoracic pressure by repeated coughing could maintain adequate systemic blood pressure and flow to maintain consciousness without precordial compression in a patient who developed ventricular fibrillation during cardiac catheterization. This observation was confirmed by Niemann et al. (14), lending further support to the notion that pressurization of the thoracic cavity could generate blood flow and pressure by forcing blood out of both the heart and thoracic vessels. Sudden increase in the intrathoracic pressure causes air trapping in the alveoli and small bronchioles during chest compression, creating a pressure gradient between the intrathoracic and extrathoracic cavities (15). According to this "thoracic pump" theory, the heart functions as a passive conduit (16). Pressurization of the thorax collapses veins at the thoracic inlet, preventing venous backflow (17). Forward flow occurs because the more muscular arteries remain open, particularly if epinephrine is administered exogenously.

The relative contributions of the cardiac and thoracic pump mechanisms have been debated (16,18–20). Transesophageal echocardiography studies during cardiopulmonary resuscitation demonstrate that both mechanisms are operative in humans (19,21–24). Sternal compression virtually always squeezes blood out of the right ventricle (cardiac pump), whereas the amount of left ventricular compression is highly variable among patients (22). Physiologic studies in experimental models (25) and humans (26) suggest a strong role for the thoracic pump. In addition, active decompression of the chest by application of negative pressure or suction to the sternum can further enhance cardiac output by improving venous inflow (27–32). Finally, interposing an abdominal compression between each pair of chest compressions has also been tried in an attempt to mimic the physiologic effects of intraaortic balloon counterpulsation (27,33–55).

Three Phases of Resuscitation

Weisfeldt and Becker postulated that there are three physiologic phases of resuscitation: electrical, circulatory, and metabolic (56). When cardiac arrest occurs due to ventricular fibrillation, myocardial cells are rich in adenosine triphosphate (ATP) for the first 3 to 4 minutes (electrical phase). During the first few minutes, prompt defibrillation may be all that is required to restore the circulation. However, fibrillating myocardial cells consume ATP at a nearly normal rate (57). After several minutes, myocardial ATP stores are reduced sufficiently so that a defibrillation shock will ablate the ventricular fibrillation but will usually result in either asystole or pulseless electrical activity (PEA). During this "circulatory phase," a brief (90 seconds to 3 minutes) period of effective CPR before defibrillation will boost myocardial ATP stores and increase the likelihood that a perfusing rhythm will result (58). This "CPR-first" strategy is now being used increasingly for patients whose cardiac arrest was not witnessed by trained health-care providers (59,60). The standard "shock-first" strategy is still advisable when a patient is witnessed to go into ventricular fibrillation and defibrillation can be accomplished within the first 3 to 4 minutes. If the patient remains in cardiac arrest from more than approximately 8 minutes, increasing ischemic cellular injury occurs that currently cannot be corrected with chest defibrillation and conventional CPR alone. This period is termed the "metabolic phase" of resuscitation, indicating that cellular-protective measures will likely be needed for successful recovery of vital organ function.

Minimal interruption of chest compression during resuscitation is important to maximize tissue oxygen delivery and, hence, myocardial ATP reserves. Unfortunately, chest compressions are not maintained for as much as 40% to 50% of the time during a typical resuscitation, particularly if automated external defibrillators (AEDs) are used (61). The odds of success increase when continuous, or nearly continuous, chest compressions are performed during resuscitation (62). Shortening the time interval from the last chest compression until a defibrillation shock is administered ("hands-off interval") can also increase the likelihood that a defibrillation shock will result in return of spontaneous circulation (ROSC) (63,64). It is important to ensure that complete chest wall decompression occurs during the upstroke on the sternum to improve venous filling (65). Finally, recent evidence suggests that hyperventilation may be harmful during resuscitation because it increases intrathoracic pressure, causing a marked decrease in venous filling. This paradoxically reduces cardiac output and tissue oxygen delivery (66,67).

CLINICAL PROFILE OF SUDDEN, UNEXPECTED CARDIAC ARREST

Most episodes of sudden, unexpected cardiac arrest in adults occur in the home or workplace (68–71). The most common victim is a man between 50 and 75 years of age (68,70). The majority of these individuals have significant underlying structural heart disease such as coronary artery atherosclerosis, hypertension, left ventricular hypertrophy, and/or congestive heart failure (69,72–75).

Most cardiac arrests occur without an obvious immediate precipitant, although many families of cardiac arrest victims report that the patient experienced a variety of nonspecific symptoms such as chest pain, dyspnea, fatigue, or malaise in the days preceding the event (69,72). On rare occasions, a dramatic emotional event can trigger cardiac arrest (76–80).

There is a definite circadian pattern to the onset of sudden, unexpected, out-of-hospital cardiac arrest. The incidence of cardiac arrest is lowest during sleep and begins to rise rapidly soon after awakening (81–83). Heart rate variability studies show that, at such times, vagal activity is relatively low and sympathetic activity is high, especially in patients with reduced left ventricular function (84).

In greater than 80% of patients who develop out-of-hospital, primary cardiac arrest during ambulatory electrocardiographic monitoring the initiating event is a ventricular tachyarrhythmia (ventricular tachycardia) degenerating rapidly to ventricular fibrillation in 62% of cases, torsades de pointes in 13%, and "primary" ventricular fibrillation in 8% (85). Fewer than 70% of patients are in ventricular tachycardia or ventricular fibrillation by the time rescue personnel arrive on the scene (typically 5 to 10 minutes after the onset of collapse in most efficient emergency medical services [EMS] systems) (86). Most of the remaining patients (31%) are in a pulseless, bradycardic rhythm or asystole.

The outcome of field resuscitation is strongly influenced by the patient's initial cardiac rhythm. In one series of 352 consecutive out-of-hospital cardiac arrest patients, 67% of the patients with ventricular tachycardia and 23% of those who were initially in ventricular fibrillation survived to hospital discharge (87). None of the patients who presented with an initial bradyarrhythmia survived to hospital discharge. Similar observations have been made by others (88). One plausible hypothesis is that pulseless bradycardia or asystole may be a marker for a prolonged downtime interval or a more severe underlying disease process (89). Because ventricular tachyarrhythmias represent the most common potentially treatable mechanism of sudden cardiac arrest in adults, the best in-hospital and out-of-hospital resuscitation programs have been designed to deliver rapid defibrillation to as many patients as possible.

PRINCIPLES OF MANAGEMENT

The "Chain of Survival" Approach to Treatment

Survival from pulseless ventricular tachycardia or ventricular fibrillation is inversely related to the time interval between its onset and termination. Each minute that a patient remains in ventricular fibrillation, the odds of survival decrease by 7% to 10% (90). Survival is highest when CPR is started within the first 4 minutes of arrest and advanced cardiac life support (ACLS), including defibrillation and drug therapy, is started within the first 8 minutes (91). The American Heart Association's Emergency Cardiovascular Care Committee and its Advanced Cardiovascular Life Support Subcommittee began to widely publicize the "chain of survival" concept in 1991. This phrase represents a sequence of events that should occur in most cardiac arrest cases to maximize the odds of successful resuscitation (90). The steps include early recognition of the problem and activation of the EMS system by a bystander, early CPR, rapid provision of defibrillation for patients who need it, and advanced cardiac life support (e.g., intubation, administration of medications). Schematically, this sequence can be depicted as a "chain of survival" (Fig. 69.1).

Early Access

The victim is rarely in a position to activate the EMS system before his or her collapse because most out-of-hospital cardiac arrests occur suddenly and without immediate premonitory symptoms. The same problem exists for in-hospital cardiac arrests that occur in unmonitored patients. Bystanders who witness the event can significantly improve the victim's chance to survive by alerting the emergency response system to the presence of the problem. All too often, an untrained bystander only further delays treatment of the out-of-hospital cardiac arrest victim by attempting to inform relatives, call the neighbors, or contact the patient's personal physician instead of calling the local community emergency telephone number (in most places it is 911) (92,93).

Before EMS rescuers can aid the victim, the bystander must recognize that there is a problem, locate a telephone, make a correct call, and give accurate and precise information to the dispatcher. Once the alarm has been sounded, rescuers must travel to the scene, arrive at the patient's side, and perform an initial, cursory assessment.

Public education can improve bystander behavior significantly when a cardiac emergency occurs in the community. Citizens can be trained to summon help quickly and to initiate lifesaving CPR. The American Heart Association and the American Red Cross have trained millions of citizens to recognize cardiac emergencies, call for help, and perform CPR.

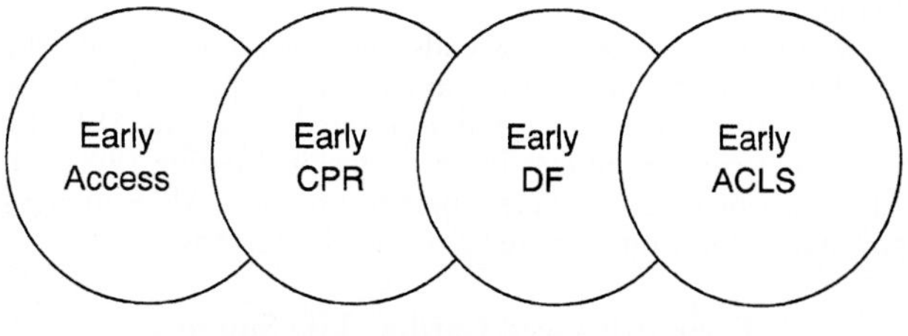

FIGURE 69.1. Chain of survival for optimizing the outcome from resuscitation. ACLS, advanced cardiac life support; CPR, cardiopulmonary resuscitation; DF, defibrillation.

Early Cardiopulmonary Resuscitation

The next link in the chain is early initiation of CPR, preferably by bystanders. One way to ensure initiation of early CPR is to educate and train a "critical mass" of the general population. The effectiveness of such training has varied widely. In Seattle, approximately 50% of the population has been trained to perform CPR (72), whereas in Minneapolis only 23% of adults surveyed have received such training (94). In smaller cities and in less affluent areas, the number of trained citizens is often much lower. What percentage of adults needs to be trained in CPR to provide reasonable protection in the community is difficult to determine with certainty. As a rule of thumb, the American Heart Association recommends that at least 20% of the adult population should be trained in basic CPR to reduce mortality from out-of-hospital cardiac arrest (95). It is also important to train a critical mass of in-hospital personnel to ensure that proper CPR can be performed on all cardiac arrest victims in all areas of the hospital while awaiting arrival of "code team" personnel.

Virtually all studies have shown that initiation of bystander CPR within 4 minutes of the patient's collapse results in up to a 12-fold improvement in the odds for survival (90). The mechanism by which early CPR improves outcome is unclear, but may be due to CPR's ability to keep coarse ventricular fibrillation from degenerating to asystole for a few extra minutes until rescuers arrive. Recent evidence suggests that a brief period (90 seconds to 2 minutes) of CPR actually improves the odds of successful defibrillation if more than several minutes elapses before defibrillation can be provided (59,60).

Early Defibrillation

The rationale for the use of early defibrillation stems from four observations: (a) ventricular tachyarrhythmias are the most common cause of sudden out-of-hospital cardiac arrest in adults; (b) defibrillation is the most effective treatment for pulseless ventricular tachyarrhythmias; (c) the effectiveness of defibrillation diminishes rapidly over time; and (d) unless treated promptly, ventricular fibrillation becomes less coarse and eventually converts to the less treatable rhythm of fine ventricular fibrillation or asystole.

The best outcomes from sudden, arrhythmic cardiac arrest in adults have been reported from cardiac rehabilitation programs, in which defibrillation can be performed within the first minute or two. In such "ideal" settings, 85% to 90% of patients are resuscitated and can be returned to their prearrest neurologic status (96–98). Survival from out-of-hospital cardiac arrest treated by EMS personnel has been considerably lower, averaging 15% or 20% or less with a maximum survival of 30%, depending on the EMS system configuration (90).

The best survival is attained in EMS systems that can provide early defibrillation to a large percentage of patients. In most cases, this is most cost-effectively accomplished by a "tiered response" system in which large numbers of rapid "first-response" firefighters or emergency medical technicians (EMTs) are trained and equipped to provide first aid, CPR, and early defibrillation using an automated external defibrillator (AED).

More novel strategies have also been tried to increase the availability of rapid defibrillation in the hospital and in the community at large. Kaye et al. pioneered the use of AEDs by non–intensive care nurses in an in-hospital setting (99,100). There has also been an increasing effort to place AEDs in high-risk public locations for use by trained laypersons.

Early Advanced Cardiac Life Support

Physicians provide prehospital ACLS by staffing specially equipped ambulances in many countries (e.g., western Europe, Scandinavia, Canada). In the United States, "intermediate"-level EMTs or paramedics provide most prehospital ACLS intervention (e.g., defibrillation or synchronized cardioversion, endotracheal intubation, intravenous fluid therapy, drug administration). Intermediate EMTs (often called cardiac technicians) typically receive several hundred hours of training; paramedics usually receive 1,000 or more hours. Adding field ACLS capability appears to favorably affect survival of out-of-hospital cardiac arrest.

The Algorithm Approach to Resuscitation

The American Heart Association's Advanced Cardiac Life Support (ACLS) algorithms provide a framework for dealing with life-threatening cardiopulmonary emergencies in a logical sequence (101,102). There are sections of the algorithm for initiating CPR and for treating patients with ventricular fibrillation or pulseless ventricular tachycardia, bradycardia, asystole, and pulseless electrical activity (PEA), which was formerly known as electromechanical dissociation (EMD). However, the algorithms are not appropriate for every clinical circumstance, and the team leader must adapt them and the general ACLS principles when necessary. Resuscitation team leaders are encouraged to function as "thinking cooks" when applying these cookbook procedures.

Ventricular Fibrillation or Pulseless Ventricular Tachycardia

Electrical countershock is the treatment of choice for ventricular fibrillation and pulseless ventricular tachycardia (VT). If an initial countershock, intubation, and epinephrine, fail to terminate the arrhythmia (refractory ventricular fibrillation or VT) or if, as in many cases, the arrhythmia rapidly recurs (recurrent ventricular fibrillation or VT), antiarrhythmic drug therapy should be considered (101). There is increasing evidence that biphasic defibrillation waveforms using lower energy (typically 125 to 175 joules) defibrillate successfully and are at least as effective as higher-energy, escalating monophasic waveforms (103–107). The American Heart Association now considers biphasic waveforms or a single 360 J monophasic shock to be preferable to the traditional escalating monophasic waveforms (108,109). Rescuers should follow the Food and Drug Administration (FDA)-approved manufacturer recommendations for energy dosing when using biphasic defibrillator devices.

Pulseless Electrical Activity

Pulseless electrical activity is present when there is organized electrical activity on the electrocardiogram but no effective circulation. There are potentially many underlying causes, but the most common denominator may involve myocardial ischemia and dysfunction due to intramyocardial increases in carbon dioxide (110). Prognosis is generally poor unless a discrete and treatable etiology for PEA can be discerned and corrected. Because of the poor prognosis when a correctable etiology cannot be defined, efforts should be directed toward detecting causes such as hypovolemia, tension pneumothorax, and pericardial tamponade (101). Normal saline or Ringer's lactate solution should be infused rapidly if there is evidence of hypovolemia. Suspected pneumothorax or pericardial tamponade should be confirmed by needle aspiration of the chest or pericardium, respectively. If confirmed, more definitive surgical management (chest tube or thoracotomy) is usually required.

Scrutiny of the neck veins may be helpful in attempting to define an etiology for PEA. Most patients with cardiac arrest have high right-sided filling pressures and distended neck veins. When neck veins are not visible in this setting and PEA is present, hypovolemia should be suspected. In the "trauma" cardiac arrest victim (such as a patient with a gunshot wound of the chest), however, prominent neck veins should lead to the suspicion of pericardial tamponade or tension pneumothorax (111).

General measures such as (a) support of ventilation, (b) properly performed closed-chest compression, and (c) frequent doses of epinephrine to maintain arterial perfusion pressure and coronary and cerebral perfusion are recommended for treatment of PEA (101). Bradycardia may be treated with atropine. Although catecholamines are frequently given, there are no data to suggest a specific benefit (other than improvement in coronary and cerebral blood flow during closed-chest compression). Calcium chloride has not been shown to affect clinical survival in controlled trials (112,113). In addition, the pathologically high serum calcium levels caused by its administration (114,115) may exacerbate reperfusion injury (116).

If penetrating cardiac trauma is present, open chest massage can be live saving (117). In other settings, open-chest massage is rarely of value, partly because it is usually initiated late after the onset of the arrest (118). Prehospital trauma victims who are pulseless and have asystole or agonal electrical cardiac activity (heart rate <40 beats per minute) have such a poor prognosis that some authors feel that they should be pronounced dead at the scene of injury (119).

Bradyasystole

Bradyasystole is one of the most common and least understood problems that can occur during resuscitation. For purposes of definition, bradyasystole refers to a cardiac rhythm that has a ventricular rate below 60 beats per minute in adults and/or periods of absent heart rhythm (asystole). Bradyasystolic states are clinical situations during which bradyasystole is the dominant heart rhythm.

Survival is poor (generally 1% to 3% or less) regardless of therapy for patients who present with bradyasystole. It is always important to exclude disconnection of a lead or monitor electrode prior to concluding that a "flat line" is the patient's rhythm. Because some patients with a "flat line" may have ventricular fibrillation (a rhythm more amenable to treatment) masquerading as asystole (120), the monitor lead configuration should be quickly switched to a second lead to confirm the diagnosis before treatment (101). Other general measures recommended for the treatment of bradyasystole include support of ventilation, properly performed closed-chest compression, and frequent doses of epinephrine to maintain arterial perfusion pressure and coronary and cerebral perfusion (101).

Treatment with atropine sulfate may improve outcome in patients with bradyasystolic cardiac arrest that is due to excessive vagal stimulation, but atropine is less effective when asystole or pulseless idioventricular rhythms are the result of prolonged ischemia or mechanical injury in the myocardium (121).

For patients with bradyasystolic cardiac arrest, a 1-mg dose of atropine is administered intravenously (IV) and is repeated every 3 to 5 minutes if asystole persists. Three milligrams (0.04 mg/kg) given IV is a fully vagolytic dose in most patients (122). The administration of a total vagolytic dose of atropine should be reserved for patients with bradyasystolic cardiac arrest. Endotracheal atropine produces a rapid onset of action similar to that observed with IV injection. The recommended adult dose of atropine for endotracheal administration is 1.0 to 2.0 mg diluted in 10 mL of sterile water or normal saline.

Pacing (transvenous, transthoracic, or transcutaneous) rarely influences survival in the unwitnessed cardiac arrest patient who is initially found with asystole or bradycardia without a pulse (123–125). However, pacing is extremely useful for bradycardic patients with a pulse and in selected patients in whom a pacemaker can be placed immediately after the development of the conduction disturbance (124,125). In such cases, a precordial thump can also stimulate ventricular complexes and a pulse ("fist pacing") (126).

Endogenous adenosine released during myocardial hypoxia and ischemia relaxes vascular smooth muscle, decreases atrial and ventricular contractility, depresses pacemaker automaticity, and impairs atrioventricular conduction (127). The cellular electrophysiologic effects of adenosine can be competitively antagonized by methylxanthines but not by atropine. A specific adenosine antagonist (BW-A1433U) has been shown to reverse and prevent postdefibrillation bradyasystole and hemodynamic depression in a domestic pig model (128).

Aminophylline, a competitive nonspecific adenosine antagonist, has been shown to restore cardiac electrical activity within 30 seconds in 12 of 15 in-hospital bradyasystolic cardiac arrest patients who were refractory to atropine and epinephrine (129). Other anecdotal case reports seem to indicate that adenosine blockade may restore normal sinus rhythm in some bradyasystole patients who do not respond to conventional therapy (130). In a relatively small randomized, prospective clinical trial on adults with asystole refractory to epinephrine and atropine there was a trend towards improved ROSC in patients who received aminophylline versus placebo, but the results did not reach statistical significance (131). Forty-five patients were assigned to the placebo group and 37 received aminophylline. Nine of 45 controls (20%; 95% confidence interval [CI] 10% to 35%) achieved ROSC compared to 10 of 37 (27%; 95% CI 14% to 44%) in the aminophylline group. Although further clinical research will be necessary to determine the potential value of adenosine blockade for bradyasystolic cardiac arrest, it is clear that these agents should not be used when ventricular fibrillation is present because they may make it more difficult to terminate this arrhythmia (132).

PHYSIOLOGIC MONITORING DURING RESUSCITATION

Real-time hemodynamic data can provide the team leader with a sound physiologic basis for altering the approach to clinical resuscitation when the standard algorithms either fail or do not apply.

Arterial Pressure Measurement During Cardiopulmonary Resuscitation

Maintenance of both the systolic and diastolic arterial pressure is vital during CPR. Because flow to most vital organs (except the heart) occurs during systole, a minimal systolic arterial pressure of 50 to 60 mm Hg is usually required to resist arteriolar collapse (133). Diastolic pressure is also important because it is a critical determinant of the coronary perfusion pressure (CPP = aortic diastolic − right atrial pressure) during CPR. CPP is one of the best hemodynamic predictors of ROSC in both animal models (20,134–144) and humans (145). A minimal threshold gradient for CPP of approximately 15 mm Hg (usually corresponding to an aortic diastolic pressure of 30 to 40 mm Hg) provides a level of myocardial blood flow that is necessary to meet the metabolic needs of the arrested myocardium (146) and to achieve ROSC (145).

A cuff manometer can be used to estimate the systolic arterial pressure during CPR by palpating the brachial artery or listening over it for flow with a peripheral Doppler device

TABLE 69.1

ARTERIAL PRESSURE MEASUREMENTS DURING CARDIOPULMONARY RESUSCITATION IN HUMANS

Authors	N	Systolic pressure (mm Hg)	Diastolic pressure (mm Hg)	CPP
Chandra et al.	8	60 ± 4	23 ± 2	11 ± 2
Gonzalez et al.	10	47 ± 5	18 ± 2	NR
McDonald	15	104 ± 51	NR	NR
Ornato et al.	12	55 ± 5	22 ± 5	NR
Ornato et al.	18	NR	NR	NR
Paradis et al.	76	NR	NR	2 ± 9 (no ROSC)
	24	NR	NR	13 ± 9 (with ROSC)
Sanders et al.	6	27 ± 18	11 ± 10	0 ± 8
Swenson et al.	9	61 ± 29	13 ± 10	9 ± 11
Taylor et al.	8	60 ± 14	NR	NR

CPP, coronary perfusion pressure (= aortic diastolic − right atrial pressure); NR, not reported; ROSC, return of spontaneous circulation.
From Ornato JP. Hemodynamic monitoring during CPR. *Ann Emerg Med* 1993;22(2 Pt 2):289–295.

(147). More accurate, invasive measurements of systolic and diastolic pressure can be obtained by inserting an arterial line into the radial, brachial, or femoral artery (26,148–155). Table 69.1 summarizes recent published invasive arterial pressure measurements during resuscitation in adult humans. Conventional CPR generates systolic, diastolic, and coronary perfusion pressures that are inadequate to sustain blood flow and function in vital organs (e.g., the brain). These measurements explain why cardiac arrest patients are rarely conscious during CPR.

Pulmonary Artery Catheter Recordings

Generation of a satisfactory arterial pressure is a prerequisite for adequate flow to vital organs; however, the presence of a reasonable arterial pressure does not ensure that there will be sufficient flow to meet metabolic needs. Pulmonary artery catheters are inserted infrequently during resuscitation because they are time consuming to set up and technically difficult to position. The low flows generated by CPR do not favor ready passage of the balloon-flotation catheter through the right heart. In addition, it is difficult to determine the catheter tip's position from pressure recordings because the pressures in the intracardiac chambers and great vessels are similar to each other during closed-chest CPR (25,156–160). Fluoroscopy is of little value during CPR, even if it is available, because it is not easy to continue chest compression impeded by the machine's C-arm. Transesophageal echocardiography (TEE) offers the greatest promise as a means of visualizing and helping to position intracardiac catheters successfully during CPR.

Despite these technical limitations, there have been several published reports of intracardiac pressure and flow measurements in humans who were already being monitored invasively in an intensive care unit at the time of their cardiac arrest (161–164). Conventional, closed-chest CPR in adult humans produces a hemodynamic state resembling profound cardiogenic shock, with a low systemic arterial pressure, markedly reduced cardiac output, and high intravascular filling pressures. Hemodynamic monitoring post-CPR may be useful for managing selected patients who survive resuscitation, but the risks, potential benefits, and cost implications must be weighed on a case-by-case basis (164).

End-Tidal Carbon Dioxide Monitoring During Resuscitation

The percentage of carbon dioxide contained in the last few milliliters of gas exhaled from the lungs with each breath is known as the end-tidal carbon dioxide concentration ($P_{et}CO_2$) (165,166). It can be measured by passing an infrared beam through exhaled gases and measuring the decrease in voltage output from a photoelectric cell calibrated to the wavelength at which carbon dioxide absorbs light. It can also be estimated by attaching an inexpensive disposable plastic, colorimetric device in-line between the endotracheal (ET) tube and the ventilation device. Color indicators on the device change hue as the exhaled gases pass through the monitor's pH-sensitive membranes. The membrane's color can be compared with the adjacent color chart on the device, thus indicating the percentage $P_{et}CO_2$.

Two important terms need to be defined with respect to end-tidal carbon dioxide monitoring. *Capnography* refers to any technology that displays and/or prints the actual capnographic waveform. If an unmistakable capnographic waveform is detected when a capnographic probe is attached to a patient who is being ventilated, then the airway device is unequivocally ventilating the lungs. *Capnometry* refers to the measurement or estimation of the end-tidal carbon dioxide concentration. It can be displayed in analogue or digital format, or it can be approximated using a colorimetric detection device. Capnometry often provides useful information on the anatomic location of an airway device (e.g., ET tube); however, it does not provide the degree of definitive certainty that the presence of a capnographic waveform does.

During normal respiration and circulation, the $P_{et}CO_2$ averages 4% to 5%. Two units of measure are popularly used in reporting the $P_{et}CO_2$: percent and mm Hg (1% is approximately 7 mm Hg). There is a logarithmic relationship between the $P_{et}CO_2$ and the cardiac output (167). At normal or elevated levels of cardiac output, ventilation is the rate-limiting factor responsible for eliminating the large amount of carbon dioxide traversing the pulmonary circuit (e.g., hyperventilation lowers, and hypoventilation raises, the $P_{et}CO_2$). In this range, if blood flow and arterial pressure are kept reasonably constant, the $P_{et}CO_2$ closely approximates arterial carbon dioxide tension (P_aCO_2) and can be used as a "real-time" guide to the adequacy of ventilation (the $P_{et}CO_2$ actually lags behind real-time events by a few seconds, the amount of time it takes for exhaled gas to be drawn into the machine and analyzed) (168).

The $P_{et}CO_2$ can also be used to confirm ET airway placement, particularly in the non–cardiac arrest patient who has a pulse and an adequate blood pressure (where the sensitivity and specificity of the $P_{et}CO_2$ for detecting correct ET tube placement approach 100% and 90%, respectively) (154,169–173). The ET tube cuff should be inflated when the $P_{et}CO_2$-monitoring device is attached to ensure that the gas being sampled is from the structure (i.e., trachea or esophagus) in which the tube resides. Ventilation through an ET tube that has been properly inserted in the trachea yields a $P_{et}CO_2$ of 4% to 5% in a patient with a normal cardiac output and no significant ventilation/perfusion gradient; ventilation through an ET tube that has been inadvertently inserted into the esophagus results in a $P_{et}CO_2$ of less than 0.5%. The only important exception occurs when the ET tube is inserted into the esophagus of a patient who has recently ingested a carbonated beverage (e.g., beer, soda pop). In such a case, the initial $P_{et}CO_2$ will appear to be normal or high on the first few ventilations but will typically decrease rapidly to less than 0.5% by the sixth or seventh ventilation (174).

At low levels of cardiac output (below approximately 50% of normal in animal models), ventilation has much less effect on the $P_{et}CO_2$. Instead, the pulmonary blood flow (and the subsequent ventilation/perfusion mismatch) is the rate-limiting factor determining the $P_{et}CO_2$. If ventilation is kept relatively constant in this range, an increase or a decrease in the cardiac output will usually be reflected by a rise or fall in the $P_{et}CO_2$, respectively.

During CPR the cardiac output falls typically to between one fourth and one third of normal (162,175–177). The $P_{et}CO_2$ also decreases to between one fourth and one third of normal as the reduced cardiac output and pulmonary blood flow present less blood and carbon dioxide to the lung for exchange with oxygen in the pulmonary capillary (178–185). As carbon dioxide builds up in venous blood, hyperventilation cleanses the reduced quantity of venous blood traversing the lungs of carbon dioxide. The result is a low arterial (P_aCO_2) and a high central venous ($P_{cv}CO_2$) carbon dioxide concentration (a venoarterial carbon dioxide and pH gradient) (186). Within seconds after ROSC, the improved cardiac output returns large quantities of carbon dioxide–rich venous blood to the lungs, and the $P_{et}CO_2$ suddenly climbs to normal or above-normal levels (178,186). The dramatic change from a low to a high $P_{et}CO_2$ due to venous carbon dioxide washout is often the first clinical indicator that ROSC has occurred (178). The $P_{et}CO_2$ typically returns to normal (4% to 5%) within 2 to 5 minutes after ROSC if the patient maintains a good cardiac output.

Knowledge of the physiologic relationship between $P_{et}CO_2$ and the cardiac output can guide clinicians during low-blood-flow states such as CPR. There are several important clinical corollaries and pitfalls. For example, inadequate chest compression is usually accompanied by a very low (i.e., <1%) $P_{et}CO_2$ that increases linearly with increasing sternal compression depth and force (150,167). Administration of sodium bicarbonate IV causes a transient rise in $P_{et}CO_2$ (167). Epinephrine causes a dose-dependent decrease in $P_{et}CO_2$ (154, 187–189). Disorders that cause significant ventilation/perfusion mismatch (e.g., pulmonary embolization) or decrease in production of carbon dioxide (e.g., hypothermia) are accompanied by a low $P_{et}CO_2$ (190). Disorders that increase the production of carbon dioxide (e.g., fever) increase the $P_{et}CO_2$ (167).

The $P_{et}CO_2$ can also be used to help confirm whether an ET tube has been positioned in the trachea or the esophagus in the cardiac arrest patient. If the $P_{et}CO_2$ during CPR is very low (<0.5%) on at least the seventh breath following intubation, it is highly likely that esophageal insertion has occurred (174). Conversely, a moderately low (>0.5% but <2.0%) $P_{et}CO_2$ does not necessarily indicate esophageal placement of the ET tube because there are many other causes for this finding during CPR (Table 69.2). Thus, a low $P_{et}CO_2$ during resuscitation should alert the rescuers that something is wrong with ventilation, perfusion, and/or carbon dioxide production and should prompt a search for correctable causes (191).

TABLE 69.2

COMMON CAUSES OF A LOW (<2%) END-TIDAL CARBON DIOXIDE CONCENTRATION ($P_{et}CO_2$) DURING CARDIOPULMONARY RESUSCITATION

Inadequate ventilation
Unrecognized esophageal intubation
Airway obstruction
Inadequate blood flow
Inadequate chest compression
Tension pneumothorax
Pericardial tamponade
Ventilation/perfusion mismatch
Pulmonary embolism
Decreased metabolic production of carbon dioxide
Hypothermia

The American Heart Association recommends secondary confirmation of ET tube location immediately after intubation in all patients using either an end-tidal carbon dioxide detector device and/or an esophageal detector device (192). The latter devices create a suction force at the tracheal end of the ET tube, either from pulling back a plunger on a large syringe or compressing a flexible bulb. If the ET tube is in the esophagus, the suction will pull the esophageal mucosa against the distal end of the detector and prevent movement of the device plunger or reexpansion of the suction bulb.

The initial $P_{et}CO_2$ has prognostic value in animal models and humans (173,184,185,193–199). Patients or animal models that attain ROSC tend to have a higher initial $P_{et}CO_2$ before the use of agents that can significantly affect its value such as high-dose adrenergic agents than those who never attain ROSC (approximately 2% vs. 1% $P_{et}CO_2$, respectively). (154, 179,188,189,200–203). In prehospital cardiac arrest patients, there is suggestive evidence that the $P_{et}CO_2$ is lower in patients who have a prolonged "downtime interval" prior to initiation of resuscitation (173). Further clinical research is needed to determine whether it is appropriate to consider the $P_{et}CO_2$ as a factor in the decision to continue resuscitative efforts.

Echocardiographic Monitoring During Resuscitation

Echocardiography is one of the most promising of the technologies that have recently been applied as a research tool during resuscitation (19,21–24,204–215). Conventional transthoracic echocardiography (TTE) is of limited value because it is difficult to image the heart from a chest wall that is in motion during closed-chest compression. In contrast, transesophageal echocardiography (TEE) can provide high-resolution, real-time images of all four cardiac chambers and the great vessels by positioning a single or biplane Doppler ultrasound probe in the esophagus. Clinical experience indicates that TEE provides a stable platform for imaging during CPR. So far, TEE has been used to better define the mechanisms of blood flow during chest compression. It has also been helpful during resuscitation for

(a) determining the presence of pericardial effusion, intracardiac tumor, chamber enlargement or hypertrophy, severe volume depletion, pneumothorax, and thoracic aortic dissection; (b) better defining the cause of pulseless electrical activity; (c) evaluating global and regional wall motion after ROSC; and (d) providing a visual guide for positioning intracardiac catheters and pacemaker wires.

CONTROVERSIES AND PERSONAL PERSPECTIVES

The Need for Mouth-to-Mouth Ventilation during the First Few Minutes of Cardiopulmonary Resuscitation

In the United States the fear of contracting infectious diseases has given rise to debate about the need to provide artificial ventilation during the first few minutes of CPR. Surveys of CPR instructors and other health care providers indicate great reluctance on the part of many rescuers to perform mouth-to-mouth ventilation on strangers (216–224).

It is not clear that it is necessary to provide mouth-to-mouth ventilation for the first several minutes of resuscitation as long as chest compression is performed and the airway is patent. Chandra et al. (225) assessed the time course of change in arterial blood gases during resuscitation in a canine experimental model during ventricular fibrillation. The dogs had no endotracheal tube in place during CPR and received only chest compression (no ventilation). Prearrest arterial pH, PCO_2, and O_2 saturation were 7.39 ± 0.02, 27.0 ± 1.5 mm Hg, and $97 \pm 11.5\%$, respectively. After 4 minutes of chest compression alone, the respective values were 7.39 ± 0.03, 24.3 ± 3.1 mm Hg, and $93.9 \pm 3.0\%$. Mean minute ventilation during the fourth minute of CPR, measured with a face mask-pneumotachometer, was 5.2 ± 1.1 liters/minute. These findings suggest that, in the dog model of witnessed arrest, chest compression alone during CPR can maintain adequate gas exchange to sustain the oxygen saturation above 90% for at least 4 minutes. These findings appear to be confirmed by the observation that survival from cardiac arrest is almost as good in humans when bystanders perform only chest compressions as occurs when bystanders perform both chest compressions and mouth-to-mouth ventilation (226). Some investigators believe that mouth-to-mouth ventilation may not be essential during the first few minutes of CPR because chest compression alone with a patent airway generates significant minute ventilation and the quantity of oxygen needed is reduced significantly during low-blood-flow states (220). Some investigators have even asked whether mouth-to-mouth ventilation with exhaled gas containing as much as 4% carbon dioxide and less oxygen than air might even have adverse effects during CPR (219).

The American Heart Association recommends that rescuers perform mouth-to-mouth ventilation along with chest compressions because clinical data indicate that this combination results in the highest rate of neurologically intact survival (226,227). If rescuers are unwilling to perform mouth-to-mouth ventilation, bystanders should activate the emergency medical services system immediately and initiate chest compressions (227).

In a recent prospective clinical trial in Seattle, telephone EMS dispatchers gave bystanders at the scene of apparent cardiac arrest instructions for performing chest compressions alone or chest compressions plus mouth-to-mouth ventilation (228). Data were analyzed for 241 patients randomly assigned to receive chest compression alone and 279 assigned to chest compression plus mouth-to-mouth ventilation. Complete instructions were delivered in 62% of episodes for the group receiving chest compression plus mouth-to-mouth ventilation and 81% of episodes for the group receiving chest compression alone ($p = .005$). Instructions for compression required 1.4 minutes less to complete than instructions for compression plus mouth-to-mouth ventilation. Survival to hospital discharge was better among patients assigned to chest compression alone than among those assigned to chest compression plus mouth-to-mouth ventilation (14.6% vs. 10.4%), but the difference was not statistically significant ($p = .18$). The authors concluded that the outcome after CPR with chest compression alone is similar to that after chest compression with mouth-to-mouth ventilation, and chest compression alone may be the preferred approach for bystanders inexperienced in CPR.

Spontaneous agonal respirations often contribute to respiratory exchange of gases. In one case series, agonal respirations occurred in 40% of 445 out-of-hospital cardiac arrests (229). Agonal respirations were present in 46% of arrests caused by a cardiac etiology compared with 32% in other etiologies ($p < .01$). Fifty-five percent of witnessed arrest patients had agonal activity compared with 16% of unwitnessed arrest patients ($p < .001$). Agonal respirations occurred in 56% of arrests due to ventricular fibrillation compared with 34% of cases with a non–ventricular fibrillation rhythm ($p < .001$). Twenty-seven percent of patients with agonal respirations were discharged alive compared to 9% without them ($p < .001$). These findings suggest that there is a high incidence of agonal respiratory activity associated with out-of-hospital cardiac arrest, and the presence of agonal respirations appears to be associated with increased survival.

Assisted ventilation, particularly when performed with supplemental oxygen through a properly inserted endotracheal tube, is clearly beneficial during CPR if resuscitation efforts continue beyond the first few minutes (217). Until the airway is protected by a properly inserted and secured endotracheal tube, each mouth-to-mouth or bag-valve-mask ventilation must be delivered with a slow inspiratory flow rate to allow adequate time for lung inflation and to prevent gastric insufflation (227). This is necessary because the lungs become very stiff during resuscitation due to decreased compliance (230). Forceful efforts to inflate the lungs rapidly will only result in elevation of the pharyngeal pressure effect, which will be transmitted down the esophagus to the esophageal-gastric sphincter, causing it to open and allow passage of air into the stomach (231). Hyperventilation appears to be harmful during resuscitation because it increases intrathoracic pressure, blocking venous return and paradoxically decreasing cardiac output and tissue oxygen delivery (66,67).

Use of Epinephrine During Resuscitation

Epinephrine, an endogenous catecholamine with both α- and β-adrenergic activity, is the vasopressor of choice for use during resuscitation. Epinephrine's potent α1- and α2-adrenergic effects improve cerebral blood flow by preventing arterial collapse and by increasing peripheral vasoconstriction (134, 137–141,232,233). Epinephrine also enhances coronary perfusion pressure, which is the major determinant of the ROSC after cardiac arrest (135,138,234). An aortic diastolic blood pressure of 30 to 40 mm Hg markedly improves survival during resuscitation in animal models (38,135,138,142,144,187,234–238). Restoration of myocardial blood flow facilitates the resynthesis of high-energy phosphates within myocardial mitochondria and enhances cellular viability and contractile force. However, the increased myocardial blood flow is at least partially antagonized by the increased myocardial oxygen consumption caused by epinephrine's β-adrenergic actions (239,240).

Despite several anecdotal case series and retrospective studies published in the late 1980s and early 1990s (154,241–249), a number of prospective, randomized clinical trials failed to show that higher doses of epinephrine than those that are used customarily (1 mg) are associated with any better survival to hospital discharge in adults or children (250–259). One of the high-dose-epinephrine trials showed a threefold increase in hospital discharge rates in patients presenting with electromechanical dissociation and asystole when treated with 5.0 mg versus 1.0 mg of epinephrine as the initial dose, but this difference did not reach statistical significance (260). Another study showed that patients older than the age of 65 and those in ventricular fibrillation did better with standard doses of epinephrine (255). However, additional clinical trials failed to show benefit from the use of high versus standard doses of epinephrine in adults (257,259,261) or in children (253,258).

Based on clinical data, the American Heart Association continues to recommend an IV epinephrine dose of 1 mg (10 mL of a 1:10,000 solution) every 3 to 5 minutes during resuscitation in adults (262). If the dose is given by peripheral injection, it should be followed by a 20-mL flush of IV fluid to ensure drug delivery into the central compartment. Higher doses of epinephrine are not recommended for routine use but can be considered if 1-mg doses fail.

The recommended pediatric epinephrine dose for bradycardia, asystolic, or pulseless arrest is 0.01 mg/kg (0.1 mL/kg of 1:10,000 solution) by the IV or intraosseous route, or 0.1 mg/kg (0.1 mL/kg of 1:1,000 solution) by the ET route (101). Repeated doses are recommended every 3 to 5 minutes for ongoing arrest. The same dose of epinephrine is recommended for second and subsequent doses for unresponsive asystolic and pulseless arrest, but higher doses of epinephrine (0.1 to 0.2 mg/kg; 0.1 to 0.2 mL/kg of 1:1,000 solution) by any intravascular route may be considered. If high-dose epinephrine is used, extra care should be taken to avoid dosing errors because two different dilutions of epinephrine are needed. The recommended pediatric ET dose of epinephrine is 0.1 mg/kg (0.1 mL/kg of a 1:1,000 solution).

Intracardiac administration should be used only during open cardiac compression or when other routes of administration are unavailable. Intracardiac injections increase the risk of coronary artery laceration, cardiac tamponade, and pneumothorax and cause interruption of external chest compression and ventilation.

During cardiac arrest epinephrine also may be administered by continuous IV infusion. The dose should be comparable to the standard IV dose of epinephrine (1 mg every 3 to 5 minutes). This is accomplished by adding 1 mg of epinephrine hydrochloride to 250 mL of normal saline or dextrose 5% in water (D5W) to run at 1 μg/minute and increased to 3 to 4 μg/minute (262). A continuous infusion of epinephrine should be administered by central venous access to reduce the risk of extravasation and to ensure good bioavailability.

Autooxidation of catecholamines and related sympathomimetic compounds is pH dependent. Contact of epinephrine with other drugs that have an alkaline pH (such as sodium bicarbonate) can cause autooxidation, but the reaction rate is too slow to be clinically important when epinephrine is given by bolus injection or when it is infused rapidly. Epinephrine should not be added to infusion bags or bottles that contain alkaline solutions.

Use of Vasopressin During Resuscitation

Vasopressin produces significantly higher coronary perfusion pressure and myocardial blood flow than epinephrine during closed-chest CPR in a pig model of ventricular fibrillation (263) and in humans during CPR (264). Both vasopressin and adrenocorticotropin concentrations are higher during CPR in patients in whom resuscitation is successful compared to those in whom it fails (265). Because of these observations, there has been considerable interest in the use of vasopressin for supporting coronary perfusion pressure during CPR in humans.

In a small blinded, randomized clinical study, 40 patients with out-of-hospital ventricular fibrillation resistant to electrical defibrillation were treated with either epinephrine (1 mg IV; $n = 20$) or vasopressin (40 U IV; $n = 20$) during resuscitation (266). Seven (35%) patients in the epinephrine group and 14 (70%) in the vasopressin group survived to hospital admission ($p = .06$). At 24 hours, 4 (20%) epinephrine-treated patients and 12 (60%) vasopressin-treated patients were alive ($p = .02$). Three (15%) patients in the epinephrine group and 8 (40%) in the vasopressin group survived to hospital discharge ($p = .16$). Neurologic outcomes were similar in both groups. In a larger study, Stiell et al. randomized 200 adult cardiac arrest patients treated in the emergency departments, critical care units, and wards of three Canadian teaching hospitals to receive either vasopressin 40 U or epinephrine 1 mg IV as the initial vasopressor. There was no difference in survival to hospital discharge between treatment groups (12% vs. 14% for vasopressin vs. epinephrine, respectively). There was also no difference in neurologic outcomes between groups (267). Finally, Wenzel et al. (268) randomized 1,186 patients with out-of-hospital cardiac arrest to receive vasopressin 40 units versus epinephrine 1 mg IV every 3 min for up to two doses. The two treatment groups had similar clinical profiles. There were no significant differences in the rates of hospital admission between the vasopressin group and the epinephrine group either among patients with ventricular fibrillation (46.2% vs. 43.0%, $p = .48$) or among those with pulseless electrical activity (33.7% vs. 30.5%, $p = .65$). In patients with asystole, vasopressin use was associated with significantly higher rates of hospital admission (29.0% vs. 20.3% in the epinephrine group; $p = .02$) and hospital discharge (4.7% vs. 1.5%, $p = .04$). Among 732 patients in whom spontaneous circulation was not restored with the two doses of the study drug, additional treatment with epinephrine resulted in significant improvement in the rates of survival to hospital admission and hospital discharge in the vasopressin group but not in the epinephrine group (hospital admission rate, 25.7% vs. 16.4%; $p = .002$; hospital discharge rate, 6.2% vs. 1.7%; $p = .002$). Cerebral performance was similar in the two groups. These findings suggest that there may be a synergistic effect between vasopressin and epinephrine during resuscitation.

The American Heart Association guidelines consider vasopressin to be an effective vasopressor and recommend it as an alternative to the first or second dose of epinephrine (Fig. 69.2). The recommended dose is 40 units IV in place of the first or second dose of epinephrine in the pulseless ventricular tachycardia/ventricular fibrillation algorithm. Although its pharmacokinetics is not fully understood, it is generally felt that this single dose should last approximately 10 to 20 minutes, after which epinephrine should be resumed if ROSC has not occurred.

It is not clear whether vasopressin should be used at all in children or infants. Unfortunately, vasopressin was less effective than epinephrine in a piglet model of prolonged asphyxial cardiac arrest (269). At this time, the American Heart Association does not recommend the use of vasopressin in infants or children because data are inadequate for evaluating its efficacy and safety (270).

The Use of Buffers During Resuscitation

The marked fall in cardiac output during closed-chest compression critically reduces tissue oxygen delivery. Cells shift to anaerobic metabolism, gradually building up lactic acid as a waste product (271–274). During anaerobic metabolism,

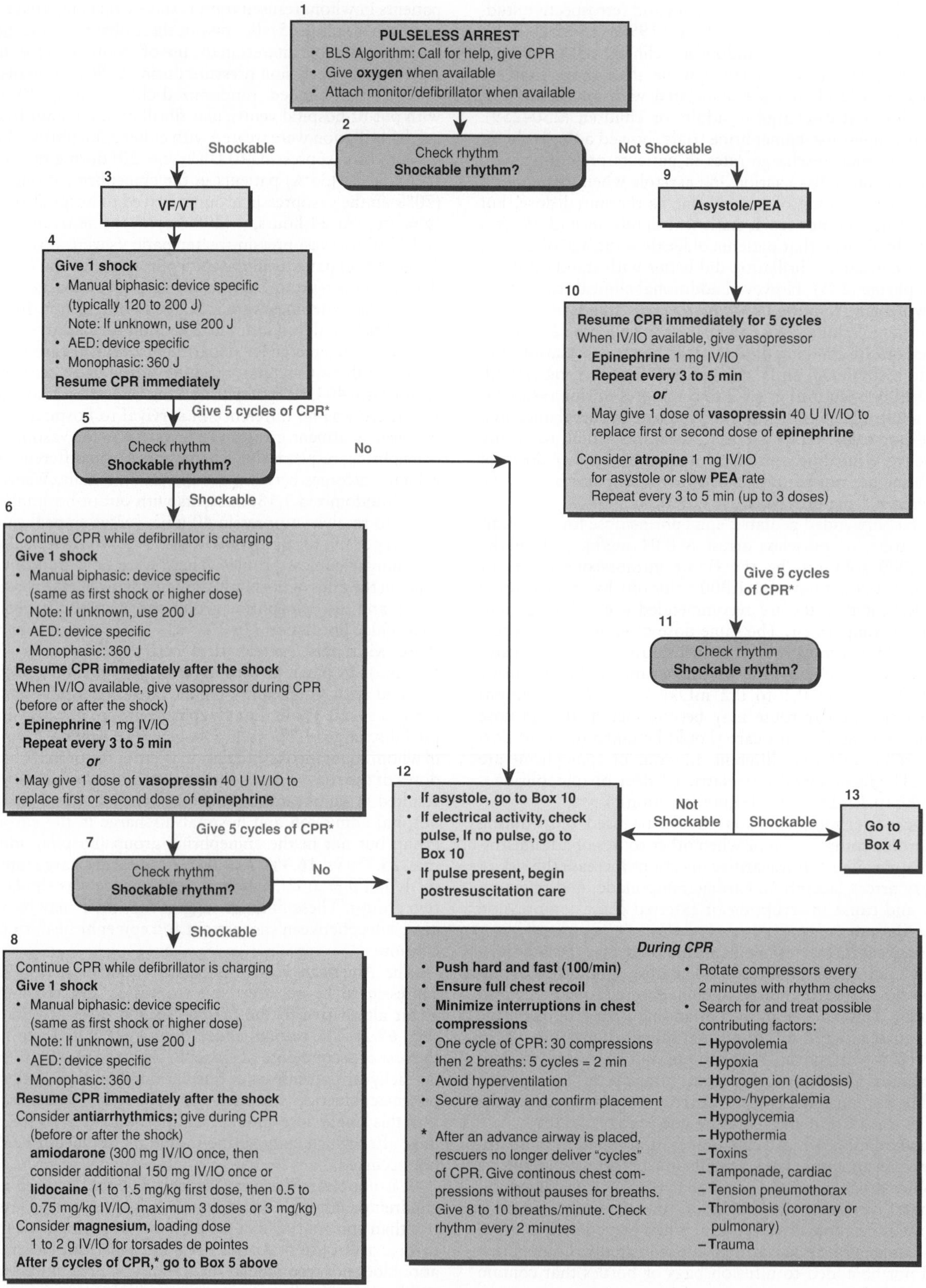

FIGURE 69.2. Comprehensive emergency cardiovascular care algorithm for cardiac arrest. ACS, acute coronary syndrome; BLS, basic life support; CPR, cardiopulmonary resuscitation; IV, intravenous; OD, overdose; VF, ventricular fibrillation; VT, ventricular tachycardia. (Reproduced with permission. *2005 American Heart Association Guidelines for Cardiopulmonary Resuscitation and Emergency Cardiovascular Care.* © 2005, *American Heart Association.*)

the carbon dioxide concentration increases rapidly inside cells. Anoxic arrest of the heart causes a progressive increase in the concentration of PCO_2 inside heart muscle cells that may reach very high levels (90 to 475 Torr) (275). Above an intramyocardial PCO_2 of approximately 475 Torr, pulseless electrical activity is present and the heart cannot be resuscitated (275). Intracellular carbon dioxide eventually diffuses into capillary blood and returns to the heart and lungs in venous blood.

Central (mixed) venous blood during closed chest compression is acidotic (pH approximately 7.15) and hypercarbic (P_vCO_2 approximately 74 Torr) (186). With hyperventilation, carbon dioxide is removed as blood flows through the lungs. Accordingly, arterial blood is less acidotic. Arterial blood pH during well-performed closed-chest compression is usually normal, slightly acidotic, or mildly alkalotic (152,154–156,186,274,276,277). Arterial blood can be slightly alkalotic while the venous blood is acidotic because pulmonary blood flow is only one fourth to one third of the normal amount during closed-chest compression, a phenomenon that has been termed the "venous paradox" (186). It is in fact not a paradox but part of normal physiology that occurs when anaerobic metabolism is required (e.g., during strenuous exercise), at which time the intramyocardial pH is much closer to the venous than the arterial pH.

Severe arterial acidosis during closed-chest compression is usually due to inadequate ventilation (278). The best solution is usually to improve the technique of closed-chest compression and to increase ventilation, if possible. If severe acidosis is present despite hyperventilation, correct intubation, and properly performed external chest compression, an alternate method for providing assisted circulation (e.g., open-chest compressions or venoarterial bypass) may need to be considered.

In the past, administration of sodium bicarbonate ($NaHCO_3$) was recommended during closed-chest compression because of the belief that bicarbonate would buffer the H^+ ion produced during anaerobic metabolism. However, sodium bicarbonate itself contains a high concentration of carbon dioxide (260 to 280 Torr) (279). In plasma, the carbon dioxide is released and diffuses into cells more rapidly than HCO_3^-, causing a paradoxical rise in intracellular PCO_2 and a fall in intracellular pH. The increases in intracellular PCO_2 in heart muscle cells decrease cardiac contractility, cardiac output, and blood pressure (280,281). Paradoxical acidosis of cerebrospinal fluid also can occur after the use of sodium bicarbonate (282) and may be responsible for prolonged confusion after a successful resuscitation as the venous acidosis increases. Sodium bicarbonate causes other potentially harmful effects, including hyperosmolality, alkalemia, and sodium overload.

There is no convincing data proving that treatment with sodium bicarbonate is of benefit during closed-chest compression, and it does not improve survival in experimental animals (137,283–285). Sodium bicarbonate should not be given during a routine cardiac arrest because it provides minimal if any benefit and adds significant risk. If used at all, bicarbonate should not be used until proven interventions such as defibrillation, cardiac compression, support of ventilation including intubation, and pharmacologic therapies such as epinephrine and antiarrhythmic agents have been used (101). If it is used, the initial dose of sodium bicarbonate is 1 mEq/kg. No more than half of the original dose should be given every 10 minutes thereafter.

Measurement of arterial pH during closed-chest compression is rarely helpful because of the markedly reduced cardiac output and the venous paradox in pH. End-tidal carbon dioxide will increase in keeping with the delivered load of carbon dioxide and will no longer reflect pulmonary perfusion (286). Ready-to-use, prefilled injection syringes containing 8.4% sodium bicarbonate (50 mEq/50 mL) are recommended for use during CPR. The administration of sodium bicarbonate may help to buffer hydrogen ions washed out after reestablishment of spontaneous circulation. In this situation, the use of bicarbonate should be guided by arterial blood gas measurement. However, bicarbonate in this situation may still depress cardiac function (287,288). In certain circumstances, such as patients with preexisting metabolic acidosis, hyperkalemia, or tricyclic or phenobarbital overdose, bicarbonate is beneficial. Sodium bicarbonate can be administered by continuous infusion when the therapeutic goal is gradual correction of acidosis or alkalinization of blood (i.e., tricyclic antidepressant overdose) or urine (e.g., barbiturate overdose). A 5% sodium bicarbonate solution (297.5 mEq/500 mL) can be used to administer a sodium bicarbonate infusion. The infusion rate should be guided by arterial blood gas monitoring. One should avoid the attempt to completely correct the base deficit to minimize the risk of alkalosis.

Alternate buffer agents also do not improve survival during cardiac resuscitation. In a Scandinavian study, 502 adults with asystole or ventricular fibrillation with failure of the first defibrillation attempt were entered into a prospective, randomized, double-blind, controlled trial comparing the use of a combination buffer agent (tribonat, containing 250 mL of a sodium bicarbonate-trometamol-phosphate mixture with a buffering capacity of 500 mmol/liter) and 250 mL of 0.9% saline placebo (289). Eighty-seven patients (36%) receiving buffer were admitted to the hospital and 24 (10%) were discharged from the hospital alive versus 92 (36%) and 35 (14%) receiving saline (no significant difference between groups). Thus, this landmark clinical trial lends further evidence to the belief that buffer therapy does not improve patient outcome after routine cardiac arrest.

The Use of Antiarrhythmic Drugs for Recurrent and/or Refractory Ventricular Fibrillation

Frequently used agents for treatment of recurrent and/or refractory ventricular fibrillation or pulseless ventricular tachycardia include lidocaine, procainamide, β-blockers, magnesium sulfate, and IV amiodarone. With the exception of IV amiodarone, there are no randomized, controlled clinical trial data confirming whether any of the other agents are any better than just repeated electrical countershocks.

The American Heart Association has long considered lidocaine to be acceptable therapy for pulseless ventricular tachycardia/ventricular fibrillation that persists after defibrillation and administration of a vasopressor agent (epinephrine or vasopressin). The primary basis for this recommendation is historical precedent and no evidence of significant harm (290). An initial dose of 1.0 to 1.5 mg/kg is suggested. For refractory ventricular fibrillation and pulseless VT, an additional bolus of 0.5 to 0.75 mg/kg can be given over 3 to 5 minutes if necessary. The total dose should not exceed 3 mg/kg (or >200 to 300 mg during a 1-hour period). Administration of antiarrhythmic agents after ROSC is controversial, but it is common to initiate a lidocaine IV infusion at a rate of 1 to 4 mg/minute. Recurrence of ventricular tachyarrhythmias during a constant infusion should be treated with a small bolus dose (0.5 mg/kg) and an increase in the infusion rate in incremental doses (maximal infusion rate of 4 mg/minute). The dose should be reduced and/or blood levels monitored if the patient remains on lidocaine for 24 hours or more because the half-life of the drug increases after 24 to 48 hours of continuous therapy.

Procainamide, a class 1A antiarrhythmic agent, is a presynaptic ganglionic blocker; it vasodilates and induces modest negative inotropic effects, especially in patients with left ventricular dysfunction. Procainamide-induced hypotension is most pronounced after rapid IV injection or when high plasma concentrations of procainamide are present. During resuscitation, procainamide is usually given by infusion at 20 mg/minute until the tachyarrhythmia is suppressed, hypotension and/or QRS prolongation by 50% from its original duration in msec, or 17 mg/kg has been given (290). Bolus administration can result in significant hypotension and toxicity. In urgent situations, up to 50 mg/minute can be given up to a total of 17 mg/kg. The maintenance infusion dose of procainamide is 1 to 4 mg/minute. Blood levels should be monitored in renal failure patients or in those receiving more than a 3-mg/minute IV infusion for more than 24 hours.

Occasionally, ventricular fibrillation or ventricular tachycardia without a pulse will remain "refractory" to, or will recur incessantly despite, repeated electrical countershocks and conventional pharmacologic treatment. In such cases, additional treatment options should be considered. The use of intravenous β-blockers, traditionally with IV propranolol (1 mg every 5 minutes IV up to a total dose of 0.1 mg/kg) or esmolol, is worthy of consideration.

Underlying metabolic derangements should also be sought and corrected. Arterial hypoxemia should be reversed or minimized by endotracheal intubation and ventilation with 100% oxygen. Acidosis is prevented (or treated) best by improving blood flow during resuscitation. Electrolyte abnormalities are common during resuscitation, either as primary disturbances that may have triggered the arrest or as secondary phenomena due to intracellular shifts and therapeutic interventions; such electrolyte abnormalities should be corrected if present.

Resuscitation from refractory ventricular fibrillation is less likely to be successful if hypokalemia and/or hypomagnesemia are present. Hypokalemia is common in cardiac patients and occurs in 23% to 40% of individuals treated with thiazide diuretics (291). When loop and thiazide diuretics are used in combination, the incidence approaches 100% (291,292). Hypokalemia can trigger ventricular fibrillation in experimental animal models and in patients with heart disease (especially acute myocardial infarction) (292,293). Hypokalemia is also common (up to 50%) in survivors of out-of-hospital ventricular fibrillation (294,295). Hypokalemia after resuscitation may be due to a shift in the distribution of potassium between the extracellular and the intracellular space induced by metabolic events during resuscitation. Many patients (55% in one study) have predisposing risk factors for the development of hypokalemia prior to cardiac arrest (295). Hypokalemia in the patient with cardiac arrest and refractory ventricular fibrillation must be treated aggressively.

Hypomagnesemia should be corrected if present because it can precipitate ventricular fibrillation in experimental models in association with hypokalemia and can hinder the replenishment of intracellular potassium (296,297). Magnesium sulfate is no longer recommended for routine management of pulseless ventricular tachycardia or ventricular fibrillation unless hypomagnesemia is suspected or present or the patient has torsades de pointes because two clinical in-hospital trials have not shown benefit (290,298).

For acute administration during ventricular tachycardia or fibrillation with known or suspected hypomagnesemia or for torsades de pointes, 1 or 2 g of magnesium sulfate (2 to 4 mL of a 50% solution) is diluted in 50 to 100 mL of D5W and administered over 5 to 60 minutes. Caution should be used when magnesium is administered to safeguard against clinically significant hypotension or asystole. A 24-hour magnesium infusion (8 g $MgSO_4$ in 500 mL of D5W at 8 drops/minute) should be considered in patients with documented magnesium deficiency. Magnesium toxicity is rare, but side effects from rapid administration include flushing, sweating, mild bradycardia, and hypotension. Hypermagnesemia can produce depressed reflexes, flaccid paralysis, circulatory collapse, respiratory paralysis, or diarrhea.

Other treatment strategies can also be used in managing incessant or recurrent ventricular fibrillation or pulseless VT. The possibility that there has been a proarrhythmic drug effect that may be exacerbating the arrhythmia must be considered. Proarrhythmic drug effects, hypokalemia, and/or hypomagnesemia can induce ventricular arrhythmias such as torsades de pointes. Torsades de pointes should be treated by stopping medications known to prolong the QT interval and correcting any electrolyte abnormalities. Other interventions can be tried including administration of magnesium sulfate or the use of pacing or other forms of overdrive suppression (including the cautious use of isoproterenol if there are no contraindications) (299).

IV amiodarone is the preferred antiarrhythmic drug used to treat patients with recurrent or refractory VF. In a randomized, controlled clinical prehospital trial (Amiodarone in the Out-of-Hospital Resuscitation of Refractory Sustained Ventricular Tachyarrhythmia [ARREST]) conducted on 504 cardiac arrest patients with recurrent and/or refractory VF, the administration of a single 300-mg bolus of IV amiodarone at the time of the first IV epinephrine administration resulted in 26% greater survival to hospital admission compared to standard ACLS therapy (300,301). There was no significant difference between the amiodarone and placebo groups in the duration of the resuscitation attempt (42 $\pm$ 16.4 and 43 $\pm$ 16.3 minutes, respectively), the number of shocks delivered (4 $\pm$ 3 and 6 $\pm$ 5, respectively), or the proportion of patients who required additional antiarrhythmic drugs after the administration of the study drug (66% and 73%, respectively). More patients in the amiodarone group than in the placebo group had hypotension (59% vs. 48%, $p = .04$) or bradycardia (41% vs. 25%, $p = 0.004$) after receiving the study drug. These side effects usually respond readily to therapy (volume infusion and vasopressors; atropine and/or electrical pacing). Recipients of amiodarone were more likely to survive to hospital admission (44% vs. 34% of the placebo group; $p = .03$). The adjusted odds ratio for survival to admission to the hospital in the amiodarone group as compared with the placebo group was 1.6 (95% CI 1.1 to 2.4; $p = .02$). The trial did not have sufficient statistical power to detect differences in survival to hospital discharge, which differed only slightly between the two groups. In the Amiodarone versus Lidocaine In Ventricular fibrillation Evaluation (ALIVE) trial, 347 out-of-hospital cardiac arrest patients with recurrent VF or VF resistant to three shocks were randomly assigned to receive IV amiodarone versus lidocaine. Survival to hospital admission was significantly higher in amiodarone- versus lidocaine-treated patients (22.8% vs. 12%, $p = .009$; odds ratio 2.17; 95% CI 1.21 to 3.83). Unfortunately, neither the ARREST nor the ALIVE trial had adequate statistical power to determine whether survival to hospital discharge is better with amiodarone than lidocaine.

The manufacturer adds polysorbate-80 to the IV amiodarone preparation to keep the latter in solution (amiodarone is relatively insoluble in water). Because diluent is a "soapy" compound, it can create bubbles if the vial is shaken before the amiodarone is drawn up into the syringe. It is recommended that the vial *not* be shaken. The bubbling phenomenon can usually be kept to a minimum by drawing up the drug with a large needle (18 gauge or larger). If bubbles do appear in the syringe, it should be held vertically as it is being injected into the IV tubing and the bubbles should not be injected into the patient.

The American Heart Association recommends the use of amiodarone after defibrillation and a vasopressor (either epinephrine or vasopressin) in cardiac arrest with persistent or recurrent pulseless ventricular tachycardia or ventricular fibrillation (290). In this setting, it is usually administered as a 300-mg rapid infusion diluted to 20 to 30 mL with saline or D5W followed by a supplemental dose of 150 mg by rapid infusion if needed for recurrent or refractory pulseless ventricular tachycardia or ventricular fibrillation (290,301). For patients not in cardiac arrest, IV amiodarone is usually diluted and administered as 150 mg over 10 minutes followed by a 1-mg/min infusion for 6 hours and then 0.6 mg/min.

New Experimental Cardiopulmonary Resuscitation Techniques

Investigators have begun to exploit the physiologic opportunities afforded by understanding the mechanisms of blood flow during CPR in an attempt to overcome the hemodynamic shortcomings of conventional chest compression. Standard chest compression of the sternum to a depth of 1 1/2 to 2 inches at a rate of 80/minute as recommended by the American Heart Association produces only about one fourth to one third of the normal cardiac output and less than one half of the normal arterial perfusion pressure (191,302). This is usually inadequate to generate the 25- to 35-mm Hg aortic diastolic pressure needed to restart the arrested heart (155,236).

Applying higher compression force to displace the sternum farther than the 1 1/2 to 2 inches recommended by the American Heart Association can improve arterial systolic pressure and cardiac output significantly (150). However, there is a practical limit to the amount of extra force that can be applied safely without causing physical injury to the chest and underlying structures. Computer modeling indicates that substantially greater force is required to generate adequate coronary and cerebral pressure and flow than that which can be provided safely by conventional sternal compression (303).

Circumferential Chest Compression Cardiopulmonary Resuscitation

Circumferential application of force to the chest using a pneumatic vest can generate enough intrathoracic pressure to provide virtually normal systemic arterial pressure and flow in animals and humans during cardiac arrest (304–307). The device looks like a large blood pressure cuff that is wrapped around the patient's thorax. It contains a bladder that can be inflated and deflated in cycles by a pneumatic pump. The device controls compression duration, inflation pressure, and rate. Typical inflation pressure is 250 mm Hg, and the chest compression rate is 60/minute. A small positive pressure is maintained between the chest and the vest to provide a tight fit between the two, but the device totally deflates during ventilation to provide for chest expansion. The total force applied to the chest with "vest CPR" is much greater than that which can be applied safely with conventional CPR. Despite this, vest CPR is much less traumatic than standard CPR because it distributes force over a much larger surface area (the entire chest).

When the pneumatic vest was applied to 29 patients who repeatedly failed to respond to conventional CPR, defibrillation, and drug therapy for 42 ± 16 minutes, vest CPR increased the peak aortic pressure from 78 ± 26 mm Hg to 138 ± 28 mm Hg ($p < .001$) and the coronary perfusion pressure from 15 ± 8 mm Hg to 23 ± 11 mm Hg ($p < .003$) (306). Despite prolonged unsuccessful manual CPR, spontaneous circulation returned with vest CPR in 4 of the 29 patients. An additional 34 patients were randomly assigned to undergo vest CPR (17 patients) or continued manual CPR (17 patients) after initial manual CPR (mean duration, 11 ± 4 minutes) was unsuccessful. Spontaneous circulation returned in 8 of the 17 patients who underwent vest CPR as compared with only 3 of the 17 patients who received continued manual CPR ($p = .14$) (306). More patients in the vest-CPR group than in the manual-CPR group were alive 6 hours after attempted resuscitation (6 of 17 vs. 1 of 17) and 24 hours after attempted resuscitation (3 of 17 vs. 1 of 17) but none survived to leave the hospital.

The original pneumatic-powered vest CPR device never made it into clinical use because its electrical current requirements prohibited development of a portable device. A second-generation vestlike device (AutoPulse, Revivant Corp., Sunnyvale, CA) that uses an electrical motor–driven circumferential chest compression band instead of a pneumatic bladder is now FDA approved and marketed in the United States. In a porcine cardiac arrest model, the AutoPulse device produced higher myocardial and cerebral perfusion pressure and flow than standard CPR (308). AutoPulse CPR with epinephrine generated prearrest levels of myocardial and cerebral flow (308). The AutoPulse CPR device increased coronary perfusion pressure over manual chest compression during CPR in an intensive care unit study performed on terminally ill, hemodynamically monitored, patients (309). Although clinical experience with the AutoPulse device is limited, the San Francisco Fire Department deployed the device on 69 patients and compared the results to 93 matched manual-CPR-only cases. AutoPulse CPR patients had a higher rate of ROSC than patients treated with manual CPR (39% vs. 29%, $p = .003$) (310). Although it is still too early to judge the true clinical value of this technology, the American Heart Association considers circumferential chest compression CPR to be an acceptable alternative to standard CPR in hospital or during ambulance transport (311).

Active Compression-Decompression Cardiopulmonary Resuscitation

Active compression-decompression CPR (ACD-CPR) is similar to conventional CPR, but it also provides negative intrathoracic pressure during the relaxation phase using a device that resembles a toilet plunger. ACD-CPR is performed with a suction-cup device called the Ambu Cardio-Pump (Ambu Inc., Ballerup, Denmark).

The ACD-CPR device consists of three parts: (a) a Neoprene suction cup, (b) a plastic circular handle with an undercut handgrip, and (c) a force gauge. The gauge can be calibrated to a fixed depth, which usually is similar to standard CPR (1.5 to 2 inches). To ensure proper function by the operator, the decompression force is also measured up to −30 pounds by the gauge. The device is positioned at the midsternum in alignment with the nipples.

Initial studies on ACD-CPR in both experimental animal models and human patients late after cardiac arrest demonstrated improved cardiopulmonary hemodynamics when compared to standard manual CPR (28,31,312–315). In one clinical study, conventional CPR was compared to ACD-CPR in 21 patients undergoing routine induction of ventricular fibrillation as part of a transvenous lead cardioverter-defibrillator implantation procedure (313). Mean coronary perfusion pressure was increased throughout the entire CPR cycle with ACD-CPR (compression, 21.5 ± 9.0 mm Hg; decompression, 21.9 ± 8.7 mm Hg) compared with conventional CPR (compression, 17.9 ± 8.2 mm Hg; decompression, 18.5 ± 6.9 mm Hg; $p < .02$ and $p < .02$, respectively). Unfortunately, despite initial promising clinical results (29), several recent randomized clinical trials have not shown any superiority of ACD-CPR over conventional CPR (316–319). However, one trial reported benefit in short-term survival with this technique (320).

The American Heart Association considers ACD-CPR to be an acceptable alternative to standard CPR when rescue personnel adequately trained in use of the device are available (311). However, the device is not FDA approved for sale in the United States.

Interposed Abdominal Compression

Interposed abdominal compression CPR (IAC-CPR), also known as abdominal counterpulsation CPR, attempts to mimic intraaortic balloon counterpulsation. Two rescuers are needed to perform this technique: one compresses the sternum and the other interposes abdominal compressions between each pair of chest compressions. Several investigators have demonstrated improvements in coronary perfusion, carotid and cerebral blood flows, and augmented venous return using IAC-CPR compared with standard CPR (33,35,45).

An early prehospital clinical trial in the mid-1980s failed to demonstrate any improvement in survival when IAC-CPR was compared to conventional CPR (321). Recently, IAC-CPR was shown to improve survival in 143 consecutive patients experiencing in-hospital cardiac arrest with an initial arrest rhythm of asystole or electromechanical dissociation (51). Patients were randomized to receive either IAC-CPR or conventional CPR. The rate of ROSC was significantly higher in the group receiving IAC-CPR than in the group receiving conventional CPR (49% vs. 28%, $p = .01$). At 24 hours, there were significantly more patients alive in the IAC-CPR group than in the conventional CPR group (33% vs. 13%, $p = .009$). No complications were demonstrated in a small subset of patients who died and underwent autopsy.

Similar findings were noted in another randomized clinical trial, one involving 135 resuscitation attempts in 103 patients (53). The rate of ROSC was significantly greater in the group receiving IAC-CPR than in the group receiving conventional CPR (51% vs. 27%, $p = .007$). At hospital discharge, a significantly greater proportion of patients were alive in the IAC-CPR group than in the conventional CPR group (25% vs. 7%, $p = .02$). Eight (17%) of 48 patients who received IAC-CPR survived to hospital discharge neurologically intact compared with only 3 (6%) of 55 patients from the conventional CPR group (not significant). Thus, IAC-CPR appears to be a promising technique that may improve survival in selected cardiac arrest patients. The American Heart Association recommends the use of IAC-CPR for in-hospital resuscitation as an alternative to standard CPR whenever sufficient personnel trained in the technique are available (311).

Cough Cardiopulmonary Resuscitation

Cough CPR has been shown to be of value in experimental animals and in clinical use (14,322–325). At the onset of lethal arrhythmias such as asystole, profound bradycardia, ventricular tachycardia, or fibrillation, coughing may assist in maintaining consciousness and an adequate systolic blood pressure. In some cases, it may also play a role in terminating the arrhythmia. The simplicity and effectiveness of this technique warrant its consideration for greater clinical use by health care providers. Similarly, "high-impulse CPR" using a rapid downstroke velocity may, in some circumstances, improve blood flow by transferring greater energy into the thorax and perhaps by enhancing the "cardiac pump" mechanism (18,19).

Impedance Threshold Valve Device

An impedance threshold device (ITD) has been developed to enhance the return of blood to the thorax during the chest decompression phase (326). This new device enhances negative intrathoracic pressure during chest wall recoil or the decompression phase, leading to improved vital organ perfusion during both standard CPR and active compression-decompression CPR (326–331). The ITD shows promise for patients in asystole or shock-refractory ventricular fibrillation, when enhanced return of blood flow to the chest is needed to "prime the pump."

In the Milwaukee EMS system, 12 patients were treated with a sham ITD versus 10 patients with an active ITD. Systolic blood pressure (BP) (mean ± standard deviation) was 85 ± 29 in the group receiving an active ITD compared with 43 ± 15 in patients treated with a sham ITD ($p < .01$). Diastolic BP was 20 ± 12 in the group receiving an active ITD compared with 15 ± 9 in patients treated with a sham ITD (p = NS). No significant adverse device events were reported (332). Thus, ITD appears to increase systolic pressures safely and significantly in cardiac arrest patients compared with sham controls. In another trial, Plaisance et al. (333) randomized patients to receive either a sham ($n = 200$) or an active ITD ($n = 200$) in combination with ACD-CPR. The 24-hour survival rate was 22% with the sham valve and 32% with the active valve ($p = .02$). Six of 10 survivors in the active ITD group and 1 of 8 survivors in the sham group had normal neurologic function at hospital discharge ($p = .1$).

The ITD appears to improve hemodynamics and, at least, short-term outcome during resuscitation. Further studies are under way to determine whether the device alone, or in combination with other techniques, improves long-term, neurologically intact survival compared to standard CPR techniques. The American Heart Association considers this device to be acceptable as an adjunct to be used with ACD-CPR (311).

Rapid Response Systems in the Hospital

Mortality from in-hospital cardiac arrest remains high, with an average survival of approximately 17%, despite significant advances in treatments (334). Survival is particularly poor for nonprimary VT/VF rhythms, which constitute over 75% of arrests in the hospital. These arrests are commonly preceded by easily recognizable physiologic changes. Nearly 80% of hospitalized patients with cardiorespiratory arrest have abnormal vital signs documented for up to 8 hours BEFORE the actual arrest (335–342). Of the small percentage of patients who experience return of spontaneous circulation and get admitted to the intensive care unit, 80% ultimately die before discharge compared to 44% mortality for nonarrest patients admitted urgently from the floor who have not yet suffered an arrest. Cardiac arrest teams have been ineffective in preventing arrests because their focus has traditionally been to respond only after the arrest has occurred. There has been a major shift in the focus regarding in-hospital cardiac arrest over the last few years to one of patient safety and prevention. The best way to improve survival from a cardiorespiratory arrest is to prevent it from happening. Rather than focusing solely on responses to cardiac arrest, the importance of recognizing clinical deterioration and intervening immediately to prevent the arrest is now being stressed. The majority of cardiorespiratory arrests in the hospital should be considered a "failure to rescue" rather than an isolated, unexpected, random occurrence.

A specifically designed rapid response system for identifying and treating early clinical deterioration in hospitalized patients has been developed in several countries over the last decade. Several names, such as medical emergency team (MET), rapid response team, and rapid assessment team, have been used to describe this system-wide approach to bringing critical care expertise to ward patients with deteriorating conditions (343–350). The MET typically comprises health care providers with critical or emergency care experience and a skill set that supports immediate intervention for numerous critical care issues. The entire system depends on appropriate activation of the team by the floor nurse based on certain previously identified physiologic criteria, including a subjective component from the treating nurse. Examples of such "calling criteria" include patients with a threatened airway, respiratory rate less than 6 or greater than 30 beats per minute, heart rate less than 40 or greater than 140 beats per minute, systolic blood pressure less than

90 mm Hg, symptomatic hypertension, sudden decrease in level of consciousness, unexplained agitation, seizure, significant fall in urine output, and nurse provider concerned about the patient. The system is critically dependent on the primary nurse identifying and acting on these specified criteria to immediately summon the team to the patient's bedside. The experienced critical care team performs a rapid assessment and begins appropriate treatment.

The majority of published studies of "before and after" MET implementation document a 17% to 65% drop in cardiac arrest rate after the MET intervention (351–355). Other documented benefits of MET are a decrease in unplanned emergency transfers to the intensive care unit, decreased intensive care unit and total hospital length of stay, postoperative reductions in morbidity and mortality, and improved survival from cardiac arrest when it does occur (351,352,356–358). The recently published Medical Emergency Response Improvement Team (MERIT) trial is the only randomized, controlled trial evaluating hospitals with a MET versus those without one (357). The study unfortunately lacked sufficient power to detect a difference between the two groups and was therefore a neutral trial.

Implementation of this type of system requires a significant cultural change in most current hospital environments. Particular attention needs to be paid to issues that may prevent the system from being used effectively, such as insufficient resources, poor education, fear of calling the team, fear of losing control over patient care, and fear of possible retribution or comments from team members.

The implementation of a rapid response system requires ongoing education, impeccable data collection and review, and feedback. The development and maintenance of these programs require a long-term cultural and financial commitment from hospital administration along with the understanding that their potential benefits in terms of decreased resource utilization and improved survival may have independent positive financial ramifications. Hospital administrators, physicians, and nurses need to reorient their approach to emergency medical events and develop a patient safety culture with a primary goal of decreasing morbidity and mortality.

Induced Hypothermia Postresuscitation

Only a small percentage of those who obtain ROSC during resuscitation efforts ultimately survive to hospital discharge, and many of them have significant neurologic dysfunction (359). The effect of transient global ischemia on the heart, brain, and other vital organs is a prominent feature in the metabolic phase of resuscitation. New therapies are needed to optimize and improve the care delivered to victims of cardiopulmonary arrest after ROSC has occurred. The induction of mild hypothermia in comatose survivors of cardiac arrest has emerged as a mechanism for improving neurologic recovery in these patients. Two large trials evaluating the effects of mild hypothermia on comatose survivors of out-of-hospital VF arrest found a significant improvement in neurologically intact survival in those patients whose core temperatures were decreased to 32°C to 34°C for a period of up to 24 hours after ROSC. The Hypothermia After Cardiac Arrest Study Group found that only six patients need to be treated with hypothermia to prevent one unfavorable neurologic outcome and only seven need to be treated to prevent one death (360). Bernard et al. found that 49% of patients treated with hypothermia survived to discharge with good neurologic outcome versus only 26% of normothermic patients (361). These data, in combination with numerous smaller animal and human studies, led to an American Heart Association/International Liaison Committee on Resuscitation interim guideline scientific statement recommending that mild hypothermia be delivered to comatose survivors of out-of-hospital cardiac arrest in cases in which VF was the initial rhythm (362).

The mechanisms of benefit from hypothermia are likely multifactorial and not yet understood completely. Hypothermia decreases the free radical production that accompanies ischemic reperfusion and lowers intracellular calcium, thus preventing the propagation of cell death. It also decreases oxygen consumption, intracellular acidosis, excitatory neurotransmitter synthesis, cerebral edema, intracranial pressure and protects membrane fluidity (363–366). Further research is needed to determine the optimal way to deliver this therapy as well as its mechanisms of benefit. However, therapeutic hypothermia is one of the first major breakthroughs in clinical postresuscitation management that has been shown to significantly improve outcomes.

Public Access Defibrillation

Another innovative idea is termed "public access defibrillation," so named because the intent is to have non–health care providers perform early defibrillation. Encouraging results were obtained when community first responders were trained to use automated external defibrillators (AEDs). In Las Vegas casinos, security officers are trained and equipped to use AEDs on suspected cardiac arrest victims (367). AEDs are placed in the casinos at strategic locations to permit rapid defibrillation in 3 minutes or less after collapse. Of 105 patients whose initial cardiac rhythm was ventricular fibrillation, 56 (53%) survived to hospital discharge. Among the 90 patients whose collapse was witnessed (86%), the clinically relevant time intervals were (mean ± standard deviation) 3.5 ± 2.9 minutes from collapse to attachment of the defibrillator, 4.4 ± 2.9 minutes from collapse to the delivery of the first defibrillation shock, and 9.8 ± 4.3 minutes from collapse to the arrival of the paramedics. The survival rate was 74% for patients who received their first defibrillation no later than 3 minutes after a witnessed collapse and 49% for those who received their first defibrillation after more than 3 minutes.

AEDs are now found on virtually all larger commercial aircraft (368–371). For example, American Airlines reported that AEDs were attached to 200 patients (191 on the aircraft and 9 in the terminal), including 99 with documented loss of consciousness (370). Electrocardiographic data were available for 185 patients. A shock was advised in all 14 patients who had electrocardiographically documented ventricular fibrillation, and no shock was advised in the remaining patients (sensitivity and specificity of the defibrillator in identifying ventricular fibrillation, 100%). The first shock successfully defibrillated the heart in 13 patients (defibrillation was withheld in 1 case at the family's request). The rate of survival to discharge from the hospital after shock with the automated external defibrillator was 40%. A total of 36 patients either died or were resuscitated after cardiac arrest. No complications arose from use of the AED as a monitor in conscious passengers.

The National Heart, Lung, and Blood Institute and the American Heart Association have taken the lead in sponsoring research into the safety, efficacy, and potential cost–benefit tradeoff of this interesting concept (372–376). The Public Access Defibrillation (PAD) study was a prospective, community-based, multicenter clinical trial that randomly assigned community units to a structured and monitored emergency response system involving lay volunteers trained in CPR alone or CPR plus the use of AEDs. The primary outcome was survival to hospital discharge. More than 19,000 volunteer responders from 993 community units in 24 North American regions participated. The two study groups had similar unit and volunteer characteristics. No inappropriate shocks were delivered. There were more survivors to hospital discharge in the units assigned to have volunteers trained in CPR plus the use of AEDs (30 survivors among 128 arrests) than there were in the units assigned to have volunteers trained only in CPR (15 among 107; $p = .03$; relative risk 2.0; 95% CI 1.07 to 3.77). Functional status at hospital discharge did not differ between the two groups. This study suggests that training and equipping volunteers to attempt early defibrillation within a structured response system does not result in inappropriate delivery of defibrillation shocks and can approximately double the number of survivors to hospital discharge after out-of-hospital cardiac arrest in public locations (376,377).

THE FUTURE

Better understanding of the mechanisms responsible for blood flow during closed-chest compression are leading to new CPR devices and techniques. It is highly probable that one or more of these innovations will result in significant improvement in the likelihood of successful resuscitation. If this occurs, the greatest challenge will be to better define from a medical and ethical perspective who should or should not receive such intervention. More emphasis will be placed on prevention of cardiac arrest and on neuroprotection after successful resuscitation. In addition, there will likely be much broader implementation of public access defibrillation.

References

1. Hermreck AS. The history of cardiopulmonary resuscitation. *Am J Surg* 1988;156(6):430–436.
2. Gordon AS, Raymon F, Sadove M, et al. Manual artificial respiration. *JAMA* 1950;14:1447–1452.
3. Wright-St Clair RE. The development of resuscitation. *N Z Med J* 1985;8: 339–341.
4. Dill DB. Symposium on mouth-to-mouth resuscitation (expired air inflation). *Council Med Phys* 1958;167:317–319.
5. Roth N. First stammering of the heart: Ludwig's kymograph. *Med Instrum* 1978;13:226.
6. McWilliam JA. Cardiac failure and sudden death. *Br Med J* 1889;5:6–8.
7. Beck CS. Prevost and Battelli. *Ariz Med* 1965;22:691–694.
8. Kouwenhoven WB, Hooker RD. Resuscitation by countershock. *Electr Engin* 1922;475–477.
9. Zoll PM, Linenthal AJ, Gibson W, et al. Termination of ventricular fibrillation in man by externally applied electrical countershock. *N Engl J Med* 1956;254:727–732.
10. Jude JR, Kouwenhoven WB, Knickerbocker GG. External cardiac resuscitation. *Monograph Surg Sci* 1964;1:59–117.
11. Jude JR, Kouwenhoven WB, Knickerbocker GG. Closed chest cardiac massage. *JAMA* 1960;173:1064–1067.
12. Ad hoc Committee on Cardiopulmonary Resuscitation of the Division of Medical Sciences National Academy of Sciences–National Research Council. Cardiopulmonary resuscitation. *JAMA* 1966;198:372–379.
13. Criley JM, Blaufuss AH, Kissel GL. Self-induced form of cardiopulmonary resuscitation. *JAMA* 1976;236:1246–1250.
14. Niemann JT, Rosborough JP, Ung S, et al. Cough CPR. Documentation of systemic perfusion in man and in an experimental model: a "window" to the mechanism of blood flow in external CPR. *Crit Care Med* 1980;8:141–146.
15. Halperin HR, Brower R, Weisfeldt ML, et al. Air trapping in the lungs during cardiopulmonary resuscitation in dogs. A mechanism for generating changes in intrathoracic pressure. *Circ Res* 1989;65(4):946–954.
16. Weisfeldt ML, Halperin HR. Cardiopulmonary resuscitation: beyond cardiac massage. *Circulation* 1986;74(3):443–448.
17. Fisher J, Vaghaiwalla F, Tsitlik J, et al. Determinants and clinical significance of jugular venous valve competence. *Circulation* 1982;65:188.
18. Maier GW, Newton Jr JR, Wolfe JA, et al. The influence of manual chest compression rate on hemodynamic support during cardiac arrest: high-impulse cardiopulmonary resuscitation. *Circulation* 1986;74(6 Pt 2):IV51–IV59.
19. Feneley MP, Maier GW, Gaynor JW, et al. Sequence of mitral valve motion and transmitral blood flow during manual cardiopulmonary resuscitation in dogs. *Circulation* 1987;76(2):363–375.
20. Wolfe JA, Maier GW, Newton Jr JR, et al. Physiologic determinants of coronary blood flow during external cardiac massage. *J Thorac Cardiovasc Surg* 1988;95(3):523–532.
21. Deshmukh HG, Weil MH, Rackow EC, et al. Echocardiographic observations during cardiopulmonary resuscitation: a preliminary report. *Crit Care Med* 1985;13(11):904–906.
22. Porter TR, Ornato JP, Guard CS, et al. Transesophageal echocardiography to assess mitral valve function and flow during cardiopulmonary resuscitation. *Am J Cardiol* 1992;70(11):1056–1060.
23. Pell ACH, Guly LM, Sutherland YR, et al. Mechanism of closed chest cardiopulmonary resuscitation investigated by transoesophageal echocardiography. *J Accid Emerg Med* 1994;11(3):139–143.
24. Kuhn C, Juchems R, Frese W. Transoesophageal echocardiography during cardiopulmonary resuscitation in man: proof of the cardiac pump theory? *Intensiv- Notfallbehandlung* 1994;19(1):1–7.
25. Halperin HR, Tsitlik JE, Guerci AD, et al. Determinants of blood flow to vital organs during cardiopulmonary resuscitation in dogs. *Circulation* 1986;73(3):539–550.
26. Ornato JP, Gonzalez ER, Garnett AR, et al. Effect of cardiopulmonary resuscitation compression rate on end-tidal carbon dioxide concentration and arterial pressure in man. *Crit Care Med* 1988;16(3):241–245.
27. Tucker KJ, Savitt MA, Idris A, et al. Cardiopulmonary resuscitation. Historical perspectives, physiology, and future directions. *Arch Intern Med* 1994;154(19):2141–2150.
28. Chang MW, Coffeen P, Lurie KG, et al. Active compression-decompression CPR improves vital organ perfusion in a dog model of ventricular fibrillation. *Chest* 1994;106(4):1250–1259.
29. Lurie KG, Shultz JJ, Callaham ML, et al. Evaluation of active compression-decompression CPR in victims of out-of-hospital cardiac arrest. *JAMA* 1994;271(18):1405–1411.
30. Cohen TJ, Tucker KJ, Lurie KG, et al. Active compression-decompression. A new method of cardiopulmonary resuscitation. *JAMA* 1992;267(21): 2916–2923.
31. Lindner KH, Pfenninger EG, Lurie KG, et al. Effects of active compression-decompression resuscitation on myocardial and cerebral blood flow in pigs. *Circulation* 1993;88(3):1254–1263.
32. Lindner KH, Brinkmann A, Pfenninger EG, et al. Effect of vasopressin on hemodynamic variables, organ blood flow, and acid–base status in a pig model of cardiopulmonary resuscitation. *Anesth Analg* 1993;77(3):427–435.
33. Einagle V, Bertrand F, Wise RA, et al. Interposed abdominal compressions and carotid blood flow during cardiopulmonary resuscitation. Support for a thoracoabdominal unit. *Chest* 1988;93(6):1206–1212.
34. Babbs CF, Tacker Jr WA. Cardiopulmonary resuscitation with interposed abdominal compression. *Circulation* 1986;74(6 Pt 2):IV37–IV41.
35. McDonald JL. Effect of interposed abdominal compression during CPR on central arterial and venous pressures. *Am J Emerg Med* 1985;3(2):156–159.
36. Hoekstra OS, Van Lambalgen AA, Groeneveld ABJ, et al. Abdominal compressions increase vital organ perfusion during CPR in dogs: relation with efficacy of thoracic compressions. *Ann Emerg Med* 1995;25(3):375–385.
37. Babbs CF, Blevins WE. Abdominal binding and counterpulsation in cardiopulmonary resuscitation. *Crit Care Clin* 1986;2(2):319–332.
38. Kern KB, Carter AB, Showen RL, et al. Twenty-four hour survival in a canine model of cardiac arrest comparing three methods of manual cardiopulmonary resuscitation. *J Am Coll Cardiol* 1986;7(4):859–867.
39. Babbs CF, Thelander K. Theoretically optimal duty cycles for chest and abdominal compression during external cardiopulmonary resuscitation. *Acad Emerg Med* 1995;2(8):698–707.
40. Hoekstra OS, van Lambalgen AA, Groeneveld AB, et al. Abdominal compressions increase vital organ perfusion during CPR in dogs: relation with efficacy of thoracic compressions. *Ann Emerg Med* 1995;25(3):375–385.
41. Babbs CF. The evolution of abdominal compression in cardiopulmonary resuscitation. *Acad Emerg Med* 1994;1(5):469–477.
42. Hillman H. Abdominal pumping. *Acad Emerg Med* 1994;1(5):478–481.
43. Ward KR. Possible reasons for the variability of human responses to IAC-CPR. *Acad Emerg Med* 1994;1(5):482–489.
44. Sack JB, Kesselbrenner MB. Hemodynamics, survival benefits, and complications of interposed abdominal compression during cardiopulmonary resuscitation. *Acad Emerg Med* 1994;1(5):490–497.
45. Adams CP, Martin GB, Rivers EP, et al. Hemodynamics of interposed abdominal compression during human cardiopulmonary resuscitation. *Acad Emerg Med* 1994;1(5):498–502.
46. Inchiosa Jr MA, Frost EA. Interposed abdominal compression-CPR: which patients are benefited? Why? *Circulation* 1994;90(2):1113–1114.
47. Babbs CF, Sack JB, Kern KB. Interposed abdominal compression as an adjunct to cardiopulmonary resuscitation. *Am Heart J* 1994;127(2):412–421.
48. Babbs CF. Interposed abdominal compression-cardiopulmonary resuscitation: are we missing the mark in clinical trials? *Am Heart J* 1993;126 (4):1035–1041.
49. Salgo IS. Interposed abdominal compression-cardiopulmonary resuscitation. *Circulation* 1993;88(2):806–807.
50. Babbs CF. Interposed abdominal compression-CPR: a case study in cardiac arrest research. *Ann Emerg Med* 1993;22(1):24–32.
51. Sack JB, Kesselbrenner MB, Jarrad A. Interposed abdominal compression-cardiopulmonary resuscitation and resuscitation outcome during asystole and electromechanical dissociation. *Circulation* 1992;86(6):1692–1700.
52. Babbs CF. Interposed abdominal compression-CPR. Low technology for the clinical armamentarium. *Circulation* 1992;86(6):2011–2012.

53. Sack JB, Kesselbrenner MB, Bregman D. Survival from in-hospital cardiac arrest with interposed abdominal counterpulsation during cardiopulmonary resuscitation. *JAMA* 1992;267(3):379–385.
54. Barranco F, Lesmes A, Irles JA, et al. Cardiopulmonary resuscitation with simultaneous chest and abdominal compression: comparative study in humans. *Resuscitation* 1990;20(1):67–77.
55. Lindner KH, Ahnefeld FW, Bowdler IM. Cardiopulmonary resuscitation with interposed abdominal compression after asphyxial or fibrillatory cardiac arrest in pigs. *Anesthesiology* 1990;72(4):675–681.
56. Weisfeldt ML, Becker LB. Resuscitation after cardiac arrest: a 3-phase time-sensitive model. *JAMA* 2002;288(23):3035–3038.
57. Brown CG, Taylor RB, Werman HA, et al. Myocardial oxygen delivery/consumption during cardiopulmonary resuscitation: a comparison of epinephrine and phenylephrine. *Ann Emerg Med* 1988;17(4):302–308.
58. Niemann JT, Cairns CB, Sharma J, et al. Treatment of prolonged ventricular fibrillation. Immediate countershock versus high-dose epinephrine and CPR preceding countershock. *Circulation* 1992;85(1):281–287.
59. Cobb LA, Fahrenbruch CE, Walsh TR, et al. Influence of cardiopulmonary resuscitation prior to defibrillation in patients with out-of-hospital ventricular fibrillation. *JAMA* 1999;281(13):1182–1188.
60. Wik L, Hansen TB, Fylling F, et al. Delaying defibrillation to give basic cardiopulmonary resuscitation to patients with out-of-hospital ventricular fibrillation: a randomized trial. *JAMA* 2003;289(11):1389–1395.
61. van Alem AP, Sanou BT, Koster RW. Interruption of cardiopulmonary resuscitation with the use of the automated external defibrillator in out-of-hospital cardiac arrest. *Ann Emerg Med* 2003;42(4):449–457.
62. Kern KB, Hilwig RW, Berg RA, et al. Importance of continuous chest compressions during cardiopulmonary resuscitation: improved outcome during a simulated single lay-rescuer scenario. *Circulation* 2002;105(5):645–649.
63. Koster RW. Limiting 'hands-off' periods during resuscitation. *Resuscitation* 2003;58(3):275–276.
64. Eftestol T, Sunde K, Steen PA. Effects of interrupting precordial compressions on the calculated probability of defibrillation success during out-of-hospital cardiac arrest. *Circulation* 2002;105(19):2270–2273.
65. Aufderheide TP, Pirrallo RG, Yannopoulos D, et al. Incomplete chest wall decompression: a clinical evaluation of CPR performance by EMS personnel and assessment of alternative manual chest compression-decompression techniques. *Resuscitation* 2005;64(3):353–362.
66. Aufderheide TP, Lurie KG. Death by hyperventilation: a common and life-threatening problem during cardiopulmonary resuscitation. *Crit Care Med* 2004;32(9 Suppl):S345–S351.
67. Aufderheide TP, Sigurdsson G, Pirrallo RG, et al. Hyperventilation-induced hypotension during cardiopulmonary resuscitation. *Circulation* 2004;109(16):1960–1965.
68. Bossaert L, Van Hoeyweghen R. Bystander cardiopulmonary resuscitation (CPR) in out-of-hospital cardiac arrest. *Resuscitation* 1989;17:S55–S69.
69. Cobb LA, Hallstrom AP. Community-based cardiopulmonary resuscitation: What have we learned? *Ann N Y Acad Sci* 1982;382:330–342.
70. Litwin PE, Eisenberg MS, Hallstrom AP, et al. The location of collapse and its effect on survival from cardiac arrest. *Ann Emerg Med* 1987;16:787–791.
71. Dracup K, Heaney DM, Taylor SE, et al. Can family members of high-risk cardiac patients learn cardiopulmonary resuscitation? *Arch Intern Med* 1989;149(1):61–64.
72. Cobb LA, Werner JA, Trobaugh GB. Sudden cardiac death: A decade's experience with out-of-hospital resuscitation. *Mod Concepts Cardiovasc Dis* 1980;49:31.
73. Messerli FH, Soria F. Hypertension, left ventricular hypertrophy, ventricular ectopy, and sudden death. *Am J Med* 1992;93(2A):21S–26S.
74. Jimenez RA, Myerburg RJ. Sudden cardiac death. Magnitude of the problem, substrate/trigger interaction, and populations at high risk. *Cardiol Clin* 1993;11(1):1–9.
75. Fornes P, Lecomte D, Nicolas G. [Sudden coronary death outside of hospital; an comparative autopsy study of subjects with and without previous cardiovascular diseases]. *Arch Mal Coeur Vaiss* 1994;87(3):319–324.
76. Cas LD, Metra M, Nodari S, et al. Stress and ischemic heart disease. *Cardiologia* 1993;38(12 Suppl 1):415–425.
77. Kaada B. An emotional trigger mechanism for sudden infant death. *Arch Dis Child* 1991;66(2):274.
78. Bairey CN, Krantz DS, Rozanski A. Mental stress as an acute trigger of ischemic left ventricular dysfunction and blood pressure elevation in coronary artery disease. *Am J Cardiol* 1990;66(16):28G–31G.
79. Adler SR. Refugee stress and folk belief: Hmong sudden deaths. *Soc Sci Med* 1995;40(12):1623–1629.
80. Leor J, Poole WK, Kloner RA. Sudden cardiac death triggered by an earthquake. *N Engl J Med* 1996;334(7):413–419.
81. Muller JE, Abela GS, Nesto RW, et al. Triggers, acute risk factors and vulnerable plaques: the lexicon of a new frontier. *J Am Coll Cardiol* 1994;23(3):809–813.
82. Arntz HR, Willich SN, Stern R, et al. Circadian variation of cardiopulmonary disease onset in the general population: an emergency care system perspective from Berlin. *Ann Emerg Med* 1994;23(2):281–285.
83. Willich SN. Epidemiologic studies demonstrating increased morning incidence of sudden cardiac death. *Am J Cardiol* 1990;66(16):15G-17G.
84. Hohnloser SH, Klingenheben T. Insights into the pathogenesis of sudden cardiac death from analysis of circadian fluctuations of potential triggering factors. *Pacing Clin Electrophysiol* 1994;17(3 Pt 2):428–433.
85. Bayes de Luna A, Coumel P, Leclercq JF. Ambulatory sudden cardiac death: Mechanisms of production of fatal arrhythmia on the basis of data from 157 cases. *Am Heart J* 1989;117:151–159.
86. Myerburg RJ, Conde CA, Sung RJ, et al. Clinical, electro-physiologic and hemodynamic profile of patients resuscitated from prehospital cardiac arrest. *Am J Med* 1980;68(4):568–576.
87. Weaver WD, Cobb LA, Hallstrom AP, et al. Factors influencing survival after out-of-hospital cardiac arrest. *J Am Coll Cardiol* 1986;7:754.
88. Hinkle LE, Argyros DC, Hayes JC, et al. Pathogenesis of an unexpected sudden death: role of early cycle ventricular contractions. *Am J Cardiol* 1977;39:873.
89. Schaffer WA, Cobb LA. Recurrent ventricular fibrillation and modes of death in survivors of out-of-hospital ventricular fibrillation. *N Engl J Med* 1975;293(6):259–262.
90. Cummins RO, Ornato JP, Thies WH, et al. Improving survival from sudden cardiac arrest: the "chain of survival" concept. A statement for health professionals from the Advanced Cardiac Life Support Subcommittee and the Emergency Cardiac Care Committee, American Heart Association. *Circulation* 1991;83(5):1832–1847.
91. Eisenberg MS, Bergner L, Hallstrom A. Cardiac resuscitation in the community. Importance of rapid provision and implications for program planning. *JAMA* 1979;241:1905–1907.
92. Walters G, Gluckman F. Planning a pre-hospital cardiac resuscitation programme: An analysis of community and system factors in London. *J R Coll Physicians Lond* 1989;23:107.
93. Stults KR. Phone first. *J Emerg Med Services* 1987;12:78.
94. Murphy RJ, Luepker RV, Jacobs DRJ, et al. Citizen cardiopulmonary resuscitation training and use in a metropolitan area: The Minnesota Heart Survey. *Am J Public Health* 1984;74:513–515.
95. Selby ML, Kautz JA, Moore TJ, et al. Indicators of response to a mass media CPR recruitment campaign. *Am J Public Health* 1982;72:1039.
96. Van Camp SP, Peterson RA. Cardiovascular complications of outpatient cardiac rehabilitation programs. *JAMA* 1986;256(9):1160–1163.
97. Haskell WL. Cardiovascular complications during exercise training in cardiac patients. *Circulation* 1978;57:920.
98. Hossack KF, Hartwig R. Cardiac arrest associated with supervised cardiac rehabilitation. *J Cardiac Rehab* 1982;2:402.
99. Kaye W, Mancini ME, Giuliano KK, et al. Strengthening the in hospital chain of survival with rapid defibrillation by first responders using automated external defibrillators: training and retention issues. *Ann Emerg Med* 1995;25(2):163–168.
100. Barnes TA, Aufderheide TP, Mathews, et al. Clinical practice guidelines for resuscitation in acute care hospitals. *Respir Care* 1995;40(4):346–363.
101. 2005 American Heart Association Guidelines for Cardiopulmonary Resuscitation and Emergency Cardiovascular Care. *Circulation.* 2005;112 (Suppl IV):W-58–W-66.
102. The American Heart Association in collaboration with the International Liaison Committee on Resuscitation. Guidelines 2000 for cardiopulmonary resuscitation and emergency cardiovascular care. Part 6: Advanced cardiovascular life support: 7B: Understanding the algorithm approach to ACLS. *Circulation* 2000;102(8 Suppl):I140–II141.
103. Schneider T, Martens PR, Paschen H, et al. Multicenter, randomized, controlled trial of 150-J biphasic shocks compared with 200- to 360-J monophasic shocks in the resuscitation of out-of-hospital cardiac arrest victims. *Circulation* 2000;102(15):1780–1787.
104. Gliner BE, White RD. Electrocardiographic evaluation of defibrillation shocks delivered to out-of-hospital sudden cardiac arrest patients. *Resuscitation* 1999;41(2):133–144.
105. White RD, Blanton DM. Biphasic truncated exponential waveform defibrillation. *Prehosp Emerg Care* 1999;3(4):283–289.
106. Gliner BE, Jorgenson DB, Poole JE, et al. Treatment of out-of-hospital cardiac arrest with a low-energy impedance-compensating biphasic waveform automatic external defibrillator. The LIFE Investigators. *Biomed Instrum Technol* 1998;32(6):631–644.
107. Bardy GH, Marchlinski FE, Sharma AD, et al. Multicenter comparison of truncated biphasic shocks and standard damped sine wave monophasic shocks for transthoracic ventricular defibrillation. Transthoracic Investigators. *Circulation* 1996;94(10):2507–2514.
108. Cummins RO, Hazinski MF, Kerber RE, et al. Low-energy biphasic waveform defibrillation: evidence-based review applied to emergency cardiovascular care guidelines: a statement for healthcare professionals from the American Heart Association Committee on Emergency Cardiovascular Care and the Subcommittees on Basic Life Support, Advanced Cardiac Life Support, and Pediatric Resuscitation. *Circulation* 1998;97(16):1654–1667.
109. The American Heart Association in collaboration with the International Liaison Committee on Resuscitation. Guidelines 2000 for cardiopulmonary resuscitation and emergency cardiovascular care. Part 6: Advanced cardiovascular life support: Section 7: Algorithm approach to ACLS emergencies: Section 7A: principles and practice of ACLS. *Circulation* 2000;102(8 Suppl):I136–I139.
110. Ewy GA. Defining electromechanical dissociation. *Ann Emerg Med* 1984; 13:830–832.
111. Ornato JP. Special resuscitation situations: near drowning, traumatic injury, electric shock, and hypothermia. *Circulation* 1986;74(6 Pt 2):IV23–IV26.

112. Harrison EE, Amey BD. Use of calcium in electromechanical dissociation. *Ann Emerg Med* 1984;13:944–945.
113. Stueven H, Thompson BM, Aprahamian C, et al. Use of calcium in prehospital cardiac arrest. *Ann Emerg Med* 1983;12:136–139.
114. Dembo DH. Calcium in advanced life support. *Crit Care Med* 1981;9:358–359.
115. Carlon GC, Howland WS, Kahn RC, et al. Calcium chloride administration in normocalcemic critically ill patients. *Crit Care Med* 1980;8:209–212.
116. Schanne FAX, Kane AB, Young EE, et al. Calcium dependence of toxic cell death: a final common pathway. *Science* 1979;206:700–702.
117. Bodai BI, Smith JPT, Ward RE, et al. Emergency thoracotomy in the management of trauma. A review. *JAMA* 1983;249:1891–1896.
118. Paradis NA, Martin GB, Rivers EP. Use of open chest cardiopulmonary resuscitation after failure of standard closed chest CPR: illustrative cases. *Resuscitation* 1992;24(1):61–71.
119. Battistella FD, Nugent W, Owings JT, et al. Field triage of the pulseless trauma patient. *Arch Surg* 1999;134(7):742–745; discussion, 745–746.
120. Ewy GA, Dahl CF, Zimmerman M, et al. Ventricular fibrillation masquerading as ventricular standstill. *Crit Care Med* 1981;9:841–844.
121. Iseri LT, Humphrey SB, Siner EJ. Prehospital bradyasystolic cardiac arrest. *Ann Intern Med* 1978;88:741–745.
122. O'Rourke GW, Greene NM. Autonomic blockade and the resting heart rate in man. *Am Heart J* 1970;80:469–474.
123. Ornato JP, Carveth WL, Windle JR. Pacemaker insertion for prehospital bradyasystolic cardiac arrest. *Ann Emerg Med* 1984;13(2):101–103.
124. Zoll PM, Zoll RH, Falk RH, et al. External noninvasive temporary cardiac pacing. *Circulation* 1985;71:937–944.
125. Falk RH, Jacobs L, Sinclair A, et al. External noninvasive cardiac pacing in out-of-hospital cardiac arrest. *Crit Care Med* 1983;11:779–782.
126. Tucker KJ, Shaburihvili TS, Gedevanishvili AT. Manual external (fist) pacing during high-degree atrioventricular block: a lifesaving intervention. *Am J Emerg Med* 1995;13(1):53–54.
127. Belardinelli L, Linder J, Berne RM. The cardiac effects of adenosine. *Prog Cardiovasc Dis* 1989;32:73–97.
128. Clemo HF, Belardinelli L. Effect of adenosine on atrioventricular conduction. I. Site and characterization of adenosine action in the guinea pig atrioventricular node. *Circ Res* 1986;59:427–436.
129. Viskin S, Belhassen B, Roth A, et al. Aminophylline for bradyasystolic cardiac arrest refractory to atropine and epinephrine. *Ann Intern Med* 1993; 118:279–281.
130. Gareis R, Stork T, Mockel M, et al. Theophylline in rhythm asystole and pulse-less bradyarrhythmia. *Intensiv Notfallbehandlung* 1995;32(2):147–154.
131. Mader TJ, Smithline HA, Gibson P. Aminophylline in undifferentiated out-of-hospital asystolic cardiac arrest. *Resuscitation* 1999;41(1):39–45.
132. Littmann L, Ashline PT, Hayes WJ, et al. Aminophylline fails to improve the outcome of cardiopulmonary resuscitation from prolonged ventricular fibrillation: a placebo-controlled, randomized, blinded experimental study. *J Am Coll Cardiol* 1994;23(7):1708–1714.
133. Kovach AGB, Sandor P. Cerebral blood flow and brain function during hypotension and shock. *Annu Rev Physiol* 1976;38:571.
134. Michael JR, Guerci AD, Koehler RC, et al. Mechanisms by which epinephrine augments cerebral and myocardial perfusion during cardiopulmonary resuscitation in dogs. *Circulation* 1984;69:822–835.
135. Crile G, Dolley DH. An experimental research into the resuscitation of dogs killed by anesthetics and asphyxia. *J Exp Med* 1906;8:713–725.
136. Crile GW. Preliminary note on a method of resuscitation of apparently recently dead animals. *Cleve Med J* 1903;2:35.
137. Redding JS, Pearson JW. Resuscitation from ventricular fibrillation. *JAMA* 1969;203:255–260.
138. Pearson JW, Redding JS. Influence of peripheral vascular tone on cardiac resuscitation. *Anesth Analg* 1967;46:746–752.
139. Pearson JW, Redding JS. Peripheral vascular tone in cardiac resuscitation. *Anesth Analg* 1965;44:746–762.
140. Pearson JW, Redding JS. The role of epinephrine in cardiac resuscitation. *Anesth Analg* 1963;42:599–606.
141. Pearson JW, Redding JS. Epinephrine in cardiac resuscitation. *Am Heart J* 1963;66:210–214.
142. Kern KB, Ewy GA, Voorhees WD, et al. Myocardial perfusion pressure: a predictor of 24-hour survival during prolonged cardiac arrest in dogs. *Resuscitation* 1988;16(4):241–250.
143. Niemann JT. Differences in cerebral and myocardial perfusion during closed-chest resuscitation. *Ann Emerg Med* 1984;13:849–853.
144. Sanders AB, Ewy GA, Taft TV. Prognostic and therapeutic importance of the aortic diastolic pressure in resuscitation from cardiac arrest. *Crit Care Med* 1984;12:871–873.
145. Paradis NA, Martin GB, Rivers EP, et al. Coronary perfusion pressure and the return of spontaneous circulation in human cardiopulmonary resuscitation. *JAMA* 1990;263(8):1106–1113.
146. Ralston SH, Voorhees WD, Babbs CF. Intrapulmonary epinephrine during prolonged cardiopulmonary resuscitation: improved regional blood flow and resuscitation in dogs. *Ann Emerg Med* 1984;13:79–86.
147. Grunau CFV. Doppler ultrasound monitoring of systemic blood flow during CPR. *JACEP* 1978;1978:180–185.
148. Taylor GJ, Tucker WM, Greene HL, et al. Importance of prolonged compression during cardiopulmonary resuscitation in man. *N Engl J Med* 1977;296:1515–1517.
149. McDonald JL. Systolic and mean arterial pressures during manual and mechanical CPR in humans. *Ann Emerg Med* 1982;11:292–295.
150. Ornato JP, Levine RL, Young DS, et al. The effect of applied chest compression force on systemic arterial pressure and end-tidal carbon dioxide concentration during CPR in human beings. *Ann Emerg Med* 1989;18(7):732–737.
151. Chandra NC, Tsitlik JE, Halperin HR, et al. Observations of hemodynamics during human cardiopulmonary resuscitation. *Crit Care Med* 1990;18(9):929–934.
152. Sanders AB, Oble M, Ewy GA. Coronary perfusion pressure during cardiopulmonary resuscitation. *Am J Emerg Med* 1985;3:11–14.
153. Swenson RD, Weaver WD, Niskanen RA, et al. Hemodynamics in humans during conventional and experimental methods of cardiopulmonary resuscitation. *Circulation* 1988;78(3):630–639.
154. Gonzalez ER, Ornato JP, Garnett AR, et al. Dose-dependent vasopressor response to epinephrine during CPR in human beings. *Ann Emerg Med* 1989;18(9):920–926.
155. Paradis NA, Martin GB, Goetting MG, et al. Aortic pressure during human cardiac arrest. Identification of pseudo-electromechanical dissociation. *Chest* 1992;101(1):123–128.
156. Thomsen JE, Stenlund RR, Rowe GG. Intracardiac pressures during closed-chest cardiac massage. *JAMA* 1968;205:116–118.
157. Paradis NA, Martin GB, Goetting MG, et al. Simultaneous aortic, jugular bulb, and right atrial pressures during cardiopulmonary resuscitation in humans. Insights into mechanisms. *Circulation* 1989;80(2):361–368.
158. Chandra N, Guerci A, Weisfeldt ML, et al. Contrasts between intrathoracic pressures during external chest compression and cardiac massage. *Crit Care Med* 1981;9:789–792.
159. Rudikoff MT, Maughan WL, Effron M, et al. Mechanism of blood flow during cardiopulmonary resuscitation. *Circulation* 1980;61:345–352.
160. Newton Jr JR, Glower DD, Wolfe JA, et al. A physiologic comparison of external cardiac massage techniques. *J Thorac Cardiovasc Surg* 1988;95(5): 892–901.
161. Ornato JP, Ryschon TW, Gonzalez ER, et al. Rapid change in pulmonary vascular hemodynamics with pulmonary edema during cardiopulmonary resuscitation. *Am J Emerg Med* 1985;3(2):137–142.
162. Dohi S, Ujike Y, Nishikawa T, et al. Pulmonary hemodynamics during external cardiac massage in humans. *Jpn Heart J* 1982;31:222–228.
163. Dohi S. Post-cardiopulmonary resuscitation pulmonary edema. *Crit Care Med* 1983;11:434–437.
164. Paidipaty BBT, Kyff J, Vaughn S, et al. Pulmonary artery catheterization and hemodynamic monitoring after cardiopulmonary resuscitation. *Acute Care* 1984;10:189–193.
165. Ward KR, Yealy DM. End-tidal carbon dioxide monitoring in emergency medicine, Part 1: Basic principles. *Acad Emerg Med* 1998;5(6):628–636.
166. Ward KR, Yealy DM. End-tidal carbon dioxide monitoring in emergency medicine, Part 2: Clinical applications. *Acad Emerg Med* 1998;5(6):637–646.
167. Ornato JP, Garnett AR, Glauser FL. Relationship between cardiac output and the end-tidal carbon dioxide tension. *Ann Emerg Med* 1990;19(10): 1104–1106.
168. Phan CQ, Tremper KK, Lee SE, et al. Noninvasive monitoring of carbon dioxide: A comparison of the partial pressure of transcutaneous and end-tidal carbon dioxide with the partial pressure of arterial carbon dioxide. *J Clin Monit* 1987;3:149–154.
169. Goldberg JS, Rawle PR, Zehnder JL, et al. Colorimetric end-tidal carbon dioxide monitoring for tracheal intubation. *Anesth Analg* 1990; 70:191–194.
170. Strunin L, Williams T. The FEF end-tidal carbon dioxide detector. *Anesthesiology* 1989;71:621–622.
171. MacLeod BA, Heller MB, Gerard J, et al. Verification of endotracheal tube placement with colorimetric end-tidal CO2 detection. *Ann Emerg Med* 1991;20(3):267–270.
172. Menegazzi JJ, Heller MB. Endotracheal tube confirmation with colorimetric CO2 detectors. *Anesth Analg* 1990;71:440–446.
173. Ornato JP, Shipley JB, Racht EM, et al. Multicenter study of a portable, hand-size, colorimetric end-tidal carbon dioxide detection device. *Ann Emerg Med* 1992;21(5):518–523.
174. Garnett AR, Gervin CA, Gervin AS. Capnographic waveforms in esophageal intubation: effect of carbonated beverages. *Ann Emerg Med* 1989;18:387–390.
175. MacKenzie GJ, Taylor SH. Haemodynamic effects of external cardiac compression. *Lancet* 1964;1:1342–1345.
176. Del Guercio LRM, Feins NR, Cohn JD, et al. Comparison of blood flow during external and internal cardiac massage in man. *Circulation* 1965;31 (Suppl 1):171–180.
177. Del Guercio LRM, Coomaraswamy RP, State D. Cardiac output and other hemodynamic variables during external cardiac massage in man. *N Engl J Med* 1963;269:1398–1404.
178. Garnett AR, Ornato JP, Gonzalez ER, et al. End-tidal carbon dioxide monitoring during cardiopulmonary resuscitation. *JAMA* 1987;257(4): 512–515.
179. Falk JL, Rackow EC, Weil MH. End-tidal carbon dioxide concentration during cardiopulmonary resuscitation. *N Engl J Med* 1988;318(10):607–611.

180. Gudipati CV, Weil MH, Bisera J, et al. Expired carbon dioxide: a noninvasive monitor of cardiopulmonary resuscitation. *Circulation* 1988;77:234–239.
181. Weil MH, Bisera J, Trevino RP, et al. Cardiac output and end tidal carbon dioxide. *Crit Care Med* 1985;13:907–909.
182. Kalenda Z. The capnogram as a guide to the efficacy of cardiac massage. *Resuscitation* 1978;6:259–263.
183. Sanders AB, Atlas M, Ewy GA, et al. Expired PCO2 as an index of coronary perfusion pressure. *Am J Emerg Med* 1985;3(2):147–149.
184. Kern KB, Sanders AB, Voorhees WD, et al. Changes in expired end-tidal carbon dioxide during cardiopulmonary resuscitation in dogs: a prognostic guide for resuscitation efforts. *J Am Coll Cardiol* 1989;13(5):1184–1189.
185. Sanders AB, Kern KB, Otto CW, et al. End-tidal carbon dioxide monitoring during cardiopulmonary resuscitation. A prognostic indicator for survival. *JAMA* 1989;262(10):1347–1351.
186. Weil MH, Rackow EC, Trevino R, et al. Difference in acid–base state between venous and arterial blood during cardiopulmonary resuscitation. *N Engl J Med* 1986;315(3):153–156.
187. Chase PB, Kern KB, Sanders AB, et al. Effects of graded doses of epinephrine on both noninvasive and invasive measures of myocardial perfusion and blood flow during cardiopulmonary resuscitation. *Crit Care Med* 1993;21(3):413–419.
188. Angelos MG, DeBehnke DJ. Epinephrine-mediated changes in carbon dioxide tension during reperfusion of ventricular fibrillation in a canine model. *Crit Care Med* 1995;23(5):925–930.
189. Callaham M, Barton C, Matthay M. Effect of epinephrine on the ability of end-tidal carbon dioxide readings to predict initial resuscitation from cardiac arrest. *Crit Care Med* 1992;20(3):337–343.
190. Chopin C, Fesard P, Mangalaboyi J, et al. Use of capnography in diagnosis of pulmonary embolism during acute respiratory failure of chronic obstructive pulmonary disease. *Crit Care Med* 1990;18:353–357.
191. Ornato JP. Hemodynamic monitoring during CPR. *Ann Emerg Med* 1993; 22(2 Pt 2):289–295.
192. The American Heart Association in collaboration with the International Liaison Committee on Resuscitation. Guidelines 2000 for cardiopulmonary resuscitation and emergency cardiovascular care. Part 6: Advanced cardiovascular life support: Section 3: Adjuncts for oxygenation, ventilation and airway control. *Circulation* 2000;102(8 Suppl):I95–I104.
193. Klausner JM, Lelcuk S, Gutman M, et al. Expired carbon dioxide: a noninvasive monitor of cardiopulmonary resuscitation. *Circulation* 1988; 77(1):234–239.
194. Domsky M, Wilson RF, Heins J. Intraoperative end-tidal carbon dioxide values and derived calculations correlated with outcome: prognosis and capnography. *Crit Care Med* 1995;23(9):1497–1503.
195. Asplin BR, White RD. Prognostic value of end-tidal carbon dioxide pressures during out-of-hospital cardiac arrest. *Ann Emerg Med* 1995;25(6): 756–761.
196. Cantineau JP, Lambert Y, Merckx P, et al. End-tidal carbon dioxide during cardiopulmonary resuscitation in humans presenting mostly with asystole: a predictor of outcome. *Crit Care Med* 1996;24(5):791–796.
197. von Planta M, von Planta I, Bisera J, et al. Determinants of survival in cardiopulmonary resuscitation. *Med Klin* 1990;85(4):181–186, 228.
198. Herschman Z, Lorbert J, Rahal W, et al. End-tidal CO2 and prognosis. *Crit Care Med* 1996;24(6):1093.
199. Levine RL, Wayne MA, Miller CC. End-tidal carbon dioxide and outcome of out-of-hospital cardiac arrest. *N Engl J Med* 1997;337(5):301–306.
200. Martin GB, Gentile NT, Paradis NA, et al. Effect of epinephrine on end-tidal carbon dioxide monitoring during CPR. *Ann Emerg Med* 1990;19(4):396–398.
201. Lindner KH, Ahnefeld FW, Bowdler IM, et al. Influence of epinephrine on systemic, myocardial, and cerebral acid–base status during cardiopulmonary resuscitation. *Anesthesiology* 1991;74(2):333–339.
202. Cantineau JP, Merckx P, Lambert Y, et al. Effect of epinephrine on end-tidal carbon dioxide pressure during prehospital cardiopulmonary resuscitation. *Am J Emerg Med* 1994;12(3):267–270.
203. Berg RA, Otto CW, Kern KB, et al. High-dose epinephrine results in greater early mortality after resuscitation from prolonged cardiac arrest in pigs: a prospective, randomized study. *Crit Care Med* 1994;22(2):282–290.
204. Werner JA, Greene HL, Janko CL, et al. Two-dimensional echocardiography during CPR in man: implications regarding the mechanism of blood flow. *Crit Care Med* 1981;9:375–376.
205. Werner JA, Greene HL, Janko CL, et al. Visualization of cardiac valve motion in man during external chest compression using two-dimensional echocardiography: implications regarding the mechanism of blood flow. *Circulation* 1981;63:1417–1421.
206. Higano ST, Oh JK, Ewy GA, et al. The mechanism of blood flow during closed chest cardiac massage in humans: transesophageal echocardiographic observations. *Mayo Clin Proc* 1990;65(11):1432–1440.
207. Hackl W, Simon P, Mauritz W, et al. Echocardiographic assessment of mitral valve function during mechanical cardiopulmonary resuscitation in pigs. *Anesth Analg* 1990;70(4):350–356.
208. Halperin HR, Weiss JL, Guerci AD, et al. Cyclic elevation of intrathoracic pressure can close the mitral valve during cardiac arrest in dogs. *Circulation* 1988;78(3):754–760.
209. Deshmukh HG, Weil MH, Gudipati CV, et al. Mechanism of blood flow generated by precordial compression during CPR. I. Studies on closed chest precordial compression. *Chest* 1989;95(5):1092–1099.
210. Rich S, Wix HL, Shapiro EP. Clinical assessment of heart chamber size and valve motion during cardiopulmonary resuscitation by two-dimensional echocardiography. *Am Heart J* 1981;102:368–373.
211. Ma MHM, Huang GT, Wang SM, et al. Aortic valve disruption and regurgitation complicating CPR detected by transesophageal echocardiography [1]. *Am J Emerg Med* 1994;12(5):601–602.
212. Nomura T, Shinzawa M, Hashimoto K, et al. Usefulness of transesophageal echocardiography in a case of cardiac arrest during anesthesia. *Anesth Resusc* 1994;30(3):243–246.
213. Ma MH, Hwang JJ, Lai LP, et al. Transesophageal echocardiographic assessment of mitral valve position and pulmonary venous flow during cardiopulmonary resuscitation in humans. *Circulation* 1995;92(4):854–861.
214. Pell AC, Guly UM, Sutherland GR, et al. Mechanism of closed chest cardiopulmonary resuscitation investigated by transoesophageal echocardiography. *J Accid Emerg Med* 1994;11(3):139–143.
215. Redberg RF, Tucker K, Schiller NB. Transesophageal echocardiography during cardiopulmonary resuscitation. *Cardiol Clin* 1993;11(3):529–535.
216. Ornato JP. Should bystanders perform mouth-to-mouth ventilation during resuscitation? *Chest* 1994;106(6):1641–1642.
217. Idris AH. Is mouth-to-mouth ventilation necessary for successful resuscitation? *Chest* 1995;108(6):1490–1491.
218. Locke CJ, Berg RA, Sanders AB, et al. Bystander cardiopulmonary resuscitation: concerns about mouth-to-mouth contact. *Arch Intern Med* 1995;155(9):938–943.
219. Wenzel V, Idris AH, Banner MJ, et al. The composition of gas given by mouth-to-mouth ventilation during CPR. *Chest* 1994;106(6):1806–1810.
220. Idris AH. Reassessing the need for ventilation during CPR. *Ann Emerg Med* 1996;27(5):569–575.
221. Ornato JP, Hallagan LF, McMahon SB, et al. Attitudes of BCLS instructors about mouth-to-mouth resuscitation during the AIDS epidemic. *Ann Emerg Med* 1990(19):151–156.
222. Safar P. Initiation of closed-chest cardiopulmonary resuscitation basic life support. A personal history. *Resuscitation* 1989;18(1):7–20.
223. Lawrence PJ, Sivaneswaran N. Ventilation during cardiopulmonary resuscitation: which method? *Med J Aust* 1985;143(10):443–446.
224. Brenner BE, Kauffmann J. Response to cardiac arrests in a hospital setting: delays in ventilation. *Resuscitation* 1996;31(1):17–23.
225. Chandra NC, Gruben KG, Tsitlik JE, et al. Observations of ventilation during resuscitation in a canine model. *Circulation* 1994;90(6):3070–3075.
226. Van Hoeyweghen RJ, Bossaert LL, Mullie A, et al. Quality and efficiency of bystander CPR. Belgian Cerebral Resuscitation Study Group. *Resuscitation* 1993;26(1):47–52.
227. The American Heart Association in collaboration with the International Liaison Committee on Resuscitation. Guidelines 2000 for cardiopulmonary resuscitation and emergency cardiovascular care. Part 3: Adult basic life support. *Circulation* 2000;102(8 Suppl):I22–I59.
228. Hallstrom A, Cobb L, Johnson E, et al. Cardiopulmonary resuscitation by chest compression alone or with mouth-to-mouth ventilation. *N Engl J Med* 2000;342(21):1546–1553.
229. Clark JJ, Larsen MP, Culley LL, et al. Incidence of agonal respirations in sudden cardiac arrest. *Ann Emerg Med* 1992;21(12):1464–1467.
230. Ornato JP, Bryson BB, Donovan PJ, et al. Measurement of ventilation during cardiopulmonary resuscitation. *Crit Care Med* 1983;11(2):79–82.
231. Melker RJ. Recommendations for ventilation during cardiopulmonary resuscitation: time for change? *Crit Care Med* 1985;13(11):882–883.
232. Koehler RC, Michael JR, Guerci AD, et al. Beneficial effect of epinephrine infusion on cerebral and myocardial blood flow during CPR. *Ann Emerg Med* 1985;14:744–749.
233. Otto CW, Yakaitas RW. The role of epinephrine in CPR: a reappraisal. *Ann Emerg Med* 1984;13:840–843.
234. White RD. Defining the pressure needs of the fibrillating heart during prolonged arrest: identification and application. *Ann Emerg Med* 1985;14: 587–588.
235. Niemann JT, Criley JM, Rosborough JP, et al. Beneficial effect. Predictive indices of successful cardiac resuscitation after prolonged arrest and experimental cardiopulmonary resuscitation. *Ann Emerg Med* 1985;14(6):521–528.
236. Sanders AB, Ogle M, Ewy GA. Coronary perfusion pressure during cardiopulmonary resuscitation. *Am J Emerg Med* 1985;3(1):11–14.
237. Raessler KL, Kern KB, Sanders AB, et al. Beneficial effect. Aortic and right atrial systolic pressures during cardiopulmonary resuscitation: a potential indicator of the mechanism of blood flow. *Am Heart J* 1988;115(5):1021–1029.
238. Lindner KH, Ahnefeld FW, Bowdler IM. The effect of epinephrine on hemodynamics, acid-base status and potassium during spontaneous circulation and cardiopulmonary resuscitation. *Resuscitation* 1988;16(4):251–261.
239. Ditchey RV, Lindenfeld J. Failure of epinephrine to improve the balance between myocardial oxygen supply and demand during closed-chest resuscitation in dogs. *Circulation* 1988;78(2):382–389.
240. Ditchey RV, Goto Y, Lindenfeld J. Myocardial oxygen requirements during experimental cardiopulmonary resuscitation. *Cardiovasc Res* 1992;26(8): 791–797.
241. Paradis NA, Brown CG. High-dose adrenaline and cardiac arrest [Letter]. *Lancet* 1988;2(8613):749.

242. Goetting MG, Paradis NA. High dose epinephrine in refractory pediatric cardiac arrest. *Crit Care Med* 1989;17(12):1258–1262.
243. Callaham M. Epinephrine doses in cardiac arrest: Is it time to outgrow the orthodoxy of ACLS? *Ann Emerg Med* 1989;18:1011–1012.
244. Martin D, Werman HA, Brown CG. Four case studies: high-dose epinephrine in cardiac arrest. *Ann Emerg Med* 1990;19(3):322–326.
245. Paradis NA, Koscove EM. Epinephrine in cardiac arrest: a critical review. *Ann Emerg Med* 1990;19(11):1288–1301.
246. Callaham ML. High-dose epinephrine therapy and other advances in treating cardiac arrest. *West J Med* 1990;152(6):697–703.
247. Cipolotti G, Paccagnella A, Simini G. Successful cardiopulmonary resuscitation using high doses of epinephrine. *Int J Cardiol* 1991;33(3):430–431.
248. Paradis NA, Martin GB, Rosenberg J, et al. The effect of standard- and high-dose epinephrine on coronary perfusion pressure during prolonged cardiopulmonary resuscitation. *JAMA* 1991;265(9):1139–1144.
249. Goetting MG, Paradis NA. High-dose epinephrine improves outcome from pediatric cardiac arrest. *Ann Emerg Med* 1991;20(1):22–26.
250. Brown CG, Martin DR, Pepe PE, et al. A comparison of standard dose epinephrine and high dose epinephrine in cardiac arrest outside the hospital. *N Engl J Med* 1992;327:1051–1055.
251. Achleitner U, Wenzel V, Strohmenger HU, et al. The effects of repeated doses of vasopressin or epinephrine on ventricular fibrillation in a porcine model of prolonged cardiopulmonary resuscitation. *Anesth Analg* 2000;90(5):1067–1075.
252. Berg RA, Otto CW, Kern KB, et al. A randomized, blinded trial of high-dose epinephrine versus standard-dose epinephrine in a swine model of pediatric asphyxial cardiac arrest. *Crit Care Med* 1996;24(10):1695–1700.
253. Dieckmann RA, Vardis R. High-dose epinephrine in pediatric out-of-hospital cardiopulmonary arrest. *Pediatrics* 1995;95(6):901–913.
254. Stiell IG, Hebert PC, Weitzman BN, et al. A study of high-dose epinephrine in human CPR. *N Engl J Med* 1992;327:1047–1050.
255. Callaham M, Madsen CD, Barton CW, et al. A randomized clinical trial of high-dose epinephrine and norepinephrine vs standard-dose epinephrine in prehospital cardiac arrest. *JAMA* 1992;268(19):2667–2672.
256. Lipman J, Wilson W, Kobilski S, et al. High-dose adrenaline in adult in-hospital asystolic cardiopulmonary resuscitation: a double-blind randomised trial. *Anaesth Intensive Care* 1993;21(2):192–196.
257. Choux C, Gueugniaud PY, Barbieux A, et al. Standard doses versus repeated high doses of epinephrine in cardiac arrest outside the hospital. *Resuscitation* 1995;29(1):3–9.
258. Carpenter TC, Stenmark KR. High-dose epinephrine is not superior to standard-dose epinephrine in pediatric in-hospital cardiopulmonary arrest. *Pediatrics* 1997;99(3):403–408.
259. Gueugniaud PY, Mols P, Goldstein P, et al. A comparison of repeated high doses and repeated standard doses of epinephrine for cardiac arrest outside the hospital. European Epinephrine Study Group. *N Engl J Med* 1998;339(22):1595–1601.
260. Lindner KH, Ahnefeld FW, Prengel AW. Comparison of standard and high-dose adrenaline in the resuscitation of asystole and electromechanical dissociation. *Acta Anaesthesiol Scand* 1991;35(3):253–256.
261. Sherman BW, Munger MA, Foulke GE, et al. High-dose versus standard-dose epinephrine treatment of cardiac arrest after failure of standard therapy. *Pharmacotherapy* 1997;17(2):242–247.
262. The American Heart Association in collaboration with the International Liaison Committee on Resuscitation. Guidelines 2000 for cardiopulmonary resuscitation and emergency cardiovascular care. Part 6: Advanced cardiovascular life support: Section 6: Pharmacology II: Agents to optimize cardiac output and blood pressure. *Circulation* 2000;102(8 Suppl):I129–I135.
263. Lindner KH, Prengel AW, Pfenninger EG, et al. Vasopressin improves vital organ blood flow during closed-chest cardiopulmonary resuscitation in pigs. *Circulation* 1995;91(1):215–221.
264. Morris DC, Dereczyk BE, Grzybowski M, et al. Vasopressin can increase coronary perfusion pressure during human cardiopulmonary resuscitation. *Acad Emerg Med* 1997;4(9):878–883.
265. Lindner KH, Haak T, Keller A, et al. Release of endogenous vasopressors during and after cardiopulmonary resuscitation. *Heart* 1996;75(2):145–150.
266. Lindner KH, Dirks B, Strohmenger HU, et al. Randomised comparison of epinephrine and vasopressin in patients with out-of-hospital ventricular fibrillation. *Lancet* 1997;349(9051):535–537.
267. Stiell IG, Hebert PC, Wells GA, et al. Vasopressin versus epinephrine for inhospital cardiac arrest: a randomised controlled trial. *Lancet* 2001;358(9276):105–109.
268. Wenzel V, Krismer AC, Arntz HR, et al. A comparison of vasopressin and epinephrine for out-of-hospital cardiopulmonary resuscitation. *N Engl J Med* 2004;350(2):105–113.
269. Voeckel WG, Lurie KG, Lindner KH, et al. Comparison of epinephrine and vasopressin in a pediatric porcine model of asphyxial cardiac arrest [Abstract]. *Circulation* 1999;100(Suppl I):I-316/1654.
270. The American Heart Association in collaboration with the International Liaison Committee on Resuscitation. Guidelines 2000 for cardiopulmonary resuscitation and emergency cardiovascular care. Part 10: Pediatric advanced life support. *Circulation* 2000;102(8 Suppl):I291–I342.
271. Weil MH, Trevino RP, Rackow EC. Sodium bicarbonate during CPR. Does it help or hinder? *Chest* 1985;88(4):487.
272. Weil MH, Ruiz CE, Michaels S, et al. Acid–base determinants of survival after cardiopulmonary resuscitation. *Crit Care Med* 1985;13(11):888–892.
273. Bishop RL, Weisfeldt ML. Sodium bicarbonate administration during cardiac arrest. *JAMA* 1976;235:506–509.
274. Grundler W, Weil MH, Yamaguchi M, et al. The paradox of venous acidosis and arterial alkalosis during CPR. *Chest* 1984;86:282.
275. MacGregor DC, Wilson GJ, Holmes DE, et al. Intramyocardial carbon dioxide tension: a guide to the safe period of anoxic arrest of the heart. *J Thorac Cardiovasc Surg* 1974;68:101–107.
276. Jaffe AS. New and old paradoxes. Acidosis and cardiopulmonary resuscitation. *Circulation* 1989;80(4):1079–1083.
277. Kette F, Weil MH, von Planta M, et al. Buffer agents do not reverse intramyocardial acidosis during cardiac resuscitation. *Circulation* 1990;81(5):1660–1666.
278. Ornato JP, Gonzalez ER, Coyne MR, et al. Arterial pH in out-of-hospital cardiac arrest: response time as a determinant of acidosis. *Am J Emerg Med* 1985;3(6):498–502.
279. Niemann JT, Rosborough JP. Effects of acidemia and sodium bicarbonate therapy in advanced cardiac life support. *Ann Emerg Med* 1984;13:781–784.
280. Clancy RL, Cingolani HE, Taylor RR, et al. Influence of sodium bicarbonate on myocardial performance. *Am J Physiol* 1967;212:917–923.
281. Graf H, Leach W, Arieff AI. Evidence for a detrimental effect of bicarbonate therapy in hypoxic lactic acidosis. *Science* 1985;227:754–756.
282. Berenyi KJ, Wolk M, Killip T. Cerebrospinal fluid acidosis complicating therapy of experimental cardiopulmonary arrest. *Circulation* 1975;52:319–324.
283. Redding JS, Pearson JW. Metabolic acidosis: a factor in cardiac resuscitation. *South Med J* 1967;60:926–932.
284. Yakaitas RW, Thomas JD, Mahaffey JE. Influence of pH and hypoxia on the success of defibrillation. *Crit Care Med* 1975;3:139–142.
285. Guerci AD, Chandra N, Johnson E, et al. Failure of sodium bicarbonate to improve resuscitation from ventricular fibrillation in dogs. *Circulation* 1986;74(6 Pt 2):IV75–IV79.
286. Gazmuri RJ, von Planta M, Weil MH, et al. Cardiac effects of carbon dioxide–consuming and carbon dioxide–generating buffers during cardiopulmonary resuscitation. *J Am Coll Cardiol* 1990;15(2):482–490.
287. Bersin RM, Chatterjee K, Arieff AI. Metabolic and hemodynamic consequences of sodium bicarbonate administration in patients with heart disease. *Am J Med* 1989;87:7–14.
288. Cooper DJ, Walley KR, Wiggs BR, et al. Bicarbonate does not improve hemodynamics in critically ill patients who have lactic acidosis. A prospective, controlled clinical study. *Ann Intern Med* 1990;112:492–498.
289. Dybvik T, Strand T, Steen PA. Buffer therapy during out-of-hospital cardiopulmonary resuscitation. *Resuscitation* 1995;29(2):89–95.
290. The American Heart Association in collaboration with the International Liaison Committee on Resuscitation. Guidelines 2000 for cardiopulmonary resuscitation and emergency cardiovascular care. Part 6: Advanced cardiovascular life support: Section 5: pharmacology I: Agents for arrhythmias. *Circulation* 2000;102(8 Suppl):I112–II128.
291. Morgan DB, Davidson C. Hypokalemia and diuretics: an analysis of publications. *Br Med J* 1980;280:905–909.
292. Hollifield JW. Potassium and magnesium abnormalities: diuretics and arrhythmias in hypertension. *Am J Med* 1984;77:28–32.
293. Nordrehaug JE, von der Lippe G. Hypokalemia and ventricular fibrillation in acute myocardial infarction. *Br Heart J* 1983;50:525–529.
294. Thompson RG, Cobb LA. Hypokalemia after resuscitation from out-of-hospital ventricular fibrillation. *JAMA* 1982;248(21):2860–2863.
295. Ornato JP, Gonzalez ER, Starke H, et al. Incidence and causes of hypokalemia associated with cardiac resuscitation. *Am J Emerg Med* 1985; 3(6):503–506.
296. Vobruba V, Cerna O. The role of magnesium in acute condition. *Cesko-Slov Pediatr* 1995;50(1):33–35.
297. Craddock L, Miller B, Clifton G, et al. Resuscitation from prolonged cardiac arrest with high-dose intravenous magnesium sulfate. *J Emerg Med* 1991;9(6):469–476.
298. Thel MC, Armstrong AL, McNulty SE, et al. Randomised trial of magnesium in in-hospital cardiac arrest. Duke Internal Medicine Housestaff. *Lancet* 1997;350(9087):1272–1276.
299. Kowey PR, Engel TR. Overdrive pacing for ventricular tachyarrhythmias: a reassessment. *Ann Int Med* 1983;99:651–656.
300. Kudenchuk PJ, Cobb LA, Copass MK, et al. Amiodarone for resuscitation after out-of-hospital cardiac arrest due to ventricular fibrillation. *N Engl J Med* 1999;341(12):871–878.
301. Gonzalez ER, Kannewurf BS, Ornato JP. Intravenous amiodarone for ventricular arrhythmias: overview and clinical use. *Resuscitation* 1998;39(1–2):33–42.
302. American Heart Association. Standards and guidelines for cardiopulmonary resuscitation (CPR) and emergency cardiac care (ECC). *JAMA* 1986;255:2841–3044.
303. Talley DB, Ornato JP, Clarke AM. Computer-aided characterization and optimization of the Thumper compression waveform in closed-chest CPR. *Biomed Instrum Technol* 1990;24(4):283–288.
304. Halperin HR, Guerci AD, Chandra N, et al. Vest inflation without simultaneous ventilation during cardiac arrest in dogs: improved survival from

prolonged cardiopulmonary resuscitation. *Circulation* 1986;74(6):1407–1415.
305. Halperin HR, Weisfeldt ML. New approaches to CPR. Four hands, a plunger, or a vest. *JAMA* 1992;267(21):2940–2941.
306. Halperin HR, Tsitlik JE, Gelfand M, et al. A preliminary study of cardiopulmonary resuscitation by circumferential compression of the chest with use of a pneumatic vest. *N Engl J Med* 1993;329(11):762–768.
307. Halperin HR, Chandra NC, Levin HR, et al. Newer methods of improving blood flow during CPR. *Ann Emerg Med* 1996;27(5):553–562.
308. Halperin HR, Paradis N, Ornato JP, et al. Cardiopulmonary resuscitation with a novel chest compression device in a porcine model of cardiac arrest: improved hemodynamics and mechanisms. *J Am Coll Cardiol* 2004;44(11):2214–2220.
309. Timerman S, Cardoso LF, Ramires JA, et al. Improved hemodynamic performance with a novel chest compression device during treatment of in-hospital cardiac arrest. *Resuscitation* 2004;61(3):273–280.
310. Casner M, Andersen D, Isaacs SM. The impact of a new CPR assist device on rate of return of spontaneous circulation in out-of-hospital cardiac arrest. *Prehosp Emerg Care* 2005;9(1):61–67.
311. The American Heart Association in collaboration with the International Liaison Committee on Resuscitation. Guidelines 2000 for cardiopulmonary resuscitation and emergency cardiovascular care. Part 6: Advanced cardiovascular life support: Section 4: devices to assist circulation. *Circulation* 2000;102(8 Suppl):I105–I111.
312. Orliaguet GA, Carli PA, Rozenberg A, et al. End-tidal carbon dioxide during out-of-hospital cardiac arrest resuscitation: comparison of active compression-decompression and standard CPR. *Ann Emerg Med* 1995; 25(1):48–51.
313. Shultz JJ, Coffeen P, Sweeney M, et al. Evaluation of standard and active compression-decompression CPR in an acute human model of ventricular fibrillation. *Circulation* 1994;89(2):684–693.
314. Tucker KJ, Idris A. Clinical and laboratory investigations of active compression-decompression cardiopulmonary resuscitation. *Resuscitation* 1994;28(1):1–7.
315. Tucker KJ, Khan J, Idris A, et al. The biphasic mechanism of blood flow during cardiopulmonary resuscitation: A physiologic comparison of active compression-decompression and high-impulse manual external cardiac massage. *Ann Emerg Med* 1994;24(5):895–906.
316. Luiz T, Ellinger K, Denz C. Active compression-decompression cardiopulmonary resuscitation does not improve survival in patients with prehospital cardiac arrest in a physician-manned emergency medical system. *J Cardiothorac Vasc Anesth* 1996;10(2):178–186.
317. Lurie KG. Active compression-decompression CPR: a progress report. *Resuscitation* 1994;28(2):115–122.
318. Schwab TM, Callaham ML, Madsen CD, et al. A randomized clinical trial of active compression-decompression CPR vs standard CPR in out-of-hospital cardiac arrest in two cities. *JAMA* 1995;273(16):1261–1268.
319. Stiell IG, Hebert PC, Wells GA, et al. The Ontario trial of active compression-decompression cardiopulmonary resuscitation for in-hospital and prehospital cardiac arrest. *JAMA* 1996;275(18):1417–1423.
320. Plaisance P, Adnet F, Vicaut E, et al. Benefit of active compression-decompression cardiopulmonary resuscitation as a prehospital advanced cardiac life support. A randomized multicenter study. *Circulation* 1997; 95(4):955–961.
321. Mateer JR, Stueven HA, Thompson BM, et al. Pre-hospital IAC-CPR versus standard CPR: paramedic resuscitation of cardiac arrests. *Am J Emerg Med* 1985;3(2):143–146.
322. Schultz DD, Olivas GS. The use of cough cardiopulmonary resuscitation in clinical practice. *Heart Lung* 1986;15(3):273–282.
323. Miller B, Lesnefsky E, Heyborne T, et al. Cough-cardiopulmonary resuscitation in the cardiac catheterization laboratory: hemodynamics during an episode of prolonged hypotensive ventricular tachycardia. *Cathet Cardiovasc Diagn* 1989;18(3):168–171.
324. Miller B, Cohen A, Serio A, et al. Hemodynamics of cough cardiopulmonary resuscitation in a patient with sustained torsades de pointes/ventricular flutter. *J Emerg Med* 1994;12(5):627–632.
325. Niemann JT, Rosborough JP, Niskanen RA, et al. Mechanical "cough" cardiopulmonary resuscitation during cardiac arrest in dogs. *Am J Cardiol* 1985;55(1):199–204.
326. Lurie KG, Coffeen P, Shultz J, et al. Improving active compression-decompression cardiopulmonary resuscitation with an inspiratory impedance valve. *Circulation* 1995;91(6):1629–1632.
327. Lurie K, Voelckel W, Plaisance P, et al. Use of an inspiratory impedance threshold valve during cardiopulmonary resuscitation: a progress report. *Resuscitation* 2000;44(3):219–230.
328. Lurie K, Zielinski T, McKnite S, et al. Improving the efficiency of cardiopulmonary resuscitation with an inspiratory impedance threshold valve. *Crit Care Med* 2000;28(11 Suppl):N207–N209.
329. Lurie KG. Recent advances in mechanical methods of cardiopulmonary resuscitation. *Acta Anaesthesiol Scand Suppl* 1997;111:49–52.
330. Lurie KG, Mulligan KA, McKnite S, et al. Optimizing standard cardiopulmonary resuscitation with an inspiratory impedance threshold valve. *Chest* 1998;113(4):1084–1090.
331. Plaisance P, Lurie KG, Payen D. Inspiratory impedance during active compression-decompression cardiopulmonary resuscitation: a randomized evaluation in patients in cardiac arrest. *Circulation* 2000;101(9):989–994.
332. Pirrallo RG, Aufderheide TP, Provo TA, et al. Effect of an inspiratory impedance threshold device on hemodynamics during conventional manual cardiopulmonary resuscitation. *Resuscitation* 2005;66(1):13–20.
333. Plaisance P, Lurie KG, Vicaut E, et al. Evaluation of an impedance threshold device in patients receiving active compression-decompression cardiopulmonary resuscitation for out of hospital cardiac arrest. *Resuscitation* 2004;61(3):265–271.
334. Peberdy MA, Kaye W, Ornato JP, et al. Cardiopulmonary resuscitation of adults in the hospital: a report of 14720 cardiac arrests from the National Registry of Cardiopulmonary Resuscitation. *Resuscitation* 2003; 58(3):297–308.
335. Buist MD, Jarmolowski E, Burton PR, et al. Recognising clinical instability in hospital patients before cardiac arrest or unplanned admission to intensive care. A pilot study in a tertiary-care hospital. *Med J Aust* 1999; 171(1):22–25.
336. Hodgetts TJ, Kenward G, Vlachonikolis IG, et al. The identification of risk factors for cardiac arrest and formulation of activation criteria to alert a medical emergency team. *Resuscitation* 2002;54(2):125–131.
337. Hodgetts TJ, Kenward G, Vlackonikolis I, et al. Incidence, location and reasons for avoidable in-hospital cardiac arrest in a district general hospital. *Resuscitation* 2002;54(2):115–123.
338. Fieselmann JF, Hendryx MS, Helms CM, et al. Respiratory rate predicts cardiopulmonary arrest for internal medicine inpatients. *J Gen Intern Med* 1993;8(7):354–360.
339. Franklin C, Samuel J, Hu TC. Life-threatening hypotension associated with emergency intubation and the initiation of mechanical ventilation. *Am J Emerg Med* 1994;12(4):425–428.
340. Garrard C, Young D. Suboptimal care of patients before admission to intensive care. is caused by a failure to appreciate or apply the ABCs of life support. *BMJ* 1998;316(7148):1841–1842.
341. Schein RM, Hazday N, Pena M, et al. Clinical antecedents to in-hospital cardiopulmonary arrest. *Chest* 1990;98(6):1388–1392.
342. Smith AF, Wood J. Can some in-hospital cardio-respiratory arrests be prevented? A prospective survey. *Resuscitation* 1998;37(3):133–137.
343. Coombs M. Critical care outreach: short-term measure or long-term solution? *Nurs Crit Care* 2002;7(3):109–110.
344. Cretikos M, Hillman K. The medical emergency team: does it really make a difference? *Intern Med J* 2003;33(11):511–514.
345. Daly FF, Sidney KL, Fatovich DM. The Medical Emergency Team (MET): a model for the district general hospital. *Aust N Z J Med* 1998;28(6):795–798.
346. Goldhill DR. A new way of managing critical care? *Anaesthesia* 2002; 57(9):843–844.
347. Hillman K. Critical care without walls. *Curr Opin Crit Care* 2002;8(6): 594–599.
348. Hillman K, Chen J, Brown D. A clinical model for Health Services Research–the Medical Emergency Team. *J Crit Care* 2003;18(3):195–199.
349. Lee TH, Pearson SD, Johnson PA, et al. Failure of information as an intervention to modify clinical management. A time-series trial in patients with acute chest pain. *Ann Intern Med* 1995;122(6):434–437.
350. McArthur-Rouse F. Critical care outreach services and early warning scoring systems: a review of the literature. *J Adv Nurs* 2001;36(5):696–704.
351. Bellomo R, Goldsmith D, Uchino S, et al. A prospective before-and-after trial of a medical emergency team. *Med J Aust* 2003;179(6):283–287.
352. Bristow PJ, Hillman KM, Chey T, et al. Rates of in-hospital arrests, deaths and intensive care admissions: the effect of a medical emergency team. *Med J Aust* 2000;173(5):236–240.
353. Buist MD, Moore GE, Bernard SA, et al. Effects of a medical emergency team on reduction of incidence of and mortality from unexpected cardiac arrests in hospital: preliminary study. *BMJ* 2002;324(7334):387–390.
354. DeVita MA, Schaefer J, Lutz J, et al. Improving medical crisis team performance. *Crit Care Med* 2004;32(2 Suppl):S61–S65.
355. DeVita MA, Braithwaite RS, Mahidhara R, et al. Use of medical emergency team responses to reduce hospital cardiopulmonary arrests. *Qual Saf Health Care* 2004;13(4):251–254.
356. Bellomo R, Goldsmith D, Uchino S, et al. Prospective controlled trial of effect of medical emergency team on postoperative morbidity and mortality rates. *Crit Care Med* 2004;32(4):916–921.
357. Hillman K, Chen J, Cretikos M, et al. Introduction of the medical emergency team (MET) system: a cluster-randomised controlled trial. *Lancet* 2005;365(9477):2091–2097.
358. Salamonson Y, Kariyawasam A, van Heere B, et al. The evolutionary process of Medical Emergency Team (MET) implementation: reduction in unanticipated ICU transfers. *Resuscitation* 2001;49(2):135–141.
359. Weil MH, Becker L, Budinger T, et al. Workshop Executive Summary Report: Post-resuscitative and initial Utility in Life Saving Efforts (PULSE): June 29–30, 2000; Lansdowne Resort and Conference Center; Leesburg, VA. *Circulation* 2001;103(9):1182–1184.
360. The Hypothermia After Cardiac Arrest Study Group. Mild therapeutic hypothermia to improve the neurologic outcome of comatose survivors of out-of-hospital cardiac arrest with induced hypothermia. *N Engl J Med* 2002; 346:557–563.
361. Bernard SA, Gray TW, Buist MD, et al. Treatment of comatose survivors of out-of-hospital cardiac arrest with induced hypothermia. *N Engl J Med* 2002;346(8):557–563.

362. Nolan JP, Morley PT, Vanden Hoek TL, et al. Therapeutic hypothermia after cardiac arrest: an advisory statement by the advanced life support task force of the International Liaison Committee on Resuscitation. *Circulation* 2003;108(1):118–121.
363. Granger DN, Korthuis RJ. Physiologic mechanisms of postischemic tissue injury. *Annu Rev Physiol* 1995;57:311–332.
364. Canevari L, Console A, Tendi EA, et al. Effect of postischaemic hypothermia on the mitochondrial damage induced by ischaemia and reperfusion in the gerbil. *Brain Res* 1999;817(1-2):241–245.
365. Wilson YT, Lepore DA, Riccio M, et al. Mild hypothermia protects against ischaemia-reperfusion injury in rabbit skeletal muscle. *Br J Plast Surg* 1997; 50(5):343–348.
366. Karibe H, Zarow GJ, Graham SH, et al. Mild intraischemic hypothermia reduces postischemic hyperperfusion, delayed postischemic hypoperfusion, blood–brain barrier disruption, brain edema, and neuronal damage volume after temporary focal cerebral ischemia in rats. *J Cereb Blood Flow Metab* 1994;14(4):620–627.
367. Valenzuela TD, Roe DJ, Nichol G, et al. Outcomes of rapid defibrillation by security officers after cardiac arrest in casinos. *N Engl J Med* 2000; 343(17):1206–1209.
368. O'Rourke MF, Donaldson E, Geddes JS. An airline cardiac arrest program. *Circulation* 1997;96(9):2849–2853.
369. Donaldson E, Pearn J. First aid in the air. *Aust N Z J Surg* 1996;66(7):431–434.
370. Page RL, Joglar JA, Kowal RC, et al. Use of automated external defibrillators by a U.S. airline. *N Engl J Med* 2000;343(17):1210–1216.
371. Glazer I. Airline use of automatic external defibrillator: shocking developments. *Aviat Space Environ Med* 2000;71(5):556.
372. Weisfeldt ML, Kerber RE, McGoldrick RP, et al. Public access defibrillation: a statement for healthcare professionals from the American Heart Association Task Force on Automatic External Defibrillation. *Circulation* 1995;92:2763.
373. Weisfeldt ML, Kerber RE, McGoldrick RP, et al. American Heart Association report on the Public Access Defibrillation Conference December 8–10, 1994. *Circulation* 1995;92:2740–2747.
374. Nichol G, Hallstrom AP, Kerber R, et al. American Heart Association report on the second public access defibrillation conference, April 17–19, 1997. *Circulation* 1998;97(13):1309–1314.
375. Kern KB. Public access defibrillation: a review. *Heart* 1998;80(4):402–404.
376. Ornato JP, Hankins DG. Public-access defibrillation. *Prehosp Emerg Care* 1999;3(4):297–302.
377. Hallstrom AP, Ornato JP, Weisfeldt M, et al. Public-access defibrillation and survival after out-of-hospital cardiac arrest. *N Engl J Med* 2004;351 (7):637–646.

CHAPTER 71 ■ SYNCOPE

DAVID G. BENDITT

OVERVIEW

Syncope is a syndrome characterized by the sudden loss of consciousness (including by definition loss of postural tone) of relatively limited duration with subsequent spontaneous recovery (1). The sine qua non of "true syncope" is its specific pathophysiology, namely, transient inadequacy of cerebral nutrient flow (1). This pathophysiology distinguishes syncope from other conditions that cause temporary loss of consciousness (e.g., concussion from trauma, seizures caused by electrical disturbances in the brain).

NOMENCLATURE: WHAT IS AND WHAT IS "NOT" TRUE SYNCOPE

The term *syncope* should not be used when there is insufficient evidence that transient global cerebral hypoperfusion caused an apparent transient loss of consciousness (TLOC) episode. In such instances, it is better to use the broader descriptor TLOC. This latter designation is akin to that of syncope, but with the cerebral hypoperfusion removed. The distinctions raised here are important clinically, because TLOC keeps the physician's "radar screen" open more widely, whereas "syncope" focuses on a narrower set of causes. Unfortunately, even the modern literature is replete with examples that fail to respect these important nomenclature issues.

FREQUENCY

Syncope is a common medical problem, accounting for about 1% of emergency department visits and up to 6% of hospital admissions (1–10). In the clinic, however, patients do not usually use the term "syncope" but speak of "blacking or passing out," "collapse," or "faint."

It has been estimated that approximately one third of individuals will experience a syncopal episode during their lifetime (9), with susceptibility to syncope increasing in association with both advancing age and increasing infirmity (9,10). Furthermore, approximately 35% of patients with syncope experience recurrences by 3 years of follow-up (9–11). A history of recurrent syncope at the time of initial presentation (especially if the recurrences have been spread over a relatively long period) is a strong predictor of future recurrences. In one report, more than five lifetime syncope recurrences were associated with a 50% chance of recurrence in the following year (11).

PATHOPHYSIOLOGY

As noted earlier, syncope is defined as "a transient, self-limited loss of consciousness, usually leading to falling. The onset of syncope is relatively rapid, and the subsequent recovery is spontaneous, complete, and usually prompt. The underlying mechanism is a transient global cerebral hypoperfusion" (1).

Most true syncope events are caused by self-limited periods of arterial hypotension. Cerebral perfusion is critically dependent on systemic arterial pressure. Thus, factors that diminish systemic arterial pressure (i.e., decreased cardiac output or peripheral vascular resistance) may impair cerebral perfusion. In patients with syncope, decreased venous filling is often a major factor in triggering reduced cardiac output. Excessive pooling of blood in dependent parts of the body or diminished blood volume predisposes to systemic hypotension and syncope. Impaired cardiac output caused by other factors may also contribute to triggering faints. Thus, bradyarrhythmias or tachyarrhythmias, especially in the setting of left ventricular dysfunction, valvular heart disease, obstructive cardiomyopathies, volume depletion, or abnormal vascular reactivity (i.e., inadequate vasoconstriction or inappropriate vasodilatation), are all considerations when one is confronted with the need to establish a basis for syncope.

Inappropriate vasodilatation with inadequate venous return is the main cause of fainting in the reflex syncopal syndromes. Vasodilatation resulting in diminished cerebral perfusion also can contribute to lightheadedness and syncope in association

TABLE 71.1

SYNCOPE: DIAGNOSTIC CLASSIFICATION

NEURALLY MEDIATED REFLEX SYNCOPE
Vasovagal faint
Carotid sinus syncope
Cough/swallow syncope and related disorders
Gastrointestinal, pelvic, or urologic origin (swallowing, defecation, postmicturition status)

ORTHOSTATIC SYNCOPE
Primary autonomic failure
Secondary autonomic failure (e.g., diabetic and alcoholic neuropathy, drug effects)

CARDIAC ARRHYTHMIAS AS A PRIMARY CAUSE OF SYNCOPE
Sinus node dysfunction (including bradycardia/tachycardia syndrome)
Atrioventricular conduction system disease
Paroxysmal supraventricular tachycardias
Paroxysmal ventricular tachycardia (including torsade de pointes)
Implanted pacing system malfunction, "pacemaker syndrome"
Brugada syndrome, long/short QT syndrome

STRUCTURAL CARDIOVASCULAR OR CARDIOPULMONARY DISEASE
Cardiac valvular disease/ischemia
Acute myocardial infarction
Obstructive cardiomyopathy
Subclavian steal syndrome
Pericardial disease/tamponade
Pulmonary embolus
Primary pulmonary hypertension
Acute aortic dissection

CEREBROVASCULAR
Intracerebral steal, migraine, vertebrobasilar transient ischemic attack

TABLE 71.2

NEURALLY MEDIATED SYNCOPAL SYNDROMES

Emotional syncope (common or "vasovagal" faint, "malignant" vasovagal faint)
Carotid sinus syncope
Gastrointestinal stimulation (swallow syncope, defecation syncope)
Micturition syncope
Cough syncope
Sneeze syncope
Glossopharyngeal neuralgia
Airway stimulation
Raised intrathoracic pressure (brass wind instrument playing, weight lifting)

with thermal stress (e.g., hot environments, excessive exercise). Impaired capacity to increase vascular resistance adequately during upright posture is critical in orthostatic hypotension, whereas a similar problem may provoke syncope during or immediately after exercise or as a consequence of exposure to certain vasodilator drugs (e.g., nitrates) (12–18). On only rare occasions is cerebral hypoperfusion attributable to an abnormally high cerebral vascular resistance (e.g., vascular spasm such as may occur in the setting of low carbon dioxide tension).

CAUSES OF TRUE SYNCOPE

Causes are listed in Table 71.1.

Neurally Mediated Reflex Syncope Syndromes

The neurally mediated syncopal syndromes (Table 71.2) comprise a variety of pathophysiologically related conditions. For the most part, clinical distinctions are based on the source of the trigger for the episodes (e.g., pain, carotid sinus stimulation, cough, micturition). In this regard, the presumed triggering neural signals may arise within the central nervous system (CNS) itself (e.g., syncope associated with fear or anxiety), or from any of a number of peripheral receptors that respond to stimuli of various types (e.g., mechanical, chemical, pain). Thus, by way of example, in carotid sinus syndrome, the afferent aspect of the reflex loop is typically believed to arise from stimulation of autonomic receptors in the cervical region. However, it now seems likely that carotid sinus stimulation may need to interact with failure of parallel CNS inputs from the ipsilateral neck muscles to trigger the syndrome (19). In typical vasovagal syncope (Fig. 71.1), the location and nature of the trigger sites are usually less certain (20–26).

Vasovagal syncope may be triggered by any of a variety of situational factors. Some of the latter include unpleasant sights

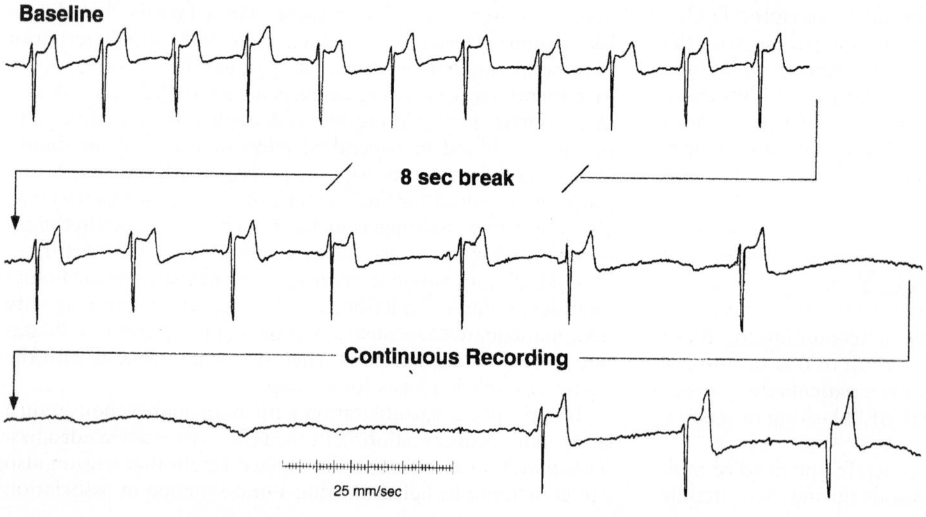

FIGURE 71.1. Recording from an in-hospital electrocardiographic monitor illustrating bradycardia associated with a spontaneous vasovagal faint accompanying an abrupt hemorrhage following an invasive cardiac procedure.

(e.g., sight of blood), pain, and extreme emotion. Common venues for fainting are churches, hospitals, queues, and restaurants. In many but not all cases, this type of faint is easy to diagnose because a clear history of preceding dizziness together with other typical phenomena is obtained (1). The patient may reports feelings of lack of air, a change in breathing pattern, sweating, loss of hearing, and nausea before partial or total loss of consciousness. Pallor is a common physical finding in association with these faints, and witnesses to the event should be queried directly regard recollection of this finding. During the recovery phase there is rapid return of orientation. However, fatigue, weakness, nausea, and headache may last from minutes to hours. Often, in older individuals, warning symptoms may be of very brief duration or nonexistent, thereby complicating establishment of the diagnosis.

When vasovagal syncope is suspected by clinical history but uncertainty remains, tilt-table testing diagnostic techniques have been of value (1,23–36). Tilt-table testing has a specificity of approximately 90% and an approximate reproducibility in the short term of 80% to 90% and in the longer term (over more than 1 year) around 60% (35). Tilt-table testing is the only investigation that provides the opportunity to precipitate a typical attack under the eyes of the investigator and allows the victim to confirm the associated symptoms.

Carotid sinus syndrome is the second most common form of the neurally mediated syncopal syndromes (1,37–40). In this setting, syncope often presents without warning (i.e., absence of premonitory symptoms). Although rare, a history suggesting that head movements trigger dizziness or syncope supports this diagnosis. As a rule, the condition almost exclusively afflicts older people, especially men.

In clinical practice, carotid sinus syndrome is often overlooked. The reasons for this include failure to perform carotid sinus massage routinely in patients with syncope and/or failure to record both blood pressure and heart rate responses when carotid massage is undertaken. Carotid massage resulting in dizziness or syncope owing to hypotension with or without bradycardia is the key diagnostic finding in patients suspected of having carotid sinus syndrome. Testing is best conducted with the patient upright on a tilt table, with continuous digital plethysmography or intraarterial pressure measurements used to record beat-to-beat arterial pressure changes (39). Firm carotid sinus massage for 5 to 10 seconds is recommended. A cardioinhibitory response is presumed to predominate when carotid sinus massage is associated with symptom reproduction in conjunction with asystole or paroxysmal atrioventricular (AV) block (37–40). However, the vasodepressor component must be assessed separately during the maneuver by beat-to-beat arterial pressure monitoring while preventing bradycardia using a temporary dual-chamber pacing system. The magnitude of this latter part of the reflex can also be estimated by examining the rate of blood pressure recovery after resumption of the native heart rate. In the absence of symptom reproduction, the demonstration of a pause of 5 seconds or longer, and/or a systolic blood pressure fall of at least 50 mmHg, is probably relevant and can be considered to support a presumptive diagnosis (1).

Among the other forms of neurally mediated reflex syncope, postmicturition syncope, swallow syncope, and cough syncope are probably the next most frequent. The medical history associated with these situational faints provides the diagnosis. The remaining conditions (Table 71.2) are only rarely encountered.

Orthostatic Syncope

Orthostatic syncope is the result of postural hypotension or orthostatic hypotension (Table 71.3). The term *orthostatic intolerance* has also come to be widely used as a descriptor of patients susceptible to recurring orthostatic syncope. Presyncopal or syncopal symptoms associated with abrupt assumption of upright posture are common occurrences (Table 71.3). Elderly persons, less physically fit individuals, or patients who are for whatever reason dehydrated or volume depleted are at greatest risk. Iatrogenic factors such as excessive diuresis or overly aggressive use of certain antihypertensive agents are important contributors. Environmental factors (e.g., excessive heat) and complications associated with certain medical conditions (e.g., hemorrhage) or diseases (e.g., diabetes insipidus, adrenal insufficiency) may also play a role in specific cases. Volume depletion (often iatrogenic) (27,28,41–44), exposure to vasodilator drugs, and neurologic disturbances of vascular control resulting from concomitant disease are the most frequent causes of orthostatic syncope. In certain cases, however, patients may be manifesting a form of primary autonomic failure with inadequate reflex adaptations to upright posture. The most important of the primary autonomic disturbances encountered in practice are pure autonomic failure, multisystem atrophy, and Parkinson disease with autonomic failure.

Specific primary autonomic nervous system dysfunctions leading to disturbances of vascular control are currently considered to be relatively infrequent causes of syncope in general medical practice. Nevertheless, as the broad spectrum of these disturbances and their potentially subtle manifestations become more widely appreciated by physicians, these diagnoses will be made more often (45–51). More commonly, neuropathies associated with chronic diseases (e.g., diabetes) or toxic agents (e.g., alcohol) are the source of the problem.

TABLE 71.3

SYNCOPE OF ORTHOSTATIC ORIGIN: A CLASSIFICATION OF CAUSES

PRIMARY AUTONOMIC FAILURE
Pure autonomic failure
Autonomic failure with multiple system atrophy
Parkinson disease with autonomic failure
SECONDARY
Diabetes mellitus
Volume/fluid depletion
Autoimmune acute and subacute dysautonomias (e.g., Guillain-Barré syndrome, myasthenia gravis)
Autonomic neuropathy associated with malignancies
Metabolic diseases (e.g., porphyria, Fabry disease)
Central nervous system infections (e.g., syphilis, Chagas disease)
Hypothalamic and midbrain lesions/tumors (e.g., craniopharyngioma)
Spinal cord lesions/tumors
DRUG/TOXIN-INDUCED
Alcohol
Diuretics
Sedatives/tranquilizers: phenothiazines, barbiturates
Vasodilators (e.g., peripheral and central sympatholytic agents)
Angiotensin-converting enzyme inhibitors
Tricyclic antidepressents

Modified from Bannister R, ed. *Autonomic failure: a textbook of clinical disorders of the autonomic nervous system*. Oxford: Oxford University Press, 1988.

In a review of 155 patients referred to a center specialized in autonomic system evaluation for assessment of suspected orthostatic hypotension, Low and colleagues (48) found that among the most severely affected symptomatic patients (n = 90; mean age, 64 years), pure autonomic failure accounted for 33%, multisystem atrophy accounted for 26%, and autonomic/diabetic neuropathy accounted for 31%. The most frequently reported symptoms in these individuals were lightheadedness (88%), weakness or tiredness (72%), cognitive difficulties (47%), blurred vision (47%), tremulousness (38%), and vertigo (37%). Patients with postural orthostatic tachycardia syndrome (POTS), conversely, tended to be symptomatic during upright posture, but they did not typically manifest sufficient hypotension to result in syncope or marked hypotension.

Cardiac Arrhythmias

Primary cardiac arrhythmias as the cause of syncope encompass those rhythm disturbances associated with intrinsic cardiac disease (e.g., sinus node dysfunction [SND], AV conduction system disease), accessory conduction pathways, or other structural abnormalities (e.g., congenital anomalies, postoperative disturbances), as well as those resulting from proarrhythmic effects of cardioactive drugs (e.g., cardiac glycosides, positive inotropic agents, antiarrhythmic drugs).

Arrhythmias resulting from intrinsic conduction system disturbances (usually acquired but occasionally congenital) are important causes of syncope. However, it is often difficult to substantiate the relationship between syncope and a suspected arrhythmia in free-living individuals (e.g., by ambulatory electrocardiographic [ECG] monitoring) resulting from the unpredictable occurrence of symptomatic events. Thus, implantable long-term loop recorders (ILRs) and mobile cardiac outpatient telemetry (MCOT) are becoming more widely applied (see later). In some cases, invasive electrophysiologic testing may be indicated (52–56).

Sinus Node Dysfunction

SND (also known as sick sinus syndrome, sinus node disease, and sinoatrial disease) encompasses an array of sinus node and/or atrial arrhythmias that result in persistent or intermittent periods of inappropriate slow or fast heart beating (57–62). The ECG manifestations of SND include sinus bradycardia (Fig. 71.2), sinus pauses, sinoatrial exit block, inexcitable atrium, chronotropic incompetence, and various atrial tachyarrhythmias (principally atrial fibrillation or atrial flutter). For the most part, SND is closely associated with underlying fibrosis or chamber enlargement). However, extrinsic factors (e.g., autonomic nervous system influences, cardioactive drugs) are also frequent contributors. Of these, drug-induced disturbances are the most important clinically.

In the patient with SND and syncope, the cause may be a transient severe bradyarrhythmia or tachyarrhythmia, or both. Most often, however, it is believed that the arrhythmias associated with syncope in patients with SND are those producing relatively long periods (≥10 to 15 seconds) of severe bradycardia (i.e., sinus pauses and sinoatrial block) with consequent inadequate cerebral blood flow (59,60,63–65).

Atrioventricular Conduction Disturbances

Although the acquired disturbances of AV conduction are most often associated with syncopal symptoms, there has been increasing concern regarding the adverse prognostic implication of syncope in congenital AV block patients (66–68). Drug effects also deserve special consideration because they are a particularly common, and a potentially reversible, cause of AV conduction disturbances. Antiarrhythmic drugs, cardiac glycosides, β-blockers, and calcium channel blockers are perhaps the most widely recognized in this regard. Patients with preexisting infranodal conduction system disease are at highest risk.

In general, the risk for syncope or dizziness is greatest at onset of AV block, prior to warmup of a subsidiary rhythm. Thereafter, the ventricular rhythm often stabilizes, and may average 35 to 40 beats per minute in acquired third-degree AV block. In fixed complete AV block, syncope may occur as a result of the unreliability of subsidiary pacemakers or because of the inability of the heart rate–limited circulation to provide sufficient cerebral blood flow during periods of exercise or stress.

The site of block in patients with congenital AV block is typically at the level of the AV node. Generally, the QRS complexes are narrow, and the block usually is associated with a reasonable subsidiary rhythm, which tends to increase in rate with exercise. Recently, however, concern has been raised regarding the supposedly benign natural history of congenital AV block (66–68), and further evaluation of this issue is needed. In the meantime, syncope and dizziness (along with exertional intolerance) are accepted indications for pacing in these patients.

Bifascicular conduction system disease is a relatively common ECG finding. However, in most cases, progression to more severe forms of AV block is slow. Susceptibility to higher-grade block (i.e., those that may be long enough to cause syncope) increases the longer the HV interval (particularly for HV intervals ≥100 milliseconds) (64,69–72) (Fig. 71.3). However, syncope in patients with evident conduction system disease may not be solely the result of bradyarrhythmias. Ventricular tachycardia (VT) is a concern in these cases owing to the usual presence of significant underlying heart disease.

Supraventricular and Ventricular Tachyarrhythmias

Supraventricular tachyarrhythmias have been reported to be the cause of syncope in about 15% of patients referred for electrophysiologic evaluation (6). When syncope does occur, it is typically at the onset of an arrhythmic episode before adequate peripheral vascular cardiovascular compensation can occur. Numerous factors determine whether syncope or dizziness occurs in patients with supraventricular tachycardia. These include the tachycardia rate, the volume status and posture of the patient at the onset of the arrhythmia, the presence of associated valvular, left ventricular, or pulmonary vascular disease,

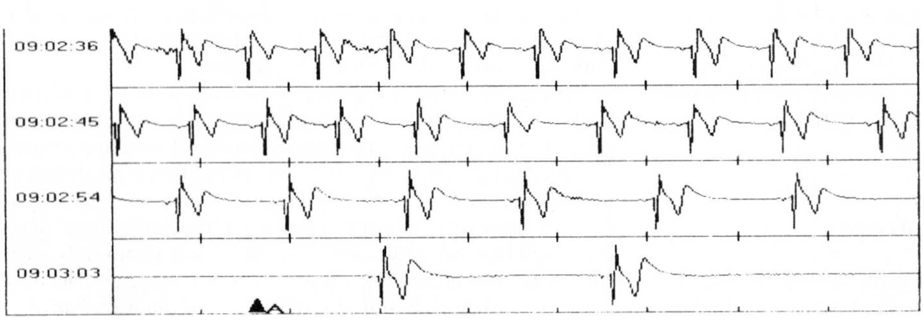

FIGURE 71.2. Symptomatic sinus bradycardia detected during ambulatory implantable loop recorder electrocardiographic monitoring in a 70-year-old woman with recurrent dizziness.

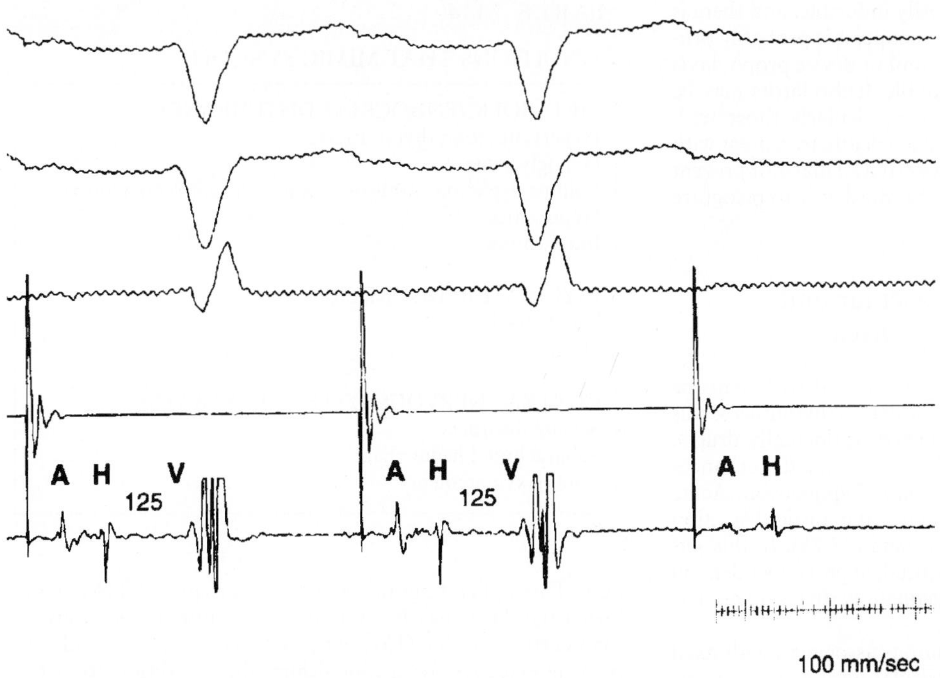

FIGURE 71.3. Electrocardiographic and intracardiac recordings illustrating a prolonged HV interval and infra-His block (Mobitz II) in a patient undergoing electrophysiologic evaluation for recurrent syncope of unknown cause.

the mechanism of the arrhythmia, and the integrity of reflex peripheral vascular compensation (73).

Sustained VT has been reported to be the cause of syncope in up to 20% of syncopal patients referred for electrophysiologic testing (6). This diagnosis is of particular concern in the setting of underlying structural heart disease or long QT syndrome (congenital or acquired). With regard to VT susceptibility, a detailed medical history should be supplemented with assessment of the status of underlying cardiac disease. Risk stratification techniques to identify syncopal patients in whom VT risk is high have been the subjects of study for many years. Methods such as signal-averaged ECG [74,75]), heart rate variability, and microvolt T-wave alternans remain in various stages of evaluation. As a rule, however, the positive predictive values have been low. A high negative predictive value may help to exclude certain patients from further VT evaluation. As has been the case for a long time, a low ejection fraction is a finding that tends to be associated with higher VT risk.

Nonsustained VT (NSVT) remains a difficult dilemma for physicians evaluating patients with syncope. NSVT is a common finding during ambulatory ECG monitoring in patients with structural heart disease. Consequently, finding NSVT in a syncopal patient is not usually very helpful in the absence of concomitant symptoms (Fig. 71.4). Similarly, induced NSVT during electrophysiologic testing (especially if polymorphic) is not a reliable diagnostic finding. However, if reproducible

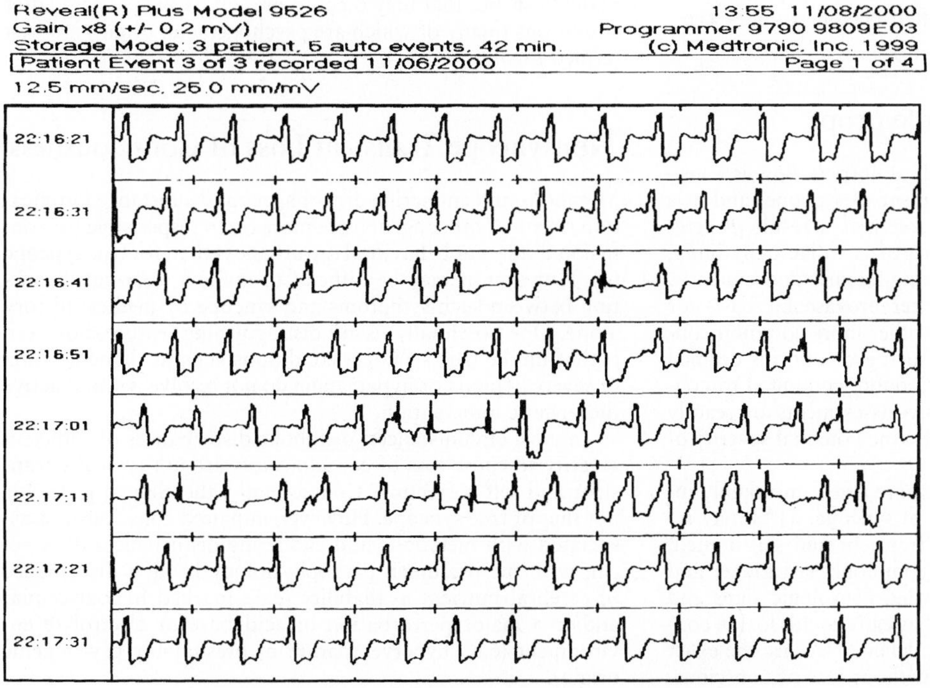

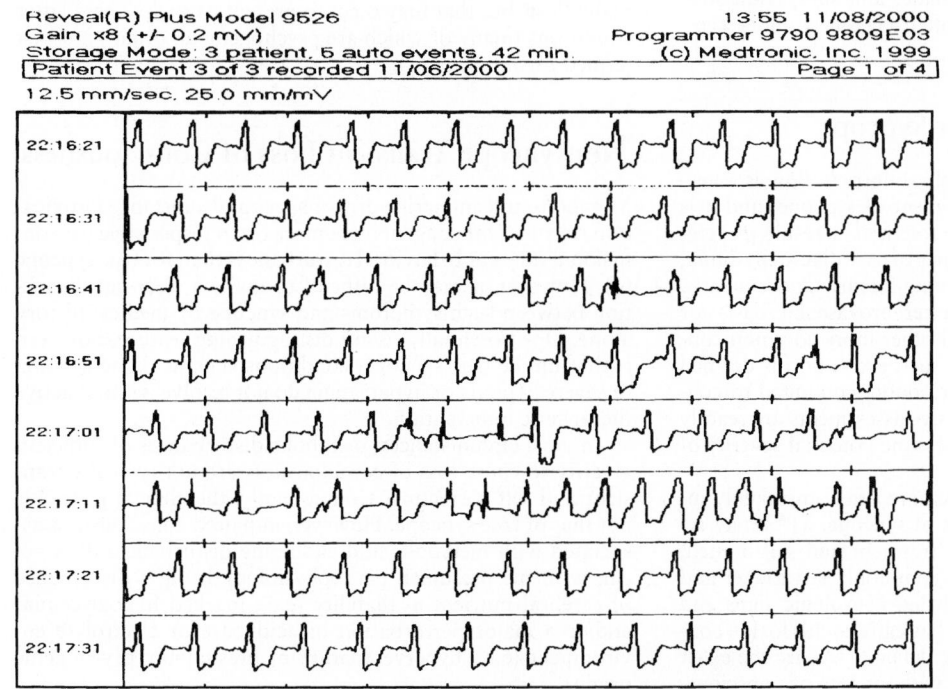

FIGURE 71.4. Recording from an implantable loop recorder. The patient complained of "lightheadedness" but had no symptoms of rapid heart action. The recording illustrates a wide-QRS nonsustained tachycardia suggestive of nonsustained ventricular tachycardia.

periods of hypotensive NSVT are easily inducible, and there is no other apparent explanation for syncope, it is probably prudent to proceed with pharmacologic and/or device prophylaxis (76,77). However, although implantable defibrillators may be indicated in many of these patients (particularly those with low ejection fractions) to prevent sudden death, treatment with implantable cardioverter-defibrillators (ICDs) may not prevent syncope (because of the time it takes for the device to recognize and treat the arrhythmia).

Structural Cardiovascular and Cardiopulmonary Disease

Structural heart disease tends to be associated with syncope most often through susceptibility to cardiac arrhythmias in this setting or as a result of iatrogenic factors (principally drugs). However, on infrequent occasion, hemodynamic disturbances may also be responsible for symptomatic hypotension. Acute myocardial ischemia or infarction and acute aortic dissection are probably the most important of these (78,79). In this setting, the basis of the faint is multifactorial, in part dependent on neural reflex effects leading to inadequate peripheral vascular compensatory response.

Syncope may also occur in conditions associated with fixed or dynamic obstruction to left ventricular outflow (e.g., aortic stenosis, hypertrophic obstructive cardiomyopathy [HOCM]) (80). Prosthetic valve disorders also require consideration as causes of syncope in patients who have previously undergone such surgery. In such cases, symptoms are often provoked by physical exertion, but they may also develop if an otherwise benign arrhythmia should occur (e.g., atrial fibrillation). The basis for the faint may be in part inadequate blood flow resulting from the mechanical obstruction. However, especially in the case of valvular aortic stenosis, ventricular mechanoreceptor-mediated bradycardia and vasodilatation are thought to be important contributors (81). Echocardiography undertaken during or immediately after exertion may provide the diagnostic evidence needed. If not, invasive study is indicated.

Noncardiac cardiovascular structural disturbances may also be associated with syncope. The most important of these conditions include primary pulmonary hypertension, acute pulmonary embolism, cardiac tamponade, and subclavian steal syndrome (this last condition is often classified under cerebrovascular disease).

Cerebrovascular Syncope

Transient global diminution of cerebral nutrient flow is a necessary requirement for the development of syncope, and it is exceedingly rare for this to occur solely as a result of cerebrovascular disease (i.e., in the absence of a cardiac arrhythmia, orthostatic stress, or other precipitating factor). Consequently, absent distinct neurologic signs, a cerebrovascular basis for syncope should not be sought until other more common conditions have been excluded. When such evaluation is deemed appropriate, both noninvasive (ultrasound, computed tomography [CT], angiography) and invasive assessments are readily available and may be needed to assess the potential severity of cerebrovascular lesions.

Transient ischemic attacks (TIAs) are often mistakenly included in the differential diagnosis of syncope. TIAs may resemble syncope in terms of being transient and self-limited, but the similarity ends there. TIAs commonly last longer and are associated with transient localizing neurologic signs and symptoms. Thus, although syncope basically entails loss of consciousness without focal neurologic deficit, TIAs are the exact opposite: focal neurologic deficits without loss of consciousness. This holds without restrictions for carotid TIAs. Vertebrobasilar TIAs may be more likely to cause unconsciousness than carotid system TIAs, but associated symptoms and signs provide evidence for distinguishing this condition from true syncope (81a). Vertebrobasilar TIAs are accompanied by focal neurologic deficits such as hemianopsia or ataxia, symptoms and signs that prove their nature as TIAs.

TABLE 71.4

CONDITIONS THAT MIMIC SYNCOPE

METABOLIC/ENDOCRINE DISTURBANCES
Hyperventilation (hypocapnia)
Hypoglycemia
Volume depletion (Addison disease, pheochromocytoma)
Hypoxemia
Intoxication
PSYCHIATRIC DISORDERS
Panic attacks
Hysteria
CENTRAL NERVOUS SYSTEM SUBSTRATES
Seizure disorders
Subarachnoid hemorrhage
Cataplexy/narcolepsy

SYNCOPE MIMICS AND PSEUDOSYNCOPE

Certain medical conditions may cause a real or apparent TLOC that may appear to be syncope but that are in fact not true syncope (82) (Table 71.4). This situation has caused considerable confusion in the literature, even in prominent journals in which the nomenclature is used in a poorly defined fashion (83,84). However, for reasons explained earlier, it is clinically important to make the distinction among true syncope, nonsyncope TLOC, and conditions in which consciousness is not really 'lost' but that may seem to present as such. These latter conditions (many of which are psychogenic in origin) are best termed *pseudosyncope*).

Nonsyncope Transient Loss of Consciousness

Metabolic and endocrine disturbances and substance intoxication (alcohol, other agents) are more often responsible for confusional states or behavioral disturbances than for true syncope (1). However, it may be difficult to make a clear-cut distinction between such symptoms and syncope by medical history alone. One potentially useful distinguishing feature, however, is that unlike true syncope, conditions such as diabetic coma or severe hypoxia or hypercapnia do not resolve without active therapeutic intervention.

In most circumstances, metabolic disturbances of sufficient severity to cause loss of consciousness are not typically transient and self-correcting. Consequently, the clinical picture is not that of true syncope. However, impaired consciousness associated with metabolic and endocrine disturbances does occur, with the presumed pathophysiology being a disturbance of cerebral nutrient availability (e.g., marked hypoglycemia) and/or a major perturbation of acid–base or electrolyte environment (e.g., hyperventilation of presumably psychogenic origin).

Epilepsy is, like syncope, clinically characterized by usually transient attacks of a self-limited nature. However, epilepsy is not syncope. There are at least two important differences from syncope. The first is that the pathophysiology is totally different, and the second is that during seizure activity consciousness need not be lost. Epilepsy is the result of aberrant functioning of neural networks, unrelated to cerebral nutrient flow in most cases. Seizures may take the form of simple movements, but sensations affecting any sense, emotions, thoughts, and complex behavior patterns may also be the result of epilepsy.

Despite the foregoing differences between syncope and epilepsy, seizures are often mistaken for syncope and vice versa (8,83,85,86). In some patients, temporal lobe seizures may so closely mimic (or induce) neurally mediated reflex bradycardia and hypotension that differentiation from true syncope is difficult. Astatic or akinetic seizures are characterized by the patient's slumping to the ground (or if the patient is supine, by a period of muscular hypotonia), combined with unresponsiveness. However, these conditions are uncommon. More often, a careful history permits differentiation of seizures from true syncope. Seizures tend to be positionally independent, whereas true syncope is most commonly associated with upright posture. Further, seizures are often preceded by an aura and occasionally sensory hallucinations, whereas true syncope is not. Seizures are often associated with convulsive activity and loss of bowel or urinary continence, whereas any abnormal motor activity in true syncope is less severe, and incontinence is unusual (85). Finally, seizures are typically followed by a confusional state, and true syncope is typically followed by prompt restoration of mental state (although fatigue may persist).

"Drop attacks" refer to a poorly defined condition in which abrupt loss of postural tone occurs, but consciousness is generally preserved. The cause of these events is unknown (87). The dramatic clinical presentation of a fall often leads to an initial diagnosis of "syncope."

With regard to primary neurologic diseases (aneurysms, tumors, seizure disorders), episodes of loss of consciousness are, once again, usually not true syncope, but more often are seizures. Nevertheless, making a clinical diagnostic distinction can prove challenging. Astatic or akinetic seizures are particularly difficult to distinguish from syncope (87). Drop attacks may also be included in this category.

Pseudosyncope

Syncope may be mimicked by a variety of psychiatric conditions (see earlier). The medical history of very frequent (e.g., daily) "faints" or of multiple events without serious injury raises suspicion. Early psychiatric consultation should be sought (87a).

The term *pseudosyncope* refers to disorders in which loss of consciousness is not present although it may appear to be so; these are most importantly cataplexy and psychiatric causes.

Cataplexy is a symptom that occurs principally only in the context of the disease narcolepsy. Although cataplexy is not widely known or recognized, it is not particularly rare. Cataplexy refers to loss of muscle tone resulting from emotions, particularly laughter. In contrast to vasovagal syncope, pain, fear and anxiety are not strong triggers. Startle may provoke cataplexy. Consciousness is not lost.

The pathophysiology of psychiatric disturbances (e.g., somatization disorders) known to mimic syncope is poorly understood. For the most part, these conditions do not result in true syncopal events but may present as pseudounconsciousness or pseudosyncope. These terms denote that patients act as if they are unconsciousness while they are not. This is not uncommon in emergency rooms. In the fourth edition of the *Diagnostic and Statistical Manual of Mental Disorders*, the standard psychiatric diagnostic manual, a distinction is made among three entities:

- In conversion disorder, patients show unexplained somatic symptoms at a time when psychologic factors are also apparent.
- Factitious disorder means that patients intentionally pretend to be ill to assume the sick role.
- Malingering is similar to factitious disorder, but with the objective of achieving some goal, such as avoiding school, work, or other some other duty.

With regard to psychiatric conditions, patients manifesting such disturbances may have a greater tendency to be subject to the emotional faint or other forms of neurally mediated syncope (see earlier). Additionally, such patients may be prescribed certain medications that increase true syncope risk (e.g., phenothiazines, tricyclic antidepressants).

The label "psychogenic" should be treated with caution. Often, the diagnosis of a psychogenic condition relies on exclusion of other causes, and the literature is replete with this diagnosis having been made without a solid diagnostic foundation provided to exclude other causes. In brief, estimates of how often attacks are "psychogenic" should be viewed with skepticism.

DIAGNOSIS AND TREATMENT

In the clinical evaluation of the syncopal patient, the principal goal should be to establish an accurate diagnosis; only after a definitive diagnosis is made can an appropriate treatment strategy be initiated (88). Given the numerous causes of syncope and the unpredictable nature of syncopal events, achieving this goal is difficult, and special testing is often essential. This is especially true when symptoms are recurrent. However, even solitary syncopal events may warrant such steps when risks to the patient or public may be excessive, such as syncope associated with substantial physical injury or motor vehicle accident, syncope in individuals with high-risk occupations such as pilots, commercial truck drivers, or competitive athletes.

Initial Evaluation

A detailed and careful medical history of the syncopal events (including eyewitness accounts) is crucial for both differentiating syncope from other conditions (especially seizures) and providing clues to possible causes. However, it is often inconclusive (1,89–91). On average, the history alone provides a sufficiently precise basis for syncope in about 40% of cases.

The comprehensive medical history (with particular attention to bystander observations) and thorough physical examination may lead the physician to suspect the basis for syncope. However, unless these findings are classic, it is usually necessary to undertake selected diagnostic studies to establish the cause with a greater degree of certainty. In all cases, testing should be carefully targeted. The ordering of "routine" hematologic and biochemical screens is not productive. Similarly, routine application of specialized neurologic studies (CT, magnetic resonance imaging [MRI]) has an exceedingly low yield and is discouraged (8). A practicable strategy for syncope evaluation is depicted in Figure 71.5. As a rule, the first step (apart from excluding a past history of seizure disorder by history) is differentiation of those individuals with normal cardiovascular status from those with evident cardiac or cardiovascular disease. Usually, physical examination and echocardiographic assessment are sufficient for this purpose, although exercise testing should also be undertaken if syncope occurred with

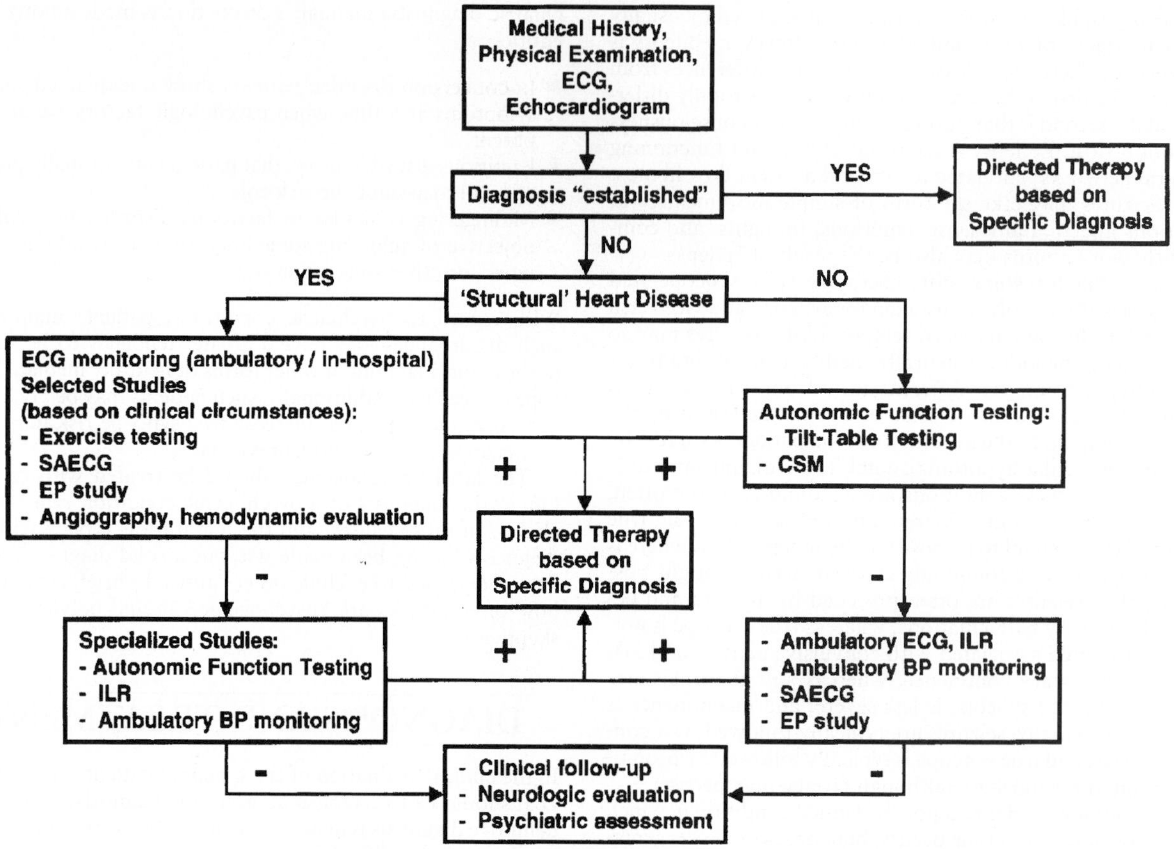

FIGURE 71.5. A proposed strategy for the syncope evaluation.

exertion, if ischemic heart disease is suspected, or if syncope occurred during physical exertion.

Specific Diagnostic Testing

Carotid Sinus Massage

One could reasonably argue that carotid massage should be part of the initial evaluation of all older (>55 years) syncopal patients (92–94). The technique for undertaking carotid sinus massage requires firm pressure for 5 to 10 seconds at a point below the angle of the mandible. Both heart rate and beat-to-beat blood pressure (e.g., noninvasive Finapres system) recordings are needed, and if the findings with the patient supine are nondiagnostic, the massage should be repeated with the patient in a head-up position on a tilt table. A cardiac pause 3 seconds or longer (some require 5 seconds) and/or a drop in systolic pressure 50 mm Hg or greater are considered abnormal. In general, the test has proved very safe, although care should be exercised in using this test in patients with carotid bruits or prior strokes or TIAs.

Electrocardiographic Recordings

ECG documentation during a spontaneous syncopal event is usually a high priority, because cardiac arrhythmias are so frequently the cause of syncope. In this regard, the 12-lead ECG is usually too brief to identify or exclude an arrhythmic cause. However, on occasion, findings such as ventricular preexcitation (e.g., Wolff-Parkinson-White syndrome) or QT interval prolongation suggest a potential mechanism. Similarly, exercise testing is usually of limited utility in the evaluation of syncope unless the events are clearly exertionally related by history. Only in rare instances does exercise testing uncover certain helpful findings (e.g., rate-dependent AV block, exertionally related tachyarrhythmias, severe degrees of chronotropic incompetence [95–99]).

For the most part, obtaining ECG documentation during spontaneous symptoms (if feasible at all) necessitates an extended period of cardiac monitoring employing ambulatory ECG recorders (52–56). The latter systems can be employed in a continuous-loop mode for patients whose symptoms preclude responding appropriately when the episode begins.

Conventional "event" recorders are external devices equipped with fixed electrodes through which an ECG can be recorded by direct application of the recorder electrodes to the chest wall (or other locations such as the wrist). Provided the patient can comply at the time of symptoms, a high-fidelity recording can be made. Recently, MCOT (Cardionet, Inc., San Diego, CA) has proven increasingly popular in the United States (56). This system can be activated by the patient due to symptom onset or automatically if a predetermined arrhythmia is detected. Wireless connection via the Internet permits the recording to be transmitted almost immediately to a central receiving station and ultimately to the appropriate physician.

The introduction of ILRs (Reveal and Reveal Plus, Medtronic Inc., Minneapolis, MN) has added a powerful new diagnostic tool. The ability of these devices to be programmed for automatic storage of rhythm strips in which heart rates fall outside a predetermined range is particularly advantageous (53–55,100). These devices are placed in a small subcutaneous pocket analogous to the technique for placement of a conventional pacemaker generator, but without the need for vascular access because there are no leads. The optimal location is usually just to the left of the sternum. However, more discreet locations in the anterior axillary region have also proven effective. The battery life is rated at 14 months, but the device often operates for 18 to 20 months.

The ILR has a solid-state loop memory, and the current version can store up to 42 minutes of continuous ECG recordings. Retrospective ECG allows activation of the device after consciousness has been restored, and the RevealPlus version is capable of both automatic recordings (based on physician-determined recording parameters) and patient-activated recordings. In one series of very symptomatic patients, symptom-ECG correlation was achieved in approximately 90% of patients within 6 months of implantation. Other studies of ILR use in syncopal patients have resulted in a diagnostic yield of 25% to 40% over an 8- to 10-month recording period. Obviously, the more prolonged the monitoring time is, the greater the chance will be of obtaining a useful recording.

As a rule, if ambulatory ECG monitoring is successful in providing a symptom–arrhythmia correlation, the need for additional diagnostic testing may be diminished but not necessarily eliminated. For example, documentation of symptomatic bradycardia does not exclude the possibility of a neurally mediated origin in which a concomitant vasodepressor element could complicate treatment.

Echocardiography and Vascular Ultrasound

Echocardiography rarely provides a definitive basis for syncope. Nevertheless, the echocardiogram has become essential for assessment of underlying structural heart disease. Furthermore, echocardiographic findings may be suggestive of a basis for syncope if evidence is obtained for HOCM, atrial myxoma, severe valvular aortic stenosis, or anomalous origin of one or more coronary arteries. Ultrasound techniques also are appropriately employed to assess vascular disturbances detected on physical examination, when these are deemed potential contributors to syncope. Thus, assessment of the carotid and/or subclavian system may be an appropriate step in selected individuals, but should not be ordered routinely.

Adenosine Triphosphate Test

Bolus injection of adenosine triphosphate (ATP) (or less desirably adenosine) has been used to unmask a propensity to AV block in older individuals with syncope of unknown origin (so-called ATP test) (101–107). Because the ATP effect is very short lasting, this test can be performed without backup pacing. The initial positive experiences reported by Flammang and colleagues should, however, be confirmed in currently ongoing larger studies before the ATP test becomes widespread. Nevertheless, the ATP test is appealing because it is safe, inexpensive, and rapid, and a positive outcome appears to bode well for cardiac pacing to prevent future syncope episodes.

Invasive Electrophysiologic Testing

In general, invasive electrophysiologic testing has proved useful for defining potential arrhythmic causes of syncope in individuals with underlying structural heart disease, including conduction system disturbances and the various forms of preexcitation syndromes. This has been especially true when tachyarrhythmias have been at fault. Conversely, such testing has proved less successful among patients without apparent structural substrate for arrhythmia (1,64).

As with any test, care must be taken in interpreting findings of invasive electrophysiologic studies. This seems to be particularly a concern when evaluating potential bradyarrhythmic causes of syncope. In this regard, Fujimura and colleagues (108) undertook such studies in patients in whom bradyarrhythmias were known to be the cause of syncope (21 syncopal patients with known symptomatic AV block or sinus pauses). Electrophysiologic testing correctly identified only 3 of 8 patients with documented sinus pauses (sensitivity, 37.5%) and 2 of 13 patients with documented AV block (sensitivity, 15.4%). Conversely, other abnormalities not known to have occurred spontaneously were often induced during electrophysiologic study. Tilt-table testing was not carried out in these patients, but had it been undertaken, the additional findings could possibly have been helpful in placing the apparently false-positive electrophysiologic findings in perspective.

Head-up Tilt-Table Testing

The importance of identifying susceptibility to vasovagal reactions in syncopal patients is readily evident, given the frequency with which vasovagal syncope appears to be responsible for patients' symptoms. To date, despite occasional criticism to the contrary (109), the head-up tilt-table test is the only diagnostic tool subjected to sufficient clinical scrutiny to assess its effectiveness in this setting (1,27–35). However, although head-up tilt-table testing may help establish a confident diagnosis, such testing is no longer advocated for predicting treatment efficacy.

Several reports have provided strong evidence that the symptomatic hypotension and bradycardia associated with a positive head-up tilt-table test are comparable to spontaneous neurally mediated vasovagal syncope (110–115). Further, tilt-table testing, especially when undertaken in the absence of provocative pharmacologic agents, appears to discriminate between symptomatic patients and asymptomatic control subjects with a level of precision considered acceptable for other clinically useful medical testing procedures (1).

The response to upright tilt-table testing in patients with suspected neurally mediated syncope differs from that observed in syncopal patients in whom other diagnostic studies have provided a firm basis for symptoms. For example, Fitzpatrick and colleagues (115) found that a 60-degree upright tilt reproduced symptoms in 53 of 71 (75%) patients with unexplained syncope; 40 patients exhibited both hypotension and bradycardia, whereas 13 manifested primarily a vasodepressor response. As a result of this and many other studies, head-up tilt-table testing has become a key component of the diagnostic strategy in patients suspected of having had neurally mediated syncope.

Neurologic Studies

Conventional neurologic laboratory studies (electroencephalography, head CT, and MRI) have had a relatively low yield in the syncopal patient. Consequently, these studies should be restricted to those situations in which other clinical observations suggest organic nervous system disease (see discussion earlier). Conversely, given the importance of orthostatic causes of syncope, tilt-table testing and other tests autonomic function have an increasingly important role to play.

Treatment

Neurally Mediated Syncopal Syndromes

In the case of neurally mediated syncopal syndromes, treatment strategies remain in evolution. Specific treatment should, when possible, be directed at relieving apparent trigger factors. Thus, alleviating or suppressing the cause of cough in cough syncope and treating esophageal abnormalities in swallow syncope are desirable approaches. However, in conditions such as carotid sinus syncope and vasovagal syncope, comparable approaches are not usually available.

In the case of vasovagal syncope, the mainstays in treatment are education and reassurance. This approach proves most effective when there is a prodrome of sufficient duration to permit the patient to take suitable evasive action. Patients whose symptoms demand more than education and reassurance are those whose attacks have minimal or no prodrome (especially if they have had resulting injury), those who cannot be taught to abort attacks, and those whose attacks are complicated by seizure-like activity or incontinence. Of particular concern are those patients with high-risk occupations or avocations in which syncope could lead to injury to themselves or others (e.g., pilots, commercial drivers, window washers, swimmers).

Increasingly, the preference for treatment of those patients in whom a more aggressive strategy is needed has focused on physical maneuvers and nonprescription volume expanders (116–119a). The former include leg crossing and/or arm tugging to abort episodes, whereas the latter focus on increased dietary salt and electrolyte intake with fluids (e.g., sport drinks, salt tablets). Moderate exercise training also appears to be among the safest initial approaches. Additionally, in highly motivated patients with recurrent vasovagal symptoms, the prescription of progressively prolonged periods of exposure to "still" upright posture (i.e., tilt training) may be beneficial (116). Tilt training requires education and a supportive environment, but it has proved a very valuable addition to the treatment armamentarium.

Beyond these measures, various pharmacologic approaches have been proposed (120–123), but few randomized clinical studies are available to confirm their utility. In this regard, fludrocortisone, β-adrenergic blocking drugs, disopyramide, and vasoconstrictor agents (e.g., midodrine) are the principal agents. Another group of drugs that appear to be useful in selected cases comprises the serotonin reuptake inhibitors. With regard to pharmacologic therapies, none (with the possible exception of midodrine) have proved particularly effective in controlled trials. However, each may have benefit in individual patients.

Cardiac pacing has proved highly successful in carotid sinus syndrome when bradycardia has been documented (124), and dual-chamber pacing is widely acknowledged to be the treatment of choice in all but the mildest forms of carotid sinus syndrome. Conversely, clinical experience with pacing in vasovagal syncope is less convincing, based on recent controlled clinical trials (125–130). Nonetheless, pacing may have a role in older individuals with refractory cardioinhibitory vasovagal faints.

Orthostatic Syncope

In orthostatic syncope, the mainstay of treatment is avoidance or removal (to the extent possible) of drugs that aggravate volume status (e.g., diuretics) and vasoconstriction (e.g., vasodilators). The desire is to favor expansion of central circulating volume. To this end, certain pharmacologic approaches are well accepted; specifically, administration of increased salt in the diet or the use of salt-retaining steroids (i.e., principally fludrocortisone) is usually the first step. Tilt training (see earlier) also may be advantageous, especially in patients with moderate dysautonomia. Other physical maneuvers such as use of counterpressure clothing (e.g., fitted stockings, abdominal compression devices) can be helpful. Unfortunately, fitted clothing is often uncomfortable (especially in hot climates), it is difficult for frail individuals to put on, and it exposes the patient to even worse symptoms when it is removed. In some cases, support hose contains latex and may thereby open the door to latex allergy.

With regard to drugs, of greatest current interest is midodrine, an agent with prominent venoconstrictor properties (120,121). Additional benefit has been reported with the use of erythropoietin, but it is not widely used for this indication.

Primary Cardiac Arrhythmias

The appropriate treatment of patients in whom bradyarrhythmias or tachyarrhythmias are the cause of syncope is relatively well understood. Patients in whom the correlation between syncope and bradycardia is well defined do very well with cardiac pacemaker therapy. However, other factors are often important contributors to the decision-making process. For instance, in the case of individuals with SND, optimal selection of treatment necessitates consideration of not only the culprit arrhythmic disturbance, but also the effects of drugs on sinus node and AV conduction properties and on ventricular function and proarrhythmic tendency. Additionally, current indications for and available modes of cardiac pacing, and the role of anticoagulation, must be incorporated in the overall treatment strategy. Finally, His bundle ablation, with placement of a permanent cardiac pacemaker, remains an important tool in treatment of selected SND patients who are symptomatic as a result of rapid ventricular rates during atrial fibrillation (131).

Many paroxysmal supraventricular tachyarrhythmias can be adequately controlled by conventional antiarrhythmic drug treatment. β-Adrenergic blockers or calcium channel blockers may be effective alone or, if necessary, in combination with class 1 antiarrhythmics (particularly class 1C drugs such as flecainide and propafenone). Rarely is amiodarone indicated, with the exception of paroxysmal refractory atrial fibrillation. More often, however, in patients with syncope resulting from paroxysmal supraventricular tachycardias, transcatheter ablation treatment options are the most highly effective and desirable option. For the most part, implantable devices for treatment of supraventricular tachycardias have fallen out of favor recently. However, the role of devices in conditions that are difficult to control may be making a resurgence with the availability of atrial implantable defibrillators and improved antitachycardia pacing systems.

In the case of syncope caused by VT, underlying heart disease (especially left ventricular dysfunction) of varying severity is usually present. The latter also increases the proarrhythmic risk associated with antiarrhythmic drug therapy, especially with class 1 agents. Consequently, pharmacologic therapeutic strategies often involve early consideration of class 3 agents (principally sotalol or amiodarone currently, but also dofetilide). However, given the difficulty of ensuring effective prophylaxis in this apparently high-risk patient population, the use of ICDs has become an important element of the overall treatment plan in many cases. In this context, Middelkauff and colleagues (132,133) noted that among patients with severe left ventricular dysfunction, the presence of a history of syncope was accompanied by a worrisome 1 year mortality (65% versus 25% in comparable patients without syncope) and a greater tendency to sudden death (45% of deaths versus 12% in comparable patients). Conversely, although ICD treatment may reduce mortality risk, syncope can still occur because of the time taken to diagnose the arrhythmia and charge the capacitors. Consequently, syncopal patients may well require concomitant antiarrhythmic drug treatment, or ablation.

Currently, ablation techniques are appropriate first choices in patients with right ventricular outflow tract tachycardia and bundle branch reentry tachycardia. The future may bring more extensive use of such techniques in a broader range of patients with VT.

Structural Cardiovascular or Cardiopulmonary Disease

In these cases, syncope is often only one of several possible types of symptoms experienced by the patient with underlying structural disease. Treatment is best directed at amelioration of the specific structural lesion or its consequences. Thus, in syncope associated with myocardial ischemia, pharmacologic therapy or revascularization is clearly the appropriate strategy. If successful, syncope susceptibility (whether the result of tachyarrhythmias or bradyarrhythmias or neural reflex effects) will be reduced. Similarly, when syncope is closely associated with surgically addressable lesions (e.g., valvular aortic stenosis, pericardial disease, atrial myxoma, congenital cardiac anomaly), a direct corrective approach is often feasible. Conversely, when syncope is caused by certain conditions that are difficult to treat such as primary pulmonary hypertension or restrictive cardiomyopathy, it is often impossible to ameliorate the underlying problem adequately. Even modifying outflow gradients in HOCM is not readily achieved surgically. In HOCM, the effectiveness of standard pharmacologic therapies remains uncertain (134,135); consequently, despite ongoing controversy, recent success with cardiac pacing techniques offers considerable promise to symptomatic individuals (136).

Cerebrovascular Conditions

Treatment of the conditions in this group is critically dependent on an accurate diagnosis. Imaging studies and neurologic and/or neurosurgical consultation assistance should be sought. For the most part, cerebrovascular disease rarely accounts for syncope, and consequently its evaluation is generally a low priority in the absence of new neurologic signs or other nervous system symptoms. Conversely, the possibility of such a cause should not be completely ignored. For example, arterial entrapment in conjunction with cervical spine disease is correctable, but it is so rare that it is hardly ever considered.

Syncope Mimics

Syncope-like states (syncope mimics, Table 71.4) occurring in the setting of conditions such as diabetic coma, intoxication, severe hypoxia, or hypercapnia obviously require urgent attention addressing the underlying problem. However, true syncope is rarely if ever solely caused by such conditions (acute hypoxia may be an exception if it reverses promptly, as can occur during high-altitude flight). From a clinical perspective, syncope resulting from psychogenic hyperventilation is the most important to consider, and over the long term it is very challenging to treat. Psychiatric assistance is essential in such cases. Pharmacotherapy, counseling, and biofeedback may be needed in combination.

Recognition of temporal lobe seizures or akinetic seizures and drop attacks requires considerable clinical acumen, appropriate laboratory testing, and expert neurologic consultation. The first two conditions are controllable with antiepileptic medications, whereas the third has proved difficult to control. Migraine is far more common, and although it is an infrequent cause of syncope, pharmacologic treatment is highly effective.

Syncope accompanying anxiety attacks and hysteria can prove to be a chronically recurring problem. A psychiatric diagnosis for symptoms has to very carefully considered before that label is applied. Subtle disturbances of autonomic control may be overlooked in this setting.

Which Patients Require Hospitalization for Assessment

Admission to hospital may be appropriate for undertaking diagnostic studies in a safe environment or for initiating therapy, or both. When the cause of syncope has been diagnosed after the initial clinical evaluation, the need for hospitalization depends in part on the immediate risk posed to the patient by the underlying problem, as well as on the treatment proposed. Thus, for example, patients with syncope accompanying an acute myocardial infarction, pulmonary embolism, or torsade de pointes VT should be admitted to hospital, preferably to a monitored unit. Patients with vasovagal syncope or orthostatic syncope (e.g., from dehydration secondary to excess diuretic therapy) usually do not need admission, and more often than not they can be treated sufficiently well in the emergency department or clinic and released after a few hours. Exceptions would be individuals in whom injury risk is a concern, usually elderly or frail patients. Similarly, in terms of therapeutic considerations, patients needing initiation of certain antiarrhythmic drugs, pacemakers, or ICDs usually need to be admitted. Conversely, for patients treated with advice to increase salt and volume, or in whom education regarding physical maneuvers such as tilt training or leg crossing is to be provided, an outpatient visit is usually adequate.

SUMMARY

Prevention of recurrent syncope is critically dependent on establishing the basis for symptoms in each patient. The principal diagnostic step is differentiation of those individuals with normal cardiovascular status from those with evident structural disease. In the former, assuming that the medical history or physical examination has not identified another systemic problem, tilt-table testing should be undertaken. In the latter group, a functional assessment of the suspected structural disturbance and an evaluation of susceptibility to tachyarrhythmias and bradyarrhythmias by conventional electrophysiologic testing are appropriate at an early stage. Tilt-table testing should follow if the diagnosis remains in doubt. In only a few instances should special neurologic studies be selected as an initial step. In all cases, the ultimate objective is to obtain a sufficiently strong correlation between the syncopal symptoms and detected abnormalities to permit both an accurate assessment of prognosis and initiation of an appropriate treatment plan.

When structural cardiac or vascular disturbances or primary cardiac arrhythmias are determined to have caused syncope, therapy is relatively well defined. Conversely, although considerable progress is being made, treatment of neurally mediated reflex syncope, orthostatic syncope, and the various neurologic and psychiatric conditions that can mimic syncope is less well established.

CONTROVERSIES AND PERSONAL PERSPECTIVES

The appropriate management of patients with syncope remains a challenge. Despite the strides that have been taken in the assessment of the syncopal patient, strategies for assessment for syncope vary widely among physicians and among hospitals and clinics. More often than not, the evaluation and treatment of syncope are haphazard. The result is a broad and largely inexplicable variance from center to center in the frequency with which various diagnostic tests are applied, in the distribution of apparent attributable causes of syncope arrived at by attending clinicians, and in the proportion of syncopal patients in whom the diagnosis remains unexplained. Clearly, the development of U.S. syncope diagnosis and treatment guidelines comparable to those pioneered by the European Society of Cardiology (1) is needed along with greater application of the syncope management unit concept. Unfortunately, the recently published American College of Cardiology/American Heart Association statement on syncope (109) is so poorly crafted as to further muddy the waters. International criticism of this statement has been dramatic, and may lead to a proper international guideline.

Still uncertain is the point at which patients with syncope should be referred for speciality evaluation. I believe that referral is warranted if any of the following are present: (a) episodes are recurrent (more than two within a 1-year period), (b) there is evidence of underlying structural heart or cardiovascular disease, (c) physical injury has occurred, (d) the patient is at risk of economic loss (e.g., job loss), (e) the public is at risk owing to the individual's occupation (e.g., pilot, bus driver), or (f) the patient or family indicates alarm regarding possible recurrences. The establishment of practice guidelines (preferably an international multi-disciplinary guideline) addressing these and related issues will be essential to ensure that all patients with syncope receive optimal care.

Recently, trends in medical care reimbursement in the United States and other countries have not been favorable to the introduction and study of new technologies. In the case of the syncope evaluation, large insurers (e.g., U.S. Medicare, Blue Cross/Blue Shield) continue to attempt to save money in the short term by denying payment for valuable ambulatory monitoring techniques, and occasionally even for well-established tools such as such as tilt-table testing, despite substantial literature documenting the value of such techniques. The ability to clarify diagnoses and to address new therapies is a long-term economic saving that these insurers have tended to ignore. One hopes that concerted efforts by physician investigators, practitioners, and professional organizations will ultimately overcome this shortsightedness.

THE FUTURE

Considerable progress has been made in understanding both the causes of syncope and the optimal approach to establishing a diagnosis. In this regard, both inpatient and outpatient improvements are needed.

In the outpatient environment, we continue to be limited in our ability to undertake long-term diagnostic monitoring in syncopal patients. The development of easy to use ECG ILRs has been important. However, documenting the ECG is only part of the problem. Next-generation devices must focus on some assessment of systemic pressure recording. Further, by utilization of wireless communication from implantable devices, it should be possible to effect more rapid recognition of symptomatic rhythm and blood pressure problems and thereby permit more efficient resolution of potentially hazardous conditions.

In the inpatient arena, we must focus on the reality that syncope is a multifaceted disorder involving many organ systems. No single specialty is competent to deal with all patients. The syncope management unit service model adopted by the Newcastle (United Kingdom) group is a multidisciplinary approach to referrals for patients with syncope or falls. All patients attend the same facility (with access to cardiovascular equipment, investigations, and trained staff) but are investigated by a geriatrician or cardiovascular physician according to the dominant symptom cited in referral correspondence (i.e., falls or syncope). Recently, this group of investigators showed that activity at the acute care hospital in which the day-case falls and syncope evaluation unit was based experienced 6,116 fewer bed-days during the course of 1 year for the International Classification of Diseases code 10 categories comprising syncope and collapse compared with peer teaching hospitals in the United Kingdom. This reduction translated into a significant saving in emergency hospital costs (about 4 million euros or 5 million U.S. dollars). The savings were attributed to a combination of factors, reduced readmission rates, rapid access to outpatient facility for accident and emergency and community patients, and implementation of effective targeted treatment strategies for syncope and falls. In the United States, such a model is exceedingly rare, and its more widespread adoption needs encouragement.

Finally, future studies need to be directed at better understanding the multiple neurotransmitters and neural pathways associated with syncopal disorders, especially the neurally mediated reflex and orthostatic syncope. Further, these studies should address both the molecular and genetic factors leading to the apparently increased susceptibility certain individuals exhibit with respect to these forms of syncope. Development of an understanding of these topics will have important implications in terms of both the treatment of individuals and, in the most severe cases, the appropriate direction for advice regarding prognosis and family counseling.

ACKNOWLEDGMENT

I would like to thank Wendy Markuson and Barry L.S. Detloff for assistance in preparation of the manuscript.

References

1. Brignole M, Alboni P, Benditt DG, et al. Guidelines on management (diagnosis and treatment) of syncope: update 2004. *Europace* 2004;6:467–537.
2. Day SC, Cook EF, Funkenstein H, et al. Evaluation and outcome of emergency room patients with transient loss of consciousness. *Am J Med* 1982; 72:15–23.
3. Silverstein MD, Singer DE, Mulley AG, et al. Patients with syncope admitted to medical intensive care units. *JAMA* 1982;248:1185–1189.
4. Gendelman HE, Linzer M, Gabelman M, et al. Syncope in a general hospital population. *NY State J Med* 1983;83:116–165.
5. Martin GJ, Adams SL, Martin HG, et al. Prospective evaluation of syncope. *Ann Emerg Med* 1984;13:499–504.
6. Camm AJ, Lau CP. Syncope of undetermined origin: diagnosis and management. *Prog Cardiol* 1988;1:139–156.
7. Wayne HH. Syncope: physiological considerations and an analysis of the clinical characteristics in 510 patient. *Am J Med* 1961;30:418–438.
8. Kapoor W. Evaluation and outcome of patients with syncope. *Medicine (Baltimore)* 1990;69:160–175.
9. Savage DD, Corwin L, McGee DL, et al. Epidemiologic features of isolated syncope: the Framingham Study. *Stroke* 1985;16:626–629.
10. Lipsitz LA, Pluchino FC, Wei JY, et al. Syncope in an elderly institutionalized population: prevalence, incidence and associated risk. *Q J Med* 1985;55:45–54.
11. Sheldon R, Rose S, Flanagan P, et al. Risk factors for syncope recurrence after a positive tilt-table test in patients with syncope. *Circulation* 1996;93: 973–981.
12. McHenry LC, Fazekas JF, Sullivan JF. Cerebral hemodynamics of syncope. *Am J Med Sci* 1961;214:173–178.
13. Gibson GE, Pulsinelli W, Blass JP, et al. Brain dysfunction in mild to moderate hypoxia. *Am J Med* 1981;70:1247–1254.
14. Rowell LB. *Human cardiovascular control.* Oxford: Oxford University Press, 1993.
15. Hainsworth R. Syncope and fainting: classification and pathophysiological basis. In: Mathias CJ, Bannister R, eds. *Autonomic failure: a textbook of clinical disorders of the autonomic nervous system,* 4th ed. Oxford: Oxford University Press, 1999:428–436.
16. Smit AAJ, Halliwill JR, Low PA, et al. Topical review: pathophysiological basis of orthostatic hypotension in autonomic failure. *J Physiol (Lond)* 1999;519:1–10.
17. Schondorf R, Wieling W. Vasoconstrictor reserve in neurally mediated syncope. *Clin Auton Res* 2000;10:53–56.
18. Mathias CJ. Autonomic diseases: clinical features and laboratory evaluation. *J Neurol Neurosurg Psychiatry* 2003;74:31–41.
19. Tea SH, Mansourati J, L'Heveder G, et al. New insights into the pathophysiology of carotid sinus syndrome. *Circulation* 1996;93:1411–1416.
20. Sharpey-Schafer EP, Hayter CJ, Barlow ED. Mechanism of acute hypotension from fear and nausea. *BMJ* 1958;2:878–880.
21. Thoren P. Role of cardiac C fibres in cardiovascular control. *Rev Physiol Biochem Pharmacol* 1979;86:1–94.
22. Oberg B, Thoren P. Increased activity in left ventricular receptors during hemorrhage or occlusion of caval veins in the cat: a possible cause of the vaso-vagal reaction. *Acta Physiol Scand* 1972;85:164–173.
23. Benditt DG, Goldstein MA, Adler S, et al. Neurally mediated syncopal syndromes: pathophysiology and clinical evaluation. In: Mandel WJ, ed. *Cardiac arrhythmias,* 3rd ed. Philadelphia: JB Lippincott, 1995:879–906.
24. Scherrer U, Vissing S, Morgan BJ, et al. Vasovagal syncope after infusion of a vasodilator in a heart-transplant recipient. *N Engl J Med* 1990;322:602–604.
25. Fitzpatrick AP, Banner N, Cheng A, et al. Vasovagal syncope may occur after orthotopic heart transplantation. *J Am Coll Cardiol* 1993;21:1132–1137.
26. Morgan-Hughes NJ, Kenny RA, Scott CD, et al. Vasodepressor reactions after orthotopic cardiac transplantation: relationship to reinnervation status. *Clin Auton Res* 1994;4:125–129.
27. Kenny RA, Bayliss J, Ingram A, et al. Head up tilt: a useful test for investigating unexplained syncope. *Lancet* 1986;1:1352–1354.

28. Abi-Samra F, Maloney JD, Fouad-Tarazi FM, et al. The usefulness of head-up tilt testing and hemodynamic investigations in the workup of syncope of unknown origin. *PACE* 1988;11:1202–1214.
29. Almquist A, Goldenberg IF, Milstein S, et al. Provocation of bradycardia and hypotension by isoproterenol and upright posture in patients with unexplained syncope. *N Engl J Med* 1989;320:346–351.
30. Benditt DG, Lurie KG, Adler SW, et al. Rationale and methodology of head-up tilt table testing for evaluation of neurally mediated (cardioneurogenic) syncope. In: Zipes DP, Jalife J, eds. *Cardiac electrophysiology: from cell to bedside,* 2nd ed. Philadelphia: WB Saunders, 1995:1115–1128.
31. Sutton R, Petersen MEV. The clinical spectrum of neurocardiogenic syncope. *J Cardiovasc Electrophysiol* 1995;6:569–576.
32. Benditt DG, Sutton R. Tilt-table testing in the evaluation of syncope. *J Cardiovasc Electrophysiol* 2005;16:1–3.
33. Fitzpatrick A, Theodorakis G, Vardas P, et al. Methodology of head-up tilt testing in patients with unexplained syncope. *J Am Coll Cardiol* 1991; 17:125–130.
34. Benditt DG, Ferguson DW, Grubb BP, et al. Tilt-table testing for assessing syncope and its treatment: an American College of Cardiology expert consensus document. *J Am Coll Cardiol* 1996;28:263–275.
35. Kapoor WN, Smith M, Miller NL. Upright tilt testing in evaluating syncope: a comprehensive literature review. *Am J Med* 1994;97:78–88.
36. Mathias CJ. Role of autonomic evaluation in the diagnosis and management of syncope. *Clin Auton Res* 2004;14(suppl 1):45–54.
37. Morley CA, Sutton R. Carotid sinus syncope. *Int J Cardiol* 1984;6:287–293.
38. Brignole M, Menozzi C, Gianfranchi L, et al. Neurally mediated syncope detected by carotid sinus massage and head-up tilt test in sick sinus syndrome. *Am J Cardiol* 1991;68:1032–1036.
39. Imholz BP, Settels JJ, van der Meiracker AH, et al. Non-invasive continuous finger blood pressure measurement during orthostatic stress compared to intra-arterial pressure. *Cardiovasc Res* 1990;24:214–221.
40. Almquist A, Gornick C, Benson DW Jr, et al. Carotid sinus hypersensitivity: evaluation of the vasodepressor component. *Circulation* 1985;71:927–936.
41. Barcroft H, Edholm OG. On the vasodilatation in human skeletal muscle during posthaemorrhagic fainting. *J Physiol (Lond)* 1945;104:161–175.
42. Oberg B, White S. The role of vagal cardiac nerves and arterial baroreceptors in the circulatory adjustments to hemorrhage in the cat. *Acta Physiol Scand* 1970;80:395–403.
43. Morita H, Vatner SF. Effects of hemorrhage on renal nerve activity in conscious dogs. *Circ Res* 1985;57:788–793.
44. Secher NH, Jensen KS, Werner J, et al. Vagal slowing of the heart during hemorrhage: observations from 20 consecutive hypotensive patients. *BMJ* 1986;292:365–366.
45. Bannister R. Chronic autonomic failure with postural hypotension. *Lancet* 1979;2:404–406.
46. Hokkins A, Neville B, Bannister R. Autonomic neuropathy of acute onset. *Lancet* 1974;2:769–771.
47. Edmonds ME, Sturrock RD. Autonomic neuropathy in the Guillian-Barre syndrome. *BMJ* 1979;2:668–670.
48. Low PA, Opfer-Gherking TL, McPhee BR, et al. Prospective evaluation of clinical characteristics of orthostatic hypotension. *Mayo Clin Proc* 1995;70: 617–622.
49. Mathias CJ, Deguchi K, Schatz I. Observations on recurrent syncope and presyncope in 641 patients. *Lancet* 2001;357:348–345.
50. Mathias CJ. To stand on one's own legs. *Clin Med* 2002;2:237–245.
51. Goldstein DS, Robertson D, Esler M, et al. Dysautonomias: clinical disorders of the autonomic nervous system. *Ann Intern Med* 2002;137:753–763.
52. Armstrong VL, Lawson J, Kamper AM, et al. The use of an implantable loop recorder in the investigation of unexplained syncope in older people. *Age Ageing* 2003;32:185–188.
53. Ermis C, Zhu AX, Pham S, et al. Comparison of automatic and patient-activated arrhythmia recordings by implantable loop recorders in the evaluation of syncope. *Am J Cardiol* 2003;92:815–819.
54. Ross PE. Managing care through the air. *IEEE Spectrum* 2004;Dec:26–31
55. Krahn AD, Klein GJ, Yee R, et al. The use of monitoring strategies in patients with unexplained syncope: role of the external and implantable loop recorder. *Clin Auton Res* 2004;14:55–61.
56. Joshi AK, Kowey PR, Prystowsky EN, et al. First experience with a mobile cardiac outpatient telemetry (MCOT) system for the diagnosis and management of cardiac arrhythmia. *Am J Cardiol* 2005;95:878–881.
57. Rubenstein JJ, Schulman CL, Yurchak PM, et al. Clinical spectrum of the sick sinus syndrome. *Circulation* 1972;46:5–13.
58. Kaplan BM, Langendorf R, Lev M, et al. Tachycardia-bradycardia syndrome (so-called "sick sinus syndrome"). *Am J Cardiol* 1973;26:497–508.
59. Scheinman MM, Strauss HC, Evans GT, et al. Adverse effects of sympatholytic agents in patients with hypertension and sinus node dysfunction. *Am J Med* 1978;64:1013–1020.
60. Sutton R, Kenny R-A. The natural history of sick sinus syndrome. *PACE* 1986;9:1110–1114.
61. Skagen K, Hansen JF. The long-term prognosis for patients with sinoatrial block treated with permanent pacemaker. *Acta Med Scand* 1975;199:13–15.
62. Sasaki S, Shimotori M, Akahane K, et al. Long-term follow-up of patients with sick sinus syndrome: a comparison of clinical aspects among unpaced, ventricular inhibited paced, and physiologically paced groups. *PACE* 1988;11:1575–1583.
63. Brignole M, Menozzi C, Moya A, et al. The mechanism of syncope in patients with bundle branch block and negative electrophysiologic test. *Circulation* 2001;104:2045–2050.
64. Fei L, Trohman RG. Advances in cardiac electrophysiology and pacing. *Crit Care Clin* 2001;17:337–364.
65. Menozzi C, Brignole M, Garcia-Civera R, et al. Mechanism of syncope in patients with heart disease and negative electrophysiologic test. *Circulation* 2002;105;2741–2745.
66. Michaelson M, Engle MA. Congenital complete heart block: an international study of the natural history. *Cardiovasc Clin* 1972;4:86–101.
67. Pordon CM, Moodie DJ. Adults with congenital complete heart block: 25-year follow-up. *Cleve Clin J Med* 1992;59:587–590.
68. Michaelsson M, Jonzon A, Riesenfeld T. Isolated congenital complete atrioventricular block in adult life. *Circulation* 1995;92:442–449.
69. Dhingra RC, Denes P, Wu D, et al. Syncope in patients with chronic bifascicular block. *Ann Intern Med* 1974;81:302–306.
70. Scheinman MM, Peters RW, Sauve MJ, et al. Value of H-Q interval in patients with bundle branch block and the role of prophylactic permanent pacing. *Am J Cardiol* 1982;50:1316–1322.
71. Dhingra RC, Amat y Leon F, Pouget M, et al. Infranodal block: diagnosis, clinical significance and management. *Med Clin North Am* 1976;60:175–192.
72. Seidl K, Drogemuller A, Rameken M, et al. Two year follow-up in 643 patients with non-invasively unexplained syncope and therapy guided by electrophysiologic study. *Z Kardiol* 2003;92:852–861.
73. Leitch JW, Klein GJ, Yee R, et al. Syncope associated with supraventricular tachycardia: an expression of tachycardia or vasomotor response. *Circulation* 1992;85:1064–1071.
74. Simson MB. Signal-averaged electrocardiography. In: Zipes DP, Jalife J, eds. *Cardiac electrophysiology: from cell to bedside,* 2nd ed. Philadelphia: WB Saunders, 1995:1038–1048.
75. Kuchar DL, Thorburn CW, Sammel NL. Signal-averaged electrocardiogram for evaluation of recurrent syncope. *Am J Cardiol* 1986;58:949–953.
76. Buxton AE, Lee KL, Fisher JD, et al., for the Multicenter Unsustained Tachycardia Trial Investigators. A Randomized Study of the Prevention of Sudden Death in Patients with Coronary Artery Disease. *N Engl J Med* 1999;341:1882–1890.
77. Steinberg JS, Beckman K, Greene HL, et al. Follow-up of patients with unexplained syncope and inducible ventricular tachyarrhythmias: analysis of the AVID registry and an AVID substudy: Antiarrhythmics Versus Implantable Defibrillators. *J Cardiovasc Electrophysiol* 2001;12:996–1001.
78. Pathy MS. Clinical presentation of myocardial infarction in the elderly. *Br Heart J* 1967;29:190–199.
79. Dixon MS, Thomas P, Sheridon DJ. Syncope is the presentation of unstable angina. *Int J Cardiol* 1988;19:125–129.
80. Maron BJ. Cardiology patient pages: hypertrophic cardiomyopathy. *Circulation* 2002;106:2419–2421.
81. Johnson AM. Aortic stenosis, sudden death, and the left ventricular baroreceptors. *Br Heart J* 1971;33:1–5.
81a. Savitz SI, Caplan LR. Vertebrobasilar disease. *N Engl J Med* 2005;352: 2618–2626.
82. Thijs RD, Benditt DG, Mathias C, et al. Unconscious confusion: a literature search for definitions of syncope and related disorders. *Clin Auton Res* 2005;15:35–39.
83. Soteriades ES, Evans JC, Larson MG, et al. Incidence and prognosis of syncope. *N Engl J Med* 2002;347:878–885.
84. Chan-Scarabelli C, Scarabelli TM. Neurocardiogenic syncope. *BMJ* 2004; 329:336–348.
85. Grubb BP, Gerard G, Rousch K, et al. Differentiation of convulsive syncope and epilepsy with head up tilt table testing. *Ann Intern Med* 1991;115:871–876.
86. Zaidi A, Clough P, Cooper P, et al. Misdiagnosis of epilepsy: many seizure-like attacks have a cardiovascular cause. *J Am Coll Cardiol* 2000;36:181–184.
87. Sulg IA. Differential diagnosis in syncope and epilepsy: clinical neurophysiological and cardiological aspects. In: Refsum H, Sulg IA, Rasmussen K, eds. *Heart and brain, brain and heart.* Berlin: Springer-Verlag, 1989:202–221.
87a. Benbadis SR. The problem of psychogenic symptoms: is the psychiatric community in denial? *Epilepsy Behav* 2005;6:9–14.
88. Benditt DG, Brignole M. Syncope: is a diagnosis a diagnosis? *J Am Coll Cardiol* 2003;41:791–794.
89. Alboni P, Dinelli M. Bettiol K, et al. What is the value of clinical history in establishing the cause of syncope? In: Raviele A, ed. *Cardiac arrhythmias 1999,* vol 1. Milan: Springer-Verlag Italia, 2000:419–422.
90. Alboni P, Brignole M, Menozzi C, et al. The diagnostic value of history in patients with syncope with or without heart disease. *J Am Coll Cardiol* 2001;37:1921–1928.
91. Sheldon R, Rose S, Ritchie D, et al. Historical criteria that distinguish syncope from seizures. *J Am Coll Cardiol* 2002;40:142–148.
92. Parry SW, Richardson D, O'Shea D, et al. Diagnosis of carotid sinus hypersensitivity in older adults: carotid sinus massage in the upright position is essential. *Heart* 2000;83:22–23.

93. Kenny RA, Richardson DA, Steen N, et al. Carotid sinus syndrome: a modifiable risk factor for non-accidental falls in older adults (SAFE PACE). *J Am Coll Cardiol* 2001;38:1491–1496.
94. Richardson DA, Bexton R, Shaw FE, et al. How reproducible is the cardioinhibitory response to carotid sinus massage in fallers. *Europace* 2002;4:361–364.
95. Grubb BP, Temesy-Armos P, Samoil D, et al. Head upright tilt table testing in the evaluation and management of young athletes with recurrent exercise-induced syncope. *Med Sci Sports Exerc* 1993;25:24–28.
96. Sakaguchi S, Shultz J, Remole C, et al. Syncope associated with exercise, a manifestation of neurally-mediated syncope. *Am J Cardiol* 1995;75:476–481.
97. Calkins H, Seifert M, Morady F. Clinical presentation and long term follow-up of athletes with exercise-induced vasodepressor syncope. *Am Heart J* 1995;129:1159–1164.
98. Fox WC, Lockette W. Unexpected syncope and death during intense physical training: evolving role of molecular genetics. *Aviat Space Environ Med* 2003;74:1223–1230.
99. Colivicchi F, Ammirati F, Santini M. Epidemiology and prognostic implications of syncope in young competing athletes. *Eur Heart J* 2004;25:1749–1753.
100. Krahn AD, Klein GJ, Yee R, et al., the Reveal Investigators. Use of an extended monitoring strategy in patients with problematic syncope. *Circulation* 1999;99:406–410.
101. Flammang D, Church T, Waynberger M, et al. Can adenosine 5′ triphosphate be used to select treatment in severe vasovagal syndrome? *Circulation* 1997;96:1201–1208.
102. Brignole M, Gaggioli G, Menozzi C, et al. Adenosine-induced atrioventricular block in patients with unexplained syncope: the diagnostic value of ATP test. *Circulation* 1997;96:3921–3927.
103. Flammang D, Chassing A, Donal E, et al. Reproducibility of the 5′ triphosphate test in vasovagal syndrome. *J Cardiovasc Electrophysiol* 1998;9:1161–1166.
104. Flammang D, Erickson M, McCarville S, et al. Contribution of head-up tilt testing and ATP testing in assessing the mechanisms of vasovagal syndrome: preliminary results and potential therapeutic implications. *Circulation* 1999;99:2427–2433.
105. Donateo P, Brignole M, Menozzi C, et al. Mechanism of syncope in patients with positive adenosine tests. *J Am Coll Cardiol* 2003;41:93–98.
106. Flammang D, Benditt D, Pelleg A. Apport du test à l'adénosine-5′-triphosphate (ATP) dans l'évaluation diagnostique et l'approche thérapeutique des syncopes d'origine indéterminée (vasovagale ou neurocardiogénique). The adenosine-5′-triphosphate (ATP) test: a diagnostic tool in the management of syncope of unknown origin: basic and clinical aspects. *Ann Cardiol Angeiol* 2005;54:144–150.
107. Flammang D, Pelleg A, Benditt DG. The adenosine triphosphate (ATP) test for evaluation of syncope of unknown origin. *J Cardiovasc Electrophysiol* 2005;16:1388–1389.
108. Fujimura O, Yee R, Klein GJ, et al. The diagnostic sensitivity of electrophysiologic testing in patients with syncope caused by bradycardia. *N Engl J Med* 1989;321:1703–1707.
109. Strickberger SA, Benson DW Jr, Biaggioni MD, et al. AHA/ACCF Scientific Statement on the Evaluation of Syncope. *Am Coll Cardiol* 2006;47:473–484.
110. Fitzpatrick A, Williams T, Ahmed R, et al. Echocardiographic and endocrine changes during vasovagal syncope induced by prolonged head-up tilt. *Eur J Card Pacing Electrophysiol* 1992;2:121–128.
111. Benditt DG, Lurie KG, Adler SW, et al. Rationale and methodology of head-up tilt table testing for evaluation of neurally mediated (cardioneurogenic) syncope. In: Zipes DP, Jalife J, eds. *Cardiac electrophysiology: from cell to bedside,* 2nd ed. Philadelphia: WB Saunders, 1995:1115–1128.
112. van Lieshout JJ, Wieling W, Karemaker JM, et al. The vasovagal response. *Clin Sci* 1991;81:575–586.
113. Chen M-Y, Goldenberg IF, Milstein S, et al. Cardiac electrophysiologic and hemodynamic correlates of neurally mediated syncope. *Am J Cardiol* 1989;63:66–72.
114. Sander-Jensen K, Secher NH, Astrup A, et al. Hypotension induced by passive head-up tilt: endocrine and circulatory mechanisms. *Am J Physiol* 1986;251:R742–R748.
115. Fitzpatrick A, Theodorakis G, Vardas P, et al. The incidence of malignant vasovagal syndrome in patients with recurrent syncope. *Eur Heart J* 1991;12:389–394.
116. Ector H, Reybrouck T, Heidbuchel H, et al. Tilt training: a new treatment for recurrent neurocardiogenic syncope or severe orthostatic intolerance. *PACE* 1998;21:193–196.
117. Kerdiet CTP, van Dijk N, Linzer M, et al. Management of vasovagal syncope: controlling or aborting faints by leg crossing and muscle tensing. *Circulation* 2002;106:1684–1689.
118. Abe H, Kohshi K, Nakashima Y. Home orthostatic self-training in neurocardiogenic syncope. *Pacing Clin Electrophysiol* 2005;28(suppl 1):S246–S248.
119. van Dijk N, de Bruin IG, Gisolf J, et al. Hemodynamic effects of leg crossing and skeletal muscle tensing during free standing in patients with vasovagal syncope. *J Appl Physiol* 2005;98:584–590.
120. Sra J, Maglio C, Biehl M, et al. Efficacy of midodrine hydrochloride in neurocardiogenic syncope refractory to standard therapy. *J Cardiovasc Electrophysiol* 1997;8:42–46.
121. Benditt DG, Wilbert L, Fahy G, et al. Midodrine for treatment of vasovagal syncope. In: Raviele A, ed. *Cardiac arrhythmias 1999,* vol 1. Milan: Springer-Verlag Italia, 2000:463–468.
122. Grubb BP, Wolfe D, Samoil D, et al. Usefulness of fluoxetine hydrochloride for prevention of resistant upright tilt induced syncope. *PACE* 1993;16:458–464.
123. Kosinski D, Grubb BP, Temesy-Armos PN. The use of serotonin re-uptake inhibitors in the treatment of neurally-mediated cardiovascular disorders. *J Serotonin Res* 1994;1:85–90.
124. Benditt DG, Remole S, Asso A, et al. Cardiac pacing for carotid sinus syndrome and vasovagal syncope. In: Barold SS, Mugica J, eds. *New perspectives in cardiac pacing,* vol 3. Mount Kisco, NY: Futura, 1993:15–28.
125. Benditt DG, Peterson M, Lurie K, et al. Cardiac pacing for prevention of recurrent vasovagal syncope. *Ann Intern Med* 1995;122:204–209.
126. Benditt DG. Cardiac pacing for prevention of vasovagal syncope (editorial). *J Am Coll Cardiol* 1999;33:21–23.
127. Connolly SJ, Sheldon R, Roberts RS, et al. The North American Vasovagal Pacemaker Study (VPS): a randomized trial of permanent cardiac pacing for the prevention of vasovagal syncope. *J Am Coll Cardiol* 1999;33:16–20.
128. Sutton R, Brignole M, Menozzi C, et al., for the VASIS investigators: dual-chamber pacing is efficacious in treatment of neurally-mediated tilt-positive cardioinhibitory syncope. Pacemaker versus no therapy: a multicentre randomized study. *Circulation* 2000;102:294–299.
129. Connolly S, Sheldon R, Thorpe KE, et al. Pacemaker therapy for prevention of syncope in patients with recurrent severe vasovagal syncope: second vasovagal pacemaker study (VPSII): a randomized trial. *N Engl J Med* 2003;289:2224–2229.
130. Raviele A, Giada F, Menozzi C, et al., Vasovagal Syncope and Pacing Trial investigators. A randomized, double-blind, placebo-controlled study of permanent cardiac pacing for the treatment of recurrent tilt-induced vasovagal syncope: the Vasovagal Syncope and Pacing trial (SYNPACE). *Eur Heart J* 2004;25:1741–1748.
131. Scheinman MM, Evans-Bell T, and the Executive Committee of the Percutaneous Cardiac Mapping and Ablation Registry. Catheter ablation of the atrioventricular junction: a report of the percutaneous mapping and ablation registry. *Circulation* 1984;70:1024–1029.
132. Middelkauff HR, Stevenson WG, Stevenson LW, et al. Syncope in advanced heart failure: high risk of sudden death regardless of origin of syncope. *J Am Coll Cardiol* 1993;21:110–116.
133. Middelkauff HR, Stevenson WG, Saxon LA. Prognosis after syncope: impact of left ventricular function. *Am Heart J* 1993;125:121–127.
134. McKenna WJ, Deanfield J, Faruqui A, et al. Prognosis in hypertrophic cardiomyopathy: role of age and clinical electrocardiographic and hemodynamic features. *Am J Cardiol* 1981;47:532–538.
135. Maron BJ, Roberts WC, Epstein SE. Sudden death in hypertrophic cardiomyopathy: a profile of 78 patients. *Circulation* 1982;65:1388–1394.
136. McAreavey D, Epstein ND, Fananapazir L. Dual chamber pacing is effective therapy for hypertrophic cardiomyopathy patients with provocable LV outflow tract obstruction and symptoms refractory to medical therapy. *J Am Coll Cardiol* 1994;23:11(abst).

CHAPTER 72 ■ ANTIARRHYTHMIC DRUGS

DAN M. RODEN

OVERVIEW

Drugs used for treating cardiac arrhythmias may not be completely effective and carry substantial risks for adverse effects. These adverse effects can be grouped into three broad categories: proarrhythmia, other cardiovascular effects such as bradycardia or heart failure, and noncardiovascular effects. Despite these shortcomings, antiarrhythmic drugs retain a place in the treatment of cardiac arrhythmias. A solid understanding of the mechanisms that underlie these adverse effects and of the drugs' pharmacokinetics can help to minimize the likelihood of adverse effects during long-term treatment.

HISTORICAL PERSPECTIVE

Treatment of cardiac arrhythmias has moved from the completely empiric administration of drugs to alleviate symptoms in the mid-eighteenth century to an increasing appreciation of the diverse mechanisms that may underlie cardiac arrhythmias and of the molecular mechanisms of action of older as well as newly available compounds. We now recognize that block of the function of membrane proteins, primarily ion channels and receptors, is the major mechanism underlying both the efficacy and toxicity of available antiarrhythmic drugs. However, with rare exceptions (notably the genetic ion channelopathies; see Chapter 96), dysfunction of these drug targets is not the mechanism responsible for most arrhythmias. It seems entirely likely that as our understanding of arrhythmia mechanisms continues to expand, new compounds devoid of serious toxicity that better target specific arrhythmic mechanisms may well be developed, thereby supplanting the highly nonspecific and poorly tolerated drugs currently available.

The increasing sophistication in understanding mechanisms underlying arrhythmias and antiarrhythmic drug actions and in nonpharmacologic approaches to arrhythmia management has resulted in more focused and narrower indications for antiarrhythmic drug therapy. Antiarrhythmic drugs continue to be first-line therapy for the acute suppression of ongoing arrhythmias. They are also used to prevent recurrence of chronic arrhythmias in patients in whom ablation has not been attempted, is not feasible, or has been unsuccessful. Although patients at high risk for serious arrhythmias can be identified, multiple trials have shown a detrimental effect of primary prophylactic antiarrhythmic drug therapy in such patients. In patients with implantable cardioverter-defibrillators (ICDs), antiarrhythmic drugs are sometimes required as adjunctive therapy to prevent arrhythmias that generate device discharges (see Chapter 76).

TRIALS OF PHARMACOLOGIC THERAPY TO PREVENT SUDDEN CARDIAC DEATH

Sudden cardiac death (SCD) resulting from ventricular fibrillation (VF) accounts for about 25% of all deaths in adults in the United States (see Chapter 67). The recent history of antiarrhythmic drug development is largely focused on the issue of whether these agents alter SCD risk; this applies to settings in which they are used for symptomatic arrhythmias such as atrial fibrillation (AF), as well as to studies directly assessing their effects in patients at risk of SCD.

Large trials of β-blockers starting in the 1970s showed their value in reducing SCD incidence (1–3). Although calcium channel blockers exhibit antiarrhythmic effects in animal models, especially during myocardial ischemia (4), these drugs have produced either no change or an increase in SCD incidence in clinical trials (5,6). In the 1970s and 1980s, nonsustained ventricular arrhythmias were identified as a risk factor for SCD in patients convalescing from acute myocardial infarction (MI). Accordingly, the Cardiac Arrhythmia Suppression Trial (CAST), the first double-blind, randomized, placebo-controlled, well-powered study of antiarrhythmic drugs, was designed to test the hypothesis that suppression of nonsustained ventricular arrhythmias in patients convalescing from acute MI would reduce mortality. However, CAST and other studies of sodium channel blockers showed that therapy with these agents unexpectedly increased mortality (7–10).

As a result, drug development moved rapidly away from sodium channel blockade and toward action potential (AP) prolongation as an antiarrhythmic intervention. This approach has theoretic advantages, such as preventing ischemic VF, lowering defibrillation energy requirements, and improving cardiac contractility (11,12). However, virtually all available AP-prolonging drugs act by blocking a specific cardiac potassium current, termed I_{Kr}; a class action of I_{Kr} blockers is the occasional development of marked QT prolongation and the potentially fatal polymorphic ventricular tachycardia (VT) called *torsade de pointes* (13). Mutations in the gene that encodes the protein responsible for I_{Kr} are one cause of the congenital long QT syndrome (LQTS), also associated with torsade de pointes (14,15). Trials of d-sotalol and dofetilide, I_{Kr} blockers devoid of other pharmacologic actions, showed no effect on or an increase in mortality (16–18). Taken together, these data suggest that if AP prolongation is to be successful as an antiarrhythmic mode of drug action, I_{Kr} blockade may not be the safest means of achieving this goal.

The most widely used antiarrhythmic, amiodarone, was originally developed as a thyroid hormone analog antianginal agent, and only subsequently was it found to exert antiarrhythmic effects (19,20). Although the drug has many pharmacologic properties including antiadrenergic effects that may explain its antiarrhythmic actions, the mechanisms by which it suppresses arrhythmias are not known. Multiple trials have assessed the effects of amiodarone to prevent SCD in patients at risk (21–25). Overall, there may be a small potential for benefit after MI (26,27), but probably not in heart failure (22,25); because the benefit is small (at most), and because the drug also has the potential for serious toxicity during long-term administration, it is not generally used for primary prophylaxis of SCD.

This chapter reviews antiarrhythmic drugs, traditionally defined as agents primarily developed or used for the therapy of arrhythmias. Recent studies with other classes of drugs widely used in cardiovascular therapy, notably hepatic 3-methylglutaryl coenzyme A (HMG CoA) reductase inhibitors ("statins") and agents inhibiting the effects of activating the renin-angiotensin system (angiotensin-converting enzyme inhibitors and receptor blockers [ACE inhibitors and ARBs]) have demonstrated antiarrhythmic actions. The reduction in SCD by these agents may relate to their effects on vascular disease and so are perhaps unsurprising (28,29). However, there is increasing evidence that these agents also can reduce the incidence of AF (30–34). The mechanisms are not well understood, and antifibrotic, antiinflammatory, and antioxidant stress mechanisms have been invoked (35–39). These agents are not sufficiently well studied in arrhythmias to suggest that they be used in primary therapy, but they may be especially desirable in certain clinical settings; an example would be AF in hypertension, in which an ACE inhibitor would be a logical drug. Most importantly, the identification of such unanticipated antiarrhythmic actions points to heretofore unappreciated molecular pathways leading to arrhythmias and thus perhaps to newer therapies better targeted to underlying mechanisms.

PATHOPHYSIOLOGY

The three major mechanisms that underlie cardiac arrhythmias—enhanced automaticity, triggered activity, and reentry—are discussed in detail elsewhere (see Chapter 57). In most cases, choosing an antiarrhythmic drug for terminating ongoing arrhythmias or for suppressing recurrent episodes is based not on an understanding of specific mechanisms but rather on clinical experience. This experience includes not only determining what drug is likely to be effective against a particular arrhythmia but also estimating the risk for serious cardiac side effects from a particular drug in a particular patient, as well as estimating the risk for noncardiac side effects. This approach has proved effective because the drugs that are available are quite nonspecific (i.e., they produce a multiplicity of cardiac and noncardiac effects), and detailed characterization of the mechanisms underlying individual arrhythmic syndromes has not been considered part of routine clinical care until recently. Increasingly, precise characterization of mechanisms in individual arrhythmia syndromes may rationalize selection of antiarrhythmic drugs, to target specific "weak links" in those mechanisms, thus restoring normal rhythm. This approach, popularized as the Sicilian Gambit in the early 1990s (40), seems self-evident (Table 72.1). However, for many arrhythmias, there is insufficient information detailing the mechanisms, or in other cases appropriate drugs are not yet available to target weak links in individual arrhythmias. Conversely, an understanding of the putative mechanism underlying an individual arrhythmia in a particular patient may help the clinician to avoid using drugs that are likely to prove ineffective or to exacerbate an individual arrhythmia. Table 72.1 lists the mechanisms of the specific arrhythmias and provides clinical examples of arrhythmias caused by those mechanisms as well as drug effects that may be antiarrhythmic (or are contraindicated) in those mechanisms.

An especially appealing model for this approach is the way in which an emerging understanding of molecular mechanisms in the congenital arrhythmia syndromes has enabled identification of specific pharmacologic therapy for certain subtypes. Examples (see also Chapters 95 and 96) include variable efficacy of β-blockers as a function of molecular subtype in the congenital LQTSs (41), mexiletine or flecainide for the sodium channel–linked form of congenital LQTS (42,43), quinidine for the Brugada syndrome (44,45) and the short QT syndrome (46), and β-blockers for catecholaminergic polymorphic VT. In fact, in catecholaminergic polymorphic VT, experimental studies have identified calcium release from the sarcoplasmic reticulum as a major arrhythmogenic mechanism, and so drug therapy to prevent this arrhythmogenic phenomenon, for this rare syndrome and perhaps for more common diseases, may be a reasonable new approach (47).

Basic electrophysiologists have identified multiple ion currents in individual cardiac cells. This information allows identification not only of specific currents that are blocked by the drugs described in this chapter but also of factors such as rate and hypokalemia that can modulate this block. As described in this chapter, these data have direct implications for the clinical use of antiarrhythmic drugs. More recently, a combination of cellular electrophysiologic and molecular biologic techniques has enabled the cloning of individual genes whose protein products are responsible for individual ion currents, as well as studies of their function. Although this information could prove useful in designing new antiarrhythmic molecules, there are virtually no data attesting to the long-term safety of any drug whose primary mode of action is to block an ion channel. Thus, another implication of such advanced molecular information is that entirely new targets may be identified at which new drugs may act to modify cardiac electrophysiology in clinically effective and safe manners.

CLINICAL PROFILES

Schemes that classify antiarrhythmic drugs by their major ionic mechanisms of action are commonly used. Their usefulness lies in that they may allow clinicians to predict the therapeutic

TABLE 72.1

ANTIARRHYTHMIC DRUG THERAPIES, TARGETED TO AN UNDERSTANDING OF UNDERLYING MECHANISMS[a]

		Drug actions that may be antiarrhythmic					
		Sodium channel block					
Arrhythmia mechanism	Clinical examples	Lidocaine plus mexiletine	Others[c]	β-Blockade	Calcium channel block	↑APD[b]	Other
Enhanced normal automaticity	Sinus tachycardia			Y			
	Some "idiopathic" VT		Y				
Abnormal automaticity	Ectopic atrial tachycardia		Y		Y	Y	
	suppress arrhythmia			Y	Y		
	control rate						
	Accelerated idioventricular rhythm	Y	Y				
EAD-related triggered activity	Torsades de pointes	Y				Ξ	Pacing; isoproterenol, magnesium
	shorten APD block triggering			Y	[Y]		
DAD-related triggered activity	Digitalis toxicity						Antidigoxin antibodies
	Exercise-induced VT originating in RVOT or (L) posterior fascicle			Y	Y		Adenosine
Reentry utilizing defined circuit(s)	AV nodal reentry/ AV reentry[d]		Y	Y	Y	Y	Adenosine, [digitalis], [↑vagal tone (phenylephrine, edrophonium)]
	Atrial flutter slow ventricular rate		Y?	Y	Y	Y	Digitalis: Y
	terminate tachycardia						
	prevent recurrence		Y			Y	
	VT with LV scarring (e.g. postmyocardial infarction)	Y	Ξ		Ξ	Y	
	Acute termination	Y	Ξ	Y	Ξ	Y	
	Prevent recurrence						
Reentry without defined circuit	Atrial fibrillation						
	Slow ventricular rate			Y	Y		Digitalis: Y
	Terminate tachycardia		Y?			Y	
	Prevent recurrence		Y			Y	
	Atrial fibrillation with ventricular preexcitation				Ξ		Digitalis: Ξ
	Slow ventricular rate		Y			Y	
	Terminate arrhythmia		Y			Y	
	Ventricular fibrillation						
	Acute termination	Y	Y			Y	
	Prevent recurrences	Y	Y	Y		Y	
Genetic arrhythmia syndromes	Long QT syndromes			Y			
	LQT1			Y			
	LQT3	Y	Y	Y (?)			
	Brugada syndrome						Transient outward potassium current block (?quinidine)
	Short QT syndrome					Y	
	Catecholaminergic polymorphic VT			Y			?Drugs to prevent calcium release from sarcoplasmic reticulum?

APD, action potential duration; AV, atrioventricular; DAD, delayed afterdepolarization; EAD, early afterdepolarization; LV, left ventricular; RVOT, right ventricular outflow tract; VT, ventricular tachycardia; Y, indicated; Ξ, contraindicated; [], approaches that are not widely used clinically or that are theoretic but as yet unproven.

[a]For further discussion of the choice of drugs individual arrhythmias, see specific chapters. For some arrhythmias, nonpharmacologic approaches may be the short- or long-term treatment of choice; see text and specific chapters for a fuller discussion. In addition, the mechanisms underlying isolated ectopic beats, in the atrium or ventricle, have not been established and may be multifactorial; these generally require no therapy.

[b]Includes drugs such as amiodarone, disopyramide, procainamide, quinidine, and sotalol that produce other important effects, as well as ibutilide and dofetilide, which are "pure" action potential prolonging drugs.

[c]Includes disopyramide, flecainide, procainamide, propafenone, and quinidine.

[d]Acute termination is generally accomplished with adenosine or verapamil; recurrences are prevented with verapamil (in the absence of preexcitation) or flecainide.

outcome of one drug based on the outcome of another. However, as mentioned previously, a major limitation of many currently available drugs is the likelihood of noncardiac side effects, which do not track with classification schemes. Moreover, members of the same drug class or subclass may exert subtle, or sometimes not so subtle, differences in pharmacologic actions, thus leading to different outcomes.

Sodium Channel Blockade

Although many antiarrhythmic drugs block cardiac sodium channels (Table 72.2), a class I action, their clinical electrophysiologic effects vary. A major factor that underlies this variability is the rate at which a drug dissociates from the sodium channel (48). During each AP, drug associates with the channel, and with each diastolic period, drug dissociates. If this dissociation rate is rapid, such as a time constant (τ) less than 1 second, no channels are blocked with the next AP (Fig. 72.1). Thus, substantial sodium channel blockade occurs only with a rapidly dissociating drug such as lidocaine (class Ib) at fast rates (*shorter diastole*) or under conditions in which dissociation is slowed (e.g., ischemia). Conversely, with flecainide (class Ic), dissociation is so slow that substantial sodium channel blockade occurs even at slow rates. If sodium channel blockade accumulates (with lidocaine, at fast rates; with flecainide, at any rate), the most important electrophysiologic effect in cardiac tissue is to slow conduction; this is manifested by widening of the QRS interval. Thus, drug-induced sodium channel blockade is greater at fast rates, and hence QRS prolongation is exaggerated at more rapid rates. With rapidly dissociating drugs, such as lidocaine, no widening of the QRS interval manifests at usual rates. With other drugs, such as flecainide or quinidine, QRS prolongation is the rule at therapeutic dosages. Conduction slowing is actually a *pro*arrhythmic effect in reentrant arrhythmias (see Chapter 57). The mechanisms by which sodium channel blockade suppresses arrhythmias are not completely understood but may include a bidirectional block in reentrant circuits (by effects on impulse propagation or on refractoriness) or suppression of abnormal automaticity. Sodium channel blockade can also produce clinically important increases in pacing and defibrillation energy requirements.

Proarrhythmic Effects of Sodium Channel Blockers

Therapy using sodium channel blockers such as flecainide has been associated with suppression of nonsustained ventricular

TABLE 72.2

MAJOR PHARMACOLOGIC EFFECTS OF ANTIARRHYTHMIC DRUGS

	Sodium channel block[a]			Calcium channel block	Autonomic effects		Comments/other actions
	$\tau < 1$ s	$\tau > 1$ s	↑APD		β-Blockade	Other	
Adenosine							Adenosine receptor blockade
Amiodarone	√		√	√		√[b]	Potent inhibitor of depolarization-induced automaticity
β-Blockers					√		
Calcium channel blockers				√			
Digitalis glycosides						Vagolytic	Inhibitor of sodium-potassium pump
Disopyramide		√	√			Anticholinergic	
Dofetilide			√				
Flecainide		√	[√]	[√]			
Ibutilide			√				
Lidocaine	√						
Magnesium				√?			
Mexiletine	√						
Procainamide	√		√			Ganglionic blockade (especially intravenously)	
Major metabolite: N-acetylprocainamide			√				
Propafenone		√			√		Extent of β-blockade genetically determined
Quinidine		√	√	[√]		α-Blocker	
Sotalol			√		√		

APD, action potential duration; [ ], minor effects that may not be clinically important.
[a]The clinical effects of sodium channel blockers depend in part on the time constant for recovery from block (τ), as described in the text (Fig. 72.1).
[b]The antiadrenergic effect produced by amiodarone resembles that of β-blockers, but it is "noncompetitive;" that is, it cannot be overcome by increasing doses of an agonist such as isoproterenol.

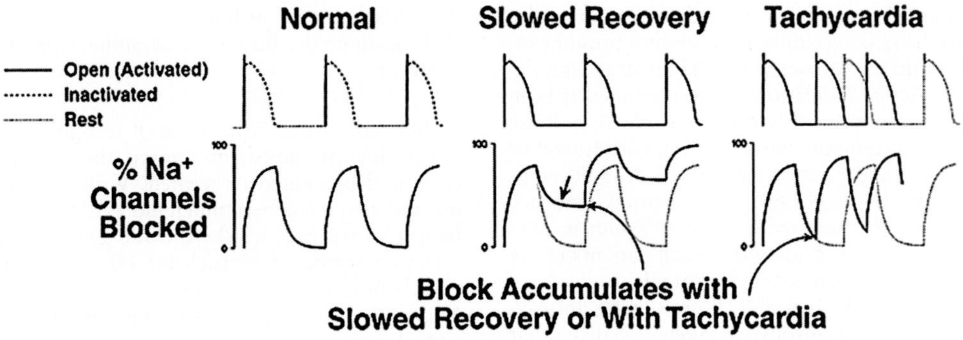

FIGURE 72.1. Rate-dependent sodium channel blockade. **Left:** A series of action potentials (APs), along with extent of sodium channel blockade (**bottom**). The sodium channel shuttles among three states during the AP: open, inactivated, and rest, as indicated in the top APs. Most sodium channel blockers that are used clinically bind to open and/or inactivated channels. Therefore, sodium channel blockade increases during the AP and decreases during each diastolic (*rest*) interval. A rapidly dissociating drug, such as lidocaine, is shown here. If the dissociation rate of the drug from the channel is decreased (**middle**), the extent of drug blockade can increase even in the absence of a change in rate. This is the case with lidocaine during ischemia or with flecainide. **Right:** Even with a rapidly dissociating drug such as lidocaine, sodium channel blockade can develop if the rate is accelerated. In the **middle** and **right panels**, the *dotted lines* indicate the data presented in the **left panel**. (From Roden DM, Echt DS, Murray KT, Lee JT. Clinical pharmacology of antiarrhythmic agents. In: Josephson ME, ed. *Sudden cardiac death*. Oxford: Blackwell Scientific, 1993:163–210.)

arrhythmias and of paroxysmal AF. However, conduction slowing in patients with known atrial flutter and in some patients with AF and no history of atrial flutter may sometimes lead to a marked slowing, but not termination, of the atrial flutter rate. With sufficient slowing, 1:1 AV conduction may ensue. To complicate the clinical picture further, because drugs such as flecainide block sodium channels more extensively at rapid than at slow rates, the ventricular complexes broaden and occasionally may even become aberrant. Thus, the clinical picture of this form of arrhythmia exacerbation is a patient with AF in whom wide, complex regular tachycardia then develops; it is therefore not a surprise that this arrhythmia is frequently misdiagnosed as VT (49,50). Management of this arrhythmia consists of recognizing the possibility of its occurrence, withdrawing the potentially offending antiarrhythmic agent, and using AV nodal blocking drugs both to establish the diagnosis as well as to control the ventricular rate. Adenosine may be useful in establishing the diagnosis.

Conduction slowing in the ventricle usually only results in QRS prolongation. However, when a reentrant circuit caused by ventricular scarring is present (e.g., in the post-MI patient), conduction slowing by sodium channel blockers can increase the frequency of VT while often slowing its rate. Such drug-facilitated VT may be very resistant to cardioversion and may prove fatal (51). Some animal and a limited number of human studies (52,53) have suggested that sodium boluses may be effective in this setting.

Another proarrhythmic effect of sodium channel blockers is the increase in mortality observed in CAST. The mechanism responsible for this finding remains unclear. However, evidence from animal studies and the CAST database (54–57) strongly suggests that in the presence of sodium channel blockade, recurrent myocardial ischemia may enhance the likelihood of fatal ventricular arrhythmias such as VF. In CAST, the relative risk of sodium channel blockers in patients with transmural MI was 1.7 compared with those given placebo. However, among those patients with non–Q-wave MIs, a group thought to be at much higher risk for subsequent ischemic events, the relative risk was much higher, 8.7 (56).

Action Potential Prolongation

The hallmark of AP prolongation, a so-called class III effect, is QT prolongation; the designation class Ia has been used to refer to drugs that both block sodium channels and prolong QT interval. As mentioned earlier, drugs that prolong QT share a number of desirable features, including decreased defibrillation energy requirement, efficacy in models of ischemic VF, and increased contractility. Their major antiarrhythmic action is probably attributable to the prolongation of refractoriness that accompanies increased AP; this, in turn, is thought to suppress reentrant arrhythmias by decreasing the likelihood of unidirectional block (see Chapter 57).

Mechanisms of QT Prolongation Drug-Induced Torsade de Pointes

Torsade de pointes resulting from QT-prolonging antiarrhythmic drugs can occur in 1% to 5% of patients (58–61), with the exception of amiodarone, in which this form of proarrhythmia is rare (62,63). Risk factors include hypokalemia, hypomagnesemia, female gender, bradycardia, left ventricular hypertrophy, congestive heart failure (CHF), recent conversion from AF, and subclinical congenital LQTS (64,65); a short-long-short series of cycle-length changes usually occurs at the initiation of an episode. Multiple in vitro electrophysiologic changes together are thought to produce torsade de pointes. *First*, APs are prolonged by decreased outward current, usually I_{Kr} block (or much less commonly increased inward current); these changes occur in a heterogeneous fashion across the ventricular wall. Second, very long APs can develop discontinuities in terminal repolarization, termed early afterdepolarizations; these may also cause triggered activity (see Chapter 57). *Third*, such triggered activity, in the setting of highly heterogeneous AP duration, generates the unstable reentry that appears as torsade de pointes on the surface ECG (13,66,67). Torsade de pointes can occur not only with exposure to QT-prolonging antiarrhythmic drugs but also with the congenital LQTS. Identification of mutations in the genes that encode I_{Kr} or other potassium channels [I_{Ks}] (to decrease outward current) or the cardiac sodium channel (to increase inward current) provides an explanation for the striking similarities between the congenital and the drug-induced syndromes (64). Many drugs not developed for cardiovascular indications have subsequently been found to block I_{Kr} and occasionally cause torsade de pointes; indeed, this has been a common cause for drug withdrawal or relabeling and has become a major issue in the drug development and approval processes (13,64). The reported incidence of torsade de pointes with "noncardiovascular" agents is quite small, but this may reflect the finding that such patients rarely have cardiac monitoring. Pharmacoepidemiologic studies have identified an excess risk of SCD with QT-prolonging antipsychotic agents (68) and with erythromycin taken with drugs that inhibit its metabolism (69).

Therapies for QT Prolongation Drug-Induced Torsade de Pointes

Torsade de pointes is recognized not simply by the presence of polymorphic VT; a markedly prolonged QT interval, often with prominent U waves, and the bradycardia-dependent onset of the tachycardia should also be present. The presence of polymorphic VT in the absence of QT changes before or after the arrhythmia suggests that other mechanisms, often acute myocardial ischemia, may be operative. Therapies such as isoproterenol infusion that are useful in torsade de pointes can be devastating in other forms of polymorphic tachycardia. Withdrawal of any QT-prolonging drugs and correction of serum potassium are the next steps in management. In vitro studies (70) have suggested that elevating extracellular potassium has two important effects in torsade de pointes: (a) it increases the magnitude of activating I_{Kr} (and thereby shortens the QT interval); and (b) it appears to reduce the potency of I_{Kr} blockers, another antiarrhythmic effect in this setting.

Strong, albeit anecdotal, evidence (71) indicates that magnesium therapy can prevent recurrences of torsade de pointes. The likely mechanism is a block of the secondary inward current (e.g., the L-type calcium current) because magnesium therapy does not generally shorten the QT interval. If torsade de pointes recurs after magnesium, the next step is to increase the heart rate, either with isoproterenol infusion or with external or transvenous pacing.

PRINCIPLES OF DRUG USE

The risks of antiarrhythmic therapy, particularly with long-term treatment, can be high, and the benefits of treatment in many cases are at least partially illusory. Management guidelines for major arrhythmia syndromes contain detailed discussion and extensive references to evidence supporting specific therapies in defined clinical settings (72–75). It is especially important to adhere to the following fundamental principles of drug therapy:

1. Define a benefit for therapy.
2. Define an end point for therapy.
3. Minimize the risks (and ensure that these do not outweigh the expected benefits).
4. Define the need for therapy.
5. Consider alternative therapies.

Intravenous antiarrhythmic drugs can be highly effective in acutely terminating ongoing sustained arrhythmias:

1. Adenosine or verapamil for most forms of reentrant supraventricular tachycardia
2. Lidocaine, procainamide, amiodarone, or sotalol (in Europe) for sustained VT
3. Ibutilide for AF or flutter
4. Procainamide, lidocaine, or amiodarone for recurrent VT or VF

In each setting, risks are well recognized, but because the patient is continuously monitored, these risks can be identified early and prevented or treated. With long-term antiarrhythmic therapy, it has been much more difficult to establish a clear benefit for treatment; risks, including proarrhythmia, other cardiovascular side effects such as CHF or bradyarrhythmias, and noncardiovascular toxicities, become a much greater concern. Many clinicians suggest in-hospital monitoring during initiation of antiarrhythmic therapy in patients thought to be at risk for serious adverse effects such as proarrhythmia, bradycardia, or heart failure (76).

A specific arrhythmia diagnosis should be established before therapy is initiated. For example, verapamil is effective for VT that arises in the right ventricular outflow tract in patients with a structurally normal heart, whereas it is dangerous to use in reentrant VT in patients with remote MI (77,78).

For long-term therapy of paroxysmal arrhythmias, it is important to recognize the phenomenon of ascertainment bias. Patients with symptomatic arrhythmias, such as paroxysmal AF or frequent ICD discharges owing to sustained VT, frequently display spontaneous unexplained variability in arrhythmia events. Such symptomatic patients are most likely to present to a physician during a period of high arrhythmia event frequency. Thus, institution of even ineffective therapy can appear to lower the frequency of arrhythmic events. In the case of AF, it is useful to establish some sense of the frequency of the arrhythmic episodes before initiating therapy. This approach is not usually possible for patients with very frequent ICD discharges that cannot be controlled in other ways (e.g., device reprogramming). However, even here, the physician should remain vigilant to the possibility that apparently effective antiarrhythmic therapy may, in fact, play very little role in reducing the frequency of arrhythmic episodes, and if drug side effects develop, discontinuation of the antiarrhythmic can still be considered.

Pharmacokinetic Principles

Because there is a small margin between dosages of antiarrhythmic drugs that may suppress arrhythmias and dosages that can produce serious or even life-threatening toxicities, an understanding of the principles that determine drug disposition is useful in guiding therapy. The processes that determine drug disposition, absorption, distribution, metabolism, and elimination are generally first order; that is, the rate of each process is determined by the amount of drug present. A characteristic of any first-order process is that it occurs exponentially as a function of time and is therefore conveniently described using half-lives. In one half-life, 50% of a given process is complete; in two half-lives, 75%; in three half-lives, 87.5%; in four half-lives, 93.75%; and so forth. Thus, any first-order process is near complete in four to five half-lives.

When drugs are administered intravenously, the time course of drug disappearance from plasma is often biexponential (Fig. 72.2). The usual explanation is that distribution occurs rapidly (accounting for a first exponential term), whereas elimination occurs more slowly (accounting for the slower exponential terms). For example, when a bolus of lidocaine is administered intravenously, plasma concentrations drop precipitously, with a half-life of 8 minutes. This reflects distribution of lidocaine into peripheral sites. As the drug is distributed, elimination, a second, slower process that occurs with a half-life of 2 hours becomes more important (Fig. 72.2).

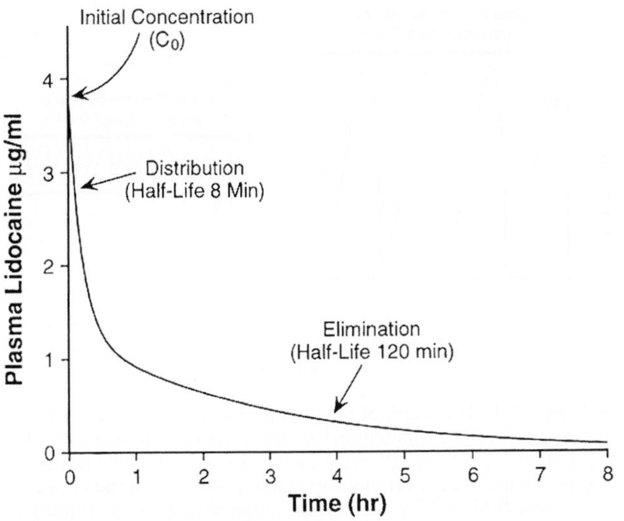

FIGURE 72.2. Plasma concentration time profile following a rapid bolus of lidocaine. Plasma concentrations decline biexponentially. The first phase of very rapid decreases in plasma lidocaine corresponds to distribution, with a half-life of 8 minutes. The terminal phase corresponds to elimination by metabolism, with a half-life of 2 hours. The plasma concentration directly after the bolus (C_0) can be used to estimate the central volume of distribution (dose/C_0).

Absorption and Metabolism

Distribution processes are generally most apparent with intravenously administered drugs. When a drug is given orally, absorption usually occurs sufficiently slowly to mask any rapid distribution. The amount of drug that actually reaches the systemic circulation, expressed as a percentage of total administered dose, is referred to as *bioavailability*. Bioavailability is commonly less than 100% following administration of a drug for two major reasons. First, the physicochemical characteristics of some drugs may not permit the gastrointestinal (GI) tract to absorb 100% of the drug. Amiodarone is only 30% to 50% bioavailable (79), probably for this reason; as a result, lower doses are used intravenously than orally. Second, some drugs are completely absorbed but undergo extensive metabolism, usually in the liver (or gut wall), before reaching the systemic circulation (80). The extent of this first-pass metabolism can be quite large and accounts for the finding that for some drugs, much greater dosages must be given orally rather than intravenously to achieve therapeutic effects. Verapamil and propranolol are excellent examples; several hundred milligrams must be given orally to achieve the same plasma concentrations as an intravenous dose of 10 mg or less.

Protein Binding

Another factor that can determine drug effect is protein binding. Many drugs are bound to plasma proteins, usually albumin. Another common ligand for many antiarrhythmic drugs is α_1-acid glycoprotein, an acute-phase reactant whose plasma concentrations are elevated with stresses such as acute MI or trauma. When α_1-acid glycoprotein is elevated, the amount of unbound drug that is available to exert pharmacologic effects is reduced. Thus, for example, some patients require (and tolerate) higher than usual lidocaine or quinidine concentrations to suppress arrhythmias shortly after MI (81).

Elimination Half-Life

Loading doses can be used to achieve a desired therapeutic drug effect rapidly. The magnitude of a loading dose can be estimated from the central volume of distribution (Fig. 72.2). However, the eventual steady-state plasma concentration that is achieved is determined by the elimination rate. Steady state is approached in four to five elimination half-lives, and this time is not abbreviated by the use of loading regimens (Fig. 72.3). Therefore, loading regimens are appropriate when a rapid drug effect is desired (e.g., to terminate an arrhythmia acutely) or when the elimination half-life of the drug is so long that no

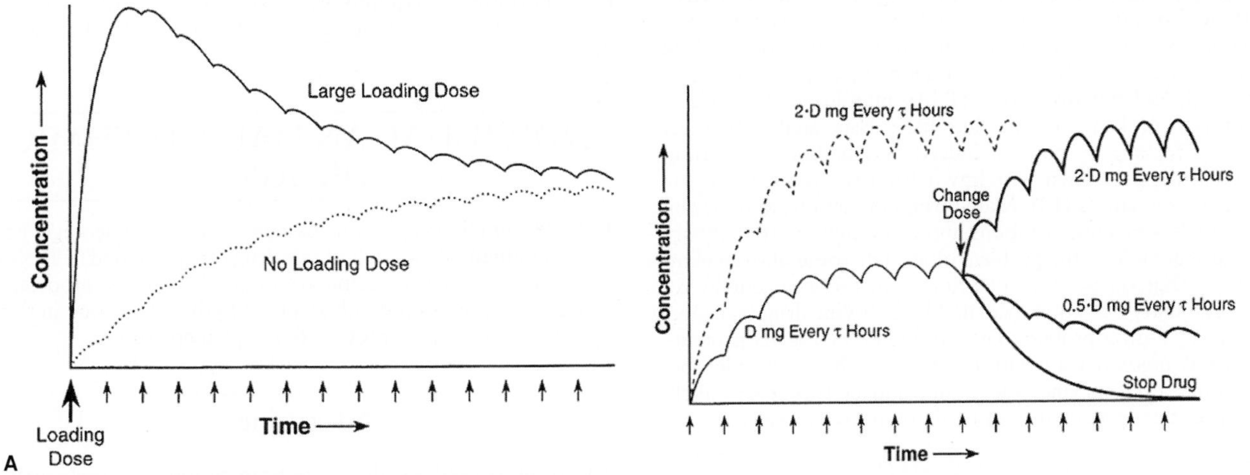

FIGURE 72.3. Effect of loading doses and of dose changes during long-term oral therapy. **A:** Hypothetic plasma concentrations are plotted as a function of time during long-term oral therapy. The *arrows* on the abscissa indicate the times at which a dose is administered, and the *heavy arrow* at the intercept indicates a loading dose. The administration of a loading dose does not abbreviate the time required to achieve steady-state concentrations, nor does it alter the steady state achieved. **B:** Concentration time profiles in the absence of a loading dose. The tracings (**left**) show the time course of drug accumulation to steady state. The steady state achieved is twice as great when the dosage is doubled (*dashed line*), but the time course of accumulation to steady state remains the same. Following a change in dosing regimen (or discontinuation of the drug), the time required to achieve the new steady state is similarly four to five elimination half-lives. (From Roden DM, Echt DS, Murray KT, Lee JT. Clinical pharmacology of antiarrhythmic agents. In: Josephson ME, ed. *Sudden cardiac death*. Oxford: Blackwell Scientific, 1993:163–210.)

therapeutic effect would occur in a reasonable time with the institution of maintenance dosages only (e.g., amiodarone). In the absence of these two situations, the use of loading dosages carries some increased risk for side effects (and little added benefit) and therefore is not recommended.

Clearance

Although the time to steady state is determined by the elimination half-life, the actual steady state achieved is determined by the dose administered (Fig. 72.3) and by *clearance,* most readily defined as dose per unit time divided by mean plasma concentration at steady state. Clearance and elimination half-life are not synonymous, because elimination half-life is determined not only by clearance but also by volume of distribution. For example, in the case of lidocaine, volume of distribution and clearance are reduced in CHF, thus leaving elimination half-life unchanged (82). Therefore, loading regimens must be reduced in CHF (*volume of distribution effect*), and maintenance infusions should be reduced to avoid toxicity (*clearance effect*). However, the time required to achieve steady state, four to five elimination half-lives (8 to 10 hours), is unchanged in CHF.

Drug Elimination in the Face of Organ Dysfunction

It is self-evident that if there is dysfunction (resulting from disease or from administration of other drugs) of a route of drug elimination, such as hepatic metabolism or renal excretion, the drug may accumulate in plasma and tissues, and toxicity may ensue. Specific hepatic enzymes are responsible for the biotransformation of antiarrhythmic (and other) drugs. It is increasingly well recognized that these enzymes are not expressed in a uniform fashion in all individuals and that such variability in enzyme activity can account for some of the clinically observed variability in response to therapy. This variability in enzyme activity can be genetically determined or can be the result of coadministration of enzyme inhibitors.

The greatest risk for highly variable drug elimination and toxicity occurs when a drug has only a single major route of elimination. The examples of propafenone and procainamide are discussed in this chapter. Drug interactions can also block the only route of elimination of a drug whose accumulation is toxic. Torsade de pointes caused by the antihistamine terfenadine is determined by just this mechanism (83): the drug is a potent I_{Kr} blocker that is eliminated by a specific enzyme, CYP3A4, and therapy with CYP3A4 inhibitors, such as erythromycin or ketoconazole, has been associated with most cases of torsade de pointes. Indeed, terfenadine and certain other drugs have been withdrawn from the market because of such interactions (13). Many drug interactions that elevate digoxin plasma concentrations and cause digoxin toxicity are also attributable to the problem of a single route of drug elimination. Digoxin is eliminated not by metabolism but by renal and biliary excretion mediated by a specific drug transport molecule, P-glycoprotein. The inhibition of P-glycoprotein–mediated digoxin transport by drugs such as amiodarone, quinidine, cyclosporine, verapamil, and erythromycin likely underlies their potential to cause digoxin toxicity (84).

Monitoring Plasma Drug Concentrations

For some drugs, monitoring plasma drug concentrations and maintaining these in a "therapeutic range" are useful adjuncts to minimizing the risk for adverse effects and maximizing potential benefits of therapy; lidocaine, digoxin, and procainamide are examples. Unfortunately, many adverse reactions to antiarrhythmic therapy are not clearly related to high plasma drug concentrations but rather occur at usual drug concentrations in patients with advanced underlying heart disease

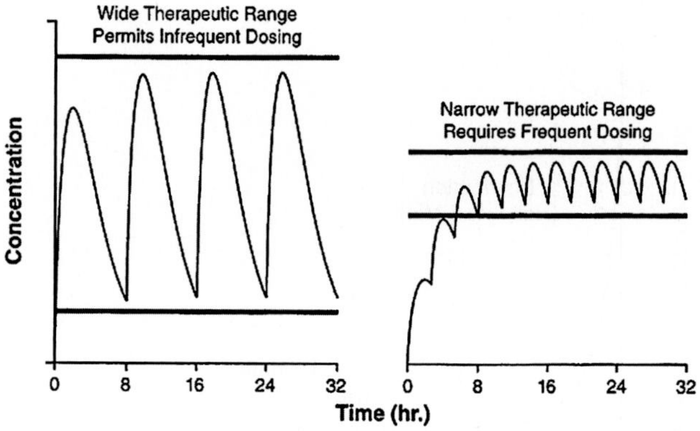

FIGURE 72.4. The width of the therapeutic range of plasma concentrations, and not the elimination half-life, determines frequency of dosing. Two therapeutic ranges are shown, one wide (**left**) and one narrow (**right**). Plasma concentrations during administration of the same drug are shown. With a wide therapeutic range, dosing every 8 hours allows plasma concentrations to remain within the therapeutic range. In contrast, dosing every 2.7 hours is required to maintain plasma concentrations within the narrow therapeutic range (**right**). (From Roden DM, Echt DS, Murray KT, Lee JT. Clinical pharmacology of antiarrhythmic agents. In: Josephson ME, ed. *Sudden cardiac death.* Oxford: Blackwell Scientific, 1993:163–210.)

or other predisposing factors (e.g., hypokalemia). In addition, the elimination of some drugs is highly variable, with an additional variable contribution to clinical effects by active metabolites (e.g., propafenone); plasma concentration measurements are virtually impossible to interpret under these conditions. Monitoring plasma drug concentrations can be especially useful when adjusting dosages in the presence of fluctuating renal or hepatic function and to establish whether a patient is compliant with therapy. It is a common misconception that long-term drug therapy should be administered once every half-life. In fact, the minimum time between doses is determined by the rate of drug elimination and by the margin between maximally tolerated and minimally effective plasma concentrations (Fig. 72.4). If this margin is small and the drug is eliminated rapidly, frequent dosing is required. If, conversely, the margin is large, infrequent dosing may suffice even for a rapidly eliminated drug.

INDIVIDUAL ANTIARRHYTHMIC DRUGS

The relevant clinical pharmacokinetics and pharmacologic actions of individual antiarrhythmic drugs are presented in Tables 72.2 and 72.3. A brief summary of issues that are important in the clinical use of individual antiarrhythmics is given in this section. The drugs are presented in alphabetic order.

Adenosine

Adenosine is used for the acute termination of supraventricular tachycardias that use the AV node as part of their circuit (e.g., AV nodal reentry, AV reentry; see Chapter 57) (85). Adenosine can also be used deliberately to create transient AV block to diagnose arrhythmias such as VT. Unlike virtually any other drug, adenosine must be administered in as rapid a fashion as possible, because the drug undergoes very rapid elimination from the circulation, primarily by cellular uptake. Uptake is inhibited by dipyridamole, which therefore potentiates effects of the adenosine. Adenosine receptors are blocked by methylxanthines, such as caffeine and theophylline,

TABLE 72.3

DISPOSITION CHARACTERISTICS OF ANTIARRHYTHMIC DRUGS

	Elimination half-life			Elimination route			Dosage adjustments	Drug interactions			
	Seconds-minutes	Hours	>12 h	Hepatic	Renal	Other	Heart failure	Decreased antiarrhythmic dose	Increased antiarrhythmic dose	Impairing the disposition of other drugs	Therapeutic plasma concentrations[a]
Adenosine	<10 s					Y		Dipyridamole	Methylxanthines		
Amiodarone			Weeks–Months	Y						Digoxin	0.5–2 μg/mL
										Flecainide	
										Procainamide	
β-Blockers										Warfarin	
Esmolol	5–10 min					Y				Lidocaine	
Propranolol		4–6		Y						Lidocaine	
Digoxin			36 h		Y			Amiodarone Cyclosporine Quinidine Verapamil			0.5–2 ng/mL
Diltiazem		4		Y							
Disopyramide		4–10		Y	Y		Ψ[b]				2–5 μg/mL
Dofetilide		8–10			Y			Verapamil Cimetidine			
Flecainide			10–18 h	Y	Y		Ψ	Amiodarone			<1 μg/mL
Ibutilide		6[a]		Y[c]							
Lidocaine	120 min			Y			↓ Load ↓ Maintenance rate	β-Blockers Cimetidine			1.5–5 μg/mL
Magnesium											
Mexiletine			11–15 h	Y					Phenytoin		0.5–2 μg/mL
Procainamide		3–4		Y	Y		↓ Dose (IV)	Amiodarone			4–10 μg/mL
N-Acetylprocainamide		6–8			Y						10–20 μg/mL
Propafenone		2–32		Y			Ψ	Fluoxetine Quinidine Tricyclics			
Quinidine		4–10		Y				Amiodarone	Phenytoin	Propafenone	2–5 μg/mL
Sotalol		8			Y						<3 μg/mL
Verapamil		6–12		Y			Ψ				

[a] As discussed in the text, monitoring plasma drug concentrations and maintaining them in a therapeutic range may be useful adjuncts to managing therapy with some drugs. Where no therapeutic range is presented, plasma concentration monitoring is of no value.
[b] Ψ, Avoid or use with caution.
[c] The arrhythmia-terminating actions of ibutilide depend on transient achievement of high concentrations; the dissipation of pharmacologic effects may result from rapid distribution, rather than from drug elimination.

which can therefore inhibit adenosine action. Most patients who receive adenosine complain of an uncomfortable feeling of chest tightness, the mechanism for which is not entirely explained. The absence of such symptoms with an adenosine bolus suggests that the drug may have been given too slowly or that a receptor blocker is present. Adenosine shortens atrial APs and can precipitate AF (86).

Amiodarone

Intravenous Amiodarone

Amiodarone given intravenously can be effective in patients with recurrent episodes of sustained VT or VF (87,88). Because intravenous amiodarone is administered for short periods, the toxicity that can characterize long-term oral therapy (see the section on oral amiodarone) is not a problem. Rather, hypotension, exacerbation of CHF, bradyarrhythmias, and phlebitis (if the drug is not given by central line) can occur. The mechanism whereby intravenous but not oral amiodarone exerts a prompt antiarrhythmic effect is not well understood but may involve a prominent sympatholytic action. In patients with out-of-hospital cardiac arrest and refractory ventricular tachyarrhythmias, intravenous amiodarone was superior to lidocaine in improving survival to the hospital, but there was no change in hospital discharge rates with intravenous amiodarone (89,90); it is first-line therapy in the most recent guidelines (72). In Europe, intravenous amiodarone has been used to control ventricular rate in AF; it is not very effective to convert AF to sinus rhythm.

Oral Amiodarone

One of the most important pharmacologic features of amiodarone is its very long elimination half-life (91,92). This necessitates the use of oral loading regimens to abbreviate the time from initiation of therapy to achievement of an antiarrhythmic effect. Another result of the slow elimination is that the minimum dose required to maintain an antiarrhythmic effect during long-term therapy is poorly defined. An advantage of very slow elimination is that missing a dose does not generally result in arrhythmia recurrence.

Randomized clinical trials examining mortality have shown that amiodarone is superior to other antiarrhythmics, and inferior to ICD therapy, in patients who have survived a cardiac arrest (93,94), and it is neutral to slightly beneficial in patients surviving MI (23,24). One trial in patients with heart failure showed a mortality benefit (21), but others have shown no difference compared with placebo (22,25). In paroxysmal AF, amiodarone has been superior to propafenone and sotalol in reducing symptoms and in maintaining sinus rhythm (95,96); in one of these trials, amiodarone and sotalol were equally effective in patients with underlying ischemic heart disease (95). Amiodarone therapy before bypass surgery reduced the incidence of postoperative AF (97).

Long-Term Use of Amiodarone: Side Effects

Side effects can be a major problem during long-term therapy with amiodarone, with dropout rates in large trials approaching 40% in 2 years (24,93,96). The most serious side effect during long-term amiodarone therapy is pulmonary fibrosis (98). The incidence appears higher with longer duration of therapy, higher dosages (especially >400 mg/day during chronic therapy), and the presence of pulmonary disease (99,100). With total daily dosages of 200 mg/day or less, pulmonary fibrosis is unusual. Routine surveillance chest radiographs or pulmonary function studies have been advocated to detect incipient pulmonary toxicity, but their utility has not been determined; some patients present with fulminant respiratory failure (100). Monitoring plasma concentrations of amiodarone during long-term therapy has not been useful in either limiting toxicity or increasing efficacy.

Amiodarone can cause a number of relatively common adverse effects that may not be life-threatening but of which the patient should be aware. Photosensitivity is frequent, and patients should be warned to use sunscreens. Corneal microdeposits are routinely detectable after 3 months of therapy but are rarely symptomatic; the major symptom is the appearance of visual halos. Rare cases of optic neuropathy with vision loss have been associated with amiodarone use (101). Hypothyroidism and hyperthyroidism, proximal muscle weakness, and hepatic dysfunction (usually asymptomatic but rarely proceeding to cirrhosis) can occur. Unlike other drugs that prolong the QT interval, torsade de pointes is rare with amiodarone therapy. The mechanism is unknown but may relate to the drug's sympatholytic or direct calcium channel-blocking actions. Drug interactions are also frequent with amiodarone: warfarin and digoxin requirements should be monitored closely because they may require downward adjustments in dosages.

Digoxin and Other Digitalis Glycosides

Digoxin and other digitalis glycosides are used to control ventricular response in AF or atrial flutter. Rate control can generally be achieved while the patient is at rest but is frequently lost during even modest exertion. The symptoms of digoxin toxicity include confusion, visual scotomata, and arrhythmias. The last include atrial arrhythmias (often with AV block), bigeminy, bidirectional VT, and bradyarrhythmias caused by suppression of sinus node function and AV block. With suicidal digoxin overdose, poisoning with sodium-potassium adenosine triphosphatase can result in extraordinary degrees of hyperkalemia. When arrhythmias are sufficiently serious to warrant specific therapy, the treatment of choice is antidigoxin antibodies (102). Lesser degrees of arrhythmias (e.g., asymptomatic slow ventricular rates in patients with AF) can be treated with discontinuation of the drug and monitoring.

Disopyramide

Disopyramide exerts quinidine-like electrophysiologic effects (sodium channel block, AP prolongation). Its major side effects relate to its anticholinergic actions (constipation, urinary retention, glaucoma, and dry mouth), and the drug can also exacerbate heart failure (103).

Dofetilide

Dofetilide is a high-potency blocker of I_{Kr} and does not exert significant other pharmacologic effects (61). Double-blind placebo-controlled trials have shown that it is effective in preventing recurrences of AF after cardioversion (104–106), but no significant effect was demonstrated in patients with paroxysmal AF or with VT. In two large placebo-controlled trials in patients with advanced heart failure or recent MI, dofetilide did not alter mortality, and a trend to decreased hospitalization for recurrent heart failure was found, possibly owing to decreased AF (16,17,104). Torsade de pointes is the major toxicity of dofetilide. In all clinical trials, dofetilide was initiated in monitored inpatients because of the concern for this proarrhythmia. The incidence was 0.8% to 3.3% and was highest in patients with heart failure. In the United States, dofetilide is currently available only to practitioners who have taken a short course in the drug's use, and the labeling mandates inpatient initiation. Because of the drug's specificity of action, other side effects are unusual.

Flecainide

Flecainide defined the class Ic drug. It is a potent suppressor of chronic ventricular ectopic activity, it routinely prolongs PR and QRS intervals by approximately 25% during long-term oral therapy, and it produces remarkably few "nuisance" side effects during long-term treatment (unlike drugs such as quinidine or procainamide) (107). It increased mortality in CAST (7). Atrial flutter with 1:1 AV conduction can occur, and flecainide can exacerbate CHF and can increase the severity or symptoms of sustained VT resulting from advanced myocardial scarring. Conversely, among patients with no structural heart disease and supraventricular arrhythmias (including AF, atrial flutter, and reentrant supraventricular tachycardias), mortality during flecainide therapy is virtually unknown (108). From a practical point of view, it is only in the latter group of patients that flecainide is currently used.

Ibutilide

Ibutilide is used for acute termination of AF or flutter (60,109–111). It is somewhat more effective in terminating atrial flutter (~60% of cases) versus AF (~30%). In AF, it is more effective if the arrhythmia has not been long standing (e.g., months) and if the left atrium is not dilated. Ibutilide pretreatment can enhance the efficacy of direct current cardioversion in AF (112). Ibutilide acts by prolonging AP, and torsade de pointes occurs in 3% to 8% of patients. Other side effects are unusual.

Lidocaine

Lidocaine is useful for the acute suppression of recurrent VF or sustained VT, although amiodarone is increasingly viewed as the drug of first choice in these settings (72). Its efficacy, especially in sustained VT that is unrelated to ongoing myocardial ischemia, is not well established. In a head-to-head comparison, it was less effective than intravenous sotalol for sustained monomorphic VT (113).

Understanding the pharmacokinetics of lidocaine is helpful in minimizing toxicity and maximizing efficacy with the drug, and the principles apply equally to other drug therapy. After a bolus of lidocaine, plasma concentrations of the drug (that correlate with its antiarrhythmic activity) drop precipitously, not as a result of elimination but as a result of distribution. Therefore, an appropriate loading regimen of lidocaine is approximately 3 to 4 mg/kg (200 to 300 mg total in an adult), either as a series of divided boluses or a rapid infusion over 20 to 30 minutes. Reduction in the size of this loading regimen is required in patients with advanced CHF (68). After loading, plasma concentrations approach true steady state in four to five elimination half-lives. Lidocaine elimination half-life is approximately 2 hours in normal individuals and in subjects with CHF and longer in those with liver disease. Thus, steady-state concentrations of lidocaine are achieved only many hours (≤ 8 to 10 hours) after the initiation of therapy (Fig. 72.5). If the maintenance dosage is too low, the steady state may be subtherapeutic, with a late recurrence of arrhythmia. If, conversely, the rate of the maintenance infusion is too high, plasma concentrations rise slowly into the toxic range hours after initiation of apparently successful therapy. Under these circumstances, lidocaine toxicity is frequently characterized by relatively non-

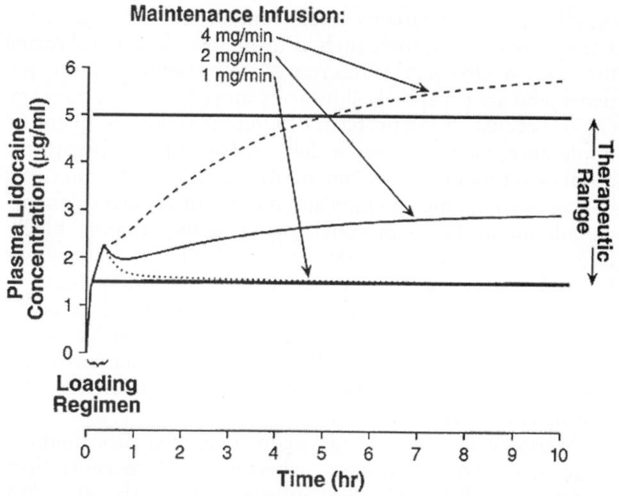

FIGURE 72.5. Plasma lidocaine concentrations during maintenance infusions. Following administration of a loading regimen, plasma concentration time profiles during approach to steady state over four to five elimination half-lives (8 to 10 hours) are shown. If the maintenance infusion is excessive, high plasma concentrations can develop many hours after institution of effective therapy (*dashed line*). Conversely, if the maintenance infusion chosen is insufficient, plasma concentrations of lidocaine may drop to subtherapeutic levels many hours after institution of what was anticipated to be effective therapy. (From Roden DM. Treatment of cardiovascular disorders: arrhythmias. In: Melamine KL, Morrelli HF, Hoffman BB, Nierenberg DW, eds. *Clinical pharmacology: basic principles in therapeutics*. New York: McGraw-Hill, 1992:151–185.)

specific symptoms such as dysarthria or disorientation (common among patients in intensive care units). Plasma lidocaine concentrations should be measured when steady state is approached, when arrhythmia recurs, or with suspected toxicity. Doses should be adjusted to maintain concentrations in the therapeutic range of 1.5 to 5.0 µg/mL.

Magnesium

Case series (71,114) suggest that magnesium infusions may have a role in suppressing torsade de pointes and atrial arrhythmias characteristic of digoxin toxicity. When it is used to treat long QT–related arrhythmias, the arrhythmia may resolve without marked shortening of the QT interval. No evidence has been found that magnesium is useful in treating other arrhythmias.

Mexiletine

Mexiletine (115) is a structural analog of lidocaine developed to permit long-term oral therapy. It is occasionally useful in the treatment of ventricular arrhythmias (e.g., to manage recurrent ICD shocks owing to VT), and it has been successfully used in combination with sotalol or quinidine. The drug is sometimes used in the sodium channel–linked form of the congenital LQTS (116).

Procainamide

Procainamide produces electrophysiologic effects that are similar to those of quinidine and disopyramide. When administered intravenously, it exerts ganglionic blocking effects that may result in hypotension. When procainamide is used for long-term oral therapy, most patients develop antinuclear antibodies, and a few develop symptoms such as arthralgia or rash indicating the lupus syndrome; this reaction is more common among patients who are genetically slow acetylators (~50% of patients) (117). Because of the problem of lupus as well as frequent GI intolerance, the drug is not widely used as primary therapy for atrial or ventricular arrhythmias. Torsade de pointes can occur during procainamide therapy and is most often the result of accumulation of the AP-prolonging (non–sodium channel blocking) metabolite *N*-acetylprocainamide (NAPA). Procainamide is eliminated by hepatic metabolism to NAPA and by direct renal excretion, whereas NAPA is eliminated by renal excretion alone. Thus, the most frequent setting in which NAPA accumulation occurs is renal failure. Bone marrow aplasia may occur in 0.2% of patients and does not appear to be related to high plasma concentrations.

At concentrations of 8 to 10 μg/mL or greater, procainamide frequently produces GI upset, whereas NAPA concentrations associated with torsade de pointes are frequently 30 μg/mL or greater. It is common practice to add procainamide and NAPA concentrations together to develop a single plasma drug concentration for monitoring purposes. However, because the drugs exert different electrophysiologic effects, produce different toxicities, and use different elimination mechanisms, this approach is inappropriate. Rather, concentrations of the compounds should be considered individually with regard to their potential toxicity.

Propafenone

Propafenone (118) has sodium channel-blocking properties that are similar to those of flecainide and quinidine in vitro. Propafenone can exacerbate VT and produces electrocardiographic changes similar to those of flecainide; therefore, although it was not evaluated in CAST, most clinicians avoid its use in patients with significant structural heart disease because its effects so closely resemble those of flecainide.

The major route of propafenone elimination is metabolism by CYP2D6, a hepatic enzyme that oxidizes the drug to an active metabolite, 5-hydroxypropafenone (119). Propafenone exerts β-blocking activity in vitro, whereas its metabolite does not. In patients who are genetically deficient in this elimination pathway (~7% of the white and black populations), propafenone elimination is impaired, and high plasma concentrations of the drug can be measured. It is in these patients that symptoms such as bradycardia or bronchospasm referable to β-blockade can occur. Some drugs, notably quinidine, tricyclic antidepressants, and some selective serotonin reuptake inhibitors such as fluoxetine, can inhibit propafenone biotransformation, elevate its plasma concentrations, and thus increase the risk for adverse effects.

Propafenone is most frequently used in the suppression of AF or flutter. In this setting, propafenone, like flecainide and quinidine, can cause atrial flutter with 1:1 conduction and wide complexes, which can be misdiagnosed as VT.

Quinidine

Quinidine has been used for antiarrhythmic therapy since the 1920s. Side effects, including proarrhythmia, are major concerns with quinidine therapy. Very high concentrations generated by aggressive quinidine dosing regimens that were formerly used to convert AF can result in sustained VT similar to that seen with flecainide intoxication. The drug blocks multiple cardiac ion channels, and even low concentrations of quinidine can produce torsade de pointes (58), likely reflecting the drug's potent ability to block I_{Kr} (70,120). Some analyses (121,122) have suggested that mortality may be increased with long-term use of quinidine in patients with atrial arrhythmias, perhaps resulting from torsade de pointes. Other side effects, notably diarrhea, are very common. With high plasma quinidine concentrations, a syndrome known as *cinchonism*, which includes tinnitus and headache, can occur. Immunologic reactions have also been reported with quinidine and include thrombocytopenia and occasionally the lupus syndrome. Most side effects from quinidine therapy, with the exception of cinchonism, are unrelated to high drug concentrations or any known metabolites.

Quinidine is an inhibitor of CYP2D6, responsible for the metabolism of propafenone and of other drugs, such as timolol, metoprolol, and carvedilol that use the same enzyme for their elimination. Quinidine blocks P-glycoprotein (84), so digoxin and digitoxin concentrations predictably double during quinidine therapy, with a corresponding rise in symptoms of toxicity.

At the beginning of the 1990s, quinidine was the most widely prescribed antiarrhythmic in North America. Because side effects are so common and the awareness of torsade de pointes is increasing, quinidine has assumed an increasingly minor role in antiarrhythmic therapy. Currently, it is probably best reserved for patients with depressed left ventricular performance and recurrent symptomatic arrhythmias (e.g., AF or frequent ICD shocks for VT) in whom other therapies such as amiodarone are deemed undesirable.

Sotalol

Sotalol is a nonselective β-blocker with prominent AP-prolonging characteristics (123). It is useful in the treatment of ventricular and supraventricular arrhythmias. Side effects are confined to those related to β-blockade and to torsade de pointes, which is dose related and occurs in 1% to 5% of patients treated for ventricular arrhythmias (59). Unlike other β-blockers, sotalol has not been shown to reduce the incidence of mortality among patients who are recovering from MI. However, the major trial (124) in which it was studied used a relatively high single dose of 320 mg once a day. Thus, it is conceivable that the lack of a significant effect on mortality reflects a trade-off between a mortality-sparing effect owing to β-blockade and a torsade de pointes–inducing effect. In support of this idea, the use of sotalol in patients with ICDs has been shown to reduce the incidence of device discharges or death (125).

CONTROVERSIES AND PERSONAL PERSPECTIVES

Antiarrhythmic drug use is declining because effective nonpharmacologic therapies are becoming more widely available and because of an increasing recognition of the limited efficacy and the potential for serious side effects during antiarrhythmic therapy, particularly during long-term treatments. Much of the long-term antiarrhythmic therapy has now devolved to amiodarone, a drug that I believe is neither as effective or as safe as its most ardent proponents think. Nevertheless, among therapies that are available for long-term antiarrhythmic treatment, amiodarone and sotalol have been shown to be more effective and probably no more dangerous than drugs such as quinidine or procainamide, which were "conventional" until the 1990s.

All available antiarrhythmic drugs were developed at a time when the mechanisms that underlie the target arrhythmias and the antiarrhythmic drug effects were incompletely defined at best; indeed, this is still the case. Catheter ablation is a superb example of a therapy that has evolved to become an effective modality from an understanding of the underlying disease mechanisms. During the past decade, our understanding of the molecular and cellular events that underlie arrhythmogenesis has grown tremendously. Thus, we are in the paradoxical position of understanding better the mechanisms underlying the proarrhythmic effects of antiarrhythmic drugs than those on which the antiarrhythmic effects of these same agents are based. It seems clear that the molecular entities targeted by many of the antiarrhythmic drugs, notably the sodium channel and the rapidly activating component of the cardiac-delayed rectifier, I_{Kr}, may not be the best targets for suppressing atrial or ventricular arrhythmias. I remain hopeful that better understanding of the mechanisms of arrhythmias may well allow identification of molecular and cellular targets for new antiarrhythmic entities that may prove to be highly effective and safe in treating common arrhythmia scenarios such as AF or patients at risk for VT or VF (126–128). In addition, progress in understanding the genetic determinants of drug response may enable "personalized medicine" approaches, in which drugs and doses are selected for a specific patient's genetic makeup (129,130).

THE FUTURE

Use of antiarrhythmic drugs will continue to decline because of their recognized limited efficacy and serious side effects, especially during long-term therapy. Continuing research resulting in an improved understanding of the mechanisms of arrhythmias will allow identification of molecular and cellular targets for new antiarrhythmic entities. Such new entities may well provide highly effective and safe treatment of common arrhythmias.

References

1. Norwegian Multicenter Study Group. Timolol-induced reduction in mortality and reinfarction in patients surviving acute myocardial infarction. *N Engl J Med* 1981;304:801–807.
2. Beta-Blocker Heart Attack Trial Research Group. A randomized trial of propranolol in patients with acute myocardial infarction. I. Mortality results. *JAMA* 1982;247:1707–1714.
3. Hjalmarson A, Herlitz J, Malek I, et al. Effect on mortality of metoprolol in acute myocardial infarction: A double-blind randomized trial. *Lancet* 1981;2:823–827.
4. Billman GE. The antiarrhythmic and antifibrillatory effects of calcium antagonists. *J Cardiovasc Pharmacol* 1991;18(suppl 10):S107–S117.
5. Multicenter Diltiazem Post-Infarction Trial Research Group. The effect of diltiazem on mortality and reinfarction after myocardial infarction. *N Engl J Med* 1988;319:385–391.
6. Teo KK, Yusuf S, Furberg CD. Effects of prophylactic antiarrhythmic drug therapy in acute myocardial infarction: an overview of results from randomized controlled trials. *JAMA* 1993;270:1589–1595.
7. CAST Investigators. Preliminary report: effect of encainide and flecainide on mortality in a randomized trial of arrhythmia suppression after myocardial infarction. *N Engl J Med* 1989;321:406–412.
8. IMPACT Research Group. International mexiletine and placebo antiarrhythmic coronary trial: I. Report on arrhythmia and other findings. *J Am Coll Cardiol* 1984;4:1148–1163.
9. UK Rythmodan Multicentre Study Group. Oral disopyramide after admission to hospital with suspected acute myocardial infarction. *Postgrad Med J* 1984;60:98–107.
10. Cardiac Arrhythmia Suppression Trial II Investigators. Effect of the antiarrhythmic agent moricizine on survival after myocardial infarction. *N Engl J Med* 1991;327:227–233.
11. Echt DS, Black JN, Barbey JT, et al. Evaluation of antiarrhythmic drugs on defibrillation energy requirements in dogs: sodium channel block and action potential prolongation. *Circulation* 1989;79:1106–1117.
12. Singh BN. Current antiarrhythmic drugs: an overview of mechanisms of action and potential clinical utility. *J Cardiovasc Electrophysiol* 1999;10:283–301.
13. Roden DM. Drug-induced prolongation of the QT Interval. *N Engl J Med* 2004;350:1013–1022.
14. Curran ME, Splawski I, Timothy KW, et al. A molecular basis for cardiac arrhythmia: *HERG* mutations cause long QT syndrome. *Cell* 1995;80:795–803.
15. Sanguinetti MC, Jiang C, Curran ME, Keating MT. A mechanistic link between an inherited and an acquired cardiac arrhythmia: HERG encodes the IKr potassium channel. *Cell* 1995;81:299–307.
16. Kober L, Bloch Thomsen PE, Moller M, et al. Effect of dofetilide in patients with recent myocardial infarction and left-ventricular dysfunction: a randomised trial. Danish Investigations of Arrhythmia and Mortality on Dofetilide (DIAMOND) Study Group. *Lancet* 2000;356:2052–2058.
17. Torp-Pedersen C, Moller M, Bloch-Thomsen PE, et al. Dofetilide in patients with congestive heart failure and left ventricular dysfunction: Danish Investigations of Arrhythmia and Mortality on Dofetilide Study Group. *N Engl J Med* 1999;341:857–865.
18. Waldo AL, Camm AJ, DeRuyter H, et al. Effect of d-sotalol on mortality in patients with left ventricular dysfunction after recent and remote myocardial infarction. *Lancet* 1996;348:7–12.
19. Singh BN, Vaughan Williams EM. The effect of amiodarone, a new antianginal drug, on cardiac muscle. *Br J Pharmacol* 1970;39:657–667.
20. Rosenbaum MB, Chiale PA, Halpern MS. Clinical efficacy of amiodarone as an antiarrhythmic agent. *Am J Cardiol* 1976;38:934–944.
21. Doval HC, Nul DR, Grancelli HO, et al. Randomised trial of low-dose amiodarone in severe congestive heart failure: Grupo de Estudio de la Sobrevida en la Insuficiencia Cardiaca en Argentina (GESICA). *Lancet* 1994;344: 493–498.
22. Singh SN, Fletcher RD, Fisher SG, et al. Amiodarone in patients with congestive heart failure and asymptomatic ventricular arrhythmia. *N Engl J Med* 1995;333:77–82.
23. Julian DG, Camm AJ, Frangin G, et al. Randomised trial of effect of amiodarone on mortality in patients with left-ventricular dysfunction after recent myocardial infarction: EMIAT. *Lancet* 1997;349:667–674.
24. Cairns JA, Connolly SJ, Roberts R, Gent M, the Canadian Amiodarone Myocardial Infarction Arrhythmia Trial Investigators. Randomised trial of outcome after myocardial infarction in patients with frequent or repetitive ventricular premature depolarisations: CAMIAT. *Lancet* 1997;349:675–682.
25. Bardy GH, Lee KL, Mark DB, et al. Amiodarone or an implantable cardioverter-defibrillator for congestive heart failure. *N Engl J Med* 2005; 352:225–237.
26. Connolly SJ, Cairns J, Gent M, et al. Effect of prophylactic amiodarone on mortality after acute myocardial infarction and in congestive heart failure: meta-analysis of individual data from 6500 patients in randomised trials. *Lancet* 1997;350:1417–1424.
27. Connolly SJ. Evidence-based analysis of amiodarone efficacy and safety. *Circulation* 1999;100:2025–2034.
28. Maisel WH, Stevenson WG. Sudden death and the electrophysiological effects of angiotensin-converting enzyme inhibitors. *J Card Fail* 2000;6:80–82.
29. Teo KK, Mitchell LB, Pogue J, et al. Effect of ramipril in reducing sudden deaths and nonfatal cardiac arrests in high-risk individuals without heart failure or left ventricular dysfunction. *Circulation* 2004;110:1413–1417.
30. Vermes E, Tardif JC, Bourassa MG, et al. Enalapril decreases the incidence of atrial fibrillation in patients with left ventricular dysfunction. insight from the Studies Of Left Ventricular Dysfunction (SOLVD) trials. *Circulation* 2003;107:2926–2931.
31. Pedersen OD, Bagger H, Kober L, Torp-Pedersen C. Trandolapril reduces the incidence of atrial fibrillation after acute myocardial infarction in patients with left ventricular dysfunction. *Circulation* 1999;100:376–380.
32. Madrid AH, Bueno MG, Rebollo JM, et al. Use of irbesartan to maintain sinus rhythm in patients with long-lasting persistent atrial fibrillation: a prospective and randomized study. *Circulation* 2002;106:331–336.
33. Young-Xu Y, Jabbour S, Goldberg R, et al. Usefulness of statin drugs in protecting against atrial fibrillation in patients with coronary artery disease. *Am J Cardiol* 2003;92:1379–1383.
34. Siu CW, Lau CP, Tse HF. Prevention of atrial fibrillation recurrence by statin therapy in patients with lone atrial fibrillation after successful cardioversion. *Am J Cardiol* 2003;92:1343–1345.
35. Rucker-Martin C, Pecker F, Godreau D, et al. Dedifferentiation of atrial myocytes during atrial fibrillation: role of fibroblast proliferation in vitro. *Cardiovasc Res* 2002;55:38–52.
36. Kumagai K, Nakashima H, Saku K. The HMG-CoA reductase inhibitor atorvastatin prevents atrial fibrillation by inhibiting inflammation in a canine sterile pericarditis model. *Cardiovasc Res* 2004;62:105–111.
37. Shiroshita-Takeshita A, Schram G, Lavoie J, Nattel S. Effect of simvastatin and antioxidant vitamins on atrial fibrillation promotion by atrial-tachycardia remodeling in dogs. *Circulation* 2004;110:2313–2319.
38. Verheule S, Sato T, Everett T, et al. Increased vulnerability to atrial fibrillation in transgenic mice with selective atrial fibrosis caused by overexpression of TGF-beta1. *Circ Res* 2004;94:1458–1465.
39. Li D, Shinagawa K, Pang L, et al. Effects of Angiotensin-converting enzyme inhibition on the development of the atrial fibrillation substrate in dogs with ventricular tachypacing-induced congestive heart failure. *Circulation* 2001;104:2608–2614.
40. Members of the Sicilian Gambit. New approaches to antiarrhythmic therapy: emerging therapeutic applications of the cell biology of cardiac arrhythmias. *Cardiovasc Res* 2001;52:345–360.
41. Priori SG, Napolitano C, Schwartz PJ, et al. Association of long QT syndrome loci and cardiac events among patients treated with beta-blockers. *JAMA* 2004;292:1341–1344.
42. Benhorin J, Taub R, Goldmit M, et al. Effects of flecainide in patients with new SCN5A mutation: mutation-specific therapy for long-QT syndrome? *Circulation* 2000;101:1698–1706.

43. Shimizu W, Antzelevitch C. Cellular basis for long QT, transmural dispersion of repolarization, and torsade de pointes in the long QT syndrome. *J Electrocardiol* 1999;32(suppl):177–184.
44. Alings M, Dekker L, Sadee A, Wilde A. Quinidine induced electrocardiographic normalization in two patients with Brugada syndrome. *Pacing Clin Electrophysiol* 2001;24:1420–1422.
45. Belhassen B, Glick A, Viskin S. Efficacy of quinidine in high-risk patients with Brugada syndrome. *Circulation* 2004;110:1731–1737.
46. Gaita F, Giustetto C, Bianchi F, et al. Short QT syndrome: pharmacological treatment. *J Am Coll Cardiol* 2004;43:1494–1499.
47. Wehrens XH, Lehnart SE, Reiken SR, et al. Protection from cardiac arrhythmia through ryanodine receptor-stabilizing protein calstabin2. *Science* 2004;304:292–296.
48. Hondeghem LM. Antiarrhythmic agents: modulated receptor applications. *Circulation* 1987;75:514–520.
49. Falk RH. Flecainide-induced ventricular tachycardia and fibrillation in patients treated for atrial fibrillation. *Ann Intern Med* 1989;111:107–111.
50. Crijns HJ, van Gelder IS, Lie KI. Supraventricular tachycardia mimicking ventricular tachycardia during flecainide treatment. *Am J Cardiol* 1988;62: 1303–1306.
51. Winkle RA, Mason JW, Griffin JC, Ross D. Malignant ventricular tachyarrhythmias associated with the use of encainide. *Am Heart J* 1981;102: 857–864.
52. Chouty F, Funck-Brentano C, Landau JM, Lardoux H. Efficacité de fortes doses de lactate molaire par voie veineuse lors des intoxications au flecainide. *La Press Med* 1987;16:808–810.
53. Turgeon J, Wisialowski TA, Wong W, et al. Suppression of longitudinal versus transverse conduction by sodium channel block: effects of sodium bolus. *Circulation* 1992;85:2221–2226.
54. Nattel S, Pedersen DH, Zipes DP. Alterations in regional myocardial distribution and arrhythmogenic effects of aprindine produced by coronary artery occlusion in the dog. *Cardiovasc Res* 1981;15:80–85.
55. Greenberg HM, Dwyer EM Jr, Hochman JS, et al. Interaction of ischaemia and encainide/flecainide treatment: a proposed mechanism for the increased mortality in CAST I. *Br Heart J* 1995;74:631–635.
56. Akiyama T, Pawitan Y, Greenberg H, et al., the CAST Investigators. Increased risk of death and cardiac arrest from encainide and flecainide in patients after non–Q-wave acute myocardial infarction in the Cardiac Arrhythmia Suppression Trial. *Am J Cardiol* 1991;68:1551–1555.
57. Lukas A, Antzelevitch C. Differences in the electrophysiological response of canine ventricular epicardium and endocardium to ischemia: role of the transient outward current. *Circulation* 1993;88:2903–29015.
58. Roden DM, Woosley RL, Primm RK. Incidence and clinical features of the quinidine-associated long QT syndrome: implications for patient care. *Am Heart J* 1986;111:1088–1093.
59. Soyka LF, Wirtz C, Spangenberg RB. Clinical safety profile of sotalol in patients with arrhythmias. *Am J Cardiol* 1990;65:74A–81A.
60. Murray KT. Ibutilide. *Circulation* 1999;97:493–497.
61. Mounsey JP, DiMarco JP. Dofetilide. *Circulation* 2000;102:2665–2670.
62. van Opstal JM, Schoenmakers M, Verduyn SC, et al. Chronic amiodarone evokes no torsade de pointes arrhythmias despite QT lengthening in an animal model of acquired long-QT syndrome. *Circulation* 2001;104:2722–2727.
63. Lazzara R. Amiodarone and torsades de pointes. *Ann Intern Med* 1989; 111:549–551.
64. Fenichel RR, Malik M, Antzelevitch C, et al. Drug-induced torsades de pointes and implications for drug development. *J Cardiovasc Electrophysiol* 2004;15:475–495.
65. Viskin S, Justo D, Halkin A, Zeltser D. Long QT syndrome caused by noncardiac drugs. *Prog Cardiovasc Dis* 2003;45:415–427.
66. Belardinelli L, Antzelevitch C, Vos MA. Assessing predictors of drug-induced torsade de pointes. *Trends Pharmacol Sci* 2003;24:619–625.
67. Akar FG, Yan GX, Antzelevitch C, Rosenbaum DS. Unique topographical distribution of M cells underlies reentrant mechanism of torsade de pointes in the long-QT syndrome. *Circulation* 2002;105:1247–1253.
68. Hennessy S, Bilker WB, Knauss JS, et al. Cardiac arrest and ventricular arrhythmia in patients taking antipsychotic drugs: cohort study using administrative data. *BMJ* 2002;325:1070.
69. Ray WA, Murray KT, Meredith S, et al. Oral erythromycin and the risk of sudden death from cardiac causes. *N Engl J Med* 2004;351:1089–1096.
70. Yang T, Roden DM. Extracellular potassium modulation of drug block of IKr: implications for torsades de pointes and reverse use-dependence. *Circulation* 1996;93:407–411.
71. Tzivoni D, Banai S, Schugar C, et al. Treatment of torsade de pointes with magnesium sulfate. *Circulation* 1988;77:392–397.
72. Cummins RO, Hazinski MF. The most important changes in the international ECC and CPR guidelines 2000. *Circulation* 2000;102(suppl I):I371–I376.
73. Fuster V, Ryden LE, Asinger RW, et al. ACC/AHA/ESC guidelines for the management of patients with atrial fibrillation: executive summary a report of the American College of Cardiology/American Heart Association Task Force on Practice Guidelines and the European Society of Cardiology Committee for Practice Guidelines and Policy Conferences (Committee to Develop Guidelines for the Management of Patients with Atrial Fibrillation) developed in collaboration with the North American Society of Pacing and Electrophysiology. *Circulation* 2001;104:2118–2150.
74. Blomstrom-Lundqvist C, Scheinman MM, Aliot EM, et al. ACC/AHA/ESC guidelines for the management of patients with supraventricular arrhythmias—executive summary: a report of the American College of Cardiology/American Heart Association Task Force on Practice Guidelines and the European Society of Cardiology Committee for Practice Guidelines (Writing Committee to Develop Guidelines for the Management of Patients with Supraventricular Arrhythmias). *Circulation* 2003;108:1871–1909.
75. Priori SG, Aliot E, Blomstrom-Lundqvist C, et al. Update of the guidelines on sudden cardiac death of the European Society of Cardiology. *Eur Heart J* 2003;24:13–15.
76. Maisel WH, Kuntz KM, Reimold SC, et al. Risk of initiating antiarrhythmic drug therapy for atrial fibrillation in patients admitted to a university hospital. *Ann Intern Med* 1997;127:281–284.
77. Stewart RB, Bardy GH, Greene HL. Wide complex tachycardia: misdiagnosis and outcome after emergent therapy. *Ann Intern Med* 1986;104:766–771.
78. Iwai S, Lerman BB. Management of ventricular tachycardia in patients with clinically normal hearts. *Curr Cardiol Rep* 2000;2:515–521.
79. Pourbaix S, Berger Y, Desager JP, et al. Absolute bioavailability of amiodarone in normal subjects. *Clin Pharmacol Ther* 1985;37:118–123.
80. Wilkinson GR, Shand DG. A physiological approach to hepatic drug clearance. *Clin Pharmacol Ther* 1975;18:377–390.
81. Kessler KM, Kissane B, Cassidy J, et al. Dynamic variability of binding of antiarrhythmic drugs during the evolution of acute myocardial infarction. *Circulation* 1984;70:472–478.
82. Thompson PD, Melmon KL, Richards JA, et al. Lidocaine pharmacokinetics in advanced heart failure, liver disease and renal failure in man. *Ann Intern Med* 1973;78:499.
83. Woosley RL, Chen Y, Freiman JP, Gillis RA. Mechanism of the cardiotoxic actions of terfenadine. *JAMA* 1993;269:1532–1536.
84. Fromm MF, Kim RB, Stein CM, et al. Inhibition of P-glycoprotein–mediated drug transport: a unifying mechanism to explain the interaction between digoxin and quinidine. *Circulation* 1999;99:552–557.
85. Camm AJ, Garratt CJ. Adenosine and supraventricular tachycardia. *N Engl J Med* 1991;325:1621–1629.
86. Israel C, Klingenheben T, Gronefeld G, Hohnloser SH. Adenosine-induced atrial fibrillation. *J Cardiovasc Electrophysiol* 2000;11:825.
87. Scheinman MM, Levine JH, Cannom DS, et al. Dose-ranging study of intravenous amiodarone in patients with life-threatening ventricular tachyarrhythmias. *Circulation* 1995;92:3264–3272.
88. Kowey PR, Levine JH, Herre JM, et al. Randomized, double-blind comparison of intravenous amiodarone and bretylium in the treatment of patients with recurrent, hemodynamically destabilizing ventricular tachycardia or fibrillation. *Circulation* 1995;92:3255–3263.
89. Kudenchuk PJ, Cobb LA, Copass MK, et al. Amiodarone for resuscitation after out-of-hospital cardiac arrest due to ventricular fibrillation. *N Engl J Med* 1999;341:871–878.
90. Dorian P, Cass D, Schwartz B, et al. Amiodarone as compared with lidocaine for shock-resistant ventricular fibrillation. *N Engl J Med* 2002;346: 884–890.
91. Mason JW. Amiodarone. *N Engl J Med* 1987;316:455–466.
92. Dorian P, Mangat I. Role of amiodarone in the era of the implantable cardioverter defibrillator. *J Cardiovasc Electrophysiol* 2003;14:S78–S81.
93. Greene HL, the CASCADE Investigators. The CASCADE Study: randomized antiarrhythmic drug therapy in survivors of cardiac arrest in Seattle. *Am J Cardiol* 1993;72:70F–74F.
94. Mcanulty J, Halperin B, Kron J, et al. A comparison of antiarrhythmic-drug therapy with implantable defibrillators in patients resuscitated from near-fatal ventricular arrhythmias. *N Engl J Med* 1997;337:1576–1583.
95. Singh BN, Singh SN, Reda DJ, et al. Amiodarone versus sotalol for atrial fibrillation. *N Engl J Med* 2005;352:1861–1872.
96. Roy D, Talajic M, Dorian P, et al. Amiodarone to prevent recurrence of atrial fibrillation. Canadian Trial of Atrial Fibrillation Investigators. *N Engl J Med* 2000;342:913–920.
97. Daoud EG, Strickberger SA, Man KC, et al. Preoperative amiodarone as prophylaxis against atrial fibrillation after heart surgery. *N Engl J Med* 1997;337:1785–1791.
98. Camus P, Martin WJ, Rosenow EC III. Amiodarone pulmonary toxicity. *Clin Chest Med* 2004;25:65–75.
99. Weinberg BA, Miles WM, Klein LS, et al. Five-year follow-up of 589 patients treated with amiodarone. *Am Heart J* 1993;125:109–120.
100. Goldschlager N, Epstein AE, Naccarelli G, et al. Practical guidelines for clinicians who treat patients with amiodarone: Practice Guidelines Subcommittee, North American Society of Pacing and Electrophysiology. *Arch Intern Med* 2000;160:1741–1748.
101. Johnson LN, Krohel GB, Thomas ER. The clinical spectrum of amiodarone-associated optic neuropathy. *J Natl Med Assoc* 2004;96:1477–1491.
102. Antman EM, Wenger TL, Butler VPJ, et al. Treatment of 150 cases of life-threatening digitalis intoxication with digoxin-specific Fab antibody fragments: final report of a multicenter study. *Circulation* 1990;81:1744–1752.
103. Morady F, Scheinman MM, Desia J. Disopyramide. *Ann Intern Med* 1982; 96:337–343.
104. Pedersen OD, Bagger H, Keller N, et al. Efficacy of dofetilide in the treatment of atrial fibrillation-flutter in patients with reduced left ventricular

function: a Danish investigations of arrhythmia and mortality on dofetilide (DIAMOND) substudy. *Circulation* 2001;104:292–296.
105. McClellan KJ, Markham A. Dofetilide: a review of its use in atrial fibrillation and atrial flutter. *Drugs* 1999;58:1043–1059.
106. Singh S, Zoble RG, Yellen L, et al. Efficacy and safety of oral dofetilide in converting to and maintaining sinus rhythm in patients with chronic atrial fibrillation or atrial flutter: the Symptomatic Atrial Fibrillation Investigative Research on Dofetilide (SAFIRE-D) study. *Circulation* 2000;102:2385–2390.
107. Roden DM, Woosley RL. Flecainide. *N Engl J Med* 1986;315:36–41.
108. Anderson JL. Summary of efficacy and safety of flecainide for supraventricular arrhythmias. *Am J Cardiol* 1988;62:62D–66D.
109. Stambler BS, Wood MA, Ellenbogen KA. Antiarrhythmic actions of intravenous ibutilide compared with procainamide during human atrial flutter and fibrillation: electrophysiological determinants of enhanced conversion efficacy. *Circulation* 1997;96:4298–4306.
110. Stambler BS, Wood MA, Ellenbogen KA, et al. Efficacy and safety of repeated intravenous doses of ibutilide for rapid conversion of atrial flutter or fibrillation. *Circulation* 1996;94:1613–1621.
111. Ellenbogen KA, Stambler BS, Wood MA, et al. Efficacy of intravenous ibutilide for rapid termination of atrial fibrillation and atrial flutter: a dose-response study. *J Am Coll Cardiol* 1996;28:130–136.
112. Oral H, Souza JJ, Michaud GF, et al. Facilitating transthoracic cardioversion of atrial fibrillation with ibutilide pretreatment. *N Engl J Med* 1999; 340:1849–1854.
113. Ho DS, Zecchin RP, Richards DA, et al. Double-blind trial of lignocaine versus sotalol for acute termination of spontaneous sustained ventricular tachycardia. *Lancet* 1994;344:18–23.
114. Seller RH. The role of magnesium in digitalis toxicity. *Am Heart J* 1971; 82:551–556.
115. Campbell RWF. Mexiletine. *N Engl J Med* 1987;316:29–34.
116. Schwartz PJ, Priori SG, Locati EH, et al. Long QT syndrome patients with mutations of the *SCN5A* and *HERG* genes have differential responses to Na^+ channel blockade and to increases in heart rate: implications for gene-specific therapy. *Circulation* 1995;92:3381–3386.
117. Woosley RL, Drayer DE, Reidenberg MM, et al. Effect of acetylator phenotype on the rate at which procainamide induces antinuclear antibodies and the lupus syndrome. *N Engl J Med* 1978;298:1157–1159.
118. Funck-Brentano C, Kroemer HK, Lee JT, Roden DM. Propafenone. *N Engl J Med* 1990;322:518–525.
119. Lee JT, Kroemer HK, Silberstein DJ, et al. The role of genetically determined polymorphic drug metabolism in the beta-blockade produced by propafenone. *N Engl J Med* 1990;322:1764–1768.
120. Antzelevitch C, Shimizu W, Yan GX, et al. The M cell: its contribution to the ECG and to normal and abnormal electrical function of the heart. *J Cardiovasc Electrophysiol* 1999;10:1124–1152.
121. Flaker GC, Blackshear JL, McBride R, et al. Antiarrhythmic drug therapy and cardiac mortality in atrial fibrillation. *J Am Coll Cardiol* 1992;20:527–532.
122. Coplen SE, Antman EM, Berlin JA, et al. Efficacy and safety of quinidine therapy for maintenance of sinus rhythm after cardioversion. *Circulation* 1990;82:1106–1116.
123. Hohnloser SH, Woosley RL. Sotalol. *N Engl J Med* 1994;331:31–38.
124. Julian DG, Jackson FS, Prescott RJ, Szekely P. Controlled trial of sotalol for one year after myocardial infarction. *Lancet* 1982;1:1142–1147.
125. Pacifico A, Hohnloser SH, Williams JH, et al. Prevention of implantable-defibrillator shocks by treatment with sotalol. *N Engl J Med* 1999;340: 1855–1862.
126. Roden DM. Antiarrhythmic drugs: past, present and future. *J Cardiovasc Electrophysiol* 2003;14:1389–1396.
127. Page RL, Roden DM. New drug therapy for atrial fibrillation. *Nat Rev Drug Discov* (in press).
128. Nattel S. New ideas about atrial fibrillation 50 years on. *Nature* 2002; 415:219–226.
129. Roden DM. Cardiovascular pharmacogenomics. *Circulation* 2003;108: 3071–3074.
130. Roden DM. Genetic polymorphisms, drugs, and proarrhythmia. *J Interv Card Electrophysiol* 2003;9:131–135.

CHAPTER 73 ■ CATHETER ABLATION THERAPY FOR ARRHYTHMIAS

DAVID E. HAINES

OVERVIEW

The rationale behind ablative therapy is that, for any arrhythmia, a critical anatomic substrate allows propagation of that arrhythmia. If that substrate is irreversibly damaged or destroyed, then the arrhythmia should no longer occur spontaneously or with provocation.

Numerous methods of catheter ablation have been attempted experimentally and clinically, but radiofrequency catheter ablation is still accepted as the safest and most effective modality. Radiofrequency energy heats myocardium by the passage of the radiofrequency electrical current through the tissue, with consequent resistive tissue heating. Deeper tissue heating results in larger lesions. Larger electrodes, higher temperatures, and very high-power deliveries coupled with irrigated-tip or cooled-tip catheters will increase lesion size. Radiofrequency ablative lesions are thermally mediated. Temperatures exceeding 50°C result in breakdown of the sarcolemmal membrane and cell death.

The mechanisms of paroxysmal supraventricular tachycardia (SVT) are varied and include atrioventricular (AV) reciprocating tachycardia, AV nodal reentrant tachycardia, atrial fibrillation (AF), atrial flutter, and atrial tachycardia of focal automatic or reentrant mechanisms. Catheter ablation of accessory pathways responsible for the Wolff-Parkinson-White syndrome and AV reciprocating tachycardias may be accomplished at either the atrial or the ventricular insertion sites of the pathway, with a very high (>95% at experienced centers) success rate. Catheter modification of the AV node is highly successful in eliminating AV nodal reentrant tachycardia. In most cases, ablation in the low septal region results in elimination or marked modification of the slow AV nodal pathway and prevents tachycardia recurrence.

Atrial flutter is a macroreentrant rhythm that travels around the tricuspid valve annulus and through the isthmus between the valve and the inferior vena caval inlet. A linear ablative lesion placed across this isthmus results in successful ablation of the atrial flutter. AF may have a reentrant mechanism or, particularly in patients with frequent paroxysmal AF and normal atrial size, may originate from rapid firing from a pulmonary vein focus. Ablation of focal origins of AF initiation is relatively successful in eliminating this arrhythmia in highly selected patients. Combinations of pulmonary vein isolation, linear atrial ablation, atrial substrate modification, and atrial denervation have been employed with varying success as curative therapy for paroxysmal or persistent AF in patients with structural heart disease.

Ventricular tachycardia (VT) may be idiopathic or may result from the presence of underlying structural heart disease. Idiopathic VT from the outflow tract (most often right ventricle) is usually focal in origin, with a likely mechanism of abnormal automaticity or triggered activity. It may be ablated with a high likelihood of success. Idiopathic left VT is usually caused by reentry involving the fascicular network and may be cured with ablation of the fascicular insertion into the myocardium. VT in the setting of structural heart disease is usually the result of a reentrant mechanism in regions of patchy fibrosis. Ablation may be accomplished at sites within the zone of slowed electrical conduction that is identified with techniques such as activation and entrainment mapping.

GLOSSARY

Accessory pathway: This anomalous bridge of electrically conducting tissue between the atrium and ventricle, which is responsible for Wolff-Parkinson-White syndrome and AV reciprocating tachycardias, is also known as a bundle of Kent or bypass tract.

Activation mapping: Multipoint electrogram acquisition during ongoing tachycardia demonstrates sites where the local electrical activity precedes the onset of the surface QRS complex. These sites represent exit points from the slow conduction zone (SCZ) for reentrant tachycardias or sites of arrhythmia origin for automatic or triggered tachycardias.

AV nodal modification: This consists of (a) ablation of the slow AV nodal pathway to treat AV nodal reentrant tachycardia and (b) nonspecific ablation of the AV node to impair anterograde conduction and to decrease the ventricular response rate to AF.

Coagulum: When boiling occurs at the electrode tip, coagulated protein from tissue and blood adheres to the tip of the electrode.

Convective cooling: This is the process by which thermal energy is removed by circulating blood flow through the heart.

Dispersive electrode: This electrode with a large surface area is placed in contact with the patient's skin (usually with electrically conductive gel) to complete the electrical circuit during ablation with radiofrequency electrical current.

Electrical impedance: The resistance and capacitance of the radiofrequency electrical circuit; this includes the electronic components, the conducting wires, the point of conduction between the ablation electrode and the heart, the tissue between the heart and the skin, and the junction between the skin and the dispersive electrode.

Entrainment mapping: Pacing slightly faster than ongoing reentrant VT from various sites in the ventricle; when one is in or near the SCZ, the morphology of the resulting complex matches the tachycardia morphology exactly, and the time from the stimulus to the QRS complex is prolonged (concealed entrainment).

Focal initiation or focal site of origin: Some specific arrhythmias originate from a point source and emanate in a centripetal fashion from that point. The mechanisms of focal tachycardias are probably abnormal automaticity of triggered activity. Typical examples are some types of AF and idiopathic VT.

Impedance rise: If boiling and coagulum adherence occur, the available surface area for radiofrequency current conduction decreases, resulting in a sudden increase in system impedance.

Pace mapping: During sinus rhythm, pacing is performed from a variety of ventricular sites. For VTs of focal origin, the electrocardiograms (ECGs) during pacing should be almost identical to those during tachycardia if the pacing site is in close proximity to the arrhythmia origin.

Radiofrequency energy: High-frequency alternating electrical current; when passed through a resistive medium, it creates heat.

Slow and fast AV nodal pathways: The AV node has multiple atrial inputs that have varying properties, including conduction time. In typical AV nodal reentrant tachycardia, electrical activation travels in an anterograde fashion down a slowly conducting AV nodal pathway, and in a retrograde fashion up a fast conducting pathway.

Tricuspid–inferior vena cava isthmus: This is the narrow anatomic region between the tricuspid annulus and the inferior vena caval orifice in the right atrium through which atrial flutter reentrant circuits conduct. It is the usual site targeted for atrial flutter ablation.

Ventricular preexcitation: This pattern, seen on surface ECGs, is characterized by δ waves (slurred QRS upstrokes) and results from the presence of an accessory pathway that conducts in an anterograde fashion. Wolff-Parkinson-White syndrome is the most common form of preexcitation syndrome.

Ventricular tachycardia slow conduction zone (VT SCZ): This region in the border zone of scar in the ventricle is bounded by areas of anatomic or physiologic conduction block, which has a slow conduction velocity. Conduction through this region accounts for the diastolic period of electrical silence on the surface ECG during ongoing reentrant VT.

Volume heating: This form of heating from radiofrequency energy or another energy source is direct and is not a result of heat conduction from a contiguous region of heated tissue.

GENERAL PRINCIPLES

Ablative therapy for the management of arrhythmias is based on the observation that most arrhythmias arise from a focal origin or are critically dependent on conduction through a defined anatomic structure. If those critical regions are irreversibly damaged or destroyed, then the arrhythmia should no longer occur spontaneously or with provocation. Traditionally, ablation was performed with open surgical techniques. It was discovered, however, that focal endocardial injury could also be achieved by a controlled delivery of destructive energy through a catheter. Since the early 1990s, catheter designs have evolved to improve site access dramatically, and our knowledge and understanding of the anatomy of the heart and the sources of arrhythmia origin have significantly expanded. In response to this progress, the indications for catheter ablation have continued to broaden, and it is now the therapy of choice for a number of arrhythmias.

HISTORY OF CATHETER ABLATION

The concept of ablative therapy for the treatment of arrhythmias was well established in the surgical literature throughout the 1970s. Since the original description of the surgical division of an accessory pathway by Sealey in 1969 (1), there had been several reports of surgical treatment of the Wolff-Parkinson-White syndrome (2,3) and VT (4,5). In these series, the concept of curative ablative therapy was proved. However, the obvious limitation to this approach was that open thoracotomy and, in most cases, cardiopulmonary bypass were required. Although researchers were pursuing a variety of approaches to decrease surgical morbidity and mortality, it was not thought possible to eliminate these arrhythmic substrates without direct visualization.

In 1979, a complication of transthoracic cardioversion was reported. Catheters had been placed for recording in the bundle of His position, and multiple direct current (DC) shocks were administered transthoracically to terminate an episode of VT. At the conclusion of the cardioversion, complete heart block was observed. It was hypothesized that shunting of defibrillator current through the His bundle catheter caused irreversible damage to the AV conduction system (6). After this report, Scheinman et al. (7) and Gallagher et al. (8) published the first series of catheter ablation of the AV junction in patients with AF and a rapid ventricular response rate that could not be controlled with drugs. In these patients, high-voltage DC electrical energy was intentionally delivered between the tip of an electrode catheter placed contiguous to the bundle of His, and a dispersive patch electrode was placed on the skin. The field of catheter ablation was born. Subsequently, investigators reported successful catheter ablation of accessory pathways (9,10) and VT (11) with this approach. Unfortunately, a relatively high complication rate was also reported, including pericardial tamponade, cardiogenic shock, and death (12).

The technique of high-energy DC shock catheter ablation was effective, but it was extremely difficult to control. An alternative energy source for controlled ablation of myocardium was needed. In 1985, Huang and associates described their use of radiofrequency electrical energy for controlled catheter ablation of the AV junction in dogs. Radiofrequency catheter ablation resulted in very controllable, well-circumscribed endocardial lesions (13). It was discovered that lesion formation could be nicely controlled by either titrating power (14) or temperature measured at the catheter tip (15). Efficacy of radiofrequency catheter ablation in the clinical setting was increased with improvements in the catheter design. Larger ablation electrodes increased lesion size (16), and an increase in the electrode tip size from 2 to 4 mm increased procedure efficacy (17). Catheter design pioneers such as Will Webster constructed catheters that had a distal segment that could be deflected by manipulation of the control handle. This advance greatly improved site access and catheter stability.

The first report of successful catheter ablation of an accessory pathway with high-frequency alternating (radiofrequency) electrical current by Borggrefe et al. brought us into the modern era of radiofrequency catheter ablation (18). Based on the important work of Jackman, Kuck, Haissaguerre, Morady, and others, the correlations among electrogram patterns, anatomic locations of accessory pathways, and access to those sites with ablation catheters were elucidated (19–21). Success rates exceeding 90% were reported by investigators in the treatment of paroxysmal SVT (22–24). In the present day, experienced operators achieve greater than 95% success rates in the ablation of these arrhythmias. The indications for radiofrequency catheter ablation continue to expand, and it has become a dominant therapeutic modality for many varieties of symptomatic tachycardia.

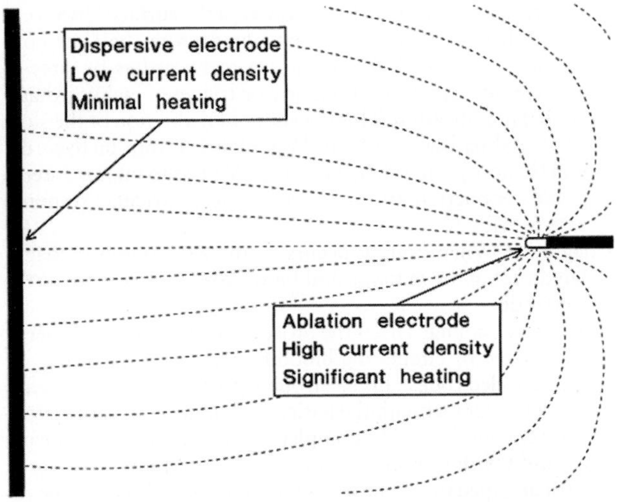

FIGURE 73.1. Schematic representation of a catheter ablation electrode and a skin dispersive electrode during radiofrequency energy delivery. The *dashed lines* represent the electrical field. Because the available electrode surface area of the ablation electrode is much smaller than that of the dispersive skin electrode, the current density and its associated tissue heating of the former are much greater. In addition, the electrical field around the ablation electrode is relatively uniform, irrespective of the location of the dispersive electrode.

BIOPHYSICS OF RADIOFREQUENCY CATHETER ABLATION

Radiofrequency electrical energy is employed to create thermal lesions in the heart. The frequencies generally employed are 300 to 1,000 kHz. Although this energy is similar to that employed for broadcast radio, the radiofrequency energy is electrically conducted, not radiated, during catheter ablation. The radiofrequency current is similar to low-frequency alternating current or DC with regard to its ability to heat tissue and create a lesion, but it oscillates so rapidly that cardiac and skeletal muscles are not stimulated, thereby avoiding induction of arrhythmias and decreasing the pain perceived by the patient. Electrical energy dissipates as heat within the first 2 mm of the tissue (direct resistive or volume heating) (15). Heating to deeper tissue layers occurs by heat conduction from the region of volume heating.

The radiofrequency current is generally delivered in a unipolar fashion between the tip of the ablation electrode and a dispersive electrode applied to the patient's skin. Because the surface area of the ablation electrode is much smaller than that of the dispersive electrode, the current density is higher at the ablation site, and heating occurs preferentially at that site (Fig. 73.1). If, however, ablation is performed with a high-amplitude current, and skin contact by the dispersive electrode is poor, it is possible to cause skin burns (25). Nath et al. (26) demonstrated that the position of the dispersive electrode has little effect on the geometry of the resulting lesion. However, sometimes it is advantageous to increase the surface area of the dispersive electrode, particularly if the ablation is power limited. With lower impedance at the dispersive electrode-skin interface, a greater proportion of the available electrical energy will be available for heating at the tip of the ablation catheter. In patients who had a baseline system impedance of greater than 100 ohm, using two dispersive electrodes resulted in more effective heating than using a single electrode.

It has been demonstrated in vitro that, at steady state, the tissue temperature decreases radially in proportion to the distance from the ablation electrode and that, at steady state, the lesion size is proportional to the temperature measured at the interface between the tissue and the electrode (14). In addition, lesion size has also been shown to be proportional to the radiofrequency power amplitude. Using higher powers and achieving higher tissue temperatures may increase lesion size. However, once the peak tissue temperature exceeds the threshold of 100°C, boiling at the electrode-tissue interface may ensue (27). When boiling occurs, denatured serum proteins and charred tissue adhere to the electrode to form an electrically insulating "coagulum," which is accompanied by a sudden rise in electrical impedance that prevents further current flow into the tissue and further heating. The consequences of this adverse event could include char embolism or excess disruption of the endocardium with subsequent thrombus formation and associated risk of thromboembolism. Conventional electrode catheters with temperature monitoring underestimate peak tissue temperature, so it is best if target temperatures not exceeding 70°C to 80°C are selected in the clinical setting. Because the rate of temperature rise at deeper sites within the myocardium is slow (28), a continuous energy delivery of at least 60 seconds is often warranted to maximize depth of lesion formation. Tissue temperatures continue to rise for several seconds after termination of radiofrequency energy delivery (29). This thermal latency effect can account for the observation that patients undergoing AV modification procedures and demonstrating transient heart block during radiofrequency energy delivery may progress to persisting complete heart block even if radiofrequency energy delivery is terminated immediately.

The dominant factor opposing effective heating of myocardium is the convective cooling from the circulating blood pool. If the catheter position is not stable, or if it is positioned in region of high blood flow, the magnitude of convective cooling is increased (30). Efficiency of energy delivery to the tissue may vary from approximately 70% to 10% in vivo. The effects of convective cooling have been exploited to increase the size of catheter ablative lesions. To eliminate the risk of

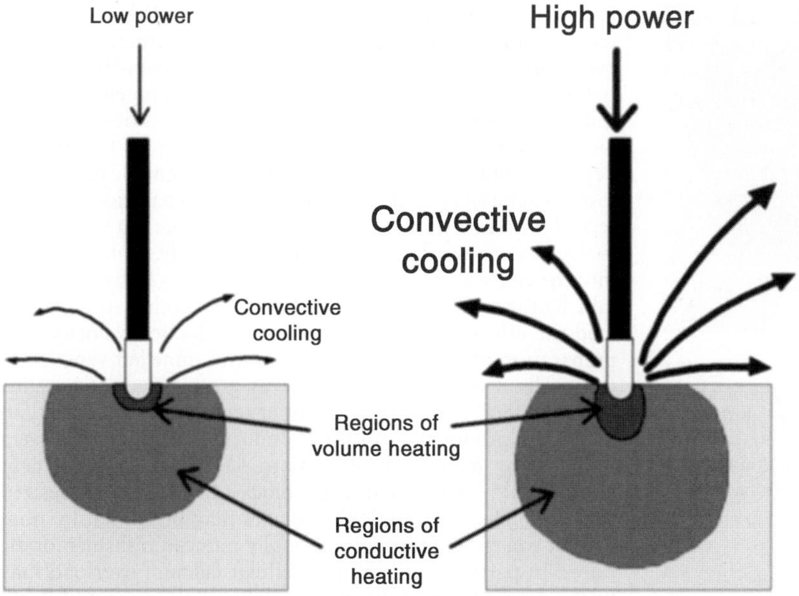

FIGURE 73.2. Schematic representation of two conditions during radiofrequency catheter ablation. On the **left** is depicted conventional conditions with a moderate degree of convective cooling. A low magnitude of radiofrequency power is applied to achieve heating at the electrode-tissue interface. This results in a small depth of volume heating and a moderate depth of conductive heating that creates the final pathologic lesion. On the **right** is depicted radiofrequency ablation in the setting of increased convective cooling, either by active tip cooling with perfused or circulating saline or by unstable catheter-tissue contact. A high magnitude of radiofrequency power is applied, but the electrode-tissue interface does not exceed 100°C because of convective dissipation of heat at the tissue surface. The higher applied power results in a greater depth of volume heating and a larger overall lesion size.

overheating at the electrode-tissue contact point but increase the magnitude of power delivery and the depth of volume heating, investigators have employed porous-tipped electrodes for open irrigation of the electrode tip or closed irrigation systems for electrode tip cooling (Fig. 73.2). Nakagawa et al. achieved temperatures of 95 ± 9°C at depths of 3.5 mm and lesion dimensions of 10 ± 1 mm depth by 14 ± 2 mm diameter with ablation through an irrigated-tip electrode in a superfused canine thigh muscle preparation. However, superheating within the tissue with a resulting sudden explosive release of the expanding steam to the surface (the so-called pop lesion) was observed in 7.5% of the ablations (31). Cooled-tip catheters have now been used extensively in the clinical setting. The larger lesions generated have yielded increased procedure success rates or decreased procedure times, particularly with ablation of difficult substrates such as atrial flutter (32,33).

Because the success of radiofrequency catheter ablation in the clinical setting is sometimes limited by the relatively small size of the lesion, attempts have been made to increase the size of those lesions reliably and safely. One approach toward this end is to increase the size and surface area of the electrode. The radiofrequency power needs to be increased comparably to achieve a similar current density and temperature at the electrode-tissue interface, and the result is a greater depth of volume heating and a larger lesion (16). Conventional ablation catheters employ 4- and 5-mm electrode tips, but catheters with 8 and 10-mm tips are now being used for difficult ablation sites where larger lesion size and depth are required (34). It is not clear that one large lesion technology is better than another (35), but each method has its advantages and disadvantages (36).

MECHANISMS OF MYOCARDIAL INJURY CAUSED BY RADIOFREQUENCY CATHETER ABLATION

It is likely that the major mechanism of tissue injury from radiofrequency catheter ablation is thermal. Heating of the myocardium occurs reproducibly during radiofrequency energy delivery, and the association of clinical effect and temperature measured at the electrode catheter interface has been established. Experimentally, lesions created from a radiofrequency or microwave source have a reliable isotherm of irreversible tissue injury of 52°C to 55°C (37). In the clinical setting, successful ablations were associated with a mean temperature measured at the electrode-tissue interface of 62 ± 15°C (38). During ablation of the AV junction, the reversible physiologic effect of an accelerated junctional rhythm was observed at temperatures of 51 ± 4°C, whereas temperatures of 58 ± 6°C were required to achieve heart block (39). These findings are consistent with an anatomic position of the ablation target that may several millimeters from the electrode-tissue contact point.

Tissue Effects of Radiofrequency Catheter Ablation

Changes in myocardial tissue are apparent immediately on completion of the radiofrequency lesion. Pallor of the central zone of the lesion is attributable to myoglobin denaturation with an associated color change. Some volume loss in the central region of lesion formation is apparent, as evidenced by a slight deformation at the point of catheter contact. Fibrin usually adheres to the endocardial surface, and if a temperature of 100°C has been exceeded, adherent char and thrombus are often apparent. On sectioning, the central portion of the lesion shows desiccation, with a surrounding region of hemorrhagic tissue, then normal-appearing tissue (Fig. 73.3) (40). Histologic examination of an acute lesion shows typical coagulation necrosis with basophilic stippling consistent with intracellular calcium overload. Immediately surrounding the central lesion is a region of hemorrhage and acute monocellular and neutrophilic inflammation. The progressive changes seen in the evolution of a radiofrequency lesion are typical of healing after any acute injury. Within 2 months of the ablation, the lesions show fibrosis, granulation tissue, chronic inflammatory infiltrates, and significant volume contraction (40). The lesion border is well demarcated from the surrounding viable myocardium without evidence of patchy fibrosis. This finding likely accounts for the absence of proarrhythmia side effects with radiofrequency catheter ablation. Because of the high-velocity blood flow within the epicardial coronary arteries,

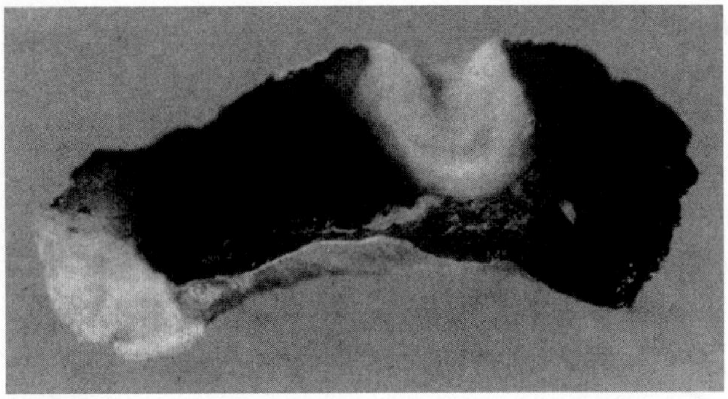

FIGURE 73.3. Example of a typical radiofrequency lesion created in an experimental preparation and stained with the histochemical dye nitro blue tetrazolium. The electrode-tissue contact point shows volume loss and dimpling. The viable myocardium (*dark stain*) is sharply demarcated from the nonviable lesion (*light stain*). The lesion width is narrower at the endocardial surface than at a 2-mm depth because of surface convective cooling from endocardial blood flow.

these vessels are continuously cooled and are spared from injury despite nearby delivery of radiofrequency energy (41). However, high-power radiofrequency delivery in small hearts, such as in pediatric patients, may potentially cause coronary arterial injury, so caution is warranted (42).

The border zone around the acute pathologic lesion is a region that can demonstrate initial stunning and then early or late recovery of function, or it can show late progression of physiologic block, resulting in a "delayed cure" in some cases (43). Significant diminution in microvascular blood flow is observed in this region. Electron microscopic examination of the border zone has demonstrated marked ultrastructural abnormalities in tissue that appears to be viable by routine histologic examination. The microvessels appear severely damaged with loss of the basement membrane, disruption of the endothelial cell plasma membrane, and erythrocyte stasis (44). The myocytes show significant ultrastructural injury of the plasma membrane, mitochondria, sarcomeres, sarcoplasmic reticulum, and gap junctions. The most thermally sensitive structures appear to be the plasma membrane and gap junctions, which show morphologic changes as far as 6 mm from the edge of the histologic lesion (45). It has therefore been documented that the effects of radiofrequency lesion formation extend well beyond the acute pathologic lesion and are characterized by marked ultrastructural abnormalities of the microvascular and myocytes acutely and a typical inflammatory response later. Therefore, the recovery of electrophysiologic function after successful catheter ablation in the clinical setting may result from healing of the damaged but surviving myocardium. Moreover, the progression of the electrophysiologic effects after completion of the ablation procedure may result from further inflammatory injury and necrosis in the border zone region.

Cellular Effects of Radiofrequency Ablation

Hyperthermic injury to the cell is both time and temperature dependent. This injury to the myocyte may be caused by changes in the membrane, protein inactivation, cytoskeletal disruption, nuclear degeneration, or a number of other potential mechanisms. Experimentally, brief duration of exposure to heat results in prominent changes in the electrophysiology of the myocyte. In one study, guinea pig papillary muscles were exposed to temperatures between 37°C and 55°C, and transmembrane potentials were measured. In the low hyperthermic range (37°C to 45°C), a minor change was seen in the resting membrane potential and action potential amplitude, and the action potential duration shortened significantly. In the intermediate hyperthermic range (45°C to 50°C), progressive depolarization of the resting membrane potential, loss of action potential amplitude, abnormal automaticity, and reversible loss of excitability were seen. In the high temperature ranges (>50°C), marked depolarization of the resting membrane potential, permanent loss of excitability, and contracture of the preparation were observed (46). In a similar preparation, hyperthermia was shown to increase intracellular calcium significantly. Calcium entry into the cell was not channel specific and was buffered by uptake by the sarcoplasmic reticulum (47). Another study examined the effects of hyperthermia on conduction velocity of a preparation of epicardial shavings from canine left ventricular free walls. Conduction velocity was greater than at baseline between 38.5°C and 45.4°C, but at temperatures higher than 45.4°C, a progressive drop in conduction velocity was seen, followed by temporary (49.5°C to 51.5°C) then permanent (51.7°C to 54.4°C) conduction block (48). It is hypothesized that these electrophysiologic changes may be caused by nonspecific ion transit through thermally induced transmembrane pores. In particular, acute intracellular calcium overload may be the dominant mechanism of cellular contracture and death at temperatures higher than 50°C.

ABLATION OF SPECIFIC SUPRAVENTRICULAR ARRHYTHMIAS

Accessory Pathway–Mediated Arrhythmias

A giant step forward was achieved with the first successful catheter ablations of accessory pathways (18). Before the catheter ablation era, patients with Wolff-Parkinson-White syndrome and concealed accessory pathways frequently required open surgical ablation of their extranodal pathways. The ability to map the location of accessory pathways precisely and to deliver a very precise ablative lesion with radiofrequency energy not only proved to be a valuable therapeutic modality, but also greatly enhanced the understanding of the physiologic-anatomic correlates of this relatively common abnormality. Important preliminary work by Jackman et al. identified electrogram patterns that correlated precisely with accessory pathway insertions in the atria and ventricles (19). The ultimate validation of the origin of these potentials arrived when small, discrete radiofrequency lesions placed at those locations resulted in elimination of both anterograde and retrograde accessory pathway conduction (Fig. 73.4) (22–24,49). Most accessory pathways have a discrete and narrow ventricular and atrial insertion, but they sometimes branch and often have a slanting course (19). The high success rate of radiofrequency catheter ablation delivered from the endocardial approach implies that most pathways are situated close to the endocardial surface. However, a small proportion of left free wall accessory pathways (1% to 4%) can be ablated successfully only from the epicardial approach via the coronary sinus and probably represent true epicardial pathways (50).

The successful catheter ablation of accessory pathways is directly related to the skill and experience of the operator (51). Careful mapping of the accessory pathway atrial and ventricular insertion points before any radiofrequency energy delivery greatly enhances the efficiency of the ablation procedure and minimizes the risk of distortion of local electrograms by poorly placed ablative lesions. In patients with manifest ventricular preexcitation (Wolff-Parkinson-White syndrome), mapping is best performed in the anterograde direction during sinus or

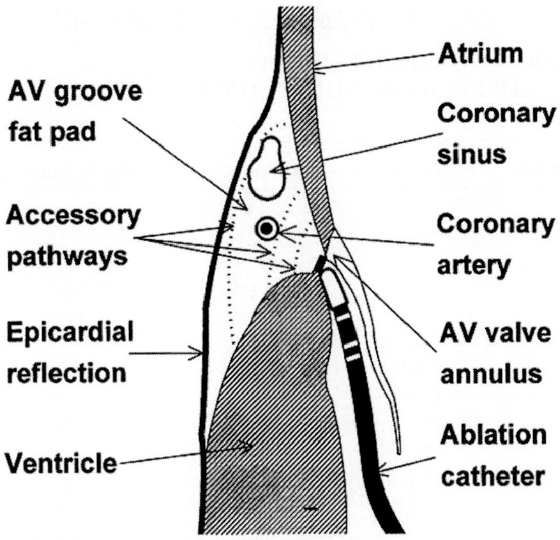

FIGURE 73.4. Schematic representation of a cross section of the left atrioventricular (AV) groove with the position of a typical ablation catheter relative to the anatomic structures in this region. The possible courses of three accessory pathways are diagrammed. One accessory pathway follows a subepicardial course and can be successfully ablated only via the coronary sinus. Another pathway passes close to the coronary artery. Fortuitously, the convective cooling of intracoronary blood flow protects the vascular endothelium from thermal injury by endocardial ablation with conventional ablation catheters.

atrial-paced rhythm. The local ventricular activation recorded from the mapping/ablation catheter should precede the onset of the δ wave on the surface ECG by at least 10 to 20 milliseconds, and the electrogram pattern should be stable, indicating stable catheter-tissue contact (Fig. 73.5). An excellent ablation site will show the presence of a high-frequency accessory pathway potential immediately preceding the local ventricular activation and a short atrial to ventricular electrogram interval (52,53). When the accessory pathway is concealed (absent anterograde but intact retrograde conduction), mapping of retrograde activation during ventricular pacing or ongoing orthodromic AV reciprocating tachycardia must be pursued. Discrimination between retrograde AV nodal conduction and conduction up the accessory pathway may be enhanced by pacing near the pathway's ventricular insertion site. The atrial insertion of the accessory pathway is determined by identifying the site with the shortest interval from the reference ventricular electrogram to the local atrial activation from the mapping/ablation electrode. One must be cautious not to mistake late components of the local ventricular electrogram for early atrial signals. As with anterograde mapping, the presence of a local high-frequency accessory pathway potential is an excellent marker for successful ablation sites.

Using electrogram criteria as described earlier, Jackman and colleagues reported an initial accessory pathway catheter ablation success rate of 99% using a median of three radiofrequency energy deliveries (22). In a comparison of the electrograms from 49 successful versus 462 failed ablation sites, an interval of the local ventricular electrogram to δ-wave onset of greater than 10 milliseconds had a sensitivity of 98% for successful ablation, but only a positive predictive value of 11% (53). The low specificity of this finding may have been caused, in part, by inadequate tissue heating by the ablation catheter despite optimal site selection. The presence of ongoing AF can complicate and prolong mapping of accessory pathways because of the absence of consistent atrial electrograms and an inability to measure the AV times. However, if the same criteria of local ventricular electrogram to δ-wave interval and presence of accessory pathway potentials are employed, a high (95%) success rate can still be achieved (54). The characteristic of the local unipolar electrogram is also useful in identifying successful ablation sites. If the recording electrode is placed directly on the accessory pathway insertion site, all conduction into the ventricle (during anterograde mapping) or atrium (during retrograde mapping) will follow a vector away from the electrode. Thus, a "QS" unipolar electrogram pattern should be more favorable than an electrogram pattern with any initial positive deflection. The positive predictive value of this feature reviewing 186 separate ablation sites in 56 patients was 86% and 92% for ventricular and atrial mapping, respectively. The negative predictive value overall was 92% (55).

Catheter placement for ablation of accessory pathways on the left free wall may be accomplished by two approaches. The catheter may be passed across a small puncture hole in the fossa ovalis (transseptal) (56), or it may be prolapsed across the

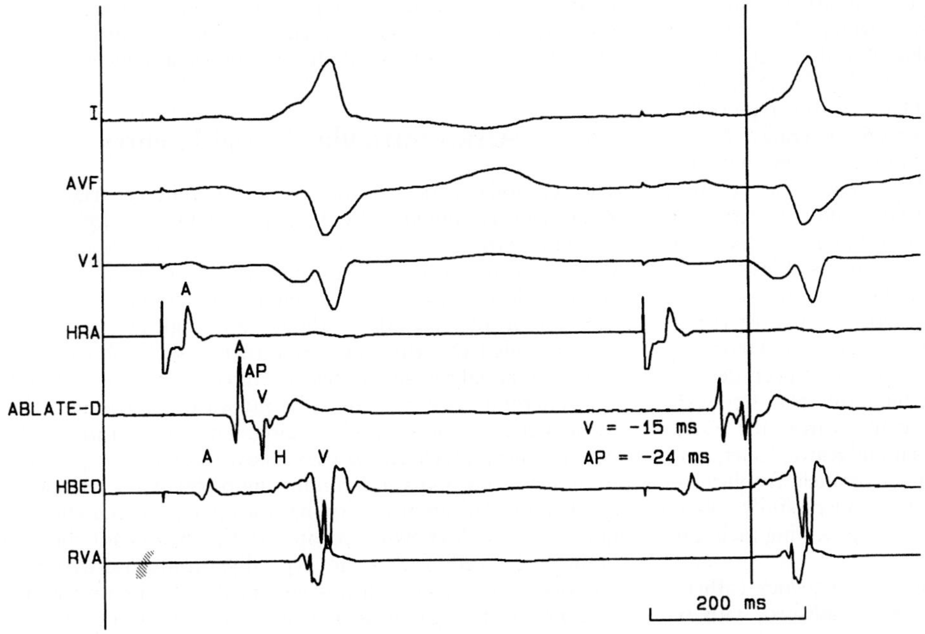

FIGURE 73.5. Surface electrocardiogram tracings I, aVF, and V_1 and intracardiac recordings from the high right atrium (HRA), distal ablation catheter bipole (ABLATE-D), the distal His bundle bipole (HBED), and the right ventricular apex (RVA) in a patient with the Wolff-Parkinson-White syndrome. The *vertical line* indicates the onset of the δ wave on the surface electrocardiogram. The recording from the ablation electrode shows a discrete atrial (A) and ventricular (V) potential with an interposed high-frequency negative deflection that arises from the accessory pathway (AP). The local accessory pathway activation precedes the δ-wave onset by 24 milliseconds, and the local ventricular activation precedes the δ wave by 15 milliseconds. H, bundle of His.

TABLE 73.1

CLINICAL RESULTS OF RADIOFREQUENCY CATHETER ABLATION OF PATIENTS WITH WOLFF-PARKINSON-WHITE SYNDROME OR ATRIOVENTRICULAR RECIPROCATING TACHYCARDIA RESULTING FROM CONCEALED ACCESSORY PATHWAYS

Authors	Year	No. of patients	Location of pathways	Acute success	Complications	Recurrence rate
Jackman, et al. (22)	1991	166	All	99%	3%	9%
Calkins, et al. (23)	1991	56	All	93%	2%	2%
Schluter, et al. (49)	1991	92	All	86%	3%	3%
Kay, et al. (24)	1993	363	All	95%	1%	—
Swartz, et al. (56)	1993	114	LFW	95%	2%	9%
Lesh, et al. (58)	1993	106	LFW	96%	8%	3%
Deshpande, et al. (57)	1994	100	LFW	100%	6%	7%
Schluter, et al. (60)	1992	12	AS	100%	0%	8%
Haissaguerre, et al. (63)	1994	8	AS	100%	0%	8%
Xie, et al. (59)	1994	48	PS	92%	4%	—
Dhala, et al. (62)	1994	50	PS	100%	6%	12%
Calkins, et al. (51)	1999	500	All	93%	3%[a]	8%

AS, anteroseptal; LFW, left free wall; PS, posteroseptal.
[a]Total major complication rate for all patients, including atrioventricular nodal modification, accessory pathway ablation, and atrioventricular nodal ablation.

aortic valve and manipulated in the left ventricle back to the mitral annulus (retrograde) (22,23). Direct comparisons of the two techniques have yielded similar success rates (57), although in children and in patients older than 65 years, complications and failure rates may be higher with retrograde versus transseptal catheter placement (58). Catheter ablation of right free wall pathways is technically challenging and has a lower success rate than ablation of left free wall pathways (51), because it is difficult to stabilize the catheter position on the tricuspid annulus. Multiple accessory pathways are more frequently found in association with right free wall pathways than other locations (≤10% of cases). A subset of patients with Ebstein anomaly has a high prevalence of Wolff-Parkinson-White syndrome, often with multiple accessory pathways. Catheter ablation in this group of patients is made more difficult by the finding that the tricuspid valve (the normal anatomic landmark for catheter placement) is displaced downward from the true anatomic annulus where the accessory pathways are located. Septal accessory pathways may be divided into anteroseptal, midseptal, and posteroseptal locations. Anteroseptal and midseptal pathways are located in close contiguity to the normal AV conduction system. Radiofrequency catheter ablation in these region may be associated with a higher than normal risk of complete heart block (59,60). Use of cryothermic ablation in this region may improve catheter stability and may be safer overall (61). The posteroseptal space is a complex anatomic region characterized by a broad region where the AV valve annuli are offset and diverge, resulting in a region of fatty and connective tissue that is not immediately accessible from endocardial ablation electrode positions and frequently requires ablation from within the coronary sinus (22,50,62). The anatomic courses of slowly and decrementally conducting accessory pathways that activate the ventricle with a left bundle branch block configuration (also known as Mahaim pathways) have been demonstrated commonly to originate from the right atrial free wall. Discrete pathway potentials may be mapped from the tricuspid annulus, along the right ventricular endocardial surface to arborized insertions into the right bundle branch. Application of radiofrequency energy along this course successfully ablates the pathways and prevents further AV reciprocating tachycardia (63–65).

Numerous large clinical series of radiofrequency catheter ablation of accessory pathways have been published, with excellent overall results (Table 73.1). At presently, experienced electrophysiology laboratories routinely achieve acute procedure success rates in the ablation of accessory pathways of greater than 95%, with recurrence rates of less than 5%. The procedure duration and fluoroscopic exposure have shortened dramatically with increasing knowledge and experience in this field. Accordingly, the indications for catheter ablation of accessory pathways have broadened to include all patients with symptomatic arrhythmias who are refractory to suppressive drug therapy or who prefer a drug-free lifestyle (66). There is little rationale for performing catheter ablation on older asymptomatic patients with ventricular preexcitation, but management of younger asymptomatic patients is controversial. A randomized trial of prophylactic ablation versus no therapy was performed in 72 young patients with induced tachycardia at invasive electrophysiologic study. The arrhythmic event rate in the ablation arm of the trial was 5% compared with 60% in the control arm. One control patient presented with ventricular fibrillation as his first symptom (67). Prophylactic catheter ablation also may be pursued in patients with high-risk or special occupations (e.g., commercial airline pilots) in whom a single arrhythmic occurrence could have serious consequences.

Atrioventricular Nodal Reentry

The AV node is located anatomically within the triangle of Koch, which is bounded by the tricuspid annulus, by the tendon of Todaro, and by the coronary sinus os. The compact AV node is located at the apex of the triangle and makes its transition with NH cells to the common bundle of His. Spreading throughout the remainder of the Koch triangle are atrial transitional cells (AN cells) and atrial myocytes. Anatomic study of the AV nodal region has demonstrated the presence of multiple anatomic insertions of atrial myocardium into the transitional cells of the AV nodal region. The typical form of AV nodal reentrant tachycardia uses a slowly conducting pathway for anterograde and a fast conducting pathway for retrograde conduction. The atypical form has the opposite conduction sequence or employs two separate slow pathways for the two limbs of the reentrant circuit. Typically, the atrial insertion of the slowly conducting pathway is located at the inferoposterior extent of the triangle of Koch, near the coronary sinus os (68).

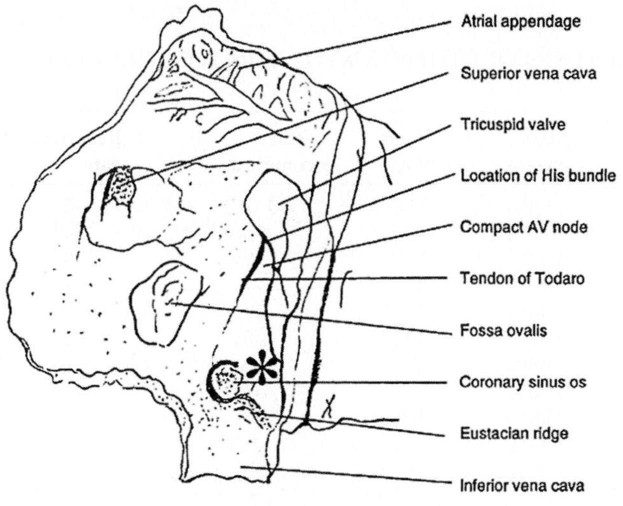

FIGURE 73.6. Drawing of the right atrium from a right anterior oblique projection with the anterolateral atrial wall cut away. The triangle of Koch is bounded by the tricuspid annulus anteriorly, the tendon of Todaro posteriorly, and the coronary sinus inferiorly. The His bundle is located at the apex of the triangle. The typical site for mapping and ablation of the slow atrioventricular (AV) nodal pathway is indicated by the *asterisk*.

The fast conducting pathway (which is thought to account for "normal" anterograde AV nodal conduction in most cases) is located in the anterosuperior region of the triangle, very close to the compact node (Fig. 73.6). It is likely that part of the atrium participates in the reentrant circuit.

Initially, the fast pathway was targeted for ablation, but lower success rates and high rates of symptomatic heart block have led most operators away from this approach and toward slow-pathway ablation (69). The technique for slow-pathway ablation involves positioning the catheter in the inferoposterior position of the triangle of Koch at a site where a pattern of fractionated atrial potentials is observed (Fig. 73.7). Subsequent catheter movement can be guided anatomically (70) or by mapping (71). Similar success rates and complication rates between the two approaches have been observed (72). During radiofrequency energy delivery at successful sites, one may observe an accelerated junctional rhythm and 1:1 junctional-to-atrial conduction. The earliest site of retrograde atrial activation in this setting is superior to the tendon of Todaro, a finding suggesting that the automaticity arises distal to the ablation site with conduction through the compact AV node and in a retrograde fashion up the fast pathway (73). Cryoablation has been proposed as a safer method of catheter ablation because cryoadhesion results in very stable catheter-tissue contact, and transient heart block occurring when the catheter is positioned too close to the compact AV node is fully reversible (74). However, long-term efficacy may be lower if a 4-mm tip catheter is employed (75).

The clinical success rates for catheter ablation of AV nodal reentrant tachycardia that have been generally reported are high (>95%), and the complication rates are low (<2%). The results of clinical series are shown in Table 73.2. The major complication reported in conjunction with this procedure is symptomatic heart block, with a prevalence of 0% to 4%. The lower prevalence of heart block in later clinical series compared with earlier series may be attributable to an increased use of the posterior (slow-pathway) approach, an increased understanding of the electrophysiology and anatomy of the AV nodal region, and improved skills of the individual operators (76). Some patients show evidence of impaired anterograde conduction before the ablation procedure. Although this may suggest the presence of fast-pathway pathologic features, slow-pathway ablation may still be pursued with a low risk of complete heart block (77). The reported recurrence rates of AV nodal reentrant tachycardia after initial successful AV nodal modification procedures are 2% to 15%. Most recurrences are reported within the first 2 months of the procedure. Some authors have found an association of persisting dual AV nodal physiology (presence of single AV nodal echo beats or evidence of a shift in anterograde conduction from a fast to a slow pathway) and late clinical recurrence of tachycardia (78), but this finding is in contrast to the experience of other operators who have not observed that association (79,80). The common practice among most operators is to terminate the ablation procedure once tachycardia can no longer be initiated at baseline

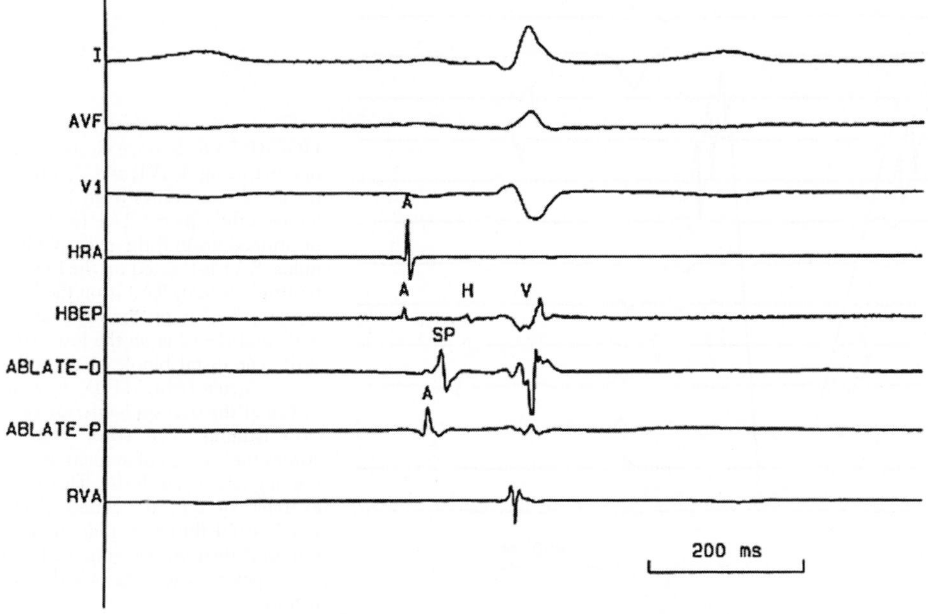

FIGURE 73.7. Surface electrocardiogram tracings I, aVF, and V_1 and intracardiac recordings from the high right atrium (HRA), the proximal His bundle bipole (HBEP), distal and proximal ablation catheter bipoles (ABLATE-D, ABLATE-P), and the right ventricular apex (RVA) in a patient with typical atrioventricular nodal reentrant tachycardia. The atrial (A), His bundle (H), and ventricular (V) deflections are labeled. On the distal bipolar tracing from the ablation electrode, a discrete high-frequency potential is observed 25 milliseconds after the contiguous atrial potential measured on the proximal bipole. This electrogram pattern is a marker for local slow-pathway (SP) activation.

TABLE 73.2

CLINICAL RESULTS OF RADIOFREQUENCY CATHETER ABLATION OF PATIENTS WITH ATRIOVENTRICULAR NODAL REENTRANT TACHYCARDIA

Authors	Year	No. of patients	Primary approach[a]	Acute success	Heart block	Other complication	Recurrence rate
Jackman, et al. (71)	1992	80	SP	99%	1%[b]	1.3%	0
Jazayeri, et al. (70)	1992	49	FP/SP	98%	4%[c]	0%	4[d]
Kay, et al. (79)	1992	34	SP	100%	3%[b]	6%	9
Wu, et al. (80)	1993	100	FP/SP	97%	3%[c]	—	1
Langberg, et al. (81)	1993	50	FP/SP	100%	2%[b]	0%	10[d]
Lindsay, et al. (82)	1993	59	SP	100%	2%[b]	0%	2
Baker, et al. (78)	1994	143	SP	99%	4%[c]	—	7
Manoli, et al. (83)	1994	55	SP	100%	0%	0%	13
Kottkamp, et al. (84)	1995	53	FP	96%	0%	0%	6
Calkins, et al. (51)	1999	373	SP	97%	1%	3%[e]	5

FP, fast pathway; SP, slow pathway.
[a]Crossovers from slow- to fast-pathway ablation approach reported in 0% to 10% of slow pathway ablations.
[b]Heart block occurred during slow-pathway ablation (either as primary approach or after crossover).
[c]Heart block occurred during fast-pathway ablation (either as primary approach or after crossover).
[d]Tachycardia induced at electrophysiologic study.
[e]Total major complication rate for all patients including atrioventricular (AV) nodal modification, accessory pathway ablation, and AV nodal ablation.

or during infusion of isoproterenol and to accept the presence of persisting but impaired slow-pathway function.

Atrial Flutter

Investigators have observed that the dominant activation wave front during atrial flutter is cranial to caudal along the lateral atrial wall and caudal to cranial up the septum. Cosio et al. originally determined that the mechanism of this rhythm was macroreentry using the tricuspid annulus as an anatomic barrier. It was hypothesized that the difference between "typical" type I atrial flutter and "atypical" type I atrial flutter was that the former had reentrant activation sequence in a counterclockwise direction around the tricuspid valve in the frontal plane (viewed from apex to base), whereas the latter had a clockwise activation pattern (Fig. 73.8). Cosio et al. also observed that the necessary prerequisite for this arrhythmia was a region of physiologic conduction block between the posterior and lateral atrial walls (85). Without this region of block, the reentrant wave front would conduct rapidly from the septum around the posterior wall of the atrium and render the lateral wall of the atrium refractory, thus preventing propagation of the subsequent reentrant wave front. Subsequent mapping studies in humans utilizing intracardiac ultrasound and careful entrainment mapping techniques demonstrated physiologic conduction block in the posteromedial (sinus venosa) region of the right atrium during atrial flutter (86).

Understanding the path of reentry of atrial flutter led researchers to identify critical sites of conduction that would be

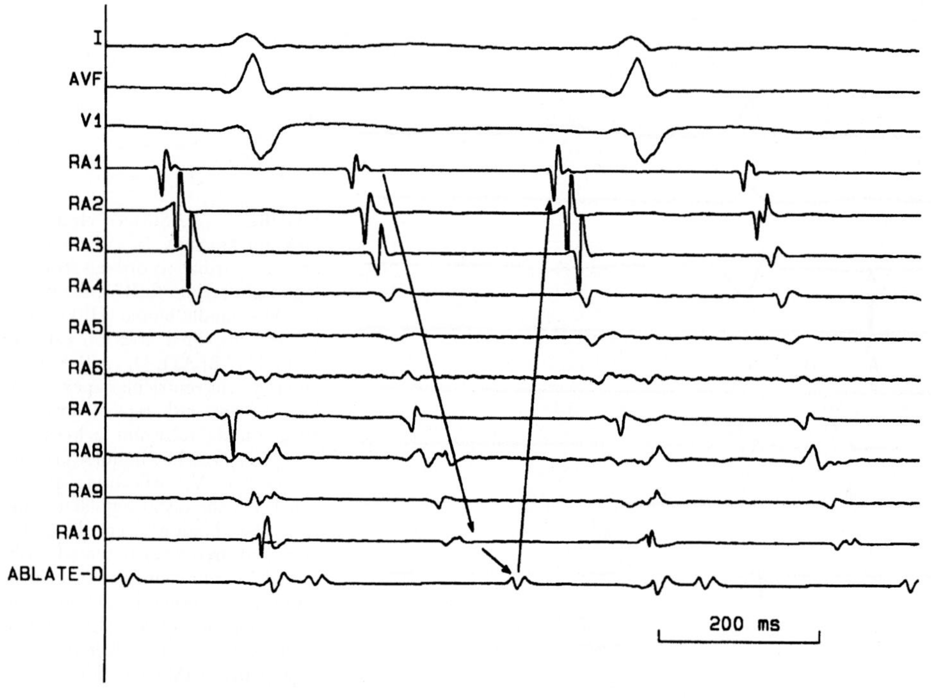

FIGURE 73.8. Surface electrocardiogram tracings I, aVF, and V_1 and intracardiac recordings from 10 bipolar recording pairs (RA1 to RA10) positioned around the tricuspid annulus. RA1 is located on the low interatrial septum, RA3 is on the high septum, RA7 is on the high lateral wall, and RA10 is on the low atrial wall. The distal bipole of the ablation catheter (ABLATE-D) is positioned at the tricuspid–inferior vena cava isthmus. The *arrow* demonstrates the pattern of activation during ongoing atrial flutter. This is an example of typical "counterclockwise" atrial flutter in that the pattern of activation (viewing the heart from apex to base) rotates in that direction.

amenable to catheter ablation to cure this arrhythmia (87,88). Cosio et al. pioneered the current approach of anatomically guided catheter ablation of atrial flutter. They reasoned that the reentrant circuit should always uses the subeustachian isthmus between the inferior vena cava orifice and the tricuspid annulus as a requisite limb of the reentrant circuit. They then demonstrated that a line of radiofrequency ablative lesions traversing this isthmus was successful in terminating atrial flutter (89).

The anatomically guided techniques that are employed today in radiofrequency ablation of typical atrial flutter place the ablation catheter across the subeustachian isthmus on the tricuspid valve. Radiofrequency power is turned on, and the electrode is pulled back in a line until the catheter crosses the eustachian valve. Persisting conduction across the subeustachian isthmus can be discerned by identification of a site where double potentials (indicating electrical activation on either side of a line of conduction block) merge to a single breakthrough potential (90). Useful indicators of conduction block include a reversal of activation sequence through the isthmus or a change in bipolar electrogram polarity beyond the line of ablation (91,92). If conduction across the isthmus persists, further radiofrequency applications may be made to those sites. Advanced mapping systems with global positioning systems, anatomic rendering, and three-dimensional mapping have increased our understanding of the path of typical and atypical atrial flutters (93). Wide variability of the anatomy of the subeustachian isthmus among patients has been observed, including width of the isthmus and its position and angle relative to the inferior vena cava (94). Thus, patients with significant right atrial hypertrophy or enlargement have thicker, wider, and more greatly angled geometries in the isthmus region, they have a higher arrhythmia recurrence rate (95), and they require a greater number of ablative application to achieve procedure success (94,96).

The results of clinical series are presented in Table 73.3. The acute success rate of this procedure now exceeds 90% when performed by experienced operators, and the late atrial flutter recurrence rate is 10% to 20%. Confirmation of bidirectional block of electrical conduction through the isthmus between the tricuspid valve and the inferior vena cava has been demonstrated to be an important criterion for the procedure's success. Despite successful termination and prevention of reinduction of atrial flutter by ablative lesions, some patients will still have residual conduction through the isthmus that can result in clinical arrhythmia recurrence (Fig. 73.9) (95,97). Success rates may also be improved with the use of irrigated-tip ablation catheters (98) or 8-mm or 10-mm tipped catheters with high-power amplitude (99), although outcomes are similar between these two technologies (96,100). Despite successful ablation of atrial flutter, the patient will likely have clinical recurrence of AF or type II atrial flutter if these arrhythmias were observed clinically before the ablation procedure (94,101–103). After initiation of antiarrhythmic drugs, particularly class 1C agents, some patients with AF or a combination of AF and atrial flutter will convert to pure type 1 atrial flutter. In these cases, a combination of drug and atrial flutter ablation therapy may be effective in preventing arrhythmia recurrence (104).

Atrial Fibrillation

AF is the most common sustained arrhythmia in the world, with a reported prevalence of 1.9% for patients less than 65 years of age and 5% to 6% for the population of patients older than 65 years (110). The morbidity and mortality of this arrhythmia may be attributed primarily to three factors: the propensity of the fibrillating atria for thrombus formation with the sequela of systemic thromboembolism including stroke, the loss of atrial systolic function as a contributor to ventricular filling, and the irregular and rapid ventricular rate response leading to symptoms of palpitations and reduction of diastolic filling time. Warfarin has been proven in a number of trials to be effective in reducing the risk of stroke with AF, but other strategies to improve overall outcomes have been pursued over the years. The Atrial Fibrillation Follow-Up Investigation of Rhythm Management (AFFIRM) study demonstrated that AF management with rate-control strategies was associated with a borderline significant reduction in mortality and no difference in stroke prevalence compared with strategies of rhythm control with suppressive antiarrhythmic drugs (111). Furthermore, subsequent multivariate analysis predicting all-cause mortality showed that the hazard ratio was 0.53 for sinus rhythm versus AF, but it was 1.49 for use of suppressive antiarrhythmic drugs (112). This finding suggests that the benefit of sinus rhythm maintenance was outweighed by the risk of drugs. Thus, nonpharmacologic approaches for the management of AF may not only reduce morbidity, but they also show the possibility

TABLE 73.3

CLINICAL RESULTS OF RADIOFREQUENCY CATHETER ABLATION OF PATIENTS WITH ATRIAL FLUTTER

Authors	Year	No. of patients	Acute success	Isthmus block confirmed	Complication	Recurrence rate	
						A flut	A fib
Feld, et al. (88)	1992	12	83%	No	0%	17%	0%
Cosio, et al. (89)	1993	9	78%	No	0%	0%	9%
Poty, et al. (95)	1995	12	100%	Yes	—	8%	—
Fischer, et al. (105)	1995	80	90%	No	8%	17%	5%
Paydak, et al. (102)	1998	110	98%	Yes[a]	—	5%	25%
Heidbuchel, et al. (94)	2000	100	99%	Yes	1%	0%	30%
Da Costa, et al. (106)	2004	185	99%	Yes	—	2%	13%
Calkins, et al. (107)	2004	150	88%[b]	Yes	3%	13%	30%
Feld, et al. (108)	2004	158	93%	Yes	4%	3%	—
Bertaglia, et al. (109)	2004	383	96%	Yes	2%	11%	42%

A Fib, atrial fibrillation; A Flut, atrial flutter.
[a]Isthmus block confirmed in a subgroup of 90 patients.
[b]Successful ablation defined as achieving isthmus block with investigational device only.

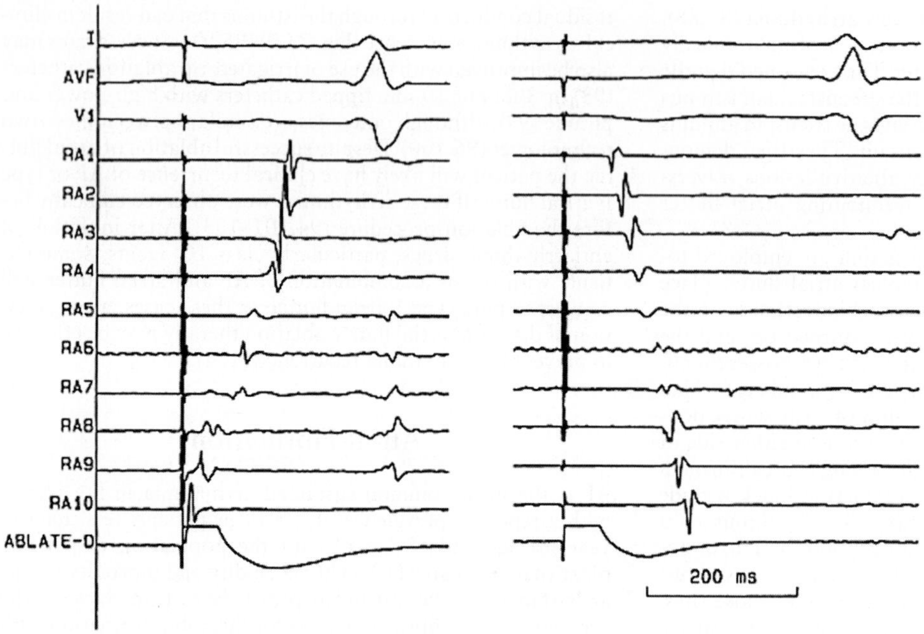

FIGURE 73.9. Surface electrocardiogram tracings I, aVF, and V_1 and intracardiac recordings from 10 bipolar recording pairs (RA1 to RA10) positioned around the tricuspid annulus as described in Figure 73.8. The roving ablation/pacing catheter (ABLATE-D) is used for pacing after completion of a linear ablation in the isthmus between the tricuspid valve annulus and the inferior vena cava. **Left:** Pacing from a site that is lateral to the line of block. The atrial activation sequence is in a clockwise direction, up the lateral wall and down the interatrial septum. **Right:** Pacing on the low interatrial septum, with the opposite (counterclockwise) atrial activation sequence. These sequences indicate complete bidirectional conduction block at the line of ablation.

of improving survival compared with suppressive drug therapies.

Atrioventricular Junctional Ablation for Rate Control in Atrial Fibrillation

Rate control of AF is typically accomplished with digitalis, β-sympathetic blockers, or calcium channel blockers. Unfortunately, these drugs are sometimes poorly tolerated, do not achieve adequate rate control, or cause intermittent symptomatic bradycardia. The nonpharmacologic strategies for rate control AF are AV junctional ablation and AV nodal modification. To produce complete block of AV conduction, an ablation catheter is positioned across the high septal portion of the tricuspid annulus contiguous to the His bundle recording and then is withdrawn to the atrial side of the tricuspid annulus, where the lesion is created. In about 10% of cases, the AV junction needs to be approached from the left-sided circulation, with ablation performed immediately inferior to the aortic valve (113). After achieving complete heart block, the patient typically has a slow but tolerable junctional escape rhythm. Implantation of a rate-responsive permanent pacemaker is necessary to maintain a normal heart rate at rest or with activity. If the patient has a pattern of paroxysmal AF, a dual-chamber rate-responsive pacemaker with mode-switching capabilities is selected. These devices will maintain AV synchrony when the patient is in sinus rhythm (thus avoiding symptoms of pacemaker syndrome) but automatically switch to ventricular pacing only at the onset of AF (Fig. 73.10). Rarely, the goal of ablation will be modification of AV nodal conduction to achieve a blunted heart rate response to AF but to maintain AV conduction so permanent pacing is not required. After AV nodal ablation or modification, the atria continue to fibrillate; despite resolution of symptoms, patients are still at risk for thromboembolic events, and ongoing treatment with warfarin is mandatory.

The technical success rate of AV junctional ablation is excellent, ranging from 95% to 100%, when performed by experienced operators (26,39,108,110). In appropriately selected patients, marked improvement in symptoms can be anticipated, with decreases in palpitations and effort dyspnea, asthenia, and exertional intolerance. Improvements in exercise time and ventricular function have been measured 3 months after ablation (114). In one study of patients with AF and reduced left

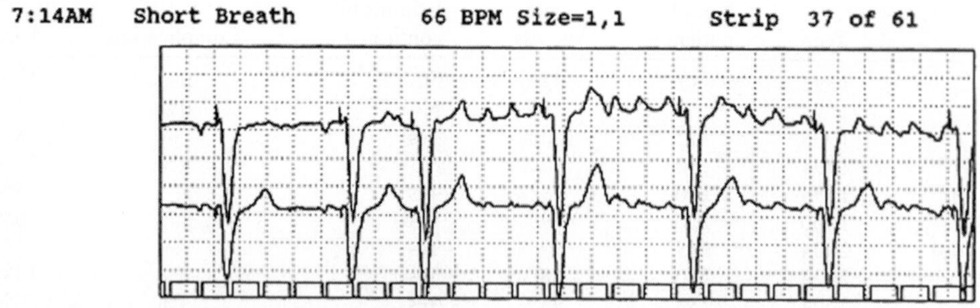

FIGURE 73.10. A monitor strip is shown from a patient with paroxysmal atrial fibrillation/flutter, complete heart block after catheter ablation of the atrioventricular junction, and implantation of a mode-switching dual-chamber pacemaker. The initial rhythm is normal sinus with appropriate atrial sensing and ventricular pacing by the pacemaker (DDD mode). There is onset of atrial flutter, but after 1 second of tachycardia, mode-switching criteria are met, and the pacemaker switches to single-chamber pacing (VVI), maintaining a regular rhythm at 60 beats per minute.

ventricular function, 90% of patients had improvement in their left ventricular ejection fractions and a decrease in left ventricular and atrial dimensions (115). The overall survival after AV junctional ablation and pacemaker implantation is similar to that in a matched population, a finding indicating that long-term pacing does not adversely affect prognosis (116). A concern about AV junctional ablation and pacing is that one necessarily converts the patient from native ventricular activation employing the His-Purkinje system to an iatrogenic left bundle branch block with right ventricular pacing, thus worsening synergy of left ventricular contraction (117). Aggressive brady pacemaker programming in a population of patients receiving implantable defibrillators was shown to decrease the 1-year survival free of heart failure hospitalization to 73.3% compared with 83.9% for patients with backup pacing at 40 beats per minute only (118). Thus, patients with left ventricular dysfunction who undergo AV junctional ablation and pacemaker implantation may benefit from implantation of a biventricular pacing device prospectively.

Curative Atrial Fibrillation Ablation

The understanding of the pathophysiology of AF has advanced considerably in recent years and has ushered in the era of curative AF ablation. In most cases, AF is initiated by bursts of rapid atrial tachycardia that are focal in origin. These arrhythmogenic foci are mapped most frequently to the myocardial sleeve tissue that extends from the atrial body into the proximal portions of the pulmonary veins (119–121). It is likely that the cellular mechanism of arrhythmogenesis in these cases is triggered activity. In contrast, persistent and chronic AF may initially be started with focal arrhythmic activity, but it propagates with ongoing reentrant spiral waves. These spiral waves act as drivers for AF, and the disorganized electrical propagation emanating from the drivers produces the irregularly irregular pattern characteristic of AF, as well as the reactivation wave fronts that cause the arrhythmia to persist (122). Vagal stimulation of atrial myocardium alters atrial electrophysiology and facilitates AF propagation (123). Therefore, within the clinical spectrum of atrial fibrillation, some patients have a predominantly focal triggered AF pattern (typically young patients with normal hearts and short paroxysms of AF), patients with a predominantly reentrant pattern of AF (typically those with structural heart disease and chronic AF), and a broad middle ground of patients who have focal initiation of the arrhythmia and reentrant propagation (those patients with mild or moderate structural heart disease and persistent AF or paroxysmal AF with prolonged episode duration). The initiation and propagation of AF may be facilitated by vagal stimulation.

The present art of curative catheter ablation has focused on eliminating conduction from the pulmonary vein musculature to the atrial body and disruption of the normal pathways of intraatrial conduction that can allow AF to propagate. Three dominant strategies are currently employed alone or in combination: pulmonary vein isolation, linear atrial ablation, and substrate modification. The rationale behind pulmonary vein isolation is that electrical disconnection of pulmonary vein musculature from the left atrial body should prevent pulmonary vein triggers from initiating AF (Fig. 73.11) (120,121). Supporting the causal relationship of pulmonary vein ectopy and clinical AF is the observation in patients who have clinical recurrence of AF after attempted curative ablation that electrical reconnection of the left atrium to the pulmonary vein is very frequently observed (124,125). Most operators now perform extraostial ablation around the atrial cuff tissue contiguous to the pulmonary veins to avoid pulmonary vein stenosis (caused by excess heating within the vein) and because the periostial atrial tissue may be an additional arrhythmic source. This approach is popular because it appears to be safer, and definitive end points (electrical conduction block in and out of the veins) can be tested during the course of the ablation procedure (126). Efficacy of this technique is high in younger patients with paroxysmal AF and normal atrial size, but efficacy data are conflicting regarding wide area circumferential ablation versus more targeted ostial pulmonary ablation (127,128).

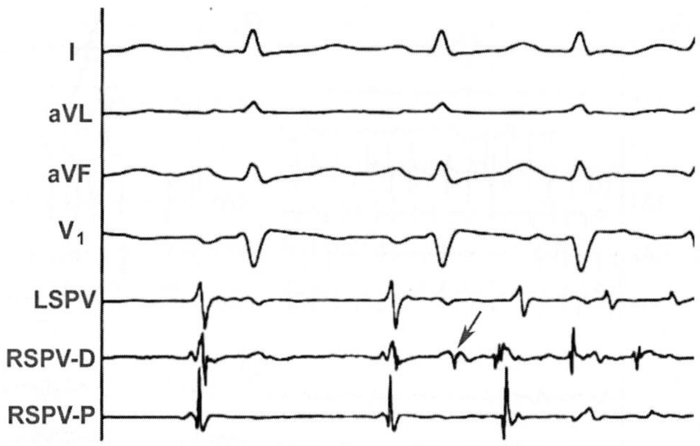

FIGURE 73.11. Surface leads 1, aVF, and V_1 and intracardiac tracings from catheters in the right superior pulmonary vein (RSPV) and left superior pulmonary vein (LSPV). The normal sinus beats show activation at the proximal RSPV bipolar electrode (RSPV-P) positioned near the venous junction with the left atrial body, followed by activation at the distal RSPV electrode (RSPV-D) positioned deeper in the vein. At the onset of a spontaneous episode of atrial fibrillation, very early activation is noted at RSPV-D (*arrow*), followed by activation at RSPV-P. This indicates focal initiation of AF from within the RSPV distal to the catheter.

When patients have structural heart disease or persistent AF, pulmonary vein isolation alone is not adequate. One prevalent approach is to supplement pulmonary vein isolation with linear atrial ablation, thus emulating the surgical maze III procedure (129). Most operators create linear ablations between the left inferior pulmonary vein and the mitral annulus (the so-called mitral isthmus) and a roof line between the right and left superior pulmonary veins (Fig. 73.12). In a similar fashion, some operators propose atrial substrate modification as a solution to more refractory forms of AF (130). The rationale for substrate modification is that AF propagation is not dependent on specific conduction pathways (e.g., the mitral isthmus) but instead depends on rotor propagation in regions of the atrium that offers a favorable electrophysiologic milieu. In addition, ablation around the base of the pulmonary veins and in regions of fractionated atrial activity may have a salutary effect by ablation of the underlying parasympathetic pathways, thereby reducing vagal stimulation of the atria (131).

The techniques employed for ablation of AF are varied and are in evolution. Transseptal catheterization is required for access to the left atrium. Either a single puncture or a double puncture is performed. Multiple sites can be mapped simultaneously using multielectrode catheter arrays or noncontact mapping so sites of arrhythmia origin can be mapped with a single spontaneous beat (132,133). Although mapping offers some incremental value, particularly when arrhythmia site of origin is outside the pulmonary vein, most cases are anatomically guided. Hence, technologies that improve the operator's understanding of anatomic relationships are useful. Fluoroscopy has traditionally been the imaging method used to guide ablation. More recently, operators have employed nonfluoroscopic electrical anatomic mapping systems to create a three-dimensional rendering of the left atrial chamber surface in space. Movement of the ablation catheter can be tracked in real time, the anatomic location of ablation targets (e.g., pulmonary veins)

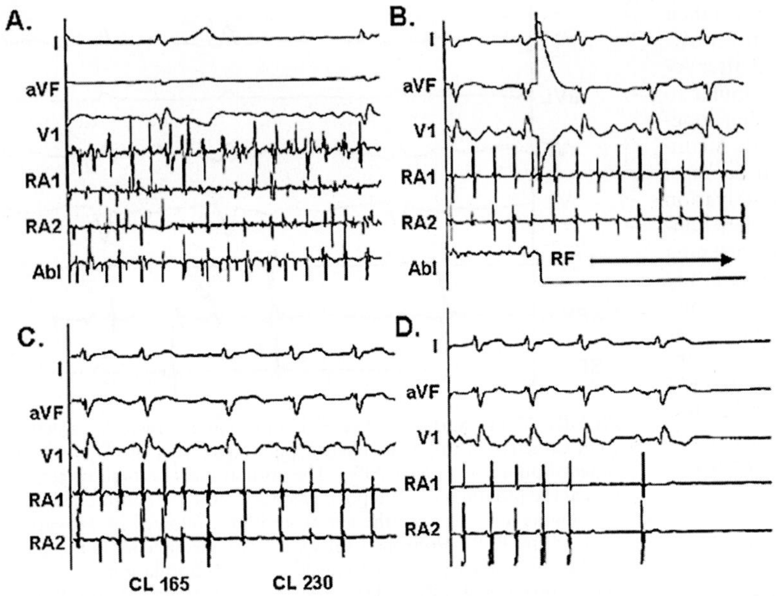

FIGURE 73.12. Surface leads I, II, and aVF and intracardiac tracings from two right atrial (RA) sites and an ablation catheter (Abl) during linear atrial ablation for persistent atrial fibrillation. **A:** The rhythm at baseline before any linear ablations. The atrial fibrillation is disorganized and rapid. **B:** The onset of radiofrequency energy delivery (RF) after completion of a partial set of linear atrial ablations. The atrial fibrillation has been organized to a type II atrial flutter by the previous lesions. **C:** Transition from fast to slower atrial reentrant tachycardia during ongoing radiofrequency energy delivery. This suggests that the remaining reentrant circuit size was suddenly increased as conduction through a residual gap in the linear lesions was blocked and the reentrant circuit increased in length. With ongoing radiofrequency energy delivery in **D**, the slower tachycardia is ultimately terminated.

can be approximated, and the locations of the ablative lesions can be recorded (129,134). An enhanced understanding of the individual's anatomy with computed tomography (CT) or magnetic resonance imaging can further guide catheter manipulation and can assist the operator in lesion placement (135–138). To take advantage of real-time monitoring of catheter position in the heart and the detailed anatomy that can be achieved with CT, systems now have can merge those images so the computer rendering of the catheter is moving within real anatomy. The limitations of these technologies are that the accuracy of registration of one three-dimensional image to another and the finding that the CT image is static, whereas the heart is moving in the chest with each heartbeat and respiration. Real-time imaging of the ablation catheter within the heart can be accomplished with intracardiac echocardiography. Intracardiac echocardiography uses either a phased-array system that produces a sector scan with a narrow near field but good far-field resolution (139) or a mechanical transducer that provides a cross-sectional tomographic view of the plane perpendicular to the transducer (140). Future technologies for visualization include direct angioscopy with a system that uses low-infrared wavelengths so blood is invisible (141). In addition to computer-enhanced mapping systems, catheter manipulation can now be performed remotely using a computer-controlled external magnet system and magnetic-tip catheters. Ultimately, the remote control system will be integrated with the mapping system such that mapping and ablation may be entirely automated.

New technologies are becoming available for clinical catheter ablation. Most systems are designed to isolate conduction effectively from pulmonary veins to the left atrium. The ideal system should create consistent circumferential extraostial pulmonary vein lesions with minimal catheter manipulation and minimal time. The lesions should be deep enough to be consistently transmural, yet not so deep that they risk collateral injury to extracardiac structures such as phrenic nerve or esophagus. One system employs an array of fine wires with 36 ablation elements that collapse for venous insertion then expand to ablate in a cuff around the base of the pulmonary vein (Bard mesh catheter, Bard EP, Lowell, MA). High-intensity focused ultrasound is employed in another design to project a ring of focused ultrasound energy forward from a balloon catheter and ablate tissue in a ring around the base of the vein (ProRhythm, Inc., Ronkonkoma, NY). Diode laser ablation is being tested to create a circular lesion around the base of pulmonary veins through an occlusive balloon catheter (Cardiofocus, Inc., Norton, MA). Another type of hyperthermic ablation employs a saline-filled balloon that is heated with radiofrequency current. The hot balloon creates a highly controlled thermal lesion with minimal risk of excess tissue heating (Toray Industries, Tokyo, Japan). In contrast to hyperthermic ablation technologies, cryothermic ablation is being employed with linear catheter designs and with a cryo balloon. The cryo balloon occludes the pulmonary vein as in other balloon technologies, but then it circulates refrigerant through the inflated balloon to create a large ice ball that freezes the perimeter of the base of the vein (Cryocath, Inc., Montreal, Canada). Clinical trials with these devices are under way. The emergence of a dominant technology will ultimately depend on efficacy, procedure speed, and safety.

Clinical series of AF ablation are listed in Table 73.4. Acute success rates of pulmonary vein isolation procedures are high (>95%), but overall reported success rates are generally lower (63% to 93%). Success rates used to be lower when map-guided focal or single vein ablation was employed because it is difficult to initiate and map all possible triggering sites of origin reliably. The accepted approach at present is to ablate around the base of all four pulmonary veins. The prevalent end point employed is bidirectional conduction block across the ablation line (142). For the most part, pulmonary vein isolation alone is used in patients with paroxysmal AF and relatively normal hearts. Patients with persistent AF and atrial enlargement require linear atrial ablation in addition to pulmonary vein isolation or some form of substrate modification. The reported success rates vary wildly from 6% to 86%, although the procedure has evolved considerably over the course of reporting. The first small multicenter randomized series of AF ablation versus drug therapy has been reported. Seventy patients were randomized to receive radiofrequency pulmonary vein isolation ($n = 33$) or suppressive antiarrhythmic drug therapy ($n = 37$). After a 1-year follow-up, AF recurrence rate was 13% in the ablation group compared with 63% in the drug-treated group ($p < .001$). Hospitalizations were reduced, and quality of life scores were improved with ablation, but the study was too small to address the issue of complications from the competing therapies (143). One important observation by Hsu et al. (144) was that patients with congestive heart failure who underwent AF ablation demonstrated improvement in left

TABLE 73.4

CLINICAL RESULTS CATHETER ABLATION OF PATIENTS WITH ATRIAL FIBRILLATION

Authors	Year	No. of patients	Structural heart disease	Paroxysmal AF	Principal technique	Non-fluoroscopic imaging	Percentage cured (no AADs)	Percentage improved (+AADs)	Percentage of multiple procedures	Complications	Follow-up duration (mo)
Chen, et al. (121)	1999	79	8%	100%	Focal ablation		86%[a]	99%[a]	9%	4%	6
Shah, et al. (145)	2001	182	30%	100%	Isolation of arrhythmogenic PV only + focal ablation		74%	—	54%	3%	16
Mangrum, et al. (146)	2002	64	47%	100%	Isolation of arrhythmogenic PV only	ICE	66%	79%	11%	9%	13
Oral, et al. (147)	2002	70	7%	83%	Nonselective isolation of all PV		<63%[b]	63%[b]	9%	1%	5
Marrouche, et al. (148)	2003	315	24%	51%	Nonselective isolation of all PV	ICE	<86%[b]	86%[b]	—	3%	14
Macle, et al. (149)	2002	136	17%	90%	Nonselective isolation of all PV + focal ablation + RA isthmus line		66%	81%	49%	1%	9
Lin, et al. (150)	2003	68	34%	100%	Mapping and ablation of non-PV foci	ICE	63%	—	—	—	22
Jais, et al. (151)	2003	100	22%	—	Nonselective isolation of all PV + LA isthmus line	CARTO	87%	0%	32%	4%	12
Pappone, et al. (152)	2003	589	37%	69%	Extraostial isolation of all PV	CARTO	<78%[b]	78%[b]	—	—	36
Kottkamp, et al. (153)	2004	100	25%	80%	Extraostial isolation of all PV + LA isthmus line	CARTO	34%	40%	22%	0%	12
Nademanee, et al. (130)	2004	121	65%	47%	Target complex fractionated atrial electrograms	CARTO	83%	8%	23%	5%	12
Hsu, et al.[c] (144)	2004	58	100%	9%	Nonselective isolation of all PV + LA isthmus line		69%	9%	50%	3%	12
Della Bella, et al. (154)	2005	234	47%	78%	Nonselective isolation of all PV		<65%[b]	65%[b]	13%	6%	12
Herweg, et al. (155)	2005	170	59%	82%	Nonselective isolation of all PV	ICE	80%	14%	16%	—	18
Cappato, et al.[d] (156)	2005	8745	—	—	All techniques	All systems	52%	24%	27%	6%	11.6

AADs, antiarrhythmic drugs; AF, atrial fibrillation; ICE, intracardiac echocardiography; LA, left atrial; PV, pulmonary vein; RA, right atrial.
[a]Brief AF episodes identified on ambulatory monitor in 15% of patients, and were not defined as recurrence
[b]Prevalence of concomitant suppressive antiarrhythmic drug use among patients with successful AF ablation not reported.
[c]Case-control trial of patients with congestive heart failure undergoing atrial fibrillation ablation.
[d]Survey of 777 centers with response from 181 (23.9%).

ventricular function with restoration of normal sinus rhythm. This improvement was observed both in patients groups with and without adequate heart rate control with AV nodal blocking drugs (144). The outcomes of clinical trials are affected by a great number of factors, foremost being patient selection. Patients who are younger and who have structurally normal hearts, normal atrial sizes, and a paroxysmal pattern of AF have a high likelihood of cure with a variety of techniques. However, patients who are older and who have structural heart disease with atrial enlargement and persistent or chronic AF require more extensive ablation and have a higher procedure-related complication rate and a lower success rate. A true arrhythmia cure can be claimed only if patients are arrhythmia free and not taking any suppressive antiarrhythmic drugs, and yet many success rates reported by operators include patients receiving agents such as amiodarone. Studies that depend on patient self-reporting are bound to underestimate arrhythmia recurrences, because many AF episodes are asymptomatic, particularly after an ablation procedure (157). Many studies do not quote the prevalence of multiple procedures to achieve their end point. Obviously, centers that perform three or more ablation procedures on patients with AF recurrence are ultimately going to achieve a better cure rate than those that limit the numbers of repeat procedures. Finally, single-center reports are always suspect because of an inherent conflict of interest in end point definition, as well as intensity of follow-up. Only when multicenter controlled trials are performed will we begin to understand the true response rate to these procedures, although even those trials will be biased because it will be impossible to blind patients or investigators to the treatment modality.

Other Atrial Arrhythmias

Tachycardias that arise from the sinus node region include sinoatrial reentrant tachycardia and inappropriate sinus tachycardia. The former is characterized by its paroxysmal nature, the ability to initiate and terminate the rhythm with programmed atrial stimulation, and a P-wave morphology and intraatrial activation sequence that are indistinguishable from normal sinus rhythm. This is an uncommon arrhythmia, and therefore the experience with ablative therapy is somewhat limited. It typically has its origin in the high atrial region at the junction between the atrium and the superior vena cava in the classical sinus node anatomic region. The optimal site of ablation may be identified by searching for the earliest site of atrial activation relative to the P-wave onset. Ablation in this region results in termination of the tachycardia and frequently results in a slight shift of sinus node activation to a lower site along the crista terminalis (158,159). Although most patients have normal sinus node function after ablation, sinus node dysfunction requiring pacemaker implantation is a potential risk. The reported clinical series are limited, but they include a description of 11 patients that were identified out of a cohort of 343 consecutive patients referred for electrophysiologic evaluation of SVT. Nine of the 11 patients had additional tachycardia mechanisms identified. Radiofrequency catheter ablation was successful in all 10 patients in whom it was attempted, and no complications were noted (159).

"Inappropriate" sinus tachycardia is similar in P-wave morphology and atrial activation sequence to sinoatrial reentry and normal sinus rhythm, but it does not follow a paroxysmal pattern and sometimes occurs incessantly. Patients with this arrhythmia have an exaggerated heart rate response to minor physiologic stresses and often have heart rates greater than 100 beats per minute at rest. It is important to confirm that patients presenting with apparent inappropriate sinus tachycardia do not have the postural orthostatic tachycardia syndrome (POTS)

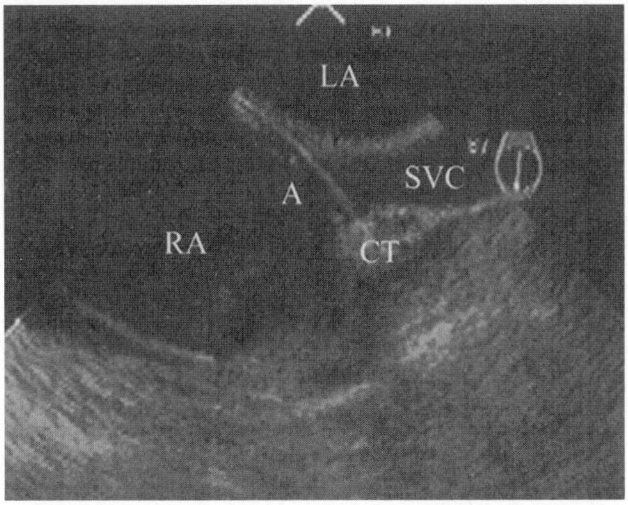

FIGURE 73.13. Transesophageal echocardiogram of a patient undergoing modification of the sinoatrial node. The image is oriented as follows: superior to the right, inferior to the left, posterior on the top, and anterior on the bottom. A longitudinal sector through the left atrium (LA), right atrium (RA), and superior vena cava (SVC) is seen. The ablation catheter (A) is positioned in contact with the superior aspect of the crista terminalis (CT). Earliest atrial activations during episodes of inappropriate sinus tachycardia were mapped to this site.

(160). These patients have a marked compensatory sinus tachycardia because of failure of peripheral autonomic vascular response to orthostatic stress. "Successful" sinus node ablation in these patients may result in crippling hypotension. For patients with true "inappropriate" sinus tachycardia, catheter ablation has been successfully performed by targeting a relatively broad region of the superior crista terminalis for radiofrequency energy delivery (Fig. 73.13). Three-dimensional electroanatomic mapping has been employed to guide ablation. In a series of 39 patients, acute success was achieved in all patients and was associated with a shift of atrial activation to a more caudal focus (161). Ablation of the sinoatrial node may be facilitated by intracardiac echocardiographic guidance as well (162). Complications of this procedure include postprocedure sinus node dysfunction requiring permanent pacing and phrenic nerve palsy. Catheter ablation for "inappropriate" sinus tachycardia may be useful in the management of these challenging patients, but it should not be considered as first-line therapy.

Atrial tachycardia is a rhythm that may originate from either the left or right atrium and may result from reentry or triggered or abnormal automaticity. In the right atrium, it commonly arises from the crista terminalis, although its origin may also be the low atrial septum or right atrial appendage. In a series of 172 patients with focal atrial tachycardia who underwent mapping and ablation, a pulmonary vein site of origin was found in 28 (16%) (163). The surface ECG can be useful to determine the arrhythmia site of origin. A positive or biphasic P-wave in surface lead aVL suggests a right atrial origin, whereas a positive P wave in V_1 and a negative P wave in aVL imply a left atrial arrhythmia origin. Mapping of atrial tachycardia is best achieved with activation mapping to identify local atrial activity before the onset of the surface P wave, pace mapping to identify a site where the paced P wave is identical to the spontaneous tachycardia P wave, and paced activation sequence mapping where the relative activation timing from multiple atrial recording sites is identical between pacing and spontaneous tachycardia. One series of catheter ablation in 91 patients with atrial tachycardia reported procedure success in 80 patients (77%). A repetitive atrial tachycardia pattern and multifocal sites of origin predicted ablation failure (164).

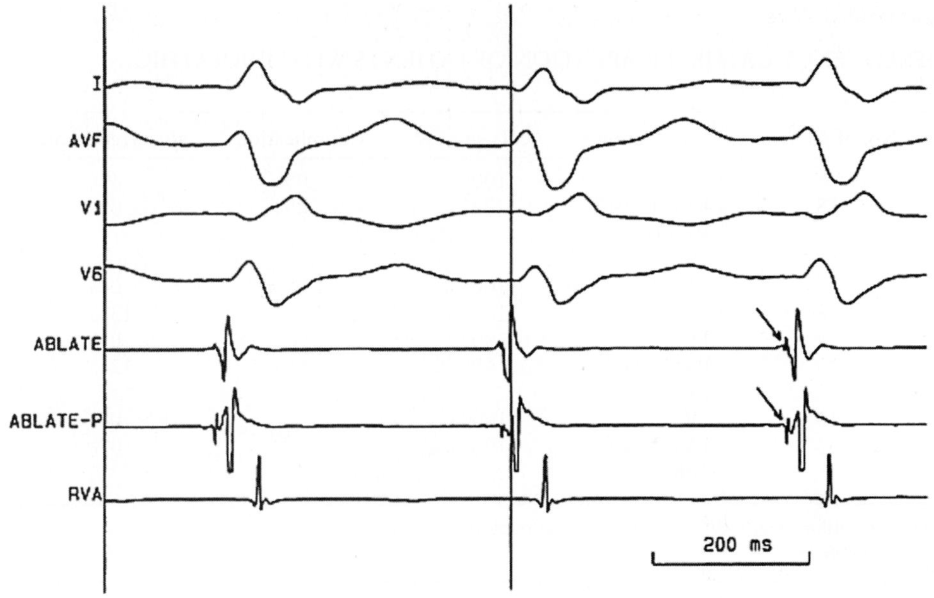

FIGURE 73.14. Surface electrocardiographic leads I, aVF, and V_1 and intracardiac electrograms from the distal (ABLATE) and proximal (ABLATE-P) poles of the mapping/ablation catheter and from the right ventricular apex (RVA). The rhythm is idiopathic left ventricular tachycardia. The *vertical line* corresponds to the onset of the surface QRS complex and is preceded by local ventricular activity recorded by the ablation electrode. The *arrows* represent Purkinje potentials, which precede local ventricular activation at this site. Catheter ablation at this location terminated this ventricular tachycardia.

ABLATION OF SPECIFIC VENTRICULAR ARRHYTHMIAS

Idiopathic Ventricular Tachycardia

Patients with structurally normal hearts may have VT with a variety of underlying arrhythmia mechanisms. Idiopathic VT most commonly arises from the right ventricle in the outflow tract below the pulmonic valve, although significant numbers of foci arise from the left ventricular outflow tract or other less common sites (43,165). These arrhythmias tend to fall into two main categories. Repetitive monomorphic VT is characterized by multiple repeating bursts of nonsustained VT and very high-density premature ventricular beats. These arrhythmias may be increased in the setting of catecholamine stress, but frequently they are suppressed in the setting of catecholamine-induced increases in sinus rate. It is hypothesized that the mechanism for repetitive monomorphic VT is abnormal automaticity (166). Catecholamine-sensitive VT may be nonsustained or sustained. Because these arrhythmias are catecholamine sensitive, they are frequently exercise induced. They should terminate in response to intravenous adenosine or verapamil bolus infusions. It is hypothesized that the mechanism for these arrhythmias is triggered automaticity. The typical features of these arrhythmias on 12-lead ECGs include left bundle branch block morphology, an inferior frontal plane axis, and a relatively isoelectric complex in surface lead (167,168). Another type of idiopathic VT of left ventricular origin has a reentrant mechanism that utilizes the Purkinje network as part of its circuit (169). The site of slowed conduction in the reentry circuit is typically sensitive to verapamil and not to adenosine (170,171).

The mapping techniques used to ablate idiopathic VTs of focal origin include activation mapping, pace mapping, electroanatomic mapping, and body surface ECG mapping. Episodes of sustained or nonsustained VT should be initiated with rapid ventricular pacing or isoproterenol infusion. During ongoing tachycardia, the local ventricular activation should precede the onset of the surface QRS complex by 20 to 80 milliseconds. Pacing from that site should result in a 12-lead or body surface ECG that is identical in all leads to that recorded during tachycardia (167,172–177). If sustained VT cannot be reproduced in the procedure laboratory, unifocal premature ventricular contractions with the same morphology can be used to map the site of origin. A marker for successful site selection for catheter ablation is immediate acceleration then termination of the VT coincident with the delivery of radiofrequency current. The site of origin of idiopathic verapamil-sensitive left VT may be best identified by activation mapping during ongoing tachycardia. Discrete high-frequency Purkinje potentials precede the site of earliest ventricular activation during tachycardia by 15 to 42 milliseconds. These potentials are identified in the medial or distal inferior septum or free wall, and they also precede local ventricular activation during sinus rhythm. Catheter ablation at the site of fusion of the Purkinje potential into the early ventricular potential yields a high success rate of arrhythmia termination and cure (Fig. 73.14) (178).

The reported clinical success rate of catheter ablation of idiopathic VT is 76% to 100%, and it is generally greater than 90% for those arrhythmias arising from the right ventricular outflow tract (Table 73.5). Reported complications with this procedure have been infrequent. Two cases of pericardial effusion (one requiring pericardiocentesis) were observed in a series of 44 patients undergoing radiofrequency ablation of VT in the right and left ventricles (179). One case of catheter-induced mitral regurgitation was reported as a consequence of catheter manipulation in the left ventricle (178).

Reentrant Ventricular Tachycardia with Structural Heart Disease

Patients with structural heart disease have varying degrees of fibrosis interspersed among bundles of surviving myocardial bundles. The most common arrhythmogenic substrate among patients with reentrant VT is chronic ischemic heart disease. The central portion of a complete transmural scar from prior infarction is commonly electrically inactive, but some broad wave fronts of slowed conduction can occur across this region in a thin surviving endocardial layer (180). The border zone of the scar is extremely heterogeneous, thus making it an ideal substrate for reentry. A typical reentrant circuit uses these small myocardial bundles at the scar border zone as regions of slowed conduction (181). Conduction through these regions accounts for the isoelectric period between QRS complexes on the surface ECG, particularly with slower tachycardias. The return

TABLE 73.5

CLINICAL RESULTS OF RADIOFREQUENCY CATHETER ABLATION OF PATIENTS WITH IDIOPATHIC VENTRICULAR TACHYCARDIA

Authors	Year	No. of patients	VT location	Acute success	Complication	Recurrence rate
Klein, et al. (172)	1992	16	RVOT	100%	0%	6%
Calkins, et al. (173)	1993	18	RVOT (10)[a] RV (5)[a] LV (5)[a]	72%	0%	0%
Wilber, et al. (167)	1993	7	RVOT	100%	0%	0%
Nakagawa, et al. (178)	1993	8	LV	100%	13%	13%
Wen, et al. (174)	1997	7	LV	100%	—	0%
Peeters, et al. (176)	1999	19	RVOT (10) LV (9)	89%	5%	12%
Tsuchiya, et al. (177)	1999	16	LV	100%	—	0%
Tanner, et al. (165)	2005	33	RVOT (20) Other (13)	100%	—	0%

LV, left ventricle; RV, right ventricle (excluding outflow tract); RVOT, right ventricular outflow tract.
[a]Two tachycardias identified in each of two patients.

circuit is complex and uses the surrounding myocardium on one or both sides of the central conduction zone, thereby creating a circular or a figure-of-eight conduction pattern (182,183). The precise courses of the reentrant wave fronts in the VTs of patients with nonischemic myopathies are not as well characterized, but they probably utilize regions of fibrosis interposed with normal or hypertrophied myocytes as the zones of slowed conduction and block (184). An interesting variant of VT found predominantly in patients with dilated cardiomyopathy is bundle branch reentrant tachycardia. This macroreentrant tachycardia uses one limb of the bundle branches in an anterograde fashion and another limb in a retrograde fashion (185). It is important to recognize this arrhythmia mechanism because bundle branch reentrant tachycardia is easily treated by ablation of the right or left bundle branch (186–188). An uncommon but important subset of patients with reentrant VT caused by scar is the group with arrhythmogenic right ventricular cardiomyopathy. A clinical presentation of a patient with normal left ventricular size and function and a tachycardia with a left bundle branch block morphology may suggest the diagnosis of idiopathic VT. Careful evaluation of these patients with magnetic resonance imaging will identify fibrofatty infiltration of the right ventricle, and electrophysiologic testing will confirm a reentrant arrhythmia mechanism in most cases (189). Mapping and entrainment studies of VT in these patients have demonstrated that the common locations of the reentrant circuit sites were around the tricuspid annulus and in the right ventricular outflow tract (173,190).

Mapping and ablation of reentrant VT are challenging, associated with a lower overall success rate than those of other tachycardias, and currently limited to a selected subset of patients. Ideally, the operator will identify the path of the SCZ that accounts for the diastolic interval on the surface ECG. Point-by-point activation mapping seeks to identify middiastolic (presystolic) activation sites that correspond to the SCZ. Entrainment mapping has superseded this technique. Pacing is performed at a rate that is slightly faster than the ongoing tachycardia from a mapping catheter positioned on or near the reentry circuit, and each paced beat advances the tachycardia slightly by entering the excitable gap between the depolarizing wave front of reentry and the tail of refractoriness of the previous beat. If pacing is performed directly on the SCZ, then the surface QRS complex during entrainment will exactly match that of the tachycardia. These sites of *concealed entrainment* are optimal sites for attempted catheter ablation (Fig. 73.15). Stevenson et al. (191) reported that sites of successful VT termination by radiofrequency energy were more likely to fulfill criteria for concealed entrainment than unsuccessful sites. Optimal sites also had intervals measured from the last paced beat to the next tachycardia that were nearly identical to the tachycardia cycle lengths, were near the middle of the SCZ, and showed electrogram patterns of isolated diastolic potentials or continuous electrical activity recorded from the ablation catheter (191). Other criteria for successful ablation site selection include an exact QRS match between entrained and spontaneous VT and an activation time between the local electrogram to the onset of the surface QRS almost identical to the stimulus to QRS interval during spontaneous VT (192,193). Nonfluoroscopic mapping systems employ real-time catheter location technologies and provide a three-dimensional anatomic map as well as an electrical map of the ventricle (194). A high-resolution noncontact mapping system rapidly localizes the tachycardia site of origin with acquisition of complete mapping data from only two or three beats of tachycardia, thereby allowing mapping in some patients with tachycardias that are poorly tolerated hemodynamically (195,196). If tachycardias are too fast and hemodynamically unstable to perform activation or entrainment mapping, alternative techniques may be employed during sinus rhythm. Substrate mapping by measuring local electrogram voltage can identify isthmuses of conduction between regions of scar that represent the SCZ. Linear ablation across the isthmus can block the VT (197,198).

The clinical series of radiofrequency catheter ablation of reentrant VT are small and comprise a highly selected subset of patients. Because patients must be able to tolerate their tachycardia hemodynamically to allow for mapping, patients with rapid, life-threatening tachycardias are not included in these series. The mean cycle lengths of the tachycardias in the reported clinical series of ablations were greater than 350 milliseconds (<171 beats per minute), and patients undergoing ablative therapy comprised only 10% to 20% of the overall population with VT. The results of the largest clinical series are summarized in Table 73.6. The reported success rates on the suppression of "clinical" tachycardias with radiofrequency catheter ablation range from 64% to 81%. Patients frequently have "nonclinical" tachycardias, defined as sustained monomorphic VTs with morphologies that have not been observed to occur spontaneously in the clinical setting but that can

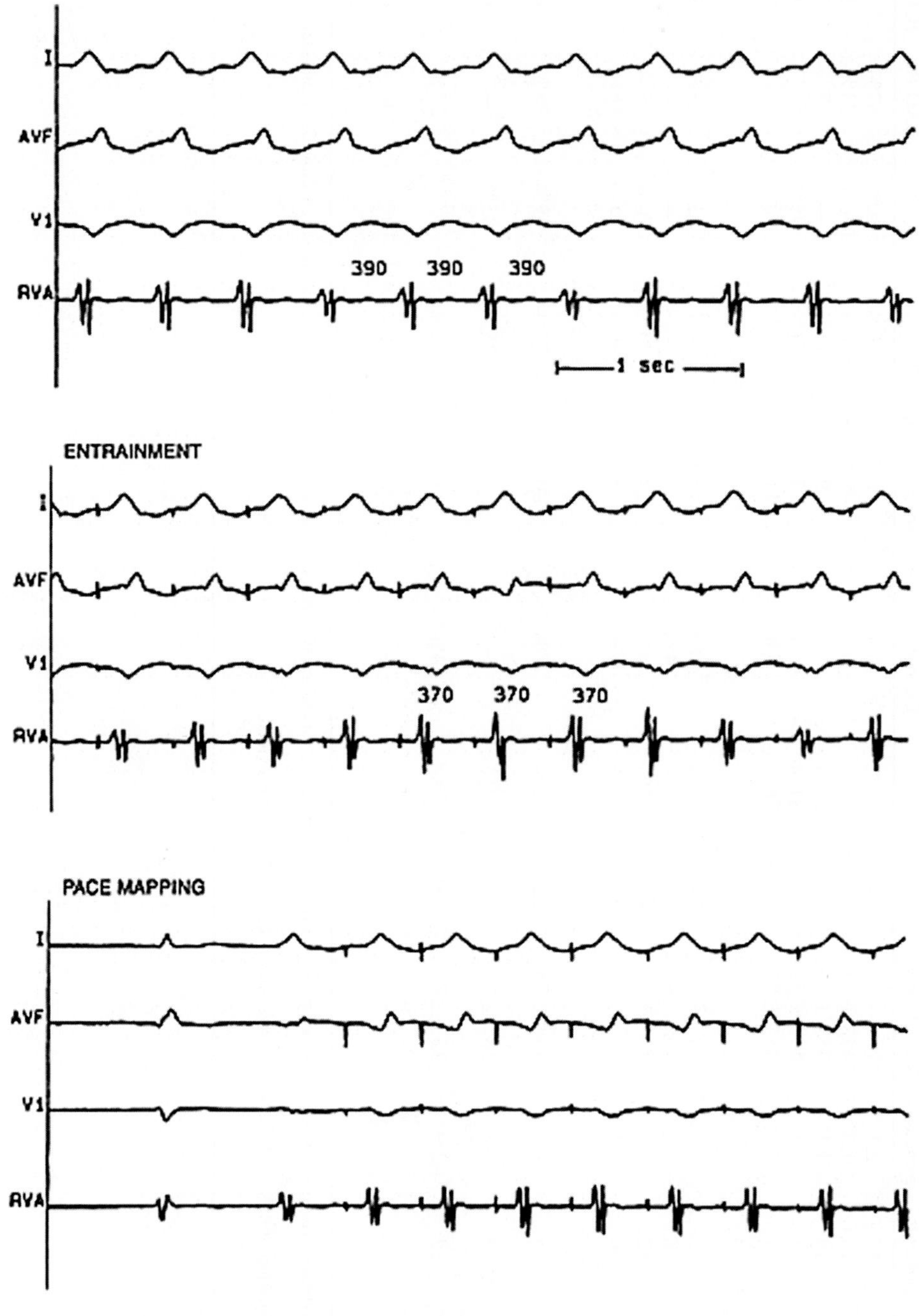

FIGURE 73.15. Surface electrocardiographic leads I, aVF, and V_1 and intracardiac electrograms from the right ventricular apex (RVA) in a patient with sustained ventricular tachycardia and a history of prior myocardial infarction. **Top:** Ongoing tachycardia with a cycle length of 390 milliseconds. **Middle:** Entrainment pacing at a cycle length of 370 milliseconds during ongoing tachycardia. The QRS morphology during pacing is identical to that of ventricular tachycardia (concealed entrainment), and a delay occurs between the pacing artifact and the QRS onset, a finding indicating that the pacing site is within the zone of slow conduction in the reentrant circuit. **Bottom:** Pace mapping during sinus rhythm from the same site. The QRS morphology similar to that of ventricular tachycardia suggests that this site is near the exit point of the slow conduction zone, thereby resulting in a similar spread of ventricular activation during pace mapping as is seen during tachycardia.

be induced by programmed ventricular stimulation. In these cases, adjunctive therapy with an implantable defibrillator is usually warranted. An expanding indication for VT ablation is for patients in whom an implantable defibrillator was previously implanted, but who are now suffering frequent or incessant runs of slower VT, resulting in multiple device discharges. Radiofrequency catheter ablation can successfully palliate this condition in a significant number of these patients (199,200).

COMPLICATIONS OF CATHETER ABLATION

The field of radiofrequency catheter ablation has been met with tremendous enthusiasm by physicians and patients alike, and both the numbers of procedures performed and the indications for the procedure have grown (201). A natural consequence of this phenomenon is that the number of interventional electrophysiologists has also dramatically increased. The time and intensity of training required to become proficient in this field are considerable. It is necessary that the physician have a detailed understanding of electrophysiologic mechanisms of arrhythmias, an excellent three-dimensional conceptualization of the anatomy of the cardiac chambers in which the ablation catheters are manipulated, and exceptional technical skill in catheter manipulation. For these reasons, success rates and complication rates of catheter ablation are first and foremost related to the skill and experience of the primary operator (202, 203).

The overall reported complication rate from radiofrequency catheter ablation (excluding risks associated with outmoded techniques or tools) is low, ranging from 1.8% to 4% (197). The risks of major, irreversible complications is approximately 0.5% to 1.0% and includes events such as complete heart block, myocardial infarction, valvular injury, irreversible stroke, and death. Early in the ablation era, the Multicentre

TABLE 73.6

CLINICAL RESULTS OF RADIOFREQUENCY CATHETER ABLATION OF PATIENTS WITH VENTRICULAR TACHYCARDIA IN PATIENTS WITH STRUCTURAL HEART DISEASE

Authors	Year	Patients studied	No. of patients	No. of VTs per patient	VT CL (ms)	Success rate all VTs	Success rate clinical VTs	Complication	Follow-up duration (mo)	VT recurrence (%)	Late survival (%)	Patients with AAD Rx	Patients with ICD Rx
Stevenson, et al. (191)	1993	Ischemic CM	15	2.1	—	—	66%	0%	8.7	0%	80%	67%	7%
Morady, et al. (204)	1993	Ischemic CM	15	1.3	438 ± 82	—	73%	0%	9.1	18%	100%	93%	20%
Gursoy, et al. (205)	1993	Ischemic CM	14	1.1	357 ± 56	—	57%	—	9	13%	—	7%	50%
Kim, et al. (206)	1994	Ischemic CM	21	1.1	445 ± 52	43%	81%	0%	13.2	31%	95%	57%	43%
Strickberger, et al. (199)	1997	Ischemic CM, frequent ICD shocks	21	2.2	455 ± 93	—	76%	5%	11.8	43%	90%	—	100%
Rothman, et al. (207)	1997	Ischemic CM	35	3.0	345 ± 74	31%	86%	11%	14.1	34%	80%	23%	51%
Callans, et al. (208)	1998	Ischemic CM	66	1.2	406 ± 63	35%	71%	4%	—	—	—	—	—
Stevenson, et al. (200)	1998	Ischemic CM	52	3.6	433 ± 108	40%	71%	10%	18	33%	70%	59%	45%
Calkins, et al. (209)	2000	Ischemic CM, Multicenter trial	146	3.1	—	41%	75%	8%	8	46%	75%	66%	79%
O'Callaghan, et al. (210)	2001	Ischemic CM	55	1.1	454 ± 75	22%	82%	7%	60	72%	49%	78%	69%
Arenal, et al. (211)	2003	Unmappable VTs	24	1.3	382 ± 51	—	84%	—	9	25%	83%	—	63%
Soejima, et al. (212)	2004	Nonischemic dilated CM	22	2.9	333 ± 81	55%	73%[a]	4%	11	46%	87%[b]	27%	93%
Szumowski, et al. (213)	2004	Polymorphic VT	5		—	100%	—	—	16	0%	100%	100%	100%

AAD Rx, concomitant therapy with suppressive antiarrhythmic drug therapy; CL, cycle length; CM, cardiomyopathy; FU, follow-up; ICD Rx, concomitant therapy with an implantable cardioverter defibrillator; VT, ventricular tachycardia.

[a]A total of 73% of patients had complete or partial elimination of induced VTs. Specific reference to clinical VTs not provided.

[b]Survival free of heart transplantation is reported.

European Radiofrequency Survey (MERFS) documented complications from a total of 4,398 catheter ablation procedures from 68 European institutions. The significant complications included the following: complete heart block (fast-pathway ablations excluded), 0.66%; significant vascular injury, 0.63%; pericardial tamponade, 0.60%; 0.53%; pulmonary embolism, 0.13%; systemic embolism, 0.44%; irreversible stroke, 0.06%; and death, 0.06% (214). Another study reported a single-center experience from 1,400 patients. The complication rate was 3.1%, including the following: systemic embolism, 0.21%; stroke 0.14%; valve trauma, 0.07%; tamponade, 0.21%; vascular injury, 0.62%; and complete heart block, 0.05%. There were no deaths. These complication rates certainly underestimate true overall complication rates because of self-reporting bias and anticipated better outcomes from high-volume centers.

With the proliferation of AF ablation, complication rates have increased. This is probably because of prolonged procedure duration and the high number of ablative lesions in the systemic circulation. Stroke and systemic thromboembolism are uncommon (0.5%) but severe complications that occur more frequently in older patients (215,216). To avoid these complications, aggressive anticoagulation is employed during and after the procedure. Anticoagulation, in turn, predisposes patients to bleeding complications such as pericardial tamponade and groin hematoma. In the early experience with pulmonary vein isolation procedures in which operators were ablating within the vein, pulmonary vein stenosis was a common problem. In a review of 608 patients, severe pulmonary vein narrowing was detected in 3.4%, and symptom development correlated with severe stenosis of more than one pulmonary vein. Lung perfusion (V/Q) scans were the best noninvasive test for diagnosis (217). With a shift to extraostial pulmonary vein ablation, pulmonary vein stenosis is no longer a major concern, but other collateral damage to extracardiac structures contiguous to the atrium has been reported. Of greatest concern is esophageal injury that can lead to esophageal perforation and death (218). At present, most operators employ some imaging of the esophagus during ablation so energy delivery directly over closely opposed esophagus can be avoided.

The final risk assumed by the patient and laboratory staff during catheter ablation procedures is radiation exposure. Unlike diagnostic procedures, in which the total fluoroscopy time is usually less than 10 minutes, exposures longer than 30 minutes occur frequently with ablation procedures. A 1999 study of fluoroscopic exposure in 31 unselected ablation patients found that median radiation doses to the thyroid, the ninth vertebral body, and the iliac crest were 0.46 rem, 7.26 rem, and 2.43 rem, respectively. This translated into a lifetime risk of radiation-induced fatal malignancy of 0.1% for every hour of fluoroscopic exposure and a risk of genetic defects of 20 per 1 million births (219). A 2005 study of patients undergoing ablation therapy for AF showed substantial fluoroscopy usage, but with improved fluoroscopy equipment, the lifetime risk of excess fatal malignancies normalized to 60 minutes of fluoroscopy was very low (women, 0.07%; men, 0.1%) (220). New fluoroscopy units that use pulsed energy delivery and improved ablation tools that decrease the time of ablation site access have significantly decreased radiation exposure in recent years, but it still remains a point of significant concern.

CONTROVERSIES AND PERSONAL PERSPECTIVES

Since the early 1990s, radiofrequency catheter ablation has become a dominant modality in the treatment of several symptomatic arrhythmias. The popularity of catheter ablation is in large part the result of the extremely low complication rate observed by practitioners. The major factors that have limited the number and severity of complications are that the operators are skilled and the sizes of the radiofrequency catheter ablation lesions are small. Small lesions are associated with minimal endocardial disruption, a low prevalence of significant thrombus formation, and a low rate of collateral injury to contiguous structures such as coronary arteries (even though most accessory pathway ablations are performed in close proximity to the epicardial coronary arteries). Small lesions require high catheter manipulation skills. New ablation technologies that result in increased lesion size are now readily available. With increased lesion size comes increased collateral injury and complication rates. It is my concern that less experienced or time-stressed operators will trade careful mapping and ablation site selection for "carpet bombing," using large lesion catheters. The patients will not be best served by this approach. In addition, the growth of our field (driven primarily by the need for more device implanters) has led to a reduction of complex catheter ablation cases performed by individual operators. If operators do not maintain their skills and take the time required for proper diagnosis arrhythmia mechanisms, patients will have a higher likelihood of suffering adverse consequences from these interventions.

Catheter ablation can and often should be considered first-line therapy for patients with symptomatic SVT and idiopathic VT. Management of asymptomatic patients with catheter ablation, however, is more controversial. Whereas it is undisputed that ablation of symptomatic arrhythmias will eliminate the symptoms caused by those arrhythmias, it is more difficult to prove that ablation of non–life-threatening arrhythmias confers any benefit to the patient aside from symptom reduction. There are clear cases of incessant SVT that lead to tachycardia-related myopathy (221). With ablation of those arrhythmias, the heart function usually normalizes. This is also observed when patients with very high-density premature ventricular beats undergo successful ablation of the arrhythmogenic focus (222). One can presume that this will translate into greater longevity, but that is unproven. Less clear is the patient with ventricular preexcitation who is entirely asymptomatic. Could their very first arrhythmia be life-threatening? The natural history of asymptomatic adult patients with preexcitation suggests otherwise, but these data to not apply to the pediatric population. It is now accepted practice for asymptomatic adolescents with a Wolff-Parkinson-White pattern on ECG to undergo prophylactic ablation, with the justification that the risk of not doing the procedure may exceed the very low risk of the procedure. In some cases, normalizing the ECG with catheter ablation is a prerequisite to joining certain activities such as piloting commercial airplanes or deep sea diving. Ultimately, all medical and nonmedical factors need to be considered, and the final decision made by the patient and his or her physician.

At present, the greatest area of interest, energy, and unknowns is catheter ablation of AF. The risk-to-benefit analysis of various treatment options in patients with AF is exceedingly complex because the risks of various treatments are all low, but all options carry some real risk. The AFFIRM trial educated us to the possibility that antiarrhythmic drugs, in addition to their well-described proarrhythmic side effects, may exacerbate other life-threatening conditions such as cancer and lung disease (223). Maintaining sinus rhythm improves survival (or is a marker for other life-prolonging factors), but not if suppressive antiarrhythmic drugs are required to achieve that goal (112). AF ablation is more complicated, time-consuming, and risky than conventional ablation of SVT. The challenge therefore lies with a subtle balance of the procedural risk versus the possible survival benefit of reestablishing sinus rhythm in the long term. Operators may present the benefit of stroke prevention as a justification for AF ablation to their patients. However, no long-term or controlled data exist regarding stroke risk with or without ablation. It is likely that restoration of electrical sinus rhythm has a salutary effect on preventing left atrial thrombus formation in these patients, but it is possible that other factors increase stroke risk independent of the rhythm documented on the ECG. So, even though it is common practice for patients to discontinue warfarin anticoagulation after apparent successful catheter ablation, the only proven strategy in the long term is chronic warfarin anticoagulation. On a positive note, preliminary evidence indicates that restoration of sinus rhythm with catheter ablation improves left ventricular function, exercise capacity, and quality of life in patients with heart failure (144). It may also be discovered that pulmonary vein isolation earlier in life may prevent the occurrence of the typical AF found among elderly patients. Ultimately, only long-term follow-up and multicenter controlled trials will address these questions.

THE FUTURE

Curative catheter ablation of common forms of SVT has exceeded most expectations with regard to both safety and efficacy. Although catheter designs and ablation techniques may evolve, it is likely that the overall outcome statistics will not change significantly. The main frontiers remaining in catheter ablation are curative therapy for AF and reentrant VT. Many different tools are being developed for ablation of complex arrhythmias. More importantly, however, advanced imaging, mapping, and ablation technologies will help us understand the pathophysiology of these complex arrhythmias and will direct us to the optimal ablation targets to achieve arrhythmia cure. Ablation successes have always depended on a clear understanding of the electrophysiology and anatomy of the arrhythmic substrate, but the next big step will be fusion of all anatomic and mapping information into integrated systems and automatic targeting by robotic systems. At present, two systems are available (Stereotaxis, Inc., St. Louis, MO) or in development (Hansen Medical, Inc., Mountain View, CA) to provide remote control of catheter movement in the heart. These systems will be merged with high-resolution cardiac images from multidetector CT scans or three-dimensional intracardiac echocardiographs. Mapping and catheter location information from three-dimensional catheter positioning systems will be registered with the anatomic imagery. At this point, catheter ablation will become completely automated. The operator will interpret the mapping and anatomic information, and the computer will then direct the movement of the catheter to the desired point or line of ablation. Such a system should allow less experienced operators to achieve ablation results commensurate with those who have more expertise. Whether it will ultimately result in improved outcomes or decreased overall procedure times remains to be seen.

References

1. Sealy WC, Hattler BG Jr, Blumenschein SD, et al. Surgical treatment of Wolff-Parkinson-White syndrome. *Ann Thorac Surg* 1969;8:1–11.
2. Guiraudon GM, Klein GJ, Sharma AD, et al. Surgery for Wolff-Parkinson-White syndrome: further experience with an epicardial approach. *Circulation* 1986;74:525–529.
3. Cox JL, Gallagher JJ, Cain ME. Experience with 118 consecutive patients undergoing operation for the Wolff-Parkinson-White syndrome. *J Thorac Cardiovasc Surg* 1985;90:490–501.
4. Horowitz LN, Harken AH, Kastor JA, et al. Ventricular resection guided by epicardial and endocardial mapping for treatment of recurrent ventricular tachycardia. *N Engl J Med* 1980;302:589–593.
5. Haines DE, Lerman BB, Kron IL, et al. Surgical ablation of ventricular tachycardia with sequential map-guided subendocardial resection: electrophysiologic assessment and long-term follow-up. *Circulation* 1988;77:131–141.
6. Vedel J, Frank R, Fontaine G, et al. [Permanent intra-hisian atrioventricular block induced during right intraventricular exploration]. [French]. *Arch Mal Coeur Vaiss* 1979;72:107–112.
7. Scheinman MM, Morady F, Hess DS, et al. Catheter-induced ablation of the atrioventricular junction to control refractory supraventricular arrhythmias. *JAMA* 1982;248:851–855.
8. Gallagher JJ, Svenson RH, Kasell JH, et al. Catheter technique for closed-chest ablation of the atrioventricular conduction system. *N Engl J Med* 1982;306:194–200.
9. Weber H, Schmitz L. Catheter technique for closed-chest ablation of an accessory atrioventricular pathway. *N Engl J Med* 1983;308:653–654.
10. Morady F, Scheinman MM. Transvenous catheter ablation of a posteroseptal accessory pathway in a patient with the Wolff-Parkinson-White syndrome. *N Engl J Med* 1984;310:705–707.
11. Belhassen B, Miller HI, Geller E, Laniado S. Transcatheter electrical shock ablation of ventricular tachycardia. *J Am Coll Cardiol* 1986;7:1347–1355.
12. Evans GT Jr, Scheinman MM, Scheinman MM, et al. The Percutaneous Cardiac Mapping and Ablation Registry: final summary of results. *Pacing Clin Electrophysiol* 1988;11:1621–1626.
13. Huang SK, Jordan N, Graham AR. Closed-chest catheter desiccation of atrioventricular junction using radiofrequency energy: a new method of catheter ablation. *Circulation* 1985;72(suppl III):III389.
14. Wittkampf FH, Hauer RN, Robles de Medina EO. Control of radiofrequency lesion size by power regulation. *Circulation* 1989;80:962–968.
15. Haines DE, Watson DD. Tissue heating during radiofrequency catheter ablation: a thermodynamic model and observations in isolated perfused and superfused canine right ventricular free wall. *Pacing Clin Electrophysiol* 1989;12:962–976.
16. Haines DE, Watson DD, Verow AF. Electrode radius predicts lesion radius during radiofrequency energy heating: validation of a proposed thermodynamic model. *Circ Res* 1990;67:124–129.
17. Jackman WM, Wang XZ, Friday KJ, et al. Catheter ablation of atrioventricular junction using radiofrequency current in 17 patients: comparison of standard and large-tip catheter electrodes. *Circulation* 1991;83:1562–1576.
18. Borggrefe M, Budde T, Podczeck A, Breithardt G. High frequency alternating current ablation of an accessory pathway in humans. *J Am Coll Cardiol* 1987;10:576–582.
19. Jackman WM, Friday KJ, Yeung-Lai-Wah JA, et al. New catheter technique for recording left free-wall accessory atrioventricular pathway activation: identification of pathway fiber orientation. *Circulation* 1988;78:598–611.
20. Jackman WM, Kuck KH, Naccarelli GV, et al. Radiofrequency current directed across the mitral anulus with a bipolar epicardial-endocardial catheter electrode configuration in dogs. *Circulation* 1988;78:1288–1298.
21. Haissaguerre M, Fischer B, Warin JF, et al. Electrogram patterns predictive of successful radiofrequency catheter ablation of accessory pathways. *Pacing Clin Electrophysiol* 1992;15:2138–2145.
22. Jackman WM, Wang XZ, Friday KJ, et al. Catheter ablation of accessory atrioventricular pathways (Wolff-Parkinson-White syndrome) by radiofrequency current. *N Engl J Med* 1991;324:1605–1611.
23. Calkins H, Sousa J, el Atassi R, et al. Diagnosis and cure of the Wolff-Parkinson-White syndrome or paroxysmal supraventricular tachycardias during a single electrophysiologic test. *N Engl J Med* 1991;324:1612–1618.
24. Kay GN, Epstein AE, Dailey SM, Plumb VJ. Role of radiofrequency ablation in the management of supraventricular arrhythmias: experience in 760 consecutive patients. *J Cardiovasc Electrophysiol* 1993;4:371–389.
25. Goette A, Reek S, Klein HU, Geller JC. Case report: severe skin burn at the site of the indifferent electrode after radiofrequency catheter ablation of typical atrial flutter. *J Intervent Card Electrophysiol* 2001;5:337–340.
26. Nath S, DiMarco JP, Gallop RG, et al. Effects of dispersive electrode position and surface area on electrical parameters and temperature during radiofrequency catheter ablation. *Am J Cardiol* 1996;77:765–767.
27. Haines DE, Verow AF. Observations on electrode-tissue interface temperature and effect on electrical impedance during radiofrequency ablation of ventricular myocardium. *Circulation* 1990;82:1034–1038.
28. Wittkampf FH, Simmers TA, Hauer RN, et al. Myocardial temperature response during radiofrequency catheter ablation. *Pacing Clin Electrophysiol* 1995;18:307–317.
29. Wittkampf FH, Nakagawa H, Yamanashi WS, et al. Thermal latency in radiofrequency ablation. *Circulation* 1996;93:1083–1086.
30. Haines DE. Determinants of lesion size during radiofrequency catheter ablation: the role of electrode tissue contact pressure and duration of energy delivery. *J Cardiovasc Electrophysiol* 1991;2:509–515.
31. Nakagawa H, Yamanashi WS, Pitha JV, et al. Comparison of in vivo tissue temperature profile and lesion geometry for radiofrequency ablation with a saline-irrigated electrode versus temperature control in a canine thigh muscle preparation. *Circulation* 1995;91:2264–2273.
32. Atiga WL, Worley SJ, Hummel J, et al. Prospective randomized comparison of cooled radiofrequency versus standard radiofrequency energy for ablation of typical atrial flutter. *Pacing Clin Electrophysiol* 2002;25:1172–1178.
33. Scavee C, Jais P, Hsu LF, et al. Prospective randomised comparison of irrigated-tip and large-tip catheter ablation of cavotricuspid isthmus-dependent atrial flutter. *Eur Heart J* 2004;25:963–969.
34. Tsai CF, Tai CT, Yu WC, et al. Is 8-mm more effective than 4-mm tip electrode catheter for ablation of typical atrial flutter? *Circulation* 1999;100: 768–771.

35. Schreieck J, Zrenner B, Kumpmann J, et al. Prospective randomized comparison of closed cooled-tip versus 8-mm-tip catheters for radiofrequency ablation of typical atrial flutter. *J Cardiovasc Electrophysiol* 2002;13:980–985.
36. McGreevy KS, Hummel JD, Zou J, et al. Comparison of a saline irrigated cooled-tip catheter to large electrode catheters with single and multiple temperature sensors for creation of large radiofrequency lesions. *J Intervent Card Electrophysiol* 2005;1:299–303.
37. Whayne JG, Nath S, Haines DE. Microwave catheter ablation of myocardium in vitro: assessment of the characteristics of tissue heating and injury. *Circulation* 1994;89:2390–2395.
38. Langberg JJ, Calkins H, el Atassi R, et al. Temperature monitoring during radiofrequency catheter ablation of accessory pathways. *Circulation* 1992;86:1469–1474.
39. Nath S, DiMarco JP, Mounsey JP, et al. Correlation of temperature and pathophysiological effect during radiofrequency catheter ablation of the AV junction. *Circulation* 1995;92:1188–1192.
40. Huang SK, Bharati S, Lev M, Marcus FI. Electrophysiologic and histologic observations of chronic atrioventricular block induced by closed-chest catheter desiccation with radiofrequency energy. *Pacing Clin Electrophysiol* 1987;10:805–816.
41. Solomon AJ, Tracy CM, Swartz JF, et al. Effect on coronary artery anatomy of radiofrequency catheter ablation of atrial insertion sites of accessory pathways. *J Am Coll Cardiol* 1993;21:1440–1444.
42. Bokenkamp R, Wibbelt G, Sturm M, et al. Effects of intracardiac radiofrequency current application on coronary artery vessels in young pigs. *J Cardiovasc Electrophysiol* 2000;11:565–571.
43. DeLacey WA, Nath S, Haines DE, et al. Adenosine and verapamil-sensitive ventricular tachycardia originating from the left ventricle: radiofrequency catheter ablation. *Pacing Clin Electrophysiol* 1992;15:2240–2244.
44. Nath S, Whayne JG, Kaul S, et al. Effects of radiofrequency catheter ablation on regional myocardial blood flow: possible mechanism for late electrophysiological outcome. *Circulation* 1994;89:2667–2672.
45. Nath S, Redick JA, Whayne JG, Haines DE. Ultrastructural observations in the myocardium beyond the region of acute coagulation necrosis following radiofrequency catheter ablation. *J Cardiovasc Electrophysiol* 1994;5:838–845.
46. Nath S, Lynch C III, Whayne JG, Haines DE. Cellular electrophysiological effects of hyperthermia on isolated guinea pig papillary muscle: implications for catheter ablation. *Circulation* 1993;88:1826–1831.
47. Everett TH, Nath S, Lynch C III, et al. Role of calcium in acute hyperthermic myocardial injury. *J Cardiovasc Electrophysiol* 2001;12:563–569.
48. Simmers TA, de Bakker JM, Wittkampf FH, et al. Effects of heating on impulse propagation in superfused canine myocardium. *J Am Coll Cardiol* 1995;25:1457–1464.
49. Schluter M, Geiger M, Siebels J, et al. Catheter ablation using radiofrequency current to cure symptomatic patients with tachyarrhythmias related to an accessory atrioventricular pathway. *Circulation* 1991;84:1644–1661.
50. Morady F, Strickberger A, Man KC, et al. Reasons for prolonged or failed attempts at radiofrequency catheter ablation of accessory pathways. *J Am Coll Cardiol* 1996;27:683–689.
51. Calkins H, Yong P, Miller JM, et al. Catheter ablation of accessory pathways, atrioventricular nodal reentrant tachycardia, and the atrioventricular junction: final results of a prospective, multicenter clinical trial. The Atakr Multicenter Investigators Group. *Circulation* 1999;99:262–270.
52. Calkins H, Kim YN, Schmaltz S, et al. Electrogram criteria for identification of appropriate target sites for radiofrequency catheter ablation of accessory atrioventricular connections. *Circulation* 1992;85:565–573.
53. Bashir Y, Heald SC, Katritsis D, et al. Radiofrequency ablation of accessory atrioventricular pathways: predictive value of local electrogram characteristics for the identification of successful target sites. *Br Heart J* 1993;69:315–321.
54. Hindricks G, Kottkamp H, Chen X, et al. Localization and radiofrequency catheter ablation of left-sided accessory pathways during atrial fibrillation: feasibility and electrogram criteria for identification of appropriate target sites. *J Am Coll Cardiol* 1995;25:444–451.
55. Barlow MA, Klein GJ, Simpson CS, et al. Unipolar electrogram characteristics predictive of successful radiofrequency catheter ablation of accessory pathways. *J Cardiovasc Electrophysiol* 2000;11:146–154.
56. Swartz JF, Tracy CM, Fletcher RD. Radiofrequency endocardial catheter ablation of accessory atrioventricular pathway atrial insertion sites. *Circulation* 1993;87:487–499.
57. Deshpande SS, Bremner S, Sra JS, et al. Ablation of left free-wall accessory pathways using radiofrequency energy at the atrial insertion site: transseptal versus transaortic approach. *J Cardiovasc Electrophysiol* 1994;5:219–231.
58. Lesh MD, Van Hare GF, Scheinman MM, et al. Comparison of the retrograde and transseptal methods for ablation of left free wall accessory pathways. *J Am Coll Cardiol* 1993;22:542–549.
59. Xie B, Heald SC, Bashir Y, et al. Radiofrequency catheter ablation of septal accessory atrioventricular pathways. *Br Heart J* 1994;72:281–284.
60. Schluter M, Kuck KH. Catheter ablation from right atrium of anteroseptal accessory pathways using radiofrequency current. *J Am Coll Cardiol* 1992;19:663–670.
61. Gaita F, Haissaguerre M, Giustetto C, et al. Safety and efficacy of cryoablation of accessory pathways adjacent to the normal conduction system. *J Cardiovasc Electrophysiol* 2003;14:825–829.
62. Dhala AA, Deshpande SS, Bremner S, et al. Transcatheter ablation of posteroseptal accessory pathways using a venous approach and radiofrequency energy. *Circulation* 1994;90:1799–1810.
63. Haissaguerre M, Marcus F, Poquet F, et al. Electrocardiographic characteristics and catheter ablation of parahissian accessory pathways. *Circulation* 1994;90:1124–1128.
64. Haissaguerre M, Cauchemez B, Marcus F, et al. Characteristics of the ventricular insertion sites of accessory pathways with anterograde decremental conduction properties. *Circulation* 1995;91:1077–1085.
65. McClelland JH, Wang X, Beckman KJ, et al. Radiofrequency catheter ablation of right atriofascicular (Mahaim) accessory pathways guided by accessory pathway activation potentials. *Circulation* 1994;89:2655–2666.
66. Zipes DP, DiMarco JP, Gillette PC, et al. Guidelines for clinical intracardiac electrophysiological and catheter ablation procedures: a report of the American College of Cardiology/American Heart Association Task Force on Practice Guidelines (Committee on Clinical Intracardiac Electrophysiologic and Catheter Ablation Procedures), developed in collaboration with the North American Society of Pacing and Electrophysiology. *J Am Coll Cardiol* 1995;26:555–573.
67. Pappone C, Manguso F, Santinelli R, et al. Radiofrequency ablation in children with asymptomatic Wolff-Parkinson-White syndrome. *N Engl J Med* 2004;351:1197–1205.
68. Inoue S, Becker AE, Riccardi R, Gaita F. Interruption of the inferior extension of the compact atrioventricular node underlies successful radio frequency ablation of atrioventricular nodal reentrant tachycardia. *J Intervent Card Electrophysiol* 1999;3:273–277.
69. Langberg JJ, Harvey M, Calkins H, et al. Titration of power output during radiofrequency catheter ablation of atrioventricular nodal reentrant tachycardia. *Pacing Clin Electrophysiol* 1993;16:465–470.
70. Jazayeri MR, Hempe SL, Sra JS, et al. Selective transcatheter ablation of the fast and slow pathways using radiofrequency energy in patients with atrioventricular nodal reentrant tachycardia. *Circulation* 1992;85:1318–1328.
71. Jackman WM, Beckman KJ, McClelland JH, et al. Treatment of supraventricular tachycardia due to atrioventricular nodal reentry, by radiofrequency catheter ablation of slow-pathway conduction. *N Engl J Med* 1992;327:313–318.
72. Kalbfleisch SJ, Strickberger SA, Williamson B, et al. Randomized comparison of anatomic and electrogram mapping approaches to ablation of the slow pathway of atrioventricular node reentrant tachycardia. *J Am Coll Cardiol* 1994;23:716–723.
73. Thakur RK, Klein GJ, Yee R, et al. Junctional tachycardia: a useful marker during radiofrequency ablation for atrioventricular node reentrant tachycardia. *J Am Coll Cardiol* 1993;22:1706–1710.
74. Friedman PL, Dubuc M, Green MS, et al. Catheter cryoablation of supraventricular tachycardia: results of the multicenter prospective "Frosty" Trial. *Heart Rhythm* 2004;1:129–138.
75. Zrenner B, Dong J, Schreieck J, et al. Transvenous cryoablation versus radiofrequency ablation of the slow pathway for the treatment of atrioventricular nodal re-entrant tachycardia: a prospective randomized pilot study. *Eur Heart J* 2004;25:2226–2231.
76. Mitrani RD, Klein LS, Hackett FK, et al. Radiofrequency ablation for atrioventricular node reentrant tachycardia: comparison between fast (anterior) and slow (posterior) pathway ablation. *J Am Coll Cardiol* 1993;21:432–441.
77. Sra JS, Jazayeri MR, Blanck Z, et al. Slow pathway ablation in patients with atrioventricular node reentrant tachycardia and a prolonged PR interval. *J Am Coll Cardiol* 1994;24:1064–1068.
78. Baker JH, Plumb VJ, Epstein AE, et al. Predictors of recurrent atrioventricular nodal reentry after selective slow pathway ablation. *Am J Cardiol* 1994;73:765–769.
79. Kay GN, Epstein AE, Dailey SM, et al. Selective radiofrequency ablation of the slow pathway for the treatment of atrioventricular nodal reentrant tachycardia: evidence for involvement of perinodal myocardium within the reentrant circuit. *Circulation* 1992;85:1675–1688.
80. Wu D, Yeh SJ, Wang CC, et al. A simple technique for selective radiofrequency ablation of the slow pathway in atrioventricular node reentrant tachycardia. *J Am Coll Cardiol* 1993;21:1612–1621.
81. Langberg JJ, Leon A, Borganelli M, et al. A randomized, prospective comparison of anterior and posterior approaches to radiofrequency catheter ablation of atrioventricular nodal reentry tachycardia. *Circulation* 1993;87:1551–1556.
82. Lindsay BD, Chung MK, Gamache MC, et al. Therapeutic end points for the treatment of atrioventricular node reentrant tachycardia by catheter-guided radiofrequency current. *J Am Coll Cardiol* 1993;22:733–740.
83. Manolis AS, Wang PJ, Estes NA III. Radiofrequency ablation of slow pathway in patients with atrioventricular nodal reentrant tachycardia: do arrhythmia recurrences correlate with persistent slow pathway conduction or site of successful ablation? *Circulation* 1994;90:2815–2819.
84. Kottkamp H, Hindricks G, Willems S, et al. An anatomically and electrogram-guided stepwise approach for effective and safe catheter ablation of the fast pathway for elimination of atrioventricular node reentrant tachycardia. *J Am Coll Cardiol* 1995;25:974–981.
85. Cosio FG, Goicolea A, Lopez-Gil M, et al. Atrial endocardial mapping in the rare form of atrial flutter. *Am J Cardiol* 1990;66:715–720.
86. Friedman PA, Luria D, Fenton AM, et al. Global right atrial mapping of human atrial flutter: the presence of posteromedial (sinus venosa region)

functional block and double potentials: a study in biplane fluoroscopy and intracardiac echocardiography. *Circulation* 2000;101:1568–1577.
87. Saoudi N, Atallah G, Kirkorian G, et al. Catheter ablation of the atrial myocardium in human type I atrial flutter. *Circulation* 1990;81:762–771.
88. Feld GK, Fleck RP, Chen PS, et al. Radiofrequency catheter ablation for the treatment of human type 1 atrial flutter: identification of a critical zone in the reentrant circuit by endocardial mapping techniques. *Circulation* 1992;86:1233–1240.
89. Cosio FG, Lopez-Gil M, Goicolea A, et al. Radiofrequency ablation of the inferior vena cava-tricuspid valve isthmus in common atrial flutter. *Am J Cardiol* 1993;71:705–709.
90. Takahashi A, Shah DC, Jais P, et al. Partial cavotricuspid isthmus block before ablation in patients with typical atrial flutter. *J Am Coll Cardiol* 1999;33:1996–2002.
91. Chen J, de Chillou C, Basiouny T, et al. Cavotricuspid isthmus mapping to assess bidirectional block during common atrial flutter radiofrequency ablation. *Circulation* 1999;100:2507–2513.
92. Yamabe H, Okumura K, Misumi I, et al. Role of bipolar electrogram polarity mapping in localizing recurrent conduction in the isthmus early and late after ablation of atrial flutter. *J Am Coll Cardiol* 1999;33:39–45.
93. Tai CT, Liu TY, Lee PC, et al. Non-contact mapping to guide radiofrequency ablation of atypical right atrial flutter. *J Am Coll Cardiol* 2004;44:1080–1086.
94. Heidbuchel H, Willems R, van Rensburg H, et al. Right atrial angiographic evaluation of the posterior isthmus: relevance for ablation of typical atrial flutter. *Circulation* 2000;101:2178–2184.
95. Poty H, Saoudi N, Abdel AA, et al. Radiofrequency catheter ablation of type 1 atrial flutter: prediction of late success by electrophysiological criteria. *Circulation* 1995;92:1389–1392.
96. Da Costa A, Faure E, Thevenin J, et al. Effect of isthmus anatomy and ablation catheter on radiofrequency catheter ablation of the cavotricuspid isthmus. *Circulation* 2004;110:1030–1035.
97. Cauchemez B, Haissaguerre M, Fischer B, et al. Electrophysiological effects of catheter ablation of inferior vena cava-tricuspid annulus isthmus in common atrial flutter. *Circulation* 1996;93:284–294.
98. Jais P, Haissaguerre M, Shah DC, et al. Successful irrigated-tip catheter ablation of atrial flutter resistant to conventional radiofrequency ablation. *Circulation* 1998;98:835–838.
99. Feld G, Wharton M, Plumb V, et al. Radiofrequency catheter ablation of type 1 atrial flutter using large-tip 8- or 10-mm electrode catheters and a high-output radiofrequency energy generator: results of a multicenter safety and efficacy study. *J Am Coll Cardiol* 2004;43:1466–1472.
100. Schreieck J, Zrenner B, Kumpmann J, et al. Prospective randomized comparison of closed cooled-tip versus 8-mm-tip catheters for radiofrequency ablation of typical atrial flutter. *J Cardiovasc Electrophysiol* 2005;13:980–985.
101. Nath S, Mounsey JP, Haines DE, et al. Predictors of acute and long-term success after radiofrequency catheter ablation of type 1 atrial flutter. *Am J Cardiol* 1995;76:604–606.
102. Paydak H, Kall JG, Burke MC, et al. Atrial fibrillation after radiofrequency ablation of type I atrial flutter: time to onset, determinants, and clinical course. *Circulation* 1998;98:315–322.
103. Philippon F, Plumb VJ, Epstein AE, et al. The risk of atrial fibrillation following radiofrequency catheter ablation of atrial flutter. *Circulation* 1995;92:430–435.
104. Schumacher B, Jung W, Lewalter T, et al. Radiofrequency ablation of atrial flutter due to administration of class IC antiarrhythmic drugs for atrial fibrillation. *Am J Cardiol* 1999;83:710–713.
105. Fischer B, Haissaguerre M, Garrigues S, et al. Radiofrequency catheter ablation of common atrial flutter in 80 patients. *J Am Coll Cardiol* 1995;25:1365–1372.
106. Da Costa A, Faure E, Thevenin J, et al. Effect of isthmus anatomy and ablation catheter on radiofrequency catheter ablation of the cavotricuspid isthmus. *Circulation* 2004;110:1030–1035.
107. Calkins H, Canby R, Weiss R, et al. Results of catheter ablation of typical atrial flutter. *Am J Cardiol* 2004;94:437–442.
108. Feld G, Wharton M, Plumb V, et al. Radiofrequency catheter ablation of type 1 atrial flutter using large-tip 8- or 10-mm electrode catheters and a high-output radiofrequency energy generator: results of a multicenter safety and efficacy study. *J Am Coll Cardiol* 2004;43:1466–1472.
109. Bertaglia E, Zoppo F, Bonso A, et al. Long term follow up of radiofrequency catheter ablation of atrial flutter: clinical course and predictors of atrial fibrillation occurrence. *Heart* 2004;90:59–63.
110. Kannel WB, Abbott RD, Savage DD, et al. Epidemiologic features of chronic atrial fibrillation: the Framingham study. *N Engl J Med* 1982;306:1018–1022.
111. Wyse DG, Waldo AL, DiMarco JP, et al. A comparison of rate control and rhythm control in patients with atrial fibrillation. *N Engl J Med* 2002;347:1825–1833.
112. Corley SD, Epstein AE, Dimarco JP, et al. Relationships between sinus rhythm, treatment, and survival in the Atrial Fibrillation Follow-Up Investigation of Rhythm Management (AFFIRM) Study. *Circulation* 2004;109:1509–1513.
113. Kalbfleisch SJ, Williamson B, Man KC, et al. A randomized comparison of the right- and left-sided approaches to ablation of the atrioventricular junction. *Am J Cardiol* 1993;72:1406–1410.
114. Brignole M, Gianfranchi L, Menozzi C, et al. Influence of atrioventricular junction radiofrequency ablation in patients with chronic atrial fibrillation and flutter on quality of life and cardiac performance. *Am J Cardiol* 1994;74:242–246.
115. Rodriguez LM, Smeets JL, Xie B, et al. Improvement in left ventricular function by ablation of atrioventricular nodal conduction in selected patients with lone atrial fibrillation. *Am J Cardiol* 1993;72:1137–1141.
116. Ozcan C, Jahangir A, Friedman PA, et al. Sudden death after radiofrequency ablation of the atrioventricular node in patients with atrial fibrillation. *J Am Coll Cardiol* 2002;40:105–110.
117. Simantirakis EN, Vardakis KE, Kochiadakis GE, et al. Left ventricular mechanics during right ventricular apical or left ventricular-based pacing in patients with chronic atrial fibrillation after atrioventricular junction ablation. *J Am Coll Cardiol* 2004;43:1013–1018.
118. Wilkoff BL, Cook JR, Epstein AE, et al. Dual-chamber pacing or ventricular backup pacing in patients with an implantable defibrillator: the Dual Chamber and VVI Implantable Defibrillator (DAVID) Trial. *JAMA* 2002;288:3115–3123.
119. Jais P, Haissaguerre M, Shah DC, et al. A focal source of atrial fibrillation treated by discrete radiofrequency ablation. *Circulation* 1997;95:572–576.
120. Haissaguerre M, Jais P, Shah DC, et al. Spontaneous initiation of atrial fibrillation by ectopic beats originating in the pulmonary veins. *N Engl J Med* 1998;339:659–666.
121. Chen SA, Hsieh MH, Tai CT, et al. Initiation of atrial fibrillation by ectopic beats originating from the pulmonary veins: electrophysiological characteristics, pharmacological responses, and effects of radiofrequency ablation. *Circulation* 1999;100:1879–1886.
122. Mandapati R, Skanes A, Chen J, et al. Stable microreentrant sources as a mechanism of atrial fibrillation in the isolated sheep heart. *Circulation* 2000;101:194–199.
123. Liu L, Nattel S. Differing sympathetic and vagal effects on atrial fibrillation in dogs: role of refractoriness heterogeneity. *Am J Physiol* 1997;273:H805–H816.
124. Cappato R, Negroni S, Pecora D, et al. Prospective assessment of late conduction recurrence across radiofrequency lesions producing electrical disconnection at the pulmonary vein ostium in patients with atrial fibrillation. *Circulation* 2003;108:1599–1604.
125. Ouyang F, Antz M, Ernst S, et al. Recovered pulmonary vein conduction as a dominant factor for recurrent atrial tachyarrhythmias after complete circular isolation of the pulmonary veins: lessons from double Lasso technique. *Circulation* 2005;111:127–135.
126. Gerstenfeld EP, Dixit S, Callans D, et al. Utility of exit block for identifying electrical isolation of the pulmonary veins. *J Cardiovasc Electrophysiol* 2002;13:971–979.
127. Oral H, Scharf C, Chugh A, et al. Catheter ablation for paroxysmal atrial fibrillation: segmental pulmonary vein ostial ablation versus left atrial ablation. *Circulation* 2003;108:2355–2360.
128. Karch MR, Zrenner B, Deisenhofer I, et al. Freedom from atrial tachyarrhythmias after catheter ablation of atrial fibrillation: a randomized comparison between 2 current ablation strategies. *Circulation* 2005;111:2875–2880.
129. Ernst S, Ouyang F, Lober F, et al. Catheter-induced linear lesions in the left atrium in patients with atrial fibrillation: an electroanatomic study. *J Am Coll Cardiol* 2003;42:1271–1282.
130. Nademanee K, McKenzie J, Kosar E, et al. A new approach for catheter ablation of atrial fibrillation: mapping of the electrophysiologic substrate. *J Am Coll Cardiol* 2004;43:2044–2053.
131. Schauerte P, Scherlag BJ, Pitha J, et al. Catheter ablation of cardiac autonomic nerves for prevention of vagal atrial fibrillation. *Circulation* 2000;102:2774–2780.
132. Michael MJ, Haines DE, DiMarco JP, et al. Elimination of focal atrial fibrillation with a single radiofrequency ablation: use of a basket catheter in a pulmonary vein for computerized activation sequence mapping. *J Cardiovasc Electrophysiol* 2000;11:1159–1164.
133. Hindricks G, Kottkamp H. Simultaneous noncontact mapping of left atrium in patients with paroxysmal atrial fibrillation. *Circulation* 2001;104:297–303.
134. Pappone C, Rosanio S, Oreto G, et al. Circumferential radiofrequency ablation of pulmonary vein ostia: a new anatomic approach for curing atrial fibrillation. *Circulation* 2000;102:2619–2628.
135. Scharf C, Sneider M, Case I, et al. Anatomy of the pulmonary veins in patients with atrial fibrillation and effects of segmental ostial ablation analyzed by computed tomography. *J Cardiovasc Electrophysiol* 2003;14:150–155.
136. Wood MA, Wittkamp M, Henry D, et al. A comparison of pulmonary vein ostial anatomy by computerized tomography, echocardiography, and venography in patients with atrial fibrillation having radiofrequency catheter ablation. *Am J Cardiol* 2004;93:49–53.
137. Kistler PM, Sanders P, Fynn SP, et al. Electrophysiological and electrocardiographic characteristics of focal atrial tachycardia originating from the pulmonary veins: acute and long-term outcomes of radiofrequency ablation. *Circulation* 2003;108:1968–1975.
138. Kato R, Lickfett L, Meininger G, et al. Pulmonary vein anatomy in patients undergoing catheter ablation of atrial fibrillation: lessons learned by use of magnetic resonance imaging. *Circulation* 2003;107:2004–2010.

139. Martin RE, Ellenbogen KA, Lau YR, et al. Phased-array intracardiac echocardiography during pulmonary vein isolation and linear ablation for atrial fibrillation. *J Cardiovasc Electrophysiol* 2002;13:873–879.
140. Mangrum JM, Mounsey JP, Kok LC, et al. Intracardiac echocardiography-guided, anatomically based radiofrequency ablation of focal atrial fibrillation originating from pulmonary veins. *J Am Coll Cardiol* 2002;39:1964–1972.
141. Knight BP, Burke MC, Hong TE, et al. Direct imaging of transvenous radiofrequency cardiac ablation using a steerable fiberoptic infrared endoscope. *Heart Rhythm* 2005;2:1116–1121.
142. Haissaguerre M, Jais P, Shah DC, et al. Electrophysiological end point for catheter ablation of atrial fibrillation initiated from multiple pulmonary venous foci. *Circulation* 2000;101:1409–1417.
143. Wazni OM, Marrouche NF, Martin DO, et al. Radiofrequency ablation vs antiarrhythmic drugs as first-line treatment of symptomatic atrial fibrillation: a randomized trial. *JAMA* 2005;293:2634–2640.
144. Hsu LF, Jais P, Sanders P, et al. Catheter ablation for atrial fibrillation in congestive heart failure. *N Engl J Med* 2004;351:2373–2383.
145. Shah DC, Haissaguerre M, Jais P, et al. Curative catheter ablation of paroxysmal atrial fibrillation in 200 patients: strategy for presentations ranging from sustained atrial fibrillation to no arrhythmias. *Pacing Clin Electrophysiol* 2001;24:1541–1558.
146. Mangrum JM, Mounsey JP, Kok LC, et al. Intracardiac echocardiography-guided, anatomically based radiofrequency ablation of focal atrial fibrillation originating from pulmonary veins. *J Am Coll Cardiol* 2002;39:1964–1972.
147. Oral H, Knight BP, Tada H, et al. Pulmonary vein isolation for paroxysmal and persistent atrial fibrillation. *Circulation* 2002;105:1077–1081.
148. Marrouche NF, Martin DO, Wazni O, et al. Phased-array intracardiac echocardiography monitoring during pulmonary vein isolation in patients with atrial fibrillation: impact on outcome and complications. *Circulation* 2003;107:2710–2716.
149. Macle L, Jais P, Weerasooriya R, et al. Irrigated-tip catheter ablation of pulmonary veins for treatment of atrial fibrillation. *J Cardiovasc Electrophysiol* 2002;13:1067–1073.
150. Lin WS, Tai CT, Hsieh MH, et al. Catheter ablation of paroxysmal atrial fibrillation initiated by non-pulmonary vein ectopy. *Circulation* 2003;107:3176–3183.
151. Jais P, Hocini M, Hsu LF, et al. Technique and results of linear ablation at the mitral isthmus. *Circulation* 2004;110:2996–3002.
152. Pappone C, Rosanio S, Augello G, et al. Mortality, morbidity, and quality of life after circumferential pulmonary vein ablation for atrial fibrillation: outcomes from a controlled nonrandomized long-term study. *J Am Coll Cardiol* 2003;42:185–197.
153. Kottkamp H, Tanner H, Kobza R, et al. Time courses and quantitative analysis of atrial fibrillation episode number and duration after circular plus linear left atrial lesions: trigger elimination or substrate modification: early or delayed cure? *J Am Coll Cardiol* 2004;44:869–877.
154. Della Bella P, Riva S, Fassini G, et al. Long-term follow-up after radiofrequency catheter ablation of atrial fibrillation: role of the acute procedure outcome and of the clinical presentation. *Europace* 2005;7:95–103.
155. Herweg B, Sichrovsky T, Polosajian L, et al. Anatomic substrate, procedural results, and clinical outcome of ultrasound-guided left atrial-pulmonary vein disconnection for treatment of atrial fibrillation. *Am J Cardiol* 2005;95:871–875.
156. Cappato R, Calkins H, Chen SA, et al. Worldwide survey on the methods, efficacy, and safety of catheter ablation for human atrial fibrillation. *Circulation* 2005;111:1100–1105.
157. Senatore G, Stabile G, Bertaglia E, et al. Role of transtelephonic electrocardiographic monitoring in detecting short-term arrhythmia recurrences after radiofrequency ablation in patients with atrial fibrillation. *J Am Coll Cardiol* 2005;45:873–876.
158. Sanders WE Jr, Sorrentino RA, Greenfield RA, et al. Catheter ablation of sinoatrial node reentrant tachycardia. *J Am Coll Cardiol* 1994;23:926–934.
159. Kay GN, Chong F, Epstein AE, et al. Radiofrequency ablation for treatment of primary atrial tachycardias. *J Am Coll Cardiol* 1993;21:901–909.
160. Grubb BP, Kosinski DJ, Boehm K, et al. The postural orthostatic tachycardia syndrome: a neurocardiogenic variant identified during head-up tilt table testing. *Pacing Clin Electrophysiol* 1997;20:2205–2212.
161. Marrouche NF, Beheiry S, Tomassoni G, et al. Three-dimensional nonfluoroscopic mapping and ablation of inappropriate sinus tachycardia: procedural strategies and long-term outcome. *J Am Coll Cardiol* 2002;39:1046–1054.
162. Ren JF, Marchlinski FE, Callans DJ, et al. Echocardiographic lesion characteristics associated with successful ablation of inappropriate sinus tachycardia. *J Cardiovasc Electrophysiol* 2001;12:814–818.
163. Kistler PM, Sanders P, Fynn SP, et al. Electrophysiological and electrocardiographic characteristics of focal atrial tachycardia originating from the pulmonary veins: acute and long-term outcomes of radiofrequency ablation. *Circulation* 2003;108:1968–1975.
164. Anguera I, Brugada J, Roba M, et al. Outcomes after radiofrequency catheter ablation of atrial tachycardia. *Am J Cardiol* 2001;87:886–890.
165. Tanner H, Hindricks G, Schirdewahn P, et al. Outflow tract tachycardia with R/S transition in lead V_3: six different anatomic approaches for successful ablation. *J Am Coll Cardiol* 2005;45:418–423.
166. Rahilly GT, Prystowsky EN, Zipes DP, et al. Clinical and electrophysiologic findings in patients with repetitive monomorphic ventricular tachycardia and otherwise normal electrocardiogram. *Am J Cardiol* 1982;50:459–468.
167. Wilber DJ, Baerman J, Olshansky B, et al. Adenosine-sensitive ventricular tachycardia: clinical characteristics and response to catheter ablation. *Circulation* 1993;87:126–134.
168. Lerman BB, Belardinelli L, West GA, et al. Adenosine-sensitive ventricular tachycardia: evidence suggesting cyclic AMP-mediated triggered activity. *Circulation* 1986;74:270–280.
169. Chen M, Yang B, Zou J, et al. Non-contact mapping and linear ablation of the left posterior fascicle during sinus rhythm in the treatment of idiopathic left ventricular tachycardia. *Europace* 2005;7:138–144.
170. Ohe T, Shimomura K, Aihara N, et al. Idiopathic sustained left ventricular tachycardia: clinical and electrophysiologic characteristics [erratum appears in Circulation 1988;78:A5]. *Circulation* 1988;77:560–568.
171. Okumura K, Yamabe H, Tsuchiya T, et al. Characteristics of slow conduction zone demonstrated during entrainment of idiopathic ventricular tachycardia of left ventricular origin. *Am J Cardiol* 1996;77:379–383.
172. Klein LS, Shih HT, Hackett FK, et al. Radiofrequency catheter ablation of ventricular tachycardia in patients without structural heart disease. *Circulation* 1992;85:1666–1674.
173. Calkins H, Kalbfleisch SJ, el Atassi R, et al. Relation between efficacy of radiofrequency catheter ablation and site of origin of idiopathic ventricular tachycardia. *Am J Cardiol* 1993;71:827–833.
174. Wen MS, Yeh SJ, Wang CC, et al. Successful radiofrequency ablation of idiopathic left ventricular tachycardia at a site away from the tachycardia exit. *J Am Coll Cardiol* 1997;30:1024–1031.
175. Kamakura S, Shimizu W, Matsuo K, et al. Localization of optimal ablation site of idiopathic ventricular tachycardia from right and left ventricular outflow tract by body surface ECG. *Circulation* 1998;98:1525–1533.
176. Peeters HA, SippensGroenewegen A, Wever EF, et al. Clinical application of an integrated 3-phase mapping technique for localization of the site of origin of idiopathic ventricular tachycardia. *Circulation* 1999;99:1300–1311.
177. Tsuchiya T, Okumura K, Honda T, et al. Significance of late diastolic potential preceding Purkinje potential in verapamil-sensitive idiopathic left ventricular tachycardia. *Circulation* 1999;99:2408–2413.
178. Nakagawa H, Beckman KJ, McClelland JH, et al. Radiofrequency catheter ablation of idiopathic left ventricular tachycardia guided by a Purkinje potential. *Circulation* 1993;88:2607–2617.
179. Klein LS, Miles WM, Mitrani RD, et al. Ablation of ventricular tachycardia in patients with structurally normal hearts. In: Zipes DP, Jalife J, eds. *Cardiac electrophysiology: from cell to bedside*. Philadelphia: WB Saunders, 1995:1518–1523.
180. Downar E, Kimber S, Harris L, et al. Endocardial mapping of ventricular tachycardia in the intact human heart. II. Evidence for multiuse reentry in a functional sheet of surviving myocardium. *J Am Coll Cardiol* 1992;20:869–878.
181. de Bakker JM, Coronel R, Tasseron S, et al. Ventricular tachycardia in the infarcted, Langendorff-perfused human heart: role of the arrangement of surviving cardiac fibers. *J Am Coll Cardiol* 1990;15:1594–1607.
182. Harris L, Downar E, Mickleborough L, et al. Activation sequence of ventricular tachycardia: endocardial and epicardial mapping studies in the human ventricle. *J Am Coll Cardiol* 1987;10:1040–1407.
183. Downar E, Saito J, Doig JC, et al. Endocardial mapping of ventricular tachycardia in the intact human ventricle. III. Evidence of multiuse reentry with spontaneous and induced block in portions of reentrant path complex. *J Am Coll Cardiol* 1995;25:1591–1600.
184. de Bakker JM, van Capelle FJ, Janse MJ, et al. Fractionated electrograms in dilated cardiomyopathy: origin and relation to abnormal conduction. *J Am Coll Cardiol* 1996;27:1071–1078.
185. Caceres J, Jazayeri M, McKinnie J, et al. Sustained bundle branch reentry as a mechanism of clinical tachycardia. *Circulation* 1989;79:256–270.
186. Tchou P, Jazayeri M, Denker S, et al. Transcatheter electrical ablation of right bundle branch: a method of treating macroreentrant ventricular tachycardia attributed to bundle branch reentry. *Circulation* 1988;78:246–257.
187. Cohen TJ, Chien WW, Lurie KG, et al. Radiofrequency catheter ablation for treatment of bundle branch reentrant ventricular tachycardia: results and long-term follow-up. *J Am Coll Cardiol* 1991;18:1767–1773.
188. Blanck Z, Dhala A, Deshpande S, et al. Bundle branch reentrant ventricular tachycardia: cumulative experience in 48 patients. *J Cardiovasc Electrophysiol* 1993;4:253–262.
189. O'Donnell D, Cox D, Bourke J, et al. Clinical and electrophysiological differences between patients with arrhythmogenic right ventricular dysplasia and right ventricular outflow tract tachycardia. *Eur Heart J* 2003;24:801–810.
190. Marchlinski FE, Zado E, Dixit S, et al. Electroanatomic substrate and outcome of catheter ablative therapy for ventricular tachycardia in setting of right ventricular cardiomyopathy. *Circulation* 2004;110:2293–2298.
191. Stevenson WG, Khan H, Sager P, et al. Identification of reentry circuit sites during catheter mapping and radiofrequency ablation of ventricular tachycardia late after myocardial infarction. *Circulation* 1993;88:1647–1670.
192. Bogun F, Bahu M, Knight BP, et al. Comparison of effective and ineffective target sites that demonstrate concealed entrainment in patients with

coronary artery disease undergoing radiofrequency ablation of ventricular tachycardia. *Circulation* 1997;95:183–190.
193. El Shalakany A, Hadjis T, Papageorgiou P, et al. Entrainment/mapping criteria for the prediction of termination of ventricular tachycardia by single radiofrequency lesion in patients with coronary artery disease. *Circulation* 1999;99:2283–2289.
194. Stevenson WG, Delacretaz E, Friedman PL, et al. Identification and ablation of macroreentrant ventricular tachycardia with the CARTO electroanatomical mapping system. *Pacing Clin Electrophysiol* 1998;21:1448–1456.
195. Greenspon AJ, Hsu SS, Datorre S. Successful radiofrequency catheter ablation of sustained ventricular tachycardia postmyocardial infarction in man guided by a multielectrode "basket" catheter. *J Cardiovasc Electrophysiol* 1997;8:565–570.
196. Strickberger SA, Knight BP, Michaud GF, et al. Mapping and ablation of ventricular tachycardia guided by virtual electrograms using a noncontact, computerized mapping system. *J Am Coll Cardiol* 2000;35:414–421.
197. Soejima K, Stevenson WG, Maisel WH, et al. Electrically unexcitable scar mapping based on pacing threshold for identification of the reentry circuit isthmus: feasibility for guiding ventricular tachycardia ablation. *Circulation* 2002;106:1678–1683.
198. Arenal A, del Castillo S, Gonzalez-Torrecilla E, et al. Tachycardia-related channel in the scar tissue in patients with sustained monomorphic ventricular tachycardias: influence of the voltage scar definition. *Circulation* 2004;110:2568–2574.
199. Strickberger SA, Man KC, Daoud EG, et al. A prospective evaluation of catheter ablation of ventricular tachycardia as adjuvant therapy in patients with coronary artery disease and an implantable cardioverter-defibrillator. *Circulation* 1997;96:1525–1531.
200. Stevenson WG, Friedman PL, Kocovic D, et al. Radiofrequency catheter ablation of ventricular tachycardia after myocardial infarction. *Circulation* 1998;98:308–314.
201. Scheinman MM. NASPE survey on catheter ablation. *Pacing Clin Electrophysiol* 1995;18:1474–1478.
202. Danford DA, Kugler JD, Deal B, et al. The learning curve for radiofrequency ablation of tachyarrhythmias in pediatric patients: participating members of the Pediatric Electrophysiology Society. *Am J Cardiol* 1995;75:587–590.
203. Rosenheck S, Rose M, Sharon Z, et al. The ongoing influence of staff training on the performance of radiofrequency catheter ablation. *Pacing Clin Electrophysiol* 1997;20:1312–1317.
204. Morady F, Harvey M, Kalbfleisch SJ, et al. Radiofrequency catheter ablation of ventricular tachycardia in patients with coronary artery disease. *Circulation* 1993;87:363–372.
205. Gursoy S, Chiladakis I, Kuck KH. First lessons from radiofrequency catheter ablation in patients with ventricular tachycardia. *Pacing Clin Electrophysiol* 1993;16:687–691.
206. Kim YH, Sosa-Suarez G, Trouton TG, et al. Treatment of ventricular tachycardia by transcatheter radiofrequency ablation in patients with ischemic heart disease. *Circulation* 1994;89:1094–1102.
207. Rothman SA, Hsia HH, Cossu SF, et al. Radiofrequency catheter ablation of postinfarction ventricular tachycardia: long-term success and the significance of inducible nonclinical arrhythmias. *Circulation* 1997;96:3499–3508.
208. Callans DJ, Zado E, Sarter BH, et al. Efficacy of radiofrequency catheter ablation for ventricular tachycardia in healed myocardial infarction. *Am J Cardiol* 1998;82:429–432.
209. Calkins H, Epstein A, Packer D, et al. Catheter ablation of ventricular tachycardia in patients with structural heart disease using cooled radiofrequency energy: results of a prospective multicenter study. Cooled RF Multi Center Investigators Group. *J Am Coll Cardiol* 2000;35:1905–1914.
210. O'Callaghan PA, Poloniecki J, Sosa-Suarez G, et al. Long-term clinical outcome of patients with prior myocardial infarction after palliative radiofrequency catheter ablation for frequent ventricular tachycardia. *Am J Cardiol* 2001;87:975–979.
211. Arenal A, Glez-Torrecilla E, Ortiz M, et al. Ablation of electrograms with an isolated, delayed component as treatment of unmappable monomorphic ventricular tachycardias in patients with structural heart disease. *J Am Coll Cardiol* 2003;41:81–92.
212. Soejima K, Stevenson WG, Sapp JL, et al. Endocardial and epicardial radiofrequency ablation of ventricular tachycardia associated with dilated cardiomyopathy: the importance of low-voltage scars. *J Am Coll Cardiol* 2004;43:1834–1842.
213. Szumowski L, Sanders P, Walczak F, et al. Mapping and ablation of polymorphic ventricular tachycardia after myocardial infarction. *J Am Coll Cardiol* 2004;44:1700–1706.
214. Hindricks G. The Multicentre European Radiofrequency Survey (MERFS): complications of radiofrequency catheter ablation of arrhythmias: the Multicentre European Radiofrequency Survey (MERFS) investigators of the Working Group on Arrhythmias of the European Society of Cardiology. *Eur Heart J* 1993;14:1644–1653.
215. Kok LC, Mangrum JM, Haines DE, et al. Cerebrovascular complication associated with pulmonary vein ablation. *J Cardiovasc Electrophysiol* 2002;13:764–767.
216. Ren JF, Marchlinski FE, Callans DJ. Left atrial thrombus associated with ablation for atrial fibrillation: identification with intracardiac echocardiography. *J Am Coll Cardiol* 2004;43:1861–1867.
217. Saad EB, Rossillo A, Saad CP, et al. Pulmonary vein stenosis after radiofrequency ablation of atrial fibrillation: functional characterization, evolution, and influence of the ablation strategy. *Circulation* 2003;108: 3102–3107.
218. Pappone C, Oral H, Santinelli V, et al. Atrio-esophageal fistula as a complication of percutaneous transcatheter ablation of atrial fibrillation. *Circulation* 2004;109:2724–2726.
219. Rosenthal LS, Mahesh M, Beck TJ, et al. Predictors of fluoroscopy time and estimated radiation exposure during radiofrequency catheter ablation procedures. *Am J Cardiol* 1998;82:451–458.
220. Lickfett L, Mahesh M, Vasamreddy C, et al. Radiation exposure during catheter ablation of atrial fibrillation. *Circulation* 2004;110:3003–3010.
221. Lashus AG, Case CL, Gillette PC. Catheter ablation treatment of supraventricular tachycardia-induced cardiomyopathy. *Arch Pediatr Adolesc Med* 1997;151:264–266.
222. Takemoto M, Yoshimura H, Ohba Y, et al. Radiofrequency catheter ablation of premature ventricular complexes from right ventricular outflow tract improves left ventricular dilation and clinical status in patients without structural heart disease. *J Am Coll Cardiol* 2005;45:1259–1265.
223. Steinberg JS, Sadaniantz A, Kron J, et al. Analysis of cause-specific mortality in the Atrial Fibrillation Follow-up Investigation of Rhythm Management (AFFIRM) study. *Circulation* 2004;109:1973–1980.

CHAPTER 74 ■ CARDIAC PACEMAKERS

MANDEEP BHARGAVA AND BRUCE L. WILKOFF

HISTORY AND OVERVIEW

The cardiac conduction system possesses the unique capability of generating its own electrical rhythm. The sinoatrial (SA) node, located at the junction of the right atrium and the superior vena cava, possesses the fastest rate of spontaneous depolarization and governs the pace of the heart under normal conditions. After traversing the atrial tissue and then the atrioventricular (AV) node, this impulse reaches the ventricles through the specialized conduction fibers of the His bundle, the right and left bundle branches, and the Purkinje fibers. Disorders of the cardiac conduction system at most of these levels can give rise to significant, symptomatic, and often life-threatening bradyarrhythmias. Collaborative efforts of biomedical engineers and clinicians led to the advent of cardiac pacemakers. Initially designed as asynchronous pacing devices for Stokes-Adams attacks, these devices now are fine microprocessors that transmit electrical information back and forth to the heart, store vast amounts of diagnostic and therapeutic information, monitor and regulate their own performance and function, prevent and pace-terminate tachyarrhythmias, and raise alarms when doubts about their malfunction arise.

Pacemakers are an important therapy not only of bradyarrhythmias, but also of other clinical situations based on newly defined roles. Before implantation, the clinician should justify its indication and define the immediate and long-term pacing needs of the patient. With the availability of a wide variety of pacemakers, pacing modes, diagnostic and therapeutic tools, and programming options, a thorough and updated knowledge is important to achieve maximum clinical benefit for the patient.

Pacemakers can be single- or dual-chamber devices. Dual-chamber devices have capabilities for biventricular or biatrial pacing. The expanding role of biventricular devices is considered in greater detail in the chapter on cardiac resynchronization therapy. When determining the most appropriate pacing mode for a patient, the clinician should consider the patient's activity level, need for AV synchrony, need for chronotropic support, need and possibility for preservation of intrinsic AV node conduction, presence of atrial or ventricular arrhythmias, and associated medical conditions.

PACEMAKER NOMENCLATURE

A three-letter code describing the basic function of the various pacing systems was first proposed in 1974 and updated in 2002. Designated the NBG code for pacing nomenclature (1) (Table 74.1), the code has five positions and is generic rather than pertaining to a specific device.

TABLE 74.1

PACEMAKER NOMENCLATURE

Position 1: chamber(s) paced	Position 2: chamber(s) sensed	Position 3: response to sensing	Position 4: rate modulation	Position 5: multisite pacing
O = None	O = None	O = None	O = None	O = None
A = Atrium	A = Atrium	T = Triggered	R = Rate modulation	A = Atrium
V = Ventricle	V = Ventricle	I = Inhibited		V = Ventricle
D = Dual (A + V)	D = Dual (A + V)	D = Dual (T + I)		D = Dual (A + V)
S = Single (A or V)[a]	S = Single (A or V)[a]			

[a] Manufacturer's designation only.
From Bernstein AD, Daubert JC, Fletcher RD, et al, and North American Society of Pacing and Electrophysiology/British Pacing and Electrophysiology Group: the revised NASPE/BPEG generic code for antibradycardia, adaptive-rate, and multisite pacing. *Pacing Clin Electrophysiol* 2002;25:260–264.

The *first position* refers to the chamber(s) in which stimulation occurs: A, atrium; V, ventricle; O, none; and D, dual chamber, that is, both A and V. The *second position* refers to the chamber(s) in which sensing occurs. The letters are the same as those for the first position. Manufacturers may also use S in both the first and second positions to indicate that the device is capable of pacing or sensing only a single cardiac chamber. The *third position* refers to how the pacemaker responds to a sensed event. An I indicates that a sensed event inhibits the output pulse and causes the pacemaker to recycle for one or more timing cycles. A T means that an output pulse is triggered in response to a sensed event. A D means that both T and I responses can occur. This designation is restricted to dual-chamber systems. An event sensed in the atrium inhibits the atrial output but triggers a ventricular output. Unlike a single-chamber–triggered mode (VVT or AAT), in which an output pulse is triggered immediately on sensing, there is a delay between the sensed atrial event and the triggered ventricular output to mimic the normal PR interval. If a native ventricular signal or R wave is sensed, it inhibits the ventricular output and possibly even the atrial output, depending on where sensing occurs.

The *fourth position* of the code reflects both programmability and rate modulation. An R in the fourth position indicates that the pacemaker incorporates a sensor to control the rate independent of intrinsic cardiac activity. Practically, R is the only indicator used in the fourth position, but other indicators described are shown in Table 74.1. The *fifth position* of the code has been changed and is used to describe whether multisite pacing is present in none of the chambers (O), in the atria (A), or in the ventricles (V). Hence, for a patient with multisite ventricular pacing available with rate responsiveness, the code is DDDRV.

GLOSSARY OF PACING MODES AND TIMING CYCLES

AAI/AAIR: Single-chamber atrial pacing modes, with R denoting the capability of rate adaptation.

Atrioventricular interval (AVI): The atrioventricular interval in a dual-chamber pacemaker is the programmed duration following a sensed or paced atrial beat that is allowed before a ventricular pacing impulse is delivered. The initial portion of this interval is the *atrial blanking period*. This is immediately followed by the *cross-talk sensing window*, which is the timing during which cross-talk can occur due to afterpotentials from an atrial output (Fig. 74.1).

Blanking period: An interval during which the sensing circuit of the pacemaker is temporarily disabled following the delivery of an output pulse. This prevents inappropriate sensing of residual energy from the pacemaker output pulse and, in dual-chamber pacemakers, prevents sensing of pacemaker output pulses or intrinsic events in the chamber other than that in which the event occurs. Hence, there could be an *atrial* or a *ventricular blanking period* in response to an atrial or ventricular output, respectively. In a dual-chamber pacemaker, the *postventricular atrial blanking period (PVAB)* refers to the period during which the atrial circuit is disabled after a ventricular sensed or paced event.

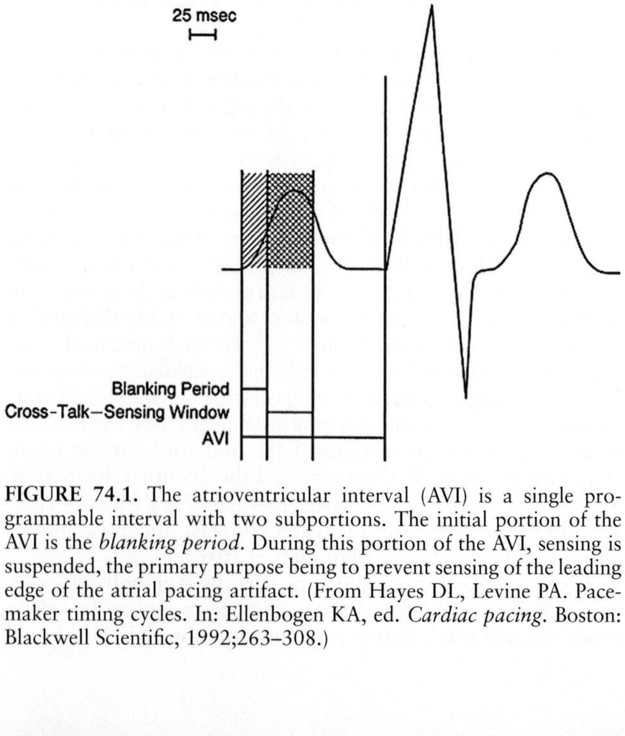

FIGURE 74.1. The atrioventricular interval (AVI) is a single programmable interval with two subportions. The initial portion of the AVI is the *blanking period*. During this portion of the AVI, sensing is suspended, the primary purpose being to prevent sensing of the leading edge of the atrial pacing artifact. (From Hayes DL, Levine PA. Pacemaker timing cycles. In: Ellenbogen KA, ed. *Cardiac pacing*. Boston: Blackwell Scientific, 1992;263–308.)

Cross-talk: In dual-chamber pacemakers, after delivery of a pacing impulse in one chamber, the afterpotentials may be of sufficient strength and duration to be sensed in the other chamber. This is referred to as cross-talk. It can rarely be seen in the ventricles after an atrial impulse but is less likely to occur in the atrium because it may be buffered by the PVAB or the PVARP.

DDD/DDDR: Dual-chamber pacing modes, with R denoting the capability of rate adaptation.

Functional pacing abnormalities (e.g., functional undersensing or functional failure to capture): Failure to sense or capture that is appropriate because of imposed pacemaker refractory periods or myocardial refractoriness due to a previous intrinsic atrial or ventricular event.

Refractory period: The interval during which a given sensing circuit detects but does not respond to any sensed event in that chamber, that is, *the atrial or ventricular refractory periods*. During the *postventricular atrial refractory period (PVARP),* the atrial-sensing circuit is refractory following a sensed or paced ventricular event. The purpose of this is to avoid sensing of retrograde atrial activity after ventricular activation that could initiate an endless-loop tachycardia.

Total atrial refractory period: The period during which the atrial channel of a dual-chamber or VDD pacemaker ignores intrinsic atrial activity or other activity sensed on the atrial-sensing circuit. This is usually a combination of the atrioventricular interval and the postventricular atrial refractory period.

Ventricular safety pacing: The delivery of a ventricular output pulse, following atrial pacing, if a signal is sensed by the ventricular channel during the early portion of the AV interval (AVI), which is the *cross-talk window*. This is to ensure that ventricular depolarization is not inhibited by cross-talk and occurs even if the sensed event was something other than an intrinsic ventricular depolarization (Fig. 74.2).

VVI/VVIR: Single-chamber ventricular pacing modes, with R referring to the capability of rate adaptation.

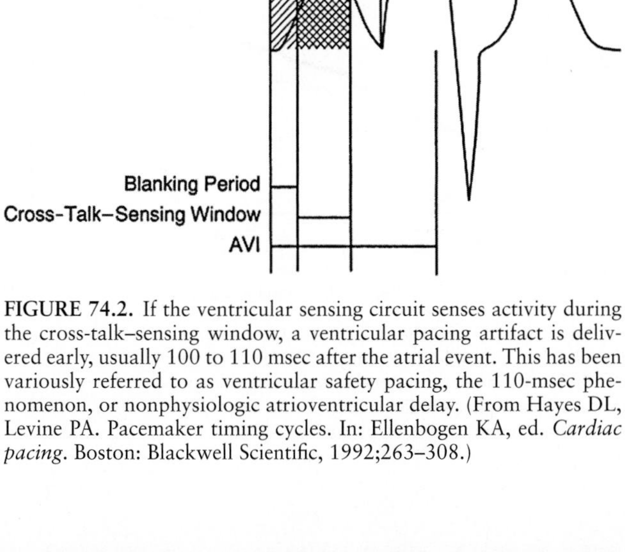

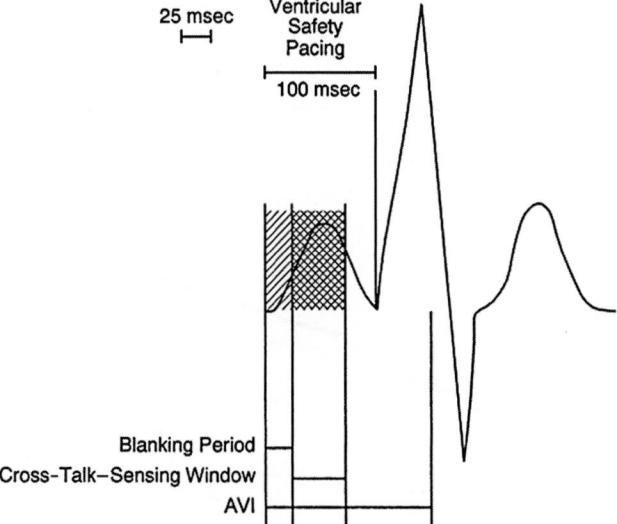

FIGURE 74.2. If the ventricular sensing circuit senses activity during the cross-talk–sensing window, a ventricular pacing artifact is delivered early, usually 100 to 110 msec after the atrial event. This has been variously referred to as ventricular safety pacing, the 110-msec phenomenon, or nonphysiologic atrioventricular delay. (From Hayes DL, Levine PA. Pacemaker timing cycles. In: Ellenbogen KA, ed. *Cardiac pacing*. Boston: Blackwell Scientific, 1992;263–308.)

INDICATIONS OF CARDIAC PACING

The American Heart Association/American College of Cardiology (AHA/ACC) guidelines classify pacing indications into three categories, namely those in which pacing is generally indicated, may be indicated, and is not indicated (2). The most common are bradyarrhythmic causes such as those from sinus node dysfunction, neurocardiogenic syncope, acquired or congenital AV block, chronic bifascicular, and trifascicular block. The nonbradycardic causes of pacing such as atrial fibrillation, hypertrophic and dilated cardiomyopathy, congestive heart failure, and long-QT syndrome are discussed separately.

Sinus Node Dysfunction

Significant sinus bradycardia is generally accepted as rate less than 40 beats per minute during waking hours. Pacing is indicated in patients with symptomatic or significant sinus node dysfunction. Sinus bradycardia, sinus pauses or arrest, and sinoatrial exit block are the usual variants of sinus node dysfunction. The rate at which pacing is indicated is debatable, but in general it is considered beneficial in patients with symptoms consistent with bradycardia. Although every patient needs to be considered individually, most clinicians agree that sinus pauses of 3 seconds or more during waking hours should be considered abnormal and may warrant pacing. Pauses that occur during sleep are more difficult to categorize. Because of vagal influences, many healthy persons may have pauses longer than 3 seconds during sleep. In the absence of symptoms or rhythm disturbances during waking hours, this should not require treatment. Permanent pacing should be considered for any patient who has symptomatic bradyarrhythmia when the cause is not reversible. Reversible sinus node dysfunction can be noted in situations such as the postoperative stages of cardiac surgery, rarely after an acute myocardial infarction, or a myocarditis.

Permanent pacing for patients with sinus node dysfunction after myocardial infarction is reserved for those who have symptoms. If drug therapy results in symptomatic bradycardia, criteria for permanent pacing should follow the guidelines given for sinus node dysfunction in Table 74.2. Paroxysmal episodes of atrial arrhythmias, most commonly atrial fibrillation and atrial flutter, can be interspersed with periods of significant sinus node dysfunction, the commonly noted diagnosis of tachycardia-bradycardia syndrome. This is most notable in the postconversion phase after either a spontaneous or an electrical cardioversion. Apart from producing symptoms, it makes drug therapy a more challenging task. Such patients are often best managed with conjunctive pacemaker therapy. Patients with chronic atrial fibrillation could also have slow ventricular rates due to AV nodal–blocking drugs or complete AV block, in either situation requiring a pacemaker.

Another manifestation of sinus node dysfunction could be the inability to achieve at least 80% of the predicted heart rate with exercise, leading to chronotropic incompetence. In such situations the resting heart rates may be normal, but patients become symptomatic with effort and can improve significantly with rate-responsive pacing.

Various clinical trials studied the relative benefits of single- and dual-chamber pacemakers in patients with sinus node dysfunction. Some of these trials also included patients with AV block. In a small study of 225 patients, Andersen et al. (3) were the first to suggest that atrial pacing may be superior to ventricular pacing in patients with sinus node dysfunction. They showed a reduction in atrial fibrillation, thromboembolism,

TABLE 74.2

RECOMMENDATIONS FOR PERMANENT PACING IN PATIENTS WITH SINUS NODE DYSFUNCTION

Class I

1. Sinus node dysfunction with symptomatic sinus bradycardia or frequently symptomatic sinus pauses. This includes iatrogenic sinus bradycardia from essential long-term drug therapy without acceptable alternatives.
2. Symptomatic chronotropic incompetence.

Class IIa

1. Sinus node dysfunction occurring spontaneously or as a result of necessary drug therapy with heart rates less than 40 beats per minute when a clear association between significant symptoms consistent with bradycardia and actual presence of bradycardia has not been documented.
2. Recurrent syncope of unexplained origin when major abnormalities of sinus node dysfunction are discovered or provoked during an electrophysiologic study.

Class IIb

1. Minimally symptomatic patients with chronic heart rates of less than 40 beats per minute when awake.

Class III

1. Sinus node dysfunction in asymptomatic patients including those in whom substantial sinus bradycardia (heart rates <40 beats per minute) is a consequence of long-term drug therapy.
2. Sinus node dysfunction in patients with symptoms suggestive of bradycardia that are clearly documented as not associated with a slow heart rate.
3. Sinus node dysfunction with symptomatic bradycardia due to nonessential drug therapy.

Adapted from ACC/AHA/NASPE Guidelines for Pacing, 2002 (2).

and cardiovascular mortality in patients with atrial pacing compared with ventricular pacing. However, larger trials, like the Canadian Trial of Physiologic Pacing (CTOPP) (4) and the MOde Selection Trial in sinus node dysfunction (MOST) (5), did show a lower incidence of atrial fibrillation with atrial or dual-chamber pacing but failed to show any significant benefit in terms or cardiovascular mortality or the risk of stroke. These effects were sustained even on longer follow-up (6) (Fig. 74.3). In patients older than the age of 65 years, the PASE (Pacemaker Selection in the Elderly) trial showed no change in the quality of life, mortality, atrial fibrillation (AF), or stroke (7). In the ongoing Danish Pacing Trial (DANPACE) (8), patients with tachycardia-bradycardia syndrome with normal AV conduction are being assessed for any differences in all-cause and cardiovascular mortality, AF, quality of life, incidence of atrial fibrillation and thromboembolism, and cost-effectiveness with AAIR versus DDDR pacing.

With the recent recognition of the importance of dyssynchrony in patients with heart failure and the benefits of resynchronization therapy (9,10), electrophysiologists have become increasingly aggressive in avoiding inadvertent ventricular pacing in patients with intact AV node function. This is especially true for patients with existing left ventricular dysfunction, in whom the reasons for avoiding pacing-induced dyssynchrony are more obvious. The increased mortality associated with the DDDR mode in implantable cardioverter-defibrillator (ICD) patients, most likely from ventricular pacing, has been established in the DAVID trial (11). When patients with left ventricular dysfunction are given dual-chamber devices for sinus node dysfunction, aggressive efforts are made to prolong the AV

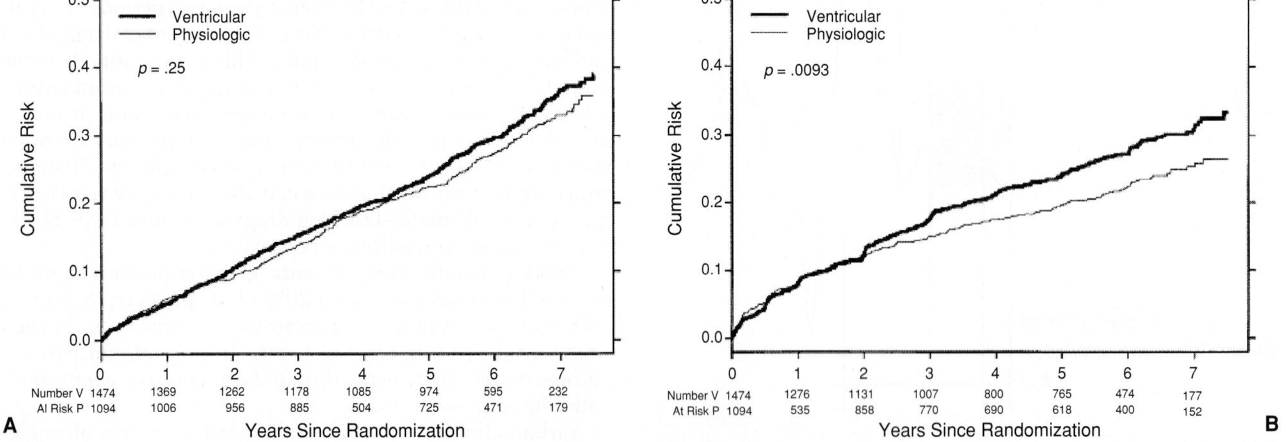

FIGURE 74.3. Cumulative risk of cardiovascular death and stroke (**A**) and the risk of atrial fibrillation (**B**) over a mean of 6.4 years follow-up in the Canadian Trial of Physiologic Pacing (CTOPP) trial in patients with ventricular pacing (V) versus physiologic pacing (P). Although the latter showed no significant difference, the risk of atrial fibrillation was significantly reduced with physiologic pacing. (From Kerr CR, Connolly SJ, Abdollah H, et al. Canadian Trial of Physiologic Pacing: effects of physiologic pacing on long term follow up. *Circulation* 2004;109:357–362.)

TABLE 74.3

INDICATIONS FOR CARDIAC PACING IN PATIENTS WITH CAROTID SINUS HYPERSENSITIVITY AND NEUROCARDIOGENIC SYNCOPE

Class I
1. Recurrent syncope caused by carotid sinus stimulation; minimal carotid sinus pressure induces ventricular asystole of duration more than 3 seconds in the absence of any medication that depresses the sinus node or atrioventricular conduction.

Class IIa
1. Recurrent syncope without clear, provocative events and with a hypersensitive cardioinhibitory response.
2. Significantly symptomatic and recurrent neurocardiogenic syncope associated with bradycardia documented spontaneously or at the time of tilt-table testing.

Class III
1. Hyperactive cardioinhibitory response to carotid sinus stimulation in the absence of symptoms or in the presence of vague symptoms such as dizziness, lightheadedness, or both.
2. Recurrent syncope, lightheadedness, or dizziness in the absence of a hyperactive cardioinhibitory response.
3. Situational vasovagal syncope in which avoidance behavior is effective.

Adapted from ACC/AHA/NASPE Guidelines for Pacing, 2002 (2).

delay enough to promote intrinsic conduction in patients with normal AV node function. Even in patients with borderline AV node function, newer devices use algorithms like AV search hysteresis, auto-intrinsic search, and managed ventricular pacing (MVP) to avoid ventricular pacing as much as possible.

Carotid Sinus Hypersensitivity and Neurocardiogenic Syncope

Although they are not related to any intrinsic sinus node dysfunction, these two syndromes could result in profound inhibition of the SA node. Both are characterized by a variable degree of cardioinhibitory and vasodepressor response, and most often a combination of the two. Permanent pacemakers may be indicated in patients with such neurally mediated syncope (12) and are especially useful in patients with a cardioinhibitory response.

In patients with carotid sinus hypersensitivity (CSH), carotid stimulation could produce sinus arrest, sinus pauses of 5 to 10 seconds, or even AV block lasting for greater than 3 seconds. In patients with a vasodepressor response, there could be a symptomatic fall in the systolic blood pressure by more than 50 mm Hg. Many patients may have a mixed response. For patients with a cardioinhibitory response, a permanent pacemaker could be beneficial (13) if they do not have improvement after removal of precipitating factors such as shaving, wearing tight collars, looking up, being subjected to the Valsalva maneuver, and so on. Because the intense vagal output may often cause AV block, the backup of ventricular pacing is essential, and hence these patients need a dual-chamber pacemaker.

The recommendations for pacing in patients with neurocardiogenic syncope have undergone significant evolution. As discussed in other chapters, patients with neurocardiogenic syncope can also have a cardioinhibitory, vasodepressor, or mixed response. In the initial North American Vasovagal Pacemaker Study I (VPS-I) (14), the trial had to be prematurely terminated due to the significantly lower incidence of syncope in patients with pacemakers versus those without pacing (17% vs. 59%). The Vasovagal Syncope International Study (VASIS) (15) also showed reduced syncopal episodes in patients with pacemakers (5% vs. 61%). Even when compared with β-blockers, which are often considered the first-line therapy, pacemakers were shown to be superior in the Syncope Diagnosis and Treatment Study (16). In contrast, the Vasovagal Syncope and Pacing study (SYNPACE) (17) and the more recent Vasovagal Pacemaker Study II (VPS II) (18) failed to show any superiority of the pacemaker therapy. Unlike the other trials, in these two trials, pacemakers were implanted even in the control group of patients but were essentially programmed to a nonpacing mode. This suggests that part of the benefit in the other trials may have been a placebo effect. The ongoing Syncope and Falls in the Elderly Pacing and Carotid Sinus Evaluation (SAFE-PACE 2) study is also looking for the possible benefits of permanent pacing in patients with neurocardiogenic syncope (19).

The recommendations for pacing in these two syndromes are summarized in Table 74.3. Because these patients have a sudden drop in heart rate, algorithms such as "rate drop," "rate hysteresis," "rate smoothing," "flywheel," and so on are useful in enhancing the benefits of a pacemaker in these situations. These options prevent a sudden drop in heart rate to the lower rate of the pacemaker and can prevent symptoms not only of absolute, but also of relative bradycardia.

Chronic Bifascicular or Trifascicular Block

Disorders of conduction at the level of the branches of the His-Purkinje system are referred to as bundle branch blocks or intraventricular conduction defects. In patients with isolated right- or left-bundle-branch block (RBBB or LBBB, respectively), the risk of progression to advanced AV block is rare and pacing is not usually indicated. Patients with a bifascicular block (RBBB with a left anterior or posterior hemiblock or a LBBB with a left-axis deviation) have a 6% incidence of progression to complete heart block (20). If such patients have intermittent advanced AV block, alternating RBBB and LBBB, or complete heart block, pacing is indicated even if they are asymptomatic. If these patients have symptoms like presyncope/syncope without a demonstrable cause, it continues to be a class II indication for pacing. Permanent pacing may also be beneficial for patients with evidence of His-Purkinje disease on electrophysiologic study [e.g., an HV interval $\geq$100 msec, or infra His block with atrial pacing (21)]. The recommendations for pacing in patients with fascicular block as per the 2002 guidelines are summarized in Table 74.4.

The development of a new intraventricular conduction disturbance with a first-degree AV block in a patient with acute myocardial infarction (MI) has a 40% risk of progression to complete heart block. In such patients, temporary pacing is certainly indicated, and many believe that permanent pacing is also needed (22). Intraventricular conduction disturbances

TABLE 74.4

RECOMMENDATIONS FOR PERMANENT PACING IN PATIENTS WITH CHRONIC BIFASICULAR AND TRIFASCICULAR BLOCK

Class I
1. Intermittent third-degree atrioventricular (AV) block.
2. Type II second-degree AV block.
3. Alternating bundle-branch block.

Class IIa
1. Syncope not demonstrated to be due to AV block when other likely causes have been excluded, specifically ventricular tachycardia.
2. Incidental finding at electrophysiologic study of markedly prolonged HV interval ($\geq$100 msec) in asymptomatic patients.
3. Incidental finding at electrophysiologic study of pacing-induced infra-His block that is not physiologic.

Class IIb
1. Neuromuscular diseases such as myotonic muscular dystrophy, Kearns-Sayre syndrome, Erb's dystrophy (limb-girdle), and peroneal muscular atrophy with any degree of fascicular block with or without symptoms because there may be unpredictable progression of AV conduction disease.

Class III
1. Fascicular block without AV block or symptoms.
2. Fascicular block with first-degree AV block without symptoms.

Adapted from ACC/AHA/NASPE Guidelines for Pacing, 2002 (2).

carry a poor prognosis in the presence of neuromuscular dystrophies or with structural heart disease such as ischemic or dilated cardiomyopathy. In a large majority of these patients, ICD or cardiac resynchronization therapy (CRT) may be indicated (as discussed in other chapters). In others, a close watch may be warranted due to the unpredictable rate or progression of the disease. For fascicular blocks in asymptomatic patients with normal hearts, pacing is not indicated. The recommendations for permanent pacing in patients with an acute MI are summarized in Table 74.5.

Congenital Complete Heart Block

There are various reasons for the gradual decline in the threshold used to decide whether to pace patients with congenital complete heart block even if they are asymptomatic. They have been shown to have unpredictable syncope, significant mortality, gradual decline in heart rates, and a high incidence of acquired mitral regurgitation. The timing for pacemaker insertion has always been a question.

In pediatric patients with congenital complete heart block, pacemaker implantation is recommended for patients with congestive heart failure, patients with an average heart rate less than 50 beats per minute while awake, and patients with a history of syncope or presyncope, significant ventricular ectopy, or exercise intolerance (23). In adults, we recommend pacing in all patients with congenital complete heart block due to the foregoing factors. The other indications for pacing in patients with congenital heart disease as per the ACC guidelines are summarized in Table 74.6.

Acquired Atrioventricular Block

Traditionally, AV block is classified as first-, second,- or third-degree (also complete) heart block. Alternatively, it can be defined anatomically/physiologically as supra-, intra-, or

TABLE 74.5

RECOMMENDATIONS FOR PERMANENT PACING AFTER THE ACUTE PHASE OF MYOCARDIAL INFARCTION

Class I
1. Persistent second-degree atrioventricular (AV) block in the His-Purkinje system with bilateral bundle-branch block or third-degree AV block within or below the His-Purkinje system after acute myocardial infarction.
2. Transient advanced (second- or third-degree) infranodal AV block and associated bundle-branch block. If the site of block is uncertain, an electrophysiologic study may be necessary.
3. Persistent and symptomatic second- or third-degree AV block.

Class IIb
1. Persistent second- or third-degree AV block at the AV node level.

Class III
1. Transient AV block in the absence of intraventricular conduction defects.
2. Transient AV block in the presence of isolated left anterior fascicular block.
3. Acquired left anterior fascicular block in the absence of AV block.
4. Persistent first-degree AV block in the presence of bundle-branch block that is old or age indeterminate.

Adapted from ACC/AHA/NASPE Guidelines for Pacing, 2002 (2).

TABLE 74.6

RECOMMENDATIONS FOR PERMANENT PACING IN PATIENTS WITH CONGENITAL HEART DISEASE

Class I
1. Advanced second- or third-degree atrioventricular (AV) block associated with symptomatic bradycardia, ventricular dysfunction, or low cardiac output.
2. Sinus node dysfunction with correlation of symptoms during age-inappropriate bradycardia. The definition of bradycardia varies with the patient's age and expected heart rate.
3. Postoperative advanced second- or third-degree AV block that is not expected to resolve or persists at least 7 days after cardiac surgery.
4. Congenital third-degree AV block with a wide QRS escape rhythm, complex ventricular ectopy, or ventricular dysfunction.
5. Congenital third-degree AV block in an infant with a ventricular rate less than 50 to 55 beats per minute or with congenital heart disease and a ventricular rate less than 70 beats per minute.
6. Sustained pause-dependent VT, with or without prolonged QT, in which the efficacy of pacing is thoroughly documented.

Class IIa
1. Bradycardia-tachycardia syndrome with the need for long-term antiarrhythmic treatment other than digitalis.
2. Congenital third-degree AV block beyond the first year of life with an average heart rate less than 50 beats per minute, abrupt pauses in ventricular rate that are two or three times the basic cycle length, or associated with symptoms due to chronotropic incompetence.
3. Long-QT syndrome with 2:1 AV or third-degree AV block.
4. Asymptomatic sinus bradycardia in a child with complex congenital heart disease with resting heart rate less than 40 beats per minute or pauses in ventricular rate more than 3 seconds.
5. Patients with congenital heart disease and impaired hemodynamics due to sinus bradycardia or loss of AV synchrony.

Class IIb
1. Transient postoperative third-degree AV block that reverts to sinus rhythm with residual bifascicular block.
2. Congenital third-degree AV block in an asymptomatic infant, child, adolescent, or young adult with an acceptable rate, narrow QRS complex, and normal ventricular function.
3. Asymptomatic sinus bradycardia in an adolescent with congenital heart disease with resting heart rate less than 40 beats per minute or pauses in ventricular rate more than 3 seconds.
4. Neuromuscular diseases with any degree of AV block (including first-degree AV block), with or without symptoms, because there may be unpredictable progression of AV conduction disease.

Class III
1. Transient postoperative AV block with return of normal AV conduction.
2. Asymptomatic postoperative bifascicular block with or without first-degree AV block.
3. Asymptomatic type I second-degree AV block.
4. Asymptomatic sinus bradycardia in an adolescent with longest RR interval less than 3 seconds and minimum heart rate more than 40 beats per minute.

Adapted from ACC/AHA/NASPE Guidelines for Pacing, 2002 (2).

infra-Hisian. If the QRS is wide and the conducted P waves have a normal PR interval, there is a greater probability that the conduction disturbance is infra-Hisian. Most commonly, acquired AV block is idiopathic and related to aging, but it has many potential causes, as discussed in other chapters. The recommendations for permanent pacing in acquired AV block are listed in Table 74.7. In general, pacing is indicated in all patients with complete heart block, symptomatic patients with second-degree AV block, and asymptomatic patients with advanced second-degree AV block if the pauses are greater than 3 seconds or the escape rates are less than 40 beats per minute when awake.

Indications for permanent pacing for AV block that occurs with acute myocardial infarction are more controversial. Generally, a pacemaker is indicated for complete AV block, Mobitz II AV block, or bilateral and alternating bundle branch blocks that persist longer than 72 hours after the acute event. Some clinicians consider new and persistent bifascicular block an indication for pacing, whether or not it is associated with transient supra- or infra-Hisian AV block. Such criteria may be more lenient after an anterior wall MI because conduction disturbances after an inferior wall MI have a better prognosis. An isolated hemiblock of one of the left-sided fascicles, an isolated transient AV conduction disturbance without a residual intraventricular conduction disturbance, transient AV conduction disturbance with new-onset left anterior or left posterior hemiblock, or a first-degree or Mobitz I block with a preexisting bundle branch block are more gray areas, but would generally not be strong indications for a pacemaker in an asymptomatic patient.

It would appear that dual-chamber pacing is the most physiologic mode of pacing in patients with AV block. With the known adverse effects of right ventricular pacing, it may be wise to consider options to avoid ventricular pacing as much as possible in patients with left ventricular dysfunction if they have intermittent AV block. In patients with class III and IV heart failure, it may be reasonable to consider a biventricular pacemaker if they have a left ventricular ejection fraction (LVEF) of 35% or less and a left ventricular end-diastolic dimension (LVEDD) of greater than 55 mm.

Even in patients with a normal LV systolic function, dual-chamber pacing appears to be most physiologic. The CTOPP (6) and PASE (7) trials discussed earlier included patients with sick sinus syndrome and AV block. Although these trials failed to show any benefit in survival, there were significant improvements with regard to quality of life and incidences of atrial fibrillation and thromboembolism. The United Kingdom Pacing and Cardiovascular Events (UKPACE) trial (24) included patients with AV block older than the age of 70 years and studied the effect of dual-chamber versus single-chamber pacemakers

TABLE 74.7

RECOMMENDATIONS FOR PERMANENT PACING IN PATIENTS WITH ACQUIRED BLOCK IN ADULTS

Class I
1. Third-degree and advanced second-degree atrioventricular (AV) block at any anatomic level, associated with any one of the following conditions:
   a. Bradycardia with symptoms (including heart failure) presumed to be due to AV block.
   b. Arrhythmias and other medical conditions that require drugs that result in symptomatic bradycardia.
   c. Documented periods of asystole greater than or equal to 3.0 seconds or any escape rate less than 40 beats per minute in awake, symptom-free patients.
   d. After catheter ablation of the AV junction.
   e. Postoperative AV block not expected to resolve after cardiac surgery.
   f. Neuromuscular diseases with AV block, such as myotonic muscular dystrophy, Kearns-Sayre syndrome, Erb's dystrophy (limb-girdle), and peroneal muscular atrophy, with or without symptoms, because there may be unpredictable progression of AV conduction disease.
2. Second-degree AV block regardless of type or site of block, with associated symptomatic bradycardia.

Class IIa
1. Asymptomatic third-degree AV block at any anatomic site with average awake ventricular rates of 40 beats per minute or faster especially if cardiomegaly or left ventricular dysfunction is present.
2. Asymptomatic type II second-degree AV block with a narrow QRS. When type II second-degree AV block occurs with a wide QRS, pacing becomes a class I recommendation.
3. Asymptomatic type I second-degree AV block at intra- or infra-His levels found at electrophysiologic study performed for other indications.
4. First- or second-degree AV block with symptoms similar to those of pacemaker syndrome.

Class IIb
1. Marked first-degree AV block (>0.30 seconds) in patients with LV dysfunction and symptoms of congestive heart failure in whom a shorter AV interval results in hemodynamic improvement, presumably by decreasing left atrial filling pressure.
2. Neuromuscular diseases such as myotonic diseases such as myotonic muscular dystrophy, Kearns-Sayre syndrome, Erb's dystrophy (limb-girdle), and peroneal muscular atrophy with any degree of AV block (including first-degree AV block), with or without symptoms, because there may be unpredictable progression of AV conduction disease.

Class III
1. Asymptomatic first-degree AV block.
2. Asymptomatic type I second-degree AV block at the supra-His (AV node) level or not known to be intra- or infra-Hisian.
3. AV block expected to resolve and/or unlikely to recur (e.g., drug toxicity, Lyme disease, or during hypoxia in sleep apnea syndrome in absence of symptoms).

Adapted from ACC/AHA/NASPE Guidelines for Pacing, 2002 (2).

on all-cause mortality and the composite endpoints of cardiovascular deaths, heart failure hospitalizations, atrial fibrillation, strokes, and reoperations. No difference was observed in any of the endpoints in the two groups.

One could argue that most of the patients enrolled in these trials were of a much older age. Our policy is to offer a dual-chamber pacemaker to all patients with complete heart block unless they have underlying chronic atrial fibrillation with no plans to pursue a rhythm control strategy. This is especially true for younger patients. The atrial lead could be beneficial in providing an additional atrial boost, avoiding pacemaker syndrome, and also taking care of any accompanying sinus node dysfunction. In addition to physiologic pacing, it also monitors the rhythm disturbances in the atrium.

Nonbradyarrhythmic Indications for Pacing

Hypertrophic Obstructive Cardiomyopathy

Dynamic left ventricular outflow obstruction occurs in 25% patients with hypertrophic cardiomyopathy. This occurs as a result of a Venturi effect created from a combination of asymmetric septal hypertrophy and a systolic anterior motion of the mitral valve. Dual-chamber pacing with a negative AV hysteresis has been used to alter the sequence of activation of the ventricles. Right ventricular apical pacing results in preexcitation of the interventricular septum, causing it to move away from the left ventricular outflow tract. This results in a reduction of the gradient and improvement in symptoms (Fig. 74.4). A short AV timing is critical to the achievement of an optimal hemodynamic improvement. Although some patients with hypertrophic obstructive cardiomyopathy have optimal improvement with a very short AV interval, others may have hemodynamic deterioration if the AV interval is too short. Some authors have even advocated AV nodal ablation to ensure ventricular depolarization via the pacing stimulus (25).

Fananapazir et al. were the first to show short- and long-term benefits of dual-chamber pacing in patients with hypertrophic obstructive cardiomyopathy (26,27). In the Pacing in Cardiomyopathy (PIC) study, a multicenter, randomized, crossover study, dual-chamber pacing resulted in a 50% decrease of the left ventricular outflow tract gradient, a 21% increase in exercise duration, and improvement in New York Heart Association (NYHA) functional class compared with baseline status (28).

In another randomized, double-blinded, crossover study, the Multicenter Study of Pacing Therapy for Hypertrophic Cardiomyopathy (M-PATHY) trial, no significant differences were evident with randomization between pacing and no pacing,

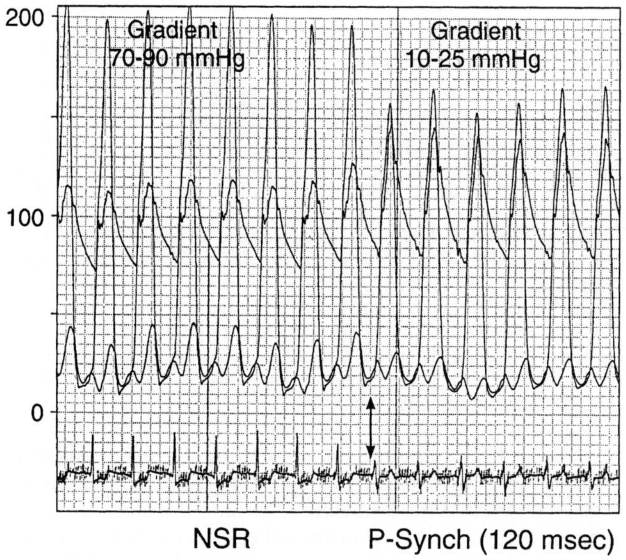

FIGURE 74.4. Hemodynamic tracing demonstrating left ventricular outflow gradient reduction during a temporary pacing study. During normal sinus rhythm (NSR), the patient exhibits marked left ventricular outflow obstruction, with a gradient of 70 to 90 mm Hg. With initiation of P-synchronous pacing (P-Synch) at an atrioventricular interval of 120 msec, the gradient is decreased to 10 to 25 mm Hg. (From Symanski JD, Nishimura RA. The use of pacemakers in the treatment of cardiomyopathies. *Curr Probl Cardiol* 1996;21:385–443.)

either subjectively or objectively, when exercise capacity, quality-of-life score, treadmill exercise time, and peak oxygen consumption were compared (29). The investigators concluded that pacing should not be regarded as a primary treatment for hypertrophic obstructive cardiomyopathy (HOCM), and subjective benefit without objective evidence of improvement should be interpreted cautiously. At our institute, surgical myectomy and septal ablation remain the preferred treatment for symptomatic patients with HOCM, and pacing may only be used as an ACC recommended class IIb indication for patients with a significant gradient who are refractory to other therapies.

Dilated Cardiomyopathy

Dual-chamber pacing has been tried in patients with dilated cardiomyopathy with the aim of optimizing the AV delay to improve the cardiac output. In addition, it was hypothesized that correction of intraventricular conduction disturbances might result in clinical improvement. However, the DAVID trial established that the DDDR mode in ICD patients, presumably from the RV pacing in patients with dilated cardiomyopathy, may not only be unnecessary, but also could rather be detrimental (11).

Permanent pacing in these patients is now restricted to conduction system defects of the sinus and AV node. However, patients with dilated cardiomyopathy often have a wide QRS causing conduction delay, which has been attributed to causing intraventricular dyssynchrony. Resynchronizing myocardial contraction using biventricular pacing has been shown to benefit such patients, not only through symptomatic improvement (30), but also by reducing heart failure hospitalization and reducing overall and cardiovascular mortality (10). The benefits are further enhanced by combining this therapy with defibrillators (9). Studies are ongoing to assess the benefit of such therapy in patients with a normal QRS duration but with echocardiographic evidence of mechanical dyssynchrony.

Pacing for the Prevention of Atrial Fibrillation

Overdriving the sinus rate with atrial pacing has been the subject of multiple investigations. This is done by increasing the base rate of a dual-chamber pacemaker, using a sensor to increase the percentage of atrial-paced versus sensed rhythm or a special algorithm that consistently maintains sinus rhythm. This concept has been supported by the Danish (3) and CTOPP trials (6).

Multisite and alternate-site pacing are under investigation for the prevention of recurrence of atrial fibrillation, presumably by reducing the dispersion of refractoriness in the atrium. For dual-site pacing, one lead is placed in the right atrium and the other at the ostium of the coronary sinus. Standard dual-chamber pacemakers are used with atrial leads that feed into a Y-adapter and are connected to the atrial port of the generator. Dual-site atrial pacing may offer some additional benefits over single-site atrial pacing as shown in the study by the Design and Implementation of the Dual Site Atrial Pacing to Prevent Atrial Fibrillation (DAPPAF) investigators (31).

Active single-site pacing also shows some promise for reducing atrial fibrillation burden. Both pacing at specific locations such as the Bachman's bundle and overdrive pacing techniques have been effective. Multiple algorithms have been used in contemporary pacemakers, with up to four different algorithms in certain pacemakers. Clinical benefit has been shown in the Atrial Dynamic Overdrive Pacing Trial (ADOPT) (32) and the Atrial Fibrillation Therapy (AFT) trial (European Society of Cardiology, 2002). Other studies have not shown such significant benefit (33). Although clinical trials are ongoing (34,35), pacing to prevent atrial fibrillation needs to be considered an adjunctive therapy in most patients, particularly with the promising results of ablation therapies for atrial fibrillation.

Long-QT Syndrome

This syndrome is characterized by genetic ion-channel pathologies that prolong ventricular repolarization. This causes QTc prolongation and puts patients with these conditions at risk of developing life-threatening ventricular arrhythmias. These are often triggered by periods of significant bradycardia, and such patients have been shown to benefit from therapeutic options like permanent pacemakers and cervical sympathectomy.

PACING MODES AND TIMING CYCLES

In selecting the optimal pacing mode, the patient's overall physical condition, associated medical problems, exercise capacity, and chronotropic response to exercise must be considered in conjunction with the underlying rhythm disturbance. Due consideration should be given to the effect of the pacing mode on the long-term morbidity and mortality. Although some of the data are retrospective, the benefits of physiologic pacing with DDD and AAI pacing are difficult to ignore when compared with the VVI mode. Accompanying this is the lower incidence of atrial fibrillation and possibly thromboembolism. The various pacing modes and their respective timing cycles are discussed in what follows, including their advantages and disadvantages in various clinical situations.

Single-Chamber–Triggered Pacing (AAT or VVT)

Single-chamber–triggered pacing (AAT and VVT) releases an output pulse every time a native event is sensed. This feature

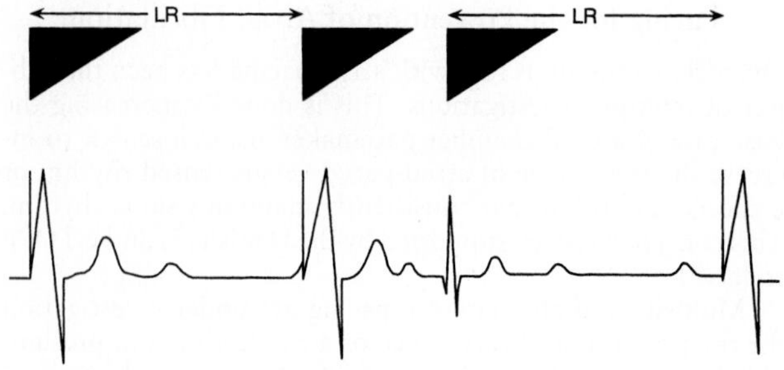

FIGURE 74.5. The VVI timing cycle consists of a defined lower-rate (LR) limit and a ventricular refractory period (*black triangle*). When the LR-limit timer is complete, a pacing artifact is delivered in the absence of a sensed intrinsic ventricular event. If an intrinsic QRS occurs, the LR-limit timer is started from that point. A ventricular refractory period begins with any sensed or paced ventricular activity. (From Hayes DL, Levine PA. Pacemaker timing cycles. In: Ellenbogen KA, ed. *Cardiac pacing*. Boston: Blackwell Scientific, 1992:263–308.)

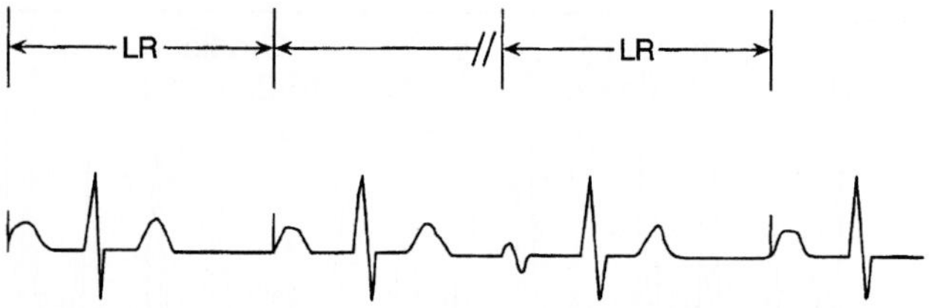

FIGURE 74.6. The AAI timing cycle consists of a defined lower-rate (LR) limit and an atrial refractory period. When the LR-limit timer is complete, a pacing artifact is delivered in the atrium in the absence of a sensed atrial event. If an intrinsic P wave occurs, the LR-limit timer is started from that point. An atrial refractory period begins with any sensed or paced atrial activity. (From Hayes DL, Levine PA. Pacemaker timing cycles. In: Ellenbogen KA, ed. *Cardiac pacing*. Boston: Blackwell Scientific, 1992:263–308.)

increases the current drain on the battery, accelerates its rate of depletion, and deforms the native signal, thus compromising interpretation of the electrocardiogram. However, it can serve as an excellent marker for the site of sensing within an intrinsic complex and can prevent inappropriate inhibition from oversensing when the patient does not have a stable native escape rhythm. In addition, it can be used for noninvasive electrophysiologic studies, with the already implanted pacemaker tracking chest wall stimuli created by a programmable stimulator. It is infrequently used in clinical situations.

Ventricular-Inhibited Pacing (VVI)

Ventricular-inhibited pacing (VVI) incorporates pacing and sensing on the ventricular channel, and pacemaker output is inhibited by a sensed ventricular event (Fig. 74.5). The *lower-rate interval* corresponds to the programmed pacing rate. The *ventricular refractory period* is a programmable interval during which ventricular events do not reset the ventricular timer. If there is no sensed event after the VRP, a pacing output is delivered after the lower rate interval.

The VVI pacing mode is protective against lethal bradycardias, and its economy makes it the most commonly used mode worldwide. As in the UKPACE trial (24), it has been shown to be an equivalent mode of pacing in elderly patients, but in many patients it does have limitations. It fails to restore AV synchrony, and there is no rate responsiveness with activity. Although the results of AV dyssynchrony may be apparent in only a few patients, the adverse hemodynamics can result in overt symptoms or limit the patient's ability to achieve optimal functional status, referred to as *pacemaker syndrome* (discussed later). The VVI pacing mode, especially when equipped with rate responsiveness, is adequate for patients with chronic atrial fibrillation and need for pacing.

Atrial-Inhibited Pacing (AAI)

Atrial-inhibited pacing (AAI) incorporates the same timing cycles as VVI, with the obvious difference that pacing and sensing occur from the atrium, and pacemaker output is inhibited by a sensed atrial event (Fig. 74.6). An atrial-paced or sensed event initiates an *atrial refractory period* during which atrial pacing is not reset by any sensed signals in the atrium. Confusion can arise when multiple ventricular events occur while there is atrial pacing. For example, in addition to the intrinsic QRS that occurs in response to the paced atrial beat, if a premature ventricular beat follows, it does not inhibit an atrial-pacing artifact from being delivered. When the *atrial lower rate interval* ends, the atrial pacing artifact is delivered regardless of ventricular events because an AAI pacemaker does not sense events in the ventricle. The single exception to this rule is far-field sensing, that is, the ventricular signal is large enough to be sensed inappropriately by the atrial lead. In this situation, the atrial timing cycle is reset. This anomaly can often be corrected by making the atrial channel less sensitive or by lengthening the refractory period.

AAI pacing is appropriate for patients with sinus node dysfunction. The advantage is that it preserves intrinsic conduction and obviates the risk of producing any pacing-induced dyssynchrony. The disadvantage of atrial pacing is lack of ventricular support should AV block occur. If the patient with sinus node dysfunction is evaluated carefully for the presence of AV nodal disease at the time of pacemaker implantation, the occurrence of clinically significant AV nodal disease is low, about 2%/year (35). The evaluation before the use of an AAI system should include incremental atrial pacing at the time of pacemaker implant. Usually adult patients should be capable of 1:1 AV nodal conduction up to rates of 120 to 140 beats per minute.

Atrioventricular Sequential Ventricular-Inhibited Pacing (DVI)

This mode is rarely used as the preimplantation pacing mode of choice. By definition, DVI provides pacing in both the atrium and the ventricle (D) but provides sensing only in the ventricle (V). The pacemaker is inhibited and reset by sensed ventricular activity, but it ignores all intrinsic atrial complexes.

Atrial Synchronous P-Tracking Pacing (VDD)

These devices pace only in the ventricle, sense both the atrium and ventricle, and respond both by inhibition of ventricular output by intrinsic ventricular activity and by ventricular tracking of sensed atrial activity (P waves). The VDD mode has increasingly become available as a single-lead pacing system. In this system, a single lead is capable of pacing in the ventricle in response to sensing atrial activity by way of a remote electrode situated on the intraatrial portion of the ventricular pacing lead (36).

A sensed atrial event initiates the *AV interval* (AVI). If an intrinsic ventricular event occurs before the termination of the AVI, ventricular output is inhibited and the lower-rate timing cycle is reset (Fig. 74.7). If a paced ventricular beat occurs at the end of the AVI, this beat resets the lower rate. If no atrial event occurs, the pacemaker escapes with a paced ventricular event

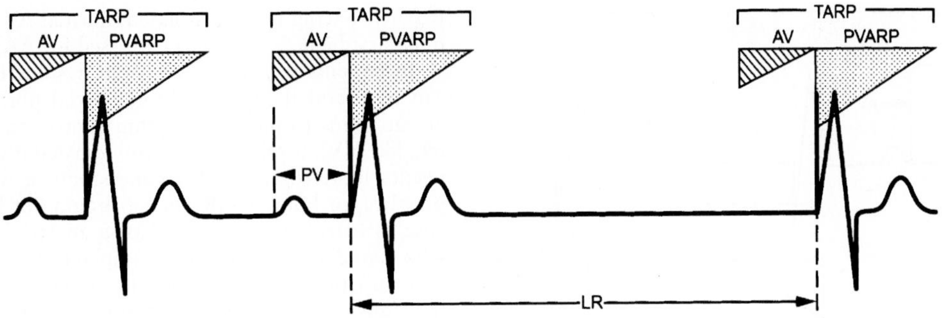

FIGURE 74.7. The timing cycle of VDD consists of a lower-rate (LR) limit, an atrioventricular (AV) interval, a ventricular refractory period, a postventricular (PV) atrial refractory period (PVARP), and an upper-rate limit. A sensed P wave initiates the AV interval (during this interval, the atrial-sensing channel is refractory). At the end of the AV interval, a ventricular pacing artifact is delivered if no intrinsic ventricular activity has been sensed (i.e., P-wave tracking). Ventricular activity, paced or sensed, initiates the PVARP and the ventriculoatrial interval (the LR-limit interval minus the AV interval). If no P-wave activity occurs, the pacemaker escapes with a ventricular pacing artifact at the LR limit. TARP, total atrial refractory period. (From Hayes DL, Zipes DP. Cardiac pacemakers and cardioverter-defibrillators. In: Braunwald E, Zipes DP, Libby P, eds. *Heart disease: a textbook of cardiovascular medicine*, 6th ed. Philadelphia: WB Saunders, 2001:775–814.)

at the lower-rate limit (i.e., the pacemaker displays VVI activity in the absence of a sensed atrial event). Hence, this mode can be a very economical dual-chamber pacemaker for patients with isolated AV nodal disease and normal sinus node function. However, doubts on the consistency of sensing of atrial activity by a remote floating electrode and the unpredictability of sinus node dysfunction in some of these patients make this an inferior choice to the DDD mode.

Dual-Chamber Pacing (DDD)

In this mode, there is pacing and sensing in both the atrium and the ventricle with inhibition and tracking (DDD). The basic timing circuit associated with lower-rate pacing is divided into two sections: the *ventriculoatrial* (VA) *interval* and the AVI. The AVI may be initiated by an atrial-paced beat or by a native P wave (Fig. 74.8). The *total atrial refractory period*, which consists of the AVI and the postventricular atrial refractory period (PVARP), defines the maximal tracking rate of the pacemaker.

In summary, four different rhythms can occur as a result of normal DDD function: *normal sinus rhythm*, with atrial sensing and intrinsic conduction; *atrial pacing* with subsequent intrinsic conduction of this impulse to the ventricles; *P-synchronous pacing*, with atrial-sensed beats being tracked by the pacemaker in the ventricle; and *AV sequential pacing*, in which an atrial-paced event is followed by a ventricular-paced event. The DDD pacing mode is most appropriate for patients with normal sinus node function and AV block. Some experts consider DDD the mode of choice in neurocardiogenic syndromes with symptomatic cardioinhibition.

DDD pacing has limitations in patients with sinus node dysfunction because it is not able to restore rate response in a patient with chronotropic incompetence. P-synchronous pacing is not possible in the presence of chronic atrial fibrillation or in patients with a paralyzed or nonexcitable atrium.

Asynchronous Pacing Modes (AOO, VOO, DOO)

In these modes, there is uninhibited, asynchronous pacing at a fixed lower-rate interval, without any sensing in the chamber involved. Because there is no sensing, there are no refractory periods. The mode is used in situations in which there is a need to avoid inhibition of pacing, as in the continuous use of electrocautery in the vicinity of the device, or with the use of a magnet over the device, which switches it to an asynchronous mode. One could temporarily switch to this mode in pacemaker-dependent patients with sensing malfunction, especially oversensing inhibition.

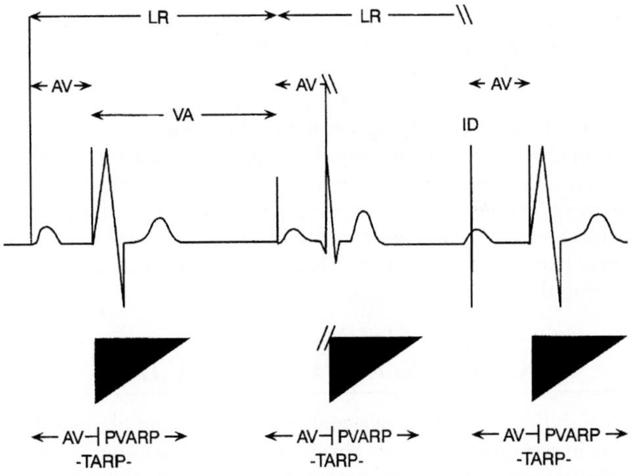

FIGURE 74.8. The timing cycle in DDD consists of a lower-rate (LR) limit, an atrioventricular (AV) interval, a postventricular atrial refractory period (PVARP), and an upper-rate limit. The AV interval and PVARP together constitute the total atrial refractory period (TARP). There are four variations of the DDD timing cycle. If intrinsic atrial and ventricular activity occurs before the LR limit times out, both channels are inhibited and no pacing occurs. If no intrinsic atrial or ventricular activity occurs, there is AV sequential pacing (first sequence). If no atrial activity is sensed before the ventriculoatrial (VA) interval is completed, an atrial pacing artifact is delivered, which initiates the AV interval. If intrinsic ventricular activity occurs before the termination of the AV interval, the ventricular output from the pacemaker is inhibited [i.e., atrial pacing (second sequence)]. If a P wave is sensed before the VA interval is completed, output from the atrial channel is inhibited. The AV interval is initiated, and if no ventricular activity is sensed before the AV interval terminates, a ventricular pacing artifact is delivered [i.e., P-synchronous pacing (third sequence)]. ID, intrinsic deflection. (From Hayes DL, Levine PA. Pacemaker timing cycles. In: Ellenbogen KA, ed. *Cardiac pacing*. Boston: Blackwell Scientific, 1992: 263–308.)

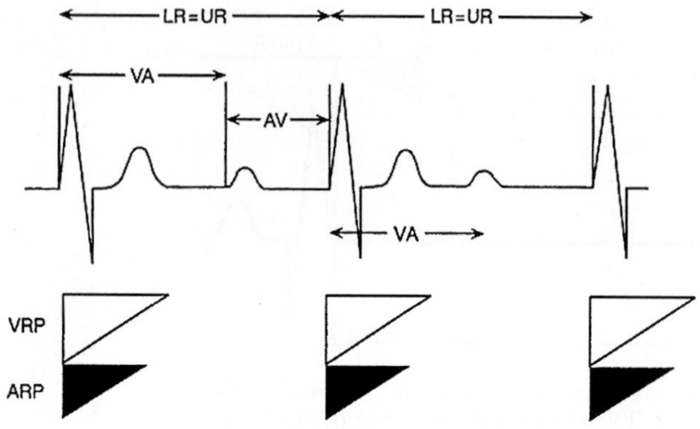

FIGURE 74.9. The timing cycle in DDI consists of a lower-rate (LR) limit, an atrioventricular (AV) interval, a ventricular refractory period (VRP), and an atrial refractory period (ARP). The VRP and ARP are initiated by any sensed or paced activity in the respective chambers. DDI can be thought of as DDD pacing without the capability of P-wave tracking. The LR limit cannot be violated even if the sinus rate is occurring at a faster rate. Hence, in a patient with DDI mode set to an LR limit of 60 beats per minute (1,000 msec) with an AV interval of 200 msec, if a P wave occurs at 500 msec, the AV interval is initiated with this beat. With the end of this AV interval, it would be only 700 msec from the previous paced ventricular beat, and the next ventricular pacing artifact would not be delivered for another 300 msec to avoid violation of the LR limit. UR upper rate; VA ventriculoatrial (From Hayes DL, Levine PA. Pacemaker timing cycles. In: Ellenbogen KA, ed. Cardiac pacing. Boston: Blackwell Scientific, 1992;263–308.)

Dual-Chamber Inhibition Mode (DDI)

In this mode, there is pacing and sensing in both chambers. However, the response of sensing in either chamber is inhibition. Hence, the atrial sensing inhibits tracking or the initiation of an AV interval, and ventricular sensing prevents pacing. However, in the absence of any sensed atrial or ventricular event, there is appropriate pacing at the lower-rate interval in either chamber, with an appropriate AV interval after an atrial-paced event (Fig. 74.9). The importance of this mode is that it prevents P-synchronous ventricular tracking in patients with atrial tachyarrhythmias. This avoids rapid ventricular rates in these patients, making it the fallback mode of choice in patients during the arrhythmia.

RATE-ADAPTIVE PACING

The ability of modern pacemakers to adapt and change their rate in response to various physiologic stimuli is known as rate-adaptive pacing. Hence, pacemakers can be potentially programmed to have a lower-rate interval and also an upper-rate interval. The pacemakers use different sensors, in response to which their rates can fluctuate between the lower-rate interval (LRI) and the upper-rate interval (URI), similar to the normal physiologic autonomic responses. The maximum rate at which a dual-chamber pacemaker is programmed to deliver P-synchronous pacing is called the upper tracking rate. The maximum rates at which an AAIR, a VVIR, or a DDDR pacemaker are programmed to pace in the respective chamber when driven by the appropriate sensor is called the upper sensor rate. The sensitivity of the sensors can be programmed to different levels depending upon the needs of an individual patient.

Single-chamber rate-adaptive pacing modes (AAIR, VVIR) have timing cycles that are not significantly different from those of their non–rate-adaptive counterparts. AAIR pacing can be considered in patients with sinus node dysfunction and normal AV node function because this mode restores rate responsiveness and maintains AV synchrony and intrinsic conduction. If AAIR pacing is contemplated, normal AV node conduction must first be determined as discussed for AAI pacing.

In patients who have AV nodal dysfunction, VVIR pacing can be useful if there is chronic atrial fibrillation and there are no plans to pursue a rhythm control strategy. VVIR pacing, like VVI, is relatively contraindicated if ventricular pacing results in retrograde (VA) conduction, a decrease in blood pressure, or both. VVIR pacing should not be used as an excuse to forego attempts at placing an atrial lead in a patient who is undergoing pacemaker implantation, has normal sinus node function, and would benefit from rate-adaptive pacing. If the sinus node is intact, P-synchronous pacing should still be considered the optimal rate-adaptive parameter and be used when possible. Although the UKPACE trial showed equivalent benefits with single-chamber pacemakers in patients older than the age of 70 years, multiple previous trials have shown benefit of dual-chamber pacing in reducing atrial fibrillation, thromboembolism, congestive heart failure, and, rarely, even mortality. This is important to take into account, especially when considering the management of younger patients.

DDDR pacemakers are also similar to their counterpart DDD pacemakers with the additional feature of rate responsiveness. It allows for rate responsiveness, which is either governed by the sinus node (as in P-synchronous pacing) or by the pacemaker sensor. In patients who have only transient dysfunction of the AV node, newer features in pacemakers allow search for intrinsic conduction by various complex algorithms intended to avoid inadvertent RV pacing, especially in patients with left ventricular dysfunction and heart failure.

The various timing cycles in dual-chamber pacemakers govern the upper tracking rate (maximum rate allowed for P-synchronous pacing) and the upper sensor rate (the maximum rate allowed for pacing with the pacemaker sensor). The sum of the AV interval and the PVARP is the *total atrial refractory period* (TARP). If the sinus rate exceeds the maximum allowable tracking rate, the pacemaker may show evidence of Wenckebach phenomenon or even 2:1 AV block (if every alternate P wave falls in the PVARP and is not sensed). Hence, the pacemaker has to be elegantly programmed for every individual according to age, physiologic requirements, exercise capacity, and intrinsic conduction system function.

MODE SWITCH

In patients with paroxysmal atrial tachyarrhythmias (atrial tachycardia, atrial flutter, atrial fibrillation) and AV block, the atrial rate clearly accelerates beyond the upper-rate interval. Sensing of such rapid rates in the atrium would lead to appropriate tracking of the atrial rhythm with the DDD or the DDDR mode. Hence, the pacemaker would exhibit ventricular pacing at rates close to the programmed upper rate. Most modern pacemakers allow programming of the pacemaker automatically during such situations to a DDI/DDIR or a VVI/VVIR mode, as may be desired for an individual patient. This feature is called "automatic mode switching." Once the tachycardia stops, the pacemaker switches back to the DDD/DDDR mode. The usefulness of this feature is not only in preventing unnecessary high-rate ventricular pacing, but also in measuring the burden and type of atrial arrhythmias in these patients. This has proven to be a very useful diagnostic tool and also helps in guiding the effectiveness of therapy of the atrial arrhythmias, even in asymptomatic patients.

RATE-RESPONSIVE SENSORS

An ideal sensor would be one that is able to provide appropriate and proportionate increase in the heart rate with exercise or with the increasing metabolic demands of the body. This acceleration should ideally start from the onset of exercise and should be followed by appropriate and gradual slowing of the heart rate once activity is terminated. A number of sensors have been developed, but there are only a few that have stood the test of time and continue to be clinically used.

Activity sensors are the most commonly used. They work on the principle of detecting vibrations that result from body motion. The piezoelectric crystals sense up-and-down motion, and the accelerometer-based sensors detect anteroposterior motion. With accelerometer-based pacemakers, heart-rate response tends to be more physiologic and heart rate less responsive to local pressure and tapping than with piezoelectric crystal–based pacemakers, making them more popular than the piezoelectric crystals. The disadvantage of accelerometer-based sensors is that they do not respond to emotional stress or isometric exercises.

Minute-ventilation sensors have a higher sensitivity and specificity with regard to metabolic demand. Minute ventilation is measured by emitting a small charge of known current from the pacemaker and measuring the resulting voltage at the lead tip. With this information, transthoracic impedance can be measured between the ring electrode and the pacemaker generator. As transthoracic impedances vary with respiration and its amplitude varies with tidal volume, the impedance measurement can be used to determine respiratory rate and tidal volume. A pacing algorithm uses the minute-volume measurements to alter pacing rate. Long-term reliability of the minute-volume sensor is excellent (37), and this sensor is increasingly being used. Although this sensor provides appropriate response to emotional stimuli and isometric exercise, it can cause inappropriate rise in the pacing rates with coughing, hyperventilation, or mechanical ventilation.

QT-interval sensors have also been used. These sensors work on the principle that the stimulus-T interval (as measured from the onset of a paced QRS complex to the end of the T wave) is affected by autonomic activity and heart rate. The response characteristics of such a sensor make it a reasonable partner for activity sensors in dual-sensor systems.

Many other sensors have either been available or are under development. Variables like temperature, preejection interval, *dP/dT* in the ventricular chamber, paced depolarization integral, and mixed venous oxygen saturation have been used. Some of these sensors need special leads and have been unable to surpass the popularity of the aforementioned sensors.

Dual-sensor pacemakers have been very useful. The combination of sensors works either by having one sensor cross-check the response of the other sensor or by having the two sensors complement for one another's deficiencies. Hence, one sensor could work better at the start of exercise (activity sensor), whereas the other could take over during the steady state, as achieved during the peak of exercise (QT, minute ventilation). Popular combinations include the activity and the QT sensor, and the activity and the minute-ventilation sensor.

PACEMAKER IMPLANTATION

It is important to undertake appropriate training before implanting pacemakers. Guidelines have been outlined by the North American Society of Pacing and Electrophysiology (NASPE) (38). Detailed descriptions of implantation techniques are beyond the scope of this chapter, but certain aspects are important. Almost all devices are placed in the right or left prepectoral area in a subcutaneous pocket. For very thin individuals, a submuscular pocket could be considered. Most leads are placed transvenously using either subclavian or cephalic venous access. The leads may be available with either tines for passive fixation or with fixed or retractable screws for active fixation. Although it appears that the active-fixation leads may be more stable and give more versatility in terms of the sites at which they can be implanted, it is possible that this may be at a slightly higher risk of perforation. In patients without reasonable venous access, an epicardial pacing lead may have to be implanted.

At our institute, we most often use the radiologically guided "first-rib approach" to cannulate the subclavian or axillary vein, lateral enough to avoid the risk of a pneumothorax or a crush injury to the lead. A cephalic cut-down may be done and usually provides enough space for at least two leads. Active-fixation leads are most often used because they provide stability, even in patients with smooth walls, large hearts, and significant valvular regurgitations. As mentioned, they also provide the flexibility of allowing the use of any site with good electrograms to fix the lead, whereas tined leads are most often placed at the RV apex and the RA appendage, respectively, because these are sites with maximum trabeculations. Mapping electrodes are used to monitor the electrograms and the injury current to choose the site of implantation and to confirm good contact with the tissue surface. After the leads are actively or passively fixed, the measurements for the electrograms, the lead impedances, and capture thresholds are assessed. Pacing at maximum output is done to confirm the absence of capture of the diaphragm or chest wall. The leads are anchored to the underlying tissues, and after they are connected to the device, the pocket is closed with nonabsorbable suture.

Lead impedances between 300 and 1,500 ohms are acceptable for most leads. We usually strive for an R-wave amplitude of greater than 5 mV and a P-wave amplitude of a minimum of 1 to 1.5 mV to allow good safety margins for appropriate sensing. The capture threshold is defined as the smallest amount of electrical activity that produces consistent myocardial stimulation outside the refractory period. Acceptable values are usually less than 1.0 V for the ventricle and less than 1.5 V in the atrium at a pulse width of 0.5 msec each. It can also be expressed in terms of the pulse width, as in the strength–duration curve (Fig. 74.10). The values at implantation are acute thresholds, which increase shortly after implantation and then usually decrease over the next 6 weeks. After this period, the leads achieve stable chronic thresholds. This variability occurs as a result of the inflammation and healing at the myocardial–electrode interface and can be minimized with steroid elution in most modern leads.

Although opinions conflict, it is our policy to give prophylactic antibiotic to prevent infections. Chest radiographs are done to confirm the position of the leads and to rule out any pleural injuries. The devices are rechecked the next day before discharge, and appropriate changes are made in programming. The patients are then followed up in the clinic after 6 weeks to monitor for chronic thresholds. At that time, programming changes are made to adjust outputs and sensitivity to allow optimum device performance and minimize battery consumption. Lead impedances also provide useful information. Whereas an inner insulation fracture can cause leakage of current and significant fall in the lead impedance, a fracture of the conductor coil causes a break in the circuit causing the impedance to rise dramatically with accompanying deterioration in sensing and capture function.

PACEMAKER PROGRAMMING

Although issues surrounding pacemaker programming and troubleshooting are complex, knowledge of a few principles helps in quick identification of pacemaker-related problems and faster triage for therapy.

Output programming is of immense priority in ensuring that adequate energy is always delivered to allow consistent

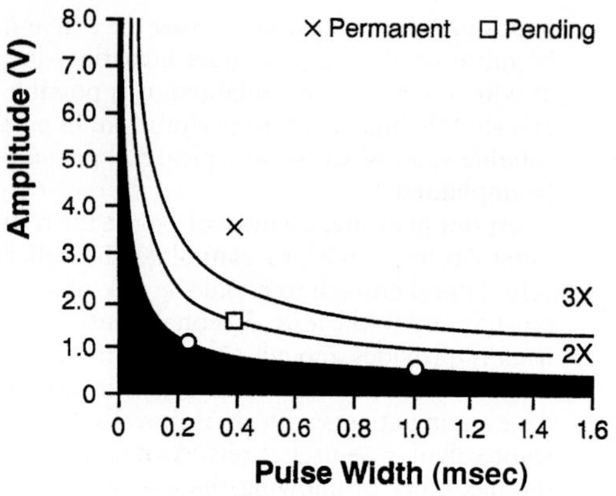

Pending Values Provide:

Safety Margin of 2.0

Estimated battery life of 78 months

	Pending	Permanent
Atrial Amplitude	1.50 V	3.50 V
Atrial Pulse Width	0.40 ms	0.40 ms
Threshold Points:	0.50 V, 1.00 ms 1.00 V, 0.25 ms	

FIGURE 74.10. Atrial strength–duration threshold curve generated by the pacemaker programmer. The voltage amplitude is represented on the y axis and the pulse width in milliseconds on the x axis. The shaded area of the graph represents amplitude/pulse width combinations that do not allow successful capture or depolarization. The upper two curves represent output combinations that result in two times and three times the safety margin, respectively (i.e., areas above the capture threshold), which is represented by the lowermost of the three curves and the open circles. Here × is the pacemaker-derived suggested point of permanent programming, in this example, 3.5 V and 0.4-msec pulse width.

stimulation of the respective cardiac chamber. The strength–duration curve allows assessment of the capture thresholds in terms of the voltage and the pulse width. A simple way to program the pacemaker is to double the voltage at chronic thresholds or triple the pulse width. Newer pacemakers have algorithms that assess capture thresholds by continuous surveillance and adjust the outputs accordingly. This ensures maximum efficacy and minimum battery drain.

Programming the *sensitivity* is important in avoiding asynchronous pacing and thereby reduce the possible risk of inducing atrial or ventricular arrhythmia. It is also important to avoid undue battery drain. The margin of safety that the device allows is governed by the appropriate P- and R-wave amplitudes that are recorded by the device during the intrinsic rhythm. At the same time, it is important for the device to be "insensitive" to far-field impulses as recorded due to the adjacent chambers or by structures like the diaphragm or chest wall.

Optimizing the *AV interval* is important achieving maximum hemodynamic benefit. This may be especially important in patients with heart failure. In all patients with biventricular pacemakers, we guide this by pulse wave Doppler as assessed on echocardiography. In other patients, it is preferred to lengthen the AVI to avoid inadvertent RV pacing in patients who have normal AV nodal function or at best transient dysfunction of the same. This not only avoids pacing-induced dyssynchrony, but also improves pacemaker longevity.

Automatic mode switching is often turned on in patients with devices with this capability. This useful diagnostic tool switches the pacemaker to an inhibitory mode during atrial arrhythmias (DDI/R or VVI/R) to avoid unnecessary tracking of fast ventricular rates. Most of the current pacemakers can keep a log of these episodes, which is a useful way to track the burden of atrial arrhythmias.

Rate adaptiveness can be programmed to optimize the patient's chronotropic response. For more objective management of the same, this has to be done with some form of exercise testing. The pacemakers have built-in algorithms with which the sensitivity of the sensor can be programmed to a low, medium, or high level as per the requirements of the patient.

Adjusting the *refractory periods* can be an important way to monitor sensing problems, and it may be used for the treatment of endless-loop tachycardia, double sensing, and so on, as discussed later in this chapter. One of the important functions of using refractory periods is avoiding response to retrograde conduction of the ventricular impulse in the atrium. Because this is a feature that can be easily affected by autonomic influences, many modern pacemakers allow programming of a dynamic PVARP to accommodate for these autonomic influences.

PACEMAKER-RELATED COMPLICATIONS

Pacemaker-related complications could be acute and related to the implantation procedure or could be subacute or chronic. Many of the complications are often related to operator experience and the volume of activity of the implanting center.

Acute Complications

Mild ecchymosis and pain around the pacemaker insertion are not uncommon. Access to the subclavian vein, commonly used for implantation of an endocardial pacemaker lead, is usually accomplished by subclavian vein puncture with a modified Seldinger technique. Due to close proximity of this vein to the lung, traumatic *pneumothorax* or *hemopneumothorax* can occur in rare cases.

Local ecchymoses that are not expanding can be treated with observation only. Discrete *hematoma* formation at the site is managed on the basis of its secondary consequences. Evacuation of the hematoma should be considered only if there is continued bleeding or potential compromise of the suture line or skin integrity or if pain from the hematoma cannot be managed with analgesics. Some people may prefer needle aspiration, but that leads to incomplete decompression and increases the risk of infection substantially. To prevent hematoma formation, it is preferable to have a normal prothrombin time and platelet count at implantation. Patients who are on heparin should have it discontinued long enough to allow a normal partial thromboplastin time. Careful attention to hemostasis before closure of the incision should prevent complications in most patients taking antiplatelet drugs. We prefer restarting Coumadin on the day of surgery and not using heparin postoperatively. For patients with mechanical valves or at high risk for thrombus formation, one may carefully start heparinization in 12 hours, or may omit the initial bolus. It is important to maintain a pressure dressing over the pocket as long as heparin is maintained. Anticoagulation at greater-than-therapeutic levels can result in late hematoma formation.

Due to its close proximity, there can be inadvertent puncture of the subclavian artery. If this is recognized promptly and the needle is removed, it is unlikely that a problem will occur. Although rare, *hemothorax* or *a supraclavicular hematoma* may occur if the artery is lacerated, but this is an extremely rare complication. To avoid mistaken entry into the artery, one should confirm the position of the wire in the superior vena cava (SVC), RV, or pulmonary artery before advancing the peel-away sheath. *Passage of a lead inadvertently in the left ventricle* can be recognized by a right-bundle-branch-block pattern during the paced beats. A pacing lead may also be placed in the left ventricle by passing it across an unsuspected atrial or ventricular septal defect. This should be avoided due to the associated risk of thromboembolism by formation of clots on the lead. Rarely, a right-bundle-branch-block pattern can be seen in patients with a pacing lead correctly placed in the right ventricle (39,40).

Lead perforation is a complication that may have very varied presentations. If it develops during the implant procedure, it could lead to pericarditis, pericardial effusion, or cardiac tamponade. Often, the only sign may be a rising capture threshold. It could also present as a right-bundle-branch-block pattern from a lead that migrates in the left ventricle, or it could lead to stimulation of the chest wall muscles or the diaphragm. Lead perforation may be confirmed by radiographic, electrocardiographic, or echocardiographic findings. After the perforation has been identified, lead withdrawal and repositioning usually are uncomplicated and rarely result in pericardial bleeding or tamponade. Rarely, delayed perforations have also been noted (Fig. 74.11), especially with active-fixation leads (41).

Lead dislodgement or damage could occur during the implant procedure. In patients with a higher risk for dislodgement, such as those with severe regurgitation or large, smooth-walled hearts, it may be reasonable to use active-fixation leads. Lead damage may occur from sharp instruments or tight sutures. It is especially important to be careful in patients undergoing a pacemaker change because portions of the lead may not be visible.

Other complications such as *air embolism*, *coronary sinus dissection*, or *perforation*, *diaphragmatic stimulation*, and *loose set-screws* have also been reported in rare cases. It is important to be aware of these possibilities for quick recognition and management.

Subacute or Chronic Complications

Venous thrombosis is a rare complication. Partial or silent inconsequential thrombosis after transvenous lead placement is not uncommon and usually is clinically insignificant, except that it may produce limitations to venous access during subsequent procedures. Complete thrombosis leading to acute insufficiency can occur, leading to the need for heparinization or anticoagulant therapy. Fortunately, major complications like *SVC syndrome* and *pulmonary thromboembolism* are rare.

Lead fractures most often occur adjacent to the generator or near the sites of venous access (stress points). Although it is uncommon, direct trauma may also damage the pacing lead or the generator. If a bipolar lead fractures and the pacemaker polarity is programmable, it may be possible to restore pacing by reprogramming to the unipolar configuration. This is a short-term solution and should not be a substitute for replacing the lead.

Insulation defects and *conductor fractures* may be caused by crush injury, specifically at the costoclavicular space, when the lead is placed via the subclavian puncture technique. In bipolar coaxial leads, the insulation defect often occurs internally (i.e., the layer of insulation between coils) as opposed to an external, outer-surface insulation defect. Thresholds, lead impedance, and electrogram noise are helpful in distinguishing an insulation defect from a conductor fracture. Although insulation

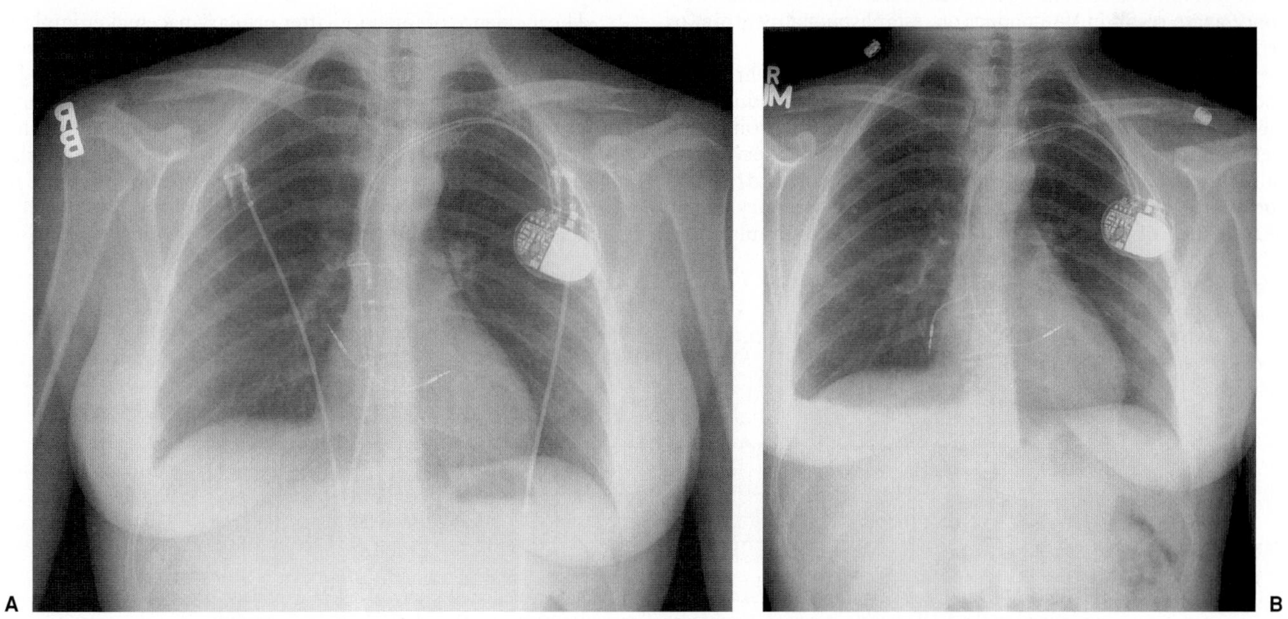

FIGURE 74.11. **A:** Chest x ray at initial presentation in a patient presenting with pleuritic chest pain 10 months after pacemaker implantation. The atrial lead is clearly seen projecting outside the border of the right atrium. **B:** Subsequently the lead migrated within the pericardial sac and shows definite change in orientation with respect to it. Note the small right-sided pleural effusion. (From Khan MN, Joseph G, Khaykin Y, et al. Delayed lead perforation: a disturbing trend. *Pacing Clin Electrophysiol* 2005;28:251–253.)

defects are often associated with very low impedances, conductor coil fractures are associated with very high impedances.

The presentation of *exit block* is progressive increase in capture thresholds that cannot be explained on the basis of radiographic dislodgment or perforation. Exit block is uncommon and appears to represent an abnormality at the interface of myocardial tissue and the electrode. Steroid-eluting leads are often effective in preventing exit block.

Lead dislodgement after the implant is a common complication. Active and passive fixation mechanisms common to current pacing leads have significantly decreased the incidence of lead dislodgment. Macrodislodgment is evident radiographically, but microdislodgment is not. Repositioning the lead is often warranted.

Pacemaker related arrhythmias have been often noted after implants. Most of them are usually inconsequential. *Tip extrasystoles* may be seen in the early postimplantation period. These are ventricular complexes with morphology similar to that of the paced beats because they originate at the same site as the paced beats, but they are not preceded by a pacemaker stimulus. Tip extrasystoles most often occur during the first 24 to 48 hours after implantation and usually resolve spontaneously. *Runaway pacemaker* refers to a sudden increase in pacing rate caused by circuit malfunction. This phenomenon is rare with current pacemakers. It has also been described as a complication of pacemaker exposure to therapeutic radiation (42). *Atrial and ventricular arrhythmias* can also occur from asynchronous pacing (VOO, AOO, DOO) if the stimulus is delivered during the vulnerable portion following intrinsic depolarization. From a practical standpoint, induction of atrial or ventricular arrhythmias during asynchronous pacing is uncommon.

Endless-loop tachycardia is another well-recognized pacemaker-related rhythm disturbance. In the presence of intact VA conduction, any event that uncouples AV synchrony may allow retrograde atrial activation. The most common stimulus for VA conduction is a premature ventricular contraction (Fig. 74.12). If the atrium is refractory at the time of VA conduction, the atrium will be depolarized and the atrial depolarization will initiate the AVI. Paced ventricular depolarization may once again result in VA conduction, establishing a reentrant or endless-loop tachycardia (43).

Extracardiac stimulation usually involves the diaphragm or pectoral muscles. Diaphragmatic stimulation may be due to direct stimulation of the diaphragm (usually stimulation of the left hemidiaphragm) or stimulation of the phrenic nerve (usually stimulation of the right hemidiaphragm from an atrial lead or the left hemidiaphragm from a lead in the coronary sinus). At the time of implantation, if any extracardiac stimulation is noted when pacing at 10 V, the pacing lead should be repositioned. Because this is usually tested with the patient supine, it does not eliminate the possibility of diaphragmatic stimulation when the patient is upright. Perforation of the myocardium by the pacing lead may also result in diaphragmatic pacing. Stimulation may be minimized or alleviated by decreasing the voltage output, the pulse width, or both. Local muscle stimulation of the pectoral muscle occurs more often with unipolar than with bipolar pacemakers and usually is noted in the early postimplantation period.

Erosion is an uncommon complication that almost always occurs because of an indolent infection. An insufficient size of the pocket could also lead to undue stress on the skin from the pacemaker, leading to pressure necrosis. This is uncommon with the small size of the current pacemakers.

Other rare complications in the postimplant phase include problems like *pacemaker allergy* or the *Twiddler syndrome*. This syndrome occurs as a result of some patients continuously manipulating their pacemaker, which results in twisting of the entire pacemaker. Although this does not have any major implications in the bipolar mode, in the older pacemakers, this can lead to malfunction of the device in the unipolar mode. The current pacemakers are all "ambidextrous" and hence this is likely to be inconsequential, except for putting the leads under stress.

Pacemaker Infection and Lead Extraction

One of the commonest concerns after any surgery is the risk of infection. This is of even bigger concern in a situation in which the surgery involves the implantation of a foreign body. With pacemakers, the foreign body is a combination of a generator in a relatively avascular space in a subcutaneous pocket and the lead in the most vascular space of the body. The former makes it vulnerable to chronic indolent infections seeding the device and difficult for antibiotics to seep through this depth. The latter gives an infection easy access to the rest of the body and a potential for rapid spread if it is not controlled in a timely way.

The incidence of infection after primary pacemaker implantation should be less than 0.5%, and in most series the overall infection rate has been less than 1%. Careful attention to surgical details and sterility during the procedure are of paramount importance. Prophylactic antibiotic therapy before implantation and in the immediate postoperative period is controversial (44). Most studies have not shown any significant difference in the rate of infection between patients who have had prophylactic antibiotic treatment and those who have not. Irrigation

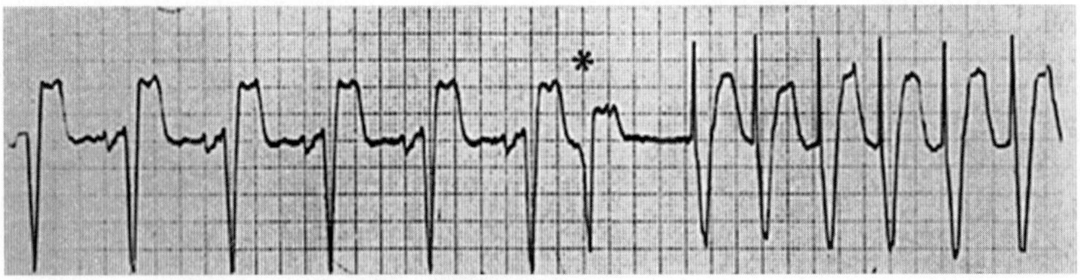

FIGURE 74.12. Electrocardiographic example of a pacemaker-mediated tachycardia in a patient programmed to the VDD pacing mode. A premature ventricular contraction *(asterisk)* results in retrograde atrial activation. The retrograde P wave must occur in the postventricular atrial refractory period. In the absence of another intrinsic atrial event, a paced ventricular event occurs at the lower-rate limit. In this example, the resulting retrograde P wave is sensed, with ventricular pacing occurring at a cycle length of approximately 500 msec, which corresponds to the upper-rate limit of 120 beats per minute. (From Hayes DL, Osborn MJ. Pacing. A. Antibradycardia devices. In: Giuliani ER, Gersh GJ, McGoon MD, et al., eds. *Mayo Clinic practice of cardiology*, 3rd ed. St. Louis: Mosby, 1996;909–976.)

of the pacemaker pocket with an antibiotic solution at the time of implantation has a similar status (45). In the absence of a large trial, it has been our standard practice to administer a dose of intravenous antibiotic during the surgery and another dose after surgery. We also use antibiotic solution to irrigate the pocket. Our incidence of infection with this practice has been below acceptable ranges, despite a high volume and multiple operators. The rate of infection after device replacement or upgrade to a dual-chamber ICD or biventricular device is about 2%, probably four times that for primary implantation.

Pacemaker infection must be recognized and treated properly. *Acute-onset infections* usually present with local inflammation and abscess formation in the area of the pacemaker pocket or as fever associated with positive blood cultures. Greater than 75% of infections are related to *Staphylococcus*. Acutely in the first month, about half of the infections are caused by *S. aureus*, can be very aggressive, and may present with or without a focus of infection elsewhere. If the infection has involved the pocket or the bloodstream, a removal of the device is usually required and a fresh implant at a different site should follow. More commonly, the infection occurs more than 1 month from implantation and is more often caused by *S. epidermidis*. *Subacute or chronic infections* are often more indolent, without fever or systemic manifestations. Such patients could also present with significant pain around the device. Not infrequently patients present with erosion of the device. Impending erosions of the lead can sometimes be treated by revising the device, but if obvious damage occurs to the integrity of the overlying skin, it is to be treated as an infection with extraction of the existing device and implantation at a different site (46). Surgery at the site of an existing device, such as for generator changes, lead revisions, and device upgrades, is particularly vulnerable to infection. In such situations and in late infections, the risks of device extraction are obviously higher and hence require additional caution. *Gram-negative bacilli and other organisms* are also responsible for infections in about 15% of the patients, particularly in those with diabetes mellitus.

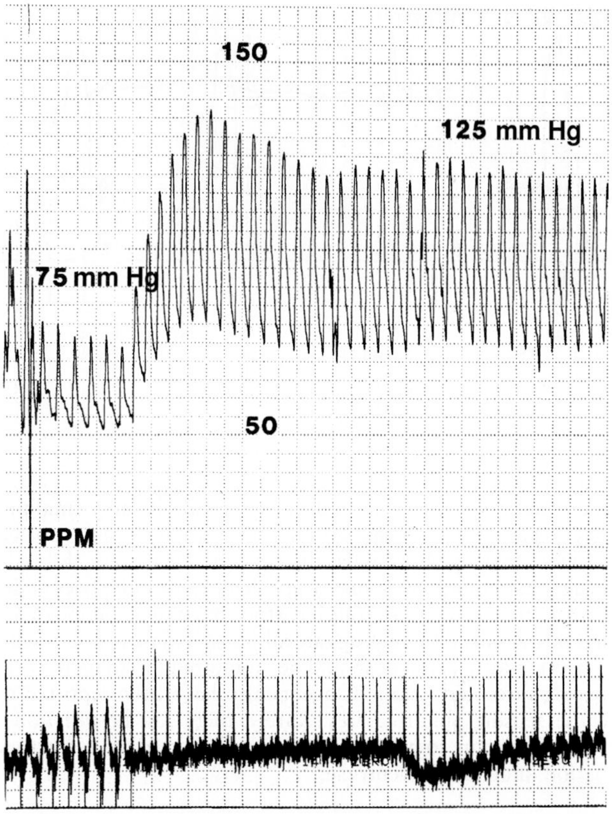

FIGURE 74.13. Hemodynamic tracing of a patient with pacemaker syndrome. In the initial portion of the tracing, there is ventricular pacing, with a systolic arterial pressure of approximately 75 mm Hg. The patient's intrinsic sinus rhythm inhibits ventricular pacing, and the arterial systolic pressure increases to approximately 125 mm Hg. PPM, pulses per minute. (From Hayes DL, Holmes Jr DR. Hemodynamics of cardiac pacing. In: Furman S, Hayes DL, Holmes Jr DR. *A practice of cardiac pacing*, 3rd ed. Mount Kisco, NY: Futura, 1993:195–218.)

Pacemaker Syndrome

This was recognized initially with VVI pacing, but it may occur with any pacing mode with AV dissociation. The incidence of pacemaker syndrome varies depending on the definition used. When defined as clinical limitation due to AV dissociation, Ausubel and Furman (47) estimated it to be in the range of 7% to 10% of patients with VVI pacing. In a crossover study by Heldman et al. (48), patients with DDD pacemakers were randomly assigned to DDD or VVI pacing mode for 1 week and subsequently to the alternate mode. Some degree of pacemaker syndrome was noted in 83% of the patients. The most common symptoms were shortness of breath, dizziness, fatigue, pulsations in the neck or abdomen, cough, and apprehension. It was concluded from the study that if patients with VVI pacing have some basis for comparison, they may be more aware of the symptoms of pacemaker syndrome.

In patients with an implantable pacemaker, a loss of AV synchrony with or without the presence of ventriculoatrial conduction can lead to deleterious hemodynamic effects. The combination of signs and symptoms that occurs as a result of this is called the pacemaker syndrome. This occurs as a consequence of a drop in the cardiac output due to loss of the atrial boost to the cardiac cycle or as a result of atrial contraction against a closed AV valve (Fig. 74.13). Milder effects leading to a drop in the blood pressure may be relatively asymptomatic or could lead to fatigue, heart failure, hypotension, or even confusional states in the more severe cases. Atrial contraction against a closed AV valve could cause palpitations, neck pulsations, cough, cannon waves, pulsatile hepatomegaly, and even gross right heart failure. The syndrome is most common in patients with VVI pacemakers, but even patients with AAI/AAIR or dual-chamber pacemakers could develop it if they have a long conduction time across the AV node, especially when associated with prolonged intraatrial conduction times. An upgrade of a VVI pacemaker and optimization of the AV delay can usually be helpful.

PACEMAKER ABNORMALITIES AND TROUBLESHOOTING

Electrocardiographic abnormalities in a patient with pacing can be grouped broadly into failure to capture, failure to output, undersensing, oversensing, and inappropriate rate change.

Failure to Capture

This usually is recognized electrocardiographically when a pacing artifact is present without subsequent cardiac depolarization (Fig. 74.14). This phenomenon can be observed if there are high thresholds with an inadequately programmed output, conductor coil fracture, lead insulation defect, lead dislodgment or perforation, impending total battery depletion, loose set-screws or incompatible connection at connector block, circuit failure, air in the pocket of a unipolar pacemaker, or

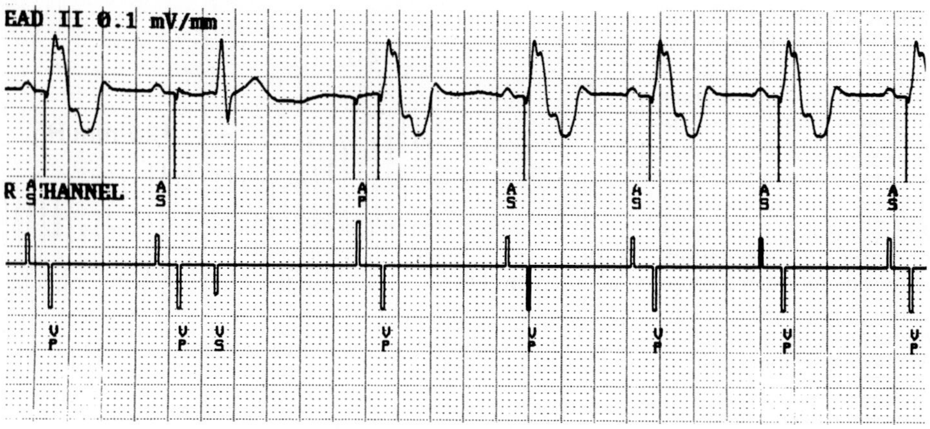

FIGURE 74.14. Electrocardiographic tracing from a patient with a DDD pacemaker. The second ventricular pacing artifact fails to result in ventricular depolarization, failure to capture, and is followed by an intrinsic ventricular escape beat after a PR interval of approximately 300 msec. AP, atrial-paced event; AS, atrial-sensed event; VP, ventricular-paced event; VS, ventricular-sensed event.

increased thresholds due to drugs or metabolic abnormalities like hyperkalemia. Although many drugs have been reported to affect pacing thresholds, the class IC agents are the only drugs that commonly cause a problem. Encainide, flecainide, propafenone, and moricizine have the potential to increase pacing thresholds. If these drugs are administered to a patient with a pacemaker, treatment should be monitored for an increase in pacing threshold. Class IC agents also have been reported to cause sensing abnormalities. Rarely, there can be *functional noncapture* due to a pacing output delivered in the refractory period of atrium or ventricle.

Failure to Output

This refers to the lack of delivery of a pacing output when there should have been one. It most often occurs as a result of oversensing inhibition, that is, the pacemaker senses an impulse in the absence of a true impulse and this results in inappropriate pauses in pacing. A failure to output can be encountered in circuit failure, complete or intermittent conductor coil fracture, intermittently or permanently loose set-screw, internal insulation failure (bipolar lead), oversensing of any noncardiac activity (lead noise, muscle potentials from diaphragm or chest wall), total battery depletion, lack of anodal connector contact, wrong programming of lead polarity, or air in the pocket of a unipolar device or when a unipolar pacemaker is not in the pocket and in patients with cross-talk.

The diagnoses of failure to capture and failure to output overlap. For example, electrocardiographic manifestations of a *conductor coil fracture* may include failure to capture due to significant leakage of current at the incomplete fracture site, leaving inadequate current for stimulation at the tip. Nonetheless, the pacemaker stimuli may appear. Alternatively, escaping current may be sensed by the pacemaker and inhibit pacemaker output. If the conductor coil is completely fractured, rendering the circuit incomplete, no pacemaker output will be detected on the electrocardiogram. In addition, secondary sensing abnormalities may be noted. *Insulation defects* may also present with oversensing and failure to output or with failure to capture, although the most common presentation of insulation failure is sensing abnormalities. Lead impedances can be helpful in such situations because they would be high in conductor coil fractures. However, if the inner insulation loses integrity, the contact of the coil with the blood pool causes easy leak of current, leading to excessively low impedances.

Electrolyte and metabolic abnormalities may also affect pacing and sensing thresholds. Hyperkalemia is the electrolyte abnormality that most commonly causes clinically significant problems, but severe acidosis or alkalosis, hypercarbia, severe hyperglycemia, hypoxemia, and myxedema should also be considered.

Sensing Abnormalities

Sensing abnormalities can be divided into true abnormalities, including undersensing (failure to recognize normal intrinsic cardiac activity; Fig. 74.15), oversensing (Fig. 74.16), unexpected sensing of intrinsic or extrinsic electrical signals, and functional sensing abnormalities. The differential diagnosis for *undersensing* includes a morphology of intrinsic event different from that measured at implantation (hence not generating enough voltage to be sensed), lead dislodgment, poor lead positioning, lead insulation failure, circuit failure, magnet application (because this puts the pacemaker in an asynchronous mode like AOO/VOO/DOO), malfunction of reed switch, electromagnetic interference, or battery depletion. Sensing abnormalities can also be noted due to local tissue changes like inflammation, ischemia, infarction, metabolic abnormalities, drugs, and change in rhythm (as in atrial fibrillation leading to a low-voltage P wave on an atrial lead). Occasionally, a normally functioning pacing system fails to detect atrial or ventricular extrasystoles because the sensing vector is different from that of the normal intrinsic beat (as during implantation), and the resulting voltage generated at the lead tip may not be large enough to be sensed by the pacemaker. It is reasonable to attempt to reprogram the sensitivity to allow sensing of extrasystoles, but if this is unsuccessful, it is rarely necessary to reposition the lead for this abnormality.

Functional undersensing is present when an intrinsic cardiac event is not sensed because it falls within a programmed refractory period. For example, if an intrinsic atrial event occurs within the PVARP, the event will not and should not be sensed. *Fusion* and *pseudofusion* beats occur as a result of superimposition of an ineffective pacemaker stimulus on a spontaneously occurring P wave or QRS complex (Fig. 74.17). Fusion is present when the morphology of the cardiac event is a hybrid of the intrinsic morphology and the paced morphology. Pseudofusion is present when the pacemaker artifact occurs late enough that the intrinsic morphology is not deformed. It usually is the consequence of pacemaker discharge during the refractory period of atrial or ventricular activity before sufficient intracardiac voltage is generated to activate the sensing circuit. This is expected to occur when the pacing rate and the intrinsic rate are similar. Pseudofusion beats also may be the result of the delayed arrival of atrial or ventricular activity at the tip of the respective lead. This is especially common in the ventricle in a patient with intraventricular conduction abnormalities.

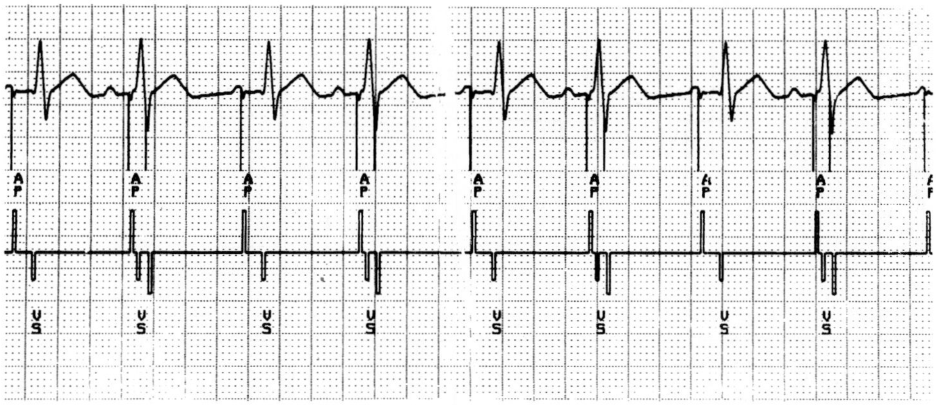

FIGURE 74.15. Electrocardiographic tracing from a patient with a DDD pacemaker programmed to a lower rate of 85 beats per minute. There is atrial failure to sense throughout the tracing. The arrow indicates an atrial-paced event (AP) that occurs immediately after an intrinsic atrial event and does not represent failure to capture but functional noncapture. When atrioventricular sequential pacing does occur, the atrioventricular interval is approximately 100 msec. This represents ventricular safety pacing that occurs because the intrinsic ventricular beat is occurring in the cross-talk–sensing window. VS, ventricular-sensed event.

Pacemaker Diagnostics and Lead Impedances

Various diagnostic functions are available in many current pacemakers and can be extremely helpful during pacemaker troubleshooting. Diagnostic capabilities vary widely and include real-time telemetry of programmed parameters and battery status, lead impedances, atrial and ventricular high-rate episodes with annotated electrocardiograms, histograms or long-term recordings of rate variations, percentage of paced and sensed beats, and so on. A full discussion of this topic is beyond the scope of this chapter. Pacemakers may also keep a log of the trends of these values. The newer pacemakers are also capable of performing automatic capture threshold assessment and can modify the outputs accordingly for safety and battery conservation.

Lead impedances can be particularly helpful in assessing lead performance and troubleshooting. Typically impedances are high with conductor fractures, loose set-screws, or myocardial scars. Impedances are typically reduced in insulation fractures due to leakage of current. Battery depletion and lead dislodgement may not affect the lead impedance significantly.

Troubleshooting

The definitive intervention for troubleshooting pacemaker problems depends on the cause. Lead dislodgement and conductor and insulation failure usually require lead revision or replacement. However, temporary care can be delivered by resetting the sensitivity and the output of the pacemaker. Battery depletion and circuit failure need timely recognition and device replacement. Loose set-screws are easy to fix, but are best avoided. Oversensing of intrinsic cardiac activity (such as T waves or far-field R or P waves) can usually be dealt with by decreasing the sensitivity; extrinsic activity such as diaphragmatic

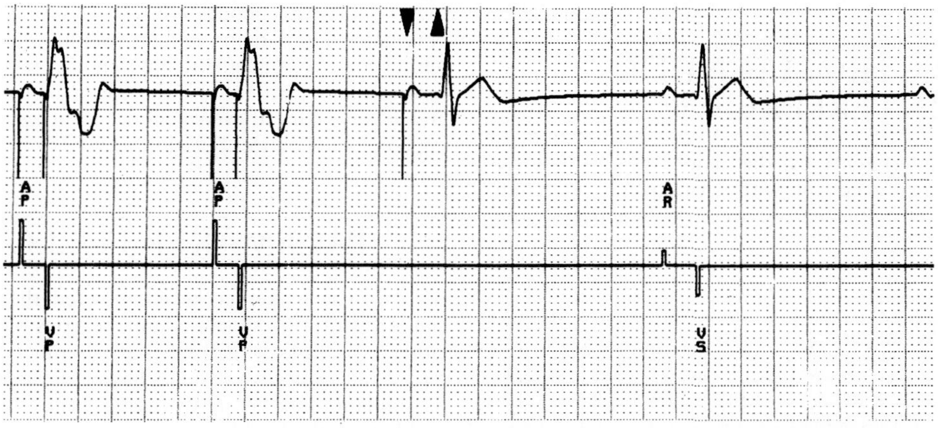

FIGURE 74.16. Electrocardiographic tracing from a patient with a DDD pacemaker with a lower rate of 55 beats per minute. The tracing begins with atrioventricular (AV) sequential pacing for two cycles. The next atrial pacing artifact results in atrial capture but is not followed by a ventricular pacing artifact at the programmed AV interval. (The programmed AV interval can be determined from the two initial paced cycles.) Following the intrinsic ventricular beat is a pause of 1,520 msec, which is greater than the programmed lower rate of 55 beats per minute, or 1,090 msec. The first event that is recognized by the pacemaker is a P wave, which is designated as an atrial beat that occurs within a refractory period (AR). Whatever extrinsic, noncardiac event that has been oversensed has initiated a refractory period(s) because there is no evidence of any intrinsic cardiac event that has initiated the refractory period. AP, atrial-paced event; VP, ventricular-paced event; VS, ventricular-sensed event.

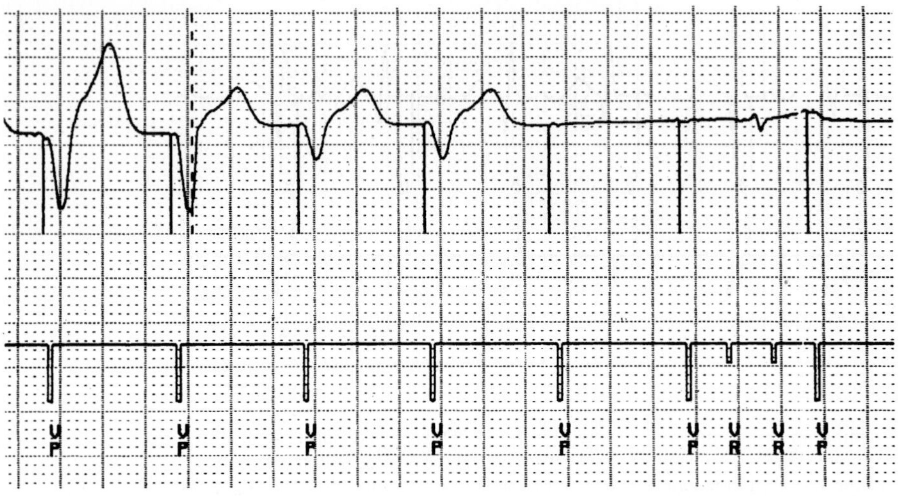

FIGURE 74.17. Electrocardiographic tracing from a patient with a VVI pacemaker. The first two complexes represent fully paced ventricular depolarizations. The third and fourth events result in different paced morphology and represent fusion beats. This is followed by failure to capture and a single ventricular escape. VP, ventricular-paced event.

interference can often be avoided by switching from a unipolar to a bipolar mode. Lead noise is best dealt with by changing the lead. Pacemaker-mediated tachycardias can immediately be taken care of by putting a magnet on the device and then changing the PVARP, followed by reassurance to the patient. Rarely, AV nodal ablation may be needed. However, it cannot be overemphasized that the best solution is to exercise maximum caution during the initial implantation and keep note of the foregoing possibilities with the intent of avoiding them.

Hysteresis

When the escape interval of a pacemaker is significantly longer than the automatic interval, the pacemaker is said to operate in the hysteresis mode. Usually the escape interval is longer (positive hysteresis) and the mode was designed to maintain sinus rhythm as long as possible (Fig. 74.18). Advanced systems may gradually lengthen the pacing cycle automatically after a fixed number of paced beats to look for an underlying intrinsic rhythm. This feature is called search hysteresis. Knowledge of this concept is important to avoid confusion during electrocardiogram interpretation of pacemaker function.

ELECTROMAGNETIC INTERFERENCE

Electromagnetic interference can be defined as any biologic or nonbiologic signal occurring within a frequency spectrum that may be detected by the sensing circuitry of the pacemaker.

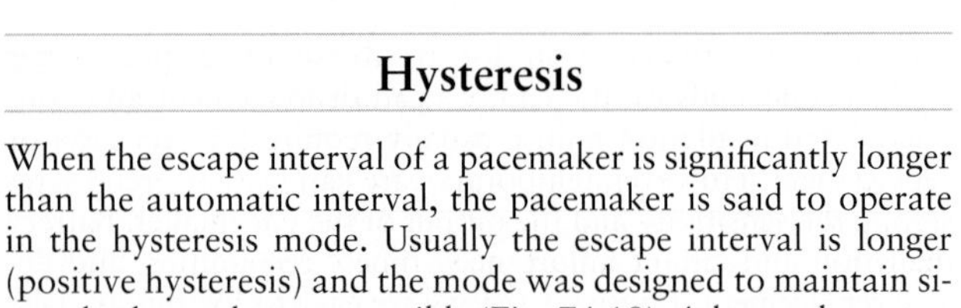

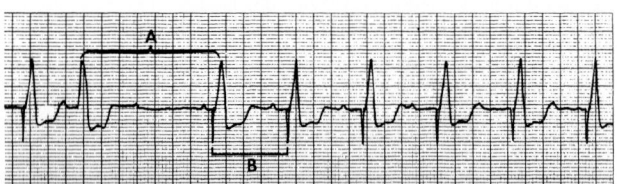

FIGURE 74.18. Electrocardiographic tracing from a patient with a VVI pacemaker programmed to a lower rate of 60 beats per minute and a hysteresis rate of 40 beats per minute. The longer cycle (escape interval; A) follows an intrinsic ventricular beat. The shorter cycle (automatic interval; B) represents the programmed lower rate of 60 beats per minute (1,000 msec). (From Hayes DL. Pacemaker electrocardiography. In: Furman S, Hayes DL, Holmes Jr DR, eds. *A practice of cardiac pacing*, 3rd ed. Mount Kisco, NY: Futura, 1993:309–359.)

It can result in rate alteration, sensing abnormalities, magnet mode response, or reprogramming. Biologic signals that may be responsible for oversensing include T waves, myopotential interference, afterpotential delay, and P waves.

Nonbiologic sources of potentially significant electromagnetic interference in the hospital include electrocautery, lithotripsy, cardioversion/defibrillation, magnetic resonance imaging, nerve stimulators, radiofrequency ablation, diathermy, and radiation therapy. Electrocautery is best used as far away from the device as possible. Preoperative and postoperative device checks are warranted. The deleterious effects of cautery can be reprogramming of the device, pacemaker inhibition or acceleration, and even myocardial thermal damage. Sometimes, pacemakers may have to be set to asynchronous modes in dependent patients. Rate responsiveness may also have to be turned off if the cautery is used close to the device. To avoid direct current shock–related damage, the paddles should be kept at least 4 inches away from the device, and the device should be interrogated before and after the procedure to ensure normal functioning.

Nonbiologic sources of interference outside the hospital include metal detectors, antitheft devices, cellular phones, high-voltage power lines, arc welding, and transformers. Analogue cellular telephones are relatively safe for patients with pacemakers, and digital cellular telephones have a greater potential for electromagnetic interference. If patients can avoid having the telephone over the pacemaker, it is unlikely that any adverse clinical event will occur; however, research is being conducted on this question.

PACEMAKER FOLLOW-UP

After the pacemaker has been implanted, the implanting physician or institution should assume responsibility for follow-up, either at the institution itself or at a commercial follow-up center. At our center, all patients have a device check the day after implantation, before discharge. Lead impedances, sensing and capture thresholds, battery measurements, and arrhythmia logs are important features that are noted during the follow-up. Other characteristics depend on individual patient requirements and device characteristics. All patients are then followed up in the device clinic in 6 to 8 weeks to assess for chronic lead thresholds and make necessary programming adjustments. Subsequently, patients may be followed up on a thrice-monthly basis via transtelephonic monitoring but at least once a year at the clinic. Initial programming for activity, AV optimization, and programming the various timing cycles are important and

TABLE 74.8

INDICATIONS FOR TEMPORARY PACING

Third-degree atrioventricular block
Symptomatic congenital, acquired, or postoperative complete heart block
Symptomatic second-degree atrioventricular block
Acute myocardial infarction with
Symptomatic bradycardia of any cause
Intermittent or sustained complete heart block
New-onset bifascicular block with or without prolonged atrioventricular conduction[a]
Alternating bundle-branch block[a]
Symptomatic sinus node dysfunction
Tachycardia prevention and treatment
Bradycardia or pause-dependent tachyarrhythmias
Long-QT syndrome with tachyarrhythmias
Ventricular tachycardia responsive to antitachycardia pacing

[a] In asymptomatic patients, observation could be considered if reliable transcutaneous pacing is available.

should be noted as the baseline for the patient. The examination of the pocket is of equal importance on every visit.

INDICATIONS FOR TEMPORARY PACING

Familiarity with temporary cardiac pacing is essential for those involved with permanent pacing and treatment of patients in coronary care units and postoperative units. Most commonly, it is used for short-term management of symptomatic bradycardias, either as a bridge to permanent pacing or for self-limited bradycardias. The decision to proceed with temporary pacing depends on assessment of the risk of developing severe symptomatic bradycardia. The indications for temporary transvenous pacing are listed in Table 74.8, but its use has considerably lessened with the advent of safe and reliable transcutaneous pacing.

CONTROVERSIES AND PERSONAL PERSPECTIVES

There is long-standing controversy regarding the optimum mode of pacing. Dual-chamber pacing has shown a reduction in the incidence of atrial fibrillation and thromboembolic phenomenon, but its impact on survival has never been definitively established. For economic reasons, VVI pacing continues to be the most commonly used mode in most parts of the world. However, in the United States, dual-chamber pacing is still most commonly used. The superiority of dual-chamber pacemakers may not have been proven, but the adverse effects of RV pacing are now evident. Newer algorithms in pacemakers that avoid RV pacing in patients with intact AV nodal function or with intermittent AV block can function only with the support of an atrial lead. Hence, even in the absence of large randomized trials, the logic of hemodynamics and currently available information seem to favor dual-chamber pacemakers. This is especially true for the younger patients, in whom the reduced incidence of pacemaker syndrome, physiologic pacing, better diagnostics and programming capabilities, and the ability to reduce RV pacing are features that make dual-chamber pacemakers a popular choice. For patients with heart failure, RV pacing has been detrimental, but the benefits of biventricular and left ventricular pacing can be best executed only in the presence of an atrial lead. For patients with sinus node dysfunction, an AAI/R pacemaker is reasonable if the normalcy of AV node function can be demonstrated.

The use of pacing in hypertrophic cardiomyopathy started off with significant enthusiasm. The surgery for myectomy is complex, and septal ablation also has limited availability. Moreover, both could have a significant risk of postprocedural heart block. The symptomatic relief from myectomy and septal ablation seems to be better and makes them the preferable option at our center. However, in patients who are not candidates for either or those who do not have access to these options, dual-chamber pacemakers may offer benefit in carefully selected patients. Pacemakers for the prevention and treatment of atrial arrhythmias and atrial fibrillation have been tried. Although there have been no randomized trials, most centers that have facilities for ablation of these complex arrhythmias are not very enthusiastic about the role of pacemakers in treating atrial fibrillation for situations other than sinus node dysfunction.

Pacemaker therapy has been the cornerstone of the management of bradyarrhythmias. The enthusiasm for its use for nonbradyarrhythmic indications such as hypertrophic cardiomyopathy, AF, sleep apnea syndrome, long-QT syndrome, vasovagal syncope, and so on has waxed and waned, but it continues to find use for these indications in patients for whom therapy can be individualized.

THE FUTURE

Pacemakers are becoming increasingly more sophisticated. The variety, complexity, and multiplicity of the algorithms offered by different vendors have made it difficult to keep abreast of the features of all of the devices. The increase in the indications and the number of eligible patients for device therapy have had a significant effect on the follow-up of these patients. Hence, one of the most significant future developments is likely to be the availability of remote monitoring of these devices. Most pacemakers are now able to check and keep a log of their battery and lead performance, sensing function, lead impedances, arrhythmia episodes, percentage of pacing, and so on. With the availability of automatic capture threshold testing, even pacing thresholds could be determined by the device. It might soon be possible to download all this information with conventional or cellular phone lines from the patient's home. This would be revolutionary in the management of these patients by limiting office visits, increasing patient compliance and satisfaction, easing the work load of busy device clinics, providing rapid access to patient information even from distant locations, and possibly even reducing emergency room visits. It would not be surprising if it is even possible to program the devices remotely by the next edition of this book.

Pacemaker algorithms for limiting RV pacing are becoming increasingly popular, although their clinical effect needs to be more objectively quantified in randomized trials. Automatic capture functions are likely to increase device reliability and prolong battery life. Device diagnostics not only store arrhythmia episodes and electrograms, but also can even store activity logs and heart failure status with the monitoring of transthoracic impedances. The joint effort of clinicians and engineers, which started as a simple solution for Stokes-Adams attacks, has led to intelligent devices and a desire for still further advances.

References

1. Bernstein AD, Daubert JC, Fletcher RD, et al. North American Society of Pacing and Electrophysiology/British Pacing and Electrophysiology Group:

Cardiac Pacemakers

The revised NASPE/BPEG generic code for antibradycardia, adaptive-rate, and multisite pacing. *Pacing Clin Electrophysiol* 2002;25:260.
2. Gregarotos G, Abrams J, Epstein AE, et al. ACC/AHA/NASPE 2002 guideline update for implantation of cardiac pacemakers and antiarrhythmia devices. Summary article: a report of the American College of Cardiology/American Heart Association Task Force on Practice Guidelines (ACC/AHA/NASPE Committee to Update the 1998 Pacemaker Guidelines). *Circulation* 2002;106:2145.
3. Andersen HR, Nielsen JC, Thomsen PE, et al. Long-term follow up of patients for a randomized trial of atrial versus ventricular pacing for sick sinus syndrome. *Lancet* 1997;350:1210–1216.
4. Connolly SJ, Kerr CR, Gent M, et al. Effects of physiologic pacing versus ventricular pacing on the risk of stroke and death due to cardiovascular causes. *N Engl J Med* 2000;342:1385–1391.
5. Lamas GA, Lee KL, Sweeney M, et al. Ventricular pacing or dual chamber pacing for sinus node dysfunction. *N Engl J Med* 2002;346:1854–1862.
6. Kerr CR, Connolly SJ, Abdollah H, et al. Canadian Trial of Physiologic Pacing: effects of physiologic pacing on long term follow up. *Circulation* 2004;109:357–362.
7. Lamas GA, Orav EJ, Stambler BS, et al. Quality of life and clinical outcomes in elderly patients treated with ventricular pacing as compared with dual chamber pacing. *N Engl J Med* 1998;338:1097–1104.
8. Andersen HR, Svendsen JH, on behalf of the DANPACE Investigators: The Danish multicenter randomized study on atrial inhibited versus dual chamber pacing in sick sinus syndrome (the DANPACE study): purpose and design of the study. *Heart Drug* 2001;1:67.
9. Bristow MR, Saxon LA, Boehmer J, et al. Cardiac-resynchronization therapy with or without an implantable defibrillator in advanced chronic heart failure. *N Engl J Med* 2004;350:2140–2150.
10. Cleland JC, Daubert JC, Erdmann E, et al. The effect of cardiac resynchronization on morbidity and mortality in heart failure. *N Engl J Med* 2005; 352:1539–1549.
11. Wilkoff BL, Cook JR, Epstein AE, et al. Dual chamber pacing or ventricular backup pacing in patients with an implantable defibrillator: the Dual Chamber and VVI Implantable Defibrillator Trial. *JAMA* 2002;288:3115–3123.
12. Bernstein AD, Irwin ME, Parsonnet V, et al. Report of the NASPE Policy Conference on Antibradycardia Pacemaker Follow-Up: effectiveness, needs and resources. *Pacing Clin Electrophysiol* 1994;17:1714–1729.
13. Katritsis D, Ward DE, Camm AJ. Can we treat carotid sinus syndrome? *PACE* 1991;14:1367.
14. Connolly SJ, Sheldon R, Roberts R, et al. The North American Vasovagal Pacemaker Study: a randomized trial of permanent cardiac pacing for the prevention of vasovagal syncope. *J Am Coll Cardiol* 1999;33:16–20.
15. Sutton R, Brignole M, Menozzi C, et al. Dual-chamber pacing in the treatment of neurally mediated tilt positive cardioinhibitory syncope. Pacemaker versus no therapy: a multicenter randomized study. *Circulation* 2000;102: 294–299.
16. Ammirati F, Colivicchi F, Santini M, et al. Permanent cardiac pacing versus medical treatment for the prevention of recurrent vasovagal syncope: A multicenter, randomized, controlled trial. *Circulation* 2001;104:52–57.
17. Raviele A, Giada F, Menozzi C, et al. A randomized, double-blind, placebo-controlled study of permanent cardiac pacing for the treatment of recurrent tilt-induced vasovagal syncope. The Vasovagal Syncope and Pacing Trial (SYNPACE). *Eur Heart J* 2004;25:1741–1748.
18. Connolly SJ, Sheldon R, Thorpe KE, et al. Pacemaker therapy for prevention of syncope in patients with recurrent severe vasovagal syncope. Second Vasovagal Pacemaker Study (VPS II): a randomized trial. *JAMA* 2003;289:2224–2229.
19. Kenny RA, Seifer C. Brief report–SAFE PACE 2 Syncope and Falls in the Elderly Pacing and Carotid Sinus Evaluation: a randomized controlled trial of cardiac pacing in older patients with falls and carotid sinus hypersensitivity. *Am J Geriatr Cardiol* 1999;8:87.
20. Smith RF, Jackson DH, Harthorne JW, et al. Acquired bundle branch block in a healthy population. *Am Heart J* 1970;80:746–751.
21. Scheinman MM, Peters RW, Suave MJ, et al. Value of the H-Q interval in patients with bundle branch block and the role of prophylactic permanent pacing. *Am J Cardiol* 1982;50:1316.
22. Antman EA, Anbe DT, Armstrong PW, et al. ACC/AHA guidelines for the management of patients with ST elevation myocardial infarction—executive summary: a report of the American College of Cardiology/American Heart Association Task Force on Practice Guidelines. *Circulation* 2004;110:588–636.
23. Serwer GA, Dorostkar PC, LeRoy SS. Pediatric pacing. In: Ellenbogen KA, Kay GN, Wilkoff BL, eds. *Clinical cardiac pacing and defibrillation*. Philadelphia: WB Saunders, 2000:953–990.
24. Toff WD, Skehan JD, De Bono DP, et al. The United Kingdom Pacing and Cardiovascular Events (UKPACE) trial: United Kingdom Pacing and Cardiovascular Events. *Heart* 1997;78;221.
25. Jeanrenaud X, Goy JJ, Kappenberger L. Effects of dual-chamber pacing in hypertrophic obstructive cardiomyopathy. *Lancet* 1992;339:1318–1323.
26. Fananapazir L, Cannon RO III, Tripodi D, et al. Impact of dual-chamber permanent pacing in patients with obstructive hypertrophic cardiomyopathy with symptoms refractory to verapamil and beta-adrenergic blocker therapy. *Circulation* 1992;85:2149–2161.
27. Fananapazir L, Epstein ND, Curiel RV, et al. Long-term results of dual-chamber (DDD) pacing in obstructive hypertrophic cardiomyopathy. Evidence for progressive symptomatic and hemodynamic improvement and reduction of left ventricular hypertrophy. *Circulation* 1994;90:2731–2742.
28. Kappenberger L, Linde C, Daubert C, et al. Pacing in hypertrophic obstructive cardiomyopathy. A randomized crossover study. PIC Study Group. *Eur Heart J* 1997;18:1249–1256.
29. Maron BJ, Nishimura RA, McKenna WJ, et al. Assessment of permanent dual-chamber pacing as a treatment for drug-refractory symptomatic patients with obstructive hypertrophic cardiomyopathy. A randomized, double-blind, crossover study (M-PATHY). *Circulation* 1999;99:2927–2933.
30. Abraham WT, Fisher WG, Smith AL, et al. Cardiac resynchronization in chronic heart failure. *N Engl J Med* 2002;36:1845–1853.
31. Saksena S, Prakash A, Ziegler P, et al. DAPPAF investigators. Improved suppression of recurrent atrial fibrillation with dual-site right atrial pacing and antiarrhythmic drug therapy. *J Am Coll Cardiol* 2002;40:1140–11450.
32. Carlson MD, Ip J, Messenger J, et al. A new pacemaker algorithm for the treatment of atrial fibrillation: results of the Atrial Dynamic Overdrive Pacing Trial (ADOPT). *J Am Coll Cardiol* 2003;42:627.
33. Hugl B, Israel CW, Unterberg C, et al. Incremental programming of atrial antitachycardia pacing therapies in bradycardia-indicted patients: effects on therapy efficacy and atrial tachyarrhythmia burden. *Europace* 2003;5:403–409.
34. Charles RG, McComb JM: Systematic Trial of Pacing to Prevent Atrial Fibrillation (STOP-AF). *Heart* 1997;224:78.
35. Hayes DL, Furman S. Stability of AV conduction in sick sinus node syndrome patients with implanted atrial pacemakers. *Am Heart J* 1984;107:644–647.
36. Lau CP, Tai YT, Leung SK, et al. Long-term stability of P wave sensing in single lead VDDR pacing: clinical versus subclinical atrial undersensing. *Pacing Clin Electrophysiol* 1994;17:1849–1853.
37. Li H, Neubauer SA, Hayes DL. Follow-up of a minute ventilation rate adaptive pacemaker. *Pacing Clin Electrophysiol* 1992;15:1826–1829.
38. Hayes DL, Naccarelli GV, Furman S, et al. NASPE policy statement: NASPE training requirements for cardiac implantable electronic devices: selection, implantation and follow up. *Pacing Clin Electrophysiol* 2003;26:1556–1562.
39. Klein HO, Beker B, Sareli P, et al. Unusual QRS morphology associated with transvenous pacemakers. The pseudo RBBB pattern. *Chest* 1985;87:517–521.
40. Yang YN, Yin WH, Young MS. Safe right bundle branch block pattern during permanent right ventricular pacing. *J Electrocardiol* 2003;36:67–71.
41. Khan MN, Joseph G, Khaykin Y, et al. Delayed lead perforation: a disturbing trend. *Pacing Clin Electrophysiol* 2005;28:251–253.
42. Souliman SK, Christie J. Pacemaker failure induced by radiotherapy. *Pacing Clin Electrophysiol* 1994;17:270–273.
43. Hayes DL. Endless-loop tachycardia: the problem has been solved? In: Barold SS, Mugica J, eds. *New perspectives in cardiac pacing*. Mount Kisco, NY: Futura, 1988:375–386.
44. Mounsey JP, Griffith MJ, Tynan M, et al. Antibiotic prophylaxis in permanent pacemaker implantation: a prospective randomized trial. *Br Heart J* 1994;72:339–343.
45. Lakkireddy D, Valasareddi S, Ryschon K, et al. The impact of povidone-iodine pocket irrigation use on pacemaker and defibrillator infections. *Pacing Clin Electrophysiol* 2005;28:789–794.
46. Chua JD, Wilkoff BL, Lee I, et al. Diagnosis and management of infections involving implantable electrophysiologic cardiac devices. *Ann Int Med* 2000; 133;604–608.
47. Ausubel K, Furman S. The pacemaker syndrome. *Ann Intern Med* 1985;103: 420–429.
48. Heldman D, Mulvihill D, Nguyen H, et al. True incidence of pacemaker syndrome. *Pacing Clin Electrophysiol* 1990;13:1742–1750.

CHAPTER 75 ■ LEFT VENTRICULAR DYSSYNCHRONY AND CARDIAC RESYNCHRONIZATION THERAPY

DAVID SPRAGG, RONALD BERGER, DAVID KASS, AND HUGH CALKINS

Congestive heart failure (CHF) is an increasingly common disorder. The incidence of CHF in the United States is more than 550,000 cases per year, with an estimated annual mortality of over 300,000 (1). The pathogenesis of CHF is complex, arising from the combined effects of compromised myocardial function, neurohormonal signaling cascades, and, in many cases, disordered mechanical ventricular activation. Left bundle branch block (LBBB), a surrogate marker for left ventricular mechanical dyssynchrony, is present in between 25% to 50% of patients with CHF and is associated with a substantial increase in morbidity, mortality, and sudden cardiac death in CHF patients (2–4).

More than 10 years ago, the first case report of multisite pacing to recoordinate a failing, dyssynchronous left ventricle (LV) was published (5). In the interim, cardiac resynchronization therapy (CRT) has become an increasingly widespread and important strategy in the treatment of patients with severe CHF. Recent large-scale, randomized clinical trials have demonstrated that CRT can reduce both morbidity and total mortality in select populations of CHF patients. This chapter reviews the pathobiology of LV dyssynchrony, as well as the acute and chronic effects of cardiac resynchronization. The major, recent trials investigating the efficacy of CRT in patients with heart failure (HF) are reviewed, as are the guidelines governing CRT implementation derived from those trials. The technical aspects of CRT device implantation are discussed briefly. Finally, unresolved issues and controversies surrounding patient selection and screening for CRT are considered.

PATHOLOGY OF LEFT VENTRICULAR DYSSYNCHRONY

LV dyssynchrony typically results from delay in the activation of the lateral LV free wall and is manifest frequently (but not necessarily) by LBBB on surface electrocardiogram (ECG). Contraction of the septum and anterior LV in early systole results in prestretch of the still-quiescent lateral wall, delaying intracavitary pressure rise and mitral valve closure. Late-systolic activation of the LV lateral free wall leads to corresponding stretch of the anteroseptal region, thereby competing with aortic ejection and reducing net cardiac output. The result is mechanical inefficiency, with transmission of the ventricular blood pool between two intracavitary sinks (the stretched lateral wall in early systole, and the anteroseptal region in late systole). Functional mitral regurgitation, which is due to delay in both the rise in LV intracavitary pressure and discoordinate papillary muscle contraction, can exacerbate this inefficiency further.

LV dyssynchrony results in an array of pathological changes (Table 75.1) Globally, systolic ventricular function is immediately compromised with the onset of disordered ventricular activation (6–8). Locally, regions of delayed myocardial activation are subject to increased fiber strain and work, with parallel increases in myocardial blood flow, metabolic activity, and tissue hypertrophy (Fig. 75.1A,B) (9–11). Electrophysiological properties of high-strain, late-activated myocardium in dyssynchronous hearts are deranged, with zones of reduced conduction velocity and reduced action potential duration and tissue refractoriness (12). Finally, late-activated myocardium in dyssynchronous, failing hearts has been shown to undergo a variety of changes in protein expression (Fig. 75.1C), including reduction in the levels of calcium-cycling proteins, including sarcoplasmic reticular calcium ATPase2a (SERCA2a) and phospholamban (PLB), reduction in expression of the gap-junction protein connexin43 (Cx43), and increased local activation of the stress response kinase extracellular-signal regulated kinase (ERK42/44) (13).

EFFECTS OF CARDIAC RESYNCHRONIZATION THERAPY

The mechanical and energetic consequences of intraventricular dyssynchrony can be mitigated by either biventricular or LV-only pacing. In both cases, early stimulation of the lateral LV free wall results in recoordination of ventricular contraction

TABLE 75.1

PATHOPHYSIOLOGICAL CONSEQUENCES OF LV DYSSYNCHRONY

Depressed LV systolic function
Reduced mechanical efficiency
Delayed MV closure and functional MR
Altered regional hypertrophy, blood flow, metabolism
Altered regional protein expression
Altered regional electrophysiology
LV, left ventricle; MV, mitral valve; MR, mitral regurgitation.

(Fig. 75.2A) (14). The effects of ventricular resynchronization on LV mechanical work are instantaneous, with appreciable increases in dP/dt_{max}, aortic systolic pressure, and cardiac output (CO) occurring within one beat of LV pacing onset (Fig. 75.2B). Stroke volume (width of the pressure-volume loop) increases acutely, with an attendant decline in end-systolic stress (Fig. 75.2C). Underlying these laudatory effects on global LV systolic function is the elimination of early- and late-systolic stretch in the lateral and anteroseptal LV walls, respectively. Rather, both territories contract throughout systole (Fig. 75.2D).

The beneficial effects of mechanical LV resynchronization appear to be independent of whether electrical synchrony is concomitantly achieved. Comparisons of LV-only to biventricular pacing have shown that although LV-only pacing did not improve (and actually worsened) electrical dyssynchrony across the LV, the mechanical effects of LV and BiV pacing schemes were essentially identical (14). Both modes increased dP/dt_{max}, CO, and stroke volume. More recent work has revealed some differences between LV and biventricular pacing, although these differences appear to be confined to diastole. In clinical studies of the two pacing strategies in patients with dyssynchronous heart failure, BiV pacing improved isovolumic relaxation rates, whereas LV-only pacing did not (15–17). This disparity may reflect differences in the duration of myocardial activation between the two pacing patterns, with BiV activation leading to more rapid contraction and earlier relaxation. When the LV alone is paced, contraction is longer in duration and thus compromises the diastolic period and relaxation rates.

Chronic ventricular resynchronization with biventricular or LV-only pacing results in further improvement of LV function and induces reverse remodeling in patients with dilated cardiomyopathy (18–22). In a study of 25 patients with class III-IV CHF and QRS widths of greater than 140 ms, for instance, Yu et al. demonstrated reductions in both end-systolic and end-diastolic volumes after 3 months of chronic biventricular pacing (18). With cessation of pacing, the investigators

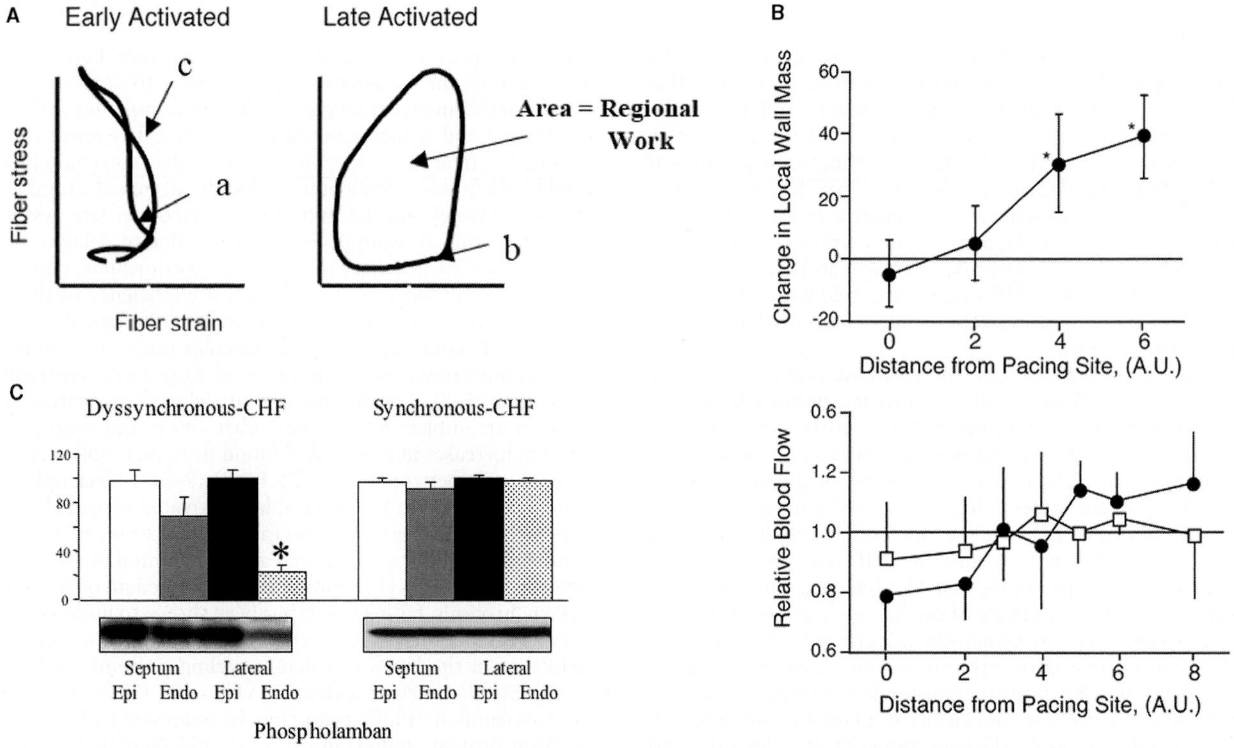

FIGURE 75.1. **A:** Stress-strain loops from early- and late-activated myocardial regions in dyssynchronous hearts (9). In early-activated regions, contraction initially occurs at low stress levels (*a*) as quiescent, late-activated regions undergo passive stretch. Later in systole, early-activated regions undergo reciprocal deformation as the late-activated territories contract (*c*). The small net area of the stress-strain loop in early-activated regions reflects reduced regional work performed. In late-activated territories, passive stretch in early systole generates increased stress before contraction (*b*). The increased stress-strain loop area reflects increased work performed by late-activated territories. **B:** Sustained ventricular pacing leads to hypertrophy at regions distant from the site of pacing and to increased myocardial blood flow (11) in regions distant from the pacing site (*solid circles*). With chronic pacing, regional changes in myocardial blood flow return equilibrate (*open squares*). **C:** Certain changes in protein expression, including downregulation of phospholamban, appear to be uniquely confined to late-activated lateral LV endocardium of dyssynchronous, failing hearts (13); similar changes in protein expression are not seen in any region of hearts with equivalent failure but preserved systolic function.

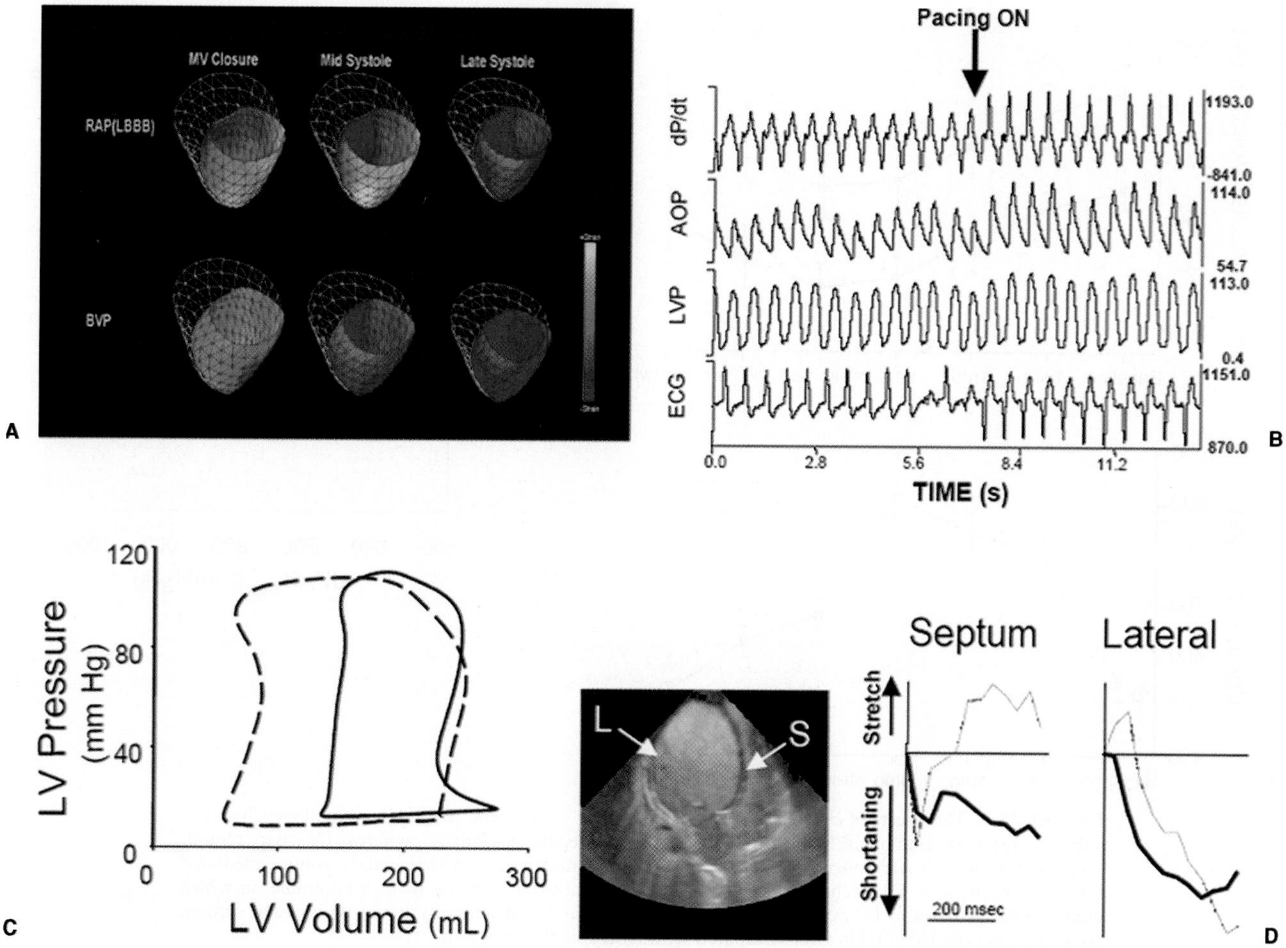

FIGURE 75.2. **A:** Tagged magnetic resonance imaging maps showing regional wall deformation during systole in an LBBB model during RA pacing (*top panel*) and BiV pacing (*bottom panel*). Transition from red to blue indicates shortening; transition from red to yellow indicates stretch (14). **B:** The acute hemodynamic effects of CRT on dP/dt_{max}, aortic pressure, and LV pressure in a dyssynchronous human LV. Onset of CRT is accompanied by instantaneous rises in all parameters, including an increase in aortic pulse pressure (consistent with enhanced cardiac output). **C:** PV loops displaying the effects of CRT. Resynchronization induces a left shift of the entire loop, with increased stroke volume and reduced end-diastolic filling pressures. **D:** Regional wall motion before (*light lines*) and during (*heavy lines*) CRT therapy. With dyssynchrony, the septum undergoes early systolic contraction and late systolic stretch (as the lateral wall contracts); the lateral LV is stretched in early systole, and then shortens. Initiation of CRT induces consistent shortening in both regions throughout systole.

found that dP/dt_{max} immediately declined (acute CRT effect), but chamber volumes were not acutely altered (Fig. 75.3A,B). This supports a remodeling effect rather than an active effect of CRT itself on chronic chamber volumes. Subsequent studies including the MIRACLE (23) and Vigor-CHF (24) trials have reported approximately 10% reductions of both end-systolic and end-diastolic volume with 6-month CRT treatment.

In contrast to therapy with positive inotropes, the increase in systolic function obtained from CRT in dyssynchronous failing hearts does not increase (and may actually reduce) myocardial oxygen consumption. Nelson et al. first reported on the energetics of a traditional inotropic treatment (dobutamine) versus CRT in dyssynchronous LV failure (25). They found that equivalent increases in dP/dt_{max} were associated with marked differences in oxygen use, with O_2 consumption (per beat) rising nearly 20% with dobutamine, but falling by 10% with CRT (Fig. 75.3C).

The impact of CRT on the electrophysiological or molecular changes reported to occur with chronic dyssynchrony is unknown. Some have expressed concern that the use of an epicardial pacemaker (i.e., the LV lead in a CRT system) is arrhythmogenic because of differences in transmural conduction and repolarization (26). However, the recent CARE-HF trial supports improved mortality both from pump function and sudden death with CRT alone (without an implantable cardioverter-defibrillator [ICD]), and would argue against CRT augmenting arrhythmia susceptibility (27). Very little remains known about the molecular changes that are induced by chronic dyssynchrony and even less about what is reversed by CRT. However, ongoing studies using controlled animal models are addressing this intriguing question.

TRIALS AND METAANALYSES OF CARDIAC RESYNCHRONIZATION THERAPY

Since 2001, a series of clinical trials has been published that have demonstrated the efficacy of CRT in reducing both morbidity and mortality in patients with moderate to severe CHF

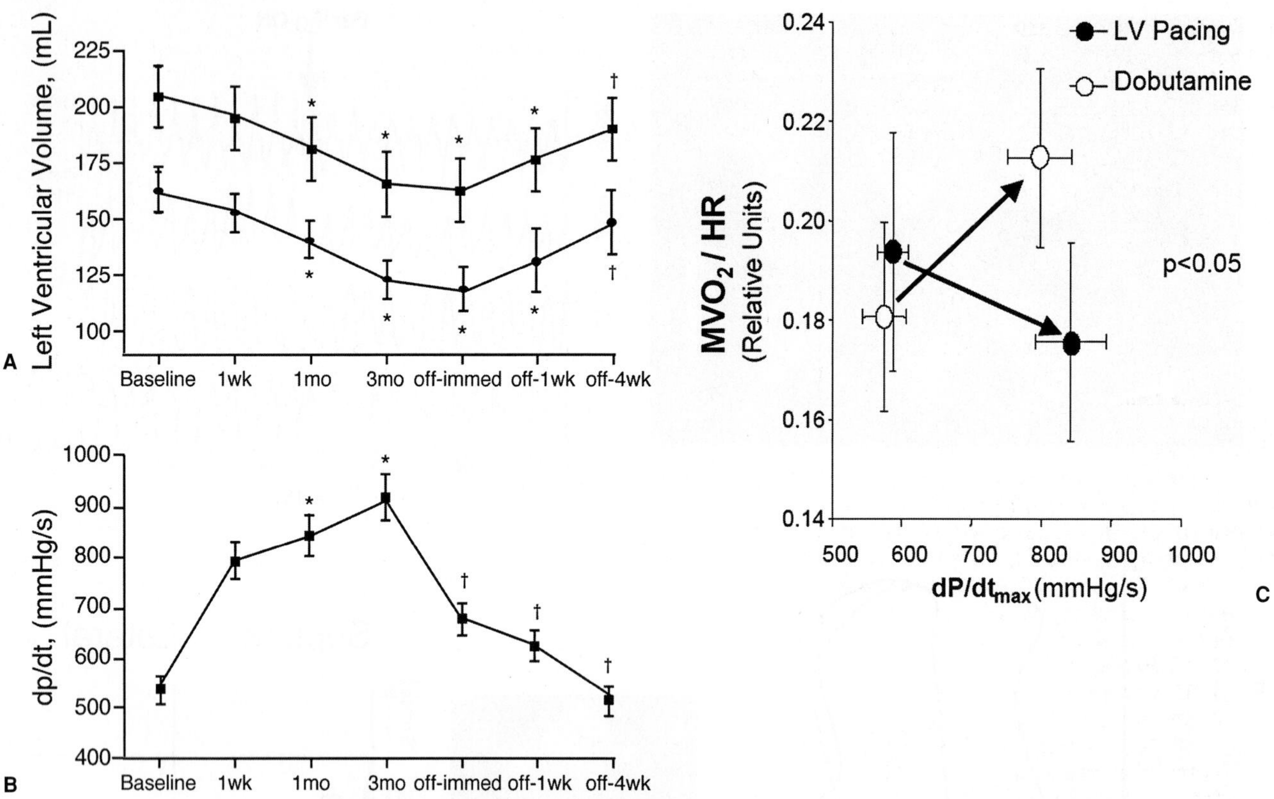

FIGURE 75.3. The effects of chronic CRT on (**A**) LV cavity volume and (**B**) dP/dt_{max} in dyssynchronous subjects (18). Cessation of CRT leads to an instantaneous decline in dP/dt_{max}, whereas LV cavity remodeling occurs more slowly, suggesting changes in tissue architecture rather than purely volume-mediated effects on cavity size. **C:** Mechanoenergetics in CRT and inotropic therapy with dobutamine, in which comparable increases in LV systolic function were achieved at substantially lower myocardial oxygen consumption rates (MVO_2) in CRT compared with inotropic therapy (25).

and LV dyssynchrony (Table 75.2). Two early studies demonstrating the feasibility of chronic multisite ventricular pacing to ameliorate HF symptoms were the MUSTIC (Multisite Stimulation in Cardiomyopathies) (28) and MIRACLE (Multicenter InSync Randomized Clinical Evaluation) (23) trials. In MUSTIC, the authors used a randomized, crossover approach to compare the effects of a 3-month period of atriobiventricular pacing versus 3 months without pacing. Study patients had class III HF despite optimal medical therapy, ejection fraction (EF) less than 35%, QRS greater than 150 ms, and LV dilation. The primary end point of the study was distance covered in the 6-minute walk test (6MWT); secondary end points included quality of life, peak 0_2 consumption during exercise, rates of death and hospitalization for CHF, and patient preference for either treatment period. In MUSTIC, CRT therapy resulted in a 23% increase in 6MWT distance and a 32% reduction (improvement) in the Minnesota quality-of-life score. Eighty-five percent of the patients preferred biventricular pacing. As such, MUSTIC was among the first trials to demonstrate that elective implantation of a multisite pacing system (or a mechanical device of any sort) could effectively treat HF symptoms in patients with moderate to severe disease.

The MIRACLE trial investigated the effects of CRT in a larger, sicker, and possibly less dyssynchronous cohort of patients compared with those studied in MUSTIC. Patients in the MIRACLE trial had class III or class IV HF symptoms, EF less than 35%, ventricular dilation, and a QRS greater than 130 ms. Of 571 patients enrolled, 453 progressed to randomization in a prospective, double-blind investigation of 6 months of atriobiventricular pacing versus no pacing. Primary end points included distance walked in the 6MWT, quality of life, and New York Heart Association (NYHA) class; secondary end points included peak 0_2 consumption during exercise, total exercise time, and reduction in hospitalizations for HF. As was the case in MUSTIC, the MIRACLE investigators found a significant increase in 6MWT distance, and a decrease in both quality of life scoring and NYHA class (both signifying improved HF symptoms). As such, the MIRACLE trial validated the results of MUSTIC in a larger, more symptomatic population treated with CRT for 6 months. Importantly, MIRACLE provided detailed information about the risks associated with implementation of CRT in a large patient population, reporting an 8% rate of unsuccessful device implantation and a 6% rate of coronary sinus or cardiac vein perforation or dissection.

MUSTIC and MIRACLE investigated the use of biventricular pacing in the treatment of heart failure, whereas more recent studies have examined the effects of combined therapy with CRT-defibrillator units. An early investigation into biventricular ICD therapy was the MIRACLE-ICD trial (29). Qualifying subjects were those meeting entry criteria for MIRACLE (EF <35%, QRS >130 ms, class III–IV HF symptoms, and LV dilation) who had either a history of aborted sudden cardiac death or a history of recurrent, hemodynamically intolerable VT. Three hundred sixty-nine such patients were enrolled in a randomized, double-blind study of CRT-defibrillator (CRT-D) therapy versus defibrillator implantation alone. Primary and secondary end points were those used in the MIRACLE trial, with analysis after 6 months of therapy. Although the investigators found no difference between the two groups in 6MWT distance (unlike the original MIRACLE trial), there were significant improvements in both quality of life and NYHA class with CRT-D therapy compared with controls. Secondary end

TABLE 75.2

CLINICAL TRIALS INVESTIGATING CARDIAC RESYNCHRONIZATION THERAPY

Trial	Duration of therapy	Number enrolled	Mean age (y)	Mean EF (%)	Major finding(s)
MUSTIC	3 m	58	64	23	Increase in 6MWT distance Improved quality-of-life assessment
MIRACLE	6 m	453	65	22	Increase in 6MWT distance Improved quality-of-life assessment Improved NYHA class
MIRACLE-ICD	6 m	369	66	22	No change in 6MWT distance Improved quality-of-life assessment Improved NYHA class No difference in arrhythmia rates
COMPANION	12 m	1,520	67	23	Reduction in all-cause death/hospitalization by CRT and CRT-D Reduction in all-cause death by CRT-D Reduction in HF-related death/hospitalization by CRT and CRT-D Improved 6MWT distance, quality-of-life assessment NYHA class by CRT and CRT-D
CARE-HF	29 m	813	67	25	Reduction in all-cause death/cardiac hospitalization Reduction in all-cause death Reduction in hospitalization caused by HF Improved NYHA class and quality-of-life assessment

EF, ejection fraction; 6MWT, 6-minute walk test; NYHA, New York Heart Association; CRT, cardiac resynchronization therapy; CRT-D, cardiac resynchronization therapy-defibrillators; HF, heart failure.

points, including total exercise duration and peak 0_2 consumption during exercise, were similarly improved with CRT-D therapy. As importantly, the authors demonstrated no significant differences in arrhythmia rates between the two study arms, arguing against either a pro- or antiarrhythmic effect of resynchronization therapy. Hospitalization and total mortality rates were similar between the two study arms.

Finally, two recent trials of CRT have reported improvement in overall mortality. The COMPANION trial (30) assessed CRT in patients with class III–IV heart failure, EF less than 35%, and QRS duration greater than 120 ms, comparing the efficacy of CRT ($\pm$ implantable defibrillator) to optimal medical therapy. The 1,520 patients were randomized in a 1:2:2 fashion to medical therapy, CRT-only, and CRT-D therapy. Follow-up ranged between 12 and 16 months. The primary end point of the trial was the composite of death or hospitalization from any cause; secondary end points included death from any cause (Fig. 75.4). Both CRT-only and CRT-D therapy reduced the primary end point by 20%. The secondary end point, death from any cause, was reduced by 24% in the resynchronization-only group ($p = .059$) and by 36% in the combined CRT-D group ($p = .003$). Similar reductions in death or hospitalizations from HF specifically were seen with both therapeutic arms. Finally, NYHA class, 6MWT distance, and quality-of-life assessments were all similarly improved with CRT-only and CRT-D therapy in COMPANION.

The CARE-HF trial (27) is the most recent large-scale investigation of CRT to be published and the first to show a clear mortality benefit from CRT alone in patients with severe, dyssynchronous HF (Fig. 75.5). Patients with class III or IV HF, EF less than 35%, and QRS greater than 120 ms were randomized to either CRT only (i.e., without defibrillator implantation) versus no device therapy. Compared with patients in COMPANION, the study population in CARE-HF was slightly more symptomatic from HF (23% of the treatment group had class IV symptoms, compared with approximately 14% in COMPANION). In addition, the selection criteria for patients with dyssynchrony were more stringent in CARE-HF; patients with QRS durations between 120 and 149 ms had to meet additional echocardiographic criteria establishing LV mechanical dyssynchrony. The primary end point was a composite of all-cause death and hospitalizations for a cardiac event; secondary end points included death from any cause, a composite of all-cause death and hospitalizations caused by HF, NYHA class, and quality of life. The 813 patients were randomized to CRT or control arms and followed for an average of 29 months. The investigators found that compared with controls, CRT reduced both the primary end point and the secondary end point of all-cause death by approximately 36%. The other secondary end points were also significantly and markedly reduced by CRT. As such, CARE-HF completes the investigative thread initiated by the MUSTIC and MIRACLE studies, demonstrating that in an ill population with a high likelihood of true mechanical LV dyssynchrony, there is a significant reduction in both morbidity and mortality from resynchronization therapy.

Two metaanalyses have investigated the effects of CRT on morbidity and mortality in patients with HF (31,32). The earlier of the two analyses included the MUSTIC, MIRACLE, MIRACLE-ICD, and CONTAK-ICD trials. In the 1,634 patients randomized to CRT therapy in these trials, there was a 51% reduction in death from progressive HF compared with controls, a trend toward reduction in all-cause mortality in CRT patients versus controls, and a significant reduction in HF hospitalizations. The second metaanalysis of CRT effects on morbidity and mortality in HF patients was published in 2004 and included nine trials (MUSTIC, MUSTIC-AF, MIRACLE, MIRACLE-ICD, CONTAK-ICD, PATH-CHF, RD-CHF, Garrigue et al., and COMPANION). In the 3,216 patients studied in the combined trials, there was a significant, 21% reduction in all-cause mortality in those patients receiving CRT versus controls. Heart failure hospitalizations were significantly reduced in patients treated with CRT by 32%, with corresponding improvements in quality of life, exercise capacity, NYHA class, and EF.

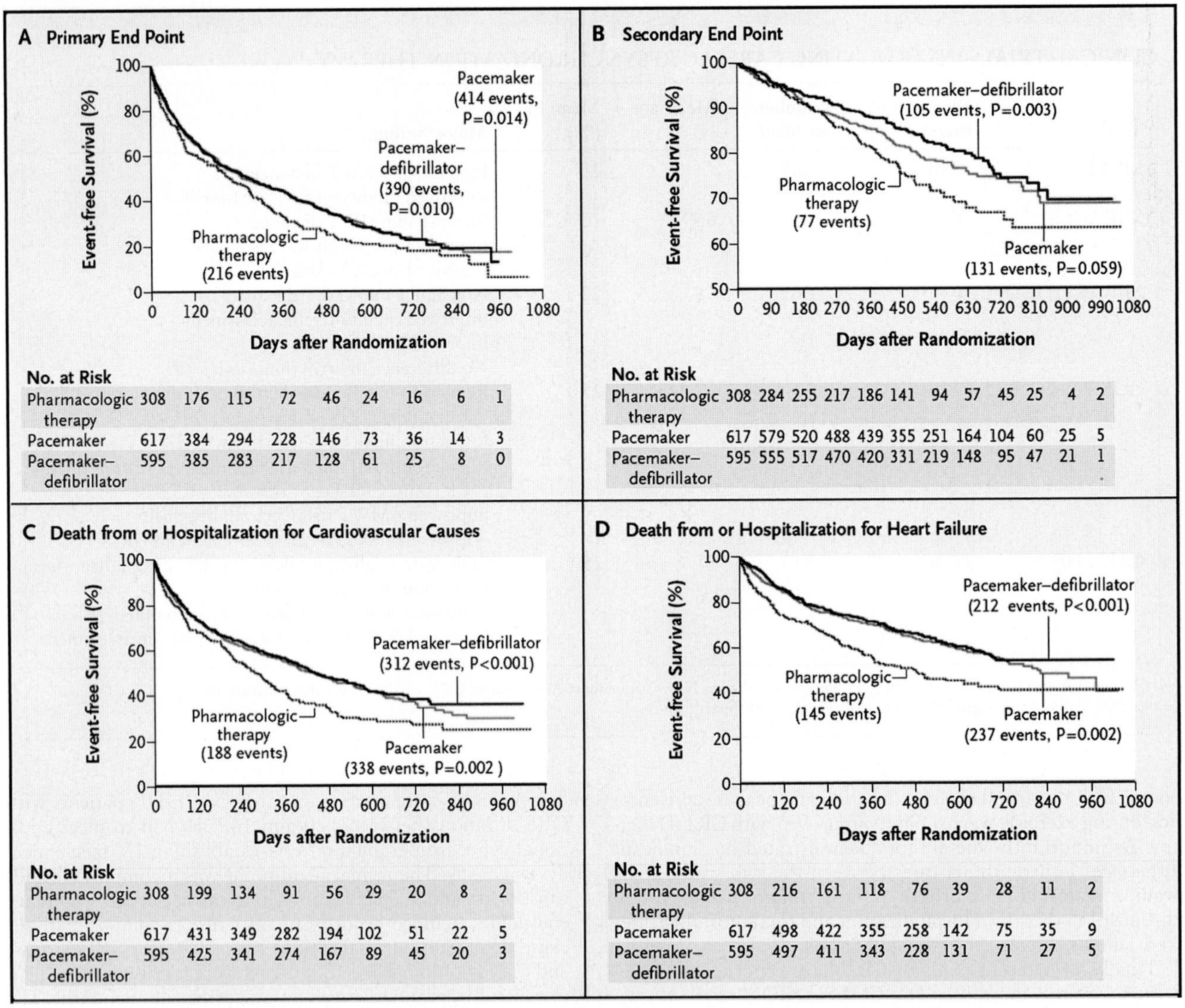

FIGURE 75.4. Primary and secondary end points in the COMPANION trial (30). With CRT and CRT-D, there was a significant reduction in the primary end point (all-cause death/hospitalization). CRT-D caused a reduction in all-cause mortality, whereas CRT alone caused a trend in mortality reduction. Both CRT and CRT-D reduced death/hospitalization from cardiac causes and specifically from HF.

CURRENT INDICATIONS

Based on the findings of these and other studies of CRT over the last 5 years, the American Heart Association and American College of Cardiology have released official guidelines for the implementation of CRT. In 2002, the American Heart Association/American College of Cardiology (AHA/ACC) listed CRT as a class IIa (supported by majority of evidence) therapy for patients with class III–IV HF, EF less than 35%, QRS greater than 120 ms, and ventricular dilation (LVIDd 55 mm or greater) (33). More recently, the AHA has released an updated set of guidelines, advocating CRT in patients with EF less than 35%, class III–IV heart failure despite maximal medical therapy, QRS greater than 120 ms, and who are in sinus rhythm (34). The appropriateness of CRT for patients in atrial fibrillation, patients with HF and sustained RV apical pacing, patients with class II HF symptoms, and patients with end-stage CHF (class IV, nonambulatory, on inotropic therapy) are explicitly recognized by the AHA advisory panel as unresolved issues (34).

TECHNICAL ASPECTS OF DEVICE INSERTION

Implementation of CRT is typically performed through the endovenous placement of pacing leads in the right atrium, right ventricle, and a tributary of the coronary sinus (CS). Access to the venous system, either at the cephalic, axillary, or subclavian veins, allows for the standard passage of leads into the RA and RV. Cannulation of the coronary sinus is usually facilitated with the use of a guiding sheath. A variety of sheaths are available for use, allowing for the selection of different curves and reaches that can be tailored to the patient's intracardiac anatomy. After CS cannulation and advancement of the guiding sheath into the body of the CS (over a guidewire or inner catheter), CS venography through an occlusive balloon-tipped catheter allows for visualization and selection of an appropriate CS tributary (Fig. 75.6) (35). An important investigation by Butter et al. explored the acute effects of LV pacing site (anterior versus free wall) on net change in global systolic function (36). In a series

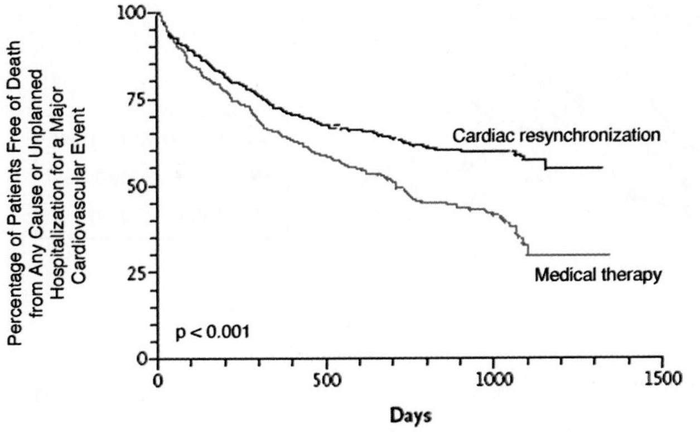

No. at Risk						
Cardiac resynchronization	409	323	273	166	68	7
Medical therapy	404	292	232	118	48	3

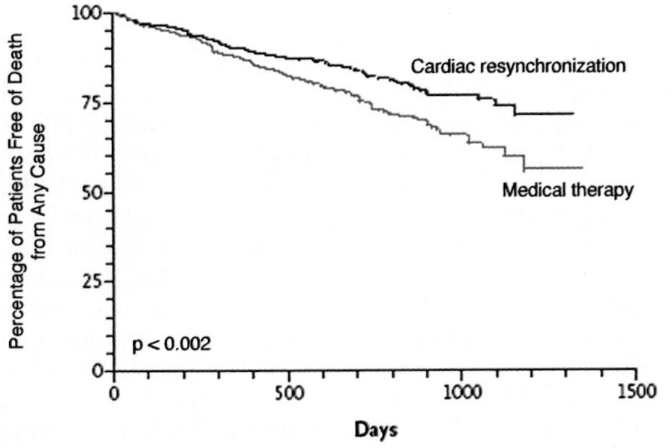

No. at Risk						
Cardiac resynchronization	409	376	351	213	89	8
Medical therapy	404	365	321	192	71	5

FIGURE 75.5. Primary (*top*) and secondary (*bottom*) end points in the CARE-HF trial (27). With CRT, there was a significant reduction in death from any cause or hospitalization for a major cardiovascular event (primary end point). There was a significant reduction in death from any cause (secondary end point).

of 30 patients with an average of class 2.7 HF, QRS width of 152 ms, and all with EF less 30%, pacing at the anterior and lateral LV was performed at a variety of AV intervals. Both LV and BiV pacing were assessed. Lateral LV pacing consistently resulted in greater increases in dP/dt_{max} and aortic pulse pressure than did anterior pacing. In one third of patients, anterior LV pacing actually reduced global LV systolic function, and deleterious effects from lateral LV pacing were never seen. Accordingly, CS pacing leads are typically placed in midlateral wall positions, frequently over a guidewire directed into the selected tributary. As is the case with introducer sheaths, a variety of pacing leads are available. All are passively fixated, relying either on tines or lead shape to assist in lead retention within the vein. Both unipolar and bipolar leads are available, allowing for multiple pacing strategies.

After successful delivery of the CS lead to the target site, LV sensing and pacing parameters should be assessed in a routine fashion. In addition, special attention should be paid to potential diaphragmatic capture, as the course of the phrenic nerve is frequently in close proximity to the lateral LV. After demonstrating acceptable lead pacing and sensing parameters, the guiding catheter is removed, and the leads are connected to a CRT or CRT-D device.

CARDIAC RESYNCHRONIZATION THERAPY OPTIMIZATION

Current biventricular pacing devices allow for modification of the AV delay during sequential atrioventricular pacing. Aurricchio et al. demonstrated that comparable mechanical benefits are achieved across a moderate range of AV delays, with optimal ventricular function at roughly half of the patient's native PR less 30 ms (Fig. 75.7A) (37). Thus, whereas some patients with particularly long intrinsic delays require customization, most will gain a similar CRT effect by using a nominal delay of roughly 120 ms. It is important to remember that all of the major clinical trials of CRT utilized a mode of pacing in which the atria were not paced. Rather, atrial sensing was used to trigger preactivation via the LV and RV leads. This is an important distinction. If an atrial pacing mode (i.e., DDD) is used, this will introduce an intraatrial conduction delay, which can alter the effective timing of the AV delay. AV delay, in turn, is important to achieving proper preexcitation of the RV and LV. Thus, optimizing AV delay is likely of far more importance if atrial pacing is utilized. Atrial pacing is suggested only in those

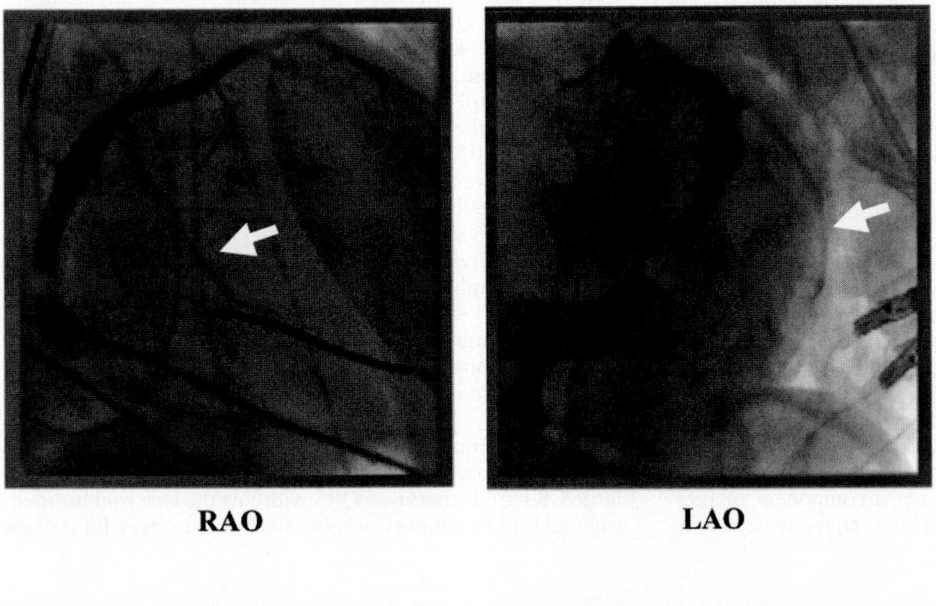

FIGURE 75.6. RAO and LAO views of CS-venography (35), showing location of a lateral LV CS tributary (*white arrow*).

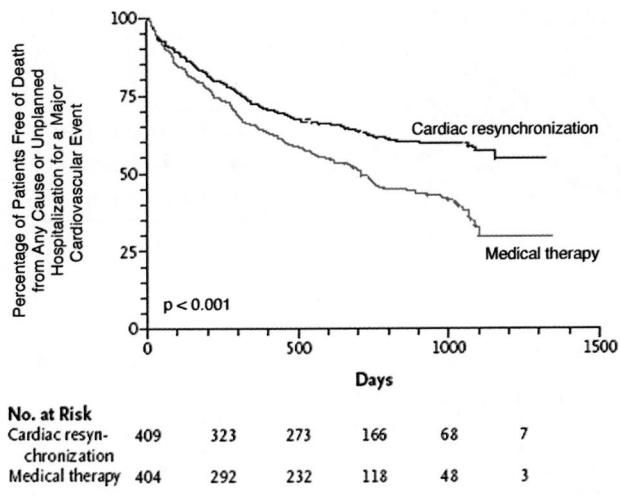

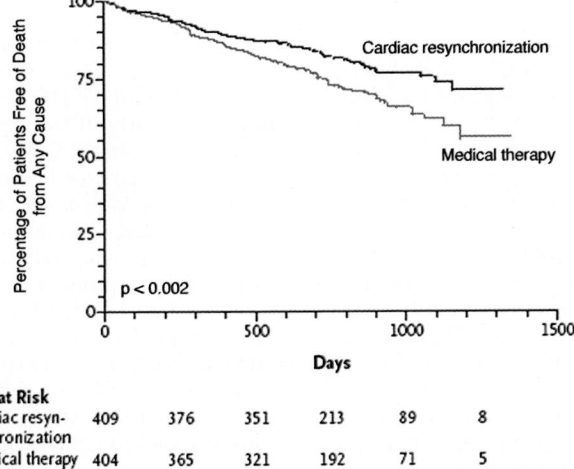

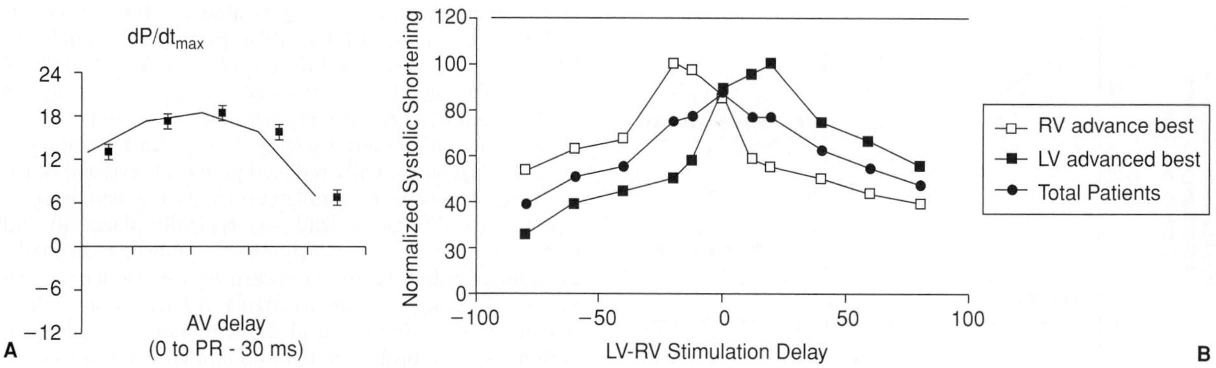

FIGURE 75.7. **A:** The influence of AV delay on systolic function in the setting of CRT. The x-axis represents a normalized AV delay (*0* indicates coincident AV contraction; *1* indicates the native PV delay less 30 ms) (37). LV systolic function is compromised at very short and very long AV delays, and is optimized across a range of intermediate values (*shaded area*). **B:** Various disparate results have been reported about the effects of varying VV timing intervals during CRT. In total, simultaneous activation of the RV and LV appears to provide maximal benefit for LV systolic function.

individuals in whom symptomatic bradycardia caused by sinus node dysfunction is present.

A more recent advance that will soon be available in all CRT devices is variable interventricular stimulation delay (i.e., RV-LV delay). Early reports have suggested that most patients will benefit from slightly premature LV activation; some patients have optimal LV systolic function with simultaneous or even premature RV activation, however (Fig. 75.7B) (38,39). In the setting of atrial fibrillation, there appears to be little benefit to preactivation of either the RV or LV (15,39). Importantly, the simultaneous RV-LV stimulation used in all the major clinical trials appears very similar (within 10%) to the best results from optimized VV delay stimulation. Presently, patients may undergo a noninvasive echocardiographic assessment of LV function and dyssynchrony at varying AV and VV delays to attempt optimization. In these studies, the effects of AV and VV timing intervals on mechanical resynchronization are assessed by tissue Doppler echocardiography. Patients' devices are programmed empirically based on echocardiographically identified optimal AV and VV delays.

FAILURE RATES AND COMPLICATIONS

A recent metaanalysis of CRT efficacy included data on both implantation success rates and peri- and postprocedural complication rates (32). Seventeen trials reported implantation success rates (3,673 patients total); biventricular pacing systems were placed successfully in 90% of attempted implant procedures. In 10 studies reporting rates of fatal complications from device implantation, there was a 0.4% risk of death associated with biventricular pacer placement. Over an average 6-month follow-up period, frequent complications included device malfunction (7%), lead dislodgement (9%), pocket infection (1.4%), and new arrhythmia (2%). In the CARE-HF study, published after this metaanalysis, two patients undergoing device implantation died, 24 had lead dislodgement, 10 had CS dissection, 8 had pocket erosion, 6 had pneumothorax, and 3 had device-related infections (27). Successful implantation on the first attempt occurred roughly 95% of the time.

PATIENT SELECTION

CRT has evolved to become a standard component of therapy for particular HF populations. However, many issues surrounding the appropriate selection of patients for CRT remain unresolved. In early trials demonstrating the clinical benefits of CRT implementation in patients with class III–IV HF, EF less than 35%, and QRS greater than 130 ms, nearly 30% of treated patients had no appreciable improvement from CRT (40). Labeling patients who failed to improve in formal exercise studies (i.e., the 6-minute-walk test) or in subjective assessments, such as NYHA functional class as "nonresponders," is admittedly problematic. These patients, while not improving relative to baseline, may have suffered worsening HF symptoms in the absence of CRT. Nevertheless, it is widely accepted that between 20% and 30% of patients with biventricular pacing do not show beneficial effects from treatment. Because of the expense of CRT devices (typically biventricular-pacing ICDs) and the risks associated with CS lead implantation, prospectively identifying patients likely to (or to not) respond to CRT is clearly important.

A likely contributor to CRT failure in nonresponders is the imperfect relationship between QRS duration on surface ECG and true mechanical LV dyssynchrony. Prolonged electrical activation, typically defined as a QRS width of greater than 120 ms, has become a standard means of identifying patients with suspected dyssynchrony. Furthermore, shortening of the QRS duration acutely at the time of CRT implementation has been correlated with long-term benefit from resynchronization (41). A number of recent investigations have shown, however, that in patients with class III–IV HF and severely impaired systolic function, QRS width is a poor predictor of LV mechanical dyssynchrony (42–44). Assessment of true mechanical dyssynchrony in these studies has typically been by tissue Doppler echocardiography, in which the relative mechanical activation times across the LV are assessed and compared (Fig. 75.8). As many as 30% of patients with marked QRS prolongation (>150 ms) have been found to have no significant intraventricular LV dyssynchrony by tissue Doppler (42,43). Interestingly, nearly 30% of patients in the same study with narrow QRS complexes were found to have marked LV dyssynchrony by echocardiography (42). This suggests that screening HF patients for CRT by QRS width alone will not only include a significant number of patients with minimal if any mechanical LV dyssynchrony, but will miss a large number of patients who may benefit from CRT.

A number of studies have examined the utility of tissue Doppler screening for CRT candidates. It appears that the rate of "nonresponders" in these studies is strikingly lower than in large CRT trials that used QRS width as the sole tool for identifying LV dyssynchrony (45,46). In these studies, CRT devices

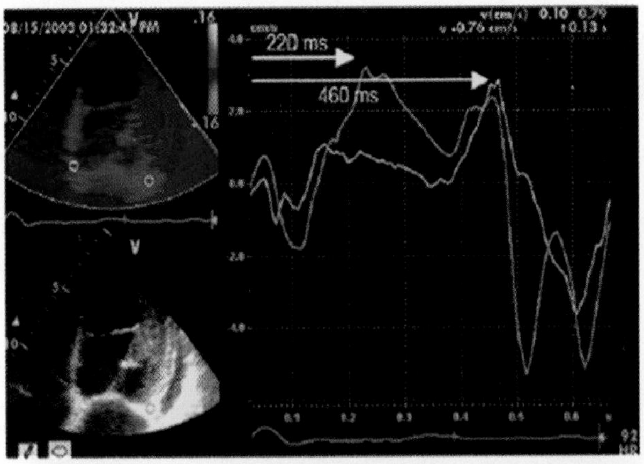

A

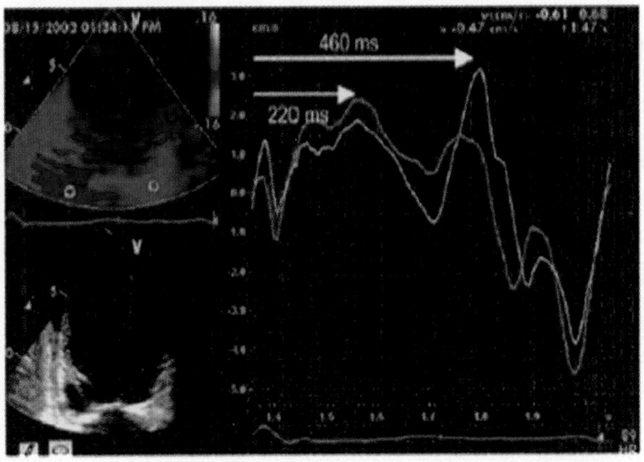

B

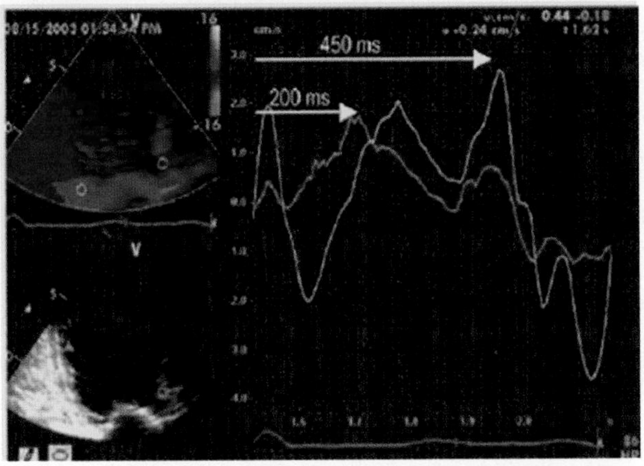

C

Septal time to peak:	460ms
Lateral time to peak:	220 ms
Inferior time to peak:	460ms
Anterior time to peak:	220ms
Posterior time to peak:	450ms
Anterospetal time to peak:	200ms
PVD	260ms

D

FIGURE 75.8. Example of tissue Doppler imaging in a patient with LV dyssynchrony (46). Images are taken in the apical four-chamber view (**A**), the apical two-chamber view (**B**), and the apical three-chamber view (**C**). In each case, time from the QRS onset to the peak velocity is assessed for each region. In the apical four-chamber view, for instance, septal activation (*yellow*) and lateral LV activation (*green*) are measured. Comparison of the earliest versus latest regions of activation provides a quantitative metric of dyssynchrony.

were implanted in patients with echocardiographic indices of dyssynchrony, regardless of QRS width. In patients with electrical synchrony (i.e., narrow QRS complexes) and echocardiographic evidence of dyssynchrony, there was a significant improvement in HF symptoms and in cardiac remodeling with CRT, providing further evidence that mechanical rather than electrical dyssynchrony is paramount to predicting CRT response.

UNRESOLVED ISSUES AND PERSONAL PERSPECTIVES

Unresolved issues surrounding CRT patient selection include HF patients not fulfilling the recommended profile for resynchronization (class III–IV HF, EF <35%, and QRS width >120 ms, sinus rhythm) but in whom CRT would logically seem beneficial. Such patients include class III–IV HF patients with chronic RV apical pacing, patients with dyssynchronous HF and atrial fibrillation, and end-stage class IV HF patients awaiting cardiac transplant. Implementation of CRT in these patients is best judged on a case-by-case basis and may certainly be warranted in appropriate circumstances. Whether patients with less symptomatic HF and evidence of LV dyssynchrony may benefit from CRT, principally by retarding the progression of HF symptoms, is an area of active investigation.

At our institution, patients meeting standard guidelines for CRT are routinely referred for and receive resynchronization devices. Almost always these devices are combined biventricular-pacing and defibrillator units, given the superimposition of patient profiles for CRT and for prophylactic ICD implantation. We also frequently implant CRT devices into otherwise qualified patients with atrial fibrillation, based on the large number of studies that have demonstrated the effectiveness of CRT in patients with dyssynchronous HF and atrial fibrillation (47–49). Furthermore, we regularly implant CRT devices into patients with class III–IV HF and chronic ventricular pacing that is unavoidable using alternate pacing strategies (i.e., DDI or DDD modes with maximum AV delays). There are substantial data demonstrating the deleterious effects of chronic RV pacing (50,51), and supporting pacing strategies designed to preserve LV mechanical synchrony (i.e., CRT) (52).

In patients with severe CHF, EF less than 35%, but without electrocardiographic evidence of LV dyssynchrony, it has become common at our institution to obtain a tissue Doppler echocardiogram to assess for mechanical dyssynchrony. Because more than 25% of patients with severe heart failure and LV systolic dysfunction may have mechanical dyssynchrony despite a narrow (<120 ms) QRS complex on ECG, we feel that these studies are well warranted. Patients with class III–IV HF and mechanical LV dyssynchrony by tissue Doppler echocardiography (regardless of QRS width) are offered CRT. Data on CRT effects in right bundle branch block (RBBB) versus LBBB patients are mixed. In the MIRACLE trial, for instance, no differences in the beneficial effects of CRT were noted between patients with right or left bundle block. In COMPANION, in contrast, reductions in mortality and hospitalizations were significant in patients with left but not right bundle block (30). Whether to implant a CRT device in patients with RBBB may be best addressed through echocardiographic assessment of mechanical ventricular dyssynchrony.

Following device implantation, our patients are referred for a "CRT optimization" session, during which the effects of different AV and VV intervals are assessed by tissue Doppler echocardiographic analysis. Long-term programming of the device is based, therefore, on empiric evidence supporting particular AV and VV delays for that patient. We feel that this multidisciplinary approach for both the screening and postimplantation management of patients, in which electrophysiologists, echocardiographers, and HF specialists play critical and complementary roles, will maximize the number of patients receiving effective and optimal CRT.

CONCLUSIONS

Left ventricular mechanical dyssynchrony has an array of deleterious consequences for patients with dilated cardiomyopathy. Principle among these is further impairment of systolic dysfunction caused by mechanical inefficiency of ventricular contraction. CRT represents an important strategy to combat the mechanical effects of LV dyssynchrony and has been shown in a number of prospective, randomized clinical trials to reduce both morbidity and mortality in patients with class III–IV HF, severe LV systolic dysfunction, and evidence of LV dyssynchrony. Accordingly, biventricular pacing is formally recommended in patients with class III–IV HF, EF less than 35%, sinus rhythm, and QRS duration greater than 120 ms. Strategies for prospectively identifying patients most likely to respond to CRT are of paramount importance and represent an active area of investigation.

THE FUTURE

As has been alluded to already, there are myriad issues surrounding CRT that can be improved greatly. These include how patients are screened for CRT implementation (i.e., identifying likely responders and nonresponders) and how CRT systems are optimized once installed. Investigations into these two difficult issues, primarily based on echocardiographic techniques both to screen and to optimize CRT patients, have already been discussed. A third area of potential development is in the area of CS lead delivery itself. A substantial portion of patients undergoing resynchronization device implantation have CS anatomy that is suboptimal for lead delivery and LV pacing. This may be due to difficult CS or side-branch access, to phrenic nerve capture, or simply to a paucity of well-positioned, lateral LV venous branches at all. There are a number of surgical delivery systems and approaches that allow for epicardial LV lead placement (53–55). Surgical access to the lateral LV remains a second-tier option for CS lead delivery (typically reserved for those patients in whom endovascular lead placement is impossible), but it may be that minimally invasive surgical lead implantation becomes a more widespread and attractive alternative as the techniques and technology improve.

References

1. Levy D, Kenchaiah S, Larson MG, et al. Long-term trends in the incidence of and survival with heart failure. *N Engl J Med* 2002;347:1397–1402.
2. Baldasseroni S, Opasich C, Gorini M, et al. Left bundle-branch block is associated with increased 1-year sudden and total mortality rate in 5517 outpatients with congestive heart failure: a report from the Italian network on congestive heart failure. *Am Heart J* 2002;143:398–405.
3. Aaronson KD, Schwartz JS, Chen TM, et al. Development and prospective validation of a clinical index to predict survival in ambulatory patients referred for cardiac transplant evaluation. *Circulation* 1997;95:2660–2667.
4. Shamim W, Francis DP, Yousufuddin M, et al. Intraventricular conduction delay: a prognostic marker in chronic heart failure. *Int J Cardiol* 1999;70: 171–178.
5. Cazeau S, Ritter P, Bakdach S, et al. 4-Chamber pacing in dilated cardiomyopathy. *Pacing Clin Electrophysiol* 1994;17:1974–1979.
6. Burkhoff D, Oikawa RY, Sagawa K. Influence of pacing site on canine left ventricular contraction. *Am J Physiol* 1986;251:H428–H435.
7. Park RC, Little WC, O'Rourke RA. Effect of alteration of left ventricular activation sequence on the left ventricular end-systolic pressure-volume relation in closed-chest dogs. *Circ Res* 1985;57:706–717.
8. Liu L, Tockman B, Girouard S, et al. Left ventricular resynchronization therapy in a canine model of left bundle branch block. *Am J Physiol Heart Circ Physiol* 2002;282:H2238–H2244.
9. McVeigh ER, Prinzen FW, Wyman BT, et al. Imaging asynchronous mechanical activation of the paced heart with tagged MRI. *Magn Reson Med* 1998;39:507–513.
10. van Oosterhout MF, Prinzen FW, Arts T, et al. Asynchronous electrical activation induces asymmetrical hypertrophy of the left ventricular wall. *Circulation* 1998;98:588–595.
11. van Oosterhout MF, Arts T, Bassingthwaighte JB, et al. Relation between local myocardial growth and blood flow during chronic ventricular pacing. *Cardiovasc Res* 2002;53:831–840.
12. Spragg DD, Akar FG, Helm RH, et al. Abnormal conduction and repolarization in late-activated myocardium of dyssynchronously contracting hearts. *Cardiovasc Res* 2005;67:77–86.
13. Spragg DD, Leclercq C, Loghmani M, et al. Regional alterations in protein expression in the dyssynchronous failing heart. *Circulation* 2003;108:929–932.
14. Leclercq C, Faris O, Tunin R, et al. Systolic improvement and mechanical resynchronization does not require electrical synchrony in the dilated failing heart with left bundle-branch block. *Circulation* 2002;106:1760–1763.
15. Hay I, Melenovsky V, Fetics BJ, et al. Short-term effects of right-left heart sequential cardiac resynchronization in patients with heart failure, chronic atrial fibrillation, and atrioventricular nodal block. *Circulation* 2004;110: 3404–3410.
16. Bordachar P, Lafitte S, Reuter S, et al. Biventricular pacing and left ventricular pacing in heart failure: similar hemodynamic improvement despite marked electromechanical differences. *J Cardiovasc Electrophysiol* 2004;15:1342–1347.
17. Kass D. Left ventricular versus biventricular pacing in cardiac resynchronization therapy: the plot in this tale of two modes. *J Cardiovasc Electrophysiol* 2004;15:1348–1349.
18. Yu CM, Chau E, Sanderson JE, et al. Tissue Doppler echocardiographic evidence of reverse remodeling and improved synchronicity by simultaneously delaying regional contraction after biventricular pacing therapy in heart failure. *Circulation* 2002;105:438–445.
19. Duncan A, Wait D, Gibson D, et al. Left ventricular remodelling and haemodynamic effects of multisite biventricular pacing in patients with left ventricular systolic dysfunction and activation disturbances in sinus rhythm: substudy of the MUSTIC (Multisite Stimulation in Cardiomyopathies) trial. *Eur Heart J* 2003;24:430–441.
20. Gras D, Leclercq C, Tang ASL, et al. Cardiac resynchronization therapy in advanced heart failure: the multicenter InSync clinical study. *Eur J Heart Fail* 2002;4:311–320.
21. Auricchio A, Stellbrink C, Butter C, et al. Clinical efficacy of cardiac resynchronization therapy using left ventricular pacing in heart failure patients stratified by severity of ventricular conduction delay. *J Am Coll Cardiol* 2003;42:2109–2116.
22. Blanc JJ, Bertault-Valls V, Fatemi M, et al. Midterm benefits of left univentricular pacing in patients with congestive heart failure. *Circulation* 2004; 109:1741–1744.
23. Abraham WT, Fisher WG, Smith AL, et al. Cardiac resynchronization in chronic heart failure. *N Engl J Med* 2002;346:1845–1853.
24. Saxon LA, De Marco T, Schafer J, et al. Effects of long-term biventricular stimulation for resynchronization on echocardiographic measures of remodeling. *Circulation* 2002;105:1304–1310.
25. Nelson GS, Berger RD, Fetics BJ, et al. Left ventricular or biventricular pacing improves cardiac function at diminished energy cost in patients with dilated cardiomyopathy and left bundle-branch block. *Circulation* 2000;102:3053–3059.
26. Fish JM, Di Diego JM, Nesterenko V, et al. Epicardial activation of left ventricular wall prolongs QT interval and transmural dispersion of repolarization: implications for biventricular pacing. *Circulation* 2004;109: 2136–2142.
27. Cleland JG, Daubert JC, Erdmann E, et al. The effect of cardiac resynchronization on morbidity and mortality in heart failure. *N Engl J Med* 2005; 352:1539–1549.

28. Cazeau S, Leclercq C, Lavergne T, et al. Effects of multisite biventricular pacing in patients with heart failure and intraventricular conduction delay. *N Engl J Med* 2001;344:873–880.
29. Young JB, Abraham WT, Smith AL, et al. Combined cardiac resynchronization and implantable cardioversion defibrillation in advanced chronic heart failure: the MIRACLE ICD Trial. *JAMA* 2003;289:2685–2694.
30. Bristow MR, Saxon LA, Boehmer J, et al. Cardiac-resynchronization therapy with or without an implantable defibrillator in advanced chronic heart failure. *N Engl J Med* 2004;350:2140–2150.
31. Bradley DJ, Bradley EA, Baughman KL, et al. Cardiac resynchronization and death from progressive heart failure: a meta-analysis of randomized controlled trials. *JAMA* 2003;289:730–740.
32. McAlister FA, Ezekowitz JA, Wiebe N, et al. Systematic review: cardiac resynchronization in patients with symptomatic heart failure. *Ann Intern Med* 2004;141:381–390.
33. ACC/AHA/NASPE 2002 Guideline update for implantation of cardiac pacemakers and antiarrhythmia devices: summary article. *Circulation* 2002;106: 2145–2161.
34. Strickberger SA, Conti J, Daoud EG, et al. Patient selection for cardiac resynchronization therapy: from the Council on Clinical Cardiology Subcommittee on Electrocardiography and Arrhythmias and the Quality of Care and Outcomes Research Interdisciplinary Working Group, in collaboration with the Heart Rhythm Society. *Circulation* 2005;111:2146–2150.
35. Mansour M, Reddy VY, Singh J, et al. Three-dimensional reconstruction of the coronary sinus using rotational angiography. *J Cardiovasc Electrophysiol* 2005;16:675–676.
36. Butter C, Auricchio A, Stellbrink C, et al. Effect of resynchronization therapy stimulation site on the systolic function of heart failure patients. *Circulation* 2001;104:3026–3029.
37. Auricchio A, Stellbrink C, Block M, et al. Effect of pacing chamber and atrioventricular delay on acute systolic function of paced patients with congestive heart failure. The Pacing Therapies for Congestive Heart Failure Study Group. The Guidant Congestive Heart Failure Research Group. *Circulation* 1999;99:2993–3001.
38. Sogaard P, Egeblad H, Pedersen AK, et al. Sequential versus simultaneous biventricular resynchronization for severe heart failure: evaluation by tissue Doppler imaging. *Circulation* 2002;106:2078–2084.
39. Van Gelder BM, Bracke FA, Meijer A, et al. Effect of optimizing the VV interval on left ventricular contractility in cardiac resynchronization therapy. *Am J Cardiol* 2004;93:1500–1503.
40. Kass DA. Predicting cardiac resynchronization response by QRS duration: the long and short of it. *J Am Coll Cardiol* 2003;42(12):2125–2127.
41. Lecoq G, Leclercq C, Leray E, et al. Clinical and electrocardiographic predictors of a positive response to cardiac resynchronization therapy in advanced heart failure. *Eur Heart J* 2005;26:1094–1100.
42. Bleeker GB, Schalij MJ, Molhoek SG, et al. Relationship between QRS duration and left ventricular dyssynchrony in patients with end-stage heart failure. *J Cardiovasc Electrophysiol* 2004;15:544–549.
43. Bleeker GB, Schalij MJ, Molhoek SG, et al. Frequency of left ventricular dyssynchrony in patients with heart failure and a narrow QRS complex. *Am J Cardiol* 2005;95:140–142.
44. Schuster P, Faerestrand S, Ohm OJ. Color Doppler tissue velocity imaging can disclose systolic left ventricular asynchrony independent of the QRS morphology in patients with severe heart failure. *Pacing Clin Electrophysiol* 2004;27:460–467.
45. Achilli A, Sassara M, Ficili S, et al. Long-term effectiveness of cardiac resynchronization therapy in patients with refractory heart failure and "narrow" QRS. *J Am Coll Cardiol* 2003;42:2117–2124.
46. Notabartolo D, Merlino JD, Smith AL, et al. Usefulness of the peak velocity difference by tissue Doppler imaging technique as an effective predictor of response to cardiac resynchronization therapy. *Am J Cardiol* 2004;94:817–820.
47. Leon AR, Greenberg JM, Kanuru N, et al. Cardiac resynchronization in patients with congestive heart failure and chronic atrial fibrillation: effect of upgrading to biventricular pacing after chronic right ventricular pacing. *J Am Coll Cardiol* 2002;39:1258–1263.
48. Hay I, Melenovsky V, Fetics BJ, et al. Short-term effects of right-left heart sequential cardiac resynchronization in patients with heart failure, chronic atrial fibrillation, and atrioventricular nodal block. *Circulation* 2004;110: 3404–3410.
49. Linde C, Leclercq C, Rex S, et al. Long-term benefits of biventricular pacing in congestive heart failure: results from the MUltisite STimulation in Cardiomyopathy (MUSTIC) study. *J Am Coll Cardiol* 2002;40:111–118.
50. Freudenberger RS, Wilson AC, Lawrence-Nelson J, et al. Permanent pacing is a risk factor for the development of heart failure. *Am J Cardiol* 2005;95:671–674.
51. Wilkoff BL, Cook JR, Epstein AE, et al. Dual-chamber pacing or ventricular backup pacing in patients with an implantable defibrillator: the Dual Chamber and VVI Implantable Defibrillator (DAVID) Trial. *JAMA* 2002; 288:3115–3123.
52. Valls-Bertault V, Fatemi M, Gilard M, et al. Assessment of upgrading to biventricular pacing in patients with right ventricular pacing and congestive heart failure after atrioventricular junctional ablation for chronic atrial fibrillation. *Europace* 2004;6:438–443.
53. Maessen JG, Phelps B, Dekker AL, et al. Minimal invasive epicardial lead implantation: optimizing cardiac resynchronization with a new mapping device for epicardial lead placement. *Eur J Cardiothorac Surg* 2004;25:894–896.
54. Koos R, Sinha AM, Markus KU, et al. Long-term comparison of the coronary venous approach and a limited lateral thoracotomy for left ventricular lead placement in patients receiving cardiac resynchronization therapy. *Circulation* 2003;108:627–628.
55. Koos R, Sinha AM, Markus K, et al. Comparison of left ventricular lead placement via the coronary venous approach versus lateral thoracotomy in patients receiving cardiac resynchronization therapy. *Am J Cardiol* 2004;94: 59–63.

[illegible]

SECTION FIVE: INVASIVE CARDIOLOGY AND SURGICAL TECHNIQUES

ERIC J. TOPOL, MD

CHAPTER 76 ■ CORONARY ANGIOGRAPHY

DEEPAK L. BHATT AND FREDERICK A. HEUPLER, JR.

OVERVIEW

Coronary angiography remains the clinical gold standard for the diagnosis of coronary artery disease. Approximately 2 million procedures are performed annually in the United States. More than 60% of cardiologists in the United States perform coronary angiography as part of their practice (1). Because it is an invasive procedure with potentially serious risks, coronary angiography should be performed only by well-trained individuals when an appropriate clinical indication exists. Physicians who perform coronary angiography must clearly understand its limitations and possess a firm grasp of the fundamental technical aspects of catheterization (2).

GLOSSARY

Caudal projection: Radiographic view with the image intensifier pointing to the inferior surface of the heart.

Conus artery: A branch that variably arises either from the right coronary artery or in close proximity to it and perfuses the right ventricular outflow tract.

Cranial projection: Radiographic view with the image intensifier pointing to the superior surface of the heart.

Crux: The intersection of the atrioventricular groove and the interatrial and interventricular septa on the inferior aspect of the heart.

Damping: Blunting of a recording of the arterial pressure waveform.

Diagonal artery: A branch of the left anterior descending artery that perfuses the left ventricular free wall.

Dominance: Reference to the vessel, either the right coronary artery or the left circumflex artery, that supplies the posterior part of the heart; in codominance, both arteries provide circulation to the posterior heart.

Image intensifier: The portion of the catheterization laboratory imaging equipment that increases the brightness of images produced by x-rays. Image intensifier units are being replaced in many catheterization laboratories with a newer technology, flat detector units.

Internal mammary artery (IMA): An artery that runs from the subclavian artery down the chest wall that can be harvested for use as a surgical conduit for bypass grafting; also called the *internal thoracic artery*.

Left anterior descending (LAD) artery: The artery that supplies the anterior surface of the heart.

Left anterior oblique (LAO) projection: Radiographic view with the image intensifier on the left side of the patient.

Left circumflex artery (LCx): The artery that supplies blood to the lateral aspect of the heart.

Left main (LM) coronary artery: The short artery that divides into the left anterior descending artery and the left circumflex artery (and sometimes the ramus intermedius) and supplies most of the left side of the heart.

Marginal artery: A branch (acute marginal) of the right coronary artery that supplies the right ventricle; also, a branch (obtuse marginal) of the left circumflex, sometimes referred to as a *lateral branch*.

Posterior descending artery (PDA): The branch of the right coronary artery, or occasionally the left circumflex artery, that provides blood flow to the posterior aspect of the interventricular septum.

Ramus intermedius (RI): A branch of the left main artery that supplies the lateral wall of the left ventricle.

Right anterior oblique (RAO) projection: Radiographic view with the image intensifier on the right of the patient.

Right coronary artery (RCA): The artery that supplies blood to the right side of the heart and usually to the posterior aspect of the left ventricle.

Saphenous vein graft: A surgical conduit harvested from the legs that is used to reroute blood from the aorta to the coronary arteries.

Scatter: Dispersion of radiation as it passes through the body; it is the source of most of the radiation exposure to the operator.

Ventricularization: Distortion of the recorded arterial pressure waveform such that the diastolic component is blunted, simulating a left ventricular pressure tracing.

GENERAL PRINCIPLES

Historical Perspective

The first selective coronary angiogram was performed in 1958 by Dr. F. Mason Sones, Jr., a cardiologist at the Cleveland Clinic Foundation in Ohio (3). When Dr. Sones and Dr. Earl K. Shirey published their results of more than 1,000 procedures in 1962, interest in coronary angiography surged. Coronary angiography as a diagnostic tool blossomed with Dr. René Favaloro's description in 1968 of his pioneering work in performing saphenous vein coronary artery bypass grafting at the Cleveland Clinic.

Radiologists played an important role in the development of catheterization techniques in the early 1960s. New preformed catheter designs, such as those by Dr. Melvin Judkins and Dr. Kurt Amplatz, enabled selective angiography to be performed with greater ease than was previously possible with the Sones catheters. Additionally, percutaneous approaches were also now possible, and arterial cutdowns were no longer required. Improvements in radiographic imaging concomitantly led to better image quality. After Dr. Andreas Grüntzig introduced percutaneous coronary angioplasty in 1977, cardiologists were able to make the transition from being diagnosticians to becoming endovascular surgeons.

Coronary Artery Anatomy

Normal Anatomy

The left main (LM) coronary artery originates from the left sinus of Valsalva and usually bifurcates into the left anterior descending artery (LAD), which supplies the left ventricle's anterior surface, and the left circumflex artery (LCx), which supplies the lateral aspect of the left ventricle (Fig. 76.1). The LAD traverses the anterior interventricular groove, giving rise to septal perforating branches to supply the interventricular septum and to diagonal branches that supply the anterolateral wall. It then bifurcates distally and tapers out as a "whale's tail" at the cardiac apex, although sometimes it wraps around the apex to supply part of the inferior wall. The LCx courses along the left atrioventricular groove and provides atrial branches to the left atrium and marginal branches that supply the lateral wall of the left ventricle. The marginal branches are sometimes referred to as *lateral branches*, with the first marginal branch called the *high lateral* and subsequent lateral branches referred to as *lateral* or *posterolateral branches*. Occasionally, the LM coronary artery trifurcates to give rise also to a ramus intermedius branch that supplies the high lateral wall of the left ventricle.

The right coronary artery (RCA) originates from the right sinus at a slightly more caudal level than the LM coronary artery and supplies the right ventricle and the inferior aspect of the left ventricle (Fig. 76.2). It traverses the right atrioventricular groove and provides small branches to the right atrium and marginal branches to the right ventricle. Approximately 60% of the time, the RCA atrial branches supply the sinus node; otherwise, the LCx atrial branches serve this function. Approximately 50% of the time, the first branch of the RCA is a conus branch, supplying the right ventricular outflow tract; the remainder of the time, the conus branch originates separately from an ostium near the RCA ostium. The dominant artery is generally defined as the one that provides the posterior descending artery (PDA) to supply the posterior wall. In approximately 85% of patients, the RCA is dominant, with the remainder of patients having either a dominant LCx or a codominant RCA and LCx. The PDA of the RCA (or the LCx) courses along the inferior interventricular groove, providing septal perforators, a feature that may aid in its identification and differentiation from the posterolateral segment of the RCA (or LCx), which gives off branches to the posterior ventricle. More than 90% of the time, the artery to the atrioventricular node originates from the atrioventricular branch of the RCA as it passes through the crux.

Coronary Anomalies

It is important for the angiographer to be alert for possible variations in normal coronary anatomy. In a series of 126,595 patients undergoing coronary angiography at the Cleveland Clinic Foundation, Yamanaka and Hobbs (4) found coronary artery anomalies in 1.3% of patients. Of the anomalies identified, 87% involved anomalies of origin or distribution, 13% involved the presence of coronary artery fistulae, and 81% were considered benign. (Table 76.1). Some anomalies may be potentially harmful, such as a coronary artery that originates from the pulmonary artery or the opposite aortic sinus. For example, most patients with an anomalous origin of the left coronary artery (LCA) from the pulmonary artery (Bland-White-Garland syndrome) die as infants unless surgical repair is undertaken.

Origin of the LCA from the right sinus may also lead to sudden death, depending in large part on the traversal of the anomalous artery. If the anomalous vessel travels intramyocardially through the septum (the most common variant of this anomaly), or anteriorly or posteriorly, symptoms of ischemia are very unlikely. If the anomalous artery courses between the pulmonary artery and aorta, however, exercise may precipitate angina or sudden death. In this latter variant, the LM coronary artery projects on end as a "dot" on the anterior surface of the aorta during a ventriculogram or aortogram in an right anterior oblique (RAO) projection. Likewise, a single coronary artery or large coronary artery fistulae may be problematic. Patients with large coronary artery fistulae may present with heart failure or ischemia, and these lesions may also cause endocarditis; therefore, endocarditis prophylaxis is recommended (5). Small coronary artery fistulae, however, are rarely problematic. These fistulae typically originate from the LAD and drain into the pulmonary artery two thirds of the time, with drainage into a cardiac chamber in the remainder of instances.

Approximately 10% of patients with coronary artery anomalies have some form of congenital heart abnormality, such as a bicuspid aortic valve (6). In tetralogy of Fallot, for example, the LAD sometimes originates from the right sinus, crossing the right ventricular outflow tract. Communication between cardiologist and cardiac surgeon is important to convey the presence of any coronary anomalies and thus prevent any accidental transection or ligation of anomalous coronary arteries (7).

Myocardial Bridging

Systolic compression of a coronary artery is referred to as *bridging*. Approximately 12% of normal angiograms demonstrate

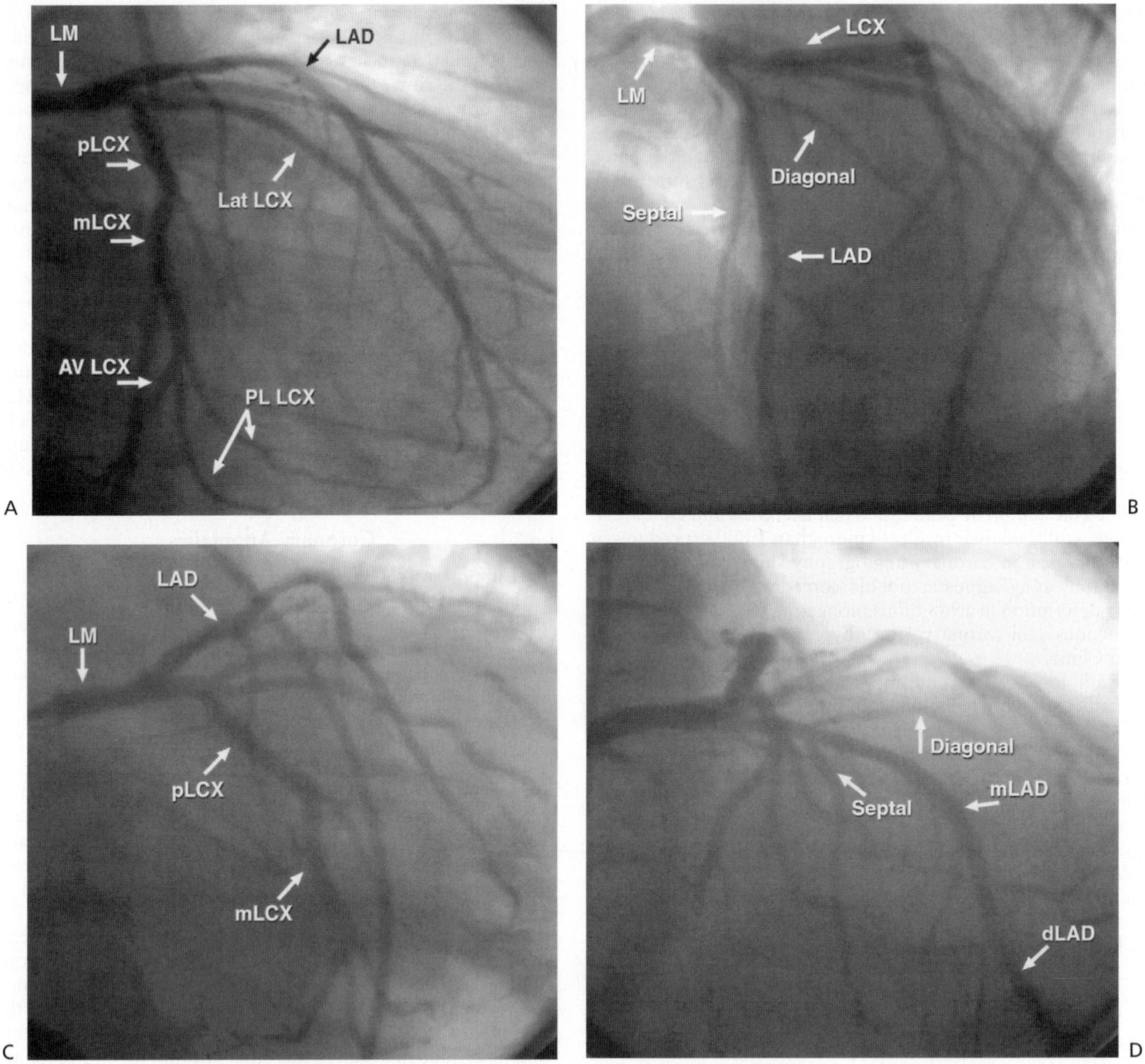

FIGURE 76.1. Normal left coronary artery with segments labeled. **A:** Shallow right anterior oblique (RAO) caudal projection. **B:** Left anterior oblique cranial projection. **C:** Posteroanterior caudal projection. **D:** RAO cranial projection. AV, atrioventricular continuation of the left circumflex artery; dLAD, distal left anterior descending artery; Lat LCX, lateral branch of the left circumflex artery; LM, left main coronary artery; mLAD, mid-left anterior descending artery; mLCX, mid-left circumflex artery; PL, posterolateral branch of the left circumflex artery; pLAD, proximal left anterior descending artery; pLCX, proximal left circumflex artery.

some degree of myocardial bridging, although only 1.7% show systolic narrowing of more than 50% (8). Bridging occurs in the mid-LAD when it courses through the septum. If this is the case, it is important to note this for the surgeon, because it makes grafting more technically challenging, especially from a minimally invasive approach. Myocardial bridging of septal perforating branches, also called *septal squeeze*, is commonly found in hypertrophic cardiomyopathy and aortic stenosis and occasionally with severe proximal LAD stenosis, but rarely in normal hearts (9). Other more unusual locations for bridging include the PDA. When a circumflex marginal branch is intramyocardial, ventricular systole usually produces little or no compression. The intramyocardial portion appears unusually straight rather than serpentine. Nitrate administration tends to make bridging more apparent angiographically. Because the majority of coronary flow occurs in diastole, the systolic phenomenon of bridging rarely leads to ischemia (8). In the few instances in which it does lead to objective signs of ischemia, stenting has been performed successfully (10–13).

Collateral Circulation

When an occlusion or severe narrowing of a coronary artery develops, collateral channels may form from a nearby artery to supply blood to the hypoperfused area of myocardium. Collaterals form between arteries that occupy adjacent areas of the heart, and such connections cannot form if a cardiac chamber is superimposed in between. For example, collateral development via septal perforators is common between the LAD and PDA when one of these vessels is occluded. Occasionally, a separate conus branch arising near the RCA supplies collaterals to the LAD; identification is important if consideration is being given

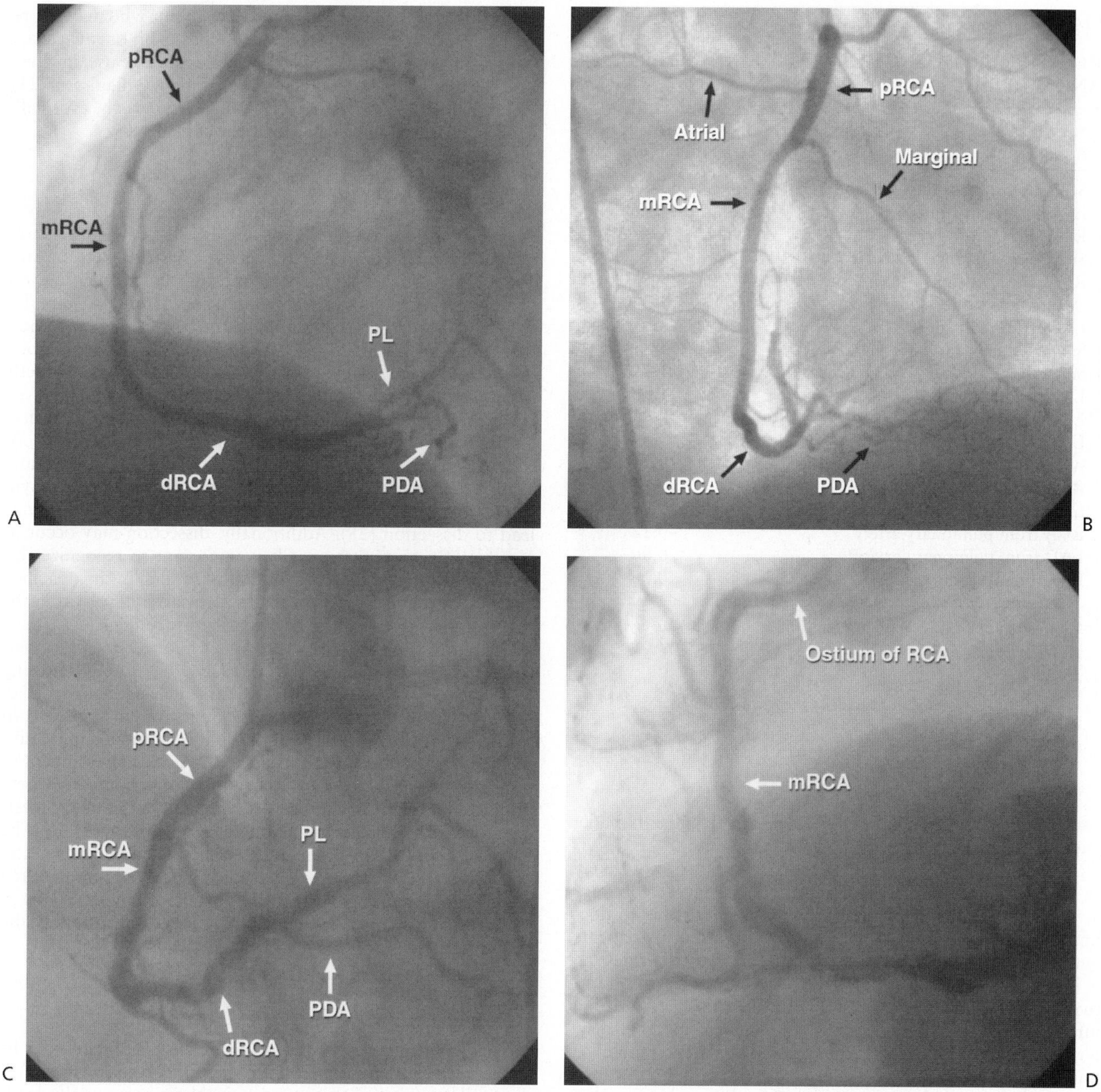

FIGURE 76.2. Normal right coronary artery with segments labeled. **A:** Left anterior oblique projection. **B:** Right anterior oblique projection. **C:** Posteroanterior cranial projection. **D:** Lateral projection. dRCA, distal right coronary artery; mRCA, mid-right coronary artery; PDA, posterior descending artery branch; PL, posterolateral branch of the right coronary artery; pRCA, proximal right coronary artery.

to bypass surgery targets. Kugel artery is a small vessel that arises from the proximal RCA or LCx, or both, and traverses the interatrial septum; it commonly terminates near the crux, where it may act as a source of collaterals to the distal RCA or LCx via the atrioventricular nodal artery. Intracoronary collaterals, so-called bridging collaterals, may form from the same coronary artery across an area of total vessel occlusion. Identification of such bridging collaterals and recognition of an underlying chronic total occlusion are important. Although rare, pericardial or bronchial arteries may provide coronary collaterals (14). When collaterals are present from more than one source, competitive flow from both sources may occur, leading to inadequate opacification of the target vessel; this may produce the false appearance of a significant luminal obstruction at the point where the two collateral flows meet.

Coronary Artery Spasm

Prinzmetal angina or *variant angina* refers to the syndrome of coronary artery spasm that causes transient ST-segment elevation during angina (15,16). This may result in anginal chest pain at rest, often in the early morning, as well as syncope from heart block or ventricular arrhythmias. The coronary arteries of these patients are predisposed to spasm, often despite the absence of angiographically severe atherosclerosis. Prinzmetal angina is rare, and it is recognized clinically even less often than in the past owing to the advent of calcium channel blockers and long-acting nitrates (17). In patients with no significant atherosclerosis but a suspicion of spasm, Holter monitoring may reveal ST-segment shifts that verify the diagnosis. If angina occurs concurrent with ST-segment elevation in a

TABLE 76.1

RELATIVE FREQUENCY OF CORONARY ARTERY ANOMALIES

Anomaly	Percentage of total (%)
Separate origin of the LAD and LCx	30.4
LCx from right sinus or RCA	27.7
RCA from aorta	11.2
Small coronary artery fistulae	9.7
RCA from left sinus[a]	8.1
Multiple or large fistulae[a]	3.7
LAD from right sinus[a]	2.3
Single left coronary artery[a]	1.85
Single right coronary artery[a]	1.46
LM from right sinus[a]	1.3
LM from aorta	0.95
LM from pulmonary artery[a]	0.59
Absent LCx (with very dominant RCA)	0.24
RCA from posterior sinus	0.24
Intercoronary communication	0.18
RCA from pulmonary artery	0.12
LAD from pulmonary artery[a]	0.06
LM from posterior sinus	0.06

LAD, left anterior descending artery; LCx, left circumflex artery; LM, left main coronary artery; RCA, right coronary artery.
[a]Potentially serious anomalies.
Source: Adapted from Yamanaka O, Hobbs RE. Coronary artery anomalies in 126,595 patients undergoing coronary angiography. *Cathet Cardiovasc Diagn* 1990;21:28–40.

patient with a "normal" catheterization, the diagnosis is made, with no need for confirmatory provocative testing.

Provocative testing for coronary artery spasm is most likely to be clinically useful in the patient with no severe coronary artery obstructions, in whom it has been impossible to document the diagnosis. It is not likely to be useful in patients with fixed severe coronary obstructions, and the risk of testing is increased in these individuals. The major risk of provocative testing is unrelenting spasm, with subsequent myocardial infarction. Therefore, when this test is performed, intraarterial nitroglycerin and calcium channel blockers should be immediately available. The method to perform provocative testing involves administration of 0.05 mg intravenous methylergonovine while monitoring a complete electrocardiogram every minute (18,19). If typical chest pain or electrocardiographic changes develop, the coronary arteries should be reimaged immediately. Five minutes after the methylergonovine has been administered, if there has been no chest pain or electrocardiographic changes, the coronary arteries should be reimaged. If there is no evidence of spasm, 0.2 mg methylergonovine should be administered and the foregoing procedure repeated. Some operators prefer to omit the 0.05-mg dose to save time. If spasm does occur, 100 to 200 μg nitroglycerin should be administered intraarterially to relieve the spasm. Intracoronary acetylcholine is another provocative agent for coronary spasm, but it probably lacks the specificity of methylergonovine.

Diffuse spasm that occurs without angina or ST-segment changes may be physiologic and is not diagnostic of Prinzmetal angina. Methylergonovine-induced severe coronary spasm may recur after immediate treatment because of the longer half-life of methylergonovine compared with nitroglycerin; therefore, the patient should be observed and treated with systemic long-acting nitrates and calcium channel blockers (20). Provocative testing should be avoided in patients with severe systemic or pulmonary hypertension, as well as in patients who may be pregnant. Spasm may also be a cause of chest pain or myocardial infarction after acute alcohol ingestion or cocaine use, in which case the clinical history is useful in making the diagnosis (21). Nonischemic, "catheter-induced" coronary spasm, especially ostial spasm, may be triggered by the catheter tip.

Coronary Artery Dissection

Rarely, spontaneous coronary artery dissection produces an ischemic syndrome or sudden death (22). Predisposing factors include pregnancy, a burst of intense physical exertion, and cocaine use (23,24). Pregnant or postpartum women are the demographic group in which spontaneous coronary artery dissection is most commonly seen, and the LAD is the vessel most frequently involved (25). Severe hypertension may also predispose to spontaneous dissection (26). Although not exactly spontaneous, blunt trauma, such as from a motor vehicle accident, may also lead to dissection (27). Aortic dissection may also extend into the coronary arteries, particularly the RCA. Marfan syndrome may be complicated by coronary dissection, as may connective tissue disorders such as Ehlers-Danlos syndrome. Arteritis, such as that seen in polyarteritis nodosa, may lead to dissection (28). Additionally, dissection may occur as a result of catheter trauma. It is important to recognize this entity, which may appear as a radiolucent flap in the opacified artery or as a linear persistent stain in the arterial wall after the contrast material has cleared from the true lumen.

Regardless of the cause, dissection can often be treated percutaneously with stent deployment (29,30). Although healing of dissection with conservative treatment has been reported, this approach is less common in the interventional era (31). In some instances of postpartum dissection, immunosuppressive therapy has been used with success (32). Eosinophils appear to be present in the dissection plane in cases of peripartum dissection, similar to peripartum cardiomyopathy, a finding suggesting an inflammatory origin in at least some instances (33). The plane of dissection is often between the media and adventitia of the vessel, although in some cases, an intimal tear is noted at autopsy. Some cases of spontaneous dissection, especially in older individuals at risk for atherosclerosis, are probably the result of plaque rupture and intimal dissection (34).

Coronary Artery Ectasia and Aneurysm

Coronary artery ectasia refers to an abnormal enlargement of the coronary arteries. Arteries that are ectatic appear to be prone to thrombus formation, dissection, and spasm (35). Additionally, prior percutaneous intervention occasionally leads to development of segments of ectasia. When the area of dilatation is more than 1.5 times the diameter of the normal portion of the artery, the enlarged portion is referred to as an *aneurysm* (36). The RCA is the vessel most frequently involved. Atherosclerosis is the most common cause of coronary ectasia and aneurysm (37). Kawasaki disease leads to formation of giant coronary artery aneurysms in approximately 20% of untreated patients (38–41). Mycotic aneurysms of the coronary arteries are rare (42). Historically, large coronary artery aneurysms have been treated conservatively with antiplatelet or anticoagulant therapy, or both, but, more recently, surgery and intracoronary stent graft deployment have been used (43,44). When there is associated stenosis, invasive treatment may be indicated.

Indications

Coronary angiography is indicated when the coronary artery anatomy needs to be delineated. The American College of Cardiology (ACC) has published guidelines to assist the clinician

TABLE 76.2

INDICATIONS FOR CORONARY ANGIOGRAPHY

Class	Indications
I	Unstable angina/ACS, refractory to medical therapy or with high/intermediate risk features Suspected Prinzmetal angina As a plan to proceed with primary PCI for ST-elevation MI Cardiogenic shock owing to acute MI Recurrent ischemia after ST-elevation MI Persistent chest pain after fibrinolysis Abnormal stress test after fibrinolysis CCS class III or IV angina with inadequate response to medical therapy Abnormal stress test with high-risk features Sudden cardiac death or ventricular arrhythmia with no obvious cause Congestive heart failure with angina or ischemia Patient requiring valve surgery or repair of a congenital defect, with angina Suspected stent thrombosis Recurrent angina within 9 mo of PCI Before repair of a mechanical complication of MI Planned vascular surgery with angina or positive stress test
II	Unstable angina/ACS controlled with medical therapy Acute ST-elevation MI after fibrinolysis when it appears that reperfusion has not occurred, to perform rescue PCI CCS class III or IV angina that improves to CCS class I or II with medical therapy Abnormal stress test without high-risk features Worsening ischemia on noninvasive testing CCS class I or II angina that is intolerant or unresponsive to medication Yearly angiography after cardiac transplantation Perioperative MI
III	Patient refusing revascularization Patient not a candidate for revascularization due to medical comorbidities Within 24 h of fibrinolysis with no evidence of ischemia Screening of asymptomatic patients

ACS, acute coronary syndrome; CCS, Canadian Cardiovascular Society; MI, myocardial infarction; PCI, percutaneous coronary intervention.
Source: Data from Scanlon PJ, Faxon DP, Audet AM, et al. ACC/AHA guidelines for coronary angiography: a report of the American College of Cardiology/American Heart Association Task Force on practice guidelines (Committee on Coronary Angiography) developed in collaboration with the Society for Cardiac Angiography and Interventions. *J Am Coll Cardiol* 1999;33:1756–1824.

in appropriate use of this invasive procedure (45) (Table 76.2). Indications are listed as class I when there is general consensus that angiography is indicated, class II when opinions diverge, and class III when the consensus is that angiography should not be performed. In a patient with anginal chest discomfort and evidence of ischemia on a functional study, coronary angiography may reveal a stenosis that is amenable to angioplasty or coronary artery bypass surgery (class I). In a patient with an acute coronary syndrome, angiography is given a class II indication. However, emerging evidence supports an invasive approach in the initial evaluation of patients with acute coronary syndromes (46,47). The development of pharmacologic adjuncts, such as the glycoprotein IIb/IIIa inhibitors, has enhanced the safety of percutaneous intervention and has broadened the indications for cardiac catheterization. Thus, the ACC guidelines provide a framework for the practice of evidence-based medicine but do not substitute for clinical judgment, and they do not necessarily incorporate the most current research.

TABLE 76.3

RELATIVE CONTRAINDICATIONS TO CORONARY ANGIOGRAPHY

Renal insufficiency
Bleeding diathesis or active bleeding
Fever or active infection
Aortic valve vegetation
Anemia
Severe dye allergy
Metabolic abnormalities
  Hyperkalemia
  Hypokalemia
Digitalis toxicity
Uncontrolled hypertension
Decompensated heart failure
Uncontrolled tachyarrhythmia
Untreated high-grade heart block

Contraindications

The only absolute contraindication to coronary angiography is patient refusal. According to the ACC classification, indications that are labeled as class III are actually situations in which coronary angiography is contraindicated (Table 76.2). Additional relative contraindications are shown in Table 76.3. *Relative* contraindications imply that in certain urgent clinical circumstances, proceeding with angiography may be appropriate, although caution must be exercised.

Operator Proficiency

The ACC has set minimum training requirements for the performance of diagnostic angiography. During cardiology fellowship, each trainee must perform 300 diagnostic coronary angiograms while serving as the primary operator on 200. Operator and institutional procedure volumes are linked to outcomes in the catheterization laboratory (48). After training is completed, a minimum yearly volume of 150 diagnostic catheterizations per year for each angiographer has been recommended, although more recently the number has been revised to 100 (49). It is desirable to have cardiac surgical backup nearby (50). Although nonphysicians may assist in coronary angiography, they should not function as independent operators (51). Additionally, performance standards for cardiac catheterization laboratories have been established. Principally, this involves monitoring of procedural outcomes to ensure some degree of internal review of complications (52,53).

Preprocedural Medication

Aspirin, 325 mg, should be given to eligible patients before the procedure in case angioplasty becomes necessary. If the probability of percutaneous intervention seems high, a loading dose of clopidogrel, 300 mg, can also be given. Metformin (Glucophage) should be discontinued on the day of the procedure, because this medication may cause lactic acidosis if renal failure results from the procedure and if metformin is continued after the onset of renal failure (54). Warfarin should be stopped before the procedure if possible until the international normalized ratio is less than 1.8. If anticoagulation is essential, warfarin can be stopped several days before the anticipated procedure, and subcutaneous injections of the low-molecular-weight heparin, enoxaparin (1 mg/kg twice daily), can be substituted; the dose of enoxaparin can then be withheld the morning of the procedure.

Radiation Principles and Safety

Most catheterization laboratories have already moved to digital image acquisition, distribution, and archiving. A major factor enabling this transition has been the widespread adoption of the Digital Imaging Communication in Medicine (DICOM) standard (55). In addition to improving image quality, digital imaging may lower radiation exposure to the operator by approximately 20%. Retrieval of angiographic information and transfer of data among physicians are also easier, because a typical catheterization study may easily fit on a single CD or be distributed rapidly on a high-bandwidth network.

Efforts to reduce radiation exposure to the angiographer and the patient are important because the cumulative doses of radiation with repeated exposures can produce direct tissue injury (deterministic effects) and neoplasms (stochastic effects). Risk reduction efforts fall into two major categories: radiation protection (usually protection of the operator from radiation exposure) and radiation production.

Radiation protection for the operator is accomplished by a variety of shielding and positioning mechanisms. A thyroid collar and lead apron provide excellent protection for the operator's thyroid (which decreases the likelihood of thyroid cancer) and trunk. Leaded glasses should be worn because radiation exposure increases the risks of cataracts; a headband may make these heavy glasses less uncomfortable. The catheterization table should be equipped with two lead shields: one for the lower body and an adjustable leaded glass shield to protect the operator's upper body and head. Doubling the distance of the operator from the x-ray entrance beam site reduces the operator's dose to one fourth. The femoral approach, in which the operator is farther away from the site of radiation, is likely to decrease the operator's exposure compared with the brachial approach. Operators should never permit repeated or prolonged exposure of their fingers in the direct field of radiation, except for extreme emergencies.

Radiation protection for the patient can be provided by avoiding unnecessary radiation exposure to body parts that are not essential to the study. For instance, in angulated views, the patient's arm commonly enters the field of view. Displacing the arm decreases the radiation dose to the patient and operator and improves image quality. If a female patient is pregnant, a lead shield placed between the x-ray source and the patient's pelvis may provide some protection, but it functions primarily as a reminder to the operator to avoid fluoroscopy in the vicinity of the pelvis. Protection of the fetus is limited because most of the radiation that the fetus receives is the result of scatter radiation, and the lead shield serves only to increase the x-ray dosage to penetrate the shield if fluoroscopy is performed directly over the shielded part of the body.

Radiation production can be reduced by a variety of methods, but care must be taken to achieve adequate image quality. A trade-off is commonly made between radiation dose and image quality. The operator should manipulate radiation dosage to produce the minimum image quality that is required for the task at hand. For instance, high image quality is generally not needed for passage or placement of catheters, whereas it is usually required for recording of diagnostic information.

Radiation dosage to the patient and operator can be reduced with no change in image quality by shortening the fluoroscopy and cine times and by using pulsed fluoroscopy. The amount of dose reduction that is obtained with pulsed fluoroscopy depends on how the manufacturer configures the equipment. Reducing the number of fluoroscopy pulses per second and the number of cine frames per second by 50% reduces dose to the patient and operator, but the former produces flicker, and the latter reduces the information content of the study by 50%. Cineangiography leads to greater radiation exposure per second than fluoroscopy. Therefore, acquiring cine images in fluoroscopy doses provides large dose reductions. Increasing the distance between the x-ray source and the patient improves image quality and reduces the x-ray intensity at the patient's skin and the likelihood of skin injury. For this reason, U.S. federal regulations mandate a spacer device mounted on the x-ray tube to maintain a minimum distance of 38 cm between the x-ray source and the end of the spacing device.

Positioning the image intensifier as close as possible to the patient reduces radiation exposure to the patient and the operator, and it improves image quality. The farther the image intensifier is positioned from the patient, the larger the image becomes, because of geometric magnification, but image quality deteriorates as a result of blurring, and the dose increases with the square of the magnification. Electronic image magnification is achieved by decreasing the field-of-view size, such as by changing from the 9-in (23-cm) or 7-in (17-cm) field to the 5-in (13-cm) field. Unless collimation is used in the larger field size, changing from the 7-in mode to the 5-in mode approximately doubles the entrance dose to the patient, has no major change on dose to the operator, and produces greater spatial resolution. The 5-in mode is usually optimal for visualizing small coronary arteries. Flat detector technology results in no change in spatial resolution with a change from 7- to 5-in mode.

Radiographic views obtained in left anterior oblique (LAO), lateral, or steeply angulated cranial or caudal projections result in decreased image quality and increased radiation exposure to the patient and operator. The same applies to any factor that increases the thickness or density of tissue being penetrated, such as obesity, large body size, cardiomegaly, and pleural effusion. If image quality is poor in any of these circumstances, the operator may wish to obtain most images in the RAO projection, switch from the 5- to 7-in mode, or perform a thoracentesis before the procedure. Use of shields to cover the bright areas of the lungs may decrease radiation exposure and enhance image quality. The use of collimators to minimize the field size improves image quality and decreases scatter radiation to the operator but produces a slight increase in entrance dose to the patient. However, the dose-area product (the entrance dose multiplied by the area of exposure) decreases with collimation, which reduces long-term (stochastic) effects for the patient.

The radiation exposure from a single catheterization is rarely significant to the patient. After prolonged fluoroscopy (usually in conjunction with prolonged or multiple interventional procedures), radiation dermatitis may rarely occur. This may manifest several hours to days after the procedure as an area of erythema, although weeks or months may pass before other effects of radiation, such as dermal atrophy or telangiectasia, are manifest.

Angiographers must consider the other important aspect—that is, image quality—as they reduce radiation dose. Subjective evaluation of angiographic image quality is unreliable. A recent testing system permits standardized objective benchmarking of cardiovascular radiographic equipment performance (56). This system permits evaluation of spatial and contrast resolution in relation to radiation dose in an anthropomorphic phantom. The clinical utility of this system remains to be validated.

Selection of Contrast Agents

Contrast agents are categorized based on their ionicity (either ionic or nonionic) and osmolality (high, low, or isosmolal). All intravascular radiopaque contrast agents contain iodine in a similar concentration. Thus, an "allergy to iodine," likely an allergy to some other component of the contrast agent, should not influence the choice of contrast agent. The ionic, high-osmolal contrast agents include diatrizoate and metrizoate. Ioxaglate is an ionic, low-osmolal agent. Iohexol, iopamidol, metrizamide, and ioversol are nonionic, low-osmolal agents. Iodixanol is a nonionic, isosmolal contrast agent. Several established factors should influence the choice of contrast agent.

The COntrast media Utilization in high Risk percutaneous Transluminal coronary angioplasty (COURT) trial compared the isosmolar nonionic dye iodixanol with the low-osmolar ionic agent ioxaglate in patients with acute coronary syndromes and found a reduction in in-hospital adverse events with the nonionic agent (57). Evidence is conflicting regarding the frequency of renal failure in relation to the type of contrast used (58,59). However, in a patient with preexisting renal insufficiency, with a serum creatinine of 2.0 mg/dL or greater before the procedure, it is reasonable to use a nonionic contrast agent. Intravenous hydration with normal saline or 0.45% saline and maintenance of adequate hydration (100 mL fluid per hour or more) during and after the procedure reduce the risk of worsening renal function in patients with baseline renal insufficiency, particularly diabetic patients at risk of renal failure (60). No convincing evidence has been found that mannitol, furosemide, or dopamine is useful in preventing renal dysfunction (61). Concomitant nephrotoxins should not be administered. When renal failure occurs, it may not manifest for 24 to 48 hours; hence, the creatinine measurement the morning after the procedure may be of limited value. The rise in creatinine may not occur until at least 24 hours after the procedure, peaking approximately 5 days after the procedure, and, commonly, resolving by the tenth day. Acetylcysteine has been shown to reduce the occurrence of contrast nephropathy in small studies (62). It is important to limit the quantity of contrast agent used in patients with chronic renal insufficiency (63). Limiting the quantity of dye to less than 30 mL markedly decreases the need for subsequent dialysis (64).

Patients, such as those with asthma, with any history of atopy are at increased risk of an allergic reaction to contrast. Allergies to seafood, such as shellfish, are no more predictive of allergy to contrast media than is a history of other allergies. Previous contrast reactions increase the risk of a subsequent reaction. Anaphylactoid reaction may occur with contrast agents, although there is no difference in the incidence among agents. In patients with previous life-threatening contrast reactions, nonionic agents should be used. The patient should be premedicated with steroids and diphenhydramine. Steroids are most useful when begun the day before the procedure (65). In severe cases, premedication may include histamine (H_2) blockers such as famotidine (Pepcid), 20 mg intravenously. When a life-threatening reaction has occurred in the past and catheterization is necessary, it is useful to give 1 or 2 mL contrast agent first, observe the patient for any reaction, and then proceed. If a reaction to a contrast agent occurs, the treatment will depend on the severity of the reaction (66). The first priority should be maintenance of the airway and hemodynamic resuscitation. Inhaled β-agonists or racemic epinephrine may be useful to alleviate bronchospasm. If severe hypotension occurs, intravenous saline should be administered rapidly for volume expansion, and epinephrine should be given subcutaneously at a dose of 0.3 mL of the 1:1,000 concentration (0.3 mg), or, for severe hypotension, 10 to 20 μg per minute of the 1:10,000 concentration should be continuously infused intravenously until the patient's condition stabilizes. Diphenhydramine and steroids should also be administered, although the steroids will not produce any effect for hours. If the patient can be stabilized, it is reasonable to continue and complete the angiographic procedure (66). When severe anaphylactoid reactions to contrast agents develop, they usually occur during the procedure. Rarely, reactions occur hours to days after contrast administration (67). These more delayed contrast reactions, unlike contrast reactions in the catheterization laboratory, may result from antibody formation (68).

Latex allergy rarely produces an anaphylactic reaction that is clinically indistinguishable from a reaction to iodinated contrast media. Patients should be questioned before catheterization regarding an allergy to latex. If a latex allergy is present, the patient should be premedicated with corticosteroids, and the catheterization should be conducted in a latex-free environment, as the first case of the day before latex particles may accumulate in the catheterization suite. If latex allergy is questionable, the patient should undergo testing.

TECHNICAL ASPECTS OF CARDIAC CATHETERIZATION

Technique

The first step in cardiac catheterization is gaining arterial access. After this, coronary angiography is performed. Next, left ventriculography and measurement of left ventricular pressures can be done. Aortography and imaging of the cerebral or peripheral vasculature can also be performed. Sterile surgical technique should be maintained throughout the procedure (69). This includes proper preparation of the access site with hair removal, skin cleaning, and sterile draping. The operator should wear a surgical cap, gown, shoe covers, and facial mask.

Anesthesia

After adequate sedation, the access site should be anesthetized with 2% lidocaine. Once the maximum pulsation of the artery is identified, an initial skin wheal can be raised with 1 to 2 mL of 2% lidocaine administered through a 25-gauge needle. Anesthesia should be administered more deeply with a 22-gauge needle, through which an additional 4 to 8 mL can be given. If a patient is allergic to lidocaine, which is an amide agent, procaine, which is an ester agent, can be used instead. Bupivacaine, a preservative-free amide agent, is another alternative, especially if the allergy is believed to result from the preservative component of the local anesthetic.

Femoral Artery Access

The most common form of arterial access for cardiac catheterization in the United States is femoral cannulation. Typically, an 18-gauge, hollow beveled needle is used. Fluoroscopy should be used to facilitate puncture of the common femoral artery at the appropriate level. Rupp and colleagues (70) identified the target site as 1 cm lateral to the most medial cortex of the femoral head as seen on an anteroposterior (AP) projection (Fig. 76.3). This increases the likelihood of infrainguinal puncture as well as the ability to compress the puncture site against the femoral head after sheath removal. Puncture of the artery more cranially may be associated with a greater risk of

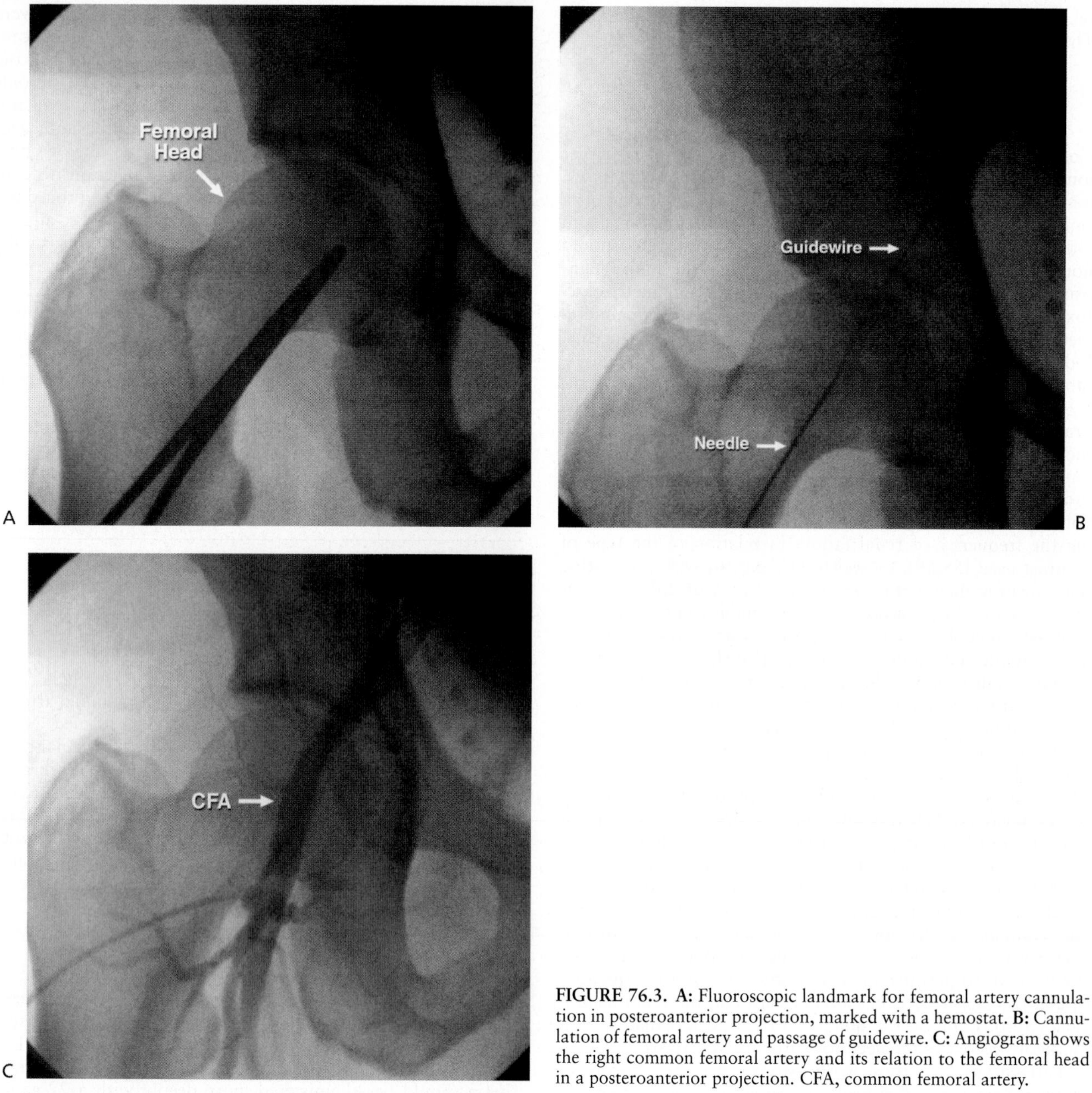

FIGURE 76.3. **A:** Fluoroscopic landmark for femoral artery cannulation in posteroanterior projection, marked with a hemostat. **B:** Cannulation of femoral artery and passage of guidewire. **C:** Angiogram shows the right common femoral artery and its relation to the femoral head in a posteroanterior projection. CFA, common femoral artery.

retroperitoneal hemorrhage, whereas a more caudal puncture is associated with arterial entry below the femoral artery bifurcation and with pseudoaneurysm formation. Use of the skin crease to determine the arterial entry site may be misleading, especially in the obese patient, in whom the skin crease is often well below the desired point of entry.

The angle of entry of the needle should be 30 to 45 degrees. A greater degree of angulation may cause problems during sheath insertion, thus leading to sheath kinking. Pulsatile blood flow should be obtained once the artery is effectively cannulated. Weaker degrees of blood flow could result from subintimal position of the needle bevel or an awkward angle of the needle, with bevel abutting the vessel wall. In these situations, gentle manipulation of the needle backward or forward, or a slight change in angulation (usually a shallower angle), usually restores blood flow. In the presence of marked hypotension or severe peripheral vascular disease, blood return may not be brisk. When the pulse is not palpable, the Smart Needle, a flow needle attached to a Doppler probe, can be used to generate acoustic signals of arterial flow and facilitate puncture of the artery (71). It is relatively easy to puncture the posterior wall of the artery with this approach. Fluoroscopy can be used to locate the medial border of the femoral head, and this facilitates locating the artery. Fluoroscopy may reveal calcification in the vessel wall, which helps to identify the location for needle entry.

Once the artery is cannulated with the needle and pulsatile flow is obtained, a guidewire is passed through the needle. If resistance is encountered, fluoroscopy should be used to ensure that the wire tip is free and that undetected subintimal wire advancement is not occurring. The wire should follow a pathway to the anatomic left of the spine, unlike with venous cannulation, in which the wire follows the inferior vena cava to the right of the spine. In patients with extensive vessel calcification or extensive scar tissue from previous procedures, resistance may be encountered during sheath advancement. Use of a small dilator, followed by progressively larger dilators, as well as a stiff wire, such as an Amplatz wire, may facilitate placement of the desired sheath size. This same technique can be used to enter Dacron grafts if they are at least 2 months old. After successful sheath placement, blood pressure measurement should be obtained and recorded from the sheath sidearm and correlated with the blood pressure cuff measurement. This approach allows detection of any aortoiliac disease and provides accurate documentation of the patient's arterial pressure.

Brachial or Radial Artery Access

Use of the radial artery for cardiac angiography has become increasingly popular. Advantages of this technique include easy compressibility and shorter times to ambulation. Catheter manipulation may be slightly more difficult from the radial artery than from the femoral artery. Before cannulation of the radial artery, it is advisable to perform an Allen test to ensure the adequacy of ulnar circulation to the hand. Another concern with radial artery cannulation is the possible need for this artery as a bypass graft conduit in the future.

Although many operators attempt to cannulate the brachial artery at the level of the elbow crease, in approximately 10% of patients the brachial artery bifurcation is more proximal than this. Therefore, it is desirable to cannulate the brachial artery more proximally, a couple of centimeters above the skin crease. After sheath placement, approximately 2,000 to 3,000 units of intraarterial heparin can be given through the sheath if no pulse is palpable distal to the sheath. Some operators also give intraarterial nitroglycerin to prevent sheath spasm around the smaller-caliber radial artery. Specially designed micropuncture kits allow use of smaller equipment with the brachial or radial arteries.

Catheter Selection

The size of the catheter is largely a matter of physician choice and the size of the coronary arteries to be visualized; 6-Fr diagnostic catheters are commonly used. They provide good opacification, with easy manual injections of contrast. A 4- or 5-Fr system creates a smaller hole at the arterial access site, but adequate coronary artery opacification may be more challenging for the operator because "streaming" (incomplete mixing of contrast and blood) may occur, resulting in overestimation or underestimation of stenosis severity. In certain circumstances, larger catheter sizes, up to 8 Fr, may be desirable, although technique this warrants a femoral approach or a brachial artery cutdown approach. Use of 6-Fr or larger catheters may be desirable for large coronary arteries, coronary ectasia, vein grafts, and any condition that leads to a state of increased coronary flow, such as aortic insufficiency, hypertrophic ventricular enlargement, dialysis, or tachycardia.

The initial catheter selected is the Judkins Left 4 (JL4) for the images of the LCA system. The Judkins Right 4 (JR4) is next used to obtain images of the RCA. The configuration of the initial catheters selected depends on the aortic root. If the aortic root is dilated or the patient is at least 6 feet tall, a JL5 or JL6 may be necessary. Similarly, if the aortic root is small, a JL3.5 may be necessary. From the left brachial or radial artery, the standard Judkins catheters are usually adequate. However, from the right arm, multipurpose or Amplatz-type catheters are most useful. In an average-sized aorta, an AL2 is often the correct size for the LM, and an AL1 or AL2 is often appropriate for the RCA. Amplatz catheters are particularly useful if the origin of LM or RCA is more anterior, posterior, or superior than usual in the aorta. The multipurpose-A catheter is well suited for coronary artery ostia that have an inferiorly directed take-off. Amplatz catheters are more likely than Judkins catheters to lead to ostial dissection owing to their ability to engage the coronary arteries deeply. This risk can be minimized by rotating the catheter counterclockwise before disengaging from the artery.

PRINCIPLES OF IMAGING

At least two orthogonal views should be obtained of each vessel (72). Adequate visualization of the LCA commonly requires five or more views. Coronary artery visualization is commonly performed in the 5-in (magnified) or 7-in image intensifier mode. In the 7-in mode, "panning" of the image intensifier is generally not necessary. The spatial resolution of coronary angiograms obtained in the 7-in mode is less than that obtained in the 5-in mode when an image intensifier is used, but there is no difference when a flat detector is used. The 7-in mode may be preferred for the steeply angulated views and for obese patients. Use of the 5-in mode usually requires panning of the image intensifier to visualize the distal vessels and collaterals. The process of panning is performed as follows. After waiting two or three systolic cycles after injection of contrast, the focus of the image should be moved from the proximal area, down the vessel of interest and then to the contralateral artery to observe for collaterals. If a stenosis is present, even a moderate one, multiple views may be necessary to delineate the severity of the stenosis, especially if it is eccentric.

Identification of coronary vessels and interpretation of angiograms may be difficult for the beginning practitioner (73). In an RAO view, a diagonal branch of the LAD, as opposed to the LAD, forms the left heart border. However, in an LAO view, the LAD usually forms the right heart border, not the diagonal branches; it is important not to overlook an occluded LAD by mistaking a well-developed septal perforator for the true LAD.

Angulated views are generally required to prevent excessive vessel overlap that may obscure an area of interest (74). It may be helpful to use 1-mL "puffs" of dye to see whether a particular view indeed adds information before filming. Obtaining images while the patient takes a deep inspiration improves image quality by moving the diaphragm.

The movement of coronary vessels provides clues to aid in differentiating them. The diagonal branches of the LAD and the marginal branches of the LCx tend to move in synchrony with cardiac contraction, because they supply the lateral aspect of the left ventricle. In the RAO projection, the LAD moves inward and the diagonal branches outward during systole if there is no anterior wall aneurysm. In patients in sinus rhythm, the portions of the RCA and LCx that lie in the atrioventricular groove move with an "atrial kick," as do the atrial branches.

Historically, the frame rate for coronary cineangiographic acquisition has been 30 frames per second to minimize flicker. Many all-digital laboratories now acquire images at 15 frames per second. This practice results in a permanent 50% loss of information—a form of "lossy compression." The clinical significance of this practice has not been established. In patients with tachycardia or high-flow states such as aortic insufficiency, and in angiographic views with multiple overlapping vessels, a rate of 30 frames per second may be necessary to visualize the coronary arteries adequately.

Hand injections of contrast should be "ramped," meaning that the injection should start slowly and increase in force; this minimizes the chance of the catheter's disengaging from the artery. The injection of contrast must be of adequate force to produce reflux into the sinus of Valsalva to visualize the ostium of the coronary artery. The artery should remain completely opacified throughout the cardiac cycle to prevent "washout" and "streaming" of contrast material. Extreme care must be taken to avoid injection of air into the coronary circulation. If this does occur, an immediate attempt should be made to aspirate the air out of the vessel with the same syringe that injected the air. Unless a very large quantity of air was injected, the patient usually has transient chest pain and ST-segment elevation. The patient should be monitored in the catheterization laboratory until the angina and electrocardiographic changes resolve.

Left Coronary Artery

Severe LM coronary artery disease is a serious finding that mandates proceeding with extreme caution. Clues to its presence include heavy calcification of the ostium, a stress test that demonstrates marked hypotension, and damping or ventricularization of the pressure waveform on catheter engagement. Alternatively, the catheter may not be coaxial to the LM coronary artery, and slight withdrawal of the catheter tip should relieve damping in this situation; forceful contrast injection through a damped, noncoaxial catheter tip pointed upward into the LM coronary artery may lead to dissection. A contrast injection in the left coronary cusp is a reasonable first step to define the ostium of the LM coronary artery. An AP view or a shallow RAO caudal view may be useful to evaluate for medial and distal LM coronary artery stenosis. A shallow LAO or LAO cranial view is usually best to visualize ostial LM stenosis. As soon as significant LM disease is identified, nonionic contrast should be used for the rest of the angiography. Limited injections of the LCA and RCA should be performed, sufficient to identify other stenoses and to delineate surgical targets. A left ventriculogram should usually not be performed in the presence of severe LM coronary artery stenosis, because the contrast load and depression in cardiac contractility may prove fatal. If the patient is hemodynamically unstable, consideration should be given to intraaortic balloon pump placement.

Initial engagement of the LM coronary artery is performed in the 30-degree LAO position. If the JL4 catheter does not line up coaxially with the LM coronary artery, slight counterclockwise rotation should move the catheter tip anteriorly and engage it. If this does not work, gentle clockwise rotation, which moves the catheter posteriorly, can be applied. In a dilated aorta, the "elbow" of the JL4 catheter curve does not rest on the aortic wall, and clockwise rotation is necessary to move the catheter tip anteriorly in the aorta.

If Amplatz catheters are being used to engage the LM coronary artery, these are pushed down into the left cusp, with the catheter tip pointing upward until the engagement is accomplished. The catheter is then withdrawn slightly, which causes the catheter to advance into the LM coronary artery. To disengage, the catheter is advanced slightly and is gently rotated counterclockwise out of the LM coronary artery. Although the JL catheters typically enable one to find the LM coronary artery with little manipulation, the Amplatz catheters are particularly useful when the orientation of this artery is unusual or anomalous. However, particular care must be used with Amplatz catheters, because the motions that are used to engage and disengage are the opposite of those of the Judkins catheters.

Isolated LM coronary artery disease occurs rarely (75). When there appears to be no other significant coronary artery disease, consideration should be given to LM coronary artery spasm, and intracoronary nitroglycerin should be administered before repeat angiography. Intravenous ultrasonography may be useful to document the severity of narrowing of the LM trunk in questionable cases.

In the setting of separate ostia of the LAD and LCx, an LAO caudal view may be particularly helpful. If the catheter first engages the LAD, engagement of the LCx may be facilitated by changing from a JL4 to a JL5, with clockwise rotation applied to the catheter. Alternatively, if the LCx is first engaged with the catheter, engaging the LAD may be facilitated by downsizing from a JL4 to a JL3.5, with counterclockwise rotation applied.

The midportion of the LAD and the origin of the diagonal branches are best evaluated by the AP cranial view, as well as by the LAO or RAO cranial views. The lateral view may further delineate the mid-LAD. The body of the LCx and the marginal-branch ostia are best evaluated by the AP caudal view and the shallow LAO or RAO views. For a ramus intermedius branch, an LAO caudal view is most useful to evaluate the ostium. An LAO cranial view is also useful for displaying a left-sided PDA.

Right Coronary Artery

The RCA should be approached in the 30-degree LAO projection. The JR4 is advanced to the aortic valve level and is slowly withdrawn approximately 2 cm while clockwise rotation is applied to rotate the catheter anteriorly to the right sinus of Valsalva. Then the catheter should sit in the RCA ostium. If this maneuver does not work, the RCA ostium can be approached from slightly above its expected level, with clockwise rotation applied to the catheter. With ostial disease of the RCA, if damping occurs with the catheter, it may sometimes be helpful to use a larger catheter, which is less likely to engage the artery deeply. Usually, two or three views of the RCA are obtained. The LAO view is useful to evaluate the proximal and mid-RCA. The AP view with 30-degree cranial angulation is often the best for evaluating the RCA bifurcation and ostia of the PDA and posterolateral branches. A shallow RAO view is useful to show the entire PDA. In the RAO view, the marginal branches point anteriorly, and the atrial branches point posteriorly; thus, this view is useful in differentiating atrial and marginal branches that may be overlapped in an LAO view. The lateral view may be useful to evaluate the mid-RCA and the ostia of RV marginal branches. If significant LM coronary artery disease has been identified, a single view of the RCA in the LAO cranial projection may be sufficient for planning bypass surgery.

Surgical Bypass Grafts

Angiographers who perform cardiac catheterization on patients with previous bypass surgery should obtain the operative report to ensure a complete catheterization with a minimal amount of contrast expenditure. It is often helpful to review any previous postoperative angiograms. If all the vein grafts were clearly documented to be occluded on a previous study (not just the report), there would be no point in searching for them again. Additionally, any unusual anatomy of the innominate or subclavian artery could be appreciated. Furthermore, review of the preoperative catheterization study is useful to ensure that all lesions were, in fact, bypassed. The relation of the patient's symptoms to the presence of lesions on consecutive angiograms may be revealing. For example, when a totally occluded bypass graft is detected in a patient with new-onset angina, knowledge that this vein graft was occluded 5 years ago would affect the management of this patient's current pain syndrome.

Sometimes information regarding the operative anatomy is not available. Fluoroscopic identification of the surgical clips along the course of the left or right internal mammary artery (IMA) and along saphenous vein grafts may be clues that these conduits were used. Finally, a 30-degree LAO aortogram can be performed, although adequate opacification must be ensured. At least a 50- to 60-mL aortogram is generally required; otherwise, it is possible to miss grafts that are, in fact, patent. A long cine run is sometimes necessary to view a late-filling, diseased vein graft.

LCA bypass grafts are best visualized in an RAO projection, whereas grafts to the RCA are best engaged in the LAO projection. If a graft is occluded, an injection should still be performed to confirm the presence of a stump and to ensure that it is not just the catheter abutting the aortic wall. Some surgeons place marker rings on the outside of the aorta at the proximal anastomosis of the graft. This facilitates engagement of the graft during subsequent catheterizations. The usual sequence of proximal anastomoses of aortocoronary bypass grafts to the LCA, going from caudal to cranial, is LAD, diagonal, ramus, first obtuse marginal, and second obtuse marginal. Grafts to the RCA are more caudal and more anterior than grafts to the LCA.

Before cannulating the IMA, the angiographer should visualize the proximal subclavian or innominate artery to provide a road map of the anatomy and to detect the presence of a subclavian stenosis proximal to the IMA. The JR4 is well suited to cannulate the subclavian or innominate artery. Measurement of a pullback gradient confirms the hemodynamic significance of an angiographic stenosis.

The contralateral oblique view is useful to evaluate the ostia of the IMA. Care must be taken on engagement of the delicate ostium of the IMA, because dissection of an IMA–LAD conduit may be catastrophic. Although a JR4 is sometimes used to cannulate the IMA, the curve on the catheter tip is often not sufficient to engage the IMA, which usually originates anteriorly from the subclavian artery. An IMA catheter has a more acute tip curve for selective IMA cannulation. One strategy is to use a JR4 to engage the subclavian artery, visualize this vessel, and then pass a 260-cm exchange-length J-wire or Glidewire into the distal subclavian artery and advance the IMA catheter over the exchange wire. In the presence of marked tortuosity, the Glidewire may be particularly useful, as may use of a Glide catheter; the hydrophilic coatings on these instruments may ease passage through curved vessels. Attempts to cannulate the IMA should be made while withdrawing the IMA catheter, not while advancing it, to prevent dissection. Counterclockwise torque is generally applied to turn the catheter anteriorly to engage the left IMA, and clockwise torque for the right IMA, while the catheter is withdrawn.

It is important to visualize precisely the distal anastomosis of the graft to the artery, because this is often the site of a culprit lesion. The lateral view is particularly useful if there is a question of a left IMA–LAD anastomosis lesion. Otherwise, the views used to visualize grafts are similar to the views required for the native vessels.

The gastroepiploic artery can be used as an in situ graft to the distal RCA. The gastroepiploic artery originates from the common hepatic artery, which arises from the celiac trunk in the abdominal aorta. It normally supplies the stomach but can be rerouted surgically to the inferior surface of the heart. Visualization of this graft involves cannulation of the celiac trunk with a curved catheter such as the Cobra catheter. If a selective injection is necessary for adequate opacification, a catheter can be advanced over a Glidewire into the origin of the gastroepiploic artery.

If left ventriculography is performed, opacification of vein grafts is sometimes observed. The contraction pattern of the left ventricle may provide a clue to the patency of coronary bypass grafts. For example, if the anterior wall is normal but the LAD is occluded and no patent graft has been found to the LAD, it is highly likely that a bypass graft has been overlooked.

Cerebral Angiography

A steep LAO arch aortogram is performed to see the great vessels (76). For cerebral angiography, nonionic contrast should be used, and images should be acquired using digital subtraction angiography. The carotid arteries should be visualized in at least two views, the ipsilateral oblique and the cross-table lateral (90-degree LAO). The ostia of the vertebral arteries are best seen in the contralateral oblique view. Often, nonselective visualization of the vertebral arteries is sufficient, with the catheter tip pointed in the direction of the vertebral and a blood pressure cuff inflated above the systolic pressure in the ipsilateral arm. If selective engagement is necessary, great care must be taken with catheter manipulation to avoid dissection. Special vertebral artery catheters are available for selective cannulation.

Renal Angiography

Although it is often possible to engage the left and right renal arteries with a JR4 catheter, an initial AP abdominal aortogram may be useful to identify the exact location of the renal arteries and allow visualization of accessory renal arteries. Philosophically, this sort of "drive-by" angiography, without clinical indications, is undesirable, because angiographic stenosis may be of little functional consequence to the patient in certain circumstances. However, in a patient with uncontrolled hypertension despite adequate doses of multiple antihypertensives, or when noninvasive imaging has suggested severe stenosis, renal angiography at the time of cardiac catheterization may be reasonable (77).

It is generally preferable to start with an abdominal aortogram. Identification of bony landmarks, such as the first lumbar vertebral body, may help to position the pigtail catheter above the renal artery ostia. Because the renal arteries tend to arise somewhat posteriorly, LAO or RAO angulation may help visualize the ostia. If an ostial stenosis is identified, recording of a pressure gradient may help to assess the severity of the angiographic stenosis. Imaging should continue for a period sufficient to view the nephrograms. An abdominal aortic aneurysm may be noted on the abdominal angiogram. Even a small angiographic aneurysm may in fact be a much larger clot-filled sac, and an ultrasound or computed tomographic (CT) scan is warranted to document the exact dimensions of the aneurysm.

Left Ventriculography

Ventriculography with a pigtail catheter remains a useful modality to assess left ventricular function. Before left ventriculography is performed, an assessment of left ventricular end-diatolic pressure should be made. If this pressure is markedly elevated (e.g., >30 mm Hg), sublingual nitroglycerin should be administered until the pressure is reduced. If left ventricular end-diatolic pressure remains elevated, consideration should be given to aborting the left ventriculogram.

The 30-degree RAO is the usual view for left ventriculography, although biplane ventriculography with an additional LAO or LAO cranial view may be preferable in some cases). If it is necessary to assess the severity of mitral regurgitation, 50 to 60 mL of dye should be used to opacify the left ventricle. The catheter must be positioned carefully to ensure that it does not trigger premature ventricular contractions or entwine the mitral valve apparatus, thereby artificially causing mitral regurgitation. The LAO cranial is the optimal view for a muscular ventricular septal defect, and the left lateral view is optimal for a membranous ventricular septal defect. The LAO cranial view is also useful to assess for mitral regurgitation and for left ventricular outflow obstruction in patients with hypertrophic cardiomyopathy.

Information obtained from fluoroscopy should not be overlooked. Pericardial calcification may be a clue for the presence of constrictive pericarditis. Fluoroscopy may also show calcification of the aortic valve or mitral annulus, perhaps indicating the presence of valvular heart disease. Fluoroscopy can also be used to assess the function of mechanical heart valve prostheses.

Aortography

Aortography is usually performed in a 60-degree LAO projection to assess the aortic root and to determine whether aortic regurgitation is present. Aortic coarctation is best seen in the lateral view. If aortic dissection is suspected, care should be taken to attempt entry into the true lumen. With a femoral approach, the stronger pulse should be used, because this also increases the likelihood of entering the true lumen if the dissection extends to involve the iliofemoral system. Entry into the true lumen may be facilitated by using a pigtail catheter or a JR4 catheter to direct the guidewire toward the medial edge of the aorta, because this increases the probability of avoiding the false lumen, which typically arises from the outer aspect of the aorta. A soft-tip exchange-length 260-cm J-wire should be used. Entry across the aortic valve into the left ventricle is desirable to confirm entry into the true lumen. Ventriculography followed by aortography can then be performed with a pigtail catheter. An aortogram at 60 degrees LAO can be performed to assess the great vessels and to ensure that these arteries are not involved. Next, over the exchange-length wire, a JL5 or 6 catheter can be used to engage the LM coronary artery in what is usually a dilatated aorta. The RCA can then be cannulated with a JR4 or JR5, although the dilatated aorta may necessitate the use of AL3 or multipurpose catheters for either the LM coronary artery or RCA. The initial aortogram may help guide the selection of catheter shapes and sizes for coronary engagement. There is no benefit to routine coronary angiography before emergency surgery for aortic dissection unless the patient has had previous coronary artery bypass surgery (78).

POSTPROCEDURAL CARE

Once it is certain that all necessary information has been obtained from the angiogram, the sheath can be pulled. If heparin was administered for a diagnostic coronary angiogram, clotting studies should be checked before the sheath is pulled. If the activated clotting time is less than 160 seconds or the activated partial thromboplastin time is less than 45 seconds, the sheath can be pulled and manual pressure applied for several minutes until hemostasis is obtained. Direct compression of the artery a few fingerbreadths above the needle insertion site in the skin with the fingertips is the most reliable method to obtain hemostasis if a closure device is not used. After a few minutes of direct manual pressure, a C-clamp can be positioned appropriately. A FemoStop is an alternative, but care must be taken to ensure correct positioning over the artery. Use of smaller sheaths may greatly decrease the time to ambulation. With the use of 5-Fr sheaths, ambulation is safe after 2 hours of bed rest.

Closure devices are commonly used to obtain hemostasis. An oblique angiogram should be performed through the sidearm of the sheath to determine the sheath insertion site. If it appears that the sheath is in the bifurcation of the common femoral artery, or in the profunda femoris or the superficial femoral artery, or if there is atherosclerotic plaque at the insertion site, it may be best not to use any closure device. Vessels 4 mm or less in diameter are not well suited to current closure devices. If a slight degree of blood oozing from the skin occurs, a 10-mL solution of lidocaine hydrochloride 1% and epinephrine 1:100,000 can be injected into the skin tract.

Various closure devices are currently available. The Perclose is a percutaneous device used to suture the hole in the artery formed by the sheath (79). The device is inserted over a wire after the sheath is removed. Then needles are deployed that pull sutures through the artery wall, and the sutures are tied to obtain hemostasis. Because the guidewire can be maintained in the artery for the entire procedure, a sheath can be reinserted if the device fails. Immediate leg movement is possible, if necessary. The technique of "preclosing" the femoral artery involves placement of a Perclose over the guidewire after its initial placement through the cannulation needle. The sutures of the Perclose are kept to the side underneath a sterile towel until the conclusion of the procedure and the removal of the sheath. The Perclose device has been used to obtain hemostasis after brachial artery cannulation as well, although care must be taken because of the smaller caliber of the brachial artery (80).

The Angio-Seal is available in an 8-Fr device for 7- or 8-Fr sheaths and in a 6-Fr device for 5- or 6-Fr sheaths (81,82). Placement involves exchange of the sheath over a guidewire for the Angio-Seal device, which places a collagen plug external to the hole in the artery, with an anchor inside the artery to hold the plug in place. Movement of the leg should be restricted for 1 to 2 hours, and repuncture is not recommended for 3 months. The VasoSeal is an external collagen plug that is placed immediately outside the hole in the artery, as well as in the skin tract that leads to the arterial cannulation site (83). The Duett device is similar in concept to the VasoSeal except that it involves injection of thrombin external to the artery. Care must be taken to avoid intraarterial injection of thrombin. Although closure devices may decrease the time to ambulation and may hasten discharge from the observation unit, there is no evidence that they decrease groin complications. Likewise, in well-trained operator hands, no evidence indicates that closure devices increase groin complications, although when complications occur, they are more often immediately apparent than when manual pressure is used (84–86).

After radial artery catheterization, if the radial pulse is lost but the hand is otherwise asymptomatic (and the ulnar supply is adequate), there is no cause for action. With loss of the brachial or radial pulse after brachial artery catheterization, vascular surgical consultation ought to be obtained. Loss of distal pulses after femoral catheterization should also prompt surgical consultation or lower extremity angiography. In patients with extensive peripheral vascular disease, if pressure is being applied to the femoral catheterization site, particular care must be given to the distal extremity to ensure that ischemia is not occurring; this is best accomplished with direct visualization of the distal extremity.

Elective diagnostic coronary angiography can be performed safely as an outpatient procedure in most circumstances. However, outpatient catheterization is not appropriate for individuals with severe aortic stenosis or LM coronary artery disease or in patients who are at risk of developing renal failure. Similarly, patients with severely impaired left ventricular function or unstable coronary artery disease should remain for observation. Individuals who live alone and have no one to watch them should be monitored overnight.

Before discharge, patients should be told to notify their physician if they subsequently have any sudden drop-off in urine quantity. Any pain or swelling at the site of the catheterization should also prompt emergency care. Patients should be counseled to avoid driving for a day to allow sedation to wear off and heavy lifting for at least 2 days to allow the catheterization site to heal. Warfarin, if necessary, can be reinitiated the night of the procedure. If more immediate anticoagulation with heparin is desired, this can be started a few hours after the

TABLE 76.4

INCIDENCE OF COMPLICATIONS WITH CARDIAC CATHETERIZATION AND CORONARY ANGIOGRAPHY

Complication	Percentage (%)
Death	0.11
Myocardial infarction	0.05
Stroke	0.07
Arrhythmia	0.38
Vascular complications	0.43
Contrast reaction	0.37
Hemodynamic complications	0.26
Perforation of cardiac chamber	0.03
Other complications	0.28
Total	1.70

Adapted from Noto TJ Jr, Johnson LW, Krone R, et al. Cardiac catheterization 1990: a report of the Registry of the Society for Cardiac Angiography and Interventions (SCA&I). *Cathet Cardiovasc Diagn* 1991;24:75–83.

sheath is removed or immediately if a closure device is used. If metformin was given, this can be resumed after 2 days if renal function appears stable.

COMPLICATIONS AND MANAGEMENT

Major complications are unusual after cardiac catheterization, but the operator must be familiar with them (87). An analysis of 59,792 patients documented the frequency of major complications with cardiac catheterization and coronary angiography (Table 76.4) (87). Although that analysis was published in 1991, the numbers have not changed significantly, although older, sicker patients are being catheterized. Death occurs in less than 1 in 1,000 cases. Patients with severe LM coronary artery stenosis or critical aortic stenosis are at particularly high risk. Myocardial infarction occurs in approximately 1 in 2,000 cases; stroke occurs in less than 1 in 1,000 cases. Thus, a major complication of death, myocardial infarction, or stroke occurs in about 1 of 500 cases.

Hypotension and Bradycardia

Vasovagal reactions may occur, especially during initial arterial access or sheath removal. Patients should be instructed not to hold their breath, because breath holding may predispose to a vagal reaction. Hypotension in the catheterization laboratory may be catastrophic in certain circumstances, and prompt treatment may be lifesaving. Norepinephrine (Levophed) should be administered to reverse rapidly hypotension that results from vasovagal reactions. Dopamine is not an ideal initial agent for serious hypotension because it takes time for blood levels to produce a pressor effect. At the initial low serum concentrations, dopamine acts primarily as a vasodilator and may transiently decrease blood pressure. Therefore, norepinephrine, not dopamine, is the agent of choice for prompt treatment of hypotension. Epinephrine is the treatment of choice for hypotension secondary to an anaphylactoid reaction. For hypotension that is unresponsive to intravenous fluids and vasopressors, placement of a Swan-Ganz catheter and an intraaortic balloon pump should be considered. With the availability of the lower profile 8-Fr intraaortic balloon pump systems, a balloon pump can often be placed through an existing sheath.

Atropine, 1.0 mg intravenously, should be administered for symptomatic bradycardia. Additionally, if bradycardia occurs with injections of ionic contrast, nonionic contrast should be substituted. Furthermore, if the bradycardia occurs with RCA injection, the minimum amount of dye to ensure opacification should be used. For sustained and symptomatic bradycardia, a transvenous pacemaker should be placed.

Vascular Complications

Bleeding from the arterial cannulation site with development of a hematoma is a risk of angiography. Retroperitoneal bleeding can be particularly sinister because of the difficulty in making the diagnosis. Although symptoms such as inguinal or abdominal tenderness, femoral neuropathy, and back pain may be clues to retroperitoneal hemorrhage, hypotension with a falling hemoglobin concentration may be the only manifestation and, if undetected, may lead to death. An abdominal CT scan can confirm the diagnosis (88). The risk of vascular complications is increased in patients who are receiving anticoagulation at the time of angiography (89). Female gender, obesity, and advanced age are other risk factors for groin complications. Color duplex ultrasound is the preferred mode of assessing groin complications (90). Pseudoaneurysm and arteriovenous fistula formation are additional risks (91). Although ultrasound-guided compression of pseudoaneurysm and arteriovenous fistula has become common, surgical therapy is still necessary in a significant minority of cases, especially when anticoagulation is administered (92). Ultrasound-guided thrombin injection has been described for the management of pseudoaneurysms that develop after catheterization (93). The success rate with this method is high, even in patients who are receiving anticoagulation, and, in experienced hands, this should likely be the first approach tried before consideration of surgical repair. Endovascular techniques have also been used successfully to treat pseudoaneurysm and arteriovenous fistula (94).

CONTROVERSIES AND PERSONAL PERSPECTIVES

In theory, improved noninvasive screening techniques may diminish the need for angiography as a diagnostic tool in the future. As magnetic resonance imaging and multislice CT scanning continue to improve, they may one day replace coronary angiography as a diagnostic tool for suspected coronary artery disease. Their major use in the future is likely to be for screening purposes, which may result in an increased need for diagnostic angiography to define the extent and severity of coronary disease. Furthermore, percutaneous coronary intervention continues to grow as a revascularization method, thus necessitating coronary angiography to define stenoses. The aging of the population may further increase the need for coronary angiography. Additionally, emerging evidence suggests that an invasive strategy incorporating angiography is the ideal approach to patients with acute coronary syndromes and that this approach is underutilized (46,47,95,96,97). Individuals with unstable angina who are treated with aggressive catheterization strategies in the United States fare better than their more conservatively treated counterparts in Canada (98). For patients with acute ST-segment elevation myocardial infarction, immediate percutaneous intervention leads to better outcomes than pharmacologic therapy (99–101). If a patient with acute myocardial infarction is in cardiogenic shock, emergency percutaneous coronary intervention may be lifesaving (102). Thus, the prominence of coronary angiography is likely to grow, as a diagnostic tool and as a prelude to percutaneous intervention.

THE FUTURE

Although the future of coronary angiography remains bright, limitations will be placed on who actually performs it. As minimum volume standards become more widely accepted and separate certification examinations are developed, coronary angiography will become part of a discrete invasive subspecialty within cardiology. The evolution and refinement of arterial closure devices will continue, allowing an even greater proportion of cases to be performed on an outpatient basis. Older patients with more medical comorbidities will undergo coronary angiography at much higher rates. Further refinements in imaging, through CT angiography and magnetic resonance, will likely reduce radiation exposure to the operator, enhance image quality, and ultimately yield "noninvasive" coronary angiography using an intravenous injection of a contrast agent. Real-time three-dimensional reconstruction of coronary arteries will become feasible. Potentially, hybrid imaging technologies will enable the identification of vulnerable atherosclerotic plaque, the ultimate goal of diagnostic angiography. Thus, although coronary angiography will probably continue to evolve, it will remain central to the evaluation of coronary artery disease.

References

1. Vetrovec GW. Optimal performance of diagnostic coronary angiography. In: Pepine CJ, Nissen SE, eds. *CathSAP*. Bethesda, MD: American College of Cardiology, 1999;5:3–19.
2. Pepine CJ, Babb JD, Brinker JA, et al. Guidelines for training in adult cardiovascular medicine: Core Cardiology Training Symposium (COCATS). Task Force 3: training in cardiac catheterization and interventional cardiology. *J Am Coll Cardiol* 1995;25:14–16.
3. Fye WB. *American cardiology: the history of a specialty and its college.* Baltimore: Johns Hopkins University Press, 1996.
4. Yamanaka O, Hobbs RE. Coronary artery anomalies in 126,595 patients undergoing coronary arteriography. *Cathet Cardiovasc Diagn* 1990;21:28–40.
5. Hobbs RE, Millit HD, Raghavan PV, et al. Coronary artery fistulae: a 10-year review. *Cleve Clin Q* 1982;49:191–197.
6. Tuzcu EM, Moodie DS, Chambers JL, et al. Congenital heart diseases associated with coronary artery anomalies. *Cleve Clin J Med* 1990;57:147–152.
7. Hobbs RE, Millit HD, Raghavan PV, et al. Congenital coronary artery anomalies: clinical and therapeutic implications. *Cardiovasc Clin* 1981;12:43–58.
8. Kramer JR, Kitazume H, Proudfit WL, Sones FM Jr. Clinical significance of isolated coronary bridges: benign and frequent condition involving the left anterior descending artery. *Am Heart J* 1982;103:283–288.
9. Kostis JB, Moreyra AE, Natarajan N, et al. The pathophysiology and diverse etiology of septal perforator compression. *Circulation* 1979;59:913–919.
10. Haager PK, Schwarz ER, vom Dahl J, et al. Long term angiographic and clinical follow up in patients with stent implantation for symptomatic myocardial bridging. *Heart* 2000;84:403–408.
11. Prendergast BD, Kerr F, Starkey IR. Normalisation of abnormal coronary fractional flow reserve associated with myocardial bridging using an intracoronary stent. *Heart* 2000;83:705–707.
12. Klues HG, Schwarz ER, vom Dahl J, et al. Disturbed intracoronary hemodynamics in myocardial bridging: early normalization by intracoronary stent placement. *Circulation* 1997;96:2905–2913.
13. Stables RH, Knight CJ, McNeill JG, Sigwart U. Coronary stenting in the management of myocardial ischaemia caused by muscle bridging. *Br Heart J* 1995;74:90–92.
14. Green CE, Kelley MJ, Higgins CB, Bookstein JJ. Acquired coronary-to-bronchial artery communication: a possible cause of coronary steal. *Cathet Cardiovasc Diagn* 1981;7:191–196.
15. Heupler FA Jr. Syndrome of symptomatic coronary arterial spasm with nearly normal coronary arteriograms. *Am J Cardiol* 1980;45:873–881.
16. Bott-Silverman C, Heupler FA Jr, Yiannikas J. Variant angina: comparison of patients with and without fixed severe coronary artery disease. *Am J Cardiol* 1984;54:1173–1175.
17. Bott-Silverman C, Heupler FA Jr. Natural history of pure coronary artery spasm in patients treated medically. *J Am Coll Cardiol* 1983;2:200–205.
18. Heupler FA Jr, Proudfit WL, Razavi M, et al. Ergonovine maleate provocative test for coronary arterial spasm. *Am J Cardiol* 1978;41:631–640.
19. Heupler FA Jr. Provocative testing for coronary arterial spasm: risk, method and rationale. *Am J Cardiol* 1980; 46:335–337.
20. Heupler FA Jr, Proudfit WL. Nifedipine therapy for refractory coronary arterial spasm. *Am J Cardiol* 1979; 44:798–803.
21. Williams MJ, Restieaux NJ, Low CJ. Myocardial infarction in young people with normal coronary arteries. *Heart* 1998;79:191–194.
22. Basso C, Morgagni GL, Thiene G. Spontaneous coronary artery dissection: a neglected cause of acute myocardial ischaemia and sudden death. *Heart* 1996;75:451–454.
23. Almahmeed WA, Haykowski M, Boone J, et al. Spontaneous coronary artery dissection in young women. *Cathet Cardiovasc Diagn* 1996;37:201–205.
24. Sherrid MV, Mieres J, Mogtader A, et al. Onset during exercise of spontaneous coronary artery dissection and sudden death. Occurrence in a trained athlete: case report and review of prior cases. *Chest* 1995;108:284–287.
25. Bucciarelli E, Fratini D, Gilardi G, Affronti G. Spontaneous dissecting aneurysm of coronary artery in a pregnant woman at term. *Pathol Res Pract* 1998;194:137–139.
26. Greenblatt JM, Kochar GS, Albornoz MA. Multivessel spontaneous coronary artery dissection in a patient with severe systolic hypertension: a possible association. A case report. *Angiology* 1999;50:509–513.
27. Masuda T, Akiyama H, Kurosawa T, Ohwada T. Long-term follow-up of coronary artery dissection due to blunt chest trauma with spontaneous healing in a young woman. *Intensive Care Med* 1996;22:450–452.
28. Chu KH, Menapace FJ, Blankenship JC, et al. Polyarteritis nodosa presenting as acute myocardial infarction with coronary dissection. *Cathet Cardiovasc Diagn* 1998;44:320–324.
29. Elming H, Kober L. Spontaneous coronary artery dissection: case report and literature review. *Scand Cardiovasc J* 1999;33:175–179.
30. Vale PR, Baron DW. Coronary artery stenting for spontaneous coronary artery dissection: a case report and review of the literature. *Cathet Cardiovasc Diagn* 1998;45:280–286.
31. Kearney P, Singh H, Hutter J, et al. Spontaneous coronary artery dissection: a report of three cases and review of the literature. *Postgrad Med J* 1993; 69:940–945.
32. Koller PT, Cliffe CM, Ridley DJ. Immunosuppressive therapy for peripartum-type spontaneous coronary artery dissection: case report and review. *Clin Cardiol* 1998; 21:40–46.
33. Borczuk AC, van Hoeven KH, Factor SM. Review and hypothesis: the eosinophil and peripartum heart disease (myocarditis and coronary artery dissection)—coincidence or pathogenetic significance? *Cardiovasc Res* 1997;33:527–532.
34. Ge J, Haude M, Gorge G, et al. Silent healing of spontaneous plaque disruption demonstrated by intracoronary ultrasound. *Eur Heart J* 1995;16:1149–1151.
35. Sorrell VL, Davis MJ, Bove AA. Current knowledge and significance of coronary artery ectasia: a chronologic review of the literature, recommendations for treatment, possible etiologies, and future considerations. *Clin Cardiol* 1998;21:157–160.
36. Syed M, Lesch M. Coronary artery aneurysm: a review. *Prog Cardiovasc Dis* 1997;40:77–84.
37. Shapira OM, Shemin RJ. Aneurysmal coronary artery disease: atherosclerotic coronary artery ectasia or adult mucocutaneous lymph node syndrome (Kawasaki's disease)? *Chest* 1997;111:796–799.
38. Rowley AH, Shulman ST. Kawasaki syndrome. *Clin Microbiol Rev* 1998; 11:405–414.
39. Kato H, Sugimura T, Akagi T, et al. Long-term consequences of Kawasaki disease: a 10- to 21-year follow-up study of 594 patients. *Circulation* 1996; 94:1379–1385.
40. Fukushige J, Takahashi N, Ueda K, et al. Long-term outcome of coronary abnormalities in patients after Kawasaki disease. *Pediatr Cardiol* 1996; 17:71–76.
41. Pongratz G, Gansser R, Bachmann K, et al. Myocardial infarction in an adult resulting from coronary aneurysms previously documented in childhood after an acute episode of Kawasaki's disease. *Eur Heart J* 1994;15:1002–1004.
42. Osevala MA, Heleotis TL, DeJene BA. Successful treatment of a ruptured mycotic coronary artery aneurysm. *Ann Thorac Surg* 1999;67:1780–1782.
43. von Rotz F, Niederhauser U, Straumann E, et al. Myocardial infarction caused by a large coronary artery aneurysm. *Ann Thorac Surg* 2000;69:1568–1569.
44. Leung AW, Wong P, Wu CW, et al. Left main coronary artery aneurysm: sealing by stent graft and long-term follow-up. *Catheter Cardiovasc Interv* 2000;51:205–209.
45. Scanlon PJ, Faxon DP, Audet AM, et al. ACC/AHA guidelines for coronary angiography: a report of the American College of Cardiology/American Heart Association Task Force on practice guidelines (Committee on Coronary Angiography) developed in collaboration with the Society for Cardiac

Angiography and Interventions. *J Am Coll Cardiol* 1999;33:1756–1824.
46. FRagmin and Fast Revascularisation during InStability in Coronary artery disease Investigators. Invasive compared with non-invasive treatment in unstable coronary-artery disease: FRISC II prospective randomised multicentre study. *Lancet* 1999;354:708–715.
47. Cannon CP, Weintraub WS, Demopoulos LA, et al. Comparison of early invasive and conservative strategies in patients with unstable coronary syndromes treated with the glycoprotein IIb/IIIa inhibitor tirofiban. *N Engl J Med* 2001;344:1879–1887.
48. Ellis SG, Weintraub W, Holmes D, et al. Relation of operator volume and experience to procedural outcome of percutaneous coronary revascularization at hospitals with high interventional volumes. *Circulation* 1997;95:2479–2484.
49. Laboratory Performance Standards Committee. Guidelines for professional staff privileges in the cardiac catheterization laboratory. *Cathet Cardiovasc Diagn* 1990;21:203–204.
50. Pepine CJ, Allen HD, Bashore TM, et al. ACC/AHA guidelines for cardiac catheterization and cardiac catheterization laboratories: American College of Cardiology/American Heart Association Ad Hoc Task Force on Cardiac Catheterization. *Circulation* 1991;84:2213–2247.
51. Marshall D, Chambers CE, Heupler F Jr. Performance of adult cardiac catheterization: nonphysicians should not function as independent operators—a position statement. *Catheter Cardiovasc Interv* 1999;48:167–169.
52. Heupler FA Jr, Chambers CE, Dear WE, et al. Guidelines for internal peer review in the cardiac catheterization laboratory: Laboratory Performance Standards Committee, Society for Cardiac Angiography and Interventions. *Cathet Cardiovasc Diagn* 1997;40:21–32.
53. Heupler FA Jr, al-Hani AJ, Dear WE. Guidelines for continuous quality improvement in the cardiac catheterization laboratory: Laboratory Performance Standards Committee of the Society for Cardiac Angiography and Interventions. *Cathet Cardiovasc Diagn* 1993;30:191–200.
54. Heupler FA Jr. Guidelines for performing angiography in patients taking metformin: members of the Laboratory Performance Standards Committee of the Society for Cardiac Angiography and Interventions. *Cathet Cardiovasc Diagn* 1998;43:121–123.
55. Holmes DR Jr, Wondrow MA, Bell MR, et al. Cine film replacement: digital archival requirements and remaining obstacles. *Cathet Cardiovasc Diagn* 1998;44:346-356; discussion 357.
56. Balter S, Heupler FA, Lin PP, Wondrow MH. A new tool for benchmarking cardiovascular fluoroscopes. *Cathet Cardiovasc Interv* 2001;52:67–72.
57. Davidson CJ, Laskey WK, Hermiller JB, et al. Randomized trial of contrast media utilization in high-risk PTCA: the COURT trial. *Circulation* 2000;101:2172–2177.
58. Parfrey PS, Griffiths SM, Barrett BJ, et al. Contrast material–induced renal failure in patients with diabetes mellitus, renal insufficiency, or both: a prospective controlled study. *N Engl J Med* 1989;320:143–149.
59. Rudnick MR, Goldfarb S, Wexler L, et al. Nephrotoxicity of ionic and nonionic contrast media in 1196 patients: a randomized trial. The Iohexol Cooperative Study. *Kidney Int* 1995;47:254–261.
60. Solomon R, Werner C, Mann D, et al. Effects of saline, mannitol, and furosemide to prevent acute decreases in renal function induced by radiocontrast agents. *N Engl J Med* 1994;331:1416–1420.
61. Stevens MA, McCullough PA, Tobin KJ, et al. A prospective randomized trial of prevention measures in patients at high risk for contrast nephropathy: results of the P.R.I.N.C.E. study. Prevention of Radiocontrast Induced Nephropathy Clinical Evaluation. *J Am Coll Cardiol* 1999;33:403–411.
62. Tepel M, van der Giet M, Schwarzfeld C, et al. Prevention of radiographic-contrast-agent-induced reductions in renal function by acetylcysteine. *N Engl J Med* 2000;343:180–184.
63. Cigarroa RG, Lange RA, Williams RH, Hillis LD. Dosing of contrast material to prevent contrast nephropathy in patients with renal disease. *Am J Med* 1989;86:649–652.
64. Manske CL, Sprafka JM, Strony JT, Wang Y. Contrast nephropathy in azotemic diabetic patients undergoing coronary angiography. *Am J Med* 1990; 89:615–620.
65. Lasser EC, Berry CC, Talner LB, et al. Pretreatment with corticosteroids to alleviate reactions to intravenous contrast material. *N Engl J Med* 1987; 317:845–849.
66. Goss JE, Chambers CE, Heupler FA Jr. Systemic anaphylactoid reactions to iodinated contrast media during cardiac catheterization procedures: guidelines for prevention, diagnosis, and treatment: Laboratory Performance Standards Committee of the Society for Cardiac Angiography and Interventions. *Cathet Cardiovasc Diagn* 1995;34:99–104; discussion 105.
67. Pedersen SH, Svaland MG, Reiss AL, Andrew E. Late allergy-like reactions following vascular administration of radiography contrast media. *Acta Radiol* 1998;39:344–348.
68. Courvoisier S, Bircher AJ. Delayed-type hypersensitivity to a nonionic, radiopaque contrast medium. *Allergy* 1998;53:1221–1224.
69. Heupler FJ, Heisler M, Keys TF, Serkey J. Infection prevention guidelines for cardiac catheterization laboratories: Society for Cardiac Angiography and Interventions Laboratory Performance Standards Committee. *Cathet Cardiovasc Diagn* 1992;25:260–263.
70. Rupp SB, Vogelzang RL, Nemcek AA Jr, Yungbluth MM. Relationship of the inguinal ligament to pelvic radiographic landmarks: anatomic correlation and its role in femoral arteriography. *J Vasc Interv Radiol* 1993;4:409–413.
71. Criado FJ, Abdul-Khoudoud O, Wellons E. Complications and troubleshooting. In: White RA, Fogarty TJ, eds. *Peripheral endovascular interventions,* 2nd ed. New York: Springer-Verlag, 1999: 445–454.
72. Bhatt DL. Left heart catheterization. In: Marso SP, Griffin BP, Topol EJ, eds. *Manual of cardiovascular medicine*. Philadelphia: Lippincott Williams & Wilkins, 1999: 700–721.
73. Bhatt DL. *Essential concepts in cardiovascular intervention.* London: Remedica, 2004.
74. Boucher RA, Myler RK, Clark DA, Stertzer SH. Coronary angiography and angioplasty. *Cathet Cardiovasc Diagn* 1988;14:269–285.
75. Kapadia SR, Martin GV, Flores JR, et al. Isolated left main trunk stenosis: how common is it? *J Am Coll Cardiol* 2001;37:375A.
76. Bhatt DL. *Guide to peripheral and cerebrovascular intervention.* London: Remedica, 2004.
77. Bhatt DL. Peripheral arterial disease in the catheterization laboratory: an underdetected and undertreated risk factor. *Mayo Clin Proc* 2004;79:1107–1109.
78. Penn MS, Smedira N, Lytle B, Brener SJ. Does coronary angiography before emergency aortic surgery affect in-hospital mortality? *J Am Coll Cardiol* 2000;35:889–894.
79. Bhatt DL, Raymond RE, Feldman T, Braden GA, Murphy B, Strumpf R, Rogers EW, Myla S, Knopf WD. Successful "pre-closure" of 7Fr and 8Fr femoral arteriotomies with a 6Fr suture-based device (the Multicenter Interventional Closer Registry). *Am J Cardiol* 2002;89:777–779.
80. Kulick DL, Rediker DE. Use of the Perclose device in the brachial artery after coronary intervention. *Catheter Cardiovasc Interv* 1999;46:111–112.
81. Ward SR, Casale P, Raymond R, et al. Efficacy and safety of a hemostatic puncture closure device with early ambulation after coronary angiography: Angio-Seal investigators. *Am J Cardiol* 1998;81:569–572.
82. Warren BS, Warren SG, Miller SD. Predictors of complications and learning curve using the Angio-Seal closure device following interventional and diagnostic catheterization. *Cathet Cardiovasc Interv* 1999;48:162–166.
83. Foran JP, Patel D, Brookes J, Wainwright RJ. Early mobilisation after percutaneous cardiac catheterisation using collagen plug (VasoSeal) haemostasis. *Br Heart J* 1993;69:424–429.
84. Chamberlin JR, Lardi AB, McKeever LS, et al. Use of vascular sealing devices (VasoSeal and Perclose) versus assisted manual compression (FemoStop) in transcatheter coronary interventions requiring abciximab (ReoPro). *Cathet Cardiovasc Interv* 1999;47:143–147; discussion 148.
85. Cura FA, Kapadia SR, L'Allier PL, et al. Safety of femoral closure devices after percutaneous coronary interventions in the era of glycoprotein IIb/IIIa platelet blockade. *Am J Cardiol* 2000;86:780–782(abst).
86. Sesana M, Vaghetti M, Albiero R, et al. Effectiveness and complications of vascular access closure devices after interventional procedures. *J Invasive Cardiol* 2000;12:395–399.
87. Noto TJ Jr, Johnson LW, Krone R, et al. Cardiac catheterization 1990: a report of the Registry of the Society for Cardiac Angiography and Interventions (SCA&I). *Cathet Cardiovasc Diagn* 1991;24:75–83.
88. Sreeram S, Lumsden AB, Miller JS, et al. Retroperitoneal hematoma following femoral arterial catheterization: a serious and often fatal complication. *Am Surg* 1993;59:94–98.
89. Omoigui NA, Califf RM, Pieper K, et al. Peripheral vascular complications in the Coronary Angioplasty versus Excisional Atherectomy Trial (CAVEAT-I). *J Am Coll Cardiol* 1995;26:922–930.
90. Paulson EK, Kliewer MA, Hertzberg BS, et al. Color Doppler sonography of groin complications following femoral artery catheterization. *AJR Am J Roentgenol* 1995;165:439–444.
91. Toursarkissian B, Allen BT, Petrinec D, et al. Spontaneous closure of selected iatrogenic pseudoaneurysms and arteriovenous fistulae. *J Vasc Surg* 1997;25:803–808; discussion 808–809.
92. Cox GS, Young JR, Gray BR, et al. Ultrasound-guided compression repair of postcatheterization pseudoaneurysms: results of treatment in one hundred cases. *J Vasc Surg* 1994;19:683–686.
93. La Perna L, Olin JW, Goines D, et al. Ultrasound-guided thrombin injection for the treatment of postcatheterization pseudoaneurysms. *Circulation* 2000;102:2391–2395.
94. Waigand J, Uhlich F, Gross CM, et al. Percutaneous treatment of pseudoaneurysms and arteriovenous fistulas after invasive vascular procedures. *Cathet Cardiovasc Interv* 1999;47:157–164.
95. Mehta SR, Cannon CP, Fox KA, et al. Routine vs selective invasive strategies in patients with acute coronary syndromes: a collaborative meta-analysis of randomized trials. *JAMA* 2005;293:2908–2917.
96. Bhatt DL. To cath or not to cath: that is no longer the question. *JAMA* 2005:2935–2937.
97. Bhatt DL, Roe MT, Peterson ED, et al. Utilization of early invasive management strategies for high-risk patients with non The Global Use of Strategies to Open Occluded Coronary Arteries in Acute Coronary Syndromes (GUSTO IIb) angioplasty substudy investigators.ST-segment elevation acute coronary syndromes: results from the CRUSADE Quality Improvement Initiative. *JAMA* 2004;292:2096–2104.
98. Fu Y, Chang WC, Mark D, et al. Canadian-American differences in the management of acute coronary syndromes in the GUSTO IIb trial: one-year follow-up of patients without ST-segment elevation. *Circulation* 2000; 102:1375–1381.

99. Grines CL, Browne KF, Marco J, et al. A comparison of immediate angioplasty with thrombolytic therapy for acute myocardial infarction: the Primary Angioplasty in Myocardial Infarction Study Group. *N Engl J Med* 1993;328:673–679.
100. Madsen JK, Grande P, Saunamaki K, et al. Danish multicenter randomized study of invasive versus conservative treatment in patients with inducible ischemia after thrombolysis in acute myocardial infarction (DANAMI): Danish trial in acute myocardial infarction. *Circulation* 1997;96:748–755.
101. Global Use of Strategies to Open Occluded Coronary Arteries in Acute Coronary Syndromes (GUSTO IIb) angioplasty substudy investigators. A clinical trial comparing primary coronary angioplasty with tissue plasminogen activator for acute myocardial infarction. *N Engl J Med* 1997; 336:1621–1628.
102. Hochman JS, Sleeper LA, Webb JG, et al. Early revascularization in acute myocardial infarction complicated by cardiogenic shock. SHOCK investigators: should we emergently revascularize occluded coronaries for cardiogenic shock. *N Engl J Med* 1999;341:625–634.

CHAPTER 77 ■ CARDIAC CATHETERIZATION AND HEMODYNAMIC ASSESSMENT

RICHARD A. LANGE AND L. DAVID HILLIS

OVERVIEW

Diagnostic cardiac catheterization is performed to establish the presence and to assess the severity of cardiac disease. Catheterization of the right and left sides of the heart can be accomplished by the introduction of catheters via several approaches. During routine right-sided heart catheterization, measurements of pressures and oxygen (O_2) saturations in the venae cavae, right atrium, right ventricle, pulmonary artery, and pulmonary capillary wedge position can be performed, and cardiac output (CO) can be quantified. The measurement of right-sided pressures helps one to evaluate the severity of tricuspid or pulmonic stenosis, to assess the presence and severity of pulmonary hypertension, and to calculate pulmonary vascular resistance. With left-sided heart catheterization, one can assess mitral and aortic valvular function, left ventricular pressures and function, systemic vascular resistance, and coronary arterial anatomy. Cardiac catheterization may be performed to assess the presence, site, and magnitude of intracardiac shunting, and injection of radiographic contrast material into various cardiac chambers (angiography) may be performed to evaluate their structure or function.

HISTORICAL PERSPECTIVE

Cardiac catheterization was first performed in the 1840s on experimental animals. In 1929, Werner Forssmann was the first to pass a catheter into the heart of a living person—himself. Guided by a fluoroscopic image projected onto a mirror, Forssmann introduced a thin urologic catheter into his left antecubital vein, advanced it to the right atrium, then climbed a flight of stairs to the radiology suite to document catheter position with a chest radiograph. Although he repeated this feat several times, concern about the utility and safety of cardiac catheterization limited its use and development until the 1940s, when Andre Cournand and Dickinson Richards systematically performed catheterization to investigate cardiac function in healthy subjects and in patients with heart disease (Table 77.1). During its early years, catheterization was performed sparingly and with substantial risk. As time has elapsed, considerable advances have been made, and the associated morbidity and mortality have fallen precipitously. Today, diagnostic cardiac catheterization is performed with minimal risk, and therapeutic catheterization (i.e., coronary angioplasty and valvuloplasty) is performed without incident in most patients. Cardiac catheterization now plays a central role in the diagnostic evaluation of the patient with suspected or known cardiac disease, and it offers percutaneous therapeutic possibilities in many individuals.

INDICATIONS AND CONTRAINDICATIONS

Diagnostic cardiac catheterization is indicated in the following situations: (a) to confirm or exclude the presence of a condition already suspected from the history, physical examination, or noninvasive evaluation; (b) to clarify a confusing or obscure clinical picture in a patient whose clinical findings and noninvasive data are inconclusive; and (c) to confirm the suspected abnormality and to exclude associated abnormalities that may require a surgeon's attention in patients for whom corrective surgery is contemplated.

TABLE 77.1

HISTORICAL HIGHLIGHTS OF CARDIAC CATHETERIZATION

1929	First cardiac (right atrial) catheterization in man: Werner Forssmann
1930	Cardiac output measured by the Fick principle: O. Klein
1940s	Right-sided heart catheterization studies: Andre Cournand and Dickinson Richards
1947	Pulmonary capillary wedge measurements: Lewis Dexter
1950	Retrograde left-sided heart catheterization: H. Zimmerman, R. Limon-Lason
1953	Percutaneous catheterization technique: S. Seldinger
1956	Nobel prize awarded to Werner Forssmann, Andre Cournand, and Dickinson Richards for their work in cardiac catheterization
1959	Transseptal catheterization: John Ross, Constantin Cope
1959	Selective coronary angiography: Mason Sones
1968	Coronary artery bypass surgery: Rene Favalaro
1970	Balloon-tipped flow-directed right-sided heart catheterization: H. Jeremy Swan and William Ganz
1977	Percutaneous transluminal coronary angioplasty: Andreas Gruentzig

Therapeutic catheterization is appropriate in several circumstances. Percutaneous coronary revascularization may be indicated in the patient with symptomatic atherosclerotic coronary artery disease whose coronary anatomy is suitable for the procedure. Valvuloplasty is indicated in the patient with symptomatic isolated pulmonic or mitral stenosis in whom valvular anatomy is suitable, and it is an acceptable alternative to surgery in the patient with aortic stenosis in whom surgery is believed to offer an unfavorable risk-to-benefit ratio.

Catheterization is absolutely contraindicated if a mentally competent individual does not consent to the procedure. It is relatively contraindicated if an intercurrent condition exists that, if corrected, would improve the safety of the procedure (Table 77.2).

TABLE 77.2

RELATIVE CONTRAINDICATIONS TO CARDIAC CATHETERIZATION

Decompensated heart failure (e.g., pulmonary edema)
Uncontrolled ventricular irritability
Uncontrolled systemic arterial hypertension
Acute or severe renal insufficiency
Difficulty with vascular access
Electrolyte imbalance (i.e., hypokalemia or hyperkalemia)
Digitalis intoxication
Active infection or febrile illness
Uncorrected bleeding diathesis
Severe anemia
Active bleeding from internal organ
Severe allergy to radiographic contrast material
Mental incompetence

RISKS AND COMPLICATIONS

As cardiac catheterization has been more frequently performed, the incidence of complications has diminished (Table 77.3) (1,2). The overall incidence of a major complication (death, myocardial infarction, or cerebrovascular accident) during or within 24 hours of diagnostic catheterization is 0.2% to 0.3%. Deaths, which occur in 0.1% to 0.2% of patients, may be caused by perforation of the heart or great vessels, cardiac arrhythmias, acute myocardial infarction, or anaphylaxis to radiographic contrast material. Individuals with an increased risk of death include those with (a) advanced (>70 years) or very young (<1 year) age, (b) marked functional impairment (class IV angina or heart failure), (c) severe left ventricular dysfunction or coronary artery disease (particularly left main disease, in which the risk of periprocedural death is 2.8% [5,6]), (d) severe valvular disease, (e) severe comorbid medical conditions (i.e., renal, hepatic, or pulmonary disease), or (f) a history of an allergy to radiographic contrast material.

Numerous minor complications may cause morbidity but exert no effect on mortality. Local vascular complications—arterial occlusion, large hematoma, pseudoaneurysm, or arteriovenous (AV) fistula—occur in 0.5% to 1.5% of patients. Compression by a large hematoma or groin clamp may cause local nerve damage. Infection may occur at the site of catheter entrance and manipulation, especially if a closure device is used to seal the arteriotomy site.

The injection of radiographic contrast material is associated with allergic reactions of varying severity, and a rare individual has anaphylaxis. Only 15% of patients with a known allergy to contrast material have another adverse reaction with repeat administration, and most of these reactions are minor (urticaria, nausea, vomiting). In most patients with a history of contrast allergy, angiography can be performed safely; however, premedication with glucocorticosteroids and antihistamines and the use of a nonionic contrast agent are generally recommended (3). Use of excessive quantities of radiographic contrast material may result in renal insufficiency, particularly in patients with preexisting renal dysfunction and diabetes mellitus. This complication can be minimized by (a) limiting the amount of contrast material used during catheterization based on the patient's body surface area and baseline serum creatinine, (b) utilizing nonionic contrast material, (c) administering *N*-acetylcysteine orally or a sodium bicarbonate infusion intravenously before catheterization, and (d) administering sufficient fluids after catheterization (4).

TABLE 77.3

COMPLICATIONS ASSOCIATED WITH DIAGNOSTIC CARDIAC CATHETERIZATION

Complications	Percentage (%)
MAJOR	
Death	0.1
Cerebrovascular accident	0.07
Myocardial infarction	0.07
Arrhythmia (life-threatening)	0.5
Vascular compromise	0.5–1.5
Anaphylaxis (to contrast material)	0.007
MINOR	
Hives	2.0–3.0
Nausea/vomiting	~5.0
Vasovagal reaction	3.0

TECHNIQUES OF CARDIAC CATHETERIZATION

Approaches

Catheterization of the right and left sides of the heart can be accomplished by the introduction of catheters (a) by direct vision into the brachial vein and artery (9) or (b) by percutaneous puncture of the radial artery or femoral or brachial vein and artery (10). The choice of approach (brachial, femoral, or radial) for venous and arterial catheterization is determined by the preference and experience of the operator as well as by the anatomic and pathophysiologic abnormalities of the patient. In general, right-sided heart catheterization is easier via the brachial approach in the patient with right ventricular or right atrial dilatation. In contrast, in the patient with a secundum atrial septal defect, a right-sided heart catheter can be passed across the defect more easily via the femoral approach. Thus, in choosing the route for right-sided heart catheterization, it is necessary to be cognizant of anatomic abnormalities and specific disease entities. In most patients, left-sided heart catheterization can be performed by the radial, brachial, or femoral approach. However, the femoral approach offers several advantages. This approach can be performed quickly and repeatedly in the same patient, allows the use of larger-lumen catheters, and has a low incidence of infection or vascular injury. Certain conditions, however, render left-sided heart catheterization by the femoral approach difficult, such as extensive peripheral vascular disease, marked obesity, severe systemic arterial hypertension, bleeding diatheses, and any disorder that results in a markedly augmented arterial pulse pressure (e.g., severe aortic regurgitation). In the patient with any of these conditions, the brachial or radial approach may be safer if performed by an operator experienced with this technique. In turn, the brachial or radial approach for left-sided heart catheterization is relatively contraindicated if there is evidence of severe brachiocephalic or ulnar arterial disease.

Brachial Approach

To use the brachial cutdown approach, local anesthetic is introduced into an area 3 to 4 cm in diameter, approximately 1 cm above the flexor crease of the arm, after which a transverse cutdown is performed. If both right- and left-sided heart catheterization is planned, the incision should be wide (2 to 3 cm in length) and located over the brachial artery; if only right-sided heart catheterization is contemplated, a small incision can be made directly over a brachial vein. Once the skin incision is made, the subcutaneous tissues are separated by blunt dissection with a curved hemostat. The vein and artery are isolated with bands, separated from adjacent tissues, and cleaned. The catheters are introduced under direct vision and are advanced into the great vessels and the heart.

After catheterization by the brachial cutdown approach, the catheters are removed, and the vein used for right-sided heart catheterization is ligated. The artery used for left-sided heart catheterization is rendered free of thrombi, and the arteriotomy is repaired. After blood flow has been successfully restored to the distal arm, the wound is flushed with saline, the incision is sutured, and the site of the cutdown is appropriately dressed. Alternatively, the brachial approach can be performed percutaneously in a manner similar to the femoral approach described in the next section.

Femoral Approach

To use the percutaneous femoral approach, local anesthetic is introduced into an area 3 to 4 cm in diameter 3 to 4 cm below the inguinal ligament (the inguinal ligament extends from the anterior superior iliac crest to the symphysis pubis). The anticipated puncture site should overlie bone, thus allowing for adequate vessel compression when the sheaths are removed. A small incision (approximately 0.5 cm in length) is made over the vessel(s) to be used for catheter introduction and passage, after which a "tunnel" is constructed (using a straight hemostat) at a 30- to 45-degree angle to the surface of the skin and to the approximate depth of the desired femoral vessel. An 18-gauge needle is introduced through the skin incision and tunnel into the lumen of the femoral artery or vein. Once blood flows freely through the needle, a Teflon-coated guidewire is advanced into the lumen of the punctured vessel. The wire is held firmly in place as the needle is removed, and the wire is wiped to remove blood and thrombi. Then a sheath with a side arm port is advanced over the wire into the vessel lumen, and the wire is removed. The side arm port allows continuous pressure monitoring and infusion as catheters are advanced through the sheath to the heart. After catheterization, the vascular sheaths are removed, and hemostasis is achieved by applying pressure over the puncture site (generally 1.0 to 1.5 cm cephalad to the skin incision) for sufficient time to ensure the cessation of bleeding. Hemostasis is generally obtained by applying direct pressure to the puncture site on the femoral vein for 5 to 10 minutes and on the femoral artery for 20 to 30 minutes. Subsequently, the patient is required to remain in bed and to immobilize the involved limb for 8 to 24 hours, depending on sheath size. The percutaneous brachial technique is performed in a similar manner by creating a tunnel 1 cm above the flexor crease of the arm.

Radial Approach

Diagnostic and interventional catheterization procedures can be performed via percutaneous cannulation of the radial artery with 5- or 6-Fr sheaths. Because of its small caliber, the radial artery may spasm during sheath placement or catheter manipulation, thus requiring treatment with intraarterial nitroglycerin or a calcium channel blocker. Bleeding is uncommon with the radial approach, but radial artery thrombosis occurs in 5% to 10% of patients, usually without sequelae provided a preprocedure Allen test result confirmed adequate perfusion of the hand through the ulnar artery. The major advantage of the radial approach is that it allows the patient to ambulate soon after catheterization, and this is conducive to the performance of outpatient diagnostic and interventional procedures.

Transseptal Approach

When access to the left atrium is necessary, transseptal catheterization is performed. With this technique, a long sheath is placed percutaneously in the right femoral vein and is advanced to the right atrium over a guidewire. A special transseptal needle is advanced through the sheath and is used to puncture the interatrial septum. The sheath is then advanced over the needle into the left atrium, and the needle withdrawn from the body. Through the sheath, left atrial pressure can be measured, and catheters can be placed for therapeutic procedures, such as mitral valvuloplasty. The transseptal approach should not be attempted in the patient with (a) severely distorted or malaligned cardiac anatomy, (b) left atrial thrombus, (c) left atrial myxoma, or (d) a bleeding diathesis. In experienced hands, significant complications (cardiac perforation, pericardial tamponade, ventricular fibrillation, cerebrovascular event, and death) occur in 1% to 2% of transseptal procedures (11).

Left Ventricular Puncture

In rare circumstances, placement of a catheter in the left ventricle across the aortic (or mitral) valve is not advisable. For example, advancement of a catheter across a tilting disk prosthetic valve may result in catheter entrapment. Accordingly, direct puncture of the left ventricle through the chest wall can be performed to measure left ventricular pressure and to perform left ventriculography. With this approach, after generous local anesthesia, an 18-gauge needle is inserted at the apical impulse and is directed toward the long axis of the left ventricle (toward the right shoulder). When heart pulsations or ventricular ectopy are noted, the needle is in contact with the ventricular epicardium, and it is slowly advanced until pulsatile blood flow is observed. Left ventricular pressure can be measured directly through the needle. If ventriculography is to be performed, the needle can be exchanged over a guidewire for a 4- or 5-Fr pigtail catheter. Significant complications (cardiac tamponade, hemothorax, pneumothorax, ventricular fibrillation) occur in 3% to 10% of these procedures, and vasovagal reactions occur in approximately 5% (12).

Endomyocardial Biopsy

Percutaneous endomyocardial biopsy may be performed to obtain pieces of myocardial tissue for microscopic examination. Most commonly, tissue is obtained from the right ventricle; however, left ventricular biopsy also can be performed. From the femoral or internal jugular vein, a long biopsy sheath with a side arm port is advanced to the right ventricle over a guidewire. Then, under fluoroscopic guidance, the bioptome is advanced through the long sheath and is directed toward the interventricular septum. After the bioptome has exited the end of the sheath, its jaws are opened, and it is advanced to the septum. The jaws are then tightly closed, and the bioptome is briskly withdrawn through the sheath to tear away a small piece of tissue. This procedure is repeated until three to five tissue specimens are obtained. Local complications related to vascular access (i.e., venous thrombosis, hemorrhage, pneumothorax, recurrent laryngeal nerve injury) are the most common problems associated with this procedure and occur in 1% to 2% of patients. Transient arrhythmias and right bundle branch block from catheter manipulation are common, but sustained rhythm abnormalities are not. Cardiac perforation is rare (13), occurring in less than 0.05% of procedures, but it may lead to pericardial tamponade and hemodynamic collapse, especially if it is not recognized promptly and treated appropriately. Other rare complications include tricuspid regurgitation (resulting from chordal tear) and formation of a fistula from the coronary artery to the right ventricle (14).

Right-Sided Heart Catheterization

During routine right-sided heart catheterization, measurements of pressures and O_2 saturations in the venae cavae, right atrium, right ventricle, pulmonary artery, and pulmonary capillary wedge position can be performed, and CO can be quantified (Table 77.4 gives normal values). The measurement of right-sided pressures helps one to evaluate the severity of tricuspid or pulmonic stenosis, to assess the presence and severity of pulmonary hypertension, and to calculate pulmonary vascular resistance. In the absence of pulmonary vein stenosis (a rare condition), the pulmonary capillary wedge pressure accurately reflects left atrial pressure. The determination of O_2 saturations from the various right-sided heart chambers is used to assess the presence, location, and magnitude of intracardiac left-to-right shunting, such as occurs with atrial or ventricular septal defect or patent ductus arteriosus. Occasionally, angiography is performed to define right-sided anatomic abnormalities or to evaluate the severity of right-sided valvular regurgitation.

TABLE 77.4

NORMAL HEMODYNAMIC VALUES

FLOWS	
Cardiac index (L/min/m^2)	2.6–4.2
Stroke volume index (mL/m^2)	35–55
PRESSURES (mm Hg)	
Aorta/systemic artery	
Peak systolic/end-diastolic	100–140/60–90
Mean	70–105
Left ventricle	
Peak systolic/end-diastolic	100–140/3–12
Left atrium (pulmonary capillary wedge)	
Mean	1–10
a wave	3–15
v wave	3–15
Pulmonary artery	
Peak systolic/end-diastolic	16–30/0–8
Mean	10–16
Right ventricle	
Peak systolic/end-diastolic	16–30/0–8
Right atrium	
Mean	0–8
a wave	2–10
v wave	2–10
RESISTANCES	
Systemic vascular resistance	
Wood units	10–20
Dynes/s/cm	770–1,500
Pulmonary vascular resistance	
Wood units	0.25–1.50
Dynes/s/cm	20–120
OXYGEN CONSUMPTION (mL/min/m^2)	110–150
AVO_2 DIFFERENCE (mL/dL)	3.0–4.5

AV, arteriovenous.

For optimal measurement of right-sided heart pressures, a relatively stiff, large-lumen, nonflotation catheter is used, which can be advanced until it "wedges" in a small pulmonary artery. The catheter's position in the pulmonary capillary wedge location is confirmed by obtaining blood with an O_2 saturation greater than 95%. Alternatively, a softer, balloon-tipped flotation catheter can be used. With this catheter, the acquisition of a blood sample to confirm the pulmonary capillary wedge position is often difficult, and the fidelity of the pressure recordings obtained with it is less ideal than that obtained with a stiffer, large-lumen catheter; however, its ease of passage and paucity of complications make it more suitable for use by operators with limited experience. Furthermore, because it is flow directed, it often can be advanced through the right side of the heart without fluoroscopic guidance. Finally, addition of a thermistor to the flotation catheter's distal portion allows one to measure CO by the thermodilution technique.

Left-Sided Heart Catheterization

With left-sided heart catheterization, one can assess (a) mitral and aortic valvular function, (b) left ventricular pressures and function, (c) systemic vascular resistance, and (d) coronary arterial anatomy. To perform angiography or to measure the pressure in the left ventricle, one usually advances a catheter in retrograde fashion across the aortic valve. In rare circumstances in which this is impossible (e.g., severe aortic stenosis or a tilting disk prosthetic valve in the aortic position), transseptal catheterization is performed, and the catheter is advanced to the left ventricle in antegrade fashion across the mitral valve.

During most catheterizations, pressures are measured directly from each of the cardiac chambers except the left atrium. The left atrial pressure is generally recorded "indirectly," that is, as the pulmonary capillary wedge pressure. To accomplish this, an end-hole catheter is placed in the pulmonary artery and is advanced into the pulmonary arterial tree until it is effectively wedged. If the catheter is wedged adequately, the resultant pressure is left atrial, and the blood withdrawn from it is fully saturated. The demonstration that fully saturated blood can be withdrawn from the catheter confirms that the pressure is indeed left atrial. When a direct left atrial pressure recording is needed, a transseptal catheterization can be performed.

HEMODYNAMIC MEASUREMENTS

Cardiac Output

The flow of blood throughout the body is known as CO and is expressed in liters per minute. Because the magnitude of CO is proportional to body surface area, one person may be compared with another by means of the cardiac index (i.e., the CO adjusted for body surface area). The normal cardiac index is 2.6 to 4.2 L per minute per m^2 of body surface area (Table 77.4). The two commonly used methods of measuring CO are the Fick method and the indicator dilution technique.

Fick Method

The measurement of CO by the Fick method is based on the hypothesis that the uptake of a substance by an organ is the product of the blood flow to that organ and the regional AV concentration difference of the substance (5). By measuring the amount of O_2 extracted from inspired air by the lungs and the AVO_2 difference across the lungs, pulmonary blood flow may be calculated, which is similar to systemic blood flow in most people. The Fick formula for the calculation of CO is as follows:

$$\text{CO (L per minute)} = O_2 \text{ consumption (mL per minute)} / AVO_2 \text{ difference across the lungs (mL/L)}$$

The normal O_2 consumption index (O_2 consumption per m^2 of body surface) is 110 to 150 mL/m^2 per minute (Table 77.4). In general, the O_2 consumption is higher for men than for women and decreases gradually with age. In many laboratories, the O_2 consumption is estimated from a nomogram, formula, or table. However, there is a poor relationship between estimated and measured O_2 consumption, in part because of the wide range of values among patients (Fig. 77.1) (6). Thus, to determine CO accurately via the Fick method, O_2 consumption should be measured directly.

The O_2 consumption can be determined directly by two methods. The most reliable method involves collecting a timed sample (usually 3 to 4 minutes) of expired air in a special receptacle called a *Douglas bag*. The volume of this collection is measured, and the difference in O_2 content between inspired and expired air is calculated. From these data, the person's O_2 consumption (in mL per minute) is determined. More commonly, O_2 consumption is determined by commercially available polarographic machines (i.e., MRM-2, Waters Instruments, Rochester, MN; MedGraphics System, Medical Graphics, St. Paul, MN), which have carbon dioxide, or O_2, or both kinds of sensors and continuously measure air flow and fractional content of carbon dioxide, O_2, or both from expired air collected through the port of a mouthpiece or tight-fitting face mask. Because of potential inaccuracies of the polarographic systems (Fig. 77.2) (18), laboratories that use them should regularly assess their reliability by comparing results obtained with them with other methods, such as a standard Douglas bag collection.

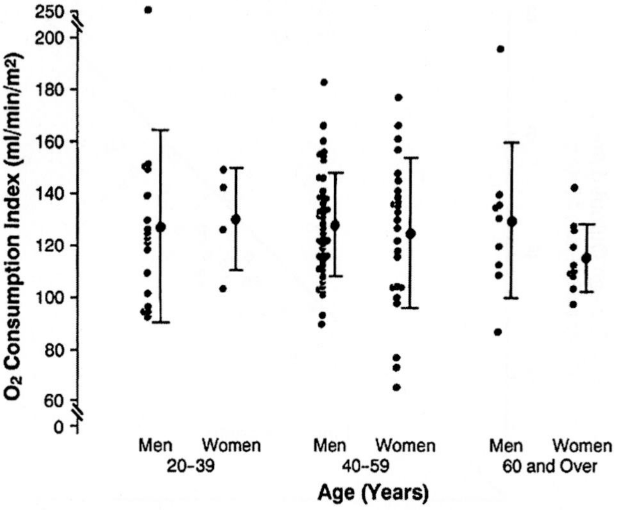

FIGURE 77.1. Oxygen (O_2) consumption (indexed to body surface area) for men and women in three age groups: 20 to 39 years, 40 to 59 years, and 60 years or older. Each symbol represents the data from one patient, and the means and standard deviations for each group are displayed. Although the mean values for oxygen consumption are similar for each of the groups, the range of values is large (65 to 250 mL/m^2 per minute), so an estimate of O_2 consumption in an individual subject may be markedly inaccurate. (From Dehmer GJ, Firth BG, Hillis LD. Oxygen consumption in adult patients during cardiac catheterization. *Clin Cardiol* 1982;5:436–440.)

Determining the AVO_2 difference across the lungs requires that blood from the vessels entering and draining the lungs be analyzed for O_2 content. Provided a right-to-left shunt is not present, systemic arterial and pulmonary arterial samples are usually obtained for the Fick determination of CO. The O_2 content of blood from these two sites may be measured directly or calculated from the O_2 saturation of the blood and its hemoglobin (Hgb) concentration:

$$O_2 \text{ content} = \text{Hgb (in g/100 mL)} \times 1.36 \text{ (mL } O_2\text{/g Hgb)} \times \text{saturation}$$

where 1.36 is the O_2-carrying capacity of 1 g of Hgb. The normal AVO_2 difference is 3.0 to 4.5 volumes percent (mL O_2/dL of blood). The following is an example of the Fick calculation of CO: (a) O_2 consumption = 250 mL per minute; (b) Hgb = 14 g/dL; (c) systemic arterial O_2 saturation = 0.95 (95%); (d) pulmonary arterial O_2 saturation = 0.65 (65%); and (e) 10 = dL/L (conversion factor).

$$\text{CO} = 250/(0.95)(14)(1.36)(10) - (0.65)(14)(1.26)(10) = 4.38 \text{ L per minute}$$

When the AVO_2 saturation difference is small, errors in measurement are magnified. Therefore, the Fick method is most accurate in the patient with a low CO (i.e., one with a relatively wide AVO_2 saturation difference) and least accurate in one with a high CO (i.e., one with a relatively narrow AVO_2 saturation difference) (Table 77.5).

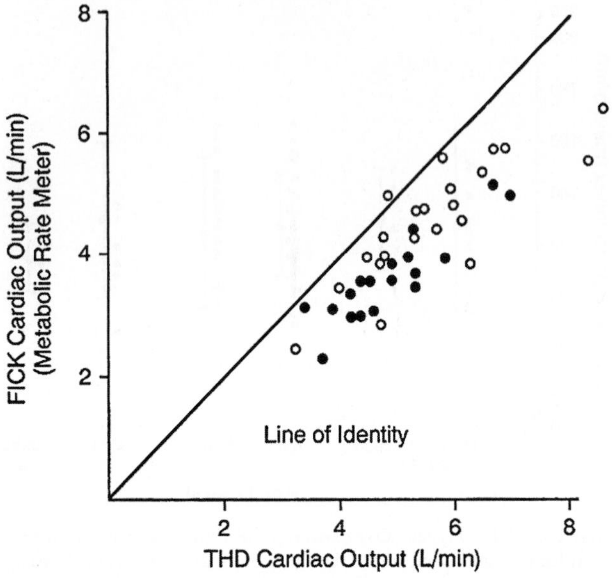

FIGURE 77.2. Comparison of thermodilution (THD) cardiac output (x-axis) and the Fick cardiac output (y-axis), with the latter calculated using oxygen consumption measured with the metabolic rate meter. *Open* and *closed circles* represent data collected at two different hospitals, and the line of identity is shown. Compared with the thermodilution technique, the results of Fick using the oxygen consumption measured with the metabolic rate meter were consistently low. (From Lange RA, Dehmer GJ, Wells PJ, et al. Measurement of oxygen consumption and cardiac output: limitations of the metabolic rate meter. *Am J Cardiol* 1989;64:783–786.)

Indicator Dilution Technique

The indicator dilution technique is based on the principle that the volume of fluid can be determined if one adds a known quantity of indicator to the fluid and then measures the concentration of the indicator over time after it has completely mixed with the fluid. A time-concentration curve is generated, and a minicomputer calculates the area of the inscribed curve.

The indicator most often used to measure CO is cold saline or 5% dextrose in water. A balloon-tipped flow-directed polyvinyl chloride catheter with a thermistor at its tip and an opening 25 to 30 cm proximal to the tip is inserted into a vein and is advanced to the pulmonary artery, so the proximal opening is located in the venae cavae or right atrium, and the thermistor is in the pulmonary artery. An amount of 5 to 10 mL of iced fluid is injected into the proximal port, and the change in temperature at the thermistor is recorded. CO via the thermodilution method is calculated with a computer via the following equation:

$$CO = \frac{(TB - TI)(vol)(60)(1.10)(0.825)}{\int \Delta TB\,(t)dt}$$

in which TB is body temperature, TI is the temperature of the injectate, vol is the volume of the injectate (in milliliters), 60 is number of seconds in 1 minute, and 1.10 is ratio of the products of specific heat and gravity for normal saline and blood; 0.825 is an empiric factor that accounts for the warming of injectate within the catheter. The denominator of the equation is the integral of the change in blood temperature during the injection of cold and is reflected by the area of the inscribed time-temperature curve. The thermodilution technique is relatively inexpensive, easy to perform, and widely available, and it does not require arterial sampling or blood withdrawal. In most patients, it accurately determines pulmonary blood flow, which (in the absence of intracardiac shunting) is similar to systemic blood flow. However, certain conditions may render the results of the thermodilution technique unreliable, including (a) tricuspid or pulmonic regurgitation (7) and (b) intracardiac shunting (Table 77.5).

To ensure an accurate assessment of CO via the indicator dilution technique, great care must be taken to (a) inject an exact amount of indicator, (b) inject the indicator as rapidly as possible (so, in fact, it is delivered as a bolus), (c) calibrate the densitometer and recorder systems precisely, and (d) ensure that the withdrawal of blood (in the case of indocyanine green) at the sampling site is uniform and is not accompanied by air bubbles. When care is taken to eliminate these potential sources of error, the indicator dilution technique is a reliable method of measuring CO. It is most accurate in individuals with a high CO and is least accurate in those with a low CO and in those with valvular regurgitation between the sites of indicator injection and sampling (24) (Table 77.5).

Angiographic Technique

From the left ventriculogram, one can determine the volume of blood ejected with each heart beat (stroke volume) and then multiply it by heart rate, thus yielding the angiographic CO. In patients with mitral or aortic regurgitation, a portion of the blood ejected from the left ventricle regurgitates into the left atrium or ventricle and does not enter the systemic circulation. In these patients, the angiographic CO exceeds the forward output. The measurement of CO by the angiographic method is potentially erroneous in patients with extensive segmental wall motion abnormalities or misshapen ventricles, in whom

TABLE 77.5

METHODS FOR DETERMINING CARDIAC OUTPUT AND CONDITIONS IN WHICH THEY ARE MOST (OR LEAST) RELIABLE

Method	Most reliable	Least reliable
Fick	Low cardiac output	High cardiac output
Thermodilution	High cardiac output	Pulmonic regurgitation
		Tricuspid regurgitation
		Intracardiac shunting
Angiographic	Normal-shaped ventricle	Extensive segmental wall motion abnormalities
		Dilated ventricle
		Aortic regurgitation[a]
		Mitral regurgitation[a]

[a] In these circumstances, angiographic output is greater than forward cardiac output (see text).

the determination of stroke volume may be inaccurate (Table 77.5).

Pressure Measurement

Fluid-Filled Systems

Among most important functions of cardiac catheterization are the accurate measurement and recording of intracardiac pressures. Once a catheter has been positioned in the desired cardiac chamber, it is connected directly or through stiff, fluid-filled tubing to a pressure transducer, which transforms a pressure signal into an electrical signal (via a Wheatstone bridge). The accurate measurement of pressures requires close attention to the details of the catheter-transducer system, including proper transducer balancing as well as removing air bubbles and blood from the catheters and connections. Errors in pressure measurement may occur in several ways. First, an accurate zero reference is essential. All manometers must be referenced to the same zero level, and their position must be adjusted if the patient's position is altered. Second, pressure transducers must be calibrated frequently, preferably before each pressure recording. To allow for meaningful interpretation of hemodynamic data, they should be collected (a) with the patient in a steady state, (b) in close temporal proximity to one another (all pressure measurements and assessments of CO should be completed within 10 to 15 minutes), and (c) before the introduction of radiographic contrast material or other agents known to alter hemodynamic variables.

Micromanometer-Tipped Catheters

With a fluid-filled recording system, distortion of the pressure waveform (Fig. 77.3) occurs as a result of (a) motion of the catheter within the heart (so-called catheter whip artifact), (b) amplification of the systolic pressure in the periphery, (c) catheter movement caused by closing or opening of valves, and (d) excessive damping or augmentation of the frequency response of the system. Despite these shortcomings, the pressure recordings obtained with a fluid-filled system provide adequate information in most clinical situations. However, when it is important to obtain precise pressure recordings with undistorted contours (e.g., in the patient with suspected constrictive or restrictive physiology), such a system may be inadequate. To improve the frequency response and to decrease distortion of the pressure recordings, micromanometer pressure chips have been mounted on the end of catheters to measure intracardiac pressures directly (Millar Instruments, Houston, TX). These catheters provide undistorted high-fidelity pressure recordings, such as are necessary to assess pressure waveform contours (especially in the tachycardic patient) and to measure accurately the rate of ventricular pressure rise (dP/dT) or other sophisticated hemodynamic variables.

Balloon-Tipped Flow-Directed (Swan-Ganz) Catheters

In 1970, the balloon-tipped flow-directed catheter was introduced for right-sided heart catheterization at the bedside, without the need for fluoroscopy (25). At present, it is widely used to monitor right-sided heart and pulmonary capillary wedge pressures in the critically ill patient in the intensive care unit. The catheter, which has an inflatable balloon at its tip, is made of polyvinylchloride and therefore is extremely soft. The standard balloon-tipped catheter has a thermistor at its tip and three lumina. One lumen allows inflation of the balloon with air; the other two lumina allow one to measure pressures and to obtain blood specimens at the catheter tip or an opening 25 to 30 cm proximal to the tip. When the catheter is inserted into a vein and is advanced to the pulmonary artery, the proximal opening is located in the vena cava or right atrium, and the distal orifice and thermistor are in the pulmonary artery.

Before one uses the balloon-tipped catheter, the balloon should be inflated in saline to exclude air leakage, and the catheter lumen should be flushed with saline. A temporary transvenous pacing catheter should be positioned in the right ventricle in patients with a preexisting left bundle branch block before passage of any catheter from the right atrium to the pulmonary artery, because such passage may induce a transient right bundle branch block. The balloon-tipped catheter may be inserted at the bedside percutaneously (via the femoral, internal jugular, subclavian, or basilic vein) or by direct exposure of the brachial vein. When the catheter is introduced without the use of fluoroscopy, it should be advanced 20 to 30 cm into the vasculature (depending on the site of introduction) before the balloon is inflated. The catheter is marked at 10-cm intervals to facilitate this procedure. Before advancing the catheter, blood should be aspirated through it to ensure that it is intravascular. The balloon is inflated gently with up to 1.5 mL of air to facilitate its flow-directed passage from the right atrium to the pulmonary artery. If there is resistance to balloon inflation, the catheter should be advanced or withdrawn carefully until the balloon can be inflated freely. The catheter is then connected to a pressure transducer to record right atrial pressure. It is also valuable to obtain a blood sample for oximetric analysis in each right-sided heart chamber or vessel where pressures are recorded to exclude left-to-right intracardiac shunting.

Once a blood sample and pressure have been obtained from the right atrium, the balloon is inflated, and the catheter is gently advanced while one observes pressure and the electrocardiogram. If the catheter does not pass easily through the right ventricle to the pulmonary artery, or if significant ventricular ectopy occurs, the catheter should be withdrawn to the right atrium and the procedure repeated. Once it has passed to the pulmonary artery and the pressure has been recorded, the catheter is advanced gently (with the balloon still inflated) until the waveform changes to that of a pulmonary capillary wedge pressure. A fully oxygenated blood specimen from this site confirms that the catheter is truly in a wedged position. When the balloon is deflated, the waveform should revert to that of pulmonary arterial pressure.

It is occasionally impossible to pass the balloon-tipped catheter without the use of fluoroscopic guidance, particularly in the patient with a large right atrium or ventricle or the patient with pulmonary hypertension. In this case, it may be necessary to introduce a 0.025-in J-tipped guidewire into the catheter to stiffen it, after which it is advanced under fluoroscopic visualization. Passage of the catheter without the use of fluoroscopy is easier when the site of vascular entry is central (i.e., internal jugular or subclavian vein) rather than peripheral.

The balloon-tipped flow-directed catheter offers several advantages over the more traditional stiff catheter used for right-sided heart catheterization; however, it also has drawbacks. Because it is unusually soft, perforation of the major vessels or heart is virtually impossible, whereas such perforation occasionally occurs with the use of a stiff catheter. As indicated, the flow-directed catheter can be inserted and advanced without fluoroscopic control, although catheter manipulation is easier with fluoroscopic assistance. Apart from its safety, the balloon-tipped flow-directed catheter is equipped with a distal thermistor to measure CO by the thermodilution technique.

The major disadvantages of the balloon-tipped flow-directed catheter stem from the same features that are responsible for its advantages. First, because the catheter is unusually soft, the pressure recordings obtained through it may contain a good deal of "catheter whip," that is, artifact introduced by the movement of the catheter itself within the heart. Second,

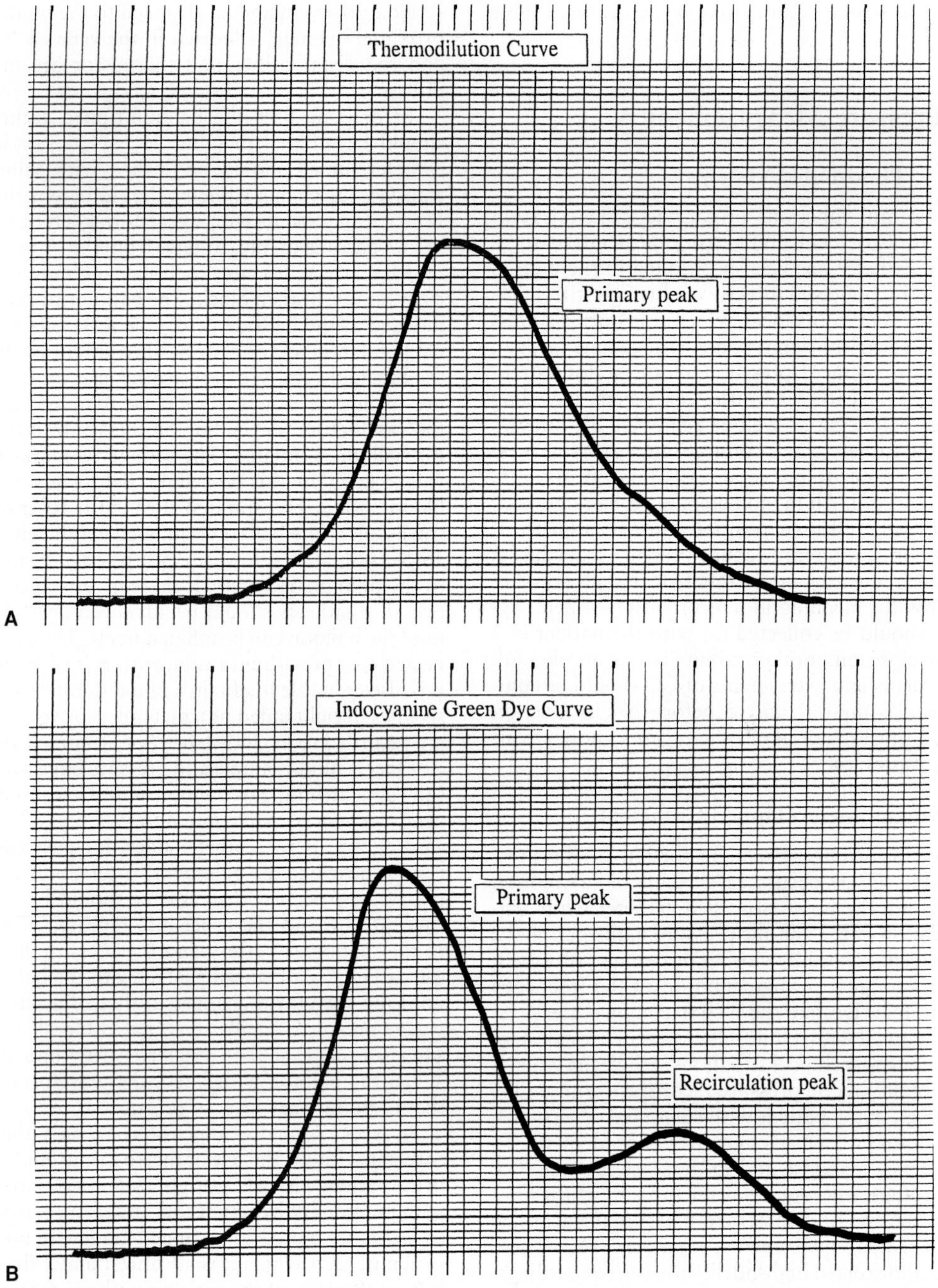

FIGURE 77.3. Time-activity curves for the indicator dilution technique for determining cardiac output: thermodilution (A) and indocyanine green (B). With indocyanine green, a primary peak and a recirculation peak are present, whereas with thermodilution, only a primary peak is observed.

because the catheter is no larger than 7 Fr and yet contains several lumina, the distal lumen is small, thus making the aspiration of blood difficult. Third, because this catheter is advanced in the direction of blood flow, its placement in the pulmonary artery may be impossible if flow within the right-sided heart chambers is bidirectional. For example, advancing a balloon-tipped flow-directed catheter to the pulmonary artery in a patient with severe tricuspid regurgitation may be difficult, because the jet of regurgitation directs the catheter from the right ventricle back into the right atrium. Despite these limitations, this catheter almost always allows one to measure right- and left-sided filling pressures and to make appropriate therapeutic decisions regarding fluid and drug administration.

The risks and complications of the balloon-tipped flow-directed catheter are similar to those of any catheter used for right-sided heart catheterization: ventricular irritability or transient right bundle branch block during passage through the right ventricle and local inflammation or infection at the site of entrance. In addition, because of its softness, the balloon-tipped catheter is easily knotted. Improper or prolonged inflation of the balloon can lead to rupture of a small pulmonary artery or to subsegmental pulmonary infarction, respectively. By and large, however, the balloon-tipped flow-directed catheter is extremely safe. Once it is positioned in the pulmonary artery, it may be left in place for 48 to 96 hours.

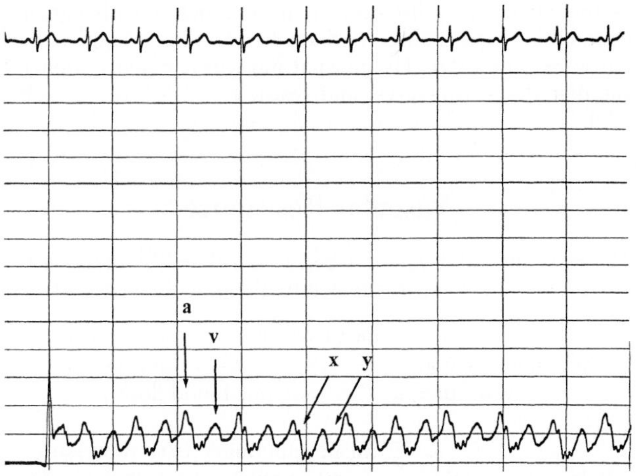

FIGURE 77.4. Typical pressure tracings from the right atrium. An a wave, x descent, v wave, and y descent are noted, and they correlate with right atrial systole, relaxation, filling, and emptying, respectively. The distance between each horizontal line represents 4 mm Hg, and the distance between each vertical time line represents 1 second.

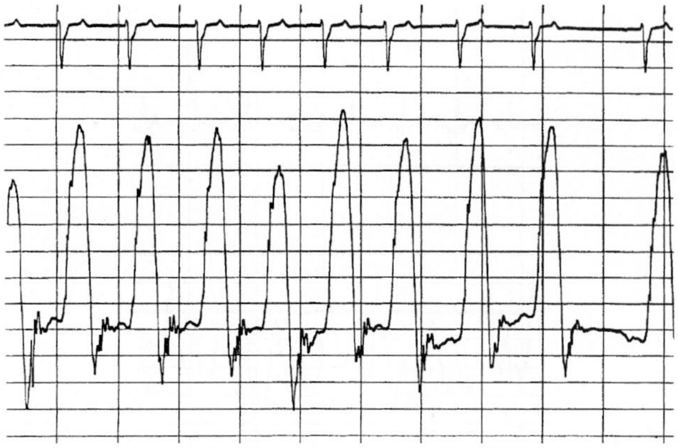

FIGURE 77.5. Simultaneous surface electrocardiogram and right ventricular pressure recordings. The right ventricular peak systolic pressure averages 45 mm Hg, and the end-diastolic pressure (measured at the R-wave peak of the QRS complex) averages 16 mm Hg. The distance between each horizontal line represents 4 mm Hg, and the distance between each vertical time line represents 1 second.

Pressure Waveforms

Right atrial systole follows the P wave of the electrocardiogram and produces the a wave of the right atrial pressure tracing (Fig. 77.4). With atrial relaxation, there is a decline in the pressure, which is known as the *x descent*. This descent may be interrupted by a slight upward deflection, the c wave, resulting from tricuspid valve closure. Filling of the right atrium from the venous circulation and retrograde movement of the tricuspid valve annulus during right ventricular systole produce the v wave, which follows the QRS complex on the electrocardiogram. When the tricuspid valve opens, blood from the right atrium empties into the right ventricle, and the right atrial pressure declines, producing the y descent. During diastole, the right ventricular and right atrial pressures are equal if tricuspid stenosis is absent. Typically, the peak a wave, v wave, and mean right atrial pressures are reported. In the normal right atrium, the peak a wave is higher than the peak v wave pressure.

In the right ventricular pressure tracing, atrial systole produces an a wave, which occurs after the P wave of the electrocardiogram (Fig. 77.5). Right ventricular systole follows the QRS complex of the electrocardiogram and gives rise to the rapidly increasing systolic pressure waveform. With ventricular relaxation, the pressure waveform declines and reaches a nadir, after which continuous filling of the chamber from the right atrium causes a slow, steady rise in the pressure waveform. The peak systolic and end-diastolic (measured at the peak of the QRS complex of the electrocardiogram) right ventricular pressures are usually reported. Similar pressures are reported for the left ventricle.

The normal pulmonary arterial pressure consists of a systolic wave that coincides with right ventricular systole and follows the QRS complex of the electrocardiogram (Fig. 77.6). The decline of this pressure wave may be interrupted by a notch, the incisura, which results from pulmonic valve closure, and the nadir of the decline represents the end-diastolic pressure. The pulmonary arterial systolic, end-diastolic, and mean pressures are usually reported. Similar pressures are reported for the aorta and peripheral arteries.

When a catheter is advanced to the pulmonary capillary wedge position and its position is confirmed oximetrically (by aspirating blood with an O_2 saturation greater than 95%), the pressure waveform obtained is a transmitted left atrial pressure (Fig. 77.7). The configuration of the waveform is similar to that of right atrial pressure, in that one sees an a wave, x descent, v wave, and y descent, which correlate to left atrial systole, relaxation, filling, and emptying, respectively. In the left atrium, however, the peak v wave pressure is typically higher than the peak a wave pressure. Transmission of the left atrial pressure through the pulmonary vasculature usually causes modest distortion of the pressure waveform. To obtain the most accurate representation of left atrial pressure, the pulmonary capillary wedge pressure should be measured through a stiff catheter with a large lumen (8). Time is required for transmission of the left atrial pressure through the pulmonary vasculature. Thus, if left atrial and pulmonary capillary wedge pressures are recorded simultaneously, a 50- to 100-millisecond time difference is noted, with the pulmonary wedge pressure occurring later.

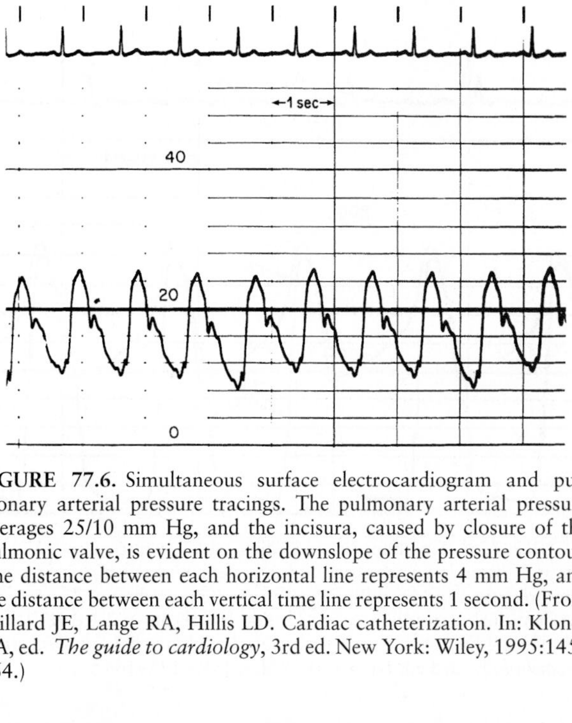

FIGURE 77.6. Simultaneous surface electrocardiogram and pulmonary arterial pressure tracings. The pulmonary arterial pressure averages 25/10 mm Hg, and the incisura, caused by closure of the pulmonic valve, is evident on the downslope of the pressure contour. The distance between each horizontal line represents 4 mm Hg, and the distance between each vertical time line represents 1 second. (From Willard JE, Lange RA, Hillis LD. Cardiac catheterization. In: Kloner RA, ed. *The guide to cardiology*, 3rd ed. New York: Wiley, 1995:145–164.)

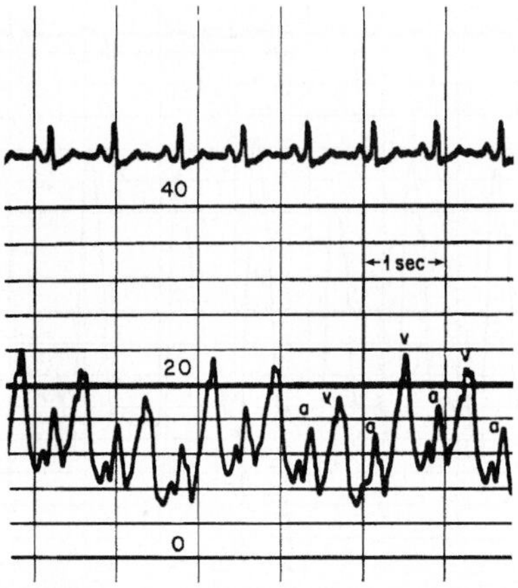

FIGURE 77.7. Pulmonary capillary wedge pressure tracing obtained through a stiff, large-lumen catheter, the position of which was confirmed oximetrically. As in the right atrial pressure tracing, one sees an a wave and v wave, which correlate with atrial systole and filling, respectively. The distance between each horizontal line represents 4 mm Hg, and the distance between each vertical time line represents 1 second. (From Willard JE, Lange RA, Hillis LD. Cardiac catheterization. In: Kloner RA, ed. *The guide to cardiology*, 3rd ed. New York: Wiley, 1995:145–164.)

In addition to the recording of pressures from each of the cardiac chambers, it is important that the pressures from certain chambers be examined simultaneously to confirm or exclude the presence of valvular abnormalities (8,9). Thus, left ventricular and left atrial (or pulmonary capillary wedge) pressures should be recorded simultaneously to ascertain whether mitral stenosis is present. Likewise, the left ventricular and systemic arterial pressures should be displayed concurrently to evaluate the presence or absence of left ventricular outflow tract obstruction (Fig. 77.8). The recording of intracardiac and peripheral vascular pressures may demonstrate hemodynamic findings consistent with valvular regurgitation. For instance, large regurgitant waves in the pulmonary capillary wedge tracing may be indicative of mitral regurgitation or other causes of left atrial pressure or volume overload (10). Conversely, a wide

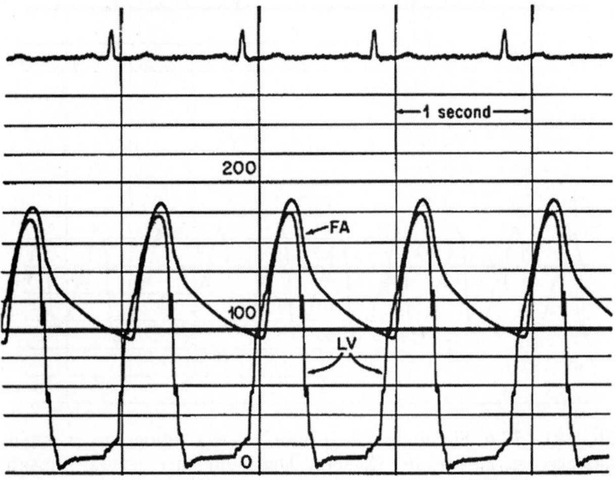

FIGURE 77.8. Simultaneous recording of left ventricular (LV) and femoral arterial (FA) pressures in a patient without aortic stenosis. The pressure scale (in millimeters of mercury) is shown. There is no gradient during systole between LV and FA. (From Willard JE, Lange RA, Hillis LD. Cardiac catheterization. In: Kloner RA, ed. *The guide to cardiology*, 3rd ed. New York: Wiley, 1995:145–164.)

peripheral arterial pulse pressure in conjunction with a greatly elevated left ventricular end-diastolic pressure is suggestive of aortic regurgitation. The normal intracardiac and peripheral vascular flows, pressures, and resistances are listed in Table 77.4.

Vascular Resistance

The resistance of a vascular bed is calculated by dividing the pressure gradient across the bed by the flow through it. Thus,

$$\text{Systemic vascular resistance} = \frac{\text{mean systemic arterial pressure} - \text{mean right atrial pressure}}{\text{systemic blood flow}}$$

and

$$\text{Pulmonary vascular resistance} = \frac{\text{mean pulmonary arterial pressure} - \text{mean pulmonary vein pressure}}{\text{pulmonary blood flow}}$$

Because pulmonary venous pressure is not usually measured, left atrial or pulmonary capillary wedge pressure is substituted for it. Resistances are expressed in (a) Woods units (millimeters of mercury per liter per minute) or (b) dynes per second per centimeter (Woods units × 80). The normal values for vascular resistances are displayed in Table 77.4.

ASSESSMENT OF VALVULAR HEART DISEASE

Valvular Stenosis

Through the application of standard fluid dynamic principles, the resistance to blood flow through a stenotic valve can be expressed as an effective valve orifice area. The data required for the calculation of a valve area may be obtained during cardiac catheterization. Specifically, the pressures on either side of a stenotic valve and the flow across it must be known. The Gorlin equation is then used to calculate the valve area:

$$\text{Valve area} = \frac{\text{CO/(DFP or SEP) (heart rate)}}{\text{(Constant)}\ (\sqrt{\text{mean pressure gradient}})}$$

where DFP is diastolic filling period and SEP is systolic ejection period. If an atrioventricular valve (mitral or tricuspid) is being evaluated, the diastolic filling period is used; if the aortic or pulmonic valve is involved, the systolic ejection period is used. The filling periods and transvalvular gradient are measured from pressure tracings obtained simultaneously from either side of the stenotic valve. The constant used is 38.0 for the mitral valve and 44.5 for the other valves. The mean pressure gradient is the average gradient throughout systole (for aortic and pulmonic valves) or diastole (for mitral or tricuspid valves).

The normal mitral valve orifice area is 4 to 6 cm^2. A mitral valve with an effective orifice area less than 1.0 cm^2 is considered severely stenotic (Fig. 77.9); 1.1 to less than 1.5 cm^2, moderately stenotic; and 1.6 to less than 2.0 cm^2, mildly stenotic. A valve area greater than 2.0 cm^2 does not usually constitute a hemodynamically significant obstruction to flow. The normal aortic valve has a cross-sectional area of 3 to 4 cm^2. An aortic valve with an effective orifice area less than 0.7 cm^2 is severely stenotic (Fig. 77.10); 0.8 to 1.0 cm^2, moderately stenotic; and 1.1 to 1.3 cm^2, mildly stenotic. The normal pulmonic valve has a cross-sectional area similar to that of the aortic valve. Although the Gorlin equation can be applied to the pulmonic valve, by convention the severity of stenosis is

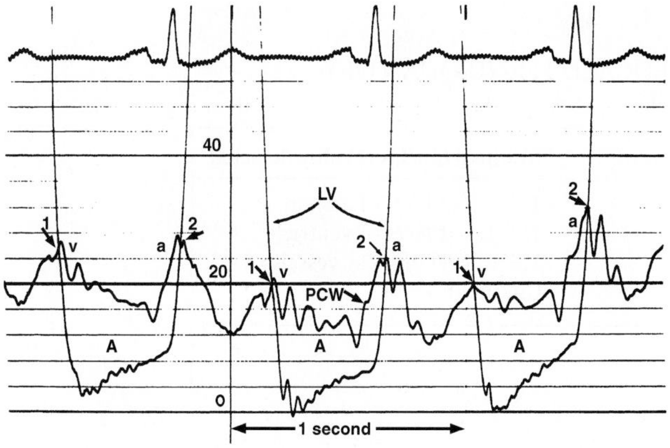

FIGURE 77.9. Simultaneous recording of left ventricular (LV) and pulmonary capillary wedge (PCW) pressures in a patient with severe mitral stenosis. Throughout diastole (from point *1* to point *2*), there is a pressure gradient (*A*) between the LV and PCW pressures. This patient had a cardiac output of 3,740 mL per minute and a heart rate of 68 beats per minute. The mean diastolic filling period was 0.49 seconds per beat, and the mean pressure gradient was 13 mm Hg. Using Gorlin's equation, the mitral valve area is as follows:

$$\frac{3{,}740/(68)(0.49)}{(38\chi\sqrt{13})} = 0.8\ \text{cm}^2$$

(From Willard JE, Lange RA, Hillis LD. Cardiac catheterization. In: Kloner RA, ed. *The guide to cardiology*, 3rd ed. New York: Wiley, 1995:145–164.)

based on the peak right ventricular systolic pressure. Pulmonic stenosis with a right ventricular peak systolic pressure of 25 to less than 50 mm Hg is termed mild; 50 to less than 100 mm Hg, moderate; and greater than 100 mm Hg, severe. Finally,

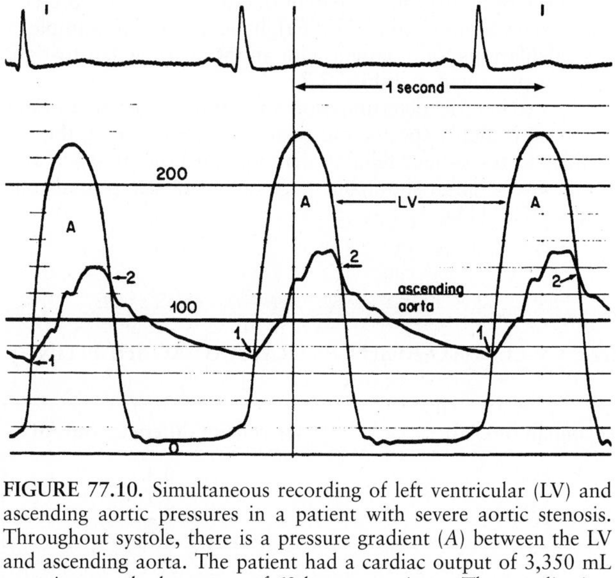

FIGURE 77.10. Simultaneous recording of left ventricular (LV) and ascending aortic pressures in a patient with severe aortic stenosis. Throughout systole, there is a pressure gradient (*A*) between the LV and ascending aorta. The patient had a cardiac output of 3,350 mL per minute and a heart rate of 62 beats per minute. The systolic ejection period (between points *1* and *2*) was 0.36 seconds per beat, and the mean systolic pressure gradient was 83 mm Hg. Thus, the aortic valve area was as follows:

$$\frac{3{,}350/(62)(0.36)}{44.5(\sqrt{83})} = 0.4\ \text{cm}^2$$

(From Willard JE, Lange RA, Hillis LD. Cardiac catheterization. In: Kloner RA, ed. *The guide to cardiology*, 3rd ed. New York: Wiley, 1995:145–164.)

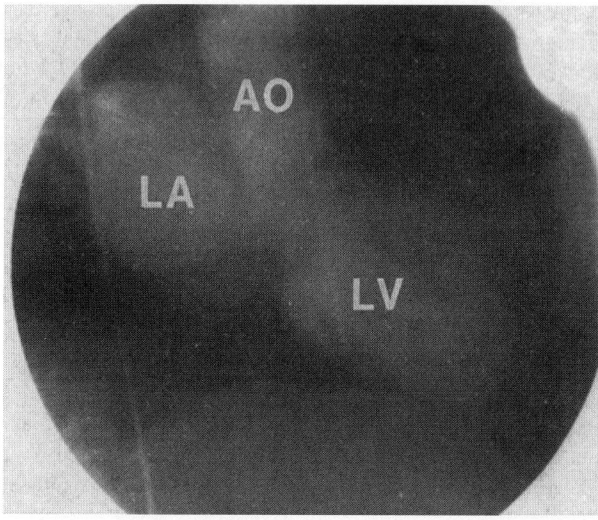

FIGURE 77.11. A single plane (30-degree right anterior oblique) left ventriculogram in a patient with severe (4+) mitral regurgitation. The left atrium (LA) is opacified with radiographic contrast material that has regurgitated through an incompetent mitral valve. Ao, aorta; LV, left ventricle.

the tricuspid valve is large, with a normal orifice area of 6 to 10 cm^2. The assessment of the severity of tricuspid stenosis is most accurate when right atrial and right ventricular pressures are recorded simultaneously. Patients with a tricuspid valve area less than 3.0 cm^2 in the presence of medically refractory right-sided heart failure should be considered for appropriate intervention (i.e., balloon valvuloplasty, open commissurotomy, or valve replacement).

Valvular Regurgitation

The presence and severity of mitral regurgitation may be evaluated qualitatively by observing the amount of radiographic contrast material that regurgitates into the left atrium during left ventricular systole on a standard left ventriculogram (Fig. 77.11). The magnitude of regurgitation is estimated as trivial (1+), mild (2+), moderate (3+), or severe (4+) (see the later discussion of left ventriculography). To obtain a quantitative assessment of the severity of mitral regurgitation, one can calculate the volume of blood that regurgitates from the left ventricle into the left atrium per minute (so-called regurgitant volume) by measuring the difference between the angiographic CO (determined by left ventriculography) and the forward CO (determined by the Fick method or thermodilution). The regurgitant fraction is the percentage of the total angiographic output that regurgitates into the left atrium: it is the quotient of the regurgitant volume and the angiographic output. Typically, valvular regurgitation with a regurgitant fraction 0.6 or greater is severe; 0.40 to 0.59, moderate; 0.20 to 0.39, mild; and less than 0.20, trivial.

The presence and severity of aortic regurgitation may be evaluated qualitatively by observing the amount of radiographic contrast material that regurgitates into the left ventricle during ventricular diastole by aortography; it is also graded as trivial (1+), mild (2+), moderate (3+), or severe (4+) (see the later discussion of aortography). As in mitral regurgitation, a quantitative assessment of the severity of aortic regurgitation can be obtained by calculating the regurgitant volume and fraction.

TABLE 77.6

COMPARISON OF METHODS TO DETECT, LOCALIZE, AND QUANTIFY INTRACARDIAC LEFT-TO-RIGHT SHUNTING

Method	Able to localize?	Able to quantify?	Minimal Qp/Qs reliably detected
Oximetry	Yes	Yes	1.5–1.9 at level of atrium 1.3–1.5 at level of ventricle 1.3 at level of great vessels
Angiography	Yes	No	Unknown

Qp/Qs, pulmonic/systemic blood flow.

ASSESSMENT OF INTRACARDIAC SHUNTING

Left-to-Right Shunting

In the patient with known or suspected congenital heart disease, as well as the patient with unexplained heart failure, cardiac catheterization may be performed to assess the presence, location, and magnitude of intracardiac shunting. Several techniques may be used (Table 77.6) (11).

Oximetric Assessment

Oxygenated blood shunted from the left side to the right side of the heart causes an abnormal increase ("step up") in the O_2 content or saturation of blood in the chamber into which shunting occurs. To detect the presence and site of the left-to-right shunt, multiple blood samples are obtained from the pulmonary artery, right ventricle, right atrium, and venae cavae, and the O_2 content or saturation of each sample is evaluated for evidence of such a step up. An abnormal step up is present when the right atrial O_2 content is greater than 1.9 mL/dL higher than that of the venae cavae, the right ventricular O_2 content is greater than 0.9 mL/dL higher than that of the right atrium, or the pulmonary arterial O_2 content is greater than 0.5 mL/dL higher than that of the right ventricle. The O_2 content of blood can be measured directly or calculated from the saturation:

saturation ? Hgb (grams per deciliter) ? 1.36 mLO_2/g of Hgb

The oximetric quantitation of shunting is accomplished by calculating pulmonic (Qp) and systemic (Qs) blood flows according to the Fick principle, where:

$$\text{Qp (L per minute)} = \frac{O_2 \text{ consumption (milliliters per minute)}}{\text{AV } O_2 \text{ content difference across the lungs (mL/L)}}$$

and

$$\text{Qs (L per minute)} = \frac{O_2 \text{ consumption (milliliters per minute)}}{\text{AV } O_2 \text{ content difference across the body (mL/L)}}$$

The AV O_2 content difference across the lungs is the difference in O_2 contents between pulmonary arterial and venous blood. The AV O_2 content difference across the body is the difference in O_2 contents between systemic arterial and mixed venous blood, with the latter obtained from the chamber immediately before (proximal to) the site of shunting. For example, if a ventricular septal defect is present, the mixed venous chamber is the right atrium; if a patent ductus arteriosus is present, the mixed venous chamber is the right ventricle. An example of the calculations for a patient with an intracardiac left-to-right shunt is presented in Table 77.7.

The oximetric determination of intracardiac left-to-right shunting is highly specific but relatively insensitive, in that an oximetric assessment reliably demonstrates the presence of a moderate or large shunt but may fail to detect a small one (Table 77.6) (11).

TABLE 77.7

OXIMETRIC ASSESSMENT OF THE PRESENCE, SITE, AND SIZE OF LEFT-TO-RIGHT INTRACARDIAC SHUNTING IN A PATIENT WITH A VENTRICULAR SEPTAL DEFECT[a]

Chamber	O_2 saturation (%)	O_2 content (mL/dL)	O_2 content difference (mL/dL)
Venae cavae	65	13.1	0.4
Right atrium	67	13.5	2.2
Right ventricle	78	15.7	0.2
Pulmonary artery	79	15.9	
Systemic artery	97		

Site of O_2 step up = right ventricle Mixed venous chamber = right atrium

$$\text{Qp} = \frac{250\,\text{mL/min}}{(0.97 - 0.79)(15\,\text{g/dL})(1.36\,\text{mL}\,O_2/\text{g hemoglobin})(10\,\text{dL/L})} = 6.81\,\text{L/min}$$

$$\text{Qp} = \frac{250\,\text{mL/min}}{(0.97 - 0.67)(15\,\text{g/dL})(1.36\,\text{mL}\,O_2/\text{g hemoglobin})(10\,\text{dL/L})} = 4.08\,\text{L/min}$$

[a]Measured oxygen (O_2) consumption, 250 mL per minute; hemoglobin, 15 g/dL; Qp/Qs (pulmonic/systemic blood flow) ratio, 6.81/4.08 = 1.7.

Angiographic Assessment

When radiographic contrast material is introduced into a left-sided chamber during angiography in a patient with left-to-right intracardiac shunting, its movement into a right-sided chamber may be visualized. The reliability of any angiographic technique for detecting or localizing intracardiac left-to-right shunting depends on the location of the defect and the obliquity in which the angiogram is performed. For example, the interventricular septum may be visualized by performing left ventriculography in a 40- to 50-degree left anterior oblique projection, thus allowing the diagnosis of a ventricular septal defect. A communication between the thoracic aorta and the pulmonary artery (i.e., patent ductus arteriosus or aortopulmonary window) may be identified by performing aortography in the left anterior oblique or left lateral projections. In contradistinction, atrial septal defects and anomalous pulmonary venous drainage are difficult to visualize angiographically. Although angiography can detect and localize certain intracardiac left-to-right shunts, it cannot measure the magnitude of shunting.

Right-to-Left Shunting

In the patient with right-to-left intracardiac shunting, passage of unoxygenated blood from the venous circulation to the systemic circulation results in arterial desaturation (less than 95%). When desaturation results from other conditions (i.e., a ventilation-perfusion mismatch or hypoventilation), it is corrected when 100% O_2 is administered, whereas this does not occur when the arterial desaturation results from right-to-left shunting. Thus, demonstration of a systemic arterial O_2 saturation less than 95% that does not correct with the administration of 100% O_2 (via face mask) is consistent with right-to-left intracardiac shunting.

ANGIOGRAPHY

Left Ventriculography

Cineangiocardiography of the left ventricle allows one to assess (a) global and segmental left ventricular function, (b) left ventricular volumes and ejection fraction, and (c) the presence and severity of mitral regurgitation. In the physiologically normal adult, 40 to 60 mL of contrast material is injected over 3 to 4 seconds (10 to 15 mL per second) into the left ventricle as cineangiography is performed. Ventriculography may be performed in one projection (single plane), which is usually performed in the 30-degree right anterior oblique projection or in two projections (biplane) 90 degrees apart in obliquity (60-degree left anterior oblique and 30-degree right anterior oblique) (Fig. 77.12).

Left ventriculography allows for calculation of left ventricular volumes and ejection fraction using a standard area-length formula. The normal values for left ventricular volumes and ejection fraction are displayed in Table 77.8. In addition to the calculation of left ventricular volumes, segmental wall motion may be assessed. A segment of the left ventricular wall with reduced systolic motion is said to be *hypokinetic*; a segment that does not move during ventricular contraction is *akinetic*; and one that moves paradoxically during ventricular systole is termed *dyskinetic*. Finally, the presence and severity of mitral regurgitation may be evaluated qualitatively during sinus beats as trivial (1+), mild (2+), moderate (3+), or severe (4+): (a) with 1+, contrast material enters the left atrium during systole and clears with each beat; (b) with 2+, contrast opacification of the left atrium does not clear with each beat and is less dense than the left ventricle; (c) with 3+, opacification of the left atrium is equal to that of the left ventricle; and (d) with 4+, the presence of one of three findings is observed—opacification of the left atrium more densely than that of the left ventricle, opacification of the left atrium in one systolic ejection period, or the presence of contrast material in a pulmonary vein.

Right Ventriculography

Cineangiography of the right ventricle allows one to assess global right ventricular function as well as the presence and severity of tricuspid regurgitation. The presence and severity of tricuspid regurgitation may be evaluated qualitatively in a manner similar to mitral regurgitation: trivial (1+), mild (2+), moderate (3+), or severe (4+). There are no reliable methods for the quantitative assessment of right ventricular volumes or ejection fraction by ventriculography.

Aortography

A proximal aortogram is performed to assess the competency of the aortic valve, to evaluate the anatomy of the proximal aorta and large vessels that supply the head and neck, or to assess the presence of bypass graft anastomoses that have been difficult or impossible to cannulate selectively. For proximal aortography, 50 to 60 mL of contrast material is injected over 2.0 to 3.0 seconds during cineangiography, typically filmed in a 45- to 60-degree left anterior oblique projection. The severity of aortic regurgitation may be evaluated qualitatively during sinus beats as trivial (1+), mild (2+), moderate (3+), or severe (4+): (a) with 1+, contrast material enters the left ventricle during diastole and clears with each beat; (b) with 2+, contrast opacification of the left ventricle does not clear with each beat and is less dense than the ascending aorta; (c) with 3+, opacification of the left ventricle is equal to that of the aorta; and (d) with 4+, opacification of the left ventricle is greater than that of the aorta, or the left ventricle is opacified in one diastolic filling period.

Analysis of the films must be meticulous because the radiographic findings associated with pulmonary embolism may be subtle. Radiographic signs diagnostic of pulmonary embolism include a large intraluminal filling defect and an abrupt pulmonary arterial cutoff. Other radiographic signs, such as localized oligemia and asymmetry of pulmonary blood flow, are suggestive but not strictly diagnostic of embolism.

CONTROVERSIES AND PERSONAL PERSPECTIVES

Routine right-sided heart catheterization in critically ill patients is associated with increased mortality (12,13). In such patients, physicians with limited catheterization experience often place an indwelling flow-directed pulmonary artery catheter. Complications associated with such indwelling catheters (i.e., pulmonary arterial perforation, sepsis, bacterial endocarditis, and large vein thrombosis) and placement by less experienced operators may account for the observed increased mortality. Conversely, when performed by physicians experienced with the technique, right-sided heart catheterization is extremely safe. Over the past 2 decades, we have performed more than 6,000 right-sided heart catheterizations with a stiff, large-lumen (e.g., 8-Fr Goodale Lubin) catheter with no major complications

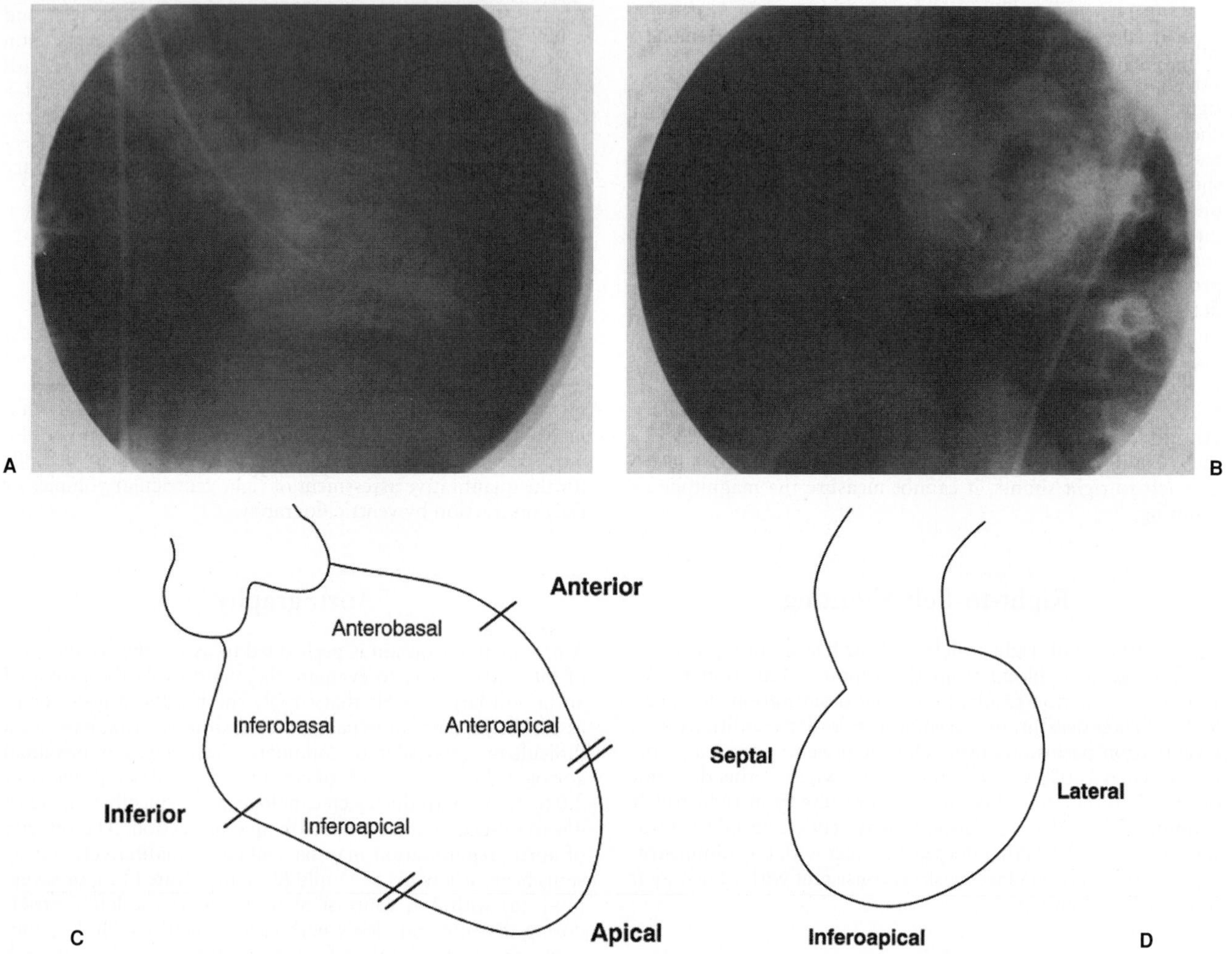

FIGURE 77.12. With biplane ventriculography, two projections 90 degrees apart in obliquity are performed: 30-degree right anterior oblique (A) and 60-degree left anterior oblique (B). The segments of the left ventricle that are visualized with each obliquity are labeled (C,D). With typical single-plane ventriculography, only the right anterior oblique projection is obtained.

(i.e., infection, hemorrhage, perforation, or death) and only one (0.02%) minor complication (femoral vein thrombosis). In our opinion, right-sided heart catheterization should not be performed in critically ill patients unless done so (a) by a physician experienced with the technique, (b) in a patient with a clear indication, or (c) for training purposes under supervision (Table 77.9).

Likewise, left-sided heart catheterization should be performed only for a proper indication (Table 77.10) and in a

TABLE 77.8

NORMAL ANGIOGRAPHIC VALUES

LV end-diastolic volume index	50–90 mL/m^2
LV end-systolic volume index	13–35 mL/m^2
LV stroke volume index	35–55 mL/m^2
LV ejection fraction	0.55%–0.70%

LV, left ventricular.

TABLE 77.9

INDICATIONS FOR RIGHT-SIDED HEART CATHETERIZATION

KNOWN OR SUSPECTED
Valvular heart disease
Congenital heart disease
Restrictive or constrictive heart disease
Pulmonary hypertension
Cardiac tamponade
HEART FAILURE
Decompensated
Origin undefined
MYOCARDIAL INFARCTION
With hypotension
With pulmonary congestion
With mechanical complication
UNEXPLAINED RIGHT-SIDED HEART FAILURE

TABLE 77.10

INDICATIONS FOR THERAPEUTIC LEFT-SIDED HEART CATHETERIZATION

ANGINA PECTORIS
Unstable or rest
With exertion
Despite medical therapy
With evidence of extensive coronary artery disease by noninvasive testing
ACUTE MYOCARDIAL INFARCTION (FOR PRIMARY ANGIOPLASTY)
AFTER MYOCARDIAL INFARCTION
Evidence of extensive coronary artery disease by noninvasive testing
Postinfarction angina
Depressed left ventricular function
Failure to reperfuse following thrombolytic therapy
Cardiogenic shock
VALVULAR STENOSIS (WITH SYMPTOMS)
VALVULAR REGURGITATION
With symptoms
With impaired left ventricular systolic function
CONGESTIVE HEART FAILURE
SUSPECTED CONGENITAL HEART DISEASE
SUDDEN CARDIAC DEATH
MAJOR NONCARDIAC SURGERY AND EVIDENCE OF EXTENSIVE CORONARY ARTERY DISEASE BY NONINVASIVE TESTING

facility capable of handling complications. Free-standing or mobile catheterization facilities without immediately available hospital and surgical support are ill equipped to handle serious catheterization-related complications. Patients with unstable symptoms or clinical features suggestive of an increased risk for cardiac or vascular complications (Table 77.4) should undergo catheterization in an inpatient setting.

THE FUTURE

As noninvasive imaging techniques (e.g., magnetic resonance imaging, multidetector computed tomographic scanning) continue to improve, they will likely reduce the need for many diagnostic catheterizations. Conversely, therapeutic catheterization will continue to increase in frequency as percutaneous techniques (e.g., coronary revascularization, valvuloplasty, valve replacement or repair, catheter closure of intracardiac defects) continue to improve.

References

1. Chandrasekar B, Doucet S, Bilodeau L, et al. Complications of cardiac catheterization in the current era: a single-center experience. *Cathet Cardiovasc Intervent* 2001;52:289–295.
2. Scanlon PJ, Faxon DP, Audet AM, et al. AHA guidelines for coronary angiography: executive summary and recommendations: a report of the American College of Cardiology/American Heart Association Task Force on Practice Guidelines (Committee on Coronary Angiography) developed in collaboration with the Society for Cardiac Angiography and Interventions. *J Am Coll Cardiol* 1999;33:1756–1824.
3. Hagan JB. Anaphylactoid and adverse reactions to radiocontrast agents. *Immunol Allergy Clin North Am* 2004;24:507–519.
4. Maeder M, Klein M, Fehr T, Rickli H. Contrast nephropathy: a review focusing on prevention. *J Am Coll Cardiol* 2004;44:1763–1771.
5. Fick A. Uber die Messung des Blutquantums in den Herzventriken. *Physmed Ges Wurzburg* July 9, 1870.
6. Kendrick AH, West J, Papouchado M, et al. Direct Fick cardiac output: are assumed values of oxygen consumption acceptable? *Eur Heart J* 1988;9:337–342.
7. Cigarroa RG, Lange RA, Williams RH, et al. Underestimation of cardiac output by thermodilution in patients with tricuspid regurgitation. *Am J Med* 1989;86:417–420.
8. Lange RA, Moore DM, Cigarroa RG, et al. Use of pulmonary capillary wedge pressure to assess severity of mitral stenosis: is true left atrial pressure needed in this condition? *J Am Coll Cardiol* 1989;13:825–829.
9. Brogan WC, Lange RA, Hillis LD. Accuracy of various methods of measuring the transvalvular pressure gradient in aortic stenosis. *Am Heart J* 1992;123:948–953.
10. Snyder RW, Glamann DB, Lange RA, et al. Predictive value of prominent pulmonary arterial wedge v waves in assessing the presence and severity of mitral regurgitation. *Am J Cardiol* 1994;73:568–570.
11. Boehrer JD, Lange RA, Willard JE, et al. Advantages and limitations of methods to detect, localize, and quantitate intracardiac left-to-right shunting. *Am Heart J* 1992;124:448–455.
12. Connors AF, Speroff T, Dawson NV, et al. The effectiveness of right heart catheterization in the initial care of critically ill patients. *JAMA* 1996;276:889–897.
13. Dalen JA, Bone RC. Is it time to pull the pulmonary artery catheter? *JAMA* 1996;276:916–918.

CHAPTER 78 ■ PERCUTANEOUS CORONARY INTERVENTION

BERNHARD MEIER

OVERVIEW

Percutaneous coronary intervention (PCI), previously called percutaneous transluminal coronary angioplasty (PTCA), has continuously gained importance since the first procedure in 1977 to become the most common major medical intervention. It can be performed using local anesthesia, even as an outpatient procedure. For optimal performance, it requires the best current radiographic and dilatation equipment as well as a properly trained operator with an experienced crew.

PCI works best for single-vessel disease, but it may be of great value for double- and triple-vessel disease, particularly in patients with discrete lesions or in those who are old, fragile, or have had prior coronary artery bypass grafting (CABG). PCI plays a dominant role in the treatment of acute coronary syndromes, in particular ST-segment elevation myocardial infarction.

Limitations of PCI are low success rates in old and long chronic total coronary occlusions, fatal outcomes in approximately 1% of cases, acute and late ischemic complications in approximately 3% and 2%, respectively, and clinically significant restenosis within the first months in approximately 10%. The strengths of PCI are a greater than 90% success rate, the possibility for a prompt return to a normal physical life, the repeatability of the procedure, and the paucity of complications after the first day or of recurrences after the first year. Stents have proved an invaluable complement to the balloon. Routine stenting (hence direct stenting) has become the standard approach, although it is unequivocally required in a minority of lesions. Drug-eluting (active) stents are about to supplant bare (passive) stents completely.

Current research is focused on technical advances in the crossing of chronic total coronary occlusions and on optimized antiplatelet and antithrombin therapy to reduce acute occlusions. The restenosis problem, already ameliorated by stenting, has been further diminished by active stents, which continue to be a main line of research and development.

GLOSSARY

Ad hoc: Performed during diagnostic catheterization.
Culprit lesion: Lesion responsible for the current event or predominant symptoms.
Fr: French, diameter unit for equipment; 1 Fr = 0.33 mm.
Guidewire: Wire over which to advance the balloon catheter.
Guiding catheter: Catheter through which to introduce the balloon catheter into the coronary artery.
PCI: Percutaneous coronary intervention.
PTCA: Percutaneous transluminal coronary angioplasty.

HISTORY

Coronary balloon angioplasty is an offspring of transluminal angioplasty of peripheral arteries initiated by Dotter and Judkins in 1964 (1). Their method of dilating stenoses by successively introducing coaxial catheters of growing diameters was crude. It required an access hole commensurate with the target lumen.

On February 12, 1974, Gruentzig performed the first balloon angioplasty in a peripheral artery at the University Hospital in Zurich, Switzerland, by using a form-constant polyvinyl chloride balloon (2,3). In 1975, he presented a double-lumen balloon catheter, introduced over a guidewire (2). In 1976, he demonstrated the feasibility of coronary balloon angioplasty in dogs. On March 22, 1976, a first human case had to be aborted before introducing the balloon catheter. The coronary ostium of a patient with inoperable end-stage coronary artery disease could not be engaged with the guiding catheter introduced through the arm because of occluded iliac arteries. On May 9, 1977, a first intraoperative balloon angioplasty procedure was accomplished in San Francisco by the cardiologists Gruentzig and Myler and the cardiac surgeon Hanna.

Gruentzig's historical first PCI case in Zurich of September 16, 1977 concerned a man his own age (38 years) who had a

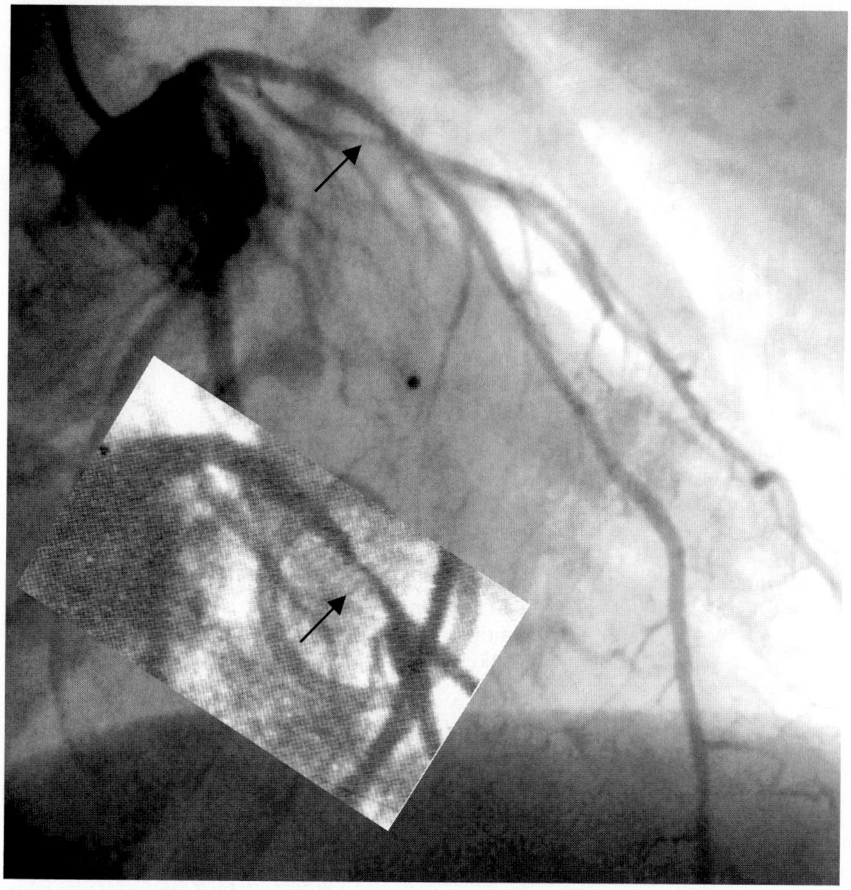

FIGURE 78.1. Coronary angiogram 23 years after the first percutaneous coronary intervention (PCI) (the patient had aged from 38 to 61 years). The *arrows* point to the dilated site at follow-up on December 7, 2000 and before PCI on September 16, 1977 (**inset**).

single discrete stenosis of the left anterior descending coronary artery (4). As the fellow in charge of the patient at the time, I have been partaking in his care ever since. He has remained free of complications and local recurrence (Fig. 78.1) for about 30 years now, a living triumph of the method (5,6). Primary success in the first 50 patients in Zurich was 64% without mortality. Emergency bypass operation was required in 14%, and infarction occurred in 6% (7,8).

The first clinical use of a coronary stent, on March 28, 1986, by Puel in Toulouse, France (9), induced a gradual change of the pattern of PCI. The stent, first a rare ally of the balloon, matured to become its conjoined twin, in contrast to the balloon's many, other mostly short-lived, companions or alternatives.

To date, PCI is thriving in spite of a tight medicoeconomic situation. With about 3 million yearly procedures performed worldwide, it tops the list of major medical interventions. In 3 decades, PCI has withstood the scrutiny of local and global peer review. It has been analyzed in numerous registries and subjected to a flurry of well-focused and meticulously monitored randomized studies. It has seen its indications expanded, cropped, and expanded again. It is far from perfect but likable and utterly useful, just as Gruentzig had presaged. He had set out for a humble 15% PCI share of the patients needing coronary revascularization. Up to his accidental death in 1985, he did not envision that PCI was ultimately going to be carried out several times more frequently than CABG.

MECHANISM

Figure 78.2 explains that dissection of intima and media, usually in thin areas of the plaque or adjacent to it, and dilatation of the vessel circumference constitute the key mechanisms for the luminal gain achieved by PCI (10). The stent prevents elastic recoil and keeps loose intimal flaps or plaque components out of the way. Reendothelialization commonly smoothes the rough surface within a few weeks. Yet it also renarrows the lumen and contributes to restenosis, together with constrictive remodeling in unstented lesions (11).

PROCEDURE

Personnel

Primary Operator

Table 78.1 lists proposed curricula to independence and activity thereafter (12–16). Minimum records are acceptable, but with a history of a more active training period and support by an experienced interventional environment (peers and team). The mortality rates decrease with the patient volume of a center, plateauing at about 600 yearly cases (17). The individual operator volume appears to affect complications less conspicuously, but further improvement beyond 75 cases per year can be demonstrated, particularly in high-risk patients (18).

Assistants

At least one person, using sterile garment, is advisable to assist the primary operator with catheter exchanges and manipulations. An additional person has to be on hand to fetch material, tend to the patient, and summon help in case of need. A single physician suffices in general, but an additional physician with advanced resuscitation skills must be available within minutes and a spare angioplasty operator within the hour. The

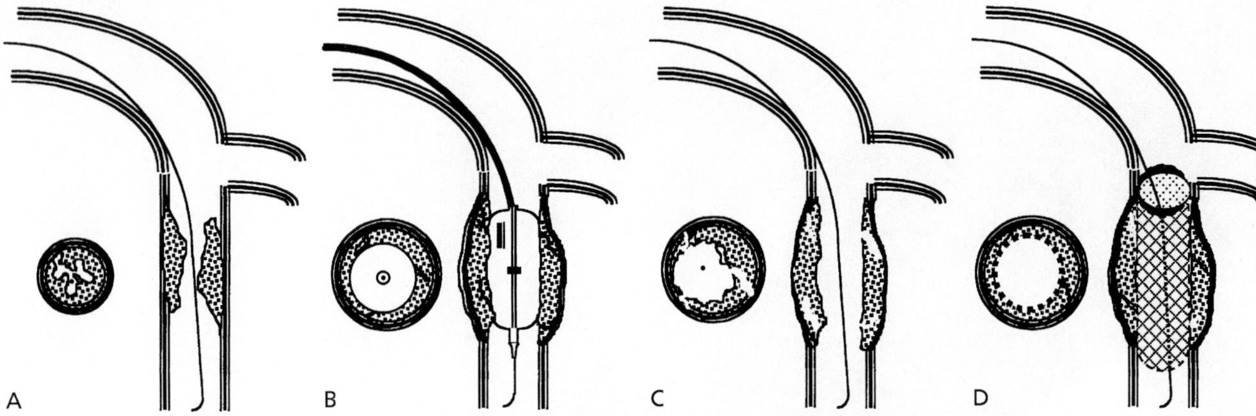

FIGURE 78.2. Schematic diagram of the primary mechanisms of balloon angioplasty and stenting. The initial gain in lumen derives from rearrangement of the noncompressible parts of the plaque made possible by an intimal dissection and vessel dilation (A–C). A stent avoids recoil and tacks tissue flaps and plaque fragments to the wall (D).

unpredictable nature of coronary artery disease in general and of freshly dilated coronary arteries in particular requires on-call 24-hour service.

Surgical Standby

A surgical standby under the same roof is ideal (15,19). However, coronary angioplasty without in-house surgery facilities is a valid option to foster ad hoc procedures and to avoid waiting lists. There are important prerequisites for PCI without in-house surgery capability (15). There should be no local legal objections, and the respective operator should be particularly well trained, the case selection adapted, the patient informed, and the institution fully equipped and staffed for advanced resuscitation and intensive care. A disaster plan with transfer options is warranted.

Material

Table 78.2 lists current standard and optional gear for PCI. Aortic counterpulsation is generally considered mandatory, albeit not helpful in hemodynamic collapse. True percutaneous left ventricular support (20,21) and replacement (20) techniques are more intricate but effective. However, the rare need for them makes their availability reasonable in high-volume centers only.

Radiographic Equipment

Catheterization laboratories have to meet high standards to be fit for interventional cardiology. Biplane fluoroscopy is helpful but less important than digital image enhancement and radiation-thrifty flat panel technology. A spare unit providing angulated fluoroscopy should be available for breakdowns during a critical phase of a case.

The storage medium is digital. Exchange is possible via data lines or various recordable disks. Still-frame hard copies are useful for the hospital chart, the patient, and the referring physician.

Monitoring Equipment

Pressure curves and electrocardiographic (ECG) tracings have to be displayed throughout the case. Pertinent ECG changes

TABLE 78.1

CURRICULUM OF INTERVENTIONAL CARDIOLOGISTS BEFORE AND AFTER INDEPENDENCE

	Minimum	Am Heart Association/ American College of Cardiology Recommendations
General (internal) medicine (y)	2	3
Clinical cardiology (y)	2.5	3
Invasive cardiology (y)	0.5	
Diagnostic catheterization (cases)		
As assistant	50	100
As operator	100	200
Interventional cardiology (y)	1	1
Therapeutic catheterization (percutaneous coronary intervention) (cases)		
As assistant	50	250
As operator	50	
Yearly cases as independent operator	50	75

TABLE 78.2

EQUIPMENT AND DRUGS FOR PERCUTANEOUS CORONARY INTERVENTION (IN 2005)

Standard	Optional
Balloons	Intravascular ultrasound
Guidewires	Angioscopy
Guiding catheters	Flow or pressure wires
Digital x-ray equipment	Atherectomy devices
Stents	Drills, grinders, lysers, softeners
Bare or coated (passive)	Clot catchers, suckers, mashers
Drug-eluting (active)	Laser (debulker catheter or penetration wire)
Covered	Local drug delivery devices
Femoral plugs or sutures	Filter devices
Aortic counterpulsation	Bifurcation stents
Acetylsalicylic acid	Brachytherapy
Thienopyridines	Percutaneous left ventricular assist device
Glycoprotein IIb/IIIa antagonists	Percutaneous cardiopulmonary support
Heparin	Low-molecular-weight heparin or bivalirudin

and symptoms, such as ST-segment alterations, malignant arrhythmia, and chest pain during balloon inflation, should be documented. A device to measure the activated clotting time is welcome but not indispensable.

Balloon Catheter

A modern balloon catheter comes in a variety of diameters and lengths, is sleek, has a slippery coating inside (minimal guidewire friction) and outside, has a low crossing profile and good "trackability" and "pushability," inflates and deflates rapidly, and tolerates pressures up to 30 bar with contained expansion (compliance).

Guiding Catheter

The coronary guiding catheters are derived from diagnostic catheters in terms of shapes and materials. Their walls are thinner but still torque true and kink resistant. Diameters of guiding catheters currently range from 5 to 10 Fr (1.7 to 3.3 mm outer diameter).

Guidewire

The guidewire has to transmit torque reliably from the stiff outside end to the floppy tip. It should provide minimal resistance during advancement but optimal support for the catheters introduced over it. A diameter of 0.014 in (0.36 mm) is standard. Hydrophilic coating reduces friction and guarantees easy advancement, but it harbors the risk of occult perforations of thin-walled healthy peripheral coronary arteries with subsequent hemopericardium. The wire tip may be equipped with a Doppler ultrasound crystal, a pressure transducer, a ball tip, a radiofrequency transmitter, or an optical lens for angioscopic tissue analysis or laser transmission.

Accessories

An adjustable Y connector prevents leaking and permits contrast medium injections and pressure monitoring through a single arterial access after the introduction of the guidewire and the balloon catheter into the guiding catheter. A wire torquer ensures controlled rotation of the wire tip. An indeflator with an incorporated pressure gauge affords effortless inflations (in fact, a misnomer for fillings with diluted contrast medium) and maintains constant negative pressure in the balloon lumen of the catheter while the balloon is not inflated.

Technique

The classic point of access is the right femoral artery. Alternatives are the left femoral artery as well as the radial, brachial, and subclavian arteries. Femoral puncture site closure devices (absorbable plugs, clips, or subcutaneous sutures) have shortened bed rest and have facilitated management of the femoral puncture site without significantly reducing complications, however (22). The radial approach features easy hemostasis and immediate mobilization. Yet it is painstaking, limits the selection of catheters and instruments, and carries a risk of radial artery occlusion (23). This condition is generally symptom free initially but may become relevant later (e.g., occlusion of ulnar artery or need for arterial grafts at subsequent CABG). The brachial and axillary routes harbor a significant risk for injury of the motor nerves of the arm.

It is useful to observe ECG and symptomatic reactions of the patient during balloon occlusions. Marked ST-segment elevation, severe pain, malignant ectopy, or a significant decrease in blood pressure mandates close monitoring after the intervention. Collaterals seen during the diagnostic study or documented by washout collaterometry (prompt washout of contrast medium distal to the balloon, injected and secluded there during the initial phase of balloon inflation) (24) project a low subsequent risk for the patient and allow for abridged and simplified aftercare.

Adjunctive Drug Therapy

Platelet inhibitors have to be administered at the latest at the inception of the procedure (16). Acetylsalicylic acid is standard. Clopidogrel, a thienopyridine, is also advocated, preferably starting a few days before the procedure or with a 600 mg or greater oral loading dose (25,26).

Intravenous direct glycoprotein IIb/IIIa receptor blockers (abciximab, tirofiban, or eptifibatide) have proved efficacious conceptually (27) and in large clinical trials (28–30). Their effect is more marked in truly acute coronary syndromes documented by troponin elevation but is not necessarily superior to that of clopidogrel (31).

Heparin is part of the standard regimen. Doses vary, but they are usually weight adjusted and are assessed by activated clotting times to be increased in lengthy procedures. Low-molecular-weight heparin has been tested in the setting of PCI; it has proved at least as effective as unfractionated heparin, and it causes less propensity to bleeding (32,33). Whether the difference in bleeding also pertains to smaller femoral catheters or to the radial approach remains to be seen.

At least equivalent efficacy and reduced bleeding were documented for the selective factor Xa antagonist fondaparinux, when it was compared with low-molecular-weight heparin in acute coronary syndromes with or without PCI (34). Of the direct thrombin antagonists, bivalirudin has proved equivalent or superior to a combination of unfractionated heparin and a glycoprotein IIb/IIIa receptor blocker in general cohorts (35–37), as well as in patients with diabetes (38) or renal failure (39).

Aftercare

The level of surveillance after the procedure depends on the clinical situation and the result of PCI. ECG monitoring for a few hours is advised but not indispensable for the routine case. Any bleeding from the puncture site is carefully assessed. Manual compression and device compression are first-choice measures. The need for duplex ultrasound examination or surgical repair remains exceptional in experienced centers. Chest pain prompts an immediate ECG for comparison with the baseline tracing. Patients with nonabating chest pain are monitored for arrhythmia and are reinvestigated by catheterization.

Hospital discharge of patients with uncomplicated cases usually occurs the morning after the intervention, but outpatient PCI is feasible in selected cases. A control ECG before discharge should be standard, and cardiac enzymes should be checked in case of problems. Performance of a stress test before discharge is rare, albeit safe (40).

INDICATIONS

The steady increase of yearly PCI cases is mainly the result of an earlier invasive diagnosis of coronary artery disease in addition to a more aggressive attitude with elderly patients regarding referral for coronary angiography. Many patients undergoing PCI today would have been treated medically 2 decades ago without invasive investigation. Triple-vessel disease involving all major arteries has largely remained the domain of CABG. The share of multivessel PCI in a single session has not increased since 1992 in Europe (41) (Fig. 78.3), despite the use of stents.

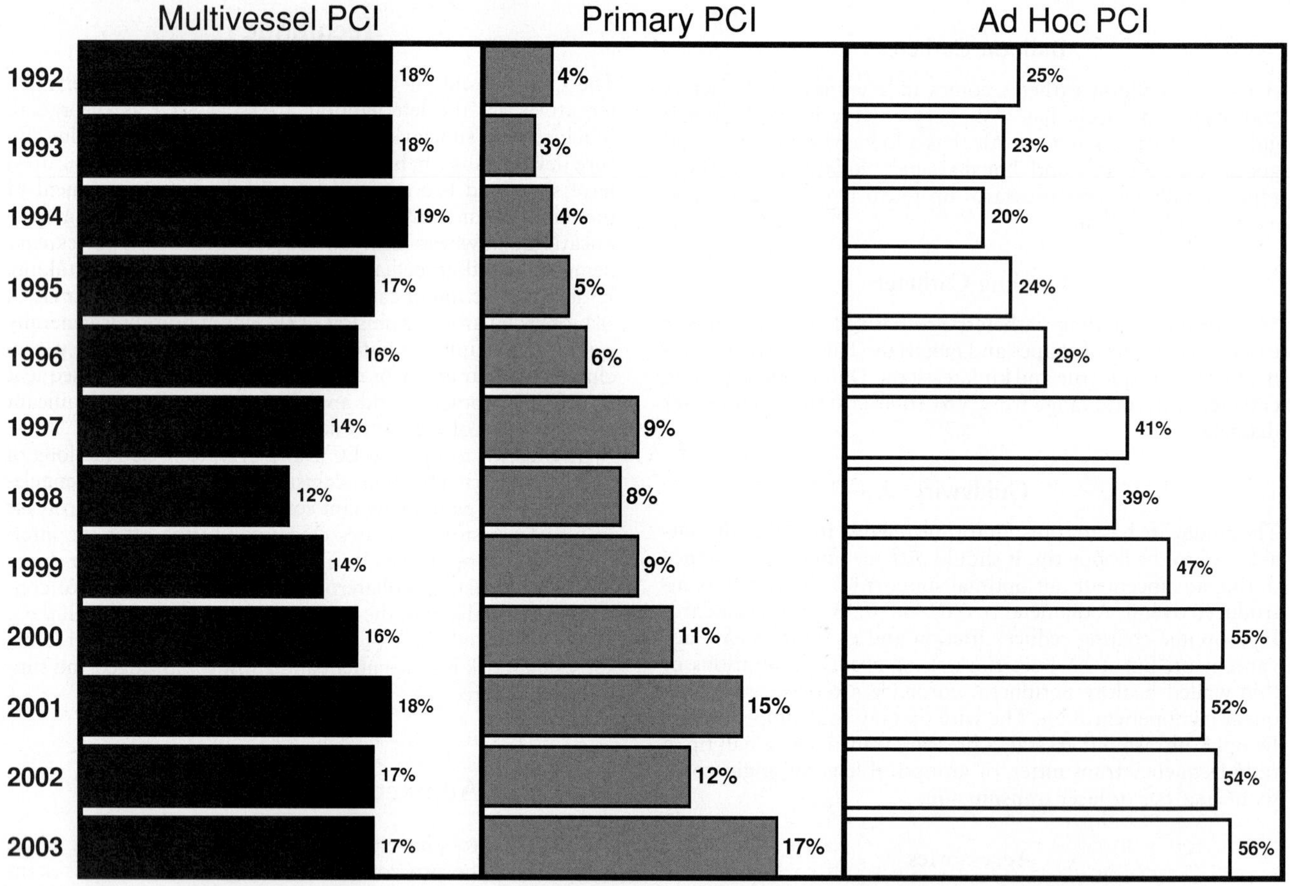

FIGURE 78.3. Percentage of percutaneous coronary intervention (PCI) procedures for more than one major vessel in a session (multivessel PCI, **left**), for acute myocardial infarction (primary PCI, **center**), and performed during the diagnostic session (ad hoc PCI, **right**) in Europe since 1992. Despite the steep increase of stent use during that period, multivessel percutaneous coronary interventions in a single session did not increase. Primary PCI quadrupled and ad hoc PCI doubled during the period. The figures are based on the official registry of the European Society of Cardiology, representing roughly 500,000 procedures per year. Data from reference 41.

TABLE 78.3

CLINICAL INDICATIONS FOR AND CONTRAINDICATIONS TO PERCUTANEOUS CORONARY INTERVENTION

INDICATIONS
- Acute coronary syndrome
  - ST-segment elevation myocardial infarction
  - Non–ST-segment elevation myocardial infarction
- Stable angina pectoris
- Angina equivalent (e.g., arrhythmia, dyspnea, dizziness)
- Multislice computer tomography with unequivocal proximal stenosis
- Objective signs of reversible ischemia
  - Resting electrocardiography
  - Ambulatory electrocardiographic monitoring
  - Stress test
  - Stress echocardiography
  - Myocardial scintigraphy
  - Positron emission tomography
  - (Functional) magnetic resonance imaging

CONTRAINDICATIONS
- Rapidly terminal cardiac or other disease (exception: uncontrollable angina)
- Prolonged cardiogenic shock after myocardial infarction (multiorgan failure)

Clinical Indications

Clinical indications and contraindications are listed in Table 78.3. They have to be customized to patients and situations, and this requires experience. Most patients undergoing coronary angiography meet the criteria. Age is not as important for PCI as it is for CABG. PCI in the elderly is feasible, but its effect is short-lived (42).

Angiographic Indications

Angiographic indications and contraindications are listed in Table 78.4.

Lesion Location and Characteristics

It is important but difficult to determine what makes a lesion significant enough to warrant PCI (43). There are different means to assess the functional significance of a stenosis. Clinical tests (e.g., exercise ECG, stress echocardiography, scintigraphy) are not very sensitive and lack specificity for the individual lesion. Quantitative coronary angiography of the lesion is imprecise almost to the degree of visual estimates (44). Intravascular ultrasound (45), flow velocity (46) or pressure measurements (47), and angioscopy (48) are more objective, but they engender additional costs and risks and have failed to gain widespread acceptance.

To restrict indications to hemodynamically significant lesions may be misguided. The ultimate threat is not the occurrence of angina (affecting only quality of life), but rather the thrombotic occlusion of the vessel, causing infarction and death. Although an individual mild stenosis has a low infarct potential, the hazard is clearly there. Besides, collaterals are rare with mild lesions, a finding that renders their occlusion particularly dangerous. Consequently, restricting PCI to flow-limiting lesions neglects its potential for plaque sealing (i.e., significantly reducing the risk of subsequent thrombotic occlusion thanks to the neoendothelium overgrowing the PCI-inflicted inner wound) (49,50). Such an effect is safely assumed based on the event-free long-term course regularly observed after uncomplicated balloon angioplasty. Restenosis after PCI for mild lesions is rare and is highly unlikely to produce infarction because of the nature of the renarrowing (smooth neoendothelium rather than rupture-prone atherosclerotic plaque). Nonetheless, the hypothesis has not been prospectively validated and may be invalidated by the use of a stent (small but significant risk of late stent thrombosis). Methods to elucidate the vulnerability of a plaque seem called for (Table 78.5) (51,52) but they provide merely a snapshot assessment. A vulnerable plaque means instability and calls for action. A stable plaque is not

TABLE 78.4

ANGIOGRAPHIC INDICATIONS FOR AND CONTRAINDICATIONS TO PERCUTANEOUS CORONARY INTERVENTION

INDICATIONS
- One to four lesions suitable for percutaneous coronary intervention
- Occlusion of any of these lesions of at least 1 minute not deemed life-threatening
- Lesion(s) subtending functional, viable, or collateral-relevant myocardium

CONTRAINDICATIONS
- Left main stem stenosis (exceptions: protected by graft or collaterals, feasible lesions, inoperable patient)
- Left main stem equivalent stenoses (exceptions: staged procedures, feasible lesions, inoperable patient)
- Last remaining vessel (exceptions: feasible lesion, inoperable patient, left ventricular support ready)
- Triple-vessel disease (exceptions: feasible lesions, secondary vessels, staged procedures, inoperable patient)
- Lesion characteristics
  - Chronic total occlusion
    - No collaterals to distal artery
    - Long and old lesion
    - No stump
    - Extensive bridging collaterals
  - Thrombotic stenosis with nonsignificant underlying lesion
  - Diffusely diseased, small-caliber coronary artery
  - Diffusely diseased or occluded old saphenous vein coronary bypass graft

TABLE 78.5

ASSESSMENT OF PLAQUE VULNERABILITY (51,52)

- Intravascular ultrasound
  - Three-dimensional reconstruction
  - Ultrasound elastography (palpography)
  - Intravascular ultrasound flow
  - Virtual histology
- Angioscopy
  - Optical coherence tomography
  - Raman (near infrared) spectroscopy
- Thermography
- Positron emission tomography
- Magnetic resonance imaging
  - Phase contrast imaging
  - Nuclear imaging
  - Intravascular imaging

particularly meaningful because it may become unstable at any time, perhaps even by the touch of the investigational device. Hence, PCI after such assessment will be the rule, rendering the assessment practically moot. Plaque passivation with statins (53) is a proved and ubiquitously applicable alternative or complement to plaque sealing by balloon angioplasty. The latter is attractive solely as an ad hoc procedure for an angiographically detected mild lesion at a strategically important site (proximal in a large vessel), and it remains clinically unproved (54).

Lesions involving branch points are technically not a particular challenge with modern equipment. However, they are fraught with a higher rate of complications and restenoses, even with active stents (55).Thrombus-containing lesions have become less ominous in the current era of stents, glycoprotein IIb/IIIa antagonists, and suction or filter devices.

RESULTS

Stenting

In contrast to the various mechanical additions or alternatives to balloon angioplasty, the stent has stood the test of time (9,56) (Table 78.2). Although stenting introduces minor procedural complications related to negotiating the slightly larger and stiffer stent balloon, it yields an immediately impeccable angiographic result that is appealing to the operator and the patient.

The potential of stenting had initially been underestimated because results were overshadowed by frequent stent thromboses, while stenting was still confined to rescue situations. Adopting elective stenting and the two-pronged antiplatelet regimen (acetylsalicylic acid and thienopyridine) changed that approach. However, subacute stent thrombosis remains a concern. Together with increased periprocedural infarctions resulting from more side branch occlusions and distal embolizations, it forfeits most of the expected advantage compared with balloon angioplasty in terms of the prognostically crucial events of myocardial infarction and death. Figure 78.4 shows that the impact of stenting on these events in the European registry was not as conspicuous as expected (41). An individual report (57) and a metaanalysis (58) of major trials comparing stenting with balloon angioplasty corroborate this finding.

Unconditional stenting curtails the stent benefit to prevention of restenosis. Most of the 2% to 3% of infarctions or lives saved acutely by stenting are lost again by late stent thromboses. Moreover, virtually all the restenosis reduction is already exploited at a stenting rate of roughly 20% (Fig. 78.5) (58). This is plausible considering that before the availability of stents, fewer than 25% of patients needed further intervention

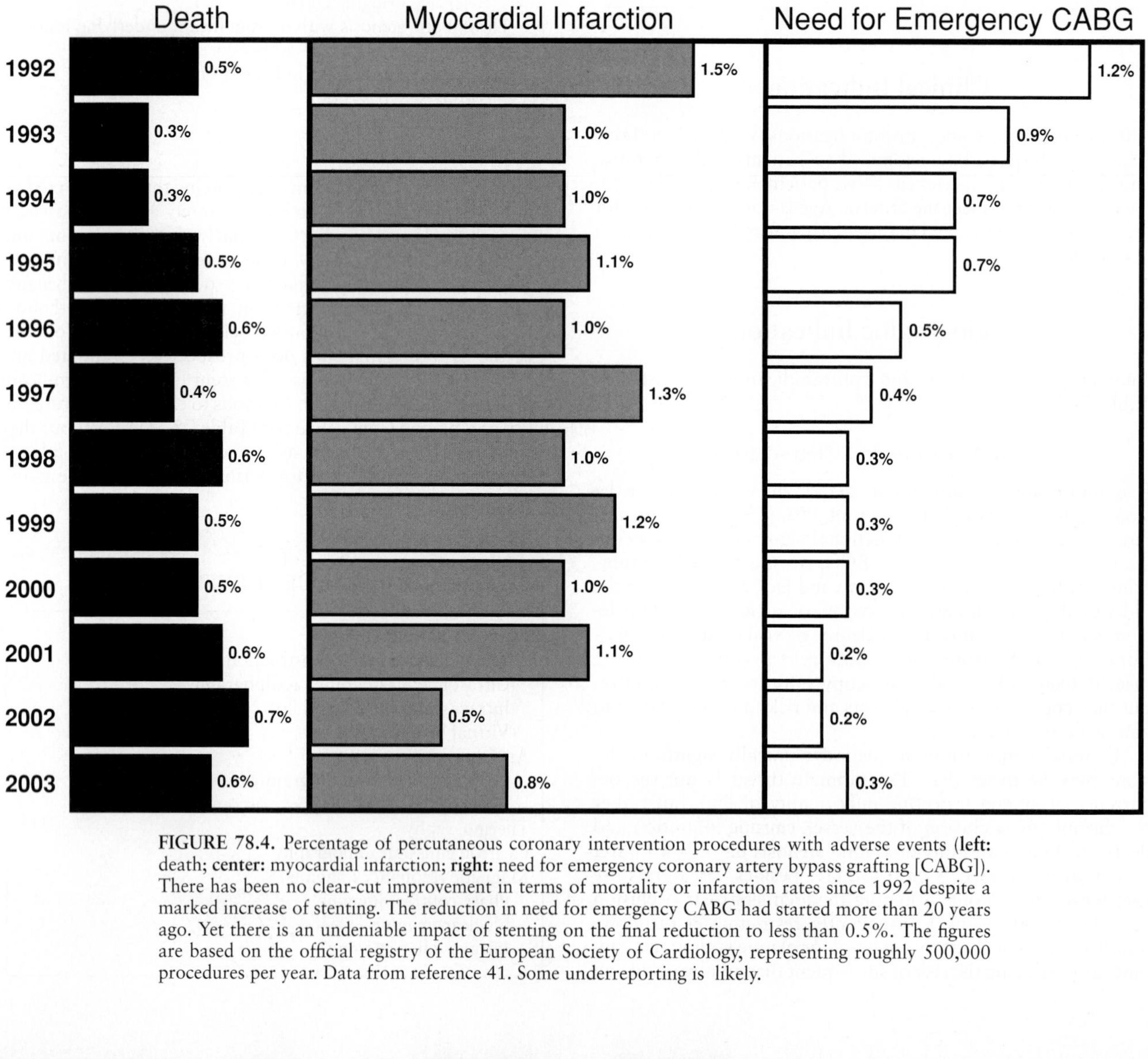

FIGURE 78.4. Percentage of percutaneous coronary intervention procedures with adverse events (**left:** death; **center:** myocardial infarction; **right:** need for emergency coronary artery bypass grafting [CABG]). There has been no clear-cut improvement in terms of mortality or infarction rates since 1992 despite a marked increase of stenting. The reduction in need for emergency CABG had started more than 20 years ago. Yet there is an undeniable impact of stenting on the final reduction to less than 0.5%. The figures are based on the official registry of the European Society of Cardiology, representing roughly 500,000 procedures per year. Data from reference 41. Some underreporting is likely.

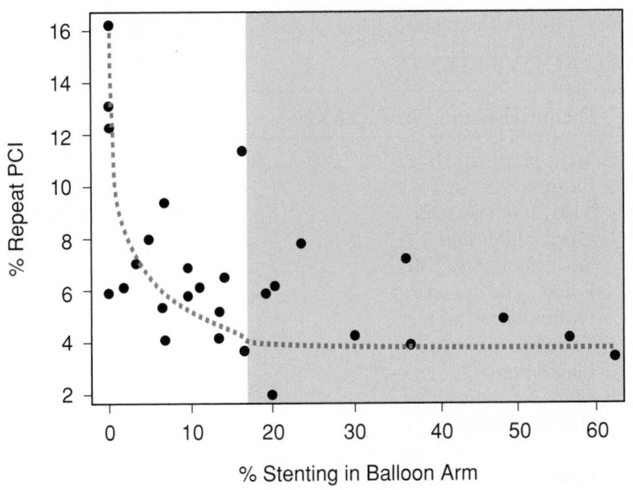

FIGURE 78.5. Metaanalysis of 29 randomized trials comparing stenting with balloon angioplasty in 9,918 patients. The need for repeat percutaneous coronary intervention (PCI) significantly shrinks with the percentage of stented patients. However, the bulk of the benefit is attained already at a stenting rate of 15% to 20%. Higher stenting rates (*gray area*) appear not warranted. Data from reference 58.

resulting from restenosis. From this total, one must deduct patients with restenosis in spite of stenting. Nonetheless, stenting is the current default procedure under the handy pretext that one cannot predict which patients constitute the roughly 20% who will benefit. The risk of acute occlusion in the first hours after balloon angioplasty is practically eliminated by the policy to stent all lesions. Conversely, occlusions are to a certain extent only deferred to the subsequent days or weeks, although they do not necessarily occur in the patients in whom the stent appeared warranted to prevent an occlusion during PCI. Some of these late problems fail to be brought to the attention of the operator. This makes them more dangerous but, paradoxically, falsely enhances the operator's perception of the benefit of stenting.

Drug-Eluting (Active) Stenting

Active stents release a compound luminally into the bloodstream and abluminally into the vessel wall during the initial days or weeks, to curb cell adhesion and proliferation. These stents reduce intimal proliferation (reason for in-stent restenosis) without affecting safety in terms of myocardial infarction or death (59). The initial concern that acute or delayed stent thrombosis could indeed be increased (thrombogenicity of the polymer drug carrier and slowed and incomplete neoendothelialization of the stent) has not materialized thus far, but the final verdict is not in yet. The trend to use more and longer active stents (in-stent restenosis considered a negligible threat) may engender an increase in late stent thromboses, in contrast to what was found as long as the total length of active stents resembled that of bare (passive) stents.

Implanting active or passive stents is technically identical. Hence, physicians and patients alike enthusiastically welcomed active stents. Active stents are about to replace passive stents as the default device, in spite of their increased cost. Some of the expenses (further increased by a globally adopted prolongation of clopidogrel as an adjunct to acetylsalicylic acid) are recompensed by less need for reinterventions. Active stents have been described cost efficient, by computing the hypothetic hospital costs saved by the avoided restenoses (fictitious rather than real savings) against the price differences between active and passive stents (60). Some clinical effects of the subtle disparities (Table 78.6) among the two current market leaders (the only active stents approved by the U.S. Food and Drug Administration in 2005) have been documented. The one eluting sirolimus (a macrolide antibiotic and immunosuppressant agent initially found in the soil on Easter Island) showed an edge in terms of a need for later reintervention over the one eluting paclitaxel (a cytostatic agent initially extracted from the Pacific yew tree) in head-to-head randomized trials (61–63), particularly in high-risk subgroups (63–65). More important, in addition to a higher restenosis probability, there may be more risk for late stent thrombosis with the paclitaxel-eluting stent (55,62,66,67).

Table 78.7 shows a nonexhaustive list of modifications of and improvements in stenting. Some have been introduced into clinical practice, some are already discarded, and some are being evaluated. A critical need exists for clinical (preferably randomized) trials to determine the ideal stent, even without considering to take full advantage of combining technologies and compounds.

Complications

The threat of a major acute complication is most relevant for the patient and haunts the operator more than the possibility of disease recurrence, but it is talked about less.

Mortality

In-hospital mortality after PCI ranges from virtually naught in young patients with single-vessel disease to more than 50% in older patients with cardiogenic shock after myocardial infarction. Overall, it lies at less than 2% and has remained stable even during the period of general adoption of stenting (Fig. 78.4) (41). Mortality reduction was achieved in randomized studies with PCI compared with fibrinolysis in acute infarction (68), even when interhospital transfer was necessary (68,69), and in younger patients with cardiogenic shock compared with conventional therapy (70,71).

Myocardial Infarction

The incidence of PCI-induced myocardial infarction varies widely according to definitions used. Yet it has remained fairly stable over time (Fig. 78.4) (41). Elevation of cardiac enzymes after PCI with active stents may be as high as 5% to 10% (72). The clinical significance of this finding remains controversial.

Side branch occlusions constitute the most prominent reason for creatine kinase elevations in otherwise successful procedures. Stents increase the incidence of this condition (73). Microemboli may also contribute, and this complication is partially preventable by the use of abciximab or a similar drug (74).

No-(Re)Flow Phenomenon

The no-(re)flow phenomenon (75) presumably originates from proximally released vasoactive substances or microembolizations producing spasm and occlusion of small intramyocardial vessels. It may be quite refractory to vasodilators and even glycoprotein IIb/IIIa antagonists and is more germane to stenting than to balloon angioplasty.

Coronary Perforation or Rupture

Coronary perforation at the site of the lesion with a guidewire may often go unnoticed, especially during recanalization attempts of chronic total occlusions. It is innocuous unless the perforation is enlarged by the balloon catheter. Distal

TABLE 78.6

CHARACTERISTICS OF THE TWO APPROVED ACTIVE STENTS

Sirolimus-Eluting Stent (Cypher)	Paclitaxel-Eluting Stent (TAXUS)
Stent platform	Stent platform
Bx Velocity	Express 2
316L stainless steel	316L stainless steel
Closed cell design	Open cell design
Strut thickness: 140 μm	Strut thickness: 130 μm
Polymer drug carrier	Polymer drug carrier
Nonbiodegradable	Nonbiodegradable
PEVA and PBMA	Translute
Elastomeric	Elastomeric
Topcoat design	Matrix design
Faster release ($t_{1/2} = 8$ days)	Slower release
Drug	**Drug**
Sirolimus	Paclitaxel
Dose density: 140 μg/cm^2	Dose density: 100 μg/cm^2
Biologic effect	Biologic effect
High affinity for intracellular FKBP12	High affinity β-tubulin binding
Upregulation of cyclin-dependent kinase p27Kip1	Stabilization of tubulin polymerization
Cell-cycle arrest at G1/S phase	Cell cycle arrest at G2/M phase
Wide therapeutic ratio: >7 times (dose-density)	Narrower therapeutic ratio: <4 times (dose-density)
Physicochemical properties	**Physicochemical properties**
Lipophilic	Lipophilic
Solubility ~6 μg/mL	Solubility ~6 μg/mL
Molecular mass 914 Da	Molecular mass <1 kDa
Protein binding characteristics	Protein binding characteristics
FKBP12 concentration in smooth muscle cells (10 to 5 M)	Microtubule concentration in arterial wall (10^{-5} M)
Distributes evenly through the artery	Remains primarily subintimal

TABLE 78.7

MODIFICATIONS OF STENTING TO REDUCE RESTENOSIS FURTHER

Reduce arterial injury	Passive stent coating	Active stent coating
Technique	Metals	Drugs
Primary stent implantation	Stainless steel	Abciximab
Stent design	(Gold)[a]	(Actinomycin D)
Strut configuration	Nitinol	(Angiopeptin)
Strut thickness	Tantalum	Batimastat
Stent geometry	Ceramics	C-*myc* antisense
Absorbable stent	Silicon-carbide	Dexamethasone
Stent surface modifications	Titanium-nitride-oxide	Estradiol
Electrochemical polishing	Biomimicry	Everolimus
Thermal processing	Phosphorylcholine	Heparin
	Fibrin	Hirudin
	Polymers	Iloprost
	>20 compounds	Methotrexate
	Durable	NO donors
	Biodegradable	Paclitaxel
		Sirolimus
		Statins
		Tacrolimus
		Zotarolimus (ABT-578)

[a]Parentheses indicate that the approach is no longer pursued.

perforations with novel hydrophilic guidewires represent a new hazard. They occur silently and perhaps repeatedly while balloons or stents are being introduced when the operator is not paying sufficient attention to the wire tip (often outside the field of vision). The tendency of these perforations to seal spontaneously is low because the walls of normal peripheral vessels are thin.

Coronary rupture by subintimal or oversized balloon inflation or debulking devices is a rare but serious complication with a mortality of approximately 10% (76). Coronary ruptures can be acutely plugged with a balloon inflation. This may permanently cover the defect with a tissue flap and solve the problem. Implantation of a (covered) stent at the ruptured site and sacrifice of the vessel by embolization or exclusion (covered stent in vessel of origin at bifurcation) are further options short of surgery (77). Cardiac tamponade is first treated by pericardiocentesis. The aspirated blood may be reinjected into a vein to avoid significant blood loss.

Results with Special Indications

Elderly Patients

Older patients are constituting a growing group of candidates for any medical intervention in light of the general aging of industrialized peoples. Coronary artery disease affects 20% of geriatric patients and is the reason for approximately 25% of their morbidity and more than 50% of their mortality (78).

Elderly patients should be spared CABG because of increased operative morbidity and mortality. Conversely, these patients typically have diffuse disease and are difficult to catheterize. Their PCI results are less favorable than those of younger PCI patients. The early results seem to be better than those with CABG. Yet geriatric patients undergoing CABG fare better during follow-up in spite of having been sicker initially (79). Compared with medical treatment, PCI showed some symptomatic advantage but no survival benefit (42).

Diabetic Patients

Diabetic patients experience increased risks with virtually any major intervention. Their propensity for complications and recurrences after PCI has been highlighted (Fig. 78.6) (80,81). The outcome with CABG has proved better than that with PCI in diabetic patients (82,83). The 7-year mortality of treated diabetic patients in the Bypass Angioplasty Revascularization Investigation trial was 44% with PCI and 24% with CABG (82). Mortality in nondiabetic patients was approximately 14% with both therapies. More brittle plaques, higher blood viscosity, enhanced platelet aggregation, increased thromboxane A_2 levels, endothelial dysfunction, and impaired endogenous fibrinolysis likely account for the problems diabetic patients have with PCI (83). Some factors explaining the high recurrence are depicted

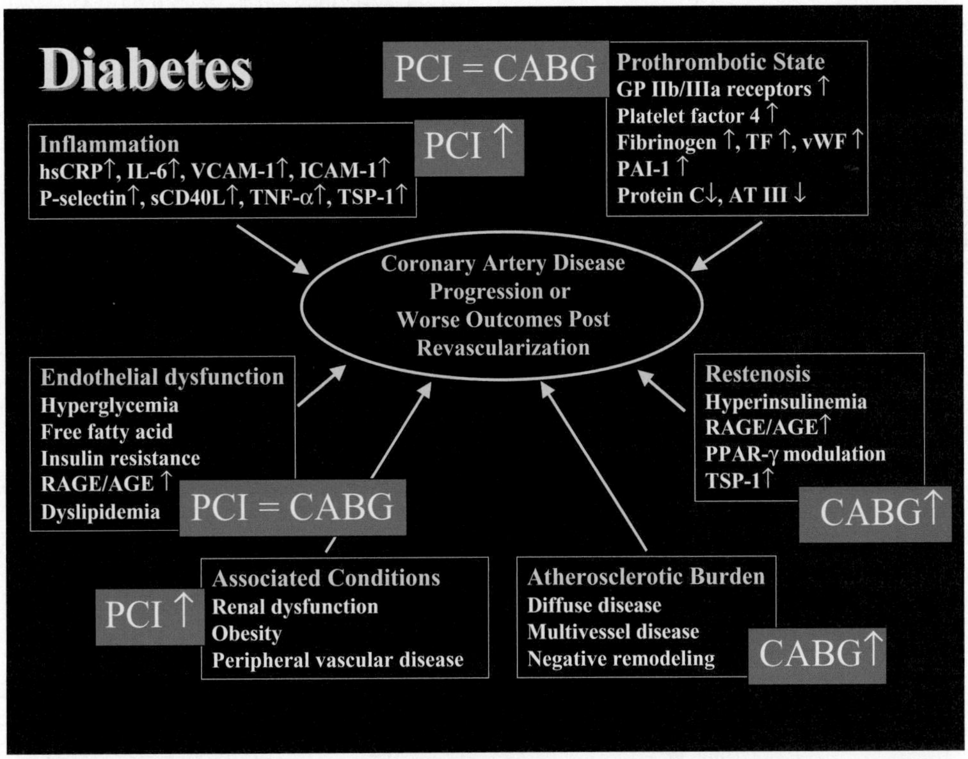

FIGURE 78.6. Diabetes mellitus and its influence on coronary revascularization procedures. The various factors have an impact both on percutaneous coronary intervention (PCI) and on coronary artery bypass grafting (CABG), some less on PCI (PCI↑) and some less on CABG (CABG↑). Overall, the factors favoring CABG prevail. AGE, advanced glycosylation end product; AT III, antithrombin III; GP IIb/IIIa, glycoprotein IIb/IIIa; hsCRP, high sensitivity C-reactive protein; ICAM-1, intercellular adhesion molecule-1; IL-6, interleukin-6; PAI-1, plasminogen activator inhibitor-1; PPAR-γ, peroxisome proliferator-activated receptor-γ; RAGE, receptors for AGE; TF, tissue factor; TNF-α, tumor necrosis factor-α; TSP-1, thrombospondin-1; VCAM-1, vascular cell adhesion molecule-1; vWF, von Willebrand factor. (Modified from reference 81.)

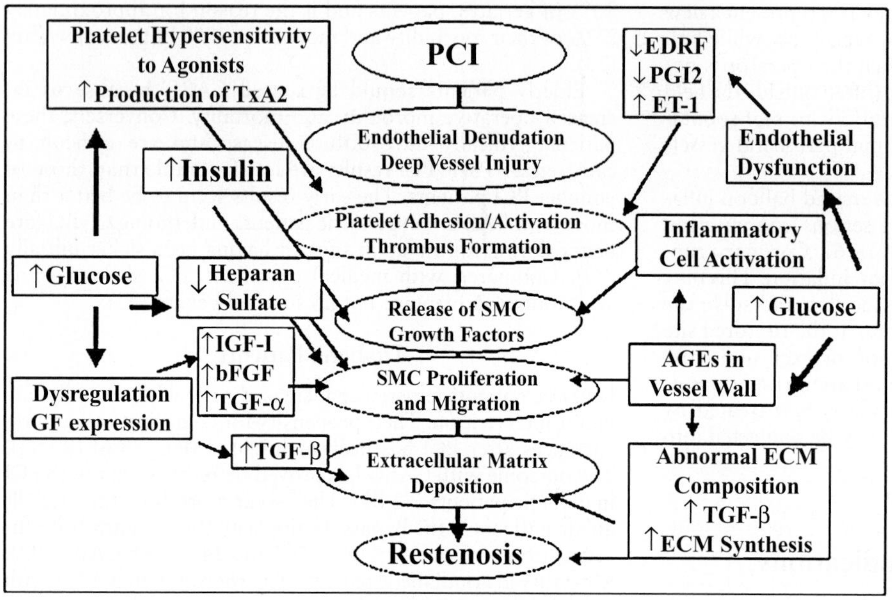

FIGURE 78.7. Mechanisms for (re-) stenosis formation in diabetes. AGEs, advanced glycosylation end products; bFGF, basic fibroblast growth factor; ECM, extracellular matrix; EDRF, endothelium-derived relaxing factor; ET-1, endothelin-1; GF, growth factor; IGF-I, insulin-like growth factor-I; PGI_2, prostacyclin; SMC, smooth muscle cell; TGF-α, transforming growth factor-α; TGF-β, transforming growth factor-β; TxA2, thromboxane A_2. (Modified from reference 84.)

in Figure 78.7 (84). Many are favorably influenced by stents and novel anticoagulant and antiaggregant compounds. Abciximab yields results in stented diabetic patients comparable with those of nondiabetic patients in terms of mortality, lumen at follow-up, or reinterventions (29).

Acute Coronary Syndromes

Non–ST-Segment Elevation Acute Coronary Syndrome. Non–ST-segment elevation acute coronary syndrome includes unstable angina and small (peripheral) infarctions and is characterized by transient ST-segment depression or troponin elevation. It hints at the vulnerability or severity of the culprit lesion, but it does not reliably inform about the extent of coronary artery disease. PCI is the preferred treatment with a long-term survival benefit over conservative therapy (85,86). This advantage is apparent in the long term only, because of intervention-induced early problems (Fig. 78.8) (86,87). Postponing PCI carries the risk of an intercurrent infarction while increasing the cost of treatment (88,89).

PCI of the unstable plaque (fissured atheroma with partial thrombosis) engenders more acute occlusions than routine PCI. The stent and new antiaggregant or antithrombotic agents mitigate this condition (28,36–39,74,90). Pretreatment with abciximab (28,36,74), eptifibatide (28,36,91), bivalirudin (28,36–39), or a combination thereof (92) is recommended before stenting. The value of tirofiban is controversial. It seemed to avoid the initial disadvantage of PCI (29) but partially failed in a randomized trial with a background of acetylsalicylic acid and clopidogrel (92). So did abciximab (31).

Acute Myocardial Infarction

Ongoing infarction is the most pressing and rewarding indication for PCI. Mortality is beneficially influenced when compared with fibrinolysis (68,69,93). Although coronary flow may be restored somewhat later with direct PCI than with fibrinolysis, particularly if the latter is initiated already at home (94) or aided by the dethrombotic effect of a glycoprotein IIb/IIIa antagonist (95–97), reperfusion is more complete and the underlying stenosis has simultaneously been treated (Fig. 78.9). This appears particularly instrumental in diabetic patients (98). PCI facilitated by a bolus of clopidogrel (99) or a glycoprotein IIb/IIIa antagonist appears as the ideal approach. The preliminary use of a fibrinolytic agent remains controversial (100).

PCI for acute myocardial infarction is an exception in many respects. It dictates an ad hoc procedure and, for most operators, is restricted to the culprit vessel in multivessel disease. Although it carries a higher overall complication rate than elective PCI, it has a smaller potential to harm. The major complication of PCI, abrupt closure of the lesion, is relatively innocuous when one starts with an occluded vessel.

There are data warranting stenting for all patients who undergo PCI for infarction (101). Although acute results are not improved (102), reinterventions are reduced (Fig. 78.9), and longevity is enhanced (101,102). However, the stent increases

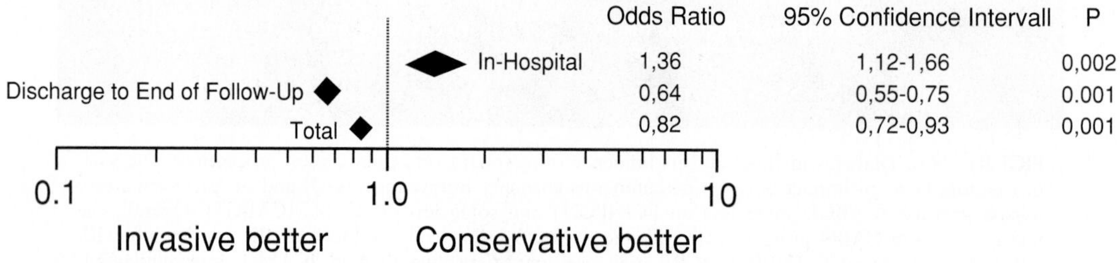

FIGURE 78.8. Odds ratios for major adverse cardiac events comparing percutaneous coronary intervention (PCI) with conservative treatment for acute coronary syndromes without ST-segment elevation. The in-hospital disadvantage of PCI is more than compensated for during follow-up after discharge in a metaanalysis of respective trials. Data from reference 86.

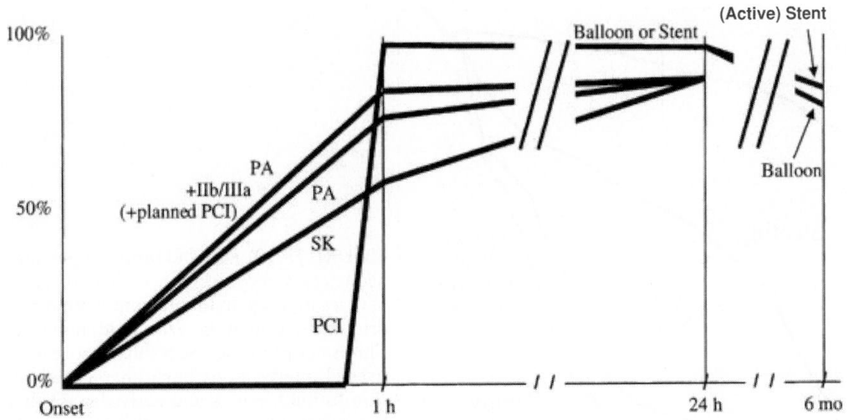

FIGURE 78.9. Percentage of normal coronary flow over time with primary percutaneous coronary intervention (PCI) or (facilitated) systemic fibrinolysis for treatment of acute myocardial infarction. The goal is to teach the highest percentage as far to the left as possible and to preserve it. Up to 1 hour, the combination of a plasminogen activator (PA) with a glycoprotein IIb/IIIa antagonist (IIb/IIIa) is preferable to PA alone or to streptokinase (SK). Meanwhile, immediate percutaneous coronary intervention should be readied. The (active) stent is superior to the balloon only during follow-up with the full benefit apparent at 6 months.

no-reflow problems, which are not preventable by current filter devices (103,104), and side branch occlusions. Both damage the myocardium; a later restenosis does not. An experienced interventional cardiologist should know to select cases not to stent (good result with crisp flow after balloon dilatation). Direct stenting is not attractive, because the extent of the lesion cannot be anticipated in totally occluded arteries typically encountered in acute myocardial infarctions.

PCI for cardiogenic shock is warranted unless the shock is too advanced or too longstanding or the patient is old (70,71). A percutaneous left ventricular assist device such as the TandemHeart may aid these patients as a bridge to recovery or cardiac transplantation (20). However, a high intrinsic complication rate annihilated a survival benefit in a randomized trial (105).

PCI should be done acutely for myocardial infarction if it can be performed within 2 hours. Otherwise (or perhaps in case of any delay), modern fibrinolysis, preferably supported by a glycoprotein IIb/IIIa antagonist, should be initiated, and PCI treatment should be appended if needed and as early as feasible. It is of note and often ignored that only sizable infarctions (greater than or equal to three ECG leads with ST-segment elevation) qualify for fibrinolysis or PCI (106).

Poor Left Ventricular Function

PCI can be performed in patients with any degree of left ventricular function. A swift introduction of the equipment and a short dilatation are tolerated by all patients even without the use of aortic counterpulsation or left ventricular assist devices. In case of problems, however, the possibility of PCI to sustain life in patients with severely compromised left ventricular function is more limited than with CABG. Therefore, markedly reduced left ventricular function tends to favor CABG as a revascularization method. Nevertheless, PCI is a valid option in inoperable cases or when only one discrete lesion is at stake, as well as when lesions are attempted in the hope of revitalizing nonfunctional myocardium. Some operators favor the prophylactic insertion of the intraaortic balloon pump, but supportive randomized data are lacking. Percutaneously insertable left ventricular assist devices requiring an oxygenator have been supplanted by simplified approaches harvesting oxygenated blood from the left atrium (TandemHeart) (20) or the left ventricle (Impella) (21).

CONTROVERSIES AND PERSONAL PERSPECTIVES

Several issues of PCI cannot be solved based on evidence and remain highly conjectural and thus controversial. They have to be seen in the light of variable geographic, economic, temperamental, and philosophical backgrounds and are also subject to change as medicine and societies evolve. It is difficult to deal with such topics in a way applicable to all situations, everywhere, and at any time.

The question of where PCI should be performed and by whom has been iteratively and hotly debated. A high-volume operator working at a high-volume institution, backed up by a high-volume cardiac surgical program, is the ideal setting. However, this means that the population with coronary artery disease will have to converge at a few megacenters to receive PCI under scientifically optimal circumstances. Approximately 1 center for 2 million people will suffice. It will perform between 2,000 and 4,000 PCIs per year with 5 to 10 primary operators. The operators will not be assisted by nonexperienced physicians because those would decrease quality while learning the trade. They would also dilute the high-volume scenario. Interventional cardiologists would be trained exclusively to replace retiring operators and to meet the growing demand for procedures.

But will the patients like that? Many of them prefer to receive treatment at their local hospital by their familiar cardiologist. There, they can find their way around. There, they know people, and people come to visit. Most patients do not care so much about the theoretic variance in the quality of PCI. First, they are unable to grasp the subtle differences, and, second, most PCI results are good, even with low-volume teams. Referring physicians like to deal with angioplasty operators they know personally, rather than sending their patients to an anonymous superinstitution. Smaller communities can use the business, too. Restriction of interventional facilities to distant PCI "hubs" hurts their economy and keeps away investors and settlers from their communities.

When respected authorities issue guidelines or when governments set regulations, they should honor these facts to a reasonable degree. It seems unwise to set limits that "outlaw" a substantial number of current operators. It is unlikely that they will abandon their practice and thereby jeopardize their professional existence. Nevertheless, guidelines should be clear regarding what is preferable, and reasonable minimal standards must be defined and followed (Table 78.1).

Indications for PCI are another topic in which science and the "real world" diverge. Data show that the risk of coronary lesions is related to the extent of ischemia they produce. Scientifically, one could deduce that it is unethical to dilate lesions for which objective proof of ischemia or at least hemodynamic significance is lacking. Yet this disregards the benefit of PCI for patients with a lesion that at the time of an "objectively unwarranted" PCI was not significant in terms of ischemia but that would have caused a lethal infarction if treated conservatively while evidence-based patients and doctors would have

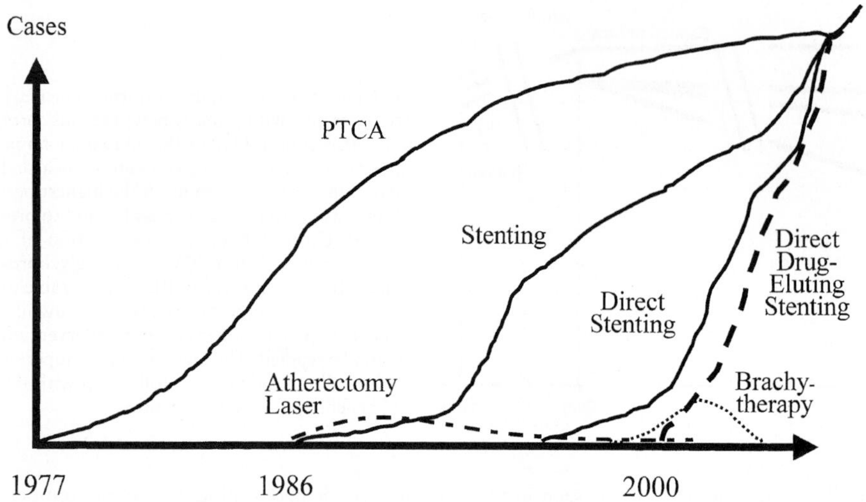

FIGURE 78.10. Past and future of percutaneous coronary intervention. The increase in cases may regain momentum, with direct drug-eluting stenting gaining dominance. This is not primarily the result of more multivessel interventions but rather of expansion to mild lesions and early disease that become more prevalent with time and improved screening for coronary artery disease in its early stage. PTCA, percutaneous transluminal coronary angioplasty.

been standing by for the lesions to attain hemodynamic significance.

Admittedly, it is currently impossible to predict these exceptions, but it is equally impossible to predict with accuracy which lesions will adhere to the rules. Intuitively, it is customary in many centers around the globe to include the eventuality of an unanticipated spontaneous occlusion of the lesion when a PCI indication is considered. An approach requiring costly assessment of the functional significance of the stenosis or the vulnerability of the plaque (Table 78.5) is difficult to enforce and may not benefit patients overall.

THE FUTURE

PCI is bound to remain a dominant asset of health care. It engenders abundant medical literature, occupies a significant segment of medical education programs, and is a remarkable economic factor. The European PCI market was assessed at 560 billion dollars in 2003 and is projected at 650 billion dollars for 2009, amounting for half of the total cardiology market. For global estimates, the multiplication factor 4 can be applied. On the bright side, these gigantic expenditures encompass tax revenue and create income, jobs, and career opportunities for countless people. Most important, PCI unequivocally benefits the well-being and perhaps even the longevity of the middle-aged and older generations of industrialized countries.

Figure 78.10 reflects the past and the future of case load and technical aspects of PCI. Stenting has been the rule for a while now, and active stents will be the rule before long. The approach will be direct active stenting to save time, spare the predilatation balloon, and reduce the restenosis risk to a minimum. New gimmicks will come and go as before, but the balloon-mounted active stent will reign.

The immediate future of PCI is bright despite some recent evidence casting doubt on its justification in multivessel disease (107) or its primacy in stable early coronary artery disease (108) and non–ST-elevation acute coronary syndrome (87). Longevity is an important aspect, but so is quality of life. If improved survival were the benchmark for all medical interventions, then orthopedic surgeons, ophthalmologists, and dentists, to name just a few, would be deprived of virtually all their indications. To rid a patient, by means of a 30-minute intervention using local anesthesia, of limiting and worrisome anginal symptoms (maybe even permanently) is quite an achievement, even if the particular ailment was unlikely to be lethal any time soon with conservative treatment.

The future of PCI is bright because coronary artery disease will remain the number 1 health problem of industrialized countries for quite some time and will become increasingly prevalent in the rest of the world. Improving technologies will expand the role of PCI for this disease, especially for its early, and perhaps for its very late, stages. The disease is increasingly discovered and documented at an early stage, and the general aging of the population creates a growing need for PCI at that end of the spectrum.

Conversely, economic constraints continue to frustrate those capable and willing to perform the procedure. Quality assurance activities take up more and more of the time of the interventional cardiologist. Finally, primary prevention will succeed in drastically reducing the need for PCI in middle age, thus stripping it of its coveted role as the most important intervention in modern medicine for people in their "best years." Then again, what can possibly be wrong with that?

References

1. Dotter CT, Judkins MP. Transluminal treatment of arteriosclerotic obstruction: description of a new technic and a preliminary report of its application. *Circulation* 1964;3:654–670.
2. Gruentzig A. Die perkutane Rekanalisation chronischer arterieller Verschlüsse (Dotter-Prinzip) mit einem neuen doppellumigen Dilatationskatheter. *Fortschr Rontgenstr* 1976;124:80–86.
3. King III SB. Angioplasty from bench to bedside to bench. *Circulation* 1996;93:1621–1629.
4. Hurst JW. The first coronary angioplasty as described by Andreas Gruentzig. *Am J Cardiol* 1986;57:185–186.
5. Meier B. The first patient to undergo coronary angioplasty: 23-year follow-up. *N Engl J Med* 2001;344:144–145.
6. Meier B, Bachmann D, Luscher T. 25 years of coronary angioplasty: almost a fairy tale. *Lancet* 2003;361:527.
7. Gruentzig AR. Transluminal dilatation of coronary-artery stenosis. *Lancet* 1978;1:263.
8. Gruentzig AR, Senning Å, Siegenthaler WE. Nonoperative dilatation of coronary-artery stenosis: percutaneous transluminal coronary angioplasty. *N Engl J Med* 1979;301:61–68.
9. Puel J, Joffre F, Rousseau H, et al. Endo-prothèses coronariennes autoexpansives dans la prévention des resténoses après angioplastie transluminale. *Arch Mal Coeur* 1987;8:1311–1312.
10. Farb A, Virmani R, Atkinson JB, et al. Plaque morphology and pathologic changes in arteries from patients dying after coronary balloon angioplasty. *J Am Coll Cardiol* 1990;16:1421–1429.
11. Mintz GS, Popma JJ, Pichard AD. Arterial remodeling after coronary angioplasty: a serial intravascular ultrasound study. *Circulation* 1996;94:35–43.
12. Hirshfeld Jr, JW, Ellis SG, Faxon DP. Recommendations for the assessment and maintenance of proficiency in coronary interventional procedures: statement of the American College of Cardiology. *J Am Coll Cardiol* 1998;31:722–743.
13. Hirshfeld Jr, JW, Banas Jr, JS Brundage BH, et al. American College of Cardiology training statement on recommendations for the structure of an

optimal adult interventional cardiology training program: a report of the American College of Cardiology task force on clinical expert consensus documents. *J Am Coll Cardiol* 1999;34:2141–2147.
14. Scanlon PJ, Faxon DP, Audet AM, et al. ACC/AHA guidelines for coronary angiography: a report of the American College of Cardiology/American Heart Association Task Force on practice guidelines (Committee on Coronary Angiography) developed in collaboration with the Society for Cardiac Angiography and Interventions. *J Am Coll Cardiol* 1999;33:1756–1824.
15. Smith Jr, SC Dove JT, Jacobs AK, et al. ACC/AHA guidelines of percutaneous coronary interventions (revision of the 1993 PTCA guidelines)—executive summary: a report of the American College of Cardiology/American Heart Association Task Force on Practice Guidelines (committee to revise the 1993 guidelines for percutaneous transluminal coronary angioplasty). *J Am Coll Cardiol* 2001;37:2215–2239.
16. Silber S, Albertsson P, Aviles FF, et al. Guidelines for percutaneous coronary interventions: the Task Force for Percutaneous Coronary Interventions of the European Society of Cardiology. *Eur Heart J* 2005;26:804–847.
17. Hannan EL, Wu C, Walford G, et al. Volume-outcome relationships for percutaneous coronary interventions in the stent era. *Circulation* 2005; 112:1171–1179.
18. Moscucci M, Share D, Smith D, et al. Relationship between operator volume and adverse outcome in contemporary percutaneous coronary intervention practice: an analysis of a quality-controlled multicenter percutaneous coronary intervention clinical database. *J Am Coll Cardiol* 2005;46:625–632.
19. Meier B. Surgical standby for percutaneous intervention. In: Topol EJ, ed. *Textbook of interventional cardiology,* 4th ed. Philadelphia: Saunders Elsevier Science, 2003:475–479.
20. Thiele H, Lauer B, Hambrecht R, et al. Reversal of cardiogenic shock by percutaneous left atrial-to-femoral arterial bypass assistance. *Circulation* 2001;104:2917–2922.
21. Lemos PA, Cummins P, Lee CH, et al. Usefulness of percutaneous left ventricular assistance to support high-risk percutaneous coronary interventions. *Am J Cardiol* 2003;91:479–481.
22. Lasic Z, Nikolsky E, Kesanakurthy S, et al. Vascular closure devices: a review of their use after invasive procedures. *Am J Cardiovasc Drugs* 2005; 5:185–200.
23. Agostoni P, Biondi-Zoccai GG, de Benedictis ML, et al. Radial versus femoral approach for percutaneous coronary diagnostic and interventional procedures: systematic overview and meta-analysis of randomized trials. *J Am Coll Cardiol* 2004;44:349–356.
24. Seiler C, Billinger M, Fleisch M, et al. Washout collaterometry, a new method of assessing collaterals using angiographic contrast clearance during coronary occlusion. *Heart* 2001;86:540–546.
25. Gurbel PA, Bliden KP, Hayes KM, et al. The relation of dosing to clopidogrel responsiveness and the incidence of high post-treatment platelet aggregation in patients undergoing coronary stenting. *J Am Coll Cardiol* 2005;45:1392–1396.
26. Patti G, Colonna G, Pasceri V, et al. Randomized trial of high loading dose of clopidogrel for reduction of periprocedural myocardial infarction in patients undergoing coronary intervention: results from the ARMYDA-2 (Antiplatelet therapy for Reduction of MYocardial Damage during Angioplasty) study. *Circulation* 2005;111:2099–2106.
27. Gurbel PA, Bliden KP, Zaman KA, et al. Clopidogrel loading with eptifibatide to arrest the reactivity of platelets: results of the Clopidogrel Loading With Eptifibatide to Arrest the Reactivity of Platelets (CLEAR PLATELETS) study. *Circulation* 2005;111:1153–1159.
28. Bhatt DL, Topol EJ. Current role of platelet glycoprotein IIb/IIIa inhibitors in acute coronary syndromes. *JAMA* 2000;284:1549–1558.
29. Cannon CP, Weintraub WS, Demopoulos LA, et al. Comparison of early invasive and conservative strategies in patients with unstable coronary syndromes treated with the glycoprotein IIb/IIIa inhibitor tirofiban. *N Engl J Med* 2001;344:1879–1887.
30. Peterson ED, Pollack Jr, CV, Roe MT, et al. Early use of glycoprotein IIb/IIIa inhibitors in non-ST-elevation acute myocardial infarction: observations from the National Registry of Myocardial Infarction 4. *J Am Coll Cardiol* 2003;42:45–53.
31. Kastrati A, Mehilli J, Schuhlen H, et al. A clinical trial of abciximab in elective percutaneous coronary intervention after pretreatment with clopidogrel. *N Engl J Med* 2004;350:232–238.
32. Borentain M, Montalescot G, Bouzamondo A, et al. Low-molecular-weight heparin vs. unfractionated heparin in percutaneous coronary intervention: a combined analysis. *Cathet Cardiovasc Interv* 2005;65:212–221.
33. Ebrahimi R, Lincoff AM, Bittl JA, et al. Bibalirudin vs heparin in percutaneous coronary intervention: a pooled analysis. *J Cardiovasc Pharmacol Ther,* 2005;10:209–216.
34. MICHELANGELO OASIS 5 Steering Committee. Design and rationale of the MICHELANGELO Organization to assess strategies in acute ischemic syndromes (OASIS-5) trial program evaluating fondaparinux, a synthetic factor Xa inhibitor, in patients with non-ST-segment elevation acute coronary syndromes. *Am Heart J.* 2005;150:1107.
35. Lincoff AM, Bittl JA, Harrington RA, et al. Bivalirudin and provisional glycoprotein IIb/IIIa blockade compared with heparin and planned glycoprotein IIb/IIIa blockade during percutaneous coronary intervention: REPLACE-2 randomized trial. *JAMA* 2003;289:853–863.
36. Kong DF, Hasselblad V, Harrington RA, et al. Meta-analysis of survival with platelet glycoprotein IIb/IIIa antagonists for percutaneous coronary interventions. *Am J Cardiol* 2003;92:651–655.
37. Lincoff AM, Kleiman NS, Kereiakes DJ, et al. Long-term efficacy of bivalirudin and provisional glycoprotein IIb/IIIa blockade vs heparin and planned glycoprotein IIb/IIIa blockade during percutaneous coronary revascularization: REPLACE-2 randomized trial. *JAMA* 2004;292:696–703.
38. Gurm HS, Sarembock IJ, Kereiakes DJ, et al. Use of bivalirudin during percutaneous coronary intervention in patients with diabetes mellitus: an analysis from the randomized evaluation in percutaneous coronary intervention linking Angiomax to reduced clinical events (REPLACE)-2 trial. *J Am Coll Cardiol* 2005;45:1932–1938.
39. Chew DP, Lincoff AM, Gurm H, et al. Bivalirudin versus heparin and glycoprotein IIb/IIIa inhibition among patients with renal impairment undergoing percutaneous coronary intervention (a subanalysis of the REPLACE-2 trial). *Am J Cardiol* 2005;95:581–585.
40. Roffi M, Wenaweser P, Windecker S, et al. Early exercise after coronary stenting is safe. *J Am Coll Cardiol* 2003;42:1569–1573.
41. Cook S, Togni M, Walpoth N, et al. Percutaneous Coronary Interventions in Europe 1992–2003. *Euro Inter* 2006;1:374–379.
42. Pfisterer M. Long-term outcome in elderly patients with chronic angina managed invasively versus by optimized medical therapy: four-year follow-up of the randomized Trial of Invasive versus Medical therapy in Elderly patients (TIME). *Circulation* 2004;110:1213–1218.
43. Kern MJ, Meier B. Evaluation of the culprit plaque and the physiological significance of coronary atherosclerotic narrowings. *Circulation* 2001; 103:3142–3149.
44. Faxon DP, Vogel R, W. Y, et al. Value of visual versus central quantitative measurements of angiographic success after percutaneous transluminal coronary angioplasty. *Am J Cardiol* 1996;77:1067–1072.
45. Nissen SE. Application of intravascular ultrasound to characterize coronary artery disease and assess the progression or regression of atherosclerosis. *Am J Cardiol* 2002;89:24B–31B.
46. Meuwissen M, Siebes M, Chamuleau SA, et al. Intracoronary pressure and flow velocity for hemodynamic evaluation of coronary stenoses. *Expert Rev Cardiovasc Ther* 2003;1:471–479.
47. Pijls NH. Optimum guidance of complex PCI by coronary pressure measurement. *Heart* 2004;90:1085–1093.
48. Emanuelsson H. Future challenges to coronary angioplasty: perspectives on intracoronary imaging and physiology. *J Intern Med* 1995;238:111–119.
49. Meier B, Ramamurthy S. Plaque sealing by coronary angioplasty. *Cathet Cardiovasc Diagn* 1995;36:295–297.
50. Weissberg PL, Clesham GJ, Bennett MR. Is vascular smooth muscle cell proliferation beneficial? *Lancet* 1996;347:305–307.
51. Naghavi M, Libby P, Falk E, et al. From vulnerable plaque to vulnerable patient: a call for new definitions and risk assessment strategies: part I. *Circulation* 2003;108:1664–1672.
52. Naghavi M, Libby P, Falk E, et al. From vulnerable plaque to vulnerable patient: a call for new definitions and risk assessment strategies: part II. *Circulation* 2003;108:1772–1778.
53. Bittl JA. Advances in coronary angioplasty. *N Engl J Med* 1996;335:1290–1302.
54. Berger A, Botman KJ, MacCarthy PA et al. Long-term clinical outcome after fractional flow reserve-guided percutaneous coronary intervention in patients with multivessel disease. *Journal of the American College of Cardiology* 2005;46:438–442.
55. Stone GW, Ellis SG, Cannon L, et al. Comparison of a polymer-based paclitaxel-eluting stent with a bare metal stent in patients with complex coronary artery disease: a randomized controlled trial. *JAMA* 2005;294: 1215–1223.
56. Meier B. New devices for coronary angioplasty: the emperor's new clothes revisited. *Am J Med* 1995;98:429–431.
57. Kiemeneij F, Serruys PW, Macaya C, et al. Continued benefit of coronary stenting versus balloon angioplasty: five-year clinical follow-up of Benestent-I trial. *J Am Coll Cardiol* 2001;37:1598–1603.
58. Brophy JM, Belisle P, Joseph L. Evidence for use of coronary stents: a hierarchical bayesian meta-analysis. *Ann Intern Med* 2003;138:777–786.
59. Babapulle MN, Joseph L, Belisle P, et al. A hierarchical bayesian meta-analysis of randomised clinical trials of drug-eluting stents. *Lancet* 2004; 364:583–591.
60. Kaiser C, Brunner-La Rocca HP, Buser PT, et al. Incremental cost-effectiveness of drug-eluting stents compared with a third-generation bare-metal stent in a real-world setting: randomised Basel Stent Kosten Effektivitats Trial (BASKET). *Lancet* 2005;366:921–929.
61. Windecker S, Remondino A, Eberli FR, et al. Sirolimus versus paclitaxel eluting stents for coronary revascularization. *N Engl J Med* 2005;353;653–662.
62. Morice MC, Colombo A, Meier B, et al. Sirolimus- vs paclitaxel-eluting stents in de novo coronary artery lesions: the REALITY trial: a randomized controlled trial. *JAMA.* 2006;295:895–904.
63. Kastrati A, Dibra A, Eberle S, et al. Sirolimus-eluting stents vs paclitaxel-eluting stents in patients with coronary artery disease: meta-analysis of randomized trials. *JAMA* 2005;294:819–825.
64. Kastrati A, Mehilli J, von Beckerath N, et al. Sirolimus-eluting stent or paclitaxel-eluting stent vs balloon angioplasty for prevention of recurrences

in patients with coronary in-stent restenosis: a randomized controlled trial. *JAMA* 2005;293:165–171.
65. Dibra A, Kastrati A, Mehilli J, et al. Paclitaxel-eluting or sirolimus-eluting stents to prevent restenosis in diabetic patients. *N Engl J Med* 2005;353: 663–670.
66. Iakovou I, Schmidt T, Bonizzoni E, et al. Incidence, predictors, and outcome of thrombosis after successful implantation of drug-eluting stents. *JAMA* 2005;293:2126–2130.
67. Bavry A. *Eur Heart J* 2006 (in press).
68. Keeley EC, Boura JA, Grines CL. Primary angioplasty versus intravenous thrombolytic therapy for acute myocardial infarction: a quantitative review of 23 randomised trials. *Lancet* 2003;361:13–20.
69. Zijlstra F. Angioplasty vs thrombolysis for acute myocardial infarction: a quantitative overview of the effects of interhospital transportation. *Eur Heart J* 2003;24:21–23.
70. Hochman JS, Sleeper LA, White HD, et al. One-year survival following early revascularization for cardiogenic shock. *JAMA* 2001;285:190–192.
71. White HD, Assmann SF, Sanborn TA, et al. Comparison of percutaneous coronary intervention and coronary artery bypass grafting after acute myocardial infarction complicated by cardiogenic shock: results from the Should We Emergently Revascularize Occluded Coronaries for Cardiogenic Shock (SHOCK) trial. *Circulation* 2005;112:1992–2001.
72. Moses JW. Head-to-head, complex DES trials highlight ACC '05. *J Interv Cardiol* 2005;18:299–302.
73. Aliabadi D, Tilli FV, Bowers TR, et al. Incidence and angiographic predictors of side branch occlusion following high-pressure intracoronary stenting. *Am J Cardiol* 1997;80:994–997.
74. Topol EJ, Mark DB, Lincoff AM, et al. Outcomes at 1 year and economic implications of platelet glycoprotein IIb/IIIa blockade in patients undergoing coronary stenting: results from a multicentre randomised trial. *Lancet* 1999;354:2019–2024.
75. Baim DS, Carrozza JP, Jr. Understanding the no-reflow problem. *Cathet Cardiovasc Diagn* 1996;39:7–8.
76. Ajluni SC, Glazier S, Blankenship L, et al. Perforations after percutaneous coronary interventions: clinical, angiographic, and therapeutic observations. *Cathet Cardiovasc Diagn* 1994;32:206–212.
77. Dorros G, Jain A, Kumar K. Management of coronary artery rupture: covered stent or microcoil embolization. *Cathet Cardiovasc Diagn* 1995;36: 148–154; discussion 155.
78. Simons LA. Epidemiologic considerations in cardiovascular diseases in the elderly: international comparisons and trends. *Am J Cardiol* 1989;63:5H–8H.
79. O'Keefe Jr, JH, Sutton MB, McCallister BD, et al. Coronary angioplasty versus bypass surgery in patients >70 years old matched for ventricular function. *J Am Coll Cardiol* 1994;24:425–430.
80. Kip KE, Faxon DP, Detre KM, et al. Coronary angioplasty in diabetic patients: the National Heart, Lung, and Blood Institute Percutaneous Transluminal Coronary Angioplasty Registry. *Circulation* 1996;94:1818–1825.
81. Roffi M, Topol EJ. Percutaneous coronary intervention in diabetic patients with non–ST-segment elevation acute coronary syndromes. *Eur Heart J* 2004; 25:190–198.
82. BARI Investigators. Seven-year outcome in the Bypass Angioplasty Revascularization Investigation (BARI) by treatment and diabetic status. *J Am Coll Cardiol* 2000;35:1122–1129.
83. Weintraub WS, Stein B, Kosinski A, et al. Outcome of coronary bypass surgery versus coronary angioplasty in diabetic patients with multivessel coronary artery disease. *J Am Coll Cardiol* 1998;31:10–19.
84. Aronson D, Bloomgarden Z, Rayfield EJ. Potential mechanisms promoting restenosis in diabetic patients. *J Am Coll Cardiol* 1996;27:528–535.
85. Fox KA, Poole-Wilson P, Clayton TC, et al. 5-year outcome of an interventional strategy in non–ST-elevation acute coronary syndrome: the British Heart Foundation RITA 3 randomised trial. *Lancet* 2005;366:914–920.
86. Mehta SR, Cannon CP, Fox KA, et al. Routine vs selective invasive strategies in patients with acute coronary syndromes: a collaborative meta-analysis of randomized trials. *JAMA* 2005;293:2908–2917.
87. de Winter RJ, Windhausen F, Cornel JH, et al. Early invasive versus selectively invasive management for acute coronary syndromes. *N Engl J Med* 2005;353:1095–1104.
88. Wallentin L, Lagerqvist B, Husted S, et al. Outcome at 1 year after an invasive compared with a non-invasive strategy in unstable coronary-artery disease: the FRISC II invasive randomised trial. FRISC II Investigators. Fast Revascularisation during Instability in Coronary artery disease. *Lancet* 2000;356:9–16.
89. Neumann FJ, Kastrati A, Pogatsa-Murray G, et al. Evaluation of prolonged antithrombotic pretreatment ("cooling-off" strategy) before intervention in patients with unstable coronary syndromes: a randomized controlled trial. *Jama* 2003;290:1593–1599.
90. Lincoff AM, Kleiman NS, Kottke-Marchant K, et al. Bivalirudin with planned or provisional abciximab versus low-dose heparin and abciximab during percutaneous coronary revascularization: results of the Comparison of Abciximab Complications with Hirulog for Ischemic Events Trial (CACHET). *Am Heart J* 2002;143:847–853.
91. ESPRIT Investigators. Enhanced Suppression of the Platelet IIb/IIIa Receptor with Integrilin Therapy. *Lancet* 2000;356:2037–2044.
92. Rasoul S. Elisa II, ESC, Stockholm, Sweden, 2005.
93. Cannon CP. Primary percutaneous coronary intervention for all? *JAMA* 2002;287:1987–1989.
94. Bonnefoy E, Lapostolle F, Leizorovicz A, et al. Primary angioplasty versus prehospital fibrinolysis in acute myocardial infarction: a randomised study. *Lancet* 2002;360:825–829.
95. Antman EM, Gibson CM, de Lemos JA, et al. Combination reperfusion therapy with abciximab and reduced dose reteplase: results from TIMI 14. *Eur Heart J* 2000;21:1944–1953.
96. Herrmann HC, Moliterno DJ, Ohman EM, et al. Facilitation of early percutaneous coronary intervention after reteplase with or without abciximab in acute myocardial infarction: results from the SPEED (GUSTO-4 Pilot) Trial. *J Am Coll Cardiol* 2000;36:1489–1496.
97. Campbell KR, Ohman EM, Cantor W, et al. The use of glycoprotein IIb/IIIa inhibitor therapy in acute ST-segment elevation myocardial infarction: current practice and future trends. *Am J Cardiol* 2000;85:32C–38C.
98. Bonnefoy E, Steg PG, Chabaud S, et al. Is primary angioplasty more effective than prehospital fibrinolysis in diabetics with acute myocardial infarction? Data from the CAPTIM randomized clinical trial. *Eur Heart J* 2005;26:1712–1718.
99. Sabatine MS, Cannon CP, Gibson CM, et al. Addition of clopidogrel to aspirin and fibrinolytic therapy for myocardial infarction with ST-segment elevation. *N Engl J Med* 2005;352:1179–1189.
100. Assessment of the Safety and Efficacy of a New Treatment Strategy with Percutaneous Coronary Intervention (ASSENT-4 PI) Investigators. Primary versus tenecteplase-facilitated percutaneous coronary intervention in patients with ST-segment elevation acute myocardial infarction (ASSENT-4 PCI): randomized trial. *Lancet* 2006;367:543–546.
101. Mehta RH, Harjai KJ, Cox DA, et al. Comparison of coronary stenting versus conventional balloon angioplasty on five-year mortality in patients with acute myocardial infarction undergoing primary percutaneous coronary intervention. *Am J Cardiol* 2005;96:901–906.
102. Stone GW, Grines CL, Cox DA, et al. Comparison of angioplasty with stenting, with or without abciximab, in acute myocardial infarction. *N Engl J Med* 2002;346:957–966.
103. Stone GW, Webb J, Cox DA, et al. Distal microcirculatory protection during percutaneous coronary intervention in acute ST-segment elevation myocardial infarction: a randomized controlled trial. *JAMA* 2005;293:1063–1072.
104. Gick M, Jander N, Bestehorn HP, et al. Randomized evaluation of the effects of filter-based distal protection on myocardial perfusion and infarct size after primary percutaneous catheter intervention in myocardial infarction with and without ST-segment elevation. *Circulation* 2005;112:1462–1469.
105. Thiele H, Sick P, Boudriot E, et al. Randomized comparison of intra-aortic balloon support with a percutaneous left ventricular assist device in patients with revascularized acute myocardial infarction complicated by cardiogenic shock. *Eur Heart J* 2005;26:1276–1283.
106. Holmvang L, Clemmensen P, Lindahl B, et al. Quantitative analysis of the admission electrocardiogram identifies patients with unstable coronary artery disease who benefit the most from early invasive treatment. *J Am Coll Cardiol* 2003;41:905–915.
107. Hannan EL, Racz MJ, Walford G, et al. Long-term outcomes of coronary-artery bypass grafting versus stent implantation. *N Engl J Med* 2005;352: 2174–2183.
108. Katritsis DG, Ioannidis JP. Percutaneous coronary intervention versus conservative therapy in nonacute coronary artery disease: a meta-analysis. *Circulation* 2005;111:2906–2912.

CHAPTER 79 ■ PERCUTANEOUS CARDIAC PROCEDURES

SAMIR R. KAPADIA AND E. MURAT TUZCU

OVERVIEW

Interventional cardiology is evolving rapidly not only to treat coronary disease but also to provide treatment options for various structural heart diseases. These include percutaneous treatment of the valvular heart diseases, atrial appendage occlusion, and treatment of congenital heart diseases. Interventional cardiologists whose patients are adults are involved with increasing frequency in treating atrial septal defect, patent foramen ovale (PFO), and ventricular septal defects.

Many exciting developments in recent years have opened up novel percutaneous avenues to treat valvular heart disease. Balloon dilatation to treat valvular stenosis has been used for many years and has been proven effective for the treatment of pulmonary stenosis (1), mitral stenosis (2), and some cases of aortic stenosis (AS) (3,4). Valvuloplasty is covered in Chapter 82. Until recently, the major limitations of percutaneous valve treatments were the lack of sustained benefit of aortic valvuloplasty and the inability to treat valvular regurgitation. In the last decade, numerous percutaneous devices have been developed for valvular heart disease through close collaboration of interventional cardiologists, cardiothoracic surgeons, and imaging specialists. Percutaneous valve prostheses have been designed for AS and pulmonary regurgitation. Many ingenious approaches that have been engineered for percutaneous repair of mitral regurgitation (MR) are under investigation. These developments have generated a phenomenal amount of interest, both in the scientific community and in the general public. Given the tremendous potential of these techniques in eliminating the need for conventional cardiothoracic surgery and its associated risks—particularly in high-risk patients—and in the treatment of patients who are currently not surgical candidates, the excitement and enthusiasm generated are understandable. In this chapter, we review the devices and approaches that are being investigated for valve treatment, PFO closure, and atrial appendage occlusion.

AORTIC VALVE REPLACEMENT

Scope of the Problem

AS is currently the most common acquired valvular disease in the industrialized nations. With the decline in rheumatic valvular disease, calcific bicuspid and senile degenerative calcific tricuspid valve diseases have emerged as the dominant causes of AS (5). The consequence of prolonged life expectancy in Western countries is a substantial increase in the number of patients surviving to develop senile calcific AS. For adult patients with severe AS, aortic valve replacement (AVR) has been the therapy of choice for more than 3 decades. Such therapy offers dramatic symptomatic relief and improved long-term survival when compared with medical therapy alone (6–8). Even though patients undergoing AVR are progressively older and less fit, clinical outcomes following AVR using contemporary surgical techniques and bioprostheses are generally good, with perioperative mortality rates of 2% to 7% (7,9–11). However, high-risk subgroups have been identified, including patients with associated coronary artery disease, higher New York Heart Association functional classifications, impaired left ventricular systolic dysfunction, and advanced age, as well as those undergoing emergency surgery. Based on the presence of one or more of these high-risk features, a significant subset of patients with severe AS is deemed ineligible for AVR (12–14).

Initial Experiments

In 1986, separate groups in France (15) and the United States (16) reported the feasibility of percutaneous balloon aortic valvuloplasty for the treatment of high-risk patients with severe AS. Valvuloplasty improves the valve area by multiple mechanisms including the fracture of valvular nodular calcification, separation of fused commissures, and plastic deformation of the rigid valve cusps (16–18). Although short-term hemodynamic results are acceptable, albeit modest, long-term clinical follow-up following percutaneous balloon aortic valvuloplasty remains disappointing, with near 100% restenosis of the aortic valve at 2 years (3,4,19,20). For this reason, the procedure is now largely restricted to use as a temporizing bridge to surgical AVR and rarely as a palliative treatment for patients with severe symptomatic AS in whom surgery is contraindicated.

The potential for percutaneous AVR was first realized in 1989, when Andersen and colleagues in Aarhus, Denmark, constructed a prosthetic aortic valve that could be successfully implanted in vivo using a transluminal catheter technique (21). The valve was constructed by suturing a dissected porcine aortic valve to a rudimentary stainless steel stent. This stent-valve was then compressed onto a carrier balloon catheter. Because the intention was to seek a percutaneous treatment for aortic regurgitation, these investigators tested the effect of placing the prostheses in both the native subcoronary position and the supracoronary position (i.e., ascending aorta), given that successful positioning in either location would be effective for the treatment of aortic regurgitation. In the initial animal (pig) studies, the large profile of the valve prosthesis necessitated delivery through the suprarenal aorta. The valve was then passed in retrograde fashion to the ascending aorta (i.e., supracoronary location) and aortic valve (subcoronary location) and was deployed by inflation and subsequent deflation of the carrier balloon catheter. Although the valves were successfully deployed, a major issue with the subcoronary position was the propensity of the prosthesis to occlude the origin of the coronary arteries. Compounding this issue was the to-and-fro movement of the carrier balloon during inflation, which made precise positioning of the stent-valve difficult.

Pavcnik and colleagues demonstrated in 1992 that a percutaneous transcatheter placement of an artificial caged-ball valve in animals is feasible, whereas Maozami and coworkers showed in 1996 that a hemodynamically acceptable prosthetic aortic valve for transluminal placement is feasible in an open chest model. Bonhoeffer and coworkers in 2000 successfully performed a percutaneous pulmonary valve implantation in five sheep. Although implantation in the descending aorta was successful, placement in the native position failed because of coronary obstruction, interference with the mitral valve, or migration. These problems were resolved with an orientation device. Sheep anatomy is such that the distance between the mitral valve and the coronary ostia is only a few millimeters, an important limitation of this model.

Cribier-Edwards Aortic Percutaneous Heart Valve (Edwards Lifesciences, Irvine, CA)

Building on these fundamental experiments, Cribier and his colleagues in Rouen, France, developed a percutaneous heart valve (PHV, Percutaneous Valve Technologies, Inc., Fort Lee, NJ) for the treatment of AS. Following animal testing in sheep (22), and ex vivo valve durability testing, the first human implantation of their PHV was performed in April 2002 and published in December 2002 (23). The initial valve was composed of three leaflets of bovine pericardium sutured to a 14-mm long stainless steel balloon expandable stent. This stent length was specifically chosen based on postmortem assessments in human subjects of the distance between the aortic annulus and both the coronary ostia and anterior mitral leaflet, which could both be impinged by the prosthesis. The stent-valve was mounted on a 30-mm long balloon valvuloplasty catheter (Z-Med II, NuMED, Inc., Hopkinton, NY) that could expand to a diameter of 23 mm. A crimping tool was used to compress the stent-valve symmetrically onto the balloon delivery catheter.

The critical elements of the technique employed by Cribier and his colleagues were as follows (Fig. 79.1) (24). The compressed stent-valve/balloon catheter assembly required a 24-Fr (8-mm) sheath for delivery. For this reason, and to facilitate accurate positioning of the PHV, Cribier and colleagues initially used an antegrade approach for delivery of the PHV. Using femoral venous access, a transseptal puncture was performed, and an 8-Fr Mullins sheath was positioned in the left atrium. A balloon-tipped catheter was then passed through the Mullins sheath and advanced across the mitral valve into the left ventricular outflow tract. Through the lumen of the balloon-tipped catheter, a straight wire was then used to cross the stenosed aortic valve. The deflated balloon-tipped catheter was then advanced across the aortic valve, reinflated, and passed into the descending aorta. A 360-cm long stiff wire was then advanced through the balloon-tipped catheter, grasped by a snare introduced from the femoral artery, and subsequently externalized. Delivery of the PHV was facilitated by dilating the interatrial septum and subsequently dilating the aortic valve with a valvuloplasty balloon (using an antegrade approach). The PHV-balloon assembly was then introduced through the venous access across the interatrial septum and the mitral valve and was finally positioned at the native aortic valve using valvular calcification as a marker. At this stage of the procedure, it was imperative to maintain a large loop of wire in the left ventricle between the mitral and aortic valves, because traction on the anterior mitral leaflet could result in severe MR and hemodynamic collapse. Rapid maximal inflation, deflation, and removal of the balloon were then performed to deploy the valvular prosthesis.

Subsequent to this first reported case description, the procedural and clinical outcomes of this patient and five others were reported in February 2004 (25). Equine pericardial valves were used in the PHV of these subsequent procedures. Some modifications to the original technique were also noted. For example, rapid right ventricular cardiac pacing (200 to 220 beats per minute) was used to decrease aortic blood flow at the time of PHV deployment, thus reducing the risk of migration of the prosthesis into the ascending aorta. In addition, the operators advanced a Sones catheter from the femoral artery access site that abutted the distal end of the delivery balloon catheter, a technique that further limited the tendency for anterograde migration of the PHV during deployment. The device was successfully deployed in five of the six patients. In the unsuccessful case, the PHV-balloon assembly migrated into the ascending aorta at the time of balloon inflation, resulting in hemodynamic collapse and death during the procedure. Among the successful procedures, the hemodynamic results were impressive, with almost complete elimination of the aortic gradient and achievement of an aortic valve area larger than 1.6 cm^2. Aortic regurgitation increased by one grade in four of the five successful procedures. In such cases, the aortic regurgitation was paravalvular in location (i.e., between the stent frame of the PHV and the native diseased aortic valve). Importantly, the coronary ostia were not compromised by the prosthesis in any of these patients.

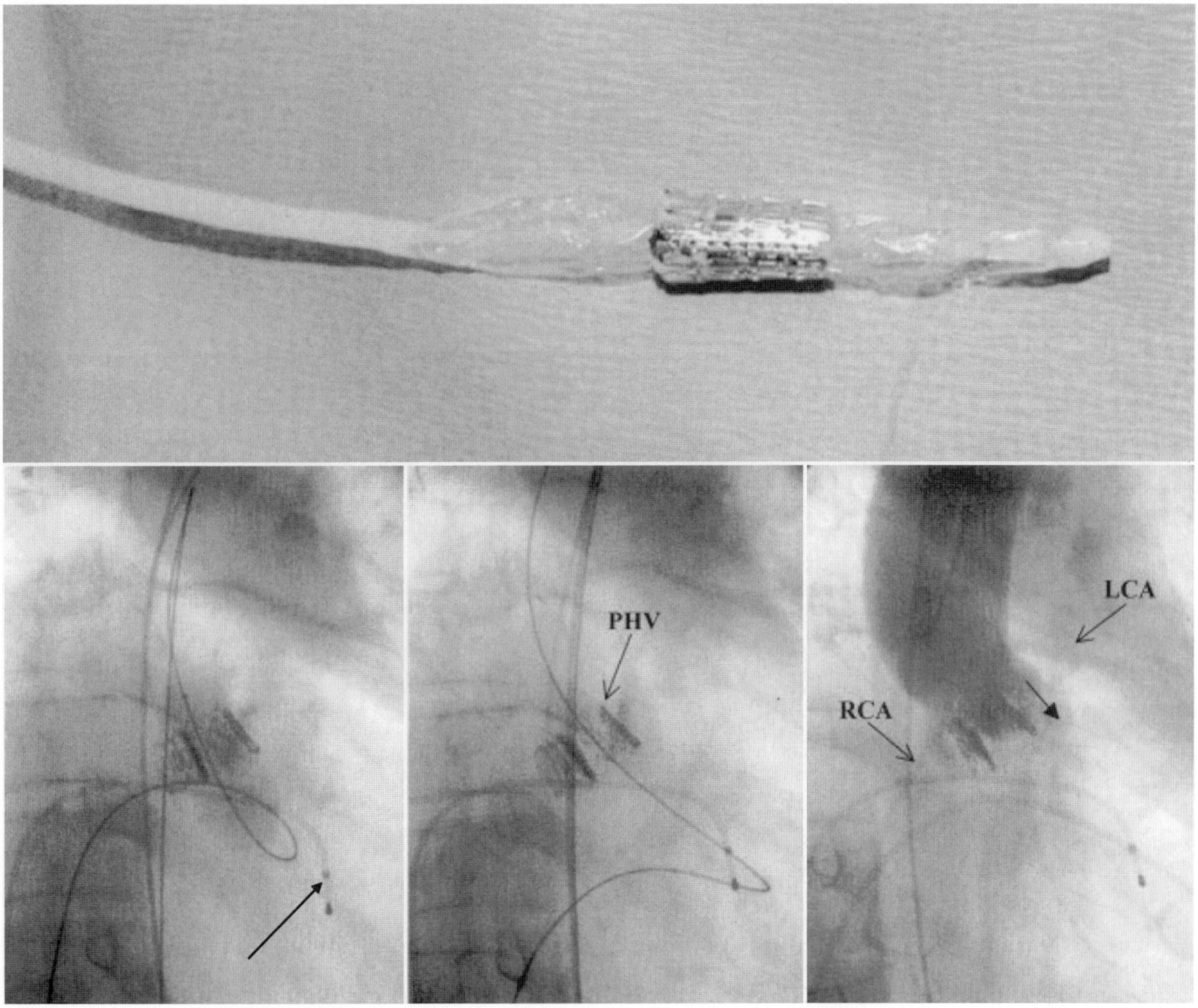

FIGURE 79.1. **Top:** An aortic valve in the stent that is mounted on the balloon. **Lower left:** The pacing wire in the left ventricle (*black arrow*) with the inflated balloon that is deploying the stent containing the aortic valve. The catheter is advanced from the inferior vena cava via the transseptal approach in an antegrade fashion. **Middle:** A well-deployed aortic valve. **Right:** Unobstructed coronary arteries and no aortic regurgitation. LCA, left coronary artery; PHV, percutaneous heart valve; RCA, right coronary artery. (Modified from Cribier A, Eltchaninoff H, Bash A, et al. Percutaneous transcatheter implantation of an aortic valve prosthesis for calcific aortic stenosis: first human case description. *Circulation* 2002;106:3006–3008.)

The longer-term clinical follow-up in this series must be interpreted with an understanding of the patient population studied. All patients had severe AS with multiple comorbidities and were deemed ineligible for surgical AVR by two independent surgeons. Most were elderly (mean age, 75 ± 12 years), and three were in cardiogenic shock. Three of the five patients who underwent successful PHV implantation died of noncardiac complications at 2, 4, and 18 weeks, whereas the remaining two patients were alive and free of heart failure at 8-week follow-up. In follow-up echocardiographic studies, the initial reduction in aortic gradient and the increase in aortic valve area were maintained, and there was a significant recovery in left ventricular systolic function.

Based on this preliminary series and on subsequent unpublished reports, the future of percutaneous AVR for the treatment of AS appears promising. The issue of obstruction of the coronary ostia appears to be less of a concern than originally envisioned. However, PHV migration at the time of deployment is a major concern. Additionally, the anterograde approach is technically very challenging and could limit the broader application of the procedure. Cribier reported using the simpler retrograde approach in about 20% of the 40 patients who have now undergone PHV implantation at the Charles Nicolle Hospital of Rouen (as of September 2005). As the profile of the PHV-delivery balloon assembly decreases, the proportion of cases in which this technically less challenging approach may be possible will likely increase. The difficulty of precise positioning of the PHV using the retrograde approach will likely be overcome by certain design modifications. It appears that the increased size of the device to 26 mm has significantly lowered the paravalvular leak problem.

CoreValve (Paris, France; Irvine, CA)

The CoreValve (Revalving) aortic valve consists of a bioprosthetic valve made of bovine pericardial tissue that is mounted and sutured in a self-expanding nitinol stent (Fig. 79.2). The

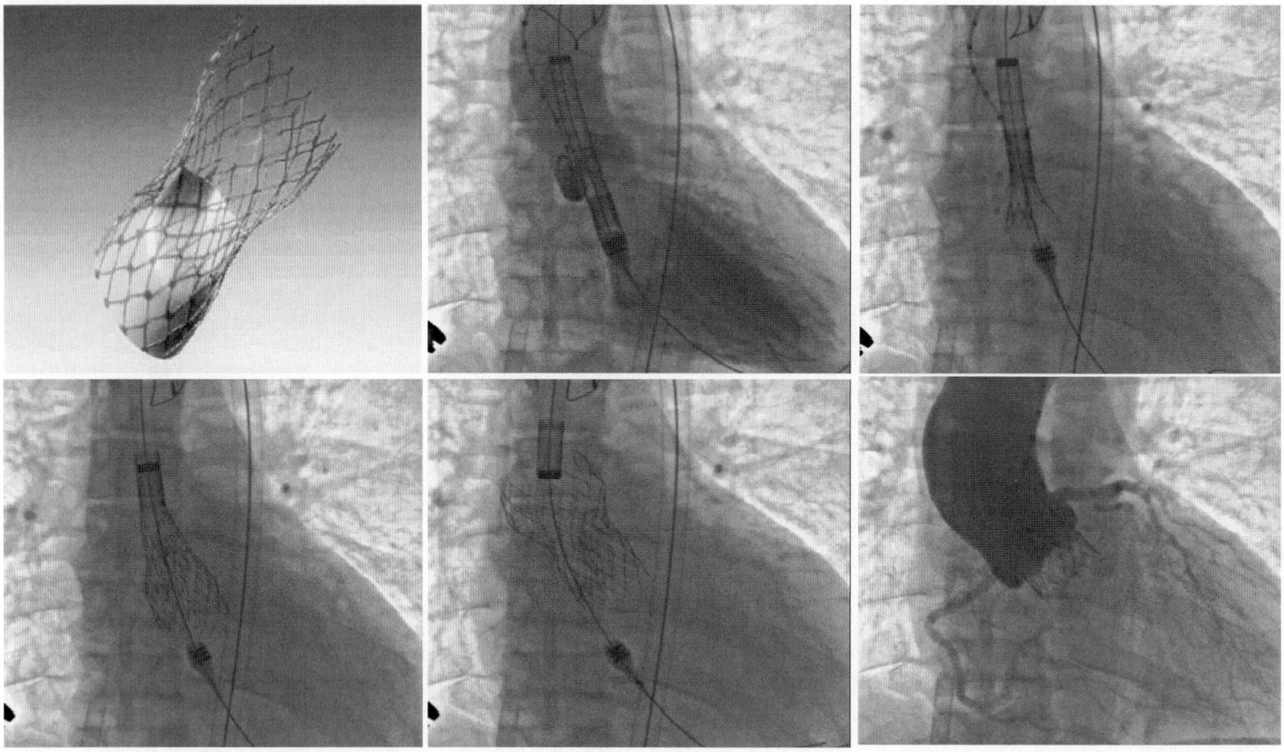

FIGURE 79.2. Upper right: The CoreValve, which is deployed in a patient with severe aortic regurgitation. The valve is deployed in retrograde fashion in the anatomic position. Coronary arteries are not jeopardized by this stent valve. There is no paravalvular leak as seen in the aortogram. (Courtesy of Dr. Vahanian)

prosthetic frame (stent) is manufactured by the laser cutting of a nitinol metal tube with a length of 50 mm. The lower part has a high radial force to push aside the calcified leaflets and avoid recoil; the middle part is constrained to avoid coronaries and carries the valve, whereas the upper part expands for fixation in the ascending aorta. The actual valve inner diameter is 21 to 22 mm. For stent deployment, the retrograde approach was used via a surgically prepared common iliac artery as the access site. The procedure was initially performed using general anesthesia with transesophageal echocardiographic (TEE) guidance and femorofemoral cardiac support. Initial results with this valve were reported from 12 patients in whom the 25-Fr system was used. The valve was successfully deployed within the diseased native aortic valve in 10 of 12 patients. One patient died of ventricular rupture before device implantation, and one patient was converted to surgical treatment because of unsuccessful device placement. During in-hospital follow-up, five patients died. Four deaths were procedure related: myocardial perforation (one), crush-syndrome (one), and multiorgan failure (two). Another patient died of lung cancer. All patients developed temporary thrombocytopenia that was persistent if antiplatelet medication was not given. The valve is now in the third generation; the delivery catheter size has been reduced to 21 Fr, and the valve has been delivered using local anesthesia via femoral artery access with a shorter procedural time.

Corazón (Menlo Park, CA)

Corazón's in situ aortic valve treatment device (Beating Heart Aortic Valve Repair [BHAVR] Demineralization System) allows for beating heart demineralization of the aortic valve to improve native valve function in moderate AS. It may also be used to aid easy implantation of a prosthetic valve with good apposition to prevent paravalvular leak. The system first isolates the aortic valve by placing a catheter into the left ventricle. This catheter has a balloon for occluding the left ventricular outflow tract below the AV. The catheter has an expandable central lumen with temporary aortic valve, thus enabling beating heart aortic valve treatment. The aortic valve is then isolated by the three foam elements molded to fit the aortic sinuses. A small pulsatile balloon proximal to this apparatus provides gentle agitation of the foam elements and AV leaflets. A low-pH solution is used for aortic mineralization. The first clinical use of Corazón's BHAVR device was on a more severely diseased aortic valve before bioprosthetic replacement, in August of 2005. No clinical adverse events were noted during the Corazón treatment.

Multiple other companies are working on the question of developing technologies to make percutaneous valve replacement a reality. Some of these include Cook, Direct Flow Medical, Edwards Lifesciences, Heart Leaflet Technologies, Medtronic, Palmaz/Baley's, Sadra Medical, Shelhigh, 3F Therapeutics, and ValveXchange.

PULMONARY VALVE REPLACEMENT

Scope of the Problem

Most pulmonary valve disease in adult patients represents untreated congenital pulmonary stenosis or pulmonary regurgitation (with or without stenosis) following reconstruction of the right ventricular outflow tract (RVOT) in patients with tetralogy of Fallot, pulmonary atresia, or transposition of the great arteries (26). These reconstructions may leave the native

RVOT intact and may include one or more of the following procedures: resection of infundibular tissue, pulmonary commissurotomy, and placement of a patch in the outflow tract, annulus, or pulmonary artery. With such repairs, the natural history is for the development of pulmonary regurgitation, which is severe in more than one third of patients (27). Alternatively, the native RVOT may be bypassed using a valved or valveless extracardiac conduit between the right ventricle and the pulmonary artery (28–30). Pulmonary regurgitation is immediate with valveless conduits. Valved conduits are associated with progressive degeneration of the conduit and valve resulting in both pulmonary regurgitation and stenosis, such that multiple surgical procedures are typically required over the lifetime of the individual. Pulmonary regurgitation produces chronic right-sided volume overload, right ventricular dilatation, and impairment of systolic and diastolic function (27,31). Clinically, these anatomic complications are manifest by heart failure, atrial and ventricular arrhythmias, and an increased risk of sudden cardiac death. Pulmonary stenosis results in right ventricular hypertension and predisposes the patient to arrhythmias.

Pulmonary valvuloplasty is well established as the primary treatment for adults with congenital pulmonary valve stenosis. The procedure is well tolerated and effective, and it provides a durable benefit (1). Percutaneous stenting of conduit stenosis has also been successfully practiced for several years (32). In contrast, until recently, the only therapeutic option for patients with severe pulmonary regurgitation was surgical valve replacement. The morbidity and mortality associated with operative replacement resulted in a tendency to perform the procedure relatively late, at a time when the degree of reversibility in right ventricular dilatation and dysfunction is likely diminished. In addition, cardiopulmonary bypass may worsen right ventricular function, thereby attenuating the potential benefit of valve replacement. A percutaneous option for valve replacement may help these patients significantly.

Devices and Initial Experience

Since 2000, Bonhoeffer and colleagues have championed the development of a percutaneous valve replacement in right ventricle to pulmonary artery prosthetic conduits and more recently in the native pulmonary position (33–37). In design, the valve consists of a piece of bovine internal jugular vein containing a bicuspid or trileaflet valve that is sutured to the interior of an 18-mm diameter balloon expandable stent composed of a soft and highly malleable alloy of platinum-iridium alloy (NuMed, Inc.). Depending on the size of the pulmonary artery or extracardiac conduit, the valve-stent is then hand-crimped onto an 18-, 20-, or 22-mm balloon catheter. With the patient under general anesthesia, and using femoral venous access, a stiff guidewire is placed in the RVOT extending into a distal pulmonary artery branch. The valve-stent balloon assembly is front-loaded into an 18- to 20-Fr (~6-mm) sheath (NuMed, Inc.) and is delivered over the guidewire to the desired location. Deployment of the prosthesis is achieved by inflation and deflation of the delivery balloon (Fig. 79.3).

Bonhoeffer and colleagues have recently reported their clinical experience with 59 consecutive patients undergoing PV replacement (38). Most of these patients had a variant of tetralogy of Fallot ($n = 36$), transposition of the great arteries, or ventricular septal defect with pulmonary stenosis ($n = 8$). The procedure was successful in 58 patients with no mortality. There was subjective and objective improvement in symptoms and exercise tolerance.

Important challenges remain in the broader application of this technology. In patients who have undergone repair of tetralogy of Fallot that maintained the native RVOT by valvotomy, valvectomy, or patch repair, there is often no secure implantation point at the site of the pulmonary annulus. This fact significantly affects the risk of immediate or delayed migration of the device. For patients with extracardiac conduits, variation in conduit size is also a limiting factor. For a conduit

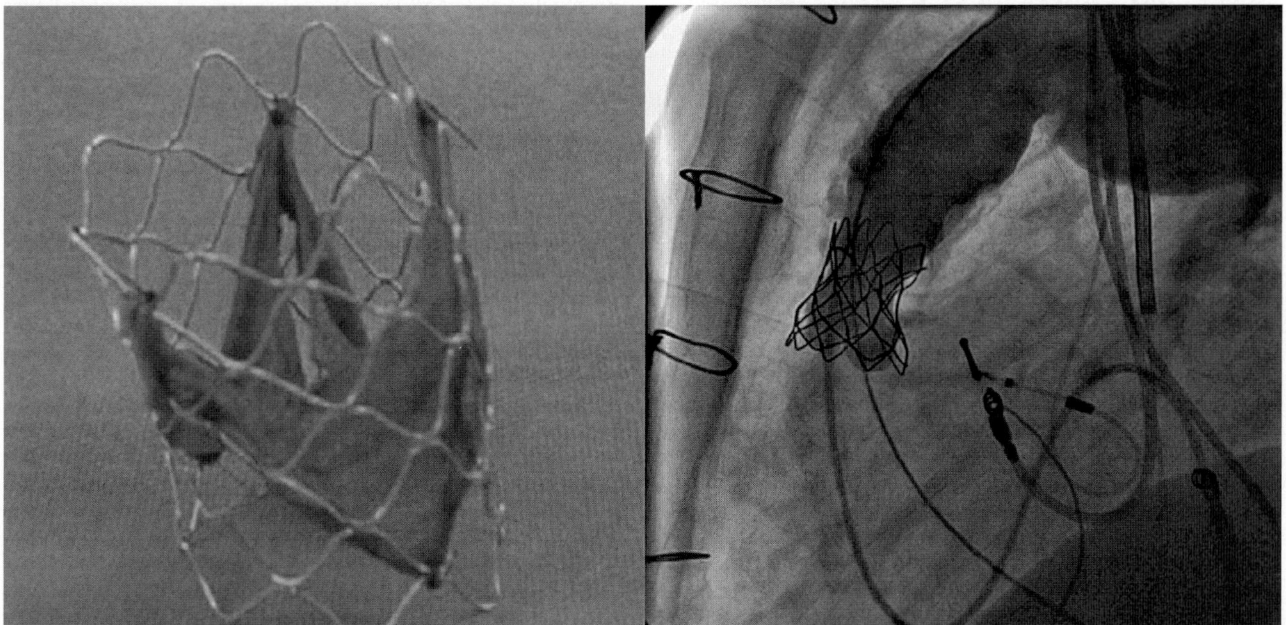

FIGURE 79.3. **Left:** One of Bonhoeffers' first trileaflet bovine jugular venous valved stents, which was used for percutaneous pulmonary implantation. **Right:** A postprocedural result from a newly implanted valve after percutaneous delivery in the one of the recent series of Bonhoeffer and colleagues. (Modified from Lutter G, Ardehali R, Cremer J, et al. Percutaneous value replacement: Current state and future prospects. *Ann Thorac Surg* 2004;79:2199–2206.)

smaller than 16 mm in diameter, there is a danger that the valve-stent assembly will be underexpanded, thus resulting in a larger profile, which may cause obstruction. Conversely, the small size of currently available bovine jugular venous valves (<22 mm) limits the use of this prosthesis for patients with a conduit exceeding this diameter because of the risk of incompetence and/or migration of the valve. Boudjemline, working with the Bonhoeffer group, described a novel pulmonary prosthesis specifically designed for patients with an enlarged conduit or RVOT (37). This device is a self-expandable nitinol stent that has a spontaneous diameter of 30 mm at the ends and a 15-mm-long central restricted area that currently has a diameter of 18 mm. The outer ends ensure fixation of the stent to the wall of an enlarged RVOT or conduit, whereas the central restricted area provides the supporting structure for the 18-mm bovine internal jugular vein valve. A polytetrafluoroethylene membrane is sutured to the outer surface of the nitinol stent to create a seal between the stent and the pulmonary artery. Animal studies with this stent have produced encouraging results that will likely form the basis for human application in the near future.

Complications from this initial experience can be classified into three categories. The first were related to balloon dilatation or stenting for conduit stenosis, including dissection, hemorrhage from conduit rupture, and residual stenosis because of external compression or undilatable conduits. The second category included issues of patient selection in which dislodgment or embolization of the valved stent occurred. In the third category, complications were thought to be related to device design, which included the "hammock" effect and stent fracture. The hammock effect was resolved with an improved design, whereby the entire length of the stent was sutured to the venous wall segment. Although stent fracture was seen in six patients, only two had clinical consequences. One was treated with another percutaneous valve replacement, whereas the second patient required surgery.

MITRAL VALVE REPAIR AND REPLACEMENT

Scope of the Problem

With the aging of the population and the declining incidence of rheumatic diseases, MR has emerged as the dominant form of mitral valve disease (39). Surgical options for severe MR include mitral valve replacement, with or without preservation of the subvalvular apparatus, and mitral valve repair. The general consensus is that, when feasible, mitral valve repair is superior to surgical replacement because it is associated with lower operative mortality, reduced rates of endocarditis, fewer thromboembolic events, and improved long-term survival (40). The survival benefits of valve repair are likely mediated by preservation of left ventricular function as a result of maintenance of the continuity between the mitral valve and its supporting structures (annulus, chordae tendineae, papillary muscles) (41). However, currently in the United States, mitral valve replacement, not repair, is performed in almost 50% patients undergoing mitral valve surgery.

Relevant Surgical Information

Various surgical techniques for the repair of acquired MR have been developed over the last 3 decades. An appreciation of the underlying mechanism of MR is of paramount importance in the decision regarding the particular surgical technique employed. This task is complicated by the finding that MR is almost always caused by multiple lesions affecting the various components of the mitral apparatus. Despite this complexity, various classification systems of MR have been proposed that serve to highlight the dominant mechanisms involved and to guide appropriate surgical therapies. An understanding of these mechanisms and of the fundamentals of surgical techniques for mitral valve repair is a necessary preamble to any discussion of the novel percutaneous approaches to mitral valve repair.

Carpentier and colleagues proposed three broad categories for the classification of the mechanism of MR (42). This classification has been embraced by the surgical community and is widely used in cardiothoracic literature. Table 79.1 summarizes the characteristic findings, underlying pathologic features, and typical surgical therapies for the various types of MR.

In type I, the dominant pathologic feature causing MR is annular dilatation resulting from left ventricular dilatation. The mitral leaflets are structurally normal and demonstrate normal mobility. This form of MR is classically seen in patients with dilated cardiomyopathy, but it accompanies any form of severe MR that causes left ventricular dilatation. Annular dilatation is typically asymmetric, predominantly occurring along the attachment of the posterior leaflet. This causes the anteroposterior diameter of the mitral orifice to be greater than the transverse diameter (normal anteroposterior/transverse diameter ratio is 3:4). These alterations in annular geometry result in failure of coaptation of the mitral leaflets and typically produce a central jet of MR. Surgical correction of annular dilatation is achieved by insertion of a flexible prosthetic ring of suitable shape and size, approximating the area of the anterior mitral leaflet with a vertical height equal to the height of the anterior leaflet. By producing a measured plication of the posterior annulus, the ring attempts to restore the normal contour and function of the valve (43,44). The flexibility of the ring is thought to be important in maintaining the normal sphincteric function and saddle shape of the mitral annulus. Despite this hypothetic advantage, rigid posterior and circumferential annuloplasty rings have also been used successfully, and there are no conclusive data proving the superiority of one method over the other.

In type II, excessive motion of the leaflets occurs such that one or both leaflets will prolapse into the left atrium during systole beyond the plane of the annulus. The dominant pathologic feature underlying this type of MR is myxomatous degeneration of the leaflets and/or chordae. Older patients may demonstrate a distinct form of degenerative mitral disease termed fibroelastic deficiency in which the leaflets are thin and translucent, as opposed to yellow and thickened. Various repair techniques specifically tailored to the site of prolapse (i.e., anterior, posterior, bileaflet) have been developed (Table 79.2) (45,46). In addition to these preparative techniques, adjunctive ring annuloplasty is almost always added to the surgical procedure (43,44,47). The best surgical results are achieved in patients with posterior leaflet prolapse, who comprise the majority of patients with mitral valve prolapse.

In type III, motion of one or both leaflets is restricted. Two major pathologic features underlie this type of MR. Restricted leaflet motion may be caused by rheumatic disease (usually affecting the posterior leaflet). Surgical repair of this condition is uncommon, and replacement is usually performed. Alternatively, restriction may occur on an ischemic basis in patients with a prior myocardial infarction (typically inferoposterior), in whom remodeling and distortion of the left ventricle and papillary muscles result in displacement of the papillary muscles away from the mitral annulus and produce tethering and restriction of the mitral leaflets (48). The optimal surgical therapy for ischemic MR is controversial (49). When utilized, repair techniques for ischemic MR generally include an undersized annuloplasty ring (50,51).

TABLE 79.1

MITRAL REGURGITATION: CLASSIFICATION AND SURGICAL TREATMENT

MR type	Anatomy of leaflets	Dominant pathologic features	Optimal surgical therapy
Type I	Normal leaflet motion	Annular dilatation and left ventricular dilatation	Annuloplasty using undersized circumferential or flexible posterior ring (112–114)
Type II	Free edges of leaflets override plane of annulus during systole	Myxomatous degeneration of mitral leaflets and chordae, resulting in prolapse of the valve leaflet from chordal rupture or elongation; less commonly, fibroelastic degeneration of mitral leaflets	a. Posterior prolapse: quadrangular resection (with or without sliding repair) (46) and annuloplasty using flexible posterior ring b. Anterior prolapse: chordal transfer (rarely chordal shortening) (46) c. Bileaflet prolapse—posterior leaflet resection and annuloplasty; posterior leaflet resection and sliding repair with triangular resection of anterior leaflet and annuloplasty: edge-to-edge Alfieri repair
Type III	Restricted leaflet motion	a. Rheumatic b. Chronic ischemic MR: Prior MI with WMA (usually inferoposterior) and PM displacement; morphologically normal mitral leaflets and subvalvular apparatus	a. Generally replacement, rarely repair (annuloplasty, leaflet debridement, commissurotomy) (115) b. Uncertain: repair (generally undersized annuloplasty ring, rarely with or without edge-to-edge repair) and CABG versus replacement (generally bioprosthesis) and CABG (49–51)

CABG, coronary artery bypass surgery; MI, myocardial infarction; MR, mitral regurgitation; PM, papillary muscle; WMA, wall motion abnormality.

In 1991, Alfieri and his colleagues reported a novel surgical technique for mitral valve repair in which the free edge of the middle scallop of the anterior leaflet of the mitral valve is approximated with the free edge of the middle scallop of the posterior leaflet (52). The result is the creation of a double orifice of the mitral valve. Generally, the technique has been reserved for more complex MR mechanisms, in which the surgical repair technique is more involved and/or is less likely to be successful. Such disorders include bileaflet prolapse, anterior leaflet prolapse, and posterior leaflet prolapse associated with extensive annular calcification. Some groups have also applied the technique to patients with ischemic cardiomyopathy with complex (i.e., eccentric) MR (53). The edge-to-edge technique is relatively straightforward and is technically less challenging than conventional nonannular techniques of mitral repair. Long-term clinical outcome studies have shown good results in the treatment of patients with severe MR secondary to degenerative mitral valve disease and dilated cardiomyopathy, especially when the procedure is combined with annuloplasty (53–55). In contrast, the recurrence rates of severe MR in patients with ischemic MR have been approximately 30% when annuloplasty is not used (53). The concern that the technique may cause mitral stenosis has not been borne out in clinical practice; surgical series have reported a mean transmitral gradient of approximately 4 mm Hg postoperatively that appears stable over time. In addition, the valve has responded to exercise physiologically with no evidence of obstruction (56).

TABLE 79.2

PERCUTANEOUS MITRAL VALVE REPAIR APPROACHES

Type	Devices
Coronary sinus approach	Edward Life Sciences Viacor Cardiac Dimensions
Shaping through ventricle	Mitralign Myocor
Edge-to-edge repair	E valve Edwards Life Sciences

Percutaneous Mitral Valve Repair

Percutaneous mitral valve repair approaches currently include reshaping the annulus through the coronary sinus (Edwards Lifesciences, Viacor, Cardiac Dimensions), reshaping the annulus through the ventricle (Mitralign, Myocor), and connecting the middle scallops of the anterior and posterior leaflets (Edwards Lifesciences, Evalve) (Table 79.2).

Reshaping of the Annulus via Coronary Sinus

Certain groups are attempting to develop an effective percutaneous annuloplasty technique by exploiting the relationship of the coronary sinus with the mitral valve (56–58) (Fig. 79.4). The coronary sinus courses from its origin in the right atrium along the atrioventricular groove, runs parallel and in direct proximity to the posterior mitral annulus, and terminates as the anterior interventricular vein in the anterior interventricular groove. Although some differences exist among the designs of individual annuloplasty devices, the basic technique and hypothesized mechanism of action are similar. Venous access may be obtained from either the jugular or the femoral vein. A sheath is inserted into the coronary sinus, and a metal

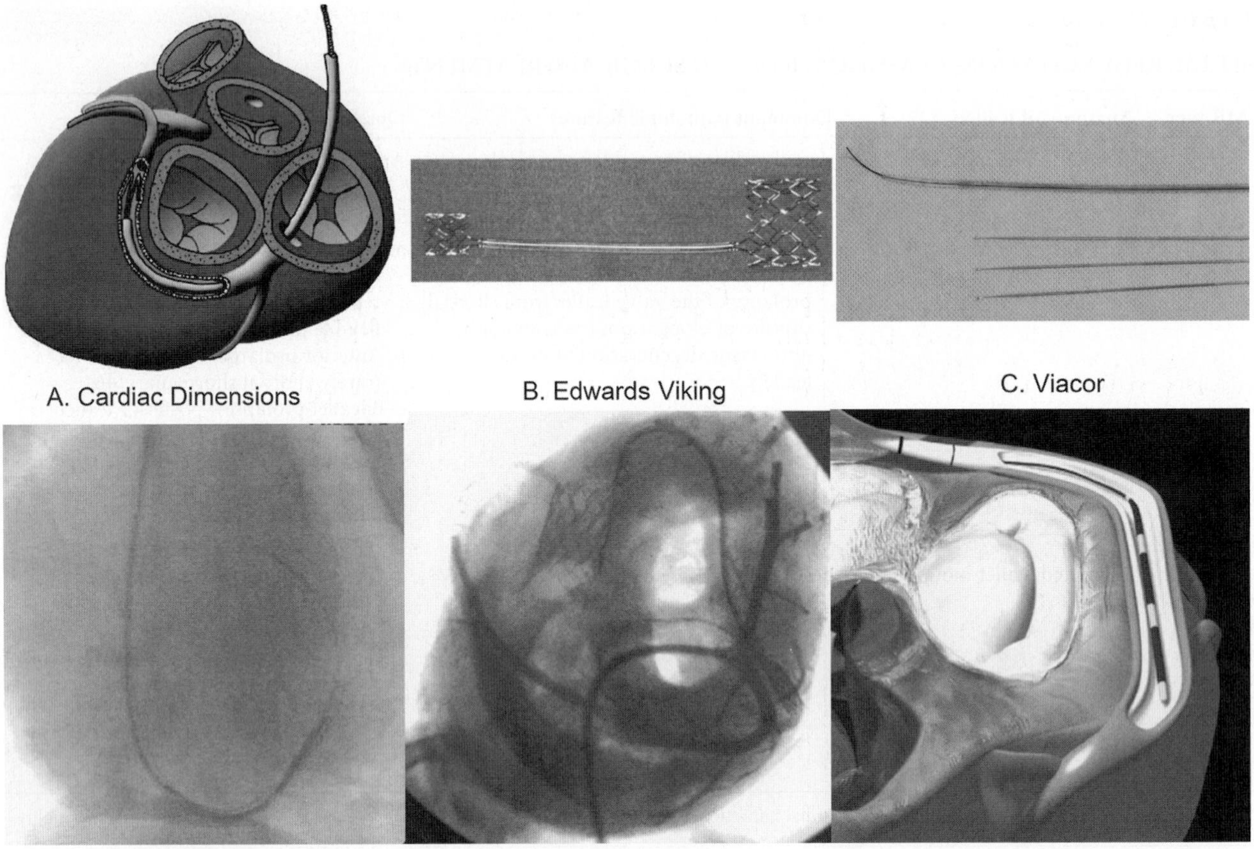

FIGURE 79.4. Different devices used via coronary sinus approach. From **left** to **right, upper** and **lower panels** show Cardiac Dimensions, Edward Viking, and Viacor devices. Courtesy of respective manufacturers.

annuloplasty device is delivered through the sheath and is positioned in the region of apposition of the coronary sinus with the posterior mitral annulus. The goal is to alter the geometry of the mitral annulus favorably and to reduce the degree of MR.

The feasibility and short-term efficacy of two percutaneous annuloplasty devices in animal models have been published (57,58). Liddicoat reported the experience with the Viacor annuloplasty device (Wilmington, MA) in an acute ischemic sheep model (58). This device consists of a nitinol and stainless steel construct, which has a rigid straight portion of variable length (35 to 85 mm) that is positioned opposite the posterior mitral annulus. The effect is to move the posterior annulus toward the anterior annulus and thus improve leaflet coaptation. In all six animals, the degree of MR decreased from 3+ to 4+ to 0 to 1+ with device deployment and returned to 3+ to 4+ with removal of the device. Permanent implants have been demonstrated to generate a sustained reduction of anteroposterior dimension for up to 6 months of chronic implantation (22 ± 2.1 to 15 ± 2.5, $n = 10$ animals). Initial human evaluation of the PTMA method has been conducted on a temporary basis in patients scheduled for surgical annuloplasty. It has demonstrated the feasibility of accessing and manipulating the mitral valve annulus with the PTMA device and approach.

In a pacemaker-induced dilated cardiomyopathy model, Kaye and colleagues reported the acute outcome following insertion of the Cardiac Dimensions device (Kirkland, WA), the CARILLON Mitral Contour System (57). This device is constructed of nitinol and has proximal and distal anchors connected by an intervening cable or shaping ribbon. The device is positioned such that the posterior mitral annulus lies between the two anchors. Application of tension results in straightening between the two anchors producing forward motion of the posterior annulus. Sufficient tension is applied to produce a reduction in the annular diameter of 25%. In the animal experiments, this resulted in a reduction in the ratio of the MR jet to the left atrial area from 40% to 4% and a significant improvement in all hemodynamic parameters (cardiac output, pulmonary artery pressure, and pulmonary capillary wedge pressure). The first human implant of the CARILLON Mitral Contour System was performed in Hamburg, Germany in July 2005 as part of the AMADEUS trial. In this patient, the implantation was successful, with significant improvement in MR and clinical status. AMADEUS (Carillon Mitral Annuloplasty Device European Union Study) is a safety and efficacy study of the CARILLON system ongoing at seven centers across Europe. The study will enroll 30 patients and assess safety and efficacy at 1-, 3- and 6-month intervals.

Although encouraging and exciting, these data are still preliminary. Several concerns have to be addressed to make these technologies become clinically applicable in a large number of patients. These include anatomic variability in relation of the coronary sinus to the mitral annulus, the risk of trauma to the coronary sinus (dissection or perforation), coronary sinus thrombosis, and circumflex artery trauma owing to the close relationship between the circumflex artery and the coronary sinus. The ventricular annuloplasty approaches potentially circumvent some of these concerns.

Ventricular Approaches for Mitral Valve Repair

Currently, the two devices that are being evaluated for this purpose are the Coapsys and the Mitralign systems. The Coapsys Device (Myocor, Inc., Maple Grove, MN) is a permanent

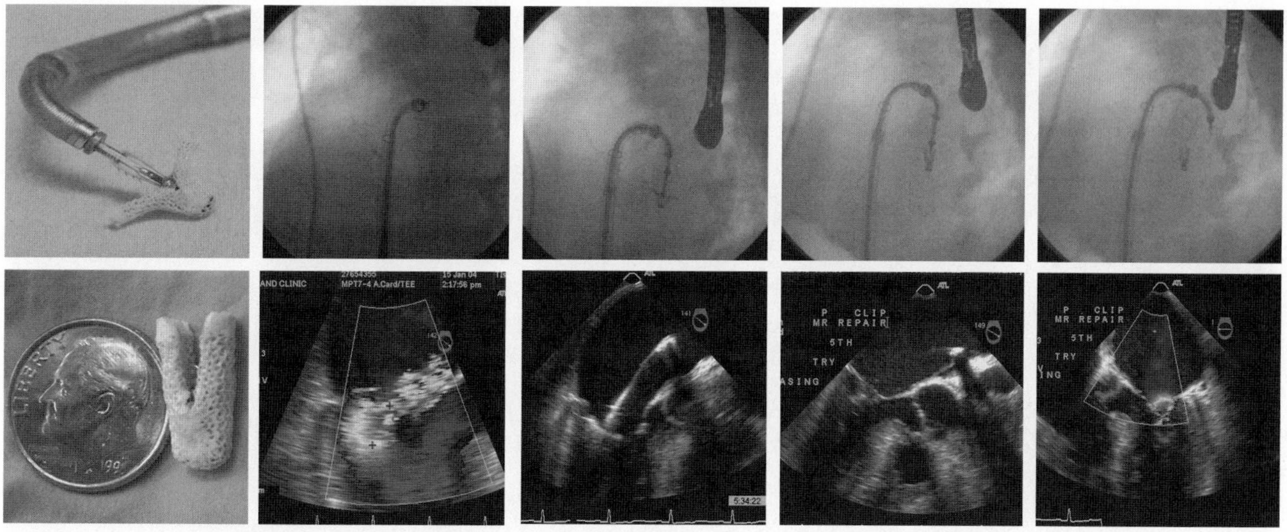

FIGURE 79.5. The clip is shown in the **left side** of the figure. **Top:** The clip advancement and deployment as seen under fluoroscopy. **Bottom:** Severe mitral regurgitation (MR) shown by transesophageal echocardiography (TEE), deployment of the clip as visualized with TEE, and postprocedural trivial MR.

implant consisting of two epicardial pads connected by a flexible subvalvular chord that is implanted during surgery in a beating heart. It is designed to reduce the anteroposterior dimension of the mitral valve while stabilizing the lateral wall of the left ventricle, thereby improving valve leaflet coaptation. The device is sized to the appropriate length during the surgical procedure while MR is evaluated via TEE. This device was tested in animal models with encouraging results in acute and chronic models. The TRACE study (Treatment of Functional Mitral Regurgitation without Atriotomy or CPB Clinical Evaluation) examined Copasys application in an off-pump setting in 30 patients with sustained MR grade 2 or more after undergoing concomitant coronary artery bypass grafting (CABG) in India. Implantation did not result in any adverse events, and all patients survived to 3 months with significant improvement in MR grade and functional class (58a). In the United States, this device is now being tested in the RESTOR-MV study that is randomizing patients with coronary artery disease and functional MR to either standard mitral annuloplasty and CABG or CABG with the Coapsys system. The initial report from this study showed that in 19 patients undergoing this device implantation, intraoperative MR was reduced in 95% (18 of 19) of patients, and 84% (16 of 19) had MR grade 1 or less after implantation. This device has been modified to be delivered percutaneously via the transpericardial approach. The epicardial pads are connected by a splint outside the heart and are tightened to reduce the annular dimension adequately. The device is designed to avoid pinching of the circumflex artery by specifically designed pads. Clinical trial of the percutaneous device has not started yet.

The Mitralign system (Mitralign, Inc., Salem, NH) involves placing multiple anchors on the mitral annulus that are plicated to reduce the annular size. The procedure involves placement of a coronary sinus catheter that carries two opposing (i.e., N-N) magnets. The catheter is positioned so the magnets are behind the middle of P_2. A left ventricular catheter with an S magnetic tip is advanced in retrograde fashion from the femoral artery and is then advanced to the lateral wall to be locked in place by the magnets in the coronary sinus. Once the initial location is secured, specialized devices are used to translate medially and laterally along the annulus to deploy other anchors. These anchors are then plicated together and are locked in position to produce annular reduction. The device had undergone animal assessment, but the data are still awaited.

Edge-to-Edge Repair

Based on the experience with the surgical Alfieri technique of mitral valve repair, percutaneous repair using a clip (MitraClip, Evalve, Menlo Park, CA) and a suture-based technique (Edward Lifesciences, Irvine, CA) has been developed. The Evalve technology has advanced to human studies with exciting results (Fig. 79.5). The system involves a 22-Fr guiding catheter that is introduced through the femoral vein and is positioned in the left atrium above the mitral valve following transseptal puncture and septal dilatation. Via this guiding catheter, a clip delivery system that contains a V-shaped clip and delivery catheter is introduced. Once it is in a proper place in the left atrium, the V clip is opened, and its position is adjusted such that the V shape is perpendicular to the medial-lateral axis of the mitral valve and the line of coaptation of the mitral leaflets. Maintaining this alignment, the clip is advanced into the left ventricle and is withdrawn in systole to grasp the appropriate scallop of both the anterior and posterior mitral leaflets. The arms of the clip are then closed to create the double orifice, and the effect on MR with the heart functioning under normal loading conditions is assessed by TEE. If a satisfactory result is achieved, the clip is released, and the delivery system and guide catheter are removed. More than one clip is necessary in some patients to achieve adequate reduction in MR.

The success of this procedure is dependent on appreciation of three-dimensional anatomy on TEE and fluoroscopic imaging. Synthesis of this information to manipulate the system to grasp the appropriate segment of the leaflets is necessary for a good result. The initial animal studies showed feasibility and safety and led to the phase I human study (59). The EVEREST 1 (Endovascular Valve Edge-to-Edge REpair STudy) trial reported the follow-up data (October 2005) from the 47 patients with moderately severe or severe MR who were experiencing symptoms or had decreased left ventricular function. Only 4% of the 47 patients enrolled experienced a significant adverse event at 30 days, and 75% of those who received a clip remain free from surgery. The first 27 patients treated have reached 1-year follow-up. Ninety-three percent of those patients who

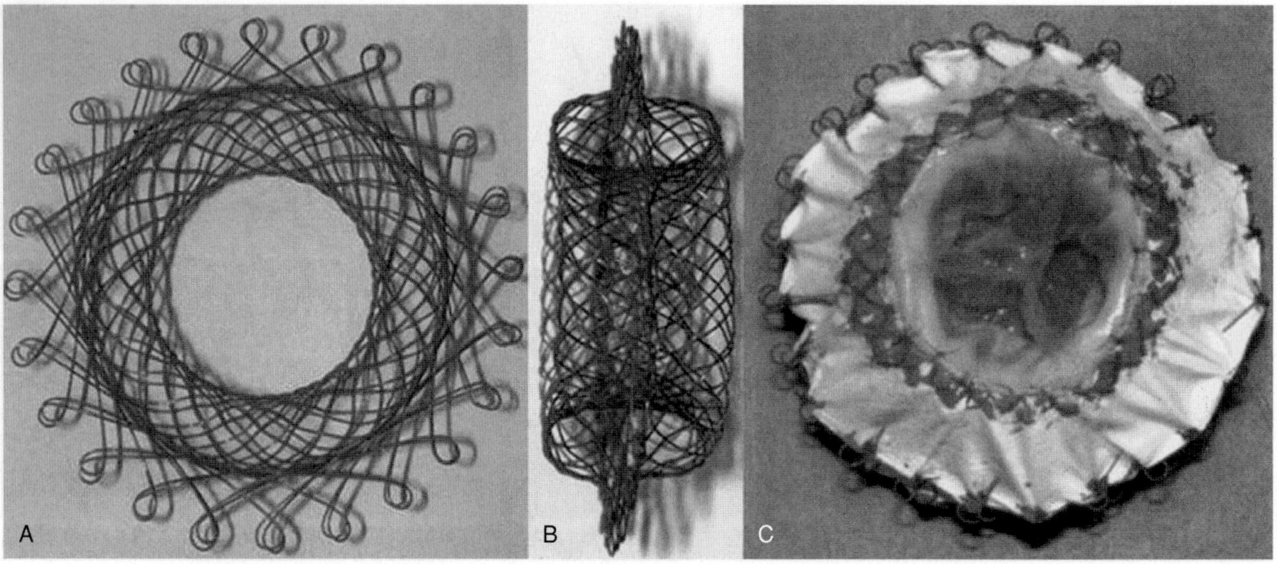

FIGURE 79.6. En face and lateral views of the tricuspid valve stent before its covering (**A, B**), after its covering by a polytetrafluoroethylene membrane and the suture of the valve in the central tubular part (**C**). The stent is shown from the ventricular side with a valve in closed position (59a).

experienced a significant reduction in MR at 1 month following treatment have maintained that improvement at 1 year. EVEREST II, a randomized, multicenter study designed to demonstrate the safety and efficacy of its MitraClip percutaneous valve repair system for patients with MR, has been recently launched. EVEREST II will compare the MitraClip technique with standard surgical mitral valve repair or replacement in patients with functional or degenerative MR in approximately 30 U.S. centers.

TRICUSPID VALVE REPLACEMENT

Despite recent advances in mitral valve repair techniques and multiple approaches, tricuspid valve–related devices are few (Fig. 79.6). Percutaneous implantation of a prosthetic valve has been envisioned, but several difficulties still remain to be resolved before these devices can be used routinely. First, the discrepancy between the size of the available transcatheter valve and that of the annulus makes the use of current stent designs impossible. Second, the valve must be anchored to the annulus not to embolize. A self-expandable stent formed of two disks separated by a tubular part has been designed and tested by Bonhoeffer's group. In animal models, this valve seemed to function reasonably well in a preliminary study. Further developments and experimental studies are necessary, however, before considering the use of such devices in humans.

PATENT FORAMEN OVALE CLOSURE

Embryology and Anatomy of Patent Foramen Ovale

PFO is a remnant of fetal cardiac development that frequently persists in adults and has been associated with stroke, migraine, platypnea-orthodeoxia, and decompression sickness (DCS) (60–62). During cardiac development, the septum primum grows from the roof of the atria and connects to the endocardial cushions to close the initial opening between the two atria (ostium primum). Communication between the atria is maintained by the ostium secundum, which is formed by the fusion of fenestrations in the septum primum. The septum secundum then grows on the right atrial side of the septum primum and covers the ostium secundum. At birth or shortly thereafter, the septum primum fuses with the septum secundum, and interatrial communication is interrupted. PFO is defined as an opening that is present when the septum primum does not fuse with the septum secundum. The two overlap to some extent, however, so there is no flow from left to right but with increased right-sided pressure there is right-to-left shunt. Primum atrial septal defects occur when the septum primum fails to fuse with endocardial cushion, and secundum defects result from excess resorption of the septum primum or inadequate development of the septum secundum.

Structural Associations with Patent Foramen Ovale

Atrial septal aneurysm (ASA) and Chiari network have been associated with PFO. ASA, as defined by at least a 10-mm excursion with a base of 15 mm or greater, is present in about 2% of the population. PFO is present in at least 50% of patients with ASA. Many times, the thin septum primum in these patients has multiple small fenestrations. Chiari network is a remnant of the septum spurium and the right valve of the sinus venosus. These fibers arise from either the eustachian or the besian valve and attach to the upper wall of right atrium or interatrial septum. Chiari network is present in 2% to 3% of the population in autopsy studies. Most patients with prominent Chiari network (83% in one study) have PFO.

Diagnosis of Patent Foramen Ovale

On autopsy, PFO can be found in about 27% of patients. PFO is diagnosed by echocardiography with detection of the passage of microbubble from the right to the left side of the heart within three to five cardiac cycles. Grading of the right-to-left shunt is somewhat arbitrary: up to 10 bubbles is trivial, more than 10 bubbles is small, and intense opacification is a large shunt. Various methods to enhance right-to-left shunts exist including cough, Valsalva maneuver (active, passive or calibrated) (63), or injection of contrast in the femoral vein (64). The relative role of each of these methods has not been well studied. Transthoracic echocardiography can detect right-to-left shunt, but the sensitivity of this test is not as good as that of TEE. TEE allows anatomic definition of PFO and allows one to measure the separation between the septum primum and secundum. It also allows for the measurement of the overlap of the two septa—"the tunnel," which is an important factor in the planning of the percutaneous closure. Intracardiac echocardiography permits detailed interrogation of the interatrial septal anatomy with high resolution similar to a TEE examination. Typically, the PFO is present in the anterior part of fossa ovales, and therefore it is seen on 60-degree view at the aortic level by TEE or by horizontal view of the interatrial septum at the aortic level by intracardiac echocardiography. Another method to detect PFO is by transcranial Doppler (TCD) interrogation of the middle cerebral artery or basilar artery. Studies have shown that TEE and TCD examination together improve sensitivity to detect PFO compared with either of these tests alone. The PFO missed by TCD examination are typically small (≤2 mm by TEE) (65). Single-gate TCD appears to be less sensitive compared with power M-mode TCD. During TCD examination, similar methods are used to generate right-to-left shunt as during echocardiography.

Association of Diseases with Patent Foramen Ovale

PFO has been associated with stroke, migraine, platypnea-orthodeoxia, and DCS.

Stroke

Of the ischemic strokes, 40% have no clear identifiable cause and are termed cryptogenic stroke (66). The recurrence rate of these cryptogenic strokes is similar to that of strokes from other causes (~10% per year) (67). A metaanalysis of nine studies investigating association of PFO with cryptogenic stroke in a young (≤55 years) population found a positive association of PFO with cryptogenic stroke (odds ratio [OR], 3.1; confidence interval [CI], 2.3 to 4.2) (68). The association was stronger for ASA (odds ratio [OR], 6.14; and 95% CI, 2.5 to 15.2) and was strongest for PFO plus ASA (15.6, 95% CI, 2.9 to 86). The size of shunt through PFO has been compared in patients with and without cryptogenic stroke by TEE and TCD. In one study, TCD determined that the severity of shunt was greater in patients with cryptogenic stroke compared with controls (69). In another study, larger shunt by omniplane TEE correlated with increased frequency of ischemic events on follow-up of about 2 years (70). In yet another study, PFO size as measured by TEE was larger in patients with neurologic events compared with controls. Further, the patients with recurrent cerebrovascular had larger PFO with greater shunt compared with controls and patients with transient ischemic attack (TIA) alone (71). TCD findings of a "shower" or "curtain" pattern have been shown to be associated with a higher risk for cryptogenic stroke (72).

Proposed mechanisms for stroke resulting from PFO include paradoxic embolism from the venous circulation and thrombus formation on the surface of the septum. Some evidence indicates increased atrial arrhythmia associated with PFO, which may contribute to stroke owing to clot formation in the left atrium. Whether there is an association of PFO with hypercoagulable state remains unknown.

Migraine

Migraine is thought to be a disorder characterized by derangement of neural influences on cranial blood vessels, predominantly arising from the brainstem. The prevalence of PFO in the population with migraine with aura is about two times higher than in the population without migraine (73–77). Further, there is an association of migraine with posterior circulation strokes, and PFO may be the missing link to explain this association (78). Although passage of microemboli or "chemokines" through PFO has been suggested as the cause for this association, the exact mechanism remains unclear. Several small retrospective studies have shown that closure of PFO leads to improvement in migraine attacks (73,76,77). An ongoing randomized trial is investigating this association in a rigorous double-blind study in Europe (MIST), and several studies are currently planned to answer this question in the United States. The association of PFO with migraines is probably one of the most exciting questions because it affects a large number of patients.

Platypnea-Orthodeoxia

The platypnea-orthodeoxia syndrome describes both dyspnea (platypnea) and arterial desaturation in the upright position with improvement in the supine position (orthodeoxia) (79,80). The mechanism of this syndrome is thought to be a distortion of the septal anatomy leading to preferential shunting of blood from right to left by stretching of a PFO in the supine position despite normal right-sided pressures. This is typically seen after right pneumonectomy, aortic aneurysm, or massive obesity (81,82). Diagnosis of a PFO with platypnea-orthodeoxia can be made with a tilt table and saline contrast transthoracic echocardiography (83) and TEE (84). A typical patient history with a significant drop in oxygen saturation while in the upright position, along with a large PFO by TEE found as the only source of a shunt, has been considered diagnostic.

Decompression Sickness

Divers with right-to-left shunt can develop serious (type II) DCS. The incidence of PFO in unexplained DCS has been reported to be as high as 70% (85,86). Multiple asymptomatic lesions on magnetic resonance imaging in asymptomatic sport divers have also been associated with the presence of right-to-left shunt detected by TCD (87). DCS is also observed in high-altitude aviators and astronauts, but no conclusive studies implicate PFO in this situation (88). However, data from a small number of instances also suggest a potential role of PFO in the generation of serious DCS in these instances (89).

Management of Patent Foramen Ovale

Percutaneous PFO closure is recommended in patients with platypnea-orthodeoxia and divers with DCS who want to continue diving. There are no specific guidelines to screen divers for primary prevention of DCS at this time because PFO is very common and severe DCS is not common. PFO closure cannot be recommended for patients with migraine until more data on this front become available. Most of the attention has been focused on PFO closure to prevent cryptogenic strokes. The main options for secondary prevention of cryptogenic stroke include medical therapy, surgical closure, and percutaneous closure of PFO. The data for efficacy of each are mainly derived from retrospective analysis of consecutively treated patients with

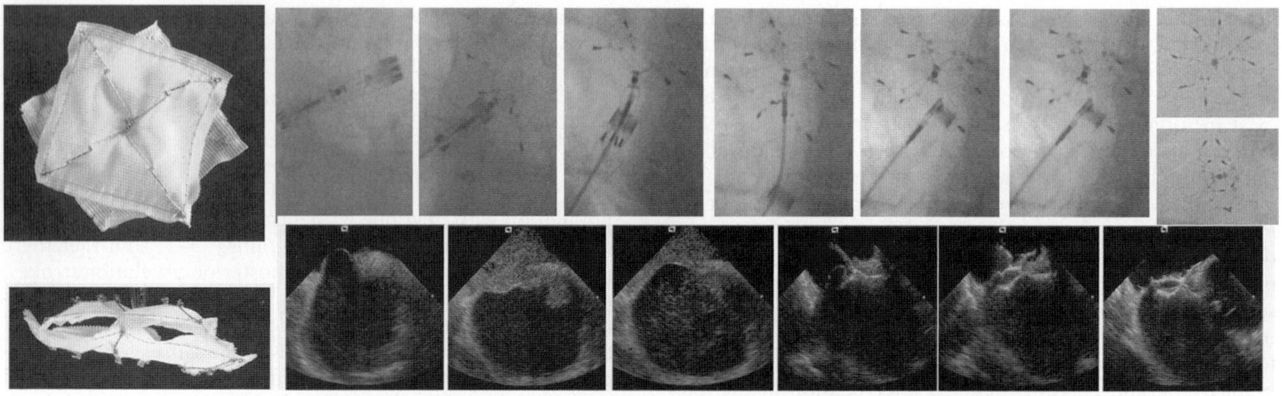

FIGURE 79.7. The CardioSEAL device. **Left:** The device en face and in lateral views. **Right:** The corresponding views on fluoroscopy. **Top:** CardioSEAL deployment under fluoroscopy. **Bottom:** Patent foramen ovale (PFO) shown by intracardiac echocardiography. Agitated saline is used to demonstrate the shunt through the PFO. The device is sequentially deployed with echocardiographic and fluoroscopic guidance.

cryptogenic stroke. Surgical closure is rarely recommended because percutaneous closure can be accomplished effectively with a minor risk.

For patients with cryptogenic stroke, medical options include antiplatelet therapy, warfarin (Coumadin), or a combination of these. The data regarding the comparative efficacy and risks of these strategies remain limited. Nonrandomized studies suggest that fewer recurrent embolic events occur with oral anticoagulants than with aspirin (90,91). However, the annual rate of bleeding complications during warfarin therapy is purported to be 1.8% to 4.8% (92–94). Moreover, primary event rates did not differ significantly in the only randomized trial of aspirin (325 mg/day) and warfarin (target international normalized ratio [INR], 1.4 to 2.8) in patients with PFO (95). However, the trial did not have a placebo-controlled arm, and this limited the assessment of treatment efficacy and was not powered to assess therapeutic equivalence (96). The choice of therapy between aspirin and warfarin should be individualized by taking into consideration the patient's age, presence or absence of prestroke ASA, bleeding risk, and psychosocial issues.

Percutaneous closure of PFO may reduce the risk of recurrent stroke and TIA in young (<55 years) patients with cryptogenic stroke, but there are no controlled studies comparing medical therapy with device closure. The average annual rate of recurrent stroke or TIA in 132 patients in the French PFO/ASA study was 1.2% and 3.4%, respectively, in which the majority of the events occurred in patients with coexistent PFO and ASA (97). However, in previous metaanalysis, the prevalence of recurrent stroke or TIA at 1 year following a first cryptogenic stroke and the presence of PFO in 895 patients who were managed medically ranged from 3.8% to 12%. The risk of recurrent TIA or stroke at 1 year in 1,355 patients treated with transcatheter septal closure ranged between 0% and 4.9%. Importantly, the major complication rate in this pooled analysis was less than 2%. These and other similar analysis suggest that closure of PFO may help to reduce recurrent event rates, but randomized trials are still ongoing to address this very important question (98). A multicenter randomized RESPECT trial is under way to test the hypothesis that transcatheter closure with the Amplatzer PFO occluder (AGA Medical Corp., Golden Valley, MN) is not inferior to medical therapy. The 1,600 patient CLOSURE trial is ongoing in the United States to determine whether closure by the Starflex device (NMT Medical, Inc., Boston, MA) is superior to medical therapy. Unfortunately, the enrollment in these trials has been slow, and therefore it remains somewhat uncertain whether we will be able to resolve the question conclusively in a reasonable time.

Percutaneous closure of PFO is becoming increasingly common in the United States. Two devices (CardioSEAL PFO device and Amplatzer PFO occluder) are approved by the U.S. Food and Drug Administration for a restricted population (Figs. 79.7 and 79.8). Humanitarian device exemption for the nonsurgical closure of a PFO allows device use only in patients with recurrent cryptogenic stroke resulting from presumed paradoxic embolism through a PFO and in whom conventional drug therapy (therapeutic INR on oral anticoagulants)

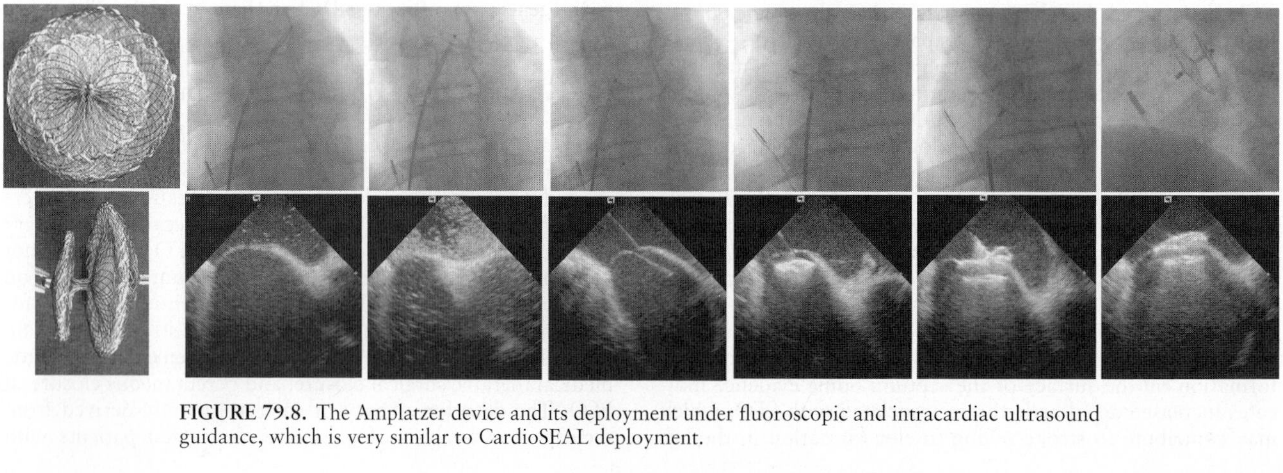

FIGURE 79.8. The Amplatzer device and its deployment under fluoroscopic and intracardiac ultrasound guidance, which is very similar to CardioSEAL deployment.

has failed. The CardioSEAL VSD device (which is similar to the PFO closure device approved under the humanitarian device exemption) and the Amplatzer septal occluder have been used with an off-label indication for closure of PFO. Patients with recurrent stroke who cannot tolerate or do not want to continue medical therapy and younger patients who have high-risk anatomic and/or functional characteristics can be considered for percutaneous closure using the latter devices.

PFO closure is typically done under fluoroscopic and intracardiac echocardiographic guidance in the catheterization laboratory. TEE guidance has been utilized in some institutions and may be less costly but more inconvenient for the patient. Transseptal puncture and septal inversion can be useful when attempting to close a PFO with long tunnel. Complete closure of the interatrial communication is considered to be the goal of any closure procedure because postprocedural shunt has been correlated in some studies with increased risk of recurrent embolic events. However, other studies have questioned this finding (99,100).

Multiple other devices are in clinical investigation including the Helex Occluder (W. L. Gore & Associates, Flagstaff, AZ), the Premere closure system (Velocimed, Inc., Minneapolis, MN), the Solysafe system (Swissimplant AG, Switzerland), the IntraSept Occluder (CARDIA, Inc., Burnsville, MN), the BioSTAR occluder (NMTMedical, Inc., Boston, MA), and the Sept Rx device (Secant Medical, Perkasie, PA). These devices have variable methods of anchoring and have different levels of flexibility in positioning and retrieval, if necessary, at different stages during delivery. The BioSTAR device is made up of biodegradable material. Many of these devices have short-term human data available from a small number of patients.

The many unknowns should caution us not to embrace a technology before establishing evidence-based indications. Cryptogenic stroke by definition is a diagnosis of elimination, limited by the thoroughness of investigation. Our current inability to differentiate between the "culprit" PFO and the "bystander" PFO may result in unnecessary implantation of closure devices in some patients. Usual investigations that help to exclude some of the commonly missed causes for cryptogenic stroke include hypercoagulation profile, Holter monitoring, and magnetic resonance angiography of the aortic arch and the carotid and vertebral arteries with intracranial evaluation. At the same time, efforts to develop safer and more effective closure devices are under way. These include devices with little or no metal component and those with biodegradable disks. Ideally, we should be able to identify the patients at risk before they sustain a stroke and should prevent it by closing the PFO with a device that would result in complete closure, would be made of material that conforms to both sides of the septum, and would have no risk of erosion, infection, arrhythmia, or thrombogenicity.

ATRIAL APPENDAGE OCCLUSION

Scope of the Problem

AF is responsible for more than 15% of all strokes (101–103). AF, whether intermittent or sustained, increases the risk for cardioembolic events leading to an overall annual stroke rate of 4.5% per year (103–105). Anticoagulation is highly effective in preventing embolic events in AF with a risk reduction of almost 70% and is superior to aspirin and aspirin in combination with low-intensity, fixed-dose warfarin treatment (104,106,107). However, warfarin therapy has many limitations including narrow therapeutic range, pharmacologic interactions, potential risk of major hemorrhage, and some restrictions in everyday life. Therefore, if stroke prevention can be achieved without anticoagulation, it would be very helpful to a large group of patients. Several surgical, echocardiographic, and autopsy studies have shown that more than 90% of all thrombi in patients with nonrheumatic AF forming in the left atrium originate in the left atrial appendage (LAA) (108–110). Consequently, either complete surgical excision/ligation or percutaneous obliteration of LAA makes intuitive sense.

Two devices are specifically designed to close the LAA that include the PLAATO (percutaneous LAA transcatheter occlusion) and the WATCHMAN device. The Amplatzer septal occluder has been used to close the LAA in a small series without long-term clinical follow-up (111).

PLAATO Device (ev3, Inc., Plymouth, MN)

The PLAATO device consists of a self-expanding nitinol cage (range of diameter, 15 to 32 mm) covered with expanded polytetrafluoroethylene to close off blood flow into the remaining part of the LAA (Fig. 79.9). Three rows of anchors along the struts help to stabilize the occluder in the appendage. This device has been tested in the safety and feasibility study in Europe and North America. This initial experience included 111 patients in 97% of whom the device was successfully implanted. Two patients, among those with a successful implant, developed ischemic stroke (173 and 215 days after the procedure). Mild leak (1- to 3-mm jet) was seen in 13% of the patients after the implant; however, both patients with stroke had trace or absent leak. TIA was seen in two additional patients. The annual stroke rate was determined to be 2.2%. This initial study demonstrated that LAA treatment could be accomplished safely with this device. However, more data are needed for long-term safety and efficacy of this intervention to prevent thromboembolic events.

WATCHMAN Device (Atritech, Inc., Plymouth, MN)

The WATCHMAN LAA system is made of nitinol with the atrial facing surface covered with a thin permeable polyester material (Fig. 79.10). This device has been tested in the feasibility study in which 66 patients were treated with this device. There is no reported stroke or systemic embolism. Two device-related embolisms occurred early in the study, but this defect has been corrected with design improvements. Seven procedural events occurred, including pericardial effusion, tamponade, or bleeding requiring transfusion.

Currently, a pivotal study of the WATCHMAN system is under way in the United States. The study is designed to demonstrate the safety and efficacy of the WATCHMAN device in patients with nonvalvular AF who require treatment for potential thrombus formation, are eligible for warfarin therapy, and who have at least one of the following risk factors: congestive heart failure, hypertension, age greater than 75 years, diabetes mellitus, and/or prior stroke or TIA. In the PROTECT AF (WATCHMAN LAA system for embolic protection in patients with AF), patients are randomized to this device or warfarin therapy.

CONTROVERSIES AND PERSONAL PERSPECTIVES

Percutaneous therapies for valvular heart disease that previously required open heart surgery have now been developed and offer tremendous promise. As with any new technology, the gap between the available animal and human trial data and

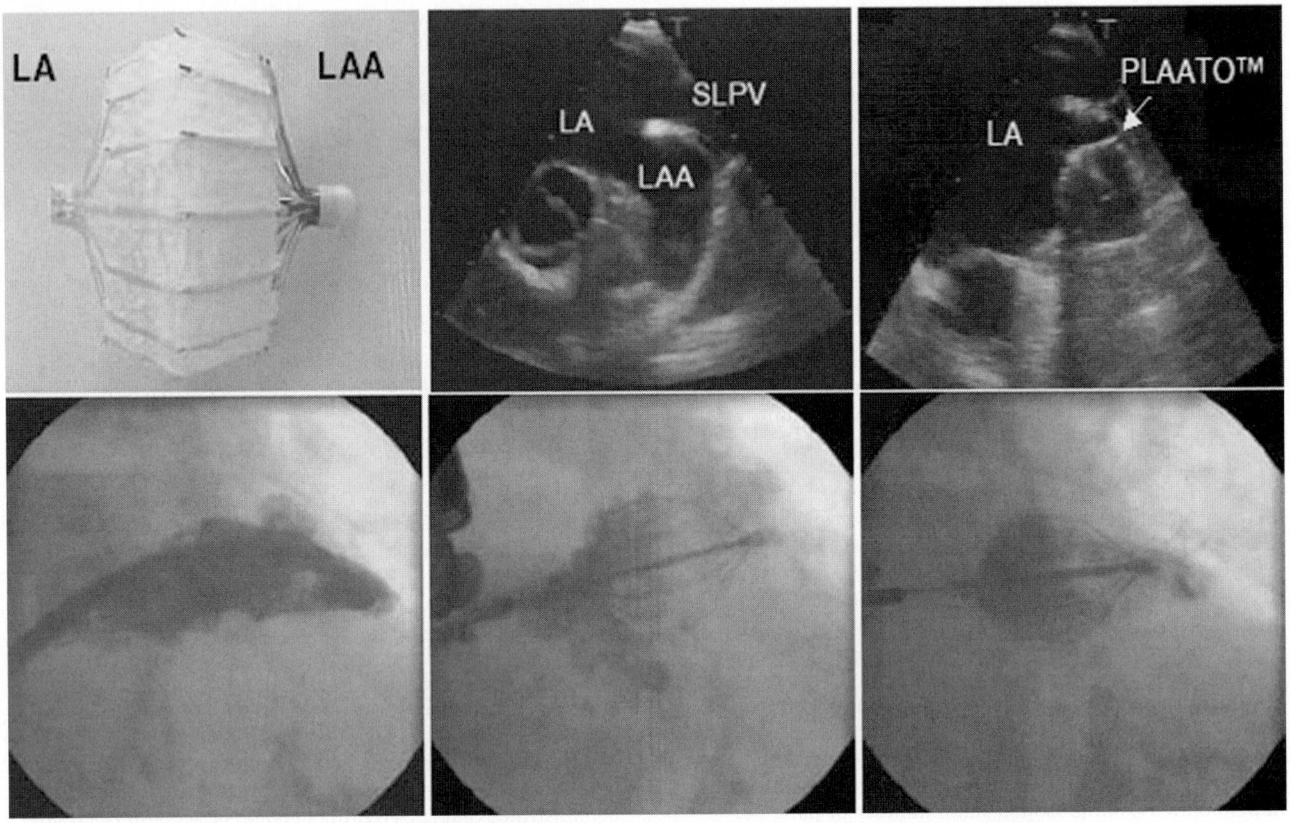

FIGURE 79.9. PLAATO device delivery under intracardiac echocardiographic and fluoroscopic guidance. LA, left atrium; LAA, left atrial appendage; SLPV, superior left pulmonary vein. Courtesy of manufacturer.

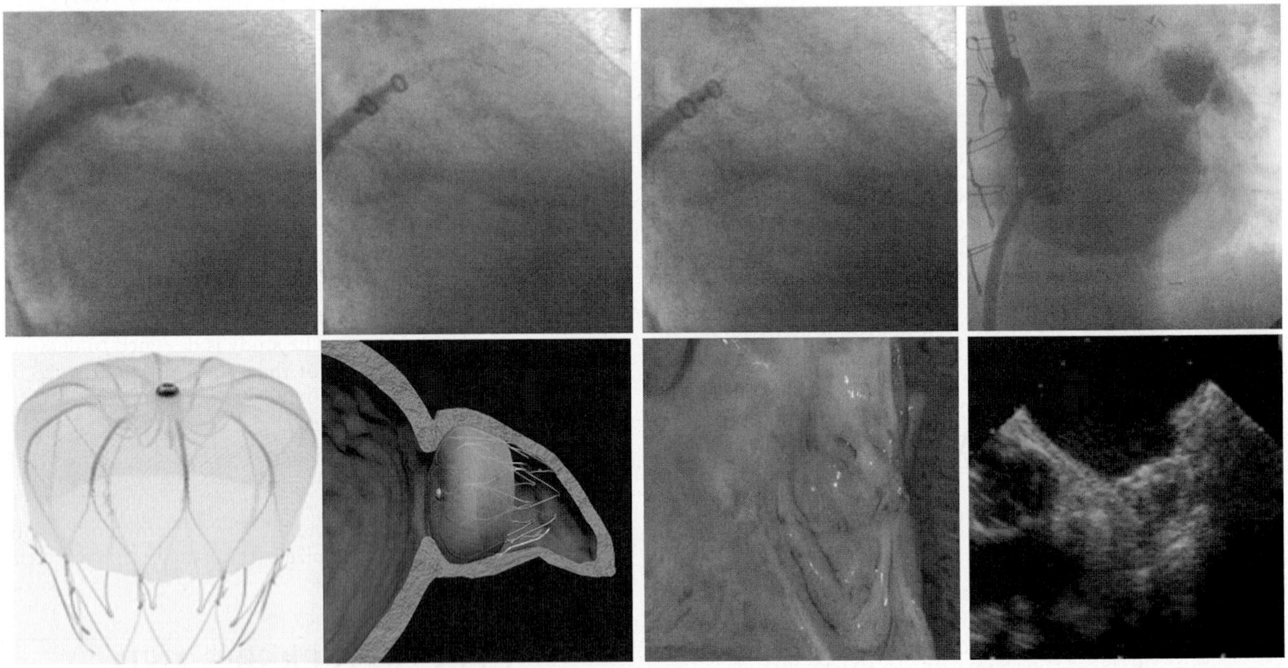

FIGURE 79.10. The WATCHMAN device. **Lower left:** The WATCHMAN Device. **Lower second panel:** It is inserted in the left atrial appendage (LAA) with filter toward the ostium of the appendage. **Lower third panel:** An endothelialized filter from an autopsy specimen 9 months after implantation. **Lower right:** Transesophageal echocardiographic (TEE) follow-up of a patient 45 days after the procedure. **Top:** Deployment under fluoroscopy. From **left** to **right** the LAA is visualized, the device is uncovered, and finally the position is confirmed with contrast injection. TEE guidance is used during deployment. Courtesy of manufacturer.

the potential application of these technologies is wide. Through dedicated investigation, this gap will likely be bridged over the coming years. Specifically, we need to demonstrate immediate feasibility and the long-term safety, durability, and efficacy of these devices in human studies. We will have to design clinical trials to compare these technologies with standard of care surgical treatments. This poses a unique challenge because there are few, if any, randomized trials to evaluate surgical techniques in valvular heart disease, and therefore study end points and methodology are debatable. The next challenge will be to disseminate the expertise required to perform these procedures in the interventional community, and this may require systematic training and collaboration of interventional and imaging specialists. However, initial studies are really promising, and the future for percutaneous treatment of valvular heart disease appears to be very bright.

On the front of PFO closure, the major challenge will be to identify the correct patient population that needs this procedure. There is a great likelihood that many patients could be subjected to unnecessary procedures if proper caution and restraint are not exercised by the scientific community. Rigorous studies with unbiased interpretation are essential in this field to characterize the need for PFO closure more definitively.

Atrial appendage closure is an evolving field with high promise. If this can be achieved safely and effectively, it will be a major help to many patients with AF. It is clear that the field of interventional cardiology is expanding at a furious pace and has a great future.

References

1. Lip GY, Singh SP, de Giovanni J. Percutaneous balloon valvuloplasty for congenital pulmonary valve stenosis in adults. *Clin Cardiol* 1999;22:733–737.
2. Cribier A, Eltchaninoff H, Letac B. Advances in percutaneous techniques for the treatment of aortic and mitral stenosis. In: Topol EJ, ed. *Textbook of interventional cardiology.* Philadelphia: WB Saunders, 2003:941–953.
3. Letac B, Cribier A, Koning R, Bellefleur JP. Results of percutaneous transluminal valvuloplasty in 218 adults with valvular aortic stenosis. *Am J Cardiol* 1988;62:598–605.
4. O'Neill WW. Predictors of long-term survival after percutaneous aortic valvuloplasty: report of the Mansfield Scientific Balloon Aortic Valvuloplasty Registry. *J Am Coll Cardiol* 1991;17:193–198.
5. Chan KL. Is aortic stenosis a preventable disease? *J Am Coll Cardiol* 2003; 42:593–599.
6. Kvidal P, Bergstrom R, Horte LG, Stahle E. Observed and relative survival after aortic valve replacement. *J Am Coll Cardiol* 2000;35:747–756.
7. Bessell JR, Gower G, Craddock DR, et al. Thirty years experience with heart valve surgery: isolated aortic valve replacement. *Aust N Z J Surg* 1996; 66:799–805.
8. Schwarz F, Baumann P, Manthey J, et al. The effect of aortic valve replacement on survival. *Circulation* 1982;66:1105–1110.
9. Anttila V, Heikkinen J, Biancari F, et al. A retrospective comparative study of aortic valve replacement with St. Jude Medical and Medtronic-Hall prostheses: a 20-year follow-up study. *Scand Cardiovasc J* 2002;36: 53–59.
10. Chiappini B, Bergonzini M, Gallieri S, et al. Clinical outcome of aortic valve replacement in the elderly. *Cardiovasc Surg* 2003;11:359–365.
11. Sharony R, Grossi EA, Saunders PC, et al. Aortic valve replacement in patients with impaired ventricular function. *Ann Thorac Surg* 2003;75:1808–1814.
12. Shanmugam G. Aortic valve replacement following previous coronary surgery. *Eur J Cardiothorac Surg* 2005;28:731–735.
13. Collart F, Feier H, Kerbaul F, et al. Valvular surgery in octogenarians: operative risks factors, evaluation of Euroscore and long term results. *Eur J Cardiothorac Surg* 2005;27:276–280.
14. Langanay T, De Latour B, Ligier K, et al. Surgery for aortic stenosis in octogenarians: influence of coronary disease and other comorbidities on hospital mortality. *J Heart Valve Dis* 2004;13:545-552; discussion 552–553.
15. Cribier A, Savin T, Saoudi N, et al. Percutaneous transluminal valvuloplasty of acquired aortic stenosis in elderly patients: an alternative to valve replacement? *Lancet* 1986;1:63–67.
16. McKay RG, Safian RD, Lock JE, et al. Balloon dilatation of calcific aortic stenosis in elderly patients: postmortem, intraoperative, and percutaneous valvuloplasty studies. *Circulation* 1986;74:119–125.
17. Letac B, Gerber LI, Koning R. Insights on the mechanism of balloon valvuloplasty in aortic stenosis. *Am J Cardiol* 1988;62:1241–1247.
18. Feldman T, Glagov S, Carroll JD. Restenosis following successful balloon valvuloplasty: bone formation in aortic valve leaflets. *Cathet Cardiovasc Diagn* 1993;29:1–7.
19. Eltchaninoff H, Cribier A, Tron C, et al. Balloon aortic valvuloplasty in elderly patients at high risk for surgery, or inoperable: immediate and mid-term results. *Eur Heart J* 1995;16:1079–1084.
20. Otto CM, Mickel MC, Kennedy JW, et al. Three-year outcome after balloon aortic valvuloplasty: insights into prognosis of valvular aortic stenosis. *Circulation* 1994;89:642–650.
21. Andersen HR, Knudsen LL, Hasenkam JM. Transluminal implantation of artificial heart valves: description of a new expandable aortic valve and initial results with implantation by catheter technique in closed chest pigs. *Eur Heart J* 1992;13:704–708.
22. Cribier A, Eltchaninoff H, Bareinstein N, et al. Trans-catheter implantation of balloon-expandable prosthetic heart valves: early results in an animal model. *Circulation* 2001;104(suppl II):552.
23. Cribier A, Eltchaninoff H, Bash A, et al. Percutaneous transcatheter implantation of an aortic valve prosthesis for calcific aortic stenosis: first human case description. *Circulation* 2002;106:3006–3008.
24. Eltchaninoff H, Tron C, Cribier A. Percutaneous implantation of aortic valve prosthesis in patients with calcific aortic stenosis: technical aspects. *J Interv Cardiol* 2003;16:515–521.
25. Cribier A, Eltchaninoff H, Tron C, et al. Early experience with percutaneous transcatheter implantation of heart valve prosthesis for the treatment of end-stage inoperable patients with calcific aortic stenosis. *J Am Coll Cardiol* 2004;43:698–703.
26. Khambadkone S, Bonhoeffer P. Nonsurgical pulmonary valve replacement: why, when, and how? *Cathet Cardiovasc Interv* 2004;62:401–408.
27. de Ruijter FT, Weenink I, Hitchcock FJ, et al. Right ventricular dysfunction and pulmonary valve replacement after correction of tetralogy of Fallot. *Ann Thorac Surg* 2002;73:1794-1800; discussion 1800.
28. Dittrich S, Vogel M, Dahnert I, et al. Surgical repair of tetralogy of Fallot in adults today. *Clin Cardiol* 1999;22:460–464.
29. Dearani JA, Danielson GK, Puga FJ, et al. Late follow-up of 1095 patients undergoing operation for complex congenital heart disease utilizing pulmonary ventricle to pulmonary artery conduits. *Ann Thorac Surg* 2003;75:399–410; discussion 410–411.
30. Park MK. Cyanotic congenital heart defects. In: Park MK, ed. *Pediatric cardiology for practitioners.* St Louis: Mosby, 2002:174–240.
31. Therrien J, Marx GR, Gatzoulis MA. Late problems in tetralogy of Fallot: recognition, management, and prevention. *Cardiol Clin* 2002;20:395–404.
32. Ovaert C, Caldarone CA, McCrindle BW, et al. Endovascular stent implantation for the management of postoperative right ventricular outflow tract obstruction: clinical efficacy. *J Thorac Cardiovasc Surg* 1999;118:886–893.
33. Bonhoeffer P, Boudjemline Y, Saliba Z, et al. Percutaneous replacement of pulmonary valve in a right-ventricle to pulmonary-artery prosthetic conduit with valve dysfunction. *Lancet* 2000;356:1403–1405.
34. Bonhoeffer P, Boudjemline Y, Saliba Z, et al. Transcatheter implantation of a bovine valve in pulmonary position: a lamb study. *Circulation* 2000;102: 813–816.
35. Bonhoeffer P, Boudjemline Y, Qureshi SA, et al. Percutaneous insertion of the pulmonary valve. *J Am Coll Cardiol* 2002;39:1664–1669.
36. Boudjemline Y, Bonhoeffer P. Steps toward percutaneous aortic valve replacement. *Circulation* 2002;105:775–778.
37. Boudjemline Y, Agnoletti G, Bonnet D, et al. Percutaneous pulmonary valve replacement in a large right ventricular outflow tract: an experimental study. *J Am Coll Cardiol* 2004;43:1082–1087.
38. Khambadkone S, Coats L, Taylor A, et al. Percutaneous pulmonary valve implantation in humans: results in 59 consecutive patients. *Circulation* 2005;112:1189–1197.
39. Enriquez-Sarano M, Schaff HV, Frye RL. Mitral regurgitation: what causes the leakage is fundamental to the outcome of valve repair. *Circulation* 2003; 108:253–256.
40. Thourani VH, Weintraub WS, Guyton RA, et al. Outcomes and long-term survival for patients undergoing mitral valve repair versus replacement: effect of age and concomitant coronary artery bypass grafting. *Circulation* 2003;108:298–304.
41. Goldman ME, Mora F, Guarino T, et al. Mitral valvuloplasty is superior to valve replacement for preservation of left ventricular function: an intraoperative two-dimensional echocardiographic study. *J Am Coll Cardiol* 1987; 10:568–575.
42. Carpentier A, Chauvaud S, Fabiani JN, et al. Reconstructive surgery of mitral valve incompetence: ten-year appraisal. *J Thorac Cardiovasc Surg* 1980;79:338–348.
43. Cosgrove DM 3rd, Arcidi JM, Rodriguez L, et al. Initial experience with the Cosgrove-Edwards annuloplasty system. *Ann Thorac Surg* 1995;60:499–503; discussion 503–4.
44. Carpentier AF, Lessana A, Relland JY, et al. The "physio-ring": an advanced concept in mitral valve annuloplasty. *Ann Thorac Surg* 1995;60: 1177–1185; discussion 1185–1186.
45. Fasol R, Mahdjoobian K. Repair of mitral valve billowing and prolapse (Barlow): the surgical technique. *Ann Thorac Surg* 2002;74:602–605.
46. Gillinov AM, Cosgrove DM. Mitral valve repair for degenerative disease. *J Heart Valve Dis* 2002;11(suppl 1):S15–S20.

47. Gillinov AM, Cosgrove DM 3rd, Shiota T, et al. Cosgrove-Edwards annuloplasty system: midterm results. *Ann Thorac Surg* 2000;69:717–721.
48. Otsuji Y, Handschumacher MD, Schwammenthal E, et al. Insights from three-dimensional echocardiography into the mechanism of functional mitral regurgitation: direct in vivo demonstration of altered leaflet tethering geometry. *Circulation* 1997;96:1999–2008.
49. Miller DC. Ischemic mitral regurgitation redux–to repair or to replace? *J Thorac Cardiovasc Surg* 2001;122:1059–1062.
50. Grossi EA, Goldberg JD, LaPietra A, et al. Ischemic mitral valve reconstruction and replacement: comparison of long-term survival and complications. *J Thorac Cardiovasc Surg* 2001;122:1107–1124.
51. Gillinov AM, Wierup PN, Blackstone EH, et al. Is repair preferable to replacement for ischemic mitral regurgitation? *J Thorac Cardiovasc Surg* 2001;122:1125–1141.
52. Alfieri O, De Bonis M, Lapenna E, et al. "Edge-to-edge" repair for anterior mitral leaflet prolapse. *Semin Thorac Cardiovasc Surg* 2004;16:182–187.
53. Bhudia SK, McCarthy PM, Smedira NG, et al. Edge-to-edge (Alfieri) mitral repair: results in diverse clinical settings. *Ann Thorac Surg* 2004;77:1598–1606.
54. Maisano F, Torracca L, Oppizzi M, et al. The edge-to-edge technique: a simplified method to correct mitral insufficiency. *Eur J Cardiothorac Surg* 1998;13:240–245; discussion 245–246.
55. Alfieri O, Maisano F, De Bonis M, et al. The double-orifice technique in mitral valve repair: a simple solution for complex problems. *J Thorac Cardiovasc Surg* 2001;122:674–681.
56. Agricola E, Maisano F, Oppizzi M, et al. Mitral valve reserve in double-orifice technique: an exercise echocardiographic study. *J Heart Valve Dis* 2002;11:637–643.
57. Kaye DM, Byrne M, Alferness C, Power J. Feasibility and short-term efficacy of percutaneous mitral annular reduction for the therapy of heart failure-induced mitral regurgitation. *Circulation* 2003;108:1795–1797.
58. Liddicoat JR, MacNeill BD, Gillinov AM, et al. Percutaneous mitral valve repair: a feasibility study in an ovine model of acute ischemic mitral regurgitation. *Cathet Cardiovasc Interv* 2003;60:410–416.
58a. Mishra YK, Mittal S, Jaguri P, et al. Coapsys mitral annuloplasty for chronic functional ischemic regurgitation: 1-year results. *Ann Thorac Surg* 2006;81:42–46.
59. St Goar FG, Fann JI, Komtebedde J, et al. Endovascular edge-to-edge mitral valve repair: short-term results in a porcine model. *Circulation* 2003;108: 1990–1993.
59a. Boudjemline Y, Agnoletti G, Bonnet D, et al. Steps toward the percutaneous replacement of atrioventricular valves: an experimental study. *J Am Coll Cardiol* 2005;46:360–365.
60. Godart F, Rey C, Prat A, et al. Atrial right-to-left shunting causing severe hypoxaemia despite normal right-sided pressures: report of 11 consecutive cases corrected by percutaneous closure. *Eur Heart J* 2000;21:483–489.
61. Wilmshurst PT. The persistent foramen ovale and migraine. *Rev Neurol (Paris)* 2005;161:671–674.
62. Horton SC, Bunch TJ. Patent foramen ovale and stroke. *Mayo Clin Proc* 2004;79:79–88.
63. Cheng TO. The proper conduct of Valsalva maneuver in the detection of patent foramen ovale. *J Am Coll Cardiol* 2005;45:1145–1146.
64. Gin KG, Huckell VF, Pollick C. Femoral vein delivery of contrast medium enhances transthoracic echocardiographic detection of patent foramen ovale. *J Am Coll Cardiol* 1993;22:1994–2000.
65. Di Tullio M, Sacco RL, Venketasubramanian N, et al. Comparison of diagnostic techniques for the detection of a patent foramen ovale in stroke patients. *Stroke* 1993;24:1020–1024.
66. Sacco RL, Ellenberg JH, Mohr JP, et al. Infarcts of undetermined cause: the NINCDS Stroke Data Bank. *Ann Neurol* 1989;25:382–390.
67. Sacco RL, Shi T, Zamanillo MC, Kargman DE. Predictors of mortality and recurrence after hospitalized cerebral infarction in an urban community: the Northern Manhattan Stroke Study. *Neurology* 1994;44:626–634.
68. Overell JR, Bone I, Lees KR. Interatrial septal abnormalities and stroke: a meta-analysis of case-control studies. *Neurology* 2000;55:1172–1179.
69. Job FP, Ringelstein EB, Grafen Y, et al. Comparison of transcranial contrast Doppler sonography and transesophageal contrast echocardiography for the detection of patent foramen ovale in young stroke patients. *Am J Cardiol* 1994;74:381–384.
70. Stone DA, Godard J, Corretti MC, et al. Patent foramen ovale: association between the degree of shunt by contrast transesophageal echocardiography and the risk of future ischemic neurologic events. *Am Heart J* 1996;131:158–161.
71. Schuchlenz HW, Weihs W, Horner S, Quehenberger F. The association between the diameter of a patent foramen ovale and the risk of embolic cerebrovascular events. *Am J Med* 2000;109:456–462.
72. Serena J, Segura T, Perez-Ayuso MJ, et al. The need to quantify right-to-left shunt in acute ischemic stroke: a case-control study. *Stroke* 1998;29:1322–1328.
73. Schwerzmann M, Wiher S, Nedeltchev K, et al. Percutaneous closure of patent foramen ovale reduces the frequency of migraine attacks. *Neurology* 2004;62:1399–1401.
74. Schwerzmann M, Nedeltchev K, Lagger F, et al. Prevalence and size of directly detected patent foramen ovale in migraine with aura. *Neurology* 2005;65:1415–1418.
75. Anzola GP, Magoni M, Guindani M, et al. Potential source of cerebral embolism in migraine with aura: a transcranial Doppler study. *Neurology* 1999;52:1622–1625.
76. Finsterer J, Sommer O, Stiskal M, et al. Closure of a patent foramen ovale: effective therapy of migraine and occipital stroke. *Int J Neurosci* 2005;115:119–127.
77. Reisman M, Christofferson RD, Jesurum J, et al. Migraine headache relief after transcatheter closure of patent foramen ovale. *J Am Coll Cardiol* 2005;45:493–495.
78. Bousser MG, Welch KM. Relation between migraine and stroke. *Lancet Neurol* 2005;4:533–542.
79. Robin ED, Laman D, Horn BR, Theodore J. Platypnea related to orthodeoxia caused by true vascular lung shunts. *N Engl J Med* 1976;294:941–943.
80. Altman M, Robin ED. Platypnea (diffuse zone I phenomenon?). *N Engl J Med* 1969;281:1347–1348.
81. Eicher JC, Bonniaud P, Baudouin N, et al. Hypoxaemia associated with an enlarged aortic root: a new syndrome?. *Heart* 2005;91:1030–1035.
82. Smeenk FW, Postmus PE. Interatrial right-to-left shunting developing after pulmonary resection in the absence of elevated right-sided heart pressures: review of the literature. *Chest* 1993;103:528–531.
83. Seward JB, Hayes DL, Smith HC, et al. Platypnea-orthodeoxia: clinical profile, diagnostic workup, management, and report of seven cases. *Mayo Clin Proc* 1984;59:221–231.
84. Herregods MC, Timmermans C, Frans E, et al. Diagnostic value of transesophageal echocardiography in platypnea. *J Am Soc Echocardiogr* 1993;6:624–627.
85. Germonpre P, Dendale P, Unger P, Balestra C. Patent foramen ovale and decompression sickness in sports divers. *J Appl Physiol* 1998;84:1622–1626.
86. Germonpre P, Hastir F, Dendale P, et al. Evidence for increasing patency of the foramen ovale in divers. *Am J Cardiol* 2005;95:912–915.
87. Knauth M, Ries S, Pohimann S, et al. Cohort study of multiple brain lesions in sport divers: role of a patent foramen ovale. *BMJ* 1997;314:701–705.
88. Saary MJ, Gray GW. A review of the relationship between patent foramen ovale and type II decompression sickness. *Aviat Space Environ Med* 2001;72:1113–1120.
89. Powell MR, Norfleet WT, Kumar KV, Butler BD. Patent foramen ovale and hypobaric decompression. *Aviat Space Environ Med* 1995;66:273–275.
90. Orgera MA, O'Malley PG, Taylor AJ. Secondary prevention of cerebral ischemia in patent foramen ovale: systematic review and meta-analysis. *South Med J* 2001;94:699–703.
91. Cujec B, Mainra R, Johnson DH. Prevention of recurrent cerebral ischemic events in patients with patent foramen ovale and cryptogenic strokes or transient ischemic attacks. *Can J Cardiol* 1999;15:57–64.
92. Hara H, Virmani R, Ladich E, et al. Patent foramen ovale: current pathology, pathophysiology, and clinical status. *J Am Coll Cardiol* 2005;46:1768–1776.
93. Sacco RL, Di Tullio MR, Homma S. Treatment of patent foramen ovale and stroke: to close or not to close, that is not yet the question. *Eur Neurol* 1997;37:205–206.
94. Nendaz M, Sarasin FP, Bogousslavsky J. How to prevent stroke recurrence in patients with patent foramen ovale: anticoagulants, antiaggregants, foramen closure, or nothing? *Eur Neurol* 1997;37:199–204.
95. Homma S, Sacco RL, Di Tullio MR, et al. Effect of medical treatment in stroke patients with patent foramen ovale: patent foramen ovale in Cryptogenic Stroke Study. *Circulation* 2002;105:2625–2631.
96. Halperin JL, Fuster V. Patent foramen ovale and recurrent stroke: another paradoxical twist. *Circulation* 2002;105:2580–2582.
97. Mas JL, Zuber M. Recurrent cerebrovascular events in patients with patent foramen ovale, atrial septal aneurysm, or both and cryptogenic stroke or transient ischemic attack: French Study Group on Patent Foramen Ovale and Atrial Septal Aneurysm. *Am Heart J* 1995;130:1083–1088.
98. Nendaz MR, Sarasin FP, Junod AF, Bogousslavsky J. Preventing stroke recurrence in patients with patent foramen ovale: antithrombotic therapy, foramen closure, or therapeutic abstention? A decision analytic perspective. *Am Heart J* 1998;135:532–541.
99. Windecker S, Wahl A, Chatterjee T, et al. Percutaneous closure of patent foramen ovale in patients with paradoxical embolism: long-term risk of recurrent thromboembolic events. *Circulation* 2000;101:893–898.
100. Schwerzmann M, Windecker S, Wahl A, et al. Percutaneous closure of patent foramen ovale: impact of device design on safety and efficacy. *Heart* 2004;90:186–190.
101. Kannel WB, Wolf PA, Benjamin EJ, Levy D. Prevalence, incidence, prognosis, and predisposing conditions for atrial fibrillation: population-based estimates. *Am J Cardiol* 1998;82:2N–9N.
102. Sandercock P, Bamford J, Dennis M, et al. Atrial fibrillation and stroke: prevalence in different types of stroke and influence on early and long term prognosis (Oxfordshire community stroke project). *BMJ* 1992;305:1460–1465.
103. Wolf PA, Benjamin EJ, Belanger AJ, et al. Secular trends in the prevalence of atrial fibrillation: the Framingham Study. *Am Heart J* 1996;131:790–795.
104. Risk factors for stroke and efficacy of antithrombotic therapy in atrial fibrillation: analysis of pooled data from five randomized controlled trials. *Arch Intern Med* 1994;154:1449–1457.

105. Hart RG, Pearce LA, Rothbart RM, et al. Stroke with intermittent atrial fibrillation: incidence and predictors during aspirin therapy: Stroke Prevention in Atrial Fibrillation Investigators. *J Am Coll Cardiol* 2000;35:183–187.
106. Hart RG, Halperin JL, Pearce LA, et al. Lessons from the Stroke Prevention in Atrial Fibrillation trials. *Ann Intern Med* 2003;138:831–838.
107. van Walraven C, Hart RG, Singer DE, et al. Oral anticoagulants vs aspirin in nonvalvular atrial fibrillation: an individual patient meta-analysis. *JAMA* 2002;288:2441–2448.
108. Aberg H. Atrial fibrillation. I. A study of atrial thrombosis and systemic embolism in a necropsy material. *Acta Med Scand* 1969;185:373–379.
109. Stoddard MF, Dawkins PR, Prince CR, Ammash NM. Left atrial appendage thrombus is not uncommon in patients with acute atrial fibrillation and a recent embolic event: a transesophageal echocardiographic study. *J Am Coll Cardiol* 1995;25:452–459.
110. Blackshear JL, Odell JA. Appendage obliteration to reduce stroke in cardiac surgical patients with atrial fibrillation. *Ann Thorac Surg* 1996;61:755–759.
111. Meier B, Palacios I, Windecker S, et al. Transcatheter left atrial appendage occlusion with Amplatzer devices to obviate anticoagulation in patients with atrial fibrillation. *Cathet Cardiovasc Interv* 2003;60:417–422.
112. Bolling SF, Deeb GM, Brunsting LA, Bach DS. Early outcome of mitral valve reconstruction in patients with end-stage cardiomyopathy. *J Thorac Cardiovasc Surg* 1995;109:676–682; discussion 682–683.
113. Calafiore AM, Gallina S, Di Mauro M, et al. Mitral valve procedure in dilated cardiomyopathy: repair or replacement? *Ann Thorac Surg* 2001;71:1146–1152; discussion 1152–1153.
114. Szalay ZA, Civelek A, Hohe S, et al. Mitral annuloplasty in patients with ischemic versus dilated cardiomyopathy. *Eur J Cardiothorac Surg* 2003;23: 567–572.
115. Piciche M, El Khoury G, D'Udekem D'akoz Y, Noirhomme P. Surgical repair for degenerative and rheumatic mitral valve disease: operative and mid-term results. *J Cardiovasc Surg (Torino)* 2002;43:327–335.

CHAPTER 80 ■ CORONARY ARTERY BYPASS SURGERY

JOSEPH F. SABIK, III

OVERVIEW

The discovery of coronary cineangiography by Mason Sones at the Cleveland Clinic in Cleveland, Ohio, in the 1960s laid the foundation for the development of coronary artery bypass surgery (1). Now in its fourth decade, coronary artery bypass surgery is one of the great success stories of medicine. It has been shown to prolong survival, relieve angina, and improve exercise tolerance in patients with coronary artery disease. Excellent early and late outcomes are the result of advances in surgical technique, myocardial protection, conduit selection, anesthesia, and postoperative care.

HISTORY

In 1951, Vineberg and Miller reported on direct implantation of an internal thoracic artery into the myocardium to improve blood flow (2). Although this operation was shown to improve myocardial blood flow, the blood flow of the implant was too limited in quantity and distribution to be effective (3). Other early approaches to improving myocardial blood flow included coronary endarterectomy by Longmire and patch grafting by Senning (4,5).

Kolessov in Leningrad, Effler and Favaloro in Cleveland, and Garrett and DeBakey in Houston, Texas, were some of the first surgeons in the 1960s to treat coronary artery disease directly with bypass grafts (6–9). With the development of selective coronary cineangiography by Mason Sones, Rene Favaloro at the Cleveland Clinic demonstrated the safety and efficacy of using saphenous vein as conduits in the treatment of left main, single-vessel, and multivessel coronary artery disease. By 1971, this group had performed more than 700 surgical myocardial revascularizations with saphenous veins (10).

The first direct left internal thoracic artery to left anterior coronary artery bypass revascularization was performed by Demikov in 1953; and in 1967, Kolessov reported performing the same procedure (11,12). Green and colleagues were early proponents of using internal thoracic arteries as bypass grafts and in the 1970s popularized its use (13). Growth of surgical myocardial revascularization exploded, and within a decade it became the most common surgical procedure performed in the United States (14).

INDICATIONS

Chronic Stable Angina

The goals of surgical myocardial revascularization are to prolong life, relieve angina, preserve myocardial function, and improve exercise capacity. Much of what is known about the indications for coronary surgery was obtained from the randomized trials of the 1970s, which compared initial surgical therapy with medical therapy for patients with mild to moderate angina and coronary artery disease. These studies were the Veterans Administration Study, the European Cooperative Surgical Study, and the Coronary Artery Surgery Study (15–22). Although patient inclusion criteria for the these trials were different, all three studies had the same objective: to determine whether initial coronary artery bypass surgery or medical therapy improved the survival of patients with surgically approachable coronary artery disease and mild to moderate angina. In applying the findings of these trials to identify patients who benefit from surgical revascularization, it is important to appreciate that only low-risk, stable, male patients were included in these trials. In addition, since the randomized studies were conducted, substantial improvements in both the surgical and medical therapy of coronary artery disease have occurred. These include lipid-lowering drugs, antiplatelet agents, β-blockers, angiotensin-converting enzyme inhibitors, internal thoracic artery grafting, better myocardial protection, and

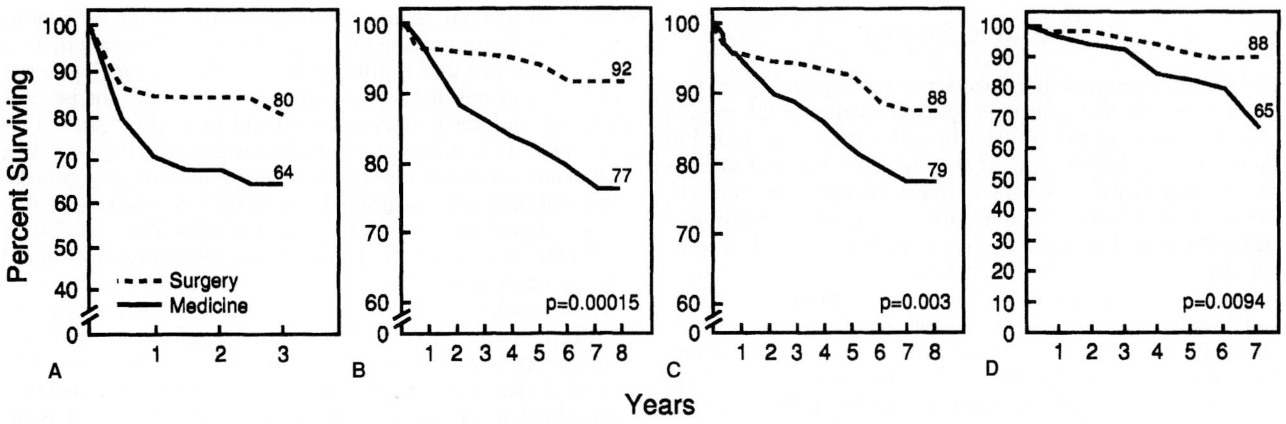

FIGURE 80.1. Survival from published randomized trials comparing coronary artery bypass surgery with medical treatment. **A:** The original Veterans Administration Coronary Arterial Disease Study, which randomly allocated 113 patients with severe left main coronary narrowing to medical or surgical treatment from 1970 to 1974. The 3-year survival was 80% for surgery and 64% for medicine. **B:** Long-term results of patients with two- and three-vessel disease from the European Coronary Surgery Study Group are depicted in this panel. Actuarial survival curves for patients with three-vessel disease who had an 8-year survival of 92% for surgery and 77% for medicine ($p = .00015$). **C:** In the subgroup of patients with more than 50% narrowing in the proximal third of the anterior descending coronary artery, there was a highly significant difference in favor of surgery in both two- and three-vessel disease subsets. **D:** Seven-year cumulative survival rates for surgery and medical patients from the randomized trial of the coronary artery surgery study. The surgical survival of 88% was significantly better ($p = .012$) than medical treatment when the left ventricular ejection fraction was less than 0.50. (Data from Takaro T, Hultgren HN, Lipton MJ, et al. The VA Cooperative randomized study of surgery for coronary arterial occlusive disease II. Subgroup with significant left main lesions. *Circulation* 1976;54(suppl III):III107–III117; European Coronary Surgery Study Group. Long-term results of prospective randomised study of coronary artery bypass surgery in stable angina pectoris. *Lancet* 1982;2;1173–1180; and Passamani E, Davis KB, Gillespie MJ, et al. A randomized trial of coronary artery bypass surgery: survival of patients with a low ejection fraction. *N Engl J Med* 1985;312:1665–1671.)

percutaneous coronary intervention. The randomized trials found both clinical and angiographic factors, such as location and extent of coronary disease, left ventricular dysfunction, severity of angina, and stress testing, useful in identifying patients in whom surgical revascularization is indicated.

Survival

Improved survival was found in patients treated with surgical revascularization who had left main disease (stenosis ≥50%), left main equivalent disease (stenosis ≥70% of the proximal left anterior descending and circumflex), three-vessel coronary artery disease (stenosis ≥50% in three epicardial coronary arteries), or one- or two-vessel disease that included the proximal left anterior descending coronary artery (stenosis ≥50% in one or two coronary arteries including the left anterior descending artery) (Fig. 80.1) (16,17,22). Patients with worse left ventricular dysfunction derived more survival benefit from surgical revascularization than patients with normal ventricular function, and similarly patients with greater clinical risk factors (severity of angina, positive stress tests, ST-segment depression at rest, history of myocardial infarction, and hypertension) derived more survival benefit from surgical revascularization than patients with few or no risk factors (16,18,22). The more severe the coronary disease, symptoms, and left ventricular dysfunction, the greater was the benefit of surgical revascularization over medical therapy on survival (15,17).

As stated earlier, these trials demonstrated the importance of left ventricular dysfunction in determining which patients obtain a survival benefit from coronary artery bypass surgery (22). However, no patients included in the randomized trials had an ejection fraction less than 35%. Observational studies have demonstrated a survival benefit of surgical revascularization in patients with coronary artery disease and ejection fractions less than 35%, particularly when the patients' primary symptom was angina (suggesting myocardial viability), and not dyspnea (suggesting myocardial scarring) (23–25). In the Coronary Artery Surgery Study Registry, patients whose primary symptom was angina derived a survival advantage with coronary surgery, whereas those whose primary symptom was dyspnea did not (23). This was an early demonstration of the importance of myocardial viability in determining which patients with ventricular dysfunction benefit from surgical revascularization. Noninvasive tests, such as positron emission tomographic scanning, radioisotope imaging, and dobutamine echocardiography, can be used to identify hibernating (viable but nonfunctioning) myocardium to help determine which patients with left ventricular dysfunction may benefit from revascularization (26–32). Observational studies have shown both a functional and a survival advantage of surgical revascularization in patients with left ventricular dysfunction and substantial myocardial viability on preoperative testing (33).

Quality of Life

In addition to prolonging life, coronary artery bypass surgery was found in the randomized trials to be more effective than medical therapy in decreasing the symptoms of ischemia and in improving quality of life. These studies demonstrated a decrease in angina, an increase in exercise capacity, and a decrease in antianginal medical therapy in patients treated surgically independent of the severity of coronary artery disease (18,21). However, the risk of subsequent myocardial infarction was not lowered in the surgically treated patients in the randomized trials, although registry studies have suggested a lower risk of subsequent myocardial infarctions in patients treated with surgical revascularization.

Unstable Angina

Early studies reported that coronary artery bypass surgery was effective in relieving ischemia in patients with unstable angina (34). However, no survival benefit with surgery was found in these early studies because of the increased hospital mortality of surgical patients with unstable angina. Not until the randomized Veterans Administration Cooperative Study was surgical revascularization found to improve survival in some subsets of patients with unstable angina (35–37). This study compared the outcomes of patients with unstable angina who were treated either medically or surgically. Patients were classified by extent of coronary artery disease, ventricular dysfunction, and severity of unstable angina. Patients with left main stenosis were excluded. Coronary revascularization was found to improve survival in patients with (a) triple-vessel coronary artery disease; (b) left ventricular dysfunction, and (c) both left ventricular dysfunction and severe angina at rest (ST-segment and T-wave changes) (36). In addition, the Veterans Administration Cooperative Study also found that quality of life was better in surgically treated patients. Patients treated with coronary revascularization were found to have less angina, to require less antianginal medication, to have increased exercise tolerance, and to have fewer hospital admissions for cardiovascular reasons than patients treated medically (36,37).

Acute Myocardial Infarction

Acute myocardial infarctions are mostly treated with thrombolytic therapy or percutaneous intervention. However, emergency surgical revascularization has been demonstrated to improve survival, especially if it can be performed within 6 hours of the onset of symptoms (38,39).

TECHNIQUE OF OPERATION

The goal of coronary artery surgery is to obtain complete revascularization by bypassing all coronary arteries of sufficient size that have proximal stenosis $\geq 50\%$. The two most commonly used bypass graft conduits are saphenous veins and internal thoracic arteries. Less commonly used arterial grafts include radial, gastroepiploic, and inferior epigastric arteries. Most coronary artery bypass operations are performed through a median sternotomy. This approach has multiple advantages: (a) access to the ascending aorta and right atrium for central cannulation during on-pump procedures, (b) access to all coronary arteries, (c) ability to harvest both internal thoracic arteries and the right gastroepiploic artery, and (d) ability to perform concomitant cardiac procedures such as valve or aortic replacement. Other approaches that are useful in specific situations of limited coronary revascularization include anterior and lateral thoracotomies, partial sternotomies, parasternotomies, and epigastric incisions (40). Conduit harvesting and preparation occur during and after completion of the median sternotomy. Today, coronary artery bypass surgery is usually performed with the assistance of cardiopulmonary bypass and cardioplegic myocardial arrest (*on-pump*) or without the assistance of cardiopulmonary bypass on a beating heart (*off-pump*).

On-Pump Procedure

After the median sternotomy has been completed and all bypass conduits have been harvested, cannulation for cardiopulmonary bypass is performed. Heparin is administered, and cannulation is attained by placing cannulas in the ascending aorta for arterial return and in the right atrium for venous drainage. Before cannulation, the aorta should be evaluated for atherosclerosis, and if atherosclerosis makes ascending aortic cannulation unsafe, the ascending aorta should not be cannulated, and the axillary artery should be used for arterial return (41,42). Cardioplegia cannulas are placed in the ascending aorta and coronary sinus for both antegrade and retrograde delivery of cardioplegia during the period of myocardial ischemia.

Cardiopulmonary bypass is begun with flows of 2.0 to 2.2 L/m^2 per minute. Systemic arterial blood pressure should be maintained between 50 and 70 mm Hg. In patients with cerebrovascular occlusive arterial disease, it may be beneficial to keep systemic arterial blood pressure higher to maintain adequate cerebral perfusion and prevent neurologic injury. The aorta is clamped proximal to the arterial cannula, thus keeping blood from perfusing the myocardium. The heart is arrested and protected with first antegrade and then retrograde cardioplegia. Cardioplegia should be administered every 15 to 30 minutes during myocardial ischemia. Construction of the coronary artery bypass grafts is then performed. The distal bypass graft to coronary artery anastomoses are constructed first, and then the proximal bypass graft to aortic anastomoses are performed. To reduce the risk of arterial embolization, it is best to perform the proximal anastomoses during the cross-clamp period, thus eliminating the need for tangential and multiple clampings of the aorta. After all bypass graft anastomoses are completed, the aorta is unclamped, allowing blood to perfuse the myocardium once again. When the heart has recovered, weaning from cardiopulmonary bypass is performed, and the cannulas are removed.

Off-Pump Procedure

During off-pump surgery, a major challenge is to be able to position the heart to permit access to all coronary arteries while maintaining adequate hemodynamics and cardiac output. After completion of the median sternotomy and harvesting of bypass conduits, the patient is placed in the Trendelenburg position. This increases preload and helps to maintain cardiac output while the heart is positioned. Next, the operating table is rotated to the right. Because of gravity, the heart rotates to the right, bringing the apex out of the chest and exposing the lateral, inferior, and posterior surfaces of the heart. As the heart is retracted to the right, the right ventricle becomes compressed against the pericardium. To avoid right ventricular compression and hemodynamic collapse, the right pleura is incised along the sternum, and the pericardium is incised posteriorly along the right diaphragm down toward the inferior vena cava. This allows the heart to move into the right side of the chest, thus assisting with exposure of the coronary arteries and preventing right ventricular compression.

To improve exposure of the coronary arteries, traction can be placed on pericardial sutures or on an apical suction device. Coronary artery stabilization is obtained with either compression or suction stabilizers. These stabilizers allow for performance of the coronary to bypass graft anastomosis in a motionless field.

To obtain a bloodless operating field and to prevent ischemia during the construction of the distal anastomosis, intravascular coronary shunts or proximal and distal silastic loops can be used. Heparin is administered before grafting.

The sequence of grafting is important when performing off-pump revascularization. The grafting sequence should be individualized for each patient, depending on anatomic patterns of coronary occlusion and collateralization. The goal is to avoid making large areas of the myocardium ischemic simultaneously. In general, perform bypass grafts to completely occluded, collateralized coronary arteries before grafting collateralizing arteries. The left internal thoracic artery graft to the left anterior descending bypass graft should be performed early, especially if the left anterior descending is occluded or there is left main stenosis. Proximal anastomosis may be constructed to in situ arterial grafts or to the aorta.

After the patient is decannulated in *on-pump* procedures and after all bypass grafts are completed in *off-pump* procedures, heparin is reversed with protamine, and the incisions are closed. Aspirin should be administered 6 to 8 hours postoperatively and continued for at least 1 year.

CONDUITS

Saphenous Vein

The first conduit used in coronary surgery was saphenous vein, and today, except for revascularization of the left anterior descending coronary artery, the most commonly used conduit in coronary surgery remains saphenous vein. Use of this vein has many benefits. Because of its relatively large diameter and wall characteristics, it is technically easy to use. In addition, patients have plenty of saphenous vein, so there is enough to perform multiple grafts, and it is also long enough to reach any coronary artery.

Early in the experience of coronary artery bypass surgery, the durability and longevity of saphenous vein grafts came into question. One year after surgery, only 80% to 90% of saphenous vein grafts are patent (43–45). Early vein graft closure results from technical errors, thrombosis, and intimal hyperplasia. One to 5 years after surgery, 1% to 2% of patent saphenous vein grafts occlude per year, and 6 to 10 years after surgery, 4% to 5% of these grafts occlude per year (46). Vein graft closure 1 year postoperatively results from development of arteriosclerosis. By 10 years, only 50% to 60% of saphenous vein grafts are patent, and only half of those are free of angiographic arteriosclerosis (46) (Fig. 80.2).

Occlusion of saphenous vein grafts in the first year after surgery is caused by both thrombosis and fibrous intimal hyperplasia. All saphenous vein grafts suffer endothelial damage during surgical manipulation and initial exposure to arterial pressure. This intimal injury results in platelet adherence. Early (<1 month) after surgery, this platelet adherence may result in thrombosis and acute vein graft occlusion. Platelet adherence to the intimal surface is also believed to be the inciting event in the development of fibrous intimal hyperplasia. When platelets adhere to the intima of saphenous vein grafts, they release mitogenic proteins that stimulate smooth muscle cell migration. This leads to intimal proliferation and hyperplasia. Administration of antiplatelet agents (aspirin) after coronary artery bypass grafting has been shown to improve both the early (<1 month) and 1-year patency of saphenous vein grafts (45,47).

After 1 year, saphenous vein graft atherosclerosis is responsible for further vein graft occlusion (46,48). Mural thrombi and intimal hyperplasia are believed to be the early stages of vein graft atherosclerosis (45,49). Lipid becomes incorporated in the areas of intimal hyperplasia, resulting in atherosclerotic plaques (47). Supporting the importance of early platelet adherence in the development of vein graft atherosclerosis is the observation that perioperative antiplatelet administration decreases the amount of lipid accumulation in the intima of vein grafts (50). Evidence supporting the importance of atherosclerosis in late vein graft occlusion has been demonstrated by the findings that atherosclerosis risk factors, such as diabetes mellitus, hypercholesterolemia, and hypertriglyceridemia, all increase the risk of late saphenous vein graft closure (51–53). In addition, risk factor modification, such as lipid-lowering therapy, has been shown to improve late saphenous vein graft patency (54).

Internal Thoracic Arteries

One of the greatest achievements in surgical myocardial revascularization has been the use of the internal thoracic artery as a bypass graft. The superiority of internal thoracic artery grafts over other conduits results from its excellent and stable long-term patency. At 10 years, 90% of internal thoracic artery grafts are patent (12,43,44,55–63) (Fig. 80.2). Unlike saphenous vein grafts, internal thoracic artery grafts very rarely develop arteriosclerosis. It has been reported that fewer than 4% of internal thoracic arteries develop arteriosclerosis, and only 1% have important luminal narrowing from atherosclerosis. The resistance of internal thoracic artery grafts to arteriosclerosis results from both their histology and their physiology. The nearly continuous internal elastic lamina of the internal thoracic artery inhibits smooth muscle cell migration and therefore prevents the early stages of arteriosclerosis. In addition, internal thoracic artery endothelium produces both prostacyclin and endothelium-derived relaxing factor. These are both are potent vasodilators and inhibitors of platelet function, and both should therefore enhance graft patency.

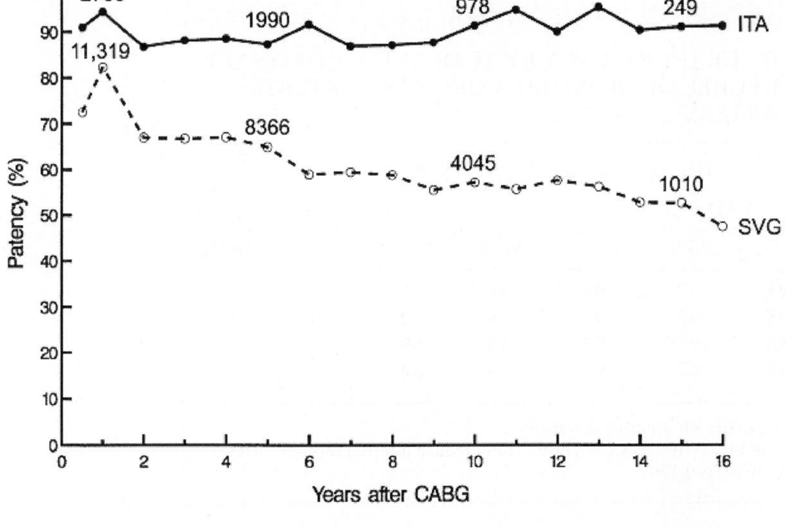

FIGURE 80.2. Internal thoracic artery (ITA) and saphenous vein graft (SVG) patency by year after coronary artery bypass grafting (CABG). Numbers represent the number of grafts studied at the corresponding year after CABG. (From Sabik JF 3rd, Lytle BW, Blackstone EH, et al. Comparison of saphenous vein and internal thoracic artery graft patency by coronary system. *Ann Thorac Surg* 2005;79:544–551.)

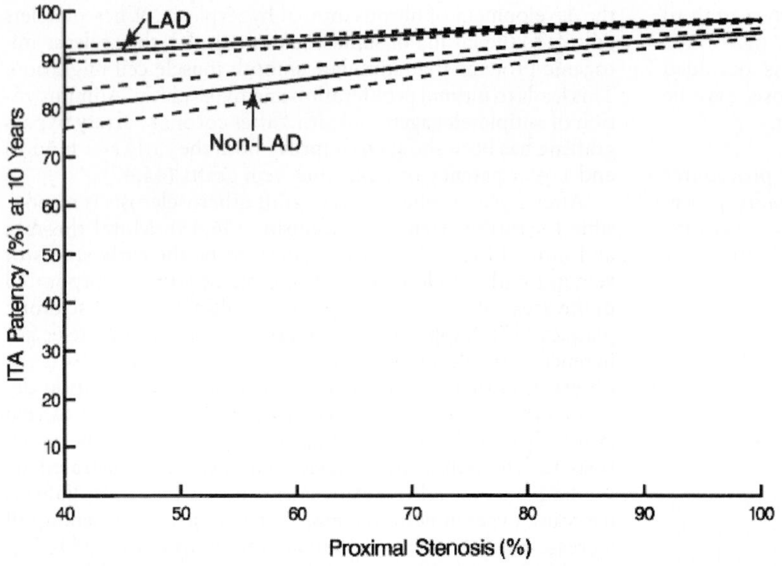

FIGURE 80.3. Internal thoracic artery (ITA) patency of left ITA to left anterior descending (LAD) and non-LAD coronary arteries at 10 years after coronary artery bypass grafting, by degree of proximal coronary artery stenosis. The *solid lines* represent estimates and the *dashed lines* 70% confidence intervals. (From Sabik JF 3rd, Lytle BW, Blackstone EH, et al. Does competitive flow reduce internal thoracic artery graft patency? *Ann Thorac Surg* 2003;76:1490–1496.)

A weakness of internal thoracic arteries is their susceptibility to spasm and possible occlusion when used to graft coronary arteries with only moderate proximal stenosis (43,55,64–72). This observation is consistent with the physiology of arteries. Unlike saphenous veins, internal thoracic arteries are muscular and can autoregulate their lumen in response to blood flow demand (67–72). When internal thoracic arteries are used to bypass coronary arteries with only moderate proximal stenosis, the need for internal thoracic artery blood flow is low, and the graft may constrict and fail. However, the decrease in internal thoracic artery patency when bypassing coronaries with lesser degrees of stenosis is gradual, and there is not a degree of proximal coronary artery stenosis below which internal thoracic artery patency declines dramatically (55) (Fig. 80.3 and Table 80.1). More importantly, for all the left-sided coronary arteries and the posterior descending coronary artery, internal thoracic artery patency appears to better than saphenous vein graft patency at all levels of coronary artery stenosis greater than 50% (43). Internal thoracic artery patency does not appear to be superior to saphenous vein patency when used to graft a right coronary artery with only moderate stenosis (43).

In addition to moderate proximal coronary artery stenosis, other factors shown to influence internal thoracic artery patency include (a) coronary artery grafted, (b) younger age, (c) diabetes, (d) female gender, (e) quality and run-off of the target coronary artery, and (f) laterality of the graft (55). Internal thoracic artery grafts to the left anterior descending have better patency than grafts to other coronary arteries (55). The risk factors of younger age, diabetes, and female gender may be surrogates for diffuse, aggressive coronary arteriosclerosis. Patients with these characteristics often have small, diffusely diseased coronary arteries, and bypass grafts to them are more likely to fail because of poor outflow and the technical difficulties of grafting small arteries.

Other Arterial Grafts

The radial, right gastroepiploic, and inferior epigastric arteries are also used as conduits for coronary artery bypass surgery (Fig. 80.4). Not as much is known about these conduits as about internal thoracic artery and saphenous vein grafts.

Radial arteries are the second most common arterial conduit. Their length and diameter make them very versatile bypass grafts. However, the radial artery is more muscular than the internal thoracic artery, and it appears to be more susceptible to

TABLE 80.1

INTERNAL THORACIC ARTERY GRAFT PATENCY BY YEAR AFTER CORONARY ARTERY BYPASS GRAFTING, DEGREE OF PROXIMAL CORONARY ARTERY STENOSIS, AND CORONARY ARTERY

	Degree of proximal coronary stenosis							
	LAD				Non-LAD			
Year after CABG	50%	70%	90%	100%	50%	70%	90%	100%
1	92	95	97	98	91	94	97	98
5	92	95	97	98	88	92	98	97
10	93	95	97	98	83	89	94	96
15	93	95	97	98	76	84	91	93

CABG, coronary artery bypass grafting; LAD, left anterior descending.
From Sabik JF 3rd, Lytle BW, Blackstone EH, et al. Does competitive flow reduce internal thoracic artery graft patency? *Ann Thorac Surg* 2003;76:1490–1496.

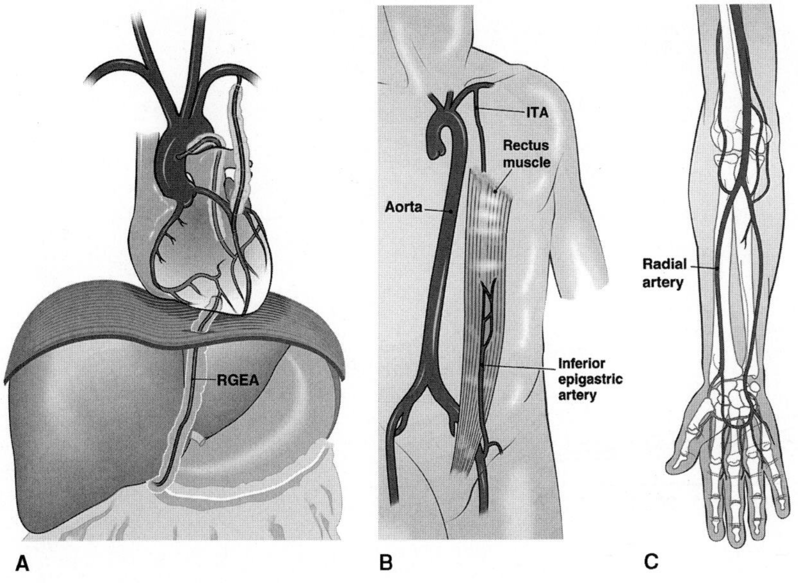

FIGURE 80.4. **A:** The gastroepiploic artery is mobilized from the greater curvature of the stomach and is generally brought anterior to the liver through the diaphragm and grafted to one of the two branches of the right coronary artery. The conduit is small and prone to spasm. Using it to graft a large coronary artery may result in hypoperfusion. RGEA, right gastroepiploic artery. **B:** The inferior epigastric artery lies behind each rectus muscle and is removed through a midline incision. This conduit is used infrequently today but may be advantageous as a Y graft sewn proximally to an arterial conduit and distally to a secondary target. ITA, internal thoracic artery. **C:** The radial artery is removed with its venae comitantes. Today, it is the second arterial graft of choice after both internal thoracic arteries, and it may be used as an aortocoronary graft or attached as a Y graft.

spasm and occlusion when used to graft coronary arteries with important competitive flow. Its patency has been demonstrated to be better when used to bypass coronary arteries with at least a 70% proximal stenosis (73,74). The 1- and 5-year patency of radial artery grafts has been reported to be about 90% and 83%, respectively (74,75).

The right gastroepiploic artery is usually used as an in situ graft to bypass the distal right coronary artery or the posterior descending coronary. On occasion, it may be long enough to graft the left anterior descending coronary artery as an in situ graft. Similar to the radial artery, this conduit is prone to spasm and should therefore be used to bypass coronary arteries with severe stenosis. Reported 1-, 5-, and 10-year patencies of gastroepiploic artery grafts are 91%, 80%, and 62% (76).

The inferior epigastric is a short conduit (8 to 10 cm in length) and must be used as a free graft. It also is prone to spasm and has better patency when used to bypass coronary arteries with severe stenosis. This graft has a 1-year patency of about 93% (77,78).

RESULTS

Coronary artery bypass surgery is probably the most thoroughly studied operation in the history of medicine. Preoperative patient characteristics, operative techniques (particularly conduit choice), and postoperative risk factor modifications all influence the outcomes of surgical revascularization.

Hospital Death

The hospital mortality for both primary and reoperative coronary artery bypass surgery has declined with surgical experience (79) (Fig. 80.5). In a review of seven large databases containing more than 172,000 patients, Jones and colleagues identified (a) older age, (b) female gender, (c) previous coronary artery bypass surgery, (d) urgency of operation, (e) increasing left ventricular dysfunction, (f) left main disease, and (g) increasing extent of coronary artery disease as patient

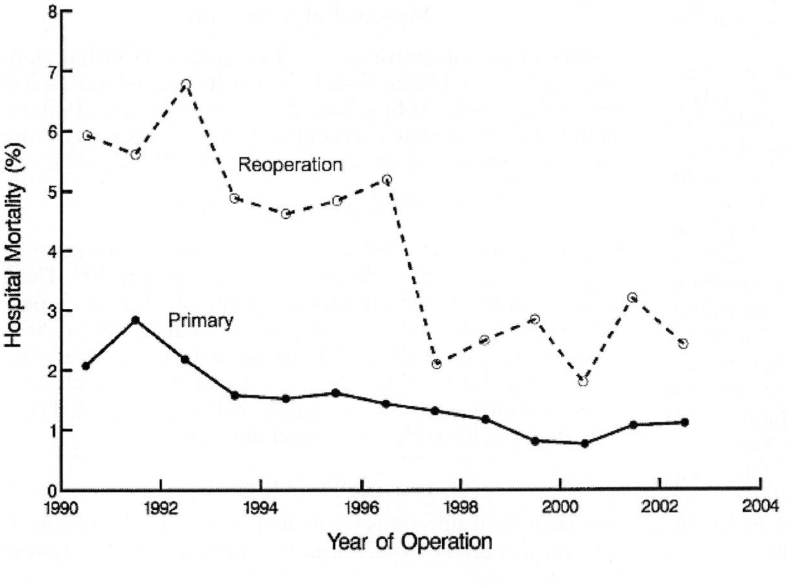

FIGURE 80.5. Hospital mortality after primary and reoperative coronary artery bypass grafting by year of operation. (From Sabik JF, Blackstone EH, Houghtaling PL. Is reoperation still a risk factor in coronary artery bypass surgery? *Ann Thorac Surg* 2005;80: 1719–1727.)

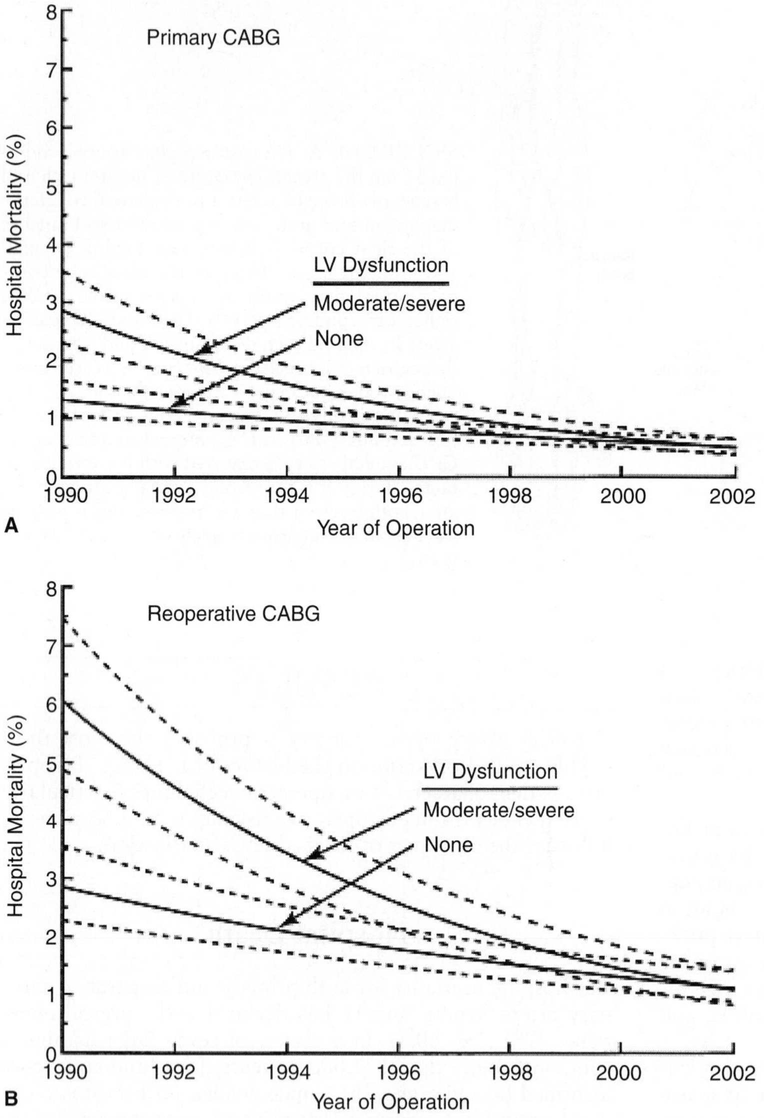

FIGURE 80.6. Hospital mortality for patients with normal left ventricular (LV) function and LV dysfunction by year of operation and by primary (**A**) and reoperative (**B**) coronary artery bypass grafting (CABG). (From Sabik JF, Blackstone EH, Houghtaling PL. Is reoperation still a risk factor in coronary artery bypass surgery? *Ann Thorac Surg* 2005;80:1719–1727.)

characteristics associated with an increased likelihood of hospital mortality (80). Other risk factors for hospital death include patient comorbidities such as diabetes, renal failure, chronic obstructive lung disease, and peripheral vascular disease (14,81).

In a recent review of more than 21,000 patients undergoing isolated coronary artery bypass surgery at the Cleveland Clinic, investigators questioned whether left ventricular dysfunction and reoperation continue to be risk factors for hospital death after coronary artery bypass surgery (Fig. 80.6). In the most recent time period of this study, both left ventricular dysfunction and reoperation were no longer risk factors for hospital mortality (79). Improved myocardial protection, better perioperative management, and revascularization of patients with hibernating (viable but dysfunctional) myocardium are believed to be the reason that left ventricular dysfunction is no longer a risk factor, and better operative techniques and surgical experience are believed to be the reason that reoperation is no longer a risk factor. Although the actual hospital mortality of patients undergoing coronary reoperations was higher than that of patients undergoing first-time surgery (Fig. 80.5), this increased risk of death was found to be attributable to the higher-risk profile of reoperative patients and not to the increased technical difficulty of coronary reoperations.

Hospital Morbidity

Myocardial Infarction

Causes of postoperative myocardial infarctions include failure of myocardial protection, technical errors, and incomplete revascularization. Although postoperative myocardial infarctions have been reported to occur in up to 5% of patients, more recent reports suggest an occurrence of only 1% (82–87).

Cerebrovascular Accidents

Important neurologic deficits have been reported to occur in 5% to 6% of patients undergoing coronary surgery (88). These adverse neurologic events appear equally divided into type 1 deficits (major focal deficits, stupor, coma) and type 2 deficits (deterioration in intellectual function or memory). Risk factors for type 1 deficits include ascending aortic atherosclerosis, prior neurologic disease, intraaortic balloon pump, diabetes, hypertension, unstable angina, and older age.

Mediastinitis

Sternal wound infections occur in 1% to 4% of patients after coronary artery bypass surgery (14,81,82,89). Risk factors

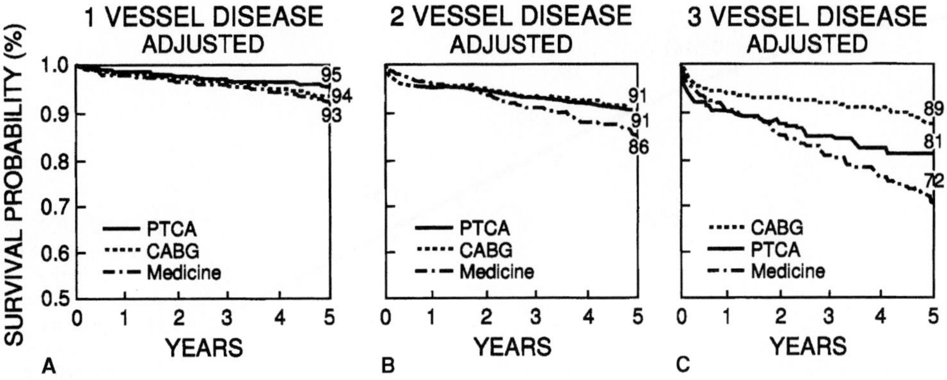

FIGURE 80.7. Survival curves for one-, two-, and three-vessel disease showing adjusted comparisons of angioplasty (percutaneous transluminal coronary angioplasty [PTCA]), coronary artery surgery (coronary artery bypass surgery [CABG]), and medicine. **A:** For one-vessel disease, there is a slight but insignificant trend toward higher survival in the angioplasty group: PTCA, 95%; CABG, 93%; and medicine, 94%. **B:** Patients with two-vessel disease showed the following adjusted 5-year survivals: PTCA, 91%; CABG, 91%; and medicine, 86%. **C:** In three-vessel disease, CABG was superior to medicine and PTCA: CABG, 89%; PTCA, 81%; and medicine, 72%. (From Mark DB, Nelson CL, Califf RM, et al. Continuing evolution of therapy for coronary artery disease: initial results from the era of coronary angioplasty. *Circulation* 1994;89:2015–2025.)

for mediastinitis include obesity, diabetes, previous coronary surgery, and duration of operation (90–92).

Late Survival

In general, the 1-, 5-, 10-, and 15-year survival of patients after coronary artery bypass surgery is 97%, 92%, 81%, and 66% respectively (93). Risk factors for late death include patient factors and operative techniques. Patient characteristics associated with an increased risk of late death include older age, obesity, severity of angina, atrial fibrillation, diabetes, hypertension, renal failure, peripheral vascular disease, elevated triglycerides, left ventricular dysfunction, and extent of coronary artery disease (93). Operative factors that influence late survival include completeness of revascularization and internal thoracic artery graft use.

Several observational studies have demonstrated improved late survival when the left internal thoracic artery is used to graft the left anterior descending artery (56,94,95) (Fig. 80.7). The survival advantage of internal thoracic artery grafting of the left anterior descending over saphenous vein grafting has been demonstrated in patients with single-vessel disease, double-vessel disease, triple-vessel disease, normal left ventricular function, and left ventricular dysfunction, in both men and woman, and in younger as well as older patients (56,94). Therefore, with the exception of emergency surgery or poor internal thoracic artery blood flow resulting from conduit damage, subclavian stenosis, radiation injury, or arteriosclerosis, left internal thoracic artery grafting to the left anterior descending is indicated in most patients undergoing coronary artery bypass surgery. An interesting observation is that the survival advantage of internal thoracic artery grafting increases with time, a finding suggesting that its choice as a bypass conduit has a greater influence on long-term survival than any postoperative factor, including arteriosclerosis progression (94,95).

Left internal thoracic artery grafting of the left anterior descending coronary artery has also been reported to decrease the risk of late myocardial infarction, hospitalization for cardiac events, need for reoperation, and return of angina when compared to a revascularization strategy using saphenous vein to bypass the left anterior descending artery (56,95).

Because of the success of single internal thoracic artery grafting, it is logical to assume that bilateral internal thoracic artery grafting should further improve the long-term outcomes of coronary revascularization. Despite this logic, bilateral internal thoracic artery revascularization has not been widely adopted. The Society of Thoracic Surgeons' Adult Cardiac National Database (Fall 2003) reports that bilateral internal thoracic arteries are used in only 3% to 4% of patients undergoing surgical coronary revascularization. There are several possible reasons for bilateral internal thoracic artery underutilization. First, bilateral internal thoracic artery grafting is more difficult and time-consuming. Second, some patients may have an increased risk of sternal wound infection with bilateral internal thoracic artery grafting. Third, there is a general lack of conviction that bilateral internal thoracic artery grafting confers any benefit over single internal thoracic artery grafting.

Although there are no randomized studies comparing single with bilateral internal thoracic artery grafting, many observational studies have used sophisticated statistical techniques to demonstrate the long-term survival and freedom from reintervention advantage of bilateral internal thoracic artery over single internal thoracic artery grafting (96–99) (Fig. 80.8). Subgroup analysis has demonstrated benefit in young patients with few or no comorbidities as well as in patients with comorbidities (96,97).

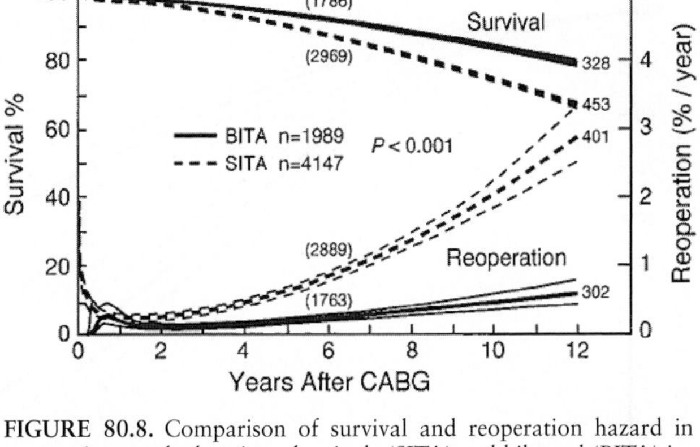

FIGURE 80.8. Comparison of survival and reoperation hazard in propensity-matched patients by single (SITA) and bilateral (BITA) internal thoracic artery grafting. CABG, coronary artery bypass grafting. (From Lytle BW, Blackstone EH, Loop FD, et al. Two internal thoracic artery grafts are better than one. *J Thorac Cardiovasc Surg* 1999;117:855–872.)

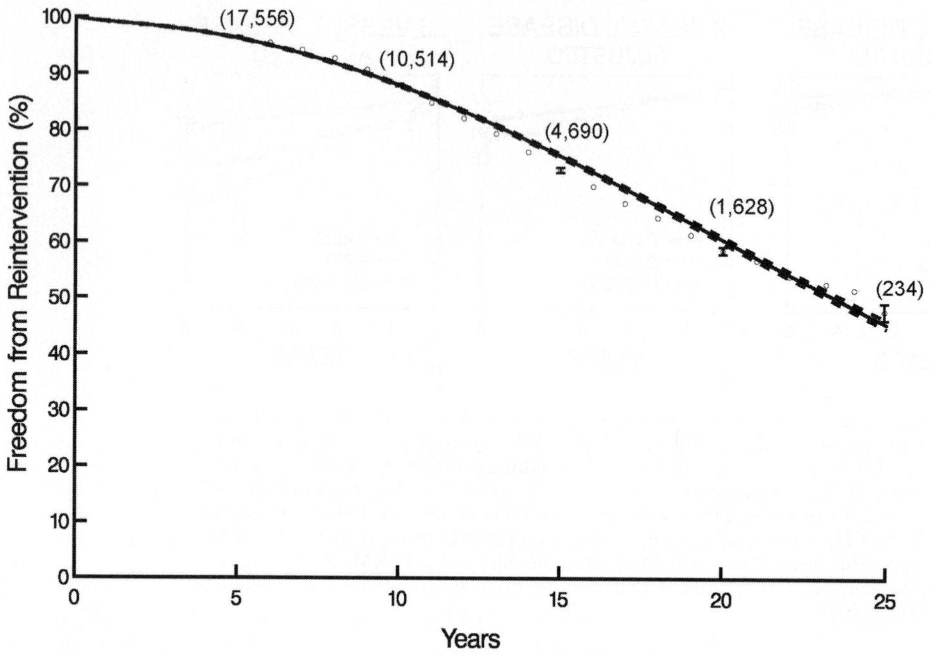

FIGURE 80.9. Predicted and actuarial estimates of freedom from reintervention (either reoperative coronary surgery or percutaneous intervention) after primary coronary artery bypass surgery (N = 27,968). The *solid line* represents predicted estimates enclosed within dashed 70% confidence limits. *Symbols* represent actuarial estimates at yearly intervals, and *error bars* represent 70% confidence limits. *Numbers in parentheses* are the number of patients remaining at risk. (From Sabik JF, Blackstone EH, Gillinov AM, et al. Occurrence and risk factors for reintervention after coronary artery bypass grafting. *Circulation* 2006;114:I-454–I-460.)

There have also been observational studies comparing single versus bilateral internal thoracic artery revascularization that have not found a clinical benefit of bilateral internal thoracic artery grafting (59,100). This finding has several possible explanations. First, single internal thoracic artery grafting of the left anterior descending results in good outcomes during the first postoperative decade, thus making it necessary to follow patients into the second postoperative decade to identify a benefit of bilateral internal thoracic artery grafting. Second, it is probably important which coronary artery is grafted with the second internal thoracic artery. Some bilateral internal thoracic artery revascularization strategies may not improve outcomes. Several studies have suggested that using the second internal thoracic artery graft to bypass the right coronary artery is not as beneficial in improving clinical outcomes as is using it to bypass a left-sided coronary artery (60,100–102).

In summary, internal thoracic artery grafting improves the long-term survival and freedom from subsequent reintervention after coronary revascularization as compared with a revascularization strategy of only saphenous vein grafts. The left internal thoracic artery should be used to bypass the left anterior descending coronary artery. A second internal thoracic artery graft appears to be beneficial in prolonging survival and decreasing coronary reintervention, especially when it is used to graft a second left-sided coronary artery.

Freedom from Coronary Reintervention

In general, the 1-, 5-, 10-, 15-, 20-, and 25-year freedom from coronary reintervention (either coronary reoperation or percutaneous intervention) after primary coronary artery bypass surgery is 99%, 96%, 88%, and 73%, 60%, and 46%, respectively (103) (Fig. 80.9). Similar to survival, both patient characteristics and conduit selection at the primary operation influence the likelihood of having a repeat coronary intervention. Patient characteristics that increase the likelihood of coronary reintervention include younger age, higher serum triglyceride, lower serum, high-density lipoprotein, diabetes mellitus, and more extensive coronary artery disease (103). Internal thoracic arterial grafting at the primary operation decreased the likelihood of having a coronary reintervention (Fig. 80.10).

Risk Factor Modification

Both smoking cessation and lipid-lowering therapy have been shown to improve the late outcomes of surgical revascularization. Smoking cessation lowered the risk of late myocardial infarction, coronary reoperation, and recurrence of angina, and

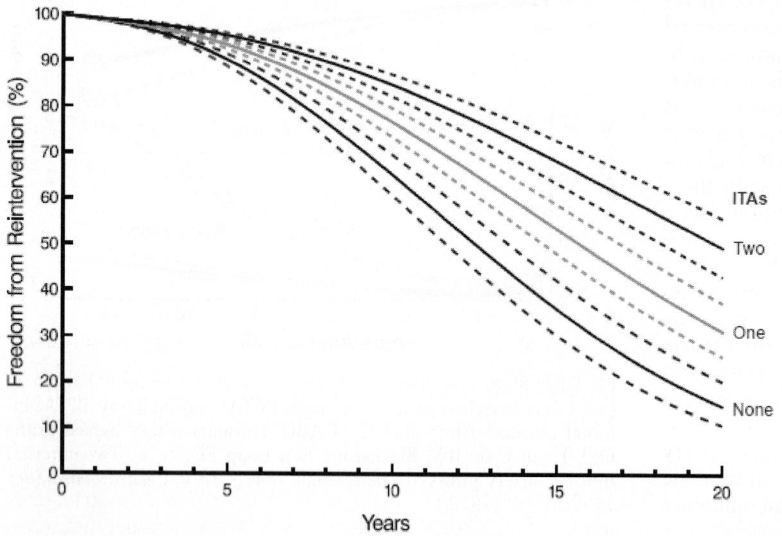

FIGURE 80.10. Freedom from reintervention after primary coronary artery bypass grafting stratified by use of single or double internal thoracic artery (ITA) grafting at primary operation. *Solid lines* represent predicted estimates and *dashed lines* 70% confidence limits. (From Sabik JF, Blackstone EH, Gillinov AM, et al. Occurrence and risk factors for reintervention after coronary artery bypass grafting. *Circulation* 2006; 114:I-454–I-460.)

aggressive lipid-lowering therapy decreased saphenous vein graft atherosclerosis progression the need for subsequent revascularization (104,105).

CONTROVERSIES AND PERSONAL PERSPECTIVES

Coronary Artery Bypass Grafting or Percutaneous Coronary Intervention in Treating Multivessel Coronary Artery Disease?

Both randomized trials and observational studies have tried to determine whether survival after initial percutaneous coronary intervention is equivalent, better, or worse than survival after initial coronary artery bypass surgery in the treatment of patients with multivessel coronary artery disease. Despite many studies, the answer remains controversial. The studies have compared coronary artery bypass surgery with angioplasty without stenting and coronary artery bypass surgery with angioplasty with stenting.

Nine randomized trials have compared initial coronary artery bypass surgery with percutaneous coronary intervention without stenting (14,106–113). Each study enrolled from 127 to 1,829 low-risk patients who had no serious comorbidities, primarily two-vessel coronary artery disease amenable to both percutaneous coronary intervention and coronary artery bypass surgery, and normal ventricular function. Patients were followed from 1 to 8 years, although in most of the studies the patients were followed for 1 to 3 years. No difference in overall survival was found in eight of the nine trials. At 8-year follow-up, the Bypass Angioplasty Revascularization Investigation (BARI) found a survival advantage in patients who underwent coronary artery bypass surgery. The survival benefit of coronary artery bypass surgery appeared to occur in patients with medically treated diabetes (Fig. 80.11). Most of the randomized trials found that coronary artery bypass surgery resulted in greater freedom from angina and need for subsequent revascularization procedures. The rate of repeat revascularization was 4 to 10 times higher in patients who underwent percutaneous coronary intervention without stenting as compared with patients who had coronary artery bypass surgery.

Six randomized trials have compared coronary artery bypass surgery with percutaneous coronary intervention with stenting (14,114–118). The largest trial, the Arterial Revascularization Therapy Study, enrolled 1,205 low-risk patients with normal left ventricular function and two- to three-vessel coronary artery disease amenable to both coronary artery bypass surgery and percutaneous coronary intervention (114). At 1 year, survival was similar. The Stent or Surgery trial included 988 patients with multivessel disease (115). At 1 year, survival was greater in patients treated with surgery. However, in the Argentine Coronary Angioplasty with Stenting versus Coronary Bypass Surgery in Patients with Multiple-Vessel Disease (ERACI II) trial, at a mean follow-up of 18 months, survival was better in patients treated with coronary stenting (116). A consistent finding of all these studies was the greater need for subsequent revascularization in patients who were treated initially with coronary stenting. Stenting, however, did reduce the rate of repeat revascularization by half compared with balloon angioplasty alone (119).

Although these randomized trials are believed to be the gold standard and have been widely cited as demonstrating survival equivalence, their multiple shortcomings make their observation of survival equivalence less than conclusive. First, for the findings of randomized trials to be generalizable, the trials needed to include patients who were similar to patients

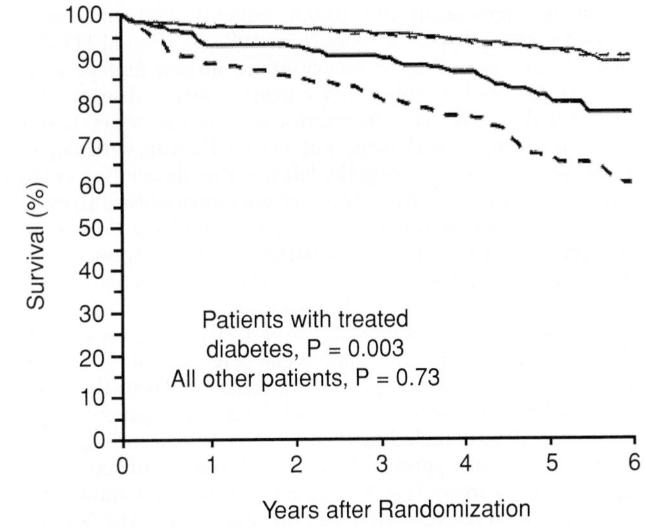

PATIENTS WITH TREATED DIABETES			
CABG	180	161	93
PTCA	173	139	69
ALL OTHER PATIENTS			
CABG	734	696	449
PTCA	742	701	408

FIGURE 80.11. Comparison of survival among medically treated diabetic patients (*heavy lines*) and nondiabetic patients (*light lines*) by treatment assignment: coronary artery bypass grafting (CABG; *solid lines*) and percutaneous transluminal coronary angioplasty (PTCA; *dashed lines*). (From Bypass Angioplasty Revascularization Investigation (BARI) Investigators. Comparison of coronary bypass surgery with angioplasty in patients with multivessel disease. *N Engl J Med* 1996;335:217–225.)

not enrolled in the studies. The randomized trials had strict entry criteria that excluded many patient subgroups, thereby limiting their applicability. In addition, the randomized trials included only a small minority of patients who were eligible for enrollment (111,112). Second, for the trials to evaluate survival benefit truly, only patient subgroups in which coronary artery bypass surgery had been demonstrated to be superior to medical therapy in prolonging survival should have been included in the trials. Most of the trials excluded these patient subgroups. Instead, the outcomes were compared in low-risk patient subgroups in which coronary artery bypass surgery did not offer a survival advantage over medical therapy. The only way coronary artery bypass surgery could have been better than percutaneous coronary intervention in prolonging survival in these low-risk groups was if percutaneous coronary intervention had been worse than medical therapy! Third, the randomized trials needed to be large enough to have adequate statistical power to detect a survival difference between coronary artery bypass surgery and percutaneous coronary intervention. To compare the outcomes of these invasive therapies adequately, 2,000 to 4,000 patients would need to be included in each arm of the individual studies (14). The technical difficulties and expense of such large trials are enormous, and none of the randomized trials had enough patients to compare survival adequately. Fourth, to detect a survival difference, the study follow-up should be at least 5 years. Except for BARI, most of the trials lacked sufficient follow-up (106).

In contrast to the randomized trials, observational studies have demonstrated a survival benefit of initial coronary artery bypass surgery over percutaneous coronary intervention (120–122). Two large New York State registry observational studies identified angiographic subgroups of patients who derive survival benefit from coronary artery bypass surgery (120,121). The first study, conducted before widespread coronary stenting, included 30,000 patients who underwent percutaneous coronary intervention and 30,000 patients who underwent coronary artery bypass surgery from 1993 to 1995 (121). Patients with triple-vessel coronary artery disease and patients with single- and double-vessel coronary artery disease that included the proximal left anterior descending artery had a survival advantage with surgery at 3 years. Patients with single-vessel disease not involving the left anterior descending coronary artery had a survival advantage with angioplasty. To evaluate the effects of coronary stenting, a second New York State registry study was performed on patients with multivessel coronary artery disease who underwent coronary revascularization from 1997 to 2000 (121). In this study, 3-year survival of 37,212 patients who underwent coronary artery bypass surgery and 22,102 patients who underwent percutaneous coronary intervention with stenting was compared. Similar to the prior study, all patients with triple-vessel disease and patients with two-vessel disease including the left anterior descending coronary artery had a survival benefit at 3 years with coronary artery bypass surgery (Fig. 80.12). Patients with left main coronary disease were excluded from both studies. Surprisingly, the findings of these observational studies are similar to the findings of randomized trials comparing coronary surgery with medical therapy. These observations support an initial strategy of surgery in patients with triple-vessel disease or stenosis of the proximal left anterior descending coronary artery. These registry studies also found that repeat revascularization was higher in patients treated with percutaneous coronary intervention. Other observational studies have also suggested the superiority of coronary artery bypass surgery in prolonging survival over percutaneous coronary intervention (122).

Similar to randomized studies, observational studies have limitations, the most important being that risk stratification will not account for selection bias related to unmeasured patient characteristics. The benefits of these observational studies are that large numbers of patients and therefore events are available for comparison, and these studies compare how coronary revascularization is actually practiced.

How will drug-eluting stents alter the outcomes of coronary intervention? Just as bare metal stenting decreased restenosis and subsequent reintervention after percutaneous coronary intervention as compared with balloon angioplasty, drug-eluting stents have decreased restenosis and subsequent revascularization after percutaneous coronary intervention compared with bare metal stenting (123,124). However, will the lower rate of restenosis found with drug-eluting stents improve the survival of patients undergoing percutaneous coronary intervention? Early results do not suggest it will. Implantation of drug-eluting stents did not lower mortality, myocardial infarction, or stroke rates (125). This finding is consistent with a previous study that failed to identify a difference in survival between patients with and without restenosis (126).

Other investigators have suggested that even if restenosis after percutaneous coronary intervention is completely eliminated, angioplasty will still not be as effective as bypass surgery (127). The explanation for this lies in the difference of how percutaneous coronary intervention and surgery differ in their treatment of coronary artery disease. Angioplasty treats only the site of the culprit lesion, whereas surgery bypasses most of the epicardial vessel, treating not only the coronary stenosis present at the time of treatment, but also any additional stenosis that may develop in the future proximal to the bypass graft.

In summary, whether initial angioplasty is equivalent to coronary artery bypass surgery in prolonging survival is controversial. Several randomized studies suggested that initial percutaneous coronary intervention is equivalent to coronary artery bypass grafting, but these studies were underpowered, lacked sufficient follow-up, and compared mostly low-risk patients who would not be expected to benefit from coronary artery bypass surgery versus medical therapy. The BARI trial with sufficient follow-up suggests that survival is better with initial

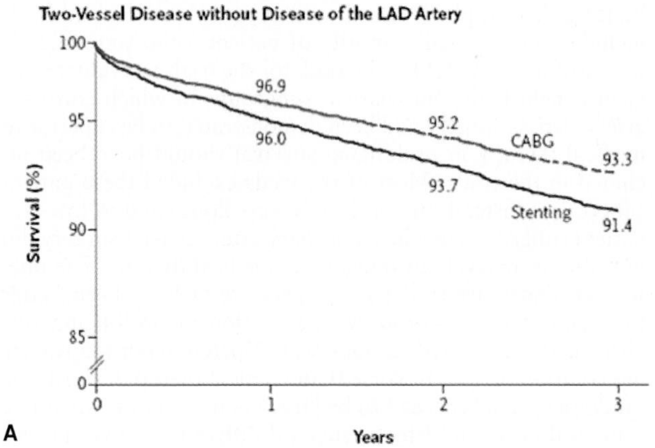

A

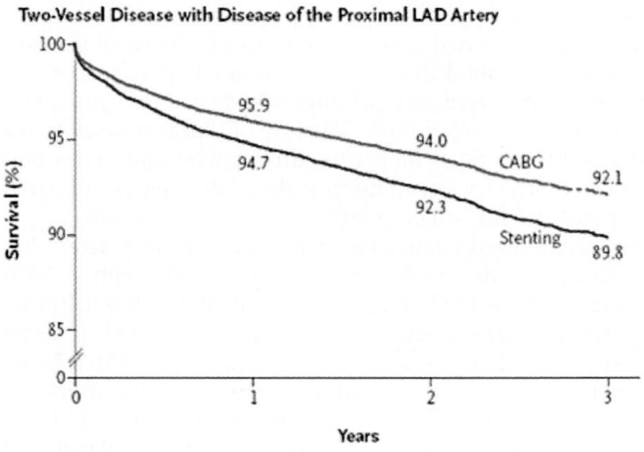

B

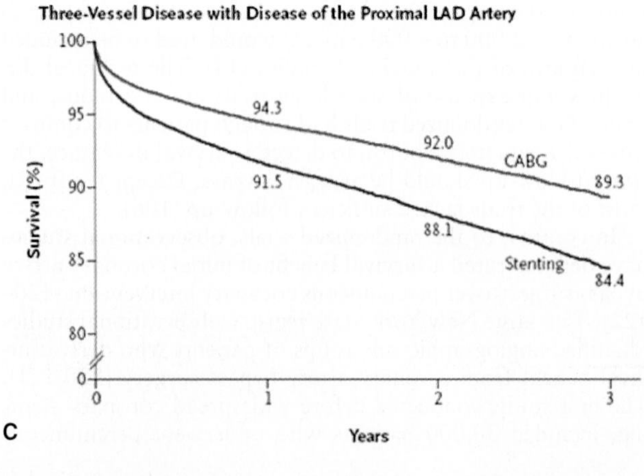

C

FIGURE 80.12. Adjusted survival among patients treated with stenting or coronary artery bypass grafting (CABG) by extent of coronary artery disease. (From Hannan EL, Racz MJ, Walford G, et al. Long-term outcomes of coronary-artery bypass grafting versus stent implantation. *N Engl J Med* 2005;352:2174–2183.)

coronary artery bypass surgery over percutaneous coronary intervention. Large, risk-adjusted observational studies find that initial coronary artery bypass surgery results in better survival than percutaneous coronary intervention in patients with high-risk angiographic characteristics. Despite improvements in percutaneous coronary intervention that have decreased restenosis, the decrease in restenosis may not improve the survival of patients after percutaneous coronary intervention.

Off-Pump Versus On-Pump Coronary Revascularization

Whether performing coronary artery bypass surgery without cardiopulmonary bypass (off-pump) results in better clinical outcomes than those obtained with cardiopulmonary bypass (on-pump) has been a highly debated and controversial issue in coronary surgery during the last decade. Although several early, observational studies suggested the superiority of off-pump revascularization in lowering the mortality and morbidity of surgical myocardial revascularization, well risk-adjusted observational studies and randomized studies have challenged the findings of these early studies (82,128–137). In patients able to undergo either procedure, off-pump or on-pump revascularization has been demonstrated to result in similar risks of mortality, serious morbidity, and neurocognitive dysfunction. Some randomized studies have suggested that there may be less blood loss, need for transfusion, and myocardial enzyme release after off-pump surgery (131–133,136). Midterm survival and freedom from reintervention have also been reported to be similar after both revascularization strategies (Fig. 80.13), and although there have been conflicting reports on whether graft patency after off-pump surgery is as good as that obtained with on-pump revascularization, studies

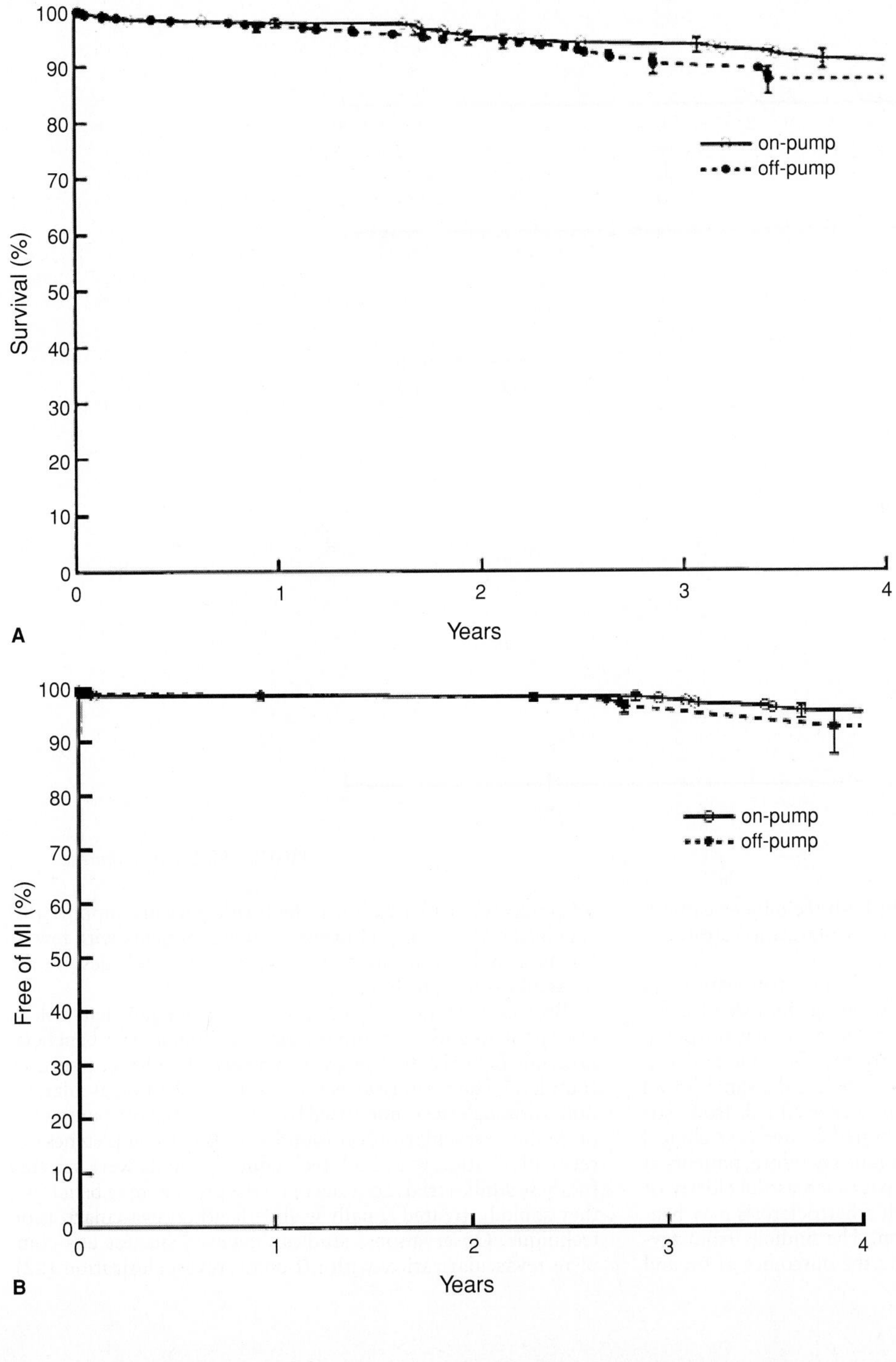

FIGURE 80.13. A–D: Survival (**A**), freedom from myocardial infarction (MI) (**B**), freedom from percutaneous coronary intervention (PCI) (**C**), and freedom from reoperative coronary artery bypass grafting (CABG) (**D**), in propensity-matched patients after on-pump and off-pump CABG. (From Sabik JF, Blackstone EH, Lytle BW, et al. Equivalent midterm outcomes after off-pump and on-pump coronary surgery. *J Thorac Cardiovasc Surg* 2004;127:142–148.)

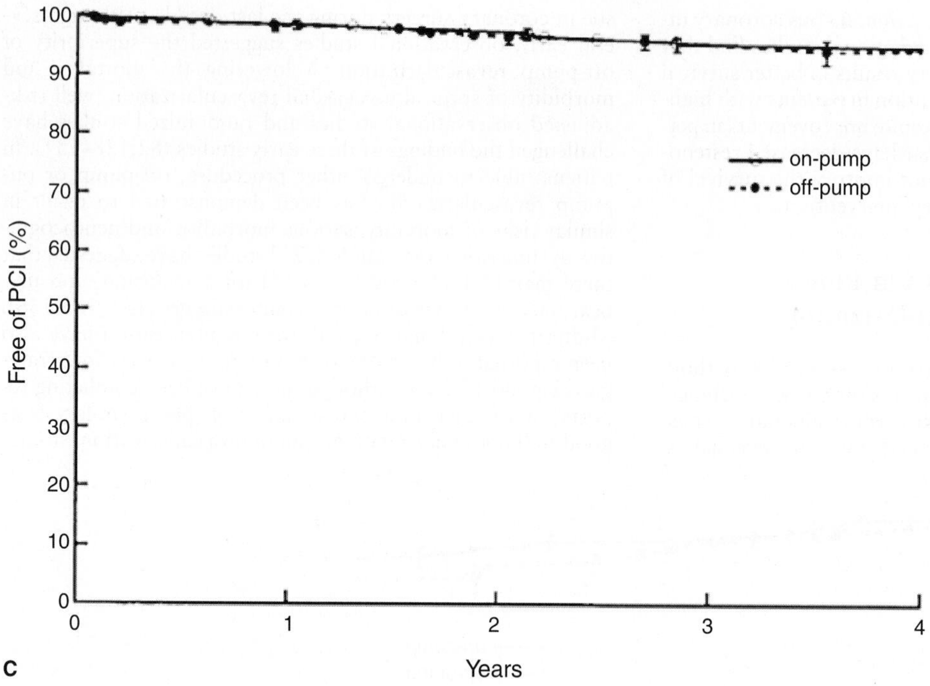

C

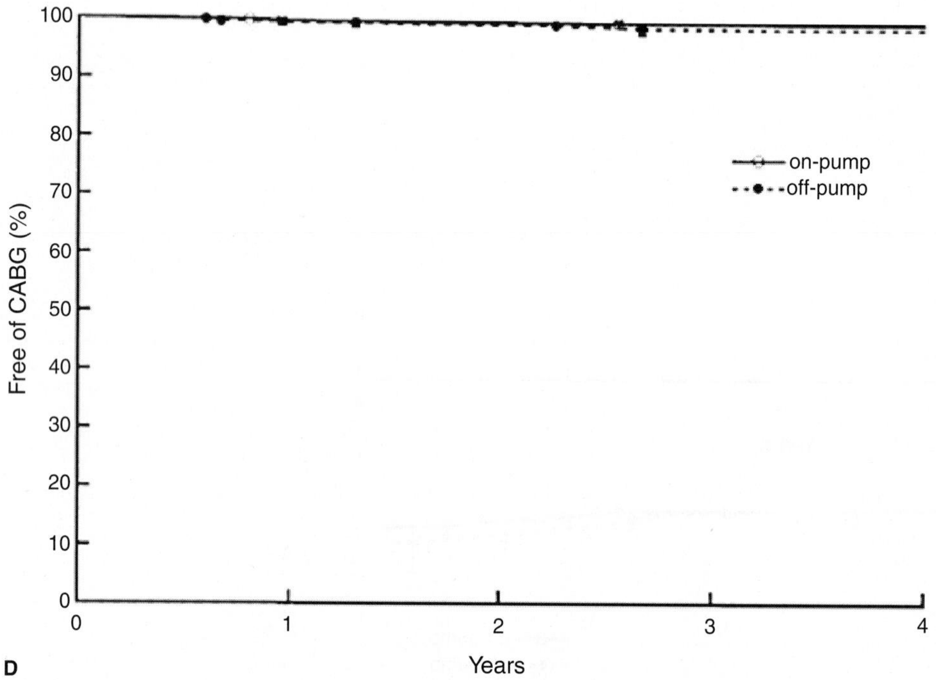

D

FIGURE 80.13. *(Continued)*

suggest that surgeons experienced in both techniques can obtain similar graft patency with both revascularization strategies (129,135–137).

Although the randomized studies did not demonstrate an advantage of off-pump surgery in lowering the risk of coronary artery bypass grafting, this does not mean that off-pump revascularization is not a superior strategy for some patients. The risks of cardiopulmonary bypass are not the same for all patients, and therefore patients at an increased risk from cardiopulmonary bypass would be expected to derive a clinical benefit from off-pump revascularization. Therefore, patients at greater risk of cardiopulmonary bypass such as the elderly or those with ascending aortic and arch atherosclerosis may benefit from off-pump revascularization. The findings from several observational studies comparing the outcomes of on-and off-pump revascularization in high-risk patients support this conclusion (138–141). However, younger patients with few or no comorbidities are likely to have a similar risk despite the revascularization technique.

Because both procedures appear to have equivalent risk in most patients and off-pump revascularization may be beneficial in certain high-risk patients, why not perform off-pump surgery routinely? The main issue is the effectiveness of revascularization. Although the randomized trials comparing off-pump with on-pump revascularization found equivalent completeness of revascularization with both techniques, patients were selected for these studies trials contingent on the preoperative belief that they could be treated equally well with either revascularization technique. Observational studies, however, suggest less complete revascularization with off-pump revascularization (82).

No study has demonstrated more grafts being performed as off-pump procedures.

An additional measure of effective revascularization is the amount of arterial grafting. The randomized trials included revascularization strategies of mostly single internal thoracic artery and saphenous vein grafting. Off-pump revascularization is not incompatible with complex arterial grafting; however, off-pump revascularization does increase the level of difficulty. Because the benefits of off-pump revascularization appear to be small in most patients, it does not appear wise to compromise the quality of revascularization just to perform the revascularization as an off-pump procedure. Instead, because cardiopulmonary bypass and cardioplegic myocardial arrest provide optimal exposure and an optimal surgical field, it may be best to perform complex arterial and difficult revascularizations with the assistance of cardiopulmonary bypass.

SUMMARY

Coronary artery bypass surgery is an effective treatment for patients with coronary artery disease. It increases life expectancy, decreases angina, and improves exercise tolerance. Patients at the greatest preoperative risk and those with extensive coronary artery disease, worse symptoms, and left ventricular dysfunction derive the greatest relative benefit from surgical myocardial revascularization. Both patient characteristics and bypass conduits influence the long-term outcomes of surgical revascularization. The left internal thoracic artery graft to the left anterior descending coronary artery improves survival and freedom from reintervention in virtually all subsets of patients with anterior wall ischemia, and it therefore should be an integral component of surgical myocardial revascularization. Recent evidence suggests that additional arterial grafting should further improve the late outcomes of coronary artery bypass surgery.

References

1. Sones FM Jr, Shirey EK. Cine coronary arteriography. *Mod Concepts Cardiovasc Dis* 1962;31:735–738.
2. Vineberg A, Miller G. Internal mammary coronary anastomosis in the surgical treatment of coronary artery insufficiency. *Can Med Assoc J* 1951; 64:204–210.
3. Effler DB, Sones FM Jr, Groves LK, Suarez E. Myocardial revascularization by Vineberg's internal mammary artery implant: evaluation of postoperative results. *J Thorac Cardiovasc Surg* 1965;50:527–533.
4. Longmire WP Jr, Cannon JA, Kattus AA. Direct-vision coronary endarterectomy for angina pectoris. *N Engl J Med* 1958;259:993–999.
5. Senning A. Strip grafting in coronary arteries: report of a case. *J Thorac Cardiovasc Surg* 1961;41:542–549.
6. Kolessov VI, Potashov LV. [Surgery of coronary arteries.] *Eksp Khir Anesteziol* 1965;10:3–8.
7. Kolessov VI. Mammary artery-coronary artery anastomosis as method of treatment for angina pectoris. *J Thorac Cardiovasc Surg* 1967;54:535–544.
8. Favaloro RG. Saphenous vein graft in the surgical treatment of coronary artery disease: operative technique. *J Thorac Cardiovasc Surg* 1969;58: 178–185.
9. Garrett HE, Dennis EW, DeBakey ME. Aortocoronary bypass with saphenous vein graft: seven-year follow-up. *JAMA* 1973;223:792–794.
10. Loop FD, Cosgrove DM, Lytle BW, et al. An 11 year evolution of coronary arterial surgery (1968–1978). *Ann Surg* 1979;190:444–455.
11. Kolessov VI. Mammary artery-coronary artery anastomosis as a method for treatment of angina pectoris. *J Thorac Cardiovasc Surg* 1967;54:535–544.
12. Tector AJ, Kress DC, Downey FX, Schmahl TM. Complete revascularization with internal thoracic artery grafts. *Semin Thorac Cardiovasc Surg* 1996;8:29–41.
13. Green GE, Stertzer SH, Reppert EH. Coronary arterial bypass grafts. *Ann Thorac Surg* 1968;5:443–450.
14. Eagle KA, Guyton RA, Davidoff R, et al. ACC/AHA 2004 guideline update for coronary artery bypass graft surgery: summary article. A report of the American College of Cardiology/American Heart Association Task Force on Practice Guidelines (Committee to Update the 1999 Guidelines for Coronary Artery Bypass Graft Surgery). *J Am Coll Cardiol* 2004;44:e213–e310.
15. Veterans Administration Coronary Artery Bypass Surgery Cooperative Study Group. Eleven-year survival in the Veterans Administration randomized trial of coronary bypass surgery for stable angina. *N Engl J Med* 1984;311:1333–1339.
16. Takaro T, Hultgren HN, Lipton MJ, Detre KM. The VA cooperative randomized study of surgery for coronary arterial occlusive disease. II. Subgroup with significant left main lesions. *Circulation* 1976;54(suppl III):III107–III117.
17. European Coronary Surgery Study Group. Prospective randomized study of coronary artery bypass surgery in stable angina pectoris: second interim report by the European Coronary Surgery Study Group. *Lancet* 1980;2: 491–495.
18. Varnauskas E. Twelve-year follow-up of survival in the randomized European Coronary Surgery Study. *N Engl J Med* 1988;319:332–337.
19. Passamani E, Davis KB, Gillespie MJ, Killip T. A randomized trial of coronary artery bypass surgery: survival of patients with a low ejection fraction. *N Engl J Med* 1985;312:1665–1671.
20. Coronary Artery Surgery Study (CASS). A randomized trial of coronary artery bypass surgery: survival data. *Circulation* 1983;68:939–950.
21. Coronary Artery Surgery Study (CASS). A randomized trial of coronary artery bypass surgery: quality of life in patients randomly assigned to treatment groups. *Circulation* 1983;68:951–960.
22. Alderman EL, Bourassa MG, Cohen LS, et al. Ten-year follow-up of survival and myocardial infarction in the randomized Coronary Artery Surgery Study. *Circulation* 1990;82:1629–1646.
23. Alderman EL, Fisher LD, Litwin P, et al. Results of coronary artery surgery in patients with poor left ventricular function. *Circulation* 1983;68:785–795.
24. Bounous E, Mark DB, Pollock BG. Surgical survival benefits from coronary disease patients with left ventricular dysfunction. *Circulation* 1988;78: 1151–1157.
25. Califf RM, Harrell F Jr, Lee K. The evolution of medical and surgical therapy for coronary artery disease: a 15-year perspective. *JAMA* 1989;261: 2077–2089.
26. Pierard LA, DeLandsheere CM, Berthe C. Identification of viable myocardium by echocardiography during dobutamine infusion in patients with myocardial infarction after thrombolytic therapy: comparison with positron emission tomography. *J Am Coll Cardiol* 1990;15:1021–1031.
27. Smart S, Sawada S, Ryan T. Low-dose dobutamine echocardiography detects reversible dysfunction after thrombolytic therapy of acute myocardial infarction. *Circulation* 1993;88:405–415.
28. Ragosta M, Beller GA, Watson DD. Quantitative planar rest-redistribution 201T1 imaging in detection of myocardial viability and prediction of improvement in left ventricular function after coronary artery bypass surgery in patients with severely depressed left ventricular function. *Circulation* 1993;87:1630–1641.
29. Ragosta M, Carmarano G, Kaul S, et al. Microvascular integrity indicates myocellular viability in patients with recent myocardial infarction: new insights using myocardial contrast echocardiography. *Circulation* 1994; 89:2562–2569.
30. Tillisch J, Brunken R, Marshall R. Reversibility of cardiac wall-motion abnormalities predicted by positron tomography. *N Engl J Med* 1986;314: 884–888.
31. Schwaiger M, Hicks R. The clinical role of metabolic imaging of the heart by positron emission tomography. *J Nucl Med* 1991;32:565–578.
32. Iskandrian AS, Hakki A, Kane SA, et al. Rest and redistribution thallium-201 myocardial scintigraphy to predict improvement in left ventricular function after coronary artery bypass grafting. *Am J Cardiol* 1983;51: 1312–1316.
33. Pagley PR, Beller GA, Watson DD. Improved outcome after coronary bypass surgery in patients with ischemic cardiomyopathy and residual myocardial viability. *Circulation* 1997;96:793–800.
34. National Cooperative Study Group to Compare Surgical and Medical Therapy. Unstable angina pectoris. II. In-hospital experience and initial follow-up results in patients with one, two and three vessel disease. *Am J Cardiol* 1978;42:839–848.
35. Parisi AF, Khuri S, Deupree RH. Medical compared with surgical management of unstable angina. *Circulation* 1989;80:1176–1189.
36. Luchi RJ, Scott SM, Deupree RH. Comparison of medical and surgical treatment for unstable angina pectoris: results of a Veterans Administration Cooperative Study. *N Engl J Med* 1987;316:977–984.
37. Sharma GV, Deupree RH, Khuri SF. Coronary bypass surgery improves survival in high-risk unstable angina: results of a Veterans Administration Cooperative Study with an 8-year follow-up. *Circulation* 1991;84(suppl III):III260–III267.
38. Coleman WS, DeWood MA, Berg R Jr, et al. Surgical intervention in acute myocardial infarction: an historical perspective. *Semin Thorac Cardiovasc Surg* 1995;7:176–183.
39. DeWood MA, Notske RN, Berg R Jr. Medical and surgical management of early Q wave myocardial infarction. I. Effects of surgical reperfusion on survival, recurrent myocardial infarction, sudden death and functional class at 10 or more years of follow-up. *J Am Coll Cardiol* 1989;14: 65–77.

40. Azoury FM, Gillinov AM, Lytle BW, et al. Off-pump reoperative coronary artery bypass grafting by thoracotomy: patient selection and operative technique. *Ann Thorac Surg* 2001;71:1959–1963.
41. Sabik JF, Lytle BW, McCarthy PM, Cosgrove DM. Axillary artery: an alternative site of arterial cannulation for patients with extensive aortic and peripheral vascular disease. *J Thorac Cardiovasc Surg* 1995;109:885–890.
42. Sabik JF, Nemeh H, Lytle BW, et al. Cannulation of the axillary artery with a side graft reduces morbidity. *Ann Thorac Surg* 2004;77:1315–1320.
43. Sabik JF 3rd, Lytle BW, Blackstone EH, et al. Comparison of saphenous vein and internal thoracic artery graft patency by coronary system. *Ann Thorac Surg* 2005;79:544–551.
44. Fitzgibbon GM, Kafka HP, Leach AJ, et al. Coronary bypass graft fate and patient outcome: angiographic follow-up of 5,065 grafts related to survival and reoperation in 1,388 patients during 25 years. *J Am Coll Cardiol* 1996;28:616–626.
45. Cheseboro JH, Fuster V, Elveback LR, et al. Effect of dipyridamole and aspirin on late vein-graft patency after coronary bypass operations. *N Engl J Med* 1984;310:209–214.
46. Bourassa MG, Fisher LD, Campeau L, et al. Long-term fate of bypass grafts: the Coronary Artery Surgery Study (CASS) and Montreal Heart Institute experience. *Circulation* 1985;72(suppl V):V71–V78.
47. Cheseboro JH, Clements IP, Fuster V, et al. A platelet inhibitor drug trial in coronary artery bypass operations: benefit of perioperative dipyridamole and aspirin on early vein graft patency. *N Engl J Med* 1982;307:73–78.
48. Campeau L, Lesperance J, Hermann J, et al. Loss of the improvement of angina between 1 and 7 years after aortocoronary bypass surgery: correlations with changes in vein grafts and in coronary arteries. *Circulation* 1979;60:1–5.
49. Fuster V, Dewanjee MK, Kaye MP, et al. Noninvasive radioisotopic technique for detection of platelet in coronary artery bypass grafts in dogs and its reduction with platelet inhibitors. *Circulation* 1979;60:1508–1512.
50. Metke MP, Lie JT, Fuster V, et al. Reduction of intimal thickening in canine coronary bypass grafts with dipyridamole and aspirin. *Am J Cardiol* 1979;43:1144–1148.
51. Lytle BW, Loop FD, Cosgrove DM, et al. Long-term (5–12 years) serial studies of internal mammary artery and saphenous vein coronary bypass grafts. *J Thorac Cardiovasc Surg* 1985;89:248–258.
52. Campeau L, Enjalbert M, Lesperance J, et al. The relation of risk factors to the development of atherosclerosis in saphenous vein bypass grafts and the progression of disease in the native circulation: a study of 10 years after aortocoronary bypass. *N Engl J Med* 1984;311:1329–1332.
53. Lie JT, Lawrie GM, Morris GC Jr. Aortocoronary bypass saphenous vein graft atherosclerosis: anatomic study of 99 vein grafts from normal and hyperlipoproteinemic patients up to 75 months postoperatively. *Am J Cardiol* 1977;40:906–914.
54. Post Coronary Artery Bypass Graft Trial Investigators. The effect of aggressive lowering of low-density lipoprotein cholesterol levels and low-does anticoagulation on obstructive changes in saphenous-vein-coronary-artery bypass grafts. *N Engl J Med* 1997;336:153–162.
55. Sabik JF 3rd, Lytle BW, Blackstone EH, et al. Does competitive flow reduce internal thoracic artery graft patency?. *Ann Thorac Surg* 2003;76:1490–1496.
56. Loop FD, Lytle BW, Cosgrove DM, et al. Influence of the internal-mammary artery graft on 10-year survival and other cardiac events. *N Engl J Med* 1986;314:1–6.
57. Grondin CM, Campeau L, Lesperance J, et al. Comparison of late changes in internal mammary artery and saphenous vein grafts in two consecutive series of patients 10 years after operation. *Circulation* 1984;70(suppl I):I208-I212.
58. Barner HB, Standeven JW, Reese J. Twelve-year experience with internal mammary artery for coronary artery bypass. *J Thorac Cardiovasc Surg* 1985; 90:668–675.
59. Fiore AC, Naunheim KS, Dean P, et al. Results of internal thoracic artery grafting over 15 years: single versus double grafts. *Ann Thorac Surg* 1990; 49:202–209.
60. Pick AW, Orszulak TA, Anderson BJ, Schaff HV. Single versus bilateral internal mammary artery grafts: 10 year outcome analysis. *Ann Thorac Surg* 1997;64:599–605.
61. Galbut DL, Traad EA, Dorman MJ, et al. Seventeen-year experience with bilateral internal mammary artery grafts. *Ann Thorac Surg* 1990;49:195–201.
62. Lytle BW, Loop FD, Thurer RL, et al. Isolated left anterior descending coronary atherosclerosis: long-term comparison of internal mammary artery and venous autografts. *Circulation* 1980;61:869–874.
63. Bjork VO, Ivert T, Landou C. Angiographic changes in internal mammary artery and saphenous vein grafts, two weeks, one year and five years after coronary bypass surgery. *Scand J Thorac Cardiovasc Surg* 1981;15:23–30.
64. Barner HB. Double internal mammary-coronary artery bypass. *Arch Surg* 1974;109:627–630.
65. Geha AS, Baue AE. Early and late results of coronary revascularization with saphenous vein and internal mammary artery grafts. *Am J Surg* 1979;137: 456–463.
66. Ivert T, Huttunen K, Landou C, Bjork VO. Angiographic studies of internal mammary artery grafts 11 years after coronary artery bypass grafting. *J Thorac Cardiovasc Surg* 1988;96:1–12.
67. Hashimoto H, Isshiki T, Ikari Y. Effects of competitive blood flow on arterial graft patency and diameter: medium-term postoperative follow-up. *Thorac Cardiovasc Surg* 1996;111:399–407.
68. Seki T, Kitamura K. A quantitative study of postoperative luminal narrowing of the internal thoracic artery graft in coronary artery bypass surgery. *J Thorac Cardiovasc Surg* 1992;104:1532–1538.
69. Pagni S, Storey J, Ballen J. ITA versus SVG: a comparison of instantaneous pressure and flow dynamics during competitive flow. *Eur J Cardiothorac Surg* 1997;11:1086–1092.
70. Shimizu T, Hirayama T, Suesada H, et al. Effect of flow competition on internal thoracic artery graft: postoperative velocimetric and angiographic study. *J Thorac Cardiovasc Surg* 2000;120:459–465.
71. Pagni S, Storey J, Ballen J. Factors affecting internal mammary artery graft survival: how is competitive flow from a patent native coronary vessel a risk factor? *J Surg Res* 1997;71:172–178.
72. Nasu M, Akasaka T, Okazaki T. Postoperative flow characteristics of left internal thoracic artery grafts. *Ann Thorac Surg* 1995;59:154–161.
73. Moran SV, Baeza R, Guarda E, et al. Predictors of radial artery patency for coronary bypass operations. *Ann Thorac Surg* 2001;72:1552–1556.
74. Royse AG., Royse CF, Tatoulis J, et al. Postoperative radial artery angiography for coronary artery bypass surgery. *Eur J Cardiothorac Surg* 2000; 17:294–304.
75. Acar C, Ramsheyi A, Pagny JY, et al. The radial artery for coronary artery bypass grafting: clinical and angiographic results at five years. *J Thorac Cardiovasc Surg* 1998;116:981–989.
76. Suma H, Isomura T, Horii T, Sato T. Late angiographic result of using the right gastroepiploic artery as a graft. *J Thorac Cardiovasc Surg* 2000; 120:496–498.
77. Buche M, Schroeder E, Gurne O. Coronary artery bypass grafting with the inferior epigastric artery: midterm clinical and angiographic results. *J Thorac Cardiovasc Surg* 1995;109:553–560.
78. Gurne O, Buche M, Chenu P, et al. Quantitative angiographic follow-up study of the free inferior epigastric coronary bypass graft. *Circulation* 1994; 90(suppl II):II148–II54.
79. Sabik JF, Blackstone EH, Houghtaling PL, et al. Is reoperation still a risk factor in coronary artery bypass surgery? *Ann Thorac Surg* 2005;80:1719–1727.
80. Jones RH, Hannan EL, Hammermeister KE, et al. Identification of preoperative variables needed for risk adjustment of short-term mortality after coronary artery bypass graft surgery: the Working Group Panel on the Cooperative CABG Database Project. *J Am Coll Cardiol* 1996;28:1478–1487.
81. Eagle KA, Guyton RA, Davidoff R, et al. ACC/AHA Guidelines for Coronary Artery Bypass Graft Surgery: a Report of the American College of Cardiology/American Heart Association Task Force on Practice Guidelines (Committee to Revise the 1991 Guidelines for Coronary Artery Bypass Graft Surgery). American College of Cardiology/American Heart Association. *J Am Coll Cardiol* 1999;34:1262–1347.
82. Sabik JF, Gillinov AM, Blackstone EH, et al. Does off-pump coronary surgery reduce morbidity and mortality? *J Thorac Cardiovasc Surg* 2002; 124:698–707.
83. Chaitman BR, Alderman EL, Sheffield LT, et al. Use of survival analysis to determine the clinical significance of new Q waves after coronary bypass surgery. *Circulation* 1983;67:302.
84. Chaitman BR, Rosen AD, Williams DO, et al. Myocardial infarction and cardiac mortality in the Bypass Angioplasty Revascularization Investigation (BARI) randomized trial. *Circulation* 1997;96:2162–2170.
85. Klatte K, Chaitman BR, Theroux P, et al. Increased mortality after coronary artery bypass graft surgery is associated with increased levels of post-operative creatine kinase-myocardial band isoenzyme release: results from the GUARDIAN trial. *J Am Coll Cardiol* 2001;38:1070–1077.
86. Oberman A, Kouchoukos NT, Makar YN, et al. Perioperative myocardial infarction after coronary bypass surgery. *Cleve Clin Q* 1978;45:172–174.
87. Schaff HV, Gersh BJ, Fisher LD, et al. Detrimental effect of perioperative myocardial infarction on late survival after coronary artery bypass: report from the Coronary Artery Surgery Study—CASS. *J Thorac Cardiovasc Surg* 1984;88:972–981.
88. Roach GW, Kanchuger M, Mangano CM, et al. Adverse cerebral outcomes after coronary bypass surgery: Multicenter Study of Perioperative Ischemia Research Group and the Ischemia Research and Education Foundation Investigators. *N Engl J Med* 1996;335:1857–1863.
89. Loop FD, Lytle BW, Cosgrove DM, et al. J. Maxwell Chamberlain memorial paper: sternal wound complications after isolated coronary artery bypass grafting: early and late mortality, morbidity, and cost of care. *Ann Thorac Surg* 1990;49:179–186.
90. Milano CA, Kesler K, Archibald N, et al. Mediastinitis after coronary artery bypass graft surgery: risk factors and long-term survival. *Circulation* 1995;92:2245–2251.
91. Nagachinta T, Stephens M, Reitz B, Polk BF. Risk factors for surgical-wound infection following cardiac surgery. *J Infect Dis* 1987;156:967–973.
92. Kouchoukos NT, Wareing TH, Murphy SF, et al. Risks of bilateral internal mammary artery bypass grafting. *Ann Thorac Surg* 1990;49:210–217.
93. Sergeant P, Blackstone E, Meyns B. Validation and interdependence with patient-variables of the influence of procedural variables on early and late

survival after CABG: K. U. Leuven Coronary Surgery Program. *Eur J Cardiothorac Surg* 1997;12:1–19.
94. Cameron A, David KB, Green G, Schaff HV. Coronary bypass surgery with internal-thoracic-artery grafts: effects of survival on a 15-year period. *N Engl J Med* 1996;334:216–219.
95. Boylan MJ, Lytle BW, Loop FD, et al. Surgical treatment of isolated left anterior descending coronary stenosis. *J Thorac Cardiovasc Surg* 1994;107: 657–662.
96. Lytle BW, Blackstone EH, Loop FD, et al. Two internal thoracic artery grafts are better than one. *J Thorac Cardiovasc Surg* 1999;117:855–872.
97. Lytle BW, Blackstone EH, Sabik JF, et al. The effect of bilateral internal thoracic artery grafting on survival during 20 postoperative years. *Ann Thorac Surg* 2004;78:2005–2012.
98. Stevens LM, Carrier M, Perrault LP. Single versus bilateral internal thoracic artery grafts with concomitant saphenous vein grafts for multivessel coronary artery bypass grafting: effects on mortality and event-free survival. *J Thorac Cardiovasc Surg* 2004;127:1408–1415.
99. Buxton BF, Komeda M, Fuller JA. Bilateral internal thoracic grafting may improve outcome of coronary artery surgery: risk adjusted survival. *Circulation* 1998;98(suppl II):II1–II6.
100. Naunheim KS, Barner HB, Fiore AC. Results of internal thoracic artery grafting over fifteen year: single versus double grafts 1992 update. *Ann Thorac Surg* 1992;53:716–718.
101. Schmidt SE, Jones JW, Thornby JI, et al. Improved survival with multiple left-sided bilateral internal thoracic artery grafts. *Ann Thorac Surg* 1997;64:9–15.
102. Carrel T, Horber P, Turina MI. Operation for two vessel coronary artery disease: midterm results of bilateral ITA grafting versus unilateral ITA and saphenous vein grafting. *Ann Thorac Surg* 1996;62:1289–1294.
103. Sabik JF, Blackstone EH, Gillinov AM, et al. Occurrence and risk factors for reintervention after coronary artery bypass grafting. *Circulation* 2006; 114:I-454–I-460.
104. Voors AA, van Brussel BL, Lokker T. Smoking and cardiac events after venous coronary bypass surgery: a 15-year follow-up study. *Circulation* 1996; 93:42–47.
105. Post Coronary Artery Bypass Graft Trial Investigators. The effect of aggressive lowering of low-density lipoprotein cholesterol levels and low-dose anticoagulation on obstructive changes in saphenous-vein-coronary-artery bypass grafts. *N Engl J Med* 1997;336:153–162.
106. Bypass Angioplasty Revascularization Investigation (BARI) Investigators. Comparison of coronary bypass surgery with angioplasty in patients with multivessel disease. *N Engl J Med* 1996;335:217–225.
107. CABRI Trial Participants. First-year results of CABRI (Coronary Angioplasty versus Bypass Revascularisation Investigation). *Lancet* 1995;346: 1179–1184.
108. King SB 3rd, Lembo NJ, Weintraub WS, et al. A randomized trial comparing coronary angioplasty with coronary bypass surgery: Emory Angioplasty versus Surgery Trial (EAST). *N Engl J Med* 1994;331:1044–1050.
109. Hamm CW, Reimers J, Ischinger T, et al. A randomized study of coronary angioplasty compared with bypass surgery in patients with symptomatic multivessel coronary disease: German Angioplasty Bypass Surgery Investigation (GABI). *N Engl J Med* 1994;331:1037–1043.
110. Rodriguez A, Boullon F, Perez-Balino N, et al. Argentine randomized trial of percutaneous transluminal coronary angioplasty versus coronary artery bypass surgery in multivessel disease (ERACI): in-hospital results and 1-year follow-up. ERACI Group. *J Am Coll Cardiol* 1993;22:1060–1067.
111. Sim I, Gupta M, McDonald K, et al. A meta-analysis of randomized trials comparing coronary artery bypass grafting with percutaneous transluminal coronary angioplasty in multivessel coronary artery disease. *Am J Cardiol* 1995;76:1025–1029.
112. Bourassa MG, Roubin GS, Detre KM, et al. Bypass Angioplasty Revascularization Investigation: patient screening, selection, and recruitment. *Am J Cardiol* 1995;75:3C–8C.
113. Coronary angioplasty versus coronary artery bypass surgery: the Randomized Intervention Treatment of Angina (RITA) trial. *Lancet* 1993;341:573–580.
114. Serruys PW, Unger F, Sousa JE, et al. Comparison of coronary-artery bypass surgery and stenting for the treatment of multivessel disease. *N Engl J Med* 2001;344:1117–1124.
115. Coronary Artery Bypass Surgery Versus Percutaneous Coronary Intervention with Stent Implantation in Patients with Multivessel Coronary Artery Disease (the Stent or Surgery trial): a randomised controlled trial. *Lancet* 2002;360:965–970.
116. Rodriguez A, Bernardi V, Navia J, et al. Argentine randomized study: Coronary Angioplasty with Stenting versus Coronary Bypass Surgery in Patients with Multiple-Vessel Disease (ERACI II): 30-day and one-year follow-up results. ERACI II Investigators. *J Am Coll Cardiol* 2001;37:51–58.
117. Morrison DA, Sethi G, Sacks J, et al. Percutaneous coronary intervention versus coronary artery bypass graft surgery for patients with medically refractory myocardial ischemia and risk factors for adverse outcomes with bypass: a multicenter, randomized trial. Investigators of the Department of Veterans Affairs Cooperative Study #385, the Angina With Extremely Serious Operative Mortality Evaluation (AWESOME). *J Am Coll Cardiol* 2001;38:143–149.
118. Goy JJ, Kaufmann U, Goy-Eggenberger D, et al. A prospective randomized trial comparing stenting to internal mammary artery grafting for proximal, isolated de novo left anterior coronary artery stenosis: the SIMA trial: Stenting vs Internal Mammary Artery. *Mayo Clin Proc* 2000;75:1116–1123.
119. Hoffman SN, TenBrook JA, Wolf MP, et al. A meta-analysis of randomized controlled trials comparing coronary artery bypass graft with percutaneous transluminal coronary angioplasty: one- to eight-year outcomes. *J Am Coll Cardiol* 2003;41:1293–1304.
120. Hannan EL, Racz MJ, Walford G, et al. Long-term outcomes of coronary-artery bypass grafting versus stent implantation. *N Engl J Med* 2005;352: 2174–2183.
121. Hannan EL, Racz MJ, McCallister BD, et al. A comparison of three-year survival after coronary artery bypass graft surgery and percutaneous transluminal coronary angioplasty. *J Am Coll Cardiol* 1999;33:63–72.
122. Brener SJ, Lytle BW, Casserly IP, et al. Propensity analysis of long-term survival after surgical or percutaneous revascularization in patients with multivessel coronary artery disease and high-risk features. *Circulation* 2004;109:2290–2295.
123. Moses JW, Leon MB, Popma JJ, et al. Sirolimus-eluting stents versus standard stents in patients with stenosis in a native coronary artery. *N Engl J Med* 2003;349:1315–1323.
124. Stone GW, Ellis SG, Cox DA, et al. A polymer-based, paclitaxel-eluting stent in patients with coronary artery disease. *N Engl J Med* 2004;350:221–231.
125. Berger PB, Sketch MH Jr. Choosing between percutaneous coronary intervention and coronary artery bypass grafting for patient with multivessel disease: what can we learn from the Arterial Revascularization Therapy Study (ARTS)? *Circulation* 2004;109:1079–1081.
126. Weintraub WS, Ghazzal ZM, Douglas JS Jr, et al. Long-term clinical follow-up in patients with angiographic restudy after successful angioplasty. *Circulation* 1993;87:831–840.
127. Yock CA, Boothroyd DB, Owens DK, et al. Cost-effectiveness of bypass surgery versus stenting in patients with multivessel coronary artery disease. *Am J Med* 2003;115:382–389.
128. Mack MJ, Pfister A, Bachand D, et al. Comparison of coronary bypass surgery with and without cardiopulmonary bypass in patients with multivessel disease. *J Thorac Cardiovasc Surg* 2004;127:167–173.
129. Sabik JF, Blackstone EH, Lytle BW, et al. Equivalent midterm outcomes after off-pump and on-pump coronary surgery. *J Thorac Cardiovasc Surg* 2004;127:142–148.
130. Racz MJ, Hannan EL, Isom OW, et al. A comparison of short- and long-term outcomes after off-pump and on-pump coronary artery bypass graft surgery with sternotomy. *J Am Coll Cardiol* 2004;43:557–564.
131. Gerola LR, Buffolo E, Jasbik W, et al. Off-pump versus on-pump myocardial revascularization in low-risk patients with one or two vessel disease: perioperative results in a multicenter randomized controlled trial. *Ann Thorac Surg* 2004;77:569–573.
132. Straka Z, Widimsky P, Jirasek K, et al. Off-pump versus on-pump coronary surgery: final results from a prospective randomized study PRAGUE-4. *Ann Thorac Surg* 2004;77:789–793.
133. Puskas JD, Williams WH, Duke PG, et al. Off-pump coronary artery bypass grafting provides complete revascularization with reduced myocardial injury, transfusion requirements, and length of stay: a prospective randomized comparison of two hundred unselected patients undergoing off-pump versus conventional coronary artery bypass grafting. *J Thorac Cardiovasc Surg* 2003;125:797–808.
134. Hart JC, Puskas JD, Sabik JF, 3rd. Off-pump coronary revascularization: current state of the art. *Semin Thorac Cardiovasc Surg* 2002;14:70–81.
135. Puskas JD, Williams WH, Mahoney EM, et al. Off-pump vs conventional coronary artery bypass grafting: early and 1-year graft patency, cost, and quality-of-life outcomes: a randomized trial. *JAMA* 2004;291:1841–1849.
136. Khan NE, De Souza A, Mister R, et al. A randomized comparison of off-pump and on-pump multivessel coronary-artery bypass surgery. *N Engl J Med* 2004;350:21–28.
137. Nathoe HM, van Dijk D, Jansen EW, et al. A comparison of on-pump and off-pump coronary bypass surgery in low-risk patients. *N Engl J Med* 2003;348:394–402.
138. Sharony R, Bizekis CS, Kanchuger M, et al. Off-pump coronary artery bypass grafting reduces mortality and stroke in patients with atheromatous aortas: a case control study. *Circulation* 2003;108(suppl II):II15–II20.
139. Sharony R, Grossi EA, Saunders PC, et al. Propensity score analysis of a six-year experience with minimally invasive isolated aortic valve replacement. *J Heart Valve Dis* 2004;13:887–893.
140. Hoff SJ, Ball SK, Coltharp WH, et al. Coronary artery bypass in patients 80 years and over: is off-pump the operation of choice? *Ann Thorac Surg* 2002;74:S1340–S1343.
141. Hirose H, Amano A, Takahashi A. Off-pump coronary artery bypass grafting for elderly patients. *Ann Thorac Surg* 2001;72:2013–2019.

CHAPTER 81 ■ APPROACHES TO THE PATIENT WITH PRIOR BYPASS SURGERY

JOHN S. DOUGLAS, JR.

OVERVIEW

The important issues in the patient who has undergone coronary artery bypass grafting (CABG) and who has recurrent angina or ischemia are providing relief with the least morbidity and cost and doing it in a manner that provides durable benefit. It takes considerable judgment to make the best decision in these patients because there are frequently many options, most of which have substantial baggage in the form of complications and short-term benefit.

HISTORICAL PERSPECTIVE

Advent and Maturation of Surgical Revascularization

As was later true of percutaneous transluminal coronary angioplasty (PTCA) (1,2), surgical coronary artery revascularization began more than 30 years ago with attempts to revascularize a single coronary artery. The result of these efforts was a dramatic change in cardiologic practice as surgical techniques adequate to palliate multivessel obstructive disease evolved. Within a decade, the growth of CABG surgery was exponential (Fig. 81.1). Hundreds of thousands of patients were operated on annually, creating a large population of several million postbypass patients in the United States alone. Owing to the progressive nature of the atherosclerotic process and the limited durability of venous conduits and in spite of widespread use of arterial grafts and antiplatelet agents, recurrent ischemia after surgical revascularization is a problem all cardiologists face with increasing frequency. Recurrence of angina in the first year alone was reported in 24% of patients in the Coronary Artery Surgery Study, and by the fifth postoperative year, almost one half of the broad spectrum of postoperative patients will have recurrent symptoms (3).

Recurrent angina sufficient to require reoperation occurred in 12% to 15% of patients within 1 decade of a first coronary operation at Emory University in Atlanta, Georgia and at the Cleveland Clinic in Cleveland, Ohio, and by the twelfth to fifteenth year, 30% required reoperation (4,5). Reoperative coronary surgery when compared with initial operation proved to be more costly, two to three times more likely to lead to in-hospital death or myocardial infarction (MI), and less effective in relieving angina. Among 2,030 patients who underwent reoperation at Emory University, in-hospital mortality was 7.0% (4.6% $<$ 60 years, 8.2% aged 60 to 69, 10.0% $\geq$ 70 years). Five- and 10-year survival was 76% and 55%, respectively (6). Reported outcome data confined to patients who underwent reoperation in the 1990s confirmed the relatively high operative mortality noted earlier (7.4%) and reported a higher rate of Q-wave infarction, a longer length of stay, and higher costs than initial operations (7). The increase in complications and reduced efficacy of reoperative coronary surgery are probably related to the more extensive disease present, the requirement to use second-line venous conduits in many cases, and the technically more difficult and operator-dependent nature of reoperative heart surgery.

Percutaneous Postbypass Intervention

Percutaneous catheter revascularization in patients who had prior CABG surgery (Fig. 81.2) was first described by Gruentzig, who treated 8 patients, 6 successfully, among the first 50 patients he reported. Seven of the 8 postbypass patients had angioplasty of saphenous vein graft (SVG) lesions, and 3 of 5 treated successfully had recurrences, findings that led Gruentzig to make the following insightful comments based on such limited observations: "The different kind of disease may explain the high incidence of recurrence in graft stenosis. Further experience will show whether we should eliminate this lesion from consideration" (8).

Among the first 1,116 patients treated with coronary angioplasty in the National Heart, Lung, and Blood Institute PTCA Registry, 62 patients had had previous bypass surgery. The in-hospital mortality rate in these patients, 8.1%, was significantly

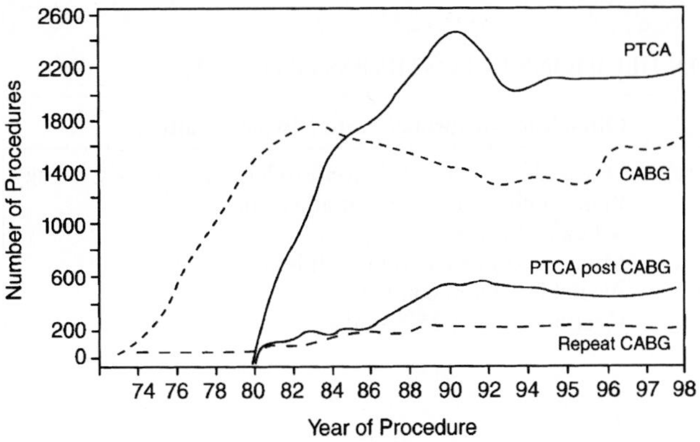

FIGURE 81.1. Coronary artery revascularization procedures at Emory University Hospitals in Atlanta, Georgia. CABG, coronary artery bypass grafting; PTCA, percutaneous transluminal coronary angioplasty.

higher than in patients without prior surgery, 0.7%, thus causing concern about the safety of the procedure in this group of patients (9). The early experience at Emory University was reassuring, however; 116 treated patients had no procedural deaths, 3 had emergency operations, and one had a Q-wave MI (Fig. 81.2). One late death occurred during an 8.3-month mean follow-up. Gruentzig's observation of higher restenosis rates for SVGs was reaffirmed for medial and proximal graft sites, but an acceptable restenosis rate for distal anastomosis lesions of 18% (4 of 22) was first reported (Fig. 81.3), as well as the initial report of attempted internal mammary artery (IMA) graft angioplasty (10). In subsequent experience with more than 34,000 coronary angioplasty procedures at Emory University, a history of prior bypass surgery was not associated with an increased risk of death or Q-wave MI and was negatively correlated with the need for in-hospital CABG surgery (11).

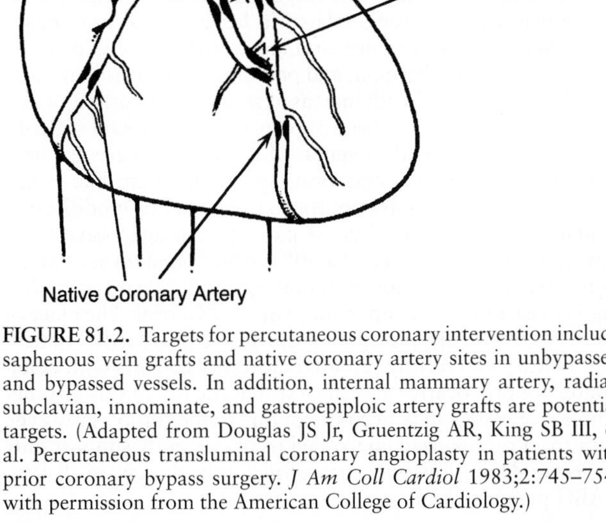

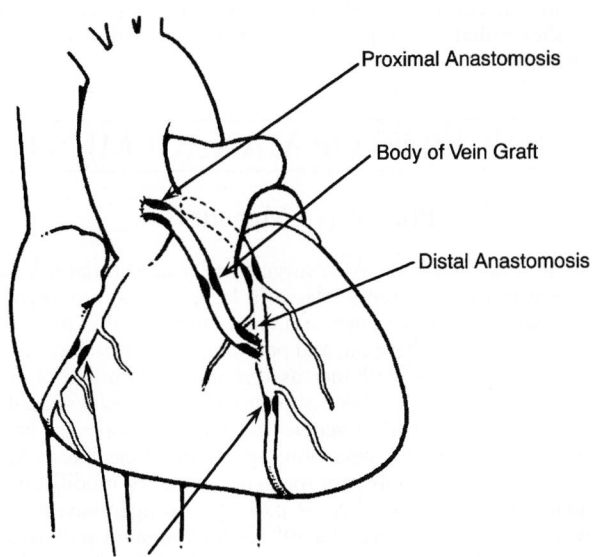

FIGURE 81.2. Targets for percutaneous coronary intervention include saphenous vein grafts and native coronary artery sites in unbypassed and bypassed vessels. In addition, internal mammary artery, radial, subclavian, innominate, and gastroepiploic artery grafts are potential targets. (Adapted from Douglas JS Jr, Gruentzig AR, King SB III, et al. Percutaneous transluminal coronary angioplasty in patients with prior coronary bypass surgery. *J Am Coll Cardiol* 1983;2:745–754, with permission from the American College of Cardiology.)

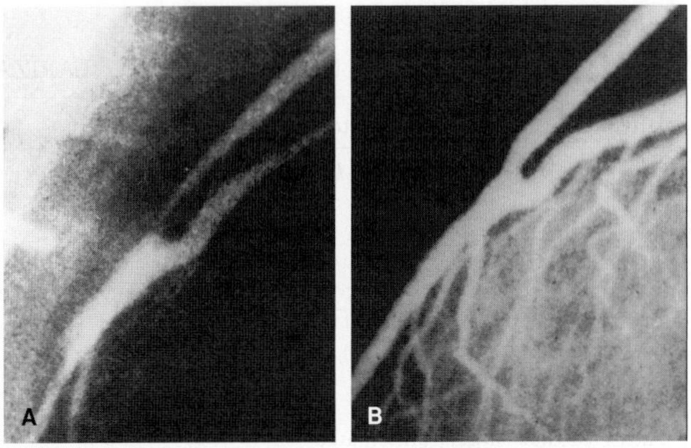

FIGURE 81.3. A 57-year-old man underwent saphenous vein bypass grafting to the distal left anterior descending (LAD) artery; coronary arteriography a few months later (**A**) revealed high-grade stenosis at the junction of the saphenous vein graft to the LAD artery (left lateral view). Percutaneous transluminal coronary angioplasty was successful (residual stenosis 13%), and recatheterization 9 months later showed a widely patent anastomosis (**B**). The patient subsequently remained completely asymptomatic, and at last follow-up 19 years later, he had a negative stress thallium scan. (From Douglas JS Jr, Gruentzig AR, King SB III, et al. Percutaneous transluminal coronary angioplasty in patients with prior coronary bypass surgery. *J Am Coll Cardiol* 1983;2:745–754, with permission from the American College of Cardiology.)

Percutaneous coronary intervention (PCI) became a less invasive revascularization alternative for many symptomatic postbypass patients, including increasing numbers who, because of contraindications (pulmonary and renal failure, old age, malignancy), were not candidates for reoperative coronary artery surgery. Patients with patent arterial grafts that would be jeopardized by reoperation, patients with relatively small amounts of ischemic, symptom-producing myocardium, and patients with no available venous or arterial conduits for grafts underwent percutaneous revascularization at an acceptable risk. At many centers, patients with prior bypass surgery account for up to 25% of the PCI procedures performed.

ANATOMIC CONSIDERATIONS

Among the anatomic factors influencing revascularization decisions (Table 81.1), the status of the left anterior descending coronary artery (LAD) and its graft are paramount. Placement of an IMA, a conduit immune to atherosclerosis, as a graft to the LAD has been shown to enhance survival and to reduce ischemic events 10 to as long as 20 years later. In a patient with a patent IMA graft to the LAD, reoperative surgery to treat non-LAD ischemia has been reported to offer no survival benefit, may jeopardize the arterial graft, and, in our experience and that of others, more frequently leads to percutaneous intervention. Multivessel involvement, small number of patent grafts, severe vein graft disease (especially if to the LAD), and a moderately impaired left ventricle are factors more likely to lead to reoperative surgery.

PATHOPHYSIOLOGY: BASIS FOR RECURRENT ISCHEMIA

Incomplete Revascularization

In many patients, complete surgical revascularization was not achieved because of the presence of distal coronary disease,

TABLE 81.1

ANATOMIC FACTORS INFLUENCING REVASCULARIZATION DECISIONS IN POSTBYPASS PATIENTS

Often leads to percutaneous intervention	Often leads to coronary artery bypass grafting
Patent arterial graft (*especially left anterior descending coronary artery*)	Diseased saphenous vein graft to left anterior descending
≥2 patent grafts	Bulky saphenous vein graft atheroma
1–3 culprit lesions	>3 culprit lesions
Difficult surgical access	Multiple saphenous vein graft lesions
Mediastinal scarring secondary to radiation, infection, or pericarditis	Available arterial conduits
Prior muscle transfer closure of unhealed sternotomy	Ejection fraction 25%–35%
Posterior lateral target vessel	
Inadequate conduits	
Near-normal left ventricle	
Future cardiac surgery anticipated	
In situ prosthetic valve	
Mild to moderate aortic or mitral valve disease	

whereas less common causes include the following: an inadequate amount of venous or arterial conduit, inadequate conduit lumen resulting from small vessel size (IMA especially) or injury, intramyocardial location of target coronary vessel, placement of grafts to wrong coronary artery or to a coronary vein, creation of an arteriovenous fistula, use of an IMA in the presence of significant stenosis of the subclavian or innominate arteries, or coronary steal phenomenon attributed to large arterial graft side branches, a cause that has been questioned. Intentional incomplete surgical revascularization is an increasingly frequent phenomenon in patients selected for "beating heart" operations because of the technical difficulty of bypassing posteriorly located coronary arteries. In some patients, this strategy has resulted in subsequent percutaneous revascularization because of inadequate relief of symptoms. In others, incomplete surgical revascularization has been dealt with up front with adjunctive percutaneous revascularization during the same hospitalization, the so-called hybrid approach. In addition to less complete revascularization with beating heart surgery, there is some evidence that less precise anastomoses may compromise graft patency, especially in the surgical learning curve (see the later discussion of venous graft attrition and arterial graft compromise).

Loss of Revascularization Benefit

Venous Graft Attrition

In patients with recurrent ischemia and infarction after bypass surgery, stenosis or occlusion of SVGs is the most common cause. Thrombotic occlusion related to surgical technical problems or slow graft flow secondary to a small or compromised distal coronary arterial bed results in closure of 10% to 15% of SVGs within the first month, and even with aspirin therapy, one report noted that 7% of vein grafts were shown to be occluded by 9 days, and up to 17% of patients had a closed graft at that time (12). Subsequently, 15% to 20% of vein grafts occluded by 1 year, 1% to 2% per year from years 1 to 6, and 4% per year from 6 to 10 years after surgery. After 10 years, a few vein grafts were free of significant occlusive disease.

Native Coronary Artery Progression

Worsening of native coronary artery disease after bypass surgery has been reported in about 5% of patients annually (13). Frequency of disease progression at native vessel sites at 5 years was reported as follows: proximal to graft insertion (70%), unbypassed artery (15%), and distal to graft insertion (0%) (14). Loop noted that progression of disease distal to grafts was uncommon, and at 2 years, progression of disease proximal to grafts was more common for SVG than for IMA grafts (67% versus 39%) (15). Progression of native coronary disease proximal to grafts has implications for coronary intervention when graft disease or occlusion occurs and is an important cause of ischemia resulting from poor retrograde perfusion of side branches (e.g., diagonal coronary arteries).

Arterial Graft Compromise

Although numerous publications attest to the excellent long-term patency of arterial grafts, several hundred patients have been reported who required IMA, radial artery, or subclavian artery intervention (16–22). In most instances, IMA interventions were needed for anastomotic lesions, but proximal and midgraft sites have been treated (see the discussion of arterial graft intervention). The technical difficulty of performing an anastomosis in beating heart surgery probably accounts for more anastomotic problems following this type of surgery. Whether radial artery grafts are superior to SVGs has been questioned.

PRINCIPLES OF MANAGEMENT

Preventive Measures

Patients who have had CABG surgery are at substantial risk for subsequent cardiac events related in large part to progressive arteriosclerosis. Recurrence of angina, angiographic progression of vein graft atheroma, and pathologic changes at autopsy have been correlated with increased serum lipids and smoking, and lipid lowering has been shown to be beneficial (23,24). Given the increased effectiveness of current strategies for lipid lowering and smoking cessation, and reduced cardiac events that accrue, an aggressive approach to risk factor modification is mandatory in all postbypass patients. An aggressive lipid-lowering strategy resulted in a 30% reduction in revascularization and a 24% reduction in a composite clinical end point during 7.5 years of follow-up in the post-CABG Trial. The place of more aggressive antiplatelet therapy in the post-CABG patient is not clear, but recently reported mortality benefits with clopidogrel are provocative and suggest that the use of this or other adjunctive agents may become routine in the future. However, data from randomized controlled trials currently support only aspirin and lipid-lowering agents for routine therapy in all post-CABG patients (25).

Treatment of Ischemia in the Postoperative Patient

Patients with recurrent symptoms or signs of ischemia after bypass surgery constitute an extremely heterogenous group (Fig. 81.2). Treatment strategies must be based on a careful analysis of multiple factors (many angiographically based) including anatomic factors (Table 81.1), the likelihood of a successful percutaneous intervention, risk of complications, probability of long-term symptomatic benefit, and resource consumption compared with other viable options. Patient preferences must be considered because reinterventions are common with percutaneous revascularization in postbypass patients and occur in about 50% of patients at 5 years. In the postbypass patient, the ability to effect ischemia relief percutaneously is influenced by the time that has lapsed since surgery, the type of conduit (SVG versus native vessel versus IMA graft), and the location of the stenotic segment.

Results of Native Coronary Intervention

The procedural outcome of angioplasty for native coronary intervention after CABG was reported for the first 372 such patients treated at Emory University in 1987 (26). Most were men (81%), and 78% had multivessel disease. Angiographic success was achieved in 91%, and in-hospital complications were infrequent: mortality, 0.3%; Q-wave MI, 2%; non–Q-wave MI, 4%; CABG surgery, 6%. At the Mid-America Heart Institute (Kansas City, MO), 1,543 postbypass patients underwent angioplasty of native coronary arteries. Angiographic success was 94%, in-hospital mortality was 0.8%, Q-wave MI was 1.5%, and emergency bypass surgery was 1.0% (27). At Emory University between 1980 and 1995, 2,246 postbypass patients underwent coronary intervention of native arteries with favorable outcome: procedural success, 89%; in-hospital mortality, 1%, Q-wave MI, 1%; non–Q-wave MI 4% (creatine kinase greater than three times normal); and emergency or elective surgery, 2.8%. Although the definitions of outcomes were slightly different in these series, the overall procedural results were favorable, with a trend toward less need for in-hospital bypass surgery for failed percutaneous intervention. These outcomes were largely that of conventional balloon angioplasty. The Mayo Clinic (Rochester, MN) experience with 937 post-CABG patients treated between 1995 and 1998 reflected a dramatic increase in stent use to 76% of patients and a reduction in use of atherectomy and laser strategies. Patients who underwent interventions in native vessels were younger, more likely female, had less severe coronary disease, and had a more favorable long-term outlook than those who underwent venous bypass graft intervention (28). Results of the use of drug-eluting stents in native coronary intervention after CABG have not been reported.

Results of Saphenous Vein Graft Intervention

Numerous reports have described the results of balloon angioplasty in SVG disease, indicating that, in selected patients, success rates of approximately 90% were achieved, with mortality of about 1%, Q-wave MI of less than 2%, and in-hospital CABG in approximately 2% of patients. Many of these patients had relatively favorable anatomy with focal lesions free of obvious thrombus. Non–Q-wave MI, the most frequent complication, occurred in 78 (13%) of 599 patients at Emory University (29,30). The length of time since surgery was an important predictor of restenosis (<6 months, 32%; 6 months to 1 year, 43%; 1 to 5 years, 61%; and 64% for >5 years; $p < .02$), as was the location of the lesion (proximal anastomosis, 68%; midgraft, 61%; distal anastomosis, 45%; $p < .06$). The lowest restenosis rate, 22%, was noted for lesions that occurred at the distal anastomosis within 1 year of surgery, and these patients had excellent, event-free survival (Fig. 81.3).

Stenting of SVGs has become the dominant percutaneous strategy (31–48). The largest early experience in vein graft stenting was with the Palmaz-Schatz stent (Johnson & Johnson Interventional Systems) (Table 81.2). Deployment success rates were very high, and in-hospital complications were low, including a lower rate of stent thrombosis than was observed in native coronary artery stenting at that time. Six-month restenosis rates in the Multicenter U.S. Palmaz-Schatz Registry were a surprisingly low 18% for de novo lesions and 46% for restenotic lesions. The 12-month actuarial event-free survival was 76% (35).

A randomized multicenter comparison of the use of balloon angioplasty and stents in SVGs (the Stent Versus Angioplasty in Saphenous Vein Graft Disease [SAVED] trial) was carried out with the Palmaz-Schatz coronary stent in 215 patients with focal de novo stenosis (36). Patients were excluded who had MI within 7 days, thrombus, ejection fraction less than 25%, or contraindications to warfarin (Coumadin) anticoagulation. Graft age (mean, 10 years), lesion characteristics, and patient characteristics in the balloon (n = 107) and stent (n = 108) groups were similar except for an increased incidence of diabetes in the balloon group (36% versus 23%, $p = .03$). Procedural technical success (<50% stenosis with assigned therapy) was higher with stenting (95% versus 75%, $p < .001$). In-hospital complications of death, Q-wave MI, bypass surgery, and abrupt closure were similar, but there was a trend toward more non–Q-wave MIs in the balloon group (7% versus 2%, $p = .10$), and more stent-treated patients required transfusions (10% versus 1%, $p = .003$). At 6 months, restenosis occurred in 36% of stent patients versus 47% of balloon patients ($p = .11$), and the minimal luminal diameter of stent patients was significantly larger (1.75 versus 1.47 mm, $p = .05$) as was the net gain in lumen diameter (0.87 versus 0.52 mm, $p = .015$). Cumulative cardiac events (death, Q-wave MI, non–Q-wave MI, CABG, and repeat PTCA) were significantly less frequent in stent patients (26% versus 38%, $p = .05$) (Fig. 81.4). Numerous single-center and multicenter observational reports of stenting in SVGs have been reported (Table 81.2). However, data are limited regarding the use of drug-eluting stents in SVGs. In the SECURE trial, sirolimus-eluting stents were deployed in patients with no other options, and outcomes in SVGs and native coronary arteries were similar (49). Hoye and colleagues treated 19 consecutive patients with de novo SVG lesions with sirolimus-eluting stents, and target lesion revascularization was needed in only one patient at 1-year mean follow-up (50). The first randomized trial comparing drug-eluting stents with bare metal stents in SVGs was reported by Vermeersch and colleagues from Antwerp, Belgium (47,48). Seventy-five patients with de novo SVG stenoses treatable with up to two stents were randomized to Cypher (Cordis, Miami Lakes, FL) or bare metal stents. The primary end point was late loss; binary restenosis and clinical events were secondary end points. Distal protection was used in 80% of patients. Late loss at 6 months was significantly lower in Cypher-treated patients (in-segment late loss 0.46 versus 0.93 mm, $p < .0005$), as was restenosis (5% versus 37%, $p = .0005$). Major adverse cardiac events (MACEs) at 6 months occurred in 16% of Cypher-treated patients and in 27% of patients treated with bare metal stents. Cypher stents appeared to be safe and effective in reducing late loss and binary restenosis.

Several studies of contemporary SVG stenting indicated that even with mostly single-lesion, single-stent procedures, the incidence of clinically important myocardial necrosis (creatine kinase levels greater than three times normal) was approximately 20%. In the Reduced Anticoagulation Vein Graft Study 22% of patients had Q-wave or non–Q-wave MI (51), and in more than 400 patients treated in two high-volume

TABLE 81.2

RESULTS OF STENTING OF AORTOCORONARY SAPHENOUS VEIN GRAFTS: SELECTED REPORTS

Author (y)	Reference	Early implantation success (%)	Thrombosis (%)	CABG (%)	Death (%)	AMI (%)	Restenosis (%)
PALMAZ-SCHATZ							
Pomerantz, et al. (1992)	31	83/84 (99%)	0	0	0	10	36
Carrozza, et al. (1992)	32	84/84 (100%)	0	0	0	8	—
Fenton, et al. (1994)	33	196/198 (99%)	0.5	—	—	—	34
Piana, et al. (1994)	34	147/150 (98%)	1	0	1	7.3	17
Wong, et al. (1995)	35	571/589 (97%)	1.4	0.9	1.7	0.3	30
Savage, et al. (1997)	36	105/108 (97%)	1	2	2	4	36
WALLSTENT							
de Scheerder, et al. (1992)	37	69/69 (100%)	10	0	1.5	7	47
Strauss, et al. (1992)	38	145/145 (100%)	8	—	—	—	34
de Jaegere[a], et al. (1996)	39	92/93 (99%)	4	5	3	3	—
WIKTOR							
Fortuna, et al. (1993)	40	101/101 (100%)	2	1	1	3	—
Hanekamp, et al. (2000)	41	77/78 (99%)	—	—	—	—	22
VARIOUS STENTS							
Safian, et al. (1998)	42						
■ Palmaz-Schatz		101/101 (100%)	—	—	—	—	32
■ Wallstent		109/114 (95%)	—	—	—	—	13
■ Wallstent (SVG >4 mm)		197/207 (95%)	—	—	—	—	39
Le May, et al. (1999)	43	103/106 (98%)	0	0	0	—	—
Dharmadhikari (2000)	44						
■ Covered stents		30	—	3	0	0	Revasc. 20
■ Noncovered stents		125	—	0	0	8.8	Revasc. 28
Baldus, et al.[b] (2000)	45	108/109 (99%)	0.9	0	0	1	26
Nishida, et al. (2000)	46	97/101 (96%)	—	2	1	10.9	TVR 21
■ Drug-eluting stents[c]	47,48	42/42 (100%)	0	0	0	—	5%

AMI, acute myocardial infarction. CABG, coronary artery bypass grafting; SVG, saphenous vein graft; TVR, target vessel revascularization.
[a]90% Wallstents.
[b]All covered stents.
[c]All sirolimus-eluting stents.

centers from 1995 to 1997, 17% had creatine kinase MB levels greater than three times normal, and among these patients the 30-day mortality was 14% (52). As the lesion complexity, length, and plaque volume increased, so did the rate of myonecrosis and procedural risks (53). Procedural MI also affected long-term outcomes. In a study of 1,056 consecutive SVG PCI procedures, procedural creatine kinase MB elevation was the strongest independent predictor of late mortality (54). A heightened appreciation of the importance of atheroembolic MI in SVG PCI dovetailed with the development of strategies for distal protection, thus generating enormous interest in its potential for improving outcomes of SVG PCI. Webb and colleagues, using the PercuSurge system (distal occlusion balloon and aspiration, Medtronic-AVE, Santa Rosa, CA) in 45 patients, reported aspiration of atherosclerotic debris in more than 80% of patients and a MI rate of less than 4% (55). In a randomized trial comparing SVG PCI outcomes with and without PercuSurge (SAFER trial) in 801 patients, in-hospital MACEs were reduced by 42% (16.5% to 9.6%, $p < .001$) with distal protection (56). MI was reduced from 14.7% to 8.6%. The PercuSurge Guardwire has a relatively low profile, an advantage in the presence of severe stenosis. Its use in SVGs has been shown to capture soluble vasoactive agents including endothelin and serotonin as well as a variety of coagulation components (tissue factor, plasminogen activator inhibitor, prothrombin fragments 1 and 2, and thrombin-antithrombin complex) (57). Benefits of PercuSurge extended to short lesions (<10 mm) where 30-day MACEs were reduced by 77% (8.1% to 2.2%) (58). Disadvantages of the PercuSurge Guardwire include the need to occlude the treated vessel completely for 3 to 5 minutes, a relatively long normal segment beyond the lesion in which to place the occlusion balloon and the complexity of the procedure.

Filter-based distal protection with the Filter-wire (Boston Scientific, Natick, MA) was tested in the FIRE trial, a 650-patient multicenter study in which patients were randomly assigned to Filter-wire or Guardwire therapy (59). Thirty-day MACEs were similar (9.9% with filter, 11.6% with Guardwire), and there were virtually identical rates of MI (9% versus 10%) and death (0.9% versus 0.9%). It seems likely that some form of distal protection will be used in many, perhaps all, SVG PCI procedures in the future. Another device for distal protection using proximal vessel occlusion, known as PROXIS, is currently being evaluated. Some theoretic advantages of proximal occlusion include side branch protection, protection during wire passage, and no requirement for a normal segment beyond the lesion for placement of the occlusion balloon, but a proximal normal segment is required.

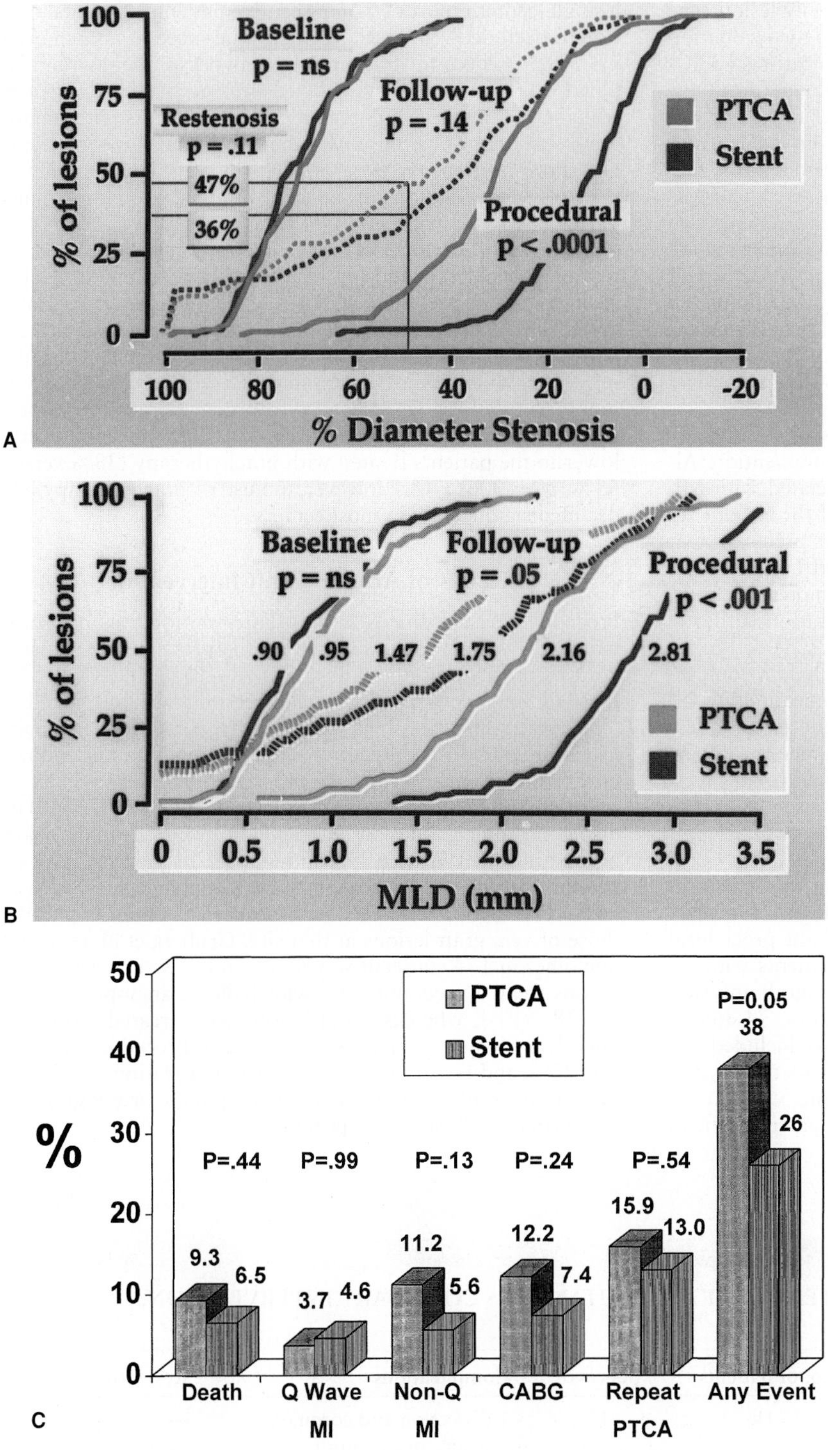

FIGURE 81.4. **A:** Cumulative frequency of percentage of diameter stenosis determined by quantitative coronary angiography before, immediately after, and at 6 months following stent or balloon angioplasty in the Stent Versus Angioplasty in Saphenous Vein Graft Disease (SAVED) Trial. **B:** Cumulative frequency of minimal luminal diameter (MLD) before, immediately after, and 6 months after stenting or balloon angioplasty in the SAVED Trial. **C:** Major cardiac events experienced by patients 6 months following randomization to balloon angioplasty or stent in the SAVED Trial. CABG, coronary artery bypass grafting; MI, myocardial infarction; PTCA, percutaneous transluminal coronary angioplasty.

Early observational reports of the use of a polytetrafluoroethylene (PTFE)-covered stent in SVG PCI suggested that both immediate and long-term outcomes were better than with conventional stents or balloon angioplasty. However, the results of two recently published trials comparing PTFE-covered stents with bare metal stents in SVGs were not encouraging. Six-month MACE rates were higher in patients receiving covered stents as a result of more MIs and late occlusion (60,61). In addition, the Barricade Trial, presented at the American College of Cardiology in 2005, a randomized prospective study testing the safety and efficacy of a PTFE-covered stent compared with a bare metal stent in SVGs, was disappointing (48,62). Analysis of the first 243 patients randomized revealed poorer outcomes in patients receiving covered stents with respect to MACE (33% versus 21%, $p = .047$), restenosis (32.5% versus 25.6%, $p = .39$), and there was a trend toward more total occlusions (20.5% versus 10.5%, $p = .09$). On the basis of these outcomes, the trial was terminated. Currently the PTFE-covered stent is available for treatment of PCI-related perforations, and its use in this setting can be lifesaving.

The large amount of atheroembolic debris filtered or aspirated during SVG stent procedures provides insight into the failure of glycoprotein (GP) IIb/IIIa platelet receptor inhibitors to reduce periprocedural ischemic events during SVG PCI.

Ellis et al. found degenerated SVG to be the only lesion type not to benefit from abciximab when data from the evaluation of c7E3 for the Prevention of Ischemic Complications (EPIC) trial and the Evaluation of PTCA to Improve Long-Term Outcome with Abciximab GPIIb/IIIa Receptor Blockade (EPILOG) trial were pooled (63). Similarly, when data from five trials of SVG PCI totalling 627 patients and the Cleveland Clinic registry of 278 patients with SVG PCI were analyzed, there was no benefit from GPIIb/IIIa inhibitors or stents with respect to 30-day outcome, and a trend was present toward increased MI with stenting ($p = .09$) (64,65). The lack of any acute benefit with SVG stent deployment is consistent with the findings of the SAVED trial (36) and the VENESTENT Study (41), each of which randomized patients to balloon angioplasty or stent implantation and demonstrated an improved MACE-free survival at 6 months, but no early difference in MACEs.

Plaque debulking strategies such as atherectomy and laser have not been shown to have benefit in SVG intervention. Although it is clear that SVG thrombus is associated with MI, no-reflow, and death, optimal management of thrombotic lesions has not been determined. Some operators prefer to treat thrombotic lesions with heparin and a GPIIb/IIIa platelet receptor inhibitor for several days; others attempt mechanical thrombectomy with a guide catheter or aspiration catheters such as Export (AVE Medtronic, Santa Rosa, CA) or Pronto (Vascular Solutions, Minneapolis, MN). Rheolytic thrombectomy with the Angiojet (Possis Medical, Minneapolis, MN) was shown in a randomized trial to be more effective and less expensive than urokinase (66). A novel dual-lumen thrombectomy catheter known as the X-Sizer (ev 3, Plymouth, MN) was tested in a randomized trial in 797 patients; its use was associated with fewer large MIs (5.4% versus 10.4%, $p = .03$), but with a similar rate of all infarctions (67).

Recanalizing totally occluded SVGs, not in the setting of acute MI, has tempted interventional cardiologists for years in spite of low long-term patency and significant procedural complications. In a multicenter trial of 107 patients with total vein graft occlusion who received an intragraft infusion of thrombolytic agent for a mean of 25 hours, 74 (69%) achieved initial patency. Adverse acute events included MI (22.0%), emergency CABG (4.0%), stroke (3.0%), transfusion (19.0%), and death (6.5%) (68). Of 40 patients who underwent recatheterization at 6 months, 16 had a patent graft. In a single-center report of 77 consecutive patients with intervention to occluded vein graft, angiographic success was achieved in 71%, 5% died, and 8% underwent bypass surgery within 30 days (69). Three-year survival, event-free survival, and freedom from severe angina were not different in patients with angiographic success and failure. Whether new strategies of mechanical thrombectomy or ultrasound thrombolysis will alter the risk-to-benefit relationship in these difficult patients remains unclear.

Intravascular radiation for the prevention of recurrence of restenosis yielded promising results in the Washington Radiation for In-Stent Restenosis Trial for Saphenous Vein Grafts (WRIST). This was a double-blind, randomized trial in 120 patients with diffuse in-stent restenosis (<47 mm in length) in SVGs, which compared iridium-192 versus placebo. At 6 months, restenosis was lower with brachytherapy (21% versus 44%, $p = .005$). At 36 months, MACEs were significantly lower in the patients treated with brachytherapy (38% versus 63%, $p = .006$) (70). However, the use of brachytherapy has declined significantly in most centers.

Results of Arterial Graft Intervention

Procedural success in IMA graft intervention was approximately 90% and was influenced by the presence of excessive graft tortuosity and lesion location (71–73) (Table 81.3). The most common complication was dissection, which occurred in 3.5%, rarely resulting in infarction or bypass surgery. In a published report of 68 consecutive patients, angiographic follow-up at a mean interval of 8 months was available in 78% of successful procedures. Restenosis occurred in 15% (6 of 40) of distal anastomotic sites and in 43% (3 of 7) in the midportion of the graft (72). At a mean follow-up of 14 months, 76% of patients had class 1 or 2 angina, and event-free survival was 86%. The favorable results at the distal anastomosis parallel those of vein graft lesions at that site. Gruberg et al. reported outcomes in 174 consecutive patients, 63% with anastomotic lesions treated predominantly with balloon angioplasty (116 of 128, 91%), whereas ostial lesions were treated more frequently with stents (11 of 16, 69%) (21). Procedural success was 97%, and 1-year target lesion revascularization was 7.4%. Long-term results of radial and gastroepiploic artery graft intervention have not been reported.

TABLE 81.3

RESULTS OF INTERNAL MAMMARY ARTERY GRAFT PERCUTANEOUS CORONARY INTERVENTION: SELECTED SERIES

Author (y)	Reference	No. of patients	Success	Complications	Restenosis
Webb, et al. (1990)	71	18	12	1 dissection and coronary artery bypass graft	—
Dimas, et al. (1991)	17	31	28	2 dissections	1
Sketch, et al. (1992)	18	14	13	—	1
Shimshak, et al. (1988)	19	26	24	3 dissections	1
Hill, et al. (1989)	16	11	9	0	2
Shimshak, et al. (1991)	20	86	81	1 Q-wave MI, 4 late deaths	
Hearne, et al. (1995)	72	68	60	2 dissections	9 (19%)
Ischizaka, et al. (1995)	73	46	34	1 spasm	30%
Gruberg, et al. (2000)	21	174	168	1 death 1 coronary artery vascularization, bypass graft, 15 non-Q-wave myocardial infarction	1-y target lesion revascularization, 7.4%

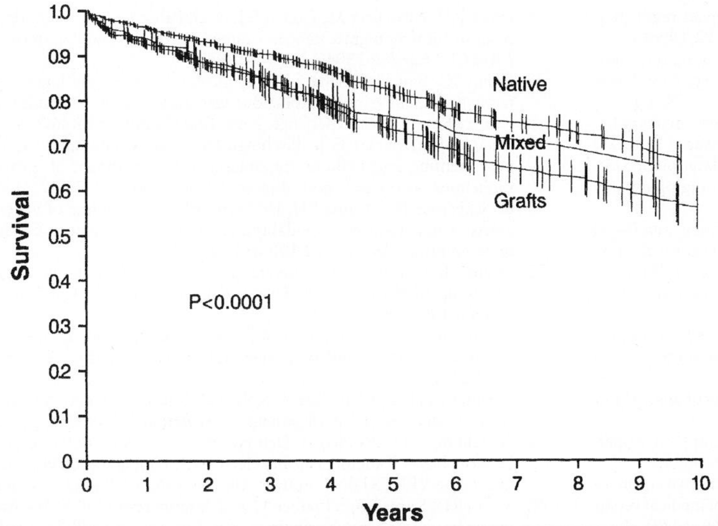

Native											
N Remaining	1502	1341	1035	833	695	556	369	290	199	125	79
Survival	1	0.956	0.925	0.897	0.862	0.813	0.773	0.745	0.719	0.699	0.658
Deaths	0	65	103	132	162	199	220	232	240	244	250
Grafts											
N Remaining	864	772	606	495	418	334	232	184	156	120	88
Survival	1	0.92	0.872	0.842	0.776	0.729	0.681	0.643	0.624	0.588	0.555
Deaths	0	69	104	123	160	184	202	214	219	227	233
Mixed											
N Remaining	197	180	140	113	102	73	39	34	24	19	11
Survival	1	0.934	0.88	0.824	0.793	0.758	0.722	0.722	0.693	0.693	0.65
Deaths	0	13	22	30	34	38	40	40	41	41	42

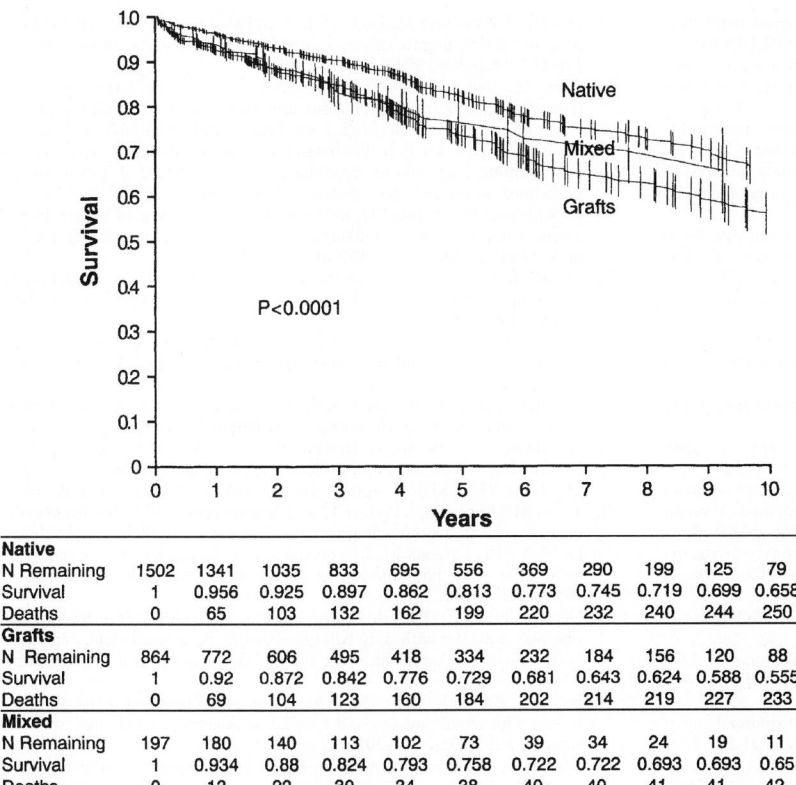

FIGURE 81.5. Ten-year survival of postbypass patients who underwent percutaneous coronary intervention of a native coronary artery (native), saphenous vein grafts (grafts), or both (mixed) at Emory University Hospitals in Atlanta, Georgia. (Kaplan-Meier method).

CONTROVERSIES AND PERSONAL PERSPECTIVES

Value of Saphenous Vein Graft Intervention

After successful SVG intervention, there is a high cardiac event rate for most patient subgroups. Distal anastomotic lesions are a possible exception. The restenotic process in vein grafts does not plateau as it does in native coronary arteries, and mild to moderate nontarget vein graft lesions are associated with recurrent ischemic events in about one third of patients (74). Even with careful selection of patients, emphasizing focal disease and absence of thrombus as was the case in the SAVED trial, the 6-month MACE rate was 26% following SVG stenting, and restenosis occurred in almost 40% of patients (36). At Emory University, 5-year event-free survival for vein graft intervention was 31% (29), and survival was less favorable than that with native coronary intervention (Fig. 81.5). If one moves from these relatively ideal candidates to the treatment of diffuse vein graft disease, recent total occlusions, or even chronic occlusions, the prospects for long-term patency and clinical stability diminish, whereas the acute risk of thromboembolic MI and bleeding and costs escalate. Although continued study is needed to develop methods to prolong the functional life of degenerating venous grafts, day-to-day application of percutaneous strategies to these difficult problems must be done with caution and should include the use of embolic protection and drug-eluting stents in most patients.

Repeat Interventions

Andreas Gruentzig envisioned coronary angioplasty as a strategy that could be used over the years to prevent patients from moving from low-risk categories (nil or single-vessel disease) to high-risk coronary disease. In the postbypass patient, percutaneous intervention is more often performed in an attempt to control symptoms and to preserve quality of life. If the patient can be palliated safely by repeat interventions, even for periods as short as a year, this may be reasonable. However, thoughtful cost-conscious consideration of risks and benefits and of resource consumption must take place.

THE FUTURE

In the next decade, increasing numbers of postbypass patients will have recurrent angina that requires hospitalization. Because of the enormous cost, morbidity, and impracticality of repeat surgical revascularization, it will be important to palliate these patients by percutaneous means as much as possible. We expect technology (especially better, coated, and perhaps covered stents) to help, but a major problem is the inadequacy of strategies to treat old, degenerated SVGs. With the development of more reliable methods of distal protection, techniques to renew (pave?) old grafts and to prevent restenosis will evolve.

References

1. Gruentzig A. Transluminal dilatation of coronary artery stenosis. *Lancet* 1978;1:263.
2. Hurst JW. History of cardiac catheterization. In: King SB III, Douglas JS Jr, eds. *Coronary arteriography and angioplasty.* New York: McGraw-Hill, 1985:19.
3. Cameron AAC, David KB, Rodgers WJ. Recurrence of angina after coronary artery bypass surgery: predictors and prognosis (CASS Registry). *J Am Coll Cardiol* 1995;26:895–899.
4. Loop FD, Lytle BW, Cosgrove DM, et al. Reoperation for coronary atherosclerosis. *Ann Surg* 1990;212:378–386.

5. Weintraub WS, Jones EL, Craver JM, et al. Incidence of repeat revascularization after coronary bypass surgery. *J Am Coll Cardiol* 1992;19:98A.
6. Weintraub WS, Jones EL, Craver JM, et al. In-hospital and long-term outcome after reoperative coronary artery bypass graft surgery. *Circulation* 1995;92(suppl II):II50–II57.
7. Jurkovitz C, Jones EL, Craver JM, et al. Update on reoperative coronary bypass surgery: results from the 1990's. *Circulation* 2000;102(suppl II):II555.
8. Gruentzig AR, Senning A, Siegenthaler WE. Nonoperative dilatation of coronary artery stenosis: percutaneous transluminal coronary angioplasty. *N Engl J Med* 1979;303:61–68.
9. Mock MB, Kent KM, Bentivoglio LG. The National Heart, Lung, and Blood Institute percutaneous transluminal coronary angioplasty registry: the first 1116 cases. In: Kaltenbach M, Gruentzig A, Rentrop K, Bussman WD, eds. *Transluminal coronary angioplasty and intracoronary thrombolysis. Coronary heart disease, IV.* New York: Springer-Verlag, 1982:1119.
10. Douglas JS Jr, Gruentzig AR, King SB III, et al. Percutaneous transluminal coronary angioplasty in patients with prior coronary bypass surgery. *J Am Coll Cardiol* 1983;2:745–754.
11. Douglas JS, Ghazzal ZMB, Morris DC, King SB. Twenty years of angioplasty at Emory University. *Circulation* 2000;102(suppl II):II753.
12. Goldman S, Copeland J, Moritz T, et al. Starting aspirin therapy after operation: effects on early graft patency. *Circulation* 1991;84:520–525.
13. Hwang MH, Meadows WR, Palac RT, et al. Progression of native coronary artery disease at 10 years: insights from a randomized study of medical versus surgical therapy for angina. *J Am Coll Cardiol* 1990;16:1066–1070.
14. Hair D, Antonescu A, Ishimori T, Michael AD. Does coronary artery bypass surgery cause native vessel occlusion? *J Am Coll Cardiol* 1996;27(suppl A):92A.
15. Loop FD. Internal-thoracic-artery grafts. *N Engl J Med* 1996;334:263–265.
16. Hill DM, McAuley BJ, Sheehan DJ, et al. Percutaneous transluminal angioplasty of internal mammary artery bypass grafts. *J Am Coll Cardiol* 1989; 13:221A.
17. Dimas AP, Arora RR, Whitlow PL, et al. Percutaneous transluminal angioplasty involving internal mammary artery grafts. *Am Heart J* 1991;122:423–429.
18. Sketch MH, Quigley PG, Perez JA, et al. Angiographic follow-up after internal mammary artery graft angioplasty. *Am J Cardiol* 1992;70:401–403.
19. Shimshak TM, Giorgi LV, Johnson WL, et al. Application of percutaneous transluminal coronary angioplasty to the internal mammary artery graft. *J Am Coll Cardiol* 1988;12:1205–1214.
20. Shimshak TM, Rutherford BD, McConahay DR, et al. PTCA of internal mammary artery (IMA) grafts procedural results and late follow-up. *Circulation* 1991;84(suppl II):II590.
21. Gruberg L, Dangas G, Mehran R, et al. Percutaneous revascularization of the internal mammary artery graft: short- and long-term outcomes. *J Am Coll Cardiol* 2000;35:944–948.
22. Kollar A, Simonton CA, Thomley AM, Selle JG. Balloon angioplasty of the internal mammary artery trunk for early postoperative ischemia: a case report. *Cathet Cardiovasc Diagn* 1996;37:49–51.
23. Knatterud GL, Rosenberg Y, Campeau L, et al. Long term effects on clinical outcomes of aggressive lowering of low density lipoprotein cholesterol levels and low dose anticoagulation in the post coronary artery bypass graft trial. *Circulation* 2000;102:157–165.
24. Domanski MJ, Borkowf CB, Campeau L, et al. Prognostic factors for atherosclerosis progression in saphenous vein grafts: the Post Coronary Artery Bypass Grafts (Post-CABG) Trial. *J Am Coll Cardiol* 2000;36:1877–1883.
25. Okrainec K, Platt B, Pilote L, et al. Cardiac medical therapy in patients after undergoing coronary artery bypass graft surgery. *J Am Coll Cardiol* 2005; 45:177–184.
26. Douglas JS Jr, King SB III, Roubin GS, et al. Native coronary artery angioplasty in patients with previous coronary bypass surgery: update of in-hospital and long-term results. *Circulation* 1987;76(suppl IV):IV465.
27. Miranda CP, Rutherford BD, McConahay DR, et al. Elective PTCA in post-bypass patients: comparison between those undergoing native artery dilatations and those undergoing bypass graft dilatations. *Circulation* 1992; 86(suppl I):I457.
28. Mathew V, Clavell AL, Lennon RJ, et al. Percutaneous coronary interventions in patients with prior coronary bypass surgery: changes in patient characteristics and outcome during two decades. *Am J Med* 2000;108:127–135.
29. Douglas JS Jr, Weintraub WS, Liberman HA, et al. Update of saphenous graft (SVG) angioplasty: restenosis and long-term outcome. *Circulation* 1991;84(suppl II):II249.
30. Douglas JS Jr, Weintraub WS, King SB III. Changing perspectives in vein graft angioplasty. *J Am Coll Cardiol* 1995;25(suppl A):78A.
31. Pomerantz RM, Kuntz RE, Carroza J, et al. Acute and long-term outcome of narrowed saphenous vein grafts treated with endoluminal stenting and directional atherectomy. *Am J Cardiol* 1992;70:161–167.
32. Carrozza JP, Kuntz RE, Levine MJ, et al. Angiographic and clinical outcome of intracoronary stenting: immediate and long-term results from a large single-center experience. *J Am Coll Cardiol* 1992;20:328–337.
33. Fenton SH, Fischman DL, Savage MP, et al. Long-term angiographic and clinical outcome after implantation of balloon-expandable stents in aortocoronary saphenous vein grafts. *Am J Cardiol* 1994;74:1187–1191.
34. Piana RN, Moscucci M, Cohen DJ, et al. Palmaz-Schatz stenting for treatment of focal vein graft stenosis: immediate results and long-term outcome. *J Am Coll Cardiol* 1994;23:1296–1304.
35. Wong SC, Baim DS, Schatz RA, et al. Acute results and late outcomes after stent implantation in saphenous vein graft lesions: the multicenter USA Palmaz-Schatz stent experience. *J Am Coll Cardiol* 1995;26:704–712.
36. Savage MP, Douglas JS Jr, Fischman DL, et al. A randomized trial of coronary stenting and balloon angioplasty in the treatment of aortocoronary saphenous vein bypass graft disease. *N Engl J Med* 1997;337:740–747.
37. de Scheerder JK, Strauss BH, De Feyter PJ, et al. Stenting of venous bypass grafts: a new treatment modality of patients who are poor candidates for reintervention. *Am Heart J* 1992;23:1296–1304.
38. Strauss BH, Serruys PW, Bertrand ME, et al. Qualitative angiographic follow-up of the coronary Wallstent in native vessel bypass grafts. *Am J Cardiol* 1992;69:475–481.
39. de Jaegere PP, Van Domburg RT, De Feyter PJ, et al. Long-term clinical outcome after stent implantation in saphenous vein grafts. *J Am Coll Cardiol* 1996;28:89–96.
40. Fortuna R, Heuser RR, Garrat KN, et al. Wiktor intracoronary stent: experience in the first 101 graft patients. *Circulation* 1993;88(suppl I):I308.
41. Hanekamp CEE, Koolen JJ, Den Heyer P, et al. A randomized comparison between balloon angioplasty and elective stent implantation in venous bypass grafts: the VENESTENT study. *J Am Coll Cardiol* 2000;35(suppl A):9A.
42. Safian RD, Kaplan B, Schreiber T, et al. Interim results of the Wallstent endoprosthesis in saphenous vein graft trial. *Circulation* 1998;98(suppl I):I662.
43. Le May MR, Labinaz M, Marquis JF, et al. Predictors of long-term outcome after stent implantation in a saphenous vein graft. *Am J Cardiol* 1999;83:681–686.
44. Dharmadhikari A, Di Mario C, Tzifos V, et al. Comparison of procedural and one-year outcome with only balloon angioplasty, covered stents, and non-covered stents in saphenous vein grafts. *J Am Coll Cardiol* 2000;35(suppl A):26A.
45. Baldus S, Koster R, Elsner M, et al. Treatment of aortocoronary vein graft lesions with membrane-covered stents: a multicenter surveillance trial. *Circulation* 2000;102:2024–2027.
46. Nishida T, Colombo A, Briguori C, et al. Contemporary percutaneous treatment of saphenous vein graft stenosis: immediate and late outcomes. *J Invasive Cardiol* 2000;12:505–512.
47. Vermeersch P, Van Langenhove G, Covens C, et al. First randomized trial comparing sirolimus-eluting stents versus bare metal stents in severely diseased saphenous vein graft treatment: six month clinical and angiographic outcome. *J Am Coll Cardiol* 2005;45(suppl A):84A.
48. Douglas JS Jr. Interventional cardiology highlights of ACC 2005. *J Am Coll Cardiol* 2005;45(suppl B):4B–8B.
49. Costa M, Gilmore P, Jacks S, et al. Sirolimus-eluting stent for the treatment of bypass graft disease: long-term results of the initial U.S. experience. *Circulation* 2003;108(suppl IV):IV390.
50. Hoye A, Lemos PA, Arampatzis CA, et al. Effectiveness of the sirolimus-eluting stent in the treatment of saphenous vein graft disease. *J Invasive Cardiol* 2004;16:230–233.
51. Leon MB, Ellis SG, Moses J, et al. Interim report from the reduced anticoagulation vein graft stent (RAVES) study. *Circulation* 1996;94(suppl I):I683.
52. Kalon KL, Carrozza JP, Popma JJ, et al. Creatine-kinase MB isoform (CK-MB) elevations following single vessel percutaneous revascularization of saphenous vein grafts. *Circulation* 1998;98(suppl I):I353.
53. Liu MW, Douglas JS Jr, King SB III, et al. Angiographic predictors of coronary embolization in the PTCA of vein graft lesions. *Circulation* 1989;80 (suppl II):II172.
54. Hong MK, Mehran R, Dangas G, Mintz GS, et al. Creatine kinase-MB enzyme elevation following successful saphenous vein graft intervention is associated with late mortality. *Circulation* 1999;100:2400–2405.
55. Webb JG, Carere RG, Virmani R, et al. Retrieval and analysis of particulate debris following saphenous vein graft intervention. *J Am Coll Cardiol* 1999;34:461–467.
56. Baim DS, Wahr D, George B, et al. Randomized trial of a distal embolic protection device during percutaneous intervention of saphenous vein aortocoronary bypass grafts. *Circulation* 2002;105:512–590.
57. Salloum J, Reddy B, Vaughan DE, et al. Elimination of soluble vasoactive factors by the PercuSurge Guardwire distal protection device during percutaneous coronary intervention of saphenous vein graft. *J Am Coll Cardiol* 2004;43:71A.
58. Giugliano GR, Prpic R, Cutlip, et al. Does the beneficial effect of distal protection in saphenous vein graft interventions vary with lesion length? A SAFER (Saphenous Vein Graft Angioplasty Free of Emboli Randomized) Substudy. *J Am Coll Cardiol* 2002;30(suppl A):9A.
59. Stone G, Rogers C, Hermiller J, et al. Randomized comparison of distal protection with filter-based catheter and a balloon occlusion and aspiration system during percutaneous intervention of diseased saphenous vein aortocoronary bypass grafts. *Circulation* 2003;108:548–553.
60. Stankovic G, Colombo A, Presbitero P, et al. Randomized evaluation of polytetrafluoroethylene-covered stent in saphenous vein grafts. *Circulation* 2003;108:37–42.
61. Schachinger V, Hamm CW, Munzel T, et al. A randomized trial of polytetrafluoroethylene-covered stents compared with conventional stents in aortocoronary saphenous vein grafts. *J Am Coll Cardiol* 2003;42:1360–1369.

62. Stone GW, Goldberg S, Mehran R, et al. A prospective, randomized U.S. trial of the PTFE covered JOSTENT for the treatment of diseased saphenous vein grafts: the BARRICADE trial. *J Am Coll Cardiol* 2005;45(suppl A):27A.
63. Ellis SG, Lincoff AM, Miller D, et al. Reduction in complications of angioplasty with abciximab occurs largely independently of baseline lesion morphology. *J Am Coll Cardiol* 1998;32:1619–1623.
64. Roffi M, Chan A, Chew DP, et al. Stents and glycoprotein IIb/IIIa inhibitors do not improve 30-day outcome in bypass graft percutaneous interventions: a retrospective registry-based analysis. *J Am Coll Cardiol* 2001;37(suppl A):77A.
65. Roffi M, Bhatt DL, Mukherjee D, et al. Stents and glycoprotein IIb/IIIa blockade have no salutory effect on 30-day outcome following percutaneous interventions of coronary bypass grafts. *J Am Coll Cardiol* 2001;37(suppl A):68A.
66. Kuntz RE, Baim DS, Cohen DJ, et al. A trial comparing rheolytic thrombectomy with intracoronary urokinase for coronary and vein graft thrombus (the Vein Graft Angiojet Study (VeGAS 2). *Am J Cardiol* 2002;89:326–330.
67. Stone GW, Cox DA, Babb J, et al. Prospective, randomized evaluation of thrombectomy prior to percutaneous intervention in diseased saphenous vein grafts and thrombus-containing coronary arteries. *J Am Coll Cardiol* 2003;42:2007–2013.
68. Hartmann JR, McKeever LS, O'Neill WW, et al. Recanalization of chronically occluded aortocoronary saphenous vein bypass grafts with long-term, low dose direct infusion of urokinase (ROBUST): A serial trial. *J Am Coll Cardiol* 1996;27:60–66.
69. Berger PB, Bell MR, Simari R, et al. Immediate and long-term clinical outcome in patients undergoing angioplasty of occluded vein grafts. *J Am Coll Cardiol* 1996;76(suppl A):180A.
70. Rha SW, Waksman R, Kuchulakanti PK, et al. Three-year follow-up after intracoronary gamma radiation for in-stent restenosis in saphenous vein grafts. *J Am Coll Cardiol* 2004;104A.
71. Webb JG, Myler RF, Shaw RE, et al. Coronary angioplasty after coronary bypass surgery: Initial results and late outcome in 422 patients. *J Am Coll Cardiol* 1990;16:812–820.
72. Hearne SE, Wilson JS, Harrington J, et al. Angiographic and clinical follow-up after internal mammary artery graft angioplasty: a 9-year experience. *J Am Coll Cardiol* 1995;25(suppl A):139A.
73. Ishizaka N, Ishizaka Y, Ikari Y, et al. Initial and subsequent angiographic outcome of percutaneous transluminal angioplasty performed on internal mammary artery grafts. *Br Heart J* 1995;74:615–619.
74. Ellis SG, Brener S, De Luca S, et al. Late myocardial ischemic events after saphenous vein graft intervention: importance of initially "non-significant" vein graft lesions. *Am J Cardiol* 1997;79:1460–1464.
75. Lehmann KG, Maas AC, Van Domberg R, et al. Repeat interventions as a long-term treatment strategy in the management of progressive coronary artery disease. *J Am Coll Cardiol* 1996;27:1398–1405.

CHAPTER 82 ■ PERCUTANEOUS VALVE DILATATIONS

ALEC S. VAHANIAN

OVERVIEW

More than 20 years of experience with percutaneous valve dilatation for acquired valve stenoses have shown the following:

- Percutaneous mitral valvuloplasty is an effective treatment in a wide range of patients with mitral stenosis. It is a low-risk procedure when it is performed by experienced teams, and follow-up at up to 15 years demonstrates excellent durability of the procedure.
- Percutaneous aortic valvuloplasty (PAV) for degenerative calcified aortic stenosis provides short-term palliation of symptoms at the cost of high periprocedural risk. Its role is in question.
- Percutaneous tricuspid or multivalve dilatation is used in exceptional cases.
- Percutaneous dilatation of a bioprosthesis has no future.

HISTORICAL PERSPECTIVE

Until the early 1980s, surgery was the only possible treatment for severe valvular stenoses. Then a new alternative appeared: percutaneous balloon valvuloplasty. The first to perform balloon valvuloplasty in the treatment of mitral stenosis was K. Inoue in 1982 (1). In the field of aortic stenosis, percutaneous valvuloplasty was used for the first time by Cribier et al. in 1985 (2).

This chapter deals with percutaneous balloon valvuloplasty for acquired valvular stenoses in patients with mitral stenosis, aortic stenosis, and the less common tricuspid, bioprosthetic, and multivalvular stenoses.

PERCUTANEOUS MITRAL VALVULOPLASTY

Rheumatic fever continues to be endemic in developing countries, where mitral stenosis is the most common valve disease. Although the prevalence of rheumatic heart disease has greatly decreased in industrialized countries, this disease continues to represent an important clinical entity because of outmigration from developing countries and the presence of restenosis after previous surgical commissurotomy (3,4).

Mechanisms

Balloon dilatation acts in the same way as surgical commissurotomy by opening the fused commissures; therefore, a more appropriate term for the procedure is probably *percutaneous mitral commissurotomy* rather than *percutaneous mitral valvuloplasty* (5) (Fig. 82.1). Balloons are also able to enlarge the valve area by fracturing nodular deposits in patients with calcified valves (6).

Technique

The *transvenous* or *antegrade approach* is the most widely used. Transseptal catheterization, which allows access to the left atrium, is the first step in the procedure and one of the most crucial. The *retrograde technique without transseptal catheterization,* in which the balloon is introduced through the femoral artery, is very seldom used today (7).

The Inoue technique (Fig. 82.2), the first to be developed (1,8), is used almost exclusively. The Inoue balloon is made

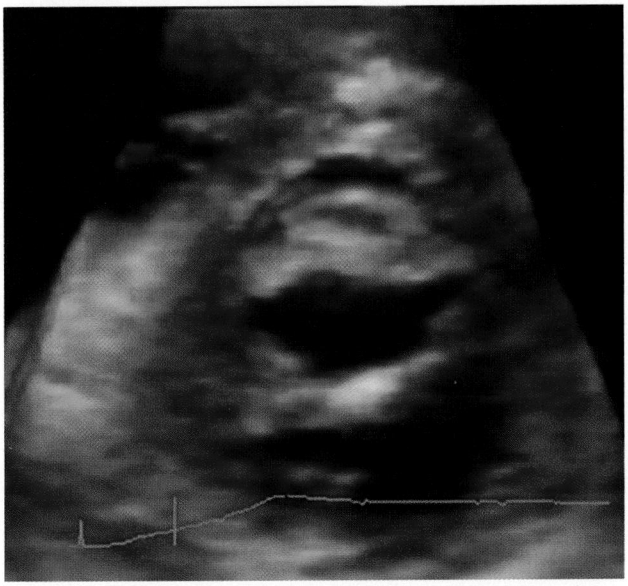

FIGURE 82.1. Transthoracic echocardiography, three-dimensional mode. This parasternal short-axis view shows a bicommissural opening. (Courtesy of Dr. Messika-Zeitoun.)

of nylon and rubber micromesh, and it is self-positioning and pressure extensible. The balloon has three distinct parts, each with a specific elasticity, which can be inflated sequentially. The Inoue balloon comes in four sizes, ranging from 24 to 30 mm, and each is pressure dependent, so its diameter can be varied by up to 4 mm as required by circumstances. Inoue recommends the use of a stepwise dilatation technique under echocardiographic guidance: the first inflation is performed to the minimal diameter of the balloon chosen. The balloon is then deflated and is withdrawn into the left atrium. If mitral regurgitation has not increased and valve area is insufficient, the balloon is readvanced across the mitral valve, and inflation is repeated with the balloon diameter increased by 1 to 2 mm.

In developing countries, economic constraints lead to a limited residual use of multitrack balloons (9), a variant of the double-balloon technique, and the use of a reusable metallic commissurotome (10). Balloon size is usually chosen according to patient characteristics: height and body surface area (8,11,12).

Monitoring of the Procedure and Assessment of Immediate Results

Two methods are used to assess immediate results in the catheterization laboratory: hemodynamic testing and echocardiography. Although echocardiography may be difficult to perform in the catheterization laboratory for logistic reasons, it

A

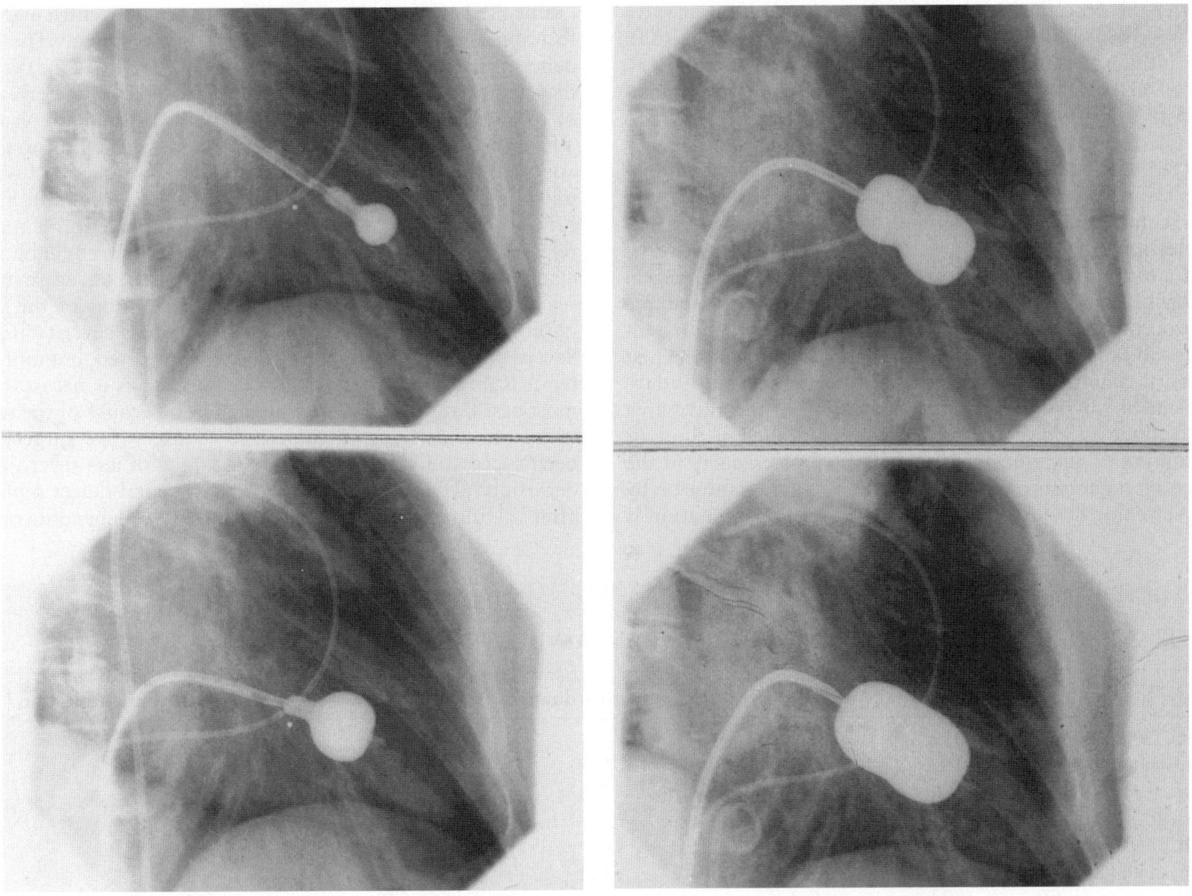

B

FIGURE 82.2. Mitral valvuloplasty: Inoue technique. **A:** Inflation of the distal portion of the balloon, which is thereafter pulled back and anchored at the mitral valve. **B:** Subsequent inflation of the proximal and middle portions of the balloon. At full inflation, the waist of the balloon in its midportion has disappeared.

TABLE 82.1

VALVE AREA AFTER PERCUTANEOUS MITRAL VALVULOPLASTY

Study	Number	Valve area (cm^2) Before PMV	After PMV
Tuzcu, et al. (16)	311	0.9	2
Ben Farhat, et al. (18)	463	1	2.1
Arora, et al. (19)	600	0.75	2.2
Chen and Cheng (20)	4,832	1.1	2.1
NHLBI (21)	738	1	2
Iung, et al. (22)	1,514	1.1	2
Stefanadis, et al. (7)	893	1	2.1
Cribier, et al. (10)	882	0.9	2.1
Bonhoeffer, et al. (9)	153	0.7	2

NHLBI, National Heart, Lung, and Blood Institute; PMV, percutaneous mitral valvuloplasty.

provides essential information on the efficacy of the procedure and also enables early detection of complications. The following criteria have been proposed for the desired end point of the procedure: (a) mitral valve area greater than 1 cm^2/m^2 body surface area, (b) complete opening of at least one commissure, or (c) appearance or increment of regurgitation greater than 1/4 classification (8).

After the procedure, the most accurate evaluation of valve area is provided by planimetry using echocardiography (13). Tailoring the strategy to the individual circumstances is vital; clinical factors as well as anatomic factors and the cumulative data of periprocedural monitoring should be taken into account. For example, balloon size, increments of size, and expected final valve area are smaller in elderly patients, in patients with very tight mitral stenosis or extensive valve and subvalvular disease, and in patients with nodular commissural calcification.

In addition, echocardiography using the transesophageal approach, or more recently intracardiac probes, may facilitate the procedure, especially transseptal puncture (14,15). To allow for the slight loss in valve area that occurs during the first 24 hours, echocardiography should be performed 1 or 2 days after mitral valvuloplasty, when calculation of the valve area may be done by planimetry, the half-pressure time method, or the continuity equation method. The final assessment of the degree of regurgitation may be made by angiography or by Doppler color flow imaging. Transesophageal examination is recommended in patients with severe mitral regurgitation to determine the mechanisms involved. The most sensitive method for the assessment of shunting is Doppler color flow imaging, especially when transesophageal examination is used, because this type of Doppler imaging shows the severity of the defect and detects shunting in a more sensitive way than does assessment of hemodynamics.

Immediate Results

The technique of mitral valvuloplasty has been evaluated in several thousand patients with different clinical conditions and valve anatomy (7,9,10,16–23).

Efficacy

The results shown in Table 82.1 demonstrate that mitral valvuloplasty usually provides an increase of more than 100% in valve area. Overall good immediate results, defined by a final valve area greater than 1.5 cm^2 without mitral regurgitation greater than 2/4, are observed in more than 80% of cases.

Failures

The failure rates range from 1% to 17% (7,9,10,16–23). Most failures occur in the early part of the investigators' experience. Others are the result of unfavorable anatomy.

Risks

Procedural mortality ranges from 0% to 3% (7,9,10,16–23) (Table 82.2). The main causes of death are left ventricular perforation and poor general condition of the patient. The incidence of hemopericardium varies from 0.5% to 12%. Pericardial hemorrhage may be related to transseptal catheterization or to apex perforation by the guidewires or the balloon itself when one uses the double-balloon technique. Embolism is encountered in 0.5% to 5% of cases. The frequency of severe mitral regurgitation ranges from 2% to 19% (24–26). Surgical findings (26,27) have shown that this condition is mostly related to noncommissural leaflet tearing, which could be associated with chordal rupture. The development of severe mitral regurgitation depends more on the distribution of the morphologic changes of the valve than on their severity (6,28). Severe mitral regurgitation may be well tolerated, but more often it is not, and surgery on a scheduled basis is necessary. In most cases, valve replacement is required because of the severity of the underlying valve disease. Conservative surgery has been successfully performed in patients with less severe valve deformity (26). The frequency of atrial septal defect reported after valvuloplasty varies from 10% to 90%, depending on the

TABLE 82.2

MAJOR COMPLICATIONS OF PERCUTANEOUS MITRAL VALVULOPLASTY

Study	Number	Mortality (%)	Hemopericardium (%)	Embolism (%)	Severe mitral regurgitation (%)
Tuzcu, et al. (16)	311	1.7	—	—	8.7 (>2+ increase)
Ben Farhat, et al. (18)	463	0.4	0.7	2	4.6
Arora, et al. (19)	600	1	1.3	0.5	1
Chen and Cheng (20)	4,832	0.12	0.8	0.5	1.4
NHLBI (21)	738	3	4	3	3
Iung, et al. (17)	2773	0.4	0.2	0.4	4.1
Stefanadis, et al. (7)	893	0.3	0	0	3.1
Cribier, et al. (10)	882	NA	1.4	NA	2.1

NA, not available; NHLBI, National Heart, Lung, and Blood Institute.

TABLE 82.3

FOLLOW-UP AFTER PERCUTANEOUS MITRAL VALVULOPLASTY

Study	Number	Mean age (y)	Length of follow-up (y)	Survival (%)	Freedom from operation (%)	NYHA class I/II (%)
Stefanadis, et al. (7)	441	44	9	—	—	75
Meneveau, et al. (39)	532	54	7.5	83	—	52
Hernandez, et al. (40)	561	53	7	95	84	69
Iung, et al. (42)	1,024	49	10	85	61	56
Orrange, et al. (37)	132	44	7	95	65	—

NYHA, New York Heart Association.

technique used for its detection (29,30). These shunts are usually small and without clinical consequences. Although urgent surgery (within 24 hours) is seldom needed for complications, it may be required for massive hemopericardium resulting from left ventricular perforation intractable to treatment by pericardiocentesis or, less frequently, for severe mitral regurgitation with poor hemodynamic tolerance (21,22,23,31).

Predictors of Immediate Results

The prediction of results is multifactorial (22,32,33). Several studies have shown that, in addition to morphologic factors (22,32–36), preoperative variables such as age, history of surgical commissurotomy, functional class, small mitral valve area, presence of mitral regurgitation before valvuloplasty, atrial fibrillation, high pulmonary artery pressure, and presence of severe tricuspid regurgitation, as well as procedural factors such as balloon type and size, are all independent predictors of the immediate results. The identification of variables linked to outcome enabled the development of predictive models, from which it appears that the sensitivity of prediction is high. Nevertheless, specificity is low, indicating insufficient prediction of poor immediate results. This latter finding is particularly true with regard to the lack of accurate prediction of severe mitral regurgitation. This low specificity is related to the intrinsic limitations of the prediction of immediate results, that is, to the possibility of good results in patients who are at high risk for poor results. The possibility of good results in theoretically unsuitable cases has been demonstrated in experimental studies and confirmed clinically.

Long-Term Results

Data from follow-up of up to 15 years can now be analyzed. In clinical terms, the overall long-term results of valvuloplasty are good (36–46) (Table 82.3). Late outcome after valvuloplasty differs according to the quality of the immediate results (Fig. 82.3).

When the immediate results are unsatisfactory, patients experience only transient or no functional improvement, and delayed surgery is usually performed when extracardiac conditions allow.

Conversely, if valvuloplasty is initially successful, then survival rates are excellent, functional improvement occurs in the majority of cases, and the need for secondary surgery is infrequent (37,42). When clinical deterioration occurs in these patients, it is late and mainly related to mitral restenosis. Determining the incidence of restenosis by echocardiography is compromised by the absence of a uniform definition. Restenosis has generally been defined as a loss of more than 50% of the initial gain, with a valve area becoming smaller than 1.5 cm^2. After a successful procedure, the incidence of echographically identified restenosis is usually low, ranging from 2% to 40% at time intervals of 3 to 5 years (36,40–44). The possibility of repeat valvuloplasty in patients with recurrent mitral stenosis is one of the potential advantages of this nonsurgical procedure. Repeated valvuloplasty can be proposed if recurrent stenosis leads to symptoms, if it occurs several years after an initially successful procedure, and if the predominant mechanism of restenosis is commissural refusion (45,46). At the moment, results of only a small number of series on revalvuloplasty are available; these show good immediate and midterm outcome in patients with favorable characteristics (45). Although the results are less favorable in patients presenting with worse characteristics, repeat valvuloplasty has a palliative role in patients who are not surgical candidates (46). These preliminary results are encouraging; however, defining the exact role of revalvuloplasty must await larger series with longer follow-up.

Predictors of Long-Term Results

Prediction of long-term results is multifactorial (37,38–44). It is based on the following: clinical variables such as age; valve anatomy as assessed by different echocardiography scores; factors related to the evolutional stage of the disease, that is, a higher New York Heart Association class before valvuloplasty; history of previous commissurotomy; severe tricuspid regurgitation; cardiomegaly; atrial fibrillation; high pulmonary

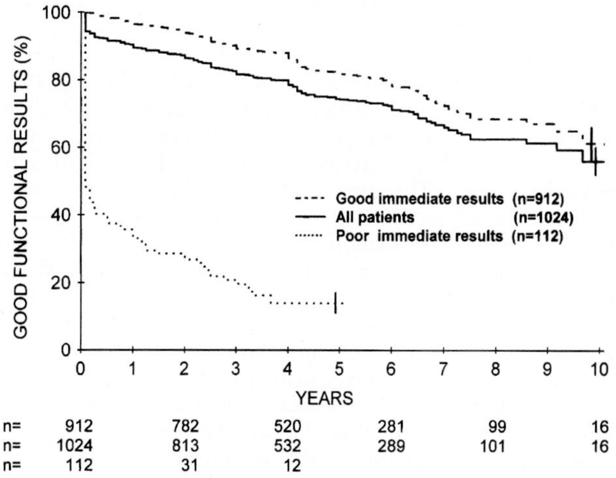

FIGURE 82.3. Long-term results of mitral valvuloplasty. "Good functional results" refers to survival considering cardiovascular-related deaths with no need for mitral surgery or repeat dilatation and in New York Heart Association functional class I or II. (Adapted from Iung B, Garbarz E, Michaud P, et al. Late results of percutaneous mitral commissurotomy in a series of 1024 patients: analysis of late clinical deterioration: frequency, anatomic findings, and predictive factors. *Circulation* 1999;99:3272–3278.)

vascular resistances; and the results of the procedure, that is, final valve area, final gradient, and degree of regurgitation. The quality of the late results is generally considered independent of the technique used. The identification of these predictors provides important information for patient selection and is relevant to follow-up: patients who have good immediate results but who are at high risk of further events must be carefully followed to detect deterioration and to allow for timely intervention.

The degree of mitral regurgitation generally remains stable or slightly decreases during follow-up. Atrial septal defects are likely to close over time in the majority of cases because of reduction in the interatrial pressure gradient. The persistence of shunts is related to their magnitude or to unsatisfactory relief of the valve obstruction (29). Finally, clinical series of surgical and balloon commissurotomy suggest that intervention reduces markers of the risk of embolism such as intensity of left atrial echocardiographic contrast and size and function of the atrium (47–52).

Indications

The decision to perform valvuloplasty must be based on both clinical and anatomic variables. Clinical evaluation of patients concentrates mainly on functional disability and the alternative risk of surgery.

For symptomatic patients, the indication for valvuloplasty is perfectly clear. Truly asymptomatic patients, however, are not usually candidates for the procedure because of the small but definite risk inherent in the technique. For patients in the latter group, balloon commissurotomy may be considered in selected cases. This group includes patients at high risk of thromboembolism: those with a previous history of embolism or with heavy spontaneous contrast in the left atrium, recurrent atrial arrhythmias, or pulmonary hypertension. Guidelines also recommend balloon valvuloplasty when systolic pulmonary pressure is higher than 50 mm Hg at rest or 60 mm Hg during exercise (53,54). However, the nature of these thresholds should be refined by the increasing experience gained in exercise echocardiography (55,56). Finally, balloon valvuloplasty can be considered for patients requiring major extracardiac surgery or to allow for pregnancy.

Conversely, valvuloplasty is the only solution when surgery is contraindicated. It is also preferable to surgery, at least as a first attempt, in patients with increased cardiac surgical risk. In patients with restenosis after surgical commissurotomy, available data (57,58) suggest that valvuloplasty may well allow selected patients to postpone reoperation, provided their anatomy is still suitable and restenosis is mainly the result of commissural refusion. The same reasoning applies to patients who have undergone aortic valve replacement. Preliminary reports have suggested that valvuloplasty can be performed safely and effectively in patients with pulmonary hypertension (59). When mitral stenosis and moderate aortic valve disease coexist (60), balloon valvuloplasty can be performed as a means of postponing the inevitable later surgical treatment of both valves.

In industrialized countries, many patients with mitral stenosis have comorbidity, which increases the risk of surgery. Valvuloplasty can be performed as a lifesaving procedure in critically ill patients (61,62), either as sole treatment in those with an absolute contraindication to surgery or as a bridge to surgery. In elderly patients, valvuloplasty results in moderate but significant improvement in valve function at an acceptable risk, although subsequent functional deterioration is frequent (63–65). In pregnant patients, the procedure is efficacious in terms of improving the mother's hemodynamic status; it is also well tolerated by the fetus if the procedure is performed after the twentieth week. Because of the ever-present risk of complication, use of valvuloplasty should be limited to patients who remain symptomatic despite appropriate medical treatment (66–68).

The assessment of anatomy has several aims with respect to establishing indications and prognostic considerations. Ensuring that no anatomic contraindications exist to use of the technique is critical (Table 82.4).

For prognostic purposes, echocardiographic assessment allows the classification of patients into anatomic groups. Most investigators use the Wilkins score (Table 82.5) for

TABLE 82.4

CONTRAINDICATIONS FOR PERCUTANEOUS MITRAL VALVULOPLASTY

Left atrial thrombosis
Mitral regurgitation greater than 2/4
Massive or bicommissural calcification
Severe aortic valve disease, or severe tricuspid stenosis and regurgitation associated with mitral stenosis
Severe concomitant coronary artery disease requiring bypass surgery

TABLE 82.5

ANATOMIC CLASSIFICATION OF THE MITRAL VALVE (MASSACHUSETTS GENERAL HOSPITAL, BOSTON): ECHOCARDIOGRAPHIC EXAMINATION

LEAFLET MOBILITY
1. Valve highly mobile, with restriction of only the leaflet tips
2. Reduced mobility of the midportion and base of the leaflets
3. Forward movement of the valve leaflets in diastole mainly at the base
4. No or minimal forward movement of the leaflets in diastole
VALVULAR THICKENING
1. Leaflets near normal (4–5 mm)
2. Midleaflet thickening, marked thickening of the margins
3. Thickening extending through the entire leaflets (5–8 mm)
4. Marked thickening of all leaflet tissue (>8–10 mm)
SUBVALVULAR THICKENING
1. Minimal thickening of chordal structures just below the valve
2. Thickening of chordae extending up to one third of chordal length
3. Thickening extending to the distal third of the chordae
4. Extensive thickening and shortening of all chordae extending down to the papillary muscle
VALVULAR CALCIFICATION
1. A single area of increased echo brightness
2. Scattered areas of brightness confined to leaflet margins
3. Brightness extending into the midportion of leaflets
4. Extensive brightness through most of the leaflet tissue

Note: The final score is found by adding the scores for each of the components.
From Wilkins GT, Gillam LD, Weyman AE, et al. Percutaneous balloon dilatation of the mitral valve: an analysis of echocardiographic variables related to outcome and the mechanism of dilatation. *Br Heart J* 1988;60:299–308.

TABLE 82.6

ANATOMIC CLASSIFICATION OF THE MITRAL VALVE

Echocardiographic group	Mitral valve anatomy
Group 1	Pliable noncalcified anterior mitral leaflet and mild subvalvular disease (i.e., thin chordae ≥10 mm long)
Group 2	Pliable noncalcified anterior mitral leaflet and severe subvalvular disease (i.e., thickened chordae <10 mm long)
Group 3	Calcification of mitral valve of any extent, as assessed by fluoroscopy, any condition of subvalvular apparatus

From Iung B, Cormier B, Ducimetiere P, et al. Immediate results of percutaneous mitral commissurotomy. *Circulation* 1996;94: 2124–2130.

TABLE 82.7

CALCULATION OF ECHOCARDIOGRAPHIC SCORE TO PREDICT MITRAL REGURGITATION AFTER PERCUTANEOUS MITRAL VALVULOPLASTY

A/B. CALCIFICATION/FIBROSIS OF LEAFLETS (SCORE ANTERIOR AND POSTERIOR LEAFLET)
1. Thickening normal (4–5 mm) or only one thick segment
2. Evenly fibrotic/calcified without thin areas
3. Uneven distribution of calcification/thickening; thinner segments mildly thickened (5–8 mm)
4. Uneven distribution of calcification /thickening; thinner segments near normal (4–5 mm)

C. FIBROSIS/CALCIFICATION OF COMMISSURES
1. Only one commissure affected
2. Both commissures mildly affected
3. Calcification of both commissures: one severely affected
4. Marked calcification of both commissures

D. SUBVALVULAR DISEASE
1. Minimal chordal thickening just below valve
2. Chordal thickening to one third of length
3. Thickening to distal one third of chordae
4. Shortening/fibrosis of all chordae to papillary muscle

Adapted from Padial LR, Abascal VM, Moreno PR, et al. Echocardiography can predict the development of severe mitral regurgitation after percutaneous mitral valvuloplasty by the Inoue technique. *Am J Cardiol* 1999;83:1210–1213.

categorization, whereas others use a more general assessment of valve anatomy (Table 82.6). In fact, of the scores available today, no one score has been shown to be superior, and all echocardiographic classifications have the same limitations: (a) technical factors; (b) difficulty of reproducibility, because they are only semiquantitative; (c) underestimation of the lesions, especially regarding the assessment of subvalvular disease; and (d) inability of scores describing the degree of overall valve deformity to identify localized changes in very specific portions of the valve apparatus (leaflets, commissures) that may increase the risk of severe mitral regurgitation. Therefore, the use of the system with which one is most familiar and at ease is recommended. More recently, scores that take into account the uneven distribution of the anatomic deformities of the leaflets or the commissural area have been developed (Table 82.7). Preliminary results for their use are promising but disputed (69–73).

In patients with favorable anatomy—that is, pliable valves and moderate subvalvular disease (echocardiographic score of 8 or less)—results of valvuloplasty are generally excellent. Results of several randomized studies with follow-up comparing valvuloplasty and surgical commissurotomy are available (74–76). They show that valvuloplasty is at least comparable to surgical commissurotomy with regard to immediate and long-term results and is no doubt more comfortable for the patient. In addition, if restenosis occurs, patients treated by valvuloplasty can undergo repeat balloon procedures or surgery without the difficulties and inherent risk resulting from pericardial adhesions and chest wall scarring (Table 82.8). Valvuloplasty thus appears to be the procedure of choice for patients in whom we expect to delay surgery further, for example, in patients who either are pregnant or are planning a pregnancy.

Conversely, much remains to be done in refining the indications for valvuloplasty in patients with unfavorable anatomy (77–80). For this group, some investigators favor immediate surgery because of the less satisfying results of valvuloplasty, whereas others prefer valvuloplasty as an initial treatment for selected candidates and reserve surgery for when this treatment fails.

TABLE 82.8

COMPARISON BETWEEN PERCUTANEOUS VALVULOPLASTY AND SURGICAL COMMISSUROTOMY

	PMV (n = 50)	Open commissurotomy (n = 50)	Closed commissurotomy (n = 50)
Age (y)	29	28	27
Echocardiographic score	6	6.1	6
Valve area (cm^2)			
Before	0.9	0.9	0.9
After	2.1	2.2	1.6
7 y	1.8	1.8	1.3
Restenosis (%)	6.6	6.6	37

PMV, percutaneous mitral valvuloplasty.
Adapted from Ben Farhat M, Ayari M, Maatouk F. Percutaneous balloon versus surgical closed and open mitral commissurotomy. *Circulation* 1998;97:245–250.

PERCUTANEOUS AORTIC VALVULOPLASTY

Severe degenerative calcified aortic stenosis is the most frequent valve disease in industrialized countries. This prevalence accounted for the initial interest in its potential treatment using interventional cardiology (3,81).

Mechanisms

Dilatation of a calcified aortic valve using a balloon results in cracking the calcified nodulus and stretching the aortic wall (81,82). These mechanisms easily explain the early loss of effects in severe degenerative aortic stenosis. In rheumatic aortic stenosis, in which commissural fusion does occur, valvuloplasty may be more effective.

Technique

Approaches

The femoral retrograde approach is most frequently used (83,84). After one crosses the aortic valve (Fig. 82.4), a stiff wire is inserted into the apex of the left ventricle to stabilize the balloon during inflation. The alternative is the anterograde approach, which necessitates a transseptal catheterization. This latter technique is a difficult procedure but constitutes a recourse in case the femoral approach is inaccessible (85).

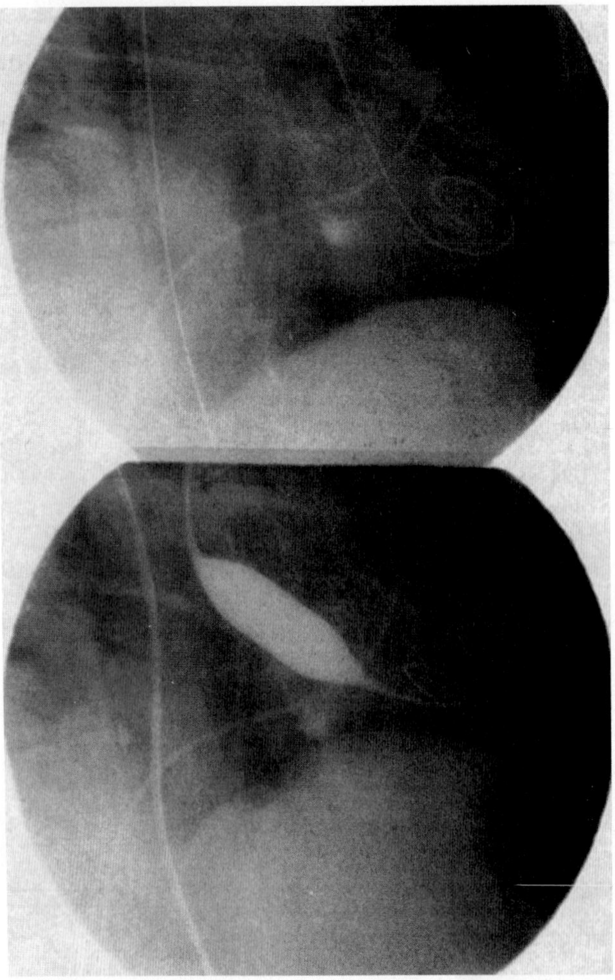

FIGURE 82.4. Aortic valvuloplasty: retrograde technique. **Upper panel:** Crossing of the valve with a stiff guidewire with a preshaped tip. **Lower panel:** Dilatation of the valve with a conventional balloon (23 mm).

Balloons

Valvuloplasty is performed with balloons 15 to 25 mm in diameter and of conventional or double size.

Monitoring of the Procedure and Assessment of Immediate Results

Methods for evaluating immediate results during the procedure include monitoring the transaortic gradient and cardiac output. Nevertheless, because of the hemodynamic instability of the patient during the procedure and the very early loss in valve area after the procedure, the most viable method is measurement of the valve area by Doppler echocardiography in the days after the procedure (86).

Immediate Results

The technique has been used in several hundred patients. Any analysis of the results must take into account the severity of the cardiac disease and comorbidities frequently found in this population of elderly patients.

Hemodynamics

Overall, PAV reduces tight stenosis to moderate stenosis (83–91) (Table 82.9).

Risks

Mortality and morbidity of the procedure are high (83–91) (Table 82.10). Hospital mortality varies from 3.5% to 13.5%, and 20% to 25% of the patients have at least one serious complication within the first 24 hours. The most frequent complications are vascular complications at the puncture site, which necessitate intervention in nearly half these patients. Ventricular perforations can lead to tamponade. Acute aortic incompetence is rare, as are embolic complications.

Predictors of Immediate Results

The immediate outcome is linked to the clinical status of the patient (age, New York Heart Association class, and presence of congestive heart failure) or to procedural complications. Depressed left ventricular function, low cardiac output, and the

TABLE 82.9

AORTIC VALVE AREA AFTER PERCUTANEOUS AORTIC VALVULOPLASTY

		Valve area (cm^2)	
Study	n	Before PAV	After PAV
Cribier, et al. (83)	506	0.6	1.0
Safian, et al. (88)	170	0.6	0.9
Mansfield Registry (90)	492	0.5	0.8
NHBLI (87)	674	0.5	0.8
Block and Palacios (91)	375	0.5	0.9

NHLBI, National Heart, Lung, and Blood Institute; PAV, percutaneous aortic valvuloplasty.

TABLE 82.10

IMMEDIATE COMPLICATIONS OF PERCUTANEOUS AORTIC VALVULOPLASTY

	NHBLI (87) (n = 674)	Mansfield registry (89) (n = 492)	Cribier, et al. (83) (n = 363)	Safian, et al. (88) (n = 170)
Hospital mortality (%)	10	7.5	4	3.5
Tamponade (%)	1.5	1.8	1	1.8
Severe aortic regurgitation (%)	1	1	0	1.2
Stroke (%)	3	2.2	1.4	0
Myocardial infarction (%)	2	0.2	0.3	0.6
Vascular events[a] (%)	7	5.5	5	10

NHLBI, National Heart, Lung, and Blood Institute.
[a]Vascular events requiring surgical treatment.

existence of diffuse coronary lesions are all important covariates associated with worse outcome (85,90,91).

Long-Term Results

Despite a relatively modest improvement in valve function, a degree of functional improvement is commonly noted during the first weeks. The benefit, however, disappears after a few months (92–95) (Table 82.11). In selected patients, aortic valve replacement has been subsequently performed with good results (95), although the prognosis of many other patients is particularly poor (Fig. 82.5). Overall, current opinion is that PAV alone does not change the natural course of the disease (96), even after repeated procedures (97). These poor long-term results are mainly related to the clinical status of the patients and to the only moderate and transient improvement in valve function obtained by PAV.

Indications

Comparison with surgical results is difficult because the patients included in the dilatation series are older, are in a more precarious clinical condition, and very frequently have associated comorbidities. The indications should take into account the excellent results of surgery when it is possible and the poor results of PAV. In practice, aortic valve replacement is the treatment of choice for symptomatic patients with tight aortic stenosis (53,98,99). Valvuloplasty can be considered only in the following circumstances (53):

1. Critically ill patients with cardiogenic shock with multivisceral organ failure. Good midterm results have been obtained in limited series when surgical intervention was possible secondarily (100). For this group of patients, valvuloplasty can be considered a bridge to surgery, thus permitting the secondary operation with less risk
2. Severe, poorly tolerated aortic stenosis requiring significant emergency noncardiac surgery
3. More rarely, patients who have an absolute, but not life-threatening, short-term contraindication to surgery and significant functional disability
4. Patients who refuse surgery

OTHER PERCUTANEOUS VALVE DILATATIONS

Unlike percutaneous valvuloplasty for mitral and aortic stenosis, other applications of percutaneous valve dilatation have been used only sparingly. Case numbers are insufficient to allow evaluation of results and establishment of clear indications.

Percutaneous Tricuspid Valvuloplasty

The procedure is reserved for symptomatic patients presenting with tight tricuspid stenosis, alone or associated with mild regurgitation (101). When tricuspid stenosis is accompanied by significant or moderate regurgitation, or when it is associated with another valvular disease necessitating surgical treatment, treatment must be surgical.

Percutaneous Dilatation of Bioprostheses

Anatomic findings and experimental dilatations lead to the conclusion that dilatation of bioprostheses does not produce good results (102–104). This procedure may give rise to severe immediate complications when it is performed at the level of the

TABLE 82.11

RESULTS OF CLINICAL FOLLOW-UP AFTER PERCUTANEOUS AORTIC VALVULOPLASTY

		Survival (%)				Survival without reintervention (%)			
Study	n	1-y	2-y	3-y	5-y	1-y	2-y	3-y	5-y
Lieberman, et al. (93)	165	60	48	35	—	40	19	6	—
Otto, et al. (94)	674	55	35	23	—	—	—	—	—
Bernard, et al. (95)	46	75	47	—	33	70	25	—	7

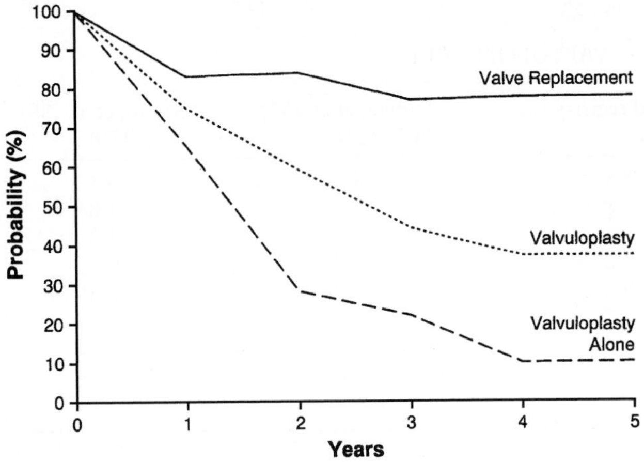

FIGURE 82.5. Long-term survival rate after aortic valve replacement or balloon valvuloplasty. (From Bernard Y, Etievent J, Mourand JL, et al. Long-term results of percutaneous aortic valvuloplasty compared with aortic replacement in patients older than 75 years. *J Am Coll Cardiol* 1992;20:796–801.)

left side of the heart (103), and it gives poor midterm results in the tricuspid position (104).

Multiple Dilatations

Current experience indicates that multiple dilations are technically feasible in selected patients (105). One application that could be imagined in the field of rheumatic pathology is in patients in whom surgery is contraindicated or for whom surgery poses a high risk, such as during pregnancy.

CURRENT USE OF PERCUTANEOUS VALVE PROCEDURES

An image of current practice can be derived from the Euro Heart Survey on Valvular Heart Disease (3), which was performed prospectively in 92 centers throughout Europe during a 4-month period in 2001. It showed that percutaneous mitral commissurotomy is now used in more than one third of cases of mitral stenosis and has virtually replaced surgical commissurotomy. Conversely, aortic valvuloplasty was not performed.

CONTROVERSIES AND PERSONAL PERSPECTIVES

Mitral valvuloplasty is the valvuloplasty technique used most frequently, if not exclusively. Further developments in its application depend on the possibilities for use in countries where mitral stenosis is still endemic but where limitations in finances restrict the use of balloon valvuloplasty or lead to reuse of balloons, with attendant risks.

In my opinion, performance of percutaneous mitral valvuloplasty should be restricted to groups whose experience with transseptal catheterization has been positive and who have been able to carry out an adequate number of procedures and thus improve their technical performance and ability to select patients. The decision to perform valvuloplasty also depends on the results of surgery at each particular institution.

Regarding indications, no problems are presented in patients in whom surgery is contraindicated or in "ideal candidates," such as young adults (106) with favorable characteristics. Conversely, much remains to be done to refine the indications in patients with minimal symptoms and/or with unfavorable anatomy.

The level of evidence for performing valvuloplasty in asymptomatic patients is low because no randomized studies exist for comparing the results of valvuloplasty and medical therapy in such patients. For these patients, the goal is not to prolong life or to decrease symptoms but rather to prevent thromboembolism. The efficacy of valvuloplasty for the specific problem of embolism is not established, but the different findings previously mentioned consistently show a beneficial effect on the causes of thromboembolism. No direct evidence indicates that valvuloplasty reduces the incidence of atrial fibrillation, even if its favorable influence on predictors of atrial fibrillation (107–110), such as atrial size or degree of obstruction, seems to indicate that this is indeed the case. In asymptomatic patients, valvuloplasty should be performed only by experienced interventionists and when valve anatomy is favorable, in which case a safe and successful procedure can be expected. Finally, it could be expected that in the future mitral valvuloplasty could be combined with percutaneous closure of the left atrial appendage (111) or catheter ablation of atrial fibrillation (112) to decrease the embolic risk further.

Among patients with less favorable valve anatomy, comparison between the results of valvuloplasty and those of surgery is also difficult. Unfortunately, no randomized study has been performed to examine this issue. Indications in this subgroup of patients must take into account heterogeneity with respect to anatomy and clinical status. An individualistic approach is favored that allows for the multifactorial nature of prediction (Fig. 82.6). Current opinion is that surgery can be considered the treatment of choice in patients with bicommissural or

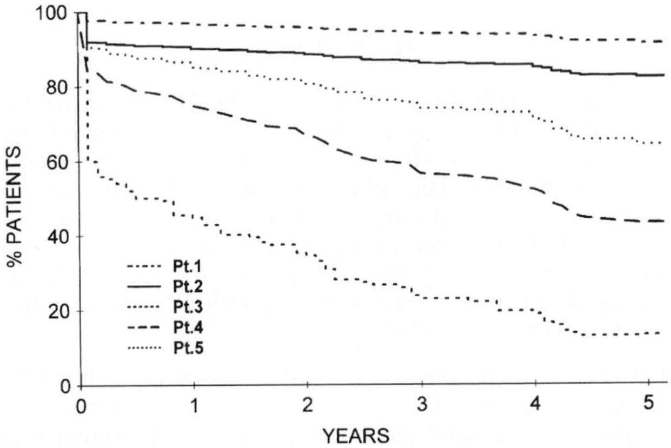

FIGURE 82.6. Multifactorial nature of the prediction of the results of mitral valvuloplasty. Predicted probability of good immediate results (valve area at least 1.5 cm^2 without regurgitation, Seller grade >2) and good late functional results (survival with no intervention and in New York Heart Association [NYHA] class I or II) according to patient characteristics. Values are given for a procedure using an Inoue balloon with an effective balloon dilating area of at least 5.5 cm^2 (i.e., a final diameter $\geq$27 mm). *Pt. 1,* less than 50 years, NYHA class II, sinus rhythm, calcium grade I, valve area 1.25 to 1.5 cm^2; *Pt. 2,* less than 50 years, NYHA class II, sinus rhythm, calcium grade 2, valve area 1 to 1.25 cm^2; *Pt. 3,* 50 to 70 years, NYHA class III, sinus rhythm, calcium grade 2, valve area 1.25 to 1.5 cm^2; *Pt. 4,* 50 to 70 years, NYHA class III, atrial fibrillation, calcium grade 2, valve area 1.25 to 1.5 cm^2; *Pt. 5,* at least 70 years, NYHA class III, atrial fibrillation, calcium grade 3, valve area 0.75 to 1 cm^2. (Adapted from Iung B, Garbarz E, Doutrelant L, et al. Late results of percutaneous mitral commissurotomy for calcific mitral stenosis. *Am J Cardiol* 2000;85:1308–1314.)

heavy calcification. Conversely, in my opinion, balloon valvuloplasty can be attempted as a first approach in patients with extensive lesions of the subvalvular apparatus or moderate or unicommissural calcification, such as in young patients, with the expectation of further delaying valve replacement with its inherent mortality and morbidity. Surgery should be considered reasonably early after unsatisfactory results or secondary deterioration. Extending knowledge regarding this group requires evaluation of predictive models that take into account the multifactorial aspect of the prediction and the fact that new anatomic scores may be developed in the future using newer echocardiographic methods such as three-dimensional imaging (113). In addition, no consensus has been reached regarding an indication for valvuloplasty in patients with left atrial thrombosis located in the left atrial appendage (114) and in patients with moderate stenosis (115).

In my opinion, in the former group the indications for valvuloplasty are limited to patients with contraindications to surgery or those without urgent need for intervention, when oral anticoagulation can be given for at least 2 months up to 6 months and provided a new transesophageal echocardiographic examination shows the disappearance of the thrombus (116,117).

The suggestion has been made that valvuloplasty be performed in patients with moderate stenosis in the hope of delaying the natural course of the disease (115). These patients are usually candidates for medical treatment, and the risks of valvuloplasty outweigh the benefits. To define a threshold of valve area above which valvuloplasty should not be performed is somewhat arbitrary because, besides measuring valve area, one must take into account functional disability and pulmonary pressures at rest and on exercise. My current practice is usually to avoid valvuloplasty in patients with a valve area larger than 1.5 cm^2.

THE FUTURE

After nearly 20 years of extensive clinical evaluation, the technique of percutaneous valve dilatation, which for practical purposes can be summed up as percutaneous mitral valvuloplasty, is now here to stay (118–121). This is because of its proven efficacy in the treatment of mitral stenosis as a substitute for surgical commissurotomy (121) and as a complement to valve replacement. Aortic valvuloplasty probably has a very limited role in isolation (122), but it may find new applications as the first step in the performance of percutaneous aortic valve replacement (123). Other percutaneous valve dilatation techniques will probably be used only in exceptional cases.

References

1. Inoue K, Owaki T, Nakamura T, et al. Clinical application of transvenous mitral commissurotomy by a new balloon catheter. *J Thorac Cardiovasc Surg* 1984;87:394–402.
2. Cribier A, Savin T, Saoudi N, et al. Percutaneous transluminal valvuloplasty of acquired aortic stenosis in elderly patients: an alternative to valve replacement? *Lancet* 1986;11:63–67.
3. Iung B, Baron G, Butchart EG, et al. A prospective survey of patients with valvular heart disease in Europe: the Euro Heart Survey on Valvular Heart Disease. *Eur Heart J* 2003;24:1231–1243
4. Shaw TRD, Sutaria N, Prendergost B. Clinical and hemodynamic profiles of young, middle aged and elderly patients with mitral stenosis undergoing mitral balloon valvotomy. *Heart* 2003;89:1430–1436.
5. Block PC, Palacios IF, Jacobs ML, et al. Mechanism of percutaneous mitral valvotomy. *Am J Cardiol* 1987;59:178–179.
6. Reifart N, Nowak B, Baykut D, et al. Experimental balloon valvuloplasty of fibrotic and calcific mitral valves. *Circulation* 1990;81:1105–1111.
7. Stefanadis CI, Stratos CG, Lambrou SG, et al. Accomplishments and perspectives with retrograde nontransseptal balloon mitral valvuloplasty. *J Interv Cardiol* 2000;13:269–280.
8. Vahanian A, Cormier B, Iung B. Percutaneous transvenous mitral commissurotomy using the Inoue balloon: international experience. *Cathet Cardiovasc Diagn* 1994;2:8–15.
9. Bonhoeffer P, Hausse A, Yonga G. Technique and results of percutaneous mitral valvuloplasty with the multi-track system. *J Interv Cardiol* 2000;13: 263–269.
10. Cribier A, Eltchaninoff H, Carlot R. Percutaneous mechanical mitral commissurotomy with the metallic valvotome: detailed technical aspect and overview of the results of the multicenter registry 882 patients. *J Interv Cardiol* 2000;13:255–262.
11. Roth BR, Block PC, Palacios IF. Predictors of increased mitral regurgitation after percutaneous mitral balloon valvotomy. *Cathet Cardiovasc Diagn* 1990;20:17–21.
12. Chen C, Wang X, Wang Y, et al. Value of two-dimensional echocardiography in selecting patients and balloon sizes for percutaneous balloon mitral valvuloplasty. *J Am Coll Cardiol* 1989;14:1651–1658.
13. Palacios IG. What is the gold standard to measure mitral valve area post-mitral balloon valvuloplasty? *Cathet Cardiovasc Diagn* 1994;33:315–316.
14. Park SH, Kim MA, Hyon MS. The advantages of on-line transesophageal echocardiography guide during percutaneous balloon mitral valvuloplasty. *J Am Soc Echocardiogr* 2000;13:26–34.
15. Green NE, Hansgen AR, Carroll JD. Initial clinical experience with intracardiac echocardiography in guiding balloon mitral valvuloplasty: technique, safety, utility, and limitations. *Cathet Cardiovasc Interv* 2004;63: 385–394.
16. Tuzcu EM, Block PC, Palacios IF, et al. Comparison of early versus late experience with percutaneous mitral balloon valvuloplasty. *J Am Coll Cardiol* 1991;17:1121–1124.
17. Iung B, Nicoud-Houel A, Fondard O, et al. Temporal trends in percutaneous mitral commissurotomy over a 15-year period. *Eur Heart J* 2004;25:701–708.
18. Ben Farhat M, Betbout F, Gamra H, et al. Results of percutaneous double-balloon mitral commissurotomy in one medical center in Tunisia. *Am J Cardiol* 1995;76:1266–1270.
19. Arora R, Singh Kalra G, Ramachandra Murty GS, et al. Percutaneous transatrial mitral commissurotomy: immediate and intermediate results. *J Am Coll Cardiol* 1994;23:1327–1332.
20. Chen CR, Cheng TO. Percutaneous balloon mitral valvuloplasty by the Inoue technique: a multicenter study of 4832 patients in China. *Am Heart J* 1995;129:1197–1202.
21. National Heart, Lung, and Blood Institute Balloon Valvuloplasty Registry. Complications and mortality of percutaneous balloon mitral commissurotomy. *Circulation* 1992;85:2014–2024.
22. Iung B, Cormier B, Ducimetiere P, et al. Immediate results of percutaneous mitral commissurotomy. *Circulation* 1996;94:2124–2130.
23. Harrison KJ, Wilson JS, Hearne SE, et al. Complications related to percutaneous transvenous mitral commissurotomy. *Cathet Cardiovasc Diagn* 1994; 2:52–60.
24. Essop MR, Wisenbaugh T, Skoularigis J, et al. Mitral regurgitation following mitral balloon valvotomy: differing mechanisms for severe versus mild-to-moderate lesions. *Circulation* 1991;84:1669–1679.
25. Herrmann HC, Lima JAC, Feldman T, et al. Mechanisms and outcome of severe mitral regurgitation after Inoue balloon valvuloplasty. *J Am Coll Cardiol* 1993;27:783–789.
26. Acar C, Jebara VA, Grare PH, et al. Traumatic mitral insufficiency following percutaneous mitral dilation: anatomic lesions and surgical implications. *Eur J Cardiothorac Surg* 1992;6:660–664.
27. Hernandez R, Macaya C, Benuelos C, et al. Predictors, mechanisms and outcome of severe mitral regurgitation complicating percutaneous mitral valvotomy with the Inoue balloon. *Am J Cardiol* 1993;70:1169–1174.
28. Padial LR, Freitas N, Sagie A, et al. Echocardiography can predict which patients will develop severe mitral regurgitation after percutaneous mitral valvulotomy. *J Am Coll Cardiol* 1996;27:1225–1231.
29. Cequier A, Bonan R, Dyrda I, et al. Atrial shunting after percutaneous mitral valvuloplasty. *Circulation* 1990;81:1190–1197.
30. Goldberg N, Roman CF, Do Cha S, et al. Right to left interatrial shunting following balloon mitral valvuloplasty. *Cathet Cardiovasc Diagn* 1989; 16:133–135.
31. National Heart, Lung and Blood Institute Balloon Valvuloplasty Registry participants. Multicenter experience with balloon mitral commissurotomy: NHLBI Balloon Valvuloplasty Registry report on immediate and 30-day follow-up results. *Circulation* 1992;85:448–461.
32. Abascal V, Wilkins GT, O'Shea JP, et al. Prediction of successful outcome in 130 patients undergoing percutaneous balloon mitral valvotomy. *Circulation* 1990;82:448–456.
33. Herrmann HC, Ramaswamy K, Isner JM, et al. Factors influencing immediate results, complications, and short-term follow-up status after Inoue balloon mitral valvotomy: a North-American multicenter study. *Am Heart J* 1992;124:160–166.
34. Feldman T, Carroll JD, Isner JM, et al. Effect of valve deformity on results and mitral regurgitation after Inoue balloon commissurotomy. *Circulation* 1992;85:180–187.
35. Nair M, Agarwala R, Kalra GS, et al. Can mitral regurgitation after balloon dilatation of the mitral valve be predicted? *Br Heart J* 1992;67:442–444.
36. Palacios IF, Sanchez PL, Harrell LC, et al. Which patients benefit from percutaneous mitral balloon valvuloplasty? Pre-valvuloplasty and

post-valvuloplasty variables that predict long-term outcome. *Circulation* 2002;105:1465–1471.
37. Orrange S, Kawanishi D, Lopez B, et al. Actuarial outcome after catheter balloon commissurotomy in patients with mitral stenosis. *Circulation* 1997;95:382–389.
38. Stefanadis C, Stratos C, Lambrou S, et al. Retrograde nontransseptal balloon mitral valvuloplasty: immediate results and intermediate long-term outcome in 441 cases—a multi-centre experience. *J Am Coll Cardiol* 1998;32:1009–1016.
39. Meneveau N, Schiele F, Seronde MF, et al. Predictors of event-free survival after percutaneous mitral commissurotomy. *Heart* 1998;80:359–364.
40. Hernandez R, Bañuelos C, Alfonso F, et al. Long-term clinical and echocardiographic follow-up after percutaneous mitral valvuloplasty with the Inoue balloon. *Circulation* 1999;99:1580–1586.
41. Wang A, Krasuski RA, Warner JJ, et al. Serial echocardiographic evaluation of restenosis after successful percutaneous mitral commissurotomy. *J Am Coll Cardiol* 2002;39:328–334.
42. Iung B, Garbarz E, Michaud P, et al. Late results of percutaneous mitral commissurotomy in a series of 1024 patients: analysis of late clinical deterioration: frequency, anatomic findings, and predictive factors. *Circulation* 1999;99:3272–3278.
43. Chen CR, Cheng T, Chen JY, et al. Long-term results of percutaneous balloon mitral valvuloplasty for mitral stenosis: a follow-up study to 11 years in 202 patients. *Cathet Cardiovasc Diagn* 1998;43:132–139.
44. Langerveld J, Thijs Plokker HW, Ernst SMPG, et al. Predictors of clinical events or restenosis during follow-up after percutaneous mitral balloon valvotomy. *Eur Heart J* 1999;20:519–526.
45. Iung B, Garbarz E, Michaud P, et al. Immediate and mid-term results of repeat percutaneous mitral commissurotomy for restenosis following earlier percutaneous mitral commissurotomy. *Eur Heart J* 2000;21:1683–1690.
46. Pathan AZ, Mahdi NA, Leon MN, et al. Is redo percutaneous mitral balloon valvuloplasty (PMV) indicated in patients with post-PMV mitral restenosis? *J Am Coll Cardiol* 1999;34:49–54.
47. Chiang CW, Lo SK, Ko YS, et al. Predictors of systemic embolism in patients with mitral stenosis: a prospective study. *Ann Intern Med* 1998;128:885–889.
48. Cormier B, Vahanian A, Iung B, et al. Influence of percutaneous mitral commissurotomy on left atrial spontaneous contrast of mitral stenosis. *Am J Cardiol* 1993;71:842–847.
49. Stefanadis C, Dernellis J, Stratos C, et al. Effects of balloon mitral valvuloplasty on left atrial function in mitral stenosis as assessed by pressure-area relation. *J Am Coll Cardiol* 1998;32:159–168.
50. Porte JM, Cormier B, Iung B, et al. Early assessment by transesophageal echocardiography of left atrial appendage function after percutaneous mitral commissurotomy. *Am J Cardiol* 1996;77:72–76.
51. Zaki A, Salama M, El Masry M, et al. Immediate effect of balloon valvuloplasty on hemostatic changes in mitral stenosis. *Am J Cardiol* 2000;85:370–375.
52. Chen MC, Wu CJ, Chang HW, et al. Mechanism of reducing platelet activity by percutaneous transluminal mitral valvuloplasty in patients with rheumatic mitral stenosis. *Chest* 2004;125:1629–1634.
53. ACC/AHA Guidelines for the management of patients with valvular heart disease. A report of the American College of Cardiology/American Heart Association: Task Force on Practice Guidelines (Committee on Management of Patients with Valvular Heart Disease). *J Am Coll Cardiol* 1998;32:1486–1588.
54. Iung B, Gohlke-Bärwolf C, Tornos P, et al. Recommendations in the management of the asymptomatic patient with valvular heart disease. *Eur Heart J* 2002;23:1253–1266.
55. Cheitlin M. Stress echocardiography in mitral stenosis: when is it useful? *J Am Coll Cardiol* 2004;43:402–404.
56. Reis G, Motta MS, Barbosa MM, et al. Dobutamine stress echocardiography for noninvasive assessment and risk stratification of patients with rheumatic mitral stenosis. *J Am Coll Cardiol* 2004;44:391–401.
57. Jang IK, Block PC, Newell JB, et al. Percutaneous mitral balloon valvotomy for recurrent mitral stenosis after surgical commissurotomy. *Am J Cardiol* 1995;75:601–605.
58. Iung B, Garbarz E, Michaud P. Percutaneous mitral commissurotomy for restenosis after surgical commissurotomy: late efficacy and implications for patient selection. *J Am Coll Cardiol* 2000;35:1295–1302.
59. Alfonso F, Macaya C, Hernandez R, et al. Percutaneous mitral valvuloplasty with severe pulmonary artery hypertension. *Am J Cardiol* 1993;72:325–330.
60. Chen CR, Cheng TO, Chen JY, et al. Percutaneous balloon mitral valvuloplasty for mitral stenosis with and without associated aortic regurgitation. *Am Heart J* 1993;125:128–137.
61. Shaw TRD, McAreavey D, Essop AR, et al. Percutaneous balloon dilatation of mitral valve in patients who were unsuitable for surgical treatment. *Br Heart J* 1992;67:454–459.
62. Goldman J, Slade A, Clague J. Cardiogenic shock to mitral stenosis treated by balloon mitral valvuloplasty. *Cathet Cardiovasc Diagn* 1998;43:195–197.
63. Tuzcu EM, Block PC, Griffin BP, et al. Immediate and long-term outcome of percutaneous mitral valvotomy in patients 65 years and older. *Circulation* 1992;85:963–971.
64. Iung B, Cormier B, Farah B, et al. Percutaneous mitral commissurotomy in the elderly. *Eur Heart J* 1995;16:1092–1099.
65. Sutaria N, Elder AT, Shaw TRD. Long term outcome of percutaneous mitral balloon valvotomy in patients aged 70 and over. *Heart* 2000;83:433–438.
66. Iung B, Cormier B, Elias J, et al. Usefulness of percutaneous balloon commissurotomy for mitral stenosis during pregnancy. *Am J Cardiol* 1994;73:398–400.
67. Presbitero P, Prever SB, Brusca A. Interventional cardiology in pregnancy. *Eur Heart J* 1996;17:182–188.
68. Mangione JA, Lourenco RM, Souza dos Santo E, et al. Long-term follow-up of pregnant women after percutaneous mitral valvuloplasty. *Cathet Cardiovasc Interv* 2000;50:413–417.
69. Cannan CR, Nishimura RA, Reeder GS, et al. Echocardiographic assessment of commissural calcium: a simple predictor of outcome after percutaneous mitral balloon valvotomy. *J Am Coll Cardiol* 1997;29:175–180.
70. Fatkin D, Roy P, Morgan JJ, et al. Percutaneous balloon mitral valvotomy with the Inoue single balloon catheter: commissural morphology as a determination of outcome. *J Am Coll Cardiol* 1993;21:390–397.
71. Padial LR, Abascal VM, Moreno PR, et al. Echocardiography can predict the development of severe mitral regurgitation after percutaneous mitral valvuloplasty by the Inoue technique. *Am J Cardiol* 1999;83:1210–1213.
72. Mezilis ME, Salame MY, Oakly DG. Predicting mitral regurgitation following percutaneous mitral valvotomy with the Inoue balloon: comparison of two echocardiographic scoring systems. *Clin Cardiol* 1999;22:453–458.
73. Sutaria N, Northridge DB, Shaw TRD. Significance of commissural calcification on outcome of mitral balloon valvotomy. *Heart* 2000;84:398–402.
74. Turi ZG, Reyes VP, Soma Raju B, et al. Percutaneous balloon surgical closed commissurotomy for mitral stenosis. *Circulation* 1991;83:1179–1185.
75. Reyes VP, Raju BS, Wynne J, et al. Percutaneous balloon valvuloplasty compared with open surgical commissurotomy for mitral stenosis. *N Engl J Med* 1994;331:961–967.
76. Ben Farhat M, Ayari M, Maatouk F. Percutaneous balloon versus surgical closed and open mitral commissurotomy: seven-year follow-up results of a randomized trial. *Circulation* 1998;97:245–250.
77. Tuzcu ME, Block PC, Griffin B, et al. Percutaneous mitral balloon valvotomy in patients with calcific mitral stenosis: immediate and long-term outcome. *J Am Coll Cardiol* 1994;23:1604–1609.
78. Ping Zhang H, Allen JW, Lau FYK, et al. Immediate and late outcome of percutaneous balloon mitral valvotomy in patients with significantly calcified valves. *Am Heart J* 1995;129:501–506.
79. Post JR, Feldman T, Isner J, et al. Inoue balloon mitral valvotomy in patients with severe valvular and subvalvular deformity. *J Am Coll Cardiol* 1995; 25:1129–1136.
80. Iung B, Garbarz E, Doutrelant L, et al. Late results of percutaneous mitral commissurotomy for calcific mitral stenosis. *Am J Cardiol* 2000;85:1308–1314.
81. Safian RD, Mandell VS, Thurer RE, et al. Post-mortem and intra-operative balloon valvuloplasty of calcific aortic stenosis in elderly patients: mechanisms of successful dilatation. *J Am Coll Cardiol* 1987;9:665–670.
82. Robicsek F, Harbold NB. Limited value of balloon dilatation in calcified aortic stenosis in adults: direct observations during open heart surgery. *Am J Cardiol* 1987;60:857–864.
83. Cribier A, Gerber LI, Letac B. Aortic valvuloplasty. In: Topol EJ, ed. *Update 3: textbook of interventional cardiology.* Philadelphia: WB Saunders, 1992: 43–58.
84. Acar J, Vahanian A, Slama M, et al. Treatment of calcified aortic stenosis: surgery or percutaneous transluminal aortic valvuloplasty. *Eur Heart J* 1988;9(suppl E):163–168.
85. Block PC, Palacios IF. Comparison of hemodynamic results of anterograde versus retrograde percutaneous balloon aortic valvuloplasty. *Am J Cardiol* 1987;60:659–662.
86. Nishimura RA, Holmes DR Jr, Reeders GS, et al. Doppler evaluation of results of percutaneous aortic balloon valvuloplasty in calcific aortic stenosis. *Circulation* 1988;78:791–799.
87. NHLBI Balloon Registry participants. Percutaneous balloon aortic valvuloplasty. Acute and 30-day follow-up results in 674 patients from the NHBLI Balloon Valvuloplasty Registry. *Circulation* 1991;84:2383–2387.
88. Safian RD, Berman AD, Diver DJ, et al. Balloon aortic valvuloplasty in 170 consecutive patients. *N Engl J Med* 1988;319:125–130.
89. McKay R. Mansfield Scientific Registry experience: overview of acute hemodynamic results and procedural complications. *J Am Coll Cardiol* 1991;17:485–491.
90. Holmes DR Jr, Nishimura RA, Reeder GS. Mansfield Scientific Registry experience: in-hospital mortality after balloon aortic valvuloplasty: frequency and associated factors. *J Am Coll Cardiol* 1991;17:189–192.
91. Block PC, Palacios IF. Aortic and mitral balloon valvuloplasty: the United States experience. In: Topol EJ, ed. *Textbook of interventional cardiology.* Philadelphia: WB Saunders, 1994:1189–1205.
92. O'Neill WW. Mansfield Scientific Registry experience: predictors of long term survival after percutaneous aortic valvuloplasty. Report of the Mansfield Valvuloplasty Registry. *J Am Coll Cardiol* 1991;17:193–198.
93. Lieberman EB, Bashore TM, Hermiller JB, et al. Balloon aortic valvuloplasty in adults: failure of procedure to improve long-term survival. *J Am Coll Cardiol* 1995;26:1522–1528.

94. Otto CM, Mickel MC, Kennedy W, et al. Three-year outcome after balloon aortic valvuloplasty: insights into prognosis of valvular aortic stenosis. *Circulation* 1994;89:642–650.
95. Bernard Y, Etievent J, Mourand JL, et al. Long-term results of percutaneous aortic valvuloplasty compared with aortic replacement in patients more than 75 years old. *J Am Coll Cardiol* 1992;20:796–801.
96. O'Keefe JTL Jr, Vliesta RE, Bailey KR, et al. Natural history of candidates for balloon aortic valvuloplasty. *Mayo Clin Proc* 1987;62:986–991.
97. Agarwal A, Kini AS, Attanti S, et al. Results of repeat balloon valvuloplasty for treatment of aortic stenosis in patients aged 59 to 104 years. *Am J Cardiol* 2005;95:43–47.
98. Freeman WK, Schaff HV, O'Brien PC, et al. Cardiac surgery in octogenarians: perioperative outcome and clinical follow-up. *J Am Coll Cardiol* 1991;18:29–35.
99. Kvidal P, Bergstöm R, Hörte L-G, et al. Observed and relative survival after aortic valve replacement. *J Am Coll Cardiol* 2000;35:747–756.
100. Moreno PR, Ik-Kyung Jang, Newell JB, et al. The role of percutaneous aortic balloon valvuloplasty in patients with cardiogenic shock and critical aortic stenosis. *J Am Coll Cardiol* 1994;23:1071–1075.
101. Shaw TRD. The Inoue balloon for dilatation of the tricuspid valve: a modified over-the-wire approach. *Br Heart J* 1992;67:263–265.
102. McKay C, Waller BF, Hong R, et al. Problems encountered with catheter balloon valvuloplasty of bioprosthetic aortic valves. *Am Heart J* 1988;115:463–465.
103. Lin PJ, Chang JP, Chu JJ, et al. Balloon valvuloplasty is contraindicated in stenotic mitral bioprosthesis. *Am Heart J* 1994;127:724–726.
104. Block PC, Smalling R, Owing RM. Percutaneous double balloon valvotomy for bioprosthetic tricuspid stenosis. *Cathet Cardiovasc Diagn* 1994;33:342–344.
105. Sobrino N, Calvo Orbe L, Merino JL. Percutaneous balloon valvuloplasty for concurrent mitral, aortic, and tricuspid rheumatic stenosis. *Eur Heart J* 1995;16:711–713.
106. Gamra H, Betbout F, Ben Hamda K, et al. Balloon mitral commissurotomy in juvenile rheumatic mitral stenosis: a ten-year clinical and echocardiographic actuarial results. *Eur Heart J* 2003;24:1349–1356.
107. Leon MN, Harrell LC, Simosa HF, et al. Mitral balloon valvotomy for patients with mitral stenosis in atrial fibrillation: immediate and long-term results. *J Am Coll Cardiol* 1999;34:1145–1152.
108. Krasuski RA, Assar MD, Wang A, et al. Usefulness of percutaneous balloon mitral commissurotomy in preventing the development of atrial fibrillation in patients with mitral stenosis. *Am J Cardiol* 2004;93:936–939.
109. Langerveld J, van Hemel NM, Kelder JC, et al. Long-term follow-up of cardiac rhythm after percutaneous mitral balloon valvotomy. Does atrial fibrillation persist? *Europace* 2003;5:47–53.
110. Fan K, Lee KL, Chow WH, et al. Internal cardioversion of chronic atrial fibrillation during percutaneous mitral commissurotomy: insight into reversal of chronic stretch-induced atrial remodeling. *Circulation* 2002;105:2746–27452.
111. Sievert H, Lesh MD, Trepels T, et al. Percutaneous left atrial appendage transcatheter occlusion to prevent stroke in high-risk patients with atrial fibrillation: early clinical experience. *Circulation* 2002;105:1887–1889.
112. Adragao P, Machado FP, Aguiar C, et al. Ablation of atrial fibrillation in mitral valve disease patients: five year follow-up after percutaneous pulmonary vein isolation and mitral balloon valvuloplasty. *Rev Port Cardiol* 2003;22:1025–1036.
113. Zamorano J, Perez de Isla L, Sugeng L, et al. Non-invasive assessment of mitral valve area during percutaneous balloon mitral valvuloplasty: role of real-time 3D echocardiography. *Eur Heart J* 2004;25:2086–2091.
114. Chen WJ, Chen MF, Liau CS, et al. Safety of percutaneous transvenous balloon mitral commissurotomy in patients with mitral stenosis and thrombus in the left atrial appendage. *Am J Cardiol* 1992;70:117–119.
115. Pan M, Medina A, Suarey de Lejo J, et al. Balloon valvuloplasty for mild mitral stenosis. *Cathet Cardiovasc Diagn* 1991;24:1–5.
116. Silaruks S, Thinkhamrop B, Tantikosum W, et al. A prognostic model for predicting the disappearance of left atrial thrombi among candidates for percutaneous transvenous mitral commissurotomy. *J Am Coll Cardiol* 2002;39:886–891.
117. Silaruks S, Thinkhamrop B, Kiatchoosakun S, et al. Resolution of left atrial thrombus after 6 months of anticoagulation in candidates for percutaneous transvenous mitral commissurotomy. *Ann Intern Med* 2004;140:101–105.
118. Feldman T. Core curriculum for interventional cardiology: percutaneous valvuloplasty. *Cathet Cardiovasc Interv* 2003;60:48–56.
119. Vahanian A, Palacios IF. Percutaneous approaches to valvular disease. *Circulation* 2004;109:1572–1579.
120. Rahimtoola SH, Durairaj A, Mehra A, et al. Current evaluation and management of patients with mitral stenosis. *Circulation* 2002;106:1183–1188.
121. Palacios IF. Farewell to surgical mitral commissurotomy for many patients. *Circulation* 1998;97:223–226.
122. Rahimtoola SH. Catheter balloon valvuloplasty for severe calcific aortic stenosis: a limited role. *J Am Coll Cardiol* 1994;203:1076–1078.
123. Cribier A, Eltchaninoff H, Bash A, et al. Percutaneous transcatheter implantation of an aortic valve prosthesis for calcific aortic stenosis: first human case description. *Circulation* 2002;106:3006–3008.

SECTION SIX: HEART FAILURE AND TRANSPLANTATION

ERIC J. TOPOL, MD

CHAPTER 84 ■ GLOBAL PANDEMIC OF HEART FAILURE

RANDALL C. STARLING

OVERVIEW

Congestive heart failure is an increasing, global epidemic, particularly in the elderly, that results in significant health care expenditure, disability, and mortality. Coronary artery disease, hypertension, and diabetes mellitus are the major etiologic risk factors. Ironically, advances in the treatment of coronary artery disease and acute ischemic syndromes, which have saved lives, have resulted in a growing population of survivors with left ventricular dysfunction who are destined to develop the heart failure syndrome. Preventive measures that have evolved over the last 25 years, including hypertension management, have not reduced the incidence of heart failure. Congestive heart failure is the leading indication for hospitalization in the United States for patients older than 65 years. Most health care dollars spent on heart failure are for inpatient care. Heart failure is a chronic disease amenable to an intensive multidisciplinary care model (disease management program) designed to prevent hospital admissions through patient education, focused outpatient initiatives, and adherence to management guidelines that should enhance cost effectiveness and improve quality of life. Patients with advanced heart failure represent approximately 10% of the total heart failure population; they have the highest short-term mortality and consume the greatest percentage of resources (labor and dollars). Cardiovascular centers with expertise in the management of patients with advanced heart failure (through pharmacotherapy, circulatory support devices, surgical procedures, and heart transplantation) are necessary to deliver sophisticated care for this expanding population.

Congestive heart failure, traditionally considered an edematous disorder, was described hundreds of years ago. Hypertension and valvular heart disease were the most frequent comorbidities (1). Physicians could only attempt to control pulmonary and peripheral congestion with diuretic therapy. Heart failure was a progressive disease culminating in biventricular dysfunction, anasarca, and finally organ failure resulting from hypoperfusion. Today, symptomatic heart failure is most often characterized by effort intolerance (dyspnea) and fatigue without frank congestion. Thus, current guidelines refer to the condition as simply "heart failure."

Heart failure is growing at epidemic proportions, particularly in the elderly. It consumes significant health care dollars and results in disability and premature death. Common illnesses, including coronary artery disease, hypertension, and diabetes mellitus, are the major etiologic risk factors. In the United States, heart failure incidence is twice as common in hypertensive patients and five times greater in persons who have had a myocardial infarction (2). The National Heart, Lung, and Blood Institute (NHLBI) estimates that 75% of patients with heart failure have antecedent hypertension. Major advances in the treatment of coronary artery disease and acute ischemic syndromes that have saved countless lives have resulted in a growing population of patients with chronic left ventricular dysfunction who may develop clinical heart failure. The NHLBI estimates that 22% of male and 46% of female myocardial infarction victims will develop heart failure within 6 years. Heart failure is the most common indication for hospitalization in the United States in patients more than 65 years of age. It is estimated that about one half of patients with heart failure are 65 years old or older. Finally, it is now recognized that the syndrome of heart failure may also occur as a consequence of diastolic dysfunction. Recent reports have shown that 40% to 50% of patients hospitalized with heart failure have normal ejection fractions.

The mainstay of heart failure therapy today is "treatment" for established and symptomatic disease. The public health impact of heart failure for our society will continue to grow until effective primary and secondary prevention strategies are adopted and employed. Recent heart failure guidelines now define patients at risk of heart failure (American College of Cardiology [ACC] stage A) as a high priority for preemptive therapy. Patients with advanced heart failure, ACC stage D, represent almost 10% of the total heart failure population, have the highest short-term mortality, and consume the greatest percentage of resources (3). The cost of treating advanced symptomatic heart failure is a growing economic burden for industrialized nations. An analysis of six countries revealed that 1% to 2% of total health care expenditures were for heart failure, and about 70% of the total heart failure cost was for hospital expenses (4). The rapidly increasing prevalence of heart failure clearly represents the most important public health problem in cardiovascular medicine (1,4,5).

EPIDEMIOLOGY

An *epidemic* is described as affecting or tending to affect a disproportionately large number of individuals within a

Population Group	Prevalence 2002	Incidence (New Cases)	Mortality 2001	Hospital Discharges 2002	Cost 2005
Total population	4,900,000 (2.3%)	550,000	52,828	970,000	$27.9 billion
Total males	2,400,000 (2.6%)	—	19,805 (37.5%)*	441,000	—
Total females	2,500,000 (2.1%)	—	33,023 (62.5%)*	529,000	—
White males	2.5%	—	17,782	—	—
White females	1.9%	—	29,942	—	—
Black males	3.1%	—	1,802	—	—
Black females	3.5%	—	2,797	—	—
Mexican-American males	2.7%	—	—	—	—
Mexican-American females	1.6%	—	—	—	—

Note: (—) = data not available.

* These percentages represent the portion of total mortality that is males vs. females.

Sources: ***Prevalence:*** *NHANES (1999–2002), CDC/NCHS and NHLBI; data for white and black males and females are for non-Hispanics; percentages are age-adjusted for Americans age 20 and older. These data are based on self reports.* ***Incidence:*** *FHS, NHLBI.* ***Mortality:*** *CDC/NCHS; data for white and black males and females include Hispanics.* ***Hospital discharges:*** *CDC/NCHS: data include people both living and dead. Cost: NHLBI; data include direct and indirect costs for 2005.*

FIGURE 84.1. Heart failure statistics. CDC/NCHS, Centers for Disease Control and Prevention/National Center for Health Statistics; NHANES, National Health and Nutrition Examination Survey; NHLBI, National Heart, Lung, and Blood Institute. (From American Heart Association. *Heart disease and stroke statistics: 2005 update.* Dallas, TX: American Heart Association, 2005; www.americanheart.org)

population, community, or region at the same time (excessively prevalent). *Pandemic* refers to a disease occurring over a wide geographic area and affecting an exceptionally high proportion of the population. Heart failure is a worldwide phenomenon that is indeed pandemic. Heart failure affects approximately 2 to 4 million U.S. residents and more than 15 million people worldwide (5) (Fig. 84.1). The American Heart Association estimates that there were 5 million U.S. residents alive in 2003 with congestive heart failure and 57,200 deaths (www.americanheart.org). Based on the 44-year follow-up of the NHLBI's Framingham Health Study, heart failure incidence approaches 10 per 1,000 population after age 65 years. Despite declining mortality rates for cardiovascular disease in the United States, hospitalizations for heart failure have increased substantially. Hospital discharges for congestive heart failure in the United States rose from 399,000 in 1979 to 1,093,000 in 2003, a 174% increase (www.americanheart.org).

The criteria for the diagnosis of the syndrome of congestive heart failure are not standardized; hence population estimates may underestimate the extent of heart failure. Measures used in population-based studies and cardiovascular drug research rely on a composite of signs, symptoms, and diagnostic findings. Attempts to validate the Framingham clinical heart failure score against a measure of ejection fraction showed that, in patients with a low left ventricular ejection fraction (LVEF <0.40), 20% met none of the criteria for congestive heart failure. A cohort of 2,000 persons aged 25 to 74 years living in Scotland underwent a detailed assessment of cardiac status including echocardiography (4). The overall prevalence of left ventricular systolic dysfunction (ejection fraction <30%) was 2.9%; concurrent symptoms of heart failure were found in 1.5%, whereas the remaining 1.4% of study subjects were asymptomatic. Prevalence was greater with age and in men, reaching 6.4% in men aged 65 to 74 years. Population estimates of heart failure have many pitfalls, and utilization of death rates and hospitalizations likely grossly underestimates the true magnitude of the heart failure pandemic. An analysis using administrative data sets to create a definition of heart failure using diagnosis codes (REACH study) confirmed the heart failure epidemic in the United States (6). The authors concluded that ninth International Classification of Diseases–Clinical Modification codes and automated sources of data can be used within health systems to describe the epidemiology of heart failure. A population survey performed in Olmsted County, Minnesota by Redfield and coworkers provided further insights into the difficulty in truly measuring the prevalence of heart failure without sensitive techniques. Using detailed echocardiographic examinations and record reviews, the prevalence of validated congestive heart failure was 2.2%, with 44% having an ejection fraction greater than 50% (15). However, among those persons with moderate or severe diastolic or systolic dysfunction, fewer than half had recognized heart failure (Fig. 84.2), and, importantly, diastolic dysfunction, often unaccompanied by clinically recognized heart failure, was associated with marked increases in all-cause mortality. It can be concluded that the true incidence

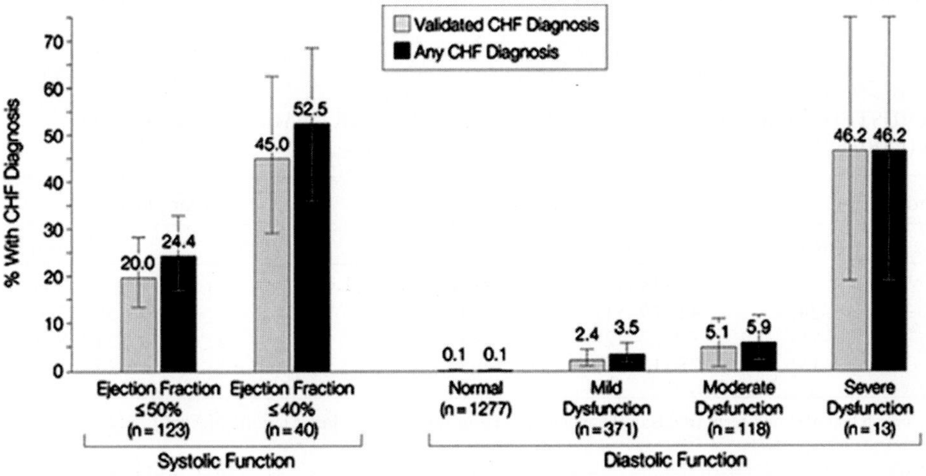

FIGURE 84.2. The frequency and 95% confidence intervals of the percentage estimate of any heart failure diagnosis among participants with systolic or diastolic dysfunction. CHF, congestive heart failure. (From Redfield MM, Jacobsen SJ, Burnett JC, et al. Burden of systolic and diastolic ventricular dysfunction in the community: appreciating the scope of the heart failure epidemic. *JAMA* 2003;289:194–202.)

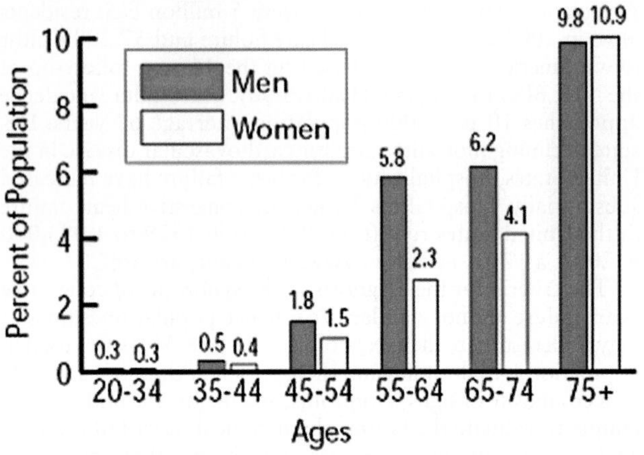

FIGURE 84.3. Prevalence of congestive heart failure by sex and age, National Health and Nutrition Examination Survey 1999 to 2002. Source: Centers for Disease Control and Prevention/National Center for Health Statistics and National Heart, Lung, and Blood Institute. (From American Heart Association. *Heart disease and stroke statistics: 2005 update*. Dallas, TX: American Heart Association, 2005.)

and prevalence of heart failure are difficult to capture; however, most likely our current estimates are conservative and underestimate the true magnitude of the pandemic.

Incidence and Prevalence

Incidence refers to the number of new cases observed in a year in a defined population. *Prevalence* refers to the number of cases observed at a specified point in time in a defined population. The crude incidence of heart failure (unadjusted for age) ranges from 1 to 5 cases per 1,000 population per year and increases sharply with advancing age to as high as 40 cases per 1,000 population more than 75 years old (7). A reflection of the incidence of heart failure in the United States is made from the Framingham Study and the Framingham Offspring Study, representing a population of more than 10,000 (8). The prevalence of heart failure rises with age in both men and women, as shown in Figure 84.3.

A recent analysis of the Framingham Heart Study cohort demonstrated over the past 50 years that the incidence of heart failure has declined among women, but not among men; however, survival after the onset of heart failure has improved in both sexes (9). When established clinical criteria are used to define heart failure, the lifetime risk for heart failure is 1 in 5 for both men and women (10). Both hypertension and antecedent myocardial infarction significantly affect the lifetime risk for heart failure between ages 40 and 80 years in both men and women. These findings highlight the importance of risk factor modification to reduce ischemic heart disease and the potential impact of antihypertensive therapy to reduce the development of overt clinical heart failure. The incidence of heart failure is 550,000 cases per year in the United States. The annual rates per 1,000 population of new and recurrent heart failure events for nonblack men are 21.5 for ages 65 to 74 years, 43.3 for ages 75 to 84 years, and a striking 73.1 for age 85 years and older. For nonblack women in the same age groups, the rates are 11.2, 26.3, and 64.9, respectively. For black men, the rates are 21.1, 52.0, and 66.7, and for black women the rates are 18.9, 35.5, and 48.4, respectively (2).

Mortality

Since 1968, heart failure as the primary cause of death has increased fourfold (8). The most dismal prognosis for patients with severe symptoms (New York Heart Association class IV) and coronary artery disease was an 18% and 43% survival rate at 1 and 3 years, respectively (11). Symptomatic patients with dilated nonischemic cardiomyopathy who are receiving medical therapy have a better prognosis compared with patients with underlying coronary artery disease (11). Various risk factors influence mortality rates including age, renal dysfunction, diabetes, and atrial fibrillation.

Survival in patients with heart failure has improved over the past 50 years (Table 84.1). The 30-day, 1-year, and 5-year age-adjusted mortality among men declined from 12%, 30%, and 70% from 1950 through 1969 to 11%, 28%, and 59% in the period from 1990 through 1999. In women, the corresponding rates were 18%, 28%, and 57% for the period 1950 through 1969 and 10%, 24%, and 45% from 1990 through 1999 (9). Overall, there was an improvement in survival rate after the onset of heart failure of 12% per decade, a significant reduction in both men ($p = .01$) and women ($p = .02$). The explanation for this is purely speculative; however, the improved survival was temporally associated with the use of both angiotensin-converting enzyme (ACE) inhibitors and β-blockers. Another analysis examined the short- and long-term mortality of patients after initial hospitalizations for heart failure using a cohort of 38,702 consecutive patients from April 1994 through March 1997 in Ontario, Canada. The crude 30-day and 1-year mortality rates were 11.6% and 33.1%, respectively (12). Complex interactions among age, sex, and comorbidities affected short- and long-term survival. In the oldest comorbidity-laden subgroup, 30-day and 1-year mortality rates were 23.8% and 60.7%, respectively. A subgroup analysis from the Digitalis Investigation Group study showed that in ambulatory patients with congestive heart failure,

TABLE 84.1

TEMPORAL TRENDS IN AGE-ADJUSTED MORTALITY AFTER THE ONSET OF HEART FAILURE: MEN AND WOMEN AGES 65 TO 74 YEARS (PERCENT; 95% CONFIDENCE INTERVAL)

	30-day mortality		1-year mortality		5-year mortality	
Period	Men	Women	Men	Women	Men	Women
1950–1969	12 (4–19)	18 (7–27)	30 (18–40)	28 (16–39)	70 (57–79)	57 (43–67)
1970–1979	15 (7–23)	16 (6–24)	41 (29–51)	28 (17–38)	75 (65–83)	59 (45–69)
1980–1989	12 (5–18)	10 (4–16)	33 (23–42)	27 (17–35)	65 (54–73)	51 (39–60)
1990–1999	11 (4–17)	10 (3–15)	28 (18–36)	24 (14–33)	59 (47–68)	45 (33–55)

Adapted from Levy D, Kenchaiah, S, Larson MG, et al. Long-term trends in the incidence of and survival with heart failure. *N Engl J Med* 2002;347:1397–1402.

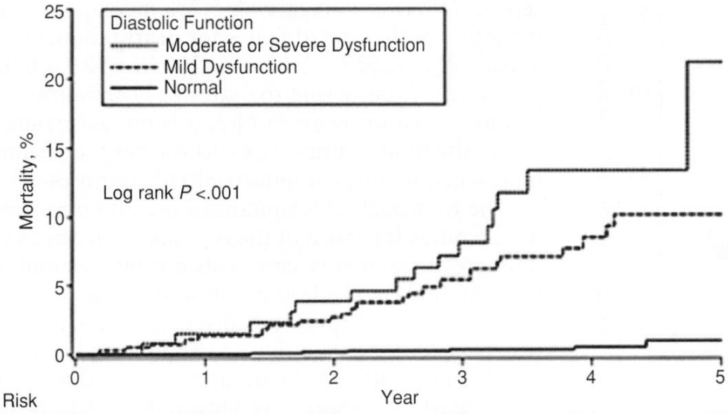

No. at Risk	0	1	2	3	4	5
Normal	1277	1277	1275	885	404	38
Mild	371	366	361	246	122	8
Moderate or Severe	131	129	126	94	39	5

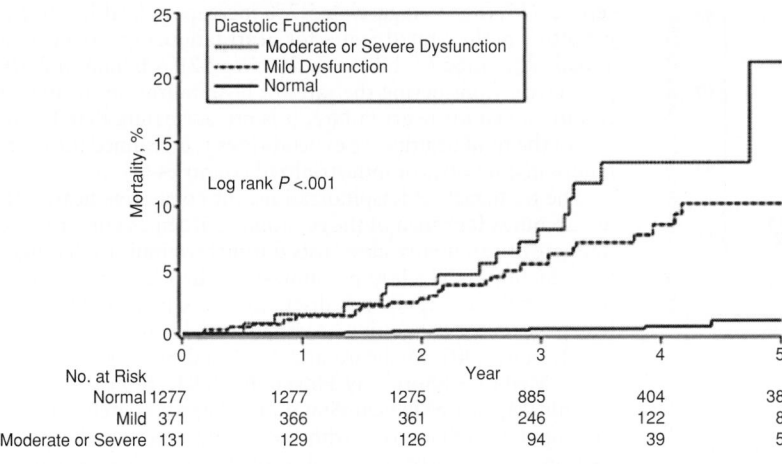

FIGURE 84.4. Kaplan-Meier mortality curves for participants with normal diastolic function compared with those with mild, moderate, or severe diastolic dysfunction. (Adapted from Redfield MM, Jacobsen SJ, Burnett JC, et al. Burden of systolic and diastolic ventricular dysfunction in the community: appreciating the scope of the heart failure epidemic. *JAMA* 2003;289:194–202.)

estimated creatinine clearance predicted all-cause mortality independently of established prognostic variables (13). In Cox regression analyses, independent predictors of mortality were estimated creatinine clearance, 6-minute walk distance of up to 262 m, ejection fraction, recent hospitalization for worsening heart failure, and need for diuretic treatment. It is obvious that, as a population ages, heart failure becomes more prevalent and the mortality rises, especially in patients with compromised renal function and comorbidities. It has been recognized that elderly persons have a substantial risk for death after a diagnosis of heart failure with normal left ventricular systolic function. A longitudinal population-based study in 5,888 persons at least 65 years of age revealed that 4.9% had congestive heart failure, and the ejection fraction was normal in 63%, borderline decreased in 15%, or impaired in 22%, as determined by a core echocardiographic laboratory (14). Forty-five percent of those with heart failure and 16% without heart failure died within 6 to 7 years (14). A cross-sectional survey was performed in Olmsted County, Minnesota to determine the prevalence of diastolic and systolic dysfunction and to ascertain whether diastolic dysfunction was predictive of all-cause mortality (15). A cohort of 2,042 randomly selected residents of Olmsted County aged 45 years or older was surveyed between June 1997 and September 2000. The prevalence of heart failure was 2.2%, and 44% had an ejection fraction greater than 50%. Among those with moderate or severe diastolic or systolic dysfunction, fewer than 50% had recognized heart failure. Both mild and moderate or severe diastolic dysfunction were predictive of all-cause mortality as shown in Figure 84.4 (hazard ratio for severe diastolic dysfunction 10.17, $p < .001$).

Despite medical advances, heart failure remains a lethal illness. Heart failure in the elderly has the highest mortality. Heart

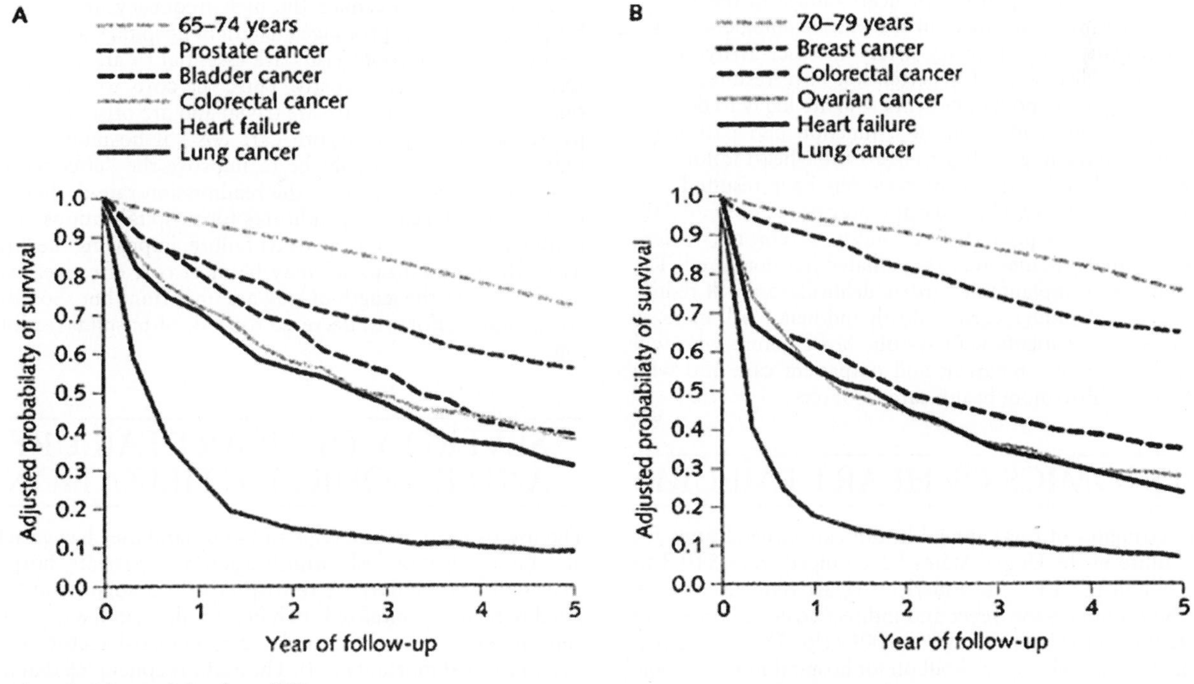

Adapted with permission from [32].

FIGURE 84.5. Five-year age-adjusted, survival curves following an incident admission for heart failure versus common types of cancer in age-matched patients. **A:** Scottish men. **B:** Scottish women. (Adapted from Stewart S. Prognosis of patients with heart failure compared with common types of cancer. *Heart Fail Monitor* 2003;3;87–94.)

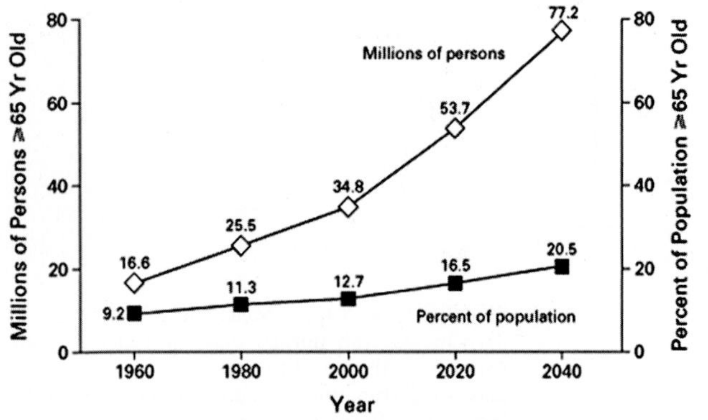

FIGURE 84.6. Projected increases in the U.S. population 65 years of age or older. Data are from the U.S. Census Bureau. (Adapted from Redfield MM. Heart failure: an epidemic of uncertain proportions. *N Engl J Med* 2002;347:1442–1444.)

failure with preserved systolic function is a growing concern and carries an ominous prognosis. Mortality from heart failure is high, and most patients and families are uninformed and unprepared for the risk of death and the need to make end-of-life decisions. A recent Scottish analysis showed that the 5-year age- and sex-adjusted mortality for heart failure is worse than for common forms of cancer (16), as depicted in Figure 84.5.

Reasons for Increasing Prevalence

The prevalence of heart failure increases with age. The U.S. Census Bureau estimates that U.S. residents age 65 years or older will increase from 34.8 million (12.7% of population) in 2000 to 77.2 million (20.5% of population) by 2040 (Fig. 84.6). Considering the high prevalence in this age cohort, we expect a continued expansion of heart failure in the United States. Furthermore, advances in the pharmacologic and surgical management of coronary artery disease, arrhythmias, valvular heart disease, and hypertension have resulted in an ever-enlarging aging pool of patients who are likely to develop worsening systolic and/or diastolic function and pathologic ventricular remodeling leading to irreversible heart failure. Effective medical and surgical interventions have resulted in a reduction in mortality. However, the prevalence of heart failure is rising because predisposing conditions (coronary artery disease and diabetes mellitus) are palliated but not cured. The increased use of implantable cardiac defibrillators will reduce the incidence of sudden cardiac death and hence will increase the longevity of patients with systolic heart failure who will subsequently require inpatient and outpatient care and who will thereby utilize more health care resources.

ECONOMICS OF HEART FAILURE

Recent estimates of total annual health care expenditures for heart failure in the United States have ranged from $10.3 to $37.8 billion (17,18). The American Heart Association estimates $29.6 billion for direct and indirect costs of congestive heart failure in the United States in 2006 (19). The breakdown includes the following: $19.3 billion for hospital/nursing home care, $2.0 billion for physician/professionals, $3.1 billion for drugs/medical durables, $2.4 billion for home health care, and $2.8 billion for lost productivity/mortality. Hence, 65.2% of the total expense is for inpatient care, very similar to the estimates on inpatient care (73% and 62%) in the other two reports (17,18). A staggering 5.7% increase in health care expenditure in the United States for heart failure occurred over a 1-year period ($27.9 billion in 2005 to $29.6 billion in 2006 projected). Considering the rates of hospitalization (including readmissions) for heart failure, it is not surprising that 1% to 2% of the total health care expenditures is consumed for heart failure in a number of industrialized countries (4).

The frequency of hospitalizations for congestive heart failure accounts for much of the economic burden. A conservative estimate of cumulative care costs during hospitalization ranges from $6,000 to $12,000 per admission. In 1999, the amount of $3.6 billion ($5,456 per discharge) was paid to Medicare beneficiaries for congestive heart failure (Health Care Financing Review, 2001 Medicare and Medicaid Statistical Supplement. Medicare Short-Stay Hospitals, 2001, Table 27. www.cms.hhs/MedicareMedicaidStatSupp). Approximately 35% of the population diagnosed with heart failure become hospitalized on an annual basis (5). Multiple hospitalizations, particularly of elderly patients with multiple comorbid conditions (50% have three or more), are especially common. Indeed, it has been found that the 3-month readmission rate after an index hospitalization for congestive heart failure was as high as 47% of discharges (20). Many factors are related to the high rates of hospitalization for heart failure, including progression of underlying disease, inappropriate treatment plans, lack of patient compliance with prescribed regimens or diet or both, and use of detrimental drug therapy in certain heart failure settings. Numerous patient- and physician-specific issues that contribute to "heart failure decompensation" culminating in hospitalization are potentially reversible (3,21). An analysis in Germany of 179 patients admitted to the hospital with acute decompensation of preexisting heart failure concluded that 54% of admissions could be regarded as preventable (22). Noncompliance with drugs or diet was the leading cause of acute decompensation, present in 42%. Practitioners should utilize pharmacologic agents proven to be effective in multicenter clinical trials at target doses when managing patients with chronic heart failure (3).

Interventions to reduce the high frequency and acuity of hospitalization, the prolonged length of hospital stays, and frequent emergency room visits are essential to attenuate costs. Outpatient care is less costly. Thus, the costs to intensify the outpatient delivery of care are trivial and are offset by the major reduction in total health care costs if hospital days are reduced. One goal should be to improve the "effectiveness" of inpatient stays such that the readmission rate declines. Up to 25% of Medicare expenditures for hospitalizations are for readmissions (23). Thus, in heart failure, improving the "quality of the hospitalization" may be most cost effective. Initiatives to reduce the length of stay are important but should not compromise efforts to decrease the risk of hospital readmission.

SEVERITY OF HEART FAILURE AND RESOURCE UTILIZATION

The use of heart failure registries and databases has enriched our knowledge of risk stratification for patients hospitalized with heart failure. A retrospective Canadian study analyzed patients hospitalized with heart failure, and a derivation and validation cohort was used to determine risk factors for 30-day and 1-year mortality (24). The authors concluded that mortality could be predicted within minutes of admission, and risk factors included older age, lower systolic blood pressure, higher respiratory rate, higher urea nitrogen level (all $p < .001$), and hyponatremia ($p < .01$). Comorbid conditions associated with mortality included cerebrovascular disease (30-day mortality

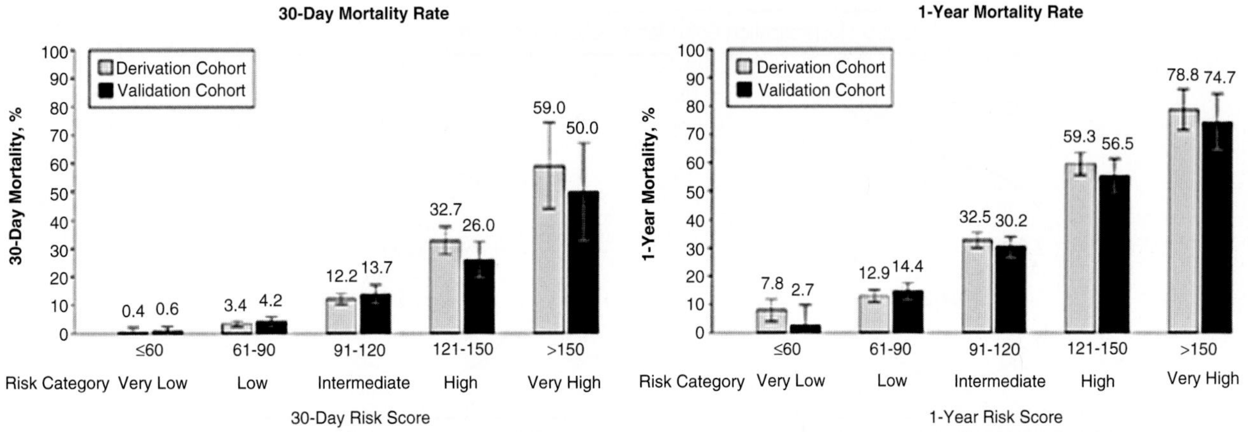

FIGURE 84.7. Mortality rates stratified by 30-day and 1-year risk scores. *Error bars* indicate 95% confidence intervals for the mortality rates in each category. (From Lee DS, Austin PC, Rouleau JL, et al. Predicting mortality among patients hospitalized for heart failure: derivation and validation of a clinical model. *JAMA* 2003;290:2581–2587.)

odds ratio [OR], 1.43; 95% confidence interval [CI], 1.03 to 1.98; $p = .03$), chronic obstructive pulmonary disease (OR, 1.66; 95% CI, 1.22 to 2.27; $p = .002$), hepatic cirrhosis (OR, 3.22; 95% CI, 1.08 to 9.65; $p = .04$), dementia (OR, 2.54; 95% CI, 1.77 to 3.65; $p < .001$), and cancer (OR, 1.86; 95% CI, 1.28 to 2.70; $p = .001$). As shown in Figure 84.7, a risk index stratified the risk of death and identified low- and high-risk individuals. Patients with very low-risk scores ($\leq$60) had a mortality rate of 0.4% at 30 days and 7.8% at 1 year. Patients with very high-risk scores (>150) had a mortality rate of 59.0% at 30 days and 78.8% at 1 year. A similar risk stratification of patients admitted with acutely decompensated heart failure was performed using data from the Acute Decompensated Heart Failure National Registry (ADHERE) (25). The best single predictor for mortality was high admission levels of blood urea nitrogen ($\geq$43 mg/dL) followed by low admission systolic blood pressure ($\geq$115 mm Hg) and then by high levels of serum creatinine ($\geq$2.75 mg/dL). A simple risk tree identified patient groups with mortality ranging from 2.1% to 21.9%, as shown in Figure 84.8. The OR for mortality between patients identified as high and low risk was 12.9 (95% CI, 10.4 to 15.9). These results suggest that patients hospitalized for acutely decompensated heart failure at low, intermediate, and high risk for in-hospital mortality can be easily identified using standard clinical information obtained on hospital admission. High-risk patients of course have the longest length of stays, have the highest readmission rates, and consume the highest percentage of resources. Now that clinicians have the knowledge to risk stratify hospitalized patients, we need to develop better treatment algorithms for evidence-based care of patients with acutely decompensated heart failure.

Patients with advanced heart failure represent about 10% of the total heart failure population, experience the highest short-term mortality, and consume tremendous resources. With improved pharmacotherapy and management, increasing numbers of patients are expected to survive with severe left ventricular dysfunction who will ultimately die of refractory heart failure. Patients with stage D or refractory heart failure are candidates for heart transplantation, mechanical circulatory support devices, outpatient infusion therapies, or hospice care (3). Patients with refractory heart failure are the consumers of expensive, technologically sophisticated therapies (open heart surgical procedures, cardiac transplantation, mechanical circulatory assist devices, automatic implantable cardiac defibrillators, biventricular pacemakers, outpatient intravenous therapy) and require frequent high-acuity admissions (intensive care unit stays and hemodynamic monitoring). A European analysis has shown that it is more expensive to treat severe heart failure than mild heart failure, primarily because of the high rate and costs of hospitalization over a 6- to 12-month period before the patient dies (26). An admission for cardiac transplantation and postoperative care averages $303,400. Costs for implantation and care associated with a left ventricular assist device average $175,000, and implantation of a cardiac defibrillator costs $50,000. Specialized regional heart failure centers will continue to play a critical role in the delivery of cost-effective high-quality care to this group of patients. The proper use of sophisticated therapies, including ventricular assist devices, biventricular pacemakers/implantable cardioverter-defibrillators, outpatient infusion therapies, and high-risk surgical procedures (coronary artery bypass grafting, mitral valve repair, surgical ventricular remodeling procedure) can improve outcomes and reduce costs. Registries required by health care payers that monitor the outcomes of procedures (e.g., Scientific Registry of Transplant Recipients, United Network of Organ Sharing, Interagency Registry for Mechanically Assisted Circulatory Support) will mandate that providers maintain benchmark standards that will optimize patient outcomes and contain costs.

HEART FAILURE GUIDELINES

Clinical practice guidelines have been developed by carefully evaluating the world's literature with emphasis on well-controlled randomized clinical trials of solid scientific validity and expert opinion from prominent clinicians. Consensus guideline documents for the evaluation and management of heart failure have been published (3,27). Heart failure experts believe that the pharmacologic treatment of patients remains suboptimal, and that both β-blockers and ACE inhibitors are underutilized. Data collected from the ADHERE registry confirm that ACE inhibitors were used in only 74% of more than 40,000 hospitalized patients examined at 260 U.S. hospitals between August 2003 and July 2004 (2). β-Blocker use at discharge for eligible patients was 73%, complete discharge instructions were given in only 47%, and smoking cessation instructions were given in 64%; these core performance indicators thus fall significantly below their benchmarks. The guidelines emphasize the importance of appropriate pharmacologic therapy (target doses and ACE inhibitor use for asymptomatic left ventricular dysfunction) and nonpharmacologic

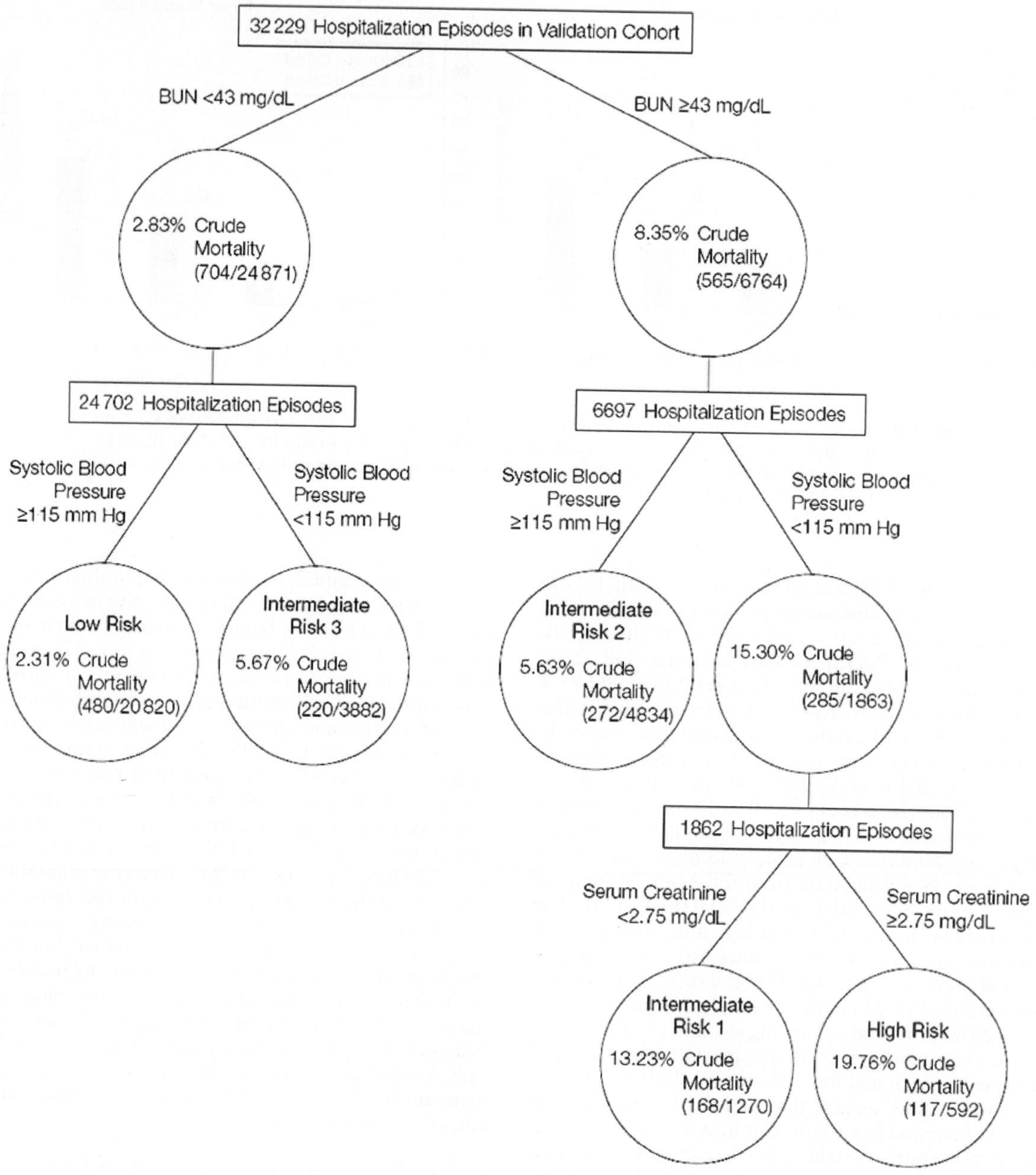

FIGURE 84.8. Predictors of in-hospital mortality and risk stratification for patients with acutely decompensated heart failure who are admitted to the hospital. BUN, blood urea nitrogen. (Adapted from Fonarow GC, Adams KF, Abraham WT, et al. Risk stratification for in-hospital mortality in acutely decompensated heart failure: classification and regression tree analysis. *JAMA* 2004;293:572–580.)

treatment (counseling, education, and lifestyle modifications) in the management of heart failure. The economic and quality of care ramifications related to the adoption and improved adherence of heart failure guidelines are enormous. The advent of published guidelines has led to the development of disease care management algorithms that can be implemented within health care systems (28,29).

Educational programs can improve quality of life for the patient and can reduce hospitalization. Multidisciplinary interventions designed to improve dietary compliance and to reduce hospital admissions in patients with heart failure have been found to be highly effective. A multidisciplinary heart failure disease management program is employed at the Cleveland Clinic Health System in Cleveland, Ohio (28). The cornerstone of a heart failure disease management program is to employ pharmacologic therapy in compliance with evidence-based heart failure guidelines and to develop a mechanism to monitor compliance both for patients and physicians. Elderly, socially deprived, recently hospitalized patients with heart failure are at increased high risk for readmission and likely will derive the greatest benefit from disease management programs (30,31). Early single-center studies showed that multidisciplinary management and education could reduce the posthospitalization readmission rate for heart failure. A metaanalysis of 18 studies representing data from 8 countries randomized 3,304 elderly patients who were hospitalized with heart failure to comprehensive discharge planning and postdischarge support or usual care (32). It was concluded that discharge planning and postdischarge support significantly reduced readmission rates (RR, 0.75 [0.64 to 0.88]; $p < .001$). A second recent metaanalysis examined 30 trials and found a reduction in all-cause admission (RR, 0.87 [0.79 to 0.95]; $p = .002$) (33). This metaanalysis also concluded that the most effective interventions were delivered at least partially in the home and that multidisciplinary interventions could reduce all-cause mortality as well. A Medicare demonstration project is currently under way to determine prospectively the effectiveness of home monitoring after hospital discharge in patients with heart failure.

CONTROVERSIES AND PERSONAL PERSPECTIVES

The a priori end point in most randomized heart failure trials is mortality. Therapies that improve quality of life and reduce hospitalizations but increase mortality are unlikely to obtain approval from the U.S. Food and Drug Administration (FDA). Initial reports on the use of outpatient dobutamine hydrochloride therapy showed that functional class improved significantly, but mortality was high. Cardiac resynchronization therapy showed improvement in functional capacity and quality of life in early clinical trials and was embraced by clinicians and approved by the FDA and Centers for Medicare and Medicaid Services (CMS). In 2005, the results of a prospective, randomized clinical trial ultimately showed a reduction in mortality, and the adoption of the therapy continues to grow. Implantable cardiac defibrillators did not receive approval for seemingly intuitive indications until painstakingly derived data were available from a randomized clinical trial that took years to complete (34). Nesiritide was approved for use in the treatment of acutely decompensated heart failure by the FDA in 2001, but no mortality data were available. Clinicians used nesiritide extensively and, with good intentions, hoped to be helping their patients symptomatically. Subsequent intriguing but flawed pooled analyses have raised concerns that nesiritide is associated with worsening renal function and increased mortality (35). Clinicians and heart failure experts now await mortality data; the use of nesiritide for hospitalized patients with acutely decompensated heart failure has fallen markedly. Heart failure must be studied in populations, and mortality data are needed before conclusions can be made. Before nesiritide, we saw the same situation played out with mibefradil, flosequinan, and vesnarinone. Seemingly innocuous treatments such as education and postdischarge follow-up require demonstration of objective efficacy data before reimbursement will be forthcoming. In a fatal chronic illness such as heart failure, the quality-of-life benefits of a therapy must be considered, because they may outweigh any mortality effects. Clinicians, however, should have all the data and should be able to make informed decisions before utilizing any therapeutic agent, device, procedure, or strategy.

The new heart failure guidelines have created stages A, B, C, and D. We have discussed that the bulk of health care dollars spent on heart failure are for stage D patients, who have refractory heart failure and very high short-term mortality. Stage A patients are those at risk of developing heart failure with comorbidities including hypertension, diabetes, atherosclerotic disease, obesity, metabolic syndrome, family history of cardiomyopathy/heart failure, or use of cardiotoxins. The guidelines encourage the treatment of hypertension, smoking cessation, exercise, and weight loss, discourage alcohol use, and include treatment of metabolic syndrome and management of lipid levels. Furthermore, the use of ACE inhibitors or adrenergic receptor blockers (ARBs) for diabetes and/or vascular disease is encouraged. One must ask: What has been the impact of statin use and ACE inhibitors and ARBs to common diseases on the subsequent development of heart failure? The greatest impact on reducing the global pandemic of heart failure will be to make therapies available to populations at risk and to facilitate widespread availability and use of lipid-lowering drugs and antihypertensives in addition to risk factor modification lifestyle changes that will reduce smoking, reduce obesity, and increase physical activity. This strategy will ultimately be the most cost-effective and influential approach to the global pandemic of heart failure.

THE FUTURE

Many patients with heart failure are treated suboptimally with pharmacotherapy (36–38). A U.S. survey showed that cardiologists are more likely to prescribe ACE inhibitors than are general practitioners and internists (35). A survey comparing the practice patterns between cardiologists and heart failure specialists showed general conformity but concluded that some patients with heart failure may be better managed by heart failure specialists (36). Few data are currently available to prove that heart failure specialists provide superior care for patients with heart failure. Perhaps the greatest impact of heart failure specialists is to evaluate patients with cryptogenic heart failure, with the goal of finding treatable components that have precipitated the heart failure syndrome (i.e., surgical coronary and/or valvular disease, dyssynchrony responding to resynchronization therapy, ablation for tachycardia-induced cardiomyopathy). A recent study concluded that cardiology participation in outpatients with new-onset heart failure was associated with improved guideline adherence and a reduction in the composite end point of death plus cardiovascular hospitalization (38). Specialized centers for heart failure can treat patients with severe decompensation, often resulting in prolonged stabilization and improved quality of life in patients originally referred expecting that cardiac transplantation was the only option (40).

Strategies to attack the epidemic of heart failure should include the following initiatives: (a) reduction of inpatient costs, (b) investment in outpatient care and development of chronic disease management programs, (c) reduction of admissions (more important than reduction in length of stay), (d) focus of efforts and resources on the high-risk patient (history of frequent readmissions), (e) utilization of specialized heart failure providers (physicians, nurses, dietitians, rehabilitation specialists), and (f) extensive patient education. Dedicated specialized heart failure centers should include the following mandates to help achieve these initiatives: (a) detailed patient evaluation to stage disease and to ensure appropriate diagnosis and treatment, (b) close patient monitoring at intervals tailored to the individual patient's needs, (c) immediate access to heart failure team staff and timely responses to patient needs, and (d) patient education concerning heart failure. Specialized heart failure centers can provide expertise in the medical and surgical management of heart failure (40). Surgical therapy for heart failure (high-risk standard cardiac surgical procedures, cardiac transplantation, mechanical circulatory assist devices, and ventricular remodeling procedures) has become an essential component and now extends far beyond cardiac transplantation (41). Many high-risk patients (ACC stage B and C) will benefit from standard surgical procedures with a safety net of mechanical support and transplantation available at specialized heart failure centers.

Primary prevention is the solution to heart failure. Emphasis should continue to be on primary prevention as the seminal solution to the increasing cost of heart failure management. The new ACC/American Heart Association guidelines emphasize prevention by creating stage A, which represents patients with risk factors and the potential to develop structural heart disease and subsequently heart failure. The guidelines emphasize the need to treat stage A patients with hypertension, diabetes, coronary artery disease, and obesity aggressively so they never progress to frank heart failure. Secondary prevention strategies to alleviate morbidity and to reduce mortality are the immediate focus to reduce the burden of this global pandemic. The role of the heart failure nursing team will continue to expand in heart failure patient management. Better patient monitoring and education and increased use of implantable monitoring devices and the Internet to manage patients with heart failure will facilitate improved patient outcomes and reduced health care expenditures.

References

1. Garg R, Packer M, Pitt B, Yusaf S. Heart failure in the 1990s: evolution of a major public health problem in cardiovascular medicine. *J Am Coll Cardiol* 1993;22(suppl A):3A–5A.
2. American Heart Association. *Heart disease and stroke statistics: 2005 update.* Dallas, TX: American Heart Association, 2005.
3. Hunt SA, Abraham WT, Chin MH, et al. ACC/AHA 2005 guideline update for the diagnosis and management of chronic heart failure in the adult—summary article: a report of the American College of Cardiology/American Heart Association Task Force on Practice Guidelines (Writing Committee to Update the 2001 Guidelines for the Evaluation and Management of Heart Failure): developed in collaboration with the American College of Chest Physicians and the International Society for Heart and Lung Transplantation: endorsed by the Heart Rhythm Society. *Circulation* 2005;112:1825–1852.
4. McMurray JJ, Stewart S. Epidemiology, aetiology, and prognosis of heart failure. *Heart* 2000;83:596–602.
5. Eriksson H. Heart failure: a growing public health problem. *J Intern Med* 1995;237:135–141.
6. McCullough PA, Philbin EF, Spertus JA, et al. Confirmation of a heart failure epidemic: findings from the Resource Utilization Among Congestive Heart Failure (REACH) study. *J Am Coll Cardiol* 2002;39:60–69.
7. Cowie MR, Mosterd A, Wood DA, et al. The epidemiology of heart failure. *Eur Heart J* 1997;18:208–225.
8. Ho KKL, Pinsky JL, Kannel WB, Levy D. The epidemiology of heart failure: the Framingham study. *J Am Coll Cardiol* 1993;22(suppl A):6A–13A.
9. Levy D, Kenchaiah, S, Larson MG, et al. Long-term trends in the incidence of and survival with heart failure. *N Engl J Med* 2002;347:1397–1402.
10. Lloyd-Jones DM, Larson MG, Leip EP, et al. Lifetime risk for developing congestive heart failure: the Framingham Heart Study. *Circulation* 2002; 106:3068–3072.
11. Smith WM. Epidemiology of congestive heart failure. *Am J Cardiol* 1985; 55(suppl A):3A–8A.
12. Jong P, Vowinckel E, Liu P, et al. Prognosis and determinants of survival in patients newly hospitalized for heart failure. *Arch Intern Med* 2002; 162:1689–1694.
13. Mahon NG, Blackstone EH, Francis GS, et al. The prognostic value of estimated creatinine clearance alongside functional capacity in ambulatory patients with chronic congestive heart failure. *J Am Coll Cardiol* 2002;40: 1106–1113.
14. Gottdiener JS, McClelland RL, Marshall R, et al. Outcome of congestive heart failure in elderly persons: influence of left ventricular systolic function. *Ann Intern Med* 2002;137:631–639.
15. Redfield MM, Jacobsen SJ, Burnett JC, et al. Burden of systolic and diastolic ventricular dysfunction in the community: appreciating the scope of the heart failure epidemic. *JAMA* 2003;289:194–202.
16. Stewart S. Prognosis of patients with heart failure compared with common types of cancer. *Heart Fail Monitor* 2003;3;87–94.
17. O'Connell JB, Bristow MR. Economic impact of heart failure in the United States: time for a different approach. *J Heart Lung Transplant* 1993;13: S107–S112.
18. Parmley WW. Cost-effective cardiology: cost-effective management of heart failure. *Clin Cardiol* 1996;19:240–242.
19. American Heart Association. *2006 heart and stroke statistical update: economic cost of cardiovascular diseases.* Dallas, TX: American Heart Association, 2006.
20. Rich MW, Beckham V, Wittenberg C, et al. A multidisciplinary intervention to prevent the readmission of elderly patients with congestive heart failure. *N Engl J Med* 1995;333:1190–1195.
21. Mudge GH, Goldstein S, Addonizio LJ, et al. 24th Bethesda conference: cardiac transplantation. Task Force 3: recipient guidelines/prioritization. *J Am Coll Cardiol* 1993;22:21–31.
22. Michalsen A, Konig MA, Thimme W. Preventable causative factors leading to hospital admission with decompensated heart failure. *Heart* 1998;80: 437–441.
23. Anderson GF, Steinberg EP. Hospital readmission in the Medicare population. *N Engl J Med* 1984;311:1349–1353.
24. Lee DS, Austin PC, Rouleau JL, et al. Predicting mortality among patients hospitalized for heart failure: derivation and validation of a clinical model. *JAMA* 2003;290:2581–2587.
25. Fonarow GC, Adams KF, Abraham WT, et al. Risk stratification for in-hospital mortality in acutely decompensated heart failure: classification and regression tree analysis. *JAMA* 2004;293:572–580.
26. Cleland JGF. Health economic consequences of the pharmacological treatment of heart failure. *Eur Heart J* 1998;19:P32–P39.
27. Adams KF, Lindenfeld J, Arnold JMO, et al. Executive summary: HFSA 2006 comprehensive heart failure practice guideline. *J Card Fail* 2006;12: 10–38.
28. Albert NM, Young JB. Heart failure disease management: a team approach. *Cleve Clin J Med* 2001;68(1):53–62.
29. Starling RC. The heart failure pandemic: changing patterns, costs, and treatment strategies. *Cleve Clin J Med* 1998;65:351–358.
30. Kornowski R, Zeeli D, Averbuch M, et al. Intensive home-care surveillance prevents hospitalization and improves morbidity rates among elderly patients with severe congestive heart failure. *Am Heart J* 1995;129:762–766.
31. Rich MW, Nease RF. Cost-effectiveness analysis in clinical practice; the case of heart failure. *Arch Intern Med* 1999;159:1690–1700.
32. Phillips CO, Wright SM, Kern DE. Comprehensive discharge planning with postdischarge support for older patients with congestive heart failure: a meta-analysis. *JAMA* 2004;291:1356–1367.
33. Holland R, Battersby J, Harvey I, et al. Systematic review of multidisciplinary interventions in heart failure. *Heart* 2005;91:899–906.
34. Bardy GH, Lee KL, Mark DB, et al. Amiodarone or an implantable cardioverter-defibrillator for congestive heart failure. *N Engl J Med* 2005; 352:225–237.
35. Topol EJ. Nesiritide: not verified. *N Engl J Med* 2005;353:113–116.
36. Jessup M, Brozena S. Heart failure. *N Engl J Med* 2003;348:2007–2018.
37. Bello D, Shah NB, Edep ME, et al. Self-reported differences between cardiologists and heart failure specialists in the management of chronic heart failure. *Am Heart J* 1999;138:100–107.
38. Ansari M, Alexander M, Tutar A, et al. Cardiology participation improves outcomes in patients with new-onset heart failure in the outpatient setting. *J Am Coll Cardiol* 2003;41:62–68.
39. Nohria A, Lewis E, Stevenson LW. Medical management of advanced heart failure. *JAMA* 2002;287:628–640.
40. Abraham WT, Bristow MR. Specialized centers for heart failure management. *Circulation* 1997;96:2755–2757.
41. O'Neill JO, Starling RC. Surgical remodeling in ischemic cardiomyopathy. *Curr Treat Option Cardiovasc Med* 2003;5:311–319.

CHAPTER 85 ■ PATHOPHYSIOLOGY OF THE HEART FAILURE CLINICAL SYNDROME

GARY S. FRANCIS

OVERVIEW

Heart failure has emerged to have a major bearing on public health: In the United States, the numbers are staggering:

- 995,000 annual hospitalizations for heart failure as a primary diagnosis
- 2.5 million annual hospitalizations for heart failure as a primary diagnosis
- 164% increase in hospitalization rate over the past 15 years
- 12 to 15 million physician visits annually
- 6.5 million hospital days per year
- In-hospital mortality of 5% to 8%
- Annual mortality for heart failure of 40% to 60% for some patients
- Average patient taking six medications
- 78% of patients with at least two hospitalizations per year
- 20% of hospitalized patients rehospitalized within 6 months
- Single highest diagnosis-related group in patients more than 65 years of age
- Estimated direct costs $23.7 billion in 2004

Two questions come to mind when one is made aware of these statistics: What is "heart failure"? What is the driving force behind this huge increase in incidence and prevalence?

The definition of heart failure is still debated among experts. This lack of clarity stems from differences between historical bedside observations (e.g., tachypnea, cardiomegaly, gallop rhythm, rales, fluid retention) and later laboratory observations regarding muscle mechanics and organ function. It is important to recognize that the historical bedside observations originally used to define heart failure were probably made in severely ill hospitalized patients and as such would represent only a fraction of today's heart failure population. Textbook signs and symptoms of advanced heart failure do not often pertain to the largest segment of the heart failure population, because most patients today are ambulatory and stable.

Measurement of contractile abnormalities at the organ and molecular levels likewise fails to provide a clear picture of what is wrong with the heart. Part of the problem is the lack of a simple laboratory test that defines heart failure, including plasma β-type natriuretic peptide (BNP). In my view, heart failure should be defined as a clinical syndrome manifested by breathlessness and fatigue at rest or during exertion with accompanying structural and/or functional myocardial disease. In this chapter, I concentrate on patients with major impairment of systolic function. Their hearts are typically remodeled to a more rounded shape, are usually dilated, are often hypertrophied, and by definition are dysfunctional. Mitral regurgitation is frequently evident.

Why are we seeing so much heart failure today when newer therapies that block the renin-angiotensin-aldosterone system (RAAS) and the sympathetic nervous system are claimed to be so effective at reducing mortality? What we are probably seeing is a medically induced delay or forestallment of severe signs and symptoms, but not an actual cure of heart failure. The progression of heart failure may slow down with modern therapy, and the end stages are typically now seen later than before. Heart failure is basically a syndrome that clusters in the elderly.

Unlike thrombolysis for acute myocardial infarction, in which the case fatality rate is reduced early after treatment, in heart failure the Kaplan-Meier survival curves diverge and then later converge. This finding indicates that the benefit is only temporary. Mortality is delayed rather than truly reduced

(1). Unlike in acute myocardial infarction, the natural history of heart failure is one of progressive decline in systolic function. Although the progressive decline may slow in response to specific drug therapy, patients with heart failure usually deteriorate with worsening symptoms, and all eventually die of the disease. Patients are now dying later in the natural history of heart failure. Angiotensin-converting enzyme (ACE) inhibitor therapy prolongs life by only 9 months on average. The addition of β-blockers confers an additional 7-month survival benefit, and spironolactone may provide 12 months of additional survival. However, toward the end of life, many patients express a desire for improved quality of life over increased quantity of life. Their survival may have been prolonged, but some patients have intolerable symptoms and multiple comorbid conditions. From a public health stand point, what we are seeing is older patients with heart failure who are "sicker" with multiple comorbidities and who are in need of multiple therapies.

WHAT IS THE HALLMARK OF CHRONIC SYSTOLIC HEART FAILURE?

The diagnosis of heart failure remains largely clinical. It is predominantly a bedside diagnosis. However, certain structural features of chronic heart failure are nearly always evident by echocardiography. Systolic heart failure is characterized by progressive left ventricular (LV) dilatative remodeling, and this is perhaps the fundamental lesion or hallmark. The LV chamber increases in size. The heart becomes more spheroidal. Wall tension increases commensurate with LV dilatation. Systolic performance worsens. Stroke volume can be maintained even when ejection fraction is markedly reduced, because end-diastolic volume is increased. It is the LV remodeling that drives the natural history of heart failure under most circumstances, and it is the remodeling that is now the prime target for therapy (2).

DIAGNOSIS AND EVALUATION OF HEART FAILURE

History and Physical Examination

Breathlessness is the paramount symptom of heart failure (3). It is sensitive but not specific for the disease. It can occur at rest or with minimal physical activity. For most patients with heart failure, feeling breathless is part of everyday life; it is also something for which they develop strategies to prevent or minimize. When the condition becomes "worsening," it often results in hospitalization (3). The mechanism of dyspnea in heart failure is complex, incompletely understood, and multifactorial (4). It also depends on the context in which it occurs. In acute pulmonary edema, hypoxemia likely contributes to a sense of dyspnea. However, patients with stable chronic heart failure are not usually hypoxemic, but they still are dyspneic. The sensation of dyspnea in the setting of chronic heart failure seems to bear little relation to pulmonary capillary wedge pressure, central hemodynamics, or dead space inhalation (4). Rather, multiple mechanisms cause dyspnea, including respiratory muscle fatigue, increased physiologic dead space, reduced pulmonary compliance, increased airway dysfunction, and perhaps efferent signals from pulmonary J receptors and respiratory muscles (5,6).

Orthopnea, paroxysmal nocturnal dyspnea, and Cheyne-Stokes respirations (7) occur in patients with more advanced heart failure. Cheyne-Stokes breathing carries a poor prognosis (8). Sleep apnea is also common in patients with heart failure and can be associated with an elevated pulmonary capillary wedge pressure (7). Sleep apnea can be central or the result of airway obstruction (9,10). Patients and their spouses should be thoroughly queried about the patient's sleeping disorder, because it can influence both prognosis and treatment of heart failure. Obstructive sleep apnea can be successfully treated with continuous positive airway pressure in perhaps 60% of cases (11), whereas the treatment of central sleep apnea

TABLE 85.1

RECOMMENDED TESTS FOR PATIENTS WITH SIGNS OR SYMPTOMS OF HEART FAILURE

Test recommendation	Finding	Suspected diagnosis
Electrocardiogram	Acute ST-T–wave changes	Myocardial ischemia
	Atrial fibrillation, other tachyarrhythmia	Thyroid disease or heart failure resulting from rapid ventricular rate
	Bradyarrhythmias rate	Heart failure resulting from low heart rate
	Previous myocardial infarction (e.g., Q waves) left ventricular performance	Heart failure resulting from reduced contractile tissue
	Low voltage	Pericardial effusion
	Left ventricular hypertrophy	Diastolic dysfunction
Complete blood cell count	Anemia	Heart failure resulting from or aggravated by decreased oxygen-carrying capacity
Urinalysis	Proteinuria	Nephrotic syndrome
	Red blood cells or cellular casts	Glomerulonephritis
Serum creatinine	Elevated failure	Volume overload resulting from renal dysfunction
Serum albumin	Decreased	Increased extravascular volume due to hypoalbuminemia
T4 and TSH (obtain only if atrial fibrillation, evidence of thyroid disease, or patient age >65 y)	Abnormal T4 or TSH	Heart failure resulting from or aggravated by hypo/hyperthyroidism

TSH, thyroid-stimulating hormone; T_4, thyroxine.
From Konstam M, Dracup K, Baker D, et al. *Heart failure: management of patients with left-ventricular systolic dysfunction. Quick reference guide for clinicians No. 11.* AHCPR Publication No. 94-0613. Rockville, MD: Agency for Health Care Policy and Research, Public Health Service, U.S. Department of Human Service, June 1994, with permission.

TABLE 85.2

ECHOCARDIOGRAPHY AND RADIONUCLIDE VENTRICULOGRAPHY COMPARED IN EVALUATION OF LEFT VENTRICULAR PERFORMANCE

Test	Advantages	Disadvantages
Echocardiogram	Permits concomitant assessment of valvular disease, left ventricular hypertrophy, and left atrial size	Difficult to perform in patients with lung disease
	Less expensive than radionuclide ventriculography in most areas	Usually only semiquantitative estimate of ejection fraction provided
	Able to detect pericardial effusion and ventricular thrombus	Technically inadequate in up to 18% of patients under optimal circumstances
	More generally available	
Radionuclide ventriculogram	More precise and reliable measurement of ejection fraction	Requires venipuncture and radiation exposure
	Better assessment of right ventricular function	Limited assessment of valvular heart disease and left ventricular hypertrophy

From Konstam M, Dracup K, Baker D, et al. *Heart failure: management of patients with left-ventricular systolic dysfunction. Quick reference guide for clinicians No. 11.* AHCPR Publication NO. 94-0613. Rockville, MD: Agency for Health Care Policy and Research, Public Health Service, U.S. Department of Human Services, June 1994.

may require more aggressive diuretic use in some cases. It is not clear whether continuous positive airway pressure is effective treatment for central sleep apnea. Referral of patients to a sleep laboratory should be considered when sleep apnea or Cheyne-Stokes breathing is suspected.

The second cardinal feature of heart failure is chronic fatigue. Unfortunately, fatigue is also common, very nonspecific, and, like dyspnea, poorly understood. Fatigue in patients with heart failure can result from low cardiac output, but the mechanism of fatigue is likely multifactorial and much more complex. Improving cardiac output does not always improve fatigue (12,13). Skeletal muscle abnormalities (14,15) can lead to general deconditioning. About 15% to 20% of patients with chronic heart failure are anemic. The mechanism of anemia in heart failure is poorly understood, and its treatment is under investigation. Nevertheless, anemia is common, can be associated with fatigue, and is a poor prognostic sign in patients with heart failure.

Tissue congestion occurs in acute and advanced heart failure and can lead to multiple signs and symptoms. These include dyspnea, right upper quadrant pain (acute passive liver congestion), abdominal discomfort from ascites, and heavy legs with difficulty walking as a result of peripheral edema.

The physical findings in heart failure, as classically described in textbooks, are not truly representative of today's patients. Resting tachycardia, tachypnea, low blood pressure, rales, a gallop rhythm, mitral regurgitation, jugular venous distention, tender hepatomegaly, ascites, and peripheral edema are signs of advanced heart failure. With the modern use of powerful diuretics, ACE inhibitors, and β-blockers, many ambulatory patients have few physical signs. Moreover, the physical findings are rather limited for estimating hemodynamic compromise (16), but they should not be abandoned. The echocardiogram and plasma BNP determination have not replaced the physical examination, but they can facilitate it. Careful examination of the patient with heart failure is particularly important. The physical examination should include inspection of the neck veins with the patient at 45 degrees, a procedure that requires some training and experience. Close inspection of the neck veins on segmental examination is particularly helpful in judging volume status.

Routine Laboratory Tests

The recommendations for laboratory testing in a "new" patient with heart failure have not changed much throughout the years (Table 85.1). Many physicians would add an echocardiogram and a chest radiography, especially for a patient with new-onset heart failure. In fact, the echocardiogram is the cornerstone of evaluation. It provides information regarding chamber size, wall thickness, ventricular performance, valvular lesions, diastolic dysfunction, and regional wall motion abnormalities. The echocardiogram is also used to distinguish systolic heart failure (dilated LV, low ejection fraction) from diastolic heart failure (preserved systolic function). Radionuclide techniques and contrast left ventriculography are still used to assess myocardial function, but echocardiography has become the standard (Table 85.2).

In recent years, plasma BNP and NT-pro-BNP (N-terminal-pro-brain natriuretic peptide) have become available as diagnostic tools for heart failure. Plasma BNP is available as a point-of-care test in most emergency departments, where it is widely used to facilitate the diagnosis of acute decompensated heart failure (ADHF). There is no question that plasma BNP measurement is useful in the evaluation of patients with dyspnea in the emergency department setting (17–19). The more important and as yet unanswered question is whether BNP should be measured routinely to guide the diagnosis and management of chronic heart failure (20). Our own data would suggest caution in this regard (21). Physicians should continue to trust their own clinical skills and judgment. Plasma BNP, which is released in response to increased wall stress in both systole and diastole (22), is not a stand-alone test for heart failure. Patients still need to be seen, questioned, and examined. It is true that it may be helpful to monitor BNP or NT-pro-BNP to help understand prognosis and response to therapy, but these strategies have not been critically tested in rigorous clinical trials. However, such studies are now under way.

FACTORS KNOWN TO PRECIPITATE ACUTE DECOMPENSATED HEART FAILURE

The natural history of heart failure is highly variable and complex (23). What is clear is that patients with chronic heart failure periodically develop ADHF. Invasive ambulatory monitoring suggests that deterioration often begins many days before presentation to the hospital. There seems to be little difference between worsening chronic systolic heart failure secondary to a precipitant factor and de novo heart failure (24). The Acute Decompensated Heart Failure National Registry (ADHERE registry) has provided some interesting observations regarding hospitalization for ADHF:

- The median age is 75.2 years.
- Twenty-five percent of patients have de novo ADHF, and 75% have a history of chronic heart failure.
- More than half these patients have been previously hospitalized for ADHF.
- Dyspnea and congestion are the dominant presenting features.
- Seventy-two percent of patients have a history of hypertension.
- Nearly 50% of patients have a systolic blood pressure higher than 140 mm Hg on presentation.
- Twenty percent of patients have atrial fibrillation.
- The median length of stay is 4.3 days.
- Only 20% are ultimately admitted to a medical or coronary intensive care unit; most are admitted to telemetry units.
- Thirty percent of patients have a history of renal insufficiency
- Twenty percent of patients have serum creatinine levels greater than 2.0 mg/dL.
- Sixty percent of patients have an ejection fraction lower than 40%.
- Fifty-eight percent of patients have coronary artery disease.
- Forty-four percent of patients have diabetes mellitus.
- Only 5% of patients have a pulmonary artery catheter inserted during hospital admission.
- The in-hospital mortality is 4%.
- Twenty percent of patients are readmitted within 30 days after discharge; 50% are readmitted for ADHF within 6 months following discharge.

Not all patients with ADHF are similar. Two distinct groups seem to emerge. One group has acute pulmonary edema that often responds quickly to therapy, and the other group manifests severe, chronic heart failure before admission that fails to improve quickly. The latter group often develops the cardiorenal syndrome, characterized by a poor response to diuretics and rising blood urea nitrogen and serum creatinine levels.

When patients deteriorate with ADHF, a search should begin for identifiable causes (Table 85.3). A 12-lead electrocardiogram should always be performed to look for myocardial ischemia or infarction. Sequential serum troponin levels are also useful. Superimposed infections, arrhythmias (i.e., rapid atrial fibrillation), and metabolic problems should be sought and aggressively treated. In general, patients with ADHF benefit from hospitalization. According to the ADHERE registry, most patients are admitted to telemetry units and stay about 4 to 5 days. Of some interest, most episodes of ADHF are associated with hypertension and congestion, a finding suggesting that vasodilators and diuretics are the mainstay of therapy, whereas correction of precipitating factors remains an important feature of treatment.

TABLE 85.3

CAUSES OF ACUTE DECOMPENSATION OF CHRONIC HEART FAILURE

Acute myocardial ischemia
Uncorrected high blood pressure
Obesity
Superimposed infection
Atrial fibrillation and other arrhythmias
Excessive alcohol consumption
Endocrine abnormalities (e.g., diabetes mellitus, hyperthyroidism, hypothyroidism)
Negative inotropic drugs (e.g., verapamil, nifedipine, diltiazem, β-adrenergic blockers)
Nonsteroidal antiinflammatory drugs
Treatment and sodium noncompliance; lack of information given to patient about diet, medications, etc.

MECHANISMS OF LEFT VENTRICULAR DYSFUNCTION

Abnormalities of Chamber Function

Because virtually any form of heart disease can lead to heart failure, the etiologic basis of heart failure is vast. Coronary artery disease, hypertension, diabetes mellitus, valvular heart disease, and dilated cardiomyopathy are frequently associated with systolic heart failure. The Framingham Study suggests that progression from hypertension to heart failure is still very common (25), and hypertension is frequently present on admission to hospital for ADHF (24). A functional abnormality of systolic heart failure is a diminished ability of the failing muscle to develop force and to shorten at a given velocity and specified loading conditions. Of course, performance may be aggravated by many factors such as noncontractile scar, valvular insufficiency or stenosis, or excessive afterload (i.e., wall stress). There is a decrease in the maximal rate of force development, but generally no major change occurs in the passive length tension or elastic element of heart muscle. However, the passive pressure-volume relation can change dramatically. The failing LV is exquisitely sensitive to afterload conditions (Fig. 85.1).

Several compensatory mechanisms are activated in the heart failure syndrome to adapt myocardial performance to altered loading conditions. Normally, as preload rises and sarcomeres stretch toward their limit of 2.2 μg, contractile force is increased, the so-called Frank-Starling mechanism (Fig. 85.2). The relation between sarcomere length and the development of tension in cardiac muscle is the basis for the Starling law of

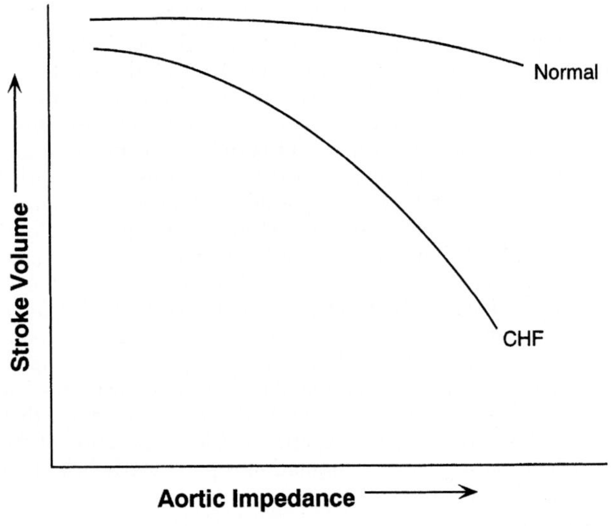

FIGURE 85.1. A hallmark of heart failure is the exquisite sensitivity of the left ventricle to an afterload stress. As impedance to ejection is raised, there is an impressive reduction in left ventricular performance. CHF, congestive heart failure.

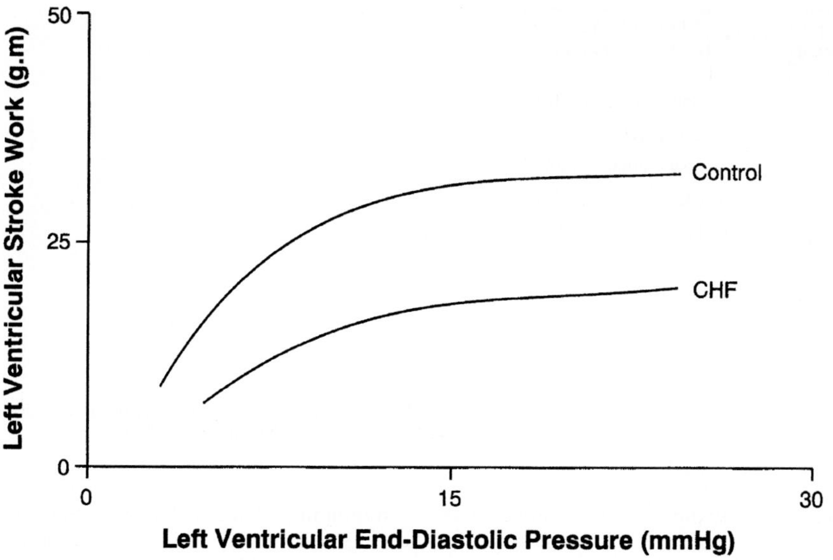

FIGURE 85.2. The Frank-Starling mechanism is altered in heart failure. The failing ventricle is unable to respond to an increase in preload with a normal increase in left ventricular stroke work. CHF, congestive heart failure.

the heart. There is a length-dependent activation of cardiac myofibrils by calcium, probably owing to a change in calcium sensitivity of the myofibrils in the extended state. In systolic heart failure, the myocardium fails to generate a normal increase in force development when preload (i.e., sarcomere stretch) is enhanced (Fig. 85.2). Thus, the Frank-Starling mechanism fails to improve myocardial performance to a normal extent in the failing heart (26). In contrast, a diuretic-induced reduction in preload in patients with heart failure does not necessarily reduce stroke volume, just as volume expansion does not raise stroke volume sufficiently. Dogs with experimental heart failure from rapid pacing are unable to mount a normal response to improved preload (27). Alterations in filament-regulatory proteins such as troponin T or troponin I or other isoform changes may play some role (28), or there may be a problem with delivery of calcium to the myofibrils. Despite decades of investigation regarding the cellular and molecular mechanisms of heart failure, there is still no clear understanding of the precise events leading to diminished LV performance (29). Undoubtedly, multiple mechanisms are operative at a cellular level, including regulation of gene expression, imprecisely understood metabolic changes, and important peripheral adaptations. The complexities inherent in the heart failure syndrome and its multiple causes suggest that no single effective therapy will emerge.

LEFT VENTRICULAR REMODELING

The hallmark of chronic systolic heart failure is progressive remodeling of the heart. Remodeling is a change in the size and shape of the heart, usually involving the LV. The increase in LV chamber size during heart failure is by definition is not attributed to acute changes in distending pressure (2). Cardiomegaly eventually occurs and leads to a dilated and thin-walled LV. Although wall thickness may vary, it generally thickens insufficiently to accommodate the increase in chamber dimension, thus further increasing wall tension and reducing LV performance. The mechanisms whereby LV remodeling occurs has been the subject of intensive study (30,31). Multiple mechanisms drive the remodeling process, including myocyte loss, replacement fibrosis, and reactive growth in remaining viable cells (Table 85.4). The early sequence of events at the molecular level are still poorly understood, but there is repeat expression of the so-called "fetal program" leading to elongation of myocytes and an increase in intramyocyte natriuretic peptide synthesis. We have known for years that LV dilation following acute myocardial infarction is an accurate predictor of an unfavorable long-term prognosis (32,33). We now understand that this same process of remodeling occurs progressively in patients with chronic systolic heart failure as a consequence of multiple causes and is linked to a poor prognosis (Fig. 85.3).

The Special Case of Remodeling Following Acute Myocardial Infarction

The classic setting of LV remodeling occurs during and following acute myocardial infarction. Although chronic enlargement of the LV cavity may help to preserve stroke volume in the presence of a very low ejection fraction, it is clear that LV enlargement has very deleterious long-term consequences (31). In acute myocardial infarction, an increase in LV chamber size affords some advantage, at least in the short term.

The extent of LV remodeling in acute myocardial infarction depends on the size of the infarction as well as the location and depth of the injury. So-called "infarct expansion" occurs within hours of a large acute anterior myocardial infarction and is associated with increased mortality (34). Infarct expansion is caused by acute dilatation and thinning of the area of infarction that is not explained by new myocardial necrosis (35).

TABLE 85.4

FACTORS THAT CONTRIBUTE TO LEFT VENTRICULAR REMODELING

Neurohormones and cytokines
Increased left ventricular volume and pressure
Myocardial cell elongation
Replacement and reactive collagen deposition (i.e., increased collagen turnover)
Myocyte slippage secondary to dissolution of collagen struts
Apoptosis
Necrosis
Myocardial infarct expansion
Dilation and reshaping of left ventricle

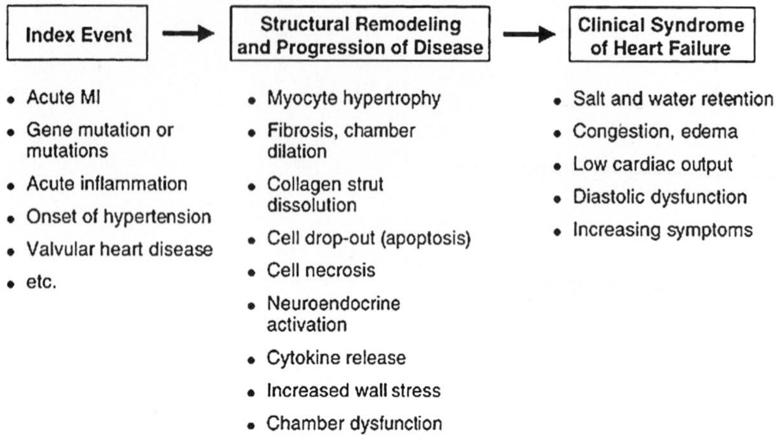

FIGURE 85.3. Progression of left ventricular remodeling in heart failure. MI, myocardial infarction.

Wall thinning may result from slippage between myocyte bundles. Infarct expansion is readily detected by echocardiogram (36). The eventual increase in end-systolic volume carries powerful prognostic power, even more than the extent of underlying coronary artery disease. Patency of the infarct-related artery is important in protecting against LV enlargement (37,38). The presence of good antegrade blood flow through the infarct-related artery, by either collateral vessels or reperfusion therapy, protects against abnormal wall motion abnormalities and progressive dilatation of the LV (39–42).

Mechanisms of Progressive Left Ventricular Remodeling

Unlike infarct expansion, progressive LV remodeling is a more gradual process that occurs months to years following an index event (Fig. 85.3) (43). The index event may be sudden loss of contractile tissue owing to acute myocardial infarction, expression of mutant genetic programs, onset of valvular heart disease, hypertension, acute myocarditis, chemotherapy, or exposure to virtually any cause of disrupted myocardial homeostasis. The index event may be clinically obvious (e.g., acute myocardial infarction) or clinically silent (e.g., the onset of hypertension). The subsequent changes in the size and shape of the heart occur as a generalized response to injury and/or altered loading conditions. Stroke volume can be preserved in the short term by augmenting cavity size, but the "adaptive" response incurs a substantial long-term cost. According to the Laplace principle, LV enlargement (change in chamber radius) is accompanied by an increase in wall stress. The increased wall stress serves as a stimulus for myocardial hypertrophy (43–46). It is clear that cardiac myocytes increase in length (eccentric hypertrophy) shortly after acute myocardial injury (47,48). It is possible that the increase in myocyte length may contribute to the dilated chamber size (49). Elongated cardiac myocytes may be structurally inadequate, although direct proof in support of this concept is lacking. Nevertheless, there is a growing recognition that structural changes in the architecture of the cardiac myocytes (and thus the LV chamber) may contribute substantially to reduced myocardial performance (50). Obviously, many changes occur in the setting of LV remodeling, and no single mechanism can be responsible for the changes in the size and shape of the heart. However, progressive remodeling in the setting of chronic systolic heart failure drives the natural history of the heart failure syndrome (23), and it can be slowed and even sometimes reversed by drugs that block the sympathetic nervous system and RAAS.

Finally, the distortion of myocardial architecture predisposes patients to ventricular and atrial arrhythmias. Sudden arrhythmic death is common in patients with heart failure and is likely related to development of scar and fibrosis, thus setting the stage for macroscopic and macroscopic reentry circuits. Hypokalemia and excessive sympathetic activity may also contribute to sudden, unexpected death in patients with heart failure. About one third of patients with heart failure die of sudden ventricular arrhythmias, and these deaths tend to cluster in patients with New York Heart Association functional class II. It is expected that implantable cardiac defibrillators will reduce this sudden death burden, now that the indications for this treatment have expanded, but the result could be more deaths related to progressive pump dysfunction.

NEUROENDOCRINE ABNORMALITIES

The neuroendocrine hypothesis of heart failure basically states that neurohormones are "released" early in the heart failure syndrome, before signs and symptoms ensue (Fig. 85.4), and they contribute importantly to progressive LV remodeling and the natural history of heart failure (23). Support for the hypothesis comes from the emergence of ACE inhibitors, angiotensin receptor blockers, and β-adrenergic receptor blockers as cornerstones for the treatment of heart failure (23). Many neurohormones and cytokines are active in heart failure (Table 85.5), some more important than others. The sympathetic nervous system and the RAAS appear to be the two dominant systems activated in heart failure, and both have been extensively studied (51–54).

BNP is synthesized and stored in cardiac myocytes. It is released in response to heightened wall stress in both systole and diastole (22). Unlike norepinephrine and angiotensin II, BNP is a counterregulatory peptide that has smooth muscle relaxation (vasodilator) properties, as well as modest natriuretic and diuretic properties (55,56). BNP also tends to reduce sympathetic nervous system activity and RAAS activity, and may it have antiremodeling and antifibrotic activity. On balance, however, most of the neurohormones and cytokines active in chronic heart failure are believed to contribute to the pathophysiology of the disease (57), including arginine vasopressin (58), endothelin (59), and tumor necrosis factor-α (TNF-α). Recent clinical trials designed to block endothelin and TNF-α have failed to improve survival in patients with heart failure. This finding suggests that simply adding drugs to block multiple neuroendocrine systems may be an oversimplified strategy. Blocking inflammatory pathways and endothelin may require drugs that target multiple sites.

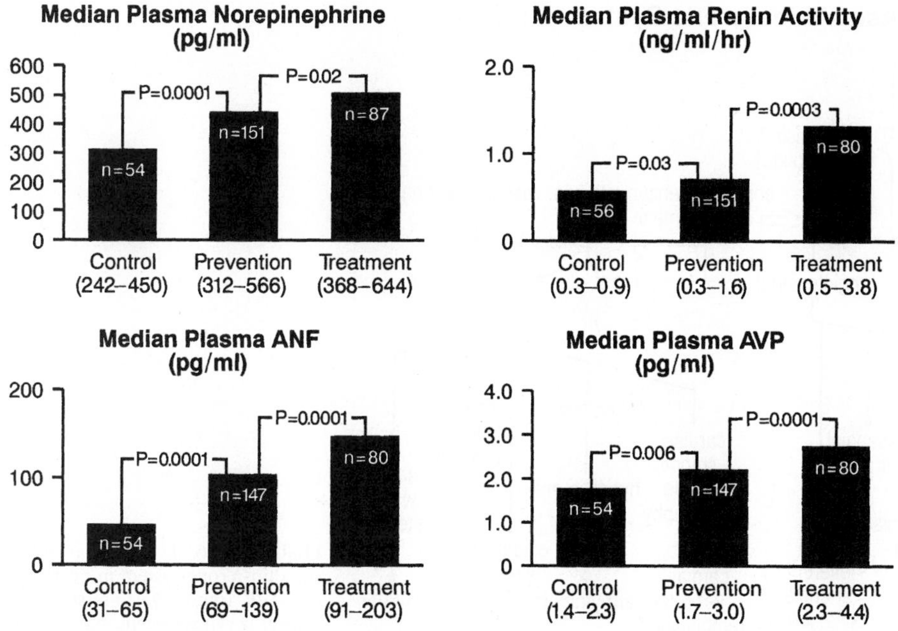

FIGURE 85.4. Data from the Studies of Left Ventricular Dysfunction substudy of baseline neurohormones. There is a progressive incremental rise in neurohormones as patients pass from the asymptomatic left ventricular dysfunction phase (prevention) to overt heart failure (treatment), a finding suggesting that neurohormone activation may precede the onset of symptomatic heart failure. ANF, atrial natriuretic factor; AVP, arginine vasopressin. (From Francis GS, Benedict C, Johnstone DE, et al. Comparison of neuroendocrine activation in patients with left ventricular dysfunction with and without congestive heart failure. *Circulation* 1990;82:1724–1729.)

Abnormalities of the Sympathetic Nervous System

How the sympathetic nervous system is activated in patients with heart failure remains unclear. Abnormal reflex control mechanisms play some role (60–65), but reflex control dysregulation does not explain the unrelenting rise in plasma norepinephrine common to the heart failure syndrome (66). Excessive norepinephrine is directly toxic to the myocardium (67), and cardiomyopathy can occur as a consequence of excessive catecholamines (68). Most of the excessive sympathetic traffic is from the central nervous system and can be directly measured in humans (69). The increased plasma norepinephrine levels are associated with a poor prognosis (Fig. 85.5) (70), but they do not correlate well with resting hemodynamic abnormalities or exercise tolerance (71). Much of the excessive sympathetic drive is directed at the heart and kidneys (72), although the failing myocardium itself is depleted of catecholamines (73).

Excessive sympathetic drive to the heart is not only directly toxic, but also is likely responsible for downregulation of β_1-receptors and uncoupling of β_2-receptors from G proteins (74). A concept has emerged that excessive norepinephrine release may be a short-term adaptive response to increase heart rate, inotropy, and myocardial mass and to protect blood pressure, all likely to enhance short-term survival. In the long-term, however, excessive norepinephrine leads to injured myocardial cells, myocardial remodeling, downregulation of β_1-receptors in the heart, excessive afterload stress, salt and water retention, and activation of RAAS, essentially all the features of chronic progressive systolic heart failure. It is no wonder that β-adrenergic blockade has been so strikingly successful in the management of chronic systolic heart failure (75–79).

TABLE 85.5

NEUROENDOCRINE FACTORS KNOWN TO BE INCREASED IN PATIENTS WITH HEART FAILURE

Norepinephrine	Endothelin
Epinephrine	β-endorphins
Renin activity	Calcitonin gene–related peptide
Angiotensin II	Growth hormone
Aldosterone	Cortisol
Arginine vasopressin	Tumor necrosis factor-α
Neuropeptide Y	Neurokinin A
Vasoactive intestinal peptide	Substance P
Prostaglandins	Adrenomedullin
Atrial natriuretic factor	Brain natriuretic peptide

Renin-Angiotensin-Aldosterone System

Similar to the sympathetic nervous system, it has been long recognized that the RAAS is activated in patients with heart failure (Fig. 85.6) (80–83). In evolutionary terms, the RAAS is

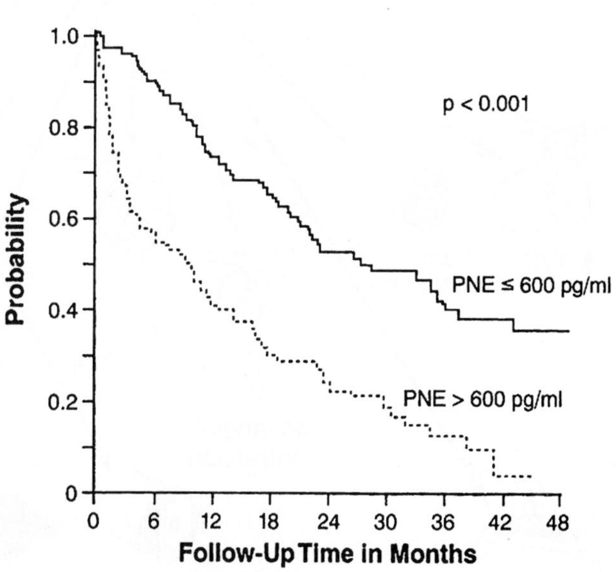

FIGURE 85.5. Correlation of plasma norepinephrine (PNE) levels with prognosis in heart failure.

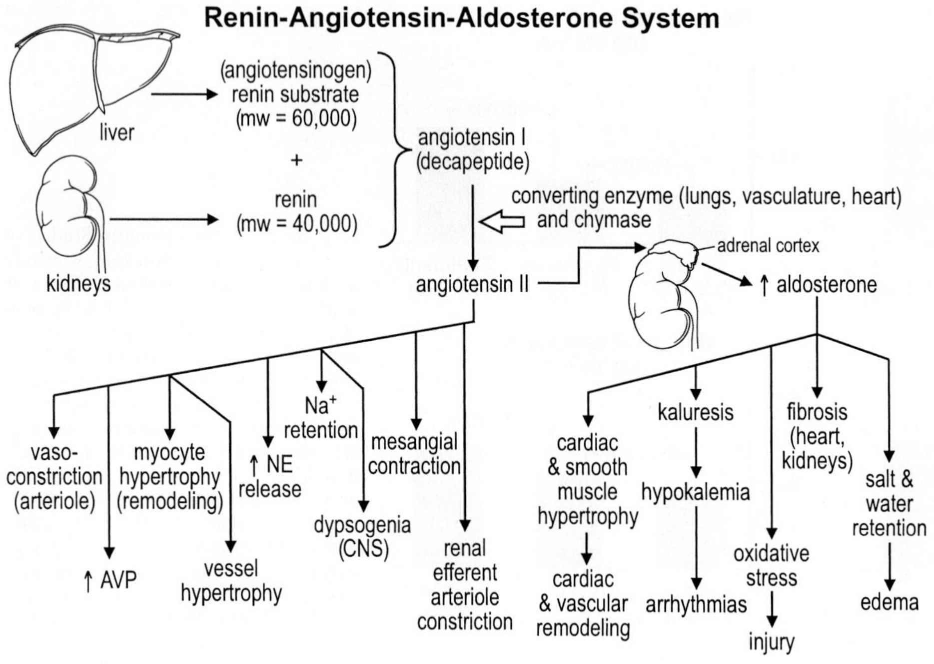

FIGURE 85.6. The renin-angiotensin-aldosterone system in heart failure. AVP, arginine vasopressin; CNS, central nervous system; NE, norepinephrine.

highly conserved, dating back some 600 million years (57). It likely served as a highly adaptive system for life forms transitioning from the sea (salt and water plentiful) to land (salt and water scarce). The RAAS is essentially a system that conserves salt and water and therefore restores circulating volume, thus helping to maintain blood pressure and cardiac output in the setting of volume depletion. There is both a circulating RAAS (endocrine) and a tissue RAAS (paracrine and autocrine). Probably both are important in circulatory homeostasis.

In addition to maintaining circulatory homeostasis in conditions of volume contraction, the RAAS has profound effects on vascular smooth muscle cells, fibroblasts, renal mesangial cells, and cardiac myocytes. Both angiotensin II and aldosterone are active proliferative and progrowth biochemicals. Wound healing in the heart, such as occurs in response to acute myocardial infarction or inflammation, has a standard "package" that includes fibrosis and hypertrophy, ultimately transitioning to cardiac remodeling. Angiotensin II and aldosterone are major participants in this package. Of course, angiotensin II has many other activities (Fig. 85.7), most of which are known to be important features of the heart failure syndrome. More recently, with the striking efficacy of spironolactone and eplerenone in the treatment of chronic heart failure and acute postmyocardial infarction heart failure, the adverse role of excessive aldosterone has become more apparent. Angiotensin II and aldosterone have important genomic targets that contribute substantially to replacement fibrosis and muscle (smooth and cardiac) hypertrophy. The tissue RAAS may be important in

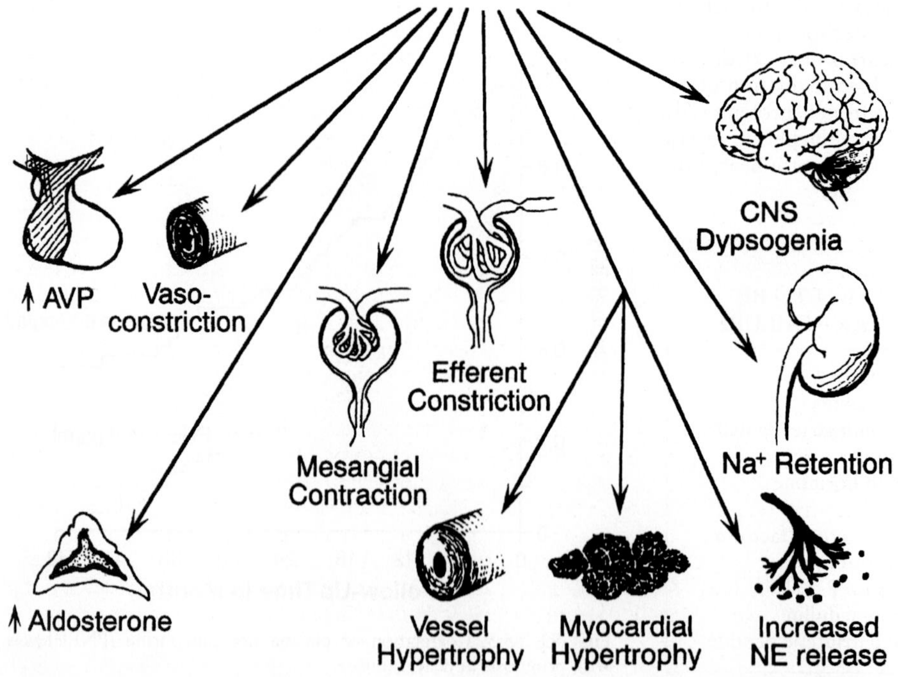

FIGURE 85.7. Angiotensin II has a wide array of biologic activities. They include release of arginine vasopressin (AVP) from the posterior pituitary, peripheral arteriole vasoconstriction, release of aldosterone from the adrenal cortex, mesangial contraction, constriction of the efferent glomerular arterioles, vascular hypertrophy, myocardial hypertrophy, facilitation of norepinephrine (NE) release from sympathetic neurons, sodium retention, and thirst sensation. CNS, central nervous system. (From Francis GS. The relationship of the sympathetic nervous system and the renin-angiotensin system in congestive heart failure. *Am Heart J* 1989;118:642–648.)

TABLE 85.6

FACTORS THAT RELEASE RENIN

Renal artery baroreceptor activity
Renal hypoperfusion
Hyponatremic perfusate to the macula densa
Volume contraction secondary to diuretics and salt restriction
Stimulation of β-adrenergic receptors in the kidney

this regard (84,85). The importance of the RAAS in the syndrome of heart failure, like that of the sympathetic nervous system, likely represents a fundamentally highly conserved short-term system to allow for adaptation of volume depletion. In heart failure, the RAAS seems permanently activated, leading to very adverse long-term effects. The pathophysiologic role of the RAAS in heart failure is difficult to overstate (86).

Multiple factors stimulate renin, a large enzyme (mw, 40,000) released from the kidney (Table 85.6). Renin interacts with a substrate, angiotensinogen (mw, 60,000), that is largely synthesized and released from the liver. These two large molecules interact to produce a small decapeptide, angiotensin I. It, in turn, is converted by ACE and in some cases chymase to angiotensin II, the major effector peptide. In addition to its multiple direct effects on organs, angiotensin II and potassium stimulate the release of aldosterone from the adrenal cortex, leading to further long-term complications common to heart failure. The sympathetic nervous system and the RAAS are very interactive. Sympathetic activity to the kidney leads to renin release, and angiotensin II facilitates norepinephrine release. Angiotensin II also sensitizes blood vessels to the vasoconstrictor activity of norepinephrine. Given what we know about the RAAS in heart failure, it is not surprising today how important the role of ACE inhibitors and angiotensin receptor blockers is in the treatment of this condition. However, when ACE inhibitors were first studied in the 1970s, it was not immediately clear how powerful this class of drugs would become (86).

Disturbances of Salt and Water Control

It has been understood by generations of physicians that heart failure is characterized by excessive sodium and water retention, but the mechanisms that underlie this observation continue to be elusive. It is unlikely that any single mechanism accounts for the maintenance of normal sodium balance. Patients with very severe heart failure have glomerular filtration reduced to approximately one half of normal and renal blood flow reduced to approximately one fifth of normal, findings suggesting considerable diversion of blood away from the kidney (Fig. 85.8). As a result of the lowered filtration rate, a smaller quantity of sodium is probably delivered to the renal tubular cells. However, glomerular filtration rate is not invariably reduced in patients with heart failure, and its preservation depends on activation of the renin-angiotensin system (87).

Vasoconstriction and sodium retention are appropriate responses to loss of circulating volume. In heart failure, the kidney is responding to a perceived loss of extracellular fluid and plasma volume. The kidney therefore is not the culprit, but the victim. Glomerular filtration may be maintained by the vasoconstrictor effects of angiotensin II on glomerular efferent arterials. In the later stages of heart failure, salt retention and water retention are enhanced by the effects of aldosterone and angiotensin II on the kidney. In some cases, vasopressin is released, leading to further reabsorption of free water. Eventually, heightened systemic resistance, circulatory congestion, edema, and hyponatremia become clinically manifest.

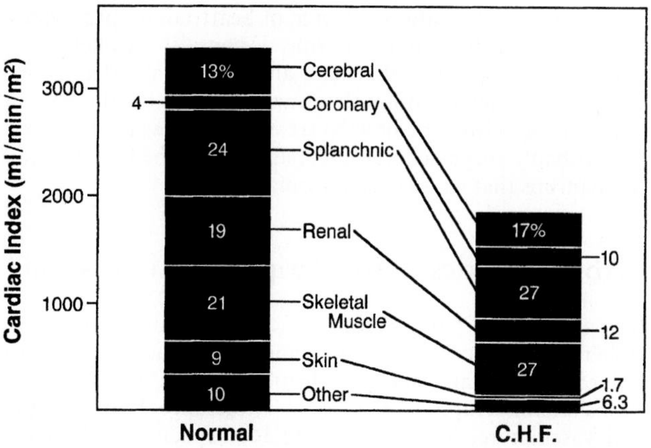

FIGURE 85.8. Cardiac output at rest. The normal distribution of cardiac index and the distribution of flow in heart rate. Renal and skin blood flow are markedly reduced in heart failure, whereas flow to the brain, heart, splanchnic bed, and skeletal muscles is preserved. CHF, congestive heart failure. (From Zelis R, Nellis SH, Longhurst J, et al. Abnormalities in the regional circulations accompanying congestive heart failure. *Prog Cardiovasc Dis* 1975;18:181–199.)

The primary signal that the kidney receives to initiate salt and water retention has remained elusive. It is not known what initiates the signal, nor is it understood where the signal is processed. Early studies by Barger observed that sodium excretion alterations are detected even in the mildest forms of experimental heart failure, before venous pressure is even changed (88). Abnormalities of cardiac output may not necessarily precede the increase in salt and water retention. These findings would suggest that sodium excretion abnormalities occur very early in the syndrome of heart failure, perhaps before a major reduction in maximal LV performance (89). Clearly, a reduction in cardiac output is not the only cause of sodium retention in patients with heart failure.

One of the major determinants of sodium retention is activation of the renin-angiotensin system. However, there is only a rough correlation among hemodynamic measurements, the renin-angiotensin system, and urinary sodium excretion in patients with heart failure. Undoubtedly, neural and humoral pathways involve physical adjustments in renal microvascular hemodynamics, tubule fluid composition, flow rate, and tubular ion gradients, but these interactions are highly complex and are difficult to measure precisely (92).

Despite the lack of a penetrating understanding of the initiation of salt and water retention in heart failure, it does seem clear that the kidney perceives, in some way, a threat to the arterial blood pressure. There is a very consistent response to this perceived threat, with activation of baroreceptor reflexes, increases in sympathetic nervous system activity, and enhanced activity of the RAAS. Ultimately, the increase in sympathetic nervous system activity may be coupled to reduced renal blood flow, thus leading to the nonosmotic release of vasopressin and other neurohormones. The net effect of these changes is an expansion of the extracellular volume, which helps to maintain blood pressure. Increased blood volume, in turn, acts as a negative feedback message to reduce the RAAS response, thus accounting for some of the observed heterogeneity in the RAAS in patients with early heart failure.

To some extent, the expanded blood volume and intracardiac pressures lead to counterregulatory steps, including the release of BNP and other natriuretic peptides that have important endogenous natriuretic and vasodilator properties. However, the effects of the various natriuretic peptides on the kidney seem to diminish as the syndrome of heart failure progresses. Ultimately, the effects of the natriuretic peptides are likely overwhelmed by opposing influences, and the overall effect is one of salt and water retention. It seems fortunate for the patient that our knowledge of how to treat salt and water retention has probably surpassed our understanding of the fundamental mechanisms that cause edema formation (91).

Abnormalities of the Peripheral Circulation

It is now recognized that the maladaptive changes in the peripheral vasculature and skeletal muscles of patients with heart failure, rather than the central hemodynamics, are largely responsible for symptoms of exercise intolerance. In the peripheral vasculature, impaired vasodilator capacity results from enhanced vessel wall stiffness, endothelial dysfunction, and other structural abnormalities. The blood vessels of patients with heart failure are generally more vasoconstricted. Initially, the vasoconstriction is minimal and somewhat selective as the body strives to redistribute blood flow among organs to maintain circulatory efficiency (Fig. 85.8) (92). However, over time, vasoconstriction becomes excessive in an attempt to protect blood pressure. Only the coronary and cerebral circulations are spared. The vasoconstriction ultimately becomes inappropriate and increases aortic impedance, thus placing a further burden on the already failing heart.

Although the cause of the heightened vasoconstrictor tone in heart failure is not entirely clear, it appears to be related to increased circulating catecholamines, particularly norepinephrine, as well as to other vasoconstrictors, including angiotensin II, vasopressin, and possibly endothelin. The abnormal redistribution of blood flow that occurs at rest is accentuated by exercise in patients with heart failure. Maximum metabolic vasodilation is significantly reduced. The increased sodium content of the vessels accounts for some of the vascular stiffness observed in heart failure. Venous tone is also heightened. Ultimately, the limited arteriolar dilator capacity results in a relative skeletal muscle hypoxia that may, through a reflex arc, lead to further sympathetic tone.

Although the increase in vascular resistance in heart failure is rather consistent, it is only partially explained by neurogenic and humoral stimuli. More recently, interest has focused on endothelial function, which is well known to be impaired in heart failure (93). Endogenous systemic nitric oxide (NO) is thought to be increased in patients with heart failure (94–96) and correlates with the severity of the syndrome as measured by the New York Heart Association functional class (96). It is believed that increased NO production in heart failure may compensate to some extent for the excessive vasoconstrictor adaptation. Despite an elevated basal release of NO and its role in depressing cardiac function, evidence suggests that the peripheral vasculature has impaired release of NO on stimulation, which may play a role in inadequate vasodilator responses to exercise (97). In support of this hypothesis, data suggest that oral L-arginine, when given in a supplemental fashion to patients with heart failure, has a beneficial effect by increasing forearm blood flow, improving the distances as walked during the 6-minute walk test and improving quality of life as measured by a questionnaire (98). Dysfunction of the endothelium may persist and worsen as heart failure progresses, as evidenced by diminished vasodilator responses to acetylcholine and attenuated hyperemic responses to exercise and ischemia, both of which are largely endothelium dependent. Heart transplantation results in some reversal of impaired vasodilation, but restoration of vasodilation is delayed and incomplete (99).

In summary, congestive heart failure is characterized by abnormal peripheral vascular blood flow distribution with diminished hepatic, renal, and limb flow. The changes in peripheral blood flow are proportional and are linearly related to the reduction in cardiac output. Vascular resistance is increased and is related to circulating catecholamines, angiotensin II, and arginine vasopressin. Additionally, there appears to be significant impairment of vascular NO release resulting from endothelial dysfunction, and this probably accounts for some of the exercise intolerance noted in patients with heart failure. A generalized inability to dilate maximally in response to various stimuli characterizes the abnormal circulatory response, which may be corrected to some extent by medical therapy and heart transplantation.

Exercise Intolerance in Heart Failure

One of the primary features of the syndrome of heart failure is exercise intolerance. Although exercise tolerance is associated with LV systolic dysfunction, numerous studies have suggested that the extent of LV dysfunction bears little correlation to it (100–103). Moreover, investigators have demonstrated that short-term administration of positive inotropic agents and vasodilators, which acutely improve LV performance, do not improve maximal exercise capacity in patients with heart failure (104). Even agents that are knowingly effective for the long-term therapy of heart failure, such as ACE inhibitors, have failed to demonstrate consistent improvement in exercise tolerance. The reasons for this are not entirely understood but may be related to inadequate methodology. The maximal exercise test may not be truly representative of the daily activities of patients suffering from advanced heart failure (105). Maximal exercise testing is also somewhat subjective in that motivational factors and the experience of the operator or investigator can influence the end point of peak oxygen consumption. Because of this, the anaerobic threshold may be a more objective end point, but it is sometimes difficult to demonstrate, even with sophisticated gas exchange techniques. The simple 6-minute walk test is highly correlated to overall prognosis and seems to be emerging as an important measurement of exercise tolerance (106). However, bias can also be introduced by patient and/or operator motivational factors.

Maximal oxygen consumption is characterized by a plateau in oxygen uptake despite an increasing work rate. It is highly reproducible in physiologically normal subjects but can be difficult to measure in patients with advanced heart failure. The regional distribution of cardiac output during exercise is regulated by a complex interaction among the sympathetic nervous system, regional vasoactive factors including metaboreceptors, and endothelial-derived vasoactive substances including NO. The extent of widening of the arteriovenous oxygen difference is determined by increasing oxygen extraction in the exercising skeletal muscles. This, in turn, is somewhat dependent on capillary density, the number of open capillaries, and the transit time of the red blood cells through the capillaries. These complexities, coupled with the notorious difficulty in making accurate measurements during maximal exercise, have hampered our resolve to understand the precise mechanism of exercise intolerance in patients with heart failure.

In contrast to physiologically normal subjects, patients with heart failure often do not achieve a plateau in oxygen uptake at the end of exercise. Rather, a "peak" oxygen uptake is determined in patients with heart failure that is somewhat less reproducible. Whereas normal subjects distribute close to 90% of their total output to exercising skeletal muscle during maximal exercise, patients with heart failure distribute only 50% to 60% of the total cardiac output to exercising muscle. It has been presumed that the maximum caliber of the resistance arterioles is decreased in patients with heart failure as a result of changes in structure or perhaps vascular remodeling. When blood flow is chronically reduced, as occurs in advanced heart failure, the maximal vasodilator capacity of the peripheral circulation is markedly diminished through a complex sequence of events. These events include neurohormonal activation, diminished endothelial function related to impaired synthesis of NO, increased synthesis of endothelin, and possibly activation of cytokines and local factors that may further reduce arteriolar diameter. Patients with heart failure compensate for the reduced perfusion by widening their arteriovenous oxygen difference. Complete oxygen extraction can occur in the exercising skeletal muscle beds of patients with heart failure. This compensatory increase in oxygen extraction by skeletal muscles is similar to that observed in highly trained athletes. The mechanism of hyperextraction of oxygen is not completely understood. Unlike in well-trained athletes, increased capillary density has not been observed in patients with heart failure. In fact, there may well be diffuse atrophy of the lower extremities with diminished oxidative skeletal muscle fibers and oxidative enzyme content. This paradox remains poorly explained.

The exercise response in heart failure is very complex. Central hemodynamics and ejection fraction are poorly related to exercise tolerance. Factors in the peripheral musculature, not the central hemodynamics, seem largely to determine shortness of breath and fatigue. These peripheral factors include endothelial function, vasodilator capacity, distribution of cardiac output, heightened chemoreceptor and ergoreceptor sensitivity, skeletal muscle histology, and oxidative enzyme activity. Minute ventilation is markedly increased. There is a higher ventilation for any given carbon dioxide production (VE/VCO_2 slope), which reflects the severity of heart failure and the prognosis. Enhanced ergoreflexes and chemoreceptor responses drive hyperventilation and heightened sympathetic outflow, leading to increased peripheral resistance and a decrease in muscle perfusion.

Reduced muscle endurance can be improved with long-term exercise training in patients with heart failure (107–109). Although drugs such as ACE inhibitors may not improve maximal exercise tolerance in patients with heart failure, they can redistribute blood flow to the skeletal muscles during exercise and can thereby improve submaximal exercise tolerance. Changes in skeletal muscle structure and function in heart failure may be related in part to deconditioning (110). Therefore, it is reasonable to recommend that all patients with heart failure continue to be physically active, at least with regard to isotonic activity. Conversely, isometric activities, such as work against gravity, are to be generally discouraged because such activities impose an immediate afterload stress on the LV, sometimes causing severe dyspnea. Reduced physical activity alone, however, does not easily explain the genesis of the skeletal muscle changes observed in heart failure (110). Clearly, we still have much to learn regarding the cause of exercise intolerance in patients with heart failure.

CONTROVERSIES AND PERSONAL PERSPECTIVES

Heart failure remains a problem of growing magnitude throughout the world. It primarily afflicts the older population and is a major drain on scarce medical resources. Although great strides have been made in the past 2 decades regarding the management of this complex syndrome, much work remains to be done.

Heart failure is a prime example whereby a clearer understanding of the basic pathophysiology has led to highly specific therapies that are uniformly effective, such as ACE inhibitors, β-blockers, angiotensin receptor blockers, and aldosterone receptor blockers. As we delve further into the neuroendocrine and cytokine disturbances in the syndrome, it becomes clear that other potential therapeutic targets are worth developing. Over the years, there has been a rather direct course away from drugs designed to stimulate the inotropic state to agents that block excessive neuroendocrine activation pathways, promote vasodilation, and reduce oxidative stress.

It will be useful, perhaps, to screen for asymptomatic LV enlargement clinically. Identification of markers in such patients could enable the early introduction of pharmaceutical interdiction. It is also possible that surgical reduction of a markedly expanded LV cavity will prove to be a valuable adjunct form of therapy. Stem cell therapy is undergoing clinical trials, mostly in Europe, with some positive preliminary data. Until such strategies are available in the clinic, it is perhaps important to recognize that most cases of heart failure result from coronary artery disease and hypertension. Many of the consequences of long-term high blood pressure can now be prevented with early identification and aggressive treatment. All physicians need to recognize that LV hypertrophy is a powerful risk factor for heart failure and premature death and should be prevented or controlled when possible. Although the prevention of coronary artery disease is still not fully within our grasp, identification and aggressive control of coronary risk factors are now certainly possible. In the long run, it is through the prevention of heart failure that measurable strides will be made in curbing what is now described as an emerging epidemic. For the most part, heart failure is a preventable disease. Despite obvious progress, many controversies and uncertainties remain. The role of anticoagulation, especially aspirin, is still debated. Tailoring therapy to polymorphic markers (pharmacogenetics) is widely discussed. The role and costs of polypharmacy remain a challenge. Controversy and uncertainty remain the driving forces behind additional study, however, and will continue to serve us well.

CONCLUSIONS

Heart failure is a complex syndrome that is still rather poorly understood. An index event occurs, such as acute myocardial infarction or onset of cardiomyopathy, and multiple "adaptations" are staged. Abnormal LV function from any cause appears to stimulate the release of certain neurohormones and cytokines in an attempt to provide presumed circulatory homeostasis. However, over time, neuroendocrine and cytokine activity may become highly maladaptive, contributing to LV remodeling, heightened systemic vascular resistance, and ultimately worsening heart failure (Fig. 85.9). To date, the most impressive long-term effective therapy has been designed to limit

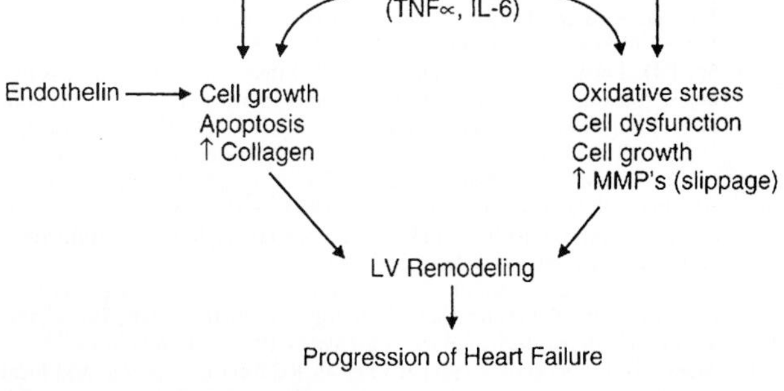

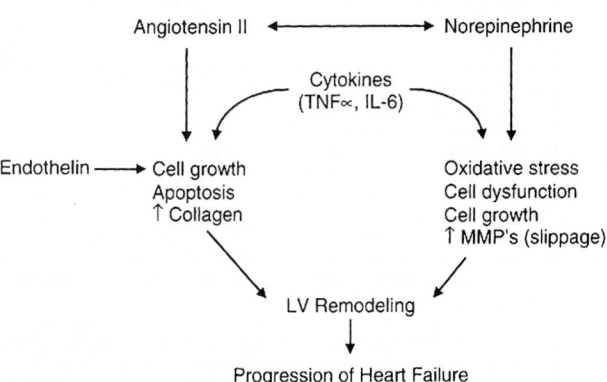

FIGURE 85.9. Neuroendocrine and cytokine activity in left ventricular (LV) remodeling in heart failure. IL, interleukin; MMP, matrix metalloproteinase; TNF, tumor necrosis factor.

excessive neuroendocrine activation, and this is likely where more imaginative therapies will also reside, at least in the near future.

THE FUTURE

Heart failure is a common and highly disabling clinical syndrome. Although advances have been made in our understanding of the pathogenesis and management of this complex disorder, we are still lacking substantial information regarding fundamental abnormalities, particularly at the cellular level. The mechanisms whereby neurohormones are activated and released are still not well explained, but we have the means to abrogate their excessive activity. The underlying myocyte contractile abnormalities that occur on a molecular level are still poorly defined. The precise mechanism leading to exercise intolerance is still debated. Despite these misgivings, it is likely that continued research at both the basic and clinical level will afford clinicians the opportunity to understand and manage this common clinical syndrome better, provided sufficient support exists for basic science as well as clinical investigation. However, clinical trials are expensive, may not be representative of most patients, and enlighten us little regarding mechanisms. We must learn new ways to study therapy other than simply counting deaths and other events. It is likely that we will be able to screen for heart failure better via biochemical markers such as BNP and abbreviated echocardiograms, thereby initiating therapy at an earlier stage and thus preventing onset of the full-blown syndrome. Stem cell therapy is just beginning clinical trials. Many new devices are currently undergoing study. The future looks bright.

References

1. Malkin CJ, Channer KS. Life-saving or life-prolonging? Interpreting trial data and survival curves for patients with congestive heart failure. *Eur J Heart Fail* 2004;7:143–148.
2. Pfeffer MA, Braunwald E. Ventricular remodeling after myocardial infarction. *Circulation* 1990;81:1161–1172.
3. Edmonds PM, Rogers A, Addington-Hall JM, et al. Patient descriptions of breathlessness in heart failure. *Int J Cardiol* 2005;98:61–66.
4. Lipkin DP, Canepa-Anson R, Stephens MR, Pool-Wilson PA. Factors determining symptoms in heart failure: comparison of fast and slow exercise tests. *Br Heart J* 1986;55:439–445.
5. Meyers J, Froelicher VF. Hemodynamic determinants of exercise capacity in chronic heart failure. *Ann Intern Med* 1991;115:377–386.
6. Meyers J, Salleh A, Buchanan N, et al. Ventilatory mechanisms of exercise intolerance in chronic heart failure. *Am Heart J* 1992;124:7–10.
7. Solin P, Bergin P, Richardson M, et al. Influence of pulmonary capillary wedge pressure on central apnea in heart failure. *Circulation* 1999;99:1574–1579.
8. Lanfranchi PA, Brahiroli A, Bosimini E, et al. Prognostic value of nocturnal Cheyne-Stokes respiration in chronic heart failure. *Circulation* 1999;99:1435–1440.
9. Javaheri S, Parker TJ, Liming JD, et al. Sleep apnea in 81 ambulatory male patients with stable heart failure. *Circulation* 1998;97:2154–2159.
10. Javaheri S. A mechanism of central sleep apnea in patients with heart failure. *N Engl J Med* 1999;341:949–954.
11. Sin DD, Logan AG, Fitzgerald FS, et al. Effects of continuous positive airway pressure on cardiovascular outcomes in heart failure patients with and without Cheyne-Stokes respiration. *Circulation* 2000;102:61–66.
12. Wilson JR, Martin JL, Ferraro N, Weber KT. Effect of hydralazine on perfusion and metabolism in the leg during upright bicycle exercise in patients with heart failure. *Circulation* 1983;68:425–432.
13. LeJemtel TH, Sonnenblick EH. Should the failing heart be stimulated? (editorial). *N Engl J Med* 1984;310:1384–1385.
14. Chati Z, Zannad F, Jeandel C, et al. Physical deconditioning may be a mechanism for the skeletal muscle energy phosphate metabolism abnormalities in chronic heart failure. *Am Heart J* 1996;131:560–566.
15. Massie BM, Simonini A, Sahgal P, et al. Relation of systemic and local muscle exercise capacity to skeletal muscle characteristics in men with congestive heart failure. *J Am Coll Cardiol* 1996;27:140–145.
16. Stevenson LW, Perloff JK. The limited reliability of physical signs for estimating hemodynamics in chronic heart failure. *JAMA* 1989;261:884–888.
17. Maisel AS, Krishnaswamy P, Nowak RM, et al. Rapid measurement of β-type natriuretic peptide in the emergency diagnosis of heart failure. *N Engl J Med* 2002;347:161–167.
18. McCullough PA, Nowak RM, McCord J, et al. β-type natriuretic peptide and clinical judgement in emergency diagnosis of heart failure: analysis from breathing not properly (BNP) multinational study. *Circulation* 2002;106:416–422.
19. Mueller C, Scholer A, Laule-Kilian K, et al. Use of β-type natriuretic peptide in the evaluation and management of acute dyspnea. *N Engl J Med* 2004;350:647–654.
20. Packer M. Should β-type natriuretic peptide be measured routinely to guide the diagnosis and management of chronic heart failure? *Circulation* 2003;108:2950–2953.
21. Tang WHW, Girod JP, Lee MJ, et al. Plasma β-type natriuretic peptide levels in ambulatory patients with established chronic symptomatic systolic heart failure. *Circulation* 2003;108:2964–2966.
22. Vanderheyden M, Goethals M, Verstreken S, et al. Wall stress modulates brain natriuretic peptide production in pressure overload cardiomyopathy. *J Am Coll Cardiol* 2004;44:2349–2354.
23. Tang WHW, Francis GS. Natural history of heart failure. In: Kukin M, Fuster V, eds. *Oxidative stress and heart failure.* Armonk, NY: Futura, 2003:3–47.
24. Adams KF Jr, Fonarow GC, Emerman CL, et al. Characteristics and outcomes of patients hospitalized for heart failure in the United States: rationale, design, and preliminary observations from the first 100,000 cases in the Acute Decompensated Heart Failure National Registry (ADHERE). *Am Heart J* 2005;149:209–216.
25. Levy D, Larson MG, Vasan RS, et al. The progression from hypertension to congestive heart failure. *JAMA* 1996;275:1557–1562.
26. Schwinger RHG, Bohm M, Koch A, et al. The failing human heart is unable to use the Frank-Starling mechanism. *Circ Res* 1994;74:959–969.
27. Komamura K, Shannon RP, Ihara R, et al. Exhaustion of Frank-Starling mechanism in conscious dogs with heart failure. *Am J Physiol* 1993;265:H1119–H1131.
28. Kitsis RN, Scheuer J. Functional significance of alterations in cardiac contractile protein isoforms. *Clin Cardiol* 1996;19:9–18.
29. Houser SR, Lakatta EG. Function of the cardiac myocyte in the conundrum of end-stage dilated human heart failure. *Circulation* 1999;99:600–604.
30. Cohn JN, Ferrari R, Sharpe N, et al. Cardiac remodeling—concepts and clinical implications: a consensus paper from an international forum on cardiac remodeling. *J Am Coll Cardiol* 2000;35:569–582.
31. St. John Sutton MG, Sharpe N. Left ventricular remodeling after myocardial infarction. *Circulation* 2000;101:2981–2988.
32. Hammermeister KE, DeRouen TA, Dodge HT. Variables predictive of survival in patients with coronary disease: selection by univariate and multivariate analysis from the clinical electrocardiographic, exercise, arteriographic, and quantitative angiographic evaluations. *Circulation* 1979;59:421–430.
33. White HD, Norris RM, Brown MA, et al. Left ventricular end-systolic volume as the major determinant of survival after recovery from myocardial infarction. *Circulation* 1987;76:44–51.
34. Weisman HF, Bush DE, Mannisi JA, et al. Cellular mechanisms of myocardial infarct expansion. *Circulation* 1988;78:186–201.
35. Eaton LW, Bulkley BH. Expansion of acute myocardial infarction: its relationship to infarct morphology in a canine model. *Circ Res* 1981;49:80–88.
36. Eaton LW, Weiss JL, Garrison JB, Bulkley BH. Regional cardiac dilatation after acute myocardial infarction: recognition by two-dimensional echocardiography. *N Engl J Med* 1979;300:57–62.
37. Kim CB, Braunwald E. Potential benefits of late reperfusion of infarcted myocardium. *Circulation* 1993;88:2426–2436.
38. Brown EJ, Swinford RD, Gadde P, Lillis O. Acute effects of delayed reperfusion on myocardial infarct shape and left ventricular volume: a potential mechanism of additional benefits from thrombolytic therapy. *J Am Coll Cardiol* 1991;17:1641–1650.
39. Hirayama A, Adachi T, Asada S, et al. Late reperfusion for acute myocardial infarction limits the dilatation of left ventricle without the reduction of infarct size. *Circulation* 1993;88:2565–2574.
40. Lamas GA, Flaker GC, Mitchell G, et al. Effect of infarct artery patency on prognosis after acute myocardial infarction. *Circulation* 1995;92:1101–1109.
41. Popvic AD, Neskovic AN, Babic R, et al. Independent impact of thrombolytic therapy and vessel patency on left ventricular dilation after myocardial infarction. *Circulation* 1994;90:800–807.
42. McKay RG, Pfeffer MA, Pasternak RC, et al. Left ventricular remodeling after myocardial infarction: a corollary to infarct expansion. *Circulation* 1986;74:693–702.
43. Francis GS, McDonald KM. Left ventricular hypertrophy: an initial response to myocardial injury. *Am J Cardiol* 1992;69:3G–9G.
44. Francis GS, McDonald KM, Cohn JN. Neurohumoral activation in preclinical heart failure. *Circulation* 1993;87(suppl IV):IV90–IV96.
45. Francis GS, Carlyle WC. Hypothetical pathways of cardiac myocyte hypertrophy: response to myocardial injury. *Eur Heart J* 1993;14:49–56.
46. Francis GS, Chu C. Post-infarction myocardial remodeling: why does it happen? *Eur Heart J* 1995;16:31–36.
47. Anversa P, Li P, Zhang X, et al. Ischaemic myocardial injury and ventricular remodelling. *Cardiovasc Res* 1993;27:145–157.

48. Beltrami CA, Finato N, Rocco M, et al. Structural basis of end-stage heart failure in ischemic cardiomyopathy in humans. *Circulation* 1994;89:151–163.
49. Gerdes AM, Capasso JM. Structural remodeling and mechanical dysfunction of cardiac myocytes in heart failure. *J Mol Cell Cardiol* 1995;27:849–856.
50. Anand IS, Liu D, Chugh SS, Prahash AJC, et al. Isolated myocyte contractile function is normal in post-infarct remodeled rat heart with systolic dysfunction. *Circulation* 1997;96:3974–3984.
51. Levine TB, Francis GS, Goldsmith SR, et al. Activity of the sympathetic nervous system and renin-angiotensin system assessed by plasma hormone levels and their relation to hemodynamic abnormalities in congestive heart failure. *Am J Cardiol* 1982;49:1659–1666.
52. Cohn JN, Levine B, Olivari MT, et al. Plasma norepinephrine as a guide to prognosis in patients with chronic congestive heart failure. *N Engl J Med* 1984;311:819–823.
53. Francis GS, Goldsmith SR, Levine TB, et al. The neurohumoral axis in congestive heart failure. *Ann Intern Med* 1984;101:370–377.
54. Francis GS, Benedict C, Johnstone DE, et al. Comparison of neuroendocrine activation in patients with left ventricular dysfunction with and without congestive heart failure. *Circulation* 1990;82:1724–1729.
55. Taemura G, Fujiwara H, Horike K, et al. Ventricular expression of atrial natriuretic polypeptide and its relations with hemodynamics and histology in dilated human hearts. *Circulation* 1989;80:1137–1147.
56. Wei C-M, Heublein DM, Perrella MA, et al. Natriuretic peptide system in human heart failure. *Circulation* 1993;88:1004–1009.
57. Harris P. Evolution and the cardiac patient. *Cardiovasc Res* 1983;17:3–22.
58. Goldsmith SR, Francis GS, Cowley AW, et al. Increased plasma arginine vasopressin levels in patients with congestive heart failure. *J Am Coll Cardiol* 1993;1:1385–1390.
59. Rodeheffer RJ, Lerman A, Heublein D, Burnett JC. Increased plasma concentrations of endothelin in congestive heart failure in humans. *Mayo Clin Proc* 1992;67:719–724.
60. Hirsch AT, Dzau VJ, Creager MA. Baroreceptor function in congestive heart failure: effect on neurohumoral activation and regional vascular resistance. *Circulation* 1987;75(suppl IV):IV36.
61. Thames MD, Kinugawa T, Smith ML, Dibner-Dunlap ME. Abnormalities of baroreflex control in heart failure. *J Am Coll Cardiol* 1993;22:56A–60A.
62. Eckberg DL, Drabinsky M, Braunwald E. Defective cardiac parasympathetic control in patients with heart disease. *N Engl J Med* 1971;265:877–883.
63. Levine TB, Francis GS, Goldsmith ST, Cohn JN. The neurohumoral and hemodynamic response to orthostatic tilt in patients with congestive heart failure. *Circulation* 1983;67:1070–1075.
64. Zucker IH, Wang W, Brandle M. Baroreflex abnormalities in congestive heart failure. *News Physiol Sci* 1993;8:87–90.
65. Creager MA, Creager SJ. Arterial baroreflex regulation of blood pressure in patients with congestive heart failure. *J Am Coll Cardiol* 1994;23:401–405.
66. Thomas JA, Marks BH. Plasma norepinephrine in congestive heart failure. *Am J Cardiol* 1978;41:233–243.
67. Mann DL, Kent RL, Parsons B, Cooper G. Adrenergic effects of the biology of the adult mammalian cardiocyte. *Circulation* 1992;85:790–804.
68. Jiang JP, Downing SE. Catecholamine cardiomyopathy: review and analysis of pathogenetic mechanisms. *Yale J Biol Med* 1990;63:581–591.
69. Leimbach WN, Wallin BG, Victor RG, et al. Direct evidence from intraneural recordings for increased central sympathetic outflow in patients with heart failure. *Circulation* 1986;73:913–919.
70. Rector TS, Olivari MT, Levine TB, et al. Predicting survival for an individual with congestive heart failure using the plasma norepinephrine concentration. *Am Heart J* 1987;114:148–152.
71. Francis GS, Goldsmith SR, Cohn JN. Relationship of exercise capacity to resting left ventricular performance and basal plasma norepinephrine levels in patients with congestive heart failure. *Am Heart J* 1982;104:725–731.
72. Eisenhofer G, Friberg P, Rundqvist B, et al. Cardiac sympathetic nerve function in congestive heart failure. *Circulation* 1996;93:1667–1676.
73. Gaffney TE, Braunwald E. Importance of the adrenergic nervous system in the support of circulatory function in patients with congestive heart failure. *Am J Med* 1963;34:320–324.
74. Bristow MR, Port JD, Sandoval AB, et al. Beta-adrenergic-receptor pathways in the failing human heart. *Heart Fail* 1989;5:77–90.
75. Eichhorn EJ, Bristow MR. Medical therapy can improve the biological properties of the chronically failing heart. *Circulation* 1996;94:2285–2296.
76. Bristow PM, Cohn JN, Colucci WS, et al. The effect of carvedilol on morbidity and mortality in patients with chronic heart failure. *N Engl J Med* 1996;23:1349–1355.
77. Bristow MR, Gilbert Em, Abraham WT, et al. Carvedilol produces dose-related improvements in left ventricular function and survival in subjects with chronic heart failure. *Circulation* 1996;94:2807–2816.
78. CIBIS II Investigators and committees. The cardiac insufficiency bisoprolol study II (CIBIS II): a randomized trial. *Lancet* 1999;353:9–13.
79. MERIT-HF Study Group. Effect of metoprolol CR/XL in chronic heart failure: metoprolol CR/XL randomized intervention trial in congestive heart failure (MERIT HF). *Lancet* 1999;353:2001–2007.
80. Merrill AJ. Edema and decreased renal blood flow in patients with chronic congestive heart failure: evidence of "forward failure" as the primary cause of edema. *J Clin Invest* 1946;25:389–400.
81. Laragh JH. Hormones and the pathogenesis of congestive heart failure: vasopressin, aldosterone, and angiotensin II. *Circulation* 1962;25:1015–1023.
82. Genest J, Granger P, DeChamplain J, Boucher R. Endocrine factors in congestive heart failure. *Am J Cardiol* 1968;22:35–42.
83. Brown JJ, Davies DL, Johnson VW, et al. Renin relationships in congestive cardiac failure, treated and untreated. *Am Heart J* 1970;80:329–342.
84. Lindpaintner K, Ganten D. The cardiac renin-angiotensin system. *Circ Res* 1991;68:905–921.
85. Grinstaed WC, Young JB. The myocardial renin-angiotensin system: existence, importance, and clinical implications. *Am Heart J* 1992;123:1039–1045.
86. Curtiss C, Cohn JN, Vrobel T, Franciosa JA. Role of the renin-angiotensin system in the systemic vasoconstriction of chronic congestive heart failure. *Circulation* 1978;58:763–776.
87. Packer M, Lee W-H, Kessler PD. Preservation of glomerular filtration rate in human heart failure by activation of the renin-angiotensin system. *Circulation* 1986;74:766–774.
88. Barger AC. The pathogenesis of sodium retention in congestive heart failure. *Metabolism* 1956;5:480–489.
89. Hostetter TH, Pfeffer JM, Pfeffer MA, et al. Cardiorenal hemodynamics and sodium excretion in rats with myocardial infarction. *Am J Physiol* 1983;245:H98–H103.
90. Skorecki KL, Brenner BM. Body fluid homeostasis in congestive heart failure and cirrhosis with ascites. *Am J Med* 1982;72:323–338.
91. Francis GS. Sodium and water excretion in heart failure: efficacy of treatment has surpassed knowledge of pathophysiology. *Ann Intern Med* 1986; 105:272.
92. Zelis R, Nellis SH, Longhurst J, et al. Abnormalities in the regional circulations accompanying congestive heart failure. *Prog Cardiovasc Dis* 1975; 18:181–199.
93. Drexler H, Hayoz D, Munzel T, et al. Endothelial function in chronic congestive heart failure. *Am J Cardiol* 1992;69:1596–1601.
94. Habib F, Dutka D, Crossman D, et al. Enhanced basal nitric oxide production in heart failure: another failed counter-regulatory vasodilator mechanism? *Lancet* 1994;344:371–373.
95. Winlaw DS, Smythe GS, Keogh AM, et al. Increased nitric oxide production in heart failure. *Lancet* 1994;344:373–374.
96. Hickey M, Fraser IS. Nitric oxide production and heart failure (letter). *Lancet* 1995;345:390–391.
97. Gilligan DM, Panza JA, Kilcoyne CM, et al. Contribution of endothelium-derived nitric oxide to exercise-induced vasodilation. *Circulation* 1994;90:2853–2858.
98. Rector RS, Bank AJ, Mullen KA, et al. Randomized, double-blind, placebo-controlled study of supplemental oral Larginine in patients with heart failure. *Circulation* 1996;93:2135–2141.
99. Sinoway LI, Minotti JR, Davis D, et al. Delayed reversal of impaired vasodilation in congestive heart failure after heart transplantation. *Am J Cardiol* 1988;61:1076–1079.
100. Franciosa JA, Ziesche S, Wilen M. Functional capacity of patients with chronic left ventricular failure. *Am J Med* 1979;67:460–466.
101. Benge W, Litchfield RL, Marcus ML. Exercise capacity in patients with severe left ventricular dysfunction. *Circulation* 1980;61:955–959.
102. Franciosa JA, Park M, Levine TB. Lack of correlation between exercise capacity and indexes of resting left ventricular performance in heart failure. *Am J Cardiol* 1981;47:33–39.
103. Litchfield RL, Kerber RE, Benge W, et al. Normal exercise capacity in patients with severe left ventricular dysfunction: compensatory mechanisms. *Circulation* 1982;66:129–134.
104. Wilson JR, Martin JL, Ferraro N, Weber KT. Effect of hydralazine on perfusion and metabolism in the leg during upright bicycle exercise in patients with heart failure. *Circulation* 1983;68:425–432.
105. Francis GS, Rector TS. Maximal exercise tolerance as a therapeutic end point in heart failure: are we relying on the right measure? *Am J Cardiol* 1994;73:304–306.
106. Bittner V, Weiner DH, Yusuf S, et al. Prediction of mortality and morbidity with a 6-minute walk test in patients with left ventricular dysfunction. *JAMA* 1993;270:1702–1707.
107. Sullivan MJ, Higginbotham MB, Cobb FR. Exercise training in patients with severe left ventricular dysfunction. *Circulation* 1988;78:506–515.
108. Coats AJS, Adamopoulos S, Radaelli A, et al. Controlled trial of physical training in chronic heart failure. *Circulation* 1992;85:2119–2131.
109. Keteyian SJ, Levine AB, Brawner CA, et al. Exercise training in patients with heart failure. *Ann Intern Med* 1996;124:1051–1057.
110. Simonini A, Long CS, Dudley GA, et al. Heart failure in rats causes changes in skeletal muscle morphology and gene expression that are not explained by reduced activity. *Circ Res* 1996;79:128–136.

CHAPTER 86 ■ ACUTE HEART FAILURE

SRINIVAS IYENGAR, GARRIE J. HAAS, AND JAMES B. YOUNG

OVERVIEW

Since the early 1980s, hospital discharges for heart failure (HF) have increased more than 150% and now represent the most common reason for hospitalization in the elderly (1). The incidence of HF approaches 10 per 1,000 population after the age of 65 years, and it was estimated that in 2005 alone, the direct and indirect costs of managing this disease process in the United States approached 28 billion dollars. This considerable economic burden is fueled by the astonishingly high early hospital readmission rate for patients with HF. It is estimated that nearly 50% of patients initially admitted with decompensated HF are readmitted within 60 to 90 days after hospital discharge (2). A seeming paradox is that most patients with HF do not die in a hospital. Although in-hospital mortality for acute HF averages 5% to 8%, the 1-year mortality following an acute HF exacerbation requiring hospitalization may be as high as 60%. Given these staggering statistics, it is essential for the clinician to recognize this syndrome early and to institute appropriate therapy in a timely fashion. Clinicians should focus on both the rapid reversal of HF symptoms and the appropriate transition to accepted long-term outpatient HF therapies.

Acutely decompensated HF (ADHF) is a complex syndrome that is most often a direct result of myocardial injury caused by underlying ischemia or infarction. Although coronary artery disease (CAD) is the most common cause of acute HF in Western societies, a broad spectrum of other potential causes exists, including such diverse conditions as acute valvular abnormalities, pericardial disease, and acute myocarditis (Table 86.1). Hypertension and HF resulting from diastolic dysfunction may precipitate as many as 50% of HF-related hospitalizations in the elderly, particularly in women, a situation not previously generally recognized (3). The management of acute HF requires rapid identification of the underlying cause, with specific treatment directed at reversing the associated abnormal pathophysiologic state. The support of patients while the diagnostic evaluation is pursued can range from urgent therapy with intravenous vasodilators and diuretics to more aggressive pharmacologic support with varying combinations of inotropic, vasodilator, and vasopressor agents. In complicated or confusing situations, hemodynamic monitoring is essential. When a reparable lesion has been identified or when cardiac transplantation is considered an option, mechanical circulatory support may be required until definitive treatment can be instituted. Because of the complexity and diverse nature of the acute HF syndrome, treatment must be individualized. Finally, unfortunately, it must be pointed out that for many different reasons, few short-term or long-term large-scale, properly powered morbidity and mortality trials have been completed in patients with acute HF or ADHF. Perhaps this explains why consensus cannot be often reached regarding the best management strategies with few definitive guidelines published.

Patients presenting with acute HF may be classified into one of three fundamental categories, based in part, on differences in pathophysiology and the chronicity of their cardiac disease (2). These categories of acute HF are new-onset HF, decompensation of previously stable chronic HF (ADHF), and advanced or "end-stage" HF that has responded poorly to standard medical therapy with a downward spiral of symptoms and physical findings.

The syndrome of new-onset HF, particularly when it is acute in presentation, represents a true medical emergency that warrants an expedient diagnostic and therapeutic approach. If appropriate treatment is not instituted within a reasonable period, irreversible cardiac decompensation may ensue, leading to a progressive syndrome of shock, multiorgan failure, and death (Fig. 86.1). New-onset acute HF is generally recognized when symptoms develop within hours to days in patients without a history of prior cardiac decompensation (4). A history of previous treatment for heart disease may be elicited because many patients will have experienced symptoms (i.e., angina or exertional dyspnea) related to myocardial ischemia. In fact, atherosclerotic heart disease and the complications of myocardial ischemia and infarction are the most common causes of acute HF in Western societies, though other conditions can precipitate this condition. Many of the conditions resulting in new-onset HF may be definitively treated, thus resulting in a favorable impact on the patient's short- and long-term course. Often, a rapid decision regarding the appropriateness of surgical intervention is necessary if the patient is to realize a favorable outcome. For example, the 1-year mortality rate for patients presenting with acute pulmonary edema, a common

TABLE 86.1

MAJOR CAUSES OF ACUTE HEART FAILURE

Myocardial ischemia or infarction
Complications of myocardial infarction
Acute mitral regurgitation (papillary muscle rupture)
Ventricular septal rupture
Cardiac free wall rupture and pericardial tamponade
Acute valvular catastrophe (mitral or aortic)
Severe, poorly controlled hypertension
Myocarditis
Sustained cardiac arrhythmias
Acute pulmonary embolism
Decompensation of chronic heart failure or cardiomyopathy
Acute aortic dissection with myocardial ischemia or infarction

clinical manifestation of new-onset HF, may exceed 50% when an underlying lesion or condition is not defined and treated (5). In certain life-threatening presentations, such as acute ischemic myocardial injury or complications thereof (i.e., acute valvular regurgitation, ventricular septal defect, cardiac tamponade), immediate evaluation and directed therapy are indicated for stabilization and treatment of the acute HF syndrome. In these emergency situations, definitive therapy should not be delayed by prolonged efforts to achieve a more stable clinical situation. Without correction of the underlying lesions, such efforts are often unsuccessful and commonly result in further clinical deterioration with the development of irreversible myocardial dysfunction. When the disorder precipitating new-onset HF does not appear to be one requiring urgent therapy, definitive diagnostic studies and consideration of specific forms of therapy can be delayed until clinical and hemodynamic stabilization has been achieved.

Patients with advanced or end-stage HF comprise only about 2% of all HF hospital admissions (6). These patients typically present with symptoms of congestion, poor peripheral perfusion, and multiorgan dysfunction, and they are often cachectic and functionally extremely limited. They have usually failed over a long period to respond to standard medical, surgical, and device therapies, and their prognosis without extreme measures is exceedingly poor. These are the patients who are classified in American College of Cardiology/American Heart Association (ACC/AHA) stage D category (Fig. 86.2; see also Chapter 87), and they may be considered and evaluated for advanced surgical therapies including cardiac transplantation and so-called destination therapy with mechanical assist devices (the destination is the patient's home). If these options are not tenable, then palliative therapy and hospice referral should be considered.

A prime focus of this chapter is the most common reason for HF hospitalization, acute decompensation in the patient

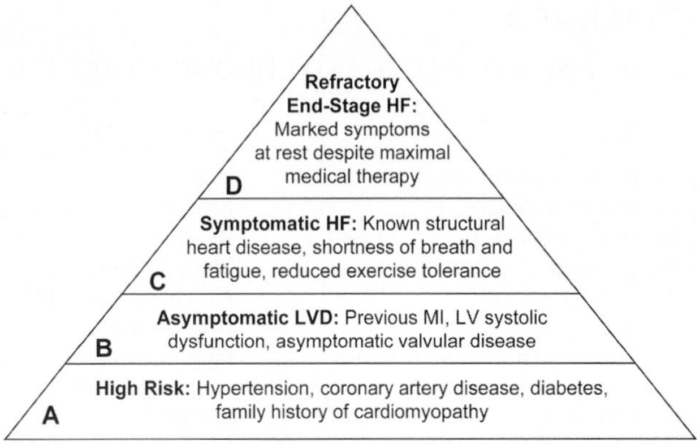

FIGURE 86.2. Disease progression of heart failure (HF): American College of Cardiology/American Heart Association HF stages. LV, left ventricular; LVD, left ventricular dysfunction; MI, myocardial infarction. (Adapted from Hunt, SA, Baker, DW, Chin, MH, et al. 2001 ACC/AHA guidelines for the evaluation and management of chronic heart failure in the adult: executive summary. A report of the American College of Cardiology/American Heart Association Task Force on Practice Guidelines Committee to Revise the 1995 Guidelines for the Evaluation and Management of Heart Failure: developed in collaboration with the International Society for Heart and Lung Transplantation, endorsed by the Heart Failure Society of America. *Circulation* 2001;104:2996–3007.)

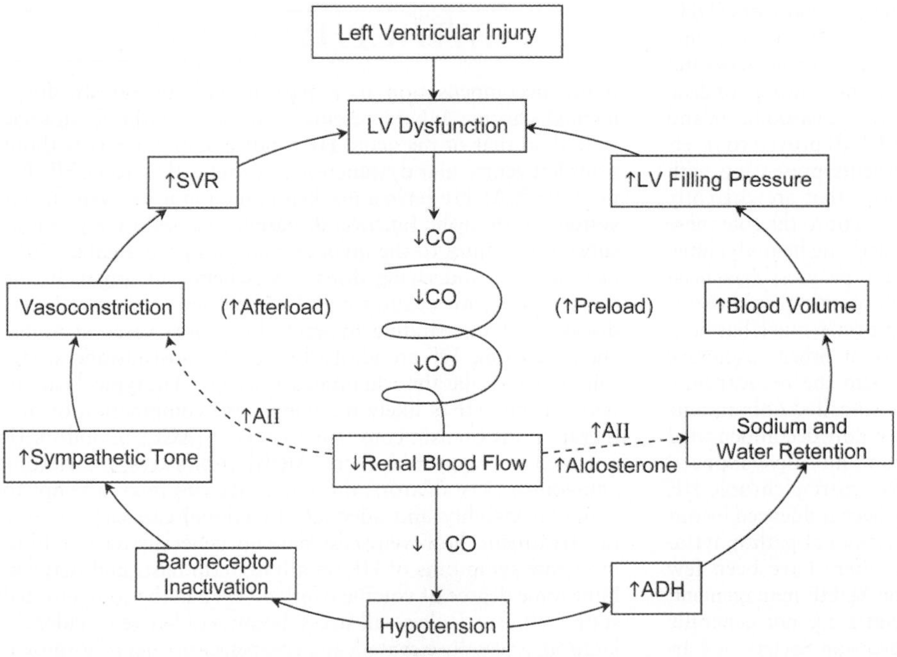

FIGURE 86.1. Depicted are the factors in cardiogenic shock perpetuating continued left ventricular (LV) dysfunction and progressive deterioration in cardiac output (CO). As CO falls, renal blood flow is reduced, which thus activates the renin-angiotensin-aldosterone system. Angiotensin II (AII) directly results in vasoconstriction and indirectly increases blood volume by enhancing aldosterone release. Hypotension resulting from a further fall in CO activates the central nervous system release of antidiuretic hormone (ADH). Inactivation of baroreceptors enhances sympathetic tone and vasoconstriction. As CO, renal blood flow, and hypotension remain reduced, preload and afterload continue to increase, and this leads to further LV dysfunction. ↑, increased; ↓, decreased; SVR, systemic vascular resistance.

TABLE 86.2

COMPARISON OF ACUTE AND CHRONIC HEART FAILURE

Feature	New onset HF	ADHF	Stable chronic HF
Symptom severity	Marked	Marked	Mild to moderate
Pulmonary edema	Frequent	Frequent	Rare
Peripheral edema	Rare	Frequent	Frequent
Weight gain	None to mild	Marked	Frequent
Total body volume	No change or mildly increased	Markedly increased	Increased
Cardiomegaly	Uncommon	Usual	Common
Left ventricular systolic function	Hypocontractile, normocontractile, or hypercontractile	Reduced	Markedly reduced
Wall stress	Elevated	Markedly elevated	Elevated
Activation of sympathetic nervous system	Marked	Marked	Mild to marked
Activation of RAAS	Acutely abnormal	Marked	Mild to marked
Acute ischemia	Common	Occasional	Rare
Hypertensive crisis	Common	Occasional	Rare
Reparable, remediable causative lesions	Common	Occasional	Occasional

ADHF, acute decompensated heart failure; HF, heart failure; RAAS, renin-angiotensin-aldosterone system. (Adapted from Leier CV. Unstable heart failure. In: Colucci WS, ed. *Heart Failure: cardiac function and dysfunction,* St. Louis. Mosby, 1995:9.2–9.15. Braunwald E, ed. *Atlas of heart disease,* vol 4.)

with previously stable HF (ADHF). Approximately 75% of HF admissions fall into this category, and unlike the conditions discussed earlier, medical management is usually the preferred therapeutic approach. Distinct clinical findings differentiating those with ADHF from new-onset and stable chronic HF are presented in Table 86.2. These patients comprise ACC/AHA stage C HF and often have a history of one or more prior hospitalizations for ADHF. These patients are usually congested with normal peripheral perfusion at presentation, and they generally respond favorably to the rapid institution of vasoactive therapy of one sort or another.

HISTORICAL PERSPECTIVE

Significant advances in the pharmacologic support of ADHF have been made over the past 4 decades. In the 1960s, only digitalis and diuretics were available for HF management, and furosemide, approved for use in 1967, was the mainstay of drug therapy for ADHF. The intravenous inotropic, vasodilator, and vasopressor therapies introduced in the 1970s proved to be effective in the stabilization of many patients presenting with ADHF. Newer forms of these medications that are currently available and/or being studied are a testament to the role these drugs have assumed in correcting the underlying hemodynamic derangements seen in ADHF. Important progress has been made toward the development of novel, more directed therapies with less toxic side effects. At the same time, much has been learned regarding important limitations of other vasoactive therapies, particularly those that stimulate the myocardium and increase inotropy. No longer is the so-called dobutamine "holiday" advocated as a "tune-up" for mildly decompensated patients, given the substantive toxicities of inotropic support. As with the pharmacologic approach for treating chronic HF, the treatment of ADHF has also recently been influenced by our newer understanding of the HF neurohormonal pathophysiologic paradigm. Unfortunately, to date there have been few randomized, controlled clinical trials in ADHF management, and thus specific evidence-based guidelines are not generally available. Only the recently released European Society of Cardiology HF Guidelines attempt to address this patient population, and these recommendations are hampered by absence of reliable clinical trial data and consensus of clinicians (especially those with ADHF treatment expertise in North America). Thus, the management of ADHF is less standardized and highly variable. Recently, the development of large acute HF registries such as the Acute Decompensated Heart Failure National Registry (ADHERE Registry) (7) has provided important observational data regarding HF demographics and therapy in more than 100,000 patients. These data promise to advance our understanding of the ADHF syndrome significantly. Certainly, ongoing clinical trials in ADHF will have a major impact in the future as standardized and evidence-based methods of managing these patients are developed.

PATHOPHYSIOLOGY

Acute decompensation in a patient with previously documented chronic HF represents a different pathophysiologic state than that of the acute HF syndrome in patients without prior left ventricular dysfunction or those with chronic HF. Patients with ADHF have a marked reduction in left ventricular systolic or diastolic function at baseline caused by a previous substantial injury to the myocardium. In approximately 50% of cases, the underlying disease is ischemic in origin. In the remainder, various causes may be identified, such as valvular disease or long-standing hypertension. Most cases of nonischemic chronic HF are idiopathic (8). In most instances, systolic and diastolic abnormalities are present. The typical patient with chronic HF is likely receiving some combination of oral therapy (angiotensin-converting enzyme [ACE] inhibitors or angiotensin-receptor blockers [ARBs], β-blockers, aldosterone antagonists, vasodilators, diuretics, digoxin) in an attempt to maintain stability and adequate functional capacity. Despite this treatment, however, these patients generally have mild to moderate symptoms of HF on a long-term basis and may exhibit some degree of volume overload even in the compensated state. Left ventricular wall stress, because of left ventricular dilatation, is usually elevated, and compensatory neurohormonal

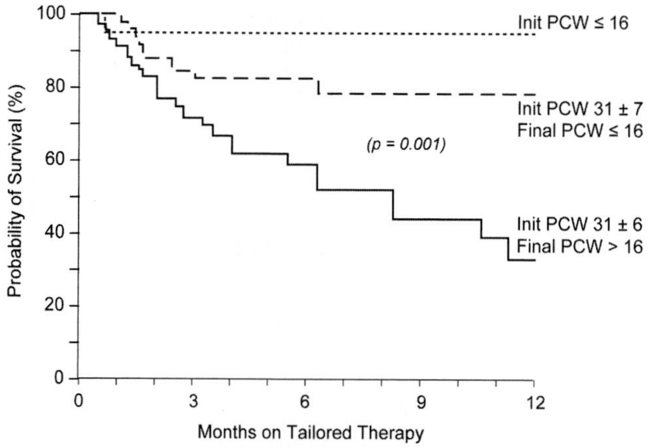

FIGURE 86.3. Relationship between pulmonary capillary wedge pressure (PCWP) and survival in 152 patients referred for heart transplantation with ejection fractions lower than 20% and receiving optimal medical therapy. Init, initial. (Adapted from Stevenson LW, Tillisch JH, Hamilton M, et al. Importance of hemodynamic response to therapy in predicting survival with ejection fraction <20% secondary to ischemic or non-ischemic dilated cardiomyopathy. *Am J Cardiol* 1990;6:1348–1354.)

mechanisms are activated (see Chapter 85). When acute decompensation occurs, these baseline abnormalities become further deranged. This is associated with a further deterioration in hemodynamic status that manifests primarily as an increase in left ventricular filling pressure. Further neurohormonal perturbation ensues, including activation of the renin-angiotensin-aldosterone axis, sympathetic nervous system, arginine vasopressin, and endothelin, leading to systemic and pulmonary vasoconstriction with sodium and water retention. Although initially compensatory, this process becomes maladaptive over time and causes disease progression. In a minority of patients with ADHF, cardiac output is reduced on presentation and is seen clinically as multiorgan hypoperfusion. Renal function must be monitored closely because the cardiorenal syndrome, reflecting poor renal perfusion with rising serum creatinine, is increasingly recognized as a predictor of poor outcome during ADHF hospitalization (9,10). The worsening of congestion and increasing left ventricular filling pressures in the patient with ADHF may lead to a progression of subendocardial ischemia, atrioventricular valvular regurgitation, alterations in extracellular matrix deposition and repair, and continued detrimental left ventricular remodeling (11). This process leads to progressive myocardial dysfunction, thereby increasing the risk of recurrent ADHF (12). In addition, the arrhythmia threshold is lowered as a result of this process, and the risk of sudden cardiac death is thus increased. Given these potential adverse effects of congestion, it is not surprising that persistent elevation of left ventricular filling pressures in patients with ADHF is an important independent predictor of survival, and the reduction of these pressures remains a major goal of pharmacologic therapy (13) (Fig. 86.3).

PRESENTATION AND EVALUATION

When patients first present to the emergency department or outpatient office with signs and symptoms suggesting ADHF, a methodical and rapid assessment should ensue. Patients with ADHF usually present with congestive symptoms and preserved cardiac output. They may describe worsening exertional dyspnea or dyspnea at rest, orthopnea, paroxysmal nocturnal dyspnea, and fatigue. According to the ADHERE registry, the most common presenting symptom is dyspnea, which occurs in 89% of patients, whereas fatigue (an indication of low cardiac output) is much less common, occurring in only 32% (Table 86.3). Because symptoms of dyspnea and edema have a broad differential diagnosis, particularly in the elderly and in those patients with multiple comorbid conditions, additional testing may be necessary before a firm diagnosis can be made. The history should explore possible precipitating factors for ADHF. These factors are presented in Table 86.4 and include such diverse causes as dietary and medical noncompliance, arrhythmias, and drugs such as nonsteroidal antiinflammatory agents. New or recurrent ischemia or infarction is a serious and potentially life-threatening cause of decompensation and should be considered in all patients even if they were previously determined to have "normal" coronary arteries.

In conjunction with the history, the patient should have a targeted physical examination with emphasis on the presence of jugular venous distention, abnormal heart and lung sounds, displaced apical impulse, and evidence of fluid retention. Evidence of low cardiac output (tachycardia, hypotension, cool extremities, mental status changes) should also be thoroughly evaluated. In most patients with ADHF, findings of the physical examination often reflect volume overload with peripheral edema and jugular venous distention. Pulmonary rales may be present but are certainly not as impressive as in the patient with acute myocardial injury and pulmonary edema. In fact, pulmonary findings may be relatively unremarkable in patients with ADHF even when cardiac filling pressure is markedly elevated. In the ADHERE registry, only 68% of patients admitted

TABLE 86.3

CLINICAL PRESENTATION OF PATIENTS HOSPITALIZED WITH HEART FAILURE

Presenting feature	Percentage (%)
Any dyspnea	89
Dyspnea at rest	34
Fatigue	32
Rales	68
Peripheral edema	66
Radiographic pulmonary congestion	75

Adapted from Fonarow GC. ADHERE. Scientific Advisory Committee. The Acute Decompensated Heart Failure National Registry (ADHERE): opportunities to improve care of patients hospitalized with acute decompensated heart failure. *Rev Cardiovasc Mes* 2003;4(suppl 7): S 21–30.)

TABLE 86.4

COMMON CAUSES OF ACUTE DECOMPENSATED HEART FAILURE IN PATIENTS WITH CHRONIC HEART FAILURE

Worsening ischemic disease
Deterioration of valvular function
Hypertensive crisis
Arrhythmias
Infections
Poor diet and/or fluid control
Medication noncompliance
Toxins (i.e., nonsteroidal antiinflammatory drugs)

with ADHF had pulmonary rales (Table 86.3). A gallop rhythm and murmur of mitral regurgitation are typically audible, and the cardiac impulse is enlarged, sustained, and laterally displaced (14). Certain findings on physical examination are prognostically important. Jugular venous distention and an S3 gallop have been reported to be independent predictors of hospitalization and all-cause mortality (15). A broad range of variability exists concerning physical findings, which often depend on the underlying lesion and duration of cardiac dysfunction.

A laboratory evaluation including complete blood count, serum electrolytes, glucose, blood urea nitrogen, creatinine, and liver function tests should all be part of the initial diagnostic protocol for a patient presenting with ADHF. Thyroid function tests and cardiac biomarkers can be performed if one suspects an underlying endocrine or ischemic condition that precipitated the event. Anemia and poorly controlled diabetes may also cause or complicate ADHF. As discussed previously, the finding of renal impairment has important implications regarding risk stratification and prognosis. The idea of risk stratification for patients with ADHF has recently come to light from an additional analysis of the ADHERE database (16). Utilizing a classification and regression tree (CART) analysis, this inquiry found that patients admitted to the hospital for ADHF could be stratified into low-, intermediate-, and high-risk groups for in-hospital mortality by means of routine blood tests and vital signs. The single best predictor for mortality was a high blood urea nitrogen level (>43 mg/dL), followed by a low systolic blood pressure on admission (<115 mm HG), and then by an elevated serum creatinine level (>2.75 mg/dL). These results are informative because they provide clinical parameters in which risk assessment can be made on an immediate basis by the clinician.

Types A, B, and C natriuretic peptides (NPs) appear to be beneficial counterregulatory hormones produced by the heart (types A and B) or the vascular endothelium (type C) in response to certain pathophysiologic events. Indeed, these hormones may play a significant role in attenuating potentially detrimental left ventricular hypertrophy, and they protect the heart during ischemic events (17–19). BNP is an endogenously secreted hormone constitutively released by the heart under conditions of increased pressure or volume overload (20). BNP has been found to have vasodilatory and natriuretic properties, as well as potentially mediating the effects of the renin-angiotensin-aldosterone pathway (21). Although several blood assays for natriuretic peptides have been developed, arguably the most experience exists with determination of BNP levels. Measurement of plasma BNP is recommended when the diagnosis based on history and physical examination remains uncertain. The introduction of a rapid, point-of-care assay method of measuring BNP levels has facilitated the use of this test in the emergency department and outpatient setting. The Breathing Not Properly (BNP) study was a prospective study of 1,586 patients who came to the emergency department with complaints of acute dyspnea (22) and who had a BNP level drawn on presentation. It was reported that BNP levels greater than 100 pg/mL were diagnostic of HF with a sensitivity of 90%, a specificity of 76%, and a predictive accuracy of 83%. The BNP test is best utilized when integrated into the entire clinical evaluation. Relying on a single BNP measurement to diagnose ADHF, in the absence of a thoughtful and complete clinical evaluation, should be discouraged. BNP levels can vary with age (increased) and sex (higher in women) and can be elevated in renal insufficiency, which is most likely the result of decreased clearance. Morbid obesity can also affect interpretation of the BNP level, resulting in a falsely low level. Because of the high negative predictive value of this test, we have found the BNP test to be most helpful when the results are low (<100 pg/mL) in a dyspneic patient in whom the cause of the problem is uncertain. In this setting, ADHF as a cause of dyspnea can be excluded with a high degree of certainty. Figure 86.4 incorporates the BNP test into a diagnostic algorithm for the patient presenting with dyspnea.

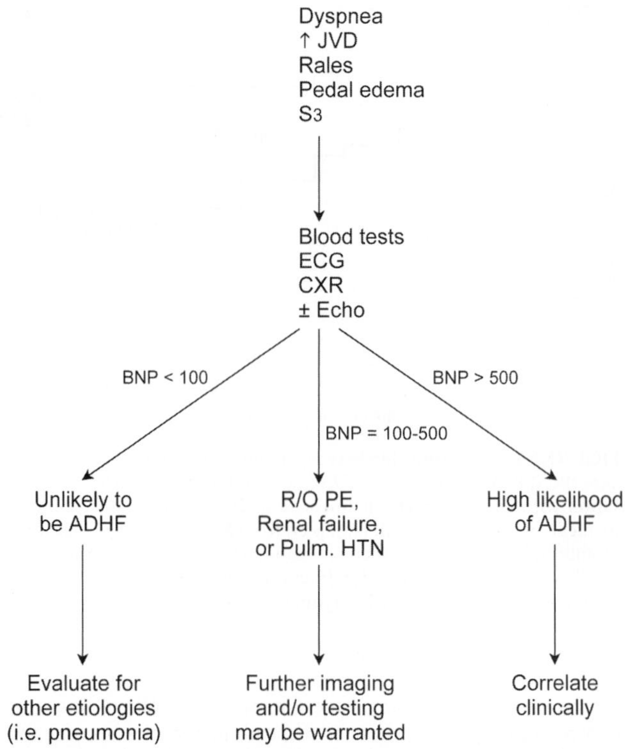

FIGURE 86.4. Ladder diagram for clinical stratification according to brain natriuretic peptide (BNP) levels. Emphasis should be placed on the history and physical examination, along with correlation with the appropriate diagnostic testing. ADHF, acutely decompensated heart failure; CXR, chest radiograph; ECG, electrocardiogram; Echo, echocardiogram; HTN, hypertension; JVD, jugular venous distention; PE, pulmonary embolism; R/O, rule out.

A chest radiograph (CXR) provides a rapid method of visualization of the heart as well the lung spaces. The presence of cardiomegaly and/or infiltrative processes in the lung fields can help better direct the clinician toward a pulmonary versus cardiac disorder. In the ADHERE database, 75% of patients admitted with ADHF had radiographic evidence of pulmonary congestion, whereas 25% had no such finding, again reinforcing the poor predictive value of a single test such as a CXR for diagnosing ADHF.

An electrocardiogram should be done to evaluate for any underlying ischemic event. Rhythm disorders such as atrial fibrillation and complete heart block can result in the signs and symptoms of ADHF. Identification of pacemaker dysfunction may also be important, particularly in the current era of cardiac resynchronization and biventricular pacing therapy for HF.

Echocardiography is an excellent tool for evaluating certain parameters including wall motion abnormalities, valvular function, and the presence of myocardial infiltrative processes. Ejection fraction and left ventricular dimensions determined from an echocardiogram have prognostic implications. All patients who have a new diagnosis of HF should have an echocardiogram as part of their initial workup. If a patient with a history of chronic HF presents with an episode of acute decompensation, we believe that another echocardiogram should be performed at the clinician's discretion.

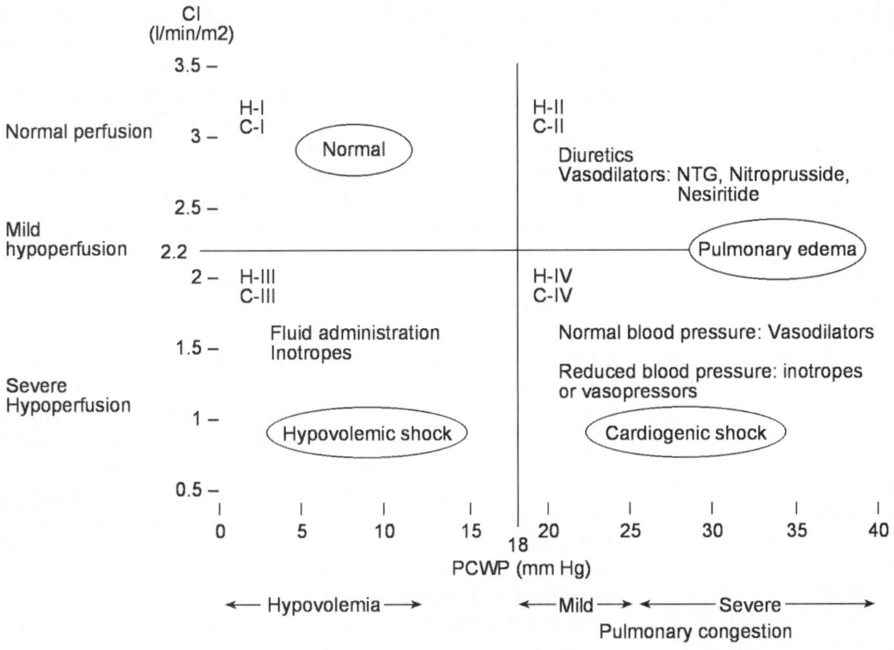

FIGURE 86.5. Four-square diagram of hemodynamic assessment of patients with heart failure (Forrester classification). H-I to H-IV refers to hemodynamic severity, with cardiac index (CI) and pulmonary capillary wedge pressure (PCWP) shown on the vertical and horizontal axes, respectively. C-I to C-IV refers to clinical severity. NTG, nitroglycerin. (Adapted from Forrester JS, Diamond GA, Swan HJ. Correlative classification of clinical and hemodynamic function after acute myocardial infarction. *Am J Cardiol* 1977;39:137–145.)

CLASSIFICATION OF HEMODYNAMIC PROFILE

Following the initial clinical evaluation of the patient with ADHF, a decision must be made regarding the therapeutic approach. Those patients with evidence of myocardial ischemia, significant volume overload, severe symptoms of dyspnea, significant renal insufficiency, hypotension, or other major comorbid conditions complicating their HF syndrome should be hospitalized for aggressive vasoactive and diuretic therapy. In some cases when symptoms and volume excess are mild, the patient may be treated in the emergency department or observation unit with close follow-up in the outpatient setting. The use of a "four-square" model (Fig. 86.5) can help to identify specific hemodynamic profiles in the patient with ADHF quickly and can aid the clinician in instituting therapy expeditiously. This diagram, initially proposed by Forrester et al. in 1977 for the clinical assessment of patients after myocardial infarction, was modified in 1999 by Lynne Warner Stevenson, now of the Brigham and Women's Hospital and Harvard University in Boston, to characterize patients admitted with ADHF better and to facilitate communication regarding prognosis and therapies for ADHF (23) (Fig. 86.6). Most patients admitted with ADHF are in profile B ("wet and warm"), whereas a much smaller number is in profile C ("wet and cold"). Hemodynamic profile L ("cold and dry") is rare and typically results from overdiuresis of a profile C patient. The prognosis is better for a profile B patient compared with profile C; the prognosis for profile L patients is unknown, but it is probably better than for profile C. Patients admitted with dyspnea who are subsequently found to have normal filling pressures (not congested) and a normal cardiac output are in profile A ("warm and dry"), which is the hemodynamic goal for all patients. In profile A patients who are hospitalized for dyspnea or edema, symptoms may be caused by conditions other than chronic HF, such as chronic pulmonary disease, arrhythmia, or transient ischemia associated with valvular dysfunction (24). The ability to determine the appropriate hemodynamic profile for any patient with ADHF is based on an accurate initial evaluation, as previously outlined.

PHARMACOTHERAPEUTICS

Goal of Acute Pharmacologic Therapy

The objectives of the pharmacologic management of ADHF are to relieve disabling symptoms and discomfort rapidly, to reverse hemodynamic derangement, to preserve myocardial blood flow and energetics, to prevent end-organ dysfunction, and to stabilize the patient while further definitive diagnostic evaluation and therapy are pursued (Table 86.5). Of course, keeping the patient alive during the hospital admission is paramount, but, as noted previously, most patients succumb to HF in a nonacute hospital setting. Acute intravenous therapy is directed toward improving overall ventricular performance by favorably affecting the major determinants of ventricular function, including ventricular preload, afterload, and myocardial

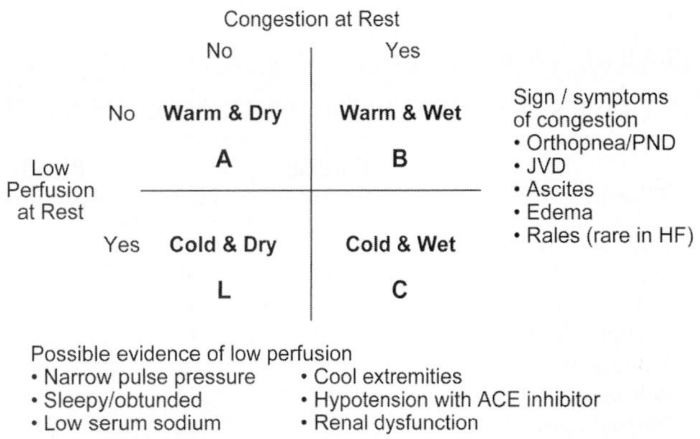

FIGURE 86.6. Modified four-square diagram of hemodynamic assessment of patients with heart failure (HF). This diagram emphasizes the bedside presentation of patients with acutely decompensated HF. ACE, angiotensin-converting enzyme; JVD, jugular venous distention; PND, paroxysmal nocturnal dyspnea. (Adapted from Stevenson LW. Tailored therapy to hemodynamic goals for advanced heart failure. *Eur J Heart Fail* 1999;1:251–257.)

TABLE 86.5

GOALS FOR PATIENTS HOSPITALIZED WITH HEART FAILURE

Relieve symptoms rapidly
Reverse hemodynamic abnormalities
Prevent end-organ dysfunction
Initiate patient education and survival-enhancing medications before discharge
Optimize survival-enhancing oral medications (angiotensin-converting enzyme inhibitor, β-blocker, aldosterone receptor antagonist)
Optimize patient education and heart failure management

contractility. As discussed previously, the ability to reduce pulmonary congestion and left ventricular filling pressure in the acute setting has important prognostic implications and is a major goal of ADHF therapy. Dyspnea in this setting, after all, is clearly related to elevated left ventricular end-diastolic pressure and pulmonary hypertension. The medications commonly used to accomplish this goal are generally administered intravenously, exhibit pharmacokinetic properties that allow for rapid titration to hemodynamic effect, and have a relatively short plasma half-life, so any untoward effect can be quickly terminated (Table 86.6). The medications commonly used to initially treat the ADHF patient are discussed in detail.

Acute Vasodilator Therapy

Nitroglycerin

Nitroglycerin is often utilized in the early management of ADHF for patients fitting the warm and wet hemodynamic profile (profile B). The major hemodynamic effect of nitrates is to evoke a reduction in ventricular filling pressure and volume by increasing venous capacitance through venodilation (25–35). This shifts central blood volume to the venous capacitance vessels, which decreases pulmonary congestion and improves the symptoms of breathlessness associated with ADHF and elevated ventricular filling pressures. This vasodilating action is mediated through relaxation of vascular smooth muscle resulting primarily from a nitrate-induced production of *S*-nitrosothiols, which cause an increase in intracellular cyclic guanosine monophosphate (cGMP) (36,37). Nitrates may also elicit vasodilation by other mechanisms, including stimulation of the endothelial production and release of prostacyclin or prostaglandin E (38–40). Although these agents are predominantly considered for venodilation, higher doses of nitrates produce arterial dilatation and therefore reduce systemic vascular resistance (SVR) and ventricular impedance, particularly in the setting of systemic vasoconstriction (41).

Nitrates are generally effective in improving dyspnea in patients with ADHF, and therapy can be instituted rapidly when it is evident that pulmonary congestion is present and requires preload reduction. Intravenous nitroglycerin is the preparation most commonly used. However, sublingual tablets and a lingual-buccal spray may occasionally be used until an intravenous preparation is available to be infused (42,43). Intravenous nitroglycerin (typically starting at a dose of 0.2 μg/kg per minute) may be rapidly titrated upward in increments of 0.1 to 0.2 μg/kg per minute to improve symptoms and to reduce pulmonary and systemic venous pressures and resistance, ventricular filling pressures, and, to a variable degree, SVR. The ability of nitrates to augment stroke volume and cardiac output by decreasing left ventricular afterload is often dose dependent and usually requires an initial intravenous dose of at least 0.4 μg/kg per minute (27). Interestingly, the only major randomized controlled trial to date assessing the efficacy of nitroglycerin for use in ADHF was the Vasodilation in the Management of Acute Congestive Heart Failure (VMAC) trial, which showed that nitroglycerin was less effective than nesiritide and not different than placebo in improving a number of clinical and hemodynamic parameters (44) (see the later discussion of nesiritide).

One must also consider the propensity for the development of pharmacodynamic tolerance during continuous intravenous infusions, which necessitates an intermittent increase in dose to maintain the desired hemodynamic effect (45,46). In the VMAC trial, those patients who underwent hemodynamic monitoring with a pulmonary artery catheter received higher doses of nitroglycerin than patients in whom hemodynamics were estimated clinically. In those monitored with a pulmonary artery catheter, there was a progressive escalation of nitroglycerin dose to achieve favorable hemodynamics over time. Another problem with infusion of nitroglycerin intravenously is that polyvinyl chloride tubing and solution bags adsorb the drug. These observations suggest that the development of nitrate tolerance and the need to escalate dosing are critical issues, and these problems may go unrecognized in the clinical setting when invasive monitoring is not utilized (44).

TABLE 86.6

INTRAVENOUS AGENTS FOR ACUTE DECOMPENSATED HEART FAILURE

Therapy	Cardiac output	PCWP	Blood pressure	Heart rate	Arrhythmia	Shorter onset	Longer offset
Dopamine (μg/kg/min)							
Low (<3)	↔	↔	↔	↔	↔	+++	0
Moderate (3–7)	↑	↔	↑	↑	↑↑	+++	0
High (7–15)	↑↑	↔	↑↑	↑↑	↑↑↑	+++	0
Dobutamine	↑↑↑	↓	↔	↑	↑↑	+++	0
Milrinone	↑↑	↓↓	↓	↑	↑↑	+	++
Nitroglycerin	↑	↓↓	↓↓	↔	↔	+++	0
Nesiritide	↑	↓↓	↓↓	↔	↔	++	++
Nitroprusside	↑	↓↓	↓↓↓	↔	↔	++++	0
Levosimendan[a]	↑↑	↓↓	↓	↑	↔	+++	+++ (metabolites)

PCWP, pulmonary capillary wedge pressure. ↑, increased; ↓, decreased; ↔; no change; +, more profound effect; 0, normal offset.
[a]Investigational.

Nitroprusside

Sodium nitroprusside is a powerful venous and arterial vasodilator with potent afterload-reducing properties (47). Nitroprusside relaxes arterial and venous smooth muscle via the production of nitric oxide and nitrosothiols, leading to an increase in cGMP and smooth muscle relaxation (29). As with nitroglycerin, nitroprusside causes preload reduction by diminishing heightened venous tone and increasing venous capacitance with a concomitant shift in central blood volume to the periphery (30). This causes a reduction in right ventricular pressure and volume. More relevant to nitroprusside is its rapid and powerful effect on afterload. This agent reduces the major components of aortic impedance (mean and hydraulic vascular load), and the results are improved and often dramatic increases in forward stroke volume and cardiac output with reductions in left ventricular filling pressure, volume, and valvular regurgitation (25,27,30,48–51). Fortunately, this decrease in afterload occurs without major changes in aortic pressure (49). This characteristic of nitroprusside enhances its efficacy in patients fitting the wet and cold profile (profile C) when the reduction in stroke volume is secondary to a high SVR.

In most patients with ADHF, judicious titration of nitroprusside can result in decreased aortic impedance, increased cardiac output, and reduced ventricular filling pressures without the undesirable effects of a decrease in systemic blood pressure or rise in heart rate. Unlike nitroglycerin, nitroprusside may cause "coronary steal" whereby arteriolar dilatation in nonischemic zones diverts coronary flow away from areas of ischemia (52,53). The frequency with which this occurs in HF is not well documented.

Nitroprusside is administered intravenously with an infusion pump and is usually initiated at a dose of 0.10 to 0.20 μg/kg per minute. Its effects are evident within 60 to 90 seconds after initiation of the infusion, and should an adverse effect such as symptomatic hypotension occur, the vasodilating properties usually abate within 20 to 30 minutes after discontinuation (25). In ADHF, insertion of an arterial catheter for continuous systemic blood pressure recording and monitoring and for frequent blood gas determinations is often recommended. One should recognize, however, that during nitroprusside infusion, the pressure measured in a peripheral artery (i.e., radial artery) may not reflect a reduction in central aortic pressure because of nitroprusside-induced changes in the amplitude and timing of reflected waves within the central aorta (54). One must remain cognizant of this when the clinical findings are consistent with systemic hypoperfusion despite a seemingly acceptable peripheral arterial pressure.

Nitroprusside can be rapidly titrated to achieve the desired clinical and hemodynamic end points, including a reduction in pulmonary capillary wedge pressure (PCWP) to 18 to 20 mm Hg, a decrease in SVR to 1,000 to 1,200 dynes/cm^5 per second, a reduction in valvular regurgitation, and an improvement in stroke volume, cardiac output, and systemic perfusion, while avoiding significant hypotension and tachycardia (Fig. 86.7). In ADHF, particularly when myocardial ischemia is present,

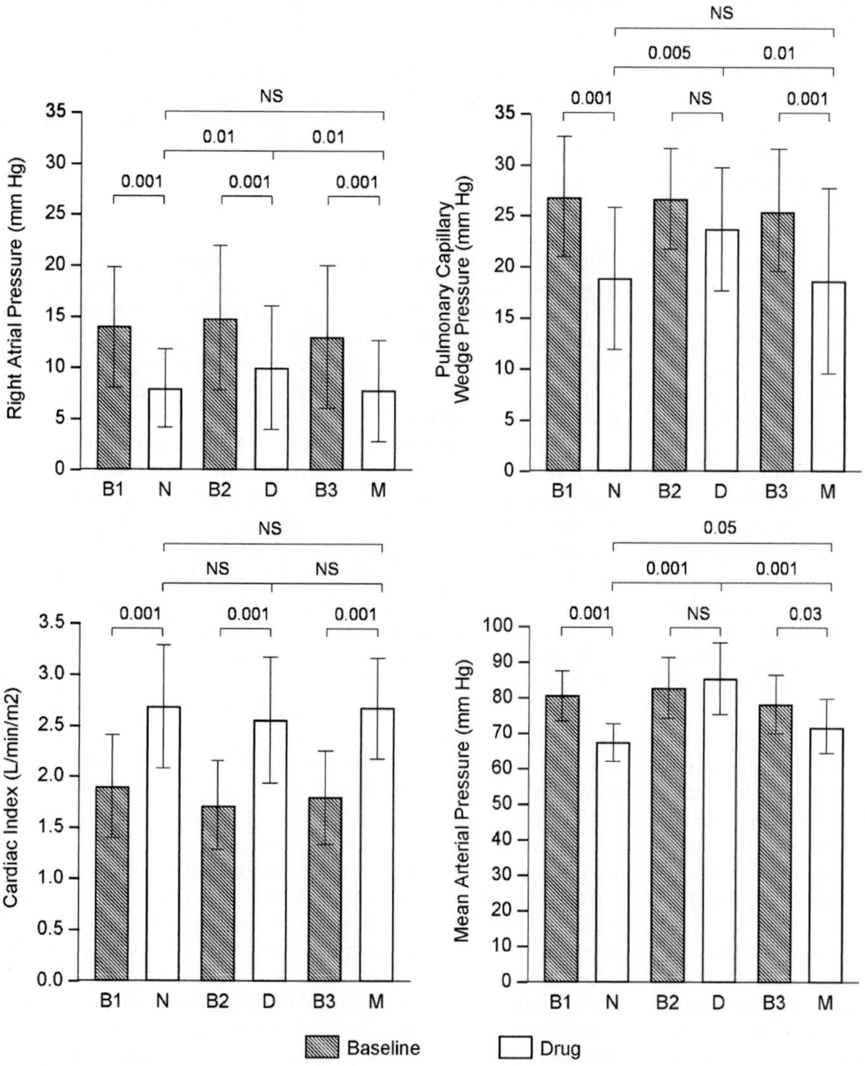

FIGURE 86.7. Effects of sodium nitroprusside (N), dobutamine hydrochloride (D), and milrinone lactate (M) on right atrial pressure, pulmonary capillary wedge pressure, cardiac index, and mean arterial pressure in patients with severe heart failure (B1, B2, and B3 represent baseline measurements). At dosages evoking a similar increase in cardiac index, all agents significantly reduced right atrial pressure, with nitroprusside and milrinone also producing a significant reduction in mean arterial pressure compared with baseline. The effect of milrinone and nitroprusside on pulmonary capillary wedge pressure was greater than that observed with dobutamine. NS, not significant. (Adapted from Monrad ES, Baim DS, Smith HS, et al. Milrinone, dobutamine, and nitroprusside: comparative effects on hemodynamics and myocardial energetics in patients with severe congestive heart failure. *Circulation* 1986;73[suppl III]:III168–III174.)

attention to Starling mechanisms with respect to preload and augmentation of stroke volume remains important. Although nitroprusside is titrated to achieve hemodynamic goals, rarely are doses greater than 4 to 5 μg/kg per minute required to maintain adequate vasodilation in the acute HF setting, and doses this high for prolonged periods (>72 hours) should generally be avoided because of the risk of thiocyanate and cyanide toxicity (55,56).

The most common serious adverse effect of nitroprusside administration in ADHF is systemic hypotension (47,53,57). One should be particularly cautious when initiating nitroprusside therapy in a patient with ischemia or infarction and a systolic arterial pressure of less than 100 mm Hg. An increase in heart rate during the infusion is an ominous finding and usually presages hypotension. This typically occurs when stroke volume has not increased appropriately, often because of ongoing or worsening ischemia, valvular regurgitation, and inadequate cardiac reserve. A reduction or cessation of the nitroprusside infusion is usually warranted. Alternatively, the addition of a positive inotropic agent such as dobutamine is often advantageous and may allow for the continuation of nitroprusside. Such a combination is commonly used to stabilize patients with particularly severe, low-output HF (stage D) until more definitive therapy can be instituted. When systemic hypotension and poor peripheral perfusion are present at the outset, nitroprusside should generally be avoided as initial treatment.

As noted earlier, thiocyanate toxicity is a potentially serious side effect of prolonged nitroprusside infusion and is manifested clinically by nausea, disorientation, psychosis, muscle spasm, and hyperreflexia when plasma thiocyanate concentrations exceed 6 mg/dL (56,57). Such toxicity is uncommon in the management of ADHF in which nitroprusside therapy is usually a temporary means of support while the patient awaits definitive therapy. Cyanide toxicity is extremely rare in HF management and occurs only during prolonged high-dose infusion, usually in the setting of significant hepatic dysfunction.

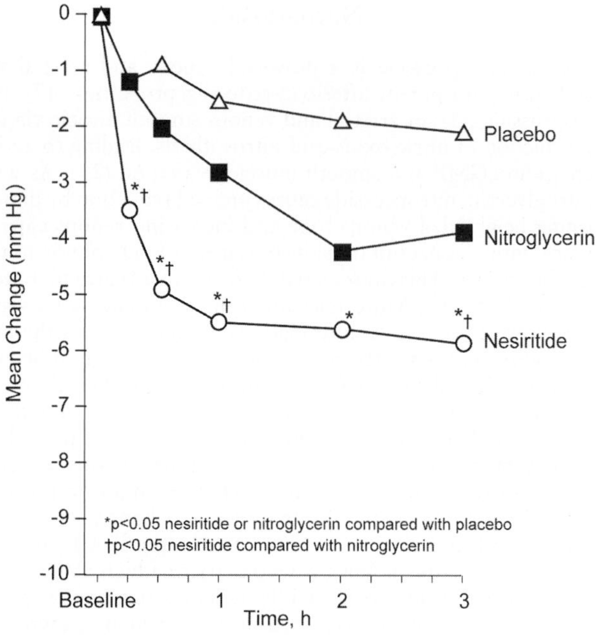

No of Patients						
Nitroglycerin	60	58	58	58	56	59
Nesiritide	124	121	122	121	118	121
Placebo	62	62	62	62	61	62

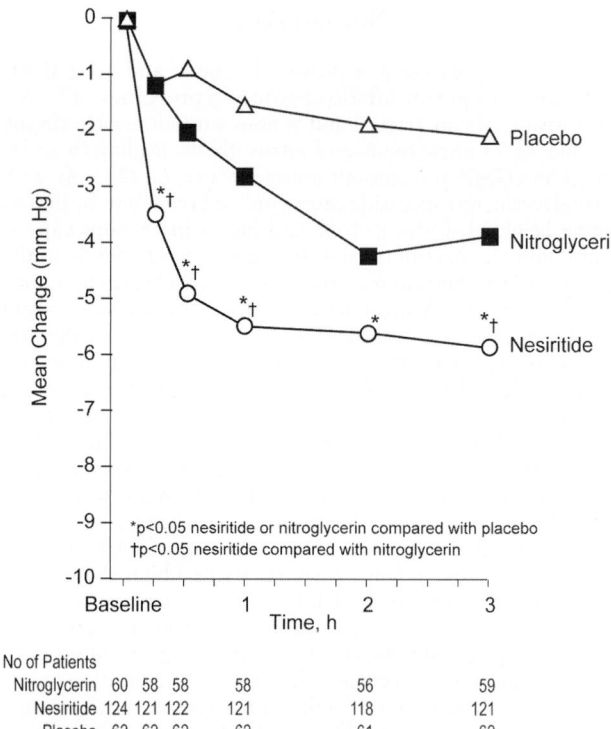

FIGURE 86.8. Three-hour changes from baseline pulmonary capillary wedge pressures (PCWP) in patients treated with intravenous therapies: nesiritide versus nitroglycerin versus placebo. Nesiritide produced a greater decrease in PCWP than nitroglycerin or placebo at 3 hours. (Adapted from the Publication committee for the VMAC investigators. Intravenous nesiritide versus nitroglycerin for treatment of decompensated congestive heart failure. *JAMA* 2002;287:1531–1540.)

Nesiritide

Nesiritide is the recombinant form of BNP and is the newest vasodilator approved for treatment of ADHF. Nesiritide is thought to function in a fashion similar to that of endogenous BNP by binding to the guanylate cyclase receptors of vascular smooth muscle and endothelial cells that activate the intracellular secondary messenger cGMP (58). This activation results in smooth muscle relaxation and in both venous and arterial dilation. In patients with HF, nesiritide has been shown to have modest effects on renal excretion of salt and water (59).

Nesiritide is administered intravenously, usually as a bolus of 2 μg/kg intravenously, followed by a continuous infusion of 0.01 μg/kg per minute. The half-life of nesiritide is approximately 18 minutes, and its side effects are primarily related to the vasodilatory properties, resulting in hypotension. Nesiritide has not been shown to cause tachyphylaxis, nor does it have toxic metabolites. In addition, nesiritide has not been demonstrated to be proarrhythmic (60).

Nesiritide has been shown to be effective in patients with ADHF by evoking a vasodilatory response that rapidly lowers ventricular filling pressures and relieves dyspnea. In one randomized controlled trial of patients hospitalized with ADHF, nesiritide caused significant dose-dependent decreases in right atrial pressure, PCWP, and SVR while increasing stroke volume (61). These favorable hemodynamic changes were associated with an improvement in HF symptoms.

The clinical effects of nesiritide compared with placebo or nitroglycerin in 498 patients with ADHF were studied in the VMAC trial (44). Patients who had a pulmonary artery catheter placed (which was determined by the investigator's discretion) were randomized to a 3-hour placebo-controlled period, in which they received either fixed-dose nesiritide, adjustable-dose nesiritide, placebo, or nitroglycerin. After 3 hours, the placebo group was crossed over to a predetermined treatment of nitroglycerin or fixed-dose nesiritide. Patients who did not have a pulmonary artery catheter underwent a similar 3-hour placebo-controlled period but without receiving the adjustable-dose nesiritide option.

The primary end points, change in PCWP and level of dyspnea, were assessed in both groups. Nesiritide decreased PCWP and improved dyspnea more rapidly and to a greater extent relative to both nitroglycerin and placebo (PCWP: −5.8 mm Hg versus −3.8 and −2 mm Hg, respectively). Interestingly, the effect of nitroglycerin on PCWP was not statistically different than that of placebo (Fig. 86.8). Nesiritide-treated patients had less acute adverse events when compared with those treated with nitroglycerin, the most common event being headache (8% in nesiritide versus 20% in nitroglycerin). The length of hospital stay for the patients receiving nesiritide, however, was longer than for those patients receiving nitroglycerin, although this was not a specified end point (10.0 ± 8.4 versus 8.1 ± 7.0 days, respectively) (44,62).

The potential for adverse effects of nesiritide on patient survival have been raised. Recently, a report suggested a nonstatistically significant increase in 30-day mortality when nesiritide therapy was compared with intravenous nitrate or placebo infusion (63). This opinion arose from a metaanalysis of three selected trials. Additional analysis of the VMAC trial in this report also pointed to an increased rate of death at 30 days for patients receiving nesiritide (8.6%) when compared with control groups (5.5%), although a nonsignificant difference in mortality between the nitroglycerin and nesiritide groups was

TABLE 86.7

EFFECT OF NESIRITIDE ON DEVELOPMENT OF WORSENING RENAL FUNCTION IN PATIENTS WITH ACUTELY DECOMPENSATED HEART FAILURE

	Events, n/N (%)		RR_{MH} (95% confidence interval)	*p*
	Nesiritide[a]	Control		
Nesiritide ≤0.03 vs non-inotrope based controls	134/610 (22)	60/389 (15)	1.52 (1.16–2.00)	.003
Nesiritide ≤0.03 vs all control therapies, including inotropes	163/772 (21)	69/472 (15)	1.54 (1.19–1.98)	.001
Nesiritide ≤0.015 vs non-inotrope based controls	100/442 (23)	60/389 (15)	1.46 (1.09–1.95)	.012
Nesiritide ≤0.015 vs all control therapies, including inotropes	99/464 (21)	69/472 (15)	1.47 (1.12–1.93)	.006
Nesiritide ≤0.06 vs non-inotrope based controls	140/635 (22)	60/389 (15)	1.53 (1.16–2.00)	.002
Nesiritide ≤0.06 vs all control therapies, including inotropes	169/797 (21)	69/472 (15)	1.54 (1.20–1.99)	.001

[a]Nesiritide doses refer to infusion rates (μg/kg/min) that followed bolus administration.
Adapted from Sockner-Bernstein JD, Skopicki HA, Aaronson KD. Risk of worsening renal function with nesiritide in patients with acutely decompensated heart failure. *Circulation* 2005;111:1487–1491.

found at 6 months (20.8% versus 25.1% respectively; $p = .32$) (44,63). Although this analysis has limitations, including qualitative heterogeneity among patient cohorts and the inability to control for background treatment with inotropes, the observations that were identified merit further inquiry.

In an additional analysis, nesiritide therapy was also associated with a dose-related increase in the risk of worsening renal function (64) (Table 86.7). This analysis was drawn from five randomized trials that included 1,269 patients, although it was not restricted to patients receiving nesiritide at the recommended dose. Although it was limited in certain ways, this analysis did provide some insight into potential cardiorenal interactions with nesiritide use. Significant increases in serum creatinine (defined as by >0.5 mg/dL) with nesiritide use were found when compared with the control groups. In some analyses, this effect was most notable as the dose increased. Given the negative prognosis of concomitant renal and cardiac disease, further evaluation of nesiritide's effect, both short- and long-term, on renal function is warranted.

Nesiritide is effective in acutely improving symptoms when it is used in patients with ADHF who are admitted to the hospital for dyspnea at rest or with minimal activity who have clinical evidence of volume overload (a left ventricular filling pressure estimated or measured to be ≥20 mm Hg) with a systolic blood pressure greater than 90 mm Hg. In this population, nesiritide infusion can be expected to quickly and significantly reduce PCWP and to improve dyspnea with fewer side effects than intravenous nitroglycerin and inotropes. It seems prudent at the present time, however, that nesiritide *not* be used to replace diuretics, to enhance diuresis, for intermittent outpatient infusion, for scheduled repetitive use, or to improve renal function or in patients presenting with clinical difficulties in whom excessive vasodilation could lead to complications (acute coronary syndromes, critical aortic stenosis, and significant renal artery stenosis). Furthermore, the recommended bolus dose for nesiritide is 2 μg/kg administered intravenously over 60 seconds and followed by an infusion of 0.01 μg/kg per minute. As was done in the clinical trials of this drug, appropriate patient monitoring, particularly of blood pressure, renal function, and urine output, is critical. Given the recent data concerning the safety of nesiritide and its possible adverse effects on renal function and mortality, larger, randomized trials directly focusing on these issues are currently under way.

Positive Inotropic Therapy

The use of routine or rudimentary inotropic support to enhance myocardial contractility in ADHF should generally be discouraged. Basically, inotropic therapy is contraindicated for routine management of the patient with ADHF who has a hemodynamic profile of warm and wet (profile B) because of documented adverse effects on myocardial function, remodeling, and arrhythmia potential. There are, however, specific situations in which positive inotropic treatment may be necessary to support a patient until more definitive therapy can be applied. The inotropes discussed in the following subsections are beneficial in the support of a hypotensive patient until the cause can be elucidated. Inotropic therapy is often utilized to improve cardiac output and renal blood flow when diuretic resistance and refractory volume overload ensue (cardiorenal syndrome) (24). Certainly, inotropic support is used commonly to bridge patients with advanced HF to either cardiac transplantation or mechanical support. Generally, the therapy discussed here is reserved for the ACC/AHA stage D patient who has a hemodynamic profile of cold and wet (profile C).

Dobutamine

Dobutamine hydrochloride is a synthetic catecholamine and positive inotropic agent that is useful in the management of ADHF when systemic hypoperfusion is evident. Along with intravenous diuretics, it is used commonly in patients with ADHF or myocardial infarction who present with pulmonary congestion and low cardiac output symptoms. Dobutamine exists as a racemic mixture of dextroisomers and levoisomers, which are potent β- and α-adrenergic agonists, respectively (65). Therefore, dobutamine produces its positive inotropic effect via stimulation of myocardial β_1 and probably α_1 receptors (66). Theoretically, the opposing forces of α_1 and β_2 stimulation on the peripheral vasculature should result in a negligible change in vascular resistance.

The safety of inotropic therapy in patients with occlusive CAD and active myocardial ischemia is of great concern and is often unpredictable. Although the positive inotropic effect of dobutamine increases mixed venous oxygen saturation (MVO_2), which could be detrimental in acute ischemia or infarction, this is balanced by other factors that decrease MVO_2 and improve coronary blood flow and myocardial perfusion (67). Dobutamine, when carefully administered to the patient with HF, systemic hypoperfusion, and elevated filling pressures, reduces MVO_2 by decreasing ventricular volume and wall tension. Dobutamine may increase coronary blood flow by increasing coronary perfusion pressure (increase in arterial diastolic pressure and decrease in ventricular diastolic pressure) and coronary perfusion time and possibly by causing mild coronary vasodilation (67–70). These factors tend to offset any increase in MVO_2 evoked by positive inotropy. Avoiding significant increases in heart rate during dobutamine infusion is imperative, however, because this would serve to increase MVO_2 and reduce coronary perfusion time (67). Also, dobutamine administration should be avoided when ventricular filling pressures are not significantly elevated. Therefore, the titration of dobutamine dosage in the patient with occlusive CAD mandates careful attention to multiple parameters, including heart rate, central hemodynamics, presence of arrhythmias, and clinical signs of improved systemic perfusion.

In ADHF, dobutamine therapy is usually initiated when an augmentation in cardiac output and systemic perfusion is desired in patients with elevated filling pressures. The infusion is started at 2.5 to 5.0 μg/kg per minute and is titrated in increments of 1 to 2 μg/kg per minute at 20- to 30-minute intervals until the desired clinical and hemodynamic response is attained. Rarely is it necessary to exceed a dose of 15 μg/kg per minute in treating ADHF, although doses this high are sometimes necessary for a brief time while more definitive therapy is pursued.

The pharmacokinetic profile of dobutamine makes this agent ideal for the critical care setting. It has an extremely short half-life (<5 minutes), and a full pharmacodynamic response to a particular dose and its steady-state phase is attained within 10 to 15 minutes (71). Importantly, any adverse effect of dobutamine is also eliminated within only 10 to 15 minutes of stopping the infusion. Additional side effects that may occur during dobutamine infusion include headache, anxiety, and tremor. Dobutamine must also be used cautiously in patients with an atrial arrhythmia such as atrial fibrillation or atrial flutter. Dobutamine has been reported to increase atrioventricular conduction in atrial fibrillation (72). Because of the excessive dosing required to achieve hemodynamic benefit in patients who are receiving long-term β-blocker therapy, dobutamine should generally not be used for inotropic support in these patients (Table 86.8), as discussed in the following section.

Milrinone

Milrinone lactate, a bipyridine analog of amrinone, is a second-generation phosphodiesterase inhibitor that exhibits both direct inotropic and vasodilator properties (67,71,73). Milrinone is approved for parenteral use in the treatment of congestive HF. The parent compound, amrinone, has largely been supplanted by milrinone because of its substantial side effect profile, including significant thrombocytopenia during more prolonged infusions.

TABLE 86.8

HEMODYNAMIC EFFECT OF MILRINONE COMPARED WITH DOBUTAMINE IN PATIENTS TREATED WITH CARVEDILOL

Parameter	Milrinone	Dobutamine
Cardiac index	↑	↑
Heart rate	→	↑
Mean arterial pressure	↓	↑
Pulmonary capillary wedge pressure	↓	→
Mean pulmonary artery pressure	↓	↑
Left ventricular stroke work, index	↑	↑↑
Left ventricular stroke volume, index	↑	→

Adapted from Bristow MR. Enhancing contractile function pharmacologically may improve natural history of heart failure. *Cardiol Rev* 2000;17(suppl):3.

Through inhibition of the phosphodiesterase III isoenzyme located primarily in cardiomyocytes and vascular smooth muscle, milrinone increases the concentration of cyclic adenosine monophosphate (cAMP) in these tissues. Elevated cAMP levels, via phosphorylation of several cellular proteins, increase intracellular calcium, which is the final common pathway to enhanced inotropy and vasodilatation. Although dobutamine and milrinone exert their effects through the cAMP-dependent pathway, important differences are found. Dobutamine actually increases cAMP production via β-receptor activation, whereas milrinone raises cAMP levels by preventing its degradation. This mechanistic difference is important with respect to the potential for both drugs to act synergistically to enhance myocardial contractility in patients with HF (74).

The acute hemodynamic effects of milrinone in patients with chronic HF have been well described (75–79). The hemodynamic profile is one that would be expected from a drug with potent inotropic and balanced vasodilator properties. Once therapeutic plasma levels are achieved, milrinone elicits a reduction in right and left ventricular filling pressures and increases cardiac output without producing significant changes in the heart rate–blood pressure product. Because of its potent vasodilator properties, however, milrinone has the potential to worsen preexisting systemic hypotension. A reduction in pulmonary vascular resistance is usually observed and is mostly secondary to the reduction in left ventricular filling pressure rather than a direct pulmonary vasodilator effect. Even though milrinone may be expected to increase MVO_2 via its direct positive inotropic effect, its substantial vasodilator properties usually offset any detrimental increase in MVO_2 (77). This favorable effect is further enhanced by mild coronary vasodilatation (80). Compared with dobutamine, milrinone tends to evoke a greater reduction in left ventricular filling pressure and SVR while producing an equivalent increase in cardiac output (78). For the same reduction in SVR, milrinone produces a greater increase in stroke work index than nitroprusside, which reflects its additional inotropic properties (78,79).

Based on its hemodynamic profile in HF, milrinone would appear to be advantageous in the treatment of the patient with acute pulmonary congestion and low cardiac output. Unfortunately, the pharmacokinetic properties of milrinone may make it less desirable as a short-term, first-line therapy in some patients. Milrinone has a long half-life (20 to 45 minutes) compared with other vasoactive agents (67,71). To achieve a therapeutic plasma level rapidly, a bolus administration of 50 μg/kg is given over a 10-minute period followed by a constant infusion at a rate of 0.375 to 0.750 μg/kg per minute. This requirement for an initial bolus or high infusion rate to elicit a significant inotropic response places the unstable patient at greater risk for hypotension. The elimination half-life of 1.7 hours is also much longer than that of other vasoactive agents, and more time would be required to eliminate the drug should an undesirable side effect occur (71).

The results of the Outcomes of a Prospective Trial of Intravenous Milrinone for Exacerbations of Chronic Heart Failure (OPTIME-CHF) trial provide additional insight concerning the clinical utility of milrinone in ADHF (81). This was a prospective, randomized, double-blind, placebo-controlled trial in which 949 patients admitted to the hospital for ADHF with systolic dysfunction and a warm and wet hemodynamic profile (profile B) were treated with either a 48- to 72-hour infusion of milrinone or saline placebo and were followed for 60 days. The results revealed that the median number of days hospitalized for cardiovascular causes within 60 days after the start of the study did not differ significantly between the milrinone and placebo groups (6 days versus 7 days, respectively; $p = .71$), nor did the rates of in-hospital mortality (3.8% versus

2.3%; $p = .19$) or 60-day mortality (10.3% versus 8.9%; $p = .92$). Importantly, the milrinone group had significantly higher rates of hypotension and new atrial arrhythmias when compared with placebo. A post hoc analysis of this trial by Felker et al. (82) revealed that patients in the milrinone group whose HF had an ischemic origin tended to have worse outcomes than those treated with placebo in terms of the primary end point (13.6 days for milrinone versus 12.4 days for placebo; $p = .055$) and the composite of death or rehospitalization (42% versus 36%; $p = .01$). The results from OPTIME-CHF confirm that inotropic therapy should not be routinely utilized in ADHF, but it should be reserved only for those patients with persistent hypotension and systemic hypoperfusion.

When inotropic therapy must be used in ADHF, the growing numbers of patients receiving long-term β-blocker therapy will likely affect the selection of the appropriate agent. β-Blockers have been shown to improve survival dramatically in chronic HF and to play an integral role in the pharmacotherapy of this condition. Therefore, patients presenting with acute decompensation are increasingly likely to be receiving some form of long-term β-blocker treatment. If inotropic support is necessary, milrinone should be considered, given that it acts beyond the level of the β-receptor and its inotropic effect is not altered by β-receptor blockade (83,84). Depending on the degree of decompensation and hemodynamic compromise, the dose of β-blocker should generally remain unchanged or be gradually reduced during institution of inotropic support. If prolonged inotropic support is likely to be necessary or an inadequate hemodynamic response is observed, then the β-blocker should be stopped.

Vasopressor Therapy

Vasopressor therapy should generally be avoided in the typical patient with ADHF. The only indication for these agents in patients with HF is to support blood pressure and to maintain organ perfusion in situations of shock or near shock. Extended therapy is rarely successful, and prognosis is extremely poor when vasopressor treatment is required for an extended duration, particularly if the origin of the hemodynamic instability is not identified and is rapidly corrected.

Dopamine

Dopamine hydrochloride is a drug that exhibits complex pharmacologic properties. This agent mediates its effects through either direct activation or indirect activation (via norepinephrine release) of multiple presynaptic and postsynaptic receptors (85,86). Receptors that are activated are extremely sensitive to dopamine concentration, and this contributes further to the complexity of drug administration (86). The positive inotropic and chronotropic effect of dopamine is mediated through activation of postsynaptic myocardial β_1 receptors. This effect is most evident clinically at doses greater than 5 μg/kg per minute. At low doses, the primary effect of dopamine is one of vascular relaxation and sodium excretion by stimulation of specific dopaminergic receptors located postsynaptically on vascular smooth muscle cells (primarily in renal and mesenteric vascular beds) and renal tubular cells (87,88). Dopamine receptors may also be found in cerebral, coronary, skeletal muscle, and cutaneous vessels (85). Low-dose dopamine (0.5 to 2.0 μg/kg per minute) is often used to treat patients with HF and renal insufficiency to activate renal dopaminergic receptors selectively, to induce renal vasodilatation and improve renal blood flow, and to provoke natriuresis (89). As the dopamine dosage is progressively increased to more than 5 μg/kg per minute, postsynaptic α_1 and α_2 receptors are activated, and this mediates vasoconstriction and produces blood pressure elevation.

Dopamine does not stimulate postsynaptic β_2 receptors, so the predominant effect of higher dosing is one of vasoconstriction. On the presynaptic membrane, dopamine activates α_2 and dopaminergic$_2$ receptors, both of which inhibit the release of norepinephrine (90). By another mechanism, however, dopamine directly increases the release of norepinephrine, which further enhances peripheral vasoconstriction via α-adrenergic receptor activation (86,88).

Because dopamine selectively affects multiple receptors in a dose-dependent manner, a variety of hemodynamic effects can be achieved with careful titration (91). In the setting of ADHF, the primary use of dopamine is to elevate systemic blood pressure and to improve renal perfusion through activation of β_1, α, and dopaminergic receptors. In patients with cardiogenic shock and significant hypotension, dopamine is usually the drug of choice and may be used either alone or in combination with dobutamine to elevate blood pressure and to improve systemic and renal perfusion (92,93).

Prolonged use at high doses, however, will ultimately worsen myocardial function because of the increase in aortic impedance and the negative influence of dopamine on ventricular-vascular coupling (94). This is reflected in significant increases in PCWP and systemic blood pressure when dopamine is administered at doses of 5 μg/kg per minute and greater (91). As the dopamine dosage is progressively increased, peripheral vasoconstriction is the predominant clinical feature similar to that seen with norepinephrine infusion. Upward titration of dopamine is usually limited by tachycardia, ischemia, and arrhythmia, particularly in the presence of occlusive CAD. At low to moderate doses, coronary blood flow increases in parallel with increased myocardial work and a mild dopamine-induced coronary vasodilator effect (80,95). At high doses, dopamine further increases MVO_2; however, coronary vascular resistance also increases because of α-mediated vasoconstriction (95).

Norepinephrine and Epinephrine

Norepinephrine is a potent α-adrenergic agonist that also possesses mild β_1-agonist properties. It elicits a cardiovascular vasopressor response through dose-related vasoconstriction (67,96,97). This drug is not used for positive inotropic therapy because any increase in myocardial contractility is offset by increased afterload. During norepinephrine infusion, the combination of high preload and afterload markedly increases MVO_2 to the point at which the ratio of myocardial oxygen demand to supply is threatened (67). Its primary indication in ADHF is to improve blood pressure and coronary perfusion in the setting of shock and persistent hypotension when dopamine and dobutamine are ineffective.

Norepinephrine can be infused starting at a rate of 0.02 to 0.04 μg/kg per minute, and the dose can be advanced every 10 to 15 minutes until the desired blood pressure response is achieved (67). The target blood pressure should be that which is considered minimally acceptable in the individual patient to maintain adequate coronary perfusion and avoid serious side effects. Dopamine or dobutamine may be used in combination with norepinephrine to allow for lower dosing.

Epinephrine, like norepinephrine, is a catecholamine with potent α- and β-agonist properties. Unlike norepinephrine, epinephrine also exhibits mild β_2-agonist properties, which offset some of the α effect and thereby mildly reduce its pressor response in comparison with norepinephrine (98). Epinephrine may be used in intensive care units for hemodynamic support in patients with severe HF and shock. It may be used in conjunction with other catecholamine inotropic and pressor drugs. Infusions of 0.1 to 1.0 μg per minute are commonly used.

The adverse effects seen during norepinephrine and epinephrine infusions are those usually observed with catecholamine administration, including ischemia and serious arrhythmia. Prolonged use may result in problems associated with reduced organ and tissue perfusion. The plasma half-life of these agents is short (<10 minutes), so undesirable pharmacologic effects generally resolve by 10 to 20 minutes after discontinuation of the infusion (67,98). As with high-dose dopamine therapy, the duration of treatment with any potent vasopressor should be as brief as possible, because prolonged use leads to continued myocardial dysfunction, decreased organ perfusion, and metabolic derangement.

Vasopressin

In the critical care setting, some centers advocate the use of vasopressin (antidiuretic hormone) for systemic pressure support when catecholamine infusions have failed to improve hemodynamics or when serious adverse responses to catecholamine infusions have occurred (98). Vasopressin, by activation of vascular smooth muscle V1 receptors, is a potent vasoconstrictor of skeletal muscle vascular beds at high dosages, but importantly, it produces less intense vasoconstriction of the renal and coronary vasculature (98).

Interestingly, vasopressin seems to produce vasodilation of the cerebral vasculature, which results in an improvement in cerebral blood flow during infusions (98–100). This selective vasodilatory response may be mediated by nitric oxide (100). In the absence of direct myocardial stimulation through β-receptor activation, vasopressin may result in lower MVO_2 compared with catecholamines. Also, unlike with catecholamines, the pressor response to vasopressin remains intact during severe metabolic acidosis.

Diuretic Therapy

Intravenous furosemide is the loop diuretic most commonly used to treat the patient presenting with ADHF and pulmonary congestion. The major objective of diuretic therapy in this circumstance is to decrease excessive lung water through natriuresis and diuresis with a reduction in intravascular volume. Intravenous administration is necessary to achieve adequate furosemide levels rapidly at its site of action, the renal tubules.

The most important effect of furosemide in the acute management of HF probably relates to its substantial hemodynamic effects. Although both vasodilatory and vasoconstrictive properties have been attributed to intravenous furosemide (101–104), most data support the view that furosemide evokes a reduction in cardiac filling pressures, and this likely results from an early vasodilatory effect. A vasoconstrictive effect with reduction in cardiac output has also been reported, however, and may be a consequence of diuretic-induced neurohormonal activation with subsequent increases in plasma aldosterone levels (103–105) (Fig. 86.9). Although diuretic agents are considered as a first-line treatment for patients with ADHF, no long-term studies have been performed to assess their effect on mortality and morbidity in this population (106). What these agents do accomplish is the decongestion of the patient with ADHF and the reduction of symptoms. Reducing mesenteric edema and increasing the perfusion across renal vascular beds by decreasing venous pressures without a drop arterial pressure will likely benefit renal function in patients with ADHF.

The effective dose of intravenous furosemide is variable but is usually in the range of 20 to 40 mg in the patient not previously receiving diuretic therapy and exhibiting normal renal function. Conversely, patients with ADHF often present with substantial volume overload and usually require much larger

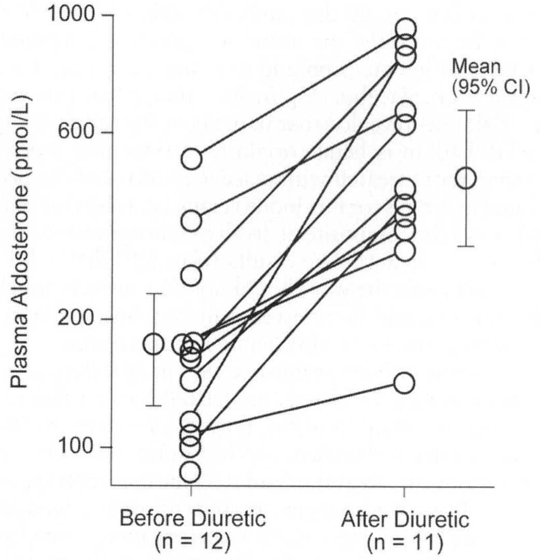

FIGURE 86.9. Plasma aldosterone levels before and after treatment with furosemide 40 mg and amiloride 5 mg orally once daily for 4 weeks. Aldosterone levels were observed to be markedly increased in patients treated with diuretic therapy, when compared with baseline values. CI, confidence interval. (Adapted from Bayliss J, Norell M, Canepa-Anson R, et al. Untreated heart failure: clinical and neuroendocrine effects of introducing diuretics. *Br Heart J* 1987;57:17–22.)

dosages to achieve an adequate diuresis. This is because of prior long-term oral diuretic use and activation of renal compensatory mechanisms to counteract natriuresis in the chronic HF milieu. As with any diuretic, hypotension and electrolyte imbalances can occur, and they are more profound with higher doses.

Increasingly higher oral diuretic doses in the outpatient setting as well as repetitive treatments with intravenous diuretics for ADHF to prevent hospital readmissions can eventually lead to some form of renal impairment. Monotherapy with intravenous furosemide has been demonstrated to worsen glomerular filtration rate when compared with placebo (107) (Fig. 86.10). Worsening of renal function during an admission for ADHF is a poor prognostic indicator and is associated with an increase in mortality and a prolonged hospital stay (108).

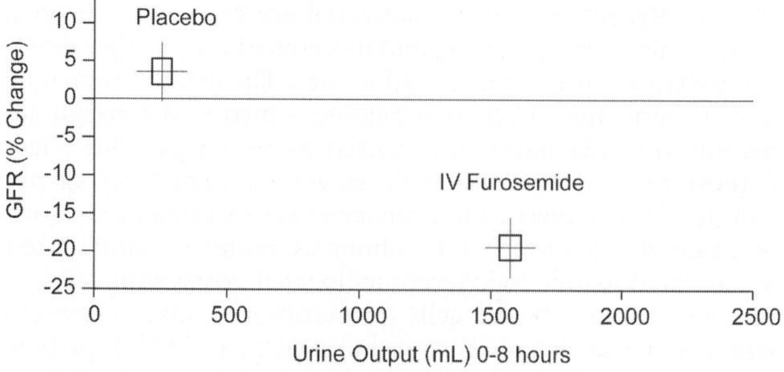

FIGURE 86.10. Changes in glomerular filtration rate (GFR) after treatment with 80 mg intravenous (IV) furosemide in patients with heart failure. Although urine output was greater in patients treated with furosemide, GFR was markedly decreased in this group when compared with placebo. (Adapted from Gottlieb SS, Brater DC, Thomas I, et al. BG9719 (CVT-124), an A1 adenosine receptor antagonist, protects against the decline in renal function observed with diuretic therapy. *Circulation* 2002;105:1348–1353.)

Although the initial insult to renal mechanics is most likely related to a diminution of renal perfusion that has a cardiovascular basis (so called "prerenal" syndrome), progression of renal disease can proceed independently, even with a compensated cardiac state. This "cardiorenal syndrome" has emerged as a two-headed beast that has plagued both renal and cardiac specialists trying to maximize the function of one organ without compromising the integrity of the other. In patients exhibiting volume overload and diuretic resistance, a continuous infusion of furosemide (5 to 20 mg per hour, as discussed earlier) may prove advantageous and less ototoxic than high-bolus dosing (109). Combination therapy with a thiazide diuretic is another option for patients demonstrating an inadequate diuresis to monotherapy with a loop diuretic, because the combination of both types of medications will block sodium reabsorption at multiple nephron sites (110). An attempt to enhance renal perfusion by increasing cardiac output (with dobutamine) or by reducing renal vascular resistance (with low-dose dopamine) may also be considered. Unfortunately, these patients often become refractory to intravenous diuretics, even when the drugs are used in conjunction with inotropic therapy, and patients not infrequently require hemodialysis for effective fluid removal, relief of congestive symptoms, and normalization of metabolic abnormalities. An alternative to traditional hemodialysis, ultrafiltration, represents an attractive treatment option in many patients deemed "diuretic resistant" (111) (see the section on ultrafiltration later in this chapter).

Investigational Agents

Although all the previous agents discussed have played a role in the management of ADHF, the search for safer, more efficacious therapies to ameliorate this process continues. The increased prevalence of HF in society has spurred the development of novel agents targeted specifically for ADHF, in the hopes of curbing the morbidity and mortality associated with it. Several promising therapies have emerged over the last few years and could potentially represent the future of ADHF treatment.

Positive Inotropic Drugs

Levosimendan is a compound that not only has positive inotropic properties, but also possesses other unique properties that set it apart from dobutamine and milrinone. It evokes a positive inotropic response primarily by increasing the sensitivity of myofilaments (specifically troponin C) to intracellular calcium (112,113). This action is independent of cAMP mechanisms and thus elicits inotropy while avoiding many of the adverse effects commonly associated with cAMP-dependent agents (114,115). Levosimendan also exhibits vasodilator properties through its mild inhibition of phosphodiesterase III and by activation of potassium-dependent adenosine triphosphate channels (115,116). In vitro, it does not impair myocardial relaxation and, in fact, has lusitropic actions in the failing myocardium (112). These multiple mechanisms of action result in the expected hemodynamic changes during short-term intravenous administration to patients with severe HF. Investigators have reported a significant improvement in cardiac index (primarily as a result of increased stroke volume), reduction in SVR and pulmonary vascular resistance, and reduced filling pressures with only a small increase (~8%) in heart rate (115). A study examining the dosing of levosimendan has revealed that its multiple effects on hemodynamic parameters are dose dependent, and as with most cardiotonic medications, increased heart rates and ventricular arrhythmias were more likely to be evident at higher infusion rates (117). Also important is the finding that a vasoactive metabolite remains measurable for several days; it perpetuates the effects of levosimendan for more prolonged periods and explains the presence of tachycardia. Recent evidence supports the hypothesis that levosimendan produces its inotropic effect mainly through a calcium-sensitization mechanism, as opposed to phosphodiesterase inhibition (118). This information may help to shed some light on the correlation of adverse effects seen with the use of inotropic agents and the underlying mechanism of how these agents function.

The Levosimendan Infusion versus Dobutamine in severe low output heart failure (LIDO) trial compared the effects of levosimendan and dobutamine on hemodynamic parameters and clinical outcomes in 203 patients with low-output HF (profile C, cold and wet) (119). The primary end point of this multicenter, randomized, double-blind study was the proportion of patients with hemodynamic improvement (defined as an increase of $\geq$30% in cardiac output and a decrease of $\geq$25% in PCWP) at 24 hours. An initial loading dose of levosimendan of 24 μg/kg was infused over 10 minutes, followed by a continuous infusion of 0.1 μg/kg per minute for 24 hours to 103 patients. Dobutamine was infused for 24 hours at an initial dose of 5 μg/kg per minute without a loading dose to 100 patients. The infusion rate was doubled if the response was inadequate at 2 hours. Results revealed that the primary hemodynamic end point was achieved in 29 (28%) of the levosimendan-group patients and in 15 (15%) of the dobutamine group ($p = .022$). At 6 months, a significant mortality benefit was observed in the levosimendan group as opposed to the dobutamine arm of the trial (26% versus 38%; $p = .029$).

The Randomized Study on Safety and Effectiveness of Levosimendan in Patients with Left Ventricular Failure After an Acute Myocardial Infarct (RUSSLAN) trial examined the use of levosimendan versus placebo in 504 patients with HF within 2 days of an acute myocardial infarction (120). The primary end point of this study was hypotension or clinically significant myocardial ischemia, with the secondary end points being risk of death and worsening HF, symptoms of HF and all-cause mortality. The incidence of ischemia and/or hypotension was similar in all treatment groups ($p = .319$). The levosimendan arm of the trial had a lower risk of death and worsening HF than patients receiving placebo, during both the 6-hour infusion (2.0% versus 5.9%; $p = .033$) and over 24 hours (4.0% versus 8.8%; $p = .044$). Mortality was lower with levosimendan compared with placebo at 14 days (11.7% versus 19.6%; $p = .031$), and the reduction was maintained at the 6-month follow-up (22.6% versus 31.4%; $p = .053$).

Two seminal clinical trials with levosimendan will soon be completed and may provide definitive information to answer the question of this drug's role in ADHF. The SURVIVE study is a multicenter, parallel-group, randomized, double-blind, double-dummy study in patients with acute HF and in need of intravenous inotropic support that compares the efficacy of levosimendan with dobutamine on mortality. The study is a European effort with a 24-hour infusion of the study drug versus control and a primary end point of 31-day mortality. The REVIVE trial is a placebo-controlled 24-hour infusion study in hospitalized patients with ADHF; the study has a combined primary end point of patient-reported symptomatic improvement, survival, and the lack of a need for an "intravenous medication bailout" to treat worsening symptoms at the 5-day mark.

Vasopressin Receptor Antagonists

The interactions of the neurohormonal cascade in HF have received a significant amount of focus over the last 10 years, as researchers have labored to find a weak link in this downward spiral that could be amenable to treatment. The hormone vasopressin is no exception, and its role in the pathogenesis of HF has made it a promising target for therapeutic research.

Vasopressin is released from the hypothalamus as a result from imbalances in the body's natural osmotic state. In HF, excess amounts of vasopressin are present, in response to the systemic inflammatory-hormonal imbalances that are present resulting in systemic vasoconstriction as well as fluid and salt retention (121). Specifically, the V1A receptors are largely responsible for the vasoconstrictive effect of vasopressin, whereas the V2 receptors are responsible for salt and water retention in the kidney. Bolstered by positive experimental data in canines (122), the development of therapies suited for clinical use is ongoing.

One agent, tolvaptan, a selective V2 vasopressin receptor antagonist, was recently examined in the Acute and Chronic Therapeutic Impact of a Vasopressin Antagonist in Congestive Heart Failure (ACTIV CHF) trial (123). This trial was a randomized, double-blind, multicenter study that enrolled 319 hospitalized patients with HF and a decreased ejection fraction who had continued symptoms despite optimal standard therapy. The patients were randomized to receive 30, 60, or 90 mg per day of tolvaptan orally or placebo in addition to standard therapy. The study drug was continued for up to 2 months. The results revealed that tolvaptan use was associated with significant weight reduction when compared with placebo ($p = .008$ for all tolvaptan groups versus placebo). There were no significant alterations in hemodynamic status, electrolyte levels, or renal function in the tolvaptan arm of the trial. Although all-cause mortality was lower in the tolvaptan group, it did not reach statistical significance. This initial examination of tolavaptan's clinical use led to the (Effects of Vasopressin antagonists in hEart failure (EVEREST) trial, which is focusing on the effects of a 30-mg oral dose of tolvaptan in conjunction with standard therapy in ADHF and is currently still active at the time of this writing.

Ultrafiltration

The use of ultrafiltration as a means to treat patients who are fluid overloaded and edematous despite high-dose diuretic treatment has emerged as an exciting alternative treatment modality. These "diuretic-resistant" patients normally would continue to retain fluid and develop worsening renal function until their only respite would be hemodialysis. Given the bleak long-term prognosis of patients with chronic renal insufficiency and HF, the ability to temporize the acute onset of this condition quickly represents a vital asset for the clinician.

As opposed to hemodialysis, the process of ultrafiltration involves creating an ultrafiltrate of plasma through hydrostatic pressure across a semipermeable membrane. This process is based on convective solute transport and results in minimal swings in electrolyte levels. Ultrafiltration has been shown to produce less hemodynamic imbalance than conventional dialysis even when removing up to 500 mL per hour (111,124). The initial concept of ultrafiltration involved arteriovenous connections but has been progressively modified to become a venous-to-venous configuration. The use of ultrafiltration as a means of mechanically unloading edematous patients has been used for nearly 3 decades, although questions about its technical issues and proper place in the treatment algorithm for ADHF have prevented widespread acceptance by cardiologists. Recent modifications to the workings of the device, namely the use of peripherally inserted lines for access, have provided a wider range of possibilities for this modality to be implemented at the clinical level (125). Numerous studies are currently ongoing and will, we hope, further delineate the role that ultrafiltration may play in the future of ADHF management.

TABLE 86.9

INDICATIONS FOR PULMONARY ARTERY CATHETERIZATION AND HEMODYNAMIC MONITORING IN ACUTE HEART FAILURE

- Acute pulmonary edema
  - After poor response to initial treatment
  - To exclude noncardiogenic pulmonary edema
- Cardiogenic shock or preshock syndrome not responsive to initial fluid challenge
- Acute decompensation of chronic heart failure to allow tailored therapy
- Questionable volume status

HEMODYNAMIC MONITORING

Catheterization with a flow-directed thermodilution pulmonary artery catheter (Swan-Ganz catheter) is often indicated for optimal management of ADHF (Table 86.9). Although hemodynamic monitoring is rarely necessary in uncomplicated cases such as the warm and wet profile B patient, it is often helpful in the patient who does not respond initially to standard therapy, and it is vital in managing those with persistent hypotension and preshock or shock syndromes (Table 86.10). These patients have evidence of hypoperfusion on examination, including a narrow pulse pressure, cool skin, reduced

TABLE 86.10

COMMON HEMODYNAMIC PATTERNS IN LOW CARDIAC OUTPUT STATES

	Cardiac output	Right atrial pressure	Pulmonary artery pressure	PCWP	Systemic vascular resistance	SVO_2
Acute pulmonary edema	Variable	→	Variable	Variable	Variable	Variable
Cardiogenic shock	↓	↑	↑or→	↑or→	↑↑	↓↓
Decompensation heart failure	↓	↑	↑↑	↑↑	↑	↓
Acute right ventricular failure	↑	↑↑	→or↓	→or↓	↑	↓
Massive pulmonary embolism	↓	↑	↑	→	↑	↓
Acute aortic/mitral valve insufficiency	↓	→	↑	↑↑	↑	↓
Tamponade	↓	↑	↑	↑	↑	↓
Hypovolemic shock	↓	↓	↓	↓	↑	↓

PCWP, pulmonary capillary wedge pressures; SVO_2 mixed venous oxygen saturation, ↑, increased; ↑↑, markedly increased; ↓, decreased; ↓↓, markedly decreased; →, normal.

urine output, and mental obtundation. Continuous assessment of cardiac output and of ventricular filling pressure is essential to guide and determine appropriately the effectiveness of pharmacologic therapy or assess the need for mechanical support. Other indications for hemodynamic monitoring include acute HF in which volume status is in question (profile L, cold and dry) and pulmonary edema in which a cardiac cause has not been definitely determined (126,127). The major parameters measured during hemodynamic monitoring are cardiac output, PCWP, systemic arterial pressure (usually measured with an indwelling arterial catheter), heart rate, and the calculated SVR (mean arterial pressure minus mean right atrial pressure, divided by cardiac output). The measurement of MVO_2 is also important (127,128), particularly when the thermodilution cardiac output may not be reliable (i.e., in cases of tricuspid regurgitation). By repeated assessment of these parameters, pharmacologic therapy using the agents previously discussed can be more effectively tailored to achieve the optimal hemodynamics for the individual patient (129). The therapeutic approach must take into account not only the presenting hemodynamics but also the cause of the underlying condition. For example, the optimal PCWP for patients with acute myocardial injury is higher (18 to 20 mm Hg) (130) than that for patients with ADHF in which a normal PCWP (10 to 12 mm Hg) is often the goal (131). Even when the underlying condition is known and general hemodynamic goals have been defined, individualization of therapy is important. Metabolic demand may be significantly different among individuals, and often significant variability exists in individual peripheral oxygen extraction ratios and oxygen use. Because of these differences, some patients tolerate a much lower cardiac output than others. Therefore, parameters in addition to hemodynamics must be considered when treating severe HF, and assessment should include a physical examination with attention to peripheral perfusion, urine output, and mentation. The blood lactate level is an important prognostic indicator in shock and is also useful in guiding therapy (132,133).

The use of hemodynamic monitoring in the management of critically ill HF patients has come under scrutiny since the publication of data from the Study to Understand Prognoses and Preferences for Outcomes and Risks of Treatment (134). In this study, patients undergoing right-sided heart catheterization had a significantly lower survival at 30 days than did those not undergoing this invasive monitoring approach. Drawing conclusions from this trial is difficult, however, because only 11% of patients had HF as the primary reason for admission to the intensive care unit, and multisystem failure was present in the majority. Recent results of the National Heart, Blood, and Lung Institute–sponsored Evaluation Study of Congestive Heart Failure and Pulmonary Artery Catheterization Effectiveness (ESCAPE) trial, which evaluated the use of Swan-Ganz catheters in patients hospitalized for ADHF who also had systolic dysfunction, revealed no significant difference in 30-day mortality between patients who received a Swan-Ganz catheter and those in the control arm (135). In addition, there were no significant differences between the groups with respect to clinical outcomes or adverse events at 6 months.

GENERAL APPROACH TO MANAGEMENT

Although the ultimate management strategy for patients presenting with ADHF is dictated by the precipitating factor or factors causing the decompensation, initial therapy must be guided by the early clinical findings until a definitive diagnostic evaluation can be completed (i.e., electrocardiography, blood tests, CXR, echocardiogram). As discussed previously, the evaluation for precipitating factors and the initial therapeutic intervention usually occur simultaneously. Following the initial evaluation process, it is helpful to identify the hemodynamic profile of the patient to direct management and drug selection more precisely. A reasonable algorithm for this process is presented in Figure 86.11.

If the patient with ADHF has congestion and an arterial pressure that is normal or elevated (warm and wet, profile B), nitroglycerin or nesiritide in combination with intravenous diuretics is a rational approach. In the patient who is extremely dyspneic, administration of nitroglycerin by the sublingual route can be utilized until intravenous therapy is available (43). If afterload reduction is the most important objective, as in a patient with severe pulmonary edema or those with hemodynamic profile C (cold and wet with an elevated SVR), nesiritide or nitroprusside should be substituted for their balanced vasodilator properties. An indwelling arterial catheter for continuous monitoring of systemic blood pressure is optimal if the patient has considerable hypotension. Generally, vasodilators such as nesiritide, nitroglycerin, or nitroprusside should not be initiated if systolic blood pressure is consistently less than 90 mm Hg.

The patient's failure to respond to these measures within a reasonable period should warrant strong consideration of hemodynamic monitoring and the addition of inotropic therapy. If both cardiac output and PCWP remain unacceptable, the option of changing to or adding milrinone should be considered (76,78). Other therapeutic considerations include the addition of low-dose dopamine to augment renal blood flow, frequent assessment of volume status, and appropriate intravenous diuretic administration.

Additionally, patients may also benefit from morphine sulfate, 2 to 6 mg given intravenously (4). This medication may have an immediate hemodynamic effect through its preload-reducing properties, which can result in hypotension. It may also alleviate anxiety and blunt the catecholamine response to the acute illness. Caution must be used, however, in patients with evidence of respiratory or metabolic acidosis or in those with significant underlying obstructive lung disease.

Supplemental oxygen is traditionally administered to patients with acute pulmonary edema regardless of arterial oxygen saturation. This is essential in the patient with hypoxemia; however, its utility in those with normal oxygen saturation is questionable, and typically therapy is empiric. Although patients may receive a subjective benefit, supplemental oxygen administration may have an adverse effect on central hemodynamics in patients with chronic HF (136). Optimally, one should obtain information from arterial blood gas analysis before administering supplemental oxygen. When severe respiratory distress or acidosis is present, the threshold for proceeding to mechanical ventilatory support should be low. This not only corrects hypoxemia but also may reduce metabolic demands and therefore favorably affect the relationship between oxygen delivery and utilization (129).

Evidence of acute myocardial infarction would warrant proceeding to cardiac catheterization with consideration of urgent reperfusion therapy. A diligent effort must be made to identify the cause of acute HF, because without correction of a reversible lesion, the long-term prognosis is poor.

Patients with acute unstable HF (preshock or shock syndromes, cold and wet, profile C) require an expedient diagnostic evaluation and therapeutic plan. They usually exhibit severe cardiac dysfunction and hemodynamic compromise and often present with symptoms and signs of organ hypoperfusion (cyanosis, cool extremities, altered mentation) (137). These patients often require initial inotropic support in addition to diuretic and vasodilator therapy.

When cardiogenic shock occurs or when standard therapy fails to stabilize ADHF, hemodynamic monitoring to guide

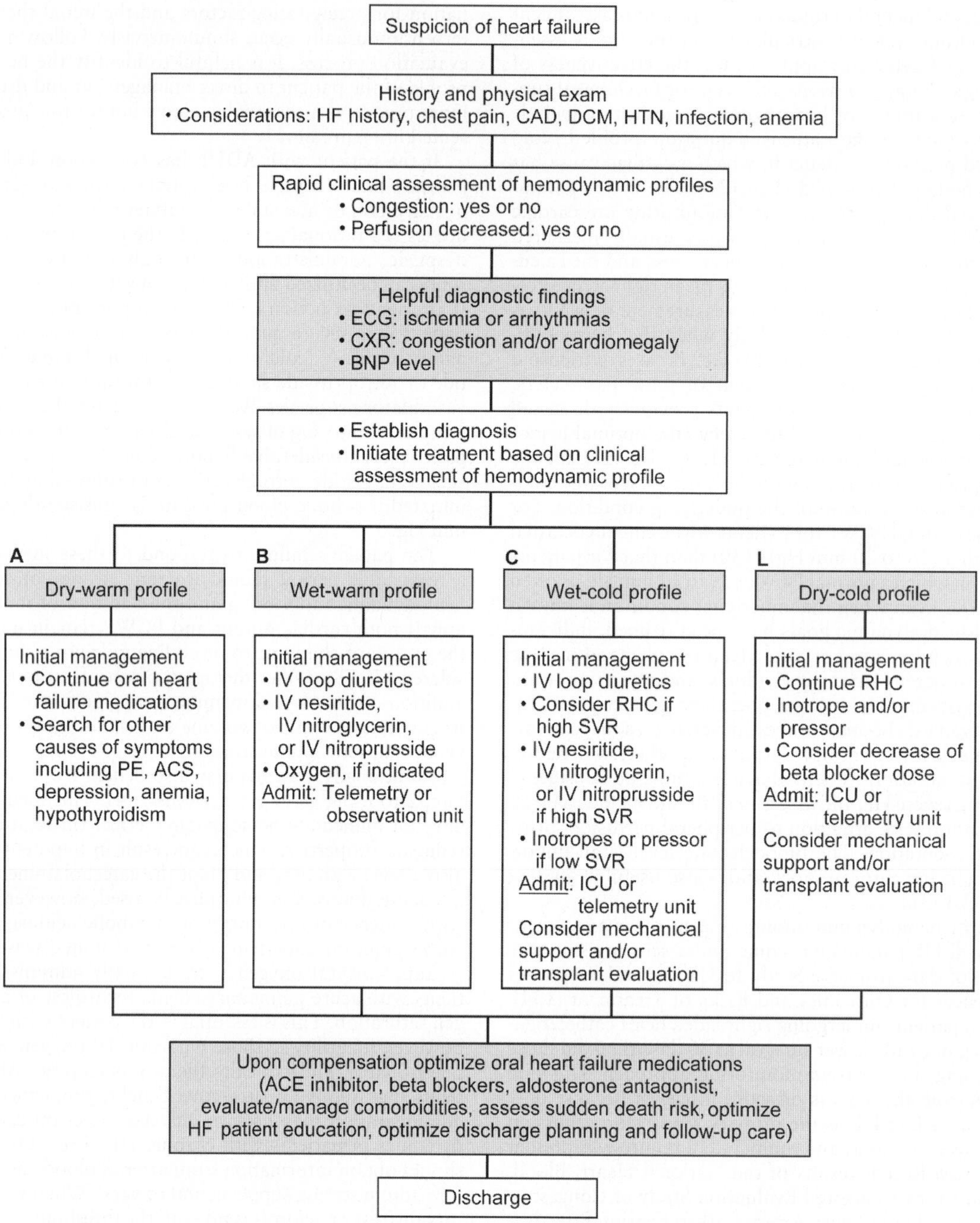

FIGURE 86.11. Assessment and treatment algorithm for acutely decompensated heart failure (ADHF). This ladder diagram expands on the concept of the four-square model (see Fig. 86.6) with emphasis on treatment options for each type of clinical presentation of ADHF. ACE, angiotensin-converting enzyme; ACS, acute coronary syndrome; BNP, brain natriuretic peptide; CAD, coronary artery disease; CXR, chest radiograph; DCM, dilated cardiomyopathy; ECG, electrocardiogram; HTN, hypertension; ICU, intensive care unit; IV, intravenous; PE, pulmonary embolism; RHC, right heart catheterization; SVR, systemic vascular resistance. (Adapted from Fonarow GC, Weber JE. Rapid clinical assessment of hemodynamic profiles and targeted treatment of patients with acutely decompensated heart failure. *Clin Cardiol* 2004;27[suppl V]:V1–V9.)

pharmacologic support is essential (127,128,130). The initial therapeutic decision is influenced primarily by systemic arterial pressure. Although the optimal systolic or mean arterial pressure for the individual patient is variable, a systolic arterial pressure of less than 80 to 85 mm Hg would be classified as significant hypotension when accompanied by evidence of organ hypoperfusion, such as renal dysfunction and altered central nervous system activity. When this clinical situation is present, arterial pressure must be rapidly augmented to the level at which myocardial perfusion is not jeopardized.

When significant systemic hypotension persists, therapy with vasopressor doses of dopamine (>5 μg/kg per minute) should be used (92,93). Failure to achieve an acceptable blood pressure response with high-dose dopamine would warrant consideration of switching to another vasopressor, such as norepinephrine or vasopressin, or adding dobutamine (67,71).

The approach to the pharmacologic support of the patient with cardiogenic shock or severely decompensated HF must be individualized. Evaluation of multiple clinical variables is often necessary for appropriate drug selection. Even then, several therapeutic trials may be required. When pharmacologic support obviously will not be sufficient to avoid progressive circulatory failure, then mechanical assistance such as the intraaortic balloon counterpulsation pump, extracorporeal membrane oxygenation systems, and univentricular and biventricular nonpulsatile and pulsatile devices must be considered as options (see Chapter 90).

TRANSITION TO OUTPATIENT THERAPY

During the acute exacerbation process of HF, oral therapy is often held in favor of intravenous medications. Depending on the hemodynamic status of the patient on presentation, the use of ACE inhibitors, ARBs, and β-blockers can be continued during the early hospitalization phase, but caution should be taken before the patient is uptitrated (for possibly creating untoward hemodynamic compromise). If the patient is newly diagnosed with HF, or has not received any of the standard chronic HF therapies before, an oral ACE inhibitor (or ARB if the patient is intolerant to an ACE inhibitor) should be initiated before discharge once the patient has obtained a euvolemic state. Diuretics and vasodilators can also be transitioned to oral regimens and should be continued in the outpatient setting until the patient has reached a compensated state with significantly decreased symptoms, in which case the doses of both drugs can be reduced as needed by the physician. The use of potassium supplementation is vital, and efforts should be made to have an assessment of serum electrolyte levels within 2 to 3 weeks after discharge.

Patients who are taking potassium-sparing diuretics, such as spironolactone, can be maintained on this therapy as long as potassium and creatinine levels are normal. If the patient has not taken spironolactone before, it should generally be given on an outpatient basis if the patient has advanced HF and only after stability has been reached with other oral HF drugs (ACE inhibitors, ARBs, β-blockers). This is because of the risk of hyperkalemia, which may manifest itself only after a few days of therapy. Again, tests for serum electrolytes and renal function should be checked in these individuals, and doses of potassium supplementation should be modified as needed.

The use of β-blockers during an acute admission is less clear. Patients who were receiving a β-blocker before admission can generally be continued on it, as long as their hemodynamic profile is stable. In patients who may require inotropic support during an admission, the use of milrinone would be facilitated in this group, because β-blocker therapy would not necessarily need to be held (pending blood pressure status). The initiation of β-blocker therapy during an admission can be considered if the patient is already on a stable oral regimen of an ACE inhibitor or ARB. Barring an acute ischemic event with subsequent HF as the cause of the hospitalization, starting both classes of medications (ACE inhibitor/ARB and β-blocker) during an admission for ADHF is generally not recommended because close hemodynamic monitoring and observation of symptoms is usually needed. If the patient is to have close follow-up after discharge, and compliance is not in question, then a low dose of a β-blocker can be started on an outpatient basis immediately after discharge once the patient is deemed tolerant of other HF therapies initiated during the hospitalization.

Patients who are discharged from the hospital for an episode of ADHF often are readmitted for the same reason. There are multiple potential explanations for this early readmission, including inadequate patient education. Patients with HF should be thoroughly informed about the causes of HF exacerbations and the ways in which they can be prevented (e.g., salt and fluid restriction, taking daily weights). Patients should also have close follow-up immediately after discharge, to ensure that they are being compliant with medications and diet. The physician and/or HF management team should strive to make patients more aware of the circumstances of their condition and the ways in which they can address any changes in their clinical status, thus possibly breaking the pattern of continuous readmissions for exacerbations in the future.

CONTROVERSIES AND PERSONAL PERSPECTIVES

As emphasized throughout this chapter, the finding of a treatable condition of ADHF has important prognostic implications, and the ability to uncover a reparable lesion in an individual with HF continues to improve. The continued advances in reperfusion strategies (angioplasty and antithrombotic therapy), as well as improved outcome after high-risk coronary bypass surgery, provide a means potentially to avoid irreversible myocardial injury and its sequela of severe HF.

The advances in technologic support and treatment options for acute HF, however, have not simplified its management. Despite new AHA/ACC guidelines for the management of chronic HF, the lack of a widely accepted consensus statement on the management of acute HF in the United States is an obvious gap in our ability to manage this patient population cohesively (138). Thus, the significance of the initial clinical assessment and treatment plan cannot be overemphasized.

Because of the complexity and diverse nature of the acute HF syndrome, diagnostic and therapeutic strategies must be individualized, and a generic approach to pharmacologic therapy or other modes of support cannot be advocated. Certainly, the patient presenting with acute pulmonary edema and hypertension is treated differently from the patient with a large anterior myocardial infarction who presents with congestion and hypotension. Within these two extremes lies a great diversity of acute HF presentations, each with subtle differences requiring a different diagnostic and therapeutic approach. Therefore, the basics of patient care cannot be ignored but must be used in conjunction with advanced therapeutic capabilities.

THE FUTURE

Therapy for ADHF has been progressively modified since the mid-1990s. Although the mainstay of therapy still revolves around the use of vasodilators, diuretics, and inotropic agents, advances in each of these classes hold promise as possible future remedies. Research in novel compounds targeted at alternate areas of the neurohormonal pathway represents an exciting avenue for potential discoveries, and these areas are continually being evaluated for their ability to be utilized in the clinical arena. Given the immense financial and emotional burden that HF currently places on society as a whole, the ability to treat this patient population with the appropriate measures is essential. With mortality rates for HF still on the rise, the combination of sound clinical skills, optimal pharmacotherapy, and viable technologic support will all be vital aspects in the treatment paradigm for ADHF over the next decade.

References

1. American Heart Association. *2005 heart and stroke statistical update*. Dallas, TX: American Heart Association, 2005.

2. Francis GS. Acute heart failure: patient management of a growing epidemic. *Am Heart Hosp J* 2004;2(suppl 1):10–14.
3. Lapu-Bula R, Ofili E. Diastolic heart failure: the forgotten manifestation of hypertensive heart disease. *Curr Hypertens Rep* 2004;6:164–170.
4. Chatterjee K, Hutchison SJ, Chou TM. Acute ischemic heart failure: pathophysiology and management. In: Poole-Wilson P, Colucci W, Chatterjee K, et al., eds. *Heart failure: scientific principles and clinical practice*. New York: Churchill Livingstone, 1996:523–549.
5. Goldberger JJ, Peled HB, Stroh JA, et al. Prognostic factors in acute pulmonary edema. *Arch Intern Med* 1986;146:489–493.
6. Fonarow GS, ADHERE Scientific Advisory Committee. The Acute Decompensated Heart Failure National Registry (ADHERE): opportunities to improve care of patients hospitalized with acute decompensated heart failure. *Rev Cardiovasc Med* 2003;4(suppl 7):S21–S30.
7. Acute Decompensated Heart Failure National Registry Web site. Available at www.adhereregistry.com.
8. Teerlink JR, Goldhaber SZ, Pfeffer MA. An overview of contemporary etiologies of congestive heart failure. *Am J Cardiol* 1991;121:1852–1853.
9. Forman DE, Butler J, Wang Y, et al. Incidence, predictors at admission, and impact of worsening renal function among patients hospitalized with heart failure. *J Am Coll Cardiol* 2004;43:61–67.
10. McAlister FA, Ezekowitz J, Tonelli M, et al. Renal insufficiency and heart failure prognostic and therapeutic implications from a prospective cohort study. *Circulation* 2004;109:1004–1009.
11. Filippatos G, Leche C, Sunga R, et al. Expression FAS adjacent to fibrotic foci in the failing human heart is not associated with increased apoptosis. *Am J Physiol* 1999;277:H445–H451.
12. Jain P, Massie BM, Gattis WA, et al. Current medical treatment for the exacerbation of chronic heart failure resulting in hospitalization. *Am Heart J* 2003;145(suppl):S3–S17.
13. Stevenson LW, Tillisch JH, Hamilton M, et al. Importance of hemodynamic response to therapy in predicting survival with ejection fraction <20% secondary to ischemic or non-ischemic dilated cardiomyopathy. *Am J Cardiol* 1990;6:1348–1354.
14. Young JB. Assessment of heart failure. In: Colucci WS, ed. *Heart failure: cardiac function and dysfunction*. St. Louis: Mosby, 1995:7.2–8.1. Braunwald E, ed. *Atlas of heart disease*, vol 4.
15. Drazner MH, Rame JE, Stevenson LW, et al. Prognostic importance of elevated jugular venous pressure and a third heart sound in patients with heart failure. *N Engl J Med* 2001;345:574–581.
16. Fonarow GC, Adams KF Jr, Abraham WT, et al. Risk stratification for in-hospital mortality in acutely decompensated heart failure: classification and regression tree analysis. *JAMA* 2005;293:572–580.
17. Holtwick R, van Eickels M, Skryabin H, et al. Pressure independent cardiac hypertrophy in mice with cardiomyocyte-restricted inactivation of the atrial natriuretic peptide receptor guanyl cyclase A. *J Clin Invest* 2003;111:1399–1407.
18. Hobbs A, Foster P, Prescott C, et al. Natriuretic peptide receptor C regulates coronary blood flow and prevents myocardial ischemia/reperfusion injury. *Circulation* 2004;110:1231–1235.
19. Molkentine JD. A friend within the heart: natriuretic peptide receptor signaling. *J Clin Invest* 2003;111:1275–1277.
20. Clerico A, Lervasi G, Mariani G. Clinical relevance of the measurement of cardiac natriuretic peptide hormones in humans. *Horm Metab Res* 1999;31:487–498.
21. Boomama F, Van der Meiracker AH. Plasma A- and B-type natriuretic peptides: physiology, methodology, and clinical use. *Cardiovasc Res* 2001;51:442–449.
22. Maisel A, Krishnaswamy P, Nowak RM, et al. Rapid measurement of B-type natriuretic in the emergency diagnosis of heart failure. *N Engl J Med* 2002;347:161–167.
23. Stevenson LW. Tailored therapy to hemodynamic goals for advanced heart failure. *Eur J Heart Fail* 1999;1:251–257.
24. Stevenson LW. Management of acute decompensation. In: Mann DL eds. *Heart failure: a companion to Braunwald's heart disease*. Philadelphia: WB Saunders, 2003:579–594.
25. Haas GJ, Leier CV. Vasodilator therapy for congestive heart failure (non-ACE inhibition). In: Hosenpud JD, Greenberg BH, eds. *Congestive heart failure: pathophysiology, differential diagnosis and comprehensive approach to therapy*. New York: Springer-Verlag, 1994:400–454.
26. Delius W, Enghoff E. Studies of the central and peripheral hemodynamic effects of amyl nitrate in patients with aortic insufficiency. *Circulation* 1970; 42:787–796.
27. Leier CV, Bambach D, Thompson MJ, et al. Central and regional hemodynamic effects of intravenous isosorbide dinitrate, nitroglycerin, and nitroprusside in patients with congestive heart failure. *Am J Cardiol* 1981;48: 1115–1123.
28. Leier CV, Magorien RD, Desch CE, et al. Hydralazine and isosorbide dinitrate: comparative central and regional hemodynamic effects when administered alone or in combination. *Circulation* 1981;63:102–109.
29. Tsai SC, Adamik R, Manganiello VC, et al. Effects of nitroprusside and nitroglycerin on cGMP content and PGI_2 formation in aorta and vena cava. *Biochem Pharmacol* 1989;38:61–65.
30. Miller RR, Vismara LA, Williams DO, et al. Pharmacological mechanisms for left ventricular unloading in clinical congestive heart failure. *Circ Res* 1976;39:127–133.
31. Leier CV, Magorien RD, Boudoulas H, et al. The effect of vasodilator therapy on systolic and diastolic time intervals in congestive heart failure. *Chest* 1982;81:723–729.
32. Flaherty JT. Comparison of intravenous nitroglycerin and sodium nitroprusside in acute myocardial infarction. *Am J Med* 1983;74:53–60.
33. Packer M. New perspectives on therapeutic application of nitrates as vasodilator agents for severe chronic heart failure. *Am J Med* 1983;74:61–72.
34. Cohn JN. Nitrates for congestive heart failure. *Am J Cardiol* 1985;56:19A–23A.
35. Cohn JN. Role of nitrates in congestive heart failure. *Am J Cardiol* 1987; 60:39H–43H.
36. Needleman P, Jakschik B, Johnson EM. Sulfhydryl requirement for relaxation of vascular smooth muscle. *J Pharmacol Exp Ther* 1973;187:324–331.
37. Ignarro LJ, Lippton H, Edwards JC, et al. Mechanism of vascular smooth muscle relaxation by organic nitrates, nitrites, nitroprusside, and nitric oxide: evidence for the involvement of *S*-nitrosothiols as active intermediates. *J Pharmacol Exp Ther* 1981;218:739–749.
38. Levin RI, Jaffe EA, Weksler BB, et al. Nitroglycerin stimulates synthesis of prostacyclin by cultured human endothelial cells. *J Clin Invest* 1981;67: 762–769.
39. DeCaterina R, Dorso CR, Tack-Goldman K, et al. Nitrates and endothelial prostacyclin production: studies in vitro. *Circulation* 1985;71:176–182.
40. Morcillio E, Reid PR, Dubin N, et al. Myocardial prostaglandin E release by nitroglycerin and modification by indomethacin. *Am J Cardiol* 1980;45:53–57.
41. Keren G, Katz S, Gage J, et al. Effect of isometric exercise on cardiac performance and mitral regurgitation in patients with severe congestive heart failure. *Am Heart J* 1989;118:973–979.
42. Baxter RH, Tait CM, McGuinness JB. Vasodilator therapy in acute myocardial infarction: use of sublingual isosorbide dinitrate. *Br Heart J* 1977;39:1067–1070.
43. Bussmann WD, Schupp D. Effects of sublingual nitroglycerin in emergency treatment of severe pulmonary edema. *Am J Cardiol* 1978;41:931–936.
44. Publication committee for the VMAC investigators. Intravenous nesiritide versus nitroglycerin for treatment of decompensated congestive heart failure. *JAMA* 2002;287:1531–1540.
45. Elkayam U, Kulick D, McIntosh N, et al. Incidence of early tolerance to hemodynamic effects of continuous infusion of nitroglycerin in patients with coronary artery disease and heart failure. *Circulation* 1987;76:577–584.
46. Elkayam U, Bitar F, Akhter MW, et al. Intravenous nitroglycerin in the treatment of decompensated heart failure: potential benefits and limitations. *J Cardiovasc Pharmacol Ther* 2004;9:227–241.
47. Cohn JN, Burke LP. Nitroprusside. *Ann Intern Med* 1979;91:752–757.
48. Laskey WK, Kussmaul WG. Arterial wave reflection in heart failure. *Circulation* 1987;75:711–722.
49. Pepine CJ, Nichols WW, Curry RC Jr, et al. Aortic input impedance during nitroprusside infusion. *J Clin Invest* 1979;64:643–654.
50. Merillon JP, Fontenier G, Lerallut JF, et al. Aortic input impedance in heart failure: comparison with normal subjects and its changes during vasodilator therapy. *Eur Heart J* 1984;5:447–455.
51. Yin FC, Guzman PA, Brin KP, et al. Effect of nitroprusside on hydraulic vascular loads on the right and left ventricle of patients with heart failure. *Circulation* 1983;67:1330–1339.
52. Hasenfuss G, Holubarsch C, Heiss W, et al. Myocardial energetics in patients with dilated cardiomyopathy. *Circulation* 1989;80:51–64.
53. Mann T, Cohn PF, Holman BL, et al. Effect of nitroprusside on regional myocardial blood flow in coronary artery disease. *Circulation* 1978;57:732–738.
54. Simkus GJ, Fitchett DH. Radial artery pressure measurements may be a poor guide to the beneficial effects of nitroprusside on left ventricular systolic pressure in congestive heart failure. *Am J Cardiol* 1990;66:323–326.
55. duCailar J, Mathier-Daude JC, Kienlen J, et al. Blood and urinary cyanide concentrations during long-term sodium nitroprusside infusions. *Anesthesiology* 1979;51:363–364.
56. Vesey CJ, Cole PV. Blood cyanide and thiocyanate concentrations produced by long-term therapy with sodium nitroprusside. *Br J Anaesth* 1985;57:148–155.
57. Chiariello M, Gold HK, Leinbach RC, et al. Comparison between the effects of nitroprusside and nitroglycerin on ischemic injury during acute myocardial infarction. *Circulation* 1976;54:766–773.
58. Mukoyama M, Nakao K, Hosoda N, et al. Brain natriuretic peptide as a novel cardiac hormone in humans: evidence for an exquisite dual natriuretic peptide system, atrial natriuretic peptide system, and brain natriuretic peptide. *J Clin Invest* 1991;87:1402–1412.
59. Marcus LS, Hart D, Packer M, et al. Hemodynamic and renal excretory effects of human brain natriuretic peptide infusion in patients with congestive heart failure. *Circulation* 1996;94:3184–3189.
60. Burger AJ, Horton DP, Lejemtel T, et al. Effect of nesiritide (β-type natriuretic peptide) and dobutamine on ventricular arrhythmias in the treatment of patients with acutely decompensated congestive heart failure: the PRECEDENT study. *Am Heart J* 2002;144:1102–1108.
61. Colucci WS, Elkayam U, Horton DP, et al. Intravenous nesiritide, a natriuretic peptide, in the treatment of decompensated congestive heart failure: Nesiritide Study Group. *N Engl J Med* 2000;343:246–253.

62. Teerlink JR, Massie BM. Nesiritide and worsening of renal function: the emperor's new clothes? *Circulation* 2005;111:1459–1461.
63. Sackner-Bernstein JD, Kowalski M, Fox M, et al. Short-term risk of death after treatment with nesiritide for decompensated heart failure: a pooled analysis of randomized controlled trials. *JAMA* 2005;293:1900–1905.
64. Sackner-Bernstein JD, Skopicki HA, Aaronson KD. Risk of worsening renal function with nesiritide in patients with acutely decompensated heart failure. *Circulation* 2005;111:1487–1491.
65. Ruffolo RR Jr, Spradlin TA, Pollack GD, et al. Alpha and beta adrenergic effects of the stereoisomers of dobutamine. *J Pharmacol Exp Ther* 1981;219:447–452.
66. Schumann HJ, Wagner J, Knorr A, et al. Demonstration in human atrial preparations of alpha-adrenoceptors mediating positive inotropic effects. *Naunyn Schmiedebergs Arch Pharmacol* 1978;302:333–336.
67. Leier CV. Acute inotropic support: intravenously administered positive inotropic drugs. In: Leier CV, ed. *Cardiotonic drugs: a clinical review*. New York: Marcel Dekker, 1991:63–105.
68. Boudoulas H, Rittgers SE, Lewis RP, et al. Changes in diastolic time with various pharmacologic agents: implications for myocardial perfusion. *Circulation* 1979;60:164–169.
69. Dubois-Rande JL, Merlet P, Duval-Moulin AM, et al. Coronary vasodilating action of dobutamine in patients with idiopathic dilated cardiomyopathy. *Am Heart J* 1983;105:176–181.
70. Vatner SF, McRitchie RJ, Braunwald E. Effects of dobutamine on left ventricular performance, coronary dynamics, and distribution of cardiac output in conscious dogs. *J Clin Invest* 1974;53:1265–1273.
71. Leier CV. Positive inotropic therapy: an update and new agents. *Curr Probl Cardiol* 1996;21:521–581.
72. Bianchi C, Diaz R, Gonzales C, et al. Effects of dobutamine on atrioventricular conduction. *Am Heart J* 1975;90:474–478.
73. Feldman AM, Massie BM. Positive inotropic therapy. In: Poole-Wilson P, Colucci W, Chatterjee K, et al., eds. *Heart failure: scientific principles and clinical practice*. New York: Churchill Livingstone, 1996:701–718.
74. Pozen RG, DiBanco R, Katz RJ, et al. Myocardial metabolic and hemodynamic effects of dobutamine in heart failure complicating coronary artery disease. *Circulation* 1981;63:1279–1285.
75. Colucci WS, Denniss AR, Leatherman GF, et al. Intracoronary infusion of dobutamine to patients with and without severe congestive heart failure: dose-response relationships, correlation with circulating catecholamines and effect of phosphodiesterase inhibition. *J Clin Invest* 1988;81:1103–1110.
76. Simonton CA, Chatterjee K, Cody RJ, et al. Milrinone in congestive heart failure: acute and chronic hemodynamic and clinical evaluation. *J Am Coll Cardiol* 1985;6:453–459.
77. Grose R, Strain J, Greenberg M, et al. Systemic and coronary effects of intravenous milrinone and dobutamine in congestive heart failure. *J Am Coll Cardiol* 1986;7:1107–1113.
78. Monrad ES, Baim DS, Smith HS, et al. Milrinone, dobutamine, and nitroprusside: comparative effects on hemodynamics and myocardial energetics in patients with severe congestive heart failure. *Circulation* 1986; 73(suppl III):III168–III174.
79. Jaski BE, Fifer M, Wright RF, et al. Positive inotropic and vasodilator actions of milrinone in patients with severe congestive heart failure. *J Clin Invest* 1985;75:643–649.
80. Monrad ES, Baim DS, Smith HS, et al. Effects of milrinone on coronary hemodynamics and myocardial energetics in patients with congestive heart failure. *Circulation* 1985;71:972–979.
81. Cuffe MS, Califf RM, Adams KF Jr, et al. Short-term intravenous milrinone for acute exacerbation of chronic heart failure: a randomized controlled trial. *JAMA* 2002;287:1541–1547.
82. Felker GM, Benza RL, Chandler AB, et al. Heart failure etiology and response to milrinone in decompensated heart failure: results from the OPTIME-CHF study. *J Am Coll Cardiol* 2003;4:997–1003.
83. Lowes BD, Simon MA, Tsvetkova TO, et al. Inotropes in the beta blocker era. *Clin Cardiol* 2000;23(suppl III):III11–III16.
84. Sigmund M, Jakob H, Becker H, et al. Effects of metoprolol on myocardial beta-adrenoreceptors and G alpha i-proteins in patients with CHF. *Eur J Clin Pharmacol* 1996;51:127–132.
85. Goldberg LI. Cardiovascular and renal actions of dopamine: potential clinical application. *Pharmacol Rev* 1972;241:1–29.
86. McDonald RH, Goldberg LI. Analysis of the cardiovascular effects of dopamine in the dog. *J Pharmacol Exp Ther* 1963;140:60.
87. Lee MR. Dopamine and the kidney. *Clin Sci* 1982;62:439–448.
88. Lokhandwala MF, Barrett RJ. Cardiovascular dopamine receptors: physiological, pharmacological, and therapeutic implications. *J Auton Pharmacol* 1982;3:189–215.
89. Beregovich J, Bianchi C, Rubler S, et al. Dose-related hemodynamic and renal effects of dopamine in congestive heart failure. *Am Heart J* 1974; 87:550–557.
90. Stoof JC, Kebabian JW. Two dopamine receptors: biochemistry, physiology, and pharmacology. *Life Sci* 1984;35:2281–2296.
91. Leier CV, Heban P, Huss P, et al. Comparative systemic and regional hemodynamic effects of dopamine and dobutamine in patients with cardiomyopathic heart failure. *Circulation* 1978;58:466–475.
92. Loeb HS, Bredakis J, Gunnar RM. Superiority of dobutamine over dopamine for augmentation of cardiac output in patients with chronic low output cardiac failure. *Circulation* 1977;55:375–381.
93. Holzer J, Karliner JS, O'Rourke RA, et al. Effectiveness of dopamine in patients with cardiogenic shock. *Am J Cardiol* 1973;32:79–84.
94. Binkley PF, VanFossen DB, Haas GJ, et al. Increased ventricular contractility is not sufficient for effective positive inotropic intervention. *Am J Physiol* 1996;271:H1635–H1642.
95. Toda N, Goldberg LI. Effects of dopamine on isolated canine coronary arteries. *Cardiovasc Res* 1975;9:384–389.
96. Cohn JN. Comparative cardiovascular effects of tyramine, ephedrine, and norepinephrine in man. *Circ Res* 1965;16:174.
97. Mueller H, Ayres SM, Giannelli S, et al. Effect of isoproterenol, L-norepinephrine, and intra-aortic counterpulsation on hemodynamics, and myocardial metabolism in shock following acute myocardial infarction. *Circulation* 1972;45:335–351.
98. American Heart Association in collaboration with the International Liaison Committee on Resuscitation (ILCOR). Agents to optimize cardiac output and blood pressure. *Circulation* 2000;102(suppl I):I129–I135.
99. Wenzel V, Lindner KH, Augenstein S. Vasopressin combined with epinephrine decreases cerebral perfusion compared with vasopressin alone during CPR in pigs. *Stroke* 1998;29:1467–1468.
100. Oyama H, Suzuki Y, Satoh S. Role of nitric oxide in the cerebral vasodilatory responses to vasopressin and oxytocin in dogs. *J Cereb Blood Flow Metab* 1993;13:285–290.
101. Cody RJ. Clinical trials of diuretic therapy in heart failure: research directions and clinical considerations. *J Am Coll Cardiol* 1993;22(suppl A): 165A–171A.
102. Lal S, Murtagh JG, Pollock AM, et al. Acute hemodynamic effects of furosemide in patients with normal and raised left atrial pressures. *Br Heart J* 1969;31:711–717.
103. Ikram H, Chan W, Espiner EA, et al. Hemodynamic and hormone response to acute and chronic furosemide therapy in congestive heart failure. *Clin Sci* 1980;59:443–449.
104. Francis GS, Siegel RM, Goldsmith SR, et al. Acute vasoconstrictor response to intravenous furosemide in patients with chronic congestive heart failure. *Ann Intern Med* 1985;103:1–6.
105. Bayliss J, Norell M, Canepa-Anson R, et al. Untreated heart failure: clinical and neuroendocrine effects of introducing diuretics. *Br Heart J* 1987;57:17–22.
106. Ravnan SL, Ravnan MC, Deedwania PC. Pharmacotherapy in congestive heart failure: diuretic resistance and strategies to overcome resistance in patients with congestive heart failure. *Congest Heart Fail* 2002;8:80–85.
107. Gottlieb SS, Brater DC, Thomas I, et al. BG9719 (CVT-124), an A1 adenosine receptor antagonist, protects against the decline in renal function observed with diuretic therapy. *Circulation* 2002;105:1348–1353.
108. Gottlieb SS, Abraham WT, Butler J, et al. The prognostic importance of different definitions of worsening renal function in congestive heart failure. *J Card Fail* 2002;8:136–141.
109. Dormans TP, VanMeyel JJ, Gerlag PG, et al. Diuretic efficacy of high dose furosemide in severe heart failure: bolus injection versus continuous infusion. *J Am Coll Cardiol* 1996;28:376–382.
110. Channer KS, Mclean KA, Lawson-Matthew P, et al. Combination diuretic treatment in severe heart failure: a randomised controlled trial. *Br Heart J* 1994;71:146–150.
111. Agostoni PG, Marenzi GC, Pepi M, et al. Isolated ultrafiltration in moderate congestive heart failure. *J Am Coll Cardiol* 1993;21:424–431.
112. Hasenfuss G, Pieske B, Castell M, et al. Influence of the novel inotropic agent levosimendan on isometric tension and calcium cycling in failing human myocardium. *Circulation* 1998;98:2141–2147.
113. Haikala H, Nissinen E, Etemadzadeh E, et al. Troponin C-mediated calcium sensitization induced by levosimendan does not impair relaxation. *J Cardiovasc Pharmacol* 1995;25:794–801.
114. Movesian MA. Beta-adrenergic receptor agonists and cyclic nucleotide phosphodiesterase inhibitors: shifting the focus from inotropy to cyclic adenosine monophosphate. *J Am Coll Cardiol* 1999;34:318–324.
115. Slawsky MT, Colucci WS, Gottlieb SS, et al. Acute hemodynamic and clinical effects of levosimendan in patients with severe heart failure. *Circulation* 2000;102:2222–2227.
116. Yokoshiki H, Katsube Y, Sunagawa M, et al. Levosimendan, a novel calcium sensitizer, activates the glibenclamide-sensitive potassium channel in rat arterial myocytes. *Eur J Pharmacol* 1997;333:249–259.
117. Nieminen MS, Akkila J, Hasenfuss G, et al. Hemodynamic and neurohumoral effects of continuous infusion of levosimendan in patients with congestive heart failure. *J Am Coll Cardiol* 2000;36:1903–1912.
118. Szilagyi S, Pollesello P, Levijoki J, et al. Two inotropes with different mechanisms of action: contractile, PDE-inhibitory and direct myofibrillar effects of levosimendan and enoximone. *J Cardiovasc Pharmacol* 2005;46:369–376.
119. Follath F, Cleland JG, Just H, et al. Efficacy and safety of intravenous levosimendan compared with dobutamine in severe low-output heart failure (the LIDO study): a randomised double-blind trial. *Lancet* 2002;360:196–202.
120. Moiseyev VS, Poder P, Andrejevs N, et al. Safety and efficacy of a novel calcium sensitizer, levosimendan, in patients with left ventricular failure due to an acute myocardial infarction: a randomized, placebo-controlled, double-blind study (RUSSLAN). *Eur Heart J* 2002;23:1422–1432.

121. Francis GS, Benedict C, Johnstone DE, et al. Comparison of neuroendocrine activation in patients with left ventricular dysfunction with and without congestive heart failure: a substudy of the Studies of Left Ventricular Dysfunction (SOLVD). *Circulation* 1990;82:1724–1729.
122. Yatsu T, Tomura Y, Tahara A, et al. Cardiovascular and renal effects of conivaptan hydrochloride (YM087), a vasopressin V1A and V2 receptor antagonist, in dogs with pacing-induced congestive heart failure. *Eur J Pharmacol* 1999;376:239–246.
123. Gheorghiade M, Gattis WA, O'Connor CM, et al. Effects of tolvaptan, a vasopressin antagonist, in patients hospitalized with worsening heart failure: a randomized controlled trial. *JAMA* 2004;291:1963–1971.
124. Dileo M, Paciti A, Bergerone S, et al. Ultrafiltration in the treatment of refractory congestive heart failure. *Clin Cardiol* 1988;11:449–452.
125. Jaski BE, Ha J, Denys BG, et al. Peripherally inserted veno-venous ultrafiltration for rapid treatment of volume overloaded patients. *J Card Fail* 2003;9:227–231.
126. Haas GJ, Leier CV. Invasive cardiovascular testing in chronic congestive heart failure. *Crit Care Med* 1990;18:S1–S4.
127. Vincent JL. Hemodynamic monitoring: pharmacologic therapy and arrhythmia management in acute congestive heart failure. In: Hosenpud JD, Greenberg BH, eds. *Congestive heart failure: pathophysiology, differential diagnosis, and comprehensive approaches to therapy*. New York: Springer-Verlag, 1994:509–521.
128. Edwards JD. Practical application of oxygen transport principles. *Crit Care Med* 1990;18:S45–S48.
129. Stevenson LW, Dracup KA, Tillisch JH. Efficacy of medical therapy tailored for severe congestive heart failure in patients transferred for urgent cardiac transplantation. *Am J Cardiol* 1989;63:461–464.
130. Crexells C, Chatterjee K, Forrester JS, et al. Optimal level of filling pressure in the left side of the heart in acute myocardial infarction. *N Engl J Med* 1973;289:1263–1266.
131. Stevenson LW, Tillisch JH. Maintenance of cardiac output with normal filling pressures in dilated heart failure. *Circulation* 1986;74:1303–1308.
132. Mavric Z, Zaputovic L, Zagar D, et al. Usefulness of blood lactate as a predictor of shock development in acute myocardial infarction. *Am J Cardiol* 1991;67:565–568.
133. Weil MW, Afifi AA. Experimental and clinical studies on lactate and pyruvate as indicators of acute circulatory failure. *Circulation* 1970;16:989–1001.
134. Connors AFJ, Speroff T, Dawson NV, et al. for the SUPPORT investigators. The effectiveness of right heart catheterization in the initial care of critically ill patients. *JAMA* 1996;276:889–897.
135. Stevenson LW. The Evaluation Study of Congestive Heart Failure and Pulmonary Artery Catheterization Effectiveness (ESCAPE) Trial: presented at 2004 AHA scientific sessions. *Rev Cardiovasc Med* 2005;6:38.
136. Hague WA, Boehmer J, Clemson BS, et al. Hemodynamic effects of supplemental oxygen administration in congestive heart failure. *J Am Coll Cardiol* 1996;27:353–357.
137. Califf RM, Bengston JR. Cardiogenic shock. *New Engl J Med* 1994;330:1724–1730.
138. Hunt SA, Abraham WT, Chin MH, et al. ACC/AHA 2005 Guideline update for the diagnosis and management of chronic heart failure in the adult–summary article: a report of the American College of Cardiology/American Heart Association Task Force on Practice Guidelines (Writing Committee to Update the 2001 Guidelines for the Evaluation and Management of Heart Failure) *Circulation* 2005;112:1825–1852.

CHAPTER 87 ■ CHRONIC HEART FAILURE MANAGEMENT

W. H. WILSON TANG AND JAMES B. YOUNG

OVERVIEW

Treatment of heart failure is a challenging task that depends on making the proper diagnosis, staging the syndrome severity, and choosing interventions that both diminish suffering and decrease an exceptionally high mortality. Contemporary insight into the pathophysiology of heart failure and a large number of recent clinical trials have given us guidance on utilizing medical and surgical therapies. Greater understanding of the molecular dynamics, humoral perturbation, and circulatory insufficiency characteristic of heart failure will some day lead to even newer and more radical heart failure treatments. Another important paradigm shift in heart failure treatment is early detection of structural heart diseases, such that "preventive" strategies can be implemented before ventricular dysfunction and clinically manifest congestive heart failure develop.

Historical Perspectives

Substantive evolution of treatment paradigms has occurred over the past centuries (Table 87.1). Therapies have evolved from crude attempts to relieve dropsy to suppression of neurohormonal perturbations using combinations of neurohormonal antagonists (1,2). Today, strategies that block or ameliorate adverse remodeling have become the primary focus when considering therapeutic options (3). Indeed, current advances in treatment of the heart failure syndrome include a wide and complicated array of surgical, electrophysiologic, and pharmacologic treatment options.

The three most representative (and "equivalent") cohorts to demonstrate this evolution are (a) Studies of Left Ventricular Dysfunction (SOLVD) in the late 1980s (4), (b) Studies of Patients Intolerant to Converting Enzyme inhibitors (SPICE) trial in the late 1990s (5), and (c) the Sudden Cardiac Death in Heart Failure Trial (SCD-HeFT) in the early 2000s (6). These data sets document the change in prescription patterns with regard to heart failure since the late 1980s, particularly with the increased use of neurohormonal antagonists such as angiotensin-converting enzyme (ACE) inhibitors/angiotensin II receptor blockers (ARBs) and/or β-adrenergic blockers (Fig. 87.1).

Clinical Trials Insights

Tables 87.2 and 87.3 present selected multicenter clinical trials that have greatly shaped our philosophy regarding best approaches to the patients with heart failure. These trials were well performed and therefore provide credible information regarding therapeutic algorithms. A wide spectrum of placebo mortality can be observed, a finding implying that different patient populations have been studied. It is also likely that, over time, patient management strategies have generally improved. The clinical trial data supporting use of specific agents for the heart failure syndrome are discussed in the sections that follow.

Consensus Guidelines

The Agency for Health Care Policy and Research (AHCPR) published the first guidelines for evaluating and treating patients with chronic heart failure in 1994 (7–11). Subsequently, guidelines emerged from several cardiology societies as our

TABLE 87.1

PROGRESS OF UNDERSTANDING OF HEART FAILURE RELATED TO THERAPIES

HEART FAILURE IS A DROPSICAL CONDITION
Lymphatic drainage tubes
Primitive diuretic therapies
Foxglove tea
HEART FAILURE IS A CENTRAL CARDIAC PUMP INADEQUACY
Cardiac glycoside preparations
Alternative inotropic therapies
Cardiac transplantation
Mechanical ventricular assist devices and total artificial heart
HEART FAILURE IS CAUSED BY DECOMPENSATED VENTRICULAR HYPERTROPHY
Antihypertensive therapy
Surgical repair of valvular defects
HEART FAILURE IS A CIRCULATORY DYSFUNCTION
Vasodilator therapy
HEART FAILURE IS AN ENDOCRINOPATHY
Angiotensin-converting enzyme inhibitors
Angiotensin II receptor blockers
Aldosterone receptor antagonists
β-Adrenergic blockers
HEART FAILURE IS A FEVER
Development of immune-modulating therapies

knowledge base increased. Recent guideline updates from the European Society of Cardiology, the American College of Cardiology/American Heart Association (12), and the Heart Failure Society of America (13) have further broadened their recommendations regarding issues pertinent to the mildly ill (prevention) or severely ill (end-of-life care) patients.

All guidelines support an aggressive approach to diagnosing and treating patients with active ischemia and left ventricular dysfunction. The guidelines are unanimous in recommending ACE inhibitors and ARBs, as well as β-adrenergic blockers in all patients with left ventricular systolic dysfunction unless these drugs are contraindicated. All guidelines suggest avoiding agents with incomplete benefit-to-risk profiles, and they remind clinicians about diagnosing and treating underlying and precipitating factors. Furthermore, most of the guidelines emphasize the importance of prescribing nonpharmacologic therapy such as exercise and salt and fluid restriction while addressing patient education about heart failure.

Indeed, many of these recommendations have been further distilled into core performance measures for regulatory agencies to determine the quality of heart failure care in clinical practice (Table 87.4) (14–16). However, implementation of guidelines into everyday clinical practice has recognized limitations, because guidelines cannot possibly address all relevant clinical situations (17).

CREATING A MANAGEMENT STRATEGY

Philosophy

The principles of managing chronic heart failure are rooted in careful evaluation by making the appropriate diagnosis, staging the syndrome, addressing diseases causing or precipitating the difficulty, and using strategies that prevent disease progression. Besides ameliorating symptoms with tailored therapeutic programs, identifying individuals with insidious hemodynamic and hormonal perturbation early on is critical, so therapy can be given early in the syndrome's course to prevent the development of symptomatic heart failure (Fig. 87.2). Underlying these important principles is the concept that rational polypharmacy is mandatory because these patients are taking multiple drugs and combinations of drugs. The fewest drugs possible should be prescribed and dispensed in such a way that the fewest side effects appear with the most benefit, and cost effectiveness and compliance can be high.

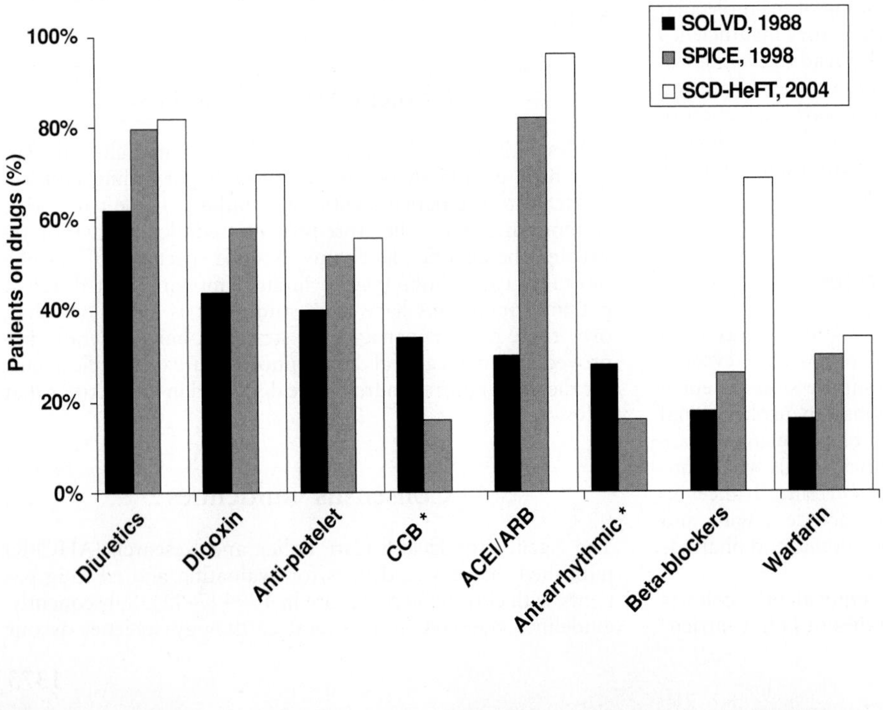

FIGURE 87.1. Evolving drug utilization patterns in heart failure. ACEI, angiotensin-converting enzyme inhibitor; ARB, angiotensin-II receptor blocker; CCB, calcium channel blocker; SOLVD, Studies of Left Ventricular Dysfunction; SPICE, Study of Patients Intolerant of Converting Enzyme Inhibitors; SCD-HeFT, Sudden Cardiac Death in Heart Failure Trial. *The asterisk* denotes statistics not reported in the literature.

TABLE 87.2

PIVOTAL CLINICAL TRIALS USING DRUGS TARGETING THE RENIN-ANGIOTENSIN-ALDOSTERONE SYSTEM IN CHRONIC HEART FAILURE

Trial (reference)	Year	Study population	Comparison and target dose	Sample size	Withdrawal	Duration (mo)	IHD	All-cause mortality	Annualized mortality[a]	Mortality reduction
Angiotensin-converting enzyme (ACE) inhibitors										
CONSENSUS (44)	1987	NYHA IV	Enalapril 20 mg BID	127	17%	12	73%	46 (36%)	36%	18%
			Placebo	126	14%			66 (52%)		RRR 31%
V-HeFT II (45)	1991	NYHA II–III	Enalapril 10 mg BID	403	22%	24	53%	132 (18%)	13%	7%
		EF <45%	HYD 75/ ISDN 40 mg QID	401	31%			153 (25%)		RRR 28%
SOLVD-T (47)	1991	NYHA II–III	Enalapril 10 mg BID	1,285	33%	41	71%	42 (35%)	10%	4.5%
		EF ≤35%	Placebo	1,284	42%			510 (40%)		RRR 16%
SOLVD-P (46)	1992	NYHA I	Enalapril 10 mg BID	2,111	24%	37	83%	313 (15%)	5%	1%
		EF ≤35%	Placebo	2,117	27%			334 (16%)		RRR 9%
SAVE (48)	1992	Post-MI	Captopril 50 mg TID	1,115	30%	42	100%	228 (20%)	6%	4.2%
		EF ≤40%	Placebo	1,116	27%			275 (25%)		RRR 19%
AIRE (49)	1993	Post-MI	Ramipril 5 mg BID	1,004	35%	15	100%	170 (17%)	16%	5.6%
		NYHA II–III	Placebo	982	32%			222 (23%)		RRR 27%
TRACE (50)	1995	Post-MI	Trandolapril	876	37%	48	100%	304 (35%)	24%	7.6%
		EF ≤35%	Placebo	873	36%			369 (42%)		RRR 22%
NETWORK (130)	1998	NYHA II–IV	Enalapril 2.5 mg BID	506	20%	6	71%	21 (4%)	7%	6%
			Enalapril 5 mg BID	510	19%			17 (3%)		NS
			Enalapril 10 mg BID	516	26%			15 (3%)		
ATLAS (57)	1999	NYHA II–III	Lisinopril 5 mg QD	1,596	31%	48	65%	717 (45%)	11%	2%
		EF ≤30%	Lisinopril 35 mg QD	1,568	27%			666 (43%)		NS
Angiotensin II receptor blockers (ARBs)										
ELITE-I (68)	1997	NYHA II–IV	Losartan 50 mg QD	352	18%	12	68%	17 (5%)	7%	4%
		EF ≤40%	Captopril 25 mg TID	370	30%			32 (9%)		RRR 46%
ELITE-II (69)	2000	NYHA II–IV	Losartan 50 mg QD	1,578	10%	18	80%	280 (18%)	11%	−2%
		EF ≤40%	Captopril 25 mg TID	1,574	15%			250 (16%)		NS
Val-HeFT (62)	2001	NYHA II–IV	Valsartan 160 mg BID	2,511	10%	23	57%	495 (20%)	10%	−1%
		EF ≤40%	Placebo	2,499	7%			484 (19%)		NS
OPTIMAAL (70)	2002	Post-MI	Losartan 50 mg QD	2,744	17%	18	100%	499 (18%)	6%	−2%
		NYHA II–III	Captopril 50 mg TID	2,733	23%			447 (16%)		NS
VALIANT (61)	2004	Post-MI	Valsartan 80 mg BID	4,909	8%	25	100%	979 (20%)	13%	0%
		NYHA II–III	Captopril 25 mg TID	4,909	7%			958 (20%)		NS
		EF ≤40%	Valsartan 40 mg BID+ Captopril 25 mg TID	4,885	8%			941 (19%)		
CHARM (71)	2004	NYHA II–III	Candesartan 32 mg QD	3,803	25%	38	53%	886 (23%)	9%	2%
			Placebo	3,796	18%			945 (25%)		RRR 9%
Aldosterone receptor antagonists										
RALES (105)	1999	NYHA III–IV	Spironolactone 25 mg QD	822	26%	24	55%	284 (35%)	20%	11%
		EF ≤35%	Placebo	841	24%			386 (46%)		RRR 30%
EPHESUS (132)	2003	Post-MI	Eplerenone 50 mg QD	3,319	15%	16	100%	478 (14%)	14%	3%
		EF ≤40%	Placebo	3,313	19%			554 (17%)		RRR 15%

BID, twice daily; EF, ejection fraction; IHD, ischemic heart disease; MI, myocardial infarction; NS, not significant; NYHA, New York Heart Association functional classification; QD, once daily; QID, four times daily; RRR, relative risk reduction; TID, three times daily.

[a] Annualized mortality, (total mortality/duration) for ACE inhibitor-treated group.

TABLE 87.3

PIVOTAL CLINICAL TRIALS USING DRUGS TARGETING THE SYMPATHETIC NERVOUS SYSTEM IN CHRONIC HEART FAILURE

Trial (reference)	Year	Study population	Comparison and target dose	Sample size	Withdrawal	Duration (mo)	IHD	All-cause mortality	Annualized mortality[a]	Mortality reduction
MDC (82)	1993	NYHA III–IV	Metoprolol T. 50 mg BID-TID	194	23%	10	0%	23 (12%)	10%	−2%
		EF ≤35%	Placebo	189	31%			19 (10%)		NS
ANZ (131)	1995	NYHA I–III	Carvedilol 25 mg BID	207	14%	18	100%	20 (10%)	7%	3%
		Post-MI	Placebo	208	6%			26 (13%)		NS
US Carvedilol (83)	1996	NYHA II–III	Carvedilol 25–50 mg BID	696	2%	6	48%	22 (3%)	16%	5%
		EF ≤35%	Placebo	398	4%			31 (8%)		RRR 65%
MERIT-HF (90)	1999	NYHA II–III	Metoprolol S. 200 mg QD	1,990	12%	12	65%	145 (7%)	11%	4%
		EF ≤45%	Placebo	2,001	13%			217 (11%)		RRR 34%
CIBIS-II (89)	1999	NYHA II–III	Bisoprolol 10 mg QD	1,327	15%	16	50%	156 (12%)	13%	5%
		EF ≤35%	Placebo	1,320	13%			228 (17%)		RRR 34%
COPERNICUS (93)	2001	NYHA III–IV	Carvedilol 25 mg BID	1,156	15%	11	67%	130 (10%)	19%	7%
		EF ≤25%	Placebo	1,133	19%			190 (17%)		RRR 35%
BEST (95)	2001	NYHA III–IV	Bucindolol 50–100 mg BID	1,354	23%	24	58%	411 (30%)	17%	3%
		EF ≤35%	Placebo	1,354	25%			449 (33%)		NS
CAPRICORN (91)	2001	Post-MI	Carvedilol 25 mg BID	975	20%	16	100%	116 (12%)	12%	3%
		EF ≤40%	Placebo	984	18%			151 (15%)		RRR 23%
COMET (99)	2003	NYHA II–III	Carvedilol 25 mg BID	1,511	32%	58	53%	512 (34%)	10%	6%
		EF <35%	Metoprolol T. 200 mg BID	1,518	32%			600 (40%)		RRR 17%
SENIORS (94)	2004	Age >70 y	Nebivolol 10 mg QD	1,067	27%	21	68%	169 (16%)	10%	2%
		EF ≤35% or CHF	Placebo	1,061	25%			192 (18%)		NS

BID, twice daily; CHF, congestive heart failure; EF, ejection fraction; IHD, ischemic heart disease; Metoprolol S., metoprolol succinate; Metoprolol T., metoprolol tartrate; MI, myocardial infarction; NS, not significant; NYHA, New York Heart Association functional classification; QD, once daily; RRR, relative risk reduction.

TABLE 87.4

CORE PERFORMANCE MEASURES FOR QUALITY OF HEART FAILURE CARE

JCAHO (135)	ACC/AHA (hospital) (136)	ACC/AHA (OPD) (136)	Performance measure
		Diagnostics	
		1	Initial laboratory tests
HF-2	1	2	Evaluation of LV systolic function
		3	Weight measurement
		4	Blood pressure measurement
		6	Assessment of clinical signs of volume overload
		Monitoring of disease status	
		5	Assessment of clinical symptoms of volume overload
		7	Assessment of activity level
		Treatment	
HF-3	2	10	ACE inhibitor or ARB for LV systolic dysfunction
		9	β-Blocker therapy for LV systolic dysfunction
	3	11	Anticoagulant at discharge for HF patients with AF
		Self-management	
HF-1	4	8	Discharge instructions/patient education
		Patient education	
HF-4	5	8	Adult smoking cessation advice/counseling

ACC/AHA, American College of Cardiology/American Heart Association; ACE, angiotensin-converting enzyme; AF, atrial fibrillation; ARB, angiotensin II receptor blocker; HF, heart failure; JCAHO, Joint Commission on Accreditation of Healthcare Organizations; LV, left ventricular; OPD, out-patient department.

A variety of injurious processes can cause acute or chronic myocardial dysfunction (diastolic or systolic and right-sided or left-sided heart dysfunction). Injured myocytes, because of inotropic and lusitropic dysfunction, are exposed to passive tension and workload demand changes that ultimately translate into increased preload and afterload. This process sets the stage for detrimental cardiac remodeling. Therapies designed to normalize these hemodynamic perturbations seem logical. Less easy to address is myocyte interstitial matrix deposition, which occurs in heart failure and causes stiffening of the myocardium, with all its diastolic dysfunction implications. Strategies (not yet clearly defined) that prevent inflammation and fibrosis may become important with respect to this issue. The aforementioned mechanical alterations produce peripheral vascular bed flow decrement in either subtle or more obvious fashion. Therein lies the attraction of using agents that increase stroke volume (e.g., vasodilators or inotropic agents). The combination of mechanical cardiovascular and peripheral vascular blood flow changes triggers a variety of humoral, neurohormonal, and inflammatory responses, which initially appear to create systemic organ flow compensation. Ultimately, these factors intertwine to precipitate detrimental remodeling of the heart (cardiac hypertrophy and chamber dilation) and to provide targets for therapies that can block molecular factors leading to this remodeling. Because these processes vary in degree from patient to patient, individuals may present without symptoms or may suffer from a variety of fatigue, dyspnea, or fluid retention states that fluctuate based on treatment protocols, diet, physical conditioning, and diseases that caused the problem in the first place. Obviously, findings of potential reversible conditions such as valvular heart disease, coronary artery stenosis, cardiac conduction disturbances, and ventricular or atrial arrhythmias important in the pathophysiology of heart failure need to be surgically or electrophysiologically addressed as well.

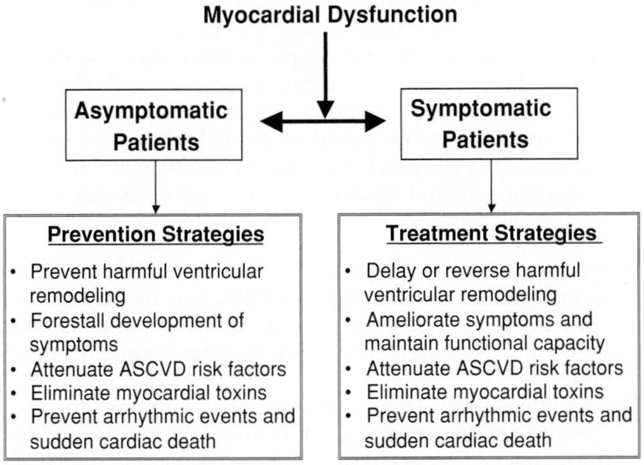

FIGURE 87.2. Philosophy of heart failure therapy focusing on prevention strategies for the asymptomatic patient and treatment strategies for the symptomatic patient. ASCVD, atherosclerotic cardiovascular disease.

Careful Evaluation of Patients

It is critical to remember that patients with heart failure have varied clinical presentations as they move from asymptomatic cardiac dysfunction to symptomatic heart failure. Complicating this issue further is that patients make this transition over highly variable time intervals. Several important questions should be kept in mind when managing patients with chronic heart failure, even before a treatment plan is formulated.

Does the patient actually suffer from heart failure, and are symptoms or physical findings related to this difficulty? Because of the nonspecific nature of clinical findings, many patients with weakness, fatigue, dyspnea, and edema do not have heart failure. Furthermore, patients with heart failure may present with these symptoms and physical findings, but the symptoms can be related to ancillary comorbidities rather than to cardiac dysfunction (e.g., poorly controlled blood pressure or glucose). Therefore, any patient with symptoms suggestive of heart failure, such as paroxysmal nocturnal dyspnea, orthopnea, dyspnea on exertion, lower extremity edema, decreased exercise tolerance, unexplained confusion, altered mental status or fatigue in an elderly patient, and abdominal complaints associated with ascites and hepatic engorgement (nausea or abdominal pain), should be evaluated at the bedside. Physical examination is essential to elicit findings supportive of congestive heart failure, such as elevated jugular venous pressure or positive abdominal jugular reflex, a third heart sound, a laterally displaced apical cardiac impulse, pulmonary rales not clearing with cough, and peripheral edema not resulting from simple venous insufficiency (7).

What is the cause of the syndrome? This question forces consideration of diseases that can be treated and eliminated or, at the least, ameliorated, such that progression of the heart failure milieu is halted. Table 87.5 outlines a common list of important clues that can be elicited from careful history or laboratory testing (12).

TABLE 87.5

EVALUATION OF THE CAUSE OF HEART FAILURE: THE HISTORY

CLINICAL HISTORY TO INCLUDE INQUIRY REGARDING THE FOLLOWING
Hypertension
Diabetes
Dyslipidemia
Valvular heart disease
Coronary or peripheral vascular disease
Myopathy
Rheumatic fever
Mediastinal irradiation
History or symptoms of sleep-disordered breathing
Exposure to cardiotoxic agents
Current or past alcohol consumption
Smoking
Hemochromatosis
Collagen-vascular diseases
Exposure to sexually transmitted diseases
Thyroid disorder
Pheochromocytoma
Obesity
FAMILY HISTORY TO INCLUDE INQUIRY REGARDING THE FOLLOWING
Predisposition to atherosclerosis (myocardial infarction, stroke, peripheral vascular disease)
Sudden cardiac death
Myopathy
Conduction system disease (need for pacemaker)
Tachyarrhythmias
Hemochromatosis
Cardiomyopathy (unexplained heart failure)
LABORATORY TESTING TO INCLUDE THE FOLLOWING
Complete blood count
Urinalysis
Serum electrolytes
Glycohemoglobin and fasting lipid panel
Thyroid function tests
Renal and liver function tests
B-type natriuretic peptide (BNP) or N-terminal pro-BNP

What evaluation is needed to confirm the diagnosis and stage the syndrome severity? In individuals with symptoms and physical findings suggestive of heart failure, determination and quantification of left ventricular function are mandated. Echocardiography can provide comprehensive assessment of cardiac structure and performance as well as valvular integrity and synchrony. Electrocardiograms and chest radiographs are also useful diagnostic tests in selected cases. Laboratory testing may reveal the presence of conditions that can lead to or exacerbate heart failure, and natriuretic peptide measurements can further aid in the diagnosis and prognostic determination. Selected patients may benefit from more advanced staging tests such as right-sided heart catheterization, metabolic stress testing, or left-sided heart catheterization and revascularization.

What precipitated the patient's deterioration? Frequently, medication noncompliance, excessive sodium or fluid consumption, worsening ischemic syndromes, atrial and ventricular arrhythmias, concurrent infection, uncontrolled chronic obstructive pulmonary disease, diabetes mellitus, and hypertension plunge patients into symptomatic congestive heart failure.

Does the patient take medications that can be detrimental in the heart failure setting? Drugs such as nonsteroidal antiinflammatory agents, certain calcium channel blockers, steroids, thiazolidinediones, and Vaughn Williams class I antiarrhythmic drugs may have deleterious effects or cause fluid retention that mimics congestive heart failure.

How should the patient be treated in the short term as well as in the long term, and what is the patient's expectation? Often, we neglect social factors that play a significant role in morbidity; we should always ask what social support mechanisms can be considered adjunctive nonpharmacologic treatments. Assessment should be made of the patient's ability to perform routine and desired activities of daily living.

Patient Counseling and Education

As in any chronic disease management, therapeutic success is highly dependent on effective communication between the health care providers and the patient. Ongoing nonpharmacologic interventions are often overlooked. Table 87.6 presents topics for patient, family, and caregiver education and counseling that have been modified from the AHCPR guidelines (11). These guidelines further highlighted the important role of family members or other caregivers in the treatment plan.

Discussion of the cause or probable cause of heart failure is important, as are expected symptoms, symptoms that herald worsening heart failure, and strategies to pursue if symptoms worsen. Furthermore, prognosis should be frankly discussed, and advanced directives should be elicited when appropriate. Advice should be given to family members with regard to resuscitation efforts should sudden cardiac death syndrome occur. The following topics should be reviewed at every visit:

- *Self-monitoring.* It is good practice to provide forms to record medication consumption, pulse rate, blood pressure, and daily weights. Instruction with regard to self-monitoring of blood glucose in patients with diabetes is equally important.
- *Diet counseling.* Patients with heart failure are often salt sensitive and frequently benefit from a 2.5 g per day sodium restriction (2.0 g per day in advanced congestive states). Fluid restriction is often recommended but controversial; it is more likely to be effective in hyponatremic states (usually ~1.5 L per day). General nutritional counseling, especially in patients with underlying diabetes or metabolic

TABLE 87.6

SUGGESTED TOPICS FOR PATIENT, FAMILY, AND CAREGIVER EDUCATION AND COUNSELING

GENERAL COUNSELING
Explanation of heart failure and the reason for symptoms
Cause or probable cause of heart failure
Expected symptoms
What to do if symptoms worsen
Self-monitoring with daily weights, blood pressure, pulse rate, blood glucose
Explanation of treatment or care plan
Clarification of patients' responsibilities
Importance of cessation of tobacco use
Role of family members or other caregivers in the treatment or care plan
Availability and value of qualified local support group
Importance of obtaining vaccinations against influenza and pneumococcus
PROGNOSIS
Life expectancy
Advance directives
Advice for family members in the event of cardiac arrest
ACTIVITY RECOMMENDATIONS
Cardiac rehabilitation programs with supervised exercise protocols
Recreations, leisure, and work activity
Exercise
Sex, sexual difficulties, and coping strategies
DIETARY RECOMMENDATIONS
Sodium restriction
Avoidance of excessive fluid intake
Alcohol restriction, if appropriate
Low-animal-fat diet, if appropriate
MEDICATIONS
Effects of medications on quality of life and survival
Dosing of drugs
Likely side effects and what to do if they occur
Coping mechanisms for complicated medical regimens
IMPORTANCE OF COMPLIANCE WITH TREATMENT OF CARE PLAN
Methods to ensure medications are taken in a timely manner
Provision of forms to record medications taken
Pulse rate, blood pressure, weight charts

abnormalities (e.g., cachexia), can be helpful. Malnutrition and malabsorption can be common, especially in congestive states. Although many patients may inquire about the role of vitamins and micronutrients in heart failure management (e.g., coenzyme-Q, carnitine, and other antioxidants), clinical data to support their use have been sparse.

- *Medication compliance and smoking and alcohol cessation.* Optimization of compliance with treatment and care plans is important. One should be specific when discussing patient responsibilities with regard to cessation of tobacco and alcohol use. However, well-controlled studies on the benefits of alcohol abstinence in patients with heart failure are few.
- *Exercise prescription.* Exercise should be encouraged in patients with heart failure, usually in a gradually progressive format. Patients should be encouraged to perform aerobic activities that are symptom limited. Activity recommendations need to focus on benefits of exercise-based cardiac rehabilitation programs.
- *Other preventive measures.* Vaccinations at appropriate intervals against influenza and pneumococcal disease should be administered. One should not ignore the importance of education with regard to atherosclerotic cardiovascular disease risk factor modification.

Pharmacotherapeutic Approaches

Table 87.7 outlines the major drug classes and commonly used drugs and their doses. At the core of therapy for systolic dysfunction are ACE inhibitors and β-adrenergic blockers. If an ACE inhibitor cannot be used because of intolerance or undesirable pharmacologic effects, one should consider ARBs or the combination of hydralazine and isosorbide dinitrate. Digoxin and diuretics can be added when signs and symptoms of congestive heart failure are present. Long-acting nitrate preparations may be important for dyspnea relief. In individuals with congestive heart failure but preserved left ventricular systolic function, the choice of drugs remains highly contentious.

SPECIFIC THERAPIES

Digitalis Glycosides (Digoxin)

Digitalis glycoside (or foxglove), often referred to as digoxin, is a competitive inhibitor of sodium/potassium/adenosine triphosphatase on the cardiac myocyte cell membranes that causes an increase in intravascular sodium and calcium. Digitalis has several pharmacologic effects that make it attractive in heart failure: (a) positive inotropic action, (b) negative chronotropic effects, (c) modulation of neurohormonal factors (by increasing baroreceptor sensitivity), (d) attenuation sympathetic nervous system tone, (e) reduction in norepinephrine concentration, and (f) diminution of renin-angiotensin levels (18). It is not clear which of these factors predominates in patients receiving low to moderate doses of digitalis (19).

Controversy about using digoxin has centered on proper patient selection and drug dosing (20–22). Little debate exists regarding its utility in patients with congestive heart failure who have atrial fibrillation (23). Higher plasma digoxin concentration has been associated with greater rate control in patients with atrial fibrillation (24), and it can be a particularly useful drug when there is a concern about the negative inotropic effects of other rate-controlling agents in congested patients. This is especially useful in the setting of rapid atrial fibrillation in patients who are significantly volume overloaded with marginal hemodynamics.

In the SOLVD Registry, 65% of patients with an ejection fraction of less than 20% were receiving digoxin compared with only 29% with ejection fractions of 36% to 45% (4). Two early, double-blind randomized studies, the Prospective Randomized Study of Ventricular Failure and the Effect of Digoxin (PROVED) (25) and the Randomized Assessment of Digoxin on Inhibitors of the Angiotensin-Converting Enzyme (RADIANCE) (26), demonstrated that digoxin therapy was related to improved ventricular performance and median exercise times regardless of serum concentrations. Pooled analysis of outcome in patients from both trials demonstrated that the lowest probability of treatment failure was seen in patients treated with the triple-drug combination of diuretics, diuretics, and ACE inhibitors (18). Furthermore, both trials suggested that withdrawal of digoxin in stable patients with heart failure was associated with higher adverse event rates, and that stopping this drug should be avoided unless the risks outweigh the benefits.

TABLE 87.7

COMMON DRUGS USED IN MANAGING CHRONIC HEART FAILURE IN THE UNITED STATES

Drug	Trade name	Heart failure indication	Post-myocardial infarction indication	Dosing
		Angiotensin-converting enzyme (ACE) inhibitors		
Benazepril	*Lotensin*	*No*	*No*	*5–40 mg QD*
Captopril	Capoten	Yes	No	6.25–150 mg TID
Enalapril	Vasotec	Yes	No	2.5–20 mg BID
Fosinopril	Monopril	Yes	No	10–80 mg QD
Lisinopril	Prinivil, Zestril	Yes	No	5–20 mg QD
Moexipril	*Univasc*	*No*	*No*	*7.5–60 mg QD*
Perindopril	*Aceon*	*No*	*No*	*2–16 mg QD*
Quinapril	Accupril	Yes	No	5–20 mg BID
Ramipril	Altace	Yes	Yes	2.5–20 mg QD
Trandolapril	*Mavik*	*No*	*Yes*	*1–4 mg QD*
Zofenopril	*Bifril*	*NA*	*NA*	*7.5–60 mg QD*
		Angiotensin II receptor blockers (ARBs)		
Candesartan	Atacand	Yes	No	8–32 mg QD/BID
Eprosartan	*Teveten*	*No*	*No*	*400–800 mg QD*
Irbesartan	*Avapro*	*No*	*No*	*150–300 QD*
Losartan	*Cozaar*	*No*	*No*	*50–100 mg QD/BID*
Telmisartan	*Micardis*	*No*	*No*	*40–80 QD*
Olmesartan	*Benicar*	*No*	*No*	*20–40 mg QD*
Valsartan	Diovan	Yes	No	80–320 mg QD
		β-Adrenergic receptor antagonists		
Carvedilol	Coreg	Yes	Yes	3.125–25 mg BID
Metoprolol succinate	Toprol XL	Yes	No	25–200 mg QD
Bisoprolol	*Zebeta*	*No*	*No*	*1.25–10 mg QD*
Nebivolol	*Nebilet*	*No*	*No*	*1.25–10 mg QD*
		Aldosterone receptor antagonists		
Spironolactone	Aldactone	Yes	No	25–50 mg QD
Eplerenone	Inspra	No	Yes	25–50 mg QD
		Others		
Amlodipine	*Norvasc*	*No*	*No*	*2.5–10 mg QD*
Hydralazine-isosorbide dinitrate	BiDil (37.5/20)	Yes	No	1–2 tablets TID
Digoxin	Digitek	Yes	No	0.125–0.25 mg QD

BID, twice daily; QD, once daily; TID, three times daily. *Italics* indicate a drug that is currently not indicated by the U.S. Food and Drug Administration for treating patients with heart failure.

When patients were divided into tertiles of serum digoxin concentration (0.5 to 0.9 ng/mL; >0.9 to 1.2 ng/mL; >1.2 ng/mL), there was a dose-dependent reduction of median exercise time after placebo was substituted for digoxin (27).

Gaining insight into the effect of digitalis on survival has been more difficult. Several postinfarction studies have indicated contrasting effects of digoxin on mortality (28–30). The Digitalis Investigation Group (DIG) trial evaluated almost 8,000 patients with digoxin added to a background of ACE inhibitor and diuretics (31). Approximately 1,000 patients had congestive heart failure but preserved left ventricular systolic function (ejection fraction >45%). The trial was relatively nonselective, with inclusion criteria being a history of clinical heart failure with current or previous evidence of low output (manifest by historic limitation of physical activity), normal sinus rhythm, chest radiograph, ejection fraction performed within 6 months of trial entry, and evidence at some time of congestion (i.e., peripheral or central edema, jugular venous distention, pulmonary rales, or chest radiographic pulmonary edema). This trial demonstrated that digoxin had a completely neutral effect on mortality. Still, digoxin reduced hospitalizations and favorably affected the combined end point of death or hospitalization resulting from worsening congestive heart failure (32). There was a trend toward increased death caused by arrhythmic events in analysis of certain subgroups, and this led some investigators to urge caution with prescription of this drug. Careful analysis of the diastolic dysfunction subset (33) demonstrated the same beneficial outcome results noted in the trial more generally (31). Contemporary use of digoxin is more prevalent in patients with a low ejection fraction, atrial fibrillation, and more advanced stages of heart failure (34).

Digoxin has a relatively narrow therapeutic window, and high doses and levels of digoxin may be unnecessary for efficacy in patients with congestive heart failure. In fact, recent post hoc analyses of the DIG trial demonstrated significantly increased mortality in women with left ventricular systolic dysfunction (ejection fraction ≤45%), possibly owing to their smaller body sizes (35), and in patients with higher serum digoxin levels (22). Therefore, in our experience, rarely do patients require more than 0.125 mg daily unless digoxin is used for better rate control in the setting of atrial fibrillation. Digitalis toxicity may lead to arrhythmias, gastrointestinal symptoms, and/or central nervous system abnormalities. The diagnosis of digoxin toxicity seems to be related to elevated plasma levels, but few data are available that link plasma levels to their physiologic effects. Although routine determination of serum digoxin levels is not necessary, serum concentrations should be measured with worsening of the heart failure syndrome, development of gastrointestinal absorption problems, patient noncompliance, or deterioration of renal function, or if toxicity is suspected. The serum concentration should be less than 1 ng/mL (35). It is important to monitor patients intermittently for serum electrolyte levels, renal function, and drug interactions (especially with coadministration of amiodarone, verapamil, or certain antibiotics that inactivate colonic bacteria). Administration of antidigoxin antibodies should be reserved for severe digitalis toxicity (36).

Diuretics

Diuretics continue to play an important role in the treatment of congestive heart failure. However, diuretics have not been properly studied to date in large-scale mortality trials in noncongested patients with heart failure (with the exception of aldosterone receptor antagonists, which are more appropriately considered a separate drug class). Diuretic therapy can be used to treat either congestion or hypertension. By reducing blood volume via renal inhibition of salt and water reabsorption, diuretics can lower cardiac filling pressures, with subsequent reduction in wall stress, pulmonary edema, and peripheral congestion, and neurohormonal activation can be suppressed (37). In the setting of hypertension, diuretics can induce effective blood pressure control and associated reduction in the incidence of stroke, congestive heart failure, coronary disease, and total mortality (38). Overzealous reduction in plasma volume with diuretics may paradoxically and adversely activate the renin-angiotensin-aldosterone system (RAAS) and the sympathetic nervous system. This may promote further sodium and water retention while increasing impedance to left ventricular ejection, eventually contributing to the progression of heart failure remodeling and worsening renal insufficiency (39).

The need for salt and fluid removal in response to fluid retention and edema is often a matter of pavlovian conditioning by patients and health care providers. Although there is no question that diuretics are essential agents to relieve volume-overload states, congestion is not always present in patients with heart failure. In fact, many patients develop congestive states that can resolve with pulsed or intermittent diuretic therapy (40). With a low-salt diet and maximal neurohormonal blockade, these patients may not require long-term diuretic therapy. Physicians' reluctance to reduce diuretic doses when patients do not complain of congestive symptoms can lead to hypovolemia, manifested as fatigue, dizziness, and azotemia, a presentation that is similar to impending decompensation. There is a broad range of diuretic requirements in patients with congestive heart failure: some patients may need intermittent, but regular, oral pulses of diuretics, whereas others may require continuous administration of diuretics in large doses or combinations. Stopping diuretics entirely or creating an interval "drug holiday" should be considered in patients who have been taking diuretics for chronic congestive heart failure but whose fluid retention state has resolved.

Generally, diuretics should be initiated at the lowest effective dose of the class chosen. Problems that may occur with short- and long-term use of diuretics include hyponatremia, hypokalemia, metabolic alkalosis, and increased uric acid levels (setting the stage for overt gout or worsening renal function). Carbohydrate metabolism is frequently disturbed, with resultant hyperglycemia, insulin resistance, and nonketotic hyperosmolar states. Lipid perturbation is also a problem, but its significance is not well understood. Diuretic-specific side effects include ototoxicity with furosemide, gynecomastia and galactorrhea with spironolactone, metabolic acidosis with carbonic anhydrase inhibitors, and hyperkalemia with potassium-sparing diuretics (triamterene, spironolactone, and amiloride).

Treatment with diuretics is often started with thiazide diuretics (e.g., hydrochlorothiazide or chlorthalidone) prescribed in the lowest dose necessary to induce effective diuresis. Thiazide and thiazide-type diuretics and the combination of thiazide diuretics with a loop diuretic can easily precipitate hyponatremia. As congestion worsens, standing doses of loop diuretics (e.g., furosemide, bumetanide, or torsemide) are often prescribed. Occasionally, for particularly refractory edematous states, combinations of diuretic classes may be necessary. However, failure to mobilize salt and water (so-called "diuretic resistance") is often the result of inadequate sodium and fluid restriction, particularly in individuals who were recently treated with diuretics and are at risk of rebound sodium retention (41). Ensuring low sodium consumption is essential to success with these compounds. Acute resistance is generally overcome with an increased single diuretic dose. Chronic resistance can be addressed with the coadministration of thiazide or potassium-sparing diuretics with a loop diuretic. Using combinations of agents active at different points of the nephron is essential. From a pharmacokinetic standpoint, overcoming diuretic resistance by simply increasing diuretic dose is important, but the consequences are variable. Altered bioavailability may account for some aspects of diuretic resistance, and there are different absorption kinetics associated with furosemide, bumetanide, and torsemide. Switching among these oral loop diuretics may be helpful in selected cases, and data from small, unblinded studies support the safety and benefits of torsemide over furosemide (42,43). Giving diuretics intravenously may overcome the absorption difficulties associated with bowel wall edema.

Angiotensin-Converting Enzyme Inhibitors

The RAAS is an established major pathway operative in the regulation of volume, salt, and water retention. ACE inhibitors have assumed the role of first-line drugs in patients with heart failure for the past 2 decades. ACE inhibitors have multifactorial benefits, including antagonism of the RAAS and balanced arterial and venous vasodilation. Furthermore, ACE inhibitors can block kininase II, a ubiquitous enzyme that degrades bradykinin and converts angiotensin I to angiotensin II. Direct ACE inhibitor effects and/or increased bradykinin levels lead to nitric oxide and prostacyclin release, which may mediate beneficial pleiotropic and antiinflammatory effects.

ACE inhibitor use has been studied in a broad spectrum of patients with heart failure. Although some of these studies are relatively small scale by today's standards, these pivotal studies have transformed heart failure from a terminal illness into a potentially treatable chronic (and sometimes reversible) condition (Table 87.2). First and foremost, the Cooperative Scandinavian Enalapril Survival Study (CONSENSUS) (44) used enalapril in severely ill patients with heart failure (New York Heart Association [NYHA] class IV). The dramatic 18% absolute mortality risk reduction is unprecedented. The observed clinical benefit with respect to mortality reduction was achieved by blocking certain aspects of neurohormonal compensatory systems characteristic of heart failure (specifically, the RAAS cascade), which spawned a new "neurohormonal hypothesis" in the treatment of heart failure (1). Subsequently, the second Veterans Administration Cooperative Vasodilator Heart Failure Trial (V-HeFT-II) (45) compared the combination of hydralazine and isosorbide dinitrate with enalapril and demonstrated that enalapril effected greater mortality reduction than did the direct-acting vasodilator combination. This finding further supported the benefits of neurohormonal blockade beyond their hemodynamic actions alone. The large-scale SOLVD program evaluated enalapril in asymptomatic or minimally symptomatic patients (the prevention trial) (46), as well as in patients with mild to moderate congestive heart failure (the treatment trial) (47). Baseline medications generally included diuretics and digoxin. In patients with ejection fraction less than 35% and symptomatic heart failure, enalapril significantly reduced mortality, morbidity, and, importantly, major ischemic events, such as acute myocardial infarction or hospital admission for unstable angina. In fact, the reduction in major ischemic events was more impressive than reduction of any other single morbid event, including hospitalization for heart failure. The SOLVD prevention trial demonstrated significant decrement in the combined end point of congestive heart failure morbidity (hospital admission for heart failure) and mortality that further points to the role of delaying disease progression with ACE inhibition. Smaller well-defined clinical trials have demonstrated the ability of ACE inhibitors to relieve dyspnea and to decrease the incidence of hospitalization for patients with mild to moderate heart failure. The role of ACE inhibitors for improving exercise tolerance is not as well defined.

Although the beneficial effects of ACE inhibitors are likely related to "class" actions, regulatory labeling has been based on the types of clinical trials performed. For example, some agents (e.g., captopril and ramipril) may be useful in the postinfarct setting (48–51), whereas other ACE inhibitors have been given labeling approbation for mortality as well as morbidity reduction in patients with heart failure. Retrospective studies have also suggested possible differences among specific agents, although these differences were statistically derived from administrative data (52). Furthermore, identification of renin-angiotensin system components and angiotensin II receptors in cardiac tissue suggests the existence of an autocrine/paracrine system with effects independent of circulating neurohormones (53). Tissue-specific ACE activity cannot be overcome by higher doses of enalapril (54). Therefore, there is an ongoing debate over the differential efficacies of tissue-specific (e.g., quinapril, ramipril, perindopril, trandolapril) versus non–tissue-specific (e.g., captopril, enalapril, lisinopril) ACE inhibitors in treating patients with heart failure. However, in vivo mechanistic evaluations have yet to demonstrate any significant differences in head-to-head comparisons (55). At this time, most experts still consider the benefits of ACE inhibition as a class effect of ACE inhibitors.

ACE inhibitors are more important than diuretics in patients with heart failure in the long term, and therefore, when congestive states are relieved, it is more appropriate to sacrifice diuretic administration so ACE inhibitors can be begun or maintained rather than continuing high diuretic doses (or continuing diuretics at all). Still, ACE inhibitors can be challenging to administer, and intolerance to ACE inhibitor titration because of cardiorenal limitations is associated with more advanced disease status and poorer prognosis (56). Nevertheless, randomized controlled trials have suggested potential morbidity benefits with high-dose ACE inhibitor compared with lower target doses (57), even though their differential effects on circulating neurohormonal levels are similar (54). Underdosing of ACE inhibitors is common. This may be fueled by fear of causing unacceptable reduction in blood pressure or worsening renal function. Defining optimal blood pressure in patients with ventricular dysfunction and heart failure is a contentious issue, and no precise target pressure can easily be identified. It appears, however, that the lowest blood pressure a patient can tolerate without significant orthostatic symptoms or renal dysfunction is the best in any specific clinical setting. The shorter-acting agent captopril can be used acutely, but it sometimes has to be held during aggressive diuretic administration. Although low doses are used initially, higher doses should be mandated (58,59). After patients have been exposed to the short-acting drug, switching to a longer-acting preparation such as enalapril or lisinopril is reasonable to improve medication compliance. Reasonable target doses are illustrated in Table 87.7. Patients who are at risk for developing orthostatic hypotension after ACE inhibitor exposure include those with hyponatremia, azotemia, volume depletion, and orthostatic dizziness or syncope (60). Problems can be avoided with simple dose adjustment techniques or reduction of aggressive diuretic therapies.

At this time, one should try to use a target-dose strategy. These ACE inhibitor doses were chosen for evaluation in the many clinical trials carried out in heart failure populations. When patients are hyponatremic, ACE inhibitor–naive, azotemic, or recently diuresed aggressively, slow upward titration of drug after starting with low doses is reasonable. Goals for electrolyte levels and renal function during ACE inhibitor therapy include the following: serum magnesium, greater than 1.8 mg/dL; potassium, 4.0 to 5.5 mEq/dL; sodium, 135 mEq/L or greater; and creatinine levels, less than 3.0 mg/dL. Administering magnesium often helps to control hypokalemia. In the SOLVD study, side effects resulted in discontinuation of blinded therapy in 15% of the treatment group compared with 9% of the placebo group. Enalapril use was associated with a higher rate of orthostatic hypotension (15% versus 7%), azotemia and worsening renal function (4% versus 2%), cough (5% versus 2%), fatigue (6% versus 4%), and hyperkalemia (1.2% versus 0.4%). These rates have been seen in similar rates in contemporary clinical trials of other ACE inhibitors. Severe renal function impairment may occur when ACE inhibitors are employed in patients with severe, bilateral renal artery stenosis or cardiogenic shock. Other common side effects of ACE inhibitors include rash and anemia (presumably because of erythropoietin suppression). Angioneurotic edema occurred in 0.4% of patients exposed to the ACE inhibitor and can be more prevalent in African Americans. A dry, harsh involuntary barking cough in the absence of congestion can be seen in up to 5% of patients taking ACE inhibitors, presumably related to bradykinin effects. One must be cautious about the inappropriate discontinuation of the ACE inhibitor, however, because many patients cough as a result of pulmonary hypertension, pulmonary congestion, or chronic obstructive pulmonary disease that accompanies the heart failure syndrome. Clinical data now support the use of ARBs such as valsartan or candesartan in patients intolerant to ACE inhibitors (61–63).

More recently, attention has been directed toward the question of differential effects of drugs based on race. Indeed, African American patients with heart failure have a seemingly worse prognosis than whites. To address this issue with respect to ACE inhibitors, an analysis of the SOLVD database has been published (64). Using a matched-cohort design in which up to four white patients were matched with each black patient, enalapril therapy, as compared with placebo, was associated with a 44% reduction (95% confidence interval, 27% to 57%) in the risk of hospitalization for heart failure among the white patients ($p < .001$), but with no significant reduction among black patients ($p = .74$). These results do not mean that ACE inhibitors should not be prescribed in this cohort. In fact, the significant benefits of hydralazine-isosorbide dinitrate combination seen in black patients with heart failure in the African American Heart Failure Trial (A-HeFT) are in addition to baseline ACE inhibition (65).

Angiotensin II Receptor Blockers

Specific ARBs are an alternative to ACE inhibitors. The hypothesis that ARBs may be beneficial in heart failure is intriguing because ACE inhibitors have been found to provide incomplete blockade of the RAAS over time and can be poorly tolerated by patients as a result of side effects. Alternative non-ACE or tissue chymase-dependent pathways may generate angiotensin II, thereby generating elevated circulating angiotensin II and aldosterone levels in patients with heart failure who are treated with long-term ACE inhibition (54). This "escape" phenomenon hypothesis is still being tested. Because ARBs do not affect potentially beneficial cyclooxygenase pathways or bradykinin production (which are activated by ACE inhibitors), ARBs give the promise of better-tolerated and more complete RAAS blockade.

Several clinical studies in patients with heart failure that used the first commercially available ARB, losartan, produced beneficial short-term hemodynamic effects similar to those of ACE inhibitors (with respect to reducing preload and afterload and increasing cardiac output) (Table 87.2) (66). Furthermore, losartan proved effective in reversing left ventricular hypertrophy over atenolol in hypertensive patients in the Losartan Intervention For Endpoint (LIFE) trial (67). In the Evaluation of Losartan in the Elderly (ELITE) study (68), 722 ACE inhibitor–naive elderly patients with mild to moderate (NYHA II to III) systolic heart failure (mean ejection fraction ~30%) were randomized to receive losartan versus captopril after a 2-week placebo regimen. The incidence of persistent renal dysfunction was the same (10.5%) in the losartan and captopril cohorts at 48 weeks of follow-up. Furthermore, the ELITE study showed an association between losartan and an unexpected survival benefit in elderly patients with heart failure compared with captopril. However, no significant differences in all-cause mortality (11.7% versus 10.4% average annual mortality rate) or sudden death or resuscitated arrests (9.0% versus 7.3%) were found between the two treatment groups in the setting of chronic heart failure, as reported in the ELITE-II trial (69), or in postinfarction cardiac dysfunction, as reported in the Optimal Trial in Myocardial Infarction with Angiotensin II Antagonist Losartan [OPTIMAAL] trial (70). Because of these data, losartan currently does not have an official indication for treatment for chronic heart failure. Nevertheless, losartan was better tolerated than captopril in these trials, a theme that has emerged across all comparison studies of ACE inhibitors and ARBs. However, the benefits of using valsartan and candesartan in ACE inhibitor–intolerant patients with heart failure have led to their current indications (62,71).

Exploring the potential for added benefit with an ARB was the Valsartan Heart Failure Trial (Val-HeFT) (62). This study was a double-blind, placebo-controlled multicenter clinical trial of valsartan generally added onto an ACE inhibitor (92% of patients concomitantly taking ACE inhibitors) with approximately 35% of the population receiving β-blockers. Valsartan significantly reduced the combined end point of mortality and morbidity (relative risk, 0.87; $p = .009$), predominantly because of a lower number of patients hospitalized for heart failure. Valsartan also improved clinical signs and symptoms in patients with heart failure when added to ACE inhibitor background therapy. However, improvement in survival was mainly seen in those without background β-blocker use (72). These results were confirmed in two other large clinical trials, the Candesartan in Heart Failure—Assessment of Reduction in Mortality and Morbidity (CHARM) program (63,71,73,74) and the Valsartan in Acute Myocardial Infarction Trial (VALIANT) (61). In particular, in the CHARM trial low ejection fraction prespecified analysis (with a high proportion of background β-blocker therapy), a 12% relative risk reduction in all-cause mortality ($p = .018$), a 16% relative risk reduction in cardiovascular deaths ($p = .005$), and a 24% relative risk reduction in heart failure hospital admissions ($p < .001$) were seen when candesartan was added to standard treatment in the 4,576 symptomatic patients with heart failure who had a left ventricular ejection fraction of 40% or less (75).

Early data from the Randomized Evaluation of Strategies for Left Ventricular Dysfunction (RESOLVD) study suggested that ARB use was not associated with any significant differences in exercise, functional class, or quality of life measurements compared with ACE inhibitors. There was a greater reduction in left ventricular volumes and in neurohormonal levels with the combination of an ACE inhibitor and ARB than with an ACE inhibitor alone (76). However, additional echocardiographic improvement with dual ACE inhibitor–ARB therapy over ACE inhibition alone has been less clear (77,78). The side effects of ARBs are similar to those of ACE inhibitors. Both classes of drugs can lead to angioedema and can impair renal function. Additional improvement of left ventricular systolic function and attenuation of detrimental remodeling with a greater decrease of angiotensin II and renin levels were noted when metoprolol was added to the ACE inhibitor–ARB combination (79).

β-Adrenergic Blocking Agents

The benefits of β-blockers in patients with heart failure were suggested as early as the early 1970s, but the evidence supporting β-blocker use in patients with heart failure has expanded rapidly over the past decade. Early data supporting β-blocker use have been confined to the positive impact with propranolol (80) and timolol (81) after myocardial infarction with respect to improvements in survival and major ischemic events. Although small clinical trials attempting to evaluate beneficial effects of β-blockers in heart failure have been published with disparate results, the Metoprolol in Dilated Cardiomyopathy (MDC) study was the first larger-scale trial to resolve some of the controversy about this strategy (82). The β_1-selective β-blocker metoprolol tartrate versus placebo was studied in patients with dilated cardiomyopathy. Compared with placebo, patients in the active drug limb of the trial had improved symptoms, with a decrement in the combined end point of survival and need for heart transplant. Although conclusions were tenuous, the observations added some support to the benefits of therapy with β-blockers in patients with heart failure.

Several important studies in the early to mid-1990s provided the basis for β-blocker therapy in chronic heart failure (Table 87.3). In a series of randomized, placebo-controlled multicenter trials of the comprehensive antiadrenergic (β_1, β_1, and α_1 receptor blocking) drug, carvedilol, pooled analysis showed a 33% risk reduction for all-cause mortality (83). The effects of carvedilol on patients' symptoms have been varied: some studies did not show an improvement in exercise tolerance (84), whereas other trials indicated that cardiac performance (85), congestive heart failure symptoms and NYHA functional classification (86), and general patient well-being were significantly improved by carvedilol (87). These individual trial results, as well as the combined analysis, suggested a significant reduction in mortality. Two other important trial networks, Cardiac Insufficiency Bisoprolol Studies (CIBIS) I (88) and II (89) using bisoprolol, and Metoprolol CR/XL Randomized Intervention Trial in Heart Failure (MERIT-HF) (90) using sustained-release metoprolol, presented positive study results around the same time period. A contemporary postinfarction heart failure study was conducted in Europe to support the theory further that β-blocker therapy remains beneficial in modern-day strategies in acute myocardial infarction. Recent data from the Carvedilol Post-Infarct Survival Controlled Evaluation Study (CAPRICORN) suggests additional benefit from carvedilol when added to ACE inhibitor treatment 48 hours after the ACE inhibitor has been initiated in postinfarction patients (left ventricular ejection fraction <40%). In particular, carvedilol reduces recurrent infarction by 41% and all-cause mortality by 23% (91), which was accompanied by evidence of reverse remodeling (92).

Perhaps the β-blocker trial comprising patients with the most severe heart failure was the Carvedilol Prospective Randomized Cumulative Survival (COPERNICUS) trial (93). This mortality end point study extended observations of benefit noted in prior trials to advanced (NYHA class IIII to IV) but euvolemic patients. Nonetheless, COPERNICUS markedly broadened the patient population likely to benefit from these agents and demonstrated that, when these agents are carefully titrated, even very ill individuals could tolerate β-blockers. These investigators found statistically significant mortality and morbidity benefits consistent with those of prior β-blocker studies. In particular, there was a 35% decrease in the risk of death with carvedilol and a 24% decrease in the combined risk of death or hospitalization. The recently presented Study of Effects of Nebivolol Intervention on Outcomes and Rehospitalization in Seniors with heart failure (SENIORS) trial also demonstrated that nebivolol reduced all-cause mortality and cardiovascular hospitalizations by a relative risk reduction of 14%, independent of age, gender, or left ventricular ejection fraction (94). However, another large clinical study with relatively ill patients, the Beta-blocker Evaluation and Survival Trial (BEST), did not find a mortality benefit when bucindolol was used (95). Perhaps important was that, in BEST, the point estimate of mortality reduction favored bucindolol, but the confidence intervals were wide and were not statistically significant compared with placebo, yet when white participants only were included in the analysis, benefits were noted (96). Some recent results from the genetic substudy suggest that polymorphic variants of the β_1-adrenergic receptor at amino acid position 389 influenced the pharmacologic effect of β-blockers (lower mortality in Arg398 compared with that of Gly398), but not the disease process itself (placebo mortality similar between two polymorphisms) (97). Apparently, the frequency of Arg389 has been found to be higher in whites than in blacks (reported as 70% versus 55%, respectively), consistent with the previous observations regarding racial differences in the reported results. Nonetheless, this observation of a potential difference between black and nonblack patients in BEST should be counterposed to a report suggesting that the benefits of carvedilol prescription in the United States carvedilol heart failure trials program were of similar magnitude in black and nonblack patients (98).

It has become more and more apparent that the drug class of β-blockers has very different properties depending on specific adrenergic receptor interactions. Additionally, some agents may have intrinsic sympathomimetic activity that may have detrimental effects. The exact underlying mechanism behind beneficial effects of β-blockers in heart failure remains unclear. A few trials comparing metoprolol with carvedilol in patients with heart failure are available. Based on these observations, some investigators have suggested that carvedilol, with its significant vasodilating and antioxidant properties, may be a superior agent. To resolve the controversy, the Carvedilol and Metoprolol Evaluation Trial (COMET) study was conducted, with a head-to-head design between carvedilol and metoprolol tartrate (short-acting agent) in patients with chronic systolic heart failure. This trial challenged the "class effect" principle and tested the hypothesis that comprehensive antiadrenergic blockade with carvedilol is superior to β_1-specific adrenergic blockade with metoprolol tartrate. Carvedilol was associated with a 17% relative risk reduction in all-cause mortality and with substantial morbidity benefits over the active control, metoprolol tartrate on a variety of end points including all-cause and cardiovascular hospitalizations, sudden death, stroke, and risk of new-onset diabetes (99,100).

In the United States, then, two β-adrenergic blocking drugs now have approval by the Food and Drug Administration for use in patients with heart failure, carvedilol (Coreg) and long-acting metoprolol succinate (Toprol-XL). It is important to consider their use in every patient who has had an acute myocardial infarction, particularly for use in combination with an ACE inhibitor when left ventricular systolic dysfunction or heart failure is present (101). β-Blocker therapy should be begun when patients are stable and are not overtly congested. Although it has been suggested that nonselective agents with vasodilating effects (e.g., carvedilol) are preferred, metoprolol succinate is one β_1-selective agent used frequently in heart failure settings and has data from MERIT-HF to support its efficacy. However, atenolol and short-acting metoprolol tartrate are no longer recommended based on the COMET results. Therapy should be begun with low drug doses (3.125 mg twice daily for carvedilol or 25 mg daily for metoprolol succinate) and a titration time period of 4 to 6 weeks. Some patients require longer time interval during uptitration doses and may benefit from stepwise titration (e.g., increasing the evening drug dose first before increasing both doses). Other patients may have the limitation of marginal blood pressures, which may necessitate less diuretic use or having a staggered drug schedule. Overall, about 70% of patients with heart failure (or $\leq$85% in clinical trial participants) may tolerate β-blockers (102). Patients with concomitant pulmonary diseases may benefit from pulmonary function testing to determine the severity of their obstructive lung diseases, and both drugs have been used in this setting.

Aldosterone Receptor Antagonists

Aldosterone is associated with salt and water retention and may lead to deposition of collagen in the cardiovascular system. Although in the past, drugs such as spironolactone were considered potassium-sparing diuretics, this drug class has established its place as a neurohormonal antagonist. Aldosterone receptor blockade is built on the same line of argument that aldosterone escape occurs as alternative pathways of RAAS lead to downstream aldosterone effects unaltered by ACE inhibition (103). Some of the proposed mechanisms of action of aldosterone antagonists include inhibition of myocardial and vascular remodeling, blood pressure reduction, decreased collagen deposition, decreased myocardial stiffness, prevention of hypokalemia and arrhythmia, modulation of nitric oxide synthesis, and immunomodulation (104).

According to the latest guidelines, aldosterone receptor antagonists are usually reserved for patients with advanced heart failure. These recommendations are based on the Randomized Aldactone Evaluation Study (RALES) trial, which enrolled patients with relatively advanced heart failure (NYHA IV, or NYHA III with previous class IV symptoms). RALES randomized 1,663 patients with heart failure (left ventricular ejection fraction $\leq$35%) who were already taking loop diuretics, ACE inhibitors, and digoxin, to receive either spironolactone or placebo. There was an astounding 30% reduction in mortality risks, as well as substantial reduction in sudden death, progressive heart failure, collagen turnover, and symptom burden in the spironolactone group (105,106).

The more selective aldosterone receptor antagonist, eplerenone, has also been studied in a phase III multicenter, double-blind, placebo-controlled trial Eplerenone Post-Acute Myocardial Infarction Heart Failure Efficacy and Survival Study (EPHESUS). In EPHESUS, eplerenone, 25 to 50 mg daily, was compared with placebo plus standard therapy in 6,644 patients with heart failure following acute myocardial infarction. The addition of eplerenone to optimal medical therapy (75% β-blocker users) reduced total all-cause mortality by 15% and reduced cardiovascular-related deaths and hospitalizations by 13%. Patients who were already optimally treated with an ACE inhibitor/ARB plus β-blocker, statin, aspirin, and reperfusion had a 26% reduction in all-cause mortality. Data on improving diastolic dysfunction with eplerenone treatment are emerging (107), although large-scale clinical trials on using aldosterone receptor antagonists in diastolic heart failure are still ongoing.

Careful patient selection and monitoring are essential in using aldosterone receptor antagonists. Aldosterone receptor antagonists are contraindicated if the serum potassium concentration is greater than 5.5 mEq/L at initiation, or if creatinine clearance is less than 30 mL per minute (in RALES, patients were excluded if they had a serum creatinine level <2.5 mg/dL). Elderly and diabetic patients are more vulnerable to adverse events, largely because of an increased risk of renal impairment. Dose adjustments of concomitant drugs, such as nonsteroidal antiinflammatory drugs or cyclooxygenase-2 inhibitors, potassium supplements, or ACE inhibitors, should be made before or during drug initiation. Indiscriminate use and poor compliance with monitoring protocols have led to serious adverse effects of spironolactone in real-world clinical practices. Several reports have highlighted the risks of hyperkalemia and worsening renal failure following treatment with aldosterone antagonists (108–111). Like other RAAS blockers, aldosterone receptor antagonists can lead to hyperkalemia and renal dysfunction, even more so than ACE inhibitors and/or ARBs. Careful monitoring of potassium and serum creatinine is advised.

Other Vasodilators

It is now well accepted that preload and afterload diminution in patients with heart failure reduces short-term morbidity and, with certain agents, long-term mortality (112). Relaxing venous capacitance vessels diminishes preload, whereas peripheral arteriolar dilation drops afterload and impedance to ventricular emptying. Venous capacitance vessels can be dilated by nitrates, such as nitroglycerin, nitroprusside, isosorbide dinitrate, and mononitrate preparations. Arterial resistance vessels are dilated by hydralazine. The combination of arterial and venous dilation occurs with ACE inhibitors and some α-adrenergic blockers (e.g., clonidine). Calcium channel blocking drugs are arteriolar dilators as well, but, as mentioned, concern exists about their use in the heart failure setting, perhaps with the exception of dihydropyridines. Dilation of the arteriolar bed alone, without concomitant venous dilation, may fail to achieve sustained morbidity and mortality benefit. Likewise, although sudden dyspnea can be alleviated with acute administration of short-acting sublingual nitroglycerin, long-term attenuation of neurohormonal or mechanical responses by the failing ventricle may not be observed. The combination of hydralazine and isosorbide dinitrate in doses that provided balanced vasodilatory effects was beneficial in the V-HeFT-I trial (113). Although isolated use of long-acting oral nitrates in patients with congestive heart failure is thought to be useful at times, there are significant issues surrounding the development of nitrate tolerance, and no current preparation has regulatory labeling for this use (114).

The nitrovasodilators, as a group, induce nitric oxide within vascular smooth muscle cells. This results in guanylate cyclase activation, which causes increases in cyclic guanosine monophosphate with subsequent vasodilation. Particularly in the setting of atherosclerosis, endothelial dysfunction is associated with decreased nitric oxide availability, and nitrate supplies exogenous nitric oxide to the vascular wall and improves the vasodilator state. Evidence also suggests that nitrites have antiplatelet effects that may be important in patients with ischemic heart disease with respect to platelet aggregation and thrombosis. Nitrate tolerance develops, however, when blood levels are constantly elevated. There is some suggestion that enhancement of vascular superoxide production secondary to exposure to nitrates may be an important mechanism in the development of tolerance (115). In vitro studies suggest that hydralazine, which has an antioxidant effect, prevents the nitrate-mediated formation of vascular superoxide and thus prevents nitrate tolerance. This observation may provide an explanation for benefits seen in V-HeFT-I with the combination of isosorbide dinitrate and hydralazine (116). By virtue of its capability to become a sulfhydryl donor, captopril is another drug that may combat nitrate tolerance. Alternatively, nitrate tolerance can be reversed after a washout period of 10 to 12 hours with thrice-daily administration patterns of isosorbide dinitrate (rather than every 4-, 6-, or 8-hour dosing schedules). Alternatively, isosorbide mononitrate preparations given once daily or in an asymmetric twice-daily fashion can obviate tolerance. If nitroglycerin patches are used, they should be limited to 8- or 12-hour administration periods, either at night to combat nocturnal dyspnea or during the day to treat exercise intolerance and dyspnea (114,115). Nitrates have also been demonstrated to have beneficial effects when they are given in conjunction with ACE inhibitors (117). In the recent A-HeFT study, when African American patients with symptomatic heart failure (NYHA III to IV and dilated ventricles) were randomized to receive a fixed dose of isosorbide dinitrate plus hydralazine or placebo in addition to standard therapy for heart failure, the treatment group was associated with lower mortality (6.2% versus 10.2%; $p = .02$), as well as reduced hospitalization and better quality of life (65).

Calcium channel blockers, as a group, may create significant problems in patients with heart failure. Although these drugs are very effective in lowering systemic vascular resistance, they generally have negative inotropic effects. Newer drugs in this class seem to have less negative inotropic activity and more potent selective peripheral vasodilatory effects. Still, to date, no overall sustained symptomatic or mortality benefit has been demonstrated for these drugs when used in patients with congestive heart failure. Indeed, in patients who have had acute myocardial infarction complicated by left ventricular systolic dysfunction, calcium channel blockers have proved detrimental more often than not, with a greater chance of adverse effects seen in patients randomized to drugs such as nifedipine and diltiazem. Nevertheless, because patients with heart failure frequently have concomitant ischemic heart disease or hypertension, calcium channel blockers are frequently found as therapies in patients with heart failure. Indeed, in the late 1980s, more patients in the SOLVD registry were taking calcium channel blockers than ACE inhibitors (4). Although this has changed somewhat more recently, it has been suggested that significant numbers of patients with heart failure (probably ~20%) are still taking these drugs. This strategy may best be reassessed on an individual patient basis. Treatment of angina pectoris with nitrates can be considered a substitute for treatment with calcium channel blockers. Patients with heart failure and angina pectoris should have aggressive attempts at percutaneous or surgical revascularization or medication therapies refocused on long-acting nitrates and β-blockers. To date, amlodipine (118) and felodipine (116) have been the only two agents studied with reasonably designed clinical trials to suggest no detriment with the drugs.

The use of non-ACE inhibitor vasodilator therapy in patients with heart failure can be particularly useful when the systemic blood pressure is elevated (sometimes despite ACE inhibitors) and in the setting of mitral regurgitation. Of course, the combination of hydralazine and isosorbide dinitrate is more frequently used because this combination was the first reported to suggest that mortality could be attenuated in heart failure populations with vasoactive compounds. When used as mortality-reducing therapies, the drugs should be combined. Pulmonary hypertension often responds well to long-acting nitrate therapy. One should be careful to administer these drugs in a fashion that does not produce continuous serum levels of nitrate such that tachyphylaxis could occur. Often, troublesome paroxysmal nocturnal dyspnea or orthopnea improves greatly when long-term, long-acting nitrates are administered at bedtime.

Chronic Inotropic Therapy

Few inotropic agents have met the challenge of both morbidity and mortality reduction in patients with heart failure. Although some of these drugs (e.g., xamoterol, milrinone, and flosequinan) have seemingly improved patients' symptoms, this effect has generally occurred in a setting of increased mortality (119). It is important to distinguish long-term therapy with these oral drugs from the use of inotropic agents, such as dobutamine and milrinone, in the acute heart failure setting (see Chapter 86) or as last-ditch attempts to control symptoms when the drugs are given parenterally to patients with advanced heart failure on a long-term basis. The recent disappointment over neutral results of the Studies of Oral Enoximone Therapy in Advanced Heart Failure (ESSENTIAL) (120) points to a lack of justification for oral inotropic therapy even for the most symptomatic patients with heart failure in contemporary management.

Anticoagulants

Routine anticoagulation in patients with heart failure in sinus rhythm has not been indicated in all clinical guidelines. Patients with substantive congestive heart failure frequently have significant hepatic congestion, and, because of this, anticoagulation can be difficult to achieve safely. Furthermore, with the large number of drugs taken by patients with heart failure, an important tenet is to continue only those medications with demonstrated effectiveness. This practice helps to ensure compliance with drug treatment regimens.

Routine anticoagulation in patients with heart failure has never been convincingly demonstrated to be beneficial in well-designed clinical trials, even though patients with heart failure have relative hypercoagulable states. Some studies have suggested a lower incidence of pulmonary and peripheral emboli in patients receiving warfarin, but, on the whole, the data are not overwhelmingly persuasive. In the open-label Warfarin/Aspirin Study in Heart Failure (WASH) study, warfarin (target international normalized ratio [INR], 2.5) was more effective in preventing stroke and hospitalization than aspirin (300 mg daily) or no antithrombotic therapy in the 279 patients with chronic heart failure, but at the cost of increased bleeding complications in the treatment arms of the trial (121). Preliminary results from the Warfarin and Antiplatelet Therapy in Heart Failure (WATCH) trial have been presented (122). Briefly, the WATCH trial randomized patients with advanced heart failure (left ventricular ejection fraction ≤35%, NYHA II to III) in sinus rhythm to open-label warfarin (target INR, 2.5 to 3.0) or double-blind aspirin plus clopidogrel. The study was terminated early because of sponsor withdrawal after 1,587 of the intended 4,500 patients had been enrolled (123). The ongoing Warfarin versus Aspirin in Reduced Ejection Fraction (WARCEF) trial, sponsored by the National Institute of Neurological Diseases and Stroke, is comparing warfarin and aspirin in 2,860 patients with heart failure with regard to the end points of death and stroke (124). This double-blind randomized controlled study will provide additional information about the relative effectiveness of these two agents in the future.

For current practice, it may be prudent to anticoagulate patients with heart failure with a history of systemic or pulmonary embolism or when left or right ventricular thrombi are noted on echocardiography. Certainly, atrial fibrillation is a clear-cut indication for careful anticoagulation. Candidates for anticoagulation should be monitored carefully, with a goal of achieving an INR of 2 to 4.

Device Therapies

Since the mid-1990s, devices have become an integral part of heart failure management, and the evaluation and monitoring of patients with heart failure now require the incorporation of the expanding considerations for device therapies such as implantable cardioverter-defibrillators and cardiac resynchronization therapy. These devices are discussed in detail in Chapters 67 and 75.

As more and more patients with heart failure have implanted devices, there has also been great interest in incorporating device information into day-to-day clinical practices. All devices can record information regarding pulse rates and incident arrhythmia, and some devices have specific information regarding activity levels, as well as sophisticated information about intrathoracic impedance. This makes true remote monitoring and telemedicine feasible, although the clinical benefits and cost effectiveness remain to be determined.

Other Comorbid Conditions

Patients with heart failure may have many comorbid conditions that can contribute to their symptoms and disease progression. Thyroid abnormalities are common, whether resulting from underlying metabolic derangements, unrecognized causes of heart failure, or medications (especially amiodarone). Patients with heart failure may have inadequate conversion of thyroxine to triiodothyronine (T_3, the active thyroid hormone) leading to an isolated "low T_3 syndrome." Many patients with heart failure have unrecognized or unexplained anemia caused by nutritional deficiencies (vitamin B deficiencies with loop diuretic use), medications, or hypervolemia.

For patients with unexplained anemia, the use of erythropoietin and its analogs for the purpose of treating anemia of chronic disease has been associated with improved symptoms and well-being, but no large-scale clinical trials have yet justified this approach.

Diabetes mellitus is a common comorbid problem related to heart failure. Insulin resistance is highly prevalent in patients with heart failure, and as many as half of the patients with dilated cardiomyopathy have some abnormalities of glucose metabolism. Poor glycemic control can lead to all the same signs and symptoms often associated with heart failure. Glycemic control can be challenging because most drugs used to treat diabetes mellitus have side effect profiles that are unsuitable for patients with heart failure. Drugs such as metformin and thiazolidinediones have been contraindicated in patients with heart failure, even though these agents may provide long-term benefits. Many dietary interventions for weight loss may also have adverse consequences with adjustments of concomitant heart failure medications.

Sleep apnea is common in patients with heart failure, and central sleep apnea is the most common form of sleep-related breathing disorder. Episodes of apnea, hypopnea, and subsequent hyperpnea cause sleep disruption, arousals, hypoxemia with reoxygenation, hypercapnia and hypocapnia, and changes in intrathoracic pressure. These pathophysiologic consequences of sleep-related breathing disorders have deleterious effects on the cardiovascular system. Also, clear evidence regarding the influence of depression in patients with heart failure is also emerging (125). There is frequently a lack of recognition of depression in patients with heart failure because many of the signs and symptoms of depression mimic those of heart failure (126). Social factors have a large role in the development of depression (127).

PITFALLS IN TREATING HEART FAILURE

Heart failure is a moving target, and patients and caregivers should be vigilant for signs and symptoms of deterioration. Starting late in a patient's disease course makes long-term morbidity and mortality more likely. A focus on preventive therapeutics is necessary. Ignoring the patient's underlying disease state and focusing only on symptomatic elements of heart failure set the stage for recurring difficulties. Treatment of ischemic heart disease should be pursued whenever possible. Atrial arrhythmias can be quite problematic, and an attempt should be made, if at all possible, to keep patients in normal sinus rhythm. Chronotropic incompetence or certain arrhythmias may respond to pacemaker therapy. Inadequate salt and water restriction can lead to hyponatremia, hypokalemia, and edematous states despite aggressive diuretic use. Concomitant use of potentially harmful medications (e.g., Vaughn Williams class I antiarrhythmic drugs and nonsteroidal antiinflammatory drugs) may be part of a therapeutic protocol and should be stopped, if possible. Use of inadequate doses or failure to start ACE inhibitor or β-blocker therapy is a major difficulty. Every attempt should be made to ensure that patients receive target ACE inhibitor and β-blocker doses; rather than sacrificing the ACE inhibitor in an aggressively diuresed patient, the diuretic dose should be decreased. Likewise, use of suboptimal doses of vasodilators because of "relative hypotension" can produce a clinical situation in which high afterload negatively affects cardiac systolic performance.

Excessive intravascular volume depletion with diuretics can be counterproductive by producing orthostatic symptoms and further activating adverse neurohumoral factors important in the pathophysiology of heart failure. On the opposite side of this spectrum is ineffective diuretic prescription (e.g., diuretic doses that are too low, combinations that are not rational, such as combining two loop diuretics, or failure to switch from oral to parenteral diuretic administration when necessary). Sometimes we see the reflex prescription of parenteral salt solutions for orthostatic hypotension or hyponatremia. A cycle of aggressive diuretic administration, low blood pressure, parenteral fluid administration, then congestion often develops in hospitalized patients. Only patients with shock and clear-cut intravascular volume depletion should have volume-expanding fluids administered. It is best to allow hyponatremia to correct with salt and water restriction and, possibly, concomitant parenteral loop diuretic administration. Orthostatic hypotension generally responds to bed rest with a reduction in diuretics or, possibly, vasodilators. When the situation becomes confusing and volume status is difficult to assess clinically, hemodynamic monitoring is advised. Because of the cytokine liberation that infections produce, not recognizing or treating intercurrent infections in patients with heart failure allows the syndrome to worsen. Furthermore, when certain conditions are treated, such as the use of theophylline preparations or nocturnal positive pressure breathing devices in hypoventilation sleep apnea syndromes, the heart failure syndrome improves dramatically. This is particularly true in individuals with pulmonary hypertension and right-sided heart failure.

STRATEGIES FOR PERSISTENT CONGESTION

One should first attempt to identify ancillary or extraneous issues that may account for this decompensation and then move toward the strategies outlined. Of course, many patients simply have progression of their disease. Placing pulmonary artery catheters and objectively measuring hemodynamics are at the root of clarifying confusing or challenging situations. With objective flow and pressure measurements, as well as the frequent determination of mixed venous oxygen saturation, tailoring therapeutics to each patient's clinical situation becomes possible. Parenteral vasodilator therapy (generally nitroglycerin and nitroprusside) alone or in combination with inotrope infusion (usually dobutamine or milrinone) can be dramatically effective. The use of continuous diuretic infusions, generally with a loop diuretic, such as furosemide, is an alternative strategy to consider in patients with refractory edema. When substantive edema persists despite all these recommendations, hemofiltration ultrafiltration or, possibly, peritoneal dialysis frequently removes substantial quantities of volume and improves symptoms rather dramatically.

TREATMENT OF ADVANCED OR REFRACTORY HEART FAILURE

When all attempts fail to create an adequate pharmacotherapeutic program that is successful in keeping patients symptom free over the long term, parenteral drug infusion protocols (which generally use dobutamine, dopamine, or milrinone or sometimes combinations of these drugs) can dramatically reduce symptoms. There is a suggestion, however, that these infusion therapies actually increase mortality. One must weigh carefully the risks and benefits of this approach. It may be an entirely acceptable trade-off in the patient with true end-stage disease who is suffering greatly from refractory congestive states. Furthermore, the necessity of placing an indwelling central venous catheter line access creates many challenges with respect to provision of skilled caregivers and support for administering the drugs. Infections and catheter malfunction are major difficulties. It is not clear whether these drugs should be administered as long-term infusions or as pulsed parenteral infusions, once weekly or monthly over shorter periods (6 to 24 hours). Also unknown is the best strategy to attempt long-term drug weaning. One practice is to infuse these drugs continuously for a 4- to 6-week period and then attempt to wean on an outpatient basis over several days or weeks.

One should always consider higher-risk standard operative or percutaneous coronary interventional procedures in the patient with advanced heart failure. Although these procedures are not always options, some patients with substantive ischemia or reparable valvular heart lesions have responded rather dramatically. Coronary artery bypass graft surgery, mitral and aortic valve repair or replacement, left ventricular aneurysmectomy, and endoaneurysmorrhaphy can all be effective options. Percutaneous coronary intervention also likely plays a role when objective evidence of ischemic myocardium related to target coronary lesions is apparent. The main challenge is to identify patients with viable and salvageable myocardium who are likely to benefit from procedures of this sort. Individuals with extensive scarring of their ventricles may not be the best candidates. Several alternative operative approaches are currently being evaluated. These include dynamic cardiomyoplasty, ventricular remodeling surgery, ventricular assist devices, and total artificial heart implantation (see Chapters 90 and 91).

CONTROVERSIES AND PERSONAL PERSPECTIVES

Clinicians who frequently manage patients with heart failure have had different experiences and interpret anecdotal or clinical trial data in many ways. It should be apparent from the foregoing discussion that heart failure treatment protocols are broad and complex. This is because the syndrome is, in fact, a difficult milieu. Much has been learned about designing heart failure treatment protocols, but perhaps most important is the necessity of beginning early to prevent deterioration to advanced stages. Taking care of patients with heart failure has become a specialty on its own, and the most difficult barrier has been the underestimation of the severity and complexity of the disease, which has led to undertreatment and missed treatment opportunities. Tailoring therapeutics to each individual's particular clinical situation seems most important. ACE inhibitors and β-blockers are now considered first-line therapy, but they are frequently underprescribed or prematurely discontinued. Device therapy has changed the landscape of heart failure therapeutics and seems to be an indispensable tool in heart failure management and sudden death prevention. Drugs and devices can do as much harm as good, and it is the caregivers' job to tailor the medical regimen to the individual patient. The "salvage" approach of heart failure care will only lead to costly hospitalizations and unnecessary suffering.

Clinical trials have guided us to a point which we have transformed heart failure from a once irreversible and terminal disease to a manageable and potentially reversible one. There is a desperate need to improve our understanding of the pathophysiologic process that underlies each individual patient so medical regimens can be tailored to minimize their adverse effects. We must learn how better to monitor our patients and to stratify them according to their needs for different medications. We often have very limited knowledge regarding adequacy of therapy, risk stratification, and prognosis, particularly when we have maximized all the medications and patients still feel symptomatic. Only until we can break away from the one-drug-for-all paradigm can we move forward with the difficult task of managing patients with chronic heart failure.

THE FUTURE

Emerging pharmacotherapeutic strategies will likely influence the direction heart failure treatment paradigms take in the future. The development of new pharmacologic therapy for the treatment of chronic heart failure has undergone substantial growth in recent years, largely driven by the increase in prevalence of cases. However, many of the novel drugs never progress beyond phase I trials. Because of the vast heterogeneity of the syndrome and the lack of a single recognizable lesion, drugs cannot be easily targeted toward a single mechanism or lesion. Although some recent clinical trials in chronic heart failure have been disappointing, the process of developing drugs to treat heart failure is long and tortuous (128,129).

Table 87.8 illustrates several drug classes currently in development for chronic heart failure. The RAAS still remains an important therapeutic target. Large-scale multicenter mortality trials of aldosterone receptor antagonists in patients with mild to moderate systolic heart failure and diastolic heart failure are under way. Renin inhibitors such as aliskiren are also emerging as the next wave of RAAS inhibitors, with the potential to provide upstream inhibition. Future treatment paradigms may include attenuation of inflammatory and metabolic processes important in the pathophysiology of heart failure and

TABLE 87.8

FUTURE CLINICAL DRUG TRIALS IN CHRONIC HEART FAILURE

Drug class	Drug	Phase	Conditions	Ongoing trials (Acronyms)
	Approved drug classes with extended indications			
Aldosterone receptor antagonist	Spironolactone	IV	Diastolic HF	TOPCAT
	Eplerenone	IV	Mild systolic HF	European study
Natriuretic peptides	Nesiritide	IV	Intermittent infusion	FUSION-II
Statins	Rosuvastatin	IV	Chronic HF	CORONA
				GISSI-Prevenzione
				UNIVERSE
Recombinant human erythropoietin	Darbepoetin-alpha	III	Chronic HF	RED-HF
	Novel drug classes with promising development			
Vasopressin receptor antagonists	Tolvaptan	III	Acute to chronic HF	EVEREST
		II	Chronic HF	
Renin inhibitors	Aliskiren	II	Chronic HF	ALOFT
Calcium transient modulators	Caldaret	II	Diastolic HF	MCC-135-G01 Study
Immunomodulation therapy	Celacade	III	Chronic HF	ACCLAIM
Xanthine oxidase inhibition	Oxypurinol	III	Chronic HF	OPT-CHF
Metabolic modulation	GLP-1 (AC2592)	II	Chronic HF	PROCLAIM
AGE crosslink breakers	Alagebrium	II	Diastolic HF	DIAMOND PEDESTAL
Hormone replacement	DITPA	II	Chronic HF	DITPA study
Adenosine A, receptor antagonist	KW-3902	III	Acute HF	PROTECT I, PROTECT II
	BG-9928	II	Acute HF	AB-CHF
Endothelin ET, receptor antagonist	Sitaxsentan	II	Diastolic HF	STRIDE-DHF

AB-CHF, adenosine blockade with BG9928 in CHF; ACCLAIM, advanced chronic heart failure clinical assessment of immune modulation therapy; AGE, advanced glycation end-product; ALOFT, aliskiren observation of heart failure treatment; CORONA, controlled rosuvastatin multinational trial in heart failure; EMPHESIS-HF, eplerenone in mild patients hospitalisation and survival study in heart failure; EVEREST, efficacy of vasopressin antagonism in heart failure: outcome study with tolvaptan; FUSION-II, follow-up serial infusions of natrecor (nesiritide) for the management of patients with heart failure–second study; GISSI-Prevenzione, gruppo italiano per lo studio della sopravvivenza nell'insufficienza cardiaca-heart failure project; HF, heart failure; OPT-CHF, oxypurinol therapy for congestive heart failure; PEDESTAL, patients with impaired ejection fraction and diastolic dysfunction: efficacy and safety trial of alagebrium; PROCLAIM, proof of concept–GLP-1 action in CHF management; PROTECT, (pending); RED-HF, reduction of events with darbepoetin alfa in heart failure; STRIDE-DHF, sitaxsentan to relieve impaired exercise in diastolic heart failure; TOPCAT, treatment of preserved cardiac function heart failure with an aldosterone antagonist.

blocking, at the molecular signaling level, necrotic or apoptotic events that lead to cell death. Despite early failures for specific anticytokine therapies with etanercept, there will likely be many antiinflammatory strategies to delay the disease progression. Immune modulation has been another major focus, and clinical studies of oxypurinol (OPT-CHF study) and Celacade (ACCLAIM) are near completion. Two large-scale mortality trials on statins (rosuvastatin) are also in progress. Renewed interests in metabolic modulation using novel compounds such as glycoprotein-like peptide-1 (GLP-1) and T_3 analog (DITPA) have also emerged. Stem cell therapies in various forms have been the newest development. It is likely that genomic medicine will become part of managing heart failure. Pharmacogenomics have led to many exciting new opportunities in risk stratification, with direct consequences to transplant evaluation or individualization of care plans. The discoveries of genetic mutations in dilated cardiomyopathy and exciting genomic-based diagnostic strategies are evolving. Finally, device therapy will be here to stay, and better and more sophisticated pacing strategies will evolve, including better positioning of leads, better pacing techniques and pacing modalities (including noncontractile pacing), new targets for electrical therapy, and new patient monitoring capabilities that allow true telemonitoring.

References

1. Packer M. The neurohormonal hypothesis: a theory to explain the mechanism of disease progression in heart failure. *J Am Coll Cardiol* 1992;20:248–254.
2. Young JB, Pratt CM. Hemodynamic and hormonal alterations in patients with heart failure: toward a contemporary definition of heart failure. *Semin Nephrol* 1994;14:427–440.
3. Cohn JN. New therapeutic strategies for heart failure: left ventricular remodeling as a target. *J Card Fail* 2004;10:S200–S201.
4. Young JB, Weiner DH, Yusuf S, et al. Patterns of medication use in patients with heart failure: a report from the Registry of Studies of Left Ventricular Dysfunction (SOLVD). *South Med J* 1995;88:514–523.
5. Bart BA, Ertl G, Held P, et al. Contemporary management of patients with left ventricular systolic dysfunction: results from the Study of Patients Intolerant of Converting Enzyme Inhibitors (SPICE) Registry. *Eur Heart J* 1999;20:1182–1190.
6. Bardy GH, Lee KL, Mark DB, et al. Amiodarone or an implantable cardioverter-defibrillator for congestive heart failure. *N Engl J Med* 2005;352:225–237.
7. Agency for Healthcare Research and Quality. Heart failure: evaluation and care of patients with left-ventricular systolic dysfunction. Clinical practice guideline no. 11. AHCPR publication no. 94-0612. Rockville, MD: Public Health Service, U.S. Department of Health and Human Services, 1994.
8. Baker DW, Konstam MA, Bottorff M, et al. Management of heart failure. I. Pharmacologic treatment. *JAMA* 1994;272:1361–1366.
9. Baker DW, Jones R, Hodges J, et al. Management of heart failure. III. The role of revascularization in the treatment of patients with moderate or severe left ventricular systolic dysfunction. *JAMA* 1994;272:1528–1534.
10. Baker DW, Wright RF. Management of heart failure. IV. Anticoagulation for patients with heart failure due to left ventricular systolic dysfunction. *JAMA* 1994;272:1614–1618.
11. Dracup K, Baker DW, Dunbar SB, et al. Management of heart failure. II. Counseling, education, and lifestyle modifications. *JAMA* 1994;272:1442–1446.
12. Hunt SA, Baker DW, Chin MH, et al. ACC/AHA guidelines for the evaluation and management of chronic heart failure in the adult: executive summary. A report of the American College of Cardiology/American Heart Association Task Force on Practice Guidelines (Committee to Revise the 2001 Guidelines for the Evaluation and Management of Heart Failure): developed in collaboration with the International Society for Heart and Lung Transplantation, endorsed by the Heart Failure Society of America. Circulation 2005;112:1825–1852.
13. Heart Failure Society of America Executive Summary: HFSA 2006 Comprehensive Heart Failure Practice Guidelines. *J Card Fail* 2006;12:10–38.
14. Landis NT. JCAHO selects core performance measures: Joint Commission on Accreditation of Healthcare Organizations. *Am J Health Syst Pharm* 2000;57:632–635.
15. Executive Council of the Heart Failure Society of America. Implications of recent clinical trials for heart failure performance measures. *J Card Fail* 2004;10:4–5.
16. Krumholz HM, Baker DW, Ashton CM, et al. Evaluating quality of care for patients with heart failure. *Circulation* 2000;101:E122–E140.
17. Parmley WW. Clinical practice guidelines: does the cookbook have enough recipes?. *JAMA* 1994;272:1374–1375.
18. Young JB. Do digitalis glycosides still have a role in congestive heart failure? *Cardiol Clin* 1994;12:51–61.
19. Slatton ML, Irani WN, Hall SA, et al. Does digoxin provide additional hemodynamic and autonomic benefit at higher doses in patients with mild to moderate heart failure and normal sinus rhythm? *J Am Coll Cardiol* 1997;29:1206–1213.
20. See S, Bruno P. Digoxin increases mortality among women with congestive heart failure. *J Fam Pract* 2003;52:106–111.
21. Adams KF Jr, Gheorghiade M, Uretsky BF, et al. Clinical benefits of low serum digoxin concentrations in heart failure. *J Am Coll Cardiol* 2002;39:946–953.
22. Rathore SS, Curtis JP, Wang Y, et al. Association of serum digoxin concentration and outcomes in patients with heart failure. *JAMA* 2003;289:871–878.
23. Dec GW. Digoxin remains useful in the management of chronic heart failure. *Med Clin North Am* 2003;87:317–337.
24. Redfors A. Plasma digoxin concentration: its relation to digoxin dosage and clinical effects in patients with atrial fibrillation. *Br Heart J* 1972;34:383–391.
25. Uretsky BF, Young JB, Shahidi FE, et al. Randomized study assessing the effect of digoxin withdrawal in patients with mild to moderate chronic congestive heart failure: results of the PROVED trial. PROVED Investigative Group. *J Am Coll Cardiol* 1993;22:955–962.
26. Packer M, Gheorghiade M, Young JB, et al. Withdrawal of digoxin from patients with chronic heart failure treated with angiotensin-converting enzyme inhibitors: RADIANCE Study. *N Engl J Med* 1993;329:1–7.
27. Young JB, Gheorghiade M, Packer M. Are serum levels of digoxin effective in chronic heart failure? Evidence challenging the accepted guidelines for a therapeutic serum level of the drug. *J Am Coll Cardiol* 1993;21:378A.
28. Moss AJ, Davis HT, Conard DL, et al. Digitalis-associated cardiac mortality after myocardial infarction. *Circulation* 1981;64:1150–1156.
29. Madsen EB, Gilpin E, Henning H, et al. Prognostic importance of digitalis after acute myocardial infarction. *J Am Coll Cardiol* 1984;3:681–689.
30. Bigger JT Jr, Fleiss JL, Rolnitzky LM, et al. Effect of digitalis treatment on survival after acute myocardial infarction. *Am J Cardiol* 1985;55:623–630.
31. Digitalis Investigation Group. The effect of digoxin on mortality and morbidity in patients with heart failure. *N Engl J Med* 1997;336:525–533.
32. Gheorghiade M, Adams KF Jr, Colucci WS. Digoxin in the management of cardiovascular disorders. *Circulation* 2004;109:2959–2964.
33. Jones RC, Francis GS, Lauer MS. Predictors of mortality in patients with heart failure and preserved systolic function in the Digitalis Investigation Group Trial. *J Am Coll Cardiol* 2004;44:1025–1029.
34. Camerini A, Griffo R, Fabbri G, et al. Use of digitalis in the treatment of heart failure: data from the Italian Network on Congestive Heart Failure (IN-CHF). *Ital Heart J* 2004;5:523–529.
35. Rathore SS, Wang Y, Krumholz HM. Sex-based differences in the effect of digoxin for the treatment of heart failure. *N Engl J Med* 2002;347:1403–1411.
36. Bateman DN. Digoxin-specific antibody fragments: how much and when? *Toxicol Rev* 2004;23:135–143.
37. Johnson W, Omland T, Hall C, et al. Neurohormonal activation rapidly decreases after intravenous therapy with diuretics and vasodilators for class IV heart failure. *J Am Coll Cardiol* 2002;39:1623–1629.
38. The Antihypertensive and Lipid-Lowering Treatment to Prevent Heart Attack Trial (ALLHAT). Major outcomes in high-risk hypertensive patients randomized to angiotensin-converting enzyme inhibitor or calcium channel blocker vs diuretic. *JAMA* 2002;288:2981–2997.
39. Butler J, Forman DE, Abraham WT, et al. Relationship between heart failure treatment and development of worsening renal function among hospitalized patients. *Am Heart J* 2004;147:331–338.
40. Grinstead WC, Francis MJ, Marks GF, et al. Discontinuation of chronic diuretic therapy in stable congestive heart failure secondary to coronary artery disease or to idiopathic dilated cardiomyopathy. *Am J Cardiol* 1994;73:881–886.
41. De Bruyne LK. Mechanisms and management of diuretic resistance in congestive heart failure. *Postgrad Med J* 2003;79:268–271.
42. Cosin J, Diez J. Torasemide in chronic heart failure: results of the TORIC Study. *Eur J Heart Fail* 2002;4:507–513.
43. Spannheimer A, Goertz A, Dreckmann-Behrendt B. Comparison of therapies with torasemide or furosemide in patients with congestive heart failure from a pharmacoeconomic viewpoint. *Int J Clin Pract* 1998;52:467–471.
44. CONSENSUS Trial Study Group. Effects of enalapril on mortality in severe congestive heart failure: results of the Cooperative North Scandinavian Enalapril Survival Study (CONSENSUS). *N Engl J Med* 1987;316:1429–1435.
45. Cohn JN, Johnson G, Ziesche S, et al. A comparison of enalapril with hydralazine-isosorbide dinitrate in the treatment of chronic congestive heart failure. *N Engl J Med* 1991;325:303–310.
46. SOLVD Investigators. Effect of enalapril on mortality and the development of heart failure in asymptomatic patients with reduced left ventricular ejection fractions. *N Engl J Med* 1992;327:685–691.
47. SOLVD Investigators. Effect of enalapril on survival in patients with reduced left ventricular ejection fractions and congestive heart failure. *N Engl J Med* 1991;325:293–302.

48. Pfeffer MA, Braunwald E, Moye LA, et al. Effect of captopril on mortality and morbidity in patients with left ventricular dysfunction after myocardial infarction: results of the survival and ventricular enlargement trial. The SAVE Investigators. *N Engl J Med* 1992;327:669–677.
49. Acute Infarction Ramipril Efficacy (AIRE) Study Investigators. Effect of ramipril on mortality and morbidity of survivors of acute myocardial infarction with clinical evidence of heart failure. *Lancet* 1993;342:821–828.
50. Kober L, Torp-Pedersen C, Carlsen JE, et al. Trandolapril Cardiac Evaluation (TRACE) Study Group: a clinical trial of the angiotensin-converting-enzyme inhibitor trandolapril in patients with left ventricular dysfunction after myocardial infarction. *N Engl J Med* 1995;333:1670–1676.
51. ISIS-4 (Fourth International Study of Infarct Survival) Collaborative Group. ISIS-4: a randomised factorial trial assessing early oral captopril, oral mononitrate, and intravenous magnesium sulphate in 58,050 patients with suspected acute myocardial infarction. *Lancet* 1995;345:669–685.
52. Pilote L, Abrahamowicz M, Rodrigues E, et al. Mortality rates in elderly patients who take different angiotensin-converting enzyme inhibitors after acute myocardial infarction: a class effect? *Ann Intern Med* 2004;141:102–112.
53. Dostal DE, Baker KM. The cardiac renin-angiotensin system: conceptual, or a regulator of cardiac function?. *Circ Res* 1999;85:643–650.
54. Tang WH, Vagelos RH, Yee YG, et al. Neurohormonal and clinical responses to high- versus low-dose enalapril therapy in chronic heart failure. *J Am Coll Cardiol* 2002;39:70–78.
55. Jorde UP, Vittorio TJ, Dimayuga CA, et al. Comparison of suppression of the circulating and vascular renin-angiotensin system by enalapril versus trandolapril in chronic heart failure. *Am J Cardiol* 2004;94:1501–1505.
56. Kittleson M, Hurwitz S, Shah MR, et al. Development of circulatory-renal limitations to angiotensin-converting enzyme inhibitors identifies patients with severe heart failure and early mortality. *J Am Coll Cardiol* 2003;41:2029–2035.
57. Packer M, Poole-Wilson PA, Armstrong PW, et al. Comparative effects of low and high doses of the angiotensin-converting enzyme inhibitor, lisinopril, on morbidity and mortality in chronic heart failure: ATLAS Study Group. *Circulation* 1999;100:2312–2318.
58. Packer M. Do angiotensin-converting enzyme inhibitors prolong life in patients with heart failure treated in clinical practice? *J Am Coll Cardiol* 1996;28:1323–1327.
59. Packer M, Lee WH, Yushak M, et al. Comparison of captopril and enalapril in patients with severe chronic heart failure. *N Engl J Med* 1986;315:847–853.
60. Kostis JB, Shelton B, Gosselin G, et al. Adverse effects of enalapril in the Studies of Left Ventricular Dysfunction (SOLVD): SOLVD Investigators. *Am Heart J* 1996;131:350–355.
61. Pfeffer MA, McMurray JJ, Velazquez EJ, et al. Valsartan, captopril, or both in myocardial infarction complicated by heart failure, left ventricular dysfunction, or both. *N Engl J Med* 2003;349:1893–1906.
62. Cohn JN, Tognoni G. A randomized trial of the angiotensin-receptor blocker valsartan in chronic heart failure. *N Engl J Med* 2001;345:1667–1675.
63. Granger CB, McMurray JJ, Yusuf S, et al. Effects of candesartan in patients with chronic heart failure and reduced left-ventricular systolic function intolerant to angiotensin-converting enzyme inhibitors: the CHARM-Alternative Trial. *Lancet* 2003;362:772–776.
64. Exner DV, Dries DL, Domanski MJ, et al. Lesser response to angiotensin-converting-enzyme inhibitor therapy in black as compared with white patients with left ventricular dysfunction. *N Engl J Med* 2001;344:1351–1357.
65. Taylor AL, Ziesche S, Yancy C, et al. Combination of isosorbide dinitrate and hydralazine in blacks with heart failure. *N Engl J Med* 2004;351:2049–2057.
66. Crozier I, Ikram H, Awan N, et al. Losartan in heart failure: hemodynamic effects and tolerability. Losartan Hemodynamic Study Group. *Circulation* 1995;91:691–697.
67. Dahlof B, Devereux RB, Kjeldsen SE, et al. Cardiovascular morbidity and mortality in the Losartan Intervention For Endpoint reduction in hypertension study (LIFE): a randomised trial against atenolol. *Lancet* 2002; 359:995–1003.
68. Pitt B, Segal R, Martinez FA, et al. Randomised trial of losartan versus captopril in patients over 65 with heart failure (Evaluation of Losartan in the Elderly Study, ELITE). *Lancet* 1997;349:747–752.
69. Pitt B, Poole-Wilson PA, Segal R, et al. Effect of losartan compared with captopril on mortality in patients with symptomatic heart failure: randomised trial. The Losartan Heart Failure Survival Study ELITE II. *Lancet* 2000;355:1582–1587.
70. Dickstein K, Kjekshus J. Effects of losartan and captopril on mortality and morbidity in high-risk patients after acute myocardial infarction: the OPTIMAAL randomised trial. Optimal Trial in Myocardial Infarction with Angiotensin II Antagonist Losartan. *Lancet* 2002;360:752–760.
71. Pfeffer MA, Swedberg K, Granger CB, et al. Effects of candesartan on mortality and morbidity in patients with chronic heart failure: the CHARM-Overall Programme. *Lancet* 2003;362:759–766.
72. Krum H, Carson P, Farsang C, et al. Effect of valsartan added to background ACE inhibitor therapy in patients with heart failure: results from Val-HeFT. *Eur J Heart Fail* 2004;6:937–945.
73. McMurray JJ, Ostergren J, Swedberg K, et al. Effects of candesartan in patients with chronic heart failure and reduced left-ventricular systolic function taking angiotensin-converting-enzyme inhibitors: the CHARM-Added Trial. *Lancet* 2003;362:767–771.
74. Yusuf S, Pfeffer MA, Swedberg K, et al. Effects of candesartan in patients with chronic heart failure and preserved left-ventricular ejection fraction: the CHARM-Preserved Trial. *Lancet* 2003;362:777–781.
75. Young JB, Dunlap ME, Pfeffer MA, et al. Mortality and morbidity reduction with Candesartan in patients with chronic heart failure and left ventricular systolic dysfunction: results of the CHARM Low-Left Ventricular Ejection Fraction Trials. *Circulation* 2004;110:2618–2626.
76. McKelvie RS, Yusuf S, Pericak D, et al. Comparison of candesartan, enalapril, and their combination in congestive heart failure: Randomized Evaluation of Strategies for Left Ventricular Dysfunction (RESOLVD) Pilot Study. The RESOLVD Pilot Study Investigators. *Circulation* 1999;100:1056–1064.
77. Solomon SD, Skali H, Anavekar NS, et al. Changes in ventricular size and function in patients treated with valsartan, captopril, or both after myocardial infarction. *Circulation* 2005;111:3411–3419.
78. Wong M, Staszewsky L, Latini R, et al. Valsartan benefits left ventricular structure and function in heart failure: Val-HeFT echocardiographic study. *J Am Coll Cardiol* 2002;40:970–975.
79. RESOLVD Investigators. Effects of metoprolol CR in patients with ischemic and dilated cardiomyopathy: the Randomized Evaluation of Strategies for Left Ventricular Dysfunction Pilot Study. *Circulation* 2000;101: 378–384.
80. A randomized trial of propranolol in patients with acute myocardial infarction. I. Mortality results. *JAMA* 1982;247:1707–1714.
81. Pedersen TR. Six-year follow-up of the Norwegian Multicenter Study on Timolol after Acute Myocardial Infarction. *N Engl J Med* 1985;313:1055–1058.
82. Waagstein F, Bristow MR, Swedberg K, et al. Beneficial effects of metoprolol in idiopathic dilated cardiomyopathy: Metoprolol in Dilated Cardiomyopathy (MDC) Trial Study Group. *Lancet* 1993;342:1441–1446.
83. Packer M, Bristow MR, Cohn JN, et al. The effect of carvedilol on morbidity and mortality in patients with chronic heart failure: U.S. Carvedilol Heart Failure Study Group. *N Engl J Med* 1996;334:1349–1355.
84. Packer M, Colucci WS, Sackner-Bernstein JD, et al. Double-blind, placebo-controlled study of the effects of carvedilol in patients with moderate to severe heart failure: the PRECISE Trial. Prospective Randomized Evaluation of Carvedilol on Symptoms and Exercise. *Circulation* 1996;94:2793–2799.
85. Bristow MR, Gilbert EM, Abraham WT, et al. Carvedilol produces dose-related improvements in left ventricular function and survival in subjects with chronic heart failure: MOCHA Investigators. *Circulation* 1996; 94:2807–2816.
86. Colucci WS, Packer M, Bristow MR, et al. Carvedilol inhibits clinical progression in patients with mild symptoms of heart failure: US Carvedilol Heart Failure Study Group. *Circulation* 1996;94:2800–2806.
87. Cohn JN, Fowler MB, Bristow MR, et al. Safety and efficacy of carvedilol in severe heart failure: the U.S. Carvedilol Heart Failure Study Group. *J Card Fail* 1997;3:173–179.
88. CIBIS Investigators and Committees. A randomized trial of beta-blockade in heart failure: the Cardiac Insufficiency Bisoprolol Study (CIBIS). *Circulation* 1994;90:1765–1773.
89. CIBIS II Investigators. The Cardiac Insufficiency Bisoprolol Study II (CIBIS-II): a randomised trial. *Lancet* 1999;353:9–13.
90. MERIT-HF Investigators. Effect of metoprolol CR/XL in chronic heart failure: Metoprolol CR/XL Randomised Intervention Trial in Congestive Heart Failure (MERIT-HF). *Lancet* 1999;353:2001–2007.
91. Dargie HJ. Effect of carvedilol on outcome after myocardial infarction in patients with left-ventricular dysfunction: the CAPRICORN randomised trial. *Lancet* 2001;357:1385–1390.
92. Doughty RN, Whalley GA, Walsh HA, et al. Effects of carvedilol on left ventricular remodeling after acute myocardial infarction: the CAPRICORN Echo Substudy. *Circulation* 2004;109:201–206.
93. Packer M, Coats AJ, Fowler MB, et al. Effect of carvedilol on survival in severe chronic heart failure. *N Engl J Med* 2001;344:1651–1658.
94. Flather MD, Shibata MC, Coats AJ, et al. Randomized trial to determine the effect of nebivolol on mortality and cardiovascular hospital admission in elderly patients with heart failure (SENIORS). *Eur Heart J* 2005;26:215–225.
95. BEST Investigators. A trial of the beta-blocker bucindolol in patients with advanced chronic heart failure. *N Engl J Med* 2001;344:1659–1667.
96. Braunwald E. Expanding indications for beta-blockers in heart failure. *N Engl J Med* 2001;344:1711–1712.
97. Beta1-adrenergic receptor polymorphisms and the prediction of clinical response to bucindolol in heart failure: late-breaking and recent clinical trials. Presented at the 8th Annual Scientific Meeting of the Heart Failure Society of America, Toronto, Canada, September 12–15, 2004.
98. Yancy CW, Fowler MB, Colucci WS, et al. Race and the response to adrenergic blockade with carvedilol in patients with chronic heart failure. *N Engl J Med* 2001;344:1358–1365.
99. Poole-Wilson PA, Swedberg K, Cleland JG, et al. Comparison of carvedilol and metoprolol on clinical outcomes in patients with chronic heart failure

in the Carvedilol Or Metoprolol European Trial (COMET): randomised controlled trial. *Lancet* 2003;362:7–13.
100. Torp-Pedersen C, Poole-Wilson PA, Swedberg K, et al. Effects of metoprolol and carvedilol on cause-specific mortality and morbidity in patients with chronic heart failure: COMET. *Am Heart J* 2005;149:370–376.
101. Tang WH, Francis GS. Trends and treatment of heart failure developing after acute myocardial infarction. *Am Heart Hosp J* 2003;1:216–218.
102. Gupta R, Tang WH, Young JB. Patterns of beta-blocker utilization in patients with chronic heart failure: experience from a specialized outpatient heart failure clinic. *Am Heart J* 2004;147:79–83.
103. Struthers AD. The clinical implications of aldosterone escape in congestive heart failure. *Eur J Heart Fail* 2004;6:539–545.
104. Pitt B. Effect of aldosterone blockade in patients with systolic left ventricular dysfunction: implications of the RALES and EPHESUS studies. *Mol Cell Endocrinol* 2004;217:53–58.
105. Pitt B, Zannad F, Remme WJ, et al. The effect of spironolactone on morbidity and mortality in patients with severe heart failure: Randomized Aldactone Evaluation Study Investigators. *N Engl J Med* 1999;341:709–717.
106. Zannad F, Alla F, Dousset B, et al. Limitation of excessive extracellular matrix turnover may contribute to survival benefit of spironolactone therapy in patients with congestive heart failure: insights from the Randomized Aldactone Evaluation Study (RALES). Rales Investigators. *Circulation* 2000;102:2700–2706.
107. Mottram PM, Haluska B, Leano R, et al. Effect of aldosterone antagonism on myocardial dysfunction in hypertensive patients with diastolic heart failure. *Circulation* 2004;110:558–565.
108. Bozkurt B, Agoston I, Knowlton AA. Complications of inappropriate use of spironolactone in heart failure: when an old medicine spirals out of new guidelines. *J Am Coll Cardiol* 2003;41:211–214.
109. Juurlink DN, Mamdani MM, Lee DS, et al. Rates of hyperkalemia after publication of the Randomized Aldactone Evaluation Study. *N Engl J Med* 2004;351:543–551.
110. Masoudi FA, Gross CP, Wang Y, et al. Adoption of spironolactone therapy for older patients with heart failure and left ventricular systolic dysfunction in the United States, 1998–2001. *Circulation* 2005;112:39–47.
111. Tamirisa KP, Aaronson KD, Koelling TM. Spironolactone-induced renal insufficiency and hyperkalemia in patients with heart failure. *Am Heart J* 2004;148:971–978.
112. Cohn JN. Efficacy of vasodilators in the treatment of heart failure. *J Am Coll Cardiol* 1993;22:135A–138A.
113. Cohn JN, Archibald DG, Ziesche S, et al. Effect of vasodilator therapy on mortality in chronic congestive heart failure: results of a Veterans Administration cooperative study. *N Engl J Med* 1986;314:1547–1552.
114. Elkayam U, Roth A, Mehra A, et al. Randomized study to evaluate the relation between oral isosorbide dinitrate dosing interval and the development of early tolerance to its effect on left ventricular filling pressure in patients with chronic heart failure. *Circulation* 1991;84:2040–2048.
115. Elkayam U. Prevention of nitrate tolerance with concomitant administration of hydralazine. *Can J Cardiol* 1996;12(suppl C):17C–21C.
116. Cohn JN, Ziesche S, Smith R, et al. Effect of the calcium antagonist felodipine as supplementary vasodilator therapy in patients with chronic heart failure treated with enalapril: V-HeFT III. Vasodilator-Heart Failure Trial (V-HeFT) Study Group. *Circulation* 1997;96:856–863.
117. Elkayam U, Johnson JV, Shotan A, et al. Double-blind, placebo-controlled study to evaluate the effect of organic nitrates in patients with chronic heart failure treated with angiotensin-converting enzyme inhibition. *Circulation* 1999;99:2652–2657.
118. Packer M, O'Connor CM, Ghali JK, et al. Effect of amlodipine on morbidity and mortality in severe chronic heart failure: Prospective Randomized Amlodipine Survival Evaluation Study Group. *N Engl J Med* 1996;335: 1107–1114.
119. Stevenson LW. Clinical use of inotropic therapy for heart failure: looking backward or forward? Part II. Chronic inotropic therapy. *Circulation* 2003;108:492–497.
120. Lowes BD, Shakar SF, Metra M, et al. Rationale and design of the enoximone clinical trials prognosis. *J Cardiac Fail* 2005;11:659–669.
121. Cleland JG, Findlay I, Jafri S, et al. The Warfarin/Aspirin Study in Heart failure (WASH): a randomized trial comparing antithrombotic strategies for patients with heart failure. *Am Heart J* 2004;148:157–164.
122. Massie BM, Krol WF, Ammon SE, et al. The Warfarin and Antiplatelet Therapy in Heart Failure trial (WATCH): rationale, design, and baseline patient characteristics. *J Card Fail* 2004;10:101–112.
123. Califf RM. Watching the WATCH trial: the role of sponsors and data monitoring committees. *J Card Fail* 2004;10:113–114.
124. Pullicino PM, Halperin JL, Thompson JL. Stroke in patients with heart failure and reduced left ventricular ejection fraction. *Neurology* 2000;54:288–294.
125. Gottlieb SS, Khatta M, Friedmann E, et al. The influence of age, gender, and race on the prevalence of depression in heart failure patients. *J Am Coll Cardiol* 2004;43:1542–1549.
126. Westlake C, Dracup K, Fonarow G, Hamilton M. Depression in patients with heart failure. *J Card Fail* 2005;11:30–35.
127. Havranek EP, Spertus JA, Masoudi FA, et al. Predictors of the onset of depressive symptoms in patients with heart failure. *J Am Coll Cardiol* 2004;44:2333–2338.
128. Packer M. The impossible task of developing a new treatment for heart failure. *J Card Fail* 2002;8:193–196.
129. Mehra MR, Uber PA, Francis GS. Heart failure therapy at a crossroad: are there limits to the neurohormonal model? *J Am Coll Cardiol* 2003; 41:1606–1610.
130. NETWORK Investigators. Clinical outcome with enalapril in symptomatic chronic heart failure: a dose comparison. *Eur Heart J* 1998;19:481–489.
131. Australia/New Zealand Heart Failure Research Collaborative Group. Randomised, placebo-controlled trial of carvedilol in patients with congestive heart failure due to ischaemic heart disease. *Lancet* 1997;349:375–380.
132. Pitt B, Remme W, Zannad F, et al. Eplerenone, a selective aldosterone blocker, in patients with left ventricular dysfunction after myocardial infarction. *N Engl J Med* 2003;348:1309–1321.
133. Packer M, Carver JR, Rodeheffer RJ, et al. Effect of oral milrinone on mortality in severe chronic heart failure: the PROMISE study research group. *N Engl J Med* 1991;325:1468–1475.
134. Villareal RP, Kim P, Mahmood H, et al. Meeting highlights: highlights of the 49th scientific sessions of the American College of Cardiology. *Circulation* 2000;102:E53–E60.
135. Joint Commission on Accreditation of Healthcare Organizations (JCAHO). Overview of the heart failure (HF) core measure set (3/22/2002). Accessed on August 7, 2005 at www.jcaho.org/pms/core+measures/hf_overview.htm.
136. Bonow RO, Bennett SJ, Casey DE, et al. ACC/AHA clinical performance measures for adult with chronic heart failure. *Circulation* 2005;46:1144–1178.

CHAPTER 88 ■ DIAGNOSIS AND MEDICAL TREATMENT OF INFLAMMATORY CARDIOMYOPATHY

DENNIS M. McNAMARA

OVERVIEW

Myocardial inflammation underlies cardiac dysfunction in a wide spectrum of disorders, from lymphocytic myocarditis (1,2) to idiopathic dilated cardiomyopathy (IDC) (3). Animal models and clinical studies support viral etiologies in the majority of cases, although specific infectious agents are documented in only a fraction of cases. Despite this inflammatory pathogenesis and scores of anecdotal series that suggest a therapeutic role for immunosuppression, controlled trials have consistently failed to demonstrate clinical benefit (4–6). Endomyocardial biopsy, once widely used for diagnosis, is currently not recommended for the majority of cases given the absence of specific biopsy-guided therapies (7). Giant-cell myocarditis remains one exception because biopsy confirmation of this aggressive disorder may assist in therapeutic decisions, including the consideration of immunosuppressive therapy (8). The potential future role for immune modulatory therapy is an intense area of investigation.

INTRODUCTION

Primary idiopathic dilated cardiomyopathy is a leading cause of congestive heart failure in the United States, particularly among young people (9). Myocardial inflammation, or myocarditis, is postulated as the initiating cardiac injury, which subsequently progresses to ventricular dysfunction. Despite this hypothesis, signs of systemic inflammation are rarely seen at presentation with IDC. Although myocarditis is believed to be a frequent precursor of IDC (10), it is an often suspected but infrequently diagnosed disorder. The degree to which myocarditis and IDC represent distinct disorders versus separate time points in the same inflammatory progression is a matter of significant controversy. Over the last two decades, the search for mechanistic-based therapies for primary dilated cardiomyopathy has focused on the inflammatory pathogenesis.

HISTORICAL PERSPECTIVE

Guided by introduction of the stethoscope by Laënnec, early-nineteenth-century clinicians divided cardiac disorders into valvular and nonvalvular (11). "Carditis" was a subset of nonvalvular disease that included vascular and inflammatory forms of cardiac dysfunction. The term carditis was gradually replaced by myocarditis, which continued for the remainder of the century to be a broad category of nonvalvular forms of myocardial dysfunction. In the early part of the twentieth century, coronary artery disease became recognized as an etiology for myocardial dysfunction distinct from myocardial inflammation, and the concept of "myocarditis" evolved to the modern application. By the mid-twentieth century, the search for infectious etiologies intensified, with increased recognition of the importance of viral pathogens (12–14). The introduction of transvenous endomyocardial biopsy (EMB) in the latter part of the twentieth century (15) heralded a new age of understanding for primary dilated cardiomyopathy in which an apparent heterogeneous group of disorders could now be divided into distinct pathologic subsets. With the widespread growth

TABLE 88.1

INFLAMMATORY CARDIOMYOPATHY: CLINICAL SUBSETS

Myocarditis
Biopsy defined: lymphocytic, eosinophilic
Clinically defined
Giant-cell myocarditis
Systemic autoimmune disorders with myocarditis
Systemic lupus erythematosus
Polymyositis
Sarcoid
Peripartum cardiomyopathy
Subsets of idiopathic dilated cardiomyopathy

in cardiac transplantation in the 1980s, it was recognized that the common form of cellular inflammation in native hearts, lymphocytic myocarditis, was histologically similar to cardiac allograft rejection. This supported a hypothesized autoimmune pathogenesis and led to a randomized clinical trial of immunosuppression, the Myocarditis Treatment Trial (MTT) (5). The clinical use of endomyocardial biopsy reached its zenith by the early 1990s and has subsequently declined in the absence of biopsy-guided therapeutic interventions. Molecular genetic techniques have recently been used to enhance the diagnostic power of endomyocardial biopsy (16). Systemic inflammatory mediators, including cytokines (1), chemokines (17), and autoantibodies (18), have been investigated as surrogate markers for cardiac inflammation.

INFLAMMATORY CARDIOMYOPATHY: CLINICAL AND HISTOLOGIC SUBSETS

With the increasing use of endomyocardial biopsy for diagnosis, the term myocarditis gradually became synonymous with left ventricular (LV) dysfunction with histologic evidence of cellular inflammation. As recently as 1995, the World Health Organization task force defined inflammatory cardiomyopathy as "myocarditis in association with myocardial dysfunction. Myocarditis is an inflammatory disease of the myocardium and is diagnosed by established histologic, immunologic, and immunohistochemical criteria" (19). Under current practice, endomyocardial biopsy data are not available for most subjects, and therefore reliance on strict histologic criteria is not practical. Myocarditis is commonly diagnosed as "suspected" inflammation of the myocardium; however, no clearly defined criteria exist. With this broadened clinical definition, the distinction between inflammatory myocarditis and recent onset IDC can become somewhat obscured (20–22).

Inflammatory cardiomyopathies can be subdivided into more distinct subsets based on the clinical setting of presentation (e.g., pregnancy) or diagnostic histopathology (Table 88.1). Among those patients with biopsy-proven inflammation, most have "lymphocytic myocarditis" based on lymphocyte predominance in the myocardial cellular infiltrates (23). An eosinophilic predominance can be seen in myocarditis associated with an allergic reaction or with peripheral eosinophilia (24–27). Lymphocytic myocarditis is seen in approximately 10% of biopsied patients (5), whereas 1% to 2% are diagnosed with giant-cell myocarditis, defined by the presence of multinucleated giant cells (28). The distinction between this disorder and lymphocytic myocarditis is critically important because giant-cell myocarditis is a much more aggressive pathologic process with a distinct natural history (8,28).

Myocarditis can also be seen as part of systemic autoimmune disorders such as sarcoidosis (29) and systemic lupus erythematosus (30). The histologic appearance of myocarditis in systemic disorders may be similar to that of the isolated viral myocarditis. The role of immunosupression is determined by the systemic illness because the myocardium will respond to treatment of the overall disorder. The granulomas of cardiac sarcoid in particular can be difficult to distinguish from those of its histologic mimic, giant-cell myocarditis (31). This distinction is critical because sarcoid is a less aggressive disorder and more likely to respond to corticosteroids.

PREVALENCE

The prevalence of primary idiopathic dilated cardiomyopathy has been estimated at 0.4 per 1,000, with an annual incidence of 0.08 per 1,000 (33). This corresponds to approximately 120,000 cases within the United States alone, with 24,000 new cases each year. The prevalence of histologic myocarditis varies widely in published series (Table 88.2) but can be best estimated from multicenter studies at 10% to 20% of patients with

TABLE 88.2

PREVALENCE OF MYOCARDITIS IN PUBLISHED SERIES

Author (reference)	Years	Percentage with positive biopsy	Patient group
Dec et al. (21)	1975–1983	67 (18/27)	Recent-onset cardiomyopathy with <6 mo of symptoms
Parillo et al. (4)	1982–1988	38 (38/102)	Patients referred to the National Institutes of Health for randomized trial of prednisone in idiopathic dilated cardiomyopathy
Mason et al. (5)	1986–1989	10 (214/2,233)	Patients screened for the Myocarditis Treatment Trial
McCarthy et al. (140)	1984–1997	14 (252/1,757)	Large single-center series from Johns Hopkins
McNamara et al. (6)	1996–1998	16 (10/62)	All recent-onset dilated cardiomyopathy enrolled in the IMAC trial
Drucker et al. (96)	1985–1991	51 (20/39)	Children referred with the clinical syndrome of suspected myocarditis
Midei et al. (73)	1983–1988	78 (14/18)	Patients with peripartum cardiomyopathy from a single center, Johns Hopkins
Bozkurt et al. (98)	1990–1998	9 (1/11)	Patients with peripartum cardiomyopathy from a single center, University of Pittsburgh

From Feldman AM, McNamara D. Myocarditis. *N Engl J Med* 2000;343:1388–1398.

new-onset IDC (5,6,34). The Myocarditis Treatment Trial (MTT) noted biopsies that were positive for inflammation in only 10% of 2,233 screened patients (5). In a similar fashion, the European Study of Epidemiology and Treatment of Cardiac Inflammatory Diseases reported positive biopsies in 17.2% of the first 3,055 patients screened (34). Evidence of myocarditis may be found in 1% to 9% of routine autopsy cases (35–37) and up to 20% of those that are performed for unexplained sudden cardiac death in young people (38,39). The true prevalence of these subacute forms of myocarditis is difficult to determine because the majority of cases resolve with no long-term clinical sequelae (40).

PATHOGENESIS: LESSONS FROM ANIMAL MODELS

The murine models of myocarditis initiated with the cardiotropic ribonucleic acid virus Coxsackie virus group B (41) or encephalomyocarditis virus (42) are the most extensively studied. After uptake by receptor-mediated endocytosis, viral proteins are translated, and replication of viral particles is initiated in the cytoplasm of the myocyte. Direct virally induced myocyte necrosis can be seen within 3 days, before any inflammatory infiltrates. Subsequently, macrophage activation leads to cytokine expression, including interleukin-1 (IL-1), interleukin-2 (IL-2), tumor necrosis factor-alpha (TNF-α), and interferon-γ (10). Cytokine expression, particularly IL-2, results in the activation of natural killer (NK) cells (43). Endogenous interferons likely also play a direct role in limiting viral replication.

Within 7 days of viral inoculation, infiltrates of antigen-specific T lymphocytes are seen throughout the myocardium. These cells can be subclassed based on surface antigens and function into T-helper (CD4+) cells and cytotoxic T-lymphocyte (CD8+) cells (10, 44). Viral antigens are reduced to peptides and placed in the cell membrane of target cells bound to the major histocompatibility complex (MHC) for presentation to T-cell receptors. The recognition by cytotoxic T-lymphocyte receptors of viral peptide presented by MHC class I antigens initiates myocyte damage of virally infected cells (45). The induction of intracellular adhesion molecule-1 as well as MHC class I molecules by interferon-γ and TNF-α plays an important facilitator role (46).

Of the mononuclear cells in the myocardium, 10% to 20% are B lymphocytes (47). T cell–depleted murine strains inoculated with encephalomyocarditis virus have less myocardial damage and overall less severe myocarditis than do T cell–competent strains (48). In this model, viral titers, the development of neutralizing antibody titers, and viral clearing were similar in T cell–competent and T cell–depleted strains. Although it does not participate directly in cytotoxicity, B cell–mediated humoral mechanisms play an important role in the overall elimination of viral particles.

Approximately 15 days after viral inoculation, culturable virus is no longer detected. By 90 days after inoculation, inflammatory cell infiltrates are no longer seen; however, ventricular enlargement and myocardial fibrosis become prominent (49). This chronic postviral phase closely replicates the clinical presentation of patients with IDC. Viral nucleic acid can be detected by polymerase chain reaction in only a small percentage of mice at 90 days after inoculation (50) and, in a similar fashion, is only seen in a minority of patients with dilated cardiomyopathy (51–53). The absence of detectable virus for the majority of subjects (murine or human) has powered speculation that this phase of chronic insidious myocardial injury is driven by persistent autoimmune pathologic mechanisms.

TABLE 88.3

VIRAL ETIOLOGIES OF INFLAMMATORY CARDIOMYOPATHY

Enteroviruses
Coxsackie A and B
Influenza A and B
Echovirus
Polio
Herpesviruses
Herpes simplex
Varicella-zoster
Epstein-Barr
Cytomegalovirus
Adenovirus
Mumps
Rubella
Rubeola
Vaccinia
Rabies
Hepatitis B and C
Arbovirus
Human immunodeficiency virus

ETIOLOGY

Clinical studies of myocarditis suggest that a viral trigger initiates an immune pathogenesis. Enteroviruses, in particular Coxsackie B, are the most common viral agents (54). Adenovirus, influenza A and B, and hepatitis C have also been implicated as important viral pathogens (55,56) (Table 88.3). Human immunodeficiency virus (HIV) infection has been associated with myocarditis and dilated cardiomyopathy (57–59). Additional viral genomes, cytomegalovirus and adenovirus in particular, have also been detected in the myocardium of HIV-positive patients with lymphocytic myocarditis (60).

Chagas disease is caused by parasitism with the protozoa *Trypanosoma cruzi* and is endemic in parts of South America (61). Serologic epidemiology studies indicate that between 15 and 20 million people are infected in Central and South America, with more than 60 million people at risk (62). This disorder is not seen among U.S. patients in the absence of a significant travel history to endemic areas. Among immunocompromised hosts, myocarditis associated with *Toxoplasma* (63,64) or *Aspergillus* (65,66) has been reported, but generally only with signs of other systemic infestation and only rarely as an isolated myocarditis.

Noninfectious triggers can also initiate myocardial inflammation, as demonstrated by peripartum cardiomyopathy (PPCM), the syndrome of dilated cardiomyopathy that presents in the last month of pregnancy or in the first few months postpartum (67–69). This disorder is phenotypically similar to the virally initiated syndrome; however the initiating stimulus is likely fetal or placental antigen rather than viral peptides. Modulation of maternal immunity is an important aspect of fetal tolerance during routine pregnancy (70,71). Exacerbations of autoimmune disorders such as multiple sclerosis typically decline during pregnancy, with a subsequent rebound increase noted in the postpartum period (72). The period of autoimmune "rebound" phenomenon postpartum is also the most common time for women to present with PPCM. Lymphocytic infiltrations of the myocardium can be seen in this disorder (73), particularly in patients biopsied soon after delivery. Multiparity is frequently proposed as a risk factor (74), which suggests that previous exposure to fetal paternal antigens facilitates the development of a pathologic immune response.

Toxins, namely alcohol and chemotherapeutic agents such as doxorubicin (75–77), can also initiate a progression to dilated cardiomyopathy. In contrast to the virally initiated and peripartum syndrome, these agents appear to act through direct myocardial toxicity. In these syndromes, myocardial inflammation may be more the result rather than the cause of myocardial injury. In addition, up to 25% of primary dilated cardiomyopathies may be familial in etiology (78). Responsible genetic loci have been delineated for several pedigrees and mutations identified in several cytoskeletal proteins, including dystrophin (79), cardiac actin (80), and the myosin heavy chain itself (81). Although inherited abnormalities of the inflammatory response may be important in some pedigrees (82–85), in general, the mechanism of cardiac dysfunction in familial cardiomyopathy appears quite distinct from that evident in the more common sporadic cases.

IMMUNOPATHOLOGY OF PROGRESSION

The histologic appearance of lymphocytic myocarditis is indistinguishable from acute allograft rejection in the transplanted heart (86), with a predominance of T lymphocytes. In murine models, whether the initial immune response is self-limited or results in progressive inflammation and cardiomyopathy is strain dependent (87), which supports a strong role of genetic background in determining outcome. Genetic susceptibility is equally important in clinical studies because human leukocyte antigen genotypes appear to confer an increased risk of the development of dilated cardiomyopathy (88). Perpetuation of myocardial inflammation appears to require an antigenic similarity of myocardial and viral peptides and a genetic "background" that facilitates the pathologic chronic immune response (89,90).

Cytokines play an important role in the progression of cardiomyopathy (91,92), and myocardial expression and plasma levels of TNF-α and IL-6 increase as functional status worsens (93,94). Expression of inflammatory mediators can elicit cellular infiltration of the myocardium and contribute to the decline in cardiac function. Myocardial cytokine expression plays a critical role in the progression of heart failure from the compensated to the end-stage phenotype.

IMMUNOSUPPRESSIVE AND IMMUNE MODULATORY THERAPIES

Immunosuppressive therapy has been extensively investigated in myocarditis and dilated cardiomyopathy. Multiple single-center series reported benefit of steroids, immune globulin, and other immune modulatory strategies. Given the relative infrequency of these disorders, single-center series are generally quite small, and three prospective, randomized trials of immune modulation failed to confirm the therapeutic benefits suggested by anecdotal reports (4–6) (Table 88.4).

The largest of these trials was the multicenter Myocarditis Treatment Trial (MTT), which evaluated the use of prednisone and cyclosporine for biopsy-proven lymphocytic myocarditis. Recruitment for the MTT was challenging due to the strict biopsy criteria. Local pathologists found evidence of myocarditis on endomyocardial biopsy for only 214 of 2,233 screened patients. Of these, 111 met the other entry criteria and were randomized. Overall, left ventricular (LV) function improved significantly over time from a mean of 0.25 at baseline to 0.34 at 28 weeks. No treatment effect was evident with immunosuppressive therapy because the improvement in left ventricular ejection fraction (LVEF) was similar in the two groups (0.10 with immunosuppressive therapy vs. 0.07 in the control group) (Fig. 88.1). No long-term difference in survival was seen ($p =$ .96), with an overall mortality of 20% at 1 year and 56% at 4.3 years (Fig. 88.2). In current practice, the absence of therapeutic benefit for immunosuppression in the MTT has all but eliminated its use in adults with suspected myocarditis.

Based on its use in Kawasaki disease (95), immune globulin has been used as therapy for children with myocarditis, and nonrandomized series reported improvements in LV function compared to historical controls (96). Two small series in adults with new-onset dilated cardiomyopathy and myocarditis (97) and peripartum cardiomyopathy (98) suggested enhanced improvement in LVEF compared to historical controls. The

TABLE 88.4

RANDOMIZED CLINICAL TRIALS OF IMMUNE MODULATION IN MYOCARDITIS AND DILATED CARDIOMYOPATHY

Author (reference)	Agent studied	Number randomized	Primary outcome measure	Result
Parillo et al. (4)	Prednisone	102	Change in EF at 3 mo	Modest benefit (4 EF units vs. 2 EF units in the placebo)
Mason et al. (Myocarditis Treatment Trial) (5)	Prednisone and cyclosporine	111	Change in EF at 6 mo	No significant effect (increase of 10 EF units vs. 7 EF units with placebo)
McNamara et al. (IMAC Trial) (6)	Immune globulin	62	Change in EF at 6 mo	No treatment effect (increase of 14 EF units in both groups)

EF, ejection fraction.
From Feldman AM, McNamara D. Myocarditis. *N Engl J Med* 2000;343:1388–1398.

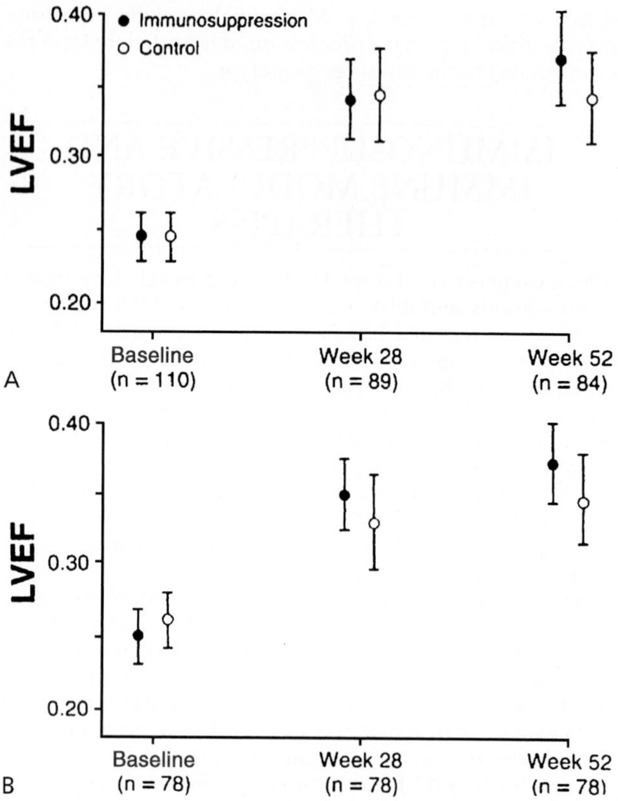

FIGURE 88.1. Serial change in left ventricular ejection fraction (LVEF) for all patients enrolled in the Myocarditis Treatment Trial (**A**) and only those who had paired studies (**B**), showing comparable improvement in LVEF in the two groups. (From Mason JW, O'Connell JB, Herskowitz A, et al. A clinical trial of immunosuppressive therapy for myocarditis. *N Engl J Med* 1995;333:269–275, with permission. Copyright © 1995 Massachusetts Medical Society. All rights reserved.)

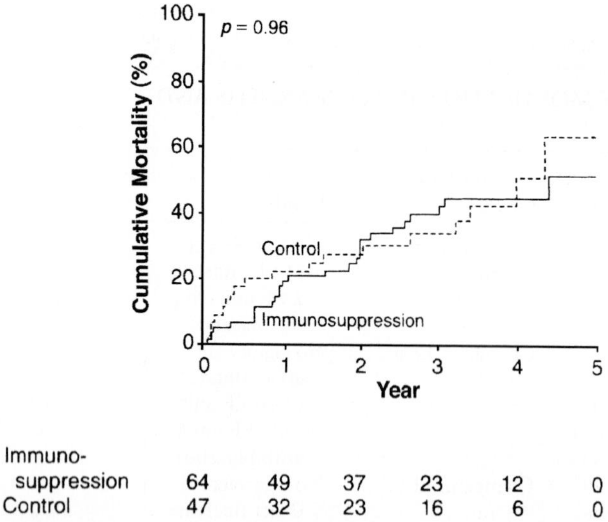

FIGURE 88.2. Cumulative mortality in subjects receiving immunosuppression and controls from the Myocarditis Treatment Trial, showing no difference between the groups. (From Mason JW, O'Connell JB, Herskowitz A, et al. A clinical trial of immunosuppressive therapy for myocarditis. *N Engl J Med* 1995;333:269–275, with permission. Copyright © 1995 Massachusetts Medical Society. All rights reserved.)

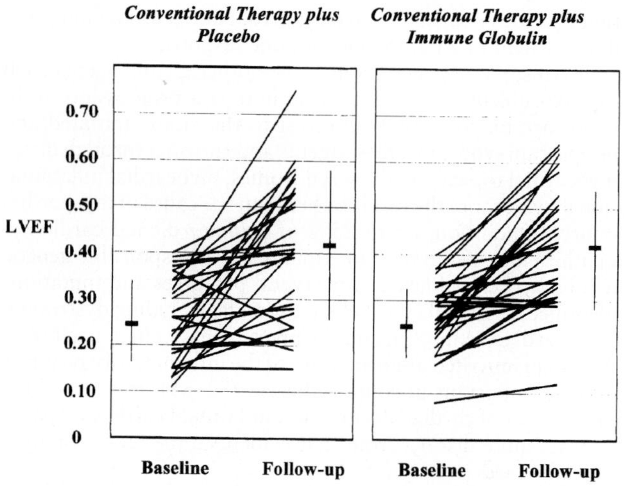

FIGURE 88.3. Left ventricular ejection fraction (LVEF) over time by treatment. LVEF by radionuclide scan at baseline and 12 months postrandomization in patients randomized to placebo and immunoglobulin. Overall, LVEF improved significantly over time (12-month LVEF significantly higher than baseline, $p < .001$). However, no differences by treatment group were evident (p = not significant for comparisons by treatment). (From McNamara DM, Holubkov R, Starling RC, et al., for the IMAC investigators. A controlled trial of intravenous immune globulin for recent onset dilated cardiomyopathy. *Circulation* 2001;103:2254–2259.)

role of intravenous immunoglobulin (IVIG) for adults with inflammatory cardiac disease was evaluated in the multicenter Intervention in Myocarditis and Acute Cardiomyopathy (IMAC) trial (6). The IMAC study randomized 62 patients to 2 g/kg IVIG or a placebo infusion. LVEF improved significantly overall from 0.25 at baseline to 0.42 at 12 months. No benefit was evident with IVIG because the improvement at 6 months was 14 EF units in both groups and at 12 months was 16 EF units with IVIG versus 15 with placebo (Fig. 88.3). Overall event-free survival (events defined as death, transplantation, or need for LV assist device [LVAD]) was 91% at 1 year and 88% at 2 years (Fig. 88.4), and there were no significant differences between treatment groups.

Spontaneous recovery of recent-onset, acute inflammatory myocarditis presents a challenge for investigative trials of innovative therapies. Many investigators have therefore shifted their focus to chronic disease, greater than 3 to 6 months in duration. Because dramatic recovery of LV function in this

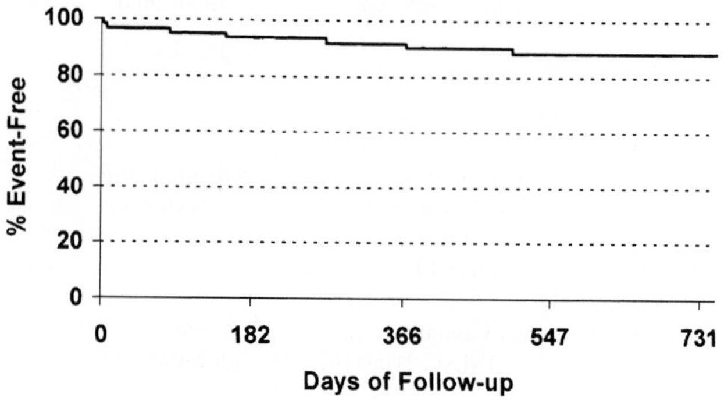

FIGURE 88.4. Event-free survival for patients with new-onset dilated cardiomyopathy and myocarditis enrolled in the Intervention in Myocarditis and Acute Cardiomyopathy trial (events defined as death, cardiac transplantation, or need for left ventricular assist device). Event-free survival was 91% at 1 year and 88% at 2 years.

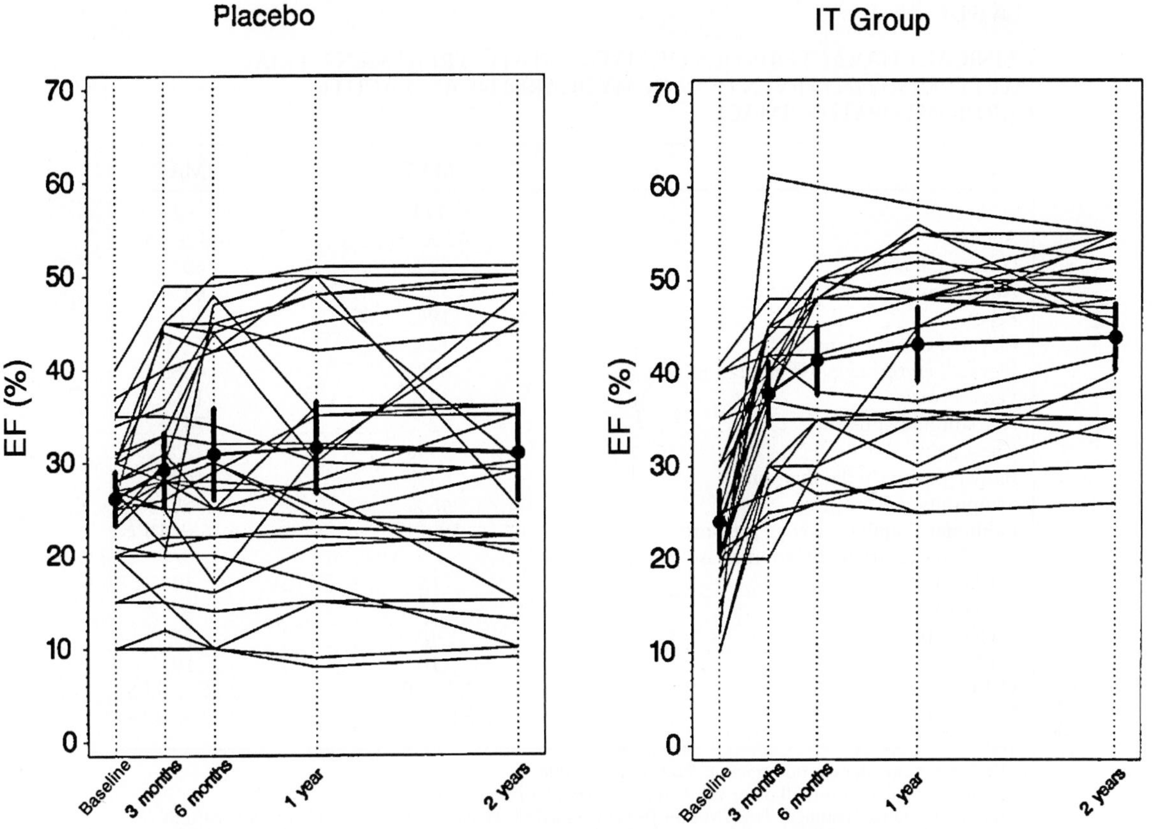

FIGURE 88.5. Serial left ventricular ejection fractions (EF) from 58 patients (all with chronic cardiomyopathy but with increased HLA expression as evidence of pathologic inflammation on biopsy) receiving either placebo ($n = 30$) or immunosuppressive therapy (IT) with azathioprine and prednisone. Thickened lines and bars delineate means and standard deviations. (From Wojnicz R, Nowalany-Kozielska E, Wojciechowska C, et al. Randomized, placebo-controlled study for immunosuppressive treatment of inflammatory dilated cardiomyopathy: two-year follow-up results. *Circulation* 2001;104:39–45.)

population is extremely rare, a positive effect of new therapies can be more easily defined. Wojnicz and colleagues (99) used HLA expression in biopsies of chronic patients to select a cohort with pathologic chronic inflammation. Treatment in these subjects with prednisone and azathioprine resulted in marked and prolonged improvements in LV function compared to controls (Fig. 88.5). Immunohistochemistry and staining for HLA expression is not routinely performed on EMB, and this single-center trial has yet to be confirmed in a larger series.

ANTIVIRAL THERAPIES

Although a viral trigger is suspected for a large subset of patients with inflammatory cardiomyopathy, the role of specific antiviral therapies is uncertain. Treatment with interferon-β is protective in murine models initiated with Coxsackie B3 (100), and case reports suggest similar improvement in clinical subjects treated with interferon-α (101). In a study of endomyocardial biopsies from 624 patients with cardiomyopathy or suspected myocarditis, viral genomes were detected by polymerase chain reaction (PCR) in 38%, with adenovirus as the predominant subtype (102). Other investigators have documented the presence of Epstein-Barr virus (103) and hepatitis C (104) as potential viral etiologies of dilated cardiomyopathy. In a series of 22 subjects with chronic LV dysfunction and PCR evidence of enteroviral or adenoviral genomes in the myocardium, prolonged treatment with interferon-β resulted in viral elimination and improvements in LV function (105). Based on these findings, a European randomized trial of interferon-β for chronic persistent viral cardiomyopathy (Betaferon in Chronic Viral Cardiomyopathy [BICC] Trial) was initiated in December 2002 (106). Although vaccination against viral etiologies has been proposed, myopericarditis has also been reported as a complication of vaccination (107). More than 50 cases were reported during a vaccination for smallpox of 450,000 military personnel, and patients with persistent progressive LV dysfunction appeared to respond to corticosteroids (108,109).

CLINICAL MANAGEMENT

Presentation

The classic presentation for a patient with myocarditis is symptoms of chest pain or dyspnea in the setting of an acute febrile illness. However, subacute myocarditis (inflammation with mild or no LV dysfunction) may present without any cardiac symptoms. Occasionally, these cases are surreptitiously diagnosed in the setting of an acute viral syndrome by the incidental finding of electrocardiographic (ECG) abnormalities (110) or elevations of cardiac enzymes (111,112). Just as cardiac symptoms are not necessarily part of the presentation with myocarditis, neither is an acute febrile illness. Fever was present in only a minority of patients in the MTT (5) (Table 88.5).

TABLE 88.5

CLINICAL CHARACTERISTICS OF MYOCARDITIS TREATMENT TRIAL (MTT) VERSUS INTERVENTION IN MYOCARDITIS AND ACUTE CARDIOMYOPATHY (IMAC)

	MTT	IMAC
n	111	62
Age	42 ± 14	43 ± 13
Gender (% male)	62%	60%
Antecedent viral syndrome	59%	62%
Fever	19%	N/A
Elevated creatine kinase	12%	N/A
Elevated erythrocyte sedimentation rate	60%	40%
Leukocytosis	24%	13%
Autoantibody present	62%	74%
Chest pain	35%	22%
Biopsy-positive inflammation	64%	16%
Symptoms at 1 mo	46%	45%
Pulmonary capillary wedge pressure	19 ± 9	16 ± 10
New York Heart Association class % entry		
Class I	15	10
Class II	35	45
Class III	40	35
Class IV	10	10
LVEF at entry	0.24 ± 0.10	0.25 ± 0.08
LVEF at 1 yr	0.34 ± 0.02[a]	0.42 ± 0.14

LVEF, left ventricular ejection fraction; N/A, not available.
[a]Mean ± standard error; all other values mean ± standard deviation.
From Myocarditis Treatment Trial (Mason JW, O'Connell JB, Herskowitz A, et al., for the Myocarditis Treatment Trial investigators. A clinical trial of immunosuppressive therapy for myocarditis. *N Engl J Med* 1995;333:269–313; and Intervention in Myocarditis and Acute Cardiomyopathy trial (McNamara DM, Holubkov R, Starling RC, et al., for the IMAC investigators. A controlled trial of intravenous immune globulin for recent onset dilated cardiomyopathy. *Circulation* 2001;103:2254–2259).

In patients who present with LV dysfunction, the most common cardiac symptoms are those of congestive heart failure (dyspnea, fatigue, and chest discomfort) (21). In general, heart failure symptoms are more left sided, although signs of right-sided failure, in particular peripheral edema, or symptoms of hepatic congestion (abdominal discomfort or nausea) can be seen. Palpitations are a common presenting complaint and may represent atrial or ventricular arrhythmias (113–115). Atrial arrhythmias generally reflect left atrial hypertension or irritation from associated pericarditis. Ventricular dysrhythmias, although usually associated with heart failure and significant LV dysfunction, are occasionally seen with relatively preserved LV function and presumably originate from an inflammatory focus within the ventricle (116).

The presentation in young children is distinctly different from that of adults, reflecting differences in the pediatric viral milieu. Children are more likely to present within days of the onset of symptoms (96) and have more systemic signs of inflammation. Because patients who present earlier generally have a higher probability of spontaneous recovery once systemic inflammation has resolved, this may lead to a higher probability of significant LV recovery in children.

Diagnostic Evaluation

The clinical examination of patients with suspected myocarditis should focus on signs of ventricular dysfunction. Although tachycardia and borderline hypotension may reflect an acute febrile syndrome, they may also be the first signs of significant hemodynamic compromise. In acute cases, rales on the pulmonary examination provide evidence of left-sided failure; however, in patients with a more insidious presentation a clear lung examination can be heard despite significant dyspnea and marked elevations in left-sided filling pressure. Elevated jugular venous pressure, hepatic tenderness, or peripheral edema is consistent with right-sided failure and suggests right ventricular involvement.

The ECG is an important clinical tool in evaluating cases of suspected myocarditis (110). Common findings are diffuse and nonspecific ST- and T-wave abnormalities. In cases of fever and acute chest pain, PR depression and diffuse global ST elevation may allow a rapid diagnosis of pericarditis. Low voltage may be evident, particularly in patients with an associated pericardial effusion. Occasionally, myocarditis presents with ECG findings suggestive of myocardial infarction in a specific vascular territory. Although this form of myocarditis that mimics the presentation of myocardial infarction has been well described (117–120), it remains important in such cases to rule out an acute ischemic event and to have a low threshold for proceeding with rapid coronary angiography.

Serum analysis for patients with a suspected myocarditis should include creatine phosphokinase (CPK) and cardiac troponin. Elevations of CPK and troponin tend to be modest even in cases of fulminant myocarditis but provide evidence of cardiac injury. In young men with dilated cardiomyopathy and chronic elevation of CPK, a detailed family history should be obtained because this may reflect not persistent myocarditis but dystrophinopathy, a familial X-linked disorder (79).

For patients who present with an acute febrile illness, acute and convalescent sera against most common viral pathogens should be performed. Such a panel should include Coxsackie B virus, influenza A and B viruses, cytomegalovirus, and appropriate adenoviral forms (59). A mild leukocytosis may be seen, particularly with a lymphocyte predominance. Marked leukocytosis should elicit a thorough evaluation for a systemic bacterial infection in which LV dysfunction may be secondary to septicemia. Peripheral eosinophilia should suggest the possibility of eosinophilic myocarditis, a syndrome that is frequently related to drug or other allergies. Serologic testing should include antinuclear antibody and rheumatoid factor, looking for occult connective tissue disease or other systemic autoimmune disease.

In young patients with chronic cough or dyspnea, chest x-ray findings of cardiomegaly or interstitial edema often initiate the cardiac consultation. Usually, marked cardiomegaly is associated with a more insidious progressive course. In these patients, as in chronic dilated cardiomyopathy, findings on chest x-ray of pulmonary edema may be minimal despite markedly elevated left-sided filling pressures. In contrast, acute fulminant myocarditis can present with florid alveolar edema and acute respiratory failure but, given the short time course, a relatively normal-sized cardiac silhouette.

Echocardiography is clinically the most useful tool for clinical management and provides information about LV size and function, right ventricular involvement, and associated pericardial effusion (121,122). The echogenicity of the myocardium does not change with inflammation, and images of the myocardium itself do not assist diagnosis. However, the presence of a pericardial effusion, relatively small chamber size with decreased systolic function, and increased LV wall thickness are essentially diagnostic of active myocardial inflammation. LV systolic dysfunction is generally global, although segmental wall motion abnormalities can be seen that can mimic the appearance of an ischemic cardiomyopathy.

In patients with LV systolic dysfunction and significant hemodynamic impairment, consideration should be given to invasive hemodynamic assessment by right heart catheterization. Persistent tachycardia may be compensatory for a decrease in stroke volume and a resultant decrease in cardiac output. Because acute myocardial inflammation can affect systolic and diastolic properties, pulmonary capillary wedge and right atrial pressures are frequently elevated out of proportion to the apparent decrease in systolic function. In addition, in any adult patient with cardiac risk factors, coronary artery disease should be ruled out either by angiography or by appropriate noninvasive evaluation, given the distinctly different treatment pathway engaged by this diagnosis.

Newer Imaging Modalities: Magnetic Resonance Imaging and Contrast Echocardiography

The limitations of conventional echocardiography for delineating myocardial inflammation have led to renewed interest in alternative, noninvasive imaging.

Cardiovascular magnetic resonance imaging (CMR) demonstrates contrast enhancement in areas of active myocarditis, with partial to complete resolution of enhancement during follow-up (123). Evaluation by CMR also reveals the segmental nature of myocarditis (Fig. 88.6). This may underlie the limited sensitivity of EMB; the inflammatory histology of enhancing lesions has been confirmed by "CMR-guided" biopsies (124). The capability of CMR to detect inflamed myocardium has the potential to vastly improve the clinical diagnosis of suspected myocarditis (125,126); however more widespread availability of cardiac magnetic resonance imaging (MRI) is required before this technology can challenge EMB as the gold standard. One significant limitation of CMR is the inability of using MRI in unstable subjects, as in the setting of the coronary care unit. Myocardial contrast echocardiography (MCE) has shown promise in animal models and has the potential of being a more useful modality for imaging myocardial inflammation in this regard (127,128).

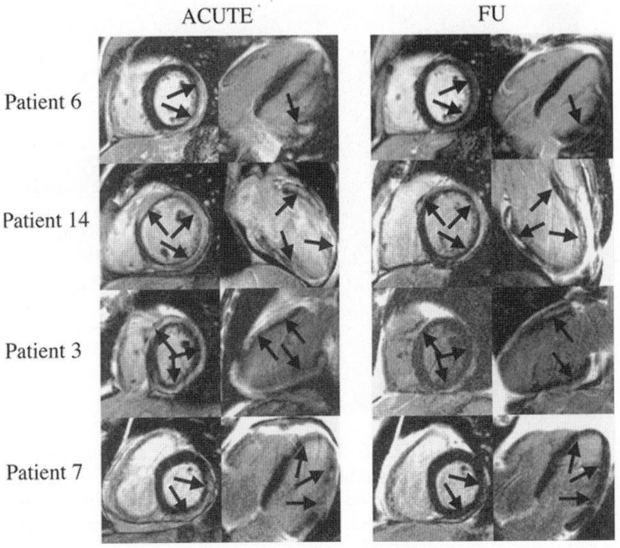

FIGURE 88.6. Evidence of enhancing lesions on cardiac magnetic resonance (CMR) imaging from subjects with acute myocarditis (ACUTE) and follow up images (FU) demonstrating significant resolution. (From Mahrholdt H, Goedecke C, Wagner A, et al. Cardiovascular magnetic resonance assessment of human myocarditis. *Circulation* 2004; 109:1250–1258.)

Endomyocardial Biopsy

In the 1960s, the development of techniques for transvenous endomyocardial right ventricular biopsy (EMB) made possible the ante mortem diagnosis of myocardial inflammation (15,129). The role of EMB in posttransplant management led to increased use in native myocardial disease (130), and histologic evidence of inflammation became the gold standard for the diagnosis of myocarditis. However, the sensitivity of EMB has historically been limited by sampling error, and autopsy studies of patients who are known to have myocarditis have estimated the sensitivity at 60% to 70% (131).

In an effort to have more consistent pathologic guidelines, a group of leading cardiac pathologists met in Dallas in 1986 to establish a consensus for the definition of myocarditis (132). The Dallas criteria defined "borderline myocarditis" as the presence of mononuclear cell infiltrates without myocyte necrosis (Fig. 88.7) and "myocarditis" as cellular infiltration with myocyte necrosis (Fig. 88.7). Despite this widely accepted consensus, interpretation is problematic and physician dependent (133). For endomyocardial biopsy in native hearts the risk of a major complication, in particular cardiac tamponade, approaches 1% (134,135), significantly higher than in cardiac transplant patients. There are few histologically guided therapies, particularly for compensated patients. For patients with more fulminant disease and hemodynamic compromise, evaluation for possible giant-cell myocarditis is frequently the rationale for EMB, given the distinct prognostic and therapeutic implications.

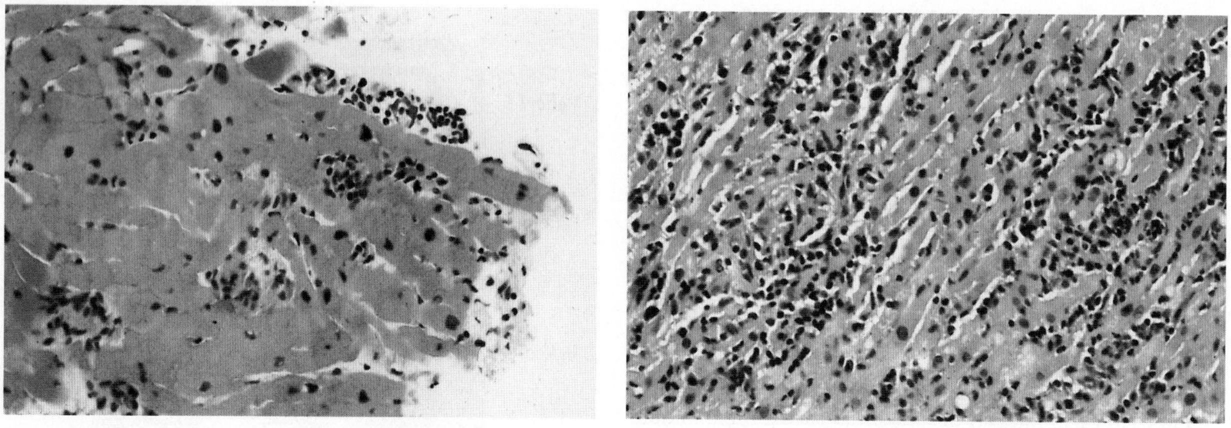

FIGURE 88.7. Histopathologic appearance of borderline myocarditis (lymphocytic infiltrates without myocyte necrosis) (A) and myocarditis (lymphocytic infiltrates with myocyte necrosis) (B) A: ×350 magnification; B: ×300 magnification. (From Feldman AM, McNamara D. Myocarditis. *N Engl J Med* 2000;343:1388–1398, with permission. Copyright © 2000 Massachusetts Medical Society. All rights reserved.)

Recently, developments in molecular diagnostics have led to increased interest in improving the prognostic utility of EMB. Analysis from the IMAC study demonstrates that gene expression on EMB of Fas, a critical cellular receptor in the initiation of apoptosis, is inversely proportional to subsequent LV recovery (136). Multiarray analysis of subjects with giant-cell myocarditis has detected patterns with immune response activation (137), which supports the anti–T cell immunosuppressive strategies generally proposed for intervention. The role of EMB may continue to evolve as newer molecular techniques are employed to increase the diagnostic information provided and improve its clinical utility.

THERAPY AND CLINICAL OUTCOMES

Despite much research and interest into the development of immune modulatory therapies, the medical therapy of patients with suspected myocarditis remains supportive. The prognosis in myocarditis depends on the degree of left ventricular systolic dysfunction at the time of presentation and the level of hemodynamic compromise. Patients presenting with myocarditis can be categorized based on LV function into those with normal systolic function, compensated LV dysfunction, and acute LV dysfunction with hemodynamic compromise (also known as fulminant myocarditis). Treatment and outcomes differ markedly in these three subgroups.

Myocarditis and Preserved Left Ventricular Systolic Function

Patients with myocarditis and normal LV function frequently present with ECG abnormalities or chest pain in a setting of an acute febrile illness. In the absence of left ventricular dysfunction there is no indication for β-adrenergic receptor antagonists or angiotensin-converting-enzyme inhibitors. In general, it is recommended that aerobic activities or heavy lifting be avoided for at least 6 to 8 weeks (139). Cardiac assessment, generally ECG and echocardiography, should be repeated roughly 6 to 8 weeks after presentation to guard against progressive cardiac involvement. Endomyocardial biopsy is of limited clinical utility and is not recommended. In general, cases of myocarditis with either mild or no left ventricular dysfunction are self-limited and carry an excellent prognosis.

Myocarditis with Left Ventricular Dysfunction

For patients presenting with left ventricular dysfunction, predicting clinical outcomes and the likelihood of myocardial recovery is difficult. From 30% to 50% of patients exhibit substantial improvement in left ventricular dysfunction in the first year after presentation (6,21,22). Routine myocardial histology does not predict the probability of recovery, and in general EMB is not recommended (7). In the most recent trial requiring myocardial biopsy, the IMAC study, routine EMB was not predictive of clinical outcomes (Table 88.6). Indeed, of the patients who normalized their LVEF (20 of 62 patients), 85% had "negative" biopsies based on routine histology.

Recommended therapy is similar to that for patients with left ventricular dysfunction in the absence of myocarditis. Angiotensin-converting-enzyme (ACE) inhibitors or angiotensin-receptor blockers and β-adrenergic antagonists are recommended for all patients. Pulmonary congestion or symptoms of fluid overload should be treated with a loop diuretic generally at the lowest effective dose. Digoxin should be added in patients with New York Heart Association class III heart failure; however, given potential proarrhythmic and proinflammatory (139) effects, it should be maintained at a low dose and avoided entirely in minimally symptomatic (class I or II) subjects. Subsequent prognosis clearly depends on the degree of ventricular recovery. Fortunately, in the age of modern heart failure therapies, the short-term prognosis in recent-onset cardiomyopathy and myocarditis has improved, with a transplant-free survival in the recent IMAC study of approximately 88% at 2 years (6).

Fulminant Myocarditis

For patients with acute lymphocytic myocarditis and severe hemodynamic compromise, long-term prognosis (and the probability of left ventricular recovery) may actually be better than for patients presenting with more insidious chronic disease (140). Dramatic and sustained recovery of left ventricular

TABLE 88.6

BASELINE, 12-MONTH LEFT VENTRICULAR EJECTION FRACTION, AND INCREASE IN LEFT VENTRICULAR EJECTION FRACTION (LVEF) AT 1 YEAR, ACCORDING TO BIOPSY STATUS

	Baseline LVEF	12-Mo LVEF	Change in LVEF at 1 yr
Cellular inflammation			
Absent ($n = 52$)	0.25 ± 0.09	0.41 ± 0.14	0.15 ± 0.14
Present ($n = 10$)	0.25 ± 0.08	0.49 ± 0.19	0.21 ± 0.14
Fibrosis			
Absent ($n = 23$)	0.26 ± 0.08	0.43 ± 0.13	0.16 ± 0.12
Present ($n = 39$)	0.25 ± 0.09	0.41 ± 0.15	0.15 ± 0.15
Myocyte hypertrophy			
Absent ($n = 31$)	0.26 ± 0.09	0.44 ± 0.14	0.17 ± 0.14
Present ($n = 31$)	0.24 ± 0.08	0.40 ± 0.15	0.13 ± 0.14

No statistically significant differences based on biopsy status were found between the subgroups with respect to LVEF at entry, at 1-year follow-up, or at the change at 1 year.
From McNamara DM, Holubkov R, Starling RC, et al., for the IMAC investigators. A controlled trial of intravenous immune globulin for recent onset dilated cardiomyopathy. *Circulation* 2001;103:2254–2259.

function has also been reported in patients with fulminant myocarditis maintained with LVAD support (141–143). In a single-center series from the University of Pittsburgh (144), subjects with acute inflammatory cardiomyopathy who normalized their LVEF on device support sustained this recovery after explantation of the device (Fig. 88.8). This supports the belief that in fulminant disease, assist device support should serve as a bridge to recovery rather than transplantation. Hemodynamic unloading should theoretically rest inflamed myocardium; however, the role of mechanical support in facilitating recovery is difficult to determine, and the use of LVADs is reserved for patients who are failing despite maximal inotropic therapy. For patients with cardiogenic shock and aggressive myocarditis, consideration should be given to referral to a tertiary center, where both cardiac transplantation and device support are more accessible.

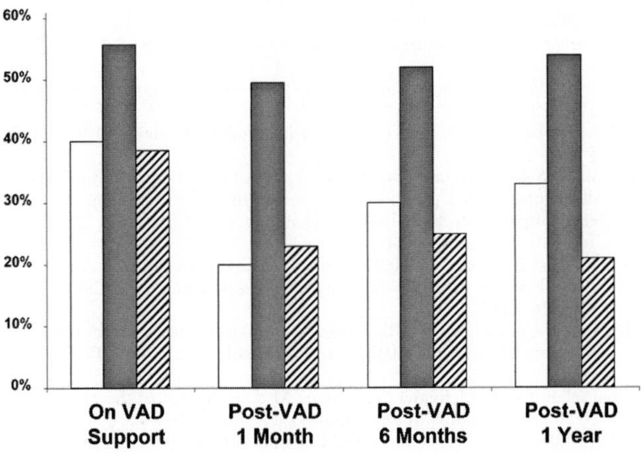

FIGURE 88.8. Mean left ventricular ejection fraction (%) in the first year postexplantation in 10 patients from the University of Pittsburgh in whom a ventricular assist device (VAD) served as a bridge to recovery. White bars indicate ischemic patients ($n = 2$), gray bars indicate patients with complete recovery on the device ($n = 6$, including 3 with acute myocarditis and 2 with acute peripartum cardiomyopathy [PPCM]), and hatched bars indicate patients with incomplete recovery on the device ($n = 2$, both with acute PPCM). (From Simon MA, Kormos RL, Murali S, et al. Myocardial recovery using ventricular assist devices. Prevalence, clinical characteristics, and outcomes. *Circulation* 2005; 112(Suppl I):I32–I36.)

Giant-Cell Myocarditis

In patients with fulminant disease, evaluation for possible giant-cell myocarditis is the primary indication for EMB. Patients with giant-cell myocarditis were excluded from the Johns Hopkins study because their prognosis and potential for recovery are significantly worse than those for patients with lymphocytic myocarditis (8,28). Anecdotal reports (145–147) and the Giant Cell Registry (8) suggest that immunosuppressive therapy, in particular the combination of cyclosporine and the anti–T-lymphocyte antibody muromonab-CD3, may improve transplant-free survival. Given the grim prognosis of giant-cell myocarditis with conventional therapy, immunosuppression should be considered. This remains investigational and is the subject of an ongoing multicenter trial.

Postrecovery Management

For patients whose left ventricular size and systolic function completely normalize, ACE-inhibitor therapy and β-receptor antagonist can potentially be discontinued with close monitoring for subsequent declines in left ventricular function. In many recovered patients, subjective limitations in functional capacity and objective limitations in metabolic stress testing may persist, potentially due to a slower recovery of diastolic function (148). Overall prognosis of such patients is excellent. Although a chance of recurrence of myocarditis exists, most investigators believe that this is seen only in a minority of patients.

Peripartum Cardiomyopathy

For women who are diagnosed with cardiomyopathy *during pregnancy*, ACE inhibitors and angiotensin-receptor antagonists are contraindicated because of the potential harmful effects to the developing fetus (149). ACE inhibitors or angiotensin-receptor antagonists are recommended for all postpartum patients. β-Blockers should be considered but used with caution in patients with small LV chamber size and reflex tachycardia. Breast-feeding is generally to be avoided because of the potential increased metabolic demands on the mother and the potential for certain therapies such as ACE inhibitors to be passed to the child through breast milk. Substantial recovery of LV function is seen in roughly 50% of cases (73,98). In patients with persistent LV dysfunction, subsequent pregnancy should clearly be avoided. In patients with recovered LV function, a risk of LV decompensation with subsequent pregnancy exists, and patients should be monitored carefully.

Pediatric Myocarditis

Children are more likely than their adult counterparts to present with an acute febrile illness and with a positive endomyocardial biopsy (96). Because they present more acutely, they appear to have a higher likelihood of ventricular recovery (150,151). ACE inhibitors are recommended for all patients with LV dysfunction (152). A study of pediatric patients with myocarditis suggests that immunoglobulin improves LV function (96). However, this study relied on historical controls, and no randomized trial has evaluated the efficacy of immunoglobulin for this indication in children. Indeed, all previous multicenter trials of immunosuppressive therapy for myocarditis have enrolled only adults, and few controlled data exist to guide therapy for the pediatric patient. In the absence of randomized, prospective data, anecdotal reports will continue to have a strong influence on practice.

CONTROVERSIES AND PERSONAL PERSPECTIVES

The absence of histologically guided therapies has limited the use of EMB in clinical practice. Recent advances in molecular diagnostics have facilitated the identification of viral nucleic acids on EMB. The question remains whether newer advances in molecular techniques, such as microarray analysis, will further increase the clinical utility and "rehabilitate" EMB as a diagnostic tool. Although technological advances will enhance the yield of biopsy, they will also facilitate the development of less invasive molecular diagnostic testing for myocarditis. Molecular expression patterning in peripheral leukocytes is being evaluated in transplant recipients as a noninvasive test for possible cardiac rejection (153). It is hoped that in patients being evaluated for possible myocarditis similar expression patterning may one day allow us to "estimate" the inflammatory state of the myocardium, limiting the need for patients to undergo the risk of EMB except in rare cases. The role of biopsy in the evaluation of myocarditis is limited and controversial. I believe that with increased noninvasive diagnostic capabilities its role will continue to diminish.

THE FUTURE

The recent advances in MRI hold great promise for the development of noninvasive imaging of inflammatory myocardium. In addition, the emergence of myocardial contrast echocardiography with molecular targeting of biomarkers will clearly enhance our ability to noninvasively diagnose myocarditis. These imaging capabilities will enable practitioners to determine which patients have chronic pathologic inflammation and are destined to have a poor outcome with conventional therapy. In addition, increasing insights into the effect of genetic background on response to inflammatory injury will allow clinicians to decipher the heterogeneous outcomes evident with acute myocarditis. Molecular diagnostic techniques will complement imaging capabilities, and together they should markedly improve our ability to predict natural history and delineate an individual's probability of spontaneous recovery. The enhanced diagnostic and prognostic tools may lead to a resurgence of interest in immune modulation because it is in patients with chronic persistent inflammation that this intervention will have the greatest impact.

References

1. Lange LG, Schreiner GF. Immune mechanisms of cardiac disease. *N Engl J Med* 1994;330:1129–1135.
2. Feldman AM, McNamara D. Myocarditis. *N Engl J Med* 2000;343:1388–1398.
3. Dec GW, Fuster V. Idiopathic dilated cardiomyopathy. *N Engl J Med* 1994;331:1564–1575.
4. Parillo JE, Cunnion RE, Epstein SE, et al. A prospective, randomized, controlled trial of prednisone for dilated cardiomyopathy. *N Engl J Med* 1989;321:1061–1068.
5. Mason JW, O'Connell JB, Herskowitz A, et al., for the Myocarditis Treatment Trial investigators. A clinical trial of immunosuppressive therapy for myocarditis. *N Engl J Med* 1995;333:269–313.
6. McNamara DM, Holubkov R, Starling RC, et al., for the IMAC investigators. A controlled trial of intravenous immune globulin for recent onset dilated cardiomyopathy. *Circulation* 2001;103:2254–2259.
7. Hunt SA, Abraham WT, Chin MH, et al., for the ACC/AHA task force report. Guidelines for the evaluation and treatment of heart failure. *J Am Coll Cardiol* 2005;46:1116–1143.
8. Cooper LT, Berry GJ, Shabetai R, et al. Idiopathic giant-cell myocarditis—natural history and treatment. *N Engl J Med* 1997;336:1860–1866.
9. Taylor DO, Edwards LB, Boucek MM, et al. The registry of the International Society for Heart and Lung Transplantation: twenty-first official report. *J Heart Lung Transplant* 2004;7:796–803.
10. Kawai C. From myocarditis to cardiomyopathy: mechanisms of inflammation and cell death. Learning from the past for the future. *Circulation* 1999;99:1091–1100.
11. Mattingly TW. Changing concepts of myocardial diseases. *JAMA* 1965; 191:127–131.
12. Kibrick S, Benirschke K. Severe generalized disease (encephalohepatomyocarditis) occurring in newborn period and due to infection with Coxsackie virus group B: evidence of intra-uterine infection with this agent. *Pediatrics* 1958;22:857–874.
13. Lerner AM. Experimental approach to virus myocarditis. *Prog Med Virol* 1965;7:97–115.
14. Smith WG. Adult heart disease due to Coxsackie virus group B. *Br Heart J* 1966;28:204–220.
15. Sakakibara S, Konno S. Endomyocardial biopsy. *Jpn Heart J* 1962;3:537–543.
16. Jin O, Sole MJ, Butany JW, et al. Detection of enterovirus RNA in myocardial biopsies from patients with myocarditis and cardiomyopathy using gene amplification by polymerase chain reaction. *Circulation* 1990;82:8–16.
17. Aukrust P, Ueland T, Muller F, et al. Elevated circulating levels of C-C chemokines in patients with congestive heart failure. *Circulation* 1998; 97:1136–1143.
18. Limas CJ, Goldenberg IF, Limas C. Autoantibodies against β-adrenoreceptors in human dilated cardiomyopathy. *Circ Res* 1989;64:97–103.
19. Richardson P, McKenna W, Bristow M et al. Report of the 1995 World Health Organization/International Society and Federation of Cardiology Task Force on the Definition and Classification of Cardiomyopathies. *Circulation* 1996;93:841–842.
20. Davies MJ. The cardiomyopathies: a review of terminology, pathology and pathogenesis. *Histopathology* 1984;8:363–393.
21. Dec GW, Palacios IF, Fallon JT, et al. Active myocarditis in the spectrum of acute dilated cardiomyopathies: clinical features, histologic correlates, and clinical outcome. *N Engl J Med* 1985;312:885–890.
22. Steimle AE, Stevenson LW, Fonarow GC, et al. Prediction of improvement in recent onset cardiomyopathy after referral for heart transplantation. *J Am Coll Cardiol* 1994;23:553–559.
23. Lieberman EB, Hutchins GM, Herskowitz A, et al. Clinicopathologic description of myocarditis. *J Am Coll Cardiol* 1991;18:1617–1626.
24. Burke AP, Saenger J, Mullick F, et al. Hypersensitivity myocarditis. *Arch Pathol Lab Med* 1991;115:764–769.

25. Fenoglio JJ, McAllister HA, Mullick FG. Drug related myocarditis. I. Hypersensitivity myocarditis. *Hum Pathol* 1981;12:900–907.
26. Galiuto L, Enriquez-Sarano M, Reeder GS, et al. Eosinophilic myocarditis manifesting as myocardial infarction: early diagnosis and successful treatment. *Mayo Clinic Proc* 1997;72:603–610.
27. Beghetti M, Wilson GJ, Bohn D, et al. Hypersensitivity myocarditis caused by an allergic reaction to cefaclor. *J Pediatr* 1998;132:172–173.
28. Davidoff R, Palacios P, Southern J, et al. Giant cell versus lymphocytic myocarditis. A comparison of their clinical features and long term outcomes. *Circulation* 1991;83(3):953–961.
29. Lorell B, Alderman EL, Mason JW. Cardiac sarcoidosis. Diagnosis with endomyocardial biopsy and treatment with corticosteroids. *Am J Cardiol* 1978;42:143–146.
30. Jolles PR, Tatum JL. SLE myocarditis. Detection by Ga-67 citrate scintigraphy. *Clin Nucl Med* 1996;21:284–286.
31. Litovsky SH, Burke AP, Virmani R. Giant cell myocarditis: an entity distinct from sarcoidosis characterized by multiphasic myocyte destruction by cytotoxic T cells and histocytic giant cells. *Mod Pathol* 1996;9:1126–1134.
32. Melvin KR, Richardson PJ, Olson EG, et al. Peripartum cardiomyopathy due to myocarditis. *N Engl J Med* 1982;307:731–734.
33. Codd MB, Sugrue DD, Gersh BJ, et al. Epidemiology of idiopathic and hypertrophic cardiomyopathy. *Circulation* 1989;80(3):564–572.
34. Hufnagal G, Pankuweit S, Schonian U, et al. The European Study of Epidemiology and Treatment of Cardiac Inflammatory Diseases (ESETCID). First epidemiology results. *Herz* 2000;25(3):279–285.
35. Saphir O. Myocarditis, a general review with an analysis of 240 cases. *Arch Pathol* 1951;32:1000.
36. Gore E, Saphir O. Myocarditis, a classification of 1402 cases. *Am Heart J* 1947;34:827–830.
37. Blankenhorn MA, Gall EA. Myocarditis and myocardosis: a clinicopathologic appraisal. *Circulation* 1956;X111:217–223.
38. Drory Y, Turetz Y, Hiss Y, et al. Sudden unexpected death in persons less than 40 years of age. *Am J Cardiol* 1991;68:1388–1392.
39. Eckart RE, Scoville SL, Campbell CL., et al. Sudden death in young adults: a 25-year review of autopsies in military recruits. *Ann Intern Med* 2004; 141:829–834.
40. D'Ambrosio A, Patti G, Manzoli A, et al. The fate of acute myocarditis between spontaneous improvement and evolution to dilated cardiomyopathy: a review. *Heart* 2001;85:499–504.
41. Huber SA. Animal models: immunological aspects. In: Banatvala JE, ed. *Viral infections of the heart*. London: Arnold, 1993:82–109.
42. Matsumori A, Kawai C. An animal model of congestive (dilated) cardiomyopathy: dilatation and hypertrophy of the heart in the chronic stage in DBA/2 mice with myocarditis caused by encephalomyocarditis virus. *Circulation* 1982;66:355–360.
43. Godeny EK, Gauntt CJ. Interferon and natural killer cell activity in Coxsackie virus B3–induced myocarditis. *Eur Heart J* 1987;8:433–435.
44. Liu CC, Young LHY, Young JDE. Mechanisms of disease: lymphocyte-mediated cytolysis and disease. *N Engl J Med* 1996;335:1651–1659.
45. Seko Y, Tsuchimochi H, Nakamura T, et al. Expression of major histocompatibility complex class I antigen in murine ventricular myocytes infected with Coxsackie virus B3. *Circ Res* 1990;69:360–367.
46. Seko Y, Matsuda H, Kato K, et al. Expression of intercellular adhesion molecule-1 in murine hearts with acute myocarditis caused by coxsackievirus B3. *J Clin Invest* 1993;91:1327–1336.
47. Kishimoto C, Kuribayashi K, Masuda T, et al. Immunological behavior of lymphocytes in experimental viral myocarditis: significance of T-lymphocytes in the severity of myocarditis and silent myocarditis in BALB/c-nu/nu mice. *Circulation* 1985;71:1247–1254.
48. Woodruff JF, Woodruff JJ. Involvement of T lymphocytes in the pathogenesis of Coxsackie B3 heart disease. *J Immunol* 1974;113:1726–1734.
49. Matsumori A, Kawai C. An animal model of congestive (dilated) cardiomyopathy: dilatation and hypertrophy of the heart in the chronic stage in DBA/2 mice with myocarditis caused by encephalomyocarditis virus. *Circulation* 1982;66:355–360.
50. Kyu B, Matsumori A, Sato Y, et al. Cardiac persistence of cardioviral RNA detected by polymerase chain reaction in a murine model of dilated cardiomyopathy. *Circulation* 1992;86:1605–1614.
51. Bowles NE, Archard LC, Olsen EGJ, et al. Detection of Coxsackie-B-virus-specific RNA sequences in myocardial biopsy sample from patients with myocarditis and dilated cardiomyopathy. *Lancet* 1986;1:1120–1123.
52. Schwaiger A, Umlauft F, Weyrer K, et al. Detection of enteroviral ribonucleic acid in myocardial biopsies from patients with idiopathic dilated cardiomyopathy by polymerase chain reaction. *Am Heart J* 1993;126:406–410.
53. Fujioka S, Koide H, Kitaura Y, et al. Molecular detection and differentiation of enteroviruses in endomyocardial biopsies and pericardial effusions from dilated cardiomyopathy and myocarditis. *Am Heart J* 1996;131:760–765.
54. Fairly CK, Ryan M, Wall PG, Weinberg J. The organisms reported to cause infective myocarditis and pericarditis in England and Wales. *J Infect Dis* 1996;32:223–225.
55. Grumbach IM, Heim A, Pring-Akerblom P, et al. Adenoviruses and enteroviruses as pathogens in myocarditis and dilated cardiomyopathy. *Acta Cardiol* 1999;54:83–88.
56. Matsumori A. Hepatitis C virus infection. *Circ Res* 2005;96:144-147.
57. Cohen IS, Anderson DW, Virmani R, et al. Congestive cardiomyopathy in association with the acquired immunodeficiency syndrome. *N Engl J Med* 1986;315:628–630.
58. Lipshultz SE, Easley KA, Orav EJ, et al. Left ventricular structure and function in children infected with human immunodeficiency virus. Group for the Pediatric Pulmonary and Cardiac Complications of Vertically Transmitted HIV Infection (P2C2 HIV) study group. *Circulation* 1998;97:1246–1256.
59. Barbaro G, DiLorenzo G, Grisorio B, et al. Incidence of dilated cardiomyopathy and detection of HIV in myocardial cells of HIV-positive patients. Gruppo Italiano per lo Studio Cardiologico dei Pazienti Affetti da AIDS. *N Engl J Med* 1998;339:1093–1099.
60. Bowles NE, Kearney DL, Ni J, et al. The detection of viral genomes by polymerase chain reaction in the myocardium of pediatric patients with advanced HIV disease. *J Am Coll Cardiol* 1999;34:857–865.
61. Dias JCP. Control of Chagas' disease in Brazil. *Parasitol Today* 1987;3:336–339.
62. World Health Organization. *Sixth program report: Chapter 6: Chagas' disease. Special program for research and training in tropical diseases* (Document TDR, PR-6, 83.6-CHA, YNDP). Geneva: World Bank, World Health Organization,1983.
63. Williams A. *Aspergillus* myocarditis. *Am J Pathol* 1974;61:247–248.
64. Walsh TJ, Hutchins GM, Buckley BH, et al. Fungal infections of the heart. Analysis of 51 autopsy cases. *Am J Cardiol* 1980;45:357–366.
65. Duffield JS, Jacob AJ, Miller HC. Recurrent, life threatening atrioventricular dissociation associated with toxoplasma myocarditis. *Heart* 1996; 76:453–454.
66. Montoya JG, Jordan R, Lingamneni S, et al. Toxoplasmic myocarditis and polymyositis in patients with acute acquired toxoplasmosis diagnosed during life. *Clin Infect Dis* 1997;24:676–683.
67. Lampert MB, Lang RM. Peripartum cardiomyopathy. *Am Heart J* 1995; 130:860–870.
68. Huerta EM, Erice A, Espino RF, et al. Post-partum cardiomyopathy and acute myocarditis. *Am Heart J* 1985;110:1079–1081.
69. Rizeq MN, Rickenbacher PR, Fowler MB, et al. Incidents of myocarditis in peripartum cardiomyopathy. *Am Heart J* 1994;74:474–477.
70. Foelich CJ, Goodwin JS, Bankhurst AD, et al. Pregnancy, a temporal fetal graft of suppressor cells in autoimmune disease. *Am J Med* 1980;69: 329–331.
71. Kovithavongs T, Dossetor JB. Suppressor cells in human pregnancy. *Transplant Proc* 1978;10:911–913.
72. Damek DM, Shuster EA. Pregnancy and multiple sclerosis. *Mayo Clin Proc* 1997;72:977–989.
73. Midei MG, DeMent SH, Feldman AM, et al. Peripartum myocarditis and cardiomyopathy. *Circulation* 1990;81:922–928.
74. Demakis JG, Rahimtoola SH. Peripartum cardiomyopathy. *Circulation* 1971;44:964–968.
75. Billingham ME. Pharmacotoxic myocardial disease: an endomyocardial study. In: Sekiguchi C, Olsen EGJ, Goodwin JF, eds. *Myocarditis and related disorders*. Tokyo: Springer-Verlag,1985:278–282.
76. Feenstra J, Grobbee DE, Remme WJ, et al. Drug-induced heart failure. *J Am Coll Cardiol* 1999;33:1152–1162.
77. Singal PK, Iliskovic N. Doxorubicin-induced cardiomyopathy. *N Engl J Med* 1998;339:900–905.
78. Michels VV, Moll PP, Miller FA, et al. The frequency of familial dilated cardiomyopathy in a series of patients with idiopathic dilated cardiomyopathy. *N Engl J Med* 1992;326:77–82.
79. Towbin JA, Hejtmancik, Brink P, et al. X-linked cardiomyopathy. Molecular evidence of linkage to the Duchenne muscular dystrophy gene at the Xp21 locus. *Circulation* 1993;87:1854–1865.
80. Olson TM, Michels VV, Thibodeau SN, et al. Actin mutations in dilated cardiomyopathy, a heritable form of heart failure. *Science* 1998;280:750–752.
81. Kamisago M, Sharma SD, DePalma SR, et al. Mutations in sarcomere protein genes as a cause of dilated cardiomyopathy. *N Engl J Med* 2000; 343:1688–1696.
82. Mestroni L, Rocco C, Gregori D, et al. Familial dilated cardiomyopathy: evidence for genetic and phenotypic heterogeneity. *J Am Coll Cardiol* 1999; 34:181–190.
83. Baig MK, Goldman JH, Caforio ALP, et al. Familial dilated cardiomyopathy: cardiac abnormalities are common in asymptomatic relative and may represent early disease. *J Am Coll Cardiol* 1998;31:195–201.
84. Michels VV, Moll PP, Rodeheffer RJ. Circulating heart autoantibodies in familial as compared to nonfamilial idiopathic dilated cardiomyopathy. *Mayo Clin Proc* 1994;69:24–27.
85. Caforio ALP, Keeling PJ, Zachara E. Evidence from family studies for autoimmunity in dilated cardiomyopathy. *Lancet* 1994;344:773–777.
86. Tazelaar HD, Billingham ME. Leukocytic infiltrates in idiopathic dilated cardiomyopathy. *Am J Surg Pathol* 1986;10:405–412.
87. Kuan AP, Chamberlain W, Malkiel S, et al. Genetic control of autoimmune myocarditis mediated by myosin-specific antibodies. *Immunogenetics* 1999;49:79–85.

88. McKenna CJ, Codd KA, McCann HA, et al. Idiopathic dilated cardiomyopathy: familial prevalence and HLA distribution. *Heart* 1197;77: 549–552.
89. Albert LJ, Inman RD. Molecular mimicry and autoimmunity. *N Engl J Med* 1999;341:2068–2074.
90. Limas C, Limas CJ, Boudoulas H. T-cell receptor gene polymorphisms in familial cardiomyopathy: correlation with anti–β-receptor autoantibodies. *Am Heart J* 1992;124:1258–1263.
91. Levine B, Kalman J, Mayer L, et al. Elevated circulating levels of tumor necrosis factor in severe chronic heart failure. *N Engl J Med* 1990;323:236–241.
92. Torre-Amione G, Kapadia S, Benedict C, et al. Proinflammatory cytokine levels in patients with depressed left ventricular ejection fraction: a report from the Studies of Left Ventricular Dysfunction (SOLVD). *J Am Coll Cardiol* 1996;27:1201–1206.
93. Kubota T, Alvarez RJ, Miyagishima M, et al. Expression of proinflammatory cytokines in the failing human heart: comparison of recent onset and endstage cardiomyopathy. *J Heart Lung Transplant* 2000;19:819–824.
94. MacGowan GA, Mann DL, Kormos RL, et al. Circulating interleukin-6 in severe heart failure. *Am J Cardiol* 1997;79:1128–1131.
95. Newberger JW, Takahashi M, Burns JC, et al. The treatment of Kawasaki syndrome with intravenous gamma globulin. *N Engl J Med* 1986;315:341–347.
96. Drucker MA, Colan SD, Lewis AB, et al. Gammaglobulin treatment of acute myocarditis in the pediatric population. *Circulation* 1994;89:252–257.
97. McNamara DM, Rosenblum WD, Janosko KM, et al. Intravenous immune globulin in the therapy of myocarditis and acute cardiomyopathy. *Circulation* 1997;95:2476–2478.
98. Bozkurt B, Villanueva FS, Holubkov R, et al. Intravenous immune globulin in the therapy of peripartum cardiomyopathy. *J Am Coll Cardiol* 1999; 34:177–180.
99. Wojnicz R, Nowalany-Kozielska E, Wojciechowska C, et al. Randomized, placebo-controlled study for immunosuppressive treatment of inflammatory dilated cardiomyopathy: two-year follow-up results. *Circulation* 2001;104:39–45.
100. Deonarain R, Cerullo D, Fuse K, et al. Protective role for Interferon-β in coxsackievirus B3 infection. *Circulation* 2004;110:3540–3543.
101. Daliento L, Calabrese F, Tona F, et al. Successful treatment of enterovirus-induced myocarditis with interferon-α. *J Heart Lung Transplant* 2003;22:214–217.
102. Bowles NE, Ni Jiyuan, Kearney DL, et al. Detection of viruses in myocardial tissues by polymerase chain reaction: evidence of adenovirus as a common cause of myocarditis in children and adults. *J Am Coll Cardiol* 2003;42:466–472.
103. Chimenti C, Russo A, Pieroni M, et al. Intramyocyte detection of Epstein-Barr virus genome by laser capture microdissection in patients with inflammatory cardiomyopathy. *Circulation* 2004;110:3534–3539.
104. Matsumori A. Hepatitis C virus infection and cardiomyopathies. *Circ Res* 2005; 96:144–147.
105. Kühl U, Pauschinger M, Schwimmbeck PL, et al. Interferon-β treatment eliminates cardiotropic viruses and improves left ventricular function in patients with myocardial persistence of viral genomes and left ventricular dysfunction. *Circulation* 2003; 107:2793–2798.
106. Pauschinger M, Chandrasekharan K, Noutsias M, et al. Viral heart disease: molecular diagnosis, clinical prognosis, and treatment strategies. *Med Microbiol Immunol* 2004; 193:65–69.
107. Centers for Disease Control and Prevention (CDC). Update: adverse events following civilian smallpox vaccination—United States, 2003. *MMWR Morb Mortal Wkly Rep* 2003;52(18):419–420.
108. Halsell JS, Riddle JR, Atwood JE, et al. Myopericarditis following smallpox vaccination among vaccinia-naïve US military personnel. *JAMA* 2003; 289(24):3283–3289.
109. Cassimatis DC, Atwood JE, Engler RM, et al. Smallpox vaccination and myopericarditis: a clinical review. *J Am Coll Cardiol* 2004;43:1503–1510.
110. Heikkila J, Karjalainen J. Evaluation of mild acute infectious myocarditis. *Br Heart J* 1982;47:381–391.
111. Smith SC, Ladenson JH, Mason JW, et al. Elevations of cardiac troponin I associated with myocarditis. Experimental and clinical correlates. *Circulation* 1996;95:163–168.
112. Lauer B, Niederau C, Kuhl U, et al. Cardiac troponin T in patients with clinically suspected myocarditis. *J Am Coll Cardiol* 1997;30:1354–1359.
113. Karjalainen J, Viitasalo M, Kala R, Heikkila J. 24-hour electrocardiographic recordings in mild acute infectious myocarditis. *Ann Clin Res* 1984; 16:34–39.
114. Tai YT, Law CP, Fong PC, et al. Incessant automatic ventricular tachycardia complicating acute Coxsackie B myocarditis. *Cardiology* 1992;30:339–344.
115. Zeppilli P, Santini C, Palmieri V, et al. Role of myocarditis in athletes with minor arrhythmias and/or echocardiographic abnormalities. *Chest* 1994;106:373–380.
116. Vignola PA, Aonuma K, Swaye PS. Lymphocytic myocarditis presenting as unexplained ventricular arrhythmias: diagnosis with endomyocardial biopsy and response to immunosuppression. *J Am Coll Cardiol* 1984;4: 812–819.
117. Frustaci A, Maseri A. Localized left ventricular aneurysms with normal global function caused by myocarditis. *Am J Cardiol* 1992;70:1221–1224.
118. Costanzo-Nordin MR, O'Connell JB, Subramanian R. Myocarditis confirmed by biopsy presenting as acute myocardial infarction. *Br Heart J* 1985; 53:25–29.
119. Dec GW, Waldman H, Southern J, et al. Viral myocarditis mimicking acute myocardial infarction. *J Am Coll Cardiol* 1992;20:85–89.
120. Pasquini JA, Gottdiener JS, Cutler DJ, et al. Myocarditis with transient left ventricular apical dyskinesis. *Am Heart J* 1985;109:371–373.
121. Gibson DG. Value and limitations of echocardiography in the diagnosis of myocarditis. *Eur Heart J* 1987;8:85–88.
122. Pinamonti B, Alberti E, Cigalotto A, et al. Echocardiographic findings in myocarditis. *Am J Cardiol* 1988;62:285–291.
123. Dill T, Ekinci O, Hansel J, et al. Delayed contrast-enhanced magnetic resonance imaging for the detection of autoimmune myocarditis and long-term follow-up. *J Cardiovasc Magn Reson* 2005;7(2):521–523.
124. Mahrholdt H, Goedecke C, Wagner A, et al. Cardiovascular magnetic resonance assessment of human myocarditis. *Circulation* 2004;109:1250–1258.
125. Abdel-Aty H, Boyé P, Zagrosek A, et al. Diagnostic performance of cardiovascular magnetic resonance in patients with suspected acute myocarditis. *J Am Coll Cardiol* 2005;45:1815–1822.
126. Liu PP, Yan AT. Cardiovascular magnetic resonance for the diagnosis of acute myocarditis. *J Am Coll of Cardiol* 2005;45(11):1823–1825.
127. Weller GER, Lu E, Csikari MM, et al. Ultrasound imaging of acute cardiac transplant rejection with microbubbles targeted to intercellular adhesion molecule-1. *Circulation* 2003;108:218–224.
128. Miller DL, Peng L, Gordon D, et al. Histological characterization of microlesions induced by myocardial contrast echocardiography. *Echocardiography* 2005;22(1):25–34.
129. Mason JW. Techniques for right and left ventricular endomyocardial biopsy. *Am J Cardiol* 1978;41:887–892.
130. Fowles RE, Mason JW. Role of cardiac biopsy in the diagnosis and management of cardiac disease. *Prog Cardiovasc Dis* 1984;27:153–172.
131. Hauk AJ, Kearney DL, Edwards WD. Evaluation of postmortem biopsy specimens from 38 patients with lymphocytic myocarditis: implications for role of sampling error. *Mayo Clin Proc* 1989;64:1235–1245.
132. Aretz HT, Billingham ME, Edwards WD. Myocarditis, a histopathologic definition and classification. *Am J Cardiovasc Pathol* 1987;1:3–14.
133. Shanes JG, Gahli J, Billingham ME, et al. Interobserver variability in the pathological interpretation of endomyocardial biopsy results. *Circulation* 1987;75:401–405.
134. Starling RC, Van Fossen DB, Hammer DF, et al. Morbidity of endomyocardial biopsy in cardiomyopathy. *Am J Cardiol* 1991;68:133–136.
135. Deckers JW, Hare JM, Baughman KL. Complications of transvenous right ventricular endomyocardial biopsy in adult patients with cardiomyopathy: a seven year survey of 546 consecutive diagnostic procedures in a tertiary referral center. *J Am Coll Cardiol* 1992;19:43–47.
136. Sheppard R, Bedi M, Kubota T, et al. Myocardial expression of Fas and recovery of left ventricular function in patients with recent-onset cardiomyopathy. *J Am Coll Cardiol* 2005;46:1036–1042.
137. Kittleson MM, Minhas KM, Irizarry RA, et al. Gene expression in giant cell myocarditis: altered expression of immune response genes. *Intl J Cardiol* 2005;102:333–340.
138. Friman G, Ilback NG. Acute infection: metabolic responses, effect on performance, interaction with exercise, and myocarditis. *Int J Sports Med* 1998;19:S172–S182.
139. Matsumori A, Igata H, Ono K, et al. High doses of digitalis increase the myocardial production of proinflammatory cytokines and worsen myocardial injury in viral myocarditis: a possible mechanism of digitalis toxicity. *Jpn Circ J* 1999;63:934–940.
140. McCarthy RE, Boehmer JP, Hruban RH, et al. Long-term outcome of fulminant myocarditis as compared with acute (nonfulminant) myocarditis. *N Engl J Med* 2000;342:690–695.
141. Reiss N, El-Banayosy A, Posival H, et al. Management of acute fulminant myocarditis using circulatory support systems. *Artif Organs* 1995;20:964–970.
142. Martin J, Sarai K, Schindler M, et al. MEDOS HIA-VAD biventricular assist device for bridge to recovery in fulminant myocarditis. *Ann Thorac Surg* 1997;63:1145–1146.
143. Marelli D, Laks H, Amsel B, et al. Temporary mechanical support with the BVS 5000 assist device during treatment of acute myocarditis. *J Cardiol Surg* 1997;12:55–59.
144. Simon MA, Kormos RL, Murali S, et al. Myocardial recovery using ventricular assist devices. Prevalence, clinical characteristics, and outcomes. *Circulation* 2005;112(Suppl I):I32–I36.
145. Menghini VV, Savcenko V, Olson LJ, et al. Combined immunosuppression for the treatment of idiopathic giant cell myocarditis. *Mayo Clin Proc* 1999;74:1221–1226.
146. Levy NT, Olson LJ, Weyand C, et al. Histologic and cytokine response to immunosuppression in giant-cell myocarditis. *Ann Intern Med* 1998; 128:648–650.

147. Singh TP, Rabah R, Cooper LT, et al. Total lymphoid irradiation: new therapeutic option for refractory giant cell myocarditis. *J Heart Lung Transplant* 2004;23:492–495.
148. Semigran MJ, Thaik CM, Fifer MA, et al. Exercise capacity and systolic and diastolic ventricular function after recovery from acute dilated cardiomyopathy. *J Am Coll Cardiol* 1994;24:462–470.
149. Philips SD, Warnes CA. Peripartum cardiomyopathy: current therapeutic perspectives. *Curr Treat Options Cardiovasc Med* 2004;6:481–488.
150. Kleinert S, Weintraub RG, Wilkinson JL, et al. Myocarditis in children with dilated cardiomyopathy: incidence and outcome after dual therapy immunosuppression. *J Heart Lung Transplant* 1997;16:1248–1254.
151. Lee KJ, McCrindle BW, Bohn DJ, et al. Clinical outcomes of acute myocarditis in childhood. *Heart* 1999;82:226–233.
152. Zales VR, Wright KL. Endocarditis, pericarditis, and myocarditis. *Pediatr Ann* 1997;26:116–121.
153. Evans RW, Williams GE, Baron HM, et al. The economic implications of noninvasive molecular testing for cardiac allograft rejection. *Am J Transplant* 2005; 5(6):1553–1558.

CHAPTER 89 ■ NONISCHEMIC CARDIOMYOPATHIES

CARMELA D. TAN, NORMAN B. RATLIFF, JAMES B. YOUNG, AND E. RENE RODRIGUEZ

OVERVIEW

Cardiomyopathies are defined by the World Health Organization as diseases of the myocardium associated with cardiac dysfunction. They are classified to reflect the recent insight gained into the pathogenesis of the heart muscle disorders. Cardiomyopathies are categorized into dilated, restrictive, hypertrophic, and unclassified based on the predominant pathophysiologic characteristics. Figure 89.1 shows that there is predominant remodeling of the left ventricle that distinguishes these categories. A new category has been added to include right ventricular abnormalities. The disorders that are associated with systemic or certain cardiac diseases are called *specific heart muscle diseases* and include ischemic cardiomyopathy, valvular, hypertensive, inflammatory, metabolic, peripartal, general systemic disease, muscular dystrophies, neuromuscular disorders, and toxic and hypersensitivity reactions. The unclassified cardiomyopathy category includes disorders such as fibroelastosis, noncompacted myocardium, and systolic dysfunction with minimal dilation. These diseases either have features that overlap the other classifications or do not readily fit any category. The identification of the etiology of any patient who presents with cardiomyopathy is very important, because specific treatment may reverse cardiac dysfunction. Endomyocardial biopsy is useful to diagnose specific diseases, as part of a clinical trial, to differentiate between restrictive and constrictive disorders, and to monitor anthracycline toxicity. Routine biopsies for idiopathic dilated cardiomyopathies (DCM) are helpful to establish specific diagnosis. Future directions in the diagnosis and management of cardiomyopathies include elucidating genetic and molecular mechanisms of their pathogenesis and the role of these mechanisms in heart failure.

HISTORICAL PERSPECTIVE

In 1891, one of the earliest descriptions of heart muscle diseases appeared (1). Unfortunately, little more about these "obscure disorders" was gleaned in the six decades that followed. In 1957, Brigden highlighted the ignorance and confusion that existed regarding "noncoronary cardiomyopathies," their terminology, and clinicians' reluctance to diagnose them (2). Since then, medical science has amassed considerable insight regarding the pathophysiology and treatment of these prevalent disorders. Although remarkable progress has been made, there is considerable need for further investigation.

To understand more fully the current nomenclature relating to myocardial failure, it is helpful to review the original working terminology of heart muscle disorders. In 1980, the World Health Organization and International Society and Federation of Cardiology task force met in Paris to clarify this area. They defined the *cardiomyopathies* as "heart muscle diseases of unknown cause" and divided them into three broad classifications based on characteristic anatomic findings of the heart: dilation, hypertrophy, and restriction (3). A fourth group, "unclassified cardiomyopathies," was also listed to include cases that did not easily fit into one of the other three general categories. Unclassified cardiomyopathies were sometimes referred to as *latent cardiomyopathies*. Completely separate from the cardiomyopathies were specific heart muscle diseases, characterized

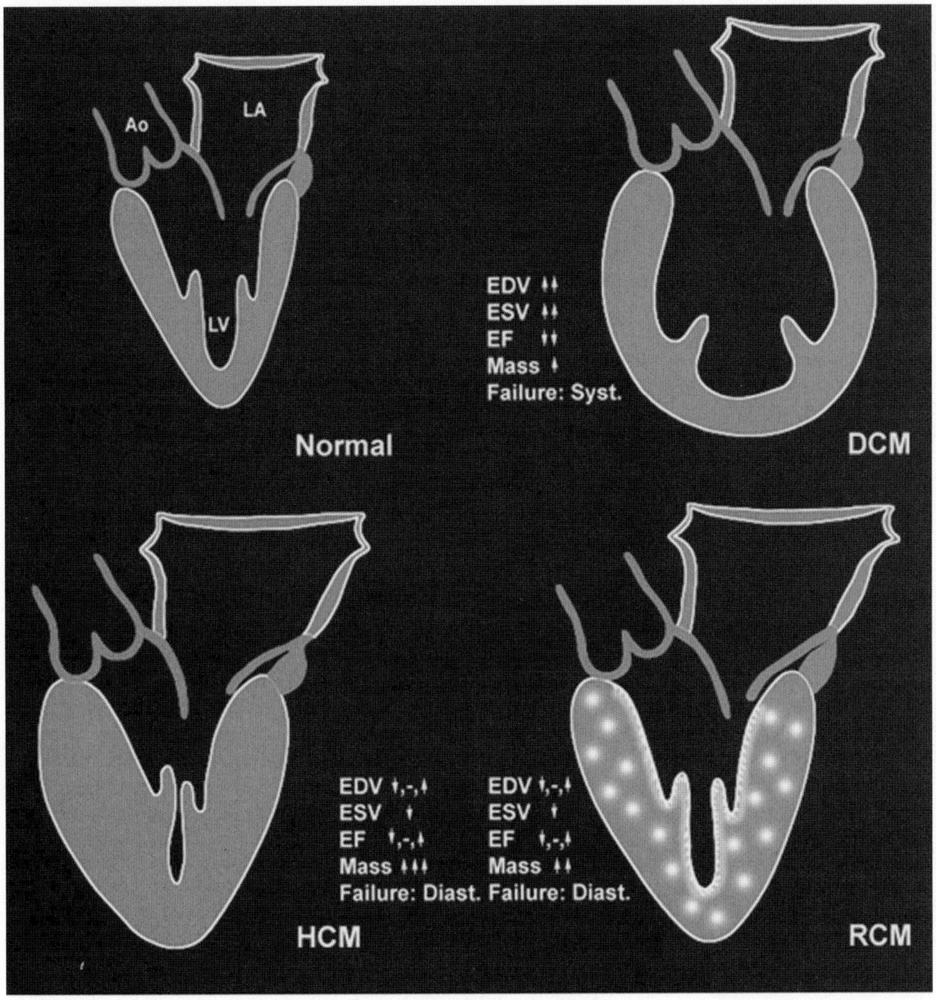

FIGURE 89.1. Morphologic features of the main types of cardiomyopathies. The normal geometry of the LV is shown. In comparison, there is enlargement and dilatation of the LV in DCM. In HCM, there is marked thickening of the LV wall, often asymmetric, with the septum being even thicker than the free wall of the LV. In restrictive cardiomyopathy (RCM), the ventricular wall may be normal, hypertrophic, or slightly dilated, but the main feature is that the restriction to diastolic compliance of the ventricle is intrinsic to the ventricle. This occurs by involvement of the endocardium or more commonly by infiltration of the interstitial space with excess collagen, amyloid, or granulomata and their ensuing fibrosis. *Abbreviations:* EDV, end-diastolic volume; ESV, end-systolic volume; EF, ejection fraction; Mass, ventricular mass; Failure, mode of failure, systolic versus diastolic.

as diseases of known cause or associated with specific disorders of other systems. They were further divided into infective, metabolic, general system diseases, heredofamilial, hypersensitivity, and toxic reactions categories. Myocardial dysfunction as a result of systemic or pulmonary hypertension, coronary artery disease, valvular heart disease, or congenital anomalies was excluded.

Etymologically, *cardiomyopathy* refers to a disease that arises from the heart itself (4). When clinical heart failure syndromes are diagnosed, it is the functional integrity of the circulatory network—including the heart—that is important for characterization of heart failure. Obviously, all cardiomyopathies have some etiologic factor. Many times, the specific reason for the cardiac malfunction and subsequent remodeling cannot be precisely characterized. The term *idiopathic* is used to describe this clinical situation. It is not a specific disease entity, but likely represents a wide spectrum of difficulties and is a term that largely reflects our ignorance regarding the etiology of heart failure in many given instances. As more became known about the individual disorders, it was apparent that new definitions and classifications were needed, and in 1996, The World Health Organizations released a revised categorization (5) (Table 89.1). Cardiomyopathies were generally more simply defined as diseases of the myocardium associated with cardiac dysfunction. As in the previous scheme, dilated, hypertrophic, restrictive, and unclassified divisions remained. However, arrhythmogenic right ventricular cardiomyopathy (ARVC) was added. Further, specific heart muscle diseases were referred to as specific cardiomyopathies that included myocardial dysfunction associated with distinct cardiac or systemic disorders.

DILATED CARDIOMYOPATHY

DCM is characterized by ventricular remodeling that produces chamber dilation, with normal or decreased wall thickness, and diminution in systolic function (Fig. 89.2). The impairment of systolic function can involve the left, right, or both ventricles, with the ejection fraction traditionally being defined as less than 40% (6). Although the total mass of the heart is increased, the ratio of left ventricular (LV) volume to ventricular wall thickness is much greater than for patients with hypertrophic cardiomyopathy (HCM) or diastolic dysfunction owing to hypertensive heart disease (7). This eccentric hypertrophy provides a unifying concept for many different disease processes, ultimately resulting in dilation of the heart. It is important to note that remodeling of this sort is caused by diseases that are, for the most part, distinct from those causing hypertrophic and restrictive cardiomyopathy, problems that generally do not result in chamber dilation. Myocardial remodeling is associated with altered hemodynamics characterized by diminished ejection fraction, reduced stroke volume, increased chamber volumes, and, therefore, increased chamber pressures. This triggers the multiple neurohormonal aberrations that are characteristic of the heart failure milieu.

Often, if the toxic or injurious agent can be identified and removed, further detrimental chamber remodeling can be

TABLE 89.1

WORLD HEALTH ORGANIZATION CLASSIFICATION OF CARDIOMYOPATHIES

DILATED
- Alcohol/toxic
- Certain specific cardiomyopathies
- Familial/genetic
- Idiopathic
- Viral and/or immune

HYPERTROPHIC

RESTRICTIVE
- Certain specific cardiomyopathies
- Endomyocardial and Löeffler endocardial fibrosis
- Idiopathic myocardial fibrosis

RIGHT VENTRICULAR
- Arrhythmogenic
- Uhl anomaly

UNCLASSIFIED
- Fibroelastosis
- Mitochondrial myopathies
- Noncompacted myocardium
- Systolic dysfunction with minimal dilatation

SPECIFIC
- General systemic disease
- Hypertensive
- Inflammatory or infectious
- Ischemic
- Metabolic
- Muscular dystrophies
- Neuromuscular disorders
- Peripartal
- Sensitivity and toxic reactions
- Valvular

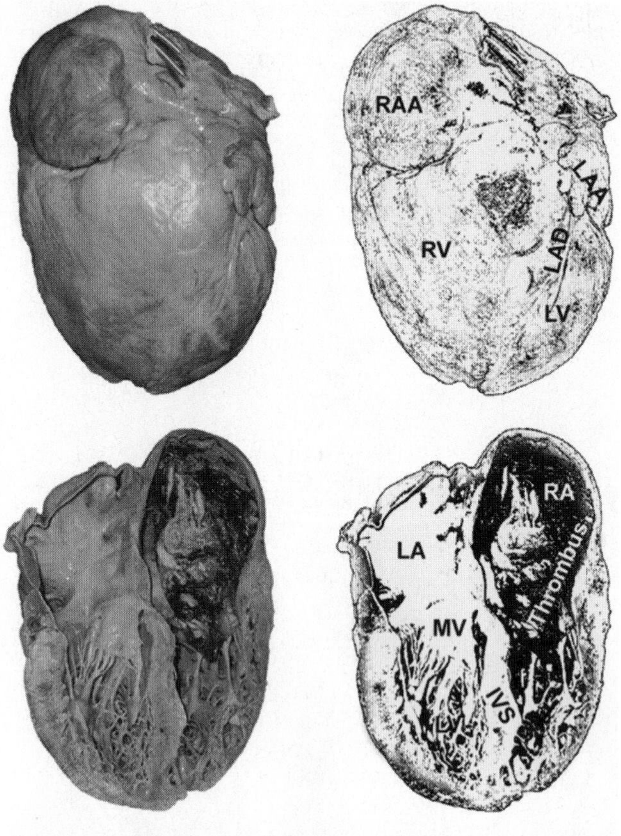

FIGURE 89.2. Dilated cardiomyopathy. There is marked global enlargement of the heart. In this case, there is enlargement of the left- and right-sided cavities as the result of severe LV failure. There is also a thrombus in the right atrium. *Abbreviations:* IVS, interventricular septum; LA, left atrium; LAA, left atrial appendage; LAD, left anterior descending coronary artery; LV, left ventricle; MV, mitral valve; RA, right atrium; RAA, right atrial appendage; RV, right ventricle.

blocked and systolic function returned to a more normal state. However, DCMs generally pass through an early and late evolutionary period. The stages parallel pathophysiologic events triggered by whatever myocardial insult initiated the heart failure process in the first place. At some point, injury produces myocyte and myocardial dysfunction that antedates clinically apparent disease. As progression occurs and decompensation develops, symptoms begin to appear that are characteristic of heart failure in general. Disease-specific cardiac and extracardiac signs and symptoms may provide insight to the etiology of the heart failure and cardiomyopathy. If the process is not interdicted, later stages will appear and manifest with profound eccentric hypertrophy and, ultimately, marked reduction in systemic flows accompanying elevation of intracardiac pressures.

DCM was previously referred to as *congestive cardiomyopathy*; however, this term is no longer applied because congestion is not consistently present, particularly in the milder and earlier stages or after therapy. DCM is the most common of the cardiomyopathies, comprising more than 90% of all cases that are referred to specialized centers (8), and represents the end result of more than 50 distinct diseases (9,10). When diagnosing DCM, it is important to review the major etiologic and pathophysiologic classes responsible for this disorder (see Table 89.1). By and large, DCMs can be familial or genetic in origin; secondary to infection or inflammation, toxic substance exposure, metabolic derangements; or idiopathic.

Some progress has been made in characterizing the molecular genetics of DCM (11). Perhaps as many as 20% of DCM cases are inherited or familial, with a significant percentage of the remaining being acquired as suggested. Inherited forms of DCM may have autosomal-dominant, autosomal-recessive, X-linked, or mitochondrial transmission. Mutations have been found in gene encoding for proteins that fall in four general classes according to their function in the cardiac myocyte: (a) force generation and propagation (sarcomere components, M-band components, Z-disc components, cytoskeletal components); (b) energy production and regulation (mitochondrial mutations, glycogen metabolism); (c) calcium cycling; and (d) transcriptional regulators (Nkx2.5, NFAT3, GATA4, HDACs, MEF2, Hop, PPARs) (12).

Idiopathic Dilated Cardiomyopathy

Background and Prevalence

Idiopathic DCM is a primary global myocardial disorder of unknown cause. Because it is the pathophysiologic model for other specific DCMs, this section focuses on the idiopathic type, with distinguishing characteristics of other specific disorders discussed subsequently. Idiopathic DCM alone accounts for 36 cases per 100,000 population, 10,000 deaths in the United States per year, and approximately 25% of all cases of cardiomyopathy.

Pathology

As shown in Figure 89.1, there are anatomic differences in the cardiomyopathies, emphasizing that DCM has marked enlargement of LV end-diastolic and end-systolic volumes, usually with profound reduction of the ejection fraction. This is in contrast to restrictive and hypertrophic cardiomyopathies, which have more normal end-diastolic volumes and, sometimes, supernormal ejection fractions. In DCM, the mitral and tricuspid annuli are frequently enlarged from ventricular dilation, with resultant valvular regurgitation. By definition, idiopathic DCM is not caused by coronary artery disease, and therefore the coronary arterial tree is usually normal. It is possible to have some plaque formation; however, the degree of systolic impairment is out of proportion to atherosclerotic involvement. The histology is usually nonspecific, but certain features are present. Under the light microscope, the myocytes are commonly quite hypertrophied. The nuclei may be very large with bizarre shapes. The areas of interstitial fibrosis are frequently underappreciated. Occasionally, small clusters of lymphocytes in the interstitium or in perivascular location can be present. By electron microscopy, the mitochondria may be abnormal, the T tubules dilated, and lipid vacuoles present.

Clinical Profile and Management

Chapters 86 and 87 discuss in detail the treatment of acute and chronic heart failure. Management options include supportive therapy (diet, sodium, toxin and fluid restriction, exercise), medications (diuretics, digoxin, angiotensin-converting enzyme [ACE] inhibitors, angiotensin II receptor blockers, inotropes, anticoagulants, antiarrhythmics, and β-blockers), ventricular assist devices, and novel surgical procedures (cardiomyoplasty, mitral and tricuspid valve repair, partial left ventriculectomy, and cardiac transplantation).

HYPERTROPHIC CARDIOMYOPATHY

Background and Prevalence

HCM is addressed in detail in Chapter 29. Since the modern description by Teare in 1958 (13), HCM has been known by a confusing array of names that largely reflect its clinical heterogeneity, relatively uncommon occurrence in cardiologic practice, and the skewed experience of early investigators. This problem in nomenclature has been an obstacle to the general recognition of the disease within the medical and nonmedical communities. *Hypertrophic cardiomyopathy* (or *HCM*) is now widely accepted as the preferred term (14) because it describes the overall disease spectrum without introducing misleading inferences that LV outflow tract obstruction is an invariable feature of the disease, such as is the case with hypertrophic obstructive cardiomyopathy, muscular subaortic stenosis, or idiopathic hypertrophic subaortic stenosis. Indeed, most patients with HCM do not demonstrate outflow obstruction under resting (basal) conditions, although many may develop dynamic subaortic gradients of varying magnitude with provocative maneuvers or agents (14). The contemporary definition of HCM focuses on the fact that this disorder is characterized by disproportionate and remarkable left, and sometimes right, ventricular hypertrophy (14,15). Typically, the septum is more involved than the free LV wall, although on occasion the hypertrophy can be completely concentric in nature (Fig. 89.3). HCM, which may develop at any age, is associated with marked LV volume reduction, and systolic LV outflow tract gradients are common. Up to 70% of cases have a familial pattern of occurrence, with autosomal-dominant inheritance. Clinically, the diagnosis of HCM is most reliably made by two-dimensional echocardiography showing left ventricular

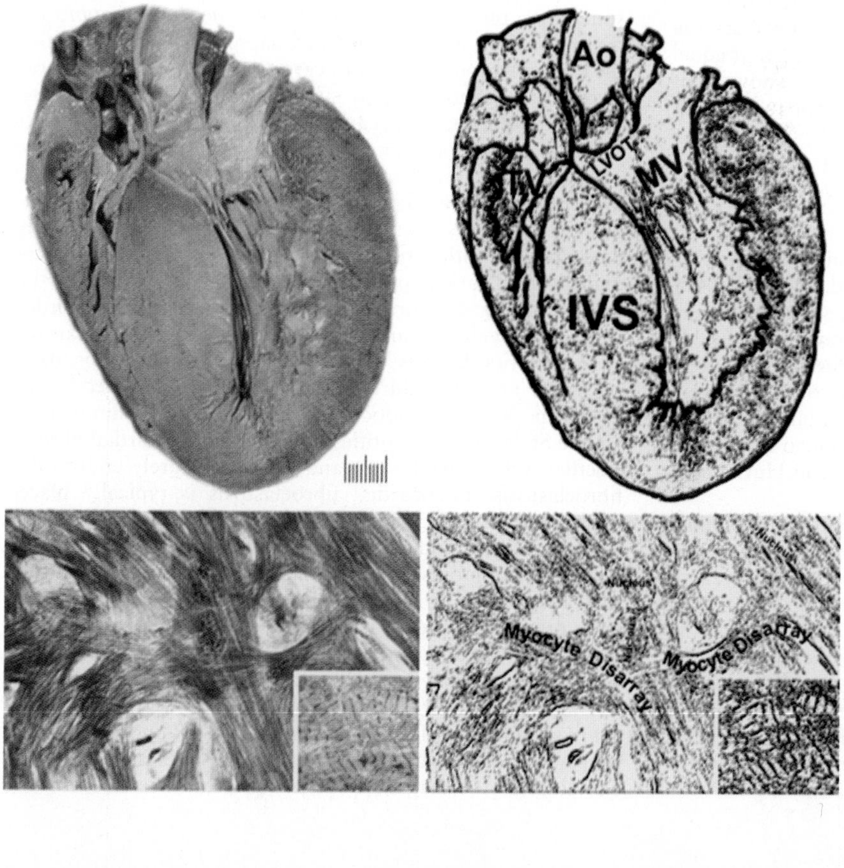

FIGURE 89.3. Hypertrophic cardiomyopathy. The gross image shows a coronal section of a heart with marked asymmetric septal hypertrophy. The interventricular septum is 2.5 times thicker than the LV free wall. The anterior leaflet of the mitral valve is in very close apposition to the LV outflow tract. The bottom panel is a light micrograph showing marked myocyte disarray, where the individual myocytes no longer have a parallel orientation with respect to each other. Instead, they have a "storiform" array of the myofibrils. The inset shows that the myofibrils themselves and the sarcomeres are disarrayed when examined by transmission electron microscopy. *Abbreviations:* Ao, aorta; IVS, interventricular septum; LVOT, left ventricular outflow tract; MV, mitral valve.

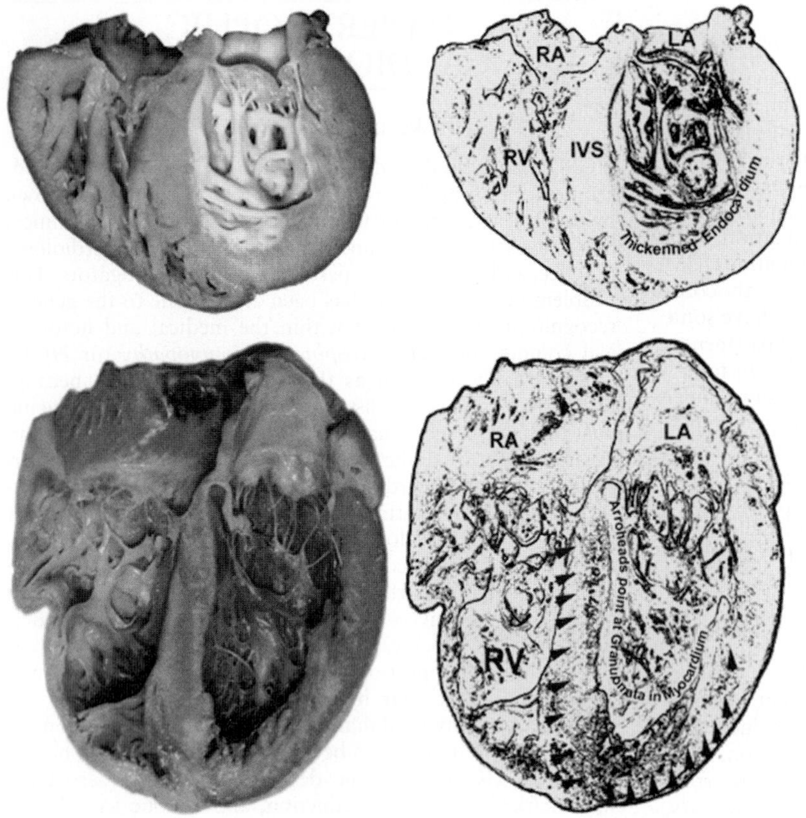

FIGURE 89.4. Restrictive/infiltrative cardiomyopathy. The gross image on top shows a heart with marked endocardial fibroelastosis which prevents diastolic compliance of the left ventricle. Note the markedly thick (*white*) endocardium. The heart in the lower part of the panel is a heart with patchy pale/white areas involving the interventricular septum from the base to the apex and continuing into the free wall of the left ventricle owing to infiltration by noncaseating granulomata in a case of sarcoidosis. *Abbreviations:* IVS, interventricular septum; LA, left atrium; RA, right atrium; RV, right ventricle.

hypertrophy (LVH) with asymmetric distribution. This LVH is associated with a nondilated and hyperdynamic chamber, which often shows systolic LV cavity obliteration in the absence of another cardiac or systemic disease such as hypertension or aortic stenosis. Although the usual clinical diagnostic criteria for HCM is a maximal LV wall thickness greater than or equal to 15 mm, genotype–phenotype correlations have shown that virtually any wall thickness is compatible with the presence of a HCM mutant gene (14,15).

Pathology

The morphologic hallmark of HCM is asymmetric septal hypertrophy (see Figure 89.3) with myocyte and myofibril disarray (16). Some reports have emphasized that variable degrees of myocyte ultrastructural, myofibrillar, and muscle bundle disorganization can be detected, often with substantial degrees of interstitial fibrosis (16). Mutations in sarcomeric protein encoding genes have been described in HCM, but other conditions can mimic the phenotype such as Noonan syndrome, Friedreich ataxia, Fabry disease, and Hunter and Hurler syndromes.

Recently, a proposal for screening patients with familial HCM suggests the use of echocardiography from the age of 12 until full growth and maturation is achieved (18–21 years). If echocardiographic abnormalities are not demonstrated, then a strong reassurance to the family can be made regarding the absence of cardiomyopathy (17). The medical therapy of HCM is discussed in Chapter 29. Other modalities of therapy for patients with outflow tract obstruction include ethanol ablation (via catheterization) and surgical resection of the outflow tract hypertrophied muscle (myectomy). This last procedure is better in terms of outcome (18).

RESTRICTIVE CARDIOMYOPATHY

The restrictive or infiltrative cardiomyopathies (Fig. 89.4), sometimes referred to as *nondilated, nonhypertrophic cardiomyopathies,* are described in Chapter 27. Generally, this is the least common of the major cardiomyopathies and is characterized by a normal or only slightly enlarged heart, decreased diastolic volumes, and, early in the disease, normal systolic function (19). The main pathologic disorder is one of impaired diastolic functioning, resulting from decreased ventricular compliance and filling. This dysfunction may result from a process that involves, primarily, the endocardium, myocardium, or both. The most commonly encountered myocardial disorder is amyloid heart disease (Fig. 89.5) and other specific myocardial forms include metabolic storage disorders such as Fabry disease and hemochromatosis, sarcoid heart disease, radiation fibrosis, and various tumor infiltrations, many of which are also addressed in the section on specific cardiomyopathies. The endocardial disorders, less common in the United States, include entities such as endomyocardial fibrosis, Löeffler endocardial fibrosis and, even more rarely, endocardial fibroelastosis. Endocardial fibroelastosis is typically placed in the unclassified cardiomyopathy category. Restrictive cardiomyopathy should be considered when patients present with signs and symptoms of myocardial failure but normal cardiac size. Frequently, right-sided findings of increased jugular venous pressure, ascites, and peripheral edema predominate, although left-sided failure does occur. The differential diagnosis includes constrictive pericarditis, which is a more readily treatable condition. Echocardiography and right heart catheterization may help to differentiate these disorders. Endomyocardial biopsy should also be considered if other historical and physical clues to the diagnosis are not present. The treatment of

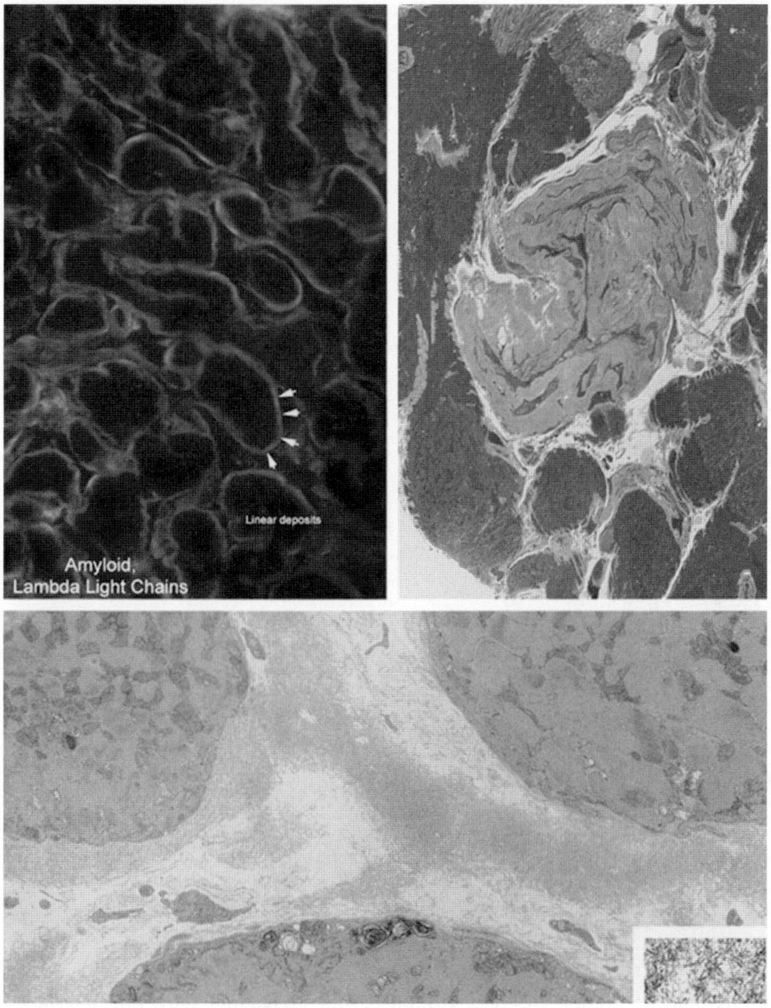

FIGURE 89.5. Amyloidosis of the heart. The left upper panel shows a thioflavin-S stain showing thick, linear, ring-like deposits of amyloid (*white arrows*) surrounding individual myocytes. In this particular example, the protein responsible for the formation of these amyloid deposits is the λ light chain. The image on the upper right side shows a "nodular deposit" of amyloid. The bottom image shows typical electron microscopic view of perimyocytic deposits of 10-nm thick amyloid fibrils in the interstitium of the heart. The lower inset shows a close up of the amyloid fibrils.

restrictive cardiomyopathy is also reviewed in Chapter 27 and generally remains quite unsatisfactory.

Endomyocardial Fibrosis

Endomyocardial fibrosis, also known as *tropical eosinophilic endomyocardial fibrosis,* is common in South and Central America and tropical and subtropical Africa. Surprisingly, it accounts for 15% to 25% of the cardiac deaths in equatorial Africa (20). Endomyocardial fibrosis is characterized by thickening and scarring of the endocardium, which can be so extensive that the ventricular cavity is obliterated. Thrombi may overlie these lesions, increasing the risk of thromboembolism. Frequently, the subendocardial myocardium is also affected. In 50% of cases, the left and the right ventricles are involved, whereas another 40% of cases have lesions isolated to the left ventricle. The mitral and tricuspid valves may become fibrotic as well, leading to valvular regurgitation. Many believe that this disease is a form of, if not the same as, Löeffler endocardial fibrosis, perhaps at a different stage (20,21). Although the overall prognosis is poor, palliative treatment with surgical endocardial resection and valvular repair/replacement may alleviate some symptoms.

Löeffler Endocardial Fibrosis

Löeffler endocardial fibrosis is also associated with eosinophilia, giving it its other names, *eosinophilic cardiomyopathy* and *nontropical eosinophilic endomyocardial fibrosis*. The severity of cardiac dysfunction seems to parallel the degree and duration of the eosinophilia, leading to the belief that the eosinophil itself is responsible for the dysfunction. The contents of the intracytoplasmic granules of the eosinophils can cause direct myocardial necrosis. It has also been observed that the eosinophils bind immunoglobulin G and increase peroxidase, which can have further direct toxic effects. The cardiac manifestations of this eosinophilic disorder are similar, if not identical to, those produced by eosinophilic leukemia and the eosinophilia–myalgia syndrome, which has been associated with tryptophan. Treatment with corticosteroids and cytotoxic agents (hydroxyurea) can improve symptoms and survival (22).

RIGHT VENTRICULAR CARDIOMYOPATHY—ARRHYTHMOGENIC RIGHT VENTRICULAR CARDIOMYOPATHY/DYSPLASIA

Background and Prevalence

ARVC, also commonly known as *arrhythmogenic right ventricular dysplasia* (ARVD), is a rare disorder that occurs in adolescence and young adulthood. It has a male : female ratio of approximately 2 to 3 : 1 (23). The true incidence of ARVC

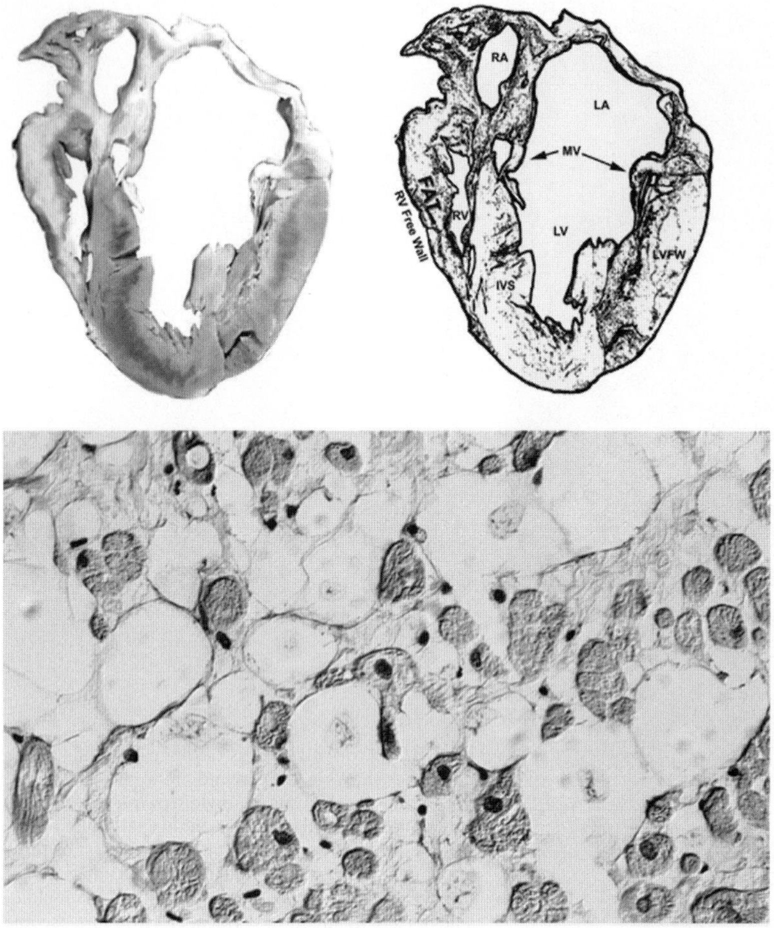

FIGURE 89.6. Arrhythmogenic right ventricular cardiomyopathy/dysplasia (ARVC/D). In this gross specimen, the right ventricular free wall has been replaced by adipose tissue, which is noticeable from the atrioventricular groove, just below the right atrium, all the way to the junction of the right ventricular free wall to the interventricular septum. The bottom panel shows a light micrograph of the adipose tissue infiltration in the right ventricular wall. *Abbreviations:* LA, left atrium; LV, left ventricle; MV, mitral valve; RA, right atrium.

remains unknown, partly because of difficulties with its diagnosis, as described below.

Pathology

The abnormalities of ARVC affect primarily the right ventricle, although in rare instances, the left ventricle is involved (24,25). Grossly, the ventricle is mildly dilated and thinned (Fig. 89.6). The characteristic feature is the segmental, progressive, noninflammatory loss of myocytes and their replacement by adipose tissue and fibrosis (26). This is in contrast to the nonfibrotic adipose tissue infiltration that normally occurs in the right ventricle and increases as a function of age (27). In ARVC/D, the fibroadipose infiltration is transmural in nature and can be confirmed either at autopsy or with surgical biopsy. Endomyocardial biopsies are sometimes helpful, but have limitations (28). Despite this, finding extensive fibrofatty replacement of myocytes in the right ventricle is concerning. But when interpreted by an experienced team including cardiologists, pathologists, and radiologists, the diagnosis of ARVD can be accurately established (29). Cinemagnetic resonance imaging has the potential to aid diagnosis by being able to differentiate normal myocardium from adipose tissue, assess morphologic alterations, and detect areas of regional and global ventricular dysfunction (30). In fact, a good correlation between imaging and tissue characterization of ARVD has been demonstrated (31).

Genetic studies from several sources have identified at least 7 loci (ARVD1-ARVD7) by linkage analysis. Furthermore, mutations in three desmosomal proteins (desmoplakin, plakoglobin with specific phenotype or Naxos disease [palm plantar keratoderma and wooly hair], and plakophilin) (32,33) have been associated with ARVC. Also, mutations in the cardiac ryanodine receptor (hRYR2), are associated with effort-induced polymorphic ventricular tachycardia and juvenile sudden death (ARVD2) (33). Last, mutations in the transforming growth factor-$\beta 3$ have been associated with an autosomal dominant inheritance (ARVD1).

Clinical Profile and Management

Because of the difficulties and risks of obtaining tissue to confirm the diagnosis of ARVC, as well as inaccuracies in assessing right ventricular structure and function with many of the noninvasive tests, a task force from the European Society of Cardiology and the International Society and Federation of Cardiology met and released criteria to assist in this process. The diagnosis can be made by meeting any of the following: two major criteria, one major plus two minor, or four minor criteria (Table 89.2) (34). A recent report of electrocardiographic (ECG) changes evaluated over time shows usefulness of the ECG in assessing progression of ARVC/D (35).

To assess the natural history of ARVC/D, a recent study of 130 patients showed a cardiovascular mortality of 16% (n = 24). Risk stratification showed that the most ominous risk factors presence of right or left ventricular dysfunction and ventricular tachycardia. However, when cause of death in these 24 patients was analyzed, 59% of the patients died of heart failure and 29% of sudden death (36).

UHL Anomaly

This entity shows marked thinning of the right ventricular wall with virtual apposition of the epicardium to the endocardium

TABLE 89.2

CRITERIA FOR DIAGNOSIS OF ARVD/C

FAMILY HISTORY
Major
Familial disease confirmed at necropsy or surgery.
Minor
Family history of premature sudden death (<35 years of age) owing to suspected ARVD/C.
Family history (clinical diagnosis based on present criteria).
ECG DEPOLARIZATION/CONDUCTION ABNORMALITIES
Major
Epsilon waves or localized prolongation (>110 ms) of QRS complex in right precordial leads (V_1–V_3).
Minor
Late potentials on signal-averaged ECG.
ECG REPOLARIZATION ABNORMALITIES
Minor
Inverted T waves in right precordial leads (V_2 and V_3) in people >12 years of age and in absence of right bundle branch block.
ARRHYTHMIAS
Minor
Sustained or nonsustained left bundle branch block–type ventricular tachycardia documented on ECG or Holter monitoring or during exercise testing.
Frequent ventricular extrasystoles (>1,000/24 hours on Holter monitoring).
GLOBAL OR REGIONAL DYSFUNCTION AND STRUCTURAL ALTERATIONS[a]
Major
Severe dilatation and reduction of RV ejection fraction with no or mild LV involvement.
Localized RV aneurysms (akinetic or dyskinetic areas with diastolic bulgings). Severe segmental dilatation of RV.
Minor
Mild global RV dilatation or ejection fraction reduction with normal LV.
Mild segmental dilatation of RV.
Regional RV hypokinesia.
TISSUE CHARACTERISTICS OF WALLS
Major
Fibrofatty replacement of myocardium on endomyocardial biopsy.

[a]Detected by echocardiography, angiography, magnetic resonance imaging, or radionuclide scintigraphy.
Abbreviations: ARVD/C, arrhythmogenic right ventricular dysplasia/cardiomyopathy; ECG, electrocardiograph; LV, left ventricular; RV, right ventricular.

without myocardium in between (37). This anomaly has been compared to ARVC/D. However, it is distinct in that it occurs in infancy and early childhood, is incessant, and results in complete destruction of the right ventricle. Furthermore, it does not show fatty infiltration of the wall (38).

UNCLASSIFIED CARDIOMYOPATHIES

Endocardial Fibroelastosis

Endocardial fibroelastosis is an abnormal thickening of the endocardium of the left ventricle and aortic and mitral valves. It occurs in infancy and early childhood. The fibrosis leads to decreased compliance of the myocardium and diastolic dysfunction. Typically, a DCM occurs frequently with significant mitral regurgitation, but a restrictive cardiomyopathy (see Fig. 89.4) can also occur. A genetic defect has not been identified; autosomal-recessive, autosomal-dominant, and X-linked recessive patterns of inheritance have been reported. The X-linked forms demonstrate mitochondrial abnormalities that are similar to those of Barth syndrome. Endocardial fibroelastosis has also been associated with tissue carnitine deficiency (39), and there is evidence that it may be related to a defect in the plasma membrane carnitine transporter (40). The ECG frequently shows features of LVH, with occasional pseudoinfarction patterns and atrioventricular block. The echocardiogram is remarkable for dense echoes along the LV endocardium. Pathologic examination shows a uniform thickening of the encodardium of the left ventricle, which is composed of a mixture of collagen and elastic fibers.

Noncompacted Myocardium

Left ventricular noncompaction (LVNC) is a rare form of cardiomyopathy believed to be a result of an arrest in cardiac

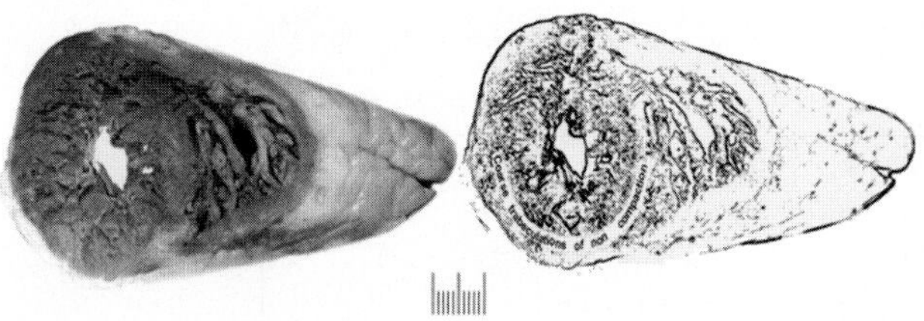

FIGURE 89.7. Left ventricular noncompaction. Note the coarse trabeculations present throughout the LV wall. These trabeculations closely resemble the trabeculation pattern of the right ventricle.

development (Fig. 89.7). It affects adults and children. In adults, it is often limited to patients without associated cardiac defects, and is thus called *isolated LVNC*. In children, it is associated with other heart defects in up to 14% of patients. In children, there are two phenotypes: (a) progressive systolic dysfunction that results in early death; and (b) an undulating type, with periods of deterioration and recovery that allow survival into adulthood. Other terms for persistent noncompacted myocardium include *spongy myocardium* and *persistence of myocardial sinusoids*; however, the *intramyocardial vessels* that communicate with the cardiac chambers are invaginations rather than sinusoids (41,42). There are associations of LVNC with mutation in the gene G4.5, which encodes tafazzin. This gene has also been associated with other myopathies and with Barth syndrome (43,44).

Mitochondrial Cardiomyopathy

Mitochondrial cardiomyopathy is defined as ventricular dysfunction caused by mitochondrial DNA mutations, which are maternally inherited. These mutations are not limited to the heart mitochondria and may also be demonstrated throughout the liver, kidney, pancreas, central nervous system, skeletal muscles, and thyroid gland. The mitochondria are typically irregular, vary in size, and have a very abnormal cristae structure (Fig. 89.8). The myocardial changes can mimic HCM. Mitochondrial cardiomyopathy may also present with signs, symptoms, and features of DCM. Progressive hypertrophy and dilation of the heart with cardiac dysrhythmias are characteristics of these mitochondrial abnormalities. DNA defects frequently result in cytochrome c oxidase deficiency and abnormalities in the mitochondrial respiratory chain. Research is active in identifying these mutations by endomyocardial biopsy (45). Several systemic diseases are associated with mitochondrial dysfunction. For example, the MELAS syndrome (*m*itochondrial *e*ncephalopathy, *l*actic *a*cidosis, and *s*troke-like episodes) is complicated by cardiomyopathy and generalized microangiopathic occlusive disease (46). The wide spectrum of mitochondrial diseases is not limited to the heart; in fact, they are commonly accompanied by manifestations in other organ systems (47,48).

SPECIFIC CARDIOMYOPATHIES

Ischemic

Ischemic cardiomyopathy, defined as an ejection fraction of less than 40%, with multifocal wall motion abnormalities owing to coronary artery diseases, is the most common DCM in the United States (Fig. 89.9). It carries with it significant disability and mortality. In the past, a 5-year survival rate of only approximately 40% has been reported (49). Adequate perfusion

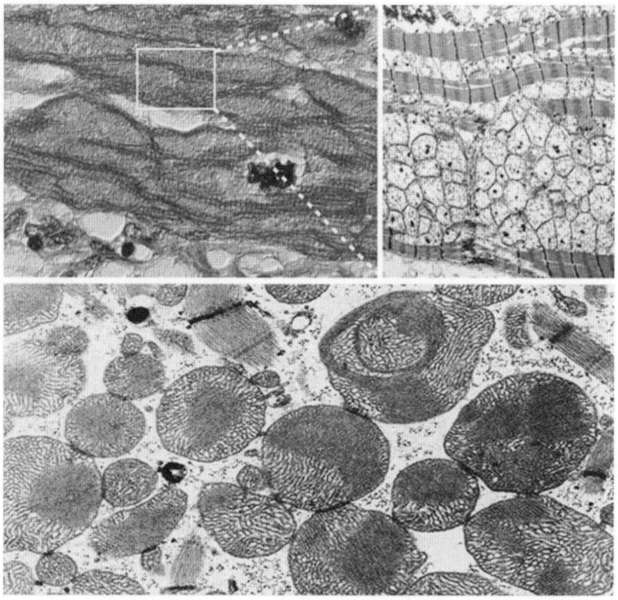

FIGURE 89.8. Mitochondrial cardiomyopathy. The top left image is a light micrograph of a cardiac myocyte in which the myofibrils (striations) are separated by granular material present throughout the sarcoplasm. The top right image is an electron micrograph from an area like the one shown in the white frame. Mitochondria are markedly increased in number and spreading apart the contractile myofibrils. The lower panel shows another case in which the mitochondria are pleomorphic in size and shape with very abnormal cristae. Some of them have "fingerprint" patterns and others show darker, electron-dense areas with paracrystalline inclusions.

of the myocardium is essential for appropriate cellular aerobic respiration, and heart failure due to ischemic cardiomyopathy is caused by at least four distinct mechanisms. Stunned and hibernating myocardial tissue are viable, with potential for improvement in functioning with better perfusion. Differentiation of ischemia, scar, and hibernating myocardial tissue is discussed in Chapters 50 and 55, and includes methods such as positron emission tomography, dobutamine and myocardial contrast echocardiography, and rest-redistribution thallium-201 scintigraphy (50). Diffuse small-vessel atherosclerosis can also produce ischemia-related malfunction of the cardiac

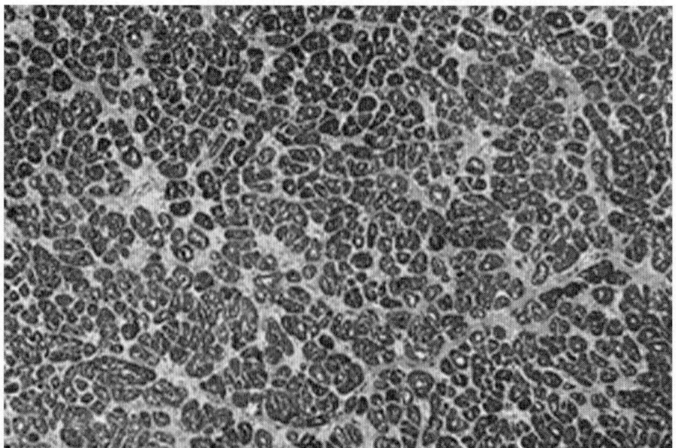

FIGURE 89.9. Chronic ischemic heart disease. This micrograph shows a cross-section of a bundle of cardiac myocytes and an increase of extracellular matrix, representing interstitial fibrosis, which surrounds and separates individual myocytes.

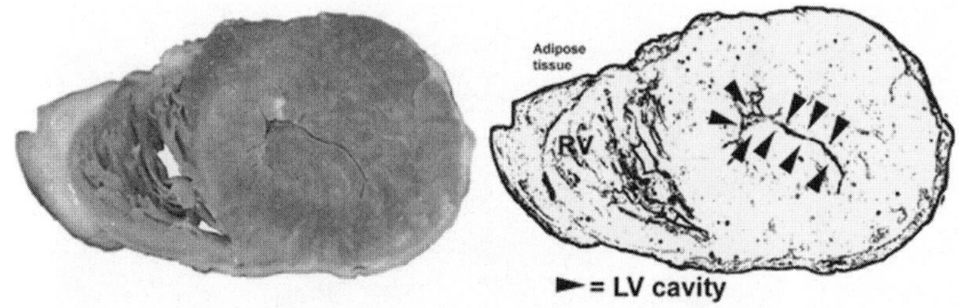

FIGURE 89.10. Marked concentric hypertrophy of the left ventricle. Notice the virtual absence of LV cavity owing to the massive hypertrophy of the wall and papillary muscles.

myocyte. Indeed, small vessel disease is involved in the pathogenesis of the cardiomyopathy of diabetes mellitus. Thus, diabetic cardiomyopathy may be due, in part, to epicardial vessel disease as well as diffuse small-vessel subendocardial atherosclerosis. Systemic lupus erythematosus and other autoimmune chronic inflammatory disease states occasionally produce similar findings.

Differentiation of ischemic cardiomyopathy from nonischemic processes is extraordinarily important. Patients with ischemic cardiomyopathy frequently, but not always, have histories of chest discomfort, myocardial infarctions, or abnormal ECGs, suggesting previous infarction. Restoring adequate perfusion to the heart is key to reversing the progression of a clinical heart failure state. Coronary angiography is key, although often lesions are seen that are not producing ischemia, and, on the other hand, diffuse small-vessel disease may not be well appreciated. Relating angiographic findings to perfusion, viability, and functional studies of the heart differentiates contributions of ischemia, scar, hibernation, and periinfarction stunning to the pathologic remodeling process of heart failure.

Valvular

Valvular cardiomyopathy is produced by valvular defects of numerous etiologies, discussed in Chapters 22 to 24. Typically, defects that produce volume-overloaded states (regurgitation) are more likely to cause cardiomyopathy than are lesions associated with pressure overload (valvular stenosis). Frequently, the issue of corrective valvular surgery in the setting of severe myocardial dysfunction is raised, with the hope of promoting myocardial recovery if the lesion is fixed. For instance, attempts at reducing mitral regurgitation have been performed in patients with severe cardiomyopathy, either as an isolated surgery or in conjunction with partial left ventriculectomy, with some symptomatic success and at least early improvement in certain cases (51,52).

Hypertensive

Hypertensive cardiomyopathy is discussed in detail in Chapter 7. Occasionally, patients with hypertensive cardiomyopathy can present with heart failure and a dilated heart. However, most patients show marked symmetric hypertrophy of the left ventricle (Fig. 89.10).

Obesity

Obesity is recognized as a specific separate disorder that can result in a cardiomyopathy. This is a condition distinct from other entities that can cause heart failure and are also associated with obesity, such as hypertension, coronary atherosclerosis, sleep apnea, and diabetes.

Inflammatory

Inflammatory cardiomyopathies are addressed specifically in Chapter 88. They are generally divided into idiopathic, autoimmune, and infectious categories (Table 89.3). Cardiomyopathies associated with systemic autoimmune disorders include the collagen-vascular disease syndromes and many of the mixed connective tissue diseases. Numerous infections are associated with DCM, including viral (enterovirus, adenovirus, cytomegalovirus, and Coxsackie virus), rickettsial, bacterial (diphtheria), mycobacterial, fungal, parasitic (toxoplasmosis, trichinosis, Chagas disease), and spirochetal (see Chapter 35). Lymphocytic myocarditis and giant cell myocarditis can readily be diagnosed by endomyocardial biopsy. It is important to remember that an accurate tissue diagnosis can support the justification of an aggressive treatment (Fig. 89.11). The one particular cardiomyopathy associated with HIV warrants further mention here because it will, unfortunately, be encountered more and more frequently in clinical practice.

TABLE 89.3

CAUSES OF INFLAMMATORY CARDIOMYOPATHY

AUTOIMMUNE
Collagen-vascular and mixed connective tissue diseases
Churg-Strauss syndrome
Systemic lupus erythematosus
Polyarteritis nodosa
Progressive systemic sclerosis
IDIOPATHIC
INFECTIOUS
Bacterial
Fungal
Parasitic
Trichinosis
Toxoplasmosis
Trypanosoma cruzi
Viral
Adenovirus
Coxsackie virus
Cytomegalovirus
Echovirus
Influenza
Human immunodeficiency virus
Parvovirus

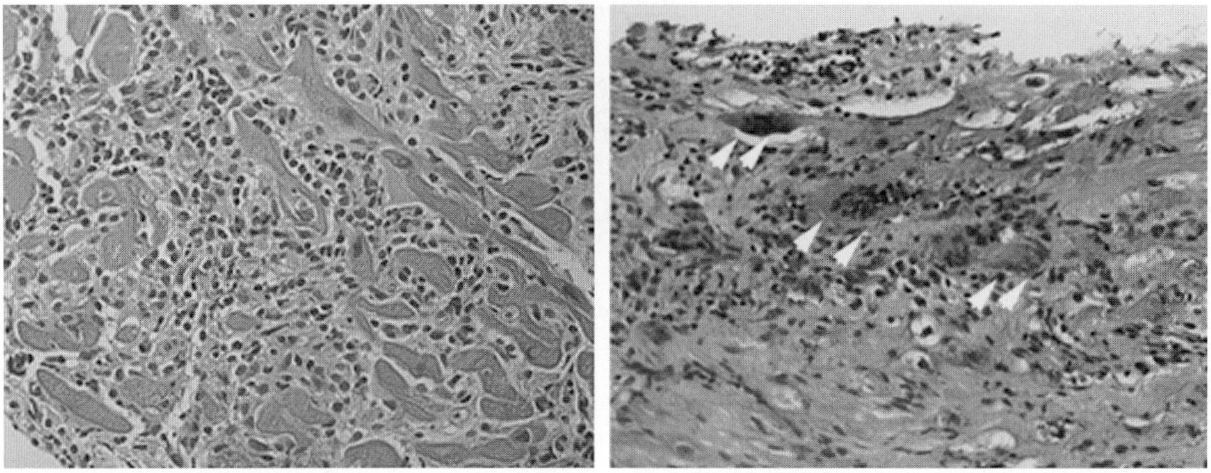

FIGURE 89.11. Myocarditis. The image on the left illustrates an aggressive case of lymphocytic myocarditis. Note the mononuclear inflammatory cells infiltrating the interstitial space of the myocardium and replacing "dropped out" myocytes. The image on the right illustrates a case of giant cell myocarditis. The giant cells (*arrows*) are present in an area of fibrosis adjacent to myocytes.

Human Immunodeficiency Virus

Background and Prevalence

The first mention of a cardiac manifestation of the acquired immunodeficiency syndrome (AIDS) occurred in 1983, when a woman with cardiac Kaposi sarcoma and heart failure was described (53). Since then, several cardiac pathologies associated with HIV infection have been identified, including pericardial diseases, valvular lesions with or without endocarditis, lymphocytic myocarditis and myocardial necrosis, neoplasms, right ventricular failure, and DCM (54,55). The actual incidence of cardiac abnormalities in HIV-infected patients remains unknown; however, it has been estimated to be approximately 50% in cases when confirmed at autopsy (56). About 20% of these had DCM, although many were not clinically apparent. The presence of a cardiomyopathy is strongly associated with low CD4 cell counts (57).

Pathophysiology

Many theories have been advanced proposing possible etiologies of HIV cardiomyopathy. The following factors may play a role: (a) underlying mononuclear cell infiltrate/myocarditis; (b) opportunistic infections, including bacterial, fungal, viral, and protozoal infections; (c) an autoimmune process; (d) the HIV virus itself, which has been shown to be present in the cardiac myocytes and in cardiac dendritic cells (58).

Many of the drugs commonly used to treat AIDS or one of its associated problems have been implicated in the cardiomyopathy, including zidovudine (AZT) and interferon.

Clinical Profile and Management

The clinical presentation of heart failure is frequently misinterpreted to be one of the other more common illnesses in HIV-positive patients. For example, shortness of breath and dyspnea with exertion immediately raise the suspicion of an opportunistic pulmonary infection. It is important to consider also the possibility of heart failure when these patients present with new complaints. Chest x-ray is insensitive, but may be helpful by demonstrating cardiomegaly or pulmonary edema. ECGs are usually nonspecific with HIV cardiomyopathy, although they could exclude other possibilities such as ischemia or infarction. The most helpful diagnostic test is an echocardiogram, which assesses ventricular size and contractility and valvular function and detects pericardial effusions.

In addition to the conventional treatment of heart failure with digoxin, diuretics, and ACE inhibitors, several other therapies have been suggested. Selenium supplementation has been documented to improve LV function in a few cases (59). If AZT or another drug is suspected of causing or contributing to the ventricular dysfunction, the risk–benefit ratio of discontinuing therapy warrants examination. Some clinicians have supported the use of immunosuppressive agents, such as corticosteroids with or without azathioprine, especially if an inflammatory or autoimmune mechanism is responsible.

Tachycardia Induced

One of the more important cardiomyopathies is that related to chronic tachyarrhythmia. If substantive ventricular dysfunction and heart failure are due to this difficulty, response to treatment can be gratifying. As electrophysiologic techniques became more sophisticated and pathophysiologic clarification of atrial tachycardias emerged, it became even more apparent that rapid heart rates alone could cause heart failure and cardiomyopathy. Restoration of systolic function, manifest by normalization of ejection fraction, has been reported for accessory pathway–reciprocating tachycardias (60,61) and atrial ventricular nodal reentry tachyarrhythmia (62,63). In children, control of incessant ventricular tachycardia has also been noted to reverse dilated myopathic ventricles (64,65).

Controlling rapid ventricular responses is, therefore, paramount in attempting to ameliorate heart failure states associated with tachycardia. Because atrial fibrillation is so common in patients with heart failure, control of the ventricular rate needs to be emphasized. Focus should first be on attempts to convert the patient, either with pharmacologic therapy or direct current cardioversion, to sinus rhythm. Should this not be possible, consideration of pharmacologic strategies to control ventricular rate is important, as might be atrioventricular junction nodal ablation with permanent ventricular pacemaker insertion. Other types of supraventricular tachycardias might respond to more focused electrophysiologic arrhythmia-track ablation techniques or insertion of electronic arrhythmia-termination pacing devices. Likewise, incessant, but not necessarily sustained, ventricular arrhythmias need to be addressed in similar fashion, with consideration of pharmacologic treatment strategies, ablation therapeutics, or use of electronic arrhythmia-termination and control devices. Finally, the Maze operation is a surgical alternative that may assist in controlling the dysrhythmia and ameliorate heart failure. The procedure involves making several intertwining incisions in the atria to interrupt the fibrillation circuits.

Metabolic

Many metabolic disorders are known to induce myocardial dysfunction and can be categorized into endocrine, familial storage disease and infiltrations, deficiency states and nutritional disorders, and amyloidosis. Endocrine diseases, such as adrenocortical insufficiency, thyrotoxicosis, hypothyroidism, acromegaly, and pheochromocytoma, are covered in detail in the endocrine section of Chapter 35. Because diabetes mellitus and diabetic heart disease are so frequently encountered, they are further explored here. Additionally, amyloidosis and its unique nature deserve additional description.

Diabetic

Heart failure in the setting of diabetes is multifactorial and can be due to epicardial atherosclerotic coronary artery disease, small subendocardial vessel disease, or diabetes itself (66). Patients with diabetes mellitus are well known to be prone to silent myocardial ischemia and infarction. Furthermore, hypertension often complicates diabetes and can also contribute to detrimental remodeling of the heart. It is disturbing to note that almost half of asymptomatic diabetics experience a reduction in LV ejection fraction during stress.

The hearts of diabetic patients at autopsy can demonstrate the characteristic findings of DCM, with widespread regions of myocardial fibrosis, intimal proliferation of small myocardial arterioles, and accumulation of interstitial glycoprotein and collagen, all leading to decreased ventricular compliance and contractility (67).

Familial Storage Disease and Infiltrations

Many of the familial storage diseases and infiltrations cause various substances to be deposited within the myocardium, either intracellularly (frequently interfering with cellular metabolism and functioning) or extracellularly (resulting in a restrictive cardiomyopathy). Many of these disorders, such as Hurler syndrome, Niemann-Pick disease, Hand-Schüller-Christian disease, and Morquio-Ullrich disease, are more fully reviewed in the neurology section of Chapter 35. A few of the more understood and common disorders are further discussed here.

Hemochromatosis. Hemochromatosis is an autosomal-recessive metabolic storage disorder caused by mutation in iron transport molecules, including HFE, HAMP/Hepcidin (68,69), ferroportin/IREG1, DMT1, Hemojuvelin, and the transferrin receptor Tfr2 (68). Hemochromatosis is associated with HLA-A3 and HLA-B14. In some patients, polymorphisms in other proteins such as the mitochondrial superoxide dismutase A16V seem to influence adversely the deposition of iron (70). Usually, the iron deposits occur in many organs. In the heart, these deposits appear in the sarcoplasm (Fig. 89.12). It results clinically in the classic description of the bronzed diabetic with heart failure due to skin, pancreatic, and cardiac iron deposition. The cardiac deposits tend to be in the subepicardial and subendocardial regions, as well as in the papillary muscles. Cardiac hemochromatosis may present as either a restrictive cardiomyopathy early on or, more commonly, a dilated one, with impressively enlarged ventricles. In addition to iron deposition, an interstitial fibrosis that is unrelated to the degree of iron overload may occur independently. Endomyocardial biopsy is extremely useful in demonstrating iron deposits and important in establishing the diagnosis because the most common form of death in hemochromatosis is cardiac. Treatment consists of repeated phlebotomy or possibly chelation therapy, with the cardiomyopathy often reversible when the iron load is decreased.

Refsum Disease. Refsum syndrome is an autosomal-recessive disorder caused by the absence of the enzyme α-hydroxylase, which metabolizes dietary phytol and phytanic acid. This results in an accumulation of intracellular phytanic acid. The syndrome is characterized by cerebellar ataxia, peripheral neuropathies, retinitis pigmentosa, and cardiac disorders. A cardiomyopathy may result and can be either dilated or hypertrophic, depending on the stage of the disease. Wide-ranging conduction disturbances may occur, as well as dysrhythmias and sudden cardiac death. Current treatment consists of dietary

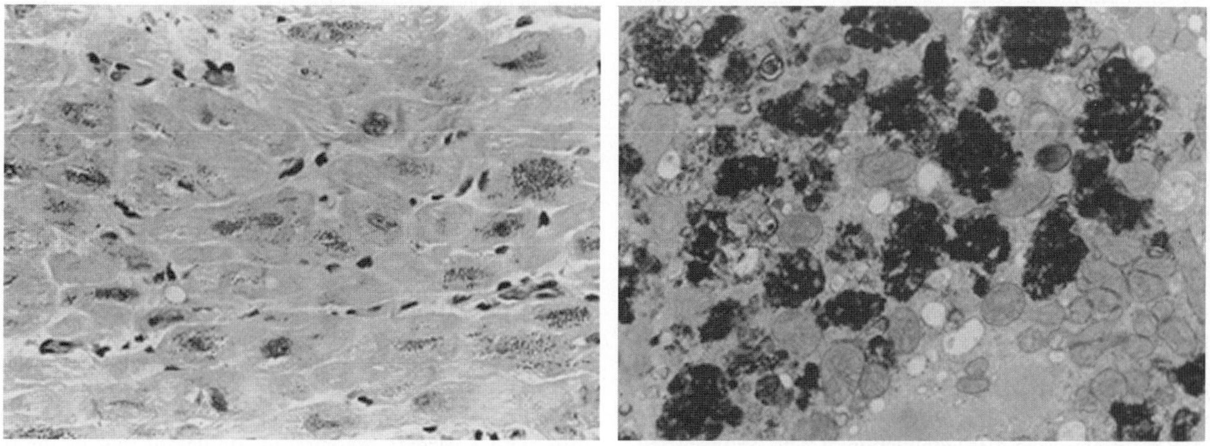

FIGURE 89.12. Hemochromatosis. The light micrograph on the left shows an endomyocardial biopsy with numerous dark granules in the sarcoplasm of the myocytes. These granules are usually located in the perinuclear region of the myocyte. The image on the left is an electron micrograph of a biopsy showing the black electron-dense iron deposits in the myocyte sarcoplasm.

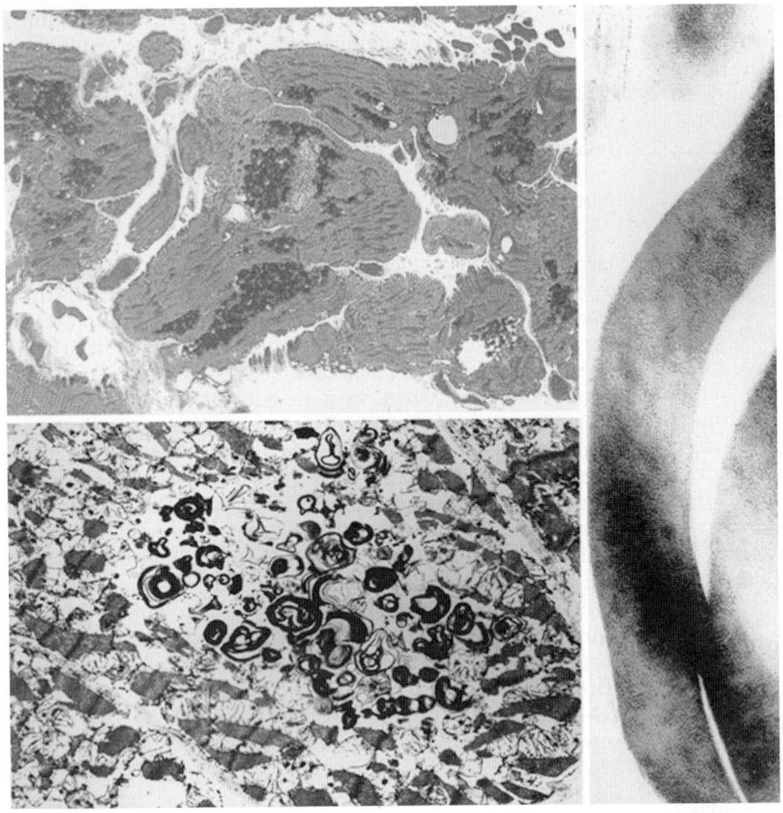

FIGURE 89.13. Fabry disease. This entity can readily be diagnosed by endomyocardial biopsy because of the typical sarcoplasmic inclusions which are detectable in endomyocardial biopsy as eosinophilic granules and mild "vacuolation." These granules can be seen in the center of the myocytes (*top left image*). On electron microscopy, they consist of numerous "myelin" figures (*bottom left image*) because of the multiple layers of electron-dense curvilinear "myelin-like" material. A high magnification of these structures is shown on the right image and shows the multiple, parallel, curvilinear, membrane-like structures.

modifications. Plasmapheresis has been shown to remove the accumulated phytanic acid.

Fabry Disease. Fabry disease or Anderson-Fabry disease, formally known as *angiokeratoma corporis diffusum universale*, is an X-linked disorder of glycosphingolipid metabolism and is present in 1 in 40,000 live births. It is due to a deficiency of the lysosomal enzyme α-galactosidase A, which normally degrades the neutral glycolipid ceramide trihexoside. The disorder is characterized by the intracellular lysosomal accumulation of this glycolipid, with prominent involvement of the skin, glomerular and tubular cells of the kidneys, and the heart (Fig. 89.13). Within the heart, the myocytes, vascular endothelium, conducting system, and valves can all be affected (71). Storage of the lipid in the blood vessels, with eventual occlusion of the small arterioles, leads to most of the clinical manifestations. Mostly males are affected; female carriers are usually asymptomatic or have only mild symptoms. Patients are generally diagnosed in childhood, when they present with burning pains, fevers, multiple angiokeratomas, corneal opacifications, and strokes; however, they do not present with renal and cardiac failure until their third or fourth decade of life. An atypical form of Fabry disease exists, in which there is retention of some residual α-galactosidase activity, probably from partial gene deletions and point mutations (72). These patients present late with a cardiomyopathy but no other systemic complaints.

Cardiovascular manifestations include renovascular and systemic hypertension, aortic root dilatation, mitral valve prolapse, and congestive heart failure. Patients may additionally have severe vasospastic angina and myocardial infarctions, perhaps from endothelial cell damage (73). The ECG may show LVH, P-wave abnormalities, conduction defects, and ventricular dysrhythmias. The echocardiogram typically shows marked increases in wall thickness and ventricular dilatation later in the disease process. The diagnosis may be confused with other disorders, such as HCM (74,75). Magnetic resonance imaging may help to differentiate this from amyloid (76). Endomyocardial biopsy is remarkable, showing the lipid deposits in the form of "myelin figures," with increased levels of ceramide trihexoside. Definitive diagnosis requires showing decreased α-galactosidase activity in leukocytes. No specific therapy exists for Fabry disease. Enzyme replacement therapy is of some use (77).

Selenium Deficiency

Selenium deficiency is a form of DCM that has been primarily reported in northeast China, where it is known as *Keshan disease*. It has, however, been demonstrated in HIV-positive patients with cardiomyopathy and in individuals receiving chronic parenteral nutrition. Selenium is an essential mineral, and deficiency results in the decreased activity of glutathione peroxidase. This causes an increase in free radicals that can be directly toxic to myocytes. Selenium replacement can reverse the ventricular dysfunction.

Thiamine Deficiency (Beriberi)

The Sinhalese word *beriberi* translates as *I cannot*, meaning the patient is too ill to do anything. Thiamine (vitamin B_1) is a necessary coenzyme for carbohydrate metabolism, and patients with this deficiency can present with edema, polyneuritis, and cardiac pathologies for at least 3 months. *Dry beriberi* refers to the constellation of flaccid paralysis, muscular atrophy, areflexia, and cardiac enlargement with tachycardia. *Wet beriberi* is similar in terms of the cardiac failure, except it has extensive edema. The extensive nervous system involvement is not present. Patients with beriberi have high-output failure, with a cardiac presentation similar to that of the other DCMs. The mechanism of this failure is uncertain. Lesions in sympathetic nuclei have been observed (78) and may lead to decreased peripheral resistance with compensatory increases in cardiac workload, eventually resulting in ventricular failure.

The cardiac dysfunction can rapidly return to near normal with thiamine replacement, although if the deficiency has been long-standing, dysfunction may be irreversible.

Carnitine Deficiency

In carnitine deficiency, the oxidation and mitochondrial transport of fatty acids are impaired, leading to lipid accumulation in the cytoplasm. The deficiency may be familial (79). Carnitine deficiency may result in a dilated or occasionally restrictive cardiomyopathy or a worsening of a preexisting cardiomyopathy of another cause. The cardiac lesions are often associated with endocardial fibroelastosis. Oral therapy with L-carnitine can be quite effective (80).

Amyloidosis

Background and prevalence. Amyloid restrictive cardiomyopathy is caused by the abnormal deposition of various proteins into the interstitium of the myocardium. The four general categories of amyloid heart disease are primary systemic, secondary, familial or hereditary, and senile (Table 89.4). Primary systemic amyloidosis is also known as *myeloma-associated* or *amyloid AL* from a monoclonal population of plasma cells. It is usually, but not always, the consequence of multiple myeloma, is more common in men, and rarely presents before age 30. Secondary amyloidosis results from the production of nonimmunoglobulin proteins. It is frequently encountered with chronic inflammatory disorders, such as rheumatoid arthritis, tuberculosis, and Crohn disease, and in familial Mediterranean fever. Familial and hereditary cardiac amyloidosis consists of six different forms. They most commonly result from the production of a prealbumin protein component known as *transthyretin*. They are autosomal-dominant disorders, unlike familial Mediterranean fever, which is autosomal recessive. Senile cardiac amyloid, also known as *amyloid SSA*, is also due to the production of an abnormal transthyretin and is seen in older individuals (81). The other two forms of age-related amyloidosis are atrial amyloidosis, which only affects the atria, and senile aortic amyloidosis limited to the aorta.

Each of the four main categories of amyloid heart disease has varying degrees of cardiac involvement, clinical significance, and survival rates. For instance, cardiac failure is the most common cause of death in primary amyloidosis. At autopsy, nearly 100% of systemic amyloid cases have demonstrable cardiac infiltration, although only 25% to 33% have clinically apparent disease (82). In contrast, fewer than 10% of secondary amyloid cases are associated with clinically significant cardiac derangement. Even when present, the deposits are typically small and perivascular in location and do not result in considerable ventricular dysfunction. Familial amyloidosis rarely has cardiac involvement, and then only very late in the disease. Senile amyloidosis is much more variable than the other types. Almost all individuals over the age of 60 have scattered deposits of amyloid in locations such as the aorta, and one fourth have some cardiac infiltration (84). This ranges from small atrial deposits to extensive ventricular involvement with severe congestive failure. Survival with senile amyloidosis is much longer than with primary amyloidosis. In one study, the median survival was 60.0 months and 5.5 months, respectively, from the time of diagnosis (85).

Pathology. The myocardium in amyloidosis is usually firm, thickened, and noncompliant, with the amyloid being present extracellularly. The deposits occur in the interstitium in a pericellular or focal nodular pattern and can result in systolic and diastolic impairment (see Figure 89.5). Nodular deposits and thick perimyocyte layers of amyloid are associated with shorter survival (83). The intramural arteries and veins can contain deposits in the media and adventitia, occasionally compromising blood flow. Rarely, deposits can also occur directly in the lumen of the vessels (84). The different types of amyloid vary in their vascular encroachment. Only 4% of senile amyloidosis has vascular involvement, whereas it is found in up to 90% of primary amyloid cases (85).

Cardiac amyloidosis can specifically be diagnosed by endomyocardial biopsy. In a series of 196 patients with restrictive ventricular function, 29% were proven to have amyloid infiltration in the heart, 51% had marked myocyte hypertrophy with or without fibrosis, and the remainder had myocarditis or nonspecific findings. Of the patients with amyloid, 12% had AL type and 10% had transthyretin infiltration (83).

Clinical profile and management. Cardiac amyloidosis can manifest one of four general ways; however, it is important to realize that by the time symptoms appear, there is generally quite extensive myocardial infiltration. The first presentation is that of a restrictive cardiomyopathy, with primarily diastolic dysfunction and right-sided heart failure findings. These include peripheral edema, jugular venous distention, and hepatic congestion. A fourth heart sound is uncommon, because atrial infiltration can decrease pumping ability. Right heart catheterization can demonstrate a restrictive physiology, including the characteristic diastolic dip and plateau in the ventricular pressure waveform. The second presentation is one of more typical congestive heart failure symptoms from systolic dysfunction. In this case, hemodynamic restriction may not be as prominent. Systolic ventricular impairment, when present, is an ominous sign, with a generally poor response to treatment and a progressive decline. Patients may have angina, either from involvement of the coronaries with amyloid deposition or from unrelated coronary atherosclerosis (86). Third, orthostatic hypotension may be the initial presenting complaint in approximately 10% of patients. Amyloid infiltration of the autonomic nervous system, blood vessels, or the adrenal glands may be partially responsible. Finally, because there may be amyloid

TABLE 89.4

CLASSIFICATION OF AMYLOIDOSIS

Name	Designation	Other names	Amyloid deposit
Primary	AL	Myeloma-associated, idiopathic[a]	Immunoglobulin light chain, κ or λ
Secondary	AA	Associated with other inflammatory disorders, familial Mediterranean fever	Nonimmunoglobulin protein A
Familial	AF	Hereditary	Transthyretin
Senile	SSA	Senile systemic amyloid	Transthyretin

[a]This term is outdated and should no longer be used.

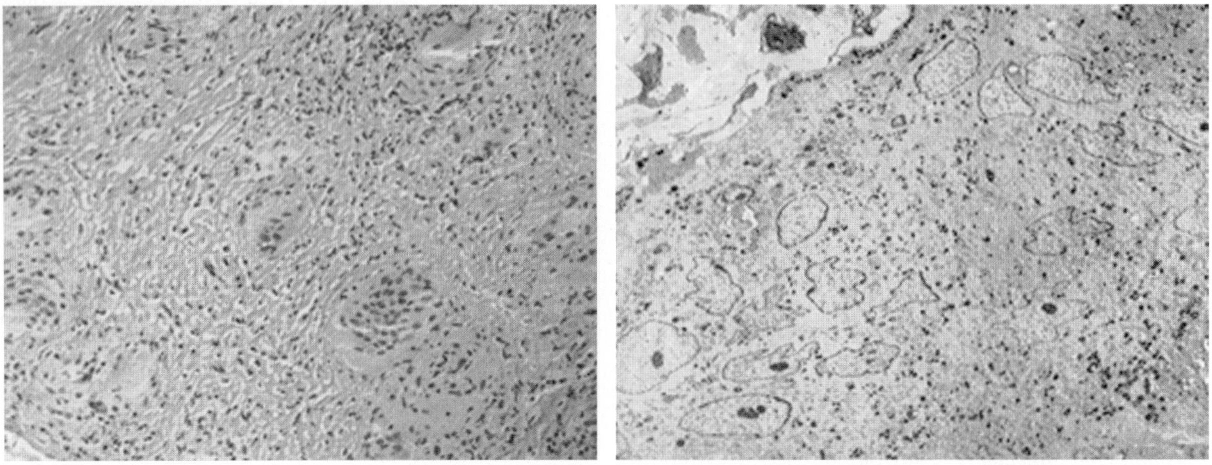

FIGURE 89.14. Cardiac sarcoidosis. The image on the left shows an endomyocardial biopsy with noncaseating granuloma. Multinucleated giant cells are present in the midst of the dense fibrous granuloma (such as shown in Figure 89.4 [*bottom*]). On the right, electron microscopy of these cells shows multiple nuclei and numerous filopodia, typical of monocyte/macrophage origin of these cells.

deposits within the conduction system, various abnormalities of impulse formation and conduction may occur. Patients may have bradycardia and varying degrees of blocks, including complete heart block and atrial and ventricular dysrhythmias. In such patients with conduction system involvement, sudden death, unfortunately, is relatively common.

Finally, endomyocardial biopsy can demonstrate amyloid if other laboratory tests and areas of biopsy are negative or equivocal. Special stains, including immunoperoxidase stains for κ and λ immunoglobulin chains and transthyrefin, may help to distinguish subtypes of the amyloid infiltrate, guiding management decisions and prognosis.

Management of amyloid cardiomyopathy is exceedingly difficult and typically ineffective. Low doses of diuretics and vasodilators are the most useful of the drug options, but require careful supervision. Patients with nephrotic syndrome from the amyloid, for example, may have a considerable amount of extravascular fluid, but they may be intravascularly depleted. Vasodilators can easily cause orthostatic symptoms, especially in patients who already have amyloid-induced autonomic dysfunction. ACE inhibitors have been reported to be of benefit, although no controlled trials have confirmed this. Unfortunately, calcium channel blockers, which have been of benefit in other disorders that cause diastolic dysfunction, have been disappointing in the treatment of amyloid cardiomyopathy. Nifedipine is bound by the amyloid fibrils and its use, as well as that of other calcium channel blockers, may exacerbate congestive heart failure symptoms by a local, enhanced, negative inotropic mechanism (87–89). Digoxin, which controls supraventricular dysrhythmias, is similarly relatively contraindicated because the drug may also be selectively bound to the fibrils, resulting in increased sensitivity and toxicity (90,91). It is unknown whether other antiarrhythmics share this same potential for toxicity. β-Blockers can be detrimental by promoting heart blocks. Pacemakers are helpful for the treatment of severe and symptomatic conduction disease.

General System Diseases

The connective tissue and collagen-vascular disorders, such as systemic lupus erythematosus, polyarteritis nodosa, and rheumatoid arthritis, are covered in Chapter 35. A few entities warrant additional description.

Sarcoidosis

Sarcoidosis is a systemic disease that is typified by noncaseating granulomas infiltrating the lungs, skin, and reticuloendothelial system. Cardiac sarcoidosis results in a restrictive cardiomyopathy, although rarely it more closely resembles a DCM. Interstitial lymphocytic inflammation and fibrosis may be present, in addition to the myocardial granulomas, which early on cause diastolic dysfunction but preserve systolic function (Fig. 89.14). Later on, further fibrosis and infiltration can lead to systolic impairment as well. Cardiac sarcoid is often present with systemic sarcoidosis, but clinically remains silent approximately 95% of the time (92). The initial cardiac presentation may be with high-degree atrioventricular blocks, syncope, or sudden cardiac death. Gallium-67, thallium-201, and Tc-99m–pyrophosphate myocardial imaging have been useful in localizing segmental myocardial involvement (93,94). Endomyocardial sampling can be helpful in confirming the diagnosis; however, the false-negative rate is high, even when numerous pieces are obtained. One explanation for this is that the granulomas have a predilection for the basal and free wall portions of the myocardium, areas where sampling does not usually occur (95). The cardiac granulomas occasionally respond to treatment with steroids. Pacemakers may help with symptomatic conduction disturbances.

Scleroderma

The cardiac manifestations of scleroderma include a slowly progressive fibrosis that involves the pericardium, myocardial interstitium, and conduction system. Small vessel coronary artery disease may also occur. These patients can present with either dilated or restrictive cardiomyopathies (96).

Muscular Dystrophies

A variety of neuromuscular diseases are associated with cardiomyopathy as part of their syndrome complex. Molecules that have been proven to have mutations associated with cardiomyopathy include dystrophin, sarcoglycans (α, β, γ, and δ), laminin $\alpha 2$, fukutin, myotilin, titin, emerin, and lamin A/C (97). Disorders of oxidative phosphorylation have been identified that are associated with these neuromuscular disorders as described under mitochondrial diseases. Many of the muscular dystrophies and neuromuscular disorders are covered in Chapter 35.

Duchenne Muscular Dystrophy

Duchenne muscular dystrophy, also known as *pseudohypertrophic muscular dystrophy*, is an X-linked, proximal muscle dystrophic disease that is frequently associated with cardiac involvement manifesting as DCM (97,98). Indeed, death usually results either from respiratory infection owing to cardiorespiratory failure or from the development of congestive heart failure with sudden cardiac death syndrome. Becker-type muscular dystrophy, similar to Duchenne, is also X-linked recessive in inheritance. Its onset is later in life, but it is slowly progressive once it manifests signs and symptoms.

Erb Limb-Girdle Dystrophy

Limb-girdle muscular dystrophy (97,98), or *Erb disease*, is an autosomal-recessive condition, with DCM as a potential complicating factor. Like myotonic dystrophy, it appears toward the middle years. It is a slowly progressive disorder that can affect either sex.

Myotonic Dystrophy

Myotonic dystrophy, also known as *Steinert disease*, is an autosomal-dominant disorder that demonstrates incomplete penetrance and variable expressiveness. The defect has been located to chromosome 19, with the production of a protein kinase that may be associated with receptor signal transduction. Myotonic dystrophy is the most common inherited dystrophy in adults. This slowly progressive and insidious dystrophic process frequently manifests symptoms between the ages of 20 and 50 years. Patients present with ptosis, cataracts, hypogonadism, and a mask-like expression from atrophy of the face and neck muscles. Cardiac involvement occurs in up to 90% of patients, and it typically presents as a DCM or with conduction disturbances. Replacement of the myocytes and Purkinje system with fibrofatty tissue occurs. Indeed, these patients are at extremely high risk of sudden cardiac death syndrome owing to either a malignant ventricular arrhythmia or sudden-onset high-degree atrioventricular heart block. Cardiac transplantation is generally not an option because of the systemic nature of the disease. Often the respiratory muscles are involved, and general anesthesia should be avoided if at all possible.

Neuromuscular Disorders

X-Linked Cardioskeletal Myopathy

Barth syndrome is the childhood form of X-linked recessive condition characterized by cardiomyopathy (43), accompanied by a variety of neuromuscular abnormalities (proportionate short stature) and recurrent neutropenia (99). Some patients exhibit carnitine deficiency, although this is an inconsistent finding. Contrary to most cardiomyopathies, this syndrome tends to improve with age. It is known that the primary defect in this disorder is in the G4.5 gene encoding the protein Tafazzin (43).

Friedreich Ataxia

Friedreich ataxia is a spinocerebellar degenerative disorder that has an autosomal-recessive form of inheritance, with the genetic defect located to chromosome 9. It is characterized by a broad-based gait; impaired vibration, position, and joint sense; dysarthria; pes cavus; and incoordination. Childhood onset has a high likelihood of also developing diabetes, although the reasons for this are unclear (100). Interestingly, Friedreich ataxia is commonly associated with HCM, either with concentric or asymmetric LVH (101). More rarely, this neuromuscular syndrome can present as a DCM, with myocardial fibrosis, at times apparently transformed from an initially hypertrophic ventricle. Death from cardiac origin occurs in 5% of cases. Histologic findings include diffuse interstitial fibrosis, myocellular hypertrophy, and necrosis. Abnormalities of large and small coronary arteries can also occur. One theory of the etiology of the dysfunction suggests that myocardial calcium overload may have a role. Verapamil treatment, effective with other forms of HCM, has had no effect on patients with established hypertrophy (102).

TABLE 89.5

TOXINS KNOWN TO CAUSE CARDIOMYOPATHY

Alcohol
Amsacrine
Antibiotics
Antipsychotics
Bleomycin
Busulfan
Carbon monoxide
Catecholamines
Chemotherapeutic agents
Chloroquine
Cisplatin
Cobalt
Cocaine
Cytosine arabinoside
Didanosine
Doxorubicin
Etoposide
5-Fluorouracil
Irradiation
Lead
Lithium
Mercury
Methotrexate
Mitomycin
Mitoxantrone
Phenothiazines
Sulfonamides
Vincristine
Zidovudine (AZT)

Sensitivity and Toxic Reactions

A variety of toxins can cause myocyte injury, with subsequent dysfunction leading to actual cell death with fibrotic replacement or, simply, more transient contractile dysfunction. Table 89.5 lists many cardiotoxic agents that have been reported to cause heart muscle disease. Discontinuing some of these drugs has led to substantive improvement in cardiac function on occasion. Specific examples of this include lithium, phenothiazines, and tricyclic antidepressants. One should always be particularly sensitive to the possibility that these drugs are producing cardiomyopathy in patients who receive them for psychiatric conditions. Therapy with specific cytokines such as α-interferon can produce profound myocardial depression, which as a pathologic substrate is detectable in endomyocardial biopsies (103). Some other specific toxins are discussed in the following sections.

Alcoholic Cardiomyopathy

Background and Prevalence

It was not until the 1950s that clinicians began to realize that alcohol and its major metabolite, acetaldehyde, could cause direct toxicity to the myocardium (104). Substantive DCM develops in only a small proportion of ethanol drinkers who meet diagnostic criteria for alcoholism. On the other hand, 60% to 80% of patients with "idiopathic" dilated congestive cardiomyopathy report a history of substantial alcohol intake. Furthermore, individuals with DCM who continue to imbibe to excess have continued and progressive ventricular function deterioration. Currently, alcoholic cardiomyopathy accounts for approximately one third of all nonischemic DCM (104). If alcohol consumption continues, 40% to 50% of patients die within 3 to 6 years (105). The effects of alcohol on the cardiovascular system are fully explored in Chapter 10.

Pathology

The pathologic findings of alcoholic cardiomyopathy are nonspecific and similar to, if not indistinguishable from, idiopathic DCM. The electron microscopic study of endomyocardial biopsies suggests that an accumulation of intracellular lipid droplets within the cardiac myocytes, too small to be seen with the light microscope, is a common finding in patients with alcoholic cardiomyopathy. Additionally, edema of the vascular wall and perivascular fibrosis of intramyocardial coronaries have been seen.

Clinical Profile and Management

The stereotyped profile of a patient with alcoholic cardiomyopathy is a man, aged 30 to 55, who has consumed whiskey, wine, or beer for more than 10 years. In reality, however, it has been virtually impossible to quantitate the amount of alcohol consumption that is required to produce cardiomyopathic effects. The diagnosis of alcoholic cardiomyopathy is likely best made in the setting of an idiopathic DCM accompanied by the traditional psychosocial characteristics of a chronic alcoholic (blackouts, marital discord, excessive work absenteeism, business failures, misdemeanor driving citations, and high blood alcohol concentrations while appearing not to be intoxicated). Besides the more common presentation of congestive heart failure with right- and left-sided findings, atrial fibrillation, and other supraventricular dysrhythmias may be the initial manifestation of the disorder. Complete abstinence may stop the progression or even allow for reversal of the failure (106–108) in early stages (usually in the first 2–6 months); however, severe heart failure may have little improvement.

Anthracycline-Induced Cardiomyopathy

Chronic anthracycline toxic cardiomyopathy is a dose-dependent DCM that is seen after therapy with agents such as doxorubicin (109). It is believed that anthracyclines cause myocyte cell death by increasing oxygen-derived free radical molecules, activating platelets, increasing histamine secretion, and producing C-13 hydroxymetabolites. This ultimately inhibits enzymatic activity within the sarcoplasmic reticulum, mitochondria, and sarcolemma such that energy production by adenosine triphosphate cleavage is altered. Myocyte destruction is associated with the characteristic histopathologic findings of marked sarcoplasmic reticulum dilatation and myofibrillar loss (Fig. 89.15). Thus, this is one of the cardiomyopathies readily diagnosed by specific electron microscopic changes noted at the time of endomyocardial biopsy sample analysis. Evaluation of anthracycline cardiotoxicity requires the evaluation of 10 blocks of plastic-embedded biopsy tissue to ensure an adequate evaluation of the severity of cardiotoxicity (110). Doxorubicin has been associated with this cardiomyopathy, with cumulative doses under 400 mg/m^2 having a trivial incidence, but dose levels over 700 mg/m^2 have resulted in a nearly 20% incidence of cardiomyopathy. Most patients who are exposed to this drug have a determination of the baseline ejection fraction with serial studies performed to follow ventricular performance indexes during treatment. Some data suggest that using continuous infusion of doxorubicin rather than bolus dosing, coadministering antioxidants or free radical scavengers, or treating patients with concomitant β-adrenergic or calcium channel blocking drugs reduces the incidence of anthracycline cardiotoxicity. Unfortunately, this form of DCM does not usually improve with time.

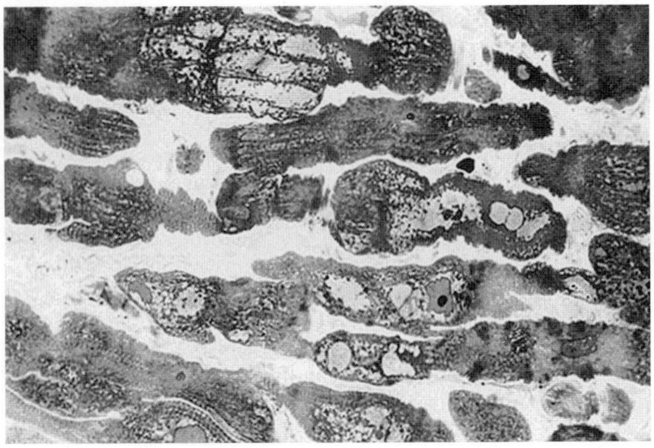

FIGURE 89.15. Anthracycline-induced cardiomyopathy. This light micrograph of a semithin plastic section illustrates the swollen sarcoplasmic reticulum, appearing as cytoplasmic vacuoles by light microscopy, and the loss of contractile elements.

Cocaine

Cocaine-related heart disease is increasing in frequency, with myocardial infarction sometimes noted after acute cocaine intoxication (111,112). An acute DCM has been described, as well as DCM occurring after long-term use of this drug. Cocaine produces central and peripheral nervous system adrenergic stimulation by inhibiting the presynaptic uptake of catecholamine. Therefore, this cardiomyopathy is likely due to excessive or excessively long myocyte exposure to adrenergic stimulation. In addition, cocaine can have direct effects on myocardial contractility and coronary resistance. Finally, vasospasm may cause chronic focal ischemia, leading to segmental wall motion abnormalities.

Irradiation

Radiation therapy, especially when used to treat Hodgkin disease, may induce acute and chronic ventricular dysfunction and is an increasingly common entity as more and more patients are receiving radiation. Acutely, radiation may cause a pancarditis and arteritis, producing a transient decrease in ventricular function, which usually resolves over 48 hours (113). Chronically, radiation may induce several cardiac disorders, each of which can lead to ventricular failure (114,115). First, endocardial and myocardial fibrosis, sometimes massive in nature, result causing a restrictive cardiomyopathy (116). The fibrosis is usually more prominent in the right ventricle, because it is more anterior and therefore receives a higher dose of radiation. The fibrosis is typically very dense, nearly acellular, and primarily perivascular in location. Second, the vascular endothelium is particularly sensitive to the effects of radiation. Third, the clinical picture may be confused by concomitant radiation-induced constrictive pericarditis, which may also be present for years after the therapy was administered. Next, radiation may also cause valvular fibrosis, resulting in either regurgitant or stenotic lesions (117). Finally, accelerated atherosclerosis usually manifests 6 to 12 years after exposure and may cause more of a DCM picture (118). If endomyocardial biopsy is performed to evaluate chemotherapeutic cardiac toxicity, radiation heart disease may complicate the interpretation. Further, radiation injury to the heart may be compounded by certain chemotherapeutic agents, especially the anthracyclines and cyclophosphamide (119). Additionally, some drugs, particularly doxorubicin, may recall the radiation effects even years after the administration of radiation. Risks for cardiac mortality from irradiation therapy increase with higher mediastinal doses, minimal protective cardiac blocking, and younger age at irradiation (120). No specific therapy is available.

Chloroquine Cardiomyopathy

Chloroquine is a 4-aminoquinoline compound, which was widely used during World War II as an antimalarial drug. It was subsequently found to be useful in the treatment of a variety of collagen-vascular diseases, including rheumatoid arthritis, systemic lupus erythematosus, and certain dermatologic disorders. Hydroxychloroquine was found to be less toxic than chloroquine and equally effective for the treatment of rheumatoid arthritis and systemic lupus erythematosus. Hydroxychloroquine contains a single hydroxyl group at the end of the side chain—-its only difference from chloroquine.

It has been known for some time that the long-term administration of chloroquine could result in a vacuolar myopathy of skeletal muscle. More recently, it has been recognized that hydroxychloroquine can produce a similar myopathy and that both drugs can also induce a severe toxic cardiomyopathy (121,122). Biventricular hypertrophy, congestive heart failure, and heart block have all been reported with chloroquine cardiomyopathy. Some, but not all, patients with chloroquine cardiomyopathy have a concomitant skeletal muscle myopathy. Biopsy findings in cardiac muscle are similar to those in skeletal muscle and are diagnostic of the disease (123). The light microscopic findings in semithin plastic sections are highly suggestive, with striking accumulation of large lysosomes and membrane profiles within the myocytes. The diagnostic changes of curvilinear bodies, which resemble myelin figures, can only be visualized in biopsies that have been fixed according to an electron microscopy protocol and embedded in plastic (Fig. 89.16). On cessation of the drug, patients begin a slow but progressive recovery over months from the skeletal and cardiac myopathies.

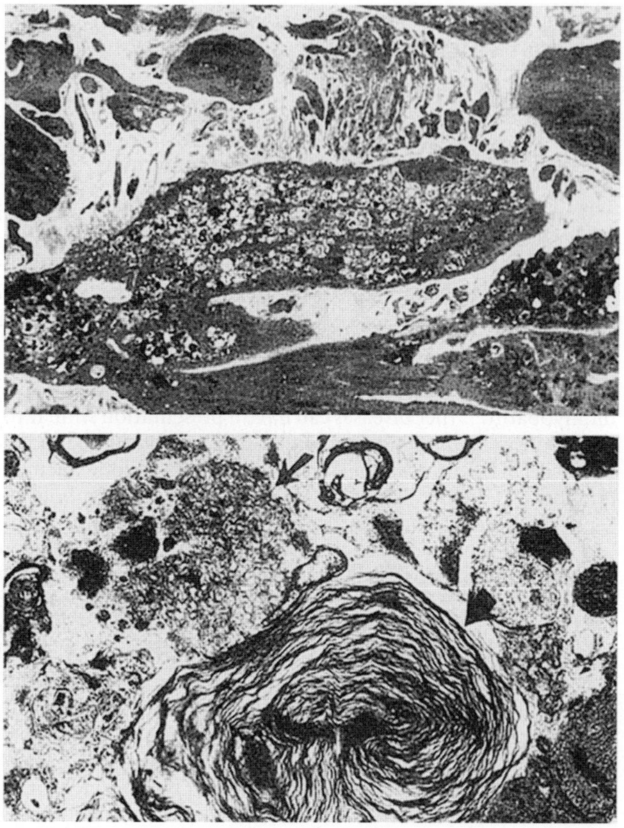

FIGURE 89.16. Chloroquine cardiomyopathy. The top image is a high-magnification light micrograph of a semithin plastic section, which has been fixed with glutaraldehyde and osmium tetroxide by an electron micrograph protocol. This preserves the secondary lysosomes that fill the cytoplasm of the myocytes. The large, complex secondary lysosomes vary in size, shape, and staining intensity, from pale gray to black. By standard light microscopy, this appears as a vacuolar myopathy, with the center of the myocytes appearing largely empty. The bottom image is an electron micrograph showing a curvilinear body (*thin arrow*), characteristic of chloroquine cardiomyopathy, and a large myelin figure (*thick arrow*), a common feature of this disease, but one that is not diagnostic.

Peripartum Cardiomyopathy

Background and Prevalence

Peripartum DCM is defined as LV systolic dysfunction without other apparent causes or underlying heart disease, occurring in the peripartum period. The onset must occur during the last month of pregnancy or within the first 5 months after delivery, although it is most common (75%) during the first 2 months postpartum (124). Because of differences in precisely defining this cardiomyopathy and aggressiveness in searching out other causes, the incidence has been reported to be anywhere between 1 in 1,300 to 1 in 15,000 pregnancies (125–127). Several risk factors have been identified, including twin pregnancy, age greater than 30, multiparity, a family history of peripartum cardiomyopathy, African descent, and prolonged therapy with tocolytic agents. The natural history differs from other forms of DCM. If recovery is going to occur, there is usually some sign of improvement within the first 6 weeks. Approximately 50% of patients spontaneously recover, usually in the first 6 months, with improvement after that time unlikely. The initial severity of heart failure or ventricular dysfunction is not predictive of long-term outcome (128). Death or deterioration to the point of requiring transplantation occurs in 25% to 50% of patients (129). Progressive congestive heart failure, dysrhythmias, and embolic events are the usual immediate causes of death. However, identifying patients who are likely to improve is not usually possible. A notable exception: In one small report, women who appeared to have peripartum cardiomyopathy associated with prolonged sympathomimetic tocolysis recovered fully (130).

Pathophysiology

The actual mechanism that causes ventricular dysfunction remains unknown. Numerous series have reported a higher incidence of myocarditis diagnosed by endomyocardial biopsy compared to idiopathic DCM (131–134). However, the incidence of myocarditis by biopsy with peripartum cardiomyopathy did not differ from age- and gender-controlled matches that had idiopathic DCM (135). Other possibilities include autoimmune disease (maternal exposure to fetal or placental antigens), viral infections, hormonal (the hormone relaxin produced by the corpus luteum), and cytokine induction of apoptosis (136).

Clinical Profile and Management

The diagnosis of heart failure in the last month of pregnancy may be difficult to make, because many of the early signs and symptoms of ventricular dysfunction mimic those of normal pregnancy. These include fatigue, dyspnea on exertion, pretibial edema, and an increase in baseline heart rate. Orthopnea, chest discomfort, cough, gallops, and rales are also suggestive of heart failure. After delivery, these findings should quickly resolve, and failure to do so may indicate an underlying cardiomyopathy. Other diseases can have a presentation similar to that of heart failure and should therefore be considered in the differential diagnosis. Some of these disorders include anemia, amniotic fluid embolism, hypertension, pulmonary embolism, sepsis, thyrotoxicosis, and toxemia of pregnancy. Echocardiography, the most helpful study, typically shows four-chamber enlargement, biventricular hypokinesia, and a small, hemodynamically insignificant pericardial effusion. Strong opposing views have been presented regarding the necessity of performing endomyocardial biopsies.

The treatment of peripartum cardiomyopathy is different from that of the more traditional DCMs in several aspects. First, ACE inhibitors are contraindicated during pregnancy because of the risks of fetal anuria and death. They are also relatively contraindicated in nursing women. Hydralazine can be safely used in place of ACE inhibitors if afterload reduction is required. It should be recalled that during pregnancy the systemic vascular resistance is already low because of the placenta, and further afterload reduction may not be necessary or may not be well tolerated. Digoxin is a U.S. Food and Drug Administration (FDA) class C drug, and its risks and benefits should be considered. Digoxin can pass into the placenta and is secreted in breast milk. Similarly, diuretics are also FDA class C drugs. Frequently, strict sodium restriction diminishes fluid overload and can avert the need for diuretics. β-Blockers may be helpful if the patient is not volume overloaded. Strong consideration for anticoagulation is important because of the marked increased incidence of thromboembolic events, which has been reported to be as high as 53% (137,138). As reviewed in Chapter 31, pregnancy is a hypercoagulable state, with demonstrated increases in coagulation factors II, VII, VIII, and X, and plasma fibrinogen. Coagulation slowly returns to normal by approximately 6 weeks postpartum (139), and after this time anticoagulation becomes less critical. Warfarin is contraindicated (FDA class D) and should not be used prenatally because of severe teratogenic effects. Short-term unfractionated or low-molecular-weight heparin use is easily stopped just before delivery. If symptoms and ventricular function do not improve or if the clinical condition deteriorates, referral for cardiac transplantation should be contemplated. Some of these patients may even require a LV assist device for stabilization while awaiting a suitable donor (140,141). A compatible donor may be more difficult to identify, because postpartum women tend to have higher panels of reactive antibodies from fetal antigen exposure. Some have advocated the use of immunosuppressants or intravenous immunoglobulin (142) for the treatment of peripartum cardiomyopathy based on small, retrospective, nonrandomized trials and observations. No large, prospective, randomized, controlled trials have demonstrated a benefit for any of these therapies.

If full recovery of LV function does not occur, the mother should be warned to avoid future pregnancies, because the rate of maternal and fetal morbidity and mortality is unacceptably high. The recommendation to the patient who is clinically completely recovered and contemplating another pregnancy is controversial. In general, the woman should be advised that recurrence is certainly possible, is usually more severe the second time, and is fatal approximately 10% of the time (143). One group has suggested performing dobutamine stress testing on apparently recovered hearts. Evidence of impaired contractile reserve may identify a subset of patients who have inducible abnormalities, which may become significant with the increased hemodynamic load of pregnancy (144). Finally, it has been demonstrated that there is increased activity of calcium-independent inducible nitric oxide synthetases (iNOS) in peripartum cardiomyopathy (145). The generation of nitric oxide by iNOS may be responsible for some of the dilation and impaired contractility of the heart. In the future, nitric oxide or iNOS antagonists may play a critical role in the early treatment of peripartum as well as some of the other DCM.

Currently, if a specific disease process is strongly suggested and cannot be diagnosed by a less invasive manner, a biopsy is reasonable. The treatment of cardiomyopathy is covered in Chapters 86 and 87.

CONTROVERSIES AND PERSONAL PERSPECTIVES

Despite its usefulness in the last 30 years, endomyocardial biopsy is still a matter of some controversy. Many studies have shown its value as a diagnostic procedure and not only a research tool. However, many cardiologists do not take advantage of this tool because they assume that an accurate diagnosis is obtained only some of the time. Further, they reason that even if one obtains an accurate diagnosis, then there is no specific therapy for the condition diagnosed. Thus, why bother with a high-risk procedure? To this question, there is an objective answer. This procedure is of paramount importance. In experienced hands the procedure carries very low risk. Proper evaluation of the biopsy specimen by an experienced cardiovascular pathologist is imperative. The recommendations from a highly successful center include considering an endomyocardial biopsy in (a) new LV dysfunction; (b) transplant candidates; (c) worsening heart failure despite therapy; (d) restrictive cardiomyopathy; (e) definition of the type of myocarditis; (f) patients who are "too ill" to undergo cardiac catheterization; (g) determination of specific heart muscle disorder; and (h) research (randomization of a patient during a trial) (146).

In patients with unexplained cardiomyopathy after standard evaluation, the clinical assessment of the etiology is inaccurate in 31% of patients. Endomyocardial biopsy establishes the final diagnosis in 75% of these patients with high specificity (147). It is our opinion that in experienced teams the complications are low and the diagnostic yields are high. Table 89.6 lists some specific cardiomyopathies that can be diagnosed by biopsy.

Another controversial point is the usefulness of ascertaining whether or not there is myocarditis present in a patient. This should not be considered appropriate justification not to perform a biopsy. The information yield provides reassurance of the etiology, evaluates the intensity of the process, and provides information about the overall status of the myocardium, for example, the presence or absence of fibrosis. This in turn correlates with reversibility of the heart failure.

THE FUTURE

As we understand the molecular basis of nonischemic cardiomyopathies, it will become clear that they indeed represent distinct disease entities which can be grouped into broad

TABLE 89.6

DISEASE ENTITIES THAT CAN BE DIAGNOSED WITH HEART BIOPSY

VASCULAR
Myocardial ischemia
Small intramural coronary artery disease
RESTRICTIVE HEART DISEASE
Amyloidosis
Endocardial fibroelastosis
Endomyocardial fibrosis without eosinophilia
Fibrosis
Hemochromatosis
Löeffler disease
PHYSICAL AGENTS
Radiation injury
INFLAMMATORY/INFECTIOUS
Allergic/hypersensitivity myocarditis (ephedra, tryptophan)
Chagas disease
Cytomegalovirus infection
Myocarditis secondary to autoimmune diseases
Giant cell myocarditis
Fungal myocarditis
Rheumatic heart disease
Sarcoidosis
Parvovirus infection
Toxoplasmosis
DRUG TOXICITY
Adriamycin
Chloroquine
Cocaine
5-Fluorouracil
IATROGENIC
Interferon-α
Zidovudine (AZT)
METABOLIC DISEASES
Fabry disease
Gaucher disease
Glycogen storage diseases
GM1 gangliosidosis
Hemochromatosis
Mucopolysaccharidosis
Wilson disease

categories according to their phenotype (dilated, hypertrophic, or restrictive). These phenotypes are useful because they are based on clinical, physiologic, and pathologic observations, and withstood the test of time. As specific genetic entities have been discovered in the last 15 years, it is clear that some genotypes are going to be expressed in more than one phenotype. For example, HCM was at one point thought to be a disease in which mutations in sarcomeric genes (148) were responsible for the phenotype. However, in the following years it became clear that mutations in sarcomeric proteins were also associated with a DCM phenotype. In a similar manner, ascertaining the etiology of the myocarditides is likely to become a required test in the clinical setting.

It follows that other, less well-characterized entities such as ARVC/D, mitochondrial diseases, and diseases that preferentially affect the endomyocardium, will require more sophisticated tests, including genotyping to fully characterize them and to properly classify individual patients. To this end, we must focus our efforts on obtaining the best phenotype of every patient possible, because this information will be the most valuable to have when the routine determination of gene expression patterns, mutations, and chromosomal abnormalities becomes close to standard of practice. Clearly, many of these mutations will behave differently in individual patients. Depending on individual factors in a given patient, the expression of a mutation or its potential treatment will vary. The systematic determination of the interaction of mutations and specific polymorphisms in patients will certainly become the ideal way to characterize and treat individuals. We are beginning to see this take place in several areas of cardiovascular medicine.

References

1. Krehl L. Beitrag zur Kentniss der idiopathischen Herz-muskelerkrankungen. *Dtsch Arch Klin Med* 1891;48:414–431.
2. Bridgen W. Uncommon myocardial diseases: the non-coronary cardiomyopathies. *Lancet* 1957;2:1179–1184.
3. Report of the WHO/ISFC task force on the definition and classification of cardiomyopathies. *Br Heart J* 1980;44:672–673.
4. Giles TD. A perspective on nosology and incidence of cardiomyopathy. In: Giles TD, Sanders GE, eds. *Cardiomyopathy*. Littleton, MA: PSG Publishing, 1988.
5. Report of the 1995 World Health Organization/International Society and Federation of Cardiology task force on the definition and classification of cardiomyopathies. *Circulation* 1996;93:841–842.
6. Feild BJ, Baxley WA, Russell Jr RO, et al. Left ventricular function and hypertrophy in cardiomyopathy with depressed ejection fraction. *Circulation* 1973;47:1022–1031.
7. Goodwin JF. Cardiac function in primary myocardial disorders. *BMJ* 1964;1:1527–1533, 1595–1597.
8. Bristow MR, O'Connell JB. Myocardial diseases. In: Kelley WN, ed. *Textbook of internal medicine,* 3rd ed. Philadelphia: Lippincott, 1997:398–405.
9. Johnson RA, Palacios I. Dilated cardiomyopathies of the adult (Pt 1). *N Engl J Med* 1982;307:1051–1058.
10. Johnson RA, Palacios I. Dilated cardiomyopathies of the adult (Pt 2). *N Engl J Med* 1982;307:1119–1126.
11. Burkett EL, Hershberger RE. Clinical and genetic issues in familial dilated cardiomyopathy. *J Am Coll Cardiol* 2005;45:969–981.
12. Morita H, Seidman J, Seidman CE. Genetic causes of human heart failure. *J Clin Invest* 2005;115:518–526.
13. Teare D. Asymmetrical hypertrophy of the heart in young adults. *Br Heart J* 1958;20:1–8.
14. Maron B, Epstein S. Hypertrophic cardiomyopathy: a discussion of nomenclature. *Am J Cardiol* 1979;43:1242–1244.
15. Maron BJ, McKenna WJ, Danielson GK, et al. Task force on clinical expert consensus documents. American College of Cardiology; Committee for Practice Guidelines. European Society of Cardiology. American College of Cardiology/European Society of Cardiology clinical expert consensus document on hypertrophic cardiomyopathy. A report of the American College of Cardiology Foundation Task Force on Clinical Expert Consensus Documents and the European Society of Cardiology Committee for Practice Guidelines. *J Am Coll Cardiol* 2003;42:1687–1713.
16. Ferrans VJ, Morrow AG, Roberts WC. Myocardial ultrastructure in idiopathic hypertrophic subaortic stenosis: a study of operatively excised left ventricular outflow tract muscle in 14 patients. *Circulation* 1972;45:769–792.
17. Maron BJ, Seidman JG, Seidman CE. Proposal for contemporary screening strategies in families with hypertrophic cardiomyopathy. *J Am Coll Cardiol* 2004;44:2125–2132.
18. Maron BJ, Dearani JA, Ommen SR, et al. The case for surgery in obstructive hypertrophic cardiomyopathy. *J Am Coll Cardiol* 2004;44:2044–2053.
19. Goodwin JF. Cardiomyopathies and specific heart muscle diseases: definitions, terminology, classifications and new and old approaches. *Postgrad Med J* 1992;68[Suppl 1]:S3–S6.
20. Spry CJ. Eosinophils in eosinophilic endomyocardial disease. *Postgrad Med J* 1986;62:609–613.
21. Fauci AS, Harley JB, Roberts WC, et al. The idiopathic hypereosinophilic syndrome: clinical, pathophysiologic, and therapeutic considerations. *Ann Intern Med* 1982;97:78–92.
22. Parillo JE, Borer JS, Henry WC, et al. The cardiovascular manifestations of the hypereosinophilic syndrome: prospective study of 26 patients, with review of the literature. *Am J Med* 1979;67:572–582.
23. Marcus FI, Fontaine GH, Guiraudon G, et al. Right ventricular dysplasia: a report of 24 adult cases. *Circulation* 1982;65:384–398.

24. Manyari D, Klein G, Gulamhusein S. Arrhythmogenic right ventricular dysplasia: generalized cardiomyopathy? *Circulation* 1983;68:251–257.
25. Pinamonti B, Sinagra G, Salvi A, et al. Left ventricular involvement in right ventricular dysplasia. *Am Heart J* 1992;123:711–724.
26. Thiene G, Nava A, Angelini A, et al. Anatomoclinical aspects of arrhythmogenic right ventricular cardiomyopathy. In: Baroldi G, Camerini F, Goodwin JF, eds. *Advances in cardiomyopathies*. Berlin: Springer-Verlag, 1990: 397–408.
27. Tansey DK, Aly Z, Sheppard MN. Fat in the right ventricle of the normal heart. *Histopathology* 2005;46:98–104.
28. Angelini A, Thiene G, Boffa GM, et al. Endomyocardial biopsy in right ventricular cardiomyopathy. *Int J Cardiol* 1993;40:274–282.
29. Bomma C, Rutberg J, Tandri H, et al. Misdiagnosis of arrhythmogenic right ventricular dysplasia/cardiomyopathy. *J Cardiovasc Electrophysiol* 2004;15:300–306.
30. Auffermann W, Wichter T, Breithardt G, et al. Arrhythmogenic right ventricular disease: MR imaging versus angiography. *AJR Am J Roentgenol* 1993;161:549–555.
31. Castillo E, Tandri H, Rodriguez ER, et al. Arrhythmogenic right ventricular dysplasia: ex vivo and in vitro fat detection with black-blood MR imaging. *Radiology* 2004;232:38–48.
32. Danieli GA, Rampazzo A. Genetics of arrhythmogenic right ventricular cardiomyopathy. *Curr Opin Cardiol* 2002;17:218–221.
33. Sen-Chowdhry S, Syrris P, McKenna WJ. Genetics of right ventricular cardiomyopathy. *J Cardiovasc Electrophysiol* 2005;16:927–935.
34. Corrado D, Fontaine G, Marcus FI, et al. Arrhythmogenic right ventricular dysplasia/cardiomyopathy: need for an international registry. Study Group on Arrhythmogenic Right Ventricular Dysplasia/Cardiomyopathy of the Working Groups on Myocardial and Pericardial Disease and Arrhythmias of the European Society of Cardiology and of the Scientific Council on Cardiomyopathies of the World Heart Federation. *Circulation* 2000;101:E101–E106.
35. Piccini JP, Nasir K, Bomma C, et al. Electrocardiographic findings over time in arrhythmogenic right ventricular dysplasia/cardiomyopathy. *Am J Cardiol* 2005;96:122–126.
36. Hulot JS, Jouven X, Empana JP, et al. Natural history and risk stratification of arrhythmogenic right ventricular dysplasia/cardiomyopathy. *Circulation* 2004;110:1879–1884
37. Uhl HSM. A previously undescribed congenital malformation of the heart: almost total absence of the myocardium of the right ventricle. *Bull Johns Hopkins Hosp* 1952;91:197–209.
38. Greer ML, MacDonald C, Adatia I: MRI of Uhl's anomaly. *Circulation* 2000;101:E230–E232.
39. Tripp ME, Katcher ML, Peters HA, et al. Systemic carnitine deficiency presenting as familial endocardial fibroelastosis: a treatable cardiomyopathy. *N Engl J Med* 1981;305:385–390.
40. Bennett MJ, Hale DE, Pollitt RJ, et al. Endocardial fibroelastosis and primary carnitine deficiency due to a defect in the plasma membrane carnitine transporter. *Clin Cardiol* 1996;19:243–246.
41. Chin TK, Perloff JK, Williams RG, et al. Isolated non-compaction of left ventricular myocardium: a study of eight cases. *Circulation* 1990;82:507–513.
42. Burke A, Mont E, Kutys R, et al. Left ventricular noncompaction: a pathological study of 14 cases. *Human Pathol* 2005;36:403–411.
43. Hughes SE, McKenna WJ. New insights into the pathology of inherited cardiomyopathy. *Heart* 2005;91:257–264.
44. Weiford BC, Subbarao VD, Mulhern KM. Noncompaction of the ventricular myocardium. *Circulation* 2004;109:2965–2971.
45. Rustin P, Chretien D, Bourgeron T, et al. Investigation of respiratory chain activity in the human heart. *Biochem Med Metab Biol* 1993;50:120–126.
46. Taylor G, Rodriguez ER. Metabolic and hereditary cardiomyopathies of childhood. In Braunwald E, McMannus BM, eds. *Atlas of cardiovascular pathology for the clinician,* Philadelphia: Current Medicine; 2001.
47. Finsterer J. Mitochondriopathies. *Eur J Neurol* 2004;11:163–186.
48. Taylor RW, Turnbull DM. Mitochondrial DNA mutations in human disease. *Nat Rev Genet* 2005;6:389–402.
49. Manley JC, King JF, Zeft HJ, et al. The "bad" left ventricle: results of coronary surgery and effect on late survival. *J Thorac Cardiovasc Surg* 1976;72:841–848.
50. Nagueh SF, Vaduganathan P, Ali N, et al. Identification of hibernating myocardium: comparative accuracy of myocardial contrast echocardiography, rest-redistribution thallium-201 tomography and dobutamine echocardiography. *J Am Coll Cardiol* 1997;29:985–993.
51. Bolling SF, Deeb M, Brunsting LA, et al. Surgery for acquired heart disease. *J Thorac Cardiovasc Surg* 1995;109:676–683.
52. Scalia PM, McCarthy PM, Starling RC. Intra-operative echocardiography in left ventricular remodeling surgery. *J Am Coll Cardiol* 1997;29[Suppl A]:66A.
53. Autran BR, Gorin I, Lerbowitch M. AIDS in a Haitian woman with cardiac Kaposi's sarcoma and Whipple's disease. *Lancet* 1983;1:767–768.
54. Cohen IS, Anderson DW, Viemani R, et al. Congestive cardiomyopathy in association with the acquired immunodeficiency syndrome. *N Engl J Med* 1986;315:628–630.
55. Kaul S, Fishbein MC, Siegel RJ. Cardiac manifestations of acquired immune deficiency syndrome: a 1991 update. *Am Heart J* 1991;122:535–544.
56. Reilly JM, Cunnion RE, Anderson DW, et al. Frequency of myocarditis, left ventricular dysfunction and ventricular tachycardia in the acquired immune deficiency syndrome. *Am J Cardiol* 1988;62:789–793.
57. Currie PF, Jacob AJ, Foreman AR, et al. Heart muscle disease related to HIV infection: prognostic implications. *BMJ* 1994;309:1605–1607.
58. Rodriguez ER, Nasim S, Hsia J, et al. Cardiac myocytes and dendritic cells harbor Human Immunodeficiency Virus: detection by multiplex, nested, polymerase chain reaction (PCR) in individually microdissected cells from right ventricular endomyocardial biopsy tissue. *Am J Cardiol* 1991; 68:1511–1520.
59. Kavanaugh-McHugh AL, Ruff A, Perlman E, et al. Selenium deficiency and cardiomyopathy in acquired immunodeficiency syndrome. *JPEN J Parenter Enteral Nutr* 1991;15:347–349.
60. McLaran CJ, Gersh BJ, Sugrue DD, et al. Tachycardia induced myocardial dysfunction: a reversible phenomenon? *Br Heart J* 1985;53:323–327.
61. Cruz FE, Cheriex EC, Smeets JL, et al. Reversibility of tachycardia-induced cardiomyopathy after cure of incessant supraventricular tachycardia. *J Am Coll Cardiol* 1990;16:739–744.
62. Rosenqvist M, Lee MA, Moulinier L, et al. Long-term follow-up of patients after transcatheter direct current ablation of the atrioventricular junction. *J Am Coll Cardiol* 1990;16:1467–1474.
63. Corey WA, Markel ML, Hoit BD, et al. Regression of a dilated cardiomyopathy after radiofrequency ablation of incessant supraventricular tachycardia. *Am Heart J* 1993;126:1469–1473.
64. Kugler JD, Baisch SD, Cheatham JP, et al. Improvement of left ventricular dysfunction after control of persistent tachycardia. *J Pediatr* 1984;105: 543–548.
65. Fyfe DA, Gillette PC, Crawford FJ, et al. Resolution of dilated cardiomyopathy after surgical ablation of ventricular tachycardia in a child. *J Am Coll Cardiol* 1987;9:231–234.
66. Starling MR. Does a clinically definable diabetic cardiomyopathy exist? *J Am Coll Cardiol* 1990;15:1518–1520.
67. Regan TJ, Wu CF, Yeh CK, et al. Myocardial composition and function in diabetes: the effects of chronic insulin use. *Circ Res* 1981;49:1268–1277.
68. Schilsky ML, Oikonomu I. Inherited metabolic liver disease. *Curr Opin Gastroenterol* 2005;21:275–282.
69. Hannuksela J, Leppilampi M, Peuhkurinen K, et al. Hereditary hemochromatosis gene (HFE) mutations C282Y, H63D and S65C in patients with idiopathic dilated cardiomyopathy. *Eur J Heart Fail* 2005;7:103–108.
70. Valenti L, Conte D, Piperno A, et al. The mitochondrial superoxide dismutase A16V polymorphism in the cardiomyopathy associated with hereditary haemochromatosis. *J Med Genet* 2004;41:946–950.
71. Sakuraba H, Yanagawa Y, Igarashi T, et al. Cardiovascular manifestations in Fabry's disease: a high incidence of mitral valve prolapse in hemizygotes and heterozygotes. *Clin Genet* 1986;29:276–283.
72. Ishii S, Kase R, Sakuraba H, et al. Characterization of a mutant alpha-galactosidase gene product for the late-onset cardiac form of Fabry disease. *Biochem Biophys Res Commun* 1993;197:1585–1589.
73. Ogawa T, Kawai M, Matsui T, et al. Vasospastic angina in a patient with Fabry's disease who showed normal coronary angiographic findings. *JnpJpn Circ J* 1996;60:315–318.
74. Arad M, Maron BJ, Gorham JM, et al. Glycogen storage diseases presenting as hypertrophic cardiomyopathy. *N Engl J Med* 2005;352:362–372.
75. Ferrans VJ, Rodriguez ER. Hypertrophic obstructive cardiomyopathy and Fabry's disease. *N Engl J Med* 1983;308:460.
76. Matsui S, Murakami E, Takekoshi N, et al. Myocardial tissue characterization by magnetic resonance imaging in Fabry's disease. *Am Heart J* 1989;117:472–474.
77. Brady RO, Schiffmann R. Enzyme-replacement therapy for metabolic storage disorders. *Lancet Neurol* 2004;3:752–756.
78. Akbarian M, Yankopoulos NA, Abelmann WH. Hemodynamic studies in beriberi heart disease. *Am J Med* 1966;41:197–212.
79. Waber LJ, Valle D, Neill C, et al. Carnitine deficiency presenting as familial cardiomyopathy: a treatable defect in carnitine transport. *J Pediatr* 1982;101:700–705.
80. Tripp ME, Katcher ML, Peters HA, et al. Systemic carnitine deficiency presenting as familial endocardial fibroelastosis: a treatable cardiomyopathy. *N Engl J Med* 1984;310:142–148.
81. Cornwell GG III, Westermark P, Natvig JB, et al. Senile cardiac amyloid: evidence that fibrils contain a protein immunologically related to prealbumin. *Immunology* 1981;44:447–452.
82. Gertz MA, Kyle RA. Primary systemic amyloidosis: a diagnostic primer. *Mayo Clin Proc* 1989;64:1505–1519.
83. Rahman JE, Helou EF, Gelzer-Bell R, et al. Noninvasive diagnosis of biopsy-proven cardiac amyloidosis. *J Am Coll Cardiol* 2004;43:410–415.
84. Roberts WC, Waller BF. Cardiac amyloidosis causing cardiac dysfunction: analysis of 54 necropsy patients. *Am J Cardiol* 1983;52:137–146.
85. Smith TJ, Kyle RA, Lie JT. Clinical significance of histopathologic patterns of cardiac amyloidosis. *Mayo Clin Proc* 1984;59:547–555.
86. Narang R, Chopra P, Wasir HS. Cardiac amyloidosis presenting as ischemic heart disease: a case report and review of literature. *Cardiology* 1993;82:294–300.
87. Pollak A, Falk RH. Left ventricular systolic dysfunction precipitated by verapamil in cardiac amyloidosis. *Chest* 1993;104:618–620.

88. Gertz MA, Falk RH, Skinner M, et al. Worsening of congestive heart failure in amyloid heart disease treated by calcium channel-blocking agents. *Am J Cardiol* 1985;55:1645.
89. Griffiths BE, Hughes P, Dowdle R, et al. Cardiac amyloidosis with asymmetrical septal hypertrophy and deterioration after nifedipine. *Thorax* 1982;37:711–712.
90. Rubinow A, Skinner M, Cohen AS. Digoxin sensitivity in amyloid cardiomyopathy. *Circulation* 1981;63:1285–1288.
91. Cassidy JT. Cardiac amyloidosis: two cases with digitalis sensitivity. *Ann Intern Med* 1961;55:989–994.
92. Perry A, Vuitch F. Causes of death in patients with sarcoidosis: a morphologic study of 38 autopsies with clinicopathologic correlations. *Arch Pathol Lab Med* 1995;119:167–172.
93. Bulkley BH, Rouleau JR, Whitaker JQ, et al. The use of ^{201}thallium for myocardial perfusion imaging in sarcoid heart disease. *Chest* 1977;72:27–32.
94. Forman MB, Sandler MP, Sacks GA, et al. Radionuclide imaging in myocardial sarcoidosis: demonstration of myocardial uptake of technetium pyrophosphate^{99m} and gallium. *Chest* 1983;83:578–580.
95. Ferrans VJ, Rodriguez ER, McAllister HA Jr. Granulomatous inflammation of the heart. *Heart Vessels Suppl* 1985;1:262–270.
96. Ferrans VJ, Rodriguez ER. Cardiovascular lesions in collagen-vascular diseases. *Heart Vessels Suppl* 1985;1:256–261.
97. Goodwin FC, Muntoni F. Cardiac involvement in muscular dystrophies: molecular mechanisms. *Muscle Nerve* 2005;32:577–588.
98. Muntoni F. Cardiomyopathy in muscular dystrophies. *Curr Opin Neurol* 2003;16:577–583.
99. Ades LC, Gedeon AK, Wilson MJ, et al. Barth syndrome. Clinical features and confirmation of gene localization to distal Xq28. *Am J Med Genet* 1993;45:327–334.
100. De Michele G, Di Maio L, Filla A, et al. Childhood onset of Friedreich's ataxia: a clinical and genetic study of 36 cases. *Neuropediatrics* 1996; 27:3–7.
101. Gunal N, Saraclar M, Ozkutlu S, et al. Heart disease in Friedreich's ataxia: a clinical and echocardiographic study. *Acta Pediatr Jpn* 1996;38:308–311.
102. Casazza F, Ferrari F, Finocchiaro G. Echocardiographic evaluation of verapamil in Friedreich's ataxia. *Br Heart J* 1986;55:400–404.
103. Khakoo AY, Halushka MK, Rame EJ, et al. Reversible cardiomyopathy caused by administration of interferon-α. *Nat Clin Prac Cardiovasc Med* 2005;2:53–57.
104. McCall D. Alcohol and the cardiovascular system. *Curr Probl Cardiol* 1987;12:349–414.
105. Schwarz F, Mall G, Zebe H, et al. Determinants of survival in patients with congestive cardiomyopathy: quantitative morphologic findings and left ventricular hemodynamics. *Circulation* 1984;70:923–928.
106. Kinney EL, Wright RJ, Caldwell JW. Risk factors in alcoholic cardiomyopathy. *Angiology* 1989;40:270–275.
107. Mrlgaard H, Kristensen BØ, Baandrup U. Importance of abstention from alcohol in alcoholic heart disease. *Int J Cardiol* 1990;26:373–375.
108. Pavan D, Nicolosi GL, Lestuzzi C, et al. Normalization of variables of left ventricular function in patients with alcoholic cardiomyopathy after cessation of excessive alcohol intake: an echocardiographic study. *Eur Heart J* 1987;8:535–540.
109. Shan K, Lincoff M, Young JB. Anthracycline-induced cardiotoxicity. *Ann Intern Med* 1996;125:47–58.
110. Billingam ME, Bristow MR. Endomyocardial biopsy for cardiac monitoring of patients receiving anthracyclines. In: Fenoglio JJ, ed. *Endomyocardial biopsy: techniques and application.* Boca Raton, FL: CRC Press, 1982: 66–77.
111. Isner JM, Estes III NAM, Thompson PD, et al. Acute cardiac events temporally related to cocaine use. *N Engl J Med* 1986;315:1438–1443.
112. Karch RA, Billingham ME. The pathology and etiology of cocaine-induced heart disease. *Arch Pathol Lab Med* 1988;112:225–230.
113. Ikaheimo MJ, Niemela KO, Linnaluoto MM, et al. Early cardiac changes related to radiation therapy. *Am J Cardiol* 1985;56:943–946.
114. Totterman KG, Pesonen E, Siltanen P. Radiation-related chronic heart disease. *Chest* 1983;83:875–878.
115. Taymor-Luria H, Kohn K, Pasternak RC. Radiation heart disease. *J Cardiovasc Surg* 1983;8:113.
116. Fajardo LF, Stewart JR. Pathogenesis of radiation-induced myocardial fibrosis. *Lab Invest* 1973;29:244–257.
117. Warda M, Khan A, Massumi A, et al. Radiation-induced valvular dysfunction. *J Am Coll Cardiol* 1983;2:180–185.
118. Simon EB, Ling J, Mendizabal RC, et al. Radiation-induced coronary artery disease. *Am Heart J* 1984;108:1032–1034.
119. Merrill J, Greco FA, Zimbler H. Adriamycin and radiation: synergistic cardiotoxicity. *Ann Intern Med* 1975;82:122–123.
120. Hancock SL, Tucker MA, Hoppe RT. Factors affecting late mortality from heart disease after treatment of Hodgkin's disease. *JAMA* 1993;270:1949–1955.
121. Estes ML, Ewing-Wilson D, Chou SM, et al. Chloroquine neuromyotoxicity: clinical and pathologic perspective. *Am J Med* 1987;82:447–455.
122. McAllister HA Jr, Ferrans VJ, et al. Chloroquine-induced cardiomyopathy. *Arch Pathol Lab Med* 1987;111:953–956.
123. Ratliff NB, Estes ML, Myles JL, et al. The diagnosis of chloroquine cardiomyopathy by endomyocardial biopsy. *N Engl J Med* 1987;316:191–193.
124. Pearson GD, Veille JC, Rahimtoola S, et al. Peripartum cardiomyopathy: National Heart, Lung, and Blood Institute and Office of Rare Diseases (National Institutes of Health) workshop recommendations and review. *JAMA* 2000;283:1183–1188.
125. Cunningham FG, Pritchard JA, Hankins GD, et al. Peripartum heart failure: idiopathic cardiomyopathy or compounding cardiovascular events? *Obstet Gynecol* 1986;67:157–168.
126. Pierce JA, Price BO, Joyce JW. Familial occurrence of postpartal heart failure. *Arch Intern Med* 1963;111:651–655.
127. Veille JC. Peripartum cardiomyopathies: a review. *Am J Obstet Gynecol* 1984;148:805–818.
128. Cole P, Cook F, Plappert T, et al. Longitudinal changes in left ventricular architecture and function in peripartum cardiomyopathy. *Am J Cardiol* 1987;60:871–876.
129. Demakis JG, Rahimtoola SH, Sutton GC, et al. Natural course of peripartum cardiomyopathy. *Circulation* 1971;44:1053–1061.
130. Lampert MB, Hibbard J, Weinert L, et al. Peripartum heart failure associated with prolonged tocolytic therapy. *Am J Obstet Gynecol* 1993;168: 493–495.
131. O'Connell JB, Costanzo-Nordin MR, Subramanian R, et al. Peripartum cardiomyopathy: clinical, hemodynamic, histologic, and prognostic characteristics. *J Am Coll Cardiol* 1986;8:52–56.
132. Melvin KR, Richardson PJ, Osen EGJ, et al. Peripartum cardiomyopathy due to myocarditis. *N Engl J Med* 1982;307:731–734.
133. Midei MG, DeMent SH, Feldman AM, et al. Peripartum myocarditis and cardiomyopathy. *Circulation* 1990;81:922–928.
134. Herskowitz A, Cambell S, Deckers J, et al. Demographic features and prevalence of idiopathic myocarditis in patients undergoing endomyocardial biopsy. *Am J Cardiol* 1993;71:982–986.
135. Rizeq MN, Rickenbacher PR, Fowler MB, et al. Incidence of myocarditis in peripartum cardiomyopathy. *Am J Cardiol* 1994;74:474–477.
136. Ardehali H, Kasper EK, Baughman KL. Peripartum cardiomyopathy. *Minerva Cardioangiol* 2003;51:41–48.
137. Walsh JJ, Burch GE, Black WC, et al. Idiopathic myocardiopathy of the puerperium: postpartal heart disease. *Circulation* 1965;32:19–31.
138. Wulsch JJ, Burch GE. Postpartal heart disease. *Arch Intern Med* 1961; 108:817–823.
139. Rutherford SE, Phelan JP. Thromboembolic disease in pregnancy. *Clin Perinatol* 1986;13:719–739.
140. Hovsepian PG, Ganzel B, Sohi GS, et al. Peripartum cardiomyopathy treated with a left ventricular assist device as a bridge to cardiac transplantation. *South Med J* 1989;82:527–529.
141. Lewis R, Mabie WC, Burlew B, et al. Biventricular assist device as a bridge to cardiac transplantation in the treatment of peripartum cardiomyopathy. *South Med J* 1997;90:955–958.
142. Bozkurt B, Villaneuva FS, Holubkov R, et al. Intravenous immune globulin in the therapy of peripartum cardiomyopathy. *J Am Coll Cardiol* 1999; 34:177–180.
143. Elkayam U, Ostrzega EL, Shotan A. Peripartum cardiomyopathy. In: Gleicher N, ed. *Principles and practice of medical therapy in pregnancy,* 2nd ed. Norwalk, CT: Appleton & Lange, 1992.
144. Lampert MB, Weinert L, Hibbard J, et al. Contractile reserve in patients with peripartum cardiomyopathy and recovered left ventricular function. *J Am Coll Cardiol* 1994;23:428A (abst).
145. De Belder AJ, Radomski MW, Why HJ, et al. Myocardial calcium-independent nitric oxide synthase activity is present in dilated cardiomyopathy, myocarditis, and postpartum cardiomyopathy but not in ischaemic or valvular heart disease. *Br Heart J* 1995;74:426–430.
146. Ardehali H, Kasper EK, Baughman KL. Diagnostic approach to the patient with cardiomyopathy: whom to biopsy. *Am Heart J* 2005;149:7–12.
147. Ardehali H, Qasim A, Cappola T, et al. Endomyocardial biopsy plays a role in diagnosing patients with unexplained cardiomyopathy. *Am Heart J* 2004;147:919–923.
148. Thierfelder L, Watkins H, MacRae C, et al. Alpha-tropomyosin and cardiac troponin T mutations cause familial hypertrophic cardiomyopathy: a disease of the sarcomere. *Cell* 1994;77:701–712.

CHAPTER 90 ■ CARDIAC TRANSPLANTATION AND MECHANICAL CIRCULATORY SUPPORT

DALE G. RENLUND, DAVID O. TAYLOR, AND NICHOLAS G. SMEDIRA

OVERVIEW

Cardiac transplantation has become the most effective treatment for selected patients with end-stage heart failure. Sound, evidence-based immunosuppressive strategies have decreased morbidity and mortality, making survival routine. Most infections and rejections are either preventable or treatable, and the temporary, pretransplant use of mechanical circulatory support (MCS) no longer portends a poor prognosis following transplantation. Although cardiac allograft vasculopathy (CAV) and malignancy limit long-term survival, approximately 50% of recipients are alive 10 years after transplantation. Because the availability of this effective treatment depends on a limited supply of donor hearts, care must be taken to ensure that individuals listed as candidates for cardiac transplantation are those who will likely benefit the most. Potentially suitable candidates should be referred early in the course of their end-stage disease to heart failure and transplant specialists so that transplantation or alternative treatment strategies can be appropriately timed and implemented. After transplantation, the care of recipients should be directed, at least in part, by transplant physicians.

HISTORICAL PERSPECTIVE

Patients with severe heart failure have a 1- to 2-year mortality approaching 50% despite appropriate and advanced medical treatment (see Chapter 83). Heart transplantation alters the course of end-stage heart disease, with 1-, 3-, and 10-year survival rates exceeding 83%, 75%, and 45%, respectively. In selected patients with end-stage heart failure, heart transplantation is the most effective treatment. More than 60,000 procedures have been performed in over 330 centers worldwide, and nearly 3,000 additional procedures are performed each year (1).

Because the propensity to reject the transplanted heart decreases over time, the first year after transplantation presents the highest risk of rejection. Because higher doses of immunosuppressive agents are used during this time, the first year also presents the highest rate of infection. After the first few years, CAV and malignancy become the leading causes of death, the former accounting for one quarter of the deaths among transplant recipients (1–3).

Although management of end-stage heart failure and cardiac transplant patients is challenging, requiring vigilance and attention to detail, the care of potential transplant patients and posttransplant patients is important to both internists and cardiologists (4). Primary care physicians provide at least some of the care for patients awaiting cardiac transplantation (>4,000 in the United States alone) and for many cardiac transplant recipients. Moreover, knowing when to refer a patient to a heart failure and transplant specialist for evaluation is of paramount importance. Early referral of any patient who has persistent significant left ventricular dysfunction (ejection fraction <25%) despite appropriate medical therapy is warranted, not only to evaluate the patient's potential need for cardiac transplantation but also to assess whether alternative therapies might delay or obviate the need for transplantation.

TABLE 90.1

INDICATIONS FOR CARDIAC TRANSPLANTATION CANDIDACY

Heart failure requiring mechanical assistance (e.g., respirator, IABP, or VAD) with, at worst, reversible end-organ damage
Refractory heart failure requiring continuous inotropic support and invasive monitoring
NYHA class III or IV symptoms with marked functional limitation and poor 12-month prognosis despite optimal medical therapy (peak oxygen consumption <12–14 mL/kg/min or marked serial decline, progression of symptoms, or clinical instability)
Recurrent or rapidly progressive medically unresponsive heart failure symptoms
Severe hypertrophic or restrictive cardiomyopathy with NYHA class IV symptoms
Severe, refractory angina pectoris despite optimal β-blocker, calcium channel blocker, and nitrate therapy, not amenable to revascularization, accompanied by evidence of myocardial ischemia within the first two stages of a standard Bruce exercise protocol
Recurrent symptomatic, life-threatening ventricular arrhythmias despite all appropriate conventional medical and surgical modalities
Cardiac tumors confined to the heart with a low likelihood of metastasis at time of transplant
Hypoplastic left heart syndrome
Complex congenital heart disease with progressive ventricular failure, not amenable to conventional surgical repair or palliation
In pediatric patients, progressive deterioration in left ventricular ejection fraction or functional status, failure to grow, or progressive rise in pulmonary vascular resistance, despite optimal medical therapy

Abbreviations: IABP, intraaortic balloon pump; VAD, ventricular assist device; NYHA, New York Heart Association.

CLINICAL PROFILE

Recipient Selection

Indications

Cardiac transplantation is indicated for any one of the many reasons listed in Table 90.1 (1,5). Before transplantation is considered, however, a thorough search for reversible or surgically repairable cardiac disease is completed and optimal medical management implemented. At the least, patients either have failed to improve with a trial of β-blocker therapy or have clear contraindications to β-blocker use. Confidence that the medical therapy is optimal is increased when the therapy is directed or administered by heart failure specialists.

Patients who require continuous intravenous inotropic support (e.g., dobutamine hydrochloride or milrinone lactate) or MCS (intraaortic balloon pump or left ventricular assist device [LVAD]) despite maximal medical therapy for heart failure are likely to benefit from transplantation and should be evaluated. Individuals whose predicted chance of survival for 1 year is less than 80% without heart transplantation warrant consideration for transplantation. Identifying all patients at high risk for death during continued medical therapy remains challenging, as does determining whether less ill, ambulatory patients with heart failure will benefit from transplantation. Most patients being considered for cardiac transplantation usually have New York Heart Association class III to IV symptoms despite receiving best medical therapy. Ambulatory candidates usually have peak oxygen consumption (Vo_2) values of 14 mL/kg/min or less when assessed by maximal exercise tolerance testing. Unless the test is terminated because of myocardial ischemia or ventricular arrhythmias, anaerobic threshold occurs at 50% to 70% of peak oxygen uptake. The effects of age, gender, and conditioning effects on maximal oxygen uptake must be considered in interpreting Vo_2 data.

Assessment of Risk of Mortality and Morbidity after Transplantation

Anecdotal experience of successfully overcoming isolated risk factors cannot justify ignoring known risks in the majority of situations (Table 90.2).

Management of the Patient Awaiting Transplantation

While the patient awaits transplantation, there should be a low threshold for hospitalization and more intensive heart failure treatment for any hemodynamic deterioration. Such deterioration may manifest as significant azotemia, refractory salt and water overload, persistent hypotension, altered mental status, or even gastrointestinal distress. Signs and symptoms of low cardiac output prompt escalation in therapy from intravenous diuretics to intravenous inotropic agents, and from intravenous inotropic agents to intraaortic balloon pump or MCS. Heart transplant candidates who nonetheless develop irreversible end-organ failure in other organ systems or who are likely to die despite transplantation are not transplanted. Therapeutic approaches to prevent sudden death, especially the use of implantable cardioverter defibrillators, are used (6).

Mechanical Circulatory Support

For patients who are unable to be stabilized on a heart failure regimen including inotropic agents, mechanical support devices have become standard. Approximately 25% to 30% of patients undergoing transplantation are bridged to transplant with a mechanical support device. The most recent LVAD registry data suggest that bridge-to-transplant survival has remained unchanged over the past 5 years (7). Approximately 65% to 70% of patients supported with an LVAD alone survive to undergo transplantation. If a right ventricular assist device is used along with an LVAD, the survival to transplant declines to 50%.

The timing of MCS deployment in a transplant candidate is challenging. Premature use of MCS is unnecessary, increases overall costs, and can potentially negate a candidate's opportunity for transplant. If MCS is used too late, overall costs again increase, lengths of hospital stays are increased, and a candidate may not sufficiently recover to become an acceptable candidate again.

As hemodynamic compromise progresses from moderate to severe in a patient awaiting heart transplantation, not only is there an increase in the risk of dying before transplantation can be performed, but the results after transplantation also worsen. The timely use of MCS halts further deterioration, decreases the likelihood of death before transplantation can occur, and reverses metabolic, cellular, and nutritional compromise. The

TABLE 90.2

MORBIDITY AND MORTALITY RISK AFTER CARDIAC TRANSPLANTATION

Characteristic	Risk
PVR >6 Wood units, unresponsive to vasodilators	Marked
PVR >6 Wood units, decreasing in response to vasodilators but not <3–4 Wood units	Moderate
Pulmonary artery systolic pressure >70 mm Hg, unresponsive to treatment	Marked
Transpulmonic gradient (mean PAP – PCWP) >15–20 mm Hg	Moderate
Active, untreated infection	Marked
Treated infection currently controlled on antibiotics	Moderate
Irreversible, severe hepatic disease	Marked
Moderate hepatic dysfunction not clearly related to cardiac congestion	Moderate
Irreversible, severe renal disease	Marked
Moderate renal dysfunction not clearly related to low cardiac output	Moderate
Irreversible, severe pulmonary disease	Marked
Irreversible, moderate pulmonary disease	Moderate
Recent pulmonary infarction	Moderate
Age 65–70 y	Moderate
Age >70 y	Marked
Diabetes mellitus with significant end-organ damage	Moderate to marked
Cerebrovascular disease, severe, symptomatic	Marked
Peripheral vascular disease, severe, symptomatic	Marked
Gastrointestinal bleeding, active	Marked
Diverticulitis, recent	Moderate
Chronic active hepatitis	Moderate to marked
Hepatitis C infection with low viral load and benign liver biopsy	Minimal
HIV	Marked
Malignancy, recent	Marked
Myocardial infiltrative disease	Marked
Myocardial inflammatory disease	Moderate
Major affective disorder or schizophrenia with poor control	Marked
Major affective disorder or schizophrenia with good control	Moderate
Personality disorders	Moderate
Cigarette abuse	Moderate
Substance abuse, active unresolved	Marked
Substance abuse, resolved albeit recently	Moderate
Medical noncompliance	Marked
Obesity, moderate (120–140% ideal body weight or BMI 30–35)	Moderate
Osteoporosis	Moderate
Lack of social support	Minimal to moderate

Abbreviations: PVR, pulmonary vascular resistance; PAP, pulmonary artery pressure; PCWP, pulmonary capillary wedge pressure; BMI, body mass index (weight in kg divided by height in m^2).

temporary use of such support thus permits heart transplant with a greater expectation of long-term survival and a better quality of life (8).

Because a variety of bridging devices are commercially available, the selection of a device depends on the type of heart failure, the size of the patient, the surgeon's experience, and the institutional preference. Implantable LVADs channel blood from the left ventricle to the pump, which then circulates blood to the aorta. The currently available implantable devices are too large for patients with a body surface area of less than 1.5 m^2, but investigations with smaller devices are ongoing. Meanwhile, paracorporeal devices, with the pump placed outside the body, provide an alternative for the support of one or both ventricles. LVADs are generally inadequate for bridging to transplantation in patients with severe biventricular heart failure, which requires the use of two paracorporeal devices (8).

When LVADs or paracorporeal devices are either difficult to use or contraindicated, the replacement of both ventricles with an implantable device such as a total artificial heart may be warranted. Such circumstances may arise in patients with severe aortic insufficiency, intractable ventricular arrhythmias, aortic prosthesis, acquired ventricular septal defect, or irreversible ventricular failure requiring a high pump output (8,9). The CardioWest artificial heart (SynCardia Systems, Tucson, AZ) provides a successful bridge to transplantation in most severely compromised patients (9). Of note, survival to transplantation of patients supported with the CardioWest artificial heart is reported to be 79% (9). Although high-flow biventricular support with the total artificial heart is theorized to improve outcomes, more experience with this Food and Drug Administration–approved device is needed for validation.

Many new devices are in clinical trials. These include inline or axial pumps such as the DeBakey (MicroMed Technology, Inc, Houston, TX), Jarvik 2000 FlowMaker (Jarvik Heart, Inc, New York, NY), HeartMate II (Thoratec Corp., Pleasanton, CA), and INCOR (Berlin Heart AG, Berlin, Germany).

Radial or centrifugal pumps include the DuraHeart (Terumo Corp., Ann Arbor, MI), VentrAssist (Ventracor Ltd, Sydney, Australia), CorAide (Arrow International, Reading, PA), HeartQuest (MedQuest Products, Inc., Salt Lake City, UT), and HeartMate III (Thoratec Corp., Pleasanton, CA). Only the CorAide and VentrAssist pumps are in clinical trials. These pumps are significantly smaller, are potentially more durable, and their thinner drivelines are associated with fewer infectious complications. However, initial survival to transplant is similar to older pulsatile pumps and pump thrombosis and thromboembolic rates appear higher than expected for devices without inflow or outflow valves.

Donor Selection

Donor selection is influenced by many factors, including ABO blood type compatibility, donor–recipient size disparity, presence of intrinsic cardiac disease, and presence of transmissible infectious or malignant diseases (10,11). The risk of using a specific donor heart is balanced against the risk with regard to a particular recipient. A decision to use a marginal donor heart may sometimes be warranted, provided that the condition of the potential recipient is sufficiently precarious and the potential recipient consents.

To identify intrinsic cardiac disease in donor hearts, electrocardiography, echocardiography, and (at times) coronary angiography are used. Electrocardiographic abnormalities that generally preclude the use of a donor heart include evidence of myocardial infarction and significant ventricular arrhythmias. Echocardiographic abnormalities that generally preclude the use of a donor heart include significant global hypokinesis, significant valvular abnormalities, and moderate to severe left ventricular hypertrophy. In addition, evidence of a significant cardiac contusion generally precludes use of the donor heart. However, far too many hearts are turned down on the basis of "poor quality." Recovery of hearts from a consented donor is around 50%. Poor cardiac function is the reason the organ is declined in 60% of the cases. To improve recovery, management recommendations include the liberal use of pulmonary artery catheters to optimize fluid resuscitation, T3 administration, corticosteroids to reduce the inflammatory state, and vasopressin to return vascular tone rather than relying on the vasoconstricting effects of high doses of dopamine (12–14). This paradigm has not been proven in a randomized clinical trial, but small series support its use. Reliance on echocardiograms to determine cardiac function has significant limitations. After brain death, the catecholamine storm often induces transient ventricular dysfunction (15). Because the echocardiogram is often not repeated, a poorly functioning heart is often turned down despite the return of normal function after resuscitation. In this setting repeating the echocardiogram or inserting a pulmonary artery catheter helps to determine if the heart has recovered. If the recovery is incomplete, careful assessment of other factors such as ischemic time, likelihood of early rejection, and high pulmonary artery pressures may impact the decision to utilize the organ for a particular recipient.

The concept of using expanded donor criteria, or marginal donors, is well established. Jeevanandum et al. (16) advanced this concept in 1996 and this group demonstrated outstanding results albeit with patients initially having a more complicated early recovery. In other reports, older donors, longer ischemic times, and undersizing by more than 50% remain risk factors for early mortality (17,18). Intracerebral bleed as the cause of donor brain death may be a risk factor or just a covariate associated with older women with hypertrophied ventricles (19). Although older donor hearts are associated with higher risks, many have been successfully used (1,20). Coronary angiography is recommended in all male donors older than 45 years and in female donors older than 50 years. If risk factors for coronary artery disease are present in younger donors, coronary angiography is also recommended.

To avoid transmitting infectious disease with the donated heart, a series of tests are performed to determine the suitability for transplantation. A history of behaviors, especially recent, that predispose to human immunodeficiency virus (HIV) infection or viral hepatitis (e.g., intravenous drug use); positivity for HIV, hepatitis B surface antigen, or hepatitis C; and uncontrolled gram-negative sepsis generally preclude donor use. Typically, if the donor has a malignancy not confined to the cranium, the donor heart is not used.

ANATOMIC CONSIDERATIONS: IMPLANTATION TECHNIQUES

Minimization of donor heart ischemic time—the time of aortic cross-clamping in the donor to release of aortic cross-clamp in the recipient—is key to successful transplantation (21). Ischemic time less than 4 hours is generally acceptable. Two orthotopic techniques are used to replace the recipient heart with the donor heart: (a) the traditional Lower and Shumway technique, in which the donor right atrium is attached directly to the recipient right atrium, and (b) the increasingly employed bicaval technique, in which superior and inferior vena cavae are attached separately. The bicaval technique results in a slightly longer donor heart ischemic time, but is associated with a more "anatomic" transplant with lower right atrial pressure, lower incidence of atrial tachyarrhythmias, and less tricuspid valve incompetence (22). Despite the increasing use of the bicaval technique, tricuspid regurgitation remains a common problem both early and late after cardiac transplantation. Often thought of as just a nuisance, a recent study suggests it may have significant hemodynamic consequences. Performing prophylactic suture annuloplasty at implant not only reduced the incidence of tricuspid regurgitation, but surprisingly and inexplicably reduced perioperative mortality from graft dysfunction (23). This study was small, but an annuloplasty of the tricuspid valve could be considered at the time of transplantation.

In heterotopic cardiac transplantation, which is rarely performed, the donor heart is placed in the right lower thorax parallel to the recipient heart, which is left in place. Anastomoses are made between donor left atrium and recipient left atrium, donor and recipient aortae, donor superior vena cava and recipient right atrium or superior vena cava, and donor pulmonary artery and recipient pulmonary artery or right atrium. The indications for heterotopic cardiac transplantation include severely elevated pulmonary hypertension, a small donor heart, or a donor heart with anticipated poor initial function.

POSTTRANSPLANT COMPLICATIONS

Most recipients experience cardiac, infectious, or other complications following cardiac transplantation. Common complications are noted in Table 90.3. Although the complications encountered after cardiac transplantation are legion, most problems can be prevented, ameliorated, or treated.

Ventricular Dysfunction

The initial function of the newly transplanted cardiac allograft is influenced by pre-explant variables (e.g., degree of inotropic support, cardiopulmonary resuscitation, and trauma), the ischemic time, effectiveness of cardioplegia, and total

TABLE 90.3

COMPLICATIONS AFTER CARDIAC TRANSPLANTATION

Cardiac	Infectious	Other
Ventricular dysfunction	Bacterial	Renal insufficiency
Arrhythmias	Viral	Hypertension
Tricuspid regurgitation	Parasitic	Hyperlipidemia
Allograft rejection	Fungal	Malignancy
Allograft vasculopathy		Psychological
		Diabetes mellitus
		Osteoporosis
		Gout

denervation. Inotropic support is usually required for 2 to 5 days. If cardiac allografts function poorly because of global ischemia, they can regain normal function after as little as 1 week. Measures of left ventricular function and resting hemodynamics normalize over time.

The cardiac allograft is totally denervated at the time of transplantation, and therefore responds differently to many common cardiovascular medicines. The response to direct β-adrenergic agonists (isoproterenol, dobutamine, epinephrine, norepinephrine) is qualitatively unchanged. The response to the sympathomimetic amines that act indirectly by releasing catecholamines from nerve terminals (e.g., dopamine) is likely diminished, and supersensitivity to adenosine is typically seen. Because of denervation, atropine sulfate, digoxin, and quinidine would not be expected to affect atrioventricular conduction. Over a period of months to years, the cardiac allograft reinnervates partially in the majority of recipients (24,25).

Cardiac Arrhythmias

Sinus node dysfunction is common early after transplantation, but only rarely requires a permanent pacemaker. Postoperative atrial tachyarrhythmias may occur and are generally treated as usual, except that cardiac allograft rejection is considered in the differential diagnosis (26). Early on, postoperative ventricular ectopy can be seen, but usually resolves. Late after transplantation, although rare, recipient remnant atrial to donor atrial conduction (across the suture line) has been reported (27). After the postoperative period, electrophysiologic disease may become manifest or develop. Generally, traditional measures are appropriate, including the use of antiarrhythmic agents, devices, or interventions.

Cardiac Allograft Rejection

Pathophysiology (The Immune System)

Transplantation of an organ between members of the same species is known as *allotransplantation*; hence, the use of the term *cardiac allograft*. Alloantigens are molecules recognized as foreign (or non-self) by the recipient immune system. In the absence of immunosuppression, destruction of the alloantigens—and the organ bearing them—occurs (2,28).

HLA antigens are serologically identified alloantigens that have been shown to correspond to the human major histocompatibility complex (MHC). These cell-surface antigens are subclassified as MHC class I (HLA-A, HLA-B, and HLA-C) or MHC class II (HLA-DP, HLA-DQ, and HLA-DR). Whereas HLA antigens have distinctly different roles in the rejection process, prospective HLA matching is generally not possible in heart transplantation. The sequence of events leading to cardiac allograft rejection encompasses antigen recognition, primary and secondary signals for T-cell activation, and T-cell proliferation and differentiation (Fig. 90.1).

After the heart is transplanted, antigen-presenting cells of recipient or donor origin migrate to secondary lymphoid organs where donor antigen is presented to T cells. Donor antigen engages T-cell receptors (primary signal), and CD80 and CD86 on the antigen-presenting cell engage CD28 on the T cell (secondary signal). The primary and secondary signals activate at least three signal transduction pathways: (a) the calcium–calcineurin pathway that activates the transcription factor, nuclear factor of activated T cells (NFAT); (b) the mitogen-activated protein kinase pathway that activates the transcription factor, activating protein 1; and (c) the protein kinase-C nuclear factor κB pathway that activates the transcription factor, NF-κB. The combined effect of these three pathways is further activation of the antigen-presenting cell, by the expression of CD154 on the T cell, which interacts with CD40 on the antigen presenting, expression of the interleukin (IL)-2 receptor α chain, CD25, and synthesis of IL-2. Activation of the IL-2 receptor delivers growth signals through the molecular-target-of-rapamycin (mTOR) pathway, which initiates the cell cycle (28–32).

T cells are activated and undergo clonal expansion and differentiation to express effector functions. Under the influence of pro-inflammatory cytokines, effector cells for cell-mediated and antibody-mediated immunity are generated. Destruction

→

FIGURE 90.1. Mechanism of action of immunosuppressive drugs. Typically, one calcineurin inhibitor (depicted in orange), one antiproliferative (depicted in green), or proliferation signal inhibitor (depicted in yellow), and a corticosteroid are used in combination. Monoclonal and polyclonal antibodies (depicted in blue) are used to delay the use of a calcineurin inhibitor or to treat rejection. The calcineurin inhibitors, cyclosporine (CsA) and tacrolimus (Tac), bind to cyclophilin (CpN) and FK-binding protein (FKBP), respectively, and then inhibit calcineurin-dependent dephosphorylation of NFAT. Mycophenolic acid (MPA), the active derivative of mycophenolate mofetil (MMF), inhibits inosine monophosphate dehydrogenase-dependent purine biosynthesis. Azathioprine (AZA) is metabolized to 6-mercaptopurine (6-MP), which inhibits cell-cycling by providing a "false" purine. Sirolimus (SRL) and everolimus (ERL) bind to FKBP and inhibit molecular target of rapamycin (mTOR), preventing cyclin-dependent kinase (CDK)-mediated cell-cycling. Antithymocyte globulins (ATG) bind to T-cell surface antigens (e.g., CD2, CD4, or CD5) enabling lymphocyte opsonization by the reticuloendothelial system (RES). Muromonab-CD3 (OKT3) binds to the CD3 surface antigen, inhibits antigen recognition by the T-cell receptor (TCR), and promotes opsonization by the RES. Anti-CD25 monoclonal antibodies (MAB) prevent IL-2 and IL-2–receptor engagement, and are not used to treat rejection. Corticosteroids act by binding to corticosteroid receptors, negatively impact glucocorticoid response elements (GRE), and decrease production and action of multiple interleukins. *Abbreviations:* CD, cluster determinant; MHC, major histocompatibility class; MAP, mitogen activated protein; AP-1, activating protein 1; NFκB, nuclear factor κB; mRNA, messenger ribonucleic acid.

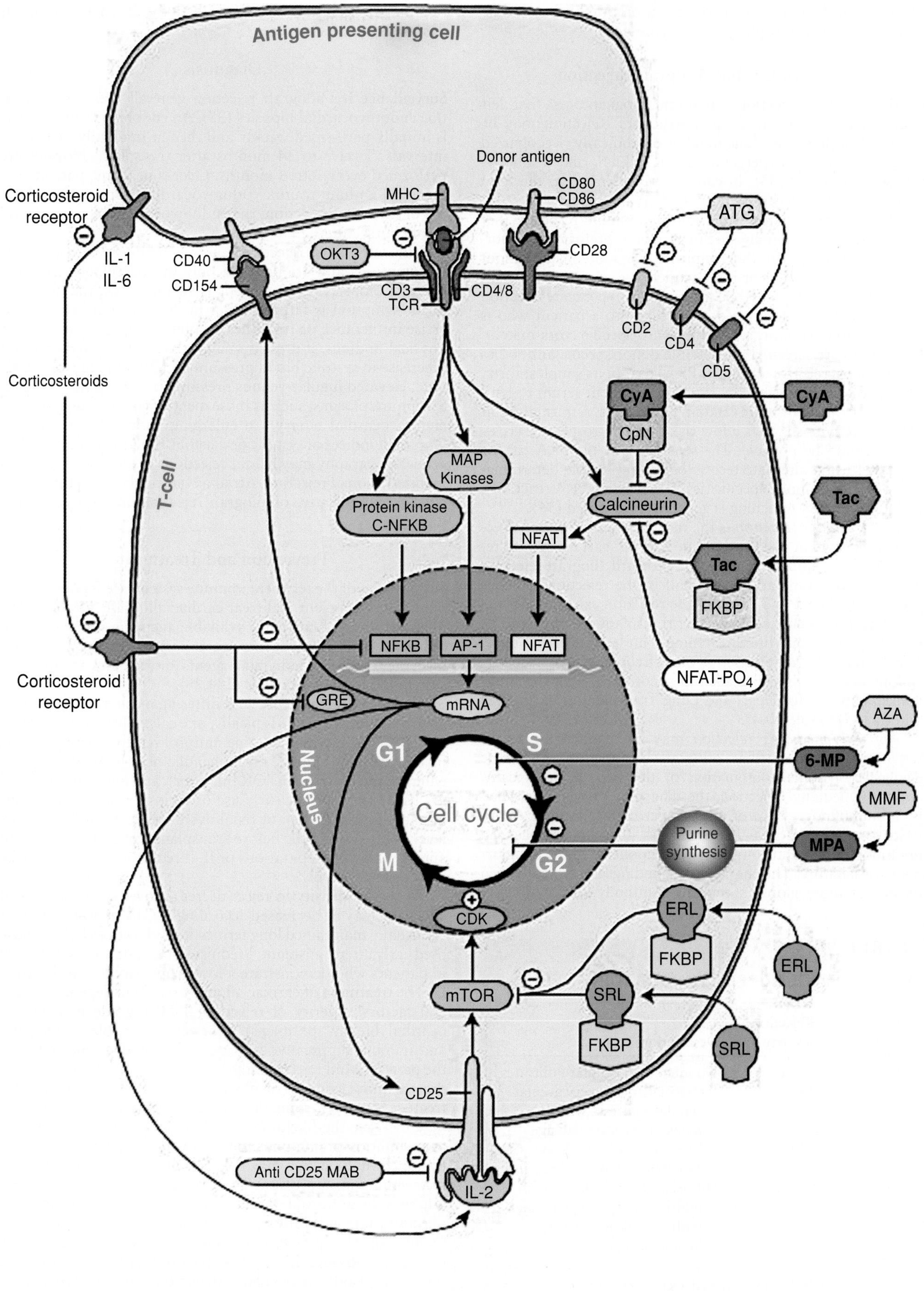
Antigen presenting cell
Donor antigen
Corticosteroid receptor
MHC
CD80
CD86
ATG
OKT3
CD28
IL-1
IL-6
CD40
CD154
CD3
TCR
CD4/8
CD2
CD4
CD5
Corticosteroids
CyA
CyA
CpN
MAP Kinases
T-cell
Protein kinase C-NFKB
Calcineurin
Tac
NFAT
Tac
FKBP
NFKB
AP-1
NFAT
NFAT-PO4
Corticosteroid receptor
GRE
mRNA
AZA
G1
S
6-MP
Nucleus
Cell cycle
MMF
M
G2
Purine synthesis
MPA
CDK
ERL
FKBP
ERL
mTOR
SRL
FKBP
SRL
CD25
Anti CD25 MAB
IL-2

of the allograft occurs via involvement of antibody, cytotoxic T lymphocytes, macrophages, and cytokines.

Types of Cardiac Allograft Rejection

Cardiac allograft rejection is an immunologic process that, left unchecked, leads to allograft destruction. Rejection may be defined histologically, functionally, or clinically. Recognized categories include hyperacute, acute cellular, and antibody-mediated rejection (33). In cardiac transplantation, the term *chronic rejection* generally refers to CAV.

Hyperacute rejection is a vigorous immune response that takes place within minutes to hours, due to preformed, donor-specific antibodies in the recipient. The outcome, without repeat transplantation or total artificial heart support, is uniformly fatal. The best method for avoiding hyperacute rejection is to avoid transplanting a donor heart into a patient who is sensitized to the donor (a positive donor-specific cross-match). Candidates are screened for possible donor-specific antibodies using a panel reactive antibody (PRA) test. In its simplest form, PRA testing is performed by exposing recipient serum to lymphocytes from 50 or more random individuals. A normal result of 0% reactivity suggests a low risk that a retrospective cross-match would be positive. The sensitivity of the PRA can be increased using alternate technologies that enable determination of HLA antibody specificities. For elevated PRA reactivity, prospective cross-matching is generally warranted (34).

Acute cellular rejection is the most common form of rejection and occurs in one third to one half of heart transplant recipients. Even though the propensity toward allograft rejection decreases over time and nearly half of the rejection episodes occur in the first 2 to 3 months, late rejection can and does occur. Rejection occurring early after transplantation tends to be more aggressive and life threatening than late-occurring rejection. Acute cellular rejection is most frequently diagnosed by endomyocardial biopsy graded in accordance with the International Society for Heart and Lung Transplantation (ISHLT) criteria (35) (Table 90.4).

Antibody-mediated rejection may be manifest by otherwise unexplained cardiac allograft dysfunction, histologic evidence, or some combination of the two. Histologically, antibody-mediated rejection, the diagnosis of which is aided by immunofluorescence or immunoperoxidase staining, manifests as a scant cellular infiltrate with abundant colocalized immunoglobulin and complement components in the allograft microvasculature. The characteristic findings are typically seen on one or more biopsy specimens. Antibody-mediated rejection may be seen only histologically in the absence of allograft dysfunction and vice versa (36,37).

TABLE 90.4

ACUTE CELLULAR REJECTION GRADING (ISHLT)

Numeric grade	Rejection severity	Description
0 R	None	No interstitial cellular infiltrates
1 R	Mild	Interstitial and/or perivascular cellular infiltrate with ≤1 focus of myocyte damage
2 R	Moderate	≥2 foci of cellular infiltrate with associated myocyte damage
3 R	Severe	Diffuse cellular infiltrate with multifocal myocyte damage, with or without edema, hemorrhage, or vasculitis

Abbreviations: ISHLT, International Society for Heart and Lung Transplantation; R, refers simply to a revision of an earlier scale.

Diagnosis

Surveillance for allograft rejection generally centers on routine endomyocardial biopsies (38). An endomyocardial biopsy is initially performed weekly and then at gradually increasing intervals. Twelve to 24 months after transplant, biopsies are performed every 3 to 6 months. Over time, some patients are managed without routine endomyocardial biopsies (39). After the diagnosis of rejection, the endomyocardial biopsy interval is, of course, altered.

Clinically, most rejection episodes manifest with no signs or symptoms and are detected only by surveillance endomyocardial biopsies. If the episode is symptomatic, the most frequent symptom is fatigue. Later in the rejection process, exercise intolerance or frank heart failure symptoms may occur. Physical findings, if present, may include relative hypotension (decrease in systolic blood pressure of >20 mm Hg from baseline), elevated jugular venous pressure, or a third heart sound. Symptoms or signs, such as those mentioned, prompt an urgent endomyocardial biopsy. An enlarging pericardial effusion or worsened indices of systolic or diastolic function determined by echocardiography may herald rejection. Fever is an infrequent manifestation of rejection. Atrial or ventricular arrhythmias are considered indicative of allograft rejection until proven otherwise.

Prevention and Treatment

Suppression of the recipient immune system (see Figure 90.1) is necessary to prevent and treat cardiac allograft rejection. The pharmacology of currently available agents is summarized in Table 90.5. Multiple agents are almost always used to minimize the toxicity of individual agents and to block the immune system in multiple locations (2–4,28).

Generally, three agents with differing mechanisms of action and toxicities are used. Typically, one calcineurin inhibitor (cyclosporine or tacrolimus), one antiproliferative (azathioprine, mycophenolate mofetil, mycophenolic acid [extended release enteric coated], or an mTOR inhibitor), and one corticosteroid are used. To avoid the early use of cyclosporine or tacrolimus in patients at high risk of renal dysfunction (serum creatinine level >2.0–3.0 mg/dL before transplant), one of a variety of antilymphocyte preparations or IL-2 receptor blockers may be used perioperatively.

As the propensity to reject decreases over time, dosages of all agents may be decreased accordingly. Calcineurin inhibitors are usually maintained long term at levels less than half of those used early after transplant. Prednisone can safely be withdrawn in patients who demonstrate a low propensity to reject (40).

The treatment of cardiac allograft rejection depends on several factors: severity of rejection (ISHLT grade of endomyocardial biopsy specimens), time since transplant, rejection and immunosuppressive history, and hemodynamic status of the patient. Mild rejection in hemodynamically stable patients, those without evidence of allograft dysfunction, is generally not treated. However, some data suggest that even mild rejection may increase the likelihood of CAV. Mild rejection warrants augmentation of immunosuppression in the setting of allograft dysfunction. Rejection may be treated by changing the maintenance immunosuppression. For instance, a different calcineurin inhibitor or antiproliferative agent could be used. In treating rejection, one generally optimizes or increases the dosages of maintenance immunosuppressants and markedly increases corticosteroid dosages. In corticosteroid-refractory rejection or in rejection episodes associated with hemodynamic instability, antilymphocyte antibodies are added. Moderate rejection in the absence of hemodynamic instability is usually treated initially

TABLE 90.5

PHARMACOLOGY OF IMMUNOSUPPRESSIVE AGENTS

Agent	Identification	Mechanism of action	Administration	Toxicity	Drug interactions and uses
Cyclosporine[a]	Cyclic undecapeptide produced by *Tolypocladium inflatum Gams*	Inhibits calcineurin	PO or IV, oral to IV dose adjustment is 3:1, oral dosage 3–6 mg/kg/d, monitor levels	Nephrotoxicity, hypertension, gingival hyperplasia, hirsutism, tremor, headache, paresthesias	Metabolism decreased by ketoconazole, diltiazem hydrochloride, verapamil hydrochloride, erythromycin, cimetidine, grapefruit; metabolism increased by phenytoin, phenobarbital, isoniazid, rifampin, carbamazepine; used in long-term maintenance
Tacrolimus	Macrolide isolate of *Streptomyces tsukubaensis*	Inhibits calcineurin	PO or IV, oral to IV dose adjustment is 5:1, oral dose 0.05–0.15 mg/kg/d, monitor levels	Nephrotoxicity, hypertension, tremor, headache, flushing, paresthesias, glucose intolerance	Metabolism decreased by ketoconazole, diltiazem, verapamil, erythromycin, cimetidine, grapefruit; metabolism increased by phenytoin, phenobarbital, isoniazid, rifampin, carbamazepine; used in long-term maintenance
Azathioprine	Prodrug of 6-mercaptopurine	Inhibits purine biosynthesis	PO or IV, 1–2 mg/kg/d, WBC to remain >4,500/mm^3	Anemia, leukopenia, pancreatitis, cholestatic jaundice, hepatitis	Metabolism decreased by allopurinol which inhibits xanthine oxidase. When used with allopurinol, azathioprine dosage is decreased by two thirds and WBC monitored; used in long-term maintenance
Mycophenolate mofetil	Morpholinoethylester of mycophenolic acid	Inhibits inosine monophosphate dehydrogenase, inhibiting purine biosynthesis	PO or IV, 2,000–6,000 mg/d.	Gastrointestinal distress, leukopenia, anemia	No significant interactions; used in long-term maintenance
Mycophenolic acid	Enteric-coated, extended-release formulation	Inhibits inosine monophosphate dehydrogenase, inhibiting purine biosynthesis.	PO only, 1,440–4,320 mg/d	Gastrointestinal distress, anemia, leukopenia	No significant interactions; used in long-term maintenance
Sirolimus	Macrocyclic triene produced by *Streptomyces hygroscopicus*	Inhibits mTOR, inhibiting cell cycling	PO only, 1–2 mg/d	Hypertriglyceridemia, thrombocytopenia, leukopenia, rash, gastrointestinal distress	Metabolism decreased by diltiazem and ketoconazole; metabolism increased by rifampin; interactions probably similar to those for cyclosporine; used in long-term maintenance
Everolimus	Derivative of sirolimus	Inhibits mTOR, inhibiting cell cycling.	PO only, 1.5–3.0 mg/d.	Hypertriglyceridemia, thrombocytopenia, leukopenia, rash, gastrointestinal distress	Metabolism decreased by diltiazem and ketoconazole; metabolism increased by rifampin; interactions probably similar to those for cyclosporine; used in long-term maintenance

(*Continued*)

TABLE 90.5

(CONTINUED) PHARMACOLOGY OF IMMUNOSUPPRESSIVE AGENTS

Agent	Identification	Mechanism of action	Administration	Toxicity	Drug interactions and uses
Corticosteroids	Synthetic or semisynthetic analogs of adrenocorticotropic hormones	Multiple; inhibits release and action of various interleukins, interferes with antigen receptor interactions	PO or IV with methylprednisolone and hydrocortisone (no significant oral to IV dose adjustment), PO with prednisone, prednisone 1 mg = hydrocortisone 4 mg = methylprednisolone 0.8 mg; maintenance dosage of prednisone is 0.0–0.1 mg/kg/d	Pituitary–adrenal suppression, cushingoid habitus, glucose intolerance, hyperlipidemia, hypertension, posterior subcapsular cataracts, myopathy, osteoporosis, skin fragility, PUD	Multiple drug interactions, none clinically significant; used in long-term maintenance and in the treatment of established rejection episodes.
Muromonab-CD3 antibody (OKT3)	IgG_{2A} murine monoclonal immunoglobulin molecule	Binds to the CD3 surface antigen of lymphocytes, inhibits antigen recognition, opsonizes lymphocytes	IV only, 2.5–5.0 mg/d	Fever, chills, gastrointestinal distress, pulmonary edema, HAMA formation	No interactions; used in early rejection prophylaxis and in the treatment of rejection
Antithymocyte globulin (ATG)	Equine polyclonal antibodies to human thymocytes	Opsonizes lymphocytes.	IV only, 10–20 mg/kg/d	Fever, chills, serum sickness, leukopenia, thrombocytopenia	No interactions; used in early rejection prophylaxis and in the treatment of rejection
Thymoglobulin	Rabbit polyclonal antibodies to human thymocytes	Opsonizes lymphocytes	IV only, 0.75–1.50 mg/kg/d	Fever, chills, serum sickness, leukopenia, thrombocytopenia	No interactions; used in early rejection prophylaxis and in the treatment of rejection
Daclizumab	Chimeric monoclonal IgG_1 antibody	Blocks the IL-2 receptor α chain (CD25)	1 mg/kg IV once at transplant, repeated, 4 times at 2-wk intervals	Gastrointestinal distress	No interactions; used in early rejection prophylaxis
Basiliximab	Chimeric monoclonal IgG_{1K} antibody	Blocks the IL-2 receptor α chain (CD25)	20 mg IV at transplant and repeated 4 d after	Gastrointestinal distress	No interactions; used in early rejection prophylaxis

[a]Cyclosporine is available in two formulations, oil based and microemulsion based. The latter is associated with better bioavailability.
Abbreviations: PO, by mouth; IV, by vein; WBC, white blood cell count; PUD, peptic ulcer disease; HAMA, human antimouse antibody; IgG, immunoglobulin G; IL, interleukin; mTOR, molecular target of rapamycin.

with a several-day course of either intravenous or high-dose oral corticosteroids. If a subsequent biopsy specimen shows resolution, the maintenance dosages are resumed. If a subsequent biopsy specimen does not show resolution, however, intravenous corticosteroids are used. Failure of a second course of corticosteroids to resolve the rejection episode generally leads to the use of antilymphocyte antibodies.

Cardiac Allograft Vasculopathy

Pathophysiology

After the first few years following transplantation, CAV is a leading cause of death and the cause of significant morbidity (1,41–43). The prevalence of angiographically detectable disease approaches 50% to 60% at 5 years, and the prevalence of disease detected by intravascular ultrasonography or at autopsy is even greater. CAV is not a homogeneous disease; rather, it changes over time. Early CAV is characterized by diffuse and distal involvement, whereas later-onset coronary artery disease is more proximal, focal, and eccentric.

Histologically, CAV is characterized by proliferation and migration of smooth muscle cells, proliferation and migration of macrophages, intact elastic lamina, increased ground substance and foam cells, and macrophage-engulfed cholesterol (44). Angiographically, several types of lesions have been described (Fig. 90.2) (45).

Various risk factors have been identified for the development of CAV diagnosed by angiography, intravascular ultrasonography, or angioscopy (1,44,46-48). Although older donor hearts are associated with an increased risk of the development of CAV, older donor hearts will likely continue to be used with even greater frequency. The more common risk factors for native coronary artery disease (e.g., hypertension, diabetes, cigarette use, hyperlipidemia, hyperhomocysteinemia, and low folate and vitamin B_6 concentrations) likely have a greater influence on the development of CAV later after transplantation (49,50).

Diagnosis

The clinical presentation of CAV early after transplant may be silent, manifesting as acute myocardial infarction, congestive heart failure, arrhythmias, wall motion abnormalities, or sudden death. Later, typical angina pectoris may occur due to partial reinnervation. Most CAV is diagnosed by routinely scheduled yearly surveillance angiography, although many noninvasive techniques have been evaluated in an attempt to decrease the need for invasive testing (42,43,51).

Regrettably, angiography is insensitive in detecting CAV. Intravascular ultrasonography is superior to angiography, detecting disease in a much larger percentage of patients. Intravascular ultrasonography predicts the development of angiographic coronary artery disease and is predictive of morbidity and mortality (42,43).

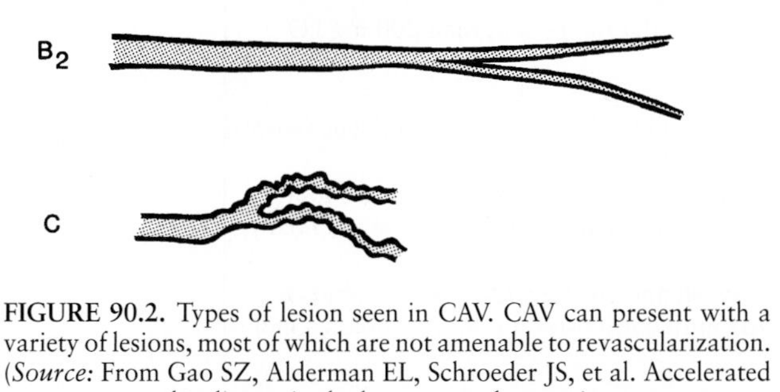

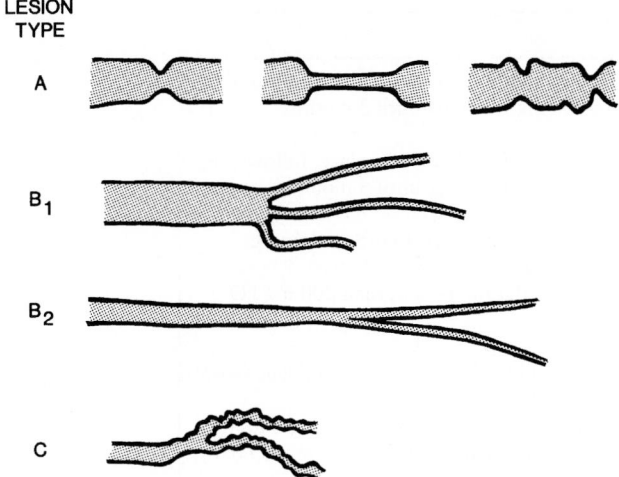

FIGURE 90.2. Types of lesion seen in CAV. CAV can present with a variety of lesions, most of which are not amenable to revascularization. (*Source:* From Gao SZ, Alderman EL, Schroeder JS, et al. Accelerated coronary vascular disease in the heart transplant patient: coronary arteriographic findings. *J Am Coll Cardiol* 1988;12:334–348, with permission.)

Prevention and Treatment

The mTOR inhibitors mitigate the development of CAV when compared to azathioprine (52,53). Further, sirolimus may decrease progression of established disease (54). Primary and secondary prevention of CAV are key; treatment of established disease appears to be limited to retransplantation and revascularization techniques. Retransplantation is the only option for patients with type B and C lesions (see Figure 90.2). Retransplantation for CAV can, if performed years after the initial transplantation, result in acceptable survival rates (1).

Infectious Complications

The types of infections expected in cardiac transplant recipients vary depending on the time from transplantation, as the intensity of immunosuppression administered varies directly with the propensity for rejection. Figure 90.3 depicts the changing frequencies of bacterial, viral, protozoal, and fungal infections after transplantation (55,56).

Bacteria and viruses account for more than 80% of infections after transplantation. The most common bacterial infections early after transplantation are nosocomial. Infected intravascular catheters or lines and pneumonias can occur. As can be seen in Figure 90.3, the risk decreases rapidly over time. The most common viral infections are caused by cytomegalovirus (CMV) and herpes simplex. Although CMV infection used to be associated with significant morbidity and mortality, the use of ganciclovir has significantly improved the prognosis (57). Patients who are CMV seronegative who receive a heart from a seropositive donor are at greatest risk for aggressive disease. Although fungi and protozoa account for less than 15% of infections after transplantation, such infections can be associated with the worst prognosis (58). Fungal infections occur in patients who require intensive treatment over a prolonged period before transplantation or who develop significant rejection in the setting of a bacterial infection that requires the use of broad-spectrum antibiotics.

Given the potential morbidity and mortality associated with infections during the first posttransplant year, infection prophylaxis is common. Prophylactic regimens are commonly used against CMV (if either recipient or donor is seropositive), toxoplasmosis (especially if the recipient tests negative and the donor tests positive), *Pneumocystis carinii*, *Candida albicans*, and herpes simplex. Strategies that have reduced the morbidity and mortality after cardiac transplantation for CMV infection, *P. carinii* pneumonia, and toxoplasmosis are shown in Table 90.6.

Renal Insufficiency

Five years after heart transplantation, 8.5% of recipients have a serum creatinine level higher than 2.5 mg/dL, and 1.9% require long-term dialysis (1). Although some renal dysfunction

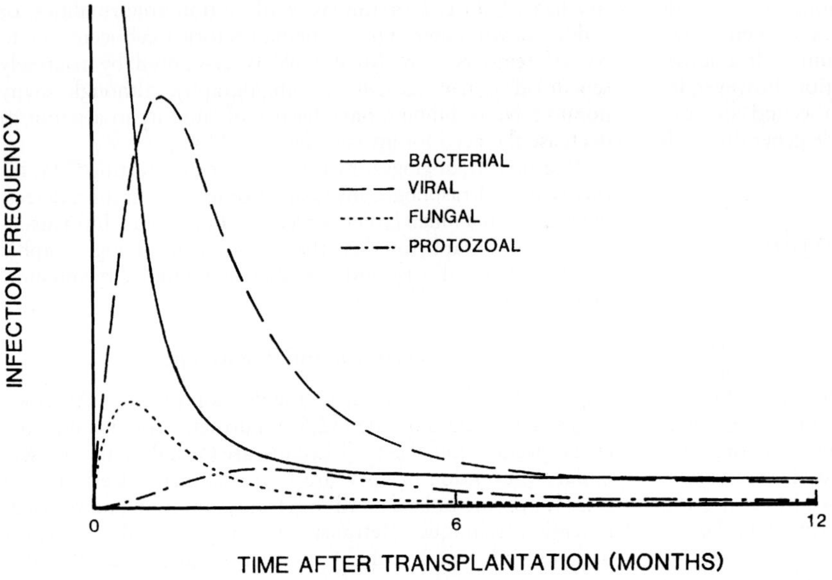

FIGURE 90.3. The risk of infection from various etiologic agents peaks at different times after cardiac transplantation. (*Source:* Adapted from Miller LW, Naftel DC, Bourge RC, et al. Infection after heart transplantation: a multi-institutional study. *J Heart Lung Transplant* 1994;13:384, with permission.)

is related to preexisting renal disease, most is acquired (59). Cyclosporine and tacrolimus are nephrotoxic and probably account for the majority of renal problems (60). Minimizing the dosages of these drugs or implementing calcineurin inhibitor-free strategies, avoiding dehydration, and searching carefully for non-immunosuppression–related reversible causes are warranted (2–4).

Hypertension

After transplantation, hypertension occurs in approximately two thirds of recipients, less frequently and less severely with tacrolimus than with cyclosporine (1). Moderate limitation of salt intake, maintenance of ideal body weight, and moderate exercise are encouraged in hypertensive cardiac transplant recipients, even though most require pharmacologic treatment. Generally, blood pressures consistently greater than 140/90 mm Hg are treated. For many patients, angiotensin-converting enzyme (ACE) inhibitors, angiotensin receptor blockers (ARB), calcium channel blockers, and β-blockers in conventional dosages are effective, alone or in combination (4). Care is taken when using ACE inhibitors or ARBs as some patients are prone to hyperkalemia due to renal effects of the calcineurin inhibitors. The use of either diltiazem or verapamil necessitates lowering of the dosages of cyclosporine or tacrolimus and, initially, monitoring cyclosporine or tacrolimus levels. Diuretics are effective in some patients, although rarely as monotherapy. Dehydration should, of course, be avoided with the concomitant use of cyclosporine or tacrolimus.

TABLE 90.6

INFECTION PROPHYLAXIS AFTER CARDIAC TRANSPLANTATION

Organism	Regimen
CMV (recipient seropositive)	Ganciclovir 5 mg/kg IV BID while IV in place, followed by valganciclovir, 900 mg PO daily until 3 months posttransplant
CMV (recipient seronegative and donor seropositive)	Ganciclovir 5 mg/kg IV BID while IV in place, followed by valganciclovir, 900 mg PO daily until 6 months posttransplant
Herpes simplex	Acyclovir 200 mg PO QID until corticosteroid dosage <20 mg prednisone/d
Epstein-Barr virus (recipient seronegative and donor seropositive)	Acyclovir 800 mg PO QID for 12 mo, then 200 mg PO QID
Toxoplasma gondii (donor or recipient seropositive)	Pyrimethamine 25 mg PO daily for 6 weeks and leucovorin calcium 5–10 mg PO daily for 6 weeks
Pneumocystis carinii	Trimethoprim maleate/sulfamethoxazole 160 mg/800 mg PO 3–7 times per week or dapsone 75–100 mg PO daily if sulfa allergic
Candida albicans	Nystatin 10 mL swish and swallow QID or clotrimazole troche PO QID until corticosteroid dosage (prednisone) <20 mg/d

Abbreviations: BID, twice daily; IV, intravenous line; PO, by mouth; QID, four times daily.

Osteoporosis

By the time most patients undergo cardiac transplantation, the risk of osteoporosis and other skeletal complications is high. Prolonged inactivity and, in some cases, prolonged heparin administration can demineralize bone and put the patient at risk for complications. Further bone loss occurs owing to high-dose corticosteroid therapy. Bone loss is rapid in the first 6 months after transplantation and is most marked in the lumbar spine. Vertebral compression fractures and aseptic necrosis of the femoral head are among the most common skeletal problems after heart transplantation. Because of the morbidity associated with osteoporosis, patients at risk are treated (61). All patients with evidence of pretransplant osteoporosis receive supplemental calcium and vitamin D while awaiting transplantation and indefinitely thereafter. Alendronate or other bisphosphonates may effectively increase bone density and can be safely added to calcium and vitamin D supplementation. Postmenopausal women are generally prescribed estrogen replacement therapy (62).

Hyperlipidemia

A 3-hydroxy-3-methylglutaryl coenzyme A (HMG-CoA) reductase inhibitor is used in the majority of transplant recipients, regardless of lipid profile (63,64). Not only do the HMG-CoA reductase inhibitors effectively treat the frequently encountered posttransplant hypercholesterolemia, they appear to decrease hemodynamically significant rejection. However, the combination of a calcineurin inhibitor and an HMG-CoA reductase inhibitor increases the risk of rhabdomyolysis over that for the HMG-CoA reductase inhibitor alone. HMG-CoA reductase inhibitors are started at low dosage and the dosage is increased periodically while levels of creatine kinase and liver enzymes are monitored.

All patients are encouraged to limit intake of cholesterol and other fats, maintain ideal body weight, and exercise. The goal for low-density lipoprotein cholesterol is less than 70 to 100 mg/dL. Whereas HMG-CoA reductase inhibitors are first-line therapy, the use of gemfibrozil or fenofibrate can be successful in some patients, particularly in the setting of hypertriglyceridemia. Combining an HMG-CoA reductase inhibitor with gemfibrozil or nicotinic acid in lipid-lowering doses ($\geq$1 g/d) can cause rhabdomyolysis, and these combinations are used cautiously in transplant patients. Bile acid sequestrants and fish oil (omega-3 free fatty acids) are infrequently used to treat hyperlipidemia after transplantation.

Malignancy

After transplantation, cardiac allograft recipients have an increased risk of malignancy compared with the general population. The overall degree of immunosuppression may be more important than any intrinsic property associated with a particular drug. Care is taken to avoid overimmunosuppression. By 5 years after transplantation, nearly 10% of survivors have experienced a malignancy (1). Fortunately, nearly half are skin cancers, occurring predominantly in those who would otherwise be at risk (65). Because locally invasive skin cancer can be fatal if not treated promptly and adequately, routine screening is performed. Posttransplant lymphoproliferative disease (PTLD) occurs in less than 2% of patients (66). PTLD can be refractory to any treatment or relatively localized and benign, responding simply to reduction in immunosuppression. The Epstein-Barr virus, a lymphotropic virus that infects more than 90% of the population by adulthood, is thought to be the etiologic agent responsible for most cases of PTLD (67–68).

Although other malignancies occur in heart transplant recipients, the behavior of prostate, breast, and cervical cancer and of other solid tumors seems no different than in the general population.

MANAGEMENT OF THE CARDIAC TRANSPLANT RECIPIENT UNDERGOING SURGERY

Because of bone complications, biliary disease, and other surgically amenable problems, many cardiac transplant recipients undergo noncardiac surgery. In general, antibiotic prophylaxis is used for dental procedures and other procedures in which the risk of septicemia is high. The risk associated with noncardiac surgery depends on the status of the allograft. In patients without ongoing rejection, significant coronary disease, or left ventricular dysfunction, the risk is low. Before elective major surgical procedures, an endomyocardial biopsy is typically performed, and the most recent angiogram is reviewed. Patients receiving corticosteroids within the preceding 9 months receive stress doses of corticosteroids. If intravenous immunosuppressants are required because of prolonged ileus, appropriate dosage adjustments must be made.

PREGNANCY

Successful pregnancies after heart transplantation have been reported (69). Maternal and fetal risk is undoubtedly higher than in the general population, and transplant recipients are so counseled. Once the recipient is pregnant, close collaboration with an obstetrician knowledgeable about high-risk cases is warranted to avoid teratogenic drugs and manage the pregnancy. Immunosuppressive drug levels are monitored frequently, as volume changes and metabolic changes occur during pregnancy. Radiation exposure can be minimized by using echocardiographically guided endomyocardial biopsies.

CONTROVERSIES AND PERSONAL PERSPECTIVES

Controversies in Recipient and Donor Selection

Since 1994, there has been a dramatic and unanticipated decline in the number of heart transplants performed in the United States. As reported by the United Network for Organ Sharing (UNOS), the number of heart transplants has been declining approximately 1% to 2% per year over the past decade from a peak of 2,528 in 1994 to 2,016 in 2004. During this period the number of patients listed annually declined from a peak of 4,079 in 1998 to 3,802 in 2002, and the median waiting time for actively listed patients decreased from 207 to 141 days. The good news is that death rates while waiting have also decreased from a high of 275 per 1,000 patient-years in 1993 to 143 in 2002. This undoubtedly reflects improvements and compliance with medical management guidelines for patients with heart failure, use of pacemakers and defibrillators, and to a lesser extent surgical alternatives for patients with advanced heart failure. However, medical advances have made it possible to successfully transplant patients who were previously considered inappropriate candidates. If we are to offer transplantation to these additional patients, we must expand the supply of suitable donor organs to prevent the donor–recipient mismatch from worsening. Nationally, the turndown rate for lack of an appropriate recipient is 8%, but there is marked regional variation. In 1992, the University of California—Los Angeles program estimated that about 40% of their donor hearts could not be matched to an appropriate candidate and this led them to develop an alternative recipient list for transplantation (70). The predominant reason for alternative listing was advanced recipient age. Once informed consent was obtained, these alternate candidates received donor hearts that were declined for younger candidates because of donor characteristics that included coronary artery disease, left ventricular hypertrophy, high doses of inotropes, intravenous drug abuse, and hepatitis C seropositivity. The hospital mortality of 18% and 4-year survival of 68% supports the use of alternate recipient list. Both recipient (older age, previous cardiac surgery) and donor (intracerebral bleed and longer ischemic times) factors increased the mortality. These outcomes are worse than in younger patients receiving healthy donor hearts, but a more accurate comparison would be the outcomes without transplantation or with permanent or destination mechanical support therapy. Currently, the 6-month mortality for patients treated with the Thoratec implantable device for permanent therapy is 30% to 40%, making an alternative list and utilization of less-than-optimal donor hearts a reasonable approach.

Although individual patient advocacy is admirable, physicians bear a responsibility in their stewardship over donor hearts. Physicians must balance two competing interests—those of individual patient advocacy and societal responsibility—to ensure that appropriate candidates are given the scarce donor hearts. One commonly advocated utilitarian view is that the greatest "societal" good is provided by allocating donor organs first to those at the greatest risk of death while waiting, assuming that the posttransplant outcomes are comparable. The current UNOS status system is essentially based on the presumed risk for mortality on the list. Surprisingly, not all patients transplanted are at the highest risk (at higher status, status 1A or 1B). At any given time only 11% of listed patients are status 1A or 1B, 43% are status 2, and 46% are inactive. Recently, Jimenez et al. (71) recommended that only patients listed as status 1 should be offered transplantation because there appeared to be no survival benefit of transplantation for status 2 patients. Status 2 patients are transplanted because the organ is not appropriate for a status 1 patient; usually, the organ is too small and current UNOS guidelines allow the organ to remain "local" before extending the offer to distant status 1 candidates. With these issues in mind, the allocation rules are undergoing reassessment, with an emphasis on more regional/national allocation rather than the current "local-first" system.

Although the success of cardiac transplantation in lowering the mortality of patients with end-stage heart failure is unquestioned, the need for transplantation generally represents a failure of heart muscle disease prevention or early detection and treatment. Viewed simplistically, decreasing the number of patients who could benefit from cardiac transplantation by preventive and early treatment measures is of greater importance than perfecting cardiac transplantation for the relative few who need it.

Cost of Transplantation: Who Should Pay?

An unstated consideration in selecting a transplant candidate is the ability to pay. Most heart transplant centers will not list a patient if he or she is uninsured, yet more than one fifth of donors come from the ranks of the uninsured. In short, many individuals donate their hearts although they themselves would not have been eligible to receive a transplant had they needed one (72). Surely a remedy should be available for such a shameful inequity.

THE FUTURE

During the next decade, as permanent MCS systems become clinically feasible, the decisions regarding transplant candidacy will become more complex. Less toxic and more effective immunosuppressive strategies will evolve even as the induction of donor-specific tolerance decreases the need for pharmacologic immunosuppression. The socioeconomic inequities in heart transplantation will be mitigated.

References

1. Taylor DO, Edwards LB, Boucek MM, et al. The Registry of the International Society for Heart and Lung Transplantation: Twenty-first official adult heart transplant report—2004. *J Heart Lung Transplant* 2004;23:796–803.
2. Lindenfeld J, Miller GG, Shakar SF, et al. Drug therapy in the heart transplant recipient. Part I: cardiac rejection and immunosuppressive drugs. *Circulation* 2004;110:3734–3740.
3. Lindenfeld J, Miller GG, Shakar SF, et al. Drug therapy in the heart transplant recipient. Part II: immunosuppressive drugs. *Circulation* 2004;110:3858–3865.
4. Lindenfeld J, Page RL, Zolty R, et al. Drug therapy in the heart transplant recipient. Part III: common medical problems. *Circulation* 2005;111:113–117.
5. Miller LW. Criteria for selection of recipients and donors for cardiac transplantation. *Graft* 1999;2:S49–S53.
6. Bardy GH, Lee KL, Mark DB, et al., for the Sudden Cardiac Death in Heart Failure Trial (SCD-HeFT) Investigators. Amiodarone or an implantable cardioverter-defibrillator for congestive heart failure. *N Engl J Med* 2005;352:225–237.
7. Deng MC, Edwards LB, Hertz MI, et al. Mechanical circulatory support device database of the International Society for Heart and Lung Transplantation: Second annual report—2004. *J Heart Lung Transplant* 2004;23:1027–1034.
8. Renlund DG. Building a bridge to heart transplantation. *N Engl J Med* 2004;351:849–851.
9. Copeland JG, Smith RG, Arabia FA, et al. Cardiac Replacement with a Total Artificial Heart as a Bridge to Transplantation. *N Engl J Med* 2004;351:859–867.
10. Gridelli B, Remuzzi G. Strategies for making more organs available for transplantation. *N Engl J Med* 2000;343:404–410.
11. Delmonico FL, Snydman DR. Organ donor screening for infectious diseases: review of practice and implications for transplantation. *Transplantation* 1998;65:603–610.
12. Zaroff JG, Rosengard BR, Armstrong WF, et al. Consensus Conference Report: maximizing use of organs recovered from a cadaver: Cardiac recommendations. *Circulation* 2002;106:836–841.
13. Stoica SC, Satchithananda DK, Charman S, et al. Swanz-Ganz catheter assessment of donor hearts: Outcomes of organs with borderline hemodynamics. *J Heart Lung Transplant* 2002;21:615–622.
14. Hauptman PJ, O'Connor KJ. Procurement and allocation of solid organs for transplantation. *N Engl J Med* 1997;336:422–431.
15. Pratschke J, Wilhelm MJ, Kusaka M, et al. Brain death and its influence on donor organ quality and outcome after transplantation. *Transplantation* 1999;67:343–348.
16. Jeevanandum V, Furukawa S, Prendergast TW, et al. Standard criteria for an acceptable donor heart are restricting heart transplantation. *Ann Thorac Surg* 1996;62:1268–1275.
17. Kirklin JK, Naftel DC, Bourge RC, et al. Evolving trends in risk profiles and causes of death after heart transplantation: a ten year multi-institutional study. *J Thorac Cardiovasc Surg* 2003;125:881–890.
18. Gupta D, Piacentino V, Macha M, et al. Effect of older donor age on risk for mortality after heart transplantation. *Ann Thorac Surg* 2004;78:890–899.
19. Ganesh JS, Rogers CA, Banner NR, et al., on behalf of the Steering Group. Donor cause of death and medium-term survival after heart transplantation: a United Kingdom national study. *J Thorac Cardiovasc Surg* 2005;126:1153–1159.
20. Young JB. Age before beauty: the use of "older" donor hearts for cardiac transplantation. *J Heart Lung Transplant* 1999;18:488–491.
21. Adams DH. Surgical techniques in heart transplantation. *Graft* 1999;2:119–122.
22. Bainbridge AD, Cave M, Roberts M, et al. A prospective randomized trial of complete atrioventricular transplantation versus ventricular transplantation with atrioplasty. *J Heart Lung Transplant* 1999;18:407–413.

23. Jeevanandam V, Russell H, Mather P, et al. A one-year comparison of prophylactic donor tricuspid annuloplasty in heart transplantation. *Ann Thorac Surg* 2004;78:759–766.
24. Bengel FM, Ueberfuhr P, Ziegler SI, et al. Serial assessment of sympathetic reinnervation after orthotopic heart transplantation: a longitudinal study using PET and C-11 hydroxyephedrine. *Circulation* 1999;99:1866–1871.
25. Schwaiblmair M, von Scheidt W, Uberfuhr P, et al. Functional significance of cardiac reinnervation in heart transplant recipients. *J Heart Lung Transplant* 1999;18:838–845.
26. Cui G, Kobashigawa J, Chung T, et al. Atrial conduction disturbance as an indicator of rejection after cardiac transplantation. *Transplantation* 2000;70:223–227.
27. Lefroy DC, Fang JC, Stevenson LW, et al. Recipient-to-donor atrioatrial conduction after orthotopic heart transplantation: surface electrocardiographic features and estimated prevalence. *Am J Cardiol* 1998;82:444–450.
28. Halloran PF. Immunosuppressive drugs for kidney transplantation. *N Engl J Med* 2004;351:2715–2729.
29. Sayegh MH, Turka LA. The role of T-cell costimulatory activation pathways in transplant rejection. *N Engl J Med* 1998;338:1813–1821.
30. Delves PJ, Roitt IM. The immune system: first of two parts. *N Engl J Med* 2000;343:37–49.
31. Delves PJ, Roitt IM. The immune system: second of two parts. *N Engl J Med* 2000;343:108–117.
32. von Andrian UH, MacKay CR. Advances in immunology: T-cell function and migration—two sides of the same coin. *N Engl J Med* 2000;343:1020–1034.
33. Dallman MJ. Immunobiology of graft rejection. In: Ginns LC, Cosimi AB, Morris PJ, eds. *Transplantation*. Cambridge, MA: Blackwell Science, 1999: 23–42.
34. Tambur AR, Bray RA, Takemoto SK, et al. Flow cytometric detection of HLA-specific antibodies as a predictor of heart allograft rejection. *Transplantation* 2000;70:1055–1059.
35. Stewart S, Winters GL, Fishbein MC, et al. Revision of the 1990 working formulation for the standardization of nomenclature in the diagnosis of heart rejection: The International Society for Heart and Lung Transplantation. *J Heart and Lung Transplant* 2005;24:1710–1720.
36. Ma H, Hammond EH, Taylor DO, et al. The repetitive histologic pattern of vascular cardiac allograft rejection: increased incidence associated with longer exposure to prophylactic murine monoclonal anti-CD3 antibody (OKT3). *Transplantation* 1996;62:205–210.
37. Reed EF, Demetris AJ, Hammond E, et al. , and the International Society for Heart and Lung Transplantation. Acute antibody-mediated rejection of cardiac transplants. *J Heart Lung Transplant* 2006;25:153–159.
38. Baughman, KL. History and current techniques of endomyocardial biopsy. In: Baumgartner WA, Reitz BA, Achuff SA, eds. *Heart and heart-lung transplantation*. Philadelphia: WB Saunders, 1990.
39. Brunner-La Rocca HP, Kiowski W. Identification of patients not requiring endomyocardial biopsies late after cardiac transplantation. *Transplantation* 1998;65:533–538.
40. Taylor DO, Bristow MR, O'Connell JB, et al. Improved long-term survival after heart transplantation predicted by successful early withdrawal from maintenance corticosteroid therapy. *J Heart Lung Transplant* 1996;15:1039–1046.
41. Weis M, von Scheidt W. Cardiac allograft vasculopathy: a review. *Circulation* 1997;96:2069–2077.
42. Kobashigawa JA, Tobis JM, Starling RC, et al. Multicenter intravascular ultrasound validation study among heart transplant recipients: outcomes after five years. *J Am Coll Cardiol* 2005;45:1532–1537.
43. Tuzcu EM, Kapadia SR, Sachar R, et al. Intravascular ultrasound evidence of angiographically silent progression in coronary atherosclerosis predicts long-term morbidity and mortality after cardiac transplantation. *J Am Coll Cardiol* 2005;45:1538–1542.
44. Gao SZ, Hunt SA, Schroeder JS, et al. Early development of accelerated graft coronary artery disease: risk factors and course. *J Am Coll Cardiol* 1996; 28:673–679.
45. Gao SZ, Alderman EL, Schroeder JS, et al. Accelerated coronary vascular disease in the heart transplant patient: coronary arteriographic findings. *J Am Coll Cardiol* 1988;12:334–348.
46. Hornick P, Smith J, Pomerace A, et al. Influence of acute rejection episodes, HLA matching, and donor/recipient phenotype on the development of "early" transplant-associated coronary artery disease. *Circulation* 1997;96[Suppl II]:II-148–II-153.
47. Benza RL, Grenett HE, Bourge RC, et al. Gene polymorphisms for plasminogen activator inhibitor-1/tissue plasminogen activator and development of allograft coronary artery disease. *Circulation* 1998;98:2248–2254.
48. Labarrere CA. Anticoagulation factors as predictors of transplant-associated coronary artery disease. *J Heart Lung Transplant* 2000;19:623–633.
49. Gupta A, Moustapha A, Jacobsen DW, et al. High homocysteine, low folate, and low vitamin B_6 concentrations: prevalent risk factors for vascular disease in heart transplant recipients. *Transplantation* 1998;65:544–550.
50. Cooke GE, Eaton GM, Whitby G, et al. Plasma atherogenic markers in congestive heart failure and posttransplant (heart) patients. *J Am Coll Cardiol* 2000;36:509–516.
51. Spes CH, Klauss V, Mudra H, et al. Diagnostic and prognostic value of serial dobutamine stress echocardiography for noninvasive assessment of cardiac allograft vasculopathy: a comparison with coronary angiography and intravascular ultrasound. *Circulation* 1999;100:509–515.
52. Keogh A, Richardson M, Ruygrok P, et al. Sirolimus in de novo heart transplant recipients reduces acute rejection and prevents coronary artery disease at 2 years: a randomized clinical trial. *Circulation* 2004;110:2694–2700.
53. Eisen JH, Tuzcu EM, Dorent R, et al. Everolimus for the prevention of allograft rejection and vasculopathy in cardiac transplant recipients. *N Engl J Med* 2003;349:847–858.
54. Mancini D, Pinney S, Burkhoff D, et al. Use of rapamycin slows progression of cardiac transplantation vasculopathy. *Circulation* 2003;108:48–53.
55. Fishman JA, Rubin RH. Infection in organ-transplant recipients. *N Engl J Med* 1998;338:1741–1751.
56. Miller LW, Naftel DC, Bourge RC, et al. Infection after heart transplantation: a multiinstitutional study. *J Heart Lung Transplant* 1994;13:381–393.
57. Rubin RH. Prevention and treatment of cytomegalovirus disease in heart transplant patients. *J Heart Lung Transplant* 2000;19:731–735.
58. Grossi P, Farina C, Fiocchi R, et al. Prevalence and outcome of invasive fungal infections in 1,963 thoracic organ transplant recipients. *Transplantation* 2000;70:112–116.
59. Campistol JM, Sacks SH. Mechanisms of nephrotoxicity. *Transplantation* 2000;69:SS5–SS10.
60. Parry G, Meiser B, Rbago G. The clinical impact of cyclosporine nephrotoxicity in heart transplantation. *Transplantation* 2000;69:SS23–SS26.
61. Stempfle H-U, Werner C, Echtler S, et al. Prevention of osteoporosis after cardiac transplantation: a prospective, longitudinal, randomized, double-blind trial with calcitriol. *Transplantation* 1999;68:523–530.
62. Shane E, Rodino MA, McMahon DJ, et al. Prevention of bone loss after heart transplantation with antiresorptive therapy: a pilot study. *J Heart Lung Transplant* 1998;17:1089–1096.
63. Kobashigawa JA, Kasiske BL. Hyperlipidemia in solid organ transplantation. *Transplantation* 1997;63:331–338.
64. Magnani G, Carinci V, Magelli C, et al. Role of statins in the management of dyslipidemia after cardiac transplant: randomized controlled trial comparing the efficacy and safety of atorvastatin with pravastatin. *J Heart Lung Transplant* 2000;19:710–715.
65. Lampros TD, Cobanoglu A, Parker F, et al. Squamous and basal cell carcinoma in heart transplant recipients. *J Heart Lung Transplant* 1998;17:586–591.
66. Mihalov ML, Gattuso P, Abraham K, et al. Incidence of post-transplant malignancy among 674 solid-organ-transplant recipients at a single center. *Clin Transplant* 1996;10:248–255.
67. Paya CV, Fung JJ, Nalesnik MA, et al. Epstein-Barr virus–induced post-transplant lymphoproliferative disorders. *Transplantation* 1999;68:1517–1525.
68. Darenkov IA, Marcarelli MA, Basadonna GP, et al. Reduced incidence of Epstein-Barr virus–associated posttransplant lymphoproliferative disorder using preemptive antiviral therapy. *Transplantation* 1997;64:848–852.
69. Branch KR, Wagoner LE, McGrory CH, et al. Risks of subsequent pregnancies on mother and newborn in female heart transplant recipients. *J Heart Lung Transplant* 1998;17:698–702.
70. Laks H, Marelli D, Fonarow GC, et al., for the UCLA Heart Transplant Group. Use of two recipient lists for adults requiring heart transplantation. *J Thorac Cardiovasc Surg* 2003;125:49–59.
71. Jimenez J, Bennett Edwards L, et al. Should stable UNOS status 2 patients be transplanted? *J Heart Lung Transplant* 2005;24:178–183.
72. King LP, Siminoff LA, Meyer DM, et al. Health insurance and cardiac transplantation: a call for reform. *J Am Coll Cardiol* 2005;45:1388–1391.

CHAPTER 91 ■ SURGICAL APPROACHES FOR HEART FAILURE

NICHOLAS G. SMEDIRA, KATHERINE J. HOERCHER, AND RANDALL C. STARLING

Heart failure surgery has been called "high-risk" conventional or nontransplant surgery. These procedures represent the evolution of well-known operations such as coronary bypass grafting, valve interventions, and left ventricular (LV) reconstruction now applied to patients with severe LV dysfunction. Perceived as incurring a substantial early risk, many patients in the past were not offered a surgical alternative other than transplantation. An increasing body of evidence has demonstrated that surgical procedures and devices to arrest or reverse remodeling are safely performed in the failing heart, improve LV function, and may play a key role in providing lasting benefit for patients with heart failure. Surgery for advanced heart failure has become a common treatment of choice for many patients. A key ingredient to the success of any surgery for heart failure is the combination of state-of-the-art pharmacologic therapy. When used together, medical and surgical therapies offer marked improvement in both quantity and quality of life for the many patients suffering from end-stage heart failure.

At the time the first edition was being written, we were assessing the use of conventional surgical therapies and beginning to explore multiple new surgical options to address the problem of heart failure with the belief that symptoms would be reduced and survival improved with an acceptably low operative mortality. Many studies have confirmed the low operative risks and two eagerly awaited randomized trials—Randomized Evaluation of Mechanical Assistance for the Treatment of Congestive Heart Failure (REMATCH) and Acorn CorCap—provide insight into the utility of surgical therapy for advanced heart failure. This chapter reviews the current status of surgical treatments for heart failure, focusing on results that have been published since the last edition and highlighting changes in our understanding of how surgery impacts survival and quality of life.

RISK ASSESSMENT

The risk of all cardiac surgery has declined over the past decade. Perioperative risks have diminished owing to improvements in intraoperative myocardial protection, increased surgeon experience, and more consistent postoperative care strategies. For example, hospital death after reoperative coronary artery bypass grafting (CABG) is now less than 2%. This is clinically indistinguishable from the 1% mortality of patients undergoing primary CABG (Fig. 91.1). This must be interpreted with caution, however; we have found that older age, smoking, renal dysfunction, and poor LV dysfunction decreased the likelihood of undergoing reoperation (1). All these factors have been shown to increase the morbidity and mortality associated with reoperation and may have biased the decision against surgery in favor of medical therapy or percutaneous intervention (1).

Many small series have described operative mortalities of less than 2% in patients with severe heart failure and reduced LV function. The Cleveland Clinic experience from the early 1990s demonstrated reduced ejection fraction (EF) was associated with a marked increase in mortality in patients undergoing primary or reoperative CABG. This risk factor was eliminated by 2002 (Figs. 91.2 and 91.3) (1). This statistic is further underscored by a recent study of contemporary outcomes of nontransplant surgical strategies for managing ischemic cardiomyopathy. From January 1997 to July 2003, 1,108 patients at the Cleveland Clinic with ischemic cardiomyopathy and an EF of less than 35% underwent CABG alone ($n = 760$), CABG plus mitral valve (MV) repair ($n = 191$), or LV reconstruction ($n = 167$). All three strategies demonstrated a hospital mortality of less than 5% and an excellent 5-year survival (Fig. 91.4). Rather than a low EF, we found the presence of comorbidities, especially renal dysfunction, chronic obstructive pulmonary disease, and vascular disease, to be more powerful predictors of early death. Other studies have repeatedly shown that parameters of LV function reflecting a reduced EF have little impact on early surgical mortality. Although there remains an incremental risk during bypass surgery produced by abnormal LV function, with modern myocardial protection that increment is small and represents a relatively small proportion of the total risk for patients with ischemic cardiomyopathy. A review of 14,075 Cleveland Clinic patients undergoing primary

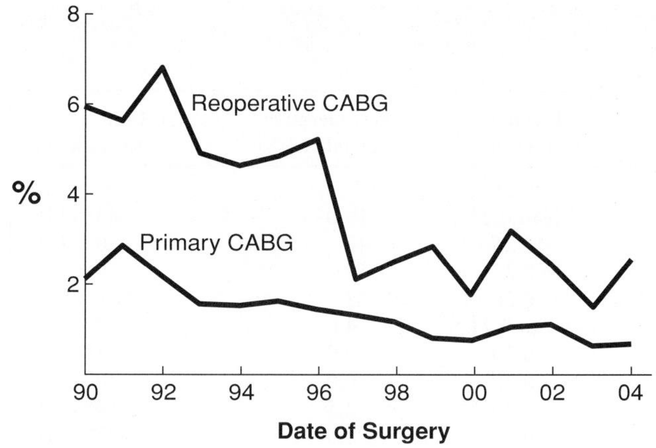

FIGURE 91.1. Operative mortality for all primary and reoperative CABG at The Cleveland Clinic Foundation.

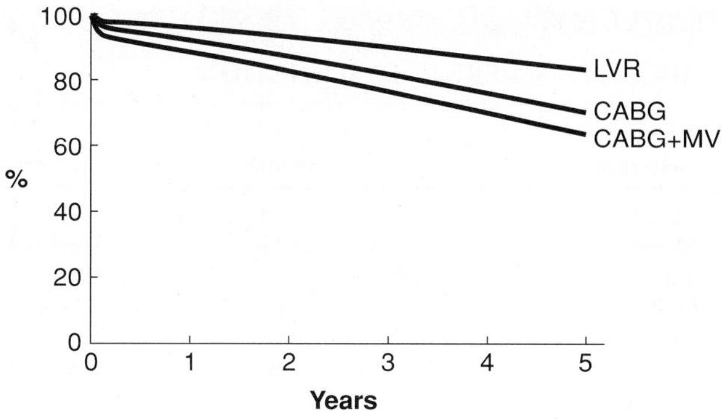

FIGURE 91.4. At The Cleveland Clinic, 1,108 patients with ischemic cardiomyopathy and LVEF of less than 35% underwent CABG alone (n = 760), CABG plus MV repair (n = 191), or LV reconstruction (n = 167). All three strategies demonstrated a hospital mortality of less than 5% and an excellent 5-year survival.

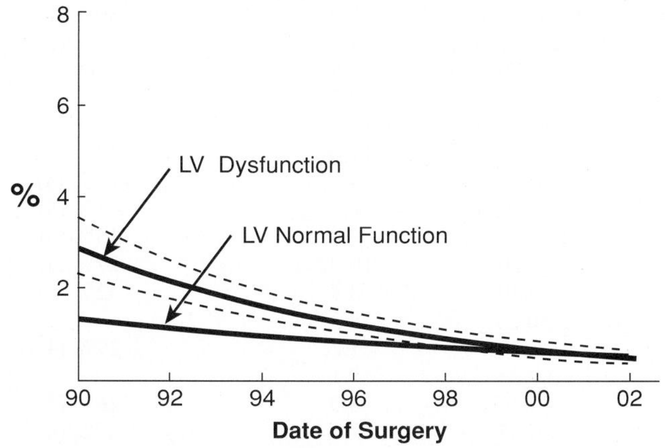

FIGURE 91.2. The Cleveland Clinic experience from the early 1990s demonstrated that LV dysfunction was associated with a marked increase in hospital mortality in patients undergoing primary or reoperative CABG. By 2002, this risk factor was eliminated.

isolated bypass surgery from 1990 to 1999 showed in-hospital mortality rates when preoperative LV function was normal (n = 7,203) of 1.5%, mild impairment (n = 3,378) of 0.8%, moderate impairment (n = 2,132) of 2.5%, and severe impairment (n = 1,362) of 3.2%.

The Cleveland Clinic Risk Score was developed in 1988 and is still in use today. It determines preoperative risk factors for patients undergoing coronary artery bypass surgery (2). Compared with the 1980s, patients undergoing surgery in this decade are at much higher estimated risk as a result of an older population, higher number of reoperations, emergency operations, the incidence of LV dysfunction, and the presence of comorbidities, such as diabetes and renal dysfunction. Yet despite this, these patients have a significantly lower incidence of morbidity and hospital mortality (Fig. 91.5) (2,3).

We now have solid data to demonstrate that surgical risk has been substantially reduced for even the patients at highest risk, but therein lies the quandary. Given that the vast majority of patients will survive the operation, the much more difficult question is this: Do these procedures improve symptoms and prolong survival? The remainder of this chapter addresses these concerns.

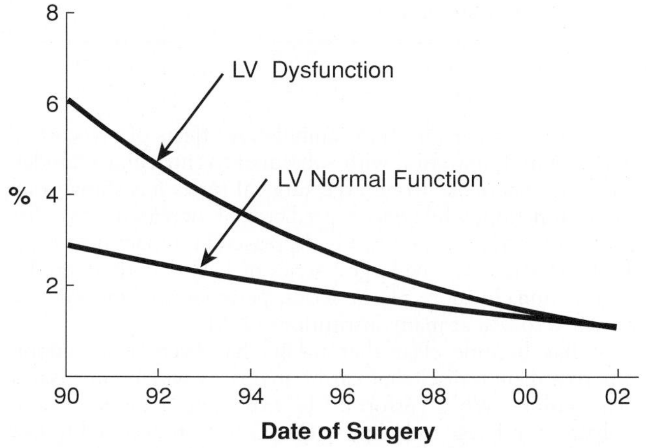

FIGURE 91.3. The Cleveland Clinic experience from the early 1990s demonstrated that LV dysfunction was associated with a marked increase in hospital mortality in patients undergoing primary or reoperative CABG. By 2002, this risk factor was eliminated.

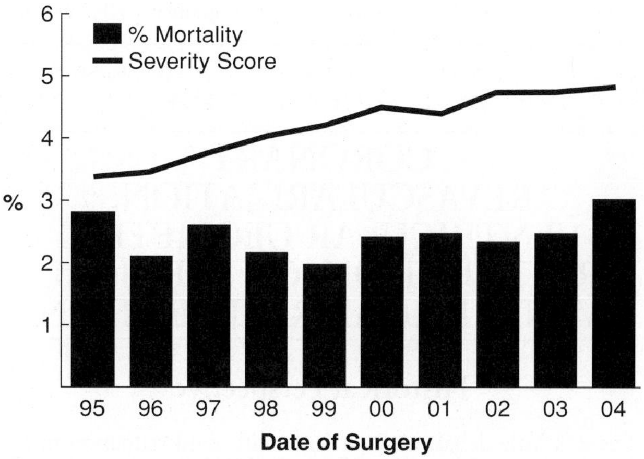

FIGURE 91.5. Compared with the 1980s, patients undergoing CABG in this decade are at much higher risk. Yet despite this, these patients have a significantly lower incidence of morbidity and hospital mortality.

TABLE 91.1

CABG WITH SEVERE LV DYSFUNCTION

First author	Points	Years	Ejection fraction	Perioperative mortality (%)	Late mortality (y)
Vlietstra	10	1966–1972	<0.25	—	60% (2)
Manley	183	1968–1971	Mean 0.22	16.0	43% (5)
Yatteau	24	1968–1972	<0.25	42	50% (2)
Oldham	11	1969–1972	≤0.25	55	—
Zubiate	140	1969–1975	<0.20	22	41.6% (6)
Faulkner	46	1969–1975	Mean 0.21	4.0	17% (2)
Mitchel	9	—	<0.20	0.0	11% (1)
Fox	7	1971–1974	<0.20	0.0	14%
Jones	41	1973–1977	<0.20	2.5	10% (1)
Alderman	82	1975–1979	≤0.25	8.0	37% (5)
Mochtar	62	1975–1983	Mean 0.25	4.8	30% (5)
Zubiate	93	1976–1981	<0.20	5.0	50% (5)
Hochberg	51	1976–1982	0.20–0.24	12.0	42% (3)
Hochberg	41	1976–1982	<0.20	37.0	85% (3)
Sanchez	23	1982–1989	Mean 0.28	9.0	24% (2)
Kron et al.	39	1983–1988	<0.20	2.6	17% (3)
Blakeman	20	1984–1988	Mean 0.18	15.0	30% (1)
Wong	22	1986–1989	Mean 0.25	9.0	23% (3)
Christakis	487	1982–1990	<0.20	9.8	—
Hammermeister	251	1987–1990	<0.20	9.2	—
Louie	22	1984–1990	Mean 0.23	13.6	28% (3)
Milano et al.	118	1981–1991	<0.25	11.0	42% (5)
Shapira et al.	74	1986–1991	<0.30	—	13.5% (5)
Anderson et al.	203	1983–1992	Mean 0.34	6.0	41% (5)
Hausmann et al.	265	1986–1992	Mean 0.24	7.6	13% (3)
Kaul et al.	210	1987–1992	≤0.20	10.0	27% (5)
Mickleborough et al.	79	1982–1993	<0.20	3.8	32% (5)
Langenburg et al.	96	1983–1993	≤0.25	8.3	—
Elefteraides et al.	135	1986–1994	≤0.30	5.2	29% (4.5)
Iskandrian et al.	269	1991–1994	≤0.35	7.1	—
Kawachi et al.	50	1982–1995	≤0.30	8.0	26% (5)
Moshkovitz et al.	75	1991–1994	≤0.35	2.7	27% (4)
Trachiotis et al.	156	1981–1995	<0.25	3.8	35% (5)
Baumgartner et al.	61	1990–1996	<0.25	8.0	—
Cimochowski et al.	111	1992–1996	<0.35	1.8	—
Argenziano et al. (CABG Patch)	454 no CHF 443 CHF	1993–1996	≤0.35	3.5 no CHF 7.7 CHF	—
DeCarlo et al.	80	1994–1996	≤0.30	6.3	18% (2)
Luciani et al.	116	1991–1998	≤0.30	1.7	25% (5)

Abbreviations: CABG, coronary artery bypass grafting; CHF, congestive heart failure; LV, left ventricular.

CORONARY REVASCULARIZATION, VENTRICULAR GEOMETRIC RESTORATION, OR SURGICAL VENTRICULAR RESTORATION

Historical Perspective

There is little debate that patients with mild reduction in LV function and severe triple vessel disease benefit from surgical revascularization. On the other hand, in a busy heart failure surgery practice, the question of revascularization in a patient with severe LV dysfunction arises daily. In the current era, the most common operation performed for patients with ischemic cardiomyopathy continues to be CABG. Ischemic cardiomyopathy stems from the cumulative effects of myocardial ischemia and infarction with subsequent ventricular remodeling. The experience from large surgical series has shown that LV dysfunction, while once a predictor of increased morbidity and mortality, has significantly decreased in impact over time. Table 91.1 reviews the largest series of CABG with severe LV dysfunction. In more recent series, perioperative mortality is now 2% to 8% at many institutions (3–8).

It has become clear that CABG has become an important treatment for ischemic cardiomyopathy with compensated heart failure. When performed by experienced surgical teams utilizing the latest techniques, CABG has an acceptably low mortality and morbidity and appears to justify surgical revascularization for this high-risk group of patients. Kron and others advocate revascularization in all patients with graftable coronary arteries and EF of less than 20% (9–11). Hospital mortality was very low in these series, particularly if evidence of ischemia was present. However, Kron has shown that poor

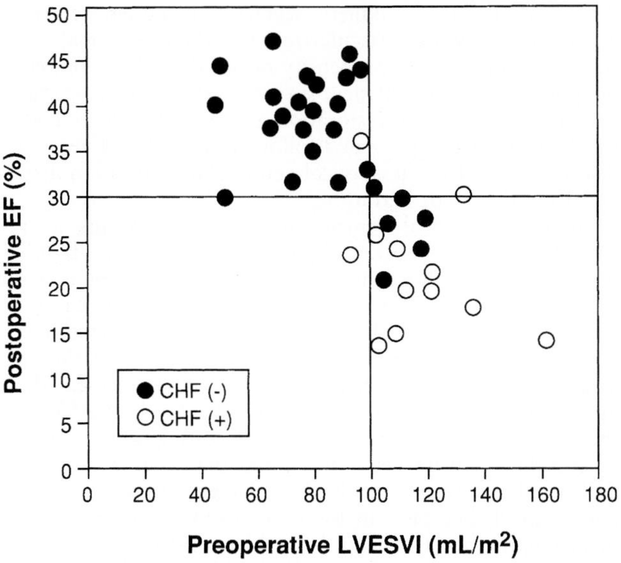

FIGURE 91.6. For patients with ischemic cardiomyopathy, EF less than 30% and LVESVI greater than 100 mL/m^2, functional recovery was unlikely after revascularization. *Abbreviations:* CHF, congestive heart failure; EF, ejection fraction; LVESVI, left ventricular end-systolic volume index. (*Source:* From Yamaguchi A, Takashi I, Adachi H. Left ventricular volume predicts postoperative course in patients with ischemic cardiomyopathy. *Ann Thorac Surg* 1998;65:434–438, with permission.)

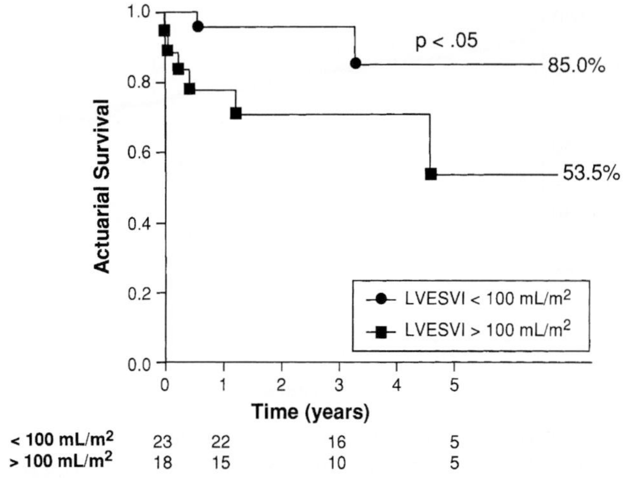

FIGURE 91.7. Ischemic cardiomyopathy and ventricular enlargement greater than 100 mL/m^2 is associated with reduced survival after revascularization. *Abbreviation:* LVESVI, left ventricular end-systolic volume index. (*Source:* From Yamaguchi A, Takashi I, Adachi H. Left ventricular volume predicts postoperative course in patients with ischemic cardiomyopathy. *Ann Thorac Surg* 1998;65:434–438, with permission.)

distal coronary vasculature, even in the presence of angina, yields poor outcomes following revascularization (12).

Overall, published results have been uniformly outstanding and have supported the wider application of these procedures. Thus in 1999, consensus panels from the American Heart Association/American College of Cardiology (AHA/ACC) established the principal that abnormal LV function combined with left main or multivessel coronary artery disease represents an indication for bypass surgery regardless of the severity of symptoms (13).

An increasing body of evidence has shown that patients with high end-systolic volumes secondary to LV remodeling have a decreased likelihood of improvement in global function with myocardial revascularization alone (14,15). Yamaguchi et al. (16) showed that in patients undergoing revascularization with an EF of less than 30% and a left ventricular end-systolic volume index (LVESVI) of more than 100 mL/m^2, 5-year survival was significantly worse than those patients with an LVESVI of less than 100 mL (Figs. 91.6 and 91.7). In patients with ICMP, anterior myocardial infarction is a common initiating event, leading to loss of function of the anterior LV and parts of the interventricular septum, and subsequent LV remodeling. Based on imaging, infarcted areas have two general morphologic types: dyskinesia/LV aneurysm–transmural LV infarct with subsequent wall thinning, leading to paradoxical segmental outward bulging during LV systole; and akinesia–LV infarct with a thin rim of viable myocardium, leading to no movement during systole (but with enough myocardium to prevent paradoxical bulging). Surgical treatment of ischemic cardiomyopathy has long included excision of dyskinetic ventricular scar at the time of revascularization. However, with the advent of early coronary reperfusion following acute infarction, there is a decreasing incidence of the classic thin-walled dyskinetic aneurysm, but an increasing presentation of an akinetic myocardium, which left untreated results in ventricular remodeling, global systolic deterioration, and ultimately heart failure. Hence, treatment of the index event following acute MI may not result in a cure; it is estimated that 20% of patients will present with LV dilation at 6 months postintervention (17). Yet many surgeons are hesitant to exclude the normal appearing akinetic segments when LV shape is not seriously distorted.

More than a decade ago, Dor et al., recognizing the deleterious effects of reverse remodeling on the noninfarcted areas remote from the akinetic area, argued for early and aggressive operative intervention. Although often asymptomatic, patients with akinetic segments are more likely to have worse baseline hemodynamics with elevated pulmonary artery pressures, severely depressed EFs, and high systolic and diastolic indices. Dor's technique of endoventricular circular patch plasty in patients with anterior akinetic or dyskinetic scar excludes the infarcted distal interventricular septum from the reconstructed LV, restoring overall LV shape. Utilizing a true surgical reconstruction of the dysfunctional LV has yielded an improvement in global LV EF and New York Heart Association (NYHA) class. Importantly, the results of this technique demonstrate that early outcomes in patients with akinetic regions were similar to patients with dyskinesia. In a retrospective, noncontrolled study of 100 patients, 51 with akinetic and 49 with dyskinetic scars, in-hospital mortality in akinetic and dyskinetic cases was 10% and 14%, respectively. Nineteen late deaths occurred, 13 in the akinetic group at 5 years. Overall mortality was similar between the two groups (18). Dor reported his largest series in 2001 (19). In a cohort of 1,011 patients operated on since 1984, hospital mortality was 7.5%. Dor emphasized the concept of using a balloon to adequately size the LV cavity to avoid making it too small. This approach resulted in a hospital mortality of 4.8% in the 187 cases from 1998 to 2000. Long-term survival in Dor's cohort is 80% at 10 years in patients with preoperative LVESI of less than 90 mL/m^2. Ten-year survival falls to 50% when the preoperative LVESI is greater than 120 mL/m^2.

The objective of the Reconstructive Endoventricular Surgery, Returning Torsion Original Radius Elliptical Shape to the LV (RESTORE) group was to validate Dor's concept of surgical intervention in patients with post infarction akinetic and dyskinetic scars. A nonrandomized registry of 1,198 patients undergoing surgical ventricular restoration was analyzed to determine early and late outcomes and establish risk factors for poor outcomes (20). Overall, 30 day mortality after

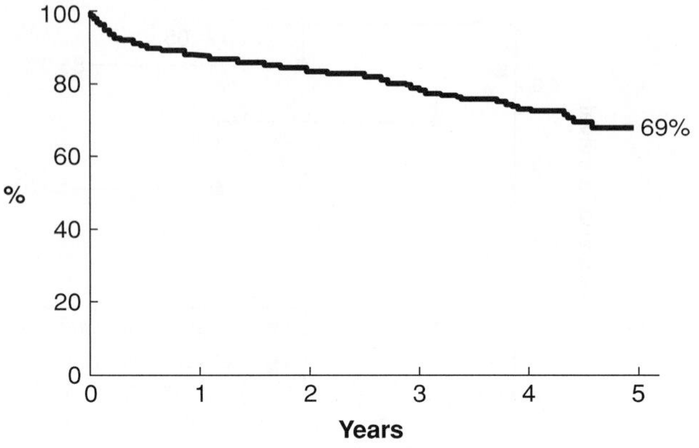

FIGURE 91.8. The RESTORE registry demonstrated an overall 5-year survival of 68.6%. Survival at 5 years was better in the group of patients who had dyskinetic as compared with akinetic morphology (80% versus 65%; $P < .001$).

surgical ventricular restoration was 5.3% and 5-year survival was 68.6% with improved survival in the dyskinetic group as compared to akinetic morphology (80% versus 65%) (Figs. 91.8 and 91.9). Patients experienced an improvement in NYHA functional class from a mean of 2.9 preoperatively to 1.7 postoperatively and a freedom from rehospitalization for heart failure of 78%. There have, however, been some questions raised about these results following a presentation by Smith at the AHA meetings in 2003. He found that outcomes of the surgical ventricular restoration operation as reported in the STS database showed a 10% 30-day mortality, which was much higher than reported by the RESTORE group (21).

Although published outcomes from the RESTORE registry have been promising, the absence of a control group has made it difficult to draw any conclusions regarding the efficacy of surgical ventricular restoration relative to CABG. At the Cleveland Clinic, we analyzed 140 patients who underwent surgical ventricular restoration and CABG who were propensity matched with 140 patients who underwent CABG without Surgical Ventricular Restoration (SVR). Both groups were comparable with respect to the variables used for the propensity matching. LV function was severely depressed with a mean LV EF of 24 ± 8% in the surgical ventricular restoration group and 23 ± 9% in the control group. We were unable to demonstrate a survival benefit when surgical ventricular restoration was performed in patients with ischemic cardiomyopathy and discrete dyskinetic or akinetic segments of the left ventricle, in conjunction with revascularization and conventional valve surgery, compared to a propensity-matched, CABG-alone contemporaneous cohort. Patient survival was excellent—92% at 1 year for the surgical restoration group, and 93% at 1 year for the control group. Over a follow-up period of 4 years, 14 deaths occurred in the surgical ventricular restoration group and 15 in the control group.

Similarly, surgical ventricular restoration results as reported by the RESTORE group have been challenged by Elefteriades (6,22), who demonstrated excellent outcomes with isolated CABG. In addition, decision making in cases of Ischemic Cardiomyopathy (ICMP) have become further complicated by the major advances in pharmaceutical therapy. Trials comparing a strategy of CABG versus medical therapy such as the Coronary Artery Surgery Study (CASS) and the Veterans Affairs study, although considerable in terms of enrollment, were performed more than two decades ago and we have seen considerable changes in both medical and surgical therapies. In the current era of evidence-based medicine, the best treatment for ischemic cardiomyopathy remains controversial, without clear evidence of benefit from either medical or surgical therapy for the vast majority of patients. All of these issues have led to the development of the National Heart, Lung, and Blood Institute–sponsored Surgical Treatment for Ischemic Heart Failure (STICH) trial, which in many respects revisits the nonrandomized arm of CASS, but with the important advantage of modern medical and surgical therapies (23–25). This multicenter international randomized trial will address two hypotheses. The first is that surgical restoration with revascularization and medical therapy will improve survival free of cardiac hospitalizations compared to revascularization and medical therapy alone (Fig. 91.10). This trial will be the first randomized trial that looks closely at a surgical therapy that actively alters LV geometry. It will try to answer whether active geometric changes add significantly to revascularization and intensive medical and device (Internal Cardiac Defibrilator [ICD] and biventricular pacing) therapies. Success will require low surgical mortality, consistent surgical remodeling (not too much or too little), and complete follow-up of the patients.

The second hypothesis is that coronary revascularization with intensive medical therapy improves long-term survival compared to medical therapy alone (Fig. 91.11). This is the more controversial arm of the trial; some feel it is unethical to

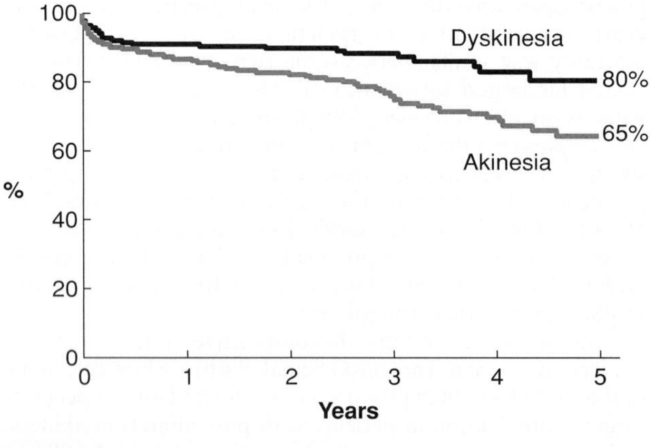

FIGURE 91.9. The RESTORE registry demonstrated an overall 5-year survival of 68.6%. Survival at 5 years was better in the group of patients who had dyskinetic as compared with akinetic morphology (80% versus 65%; $P < .001$).

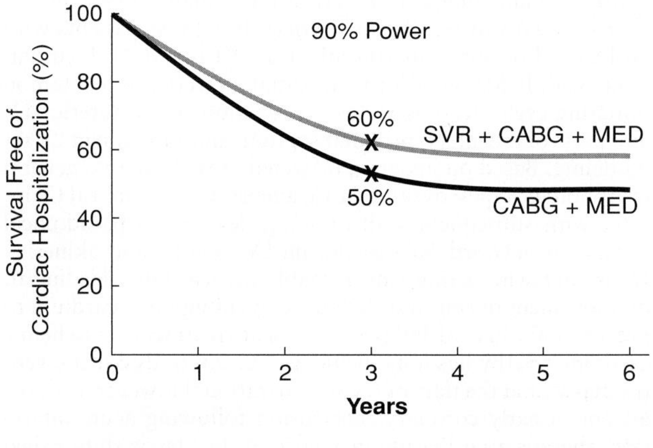

FIGURE 91.10. The multicenter international randomized STICH trial will address two hypotheses. The first is that surgical restoration with revascularization and medical therapy will improve survival, free of cardiac hospitalizations compared to revascularization and medical therapy alone. *Abbreviations:* CABG, coronary artery bypass grafting; MED, medical therapy; SVR, surgical ventricular restoration.

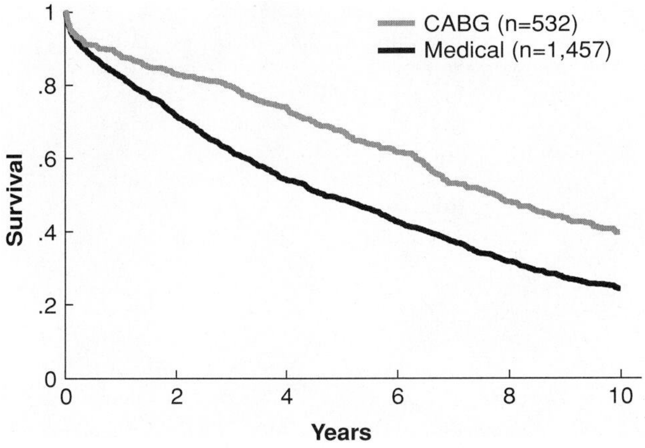

FIGURE 91.11. The second hypothesis of the STICH trial is that coronary revascularization with intensive medical therapy improves long-term survival compared to medical therapy alone. *Abbreviations:* CABG, coronary artery bypass grafting; SVR, surgical ventricular restoration.

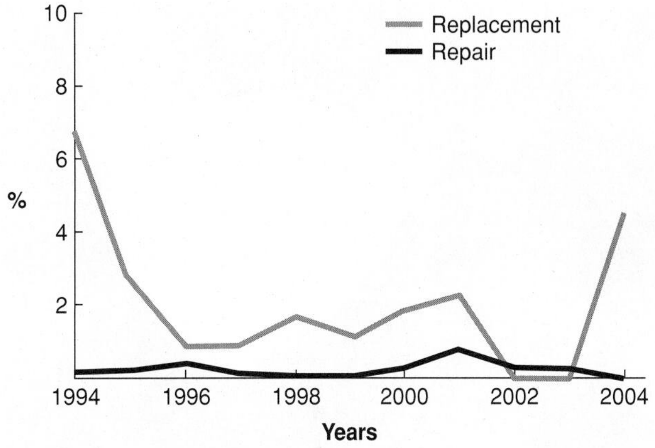

FIGURE 91.12. Operative mortality for isolated MV operations at The Cleveland Clinic Foundation.

not offer surgery to patients with multivessel disease and LV dysfunction. The authors feel there are many patients with severe LV dysfunction and very large ventricles, without angina and well-controlled heart failure symptoms in which the optimal therapy remains uncertain. Imaging studies may provide some guidance by identifying hibernating regions of the LV or percentage of scarring but in general these studies have involved small numbers of patients and looked at surrogate endpoints like global or regional improvement in LV function. Survival and symptomatic improvement have not been systematically assessed and will be part of the STICH results.

Over a 3-year period, 2,800 patients with heart failure, EF of less than 35%, and coronary artery disease amenable to revascularization will be enrolled. At the time of writing, it is disappointing that only 1,181 of the 2,800 patients have been enrolled as a result of unanticipated difficulties with recruitment and many believe the reluctance to enroll patients is a result of the possibility of randomization into the medicine-only arm of the study. The ischemic heart failure population is escalating and the STICH trial is the first trial designed and powered to yield important information about the applicability of surgical options for this group.

MITRAL VALVE SURGERY IN CONGESTIVE HEART FAILURE

A common complication of ischemic and nonischemic cardiomyopathy is severe mitral regurgitation (MR). Historically, MV surgery in these patients was long thought to be associated with a prohibitive operative mortality, with previous reports identifying severe LV dysfunction as highly significant for adverse outcomes. For the patient with ischemic MR, the results reported were even more dismal, as ischemic MR is usually caused by LV and/or papillary muscle dysfunction. However, these observations were largely based on the use of traditional MV replacement with disruption of the subvalvular apparatus, which resulted in immediate worsening of LV function. Significant advances have been made since those early series both in our understanding of the importance of conservation of the subvalvular apparatus and improvements in surgical techniques. An increasing body of evidence now demonstrates low surgical mortality and good intermediate-term survival for MV surgery in patients with severe LV dysfunction (Fig. 91.12).

Operative Risks

Concern about the high perioperative risk after MV surgery in patients with severe LV dysfunction was put to rest with the presentation of the ACORN CorCap cardiac support device (CSD) trial at the 2005 meeting of the American Association of Thoracic Surgeons (26). This prospective randomized multicenter trial evaluated outcomes following MV surgery with and without the Acorn CorCap (discussed below) in patients with NYHA Class II to IV symptoms, dilated cardiomyopathy, and mitral insufficiency. In this trial, a subgroup of 193 patients in the larger study of 300 were assigned to MV repair or replacement, 91 of whom concomitantly received the CorCap. These patients had advanced cardiac dysfunction and heart failure: 77% NYHA Class III or IV, average LVEF 23%, and mean LV end-diastolic volume of 70 mm. MV repair was possible in 155 (84%) patients and replacement in 29 (16%). Three patients (1%) died within 30 days. All MV replacements survived hospitalization. These results are outstanding and unequivocally show MV interventions in patients with cardiomyopathy are safe, and importantly suggest that MV replacement does not substantially increase perioperative risk.

Long-Term Outcomes

Confident that MV interventions are safe, uncertainty remains about whether these interventions impact long-term survival. Gillinov et al. (27) reported that for both degenerative and ischemic MV disease, the severity of LV dysfunction is the major determinant of survival after MV intervention and the greater the LV dysfunction, the less obvious the benefit of MV repair over replacement; some would advocate cardiac transplantation for certain subsets of patients. Wu et al. (28) have tried to answer the question of the endpoint of long-term mortality with a propensity matched analysis from a single institution experience with MV repair in patients with cardiomyopathy. Several published series from this same institution had previously shown a low operative mortality and a good intermediate-term outcome, and in many cases advocated for surgical intervention as an alternative to transplantation (29,30). Although there are limitations to this study published in the *Journal of the American College of Cardiology* in 2005, they were unable to demonstrate a late survival advantage of MV intervention over that of medical therapy in patients with MR and LV dysfunction; however, the important issue of possible symptomatic improvement was not studied. From the Cleveland Clinic, in a small series of

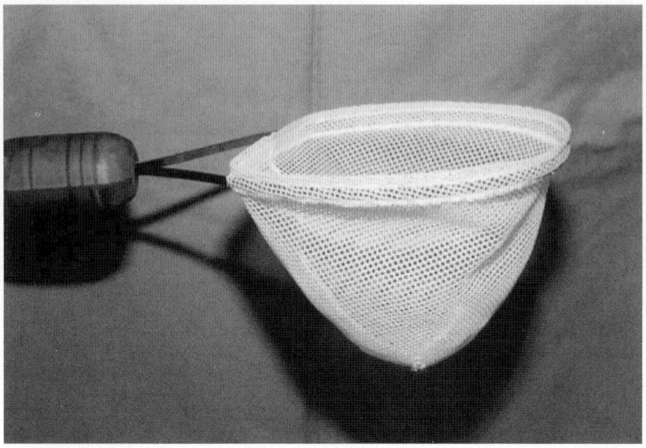

FIGURE 91.13. Acorn mesh.

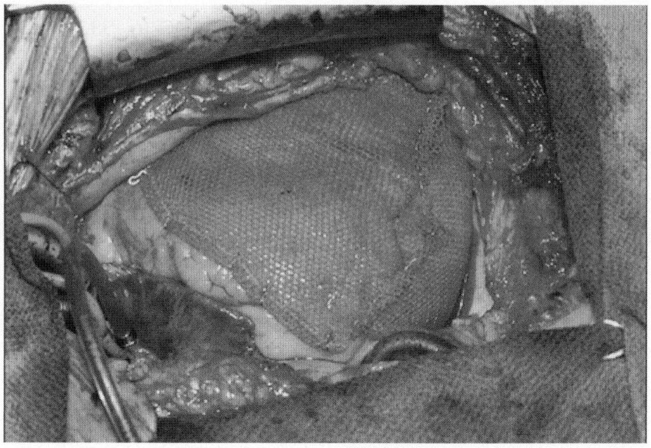

FIGURE 91.14. Acorn CorCap after placement around the left ventricle and right ventricle.

44 patients with a LV EF of less than 35% undergoing isolated MV surgery, we found the NYHA Class improved for survivors from 2.8 ± 0.8 preoperatively to 1.2 ± 0.5 at follow-up. In the CorCap trial, patients had a significant 18- to 22-point reduction in their Minnesota Living with Heart Failure Questionnaire, suggesting that the MV intervention significantly improves symptoms; however, it should be noted that these results were in patients with predominantly dilated cardiomyopathy and it is not certain that these results can be applied to ischemic MR (31).

Overall, the heart failure community applauds the honest assessment from the University of Michigan of what is perhaps the largest experience of MV repair in patients with severe LV dysfunction. This paper has resulted in serious questions on what many clinicians refer to as an "alternative to transplantation" strategy and certainly suggests a need for a prospective randomized controlled trial that will provide answers.

DEVICE THERAPY: CorCap, CoApsys, PERMANENT DEVICES

Restraining Device: CorCap Trial

The previous edition reviewed the history of restraining devices developed from the earlier work with dynamic cardiomyoplasty, which demonstrated that the benefit gained from the procedure may have been as a consequence of the girdling effect from the latissimus dorsi muscle. From the original, complex latissimus dorsi cardiomyoplasty procedure evolved a simple synthetic mesh developed by the Acorn Company called the CorCap CSD (Figs. 91.13 and 91.14). Konertz (32) conducted the initial preclinical study on a cohort of 29 patients treated with the CorCap CSD alone or concomitant MV surgery. This preclinical experiment demonstrated improved LV function and reverse remodeling initially noted at 3 months and sustained at 1 year. This early work provided the basis and selection criteria for the worldwide trial, which randomized 300 patients at 29 centers in North America treated with the device alone and those undergoing MV interventions (Fig. 91.15) (33). All patients were followed for a minimum of 12 months with a median follow-up of 22 months. Compliance with optimal medical therapy was excellent. Compared to the control group, the Acorn CSD patients experienced fewer major cardiac procedures defined as LVAD or transplant, demonstrated a greater reduction in LV volumes, and a greater improvement in LV shape. Patients in the Acorn CSD group significantly improved their quality of life as measured by the Minnesota Living with Heart Failure and SF36. Despite these positive results, the device failed to receive endorsement from an FDA advisory panel. Reasons may include failure to show a survival advantage and concerns about difficulties with reoperations after placement of the device. The primary endpoint also required a core laboratory assessment of NYHA functional class; however, the baseline value was imputed in over 50% of the patients. These factors raised significant concern and the data are still under review by the FDA.

Unfortunately, this is the second restraining device trial showing early promise that either failed to complete the trial (cardiomyoplasty) or to date has not been approved (CorCap CSD). This highlights the expensive and extremely complex nature of surgical device trials in patients with advanced heart failure.

CoApsys System

It quickly became apparent that external device-based ventricular remodeling would be extremely difficult. Simultaneous with this realization was the disappointing cumulative experience with MV repair for cardiomyopathy. Recurrent MR occurred in 20% to 30% of patients after repair. It was suggested that part of the reason was that "valvular" repair alone was

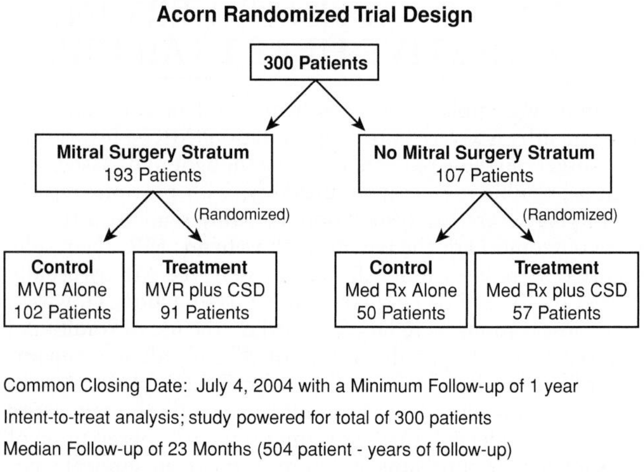

FIGURE 91.15. Acorn CorCap randomized trial design. *Abbreviations:* CSD, cardiac support device; Med Rx, medical treatment; MVR, mitral valve repair.

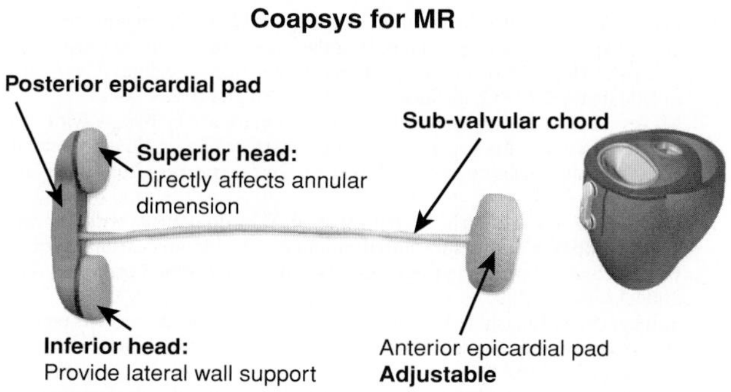

FIGURE 91.16. Modifying the Myocor Myosplint ventricular shape change concept (originally described in the first edition), a transventricular MV repair device has been developed. Currently in clinical trials, the Coapsys technology is designed to geometrically reshape the MV and to improve valve function using a less invasive approach compared to current therapies.

inadequate for a "ventricular" problem. Modifying the Myocor Myosplint ventricular shape change concept (originally described in the first edition), a transventricular MV repair device has been developed (34). Currently in clinical trials, the Coapsys technology is designed to geometrically reshape the MV and to improve valve function using a less invasive approach compared to current therapies (Fig. 91.16). The Coapsys device is implanted on a closed, beating heart without the use of cardiopulmonary bypass. Similar to the Myocor Myosplint ventricular remodeling approach, the CoApsys device pulls the basilar section of the left ventricle anteriorly reducing the tethering of the posterior valvular leaflet. As with the CorCap, the CoApsys system will still need to prove clinical utility.

PERMANENT DEVICE SUPPORT

Since publication of the last edition of this textbook the REMATCH Trial comparing the Heartmate VE device to best medical therapy in patients with very advanced heart failure was published (35). The results have received mixed reviews. On the one hand the devices did show a survival advantage at 1 and 2 years, but by $2\frac{1}{2}$ years most patients in both arms were dead (Fig. 91.17). It is of interest that a follow-up analysis of

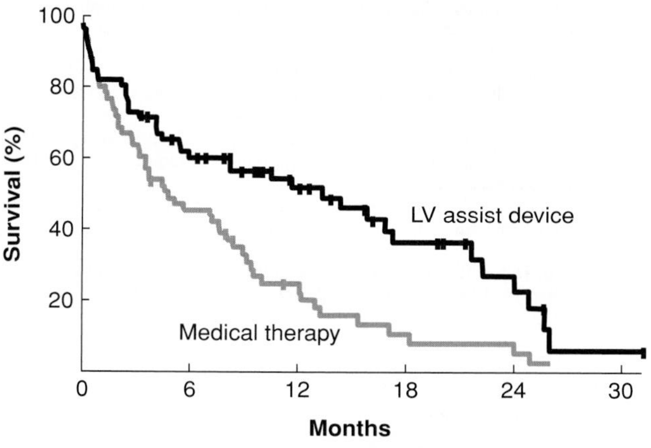

FIGURE 91.17. The REMATCH Trial compared the Heartmate VE device to best medical therapy in patients with very advanced heart failure. The devices did show a survival advantage at 1 and 2 years, but by $2\frac{1}{2}$ years most patients in both arms were dead.

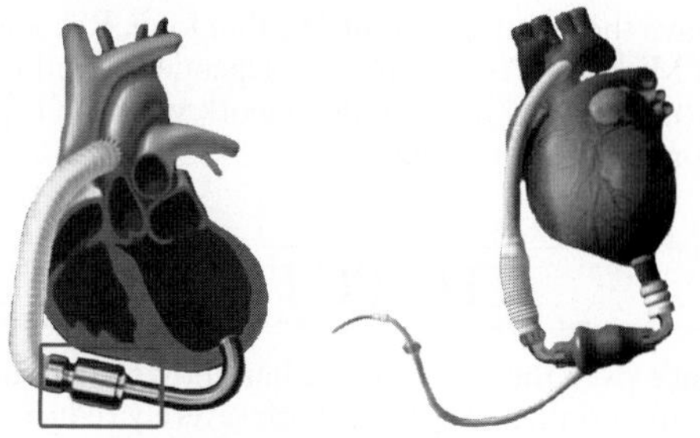

FIGURE 91.18. The Heartmate II and the Debakey pumps represent the second-generation of mechanical ventricular support, are much smaller than the earlier technology, and are nonpulsatile continuous flow pumps.

this same data found that time of enrollment was a significant factor in determining mortality with a 15% improvement in survival at both 1 and 2 years for patients enrolled during the latter half of the trial and may be explained by the learning curve associated with destination therapy (36). Patients supported with the Heartmate VE frequently died of sepsis and device failures were common. Finally, device durability was limited to 12 to 18 months. These device capabilities generated concern about wider application of these technologies. The device received FDA and CMS approval for permanent therapy in late 2002 with 310 devices utilized since. Recent reports have suggested that only inotrope dependent patients receive true benefit from device support, but at the same time recent results in patients supported with the latest generation of the Heartmate, the XVE, also show reduced infections, better early survival, and decreased pump failures.

We believe that the best way to determine if device therapy has improved is to enroll most patients being considered for permanent support into one of three ongoing clinical trials. This will serve two important goals: (a) to determine if device therapy has improved since the REMATCH trial and (b) to compare the outcomes of patients supported with low pulsatility continuous flow pumps to the larger pulsatile devices (Fig. 91.18).

The RELIANT trial compares two pulsatile devices, the Novacor LVAS and the Heartmate XVE. This is a reasonable comparison because the Novacor system is considered more durable with probably fewer infections, but has been troubled with high rates of thromboemboli.

The DELTA Trial and the Heartmate II Trial compares two continuous flow pumps, the DeBakey Micromed and the Heartmate II to the larger pulsatile flow Heartmate XVE. The smaller pumps have several advantages, namely, small to no pump pockets, thus fewer infections; potentially greater durability without valves; and utility in patients of small stature. Concerns raised about these devices are higher thromboembolic and pump thrombosis rates, lack of an intrinsic Frank Starling mechanism to augment flow during exercise, and tolerability of low or reduced pulsatility for extended periods of time.

CONTROVERSIES AND PERSONAL PERSPECTIVES

By far the greatest limitation is the availability of patients to enroll in these trials, this despite the fact that there are over 5 million patients in the United States with a diagnosis of heart failure. Each trial is planning to randomize 300 to 350 patients. Extrapolating from the REMATCH Trial, nearly 10,000 potential permanent LVAD candidates will need to be screened to enroll 1,000 patients and at the current rate, this will take well over 5 years. It well may be that many of these device companies do not have the resources to survive that long. Recognizing this fact, the Micromed company has suspended enrollment in the DELTA trial while they attempt to work with the FDA to ease restrictions on trial participation.

THE FUTURE

Experience over the past 5 years has shown that surgery can be safely undertaken in patients with severely reduced LV function. Now an effort is being made to show that these interventions improve quality of life and prolong survival. Creeping into the world of heart failure surgery is doubt that "conventional" surgical therapies are enough to reverse the deleterious effects of LV remodeling and advanced LV dysfunction. Adjunct therapies like stem cells and myoblasts or more advanced devices such as the Coapsys system are felt to be necessary to make a significant impact on the disease process. Undoubtedly, future therapy for patients with heart failure will include intensive medical therapy, conventional and "unconventional" surgical procedures, cellular replacement, and devices. As mechanical circulatory support devices become increasingly durable and safe, we will begin to struggle with the timing of abandonment of the native heart and proceeding directly to mechanical support.

References

1. Sabik JF, Blackstone EH, Gillinov AM, et al. Influence of patient characteristics and arterial grafts on freedom from coronary reoperation. Presented at the 85th Annual Meeting of the American Association for Thoracic Surgery, San Francisco, April 10–13, 2005.
2. Estafanous FG, Lloyd FD, Higgins TL, et al. Increased risk and decreased morbidity of coronary artery bypass grafting between 1986 and 1994. *Ann Thorac Surg* 1998;65:383–389.
3. Anderson WA, Ilkowski DA, Mahan VL, et al. Coronary artery bypass grafting in patients with chronic congestive heart failure: a 10 year experience with 203 patients. *J Cardiac Surg* 1997;12:167–175.
4. Argenazio M, Spotnitz HM, Whang W, et al. Risk stratification for coronary bypass surgery in patients with left ventricular dysfunction: analysis of the coronary artery bypass grafting patch trial database. *Circulation* 1999;100[Suppl 19]:III:19–24.
5. Baumgartner FJ, Omari BO, Goldberg S, et al. Coronary artery bypass grafting in patients with profound ventricular dysfunction. *Tex Heart Inst J* 1998;25:125–129.
6. Elefteriades JA, Morales DL, Gradel C, et al. Results of coronary artery bypass grafting by a single surgeon in patients with left ventricular ejection fractions < or =30%. *Am J Cardiol* 1997;79:1573–1578.
7. Kaul TK, Agnihotri AK, Fields BL, et al. Coronary artery bypass grafting in patients with an ejection fraction of 20% or less. *J Thorac Cardiovasc Surgery* 1996;111:1001–1012.
8. Kawachi K, Kitamura S, Hasegawa J, et al. Increased risk of coronary artery bypass grafting for left ventricular dysfunction with dilated left ventricle. *J Cardiovasc Surg* 1997;38:501–505.
9. Ascione R, Narayan P, Rogers CA, et al. Early and midterm clinical outcome in patients with severe left ventricular dysfunction undergoing coronary artery surgery. *Ann Thorac Surg* 2003;76:793–800.
10. Kron IL, Flanagan TL, Blackbourne LH, et al. Coronary revascularization rather than cardiac transplantation for chronic ischemic cardiomyopathy. *Ann Surg* 1989;210:348–354.
11. Luciani GB, Faggian G, Razzolimi R, et al. Severe ischemic left ventricular failure: coronary operation or heart transplantation. *Ann Thorac Surg* 1993;55:719–723.
12. Langenburg SE, Buchanan SA, Blackbourne LH, et al. Predicting survival after coronary revascularization for ischemic cardiomyopathy. *Ann Thorac Surg* 1995;60:1193–1196.
13. Eagle KA, Guyton RA, Davidoff R, et al. ACC/AHA Guidelines for coronary artery bypass graft surgery: a report of the American College of Cardiology/American Heart Association Task Force on Practice Guidelines (Committee to Update the 1999 Guidelines). *Circulation* 2004;110:e340–437.
14. Maxey TS, Reece TB, Ellman PI, et al. Coronary artery bypass with ventricular restoration is superior to coronary artery bypass alone in patients with ischemic cardiomyopathy. *J Thorac Cardiovasc Surg* 2004;127:428–434.
15. Schinkel AF, Polderman S, Rizzello V, et al. Why do patients with ischemic cardiomyopathy and a substantial amount of viable myocardium not always recover in function after revascularization? *J Thorac Cardiovasc Surg* 2004;1276:385–390.
16. Yamaguchi A, Takashi I, Adachi H. Left ventricular volume predicts postoperative course in patients with ischemic cardiomyopathy. *Ann Thorac Surg* 1998;65:434–438.
17. Gaudron P, Eilles C, Kugler I. Progressive left ventricular dysfunction and remodeling after MI. Potential mechanisms and early predictors. *Circulation* 1993;87:755–763.
18. Dor V, Sabatier M, DiDonato M. Efficacy of endoventricular patch plasty in large postinfarction akinetic scar and severe left ventricular dysfunction comparison with a series of large dyskinetic scars. *J Thorac Cardiovasc Surg* 1998;116:50–59.
19. Dor V, Di Donato M, Sabatier M, et al. Left ventricular reconstruction of endoventricular circular patch plasty repair: a 17 year experience. *Semin Thorac Cardiovasc Surg* 2001;13:435–447.
20. Athanasuleas CL, Buckberg GD, Stanley AWH, et al. Surgical ventricular restoration in the treatment of congestive heart failure due to post-infarction ventricular dilatation. *J Am Coll Cardiol* 2004;44:1439–1445.
21. Smith. American Heart Association Annual Scientific Sessions 2003. Invited lecture.
22. Elefteriades JA, Tolis G, Levi E, et al. Coronary artery bypass grafting in severe left ventricular dysfunction: excellent survival with improved ejection fraction and functional state. *J Am Coll Cardiol* 1993;22:1411–1417.
23. Menicante L, Di Donato M. Surgical left ventricle reconstruction, pathophysiologic insights, results and expectations from the STICH trial. *Eur J Cardiothorac Surg* 2004;26:S42–47.
24. Doenst T, Velazquez EJ, Beyersdorf F, et al. To STICH or not to STICH: We know the answer but do we understand the question? *J Thorac Cardiovasc Surg* 2005;129:246–249.
25. Buckberg G. Questions and answers about the STICH trial: a different perspective. *J Thorac Cardiovasc Surg* 2005;130:245–249.
26. Acker MA, Bolling SF, Mann DL, et al. Mitral valve surgery in heart failure: results of the Acorn Corcap randomized trial. Presented at the 85th Annual Meeting of the American Association for Thoracic Surgery, San Francisco, California, April 11, 2005. *J Thorac Cardiovasc Surg* (In press).
27. Gillinov AM, Wierup PN, Blackstone EH, et al. Is repair preferable to replacement for ischemic mitral regurgitation? *J Thorac Cardiovasc Surg* 2001;122:1125–1141.
28. Wu AH, Aaronson KD, Bolling SF, et al. Impact of mitral valve anuloplasty on mortality risk in patients with mitral regurgitation and left ventricular dysfunction. *J Am Coll Cardiol* 2005;45:381–387.
29. Bolling SF, Pagani FD, Deeb GM, et al. Intermediate-term outcome of mitral reconstruction in cardiomyopathy. *J Thorac Cardiovasc Surg* 1998;115:381–386.
30. Bach DS, Bolling SF. Improvement following correction of secondary mitral regurgitation in end-stage cardiomyopathy with mitral annuloplasty. *Am J Cardiol* 1996;78:966–969.
31. Bishay ES, McCarthy PM, Cosgrove DM, et al. Mitral valve surgery in patients with left ventricular dysfunction. *Eur J Cardiothorac Surg* 2000;17:213–221.
32. Konertz W. Initial efficacy trends with the Acorn cardiac support device in patients with advanced heart failure. *J Am Coll Cardiol* 2001;37[Suppl A]:143A.
33. Mann DL. Clinical evaluation of the Corcap cardiac support device in patients with dilated cardiomyopathy. Presented at the American Heart Association Scientific Sessions, November 7, 2004.
34. Inoue M, McCarthy PM, Popocic ZB, et al. The Coapsys device to treat functional mitral regurgitation: In vivo long-term canine study. *J Thorac Cardiovasc Surg* 2004;127:1068–1077.
35. Rose E, Gelijns A, Moskowitz A, et al. Long-term mechanical left ventricular assistance for end-stage heart failure. *N Engl J Med* 2001;345:1435–1443.
36. Park SJ, Tector A, Piccioni W, et al. Left ventricular assist devices as destination therapy: A new look at survival. *J Thorac Cardiovasc Surg* 2005;129:9–17.

CHAPTER 92 ■ PREVENTION OF HEART FAILURE

W. H. WILSON TANG AND ANJLI MAROO

OVERVIEW

Heart failure accounts for a substantial proportion of hospitalizations and mortality, particularly in patients over 65 years of age (1). The incidence of the heart failure syndrome continues to increase because of the expansion of the aging population and therapeutic advances in the management of cardiovascular diseases. Recent estimates indicate that one out of five persons will be at risk of developing heart failure over the course of his or her lifetime (Fig. 92.1) (2). As more drugs become available, our attention has been directed toward the escalation of various "salvage therapies" to reduce morbidity and mortality in patients with advanced heart failure (such as destination left ventricular [LV] assist device therapy, internal cardioverter defibrillator, and cardiac resynchronization therapy; see Chapter 86). In the grand scheme of heart failure management, it has become more and more apparent that this costly strategy is providing only modest incremental benefits and is not geared to reduce disease burden or improve public health.

STAGING OF HEART FAILURE

The concept of "heart failure prevention" generally has been lumped into the category of primary prevention of cardiovascular risk factors. Because of the segregation of specialty "silos," patients with early heart failure (especially following an acute myocardial infarction or chemotherapeutic insult) frequently escape detection until they develop signs and symptoms of heart failure. It is conceivable that multiple factors may contribute to the pathogenesis of symptomatic heart failure; early initiation of pharmacologic therapy may help to prevent disease progression. There are certain known risk factors and structural prerequisites that lead to the development of LV systolic and/or diastolic dysfunction and the clinical syndrome of heart failure. To emphasize that "heart failure" represents a continuum of disease, the latest guidelines from the American College of Cardiology and American Heart Association categorize patients with chronic heart failure into four stages (3) (Table 92.1):

- **Stage A** encompasses patients at risk for development of symptomatic heart failure. Risk factors include hypertension, atherosclerotic coronary artery disease, diabetes, obesity, metabolic syndrome, familial predisposition for dilated cardiomyopathy, and cardiotoxic drug exposure (e.g., adriamycin chemotherapy or alcohol). If left unchecked, these patients are likely to develop structural abnormalities of the heart.
- **Stage B** is defined by the development of structural abnormalities of the heart without (or with minimal) symptoms of heart failure. This is a poorly understood category because these patients are often identified serendipitously. Examples of stage B heart failure include (a) a hypertensive patient who develops left ventricular hypertrophy (LVH), (b) the onset of a LV wall motion abnormality in a patient with prior myocardial infarction, or (c) patients with asymptomatic valvular diseases. Because these patients do not have overt symptoms, only large epidemiologic studies have been able to describe the prevalence and incidence of asymptomatic left ventricular dysfunction (ALVD).
- **Stages C and D** are the commonly recognized forms of congestive heart failure where patients may develop progressive degrees of symptomatic heart failure. By definition, stage C patients have either ongoing symptomatic heart failure, or have had symptoms of heart failure in the past. Most clinical trials in heart failure have focused on treating symptomatic patients in these categories because they can be easily identified.

These "stages" are largely descriptive. In fact, our understanding of the pace at which the signs and symptoms of heart failure

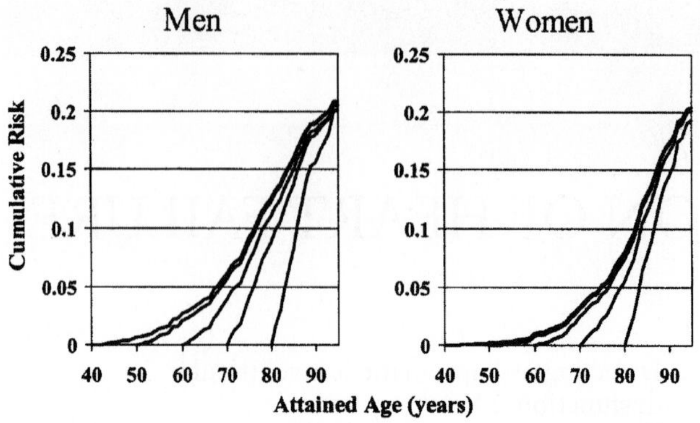

FIGURE 92.1. Lifetime risk of developing heart failure. (*Source:* reproduced with permission from Lloyd-Jones DM, Larson MG, Leip EP, et al. Lifetime risk for developing congestive heart failure: the Framingham Heart Study. *Circulation* 2002;106:3068–3072.)

progress is rudimentary. The prevention of heart failure exacerbations in patients with stages C and D were discussed in Chapter 86. This chapter focuses our current knowledge in detecting and preventing heart failure in patients at stages A and B.

DETECTION AND MANAGEMENT OF STAGE A HEART FAILURE

Like any disease screening recommendations, determining the "population at risk" is the most difficult task. Table 92.2 outlines the population-attributable risks of various risk factors for the development of heart failure in three large-scale epidemiologic studies. It is very important to recognize that these variables have been documented as binomial variables, and there is large heterogeneity among patients with the same risk factor.

Age

Like all chronic diseases, advancing age is an important risk factor. Increasing age has been consistently associated with increased risk of developing heart failure and ventricular dysfunction, and carries an increased risk of morbidity and mortality. In the Olmsted County database, 88% of the 216 incident heart failure cases identified in 1991 and 1992 were over 65 years of age (4). Data across almost all large epidemiologic databases indicate that heart failure is present in about 1% of adults in their 50s and in as many as 10% of those in their 80s (5). Although this association between advancing age and heart failure may relate to "normal" aging of the human heart, it is more likely the result of decades of inadequate treatment of other underlying risk factors. Because of age-related changes in the cardiovascular system, elderly patients are more likely to have advanced heart failure at the time of initial presentation, and may be less likely to receive effective medial therapies.

Family History

Up to 30% to 50% of patients with dilated cardiomyopathy may have family members that have similar conditions, a process known as *familial dilated cardiomyopathy* (FDC) (6,7). Discovery of complex genetic predispositions are ongoing. Mutation patterns of FDC bear a close resemblance to the mutation patterns of hypertrophic cardiomyopathy (7) (see Chapter 84). The latest figures indicate that treatable asymptomatic dilated cardiomyopathy can be identified in as many as 4.6% of asymptomatic relatives of patients with dilated cardiomyopathy (8). Although there have been no solid standardized criteria to determine the diagnosis of FDC, echocardiographic, electrocardiographic, and metabolic screening has been advocated to detect ALVD in all first-degree relatives (8,9). Patients who have familial ALVD may require aggressive treatment and careful monitoring, because their prognosis can be relatively poor (10).

Hypertension

Up to 76% of men and 79% of women with symptomatic heart failure at Framingham had preexisting hypertension (11,12). Numerous randomized controlled trials have consistently demonstrated that optimal blood pressure control decreases the risk of incident heart failure by approximately 50%. The benefits of treating hypertension in heart attack survivors can lead to an 81% reduction in incident heart failure. Hypertension may lead to heart failure via one of two major

TABLE 92.1

STAGES OF HEART FAILURE

Stage	Definition	Examples	Functional Class
A	At high risk of HF, but no structural heart disease or symptoms of HF	Patients with hypertension, coronary artery disease, diabetes mellitus, or patients with cardiotoxin or family history of cardiomyopathy	N/A
B	Structural heart disease but without symptoms of HF	Patients with previous MI, LV systolic dysfunction, and valvular diseases	I
C	Structural heart disease but prior or current symptoms of HF	Patients with known structural heart disease, shortness of breath and fatigue, reduced exercise tolerance	II–III
D	Refractory HF requiring specialized intervention	Patients with marked symptoms at rest despite maximal medical therapy	III–IV

Abbreviations: HF, heart failure; MI, myocardial infarction; LV, left ventricular.

TABLE 92.2

POPULATION-ATTRIBUTABLE RISKS IN DEVELOPING HEART FAILURE FROM POPULATION-BASED STUDIES

	Framingham (60)	CHS (61)	NHANES (62)
Hypertension (%)	39–59	13	9–12
Coronary artery disease (%)	13–34	13	56–68
Angina (%)	5	—	—
Diabetes mellitus (%)	6–12	8	3
LVH (ECG) (%)	4–5	6	—
Valvular heart disease (%)	7–8	—	2–3
Renal insufficiency (%)	—	6	—
Low FEV_1 (%)	—	3	—
Peripheral vascular disease (%)	—	9	—
Atrial fibrillation (ECG) (%)	—	2	—
Cigarette smoking (%)	—	—	16–22
Low physical activity (%)	—	—	9–13
Male sex (%)	—	—	9
Overweight (%)	—	—	6–10
<High-school education (%)	—	—	9–10

Abbreviations: CHS, Cardiovascular Health Study; ECG, electrocardiograph; LVH, left ventricular hypertrophy; NHANES, National Health and Nutrition Examination Survey; FEV_1, forced expiratory volume in 1 second.

pathways, both mediated by the development of a structural abnormality of the heart: LVH and the development of atherosclerotic heart disease. LVH is a strong, independent risk factor for developing heart failure. In general, data support a lower ideal or target blood pressure goal in patients with associated major cardiovascular risk factors, especially diabetes mellitus. Treatment to target blood pressure should remain the primary goal of antihypertensive treatment. The choice of a particular agent is less straightforward. The presence of certain comorbidities may favor initiation of specific agents (e.g., use of drugs blocking the renin–angiotensin–aldosterone system in patients with diabetes, coronary artery disease, or LV dysfunction). However, to date there have been no specific recommendations (see Chapter 7).

Diabetes Mellitus, Obesity, and the Metabolic Syndrome

Obesity and insulin resistance are established risk factors for the development of heart failure. Obesity alone has been shown to be an independent risk factor for new-onset heart failure (13). There are many ways by which obesity may contribute to the development of structural abnormalities of the heart. Many of these appear to be mediated by the proliferative milieu associated with insulin resistance (or hyperinsulinemia) and overt diabetes. In this regard, the metabolic syndrome may also play a major role in elevating the risk of heart failure (14,15). The presence of diabetes mellitus substantially increases the risk of heart failure in patients without preexisting structural heart disease, especially for women (16). Many diabetic patients exhibit angiographically normal epicardial coronary arteries with a presumed "nonischemic" dilated cardiomyopathy. Often with LVH, "diabetic cardiomyopathy" has been associated with fatty depositions, small vessel coronary disease, and endothelial dysfunction (17,18). These structural and functional changes in the microvasculature may represent an ischemic form of heart failure. Silent ischemia is highly prevalent in asymptomatic diabetic patients (up to 39% in one study) (19). Recent data from the Mayo Clinic have identified a prevalence of 16.7% for LV dysfunction (left ventricular ejection fraction [LVEF] <50%) in 1,064 consecutive asymptomatic diabetic patients without known coronary artery disease who underwent nuclear stress testing between 1986 and 2000. In this cohort, a relatively high unadjusted annual mortality of 7% has been documented despite the lack of symptoms and "known" coronary artery disease (20). Alternatively, hyperinsulinemia, hyperglycemia, and other growth-promoting hormones may mediate the pathologic myocyte remodeling seen in these patients.

Coronary Artery Disease

Coronary artery disease appears to account for 60% to 70% of the incidence of systolic heart failure in developed countries. Annually in the United States, approximately 1.1 million individuals suffer a myocardial infarction and about 40% of them may be left with a reduced LVEF (21). Data from clinical trial registries such as the Studies of Left Ventricular Dysfunction (SOLVD) Registry identified over two thirds of patients with ischemic heart disease as underlying cause of heart failure (22). This is not entirely representative of the broader heart failure population as subjects were predominantly middle-aged white men. In the African-American Heart Failure study, most subjects had nonischemic heart failure in association with hypertension, diabetes, and obesity (23). Interestingly, the prevalence of hypertension in black subjects enrolled in the SOLVD registry was 32%, compared to 4% in white subjects (22). Nevertheless, therapies aimed at reducing ischemic events should be aggressively pursued, including potential revascularization strategies (see Chapter 17).

Cardiotoxic Chemotherapy

Cardiotoxic effects of chemotherapy have been well established, but the majority of our experience has focused on detection, management, and prevention of dose-dependent early compromise of cardiac function (24). The best-known cardiotoxic drugs include anthracyclines/anthraquinones and many alkylating agents; recent concerns of cardiotoxicity with the use of trastuzumab (Herceptin) and paclitaxel (Taxol) for breast cancer, imatinib (Gleevec) for chronic myelogenous leukemia, alemtuzumab (CamPath) for chronic lymphocytic leukemia, and bevacizumab (Avastin) for colorectal cancer have been reported in the literature (24). Early detection of anthracycline-induced cardiotoxicities has been evaluated in several small-scale studies. Reports of a subacute form of toxicity have been reported between 3 to 8 months from the last chemotherapy dose. Late onset can occur as many as 6 to 25 years after therapy with no prior symptoms. Risk factors for chemotherapy cardiotoxicity include advanced age, male gender, being overweight, history of combination therapy or mediastinal radiotherapy, prior cardiac diseases or hypertension, history of liver disease, and dosage and schedule of drugs administered. Much less is known about the long-term cardiotoxicity risks of newer agents, particularly with respect to drug combinations.

Currently, there are no guidelines for long-term clinical monitoring for cardiovascular toxicities in patients who have received chemotherapy, and little is known regarding the epidemiology of cardiomyopathy in long-term cancer survivors. Cardiac imaging remains the gold standard for detecting chemotherapy-induced cardiotoxicity; however, most studies have focused on early or subacute manifestations of heart failure (25). In a study of 141 lymphoma survivors who had previously received doxorubicin-based chemotherapy and underwent echocardiography screening at least 5 years later (one had clinical heart failure signs and symptoms), subclinical reduction in fractional shortening was found in 39 patients (28%) (26). To date, there has been no large-scale screening study performed in cancer survivors because late cardiomyopathy has been considered "rare," despite a potentially large cohort of at-risk patients. Optimal timing and diagnostic value of biomarker screening and the incremental value over screening echocardiography have yet to be determined.

DETECTION AND MANAGEMENT OF STAGE B HEART FAILURE

It is estimated that the number of patients with stage B heart failure may be up to fourfold greater than the number of patients with clinically overt heart failure (27). Identification of a cohort of asymptomatic (or minimally symptomatic) patients with structural heart disease at risk for heart failure disease progression will theoretically focus resource utilization to those who would benefit most from preventive therapeutic intervention and long-term follow-up.

There has been no uniform and precise definition of stage B heart failure, and the guidelines have been purposefully nonspecific. Therefore, the true prevalence of unrecognized patients with stage B heart failure in the primary care setting has not been well described in the literature. For the purpose of this discussion, we have distinguished two main subcategories: ALVD and LVH. Asymptomatic valvular disorders are briefly discussed in Chapters 22, 23, and 24. In population studies, up to 90% of patients with LV dysfunction (LVEF $\leq$ 35%) have underlying cardiovascular disease, hypertension, or diabetes. However, the onset of symptoms of heart failure may occur at all levels of ventricular dysfunction. Furthermore, the time course of the natural progression is highly variable. Some patients with deteriorating ventricular function may even die before developing any symptoms of overt heart failure. Relying on self-reporting is therefore inadequate. This point is highlighted in the findings from the SOLVD Registry, in which patients with ventricular dysfunction (LVEF <45%) were recruited to participate in clinical trials to determine the efficacy of enalapril in heart failure (22). In 6,273 consecutive patients with LV dysfunction identified from echocardiographic screening, approximately 80% had mild or no symptoms (New York Heart Association functional class I or II). Only 32% of patients had pulmonary rales, 26% had edema, and 20% had elevated jugular venous distension on clinical examination at the time of enrollment.

Detecting Asymptomatic Left Ventricular Dysfunction

When characteristics of ALVD patients are explored, patients are found to be more underrecognized than asymptomatic; many patients have subtle symptoms following detailed assessment. When comparing patients with ALVD to healthy, age-matched control subjects, ALVD is associated with shorter exercise times on treadmill testing and lower questionnaire scores for assessing physical functioning.

The number of asymptomatic patients with structural heart abnormalities is not inconsequential. Despite the wide variation of definitions, it is estimated that the prevalence of ALVD in the community is at least the same if not higher than that of overt heart failure. Several large epidemiologic projects (such as the Framingham Heart Study [28], the Rochester Epidemiology Project [29], the Strong Heart Study [30], the Glasgow Clinical Research Initiative [31], and the Cardiovascular Health Study [32]) have provided highly valuable information regarding the general incidence, prevalence, and characteristics of heart failure and cardiac dysfunction in the general population (Table 92.3). In particular, the 4,257 unselected individuals in the Framingham Offsprings' Study showed 6.0% of men and 0.8% of women had an LV ejection fraction of less than 50%, with an unadjusted incidence rate for congestive heart failure ranging from 3.9 per 100 person-years (mild ALVD) to 9.6 per 100 person-years (moderate-to-severe ALVD) (28). Furthermore, an increase in LV dimension itself has been identified as the most important risk factor for development of heart failure in patients without myocardial infarction (when compared to other variables such as fractional shortening, LV mass, or LV wall thickness) (33). However, large-scale cohort programs were not designed to study mechanisms that underlie the progression of heart failure. Because the incidence of heart failure in the general population is relatively low (2% to 5% per year depending on age and risk factors), these large epidemiology programs have insufficient number of patients to allow for further, more focused investigations of the natural history (particularly regarding how various biomarkers and clinical predictors unfold as the disease progresses). This creates a large knowledge gap in heart failure prevention, allowing many opportunities for intervention to be missed. Specifically, the pace of progression, relative contributions of various precipitating factors, and the impact of monitoring and therapy remain largely unknown.

Recent population-based studies of ALVD have demonstrated that ischemic heart disease may accompany ventricular dysfunction by echocardiography in up to 78% of these cases. A lower prevalence of asymptomatic ventricular dysfunction seen in the Rotterdam study may also be explained by a lower percentage of patients with ischemic diseases (34). Following a myocardial infarction, the development of LV systolic dysfunction and dilation is the most potent predictor of subsequent heart failure and all-cause mortality. Once LV injury has occurred, progressive LV dysfunction and dilation ensues unless attenuated by medical and/or surgical therapy. An analysis from the placebo arm of the Danish Trandolapril Cardiac Evaluation (TRACE) study revealed a total of 2,606 out of 6,676

TABLE 92.3

PREVALENCE OF ASYMPTOMATIC LV DYSFUNCTION IN POPULATION-BASED STUDIES

			Prevalence (per 1,000)			
Study (start year)	Population	Definition	Male	Female	Total	% ALVD
Cardiovascular Health Study, U.S.A. (1989) (63)	N = 5,201, Ages 65–100 y	Subjective	63	18	37	25
Rotterdam, The Netherlands (1990) (34)	N = 1,698, Ages 55–95 y	FS ≤25%	55	22	37	60
Augsburg, Germany (1992) (64)	N = 1,866, Ages 25–75 y	EF <48%	32	23	28	42
Glasgow, UK (1992) (65)	N =1,640, Ages 25–74 y	EF ≤30%	—	—	29	48
Strong Heart Study, U.S.A. (1993) (30)	N = 3,184, Ages 45–74 y	EF <40%	47	18	29	72
Copenhagen, Denmark (1993) (66)	N = 2,158, Ages ≥50 y	LWMI ≤1.5 or FS <26%	—	—	29	34
Birmingham, UK (1995) (67)	N = 3,960, Ages 45–84 y	EF <40%	—	—	18	47
Olmsted County, Minnesota, USA (1997) (29)	N = 2,042, Ages >45y	EF <40%	36	11	22	61
Vasterås, Sweden (1997) (68)	N = 433, Age 75	LWMI <1.7	102	34	68	46

Abbreviations: ALVD, asymptomatic left ventricular dysfunction; EF, left ventricular ejection fraction; FS, fractional shortening; LVSD, left ventricular systolic dysfunction; LWMI, left ventricular wall motion index.

recent (2–6 days) postinfarction patients (39%) had definite LV impairment (LV ejection fraction (35%), and among those with LV dysfunction, 31% had no overt heart failure symptoms (or 8% of total population) (35). More alarming is the continuing loss of myocardium owing to reinfarction in other arterial distributions (up to 12% new infarctions at follow-up in TRACE). These figures were consistent when unselected echocardiography was performed in non–heart failure hospitalized patients, where the prevalence of ALVD was as high as 12% in postinfarction patients in a tertiary care hospital.

The natural history of postinfarction ALVD has been further explored in the Survival and Ventricular Enlargement trial (36). In this study, 2,231 postinfarction subjects with ALVD (LV ejection fraction ≤40%, mean 31%) were randomized to captopril or placebo. After an average of 3.5 years of follow-up, a total of 16% in the placebo group noted deterioration of cardiac structure and performance (reduction of LV ejection fraction ≥9%), with an annualized mortality of 12% if untreated. Indeed, hibernating myocardium may be present in up to 50% of patients with myocardial infarction, and persistent severe ischemia may also irreversibly injure remaining myocytes.

Biomarker Screening Modalities for Stage B Heart Failure

There has been an ongoing debate regarding the merits and limitations of applying specific screening tests to the general population. To address the accruing morbidity, mortality, and cost of advanced heart failure, effective screening strategies are desperately needed to specifically target asymptomatic patients who have stage B heart failure. Indeed, data from large-scale epidemiologic studies indicate a substantial population at risk of disease progression. The presence of a long "latent phase" for heart failure laid the foundation for the concept that early identification and treatment of factors (both pharmacologic and nonpharmacologic) that lead to myocardial dysfunction may abrogate progression to symptomatic advanced heart failure.

The use of natriuretic peptides as screening biomarkers for heart failure has been tested in several studies, with varying results (Table 92.4). The diagnostic utility of BNP and aminoterminal-proBNP (NT-proBNP) in the acute setting has prompted interest in evaluation of these biomarkers as effective screening tools for ALVD. There have been two major approaches to determining the utility of BNP and NT-proBNP in this setting. First, plasma BNP may be useful in the setting of acute myocardial infarction in the absence of overt heart failure, where plasma BNP levels have been inversely associated with postinfarction LVEF (37). However, because of the heterogeneity of study population and the timing of sampling, the accuracy of BNP screening has been variable. There were limitations in detecting those with marginally impaired LV abnormalities in the general population, and the cutoff value is highly dependent on the population being screened and the assay being used. This may also be due to the relatively nonspecific association with LV systolic dysfunction at lower levels of plasma BNP or NT-proBNP. Therefore, echocardiography is likely to remain the main method of assessing LV structural and functional abnormalities after a myocardial infarction, with BNP testing playing a potential adjunctive role.

Some investigators have suggested increasing the yield by focusing on high-risk subgroups, which may be more cost effective. A high prevalence of elevated plasma BNP levels has been observed in a patient population at risk of developing heart failure, particularly in those with a history of diabetes mellitus and in the elderly. It is conceivable that plasma BNP and NT-proBNP may be useful to screen for these high-risk populations who may be referred for further echocardiographic screening for ALVD (38). There are also promising data suggesting the use of urinary NT-proBNP measurements, which parallel the results obtained from measuring plasma NT-proBNP levels (39). However, at this time routine BNP testing is not appropriate for screening large asymptomatic patient populations for LV systolic dysfunction.

TABLE 92.4

NATRIURETIC PEPTIDE SCREENING FOR ASYMPTOMATIC LV DYSFUNCTION

Study	*n*	Define	Limit (ng/L)	Sensitivity	Specificity	ROC
Framingham Offsprings (69)	men 1,470	FS <29%	>21	53%	84%	0.72
	women 1,707	FS <29%	>21	26%	89%	0.56
Luchner et al. (70)	479	FS <28%	>34	28%	86%	0.61
Landray et al. (71)	126	Visual	>17.9	88%	34%	—
Smith et al. (72)	155	Visual	>64.7	92%	65%	0.85
Hetmanski et al. (73)	653	FS <40%	"positive"	—	—	0.59
McDonagh et al. (31)	1,252	EF ≤35%	>17.9	43%	88%	—
		EF ≤30%	>17.9	77%	87%	0.88
Yamamoto et al. (74)	466	EF <45%	>37	79%	64%	0.79
Krishnaswamy et al. (75)	400	EF <50%	>87	90%	67%	0.82
Friedl et al. (76)	75	EF ≤55%	>30	58%	76%	0.7
Omland et al. (77)	254	EF ≤45%	"positive"	—	—	0.74
Ng et al. (39)	1,360	EF ≤45%	>19.2	—	44%	0.94

Abbreviations: ROC, receiver operator characteristic; FS, fractional shortening; LVEF, left ventricular ejection fraction.

Echocardiographic Screening Modalities for Stage B Heart Failure

Echocardiography is the gold standard for detecting structural abnormalities in patients at risk of developing heart failure. Targeted screening by limited echocardiography has been considered as an option. For example, Baker et al. (40) evaluated 482 patients admitted to a tertiary care hospital for noncardiac reasons and found a total of 7.9% of patients with LV ejection fraction of 45% or less (40). The prevalence was 15.4% among those with a prior MI (particularly if MI occurred >5 years ago), with lower (but still substantial) prevalence in patients with history of coronary artery disease and diabetes mellitus. However, the expenses of obtaining formal two-dimensional echocardiography for routine screening cannot be justified at this time, except in cases of FDC (where first-degree relatives should be routinely screened) and in patients with known asymptomatic valvular diseases (1).

Portable ultrasonography in screening for ALVD has been an attractive and potentially affordable option, and the increasing versatility and improving quality of images obtained from these compact devices can be useful screening tools even when performed by noncardiologists (41). In a recent study using a miniaturized portable ultrasound system, cardiac structures and performances were reliably diagnosed in a blinded manner (42). In a heart failure screening study, of the 562 consecutive patients screened by experienced sonographers using portable ultrasound systems 97% were possible, and the decision statistics were excellent (sensitivity, specificity, and negative predictive value for LV systolic dysfunction of 96%, 98%, and 99.6%, respectively) (43). Furthermore, LVH screening for hypertensive patients also yields good accuracies (sensitivity, specificity, and negative predictive values for predicting LVH were 72%, 91%, and 90%, respectively) (44).

Cost-Effectiveness of Screening for Stage B Heart Failure

The major limitation for screening protocols for ALVD has been the issue of cost. Two retrospective analyses have contributed to this area. In the post hoc analysis from the North Glasgow MONICA Risk Factor Survey, BNP was only associated with LV systolic dysfunction in ischemic heart disease patients and those with high-risk clinical profiles, but BNP testing did reduce the number of screening echocardiograms needed by 26% (with BNP being only 5% of the cost of an echocardiogram) (45). Heidenreich et al. (46) further developed a decision model to estimate the estimated economics and health outcomes with decade-old assumptions, and identified over 1% prevalence of LV dysfunction is needed to demonstrate cost effectiveness of a BNP-based screening protocol followed by echocardiographic confirmation. Multimarker approaches in the postinfarction setting have yielded greater diagnostic accuracies, and there is potential for a combined biomarker approach, if the costs can be justified.

Treatment Strategy for Stage B Heart Failure

The only large-scale clinical trial to address the issue of treatment for ALVD was performed almost two decades ago. Patients with stage B were part of the SOLVD Prevention trial, where the use of enalapril was associated with reversal of LV remodeling. The SOLVD Prevention trial demonstrated significant decrement in the combined endpoint of congestive heart failure morbidity (hospital admission for heart failure) and mortality (Fig. 92.2) (47). This trial was the first to suggest that a preventive intervention strategy with angiotensin-converting enzyme (ACE) inhibitors could attenuate progression toward clinically manifest heart failure when used as first-line drug therapy in asymptomatic or minimally symptomatic patients with systolic LV dysfunction. Observations from SOLVD shifted the paradigm of therapy from simply a diuretic and digoxin prescription, begun when patients develop congestive heart failure, to instituting ACE inhibitor therapy first even in noncongested, asymptomatic, or minimally symptomatic patients. Moreover, patients with ALVD randomly allocated to enalapril had lower mortality rates when compared to that of placebo when the follow-up was extended to 12 years (48). These data suggest that there is benefit to treating minimally symptomatic or even asymptomatic patients with structural heart disease who are at risk of developing overt heart failure. Such therapy not only may reverse the underlying structural abnormality, but may also forestall the onset of symptomatic heart failure.

Other primary and secondary preventive strategies have also been shown to reduce the risk of incident heart failure. For example, lipid-lowering therapy results in a significant reduction

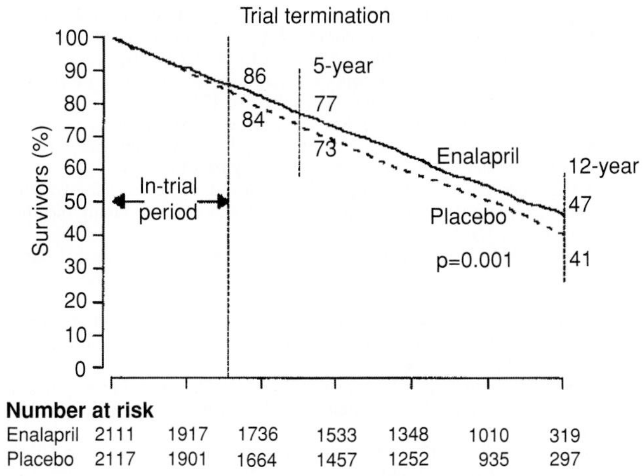

FIGURE 92.2. Studies of Left Ventricular Dysfunction (SOLVD) Prevention Arm: 12-year follow-up. (*Source:* Reproduced with permission from Jong P, Yusuf S, Rousseau MF, et al. Effect of enalapril on 12-year survival and life expectancy in patients with left ventricular systolic dysfunction: a follow-up study. *Lancet* 2003;361:1843–1848.)

in new-onset heart failure in postinfarction patients (49). There have also been interests in using statin therapy for heart failure independent of their lipid-lowering properties, and there are circumstantial evidence from post hoc analyses (50–52) to justify the ongoing rosuvastatin heart failure trials.

Regression of structural heart disease has been used as a surrogate marker in these studies. For example, pharmacologic regression of LVH (or "reverse remodeling") (53), as reported in a recent metaanalysis, suggested that ACE inhibitors, angiotensin receptor blockers (ARBs), and calcium channel blockers were more potent in reducing LV mass when compared to that of β-blockers (with the effect of diuretics being intermediate) (54). Results from the Heart Outcomes Prevention Evaluation study (55), the Ramipril Cardioprotective Evaluation Study (56), Prospective Randomized Enalapril Study Evaluating Regression of Ventricular Enlargement Study (57), the Losartan Intervention For Endpoint Reduction in Hypertension Study (58), and the Eplerenone, Enalapril, and Eplerenone/Enalapril Combination Therapy in Patients with Left Ventricular Hypertrophy Study (59) all confirm the important role of renin–angiotensin–aldosterone system inhibition on LVH regression.

Most antihypertensive medications promote regression of LVH, although some appear more potent than others, when indexed to the degree of blood pressure lowering. In subjects with ALVD, use of ACE inhibitors, β-adrenergic receptor blockers, and ARBs has been shown to be particularly effective in promoting reverse remodeling and attenuating clinical events. Aldosterone receptor antagonists may also be useful, but there are limited data to support their use in minimally symptomatic patients at this time. At present, this class of drugs has been studied in symptomatic patients with reduced ejection fractions and in those who had symptoms of heart failure immediately following myocardial infarction. Despite the lack of randomized controlled trials evaluating ARBs or aldosterone antagonists in truly asymptomatic LV dysfunction, ARBs represent acceptable alternatives in ACE inhibitor intolerant patients, and the addition of an aldosterone antagonist to an ACE inhibitor/β-blocker–based regimen may optimize the reverse remodeling process. As mentioned, mechanical interventions such as coronary revascularization following myocardial infarction may also improve heart function and thus attenuate heart failure. Other therapies resulting in reverse remodeling in patients with established advanced heart failure (e.g., cardiac resynchronization therapy, aldosterone receptor antagonists) are currently being evaluated in minimally symptomatic patients with cardiac dysfunction.

CONTROVERSIES AND PERSONAL PERSPECTIVES

The majority of discussions regarding heart failure prevention have focused on risk factor modification in patients at risk of developing heart failure (stage A intervention), but often ignores the potential benefits of better strategies to identify those with asymptomatic structural heart diseases (stage B detection) and better initiate appropriate medical therapy and counseling (stage B intervention). The biggest controversy regarding the prevention of heart failure is the cost effectiveness of "proactive" screening strategies in patients at risk, similar to current proactive cancer screening protocols. After all, the cost, disease burden, and mortality of heart failure can be as high (if not more) than that of many cancers, but many prerequisites have to be met before screening can become a reality (Table 92.5).

TABLE 92.5

PREREQUISITES FOR POPULATION SCREENING AND THE CASE FOR SCREENING IN HEART FAILURE

Prerequisites for screening	Case for screening in heart failure
The condition is of public health importance.	Heart failure is costly and leads to significant morbidity and mortality if treatment is delayed.
The natural history is understood, and there is an unsuspected but detectable preclinical stage.	There are data from postinfarction studies to suggest general progression of cardiac dysfunction and heart failure.
There is an ethical, acceptable, safe and accurate screening test for early detection and intervention.	Echocardiogram and plasma biomarkers are acceptable, safe screening tests, but their accuracies and cost effectiveness are still unclear. Handheld echocardiogram is increasingly accepted.
Consensus is reached on the frequency, screening ages, quality control and monitoring of screening program, and mechanisms of referral and treatment of positive tests.	No consensus has been reached. There is currently no formal recommendation regarding screening except for first-degree relatives for familial cardiomyopathy and patients with asymptomatic valve diseases.
There is sufficient political will, resources, and strategies to adopt and implement screening practice.	There is still a large emphasis on "salvage" therapies rather than preventive strategies in heart failure, and there have not been any clinical trials.

Meanwhile, the assumption of a continuum across the proposed "stages" of heart failure, although logical and plausible, is by no means universal. The heart failure phenotype is heterogeneous, and this staging classification is purely arbitrary. Not all hypertrophy will lead to ventricular failure; some progress to dilation whereas others remain relatively stable. There is far more to understand regarding how heart failure and cardiomyopathy progress, particularly in the earliest stages. The most important message is to consider the presence of underlying structural heart disease in every at-risk patient being evaluated, or vigilant monitoring and aggressive therapy in those with known stage B heart failure, because treatment will likely be far less successful and far more expensive if given later in the disease process.

THE FUTURE

The inability to identify this patient population in the earliest stages has limited our ability to better understand the pathophysiology of disease progression in heart failure. There are several features of stage B heart failure that deserve further understanding. It is increasingly apparent that cardiac dyssynchrony contributes to the pathogenesis of heart failure, and is now the target of widespread use of cardiac resynchronization therapy in the late stages of heart failure. However, it is unclear where in the natural history of heart failure that dyssynchrony occurs, or how it drives the progression of the syndrome. Despite the fact that neurohormones are activated in patients with stage B heart failure and precede the onset of symptoms, there are few longitudinal data that characterize the change in neurohormonal activation, endothelial dysfunction, and inflammation throughout the progression of heart failure from stage B to stages C and D. There are substantial data to indicate that cardiac remodeling is one of the central features of the heart failure syndrome. However, there are very few data that track LV remodeling from stage B through stages C and D, particularly in the non–myocardial infarction population. Last, the remodeling process is characterized by high matrix turnover within the myocardium with the deposition of reparative and replacement fibrosis.

The candidate gene approach for early detection of cardiomyopathy will likely involve only a subset of patients. In the future, proteomic approaches may have the greatest potential to develop effective screening strategies in a similar manner as using prostate specific antigen to screen for prostate cancer. The acceptance and availability of easy-to-use and affordable handheld ultrasound systems will be the ultimate revolution, so that these "ultrasonic stethoscopes" can be used in everyday clinical practice for early detection of structural heart diseases.

References

1. American Heart Association. *Heart disease and stroke statistics—2005 update*. Dallas, TX: American Heart Association, 2005.
2. Lloyd-Jones DM, Larson MG, Leip EP, et al. Lifetime risk for developing congestive heart failure: the Framingham Heart Study. *Circulation* 2002; 106:3068–3072.
3. Hunt SA, Abraham WT, Chin MH, et al. ACC/AHA 2005 guideline update for the diagnosis and management of chronic heart failure in the adult: a report of the American College of Cardiology/American Heart Association Task Force on Practice Guidelines (Writing Committee to update the 2001 Guidelines for the Evaluation and Management of Heart Failure). American College of Cardiology Web Site. Available: www.acc.org/clinical/guidelines/failure//index.pdf. 2005.
4. Rodeheffer RJ, Jacobsen SJ, Gersh BJ, et al. The incidence and prevalence of congestive heart failure in Rochester, Minnesota. *Mayo Clin Proc* 1993;68:1143–1150.
5. Ho KK, Pinsky JL, Kannel WB, et al. The epidemiology of heart failure: the Framingham Study. *J Am Coll Cardiol* 1993;22:6A–13A.
6. Baig MK, Goldman JH, Caforio AL, et al. Familial dilated cardiomyopathy: cardiac abnormalities are common in asymptomatic relatives and may represent early disease. *J Am Coll Cardiol* 1998;31:195–201.
7. Murphy RT, Starling RC. Genetics and cardiomyopathy: where are we now? *Cleve Clin J Med* 2005;72:465–466, 469–470, 472–473 passim.
8. Mahon NG, Murphy RT, MacRae CA, et al. Echocardiographic evaluation in asymptomatic relatives of patients with dilated cardiomyopathy reveals preclinical disease. *Ann Intern Med* 2005;143:108–115.
9. Hershberger RE, Ni H, Crispell KA. Familial dilated cardiomyopathy: echocardiographic diagnostic criteria for classification of family members as affected. *J Card Fail* 1999;5:203–212.
10. Valantine HA, Hunt SA, Fowler MB, et al. Frequency of familial nature of dilated cardiomyopathy and usefulness of cardiac transplantation in this subset. *Am J Cardiol* 1989;63:959–963.
11. Kannel WB, Castelli WP, McNamara PM, et al. Role of blood pressure in the development of congestive heart failure. The Framingham study. *N Engl J Med* 1972;287:781–787.
12. McKee PA, Castelli WP, McNamara PM, et al. The natural history of congestive heart failure: the Framingham study. *N Engl J Med* 1971;285:1441–1446.
13. Kenchaiah S, Evans JC, Levy D, et al. Obesity and the risk of heart failure. *N Engl J Med* 2002;347:305–313.
14. Ingelsson E, Sundstrom J, Arnlov J, et al. Insulin resistance and risk of congestive heart failure. *JAMA* 2005;294:334–341.
15. Witteles RM, Tang WH, Jamali AH, et al. Insulin resistance in idiopathic dilated cardiomyopathy: a possible etiologic link. *J Am Coll Cardiol* 2004;44:78–81.
16. Kannel WB, Hjortland M, Castelli WP. Role of diabetes in congestive heart failure: the Framingham study. *Am J Cardiol* 1974;34:29–34.
17. Hayat SA, Patel B, Khattar RS, et al. Diabetic cardiomyopathy: mechanisms, diagnosis and treatment. *Clin Sci (Lond)* 2004;107:539–557.
18. Fang ZY, Prins JB, Marwick TH. Diabetic cardiomyopathy: evidence, mechanisms, and therapeutic implications. *Endocr Rev* 2004;25:543–567.
19. Zellweger MJ, Hachamovitch R, Kang X, et al. Prognostic relevance of symptoms versus objective evidence of coronary artery disease in diabetic patients. *Eur Heart J* 2004;25:543–550.
20. Chareonthaitawee P, Sorajja P, Miller TD, et al. Prevalence and prognosis of left ventricular systolic dysfunction in asymptomatic diabetics without known coronary artery disease. *J Am Coll Cardiol* 2005;45(3 suppl):279A.
21. Hellermann JP, Jacobsen SJ, Gersh BJ, et al. Heart failure after myocardial infarction: a review. *Am J Med* 2002;113:324–330.
22. Bourassa MG, Gurne O, Bangdiwala SI, et al. Natural history and patterns of current practice in heart failure. The Studies of Left Ventricular Dysfunction (SOLVD) Investigators. *J Am Coll Cardiol* 1993;22:14A–19A.
23. Taylor AL, Ziesche S, Yancy C, et al. Combination of isosorbide dinitrate and hydralazine in blacks with heart failure. *N Engl J Med* 2004;351:2049–2057.
24. Yeh ET, Tong AT, Lenihan DJ, et al. Cardiovascular complications of cancer therapy: diagnosis, pathogenesis, and management. *Circulation* 2004;109: 3122–3131.
25. Shan K, Lincoff AM, Young JB. Anthracycline-induced cardiotoxicity. *Ann Intern Med* 1996;125:47–58.
26. Hequet O, Le QH, Moullet I, et al. Subclinical late cardiomyopathy after doxorubicin therapy for lymphoma in adults. *J Clin Oncol* 2004;22:1864–1871.
27. Frigerio M, Oliva F, Turazza FM, et al. Prevention and management of chronic heart failure in management of asymptomatic patients. *Am J Cardiol* 2003;91:4F–9F.
28. Wang TJ, Evans JC, Benjamin EJ, et al. Natural history of asymptomatic left ventricular systolic dysfunction in the community. *Circulation* 2003;108:977–982.
29. Redfield MM, Jacobsen SJ, Burnett JC Jr, et al. Burden of systolic and diastolic ventricular dysfunction in the community: appreciating the scope of the heart failure epidemic. *JAMA* 2003;289:194–202.
30. Devereux RB, Roman MJ, Paranicas M, et al. A population-based assessment of left ventricular systolic dysfunction in middle-aged and older adults: the Strong Heart Study. *Am Heart J* 2001;141:439–446.
31. McDonagh TA, Robb SD, Murdoch DR, et al. Biochemical detection of left-ventricular systolic dysfunction. *Lancet* 1998;351:9–13.
32. Aurigemma GP, Gottdiener JS, Shemanski L, et al. Predictive value of systolic and diastolic function for incident congestive heart failure in the elderly: the cardiovascular health study. *J Am Coll Cardiol* 2001;37:1042–1048.
33. Vasan RS, Larson MG, Benjamin EJ, et al. Left ventricular dilatation and the risk of congestive heart failure in people without myocardial infarction. *N Engl J Med* 1997;336:1350–1355.
34. Mosterd A, Hoes AW, de Bruyne MC, et al. Prevalence of heart failure and left ventricular dysfunction in the general population: The Rotterdam Study. *Eur Heart J* 1999;20:447–455.
35. Kober L, Torp-Pedersen C, Carlsen JE, et al. A clinical trial of the angiotensin-converting-enzyme inhibitor trandolapril in patients with left ventricular dysfunction after myocardial infarction. Trandolapril Cardiac Evaluation (TRACE) Study Group. *N Engl J Med* 1995;333:1670–1676.
36. Pfeffer MA, Braunwald E, Moye LA, et al. Effect of captopril on mortality and morbidity in patients with left ventricular dysfunction after myocardial infarction. Results of the survival and ventricular enlargement trial. The SAVE Investigators. *N Engl J Med* 1992;327:669–677.

37. Richards AM, Nicholls MG, Yandle TG, et al. Plasma N-terminal pro-brain natriuretic peptide and adrenomedullin: new neurohormonal predictors of left ventricular function and prognosis after myocardial infarction. *Circulation* 1998;97:1921–1929.
38. Hobbs FD, Davis RC, Roalfe AK, et al. Reliability of N-terminal proBNP assay in diagnosis of left ventricular systolic dysfunction within representative and high risk populations. *Heart* 2004;90:866–870.
39. Ng LL, Loke IW, Davies JE, et al. Community screening for left ventricular systolic dysfunction using plasma and urinary natriuretic peptides. *J Am Coll Cardiol* 2005;45:1043–1050.
40. Baker DW, Bahler RC, Finkelhor RS, et al. Screening for left ventricular systolic dysfunction among patients with risk factors for heart failure. *Am Heart J* 2003;146:736–740.
41. DeCara JM, Lang RM, Koch R, et al. The use of small personal ultrasound devices by internists without formal training in echocardiography. *Eur J Echocardiogr* 2003;4:141–147.
42. Scholten C, Rosenhek R, Binder T, et al. Hand-held miniaturized cardiac ultrasound instruments for rapid and effective bedside diagnosis and patient screening. *J Eval Clin Pract* 2005;11:67–72.
43. Galasko GI, Lahiri A, Senior R. Portable echocardiography: an innovative tool in screening for cardiac abnormalities in the community. *Eur J Echocardiogr* 2003;4:119–127.
44. Senior R, Galasko G, Hickman M, et al. Community screening for left ventricular hypertrophy in patients with hypertension using hand-held echocardiography. *J Am Soc Echocardiogr* 2004;17:56–61.
45. Nielsen OW, McDonagh TA, Robb SD, et al. Retrospective analysis of the cost-effectiveness of using plasma brain natriuretic peptide in screening for left ventricular systolic dysfunction in the general population. *J Am Coll Cardiol* 2003;41:113–120.
46. Heidenreich PA, Gubens MA, Fonarow GC, et al. Cost-effectiveness of screening with B-type natriuretic peptide to identify patients with reduced left ventricular ejection fraction. *J Am Coll Cardiol* 2004;43:1019–1026.
47. The SOLVD Investigators. Effect of enalapril on mortality and the development of heart failure in asymptomatic patients with reduced left ventricular ejection fractions. *N Engl J Med* 1992;327:685–691.
48. Jong P, Yusuf S, Rousseau MF, et al. Effect of enalapril on 12-year survival and life expectancy in patients with left ventricular systolic dysfunction: a follow-up study. *Lancet* 2003;361:1843–1848.
49. Kjekshus J, Pedersen TR, Olsson AG, et al. The effects of simvastatin on the incidence of heart failure in patients with coronary heart disease. *J Card Fail* 1997;3:249–254.
50. Ray JG, Gong Y, Sykora K, et al. Statin use and survival outcomes in elderly patients with heart failure. *Arch Intern Med* 2005;165:62–67.
51. Mozaffarian D, Nye R, Levy WC. Statin therapy is associated with lower mortality among patients with severe heart failure. *Am J Cardiol* 2004;93:1124–1129.
52. Horwich TB, MacLellan WR, Fonarow GC. Statin therapy is associated with improved survival in ischemic and non-ischemic heart failure. *J Am Coll Cardiol* 2004;43:642–648.
53. Verdecchia P, Angeli F. Reversal of left ventricular hypertrophy: what have recent trials taught us? *Am J Cardiovasc Drugs* 2004;4:369–378.
54. Klingbeil AU, Schneider M, Martus P, et al. A meta-analysis of the effects of treatment on left ventricular mass in essential hypertension. *Am J Med* 2003;115:41–46.
55. Arnold JM, Yusuf S, Young J, et al. Prevention of Heart Failure in Patients in the Heart Outcomes Prevention Evaluation (HOPE) Study. *Circulation* 2003;107:1284–1290.
56. Agabiti-Rosei E, Ambrosioni E, Dal Palu C, et al. ACE inhibitor ramipril is more effective than the beta-blocker atenolol in reducing left ventricular mass in hypertension. Results of the RACE (ramipril cardioprotective evaluation) study on behalf of the RACE study group. *J Hypertens* 1995;13:1325–1334.
57. Devereux RB, Palmieri V, Sharpe N, et al. Effects of once-daily angiotensin-converting enzyme inhibition and calcium channel blockade-based antihypertensive treatment regimens on left ventricular hypertrophy and diastolic filling in hypertension: the prospective randomized enalapril study evaluating regression of ventricular enlargement (PRESERVE) trial. *Circulation* 2001;104:1248–1254.
58. Dahlof B, Devereux RB, Kjeldsen SE, et al. Cardiovascular morbidity and mortality in the Losartan Intervention For Endpoint reduction in hypertension study (LIFE): a randomised trial against atenolol. *Lancet* 2002;359:995–1003.
59. Pitt B, Reichek N, Willenbrock R, et al. Effects of eplerenone, enalapril, and eplerenone/enalapril in patients with essential hypertension and left ventricular hypertrophy: the 4E-left ventricular hypertrophy study. *Circulation* 2003;108:1831–1838.
60. Levy D, Larson MG, Vasan RS, et al. The progression from hypertension to congestive heart failure. *JAMA* 1996;275:1557–1562.
61. Gottdiener JS, Arnold AM, Aurigemma GP, et al. Predictors of congestive heart failure in the elderly: the Cardiovascular Health Study. *J Am Coll Cardiol* 2000;35:1628–1637.
62. He J, Ogden LG, Bazzano LA, et al. Risk factors for congestive heart failure in US men and women: NHANES I epidemiologic follow-up study. *Arch Intern Med* 2001;161:996–1002.
63. Gardin JM, Siscovick D, Anton-Culver H, et al. Sex, age, and disease affect echocardiographic left ventricular mass and systolic function in the free-living elderly. The Cardiovascular Health Study. *Circulation* 1995;91:1739–1748.
64. Schunkert H, Broeckel U, Hense HW, et al. Left-ventricular dysfunction. *Lancet* 1998;351:372.
65. McDonagh TA, Morrison CE, Lawrence A, et al. Symptomatic and asymptomatic left-ventricular systolic dysfunction in an urban population. *Lancet* 1997;350:829–833.
66. Nielsen OW, Hilden J, Larsen CT, et al. Cross sectional study estimating prevalence of heart failure and left ventricular systolic dysfunction in community patients at risk. *Heart* 2001;86:172–178.
67. Davies M, Hobbs F, Davis R, et al. Prevalence of left-ventricular systolic dysfunction and heart failure in the Echocardiographic Heart of England Screening study: a population based study. *Lancet* 2001;358:439–444.
68. Hedberg P, Lonnberg I, Jonason T, et al. Left ventricular systolic dysfunction in 75-year-old men and women; a population-based study. *Eur Heart J* 2001;22:676–683.
69. Vasan RS, Benjamin EJ, Larson MG, et al. Plasma natriuretic peptides for community screening for left ventricular hypertrophy and systolic dysfunction: the Framingham heart study. *JAMA* 2002;288:1252–1259.
70. Luchner A, Burnett JC Jr, Jougasaki M, et al. Evaluation of brain natriuretic peptide as marker of left ventricular dysfunction and hypertrophy in the population. *J Hypertens* 2000;18:1121–1128.
71. Nielsen OW, Hansen JF, Hilden J, et al. Risk assessment of left ventricular systolic dysfunction in primary care: cross sectional study evaluating a range of diagnostic tests. *BMJ* 2000;320:220–224.
72. Smith H, Pickering RM, Struthers A, et al. Biochemical diagnosis of ventricular dysfunction in elderly patients in general practice: observational study. *BMJ* 2000;320:906–908.
73. Hetmanski DJ, Sparrow NJ, Curtis S, et al. Failure of plasma brain natriuretic peptide to identify left ventricular systolic dysfunction in the community. *Heart* 2000;84:440–441.
74. Yamamoto K, Burnett JC Jr, Bermudez EA, et al. Clinical criteria and biochemical markers for the detection of systolic dysfunction. *J Card Fail* 2000;6:194–200.
75. Krishnaswamy P, Lubien E, Clopton P, et al. Utility of B-natriuretic peptide levels in identifying patients with left ventricular systolic or diastolic dysfunction. *Am J Med* 2001;111:274–279.
76. Friedl W, Mair J, Thomas S, et al. Natriuretic peptides and cyclic guanosine 3′,5′-monophosphate in asymptomatic and symptomatic left ventricular dysfunction. *Heart* 1996;76:129–136.
77. Omland T, Aakvaag A, Vik-Mo H. Plasma cardiac natriuretic peptide determination as a screening test for the detection of patients with mild left ventricular impairment. *Heart* 1996;76:232–237.

SECTION EIGHT
VASCULAR BIOLOGY AND MEDICINE

ERIC J. TOPOL, MD

CHAPTER 103 ■ THERAPEUTIC ANGIOGENESIS

G. CHAD HUGHES AND BRIAN H. ANNEX

Atherosclerosis is the leading cause of morbidity and mortality in the Western world (1). The term *therapeutic angiogenesis* describes the field of cardiovascular medicine whereby new blood vessels are induced to grow to supply oxygen and nutrients to cardiac or skeletal muscle rendered ischemic as a result of progressive atherosclerosis (2). This chapter focuses on therapeutic angiogenesis as it applies to the treatment of patients with ischemic heart disease and peripheral arterial obstructive disease (PAD).

SCOPE OF CLINICAL PROBLEM

Coronary artery disease (CAD) continues to be the leading cause of mortality in the industrialized world, with more than 13 million Americans alive today with a history of angina pectoris, myocardial infarction, or both (3). Despite advances in pharmacologic therapies as well as catheter-based and surgical revascularization, significant numbers of these patients have diffuse CAD, small distal vessels, or other comorbidities that make them poor candidates for traditional methods of treatment. This number may represent as many as 12% of all patients with symptomatic CAD (4). As the average age of the population increases, the proportion of patients who are ineligible for traditional therapies will likely increase. Consequently, alternative means of improving blood flow to the heart such as therapeutic angiogenesis may take on a larger role in the treatment of CAD.

To date, clinical trials of therapeutic angiogenesis in CAD have generally been restricted to patients with refractory angina pectoris and so-called "end-stage" CAD (2). This term refers to patients with the persistence of severe anginal symptoms (Canadian Cardiovascular Society [CCS] class III and IV) despite maximal conventional antianginal combination therapy and coronary atherosclerosis not amenable to revascularization by percutaneous means or surgical bypass. Most of these "no-option" patients have multivessel CAD and have undergone one or more prior revascularization procedures (5). However, even though they typically have long-standing and diffuse disease, the patients selected for study of these alternative therapies generally have only mildly to, at worse, moderately impaired left ventricular function. Consequently, heart transplantation is not an option, and the goals of early trials have been targeted toward softer end points such as exercise time or quality of life measures. On the contrary, patients with large areas of prior myocardial infarction and its attendant necrosis and scar formation are typically excluded because these changes are considered not reversible with improvements in myocardial perfusion (6). Rather, patients should have ischemic yet viable myocardium as demonstrated by positron emission tomography, thallium or technetium (^{99m}Tc)-sestamibi scintigraphy, dobutamine echocardiography, or magnetic resonance imaging (MRI), because this situation is reversible with increases in myocardial blood flow (6).

The other major manifestation of atherosclerosis is PAD, which itself encompasses a spectrum of clinical syndromes with an incidence and prevalence nearly equal to that of CAD. Approximately 15% of adults who are more than 55 years old have detectable hemodynamic impairments attributed to PAD, and, similar to the incidence of CAD, the number of patients with PAD can be expected to increase as the population ages (7,8). The two major clinical presentations of PAD are intermittent claudication and critical limb ischemia. In patients with intermittent claudication, arterial occlusive disease is manifested by insufficient blood flow during exercise, whereas in critical limb ischemia, blood flow is inadequate to meet the demands of the limb even at rest. Consequently, the goals of therapy for claudication are quite different from those of critical limb ischemia.

Standard therapy for PAD manifest as intermittent claudication includes atherosclerotic risk factor modification, smoking cessation, exercise, and pharmacologic therapy. Surgical revascularization, although effective, is generally not indicated except in lifestyle-limiting, medically refractory claudication. Percutaneous therapy is another option, although long-term results are poor except in proximal aortoiliac disease (9). For critical limb ischemia presenting as rest pain or tissue loss, mechanical revascularization with surgery or percutaneous intervention is the treatment of choice (9). However, these patients typically have significant comorbidities as well as diffuse, distal atherosclerosis that make mechanical revascularization both higher risk in the short term and less successful in the long term as a result of graft loss from small target vessels and poor runoff. Consequently, a search for new and more efficacious treatment options for PAD, including therapeutic angiogenesis, is ongoing (Fig. 103.1).

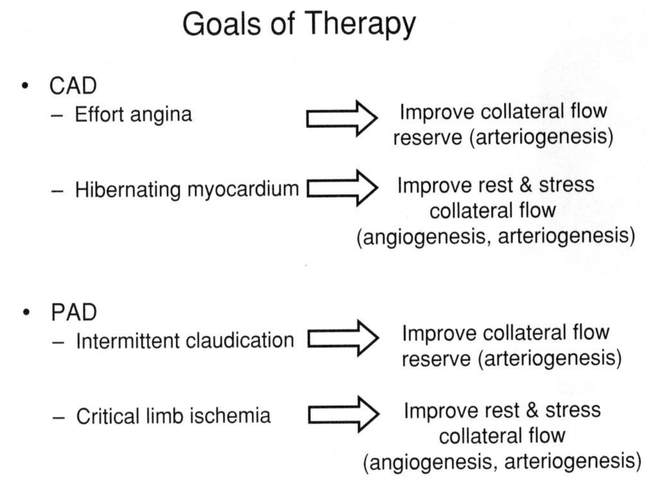

Goals of Therapy
• CAD
– Effort angina
Improve collateral flow reserve (arteriogenesis)
– Hibernating myocardium
Improve rest & stress collateral flow (angiogenesis, arteriogenesis)
• PAD
– Intermittent claudication
Improve collateral flow reserve (arteriogenesis)
– Critical limb ischemia
Improve rest & stress collateral flow (angiogenesis, arteriogenesis)

FIGURE 103.1. The goals of therapeutic neovascularization may vary depending on the disease process treated. Both coronary artery disease (CAD) and peripheral arterial disease (PAD) may be divided into subcategories. In the first (effort angina, intermittent claudication), regional perfusion is adequate at rest but is unable to meet tissue demands during stress. The goal of therapy in this situation is primarily to increase flow during periods of increased demand via conductance arterioles (i.e., arteriogenesis). The other category of disease includes situations in which regional perfusion is inadequate both at rest and during stress (i.e., chronic myocardial ischemia with hibernating myocardium and chronic limb ischemia with rest pain or tissue loss). In this situation, more significant increases in blood flow are necessary and will likely require increased numbers of capillaries (angiogenesis) as well as conductance vessels (angiogenesis). Although not listed, the exact contribution of vasculogenesis to each of these processes is unclear, but it is almost certainly necessary for sustained improvements in regional flow in the latter conditions and may play a role in the former as well.

POSTNATAL REVASCULARIZATION VIA BLOOD VESSEL GROWTH

Neovascularization in ischemic adult cardiac and skeletal muscle is now recognized to result from the processes of angiogenesis, arteriogenesis, and vasculogenesis (Fig. 103.2). Angiogenesis refers to the sprouting of new capillaries lacking a developed tunica media from preexisting ones (10). In the adult, this process is mainly caused by hypoxia and is mediated via activation of hypoxia-inducible factor (HIF-1α), which serves to increase transcription of vascular endothelial growth factor (VEGF) and its receptors and to stabilize VEGF mRNA (11).

Arteriogenesis describes the type of vascular growth responsible for the production of vessels with a fully developed tunica media and capable of carrying significant blood flow as well as being visualized with angiography (10–12). This process may involve the maturation of preexisting collateral vessels or may reflect do novo formation of mature vessels (10). Preexisting coronary collateral vessels have been demonstrated even in patients with angiographically normal coronary arteries (13). These collateral vessels may be important for the process of arteriogenesis. Unlike angiogenesis, ischemia is not a prerequisite for arteriogenesis (14). Rather, primary arteriogenic stimuli include shear stress and inflammation in which an invasion of monocytes and other white blood cells leads to the production of growth factors such as the fibroblast growth factors (FGFs) and tumor necrosis factor-α (TNF-α) with subsequent vascular growth (15–17). Following arterial occlusion, monocytes/macrophages, in particular, accumulate in the tissue surrounding collateral vessels via ICAM-1/Mac-1 dependent mechanisms (18). Moreover, a recent study in the rabbit hind limb model clearly demonstrated that monocytes, and not granulocytes or T lymphocytes, are the key cellular mediators of arteriogenesis (17).

Vasculogenesis (19,20) describes the in situ formation of blood vessels from endothelial progenitor cells (EPCs) termed angioblasts (12,21). Angioblasts are CD34$^+$ stem cells recruited from the bone marrow that are thought to migrate and fuse with other EPCs and capillaries to form a primitive network of vessels known as the primary capillary plexus. After this primary capillary plexus is formed, it is remodeled by sprouting and branching via the process of angiogenesis. However, some investigators have questioned the origin of these EPCs as well as whether EPCs truly incorporate into vessel walls in areas of vascular growth (22–25). Schmeisser et al. demonstrated that CD34$^-$ monocytes may develop an endothelial phenotype and even form tube-like structures in vitro, a finding suggesting a potential role for non–stem cell monocytes in vasculogenesis (22). Further, Rehman et al. (23) found that most so-called EPCs are actually derived from the monocyte/macrophage lineage, with only a small population of true CD34$^+$ stem cells/progenitor cells that originate from hematopoietic stem cells/angioblasts. These monocyte/macrophage–derived "circulating angiogenic cells" secrete multiple angiogenic growth factors that likely mediate their angiogenic effects. Finally, Ziegelhoeffer (24) published a study suggesting that, in the adult organism, bone marrow–derived stem cells do not promote vascular growth by incorporating into vessel walls but rather via paracrine effects from the production of multiple angiogenic cytokines. Regardless of the true mechanism, however, vasculogenesis appears to be a real phenomenon in the postnatal organism, and vasculogenesis, angiogenesis, and arteriogenesis all potentially contribute to neovascularization in adult cardiac and skeletal muscle (12,26), although some authors (16,27) have suggested that arteriogenesis is necessary for significant improvements in blood flow.

THERAPEUTIC ANGIOGENESIS

The endothelium in adults normally exists in a quiescent state. Only when provoked by stress or pathologic conditions does the vascular bed expand via the processes of vasculogenesis, angiogenesis, and arteriogenesis (26). This neovascularization represents a highly ordered physiologic mechanism under tight regulation with many factors active at the molecular level to influence the process including numerous soluble polypeptides such as the VEGFs, the angiopoietins, FGFs, platelet-derived growth factors (PDGFs), transforming growth factor-β (TGF-β), TNF-α, the colony-stimulating factors, and many others (21) (Table 103.1). In addition, several membrane-bound proteins play prominent roles in angiogenesis including various members of the integrin, cadherin, syndecan, and ephrin families (21,28). Finally, mechanical forces acting on the endothelium also contribute to the regulation of neovascularization via shear-stress induced upregulation of angiogenic and inflammatory mediators, primarily serving to stimulate adaptive arteriogenesis (21,26). However, even though the myocardial and skeletal muscle vascular beds can expand via the neovascularization process, this expansion is typically limited, and regional ischemia results. This fact has provided a rationale for the administration of angiogenic growth factors or their genes to rescue ischemic cardiac or skeletal muscle (26).

Theoretically, neovascularization in the heart or extremities could be achieved via a process whereby all the elements necessary for the angiogenic response could be derived from

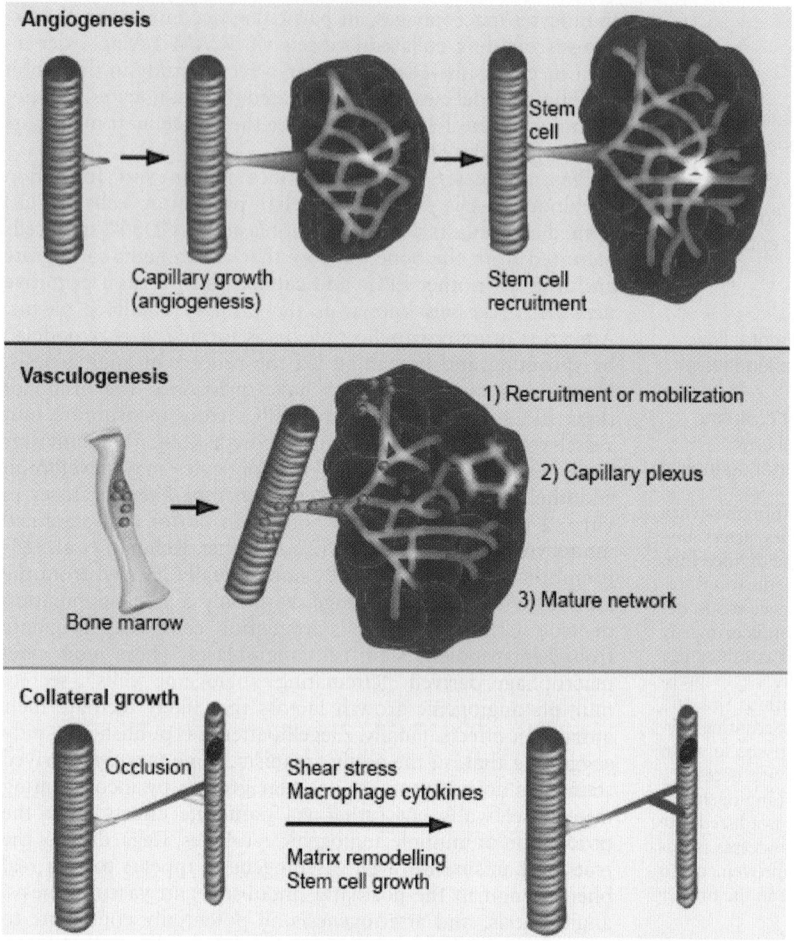

FIGURE 103.2. Vascular expansion in adult cardiac and skeletal muscle may involve three different mechanisms, possibly driven by distinct signals: (1) angiogenesis, which is the growth of new blood vessels from preexisting ones; (2) vasculogenesis, which refers to the formation of new blood vessels by fusion and differentiation of endothelial progenitor cells originating in the bone marrow; and (3) arteriogenesis (collateral growth), which is the growth of arteries from preexisting arterioles. (From Hughes GC, Annex BH. Angiogenic therapy for coronary artery and peripheral arterial disease. *Exp Rev Cardiovasc Ther* 2005;3:521–535.)

TABLE 103.1

COMMON ANGIOGENIC GROWTH FACTORS: THEIR RECEPTORS AND UNIQUE PROPERTIES

Growth factor	Full name	Receptor	Properties
VEGF-A (VEGF,VEGF-1)	Vascular endothelial growth factor-A	VEGFR-1 (*flt-1*), VEGFR-2 (*flk-1, kdr*), VEGFR-3	Endothelial cell mitogen; required for angiogenesis/vasculogenesis; multiple isoforms
VEGF-B	Vascular endothelial growth factor-B	VEGFR-1 (*flt-1*)	Forms dimers with VEGF-A; preferentially expressed in heart and skeletal muscle
VEGF-C	Vascular endothelial growth factor-C	VEGFR-2 (*flk-1*, (*kdr*) VEGFR-3	May play a role in lymphangiogenesis; not regulated by hypoxia
aFGF (FGF-1)	Acidic fibroblast growth factor	FGF receptor	Endothelial cell, fibroblast, smooth muscle cell mitogen; isoelectric point 5.6
bFGF (FGF-2)	Basic fibroblast growth factor	FGF receptor	Endothelial cell, fibroblast, smooth muscle cell mitogen; isoelectric point 9.6
HIF-1α	Hypoxia inducible factor-1α		Constitutively expressed; binds VEGF promoter, thus inducing VEGF transcription
HGF (scatter factor, SF)	Hepatocyte growth factor	*c-met* tyrosine kinase	
PGF (PIGF)	Placental growth factor	Neuropilin	
Ang-1	Angiopoietin-1	*tie-2*	Vascular branching morphogenesis; potentiates effect of VEGF
Ang-2	Angiopoietin-2	*tie-2*	Inhibition of vascular stabilization

the muscle itself. In their seminal work, Asahara et al. (19,20) demonstrated that cells derived from the peripheral circulation and bone marrow were present in the angiogenic response occurring after experimentally induced hind-limb ischemia. This work established that postnatal neovascularization involves circulating EPCs that home to sites of neovascularization and contribute to vasculogenesis. These circulating EPCs derive from hematopoietic stem cells and contribute to reparative processes such as neovascularization after ischemia.

Studies subsequent to those of Asahara et al. demonstrated that the exogenous administration of angiogenic growth factors leads to increases in EPCs and that these cells may contribute to the effects of therapeutic angiogenesis (29). Patient risk factors such as diabetes, aging, and hypercholesterolemia that are associated with an impaired "endogenous" response to ischemia are also associated with reduced numbers of circulating EPCs (26). Thus, lack of sufficient availability of angiogenic growth factors may not be the only reason for these patients to develop cardiac or skeletal muscle ischemia because underlying conditions may prevent the adult endothelium from responding normally to angiogenic stimuli (26). Furthermore, therapies designed to modify these risk factors (e.g., statin medications) lead to increases in circulating EPC numbers (30). If stem cells contribute or are even essential for therapeutic angiogenesis, it follows that stem cell–based therapies for angiogenesis may be sufficient to produce the desired angiogenic response and may reduce or even reverse the sequelae of CAD and PAD.

Mechanical Therapies

Mechanical means of producing neovascularization have been investigated much more extensively for CAD than for PAD and have generally involved using some mechanical means to injure ischemic muscle, thus producing an inflammatory response and subsequent neovascularization (31). Although many techniques have been utilized including needles (32), mechanical drills (33), and transmyocardial implant devices (34), among others, most work has focused on the use of laser energy (31) for this application. This technique, known as transmyocardial laser revascularization (TMR), involves using a laser to create channels through the walls of the left ventricle of the beating heart. TMR may be performed surgically through a small left anterior thoracotomy or via a percutaneous approach (PMR). PMR creates channels via advancement of a fiberoptic catheter against the endocardial surface from the left ventricular cavity. Unlike surgical TMR, complete transmural penetration of the left ventricular myocardium is avoided. At the present time, two laser systems, the carbon dioxide and the holmium:yttrium-aluminum-garnet (YAG), are currently approved by the U.S. Food and Drug Administration (FDA) for clinical use for surgical TMR. No PMR devices have as yet obtained FDA approval. However, despite FDA approval, TMR has not established itself as a mainstay of angiogenic therapy, and there is no evidence that its use as a stand-alone modality will increase in the future.

Nonetheless, the original rationale behind TMR provides important background information on the field of angiogenesis. TMR was a surgical attempt to mimic the pattern of myocardial circulation of reptiles, in which blood flows directly into the myocardial tissue from the ventricular cavity. Numerous experimental and clinical studies have disproved this concept that patent channels perfuse the left ventricular myocardium by demonstrating that the laser channels become occluded in the early postoperative period (31). The mechanism of action of TMR appears to involve at least some degree of improved blood flow via laser injury induced neovascularization. Numerous groups (32,34–43) have investigated changes in regional myocardial perfusion and function in long-term follow-up after experimental TMR. Chronic myocardial ischemia models in rats (43), dogs (35), sheep (36), and pigs (32,34,37–42) have all demonstrated improved myocardial perfusion weeks to months after TMR using various techniques including radioactive (38) and colored (35,36) microspheres, ^{99m}Tc-sestamibi perfusion scanning (39), MRI (40,43), and positron emission tomography (34,41,42) to measure regional myocardial blood flow directly. These studies have generally demonstrated some degree of improvement in either rest or stress function concomitant with the increased perfusion. In addition, the changes in regional perfusion and function have been associated with histologic evidence for neovascularization in regions of the myocardium treated with laser therapy.

Although conceptually similar, very little work has been done investigating mechanical means of producing neovascularization in peripheral skeletal muscle for the treatment of PAD. A single small study utilizing the rabbit hind limb model found no evidence for therapeutic angiogenesis 6 weeks after laser therapy of skeletal muscle in the distribution of a ligated femoral artery (44). Given the capacity of skeletal muscle for self-repair, further work in this area is clearly needed to determine whether mechanical therapies may play a role in the treatment of PAD.

Growth Factor–Based Therapies

Numerous growth factor based treatment options are available for the induction of new blood vessel growth in skeletal and cardiac muscle. The explosive growth of the therapeutic angiogenesis field since the mid-1990s was a direct result of the development of recombinant growth factors, the best characterized of which are ligands of the FGF and VEGF families. A large body of preclinical evidence (45–58) supports the efficacy of both VEGF and FGF as angiogenic agents, and these latter two cytokines serve as the focus of this discussion.

The VEGFs are a family of glycoproteins of which VEGF-1 (or VEGF-A) has been studied most extensively with regard to its use as a proangiogenic agent. The other VEGFs, which are structurally similar to VEGF-1, include VEGF-2 (VEGF-C), VEGF-3 (VEGF-B), VEGF-D, VEGF-E, and placental growth factor (12). As a result of alternative splicing, at least four isoforms of VEGF-1 are produced, containing 121 ($VEGF_{121}$), 165 ($VEGF_{165}$), 189 ($VEGF_{189}$), and 206 ($VEGF_{206}$) amino acids. The isoforms, which differ in their heparin binding capacity, appear to have similar angiogenic potency (12,21). $VEGF_{121}$ and $VEGF_{165}$ are secreted into the extracellular environment, whereas $VEGF_{189}$ and $VEGF_{206}$ remain cell- or matrix-associated via their affinity for heparan sulfates (12,21). VEGF binds to at least three known tyrosine kinase receptors (Fig. 103.3): Flt-1 (VEGFR-1), KDR/Flk-1 (VEGFR-2), and Flt-4 (VEGFR-3) (21). VEGFR-2 is thought to transduce angiogenic signals, whereas the role of VEGFR-1 is less well defined, and VEGFR-3 is involved in lymphangiogenesis (12,21). Endothelial cells were once considered the sole cellular target of VEGF, although functional VEGF receptors are now known to be present on vascular smooth muscle cells and monocytes/macrophages. Consequently, VEGF may utilize endothelial as well as other cell types as effectors and may exert effects on proliferation and survival (12,21).

VEGF exerts several effects on endothelial cells including enhanced migration, increased permeability, and increased production of plasminogen activators, plasminogen activator inhibitor-1, and interstitial collagenase, all of which contribute to angiogenesis (21). VEGF can also stimulate endothelial cell proliferation, an effect specific to vascular endothelial cells because VEGF does not induce proliferation of other cells types such as smooth muscle cells or fibroblasts (21). VEGF production is regulated by local oxygen concentration; hypoxia

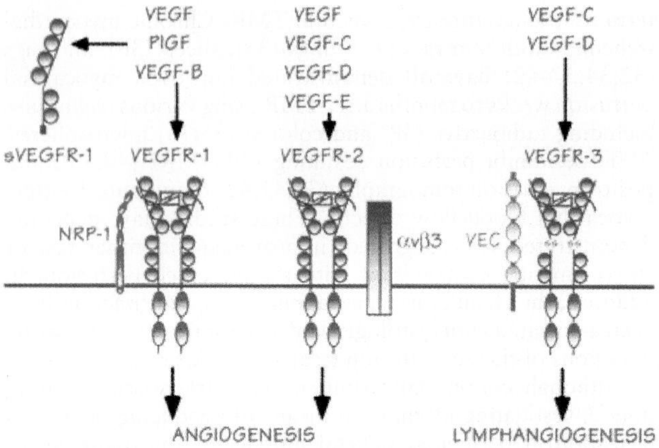

FIGURE 103.3. Currently known vascular endothelial growth factors (VEGFs) and their receptors: VEGFR-1 and VEGFR-2 have seven extracellular immunoglobulin homology domains, but in VEGFR-3, the fifth immunoglobulin domain is cleaved on receptor processing into disulfide-linked subunits. VEGFR-1 and VEGFR-2 mediate angiogenesis, whereas VEGFR-3 is also involved in lymphangiogenesis. Neuropilin (NRP)-1 binds to specific COOH-terminal sequences present only in certain VEGFs that bind to VEGFR-1 and/or VEGFR-2. $\alpha_V\beta_3$ integrin and VE-cadherin have been found in complexes with activated VEGFR-2, and the latter also associates with an activated VEGFR-3 complex. *sVEGFR-1*, soluble VEGFR-1;*VEC*, VE-Cadherin. (From Veikkola T, Karkkainen M, Claesson-Welsh L, Alitalo K. Regulation of angiogenesis via vascular endothelial growth factor receptors. *Cancer Res* 2000;60:203–212.)

stimulates VEGF production via the binding of HIF-1α to the VEGF promoter with subsequent increased VEGF gene transcription and mRNA stability, as mentioned earlier (12,21). Thus, low oxygen tension acts to stimulate angiogenesis via VEGF.

Acidic FGF (FGF-1) and basic FGF (FGF-2) are members of a large family of structurally related polypeptide growth factors (FGF-1 to FGF-23) (59). Both FGF-1 and 2 are potent endothelial cell mitogens and, similar to VEGF, induce processes in endothelial cells critical to angiogenesis (12,21). The biologic functions of FGFs are mediated primarily by specific cell surface receptors of the tyrosine kinase family (59). Like VEGF, FGF is involved in endothelial cell proliferation, migration, and production of plasminogen activator and collagenase (21,59). Unlike VEGF, which is mitogenic primarily for endothelial cells, FGF stimulates proliferation of most cells derived from embryonic mesoderm and neuroectoderm including pericytes, fibroblasts, myoblasts, chrondrocytes, and osteoblasts (21). Also unlike VEGF, FGFs lack a signal sequence and are not secreted proteins (12,21). Thus, FGF does not appear to play a general role in all angiogenic processes, but rather is normally involved in blood vessel remodeling associated with tissue repair (21).

Angiogenic cytokines utilized for therapeutic angiogenesis may be administered as recombinant human protein, or the gene encoding the protein may be transferred into target tissue with subsequent protein production by transfected cells. Each approach has inherent advantages and disadvantages. With protein therapy, a known quantity of protein is administered, and thus a more precise dose-response relationship can be attained (12). Unlike gene therapy, protein therapy avoids the need for transfection, transcription, and translation and assumes that the presence of the protein in a therapeutic concentration is sufficient to induce the desired angiogenic response. The major disadvantage of protein therapy is the short tissue half-life of angiogenic proteins, which may be insufficient for the sustained stimulation and multiple cell cycling required for the growth and remodeling of new collateral vessels (60). Conversely, the advantage of gene therapy techniques is that sustained local production may lead to prolonged elevation of tissue protein levels beyond that which may be obtained using protein-based approaches. Gene therapy techniques utilized to date generally involve either plasmid DNA or replication defective adenovirus containing the gene of interest. These vectors have a limited duration of expression on the order of 1 to 2 weeks as a result of neutralization by cytotoxic T lymphocytes (60). Proponents of gene therapy techniques have suggested that this limited duration of expression may be ideal for therapeutic angiogenesis in which prolonged exposure to elevated levels of angiogenic protein raises concern over promotion of malignancy and pathologic neovascularization, as well as acceleration of atherosclerosis. However, a recent study (61) utilizing Ad-VEGF$_{165}$ in the rabbit hind limb model found that collateral vessels were formed primarily in the first week after treatment. Immunostaining techniques demonstrated that activation of endothelial nuclear cycling peaked in the first few days after Ad-VEGF$_{165}$ treatment, a time course that coincided with the peak in systemic serum VEGF levels. No further endothelial cell proliferation took place after 1 week, a finding suggesting that angiogenesis is confined to the short period of VEGF expression produced by the adenoviral vector, and early gains in collateralization rapidly regress to control levels when VEGF production ceases. If confirmed, these findings have very important potential ramifications regarding the use of growth factors for therapeutic angiogenesis.

The main disadvantages of gene therapy techniques include the inflammatory response to adenoviral proteins and the inconsistent level of gene expression in different patients with a given dose of vector (60). In addition, adenoviral vectors are generally not suitable if treatment needs to be repeated because transduction efficiency is limited by prior viral exposure, and therapeutic results have been negatively correlated with anti-adenoviral titers. Other viral vectors have been utilized for gene therapy including adeno-associated virus and lentiviral vectors, both of which may integrate into the host genome with a presumably low risk of insertional mutagenesis (62). Concerns regarding the safety of long-term gene expression, as noted earlier, have limited the use of these alternative vectors with regard to promoting angiogenesis, although given the findings of only transient upregulation of angiogenesis after Ad-VEGF$_{165}$ administration (61), further investigation into the use of these alternative vectors seems warranted. In particular, sustained growth factor expression using an adeno-associated viral delivery system with VEGF expression regulated by a HIF-1α responsive promoter may promote stable conducting vessels (61).

Another novel growth factor–based approach involves using engineered transcription factors to regulate a patient's endogenous genetic loci for upregulation of angiogenic growth factor production (63). Two engineered transcription factors currently under development target a constitutive activation module to a defined sequence in the promoter region of VEGF-A via linkage to a specific DNA-binding domain, either the basic helix-loop-helix motif of HIF-1α or a designed zinc finger protein. Both factors activate the expression of VEGF-A and stimulate angiogenesis in animal models. Phase I trials in humans are under way for the HIF-1α based factor and expected to begin in the near future for the zinc finger protein–based factor (63).

Consideration of the route of administration is important with angiogenic therapies. Angiogenic proteins may be administered systemically (i.e., intravenously through a peripheral vein), intraarterially, or via direct intramuscular injection. Intramuscular injection is required in the case of naked plasmid DNA because the plasmid undergoes prompt degradation if it is delivered into circulating blood. In addition, plasmid DNA gene transfer is less efficient than with adenoviral vectors, although the clinical differences are uncertain. Viral vectors are not subject to similar intravascular degradation and may be delivered either via an intraarterial route or intramuscular injection. One theoretic disadvantage of systemic versus local delivery is that growth factors administered to specific regions of muscle may provide critical directional clues for new vessels to grow into the ischemic region rather than promoting disorganized growth (61).

Trials of single angiogenic growth factor therapy have established the safety of this approach. However, despite the apparent safety, several theoretic concerns do exist. Plaque angiogenesis following angiogenic growth factor administration may precipitate plaque growth or destabilization, potentially leading to adverse cardiovascular events (10). Proliferative retinopathy resulting from angiogenic growth factors in orbital fluid is another concern. Finally, accelerated tumor growth or metastasis may theoretically be stimulated by proangiogenic therapy. To date, clinical experience with the various growth factors tested has not substantiated these fears, and these adverse effects appear unlikely with short-term administration, appropriate patient selection, and local drug delivery (10).

Cellular-Based Therapies

Stem cells are defined as undifferentiated cells with the capacity for proliferation and self-renewal as well as an ability to regenerate multiple cell types and tissues (64–66). Embryonic stem cells are derived from mammalian embryos in the blastocyst stage and have the ability to generate any terminally differentiated cell in the body. Adult stem cells are part of the tissue-specific cells of the postnatal organism into which they are committed to differentiate (64–66). Stem cells are capable of maintaining, generating, and replacing terminally differentiated cells lost as a result of physiologic cell turnover or tissue injury. Stem cells have clonogenic and self-renewing capabilities and may differentiate into multiple cell lineages, a phenomenon known as *stem cell plasticity*. The means by which circulating stem cells are recruited into various solid organ tissues and differentiate into the tissue-specific cells subsequently generated are not fully understood (64,66). Tissue injury results in changes in the microenvironment, and this may play an important role in stem cell recruitment. After tissue injury in organs such as the liver, skin, or intestine, which have their own supply of intrinsic stem cells, resident stem cells at the site of tissue damage contribute to tissue repair. If the pool of endogenous stem cells is exhausted, exogenous circulating stem cells are then signaled to replenish the pool and participate in tissue repair, thus serving as a backup rescue system (66). However, in organs such as the heart, which appear to lack resident stem cells, the release of chemokines such as VEGF following ischemic injury stimulate mobilization of bone marrow–derived stem cells. These mobilized stem cells are then attracted to ischemic areas by locally elevated VEGF or stromal cell–derived factor-1 levels (29,66). Thus, neovascularization in ischemic tissue depends on the mobilization and integration of stem cells. It has been estimated that 10% of endothelial cells involved in neovascularization are derived from EPCs (67). In addition, stem cells have also been demonstrated to differentiate into cardiac muscle, and there is intense interest in their use for promoting myogenesis (64), although this use is outside the scope of this chapter.

The clinical use of embryonic stem cells is currently limited by practical issues such as immunologic rejection following embryonic stem cell derived cell transplantation and possible teratoma formation (68). Ethical issues surrounding the use of human embryos may also limit their use, and consequently widespread utilization of embryonic stem cells for cardiovascular therapy in the near future is unlikely (64–66).

Adult stem cells, conversely, are present within the adult organism and present an attractive option for clinical use. These cells retain the ability to differentiate beyond their own tissue boundaries and are found within multiple organs including bone marrow, peripheral blood, brain, liver, and skeletal muscle, among others, where they normally participate in tissue repair (64–66). Multipotent adult progenitor cells are similar to embryonic stem cells in that they can be extensively expanded in vivo and form cells of all three germ cell layers. In contrast to embryonic stem cells, autologous adult stem cells avoid the rejection resulting from the expression of major histocompatability complex proteins in human embryonic stem cells (66). Also unlike embryonic stem cells, tumorigenicity has not been observed with adult stem cells. However, as with growth factor–based therapies, concerns exist regarding the use of stem cell approaches. For example, Sata et al. (69) demonstrated that bone marrow–derived hematopoietic stem cells give rise to most of the smooth muscle cells involved in neointimal hyperplasia, transplant graft vasculopathy, and atherosclerosis. Consequently, acceleration of these processes of pathologic arterial remodeling by stem cell therapy is a theoretic possibility.

A new approach to therapeutic angiogenesis involves combining stem cell and gene therapy, whereby ex vivo engineered EPCs are genetically manipulated for use as vectors producing angiogenic proteins of interest (70). This combination may overcome the limitations of these individual therapies in patients with CAD and PAD who have impaired neovascularization in part from diminished angiogenic growth factor production and also from endothelial cell dysfunction and diminished numbers of EPCs (70). Thus, combination therapy provides additional growth factors to overcome the endogenous deficit as well as supplemental EPCs necessary for vascular growth.

With regard to cardiovascular therapeutics, the adult stem cells most likely to be useful for therapeutic angiogenesis are bone marrow–derived and peripheral blood–derived stem cells, which are thought to be the source of EPCs, although this topic remains controversial, as discussed earlier. Experimental transplantation of stem cells has been carried out via percutaneous means using an intraarterial or coronary sinus route, direct intramuscular injection, or systemically. The preferable route of delivery at the present time remains unclear and awaits further study (64). Finally, evidence of efficacy of stem cell therapy is indirect because there is currently no available method to determine engraftment in the living patient.

Clinical Trials in Coronary Artery Disease

Mechanical Therapies

To date, seven prospective, randomized, controlled trials of surgical TMR versus best medical therapy have been conducted (71–77). These studies have randomized patients with CCS class III or IV angina to either TMR or continued medical management. The studies have consistently demonstrated significant improvements in anginal class and exercise time in TMR versus medically treated patients at 12-month follow-up. However, improvements in myocardial perfusion as measured using single-photon emission computed tomography (SPECT) have not been consistently observed. Of the five studies (71–75) measuring myocardial perfusion with SPECT, only one (71) reported a significant improvement in the TMR-treated patients as compared with medically managed controls. In none of the trials was TMR associated with a survival benefit at 1-year follow-up.

Three of these trials have now published follow-up data out to 5 years (78–80). All three trials demonstrated that the angina relief after TMR was sustained throughout the period of follow-up and continued to be superior to that of medical management. No survival benefit was seen at 5 years in either of the carbon dioxide laser trials (78,79). However, in the recently published follow-up of patients treated with holmium:YAG TMR, a significant improvement in survival was seen at 5 years in the patients randomized to TMR (80). This trial represents the only published data to suggest a survival benefit with TMR.

There are currently three published prospective, randomized, controlled trials of PMR versus medical therapy (81–83). Two of the three trials (81,83) found a significant benefit at 12-month follow-up with regard to both exercise tolerance time and anginal scores in patients randomized to PMR. The third trial (82), however, found no significant differences in either anginal scores or exercise tolerance at 6-month follow-up. No assessment of myocardial perfusion was performed as part of any of the published PMR trials.

A recent study (84) on the use of surgical TMR in "real-world" community practice analyzing data from the Society of Thoracic Surgeons National Cardiac Database found a 30-day mortality rate of 3.7% for patients with class III to IV angina and ischemic, viable (hibernating) myocardium in regions to be treated. No such data are currently available for PMR owing to lack of FDA approval.

Growth Factor–Based Therapies

To date, there have been seven prospective, randomized, double-blind, placebo-controlled trials of cytokine growth factor therapy for the induction of therapeutic angiogenesis in the heart (85–91), including one trial of granulocyte-macrophage colony-stimulating factor (GM-CSF) (85), three of VEGF (88,89,91), and three of FGF (86,87,90). Seiler et al. (85) randomized 21 patients with advanced two- and three-vessel CAD to a single intracoronary dose of GM-CSF or placebo followed by a 2-week period of subcutaneous GM-CSF or placebo administration. The rationale behind using GM-CSF is an attempt to increase circulating monocyte numbers, which via their production of multiple angiogenic growth factors stimulate arteriogenesis (27). In addition, GM-CSF can increase the number of circulating EPCs (27). The major finding of the study was a significant increase in recruitable coronary collateral flow 2 weeks after treatment in GM-CSF group.

Losordo et al. (88) investigated the use of percutaneous catheter-based gene transfer via direct endocardial injection of naked plasmid DNA encoding for VEGF-2 in no-option patients ($n = 19$) with CCS class III or IV angina. Twelve-week follow-up demonstrated a statistically significant improvement in CCS angina class in VEGF-2–treated versus placebo-treated patients. VEGF-2–treated patients also had a statistically significant increase in their mean duration of exercise tolerance over the 12-week period, whereas no change occurred in the placebo group. Left ventricular electromechanical mapping using the NOGA system demonstrated a significant reduction in the area of myocardial ischemia at 90 days after treatment in the VEGF-2 patients, whereas no change was seen in controls. Similarly, a trend toward improved perfusion was observed in a subset of VEGF-2 patients undergoing SPECT myocardial perfusion imaging at 90 days.

The Vascular Endothelial Growth Factor in Ischemia for Vascular Angiogenesis (VIVA) trial (89) randomized 178 no-option patients to placebo, low-dose $VEGF_{165}$, or high-dose $VEGF_{165}$ protein with follow-up out to 120 days. Patients in the VEGF groups received an intracoronary infusion on day 0 followed by intravenous infusions on days 3, 6, and 9. There was no significant improvement in exercise treadmill time (ETT), the primary end point of the study, from baseline to 60 days in VEGF-treated patients. By 120 days, there was a trend toward improved ETT in the high-dose VEGF group versus placebo. Similarly, 60 days after treatment, no difference in angina class improvement from baseline was noted in VEGF-treated versus control patients, whereas at 120 days a statistically significant improvement in angina class for high-dose VEGF-treated patients compared with placebo was present. Myocardial perfusion studies performed at day 60 demonstrated no significant improvement in VEGF-treated versus placebo-treated patients.

The Euroinject One phase II multicenter, double-blind trial randomized 80 no-option patients with severe stable ischemic heart disease to direct intramyocardial injection of either 0.5 mg of phVEGF-A_{165} or placebo plasmid administered percutaneously using NOGA guidance (91). The primary study end point was change in myocardial perfusion during rest and stress, as measured using SPECT at 3-month follow-up. Secondary end points included regional wall motion assessed by NOGA and left ventriculography, CCS angina class, Seattle angina scores, nitroglycerin usage, and exercise capacity. There was no difference between the phVEGF-A_{165} or placebo groups in the primary end point of number of severe or moderate perfusion defects by SPECT at rest or during stress at 3-month follow-up. However, when both moderate and severe defects were analyzed together as an indicator of global perfusion, there was a significant improvement from baseline during stress in the phVEGF-A_{165} group that was not seen in patients receiving placebo plasmid. In addition, evidence indicated improved wall motion by both NOGA and left ventriculography in phVEGF-A_{165} versus placebo groups at 3-month follow-up. No difference between groups was seen regarding CCS angina class or Seattle angina score improvement, exercise capacity, or nitroglycerin consumption. Interestingly, there was no difference in peak plasma VEGF-A values between groups, although a trend toward increased numbers of $CD34^+$ stem cells was noted in the patients who received phVEGF-A_{165}.

The FGF Initiating Revascularization Trial (FIRST) randomized 337 patients considered to be suboptimal candidates for standard surgical or catheter-based revascularization to a single intracoronary infusion of placebo or one of three escalating doses of recombinant FGF-2 with 180-day follow-up (86). There was no significant improvement in ETT in FGF-2–treated versus placebo-treated patients at 90-day follow-up, the primary study end point. Likewise, no evidence indicated a treatment effect on ETT at 180 days. Angina frequency and CCS angina scores were significantly improved in FGF-2–treated versus placebo-treated patients at 90-day follow-up, although this difference was lost at 180 day follow-up. The improvements in anginal scores were more pronounced in highly symptomatic (CCS class III to IV) patients. Nuclear perfusion imaging demonstrated no significant changes in rest or stress perfusion at 90 or 180 days.

The Angiogenic Gene Therapy (AGENT) trial (87) examined the effects of single intracoronary administration of placebo or five escalating doses of replication defective adenovirus containing the human FGF-4 gene in 79 patients with CCS class II to III angina with 12-week follow-up. Unlike the other six randomized, placebo-controlled angiogenesis trials (85,86,88–91), the AGENT trial did not enroll no-option patients, but rather patients with one-, two-, or three-vessel CAD, the majority of whom had anatomy suitable for coronary artery bypass grafting or percutaneous transluminal coronary angioplasty. There was a trend toward improved ETT in FGF versus placebo-treated patients at both 4-week and 12-week follow-up, although the differences did not reach statistical significance. Post hoc analysis revealed that when patients with a baseline ETT time longer than 10 minutes were excluded, ETT improvement was significantly greater for FGF patients at both 4 and 12 weeks. There was no difference in time to angina during ETT for FGF versus placebo. However, as with the ETT time data, when patients with ETT longer than 10 minutes were excluded, investigators noted an overall significant improvement in time to angina in FGF-treated patients. A follow-up study from this same group (AGENT-2 trial) (90) randomized 52 patients to intracoronary infusion of 10^{10} adenoviral particles containing the human FGF-4 gene or placebo. The dose of adenovirus used was based on the dose escalation results from the preceding AGENT trial (87). Unlike in the AGENT trial, patients enrolled were not optimal candidates for revascularization by surgical or percutaneous means. The primary end point was change in myocardial perfusion as assessed using stress adenosine SPECT 8 weeks after treatment. There was a strong trend toward greater reduction in the size of reversible perfusion defect by SPECT in the FGF-4–treated patients versus controls. Likewise, there was a trend toward greater angina reductions and less nitroglycerin use in the FGF-4 group. These encouraging results, however, were not borne out in a large placebo-controlled trial that has been completed but not yet published.

Cellular-Based Therapies

The published clinical experience to date with stand-alone stem cell–based therapies consists mainly of small, mostly uncontrolled, phase I clinical series (92–95). These trials have generally used autologous bone marrow derived EPCs originating from $CD34^+$ mononuclear cells. These EPCs promote neovascularization via incorporation into active sites of angiogenesis as well as through paracrine effects such as the release of multiple angiogenic cytokines (96,97). Assmus et al. (95) treated a total of 20 patients with intracoronary infusion of either autologous bone marrow– or peripheral blood–derived progenitor cells into the infarct-related artery several days after reperfused acute myocardial infarction and found evidence for improved regional and global function 4 months after treatment. There did not appear to be any difference between patients treated with bone marrow–derived cells and those given peripheral blood–derived cells. Tse et al. (92) injected autologous bone marrow cells into regions of chronic myocardial ischemia using a catheter-based technique with NOGA guidance in eight patients with medically refractory angina pectoris and found a reduction in angina along with small improvements in regional function and myocardial perfusion by MRI in an uncontrolled study with 3-month follow-up. Similar results were reported by Fuchs et al. (94) in 10 no-option patients receiving transendocardial injections of autologous bone marrow. In the only study to date of cellular therapy in CAD with a control group (although not concurrently enrolled), Perin et al. enrolled 21 no-option patients with ischemic cardiomyopathy (mean ejection fraction, 20%) in a prospective, nonrandomized study of NOGA-guided transendocardial injection of autologous bone marrow cells. These investigators found a significant reduction in myocardial ischemia and improved function by SPECT in treated versus control patients at 2-month follow-up (93).

Clinical Trials in Peripheral Arterial Disease

Growth Factor–Based Therapies

To date, there have been fewer prospective, randomized, clinical studies investigating the use angiogenic growth factor–based therapies in PAD as compared with CAD. In a small phase I randomized, double-blind, placebo-controlled, dose-escalation trial of FGF-2 performed at the National Institutes of Health (98), intraarterial FGF-2 was administered to patients with intermittent claudication and an ankle-brachial index (ABI) of less than 0.8. The study demonstrated that FGF-2 was safe and well tolerated, even at the highest doses. In addition, plethysmographic evidence of a significant improvement in calf blood flow was seen in the treatment group at 1- and 6-month follow-up, whereas no change in blood flow was seen in placebo-treated patients.

The Therapeutic Angiogenesis with Recombinant Fibroblast Growth Factor-2 for Intermittent Claudication (TRAFFIC) study was a phase II randomized, double-blind, placebo-controlled study comparing intraarterial recombinant FGF-2 (rFGF-2) with placebo (99). In this study, 190 patients with moderate to severe intermittent claudication, infrainguinal obstructive atherosclerosis, and a resting ABI of less than 0.8 were randomly assigned to receive bilateral infusions of placebo, single-bolus, or double-bolus rFGF-2. All groups demonstrated an increase in the primary end point of change in peak walking time at 90 days, with the increase in rFGF-2–treated patients significantly greater than in the placebo group. Interestingly, the addition of a second bolus did not provide further benefit. The secondary end points included encouraging results regarding changes in ABI and some quality of life measures. Claudication onset time did not differ significantly between the groups. TRAFFIC remains the only phase II trial of therapeutic angiogenesis in either CAD or PAD to show benefit in its primary efficacy measure.

The Regional Angiogenesis with Vascular Endothelial Growth Factor in Peripheral Arterial Disease (RAVE) trial was a phase II, double-blind, placebo-controlled trial comparing intramuscular injections of $VEGF_{121}$ adenovirus ($AdVEGF_{121}$) with placebo (100). One hundred five patients with chronic, stable, predominately unilateral, intermittent claudication and a resting ABI of less than 0.8 were randomly assigned to receive intramuscular injections of low-dose $AdVEGF_{121}$, high-dose $AdVEGF_{121}$, or placebo. Although all groups demonstrated an increase in the primary end point of change in peak walking time at 12 weeks, this change did not differ among the placebo, low-dose, and high-dose groups. Furthermore, the secondary end points of peak walking time at 26 weeks, quality of life measures, claudication onset time, and ABI also did not differ among groups.

Given the success reported with the use of GM-CSF in CAD (83), the START trial (Stimulation of Arteriogenesis Using Subcutaneous Application of GM-CSF as a New Treatment for Peripheral Vascular Disease) (101) will randomize 40 patients with PAD to subcutaneous only GM-CSF versus placebo. The primary end point will be change in walking distance assessed by an exercise treadmill test with secondary end points of ABI, pain-free walking distance, cutaneous microcirculatory alterations, and measurements of blood flow. The results of this study are awaited to determine the utility of GM-CSF for the treatment of PAD.

Another PAD study on the horizon is the HGF-STAT trial (102), which aims to determine whether perfusion can be improved by gene transfer of plasmid DNA containing hepatocyte growth factor (HGF) in the affected limb of patients with unreconstructable critical hind limb ischemia. A total of 100 patients will be randomized to placebo or one of three escalating doses of HGF plasmid DNA. Outcome measures will be assessed at 30month follow-up to help determine whether therapeutic angiogenesis with HGF is a viable option in the treatment of patients with critical limb ischemia.

Cellular-Based Therapies

In the only randomized, controlled trial of cellular therapy to date, Tateishi-Yuyama et al. (97), following a pilot study in 25 patients, randomized 22 patients with bilateral ischemic rest pain or nonhealing ulcers and an ABI of less than 0.6 to intramuscular injection of bone marrow mononuclear cells (active treatment) in one leg and peripheral blood mononuclear cells in the other (placebo). The results of this Therapeutic Angiogenesis by Cell Transplantation (TACT) study were a significant improvement in ABI, transcutaneous oxygen pressure, rest pain, and pain-free walking time at 4 weeks after injection with bone marrow–derived mononuclear cells. These results were sustained out to 24-week follow-up. No improvement was seen in legs injected with peripheral blood mononuclear cells. Higashi et al. (103) demonstrated that bone marrow mononuclear cell therapy improves endothelial cell function in patients with PAD. Because endothelial dysfunction is the initial step in the pathogenesis of atherosclerosis (1), bone marrow mononuclear cell therapy may prevent the development of atherosclerosis via an improvement in endothelial function (103,104).

CONTROVERSIES AND PERSONAL PERSPECTIVES

The field of therapeutic angiogenesis is now approximately a decade old, and the area remains one of great potential and excitement. Led most notably by the late Jeffery M. Isner, M.D. and others, few areas of cardiovascular medicine were met with such exuberance and excitement. Unfortunately, the field did not live up to the lofty early expectations. For example, when the results of randomized, placebo-controlled trials became available and primary end points were not met, the field was quickly written off by some as a passing fad. In many ways, therapeutic angiogenesis was probably not quite as good as its early expectations, but, certainly, not as bad as often portrayed.

The field of therapeutic angiogenesis highlights many of the issues that need to be considered regarding gaps that limit the translation of solid preclinical investigation into the clinical world. For the area of therapeutic angiogenesis, the potential pitfalls are many. Is the therapeutic agent chosen the correct agent? What endogenous changes are occurring in the levels of a chosen angiogenic agent in the human pathologic condition, and how will pharmacologic administration affect these changes? Strikingly, almost all the angiogenic agents administered in early human studies were utilized in situations in which their expression was thought to be already upregulated. Possibly our targets should be those that are downregulated. The administration of HGF is an example of such a paradigm, because this cytokine may be downregulated in the setting of ischemia.

The next step, assuming one has the right therapeutic agent, concerns the route, vector, and method of delivery. Too often, this critical step is overlooked in the rush to human studies. What are the differences between plasmid and adenoviral vectors for gene transfer? Are the differences between the myocardium and peripheral skeletal muscle important in these regards? Within the group of plasmids, a potential exists to employ more advanced gene designs and tissue specific targeting. However, to date, these potentially beneficial approaches have not been utilized.

The duration of growth factor expression in the target tissue is another critical factor. One may design elegant preclinical studies to determine the duration of cytokine growth factor expression that yields durable effects in developmental models, but how do these apply to the complex human situation? Do these models of development apply to ischemic human tissue at all? Is the expression of a single cytokine in a differential amount capable of inducing a cascade of downstream effects which can invoke long-term beneficial effects? One must consider that in preclinical models the duration of therapeutic effects often extends beyond the period of measurable upregulation in cytokine growth factor expression.

To date, therapeutic angiogenesis has generally focused on the supply side, with the stimulation of endothelial proliferation as its goal. However, the growth of blood vessels is clearly a process subject to both stimulatory and inhibitory effects. Consequently, understanding how various therapeutic strategies alter this balance may eventually provide new insights into approaches to induce angiogenesis.

The field of therapeutic angiogenesis was barely recognized when, in parallel, it became clear that the physiologic process of angiogenesis likely involved critical contributions from cells outside the target blood vessel. Therefore, therapeutic angiogenesis is unlikely to result solely from a sheer proliferation and remodeling of blood vessels and endothelial cells in an ischemic bed. Rather, this process likely requires the contribution of cells homing to the target tissue. The ability of angiogenic cytokines to mobilize endothelial and other vascular progenitor cells has rapidly emerged as an important area of study. Likewise, although the field of cellular therapy initially began as independent from therapeutic angiogenesis, it has become increasingly clear that many of the beneficial effects of cell therapy may indeed be attributed to their therapeutic angiogenic effect.

Finally, even if one is capable of solving all the aforementioned problems, the difficulties in the complex heterogeneity that is part of any human pathophysiologic disease state remain. Appropriate and targeted clinical trial design is absolutely essential to ensure patient safety and to maximize the probability of successful outcomes and advancement of the field. The selection of patient populations that are markedly heterogeneous or minimally affected by their disease is likely to result in poor clinical trial outcomes even if the best of agents and delivery strategies are utilized. Far too often, trials begin with the best of intentions regarding enrollment but are subsequently forced to alter inclusion and exclusion criteria that, over the course of the study, lead to heterogeneity among the trial population. In addition, the constraints of a clinical trial often force one to enroll a patient population that may be different from that for whom the drug will ultimately be used. In no case has this been more apparent than in the critical limb ischemia clinical trials in which the devastating short-term outcomes for these patients run counter to the long inclusion and study-specific tests required for entry. Clearly, partnering among sponsors, regulatory agencies, and investigators is required in this complex area.

THE FUTURE

The field of therapeutic angiogenesis has thus far yielded some critical observations regarding physiologic and therapeutic neovascularization, and the short- and long-term future continues to appear bright. Currently, the realistic goal of successful therapeutic angiogenesis in humans within a decade appears in reach. The first generation of "simple" growth factors is being replaced by more complex transcription factors that alter multiple cytokines in a manner more analogous to what nature can create. The recognition of the overlap between "therapeutic angiogenesis" and "cell therapy" also has great potential to advance our understanding of both fields. The discovery that endothelial cells interact and communicate with surrounding cells within the organ also offers enormous potential for future investigation. For example, can angiogenic growth factors affect cell survival independent of angiogenesis to bestow clinical benefit? Can angiogenic growth factors targeting endothelial cells improve the structure and function of nervous tissue? Can angiogenic growth factors improve endothelial function leading to clinical benefit apart from the angiogenic process? The field of therapeutic angiogenesis has moved at a great pace in its first decade, and the potential for advancement over its next decade and beyond is even greater. This exciting field continues to warrant close monitoring.

References

1. Ross R. Atherosclerosis: an inflammatory disease. *N Engl J Med* 1999;340:115–126.
2. Hughes GC, Annex BH. Angiogenic therapy for coronary artery and peripheral arterial disease. *Exp Rev Cardiovasc Ther* 2005;3:521–535.
3. American Heart Association. *Heart disease and stroke statistics: 2005 update.* Dallas, TX: American Heart Association, 2005.
4. Mukherjee D, Bhatt DL, Roe MT, et al. Direct myocardial revascularization and angiogenesis: how many patients might be eligible? *Am J Cardiol* 1999;84:598–600.
5. Schoebel FC, Frazier OH, Jessurun GAJ, et al. Refractory angina pectoris in end-stage coronary artery disease: evolving therapeutic concepts. *Am Heart J* 1997;134:587–602.
6. DiCarli MF. Predicting improved function after myocardial revascularization. *Curr Opin Cardiol* 1998;13:415–424.
7. Criqui MH, Fronek A, Barrett-Connor E, et al. The prevalence of peripheral arterial disease in a defined population. *Circulation* 1985;71:510–515.
8. Hirsch AT, Criqui MH, Treat-Jacobson D, et al. Peripheral arterial disease detection, awareness, and treatment in primary care. *JAMA* 2001;286:1317–1324.
9. Hughes GC, Gray JL. Aortoiliac disease. In: Pappas TN, Purcell GP, eds. *Unbound surgery.* Charlottesville, VA: Unbound Medicine, 2004, available at www.unboundsurgery.com.
10. Simons M, Bonow RO, Chronos NA, et al. Clinical trials in coronary angiogenesis: issues, problems, consensus. *Circulation* 2000;102:e73–e86.
11. Schaper W, Buschmann I. Arteriogenesis: the good and bad of it. *Cardiovasc Res* 1999;43:835–837.
12. Freedman SB, Isner JM. Therapeutic angiogenesis for coronary artery disease. *Ann Intern Med* 2002;136:54–71.
13. Wustmann K, Zbinden S, Windecker S, et al. Is there functional collateral flow during vascular occlusion in angiographically normal coronary arteries? *Circulation* 2003;107:2213–2220.
14. Ito WD, Arras M, Winkler B, et al. Angiogenesis but not collateral growth is associated with ischemia after femoral artery occlusion. *Am J Physiol* 1997;273:H1255–H1265.
15. Schaper W, Ito WD. Molecular mechanisms of coronary collateral vessel growth. *Circ Res* 1996;79:911–919.
16. Schaper W. Quo vadis collateral blood flow? A commentary on a highly cited paper. *Cardiovasc Res* 2000;45:220–223.
17. Hoefer IE, Grundmann S, van Royen N, et al. Leukocyte subpopulations and arteriogenesis: specific role of monocytes, lymphocytes, and granulocytes. *Atherosclerosis* 2005;181:285–293.
18. Hoefer IE, van Royen N, Rectenwald JE, et al. Arteriogenesis proceeds via ICAM-1/Mac-1-mediated mechanisms. *Circ Res* 2004;94:1179–1185.
19. Asahara T, Murohara T, Sullivan A, et al. Isolation of putative progenitor endothelial cells for angiogenesis. *Science* 1997;275:964–967.
20. Asahara T, Masuda H, Takahashi T, et al. Bone marrow origin of endothelial progenitor cells responsible for postnatal vasculogenesis in physiological and pathological neovascularization. *Circ Res* 1999;85:221–228.
21. Papetti M, Herman IM. Mechanisms of normal and tumor-derived angiogenesis. *Am J Physiol* 2002;282:C947–C970.
22. Schmeisser A, Garlichs CD, Zhang H, et al. Monocytes coexpress endothelial and macrophagocytic lineage markers and form cord-like structures in Matrigel under angiogenic conditions. *Cardiovasc Res* 2001;49:671–680.
23. Rehman J, Li J, Orschell CM, March KL. Peripheral blood "endothelial progenitor cells" are derived from monocyte/macrophages and secrete angiogenic growth factors. *Circulation* 2003;107:1164–1169.
24. Ziegelhoeffer T, Fernandez B, Kostin S, et al. Bone marrow-derived cells do not incorporate into the adult growing vasculature. *Circ Res* 2004;94:230–238.
25. Heil M, Ziegelhoeffer T, Mees B, Schaper W. A different outlook on the role of bone marrow stem cells in vascular growth. *Circ Res* 2004;94:573–574.
26. Luttun A, Carmeliet P. De novo vasculogenesis in the heart. *Cardiovasc Res* 2003;58:378–389.
27. Schaper W. Therapeutic arteriogenesis has arrived. *Circulation* 2001;104:1994–1995.
28. Annex BH, Simons M. Growth factor-induced therapeutic angiogenesis in the heart: protein therapy. *Cardiovasc Res* 2005;65:649–655.
29. Dimmeler S, Vasa-Nicotera M. Aging of progenitor cells: limitation for regenerative capacity? *J Am Coll Cardiol* 2003;42:2081–2082.
30. Rupp S, Badorff C, Koyanagi M, et al. Statin therapy in patients with coronary artery disease improves the impaired endothelial progenitor cell differentiation into cardiomyogenic cells. *Basic Res Cardiol* 2004;99:61–68.
31. Hughes GC, Abdel-aleem S, Biswas SS, et al. Transmyocardial laser revascularization: experimental and clinical results. *Can J Cardiol* 1999;15:797–806.
32. Horvath KA, Belkind N, Wu I, et al. Functional comparison of transmyocardial revascularization by mechanical and laser means. *Ann Thorac Surg* 2001;72:1997–2002.
33. Malekan R, Reynolds C, Narula N, et al. Angiogenesis in transmyocardial laser revascularization: a nonspecific response to injury. *Circulation* 1998;98(suppl II):II62–II65.
34. Hughes GC, Biswas SS, Yin B, et al. A comparison of mechanical and laser transmyocardial revascularization for induction of angiogenesis and arteriogenesis in chronically ischemic myocardium. *J Am Coll Cardiol* 2002;39:1220–1228.
35. Yamamoto N, Kohmoto T, Gu A, et al. Angiogenesis is enhanced in ischemic canine myocardium by transmyocardial laser revascularization. *J Am Coll Cardiol* 1998;31:1426–1433.
36. Ozaki S, Meyns B, Racz R, et al. Effect of transmyocardial laser revascularization on chronic ischemic hearts in sheep. *Eur J Cardiothorac Surg* 2000;18:404–410.
37. Horvath KA, Greene R, Belkind N, et al. Left ventricular functional improvement after transmyocardial laser revascularization. *Ann Thorac Surg* 1998;66:721–725.
38. Martin JS, Sayeed-Shah U, Byrne JG, et al. Excimer versus carbon dioxide transmyocardial laser revascularization: effects on regional left ventricular function and perfusion. *Ann Thorac Surg* 2000;69:1811–1816.
39. Hamawy AH, Lee LY, Samy SA, et al. Transmyocardial laser revascularization dose response: enhanced perfusion in a porcine ischemia model as a function of channel density. *Ann Thorac Surg* 2001;72:817–822.
40. Mühling OM, Wang Y, Panse P, et al. Transmyocardial laser revascularization preserves regional myocardial perfusion: an MRI first pass perfusion study. *Cardiovasc Res* 2003;57:63–70.
41. Hughes GC, Kypson AP, St. Louis JD, et al. Improved perfusion and contractile reserve after transmyocardial laser revascularization in a model of hibernating myocardium. *Ann Thorac Surg* 1999;67:1714–1720.
42. Hughes GC, Kypson AP, Annex BH, et al. Induction of angiogenesis after TMR: a comparison of holmium: YAG, CO_2, and excimer lasers. *Ann Thorac Surg* 2000;70:504–509.
43. Nahrendorf M, Hiller K-H, Theisen D, et al. Effect of transmyocardial laser revascularization on myocardial perfusion and left ventricular remodeling after myocardial infarction in rats. *Radiology* 2002;225:487–493.
44. Buckwalter JB, Curtis VC, Ruble SB, et al. Laser revascularization of ischemic skeletal muscle. *J Surg Res* 2003;115:257–264.
45. Harada K, Grossman W, Friedman M, et al. Basic fibroblast growth factor improves myocardial function in chronically ischemic porcine hearts. *J Clin Invest* 1994;94:623–630.
46. Unger EF, Banai S, Shou M, et al. Basic fibroblast growth factor enhances myocardial collateral flow in a canine model. *Am J Physiol* 1994;266:H1588–H1595.
47. Lopez JJ, Edelman ER, Stamler A, et al. Basic fibroblast growth factor in a porcine model of chronic myocardial ischemia: a comparison of angiographic, echocardiographic and coronary flow parameters. *J Pharmacol Exp Ther* 1997;282:385–390.
48. Lazarous DF, Shou M, Stiber JA, et al. Pharmacodynamics of basic fibroblast growth factor: route of administration determines myocardial and systemic distribution. *Cardiovasc Res* 1997;36:78–85.
49. Laham RJ, Rezaee M, Post MJ, et al. Intrapericardial delivery of fibroblast growth factor-2 induces neovascularization in a porcine model of chronic myocardial ischemia. *J Pharmacol Exp Ther* 2000;292:795–802.
50. Rajanayagam MAS, Shou M, Thirumurti V, et al. Intracoronary basic fibroblast growth factor enhances myocardial collateral perfusion in dogs. *J Am Coll Cardiol* 2000;35:519–526.
51. Banai S, Shou M, Lazarous DF, et al. Angiogenic-induced enhancement of collateral blood flow to ischemic myocardium by vascular endothelial growth factor in dogs. *Circulation* 1994;89:2183–2189.
52. Pearlman JD, Chuang ML, Harada K, et al. Magnetic resonance mapping demonstrates benefits of VEGF-induced myocardial angiogenesis. *Nat Med* 1995;1:1085–1089.
53. Lazarous DF, Scheinowitz M, Hodge E, et al. Comparative effects of basic fibroblast growth factor and vascular endothelial growth factor on coronary collateral development and the arterial response to injury. *Circulation* 1996;94:1074–1082.
54. Harada K, Friedman M, Lopez JJ, et al. Vascular endothelial growth factor administration in chronic myocardial ischemia. *Am J Physiol* 1996;270:H1791–H1802.
55. Hariawala M, Horowitz J, Esakof D, et al. VEGF improves myocardial blood flow but produces EDRF-mediated hypotension in porcine hearts. *J Surg Res* 1996;63:77–82.
56. Lopez JJ, Stamler A, Pearlman JD, et al. VEGF administration in chronic myocardial ischemia in pigs. *Cardiovasc Res* 1998;40:272–281.
57. Hughes GC, Biswas SS, Yin B, et al. Therapeutic angiogenesis in chronically ischemic porcine myocardium: comparative effects of bFGF and VEGF. *Ann Thorac Surg* 2004;77:812–818.
58. Biswas SS, Hughes GC, Scarborough JE, et al. Intramyocardial and intracoronary basic fibroblast growth factor in porcine hibernating myocardium: a comparative study. *J Thorac Cardiovasc Surg* 2004;127:34–43.
59. Detillieux KA, Sheikh F, Kardami E, Cattini PA. Biological activities of fibroblast growth factor-2 in the adult myocardium. *Cardiovasc Res* 2003;57:8–19.
60. Post MJ, Laham R, Sellke FW, Simons M. Therapeutic angiogenesis in cardiology using protein formulations. *Cardiovasc Res* 2001;49:522–531.

61. Gounis MJ, Spiga M-G, Graham RM, et al. Angiogenesis is confined to the transient period of VEGF expression that follows adenoviral gene delivery to ischemic muscle. *Gene Ther* 2005;12:762–771.
62. Isner JM. Myocardial gene therapy. *Nature* 2002;415:234–239.
63. Rebar EJ. Development of pro-angiogenic engineered transcription factors for the treatment of cardiovascular disease. *Expert Opin Invest Drugs* 2004;13:829–839.
64. Abbott JD, Giordano FJ. Stem cells and cardiovascular disease. *J Nucl Cardiol* 2003;10:403–412.
65. Perin EC, Geng Y-J, Willerson JT. Adult stem cell therapy in perspective. *Circulation* 2003;107:935–938.
66. Körbling M, Estrov Z. Adult stem cells for tissue repair: a new therapeutic concept? *N Engl J Med* 2003;349:570–582.
67. Crosby JR, Kaminski WE, Schatteman G, et al. Endothelial cells of hematopoietic origin make a significant contribution to adult blood vessel formation. *Circ Res* 2000;87:728–730.
68. van der Heyden MAG, Hescheler J, Mummery CL. Spotlight on stem cells: makes old hearts fresh. *Cardiovasc Res* 2003;58:241–245.
69. Sata M, Saiura A, Kunisato A, et al. Hematopoietic stem cells differentiate into vascular cells that participate in the pathogenesis of atherosclerosis. *Nat Med* 2002;8:403–409.
70. Alessandri G, Emanueli C, Madeddu P. Genetically engineered stem cell therapy for tissue regeneration. *Ann NY Acad Sci* 2004;1015:271–284.
71. Frazier OH, March RJ, Horvath KA. Transmyocardial revascularization with carbon dioxide laser in patients with end-stage coronary artery disease. *N Engl J Med* 1999;341:1021–1028.
72. Allen KB, Dowling RD, Fudge TL, et al. Comparison of transmyocardial revascularization with medical therapy in patients with refractory angina. *N Engl J Med* 1999;341:1029–1036.
73. Schofield PM, Sharples LD, Caine N, et al. Transmyocardial laser revascularization in patients with refractory angina: a randomized controlled trial. *Lancet* 1999;353:519–524.
74. Burkhoff D, Schmidt S, Schulman SP, et al. Transmyocardial laser revascularization compared with continued medical therapy for treatment of refractory angina pectoris: a prospective randomized trial. ATLANTIC investigators: Angina Treatments: Lasers and Normal Therapies in Comparison. *Lancet* 1999;354:885–890.
75. Jones JW, Schmidt SE, Richman BW, et al. Holmium:YAG laser transmyocardial revascularization relieves angina and improves functional status. *Ann Thorac Surg* 1999;67:1596–1602.
76. Aaberge L, Nordstrand K, Dragsund M, et al. Transmyocardial revascularization with CO_2 laser in patients with refractory angina pectoris: clinical results from the Norwegian randomized trial. *J Am Coll Cardiol* 2000;35:1170–1177.
77. Huikeshoven M, van der Sloot JAP, Tukkie R, et al. Improved quality of life after XeCl excimer transmyocardial laser revascularization: results of a randomized trial. *Lasers Surg Med* 2003;33:1–7.
78. Horvath KA, Aranki SF, Cohn LC, et al. Sustained angina relief 5 years after transmyocardial laser revascularization with a CO_2 laser. *Circulation* 2001;104(suppl I):I-81–I-84.
79. Aaberge L, Rootwelt K, Blomhoff S, et al. Continued symptomatic improvement three to five years after transmyocardial revascularization with CO_2 laser: a late clinical follow-up of the Norwegian randomized trial with transmyocardial revascularization. *J Am Coll Cardiol* 2002;39:1588–1593.
80. Allen KB, Dowling RD, Angell WW, et al. Transmyocardial revascularization: 5-year follow-up of a prospective, randomized multicenter trial. *Ann Thorac Surg* 2004;77:1228–1234.
81. Oesterle SN, Sanborn TA, Ali N, et al. Percutaneous transmyocardial laser revascularization for severe angina: the PACIFIC randomised trial. *Lancet* 2000;356:1705–1710.
82. Stone GW, Teirstein PS, Rubenstein R, et al. A prospective, multicenter, randomized trial of percutaneous transmyocardial laser revascularization in patients with nonrecanalizable chronic total occlusions. *J Am Coll Cardiol* 2002;39:1581–1587.
83. Gray TJ, Burns SM, Clarke SC, et al. Percutaneous myocardial laser revascularization in patients with refractory angina pectoris. *Am J Cardiol* 2003;91:661–666.
84. Peterson ED, Kaul P, Kaczmarek RG, et al. From controlled trials to clinical practice: monitoring transmyocardial revascularization use and outcomes. *J Am Coll Cardiol* 2003;42:1611–1616.
85. Seiler C, Pohl T, Wustmann K, et al. Promotion of collateral growth by granulocyte-macrophage colony-stimulating factor in patients with coronary artery disease: a randomized, double-blind, placebo-controlled study. *Circulation* 2001;104:2012–2017.
86. Simons M, Annex BH, Laham RJ, et al. Pharmacological treatment of coronary artery disease with recombinant fibroblast growth factor-2: double-blind, randomized, controlled clinical trial. *Circulation* 2002;105: 788–793.
87. Grines CL, Watkins MW, Helmer G, et al. Angiogenic Gene Therapy (AGENT) trial in patients with stable angina pectoris. *Circulation* 2002;105:1291–1297.
88. Losordo DW, Vale PR, Hendel RC, et al. Phase 1/2 placebo-controlled, double-blind, dose-escalating trial of myocardial vascular endothelial growth factor 2 gene transfer by catheter delivery in patients with chronic myocardial ischemia. *Circulation* 2002;105:2012–2018.
89. Henry TD, Annex BH, McKendall GR, et al. The VIVA trial: Vascular Endothelial Growth Factor in Ischemia for Vascular Angiogenesis. *Circulation* 2003;107:1359–1365.
90. Grines CL, Watkins MW, Mahmarian JJ, et al. A randomized, double-blind, placebo-controlled trials of Ad5FGF-4 gene therapy and its effect on myocardial perfusion in patients with stable angina. *J Am Coll Cardiol* 2003;42:1339–1347.
91. Kastrup J, Jørgensen E, Rück A, et al. Direct intramyocardial plasmid vascular endothelial growth factor-A_{165} gene therapy in patients with stable severe angina pectoris. *J Am Coll Cardiol* 2005;45:982–988.
92. Tse H-F, Kwong Y-L, Chan JKF, et al. Angiogenesis in ischaemic myocardium by intramyocardial autologous bone marrow mononuclear cell implantation. *Lancet* 2003;361:47–49.
93. Perin EC, Dohmann HFR, Borojevic R, et al. Transendocardial, autologous bone marrow cell transplantation for severe, chronic ischemic heart failure. *Circulation* 2003;107:2294–2302.
94. Fuchs S, Satler LF, Kornowski R, et al. Catheter-based autologous bone marrow myocardial injection in no-option patients with advanced coronary artery disease. *J Am Coll Cardiol* 2003;41:1721–1724.
95. Assmus B, Schächinger V, Teupe C, et al. Transplantation of Progenitor Cells and Regeneration Enhancement in Acute Myocardial Infarction (TOPCARE-AMI). *Circulation* 2002;106:3009–3017.
96. Losordo DW, Dimmeler S. Therapeutic angiogenesis and vasculogenesis for ischemic disease. II. Cell based therapies. *Circulation* 2004;109:2692–2697.
97. Tateishi-Yuyama E, Matsubara H, Murohara T, et al. Therapeutic angiogenesis for patients with limb ischaemia by autologous transplantation of bone-marrow cells: a pilot study and a randomized controlled trial. *Lancet* 2002;360:427–435.
98. Lazarous DF, Unger EF, Epstein SE, et al. Basic fibroblast growth factor in patients with intermittent claudication: results of a phase I trial. *J Am Coll Cardiol* 2000;36:1239–1244.
99. Lederman RG, Mendelsohn FO, Anderson RD, et al. Therapeutic Angiogenesis with Recombinant Fibroblast Growth Factor-2 for Intermittent Claudication (the TRAFFIC study): a randomised trial. *Lancet* 2002;359: 2053–2058.
100. Rajagopalan S, Mohler ER, Lederman RJ, et al. Regional angiogenesis with vascular endothelial growth factor in peripheral arterial disease: a phase II randomized, double-blind, controlled study of adenoviral delivery of vascular endothelial growth factor 121 in patients with disabling intermittent claudication. *Circulation* 2003;108:1933–1938.
101. van Royen N, Piek JJ, Legemate DA, et al. Design of the START-trial: Stimulation of Arteriogenesis Using Subcutaneous Application of GM-CSF as a New Treatment for Peripheral Vascular Disease: a randomized, double-blind, placebo-controlled trial. *Vasc Med* 2003;8:191–196.
102. Powell RJ, Dormandy J, Simons M, et al. Therapeutic angiogenesis for critical limb ischemia: design of the Hepatocyte Growth Factor Therapeutic Angiogenesis clinical trial. *Vasc Med* 2004;9:193–198.
103. Higashi Y, Kimura M, Hara K, et al. Autologous bone-marrow mononuclear cell implantation improves endothelium-dependent vasodilation in patients with limb ischemia. *Circulation* 2004;109:1215–1218.
104. Veikkola T, Karkkainen M, Claesson-Welsh L, Alitalo K. Regulation of angiogenesis via vascular endothelial growth factor receptors. *Cancer Res* 2000;60:203–212.

CHAPTER 105 ■ DISEASES OF THE AORTA

HEATHER L. GORNIK AND MARK A. CREAGER

INTRODUCTION

The aorta is the largest and most important blood vessel of the body, serving as the initial conduit for the perfusion of all organs and tissues. The spectrum of pathology of the aorta is wide reaching and includes congenital anomalies, degenerative abnormalities, atherosclerosis, and inflammation. Some aortic disorders present in childhood and young adulthood, whereas others generally occur among the elderly. In this chapter, we provide an overview of diseases of the aorta. Throughout the text, we emphasize recent advances in diagnostic modalities and endovascular and surgical technologies that have revolutionized the approach to the patient with aortic disease.

ANATOMY OF THE AORTA

The aorta is the largest artery of the body, delivering oxygenated blood from the left ventricle to organs and tissues through its arterial branches. The aorta is divided into thoracic and abdominal segments based on the location relative to the diaphragm (Fig. 105.1). The thoracic aorta is further divided into the ascending aorta (containing the aortic root, the sinuses of Valsalva, and a tubular segment), the aortic arch (containing the great vessels), and the descending thoracic aorta. The aortic isthmus is a narrow region of the aorta located between the origin of the left subclavian artery and the ligamentum arteriosum. The thoracic aorta begins as an anterior structure, coursing superiorly to the right of the sternum, ultimately moving posteriorly into the mediastinum, and running along the left of the vertebral column. The descending thoracic aorta travels posterior to the esophagus and anterior to the vertebral column and gives rise to a number of branches, including small pericardial branches, bronchial and esophageal arteries, and the posterior intercostal arteries. The abdominal aorta begins at the diaphragm and ends at the aortoiliac bifurcation, giving off major visceral and mesenteric branches, including the celiac axis, superior and inferior-mesenteric arteries, and the paired renal arteries. The abdominal aorta also gives rise to paired lumbar branches, which supply the musculature of the back.

CONGENITAL ANOMALIES OF THE AORTA

Although there are dozens of anatomic variations of the aorta and its major branches, only a small number of anomalies are associated with clinical consequences. The most common anomaly of the aortic arch is the so-called bovine variant, which is present in up to 10% to 20% individuals and is characterized by the origin of the left common carotid artery arising from the brachiocephalic (innominate) trunk. Other common aortic arch anomalies include a four-vessel arch with separate origins of the right common carotid and right subclavian arteries (2.5%), symmetric right and left brachiocephalic trunks forming a two-vessel aortic arch (1.2%), and origin of the left vertebral artery directly from a four-vessel aortic arch, typically between the ostia of the left common carotid and left subclavian arteries (2.4% to 5.8%) (1). None of these anomalies is typically associated with symptoms, although each is of potential importance in planning a catheter-based or open surgical procedure for another indication, such as occlusive disease of a carotid or subclavian vessel (2).

The rare aortic arch anomalies that are associated with clinical symptoms typically form a compressive vascular ring around the esophagus and the tracheal-bronchial tree, causing bronchospasm, stridor, chronic cough, or dysphagia. The most common vascular ring anomalies are double aortic arch and right-sided aortic arch with aberrant left subclavian artery and ligamentum arteriosum (Fig. 105.2) (3–5). Although it does not cause a true vascular ring, aberrant origin of the right subclavian artery distal to the left subclavian artery of a normal left-sided aortic arch is an anatomic aortic variant that is present in approximately 1% of the population (6). This anomaly is associated with marked dilation of the right subclavian artery,

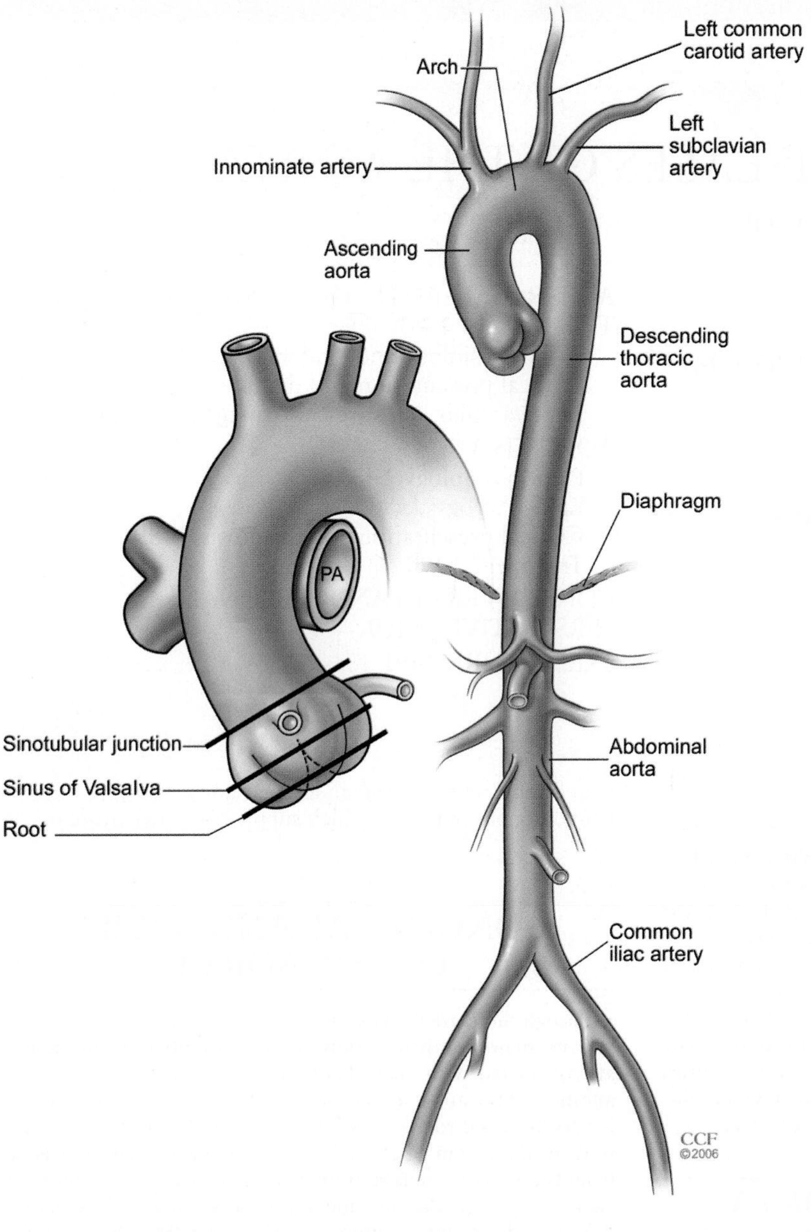

FIGURE 105.1. Anatomy of the aorta. Diseases of the aorta are classified according to the anatomic segment in which they occur. The thoracic aorta becomes the abdominal aorta on passing through the crura of the diaphragm. The abdominal aorta is divided into suprarenal, juxtrarenal, and infrarenal segments before bifurcating into two common iliac arteries approximately 1 cm above the umbilicus.

often causing dysphagia as it passes retrograde to the esophagus toward the right arm. Such dysphagia due to a vascular ring is known as dysphagia lusoria (7). Aortic arch anomalies, particularly those with aberrance of one of the subclavian arteries, are also associated with an anatomic remnant of the persistent right aortic arch known as a Kommerell's diverticulum (7–9). Kommerell's diverticula may become aneurysmal.

Symptomatic aortic arch anomalies are extremely rare, and the index of suspicion of the clinician must be high to make the diagnosis. An aortic arch anomaly may be suspected in a patient with classical symptoms and an abnormal chest radiograph demonstrating enlargement or abnormal configuration of the aortic shadow. Arch anomalies may also be detected by transthoracic or transesophageal echocardiography (10). Diagnosis is confirmed by a noninvasive imaging study of the thoracic aorta and arch vessels, such as computed tomography (CT) or magnetic resonance angiography (MRA). Treatment of symptomatic vascular ring anomalies and aberrant subclavian arteries typically involves surgical correction. Procedural outcome depends on the age and comorbidities of the patient at the time of surgery. Outcomes of vascular ring surgery in the pediatric population are typically excellent, and small case series of successful surgery in adults have also been reported (3–5,11). Aneurysms of anomalous subclavian arteries or of Kommerell's diverticula may spontaneously rupture or dissect, and prophylactic surgical correction is generally recommended, even in the absence of symptoms (9,12,13).

AORTIC ANEURYSMS

The term aortic aneurysm, derived from the Greek word *aneurysmos* for "dilation," refers to enlargement of the aorta beyond its normal diameter. A segment of the aorta is called aneurysmal if its maximal diameter is greater than 1.5 times that of the adjacent proximal normal segment. As general guidelines, the normal diameter of the thoracic aorta is approximately 2.5 cm at the aortic annulus, 3 cm at the tubular ascending portion, 2.5 cm at the descending thoracic aorta, and 2 cm in the infrarenal abdominal aorta (14,15). Aortic dimension varies by body surface area, age, and gender, with men typically having larger aortic dimensions than women (15). An

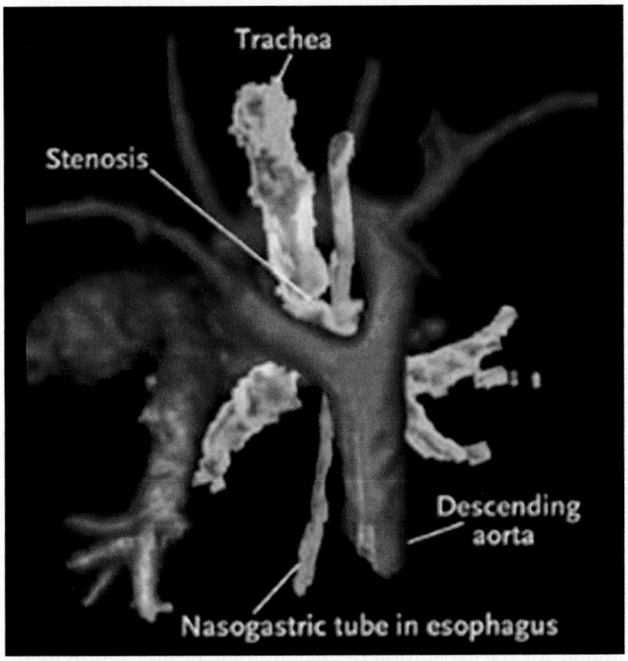

FIGURE 105.2. Double aortic arch causing vascular compression syndrome. Three-dimensional reconstructed image of a magnetic resonance angiogram obtained of an infant with acute respiratory failure. The double aortic arch is seen encircling the trachea and the esophagus. The child ultimately underwent surgical correction. (From Lotz J, Macchiarini P. Images in clinical medicine. Double aortic arch diagnosed by magnetic resonance imaging. *N Engl J Med* 2004;351:e20.)

aneurysm is described as fusiform if it symmetrically involves the entire circumference of the aorta. In contrast, a saccular aneurysm involves a focal outpouching of an area of the vessel wall. Aortic aneurysm must also be differentiated from aortic pseudoaneurysm, a contained rupture of the vessel into the adventitial space. Aortic pseudoaneurysms are typically posttraumatic (Chapter 38) or due to penetrating atherosclerotic ulcer or infectious aortitis. The epidemiology, pathophysiology, and management of aortic aneurysm are highly dependent on the anatomic location of the lesion, as discussed later. For aortic aneurysms at all locations, the objective of management is to avoid the potentially lethal complications of aortic rupture or dissection.

Thoracic Aortic Aneurysms

Thoracic aortic aneurysms (TAAs) encompass all aneurysms that involve the aorta from the level of the aortic root to the crura of the diaphragm. Thoracic aortic aneurysms are categorized by whether they involve the aortic root and/or ascending aorta, aortic arch, or descending thoracic aorta. The subset of TAAs that extend directly into the abdominal cavity are called thoracoabdominal aneurysms (TAAAs). Approximately 60% of TAAs involve the aortic root or the ascending thoracic aorta, 40% involve the descending thoracic aorta, and 10% involve the aortic arch (16). Thoracoabdominal aneurysms are relatively rare (10%) (16).

Pathophysiology

The most common causes of TAA are listed in Table 105.1. The final common pathway and underlying histopathology of most ascending aortic aneurysms is degeneration of the medial layer of the aortic wall known as cystic medial necrosis. Thus, the risk factors for the development of ascending aortic aneurysm are primarily those conditions that are associated with cystic medial necrosis of the ascending aorta. Histologically, there is loss of elastin fibers and smooth muscle cells within the medial layer as well as accumulation of ground substance, leading to cystic-appearing spaces within the media (17,18). Cystic medial necrosis weakens the aortic wall and is an important underlying factor in both aneurysmal dilation of the aorta and aortic dissection. Cystic medial necrosis has been reported as a common pathologic finding among ascending aortic aneurysms related to Marfan syndrome, congenital bicuspid aortic valves, and in the familial TAA syndromes among others (18,19). Marfan syndrome is an autosomal dominant disorder associated with mutations in the genes for fibrillin-1, a key component of myofibrils of elastin. The type IV variant of Ehlers-Danlos is an autosomal disorder due to mutations in genes for type III procollagen (20). Three specific loci for distinct familial TAA and dissection syndromes have been reported (21–23). Cystic medial necrosis may also occur in the setting of longstanding hypertension, particularly in elderly patients (24). A variant of cystic medial necrosis, annuloaortic ectasia, or dilation of the aorta at the level of the annulus, may cause isolated aortic insufficiency in association with TAA. Annuloaortic ectasia may occur in association with Marfan syndrome or other genetic disorders or may occur as an idiopathic variant. The cause of cystic medial necrosis is not known, although it appears that genetically programmed premature apoptosis of smooth muscle cells in media may play a role (18).

TABLE 105.1

ETIOLOGY OF THORACIC AORTIC ANEURYSMS

Cystic medial necrosis
Marfan syndrome
Bicuspid aortic valve
Familial thoracic aortic syndromes (5q13–14, 11q23.2–q24, 3p24–25)
Turner syndrome
Ehlers-Danlos syndrome, type IV variant
Hypertension
Advanced age
Atherosclerosis/degenerative (especially descending thoracic and thoracoabdominal aneurysms)
Chronic aortic dissection
Spontaneous
Iatrogenic (cannulation of aorta during bypass surgery, post cardiac catheterization)
Infection
Bacterial (e.g., *Salmonella*, *Staphylococcus*)
Syphilitic/luetic
Mycobacterial (*Mycobacterium tuberculosis*)
Vasculitis
Posttraumatic
Congenital (e.g., sinus of Valsalva aneurysm)

Aneurysms of the descending thoracic aorta and thoracoabdominal aneurysms are degenerative and often have pathologic characteristics of atherosclerosis. These include distortion of the arterial intima and media leading to weakening of the aortic wall and subsequent aneurysmal dilation. Recent clinical investigation, however, has challenged the notion that descending TAAs are causally related to systemic atherosclerosis (25). In addition to atherosclerosis and cystic medial necrosis, TAA may occur as a consequence of chronic aortic dissection or in response to the inflammation of a large-vessel vasculitis. Infectious, or mycotic, TAAs are related to chronic syphilis or caused by select bacterial or mycobacterial infections. Mycotic aneurysms are often saccular in appearance and are associated with a high rate of rupture or contained rupture with pseudoaneurysm formation (26,27). Sinus of Valsalva aneurysm is a rare anomaly that involves aneurysmal dilation of one of the coronary sinuses, typically the right coronary sinus (28). Sinus of Valsalva aneurysms are usually congenital, but they may also occur as a complication of aortic trauma (i.e., cardiac catheterization with aortic injury), infection, or inflammation. These lesions are prone to spontaneous rupture, including fistulization into a cardiac chamber, particularly the right ventricle (28).

Epidemiology and Prognosis

The estimated incidence of TAA is between 5.9 and 10.4 new aneurysms per 100,000 person-years (29,30). Among patients with degenerative (non–Marfan associated) TAA, diagnosis is most commonly made in the sixth or seventh decades of life, with women typically presenting up to a decade later than men (29,30). Natural history studies have estimated that the average expansion of degenerative TAA is 0.1 cm/year, with descending or thoracoabdominal aneurysms growing at a more rapid rate (0.19 cm/year) than aneurysms of the ascending aorta or aortic arch (0.07 cm/year) (31). Marfan disease–associated TAA and chronic dissecting aneurysms also grow at an increased rate (31). According to the law of Laplace, wall stress is directly proportional to the radius of the vessel. As aneurysms enlarge, there is increased wall stress, accelerated rate of expansion, and an increased risk of dissection or rupture. For TAAs less than 4 cm in diameter, the mean rate of rupture or dissection is less than 3%/year (31). For aneurysms larger than 6 cm in diameter, the estimated rate of rupture or dissection is 6.9%/year with overall mortality of 11.8%/year (31). Whereas aortic dissection and rupture are the leading causes of death among patients with degenerative TAA, cardiovascular events account for one fourth of deaths, which likely reflects the age of the population and extensive systemic burden of atherosclerosis (30,31). In addition to increasing aneurysm size, risk factors for aortic dissection, rupture, or death among patients with TAA include Marfan syndrome, history of a prior cerebrovascular event, and female gender (31). Pregnancy is also strongly associated with adverse outcomes among women with TAA due to Marfan syndrome or bicuspid aortic valve, and there are case reports of rapid aneurysmal expansion, rupture, and dissection during pregnancy (32,33).

Clinical Presentation and Diagnosis

The role of the history and physical examination in the diagnosis of TAA is limited. Most patients with TAA are asymptomatic and are diagnosed on the basis of a noninvasive imaging study that has been obtained for another indication. When present, symptoms are generally due to direct compression of surrounding intrathoracic structures, such as the superior vena cava (facial swelling), esophagus (dysphagia), trachea or bronchi (wheezing, dyspnea, chronic cough), or recurrent laryngeal nerve (hoarseness) (34). Chest or back discomfort is also a common symptom among patients with large TAA, particularly in association with rapid expansion of the aneurysm.

Among asymptomatic patients, a family history of Marfan syndrome or type IV Ehlers-Danlos syndrome should alert the clinician to the possibility of occult TAA. A dedicated imaging study of the aorta should be performed in these patients, particularly in the presence of physical findings suggestive of a genetic disorder. Physical findings of TAA, such as a visible bulge or a parasternal heave, occur rarely. Diagnostic clues for TAA relate to the underlying etiology, including signs of Marfan syndrome (i.e., tall stature, arachnodactyly, pectus deformity, and ectopia lentis). Cardiac murmurs of aortic insufficiency or aortic stenosis may be appreciated among patients with ascending TAA, particularly those with bicuspid aortic valve, who may also have a systolic ejection click. Multiple imaging modalities are used to diagnose TAA. Chest radiography, though too insensitive to be used as the sole diagnostic modality, may demonstrate widening of the aortic knob or mediastinal silhouette. In general, if there is any clinical suspicion of TAA, a dedicated imaging study of the aorta should be obtained. Magnetic resonance angiography (MRA) and computed tomographic angiography (CTA) are both excellent imaging modalities for the diagnosis and surveillance of TAA (35). The latest generation of multidetector CT scanners allow for excellent spatial resolution and sizing of the aneurysm as well as visualization of branch vessels and vascular calcification. CTA also readily diagnoses complications associated with aortic aneurysm, particularly aortic rupture or dissection. Cross-sectional CTA images can be used to generate three-dimensional reconstructions that mimic conventional aortography. CT angiography is the imaging modality of choice for follow-up after surgical or endovascular repair of a TAA. To prevent excessive interreader variability, orthogonal measurements of maximal aortic diameter, as measured from outer wall to outer wall of the aorta, should be taken using standardized protocols (36). Magnetic resonance angiography with gadolinium enhancement and a breath-hold is superior to time-of-flight magnetic resonance imaging for the sizing and characterization of TAA and also allows for the generation of angiographic projections in many planes of view (Fig. 105.3). Transthoracic echocardiography (TTE) is an excellent imaging modality for diagnosis of TAA located at or near the aortic root. Echocardiography is also able to diagnose cardiac pathologies associated with TAA, particularly bicuspid aortic valve. Transthoracic echocardiography may fail to detect aortic dilation in the tubular portion of the ascending aorta and is unable to adequately visualize the aortic arch and the descending thoracic aorta. Transesophageal echocardiography (TEE) is able to visualize the entire thoracic aorta, with the exception of a segment of the distal ascending aorta, which is obscured by tracheal shadowing.

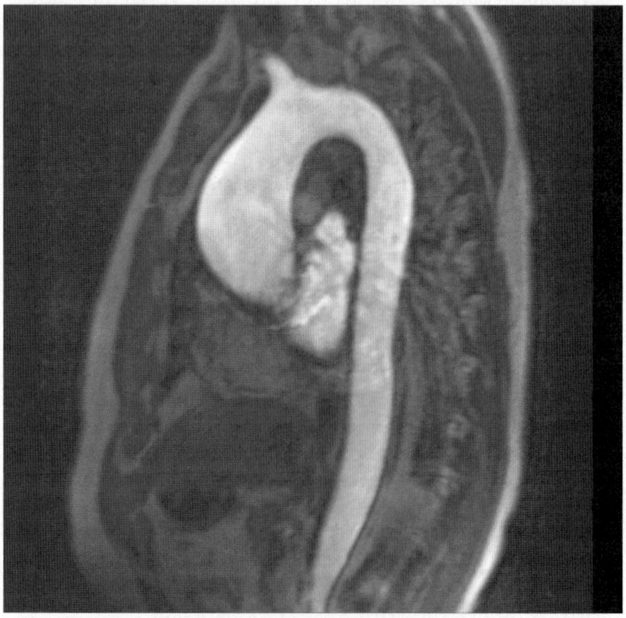

FIGURE 105.3. Thoracic aortic aneurysm (TAA). Shown is a gadolinium-enhanced magnetic resonance angiogram in the saggital plane. There is an aneurysm of the tubular portion of the ascending aorta that spares the sinuses of Valsalva and aortic arch. This is a common location for ascending TAA among patients without Marfan syndrome, such as those with bicuspid aortic valve. (Image courtesy of Dr. Srikanth Sola, the Cleveland Clinic Foundation.)

Screening for TAA is not recommended in the general population due to the infrequent occurrence of this disorder. However, patients with established or suspected Marfan syndrome, Turner syndrome, and Ehlers-Danlos type IV syndrome should undergo an imaging study to screen for TAA. Patients with suspected familial thoracic aortic disease syndromes should also be screened for TAA. It is also advisable that patients with documented bicuspid aortic valve undergo an additional imaging study to exclude concomitant TAA, particularly if the tubular ascending aorta is not well visualized by echocardiography.

Surveillance and Medical Management

Few medical therapies have been proven to slow the rate of expansion of TAA, aside from β-blockers. β-Blockers lower blood pressure and reduce the rate of rise of central arterial pressure over time (*dP/dt*), measures that reduce the likelihood of aortic dissection. In one small randomized trial of 70 patients with Marfan syndrome, long-term treatment with propranolol was associated with a slower rate of aortic root dilation and a decreased rate of death, congestive heart failure, aortic insufficiency, aortic dissection, and cardiovascular surgery (37). On the basis of this single study, β-blockers are generally recommended for all patients with TAA without contraindication, including those without Marfan syndrome. Investigators have recently begun to study the use of angiotensin-converting-enzyme inhibitors in Marfan syndrome patients for improving aortic distensibility and slowing the rate of aortic expansion, although no randomized trials have been published with this treatment (38). In addition to pharmacologic therapy with β-blockers, patients with TAA should generally be cautioned to avoid strenuous isometric exercise, such as weight lifting. Gentle aerobic exercise is acceptable. It is recommended that patients with TAA who wish to participate in vigorous aerobic exercise, such as long-distance running or aerobic dance, should undergo treadmill exercise testing while on β-blocker therapy to ensure that there is not extreme hypertension with exercise (i.e., >180 mm Hg systolic pressure) and that the pulse is well controlled (16).

Once the diagnosis of TAA has been made, a careful surveillance plan must be instituted to follow the diameter of the aneurysm and its rate of expansion. It is reasonable to obtain a second imaging study 6 months after the initial diagnosis of TAA to ensure that there is not a trajectory of rapid expansion. For patients with TAA without chronic aortic dissection, yearly imaging studies using MRA or CTA are generally adequate until the size of the aneurysm approaches the critical value at which repair is considered. Patients with chronic dissecting aortic aneurysms should be followed with an intensive imaging surveillance program for the first 2 years after the initial event, and then annually if the aneurysm is stable in size. For patients with Marfan syndrome–associated TAA, imaging studies should be performed at 6-month intervals or more frequently as the aneurysm approaches the size at which repair is needed (39). Patients with known TAA who become pregnant, particularly patients with Marfan syndrome, should be followed closely for rapid aneurysm expansion. Among pregnant patients with Marfan syndrome and TAA greater than 4 cm, consideration of Caesarian section is generally recommended (39).

Surgical and Endovascular Treatment of Thoracic Aortic Aneurysms

The goal of management of TAA is to pursue definitive correction at the point at which the risk of rupture exceeds the risk of the corrective procedure. General guidelines for referral for TAA repair are provided in Table 105.2 (14,16,40). Of note, due to the high risk of dissection or rupture among patients with Marfan syndrome, bicuspid aortic valve, or aortic aneurysm with a familial syndrome, there is a lower-diameter threshold for repair. Women with Marfan syndrome contemplating pregnancy should be considered for surgical repair before conception if the aortic root is greater than 4 to 4.5 cm.

TABLE 105.2

INDICATIONS FOR REPAIR OF AORTIC ANEURYSMS

Thoracic aortic aneurysm	
Ascending	≥5.5–6 cm
Ascending plus high-risk features[a]	≥5 cm
Ascending at time of AVR for bicuspid valve	≥4 cm
Descending	≥6.5–7 cm
Descending with dissection or Marfan syndrome	≥6 cm
Thoracoabdominal aneurysm	≥5.5–6 cm, variable
Abdominal aortic aneurysm (AAA)	≥5.5 cm or expansion >1.0 cm/y
Female patients with AAA	Consider referral at 4.5–5.0 cm

[a]High-risk features: Marfan syndrome, bicuspid aortic valve, family history of aortic dissection, rapid expansion of aneurysm.
AVR, aortic valve replacement.

The specific procedures undertaken for repair of TAA depend on the location of the aneurysm (i.e., whether it involves the aortic root or sinuses of Valsalva) and whether the aortic valve must be replaced. The Bentall procedure involves placement of a synthetic composite aortic tube graft with a built-in prosthetic aortic valve. The coronary artery ostia are directly reimplanted onto the graft. The original Bentall procedure was associated with the development of anastomotic coronary arterial stenotic lesions and pseudoaneurysms (41). The modified Bentall procedure (Fig. 105.4A), which involves mobilization of the proximal segments of the coronary artery and reimplantation of ostial buttons onto the composite graft, is associated with improved outcomes and is generally employed (42). The Cobrol technique, which is less commonly employed, involves placement of separate tube grafts to each coronary ostium. A cryopreserved aortic homograft may also be placed, with reimplantation of the coronary arteries, for patients requiring both aortic valve replacement and aortic aneurysm repair, although the long-term durability outcome of these grafts may be inferior to that of prosthetic materials, particularly for pediatric patients with Marfan syndrome (43,44). In the case of ascending aortic aneurysms that do not involve the aortic root, valve-sparing procedures have been developed. The David technique involves reimplantation of the aortic annulus and the coronary arteries into the tube graft (Fig. 105.4B) (45). Repair of aortic arch aneurysms is accomplished by replacement of the arch with a prosthetic tube graft and reattachment of the arch vessels either en bloc, with short interposition grafts, or with the use of a multilimbed prosthetic graft (41). The morbidity associated with ascending aorta and aortic arch aneurysm repair is substantial. All procedures require deep hypothermic circulatory arrest and cardiopulmonary bypass. Proximal aortic surgery is associated with a substantial risk of a periprocedural neurologic event. Recent advances have focused on blood conservation methods and the prevention of stroke during aortic arch surgery, including retrograde and antegrade cerebral perfusion (46–49). The mortality risk of elective surgery for ascending aorta and aortic arch aneurysms is approximately 2% to 3% in the most experienced centers (40,43,49). The risk of neurologic deficits following repair of aneurysms of the ascending and aortic arch varies by case series (2% to 9%), with highest

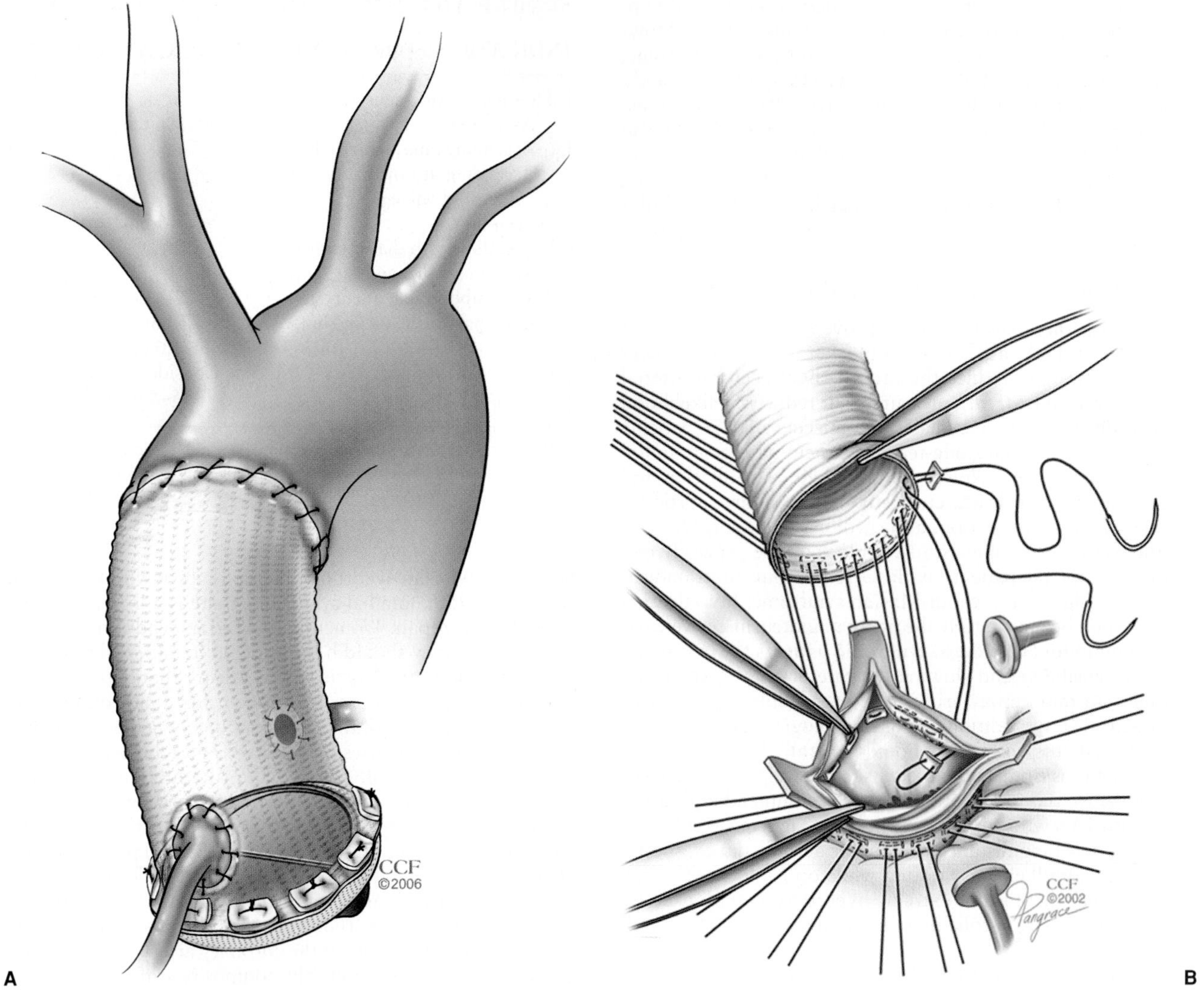

FIGURE 105.4. Surgical procedures for repair of ascending thoracic aortic aneurysm. **A:** The modified Bentall procedure. **B:** The aortic valve–sparing David procedure.

risk associated with surgical repair of aortic arch aneurysms, repair of aneurysms related to aortic dissection, and repair of aneurysms in elderly patients (40,46,49).

Surgical repair of descending TAA and TAAA carries a substantial risk of perioperative mortality, with rates ranging from 8% to 19% in published series (50–53). The perioperative risk reflects the high-risk nature of the patient population undergoing these procedures, particularly the association of these aneurysms with extensive atherosclerosis and coronary artery disease. Beyond perioperative mortality, the dreaded complication of descending thoracic or thoracoabdominal aortic surgical repair is the risk of paraplegia associated with disruption of blood supply to the spinal cord via the intercostal arteries, which supply the anterior and posterior spinal artery and the artery of Adamkiewicz. Historically, the rate of paraplegia associated with descending thoracic aorta or thoracoabdominal aneurysm surgery had been greater than 15%. Risk factors for the development of paraplegia include extent of the aneurysm repair (with thoracoabdominal aneurysms having higher risk), high aortic cross-clamp time, advanced age, emergency surgery, and postoperative renal and gastrointestinal complications (52,54). Due to advances in surgical technique, including cerebrospinal fluid drainage and reattachment of the intercostal and lumbar arteries, the rate of paraplegia associated with modern descending aortic surgery ranges from 2.3% to 8% (51,53–57).

There have been recent advances in the use of endovascular stent grafting for the repair of descending thoracic and thoracoabdominal aneurysms. Selection of optimal patients for stent grafting is critical, including consideration of anatomic features such as the length of the aneurysm and its proximal and distal aortic necks, the location of the aneurysm relative to the subclavian artery and celiac axis (for thoracoabdominal aneurysms), and the angle of the descending aorta off of the aortic arch. Early clinical experience indicates that endovascular grafting for descending thoracic aneurysms is an acceptable alternative to open surgical repair in carefully selected patients. The short-term mortality rate associated with endovascular repair of TAA is 4% to 6%, and there is a trend toward decreased aneurysm-related mortality when compared to open surgery at 2 years of follow-up (58–60). Spinal cord ischemia and paralysis have also been reported in patients undergoing thoracic stent-graft repair, with reported rates ranging from 0% to 4.3% (58–60). Patients undergoing endograft repair of thoracic or thoracoabdominal aneurysms require intensive postprocedural surveillance, typically with serial contrast CT scans, to detect leaking around the graft (endoleak) or enlarging aneurysm. In published case series, procedure-related or device-related complications occurred in as many as 38% of patients, including attachment failures requiring repeat intervention (60). Thoracic stent grafting is considered an emerging alternative to open surgical repair for descending thoracic aortic aneurysms, particularly for patients with optimal anatomy in highly experienced centers.

Thoracoabdominal Aneurysm

Thoracoabdominal aortic aneurysms begin in the descending thoracic aorta and extend into the abdominal cavity. These aneurysms are typically associated with extensive atherosclerosis, although aneurysms related to other diseases, including Marfan disease and aortitis, have been reported. TAAAs are classified according to the Crawford system, which divides these aneurysms into four categories based on their extent above and below the diaphragm, and is useful in planning operative repair (61). Guidelines for repair of TAAA vary with the type of lesion, but it is generally suggested that repair of a TAAA be undertaken at a maximal dimension of 5.5 to 6.0 cm (Table 105.2). Repair of TAAA involves an extensive open surgical procedure with placement of a synthetic graft. Morbidity of surgical repair is similar to that of TAAs. As with TAA repair, the risk of postoperative paraplegia has improved with modern surgical techniques, although it remains substantial, approximating 4.5% in recent case series (55). Renal failure is also a common complication of TAAA repair because suprarenal aortic cross clamping is typically required. The incidence of renal failure requiring hemodialysis in one large series of TAAA repair was 5.9% (55). The use of endovascular stent grafting techniques for TAAA is in its infancy and is particularly complex given the branch vessel involvement common to most of these lesions.

Abdominal Aortic Aneurysm

Although abdominal aortic aneurysms (AAA) may occur at any location from the diaphragm to the aortic bifurcation, the infrarenal aorta is by far the most common location. Suprarenal and juxtarenal AAAs are less common. An AAA is generally defined as an aortic diameter of greater than 3 cm within the abdominal cavity, although the threshold for diagnosis of AAA should be lower for certain subgroups of patients, particularly women and patients of short stature. An alternative definition is an increase the aortic diameter to 1.5 times the size of a contiguous normal segment.

Pathophysiology

Abdominal aortic aneurysms have traditionally been considered degenerative in nature and related to atherosclerosis and the aging process. More recently, the paradigm for the pathophysiology of AAA has shifted toward recognition of an active inflammatory process involving the aortic wall. There appears to be upregulation of local production of matrix metalloproteinases by the smooth muscle cells, leading to degradation of the extracellular matrix of the aortic wall with subsequent remodeling and dilation (62). Marfan syndrome and Ehlers-Danlos type IV syndrome have also been associated with AAA, although to a lesser extent than with TAA.

Epidemiology and Prognosis

Mild dilation and ectasia of the abdominal aorta commonly occur with advanced age, although true aneurysm of the aorta is less frequent (63,64). The overall prevalence of AAA among asymptomatic subjects in large screening studies is approximately 4.3% to 4.9%, although participants in these studies were primarily men with a high prevalence of tobacco use (65–67). The prevalence of AAA is substantially lower in women, with a prevalence of 1.0% to 2.2% in community-based studies compared to a prevalence of 4.3% to 8.9% in men, depending on the population studied and the specific diameter criteria used to diagnose AAA (64,68). In the Olmstead County, Minnesota, population, the incidence of AAA was 36.5 per 100,000 person-years, with analysis of epidemiologic trends demonstrating a sevenfold increase in reported incidence over the period 1951 to 1980, likely due to widespread availability of noninvasive imaging techniques (69). In addition to male gender, risk factors strongly associated with the presence of AAA are age (typically >65 years), current or past history of tobacco use, first-degree relative with AAA, atherosclerosis in other vascular beds (especially coronary artery disease), and hypertension (64,65). Smoking is the strongest risk factor for the development of AAA. The presence of diabetes mellitus seems to be protective against the development of AAA, perhaps due to the association of diabetes mellitus with vascular calcification and negative remodeling (65). Through mechanisms that are not understood, the prevalence of AAA among African Americans is approximately one half of that among whites (70). Recent data have established an association between elevated markers of inflammation, particularly C-reactive protein, and the presence and size of AAA (71,72). These findings support the paradigm of the inflammatory pathogenesis of AAA.

Rupture of an AAA is a potentially lethal occurrence, typically associated with acute abdominal pain and abrupt hemodynamic collapse. It has been estimated that 25% of patients with ruptured AAA die before reaching the hospital, with overall operative mortality approaching 50% (73,74). Ruptured AAA accounts for approximately 15,000 deaths in the United States each year. As is the case for TAA, the risk of AAA rupture increases substantially with increasing aortic diameter. Abdominal aortic aneurysms expand at an average rate of approximately 2.6 mm/year (75). Aneurysm expansion accelerates as diameter increases. In addition to aneurysm size, ongoing tobacco use is associated with an increased rate of aortic expansion, and diabetes mellitus seems to be protective (75). Rupture of an AAA is unlikely at a dimension of less than 5.0 cm (2.5% over 7-year-follow-up) (76). Beyond 5.5 cm in size, the risk of aneurysm rupture increases dramatically. In one study, the annual rate of rupture was 9.4% for an AAA of 5.5 to 5.9 cm, 10.2% for a AAA of 6.0 to 6.9 cm, and 32.5% for an AAA of 7.0 cm or more (77). In addition to aneurysm size, additional independent risk factors for rupture of an AAA include active smoking, high blood pressure, chronic obstructive pulmonary disease, and female gender (78). Although men are roughly three times as likely to have AAA as women, the risk of rupture among women with AAA appears to be 4.5 times that of men (78).

Clinical Presentation and Diagnosis

Patients with unruptured AAA are typically asymptomatic, although patients may present with back or abdominal pain or gastrointestinal symptoms as aneurysms enlarge and compress adjacent structures. Rarely, patients with AAA may present with peripheral emboli from thrombus lining the aneurysm wall. Patients with ruptured AAA are typically critically ill, with approximately one half presenting with the classic triad of abdominal pain, pulsatile abdominal mass, and hypotension. The physical examination is insensitive for the diagnosis of AAA, although in some patients, particularly thin, younger subjects, the abdominal aortic impulse can be readily palpated. Overall, the sensitivity of the physical examination for the diagnosis of a 3- to 3.9-cm AAA is 29%, increasing to 76% for an AAA of greater than 5 cm (78). Femoral and popliteal pulses should be palpated in all patients with documented AAA

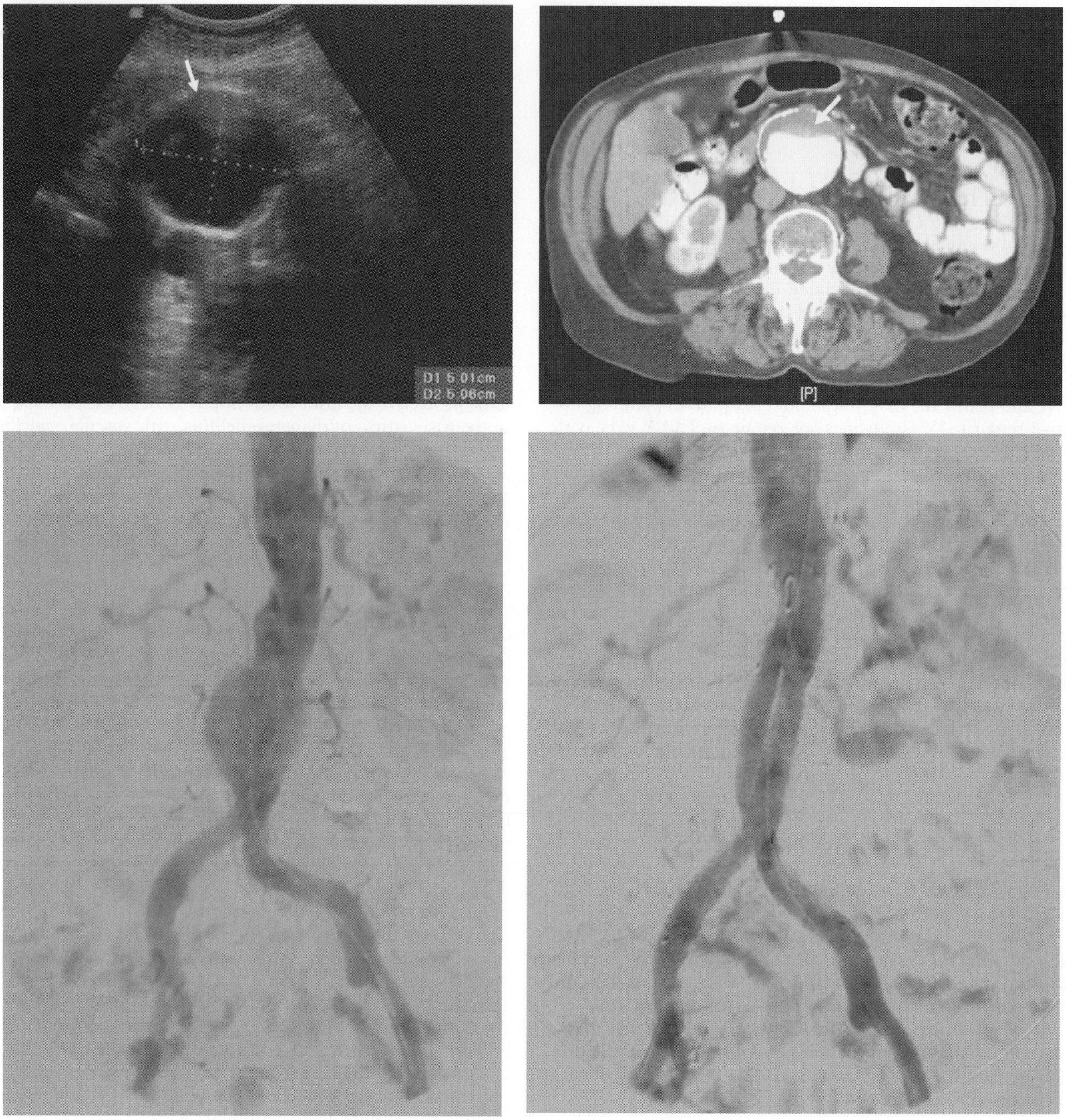

A B C D

FIGURE 105.5. Abdominal aortic aneurysm (AAA). Shown are (A) ultrasound and (B) computed tomogram images of an 84-year old woman with a 5-cm infrarenal AAA. There is mural thrombus seen on both the ultrasound and the computed tomography images (*white arrows*). Given the expansion of the aneurysm, she was referred for endovascular repair using a bifurcated aortic stent graft. Also shown are aortograms (C) before and (D) after placement of the stent graft.

for detection of concomitant aneurysms, which are common among patients with AAA. If a peripheral arterial aneurysm is suspected, an ultrasound study should be obtained for confirmation.

B-mode ultrasonography has become the standard tool for diagnosing AAA in most clinical situations (Fig. 105.5A). Compared to the gold standard of aortography, it has excellent sensitivity and specificity for the diagnosis of AAA. Computed tomography (Fig. 105.5B) and magnetic resonance imaging may also be used to diagnose AAA, but these modalities are typically reserved for follow-up of known AAA, to define the anatomic location of the aneurysm with regard to branch vessels, and to plan for aneurysm repair. The use of screening ultrasonography for the diagnosis of AAA in the general population remains controversial, but targeted screening is generally recommended. The Multicentre Aneurysm Screening Study (MASS), the largest study of screening for AAA, enrolled nearly 68,000 male patients between the ages of 65 and 74 years and randomized them to abdominal ultrasound screening or a noninterventional group (66). Among patients who were ultimately screened, there was a 4.9% prevalence of AAA. Overall, among patients invited for screening, there was a 42% reduction in the risk of AAA-related mortality compared to patients in the nonscreening group (0.19% vs. 0.33%), which became apparent after approximately 1 year of follow-up and was sustained throughout the 4-year follow-up period. In contrast, there was no difference in all-cause mortality between the two groups. Three other randomized clinical trials confirmed these findings of a moderate reduction in AAA-associated mortality with ultrasound screening and no benefit on all-cause mortality (79). Of note, only one of these fours studies randomized female patients. On the basis of these findings, the U.S. Preventive Services Task Force recently recommended one-time screening of all men ages 65 to 75 years with abdominal ultrasonography, although no recommendation for or against screening was made for women (79). Various subspecialty professional studies have also recommended screening for AAA, with extension of screening recommendations to older women and patients with a family history of AAA (80,81).

Surveillance and Medical Management

Once a diagnosis of AAA has been established, a careful surveillance plan must be instituted to monitor for AAA expansion and refer the patient for repair at the point when the risk of rupture exceeds the risk of repair. Ultrasonography is generally adequate for surveillance of AAA, although there is slight variability in measurement of AAA dimensions from study to study. CT angiography is superior for the assessment of suprarenal AAA. Compared to ultrasonography, measurements of aortic dimension on CT angiography tend to be larger, and this must be considered when comparing serial studies obtained by different modalities to avoid interpreting findings as a rapidly expanding aneurysm (82). As a general rule, AAAs less than 4.5 cm in size should be followed with annual surveillance ultrasound. Aneurysms greater than 4.5 cm in size should be reimaged every 6 months. It is also reasonable to obtain an ultrasound 6 months after the initial diagnosis of a small (<4.5 cm) AAA to exclude the possibility of rapid aneurysmal expansion.

Recently, there has been great interest in the development of targeted therapies to slow the expansion of AAA. A number of modalities have been investigated in preclinical and early clinical studies. These studies have particularly emphasized interrupting the inflammation and proteolysis of connective tissue, which seem to play a key role in the pathogenesis of AAA (83). Compounds under development as medical therapies for AAA include doxycycline, macrolide antibiotics, and statin drugs (84–88). β-Adrenergic blockers have not been shown to slow the expansion of AAA, unlike the single study of propranolol in patients with Marfan syndrome and TAA, although these agents are often prescribed for other indications (i.e., hypertension, prior myocardial infarction [MI]). Patients with AAA often have systemic atherosclerosis including concomitant coronary artery disease, and the leading cause of death in these patients is myocardial infarction rather than complications of the aneurysm. Thus, all patients with AAA should be treated with aggressive secondary preventive efforts, including smoking cessation, lipid-lowering therapy, and antihypertensive therapy. Among patients with large AAA referred for surgical correction, use of statins and β-blockers has been associated with decreased perioperative morbidity and cardiovascular mortality, and these drugs are particularly important for patients undergoing surgical intervention (89).

Two large randomized clinical trials, the United Kingdom Small Aneurysm Trial and the Aneurysm Detection and Management (ADAM) trial, each enrolling approximately 1,100 patients with small AAA less than 5.5 cm, have addressed the optimal management of patients with AAA and the timing of surgical repair for these patients (90–92). In each trial, patients were randomized to undergo early elective open surgery or to a surveillance regimen, and in both trials there was no difference in all-cause mortality among patients randomized to either management strategy during follow-up of approximately 4.5 years. In long-term follow-up of patients in the U.K. study, there was slightly improved survival at 8 years of follow-up among patients randomized to early surgery (92). On the basis of these two studies, it is recommended that patients with AAA less than 5.5 cm undergo careful surveillance and be referred for AAA repair when the diameter is 5.5 cm or greater (81). In addition, patients with rapidly expanding or symptomatic aneurysms should be referred for repair. Consideration may also be given to earlier referral for AAA repair for smaller aneurysm in patients at acceptable perioperative risk who have a smaller body surface area and women with aneurysms 5.0 cm or greater (81,93).

Surgical and Endovascular Treatment of Abdominal Aortic Aneurysms

Recently, there have been exciting advances in the use of endovascular technologies for minimally invasive repair of AAA. Repair of AAA by endovascular techniques involves the placement of an aortic stent graft under fluoroscopic guidance (Figs. 105.5C and 105.5D). The stent graft is fixed to normal aorta above and below the aneurysm (tube graft) or into each of the iliac arteries below (bifurcated stent graft), depending on the anatomy and distal extent of the aneurysm. Selection of optimal candidates for endovascular repair is based on the anatomic features of the aneurysm, including the absence of critical vessels arising from the segment to be grafted and adequate landing zones for the proximal and distal anchors of the graft. In general, approximately one half of infrarenal AAAs are suitable for endovascular repair (94). One of the most common complications of endovascular repair of AAA is endoleak. Endoleak is persistent flow within the aneurysm sac, increasing the potential for continued aneurysm expansion and rupture. There are a number of mechanisms by which endoleak occurs, the most common of which is by filling of the aneurysm sac by a branch vessel that was not ligated at the time of surgery. Endoleak may also be caused by attachment failure, either at the proximal or distal attachments of the endograft or due to a defect within modular components of the endograft. Endoleak that occurs due to graft failure typically requires immediate repair, often with an open surgical procedure. Small endoleak due to a branch vessel may often be followed expectantly, with reintervention required only if the aneurysm sac expands. Because of the high prevalence of endoleaks, all patients undergoing endovascular repair of AAA require intensive surveillance, typically with serial CT scans.

Two large randomized clinical trials have directly compared elective open surgery with endovascular repair for AAAs greater than 5.0 to 5.5 cm in diameter. In each of these trials, short-term outcomes in the group randomized to endovascular repair were favorable compared to the conventional surgery group (operative mortality 1.2% to 1.7% endovascular group vs. 4.6% to 4.7% open group) (95,96). Estimated blood loss, percentage of patients requiring blood transfusion, and pulmonary complications were substantially less in the endovascular repair group (95). Long-term follow-up of patients in these studies found that the initial perioperative survival advantage of endovascular repair is not sustained after the first postoperative year, with probability of survival equivalent in the two groups at 2 to 4 years of follow-up (97,98). In addition, among patients randomized to endovascular repair, the percentage of patients who required at least one reintervention within 4 years of follow-up was 20%, compared to 6% of patients randomized to open repair (98). In cost efficacy analysis, estimated procedural and follow-up costs for AAA repair were greater among patients randomized to endovascular repair, including cost of surveillance imaging studies and repeat procedures (98). Given these data, it appears that endovascular repair is a viable alternative to open repair for AAA, particularly for patients with increased perioperative risk, although these procedures are clearly associated with a need for increased and intensive postoperative surveillance and a higher rate of repeat procedures.

THE ACUTE AORTIC SYNDROMES

The acute aortic syndromes (Table 105.3) are life-threatening disorders that may occur in the setting of preexisting aortic disease, such as aortic aneurysm or aortic atherosclerosis, or may occur without warning in a patient with no known history of aortic disease. The acute aortic syndromes, particularly aortic dissection and aortic rupture, were the seventeenth-leading cause of death in the United States in 2002 (99). This section focuses on the three major acute aortic syndromes: aortic dissection, intramural hematoma of the aorta, and penetrating atherosclerotic ulcer. Ruptured aortic aneurysm has been discussed earlier. Aortic trauma is discussed in detail in Chapter 38.

Aortic Dissection

Pathophysiology

Aortic dissection occurs as the result of a tear within the intimal lining of the aorta, leading to exposure of the intima to elevated aortic pressures with resultant separation of the intima from the aortic wall to form a false lumen (100,101). Exposure of the intima to elevated aortic pressures ultimately results in propagation of the dissection antegrade, retrograde, or in both directions from the site of the initial aortic tear. Acute aortic dissection typically occurs in the setting of an underlying pathologic defect of the aortic wall, such as cystic medical necrosis, atherosclerosis, or inflammation. The clinical sequelae of acute aortic dissection occur either as a result of the dissection itself (e.g., back or chest pain), compromise of branch vessels of the aorta (e.g., stroke, renal failure, acute limb ischemia), aortic regurgitation due to disruption of the aortic valve, or cardiac tamponade if hemopericardium should occur. Chronic aortic dissection is associated with aneurysmal remodeling of the aorta over time. Standardized classification systems have been developed to describe the anatomic location of an aortic dissection (Fig. 105.6). These classification systems are useful for determining prognosis and the approach to management for patients with aortic dissection (102,103). In the DeBakey system, a type I dissection originates in the ascending aorta and extends into the aortic arch or beyond and may extend into the abdominal aorta or iliac arteries. Type II aortic dissection originates within, and is confined to, the ascending aorta. Type III aortic dissection originates distal to the left subclavian artery and propagates distally into the descending thoracic (IIIa) or the abdominal (IIIb) aorta. In the Stanford, or Daily, classification system, aortic dissections are classified as those involving the ascending aorta (type A) and those that do not involve the ascending aorta (type B). Type A aortic dissections are referred to as "proximal" aortic dissections and type B as "distal" aortic dissections.

TABLE 105.3

THE ACUTE AORTIC SYNDROMES

Aortic dissection
Intramural hematoma
Intimal tear without hematoma
Penetrating atherosclerotic ulcer
Rupture of aortic aneurysm
Aortic trauma

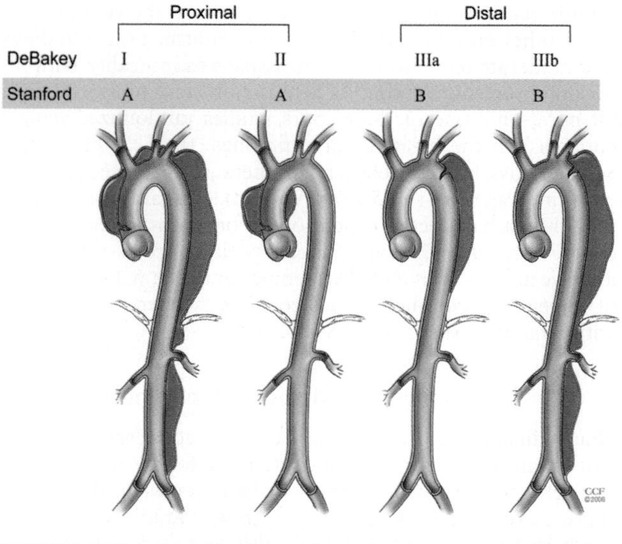

FIGURE 105.6. Classification systems for acute aortic dissection. Shown are the DeBakey and Stanford (Daily) classification systems (102,103).

Epidemiology

The estimated annual incidence of aortic dissection is 2.9 to 3.5 per 100,000 people (104,105). Multiple risk factors for the development of acute aortic dissection have been identified, the most important of which is hypertension. A history of hypertension is present in 71.8% of patients presenting with acute dissection in the largest case series of nearly 1,100 patients within the International Registry of Acute Aortic Dissection (IRAD) database (106). There is overlap of the risk factors for acute aortic dissection and for aortic aneurysm, particularly the hereditary connective tissue disorders associated with cystic medical necrosis (Marfan syndrome, Ehlers-Danlos type IV syndrome), bicuspid aortic valve, aortitis, atherosclerosis of the aortic wall, prior aortic manipulation (either during catheter-based procedure or from aortic cross-clamping at the time of cardiac or vascular surgery), and aortic trauma (101,107–110). Preexisting aneurysms of both the thoracic and abdominal aorta are associated with an increased risk of aortic dissection. Aortic dissection has been reported among families with hereditary TAA syndromes (21–23). An association with aortic dissection and pregnancy has also been reported, particularly among women with Marfan syndrome, Ehlers-Danlos syndrome, or bicuspid aortic valve with dilation of the aortic root and ascending thoracic aorta (33). Cases of pregnancy-associated aortic dissection in the absence of connective tissue disease or bicuspid aortic valve have also been reported (33). Due to catecholamine surge and hypertensive urgency, cocaine abuse is also associated with aortic dissection and accounted for 0.5% of all dissections in the IRAD registry (106). Approximately two thirds of patients with acute aortic dissection are male, and mean age at presentation ranges between 62 and 67 years (104–106). Among patients less than 40 years of age with aortic dissection, risk factors such as Marfan syndrome, previous aortic aneurysm, and bicuspid aortic valve are common (108). Type A dissection accounted for 63% of cases of aortic dissection in the IRAD registry (106). Within the IRAD registry, 87% of patients were white (106). Among patients with aortic dissection, up to 14% of patients had preexisting aortic aneurysm, and 22% had undergone cardiac surgery in the past (106).

Clinical Presentation and Diagnosis

The most common presenting symptom among patients with aortic dissection is chest or back pain, which is reported in at least 90% of patients (107,111–112). The discomfort of acute aortic dissection is classically of abrupt onset and is often described as sharp in quality or the worst pain the patient has felt in his or her lifetime (107,112). The pain is migratory in nature in 17% to 31% of cases, with migration of the pain possibly related to the propagation of the dissection (107,112). According to IRAD data, only one half of patients with acute aortic dissection give the classic descriptor of "tearing" or "ripping" pain (107). Abdominal pain may also be the primary presenting symptom among patients with aortic dissection (113). Approximately 5% to 10% of patients may not report any chest, back, or abdominal pain (107,112). Syncope is the presenting symptom of aortic dissection in up to 9% of cases (112). The precise prevalence of aortic dissection as a cause of sudden death is not known.

The most common presenting sign among patients with aortic dissection is hypertension, with approximately half of all patients with aortic dissection hypertensive at the time of presentation (107,112). The physical examination of a patient with suspected aortic dissection should include evaluation of the general appearance of the patient, with emphasis on recognition of the signs of predisposing disorders such as Marfan or Turner syndrome. Proximal aortic dissections may cause severe hypotension due to hemopericardium and cardiac tamponade (8%), aortic regurgitation (32%), or acute myocardial infarction, due to involvement of the ostium of one of the coronary arteries (typically the right coronary artery) (107). Patients with aortic dissection may present with pulse deficits, and a careful vascular examination and documentation of the blood pressures in all extremities is an important part of the evaluation. Patients with aortic dissection may develop acute limb ischemia due to compromise of the upper- or lower-extremity vessels. Stroke may occur in the setting of compromise of flow to the aortic arch vessels, and neurologic deficits are reported in up to 5% of cases (107).

Once the possibility of an acute aortic syndrome is considered, a diagnostic imaging study must be obtained in an expedient fashion. Plain chest radiography may demonstrate mediastinal widening, an abnormal aortic contour, or a left pleural effusion, but is neither adequately sensitive nor specific for the diagnostic of aortic dissection (112,114,115). Computed tomography of the chest (Fig. 105.7B), transesophageal echocardiography (TEE), and magnetic resonance angiography each has excellent sensitivity for the diagnosis of acute aortic dissection, with reported estimates of sensitivity ranging from 88% to 100%, and typically greater than 95% in reported series (116–118). The specificity of these noninvasive imaging modalities for aortic dissection is also high, with CT scanning and MRI likely slightly better than TEE (116,117). CT may have the greatest ability to detect involvement of aortic arch vessels when compared to MRI and TEE (117). TEE has the advantage of allowing for real-time physiologic evaluation of the heart, including evaluation of aortic regurgitation, pericardial tamponade, and left ventricular wall motion in the case of suspected coronary artery involvement in type A dissection. Transthoracic echocardiogram is inadequately sensitive for the diagnosis of aortic dissection (59%) (116). However, it may be used in combination with another imaging modality to evaluate the aortic valve and pericardial space. On rare occasions, a type A dissection involving the proximal ascending aorta may be visualized by TTE (Fig. 105.7A). Aortography, once considered the gold standard in the diagnosis of acute aortic dissection, is now rarely necessary. In a report of 628 patients in the IRAD registry, 98% of patients underwent a diagnostic imaging study, and 66% of patients underwent more than one imaging study (118). Computed tomography was the initial imaging study obtained in 63% of cases, followed by TTE or TEE in 32% of cases, aortography in 4% of cases, and MRI in only 1% of cases (118).

Within the last decade, there has been exploration of the use of intravascular ultrasound, in combination with aortography, for the evaluation of suspected or confirmed aortic dissection (119). Intravascular ultrasound (IVUS) allows for outstanding characterization of the dissection, including the origin of the intimal flap, the anatomy of branch vessels in relation to the true and false lumen, and the presence of intramural hematoma. Intravascular ultrasound has not become widely used as a diagnostic modality for aortic dissection because of its invasive nature and the excellent diagnostic capabilities of noninvasive imaging modalities. However, IVUS has been used for catheter-based procedures that treat branch vessel complications of type B aortic dissection with fenestration or for deployment of aortic stent grafts (120,121).

Recently, a number of investigators have sought biomarkers that may be useful in diagnosis of aortic dissection, particularly

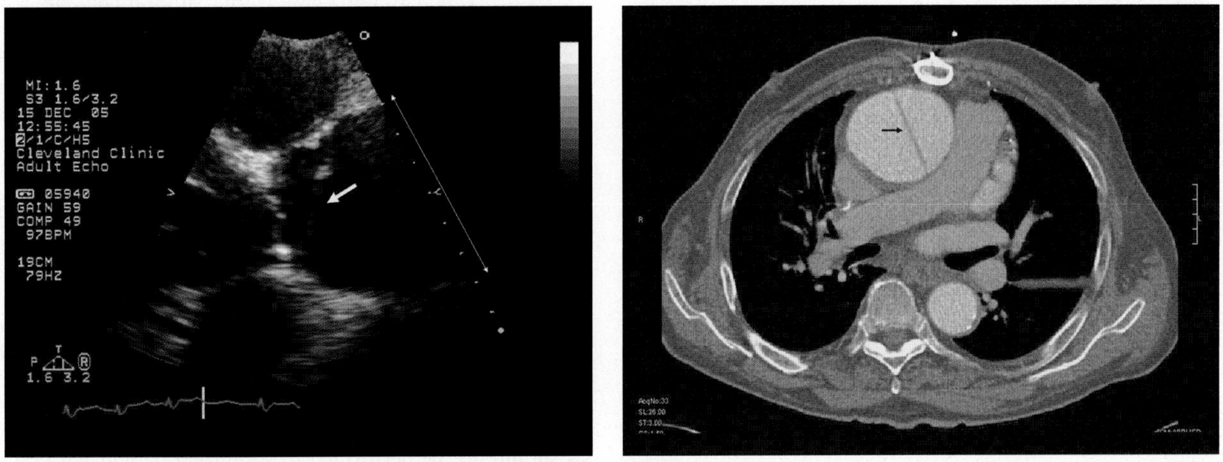

A B

FIGURE 105.7. Type A aortic dissection. Shown are images from (**A**) transthoracic echo, parasternal long-axis view, and (**B**) contrast-enhanced computed tomogram of the thoracic aorta. A dissection flap (*white arrow*) is visualized within the proximal aorta above the aortic valve leaflets. The tubular ascending aorta is 6.2 cm in diameter, consistent with prior thoracic aortic aneurysm. The computed tomogram (panel B) demonstrates a dissection flap (*black arrow*) with two separate lumens in the aneurysmal ascending thoracic aorta.

in the emergency room setting. Increased plasma d-dimer levels and increased soluble elastin fragments have been associated with acute aortic dissection, and these biomarkers are ongoing areas of clinical research (122–125).

Prognosis

Aortic dissection is a life-threatening disorder. It is estimated that up to 20% of patients with aortic dissection die before receiving medical care, and mortality estimates within the first 48 hours of treatment have been as high as 1% to 1.4% per hour (14,104). Among patients with aortic dissection, the majority of deaths occur within the first 7 days of presentation, if not within the first 48 hours (107). The prognosis of a patient with aortic dissection is largely determined by the location of the dissection and the management approach. Prognosis for type A aortic dissection is worse than for type B aortic dissection, with in-hospital mortality of 32% to 35% for type A dissection and 13% to 15% for type B dissection in the IRAD registry (107,126,127). Among patients with type A aortic dissection, prognosis is much better among those who undergo surgical repair. In the IRAD registry, in-hospital mortality is twice as high among patients who are deemed not to be candidates for surgery (26% surgical management vs. 58% medical management) (Fig. 105.8) (107). In other reports, in-hospital mortality among patients with type A aortic dissection who undergo surgical repair has ranged from 15% to 25%, with most case series reporting a mortality rate between 22% and 25% (128–132). In contrast to type A dissections, patients with type B aortic dissection have markedly better outcome if managed with medical therapy rather than a surgical approach (in-hospital mortality 31% surgical management vs. 11% medical management in IRAD) (107).

Among patients with type A dissection, risk factors for death include advanced age, hypotension at presentation, abnormal electrocardiogram (ECG), abrupt onset of chest pain, renal failure, prior aortic valve surgery, and the presence of pulse deficits (126,129,131). Among patients with type B dissection, risk factors for in-hospital death include the lack of chest or back pain on presentation (perhaps resulting in delayed diagnosis), hypotension or shock, and branch vessel involvement causing renal failure, mesenteric ischemia, or limb ischemia (127). The presence of periaortic hematoma on diagnostic imaging studies has also been associated with inferior outcome among patients with type B dissection (127,133). Women with acute aortic dissection, regardless of location of dissection, have worse outcomes than men, including increased in-hospital and perioperative mortality (106). This gender-related difference is possibly related to advanced age and delayed presentation of female patients (106). Among patients with type A aortic dissection who survive surgery and the postoperative period to hospital discharge, prognosis is favorable, with an estimated 5 year-survival of 80% to 89% and 10-year survival of 64% to 68% (128,129,132). Among patients with type B aortic dissection surviving to hospital discharge, long-term prognosis and freedom from dissection-associated complications (i.e., need for aortic surgery, dissection-related death, aortic rupture, visceral or limb ischemia) largely depend on comorbidities as well as dissection-associated factors such as patency of the false lumen (associated with worse prognosis), size and rate of expansion of the aorta, and blood pressure control during the follow-up period (134–136). The presence of Marfan syndrome has been associated with adverse outcome among survivors of type B dissection (137).

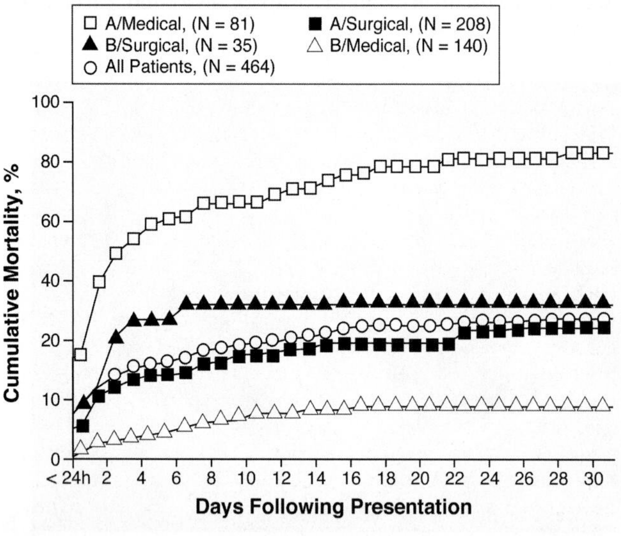

FIGURE 105.8. International Registry of Acute Aortic Dissection (IRAD) results for 30-day mortality of patients with acute aortic dissection, by type of dissection and treatment strategy. [Adapted from Hagan PG, Nienaber CA, Isselbacher EM, et al. The International Registry of Acute Aortic Dissection (IRAD): new insights into an old disease. *JAMA* 2000;283:897–903.] Copyright © 2000, American Medical Association. All rights reserved.

Management

The goal of initial therapy for the treatment of suspected aortic dissection is stabilization of the patient while obtaining a definitive diagnostic test. Guidelines have been published for the initial management of patients with suspected aortic dissection, including intensive care unit level of care, obtaining an ECG early in the hospital course, continuous heart rate and blood pressure monitoring, and aggressive control of blood pressure using parenteral agents (14). Intravenous β-blockers, such as metoprolol, labetalol, or esmolol, are first-line agents for blood pressure control, particularly given their salutary effects on decreasing the force of left ventricular contraction (*dP/dt*). Intravenous non-dihydropyridine calcium channel blockers (i.e., verapamil or diltiazem) should be considered among patients with suspected or confirmed aortic dissection and contraindication to β-blockers (e.g., asthma). For patients with persistent hypertension, additional intravenous agents should be given, such as sodium nitroprusside, labetalol (in addition to a pure β-receptor antagonist), or hydralazine. Blood pressure should be targeted to less than 120/80 mm Hg (14).

Once the diagnosis of aortic dissection has been established with a noninvasive imaging modality, management is dictated by the location of the dissection. Immediate cardiothoracic surgical consultation should be obtained for patients with type A aortic dissection. Patients with type A dissection should be monitored in an intensive care unit setting until emergent surgical repair is performed. Among patients with type A dissection presenting with hemodynamic compromise, initial supportive care should include intubation, mechanical ventilation, fluid resuscitation, and vasopressors. Transesophageal echocardiography may be the diagnostic modality of choice among patients with suspected type A aortic dissection and hypotension due to pericardial tamponade because it can be performed readily at the bedside in an intubated patient. Due to the potential for fatal bleeding into the pericardial space, pericardiocentesis should not be performed to stabilize a patient with type A aortic dissection awaiting surgical therapy (138). Intravenous fluids and immediate cardiac surgery are warranted. If pericardiocentesis must be performed in the case of a patient who develops full cardiac arrest associated with pulseless electrical activity, only the smallest amount of fluid necessary should be withdrawn to resuscitate the patient, and the patient should be taken for immediate cardiac surgery. Among patients with type A aortic dissection presenting with ECG changes suggestive of acute myocardial infarction, there is typically involvement of one of the coronary ostia by the dissection. Coronary angiography, which would delay emergent surgery, is not recommended. In some patients with type B aortic dissection who are referred on an urgent or elective basis for surgical correction, coronary angiography may be performed, particularly given the high prevalence of concomitant coronary artery disease in these patients (14).

Once the diagnosis of type B aortic dissection is confirmed, the patient should be admitted to an intensive care unit with the goal of intensive medical therapy to prevent dissection-related complications. In the absence of branch vessel compromise or propagation to involve the proximal aorta, type B dissections are typically managed with intensive medical therapy. An intraarterial catheter should be placed for continuous blood pressure monitoring. β-Blockers and vasodilators are given, initially parentally, and then orally to target a goal systolic blood pressure of 100 to 120 mm Hg (14). Severe hypertension, initially requiring four or more antihypertensive agents, is common among patients with type B aortic dissection, although such refractory hypertension typically improves by the time of hospital discharge and does not seem to be associated with aneurysm-related adverse events (139). Recurrent pain is also a common occurrence among patients with type B aortic dissection managed medically. It does not seem to be associated with adverse clinical outcome, and should be managed conservatively unless there is objective evidence of the development of a dissection-related complication (140). Patients with type B aortic dissection should be carefully followed for evidence of branch vessel compromise, including the development of acute limb ischemia, acute renal failure due to renovascular compromise, acute mesenteric ischemia, or paraplegia due to compromise of the spinal vessels.

After an initial period of parenteral blood pressure control in an intensive care unit setting, patients with aortic dissection are transitioned to a regimen of oral agents, with a target blood pressure of less than 135/80 mm Hg. β-Blockers are a critical component of maintenance therapy for chronic type B aortic dissections. The establishment of careful follow-up with a cardiovascular specialist is critical for these patients. Guidelines for management and imaging surveillance in the chronic phase have recently been published (14). Patients are followed for the development of dissecting aneurysm, rapid expansion of aortic size, evidence of branch vessel compromise, or peripheral malperfusion syndromes. After initial hospital discharge, repeat imaging should be performed at 1, 3, 6, and 12 months after the initial dissection and then at least annually thereafter (14). MRI or CT is acceptable for surveillance imaging studies, with MRI perhaps preferable because it does not require iodinated contrast or radiation exposure. Among patients with type B aortic dissection, average growth rate tends to be greater in the thoracic aorta than in the abdominal aorta (4.1 mm/year vs. 1.2 mm/year) (141). A patent false lumen is associated with more rapid expansion in the diameter of the aorta, and these patients warrant particularly close imaging surveillance (141). In general, patients with aortic aneurysm due to chronic dissection should be referred for aortic surgery at a lesser diameter than patients with aneurysm from other causes (Table 105.2).

Surgical or endovascular repair of type B aortic dissection is generally reserved for the management of complications of dissection, specifically aneurysmal dilation of the aorta or peripheral, spinal, or visceral malperfusion syndromes due to inadequate blood flow to branch vessel. Traditionally, management of the ischemic complications of type B aortic dissection was managed with open surgical procedures, including placement of aortic grafts, arterial bypass grafting (e.g., to the renal arteries), or open surgical fenestration. Recently, there have been advances in endovascular therapies for aortic dissection, including percutaneous aortic fenestration and aortic stent grafting (58,142,143). Fenestration procedures are performed in the case of clinically significant branch vessel occlusion, either due to the dissection membrane itself, as a result of the branch vessel arising from the false lumen, or due to critical compression of blood-supplying true lumen by the high-pressure false lumen. A variety of techniques has been developed to create a communication between the true and false lumen, typically involving direct puncture through the dissection flap using a needle, followed by balloon dilation. Endovascular fenestration procedures may be performed with IVUS guidance in addition to conventional aortography. Endovascular treatment of complicated type B aortic dissection involves highly specialized procedures, which should be performed by experienced vascular interventionalists in tertiary referral centers with a high volume of patients with acute aortic syndromes.

Intimal Flap without Hematoma

Intimal tear of the aorta without hematoma is a rare variant of aortic dissection in which there is an intimal aortic tear but no separation of the intima from the aortic wall (144). Clinical presentation is nearly identical to that of aortic dissection, although noninvasive imaging techniques typically fail to identify the aortic pathology. Almost all reported cases of this phenomenon have occurred among patients with ascending aortic aneurysm, and in most of these cases there was a bulge of the aortic contour seen on aortography (144). Because of the existence of this variant, conventional aortography should be considered for patients with ascending aortic aneurysm and clinical symptoms highly suggestive of dissection or intramural hematoma without diagnostic noninvasive studies. The management of this acute aortic syndrome variant is identical to that of aortic dissection.

Acute Intramural Hematoma

Acute intramural hematoma (IMH) is an acute aortic syndrome that is believed to be due to rupture of the vasa vasorum of the aorta with subsequent hemorrhage into the aortic wall. Whereas intramural hematoma may progress to become a frank dissection in a subset of patients (<20%), in pure IMH there is no identifiable dissection flap and no false lumen (145). Patients with IMH are older than patients with typical aortic dissection (145). Intramural hematomas are more commonly located in the descending thoracic aorta and are often associated with atherosclerotic plaque (145,146). Acute intramural hematoma of the aorta is diagnosed with the same noninvasive imaging modalities as aortic dissection, namely CT, TEE, and MRI. A crescentic collection of blood within the aortic wall is typically seen (Fig. 105.9). The natural history of type A IMH is a somewhat controversial topic. Nonetheless, acute IMH is generally managed in the same fashion as acute aortic dissection, with surgical referral for type A lesions and medical management for type B lesions. Some natural history series have suggested that the prognosis of type A IMH is far less lethal than that of type A aortic dissection and have suggested that medical therapy may be a viable treatment option for these (147,148). Other series have refuted this finding (145,149). As is the case of acute aortic dissection, patients with type B IMH should be monitored in an intensive care setting with parenteral medications to control blood pressure. Patients should be followed closely for the development of vascular complications. Intramural hematoma may evolve into frank aortic dissection or cause aortic remodeling to form an aortic aneurysm.

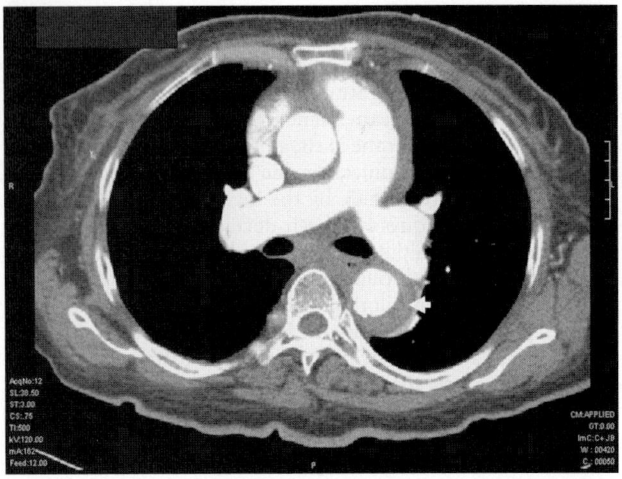

FIGURE 105.9. Acute intramural hematoma of the aorta. Contrast-enhanced computed tomogram of the thoracic aorta. Shown is a crescentic collection of blood within the wall of the descending thoracic aorta (*arrow*). No dissection flap is visualized.

Frequent imaging surveillance during the first year after the initial event should be performed according to a schedule similar to that for aortic dissection. The long-term prognosis among patients with type B IMH is at least as favorable as, if not better than, that for patients with type B aortic dissection (145,150,151). Regression of type B IMH has been reported and may occur in up to half of patients on serial imaging studies (147,152,153).

Penetrating Atherosclerotic Ulcer

Penetrating atherosclerotic ulcer (PAU) is caused by erosion of an atherosclerotic plaque through the internal elastic lamina and into the aortic media. It may occur in association with IMH or aortic aneurysms or it may be an isolated outpouching into the aortic wall (146,154). The typical patient with PAU is elderly and has extensive atherosclerosis of the aorta. The descending thoracic aorta is the most common location for PAU (Fig. 105.10), although lesions have been reported at all levels of the aorta. The range of clinical presentation among patients with PAU varies, from acute back and chest pain, which is indistinguishable from that of the other acute aortic syndromes, to the asymptomatic patient with a PAU diagnosed as an incidental finding on an imaging study that had been obtained for an unrelated indication. Computed tomography, MRI, and TEE may be used to diagnose and characterize PAU. Penetrating atherosclerotic ulcers may progress to aortic rupture or pseudoaneurysm formation (contained ruptured), although the incidence of these dangerous complications is not known. The natural history and prognosis of PAU are not well established, and there are widely variable reports of outcome (154–160). The depth of penetration of the PAU into the aortic wall, presentation with symptoms of acute aortic syndrome, and the presence of IMH seem to be associated with worse outcome (146). Both open surgical and endovascular techniques have been used to treat PAU, although published case series are small. Overall, it is not known to what extent intervention alters outcome among patients with PAU, particularly among those patients in whom the lesion was as an incidental radiologic finding. Patients with PAU, particularly those presenting as an acute aortic syndrome, are generally referred for surgical

A

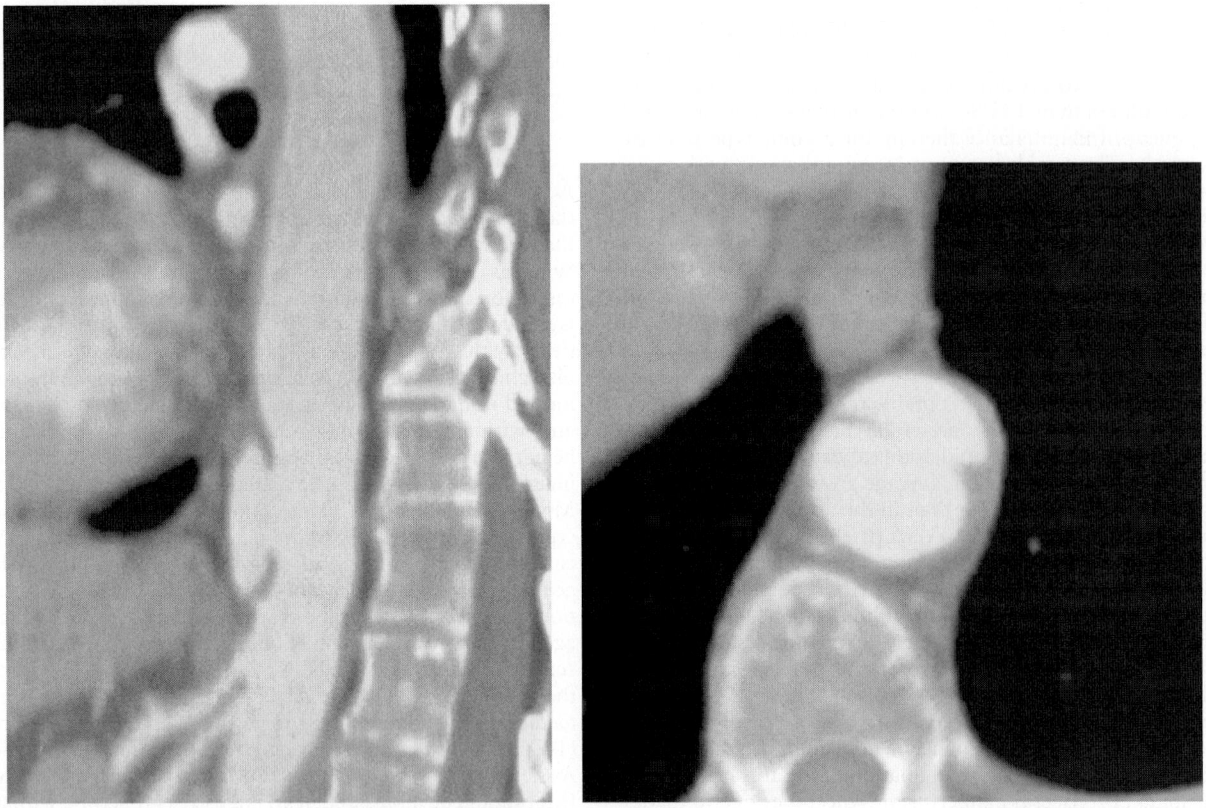

B

FIGURE 105.10. Penetrating atherosclerotic ulcer of the descending thoracic aorta. Contrast-enhanced computed tomogram of the thoracic aorta in (**A**) sagittal and (**B**) transverse planes. There is a focal outpouching of the distal descending thoracic aorta, consistent with penetrating atherosclerotic ulcer. Image courtesy of Dr. Paul Schoenhagen, the Cleveland Clinic Foundation.

or endovascular treatment, although standardized practice guidelines for the management of PAU are not available.

ATHEROSCLEROTIC OCCLUSIVE DISEASE OF THE AORTA

Pathophysiology and Epidemiology

Peripheral arterial disease (PAD) is a common condition within the elderly population, with an estimated prevalence as high as 14.5% of the population older than the age of 70 years (161). A detailed discussion of the pathogenesis and management of peripheral arterial disease is beyond the scope of this chapter and is presented in detail in Chapter 108. Though the classic lesion of symptomatic PAD is long-segment occlusion of the superficial femoral artery, atherosclerotic plaques of varying severity is a common finding at each anatomic level of the aorta. Atherosclerosis with the aorta may be asymptomatic or may be associated with clinical sequelae, such as PAU, atheroembolism, aortic aneurysm, and aortic stenosis or occlusion. When aortic stenosis or occlusion occurs as a result of atherosclerosis, the distal abdominal aorta, near the aortic bifurcation, is the most common site, likely related to local alterations of shear stress and flow dynamics (162,163). Extension of plaque and stenosis into the common iliac arteries is also common. Patients with arterial occlusive disease of the aorta often have evidence of PAD within multiple arterial segments, although aortoiliac disease may be the sole manifestation of PAD, particularly in younger patients (164). Risk factors associated with the development of aortoiliac occlusive disease relative to femoropopliteal arterial occlusive disease include more extensive tobacco histories, younger age at presentation, the absence of diabetes mellitus, and female gender (164–166). A number of investigators have suggested the possibility of a separate clinical syndrome to describe premenopausal women who present with distal aortic and iliac occlusive disease, known as the small, or hypoplastic, aorta syndrome (167–169). Typical atherosclerotic risk factors, particularly smoking, as well as short stature seem to be a commonality among patients with this entity (170). The precise nature of the hypoplastic aorta syndrome is controversial, particularly with regard to whether it represents a variant of accelerated atherosclerosis or a congenital abnormality of vascular hypoplasia (171).

In addition to atherosclerotic arterial occlusive disease, acute occlusion of the aorta may occur as a result of embolism from a cardiac source or as a result of thrombosis at the site of an existing atherosclerotic stenosis. Though rare, in situ thrombosis of the nondiseased abdominal aorta has been reported in the setting of severe hypercoagulable states, including underlying malignancy and the antiphospholipid antibody syndrome (172,173).

Clinical Presentation and Diagnosis

The classic presentation of aortoiliac occlusive disease is described by the Leriche syndrome of intermittent claudication, often involving the thighs or buttocks, and erectile dysfunction. The syndrome is named for Dr. René Leriche, the French surgeon generally considered to be the father of modern vascular surgery. Leriche described the case of a truck driver with classic symptoms who ultimately underwent the first successful aortoiliac reconstructive surgery for symptomatic occlusive disease of the aorta (174–175).

Atherosclerosis of the aorta may present with embolic events of varied clinical presentation. Atheroembolism from the aortic arch is believed to play an important role in the pathogenesis of ischemic stroke in older patients without carotid artery disease or a cardiac source of embolism (176,177). Atheroembolism from a suprarenal source may cause renal insufficiency, particularly among patients undergoing a catheter-based procedure, such as coronary angiography. Atheroembolism to the lower extremities from any site in the aorta may result in digital ischemia ("blue toe syndrome") and, in rare cases, critical limb ischemia or gangrene (178).

The diagnosis of aortoiliac arterial occlusive disease is made from clinical history, physical examination, and noninvasive diagnostic testing (see Chapters 106 and 108). For isolated aortoiliac disease, the ankle–brachial index may be normal at rest. For all patients with claudication and suspected aortoiliac occlusive disease, repeat measurement of ankle pressures after a treadmill exercise test is strongly recommended. Noninvasive cross-sectional imaging techniques, such as magnetic resonance angiography and computed tomography, have emerged as alternatives to conventional angiography for the diagnosis of aortoiliac occlusive disease, as has duplex ultrasonography.

Endovascular and Surgical Management

Catheter-based technologies have revolutionized the approach to patients with PAD in the aortoiliac segment. Five-year patency rates with surgical reconstruction, typically with aortobifemoral bypass grafting, are very good, on the order of 80% to 90% in published case series (179,180). In recent years, endovascular treatment of aortoiliac disease with balloon angioplasty and stenting has emerged as the treatment of choice for patients with favorable anatomy (Fig. 105.11). Long-term durability of endovascular treatment rivals that of open surgery, with less procedural morbidity and mortality (181). The approach to revascularization for patients with symptomatic aortoiliac occlusive disease is discussed in Chapter 108.

AORTITIS

Pathophysiology

Aortitis is the term used to describe vasculitis of the aorta. Multiple vasculitis syndromes have been associated with aortic inflammation, most notably giant cell arteritis, also known as temporal arteritis, and Takayasu arteritis (Table 105.4). Aortitis has also been associated with other rheumatologic disorders, including the HLA B27–associated spondyloarthropathies, Reiter syndrome, and ankylosis spondylitis, Behçet disease, systemic lupus erythematosus, and certain antineutrophil cytoplasmic antibodies (ANCA)-associated vasculitides (182–185). Cogan syndrome is an unusual idiopathic disorder of large- and medium-vessel vasculitis in the setting of interstitial keratitis and vestibuloauditory symptoms (186,187). There are published case reports of aortitis occurring among patients with sarcoidosis and among patients with idiopathic retroperitoneal fibrosis (188–190).

As is the case for most autoimmune disorders, the exact etiology of aortitis has not been established. Although theories continue to evolve, both giant cell and Takayasu arteritis are believed to be antigen-driven processes that are mediated by T-cell and monocyte/macrophage activation. Certain MHC subtypes and activation of matrix metalloproteinases show promise as areas of investigation (191–194). Due to the presence of granulomas in pathologic specimens as well as the epidemiology of the disease, a link between Takayasu arteritis and tuberculosis has also been postulated, with the possibility that chronic tuberculous infection may provide the antigenic stimulus for the autoimmune process (195).

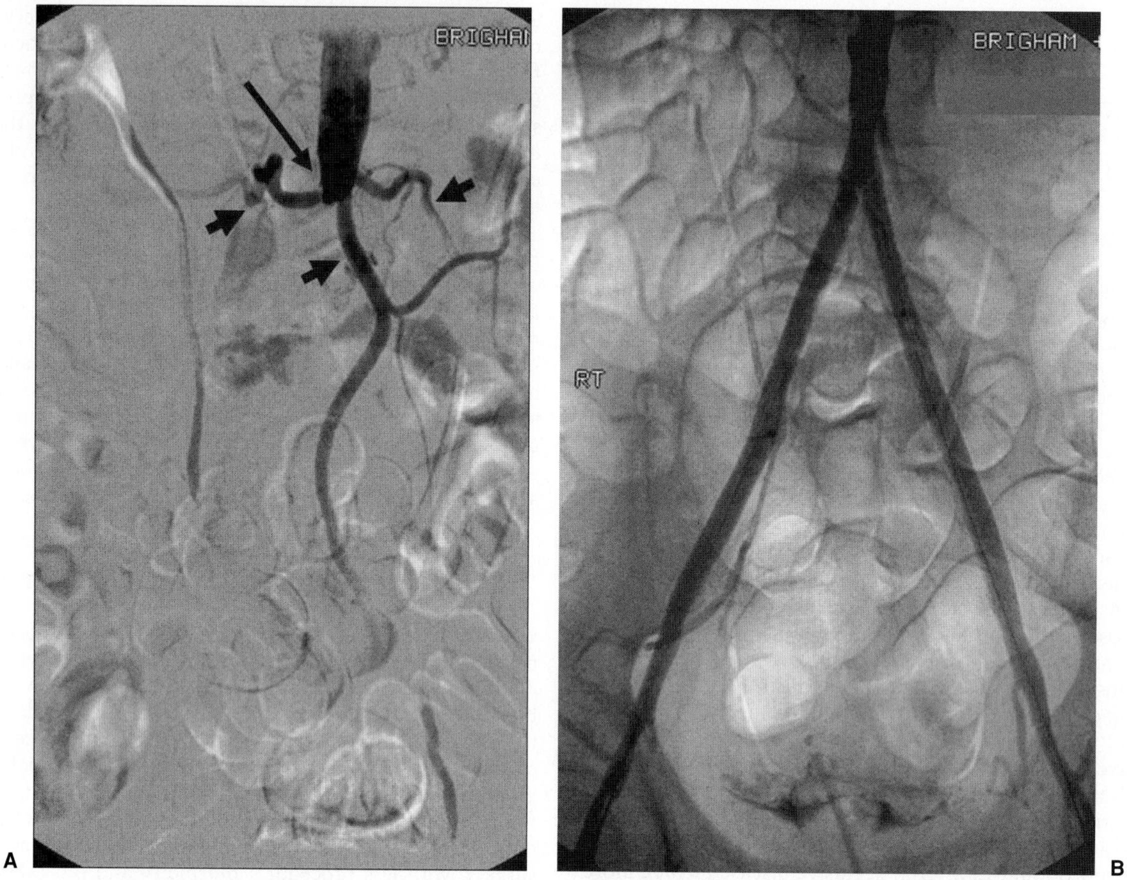

FIGURE 105.11. Distal aortic occlusion causing the Leriche syndrome. Shown are aortogram images taken (A) before and (B) after catheter-based intervention performed on an elderly man with severe intermittent claudication and erectile dysfunction. There was occlusion of the distal abdominal aorta (*long arrow*) with extensive collaterals arising from the lumbar and sacral arteries (*short arrows*). The lesion was treated with sequential balloon dilations and ultimately with stenting of the distal aorta and bilateral common iliac arteries (B). (Images courtesy of Drs. Piotr Sobieszczyk and Andrew Eisenhauer, Brigham and Women's Hospital, Boston.)

In the acute phase, both giant cell arteritis and Takayasu arteritis are associated with inflammation and edema with an inflammatory cellular infiltrate that has predilection for the internal elastica lamina and media of the vessel wall (193,196). Multinucleated giant cells and granulomas are common in both giant cell and Takayasu arteritis, as is nodular thickening and skip lesions along the arterial wall, destruction of the internal elastic lamina, and reduction of the vessel lumen (193). In the chronic phase of Takayasu arteritis, there is typically extensive fibrosis of the arterial wall with lumen obliteration. Histologically, giant cell and Takayasu arteritis are often indistinguishable and must be differentiated on the basis of clinical presentation (197). The underlying mechanisms for the disparate clinical presentations of giant cell arteritis and Takayasu arteritis have yet to be determined.

TABLE 105.4

AORTITIS AND THE LARGE-VESSEL VASCULITIDES

- Giant cell arteritis
- Takayasu arteritis
- HLA B27–associated spondyloarthropathies
  - Ankylosing spondylitis
  - Reiter syndrome
  - Relapsing polychondritis
- Other
  - Cogan syndrome
  - Behçet disease
  - Systemic lupus erythematosus
  - Antineutrophil cytoplasmic antibodies (ANCA)-associated vasculitides (Wegener, microscopic polyangiitis)
  - Sarcoidosis associated
  - Idiopathic retroperitoneal fibrosis (Ormond disease)

Epidemiology

Compared to atherosclerosis or aneurysmal disease, aortitis is a rare aortic disorder, and there are few data on its prevalence within the general population. Giant-cell arteritis is primarily a disorder of the elderly. It is more common among whites, particularly those of Nordic dissent (198). Among residents of Olmstead County, Minnesota, the age-adjusted incidence of giant cell arteritis was 18.8 per 100,000 individuals, with more than twofold incidence among women compared to men (199–200). Little is known about the epidemiology of Takayasu arteritis. It is most commonly a disease of young women, with a mean age of age at presentation of 25 years in case series

(195,198,201). The prevalence of this disorder seems to be highest in Asia, and especially in Japan, where it was initially described, although there is low-level prevalence worldwide.

Clinical Presentation and Diagnosis

The clinical presentation of aortitis varies, depending on the underlying etiology and the pattern of vessels involved, and includes the spectrum of aortic syndromes: chronic arterial occlusive disease, aortic aneurysm, acute aortic syndrome, and an acute systemic inflammatory process with aortic valvulitis.

The diagnosis of the most common aortitis syndromes, giant cell arteritis and Takayasu arteritis, is generally made on the basis of clinical features. Strict diagnostic criteria have been published for both of these disorders (202,203). Giant cell arteritis classically involves the arteries of the head, particularly the superficial temporal artery, a branch vessel of external carotid artery, and commonly presents with headache or jaw claudication. The ophthalmic arteries may also be involved, with a risk of subsequent blindness. Visual changes in the setting of suspected giant cell arteritis is a true medical emergency. Patients with giant cell arteritis may also present with arterial occlusive disease of the upper or lower extremities. Diagnostic criteria for giant cell arteritis are patient age of at least 50 years, headache, temporal artery tenderness or decreased pulsation, elevation of the erythrocyte sedimentation rate, and abnormal arterial biopsy specimen (202). The presence of three or more of these criteria is 94% sensitive and 91% specific for the diagnosis of giant cell arteritis (202). Giant cell arteritis may present with large-muscle aches and stiffness due to polymyalgia rheumatica, which occurs along with the vasculitis in up to 30% to 50% of cases. Some patients with giant cell arteritis may present with atypical features, such as fever of unknown origin or unexplained weight loss. The prevalence of aortitis in association with giant cell arteritis is not clear, but may be as high as 18%, as reported in the Olmsted County, Minnesota, population (109,204). Giant cell arteritis has also been associated with thoracic and abdominal aneurysms as well as aortic dissection (Fig. 105.12A) (109,204). Aortitis due to giant cell arteritis typically presents as a late manifestation, occurring approximately 5 years after the initial diagnosis (109,204). Among patients with giant cell arteritis, there is a 17.3-fold increase in the relative risk of TAA and a 2.4-fold increase in the relative risk of AAA compared to age and gender-matched control patients (109). Aortitis has also been diagnosed strictly on the basis of surgical pathology specimens among patients with no known history of vasculitis undergoing surgery for aortic aneurysms (205).

Takayasu arteritis has a predilection for the large vessel branches of the aortic arch, particularly the carotid and subclavian arteries (201). It is also known as "pulseless disease" for its classic presentation of severe upper-extremity arterial occlusive disease in young female patients. Diagnostic criteria for the diagnosis of Takayasu arteritis include young age at onset (<40 years of age), upper- or lower-extremity claudication, abnormalities of the brachial arterial pulse, subclavian or aortic bruits, discrepancy in arm blood pressures consistent with subclavian stenosis, and angiographic stenoses or occlusion of the aorta, its primary branches, or large arteries of the extremities (203). The presence of at least three of these criteria has a sensitivity of 91% and a specificity of 98% for the diagnosis of Takayasu arteritis (203). Stenosis of the suprarenal abdominal aorta and renal arteries is common, and hypertension is a common finding in young patients presenting with Takayasu arteritis (prevalence 33% to 77%) (195,201). Arterial occlusive disease seems to be a more common manifestation of Takayasu arteritis than giant cell arteritis. Aortic aneurysm, aortic dissection, and aortic insufficiency may occur. One rather unique feature of Takayasu arteritis is its tendency for involvement of the pulmonary arteries (201). Takayasu arteritis may also involve the coronary arteries, typically the aortoostial segments of the vessels.

Given the rare nature of aortitis, the diagnosis greatly relies on the clinical acumen of the evaluating physician. Patients may present with evidence of aortic involvement late in the course of the vasculitis, particularly in the case of giant cell arteritis, which may have been diagnosed years before the aortic pathology becomes evident. Aortitis should always be considered as a potential diagnosis among patients presenting with TAA, particularly aneurysms with rapid expansion and no other underlying etiology. Aortitis must also be suspected among young patients, particularly those without atherosclerotic risk factors

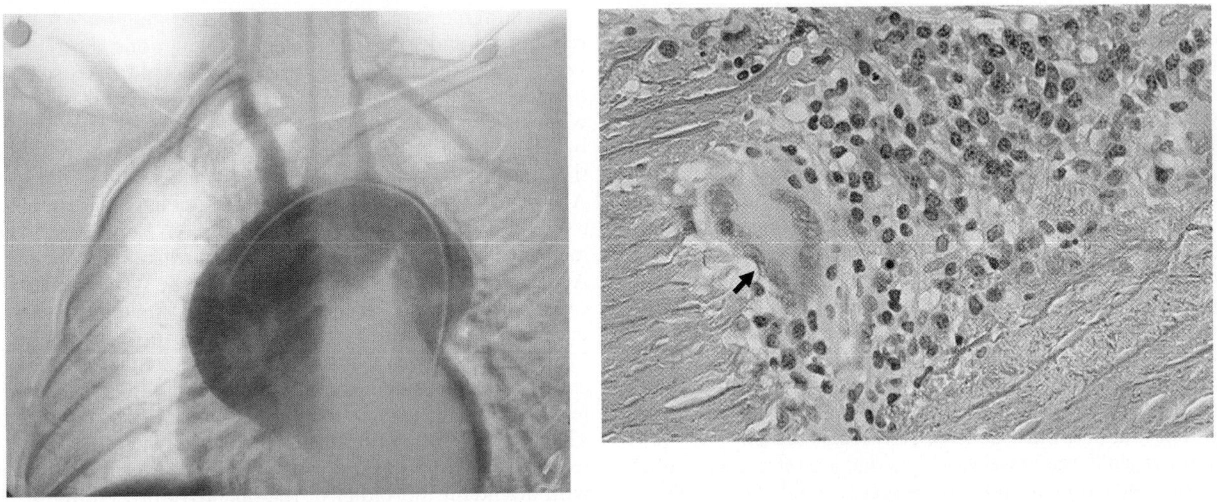
A B

FIGURE 105.12. Takayasu arteritis with aortitis and thoracic aneurysm. **A:** Thoracic aortogram of a 32-year-old woman with thoracic aortic aneurysm and aortic insufficiency. **B:** Surgical pathology revealed granulomatous inflammation with prominent giant cells (*arrow*); hematoxylin and eosin, 400×. (Adapted from Hoffman GS. Large-vessel vasculitis: unresolved issues. *Arthritis Rheum* 2003;48:2406–2414.)

Diseases of the Aorta

presenting with arterial occlusive disease, particularly arterial occlusive disease of the arch vessels or upper extremities. Inflammatory markers may be normal in cases of both giant cell and Takayasu arteritis, and care should be taken to not dismiss the possibility of this diagnosis even in the setting of normal erythrocyte sedimentation rate and C-reactive protein (206, 207). Other markers of inflammation, particularly cytokines such as interleukin-6 and interleukin-18, have shown promise as markers of disease activity in patients with Takayasu arteritis (206,208).

Historically, invasive angiography was used to diagnose and clinically monitor patients with large-vessel arteritis, particularly Takayasu disease. Recently, there has been great interest in the use of noninvasive imaging techniques for the diagnosis of large-vessel arteritis and for monitoring response to treatment. Gadolinium-enhanced magnetic resonance angiography and positive emission tomography (PET) using 18-fluorodeoxyglucose (18-FDG) have emerged as new diagnostic techniques for large-vessel vasculitis, with FDG-PET demonstrating the greatest promise in this regard. Investigators have begun to explore the use of these imaging tools to follow disease activity and monitor response to therapy, although this use remains strictly investigational (209,210). It is not clear how well findings of arterial wall edema (on magnetic resonance imaging) or increased arterial uptake of glucose (on PET imaging) correlate with disease activity (211). In one case series, evidence of vessel wall edema on MRI was found in 56% of patients with Takayasu arteritis believed to have quiescent disease (211).

Biopsy is rarely obtained to confirm the diagnosis of aortitis, which is generally made on the basis of clinical and laboratory findings. In rare cases, a patient with suspected aortitis may present with symptoms suspicious for concomitant temporal arteritis, in which case temporal artery biopsy may prove diagnostic. In general, temporal artery biopsy is not recommended for patients without evidence of temporal arterial involvement because these tend to have very low diagnostic yield. It is not uncommon for the diagnosis of aortitis to be made by analysis of histopathology from an aortic aneurysm repair procedure (Fig. 105.12B).

Treatment

Corticosteroids are the mainstay of treatment for patients with aortitis due to large-vessel vasculitis. Typical starting doses of oral prednisone range from 40 to 60 mg daily. Daily dosing of steroids has been shown to be more efficacious than alternate-day dosing among patients with giant cell arteritis (212). After achieving an acceptable clinical response at the starting steroid dose, the dose is decreased incrementally over a period of many months while inflammatory markers are closely followed. Patients with giant cell arteritis and visual symptoms are treated with intravenous pulse steroids followed by oral prednisone, although this recommendation is based upon small case series rather than randomized clinical trials (213,214). Careful clinical follow-up is critical among patients with Takayasu arteritis, with emphasis on surveillance for the development of new symptoms (i.e., upper- or lower-extremity claudication, neurologic symptoms) or worrisome signs such as new-onset hypertension, new pulse deficits, or vascular bruits.

For cases of large-vessel vasculitis that are refractory to glucocorticoids, a more common occurrence for Takayasu arteritis than giant cell arteritis, additional immunosuppressive therapy is prescribed. Multiple agents have been successfully used in combination with steroids in published case series, including methotrexate, azathioprine, and anti–tumor necrosis factor agents (215–217). The use of immunosuppressive agents in combination with steroid therapy for primary treatment of arteritis is not recommended (218). Relapse is common among patients with large-vessel vasculitis, with reported relapse rates of up to 29% to 45% for Takayasu arteritis and 48% for giant cell arteritis (201,219–221). Relapse is generally treated with more intensive steroid therapy and immunosuppressive agents. Patients with arteritis who require prolonged treatment with glucocorticoids should be treated with agents to prevent osteoporosis, *Pneumocystis carinii* pneumonia, and stress ulceration of the gastrointestinal tract (222).

Patients with aneurysm of the thoracic or abdominal aorta due to aortitis should be closely followed for expansion of the aneurysm to a size that would warrant repair. The indications for surgery for aortitis-associated aneurysm are the same as those for aneurysms of all other etiologies (Table 105.2). As a general rule, patients with aortitis should be treated with glucocorticoids, until a remission has been achieved, before referral for elective aortic surgery for aneurysmal disease. There has been recent enthusiasm for endovascular techniques for the treatment of aortitis-associated aortic aneurysm and dissection, although such procedures are in their infancy (223,224). Endovascular repair theoretically offers the advantage of avoiding operation on potentially inflamed, friable aortic tissue. Balloon angioplasty with endovascular stenting has been used to treat stenoses of the aorta among patients with Takayasu arteritis, particularly children and young adults presenting with hypertension (225–227). Patients with Takayasu arteritis seem to have a high rate of restenosis or occlusion at sites of aortic or arterial angioplasty and stenting, and this factor must be taken into account when planning revascularization and a postprocedural surveillance strategy (228).

CONTROVERSIES AND PERSONAL PERSPECTIVES

The majority of the hot topics within the field of aortic disease relate to the diagnosis and management of AAA, one of the more common aortic disorders. At the center of the controversy has been whether to screen the general population for AAA, particularly given that published studies of large screening programs have never demonstrated a reduction in all-cause mortality (only AAA-associated mortality) (66,67,79,80). A number of vascular professional societies have endorsed one-time ultrasound screening for AAA (80,81). Screening for AAA is not reimbursed under current Medicare regulations. The U.S. Preventive Services Task Force recently endorsed AAA screening for elderly men but recommended against screening for AAA in women, sparking even greater controversy (79). Political lobbying by patients and professional societies ultimately led to the bipartisan introduction of the Screening Abdominal Aortic Aneurysms Very Efficiently (SAAAVE) Act in Congress in 2005 to create a Medicare benefit for one-time AAA screening in both men and women. As of January, 2007, ultrasound screening for AAA will be available as a component of the Welcome to Medicare examination for men who have ever smoked tobacco and men and women with a family history of aortic aneurysm.

The other aspect of management of AAA that has generated controversy is the diameter at which small AAAs should be referred for repair, particularly in an era of endovascular stenting. The two large randomized clinical trials of surveillance versus treatment of small AAAs used an entirely surgical approach, with attendant morbidity of the operative procedure (90,91). These studies also randomized very few women, who tend to have smaller baseline aortic dimensions and higher relative rate of AAA rupture. There is great interest in evaluating the role of endovascular stent grafting of small aortic aneurysms (<4 to 5.5 cm) compared to surveillance, and randomized clinical trials are ongoing.

Although less controversial than the management of AAA, a number of aspects of the acute aortic syndromes are the subject of medical debate. These controversial areas include the natural history and optimal management among patients with the nondissecting variants of intramural hematoma and penetrating atherosclerotic ulcer. Some physicians feel that the management of type B aortic dissection should be more aggressive to prevent long-term complications, particularly dissecting aneurysm. The INSTEAD trial randomized 125 patients with type B aortic dissection to conventional therapy or aortic stent grafting. Results of this study are expected in 2006 (229).

THE FUTURE

The future holds advances in diagnostic modalities for the acute aortic syndromes, particularly the development of new biomarkers and point-of-care blood testing for the diagnosis of aortic dissection and the other acute aortic syndromes. New medical therapies will be developed for preventing expansion of aortic aneurysms as new insights into the pathobiology of these lesions are developed. Advances in endovascular technologies will continue to revolutionize the approach to management of the patient with aortic disease. One can anticipate a time when open surgery for aortic diseases will be a rare occurrence, analogous to the catheter-based revolution in the management of patients with coronary artery disease. The development of highly effective and safe endovascular treatments for thoracic aortic disease will be particularly vital, particularly given the substantial morbidity associated with open surgical procedures for these disorders. In addition to development of new catheter-based systems for endovascular treatment of aortic disease, there will be advances in novel adjunctive devices for long-term surveillance of endografts. Medical device companies are developing implantable aortic devices that will monitor endotension in the aneurysm sac of a grafted AAA, which, it is hoped, will avoid the need for high levels of cumulative radiation exposure required by long-term intensive surveillance with serial CT scans (230).

References

1. Uflacker R. *Atlas of vascular anatomy: an angiographic approach.* Baltimore: Williams & Wilkins, 1997.
2. Shaw JA, Gravereaux EC, Eisenhauer AC. Carotid stenting in the bovine arch. *Catheter Cardiovasc Interv* 2003;60:566–569.
3. Grathwohl KW, Afifi AY, Dillard TA, et al. Vascular rings of the thoracic aorta in adults. *Am Surg* 1999;65:1077–1083.
4. Backer CL, Mavroudis C, Rigsby CK, et al. Trends in vascular ring surgery. *J Thorac Cardiovasc Surg* 2005;129:1339–1347.
5. Sebening C, Jakob H, Tochtermann U, et al. Vascular tracheobronchial compression syndromes—experience in surgical treatment and literature review. *Thorac Cardiovasc Surg* 2000;48:164–174.
6. Bisognano JD, Young B, Brown JM, et al. Diverse presentation of aberrant origin of the right subclavian artery: two case reports. *Chest* 1997;112: 1693–1697.
7. Kommerell B. Verlagerung des osophagus durch eine abnorm verlaufende arteria subclavia dextra (arteria lusoria). *Fortschr Geb Roentgenstr Nuklearmed* 1936;54:590–595.
8. van Son JA, Konstantinov IE, Burckhard F. Kommerell and Kommerell's diverticulum. *Tex Heart Inst J* 2002;29:109–112.
9. Cina CS, Althani H, Pasenau J, et al. Kommerell's diverticulum and right-sided aortic arch: a cohort study and review of the literature. *J Vasc Surg* 2004;39:131–139.
10. Rebecca, A. Congenital anomalies of the aortic arch. *Echocardiography* 1996;13:167–182.
11. Bonnard A, Auber F, Fourcade L, et al. Vascular ring abnormalities: a retrospective study of 62 cases. *J Pediatr Surg* 2003;38:539–543.
12. Fisher RG, Whigham CJ, Trinh C. Diverticula of Kommerell and aberrant subclavian arteries complicated by aneurysms. *Cardiovasc Interv Radiol* 2005;28:553–560.
13. Kiernan PD, Dearani J, Byrne WD, et al. Aneurysm of an aberrant right subclavian artery: case report and review of the literature. *Mayo Clin Proc* 1993;68:468–474.
14. Erbel R, Alfonso F, Boileau C, et al. Diagnosis and management of aortic dissection. *Eur Heart J* 2001;22:1642–1681.
15. Lederle FA, Johnson GR, Wilson SE, et al. Relationship of age, gender, race, and body size to infrarenal aortic diameter. The Aneurysm Detection and Management (ADAM) Veterans Affairs Cooperative Study Investigators. *J Vasc Surg* 1997;26:595–601.
16. Isselbacher EM. Thoracic and abdominal aortic aneurysms. *Circulation* 2005;111:816–828.
17. Schoen F. Blood vessels. In: Kumar V, Abbas A, Fausto N, eds. *Robbins & Cotran Pathologic basis of disease.* Philadelphia: Saunders/Elsevier, 2005.
18. Bonderman D, Gharehbaghi-Schnell E, Wollenek G, et al. Mechanisms underlying aortic dilatation in congenital aortic valve malformation. *Circulation* 1999;99:2138–2143.
19. Saruk M, Eisenstein R. Aortic lesion in Marfan syndrome: the ultrastructure of cystic medial degeneration. *Arch Pathol Lab Med* 1977;101:74–77.
20. Pepin M, Schwarze U, Superti-Furga A, et al. Clinical and genetic features of Ehlers-Danlos syndrome type IV, the vascular type. *N Engl J Med* 2000;342:673–680.
21. Guo D, Hasham S, Kuang SQ, et al. Familial thoracic aortic aneurysms and dissections: genetic heterogeneity with a major locus mapping to 5q13–14. *Circulation* 2001;103:2461–2468.
22. Vaughan CJ, Casey M, He J, et al. Identification of a chromosome 11q23.2–q24 locus for familial aortic aneurysm disease, a genetically heterogeneous disorder. *Circulation* 2001;103:2469–2475.
23. Hasham SN, Willing MC, Guo DC, et al. Mapping a locus for familial thoracic aortic aneurysms and dissections (TAAD2) to 3p24–25. *Circulation* 2003;107:3184–90.
24. Schlatmann TJ, Becker AE. Histologic changes in the normal aging aorta: implications for dissecting aortic aneurysm. *Am J Cardiol* 1977;39:13–20.
25. Agmon Y, Khandheria BK, Meissner I, et al. Is aortic dilatation an atherosclerosis-related process? Clinical, laboratory, and transesophageal echocardiographic correlates of thoracic aortic dimensions in the population with implications for thoracic aortic aneurysm formation. *J Am Coll Cardiol* 2003;42:1076–1083.
26. Muller BT, Wegener OR, Grabitz K, et al. Mycotic aneurysms of the thoracic and abdominal aorta and iliac arteries: experience with anatomic and extra-anatomic repair in 33 cases. *J Vasc Surg* 2001;33:106–113.
27. Chen IM, Chang HH, Hsu CP, et al. Ten-year experience with surgical repair of mycotic aortic aneurysms. *J Chin Med Assoc* 2005;68:265–271.
28. Choudhary SK, Bhan A, Sharma R, et al. Sinus of Valsalva aneurysms: 20 years' experience. *J Card Surg* 1997;12:300–308.
29. Bickerstaff LK, Pairolero PC, Hollier LH, et al. Thoracic aortic aneurysms: a population-based study. *Surgery* 1982;92:1103–1108.
30. Clouse WD, Hallett Jr JW, Schaff HV, et al. Improved prognosis of thoracic aortic aneurysms: a population-based study. *JAMA* 1998;280:1926–1929.
31. Davies RR, Goldstein LJ, Coady MA, et al. Yearly rupture or dissection rates for thoracic aortic aneurysms: simple prediction based on size. *Ann Thorac Surg* 2002;73:17–27; discussion, 27–28.
32. Elkayam U, Ostrzega E, Shotan A, et al. Cardiovascular problems in pregnant women with the Marfan syndrome. *Ann Intern Med* 1995;123:117–122.
33. Immer FF, Bansi AG, Immer-Bansi AS, et al. Aortic dissection in pregnancy: analysis of risk factors and outcome. *Ann Thorac Surg* 2003;76:309–314.
34. Evangelista A, Soler-Soler J, Castillo HGD, et al. Aortic aneurysm. In: Nienaber CA, Fattori R, eds. *Diagnosis and treatment of aortic diseases.* Dordrecht, Netherlands: Kluwer Academic, 1999.
35. Hartnell GG. Imaging of aortic aneurysms and dissection: CT and MRI. *J Thorac Imaging* 2001;16:35–46.
36. Cayne NS, Veith FJ, Lipsitz EC, et al. Variability of maximal aortic aneurysm diameter measurements on CT scan: significance and methods to minimize. *J Vasc Surg* 2004;39:811–815.
37. Shores J, Berger KR, Murphy EA, et al. Progression of aortic dilatation and the benefit of long-term beta-adrenergic blockade in Marfan's syndrome. *N Engl J Med* 1994;330:1335–1341.
38. Yetman AT, Bornemeier RA, McCrindle BW. Usefulness of enalapril versus propranolol or atenolol for prevention of aortic dilation in patients with the Marfan syndrome. *Am J Cardiol* 2005;95:1125–1127.
39. Milewicz DM, Dietz HC, Miller DC. Treatment of aortic disease in patients with Marfan syndrome. *Circulation* 2005;111:e150–e157.
40. Elefteriades JA. Natural history of thoracic aortic aneurysms: indications for surgery, and surgical versus nonsurgical risks. *Ann Thorac Surg* 2002;74:S1877–S1880; discussion, S1892–S1898.
41. Svensson L, Crawford E. *Cardiovascular and vascular disease of the aorta.* Philadelphia: WB Saunders, 1997.
42. Milano AD, Pratali S, Mecozzi G, et al. Fate of coronary ostial anastomoses after the modified Bentall procedure. *Ann Thorac Surg* 2003;75:1797–1801; discussion, 1802.
43. Gott VL, Geene PS, Alejo DE, et al. Replacement of the aortic root in patients with Marfan's Syndrome. *N Engl J Med* 1999;340:1307.
44. Anttila V, Piaszczynski M, Mora B, et al. Improved outcome with composite graft versus homograft root replacement for children with aortic root aneurysms. *Eur J Cardiothorac Surg* 2005;27:420–424.
45. David TE, Feindel CM. An aortic valve–sparing operation for patients with aortic incompetence and aneurysm of the ascending aorta. *J Thorac Cardiovasc Surg* 1992;103:617–621; discussion, 622.

46. Hagl C, Ergin MA, Galla JD, et al. Neurologic outcome after ascending aorta-aortic arch operations: effect of brain protection technique in high-risk patients. *J Thorac Cardiovasc Surg* 2001;121:1107–1121.
47. Di Eusanio M, Schepens MA, Morshuis WJ, et al. Antegrade selective cerebral perfusion during operations on the thoracic aorta: factors influencing survival and neurologic outcome in 413 patients. *J Thorac Cardiovasc Surg* 2002;124:1080–1086.
48. Okita Y, Minatoya K, Tagusari O, et al. Prospective comparative study of brain protection in total aortic arch replacement: deep hypothermic circulatory arrest with retrograde cerebral perfusion or selective antegrade cerebral perfusion. *Ann Thorac Surg* 2001;72:72–79.
49. Svensson LG. Progress in ascending and aortic arch surgery: minimally invasive surgery, blood conservation, and neurological deficit prevention. *Ann Thorac Surg* 2002;74:S1786–S1788; discussion, S1792–S1799.
50. Fann J, Miller D. Surgical treatment of aortic aneurysms. In: Nienaber C, Fattori R., eds. *Diagnosis and treatment of aortic diseases*. Dordrecht, Netherlands: Kluwer Academic, 1999.
51. Brandt M, Hussel K, Walluscheck KP, et al. Early and long-term results of replacement of the descending aorta. *Eur J Vasc Endovasc Surg* 2005;30:365–369.
52. Svensson LG, Crawford ES, Hess KR, et al. Experience with 1509 patients undergoing thoracoabdominal aortic operations. *J Vasc Surg* 1993;17:357–368; discussion, 368–370.
53. Estrera AL, Miller 3rd CC, Chen EP, et al. Descending thoracic aortic aneurysm repair: 12-year experience using distal aortic perfusion and cerebrospinal fluid drainage. *Ann Thorac Surg* 2005;80:1290–1296; discussion, 1296.
54. Svensson LG, Crawford ES, Hess KR, et al. Variables predictive of outcome in 832 patients undergoing repairs of the descending thoracic aorta. *Chest* 1993;104:1248–1253.
55. Coselli JS, Conklin LD, LeMaire SA. Thoracoabdominal aortic aneurysm repair: review and update of current strategies. *Ann Thorac Surg* 2002;74:S1881–S1884; discussion, S1892–S1898.
56. Estrera AL, Miller 3rd CC, Huynh TT, et al. Neurologic outcome after thoracic and thoracoabdominal aortic aneurysm repair. *Ann Thorac Surg* 2001;72:1225–1230; discussion, 1230–1231.
57. Svensson LG. Paralysis after aortic surgery: in search of lost cord function. *Surgeon* 2005;3:396–405.
58. Bortone AS, De Cillis E, D'Agostino D, et al. Endovascular treatment of thoracic aortic disease: four years of experience. *Circulation* 2004;110:II262–II267.
59. Criado FJ, Abul-Khoudoud OR, Domer GS, et al. Endovascular repair of the thoracic aorta: lessons learned. *Ann Thorac Surg* 2005;80:857–863; discussion, 863.
60. Ellozy SH, Carroccio A, Minor M, et al. Challenges of endovascular tube graft repair of thoracic aortic aneurysm: midterm follow-up and lessons learned. *J Vasc Surg* 2003;38:676–683.
61. Crawford ES, Crawford JL, Safi HJ, et al. Thoracoabdominal aortic aneurysms: preoperative and intraoperative factors determining immediate and long-term results of operations in 605 patients. *J Vasc Surg* 1986;3:389–404.
62. Liapis CD, Paraskevas KI. The pivotal role of matrix metalloproteinases in the development of human abdominal aortic aneurysms. *Vasc Med* 2003;8:267–271.
63. Liddington MI, Heather BP. The relationship between aortic diameter and body habitus. *Eur J Vasc Surg* 1992;6:89–92.
64. Singh K, Bonaa KH, Jacobsen BK, et al. Prevalence of and risk factors for abdominal aortic aneurysms in a population-based study: The Tromso Study. *Am J Epidemiol* 2001;154:236–244.
65. Lederle FA, Johnson GR, Wilson SE, et al. Prevalence and associations of abdominal aortic aneurysm detected through screening. Aneurysm Detection and Management (ADAM) Veterans Affairs Cooperative Study Group. *Ann Intern Med* 1997;126:441–449.
66. Ashton HA, Buxton MJ, Day NE, et al. The Multicentre Aneurysm Screening Study (MASS) into the effect of abdominal aortic aneurysm screening on mortality in men: a randomised controlled trial. *Lancet* 2002;360:1531–1539.
67. Scott RA, Ashton HA, Kay DN. Abdominal aortic aneurysm in 4237 screened patients: prevalence, development and management over 6 years. *Br J Surg* 1991;78:1122–1125.
68. Lederle FA, Johnson GR, Wilson SE. Abdominal aortic aneurysm in women. *J Vasc Surg* 2001;34:122–126.
69. Melton 3rd LJ, Bickerstaff LK, Hollier LH, et al. Changing incidence of abdominal aortic aneurysms: a population-based study. *Am J Epidemiol* 1984;120:379–386.
70. Lederle FA, Johnson GR, Wilson SE, et al. The Aneurysm Detection and Management Study Screening Program: validation cohort and final results. Aneurysm Detection and Management Veterans Affairs Cooperative Study Investigators. *Arch Intern Med* 2000;160:1425–1430.
71. Vainas T, Lubbers T, Stassen FR, et al. Serum C–reactive protein level is associated with abdominal aortic aneurysm size and may be produced by aneurysmal tissue. *Circulation* 2003;107:1103–1105.
72. Wanhainen A, Bergqvist D, Boman K, et al. Risk factors associated with abdominal aortic aneurysm: a population-based study with historical and current data. *J Vasc Surg* 2005;41:390–396.
73. Brown MJ, Sutton AJ, Bell PRF, et al. A Meta-Analysis of 50 Years of Ruptured Abdominal Aortic Aneurysm Repair. *Br J Surg* 2002;89:714.
74. Brown LC, Powell JT. Risk factors for aneurysm rupture in patients kept under ultrasound surveillance. UK Small Aneurysm Trial Participants. *Ann Surg* 1999;230:289–296; discussion, 296–297.
75. Brady AR, Thompson SG, Fowkes FG, et al. Abdominal aortic aneurysm expansion: risk factors and time intervals for surveillance. *Circulation* 2004;110:16–21.
76. Glimaker H, Holmberg L, Elvin A, et al. Natural history of patients with abdominal aortic aneurysm. *Eur J Vasc Surg* 1991;5:125–130.
77. Lederle FA, Johnson GR, Wilson SE, et al. Rupture rate of large abdominal aortic aneurysms in patients refusing or unfit for elective repair. *JAMA* 2002;287:2968–2972.
78. Lederle FA, Simel DL. The rational clinical examination. Does this patient have abdominal aortic aneurysm? *JAMA* 1999;281:77–82.
79. Fleming C, Whitlock EP, Beil TL, et al. Screening for abdominal aortic aneurysm: a best-evidence systematic review for the U.S. Preventive Services Task Force. *Ann Intern Med* 2005;142:203–211.
80. Kent KC, Zwolak RM, Jaff MR, et al. Screening for abdominal aortic aneurysm: a consensus statement. *J Vasc Surg* 2004;39:267–269.
81. Hirsch A, Haskal Z, Hertzer N, et al. ACC/AHA guidelines for the management of patients with peripheral arterial disease (lower extremity, renal, mesenteric, and abdominal aortic). A collaborative report from the American Association for Vascular Surgery/Society for Vascular Surgery, Society for Cardiovascular Angiography and Interventions, Society for Vascular Medicine and Biology, Society of Interventional Radiology, and the ACC/AHA Task Force on Practice Guidelines (Writing Committee to Develop Guidelines for the Management of Patients With Peripheral Arterial Disease). 2006. American College of Cardiology Web Site. Available at http://www.acc.org/clinical/guidelines/pad/index.pdf.
82. Sprouse 2nd LR, Meier 3rd GH, Lesar CJ, et al. Comparison of abdominal aortic aneurysm diameter measurements obtained with ultrasound and computed tomography: Is there a difference? *J Vasc Surg* 2003;38:466–471; discussion, 471–472.
83. Powell JT, Brady AR. Detection, management, and prospects for the medical treatment of small abdominal aortic aneurysms. *Arterioscler Thromb Vasc Biol* 2004;24:241–245.
84. Baxter BT, Pearce WH, Waltke EA, et al. Prolonged administration of doxycycline in patients with small asymptomatic abdominal aortic aneurysms: report of a prospective (phase II) multicenter study. *J Vasc Surg* 2002;36:1–12.
85. Mosorin M, Juvonen J, Biancari F, et al. Use of doxycycline to decrease the growth rate of abdominal aortic aneurysms: a randomized, double-blind, placebo-controlled pilot study. *J Vasc Surg* 2001;34:606–610.
86. Wilson WR, Evans J, Bell PR, et al. HMG-CoA reductase inhibitors (statins) decrease MMP-3 and MMP-9 concentrations in abdominal aortic aneurysms. *Eur J Vasc Endovasc Surg* 2005;30:259–262.
87. Nagashima H, Aoka Y, Sakomura Y, et al. A 3-hydroxy-3-methylglutaryl coenzyme A reductase inhibitor, cerivastatin, suppresses production of matrix metalloproteinase-9 in human abdominal aortic aneurysm wall. *J Vasc Surg* 2002;36:158–163.
88. Vammen S, Lindholt JS, Ostergaard L, et al. Randomized double-blind controlled trial of roxithromycin for prevention of abdominal aortic aneurysm expansion. *Br J Surg* 2001;88:1066–1072.
89. Kertai MD, Boersma E, Westerhout CM, et al. A combination of statins and beta-blockers is independently associated with a reduction in the incidence of perioperative mortality and nonfatal myocardial infarction in patients undergoing abdominal aortic aneurysm surgery. *Eur J Vasc Endovasc Surg* 2004;28:343–352.
90. The UK Small Aneurysm Trial Participants. Mortality results for randomised controlled trial of early elective surgery or ultrasonographic surveillance for small abdominal aortic aneurysms. *Lancet* 1998;352:1649–1655.
91. Lederle FA, Wilson SE, Johnson GR, et al. Immediate repair compared with surveillance of small abdominal aortic aneurysms. *N Engl J Med* 2002;346:1437–1444.
92. United Kingdom Small Aneurysm Trial Participants. Long-term outcomes of immediate repair compared with surveillance of small abdominal aortic aneurysms. *N Engl J Med* 2002;346:1445–1452.
93. Brewster DC, Cronenwett JL, Hallett Jr JW, et al. Guidelines for the treatment of abdominal aortic aneurysms. Report of a subcommittee of the Joint Council of the American Association for Vascular Surgery and Society for Vascular Surgery. *J Vasc Surg* 2003;37:1106–1117.
94. Simons P, van Overhagen H, Nawijn A, et al. Endovascular aneurysm repair with a bifurcated endovascular graft at a primary referral center: influence of experience, age, gender, and aneurysm size on suitability. *J Vasc Surg* 2003;38:758–761.
95. Prinssen M, Verhoeven EL, Buth J, et al. A randomized trial comparing conventional and endovascular repair of abdominal aortic aneurysms. *N Engl J Med* 2004;351:1607–1618.
96. Greenhalgh RM, Brown LC, Kwong GP, et al. Comparison of endovascular aneurysm repair with open repair in patients with abdominal aortic aneurysm (EVAR trial 1), 30-day operative mortality results: randomised controlled trial. *Lancet* 2004;364:843–848.
97. Blankensteijn JD, de Jong SE, Prinssen M, et al. Two-year outcomes after conventional or endovascular repair of abdominal aortic aneurysms. *N Engl J Med* 2005;352:2398–405.

98. Endovascular aneurysm repair versus open repair in patients with abdominal aortic aneurysm (EVAR trial 1): randomised controlled trial. *Lancet* 2005;365:2179–2186.
99. National Center for Health Statistics, Centers for Disease Control and Prevention. *Deaths, percent of total deaths, and rank order for 113 selected causes of death, by race and sex: United States, 2001–02*. Hyattsville, MD: U.S. Department of Health and Human Services, 2002.
100. Wilson SK, Hutchins GM. Aortic dissecting aneurysms: causative factors in 204 subjects. *Arch Pathol Lab Med* 1982;106:175–80.
101. Tsai TT, Nienaber CA, Eagle KA. Acute aortic syndromes. *Circulation* 2005;112:3802–3813.
102. Debakey ME, Henly WS, Cooley DA, et al. Surgical management of dissecting aneurysms of the aorta. *J Thorac Cardiovasc Surg* 1965;49:130–149.
103. Daily PO, Trueblood HW, Stinson EB, et al. Management of acute aortic dissections. *Ann Thorac Surg* 1970;10:237–247.
104. Meszaros I, Morocz J, Szlavi J, et al. Epidemiology and clinicopathology of aortic dissection. *Chest* 2000;117:1271–1278.
105. Clouse WD, Hallett Jr JW, Schaff HV, et al. Acute aortic dissection: population-based incidence compared with degenerative aortic aneurysm rupture. *Mayo Clin Proc* 2004;79:176–180.
106. Nienaber CA, Fattori R, Mehta RH, et al. Gender-related differences in acute aortic dissection. *Circulation* 2004;109:3014–3021.
107. Hagan PG, Nienaber CA, Isselbacher EM, et al. The International Registry of Acute Aortic Dissection (IRAD): new insights into an old disease. *JAMA* 2000;283:897–903.
108. Januzzi JL, Isselbacher EM, Fattori R, et al. Characterizing the young patient with aortic dissection: results from the International Registry of Aortic Dissection (IRAD). *J Am Coll Cardiol* 2004;43:665–669.
109. Evans JM, O'Fallon WM, Hunder GG. Increased incidence of aortic aneurysm and dissection in giant cell (temporal) arteritis. A population-based study. *Ann Intern Med* 1995;122:502–507.
110. Januzzi JL, Sabatine MS, Eagle KA, et al. Iatrogenic aortic dissection. *Am J Cardiol* 2002;89:623–626.
111. Park SW, Hutchison S, Mehta RH, et al. Association of painless acute aortic dissection with increased mortality. *Mayo Clin Proc* 2004;79:1252–1257.
112. Klompas M. Does this patient have an acute thoracic aortic dissection? *JAMA* 2002;287:2262–2272.
113. Upchurch Jr GR, Nienaber C, Fattori R, et al. Acute aortic dissection presenting with primarily abdominal pain: a rare manifestation of a deadly disease. *Ann Vasc Surg* 2005;19:367–373.
114. Gregorio MC, Baumgartner FJ, Omari BO. The presenting chest roentgenogram in acute type A aortic dissection: a multidisciplinary study. *Am Surg* 2002;68:6–10.
115. von Kodolitsch Y, Nienaber CA, Dieckmann C, et al. Chest radiography for the diagnosis of acute aortic syndrome. *Am J Med* 2004;116:73–77.
116. Nienaber CA, von Kodolitsch Y, Nicolas V, et al. The diagnosis of thoracic aortic dissection by noninvasive imaging procedures. *N Engl J Med* 1993;328:1–9.
117. Sommer T, Fehske W, Holzknecht N, et al. Aortic dissection: a comparative study of diagnosis with spiral CT, multiplanar transesophageal echocardiography, and MR imaging. *Radiology* 1996;199:347–352.
118. Moore AG, Eagle KA, Bruckman D, et al. Choice of computed tomography, transesophageal echocardiography, magnetic resonance imaging, and aortography in acute aortic dissection: International Registry of Acute Aortic Dissection (IRAD). *Am J Cardiol* 2002;89:1235–1238.
119. Weintraub AR, Erbel R, Gorge G, et al. Intravascular ultrasound imaging in acute aortic dissection. *J Am Coll Cardiol* 1994;24:495–503.
120. Chavan A, Hausmann D, Dresler C, et al. Intravascular ultrasound-guided percutaneous fenestration of the intimal flap in the dissected aorta. *Circulation* 1997;96:2124–2127.
121. Koschyk DH, Nienaber CA, Knap M, et al. How to guide stent-graft implantation in type B aortic dissection? Comparison of angiography, transesophageal echocardiography, and intravascular ultrasound. *Circulation* 2005;112:I260–I264.
122. Akutsu K, Sato N, Yamamoto T, et al. A rapid bedside D-dimer assay (cardiac D-dimer) for screening of clinically suspected acute aortic dissection. *Circ J* 2005;69:397–403.
123. Eggebrecht H, Naber CK, Bruch C, et al. Value of plasma fibrin D-dimers for detection of acute aortic dissection. *J Am Coll Cardiol* 2004;44:804–809.
124. Shinohara T, Suzuki K, Okada M, et al. Soluble elastin fragments in serum are elevated in acute aortic dissection. *Arterioscler Thromb Vasc Biol* 2003; 23:1839–1844.
125. Weber T, Hogler S, Auer J, et al. D-dimer in acute aortic dissection. *Chest* 2003;123:1375–1378.
126. Mehta RH, Suzuki T, Hagan PG, et al. Predicting death in patients with acute type A aortic dissection. *Circulation* 2002;105:200–206.
127. Suzuki T, Mehta RH, Ince H, et al. Clinical profiles and outcomes of acute type B aortic dissection in the current era: lessons from the International Registry of Aortic Dissection (IRAD). *Circulation* 2003;108(Suppl 1):II312–II317.
128. Tan ME, Morshuis WJ, Dossche KM, et al. Long-term results after 27 years of surgical treatment of acute type A aortic dissection. *Ann Thorac Surg* 2005;80:523–529.
129. Ehrlich MP, Ergin MA, McCullough JN, et al. Results of immediate surgical treatment of all acute type A dissections. *Circulation* 2000;102:III248–II252.
130. Apaydin AZ, Buket S, Posacioglu H, et al. Perioperative risk factors for mortality in patients with acute type A aortic dissection. *Ann Thorac Surg* 2002;74:2034–2039; discussion, 2039.
131. Trimarchi S, Nienaber CA, Rampoldi V, et al. Contemporary results of surgery in acute type A aortic dissection: the International Registry of Acute Aortic Dissection experience. *J Thorac Cardiovasc Surg* 2005;129:112–122.
132. Kallenbach K, Oelze T, Salcher R, et al. Evolving strategies for treatment of acute aortic dissection type A. *Circulation* 2004;110:II243–II249.
133. Mehta RH, Bossone E, Evangelista A, et al. Acute type B aortic dissection in elderly patients: clinical features, outcomes, and simple risk stratification rule. *Ann Thorac Surg* 2004;77:1622–1628; discussion, 1629.
134. Onitsuka S, Akashi H, Tayama K, et al. Long-term outcome and prognostic predictors of medically treated acute type B aortic dissections. *Ann Thorac Surg* 2004;78:1268–1273.
135. Akutsu K, Nejima J, Kiuchi K, et al. Effects of the patent false lumen on the long-term outcome of type B acute aortic dissection. *Eur J Cardiothorac Surg* 2004;26:359–366.
136. Juvonen T, Ergin MA, Galla JD, et al. Risk factors for rupture of chronic type B dissections. *J Thorac Cardiovasc Surg* 1999;117:776–786.
137. Umana JP, Lai DT, Mitchell RS, et al. Is medical therapy still the optimal treatment strategy for patients with acute type B aortic dissections? *J Thorac Cardiovasc Surg* 2002;124:896–910.
138. Isselbacher EM, Cigarroa JE, Eagle KA. Cardiac tamponade complicating proximal aortic dissection. Is pericardiocentesis harmful? *Circulation* 1994;90:2375–2378.
139. Januzzi JL, Sabatine MS, Choi JC, et al. Refractory systemic hypertension following type B aortic dissection. *Am J Cardiol* 2001;88:686–688.
140. Januzzi JL, Movsowitz HD, Choi J, et al. Significance of recurrent pain in acute type B aortic dissection. *Am J Cardiol* 2001;87:930–933.
141. Sueyoshi E, Sakamoto I, Hayashi K, et al. Growth rate of aortic diameter in patients with type B aortic dissection during the chronic phase. *Circulation* 2004;110:II256–II261.
142. Beregi JP, Haulon S, Otal P, et al. Endovascular treatment of acute complications associated with aortic dissection: midterm results from a multicenter study. *J Endovasc Ther* 2003;10:486–493.
143. Vedantham S, Picus D, Sanchez LA, et al. Percutaneous management of ischemic complications in patients with type-B aortic dissection. *J Vasc Interv Radiol* 2003;14:181–194.
144. Svensson LG, Labib SB, Eisenhauer AC, et al. Intimal tear without hematoma: an important variant of aortic dissection that can elude current imaging techniques. *Circulation* 1999;99:1331–1336.
145. Evangelista A, Mukherjee D, Mehta RH, et al. Acute intramural hematoma of the aorta: a mystery in evolution. *Circulation* 2005;111:1063–1070.
146. Ganaha F, Miller DC, Sugimoto K, et al. Prognosis of aortic intramural hematoma with and without penetrating atherosclerotic ulcer: a clinical and radiological analysis. *Circulation* 2002;106:342–348.
147. Kaji S, Akasaka T, Horibata Y, et al. Long-term prognosis of patients with type A aortic intramural hematoma. *Circulation* 2002;106:I248–I252.
148. Moizumi Y, Komatsu T, Motoyoshi N, et al. Management of patients with intramural hematoma involving the ascending aorta. *J Thorac Cardiovasc Surg* 2002;124:918–924.
149. von Kodolitsch Y, Csosz SK, Koschyk DH, et al. Intramural hematoma of the aorta: predictors of progression to dissection and rupture. *Circulation* 2003;107:1158–1163.
150. Kaji S, Akasaka T, Katayama M, et al. Long-term prognosis of patients with type B aortic intramural hematoma. *Circulation* 2003;108(Suppl 1):II307–II311.
151. Sueyoshi E, Sakamoto I, Fukuda M, et al. Long-term outcome of type B aortic intramural hematoma: comparison with classic aortic dissection treated by the same therapeutic strategy. *Ann Thorac Surg* 2004;78:2112–2117.
152. Song JK, Kim HS, Kang DH, et al. Different clinical features of aortic intramural hematoma versus dissection involving the ascending aorta. *J Am Coll Cardiol* 2001;37:1604–1610.
153. Evangelista A, Dominguez R, Sebastia C, et al. Long-term follow-up of aortic intramural hematoma: predictors of outcome. *Circulation* 2003;108: 583–589.
154. Coady MA, Rizzo JA, Hammond GL, et al. Penetrating ulcer of the thoracic aorta: What is it? How do we recognize it? How do we manage it? *J Vasc Surg* 1998;27:1006–1015; discussion, 1015–1016.
155. Absi TS, Sundt 3rd TM, Camillo C, et al. Penetrating atherosclerotic ulcers of the descending thoracic aorta may be managed expectantly. *Vascular* 2004;12:307–311.
156. Batt M, Haudebourg P, Planchard PF, et al. Penetrating atherosclerotic ulcers of the infrarenal aorta: life-threatening lesions. *Eur J Vasc Endovasc Surg* 2005;29:35–42.
157. Cho KR, Stanson AW, Potter DD, et al. Penetrating atherosclerotic ulcer of the descending thoracic aorta and arch. *J Thorac Cardiovasc Surg* 2004;127:1393–1399; discussion 1399–1401.
158. Stanson AW, Kazmier FJ, Hollier LH, et al. Penetrating atherosclerotic ulcers of the thoracic aorta: natural history and clinicopathologic correlations. *Ann Vasc Surg* 1986;1:15–23.
159. Hussain S, Glover JL, Bree R, et al. Penetrating atherosclerotic ulcers of the thoracic aorta. *J Vasc Surg* 1989;9:710–717.
160. Coady MA, Rizzo JA, Elefteriades JA. Pathologic variants of thoracic aortic dissections. Penetrating atherosclerotic ulcers and intramural hematomas. *Cardiol Clin* 1999;17:637–657.

161. Selvin E, Erlinger TP. Prevalence of and risk factors for peripheral arterial disease in the United States: results from the National Health and Nutrition Examination Survey, 1999–2000. *Circulation* 2004;110:738–743.
162. Glagov S, Zarins C, Giddens DP, et al. Hemodynamics and atherosclerosis. Insights and perspectives gained from studies of human arteries. *Arch Pathol Lab Med* 1988;112:1018–1031.
163. Nguyen ND, Haque AK. Effect of hemodynamic factors on atherosclerosis in the abdominal aorta. *Atherosclerosis* 1990;84:33–39.
164. Cacoub P, Godeau P. Risk factors for atherosclerotic aortoiliac occlusive disease. *Ann Vasc Surg* 1993;7:394–405.
165. Barretto S, Ballman KV, Rooke TW, et al. Early-onset peripheral arterial occlusive disease: clinical features and determinants of disease severity and location. *Vasc Med* 2003;8:95–100.
166. Smith FB, Lee AJ, Fowkes FG, et al. Variation in cardiovascular risk factors by angiographic site of lower limb atherosclerosis. *Eur J Vasc Endovasc Surg* 1996;11:340–346.
167. Jongkind V, Linsen MA, Diks J, et al. Aortoiliac steno-occlusion in young women: a single center experience and review of the literature. *Acta Chir Belg* 2004;104:641–646.
168. Jernigan WR, Fallat ME, Hatfield DR. Hypoplastic aortoiliac syndrome: An entity peculiar to women. *Surgery* 1983;94:752–757.
169. Johnson TE. Small blood vessel syndrome. Constitutional arterial narrowing. *Minn Med* 1969;52:1903–1905.
170. Caes F, Cham B, Van den Brande P, et al. Small artery syndrome in women. *Surg Gynecol Obstet* 1985;161:165–170.
171. Raso AM, Varetto G, Bellan A, et al. Small aorta syndrome: hypothesis or reality? *Minerva Cardioangiol* 2001;49:211–220.
172. Poiree S, Monnier-Cholley L, Tubiana JM, et al. Acute abdominal aortic thrombosis in cancer patients. *Abdom Imaging* 2004;29:511–513.
173. McGee GS, Pearce WH, Sharma L, et al. Antiphospholipid antibodies and arterial thrombosis. Case reports and a review of the literature. *Arch Surg* 1992;127:342–346.
174. Kieny R. Rene Leriche and his work. As time goes by. *Ann Vasc Surg* 1990; 4:105–111.
175. Leriche R. De la résection du carrefour aortico-iliaque avec double sympathectomie lombaire pour thrombose artéritique de l'aorte: le syndrome de l'oblitération termino-aortique par artérite. *Presse Med* 1940;48:601–607.
176. Amarenco P, Cohen A, Tzourio C, et al. Atherosclerotic disease of the aortic arch and the risk of ischemic stroke. *N Engl J Med* 1994;331:1474–1479.
177. The French Study of Aortic Plaques in Stroke Group. Atherosclerotic disease of the aortic arch as a risk factor for recurrent ischemic stroke. *N Engl J Med* 1996;334:1216–1221.
178. Karmody AM, Powers SR, Monaco VJ, et al. "Blue toe" syndrome. An indication for limb salvage surgery. *Arch Surg* 1976;111:1263–1268.
179. Zannetti S, L'Italien GJ, Cambria RP. Functional outcome after surgical treatment for intermittent claudication. *J Vasc Surg* 1996;24:65–73.
180. Onohara T, Komori K, Kume M, et al. Multivariate analysis of long-term results after an axillobifemoral and aortobifemoral bypass in patients with aortoiliac occlusive disease. *J Cardiovasc Surg (Torino)* 2000;41:905–910.
181. Murphy TP, Ariaratnam NS, Carney Jr WI, et al. Aortoiliac insufficiency: long-term experience with stent placement for treatment. *Radiology* 2004; 231:243–249.
182. Morgan SH, Asherson RA, Hughes GR. Distal aortitis complicating Reiter's syndrome. *Br Heart J* 1984;52:115–116.
183. Lautermann D, Braun J. Ankylosing spondylitis–cardiac manifestations. *Clin Exp Rheumatol* 2002;20:S11–S15.
184. Guard RW, Gotis-Graham I, Edmonds JP, et al. Aortitis with dissection complicating systemic lupus erythematosus. *Pathology* 1995;27:224–228.
185. Chirinos JA, Tamariz LJ, Lopes G, et al. Large vessel involvement in ANCA-associated vasculitides: report of a case and review of the literature. *Clin Rheumatol* 2004;23:152–159.
186. Vollertsen RS, McDonald TJ, Younge BR, et al. Cogan's syndrome: 18 cases and a review of the literature. *Mayo Clin Proc* 1986;61:344–361.
187. Haynes BF, Kaiser-Kupfer MI, Mason P, et al. Cogan syndrome: studies in thirteen patients, long-term follow-up, and a review of the literature. *Medicine (Baltimore)* 1980;59:426–441.
188. Weiler V, Redtenbacher S, Bancher C, et al. Concurrence of sarcoidosis and aortitis: case report and review of the literature. *Ann Rheum Dis* 2000;59: 850–853.
189. Maeda S, Murao S, Sugiyama T, et al. Generalized sarcoidosis with "sarcoid aortitis." *Acta Pathol Jpn* 1983;33:183–188.
190. Kuwana M, Wakino S, Yoshida T, et al. Retroperitoneal fibrosis associated with aortitis. *Arthritis Rheum* 1992;35:1245–1247.
191. Tomita T, Imakawa K. Matrix metalloproteinases and tissue inhibitors of metalloproteinases in giant cell arteritis: an immunocytochemical study. *Pathology* 1998;30:40–50.
192. Moriuchi J, Wakisaka A, Aizawa M, et al. HLA-linked susceptibility gene of Takayasu disease. *Hum Immunol* 1982;4:87–91.
193. Gravanis MB. Giant cell arteritis and Takayasu aortitis: morphologic, pathogenetic and etiologic factors. *Int J Cardiol* 2000;75(Suppl 1):S21–S33; discussion, S35–S36.
194. Volkman DJ, Mann DL, Fauci AS. Association between Takayasu's arteritis and a B-cell alloantigen in North Americans. *N Engl J Med* 1982;306:464–465.
195. Mwipatayi BP, Jeffery PC, Beningfield SJ, et al. Takayasu arteritis: clinical features and management: report of 272 cases. *Aust N Z J Surg* 2005;75: 110–117.
196. Schoen F. Blood vessels. In: Kumar V, Abbas A, Fausto N, eds. *Robbins and Cotran Pathologic basis of disease*. Philadelphia: Saunders/Elsevier, 2005.
197. Weyand CM, Goronzy JJ. Medium- and large-vessel vasculitis. *N Engl J Med* 2003;349:160–169.
198. Lane SE, Watts R, Scott DG. Epidemiology of systemic vasculitis. *Curr Rheumatol Rep* 2005;7:270–275.
199. Huston KA, Hunder GG, Lie JT, et al. Temporal arteritis: a 25-year epidemiologic, clinical, and pathologic study. *Ann Intern Med* 1978;88:162–167.
200. Salvarani C, Crowson CS, O'Fallon WM, et al. Reappraisal of the epidemiology of giant cell arteritis in Olmsted County, Minnesota, over a fifty-year period. *Arthritis Rheum* 2004;51:264–268.
201. Kerr GS, Hallahan CW, Giordano J, et al. Takayasu arteritis. *Ann Intern Med* 1994;120:919–929.
202. Hunder GG, Bloch DA, Michel BA, et al. The American College of Rheumatology 1990 criteria for the classification of giant cell arteritis. *Arthritis Rheum* 1990;33:1122–1128.
203. Arend WP, Michel BA, Bloch DA, et al. The American College of Rheumatology 1990 criteria for the classification of Takayasu arteritis. *Arthritis Rheum* 1990;33:1129–1134.
204. Nuenninghoff DM, Hunder GG, Christianson TJ, et al. Incidence and predictors of large-artery complication (aortic aneurysm, aortic dissection, and/or large-artery stenosis) in patients with giant cell arteritis: a population-based study over 50 years. *Arthritis Rheum* 2003;48:3522–3531.
205. Rojo-Leyva F, Ratliff NB, Cosgrove 3rd DM, et al. Study of 52 patients with idiopathic aortitis from a cohort of 1,204 surgical cases. *Arthritis Rheum* 2000;43:901–907.
206. Salvarani C, Cantini F, Boiardi L, et al. Laboratory investigations useful in giant cell arteritis and Takayasu's arteritis. *Clin Exp Rheumatol* 2003; 21:S23–S28.
207. Hoffman GS, Ahmed AE. Surrogate markers of disease activity in patients with Takayasu arteritis. A preliminary report from the International Network for the Study of the Systemic Vasculitides (INSSYS). *Int J Cardiol* 1998;66(Suppl 1):S191–S194; discussion, S195.
208. Park MC, Lee SW, Park YB, et al. Serum cytokine profiles and their correlations with disease activity in Takayasu's arteritis. *Rheumatology (Oxford)* 2005.
209. Meller J, Strutz F, Siefker U, et al. Early diagnosis and follow-up of aortitis with [(18)F]FDG PET and MRI. *Eur J Nucl Med Mol Imaging* 2003;30: 730–736.
210. Webb M, Chambers A, Al-Nahhas A, et al. The role of 18F-FDG PET in characterising disease activity in Takayasu arteritis. *Eur J Nucl Med Mol Imaging* 2004;31:627–34.
211. Tso E, Flamm SD, White RD, et al. Takayasu arteritis: utility and limitations of magnetic resonance imaging in diagnosis and treatment. *Arthritis Rheum* 2002;46:1634–1642.
212. Hunder GG, Sheps SG, Allen GL, et al. Daily and alternate-day corticosteroid regimens in treatment of giant cell arteritis: comparison in a prospective study. *Ann Intern Med* 1975;82:613–618.
213. Chan CC, Paine M, O'Day J. Steroid management in giant cell arteritis. *Br J Ophthalmol* 2001;85:1061–1064.
214. Danesh-Meyer H, Savino PJ, Gamble GG. Poor prognosis of visual outcome after visual loss from giant cell arteritis. *Ophthalmology* 2005;112:1098–1103.
215. Hoffman GS, Leavitt RY, Kerr GS, et al. Treatment of glucocorticoid-resistant or relapsing Takayasu arteritis with methotrexate. *Arthritis Rheum* 1994;37:578–582.
216. Valsakumar AK, Valappil UC, Jorapur V, et al. Role of immunosuppressive therapy on clinical, immunological, and angiographic outcome in active Takayasu's arteritis. *J Rheumatol* 2003;30:1793–1798.
217. Hoffman GS, Merkel PA, Brasington RD, et al. Anti-tumor necrosis factor therapy in patients with difficult to treat Takayasu arteritis. *Arthritis Rheum* 2004;50:2296–2304.
218. Hoffman GS, Cid MC, Hellmann DB, et al. A multicenter, randomized, double-blind, placebo-controlled trial of adjuvant methotrexate treatment for giant cell arteritis. *Arthritis Rheum* 2002;46:1309–1318.
219. Park MC, Lee SW, Park YB, et al. Clinical characteristics and outcomes of Takayasu's arteritis: analysis of 108 patients using standardized criteria for diagnosis, activity assessment, and angiographic classification. *Scand J Rheumatol* 2005;34:284–292.
220. Proven A, Gabriel SE, Orces C, et al. Glucocorticoid therapy in giant cell arteritis: duration and adverse outcomes. *Arthritis Rheum* 2003;49:703–708.
221. Hachulla E, Boivin V, Pasturel-Michon U, et al. Prognostic factors and long-term evolution in a cohort of 133 patients with giant cell arteritis. *Clin Exp Rheumatol* 2001;19:171–176.
222. American College of Rheumatology Ad Hoc Committee on Glucocorticoid-Induced Osteoporosis. Recommendations for the prevention and treatment of glucocorticoid-induced osteoporosis: 2001 update. *Arthritis Rheum* 2001;44:1496–1503.
223. Engelke C, Sandhu C, Morgan RA, et al. Endovascular repair of thoracic aortic aneurysm and intramural hematoma in giant cell arteritis. *J Vasc Interv Radiol* 2002;13:625–629.
224. Krohg-Sorensen K, Hafsahl G, Fosse E, et al. Acceptable short-term

results after endovascular repair of diseases of the thoracic aorta in high risk patients. *Eur J Cardiothorac Surg* 2003;24:379–387.
225. Tyagi S, Kaul UA, Arora R. Endovascular stenting for unsuccessful angioplasty of the aorta in aortoarteritis. *Cardiovasc Interv Radiol* 1999;22:452–456.
226. Bali HK, Jain S, Jain A, et al. Stent supported angioplasty in Takayasu arteritis. *Int J Cardiol* 1998;66(Suppl 1):S213–S217; discussion, S219–S220.
227. D'Souza SJ, Tsai WS, Silver MM, et al. Diagnosis and management of stenotic aorto-arteriopathy in childhood. *J Pediatr* 1998;132:1016–1022.
228. Liang P, Tan-Ong M, Hoffman GS. Takayasu's arteritis: vascular interventions and outcomes. *J Rheumatol* 2004;31:102–106.
229. Nienaber CA, Zannetti S, Barbieri B, et al. INvestigation of STEnt grafts in patients with type B Aortic Dissection: design of the INSTEAD trial—a prospective, multicenter, European randomized trial. *Am Heart J* 2005;149:592–599.
230. Ohki T, Ouriel K, Stern D, et al. *Preliminary outcome of wireless pressure sensing for EVAR (the Apex Trial)*. Presented at the 2005 Society for Vascular Surgery Annual Meeting, Chicago.

CHAPTER 106 ■ NONINVASIVE ASSESSMENT OF PERIPHERAL VASCULAR DISEASE

MICHAEL R. JAFF AND STEVEN DEITELZWEIG

OVERVIEW

With the rapid proliferation of effective, safe, and minimally invasive alternatives to treat patients with a myriad of noncoronary vascular disorders, it is no surprise that interest in understanding the intricacies of vascular testing has risen to previously unmatched levels among cardiovascular specialists. As many interventional cardiologists gain experience in the endovascular treatment of peripheral vascular disease (PVD), the need to develop testing algorithms for the diagnosis and surveillance of these disorders is critical. In addition, the Core Curriculum in Cardiology for Adult Cardiovascular Training Programs (COCATS-2) recently described mandatory training for all fellow candidates in adult cardiovascular training programs in vascular medicine, including knowledge of vascular diagnostic testing (1). This chapter is designed to provide a broad overview of the available tests, including advantages, limitations, and alternatives. Obviously, there is insufficient space to provide a level of detail that would allow for the development of expertise solely by reviewing this chapter. However, the information provided will allow for an assessment of areas of interest and need for further study.

HISTORY AND PHYSICAL EXAMINATION IN THE DIAGNOSIS OF PERIPHERAL VASCULAR DISEASE

Contrary to many other disorders in which diagnostic testing is often the most important component in the evaluation of patients, the history and physical examination is critical. Peripheral arterial disease (PAD) is the optimal example. Without a thorough understanding of the symptoms and physical findings, diagnostic testing will only provide an anatomic assessment, but will not assist in determining optimal therapy. If a patient has minimal symptoms of intermittent claudication which does not particularly limit physical functioning, the finding of a 30-cm occlusion of the superficial femoral artery is superfluous.

In addition, cardiovascular specialists, already possessing skills in the physical examination of the heart, must gain expertise in the peripheral vascular examination. Auscultation for bruits over the cervical, abdominal, flank, and femoral regions must be routinely performed. Palpation of all pulses, including superficial temporal (a diminished superficial temporal pulse may suggest an important carotid bifurcation stenosis), carotid, subclavian, axillary, brachial, radial, ulnar, femoral, popliteal, dorsalis pedis, and posterior tibial pulses, is important to perform and record. Grading of pulse intensity is commonly noted as follows: absent (grade 0); diminished (grade 1); and normal (grade 2). An aneurysm of the popliteal artery should be noted as such and not as grade 2 + or grade 4. Examination of the feet and toes must become a routine component of the physical examination. Subtle findings of tinea pedis in the intertriginous regions of the toes may result in ischemic ulcerations in patients with PAD and diabetes mellitus, for example (Fig. 106.1).

VASCULAR DIAGNOSTIC LABORATORY: BASIC COMPONENTS

Once the suspicion for PVD has been raised, the initial objective diagnostic testing commonly begins in the vascular diagnostic

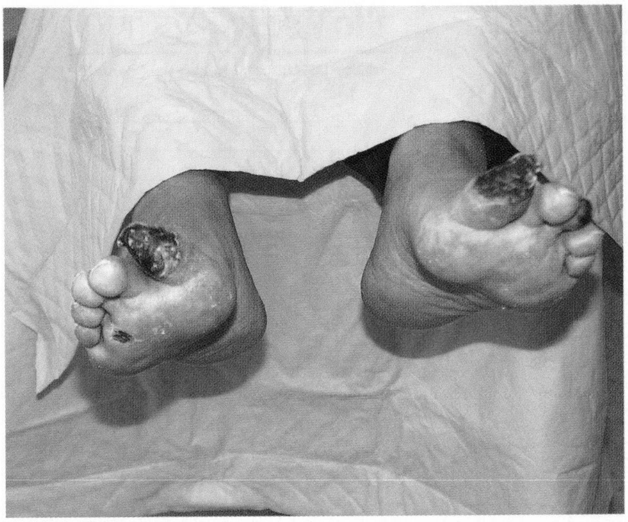

FIGURE 106.1. Patient with diabetes mellitus, dense peripheral sensory neuropathy, and advanced peripheral arterial disease with critical limb ischemia.

laboratory. Although ranging in size and scope of services, a comprehensive vascular diagnostic laboratory provides objective testing for physiologic evaluation of lower and upper extremity arterial disease, as well as of cerebrovascular, aortic, renal mesenteric, and venous diseases. Current commercially available equipment includes limb blood pressure cuff devices continuous wave hand-held Doppler units, color duplex ultrasonography (DUS) units, and, more recently, portable DUS devices.

Tests are performed by trained vascular technologists, preferably possessing the registered vascular technologist (RVT) certification demonstrating a minimum level of training, expertise, and experience. Physicians who interpret these studies commonly receive formal training during fellowship, or they must receive training in an accredited vascular diagnostic laboratory, proctored by physicians with appropriate credentials. Images are commonly stored on Picture Archiving Computerized Systems in digital format that provide the highest-quality images for evaluation and interpretation.

ACCREDITATION OF VASCULAR DIAGNOSTIC LABORATORIES

Vascular diagnostic laboratories may be found in large tertiary urban medical centers, rural community hospitals, multispecialty physician outpatient facilities, and single physician offices. Despite the variability in location and scope of services, certain components of organization, credentialing, testing algorithms, quality assurance, accuracy, and continuing education must be constant from laboratory to laboratory. Although compliance is still voluntary, many vascular laboratories around the United States submit comprehensive applications for credentialing by either the American College of Radiology (www.acr.org/s_acr/sec.asp?CID=594&DID=14258) or the Intersocietal Commission for the Accreditation of Vascular Laboratories (ICAVL) (www.icavl.org). The ICAVL is sponsored by multiple professional vascular organizations and provides a rigorous application process to ensure the public and physicians of a minimum degree of accuracy and quality. There is a trend among many state legislators to require accreditation for full reimbursement of vascular laboratory tests.

TESTING IN PERIPHERAL ARTERIAL DISEASE

Physiologic Testing

Ankle-Brachial Index, Segmental Limb Pressures, Pulse Volume Recordings, and Exercise Testing

The ankle-brachial index (ABI) is the easiest, most widely reproducible, and most accurate method of determining the degree of diminished arterial circulation in a limb. Using a standard sphygmomanometer and a hand-held continuous wave Doppler probe, the higher of the two pedal pressures (dorsalis pedis or posterior tibial artery) is compared with the higher of the two brachial blood pressures, and a ratio is obtained. Given that the systolic pressure normally increases in the peripheral arteries (predominantly owing to increased resistance of these vessels), a normal ABI is 0.9 or greater. An ABI less than 0.5 suggests significant arterial disease and likely represents multisegmental involvement (Table 106.1). Although there is variability in sequential ABI measurements (2), the ABI can objectively demonstrate improvement in lower limb circulation at rest.

In addition to the utility of the ABI in determining the presence of PAD, the ABI has also been used to identify the prevalence of PAD in populations at risk (3), and it defines risk for major adverse cardiovascular events (myocardial infarction, stroke) and cardiovascular death (4).

The addition of segmental limb pressures can aid in localizing segments of disease involvement. A series of limb pressure cuffs is placed on the thigh (some centers prefer high- and low-thigh cuffs), calf, ankle, transmetatarsal region of the foot, and digit. The ABI is calculated, and then the pressure is sequentially inflated in each cuff to approximately 20 to 30 mm Hg above systolic pressure. Utilizing a continuous wave Doppler probe placed at a pedal vessel, the pressure in the cuff is gradually released, and the pressure at each segment is measured. If a decrease in pressure between two consecutive levels greater than 30 mm Hg is identified, this suggests arterial disease of the artery proximal to the cuff. In addition, comparing the two limbs, a 20- to 30-mm Hg discrepancy from one limb to the other at the same cuff level also suggests significant arterial stenosis or occlusion proximal to the cuff (5) (Fig. 106.2).

The ABI can be a highly accurate method of determining the presence of PAD and its severity. However, if the ankle vessel is calcified, as is commonly seen in patients with diabetes mellitus or end-stage renal disease, an accurate ankle pressure cannot be obtained. The pressure in these calcified arteries is often greater than 200 mm Hg. If this result is not recognized as artifactually high, the physician may falsely conclude that arterial circulation is adequate or even normal, in these patients. In

TABLE 106.1

ANKLE-BRACHIAL INDEX AND PERIPHERAL ARTERIAL DISEASE

ABI	PAD severity
≥0.9	Normal
≥0.7–0.9	Mild
≥0.4–0.7	Moderate
<0.4	Severe (critical limb ischemia)

ABI, ankle-brachial index; PAD, peripheral arterial disease.

Noninvasive Assessment of Peripheral Vascular Disease

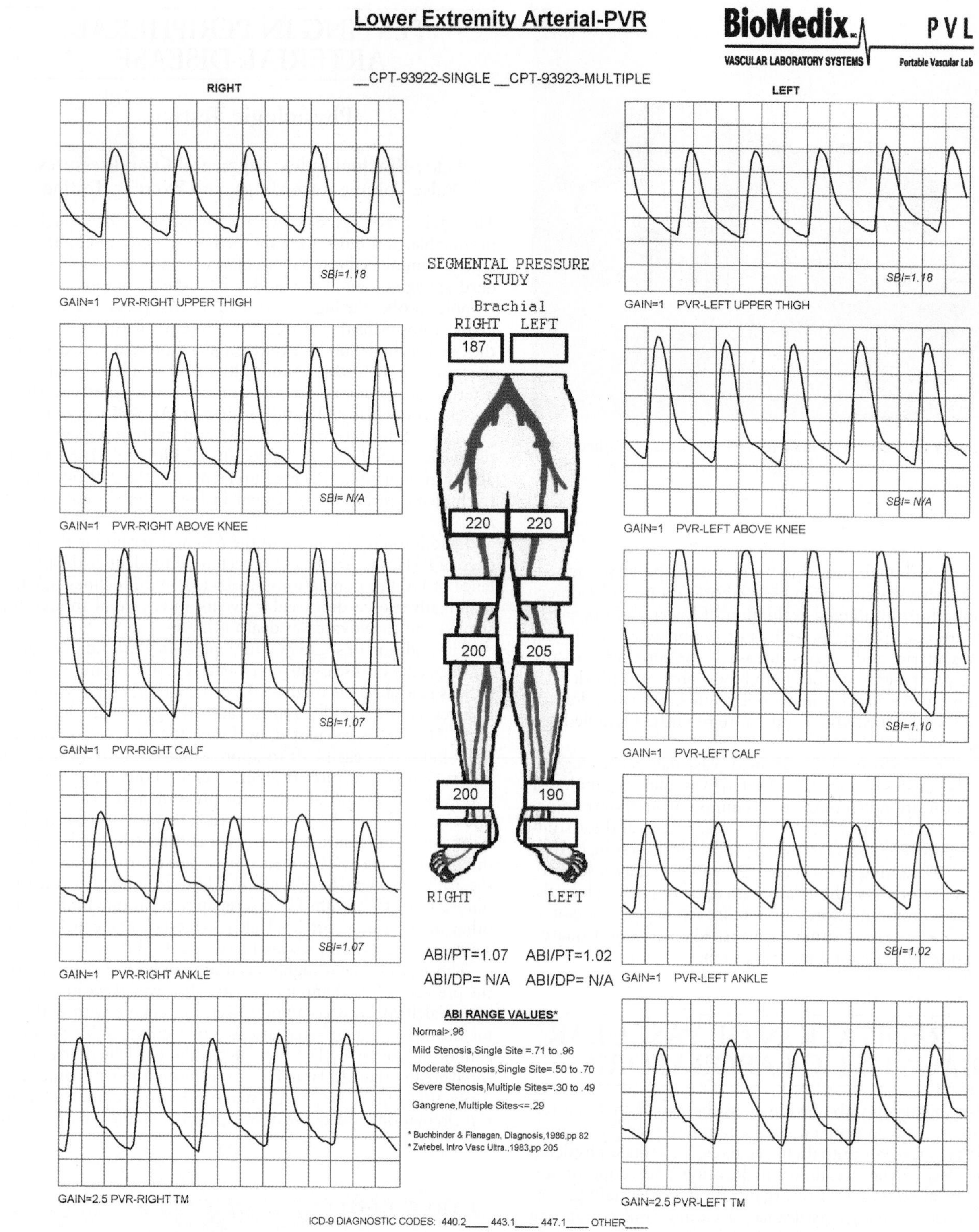

FIGURE 106.2. Report of a study including ankle-brachial index (ABI), segmental limb pressures, and pulse volume recordings (PVR) at rest. This represents a normal study. Note the normal ABIs bilaterally. DP, dorsalis pedis artery; PT, posterior tibial artery.

this situation, other tests are available in the vascular diagnostic laboratory, including photoplethysmography, digital pressures, arterial DUS, and even assessments of wound healing potential utilizing transcutaneous oximetry. Digital pressures are most commonly utilized in this situation (6). Absolute measurements of digital pressures (using photoplethysmography) lower than 30 mm Hg in association with diminished pulse wave amplitudes in the digit suggest inadequate arterial circulation to promote wound healing (7).

Pulse volume recordings (PVRs) are plethysmographic tracings that detect the changes in the volume of blood flowing through a limb. Using similar equipment as described previously, the cuffs are inflated to 65 mm Hg, and a plethysmographic tracing is recorded at various levels (8). The normal

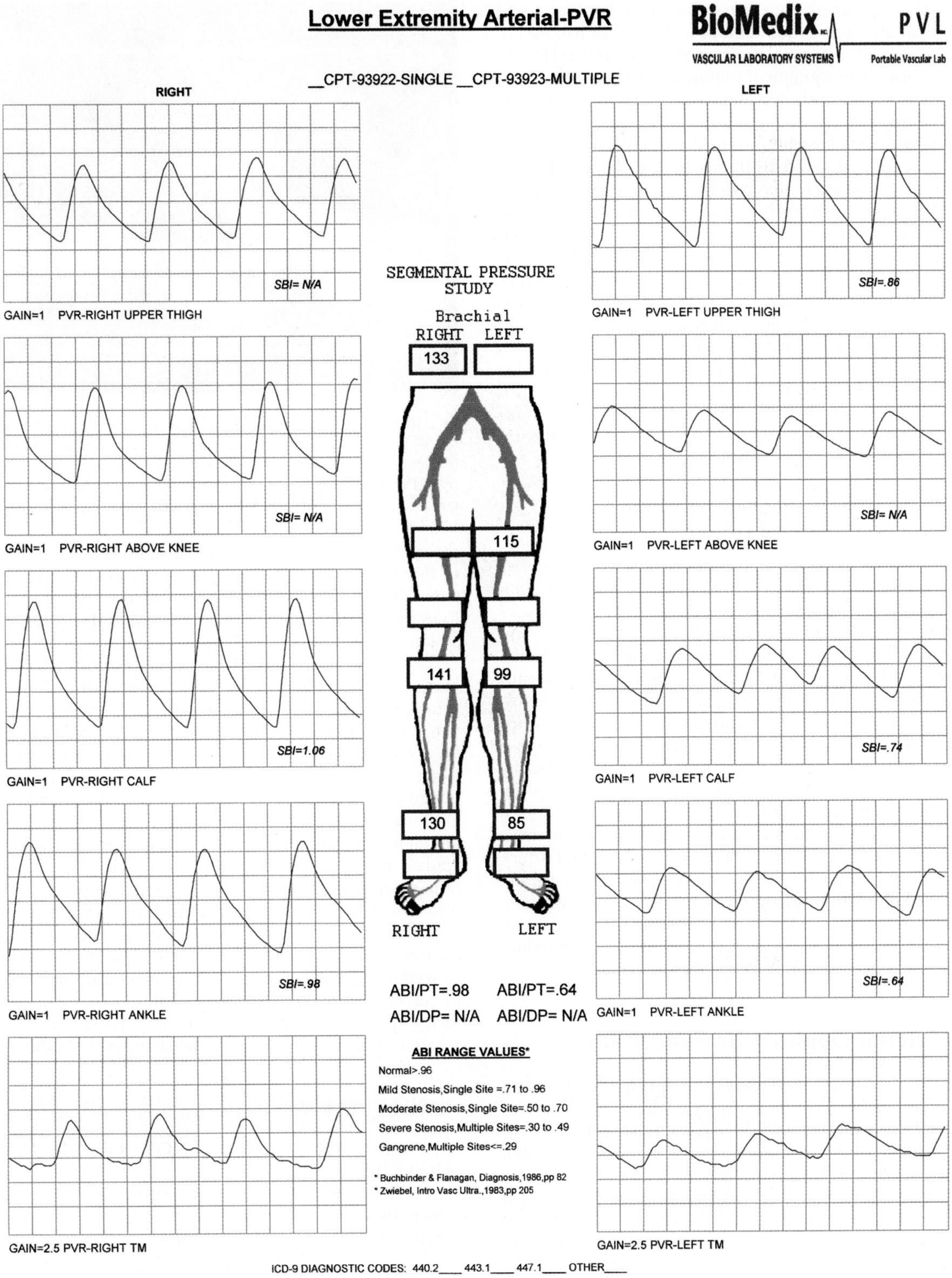

FIGURE 106.3. Report of a physiologic lower extremity arterial circulation test. The right leg ankle-brachial index (ABI) is normal. The left leg ABI is 0.64, representing moderate arterial disease. Segmental pressures and pulse volume waveforms (PVR) demonstrate left superficial femoral artery disease, with abnormal thigh and calf waveforms and a reduction in arterial pressure on the left calf compared with the right calf (99 versus 141 mmHg). DP, dorsalis pedis artery; PT, posterior tibial artery.

PVR is similar to the normal arterial pulse wave tracing and consists of a rapid systolic upstroke and rapid downstroke, with a prominent dicrotic notch. With increasing severity of disease, the waveform becomes more attenuated, with a wide downslope and, ultimately, virtually absent waveforms. An example of normal right leg PVR and segmental pressure tracings and abnormal left leg tracings suggestive of left superficial femoral artery disease is shown (Fig. 106.3).

ABIs, segmental pressures, and PVRs are useful objective tests in patients with suspected PAD, in those with limb discomfort without an obvious cause, as a method of evaluating the success of an intervention, and as a method of follow-up. The test is inexpensive, painless, reproducible, and relatively easy to perform. The equipment required to perform these examinations is significantly less expensive than modern color flow DUS units.

Patients with classic symptoms of PAD may have a normal physical examination and ABI. In this setting, the astute clinician must pursue an exercise physiology study performed in a vascular diagnostic laboratory. Resting pressures are measured, and the patient is then placed on a treadmill at a constant speed and constant grade of incline (commonly 2.0 miles per hour at an incline of 12.0%). The patient is asked to report initial symptoms of limb discomfort, and then the exercise is terminated when the discomfort is limiting. Following exercise, ankle and arm pressures are again measured. A significant decrease in postexercise pressure confirms the diagnosis of PAD and also characterizes the functional limitation of the symptoms (9). When treadmill testing is unavailable, or if the patient is unable to perform treadmill walking, active pedal plantarflexion is a reliable surrogate exercise test (10).

Provocative Testing in Upper Extremity Arterial Disease

Atherosclerosis is uncommon in the upper extremity arteries other than at the origin and proximal aspect of the subclavian artery. Thoracic outlet syndrome is a common nonatherosclerotic upper extremity vascular disorder. Although there are several pathophysiologic types, the most common syndrome occurs when a cervical rib or ligament compresses the sheath encompassing the subclavian artery, vein, and brachial plexus. Although most patients present with vague neurologic symptoms, approximately 10% of patients may present with upper extremity venous thrombosis, and 2% present with arterial ischemia, either from direct compression or as a result of emboli from a proximal aneurysm (11).

The physical diagnostic test known as the Adson maneuver may detect some qualitative alteration in the radial artery pulse when compared with the neutral position. However, using digital photoplethysmography in the vascular diagnostic laboratory, arterial waveforms can be assessed in the neutral and provocative positions to demonstrate an objective reduction in arterial circulation during the Adson maneuver.

Arterial Duplex Ultrasonography

Ultrasound is the use of sound waves at frequencies higher than those that can be heard by humans (typically >20,000 cycles per second [Hz]). Commercially available ultrasound units generate frequencies of 2 to 10 million cycles per second (MHz). When an electronic voltage is transmitted to an oscillator, a crystal vibrates and emits an ultrasound beam with a defined frequency in the range of 2 to 10 MHz. The ultrasound beam hits various targets in its path (i.e., soft tissue, bone, and flowing blood) and is reflected back to the crystal (12).

Ultrasound units available today use B-mode ("brightness") technology to provide a real-time, gray-scale image. High-frequency probes (i.e., 10 MHz) provide excellent image resolution; however, the beam attenuates rapidly and cannot penetrate depths. Low-frequency probes (i.e., 2 MHz) penetrate to visualize deeper structures, while sacrificing image resolution. DUS refers to B-mode real-time imaging and focused analysis of the velocity of flowing blood in arteries and veins.

Christian Doppler described the physics of ultrasonography by identifying the Doppler shift (13). Using variables of velocity of flowing blood, velocity of sound in tissue, the difference between the frequency of transmitted and reflected sound, and the cosine of the angle of the ultrasound beam to the direction of flowing blood, the velocity of blood in vessels can be measured. This is the basis for all vascular ultrasonography and allows modern ultrasonographers to quantitate degrees of stenosis based on the velocity of blood in various segments of vessels.

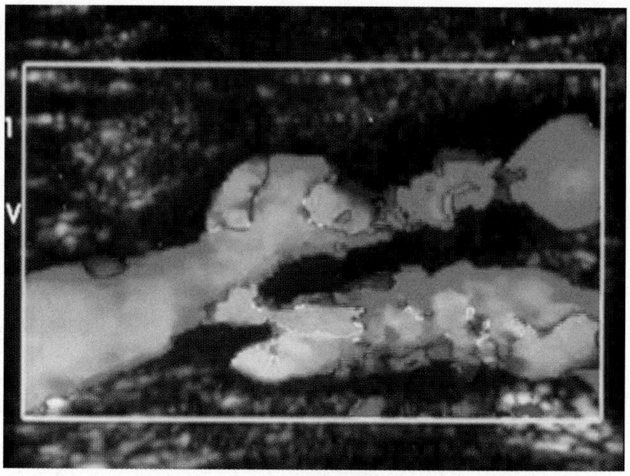

FIGURE 106.4. Color duplex ultrasonography of the bifurcation of the right common femoral into the superficial femoral and profunda femoris artery. Note the significant atherosclerotic plaque extending from the distal common femoral into the origin and proximal superficial femoral and profunda femoris arteries.

Native vessel arterial DUS is widely performed. This examination is generally accepted as a method of defining arterial stenoses or occlusions (Fig. 106.4). The sensitivity of DUS to detect occlusions and stenoses has been reported to be 95% and 92%, with specificities of 99% and 97%, respectively (14). Limitations have included tandem stenoses (15), tibial vessel imaging (16), and difficulty imaging the inflow arteries (17).

Using a 5.0- to 7.5-MHz transducer, imaging of the suprainguinal and infrainguinal arteries is performed. The vessels are studied in the sagittal plane, and Doppler velocities are obtained using a 60-degree Doppler angle. Vessels are classified into one of five categories: normal; 1% to 19% stenosis, 20% to 49% stenosis, 50% to 99% stenosis, and occlusion. The categories are determined by alterations in the Doppler waveform, as well as increasing peak systolic velocities. For a stenosis to be classified as 50% to 99%, for example, the peak systolic velocity must increase by 100% in comparison with the normal segment of artery proximal to the stenosis (18) (Table 106.2).

TABLE 106.2

DUPLEX ULTRASOUND STENOSIS OF PERIPHERAL ARTERIES

Stenosis category (%)	Doppler waveform	Doppler velocities
Normal	Triphasic	PSV <200 cm/s
1–19	Triphasic with spectral broadening	PSV <200 cm/s
20–49	Spectral broadening	PSV <200 cm/s +SVR[a] >30%
50–99	Spectral broadening	SVR >100% PSV >200 cm/s
Occluded	Absent waveform	N/A

PSV, peak systolic velocity; SVR, systolic velocity ratio.
[a]Systolic velocity ratio: PSV in area of stenosis compared with PSV in normal arterial segment proximal to stenosis.

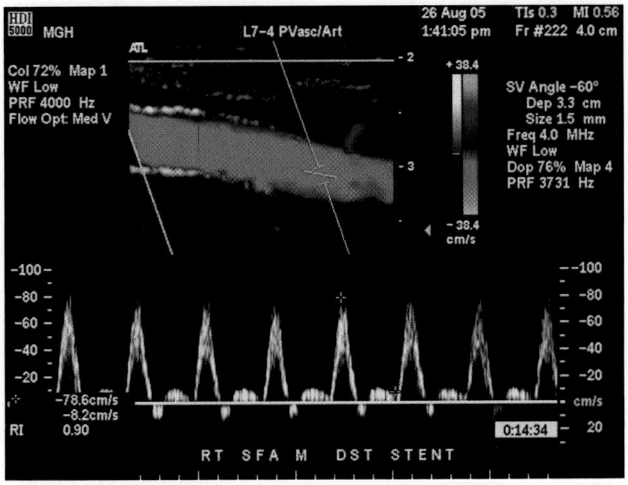

FIGURE 106.5. Duplex ultrasonography of a superficial femoral artery stent. Note the normal triphasic Doppler waveform within the stent, with a normal peak systolic velocity (78.6 cm per second). The *bright white parallel lines* represent the margins of the stent. DST, distal; M, mid; RT, right; SFA, superficial femoral artery.

Arterial DUS has been used to guide the interventionist toward appropriate access to a lesion potentially amenable to endovascular therapy (19). This technology has also been used after endovascular therapy to determine technical success (20) and durability of the procedure (21) (Fig. 106.5). Unfortunately, it appears that DUS soon after balloon angioplasty may overestimate residual stenosis, and it may be a limitation of this technology after endovascular therapy (22).

In patients who have undergone surgical bypass graft revascularization, particularly with saphenous vein, stenoses will develop in 21% to 33% of cases. Once the graft becomes thrombosed, secondary patency rates are dismal. If the stenosis is detected and repaired before graft thrombosis, it is estimated that 80% of grafts will be salvaged (23). A well-organized graft surveillance program is crucial in preserving patency of the bypass graft (Fig. 106.6). In one series of 170 saphenous vein bypass grafts, 110 stenoses were detected over a 39-month period. In those patients with grafts who underwent surgical revision once a stenosis was detected, the 4-year patency was 88%, whereas in those patients with grafts who did not undergo surgical revision despite the detection of a stenosis, the 4-year patency was 57% (24). The use of an intensive surveillance program has been less beneficial in patients with prosthetic grafts (25).

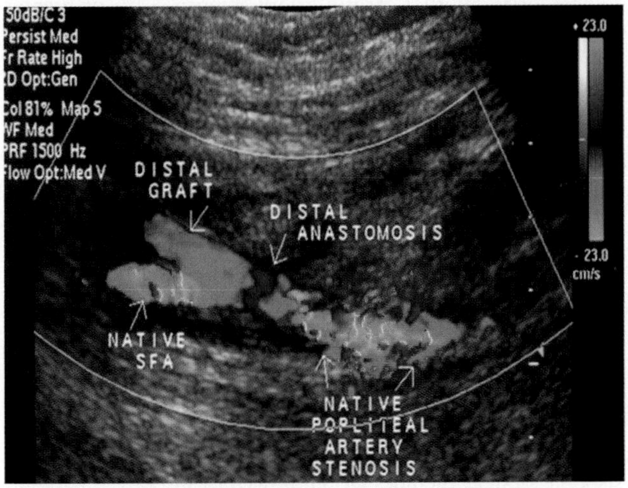

FIGURE 106.6. Surveillance color duplex ultrasonography of the distal aspect of a femoral-popliteal bypass graft. Note the marked turbulence within the distal native popliteal artery, suggestive of significant stenosis distal to the bypass graft. SFA, superficial femoral artery.

The procedure for graft surveillance resembles that used in native vessel arterial DUS. The inflow artery to the bypass graft is initially imaged using a 5.0- to 7.5-MHz transducer and a Doppler angle of 60 degrees. Subsequently, the proximal anastomosis, proximal, medial, and distal graft, distal anastomosis, and outflow artery are interrogated. Peak systolic and end-diastolic velocities are obtained at each segment and are compared with the segment of graft proximal to the area being studied. If the ratio of the peak systolic velocity within a stenotic segment relative to the normal segment proximal to the stenosis is greater than 2, this suggests a 50% to 75% diameter reduction. The addition of end-diastolic velocities faster than 100 cm per second suggests greater than 75% stenosis (26).

Vein bypass grafts should be studied within 7 days of formation and then in 1 month, followed by 3-month intervals for the first year. If the graft remains normal after year 1, follow-up surveillance should be done every 6 months thereafter. Ankle pressures and waveforms should be performed at the time of each surveillance study. The development of a stenosis during a surveillance examination should prompt consideration of arteriography, either with contrast or utilizing magnetic resonance (MR) technology (27). Arterial DUS has recently demonstrated utility in determining patency of endovascular devices and procedures in multicenter clinical trials (28).

TESTING IN CAROTID ARTERY DISEASE

Carotid Duplex Ultrasonography

Although physicians have known that significant stenosis of the internal carotid artery can lead to transient cerebral ischemia and stroke, and that fully one third of all strokes are the result of extracranial carotid stenosis, it was not known until recently that surgical endarterectomy of carotid stenosis decreases the incidence of these neurologic events in symptomatic and asymptomatic patients (29,30). It is now generally accepted that patients with symptoms of cerebral ischemia referable to a 70% to 99% internal carotid stenosis have lower subsequent stroke risk after carotid endarterectomy than with medical therapy alone. There remains some controversy over asymptomatic patients with 60% to 99% internal carotid artery stenosis (31).

To add to the debate, more recently, carotid artery stenting with embolic protection devices have demonstrated similar safety and efficacy when compared with patients with high-grade carotid stenosis, either with or without symptoms (32).

Carotid DUS (CDUS) is widely accepted as the initial diagnostic test for patients suspected of having extracranial carotid artery disease. Initially performed using real-time B-mode imaging with pulsed Doppler, accuracy was excellent (97%) (33). With the addition of color-coded imaging, CDUS is now widely used and reproducible from site to site. CDUS has clarified the natural history of cervical bruits (34) and has defined restenosis rates after carotid endarterectomy (35) and carotid artery stenting (36).

The technique of CDUS has been standardized. Using a 5.0- or 7.5-MHz linear-array transducer in most cases, the common carotid artery is identified in both the transverse and

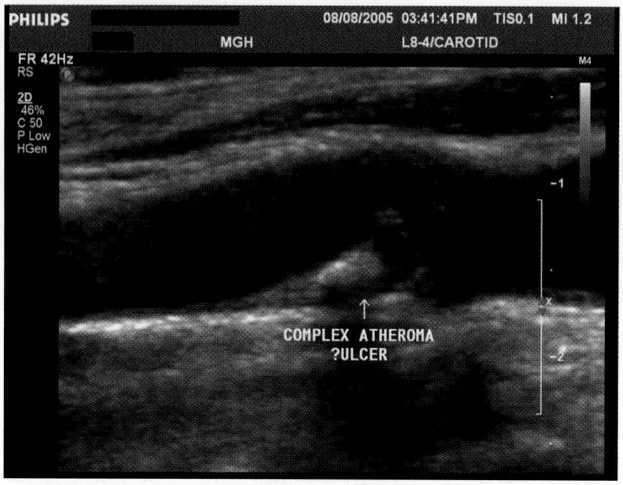

FIGURE 106.7. Gray-scale duplex ultrasound examination of a complex heterogeneous plaque in the origin of the internal carotid artery. There is evidence of a ruptured fibrous cap with an echolucent central region, suggestive of a lipid-rich core and ulceration. 2D, two-dimensional; SFA, superficial femoral artery.

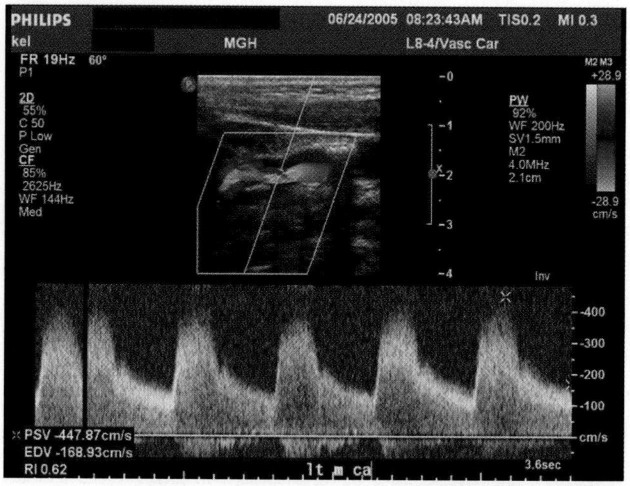

FIGURE 106.9. Color duplex ultrasound image of a critical (80% to 99%) internal carotid artery stenosis. Note the following: peak systolic velocity (PSV), 448 cm per second; end-diastolic velocity (EDV), 169 cm per second. There is marked color turbulence within the area of maximal stenosis. 2D, two-dimensional; lt ca, left carotid; RI, resistive index.

sagittal planes. The location and quantity of plaque are documented in each segment of the common, internal, and external carotid arteries (Fig. 106.7). Attempts at discerning varying types of plaque morphology and identifying plaque ulceration have been suggested as being reliable utilizing DUS; however, this remains controversial (37).

Determination of the plaque composition using high-resolution gray-scale imaging correlates well with histopathologic findings and may assist in predicting "vulnerable plaque" in the future (38). In addition, in a very large prospective CDUS study performed in more than 1,200 patients followed for a median of 7.5 months, progressive carotid stenosis found on CDUS correlated well with serologic markers of atherosclerosis (39).

An emerging role of CDUS is the measurement of carotid intima-media thickness (IMT). The methodology of carotid IMT has been described and utilizes the gray-scale appearance of the "double-line density" of the intima-media complex and the adventitia of the artery (40) (Fig. 106.8). The carotid IMT has correlated in multiple prospective multicenter epidemiology and natural history studies with an increased risk of major

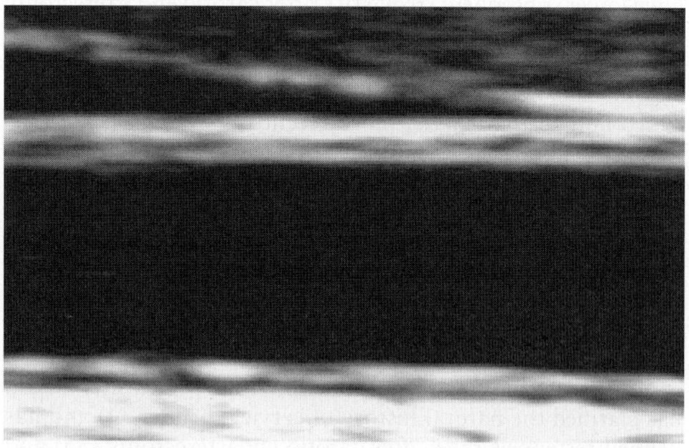

FIGURE 106.8. Gray-scale duplex ultrasound image of the common carotid artery demonstrating the intima-media interface. This is the image commonly used for measurement of carotid intima-media thickness.

cardiovascular events and cardiovascular mortality (41). Although not currently reimbursed in the United States for clinical risk prediction, the emergence of automated acquisition software will facilitate reliable data and interpretation and will likely result in the utility of carotid IMT as a useful predictor of cardiovascular risk (42).

Real-time gray-scale, B-mode imaging, and Doppler analysis of the carotid bifurcation, proximal, medial, and distal internal carotid artery, the proximal external carotid artery, and the vertebral artery is performed. The addition of color imaging facilitates identification of stenotic segments of a vessel and shortens the examination time. Using a Doppler angle optimized to 60 degrees, and parallel to the direction of arterial flow, Doppler waveforms, peak systolic, and end-diastolic velocities are obtained in each segment (Fig. 106.9). Degrees of stenosis are based on these velocities and on waveform analysis (Table 106.3).

Since publication of the Asymptomatic Carotid Atherosclerosis Trial (43), criteria devised to improve the accuracy of DUS to categorize internal carotid artery stenosis 60% or greater have been proposed. These criteria emphasize the peak systolic and end-diastolic velocity within the internal carotid artery, and calculating ratios within the internal carotid artery and ipsilateral distal common carotid artery, yielding 100% accuracy for determining this degree of stenosis if all criteria are met (44). Carotid duplex is also quite accurate for diagnosing carotid occlusion, with a positive predictive value of 92.5% (45).

A multispecialty consensus panel of experts reviewed the entire published body of literature and developed a series of recommendations for the performance and interpretation of CDUS examinations (46). Although there may be some disagreement in specific ultrasound criteria, this document provides important recommendations for standardization techniques for CDUS.

There is some disagreement about the appropriate algorithm for the diagnosis of extracranial carotid artery stenosis. One strategy includes DUS followed by intraarterial digital subtraction arteriography (IADSA). Other algorithms suggest that DUS be followed by MR arteriography (MRA), with IADSA saved for those studies which do not correlate (47) (Fig. 106.10). Still other investigators suggest that DUS alone

TABLE 106.3

GRADING OF CAROTID ARTERY STENOSIS WITH DUPLEX ULTRASONOGRAPHY

Stenosis severity (%)	Doppler waveform	PSV (cm/s)	EDV+ (cm/s)
0–19	Normal low resistant	<105	—
20–39	Spectral broadening	<105	—
40–59	Spectral broadening	≥105, ≤150	—
60–79	Spectral broadening	>150, ≤220[a]	—
80–99	Spectral broadening	>220	>135
Occluded	No waveform; preocclusive wall "thump"		

EDV, end-diastolic velocity; PSV, peak systolic velocity.
[a]Some use the ratio of the PSV in the internal carotid artery (ICA) compared with the distal common carotid artery (CCA) to subdivide this category into >70% stenosis (ICA/CCA PSV ratio >4.0).

can accurately determine the degree of carotid stenosis (47). With the inclusion of carotid artery stenting into the therapeutic milieu, the current strategy will likely evolve to CDUS followed by cerebral angiography. Every diagnostic algorithm assumes, however, that the examination is performed by a qualified ultrasonographer in a vascular laboratory that continues to monitor accuracy (49).

CDUS is the initial examination of choice in patients with hemispheric neurologic symptoms, a cervical bruit, and previous carotid revascularization. Patients with suspected carotid dissection or trauma or who have symptoms suggested of vertebrobasilar insufficiency or subclavian steal phenomena should be evaluated with DUS. With increasing interest in endovascular therapy for carotid stenosis, DUS is an ideal method of studying stent patency (Fig. 106.11).

Limitations of carotid duplex includes acoustic shadowing from calcific atherosclerotic plaque, which inhibits Doppler spectral waveform interrogation, false elevation in peak systolic velocity with contralateral internal carotid artery occlusion, and artifactually increased peak systolic velocities in tortuous internal carotid arteries.

There are no well-studied duplex criteria to grade stenosis within carotid stents during surveillance. In a recent report of the Carotid and Vertebral Transluminal Angioplasty Study (CAVATAS) trial, a prospective randomized trial of endovascular therapy versus surgery for extracranial carotid artery disease, restenosis was defined with identical criteria used for native vessel carotid arteries (43).

Transcranial Carotid Doppler Analysis

Neurologists have long appreciated the role of transcranial Doppler (TCD) analysis in the evaluation of intracerebral vasoconstriction after subarachnoid hemorrhage and the assessment of brain death in critically ill patients. This has now become standard practice. However, the utility of TCD analysis in the evaluation of large artery extracranial carotid artery stenosis and its impact in therapeutic decision making have remained controversial. Many vascular diagnostic laboratories routinely perform TCD analysis when a significant extracranial carotid artery stenosis has been identified on CDUS. TCD analysis provides relevant hemodynamic information on the direction of major branches arising from the circle of Willis, thereby reflecting the significance of a bifurcation internal carotid artery stenosis. In addition, TCD analysis reliably detects cerebral emboli (high-intensity transient signals) (50). High-intensity

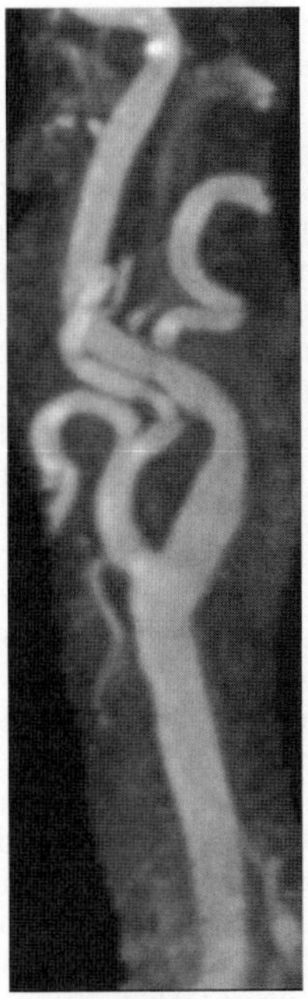

FIGURE 106.10. Magnetic resonance arteriogram of a normal carotid artery bifurcation. This was gadolinium enhanced.

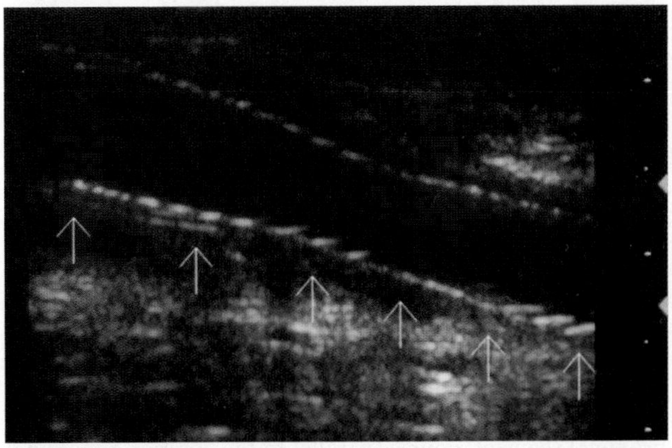

FIGURE 106.11. Gray-scale duplex ultrasound image of a carotid artery stent. The *bright parallel lines (arrows)* represent the struts of the stent.

transient signals have been shown to predict stroke and transient ischemic attacks reliably in patients with symptomatic extracranial carotid artery stenosis (51). Recently, TCD analysis has been utilized to assess the necessity for embolic protection devices during carotid artery stent deployment (52).

TCD analysis is performed with a low-frequency Doppler probe and is successful when an "acoustic bone window" is identified. For example, the transtemporal window allows for reliable interrogation of the middle cerebral artery. Doppler spectral analysis is performed at a 0-degree Doppler angle, because visualization of the flow jet is rarely possible. There are multiple grading scales for interpretation of intracranial artery stenosis; however, in many cases, retrograde flow in an ophthalmic artery, for example, confirms the hemodynamic relevance of a bifurcation internal carotid artery stenosis.

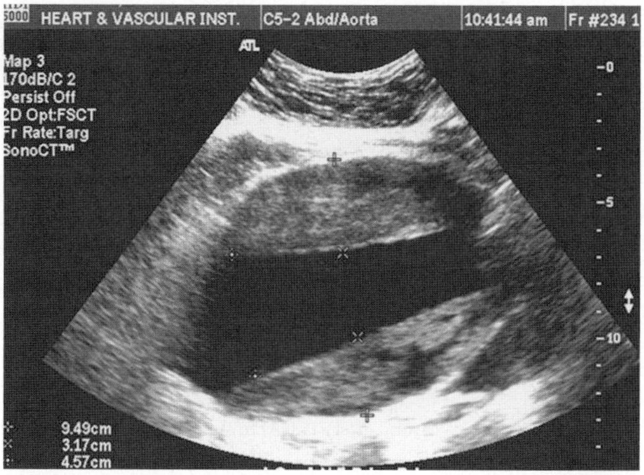

FIGURE 106.12. Gray-scale longitudinal duplex ultrasound image of a large abdominal aortic aneurysm. The maximal diameter of the abdominal aortic aneurysm is 9.49 cm. There is extensive thrombus formation within the aneurysm.

ABDOMINAL AORTIC DUPLEX ULTRASONOGRAPHY

Although atherosclerotic plaque in the abdominal aorta is common, the finding of a significant abdominal aortic stenosis is uncommon. There are no well-defined Doppler-derived velocity criteria that reliably predict the severity of an abdominal aortic stenosis.

The more common pathologic process studied by vascular diagnostic laboratories in the abdominal aorta is aneurysm formation. Abdominal aortic aneurysms (AAAs) represent a major cause of mortality in the United States. A recent consensus document suggested the role of DUS in the screening of patients at risk for AAA (53).

Most vascular diagnostic laboratories perform abdominal aortic DUS after an overnight fast to reduce overlying bowel gas. A low-frequency ultrasound transducer (2.4 MHz) is needed to improve depth of penetration. Commonly, curved deep abdominal probes are used to facilitate complete visualization of the abdominal aorta. A midrange transducer (4 to 8 MHz) is typically used for femoral or popliteal aneurysms. The examination of an aneurysm should be focused on determining the aneurysmal size, shape, location (suprarenal, juxtarenal, or infrarenal), and distance from other arterial segments.

Ultrasound scanning of the abdominal aorta begins in the supine position. To facilitate accurate measure of its size, two sonographic views are usually obtained of the abdominal aorta: the sagittal (anteroposterior diameter) and coronal planes (longitudinal and transverse diameters) (Fig. 106.12). The transducer must be oriented so the maximal length of the segment is visualized. By design, in the sagittal view, the cephalad portion is oriented to the left of the imaging screen. Once one has obtained sagittal images identifying the location of the abdominal aorta, the presence or absence of atherosclerotic plaque and aneurysm formation, and the location of the mesenteric and renal arterial branches, the transducer is then rotated 90 degrees to achieve a coronal view. If overlying bowel gas obstructs the aorta from view, patients are instructed to lie in the lateral decubitus position, and the aorta is visualized via either flank.

The celiac artery arises in an anterior orientation from the aorta as the first abdominal aortic branch, and is a very short vessel. It immediately branches into the common hepatic and splenic arteries. The superior mesenteric artery (SMA) arises as the second major abdominal aortic arterial branch and, in its proximal segment, courses parallel to the anterior abdominal aorta. Just caudal to the SMA, the right renal artery arises and, after a brief anterior course, dives in a posterior orientation to the inferior vena cava.

An AAA is defined as an aortic diameter of at least 1.5 times the diameter of the aorta measured at the level of the renal arteries. A normal diameter of the abdominal aorta is approximately 2.0 cm (range, 1.4 to 3.0 cm) in most individuals; a diameter larger than 3.0 cm is considered aneurysmal. A mildly dilated abdominal aorta is described as ectatic.

AAAs are described as saccular, fusiform, or cylindric. Most AAAs are fusiform in shape, are located in the infrarenal position, and may involve one or both iliac arteries. Atherosclerotic changes and/or mural thrombus commonly line the aneurysm sac. Dissection has been reported with an AAA, but it is less common. The typical growth rate reported in the literature of AAAs measuring 3 to 5.9 cm is approximately 0.3 to 0.4 cm per year. However, larger AAAs may progress more quickly than smaller AAAs, whereas some AAAs may remain dormant and then expand rapidly.

Repair of AAA commonly is considered when the maximal outer wall diameter of the AAA exceeds 4.9 cm (54). Some investigators have suggested lack of benefit until the AAA exceeds 5.5 cm (55).

Given the evolving role of endoluminal abdominal aortic stent graft therapy as an alternative to standard vascular surgical repair of AAA (56), other components of DUS must be provided. Aside from the location of the AAA in relation to the renal arteries, attempts at measuring the distance from the renal artery axis to the proximal aspect of the AAA are important. The patency and tortuosity of the iliac arteries need to be noted because currently available endoluminal devices are deployed via surgical exposure of the common femoral artery and passage in retrograde fashion into the AAA.

Ultrasound surveillance of AAA is commonly performed. Patients whose aneurysms are deemed not of the size for repair are enrolled in surveillance DUS programs at a frequency of 6 to 12 months to observe growth of the aneurysm. After surgical repair, surveillance is not routinely performed, given the excellent durability of this procedure. However, following endoluminal grafting of AAA, surveillance is required to ensure regression of the aneurysm sac and to detect endoleak, with the development of systemic arterial pressure within the native aneurysm sac. Although helical computed tomography (CT) is the common method of surveillance for endografts, some centers have adopted DUS because this avoids iodinated contrast and significant external-beam radiation exposure to patients (57). The addition of ultrasound contrast agents via

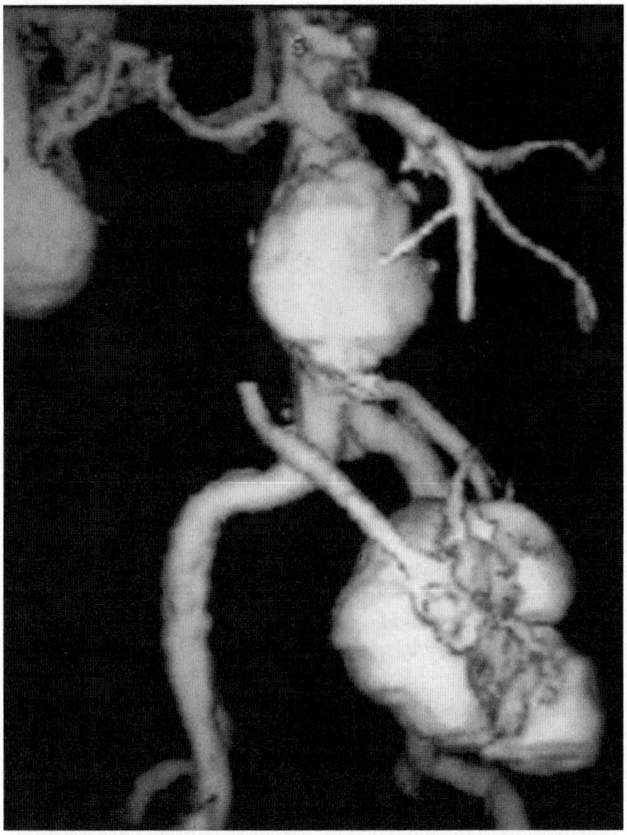

FIGURE 106.13. Surface shaded three-dimensional computed tomographic arteriogram of an infrarenal abdominal (Abd) aortic aneurysm.

a peripheral vein may improve the accuracy of DUS in this clinical situation (Fig. 106.13).

RENAL ARTERY DUPLEX ULTRASONOGRAPHY

Atherosclerotic renal artery stenosis has become increasingly recognized as a contributing factor to resistant hypertension (58), and it may promote deterioration in renal function. Patients with severe bilateral renal artery stenosis, or stenosis to a solitary functioning kidney, are at risk for the development of end-stage renal disease (59). Long-term survival of patients with atherosclerotic renal artery stenosis requiring dialysis support is dismal (60). Although numerous noninvasive methods of diagnosis in renal artery stenosis have been proposed, none have obviated the role of the "gold standard," renal arteriography. Each screening test has significant limitations that prevent widespread acceptance. Renal artery DUS has significant advantages that make it an excellent diagnostic test.

Current reimbursement rules provide payment if a renal artery DUS examination is performed for the indication of renal artery stenosis. DUS is the ideal method of determining the adequacy of revascularization (61). Given the proliferation of endovascular therapy (percutaneous angioplasty with stent deployment) (62), DUS is helpful in detecting important areas of restenosis. Appropriate indications for performance of this test include the following:

- Sudden exacerbation of previously well-controlled hypertension
- New-onset hypertension at a young age
- Malignant hypertension
- Unexplained azotemia
- Hypertension and aortoiliac or infrainguinal atherosclerosis
- Azotemia after administration of an angiotensin converting enzyme inhibitor
- An atrophic kidney
- Recurrent flash pulmonary edema without cardiac explanation

Renal artery DUS requires a vascular technologist who has demonstrated dedication to perfecting the procedure, as well as the best current ultrasound equipment. Patients are instructed to fast from midnight before the examination. Each study must be performed in the early morning, and patients are instructed to take their morning medications with small sips of liquid. If significant bowel gas is identified, the study is terminated, the patient is given simethicone, and the examination is rescheduled for another morning. A low-frequency (2.25- to 3.5-MHz) pulsed Doppler transducer is required for adequate deep abdominal imaging. The addition of color imaging will increase the ease with which the renal arteries are identified.

The examination is started with the patient supine and in reverse Trendelenburg positioning. The aorta is scanned in the longitudinal view from the diaphragm to the aortic bifurcation. The presence of atherosclerotic plaque and aneurysmal dilation is noted. The origin of the celiac, superior, and inferior mesenteric arteries is defined. A Doppler velocity is obtained at the level of the SMA, in the center stream of arterial flow, and at a 60-degree angle. This velocity is recorded and will be used as the denominator for renal-to-aortic velocity ratio calculations (Fig. 106.14).

The transducer is then reoriented into the transverse plane, and the celiac artery and SMA are noted arising from the anterior aspect of the aorta. In 75% of patients, the left renal vein crosses anterior to the abdominal aorta as it enters the inferior vena cava. These two ultrasound landmarks (origin of the SMA and left renal vein crossing anterior to the aorta) are important for the identification of the right renal artery. The right renal artery arises from the anterior aorta and then courses in posterior fashion as it enters the hilum of the kidney. The left renal artery generally arises inferior to the right and takes a posterior course. The Doppler cursor, at a 60-degree angle (or less), is placed within the aorta and is then "walked" into the ostium of the right renal artery. Peak systolic and end-diastolic velocities are obtained in the origin, proximal, medial, and, if possible from this orientation, distal renal artery

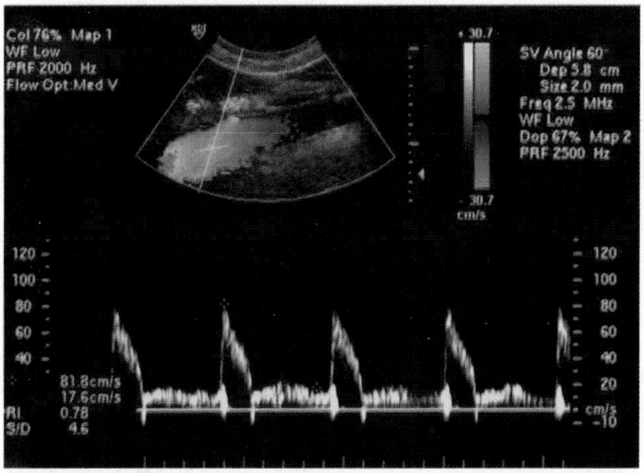

FIGURE 106.14. Color duplex ultrasound image of normal Doppler velocities within the abdominal aorta. RI, resistive index; SV, systolic velocity.

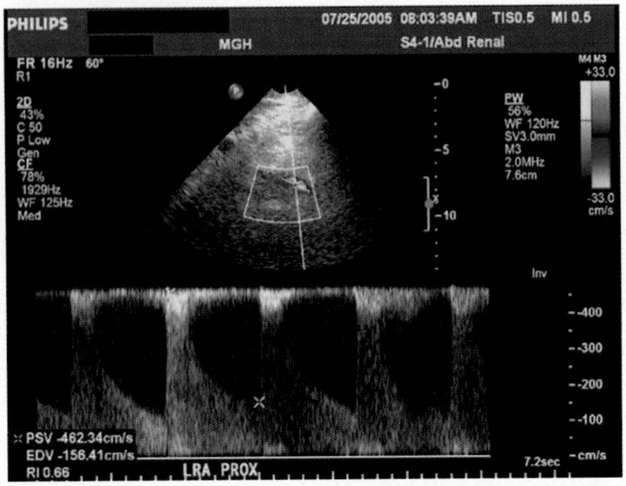

FIGURE 106.15. Color duplex ultrasound image of 60% to 99% left renal artery (LRA) stenosis. Note the following: peak systolic velocity (PSV), 462 cm per second; end-diastolic velocity (EDV), 156 cm per second. 2D, two-dimensional; Abd, abdominal; PROX, proximal; RI, resistive index; SV, systolic velocity.

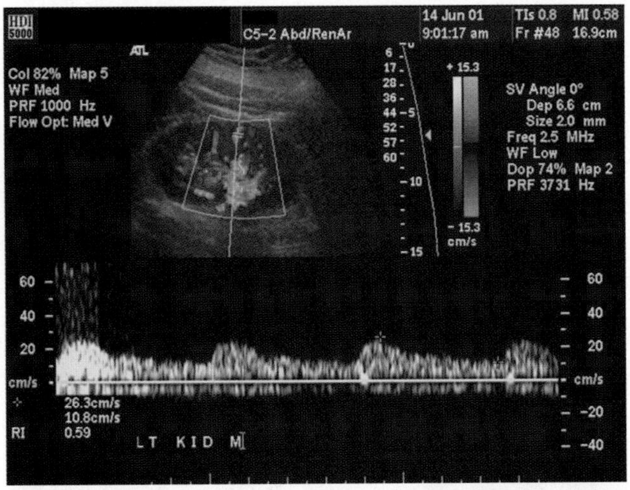

FIGURE 106.16. Color duplex ultrasound image of the kidney (KID) demonstrating a normal renal resistive index (RI). The renal RI is 0.59. Abd, abdominal; LT, left; SV, systolic velocity.

(Fig. 106.15). The renal artery Doppler waveform has a characteristic low-resistance signal, with significant forward diastolic flow. Similar measurements are obtained from the left renal artery. It is critical that the entire renal artery is visualized, so a focal stenosis or web (in the case of fibromuscular dysplasia) is not overlooked. Both renal veins are noted to be patent or occluded.

The patient is then placed in the left lateral decubitus position, and the right kidney is visualized from the flank. Three discrete measurements of the pole-to-pole length of the kidney are recorded, in centimeters. Doppler velocities in the cortex, medulla, and hilum of the kidney are recorded at a 0-degree angle, with a large sample volume, because discrete parenchymal vessels are difficult to identify. The Doppler transducer is then moved slightly anteriorly, and attempts are made to visualize the entire right renal artery from the aorta to the hilum of the right kidney. This "banana-peel" technique can be particularly helpful in imaging and analyzing the entire renal artery. A limitation of the banana peel approach on the right is the presence of the overlying inferior vena cava, a problem that does not occur on the contralateral side. This process is then repeated with the patient in the right lateral decubitus position, in an effort to interrogate the left kidney and the entire left renal artery.

A greater than 60% renal artery stenosis is characterized by a renal-to-aortic peak velocity ratio of more than 3.5, with a peak systolic velocity within the stenosis faster than 180 cm per second. End-diastolic velocities faster than 150 cm per second suggest a subgroup of stenoses ranging from 80% to 99%. A critical renal artery stenosis may actually reveal low systolic flow, with significant poststenotic turbulence, and a color mosaic appearance on the two-dimensional color image. An occluded renal artery demonstrates no flow in the affected vessel, a patent ipsilateral renal vein, and low parenchymal Doppler velocities in the ipsilateral kidney. In addition, the ipsilateral kidney is often small, less than 9 cm in length. Measurement of the resistive index (RI) may be helpful in determining renal parenchymal disease. At least three Doppler spectra are obtained from the various regions of each kidney. The RI is calculated using the formula, RI = systolic Vmax − diastolic Vmin/Vmax, where Vmax is maximum and Vmin is minimum velocity. Some investigators have postulated that in severe renal artery stenosis, if there is significant concomitant renal parenchymal disease, the end-diastolic velocity may not rise (63). Therefore, an RI greater than 0.80 suggests significant parenchymal renal disease (Fig. 106.16).

Obese patients, and patients with significant overlying bowel gas, pose the greatest difficulty for the sonographer. Multiple positions and aggressive preparation of the patient, along with breath holding, if possible, may facilitate a more accurate examination.

It is estimated that 30% of patients will have accessory or "polar" renal arteries, which are very difficult to identify on DUS. These arteries are often smaller in diameter than main renal arteries and may arise from any level of the abdominal aorta, as well as the iliac arteries. If these vessels are not obvious on color and Doppler imaging of the aorta, one other method of identifying accessory renal arteries is to compare the parenchymal waveforms obtained at different locations within the kidney. There may be changes in the contour of one Doppler spectral waveform compared with a waveform in a different segment of the kidney. This finding should prompt the ultrasonographer to look more aggressively for an accessory renal artery.

MESENTERIC ARTERY DUPLEX ULTRASONOGRAPHY

Mesenteric artery disease is an uncommon but potentially catastrophic disorder. In its acute form, most often as a result of an embolic event originating from a cardiac source, there is limited time for diagnosis and restoration of arterial flow before necrosis of bowel and death occurs. In the chronic form, patients may have postprandial abdominal pain, resulting in weight loss, failure to thrive, and malnutrition.

Vascular diagnostic laboratories are most often asked to diagnose the patency of the major arteries supplying circulation to the gut, including the celiac artery, SMA, and inferior mesenteric artery. Although many investigators have resorted to MRA and CT arteriography (CTA), DUS has demonstrated accuracy in confirming the status of the arterial supply to the gut.

Patients are asked to fast before the examination, commonly not a concern given the inability of these patients to eat. Low-frequency curved, phased-array (2- to 4-MHz) transducers are commonly used. Patients are examined while they are in the supine position, commonly using reverse Trendelenburg positioning. Initially, longitudinal gray-scale imaging of the abdominal aorta is performed to assess for the presence of atherosclerotic plaque and AAAs. With a Doppler angle correction of up to 60 degrees, Doppler waveforms at the origin and several centimeters into the proximal segments of the celiac artery and the SMA are obtained. Because of the small size of these arteries and the depth, color-coded DUS can be very helpful. The peak systolic and end-diastolic velocities are measured. Although challenging, attempts to identify the inferior mesenteric artery should be made. This artery arises a few centimeters proximal to the aortic bifurcation, often posterolaterally. The inferior mesenteric artery is smaller in diameter than the celiac artery and the SMA.

In the fasting state, the celiac artery supplies a low-resistant vascular bed, with preserved end-diastolic flow. The SMA supplies a high-resistant vascular bed, and therefore, fasting Doppler waveforms are high resistant. In the postprandial state, the gut becomes a low-resistant vascular bed, and the waveforms commonly demonstrate greater end-diastolic flow.

Several validated studies have established diagnostic criteria for mesenteric artery DUS. The most widely utilized, published by Moneta and colleagues, indicates that a peak systolic velocity faster than 275 cm per second in the SMA and faster than 200 cm per second in the celiac artery is abnormal, a finding suggesting a stenosis greater than 70% (64). Some investigators have suggested that an end-diastolic velocity faster than 45 cm per second is a more reliable predictor of greater than 50% stenosis, with sensitivities of 90% and specificity of 91% (65). Future use of ultrasound contrast agents may improve the accuracy of DUS of the mesenteric arteries (66).

VENOUS DUPLEX ULTRASONOGRAPHY

Deep vein thrombosis (DVT) is a common medical problem and a major cause of morbidity and mortality in the United States. It is estimated that 6 million U.S. residents suffer from venous thromboembolic disease annually. Unfortunately, relying on the symptoms or physical examination findings to secure the diagnosis of DVT will result in misdiagnosis in 50% of patients. The consequences of DVT include propagation of thrombus, embolization to the pulmonary vasculature (pulmonary embolus [PE]), and chronic obstruction of the deep veins with loss of venous valvular function, resulting in the postthrombosis syndrome (PTS) from chronic venous insufficiency (CVI). PE causes sudden death in 10% of patients within the first hour and may result in chronic thromboembolic pulmonary hypertension, a serious condition with limited therapeutic options. PTS is characterized by chronic lower extremity pain, edema, and ulceration of the lower extremities. PTS can develop in 30% of patients within 8 years of an initial thrombotic event (67).

Given effective pharmacotherapy to prevent propagation of thrombi and ultimate PE, early and reliable diagnosis of DVT is critical. Several imaging and laboratory modalities exist for diagnosing DVT: venous DUS, ascending venography, CT venography, D-dimer, nuclear medicine–based thrombus scanning, and MR venography.

Contrast venography remains the gold standard technique for the diagnosis of DVT, but it is infrequently performed since the advent of DUS (68). Venography remains an option when noninvasive testing is nondiagnostic or impossible to perform. It is accurate and generally safe, but it is an invasive and painful procedure that requires administration of iodinated contrast and carries a 1.3% risk of actually causing DVT (69).

DUS combines real time B-mode ("brightness mode") gray-scale, color-enhanced Doppler, and focused Doppler methods. The gray-scale B-mode image provides detailed imaging of the deep and superficial venous systems to visualize the direction of venous flow and to note the presence or absence of thrombus. DUS is routinely performed with medium frequency, linear-array transducers of 4 to 7 MHz. In morbidly obese patients, and for imaging of the pelvic veins and the inferior vena cava, a low-frequency phased- or curvilinear-array transducer of lower frequency (i.e., 4 MHz) is required.

The venous segments are visualized in the transverse plane proximal to the inguinal crease distally through the deep veins of the calf. Using the B-mode gray-scale image, segments of deep vein are gently compressed. If the walls of the vein coapt, this confirms a patent segment of vein. This process continues distally.

The venous DUS examination is positive for DVT if a segment of vein demonstrates noncompressibility. This is the most accurate finding predictive of DVT on DUS. Other findings suggestive of DVT include visualization of echogenic material in the lumen, a defect on color imaging with incomplete venous filling, and the absence of normal venous Doppler physiology. The results of 18 studies that included 1,189 patients in whom DUS was compared with venography for occlusive thrombi proximal to the calf revealed a sensitivity of 83% and a specificity of 88% (70,71). Studies have reported that DUS detects DVT with a sensitivity of 88% to 100% and a specificity of 86% to 100% (72,73).

Another advantage of DUS is its ability to detect other nonvascular causes of limb pain and edema, such as popliteal synovial ("baker's cysts"), native arterial aneurysms, tumors, and pseudoaneurysms that may explain a patient's clinical presentation.

A common, yet challenging clinical question is the ability of venous DUS to discern between acute and remote ("chronic") DVT. Several criteria have been suggested with DUS to aid in this determination. Acute DVT often results in dilation of the venous segment. Remote DVT commonly causes atresia of the vein and results in a contracted venous segment. In addition, remote or "old" thrombus produces bright echoes within the lumen. Acute DVT is commonly echolucent. The lumen and wall characteristics in remote DVT often show partial recanalization of flow within the venous thrombus itself. In cases of acute DVT, the venous flow is either completely obstructed or streams around the margins of the thrombus. Collateral veins are commonly seen around obstructed venous segments. It has been reported that 6 months after acute DVT, 48% of veins still have demonstrable abnormalities, and 14% of veins remain completely occluded (74).

A second common clinical question is that of recurrence of DVT. The optimal method of determining this recurrence is comparison with a previously performed DUS study. Recurrent DVT may occur in a previously affected vein, in the contralateral limb, or in a different venous segment entirely. An increase of more than 2 mm in the compressed lumen of a previously thrombosed vein has been reported to be diagnostic of recurrent DVT, but this criterion remains highly controversial and is not widely accepted by many vascular diagnostic laboratories (75). Recent data do suggest, however, that reduction in the "thrombus burden" is an independent predictor of future events and may be an important guide to the length of anticoagulant therapy (76).

The major limitations of venous DUS include decreased accuracy as a screening modality in asymptomatic patients, in identifying isolated calf vein thrombus, or in assessing the pelvic veins. Given that the treatment of isolated calf vein thrombus remains very controversial, many laboratories do not study these venous segments. However, because of the risk of propagation of an isolated calf vein thrombus to the popliteal vein, we suggest routine imaging of the calf veins with every study. For the inferior vena cava and pelvic veins, many investigators have turned to other imaging modalities including CT (77) and MR venography.

A non–image-based strategy for the diagnosis of venous thrombus is the use of D-Dimer assays. D-dimer represents a specific derivative of cross-linked fibrin and has been extensively evaluated in the setting of suspected DVT. In patients with a low clinical probability for DVT, the prevalence of DVT has been reported in 5% of cases by use of the D-dimer test. A negative quantitative D-dimer test can reliably exclude DVT without additional imaging because of its high negative predictive value. In patients with a high clinical probability for DVT, D-dimer testing may reduce the number of DUS procedures required. A positive D-dimer is present in almost all patients with venous thromboembolic disease (78). Clinicians must be aware that a positive D-dimer is also found in pregnancy, cancer, vasculitis, infection, advanced age, inflammation, trauma, and in the postoperative state (79). These are common situations in patients suspected of having DVT.

Given the advances in endoluminal therapy for saphenous vein reflux and venous varicosities, DUS imaging in patients with CVI is valuable. CVI results from venous outflow obstruction created by the DVT as well as from venous valvular reflux, either as a primary event, or in the case of DVT, from destruction of the one-way valves from the thrombus. Loss of valvular function results in valvular incompetence compromising the integrity of the superficial and deep valves at all levels of the limb (80).

Although physiologic tests (air plethysmography) will reliably confirm the presence of CVI (81), venous DUS is an excellent method of determining the presence, location, and severity of CVI (82). The goal is to demonstrate the duration of flow reversal following the release of limb compression distal to the ultrasound probe. There is a direct correlation between the duration of flow reversal and the severity of venous reflux. This study is performed with the patient in the standing position, except when testing for incompetent venous perforators is performed, during which the patient should be seated.

Imaging should be performed at the groin level of the patient's common femoral vein, saphenofemoral junction, and greater saphenous vein. The entire greater saphenous vein is then imaged throughout its length.

Following this, the limb is compressed distal to the location of the probe. With release of compression, there should be very little reversal of flow into the limb. The duration of reflux can be measured by the Doppler technique. Valve closure time of 0.5 seconds or less at the popliteal vein is normal, as is a time of 1 second or less in the thigh. If reflux lasts longer than 2 seconds, this is clearly abnormal (83).

CONTROVERSIES AND PERSONAL PERSPECTIVES

Although the growth of vascular noninvasive testing has continued to proliferate, with more sophisticated equipment, miniaturized computer chips resulting in portable DUS scanners, and algorithms utilizing vascular laboratory testing, challenges face all vascular laboratories. The two major criteria for the success of any vascular diagnostic laboratory are technical proficiency by the examiner and economic viability.

There are insufficient numbers of qualified vascular technologists to provide diagnostic services to the aging U.S. population. Given the aging of the "baby boomers," this situation is approaching crisis proportions. Professional societies must launch a coordinated marketing program to demonstrate the advantages of studying vascular technology. In addition, undergraduate and graduate programs providing bachelors and masters programs in vascular technology must proliferate throughout the United States.

Third-party payers must provide differential reimbursement to vascular laboratories staffed by RVTs and accredited by national accrediting organizations. Currently, the reimbursement for noninvasive vascular diagnostic procedures is insufficient to keep most laboratories operational. Technologists, being in such great demand, require significant salaries and benefits. Equipment remains expensive, as is the support to run them (electricity, space, digital archiving, administrative assistants). This overhead is currently not supported by reimbursement unless the volume of testing is sufficient. This constraint, of course, adds additional pressure to technical staff to perform rapid tests, thus potentially sacrificing accuracy. Given the cost effectiveness of noninvasive vascular testing in the diagnostic algorithm of PVDs, reimbursement must be modified to allow accredited vascular laboratories to function.

One evolving area of controversy is the skill set required for physicians to interpret vascular diagnostic tests. Many different specialties participate as members of the medical staff interpretation panel in vascular diagnostic laboratories, including radiologists, vascular surgeons, vascular medicine specialists, cardiologists, general internists, neurologists, and podiatrists. Currently, the only certification available for physicians to demonstrate expertise in examination interpretation has been the RVT certification. However, this registry is really designed to demonstrate skills in performance of vascular diagnostic tests and a basic understanding of the clinical aspects of vascular disease. This registry was not designed for physician interpreters.

Beginning in 2006, the American Registry of Diagnostic Medical Sonographers will launch the first certification program for physicians interested in demonstrating expertise in the interpretation of vascular diagnostic tests. Successful completion of this certification examination will result in the designation of registered physician vascular interpreter (RPVI). All physicians who currently interpret vascular noninvasive studies should obtain this certification.

Finally, it is our opinion that two specific "screening tests" should receive reimbursement codes by the U.S. government: the ABI and carotid IMT. There is a preponderance of data demonstrating the ability of each test to provide invaluable risk stratification for future cardiovascular events and mortality in populations at risk (84). Many unfounded arguments have been levied against reimbursement for these two examinations. However, large-scale published epidemiologic data have repeatedly documented the utility of these tests in providing risk assessment with virtually no risk and minimal cost. We certainly do not recommend indiscriminate testing; however, when the test outcomes will change therapy, there is no better testing strategy than the use of the ABI and carotid IMT testing. For example, in a 55-year-old man without known atherosclerosis whose low-density lipoprotein (LDL) cholesterol level on pharmacologic therapy is 100 mg/dL, the finding of PAD (abnormal ABI or fifth quintile carotid IMT scores) would suggest the need for more aggressive LDL cholesterol reduction based on the latest National Cholesterol Education Program guidelines (85).

THE FUTURE

Many alternate imaging modalities are emerging in clinical use, including MRA, CTA, and positron emission tomography (PET). Although data suggest that these modalities, depending on the vascular bed evaluated, are superior to noninvasive vascular testing, it is our opinion that these tests are additive, not exclusive.

MRA is a useful test to determine the vascular anatomy, but it has several limitations:

- Cost
- Need for peripheral intravenous access
- Inability to perform in patients with
  - Pacemakers
  - Implantable defibrillators
  - Claustrophobia
- Tendency to overestimate severe stenosis as occlusion and moderate stenosis as severe
- Inability to visualize the arterial lumen with endoluminal stents in place (this limitation may be less significant with cobalt chromium metallic alloy stents)
- Inability to visualize arterial calcification

CTA has emerged as a very useful tool for determining the vascular anatomy. With improving hardware and software, CTA may become the test of choice for mapping the vascular tree. However, CTA also has significant limitations:

- Cost
- Need for peripheral intravenous access
- Administration of iodinated contrast media
- Significant exposure to external-beam radiation
- Difficulty in determining the severity of stenosis in the presence of calcification

PET scanning is a fascinating technology that utilizes glucose metabolism in cells to determine disease activity. PET scanning has been utilized extensively in cancer evaluation (86). More recently, PET scanning has been correlated with plaque vulnerability and activity (87). The future will provide expanding information on the concept of "vulnerable plaque" in both the coronary and peripheral arteries.

The future of contrast enhancement for vascular imaging remains unclear. Although it has many potential applications (renal and visceral artery DUS, endoleak assessment after endoluminal stent-graft repair of AAAs, TCD ultrasonography) (88–90), the added cost, time, lack of reimbursement, and the need for peripheral intravenous access remain significant obstacles.

References

1. Creager MA, Cooke JP, Olin JW, et al. ACC revised recommendations for training in adult cardiovascular medicine. Core Cardiology Training II (COCATS-2). Task Force 11: training in vascular medicine and peripheral vascular catheter-based interventions. American College of Cardiology. Available at www.acc.org/clinical/training/COCATS2.pdf.
2. Fisher CM, Burnett A, Makeham V, et al. Variation in measurement of ankle-brachial pressure index in routine clinical practice. *J Vasc Surg* 1996;24:871–875.
3. Hirsch AT, Criqui MT, Treat-Jacobson D, et al. Peripheral arterial disease detection, awareness, and treatment in primary care. *JAMA* 2001;286:1317–1324.
4. Diehm C, Schuster A, Allenberg JR, et al. High prevalence of peripheral arterial disease in 6880 primary care patients: A cross sectional study. *Atherosclerosis* 2004;172:95–105.
5. Strandness DE. Noninvasive vascular laboratory and vascular imaging. In: Young JR, Olin JW, Bartholomew JR, eds. *Peripheral vascular diseases,* 2nd ed. St. Louis: Mosby, 1996:33–64.
6. Gensler SW, Haimovici H, Hoffert P, et al. Study of vascular lesions in diabetic, non-diabetic patients. *Arch Surg* 1965;617–622.
7. Carter SA, Tate RB. Value of toe pulse waves in addition to systolic pressures in the assessment of the severity of peripheral arterial disease and critical limb ischemia. *J Vasc Surg* 1996;24:258–265.
8. MacDonald NR. Pulse volume plethysmography. *J Vasc Tech* 1994;18:241–248.
9. Feinglass J, McCarthy WJ, Slavensky R, et al. Effect of lower extremity blood pressure on physical functioning in patients who have intermittent claudication. *J Vasc Surg* 1996;24:503–512.
10. McPhail IR, Spittell PC, Weston SA, Bailey KR. Intermittent claudication: An objective office-based assessment. *J Am Coll Cardiol* 2001;37:1381–1385.
11. Degeorges R, Reynaud C, Becquemin JP. Thoracic outlet syndrome surgery: Long-term functional results. *Ann Vasc Surg* 2004;18:558–565.
12. Stewart JH, Grubb M. Understanding vascular ultrasonography. *Mayo Clin Proc* 1992;67:1186–1196.
13. Nelson TR, Pretorius DH. The Doppler signal: Where does it come from and what does it mean? *AJR Am J Roentgenol* 1988;151:439–447.
14. Whelan JF, Barry MH, Moir JD. Color flow Doppler ultrasonography: Comparison with peripheral arteriography for the investigation of peripheral vascular disease. *J Clin Ultrasound* 1992;20:369–374.
15. Allard L, Cloutier G, Durand LG, et al. Limitations of ultrasonic duplex scanning for diagnosing lower limb arterial stenoses in the presence of adjacent segment disease. *J Vasc Surg* 1994;19:650–657.
16. Larch E, Minar E, Ahmadi R, et al. Value of color duplex sonography for evaluation of tibioperoneal arteries in patients with femoropopliteal obstruction: A prospective comparison with anterograde intraarterial digital subtraction angiography. *J Vasc Surg* 1997;25:629–636.
17. Lewis WA, Bray AE, Harrison CL, et al. A comparison of common femoral waveform analysis with aorto-iliac duplex scanning in assessment of aorto-iliac disease. *J Vasc Tech* 1994;18:337–344.
18. Kohler TR, Nance DR, Cramer MM, et al. Duplex scanning for diagnosis of aortoiliac and femoropopliteal disease: A prospective study. *Circulation* 1987;76:1074–1080.
19. Elsman BHP, Legemate DA, van der Heyden FWHM, et al. The use of color-coded duplex scanning in the selection of patients with lower extremity arterial disease for percutaneous transluminal angioplasty: A prospective study. *Cardiovasc Interv Radiol* 1996;19:313–316.
20. Silke CM, Grouden MC, Nicholls S, et al. Noninvasive follow-up of peripheral angioplasty: A prospective study. *J Vasc Tech* 1997;21:23–25.
21. Mewissen MW, Kinney EV, Bandyk DF, et al. The role of duplex scanning versus angiography in predicting outcome after balloon angioplasty in the femoropopliteal artery. *J Vasc Surg* 1992;15:860–866.
22. Sacks D, Robinson ML, Marinelli DL, Perlmutter GS. Evaluation of the peripheral arteries with duplex US after angioplasty. *Radiology* 1990;176:39–44.
23. Bandyk DF. Ultrasonic duplex scanning in the evaluation of arterial grafts and dilatations. *Echocardiography* 1987;4:251–264.
24. Mattos MA, van Bemmelen PS, Hodgson KJ, et al. Does correction of stenoses identified with color duplex scanning improve infrainguinal graft patency? *J Vasc Surg* 1993;17:54–66.
25. Lalak NJ, Hanel KC, Hunt J, Morgan A. Duplex scan surveillance of infrainguinal prosthetic bypass grafts. *J Vasc Surg* 1994;20:637–641.
26. Bandyk DF. Postoperative surveillance of infrainguinal bypass. *Surg Clin North Am* 1990;70:71–85.
27. Jaff MR, Breger R, Deshur W, Pipia J. Detection of an arterial bypass graft threatening lesion by use of duplex ultrasonography and magnetic resonance angiography in an asymptomatic patient. *Vasc Surg* 1998;32:109–114.
28. Laird J, Jaff MR, Biamino G, et al. Cryoplasty for the treatment of femoropopliteal arterial disease: Results of a prospective, multicenter trial. *J Vasc Interv Radiol* 2005;16:1067–1073.
29. North American Symptomatic Carotid Endarterectomy Trial Collaborators. Beneficial effect of carotid endarterectomy in symptomatic patients with high-grade carotid stenosis. *N Engl J Med* 1991;325:445–453.
30. Executive Committee for the Asymptomatic Carotid Atherosclerosis Study. Endarterectomy for asymptomatic carotid artery stenosis. *JAMA* 1995;73:1421–1428.
31. Perry JR, Szalai JP, Norris JW. Consensus against both endarterectomy and routine screening for asymptomatic carotid artery stenosis. *Arch Neurol* 1997;54:25–28.
32. Yadav JS, Wholey MH, Kuntz RE, et al. Protected carotid-artery stenting versus endarterectomy in high-risk patients. *N Engl J Med* 2004;351:1493–1501.
33. Fell G, Phillips DJ, Chikos PM, et al. Ultrasonic duplex scanning for disease of the carotid artery. *Circulation* 1981;64:1191–1195.
34. Roederer GO, Langlois YE, Jager KA, et al. The natural history of carotid arterial disease in asymptomatic patients with cervical bruits. *Stroke* 1984;15:605–613.
35. Roederer GO, Langlois Y, Chan ATW, et al. Post-endarterectomy carotid ultrasonic duplex scanning: Concordance with contrast angiography. *Ultrasound Med Biol* 1983;9:73–78.
36. McCabe DJH, Pereira AC, Clinton A, et al. Restenosis after carotid artery angioplasty, stenting, or endarterectomy in the Carotid and Vertebral Artery Angioplasty Study (CAVATAS). *Stroke* 2005;36:281–286.
37. Hayward JK, Davies AH, Lamont PM. Carotid plaque morphology: A review. *Eur J Vasc Endovasc Surg* 1995;9:368–374.
38. Sztajzel R, Momjian S, Momjian-Mayor I, et al. Stratified gray-scale median analysis and color mapping of the carotid plaque: Correlation of endarterectomy specimen histology of 28 patients. *Stroke* 2005;36(4):1–5.
39. Schillinger M, Exner M, Mlekusch W, et al. Inflammation and Carotid Artery—Risk for Atherosclerosis Study (ICARAS). *Circulation* 2005;111:2203–2209.
40. Touboul PJ, Hennerici MG, Meairs S, et al. Mannheim intima-media thickness consensus. *Cerebrovasc Dis* 2004;18:346–349.
41. O'Leary DH, Polak JF, Kronmal RA, et al. The cardiovascular health study collaborative research group: Carotid-artery intima and media thickness as a risk factor for myocardial infarction and stroke in older adults. *N Engl J Med* 1999;340:14–22.
42. Secil M, Altay C, Gulcu A, et al. Automated measurement of intima-media thickness of carotid arteries in ultrasonography by computer software. *Diagn Interv Radiol* 2005;11:105–108.

43. McCabe DJH, Pereira AC, Clifton A, et al. Restenosis after carotid angioplasty, stenting, or endarterectomy in the Carotid and Vertebral Transluminal Angioplasty Study. *Stroke* 2005;36:281–286.
44. Carpenter JP, Lexa FJ, Davis JT. Determination of sixty percent or greater carotid artery stenosis by duplex Doppler ultrasonography. *J Vasc Surg* 1995;22:697–705.
45. Kirsch JD, Wagner LR, James EM, et al. Carotid artery occlusion: Positive predictive value of duplex sonography compared with arteriography. *J Vasc Surg* 1994;19:642–649.
46. Grant EG, Benson CB, Moneta GL, et al. Carotid artery stenosis: Gray-scale and Doppler US diagnosis—Society of Radiologists in Ultrasound Consensus Conference. *Radiology* 2003;229:340–346.
47. Kent KC, Kuntz KM, Patel MR, et al. Perioperative imaging strategies for carotid endarterectomy: An analysis of morbidity and cost-effectiveness in symptomatic patients. *JAMA* 1995;274:888–893.
48. Smith LL, Anderson DC, Gramith F. A step-by-step guide for validation of carotid duplex studies. *J Vasc Tech* 1993;17:17–22.
49. Muto PM, Welch HJ, Mackey WC, O'Donnell TF. Evaluation of carotid artery stenosis: Is duplex ultrasonography sufficient? *J Vasc Surg* 1996;24: 17–24.
50. Ringelstein EB, Droste EW, Babikian DL, et al. Consensus on microemboli detection with TCD: International Consensus Group on Microembolus Detection. *Stroke* 1998;29:725–829.
51. Markus HS, MacKinnon A. Asymptomatic embolization detected by Doppler ultrasound predicts stroke risk in symptomatic carotid artery stenosis. *Stroke* 2005;36:971–975.
52. Vos JA, van den Berg JC, Ernst SMPG, et al. Carotid angioplasty and stent placement: Comparison of transcranial Doppler US data and clinical outcome with and without filtering cerebral protection devices in 509 patients. *Radiology* 2005;234:493–499.
53. Kent KC, Zwolak RM, Jaff MR, et al. Screening for abdominal aortic aneurysm: A consensus statement. *J Vasc Surg* 2004;39:267–269.
54. Lederle FA, Wilson SE, Johnson GR, et al. Immediate repair compared with surveillance of small abdominal aortic aneurysms. *N Engl J Med* 2002;346: 1437–1444.
55. United Kingdom Small Aneurysm Trial Participants. Long-term outcomes of immediate repair compared with surveillance of small abdominal aortic aneurysms. *N Engl J Med* 2002;346:1445–1452.
56. Blankensteijn JD, de Jong SECA, Prinssen M, et al. Two-year outcomes after conventional or endovascular repair of abdominal aortic aneurysms. *N Engl J Med* 2005;352:2398–2405.
57. Bargellini I, Napoli V, Petruzzi P, et al. Type II lumbar endoleaks: Hemodynamic differentiation by contrast-enhanced ultrasound scanning and influence on aneurysm enlargement after endovascular aneurysm repair. *J Vasc Surg* 2005;41:10–18.
58. Hollenberg NK. Medical therapy for renovascular hypertension: A review. *Am J Hypertens* 1988;1:338–1343.
59. Mailloux LU, Napolitano B, Bellucci AG, et al. Renal vascular disease causing end-stage renal disease, incidence, clinical correlates, and outcomes: A 20-year clinical experience. *Am J Kidney Dis* 1994;24:622–629.
60. Scoble JE, Maher ER, Hamilton G, et al. Atherosclerotic renovascular disease causing renal impairment: A case for treatment. *Clin Nephrol* 1989;31:119–122.
61. Eidt JF, Fry RE, Clagett GP, et al. Postoperative follow-up of renal artery reconstruction with duplex ultrasound. *J Vasc Surg* 1988;8:667–673.
62. Dorros G, Jaff M, Mathiak L, et al. Four-year follow-up of Palmaz-Schatz stent revascularization as treatment for atherosclerotic renal artery stenosis. *Circulation* 1998;98:642–647.
63. Olin JW, Piedmonte MR, Young JR, et al. The utility of duplex ultrasound scanning of the renal arteries for diagnosing significant renal artery stenosis. *Ann Intern Med* 1995;122:833–838.
64. Moneta GL, Lee RW, Yeager RA, et al. Mesenteric duplex scanning: A blinded prospective study. *J Vasc Surg* 1993;17:79–86.
65. Zwolak RM, Fillinger MF, Walsh DB, et al. Mesenteric and celiac duplex scanning: A validation study. *J Vasc Surg* 1998;27:1078–1087.
66. Blebea J, Volteas N, Neumyer M, et al. Contrast enhanced duplex ultrasound imaging of the mesenteric arteries. *Ann Vasc Surg* 2002;16:77–83.
67. PIOPED Investigators. Value of the ventilation/perfusion scan in acute pulmonary embolism: Results of the Prospective Investigation of Pulmonary Embolism Diagnosis (PIOPED). *JAMA* 1990;263:2753–2759.
68. Killewich LA, Bedford GR, Beach KW, Strandness DE Jr. Diagnosis of deep venous thrombosis: A prospective study comparing duplex scanning to contrast venography. *Circulation* 1989;79:810–814.
69. Hull R, Hirsh J, Sackett DL, et al. Clinical validity of a negative venogram in patients with clinically suspected venous thrombosis. *Circulation* 1981; 64:622–625.
70. Aitkon AGF, Godden DJ. Real-time ultrasound diagnosis of deep vein thrombosis: A comparison with venography. *Clin Radiol* 1987;38:309–313.
71. Weinmann EE, Salzman EW. Deep-vein thrombosis. *N Engl J Med* 1994;331: 1630–1641.
72. Appleman PT, De John TE, Lampmann LE. Deep venous thrombosis of the leg: US findings. *Radiology* 1987;163:743–746.
73. Lensing AW, Prandoni P, Brandjes D, et al. Detection of deep-vein thrombosis by real-time B-mode ultrasonography. *N Engl J Med* 1989;320:342–345.
74. Cronan JJ. Venous thromboembolic disease: The role of US. *Radiology* 1993;186:619–630.
75. Prandoni P, Cogo A, Bernardi E, et al. A simple ultrasound approach for detection of recurrent proximal vein thrombosis. *Circulation* 1993;88:1730–1735.
76. Hull RD, Marder VJ, Mah AF, et al. Quantitative assessment of thrombus burden predicts the outcome of treatment for venous thrombosis: A systematic review. *Am J Med* 2005;118:456–464.
77. Begemann PG, Bonacker M, Kemper J, et al. Evaluation of the deep venous system in patients with suspected pulmonary embolism with multi-detector CT: A prospective study in comparison to Doppler sonography. *J Comput Assist Tomogr* 2003;27:399–409.
78. Bockenstedt P. D-dimer in venous thromboembolism. *N Engl J Med* 2003; 349:1203–1204.
79. Wells PS, Anderson DR, Rodger M, et al. Evaluation of D-dimer in the diagnosis of suspected deep vein thrombosis. *N Engl J Med* 2003;349:1227–1235.
80. Van Bemmelen PS, Bedford G, Beach K, Strandness DE Jr. Status of the valves in superficial and deep venous system in chronic venous disease. *Surgery* 1991;109:730–734.
81. Nicolaides AN, Christopoulos D, Vasdekis S. Progress in the evaluation of chronic venous insufficiency. *Ann Vasc Surg* 1989;3:278–292.
82. Vasdekis SN, Clarek GH, Nicolaides AN. Quantification of venous reflux testing by means of duplex scanning. *J Vasc Surg* 1989;10:670–677.
83. Needham T. Assessment of lower extremity venous valvular insufficiency examinations. *J Vasc Ultrasound* 2005;29:123–129.
84. Sankatsing RR, de Groot E, Jukema JW, et al. Surrogate markers for atherosclerotic disease. *Curr Opin Lipidol* 2005;16:434–441.
85. Grundy SM, Cleeman JI, Merz CN, et al. Implications of recent clinical trials for the National Cholesterol Education Program Adult Treatment Panel III guidelines. *Circulation* 2004;110:227–239.
86. Antoch G, Vogt FM, Freudenberg LS, et al. Whole-body dual-modality PET/CT and whole-body MRI for tumor staging in oncology. *JAMA* 2003; 290:3199–3206.
87. Rudd JH, Warburton EA, Fryer TD, et al. Imaging atherosclerotic plaque inflammation with [18F]fluorodeoxyglucose positron emission tomography. *Circulation* 2002;105:2708–2711.
88. Viguier A, Petit R, Rigal M, et al. Continuous monitoring of middle cerebral artery recanalization with transcranial color-coded sonography and Levovist. *J Thromb Thrombolysis* 2005;19:55–59.
89. Ohm C, Bendick PJ, Monash J, et al. Diagnosis of total internal carotid occlusions with duplex ultrasound and ultrasound contrast. *Vasc Endovasc Surg* 2005;39:237–243.
90. Napoli V, Bargellini I, Sardella SG, et al. Abdominal aortic aneurysm: Contrast-enhanced US for missed endoleaks after endoluminal repair. *Radiology* 2004;233:217–225.

CHAPTER 107 ■ CEREBROVASCULAR DISEASE

CATHY A. SILA, ANTHONY J. FURLAN, AND JAY S. YADAV

OVERVIEW

The term *stroke* encompasses a heterogeneous group of cerebrovascular disorders, each with distinctive clinical presentations, underlying causes, and management strategies. Stroke prevention targets high-risk patients with prior cerebrovascular events, atherosclerotic risk factors, nonvalvular atrial fibrillation, severe carotid stenosis or intracranial atherosclerosis, and saccular aneurysms. Therapeutic strategies focus on the identification and management of risk factors, antithrombotic drugs for ischemic stroke, revascularization procedures for occlusive disease, and emerging endovascular procedures for complementing or replacing surgery for both ischemic and hemorrhagic stroke. Although intervention in acute ischemic stroke is modeled after strategies for acute myocardial infarction, the diversity of ischemic stroke mechanisms and the increased risk for brain hemorrhage remain formidable challenges.

HISTORICAL PERSPECTIVE

400 BC Hippocrates: aphorism on apoplexy; Greek *apo* ("from"), *pleso* ("thunderstruck"), *ia* ("condition")
1664 Willis: contributed the word *neurology*, anastomotic "circle" at the base of the brain
1658 Wepfer, 1832 Rostan: apoplexy is caused by cerebral hemorrhage and cerebral infarction
1802 Heberden, 1820 Cheyne, 1872 Kussmaul: described transient ischemic attacks
1875 Gowers: described embolism with mitral stenosis, differentiated embolism from thrombosis
1905 Chiari, 1914 Hunt: described emboli from carotid bifurcation, syndrome of internal carotid artery occlusion
1927 Moniz, 1936 Loman and Myerson, 1960s Seldinger: carotid arteriography
1950s: carotid artery surgery, use of oral anticoagulants and aspirin

1960s: definitions of ischemic events, clinical trials of intracerebral hemorrhage management

1970s: computed tomography brain scans redefine the "cerebrovascular accident," epidemiology of atrial fibrillation, first clinical trials of aspirin therapy for stroke prevention

1980s: U.S. Food and Drug Administration approval of aspirin for stroke prevention, clinical trials of carotid endarterectomy, warfarin for atrial fibrillation and acute myocardial infarction, and management of aneurysmal subarachnoid hemorrhage, magnetic resonance imaging, angioplasty of cerebral arteries

1990s: intraarterial thrombolysis and Food and Drug Administration approval of intravenous tissue-type plasminogen activator for acute ischemic stroke, redefining systems for acute stroke care, diffusion/perfusion magnetic resonance imaging (MRI), carotid stenting, endovascular therapy of cerebral aneurysms

ANATOMIC CONSIDERATIONS

THE HETEROGENEITY OF CEREBROVASCULAR DISORDERS

Cerebrovascular disorders are a heterogeneous group of neurologic symptoms, signs, and mechanisms of injury (1). *Ischemic stroke*, or *cerebral infarction*, accounts for 80% to 85% of all strokes and typically presents as a sudden, painless, focal neurologic deficit with preserved consciousness. *Hemorrhagic stroke* accounts for 15% to 20% of all strokes, 10% to 15% due to *intracerebral hemorrhage* and 5% to 8% due to *subarachnoid hemorrhage*. Cerebral hemorrhage presents as an acute, focal neurologic deficit but continues to worsen as the hematoma expands manifest as a progressive deficit with headache and altered consciousness. Subarachnoid hemorrhage presents as a sudden, severe headache and altered consciousness when severe, but early focal findings only occur in the presence of aneurysmal compression of cranial nerves or concomitant intracerebral hemorrhage.

EPIDEMIOLOGY

Each year, approximately 700,000 strokes occur, with 200,000 representing a recurrent stroke. There are approximately 5.5 million stroke survivors in the United States, and it is estimated that 13 million individuals have sustained a silent stroke. The risk of stroke doubles with each decade over the age of 55 years. The 10- to 20-year gender lag that is observed for myocardial infarction is not seen with stroke; and the ratio of strokes suffered by men and women is stable over different age groups. Overall, the stroke risk is 19% to 33% greater in men than women, but because women live longer, they account for 46,000 more strokes each year. Stroke prevalence varies by race, affecting 3.6% of American Indians/Alaskan Natives, 3% of blacks/African Americans, 2.2% of whites, and 2% of Asians. Blacks have twice the rate of stroke as whites, with the highest prevalence in the 10 southeastern U.S. states, known as the "Stroke Belt." About 10% of ischemic strokes and greater than one third of hemorrhagic strokes are fatal, and although cerebrovascular mortality has declined since the 1920s, stroke remains the third-leading cause of death in the United States and is second worldwide. Women account for 60% of stroke fatalities, which may be related to a greater ischemic stroke severity in the setting of atrial fibrillation and older age and the higher rates of subarachnoid hemorrhage.

TABLE 107.1

STROKE RISK FACTORS

Age	Hypertension	Cigarette smoking
Gender	Transient ischemic attack/prior stroke	Alcohol abuse
Race/ethnicity	Atrial fibrillation	Physical inactivity, obesity
	Cardiac diseases	Sickle cell disease
	Carotid artery stenosis	Polycythemia, hyperfibrinogenemia
	Hyperlipidemia	Inflammatory markers
	Diabetes mellitus	Metabolic syndrome

STROKE RISK FACTORS AND TREATMENT FOR PRIMARY AND SECONDARY STROKE PREVENTION

Stroke risk factors define populations at risk and provide a framework for individual patient management (Tables 107.1 and 107.2). Patient education should include the warning symptoms of stroke, foster an understanding of individual risk factors and the target goal of treatment, and provide follow-up for adherence to the treatment plan.

Transient Ischemic Attacks

The classic definition of a transient ischemic attack (TIA) is a sudden focal neurologic deficit, referable to a specific arterial distribution and of presumed vascular origin that resolves within 24 hours. However, the majority resolve within 1 hour, and only 15% of those persisting beyond 1 hour resolve within 24 hours. Neuroimaging evidence of cerebral infarction can be demonstrated in 15% to 20% of computed tomography (CT) scans and 50% to 71% of diffusion-weighted magnetic resonance imaging (DWI) with symptoms of duration greater than 6 hours but less than 24 hours. The perception that TIAs are benign whereas strokes are more serious results in inadequate patient reporting and physician treatment (2). In two recent studies of patients presenting with TIAs, 8% to 10% suffered a stroke. However, there is a high-risk subset of patients with TIAs whose risk of stroke is 10% within the first week, and for these patients, emergent evaluation and treatment is essential, particularly because less than 20% of strokes are forewarned by TIA symptoms (3). High-risk features that were identified include older age, hypertension, focal symptoms consisting of unilateral weakness or speech disturbance, symptom duration, and diabetes. The "ABCD" risk scoring system separated those patients who did not go on to have an early recurrent stroke from a group consisting of 95% of the patients who had a 30% risk of having a stroke within the first week (4). These data can be used to determine which patients may require hospital admission for urgent evaluation and treatment (Table 107.3).

Hypertension

Hypertension is the most important risk factor for both ischemic and hemorrhagic stroke, and given its prevalence, it should be a major focus of therapy. The risk of stroke is directly related to the magnitude of elevation of both the systolic and

TABLE 107.2

STROKE RISK ACCORDING TO STROKE SUBTYPE

Stroke subtype	Risk
Large-artery atherosclerosis	
Symptomatic ≥70% carotid stenosis	26% ipsilateral stroke at 2 y
Symptomatic 50%–69% carotid stenosis	22% ipsilateral stroke at 5 y
Symptomatic <50% carotid stenosis	18% ipsilateral stroke at 5 y
Asymptomatic ≥60% carotid stenosis	11% ipsilateral stroke at 5 y
Asymptomatic >80% carotid stenosis	9%–14% ipsilateral stroke at 3 y
Symptomatic ≥50% intracranial stenosis	19% ipsilateral stroke at 1.7 y
Lacunar stroke	15%–17% recurrent stroke at 2 y
Cryptogenic stroke	15%–16% recurrent stroke at 2 y
Cardioembolism	
Recent cardioembolic stroke	2%–4% recurrent stroke within 30 d
AF, age <65 y, no risk factors	1%/y
AF, age >75 y, ≥1 risk factors	8.1%/y
AF, others	3%–6%/y
AMI overall	1%–3% within 3 mo
AMI, anterior wall	2%–6% within 3 mo
AMI, with LV thrombus	15% within 3 mo
Dilated cardiomyopathy	1%–3%/y
Rheumatic mitral stenosis	5%/y
Bioprosthetic aortic valve	0.2%–2.9%/y
Bioprosthetic mitral valve	0.4%–1.9%/y
Mechanical aortic valve, not anticoagulated	12.3%/y
Mechanical aortic valve, anticoagulated	1.4%–3.9%/y
Mechanical mitral valve, not anticoagulated	22.2%/y
Mechanical mitral valve, anticoagulated	1.1%–6.5%/y
Symptomatic PFO	1%–2%/y
Symptomatic PFO + atrial septal aneurysm	2%–4%/y
High-risk transient ischemic attack	30% stroke within 1 wk
Cerebrovascular disease	2%–3.5% cardiovascular mortality/y

AF, atrial fibrillation; AMI, acute myocardial infarction; LV, left ventricular; PFO, patent foramen ovale.

diastolic blood pressures for both genders and all age groups. The lifetime stroke risk for those with normal blood pressure (<120/80 mm Hg) is half of that for individuals with hypertension. Isolated systolic hypertension increases stroke risk two to four times even after controlling for age and diastolic blood pressure.

The decline in stroke mortality has been credited to the effective treatment of hypertension. From a meta-analysis of 14 trials of hypertension therapy, a 35% to 40% reduction in stroke risk over 5 years was obtained with a 5- to 6-mm Hg reduction in diastolic blood pressure. The guidelines of the Joint National Committee on Prevention, Detection, Evaluation, and Treatment of High Blood Pressure (JNC 7) define normal blood pressure as less than 120/80 mm Hg, but only 1/2 of hypertensive individuals even achieve the treatment goal of less than 140/90 mm Hg. The Perindopril Protection Against Recurrent Stroke Study (PROGRESS) compared perindopril versus placebo in 6,102 patients with TIA or stroke within the prior 5 years (5). Of note, more than half of the patients had blood pressure (BP) less than 130/85 mm Hg at entry. Combination therapy with indapamide was administered with physician discretion, and nearly half of the patients were taking additional antihypertensive therapies. In follow-up averaging 4.2 years, combination therapy significantly reduced the risk of cerebral hemorrhage by 50% and ischemic stroke by 24%, with average BP lowering of 12 mm Hg systolic and 5 mm Hg diastolic, suggesting that a more aggressive target is warranted. Because the stroke risk reduction varies by stroke subtype, it is likely that different BP targets will be appropriate for different stroke subtypes. Along the lines of the more aggressive JNC 7 target for patients with small-vessel disease with diabetes or renal insufficiency, the Stroke Prevention in Small Subcortical Strokes trial (SPS-3) is investigating a systolic BP target of less than 130 mm Hg versus 130 to 149 mm Hg in patients with a prior lacunar stroke due to small-vessel disease.

TABLE 107.3

HIGH STROKE RISK AFTER TRANSIENT ISCHEMIC ATTACK: THE ABCD SCORE

Age	≥60 y (1 point)
Blood pressure	>140 mm Hg systolic and/or ≥90 mm Hg diastolic (1 point)
Clinical symptoms	Unilateral weakness (2 points)
	Speech disturbance without weakness (1 point)
Duration	≥60 min (2 points)
	10–59 min (1 point)

Score of 5 or 6: 30% risk of stroke within 1 week, captures 95% of the high-risk patients.

Hyperlipidemia

The confusion regarding hyperlipidemia as a risk factor for stroke lies in the heterogeneity of stroke subtypes.

Hypercholesterolemia is a powerful risk factor for ischemic stroke due to atherothrombosis; however an increase in fatal hemorrhage stroke is related to low cholesterol levels (6). In clinical trials of secondary prevention of coronary heart disease (CHD) in which stroke was a prespecified endpoint, statin therapy reduces stroke by 23% to 31%. In trials of primary prevention and those including patients with cerebrovascular disease without established coronary heart disease, the low event rate for stroke underpowered an analysis. In a meta-analysis of more than 200,000, largely low-risk, patients, statin therapy reduced the risk of stroke by 25% in patients with or without CHD, which translates into a number needed to treat (NNT) of 2,778 patients for 1 year to prevent 1 stroke. Benefit was not identified for other lipid-lowering strategies, including diet (7). In a higher-risk subgroup of patients with a prior TIA or ischemic stroke but without CHD from the Heart Protection Study, statin therapy reduced the risk of recurrent stroke by 21, which translates into an NNT of 102 patients for 1 year to prevent 1 stroke. Current recommendations are to initiate statin therapy in patients with symptomatic carotid atherosclerosis as a high CHD risk-equivalent and after a recent TIA or ischemic stroke. The Stroke Prevention by Aggressive Reduction in Cholesterol Levels (SPARCL) trial comparing atorvastatin 80 mg/day versus placebo initiated 1 to 6 months after a TIA or ischemic stroke should address the role of intensive therapy in this targeted population (8).

Diabetes Mellitus

The incidence of type 2 diabetes has increased dramatically and is a major risk factor for stroke, and hyperglycemia in the setting of an acute stroke is associated with poorer outcome with increased infarct size. Strict blood sugar control has been shown to reduce microvascular complications, although it is not clear that this extends to lacunar infarction of the brain from small-vessel disease. Although aggressive treatment of hypertension among type 2 diabetics has been shown to reduce stroke risk, tight diabetic control has not. Hyperglycemia in the setting of acute stroke is associated with poorer outcome related to increased infarct size. Insulin resistance and the metabolic syndrome have been demonstrated to have an intermediate risk for stroke when compared to diabetes or controls. The ongoing Insulin Resistance Intervention after Stroke (IRIS) trial will test the efficacy of insulin sensitizer therapy with pioglitazone to prevent recurrent stroke and other vascular events in nondiabetic patients with insulin resistance who have had a recent ischemic stroke.

Carotid Artery Stenosis

The risk of stroke increases with the severity of stenosis from 1%/year to 2%/year for less than 75% stenosis to 3.3%/year for greater than 75% stenosis, of which 2.5% represent infarcts within the territory of the stenotic artery (9). However, carotid bruits and carotid plaque thickness are stronger indicators of the risk of myocardial ischemia and vascular death, at 8%/year to 10%/year. In the 1980s, a Rand report suggested that one third of carotid endarterectomies were performed for inappropriate indications, and an additional one third were questionable. This prompted the organization of multiple randomized clinical trials to investigate the role of carotid revascularization procedures versus medical therapy for stroke prevention (Table 107.4).

The Carotid Artery Stenosis with Asymptomatic Narrowing: Operation Versus Aspirin (CASANOVA) study (11), the Veterans Administration Asymptomatic Carotid Stenosis Trial

TABLE 107.4

CAROTID ENDARTERECTOMY TRIALS

Clinical trial subset	Surgery would need to be done on:	To spare one:	Over:
Symptomatic carotid stenosis			
NASCET 70%–99%	6 patients	ipsilateral stroke	2 y
	10 patients	major stroke or death	2 y
NASCET 50%–69%	12 men or 67 women	ipsilateral stroke	5 y
	16 men or 125 women	major stroke	5 y
NASCET <50%	No benefit	any ipsilateral stroke	5 y
VA >50%	No benefit	any stroke or death	Terminated
	26 men	crescendo TIA or stroke	1 y
Asymptomatic carotid stenosis			
CASANOVA 50%–99%	No benefit	any stroke or death	3 y
VA >50%	No benefit	any stroke or death	4 y
MACE[a]			
ACAS ≥ 60%	17 patients	ipsilateral stroke or any perioperative stroke or death	5 y
	9 patients	TIA, stroke or death	5 y
	No benefit	any stroke or death	5 y
	No benefit	major stroke or death	5 y

ACAS, Asymptomatic Carotid Atherosclerosis Study (14); CASANOVA, Carotid Artery Stenosis with Asymptomatic Narrowing: Operation Versus Aspirin study (11); MACE, Mayo Asymptomatic Carotid Endarterectomy trial (13); NASCET, North American Carotid Endarterectomy Trial (15); TIA, Transient ischemic attack; VA, Veterans Administration Asymptomatic Carotid Stenosis Trial (12).
[a]Terminated, excessive myocardial infarctions.

(12), and the Mayo Asymptomatic Carotid Endarterectomy (MACE) trial (13) were negative or inconclusive, and the MACE trial was halted due to an excess of myocardial infarctions (MIs) in patients not on aspirin therapy. The Asymptomatic Carotid Atherosclerosis Study (ACAS) (14), which randomized 1,662 patients with greater than 60% internal carotid artery stenosis (determined by ultrasound or angiography), was stopped after 2.7 years when the projected 5-year stroke rate was significantly reduced from 11.3% to 5.6% with surgery performed at a low, 3% morbidity and mortality rate. Women did not benefit from the procedure, partly due to their higher rate of angiographic complications.

The North American Carotid Endarterectomy Trial (NASCET) randomized patients with a recent (within 3 months) ipsiterritory TIA or nondisabling ischemic stroke and 30% to 99% stenosis defined by angiographic measurements of the internal carotid artery (15). The "NASCET method" of measurement has become the standard for describing carotid stenosis and predicting a clinical benefit with therapy as described by these outcomes-driven clinical trials.

As the severity of carotid stenosis increased, so did the risk of having a stroke; as stroke risk increased, so did the benefits of surgery. Factors that identified those at high risk of stroke with medical therapy alone include age greater than 70 years, male gender, systolic BP greater than 160 mm Hg, diastolic BP greater than 90 mm Hg, symptoms within 31 days, history of stroke, stenosis greater than 80%, plaque ulceration, and a history of either smoking, hypertension, MI, congestive heart failure, diabetes mellitus, claudication, or hyperlipidemia. Those with six or more risk factors had a 39% risk of ipsilateral stroke within 2 years.

The severe (70% to 99%) stenosis subgroup was prematurely terminated when surgery significantly reduced the risk of any ipsilateral stroke at 2 years from 26% to 9% (65% relative risk reduction) and major or fatal ipsilateral stroke from 13.1% to 2.5% (81% relative risk reduction). For those with 50% to 69% stenosis, surgery also reduced the rate of any ipsilateral stroke from 22.2% to 15.7% (29% relative risk reduction) at 5 years, but the benefit was marginal (p = .045). Within this subgroup, characteristics that were associated with a greater benefit from surgery included male gender, a recent stroke (rather than a TIA), recent hemispheric symptoms (rather than retinal symptoms), and failing aspirin at 650 mg or more daily. For those with 30% to 49% stenosis, there was no significant benefit in reducing ipsilateral stroke at 5 years with surgery (14.9%) compared to medical therapy alone (18.7%). The highest risk for stroke was immediately after the index ischemic event and declined to 3%/year within 2 to 3 years; if the patient escaped recurrent symptoms during that time, he or she had little to gain from having delayed surgery. These results were confirmed in the European Carotid Surgery Trial (ECST) (16).

The benefits of carotid endarterectomy surgery were realized when the perioperative morbidity and mortality was 5.8%, which included a major stroke and death rate of 2% and a mortality rate of less than 1%. Characteristics that doubled the risk of perioperative stroke or death included contralateral carotid occlusion, evidence of an ipsilateral cerebral infarct on CT/MRI, left-sided carotid disease, diabetes, diastolic blood pressure above 90 mm Hg, absence of a history of myocardial infarction or angina, and taking less than 650 mg of aspirin per day, but not age or gender.

Guidelines for endarterectomy advise that the best indication for carotid endarterectomy is for the prevention of ipsilateral carotid territory ischemic stroke in patients with a recent transient ischemic attack or minor ischemic stroke due to greater than 70% ipsilateral carotid stenosis and is also beneficial for those with 50% to 69% stenosis if they have a good 5-year life expectancy and the procedure can be performed with a combined morbidity and mortality of less than 6%. For asymptomatic patients with greater than 60% stenosis, surgery should be recommended if the patient has a good 5-year life expectancy and the procedure can be performed with a combined morbidity and mortality rate of less than 3%. All patients should receive treatment of risk factors, patient education about TIAs, and antiplatelet therapy.

Endovascular approaches to carotid revascularization were developed in part because the low perioperative risks demonstrated in the randomized trials did not reflect clinical practice, with mortality rates of 1.4% for patients not randomized at trial hospitals to 2.5% for patients treated at low-volume, nontrial hospitals (17).

The Carotid and Vertebral Artery Transluminal Angioplasty Study (CAVATAS) was the first large-scale trial comparing carotid angioplasty, 26% with stents, to carotid endarterectomy (18). At 30 days, the 10% risk of death or stroke did not differ between the endarterectomy and angioplasty groups, but the 5.9% risk of death or disabling stroke with endarterectomy was substantially higher than the rate of less than 3% reported by NASCET and ECST. Registry data tracked the improvements in endovascular revascularization with carotid stenting, particularly with emboli protection devices. In a report of 11,243 patients entered into a global stenting registry, the 30-day rate of stroke rate was 5.3% without and 2.2% with emboli protection (19).

The Stenting and Angioplasty with Protection in Patients at High Risk for Endarterectomy (SAPPHIRE) trial was a multicenter, randomized trial of carotid stenting versus endarterectomy in asymptomatic greater than 80% or symptomatic greater than 50% carotid stenosis in patients deemed to be of high surgical risk but eligible for either procedure, with a companion registry when patients were not (20). All patients had at least one high-risk feature consisting of age greater than 80 years, significant cardiac or pulmonary disease, contralateral carotid occlusion or laryngeal-nerve palsy, prior neck surgery or radiation, or restenosis after carotid endarterectomy. All stenting patients had emboli protection (Angioguard or Angioguard XP; Cordis, Miami Lakes, FL) before deployment of a nitinol stent (Precise or Smart stent; Cordis). The study enrolled 747 patients, 334 randomized, 406 in the stent registry, and only 7 in the surgical registry. The primary endpoint of death, MI or stroke at 30 days plus death from neurologic causes or ipsilateral stroke from 31 days to 1 year, was significantly lower for carotid stenting compared to endarterectomy (12.2% vs. 20.1%, $p = .05$), with trends to decreased myocardial infarction (3.0% vs. 7.5%, $p = .07$) and death (7.4% vs. 13.5%, $p = .08$). Target vessel revascularization was significantly lower for carotid stent patients (0.6% vs. 4.3%, $p = .04$), as was cranial nerve palsy (0% vs. 4.9%, $p = .004$).

Multiple additional device registries have reported similar risks of death, MI, or stroke at 1 year from 4.5% to 9.1% by various specialties and including community hospitals. On March 17, 2005, the Centers for Medicare and Medicaid Services (CMS) expanded the reimbursement of carotid stenting to high-risk patients with symptomatic greater than 70% carotid artery stenosis. CMS will also reimburse carotid stenting for high-risk patients with greater than 80% stenosis if they are enrolled in clinical trials pending the results of several ongoing randomized trials comparing stenting to endarterectomy that have agreed to combine data for a meta-analysis. In the United States, the National Institutes of Health (NIH)-sponsored Carotid Revascularization Endarterectomy Versus Stent (CREST) trial is enrolling symptomatic and asymptomatic patients, and the Asymptomatic Carotid Stenosis Stenting Versus Endarterectomy Trial (ACT-I) is randomizing asymptomatic patients with severe carotid artery stenosis to either stenting or endarterectomy in a 3 : 1 ratio.

Intracranial Stenosis

Intracranial atherosclerosis accounts for about 10% of all ischemic stroke and is a high-risk condition. The risk of recurrent stroke with symptomatic greater than 50% stenosis is 19%, with 1/4 occurring in territory of the symptomatic artery, often early within the first year, and at similar rates regardless of oral anticoagulant or antiplatelet therapy (21). The risk of stroke with intracranial stenting was 11.5% within the first year in 61 patients treated with Neurolink stent in the Stenting of Symptomatic Atherosclerotic Lesions in the Vertebral or Intracranial Arteries (SSYLVIA) registry (22) and 7.1% within 6 months in 45 patients treated with the Wingspan stent (23). Because the rate of restenosis greater than 50% at 6 months was lower with the Wingspan stent (7.5% vs. 35%), it was chosen for an NIH phase I safety trial in patients with symptomatic 70% to 99% intracranial stenosis. Symptomatic intracranial atherosclerosis is also a predictor of high CHD risk, and the rate of MI or sudden death within 2 years was significantly higher in warfarin-treated versus aspirin-treated patients in the Warfarin-Aspirin Symptomatic Intracranial Disease (WASID) trial, 7.3% versus 2.9% (21).

Cardiac Disease

The presence of cardiac disease doubles the risk for stroke. Concomitant coronary heart disease (CAD) is frequent in patients with cerebrovascular disease; 86% have angiographic evidence, of which 40% are severe, and for patients with atherothrombotic stroke, MI is the most frequent cause of death. Cardiogenic embolism accounts for approximately 15% to 20% of all ischemic strokes. The common clinical syndromes are those involving the middle cerebral artery, posterior cerebral artery, or top of the basilar and reflect cerebral blood flow patterns. Some causes of cardiogenic cerebral embolism are well established; other more commonly encountered cardiac conditions are less well established. More detailed discussions are given elsewhere in this text.

Nonvalvular Atrial Fibrillation

Overall, 1/2 of all cardioembolic strokes and one-third of strokes occurring in the elderly are in the setting of atrial fibrillation (AF). One-third of patients with AF sustain a stroke during their lifetime, and one third have evidence of a silent stroke. The perception that oral anticoagulation was hazardous limited its use until pivotal clinical trials in the 1980s and the development and widespread adoption of the International Normalized Ratio (INR) method of anticoagulant monitoring. Stroke risk reduction with warfarin was 68% (range 50% to 79%), which increased to 83% when target anticoagulation of INR 2 to 3 was achieved. Failure of anticoagulation to prevent stroke was associated with an INR close to 1.0 in 60% of patients. The stroke risk reduction with aspirin alone, particularly 325 mg/day, was 20% to 25% when compared to placebo. Recommendations for antithrombotic therapy balance the expected benefit of protection from thromboembolic stroke and systemic embolism against the risk of intracranial hemorrhage and systemic bleeding.

The nonvalvular atrial fibrillation (NVAF) trials represent the most extensive data set for stroke prevention focused on a very specific stroke subtype, in contrast to most of the stroke prevention literature, which include many stroke subtypes with variable natural histories. As a result of these outcomes studies, calculators have been developed to further subclassify patients by risk and guide recommendations for antithrombotic therapies. The recommended therapy for patients at high risk and most patients at intermediate risk is warfarin with an INR range 2.0 to 3.0 for low-risk aspirin. Combination therapy adding low-dose aspirin to standard warfarin therapy should be considered for those with significant coronary heart disease risk, again balancing potential benefits against the increased risks of bleeding with combination therapy (24).

Despite these data, 50% to 75% of patients with atrial fibrillation do not receive appropriate treatment. The most frequently cited reasons are the fear of hemorrhagic complications, particularly hemorrhagic stroke, and the requirement for regular monitoring and adjustment of therapy. Aggregate data on the complications of oral anticoagulant therapy for NVAF included intracerebral hemorrhage at an overall rate of 0.3%/year, although patients were excluded from the trials if they were at risk for bleeding including prior intracranial hemorrhage, predisposition to trauma, inability for adequate follow-up, uncontrolled hypertension, or alcohol abuse. In warfarin-eligible patients, standard warfarin therapy was superior to the combination therapy of aspirin with low-intensity, fixed-dose warfarin (INR 1.2 to 1.5) in the Stroke Prevention in Atrial Fibrillation III (SPAF III) trial and combination aspirin with clopidogrel 75 mg/day in the Atrial Fibrillation Clopidogrel Trial with Irbesartan for Prevention of Vascular Events (ACTIVE-W), resulting in the halting of those trials.

Alternative approaches for stroke prevention in AF are sorely needed. For warfarin-ineligible patients, the combination of aspirin and clopidogrel remains under study in the ACTIVE-I trial. Because the left atrial appendage (LAA) is thought to be the primary source of emboli, endovascular closure of the LAA is under study in a randomized clinical trial comparing the Watchman device to adjusted-dose warfarin in warfarin-eligible patients. Endovascular ablation procedures have also been posed as an alternative, although one of the risks of the procedure is cardioembolic stroke, and the risk of AF relapse would still warrant long-term anticoagulation for stroke prevention. There are no pivotal randomized clinical trials comparing ablation to standard medical therapies, but aggregate case series have reported reductions in stroke (25).

In the Atrial Fibrillation Follow-up Investigation of Rhythm Management (AFFIRM) trial comparing a rate versus rhythm control strategy, all patients were initially anticoagulated, but this was discontinued in some patients who were believed to remain in sinus rhythm (26). The risk of stroke was related to the recurrence of AF as well as age, prior TIA or stroke, and diabetes but was not related to the rate or rhythm control strategy. Because warfarin therapy reduced stroke risk by 68%, the authors hypothesized that episodes of occult AF continue, and they recommended that anticoagulation be continued lifelong in eligible patients (27).

Acute Myocardial Infarction

Prior to thrombolytic therapy, stroke complicated 0.8% to 5.5% of acute MIs. For most patients, the stroke risk continues for 4 to 6 months, although 90% occur within the first 2 weeks. Risk factors for stroke include older age, prior history of stroke, paroxysmal AF, anterior or apical location, impaired left ventricular (LV) function, and severity of MI. Mural thrombi have been identified in 38% to 67% of pathologic studies, but embolization often occurs in the absence of detectable thrombus on echocardiography. Three large randomized clinical trials have demonstrated stroke reduction from 2.3% to 5% to 0.8% to 1.7% with short-term anticoagulant therapy. Long-term anticoagulant therapy after acute MI has also been shown to reduce embolic stroke but with an increased risk for intracerebral hemorrhage (ICH); such therapy is recommended in patients at increased risk for embolic stroke such as those with AF, prior systemic embolism, CHF, echo evidence of mural thrombus, or persistent LV dysfunction.

Valvular Heart Disease

Embolism occurs with all degrees of rheumatic mitral valve disease but is more frequently a complication of mitral stenosis, in which stroke risk is increased 6-fold without and 18-fold with concomitant atrial fibrillation. Long-term anticoagulation is recommended with AF as well as mitral stenosis associated with enlargement of the left atrium greater than 5.5 cm, presence of left atrial spontaneous echo contrast, and prior to balloon valvuloplasty. The risk for prosthetic valve thromboembolism is higher with valves in the mitral than in the aortic position, with multiple than with single valves, and with caged-ball than with tilting-disc or bileaflet valves. Additional risk factors for thromboembolism include prior thromboembolism, AF, CAD, an enlarged left atrium, and left atrial thrombus. Recommendations for antithrombotic therapy mirror these risk factors.

Mitral valve prolapse was commonly invoked as a cause of cryptogenic stroke in young adults several decades ago. Although pathologic documentation of platelet-fibrin aggregates on the valvular surface confirm its causal potential, it is more likely to be the cause of stroke when other risk factors are present, such as AF, an atrial septal abnormality, or hypercoagulable state. Antiplatelet therapy with aspirin 160 to 325 mg/day is recommended for secondary stroke prevention, with anticoagulation reserved for those failing antiplatelet therapy.

Embolization of calcific debris can complicate valvuloplasty or replacement of calcific aortic stenosis, but spontaneous embolization is uncommon. Mitral annual calcification is identified in 20% to 30% of elderly patients and is more a marker of vascular risk factors than a source of embolism.

Cardiomyopathy, Left Ventricular Dysfunction

Greater than 90% of all cases of chronic heart failure are due to dilated cardiomyopathy, which encompasses nearly 50 distinct diseases. Anticoagulation with an INR range of 2.0 to 3.0 (target 2.5) is recommended when chronic heart failure becomes complicated by atrial fibrillation or pulmonary or systemic embolism. The risk of ischemic stroke correlates better with the ejection fraction (EF) than clinical symptoms and increases with worsening LV from 1.5%/year to 2%/year at EF less than 30% to 35% to 2%/year to 4%/year with EF less than 10%. In the absence of atrial fibrillation, the optimum antithrombotic therapy for patients with poor LV function remains controversial.

The VA Heart Failure Trial (WATCH) was prematurely terminated due to poor enrollment. There was no difference in the primary endpoint of stroke, MI, or death among those treated with warfarin (INR 2.5 to 3), aspirin 160 mg daily, or clopidogrel 75 mg daily, although warfarin-treated patients had less stroke but more bleeding complications, and aspirin-treated patients had more hospitalizations for heart failure. The ongoing NIH-funded Warfarin vs Aspirin in Reduced Cardiac Ejection Fraction (WARCEF) trial is studying warfarin versus aspirin 325 mg daily in 2,860 patients, with prespecified plans to combine the data with the WATCH results.

Patent Foramen Ovale, Atrial Septal Aneurysm

Atrial septal abnormalities have become increasingly recognized as a potential cause of cryptogenic stroke in young adults, particularly within the last decade with the development of endovascular closure devices for treatment. Although paradoxical embolism is implied, rarely is a thrombus found straddling the atria. Patent foramen ovale (PFO) is found with a greater frequency in young patients with cryptogenic cause (50% to 60%) than in those with known cause (30% to 50%) or controls (10% to 30%). The risk of recurrent ischemic stroke is low at 0% to 4% and may be increased by large PFO size, associated atrial septal aneurysm, mitral valve prolapse, associated atrial arrhythmias, or underlying coagulopathy. The inclusion of atrial septal aneurysm, a bulging of the interatrial septum identified on echocardiography, as a potential cardioembolic source of stroke stems from its identification in 10% to 20% of those with cryptogenic stroke compared to 1% to 4% of normal controls. Risk appears to be increased with large size (>1 cm of bulging) as well as associated abnormalities such as septal fenestrations, atrial septal defects, patent foramen ovale, and mitral valve prolapse.

Case series of endovascular PFO closure support the safety and feasibility of treatment, although recurrent ischemic events are not eliminated and no data are available demonstrating superiority to medical therapy with either aspirin or warfarin alone (28). Clinical trials are underway to determine whether endovascular PFO closure with septal repair implants offers superior protection against stroke and systemic embolism compared to medical therapy with warfarin or aspirin. Trials include the CLOSURE trial (Prospective, Multicenter, Randomized Controlled Trial to Evaluate the Safety and Efficacy of the STARFlex® Septal Closure System Versus Best Medical Therapy in Patients with a Stroke and/or Transient Ischemic Attack Due to Presumed Paradoxical Embolism through a Patent Foramen Ovale) of 1,600 patients using the STARFlex device (NMT Medical, Boston), the RESPECT (Randomized Evaluation of Recurrent Stroke Comparing PFO Closure to Established Current Standard of Care Treatment) trial of 500 patients using the Amplatzer PFO occluder (AGA Medical Corporation, Golden Valley, MN), and the CARDIA-Star trial of 300 patients using the CARDIA-Star PFO closure device (Cardia, Burnsville, MN). Because the effectiveness of these devices compared to standard medical therapies has not been demonstrated, endovascular closure outside of a clinical trial in the United States should be restricted to the clinical scenario outlined in the Food and Drug Administration (FDA) Human Device Exemption statement, which specifies patients with a recurrent cryptogenic stroke presumed to be due to paradoxical embolism failing therapeutic levels of anticoagulant therapy.

Hypercoagulable States

Hypercoagulable states are linked to stroke by several mechanisms. Inherited or acquired prothrombotic disorders such as antithrombin III deficiency, factor V Leiden, protein C deficiency, protein S deficiency, prothrombin gene 20210A mutation, paroxysmal nocturnal hemoglobinuria, and the nephrotic syndrome are more likely to produce venous thromboses. Cerebral venous thrombosis can produce venous infarction and cerebral hemorrhage, and systemic venous thrombosis can serve as a source of cerebral embolism if a concomitant intracardiac defect permitting right-to-left shunting is present (29).

In a heterogeneous group of ischemic stroke patients, antiphospholipid antibodies, often of low titer, can be identified in 41%, may be transient, and neither increase the risk of recurrent stroke or other thromboembolic events nor predict a differential response to aspirin or warfarin therapy (30). Routine screening for these antibodies is not warranted. This should be distinguished from the rarer antiphospholipid syndrome, with medium to high titers of anticardiolipin antibodies and manifest as unexplained systemic venous and arterial thrombosis, thrombocytopenia, and fetal loss as well as seizures, migraine, chorea, transverse myelitis, multiinfarct dementia, livedo reticularis, and rheumatic symptoms. Rare cases of chronic, organized atrial thrombus mimicking an atrial myxoma have also been reported. Although recommendations for antithrombotic therapy are controversial, one reasonable approach is to treat most patients with aspirin and reserve long-term oral anticoagulation for patients with persistent antibody positivity and either a cardioembolic mechanism for stroke or venous thrombosis.

Although the results of individual population studies have reported conflicting results on the risk of oral contraceptive pills (OCPs) in young women, meta-analysis have reported small but significantly increased risks of ischemic stroke by 1.93 times and subarachnoid hemorrhage of 1.55 times when controlled for smoking and hypertension. When OCP use produces activated protein C resistance, the risk of deep vein thrombosis increases by 3 to 4 times in patients without, by 35 times in patients heterozygous for, and by 50 to 100 times in patient homozygous for the Leiden V mutation, which could be pertinent in young women with an associated intraatrial septal abnormality (31).

Nonbacterial thrombotic endocarditis is rare and usually is a complication of a mucin-producing malignancy, but it has also been described with autoimmune disease and AIDS and postpartum. It is often not diagnosed until autopsy, and the clinical presentation includes arterial and venous thromboses, disseminated intravascular coagulation, and multiorgan failure. Treatment includes therapy of the underlying disease, and heparins, but not warfarin, have been shown to reduce thromboembolic risk.

Genetic Factors

Most genetic influence is multifactorial, involving the interplay of genetic variants and environmental factors (32). Family studies have shown an overall 1.5- to 2.5-fold increase risk with a history of stroke in a first-degree relative, and the large, computerized Icelandic database has recently identified a potential gene on the long arm of chromosome 5 (5q12). The NIH is performing genetic linkage studies for the 15% of intracranial aneurysms that are familial and can be associated with polycystic kidney disease, Ehlers-Danlos syndrome type IV, and Marfan syndrome.

In addition, there are more than 50 uncommon causes of stroke as part of or the predominant feature due to specific monogenic mutations. Mutations of the *NOTCH3* gene cause cerebral autosomal dominant arteriopathy with subcortical infarcts and leukoencephalopathy (CADASIL), manifest as migraine headaches, seizures, and multiple small subcortical infarcts prominently displayed on MRI scans, and progressing to vascular dementia. Mutations of the *APP*, *CST3*, and *BRI* genes cause cerebral amyloid angiopathy, which is an important cause of cerebral hemorrhage, particularly complicating thrombolytic therapy, and mutation of the *KRIT1* gene causes cavernous malformations.

For some disorders, specific therapy is guided by recognizing the genetic defect. Transcranial Doppler monitoring of patients with sickle cell disease identifies those at high risk for stroke, which can be reduced with long-term infusion therapy. Sickle cell disease is an autosomal recessive disorder associated with thrombotic occlusions and stroke in young adults. Transcranial Doppler monitoring identifies high-risk patients requiring transfusion therapy for stroke prevention. Fabry disease, an X-linked lysosomal storage disease causing lacunar infarcts in young adults, skin angiokeratomas, renal disease, and painful neuropathy, can be treated by replacement of the defective α-galactosidase A enzyme. Homocystinuria, an autosomal recessive disease caused by a defect in the cystathionine β-synthase enzyme–encoding gene, causes thromboembolism and premature atherosclerosis and can be treated with a combination of pyridoxine, folic acid, vitamin B12, and dietary restriction. Mitochondrial encephalopathy, lactic acidosis, and stroke-like episodes (MELAS), caused by defects in respiratory-chain enzymes from mutations in the maternal mitochondrial DNA, produces cerebral infarctions not conforming to specific arterial distributions, short stature, seizures, dementia, and myopathy and can be suspected by elevated levels of lactate and pyruvate during an attack. Treatment with diet and nutritional supplements can be helpful.

Alcohol and Tobacco

Modest amounts of alcohol (<2 oz daily) seem to reduce the risk for stroke, possibly through antiplatelet or lipid-lowering effects. High intake of alcohol increases the risk for stroke especially hemorrhagic stroke. However, hypertension, cigarette smoking, paroxysmal AF with alcoholic cardiomyopathy (CM), and trauma are confounding factors that make the role of alcohol as an independent risk factor unclear. Cigarette smoking increases the risk of stroke relative to the degree of smoking both for thromboembolic stroke from atherosclerotic disease and subarachnoid hemorrhage, particularly in women (33).

Other Specific Considerations in Stroke Related to Cardiac Disease

Cerebrovascular Complications of Cardiovascular Procedures

Stroke complicates 2% to 5% of coronary artery bypass surgeries and up to 15% of those operations that require opening of the cardiac chambers. Risk factors include atherosclerosis of the proximal aorta, hypertension, diabetes mellitus, prior TIA or stroke, history of neurologic disease, age greater than 70 years, history of pulmonary disease, and postoperative atrial fibrillation (34). Procedural risks include embolization from the aorta during cross-clamping or aortotomy, increased complexity and length of the surgery, valvular surgery, and open-chamber procedures in which embolism of air and particulates can occur during mechanical de-airing of the heart. "Off-pump" coronary artery bypass surgery or the use of emboli capture devices has been reported to reduce these risks. Postoperative encephalopathy or confusional states is evident in about 10% of patients, although careful neuropsychologic testing discloses impairments in 35% to 75%, of which 20% are severe within the first week and 10% to 30% persist to 3 to 6 months. Risk factors for postoperative encephalopathy also include advanced age, baseline cognitive impairment, a history of excessive alcohol consumption, and the other stroke risk factors.

Cerebral embolism complicates 0.1% to 1.0% of cardiac catheterizations and 0.2% to 0.3% of coronary interventions, with a predominance for the vertebrobasilar circulation manifest as confusional states, cortical blindness or hemianoptic visual field defects, and intrinsic brain stem signs (Fig. 107.1). Angiographic procedures rarely produce a transient breakdown of the blood–brain barrier with contrast enhancement on CT, which manifests as a vascular headache with confusion and cortical blindness with contrast enhancement that resolves in 1 to 2 days with antihypertensive therapy. Cerebral embolism also complicates 1.4% to 11% of aortic valvuloplasty and 3.2% to 4.2% of mitral valvuloplasty procedures.

Ischemic complications of intraaortic balloon counterpulsation catheters include an ischemic monomelic neuropathy of

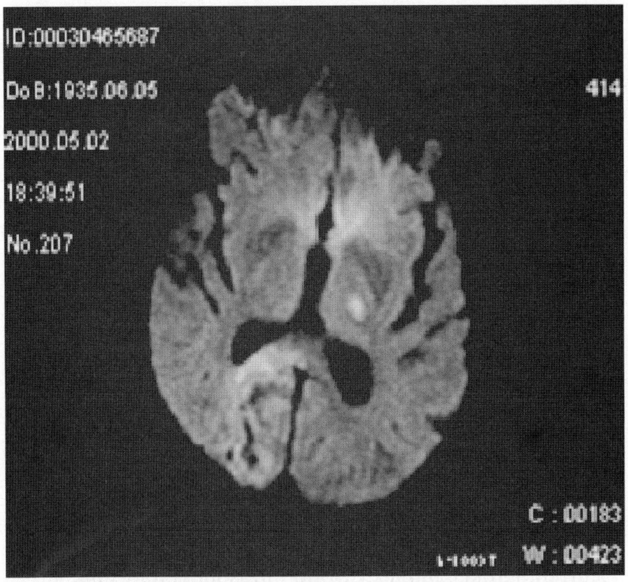

FIGURE 107.1. Diffusion-weighted magnetic resonance imaging of bilateral posterior cerebral artery embolism after cardiac catheterization.

the involved limb manifest as distal weakness and causalgic pain as well as paraplegia from spinal cord infarction. The frequency of hypoxic–ischemic encephalopathy or stroke due to hypotension before insertion of a left ventricular assist device varies in surgical series up to 25%. Subsequent stroke from embolism of air or thrombus or coagulopathy-related hemorrhage occurs in an additional 10% to 20% and is greater with longer durations of pump assist and during manipulation of the pump.

Infectious Endocarditis

The risk of stroke is greatest before the institution of appropriate antibiotic therapy at 6%/day and rapidly declines after 2 to 3 weeks. Anticoagulation in the acute period of endocarditis affecting a native or bioprosthetic valve should be avoided because the risk of serious or fatal hemorrhage is increased in the event of a mycotic aneurysm rupture and there is no evidence that it decreases the risk of embolism. For patients with anticoagulated mechanical valves, anticoagulation is typically continued except after embolism from *Staphylococcus aureus* prosthetic valve endocarditis, in which case the bleeding risk is sufficiently increased to warrant discontinuation of all anticoagulation for the first 2 weeks of antibiotic therapy.

Cerebral mycotic aneurysms are more common than peripheral aneurysms and occur in 2% of clinical and 5% to 10% of autopsy cases. With antibiotic therapy, about 1/2 of mycotic aneurysms will resolve and 30% will improve, but 20% will enlarge, and there are no clear radiographic features that predict the risk of rupture (35). Usually angiography is performed in symptomatic patients after 2 to 3 weeks of antibiotic therapy, and historically, surgical excision was reserved for cerebral mycotic aneurysms that enlarge or persist. However, patients with cerebral mycotic aneurysms are a high-risk subset; overall mortality is 60%, ranging from 30% if unruptured to nearly 80% if ruptured. Endovascular therapy has been shown in small series to be effective in obliterating proximal and distal mycotic aneurysms with low risk in experienced hands (36). Although initially recommended as preventive therapy for patients who require early cardiac surgery, it has also been advocated for definitive nonsurgical treatment at the time of diagnosis.

ISCHEMIC STROKE

Interpreting the Clinical Presentation and Determining a Diagnostic Evaluation

The neurologic history and examination elicit a pattern of symptoms and signs that are used to localize the lesion within the nervous system. Through an understanding of the cerebral vasculature supplying this region, diagnostic testing can be selected to determine a specific stroke subtype and mechanism of stroke, which, in turn, determine the treatment plan. The signs and symptoms of cerebral ischemia and infarction are determined by both the location and the extent of brain tissue injured (Table 107.5). The major causes of ischemic stroke are thrombotic occlusion or thromboembolism due to large-artery atherosclerosis from the extracranial or intracranial vessels (20%), lacunar infarcts due to small-vessel disease (20% to 25%), and cardioembolism (15% to 20%), which together account for two thirds of all ischemic strokes. Other, rarer causes (5%) include cervicocephalic dissection, nonatherosclerotic

TABLE 107.5

CLINICAL SYNDROMES OF CEREBRAL ARTERY OCCLUSIONS

Carotid system	
Ophthalmic artery	Total or partial monocular blindness, usually altitudinal
Anterior cerebral artery	Contralateral weakness leg > proximal arm, urinary incontinence, behavioral changes
Middle cerebral artery	
Anterior division	Contralateral motor and sensory loss, maximal for face, hand, and arm; if dominant hemisphere, nonfluent (Broca) aphasia
Posterior division	Contralateral hemisensory loss and homonymous hemianopsia; if dominant hemisphere, fluent (Wernicke) aphasia
Deep perforators	Contralateral hemiparesis affecting face, arm, and leg about equally
Vertebrobasilar system	
Posterior cerebral artery	Hemianopsia, cortical blindness, alexia without agraphia, agitated delirium, memory deficit
Basilar branches	Crossed cranial nerve/contralateral limb deficits, bilateral bulbar weakness with dysarthria, dysphagia and loss of airway protection, diplopia, quadriparesis, limb ataxia, vertigo, nausea, vomiting
Vertebral artery	Ipsilateral sensory/contralateral weakness, dysarthria, diplopia, dysphagia, hiccups, nausea, vomiting

TABLE 107.6

LACUNAR SYNDROMES AND THEIR TYPICAL LOCATIONS

Pure motor hemiparesis (PMH)	Internal capsule, pons
PMH with crossed III nerve palsy	Midbrain
PMH with crossed VI nerve palsy	Pons
Ataxic demiparesis	Pons
Dysarthria-clumsy hand syndrome	Pons or capsule
Pure sensory syndrome	Posterior-lateral thalamus
Lateral medullary syndrome (Wallenberg)	Lateral medulla
Sensorimotor stroke	Thalamocapsular
Thalamic dementia	Anterior thalamus

arteriopathies, coagulopathies, metabolic disorders, migraine, vasculitis, and drug abuse. The remaining cases are cryptogenic (30%) either because an adequate diagnostic evaluation was not performed (e.g., a contrast-enhanced transesophageal echocardiogram for PFO or hematologic testing for a hypercoagulable disorder) or the condition was not documented at the time of the evaluation (e.g., paroxysmal atrial fibrillation).

Lacunar infarction from occlusive disease of the small vessels produces characteristic syndromes determined by the subcortical anatomy of the arterial penetrators (37). The most common are pure-motor hemiparesis, pure-sensory syndrome, ataxic hemiparesis, sensorimotor syndrome, and dysarthria-clumsy hand syndrome (Table 107.6).

Cortical involvement including aphasia, visual field defects, inattention, neglect, and other cognitive or behavioral disorders as well as seizures implies involvement of other large arteries. Symptoms isolated to a specific arterial distribution suggest thrombosis or embolism from *large-artery atherosclerosis* or other nonatherosclerotic arteriopathies. When symptoms are confined to an arterial distribution, the more stereotyped symptoms suggest a more distal, or intracranial, source, whereas the less stereotyped symptoms suggest an extracranial source.

Cardioembolism is suggested by nonstereotyped, nonlacunar involvement of the cortex or cerebellum in multiple vascular territories including systemic embolism, cardiac symptoms of syncope or palpitations, or the profile of cryptogenic stroke in a young patient without risk factors for premature atherosclerosis. Because platelet-fibrin emboli can lyse, resulting in spontaneous reperfusion, rapid clinical recovery, seizures at onset, or hemorrhagic conversion of the infarct also suggests an embolic mechanism. Reflecting the patterns of cerebral blood flow, proximal emboli are more likely to lodge in the middle cerebral artery or the posterior cerebral artery, and thus certain clinical syndromes are overrepresented, such as Wernicke aphasia, ideomotor apraxia, isolated hemianopia, and top-of-the-basilar syndrome. Although these clinical patterns serve as a guide, it is important to remember that cardioembolism can repeatedly affect the middle cerebral artery or manifest only as transient retinal ischemia and can occur at any time regardless of physical activity. Although 90% of embolic strokes are maximal at onset, the remainder can have a stuttering onset reflecting stagnant flow with a partially occluding embolus. Alternatively, a cardioembolic mechanism cannot always be inferred by the mere presence of a potential cardioembolic source because an estimated 30% of patients have concomitant cerebrovascular atherosclerosis that may be the true cause.

The evaluation begins with a complete history, including vascular risk factors, followed by a complete physical and neurologic examination with attention to the vascular system. In an acutely symptomatic patient, the first evaluation should include a fingerstick measurement of glucose because significant hyper- and hypoglycemia can mimic an acute stroke. Additional basic evaluation includes laboratory testing of electrolytes, complete blood count, and coagulation studies. For most acute patients, neuroimaging with a CT scan of the brain without contrast is performed to differentiate hemorrhagic from ischemic stroke and exclude other structural lesions that may present in a similar fashion, such as a primary or metastatic tumor or subdural hematoma. For patients with major deficits, early infarct signs can be identified within several hours, but small cortical infarcts may not be evident for several days, and infarcts within the posterior fossa may not be evident at all due to bony artifacts within this region. MRI offers superior resolution within the posterior and temporal fossa, and, compared to CT, DWI, and T2-weighted, fluid-attenuated inversion recovery (T2/FLAIR), MRI scans are more sensitive for infarction and gradient echo MRI scans are more sensitive for iron deposition in a recent or remote hemorrhage.

Vascular imaging of the symptomatic territory is an important element of the evaluation because patients with severe extracranial or intracranial stenoses have the greatest risk of early recurrent stroke. Duplex carotid ultrasonography combines a B-mode anatomic image with a Doppler assessment of blood flow and is the preferred noninvasive study (85% sensitivity, 90% specificity), with the caveat that critical stenoses with low flow can be mistaken for an occlusion. Transcranial Doppler (TCD) ultrasonography can be used to evaluate the intracranial vasculature (38). Magnetic resonance angiography (MRA) provides an evaluation of the extracranial carotid circulation with comparable sensitivity and specificity to Duplex carotid ultrasonography but has the advantage of evaluating the vertebrobasilar system and the intracranial circulation as well. The major limitations of MRA include patient intolerance due to claustrophobia and increased cost, and it is contraindicated in patients with implanted metal devices such as pacemakers, defibrillators, certain aneurysm clips, and other intracranial or intraocular metal foreign bodies.

The electrocardiogram (ECG) is an important part of the basic evaluation because the identification of AF or a recent MI has a significant effect on further testing and choice of antithrombotic therapy. Continuous ECG is indicated for patients with hemorrhagic stroke and selected patients with temporal lobe ischemia who are at increased risk for a variety of dysrhythmias, but it should also be performed in patients with syncope or palpitations at onset, unexplained stroke, and other cardiac symptoms or signs.

Transthoracic echocardiography (TTE) provides information about LV function and is indicated in all patients with symptoms or signs of heart disease or cryptogenic stroke, but it is of limited usefulness in elderly patients with no evidence of heart disease. The diagnostic sensitivity for right-to-left shunting is highest when a Valsalva maneuver is combined with microbubble contrast during TCD monitoring (Fig. 107.2). Transesophageal echocardiography (TEE) is most helpful in patients with cryptogenic stroke in evaluating structural causes of shunting and aortic arch atheromatous disease. However, because these are highly prevalent conditions in the young and the elderly, respectively, their etiologic role should be carefully considered (39).

Carotid angiography is most useful in evaluating for vasculitis, mycotic aneurysm, and intracranial stenosis and is the reference diagnostic test for determining the severity of carotid artery stenosis. The identification of an intracranial branch occlusion or delayed perfusion of distal arterial branches in the absence of a more proximal arterial source of embolism implies a proximal source of embolism, such as the heart. However, angiography performed after 24 hours of symptom onset frequently proves normal due to spontaneous lysis of platelet-fibrin emboli. As an invasive test, serious complications occur

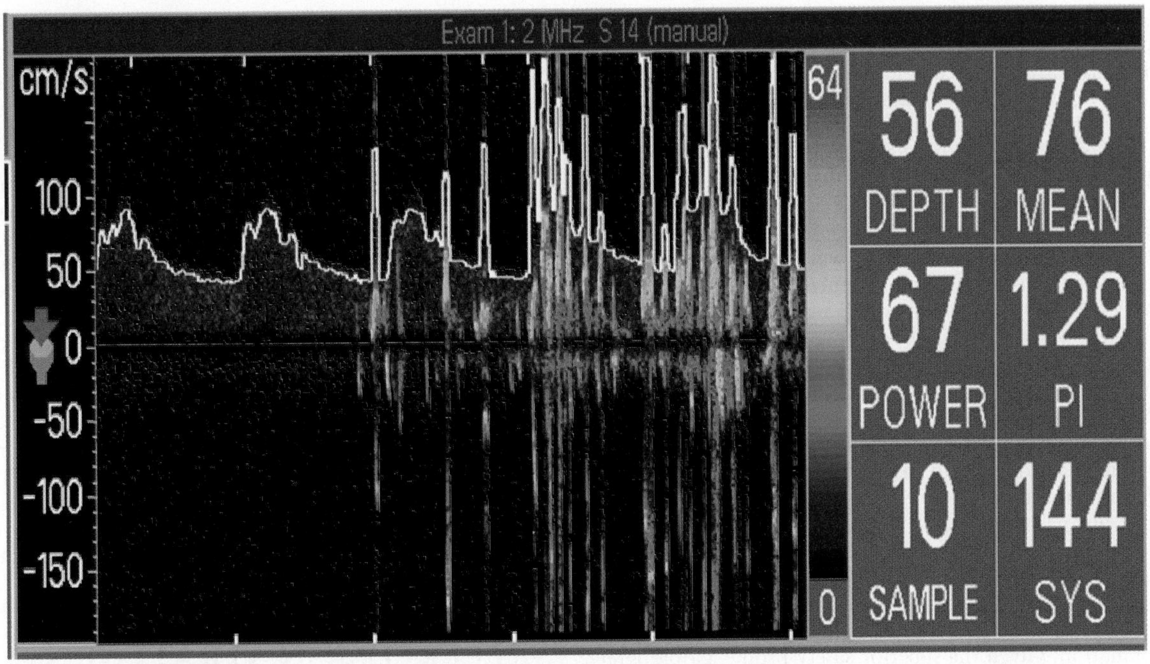

FIGURE 107.2. Transcranial Doppler with microbubble contrast and Valsalva maneuver demonstrating right-to-left shunting.

in less than 1% to 3% of patients; these include cerebral embolism, bleeding complications, and contrast-related reactions or renal insufficiency. With intraarterial digital subtraction techniques and arterial closure devices, the procedure can be performed on an outpatient basis.

Additional laboratory testing for the rarer causes of stroke, coagulopathies, metabolic disorders, and vasculitis are performed on an individual basis, particularly in young patients with cryptogenic stroke.

Antithrombotic Therapies

Antiplatelet Therapy

For 25 years, aspirin has been the standard preventive therapy for patients at risk for stroke, although the optimum dose for stroke prevention is controversial. For primary prevention in men, aspirin doses in the range of 75 to 325 mg/day significantly reduce the risk of vascular events by 12%, primarily from the 32% reduction in myocardial infarction (40). For primary prevention in women in the Women's Health Study of more than 39,000 women, aspirin 100 mg every other day significantly reduces the risk of stroke by 17%, mainly by reducing ischemic stroke by 24% (41). However, there is no significant reduction in stroke among men or myocardial infarction among women, and for neither gender is cardiovascular mortality reduced. In addition, aspirin significantly increases the relative risk of bleeding by one third, which includes hemorrhagic stroke. The risk of hemorrhagic stroke is increased by 16% with aspirin use, which translates into an absolute risk of 12 events per 10,000 persons treated for 3 years, or 0.04%/year (42). To balance the benefit-to-risk ratio for primary prevention in individual patients, the CHD calculator is most useful for men, and the Women's Health Study recommends limiting aspirin use in low-risk women to those older than the age of 60 years.

For secondary stroke prevention, the current American College of Chest Physicians guidelines recommend "aspirin, 50 to 325 mg daily, the combination of aspirin 25 mg and extended-release dipyridamole 200 mg twice daily, or clopidogrel 75 mg daily are all acceptable options for initial therapy." Aspirin was approved by the FDA in 1980, originally for "men with TIAs due to fibrin platelet emboli" based on a trial using 1,300 mg/day (43). The Antithrombotic Trialists' Collaboration meta-analysis of 287 trials of more than 130,000 patients reported that for patients with prior TIA or stroke, the significant risk reduction of 25% for the combined endpoint of vascular events was driven by the 22% reduction of a recurrent nonfatal stroke (44). Treatment was effective regardless of gender, middle or older age, or presence of hypertension or diabetes mellitus. Subgroup analyses showed no significant differences in reduction of vascular events for daily doses of 75 to 150 mg (26%), 160 to 325 mg (28%), or 500 to 1,500 mg (21%), with most individuals receiving 100 to 325 mg/day.

Aspirin at 900 to 1,300 mg/day with dipyridamole 150 to 300 mg/day was not demonstrated to be superior to aspirin alone in several trials; thus combination therapy was largely abandoned for stroke prevention until the European Stroke Prevention Study (ESPS II) evaluated aspirin 50 mg or 400 mg of extended-release dipyridamole alone or in the combination versus placebo in a factorial design (45). There were significant reductions in the relative risk of recurrent stroke at 18% for low-dose aspirin alone, 16% for dipyridamole alone, 37% for the combination versus placebo, and 23% with the combination over aspirin alone. None of the treatments reduced the risk of myocardial infarction or vascular death, but there were very few cardiovascular events in the trial overall. The predominant side effects include gastrointestinal complaints with aspirin and headache with dipyridamole.

Clopidogrel and ticlopidine are thienopyridine derivatives that inhibit platelet aggregation by selectively and irreversibly inhibiting the ADP-dependent activation of fibrinogen binding via the glycoprotein IIb/IIIa complex. The Ticlopidine Aspirin Stroke Study (TASS) (46) compared ticlopidine 500 mg/day to aspirin 1,300 mg/day in patients with TIAs or minor strokes. Ticlopidine significantly reduced the risk for fatal or nonfatal stroke by 19% compared with aspirin, 48% within the first year. Serious adverse events occurred in 2% of both agents, but ticlopidine was associated with a 1% risk of significant neutropenia, warranting complete blood count (CBC) monitoring every 2 weeks for the first 3 months of therapy. This safety and efficacy profile largely limited its use in stroke patients to aspirin failures and was replaced with other agents when postmarketing surveillance also disclosed a risk of thrombotic thrombocytopenic purpura (TTP) in 200 to 625 cases per million ticlopidine-treated patients.

Clopidogrel 75 mg once daily was approved after the Clopidrogrel versus Aspirin in Patients at Risk of Ischemic Events (CAPRIE) study demonstrated a significant but modest 9% relative risk reduction in the combined endpoint of stroke, MI, or vascular death for clopidogrel 75 mg/day over aspirin 325 mg/day in 19,185 patients with a recent vascular event (47). Although the majority of the events in the trial were recurrent strokes in patients with cerebrovascular disease, the benefit was driven by a reduction in vascular events for those patients with peripheral arterial disease. Rash and diarrhea were more frequent, but gastrointestinal intolerance and bleeding were less with clopidogrel, and no CBC monitoring was required. In postmarketing surveillance, the incidence of TTP is estimated to be 3.7 cases per million clopidogrel-treated patients against a background rate of 4 cases per million person-years in the general population. Given the superior safety profile, clopidogrel has essentially replaced ticlopidine as an aspirin alternative.

Given the superiority of aspirin with clopidogrel in acute coronary syndromes, the MATCH (Management of ATherothrombosis with Clopidogrel in High-Risk Patients with Recent Transient Ischemic Attack or Ischemic Stroke) trial evaluated the combination against clopidogrel alone in 7,599 high-risk patients with TIA or ischemic stroke within the preceding 3 months (48). The reduction in the combined vascular endpoint was not statistically significant, and subgroup analyses did not indicate a promising subset. Of concern, the statistically significant increase in major and life-threatening bleeding events, 4.49% in the combination group versus 1.88% in the clopidogrel-only group, included an increased risk of intracranial bleeding, 1.1% versus 0.07%. This trial does not support the use of combination aspirin and clopidogrel therapy over clopidogrel alone. However, there are several trials in progress evaluating this combination for specific stroke populations, such as lacunar stroke in the SPS-3 trial, aortic arch atheromatous disease in the ARCH (Aortic Arch Related Cerebral Hazard) study, and acute ischemic stroke in the FASTER (Fast Assessment of Stroke and Transient Ischemic Attack to Prevent Early Recurrence) and CASTIA (Clopidogrel in Acute Stroke and TIA) trials.

Oral Anticoagulant Therapy

Although selected cardioembolic causes of stroke are the only indications for oral anticoagulant therapy in primary or secondary stroke prevention established by proper clinical trials, there are many situations in which it is commonly used. including cerebral venous thrombosis, a recent cervicocephalic artery dissection or atherosclerotic carotid occlusion, severe aortic arch atheromatous disease, cryptogenic stroke with a patent foramen ovale, and hypercoagulable disorders. The Warfarin-Aspirin Recurrent Stroke Study (WARSS) trial compared warfarin, adjusted to an INR range of 1.4 to 2.8, with aspirin 325 mg/day for secondary stroke prevention in 2,206 patients with a recent ischemic stroke. The mechanism of the qualifying event was a lacunar infarct in 56% of patients, cryptogenic in 26% (41% of whom had a PFO), and large-vessel atherosclerosis of the extracranial or intracranial vessels in 12% (49). The 2-year rates of stroke and death were not different between warfarin and aspirin (17.8% vs. 16.0%, respectively) nor were there differences in the rate of major hemorrhage (1.92% vs. 1.49%, respectively), demonstrating no benefit of warfarin for lacunar, cryptogenic, and large-vessel atherosclerotic subtypes. Although patients on aspirin at the time of their qualifying event had a higher rate of recurrent events, there was also no difference due to whether they were randomized to aspirin or warfarin. The Patent Foramen Ovale in Cryptogenic Stroke Study (PICSS) was a subset 265 patients with cryptogenic stroke and PFO entered into the WARSS trial. As the only randomized, double-blind data on medical therapy for PFO, PICSS also did not demonstrate any significant difference in the 2-year rates of stroke and death between those treated with warfarin and those treated with aspirin, nor was there an excess risk of recurrent strokes in patients with a PFO compared to other cryptogenic patients without a PFO (28).

The WASID trial compared warfarin (INR range 2 to 3) to aspirin 1,300 mg/day in patients with a recent TIA or ischemic stroke due to 50% or greater stenosis of an intracranial internal carotid, middle cerebral, basilar, or vertebral artery (21). This trial was prematurely terminated when there was an excess of systemic bleeding events in the warfarin group and a futility analysis excluded the possibility of showing a significant difference between the two treatments.

REPERFUSION STRATEGIES FOR ACUTE ISCHEMIC STROKE

Intravenous Thrombolysis

The only FDA-approved thrombolytic therapy for acute ischemic stroke is based on the National Institute of Neurological Disorders and Stroke (NINDS) trial of intravenous tissue-type plasminogen activator (IV t-PA) limited to patients within 3 hours of symptom onset. This pivotal trial introduced a rapid stroke examination scoring tool and was the impetus for approaching stroke patients in an emergent fashion (50) (Table 107.7). However, the narrow therapeutic window and the risk of hemorrhage has limited its use, and it is one of the most controversial issues in neurology (51). The NINDS t-PA trial was a placebo-controlled, randomized trial of 0.9 mg/kg t-PA given intravenously within 3 hours of symptom onset in 624 patients with severity and subtype of ischemic stroke. Patients treated according to protocol were 30% more likely to have minimal or no disability at 3 months than patients receiving placebo, with the magnitude of improvement less at longer time to treatment, advanced age, and more severe strokes. There was a significant tenfold increased risk of symptomatic brain hemorrhage within the first 36 hours: 6.4% in the t-PA group versus 0.6% in the placebo group. Although half of the brain hemorrhages were fatal, there was no difference in overall mortality between the two treatment groups. Early signs of infarction on CT and National Institutes of Health Stroke Scale (NIHSS) score greater than 20 were associated with an increased risk of symptomatic brain hemorrhage (52). Clinical trials investigating IV therapy up to 6 hours have overall been negative, with ICH risks of 7% to 20%, but similar benefits could be demonstrated in those patients early, within 3 hours. Because the benefit-to-risk ratio is narrow, the NINDS protocol should be followed carefully; protocol deviations have been linked to increased rates of ICH (Table 107.8) (53).

Intraarterial Thrombolysis

The pivotal trial of intraarterial therapy was the Prolyse in Acute Cerebral Thromboembolism Trial (PROACT II) (54), which demonstrated clinical efficacy with intraarterial (IA) recombinant prourokinase (proUK) in patients with middle

TABLE 107.7

NATIONAL INSTITUTES OF HEALTH STROKE SCALE (NIHSS)

1a. Level of consciousness (LOC)
- (0) Alert, keenly responsive
- (1) Not alert, aroused by minor stimulation
- (2) Not alert, requires repetitive stimulation
- (3) Comatose or reflex motor to noxious stimulation

1b. LOC questions
- (0) Answers both age and month
- (1) Answers one correctly or unable to speak not due to aphasia
- (2) Answers neither correctly or is aphasic, stuporous, or comatose

1c. LOC commands
- (0) Performs both correctly
- (1) Performs one correctly
- (2) Performs neither or comatose

2. Gaze
- (0) Normal
- (1) Partial gaze, not forced or total, can overcome by doll's head maneuver, cranial nerve palsy
- (2) Forced deviation, gaze palsy not overcome by doll's head maneuver

3. Visual fields
- (0) Full, looks at side or threat
- (1) Partial hemianopia documented or extinction revealed by double simultaneous stimulation
- (2) Complete hemianopia
- (3) Bilateral hemianopia or blind from any cause

4. Facial weakness
- (0) Normal
- (1) Minor, asymmetry, flattening of nasolabial fold
- (2) Partial, weakness of lower face
- (3) Complete, total upper plus lower facial weakness

5 and 6. Motor scale: a, left; b, right
- (0) No drift (arm for 10 s, leg for 5 s)
- (1) Drift, but does not hit bed
- (2) Some antigravity but hits bed
- (3) No antigravity
- (4) No voluntary motion, comatose
- (X) Amputee/joint fusion

7. Ataxia
- (0) Absent, or untestable due to paralysis or coma
- (1) One limb
- (2) Two limbs

8. Sensory
- (0) Normal to testing or noxious
- (1) Mild to moderate
- (2) Severe, total, or comatose

9. Aphasia
- (0) None
- (1) Mild to moderate
- (2) Severe, fragmentary
- (3) Mute, global, or comatose

10. Dysarthia
- (0) Absent
- (1) Mild to moderate
- (2) Severe, mute, anarthric, coma
- (X) Intubated or other barrier

11. Neglect
- (0) None
- (1) One sensory modality
- (2) More than one modality, coma

NIHSS total (0–42): ....
Coma = 35 + score on items 2 (gaze) and 3 (visual fields)

cerebral artery (MCA) occlusion of less than 6 hours duration. Although proUK did not receive FDA approval, the principle of IA thrombolysis has been endorsed as a reasonable option for selected patients. Unfortunately, neither IV nor IA thrombolysis is an efficient way to rapidly recanalize occluded major brain arteries, and large-volume thromboses, such as those involving the internal carotid or basilar artery, are resistant to therapy. TCD monitoring of MCA occlusion suggests that IV t-PA leads to complete recanalization in only 30% of patients, with 48% partial recanalization and a 27% reocclusion rate. The MCA recanalization with IA proUK was complete in only 20% of patients after 2 hours, with 63% partial recanalization and a 10% reocclusion rate within the first hour of treatment, which could be improved with the use of heparin but at higher risk of hemorrhage. The low rate of complete recanalization and the high rate of reocclusion with stroke thrombolysis is not surprising considering that no aspirin or heparin is allowed for 24 hours after the administration of the thrombolytic agent.

Combination Intravenous–Intraarterial Thrombolysis

The only clinical trials of combination reperfusion therapy in acute stroke are the Emergency Management of Stroke (EMS) and Interventional Management of Stroke (IMS I) studies (55,56). The EMS study investigated a reduced dose (0.6 mg/kg) of IV t-PA combined with up to 20 mg IA t-PA in 35 patients with stroke of less than 3 hours duration. Recanalization was achieved in 54% of the IV/IA group and 10% of the IA group. There was no significant difference in the rate of symptomatic brain hemorrhage between the two groups at 72 hours (11.8% IV/IA vs. 5.5% placebo/IA) or in 90-day clinical outcome. The follow-up IMS I study treated 80 patients with stroke durations less than 3 hours with 0.6 mg/kg of IV t-PA combined with up to 22 mg of IA t-PA. The IMS I patients had a similar rate of symptomatic brain hemorrhage, 6.3%, but a significantly better clinical outcome at 90 days compared to historical controls from the NINDS IV t-PA trial.

Intraarterial Mechanical Reperfusion Strategies

Stroke thrombectomy devices have been developed with the goal of improving the speed and completeness of recanalization compared to thrombolytic agents alone. The MERCI (Mechanical Embolus Removal in Cerebral Ischemia) trial was a prospective, nonrandomized trial with historical controls that investigated the safety and efficacy of the Merci Retriever device

TABLE 107.8

INCLUSION AND EXCLUSION CRITERIA, NINDS INTRAVENOUS TISSUE-TYPE PLASMINOGEN ACTIVATOR ACUTE STROKE STUDY

Inclusion criteria
1. Ischemic stroke within 180 min of onset, with clearly defined time of onset
2. Neurologic deficit measurable on the National Institutes of Health Stroke Scale (NIHSS)
3. Computed tomography scan of the brain showing no evidence of intracranial hemorrhage

Exclusion criteria
1. Stroke or serious head trauma within the preceding 3 mo
2. Major surgery within 14 d
3. History of intracranial hemorrhage
4. Systolic blood pressure >185 mm Hg or diastolic blood pressure >110 mm Hg
5. Aggressive treatment required to reduce blood pressure to the specified limits
6. Rapidly improving or minor neurologic symptoms
7. Symptoms suggestive of subarachnoid hemorrhage
8. Gastrointestinal hemorrhage or urinary tract hemorrhage within the previous 21 d
9. Arterial puncture at a noncompressible site within the previous 7 d
10. Seizure at the onset of the stroke
11. On oral anticoagulants
12. Prothrombin time >15 s
13. Having received heparin within the 48 h preceding the onset of the stroke with an elevated partial thromboplastin time
14. Platelet count <100,000/mm^3
15. Glucose concentration <50 mg/dL or >400 mg/dL

Relative contraindications from the Food and Drug Administration hearings:
1. Severe neurologic deficit, with a NIHSS score >22, especially in an elderly patient
2. Early infarct signs on computed tomography including tissue hypodensity, blurring of the gray-white margins, loss of the insular ribbon, sulcal effacement in greater than one third of the middle cerebral artery territory

NINDS, National Institute of Neurological Disorders and Stroke (50).

(Concentric Medical, Mountain View, CA) to open occluded intracranial arteries in 151 patients ineligible for IV t-PA within 8 hours of an acute ischemic stroke (57). After angiography, eligible patients had to have occlusion of a treatable vessel that included the intracranial vertebral artery, basilar artery, intracranial carotid artery, or the middle cerebral artery (M1 or M2) divisions. If the device did not achieve recanalization or for significant distal emboli, concomitant thrombolytic therapy was used in 17 patients, but they were not included in the main analysis. Recanalization was achieved in 46% (69/151) of patients on an intent-to-treat analysis and in 48% (68/141) of patients in whom the device was deployed, which was significantly better than the historical control rate of 18%. Symptomatic intracranial hemorrhage occurred in 7.8% (11/141) of patients, and clinically significant procedural complications occurred in 7.1% (10/141). Good neurologic outcome, defined as a modified Rankin score of 2 or less at 90 days, was more frequent in patients with successful recanalization versus unsuccessful recanalization (46% vs. 10%, respectively; relative risk 4.4), and mortality was less (32% vs. 54%, respectively; relative risk 0.59). In August 2004, the FDA approved the MERCI clot retrieval system "to restore blood flow in the neurovasculature by removing thrombus in patients experiencing ischemic stroke... who are ineligible for IV t-PA or who fail IV t-PA therapy." The FDA approval of the MERCI Retriever raised concerns regarding the approval pathways for drugs versus devices for the indication of acute ischemic stroke therapy (58). Although vessels were opened faster with the MERCI Retriever system, the recanalization efficacy and safety was very similar to the results achieved with proUK, which did not achieve approval. Clinical efficacy studies to better define the optimal patient population and improvements to the device are being done in the Multi-MERCI registry and the MR-Rescue Trial.

There are numerous anecdotal reports of the use of other IV and IA drugs and devices in acute ischemic stroke (59). The ongoing IMS II study uses reduced-dose IV t-PA combined with IA t-PA delivered through an ultrasonic EKOS catheter in an attempt to accelerate thrombolysis (60). Transcranial ultrasound therapy combined with IV t-PA in MCA occlusion improved complete recanalization, with dramatic clinical recovery occurring in 49% of patients versus 30% in patients receiving IV t-PA only (61). Although a trial of abciximab in acute ischemic stroke of duration less than 6 hours was halted due to excessive bleeding events, there are ongoing trials of combination thrombolytics and glycoprotein IIB/IIIA inhibitors, some selecting patients based on perfusion brain imaging (Reperfusion Of Stroke-Imaging Evaluation [ROSIE]; Combination Approach to Thrombolysis Utilizing Eptifibatide and rt-PA [CLEAR]).

If we are to improve the efficiency of acute stroke thrombolysis, we will also need to develop multimodal combination therapies such as approaches for percutaneous coronary intervention. However, these will need to be modified to reduce the risk of hemorrhagic infarction, which is related to the extent of ischemic damage, which can be predicted by the presence of early infarct changes on CT as well as the severity of the initial clinical deficit, aggressiveness of thrombolytic dosing, blood pressure, advanced age, and prior head injury (51,53,62). Intracranial bleeding can also occur at sites distant from the ischemic region and are thought to indicate the presence of amyloid angiopathy, which is more prevalent in the demented elderly.

TABLE 107.9

JOINT COMMISSION ON ACCREDITATION OF HEALTHCARE ORGANIZATIONS PRIMARY STROKE CENTER QUALITY INDICATORS

Intravenous tissue-type plasminogen activator considered for treatment of acute ischemic stroke[a]
Antithrombotic therapy initiated within 48 h of admission
Institution of deep vein thrombosis prophylaxis[a]
Screen for dysphagia
Lipid profile during hospitalization
Smoking cessation counseling/therapy
Stroke education
Plan for rehabilitation considered
Anticoagulation for atrial fibrillation[a]
Discharged on antithrombotic therapy[a]
[a]In patients with no contraindication to such therapy.

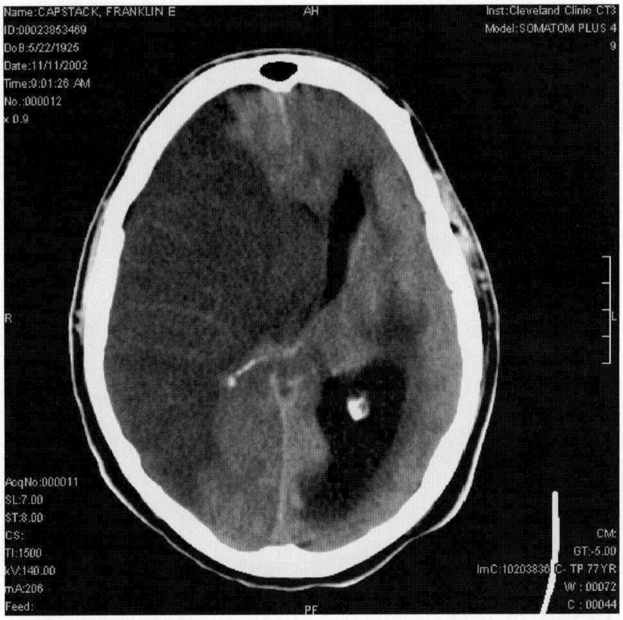

FIGURE 107.3. Computed tomography scan of fatal middle cerebral artery infarction with herniation.

Patient Stabilization and Prevention of Medical Complications after Stroke

Standard acute stroke management includes hemodynamic stabilization and respiratory and nutritional support with prevention of aspiration pneumonia and deep vein thrombosis in the high-risk plegic patient. Key interventions have been selected for quality indicators for Primary Stroke Center designation (Table 107.9). One of the most important issues in acute stroke is hemodynamic management. If a patient has sustained hypertension (>185/110 mm Hg) or requires aggressive, that is, multiple, IV doses of antihypertensive agents or an IV drip, he or she is not a candidate for thrombolysis due to the increased risk of cerebral hemorrhage. Therapeutic agents should allow for rapid titration and have a low risk of overtreatment that may compromise cerebral blood flow to the ischemic brain, which is most vulnerable within the first days after a stroke.

Hyperglycemia at stroke onset is a risk factor for poor outcome and is attributed to aggravation of tissue acidosis from excessive anaerobic metabolism within the region of ischemia. Strict control with target blood glucose levels of 80 to 100 mg/dL is recommended, avoiding IV solutions containing glucose and delaying oral nutrition for 1 to 2 days until a swallowing evaluation can be performed. The role of intensive insulin therapy is controversial; one compromise approach is to use exogenous insulin to achieve target glucose values of less than 150 mg/dL in the first 3 days, and if a critical illness persists despite therapy, to employ more aggressive insulin therapy to target blood glucose of 80 to 110 mg/dL. Cerebral edema is usually maximal 3 to 7 days after cerebral infarction. Cerebral edema is best treated in an intensive care unit with ICP monitoring and osmotic dehydration.

Neuroprotective agents shown to be promising in animal models have been uniformly disappointing in clinical trials (63). Moderate to profound hypothermia, in routine use during cardiopulmonary bypass, has also been shown to improve outcomes after cardiac arrest and acute ischemic stroke but not during aneurysm surgery after subarachnoid hemorrhage (64,65). Complications include cardiac arrhythmias, pneumonia, and sepsis, and in patients with large hemispheric infarcts, the cerebral edema may just be delayed only to recur during rewarming. Hemicraniectomy is an option for life-threatening brain swelling, but this is a difficult decision because patients who survive are left with a severe neurologic disability (66) (Fig. 107.3).

Anticoagulation and Antiplatelet Therapy

The International Stroke Trial (IST) (67) compared subcutaneous heparin at high (25,000 U/day) and low doses (10,000 U/day), with or without aspirin 300 mg/day, to placebo for 14 days in 19,436 patients with acute thrombotic or embolic stroke of duration less than 48 hours (67). There were significantly fewer in-hospital deaths and recurrent strokes among patients treated with aspirin. No early benefit was found for heparin, in part because the 0.9% reduction in recurrent ischemic stroke was offset by a 0.8% increase in symptomatic hemorrhagic stroke, mostly in those who received the higher heparin dose. However, CT scans before beginning heparin and coagulation monitoring were not required, which has sparked debate in the interpretation of the results. Aspirin begun within 48 hours of acute ischemic stroke offers a significant but modest absolute reduction of early mortality (0.5% to 0.6%) and recurrent ischemic stroke (0.5% to 1.1%) with a nonsignificant increase in symptomatic hemorrhagic stroke (0.1% to 0.2%).

The American Heart Association (AHA) guidelines strongly recommend initiating oral antithrombotic therapy within 48 hours of ischemic stroke as well as the prophylactic administration of low-dose heparin or low-molecular-weight heparins or heparinoids to prevent deep vein thrombosis in immobilized patients with no contraindication to therapy. However, because there is no evidence to support the routine use of anticoagulants for acute ischemic stroke, they state "until more data are available, the use of heparin remains a matter of preference of the treating physician. It should be understood that the use of heparin (or the lack of its administration) may not alter the outcome of a patient with acute ischemic stroke." However, anticoagulation continues to be selectively used for certain high-risk patients, including those with a symptomatic severe stenosis or progressing stroke from occlusion, reembolization, or reduced collateral perfusion, but it should be weighed against the risk of hemorrhagic transformation of the infarct. Heparin is contraindicated for 24 hours after IV t-PA for acute stroke, and risk factors for hemorrhagic transformation include advanced age, hypertension, embolic mechanism, size of infarct on CT or clinical deficit, early anticoagulant therapy for large infarcts, use of a heparin loading bolus, and

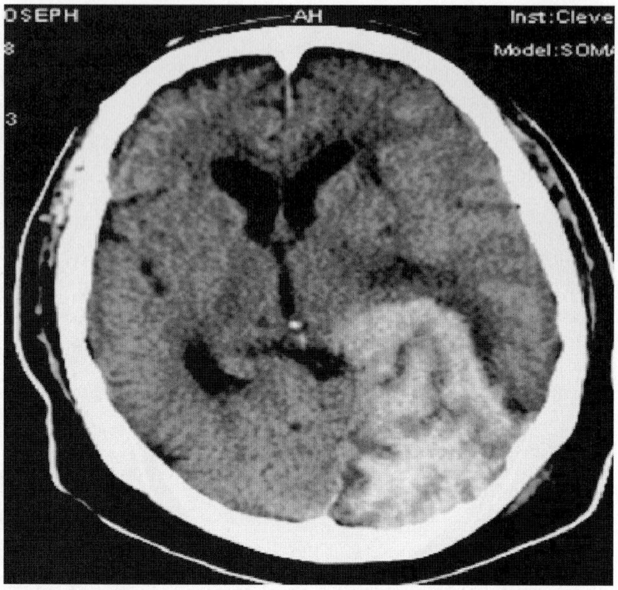

FIGURE 107.4. Computed tomography scan of hemorrhagic posterior cerebral artery infarction complicating heparin therapy for atrial fibrillation.

excessive prolongation of the activated partial thromboplastin time (Fig. 107.4).

INTRACEREBRAL HEMORRHAGE

Nontraumatic ICHs are referred to as *primary or spontaneous* when there is no evidence of an underlying cause and as *secondary* when they are due to a vascular malformation or aneurysm, coagulopathy, primary or metastatic tumor, or granuloma. Although early diagnosis and overall mortality have improved with neuroimaging techniques and hypertension therapy, early mortality remains high at 30% to 40%. Intracerebral hemorrhages exceeding 30 cm^3 are associated with a high 30-day mortality and neurologic disability rate. Significant hematoma expansion within the first 24 hours occurs in at least 33% of patients and is a significant cause of morbidity (Fig. 107.5). The sites of bleeding are related to etiology. For primary ICH, 50% occur in the deep nuclei (putamen, 35%; thalamus, 10%; caudate, 5%), 30% occur in the lobar white matter, and 20% occur in the posterior fossa (cerebellum, 15%; brain stem, 5%). Although ICHs related to coagulopathies are more frequently confluent, single, and lobar in location, there can be tremendous variability with multiple hemorrhages and blood-fluid levels within the hematomas.

Pathophysiology of Intracerebral Hemorrhage

Arterial hypertension is blamed for 70% to 90% of primary ICHs related to rupture of small perforating arteries damaged by lipohyalinosis and microaneurysm formation. Most ICHs are surrounded by an area of hypointensity on CT scanning that represents vasogenic edema; however, edema out of proportion to the size of the hematoma suggests hemorrhage into an underlying tumor such as glioblastoma multiforme or oligodendroglioma or a metastatic adenocarcinoma, melanoma, choriocarcinoma, or hypernephroma. Abnormal vascular patterns on enhanced CT or MRI or areas of calcification suggest an underlying vascular malformation. Recreational drugs associated with ICH include the sympathomimetics, most commonly cocaine, amphetamines, and phencyclidine and other over-the-counter diet aids.

Amyloid angiopathy is the most common cause of ICH in the nonhypertensive elderly and is implicated in ICH, complicating thrombolytic and antithrombotic therapy. Anticoagulant-related ICH accounts for 9% of all ICHs, with additional risk factors of long-term or excessive oral anticoagulation with advanced age or poorly controlled hypertension. ICH is the most feared complication of thrombolytic therapy; although hemorrhages are most commonly confluent, solitary, and lobar, the spectrum includes multiple, deep, or infratentorial hemorrhages and associated subdural, intraventricular, and subarachnoid bleeding.

SUBARACHNOID HEMORRHAGE

Despite major advances in neurosurgical techniques over the last two decades, mortality for subarachnoid hemorrhage

A

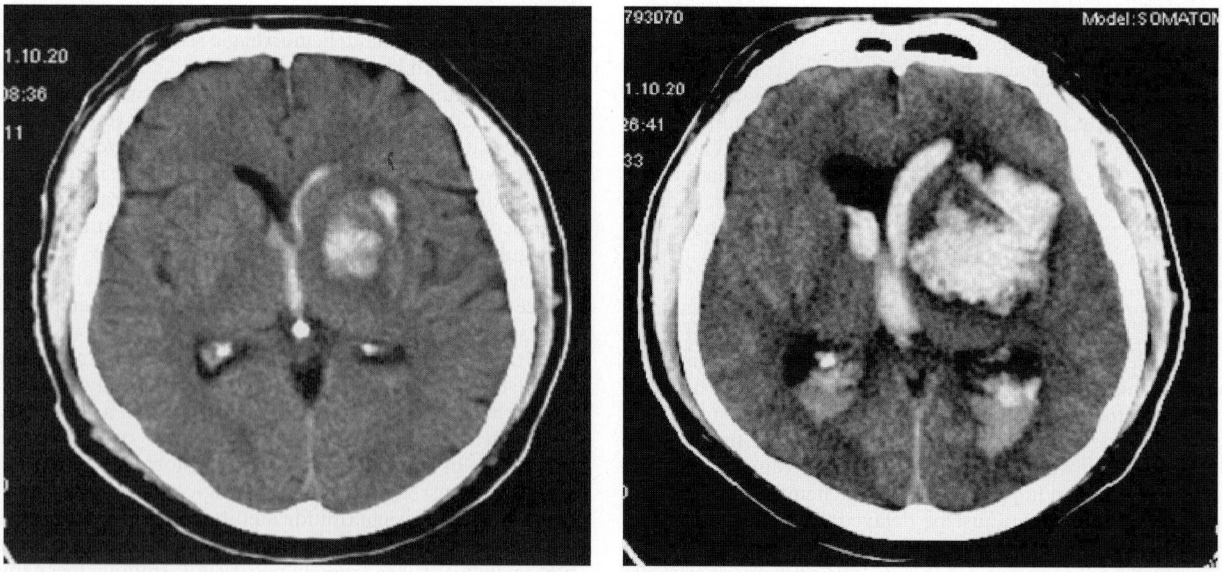

B

FIGURE 107.5. Computed tomography of hypertensive striatal intracerebral hemorrhage with intraventricular extension expanding over 6 hours.

TABLE 107.10

HUNT AND HESS CLASSIFICATION OF SUBARACHNOID HEMORRHAGE

Grade I	Asymptomatic or minimal headache and slight nuchal rigidity
Grade II	Moderate to severe headache, nuchal rigidity, no neurologic deficit other than cranial nerve palsy
Grade III	Drowsiness, confusion, or mild focal deficit
Grade IV	Stupor, moderate to severe hemiparesis, possible early decerebrate rigidity and vegetative disturbance
Grade V	Deep coma, decerebrate rigidity, moribund appearance

remains high, 10% acutely and an additional 50% within 3 months, and of those who survive, more than half are left with a major neurologic or neurocognitive disability with a diminished quality of life. Clinical grading of the patient based on headache and mental status is important in predicting prognosis and chance of recovery (Table 107.10).

A CT scan of the brain without contrast performed within 24 hours is positive in 92% of cases, but by 48 hours it bears only a 75% chance of demonstrating cisternal or subarachnoid blood. If no hemorrhage is seen, a lumbar puncture is recommended to establish the diagnosis. Selective intraarterial cerebral angiography is the standard for diagnosis and planning a therapeutic surgical or endovascular approach.

Pathophysiology of Subarachnoid Hemorrhage

Most SAHs are due to saccular intracranial aneurysms that most frequently occur at bifurcations and branch points, with most about the circle of Willis. They are associated with polycystic kidney disease, coarctation of the aorta, Ehlers-Danlos syndrome, neurofibromatosis, fibromuscular dysplasia, and arteriovenous malformations. The risk for rupture for incidental or asymptomatic unruptured aneurysms is 1%/year to 2%/year (69). Factors that increase this risk include aneurysm size, multiplicity, location, and the patient's age. The median diameter of a ruptured aneurysm is 7 mm, with most being 5 to 10 mm, which translates into the common practice of considering surgery for any aneurysm greater than 5 mm.

Mycotic aneurysms occur with bacterial, fungal, or, rarely, tumor embolism such as with an atrial myxoma. Their location at peripheral cerebral branch sites and their small size typically require angiography and are not reliably demonstrated on noninvasive MRA or CT angiography imaging. Atherosclerotic aneurysms are tortuous vessels that are most frequently located in the vertebrobasilar system; however, they can affect the major intracranial internal carotid branches. Symptoms are produced by mass effect, ischemia from branch artery occlusions, and obstructive hydrocephalus but rarely from rupture.

MANAGEMENT OF THE PATIENT WITH HEMORRHAGIC STROKE

In addition to the management strategies discussed for acute ischemic stroke, patients with hemorrhagic stroke require additional attention. The management of hypertension is much more aggressive because elevated blood pressure is an important risk factor for hemorrhage expansion and rehemorrhage. SAH patients are the most critical; 30% rebleed, most within the first few weeks, with much higher morbidity and mortality with higher rates of rebleeding. Target blood pressures for elderly or hypertensive patients (systolic, 150 mm Hg) are more liberal than those for young or nonhypertensive patients (systolic, <120 mm Hg), but in the setting of increased ICP, should be individualized to maintain cerebral perfusion pressure at levels greater than 45 to 50 mm Hg.

Blood should immediately be drawn for coagulation parameters, including platelet count, prothrombin time, partial thromboplastin time, and bleeding time and defects corrected rapidly because hemorrhage expansion can continue over the first 8 to 24 hours (70). If it is a complication of thrombolytic therapy, the event should be presumed to be an intracranial hemorrhage until proven otherwise and warrants immediately stopping all therapies, stabilizing the patient, obtaining laboratory coagulation tests, and reversing the therapies while awaiting emergency CT scanning.

Cardiac arrhythmias, usually supraventricular tachyarrhythmias, and subendocardial ischemia more commonly complicate SAH or ICH within the first several days, warrant continuing ECG monitoring and assessment of cardiac enzymes, and can lead to QT_c prolongation or sudden death. The surge in catecholamines can also lead to neurogenic pulmonary edema and diabetes. Seizures are more frequent as well, and most clinicians recommend prophylactic anticonvulsant therapy in critically ill patients.

Vasospasm with clinical deterioration complicates about 30% of SAHs, usually occurring after several days and resolving over a period of weeks. Transcranial Doppler is useful in diagnosis and helps to guide hemodynamic and fluid management. Hyponatremia with cerebral salt wasting and volume contraction mediated by atrial natriuretic factor (ANF) parallels the time course of vasospasm and is managed with intravascular administration of isotonic fluids. Hemorrhagic stroke is more likely to be complicated by increased intracranial pressure. Hydrocephalus requiring ventricular drainage complicates 20% of cases and often develops insidiously with impaired consciousness, lower limb spasticity, and significantly increases mortality.

Corticosteroids have not been shown to be of benefit in patients with hemorrhagic or ischemic stroke (71). For SAH, oral nimodipine, 60 mg every 4 hours started within 4 days of the hemorrhage and continuing for 21 days, has been shown to reduce poor outcome due to vasospasm for patients of good neurologic condition after the ictus (72). Recombinant factor VIIa was tested in a randomized fashion in 399 patients with ICH diagnosed within 3 hours of symptom onset. ICH volume expansion and 90-day rates of disability or death were significantly less with various doses of recombinant factor VIIa compared to placebo. Serious thromboembolic events, mainly MI or ischemic stroke, were nonsignificantly increased in 7% of treated versus 2% of placebo patients (73). Based on these data, an efficacy trial of NovoSeven in acute ICH is ongoing.

SURGICAL AND ENDOVASCULAR THERAPIES FOR HEMORRHAGIC STROKE

Surgical evacuation for symptomatic cerebellar ICH should be considered before neurologic deterioration because of the unpredictable course and risk for rapid and progressive brain stem compression, producing respiratory arrest and death. Accessible subcortical ICHs, particularly those involving the nondominant hemisphere or noneloquent areas of the brain, are also amenable to surgical evacuation, and should be considered in patients who present with relatively preserved neurologic function who subsequently begin to deteriorate. However, surgical evacuation was not demonstrated to improve neurologic outcome compared to medical therapy in the Surgical Trial in Intracerebral Hemorrhage (STITCH) trial (74).

Endovascular coiling is an option to surgical clipping in many patients with ruptured intracranial aneurysm. The International Subarachnoid Aneurysm Trial (ISAT) compared endovascular coiling to surgical clipping in 2,143 patients with ruptured intracranial aneurysm who were eligible for either approach (75,76). Greater than 90% of the randomized patients were Hunt and Hess grades 1 or 2. The dome of the aneurysm was less than 9 mm in greater than 80% of patients, with the most frequent location being the anterior communicating artery. A good clinical outcome (modified Rankin Scale score of 0 to 2) was achieved in significantly more coiled than clipped patients at 2 months (74.8% vs. 63.6%, respectively) and 1 year (76.5% vs. 68.2%, respectively), with a relative risk reduction of 24.3%. The risk of rebleeding in coiled patients was 0.12%/year.

CONTROVERSIES AND PERSONAL PERSPECTIVES

Properly conducted, randomized clinical trials to establish efficacy and risks in comparison to available therapies should be required of devices as they are for drugs. In addition, a nationwide mechanism for uniform reporting of outcomes and adverse events of new, and old, therapies needs to be established. Although the treatments for acute ischemic stroke in many ways parallel those for acute myocardial infarction, stroke is far more heterogeneous, both in terms of etiology and outcomes assessment, and the increased risk of brain hemorrhage has hampered the development of aggressive multimodal reperfusion strategies. Major unmet needs continue to be prevention of hemorrhagic conversion of infarcts and neuroprotective therapies to "keep the window open" because a 3-hour window means that we will never treat more than 10% of stroke patients with IV t-PA.

THE FUTURE

Optimum strategies for stroke prevention will be determined by many factors including genetic markers, responsiveness to antiplatelet therapies, and mechanism. Stroke subtype–specific recommendations for AF and carotid stenosis are available, and focused trials of intracranial atherosclerosis, lacunar stroke, PFOs, heart failure, and aortic arch atheromatous are ongoing, but orphans such as cerebral venous thrombosis and dissection also warrant specific study. Systems approaches to stroke care that link outlying community-based "primary stroke centers" with regional "comprehensive stroke centers" is rapidly evolving. Traditional boundaries based on specialty are giving way to disease-oriented "product lines" in which multidisciplinary specialists trained in vascular disorders will work together in regional vascular centers. Therapies for acute stroke will rely on new imaging technology that will offer a rapid physiologic assessment of etiology and tissue at risk. Neuroprotection for both ischemic and hemorrhagic stroke will be available for use in the field by highly trained emergency medical services personnel. Innovative anecdotes will rapidly translate into proper clinical trials to clearly define their role. Finally, all patients will be followed with uniform assessments of outcomes and complications to define the optimum health care practices for all.

Selected Guidelines, Scientific Statements and Advisories

Stroke Prevention

Guidelines for prevention of stroke in patients with ischemic stroke or transient ischemic attack. AHA/ ASA scientific statement. *Stroke* 2006;37:577.

Carotid endarterectomy. An evidence-based review. Report of the Therapeutics and Technology Assessment Subcommittee of the American Academy of Neurology. *Neurology* 2005;65:794–801.

Evidence-based guideline for cardiovascular disease prevention in women. AHA scientific statement. *Stroke* 2004;109:672.

Statins after ischemic stroke and transient ischemic attack. AHA/ASA scientific advisory. *Stroke* 2004;35:1023.

Recurrent stroke with patent foramen ovale and atrial septal aneurysm: report of the Quality Standards Subcommittee of the American Academy of Neurology. Practice parameter. *Neurology* 2004;62:1042.

Coronary risk evaluation in patients with transient ischemic attack and ischemic stroke. AHA/ASA scientific statement. *Circulation* 2003;108:1278.

AHA guidelines for primary prevention of cardiovascular disease and stroke: 2002 update. *Circulation* 2002;106:388.

ACC/AHA/ESC guidelines for the management of patients with atrial fibrillation. *J Am Coll Cardiol* 2001;38:1266.

Carotid stenting and angioplasty. AHA advisory. *Circulation* 1998;97:121.

Stroke prevention in patients with nonvalvular atrial fibrillation. Practice parameter of the American Academy of Neurology. *Neurology* 1998;51:671.

Stroke Management

Guidelines for the early management of patients with ischemic stroke. 2005 guidelines update. AHA/ASA scientific statement. *Stroke* 2005;36:916.

Management of adult stroke rehabilitation care. AHA/ASA-endorsed practice guideline. *Stroke* 2005;36:e100.

Infective endocarditis: diagnosis, antimicrobial therapy and management of complications. *Circulation* 2005;111:3167–3184.

Physical activity and exercise recommendations for stroke survivors. AHA scientific statement. *Circulation* 2004;109:2031.

Guidelines and recommendations for perfusion imaging in cerebral ischemia. AHA scientific statement. *Stroke* 2003;34:1084.

Anticoagulants and antiplatelet agents in acute ischemic stroke. ASA/AAN scientific statement. *Stroke* 2002;33:1934; also *Neurology* 2002;59:13.

Recommendations for the endovascular treatment of intracranial aneurysms, AHA scientific statement. *Stroke* 2002;33:2536.

Emergency interventional stroke therapy: A statement from the American Society of Interventional and Therapeutic Neuroradiology and Society of Cardiovascular and Interventional Radiology. *Am J Neuroradiol* 2001;22:54.

Recommendations for the management of intracranial arteriovenous malformations. AHA scientific statement. *Stroke* 2001;32:1458.

Recommendations for the management of patients with unruptured intracranial aneurysms, AHA scientific statement. *Circulation* 2000;102:2300.

Guidelines for the management of spontaneous intracerebral hemorrhage. AHA scientific statement. *Stroke* 1999;30:905.

Practice guidelines for the use of imaging in transient ischemic attacks and acute stroke. *Stroke* 1997;28:1480.

Thrombolytic therapy for acute ischemic stroke. Practice advisory of the American Academy of Neurology. *Neurology* 1996;47:835.

Stroke Systems

Heart disease and stroke statistics—2006 update. A report from the American Heart Association Statistics Committee and Stroke Statistics Subcommittee. *Circulation* 2006;113:e85–e151.

Recommendations for the establishment of stroke systems of care. AHA scientific statement. *Stroke* 2005;36:690.

The American Heart Association Stroke Outcome Classification. AHA scientific statement. *Stroke* 1998;29:1274.

References

1. Special report from the National Institute of Neurological Disorders and Stroke. Classification of cerebrovascular diseases III. *Stroke* 1990;21:637–676.
2. Albers GW, Caplan LR, Easton JD, et al., for the TIA Working Group. Transient ischemic attack—proposal for a new definition. *N Engl J Med* 2002;347:1713–1716.
3. Johnston SC, Gress DR, Browner WS, Sidney S. Short-term prognosis after emergency department diagnosis of TIA. *JAMA* 2000;284:2901–2906.
4. Rothwell PM, Giles MF, Flossmann E, et al. A simple score (ABCD) to identify individuals at high early risk of stroke after transient ischemic attack. *Lancet* 2005;366:29–36.
5. PROGRESS Collaborative Group. Randomised trial of a perindopril-based blood-pressure-lowering regimen among 6,105 individuals with a previous stroke or transient ischaemic attack. *Lancet* 2001;358:1033–1041.

6. Hachinski V, Graffagnino C, Beaudry M, et al. Lipids and stroke: A paradox resolved. *Arch Neurol* 1996;53:303–308.
7. Briel M, Studer M, Glass TR, Bucher HC. Effects of statins on stroke prevention in patients with and without coronary heart disease: a meta-analysis of randomized controlled trials. *Am J Med* 2004;117:596–606.
8. Design and baseline characteristics of the Stroke Prevention by Aggressive Reduction in Cholesterol Levels (SPARCL) study. *Cerebrovasc Dis* 2003; 16:389–395.
9. Chambers BR, Norris JW. Outcome in patients with asymptomatic neck bruits. *N Engl J Med* 1986;15:860–865.
11. CASANOVA Study Group. Carotid surgery versus medical therapy in asymptomatic carotid stenosis. *Stroke* 1991;22:1229–1235.
12. Hobson RW, Weiss DG, Fields WS, et al., for the Veterans Cooperative Study Group. Efficacy of carotid endarterectomy for asymptomatic carotid stenosis. *N Engl J Med* 1993;328:221–227.
13. Mayo Asymptomatic Carotid Endarterectomy Study Group. Results of a randomized controlled trial of carotid endarterectomy for asymptomatic carotid stenosis. *Mayo Clin Proc* 1992;67:513–518.
14. Executive Committee for the Asymptomatic Carotid Atherosclerosis Study. Endarterectomy for asymptomatic carotid artery stenosis. *JAMA* 1995;273:1421–1428.
15. Barnett H, Taylor W, Eliasziw M, et al. (1998): Benefit of endarterectomy in patients with symptomatic moderate or severe stenosis. *N Engl J Med* 1998;339:1415–1425.
16. European Carotid Surgery Trialists' Collaborative Group (1991): MRC European Carotid Surgery Trial: interim results for symptomatic patients with severe (70–99%) or with mild (0–29%) carotid stenosis. *Lancet* 1991; 337:1235–1243.
17. Wennberg DE, Lucas FL, Birkmeyer JD, et al. Variation in carotid endarterectomy mortality in the Medicare population: trial hospitals, volume, and patient characteristics. *JAMA* 1998;279(16): 1278–1281.
18. Endovascular versus surgical treatment in patients with carotid stenosis in the Carotid and Vertebral Artery Transluminal Angioplasty Study (CAVATAS): a randomised trial. *Lancet* 2001;357(9270):1729–1737.
19. Wholey MH, Al-Mubarek N. Updated review of the Global Carotid Artery Stent Registry. *Catheter Cardiovasc Interv* 2003;60(2):259–266.
20. Yadav JS, Wholey MH, Kuntz RE, et al. Protected carotid-artery stenting versus endarterectomy in high-risk patients. *N Engl J Med* 2004;351(15):1493–1501.
21. Chimowitz MI, Lynn MJ, Howlett-Smith H, et al. Comparison of warfarin and aspirin for symptomatic intracranial arterial stenosis. *N Engl J Med* 2005;352:1305–1316.
22. SYLVIA trial. *Stroke* 2004;35:1388.
23. Wingspan European/Asian pilot.
24. Atrial Fibrillation Investigators. Risk factors for stroke and efficacy of antithrombotic therapies in atrial fibrillation: analysis of pooled data from five randomized controlled trials. *Arch Intern Med* 1994;154:1449–1457.
25. Cappato R, Calkins H, Chen SA, et al. Worldwide survey on the methods, efficacy, and safety of catheter ablation for human atrial fibrillation. *Circulation* 2005;111:1100–1105.
26. The Atrial Fibrillation Follow-up Investigation of Rhythm Management (AFFIRM) Investigators. A comparison of rate control and rhythm control in patients with atrial fibrillation. *N Engl J Med* 2002;347:1825–1833.
27. Sherman DG, Kim SG, Boop BS et al. Occurrence and characteristics of stroke events in the Atrial Fibrillation Follow-up Investigation of Sinus Rhythm Management AFFIRM study. *Arch Int Med* 2005;165:1185–1191.
28. Homma S, Sacco RL, DiTullio MR, et al., for the PFO in Cryptogenic Stroke Study (PICSS) Investigators. Effect of medical treatment in stroke patients with patent foramen ovale. *Circulation* 2002;105:2625–2631.
29. Bushnell CD, Goldstein LB. Diagnostic testing for coagulopathies in patients with ischemic stroke. *Stroke* 2000;31:3067–3078.
30. Levine SR, Brey RL, Tilley BC, et al. Antiphospholipid antibodies and subsequent thrombo-occlusive events in patients with ischemic stroke. *JAMA* 2004;291:576–584.
31. Gillum LA, Mamadipudi SK, Johnston SC. Ischemic stroke risk with oral contraceptives: a meta-analysis. *JAMA* 2000;284:72–78.
32. Tournier-Lasserve E. New players in the genetics of stroke. *N Engl J Med* 2002;347:1711–1712.
33. Shinton R, Beevers G. Meta-analysis of relation between cigarette smoking and stroke. *Br Med J* 1989;298:789–794.
34. Roach GW, Kanchuger M, Mangano CM, et al. Adverse cerebral outcomes after coronary bypass surgery. *N Engl J Med* 1996;335:1857–1863.
35. Salgado AV, Furlan AJ, Keys TF et al., Neurologic complications of endocarditis; a 12 year experience. *Neurology* 1989;39:173–178.
36. Chapot R, Houdart E, Saint-Maurice JP, et al. Endovascular treatment of cerebral mycotic aneurysms. *Radiology* 2002;222:389–396.
37. Fisher CM. Lacunar strokes and infarcts: A review. *Neurology* 1982;32:871–876.
38. Bogdahn U, Becker G, Winkler J, et al. Transcranial color-coded real-time sonography in adults. *Stroke* 1990;21:1680–1688.
39. Amerenco P, Cohen A, Tzourio C, et al. Atherosclerotic disease of the aortic arch and the risk of ischemic stroke. *N Engl J Med* 1994;331:1474–1479.
40. Hayden M, Pignone M, Phillips C, Mulrow C. Aspirin for the primary prevention of cardiovascular events, a summary of the evidence. *Ann Intern Med* 2002;136:161–172.
41. Ridker PM, Cook NR, Lee Im et al. A randomized trial of low-dose aspirin in the primary prevention of cardiovascular disease in women *N Engl J Med* 2005;7:1293–1304.
42. Gorelick PB, Weisman SM. Risk of hemorrhagic stroke with aspirin use. *Stroke* 2005;36:1801–1807.
43. Canadian Cooperative Study Group. A randomized trial of aspirin and sulfinpyrazone in threatened stroke. *N Engl J Med* 1978;299:53–59.
44. Collaborative meta-analysis of randomised trials of antiplatelet therapy for prevention of death, myocardial infarction, and stroke in high risk patients. *BMJ* 2002;324:71–86.
45. Diener HC, Cunha L, Forbes C, et al. European Stroke Prevention Study 2. Dipyridamole and acetylsalicylic acid in the secondary prevention of stroke. *J Neurol Sci* 1996;143:1–13.
46. Hass WK, Easton JD, Adams HP, et al., for the Ticlopidine Aspirin Stroke Study Group. A randomized trial comparing ticlopidine hydrochloride with aspirin for the prevention of stroke in high-risk patients. *N Engl J Med* 1989; 321:501–507.
47. CAPRIE Steering Committee. A randomized, blinded, trial of Clopidogrel versus Aspirin in Patients at Risk of Ischemic Events (CAPRIE). *Lancet* 1996; 348:1329–1339.
48. Diener HC, Bogousslavsky J, Brass L, et al. Aspirin and clopidogrel compared with clopidogrel alone after recent ischemic stroke or transient ischemic attack in high-risk patients (MATCH): a randomized double-blind placebo-controlled trial. *Lancet* 2004;364:331–337.
49. Mohr JP, Thompson JLP, Lazar RM, et al. A comparison of warfarin and aspirin for the prevention of recurrent ischemic stroke. *N Engl J Med* 2001; 345:1444–1451.
50. The National Institute of Neurological Disorders and Stroke rt-PA Stroke Study Group. Tissue plasminogen activator for acute ischemic stroke. *N Engl J Med* 1995;333:1581–1587.
51. Wardlaw JM, Warlow CP, Counsell C. Systematic review of evidence on thrombolytic therapy for acute ischaemic stroke. *Lancet* 1997;350:607–614.
52. Schirger DL, Kalafut M, Starkman M, et al. Cranial CT interpretation in acute stroke. *JAMA* 1998;279:1293–1297.
53. Buchan AM, Barber PA, Newcommon N, et al. Effectiveness of t-PA in acute ischemic stroke outcome relates to appropriateness. *Neurology* 2000; 54:679–684.
54. Furlan A, Higashida R, Weschler L, et al. Intraarterial prourokinase for acute ischemic stroke-the PROACT II study. *JAMA* 1999;282;2003–2111.
55. Lewandowski CA, Frankel M, Tomsick TA, et al. Combined IV and IA t-PA vs IA therapy for acute ischemic stroke. The Emergency Management of Stroke (EMS) Bridging Trial. *Stroke* 1999;30:2598–2605.
56. The IMS Study Investigators. Combined intravenous and intra-arterial recanalization for acute ischemic stroke: The Interventional Management of Stroke Study. *Stroke* 2004;35:904.
57. Smith WS, Sung G, Starkman S, et al. Safety and efficacy of mechanical embolectomy in acute ischemic stroke: results of the MERCI trial. *Stroke* 2005;36:1432–1438.
58. Furlan AJ, Fisher M. Devices, drugs, and the Food and Drug Administration: increasing implications for ischemic stroke. *Stroke* 2005;36:398.
59. Quershi AI, Siddiqui AM, Suri MFK, et al. Aggressive mechanical clot disruption and low-dose intra-arterial third generation thrombolytic agent for ischemic stroke: a prospective study. *Neurosurgery* 2002;51:1319–1329.
60. Mahon BR, Nesbit GM, Barnwell SL, et al. North American clinical experience with the EKOS MicroLysUS infusion catheter for the treatment of embolic stroke. *Am J Neuroradiol* 2003;24:534–538.
61. Alexandrov AV, Molina CA, Grotta JC, et al. Ultrasound-enhanced systemic thrombolysis for acute ischemic stroke *N Engl J Med* 2004;351(21):2170–2178.
62. Bozzao L, Angeloni U, Bastianello S, et al. Early angiographic and CT findings in patients with hemorrhagic infarction in the distribution of the middle cerebral artery. *AJNR* 1991;12:1115–1121.
63. James A. Stroke treatment trials yield disappointing results. *Lancet* 1997; 349:1673.
64. Krieger DW, De Georgia MA, Abou-Chebl A, et al. Cooling for Acute Ischemic Brain Damage (COOL AID): feasibility and safety of induced hypothermia for severe acute ischemic stroke. *Neurology* 2004;63:312–317.
65. Todd MM, Hindman BJ, Clarke WR, et al. Mild intraoperative hypothermia during surgery for intracranial aneurysm. *N Engl J Med* 2005;352:135–145.
66. Manno EM. The management of large hemispheric cerebral infarcts. *Contemp Ther* 2005;31:124–130.
67. International Stroke Trial Collaborative Group. The International Stroke Trial (IST): a randomized trial of aspirin, subcutaneous heparin, both or neither, among 19,435 patients with acute ischemic stroke. *Lancet* 1997;349: 1569–1581.
69. Wiebers DO, Whisnant JP, Huston 3rd J, et al. Unruptured intracranial aneurysms: natural history, clinical outcome, and risks of surgical and endovascular treatment. *Lancet.* 2003;362:103–110.
70. Broderick J, Brott T, Tomsick T. Ultra-early evaluation of intracerebral hemorrhage (ICH). *Stroke* 1989;20:158.
71. Tellez H, Bauer RB. Dexamethasone as treatment in cerebrovascular disease. I. A controlled study in intracerebral hemorrhage. *Stroke* 1973;4:541–546.
72. Allen G, Ahn H, Preziosi T, et al. Cerebral arterial spasm: a controlled trial of nimodipine in patients with subarachnoid hemorrhage. *N Engl J Med* 1983;308:619–624.

73. Mayer SA, Brun NC, Begtrup K, et al. Recombinant activated factor VII for acute intracerebral hemorrhage. *N Engl J Med* 2005;352:777–785.
74. Mendelow AD, Gregson BA, Fernandes, et al. Early surgery versus initial conservative treatment in patients with spontaneous supratentorial intracerebral hematomas in the international Surgical Trial in Intracerebral Hemorrhage (STITCH): a randomized trial. *Lancet* 2005;365:387–397.
75. International Subarachnoid Aneurysm Trial (ISAT) Collaborative Group. International Subarachnoid Aneurysm Trial (ISAT) of neurosurgical clipping versus endovascular coiling in 2143 patients with ruptured intracranial aneurysms: a randomised trial. *Lancet* 2002;360:1267–1274.
76. Sacco RL, Mohr JP, Tatemichi TK, et al. Infarction of undetermined cause: The NINCDS stroke data bank. *Ann Neurol* 1989;25:382–390.

CHAPTER 108 ■ DISEASE OF PERIPHERAL VESSELS

AMJAD AL MAHAMEED AND JOHN R. BARTHOLOMEW

INTRODUCTION

Peripheral arterial disease (PAD) refers to occlusive atherosclerotic disease of the aorta and the lower extremities. It is common in the elderly and among those with risk factors for atherosclerosis, particularly smoking and diabetes mellitus (DM). The classical symptom of PAD is *intermittent claudication* (IC), defined as pain, aching, cramping, or fatigue in the leg that is triggered by walking, relieved with rest, and reproduced by resuming activity. Patients with PAD may develop ischemic ulcers or rest pain, often referred to as critical limb ischemia (CLI), or an acutely threatened limb, also known as acute limb ischemia (ALI). Recent studies, however, indicate that a significant proportion of individuals with PAD may be *asymptomatic* or present with *atypical* leg symptoms that often go unrecognized or are mistaken as part of growing old.

PAD is associated with an increased risk of cardiovascular morbidity and mortality in both symptomatic and asymptomatic individuals. Whereas endovascular interventions and surgical procedures aim at limb salvage or seek to improve functional status and prevent disability, integration of global cardiovascular risk reduction strategies into the care plan is critical to slowing progression, reducing recurrence, and decreasing adverse cardiovascular events and improving survival in this population.

PREVALENCE

The reported prevalence of PAD varies and is largely dependent on the demographic factors of the population under evaluation and the method of diagnosis. Although earlier accounts based on patients with IC reported prevalence rates of 1.8% to 7% (1–3), it is now well recognized that only 10% to 30% of all PAD patients present with this classic symptom (4). Thus, IC is a useful clinical indicator but may underestimate the prevalence of this disease. More recently, the ankle–brachial index (ABI) (the ratio of the systolic blood pressure measured at the ankle arteries to the highest systolic pressure of the brachial arteries) has become the diagnostic test of choice for establishing the presence of PAD (Fig. 108.1). Several recent epidemiologic studies used this method to evaluate the prevalence of PAD in community members of different ages. The National Health and Nutrition Examination Survey (NHANES) enrolled a representative sample of the U.S. population aged 40 years and older and reported an increased prevalence with advancing age (0.9% and 14.5% among individuals aged 40 to 49 years and 70 years and older, respectively) (5). Similarly, an ABI of 0.9 or less was uncommon (2.3% to 4%) in middle-aged (45 to 64 years) individuals enrolled in the Atherosclerosis Risk in Communities Study (ARIC) (6), whereas a relatively higher prevalence (13.4%) was seen in the Cardiovascular Health Study (CHS), which recruited older, Medicare-eligible adults (7). In the PARTNERS program, the prevalence of PAD in 6,979 at-risk individuals (age >70 or 50 to 69 years with a history of smoking or DM) attending primary care practices was also high (29%) (8). Although no difference has been detected in the prevalence of PAD between men and women (1,5,6,7,9) or among whites and Hispanics (8,10), several studies have reported an excess prevalence among non-Hispanic blacks (5,11,12). In the NHANES study, non-Hispanic blacks were at a higher risk for PAD [odds ratio (OR) 2.39] independent of age, gender, smoking status, weight, hypertension (HTN), hypercholesterolemia, DM, and renal function (5).

When both symptomatic and asymptomatic patients are considered, it is estimated that at least 10 million Americans have PAD and 4 million have IC (13). Given the reported annual incidence of IC of approximately 20 per 1,000 in American men and women older than 65 years (14), up to 1.3 million elderly persons are expected to develop disabling IC every 2 years for the next 50 years (15). Consequently, PAD should be recognized as a leading cause of morbidity and an increasing cause of disability in the United States (16). These compelling epidemiologic facts emphasize the importance of awareness, detection, treatment, and prevention of this noncardiac vascular disease (7,8,17,18), and several recent publications have called for better dissemination of this information to the medical community and the public at large (19–22).

ABI	Severity of Disease
0.9 - 1.0	Normal
0.70 - 0.89	Mild disease
040 - 0.69	Moderate disease
< .040	Severe disease

ABI is 95% sensitive and 99% specific for PAD

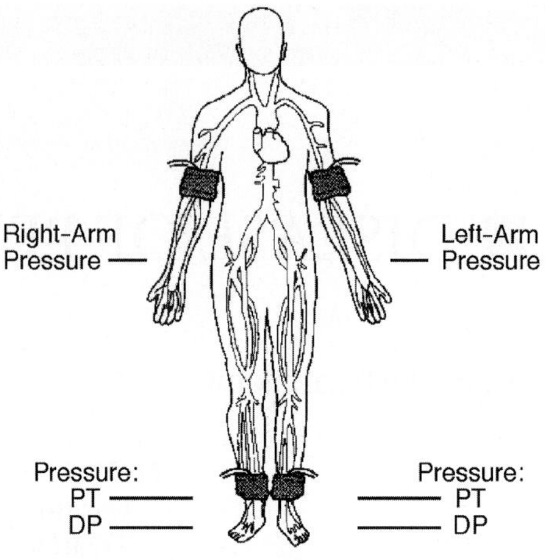

$$\textbf{ABI} = \frac{\text{Lower extremity systolic pressure}}{\text{Brachial artery pressure}}$$

FIGURE 108.1. How to measure the ankle–brachial index (ABI). DP, dorsal pedis artery; PAD, peripheral arterial disease; PT, posterior tibial artery.

PATHOPHYSIOLOGY

Atherosclerosis accounts for the vast majority of PAD, whereas uncommon vascular syndromes, such as vasculitis, thromboangiitis obliterans, popliteal entrapment syndrome, and fibromuscular dysplasia, account for less than 10% of cases. Atherosclerotic plaques frequently develop at arterial bifurcations, presumably due to both impaired atheroprotective mechanisms and the effects of disturbed blood flow on endothelial cells (23,24). These plaques are highly cellular and contain intrinsic vascular wall cells (endothelial and smooth muscle cells) and inflammatory cells (monocytes, macrophages, and lymphocytes) in addition to a thrombogenic lipid core that is covered by a fibrous cap (24–26). Once the fibrous cap is disrupted, the resultant exposure of the prothrombogenic lipid core can lead to thrombus formation and flow occlusion (24). This and other complex interactions between systemic and local factors at the atherosclerotic lesion site can lead to progression from asymptomatic PAD to IC, CLI, or ALI (24).

The pathophysiology of IC extends beyond an exercise-induced supply–demand mismatch that is caused by hemodynamic abnormalities imposed by arterial luminal stenosis. Metabolic changes also occur in chronically ischemic skeletal muscle groups (Table 108.1) (27,28) and are consistent with an "acquired metabolic myopathy" that manifests clinically as muscle weakness, functional impairment, and walking limitation.

RISK FACTORS FOR PERIPHERAL ARTERIAL DISEASE

Risk factors for PAD are similar to those for atherosclerosis in other vascular beds. Three major factors most strongly associated with PAD are advanced *age* (>60 years), *cigarette smoking*, and *DM* (29). Although the prevalence increases by 1.5- to 2.0 fold for every 10-year increase in age, DM and smoking increase the risk independently by approximately 2- to 4-fold each (9,12,29–31). Smoking also results in earlier onset of symptoms (by almost a decade) with an apparent dose–response relationship between the pack/year history and PAD risk (32–35). For example, in the Framingham Study, the likelihood for PAD increased by 40% for every 10 cigarettes smoked daily, and further analysis revealed that smoking accounts for approximately 75% of all PAD patients (36–38). Smokers are also more likely to have poorer survival rates and progress to CLI or amputation compared to nonsmokers (39–44). Of significance, the association between smoking and PAD is about twice as strong as that for coronary artery disease (CAD) (35, 36,45).

DM accounts for 45% to 70% of all nontraumatic amputations in the United States (46) and is a stronger risk factor for PAD in women than men (26,47,48). The risk of developing IC in DM in the Framingham cohort increased by 3.5-fold in men and 8.6-fold in women (47), and the 5-year incidence of IC in middle-aged men and women with newly diagnosed DM increased by 2.5- and 5.2-fold, respectively, compared to controls in another study (49). PAD is also more prevalent in individuals with an impaired glucose tolerance test (50), and a significant increase in its risk exists with higher glycosylated hemoglobin (Hgb) A1C levels even among individuals with non–diabetic range dysglycemia (HgbA1C <6%) (51). Finally,

TABLE 108.1

METABOLIC CHANGES IN CHRONICALLY ISCHEMIC SKELETAL GROUPS

- Altered mitochondrial (mt) expression
  - Increase in muscle mitochondrial enzyme activity
  - Increase in nuclear-encoded versus mtDNA-encoded mitochondrial enzyme activities
- Accumulation of metabolic intermediates
  - Increased plasma and skeletal muscle acylcamitine content
  - Resting muscle acylcamitine content inversely correlated with claudication-limited peak oxygen consumption
  - Exercise training induces changes in acylcamitine content that correlate with functional improvement
  - Accelerated accumulation of lactate in muscle with exercise
- Altered control of mitochondrial respiration
  - Altered ^{31}P magnetic resonance spectroscopy response to exercise analogous to mitochondrial myopathies
  - Slowed systemic oxygen uptake kinetics
- Increased systemic oxidative stress
- Accumulation of somatic mtDNA mutations
  - Muscle mtDNA injury not limited to hemodynamically affected muscle beds

the severity of PAD appears to be related to both the duration of hyperglycemia and glycemic control as demonstrated by a recent meta-analysis (52). Selvin and others proposed that PAD risk increased by 28% to 32% for every 1% increase in HgbA1C (52,53).

Hyperlipidemia is another risk factor, with an expected increase in the adjusted likelihood of developing PAD by 10% for every 10-mg/dL rise in total cholesterol (9). Although it was not previously considered a major risk factor, several studies now support the concept that total cholesterol, low-density lipoprotein (LDL), very low density lipoprotein (VLDL), triglycerides (TG), and lipoprotein (a) [Lp(a)] are all independent risk factors for PAD, whereas higher high-density lipoprotein (HDL) and apolipoprotein A1 appear to be protective (9,29,47,54,55). Moreover, a recent report showed that the coexistence of increased levels of Lp(a) and another metabolic risk factor (dyslipidemia or hyperhomocysteinemia) increased the likelihood of PAD symptoms (56).

There also exists a strong association between HTN and PAD. Data from the Framingham Study demonstrated a 2.5- to 4-fold increased risk of developing IC in both men and women with HTN; several other studies confirmed that as many as 50% to 92% of all PAD patients have this risk factor (47,57,58).

A number of novel risk factors for PAD have also been identified (Fig. 108.2). Elevated high-sensitivity C-reactive protein (hs-CRP) levels are found in patients with PAD, and in the Physician's Health Study, it was the strongest nonlipid predictor of incident PAD (relative risk for the highest vs. lowest quartile, 2.8; 95% confidence interval [CI], 1.3 to 5.9) (59). *Hyperfibrinogenemia,* another risk factor for PAD, is associated with worsening symptoms (59–65). Higher fibrinogen levels are seen in patients with DM, HTN, obesity, those who lead sedentary lifestyles, and smokers, with a dose–response relationship between the number of cigarettes smoked and the fibrinogen level (66,67). *Hyperhomocysteinemia* (HHcy), another novel risk factor, is associated with premature atherosclerosis and appears to be a stronger risk for PAD than CAD (59,68–71). It has also been implicated in disease progression and as a risk factor for failure of peripheral interventions (72,73), although not all studies have shown such a relationship (59,72).

A more recently recognized risk factor for PAD is *chronic kidney disease* (CKD) (74–77). Based on clinical parameters

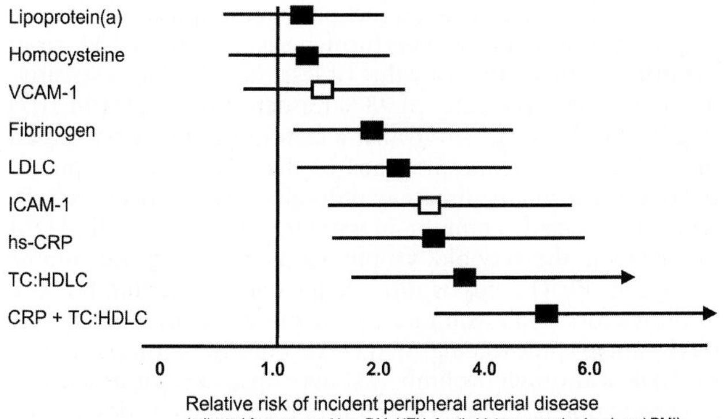

FIGURE 108.2. Novel risk factors as predictors of peripheral arterial disease. BMI, body mass index; CRP, C-reactive protein; DM, diabetes mellitus; HDLC, high-density-lipoprotein cholesterol; hs-CRP, high-sensitivity C-reactive protein; HTN, hypertension; ICAM-1, intercellular adhesion molecule-1; LDLC, low-density-lipoprotein cholesterol; TC, total cholesterol; VCAM-1, vascular cell adhesion molecule-1. (From Smith Jr SC, Milani RV, Arnett DK, et al. Atherosclerotic Vascular Disease Conference: Writing Group II: Risk factors. *Circulation* 2004;109:2613–2616.)

alone, including a prior diagnosis of PAD, history of amputation, previous revascularization procedure, IC, tissue gangrene, or decrease in peripheral pulses on physical exam, the overall prevalence of PAD in the United States Renal Data System in 1999 was 15% (77). Other studies have confirmed this relationship, and a report from the ARIC review found that a low ABI was associated with an increase in the serum creatinine level over time (OR 2.5) (78).

Genetic predisposition to PAD is supported by the observations of increased rates of cardiovascular disease (including PAD) in "healthy" relatives of patients with IC. Although the relative contributions of genes and environment to the pathogenesis of premature PAD are difficult to discern, one study found that one in four siblings of patients with premature PAD will have a vascular event before age 55 years, and up to half of asymptomatic siblings will develop occult disease at a young age (79). *Hypercoagulable states* or *thrombophilia* is an uncommon risk factor for PAD because most patients present with venous thrombosis. In select patients, however, an evaluation for an underlying hypercoagulable condition should be considered, especially younger individuals who lack traditional risk factors or when there is a strong family history of premature atherosclerosis, and in those individuals who fail arterial revascularization where no technical reason can be found. Several recent studies have suggested an independent association between altered levels of important *thrombophilic*, *hemostatic*, and *inflammatory factors* (56,80–85). In particular, D-dimer levels appear to be inversely related to the ABI and have been associated with a greater decline in walking and poorer physical functioning scores (81–85).

CLINICAL PRESENTATION

The term *claudication*, from the Latin word *claudicare* meaning "to limp," was first applied to humans in 1858 by Charcot (86,87). In the mid 1960s, physicians used the Rose Questionnaire, a test specifically designed to detect patients with PAD, which defined IC as leg pain that does not occur at rest, does not resolve with walking, prompts the patient to stop walking, and disappears within 10 minutes of rest (88). Although the Rose Questionnaire has been very useful, it has recently been recognized that it has a low sensitivity and a low positive predictive value for identifying PAD because most patients are either asymptomatic or have atypical symptoms (8,89–93). More recently, the ABI has been used as a clinical indicator to identify patients with PAD. Based on the use of this method at the bedside or at the office, the true prevalence of PAD is expected to be two to five times higher than has been previously recognized based on the presence of IC (1,4, 8,17,89,94,95).

There are other objective measures of lower-extremity function that have been used clinically to identify patients with PAD. These include the 6-minute walk test, the 4-meter walking velocity, repeated chair raises, standing balance, the San Diego Claudication Questionnaire, the Geriatric Depression Score Short-Form, and the Walking Impairment Questionnaire (4,28,96,97).

Patients with IC may complain of activity-induced aching, tightness, cramping, or sense of fatigue in the affected leg. Their walking distance seldom varies, and stopping or slowing the pace often relieves their symptoms. Inactive patients may not report symptoms until they are asked to perform specific tasks such as the 6-minutes walk test or the treadmill exercise test. The claudicating muscle group is usually located distal to the stenotic or obstructive lesion. Symptoms involving the buttock, hip, and thigh are typically seen with aortoiliac (AI) disease, whereas calf claudication is found with femoropopliteal involvement. Calf claudication presents in greater than 60% to 70% of patients and is the most common clinical presentation

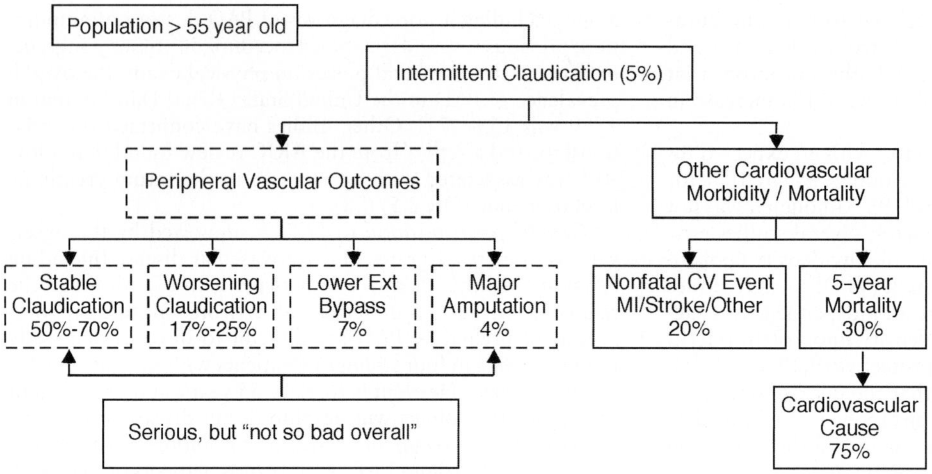

FIGURE 108.3. Proposed natural history of peripheral arterial disease. CV, cardiovascular; Ext, extremity; MI, myocardial infarction.

for PAD. Rest pain and ischemic leg ulcers are typically seen with multilevel disease and when the ABI is less than 0.4.

The natural history of lower-extremity functioning in PAD does not appear to be as benign as was once implied (Fig. 108.3 shows the proposed natural history of PAD). Although worsening IC is described in a minority of patients (98–101), when objective measures are used, self-imposed limitations on physical activity is common among patients to avoid painful symptoms (4). Furthermore, the PAD-associated disability for reportedly asymptomatic individuals, including the limitations in work-related and leisurely activities, is similar to that seen in those with IC (4).

Findings of CLI include rest pain, ischemic ulcers, and gangrene (Fig. 108.4), and clinical categories are outlined in Table 108.2 (94). Patients tend to keep their affected leg dependent to relieve their rest pain, which occasionally results in secondary edema and dependent rubor. Elevation pallor should also be sought when evaluating for CLI (Fig. 108.5 shows dependent rubor/edema). The clinical features of ALI include some or all of the six "Ps," pain, pallor, paresthesia, paralysis, pulselessness, and poikilothermia (Table 108.3). Paresthesias and paralysis are the most ominous signs and generally indicate irreversible ischemic injury, and in extreme cases, the presence of muscle rigidity and woodiness indicates a nonsalvageable limb.

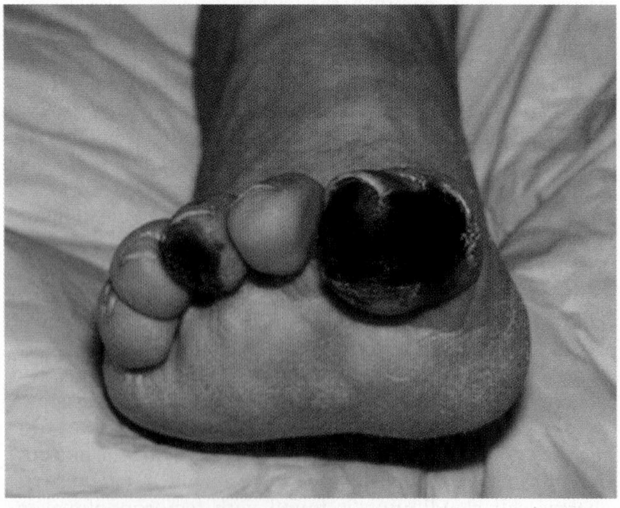

FIGURE 108.4. Ischemic ulcers and gangrene in a patient with critical limb ischemia.

The physical exam should include palpation of the pulses and auscultation for bruits in the entire vascular system along with assessment for aneurysmal disease. It is important to remember that patients with IC may have a completely normal physical examination at rest, including peripheral pulses, and that the presence of thickened nails, poor hair growth, and cold hands and feet are not reliable indicators of arterial insufficiency.

DIAGNOSIS

Screening at-risk patients for PAD is essential because most are asymptomatic and few symptomatic patients report their symptoms to their health care provider (8,94). High-risk patients include those with known cardiac disease, DM, age greater than 70 years, or age 50 years or older with one or more cardiovascular risk factors such as active or remote smoking history, dyslipidemia, dysglycemia (elevated glucose in a nondiabetic range), HTN, or a family history of atherosclerotic vascular disease (8,102,103). It is important to note that the risks of cardiovascular events, including mortality, in asymptomatic individuals are comparable to those encountered in symptomatic patients (13,94,104,105).

The ABI is a noninvasive, inexpensive, simple, and effective diagnostic test that can be performed easily at the bedside or in the office setting. An ABI value of less than 0.9 has a sensitivity of 90% and specificity of 98% for detecting PAD (106,107) (Fig. 108.6 shows the survival as a factor of PAD severity based on ABI values). The limitations of the ABI include a potential to underestimate disease in individuals with calcific vessels, which is especially common in patients with longstanding DM or CKD and the very old. Obtaining a complete pulse volume recording (PVR) study is more helpful in this setting because it allows for visual examination of the waveforms. PVRs are plethysmographic tracings that detect changes in the volume of blood flow through the limb. A slower upstroke, the absence of a dicrotic notch, decreased amplitude, and slower descending waveforms are considered abnormal (Fig. 108.7 demonstrates findings seen on an abnormal PVR). An exercise ABI can be performed as an extension of PVR testing when the clinical suspicion of PAD is high but the resting ABI is normal or in question. Patients are instructed to walk 2 miles per hour on a constant-graded treadmill for a maximum of 5 minutes and their ABI is measured both before and after exercise. A reduction in blood pressure or a decrease in the waveform after exercise is suggestive of PAD.

TABLE 108.2

CLINICAL CATEGORIES OF CHRONIC LIMB ISCHEMIA: RUTHERFORD CLASSIFICATION

Grade	Category	Clinical description	Objective criteria
0	0	Asymptomatic	Normal TM
	1	Mild Claudication	Complete TM, Post exercise AP >50 but ≤20 mm Hg resting value
I	2	Moderate Claudication	Between 1 and 3
	3	Severe Claudication	Can NOT Complete TM Post exercise AP <50 mm Hg
II	4	Ischemic Rest Pain	Resting AP <40 mm Hg, Flat PVR TP <30 mm Hg
III	5	Minor Tissue Loss	Resting AP <60 mm Hg, Flat PVR TP <40 mm Hg
	6	Major Tissue Loss (non-salvageable)	Same as Category 5

Other useful tests include arterial duplex ultrasonography (DUS), magnetic resonance angiography (MRA), computed tomography angiography (CTA), and conventional angiography. The DUS measures flow velocities and identifies stenotic or obstructive lesions. It is particularly valuable in patients with noncompressible (i.e., calcific) vessels. MRA provides better details than the DUS and may be most useful for assistance in determining bypass surgery options in patients with severe disease without the risks of contrast-induced nephropathy seen with conventional contrast media (108). CTA is gaining rapid acceptance as another noninvasive imaging method capable of delineating vascular structures, particularly the thoracoabdominal aorta (109). Although angiography remains the gold standard for evaluating the anatomy of the peripheral arterial system, it is invasive and carries a potential for nephrotoxicity. As such, it should be used only when the diagnosis of PAD is in question or an endovascular or surgical procedure is planned.

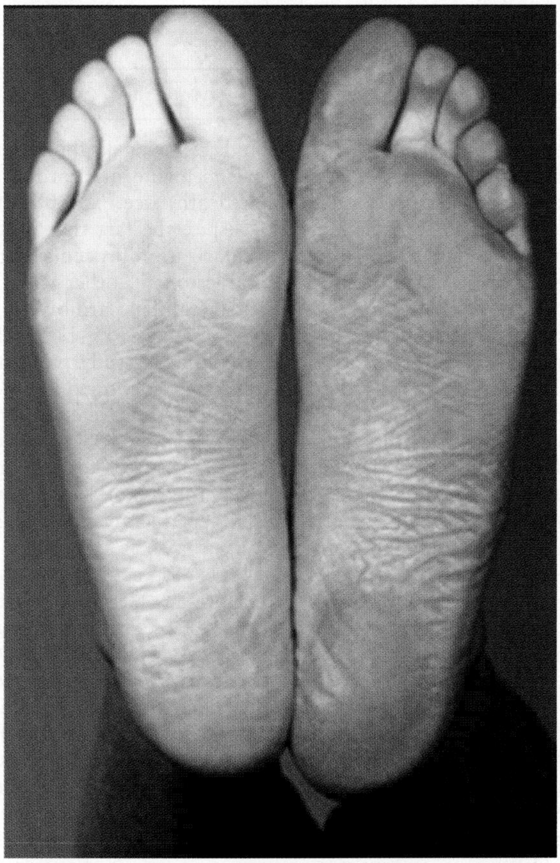

FIGURE 108.5. Elevation pallor in a patient with chronic critical limb ischemia.

Laboratory studies are nonspecific for diagnosing PAD but detect associated risk factors and are important for proper selection of pharmacologic therapies. A complete blood count, fasting blood glucose, lipid profile, measurement of HgbA1c, complete metabolic panel, and quantitative urinalysis are recommended. A baseline electrocardiogram is recommended at the time of diagnosis and in selected patients; cardiac stress testing may be indicated. Occasionally, other tests such as a sedimentation rate, fibrinogen, Lp(a), plasma homocysteine, hypercoagulable profile, and even heparin antibodies may be necessary in selected patients.

DIFFERENTIAL DIAGNOSIS

Cardiovascular physicians need to be aware of several important uncommon diseases that mimic PAD.

Thromboangiitis obliterans (*Buerger's disease*) is a nonatherosclerotic segmental inflammatory disease that affects the small and medium-sized arteries, veins, and nerves of the arms, legs, and rarely elsewhere. It is traditionally seen in smokers younger than the age of 40 years but also occurs with any type of tobacco use including smokeless tobacco or cannabis (110). It presents with digital ischemia or claudication of the arch or foot, and superficial thrombophlebitis or Raynaud's phenomenon is reported in as many as 40% of patients (111). Arteriography reveals segmental occlusions in the distal arteries without evidence for atherosclerosis. The *popliteal artery entrapment syndrome* is a rare and frequently overlooked condition. It should be suspected in any young athletic individual without conventional risk factors for atherosclerosis who presents with calf or foot claudication at high levels of exertion. On occasion the patient may also present with limb-threatening ischemia or distal thromboemboli. Symptoms are due to compression of the popliteal artery by the medial head of the gastrocnemius muscle. Pedal pulses are generally normal at rest

TABLE 108.3

CLINICAL CATEGORIES OF ACUTE LIMB ISCHEMIA

Category	Description/ prognosis	Findings		Doppler signals	
		Sensory loss	Muscle weakness	Arterial	Venous
I. Viable	Not immediately threatened	None	None	Audible	Audible
II. Threatened					
a. Marginally	Salvageable if promptly treated	Minimal (toes) or none	None	Inaudible	Audible
b. Immediately	Salvageable with immediate revascularization	More than toes, rost pain	Mild, moderate	Inaudible	Audible
III. Inevitable	Major tissue loss or permanent nerve damage inevitables	Profound, anesthetic	Profound, paralysis (rigor)	Inaudible	Inaudible

Rutherford J. *Vasc Surgery* 1997;26:517–538.

but disappear with active plantar flexion against resistance, and angiography (or MRA) demonstrates medial displacement of the popliteal artery in the neutral or flexed position (112). *Fibromuscular dysplasia* (FMD) affects small to medium-sized vessels, predominately the renal and internal carotid arteries, but rarely lead to IC, aneurysmal formation, or spontaneous arterial dissection. It is a nonatherosclerotic, noninflammatory disease usually seen in young to middle-aged women (113). *Vasculitis* can also present with symptoms of IC, and Takayasu arteritis and giant cell arteritis (GCA) can both affect the lower extremities. Takayasu arteritis, also called "pulseless disease" or "reverse coarctation," is predominately seen in younger women, whereas GCA affects older individuals and is rare before age 50 years. An infrequent condition, *exercise-induced endofibrosis of the iliac arteries*, is seen in competition cyclists, and patients present with a sensation of a swollen thigh in one or both (15%) legs that only occurs during cycling. The ABI is usually normal at rest but drops significantly (to <0.5 in 85% of cases) with maximal exercise. The histologic lesion is fibrosis of the intimal wall with stenosis affecting the first few centimeters of the external iliac artery or, less commonly, the common femoral artery without evidence for atherosclerotic lesions or focal inflammation (114). Consideration must also be given to *venous claudication*, a condition seen in patients with a history of deep vein thrombosis who develop the postphlebitic syndrome. These individuals usually describe exertional leg heaviness in the setting of a normal exercise ABI. Edema, varicose veins, and skin changes of stasis dermatitis are typically seen. A more common condition, *neurogenic claudication* (commonly referred to as *pseudoclaudication*), is seen in patients with lumbar canal stenosis or disc disease. Leg symptoms including tingling, weakness, heaviness, tightness, tiredness, or clumsiness are generally exacerbated by standing or walking and improve with leaning forward or sitting. A lumbar spine MRI or CT scan usually establishes the diagnosis.

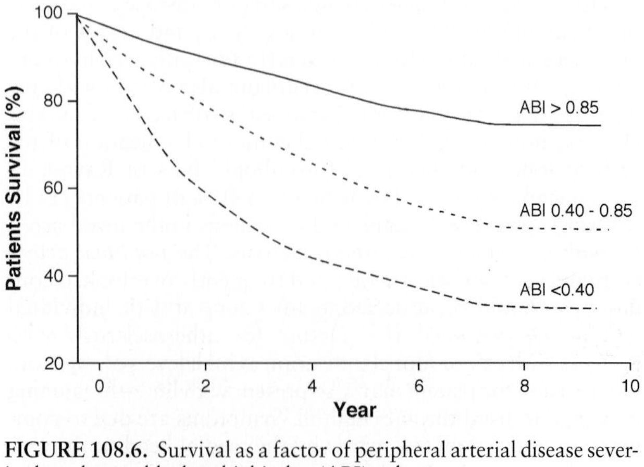

FIGURE 108.6. Survival as a factor of peripheral arterial disease severity based on ankle–brachial index (ABI) values.

THERAPY AND OUTCOMES

The goals of PAD management include reducing disability, limb loss, and future cardiovascular events (acute myocardial infarction [MI], stroke, and vascular death) (see Fig. 108.8 for the goals of PAD management). Despite the fact that only a minority of patients require revascularization procedures, the likely coexistence of atherosclerotic lesions in other vascular territories mandates applying intensive global cardiovascular risk reduction strategies to all PAD patients (115–117). This concept was well emphasized in a landmark study published in 1984 by Hertzer and coworkers. They identified a strong association between PAD and CAD (118) and reported that among patients with symptomatic PAD, only 10% had normal coronary arteries, whereas 28% had severe disease documented by coronary angiography. Other studies have since confirmed that symptomatic PAD independently predicts adverse outcomes in patients presenting with CAD, including those with chronic stable angina (119) or acute MI (AMI) (120–122) and in survivors of recent MI (123), coronary artery bypass grafting surgery (CABG) (124–126), or percutaneous coronary angioplasty (PCI) (127–130). Asymptomatic PAD is also associated with future adverse cardiovascular events (even in individuals without evidence of cardiac disease at baseline), and it has been shown to predict poor outcomes after CABG including cardiovascular mortality (131–133). Despite these compelling data, patients with IC and known CAD are still less likely to receive β-blockers (123) and adequate antithrombotic therapy (8) or have their risk factors properly controlled (8,19, 134–138).

Individuals with premature PAD (<40 years of age) represent a special population. These individuals usually present

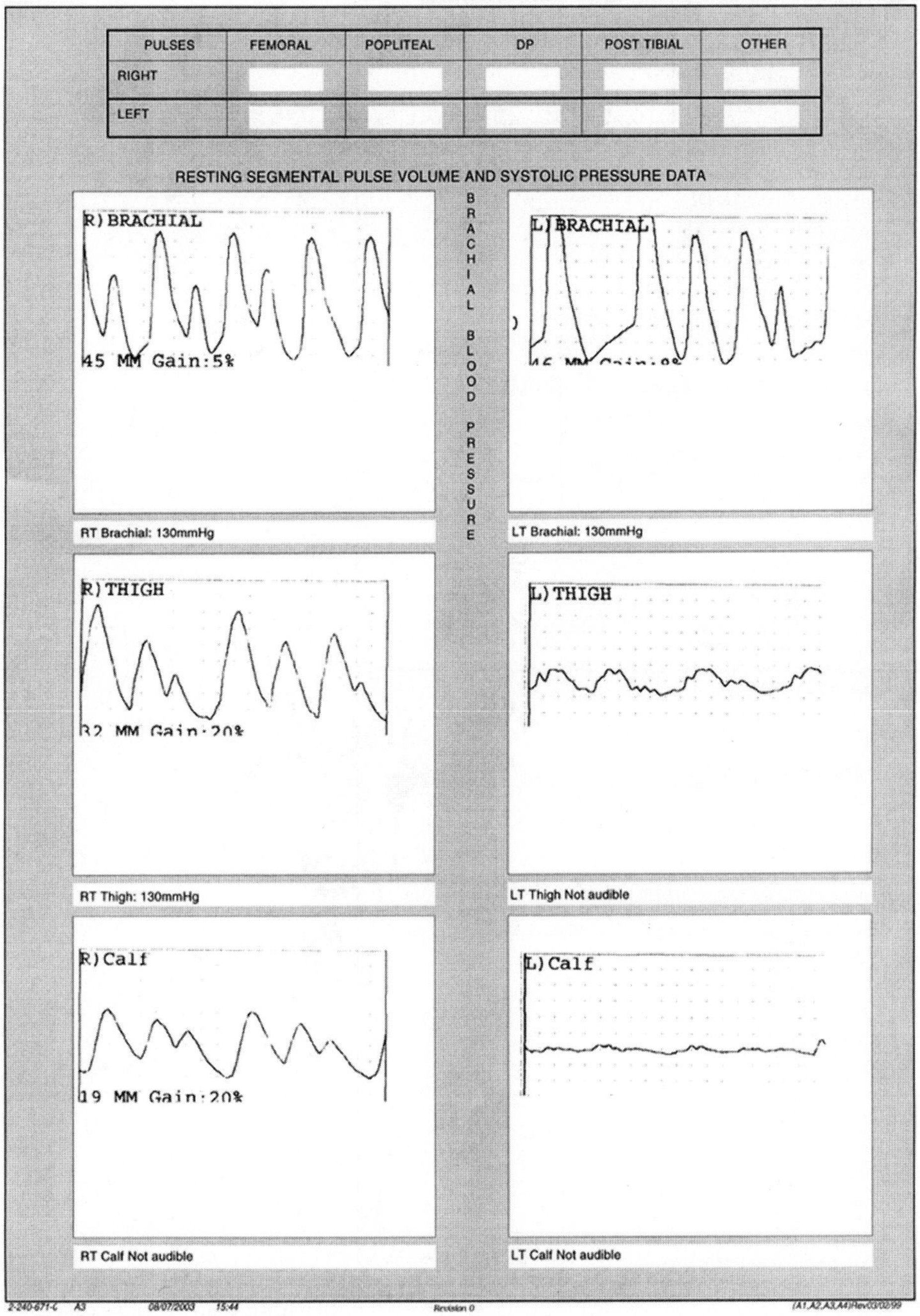

FIGURE 108.7. Pulse volume recordings in a patient with severe peripheral arterial disease.A/B, ankle–brachial; DP, dorsal pedis artery; L, left; LT, left; R, right; RT,right; PT, posterior tibial artery. (Continued)

with diffuse involvement of their aorta and iliac arteries and carry an exceptionally poor prognosis (139–147). As many as 50% will eventually require major amputations (142,145–149), and their 5-year mortality rate exceeds 60% (150).

Cardiovascular Risk Factor Reduction

Smoking Cessation

Smoking is the most important avoidable, and reversible, risk factor for the development of PAD and its complications (35–44,47,151). Up to 80% of patients report a current or prior history of cigarette smoking (39,45,152). It is significant that smoking cessation favorably changes the natural history of PAD and leads to marked improvement in limb and systemic outcomes in those who are able to quit. For example, those who stop smoking have an equivalent risk for developing future IC as nonsmokers within only 1 year of quitting (153,154), and the severity of their IC may also be reduced (41). Moreover, abstinence from smoking is also associated with a reduced risk for developing CLI (16% vs. 0% for nonsmokers over a 7-year follow-up) or major amputation (40,155–157).

Smokers must also be made aware that smoking cessation is associated with better results with endovascular and surgical procedures. A recent meta-analysis found a threefold increased risk of graft failure among those individuals who continued smoking after lower limb bypass surgery regardless of the type of graft used (autogenous or polyester grafts) (158). In this study a clear dose–response relationship was evident, with a stronger inverse relationship between the numbers of cigarettes smoked and graft patency. The patency rates in

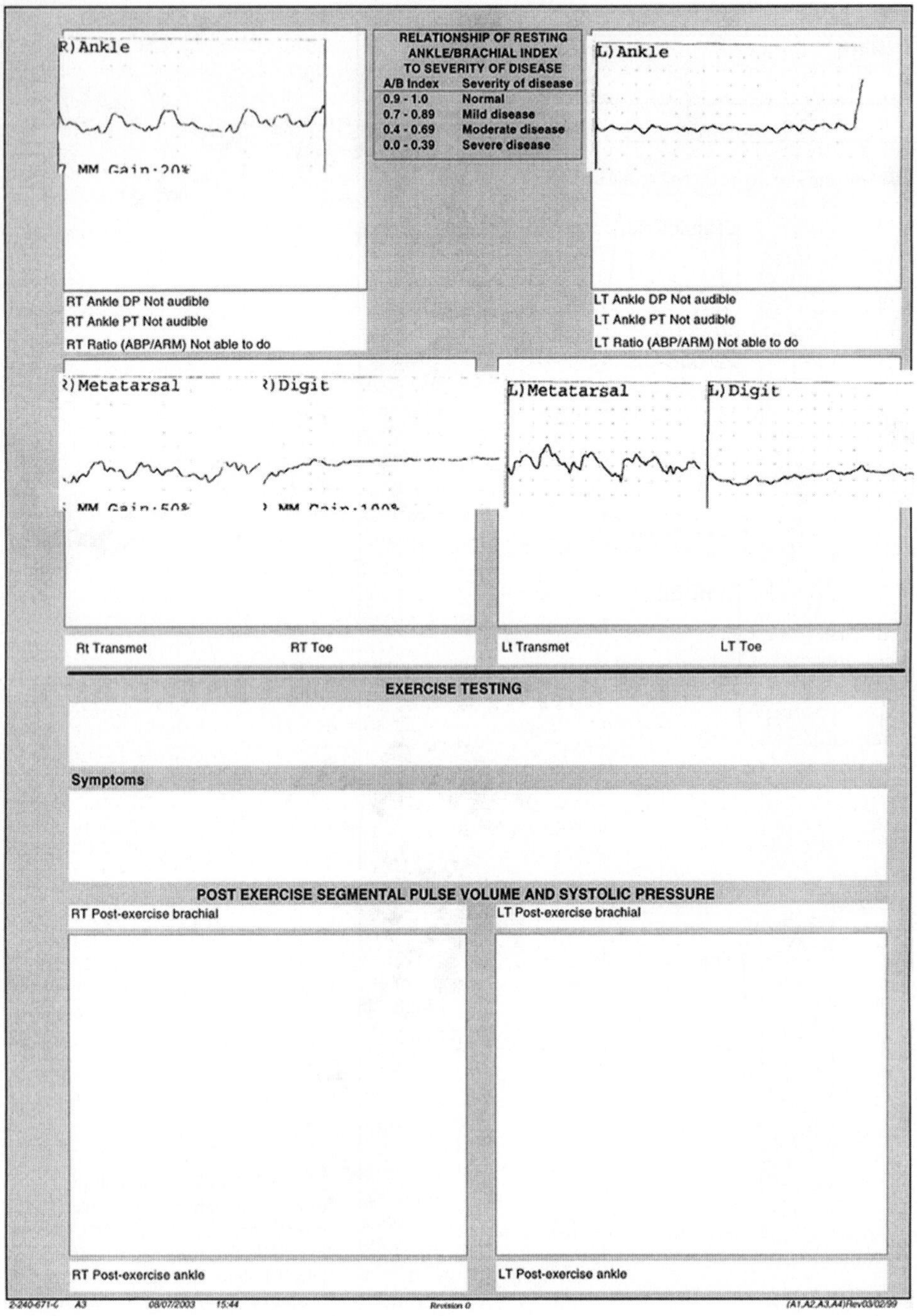

FIGURE 108.7. (Continued)

former smokers were comparable to those who had never smoked even if smoking cessation was instigated after their operation (158). Smoking cessation also has a positive impact on survival. Faulkner et al. found that individuals who quit smoking had almost twice the chance of surviving 5 years as those who continued to smoke (159). Hence, complete and permanent smoking cessation is by far the most clinically effective and cost-effective intervention in patients with PAD (36,38,39,45,160–162) and must be made a top priority. Unfortunately, most patients receive little or no treatment for their nicotine addiction, as recently demonstrated in the PARTNERS study, in which only 50% of participants received any such

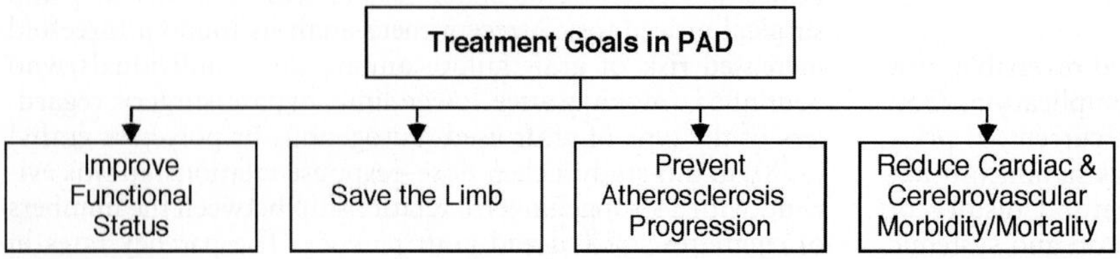

FIGURE 108.8. Treatment goals in peripheral arterial disease (PAD) patients.

advice from their physician (17). A low rate of counseling, along with the fact that the addictive characteristics of nicotine are comparable to those of heroin may explain the unacceptably low quitting rate (only 2%/year) among those who attempt to stop smoking (160,163). Clinicians caring for these individuals must identify smokers, motivate them to quit, and be prepared to provide smoking cessation strategies at each clinical encounter (160,163,164). Prescriptions for conjunctive therapies, such as nicotine replacement and bupropion (Zyban), along with referrals to smoking cessation programs are effective particularly when prescribed to patients prepared to quit within the next few weeks. In addition, there are a number of evidence-based practice guidelines available for tobacco cessation, with practical algorithms geared to improving initial success as well as long-term abstinence rates (164).

Managing Diabetes Mellitus

In addition to increasing the risk of developing PAD by two- to fourfold (47,165,166), DM also leads to a two- to fourfold increase in the risk of cardiovascular events and a 60% increase in early mortality relative to those without this risk factor (166–171). In addition, the prevalence and extent of PAD appear to correlate with the duration and severity of DM (52,53,172).

Diabetic patients develop occlusive disease in the profunda femoris and infrapopliteal arteries more commonly than nondiabetic subjects (173). They are also more likely to develop microangiopathy, neuropathy with loss of protective sensation, and impaired wound healing. These abnormalities may help to explain the 10- to 16-fold higher lifetime risk of lower-extremity amputation in DM compared to nondiabetic individuals (174) as well as the 24-fold higher risk among older individuals (aged 65 to 74 years) who have both DM and PAD (46). Arterial calcifications and pulse deficits are also common in diabetics (175,176). In one study, approximately 35% of patients had detectable pulse deficits (177) and this, combined with the presence of arterial calcifications, increased their risk for cardiovascular mortality (177,178).

Although it is accepted that stringent glycemic control favorably effects microvascular disease, particularly retinopathy (179,180), its effect on the development of PAD and its complications (such as progression to IC, CLI, or amputation) has not been convincingly demonstrated (179–181). Nevertheless, achieving a target HgbA1C of less than 6.5% to 7.0% is recommended for all patients with DM and PAD (182). Optimal management should also take into account that DM is a prothrombotic and proinflammatory state (172,183,184). Diabetic patients, for example, have been shown to have increased platelet aggregability, which may potentially contribute to their higher incidence of atherothrombotic events, such as AMI, ischemic stroke, and ALI (52,174,176,177,185). Thus, adopting an intensive multifaceted strategy that addresses hyperglycemia in addition to other cardiovascular risk factors has been found to decrease cardiovascular events by up to 50% (186).

Treatment of Dyslipidemia

Lipid-lowering therapy using hydroxymethylglutaryl-coenzyme A (HMG-CoA) reductase inhibitors (statins) in patients with CAD has produced major reductions in cardiac morbidity and mortality, as several large randomized, controlled trials have demonstrated (187,188). The 2001 National Cholesterol Education Program Adult Treatment Panel (NCEP) III considered PAD, whether diagnosed by ABI, lower-limb blood flow studies, or clinical symptoms, a CAD risk equivalent and recommended targeting the same lipid levels as sought for CAD patients (LDL-cholesterol <100 mg/dL and TG <150 mg/dL) (189). Several newer clinical trials, however, have provided a rationale for even more intensive LDL-lowering, particularly in high-risk patients. A recent consensus panel statement proposed that an LDL-cholesterol goal of less than 70 mg/dL (using combination therapy) for high-risk patients and those with other dyslipidemias such as elevated triglycerides or low HDL levels be employed (190). The Heart Protection Study recently added another paradigm to the use of statin drugs in this population, supporting their routine use regardless of the cholesterol level. In this trial, PAD patients who received simvastatin had a significantly lower cardiovascular ischemic event rate than those who did not (24.7 vs. 30.5%, $p < .0001$) irrespective of the presence of CAD or the pretreatment cholesterol or triglyceride concentrations or the sex or age of the participants (191). In addition to improving cardiovascular outcomes, statins have also been shown in several studies to have a beneficial effect on leg symptoms. A post hoc analysis of the Scandinavian Simvastatin Survival Study (4S) reported that statin therapy reduced the risk of new or worsening IC by 38% (192), and another study proposed an association between statins and improved functional outcomes, including better performance on the 6-minute walk test, faster walking capacity, and higher summary performance score (193). Two other randomized trials evaluated the effect of statin use on leg functioning (194,195). Mondillo et al. reported an increase in pain-free and total walking distance by 90 and 126 meters, respectively, as well as improvement in IC symptoms in patients randomized to simvastatin (40 mg/day for 6 months) for hypercholesterolemia compared to placebo (194), and Mohler et al. found that atorvastatin (80 mg/day for 12 months) improved the mean pain-free walking time (PFWT) by 63% (81 $\pm$ 15 seconds) compared with 38% (39 $\pm$ 8 seconds, $p = .025$) in the placebo group and also enhanced community-based physical activity (195). Mohler et al. (195) and Regensteiner et al. (196) also noted improvement in the PFWT with statin use, finding it comparable to that achieved with cilostazol, a drug marketed exclusively for IC. Although the exact mechanism for the effects of statins on leg function is unclear, it has been proposed that they induce endothelium-dependent vasodilation, which may result in reduced vascular resistance and subsequent improvement in blood flow through collateral blood vessels. They also appear to have a proangiogenic effect that may allow for new blood vessel development (195,197,198).

Treatment of Hypertension

The association between HTN and cardiovascular disease (CVD) is well established. In a robust meta-analysis of 61 prospective studies that enrolled more than 1 million individuals, Lewington and colleagues demonstrated a doubling in CVD risk for each 20-mm Hg increment in systolic blood pressure or 10 mm Hg in diastolic blood pressure in middle-aged and elderly persons (40 to 70 years) beginning at a level of 115/75 mm Hg (199). The relationship between hypertension and PAD, however, had not been as well established until recently when the PARTNERS program observed that PAD and HTN were encountered together in about 92% of enrolled individuals (8,57,58).

Despite the proven efficacy of antihypertensive therapy in reducing the risk of stroke, MI, and vascular death in most patients (200), large trials on its effect on PAD progression and specific recommendations on its use in this patient population are lacking (201). Although the choice of antihypertensive agents should be individualized, blood pressure targets are similar to those dictated for patients with atherothrombosis elsewhere (201). Although the use of β-blockers for treatment of hypertension in PAD patients was initially considered contraindicated for fear of worsening IC (202–204), a rigorous meta-analysis critically reviewed data from 11 randomized, controlled studies and found them safe in patients with stable mild to moderate disease (205). Furthermore, β-blocker therapy reduced the incidence of new coronary events in patients with CAD and concurrent symptomatic PAD by about 50% in one study and should be considered for this patient population (206). In the Heart Outcomes Prevention Evaluation (HOPE) trial (207), the PAD subgroup who received the angiotensin-converting-enzyme (ACE) inhibitor ramipril had a 22% relative risk reduction in the composite endpoints of MI, stroke, or cardiovascular death. A more recent analysis of this trial proposed that the benefits of ramipril extended to both symptomatic and asymptomatic PAD patients (the number needed to treat to prevent 1 ischemic event during the study treatment period of 4.5 years was 18 and 17 for symptomatic and asymptomatic patients, respectively) (208,209). In addition to reducing the risk of fatal and nonfatal ischemic events, an ACE inhibitor may also increase peripheral perfusion and lead to improvement in walking distance (210–212). Thus, an ACE inhibitor should be considered in all patients with PAD, particularly those with DM, documented microalbuminuria, or CKD. Although the benefits of intensive lowering of blood pressure in patients with PAD have not been systematically studied, emerging data suggest that intensive blood pressure–lowering strategies appear to be highly effective in improving cardiovascular outcomes (213).

Treatment of Nontraditional Risk Factors

Evaluation for HHcy and elevated Lp(a) levels is particularly important in individuals with diffuse PAD who lack traditional risk factors. Besides being a risk factor for PAD, HHcy is also associated with increased cardiac mortality (214). However, no large studies have evaluated whether lowering homocysteine levels leads to decreased event rates in the PAD population. There are also no controlled trials on Lp(a) reduction and cardiovascular outcomes. The challenge of lowering Lp(a) lies in the fact that the most commonly used medications (statins) and lifestyle modifications (exercise and diet) are relatively ineffective in modifying Lp(a) concentration (215–217). Nicotinic acid (3 to 4 g/day), however, has been reported in small studies to be somewhat effective as an Lp(a)-modifying agent (218).

Antiplatelet Therapy

Antiplatelet therapy should be offered to all PAD patients unless contraindicated. In a meta-analysis of 42 trials of antiplatelet therapy (primarily aspirin [ASA] at doses of 80 to 325 mg/day0 for patients with cardiovascular disease, the Antiplatelet Trialists' Collaboration Group reported a 23% risk reduction in cardiovascular ischemic events (nonfatal MI, stroke, and vascular death) (219). An earlier meta-analysis from the same group and a recent Cochrane review also found ASA to be effective in preventing peripheral arterial occlusion after revascularization procedures (220,221). The Clopidogrel versus Aspirin in Patients at Risk of Ischemic Events (CAPRIE) trial compared the efficacy of daily doses of clopidogrel (75 mg) to ASA (325 mg) in 19,185 patients with a history of atherosclerotic vascular disease (133). In the PAD subgroup, clopidogrel provided a 23.8% relative risk reduction in the composite endpoints of fatal or nonfatal MI, ischemic stroke, or vascular death compared to ASA, which was almost three times greater than the overall trial reduction of 8.7%. Although dual antiplatelet therapy appears to provide more effective platelet inhibition, the effect of this strategy on outcomes in patients with vascular disease is undergoing prospective evaluation in the Clopidogrel for High Atherothrombotic Risk and Ischemic Stabilization, Management, and Avoidance (CHARISMA) multicenter trial (222).

Another antiplatelet agent, ticlopidine, has also favorably affected outcomes in PAD patients including improvement in IC and long-term patency of autologous vein grafts (223–225) and reduction in the need for vascular surgery and overall cardiac morbidity (226,227). Although it was approved for use earlier than clopidogrel, ticlopidine has fallen out of favor due to its rare but serious side effects including neutropenia (occurring in 2% to 3% of patients) and thrombotic thrombocytopenic purpura, both of which have led to fatalities (228,229).

Treatment of Peripheral Arterial Disease Symptoms

In addition to preventing tissue and limb loss, the goals of treatment for the patient with IC are relieving exertional symptoms so patients can increase their walking capacity and quality of life. Besides walking exercise rehabilitation programs, two pharmacologic agents have been used to try to achieve these goals.

Pharmacotherapy

Cilostazol (Pletal) is a phosphodiesterase type 3 (PDE-3) inhibitor that inhibits platelet aggregation, impedes thrombin formation and vascular smooth muscle proliferation, causes vasodilation, increases HDL, and reduces triglyceride levels (230–232). In randomized, placebo-controlled trials cilostazol improved pain-free and maximal treadmill walking distance, community-based ambulation, and quality of life in patients with symptomatic PAD when compared to placebo. It has also been shown to increase maximal walking distance compared to pentoxifylline and placebo in several randomized, controlled trials (233). The recommended dose of 100 mg twice a day is essential to ensuring its effect in improving IC, and patients must be instructed that it may take up to 4 months to get the full benefit. Common side effects include headache, diarrhea, gastric upset, palpitations, and dizziness, although a temporary reduction in the dose to 50 mg twice per day may alleviate these problems. As with other PDE inhibitors (milrinone, vesnarinone), a decreased survival in patients with severe congestive heart failure has been reported, and therefore cilostazol should not be used in this patient population (234,235).

Pentoxifylline (Trental), a methylxanthine derivative that increases cyclic adenosine monophosphate, decreases blood viscosity and improves erythrocyte flexibility and has both anti-inflammatory and antiproliferative effects. Although the mechanism of action of pentoxifylline in PAD is unclear, two meta-analyses and two systematic reviews have concluded that it has only a minor effect on improving walking capacity and the current data are insufficient to support its widespread use (236,237).

Supervised Exercise Rehabilitation Program

Reduced walking capacity due to IC is associated with restrictions in an individual's activities of daily living and results in a significant reduction in quality of life. The first randomized, controlled trial of exercise training in persons with PAD reported a marked improvement in treadmill-walking ability (238), and numerous studies since then have supported its efficacy as one of the most efficient strategies for improving symptoms. Although the use pentoxifylline and cilostazol has led to only modest improvement in maximal walking ability (40% to 60% with cilostazol) (239–240), exercise-induced improvement in maximal walking time has ranged from 25% to 442% (241). In a meta-analysis of 21 nonrandomized and randomized studies, exercise increased pain-free walking time in patients with claudication by almost 180% (from 125.9 ± 57.3 meters to 351.2 ± 188.7 meters) and the maximal walking time by approximately 120% (from 325.8 ± 148.1 meters to 723.3 ± 591.5 meters) (15). Another meta-analysis included 10 randomized trials and also demonstrated an increase in maximal walking time (by 150%), an improvement that exceeded that of angioplasty and antiplatelet therapy at 6 months but did not differ considerably from that of surgical treatment (242). The greatest benefit of exercise rehabilitation is obtained when the walking sessions are 35 to 50 minutes long, occur at a frequency of three to five times per week, near-maximal pain is reached in each session, and the program lasts at least 6 months.

In addition to improving the functional capacity in PAD (as assessed by community-based walking ability and health-related quality-of-life questionnaires) (241,243), exercise training increases the benefits from revascularization procedures on claudication distance and enhances the cardiovascular risk profile of these patients (244–246). Therefore, maintenance of exercise programs should be considered indefinitely or the functional and cardiovascular benefit may eventually be lost. Unfortunately, there are limitations to exercise rehabilitation programs including cost, lack of availability, and lack of insurance coverage. Overall, supervised exercise rehabilitation programs should be implemented in all medically fit patients with IC.

Revascularization

The indications for more invasive treatment (endovascular or surgery) in PAD are limb salvage, rest pain, nonhealing ulceration, and tissue necrosis and the need to improve the functional capacity in patients with lifestyle-limiting IC.

Endovascular Interventions. Since Dotter and Judkins first described percutaneous catheter-based angioplasty for the treatment of symptomatic PAD in 1964 (247), peripheral interventional procedures have increased substantially. The annual rate of percutaneous transluminal angioplasty (PTA) for lower-extremity PAD, adjusted for age and sex, was found to have increased from 1 to 24 per 100,000 Maryland residents when data on hospital discharges between 1979 and 1989 were analyzed (248). More recent estimates imply that peripheral interventions have increased even more, from 90,000 in 1994 to more than 200,000 in 1997, making it the fastest-growing area in vascular medicine (249). This growth far exceeds that of coronary procedures and is expected to continue as many vascular diseases that traditionally have required open surgical repair become more amenable to endovascular techniques.

The lower-extremity arterial system has three distinct anatomic territories: aortoiliac (AI), femoropopliteal, and infrapopliteal or crural. Due to differences in structural and anatomic characteristic among these arteries, the indications and outcomes of endovascular procedures differ depending on the segment involved. PTA is optimally offered for short-segment stenosis of large-bore vessels, whereas surgical methods are best applied to multilevel occlusions involving smaller and more distant vessels. More favorable immediate and long-term outcomes are also achieved with lesions that are concentric and noncalcific, particularly in the presence of a good distal run-off, in the absence of postprocedure residual stenosis, and when the indication for the procedure is treatment of IC rather than CLI or ALI.

Iliac Artery Disease. The iliac arteries are most amenable to endovascular therapy and if disease is present, require intervention first. In addition to being of larger caliber, they are readily accessible, and successful PTA (with or without stent placement) achieves several important goals including improved inflow, collateral blood flow amplification, and more durable results (249). Use of PTA techniques has led to an 88% success rate for recanalization of occluded common or external iliac arteries (250,251) with a 5-year cumulative patency rate as high as 66% (252). Even better results have been attained with stents. A meta-analysis of eight angioplasty and six stent series included more than 2,116 patients and showed a higher initial success rate and an overall 42% reduction in failure at 4 years in patients who received iliac stents (253). In a randomized study of 279 patients, provisional stenting (using stents only when translesional gradient pressure was >10 mm Hg) of short (≤5-cm occlusive or ≤10-cm stenotic) lesions of the iliac arteries showed similar short- and long-term outcomes including initial success, procedural complications, patency at 2 years, and the number of reinterventions at 5 years (254). Thus, despite the clinical benefits of iliac stent placement as demonstrated by Bosch and Hunink's meta-analysis (253), many endovascular specialists favor selective stent use for distinctly complex lesions, those with flow-limiting dissections, or when PTA results are unsatisfactory.

The availability, ease, and favorable short- and long-term outcomes of AI endovascular therapy have also made it the preferred option for common or external iliac artery stenosis (up to 10 cm in length), double stenosis (each <5 cm in length) not extending into the common femoral artery, and short unilateral occlusions of the common iliac artery (94). Furthermore, iliac artery PTA (with and without stents) offers an excellent adjunctive procedure that preserves inflow to surgical bypass grafts in patients with coexistent infrainguinal disease. In a study of 70 consecutive patients undergoing femorofemoral bypass grafting, iliac interventions provided adequate inflow for the graft (for >14 years) postprocedure, granting an alternative to aortofemoral bypass surgery (255). Relative contraindications for endovascular therapy of occlusive iliac disease include long occlusions (>5 cm), AI aneurysmal disease, atheroembolic disease, and long-segment, severe diffuse bilateral AI disease (256).

Femoropopliteal Disease. Atherosclerotic involvement of the femoropopliteal system is the most common cause of IC (257). Compared to the iliac system, in which stenosis dominates, occlusions are more common in the femoropopliteal system by a factor of at least three. This system has unique anatomic and physiologic properties; the arteries are smaller, have lower blood flow rates, have higher resistance, and are more susceptible to spasm. Furthermore, the lesions are often very long, and even a mild degree of postintervention intimal hyperplasia or elastic recoil may lead to recurrence of symptoms. Although the distal segment of the superficial femoral artery (SFA) within the adductor (Hunter's) canal is a common site for occlusive PAD, SFA involvement is usually diffuse with several calcific lesions present. These factors, combined with the distinct extrinsic forces exerted on this artery and the effect of both inflow and outflow status on procedural outcome, explain the higher rate of restenosis (>50% to 80% in some reports) after PTA (257). Stent placement does not seem to improve late patency rates due to a higher incidence of in-stent restenosis but increases the initial treatment costs by as much as $3,000 compared to PTA (258). Given these findings, provisional stent utilization, in which stent placement is limited to suboptimal PTA results (residual gradient >15 mm Hg, residual stenosis >30%), flow-limiting dissections, and failure to maintain initial procedural patency, may be preferred.

The roles of several techniques in decreasing restenosis, including use of endovascular brachytherapy, self-expanding nitinol stents, and sirolimus (drug-eluting) stents, have recently been evaluated in the femoropopliteal segment. Despite encouraging initial results (259,260), brachytherapy did not improve patency rates of de novo femoropopliteal interventions but showed promise in recurrent restenosis of lesions previously treated with angioplasty (261). Brachytherapy was also associated with late acute thrombotic occlusions in up to 27% of treated patients (262). Nitinol stents have a 3-year patency rate as high as 76% (263), and in a recent analysis of the clinical and imaging data of 175 patients, their cumulative 24-month patency rates implanted in a nonrandomized setting were 69% compared to 34% with stainless steel self-expanding stents (264). Furthermore, when sirolimus-coated, self-expanding nitinol stents were compared to uncoated stents, a trend toward better late patency rates of SFA stenotic and occlusive lesions was seen in one small randomized trial (265).

Infrapopliteal (Tibioperoneal) Disease. In general, the presence of one patent infrapopliteal artery is sufficient to keep the limb from becoming ischemic. Infrapopliteal PTA has been increasingly applied to patients with CLI and selected patients with severe IC (walking distance <200 meters) and rarely to prevent failure of a proximal revascularization procedure such as femoropopliteal PTA or bypass surgery. Recent studies using different techniques for infrapopliteal PTA, including drug-eluting stents, biodegradable stents, different thrombectomy devices, and cool-laser techniques, have shown encouraging results.

Thrombolysis

Catheter-directed intraarterial thrombolytic therapy is an option for the initial treatment of ALI in select individuals with native artery or bypass graft thrombotic occlusions. In addition to dissolving the occlusive thrombus and restoring blood flow to an acutely ischemic limb, thrombolytic therapy offers other distinctive advantages. It may uncover an underlying hemodynamic cause of vessel or graft occlusion so that definitive therapy can be applied and converts an emergency limb-salvage surgery to an elective one, therefore reducing the perioperative mortality and morbidity associated with immediate surgical intervention. Three major trials have compared thrombolysis to surgery. They are the Rochester trial (266), the Surgery versus Thrombolysis for Ischemia of the Lower Extremity (STILE) trial (267), and the Thrombolysis or Peripheral Arterial Surgery (TOPAS) trial (268). The results of these studies support the recommendation that thrombolytic therapy can be offered to patients with less than 7 days of ischemia presenting at stages I and IIA (viable and marginally threatened limb; see Table 108.3) with ALI (269). Careful patient selection is critical because the presence of contraindications can lead to catastrophic sequelae. In one review of the hemorrhagic complications associated with catheter-directed regional thrombolytic therapy, the incidence of hemorrhagic stroke was 1%, major hemorrhage was 5.1%, and minor hemorrhage was 14.8% (270).

Surgical Procedures

The first synthetic vascular bypass graft was placed in 1952 (271), and surgical treatment of occlusive PAD has become a proven option that is commonly considered for patients with CLI. Less frequently, peripheral surgical revascularization may be offered to a minority of patients with claudication who present with severe disabling symptoms that interfere with daily activities or occupation or significantly impact the individual's quality of life. The two most common surgical options are endarterectomy and bypass grafting. Endarterectomy yields higher success rate if the disease is localized to the proximal territories (AI or, occasionally, the common femoral and profunda arteries), and bypass grafting is generally preferable for distal infrainguinal, infrapopliteal, or diffuse disease. Patients with multilevel disease may benefit from a dual procedure in which endarterectomy of proximal large-bore arteries is combined with a distal vessel bypass. The choice of autogenous graft depends on the level of disease and the availability of a healthy saphenous vein of adequate caliber. Synthetic grafts have excellent long-term patency rates when used for aortofemoral bypass, whereas autogenous vein grafts are preferred for infrainguinal bypass, although above-the-knee prosthetic grafts provide acceptable results (272). The long-term patency for reversed and in situ saphenous vein grafts to the crural vessels is about 70% to 80% at 5 years (273–275). When the greater saphenous vein is not available, the use of alternate veins from the upper or lower extremities provides far superior patency and foot preservation results compared to prosthetic grafts of the infrapopliteal vessels (276). Although the overall long-term patency rate is greater with surgery than endovascular procedures, the nature of the revascularization procedures should be individualized depending on the lesion(s) characteristics and consideration given to risks for perioperative morbidity and mortality.

Noncardiac vascular surgical patients are at high risk (reported risk of cardiac death or nonfatal MI >5%) for serious perioperative complications. In addition to AMI and stroke, complications of wound or graft infection, peripheral embolization, and sexual dysfunction secondary to autonomic nervous system injury are also frequently reported.

The need for preoperative coronary revascularization in the PAD patient population is an area of controversy. Participants in a recent randomized, controlled trial of 510 patients with known, stable CAD scheduled for elective peripheral vascular surgery (33% for abdominal aortic aneurysm repair, 67% for infrainguinal bypass) were randomly assigned to either coronary-artery revascularization (CABG 41% and PCI 59%) or no revascularization before surgery (277). The incidence of postoperative mortality and AMI at 30 days, left ventricular ejection fraction at 3 months, and survival after a median follow-up of 2.7 years were similar in the two groups, suggesting that CABG before elective vascular surgery among patients with stable cardiac symptoms is not indicated. Elective preoperative cardiac catheterization before elective cardiac surgery, however, should be pursued when a preoperative evaluation suggests significant left main- or three-vessel CAD, severe left ventricular dysfunction, or severe aortic stenosis.

Perioperative use of β-blockers and statins has been shown to significantly reduce the risk of cardiovascular events and mortality associated with noncardiac vascular surgery as well as improve graft patency (278–282). In a recent unblended, multicenter study of 112 patients with a positive preoperative stress echocardiogram, the β-blocker bisoprolol, started at least 1 week before surgery, continued for 30 days postoperatively, and titrated to a heart rate of 60 beats per minute or less resulted in a 10-fold reduction in 30-day MI and cardiac mortality (3.4 vs. 34%, $p < .001$) (278). A similarly small study, the multicenter perioperative β-blockade (POBBLE) for patients undergoing infrarenal vascular surgery, compared 50 mg of oral metoprolol twice daily given from admission until 7 days after surgery to placebo (279). Although one third of the study participants suffered from a perioperative cardiovascular event, metoprolol did not reduce the 30-day cardiac events, but it decreased the time from surgery to discharge from a median of 12 days to 10 days.

The benefit of perioperative statin therapy in patients undergoing vascular surgery was also recently reported. In a case–control study of 2,816 patients undergoing vascular surgery, perioperative mortality was significantly reduced in those receiving statin therapy (280), and Durazzo and colleagues reported fewer adverse cardiovascular events in a randomized trial comparing atorvastatin to placebo (281). Despite the small number of reported events in this latter trial (3 cardiac deaths and 22 nonfatal myocardial infarctions), the incidence of major cardiovascular events decreased from 26% in the placebo group to 8% in the atorvastatin group (281). Statins also appear to improve the patency rates of vascular bypass grafts. In a retrospective analysis of 189 autogenous infrainguinal arterial reconstructions performed in 172 consecutive patients (well matched for age, indication, and atherosclerotic risk factors), the risk of graft failure was 3.2-fold greater for the control group despite similar perioperative cholesterol levels (282). In summary, statins should be continued in the perioperative period, and unless contraindicated, β-blockers should be considered for all PAD patients, especially those undergoing surgery (191).

CONCLUSIONS

PAD is a prevalent systemic atherosclerotic disease with an associated high morbidity and mortality rate. Symptomatic PAD also significantly impairs an individual's quality of life. Unfortunately, it remains underdiagnosed and undertreated. PAD can be easily detected by an ABI that is less than 0.9. This is also an independent indicator of systemic atherosclerosis and a predictor of mortality. Risk factor modification and secondary prevention are the keys to management. Aggressive management should include a supervised walking exercise program, treatment of hypertension with a target blood pressure less than 130/85 mm Hg, a lowering of the cholesterol level to an LDL less than 100, blood sugar control, smoking cessation, and the addition of an antiplatelet agent. For PAD patients, the goal is to improve symptoms and quality of life. Endovascular intervention or surgical treatment is indicated to improve blood supply and maintain limb viability in ALI or CLI and in selected patients with symptomatic PAD whose quality of life is impaired despite optimal medical treatment.

CONTROVERSIES AND PERSONAL PERSPECTIVES

The cornerstone of treatment for the majority of patients with IC continues to include a supervised walking exercise program, aggressive risk factor modification, and pharmacologic therapies. Most physicians advise more aggressive treatment only if there is evidence for ALI, CLI, or lifestyle-limiting IC. Unfortunately, some patients are unable or are unwilling to participate in walking exercise programs, and many insurers, including Medicare, do not cover the cost. In addition, the modest benefits from medications like cilostazol are often limited by their side effects.

Traditional practice approaches for IC are now being questioned based on the limitations of current treatment options, and controversy exists on whether recent advances in endovascular interventions warrant lowering the threshold for extending these procedures to more patients. Many would argue that conservative strategies date to an era when the only alternative treatment for IC was surgery, which carried a potential for significant morbidity and mortality. Although it is also possible that many physicians caring for PAD patients are not aware of recent technological advances in the endovascular field, part of the reluctance to pursue more aggressive treatment may be related to previously reported low risks of worsening IC or loss of limb (1% to 2% over 5 years) and the perception that endovascular procedures are costly and may impose significant additional risks for the patient.

In addition, despite good outcomes, two studies have found no added benefits of PTA over exercise training (283,284). Perkins et al. compared PTA to exercise training in 56 patients with unilateral IC and found greater maximum walking distance in the exercise-trained group (283), and Whyman et al. reported no significant difference in walking performance in 62 patients with femoral artery stenosis who were randomized to PTA or conventional medical treatment and followed over a 2-year period (284).

Large prospective, randomized studies comparing improvement in leg symptoms after modern endovascular therapy are lacking. There is also a lack of studies evaluating the quality of life (QOL) and functional benefits in patients undergoing this treatment approach. Recently Murphy et al. looked at QOL using the Medical Outcomes Short Form 36 (SF 36) and Walking Impairment Questionnaire in 35 individuals with AI disease treated with balloon-expandable or self-expanding stents. Patients improved their exercise performance (walking distance by an average of 264%) and just as importantly their health-related quality of life after revascularization (285).

Most agree that endovascular therapy offers attractive alternatives to the traditional approach to IC. It is not yet known, however, whether PTA and/or stent placement will alter QOL and functional issues compared to conservative therapy and whether this approach should be routinely employed for the IC patient. This controversy will likely continue until randomized clinical trials are completed.

Angiogenesis may develop into another controversial area in the treatment of PAD. There are several different classes of drugs undergoing clinical trials including: vascular endothelial growth factor (VEGF), fibroblast growth factor-2 (FGF-2), and hypoxia-inducible factor-1 (HIF-1) (286–288).

Comerota et al. treated patients with CLI using FGF and found a modest increase in the ABI and evidence of partial or complete ulcer healing (286), whereas two larger PAD trials, the Regional Angiogenesis with Vascular Endothelial growth factor (RAVE) trial and the Therapeutic Angiogenesis with Recombinant Fibroblast Growth Factor-2 for Intermittent Claudication (TRAFFIC) trial, have demonstrated mixed results (287,288).

The RAVE trial used adenoviral VEGF gene transfer in 105 individuals with unilateral IC. No improved exercise performance or improved QOL was reported, whereas the TRAFFIC trial studied recombinant FGF-2 versus placebo in 180 patients with moderate to severe IC. An increase in peak walking times was reported.

Overall, the results of angiogenesis have been disappointing, although, there has been little evidence for clinically significant toxicity, and more trials are planned.

THE FUTURE

Further advances are expected in the endovascular field, but controversy over its use continues. It is hoped that the CLEVER trial (Claudication: Exercise Versus Endoluminal Revascularization) (not yet ready for enrollment) may help to solve part of this issue. The objectives of this National Institute of Health–sponsored trial are to optimize physical functioning, increase activity levels, and reduce cardiovascular disease in older individuals with PAD. CLEVER will look at maximum walking duration (MWD), comparing AI stenting and pharmacotherapy versus exercise rehabilitation and pharmacotherapy to usual care pharmacotherapy over a 6- month time frame. It will also look at free-living daily activity levels, patient-perceived quality of life, and cost-effectiveness over 18 months as well as demographic and biochemical risk factors for atherosclerosis.

Several new ongoing trials are in progress using angiogenesis. One of these, the WALK Study, is currently enrolling patients with severe IC from the United States and abroad. It is a phase 2, randomized, double-blind, placebo-controlled, parallel-group, multicenter, dose-selective trial using the gene transfer agent Ad2/HIF-1α/VP16. It is believed that upregulation of HIF-1 signaling in targeted tissues may result in more durable and robust blood vessel growth.

References

1. Criqui MH, Fronek A, Barrett-Connor E, et al. The prevalence of peripheral arterial disease in a defined population. *Circulation* 1985;71:510–515.

2. Fowkes FG. Epidemiology of atherosclerotic arterial disease in the lower limbs. *Eur J Vasc Surg* 1988;2:283–291.
3. McDaniel MD, Cronenwett JL. Basic data related to the natural history of intermittent claudication. *Ann Vasc Surg* 1989;3:273–277.
4. McDermott MM, Greenland P, Liu K, et al. Leg symptoms in peripheral arterial disease: associated clinical characteristics and functional impairment. *JAMA* 2001;286:1599–1606.
5. Selvin E, Erlinger TP. Prevalence of and risk factors for peripheral arterial disease in the United States: results from the national health and nutrition examination survey, 1999–2000. *Circulation* 2004;110:738–743.
6. Zheng ZJ, Sharrett AR, Chambless LE, et al. Associations of ankle–brachial index with clinical coronary heart disease, stroke and preclinical carotid and popliteal atherosclerosis: the Atherosclerosis Risk in Communities (ARIC) study. *Atherosclerosis* 1997;131:115–125.
7. Newman AB, Shemanski L, Manolio TA, et al. Ankle–arm index as a predictor of cardiovascular disease and mortality in the cardiovascular health study. The Cardiovascular Health Study Group. *Arterioscler Thromb Vasc Biol* 1999;19:538–545.
8. Hirsch AT, Criqui MH, Treat-Jacobson D, et al. Peripheral arterial disease detection, awareness, and treatment in primary care. *JAMA* 2001;286: 1317–1324.
9. Hiatt WR, Hoag S, Hamman RF. Effect of diagnostic criteria on the prevalence of peripheral arterial disease. The San Luis Valley Diabetes Study. *Circulation* 1995;91:1472–1479.
10. Aronow WS. Prevalence of atherothrombotic brain infarction, coronary artery disease and peripheral arterial disease in elderly blacks, Hispanics and whites. *Am J Cardiol* 1992;70:1212–1213.
11. Collins TC, Petersen NJ, Suarez-Almazor M, et al. The prevalence of peripheral arterial disease in a racially diverse population. *Arch Intern Med.* 2003;163:1469–1474.
12. Newman AB, Siscovick DS, Manolio TA, et al. Ankle–arm index as a marker of atherosclerosis in the cardiovascular health study. Cardiovascular Heart Study (CHS) collaborative research group. *Circulation* 1993;88: 837–845.
13. Criqui MH, Denenberg JO, Langer RD, et al. The epidemiology of peripheral arterial disease: importance of identifying the population at risk. *Vasc Med* 1997;2:221–226.
14. Kannel WB, McGee DL. Update on some epidemiologic features of intermittent claudication: the Framingham Study. *J Am Geriatr Soc* 1985;33:13–18.
15. Gardner AW, Poehlman ET. Exercise rehabilitation programs for the treatment of claudication pain. A meta-analysis. *JAMA* 1995;274:975–980.
16. Vogt MT, Wolfson SK, Kuller LH. Lower extremity arterial disease and the aging process: a review. *J Clin Epidemiol* 1992;45:529–542.
17. McDermott MM, Mehta S, Ahn H, et al. Atherosclerotic risk factors are less intensively treated in patients with peripheral arterial disease than in patients with coronary artery disease. *J Gen Intern Med* 1997;12:209–215.
18. Criqui MH, Langer RD, Fronek A, et al. Mortality over a period of 10 years in patients with peripheral arterial disease. *N Engl J Med* 1992;326:381–386.
19. Belch JJ, Topol EJ, Agnelli G, et al. Critical issues in peripheral arterial disease detection and management: a call to action. *Arch Intern Med* 2003; 163:884–892.
20. Durham JD, Darcy MD, McClenny TE. The next step in peripheral arterial disease public awareness. *J Vasc Interv Radiol* 2004;15:667–668.
21. Hirsch AT, Gloviczki P, Drooz A, et al. Mandate for creation of a national peripheral arterial disease public awareness program: an opportunity to improve cardiovascular health. *J Vasc Surg* 2004;39:474–481.
22. Faxon DP, Creager MA, Smith Jr SC, et al. Atherosclerotic Vascular Disease Conference: Executive summary: Atherosclerotic Vascular Disease Conference Proceeding for Healthcare Professionals from a special writing group of the American Heart Association. *Circulation* 2004;109:2595–2604.
23. Topper JN, Cai J, Falb D, et al. Identification of vascular endothelial genes differentially responsive to fluid mechanical stimuli: cyclooxygenase-2, manganese superoxide dismutase, and endothelial cell nitric oxide synthase are selectively up-regulated by steady laminar shear stress. *Proc Natl Acad Sci USA* 1996;93:10417–10422.
24. Libby P, Ridker PM, Maseri A. Inflammation and atherosclerosis. *Circulation* 2002;105:1135–1143.
25. Ross R. Atherosclerosis—an inflammatory disease. *N Engl J Med* 1999; 340:115–126.
26. Faxon DP, Fuster V, Libby P, et al. Atherosclerotic Vascular Disease Conference: Writing Group III: pathophysiology. *Circulation* 2004;109:2617–2625.
27. Brass EP, Hiatt WR. Acquired skeletal muscle metabolic myopathy in atherosclerotic peripheral arterial disease. *Vasc Med* 2000;5:55–59.
28. Hiatt WR, Nawaz D, Regensteiner JG, et al. The evaluation of exercise performance in patients with peripheral vascular disease. *J Cardiopulmon Rehab* 1988;8:525–532.
29. Murabito JM, D'Agostino RB, Silbershatz H, et al. Intermittent claudication. A risk profile from the Framingham Heart Study. *Circulation* 1997; 96:44–49.
30. Vogt MT, Cauley JA, Newman AB, et al. Decreased ankle/arm blood pressure index and mortality in elderly women. *JAMA* 1993;270:465–469.
31. Newman AB, Sutton-Tyrrell K, Rutan GH, et al. Lower extremity arterial disease in elderly subjects with systolic hypertension. *J Clin Epidemiol* 1991;44:15–20.
32. Kannel WB, Shurtleff D. The Framingham Study. Cigarettes and the development of intermittent claudication. *Geriatrics* 1973;28:61–68.
33. Powell JT, Edwards RJ, Worrell PC, et al. Risk factors associated with the development of peripheral arterial disease in smokers: A case–control study. *Atherosclerosis* 1997;129:41–48.
34. Cole CW, Hill GB, Farzad E, et al. Cigarette smoking and peripheral arterial occlusive disease. *Surgery* 1993;114:753–756; discussion, 756–757.
35. Price JF, Mowbray PI, Lee AJ, et al. Relationship between smoking and cardiovascular risk factors in the development of peripheral arterial disease and coronary artery disease: Edinburgh Artery Study. *Eur Heart J* 1999;20: 344–353.
36. Kannel WB, Shurtleff D. The Framingham Study. Cigarettes and the development of intermittent claudication. *Geriatrics* 1973;28:61–68.
37. Lu JT, Creager MA. The relationship of cigarette smoking to peripheral arterial disease. *Rev Cardiovasc Med* 2004;5:189–193.
38. Cole CW, Hill GB, Farzad E, et al. Cigarette smoking and peripheral arterial occlusive disease. *Surgery* 1993;114:753–756; discussion 756–757.
39. Hirsch AT, Treat-Jacobson D, Lando HA, et al. The role of tobacco cessation, antiplatelet and lipid-lowering therapies in the treatment of peripheral arterial disease. *Vasc Med* 1997;2:243–251.
40. Jonason T, Bergstrom R. Cessation of smoking in patients with intermittent claudication. Effects on the risk of peripheral vascular complications, myocardial infarction and mortality. *Acta Med Scand* 1987;221:253–260.
41. Quick CR, Cotton LT. The measured effect of stopping smoking on intermittent claudication. *Br J Surg* 1982;69(Suppl):S24–S26.
42. Stewart CP. The influence of smoking on the level of lower limb amputation. *Prosthet Orthot Int* 1987;11:113–116.
43. Jonason T, Ringqvist I. Changes in peripheral blood pressures after five years of follow-up in non-operated patients with intermittent claudication. *Acta Med Scand* 1986;220:127–132.
44. Reunanen A, Takkunen H, Aromaa A. Prevalence of intermittent claudication and its effect on mortality. *Acta Med Scand* 1982;211:249–256.
45. Fowkes FG, Housley E, Riemersma RA, et al. Smoking, lipids, glucose intolerance, and blood pressure as risk factors for peripheral atherosclerosis compared with ischemic heart disease in the Edinburgh Artery Study. *Am J Epidemiol* 1992;135:331–340.
46. Centers for Disease Control and Prevention (CDC). Diabetes-related amputations of lower extremities in the Medicare population—Minnesota, 1993–1995. *MMWR Morb Mortal Wkly Rep* 1998;47:649–652.
47. Kannel WB, McGee DL. Update on some epidemiologic features of intermittent claudication: the Framingham Study. *J Am Geriatr Soc* 1985;33:13–18.
48. Abbott RD, Brand FN, Kannel WB. Epidemiology of some peripheral arterial findings in diabetic men and women: experiences from the Framingham Study. *Am J Med* 1990;88:376–381.
49. Uusitupa MI, Niskanen LK, Siitonen O, et al. Five-year incidence of atherosclerotic vascular disease in relation to general risk factors, insulin level, and abnormalities in lipoprotein composition in non–insulin-dependent diabetic and nondiabetic subjects. *Circulation* 1990;82:27–36.
50. Beks PJ, Mackaay AJ, de Neeling JN, et al. Peripheral arterial disease in relation to glycaemic level in an elderly Caucasian population: the Hoorn Study. *Diabetologia* 1995;38:86–96.
51. Muntner P, Wildman RP, Reynolds K, et al. Relationship between HbA1c level and peripheral arterial disease. *Diabetes Care* 2005;28:1981–1987.
52. Selvin E, Marinopoulos S, Berkenblit G, et al. Meta-analysis: Glycosylated hemoglobin and cardiovascular disease in diabetes mellitus. *Ann Intern Med* 2004;141:421–431.
53. Beach KW, Strandness Jr DE. Arteriosclerosis obliterans and associated risk factors in insulin-dependent and non–insulin-dependent diabetes. *Diabetes* 1980;29:882–888.
54. Johansson J, Egberg N, Johnsson H, et al. Serum lipoproteins and hemostatic function in intermittent claudication. *Arterioscler Thromb* 1993;13: 1441–1448.
55. Ogren M, Hedblad B, Jungquist G, et al. Low ankle–brachial pressure index in 68-year-old men: Prevalence, risk factors and prognosis. Results from prospective population study "men born in 1914", Malmo, Sweden. *Eur J Vasc Surg* 1993;7:500–506.
56. Sofi F, Lari B, Rogolino A, et al. Thrombophilic risk factors for symptomatic peripheral arterial disease. *J Vasc Surg* 2005;41:255–260.
57. Makin A, Lip GY, Silverman S, et al. Peripheral vascular disease and hypertension: a forgotten association? *J Hum Hypertens* 2001;15:447–454.
58. Olin JW. Hypertension and peripheral arterial disease. *Vasc Med* 2005;10: 241–246.
59. Ridker PM, Stampfer MJ, Rifai N. Novel risk factors for systemic atherosclerosis: A comparison of C-reactive protein, fibrinogen, homocysteine, lipoprotein(a), and standard cholesterol screening as predictors of peripheral arterial disease. *JAMA* 2001;285:2481–2485.
60. Smith FB, Lee AJ, Hau CM, et al. Plasma fibrinogen, haemostatic factors and prediction of peripheral arterial disease in the Edinburgh Artery Study. *Blood Coagul Fibrinolysis* 2000;11:43–50.
61. Dormandy JA, Hoare E, Khattab AH, et al. Prognostic significance of rheological and biochemical findings in patients with intermittent claudication. *Br Med J* 1973;4:581–583.
62. Lee AJ, Lowe GD, Woodward M, et al. Fibrinogen in relation to personal history of prevalent hypertension, diabetes, stroke, intermittent claudication, coronary heart disease, and family history: the Scottish Heart Health Study. *Br Heart J* 1993;69:338–342.

63. Lowe GD, Fowkes FG, Dawes J, et al. Blood viscosity, fibrinogen, and activation of coagulation and leukocytes in peripheral arterial disease and the normal population in the Edinburgh Artery Study. *Circulation* 1993;87: 1915–1920.
64. Fowkes FG. Fibrinogen and peripheral arterial disease. *Eur Heart J* 1995; 16(Suppl A):36–40; discussion, 40–41.
65. Lee AJ, Fowkes FG, Lowe GD, et al. Fibrinogen, factor VII and PAI-1 genotypes and the risk of coronary and peripheral atherosclerosis: Edinburgh Artery Study. *Thromb Haemost* 1999;81:553–560.
66. Meade TW, Imeson J, Stirling Y. Effects of changes in smoking and other characteristics on clotting factors and the risk of ischaemic heart disease. *Lancet* 1987;2:986–988.
67. Wilkes HC, Kelleher C, Meade TW. Smoking and plasma fibrinogen. *Lancet* 1988;1:307–308.
68. Welch GN, Loscalzo J. Homocysteine and atherothrombosis. *N Engl J Med* 1998;338:1042–1050.
69. Boushey CJ, Beresford SA, Omenn GS, et al. A quantitative assessment of plasma homocysteine as a risk factor for vascular disease. Probable benefits of increasing folic acid intakes. *JAMA* 1995;274:1049–1057.
70. Molgaard J, Malinow MR, Lassvik C, et al. Hyperhomocyst(e)inaemia: an independent risk factor for intermittent claudication. *J Intern Med* 1992; 231:273–279.
71. Aronow WS, Ahn C. Association between plasma homocysteine and peripheral arterial disease in older persons. *Coron Artery Dis* 1998;9: 49–50.
72. Taylor Jr LM, DeFrang RD, Harris Jr EJ, et al. The association of elevated plasma homocyst(e)ine with progression of symptomatic peripheral arterial disease. *J Vasc Surg* 1991;13:128–136.
73. Currie IC, Wilson YG, Scott J, et al. Homocysteine: an independent risk factor for the failure of vascular intervention. *Br J Surg* 1996;83:1238–1241.
74. O'Hare AM, Vittinghoff E, Hsia J, et al. Renal insufficiency and the risk of lower extremity peripheral arterial disease: results from the Heart and Estrogen/Progestin Replacement Study (HERS). *J Am Soc Nephrol* 2004;15: 1046–1051.
75. O'Hare AM, Glidden DV, Fox CS, et al. High prevalence of peripheral arterial disease in persons with renal insufficiency: results from the National Health and Nutrition Examination Survey 1999–2000. *Circulation* 2004;109:320–323.
76. O'Hare AM, Bertenthal D, Shlipak MG, et al. Impact of renal insufficiency on mortality in advanced lower extremity peripheral arterial disease. *J Am Soc Nephrol* 2005;16:514–519.
77. National Institute of Diabetes and Digestive and Kidney Diseases, Division of Kidney Urologic and Hematologic Diseases. Patient characteristics. In: *United States Renal Data System, USRDS 2000 annual data report.* Bethesda, MD: National Institutes of Health, National Institute of Diabetes and Digestive and Kidney Diseases, Division of Kidney, Urologic, and Hematologic Diseases; 2000:339–348.
78. O'Hare AM, Rodriguez RA, Bacchetti P. Low ankle–brachial index associated with rise in creatinine level over time: results from the Atherosclerosis Risk in Communities study. *Arch Intern Med* 2005;165:1481–1485.
79. Valentine RJ, Verstraete R, Clagett GP, et al. Premature cardiovascular disease is common in relatives of patients with premature peripheral atherosclerosis. *Arch Intern Med* 2000;160:1343–1348.
80. Puisieux F, de Groote P, Masy E, et al. Association between anticardiolipin antibodies and mortality in patients with peripheral arterial disease. *Am J Med* 2000;109:635–641.
81. McDermott MM, Green D, Greenland P, et al. Relation of levels of hemostatic factors and inflammatory markers to the ankle brachial index. *Am J Cardiol* 2003;92:194–199.
82. McDermott MM, Greenland P, Green D, et al. D-dimer, inflammatory markers, and lower extremity functioning in patients with and without peripheral arterial disease. *Circulation* 2003;107:3191–3198.
83. McDermott MM, Greenland P, Guralnik JM, et al. Inflammatory markers, D-dimer, pro-thrombotic factors, and physical activity levels in patients with peripheral arterial disease. *Vasc Med* 2004;9:107–115.
84. McDermott MM, Guralnik JM, Greenland P, et al. Inflammatory and thrombotic blood markers and walking-related disability in men and women with and without peripheral arterial disease. *J Am Geriatr Soc* 2004;52:1888–1894.
85. McDermott MM, Ferrucci L, Liu K, et al. D-dimer and inflammatory markers as predictors of functional decline in men and women with and without peripheral arterial disease. *J Am Geriatr Soc* 2005;53:1688–1696.
86. Charcot JMC. Sur la claudication intermittente observée dans un cas d'obliteration complete de l'une des arteres iliaques primitives. *C R Soc Biol (Paris)* 1858;5:225–228.
87. Condorelli M, Brevetti G. Intermittent claudication: an historical perspective. *European Heart J Suppl* 2002;4:B2–B7.
88. Rose GA. The diagnosis of ischaemic heart pain and intermittent claudication in field surveys. *Bull World Health Org* 1962;27:645–658.
89. Novo S. Classification, epidemiology, risk factors, and natural history of peripheral arterial disease. *Diabetes Obes Metab* 2002;4(Suppl 2):S1–S6.
90. Stoffers HE, Rinkens PE, Kester AD, et al. The prevalence of asymptomatic and unrecognized peripheral arterial occlusive disease. *Int J Epidemiol* 1996;25:282–290.
91. McDermott MM, Kerwin DR, Liu K, et al. Prevalence and significance of unrecognized lower extremity peripheral arterial disease in general medicine practice. *J Gen Intern Med.* 2001;16:384–390.
92. Barzilay JI, Spiekerman CF, Kuller LH, et al. Prevalence of clinical and isolated subclinical cardiovascular disease in older adults with glucose disorders: the Cardiovascular Health Study. *Diabetes Care* 2001;24:1233–1239.
93. Criqui MH, Fronek A, Klauber MR, et al. The sensitivity, specificity, and predictive value of traditional clinical evaluation of peripheral arterial disease: results from noninvasive testing in a defined population. *Circulation* 1985;71:516–522.
94. Dormandy JA, Rutherford RB. Management of peripheral arterial disease (PAD). TASC working group. TransAtlantic Inter-Society Concensus (TASC). *J Vasc Surg* 2000;31:S1–S296.
95. Fowkes FGR. Epidemiology of occult atherosclerosis in the lower limbs. In: Salmasi A, Nicolaides AN, eds. *Occult atherosclerotic disease: diagnosis, assessment and management.* Boston: Kluwer, 1991:185–204.
96. Regensteiner JG, Steiner JF, Panzer RJ, et al. Evaluation of walking impairment by questionnaire in patients with peripheral arterial disease. *J Vasc Med Biol* 1990;2:142–152.
97. Montgomery PS, Gardner AW. The clinical utility of a six-minute walk test in peripheral arterial occlusive disease patients. *J Am Geriatr Soc* 1998; 46:706–711.
98. Boyd AM. The natural course of arteriosclerosis of the lower extremities. *Proc R Soc Med* 1962;55:591–593.
99. Imparato AM, Kim GE, Davidson T, et al. Intermittent claudication: its natural course. *Surgery* 1975;78:795–799.
100. McAllister FF. The fate of patients with intermittent claudication managed nonoperatively. *Am J Surg* 1976;132:593–595.
101. Weitz JI, Byrne J, Clagett GP, et al. Diagnosis and treatment of chronic arterial insufficiency of the lower extremities: a critical review. *Circulation* 1996;94:3026–3049.
102. Doobay AV, Anand SS. Sensitivity and specificity of the ankle–brachial index to predict future cardiovascular outcomes: a systematic review. *Arterioscler Thromb Vasc Biol* 2005;25:1463–1469.
103. Smith Jr SC, Greenland P, Grundy SM. AHA Conference Proceedings. Prevention Conference V: Beyond secondary prevention: identifying the high-risk patient for primary prevention: executive summary. American Heart Association. *Circulation* 2000;101:111–116.
104. Hooi JD, Stoffers HE, Kester AD, et al. Risk factors and cardiovascular diseases associated with asymptomatic peripheral arterial occlusive disease. The Limburg PAOD Study. Peripheral arterial occlusive disease. *Scand J Prim Health Care* 1998;16:177–182.
105. Leng GC, Lee AJ, Fowkes FG, et al. Incidence, natural history and cardiovascular events in symptomatic and asymptomatic peripheral arterial disease in the general population. *Int J Epidemiol* 1996;25:1172–1181.
106. Yao ST, Hobbs JT, Irvine WT. Ankle systolic pressure measurements in arterial disease affecting the lower extremities. *Br J Surg* 1969;56:676–679.
107. Ouriel K, McDonnell AE, Metz CE, et al. Critical evaluation of stress testing in the diagnosis of peripheral vascular disease. *Surgery* 1982;91:686–693.
108. Rofsky NM, Adelman MA. MR angiography in the evaluation of atherosclerotic peripheral vascular disease. *Radiology* 2000;214:325–338.
109. Ouwendijk R, de Vries M, Pattynama PM, et al. Imaging peripheral arterial disease: a randomized controlled trial comparing contrast-enhanced MR angiography and multi-detector row CT angiography. *Radiology* 2005;236: 1094–1103.
110. Olin JW. Thromboangiitis obliterans (Buerger's disease). *N Engl J Med* 2000;343:864–869.
111. Olin JW, Young JR, Graor RA, et al. The changing clinical spectrum of thromboangiitis obliterans (Buerger's disease). *Circulation* 1990;82:IV3–IV8.
112. Vos LD, Tielbeek AV, Vroegindeweij D, et al. Cystic adventitial disease of the popliteal artery demonstrated with intravascular US. *J Vasc Interv Radiol* 1996;7:583–586.
113. Slovut DP, Olin JW. Fibromuscular dysplasia. *N Engl J Med* 2004;350: 1862–1871.
114. Abraham P, Bouye P, Quere I, et al. Past, present and future of arterial endofibrosis in athletes: A point of view. *Sports Med* 2004;34:419–425.
115. Aronow WS, Ahn C. Prevalence of coexistence of coronary artery disease, peripheral arterial disease, and atherothrombotic brain infarction in men and women > or = 62 years of age. *Am J Cardiol* 1994;74:64–65.
116. Ness J, Aronow WS. Prevalence of coexistence of coronary artery disease, ischemic stroke, and peripheral arterial disease in older persons, mean age 80 years, in an academic hospital–based geriatrics practice. *J Am Geriatr Soc* 1999;47:1255–1256.
117. Sukhija R, Yalamanchili K, Aronow WS. Prevalence of left main coronary artery disease, of three or four-vessel coronary artery disease, and of obstructive coronary artery disease in patients with and without peripheral arterial disease undergoing coronary angiography for suspected coronary artery disease. *Am J Cardiol* 2003;92:304–305.
118. Hertzer NR, Beven EG, Young JR, et al. Coronary artery disease in peripheral vascular patients. A classification of 1000 coronary angiograms and results of surgical management. *Ann Surg* 1984;199:223–233.
119. Eagle KA, Rihal CS, Foster ED, et al. Long-term survival in patients with coronary artery disease: importance of peripheral vascular disease. The Coronary Artery Surgery Study (CASS) investigators. *J Am Coll Cardiol* 1994;23:1091–1095.

120. Krumholz HM, Chen J, Chen YT, et al. Predicting one-year mortality among elderly survivors of hospitalization for an acute myocardial infarction: results from the Cooperative Cardiovascular Project. *J Am Coll Cardiol* 2001;38:453–459.
121. Cupples LA, Gagnon DR, Wong ND, et al. Preexisting cardiovascular conditions and long-term prognosis after initial myocardial infarction: the Framingham Study. *Am Heart J* 1993;125:863–872.
122. Fournier JA, Cabezon S, Cayuela A, et al. Long-term prognosis of patients having acute myocardial infarction when </=40 years of age. *Am J Cardiol* 2004;94:989–992.
123. Narins CR, Zareba W, Moss AJ, et al. Relationship between intermittent claudication, inflammation, thrombosis, and recurrent cardiac events among survivors of myocardial infarction. *Arch Intern Med* 2004;164:440–446.
124. Magovern JA, Sakert T, Magovern GJ, et al. A model that predicts morbidity and mortality after coronary artery bypass graft surgery. *J Am Coll Cardiol* 1996;28:1147–1153.
125. Birkmeyer JD, Quinton HB, O'Connor NJ, et al. The effect of peripheral vascular disease on long-term mortality after coronary artery bypass surgery. Northern New England Cardiovascular Disease Study Group. *Arch Surg* 1996;131:316–321.
126. Birkmeyer JD, O'Connor GT, Quinton HB, et al. The effect of peripheral vascular disease on in-hospital mortality rates with coronary artery bypass surgery. Northern New England Cardiovascular Disease Study Group. *J Vasc Surg* 1995;21:445–452.
127. Rihal CS, Sutton-Tyrrell K, Guo P, et al. Increased incidence of periprocedural complications among patients with peripheral vascular disease undergoing myocardial revascularization in the bypass angioplasty revascularization investigation. *Circulation.* 1999;100:171–177.
128. Chiu JH, Topol EJ, Whitlow PL, et al. Peripheral vascular disease and one-year mortality following percutaneous coronary revascularization. *Am J Cardiol* 2003;92:582–583.
129. O'Rourke DJ, Quinton HB, Piper W, et al. Survival in patients with peripheral vascular disease after percutaneous coronary intervention and coronary artery bypass graft surgery. *Ann Thorac Surg* 2004;78:466–470; discussion, 470.
130. Nikolsky E, Mehran R, Mintz GS, et al. Impact of symptomatic peripheral arterial disease on one-year mortality in patients undergoing percutaneous coronary interventions. *J Endovasc Ther* 2004;11:60–70.
131. Nikolsky E, Mehran R, Dangas GD, et al. Prognostic significance of cerebrovascular and peripheral arterial disease in patients having percutaneous coronary interventions. *Am J Cardiol* 2004;93:1536–1539.
132. Newman AB, Shemanski L, Manolio TA, et al. Ankle–arm index as a predictor of cardiovascular disease and mortality in the cardiovascular health study. The Cardiovascular Health Study Group. *Arterioscler Thromb Vasc Biol* 1999;19:538–545.
133. CAPRIE Steering Committee. A randomised, blinded, trial of clopidogrel versus aspirin in patients at risk of ischaemic events (CAPRIE). *Lancet* 1996;348:1329–1339.
134. Belch JJ, Creager MA. A focus on risk factor management. *Vasc Med* 2004;9:169–170.
135. Cassar K, Belch JJ, Brittenden J. Are national cardiac guidelines being applied by vascular surgeons? *Eur J Vasc Endovasc Surg* 2003;26:623–628.
136. Hackam DG. Cardiovascular risk prevention in peripheral artery disease. *J Vasc Surg* 2005;41:1070–1073.
137. Henke PK, Blackburn S, Proctor MC, et al. Patients undergoing infrainguinal bypass to treat atherosclerotic vascular disease are under-prescribed cardioprotective medications: effect on graft patency, limb salvage, and mortality. *J Vasc Surg* 2004;39:357–365.
138. Ness J, Aronow WS, Newkirk E, et al. Prevalence of symptomatic peripheral arterial disease, modifiable risk factors, and appropriate use of drugs in the treatment of peripheral arterial disease in older persons seen in a university general medicine clinic. *J Gerontol A Biol Sci Med Sci* 2005;60:255–257.
139. DeBakey ME, Crawford ES, Garrett HE, et al. Occlusive disease of the lower extremities in patients 16 to 37 years of age. *Ann Surg* 1964;159:873–890.
140. Nunn DB. Symptomatic peripheral arteriosclerosis of patients under age 40. *Am Surg* 1973;39:224–228.
141. Miani S, Mingazzini P, Biasi GM, et al. Occlusive arterial disease in young patients. *J Cardiovasc Surg (Torino)* 1984;25:353–356.
142. McCready RA, Vincent AE, Schwartz RW, et al. Atherosclerosis in the young: a virulent disease. *Surgery* 1984;96:863–869.
143. Sise MJ, Shackford SR, Rowley WR, et al. Claudication in young adults: a frequently delayed diagnosis. *J Vasc Surg* 1989;10:68–74.
144. Valentine RJ, MacGillivray DC, DeNobile JW, et al. Intermittent claudication caused by atherosclerosis in patients aged forty years and younger. *Surgery* 1990;107:560–565.
145. Valentine RJ. Premature peripheral atherosclerosis. *Cardiovasc Surg* 1993; 1:473–480.
146. Levy PJ, Hornung CA, Haynes JL, et al. Lower extremity ischemia in adults younger than forty years of age: A community-wide survey of premature atherosclerotic arterial disease. *J Vasc Surg* 1994;19:873–881.
147. Valentine RJ, Jackson MR, Modrall JG, et al. The progressive nature of peripheral arterial disease in young adults: a prospective analysis of white men referred to a vascular surgery service. *J Vasc Surg* 1999;30:436–444.
148. Valentine RJ, Hansen ME, Myers SI, et al. The influence of sex and aortic size on late patency after aortofemoral revascularization in young adults. *J Vasc Surg* 1995;21:296–305; discussion, 305–306.
149. Harris LM, Peer R, Curl GR, et al. Long-term follow-up of patients with early atherosclerosis. *J Vasc Surg* 1996;23:576–580; discussion, 581.
150. Valentine RJ, Myers SI, Inman MH, et al. Late outcome of amputees with premature atherosclerosis. *Surgery* 1996;119:487–493.
151. Powell JT, Edwards RJ, Worrell PC, et al. Risk factors associated with the development of peripheral arterial disease in smokers: A case–control study. *Atherosclerosis* 1997;129:41–48.
152. Dormandy J, Heeck L, Vig S. The fate of patients with critical leg ischemia. *Semin Vasc Surg* 1999;12:142–147.
153. Ingolfsson IO, Sigurdsson G, Sigvaldason H, et al. A marked decline in the prevalence and incidence of intermittent claudication in Icelandic men 1968–1986: A strong relationship to smoking and serum cholesterol—the Reykjavik Study. *J Clin Epidemiol* 1994;47:1237–1243.
154. Dagenais GR, Maurice S, Robitaille NM, et al. Intermittent claudication in Quebec men from 1974–1986: the Quebec Cardiovascular Study. *Clin Invest Med* 1991;14:93–100.
155. McGrath MA, Graham AR, Hill DA, et al. The natural history of chronic leg ischemia. *World J Surg* 1983;7:314–318.
156. Leng GC, Papacosta O, Whincup P, et al. Femoral atherosclerosis in an older British population: prevalence and risk factors. *Atherosclerosis* 2000;152:167–174.
157. Hobbs SD, Bradbury AW. Smoking cessation strategies in patients with peripheral arterial disease: an evidence-based approach. *Eur J Vasc Endovasc Surg* 2003;26:341–347.
158. Willigendael EM, Teijink JA, Bartelink ML, et al. Smoking and the patency of lower extremity bypass grafts: A meta-analysis. *J Vasc Surg* 2005;42:67–74.
159. Faulkner KW, House AK, Castleden WM. The effect of cessation of smoking on the accumulative survival rates of patients with symptomatic peripheral vascular disease. *Med J Aust* 1983;1:217–219.
160. Hobbs SD, Bradbury AW. Smoking cessation strategies in patients with peripheral arterial disease: an evidence-based approach. *Eur J Vasc Endovasc Surg* 2003;26:341–347.
161. Hobbs SD, Wilmink AB, Adam DJ, et al. Assessment of smoking status in patients with peripheral arterial disease. *J Vasc Surg* 2005;41:451–456.
162. Willigendael EM, Teijink JA, Bartelink ML, et al. Influence of smoking on incidence and prevalence of peripheral arterial disease. *J Vasc Surg* 2004;40:1158–1165.
163. Moxham J. Nicotine addiction. *BMJ* 2000;320:391–392.
164. Anderson JE, Jorenby DE, Scott WJ, et al. Treating tobacco use and dependence: an evidence-based clinical practice guideline for tobacco cessation. *Chest* 2002;121:932–941.
165. Beach KW, Brunzell JD, Strandness Jr DE. Prevalence of severe arteriosclerosis obliterans in patients with diabetes mellitus. Relation to smoking and form of therapy. *Arteriosclerosis* 1982;2:275–280.
166. Kannel WB, McGee DL. Diabetes and glucose tolerance as risk factors for cardiovascular disease: the Framingham Study. *Diabetes Care* 1979;2:120–126.
167. Lundberg V, Stegmayr B, Asplund K, et al. Diabetes as a risk factor for myocardial infarction: population and gender perspectives. *J Intern Med* 1997;241:485–492.
168. Lotufo PA, Gaziano JM, Chae CU, et al. Diabetes and all-cause and coronary heart disease mortality among US male physicians. *Arch Intern Med* 2001;161:242–247.
169. Liao Y, Cooper RS, Ghali JK, et al. Sex differences in the impact of coexistent diabetes on survival in patients with coronary heart disease. *Diabetes Care* 1993;16:708–713.
170. Hu FB, Stampfer MJ, Solomon CG, et al. The impact of diabetes mellitus on mortality from all causes and coronary heart disease in women: 20 years of follow-up. *Arch Intern Med* 2001;161:1717–1723.
171. Miettinen H, Lehto S, Salomaa V, et al. Impact of diabetes on mortality after the first myocardial infarction. The FINMONICA Myocardial Infarction Register Study Group. *Diabetes Care* 1998;21:69–75.
172. Sobel BE, Schneider DJ. Cardiovascular complications in diabetes mellitus. *Curr Opin Pharmacol* 2005;5:143–148.
173. Jude EB, Oyibo SO, Chalmers N, et al. Peripheral arterial disease in diabetic and nondiabetic patients: a comparison of severity and outcome. *Diabetes Care* 2001;24:1433–1437.
174. Da Silva A, Widmer LK, Ziegler HW, et al. The Basle Longitudinal Study: report on the relation of initial glucose level to baseline ECG abnormalities, peripheral artery disease, and subsequent mortality. *J Chronic Dis* 1979;32:797–803.
175. Strandness Jr DE, Priest RE, Gibbons GE. Combined clinical and pathological study of diabetic and nondiabetic peripheral arterial disease. *Diabetes* 1964;13:366–372.
176. King TA, DePalma RG, Rhodes RS. Diabetes mellitus and atherosclerotic involvement of the profunda femoris artery. *Surg Gynecol Obstet* 1984;159:553–556.
177. Kreines K, Johnson E, Albrink M, et al. The course of peripheral vascular disease in non–insulin-dependent diabetes. *Diabetes Care* 1985;8:235–243.
178. Niskanen L, Siitonen O, Suhonen M, et al. Medial artery calcification predicts cardiovascular mortality in patients with NIDDM. *Diabetes Care* 1994;17:1252–1256.
179. Adler AI, Stevens RJ, Neil A, et al. UKPDS 59: hyperglycemia and other potentially modifiable risk factors for peripheral vascular disease in type 2 diabetes. *Diabetes Care* 2002;25:894–899.

180. UK Prospective Diabetes Study (UKPDS) Group. Intensive blood-glucose control with sulphonylureas or insulin compared with conventional treatment and risk of complications in patients with type 2 diabetes (UKPDS 33). *Lancet* 1998;352:837–853.
181. The effect of intensive treatment of diabetes on the development and progression of long-term complications in insulin-dependent diabetes mellitus. The Diabetes Control and Complications Trial Research Group. *N Engl J Med* 1993;329:977–986.
182. American Diabetes Association. Peripheral arterial disease in people with diabetes. *Diabetes Care* 2003;26:3333–3341.
183. Almdal T, Scharling H, Jensen JS, et al. The independent effect of type 2 diabetes mellitus on ischemic heart disease, stroke, and death: A population-based study of 13,000 men and women with 20 years of follow-up. *Arch Intern Med* 2004;164:1422–1426.
184. Lim HS, Blann AD, Lip GY. Soluble CD40 ligand, soluble P-selectin, interleukin-6, and tissue factor in diabetes mellitus: relationships to cardiovascular disease and risk factor intervention. *Circulation* 2004;109:2524–2528.
185. Vinik AI, Erbas T, Park TS, et al. Platelet dysfunction in type 2 diabetes. *Diabetes Care* 2001;24:1476–1485.
186. Gaede P, Vedel P, Larsen N, et al. Multifactorial intervention and cardiovascular disease in patients with type 2 diabetes. *N Engl J Med* 2003;348:383–393.
187. Randomised trial of cholesterol lowering in 4444 patients with coronary heart disease: the Scandinavian Simvastatin Survival Study (4S). *Lancet* 1994;344:1383–1389.
188. Sacks FM, Pfeffer MA, Moye LA, et al. The effect of pravastatin on coronary events after myocardial infarction in patients with average cholesterol levels. Cholesterol and Recurrent Events Trial investigators. *N Engl J Med* 1996;335:1001–1009.
189. National Cholesterol Education Program (NCEP) Expert Panel on Detection, Evaluation, and Treatment of High Blood Cholesterol in Adults (Adult Treatment Panel III). Third report of the National Cholesterol Education Program (NCEP) Expert Panel on Detection, Evaluation, and Treatment of High Blood Cholesterol in Adults (Treatment Panel III) final report. *Circulation* 2002;106:3143–3421.
190. Grundy SM, Cleeman JI, Merz CN, et al. Implications of recent clinical trials for the National Cholesterol Education Program Adult Treatment Panel III guidelines. *Circulation* 2004;110:227–239.
191. Heart Protection Study Collaborative Group. MRC/BHF Heart Protection Study of cholesterol lowering with simvastatin in 20,536 high-risk individuals: a randomised placebo-controlled trial. *Lancet* 2002;360:7–22.
192. Pedersen TR, Kjekshus J, Pyorala K, et al. Effect of simvastatin on ischemic signs and symptoms in the Scandinavian Simvastatin Survival Study (4S). *Am J Cardiol* 1998;81:333–335.
193. McDermott MM, Guralnik JM, Greenland P, et al. Statin use and leg functioning in patients with and without lower-extremity peripheral arterial disease. *Circulation* 2003;107:757–761.
194. Mondillo S, Ballo P, Barbati R, et al. Effects of simvastatin on walking performance and symptoms of intermittent claudication in hypercholesterolemic patients with peripheral vascular disease. *Am J Med* 2003;114:359–364.
195. Mohler 3rd ER, Hiatt WR, Creager MA. Cholesterol reduction with atorvastatin improves walking distance in patients with peripheral arterial disease. *Circulation* 2003;108:1481–1486.
196. Regensteiner JG, Ware Jr JE, McCarthy WJ, et al. Effect of cilostazol on treadmill walking, community-based walking ability, and health-related quality of life in patients with intermittent claudication due to peripheral arterial disease: meta-analysis of six randomized controlled trials. *J Am Geriatr Soc* 2002;50:1939–1946.
197. Kinlay S, Plutzky J. Effect of lipid-lowering therapy on vasomotion and endothelial function. *Curr Cardiol Rep* 1999;1:238–243.
198. Vasa M, Fichtlscherer S, Adler K, et al. Increase in circulating endothelial progenitor cells by statin therapy in patients with stable coronary artery disease. *Circulation* 2001;103:2885–2890.
199. Lewington S, Clarke R, Qizilbash N, et al. Age-specific relevance of usual blood pressure to vascular mortality: a meta-analysis of individual data for one million adults in 61 prospective studies. *Lancet* 2002;360:1903–1913.
200. Collins R, Peto R, MacMahon S, et al. Blood pressure, stroke, and coronary heart disease. Part 2. Short-term reductions in blood pressure: overview of randomised drug trials in their epidemiological context. *Lancet* 1990;335:827–838.
201. Chobanian AV, Bakris GL, Black HR, et al. The seventh report of the Joint National Committee on Prevention, Detection, Evaluation, and Treatment of High Blood Pressure: the JNC 7 report. *JAMA* 2003;289:2560–2572.
202. Schweizer J, Kaulen R, Nierade A, et al. Beta-blockers and nitrates in patients with peripheral arterial occlusive disease: Long-term findings. *Vasa* 1997;26:43–46.
203. Frohlich ED, Tarazi RC, Dustan HP. Peripheral arterial insufficiency. A complication of beta-adrenergic blocking therapy. *JAMA* 1969;208:2471–2472.
204. Solomon SA, Ramsay LE, Yeo WW, et al. Beta blockade and intermittent claudication: placebo controlled trial of atenolol and nifedipine and their combination. *BMJ* 1991;303:1100–1104.
205. Radack K, Deck C. Beta-adrenergic blocker therapy does not worsen intermittent claudication in subjects with peripheral arterial disease. A meta-analysis of randomized controlled trials. *Arch Intern Med* 1991;151:1769–1776.
206. Aronow WS, Ahn C. Effect of beta blockers on incidence of new coronary events in older persons with prior myocardial infarction and symptomatic peripheral arterial disease. *Am J Cardiol* 2001;87:1284–1286.
207. Yusuf S, Sleight P, Pogue J, et al. Effects of an angiotensin-converting-enzyme inhibitor, ramipril, on cardiovascular events in high-risk patients. The Heart Outcomes Prevention Evaluation Study investigators. *N Engl J Med* 2000;342:145–153.
208. Ostergren J, Sleight P, Dagenais G, et al. Impact of ramipril in patients with evidence of clinical or subclinical peripheral arterial disease. *Eur Heart J* 2004;25:17–24.
209. Hackam DG. Cardiovascular risk prevention in peripheral artery disease. *J Vasc Surg* 2005;41:1070–1073.
210. Breckenridge A, Roberts D, Walley T. Different vasodilating mechanisms—different peripheral effects? *J Cardiovasc Pharmacol* 1992;19(Suppl 1): S23–S26.
211. Libretti A, Catalano M. Captopril in the treatment of hypertension associated with claudication. *Postgrad Med J* 1986;62(Suppl 1):34–37.
212. Catalano M, Libretti A. Captopril for the treatment of patients with hypertension and peripheral vascular disease. *Angiology* 1985;36:293–296.
213. Mehler PS, Coll JR, Estacio R, et al. Intensive blood pressure control reduces the risk of cardiovascular events in patients with peripheral arterial disease and type 2 diabetes. *Circulation* 2003;107:753–756.
214. Graham IM, Daly LE, Refsum HM, et al. Plasma homocysteine as a risk factor for vascular disease. The European Concerted Action Project. *JAMA* 1997;277:1775–1781.
215. Stein JH, Rosenson RS. Lipoprotein lp(a) excess and coronary heart disease. *Arch Intern Med* 1997;157:1170–1176.
216. Thomas TR, Ziogas G, Harris WS. Influence of fitness status on very-low-density lipoprotein subfractions and lipoprotein(a) in men and women. *Metabolism* 1997;46:1178–1183.
217. Temme EH, Mensink RP, Hornstra G. Comparison of the effects of diets enriched in lauric, palmitic, or oleic acids on serum lipids and lipoproteins in healthy women and men. *Am J Clin Nutr* 1996;63:897–903.
218. Gurakar A, Hoeg JM, Kostner G, et al. Levels of lipoprotein lp(a) decline with neomycin and niacin treatment. *Atherosclerosis* 1985;57:293–301.
219. Antithrombotic Trialists' Collaboration. Collaborative meta-analysis of randomised trials of antiplatelet therapy for prevention of death, myocardial infarction, and stroke in high risk patients. *BMJ* 2002;324: 71–86.
220. Antiplatelet Trialists' Collaboration. Collaborative overview of randomised trials of antiplatelet therapy—I: Prevention of death, myocardial infarction, and stroke by prolonged antiplatelet therapy in various categories of patients. *BMJ* 1994;308:81–106.
221. Dorffler-Melly J, Koopman MM, Adam DJ, et al. Antiplatelet agents for preventing thrombosis after peripheral arterial bypass surgery. *Cochrane Database Syst Rev* 2003;(3):CD000535.
222. Bhatt DL, Topol EJ. Clopidogrel for High Atherothrombotic Risk and Ischemic Stabilization, Management, and Avoidance Executive Committee. Clopidogrel added to aspirin versus aspirin alone in secondary prevention and high-risk primary prevention: rationale and design of the Clopidogrel for High Atherothrombotic Risk and Ischemic Stabilization, Management, and Avoidance (CHARISMA) trial. *Am Heart J* 2004;148:263–268.
223. Balsano F, Coccheri S, Libretti A, et al. Ticlopidine in the treatment of intermittent claudication: A 21-month double-blind trial. *J Lab Clin Med* 1989;114:84–91.
224. Becquemin JP. Effect of ticlopidine on the long-term patency of saphenous-vein bypass grafts in the legs. Etude de la Ticlopidine apres Pontage Femoro-Poplite and the Association Universitaire de Recherche en Chirurgie. *N Engl J Med* 1997;337:1726–1731.
225. Castelli P, Basellini A, Agus GB, et al. Thrombosis prevention with ticlopidine after femoropopliteal thromboendarterectomy. *Int Surg* 1986;71: 252–255.
226. Bergqvist D, Almgren B, Dickinson JP. Reduction of requirement for leg vascular surgery during long-term treatment of claudicant patients with ticlopidine: Results from the Swedish Ticlopidine Multicentre Study (STIMS). *Eur J Vasc Endovasc Surg* 1995;10:69–76.
227. Boissel JP, Peyrieux JC, Destors JM. Is it possible to reduce the risk of cardiovascular events in subjects suffering from intermittent claudication of the lower limbs? *Thromb Haemost* 1989;62:681–685.
228. Janzon L, Bergqvist D, Boberg J, et al. Prevention of myocardial infarction and stroke in patients with intermittent claudication; effects of ticlopidine. Results from STIMS, the Swedish Ticlopidine Multicentre Study. *J Intern Med* 1990;227:301–308.
229. Quinn MJ, Fitzgerald DJ. Ticlopidine and clopidogrel. *Circulation* 1999; 100:1667–1672.
230. Kohda N, Tani T, Nakayama S, et al. Effect of cilostazol, a phosphodiesterase III inhibitor, on experimental thrombosis in the porcine carotid artery. *Thromb Res* 1999;96:261–268.
231. Igawa T, Tani T, Chijiwa T, et al. Potentiation of anti-platelet aggregating activity of cilostazol with vascular endothelial cells. *Thromb Res* 1990;57: 617–623.
232. Tsuchikane E, Fukuhara A, Kobayashi T, et al. Impact of cilostazol on restenosis after percutaneous coronary balloon angioplasty. *Circulation* 1999;100:21–26.

233. Dawson DL, Cutler BS, Hiatt WR, et al. A comparison of cilostazol and pentoxifylline for treating intermittent claudication. *Am J Med* 2000;109:523–530.
234. Packer M, Carver JR, Rodeheffer RJ, et al. Effect of oral milrinone on mortality in severe chronic heart failure. The PROMISE study research group. *N Engl J Med* 1991;325:1468–1475.
235. Cohn JN, Goldstein SO, Greenberg BH, et al. A dose-dependent increase in mortality with vesnarinone among patients with severe heart failure. Vesnarinone Trial Investigators. *N Engl J Med* 1998;339:1810–1816.
236. Girolami B, Bernardi E, Prins MH, et al. Treatment of intermittent claudication with physical training, smoking cessation, pentoxifylline, or nafronyl: A meta-analysis. *Arch Intern Med* 1999;159:337–345.
237. Hood SC, Moher D, Barber GG. Management of intermittent claudication with pentoxifylline: meta-analysis of randomized controlled trials. *CMAJ* 1996;155:1053–1059.
238. Larsen OA, Lassen NA. Effect of daily muscular exercise in patients with intermittent claudication. *Lancet* 1966;2:1093–1096.
239. Creager MA. Medical management of peripheral arterial disease. *Cardiol Rev* 2001;9:238–245.
240. Stewart KJ, Hiatt WR, Regensteiner JG, et al. Exercise training for claudication. *N Engl J Med* 2002;347:1941–1951.
241. Regensteiner JG. Exercise rehabilitation for the patient with intermittent claudication: a highly effective yet underutilized treatment. *Curr Drug Targets Cardiovasc Haematol Disord* 2004;4:233–239.
242. Leng GC, Fowler B, Ernst E. Exercise for intermittent claudication. *Cochrane Database Syst Rev* 2000;(2):CD000990.
243. Stewart KJ, Hiatt WR, Regensteiner JG, et al. Exercise training for claudication. *N Engl J Med* 2002;347:1941–1951.
244. Lundgren F, Dahllof AG, Lundholm K, et al. Intermittent claudication—surgical reconstruction or physical training? A prospective randomized trial of treatment efficiency. *Ann Surg* 1989;209:346–355.
245. Regensteiner JG, Steiner JF, Hiatt WR. Exercise training improves functional status in patients with peripheral arterial disease. *J Vasc Surg* 1996;23:104–115.
246. Izquierdo-Porrera AM, Gardner AW, Powell CC, et al. Effects of exercise rehabilitation on cardiovascular risk factors in older patients with peripheral arterial occlusive disease. *J Vasc Surg* 2000;31:670–677.
247. Dotter CT, Judkins MP. Transluminal treatment of arteriosclerotic obstruction. Description of a new technique and a preliminary report of its application. *Circulation* 1964;30:654–670.
248. Tunis SR, Bass EB, Steinberg EP. The use of angioplasty, bypass surgery, and amputation in the management of peripheral vascular disease. *N Engl J Med* 1991;325:556–562.
249. Krajcer Z, Howell MH. Update on endovascular treatment of peripheral vascular disease: new tools, techniques, and indications. *Tex Heart Inst J* 2000;27:369–385.
250. Ring EJ, Freiman DB, McLean GK, et al. Percutaneous recanalization of common iliac artery occlusions: an unacceptable complication rate? *AJR Am J Roentgenol* 1982;139:587–589.
251. Colapinto RF, Stronell RD, Johnston WK. Transluminal angioplasty of complete iliac obstructions. *AJR Am J Roentgenol.* 1986;146:859–862.
252. Schurmann K, Mahnken A, Meyer J, et al. Long-term results 10 years after iliac arterial stent placement. *Radiology* 2002;224:731–738.
253. Bosch JL, Hunink MG. Meta-analysis of the results of percutaneous transluminal angioplasty and stent placement for aortoiliac occlusive disease. *Radiology* 1997;204:87–96.
254. Klein WM, van der Graaf Y, Seegers J, et al. Long-term cardiovascular morbidity, mortality, and reintervention after endovascular treatment in patients with iliac artery disease: the Dutch Iliac Stent Trial Study. *Radiology.* 2004;232:491–498.
255. Perler BA, Williams GM. Does donor iliac artery percutaneous transluminal angioplasty or stent placement influence the results of femorofemoral bypass? Analysis of 70 consecutive cases with long-term follow-up. *J Vasc Surg* 1996;24:363–369; discussion, 369–370.
256. White CJ. Non-surgical treatment of patients with peripheral vascular disease. *Br Med Bull* 2001;59:173–192.
257. Martin EC. Transcatheter therapies in peripheral and noncoronary vascular disease. Introduction. *Circulation* 1991;83:I1–I5.
258. Greenberg D, Rosenfield K, Garcia LA, et al. In-hospital costs of self-expanding nitinol stent implantation versus balloon angioplasty in the femoropopliteal artery (the VascuCoil Trial). *J Vasc Interv Radiol* 2004;15:1065–1069.
259. Wolfram RM, Pokrajac B, Ahmadi R, et al. Endovascular brachytherapy for prophylaxis against restenosis after long-segment femoropopliteal placement of stents: initial results. *Radiology* 2001;220:724–729.
260. Minar E, Pokrajac B, Maca T, et al. Endovascular brachytherapy for prophylaxis of restenosis after femoropopliteal angioplasty: results of a prospective randomized study. *Circulation* 2000;102:2694–2699.
261. Wolfram RM, Budinsky AC, Pokrajac B, et al. Endovascular brachytherapy: restenosis in de novo versus recurrent lesions of femoropopliteal artery—the Vienna experience. *Radiology* 2005;236:338–342.
262. Bonvini R, Baumgartner I, Do DD, et al. Late acute thrombotic occlusion after endovascular brachytherapy and stenting of femoropopliteal arteries. *J Am Coll Cardiol* 2003;41:409–412.
263. Lugmayr HF, Holzer H, Kastner M, et al. Treatment of complex arteriosclerotic lesions with nitinol stents in the superficial femoral and popliteal arteries: A midterm follow-up. *Radiology* 2002;222:37–43.
264. Sabeti S, Schillinger M, Amighi J, et al. Primary patency of femoropopliteal arteries treated with nitinol versus stainless steel self-expanding stents: Propensity score-adjusted analysis. *Radiology* 2004;232:516–521.
265. Duda SH, Pusich B, Richter G, et al. Sirolimus-eluting stents for the treatment of obstructive superficial femoral artery disease: Six-month results. *Circulation* 2002;106:1505–1509.
266. Ouriel K, Shortell CK, DeWeese JA, et al. A comparison of thrombolytic therapy with operative revascularization in the initial treatment of acute peripheral arterial ischemia. *J Vasc Surg* 1994;19:1021–1030.
267. Results of a prospective randomized trial evaluating surgery versus thrombolysis for ischemia of the lower extremity. The STILE Trial. *Ann Surg* 1994;220:251–266; discussion, 266–268.
268. Ouriel K, Veith FJ, Sasahara AA. A comparison of recombinant urokinase with vascular surgery as initial treatment for acute arterial occlusion of the legs. Thrombolysis or Peripheral Arterial Surgery (TOPAS) investigators. *N Engl J Med* 1998;338:1105–1111.
269. Working Party on Thrombolysis in the Management of Limb Ischemia. Thrombolysis in the management of lower limb peripheral arterial occlusion—a consensus document. *Am J Cardiol* 1998;81:207–218.
270. Berridge DC, Makin GS, Hopkinson BR. Local low dose intra-arterial thrombolytic therapy: the risk of stroke or major haemorrhage. *Br J Surg* 1989;76:1230–1233.
271. Voorhees Jr AB, Jaretzki 3rd A, Blakemore AH. The use of tubes constructed from vinyon "N" cloth in bridging arterial defects. *Ann Surg* 1952; 135:332–336.
272. Veith FJ, Gupta SK, Ascer E, et al. Six-year prospective multicenter randomized comparison of autologous saphenous vein and expanded polytetrafluoroethylene grafts in infrainguinal arterial reconstructions. *J Vasc Surg* 1986;3:104–114.
273. Taylor Jr LM, Edwards JM, Porter JM. Present status of reversed vein bypass grafting: Five-year results of a modern series. *J Vasc Surg* 1990;11:193–205; discussion, 205–206.
274. Belkin M, Knox J, Donaldson MC, et al. Infrainguinal arterial reconstruction with nonreversed greater saphenous vein. *J Vasc Surg* 1996;24:957–962.
275. Ouriel K. Peripheral arterial disease. *Lancet* 2001;358:1257–1264.
276. Albers M, Romiti M, Brochado-Neto FC, et al. Meta-analysis of alternate autologous vein bypass grafts to infrapopliteal arteries. *J Vasc Surg* 2005;42:449–455.
277. McFalls EO, Ward HB, Moritz TE, et al. Coronary-artery revascularization before elective major vascular surgery. *N Engl J Med* 2004;351:2795–2804.
278. Poldermans D, Boersma E, Bax JJ, et al. The effect of bisoprolol on perioperative mortality and myocardial infarction in high-risk patients undergoing vascular surgery. Dutch Echocardiographic Cardiac Risk Evaluation Applying Stress Echocardiography Study Group. *N Engl J Med* 1999;341:1789–1794.
279. Brady AR, Gibbs JS, Greenhalgh RM, et al. Perioperative beta-blockade (POBBLE) for patients undergoing infrarenal vascular surgery: results of a randomized double-blind controlled trial. *J Vasc Surg* 2005;41: 602–609.
280. Poldermans D, Bax JJ, Kertai MD, et al. Statins are associated with a reduced incidence of perioperative mortality in patients undergoing major noncardiac vascular surgery. *Circulation* 2003;107:1848–1851.
281. Durazzo AE, Machado FS, Ikeoka DT, et al. Reduction in cardiovascular events after vascular surgery with atorvastatin: a randomized trial. *J Vasc Surg* 2004;39:967–975; discussion, 975–976.
282. Abbruzzese TA, Havens J, Belkin M, et al. Statin therapy is associated with improved patency of autogenous infrainguinal bypass grafts. *J Vasc Surg* 2004;39:1178–1185.
283. Perkins JM, Collin J, Creasy TS, et al. Exercise training versus angioplasty for stable claudication. Long and medium term results of a prospective, randomised trial. *Eur J Vasc Endovasc Surg* 1996;11:409–413.
284. Whyman MR, Fowkes FG, Kerracher EM, et al. Randomised controlled trial of percutaneous transluminal angioplasty for intermittent claudication. *Eur J Vasc Endovasc Surg* 1996;12:167–172.
285. Murphy TP, Soares GM, Kim HM, et al. Quality of life and exercise performance after aortoiliac stent placement for claudication. *J Vasc Interv Radiol* 2005;16:947–953; quiz, 954.
286. Comerota AJ, Throm RC, Miller KA, et al. Naked plasmid DNA encoding fibroblast growth factor type 1 for the treatment of end-stage unreconstructible lower extremity ischemia: preliminary results of a phase I trial. *J Vasc Surg* 2002;35:930–936.
287. Rajagopalan S, Mohler 3rd ER, Lederman RJ, et al. Regional angiogenesis with vascular endothelial growth factor in peripheral arterial disease: A phase II randomized, double-blind, controlled study of adenoviral delivery of vascular endothelial growth factor 121 in patients with disabling intermittent claudication. *Circulation* 2003;108:1933–1938.
288. Lederman RJ, Mendelsohn FO, Anderson RD, et al. Therapeutic angiogenesis with recombinant fibroblast growth factor-2 for intermittent claudication (the TRAFFIC study): a randomised trial. *Lancet* 2002;359:2053–2058.

CHAPTER 109 ■ RENAL ARTERY DISEASE

JEFFREY W. OLIN AND SUSAN M. BEGELMAN

OVERVIEW

Renal artery stenosis (RAS) is most commonly due to either fibromuscular dysplasia or atherosclerosis. The former predominates in young women, whereas the latter is almost exclusively seen in individuals older than the age of 55 years. Frequently, RAS is discovered incidentally during imaging studies for other reasons (atrophic or small kidney) or at autopsy. Incidental RAS is quite common (1,2), whereas renovascular hypertension only occurs in 1% to 5% of all patients with hypertension (3). The predominant clinical manifestation of fibromuscular dysplasia is hypertension. The hypertension can frequently be cured or significantly improved with percutaneous balloon angioplasty. The predominant clinical manifestations of atherosclerotic RAS include hypertension, renal failure (ischemic nephropathy), and recurrent episodes of congestive heart failure and flash pulmonary edema (4,5).

The presence of anatomic RAS does not necessarily establish that the hypertension or renal failure is caused by the RAS. Many patients have essential (primary) hypertension for years and then develop atherosclerotic RAS later in life. In patients with long-standing hypertension, it is unlikely that a cure of the hypertension can be achieved with surgical or percutaneous intervention. However, 50% to 80% of patients do experience improvement in blood pressure control (6–12). Ischemic nephropathy or flash pulmonary edema only occurs in the presence of bilateral renal artery disease or disease to a solitary functioning kidney. Percutaneous or surgical revascularization can lead to improvement or stabilization in renal function and improvement in heart failure if the patients are carefully selected (9,13–15).

Screening tests for RAS have improved considerably over the last decade. Whereas captopril renography was used almost exclusively in the past, direct imaging with duplex ultrasound, magnetic resonance angiography, or multidetector computed tomography (CT) angiography has replaced other modalities as the screening test of choice in most centers. Rarely does an arteriogram have to be performed for diagnostic purposes only.

Management of RAS consists of three strategies: medical management, surgical revascularization or percutaneous therapy with balloon angioplasty, and stent implantation. The treatment of choice for controlling hypertension in patients with fibromuscular disease is percutaneous angioplasty. Renal artery stenting has replaced surgical revascularization for virtually all patients with atherosclerotic disease who require a revascularization procedure.

HISTORICAL PERSPECTIVE

In 1934, Goldblatt and colleagues (16) demonstrated that hypertension could be produced in dogs by constriction of one renal artery (two-kidney, one-clip model) or both renal arteries or one renal artery if the contralateral kidney was removed (one-kidney, one-clip model). Irving Page later demonstrated that renin produced a pressor substance, which he initially called angiotonin and later named angiotensin, which was subsequently isolated by Skeggs in 1954 (17,18).

PATHOPHYSIOLOGY

Experimental Models of Renovascular Hypertension

Pickering clarified the difference between renovascular hypertension and renal artery stenosis:

> The demonstration of a RAS in a hypertensive patient does not necessarily establish a diagnosis of renovascular hypertension, because essential hypertension may accelerate the development of atheromatous plaques, which do not necessarily have any functional significance. Ideally, it is necessary to demonstrate that there is also renal ischemia, since this is thought to be the stimulus that raises the blood pressure, and leads to a decline of renal function (19).

Most investigators believe that there must be at least a 70% reduction in luminal diameter for a RAS to cause either hypertension or ischemic nephropathy (4,20,21).

Animal models for renovascular hypertension have helped to elucidate the pathophysiology of hypertension in patients with RAS (22–25). The renin–angiotensin–aldosterone system plays an important role, as shown in Figure 109.1 (26). In animals, the two-kidney, one-clip (2K-1C) model is the classic model for renin-mediated hypertension and is analogous to unilateral RAS in humans. The one-kidney, one-clip (1K-1C) model of renovascular hypertension is a model for volume-mediated hypertension and is analogous to bilateral RAS or RAS to a solitary functioning kidney in humans. Although the acute phases of both of these models are similar, different events occur in the chronic phase.

In the 2K-1C model (unilateral RAS), decreased renal blood flow stimulates the production of renin (Fig. 109.1A). Renin cleaves the proenzyme angiotensinogen to form angiotensin I and in the presence of angiotensin-converting enzyme is converted to angiotensin II. Angiotensin II has several important functions: (a) It elevates blood pressure directly by causing systemic vasoconstriction, (b) it stimulates aldosterone secretion, causing sodium reabsorption and potassium and hydrogen ion secretion in the cortical collecting duct, and (c) it changes the intrarenal hemodynamics, such as diminishing glomerular filtration, by decreasing glomerular capillary surface area and redistributing intrarenal blood flow. The salt and water retained (caused by excess aldosterone production) is rapidly excreted by the contralateral (normal) kidney by pressure natruresis. This produces a cycle of renin-dependent hypertension (23,27).

Administration of an angiotensin-converting-enzyme inhibitor (ACEI) blocks this cycle and, at least early in the course of renovascular hypertension, returns the blood pressure to normal. In the chronic phase the blood pressure remains elevated even though the plasma renin activity returns to baseline. When an ACEI or angiotensin-receptor blocker (ARB) is administered, the blood pressure does not immediately decline, but takes 5 to 7 days (28) to return to normal. The delayed blood pressure response suggests that the change in blood pressure is no longer primarily caused by the direct effects of angiotensin II, but involves some degree of salt retention as well.

In the 1K-1C model of renovascular hypertension, there is a similar decrease in blood flow to the affected kidney(s), acutely causing the secretion of renin and synthesis of angiotensin II and aldosterone (Fig. 109.1B) (26). Angiotensin II directly elevates blood pressure, and aldosterone causes salt and water retention. In this model there is not a normal kidney that can *sense* the elevated blood pressure, and therefore pressure natruresis does not occur. The increased aldosterone causes sodium and water retention and volume expansion. The expanded plasma volume suppresses plasma renin activity, thus converting the animal from renin-mediated hypertension to volume-mediated hypertension (29). During this stage, administration of an ACEI or ARB does not decrease blood pressure or change renal blood flow (30). Dietary restriction of sodium or administration of diuretics will return the subject to a renin-mediated form of hypertension and restore sensitivity to an ACEI or ARB. Functional renal insufficiency may occur in humans when ACEIs are administered to patients with bilateral RAS or RAS to a solitary kidney especially in the volume-contracted state (Fig. 109.2).

An important clinical concept is that long-standing hypertension may cause changes in intrarenal hemodynamics and structural changes in the microvasculature of the kidney leading to nephrosclerosis (30). Thus, if a patient with

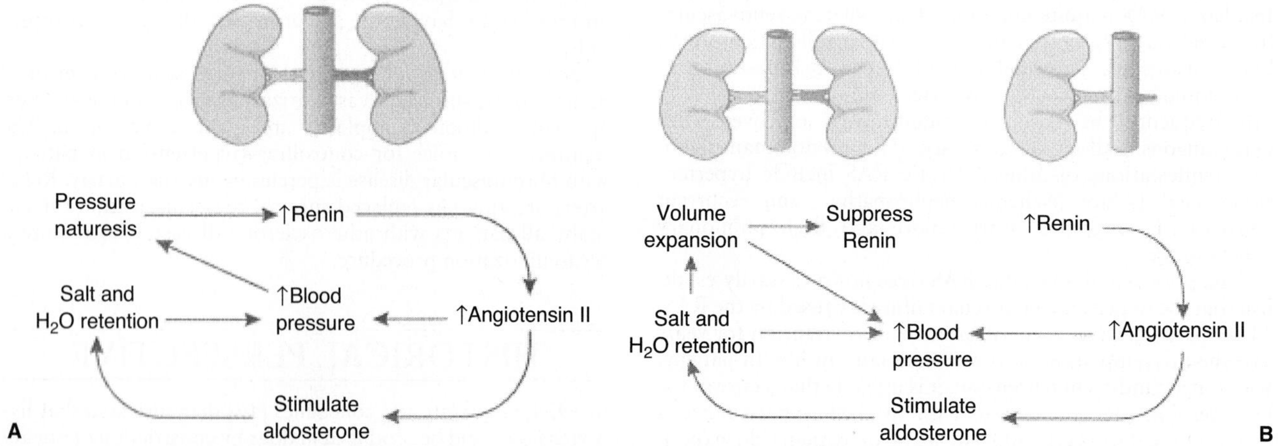

FIGURE 109.1. Pathogenesis of renovascular hypertension in (**A**) unilateral renal artery stenosis (two-kidney, one-clip) and (**B**) bilateral renal artery stenosis or renal artery stenosis to a solitary kidney (one-kidney, one-clip). (From Olin JW, Novick AC. Renovascular disease. In: Young JR, Olin JW, Bartholomew JR, eds. *Peripheral vascular diseases,* 2nd ed. St. Louis, MO: Mosby, 1996:321-342.)

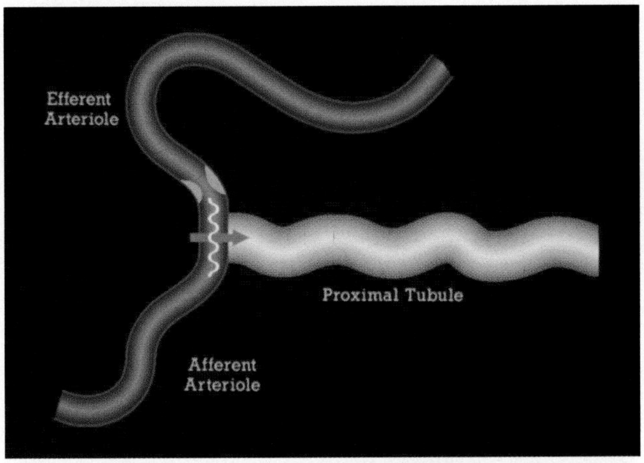

FIGURE 109.2. Patients with high-grade bilateral renal artery stenosis or renal artery stenosis to a solitary kidney may be highly dependent on the efferent arteriolar constriction caused by angiotensin II in preserving transglomerular capillary hydraulic pressure (*arrow*) and glomerular filtration rate. When an angiotensin-converting-enzyme inhibitor is given, the efferent arteriole dilates, transglomerular capillary hydraulic pressure is not maintained, and blood is shunted from the afferent arteriole to the efferent arteriole bypassing glomerular filtration.

nephrosclerosis later develops unilateral RAS, he or she may behave like a patient with bilateral disease because the contralateral kidney would no longer be able to excrete a salt load normally.

Pathophysiology of Ischemic Nephropathy

Patients who develop azotemia while receiving angiotensin-converting-enzyme inhibitors or angiotensin II–receptor blocking agents often have bilateral RAS, RAS to a solitary kidney, or decompensated congestive heart failure in the sodium-depleted state (13,21,31–34).

There are two mechanisms by which renal functional impairment may occur with the use of antihypertensive agents. The first may occur with any antihypertensive agent when a critical perfusion pressure is reached below which the kidney no longer receives adequate perfusion. This has been shown by the infusion of sodium nitroprusside in patients with high-grade bilateral RAS. When the critical perfusion pressure was reached, the urine output, renal blood flow, and glomerular filtration rate declined, and they returned to normal when the blood pressure increased above this critical perfusion pressure (35). The exact pressure necessary to perfuse a kidney with RAS varies with the degree of stenosis and is different among different patients.

The second mechanism is confined to patients receiving ACEI or ARB agents and may occur despite no significant change in blood pressure (32). Patients with severe bilateral RAS or RAS to a solitary kidney may be highly dependent on angiotensin II for glomerular filtration. This is particularly common in patients who receive a combination of ACE inhibitor and diuretic (36) or in patients who are placed on a sodium-restricted diet (37). Under these circumstances, the constrictive effect of angiotensin II on the efferent arteriole allows for the maintenance of normal transglomerular capillary hydraulic pressure, thus allowing glomerular filtration to remain normal in the presence of markedly diminished blood flow (Fig. 109.2). In this instance glomerular filtration is highly dependent on angiotensin II. When an ACEI is administered, the efferent arteriolar tone is no longer maintained and glomerular filtration is therefore decreased. A similar situation occurs in patients with decompensated congestive heart failure who are sodium depleted (34,37).

Pathology of Renovascular Disease

Shanley suggested that loss of renal mass, loss of nephrons, and renal atrophy predominate in the pathologic picture of patients with renovascular disease (38). There is a point at which many of these changes are reversible, and the goal of management is to identify the patients early and treat them to prevent progressive renal failure. Atheromatous embolization has also been associated with renovascular disease (39). The compilation of injury leads to cortical scarring, interstitial fibrosis, tubular collapse, and destruction of the renal architecture.

Systemic and glomerular pressures play important roles in renal injury in patients with renovascular disease. In the two-kidney, one-clip model of renovascular hypertension, the unclipped kidney demonstrates significantly more vascular and glomerular damage than the clipped kidney (40). It is not clear whether this is due to a direct hemodynamic effect of the elevated blood pressure or to the mitogenic and hypertrophic effects of angiotensin.

ANATOMIC CONSIDERATIONS

Atheromatous Lesions

More than 90% of all renovascular lesions are secondary to atherosclerosis (4). Although atherosclerotic RAS may occasionally be isolated to the renal artery alone, it is more commonly a manifestation of systemic atherosclerosis involving the aorta and coronary, cerebral, and peripheral vessels. Atherosclerotic RAS most often occurs at the ostium or the proximal 2 cm of the renal artery (Fig. 109.3). Distal arterial or branch involvement is distinctly uncommon (26).

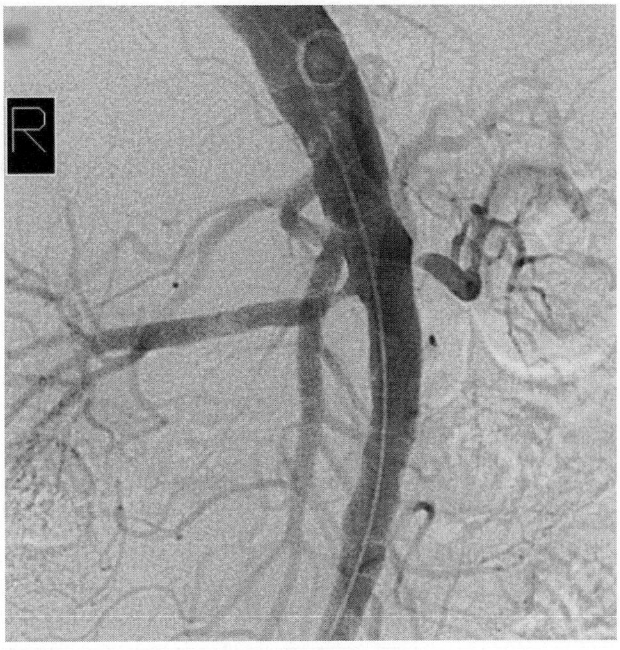

FIGURE 109.3. Aortogram showing severe bilateral renal artery stenosis. The left renal artery is nearly occluded.

Fibromuscular Dysplasia

Fibromuscular dysplasia (FMD) is a nonatherosclerotic, noninflammatory disease that most commonly affects the renal arteries and is the second-most-common cause of RAS (41). The most common clinical presentation is that of hypertension in a young woman. Fibromuscular dysplasia has been demonstrated in virtually every vascular bed. Renal artery involvement occurs in 60% to 75% of patients with FMD, followed by extracranial cerebrovascular arteries in 25% to 30%, visceral arteries in 9%, and arteries of the extremities in approximately 5% of patients (41,42). It may present as a systemic disease (affecting a combination of the carotids, mesenteric, subclavian, and/or extremity vessels) in up to 28% of patients (43). The diagnosis is rarely made pathologically but is usually determined by its typical angiographic appearance (Fig. 109.4). Whereas atherosclerosis involves the origin and proximal portion of the renal arteries, FMD characteristically involves the distal two thirds of the artery and may involve the branches (41,44).

The lesions of FMD are thought to be congenital dysplasias with maldevelopment of the fibrous, muscular, and elastic tissues of the renal artery. They are subcategorized according to the layer of the arterial wall involved (45,46). This classification is important because each type of fibrous dysplasia has distinct histologic and angiographic features and each type occurs in a different clinical setting (Table 109.1).

Medial fibromuscular dysplasia has been further divided into medial hyperplasia (the only type in which there is true smooth muscle hyperplasia), perimedial dysplasia, and medial fibroplasia. Medial fibroplasia is the histologic finding in nearly 80% of all cases of FMD. It tends to occur in 25- to 50-year-old women and often involves both renal arteries. It has a "string of beads" appearance angiographically, with the "bead" diameter larger than the proximal, unaffected artery (Fig. 109.4). The areas of stenosis are often overshadowed by contrast medium in the microaneurysms, making the degree of actual stenosis difficult to assess. This beading is due to thickening of the media, interspersed by areas of aneurysmal dilation. Microscopically, the internal elastic membrane is focally variably thinned and lost. Within the alternating thickened areas much of the muscle is replaced by collagen, hence the term medial fibroplasia. In other areas, thinning of the media occurs to the point of complete loss, and microaneurysms can be seen as saccules lined by only

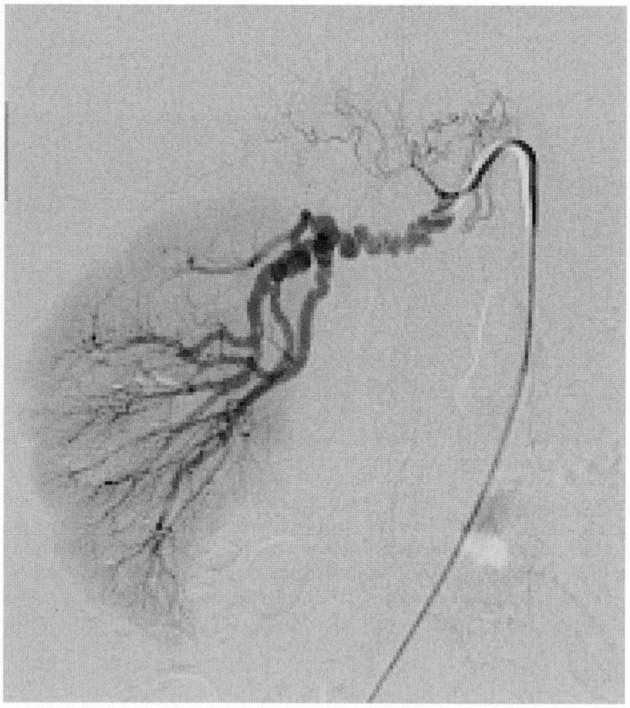

FIGURE 109.4. This renal arteriogram demonstrates typical medial fibroplasia of the renal artery. The "string of beads" appearance of the renal artery involves the distal portion of the main renal artery, and the "beads" are larger than the normal diameter of the artery. (From Slovut D, Olin JW. Fibromuscular dysplasia. *N Engl J Med* 2004;350:1862–1871.)

TABLE 109.1

CLASSIFICATION OF FIBROMUSCULAR DYSPLASIA

Classification	Frequency (%)	Pathology	Angiographic appearance
Medial dysplasia			
Medial fibroplasia	75–80	Alternating areas of thinned media and thickened fibromuscular ridges containing collagen Internal elastic membrane may be lost in some areas	"String of beads" appearance in which the diameter of the "beading" is larger than the diameter of the artery
Perimedial fibroplasia	10–15	Extensive collagen deposition in the outer half of the media	"Beading" in which the "beads" are smaller than the diameter of the artery
Medial hyperplasia	1–2	True smooth muscle cell hyperplasia without fibrosis	Concentric smooth stenosis (similar to intimal disease)
Intimal fibroplasia	<10	Circumferential or eccentric deposition of collagen in the intima No lipid or inflammatory component Internal elastic lamina fragmented or duplicated	Concentric focal band Long, smooth narrowing
Adventitial (periarterial) fibroplasia	<1	Dense collagen replaces the fibrous tissue of the adventitia and may extend into surrounding tissue	

From Begelman SM, Olin JW. Fibromuscular dysplasia. *Curr Opin Rheumatol* 2000;12:41–47.

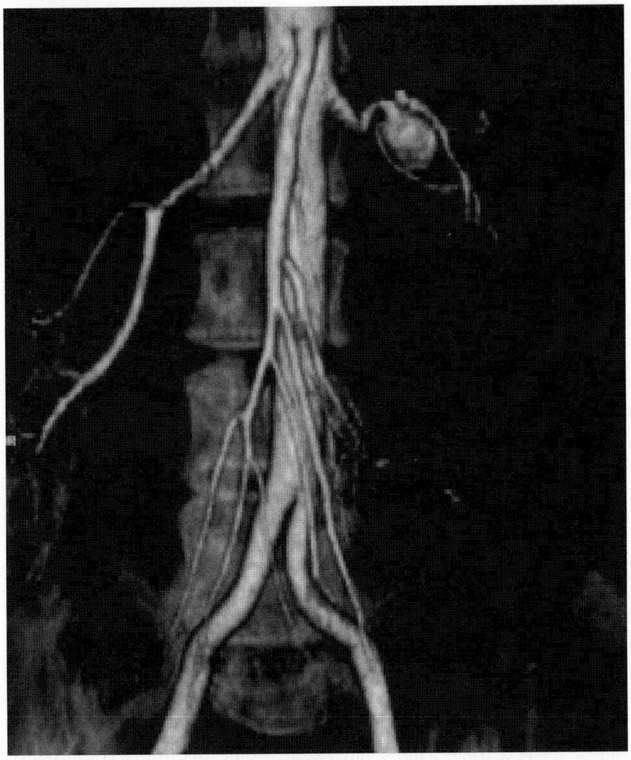

FIGURE 109.5. Computed tomography angiogram of the aorta and renal arteries. Note the "string of beads" in the right renal artery typical of medial fibroplasia. The left renal artery demonstrates a large aneurysm occasionally seen in patients with fibromusuclar dysplasia.

the external elastica. In extreme cases, giant aneurysms may be found in association with medial fibroplasia (Fig. 109.5). Progression to total occlusion is rare in this subtype. Medial fibroplasia responds very well to percutaneous balloon angioplasty. The other types of FMD are beyond the scope of this chapter and are nicely summarized in several recent reviews (41,46).

Miscellaneous Causes of Renovascular Disease

Other causes of renovascular disease include aneurysm, Takayasu arteritis, atheroemboli, thromboemboli, spontaneous renal artery dissection, arteriovenous malformations or fistulas, trauma (such as from radiation, lithotripsy, direct injury, or surgery), and neurofibromatosis. Retroperitoneal fibrosis producing external compression has also been associated with RAS.

CLINICAL ASPECTS OF RENAL ARTERY STENOSIS

Primary or essential hypertension is present in more than 60 million Americans. Renovascular disease and renal parenchymal disease are the most common secondary causes of hypertension after obesity, excess alcohol ingestion, drug abuse, and oral contraceptives are excluded. Patients with atherosclerotic RAS have the usual risk factors for atherosclerosis. Whereas the effect of atherosclerosis on the coronary and carotid arteries is well recognized, involvement of the renal arteries is frequently overlooked. Because patients with atherosclerotic RAS succumb prematurely from myocardial infarction and stroke (8,47–51), early diagnosis and treatment is of vital importance to avoid premature morbidity and mortality.

Prevalence of Renal Artery Stenosis

Although there are excellent prevalence data in specific patient populations (e.g., those with coronary artery disease, aortic aneurysm, or peripheral arterial disease), the prevalence of RAS in the general population is not known. Not all cases of RAS are clinically significant. Dustan et al. (51) reviewed 149 aortograms and found that approximately half of patients with 50% or greater RAS did *not* have hypertension.

In a recent population-based study, Hansen and colleagues reported on the prevalence of renovascular disease in a cohort of elderly patients (52). Eight hundred thirty-four participants of the Cardiovascular Health Study underwent renal duplex ultrasound. Fifty-seven (6.8%) had anatomic renal artery stenosis. There was no difference in the prevalence of RAS in whites (6.9%) and African Americans (6.7%).

Several series have looked at the prevalence of renovascular disease in patients who have atherosclerotic disease elsewhere. To determine the prevalence of atherosclerotic RAS, we studied 395 consecutive patients who had undergone arteriography as part of an evaluation for an abdominal aortic aneurysm, aortoiliac occlusive disease, and peripheral arterial disease. In addition, 78 patients had an aortogram performed for suspected renal artery stenosis (Table 109.2) (1). These patients did not have the usual clinical clues to suggest RAS. High-grade bilateral renal artery disease was present in approximately 13% of patients. In the 319 patients reported in six different studies, 44% had bilateral RAS (9). Other studies showed that 22% to 59% of patients with peripheral arterial disease have significant renal artery stenosis (53).

It has also been established that RAS is common in patients with coronary artery disease. Of 7,758 patients undergoing cardiac catheterization during a 76-month period, 3,987 underwent aortography to screen for RAS at the time of catheterization (54). One hundred ninety-one (4.8%) patients had greater than 75% renal artery stenosis and 0.8% had severe bilateral disease. In the Mayo Clinic series (55), renal arteries were studied at the time of cardiac catheterization in patients with hypertension. Ninety percent of the renal arteries were adequately visualized, and no complications occurred from the aortogram. Greater than 50% RAS was present in 19.2% of patients, greater than 70% in 7%, and bilateral RAS in 3.7%.

Natural History of Renal Artery Stenosis

Knowledge of the natural history is extremely important in the subsequent management of patients with RAS. Most natural history studies reported in the literature were retrospective studies. The rates of progression ranged from 36% to 71% (56). In Schreiber et al.'s series, only 16% of patients progressed to total occlusion over a mean follow-up of 52 months. However, the rate of progression to total occlusion occurred more frequently (39%) when there was greater than 75% stenosis on the initial renal arteriogram (56).

Zierler et al. (57,58) used renal duplex ultrasound to prospectively study anatomic progression of atherosclerotic renovascular disease. If the renal arteries were normal, only 8% progressed over 36 months. However, at 3 years, 48% of patients progressed from less than 60% stenosis to 60% or greater stenosis. All four renal arteries that progressed to occlusion had 60% or greater stenosis at the initial visit. Progression

TABLE 109.2

PREVALENCE OF ATHEROSCLEROTIC RENAL ARTERY STENOSIS

≥50% stenosis	Abdominal aortic aneurysm ($n = 109$)	Aortoiliac occlusive disease ($n = 21$)	Peripheral arterial disease ($n = 189$)	Renal artery stenosis ($n = 76$)
All patients	41 (38%)	7 (33%)	74 (39%)	53 (70%)*
Diabetic patients	6 (50%)	1 (33%)	34 (50%)**	10 (71%)
Nondiabetic patients	35 (36%)	6 (33%)	40 (33%)	43 (69%)*

*$p < .001$.
**$p < .02$.
From Olin JW, Melia M, Young JR, et al. Prevalence of atherosclerotic renal artery stenosis in patients with atherosclerosis elsewhere. *Am J Med* 1990;88:46N–51N.

of RAS occurred at an average rate of 7%/year for all categories of baseline disease combined.

The effect of RAS on kidney size has been well studied (59,60). Using duplex ultrasound, Caps and colleagues prospectively followed 204 kidneys in 122 patients with known renal artery stenosis for a mean of 33 months. The 2-year cumulative incidence of renal atrophy was 5.5%, 11.7%, and 20.8% in kidneys with a baseline renal artery disease classification of normal, less than 60% stenosis, and 60% or greater stenosis, respectively ($p = .009$, log rank test) (59).

A question that has really never been satisfactorily answered, however, is how common is atherosclerotic RAS as a cause of end-stage renal disease (ESRD)? Scoble et al. (61) found that atherosclerotic renovascular disease was the cause of ESRD in 14% of patients starting dialysis therapy. Mailloux and colleagues (50) reviewed the causes of ESRD in 683 patients over a 20-year period. Eighty-three patients (12%) had documented RAS as a cause of ESRD. Because these investigators only performed arteriography in patients in whom they highly suspected RAS, it is possible that the true incidence of RAS as a cause of ESRD was seriously underestimated. A recent study reported that 16% of 49 patients starting renal replacement therapy had greater than 50% bilateral RAS or RAS to a single functioning kidney (62). Renal artery stenosis should be searched for in every patient starting dialysis if a clear-cut etiology for the ESRD is not known (63–65).

Connolly et al. (48) showed that the 2-year actuarial *renal* survival (percentage of patients remaining off dialysis) was 97.3% for patients with unilateral RAS, 82.4% for patients with bilateral RAS, and 44.7% for patients with stenosis or occlusion to a solitary functioning kidney. Patients on dialysis have a shortened life expectancy. The average life expectancy in a patient with ESRD older than age 65 years is only 2.7 years (66,67). The survival estimates are even worse if the patient has atherosclerotic renovascular disease as the cause of ESRD. Mailloux and associates (50) showed that median survival for patients with renovascular disease was 25 months compared to 55 months in patients with malignant hypertension and 133 months for patients with polycystic kidney disease. The 2-year survival on dialysis in patients with renovascular disease was 56%, 5-year survival was 18%, and 10-year survival was only 5%. These data underscore the fact that patients with atherosclerotic RAS who progress to ESRD and require dialysis have extremely high mortality rates.

Survival in Renal Artery Stenosis

In addition, the mere presence of RAS, even prior to developing ESRD, portends a poor prognosis. Patient survival decreases as the severity of RAS increases (54), with a 2-year survival rates of 96% in patients with unilateral RAS, 74% in patients with bilateral RAS, and 47% in patients with stenosis or occlusion to a solitary functioning kidney (48). Dorros and associates (8) demonstrated that as the serum creatinine increases, the survival decreases in patients with atherosclerotic RAS. The 3-year probability of survival was 92% ± 4% for patients with a serum creatinine less than 1.4 mg/dL, 74% ± 8% for patients with a serum creatinine of 1.5 to 1.9 mg/dL, and 51% ± 8% for patients with a serum creatinine 2.0 mg/dL or greater.

Long-term survival was investigated at Duke University in a cohort of 3,987 patients who underwent aortography at the time of cardiac catheterization. In patients with 75% or greater stenosis of at least one renal artery, the 4-year survival rate was 57% compared to a 4-year survival rate of 89% in patients with less than 75% stenosis. The effect of renal artery stenosis on survival remained robust regardless of how the coronary artery disease was treated (medical, percutaneous transluminal coronary angioplasty, or coronary artery bypass grafts) (54).

Clinical Clues to the Diagnosis of Renal Artery Stenosis

The clinical clues that suggest renal artery disease are shown in Table 109.3 (5,20).

Hypertension

What was the age of onset?
Has the hypertension suddenly become more difficult to control?
Did the patient have malignant or accelerated hypertension?
Does the patient have resistant hypertension?

Individuals who develop hypertension between the ages of 30 and 55 years usually have primary (essential) hypertension. If the initial diagnosis of hypertension is made before the age of 30 years, it is usually due to fibromuscular dysplasia. Because atherosclerosis occurs in older individuals, it is usually the cause of RAS after the age of 55 years. It is not uncommon for patients to have years of primary hypertension and, as they age, develop atherosclerotic RAS. This cohort of patients may have had well-controlled blood pressure that suddenly became more difficult to control. Accelerated or malignant hypertension has also been associated with a very high prevalence of RAS. Resistant hypertension is defined as failure to reach goal blood pressure in patients who are adhering to full doses of an

TABLE 109.3

CLINICAL CLUES TO THE DIAGNOSIS OF RENAL ARTERY STENOSIS

Onset of hypertension after the age of 55 y
Exacerbation of previously well controlled hypertension
Malignant hypertension
Resistant hypertension
Epigastric bruit (systolic/diastolic)
Unexplained azotemia
Azotemia while receiving angiotensin-converting-enzyme inhibitors or angiotensin receptor–blocking agents
Atrophic kidney or discrepancy in size between the two kidneys
Recurrent congestive heart failure or "flash" pulmonary edema
Atherosclerosis elsewhere

appropriate three-drug regimen that includes a diuretic (68). The diagnosis of renovascular disease should be strongly considered in patients with resistant hypertension.

Physical Examination

Does the patient have evidence of atherosclerosis elsewhere?
Does the patient have an epigastric bruit?

In general, the physical exam is of limited help. Evidence of coronary, cerebral, or peripheral arterial disease is associated with a higher likelihood of renal artery disease due to the systemic nature of atherosclerosis. Although a systolic abdominal bruit is common and nonspecific, the presence of a systolic/diastolic bruit especially over the epigastrium may point to underlying renal artery disease. The presence of a diastolic component to the bruit indicates that the degree of narrowing of the artery is severe because there is continued flow during diastole (69). A systolic/diastolic bruit more often occurs in patients with fibromuscular disease (53%) than in patients who have atherosclerotic disease (12.5%) (70). An abdominal bruit in a young, trim person with no hypertension may be due to compression of the celiac artery by the median arcuate ligament and is often of no clinical significance. The presence of a bruit is helpful, but the absence does not exclude the diagnosis of either atherosclerotic renovascular disease or fibromuscular dysplasia.

Renal Function

Are the kidneys of differing sizes?
Has the patient ever developed azotemia associated with angiotensin-converting-enzyme inhibitors or angiotensin II–receptor blocking agents?
Does the patient have unexplained azotemia?
Is the patient receiving dialysis without a clear cause for end-stage renal disease?

Gifford et al. (71) found that 71% of patients (53 of 75) with an atrophic kidney had severe stenosis or complete occlusion of the renal artery ipsilateral to the small kidney. Several studies have shown that if there is a discrepancy in the size between the two kidneys or if one kidney is atrophic, there is a 60% chance that the *contralateral* renal artery (normal-sized kidney) is severely stenotic (1,71,72). Therefore, the presence of an atrophic kidney or a discrepancy in size between the two kidneys demands a thorough investigation for the presence of renovascular disease.

There are numerous reports suggesting that patients who develop azotemia while receiving ACE inhibitors have bilateral RAS, RAS to a solitary kidney, or decompensated congestive heart failure in the sodium-depleted state (21,32–35,73,74). The mechanisms were discussed in detail earlier in this chapter.

Congestive Heart Failure and Pulmonary Edema

Does the patient have unexplained congestive heart failure?
Has the patient had recurrent episodes of flash pulmonary edema?

Recurrent congestive heart failure and "flash" pulmonary edema not related to ischemic heart disease can result from bilateral RAS or unilateral RAS to a single functioning kidney. In our renal artery stent series, 39 patients (19% of all patients undergoing renal artery stent implantation from 1991 to 1997) had recurrent episodes of congestive heart failure or "flash" pulmonary edema as the primary indication for renal artery stenting (13). Although it is not completely understood, the mechanism of congestive heart failure may be related in part to the inability to use ACEIs or ARBs, direct toxic effects of angiotensin II on myocardial function or volume expansion, and the inability to achieve adequate diuresis (13,75).

DIAGNOSIS OF RENOVASCULAR DISEASE

The ideal imaging procedure should (a) identify the main renal arteries as well as accessory or polar vessels, (b) localize the site of stenosis or disease, (c) provide evidence for the hemodynamic significance of the lesion, and (d) identify associated pathology (i.e., abdominal aortic aneurysm, renal mass, etc.) that may affect the treatment of the renal artery disease (72,76,77). The most sensitive and specific methods of identifying RAS include the noninvasive imaging techniques such as Duplex ultrasound, CT angiography, and magnetic resonance angiography (MRA).

Arteriography

Angiography, the gold standard for arterial imaging, is rarely required to make the *diagnosis* of RAS. Usually one or more of the noninvasive modalities can accurately make the diagnosis. Exceptions to this general rule may occur in patients with fibromuscular dysplasia that primarily affects the branches of the renal arteries and in patients with renal artery aneurysms (41). Angiography or intraarterial digital subtraction angiography (IA-DSA) has several distinct advantages as an imaging modality. All portions of the renal artery including the intrarenal branches can be well visualized. In addition, accessory renal arteries can be identified and one can determine kidney size and gross function (the presence of a nephrogram). However, angiography is invasive and costly compared to other imaging modalities. Although they are not common, complications associated with angiography include access-site complications such as a hematoma, pseudoaneurysm, or arterial venous fistula, as well as acute renal failure from contrast-induced nephrotoxicity and atheromatous embolization to the kidneys, bowel, or lower extremities. Therefore, angiography is a poor *screening* test for RAS but an excellent confirmatory test once it has been decided that revascularization is indicated.

Carbon dioxide or gadolinium may be used as a contrast agent in patients with severe renal impairment (78–80).

Renal Arteriography at the Time of Cardiac Catheterization

A hotly debated and still controversial issue is the performance of renal angiography at the time of cardiac catheterization. Some cardiologists do it routinely on all patients, whereas others selectively image the renal arteries in patients who have clinical clues that suggest the presence of renal artery stenosis. In the Duke series in which 3,987 patients were screened with abdominal aortography at the time of cardiac catheterization, only 191 (4.8%) of patients had greater than 75% renal artery stenosis and only 33 (0.8%) had severe bilateral disease (54). Similarly, the Mayo Clinic (55) prospectively evaluated 297 hypertensive patients at the time of cardiac catheterization and only 19% had renal artery stenosis greater than 50%, 7% had stenosis greater than 70%, and 3.7% had bilateral disease. They did, however, demonstrate that evaluation of the renal arteries can be completed safely with the addition of only 62 cc of contrast. Therefore, although it is safe to perform angiography at the time of catheterization, the yield is low, and there is some evidence that knowing that there is renal artery stenosis present will tempt the angiographer to stent the renal artery in the absence of clear-cut indications (81,82). Therefore, we are opposed to *routine* "drive-by angiography" at the time of cardiac catheterization because it adds nothing to the overall management of the patient other than to tempt the angiographer to perform a procedure that is not indicated. However, if the patient has a clear-cut indication for intervention (inability to control the blood pressure with a good antihypertensive regimen, jeopardy of renal function, or recurrent episodes of congestive heart failure) and the clinician is prepared to perform angioplasty and stenting should significant RAS be discovered, then an aortogram at the time of cardiac catheterization should be performed.

Direct Screening Tests

Evaluation of the renal arteries is essential in acute or chronic renal failure, poorly controlled hypertension, or recurrent congestive heart failure that is not directly caused by myocardial ischemia. Imaging modalities are also useful for screening for restenosis after percutaneous or surgical revascularization of the renal arteries. Every patient who has undergone percutaneous intervention for RAS should be put in a surveillance program for detecting restenosis (5,77). Technological advances in computed tomographic angiography (CTA) and MRA provide aortic and renal artery imaging that compares well to the quality and accuracy of angiography and have virtually replaced catheter-based angiography for the evaluation of aortic, renal, and peripheral arterial disease (20). Factors such as the patient's body habitus, the degree of renal impairment, and cost may help to determine which screening test is used. However, institutional experience and expertise are perhaps the most important factors determining which of the noninvasive imaging studies is used as a screening test for renovascular disease.

Duplex Ultrasonography

Duplex ultrasonography is an excellent test for detecting RAS. It is the least expensive of the imaging modalities and provides useful information about the degree of stenosis, the kidney size, and other associated disease processes such as obstruction, and it may even predict which patients can expect an improvement in blood pressure control or renal function after renal artery angioplasty and stenting (83,84). The location and degree of stenosis can accurately be determined by duplex ultrasound of the renal artery. Duplex ultrasound can be performed without altering the antihypertensive regimen and does not require contrast agents that may have an adverse affect on renal function.

Duplex ultrasonography combines B-mode ultrasound and Doppler examination. Improvements in ultrasound hardware, software, and transducer technology are responsible for improved visualization of the arteries and more precise Doppler interrogation of the entire artery. Renal artery ultrasound should be performed from both an anterior and an oblique [or posterior (flank)] approach. In the longitudinal (long-axis) view, the peak systolic flow velocity in the aorta is recorded at the level of the renal arteries. The aortic velocity and the highest renal artery peak systolic velocity are used to calculate the renal aortic ratio.

The renal arteries are best visualized in a transverse (short-axis) view. Figure 109.6 demonstrates a high-grade stenosis of the left renal artery before and after renal artery stent implantation. With the B-mode image and a 60-degree angle of insonance the arteries are interrogated with pulse-wave Doppler. The Doppler should be swept through the artery from its origin to the renal hilum. This allows the examiner to survey the artery for velocity shifts along the entire course of the renal artery. Velocities should be recorded at the origin, proximal, mid, and distal arterial segments. From an oblique approach the renal artery can be visualized at the renal hilum and followed to the aorta. Because medial fibroplasia most often occurs in the mid to distal renal artery, the oblique approach is particularly good for identifying these entities (72,85).

Overall, when compared to angiography, duplex ultrasound has a sensitivity and specificity of 84% to 98% and 62% to 99%, respectively, when used to diagnose RAS (86–91). We performed a prospective study comparing duplex ultrasound to angiography (Table 109.4) (91).

The renal aortic ratio (RAR), the ratio of the peak systolic velocity (PSV) in the renal arteries to the PSV in the aorta, is used to classify the degree of stenosis. A three-category classification scheme is commonly used: 0% to 59% stenosis, 60% to 99% stenosis, and total occlusion (Table 109.5).

The resistive index (RI) is calculated as (peak systolic velocity–end-diastolic velocity)/peak systolic velocity and is a measure of the resistance within the renal circulation (84,92, 93). An elevated RI may be present in renal parenchymal disease, and the RI may be influenced by some antihypertensive drugs and age.

Rademacher et al. used the resistive index to predict the outcome of therapy in patients with RAS undergoing revascularization (84). One hundred thirty-eight patients with greater than 50% RAS underwent renal artery angioplasty or surgery for blood pressure control or preservation of renal function. Ninety-seven percent of patients with an increased renal resistance index demonstrated no improvement in blood pressure and 80% had no improvement in renal function. The authors suggested that the increased resistive index identifies structural abnormalities in the small vessels of the kidney. Such small-vessel disease has been seen with long-standing hypertension associated with nephrosclerosis or glomerulosclerosis. Other studies have failed to show that elevated resistive index precludes a successful endovascular result (94,95).

Renal artery duplex is an excellent test for the follow-up of RAS after percutaneous therapy or surgical bypass (Fig. 109.6C,D) (77,96,97). Unlike MRA (which may be affected by artifact or scatter produced by the stent), ultrasound transmission through the stent is not a problem. All patients who have undergone percutaneous intervention should be placed in a surveillance program in an attempt to identify restenosis and treat it before the artery occludes (5,77). After

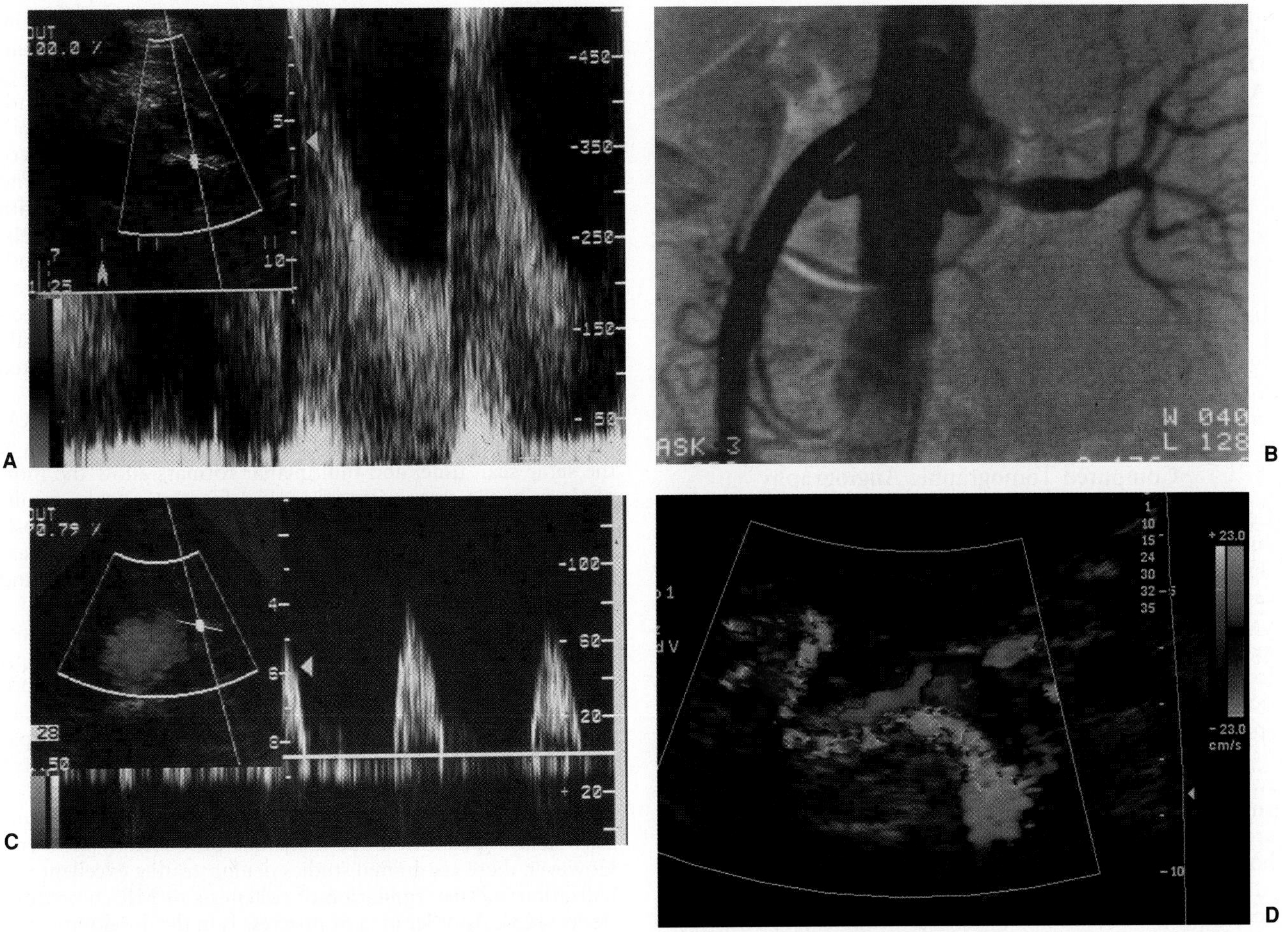

FIGURE 109.6. **A:** Renal artery duplex ultrasound from the anterior approach. The Doppler is placed in the proximal left renal artery. The peak systolic velocity is 485 cm/second and the end-diastolic velocity (*arrow*) is 210 cm/second, indicating a stenosis of greater than 80% of the left renal artery. **B:** The aortogram shows a total occlusion of the right renal artery and a severe eccentric stenosis of the left renal artery with poststenotic dilatation. **C:** Duplex ultrasound of the left renal artery after a renal artery stent was placed. Note normal velocities compared to pre-stenting. **D:** Color Doppler showing a widely patent right renal artery after renal artery stenting.

endovascular therapy a renal artery duplex should be obtained within the first few weeks to establish a baseline and then at 6 months, 12 months, and yearly thereafter.

One drawback of duplex ultrasound is that the sensitivity is lower for identifying accessory renal arteries (67%) compared to main renal arteries (98%) (87). Therefore if the patient has hypertension that cannot be adequately controlled with a good regimen and the duplex ultrasound fails to demonstrate RAS, another imaging modality may be considered to identify stenosis to an accessory renal artery.

TABLE 109.4

COMPARISON OF DUPLEX ULTRASOUND WITH ARTERIOGRAPHY

	Stenosis by arteriography				
Stenosis by ultrasound	**0%–59%**	**60%–79%**	**80%–99%**	**100%**	**Total**
0%–59%	62	0	1	1	64
60%–99%	1	31	67	0	99
100%	0	1	1	22	24
Total	63	32	69	23	187

Sensitivity, 0.98.
Specificity, 0.98.
Positive predictive value, 0.99.
Negative predictive value, 0.97.
From Olin JW, Piedmonte MR, Young JR, et al. The utility of duplex ultrasound scanning of the renal arteries for diagnosing significant renal artery stenosis. *Ann Intern Med* 1995;122:833–838.

TABLE 109.5

DUPLEX ULTRASOUND CRITERIA FOR RENAL ARTERY STENOSIS

Stenosis	Duplex criteria
<60% Stenosis	RAR <3.5
60%–99% Stenosis	RAR ≥3.5 and PSV >200 cm/s
Occlusion	No flow signal from renal artery
	Low-amplitude parenchymal signal ± small kidney

PSV, peak systolic velocity; RAR, renal to aortic ratio.

Computed Tomographic Angiography

Computed tomographic angiography can be performed safely and produce excellent images of the abdominal vasculature (Fig. 109.5). Excellent image quality with enhanced resolution can be obtained with multidetector-row CTA technology (77). Current multidetector-row scanners acquire up to 64 simultaneous interweaving helices. Thus one can visualize the anatomy from multiple angles in multiple planes after a single acquisition (98). The advantages of CTA over MRA include higher spatial resolution, absence of flow-related phenomena that may overestimate the degree of stenosis, and the ability to visualize calcification and metallic implants such as endovascular stents and stent grafts. The disadvantages of CTA compared to MRA are exposure to ionizing radiation and the need to give a large bolus of potentially nephrotoxic contrast agents.

The initial output from the CT scans consists of sets of contiguous or overlapping transverse cross sections. The angiographic representations are made from reformatting during the postprocessing of the volumetric data (99). After the initial axial images are acquired, several different software programs are commercially available to reformat the data into two-dimensional (2D) and three-dimensional (3D) reconstruction images.

Depending on the techniques used, CT angiography has a sensitivity and specificity for detecting RAS of 89% to 100% and a specificity of 82% to 100% (100–107). There are limited data on the utility of CTA in detecting restenosis after renal artery stent implantation, yet this technique appears to be a promising noninvasive method for evaluating patients after stent implantation (108–110).

In patients with renal insufficiency, CT angiography is not an ideal screening test for RAS. Patients must be able to suspend respiration during image acquisition because respiratory artifact may significantly degrade the image quality. CT angiography is generally well tolerated by most individuals. The gantry is open, and thus claustrophobia is not commonly a limiting factor.

Magnetic Resonance Angiography

Like CT angiography, MRA provides excellent imaging of the abdominal vasculature and associated anatomic structures. The examination does not require nephrotoxic contrast agents and therefore provides a good alternative to CT angiography in patients with renal insufficiency, congestive heart failure, or a contrast allergy. In general, the procedure is very similar to CT angiography. The patient must be able to cooperate and refrain from breathing during contrast-enhanced sequences; otherwise the quality of the study may be compromised.

When compared with angiography, MRA has demonstrated a sensitivity of 91% to 100% and a specificity of 71% to 100% (111–119). Contrast-enhanced MRA using gadolinium chelate improves image quality when compared with noncontrast studies and shortens imaging time, thereby eliminating some of the artifact created by gross patient movement (120). In addition, signal strength is increased, providing for better visualization of distal small-caliber vessels (121). A meta-analysis of 39 studies reported a sensitivity and specificity of 94% and 85%, respectively, for nonenhanced studies compared with a sensitivity and specificity of 97% and 93%, respectively, for contrast-enhanced studies (122). Contrast-enhanced studies also improve the visualization of accessory renal arteries. However, MRA does not have the same sensitivity and specificity in patients with fibromuscular dysplasia and is generally not a good screening test if fibromuscular dysplasia is suspected (123).

New techniques have improved the clinical utility of MRA. Parallel acquisition techniques double the spatial resolution in the same scan time, and multiplanar formats allow the morphology of the stenosis to be viewed from any angle, resulting in a more accurate interpretation of the degree of stenosis (117). The addition of cardiac-gated phase-contrast flow measurements to MRA may reduce interobserver variability and improve the accuracy of stenosis assessment (124).

MRA may not be used in patients with metallic implants such as some mechanical heart valves, cerebral aneurysm clips, and electrically activated implants (pacemakers, spinal cord stimulators). Most patients with inferior vena cava filters can be safely studied. Claustrophobia is a common problem. If patients are still apprehensive, they can usually be premedicated with a sedative hypnotic agent.

At the present time, MRA is not useful in following patients after stent implantation due to artifact produced by the stent. However, there are animal studies demonstrating excellent visualization and determination of restenosis of MR compatible stents (125). Another area of progress is in the development of interventional procedures such as stent placement under MR guidance (125–127).

Indirect Screening Tests

Other than the captopril-stimulated renal flow scan, indirect measurements such as intravenous urography, plasma renin activity, and the captopril test (plasma renin activity measured before and after the administration of oral captopril) (128–130) are not useful in the diagnosis of RAS and should not be used. In 540 patients studied by Maxwell and colleagues the false-negative and false-positive rates were extremely high at 43% and 34%, respectively (131). In addition, elevated plasma renin activity may be present in approximately 15% of patients with essential hypertension, and patients with bilateral disease or disease to a solitary functioning kidney may have normal or low plasma renin activity due to volume expansion.

Renal Vein Renin Measurements

Renal vein renin measurements are not a useful test for diagnosing RAS. However, measurement of renin produced from the renal vein of the kidney with RAS compared to the renal vein of the "normal" kidney has been used as a method for predicting which patients may benefit from revascularization. Technical factors can interfere with the interpretation of the results and therefore limit the utility of the test. Ideally patients should be off all medications that can either stimulate or suppress renin for a period of at least 5 days. Blood should be taken from the right and left renal veins and the inferior vena cava above and below the renal veins as a baseline. Either 40 mg of furosemide or 25 mg of captopril should then be administered and repeat blood samples taken 30 minutes later.

Hughes et al. (132) demonstrated that when a renal vein renin ratio greater than 1.4:1 was combined with a duration of hypertension of less than 5 years, 19 of 20 patients (95%) had a cure of their renovascular hypertension. Several reports have been published that show that renal vein renin lateralization does not predict which patient will have an *improvement* in blood pressure after revascularization (29,133–135). Renal vein renin measurements may be useful in a patient with an occluded renal artery and persistent hypertension despite good medical management. If there is lateralization of renal vein renin, a nephrectomy may help to normalize blood pressure with medications (136).

Captopril Renography

Radionuclide imaging techniques are a noninvasive and safe way of evaluating renal blood flow and excretory function. However, the renal flow scan has unacceptably high false-positive and false-negative rates. When an ACE inhibitor such as captopril is added to isotope renography, the sensitivity and specificity of the test improve considerably, especially for patients with unilateral RAS. In most instances of unilateral RAS, the glomerular filtration rate (GFR) of the stenotic kidney falls by approximately 30% after captopril administration (137–140), whereas the GFR, urine flow, and salt excretion increase in the contralateral "normal" kidney.

Captopril is administered, and a conventional radionuclide study of the kidneys is begun 60 minutes later. The Consensus Report on Captopril Renography suggested that both the scintigraphic images and computer-generated time-activity curves provide information about renal size, perfusion, and excretory capacity.

Overall, the accuracy of captopril renography in identifying patients with renovascular disease appears to be quite acceptable, with a sensitivity of approximately 85% to 90% (range 45% to 94%) and a specificity of approximately 93% to 98% (range 81% to 100%). Those patients with unilateral disease and normal renal function would be best suited for a captopril renogram. The presence of significant azotemia or bilateral RAS may adversely affect the accuracy of captopril renography.

There are no reliable data using the captopril renogram to predict whether revascularization will result in preservation or improvement in renal function.

Although the captopril renogram was once the noninvasive diagnostic test of choice for patients with RAS, it is now relegated to a secondary screening modality because the quality of the images of duplex ultrasound and MRA are so good (20).

PRINCIPLES OF MANAGEMENT

There has been a paradigm shift in management of atherosclerotic renal artery stenosis. Prior to 1990, if a patient met the criteria for intervention, surgical renal artery revascularization was almost always performed. However, since the introduction of stents, surgical revascularization is virtually never performed for the treatment of renal artery disease. Despite advances in the technical aspects of angioplasty and stent implantation, there has been a paucity of controlled clinical trials assessing the role of renal artery angioplasty and stenting in controlling hypertension or preserving renal function. Because of a lack of controlled clinical trials, there is some controversy about the most appropriate treatment of atherosclerotic renal artery disease.

The four modalities available for the treatment of RAS are medical therapy, percutaneous balloon angioplasty, angioplasty with stent placement, and surgical revascularization. For the purpose of this discussion, revascularization is defined as restoration of blood flow to the kidney. This includes both percutaneous as well as surgical techniques.

Indications for revascularization include the following (20):

- At least a 70% stenosis of one or both renal arteries *and*
- Inability to adequately control the blood pressure despite a good antihypertensive regimen *or*
- Chronic kidney disease not related to another clear-cut cause (disease should be bilateral or stenosis to a solitary functioning kidney). The treatment of an elevated serum creatinine with unilateral disease is controversial and there are no good clinical trials to help guide the clinician (20).
- Dialysis-dependent renal failure in a patient without a definite cause of ESRD (65,141,142).
- Recurrent congestive heart failure or "flash" pulmonary edema not attributable to a cardiac cause (13,75,143).

Medical Therapy

All patients with hypertension should be treated medically, even if they undergo intervention. Antiplatelet agents should be prescribed to help to lower the extremely high cardiovascular morbidity and mortality that occur in this patient population (20). Many patients have superimposed essential hypertension and still require medications long term. Despite the etiology, the guidelines of the 7th Joint National Committee on Prevention, Detection, Evaluation, and Treatment of High Blood Pressure (JNC 7) should be followed (68). Current guidelines suggest a target blood pressure of less than 130/80 mm Hg for patients with chronic kidney disease (68).

Elevated levels of angiotensin II and aldosterone may lead to effects through hypertensive injury and activation of profibrotic and atherosclerotic pathways (144). Therefore patients with renal artery disease should be placed on an ACE inhibitor or an ARB especially if they have other compelling indications such as diabetes, heart failure, and increased cardiovascular risk (145,146). There are data suggesting that survival is improved in patients with RAS who receive ACE inhibitors as part of their antihypertensive regimen (147). If goal blood pressures are achieved, survival is similar in patients receiving medical therapy alone and those receiving revascularization. In individuals with bilateral disease or disease to a solitary functioning kidney, ACE inhibitors or ARBs should be used with caution because drugs in this class may precipitate acute renal failure (5).

Patients with RAS who are treated solely with medical therapy should be carefully followed for progression of disease. This should include three important strategies:

- Follow the blood pressure closely and work to achieve a goal blood pressure within the guidelines of JNC 7 (68).
- Follow the renal function every 3 months. If the serum creatinine begins to rise and there is no other explanation, consider revascularization.
- Place the patient in a surveillance program with serial duplex ultrasound imaging. The kidney size, volume, and severity of the stenosis can be closely followed (77,148). If the patient begins to lose volume to the affected kidney, consider revascularization.

Percutaneous Balloon Angioplasty

Percutaneous transluminal angioplasty (PTA) for RAS was first performed successfully by Gruntzig et al. in 1978 (149). Although PTA is the treatment of choice for fibromuscular dysplasia, renal artery stent implantation has replaced PTA in patients with atherosclerotic renal artery stenosis (20,150).

TABLE 109.6

RESULTS OF PERCUTANEOUS TRANSLUMINAL ANGIOPLASTY OF THE RENAL ARTERIES IN PATIENTS WITH FIBROMUSCULAR RENOVASCULAR DISEASE AND HYPERTENSION

Authors	Year	No.	Technical success rate (%)	BP cured (%)	BP improved (%)	BP not improved (%)	Follow-up (mo)	Complication rate (%)
Sos et al. (151)	1983	31	87	59	34	7	16 (4–40)	6
Baert et al. (195)	1990	22	83	58	21	21	26 (6–72)	NR
Tegtmeyer et al. (209)	1991	66	100	39	59	2	39 (1–121)	13
Bonelli et al. (155)	1995	105	89	22	63	15	43 (0–168)	11 (major)
Jensen et al. (203)	1995	30	97	39	47	14	12 (NR)	3 (major) 12 (minor)
Davidson et al. (198)	1996	23	100	52	22	26	NR	13
Klow et al. (204)	1998	49	98	25	43	29	9 (1–96)	0
Birrer et al. (196)	2002	27	100	(74)[a]	(74)[a]	26	10 (NR)	7.4
Surowiec et al. (208)	2003	14	95	(79)[a]	(74)[a]	21	NR	28.5
De Fraissinette et al. (199)	2003	70	94	14	74	12	39 (1–204)	11
Alhadad et al. (154)	2005	59	95	24	39	27	84 ± 56.4	NR

NR, not reported.
[a]Reported as cured or improved.
Modified from Slovut DP, Olin JW. Fibromuscular dysplasia. *N Engl J Med* 2004;350(18):1862–1871.

Stenting is generally not indicated for patients with FMD because they respond so well to PTA alone (41). Sos et al. (151) performed PTA in 31 patients with FMD and demonstrated a technical success rate of 87.1%. Blood pressure was cured in 59.3% and improved in 33.3%. The cure or improvement in blood pressure was maintained in 93% of patients over an average follow-up of 16 months. Ramsay and Waller (152) reviewed 10 published series of patients with FMD and reported that the hypertension was cured in 50% and improved in 42%. In a series of 85 lesions in 66 patients, PTA was technically successful in 100%. The results of the use PTA to treat FMD of the renal arteries from 1983 to 2003 are shown in Table 109.6 (41).

Most studies looking at PTA in patients with FMD have concentrated on disease in the main renal artery. However, FMD may occur in the branch renal arteries as well. In the past, surgical reconstruction has been the primary therapeutic modality for treating these lesions. However, with better catheter and balloon technology, virtually all of these lesions can be treated with PTA even in the small renal artery branches (41,153,154). In 25 branch renal artery lesions, the technical success of dilation was 84%. At 6 months, stenosis recurred in only 9%, all of which were successfully redilated.

The majority of patients with RAS have underlying atherosclerosis. Unlike FMD, disease due to atherosclerosis is found in the proximal arterial segment and even more often at the ostium of the artery. Ostial lesions respond poorly to PTA alone.

The 10 case series reviewed by Ramsay and Waller (152) included 464 atherosclerotic lesions. Technically successful angioplasty was performed for 391 lesions. Overall, blood pressure was cured in 19% and improved in an additional 52%. Bonelli et al. (155) retrospectively reviewed 190 atherosclerotic renal artery lesions that had undergone PTA and reported a cure rate of only 8.4%. The technical success rate was 81.6% and was higher for those lesions that occurred in the main branch as opposed to the origin of the renal artery (82.4% vs. 60.4%).

Rimmer and Gennari (9) reviewed several studies in which angioplasty was performed in azotemic patients. Renal function improved in 25% to 53% of patients.

Comparison of Medical Therapy and Percutaneous Transluminal Angioplasty

There are three randomized, prospective trials comparing medical management to angioplasty for blood pressure control in patients with atherosclerotic RAS. Each of the three studies has significant drawbacks, precluding any definite conclusions. Plouin et al. (156) randomized 49 patients with unilateral RAS and found no significant difference in blood pressure control at 6 months (140/81 mm Hg in the PTA group vs. 141/84 mm Hg in the medical therapy–alone group). However, patients in the angioplasty group required less antihypertensive medication. In the medical group, 7 of 26 patients developed refractory hypertension and subsequently underwent PTA.

Webster et al. (157) randomized 55 of 135 eligible patients (44%) and followed them for 6 months. A significant fall in blood pressure from baseline occurred in the patients with bilateral RAS who were randomized to PTA (152/83 mm Hg in the PTA group vs. 171/91 mm Hg in the medical therapy group). This difference was not seen in patients with unilateral RAS.

The largest randomized, prospective study was recently published by van Jaarsveld et al. (158). One hundred and six patients with angiographically documented RAS were randomly assigned to PTA or medical therapy and had blood pressure and renal function assessed at 3 and 12 months. Baseline blood pressure was 179/104 and 180/103 mm Hg in the angioplasty and drug therapy groups, respectively. At 3 and 12 months there was no significant difference in blood pressure control between the two groups, but the PTA group was on less antihypertensive medications. There were several rather serious problems with this study (159). Forty-four percent of patients randomized to medical therapy crossed over to the balloon angioplasty group, resulting in dilution of the long-term outcome differences. In spite of this, the initial angioplasty group required less antihypertensive therapy than the medical group ($p = 0.002$). There was a favorable trend to all primary outcome events, and with the small sample size we calculated that the chance of a type II error was substantial. Perhaps most importantly, the authors chose a 50% diameter reduction as the

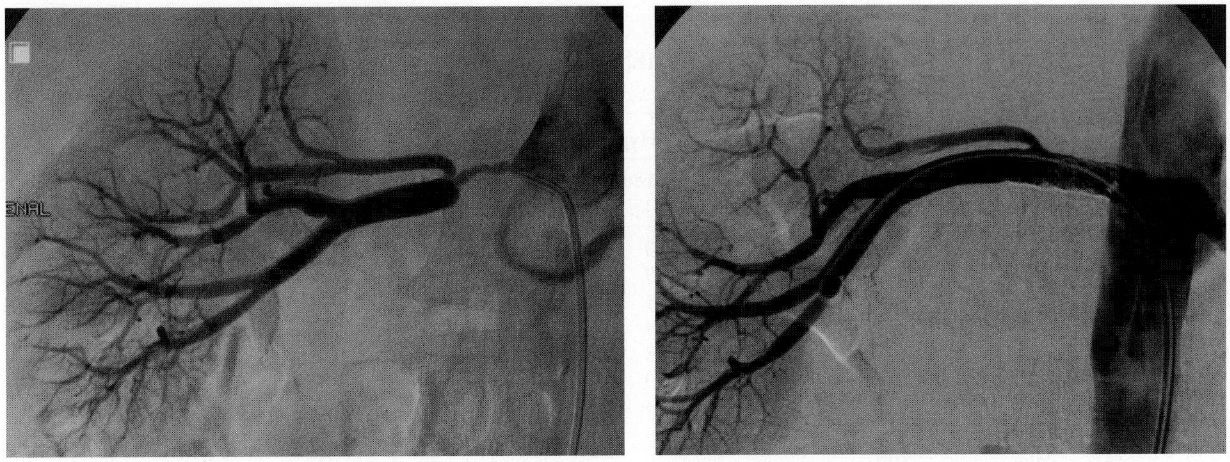
A B

FIGURE 109.7. **A:** Severe stenosis to the right renal artery. **B:** Excellent angiographic result after stent placement.

cut-off for "hemodynamically significant" renal artery lesions despite the fact that the evidence is clear that a lesion of at least 70% stenosis is required to cause significant hypertension or a decrement in renal function (160). Only 57% of patients had stenosis of greater than 70%.

The primary problems with PTA alone are (a) a good technical result is virtually impossible with ostial lesions (156) and (b) the restenosis rate is very high (156,161). PTA is no longer recommended for the treatment of atherosclerotic renal artery stenosis. Because atherosclerosis occurs at the ostium and proximal portion of the renal artery, stenting is the treatment of choice (150,162).

Renal Artery Stents

Due to the very high restenosis rate with angioplasty alone, endovascular stents offer a significant advantage over PTA in patients with atherosclerotic disease and have replaced PTA as the treatment of choice for atherosclerotic disease (10,11). The degree of stenosis after stenting approaches zero, and most dissection flaps caused by PTA alone are successfully sealed with stents (Fig. 109.7).

There are a few important technical caveats when stenting the renal arteries:

- The shortest stent to adequately cover the lesion should be used.
- The stent must extend 1 to 2 mm into the aorta in patients with ostial disease.
- The stent must be fully expanded. A common problem encountered is underdeployment or undersizing of the stent. It may be worthwhile for the novice to perform the first 10 to 15 cases with intravascular ultrasound to be certain that the stent is sized properly and adequately expanded. It is also important to make sure that no postprocedure pressure gradient exists (20,163).

White et al. (164) evaluated the safety and efficacy renal artery stent implantation in patients with lesions that did not respond well to angioplasty alone. Balloon-expandable stents were placed in 100 consecutive patients (133 renal arteries). The technical success (as assessed by quantitative angiography) was 99%. The mean blood pressure values were 173 ± 25/88 ± 17 mm Hg before stent implantation and 146 ± 20/77 ± 12 mm Hg 6 months after renal artery stenting ($p < .01$). Angiographic follow-up in 67 patients (mean 8.7 ± 5 months) demonstrated restenosis (>50%) in 15 (19%) patients.

In a multicenter registry, Dorros et al. reported on 1,058 patients who underwent renal artery stenting for either control of blood pressure or preservation of renal function (165). At 4-year follow-up, the systolic pressure decreased from 168 ± 27 mm Hg to 147 ± 21 mm Hg and diastolic pressure from 84 ± 15 mm Hg to 78 ± 12 mm Hg ($p < .05$). Patients also required less antihypertensive medication.

Blum et al. (7) prospectively placed a Palmaz stent in 68 patients (74 lesions) with ostial RAS and suboptimal percutaneous transluminal angioplasty. All patients were hypertensive and 20 had mild or severe renal dysfunction. Stents were placed due to elastic recoil (63 arteries), post-PTA dissection (1 artery), or late restenosis (10 arteries) with 100% technical success rate. Five-year patency was 84.5% (mean follow-up was 27 months). Restenosis occurred in 8 of 74 arteries (11%), but after reintervention the secondary 5-year patency rate was 92.4%. Blood pressure was cured or improved in 78% of patients. There was no significant change in the serum creatinine values after stent implantation.

Comparison of Percutaneous Transluminal Angioplasty and Endovascular Therapy with Stenting

The first randomized, prospective study comparing angioplasty alone with angioplasty and stenting was recently published (166). Eighty-five patients with ostial lesions were randomized to receive PTA alone (42 patients, 51 arteries) or PTA and stent (42 patients, 52 arteries). Secondary stent implantation was allowed if the PTA failed immediately or during the first 6 months of therapy. The primary technical success rate (individual arteries) was 57% for the PTA group and 88% for the group with PTA and stent. At 6 months the primary patency was 29% for the PTA group and 75% for the stent group. Because this was an intention-to-treat analysis and 12 patients underwent stenting in the PTA group, there were no clinical differences between the two groups.

Baumgartner et al. (167) studied 163 patients (200 arteries) with atherosclerotic RAS and evaluated the patency rates in patients undergoing PTA alone and those undergoing PTA and stent implantation. For ostial disease, the 12-month primary patency rate for PTA was 21 of 33 arteries (34%) and for PTA and stent the rate was 4 of 21 arteries (80%) ($p = .002$).

A meta-analysis of 14 studies compared the technical and clinical effect of renal artery PTA and stent implantation (Table 109.7) (168). Hypertension was improved or cured in 69% of

TABLE 109.7

CLINICAL AND ANGIOGRAPHIC FOLLOW-UP IN PATIENTS WHO UNDERWENT RENAL ARTERY STENT PLACEMENT

					Hypertension		Renal function			
Ref.	No. Pts	Stent	Technical success (%)	Follow-up (mo)	Cured (%)	Improved (%)	Improved (%)	Stable (%)	Restenosis (%)	Complications
210	11	Wallstent	83	7	30	40	0	0	29	3 (25%)
205	10	Strecker	80	11	29	43	50	NM	25	4 (40%)
206	28	Palmaz	96	7	11	54	36	36	39	5 (18%)
200	21	Wallstent	100	32	14	86	17	50	20	4 (19%)
166	24	Palmaz	100	6	68	5	36	64	13	3 (11%)
201	59	Palmaz	100	14	19	57	20	NM	9	2 (3%)
202	63	Palmaz	99	10	4	35	36	45	14	11 (13%)
7	68	Palmaz	100	27	16	62	NM	NM	11	0 (0%)
197	33	Palmaz	100	13	6	61	41	35	—	6 (17%)
169	32	Palmaz	100	6	NM	NM	34	34	13	1 (3%)
164	100	Palmaz	99	6	NM	NM	20	NM	19	2 (2%)
14	45	Palmaz	94	17	NM	NM	NM	NM	25	5 (9%)
207	21	Palmaz	100	9	NM	NM	43	29	0	2 (9%)
8	163	Palmaz	100	48	3	51	NM	NM	—	23 (11%)
Total	678	—	98[a]	16[a]	20[a]	49[a]	30	38	17	11[a]

NM, not mentioned; Pts, patients.
[a]Mean based on random-effects model.
From Leertouwer TC, Gussenhoven EJ, Bosch JL, et al. Stent placement for renal arterial stenosis: Where do we stand? A meta-analysis. *Radiology* 2000;216:78–85.

patients, and renal function improved or stabilized in 68% of patients. It should be noted that the complication rate varies considerably among centers, and high-volume centers generally can perform renal artery stenting with minimal morbidity and mortality. Although all studies reported use of an antithrombotic agent during the procedure and most patients were discharged on an antiplatelet agent, the regimens varied.

Two recent studies evaluated the effect that renal artery stent implantation had on preserving renal function (15,169). Both studies used the reciprocal of the serum creatinine to determine the rate of decline or improvement in renal function. Harden et al. (169) placed renal artery stents in 32 patients (33 arteries) and reported that renal function improved or stabilized in 22 (69%) patients. In 25 patients with complete follow-up, Watson et al. (15) demonstrated that all exhibited a negative slope to the reciprocal of the serum creatinine. After stent placement, the slopes were positive in 18 patients and less negative in 7 patients. Korsakas et al. (170) demonstrated that in patients who had progressive renal failure with a serum creatinine greater than 3.4 mg/dL, stenting significantly delayed the occurrence of end-stage renal disease. Of the 11 patients expected to become dialysis dependent within 1 year, 8 (73%) remained dialysis free.

Silva et al. (171) measured brain naturetic peptide (BNP) in 27 patients with refractory hypertension and renal artery stenosis. Clinical improvement in hypertension occurred in 77% of patients with a BNP greater than 80 pg/mL compared to 0% of patients with a baseline of 80 pg/mL or less . There was a 94% improvement rate in hypertension in patients with a greater than 30% decrease in BNP after stenting compared to 10% improvement with a lesser decrease in BNP.

Surgical Revascularization

Surgical revascularization is rarely used to treat RAS. This is due in a large part to the excellent technical results that can be achieved with angioplasty and stents. Many patients can undergo renal artery stent implantation as an outpatient procedure at a fraction of the cost of surgical revascularization.

Current indications for surgical revascularization include the following:

- Patients with branch disease from FMD that cannot be adequately treated with balloon angioplasty (20).
- Patients with recurrent stenosis after stenting (there have been no cases of this in our series of stent patients) (13).
- Patients who require simultaneous aortic surgery (abdominal aortic aneurysm repair or symptomatic aortoiliac disease). Even in this circumstance it may be advisable to stent the renal artery first and then proceed with aortic reconstruction. The mortality rate of aortic replacement and renal artery revascularization is higher than that of either procedure alone (172).

A variety of surgical revascularization techniques are available for treating patients with significant renal artery disease. These include aortorenal bypass with autogenous saphenous vein (6,134,173–176), polytetrafluoroethylene aortorenal bypass grafts, renal endarterectomy, spleenorenal bypass, hepatorenal saphenous vein bypass, and supraceliac or lower thoracic aorta-to-renal artery saphenous vein bypass. Patients with complex branch renal artery lesions can be managed with extracorporeal microvascular reconstruction and autotransplantation; however, with the use of coronary balloons, this is also not frequently required.

Reports from several large centers have demonstrated that surgical renal revascularization can be performed with operative mortality rates of 2.1% (177), 3.1% (178), 3.4% (179), and 6.1% (180) in patients with atherosclerotic RAS. The mortality rate is increased with bilateral simultaneous renal revascularizations or when renal revascularization is performed with aortic replacement (172,181,182). Most studies have indicated a high technical success rate for surgical vascular reconstruction with postoperative thrombosis or stenosis rates of less than 10% (177). In patients with fibrous dysplasia, 50% to 60% are cured, 30% to 40% are improved, and the failure rate is less than 10% (180,183). In patients undergoing revascularization for atherosclerotic renovascular hypertension the cure rate is lower.

Patient Selection for Intervention to Preserve Renal Function

Patients who are at a markedly increased risk of progressive renal dysfunction are those with greater than 75% bilateral RAS or severe stenosis to a single functioning kidney. In this patient subgroup, the risk of total occlusion of the renal artery is significant, and if this occurs, the clinical outcome is a critical decrease in functioning renal mass with resulting renal failure.

Watson et al. (15) studied 25 patients with bilateral renal artery stenosis or stenosis to a single functioning kidney and showed that in patients undergoing renal artery stenting, the slope of the reciprocal of the serum creatinine became positive (improvement in renal function) in 18 (72%) of the patients and less negative (slowed the progression of renal dysfunction) in the remaining 7 (28%) patients.

The benefit of undertaking revascularization for preservation of renal function in patients with unilateral RAS and a normal contralateral renal artery is not established. If the contralateral kidney is anatomically and functionally normal, revascularization for this purpose is clearly not warranted. If the opposite kidney is functioning but has severe parenchymal disease such as nephrosclerosis, revascularization of the ischemic kidney may be of benefit, but specific indications for this approach are not well defined.

Complete occlusion of the renal artery most often results in irreversible ischemic damage of the involved kidney. However, in some patients with gradual arterial occlusion, the viability of the kidney can be maintained through the development of collateral arterial supply. There are certain clues that may help to predict renal salvageablitity in patients with an occluded renal artery:

- Angiographic demonstration of late filling of the distal renal arterial tree by collateral vessels on the side of total arterial occlusion (184).
- Renal size of 8 to 9 cm.
- Function of the involved kidney on a renal flow scan.
- The presence of a nephrogram after a contrast arteriogram.
- A renal biopsy showing well-preserved glomeruli and an absence of significant glomerulosclerosis.

Some patients may develop acute renal failure shortly after the initiation of antihypertensive therapy (73). Acute renal failure in this setting is often a manifestation of perfusion-dependent renal function due to underlying RAS. Prompt intervention to relieve renal arterial obstruction can prevent permanent renal damage in patients with this type of severe acute renal insufficiency.

The rate of decline in overall renal function is an important determinant of the outcome after intervention in atherosclerotic ischemic renal disease. Dean et al. demonstrated that patients with a rapid deterioration in the glomerular filtration rate during the 6 months preceding surgical revascularization achieved the greatest benefit in terms of postoperative improvement in renal function (65,185).

There are several anecdotal reports showing that restoration of renal function in patients with totally occluded renal arteries with either endovascular therapy or surgical revascularization is feasible. Kaylor et al. (141) reported on 9 patients who were on dialysis from 1 week to 13 months secondary to atherosclerotic RAS. Reversal of end-stage renal failure occurred in all 9 patients with surgical revascularization. The serum creatinine at 1 month ranged from 1.1 to 4.2 mg/dL with a mean of 2.5 mg/dL. Hansen et al. (65) also showed that it is possible to restore renal function with surgical revascularization in some patients who have been on chronic hemodialysis therapy. From 1987 to 1993, 340 patients underwent surgical renal revascularization. Twenty patients were receiving hemodialysis before renal artery repair. Hemodialysis was discontinued in 16 of the 20 patients (80%). Two of the 16 patients resumed dialysis 4 and 6 months after surgery, respectively. A favorable response in this series occurred in those patients who had a relatively rapid decline in their glomerular filtration rate in the 14 weeks preceding renal revascularization. If a rapid decline occurred, there was a statistically significant likelihood of having the patient discontinue treatment. However, if there was a slow decrease in glomerular filtration rate over weeks to months, the chances of becoming dialysis independent were quite small. The long-term survival was better in those who were dialysis independent compared to those who required ongoing dialysis therapy. There were only 2 late deaths among the 14 patients not receiving dialysis, compared to 5 late deaths among the 6 patients who continued to receive dialysis after surgical revascularization ($p < .01$).

Textor (33) reported on 304 patients with renal artery stenosis and a serum creatinine greater than 2.0 mg/dL who underwent surgical revascularization. After a mean follow-up of 3 years, 83 (27.3%) patients demonstrated an improvement in renal function, 160 (50.6%) demonstrated no significant change, and 61 (20.1%) had worsening in renal function.

There are two mechanisms that can explain the worsening in renal function after renal revascularization: (a) The renal artery stenosis was not the cause of the renal impairment; for example if the patient has significant parenchymal renal disease from nephrosclerosis and most of the glomeruli are sclerotic, stenting the main renal artery will not accomplish the goal of improving glomerular filtration; or (b) the procedure itself caused atheromatous embolization, causing accelerated hypertension and progressive renal impairment often leading to end-stage renal disease (5,186). Hiramoto et al. (187) performed an elegant study ex vivo and demonstrated that each manipulation of the renal artery (guidewire passage with a 0.018-inch guidewire, angioplasty with a 3- to 5-mm balloon, and stent implantation with a 5- to 6-mm self-expanding stent) in patients with atherosclerotic renal artery stenosis resulted in the release of "thousands of fragments." This study supports the use of distal protection in an attempt to prevent this devastating complication.

Henry et al. (188) placed a distal protection device in 56 hypertensive patients undergoing renal artery stenting. They used a PercuSurge GuardWire in 38 patients, an EPI filter wire in 26 patients, and an Angioguard device in 1 patient. There were no complications related to the distal protection device, and visible debris was seen in all patients with the PercuSurge device and 80% of patients with one of the filter devices. Holden and Hill (189) retrospectively analyzed 37 patients (46 renal arteries) who underwent renal artery stenting for preservation of renal function using the Angioguard device for distal protection. There was much less renal deterioration in those patients stenting under distal protection compared to a group of patients stented before the availability of a distal protection device.

Revascularization for Control of Congestive Heart Failure or Flash Pulmonary Edema

There have been numerous reports demonstrating that surgical or endovascular revascularization is indicated for the treatment of congestive heart failure or flash pulmonary edema in some patients (13,75,143,190,191). This subgroup of patients most often has significant bilateral RAS or RAS to a single functioning kidney. The left ventricular systolic function may be normal or impaired (13). We reported 39 patients who underwent renal artery stent implantation for control of congestive heart failure (CHF) (13). This represented 19% of our renal artery stent population. In this series, 18 (46%) patients had bilateral RAS and 21 (54%) patients had stenosis to a solitary functioning kidney. Renal artery stent implantation was technically successful in all 39 patients. The blood pressure was improved in 72% of patients. Renal function was improved in 51% and was stable in 26% of patients. As has been reported in other series (33), renal function deteriorated in 23% of patients. The mean number of hospitalizations for CHF before stenting was 2.37 ± 1.42 (range 1 to 6) and after stenting was 0.30 ± 0.065 (range 0 to 3), $p < .001$. Seventy-seven percent of patients had no further hospitalizations after renal artery stenting over a mean follow-up period of 21.3 months. It was anecdotally noted that some patients were unable to be diuresed despite large doses of loop diuretics before stenting. Several patients began diuresing on the catheterization laboratory table immediately after stent placement.

The mechanism by which RAS causes CHF and pulmonary edema is not well defined. The improvement after stenting may in part be related to the ability to use ACEIs, especially for those with impaired left ventricular function and the ability to better control volume.

CONTROVERSIES AND PERSONAL PERSPECTIVES

There have been many advances in the diagnosis of RAS in the last decade. In addition, advances in catheter, balloon, and stent technology have revolutionized the treatment of renal artery disease. Whereas surgical revascularization was the treatment of choice a decade ago, endovascular stent implantation is now used to treat virtually all patients with RAS who require treatment. There is a large body of literature supporting the use of angioplasty and stent implantation for atherosclerotic RAS. However, there is a paucity of randomized, prospective trials comparing renal artery stents with medical therapy and surgical revascularization. There will probably never be a randomized trial comparing stents to surgical bypass because most clinicians now feel that that would not be ethical. Although there is compelling evidence to suggest that stent implantation can improve or at least stabilize renal function in many patients, there remain 15% to 20% of patients in whom renal function deteriorates after percutaneous intervention. Reasons for this deterioration include contrast injury and atheromatous embolization, or perhaps the renal failure was not caused by the RAS per se, but some other etiology, for example, nephrosclerosis. It is often difficult to predict which patients will exhibit a decline in renal function after percutaneous intervention. The Cardiovascular Outcomes in Renal Atherosclerotic Lesions (CORAL) trial is sponsored by the National Heart, Lung, and Blood Institute and is currently recruiting patients. The primary objective of this randomized multicenter study is to compare medical therapy with stenting of hemodynamically significant renal artery stenosis with medical therapy alone in patients with hypertension. The primary composite cardiovascular and renal endpoint is cardiovascular or renal death, myocardial infarction, hospitalization for congestive heart failure, stroke, doubling of the serum creatinine, and need for renal replacement therapy. All patients who are stented will undergo stenting with distal protection. There are a host of secondary endpoints assessing quality of life, health policy perspectives, and cost effectiveness. This is a very ambitious (goal of 1,080 randomized patients) and well-designed trial and will provide critically needed information on the utility of renal artery stenting.

Just because the renal artery obstruction can be corrected safely does not mean that it should be corrected. Despite better balloons, catheters, and stents and better training in endovascular techniques, the temptation to dilate a RAS because it is there should be suppressed. Percutaneous renal intervention should be performed for one of three indications: to better control the blood pressure in patients with suboptimal control despite a good antihypertensive regimen, preserve renal function, and/or treat congestive heart failure.

THE FUTURE

Over the last decade, renal artery angioplasty and stenting have become much safer because of better equipment and more experienced operators. However, renal function does not improve or may even worsen in 15% to 20% of patients undergoing stent implantation, and the blood pressure is not improved in 20% to 50% of patients after intervention. Even though for the first time there will be a large-scale randomized trial (CORAL), it is not designed to primarily assess whether stenting is better than medical therapy for preserving renal function. Two important advances will occur in the future: more accurate ways to predict response to therapy (i.e., identify the patient most likely to demonstrate improvement in blood pressure control and preservation of renal function) and protection of the kidneys during the procedure. The first will occur by measuring such parameters as the resistive index (83,192,193) and functional flow reserve (192–194). The second will occur with emboli protection devices similar to those used in the carotid and coronary circulations (188,189).

References

1. Olin JW, Melia M, Young JR, et al. Prevalence of atherosclerotic renal artery stenosis in patients with atherosclerosis elsewhere. *Am J Med* 1990;88:46N–51N.
2. Harding MB, Smith LR, Himmelstein SI, et al. Renal artery stenosis: prevalence and associated risk factors in patients undergoing routine cardiac catheterization. *J Am Soc Nephrol* 1992;2:1608–1616.
3. Gifford Jr RW. Evaluation of the hypertensive patient with emphasis on detecting curable causes. *Milbank Mem Fund Q* 1969;47:170–186.
4. Safian RD, Textor SC. Renal-artery stenosis. *N Engl J Med* 2001;344: 431–442.
5. Olin JW. Atherosclerotic renal artery disease. *Cardiol Clin* 2002;20:547–562.
6. Novick AC, Ziegelbaum M, Vidt DG, et al. Trends in surgical revascularization for renal artery disease. Ten years' experience. *JAMA* 1987;257: 498–501.
7. Blum U, Krumme B, Flugel P, et al. Treatment of ostial renal-artery stenoses with vascular endoprostheses after unsuccessful balloon angioplasty. *N Engl J Med* 1997;336:459–465.
8. Dorros G, Jaff M, Mathiak L, et al. Four-year follow-up of Palmaz-Schatz stent revascularization as treatment for atherosclerotic renal artery stenosis. *Circulation* 1998;98:642–647.
9. Rimmer JM, Gennari FJ. Atherosclerotic renovascular disease and progressive renal failure. *Ann Intern Med* 1993;118:712–719.
10. Nolan BW, Schermerhorn ML, Rowell E, et al. Outcomes of renal artery angioplasty and stenting using low-profile systems. *J Vasc Surg* 2005;41: 46–52.
11. Rocha-Singh K, Jaff MR, Rosenfield K. Evaluation of the safety and effectiveness of renal artery stenting after unsuccessful balloon angioplasty: the ASPIRE-2 study. *J Am Coll Cardiol* 2005;46:776–783.
12. Sivamurthy N, Surowiec SM, Culakova E, et al. Divergent outcomes after percutaneous therapy for symptomatic renal artery stenosis. *J Vasc Surg* 2004;39:565–574.
13. Gray BH, Olin JW, Childs MB, et al. Clinical benefit of renal artery angioplasty with stenting for the control of recurrent and refractory congestive heart failure. *Vasc Med* 2002;7:275–279.
14. Rundback JH, Gray RJ, Rozenblit G, et al. Renal artery stent placement for the management of ischemic nephropathy. *J Vasc Interv Radiol* 1998; 9:413–420.

15. Watson PS, Hadjipetrou P, Cox SV, et al. Effect of renal artery stenting on renal function and size in patients with atherosclerotic renovascular disease. *Circulation* 2000;102:1671–1677.
16. Goldblatt H, Lynch J, Hanzal RF, Summerville WW. Studies in experimental hypertension. I. The production of a persistent elevation of systolic blood pressure by means of renal ischemia. *J Exp Med* 1934;59:347–379.
17. Page IH, Helmer OM. Crystalline pressor substance (angiotonin) resulting from the reaction between renin and renin activator. *J Exp Med* 1940; 71:29–42.
18. Skeggs LT, Marsch WH, Kahn JR, Shumway NP. The purification of hypertensin. *J Exp Med* 1954;100:363–370.
19. Pickering TG. Renal artery disease. In: Topol EJ, Califf RM, eds. *Textbook of cardiovascular medicine*. Philadelphia: Lippincott Raven, 1997:2623–2641.
20. Hirsch AT, Haskal ZJ, Hertzer NR, et al. ACC/AHA guidelines for the management of patients with peripheral arterial disease (lower extremity, renal, mesenteric, and abdominal aortic): A collaborative report from the American Association of Vascular Surgery/Society for Vascular Surgery, Society for Cardiovascular Angiography and Interventions, Society for Interventional Radiology, Society for Vascular Medicine and Biology and the American College of Cardiology/American Heart Association Task Force on Practice Guidelines. *J Am Coll Cardiol* 2006;47:1239–1312.
21. Textor SC, Wilcox CS. Ischemic nephropathy/azotemic renovascular disease. *Semin Nephrol* 2000;20:489–502.
22. Brunner HR, Kirshman JD, Sealey JE, Laragh JH. Hypertension of renal origin: evidence for two different mechanisms. *Science* 1971;174:1344–1346.
23. Gavras H, Brunner HR, Thurston H, Laragh JH. Reciprocation of renin dependency with sodium volume dependency in renal hypertension. *Science* 1975;188:1316–1317.
24. Gavras H, Brunner HB, Vaughan ED, Laragh JH. Angiotensin–sodium interaction in blood pressure maintenance of renal hypertensive and normotensive rats. *Science* 1973;180:1369–1371.
25. Swales JD, Thurston H, Queiroz FP, et al. Dual mechanism for experimental hypertension. *Lancet* 1971;2:1181–1184.
26. Olin JW, Novick AC. Renovascular disease. In: Young JR, Olin JW, Bartholomew JR, eds. *Peripheral vascular diseases*. St. Louis: Mosby, 1996: 321–342.
27. Gross F. The renin–angiotensin system and hypertension. *Ann Intern Med* 1971;75:777–787.
28. Bengis RG, Coleman TG. Antihypertensive effect of prolonged blockade of angiotensin formation in benign and malignant, one- and two-kidney Goldblatt hypertensive rats. *Clin Sci* (London) 1979;57:53–62.
29. Vaughan Jr ED, Buhler FR, Laragh JH, et al. Renovascular hypertension: renin measurements to indicate hypersecretion and contralateral suppression, estimate renal plasma flow, and score for surgical curability. *Am J Med* 1973;55:402–414.
30. Rostand SG, Lewis D, Watkins JB, et al. Attenuated pressure natriuresis in hypertensive rats. *Kidney Int* 1982;21:331–338.
31. Textor SC, Wilcox CS. Renal artery stenosis: a common, treatable cause of renal failure? *Annu Rev Med* 2001;52:421–442.
32. Textor SC. Renal failure related to ACE inhibitors. *Semin Nephrol* 1997; 17:67–76.
33. Textor SC. Ischemic nephropathy: where are we now? *J Am Soc Nephrol* 2004;15:1974–1982.
34. Packer M, Lee WH, Medina N, et al. Functional renal insufficiency during long-term therapy with captopril and enalapril in severe chronic heart failure. *Ann Intern Med* 1987;106:346–354.
35. Textor SC, Tarazi RC, Novick AC, et al. Regulation of renal hemodynamics and glomerular filtration in patients with renovascular hypertension during converting enzyme inhibition with captopril. *Am J Med* 1984;76:29–37.
36. Watson ML, Bell GM, Muir AL, et al. Captopril/diuretic combinations in severe renovascular disease: a cautionary note. *Lancet* 1983;2:404–405.
37. Hricik DE, Browning PJ, Kopelman R, et al. Captopril-induced functional renal insufficiency in patients with bilateral renal-artery stenoses or renal-artery stenosis in a solitary kidney. *N Engl J Med* 1983;308:373–376.
38. Shanley PF. The pathology of chronic renal ischemia. *Semin Nephrol* 1996;16:21–32.
39. Vidt DG, Eisele G, Gephardt GN, et al. Atheroembolic renal disease: association with renal arterial stenosis. *Cleve Clin J Med* 1989;56:407–413.
40. Eng E, Veniant M, Floege J, et al. Renal proliferative and phenotypic changes in rats with two-kidney, one-clip Goldblatt hypertension. *Am J Hypertens* 1994;7:177–185.
41. Slovut DP, Olin JW. Fibromuscular dysplasia. *N Engl J Med* 2004;350: 1862–1871.
42. Begelman SM, Olin JW. Fibromuscular dysplasia. *Curr Opin Rheumatol* 2000;12:41–47.
43. Luscher TF, Keller HM, Imhof HG, et al. Fibromuscular hyperplasia: extension of the disease and therapeutic outcome. Results of the University Hospital Zurich Cooperative Study on Fibromuscular Hyperplasia. *Nephron* 1986;44:109–114.
44. Slovut DP, Olin JW. Fibromuscular dysplasia. *Curr Treat Options Cardiovasc Med* 2005;7:159–169.
45. Harrison Jr EG, McCormack LJ. Pathologic classification of renal arterial disease in renovascular hypertension. *Mayo Clin Proc* 1971;46:161–167.
46. Begelman SM, Olin JW. Fibromuscular dysplasia. *Curr Opin Rheumatol* 2000;12:41–47.
47. Kennedy DJ, Colyer WR, Brewster PS, et al. Renal insufficiency as a predictor of adverse events and mortality after renal artery stent placement. *Am J Kidney Dis* 2003;42:926–935.
48. Connolly JO, Higgins RM, Walters HL, et al. Presentation, clinical features and outcome in different patterns of atherosclerotic renovascular disease. *QJM* 1994;87:413–421.
49. Mailloux LU, Napolitano B, Bellucci AG, et al. Renal vascular disease causing end-stage renal disease, incidence, clinical correlates, and outcomes: a 20-year clinical experience. *Am J Kidney Dis* 1994;24:622–629.
50. Mailloux LU, Bellucci AG, Napolitano B, et al. Survival estimates for 683 patients starting dialysis from 1970 through 1989: identification of risk factors for survival. *Clin Nephrol* 1994;42:127–135.
51. Dustan HP, Humphries AW, DeWolfe VG, et al. Normal arterial pressure in patients with renal arterial stenosis. *JAMA* 1964;187:1028–1029.
52. Hansen KJ, Edwards MS, Craven TE, et al. Prevalence of renovascular disease in the elderly: a population-based study. *J Vasc Surg* 2002;36:443–451.
53. Scoble JE. The epidemiology and clinical manifestations of atherosclerotic renal artery disease. In: Novick AC, Scoble J, Hamilton G, eds. *Renal vascular disease*. London: WB Saunders, 1996:303–314.
54. Conlon PJ, Little MA, Pieper K, Mark DB. Severity of renal vascular disease predicts mortality in patients undergoing coronary angiography. *Kidney Int* 2001;60:1490–1497.
55. Rihal CS, Textor SC, Breen JF, et al. Incidental renal artery stenosis among a prospective cohort of hypertensive patients undergoing coronary angiography. *Mayo Clin Proc* 2002;77:309–316.
56. Schreiber MJ, Pohl MA, Novick AC. The natural history of atherosclerotic and fibrous renal artery disease. *Urol Clin North Am* 1984;11:383–392.
57. Zierler RE, Bergelin RO, Davidson RC, et al. A prospective study of disease progression in patients with atherosclerotic renal artery stenosis. *Am J Hypertens* 1996;9:1055–1061.
58. Zierler RE, Bergelin RO, Isaacson JA, Strandness Jr DE. Natural history of atherosclerotic renal artery stenosis: a prospective study with duplex ultrasonography. *J Vasc Surg* 1994;19:250–257.
59. Caps MT, Zierler RE, Polissar NL, et al. Risk of atrophy in kidneys with atherosclerotic renal artery stenosis. *Kidney Int* 1998;53:735–742.
60. Guzman RP, Zierler RE, Isaacson JA, et al. Renal atrophy and arterial stenosis. A prospective study with duplex ultrasound. *Hypertension* 1994; 23:346–350.
61. Scoble JE, Maher ER, Hamilton G. Atherosclerotic renovascular disease causing renal impairment—a case for treatment. *Clin Nephrol* 1989; 31:119–122.
62. van Ampting JM, Penne EL, Beek FJ, et al. Prevalence of atherosclerotic renal artery stenosis in patients starting dialysis. *Nephrol Dial Transplant* 2003;18:1147–1151.
63. Vachharajani TJ, Dacie JE, Yaqoob MM, et al. Detection of occult renovascular disease in unexplained chronic kidney disease. *Int Urol Nephrol* 2005;37:793–796.
64. O'Neil EA, Hansen KJ, Canzanello VJ, et al. Prevalence of ischemic nephropathy in patients with renal insufficiency. *Am Surg* 1992;58:485–490.
65. Hansen KJ, Cherr GS, Dean RH. Dialysis-free survival after surgical repair of ischemic nephropathy. *Cardiovasc Surg* 2002;10:400–404.
66. Eggers PW, Connerton R, McMullan M. The Medicare experience with end stage renal disease: Trends and incidence, prevalence and survival. *Health Care Finance Rev* 1984;5:69–88.
67. National Institutes of Health, National Institutes of Diabetes and Digestive Diseases. *USRDS 1993 annual data report*. Bethesda, MD: Author, 1993.
68. Chobanian AV, Bakris GL, Black HR, et al. The seventh report of the Joint National Committee on Prevention, Detection, Evaluation, and Treatment of High Blood Pressure: the JNC 7 Report. *JAMA* 2003;289:2560–2571.
69. Olin JW. Evaluation of the peripheral circulation. In: Izzo JL, Black HR, eds. *Hypertension primer*. Dallas, TX: American Heart Association, 2003: 361–365.
70. Eipper DF, Gifford Jr RW, Stewart B, et al. Abdominal bruits in renovascular hypertension. *Am J Cardiol* 1976;37:48–52.
71. Gifford Jr RW, McCormack LJ, Poutasse EF. The atrophic kidney: its role in hypertension. *Mayo Clin Proc* 1965;40:852.
72. Carman TL, Olin JW, Czum J. Noninvasive imaging of the renal arteries. *Urol Clin North Am* 2001;28:815–826.
73. Textor SC, Novick AC, Steinmuller DR, Streem SB. Renal failure limiting antihypertensive therapy as an indication for renal revascularization. A case report. *Arch Intern Med* 1983;143:2208–2211.
74. Silas JH, Klenka Z, Solomon SA, Bone JM. Captopril induced reversible renal failure: a marker of renal artery stenosis affecting a solitary kidney. *Br Med J (Clin Res Ed)* 1983;286:1702–1703.
75. Pickering TG, Herman L, Devereux RB, et al. Recurrent pulmonary oedema in hypertension due to bilateral renal artery stenosis: treatment by angioplasty or surgical revascularisation. *Lancet* 1988;2:551–552.
76. Carman TL, Olin JW. Diagnosis of renal artery stenosis: what is the optimal diagnostic test? *Curr Interv Cardiol Rep* 2000;2:111–118.
77. Olin JW, Kaufman JA, Bluemke DA, et al. Atherosclerotic Vascular Disease Conference. American Heart Association, Imaging, Writing Group IV. *Circulation* 2004;109:2626–2633.

78. Spinosa DJ, Matsumoto AH, Angle JF, et al. Renal insufficiency: usefulness of gadodiamide-enhanced renal angiography to supplement CO2-enhanced renal angiography for diagnosis and percutaneous treatment. *Radiology* 1999;210:663–672.
79. Spinosa DJ, Matsumoto AH, Angle JF, Hagspiel KD. Use of gadopentetate dimeglumine as a contrast agent for percutaneous transluminal renal angioplasty and stent placement. *Kidney Int* 1998;53:503–507.
80. Caridi JG, Stavropoulos SW, Hawkins Jr IF. Carbon dioxide digital subtraction angiography for renal artery stent placement. *J Vasc Interv Radiol* 1999;10:635–640.
81. White CJ. The renal oculosten(t)otic reflex. *Cathet Cardiovasc Diagn* 1996; 37:251.
82. Axelrod DA, Fendrick AM, Birkmeyer JD, et al. Cardiologists performing peripheral angioplasties: impact on utilization. *Eff Clin Pract* 2001;4:191–198.
83. Radermacher J, Weinkove R, Haller H. Techniques for predicting a favourable response to renal angioplasty in patients with renovascular disease. *Curr Opin Nephrol Hypertens* 2001;10:799–805.
84. Radermacher J, Chavan A, Bleck J, et al. Use of Doppler ultrasonography to predict the outcome of therapy for renal-artery stenosis. *N Engl J Med* 2001;344:410–417.
85. Olin JW. Role of duplex ultrasonography in screening for significant renal artery disease. *Urol Clin North Am* 1994;21:215–226.
86. Coen G, Calabria S, Lai S, et al. Atherosclerotic ischemic renal disease. Diagnosis and prevalence in an hypertensive and/or uremic elderly population. *BMC Nephrol* 2003;4:2.
87. Hansen KJ, Tribble RW, Reavis SW, et al. Renal duplex sonography: evaluation of clinical utility. *J Vasc Surg* 1990;12:227–236.
88. Hoffmann U, Edwards JM, Carter S, et al. Role of duplex scanning for the detection of atherosclerotic renal artery disease. *Kidney Int* 1991;39: 1232–1239.
89. Kohler TR, Zierler RE, Martin RL, et al. Noninvasive diagnosis of renal artery stenosis by ultrasonic duplex scanning. *J Vasc Surg* 1986;4:450–456.
90. Miralles M, Cairols M, Cotillas J, et al. Value of Doppler parameters in the diagnosis of renal artery stenosis. *J Vasc Surg* 1996;23:428–435.
91. Olin JW, Piedmonte MR, Young JR, et al. The utility of duplex ultrasound scanning of the renal arteries for diagnosing significant renal artery stenosis. *Ann Intern Med* 1995;122:833–838.
92. Radermacher J, Ellis S, Haller H. Renal resistance index and progression of renal disease. *Hypertension* 2002;39:699–703.
93. Radermacher J, Chavan A, Schaffer J, et al. Detection of significant renal artery stenosis with color Doppler sonography: combining extrarenal and intrarenal approaches to minimize technical failure. *Clin Nephrol* 2000; 53:333–343.
94. Zeller T, Frank U, Muller C, et al. Predictors of improved renal function after percutaneous stent-supported angioplasty of severe atherosclerotic ostial renal artery stenosis. *Circulation* 2003;108:2244–2249.
95. Garcia-Criado A, Gilabert R, Nicolau C, et al. Value of Doppler sonography for predicting clinical outcome after renal artery revascularization in atherosclerotic renal artery stenosis. *J Ultrasound Med* 2005;24:1641–1647.
96. Hudspeth DA, Hansen KJ, Reavis SW, et al. Renal duplex sonography after treatment of renovascular disease. *J Vasc Surg* 1993;18:381–388.
97. Morvay Z, Nagy E, Bagi R, et al. Sonographic follow-up after visceral artery stenting. *J Ultrasound Med* 2004;23:1057–1064.
98. Rubin GD. Techniques for performing multidetector-row computed tomographic angiography. *Tech Vasc Interv Radiol* 2001;4:2–14.
99. Addis KA, Hopper KD, Iyriboz TA, et al. CT angiography: in vitro comparison of five reconstruction methods. *AJR Am J Roentgenol* 2001;177:1171–1176.
100. Rubin GD, Alfrey EJ, Dake MD, et al. Assessment of living renal donors with spiral CT. *Radiology* 1995;195:457–462.
101. Rubin GD, Walker PJ, Dake MD, et al. Three-dimensional spiral computed tomographic angiography: an alternative imaging modality for the abdominal aorta and its branches. *J Vasc Surg* 1993;18:656–664.
102. Urban BA, Ratner LE, Fishman EK. Three-dimensional volume-rendered CT angiography of the renal arteries and veins: normal anatomy, variants, and clinical applications. *Radiographics* 2001;21:373–386.
103. Beregi JP, Elkohen M, Deklunder G, et al. Helical CT angiography compared with arteriography in the detection of renal artery stenosis. *AJR Am J Roentgenol* 1996;167:495–501.
104. Mounier-Vehier C, Lions C, Jaboureck O, et al. Parenchymal consequences of fibromuscular dysplasia renal artery stenosis. *Am J Kidney Dis* 2002;40:1138–1145.
105. Johnson PT, Halpern EJ, Kuszyk BS, et al. Renal artery stenosis: CT angiography—comparison of real-time volume-rendering and maximum intensity projection algorithms. *Radiology* 1999;211:337–343.
106. Willmann JK, Wildermuth S, Pfammatter T, et al. Aortoiliac and renal arteries: prospective intraindividual comparison of contrast-enhanced three-dimensional MR angiography and multi-detector row CT angiography. *Radiology* 2003;226:798–811.
107. Kawashima A, Sandler CM, Ernst RD, et al. CT evaluation of renovascular disease. *Radiographics* 2000;20:1321–1340.
108. Bucek RA, Puchner S, Reiter M, et al. Multidetector CT angiography with perfusion analysis in the surveillance of renal artery stents. *J Endovasc Ther* 2004;11:139–143.
109. Willoteaux S, Negawi Z, Lions C, et al. Observations from multidetector CT imaging of different types of renal artery stents. *J Endovasc Ther* 2004;11:560–569.
110. Raza SA, Chughtai AR, Wahba M, et al. Multislice CT angiography in renal artery stent evaluation: prospective comparison with intra-arterial digital subtraction angiography. *Cardiovasc Interv Radiol* 2004;27:9–15.
111. Snidow JJ, Johnson MS, Harris VJ, et al. Three-dimensional gadolinium-enhanced MR angiography for aortoiliac inflow assessment plus renal artery screening in a single breath hold. *Radiology* 1996;198:725–732.
112. Hany TF, Debatin JF, Leung DA, Pfammatter T. Evaluation of the aortoiliac and renal arteries: comparison of breath-hold, contrast-enhanced, three-dimensional MR angiography with conventional catheter angiography. *Radiology* 1997;204:357–362.
113. De Cobelli F, Vanzulli A, Sironi S, et al. Renal artery stenosis: evaluation with breath-hold, three-dimensional, dynamic, gadolinium-enhanced versus three-dimensional, phase-contrast MR angiography. *Radiology* 1997; 205:689–695.
114. De Cobelli F, Venturini M, Vanzulli A, et al. Renal arterial stenosis: prospective comparison of color Doppler US and breath-hold, three-dimensional, dynamic, gadolinium-enhanced MR angiography. *Radiology* 2000;214:373–380.
115. Rieumont MJ, Kaufman JA, Geller SC, et al. Evaluation of renal artery stenosis with dynamic gadolinium-enhanced MR angiography. *AJR Am J Roentgenol* 1997;169:39–44.
116. Bakker J, Beek FJ, Beutler JJ, et al. Renal artery stenosis and accessory renal arteries: accuracy of detection and visualization with gadolinium-enhanced breath-hold MR angiography. *Radiology* 1998;207:497–504.
117. Schoenberg SO, Rieger J, Johannson LO, et al. Diagnosis of renal artery stenosis with magnetic resonance angiography: update 2003. *Nephrol Dial Transplant* 2003;18:1252–1256.
118. Hahn U, Miller S, Nagele T, et al.Renal MR angiography at 1.0 T: three-dimensional (3D) phase-contrast techniques versus gadolinium-enhanced 3D fast low-angle shot breath-hold imaging. *AJR Am J Roentgenol* 1999; 172:1501–1508.
119. Fain SB, King BF, Breen JF, et al. High-spatial-resolution contrast-enhanced MR angiography of the renal arteries: a prospective comparison with digital subtraction angiography. *Radiology* 2001;218:481–490.
120. Saloner D. Determinants of image appearance in contrast-enhanced magnetic resonance angiography: a review. *Invest Radiol* 1998;33:488–495.
121. Thornton J, O'Callaghan J, Walshe J, et al. Comparison of digital subtraction angiography with gadolinium-enhanced magnetic resonance angiography in the diagnosis of renal artery stenosis. *Eur Radiol* 1999;9:930–934.
122. Tan KT, van Beek EJR, Brown PWG, et al. Magnetic resonance angiography for the diagnosis of renal artery stenosis: a meta—analysis. *Clin Radiol* 2002;57:617–624.
123. Vasbinder GB, Nelemans PJ, Kessels AG, et al. Accuracy of computed tomographic angiography and magnetic resonance angiography for diagnosing renal artery stenosis. *Ann Intern Med* 2004;141:674–682.
124. Schoenberg SO, Knopp MV, Londy F, et al. Morphologic and functional magnetic resonance imaging of renal artery stenosis: a multireader tricenter study. *J Am Soc Nephrol* 2002;13:158–169.
125. Buecker A, Spuentrup E, Ruebben A, et al. New metallic MR stents for artifact-free coronary MR angiography: feasibility study in a swine model. *Invest Radiol* 2004;39:250–253.
126. Yang X, Bolster Jr BD, Kraitchman DL, Atalar E. Intravascular MR-monitored balloon angioplasty: an in vivo feasibility study. *J Vasc Interv Radiol* 1998;9:953–959.
127. Buecker A, Neuerburg JM, Adam GB, et al. Real-time MR fluoroscopy for MR-guided iliac artery stent placement. *J Magn Reson Imaging* 2000;12: 616–622.
128. Thornbury JR, Stanley JC, Fryback DG. Hypertensive urogram: a nondiscriminatory test for renovascular hypertension. *AJR Am J Roentgenol* 1982; 138:43–49.
129. Maxwell MH, Marks LS, Lupu AN, et al. Predictive value of renin determinations in renal artery stenosis. *JAMA* 1977;238:2617–2620.
130. Muller FB, Sealey JE, Case DB, et al. The captopril test for identifying renovascular disease in hypertensive patients. *Am J Med* 1986;80:633–644.
131. Maxwell MH, Rudnick MR, Waks AU. New approaches to the diagnosis of renovascular hypertension. *Adv Nephrol Necker Hosp* 1985;14:285–304.
132. Hughes JS, Dove HG, Gifford Jr RW, Feinstein AR. Duration of blood pressure elevation in accurately predicting surgical cure of renovascular hypertension. *Am Heart J* 1981;101:408–413.
133. Pickering TG, Sos TA, James GD, et al. Comparison of renal vein renin activity in hypertensive patients with stenosis of one or both renal arteries. *J Hypertens Suppl* 1985;3:S291–S293.
134. Novick AC, Straffon RA, Stewart BH, et al. Diminished operative morbidity and mortality in renal revascularization. *JAMA* 1981;246:749–753.
135. Olin JW, Vidt DG, Gifford Jr RW, Novick AC. Renovascular disease in the elderly: an analysis of 50 patients. *J Am Coll Cardiol* 1985;5:1232–1238.
136. Rossi GP, Cesari M, Chiesura-Corona M, et al. Renal vein renin measurements accurately identify renovascular hypertension caused by total occlusion of the renal artery. *J Hypertens* 2002;20:975–984.
137. Nally Jr JV. Provocative captopril testing in the diagnosis of renovascular hypertension. *Urol Clin North Am* 1994;21:227–234.
138. Nally Jr JV. Renal physiology of renal artery stenosis. Implications for captopril-stimulated renography. *Am J Hypertens* 1991;4:669S–674S.

139. Prigent A. The diagnosis of renovascular hypertension: the role of captopril renal scintigraphy and related issues. *Eur J Nucl Med* 1993;20:625–644.
140. Prigent A, Cosgriff P, Gates GF, et al. Consensus report on quality control of quantitative measurements of renal function obtained from the renogram: International Consensus Committee from the Scientific Committee of Radionuclides in Nephrourology. *Semin Nucl Med* 1999;29:146–159.
141. Kaylor WM, Novick AC, Ziegelbaum M, Vidt DG. Reversal of end stage renal failure with surgical revascularization in patients with atherosclerotic renal artery occlusion. *J Urol* 1989;141:486–488.
142. Hansen KJ, Thomason RB, Craven TE, et al. Surgical management of dialysis-dependent ischemic nephropathy. *J Vasc Surg* 1995;21:197–209.
143. Diamond JR. Flash pulmonary edema and the diagnostic suspicion of occult renal artery stenosis. *Am J Kidney Dis* 1993;21:328–330.
144. Juknevicius I, Segal Y, Kren S, et al. Effect of aldosterone on renal transforming growth factor-beta. *Am J Physiol Renal Physiol* 2004;286: F1059–F1062.
145. Garovic VD, Textor SC. Renovascular hypertension and ischemic nephropathy. *Circulation* 2005;112:1362–1374.
146. Yusuf S, Sleight P, Pogue J, et al. Effects of an angiotensin-converting-enzyme inhibitor, ramipril, on cardiovascular events in high-risk patients. The Heart Outcomes Prevention Evaluation Study Investigators. *N Engl J Med* 2000;342:145–153.
147. Losito A, Gaburri M, Errico R, et al. Survival of patients with renovascular disease and ACE inhibition. *Clin Nephrol* 1999;52:339–343.
148. Olin JW, Begelman SM. Renal artery disease. In: Topol E, ed. *Textbook of cardiovascular medicine*. Philadelphia: Lippincott Raven, 2002:2139–2159.
149. Gruntzig A, Kuhlmann U, Vetter W, et al. Treatment of renovascular hypertension with percutaneous transluminal dilatation of a renal-artery stenosis. *Lancet* 1978;1:801–802.
150. Olin JW, Begelman SM. Renal artery stenosis. *Curr Treat Options Cardiovasc Med* 1999;1:55–62.
151. Sos TA, Pickering TG, Sniderman K, et al. Percutaneous transluminal renal angioplasty in renovascular hypertension due to atheroma or fibromuscular dysplasia. *N Engl J Med* 1983;309:274–279.
152. Ramsay LE, Waller PC. Blood pressure response to percutaneous transluminal angioplasty for renovascular hypertension: an overview of published series. *BMJ* 1990;300:569–572.
153. Cluzel P, Raynaud A, Beyssen B, et al. Stenoses of renal branch arteries in fibromuscular dysplasia: results of percutaneous transluminal angioplasty. *Radiology* 1994;193:227–232.
154. Alhadad A, Mattiasson I, Ivancev K, et al. Revascularisation of renal artery stenosis caused by fibromuscular dysplasia: effects on blood pressure during 7-year follow-up are influenced by duration of hypertension and branch artery stenosis. *J Hum Hypertens* 2005;19:761–767.
155. Bonelli FS, McKusick MA, Textor SC, et al. Renal artery angioplasty: technical results and clinical outcome in 320 patients. *Mayo Clin Proc* 1995;70:1041–1052.
156. Plouin PF, Chatellier G, Darne B, Raynaud A. Blood pressure outcome of angioplasty in atherosclerotic renal artery stenosis: a randomized trial. Essai Multicentrique Medicaments vs Angioplastie (EMMA) Study Group. *Hypertension* 1998;31:823–829.
157. Webster J, Marshall F, Abdalla M, et al. Randomised comparison of percutaneous angioplasty vs continued medical therapy for hypertensive patients with atheromatous renal artery stenosis. Scottish and Newcastle Renal Artery Stenosis Collaborative Group. *J Hum Hypertens* 1998;12:329–335.
158. van Jaarsveld BC, Krijnen P, Pieterman H, et al. The effect of balloon angioplasty on hypertension in atherosclerotic renal-artery stenosis. Dutch Renal Artery Stenosis Intervention Cooperative Study Group. *N Engl J Med* 2000;342:1007–1014.
159. Tan WA, Wholey MH, Olin JW. The effect of balloon angioplasty on hypertension in atherosclerotic renal-artery stenosis. *N Engl J Med* 2000;343: 438.
160. Safian RD, Textor SC. Renal-artery stenosis. *N Engl J Med* 2001;344: 431–442.
161. Plouin PF, Darne B, Chatellier G, et al. Restenosis after a first percutaneous transluminal renal angioplasty. *Hypertension* 1993;21:89–96.
162. Olin JW. Renal artery disease: diagnosis and management. *Mt Sinai J Med* 2004;71:73–85.
163. Rundback JH, Sacks D, Kent KC, et al. Guidelines for the reporting of renal artery revascularization in clinical trials. *J Vasc Interv Radiol* 2002; 13:959–974.
164. White CJ, Ramee SR, Collins TJ, et al. Renal artery stent placement: utility in lesions difficult to treat with balloon angioplasty. *J Am Coll Cardiol* 1997;30:1445–1450.
165. Dorros G, Jaff M, Mathiak L, He T. Multicenter Palmaz stent renal artery stenosis revascularization registry report: four-year follow-up of 1,058 successful patients. *Catheter Cardiovasc Interv* 2002;55:182–188.
166. van de Ven PJ, Kaatee R, Beutler JJ, et al. Arterial stenting and balloon angioplasty in ostial atherosclerotic renovascular disease: a randomised trial. *Lancet* 1999;353:282–286.
167. Baumgartner I, von Aesch K, Do DD, et al. Stent placement in ostial and nonostial atherosclerotic renal arterial stenoses: a prospective follow-up study. *Radiology* 2000;216:498–505.
168. Leertouwer TC, Gussenhoven EJ, Bosch JL, et al. Stent placement for renal arterial stenosis: where do we stand? A meta-analysis. *Radiology* 2000;216:78–85.
169. Harden PN, Macleod MJ, Rodger RS, et al. Effect of renal-artery stenting on progression of renovascular renal failure. *Lancet* 1997;349:1133–1136.
170. Korsakas S, Mohaupt MG, Dinkel HP, et al. Delay of dialysis in end-stage renal failure: prospective study on percutaneous renal artery interventions. *Kidney Int* 2004;65:251–258.
171. Silva JA, Chan AW, White CJ. Elevated brain natriuretic peptide predicts blood pressure response after stent revascularization in patients with renal artery stenosis. *Perspect Vasc Surg Endovasc Ther* 2005;17:375.
172. Tarazi RY, Hertzer NR, Beven EG, et al. Simultaneous aortic reconstruction and renal revascularization: risk factors and late results in eighty-nine patients. *J Vasc Surg* 1987;5:707–714.
173. Novick AC. Management of renovascular disease. A surgical perspective. *Circulation* 1991;83:I167–I171.
174. Novick AC, Stewart R, Hodge EE, Goldfarb D. Use of the thoracic aorta for renal arterial reconstruction. *J Vasc Surg* 1994;19:605–609.
175. Novick AC, Palleschi J, Straffon RA, Beven E. Experimental and clinical hepatorenal bypass as a means of revascularization of the right renal artery. *Surg Gynecol Obstet* 1979;148:557–561.
176. Novick AC, Banowsky LH, Stewart BH, Straffon RA. Splenorenal bypass in the treatment of renal artery stenosis. *Trans Am Assoc Genitourin Surg* 1977;69:139–145.
177. Novick AC, Ziegelbaum M, Vidt DG, et al. Trends in surgical revascularization for renal artery disease. Ten years' experience. *JAMA* 1987;257: 498–501.
178. Hansen KJ, Starr SM, Sands RE, et al. Contemporary surgical management of renovascular disease. *J Vasc Surg* 1992;16:319–330.
179. Bredenberg CE, Sampson LN, Ray FS, et al. Changing patterns in surgery for chronic renal artery occlusive diseases. *J Vasc Surg* 1992;15:1018–1023.
180. Libertino JA, Bosco PJ, Ying CY et al. Renal revascularization to preserve and restore renal function. *J Urol* 1992;147:1485–1487.
181. Lawrie GM, Morris Jr GC, Glaeser DH, DeBakey ME. Renovascular reconstruction: factors affecting long-term prognosis in 919 patients followed up to 31 years. *Am J Cardiol* 1989;63:1085–1092.
182. Hallett Jr JW, Fowl R, O'Brien PC, et al. Renovascular operations in patients with chronic renal insufficiency: do the benefits justify the risks? *J Vasc Surg* 1987;5:622–627.
183. Ernst CB, Stanley JC, Marshall FF, Fry WJ. Autogenous saphenous vein aortorenal grafts. A ten-year experience. *Arch Surg* 1972;105:855–864.
184. Olin JW, Graor RA, Young JR. Thrombolytic therapy for renal artery occlusions: a preliminary report. *Cleve Clin J Med* 1989;56:432–438.
185. Dean RH, Tribble RW, Hansen KJ, et al. Evolution of renal insufficiency in ischemic nephropathy. *Ann Surg* 1991;213:446–455.
186. Rose R, Bartholomew JR, Olin JW. Atheromatous embolization syndrome. In: Rutherford RB, ed. *Vascular surgery*, 6th edition. Philadelphia: WB Saunders, 2005;986–999.
187. Hiramoto J, Hansen KJ, Pan XM, et al. Atheroemboli during renal artery angioplasty: an ex vivo study. *J Vasc Surg* 2005;41:1026–1030.
188. Henry M, Henry I, Klonaris C, et al. Renal angioplasty and stenting under protection: the way for the future? *Catheter Cardiovasc Interv* 2003; 60:299–312.
189. Holden A, Hill A. Renal angioplasty and stenting with distal protection of the main renal artery in ischemic nephropathy: early experience. *J Vasc Surg* 2003;38:962–968.
190. Bloch MJ, Trost DW, Pickering TG, et al. Prevention of recurrent pulmonary edema in patients with bilateral renovascular disease through renal artery stent placement. *Am J Hypertens* 1999;12:1–7.
191. Messina LM, Zelenock GB, Yao KA, Stanley JC. Renal revascularization for recurrent pulmonary edema in patients with poorly controlled hypertension and renal insufficiency: a distinct subgroup of patients with arteriosclerotic renal artery occlusive disease. *J Vasc Surg* 1992;15:73–80.
192. Subramanian R, White CJ, Rosenfield K, et al. Renal fractional flow reserve: a hemodynamic evaluation of moderate renal artery stenoses. *Catheter Cardiovasc Interv* 2005;64:480–486.
193. Slovut DP, Lookstein R, Bacharach JM, Olin JW. Correlation between noninvasive and endovascular Doppler in patients with atherosclerotic renal artery stenosis: a pilot study. *Catheter Cardiovasc Interv* 2006;67:426–433.
194. Mounier-Vehier C, Cocheteux B, Haulon S, et al. Changes in renal blood flow reserve after angioplasty of renal artery stenosis in hypertensive patients. *Kidney Int* 2004;65:245–250.
195. Baert AL, Wilms G, Amery A, et al. Percutaneous transluminal renal angioplasty: initial results and long-term follow-up in 202 patients. *Cardiovasc Interv Radiol* 1990;13:22–28.
196. Birrer M, Do DD, Mahler F, et al. Treatment of renal artery fibromuscular dysplasia with balloon angioplasty: a prospective follow-up study. *Eur J Vasc Endovasc Surg* 2002;23:146–152.
197. Boisclair C, Therasse E, Oliva VL, et al. Treatment of renal angioplasty failure by percutaneous renal artery stenting with Palmaz stents: midterm technical and clinical results. *AJR Am J Roentgenol* 1997;168:245–251.
198. Davidson RA, Barri Y, Wilcox CS. Predictors of cure of hypertension in fibromuscular renovascular disease. *Am J Kidney Dis* 1996;28:334–338.
199. De Fraissinette B, Garcier JM, Dieu V, et al. Percutaneous transluminal angioplasty of dysplastic stenoses of the renal artery: results on 70 adults. *Cardiovasc Intervent Radiol* 2003;26:46–51.

200. Hennequin LM, Joffre FG, Rousseau HP, et al. Renal artery stent placement: long-term results with the Wallstent endoprosthesis. *Radiology* 1994; 191:713–719.
201. Henry M, Amor M, Henry I, et al. Stents in the treatment of renal artery stenosis: long-term follow-up. *J Endovasc Surg* 1999;6:42–51.
202. Iannone LA, Underwood PL, Nath A, et al. Effect of primary balloon expandable renal artery stents on long-term patency, renal function, and blood pressure in hypertensive and renal insufficient patients with renal artery stenosis. *Cathet Cardiovasc Diagn* 1996;37:243–250.
203. Jensen G, Zachrisson BF, Delin K, et al. Treatment of renovascular hypertension: one year results of renal angioplasty. *Kidney Int* 1995;48:1936–1945.
204. Klow NE, Paulsen D, Vatne K, et al. Percutaneous transluminal renal artery angioplasty using the coaxial technique. Ten years of experience from 591 procedures in 419 patients. *Acta Radiol* 1998;39:594–603.
205. Kuhn FP, Kutkuhn B, Torsello G, et al. Renal artery stenosis: preliminary results of treatment with the Strecker stent. *Radiology* 1991;180:367–372.
206. Rees CR, Palmaz JC, Becker GJ, et al. Palmaz stent in atherosclerotic stenoses involving the ostia of the renal arteries: preliminary report of a multicenter study. *Radiology* 1991;181:507–514.
207. Shannon HM, Gillespie IN, Moss JG. Salvage of the solitary kidney by insertion of a renal artery stent. *AJR Am J Roentgenol* 1998;171:217–222.
208. Surowiec SM, Sivamurthy N, Rhodes JM, et al. Percutaneous therapy for renal artery fibromuscular dysplasia. *Ann Vasc Surg* 2003;17:650–655.
209. Tegtmeyer CJ, Selby JB, Hartwell GD, et al. Results and complications of angioplasty in fibromuscular disease. *Circulation* 1991;83:I155–I161.
210. Wilms GE, Peene PT, Baert AL, et al. Renal artery stent placement with use of the Wallstent endoprosthesis. *Radiology* 1991;179:457–462.

CHAPTER 110 ■ VENOUS THROMBOEMBOLISM

VICTOR F. TAPSON AND RICHARD C. BECKER

HISTORICAL PERSPECTIVE

In 1846, Rudolf Virchow, then 35 years old, described the triad of stasis, vessel wall injury, and hypercoagulability and its association with the development of venous thrombosis (1). This association is perhaps one of the most enduring themes in medicine. Every scenario recognized to date that can be considered a risk factor for this disease is derived from this triad (2). The presence of risk factors may lead to suspicion of the presence of deep venous thrombosis (DVT) or pulmonary embolism (PE), collectively referred to as venous thromboembolism (VTE), as well as being critical in determining appropriate prophylaxis among patients at risk.

In 1819, Laennec wrote about "pulmonary apoplexy," stating, "The disease I call by this name is very common, but nevertheless its features are almost unknown" (3). Nine years later, Cruveilhier began his work meticulously describing thrombi in central and peripheral veins as well as describing multiple pulmonary emboli pathologically (4). Despite their important discoveries, neither Laennec nor Cruveilhier made the association between the development of DVT and PE.

In 1880, Beniamino Luzzatto described at least 160 cases of PE in a manuscript entitled "Embolism of the Pulmonary Artery," in which he emphasized the predilection for the lower lobes and the predisposing role of stasis and preexisting cardiopulmonary disease (5). Shortly after the turn of the century, Trendelenberg attempted pulmonary embolectomy (6), and in 1924, Kirschner, a student of Trendelenberg, performed the first successful embolectomy for acute PE (7). Ljungdahl described the concept of chronic PE in 1928 (8). In 1931, Moniz et al. reported the first pulmonary angiogram (although this technique did not become widely utilized for PE until decades later) (9). In 1940, Gunnar Bauer, a Swedish surgeon, diagnosed DVT by venography and investigated the natural history of untreated venous thrombosis using serial venography (10). He was also among the first to report the use of heparin therapy for this disease (11,12), although heparin had been discovered in 1916 by McLean, then a medical student (13).

The ability to diagnose PE changed dramatically after 1960 with the development and availability of new diagnostic techniques. The advantages of pulmonary angiography became more widely recognized in 1963 when Chrispin and colleagues (14) injected contrast material into the right atrium and pulmonary arteries, delineating emboli within the large pulmonary arteries. Williams, Sasahara, and their colleagues reported the utility of selective pulmonary angiography exclusively for the diagnosis of PE (15,16). Stein et al. (17) evaluated the angiographic signs of PE in 1967 and concluded that an intraluminal "filling defect" and "vessel cutoff" with a trailing edge were the only two primary angiographic criteria that could be relied on to diagnose PE. Radionuclide imaging was further explored in 1964 when Taplin et al. developed a method of generating and radiolabeling macroaggregated albumin particles (18). Wagner et al. (19) reported the diagnosis of PE in humans by radioisotope scanning the same year. These diagnostic discoveries helped to usher in a new era in the approach to VTE.

INCIDENCE

Venous thromboembolism occurs commonly in hospitalized patients seen in all specialties and subspecialties. Recent studies from the Worcester Venous Thromboembolism Study, a population-based investigation funded by the National Institutes of Health, showed an annual overall incidence rate of 200 per 100,000 population with an alarming 1,200 per 100,000 population among individuals greater than 75 years of age (F. Spencer, McMaster University, Personal communication). PE most commonly results from DVT occurring in the veins of the proximal lower extremities including and proximal to the popliteal veins. Both DVT and PE are frequently unsuspected, leading to significant diagnostic and therapeutic delays and accounting for substantial morbidity and mortality. Although there are as many as 260,000 patients in the United States in whom VTE is diagnosed and treated each year, more than half of the cases that actually occur are never diagnosed. Many patients dying from acute PE have coexisting terminal illnesses; however, this disease entity is responsible for the deaths of 50,000 to 100,000 patients with an otherwise good prognosis and, accordingly, should be diagnosed and treated aggressively (20–22). Despite advances in diagnostic technology and therapeutic approaches, VTE remains underdiagnosed, and prophylaxis is underutilized (23).

A multicenter prospective study including 5,451 patients with ultrasound-confirmed DVT found that of 1,776 patients with events while hospitalized, only 1,147 (65%) received prophylaxis within the prior 30 days (24). In the National Anticoagulation Benchmark and Outcomes report (NABOR), 15% of 928 patients undergoing high-risk orthopedic surgery received inadequate prophylaxis, and nearly 50% who were treated had a suboptimal duration of prophylaxis (25).

RISK FACTORS AND PATHOBIOLOGY

Risk Factors

The pathogenesis of DVT as proposed by Virchow is based on several potential initiating events including stasis, vessel wall injury, and hypercoagulability. Risk factors for DVT are based on these processes (Table 110.1).

Clinical Factors

Most venous thrombi arise in valve pockets, where blood flow tends to stagnate. The increased frequency of thrombosis with advanced age and associated immobilization further suggests an important relationship between stasis and thrombogenesis. Patients with acute cerebrovascular accidents commonly develop venous thrombi in the paralyzed lower extremity, but occasionally do so in the unaffected limb. Acute paraplegia is associated with a high risk of VTE, and the greatest risk occurs within the first 2 weeks after the neurologic event (26). Prolonged bed rest or long automobile or airplane trips may lead to the development of thromboemboli. The risk presented by air travel (27,28), particularly among individuals at risk, is increased. Obesity increases the risk of VTE (29), the etiology of which is likely multifactorial, with stasis and inflammatory (prothrombotic) mediators contributing. Age, in addition to increasing the risk of VTE, influences outcome after PE (30). The high mortality may be related to concomitant cardiovascular disease or malignancy (31).

Patients with prior VTE incur a substantial risk of recurrence when hospitalized, particularly in the postoperative setting (32,33) after major abdominal, spinal, or orthopedic surgery (34).

TABLE 110.1

RISK FACTORS FOR VENOUS THROMBOEMBOLISM

Clinical factors
Age greater than 40 y
Prior history of venous thromboembolism
Prior major surgical procedure/trauma
Hip fracture
Immobilization/paralysis
Varicose veins
Congestive heart failure
Myocardial infarction
Obesity
Pregnancy/postpartum
Oral contraceptive therapy
Cerebrovascular accident
Cancer
Paroxysmal nocturnal hemoglobinemia
Antiphospholipid antibody syndrome (including lupus anticoagulant)
Genetic/molecular factors
Anti–thrombin III deficiency
Factor V Leiden mutation (activated protein C resistance)
Protein C deficiency
Protein S deficiency
Prothrombin gene (G20210A) mutation
Dysfibrinogenemia
Disorders of plasminogen
Elevated factor VIII levels
Elevated factor XI levels

Venous thromboemboli are detected at autopsy in as many as 60% of patients with fractures of the lower extremities (35), and mortality has been attributed to PE in 38% to 50% of patients dying after hip fracture (36). The duration of immobility after trauma influences the development of VTE. Autopsy-confirmed incidence rates of PE in patients surviving for less than 24 hours after initial trauma is 3.3%, increasing to 5.5% in those surviving up to 7 days and up to 18.6% among those surviving for longer periods (37). Other causes of venous trauma, including central venous catheters placed in the jugular or subclavian veins, are associated with VTE. Although upper-extremity thrombosis is a potential source for PE, the overall incidence is lower than reported with lower-extremity DVT.

Autopsy series and population-based epidemiologic studies have shown that patients with cardiovascular disease and malignancies are particularly susceptible to VTE (38). A reduction in the incidence of VTE after fibrinolytic therapy for acute myocardial infarction (MI) has been demonstrated in two large-scale, placebo-controlled trials: the Gruppo Italiano per lo Studio della Streptochinasi nell'Infarto Miocardico (GISSI-1) study and the second International Study of Infarct Survival (ISIS-2) study (39,40).

Patients with malignancy have an increased risk of developing VTE (41), particularly those involving the lung, stomach, genitourinary tract, and breast. A recent analysis based on data from the Prospective Investigation of Pulmonary Embolism Diagnosis (PIOPED) trial, found that of 399 patients with PE, 73 (18.3%) had underlying malignancy (32).

Pregnancy and the postpartum period are the most common settings during which women less than 40 years of age experience VTE (42). An overwhelming majority of events involve the lower extremities, and they occur most often during the third trimester and early postpartum (first 6 weeks) period; however, the overall risk of VTE is increased throughout pregnancy. Delivery by cesarean section further increases the overall risk.

Oral contraceptives are associated with a heightened incidence of VTE (43), particularly third-generation agents (agents containing desogestrel or gestodene as the progestagen component) (44,45). In a clinical trial evaluating hormonal replacement therapy, VTE was increased among women 45 to 64 years of age. Overall, the annual incidence of VTE is 16 to 17 cases per 100,000 individuals treated (46), with the risk being greatest during the first year of exposure (47,48). Physicians must consider the potential risk for VTE before prescribing hormonal replacement therapy (49).

Systemic disease states associated with VTE include paroxysmal nocturnal hemoglobinuria, inflammatory bowel disease, homocystinuria, Behçet syndrome, polycythemia rubra vera, and primary thrombasthenia. Patients with illnesses requiring intensive care unit treatment should be considered an at-risk population. With very few exceptions, these individuals should receive VTE prophylaxis. In addition, hospitalized general medical patients, including those with congestive heart failure and/or pneumonia, should receive appropriate prophylaxis.

Atherosclerosis and Venous Thrombosis

The widely recognized triad attributed to Virchow can also be applied to arterial thrombosis in the following construct: endothelial dysfunction, atherosclerosis (abnormality of the vessel wall); increased cellular and plasma viscosity (increased shear stress, abnormality of blood flow); and heightened platelet activatability, tissue factor expression, and thrombin generation (abnormality of blood constituents). A study including 299 patients with lower-extremity VTE (50) reported at least one carotid plaque (detected by ultrasound) in 47.1% (95% confidence interval [CI] 39.1% to 55.0%) of those with spontaneous VTE; in 27.4% (95% CI 20.0% to 34.6%) of those with secondary thrombosis (recognized acquired risk factor), and in 32% (95% CI 24.5% to 39.5%) of gender- and age-matched controls. In a prospective study of 360 patients with a first PE (51), 209 with idiopathic PE and 151 with PE associated with transient risk factors, cardiovascular events occurred at a rate of 7.5% per patient-year among patients with idiopathic VTE and 3.10% per patient-year among those with transient risk factors (relative risk 2.0; 95% CI 1.71 to 30.45). The likelihood of an arterial event (MI, stroke, death) was increased sevenfold in patients with idiopathic VTE. Clearly, the association between atherosclerosis and VTE requires further investigation.

Molecular Defects

Inherited coagulopathies result in variable degrees of VTE risk (52); however, inherited traits are detectable in 40% of patients and 5% of the general population. Accordingly, knowledge of genetic predisposition may be an important stimulus for prophylaxis in high-risk settings. Patients with antithrombin III or protein C or S deficiency may remain free of thromboembolic disease until another risk factor such as immobilization, surgery, trauma, or pregnancy is superimposed. The factor V Leiden mutation, a common genetic polymorphism associated with activated protein C resistance, is detectable in 4% to 6% of the general population (53). The relative risk of a first VTE among men heterozygous for the mutation is 3 to 7-fold higher than those not affected (56). The relative risk in homozygous individuals is increased 50-fold. The prothrombin gene mutation (G20210A), like the factor V Leiden mutation, is common among healthy white individuals of eastern European descent, but rarely affects Asians and Africans. The identification of an inherited defect does not, in itself, mandate lifelong anticoagulation therapy; however, such patients should be counseled and followed carefully.

Gas Exchange and Hemodynamic Alterations in Acute Pulmonary Embolism

The hypoxemia that occurs in patients with PE can be explained through various mechanisms. In patients without previous cardiopulmonary disease, regions with low ventilation/perfusion ratios and shunting secondary to perfusion of atelectatic areas are likely predominant.

When emboli obstruct a significant portion of the pulmonary arterial bed, profound hemodynamic alterations occur. The effect of the embolic event depends on the extent of reduction of the cross-sectional area of the pulmonary vasculature as well as on the presence or absence of underlying cardiovascular disease. Submassive emboli in normal individuals may actually augment cardiac output (CO). Hypoxemia leads to an increase in sympathetic tone with systemic vasoconstriction and an increase in venous return with augmentation of stroke volume. With massive emboli, CO is diminished but may be sustained as the mean right atrial pressure increases. The ensuing increase in pulmonary vascular resistance (PVR) impedes right ventricular outflow and reduces left ventricular preload. In a patient without previous cardiopulmonary disease, occlusion of 25% to 30% of the vascular bed by emboli is associated with a significant rise in pulmonary artery pressure (PAP). With increasing vascular obstruction, hypoxemia worsens, stimulating vasoconstriction and a further rise in PAP. Greater than 50% obstruction of the pulmonary arterial bed is usually present before substantial elevation of the mean PAP evolves. When the extent of obstruction of the pulmonary circulation approaches 75%, the right ventricle must generate a systolic pressure in excess of 50 mm Hg and a mean PAP of greater than 40 mm Hg to preserve pulmonary perfusion (54). The normal right ventricle is unable to achieve this and ultimately fails (55). Patients with underlying cardiopulmonary disease are more inclined to experience more substantial deterioration in CO than normal individuals in the setting of massive PE. A depressed CO *without* elevation of the right atrial pressure suggests cardiac dysfunction superimposed upon PE. Right ventricular failure is more common in the setting of PE in patients with coronary artery disease (56). It is important to realize that although supportive measures may sustain a patient with massive embolism, any additional increment in embolic burden may be fatal.

The diagnostic technology for acute DVT has developed considerably with the evolution of convenient and inexpensive techniques such as Doppler ultrasound as well as highly accurate yet more expensive diagnostic modalities such as magnetic resonance imaging (MRI). For PE, ventilation/perfusion (VQ) scanning followed by pulmonary arteriography remains the gold standard for the diagnosis, although newer techniques such as MRI and helical computed tomography (CT) scanning are being utilized increasingly. The presence of risk factors together with the history and physical examination generally leads to further diagnostic testing in the setting of suspected VTE.

History and Physical Examination

The clinical diagnosis of both DVT and PE based on the history and physical examination are notoriously insensitive and nonspecific. Patients with lower-extremity DVT often do not exhibit erythema, warmth, pain, swelling, or tenderness. These findings, however, although not specific for DVT, merit further evaluation. Pulmonary embolism should always be considered whenever unexplained dyspnea is present. Dyspnea as well as pleuritic chest pain and hemoptysis are common in PE but are nonspecific. Anxiety, lightheadedness, and syncope are all symptoms that may be caused by PE but may also result from a number of other entities that result in hypoxemia or hypotension. Tachypnea and tachycardia are the most common signs of PE but are also nonspecific. Pulmonary embolism should always be considered in the setting of syncope or sudden hypotension. The cardiac and pulmonary physical examinations are both nonspecific. The index of clinical suspicion does, however, become a more useful parameter when considered in conjunction with V/Q scanning (56). Diagnostic efforts directed at possible VTE may be appropriate despite alternative explanations if risk factors and the clinical setting are suggestive. Dyspnea, tachypnea, clear lung fields, and hypoxemia may often be attributed to a flare of chronic obstructive disease or asthma when underlying PE is present.

Laboratory Testing

Electrocardiographic (ECG) findings in acute PE are generally nonspecific and include T-wave changes, ST-segment abnormalities, and left- or right-axis deviation. In the Urokinase Pulmonary Embolism Trial (UPET) electrocardiographic abnormalities were documented in 87% of patients who were free of underlying cardiac or pulmonary disease (57). These findings were not specific for PE, however. In this clinical trial, 26% of patients with massive or submassive PE and 32% of those with massive PE had manifestations of acute cor pulmonale such as the S1Q3T3 pattern, right-bundle-branch block, P-wave pulmonale, or right-axis deviation. Such changes are thus seen in a minority of patients. The low frequency of specific ECG changes associated with PE was confirmed in the PIOPED study (58).

Some individuals, particularly young patients without underlying lung disease, may have a normal arterial oxygen pressure (PaO_2) in the setting of acute PE. In a retrospective study of hospitalized patients with PE, the PaO_2 was greater than 80 mm Hg in 29% of patients less than 40 years old, compared with 3% in the older group (59). The alveolar-arterial (A-a) difference was elevated in all patients, however. A subset of patients participating in the PIOPED study suspected of PE with no history or evidence of preexisting cardiac or pulmonary disease was evaluated, and the PaO_2 and A-a difference values were compared (56). Patients with and without PE could not be distinguished based on either of these values. The A-a difference was elevated by more than 20 mm Hg in 76 of 88 (86%) patients with PE, however. The diagnosis of acute PE cannot be excluded based upon a normal PaO_2, and although the A-a difference is usually elevated, rarely it may be normal in patients without preexisting cardiopulmonary disease.

The utility of plasma measurements of circulating D-dimer, a specific derivative of cross-linked fibrin, as a diagnostic aid in PE has been extensively evaluated. A normal enzyme-linked immunosorbent assay (ELISA) appears to be sensitive in excluding PE. When the D-dimer level is 500 μg/liter or greater, the sensitivity and specificity for PE have been shown to be 98% and 39%, respectively (60). The sensitivity of the plasma D-dimer appears to remain high up to 1 week after presentation. In another prospective analysis, 96% of 79 patients with high-probability V/Q scans had an elevated D-dimer concentration (61). Thus, increased levels of cross-linked fibrin degradation products are an indirect but suggestive marker of intravascular thrombosis in addition to indicating fibrinolysis. A D-dimer assay together with a respiratory rate less than 20 breaths/minute and a PaO_2 greater than 80 mm Hg was shown to be very sensitive in ruling out acute pulmonary embolism (62). Although the sensitivity of the D-dimer appears to be high, the specificity is not high enough to be diagnostic. Thus, neither symptoms, signs, radiographic or electrocardiographic findings nor plasma D-dimer measurement can be considered diagnostic of PE or DVT, and when these entities are suspected, further evaluation with noninvasive or invasive testing is necessary. A recent exhaustive review of the various D-dimer assays and clinical trial results reinforces these findings (63).

Chest Radiography, Ventilation/Perfusion Scanning, and Pulmonary Arteriography

Most patients with PE have an abnormal but nonspecific chest radiograph. Common radiographic findings include atelectasis, pleural effusion, pulmonary infiltrates, and mild elevation of a hemidiaphragm (58). Classic findings of pulmonary infarction such as Hampton's hump or decreased vascularity (Westermark's sign) are suggestive but infrequent. A normal chest radiograph in the setting of severe dyspnea and hypoxemia without evidence of bronchospasm or anatomic cardiac shunt strongly suggests PE. The presence of a pleural effusion increases the likelihood of PE in young patients who present with acute pleuritic chest pain (62). Under most circumstances, however, the chest radiograph cannot be used to conclusively diagnose or exclude PE. Although exclusion of other processes, such as pneumonia, pneumothorax, or rib fracture, that may cause symptoms similar to acute PE is possible, PE may frequently coexist with other underlying lung diseases.

Ventilation/perfusion scanning should be performed when PE is suspected. Normal and high-probability scans are considered diagnostic. A normal perfusion scan rules out the diagnosis of PE with a high enough degree of certainty that further diagnostic evaluation is unnecessary. Matching areas of decreased ventilation and perfusion in the presence of a normal chest radiograph generally represent a process other than PE. However, low or intermediate probability (nondiagnostic) scans are commonly found with PE, and in such situations further evaluation with pulmonary arteriography is often appropriate. A high-probability V/Q scan is shown in Figure 110.1. The PIOPED study prospectively evaluated the utility of V/Q scanning combined with clinical assessment of patients with suspected PE (56). Patients with PE had scans that were high, intermediate, or low probability, but so did most patients without PE. Although the specificity of high-probability scans was 97%, the sensitivity was only 41%. Of interest, 33% of patients with intermediate-probability scans and 12% of patients with low-probability scans were diagnosed definitively with PE by pulmonary arteriography. When the clinical suspicion of PE was considered very high, PE was found to be present in 96% of patients with high-probability scans, 66% of patients with intermediate-probability scans, and 40% of patients with low-probability scans. The diagnosis of PE should be rigorously pursued even when the lung scan is of low or intermediate probability if the clinical scenario suggests PE (64). Therefore, although the V/Q scan may sometimes be diagnostic of PE or exclude the possibility with sufficient certainty, it is often nondiagnostic. Even in such circumstances, however, it may serve as a useful guide for limited pulmonary arteriography.

Pulmonary arteriography is the gold standard for the diagnosis of PE. It is a very sensitive, specific, and safe test. Complications of pulmonary arteriography among 1,111 patients suspected of PE in the PIOPED study included death in 0.5% and major nonfatal complications in 1% (65). An alternative to doing pulmonary arteriography is to perform lower-extremity studies when the lung scan is nondiagnostic, and if these are

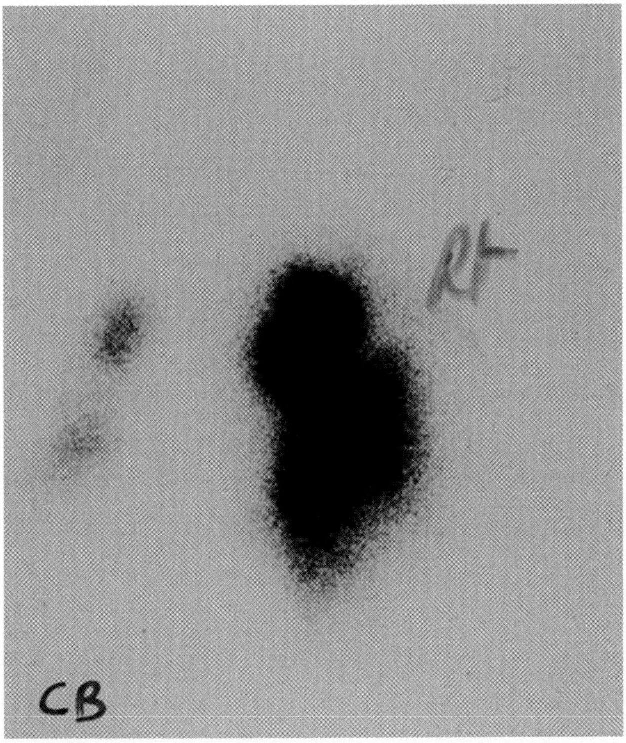

FIGURE 110.1. Perfusion scan revealing massive pulmonary embolism in a patient who presented with near-syncope and hypotension. The chest radiograph and ventilation scan were essentially normal. The patient received thrombolytic therapy with an excellent response.

negative, the chances of significant PE or morbidity from a subsequent event appears unlikely (66). This practice is gaining acceptance, and it may be appropriate in patients with cardiopulmonary stability. Finally, pulmonary angiography has been performed at the bedside using a Swan-Ganz catheter (67). This may help to avoid the need to transport critically ill patients.

Echocardiography in Acute Pulmonary Embolism

Other diagnostic techniques sometimes prove useful particularly in the setting of massive PE. Echocardiography, which can often be obtained more rapidly than either lung scanning or pulmonary arteriography, may reveal findings that strongly support hemodynamically significant PE (68) (Fig. 110.2). Studies of patients with documented PE have revealed that more than 80% of patients have imaging or Doppler abnormalities of right ventricular size or function that may suggest acute PE (69). Unfortunately, because patients with PE often have underlying cardiopulmonary disease such as chronic obstructive lung disease, neither right ventricular dilation nor hypokinesis can be reliably used even as indirect evidence of PE in such settings. Goldhaber and colleagues (70) demonstrated that echocardiography could be used to document improvement in right ventricular wall motion in patients with PE treated with recombinant tissue-type plasminogen activator (tPA). Intravascular ultrasound imaging has been shown in both the experimental and clinical settings to adequately image large emboli (71–73). This procedure may be performed at the bedside. Although the technique may be less sensitive and specific and more time consuming in the setting of smaller emboli, further investigation may be warranted.

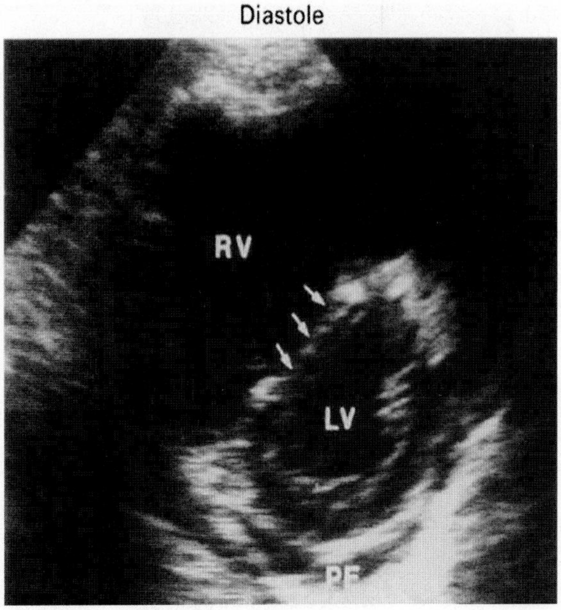

FIGURE 110.2. Echocardiography in a patient with massive pulmonary embolism. The right ventricle (RV) is markedly enlarged, flattening the intraventricular septum and compromising the left ventricle (LV).

Computed Tomography and Magnetic Resonance Imaging

The utility of computed tomography scanning and magnetic resonance imaging for diagnosing PE has recently been explored. Preliminary data suggest comparable accuracy for these techniques (74). Helical (spiral) CT has been explored in patients with both acute and chronic PE. This technique involves continuous movement of the patient through the scanner with concurrent scanning by a constantly rotating gantry and detector system that takes 1 second for a 360-degree rotation (75). A helix of raw projecting data is obtained. Continuous volume acquisitions can be obtained during a single breath, and rapid scans can be obtained, facilitating imaging in critically ill patients. Retrospective reconstructions can be performed. A contrast bolus is required for vascular imaging. Limitations of helical CT scanning include poor visualization of horizontally oriented vessels in the right middle lobe and lingula because of volume averaging. The peripheral areas of the upper and lower lobes may be inadequately scanned, and intersegmental lymph nodes may result in false-positive studies. Multiplanar reconstructions in coronal or oblique planes may aid in differentiating lymph nodes from emboli.

Helical and electron beam CT may reveal emboli in the main, lobar, or segmental pulmonary arteries with greater than 90% sensitivity and specificity (Fig. 110.3) (76–80). Others have reported very accurate results for large PE (Fig. 110.4) (81). Oser and colleagues (82) determined retrospectively that of 76 consecutive pulmonary angiograms, 23 (30%) revealed only subsegmental emboli. Nineteen studies (25%) revealed only a single PE. Thirteen of the 19 single emboli were subsegmental only. The PIOPED study, however, revealed that only 6% of patients had isolated subsegmental emboli (56). The latter prospective evaluation is likely more representative. Interestingly, however, two referee angiographers from the PIOPED agreed on the presence or absence of subsegmental emboli in only 66% of cases (52). Using selective pulmonary arteriography, Quinn and colleagues (83) emphasized

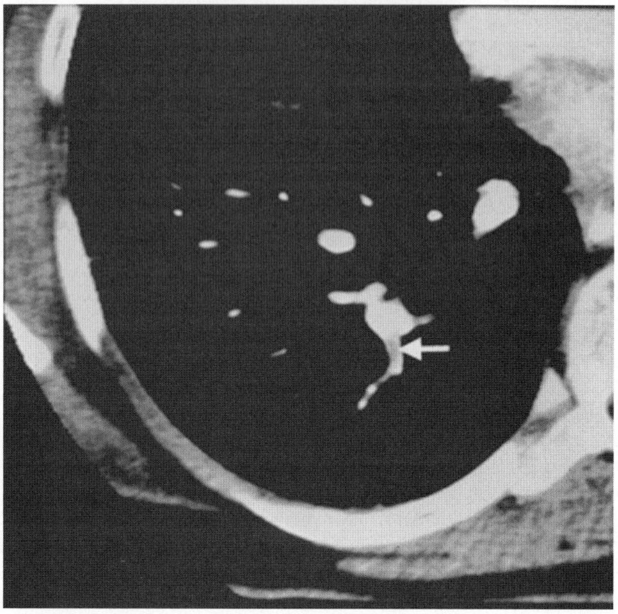

FIGURE 110.3. Contrast-enhanced single slice spiral computed tomography in a 49-year-old man shows an isolated small embolus in a subsegmental branch of the posterior basal segment of the right lower lobe (*arrow*). The other pulmonary arteries in this image are normal.

TABLE 110.2

SENSITIVITY AND SPECIFICITY FOR COMPUTED TOMOGRAPHY SCANNING FOR ACUTE PULMONARY EMBOLISM

Reference	No. patients	Sensitivity (%)	Specificity (%)
Helical computed tomography			
Goodman (77)	20	86[a]	92[a]
		63[b]	89[b]
Remy-Jardin et al. (76)	72	90	86
Van Rossum et al. (80)	124	97	98
Sostman et al. (74)	28	73	97
Remy-Jardin et al. (78)	42	100	96
Van Rossum et al. (81)	45	95	97
Drucker et al. (86)		60	81
		53	97
Electron-beam computed tomography			
Teigen et al. (79)	60	65	97
Teigen et al. (85)	25	95	80

[a]Main, lobar, and segmental emboli. Two sets of readers from different institutions were used, resulting in two sets of sensitivity and specificity values.
[b]All emboli including peripheral.

excellent agreement on main, lobar, and segmental emboli but only 13% agreement on subsegmental emboli. Thus, this apparent limitation with helical CT scanning is also a concern with angiography. Goodman and Lipchik (84) strongly endorsed the incorporation of CT scanning into diagnostic algorithms for PE. Sensitivity and specificity data from several large studies evaluating helical CT scanning for acute PE are shown in Table 110.2. Contrast-enhanced electron-beam CT also appears to be useful in diagnosing acute PE (79,85). The rapid (100 msec) scanning time makes breath-holding unnecessary, and respiratory and cardiac motion artifacts are minimized. In one comparison with pulmonary angiography, only 8 of 720 vascular zones (1.1%) were considered inadequately visualized with electron-beam CT. The entire chest examination took 10 to 15 minutes. Another potential advantage of t CT angiography includes the ability to define extrapulmonary vascular structures (Fig. 110.5), nonvascular structures such as airway abnormalities, lymphadenopathy, tumors, other lung parenchymal abnormalities, and right ventricular dimensions, as well as pleural and pericardial disease. Although a helical CT study suggested significantly lower sensitivity

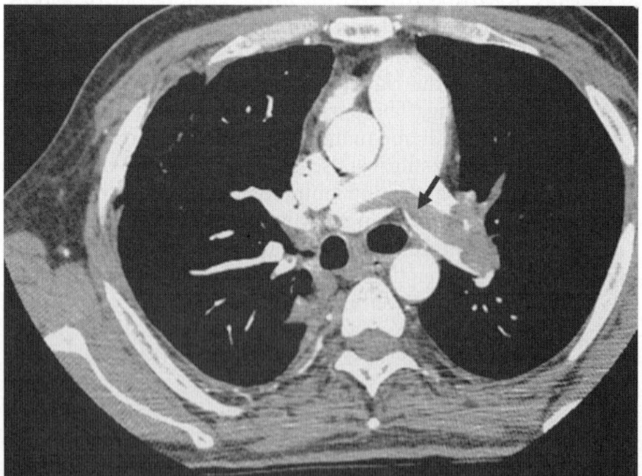

FIGURE 110.4. Massive pulmonary embolism shown by spiral computed tomography. The low-density embolus is easily visualized "saddling" the left and right main pulmonary arteries (*arrow*) surrounded by the dense white contrast. The left pulmonary artery is the one most involved.

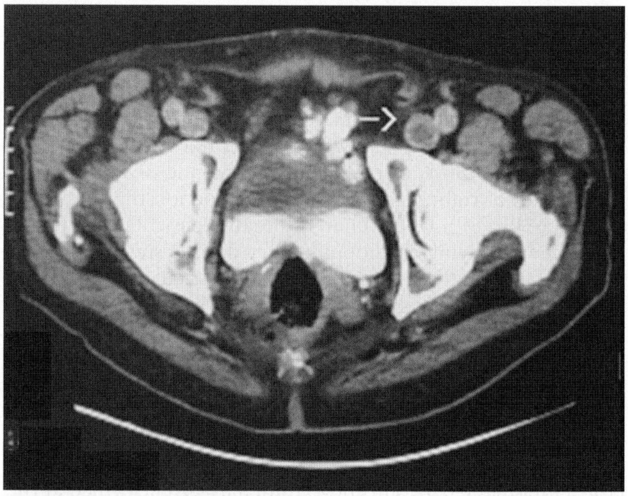

FIGURE 110.5. Contrast-enhanced computed tomography reveals a large thrombosis in the left femoral vein. Acute pulmonary embolism was also visualized in this patient.

(50% to 60%) for acute PE than previous studies (86), it is likely that interpretation of cut films instead of evaluation of the images at the computer workstation accounted for the low sensitivity. An adaptive three-dimensional voxel clustering method of CT angiography may improve the diagnostic sensitivity particularly with small and marginally (<20%) occlusive thrombi.

Magnetic resonance imaging can also be used to evaluate clinically suspected PE. In a comparison with helical CT, the average sensitivity of CT for five observers was 75% and of MRI was 46%. The average specificity of CT was 89%, compared with 90% for MRI. As expected, sensitivity and specificity were higher for expert readers (74).

Detection of Deep Venous Thrombosis

The technology for diagnosing DVT has evolved considerably over the last several decades (46,87,88).

Doppler ultrasonography is a portable and accurate diagnostic technique for proximal lower-extremity DVT. The sensitivity and specificity for symptomatic proximal DVT has been well above 90% in most recent clinical trials. Limitations include insensitivity for asymptomatic DVT, operator dependence, the inability to accurately distinguish acute from chronic DVT in symptomatic patients and the insensitivity to calf vein thrombosis (89,90). A recent prospective evaluation of the utility of bilateral color Doppler ultrasound in asymptomatic high-risk (elective unilateral hip or knee replacement) patients revealed that ultrasound was only 38% sensitive for proximal DVT (using contrast venography as the diagnostic comparator) (91). Compared to other technology, it is relatively inexpensive and represents the preferred diagnostic modality for the straightforward case of symptomatic presumed proximal DVT.

Although contrast venography remains the gold standard for diagnosing DVT in clinical trials, it is employed rarely in routine clinical practice (92). It is an invasive procedure that may result in superficial phlebitis or hypersensitivity reactions, but it is generally well tolerated.

Magnetic resonance imaging is being used increasingly for diagnosing DVT (93). A major advantage of this technique is excellent resolution of the inferior vena cava and pelvic veins (94,95). The early experience suggests that its diagnostic accuracy rivals that of contrast venography or ultrasound imaging and it is more sensitive than either for (a) detecting thrombus within the pelvic deep vein and (b) differentiating acute from chronic DVT.

At Duke University Medical Center, duplex ultrasonography represents a first-line diagnostic test in patients with suspected acute DVT. Magnetic resonance imaging is used when the ultrasound is nondiagnostic or when the clinician wishes to distinguish acute from chronic DVT. Angiography or iliofemoral venography can also be used as a second-line test and in the future may replace venous duplex scanning in conditions in which suspected PE and DVT coexist.

PRINCIPLES OF MANAGEMENT

Prophylaxis of Deep Venous Thrombosis

A significant reduction in the incidence of DVT can be achieved when patients at risk receive appropriate prophylaxis (96). Such preventive measures, appear to be grossly underused. A review of the use of prophylaxis for DVT in 16 Massachusetts hospitals (97) indicated that such therapy was administered to only 44% of high-risk patients in teaching hospitals and only 19% in nonteaching hospitals. The frequency of prophylaxis ranged from 9% to 56% among hospitals. Patients can be stratified according to DVT risk, and certain prophylactic measures are more appropriate for some patients than for others. In general medical patients at risk for DVT, subcutaneous heparin at 5,000 units every 8 to 12 hours is generally adequate. Intermittent pneumatic compression devices should be used in the unusual situation in which such prophylactic doses of heparin are contraindicated. Both methods combined would be reasonable in patients deemed to be at exceptionally high risk, but an additional reduction in risk in such patients has not been well substantiated.

In the general surgery population, a number of prophylactic methods have been employed. In a large meta-analysis, Colditz et al. (98) not only confirmed the value of prophylaxis in reducing the incidence of DVT, but also suggested that intermittent pneumatic compression plus gradient compression stockings may result in the lowest incidence of postoperative DVT. Other combined treatments were associated with lower rates than heparin alone. Another overview of the results of randomized trials in surgical patients demonstrated the benefit of DVT prophylaxis (96). In this review of more than 70 randomized trials involving 16,000 patients it was demonstrated that perioperative use of subcutaneous heparin can prevent about half of all pulmonary emboli and about two thirds of all DVT.

A number of investigators have evaluated the efficacy and safety of low-molecular-weight heparin (LMWH) for DVT prophylaxis (99). Low-molecular-weight heparin may have an advantage in producing a more predictable dose response and is administered subcutaneously once or twice per day depending on the preparation (Tables 110.3 and 110.4). The Food and Drug Administration (FDA) has approved enoxaparin for three surgical prophylaxis indications including elective total hip or knee replacement and general abdominal surgery (Table 110.5). The approved dose is either 30 mg subcutaneously twice daily or 40 mg once daily for the orthopedic indications and 40 mg once daily for abdominal surgery. Prophylaxis is generally recommended for 7 to 10 days. Longer regimens may be appropriate depending on associated additional risk factors and on whether the patient is ambulatory. A large, randomized, placebo-controlled trial in patients undergoing total hip replacement compared enoxaparin prophylaxis during hospitalization (average 10 to 11 days) with more prolonged outpatient prophylaxis (100). Blinded outpatient therapy (or placebo) was continued long enough that the total treatment period (inpatient plus outpatient) was 1 month for each patient. In the 233 patients with adequate venography, there were 43 episodes of DVT and 2 PE in the placebo group

TABLE 110.3

A COMPARISON OF LOW-MOLECULAR-WEIGHT HEPARIN (LMWH) WITH UNFRACTIONATED HEPARIN (UFH)

Characteristic	UFH	LMWH
Mean molecular weight	12,000–15,000	4,000–6,000
Protein binding	Substantial	Minimal
Anti-Xa activity	Substantial	Substantial
Anti-IIa activity	Substantial	Minimal
Platelet inhibition	Substantial	Minimal
Vascular permeability	Moderate	None
Microvascular permeability	Substantial	Minimal

TABLE 110.4

POTENTIAL ADVANTAGES OF LOW-MOLECULAR-WEIGHT HEPARIN OVER UNFRACTIONATED HEPARIN

Comparable or superior efficacy
Comparable or superior safety
Superior bioavailability
Once- or twice-daily dosing
No laboratory monitoring
Less phlebotomy
Subcutaneous administration
Earlier ambulation
Home therapy in certain patient subsets
Measurement of anti–factor Xa levels should be considered in morbidly obese patients
Low-weight/frail patients (e.g., <40 kg), and patients with severe renal insufficiency (dose adjustment should also be instituted in this patient subset if low-molecular-weight heparin is used).

compared with only 21 episodes of DVT and no PE in the group receiving 1 month of prophylaxis. The incidence of thromboembolic events was 39% and 18%, respectively ($p < .001$). Thus, more prolonged outpatient prophylaxis may be appropriate in this patient population. Further investigation in such high-risk patients appears to be warranted. A second preparation, dalteparin, has been approved for once-daily use as prophylaxis for elective abdominal surgery.

A number of other preparations are being investigated. Recent clinical trials emphasize the increased thromboembolic risk of general medical patients. Although this concept is not new, it is important to stress as the population of hospitalized patients is becoming increasingly complex. The recent MEDENOX (Prophylaxis of Medical Patients with Enoxaparin) clinical trial compared two doses of enoxaparin (20 and 40 mg) with placebo in 1,102 hospitalized medical patients at moderate risk for VTE (101). Most of these patients had acute respiratory failure, congestive heart failure, or acute infectious diseases. The primary outcome was DVT detected by venography or ultrasonography between days 6 and 14 or PE. Venous thromboembolism developed in 14.9% of the patients receiving placebo, 15% of patients on 20 mg of enoxaparin, and in only 5.5% of patients on the 40-mg enoxaparin dose ($p < .001$ for enoxaparin vs. placebo). There was no difference in major bleeding or death among the three groups. Enoxaparin is now FDA approved for prophylaxis in this commonly encountered group of patients. Results from two European studies suggest that enoxaparin is at least as effective (and as safe) as UFH for VTE prophylaxis at a dose of 5,000 units every 8 hours in medically ill patients (102,103). It is important to acknowledge that LMWH preparations are not identical, and the results of clinical trials with one agent cannot be extrapolated to another agent.

TABLE 110.5

GUIDELINES FOR USE OF ENOXAPARIN PROPHYLAXIS AFTER KNEE OR HIP REPLACEMENT

Dose: 30 mg subcutaneously twice daily or 40 mg once daily
Duration: 7–10 d (or until discharge or risk of postoperative deep venous thrombosis has diminished[a])
Initial dose: begin 12–24 h after surgery
Delivery method: deep subcutaneous administration
Monitoring: none

[a]Several randomized, prospective, placebo-controlled trials strongly suggest that extending prophylaxis in total hip replacement patients to a total of 1 mo (inpatient plus outpatient) significantly reduces the incidence of venous thromboembolism (97).

Anticoagulation

Anticoagulation has been proven to reduce mortality in acute PE. When VTE is diagnosed or strongly suspected, heparin therapy should be promptly instituted unless contraindications exist. Confirmatory testing should always be planned if anticoagulation is to be continued. Heparin exerts a prompt antithrombotic effect preventing thrombus growth. Although it does not directly prevent the development of acute PE or dissolve thrombus, it allows the fibrinolytic system to act unopposed and more readily reduces the size of the thromboembolic burden (104). Although thrombus growth can be prevented, early recurrence can develop even in the setting of therapeutic anticoagulation.

With the institution of continuous intravenous heparin, the activated partial thromboplastin time (APTT) should be aggressively followed at 6-hour intervals until it is consistently in the therapeutic range of 1.5 to 2.0 times control values (105). This range corresponds to a heparin level of 0.2 to 0.4 U/mL as measured by protamine sulfate titration. In general, heparin should be administered as an intravenous bolus of 5,000 units followed by a maintenance dose of at least 30,000 to 40,000 units per 24 hours by continuous infusion. The lower dose is administered if the patient is considered at high risk for bleeding (106). This aggressive approach decreases the risk of subtherapeutic anticoagulation, and although supratherapeutic levels are sometimes achieved initially, bleeding complications do not appear to be increased. More recent data support aggressive heparin dosing. An alternative regimen consisting of a bolus of 80 U/kg followed by 18 U/kg/hour has been recommended (107). Further adjusting of the heparin dose should also be weight based (Table 110.6). This weight-adjusted approach is recommended by the recent American College of Chest Physicians (ACCP) Consensus Conference on Antithrombotic Therapy (108). Warfarin therapy may be initiated as soon as the APTT is therapeutic, and heparin should be maintained until a therapeutic International Normalized Ratio (INR) of 2.0 to 3.0 has been overlapped with a therapeutic APTT for 3 consecutive days. Although proximal lower-extremity thrombus is more likely to result in PE, one should either follow calf thrombi for proximal extension over 10 to 14 days with noninvasive testing or institute anticoagulation (109,110). Documented proximal DVT or PE should be treated for at least 3 months. Longer treatment is appropriate when significant risk factors persist. Both short- and long-term anticoagulation guidelines are outlined in the ACCP guidelines (108).

A number of clinical trials have strongly suggested the efficacy and safety of LMWH for treatment of established acute proximal DVT using recurrent symptomatic VTE as the primary outcome measure (111–117). The incidence of DVT and recurrent bleeding in these trials indicates that LMWH preparations are at least as effective and as safe as unfractionated heparin. These agents can be administered once or twice per day subcutaneously even at therapeutic doses and do not require monitoring of the APTT. It appears to be reasonable to monitor anti–factor X levels in certain settings such as in obese patients, very small patients (<40 kg), and patients with renal insufficiency. There is no proven benefit in monitoring other patients. In two large randomized (Canadian and European) trials, therapy with LMWH was safely initiated at home or

TABLE 110.6

WEIGHT-BASED NOMOGRAM FOR HEPARIN THERAPY IN ACUTE VENOUS THROMBOEMBOLISM

Initial heparin dose = 80 U/kg bolus, then 18 U/kg/h

Subsequent modifications:

APTT		
Seconds	**Times control**	**Heparin dose adjustment after initial dose**
<35	<1.2	80-U/kg bolus, then increase by 4 units/kg/h
35–45	1.2–1.5	40-U/kg bolus, then increase by 2 units/kg/h
46–70	1.5–2.3	No change
71–90	2.3–3	Decrease infusion rate by 2 units/kg/h
>90	>3	Hold infusion 1 h, then decrease rate by 3 units/kg/h

APTT, activated partial thromboplastin time.
From Raschke RA, Reilly BM, Guidry JR, et al. The weight-based heparin dosing nomogram compared with a "standard care" nomogram. *Ann Intern Med* 1993;119:874; and The 7th ACCP Conference on Antithrombotic and Thrombolytic Therapy: Evidence-Based Guidelines. *Chest* 2004;126:163S–696S.

continued at home after a brief hospitalization (111,112). A number of outpatient studies have followed these two pivotal trials. Four meta-analyses examined the use of LMWH compared with unfractionated heparin in the initial treatment of acute proximal DVT (115,116). Although there was overlap between the analyses, they have helped to confirm the efficacy and safety of LMWH for the treatment of established DVT. The more recent of these studies suggested a reduced mortality in patients treated with LMWH, although the precise reason for this is not clear (115).

In the United States, two LMWH preparations are FDA approved for use in patients presenting with DVT with or without acute uncomplicated PE. Enoxaparin is approved for both inpatient and outpatient use at a dose of 1 mg/kg subcutaneously every 12 hours or at 1.5 mg/kg once daily for inpatient use. The latter regimens were both proven to be effective in a large study of inpatients in which both doses were as effective and as safe as unfractionated heparin (118). The second preparation, tinzaparin is administered as 175 units once daily, with the FDA approval being based upon therapy of inpatients. Neither enoxaparin nor tinzaparin is approved for use in patients presenting with acute PE, although tinzaparin has shown efficacy in a large, randomized European trial of patients with PE (119). The FDA-approved indications for the three LMWHs approved for use in the United States are shown in Table 110.7. It should be noted that the *prophylactic* doses of these agents differ from those used for treating active disease.

Novel Anticoagulants and Cell-Based Therapies

The approach to VTE has evolved in several unique and complementary directions. Anticoagulants, including direct thrombin inhibitors, direct factor Xa inhibitors, indirect, selective factor Xa inhibitors, plasminogen activator inhibitor antagonists, tissue factor pathway inhibitor (TFPI) antagonists,

TABLE 110.7

FOOD AND DRUG ADMINISTRATION-APPROVED INDICATIONS FOR SPECIFIC LOW-MOLECULAR-WEIGHT HEPARINS

	Low-molecular-weight heparin		
Indication[a]	**Enoxaparin**	**Dalteparin**	**Tinzaparin**
Patients presenting with acute DVT[b]	X		X
Prophylaxis for acute DVT in:			
Total hip replacement	X	X	
Total knee replacement	X		
General abdominal surgery	X	X	
Hospitalized medical patients	X		
Acute coronary syndromes[c]	X	X	

DVT, deep venous thrombosis.
[a]It must be recognized that prophylactic doses differ from therapeutic doses.
[b]Enoxaparin is approved for use in both inpatients with deep venous thrombosis with or without pulmonary embolism at 1 mg/kg every 12 h or 1.5 mg/kg once daily and for outpatients (1 mg/kg every 12 h). The data supporting treatment with tinzaparin (175 units once daily) are based on studies of hospitalized patients. Neither drug is approved in patients presenting with acute pulmonary embolism.
[c]Unstable angina and non–ST-segment elevation myocardial infarction.

and activated protein C are but some of the classes of drugs being actively investigated (120–122).

The oral direct thrombin inhibitor ximelagatran has been studied extensively. The potential of ximelagatran for the treatment of acute DVT was investigated in the Thrombin Inhibitor in Venous Thromboembolism (THRIVE) studies. THRIVE I was a randomized, controlled trial evaluating the safety and tolerability of ximelagatran (24, 36, 48, or 60 mg twice daily) compared with dalteparin followed by warfarin for 2 weeks. Evaluation of paired venograms from 295 of 350 patients showed regression of thrombus in 69% of patients in both groups. Change in thrombus size according to the Marder score and safety were also similar (123).

Based on the encouraging results of THRIVE I, a large, multicenter, randomized, double-blind study (THRIVE Treatment Study) was performed. A total of 2,489 patients with acute DVT (37% had confirmed PE) were assigned to receive either oral ximelagatran 36 mg twice daily for 6 months or enoxaparin 1 mg/kg subcutaneously, minimum 5 days, followed by warfarin (INR 2 to 3). Recurrent venous thromboembolism occurred in 2.1% and 2.0% of patients, respectively. Major bleeding (on treatment analyses) was experienced in 1.3% and 2.2% of patients, respectively (124).

The THRIVE III Study included 1,233 patients with confirmed venous thromboembolism who had received standard anticoagulant therapy for 6 months. They were then randomized to either ximelagatran 24 mg twice daily or placebo for another 18 months. Recurrent events occurred in 12 patients receiving ximelagatran and in 71 patients on placebo (hazard ratio 0.16; $p < .0001$). Six patients given active study drug experienced a major hemorrhagic event (some were fatal or involved the central nervous system) (125). The safety profile, hepatotoxicity in particular, will challenge the drug' s approval and clinical use. Another oral direct thrombin inhibitor, dabigatran, is under investigation.

Fondaparinux, an indirect, selective factor Xa inhibitor administered subcutaneously once daily effectively prevents VTE after orthopedic surgery and high-risk abdominal surgery and in acutely ill medical patients. It also has been shown to reduce recurrent events among patients with acute VTE (MATISSE-DVT and MATISSE-PE) (126,127). A related compound, idraparinux, which has an even longer circulating half-life permitting once weekly subcutaneous administration, was investigated in the Van Gogh-DVT and Van Gogh Extension (EXT) (DVT or PE) studies (128). Bleeding complications have challenged its development.

The role of neovascularization in the resolution of venous thrombus represents a novel means of addressing the debilitating condition known as postphlebitic syndrome (129). Similarly, the infusion of endothelial progenitor cells and/or engineered smooth muscle cells for the purpose of restoring vascular thromboresistance and venous valvular performance, respectively, represents an area of active investigation (130).

Complications of Anticoagulation

Complications of heparin include bleeding and heparin-induced thrombocytopenia (HIT). The rates of major bleeding in trials using heparin by continuous infusion or high-dose subcutaneous injection are less than 5% (111,112,114). Heparin-induced thrombocytopenia (defined as a platelet count less than 150,000/mm^3) typically develops 5 or more days after the initiation of heparin therapy, occurring in 5% to 10% of patients. The syndrome is caused by heparin-dependent immunoglobulin G (IgG) antibodies that activate platelets via their Fc receptors (131). It has been demonstrated that these antibodies recognize heparin complexed with platelet factor 4 (132). Visentin and associates (133) showed that such antibodies also react with endothelial cells coated with platelet factor 4, and such potential antibody-mediated vascular injury may help to explain the predisposition of patients with HIT to thromboembolism when challenged with heparin. Positive platelet aggregation tests for antibodies to heparin may be present in the absence of significant thrombocytopenia, and such tests may be negative despite a progressive decrease in platelet count. If a patient is placed on heparin for VTE and the platelet count progressively decreases to 100,000/mm^3 or less, heparin therapy should be discontinued. Low-molecular-weight heparins should not be considered in this setting despite the fact that formation of heparin-dependent IgG antibodies and the risk of HIT appear to be lower with this form of heparin. Heparin-induced thrombocytopenia occurred in 9 of 332 patients receiving standard unfractionated heparin compared with none of 333 patients receiving enoxaparin (134). Eight of the 9 patients receiving standard heparin developed one or more thrombotic events. However, it is important for clinicians to realize that HIT can occur with the use of either form of heparin. Platelet aggregation studies should be performed and may suggest that a LMWH preparation may be used safely in the setting of HIT caused by unfractionated heparin. Newly developed solid-phase assays that use complexes of heparin and platelet factor 4 as targets for the detection of heparin-induced antibodies are much more sensitive than the serotonin-release test. These newer assays may facilitate decisions regarding optimal treatment alternatives when thrombocytopenia develops.

Vena Cava Interruption

If heparin therapy cannot be continued, inferior vena cava (IVC) filter placement can be undertaken to prevent lower-extremity thrombus from embolizing to the lungs. These devices have been widely used for nearly two decades. The primary indications for filter placement include contraindications to anticoagulation, recurrent embolism while on adequate therapy, and significant bleeding complications during anticoagulation (135). IVC filters are sometimes placed in the setting of massive PE (with hemodynamic and/or severe respiratory compromise) when it is believed that any further emboli might be lethal (136). Potential mechanisms of IVC filter failure include migration of the filter either distally or proximally to a point that no longer protects the vena cava, improper filter position allowing thrombi to bypass the filter, venous collaterals (allowing thrombi to "bypass the filter"), and thrombosis proximal to the filter (or on the proximal tip of the filter) with subsequent embolization. Rare complications include perforation of the IVC, cephalad migration, and displacement of the filter during insertion. Inferior vena cava filters may rarely erode into the wall of the IVC. Occasionally, IVC obstruction due to thrombosis at the filter site may occur. In general, anticoagulation is initiated after an IVC filter has been placed (when the clinician determines that it is safe to do so).

Retrievable Inferior Vena Cava Filters

The development of retrievable IVC filters provides an attractive management option for patients with PE and transient contradictions to systemic anticoagulant therapy that may include recent bleeding, planned major surgery, trauma, or diagnostic testing (during which anticoagulation would be contradicted). The time of removal (according to the specific device implanted) ranges from 2 weeks to 12 weeks after insertion (137,138).

TABLE 110.8

THROMBOLYTIC THERAPY IN VENOUS THROMBOEMBOLISM: POTENTIAL INDICATIONS

Hypotension related to pulmonary embolism[a]
Severe hypoxemia
Lobar or greater perfusion defect
Right ventricular dysfunction associated with pulmonary embolism
Extensive deep vein thrombosis

[a]This indication is widely accepted. All indications require careful review of contraindications to thrombolytic therapy.

TABLE 110.9

THROMBOLYTIC THERAPY FOR ACUTE PULMONARY EMBOLISM: APPROVED REGIMENS

Streptokinase: 250,000 U intravenous (loading dose over 30 min); then 100,000 U/h for 24 h[a]
Urokinase: 2000 U/lb intravenous (loading dose over 10 min); then 2,000 U/lb/h for 12 to 24 h[b]
Tissue-type plasminogen activator: 100 mg intravenous over 2 h

[a]Streptokinase administered over 24 to 72 hr at this loading dose and rate has also been approved for use in patients with extensive DVT.
[b]Urokinase is not currently available in the United States.

Thrombolytic Therapy

The National Institutes of Health consensus guidelines for PE thrombolysis issued in 1980 recommended thrombolytic therapy for patients with obstruction of blood flow to a lobe or multiple pulmonary segments and for patients with hemodynamic compromise, regardless of the size of the PE (139). The recommendations for fibrinolytic therapy in PE have been summarized (140) (Table 110.8). We recommend thrombolytic therapy in patients with hemodynamic instability (hypotension) or severely compromised oxygenation (141). Stable patients with a significant embolic load are individualized, often receiving treatment in the absence of absolute or relative contraindications. For example, strong arguments for thrombolytic therapy can be made when the perfusion defect by lung scan or pulmonary arteriogram is extensive (defect approaching the equivalent of one half of the pulmonary vascular bed) even without clear hemodynamic instability. Another setting in which thrombolytic therapy may be considered is when extensive DVT accompanies a submassive PE. There are no clinical studies suggesting a reduction in mortality in the latter settings, and perhaps future clinical trials will clarify appropriate guidelines.

Acceleration of clot lysis in PE using thrombolytic therapy was first demonstrated several decades ago (142,143). The multicenter, prospective, randomized Urokinase Pulmonary Embolism Trial (UPET) evaluated 160 patients with arteriographically proven PE (144). Thrombolysis was accelerated in patients receiving urokinase compared with those on heparin when pulmonary arteriograms and lung perfusion scans were examined 24 hours after treatment. Thereafter, the difference between the two groups diminished, and by day 5 the improvement in each group was similar. There was no difference in the frequency of recurrent PE or mortality rate within 2 weeks of treatment. However, only 7% of the patients in the study were classified as having massive PE with shock. Although hemorrhagic complications in this trial were relatively high, further experience with thrombolytic therapy has suggested that adverse effects are reduced when venous cut-downs and unnecessary arterial phlebotomy are avoided. The second phase of this clinical trial also documented the efficacy of streptokinase administered over 24 hours. Finally, recombinant tPA is approved for use in the treatment of PE and is administered as a 100-mg intravenous infusion delivered over 2 hours (145). Thrombolytic regimens approved by the Food and Drug Administration for the treatment of PE are presented in Table 110.9. Coagulation assays are unnecessary during thrombolysis because the approved regimens are administered as fixed doses. It is recommended that heparin be withheld until the thrombolytic infusion is completed. The APTT is then determined and heparin, is initiated without a loading dose if this value is less than twice the upper limit of normal. If the APTT exceeds this value, the test is repeated every 4 hours until it is safe to proceed with heparin. The method thrombolytic delivery has also been evaluated. Although a number of investigators have employed standard or low-dose intrapulmonary arterial thrombolytic infusions as a means to deliver a high concentration of drug in close proximity to occluding thrombus (146,147), intravenous therapy appears to be adequate in most cases (148). More direct techniques, such as catheter-directed administration of intraembolic thrombolytic therapy, are discussed later.

The use of thrombolytic therapy for DVT is more controversial. A comprehensive review of the literature suggests that use of streptokinase may be associated with a reduction in postphlebitic syndrome when used for acute DVT, although bleeding is increased with thrombolytic therapy. Future studies may clarify the role of thrombolytic therapy for DVT. It is reasonable to consider systemic thrombolytic therapy in patients with proximal occlusive DVT associated with significant swelling and symptoms when there are no absolute or relative contraindications. Although agents other than streptokinase have been studied, there are no firm dosing recommendations for them. Catheter-directed techniques have been employed for the treatment of acute DVT (see the section Pulmonary Embolectomy and Catheter-Extraction Techniques).

COMPLICATIONS OF TREATMENT

Hemorrhage is the primary adverse effect associated with thrombolytic therapy and generally occurs at sites of invasive procedures such as pulmonary arteriography or arterial line placement (149). Thus, when thrombolytic therapy is administered, invasive procedures should be minimized. The most devastating complication associated with this form of treatment is the development of intracranial hemorrhage (150). Clinical trials have suggested that this occurs in significantly less than 1% of patients. Contraindications to systemic thrombolytic therapy in VTE are listed in Table 110.10. Bleeding related to thrombolytic therapy requires immediate diagnosis and management. Bleeding from vascular puncture sites should be addressed with manual compression followed by a pressure dressing. Intracranial bleeding requires immediate discontinuation of thrombolytics or heparin, and emergent neurologic and neurosurgical consultation should be obtained. A noncontrasted brain computed tomography scan should be performed. Retroperitoneal hemorrhage may result from a vascular puncture above the inguinal ligament and may be life-threatening. Patients with severe or refractory bleeding should be transfused with 10 units of cryoprecipitate (as a rich source of fibrinogen) and 2 units of fresh-frozen plasma, and unfractionated heparin can be reversed fully with protamine sulfate, whereas LMWH is only partially reversed (60%).

TABLE 110.10

THROMBOLYTIC THERAPY FOR ACUTE PULMONARY EMBOLISM: CONTRAINDICATIONS

Absolute
Intracranial tumor or hemorrhagic stroke
Recent head trauma or cranial surgery
Active or recent internal bleeding
Relative
Thrombocytopenia or coagulopathy
Uncontrolled severe hypertension
Cardiopulmonary resuscitation
Surgery or biopsy within the previous 10 d

TABLE 110.11

ACUTE MASSIVE PULMONARY EMBOLISM: CONSIDERATIONS FOR EARLY MANAGEMENT

Oxygen therapy
Intubation and mechanical ventilation
Intravenous heparin
Fluid administration
Norepinephrine or dopamine
Thrombolytic therapy
Catheter or suction cup embolectomy
Surgical embolectomy
Vena caval filter placement

PULMONARY EMBOLECTOMY AND CATHETER-EXTRACTION TECHNIQUES

Pulmonary embolectomy may be performed in the setting of acute massive PE. Although many patients die from PE before surgical embolectomy is feasible, some deteriorate hours after the initial episode, suggesting that surgery may occasionally be appropriate. In one series of 71 embolectomies performed with cardiopulmonary bypass, hospital mortality was 29% (151). The mortality in those patients who had not sustained a cardiac arrest preoperatively was only 11%, however. Transvenous embolectomy via a suction-catheter device has been employed (152) but has not received widespread acceptance. Timsit and colleagues (153) used this technique to treat 18 patients with massive PE over a 7-year period. Clot extraction was successful in 11 patients.

Although an intravenous route of administration represents the primary means of delivery, thrombolytic therapy has been delivered locally in patients with massive PE and, in some individuals, may preclude the need for surgical embolectomy (154). These studies have generally been small and uncontrolled. Although intrapulmonary arterial delivery of thrombolytic agents appears to offer no advantage over the intravenous route, *intraembolic* thrombolytic infusions may offer advantages over merely infusing the agents into the pulmonary artery. This technique has been applied in both animal models of PE and in patients with enhanced thrombolysis (155,156). Less than conventional doses of tPA or urokinase are delivered over 10 to 20 minutes via a catheter imbedded directly within the thrombus. Combining thrombolytic therapy via direct delivery (at low doses) with the possible mechanical benefits of direct intraembolic infusion may hold promise in the management of carefully selected patients with a heightened risk for bleeding. The implementation of these techniques and the catheter-directed administration of intraembolic thrombolytic therapy require an experienced radiographic/interventional team. Finally, catheter-directed techniques have been successfully employed in the setting of acute iliofemoral DVT using urokinase doses ranging from 1,400,000 to 16,000,000 U delivered over an average of 30 hours (157). Further investigation in this area is underway.

Management of Massive Pulmonary Embolism

Massive PE should always be suspected in patients with rapidly progressive hypotension or marked hypoxemia. The presence of electromechanical dissociation or sudden cardiac death should always raise the suspicion of massive PE. If the patient is stable, V/Q scanning should be performed when possible. Although PE should be proven with either a high-probability V/Q scan (helical CT or MRI may also offer proof) and when necessary pulmonary arteriography, echocardiography may support the diagnosis of massive PE and may also suggest the need for aggressive intervention including thrombolytic therapy. Once massive PE associated with hypotension and/or severe hypoxemia is suspected, supportive treatment is immediately initiated. Intravenous saline should be infused rapidly but cautiously because right ventricular function is often markedly compromised. Dopamine and norepinephrine appear to be the favored choices of vasoactive therapy in massive PE and should be administered if the blood pressure is not rapidly restored. Guidelines for the management of massive PE are summarized in Table 110.11. Because death in this setting results from right ventricular failure, dobutamine has been recommended by some as a means by which to augment right ventricular output (158,159). A vasopressor such as norepinephrine combined with dobutamine might offer optimal results, and further exploration of such combined therapy would prove enlightening. Oxygen therapy is administered, and thrombolytic therapy is considered as described earlier. Intubation and institution of mechanical ventilation are instituted as needed to support respiratory failure.

CHRONIC VENOUS THROMBOEMBOLIC DISEASE

Although the vast majority of acute PEs resolve with treatment, occasionally a substantial residual thromboembolic burden remains (160,161). In this setting, the clot becomes organized and adherent and is not amenable to thrombolysis. If the obstruction becomes extensive, pulmonary hypertension develops. This syndrome most commonly occurs in patients 40 to 70 years of age, but it can occur at any age. At least 50% of patients who develop chronic thromboembolic pulmonary hypertension have no documented history of DVT or PE. This feature greatly impedes the diagnosis. Most patients have no identifiable coagulopathy. Fatigue and dyspnea with exertion are the most common complaints. The nonspecific nature of these findings may substantially delay the correct diagnosis. The physical examination generally reveals a right ventricular heave, a loud P2, a right ventricular S3, and tricuspid regurgitation consistent with pulmonary hypertension. In 20% of patients, one or more murmurs may be auscultated over the lung fields.

Once the diagnosis is suspected, the diagnostic evaluation is generally revealing. The chest radiograph usually reveals right ventricular enlargement and enlarged main pulmonary arteries. Electrocardiographic changes are consistent with pulmonary hypertension. Arterial blood gases generally reveal hypoxemia with a widened A-a difference, although some patients may only demonstrate exercise-induced hypoxemia. Echocardiography documents pulmonary hypertension and enlargement of the right ventricle. Chest CT scanning is prudent and may reveal other rare causes of pulmonary hypertension such as mediastinal fibrosis and also may, in fact, demonstrate evidence of chronic thrombi. Helical CT scanning may be particularly useful in this regard. The VQ scan is nearly always high probability for PE, but occasionally is less impressive. Right heart catheterization and pulmonary arteriography are performed both to establish the diagnosis with certainty and to determine operability. Pulmonary angioscopy frequently has proven complementary to arteriography in assessing these patients (162).

Although anticoagulation should be instituted and IVC filters are recommended in patients with chronic thromboembolic pulmonary hypertension, the only means by which to alleviate symptoms and efficacy on survival is with surgery. The group from the University of California at San Diego has had tremendous experience with evaluation and surgical therapy of these patients. Pulmonary thromboendarterectomy is performed via median sternotomy on cardiopulmonary bypass and the overall mortality, which has continued to improve, is less than 5%. Lung transplantation can be performed in patients in whom thrombi are too distal to extract.

Venous Stenting

Endovascular management of iliofemoral occlusive disease using mechanical fibrinolysis/thrombectomy, followed by balloon angioplasty and stenting, represents an emerging technique for relieving debilitating symptoms of venous hypertension that typically include pain, swelling, and venous ulceration (163, 164).

CONTROVERSIES AND PERSONAL PERSPECTIVES

Venous thromboembolism is difficult to study in large, randomized trials because of the varying presentations of acute PE and DVT, the difficulty with diagnosis, and the institution/practice-specific approach to patient care. As a result, many relevant questions remain unanswered. In view of existing challenges facing the medical community, several groups, including the American College of Chest Physicians and the American Thoracic Society, have taken steps to form consensus guidelines for areas in which substantial data exist and opinion and position statements to address issues and plan research strategies for areas that require attention (165).

The Diagnostic Approach to Venous Thromboembolism

Critical pathways have been constructed by experts in the field for the diagnostic approach to DVT; however, these approaches suffer from institutional variability, differences in the availability of diagnostic technologies, and a lack of incorporation of newer technology such as MRI. The American Thoracic Society has recently drafted consensus guidelines for the diagnostic approach to VTE (166). These include algorithms, the role of new technologies, and account of institution-specific differences in approach. A more uniform approach to diagnosis will also support the academic community and facilitate new antithrombotic drug development. The International Cooperative Pulmonary Embolism Registry represents the largest prospective PE registry ever undertaken (167). This effort has helped to answer a number of clinical questions and contribute to future strategies in clinical investigation. It has already enhanced international communication, which should increase the number and quality of international randomized clinical trials and help to unify the approach to VTE.

The roles of newer methods for diagnosing DVT and PE such as MRI and helical CT scanning need to be clarified, and recommendations may change as the technology continues to improve. How often are venography and pulmonary arteriography still necessary? When should MRI be used in addition to, or instead of, Doppler ultrasonography?

Screening and Prophylaxis Strategies

Optimizing Treatment in Acute Pulmonary Embolism

The identification of "high-risk" patients who might potentially benefit from more aggressive treatment strategies, such as fibrinolysis, remains a topic of great clinical relevance. The combined use of biomarkers (troponin and N-terminal pro–brain natriuretic polypeptide) and echocardiography could contribute to the development of risk stratification algorithms (168); however, further investigation to include large patient cohorts and clinical outcome data will be needed for validation.

Determining a practical means by which to identify patients with recently characterized coagulopathies such as activated protein C resistance and determining their significance will facilitate the implementation of more meaningful prophylaxis and treatment protocols. Who should be screened for activated protein C resistance? Do patients with this disorder require lifelong prophylaxis? When should combined mechanical and pharmaceutical prophylaxis be applied? What *are* the differences among the different LMWH compounds? Although the ACCP guidelines are very useful, they use the term "LMWH" in a generic sense in making recommendations for prophylaxis. *At present, recommendations in specific settings must be made for specific agents that have been studied in that setting.*

Therapeutic Approaches

A number of anticoagulation issues require clarification. The duration of therapy in different subsets of patients with VTE needs to be determined. Should patients with PE and without residual DVT be treated for a shorter period of time than patients with extensive DVT? Is it beneficial to use MRI to document the extent of DVT in every patient? Is it appropriate to repeat lower-extremity studies in patients with DVT to help determine treatment duration? We will likely be treating larger numbers of outpatients, and this may be simplified with the LMWH preparations. This has already created controversy regarding which patients, if any, are truly acceptable for outpatient therapy. Which agents (and doses) are appropriate? Where do the direct thrombin inhibitors, selective factor Xa inhibitors, and tissue factor pathway inhibitor fit in?

What are appropriate guidelines for thrombolytic therapy in DVT and PE? Is one thrombolytic agent or regimen superior to others? When should acute pulmonary embolectomy be performed? Although some individuals feel that thrombolytic therapy should be reserved for patients with "hemodynamic compromise," the latter term is not clearly defined. We believe that patients with PE, hypotension, and evidence of end-organ dysfunction (from hypoperfusion) or those with hypoxemia refractory to maximal oxygen therapy should receive intravenous thrombolytic therapy if other methods such as surgical embolectomy or catheter-based therapy are not immediately accessible. It is difficult to make guidelines that address all clinical settings and patient subsets. In the end, treatment should be individualized based on existing evidence. The specific roles for systemic and local thrombolytic therapy and catheter-directed techniques, including indications, doses, duration of therapy, and delivery methods, require clarification through carefully designed clinical trials.

THE FUTURE

The future of VTE prophylaxis and treatment will address lingering questions and unmet needs, particularly among high-risk patient populations with medical illnesses and malignancy. Successfully identifying patients likely to experience recurrent events using molecular profiles, oral and selective anticoagulants, regulatable therapeutics and cell-based therapy for post-phlebitic syndrome are poised to establish patient-specific, optimal management strategies in the foreseeable future.

References

1. Virchow R von. Weitere Untersuchungen ueber die Verstopfung der Lungenarterien und ihre Folge. *Traube's Beitr Exp Path Physiol* (Berlin) 1846; 2:21–31.
2. Trousseau A. Phlegmasia alba dolens. Clinique Medicale de l'Hotel Dieu de Paris. *New Sydenham Soc* (London) 1865;3:94.
3. Laennec RHT. *De l'auscultation mediate ou Traité du diagnostic des maladies des poumons et du coeur,* Vol. I. Paris: Brosson et Chaude, 1819.
4. Cruveilhier J. *Anatomic pathologique du corps humain*. Paris, JB Ballierre, 1828.
5. Luzzatto B. *Embolia dell' arteria polmonale*. Milan: Fratelli Richiedei, 1880.
6. Trendelenberg F. Uber die Operative Behandlurig der Embolie der Lungeroarterie. *Arch Klin Chirop* 1908;24:687–700.
7. Kirschner W. Ein durch die Trendelenburgsche Operation geheilter Fall von Embolie der Art Pulmonalis. *Arch Klin Chirop* 1924;48:312–359.
8. Ljungdahl M. Gibt es eine Chronische Embolistierung der Lungen Arterie? *Dtsch Arch Klin Med* 1928;102:1–23.
9. Moniz E, Carvallio L, Limer H. Angiopneumographic. *Presse Med* 1931;53: 996–999.
10. Bauer G. A venographic study of thrombo-embolic problems. *Acta Chirop Scand* 1940;84(Suppl 65):5–75.
11. Bauer G. Thrombosis: early diagnosis and abortive treatment with heparin. *Lancet* 1946;1:447–454.
12. Clason S. Three cases of pulmonary embolism following confinement, treated with heparin. *Acta Med Scand* 1941;107:131–135.
13. McLean J. The discovery of heparin. *Circulation* 1959;19:75–78.
14. Chrispin AR, Goodwin JF, Steiner RE. The radiology of obliterative pulmonary hypertension and thromboembolism. *Br J Radiol* 1963;36:705.
15. Williams JR, Wilcox C, Andrews GJ, Burns RR. Angiography in pulmonary embolism. *JAMA* 1963;184:473.
16. Sasahara AA, Stein M, Simon M, Littman D. Pulmonary angiography in the diagnosis of thromboembolic disease. *N Engl J Med* 1964;270:1075.
17. Stein PD, O'Connor JF, Dalen JE, et al. The angiographic diagnosis of acute pulmonary embolism. Evaluation of criteria. *Am Heart J* 1967;73:730–741.
18. Taplin GV, Johnson DE, Dore EK, Kaplan HS. Suspensions of radiolabeled albumin aggregates for photoscanning the liver, spleen and other organs. *J Nucl Med* 1964;5:259–275.
19. Wagner HN, Sabiston Jr DC, McAfee JG, et al. Diagnosis of massive pulmonary embolism in man by radioisotope scanning. *N Engl J Med* 1964; 271:377–384.
20. Anderson FA, Wheeler HB. Venous thromboembolism: risk factors and prophylaxis. *Clin Chest Med* 1995;16:235–251.
21. Dalen JE, Alpert JS. Natural history of pulmonary embolism. *Prog Cardiovasc Dis* 1975;17:257–270.
22. Lindblad B, Eriksson A, Bergquist D. Autopsy-verified pulmonary embolism in a surgical department: analysis of the period from 1951 to 1988. *Br J Surg* 1991;78:849–852.
23. Bratzler DW, Raskob, GE, Murray CK, et al. Underuse of venous thromboembolism prophylaxis for general surgery patients. Physician practices in the community hospital setting. *Arch Intern Med* 1998;158:1909–1912.
24. Goldhaber SZ, Tapson VF, for the DVT FREE Steering Committee. A prospective registry of 5,451 patients with ultrasound-confirmed deep vein thrombosis. *Am J Cardiol* 2004;93:259–262.
25. Tapson VF, Hyers TM, Waldo AL, et al., for the NABOR (National Anticoagulation Benchmark and Outcomes Report) Steering Committee. Antithrombotic therapy practices in US hospitals in an era of practice guidelines. *Arch Intern Med* 2005;165:1458–1464.
26. Lamb GC, Tomski MH, Kaufman J, et al. Is chronic spinal cord injury associated with increased risk of venous thromboembolism? *J Am Paraplegia Soc* 1993;16:153–156.
27. Kraaijenhagen RA, Haverkamp D, Koopman MMW, et al. Travel and risk of venous thrombosis. *Lancet* 2000;356:1492–1493.
28. Bagshaw M. Jet "leg," pulmonary embolism, and hypoxia. *Lancet* 1996; 348:415–416.
29. Layish DT, DeLong DM, Tapson VF. Relationship between obesity and pulmonary embolism: a review of the PIOPED data. *Chest* 1996;110:53.
30. Carson JL, Kelley MA, Duffy A, et al. The clinical course of pulmonary embolism. *N Engl J Med* 1992;326:1240–1245.
31. Goldhaber SZ, Hennekens CH, Evans DA, et al. Factors associated with correct antemortem diagnosis of major pulmonary embolism. *Am J Med* 1982;73:822–826.
32. Kakkar VV, Howe CT, Nicolaides AN, et al. Deep vein thrombosis of the legs: is there a "high risk" group? *Am J Surg* 1970;120:527–530.
33. Clagett GP, Reisch JS. Prevention of venous thromboembolism in general surgical patients: results of a meta-analysis. *Ann Surg* 1988;208:227–240.
34. Fisher M, Michele A, McCann W. Thrombophlebitis and pulmonary infarction associated with fractured hip. *Clin Res* 1963;11:407.
35. Fitts Jr WT, Lehr HB, Bitner RL, et al. An analysis of 950 fatal injuries. *Surgery* 1964;56:663–668.
36. Coon WW. Risk factors in pulmonary embolism. *Surg Gynecol Obstet* 1976;143:385–390.
37. Pineo GF, Brain MC, Gallus AS, et al. Tumors, mucus production and hypercoagulability. *Ann N Y Acad Sci* 1974;230:262–270.
38. Handley AJ, Emerson PA, Fleming PR. Heparin in the prevention of deep vein thrombosis after myocardial infarction. *Br Med J* 1972;2:436–438.
39. Gruppo Italiano per lo Studio della Streptochinasi nell'Infarto Miocardico (GISSI). Effectiveness of intravenous thrombolytic treatment in acute myocardial infarction. *Lancet* 1986;1:397–402.
40. ISIS-2 Collaborative Group. Randomized trial of IV streptokinase, oral aspirin, both or neither among 17,187 cases of suspected acute myocardial infarction. *Lancet* 1988;2:349–360.
41. Rickles FR, Edwards RL. Activation of blood coagulation in cancer: Trousseau's syndrome revisited. *Blood* 1983;62:14–31.
42. Toglia MR, Weg JG. Current concepts: venous thromboembolism during pregnancy. *N Engl J Med* 1996;335:108–114.
43. Stadel BV. Oral contraceptives and cardiovascular disease. *N Engl J Med* 1981;305:672–677.
44. Weiss N. Third-generation oral contraceptives: how risky? *Lancet* 1995; 346:1570.
45. World Health Organization Collaborative Study of Cardiovascular Disease and Steroid Hormone Contraception. Venous thromboembolic disease and combined oral contraceptives: results of international multicentre case–control study. *Lancet* 1995;346:1575–1582.
46. Daly E, Vessey MP, Hawkins MM, et al. Risk of venous thromboembolism in users of hormone replacement therapy. *Lancet* 1996;348:977–980.
47. Jick H, Derby LE, Myers MW, et al. Risk of hospital admission for idiopathic venous thromboembolism among users of postmenopausal estrogens. *Lancet* 1996;348:981–983.
48. Grodstein F, Stampfer MJ, Goldhaber SZ, et al. Prospective study of exogenous hormones and risk of pulmonary embolism in women. *Lancet* 1996;348:983–987.
49. Vandenbroucke JP, Rosing J, Bloemenkamp KWM, et al. Oral contraceptives and the risk of venous thrombosis. *N Engl J Med* 2001;344:1527–1535.
50. Prandoni P, Bilora F, Marchiori A, et al. An association between atherosclerosis and venous thrombosis. *N Engl J Med* 2003(15);348:1435–1441.
51. Becattini C, Agnelli G, Prandoni P, et al. A prospective study on cardiovascular events after acute pulmonary embolism. *Eur Heart J* 2005;26:3–4.
52. Seligsohn U, Lubetsky A. Genetic susceptibility to venous thrombosis. *N Engl J Med* 2001;344:1222–1231.
53. Ridker PM, Hennekens CH, Lindpainter K, et al. Mutation in the gene coding for coagulation factor V and the risk of myocardial infarction, stroke, and venous thrombosis in apparently healthy men. *N Engl J Med* 1995;332:912.
54. Benotti JR, Dalen JE. The natural history of pulmonary embolism. *Clin Chest Med* 1984;5:403.
55. McIntyre KM, Sasahara AA. The ratio of pulmonary artery pressure to pulmonary vascular obstruction. *Chest* 1977;71:692.
56. The PIOPED investigators. Value of the ventilation/perfusion scan in acute pulmonary embolism. Results of the prospective investigation of pulmonary embolism diagnosis. *JAMA* 1990;263:2753–2759.
57. The Urokinase Pulmonary Embolism Trial; a national cooperative study. *Circulation* 1973;47(Suppl II):1–108.
58. Stein PD, Terrin ML, Hales CA, et al. Clinical, laboratory, roentgenographic, and electrocardiographic findings in patients with acute pulmonary embolism and no pre-existing cardiac or pulmonary disease. *Chest* 1991; 100:598–603.
59. Green RM, Meyer TJ, Dunn M, Glassroth J. Pulmonary embolism in younger adults. *Chest* 1992;101:1507–1511.

60. Bounameaux H, Cirafici P, DeMoerloose P, et al. Measurement of D-dimer in plasma as diagnostic aid in suspected pulmonary embolism. *Lancet* 1991;337:196.
61. Rowbotham BJ, Egerton-Vernon J, Whitaker AN, et al. Plasma cross-linked fibrin degradation products in pulmonary embolism. *Thorax* 1990;45:684–687.
62. Egermayer P, Town GI, Turner JG, et al. Usefulness of D-dimer, blood gas, and respiratory rate measurements for excluding pulmonary embolism. *Thorax* 1998;53:830–834.
63. Ahearn GS, Bounameaux H. The role of the D-dimer in the diagnosis of venous thromboembolism. *Semin Respir Crit Care Med* 2000;21:521–536.
64. McNeill BJ, Hessel SJ, Branch WT, et al. Measures of clinical efficacy: Part 3: The value of the lung scan in the evaluation of young patients with pleuritic chest pain. *J Nucl Med* 1976;17:163–164.
65. Stein PD, Athanasoulis C, Alavi A, et al. Complications and validity of pulmonary angiography in acute pulmonary embolism. *Circulation* 1992;85:462–468.
66. Hull RD, Raskob G, Ginsberg JS, et al. A noninvasive strategy for the treatment of patients with suspected pulmonary embolism. *Arch Intern Med* 1994;154:289–297.
67. Rosengarten PL, Tuxen DV, Weeks AM. Whole lung pulmonary angiography in the intensive care unit with two portable chest x-rays. *Crit Care Med* 1990;18:459–460.
68. Come PC. Echocardiographic evaluation of pulmonary embolism and its response to therapeutic interventions. *Chest* 1992;101:151S–162S.
69. Kasper W, Meinertz T, Kersting F, et al. Echocardiography in assessing acute pulmonary hypertension due to pulmonary embolism. *Am J Cardiol* 1980;45:567–572.
70. Goldhaber SZ, Haire WD, Feldstein ML, et al. Alteplase versus heparin in acute pulmonary embolism: Randomized trial assessing right ventricular function and pulmonary perfusion. *Lancet* 1993;341:507–510.
71. Tapson VF, Davidson CJ, Gurbel PA, et al. Rapid and accurate diagnosis of pulmonary emboli in a canine model using intravascular ultrasound imaging. *Chest* 1991;100:1410–1413.
72. Tapson VF, Davidson CJ, Kisslo KB, et al. Rapid visualization of massive pulmonary emboli utilizing intravascular ultrasound. *Chest* 1994;105:888–890.
73. Ricou F, Nicod PH, Moser KM, Peterson KL. Catheter-based intravascular ultrasound imaging of chronic thromboembolic pulmonary disease. *Am J Cardiol* 1991;67:749–752.
74. Sostman HD, Layish DT, Tapson VF, et al. Prospective comparison of helical CT and MR imaging in clinically suspected acute pulmonary embolism. *JMRI* 1996;6:275.
75. Touliopoulos P, Costello P. Helical (spiral) CT of the thorax. *Radiol Clin North Am* 1995;33:843–861.
76. Remy-Jardin M, Remy J, Wattinne L, Giraud F. Central pulmonary thromboembolism: Diagnosis with spiral volumetric CT with the single-breath-hold technique. Comparison with pulmonary angiography. *Radiology* 1992;185:381–387.
77. Goodman LR, Curtin JJ, Mewissen MW, et al. Detection of pulmonary embolism in patients with unresolved clinical and scintigraphic diagnosis: helical CT versus angiography. *AJR* 1995;164:1369–1374.
78. Remy-Jardin M, Remy J, Petyt L, et al. Diagnosis of acute pulmonary embolism with spiral CT: comparison with pulmonary angiography and scintigraphy [Abstract]. *Radiology* 1995;197(P):303.
79. Teigen CL, Maus TP, Sheedy PF, et al. Pulmonary embolism: diagnosis with contrast-enhanced electron-beam CT and comparison with pulmonary angiography. *Radiology* 1995;194:313–319.
80. van Rossum AB, Pattynama PM, Treurniat FE, et al. Spiral CT angiography for detection of pulmonary embolism: validation in 124 patients. *Radiology* 1995;197(P):303.
81. van Rossum AB, Treurniat FE, Kieft GJ, et al. Role of spiral volumetric computed tomographic scanning in the assessment of patients with clinical suspicion of pulmonary embolism and an abnormal ventilation perfusion scan. *Thorax* 1996;51:23–28.
82. Oser RF, Zuckerman DA, Gutirrez FR, Brink JA. Anatomic distribution of pulmonary embolism at pulmonary arteriography: implications for spiral and electron-beam CT. *Radiology* 1996;199:31–35.
83. Quinn MF, Lundell CJ, Klotz TA, et al. Reliability of selective pulmonary arteriography in the diagnosis of acute pulmonary embolism. *AJR* 1987;149:469–471.
84. Goodman LR, Lipchik RJ. Diagnosis of acute pulmonary embolism: time for a new approach. *Radiology* 1996;199:25–27.
85. Teigen CL, Maus TP, Sheedy PF, et al. Pulmonary embolism: diagnosis with electron-beam CT. *Radiology* 1993;188:839–845.
86. Drucker EA, Rivitz SM, Shepard JO. Acute pulmonary embolism: assessment of helical CT. *Radiology* 1998;209:235–241.
87. Hull R, Hirsh J, Powers P. Impedance plethysmography: the relationship between venous filling and sensitivity and specificity for proximal vein thrombosis. *Circulation* 1978;58:898–902.
88. Hull R, van Aken WG, Hirsh J, et al. Impedance plethysmography using the occlusive cuff technique in the diagnosis of venous thrombosis. *Circulation* 1976;53:696–700.
89. Patterson RB. The limitations of impedance plethysmography in the diagnosis of acute DVT. *J Vasc Surg* 1989;9:725.
90. Anderson DR, Lensing AWA, Wells PS, et al. Limitations of impedance plethysmography in the diagnosis of clinically suspected deep-vein thrombosis. *Ann Intern Med* 1993;118:25–30.
91. Lensing AW, Levi MM, Buller HR, et al. Diagnosis of deep-vein thrombosis using an objective Doppler method. *Ann Intern Med* 1990;113:9–13.
92. White R, McGahan JP, Daschbach MM, Hartling MM. Diagnosis of deep-vein thrombosis using duplex ultrasound. *Ann Intern Med* 1989;111:297–304.
93. Evans AJ, Tapson VF, Sostman HD, et al. The diagnosis of deep venous thrombosis: a prospective comparison of venography and magnetic resonance imaging. *Chest* 1992;102:120S.
94. Witty LA, Tapson VF, Evans AJ, et al. MRI versus ultrasound: a radiologic and clinical evaluation of DVT. *Am Rev Respir Dis* 1993;147:A998.
95. Burke B, Sostman HD, Carroll BA, Witty LA. The diagnostic approach to deep venous thrombosis: which technique? *Clin Chest Med* 1995;16:253–268.
96. Collins R, Scrimgeour A, Yusuf S, Peto R. Reduction in fatal pulmonary embolism and venous thrombosis by perioperative administration of subcutaneous heparin. *N Engl J Med* 1988;318:1162–1173.
97. Anderson Jr FA, Brownell W, Goldberg RJ, et al. Physician practices in the prevention of venous thromboembolism. *Ann Intern Med* 1991;115:591–595.
98. Colditz GA, Tuden RL, Oster G. Rates of venous thrombosis after general surgery: Combined results of randomised clinical trials. *Lancet* 1986;2:143.
99. Bergqvist D, Benoni G, Bjorgello XX, et al. Low-molecular-weight heparin (enoxaparin) as prophylaxis against venous thromboembolism after total hip replacement. *N Engl J Med* 1996;335:696–700.
100. Comp PC, Spiro T, Friedman, RJ, et al. Prolonged enoxaparin therapy to prevent venous thromboembolism after primary hip or knee replacement. *J Bone Joint Surg* 2001;83A:336–345.
101. Samama MM, Cohen AT, Darmon JY, et al. A comparison of enoxaparin with placebo for the prevention of venous thromboembolism in acutely ill medical patients. *N Engl J Med* 1999;341:793–800.
102. Kleber FX, Witt C, Flosbach CW, et al. Study to compare the efficacy and safety of the low-molecular-weight heparin enoxaparin and standard heparin in the prevention of thromboembolic events in medical patients with cardiopulmonary diseases. *Ann Hematol* 1998;76(Suppl 1):A93
103. Lechler E, Schramm W, Flosbach CW, et al. The venous thrombotic risk in nonsurgical patients: epidemiological data and efficacy/safety profile of a low molecular weight heparin (enoxaparin). *Haemostasis* 1996;26(Suppl 2):49–56.
104. Hirsh J, Dalen JE, Deykin D, Poller L. Heparin and low-molecular-weight heparin: mechanisms of action, pharmacokinetics, dosing, monitoring, efficacy and safety. *Chest* 2001;119(Suppl):64S–94S.
105. Hull RD, Raskob GE, Hirsh J, et al. Continuous intravenous heparin compared with intermittent subcutaneous heparin in the initial treatment of proximal vein thrombosis. *N Engl J Med* 1986;315:1109–1114.
106. Hull R, Raskob G, Rosenbloom D, et al. Optimal therapeutic level of heparin therapy in patients with venous thrombosis. *Arch Intern Med* 1992;152:1589–1595.
107. Raschke RA, Reilly BM, Guidry JR, et al. The weight-based heparin dosing nomogram compared with a "standard care" nomogram. *Ann Intern Med* 1993;119:874.
108. The 7th ACCP Conference on Antithrombotic and Thrombolytic Therapy: Evidence-Based Guidelines. *Chest* 2004;126:163S–696S.
109. Lagerstedt CI, Olsson CG, Fagher BO, Oqvist BW. Need for long-term anticoagulant treatment in symptomatic calf-vein thrombosis. *Lancet* 1985;2:515–518.
110. Moser KM, LeMoine, JR. Is embolic risk conditioned by location of deep venous thrombosis? *Ann Intern Med* 1981;94:439–444.
111. Levine M, Gent M, Hirsh J, et al. A comparison of low-molecular-weight heparin administered primarily at home with unfractionated heparin administered in the hospital for proximal deep vein thrombosis. *N Engl J Med* 1996;334:677–681.
112. Koopman MM, Prandoni P, Piovella, F et al. Low-molecular-weight heparin versus heparin for proximal deep vein thrombosis. *N Engl J Med* 1996;334:682–687.
113. Tapson VF. Treatment of acute deep venous thrombosis and pulmonary embolism: use of low molecular weight heparin. *Semin Respir Crit Care Med* 2000;21:547–553.
114. Dolovich LR, Ginsberg JS, Douketis JD, et al. A meta-analysis comparing low molecular weight heparins with unfractionated heparin in the treatment of venous thromboembolism. *Arch Intern Med* 2000;160:181–188.
115. Siragusa S, Cosmi B, Piovella F, et al. Low-molecular-weight heparins and unfractionated heparin in the treatment of patients with acute venous thromboembolism: results of a meta-analysis. *Am J Med* 1996;100:269–277.
116. Lensing AWA, Prins MH, Davidson BL, Hirsh J. Treatment of deep venous thrombosis with low-molecular-weight heparins: a meta-analysis. *Arch Intern Med* 1995;155:601–607.
117. Leizorovicz A, Simonneau G, Decousus H, Boissel JP. Comparison of efficacy and safety of low molecular weight heparins and unfractionated heparin in initial treatment of deep venous thrombosis. *BMJ* 1994;309:299–304.

118. Merli G, Spiro T, Olsson CG, et al. Subcutaneous enoxaparin once or twice daily compared with intravenous unfractionated heparin for treatment of venous thromboembolic disease. *Ann Intern Med* 2001;134:191–202.
119. Simmoneau G, Sors H, Charbonnier B, et al. A comparison of low-molecular-weight heparin with unfractionated heparin for acute pulmonary embolism. The THESEE Study Group. *N Engl J Med* 1997;337:663–669.
120. The Global Use of Strategies to Open Occluded Coronary Arteries (GUSTO) IIB investigators. A comparison of recombinant hirudin with heparin for the treatment of acute coronary syndromes. *N Engl J Med* 1996;335:775–782.
121. Antman EM, for the TIMI 9B Investigators. Hirudin in acute myocardial infarction: thrombolysis and thrombin inhibition in MI (TIMI) 9B trial. *Circulation* 1996;94:911.
122. Gustafsson D, Elg M, Lenfors S, et al. Effects of inogatran, a new low molecular weight thrombin inhibitor, in rat models of venous and arterial thrombosis, thrombolysis and bleeding time. *Blood Coagul Fibrinolysis* 1996;7:69–79.
123. Eriksson H, Wahlander K, Gustafsson D, et al. A randomized, controlled, dose-guiding study of the oral direct thrombin inhibitor ximelagatran compared with standard therapy for the treatment of acute deep vein thrombosis: THRIVE I. *J Thromb Haemost* 2003;1:41–47.
124. Huisman MV, on behalf of the THRIVE II and V Investigators. Efficacy and safety of the oral direct thrombin inhibitor ximelagatran compared with current standard therapy for the acute symptomatic deep vein thrombosis, with or without pulmonary embolism: a randomized, double blind, multinational study [Abstract]. *J Thromb Haemost* 2003;1(Suppl 1).
125. Eriksson H, Wahlander K, Lundstrom T, et al., for the THRIVE III Investigators. Extended secondary prevention with the oral direct thrombin inhibitor ximelagatran for 18 months after 6 months of oral anticoagulation in patients with venous thromboembolism: a randomized placebo-controlled trial. *J Thromb Haemost* 2003;1(Suppl 1).
126. Bauersachs RM. Fonadaparinux: an update on new study results. *Eur J Clin Invest* 2005;35(Suppl 1)27–32.
127. Robinson DM, Wellington K. Fonadaparinux sodium: a review of its use in the treatment of acute venous thromboembolism. *Am J Cardiovasc Drugs* 2005;5(5):35–46.
128. Anonymous. Idraparinux sodium: SANORG 340006. *Drugs R D* 2004; 5(3):164–165.
129. Modarai B, Burnand KG, Humphries J, et al. The role of neovascularisation in the resolution of venous thrombus. *Thromb Haemost* 2005;93(5):801–809.
130. Wakefield TW, Henke PK. The role of inflammation in early and late venous thrombosis: are there clinical implications? *Semin Vasc Surg* 2005;18(3): 118–129.
131. Kelton JG, Sheridan D, Santos A, et al. Heparin-associated thrombocytopenia: laboratory studies. *Blood* 1988;79:925–930.
132. Amiral J, Bridey F, Dreyfus M, et al. Platelet factor 4 complexed to heparin is the target for antibodies generated in heparin-induced thrombocytopenia. *Thromb Haemost* 1992;68:95–96.
133. Visentin GP, Ford SE, Scott JP, Aster RH. Antibodies from patients with heparin-induced thrombocytopenia/thrombosis are specific for platelet factor 4 complexed with heparin or bound to endothelial cells. *J Clin Invest* 1994;93:81–88.
134. Warkentin TE, Levine MN, Hirsh J, et al. Heparin-induced thrombocytopenia in patients treated with low-molecular-weight heparin or unfractionated heparin. *N Engl J Med* 1995;332:1330–1335.
135. Greenfield LJ. Vena caval interruption and pulmonary embolectomy. *Clin Chest Med* 1984;5:495–505.
136. Becker DM, Philbrick JT, Selby JB. Inferior vena cava filters: indications, safety, effectiveness. *Arch Intern Med* 1992;152:1985–1994.
137. Hann CL, Streiff MB. The role of vena caval filters in the management of venous thromboembolism. *Blood Rev* 2005;19(4):179–202.
138. Imberti D, Bianchi M, Farina A., et al. Clinical experience with retrievable vena cava filters: results of a prospective observational multicenter study. *J Thromb Haemost* 2005: 3(7):1370–1375.
139. Symposium: Thrombolytic therapy in thrombosis: a National Institutes of Health Consensus Development Conference. *Ann Intern Med* 1980;93: 141–143.
140. Goldhaber SZ. Evolving concepts in thrombolytic therapy for pulmonary embolism. *Chest* 1992(Suppl);101:183S–185S.
141. Witty LA, Steinfeld AD, Tapson VF. Thrombolytic therapy in acute pulmonary embolism: physician attitudes. *Am Rev Respir Dis* 1993;147: A1000.
142. Johnson AJ, McCarthy WR. The lysis of artificially induced intravascular clots in man by intravenous infusion of streptokinase. *J Clin Invest* 1959; 38:1627–1643.
143. Miller GAH, Gibson RV, Sutton GC. Treatment of pulmonary embolism with streptokinase. *Br Med J* 1969;1:812–815.
144. Sasahara AA, Cannilla JE, Belks JJ, et al. Urokinase therapy in clinical pulmonary embolism. *N Engl J Med* 1969;277:1168–1173.
145. Goldhaber SZ, Kessler CM, Heit J, et al. A randomized controlled trial of recombinant tissue plasminogen activator versus urokinase in the treatment of acute pulmonary embolism. *Lancet* 1988;2:293–298.
146. Leeper Jr KV, Popovich Jr J, Lesser BA, et al. Treatment of massive acute pulmonary embolism. The use of low doses of intrapulmonary arterial streptokinase combined with full doses of systemic heparin. *Chest* 1988;93: 234–240.
147. The UKEP study: multicentre clinical trial on two local regimens of urokinase in massive pulmonary embolism. *Eur Heart J* 1987;8:2–10.
148. Verstraete M, Miller GAH, Bounameaux H, et al. Intravenous and intrapulmonary recombinant tissue-type plasminogen activator in the treatment of acute massive pulmonary embolism. *Circulation* 1988;77:353–360.
149. Sane DC, Califf RM, Topol EJ, et al. Bleeding during thrombolytic therapy for acute myocardial infarction: mechanisms and management. *Ann Intern Med* 1989;111:1010–1022.
150. Gore JM. Prevention of severe neurologic events in the thrombolytic era. *Chest* 1992;101:124S–130S.
151. Gray HH, Morgan JM, Paneth M, Miller GAH. Pulmonary embolectomy: indications and results. *Br Heart J* 1987;57:572.
152. Greenfield LJ, Kimmell GO, McCurdy WC. Transvenous removal of pulmonary emboli by vacuum-cup catheter technique. *J Surg Res* 1969;9:347–352.
153. Timsit JF, Reynaud P, Meyer G, Sors H. Pulmonary embolectomy by catheter device in massive PE. *Chest* 1991;100:655–658.
154. Tapson VF, Witty LA. Massive pulmonary embolism: diagnostic and therapeutic strategies. *Clin Chest Med* 1996;16:329.
155. Tapson VF, Gurbel PA, Royster R, et al. Pharmacomechanical thrombolysis of experimental pulmonary emboli: rapid low-dose intraembolic therapy. *Chest* 1994; 106:1558–1562.
156. Tapson VF, Davidson CJ, Bauman R, et al. Rapid thrombolysis of massive pulmonary emboli without systemic fibrinogenolysis: intra-embolic infusion of thrombolytic therapy. *Am Rev Respir Dis* 1992;145:A719.
157. Semba CP, Dake MD. Iliofemoral deep venous thrombosis: aggressive therapy with catheter-directed thrombolysis. *Radiology* 1994;191:487–494.
158. Jardin F, Genevray B, Brunney D, Margairaz A. Dobutamine: a hemodynamic evaluation in pulmonary embolism shock. *Crit Care Med* 1985;13: 1009–1012.
159. Manier G, Castaing Y. Influence of cardiac output on oxygen exchange in acute pulmonary embolism. *Am Rev Respir Dis* 1992;145:130–136.
160. Shure D. Chronic thromboembolic pulmonary hypertension: diagnosis and treatment. *Sem Resp Crit Care Med* 1996;17:7.
161. Fedullo PF, Auger WR, Channick RN, et al. Chronic thromboembolic pulmonary hypertension. *Clin Chest Med* 1995;16:353–374.
162. Shure D, Gregoratos G, Moser KM. Fiberoptic angioscopy: role in the diagnosis of chronic pulmonary arterial obstruction. *Ann Intern Med* 1985; 103:844–850.
163. Hood DB, Alexander JQ. Endovascular management of iliofemoral venous occlusive disease. *Surg Clin North Am* 2004;84(5):1381–1396.
164. Robbins MR, Assi Z, Comerota AJ. Endovascular stenting to treat chronic long-segment inferior vena cava occlusion. *J Vasc Surg* 2005;41(1):136–140.
165. American College of Chest Physicians Consensus Committee on Pulmonary Embolism. Opinions regarding the diagnosis and management of venous thromboembolism. *Chest* 1996;109:233–237.
166. Tapson VF, Carroll BA, Davidson BL, et al. The diagnostic approach to acute venous thromboembolism. Clinical practice guideline. American Thoracic Society. *Am J Respir Crit Care Med* 1999;160:1043–1066.
167. Goldhaber SZ, Visani L. The International Cooperative Pulmonary Embolism Registry. *Chest* 1995;108:302.
168. Binder L, Pieske B, Olschewski M, et al. N-Terminal pro–brain natriuretic peptide or troponin testing followed by echocardiography for risk stratification of acute pulmonary embolism. *Circulation* 2005;112:1573–1579.

INDEX

NOTE: Entries showing a color CD icon for a page reference will be found by using the DVD in the back of the book. Page numbers followed by *t* indicate table; those followed by *f* indicate figure.